The Comparative Guide to American Hospitals

Volume 2

Fourth Edition

The Comparative Guide to American Hospitals

Volume 2: Southern Region

4,834 Hospitals with Key Personnel and 67 Quality Measures Relating to Heart Attack, Heart Failure, Pneumonia, Stroke, Blood Clots, Childhood Asthma, Emergency Room Care, Surgical Care, Preventative Care, Medical Imaging and Patient Experience

A SEDGWICK PRESS Book

Grey House Publishing

PUBLISHER: Leslie Mackenzie
SENIOR EDITOR: David Garoogian
EDITORIAL DIRECTOR: Laura Mars
PRODUCTION MANAGER: Kristen Thatcher
MARKETING DIRECTOR: Jessica Moody

A Sedgewick Press Book
Grey House Publishing, Inc.
4919 Route 22
Amenia, NY 12501
518.789.8700
FAX 845.373.6390
www.greyhouse.com
e-mail: books @greyhouse.com

Comparative guide to American hospitals. Vol. 2, Southern region; [ed. David Garoogian]. — 4th ed. (2014)

4 v. ; cm.

Includes index.
"4,834 Hospitals with Key Personnel and 67 Quality Measures Relating to Heart Attack, Heart Failure, Pneumonia, Stroke, Blood Clots, Childhood Asthma, Emergency Room Care, Surgical Care, Preventative Care, Medical Imaging and Patient Experience."

1. Hospitals—United States—Directories. 2. Hospitals—United States—Periodicals. 3. Hospitals—Ratings—United States—Statistics—Periodicals. 4. Myocardial infarction—Hospitals—United States—Directories. 5. Heart failure—Hospitals—United States—Directories. 6. Pneumonia—Hospitals—United States—Directories. I. Garoogian, David.

RA977 .C66
610/.025

4-Volume Set	ISBN: 978-1-61925-457-2
Volume 1	ISBN: 978-1-61925-458-9
Volume 2	**ISBN: 978-1-61925-459-6**
Volume 3	ISBN: 978-1-61925-460-2
Volume 4	ISBN: 978-1-61925-461-9

Table of Contents

Introduction

This is the fourth edition of *The Comparative Guide to American Hospitals*. It reports on how 4,834 hospitals—**141 more than last edition**—in America measure up when caring for patients with a number of specific conditions. The third edition reported on **Heart Attacks, Heart Failure, Pneumonia, Childhood Asthma, Surgical Care, Use of Medical Imaging**, and **Patients' Hospital Experiences**. This fourth edition includes new data on **Blood Clot Prevention and Treatment, Emergency Room Care, Preventative Care, Stroke,** and **Medicare Spending**. Also new are appendices on **Surgical Complication Rates** and **Best Hospitals by Category**.

This work is based on a Federal study (Hospital Compare) in which short-term acute care and critical access hospitals around the country voluntarily report on quality measures to receive an incentive payment established by the Medicare Prescription Drug, Improvement and Modernization Act of 2003. Each hospital in this edition is rated on 67 recognized quality measures—**18 more than last edition**—and is compared to both state and national averages.

In *The Comparative Guide to American Hospitals,* the data is organized, sorted and ranked by our editors. It is this organization and ranking that makes *The Comparative Guide to American Hospitals* a unique and valuable tool to the health care consumer. Data is presented in such a way as to inform and educate the user, who can then put the facts into a meaningful context as hospitals are evaluated state by state.

Due to the increased data, and the regional use of such data, this edition is again comprised of four regional volumes—**Eastern, Southern, Central** and **Western**. In addition to comprehensive **hospital rankings and profiles** for all states in the region, each volume includes four Appendices with additional information.

In addition to the data from Hospital Compare, each hospital profile in *The Comparative Guide to American Hospitals* is comprised of value-added data from Grey House's *Directory of Hospital Personnel*. This critical contact data includes fax numbers, web sites, email addresses, and number of beds plus 24,458 key contact names—**783 more names than last edition**. In addition, each state chapter includes **State Hospital Rankings**.

Section One: State Hospital Rankings & State Profiles

The first section of each regional volume of *The Comparative Guide to American Hospitals* is arranged alphabetically by state. Each state chapter starts with a ranking section, unique to Grey House, that ranks hospitals in that state on how often they meet each of the 67 accepted quality protocols. The quality measures ranked in *The Comparative Guide to American Hospitals* are based on accepted, effective treatments supported by the Centers for Medicare & Medical Services of the US Department of Health & Human Services and the Hospital Quality Alliance (HQA)—a public/private collaboration established to promote on hospital quality of care. HQA represents consumers, hospitals, doctors, employers, accrediting organizations and Federal agencies.

Following the ranking section, hospital profiles are listed first by city, then alpha within city. Profiles include name, address, phone, fax, web site, hospital type and ownership, number of beds, and whether the hospital provides emergency services. Further, each profile includes an average of five key medical contacts—representing not only the facility's top administration but also the physicians specifically responsible for the care of heart, pneumonia, and asthma patients, as well as surgical care. Again, these data points are unique to *The Comparative Guide to American Hospitals*, and complete the picture for health care consumers searching for quality care.

The remainder of each hospital profile examines the 67 quality measures in detail, comparing the hospital's score with both the state and national average: These measures include:

- **Timely and Effective Care:**
  - **Blood Clot Prevention and Treatment** ***(NEW)*** measures include anticoagulation overlap therapy, ICU venous thromboembolism prophylaxis, incidence of potentially preventable VTE, UFH with dosages/platelet count monitoring, venous thromboembolism prophylaxis, and warfarin therapy discharge instructions
  - **Chest Pain/Possible Heart Attack Care** measures include aspirin at arrival, median time to ECG, median time to transfer, and fibrinolytic medication timing
  - **Children's Asthma Care** measures include receiving systemic corticosteroids, receiving home management plan, and receiving reliever medication
  - **Emergency Department** ***(NEW)*** measures include admittance decision time, head CT results within 45 minutes of arrival, patients who left ER before being seen, time from ER arrival to admittance, time from ER arrival to discharge, time spent in ER before being evaluated, and time to pain medications for long-bone fractures
  - **Heart Attack Care** measures include aspirin given at discharge, statin prescribed at discharge, fibrinolytic medication timing, and percutaneous coronary intervention within 90 minutes of arrival
  - **Heart Failure Care** measures include angiotensin converting enzyme inhibitor or angiotensin receptor blocker for left ventricular systolic dysfunction, discharge instructions given, and evaluation of left ventricular systolic function
  - **Pneumonia Care** measures include appropriate initial antibiotic, and blood culture timing
  - **Pregnancy and Delivery Care** ***(NEW)*** measures include newborn deliveries scheduled early
  - **Preventive Care** ***(NEW)*** measures include immunization for influenza and immunization for pneumonia
  - **Stroke Care** ***(NEW)*** measures include anticoagulation therapy for atrial fibrillation, antithrombotic therapy timing, assessed for rehabilitation, discharged on antithrombotic therapy, discharged on statin medication, thrombolytic therapy timing, venous thromboembolism prophylaxis, and written stroke educational materials given
  - **Surgical Care** measures include appropriate venous thromboembolism prophylaxis within 24 hours, appropriate beta blocker usage, controlled postoperative blood glucose, perioperative temperature management ***(NEW)***, prophylactic antibiotic timing, prophylactic antibiotic selection, prophylactic antibiotic stopped, and urinary catheter removal
- **Medicare Spending** ***(NEW)*** measures include Medicare spending per beneficiary
- **Use of Medical Imaging** measures include MRI for low back pain, cardiac imaging stress test before surgery ***(NEW)***, follow-up mammogram/ultrasound, combination brain/sinus CT scan ***(NEW)***, combination abdominal CT scan, and combination chest CT scan.
- **Survey of Patients' Hospital Experiences**
  HCAHPS (Hospital Consumer Assessment of Healthcare Providers and Systems) is a national, standardized survey of hospital patients. HCAHPS (pronounced "H-caps") was created to publicly report the patient's perspective of hospital care. The survey asks a random sample of recently discharged patients about important aspects of their hospital experience. The HCAHPS results allow consumers to make fair and objective comparisons between hospitals, and of individual hospitals to state and national benchmarks, on ten important measures of patients' perspectives of care:
  - How do patients rate the hospital overall?
  - How often did doctors communicate well with patients?
  - How often did nurses communicate well with patients?
  - How often did patients receive help quickly from hospital staff?
  - How often did staff explain about medicines before giving them to patients?
  - How often was patients' pain well controlled?
  - How often was the area around patients' rooms kept quiet at night?
  - How often were the patients' rooms and bathrooms kept clean?
  - Were patients given information about what to do during their recovery at home?
  - Would patients recommend the hospital to friends and family?

Section Two: Appendixes & Index

The second section of *The Comparative Guide to American Hospitals* includes:

- **Appendix A: 30-Day Death (Mortality) Rates** Unique to Grey House, this section takes data and organize it in a helpful, informative way for the reader. It lists hospitals nationwide that are "better" or "worse" than the national average, plus a State and National Summary of Hospital Mortality Rates.
- **Appendix B: 30-Day Readmission Rates** lists hospitals nationwide that are "better" or "worse" than the national average, plus a State and National Summary of Hospital Readmission Rates.
- **Appendix C: Surgical Complication Rates** lists hospitals nationwide that are "better" or "worse" than the national average, plus a State and National Summary of Hospital Readmission Rates. Surgical complications covered include:
  - A Wound That Splits Open After Surgery on the Abdomen or Pelvis
  - Accidental Cuts and Tears From Medical Treatment
  - Collapsed Lung Due to Medical Treatment
  - Deaths Among Patients With Serious Treatable Complications After Surgery
  - Rate of Complications for Hip/Knee Replacement Patients
  - Serious Blood Clots After Surgery
  - Serious Complications
- **Appendix D: Best Hospitals by Selected Category** lists best hospitals nationwide based on their average scores in 11 categories. The categories are:
  - Blood Clot Prevention and Treatment
  - Children's Asthma Care
  - Emergency Department Care
  - Heart Care
  - Pneumonia Care
  - Preventative Care
  - Stroke Care
  - Surgical Care
  - Patient's Hospital Experiences
  - Use of Medical Imaging
  - Lowest Medicare Spending per Beneficiary
- **Appendix E: Glossary** provides a list of 87 medical terms to make the best use possible of the data in this edition.
- **Regional Hospital Profile Index** lists hospitals included in each regional volume alphabetically, including city and state.
- **National Hospital Profile Index** lists all hospitals nationwide alphabetically, including volume number, city and state. Appears in Volume 4 only.

This completely revised fourth edition of *The Comparative Guide to American Hospitals* is a valuable guide for the entire medical community, with more hospitals, more criteria measures and more key executives than the last edition. It offers an indispensable snapshot of how hospitals measure up, not only to established "best practices," but also to each other.

We welcome your comments to this edition.

User's Guide

What is the *Comparative Guide to American Hospitals*?

The *Comparative Guide to American Hospitals* (CGAH) is based on a Federal study (Hospital Compare) in which short-term acute care and critical access hospitals around the country voluntarily report on quality measures to receive an incentive payment established by the Medicare Prescription Drug, Improvement and Modernization Act of 2003. Each hospital in this edition is rated on 67 recognized quality measures and is compared to both state and national averages. The measures are grouped into four major categories: Timely and Effective Care; Survey of Patients' Experiences; Use of Medical Imaging; and Medicare Spending Per Beneficiary.

Timely and Effective Care Measures (aka "Process of Care" Measures)

Process of care measures reported under the Hospital Inpatient Quality Reporting (IQR) and Outpatient Quality Reporting (OQR) programs show: 1) The percentage of hospital patients who receive treatments known to get the best results for certain common, serious medical conditions or surgical procedures; 2) How quickly hospitals treat patients who come to the hospital with certain medical emergencies. The measures only apply to patients for whom the recommended treatment would be appropriate. By law, any measures reported on the Hospital Compare website must reflect accepted standards of care, based on current scientific evidence. The measures are regularly reviewed and revised to ensure that they are up-to-date, and new measures and types of conditions and treatments are added over time. Process of care measures include:

- Blood Clot Prevention and Treatment
- Chest Pain/Possible Heart Attack Care
- Children's Asthma Care
- Emergency Department Care
- Heart Attack Care
- Heart Failure Care
- Pneumonia Care
- Pregnancy and Delivery Care
- Preventative Care
- Stroke Care
- Surgical Care Improvment Project

Where the Information Comes From

Measures of timely and effective care come from the data that hospitals get from medical records of their eligible patients, following standards for abstracting and reporting the information. Data submissions include auditing procedures and edit checks to assess whether data submitted are consistent with CMS's defined specifications. In addition, CMS validates the data submitted to provide assurance that the hospital, or its designated agent, can accurately abstract patient medical records and accurately submit data.

What Patients the Measures Apply To

The measures of timely and effective care apply to any adult patients treated at hospitals participating in the IQR and OQR programs for whom the recommended treatments would be appropriate, including Medicare patients, Medicare managed care patients, and non-Medicare patients. Hospitals with a large number of discharges may provide data from a sample of eligible Medicare and non-Medicare patients, based CMS sampling rules.

Risk Adjustment

The measures of timely and effective care do not require risk adjustment, because patients for whom the recommended treatment would not be appropriate are not included in the calculations.

Significance Testing

CMS does not perform tests of statistical significance in reporting the measures of timely and effective care. However, the smaller the sample size, the greater the difference in rates must be in order for that difference to be statistically meaningful. Large differences between individual hospitals' rates may be significant, but small differences between hospitals are usually not significant.

Reporting Period

These 50 measures are based on a reporting period of October 1, 2012 through September 30, 2013 except for the following: Emergency Department Care—Percentage of Patients Who Left the Emergency Department Before Being Seen—January 1, 2012 through December 31, 2012; Preventative Care—Patients Assessed and Given Influenza Vaccination—October 1, 2012 through March 31, 2013; All eight Stroke Care measures—January 1, 2013 through September 30, 2013; All six Blood Clot Prevention and Treatment measures—January 1, 2013 through September 30, 2013.

Survey of Patients' Experiences

The Centers for Medicare & Medicaid Services (CMS), along with the Agency for Healthcare Research and Quality (AHRQ), developed the HCAHPS (Hospital Consumer Assessment of Healthcare Providers and Systems) Survey, also known as Hospital CAHPS®, to provide a standardized survey instrument and data collection methodology for measuring patients' perspectives on hospital care. The HCAHPS Survey is administered to a random sample of patients continuously throughout the year. CMS cleans, adjusts and analyzes the data, then publicly reports the results.

Which Patients are Included
The HCAHPS survey is administered to a random sample of adult patients across medical conditions between 48 hours and six weeks after discharge; the survey is not restricted to Medicare beneficiaries.

Where the Information Comes From
All short-term, acute care, non-specialty hospitals are invited to participate in the HCAHPS Survey. Over 4,000 hospitals participate in HCAHPS. The goal is for each hospital to get at least 300 completed patient surveys per year. In general, the more patients that respond to the survey, the more the results shown on this website will reflect the experiences of all the patients who used that hospital. HCAHPS survey data must be collected by organizations that are trained by the federal government in HCAHPS data collection procedures. Data submitted to the HCAHPS data warehouse is cleaned, adjusted and analyzed by CMS, which calculates hospitals' HCAHPS scores and publicly reports them on the Hospital Compare website.

Adjusting Rates
Preparing the data for public reporting includes taking certain factors into account to ensure fair comparisons among hospitals. For example, the mix of patients can differ from one hospital to the next, and these differences in the patient mix can affect a hospital's HCAHPS results. Patient-mix adjustment takes these differences into account so that the survey results reported on this website are what would be expected for each hospital if all hospitals had a similar mix of patients.

Reporting Period
These 10 measures are based on a reporting period of October 1, 2012 through September 30, 2013.

Use of Medical Imaging

The six measures on the use of medical imaging show how often a hospital provides specific imaging tests for Medicare beneficiaries under circumstances where they may not be medically appropriate. Lower percentages suggest more efficient use of medical imaging. The purpose of reporting these measures is to reduce unnecessary exposure to contrast materials and/or radiation, to ensure adherence to evidence-based medicine and practice guidelines, and to prevent wasteful use of Medicare resources. The measures only apply to Medicare patients treated in hospital outpatient departments. It does not include tests performed in other ambulatory care settings or hospital inpatient settings.

What Patients are Included
Outpatient imaging efficiency measures apply only to Medicare beneficiaries enrolled in Original Medicare who were treated as outpatients in hospital facilities reimbursed through the Outpatient Prospective Payment System (OPPS). They do not include Medicare managed care patients, non-Medicare patients, or patients who were admitted to the hospital as inpatients.

Where the Information Comes From
CMS calculates imaging efficiency measures using data from claims that hospitals and physicians submit for Medicare beneficiaries enrolled in Original Medicare. The data are calculated only for hospitals paid through the Outpatient Prospective Payment System (OPPS). The measures are part of the Hospital Outpatient Quality Reporting Program (OQR).

Risk Adjustment
Outpatient imaging efficiency measures are not risk adjusted. However, measures specifications do not include cases where there were clear medical reasons for performing the tests.

Significance Testing
CMS does not perform tests of statistical significance in reporting the outpatient imaging efficiency measures. Large differences between hospitals' percentages may be significant, but small differences usually are not.

Reporting Period
These six measures are based on a reporting period of July 1, 2012 through June 30, 2013.

Medicare Spending per Beneficiary

The Medicare Spending per Beneficiary (MSPB) measure assesses Medicare Part A and Part B payments for services provided to a Medicare beneficiary during a spending-per-beneficiary episode that spans from three days prior to an inpatient hospital admission through 30 days after discharge. The payments included in this measure are price-standardized and risk-adjusted. Price standardization removes sources of variation that are due to geographic payment differences such as wage index and geographic practice cost differences, as well as indirect medical education (IME) or disproportionate share hospital (DSH) payments. Risk adjustment accounts for variation due to patient health status.

By measuring cost of care through this measure, CMS hopes to increase the transparency of care for consumers and recognize hospitals that are involved in the provision of high-quality care at lower cost to Medicare.

Reporting Period
This measure is based on a reporting period of January 1, 2012 through December 31, 2012.

Sample Entry

The listing below illustrates the kind of information that is or might be included in a Hospital Profile. Each numbered item of information is described in the paragraphs following the example.

1 ▶ **Cleveland Clinic**
9500 Euclid Avenue — Phone: 216-444-2200
Cleveland, OH 44195 — Fax: 216-445-7758
URL: www.clevelandclinic.org
Type: Acute Care Hospitals — Emergency Services: Yes
Ownership: Voluntary non-profit - Private — Beds: 1,113

2 ▶ **Key Personnel:**
CEO/President. . . . . Delos M Cosgrove, MD
Chief of Medical Staff. . . . . Marc Harrison, MD
Infection Control. . . . . David L Longworth, MD
Operating Room. . . . . Allan Siperstein, MD
Pediatric Ambulatory Care . . . . . . Robert Wyllie, MD
Quality Assurance . . . . J Michael Henderson, MD
Radiology. . . . . Gregory P Borkowski, MD

	Measure	Cases	This Hosp.	State Avg.	U.S. Avg.
3 ▶					
4 ▶	**Blood Clot Prevention and Treatment**				
	Anticoagulation Overlap Therapy[2]	400	98%	93%	93%
	ICU Venous Thromboembolism Prophylaxis[2]	84	98%	93%	92%
	Incidence of Potentially Preventable VTE[2]	168	2%	6%	10%
	UFH with Dosages/Platelet Monitoring[2]	444	100%	98%	97%
	Venous Thromboembolism Prophylaxis[2]	347	96%	88%	85%
	Warfarin Therapy Discharge Instructions[2]	237	89%	79%	75%
5 ▶	**Chest Pain/Possible Heart Attack Care**				
	Aspirin Given Within 24 Hours of Arrival	190	96%	97%	96%
	Fibrinolytic Meds Within 30 Min. of Arrival[7]	-	-	44%	58%
	Median Time to ECG (minutes)	197	6	6	7
	Median Time to Transfer (minutes)[1]	-	-	58	60
6 ▶	**Children's Asthma Care**				
	Received Home Management Plan of Care	74	99%	85%	88%
	Received Reliever Medication	75	100%	100%	100%
	Received Systemic Corticosteroids	74	100%	100%	100%
7 ▶	**Emergency Department**				
	Admittance Decision Time (minutes)[2]	227	102	90	98%
	Head CT Results Within 45 Min. of Arrival	11	91%	63%	57%
	Patients Who Left ER Before Being Seen	82,229	2%	2%	2%
	Time from ER Arrival to Admit. (minutes)[2]	228	304	265	274
	Time from ER Arrival to Discharge (minutes)	294	131	128	134
	Time in ER Before Being Evaluated (minutes)	417	11	22	26
	Time to Pain Meds for Fractures (minutes)	194	46	54	57
8 ▶	**Heart Attack Care**				
	Aspirin Given at Discharge	868	100%	99%	99%
	Fibrinolytic Meds Within 30 Min. of Arrival[7]	-	-	80%	54%
	PCI Within 90 Minutes of Arrival	13	92%	97%	96%
	Statin Prescribed at Discharge	834	100%	98%	98%
9 ▶	**Heart Failure Care**				
	ACE Inhibitor or ARB for LVSD[2]	287	99%	97%	97%
	Discharge Instructions Given[2]	712	94%	96%	94%
	Evaluation of LVS Function[2]	858	100%	100%	99%
10 ▶	**Medicare Spending**				
	Medicare Hospital Spending per Patient	-	0.99	1.01	0.98
11 ▶	**Pneumonia Care**				
	Appropriate Initial Antibiotic Given	84	94%	96%	95%
	Blood Culture Timing	176	95%	98%	98%
12 ▶	**Pregnancy and Delivery Care**				
	Newborn Deliveries Scheduled Early[1]	-	-	5%	6%
13 ▶	**Preventive Care**				
	Immunization for Influenza[2]	577	96%	93%	90%
	Immunization for Pneumonia[2]	747	95%	94%	92%
14 ▶	**Stroke Care**				
	Anticoagulation Therapy for Atrial Fibrillation[2]	34	100%	95%	95%
	Antithrombotic Therapy Timing[2]	180	96%	98%	98%
	Assessed for Rehabilitation[2]	333	98%	98%	97%
	Discharged on Antithrombotic Therapy[2]	221	100%	99%	99%
	Discharged on Statin Medication[2]	152	99%	95%	94%
	Thrombolytic Therapy Timing[1,2]	-	-	65%	66%
	Venous Thromboembolism Prophylaxis[2]	349	100%	95%	94%
	Written Stroke Educational Materials Given[2]	125	98%	92%	88%
15 ▶	**Surgical Care Improvement Project**				
	Appropriate Beta Blocker Usage[2]	356	99%	98%	98%
	Appropriate VTP Within 24 Hours[2]	447	99%	98%	98%
	Controlled Postoperative Blood Glucose[2]	253	96%	97%	97%
	Perioperative Temperature Management[2]	625	100%	100%	100%
	Prophylactic Antibiotic Selection[2]	570	99%	99%	99%
	Prophylactic Antibiotic Selection (Outpatient)	1,080	100%	98%	98%
	Prophylactic Antibiotic Stopped[2]	554	97%	98%	98%
	Prophylactic Antibiotic Timing[2]	570	99%	99%	99%
	Prophylactic Antibiotic Timing (Outpatient)	563	97%	97%	98%
	Urinary Catheter Removal[2]	381	98%	97%	97%
16 ▶	**Survey of Patients' Hospital Experiences**				
	Area Around Room 'Always' Quiet at Night	300+	57%	58%	61%
	Doctors 'Always' Communicated Well	300+	82%	80%	82%
	Home Recovery Information Given	300+	90%	87%	85%
	Hospital Given 9 or 10 on 10 Point Scale	300+	84%	72%	71%
	Meds 'Always' Explained Before Given	300+	66%	64%	64%
	Nurses 'Always' Communicated Well	300+	83%	81%	79%
	Pain 'Always' Well Controlled	300+	72%	71%	71%
	Room and Bathroom 'Always' Clean	300+	78%	75%	73%
	Timely Help 'Always' Received	300+	68%	70%	68%
	Would Definitely Recommend Hospital	300+	87%	71%	71%
17 ▶	**Use of Medical Imaging**				
	Cardiac Imaging Stress Test before Surgery	4,179	6.7%	5.4%	5.3%
	Combination Abdominal CT Scan	5,813	13.0%	7.1%	10.5%
	Combination Brain/Sinus CT Scan	2,131	1.7%	2.8%	2.7%
	Combination Chest CT Scan	6,539	0.1%	1.7%	2.7%
	Follow-up Mammogram/Ultrasound	9,962	9.3%	8.7%	8.8%
	Lumbar Spine MRI for Low Back Pain	661	31.9%	34.7%	37.2%

1▶ Hospital Name and Record Header: hospital name; street address; phone; fax; e-mail; URL; hospital type; ownership; emergency services (Yes/No); and number of beds.

2▶ Key Personnel: includes the names of key personnel primarily related to the conditions covered in this publication.

3▶ Hospital Compare Data: each profile contains data covering 67 measures contained in the Centers for Medicare & Medicaid Services Hospital Compare database. There are five columns:

Measure: the 67 quality measures reported.

There are 14 possible footnotes:

(1) The number of cases/patients is too few to report
This footnote is applied: when the number of cases/patients does not meet the required minimum amount for public reporting; when the number of cases/patients is too small to reliably tell how well a hospital is performing; and/or to protect personal health information.

(2) Data submitted were based on a sample of cases/patients
This footnote indicates that a hospital chose to submit data for a random sample of its cases/patients while following specific rules for how to select the patients.

(3) Results are based on a shorter time period than required
This footnote indicates that the hospital's results were based on data from less than the maximum possible time period generally used to collect data for a measure. See Reporting Periods for more information.

(4) Data suppressed by CMS (Centers for Medicare and Medicaid Services) for one or more quarters
The results for these measures were excluded for various reasons, such as data inaccuracies.

(5) Results are not available for this reporting period
This footnote is applied when the hospital does not have data to report.

(6) Fewer than 100 patients completed the HCAHPS survey.
This footnote is applied when the number of completed surveys the hospital or its vendor provided to CMS is less than 100. Use these scores with caution, as the number of surveys may be too low to reliably assess hospital performance.

(7) No cases met the criteria for this measure
This footnote is applied when a hospital did not have any cases meet the inclusion criteria for a measure.

(8) The lower limit of the confidence interval cannot be calculated
The lower limit of the confidence interval cannot be calculated if the number of observed infections equals zero.

(9) No data are available from the state/territory for this reporting period
This footnote is applied when: too few hospitals in a state/territory had data available; or no data was reported for this state/territory.

(10) The scores shown reflect fewer than 50 completed surveys.
This footnote is applied when the number of completed surveys the hospital or its vendor provided to CMS is less than 50. Use these scores with caution, as the number of surveys may be too low to reliably assess hospital performance.

(11) There were discrepancies in the data collection process
This footnote is applied when there have been deviations from data collection protocols. CMS is working to correct this situation.

(12) This measure does not apply to this hospital for this reporting period
This footnote is applied when: there were zero device days or procedures; the hospital does not have ICU locations; the hospital is a new member of the registry and didn't have an opportunity to submit any cases; or the hospital does not report this voluntary measure.

(13) Results cannot be calculated for this reporting period
This footnote is applied when: the number of predicted infections is less than 1; the number of observed MRSA or Clostridium difficile infections present on admission (community-onset prevalence) was above a pre-determined cut-point.

(14) The results for this state are combined with nearby states to protect confidentiality
This footnote is applied when a state has fewer than 10 hospitals in order to protect confidentiality. Results are combined as follows: 1) the District of Columbia and Delaware are combined; 2) Alaska and Washington are combined; 3) North Dakota and South Dakota are combined; and 4) New Hampshire and Vermont are combined. Hospitals located in Maryland and U.S. territories are excluded from the measure calculation.

Cases: the size of the data sample (number of patients) for each hospital and quality measure. In addition, the notation "0" is applied when a hospital provided care to patients with a condition, such as pneumonia, but the cases that the hospital submitted did not meet the specific criteria for being included in the calculation of the measure.

This Hospital: the performance rate that the hospital achieved for each quality measure. This value is expressed as a percentage of the sample size that was measured. The performance rate is calculated by dividing the numerator by the denominator. The denominator is the sum of all eligible cases (as defined in the measure specifications) submitted to the QIO Clinical Data Warehouse for the reporting period. The numerator is the sum of all eligible cases submitted for the same reporting period where the recommended care was provided.

State Average: the average rate for all hospitals reporting data in the state the hospital is located in.

U.S. Average: the average rate for all hospitals reporting nationwide.

Note: Beginning in December 2010, state and national averages for the process of care measures are calculated by summing the cases in the state or nation that "passed" the measure (Numerator) and dividing that sum by the number of cases in the state or national Denominator. For the national and state averages, a simple average was constructed where the numerator was the sum of all non-excluded hospitals' scores and the denominator was the total number of hospitals, each calculated at either the national or individual state level. For the process and survey measures, the national and state averages are calculated before excluding suppressed rates and are not recalculated using only published rates as was done prior to September 2009. Acute Care-VA Medical Centers are not included in the calculation of the national and state comparison rates.

The children's asthma care national and state averages are calculated differently. The average rate for all healthcare organizations in the nation that provide results for a measure. The average rate is calculated by dividing the total number of patients who had the recommended care provided for a measure by the total number of patients who met the inclusion and exclusion criteria for that measure in the nation for the timeframe being reported.

4▸ Blood Clot Prevention and Treatment

The measures listed below show how well hospitals are providing recommended care known to prevent or treat blood clots and how often blood clots occur that could have been prevented.

Anticoagulation Overlap Therapy
Patients with blood clots who got the recommended treatment, which includes using two different blood thinner medicines at the same time.
Patients who develop blood clots in their veins (also called venous thromboembolism, or VTE) need to get treatment that can break up the clots quickly and prevent others from forming. The recommended treatment is to first give a blood thinner that can get into the bloodstream quickly through an IV or injection (heparin), then give a slower-acting oral blood thinner medicine (warfarin), and continue giving both blood thinners for 5 days or until it is safe for the patient to transition off of the IV blood thinner and use only the oral blood thinner medicine. This measure shows the percentage of hospital patients who had a confirmed diagnosis of blood clot at hospital admission or during their hospital stay, and received both medicines for at least 5 days, or were discharged from the hospital on both kinds of medicine, unless their blood work showed they no longer needed it. *Higher percentages are better.*

ICU Venous Thromboembolism Prophylaxis
Patients who got treatment to prevent blood clots on the day of or day after being admitted to the intensive care unit (ICU).
Patients in the Intensive Care Unit (ICU) are at increased risk for developing blood clots in their veins (venous thromboembolism, or VTE), because they are in bed for a long period of time. These clots can break off and travel to other parts of the body, causing serious harm. Hospitals can prevent blood clots by routinely evaluating all patients for their risk of developing blood clots and using appropriate prevention and treatment procedures. Prevention can include compression stockings, blood thinners, and/or other medicines. This measure shows the percentage of ICU patients who received treatment to prevent blood clots: on the day of or day after arrival at the hospital; or on the day of or day after transfer to the ICU; or on the day of or day after having surgery. Patients who did not receive treatment may also be included in this measure, if they had paperwork in their chart to explain why. Reasons for not receiving treatment may include having a massive wound, actively bleeding, or having an allergy to blood thinners. *Higher percentages are better.*

Incidence of Potentially Preventable VTE
Patients who developed a blood clot while in the hospital who did not get treatment that could have prevented it.
Because hospital patients often have to stay in bed for long periods of time, all patients admitted to the hospital are at increased risk of developing blood clots in their veins (also called venous thromboembolism or VTE) that can break off and travel to other parts of the body, like the heart, brain, or lung. Hospitals can prevent blood clots by routinely evaluating patients for their risk of developing blood clots and using appropriate prevention and treatment procedures. Prevention can include compression stockings, blood thinners, and/or other medicines. This measure shows the percentage of patients who developed blood clots while in the hospital who did not receive preventative treatment beforehand. *Lower percentages are better.*

UFH with Dosages/Platelet Monitoring
Patients with blood clots who were treated with an intravenous blood thinner, and then were checked to determine if the blood thinner was putting the patient at an increased risk of bleeding.
Patients who have been diagnosed with a blood clot (also called venous thromboembolism, or VTE) are usually treated with a blood thinner such as IV heparin. Some patients may be prescribed a type of IV heparin called unfractionated heparin (UFH). Unfractionated heparin carries a higher risk of increased bleeding than a different type of IV heparin (called low molecular weight heparin). Risk for bleeding increases because blood thinners increase the time it takes your blood to clot. The most common signs of increased bleeding include unusual bruising, nosebleeds, and bleeding gums. Because of their higher risk of bleeding, patients getting unfractionated heparin should be given regular blood tests to determine if they are at an increased risk of bleeding from getting the medication. This measure shows the percentage of patients who developed a blood clot at admission or during their hospital stay, treated with unfractionated IV heparin who had their blood checked using recommended procedures. *Higher percentages are better.*

Venous Thromboembolism Prophylaxis
Patients who got treatment to prevent blood clots on the day of or day after hospital admission or surgery.
Because hospital patients often have to stay in bed for long periods of time, all patients admitted to the hospital are at increased risk of developing blood clots in their veins (also called venous thromboembolism, or VTE) that can break off and travel to other parts of the body, like the heart, brain, or lung. Hospitals can prevent blood clots by routinely evaluating patients for their risk of developing blood clots and using appropriate prevention and treatment procedures. Prevention can include compression stockings, blood thinners, and/or other medicines. This measure shows the percentage of patients who received treatment to prevent blood clots: on the day of or day after arrival at the hospital; or on the day of or day after having surgery. Patients who did not receive treatment may also be included in this measure, if they had paperwork in their chart to explain why. Reasons for not receiving treatment may include having a massive wound, actively bleeding, or having an allergy to blood thinners. *Higher percentages are better.*

Warfarin Therapy Discharge Instructions
Patients with blood clots who were discharged on a blood thinner medicine and received written instructions about that medicine.
Patients who develop blood clots (also called venous thromboembolism or VTE) will usually be given blood thinner medicines to take when they leave the hospital. Educating patients about how to take the medicine and its possible side effects can help prevent problems that could bring them back to the hospital. Before leaving the hospital, patients with a blood clot, who are taking a blood thinner medicine, and their caregiver should receive information about the following topics: Compliance (how to follow medication instructions); Diet (how to eat a healthy diet and avoid foods that interfere with blood thinners); Monitoring their blood thinner medicine; Adverse drug reactions (difficulty breathing, vomiting, nausea); When to call your health care provider (dizziness or weakness, a fall, bright red bleeding). This measure shows the percentage of patients diagnosed with a blood clot (either at admission or during their hospital stay) discharged from the hospital on blood thinners (anticoagulants or anticoagulant therapy or warfarin therapy) who received written educational instructions at hospital discharge. *Higher percentages are better.*

5▶ Chest Pain/Possible Heart Attack Care

Scientific evidence shows that the following measures represent the best practices for the treatment of chest pain/possible heart attack.

Aspirin Given Within 24 Hours of Arrival
Outpatients with chest pain or possible heart attack who got aspirin within 24 hours of arrival.
Blood clots can cause heart attacks. For many patients having a heart attack, taking aspirin soon after symptoms of a heart attack begin may help break up a clot and make the heart attack less severe. If patients have not taken aspirin themselves before going to the hospital, they should get aspirin when they arrive. Standards for care say that patients should get aspirin within 24 hours of arriving at the hospital. This measure tells what percent of patients got aspirin within this time period. *Higher percentages are better.*

Fibrinolytic Meds Within 30 Minutes of Arrival
Outpatients with chest pain or possible heart attack who got drugs to break up blood clots within 30 minutes of arrival.
Blood clots can cause heart attacks. Certain patients having a heart attack should get a "clot busting" drug to help break up the blood clots and improve blood flow to the heart. Standards for care say that a clot busting drug should be given within 30 minutes of arrival at the hospital. This measure tells the percent of patients who were given a clot busting drug within this time period. *Higher percentages are better.*

Average Time to ECG (minutes)
Average number of minutes before outpatients with chest pain or possible heart attack got an ECG.
"ECG" (sometimes called EKG) stands for electrocardiogram. An ECG is a test that can help doctors know whether patients are having a heart attack. Standards of care say that patients with chest pain or a possible heart attack should have an ECG upon arrival, preferably within 10 minutes. This measure shows the average number of minutes it takes before patients had an ECG (calculated as an arithmetic median). Sometimes patients get an ECG done before they get to the hospital (for example, by the ambulance staff). This is counted as "0 minutes." *Lower numbers are better.*

Average Time to Transfer (minutes)
Average number of minutes before outpatients with chest pain or possible heart attack who needed specialized care were transferred to another hospital.
If a hospital does not have the facilities to provide specialized heart attack care, it transfers patients with possible heart attack to another hospital that can give them this care. This measure shows how long it takes, on average, for hospitals to identify patients who need specialized heart attack care the hospital cannot provide and begin their transfer to another hospital. Specifically, it shows the average (arithmetic median) number of minutes it takes from the time patients arrive in the emergency department until they are transported to a different hospital. *Lower numbers are better.*

6▶ Children's Asthma Care

Scientific evidence shows that the following measures represent best practices for treating children with asthma.

Received Home Management Plan of Care
Children and their caregivers who received a home management plan of care document while hospitalized for asthma.
This measure shows the percentage of children with asthma and their caregivers who were given a home management plan of care document while hospitalized. Because asthma is a chronic condition, controlling a child's asthma symptoms at home will help reduce the risk of further attacks. Knowledge about the disease and its treatment is the key to good asthma control. Asthma that is not managed effectively may lead to more visits to the hospital. Medications can help prevent asthma symptoms and attacks from starting in the first place and can reduce how often attacks happen and severity of the attacks. It is important for children with asthma and their caregivers to know how to prevent asthma symptoms and attacks before they happen. The home management plan of care helps children with asthma and their caregivers develop a plan to manage the child's asthma symptoms and to know when to take action. It should address all of the following: arrangements for follow-up care; environmental control and control of other triggers; method and timing of rescue actions; use of controller medications; use of reliever medications. *Higher percentages are better.*

Received Reliever Medication
Children who received reliever medication while hospitalized for asthma.
National guidelines for treating children with asthma recommend using relievers in the severe phase and gradually cutting down the dosage of medications to provide control of asthma symptoms. Although there are guidelines for medication therapy for children with asthma, there is evidence that these guidelines are not being consistently followed. Using the appropriate medications will lower the risk of severe illness and/or death. This measure shows the percentage of children with asthma who were given reliever medication (like albuterol) while hospitalized. Relievers are medications that relax the bands of muscle surrounding the airways and make breathing easier. *Higher percentages are better.*

Received Systemic Corticosteroids
Children who received systemic corticosteroid medication (oral and IV medication that reduces inflammation and controls symptoms) while hospitalized for asthma.
Oral or IV steroid medications control severe asthma well. That is why they are important for hospital care. Unfortunately, they can cause serious side effects when used long-term. That is why they are mainly used for severe episodes or chronic severe asthma, which cannot be controlled with other medications (like inhaled or oral bronchodilators and anti-inflammatory medications). This measure shows the percentage of children with asthma who were given oral or IV steroid medications while hospitalized. These medications work in the body as a whole,

rather than just on the lungs. They help reduce inflammation and control allergic reactions. *Higher percentages are better.*

7▶ Emergency Department Care

Timely and effective care in hospital emergency departments is essential for good patient outcomes. Delays before receiving care in the emergency department can reduce the quality of care and increase risks and discomfort for patients with serious illnesses or injuries. Waiting times at different hospitals can vary widely, depending on the number of patients seen, staffing levels, efficiency, admitting procedures, or the availability of inpatient beds.

Admittance Decision Time (minutes)
For patients who had to be admitted to the hospital as an inpatient, average time patients spent in the emergency department, after the doctor decided to admit them as an inpatient before leaving the emergency department for their inpatient room.
Delays in transferring emergency department patients to an inpatient unit may be a sign that there's not enough staff or there's poor coordination among hospital departments. Long delays can also create more stress for patients and families. This measure shows the average (arithmetic median) time patients spent in the emergency department—from the time the doctor decided to admit them to the time they left the emergency department for an inpatient bed. *Lower numbers are better.*

Head CT Results Within 45 Minutes of Arrival
Percentage of patients who came to the emergency department with stroke symptoms who received brain scan results within 45 minutes of arrival.
People who suffer from strokes need to receive treatment immediately to lessen the amount of brain damage that occurs with any stroke. A scan of the brain must be taken to determine the type and severity of the stroke before treatment can be provided. Long waits may be a sign that the emergency department is understaffed or overcrowded and can lead to delayed diagnosis and treatment and may lead to further brain damage. Standards of care say that patients with stroke symptoms should receive brain scan results (to diagnose whether and how severely a stroke occurred) within 45 minutes of arriving at the emergency department. This measure shows the percentage of emergency department patients with stroke symptoms who received brain scan results within that time period. *Lower numbers are better.*

Patients Who Left ER Before Being Seen
Percentage of patients who left the emergency department before being seen.
Hospital emergency departments that have high percentages of patients who leave without being seen may not have the staff or resources to provide timely and effective emergency room care. Patients who leave the emergency department without being seen may be seriously ill, putting themselves at higher risk for poor health outcomes. This measure shows the percentage of all individuals who signed into an emergency department but left before being evaluated by a healthcare professional. *Lower numbers are better.*

Time from ER Arrival to Admittance (minutes)
For patients who had to be admitted to the hospital as an inpatient, average time patients spent in the emergency department, before they were admitted to the hospital as an inpatient.
Long stays in an emergency department before a patient is admitted may be a sign that the emergency department is understaffed or overcrowded. This may result in delays in treatment or lower quality care. This measure shows the average (arithmetic median) time patients spent in the emergency department—from the time they arrived to the time they left the emergency department for an inpatient bed. This number only includes patients who were admitted to the hospital as an inpatient. It does not include those people who went home. *Lower numbers are better.*

Time from ER Arrival to Discharge (minutes)
Average time patients spent in the emergency department before being sent home.
Long stays in the emergency department before a patient is sent home may be a sign that the emergency department is understaffed or overcrowded. This may result in delays in treatment, increased suffering for those who wait, and unpleasant treatment environments. This measure shows the average (arithmetic median) time in minutes that patients spent in the emergency department—from the time they arrived to the time they were sent home. It does not include patients who were later admitted to the hospital as inpatients, admitted for observation, transferred to another acute care hospital, or who left without being seen by a licensed provider. *Lower numbers are better.*

Time in ER Before Being Evaluated (minutes)
Average time patients spent in the emergency department before they were seen by a healthcare professional.
Delays in being seen by a healthcare provider may be a sign that the emergency department is understaffed or overcrowded. This may result in delays in treatment, lower quality care, and more stress for patients and families. For patients who were later sent home, this measure shows the average (arithmetic median) time in minutes

spent in the emergency department—from the time they arrived until the time they were seen by a healthcare professional. It does not include patients who were admitted to the hospital, who died in the emergency department, or who left without being seen. *Lower numbers are better.*

Time to Pain Meds for Fractures (minutes)
Average time patients who came to the emergency department with broken bones had to wait before receiving pain medication.
Long waits before a patient is treated may be a sign that the emergency department is understaffed or overcrowded. For patients with broken bones, long waits without pain medication cause unnecessary suffering. For all patients 2 years and older who came to the emergency department with a broken arm or leg, this shows the average (arithmetic median) time they waited before receiving pain medication. *Lower numbers are better.*

8▶ Heart Attack Care

Scientific evidence shows that the following measures represent the best practices for the treatment of heart attack.

Aspirin Given at Discharge
Heart attack patients given aspirin at discharge.
Blood clots can block blood vessels. Aspirin can help prevent blood clots from forming or help dissolve blood clots that have formed. Following a heart attack, continued use of aspirin may help reduce the risk of another heart attack. Aspirin can have side effects like stomach inflammation, bleeding, or allergic reactions. Talk to your health care provider before using aspirin on a regular basis to make sure it's safe for you. This measure shows what percentage of patients were given aspirin upon leaving the hospital. *Higher percentages are better.*

Fibrinolytic Meds Within 30 Minutes of Arrival
Heart attack patients given fibrinolytic medication within 30 minutes of arrival.
The heart is a muscle that gets oxygen through blood vessels. Sometimes blood clots can block these blood vessels and the heart can't get enough oxygen. This can cause a heart attack. Fibrinolytic drugs are medicines that can help dissolve blood clots in blood vessels and improve blood flow to your heart. Standards for care say that patients should get them within 30 minutes of arrival at the hospital. This measure shows what percentage of patients got fibrinolytic drugs within this time period. *Higher percentages are better.*

PCI Within 90 Minutes of Arrival
Heart attack patients given PCI within 90 minutes of arrival.
The heart is a muscle that gets oxygen through blood vessels. Sometimes blood clots can block these blood vessels, and the heart cannot get enough oxygen. This can cause a heart attack. Percutaneous coronary interventions (PCI) are procedures that are among the most effective ways to open blocked blood vessels and help prevent further heart muscle damage. A PCI is performed by a doctor to open the blockage and increase blood flow in blocked blood vessels. Improving blood flow to your heart as quickly as possible lessens the damage to your heart muscle, and it also can increase your chances of surviving a heart attack. There are three procedures commonly described by the term PCI. These procedures all involve a catheter (a flexible tube) that is inserted, often through your leg, and guided through the blood vessels to the blockage. The three procedures are: angioplasty—a balloon is inflated to open the blood vessel; stenting—a small wire tube called a stent is placed in the blood vessel to hold it open; atherectomy—a blade or laser cuts through and removes the blockage. Standards for care say that patients should receive a PCI within 90 minutes of arriving at the hospital. This measure shows what percentage of patients got a PCI within this time period. *Higher percentages are better.*

Statin Prescribed at Discharge
Heart attack patients given a prescription for a statin at discharge.
Statins are drugs used to lower cholesterol. Cholesterol is a fat (also called a lipid) that your body needs to work properly. Cholesterol levels that are too high can increase your chance of getting heart disease, stroke, and other problems. For patients who have had one or more heart attacks and have high cholesterol, taking statins can lower the chance that they'll have another heart attack or die. This measure shows the percent of patients who had a heart attack who got a prescription for a statin upon leaving the hospital. Patients who shouldn't take statins aren't included in this measure. *Higher numbers are better.*

9▶ Heart Failure Care

Scientific evidence shows that the following measures represent the best practices for the treatment of heart failure.

ACE Inhibitor or ARB for LVSD
Heart failure patients given ACE inhibitor or ARB for left ventricular systolic dysfunction (LVSD).
ACE (angiotensin converting enzyme) inhibitors and ARBs (angiotensin receptor blockers) are medicines used to treat patients with heart failure and are particularly beneficial in those patients with decreased function of the left side of the heart. Early treatment with ACE inhibitors and ARBs in patients who have heart failure symptoms or decreased heart function after a heart attack can also reduce their risk of death from future heart attacks. ACE

inhibitors and ARBs work by limiting the effects of a hormone that narrows blood vessels, and may thus lower blood pressure and reduce the work the heart has to perform. Since the ways in which these two kinds of drugs work are different, your doctor will decide which drug is most appropriate for you. Standards for care say that if patients have a heart attack and/or heart failure, they should get a prescription for ACE inhibitors or ARBs if they have decreased heart function before leaving the hospital. *Higher percentages are better.*

Discharge Instructions Given
Heart failure patients given discharge instructions.
Heart failure is a chronic condition. It results in symptoms such as shortness of breath, dizziness, and fatigue. Before you leave the hospital, the staff at the hospital should provide you with information to help you manage the symptoms after you get home. The information should include your information about: activity level (what you can and can't do); diet (what you should, and shouldn't eat or drink); medications; your follow-up appointment; watching your daily weight; and what to do if your symptoms get worse. *Higher percentages are better.*

Evaluation of LVS Function
Heart failure patients given an evaluation of left ventricular systolic (LVS) function.
The proper treatment for heart failure depends on what area of your heart is affected. An important test is to check how your heart is pumping, called an "evaluation of the left ventricular systolic function." It can tell your health care provider whether the left side of your heart is pumping properly. Other ways to check on how your heart is pumping include: your medical history; a physical examination; listening to your heart sounds; and other tests as ordered by a physician (like an ECG (electrocardiogram), chest x-ray, blood work, and an echocardiogram) *Higher percentages are better.*

10 ▶ Medicare Spending

The Medicare Hospital Spending per Patient measure shows whether Medicare spends more, less, or about the same on an episode of care for a Medicare patient treated in a specific hospital compared to how much Medicare spends on an episode of care across all hospitals nationally. This measure includes any Medicare Part A and Part B payments made for services provided to a patient during an episode of care, which includes the 3 days prior to the hospital stay, during the stay, and during the 30 days after discharge from the hospital. This result is a ratio calculated by dividing the amount Medicare spends per patient for an episode of care initiated at this hospital by the median (or middle) amount Medicare spent per episode of care nationally.

- A ratio equal to the national average means that Medicare spends ABOUT THE SAME per patient for an episode of care initiated at this hospital as it does per episode of care across all hospitals nationally.
- A ratio that is more than the national average means that Medicare spends MORE per patient for an episode of care initiated at this hospital than it does per episode of care across all hospitals nationally.
- A ratio that is less than the national average means that Medicare spends LESS per patient for an episode of care initiated at this hospital than it does per episode of care across all hospitals nationally.

11 ▶ Pneumonia Care

Scientific evidence shows that the following measures represent the best practices for the treatment of community-acquired pneumonia.

Appropriate Initial Antibiotic Given
Pneumonia patients given the most appropriate initial antibiotic(s).
Pneumonia is a lung infection that is usually caused by bacteria or a virus. If pneumonia is caused by bacteria, hospitals will treat the infection with antibiotics. Different bacteria are treated with different antibiotics. *Higher percentages are better.*

Blood Culture Timing
Pneumonia patients whose initial emergency room blood culture was performed prior to the administration of the first hospital dose of antibiotics.
Different types of bacteria can cause pneumonia. A blood culture is a test that can help your health care provider identify which bacteria may have caused your pneumonia, and which antibiotic should be prescribed. A blood culture is not always needed, but for patients who are first seen in the hospital emergency department, it is important for the accuracy of the test that a blood culture be conducted before any antibiotics are started. It is also important to start antibiotics as soon as possible. *Higher percentages are better.*

12 ▶ Pregnancy and Delivery Care

Newborn Deliveries Scheduled Early

Percent of newborns whose deliveries were scheduled too early (1-3 weeks early), when a scheduled delivery was not medically necessary.

Guidelines developed by doctors and researchers say it's best to wait until the 39th completed week of pregnancy to deliver your baby because important fetal development takes place in your baby's brain and lungs during the last few weeks of pregnancy. Sometimes women go into early labor on their own, and early deliveries can't be prevented. Sometimes, doctors decide that inducing labor or delivering a baby early by C-section (called "elective delivery") is in the best interest of the mother and the baby. In these cases, early deliveries are medically necessary. However, doctors may also decide to induce labor or deliver babies by C-section early as a convenience to themselves or their patient. This practice is not recommended. Hospitals should work with doctors and patients to avoid early elective deliveries when they are not medically necessary. This measure shows the percent of pregnancy women who had elective deliveries 1-3 weeks early (either vaginally or by C-section) who early deliveries were not medically necessary. Higher numbers may indicate that hospitals aren't doing enough to discourage this unsafe practice. *Lower percentages are better.*

13 ▶ Preventive Care

Hospitals and other healthcare providers play a crucial role in promoting, providing and educating patients about preventive services and screenings and maintaining the health of their communities. Many diseases are preventable through immunizations, screenings, treatment, and lifestyle changes. The information below shows how well the hospitals you selected are providing preventive services.

Immunization for Influenza

Patients assessed and given influenza vaccination.

Influenza, or the "flu," is a respiratory illness that is caused by flu viruses and easily spread from person to person. There are over 200,000 hospitalizations from the flu on average every year. An average of 36,000 Americans die annually due to the flu and its complications. The best way to prevent the flu is to get a flu shot each year during the fall season. Because flu viruses change from year to year, it is important to get a flu shot each year. *Higher percentages are better.*

Immunization for Pneumonia

Patients assessed and given pneumonia vaccination.

Pneumonia is an infection of the lungs that is caused by bacteria or a virus and can spread from person to person. A cold or flu that gets worse can turn into pneumonia. Although antibiotics such as penicillin were once very effective at treating pneumonia, the disease has mutated (changed) so these treatments are not as effective. The best way to prevent pneumonia is to get a flu shot each year (as flu often leads to pneumonia) and frequently washing your hands. Those who are more at risk of getting pneumonia, such as young children, people over the age of 65, people with a chronic illness (such as heart or lung disease or diabetes), or people who have had pneumonia before, should get the pneumonia vaccine. Ask your doctor when the best time to be vaccinated is for you. *Higher percentages are better.*

14 ▶ Stroke Care

Scientific evidence shows that the following measures show some of the standards of stroke care that hospitals should follow, for adults who have had a stroke.

Anticoagulation Therapy for Atrial Fibrillation

Ischemic stroke patients with a type of irregular heartbeat who were given a prescription for a blood thinner at discharge.

Patients admitted with an ischemic stroke who have an irregular heartbeat (also called atrial fibrillation or atrial flutter) are at greater risk of having another stroke. Research suggests that medicine that thins the blood (called an anticoagulant) reduces the chance of another stroke in these patients. This measure shows the percentage of patients admitted with ischemic stroke and an irregular heartbeat (atrial fibrillation/atrial flutter) who were prescribed an anticoagulant before they were discharged from the hospital. *Higher percentages are better.*

Antithrombotic Therapy Timing

Ischemic stroke patients who received medicine known to prevent complications caused by blood clots within 2 days of arriving at the hospital.

Ischemic stroke patients should get medicine known to reduce death, disability and the risk of another stroke (known as Antithrombotic Therapy) while in the hospital. Research shows that hospitals should start this medicine within 2 days of arriving at the hospital to prevent and treat clots and reduce the risk of complications from the stroke. Serious complications caused by strokes include changes in thinking and memory; muscle, joint, and nerve problems; or difficulty swallowing or eating; or blood clots. This measure shows the percentage of patients admitted with an ischemic stroke who got antithrombotic therapy started within 2 days of arriving at the hospital. *Higher percentages are better.*

Assessed for Rehabilitation
Ischemic or hemorrhagic stroke patients who were evaluated for rehabilitation services.
Many ischemic stroke or hemorrhagic stroke patients will experience moderate or severe disability, including problems with physical, speech and mental functions. Stroke rehabilitation can help patients relearn those lost skills and regain independence. Once the stroke symptoms and related problems are under control, the hospital appropriate health care professionals should review the status of the patient and begin rehabilitation as soon as possible. Appropriate health care professionals include physicians, physical therapists, occupational therapists, speech and language therapists, and/or neuropsychologist. The earlier the patient starts rehabilitation, the better the recovery process. Patients who need stroke rehabilitation may begin while they are still at the hospital and continue in a rehabilitation setting that is right for the patient. These options include inpatient rehabilitation units (either stand-alone or part of a hospital/clinic), outpatient units (usually part of a hospital/clinic), nursing home, or home-based programs. This measure shows the percentage of patients admitted with an ischemic stroke or a hemorrhagic stroke who were evaluated for their need for rehabilitation services. *Higher percentages are better.*

Discharged on Antithrombotic Therapy
Ischemic stroke patients who received a prescription for medicine known to prevent complications caused by blood clots before discharge.
Patients admitted with an ischemic stroke are at risk for developing complications like another stroke even after discharge. These patients should get a prescription at discharge for a blood thinner that prevents complications like another stroke (called Antithrombotic Therapy.) Serious complications caused by strokes include changes in thinking and memory; muscle, joint, and nerve problems; or difficulty swallowing or eating; or blood clots. This measure shows the percentage of patients who were admitted with an ischemic stroke who were given a prescription for an antithrombotic before they were discharged from the hospital. *Higher percentages are better.*

Discharged on Statin Medication
Ischemic stroke patients needing medicine to lower cholesterol, who were given a prescription for this medicine before discharge.
Cholesterol is a fat (also called a lipid) that the body needs to work properly. Levels of bad cholesterol (LDL) that are too high can increase the chance of stroke, heart disease, and other problems. Medicines called statins can help lower LDL cholesterol levels. In patients with ischemic stroke who have high cholesterol, taking statins can help lower the chance of another stroke. This measure shows the percentage of patients admitted with an ischemic stroke who got a prescription for a statin before they were discharged from the hospital. Patients who shouldn't take statins are not included in this measure. *Higher percentages are better.*

Thrombolytic Therapy Timing
Ischemic stroke patients who got medicine to break up a blood clot within 3 hours after symptoms started.
Patients with ischemic stroke should get medicine called tissue plasminogen activator, or t-PA, to break up a blood clot within 3 hours after their symptoms start. T-PA is a kind of thrombolytic therapy. Research shows that hospitals that give t-PA within 3 hours after symptoms start can limit the damage and disability caused by an ischemic stroke. This measure shows the percentage of patients admitted with ischemic stroke who arrived in the emergency department (ED) within 2 hours of the onset of their symptoms and who got t-PA within three hours after the onset of their symptoms. *Higher percentages are better.*

Venous Thromboembolism Prophylaxis
Ischemic or hemorrhagic stroke patients who received treatment to keep blood clots from forming anywhere in the body within 2 days of arriving at the hospital.
Patients admitted to the hospital with ischemic stroke or hemorrhagic stroke are at increased risk of developing new blood clots in their veins that break off and travel to other parts of the body, like the brain or lung (also called venous thromboembolism). Research shows that hospitals should begin treatment to prevent new blood clots on the day of or day after these patients are arrived at the hospital. Treatment can include medicine, medical devices, or tightly fitting stockings designed to keep blood from clotting. This measure shows the percentage of patients admitted with an ischemic stroke or hemorrhagic stroke who either received treatment to prevent blood clots on the day of or day after arrival at the hospital or had paperwork in their chart to explain why they had not received this treatment. *Higher percentages are better.*

Written Stroke Educational Materials Given
Ischemic or hemorrhagic stroke patients or caregivers who received written educational materials about stroke care and prevention during the hospital stay.
Educating patients with ischemic stroke and hemorrhagic stroke and their caregivers about stroke care and prevention helps patients live healthier lives and reduces health care costs. During the hospital stay, hospital staff should give stroke patients and caregivers written information on: how to activate the hospital emergency system; the importance of doing follow-up after being released from the hospital; medicines prescribed at discharge;

what increases the chance of stroke; warning signs and symptoms of stroke. This measure shows the percentage of patients with an ischemic stroke or a hemorrhagic stroke or their caregivers who received written information about these topics during their hospital stay. *Higher percentages are better.*

15 ▶ Surgical Care Improvement Project

Scientific evidence shows that the following measures represent the best practices for preventing complications after certain surgeries: colon surgery, hip replacement, knee replacement, abdominal and vaginal hysterectomy, cardiac surgery- including coronary artery bypass grafts (CABG), and vascular surgery.

Appropriate Beta Blocker Usage
Surgery patients who were taking heart drugs called beta blockers before coming to the hospital, who were kept on the beta blockers during the period just before and after their surgery.
It is often standard procedure to stop taking usual medications for a while before and after surgery. But if patients who have been taking beta blockers suddenly stop taking them, they can have heart problems such as a fast heartbeat. For these patients, staying on beta blockers before and after surgery makes it less likely that they will have heart problems. This measure shows the percentage of patients who remained on beta blockers within this time period. *Higher percentages are better.*

Appropriate VTP Within 24 Hours
Patients who got treatment (venous thromboembolism prevention) at the right time (within 24 hours before or after their surgery) to help prevent blood clots after certain types of surgery.
Many factors influence a surgery patient's risk of developing a blood clot, including the type of surgery. When patients stay still for a long time after some types of surgery, they are more likely to develop a blood clot in the veins of the legs, thighs, or pelvis. A blood clot slows down the flow of blood, causing swelling, redness, and pain. A blood clot can also break off and travel to other parts of the body. If the blood clot gets into the lung, it is a serious problem that can sometimes cause death. Doctors can order treatments including blood-thinning medications, elastic support stockings, or mechanical air stockings that help with blood flow in the legs. These treatments need to be started at the right time, which is typically during the period that begins 24 hours before surgery and ends 24 hours after surgery. This measure shows the percentage of patients who received these treatments this time period. *Higher percentages are better.*

Controlled Postoperative Blood Glucose
Heart surgery patients whose blood sugar (blood glucose) is kept under good control in the days right after surgery.
Even if heart surgery patients do not have diabetes, keeping blood sugar under good control (200 mg/dL or less) after surgery lowers the risk of infection and other problems. This measure shows the percentage of patients who had their blood sugar kept under good control in the days right after surgery. *Higher percentages are better.*

Perioperative Temperature Management
Patients having surgery who were actively warmed in the operating room or whose body temperature was near normal by the end of surgery.
Hospitals can prevent surgical wound infections and other complications by keeping the patient's body temperature near normal during surgery. Medical research has shown that patients whose body temperatures drop during surgery have a greater risk of infection and their wounds may not heal as quickly. Standards of care say that patients should have their body temperature normal or near normal during the time period 30 minutes before the end of surgery to 15 minutes after anesthesia ended. This measure shows the percent of patients whose body temperature was normal or near normal within this time period. *Higher percentages are better.*

Prophylactic Antibiotic Selection
Surgery patients who were given the right kind of antibiotic to help prevent infection.
Surgical wound infections can be prevented. Medical research has shown that certain antibiotics work better to prevent wound infections for certain types of surgery. This measure shows the percentage of surgery patients who were given the right antibiotic during surgery. *Higher percentages are better.*

Prophylactic Antibiotic Selection (Outpatient)
Outpatients having surgery who got the right kind of antibiotic.
Hospitals can prevent surgical wound infections. Medical research has shown that certain antibiotics work better to prevent wound infections for certain types of surgery. Hospital staff should make sure patients get the antibiotic that works best for their type of surgery. This measure shows the percentage of patients who got the right antibiotic during surgery. *Higher percentages are better.*

Prophylactic Antibiotic Stopped
Surgery patients whose preventive antibiotics were stopped at the right time (within 24 hours after surgery).
Antibiotics are often given to patients before surgery to prevent infection. Taking these antibiotics for more than 24 hours after routine surgery is usually not necessary. Continuing the medication longer than necessary can in-

crease the risk of side effects such as stomach aches and serious types of diarrhea. Also, when antibiotics are used for too long, patients can develop resistance to them and the antibiotics won't work as well. This measure shows the percentage of patients who stopped getting preventive antibiotics within this time period. *Higher percentages are better.*

Prophylactic Antibiotic Timing
Surgery patients who were given an antibiotic at the right time (within one hour before surgery) to help prevent infection.
Surgical wound infections can be prevented. Medical research shows that surgery patients who get antibiotics within the hour before their surgery are less likely to get wound infections. Getting an antibiotic earlier, or after surgery begins, is not as effective. Hospital staff should make sure surgery patients get antibiotics at the right time. This measure shows the percentage of patients who got an antibiotic to prevent infection in this time period. *Higher percentages are better.*

Prophylactic Antibiotic Timing (Outpatient)
Outpatients having surgery who got an antibiotic at the right time (within one hour before surgery).
Hospitals can prevent surgical wound infections. Standards for care say that surgery patients who get antibiotics within an hour of their surgery are less likely to get wound infections. Getting an antibiotic earlier, or after surgery begins, is not as effective. This measure shows the percentage of patients who got an antibiotic in this time period. *Higher percentages are better.*

Urinary Catheter Removal
Surgery patients whose urinary catheters were removed on the first or second day after surgery.
Sometimes surgical patients need to have a urinary catheter, or thin tube, inserted into their bladder to help drain the urine. Catheters are usually attached to a bag that collects the urine. Surgery patients can develop infections when urinary catheters are left in place too long after surgery. Standards of care say that most surgery patients should have their urinary catheters removed within 2 days after surgery to help prevent infection. This measure shows the percent of surgery patients whose urinary catheters were removed on the first or second day after surgery. *Higher percentages are better.*

16▶ Survey of Patients' Hospital Experiences

The HCAHPS (Hospital Consumer Assessment of Healthcare Providers and Systems) Survey, also known as the CAHPS® Hospital Survey or Hospital CAHPS®, is a standardized survey instrument and data collection methodology that has been in use since 2006 to measure patients' perspectives of hospital care. A partnership of public and private organizations led by the Federal government, specifically the Centers for Medicare & Medicaid Services (CMS) and the Agency for Healthcare Research and Quality (AHRQ), created HCAHPS (pronounced "H-caps") to publicly report the patient's perspective of hospital care. The HCAHPS results posted on Hospital Compare allow consumers to make fair and objective comparisons between hospitals and with state and national averages, on important measures of patients' perspectives of care. For more on HCAHPS information, please visit the official HCAHPS website: www.hcahpsonline.org

The HCAHPS survey asks patients to give feedback about topics for which they are the best source of information. The survey asks patients to answer questions about their experiences in the hospital. To make sure the HCAHPS survey data is meaningful; patients only answer questions about topics with which they have experience. The HCAHPS survey asks patients to answer questions related to ten topics. The topics and questions are listed in the table below. Answers shown in italics are included in this publication.

Measure as it Appears in CGAH	HCAHPS Topic Text	HCAHPS Answer Description
Would Definitely Recommend Hospital	How do patients rate the hospital overall?	*Patients who gave a rating of 9 or 10 (high)*
		Patients who gave a rating of 7 or 8 (medium)
		Patients who gave a rating of 6 or lower (low)
Doctors 'Always' Communicated Well	How often did doctors communicate well with patients?	*Doctors always communicated well*
		Doctors usually communicated well
		Doctors sometimes or never communicated well
Nurses 'Always' Communicated Well	How often did nurses communicate well with patients?	*Nurses always communicated well*
		Nurses usually communicated well
		Nurses sometimes or never communicated well
Timely Help 'Always' Received	How often did patients receive help quickly from hospital staff?	*Patients always received help as soon as they wanted*
		Patients usually received help as soon as they wanted
		Patients sometimes or never received help as soon as they wanted

Measure as it Appears in CGAH	HCAHPS Topic Text	HCAHPS Answer Description
Meds 'Always' Explained Before Given	How often did staff explain about medicines before giving them to patients?	*Staff always explained*
		Staff usually explained
		Staff sometimes or never explained
Pain 'Always' Well Controlled	How often was patients' pain well controlled?	*Pain was always well controlled*
		Pain was usually well controlled
		Pain was sometimes or never well controlled
Area Around Room 'Always' Quiet at Night	How often was the area around patients' rooms kept quiet at night?	*Always quiet at night*
		Usually quiet at night
		Sometimes or never quiet at night
Room and Bathroom 'Always' Clean	How often were the patients' rooms and bathrooms kept clean?	*Room was always clean*
		Room was usually clean
		Room was sometimes or never clean
Home Recovery Information Given	Were patients given information about what to do during their recovery at home?	*YES, staff did give patients this information*
		NO, staff did not give patients this information
Would Definitely Recommend Hospital	Would patients recommend the hospital to friends and family?	*YES, patients would definitely recommend the hospital*
		YES, patients would probably recommend the hospital
		NO, patients would not recommend the hospital (they probably would not or definitely would not recommend it)

17 ▶ Use of Medical Imaging

"Medical imaging" tests create images of various parts of the body to screen for or diagnose medical conditions. Examples of medical imaging include CT scans, MRIs, and mammograms.

Cardiac Imaging Stress Test before Surgery

Outpatients who got cardiac imaging stress tests before low-risk outpatient surgery.
A cardiac stress test measures the heart's ability to respond when it is stressed, and can be useful in evaluating a patient's surgical risk. Experts agree, however, that these tests are not necessary before most low-risk outpatient surgical procedures, such as colonoscopies, cataract surgery, biopsies, or endoscopies (using an instrument to look inside the body) because these procedures put very little stress on the heart. Patients with certain risk factors that increase the likelihood of having complications are not included in the measure. This measure shows the percentage of all cardiac stress tests done in a hospital outpatient imaging department (using echocardiograms, CT scans, and MRIs) for Medicare patients who were going to have certain low-risk outpatient surgical procedures. Hospital outpatient imaging departments that have higher percentages on this measure may be giving people more tests than they need. *Hospitals that are rated well will have lower percentages.* If a percentage is high, it may mean that the facility is doing unnecessary cardiac imaging before some low-risk surgeries.

Combination Abdominal CT Scan

Outpatient CT scans of the abdomen that were "combination" (double) scans.
A CT scan (also called a CAT scan) uses multiple X-rays to produce detailed pictures of the inside of the body (bones, organs, and other body parts). For some, a substance called "contrast" is put into the patient's body before the scan begins, which help make parts of the body stand out more clearly. Contrast can be either swallowed or injected into a vein. Risks of contrast include possible harm to the kidneys or allergic reactions. Contrast shouldn't be used if it isn't needed. "Combination" CT scan means that the patient gets two CT scans—one scan without contrast, followed by a second scan with contrast. Standards of quality care say that most patients who are getting a CT scan of the chest should be given a single CT scan rather than a "combination" CT scan. Although combination CT scans are appropriate for some parts of the body and for some medical conditions, combination scans are usually not appropriate for the chest. The range for these measures is from 0% to 100%. For hospitals with higher percentages, it may mean that the facility is routinely giving patients combination CT scans of the chest or abdomen when a single scan is all they need. Giving patients two scans when they only need one needlessly doubles their exposure to radiation: Radiation exposure from a single CT scan of the chest is about 350 times higher than for an ordinary chest X-ray. For combination CT scans, radiation exposure is 700 times higher than for a chest X-ray because the patient is given two scans. For a combination CT scan, radiation exposure is 22 times higher than for an X-ray of the abdomen because the patient is given two scans. Radiation exposure from a single CT scan of the abdomen is about 11 times higher than for an ordinary X-ray of the abdomen. When contrast is used, there are risks that can include possible harm to the kidneys or allergic reactions (especially if the contrast is injected). To avoid unnecessary risk, contrast should be used only when it is needed. If you need to have a CT scan of the chest or abdomen, feel free to ask your doctor these questions to determine

what's best for your medical condition: Do you need a single scan—either with or without contrast—or is a combination scan necessary? Is using contrast appropriate for your medical condition? *Hospitals that are rated well will have lower percentages.* If a percentage is high, it may mean that the facility is doing unnecessary double/combination scans.

Combination Brain/Sinus CT Scan
Outpatients with brain CT scans who got a sinus CT scan at the same time.
Brain CTs and sinus CTs can be important tools for diagnosing problems that may be causing severe headaches or chronic sinus infections, but they also expose patients to high levels of radiation. Brain CT scans cover large parts of the sinuses, so ordering both tests may be unnecessary. For patients with chronic sinusitis, a sinus CT is usually done first before deciding if a brain CT is also needed. Experts do not recommend doing both tests at once, unless patients have head injuries or tumors. Hospital outpatient imaging departments that have higher percentages on this measure may be giving people more tests than they need, exposing them to too much radiation. This measure shows the percentage of brain CT scans done in a hospital outpatient imaging department where a sinus CT scan was done at the same time on the same Medicare patient. It does not count cases where doctors had questions about complications due to injuries, cancer, or serious infections. *Hospitals that are rated well will have lower percentages.* If a percentage is high, it may mean that the facility is doing unnecessary scans.

Combination Chest CT Scan
Outpatient CT scans of the chest that were "combination" (double) scans.
A CT scan (also called a CAT scan) uses multiple X-rays to produce detailed pictures of the inside of the body (bones, organs, and other body parts). For some, a substance called "contrast" is put into the patient's body before the scan begins, which help make parts of the body stand out more clearly. Contrast can be either swallowed or injected into a vein. Risks of contrast include possible harm to the kidneys or allergic reactions. Contrast shouldn't be used if it isn't needed. "Combination" CT scan means that the patient gets two CT scans—one scan without contrast, followed by a second scan with contrast. Standards of quality care say that most patients who are getting a CT scan of the chest should be given a single CT scan rather than a "combination" CT scan. Although combination CT scans are appropriate for some parts of the body and for some medical conditions, combination scans are usually not appropriate for the chest. The range for these measures is from 0% to 100%. For hospitals with higher percentages, it may mean that the facility is routinely giving patients combination CT scans of the chest or abdomen when a single scan is all they need. Giving patients two scans when they only need one needlessly doubles their exposure to radiation. Radiation exposure from a single CT scan of the chest is about 350 times higher than for an ordinary chest X-ray. For combination CT scans, radiation exposure is 700 times higher than for a chest X-ray because the patient is given two scans. For a combination CT scan, radiation exposure is 22 times higher than for an X-ray of the abdomen because the patient is given two scans. Radiation exposure from a single CT scan of the abdomen is about 11 times higher than for an ordinary X-ray of the abdomen. When contrast is used, there are risks that can include possible harm to the kidneys or allergic reactions (especially if the contrast is injected). To avoid unnecessary risk, contrast should be used only when it is needed. If you need to have a CT scan of the chest or abdomen, feel free to ask your doctor these questions to determine what's best for your medical condition: Do you need a single scan - either with or without contrast - or is a combination scan necessary? Is using contrast appropriate for your medical condition? *Hospitals that are rated well will have lower percentages.* If a percentage is high, it may mean that the facility is doing unnecessary double/combination scans.

Follow-up Mammogram/Ultrasound
Outpatients who had a follow-up mammogram, ultrasound, or MRI of the breast within 45 days after a screening mammogram.
A screening mammogram is an X-ray of the breast to check for possible breast cancer before it can be detected by women or health care professionals. Although mammography is a good test, it is not perfect. Some women who do not have breast cancer will have an abnormal mammogram (even though they are cancer free), and some women with breast cancer will have a normal screening mammogram (their cancer is missed). Some women may be asked to come back for follow-up testing if there are signs of possible breast cancer. A follow-up visit usually means having more tests (mammograms, an ultrasound, and/or an MRI of the breast). The numbers of women asked to follow-up varies widely among mammography facilities in the United States. There are many reasons for differences in follow-up rates including poor technique (blurry X-rays that need to be repeated), a lack of skill or experience interpreting the screening mammograms, medical history of the woman undergoing screening, and whether a woman is being screened for the first time or has previously undergone mammography screening. The follow-up rates reported here for mammography facilities include follow-up exams performed on the same day as screening mammograms, as well as those performed up to 45 days later. Medical evidence suggests that there may be a problem if a facility has either a very low or very high rate of follow-ups. *Although values for a very low follow-up rate have not been established, a follow-up rate near zero may indicate a facility that misses signs of cancer. Follow-up rates around 9% are typical. Research has established that a follow-up rate above 14% is not appropriate, and may indicate a facility doing unnecessary follow up.* If you have a screening

mammogram and you are called back for additional testing, ask your doctor why and what this additional testing means in your case for how he or she makes an accurate diagnosis.

Lumbar Spine MRI for Low Back Pain

Outpatients with low back pain who had an MRI without trying recommended treatments first, such as physical therapy.

An MRI (magnetic resonance imaging) is a test that uses a powerful magnetic field and a computer to produce detailed pictures of the inside of the body (bones, organs, and other body parts). Although MRI scans can be helpful for diagnosing low back pain, they can also be used too much. Low back pain can improve or go away within six weeks and an MRI may not be needed. Standards of care say that most patients with low back pain should start with treatment such as physical therapy or chiropractic care, and have an MRI only if the treatment doesn't help. Finding out whether treatment helps or not before having an MRI can be a safe and effective way to avoid unnecessary stress, risk, or cost of doing an MRI. For patients with certain conditions, getting an MRI right away is appropriate care. Patients with these conditions are not included in this measure. If you have low back pain, you, your doctor, and the medical imaging facility staff can talk about the best time to do an MRI if you need one. Since MRIs use magnets rather than x-rays, there is no radiation risk. However, because the magnets attract some kinds of metal, it's important for the technician to know if there are any metal objects or implants inside your body, such as pacemakers, artificial joints, screws, stents, plates, or staples. Metal objects can pose serious risk to you during the MRI and interfere with the test. For some MRIs, a substance called "contrast" is injected before the test to make parts of the body stand out more clearly on the images. Risks of contrast include possible harm to the kidneys or allergic reactions. Contrast shouldn't be used if it isn't needed. Having the test can be stressful for some people. Patients must hold still for about 15 to 45 minutes while lying on a table that moves inside a large scanning machine. While images are being taken, the machine makes loud noises. *Hospitals that are rated well will have lower percentages.* If a percentage is high, it may mean that the facility is doing unnecessary MRIs for low back pain.

Blood Clot Prevention and Treatment

Anticoagulation Overlap Therapy

Hospital Name	City	Rate	Cases
Flowers Hospital[2]	Dothan	100%	52
Saint Vincent's East[2]	Birmingham	100%	118
South Baldwin Regional Medical Center[2]	Foley	100%	110
Trinity Medical Center[2]	Birmingham	100%	74
Baptist Medical Center South[2]	Montgomery	99%	67
Huntsville Hospital[2]	Huntsville	99%	245
Crestwood Medical Center[2]	Huntsville	98%	54
Cullman Regional Medical Center[2]	Cullman	98%	43
Univ of S Alabama Med Ctr[2]	Mobile	98%	43
Vaughan Reg Med Ctr Parkway Campus[2]	Selma	98%	65
Baptist Medical Center - Princeton[2]	Birmingham	97%	99
Coosa Valley Medical Center[2]	Sylacauga	97%	39
D C H Regional Medical Center[2]	Tuscaloosa	97%	233
Brookwood Medical Center[2]	Birmingham	96%	110
Saint Vincent's Birmingham[2]	Birmingham	96%	142
Springhill Medical Center[2]	Mobile	96%	76
Marshall Medical Center South[2]	Boaz	95%	55
Shelby Baptist Medical Center[2]	Alabaster	95%	77
University of Alabama Hospital[2]	Birmingham	95%	226
Walker Baptist Medical Center[2]	Jasper	95%	44
Stringfellow Memorial Hospital[2]	Anniston	93%	29
Mobile Infirmary[2]	Mobile	92%	230
Helen Keller Memorial Hospital[2]	Sheffield	91%	32
Eliza Coffee Memorial Hospital[2]	Florence	89%	71
Providence Hospital[2]	Mobile	89%	121
Medical West[2]	Bessemer	88%	49
Thomas Hospital[2]	Fairhope	87%	91
Baptist Medical Center East[2]	Montgomery	85%	39
Southeast Alabama Medical Center[2]	Dothan	85%	117
Gadsden Regional Medical Center[2]	Gadsden	84%	80
Athens - Limestone Hospital[2]	Athens	83%	41
East Alabama Medical Center[2]	Opelika	83%	87
Saint Vincent's Saint Clair[2]	Pell City	72%	39
Jackson Hospital & Clinic[2]	Montgomery	71%	34
Decatur Morgan Hospital - Decatur Campus[2]	Decatur	62%	42
Riverview Regional Medical Center[2]	Gadsden	52%	40
Northeast Alabama Regional Medical Center[2]	Anniston	51%	85

ICU Venous Thromboembolism Prophylaxis

Hospital Name	City	Rate	Cases
Coosa Valley Medical Center[2]	Sylacauga	100%	101
Dale Medical Center[2]	Ozark	100%	66
Flowers Hospital[2]	Dothan	100%	127
Medical Center Enterprise[2]	Enterprise	100%	69
Russellville Hospital[2]	Russellville	100%	57
South Baldwin Regional Medical Center[2]	Foley	100%	74
Trinity Medical Center[2]	Birmingham	100%	181
Univ of S Alabama Med Ctr[2]	Mobile	100%	85
L V Stabler Memorial Hospital[2]	Greenville	99%	138
Vaughan Reg Med Ctr Parkway Campus[2]	Selma	99%	158
Helen Keller Memorial Hospital[2]	Sheffield	97%	62
Cullman Regional Medical Center[2]	Cullman	96%	57
Marion Regional Medical Center[2]	Hamilton	96%	27
Baptist Medical Center - Princeton[2]	Birmingham	95%	151
Dekalb Regional Medical Center[2]	Fort Payne	95%	96
Medical Center Barbour[2]	Eufaula	95%	173
Walker Baptist Medical Center[2]	Jasper	95%	106
Crestwood Medical Center[2]	Huntsville	94%	67
Southeast Alabama Medical Center[2]	Dothan	94%	85
D C H Regional Medical Center[2]	Tuscaloosa	92%	92
Lawrence Medical Center[2]	Moulton	92%	25
Shelby Baptist Medical Center[2]	Alabaster	92%	123
University of Alabama Hospital[2]	Birmingham	92%	93
George H. Lanier Memorial Hospital[2]	Valley	91%	32
Huntsville Hospital[2]	Huntsville	91%	116
Citizens Baptist Medical Center[2]	Talladega	90%	69
Troy Regional Medical Center[2]	Troy	90%	41
Andalusia Regional Hospital[2]	Andalusia	89%	61
North Baldwin Infirmary[2]	Bay Minette	89%	28
Russell Hospital[2]	Alexander City	89%	70
Springhill Medical Center[2]	Mobile	89%	101
East Alabama Medical Center[2]	Opelika	88%	88
Mobile Infirmary[2]	Mobile	88%	97
Stringfellow Memorial Hospital[2]	Anniston	88%	65
Athens - Limestone Hospital[2]	Athens	86%	71
Providence Hospital[2]	Mobile	86%	119
Saint Vincent's East[2]	Birmingham	86%	100
Atmore Community Hospital[2]	Atmore	83%	47
Decatur Morgan Hospital - Parkway Campus[2]	Decatur	83%	66
Eliza Coffee Memorial Hospital[2]	Florence	83%	129
Northeast Alabama Regional Medical Center[2]	Anniston	83%	82
Medical West[2]	Bessemer	81%	103
Thomas Hospital[2]	Fairhope	81%	78
Monroe County Hospital[2]	Monroeville	80%	40
Jack Hughston Memorial Hospital[2]	Phenix City	79%	34
Shoals Hospital[2]	Muscle Shoals	79%	42
Gadsden Regional Medical Center[2]	Gadsden	78%	147
Jackson Hospital & Clinic[2]	Montgomery	78%	93
Community Hospital[2]	Tallassee	77%	88
Brookwood Medical Center[2]	Birmingham	76%	108
D W Mcmillan Memorial Hospital[2]	Brewton	76%	83
Marshall Medical Center South[2]	Boaz	76%	85
Saint Vincent's Birmingham[2]	Birmingham	76%	99
Highlands Medical Center[2]	Scottsboro	72%	47
Decatur Morgan Hospital - Decatur Campus[2]	Decatur	71%	82
Baptist Medical Center South[2]	Montgomery	68%	107
Prattville Baptist Hospital[2]	Prattville	68%	57
Saint Vincent's Saint Clair[2]	Pell City	65%	51
Baptist Medical Center East[2]	Montgomery	61%	64
Mizell Memorial Hospital[2]	Opp	57%	46
Riverview Regional Medical Center[2]	Gadsden	51%	83
Clay County Hospital[2]	Ashland	39%	75
Jacksonville Medical Center[2]	Jacksonville	36%	25
Bryan W Whitfield Memorial Hospital[2]	Demopolis	23%	83
Wiregrass Medical Center[2]	Geneva	20%	41

Incidence of Potentially Preventable VTE

Hospital Name	City	Rate	Cases
Baptist Medical Center - Princeton[2]	Birmingham	0%	41
Saint Vincent's Birmingham[2]	Birmingham	3%	31
University of Alabama Hospital[2]	Birmingham	3%	124
Trinity Medical Center[2]	Birmingham	4%	26
Huntsville Hospital[2]	Huntsville	10%	60
Brookwood Medical Center[2]	Birmingham	13%	30
Mobile Infirmary[2]	Mobile	15%	100
Providence Hospital[2]	Mobile	18%	33
Northeast Alabama Regional Medical Center[2]	Anniston	36%	39
D C H Regional Medical Center[2]	Tuscaloosa	45%	84

UFH with Dosages/Platelet Count Monitoring

Hospital Name	City	Rate	Cases
Baptist Medical Center - Princeton[2]	Birmingham	100%	102
Brookwood Medical Center[2]	Birmingham	100%	31
D C H Regional Medical Center[2]	Tuscaloosa	100%	99
Gadsden Regional Medical Center[2]	Gadsden	100%	66
Huntsville Hospital[2]	Huntsville	100%	147
Mobile Infirmary[2]	Mobile	100%	39
Riverview Regional Medical Center[2]	Gadsden	100%	28
Saint Vincent's Birmingham[2]	Birmingham	100%	35
Saint Vincent's East[2]	Birmingham	100%	106
Shelby Baptist Medical Center[2]	Alabaster	100%	83
Trinity Medical Center[2]	Birmingham	100%	32
University of Alabama Hospital[2]	Birmingham	100%	110
Vaughan Reg Med Ctr Parkway Campus[2]	Selma	100%	53
Eliza Coffee Memorial Hospital[2]	Florence	98%	41
Saint Vincent's Saint Clair[2]	Pell City	96%	26
Northeast Alabama Regional Medical Center[2]	Anniston	3%	58

Venous Thromboembolism Prophylaxis

Hospital Name	City	Rate	Cases
Flowers Hospital[2]	Dothan	100%	344
Jackson Medical Center[2]	Jackson	100%	155
Russellville Hospital[2]	Russellville	100%	192
South Baldwin Regional Medical Center[2]	Foley	100%	414
Univ of S Alabama Med Ctr[2]	Mobile	100%	298
Coosa Valley Medical Center[2]	Sylacauga	99%	418
Cullman Regional Medical Center[2]	Cullman	98%	448
Dale Medical Center[2]	Ozark	98%	221
Dekalb Regional Medical Center[2]	Fort Payne	98%	209
L V Stabler Memorial Hospital[2]	Greenville	98%	191
Medical Center Enterprise[2]	Enterprise	98%	256
Trinity Medical Center[2]	Birmingham	98%	324
Crestwood Medical Center[2]	Huntsville	96%	356
Northwest Medical Center[2]	Winfield	96%	165
Vaughan Reg Med Ctr Parkway Campus[2]	Selma	96%	293
Crenshaw Community Hospital[2]	Luverne	95%	133
Walker Baptist Medical Center[2]	Jasper	95%	306
D C H Regional Medical Center[2]	Tuscaloosa	94%	344
Andalusia Regional Hospital[2]	Andalusia	93%	198
Jack Hughston Memorial Hospital[2]	Phenix City	92%	118
Marion Regional Medical Center[2]	Hamilton	92%	96
Lakeland Community Hospital[2]	Haleyville	91%	176
Troy Regional Medical Center[2]	Troy	91%	149
Medical Center Barbour[2]	Eufaula	90%	466
Lawrence Medical Center[2]	Moulton	89%	98
Cherokee Medical Center[2]	Centre	88%	315
Baptist Medical Center - Princeton[2]	Birmingham	87%	280
Russell Hospital[2]	Alexander City	87%	209
Highlands Medical Center[2]	Scottsboro	85%	318
Helen Keller Memorial Hospital[2]	Sheffield	83%	333
Shelby Baptist Medical Center[2]	Alabaster	83%	318
Thomas Hospital[2]	Fairhope	83%	293
University of Alabama Hospital[2]	Birmingham	83%	318
Georgiana Medical Center[2]	Georgiana	82%	116
Jackson Hospital & Clinic[2]	Montgomery	82%	334
Springhill Medical Center[2]	Mobile	82%	359
Athens - Limestone Hospital[2]	Athens	81%	320
Southeast Alabama Medical Center[2]	Dothan	81%	337
Atmore Community Hospital[2]	Atmore	79%	144
Huntsville Hospital[2]	Huntsville	79%	301
Baptist Medical Center South[2]	Montgomery	78%	255
Mobile Infirmary[2]	Mobile	78%	354
North Baldwin Infirmary[2]	Bay Minette	77%	138
Eliza Coffee Memorial Hospital[2]	Florence	75%	284
Gadsden Regional Medical Center[2]	Gadsden	75%	379
Medical West[2]	Bessemer	75%	371
Brookwood Medical Center[2]	Birmingham	74%	270
Providence Hospital[2]	Mobile	74%	307
Saint Vincent's East[2]	Birmingham	73%	263
Hale County Hospital	Greensboro	72%	178
Prattville Baptist Hospital[2]	Prattville	70%	273
Monroe County Hospital[2]	Monroeville	69%	61
Washington County Hospital[2]	Chatom	69%	111
Decatur Morgan Hospital - Parkway Campus[2]	Decatur	68%	125
Shoals Hospital[2]	Muscle Shoals	68%	142
Citizens Baptist Medical Center[2]	Talladega	65%	209
Community Hospital[2]	Tallassee	65%	231
Pickens County Medical Center[2]	Carrollton	64%	100
Saint Vincent's Birmingham[2]	Birmingham	64%	284
D W Mcmillan Memorial Hospital[2]	Brewton	63%	201
Decatur Morgan Hospital - Decatur Campus[2]	Decatur	63%	318
East Alabama Medical Center[2]	Opelika	63%	316
Fayette Medical Center[2]	Fayette	63%	131
Mizell Memorial Hospital[2]	Opp	62%	242
Stringfellow Memorial Hospital[2]	Anniston	62%	305
Baptist Medical Center East[2]	Montgomery	61%	356
Elmore Community Hospital[2]	Wetumpka	58%	204
Northeast Alabama Regional Medical Center[2]	Anniston	56%	452
George H. Lanier Memorial Hospital[2]	Valley	55%	223
Marshall Medical Center South[2]	Boaz	55%	289
Wedowee Hospital[2]	Wedowee	55%	355
Bibb Medical Center[2]	Centreville	44%	144
Saint Vincent's Saint Clair[2]	Pell City	44%	204
Grove Hill Memorial Hospital[2]	Grove Hill	43%	157
Jacksonville Medical Center[2]	Jacksonville	39%	122
Lake Martin Community Hospital[2]	Dadeville	33%	147
Riverview Regional Medical Center[2]	Gadsden	28%	388
Clay County Hospital[2]	Ashland	26%	109
Evergreen Medical Center[2]	Evergreen	26%	263
Hill Hospital of Sumter County[2]	York	18%	110
Greene County Hospital[2]	Eutaw	17%	167
Bullock County Hospital[2]	Union Springs	14%	78
J Paul Jones Hospital[2]	Camden	11%	114
Wiregrass Medical Center[2]	Geneva	10%	146
Bryan W Whitfield Memorial Hospital[2]	Demopolis	7%	236
Florala Memorial Hospital[2,3]	Florala	6%	34
Callahan Eye Hospital[3]	Birmingham	0%	30

Warfarin Therapy Discharge Instructions

Hospital Name	City	Rate	Cases
Brookwood Medical Center[2]	Birmingham	100%	75
Crestwood Medical Center[2]	Huntsville	100%	44
Cullman Regional Medical Center[2]	Cullman	100%	35
Flowers Hospital[2]	Dothan	100%	41
South Baldwin Regional Medical Center[2]	Foley	100%	88
Springhill Medical Center[2]	Mobile	100%	68
Trinity Medical Center[2]	Birmingham	100%	54
Vaughan Reg Med Ctr Parkway Campus[2]	Selma	100%	44
Athens - Limestone Hospital[2]	Athens	94%	31
Gadsden Regional Medical Center[2]	Gadsden	94%	50
Univ of S Alabama Med Ctr[2]	Mobile	93%	30
Marshall Medical Center South[2]	Boaz	92%	40
D C H Regional Medical Center[2]	Tuscaloosa	88%	165
East Alabama Medical Center[2]	Opelika	87%	62
Eliza Coffee Memorial Hospital[2]	Florence	86%	50
Riverview Regional Medical Center[2]	Gadsden	86%	28
Saint Vincent's Birmingham[2]	Birmingham	85%	103
Huntsville Hospital[2]	Huntsville	84%	183
Saint Vincent's East[2]	Birmingham	84%	63
University of Alabama Hospital[2]	Birmingham	83%	189
Baptist Medical Center - Princeton[2]	Birmingham	81%	59
Baptist Medical Center South[2]	Montgomery	80%	45
Shelby Baptist Medical Center[2]	Alabaster	80%	55
Medical West[2]	Bessemer	79%	28
Providence Hospital[2]	Mobile	58%	89
Thomas Hospital[2]	Fairhope	47%	74
Mobile Infirmary[2]	Mobile	31%	182
Northeast Alabama Regional Medical Center[2]	Anniston	20%	56
Southeast Alabama Medical Center[2]	Dothan	2%	94

Chest Pain/Possible Heart Attack Care

Aspirin Given Within 24 Hours of Arrival

Hospital Name	City	Rate	Cases
Cherokee Medical Center	Centre	100%	40
Community Hospital	Tallassee	100%	38

NOTE: Hospital profiles are in alphabetical order by state, then city, then hospital within the city; Rankings exclude hospitals with less than 25 cases except for patient surveys which excludes hospitals with less than 100 cases; (a) 100-299 cases; (1) The number of cases/patients is too few to report; (2) Data submitted were based on a sample of cases/patients; (3) Results are based on a shorter time period than required; (4) Data suppressed by CMS for one or more quarters; (5) Results are not available for this reporting period; (6) Fewer than 100 patients completed the HCAHPS survey; (7) No cases met the criteria for this measure; (8) The lower limit of the confidence interval cannot be calculated if the number of observed infections equals zero; (9) No data are available from the state/territory for this reporting period; (10) The scores shown reflect fewer than 50 completed surveys; (11) There were discrepancies in the data collection process; (12) This measure does not apply to this hospital for this reporting period; (13) Results cannot be calculated for this reporting period; (14) The results for this state are combined with nearby states to protect confidentiality; Please refer to the User's Guide for a full explanation of data.

Hospital Name	City	Rate	Cases
Coosa Valley Medical Center	Sylacauga	100%	53
Cullman Regional Medical Center	Cullman	100%	92
Dekalb Regional Medical Center	Fort Payne	100%	37
Marion Regional Medical Center	Hamilton	100%	33
Medical Center Barbour	Eufaula	100%	54
Medical West	Bessemer	100%	58
Northwest Medical Center	Winfield	100%	42
Red Bay Hospital	Red Bay	100%	43
Russellville Hospital	Russellville	100%	32
South Baldwin Regional Medical Center	Foley	100%	73
Walker Baptist Medical Center	Jasper	100%	95
Wedowee Hospital	Wedowee	100%	42
Helen Keller Memorial Hospital	Sheffield	99%	110
Medical Center Enterprise	Enterprise	99%	73
Baptist Medical Center East	Montgomery	98%	43
Fayette Medical Center	Fayette	98%	101
Highlands Medical Center	Scottsboro	98%	88
Lakeland Community Hospital	Haleyville	98%	57
Marshall Medical Center South	Boaz	98%	344
Prattville Baptist Hospital	Prattville	98%	52
Troy Regional Medical Center	Troy	98%	42
Athens - Limestone Hospital	Athens	97%	176
D W Mcmillan Memorial Hospital	Brewton	97%	59
Jackson Medical Center	Jackson	97%	33
Andalusia Regional Hospital	Andalusia	96%	47
Citizens Baptist Medical Center	Talladega	96%	49
Saint Vincent's Saint Clair	Pell City	96%	96
Dale Medical Center	Ozark	95%	39
Decatur Morgan Hospital - Decatur Campus	Decatur	95%	144
Monroe County Hospital	Monroeville	95%	99
Decatur Morgan Hospital - Parkway Campus	Decatur	94%	65
Lawrence Medical Center	Moulton	92%	39
Atmore Community Hospital	Atmore	91%	46
North Baldwin Infirmary	Bay Minette	84%	44
Clay County Hospital	Ashland	83%	69
Hale County Hospital	Greensboro	80%	25
Bryan W Whitfield Memorial Hospital	Demopolis	67%	33

Average Time to ECG (minutes)

Hospital Name	City	Min.	Cases
Dekalb Regional Medical Center	Fort Payne	0	39
Walker Baptist Medical Center	Jasper	0	99
Coosa Valley Medical Center	Sylacauga	3	54
Lakeland Community Hospital	Haleyville	3	58
Decatur Morgan Hospital - Parkway Campus	Decatur	4	65
Fayette Medical Center	Fayette	4	106
Marion Regional Medical Center	Hamilton	4	34
Saint Vincent's Saint Clair	Pell City	4	103
South Baldwin Regional Medical Center	Foley	5	77
Troy Regional Medical Center	Troy	5	44
Wedowee Hospital	Wedowee	5	44
Cherokee Medical Center	Centre	6	41
Citizens Baptist Medical Center	Talladega	6	51
Cullman Regional Medical Center	Cullman	6	94
Dale Medical Center	Ozark	6	39
Decatur Morgan Hospital - Decatur Campus	Decatur	6	145
Helen Keller Memorial Hospital	Sheffield	6	112
Marshall Medical Center South	Boaz	6	356
Russellville Hospital	Russellville	6	33
Vaughan Reg Med Ctr Parkway Campus	Selma	6	25
Athens - Limestone Hospital	Athens	7	191
Baptist Medical Center East	Montgomery	7	47
Clay County Hospital	Ashland	7	75
L V Stabler Memorial Hospital	Greenville	7	27
Lawrence Medical Center	Moulton	7	41
Medical Center Enterprise	Enterprise	7	75
Monroe County Hospital	Monroeville	7	104
Northwest Medical Center	Winfield	7	47
Andalusia Regional Hospital	Andalusia	8	51
D W Mcmillan Memorial Hospital	Brewton	8	60
Highlands Medical Center	Scottsboro	8	92
Atmore Community Hospital	Atmore	9	47
Jackson Medical Center	Jackson	9	36
North Baldwin Infirmary	Bay Minette	9	45
Prattville Baptist Hospital	Prattville	12	52
Community Hospital	Tallassee	14	36
Medical Center Barbour	Eufaula	14	59
Medical West	Bessemer	20	60
Red Bay Hospital	Red Bay	21	45
Bryan W Whitfield Memorial Hospital	Demopolis	28	34
Hale County Hospital	Greensboro	42	27

Average Time to Transfer (minutes)

Hospital Name	City	Min.	Cases
Marshall Medical Center South	Boaz	56	28
Highlands Medical Center	Scottsboro	75	25

Children's Asthma Care

Received Home Management Plan of Care

Hospital Name	City	Rate	Cases
Huntsville Hospital	Huntsville	89%	156
Univ of S AL Children's & Women's Hosp[2]	Mobile	67%	135

Received Reliever Medication

Hospital Name	City	Rate	Cases
Huntsville Hospital	Huntsville	100%	157
Univ of S AL Children's & Women's Hosp[2]	Mobile	100%	138

Received Systemic Corticosteroids

Hospital Name	City	Rate	Cases
Huntsville Hospital	Huntsville	100%	157
Univ of S AL Children's & Women's Hosp[2]	Mobile	99%	138

Emergency Department

Admittance Decision Time (minutes)

Hospital Name	City	Min.	Cases
Florala Memorial Hospital[2,3]	Florala	0	46
Greene County Hospital[2]	Eutaw	5	313
Washington County Hospital[2]	Chatom	23	56
Marion Regional Medical Center[2]	Hamilton	30	362
Hale County Hospital[2]	Greensboro	35	322
Bryan W Whitfield Memorial Hospital[2]	Demopolis	38	620
Lake Martin Community Hospital[2]	Dadeville	39	479
Medical Center Barbour[2]	Eufaula	39	667
Georgiana Medical Center[2]	Georgiana	40	322
Grove Hill Memorial Hospital[2]	Grove Hill	40	251
Andalusia Regional Hospital[2]	Andalusia	45	385
East Alabama Medical Center[2]	Opelika	45	548
Monroe County Hospital[2]	Monroeville	45	201
Citizens Baptist Medical Center[2]	Talladega	47	357
Clay County Hospital[2]	Ashland	50	131
Crenshaw Community Hospital[2]	Luverne	50	364
Dale Medical Center[2]	Ozark	50	508
Wiregrass Medical Center[2]	Geneva	50	362
Jackson Medical Center	Jackson	52	139
Lawrence Medical Center[2]	Moulton	52	297
Shoals Hospital[2]	Muscle Shoals	52	220
Bibb Medical Center[2]	Centreville	54	64
Eliza Coffee Memorial Hospital[2]	Florence	55	339
Mizell Memorial Hospital[2]	Opp	55	400
Saint Vincent's Saint Clair[2]	Pell City	55	328
Trinity Medical Center[2]	Birmingham	55	504
L V Stabler Memorial Hospital[2]	Greenville	56	371
Northeast Alabama Regional Medical Center[2]	Anniston	57	569
Northwest Medical Center[2]	Winfield	57	423
Atmore Community Hospital[2]	Atmore	60	319
D W Mcmillan Memorial Hospital[2]	Brewton	60	311
Evergreen Medical Center[2]	Evergreen	60	435
Hill Hospital of Sumter County	York	60	255
Medical West[2]	Bessemer	62	715
Medical Center Enterprise[2]	Enterprise	63	407
Marshall Medical Center South[2]	Boaz	65	1057
Fayette Medical Center[2]	Fayette	66	433
Helen Keller Memorial Hospital[2]	Sheffield	66	501
Russellville Hospital[2]	Russellville	66	341
Southeast Alabama Medical Center[2]	Dothan	66	530
Community Hospital[2]	Tallassee	67	457
Elmore Community Hospital[2]	Wetumpka	68	387
Lakeland Community Hospital[2]	Haleyville	68	232
Cherokee Medical Center[2]	Centre	69	402
Athens - Limestone Hospital[2]	Athens	70	522
Highlands Medical Center[2]	Scottsboro	72	311
Vaughan Reg Med Ctr Parkway Campus[2]	Selma	72	670
Decatur Morgan Hospital - Parkway Campus[2]	Decatur	73	476
Jack Hughston Memorial Hospital[2]	Phenix City	74	143
Stringfellow Memorial Hospital[2]	Anniston	74	487
Walker Baptist Medical Center[2]	Jasper	74	683
Decatur Morgan Hospital - Decatur Campus[2]	Decatur	75	419
Coosa Valley Medical Center[2]	Sylacauga	76	767
George H. Lanier Memorial Hospital[2]	Valley	76	255
Crestwood Medical Center[2]	Huntsville	77	579
Troy Regional Medical Center[2]	Troy	77	435
Wedowee Hospital[2]	Wedowee	77	98
North Baldwin Infirmary[2]	Bay Minette	80	288
Pickens County Medical Center[2]	Carrollton	80	343
Bullock County Hospital[2]	Union Springs	82	183
Saint Vincent's East[2]	Birmingham	85	431
D C H Regional Medical Center[2]	Tuscaloosa	86	575
Providence Hospital[2]	Mobile	88	416
Cullman Regional Medical Center[2]	Cullman	92	650
Dekalb Regional Medical Center[2]	Fort Payne	92	491
Springhill Medical Center[2]	Mobile	92	828
Jacksonville Medical Center[2]	Jacksonville	93	126
Shelby Baptist Medical Center[2]	Alabaster	95	736
Russell Hospital[2]	Alexander City	98	323
South Baldwin Regional Medical Center[2]	Foley	98	827
Brookwood Medical Center[2]	Birmingham	99	437
Huntsville Hospital[2]	Huntsville	99	622
Thomas Hospital[2]	Fairhope	101	494
Flowers Hospital[2]	Dothan	109	566
Saint Vincent's Birmingham[2]	Birmingham	115	403
Baptist Medical Center - Princeton[2]	Birmingham	117	582
Gadsden Regional Medical Center[2]	Gadsden	119	592
Baptist Medical Center East[2]	Montgomery	122	295
Riverview Regional Medical Center[2]	Gadsden	125	547
Jackson Hospital & Clinic[2]	Montgomery	139	710
Mobile Infirmary[2]	Mobile	141	612
University of Alabama Hospital[2]	Birmingham	214	320
Univ of S Alabama Med Ctr[2]	Mobile	235	951
Prattville Baptist Hospital[2]	Prattville	248	545
Baptist Medical Center South[2]	Montgomery	284	408

Head CT Results Within 45 Minutes of Arrival

Hospital Name	City	Rate	Cases
Marshall Medical Center South	Boaz	48%	31

Patients Who Left ER Before Being Seen

Hospital Name	City	Rate	Cases
Choctaw General Hospital	Butler	0%	5445
Coosa Valley Medical Center	Sylacauga	0%	31731
Eliza Coffee Memorial Hospital	Florence	0%	42353
Florala Memorial Hospital	Florala	0%	3211
Georgiana Medical Center	Georgiana	0%	3528
Grove Hill Memorial Hospital	Grove Hill	0%	8837
Lake Martin Community Hospital	Dadeville	0%	5167
Riverview Regional Medical Center	Gadsden	0%	16828
Washington County Hospital	Chatom	0%	3653
Wedowee Hospital	Wedowee	0%	9462
Bibb Medical Center	Centreville	1%	18244
Brookwood Medical Center	Birmingham	1%	42187
Bullock County Hospital	Union Springs	1%	5533
Callahan Eye Hospital	Birmingham	1%	5005
Cherokee Medical Center	Centre	1%	8842
Citizens Baptist Medical Center	Talladega	1%	22590
Clay County Hospital	Ashland	1%	5158
Crenshaw Community Hospital	Luverne	1%	6175
Cullman Regional Medical Center	Cullman	1%	47229
Dale Medical Center	Ozark	1%	16986
Dekalb Regional Medical Center	Fort Payne	1%	37985
Evergreen Medical Center	Evergreen	1%	10721
Gadsden Regional Medical Center	Gadsden	1%	41653
George H. Lanier Memorial Hospital	Valley	1%	17830
Greene County Hospital	Eutaw	1%	5202
Hill Hospital of Sumter County	York	1%	4622
J Paul Jones Hospital	Camden	1%	5276
Jack Hughston Memorial Hospital	Phenix City	1%	14580
Jacksonville Medical Center	Jacksonville	1%	14192
L V Stabler Memorial Hospital	Greenville	1%	1043
Lakeland Community Hospital	Haleyville	1%	8749
Lawrence Medical Center	Moulton	1%	9273
Marion Regional Medical Center	Hamilton	1%	9657
Medical West	Bessemer	1%	44554
Pickens County Medical Center	Carrollton	1%	11696
Russell Hospital	Alexander City	1%	24239
Shelby Baptist Medical Center	Alabaster	1%	50185
Stringfellow Memorial Hospital	Anniston	1%	24793
Trinity Medical Center	Birmingham	1%	26048
Andalusia Regional Hospital	Andalusia	2%	16364
Bryan W Whitfield Memorial Hospital	Demopolis	2%	9558
Community Hospital	Tallassee	2%	13165
D W Mcmillan Memorial Hospital	Brewton	2%	13995
Hale County Hospital	Greensboro	2%	7511
Helen Keller Memorial Hospital	Sheffield	2%	37542
Medical Center Barbour	Eufaula	2%	15009
Monroe County Hospital	Monroeville	2%	15319
Russellville Hospital	Russellville	2%	11323
Saint Vincent's Birmingham	Birmingham	2%	49943
Saint Vincent's Saint Clair	Pell City	2%	25105
South Baldwin Regional Medical Center	Foley	2%	28688
Thomas Hospital	Fairhope	2%	25360
Troy Regional Medical Center	Troy	2%	17415
Vaughan Reg Med Ctr Parkway Campus	Selma	2%	30759
Walker Baptist Medical Center	Jasper	2%	37042
Athens - Limestone Hospital	Athens	3%	33762
Atmore Community Hospital	Atmore	3%	10895
Baptist Medical Center - Princeton	Birmingham	3%	46891
Baptist Medical Center East	Montgomery	3%	43129
Crestwood Medical Center	Huntsville	3%	42713
East Alabama Medical Center	Opelika	3%	47507
Elmore Community Hospital	Wetumpka	3%	12941
Highlands Medical Center	Scottsboro	3%	18334
Jackson Medical Center	Jackson	3%	7919
Marshall Medical Center South	Boaz	3%	75338
Mizell Memorial Hospital	Opp	3%	10246

NOTE: Hospital profiles are in alphabetical order by state, then city, then hospital within the city; Rankings exclude hospitals with less than 25 cases except for patient surveys which excludes hospitals with less than 100 cases; (a) 100-299 cases; (1) The number of cases/patients is too few to report; (2) Data submitted were based on a sample of cases/patients; (3) Results are based on a shorter time period than required; (4) Data suppressed by CMS for one or more quarters; (5) Results are not available for this reporting period; (6) Fewer than 100 patients completed the HCAHPS survey; (7) No cases met the criteria for this measure; (8) The lower limit of the confidence interval cannot be calculated if the number of observed infections equals zero; (9) No data are available from the state/territory for this reporting period; (10) The scores shown reflect fewer than 50 completed surveys; (11) There were discrepancies in the data collection process; (12) This measure does not apply to this hospital for this reporting period; (13) Results cannot be calculated for this reporting period; (14) The results for this state are combined with nearby states to protect confidentiality; Please refer to the User's Guide for a full explanation of data.

Northwest Medical Center	Winfield	3%	12888
Saint Vincent's East	Birmingham	3%	52342
Wiregrass Medical Center	Geneva	3%	11061
D C H Regional Medical Center	Tuscaloosa	4%	125921
Decatur Morgan Hospital - Parkway Campus	Decatur	4%	28693
Fayette Medical Center	Fayette	4%	15025
Flowers Hospital	Dothan	4%	39118
Huntsville Hospital	Huntsville	4%	158244
Medical Center Enterprise	Enterprise	4%	29880
North Baldwin Infirmary	Bay Minette	4%	13927
Prattville Baptist Hospital	Prattville	4%	31576
Shoals Hospital	Muscle Shoals	4%	13465
Southeast Alabama Medical Center	Dothan	4%	60818
University of Alabama Hospital	Birmingham	4%	86533
Baptist Medical Center South	Montgomery	5%	62762
Decatur Morgan Hospital - Decatur Campus	Decatur	5%	44362
Northeast Alabama Regional Medical Center	Anniston	5%	42018
Providence Hospital	Mobile	5%	49564
Springhill Medical Center	Mobile	5%	34556
Jackson Hospital & Clinic	Montgomery	6%	44574
Univ of S Alabama Med Ctr	Mobile	7%	29516
Mobile Infirmary	Mobile	8%	43352

Time from ER Arrival to Being Admitted (minutes)

Hospital Name	City	Min.	Cases
Florala Memorial Hospital[2,3]	Florala	138	46
Georgiana Medical Center[2]	Georgiana	145	327
Dale Medical Center[2]	Ozark	164	508
Greene County Hospital[2]	Eutaw	165	321
Washington County Hospital[2]	Chatom	170	84
Lakeland Community Hospital[2]	Haleyville	172	233
Marion Regional Medical Center[2]	Hamilton	175	409
Wiregrass Medical Center[2]	Geneva	175	394
Bullock County Hospital[2]	Union Springs	176	191
Medical Center Barbour[2]	Eufaula	177	667
D W Mcmillan Memorial Hospital[2]	Brewton	178	331
J Paul Jones Hospital	Camden	178	106
Trinity Medical Center[2]	Birmingham	178	505
Bryan W Whitfield Memorial Hospital[2]	Demopolis	180	620
Crenshaw Community Hospital[2]	Luverne	180	364
Hill Hospital of Sumter County	York	182	259
Andalusia Regional Hospital[2]	Andalusia	184	386
Citizens Baptist Medical Center[2]	Talladega	188	358
Grove Hill Memorial Hospital[2]	Grove Hill	188	371
Lawrence Medical Center[2]	Moulton	191	321
Bibb Medical Center[2]	Centreville	192	64
L V Stabler Memorial Hospital[2]	Greenville	194	376
Helen Keller Memorial Hospital[2]	Sheffield	195	501
Stringfellow Memorial Hospital[2]	Anniston	198	510
Evergreen Medical Center[2]	Evergreen	199	458
Clay County Hospital[2]	Ashland	200	135
Mizell Memorial Hospital[2]	Opp	200	411
Hale County Hospital[2]	Greensboro	202	322
Medical Center Enterprise[2]	Enterprise	202	410
Troy Regional Medical Center[2]	Troy	203	437
Lake Martin Community Hospital[2]	Dadeville	205	532
Jackson Medical Center	Jackson	206	244
Cherokee Medical Center[2]	Centre	208	407
Fayette Medical Center[2]	Fayette	208	457
Wedowee Hospital[2]	Wedowee	210	231
Eliza Coffee Memorial Hospital[2]	Florence	214	387
Dekalb Regional Medical Center[2]	Fort Payne	218	494
Medical West[2]	Bessemer	218	744
Saint Vincent's Saint Clair[2]	Pell City	218	330
Monroe County Hospital[2]	Monroeville	220	217
Atmore Community Hospital[2]	Atmore	221	319
Northwest Medical Center[2]	Winfield	222	428
Northeast Alabama Regional Medical Center[2]	Anniston	224	591
Russellville Hospital[2]	Russellville	224	341
Springhill Medical Center[2]	Mobile	228	830
East Alabama Medical Center[2]	Opelika	229	548
Coosa Valley Medical Center[2]	Sylacauga	231	761
Decatur Morgan Hospital - Parkway Campus[2]	Decatur	235	480
Shoals Hospital[2]	Muscle Shoals	236	228
Elmore Community Hospital[2]	Wetumpka	240	421
Marshall Medical Center South[2]	Boaz	241	1140
Cullman Regional Medical Center[2]	Cullman	242	650
Pickens County Medical Center[2]	Carrollton	242	347
Crestwood Medical Center[2]	Huntsville	243	582
Vaughan Reg Med Ctr Parkway Campus[2]	Selma	243	683
Community Hospital[2]	Tallassee	245	581
Athens - Limestone Hospital[2]	Athens	248	522
George H. Lanier Memorial Hospital[2]	Valley	251	261
Highlands Medical Center[2]	Scottsboro	254	324
Russell Hospital[2]	Alexander City	260	368
Saint Vincent's East[2]	Birmingham	265	451
Jacksonville Medical Center[2]	Jacksonville	270	180
Southeast Alabama Medical Center[2]	Dothan	272	530
North Baldwin Infirmary[2]	Bay Minette	275	292
South Baldwin Regional Medical Center[2]	Foley	277	838
Flowers Hospital[2]	Dothan	278	573
Walker Baptist Medical Center[2]	Jasper	278	683
D C H Regional Medical Center[2]	Tuscaloosa	279	618
Jack Hughston Memorial Hospital[2]	Phenix City	281	143
Decatur Morgan Hospital - Decatur Campus[2]	Decatur	286	470
Providence Hospital[2]	Mobile	286	516
Riverview Regional Medical Center[2]	Gadsden	295	547
Saint Vincent's Birmingham[2]	Birmingham	296	405
Shelby Baptist Medical Center[2]	Alabaster	303	740
Baptist Medical Center - Princeton[2]	Birmingham	308	588
Brookwood Medical Center[2]	Birmingham	311	439
Thomas Hospital[2]	Fairhope	315	494
Huntsville Hospital[2]	Huntsville	318	625
Jackson Hospital & Clinic[2]	Montgomery	324	710
Baptist Medical Center East[2]	Montgomery	335	307
Gadsden Regional Medical Center[2]	Gadsden	365	595
Mobile Infirmary[2]	Mobile	384	615
University of Alabama Hospital[2]	Birmingham	395	523
Prattville Baptist Hospital[2]	Prattville	446	550
Univ of S Alabama Med Ctr[2]	Mobile	484	952
Baptist Medical Center South[2]	Montgomery	494	415

Time from ER Arrival to Discharge (minutes)

Hospital Name	City	Min.	Cases
Lakeland Community Hospital	Haleyville	70	360
Florala Memorial Hospital	Florala	78	253
Cherokee Medical Center	Centre	79	384
Dale Medical Center	Ozark	80	411
Wedowee Hospital	Wedowee	84	270
Georgiana Medical Center	Georgiana	86	388
Lawrence Medical Center	Moulton	86	384
L V Stabler Memorial Hospital	Greenville	87	393
Troy Regional Medical Center	Troy	87	385
Bullock County Hospital	Union Springs	90	337
Coosa Valley Medical Center	Sylacauga	90	381
Bibb Medical Center	Centreville	93	311
Stringfellow Memorial Hospital	Anniston	97	394
Crenshaw Community Hospital	Luverne	98	375
Russellville Hospital	Russellville	98	376
Mizell Memorial Hospital	Opp	99	278
Callahan Eye Hospital	Birmingham	100	378
Clay County Hospital	Ashland	100	341
Washington County Hospital	Chatom	100	384
D W Mcmillan Memorial Hospital	Brewton	101	559
Marion Regional Medical Center	Hamilton	101	384
Fayette Medical Center	Fayette	103	367
Trinity Medical Center	Birmingham	103	393
Jack Hughston Memorial Hospital	Phenix City	104	425
Elmore Community Hospital	Wetumpka	105	417
Helen Keller Memorial Hospital	Sheffield	105	373
J Paul Jones Hospital	Camden	106	319
Lake Martin Community Hospital	Dadeville	106	338
Saint Vincent's Saint Clair	Pell City	107	345
Medical Center Barbour	Eufaula	108	318
Russell Hospital	Alexander City	108	388
Evergreen Medical Center	Evergreen	110	520
Community Hospital	Tallassee	111	548
Monroe County Hospital	Monroeville	111	389
Andalusia Regional Hospital	Andalusia	112	388
Citizens Baptist Medical Center	Talladega	112	402
Northwest Medical Center	Winfield	113	405
Wiregrass Medical Center	Geneva	113	371
Hale County Hospital	Greensboro	115	345
Bryan W Whitfield Memorial Hospital	Demopolis	118	341
George H. Lanier Memorial Hospital	Valley	118	348
Hill Hospital of Sumter County	York	118	353
Jackson Medical Center	Jackson	118	368
Medical Center Enterprise	Enterprise	119	391
Medical West	Bessemer	119	1331
Dekalb Regional Medical Center	Fort Payne	122	398
Pickens County Medical Center	Carrollton	124	357
Cullman Regional Medical Center	Cullman	126	546
Grove Hill Memorial Hospital	Grove Hill	126	366
Eliza Coffee Memorial Hospital	Florence	127	354
Vaughan Reg Med Ctr Parkway Campus	Selma	127	377
Atmore Community Hospital	Atmore	128	363
Jacksonville Medical Center	Jacksonville	128	354
Highlands Medical Center	Scottsboro	130	578
Decatur Morgan Hospital - Parkway Campus	Decatur	131	447
Northeast Alabama Regional Medical Center	Anniston	135	472
Springhill Medical Center	Mobile	135	379
Marshall Medical Center South	Boaz	136	1900
Athens - Limestone Hospital	Athens	137	413
Greene County Hospital	Eutaw	137	388
Walker Baptist Medical Center	Jasper	140	378
Crestwood Medical Center	Huntsville	142	390
Saint Vincent's East	Birmingham	146	336
Shoals Hospital	Muscle Shoals	146	442
Riverview Regional Medical Center	Gadsden	152	888
South Baldwin Regional Medical Center	Foley	153	368
D C H Regional Medical Center	Tuscaloosa	158	416
North Baldwin Infirmary	Bay Minette	158	384
Prattville Baptist Hospital	Prattville	161	513
Thomas Hospital	Fairhope	162	378
Shelby Baptist Medical Center	Alabaster	163	405
East Alabama Medical Center	Opelika	164	446
Baptist Medical Center - Princeton	Birmingham	165	354
Decatur Morgan Hospital - Decatur Campus	Decatur	165	358
Huntsville Hospital	Huntsville	168	369
Flowers Hospital	Dothan	184	394
Jackson Hospital & Clinic	Montgomery	186	727
Gadsden Regional Medical Center	Gadsden	188	359
University of Alabama Hospital	Birmingham	190	345
Brookwood Medical Center	Birmingham	195	387
Saint Vincent's Birmingham	Birmingham	195	357
Baptist Medical Center East	Montgomery	198	257
Baptist Medical Center South	Montgomery	200	295
Southeast Alabama Medical Center	Dothan	202	361
Mobile Infirmary	Mobile	235	377
Providence Hospital	Mobile	266	358
Univ of S Alabama Med Ctr	Mobile	285	277

Time in ER Before Being Evaluated (minutes)

Hospital Name	City	Min.	Cases
Cherokee Medical Center	Centre	12	421
Eliza Coffee Memorial Hospital	Florence	13	379
Lakeland Community Hospital	Haleyville	13	417
Russell Hospital	Alexander City	16	401
Russellville Hospital	Russellville	16	422
Washington County Hospital	Chatom	16	408
Trinity Medical Center	Birmingham	17	419
Coosa Valley Medical Center	Sylacauga	18	468
Dekalb Regional Medical Center	Fort Payne	18	417
Lawrence Medical Center	Moulton	18	405
Stringfellow Memorial Hospital	Anniston	19	406
Wedowee Hospital	Wedowee	20	389
Andalusia Regional Hospital	Andalusia	21	404
Bibb Medical Center	Centreville	21	387
Fayette Medical Center	Fayette	21	393
Marion Regional Medical Center	Hamilton	21	426
Medical Center Barbour	Eufaula	21	436
Northwest Medical Center	Winfield	21	425
Clay County Hospital	Ashland	22	397
Dale Medical Center	Ozark	22	521
Helen Keller Memorial Hospital	Sheffield	22	383
Florala Memorial Hospital	Florala	23	256
Shoals Hospital	Muscle Shoals	23	431
George H. Lanier Memorial Hospital	Valley	24	371
Troy Regional Medical Center	Troy	24	404
Vaughan Reg Med Ctr Parkway Campus	Selma	24	445
Grove Hill Memorial Hospital	Grove Hill	25	361
L V Stabler Memorial Hospital	Greenville	25	423
Monroe County Hospital	Monroeville	25	349
Walker Baptist Medical Center	Jasper	25	404
Cullman Regional Medical Center	Cullman	26	596
Medical Center Enterprise	Enterprise	26	462
Medical West	Bessemer	26	1481
Citizens Baptist Medical Center	Talladega	27	422
Lake Martin Community Hospital	Dadeville	27	365
Riverview Regional Medical Center	Gadsden	27	1038
D W Mcmillan Memorial Hospital	Brewton	28	392
Jacksonville Medical Center	Jacksonville	28	315
Mizell Memorial Hospital	Opp	28	269
Crenshaw Community Hospital	Luverne	29	385
Elmore Community Hospital	Wetumpka	30	406
Saint Vincent's Saint Clair	Pell City	30	356
J Paul Jones Hospital	Camden	31	211
Baptist Medical Center South	Montgomery	32	342
Hale County Hospital	Greensboro	32	386
Athens - Limestone Hospital	Athens	33	448
Decatur Morgan Hospital - Parkway Campus	Decatur	33	469
Community Hospital	Tallassee	34	358
Bryan W Whitfield Memorial Hospital	Demopolis	35	380
South Baldwin Regional Medical Center	Foley	35	407
Thomas Hospital	Fairhope	35	384
Marshall Medical Center South	Boaz	36	1991
Shelby Baptist Medical Center	Alabaster	36	421
Baptist Medical Center - Princeton	Birmingham	37	409
Highlands Medical Center	Scottsboro	37	594
Bullock County Hospital	Union Springs	38	389
Saint Vincent's East	Birmingham	38	354
Springhill Medical Center	Mobile	38	388
Atmore Community Hospital	Atmore	39	351
Evergreen Medical Center	Evergreen	40	554
Jackson Medical Center	Jackson	41	358
Wiregrass Medical Center	Geneva	41	397
Hill Hospital of Sumter County	York	42	381
University of Alabama Hospital	Birmingham	42	368
Prattville Baptist Hospital	Prattville	43	413
D C H Regional Medical Center	Tuscaloosa	45	433
Georgiana Medical Center	Georgiana	45	397
Saint Vincent's Birmingham	Birmingham	45	383
Flowers Hospital	Dothan	46	395

NOTE: Hospital profiles are in alphabetical order by state, then city, then hospital within the city; Rankings exclude hospitals with less than 25 cases except for patient surveys which excludes hospitals with less than 100 cases; (a) 100-299 cases; (1) The number of cases/patients is too few to report; (2) Data submitted were based on a sample of cases/patients; (3) Results are based on a shorter time period than required; (4) Data suppressed by CMS for one or more quarters; (5) Results are not available for this reporting period; (6) Fewer than 100 patients completed the HCAHPS survey; (7) No cases met the criteria for this measure; (8) The lower limit of the confidence interval cannot be calculated if the number of observed infections equals zero; (9) No data are available from the state/territory for this reporting period; (10) The scores shown reflect fewer than 50 completed surveys; (11) There were discrepancies in the data collection process; (12) This measure does not apply to this hospital for this reporting period; (13) Results cannot be calculated for this reporting period; (14) The results for this state are combined with nearby states to protect confidentiality; Please refer to the User's Guide for a full explanation of data.

Baptist Medical Center East	Montgomery	47	353
Brookwood Medical Center	Birmingham	47	437
Jack Hughston Memorial Hospital	Phenix City	48	444
Pickens County Medical Center	Carrollton	48	366
North Baldwin Infirmary	Bay Minette	50	404
Huntsville Hospital	Huntsville	52	365
Callahan Eye Hospital	Birmingham	53	380
East Alabama Medical Center	Opelika	53	480
Gadsden Regional Medical Center	Gadsden	54	410
Northeast Alabama Regional Medical Center	Anniston	54	504
Decatur Morgan Hospital - Decatur Campus	Decatur	55	368
Greene County Hospital	Eutaw	57	287
Mobile Infirmary	Mobile	57	417
Southeast Alabama Medical Center	Dothan	62	381
Crestwood Medical Center	Huntsville	64	419
Jackson Hospital & Clinic	Montgomery	74	757
Univ of S Alabama Med Ctr	Mobile	76	372
Providence Hospital	Mobile	94	384

Time to Pain Meds for Bone Fractures (minutes)

Hospital Name	City	Min.	Cases
Lakeland Community Hospital	Haleyville	29	30
Troy Regional Medical Center	Troy	39	47
Fayette Medical Center	Fayette	40	51
Lawrence Medical Center	Moulton	40	49
Marion Regional Medical Center	Hamilton	40	28
Trinity Medical Center	Birmingham	42	80
Andalusia Regional Hospital	Andalusia	46	63
Dale Medical Center	Ozark	46	46
Russellville Hospital	Russellville	48	58
Clay County Hospital	Ashland	50	30
Medical Center Barbour	Eufaula	51	82
Cherokee Medical Center	Centre	52	41
Grove Hill Memorial Hospital	Grove Hill	52	38
Northwest Medical Center	Winfield	53	47
Jackson Medical Center	Jackson	54	32
Walker Baptist Medical Center	Jasper	54	162
Coosa Valley Medical Center	Sylacauga	55	125
Monroe County Hospital	Monroeville	55	41
Wedowee Hospital	Wedowee	57	32
Dekalb Regional Medical Center	Fort Payne	60	148
Elmore Community Hospital	Wetumpka	60	34
George H. Lanier Memorial Hospital	Valley	60	45
Helen Keller Memorial Hospital	Sheffield	60	154
Baptist Medical Center South	Montgomery	61	125
Citizens Baptist Medical Center	Talladega	61	92
Cullman Regional Medical Center	Cullman	62	204
Stringfellow Memorial Hospital	Anniston	62	80
South Baldwin Regional Medical Center	Foley	63	182
Eliza Coffee Memorial Hospital	Florence	64	40
L V Stabler Memorial Hospital	Greenville	64	49
Russell Hospital	Alexander City	64	78
Springhill Medical Center	Mobile	64	120
D W Mcmillan Memorial Hospital	Brewton	65	51
Shelby Baptist Medical Center	Alabaster	65	199
Thomas Hospital	Fairhope	65	165
Prattville Baptist Hospital	Prattville	66	118
East Alabama Medical Center	Opelika	68	176
Saint Vincent's Saint Clair	Pell City	68	95
Medical Center Enterprise	Enterprise	69	162
Vaughan Reg Med Ctr Parkway Campus	Selma	69	119
Community Hospital	Tallassee	70	52
Saint Vincent's East	Birmingham	70	201
Athens - Limestone Hospital	Athens	72	150
D C H Regional Medical Center	Tuscaloosa	72	236
Huntsville Hospital	Huntsville	72	425
Medical West	Bessemer	72	100
Wiregrass Medical Center	Geneva	72	42
Gadsden Regional Medical Center	Gadsden	73	150
Riverview Regional Medical Center	Gadsden	73	57
Baptist Medical Center - Princeton	Birmingham	74	70
North Baldwin Infirmary	Bay Minette	74	48
Marshall Medical Center South	Boaz	75	310
University of Alabama Hospital	Birmingham	75	151
Decatur Morgan Hospital - Parkway Campus	Decatur	76	130
Flowers Hospital	Dothan	76	103
Jack Hughston Memorial Hospital	Phenix City	76	62
Highlands Medical Center	Scottsboro	77	99
Baptist Medical Center East	Montgomery	78	130
Evergreen Medical Center	Evergreen	78	36
Decatur Morgan Hospital - Decatur Campus	Decatur	80	158
Jacksonville Medical Center	Jacksonville	80	58
Mizell Memorial Hospital	Opp	80	44
Crestwood Medical Center	Huntsville	81	101
Brookwood Medical Center	Birmingham	85	143
Saint Vincent's Birmingham	Birmingham	85	174
Bibb Medical Center	Centreville	90	30
Northeast Alabama Regional Medical Center	Anniston	90	180
Providence Hospital	Mobile	97	64
Mobile Infirmary	Mobile	98	89
Southeast Alabama Medical Center	Dothan	103	164

Pickens County Medical Center	Carrollton	104	26
Jackson Hospital & Clinic	Montgomery	113	36
Univ of S Alabama Med Ctr	Mobile	117	113

Heart Attack Care

Aspirin Given at Discharge

Hospital Name	City	Rate	Cases
Baptist Medical Center - Princeton	Birmingham	100%	399
Birmingham VA Medical Center	Birmingham	100%	54
Crestwood Medical Center	Huntsville	100%	110
Cullman Regional Medical Center[2]	Cullman	100%	70
Decatur Morgan Hospital - Decatur Campus	Decatur	100%	25
Dekalb Regional Medical Center	Fort Payne	100%	58
East Alabama Medical Center	Opelika	100%	241
Eliza Coffee Memorial Hospital[2]	Florence	100%	261
Flowers Hospital	Dothan	100%	280
Mobile Infirmary	Mobile	100%	261
Providence Hospital	Mobile	100%	275
Riverview Regional Medical Center	Gadsden	100%	69
Russell Hospital	Alexander City	100%	52
Saint Vincent's Birmingham	Birmingham	100%	271
Saint Vincent's East	Birmingham	100%	331
Shelby Baptist Medical Center	Alabaster	100%	278
Southeast Alabama Medical Center	Dothan	100%	601
Springhill Medical Center	Mobile	100%	206
Thomas Hospital	Fairhope	100%	271
Trinity Medical Center	Birmingham	100%	269
Univ of S Alabama Med Ctr	Mobile	100%	59
Vaughan Reg Med Ctr Parkway Campus	Selma	100%	155
Walker Baptist Medical Center	Jasper	100%	57
Brookwood Medical Center[2]	Birmingham	99%	288
D C H Regional Medical Center[2]	Tuscaloosa	99%	294
Gadsden Regional Medical Center	Gadsden	99%	189
Huntsville Hospital[2]	Huntsville	99%	377
Jackson Hospital & Clinic	Montgomery	99%	298
Medical West	Bessemer	99%	71
University of Alabama Hospital	Birmingham	99%	521
Baptist Medical Center South	Montgomery	98%	406
Stringfellow Memorial Hospital	Anniston	98%	51
Northeast Alabama Regional Medical Center	Anniston	97%	275
George H. Lanier Memorial Hospital	Valley	94%	36

PCI Within 90 Minutes of Arrival

Hospital Name	City	Rate	Cases
Baptist Medical Center - Princeton	Birmingham	100%	56
D C H Regional Medical Center[2]	Tuscaloosa	100%	34
Jackson Hospital & Clinic	Montgomery	100%	33
Providence Hospital	Mobile	100%	65
Saint Vincent's Birmingham	Birmingham	100%	69
Thomas Hospital	Fairhope	100%	44
Brookwood Medical Center[2]	Birmingham	98%	49
East Alabama Medical Center	Opelika	98%	52
Eliza Coffee Memorial Hospital[2]	Florence	98%	52
Huntsville Hospital[2]	Huntsville	98%	45
Shelby Baptist Medical Center	Alabaster	98%	52
Springhill Medical Center	Mobile	98%	53
Flowers Hospital	Dothan	97%	35
Gadsden Regional Medical Center	Gadsden	97%	36
Mobile Infirmary	Mobile	97%	29
Trinity Medical Center	Birmingham	97%	33
Northeast Alabama Regional Medical Center	Anniston	92%	37
Saint Vincent's East	Birmingham	92%	48
Southeast Alabama Medical Center	Dothan	91%	35
University of Alabama Hospital	Birmingham	91%	64
Baptist Medical Center South	Montgomery	88%	41

Statin Prescribed at Discharge

Hospital Name	City	Rate	Cases
Baptist Medical Center - Princeton	Birmingham	100%	393
Birmingham VA Medical Center	Birmingham	100%	54
Crestwood Medical Center	Huntsville	100%	103
Dekalb Regional Medical Center	Fort Payne	100%	57
East Alabama Medical Center	Opelika	100%	240
Eliza Coffee Memorial Hospital[2]	Florence	100%	254
Flowers Hospital	Dothan	100%	260
Medical West	Bessemer	100%	64
Mobile Infirmary	Mobile	100%	250
Providence Hospital	Mobile	100%	264
Riverview Regional Medical Center	Gadsden	100%	61
Saint Vincent's Birmingham	Birmingham	100%	265
Saint Vincent's East	Birmingham	100%	327
Trinity Medical Center	Birmingham	100%	249
Univ of S Alabama Med Ctr	Mobile	100%	62
Vaughan Reg Med Ctr Parkway Campus	Selma	100%	147
Walker Baptist Medical Center	Jasper	100%	50
Huntsville Hospital[2]	Huntsville	99%	340
Jackson Hospital & Clinic	Montgomery	99%	243
Shelby Baptist Medical Center	Alabaster	99%	258

Thomas Hospital	Fairhope	99%	261
University of Alabama Hospital	Birmingham	99%	503
Cullman Regional Medical Center[2]	Cullman	98%	64
Gadsden Regional Medical Center	Gadsden	98%	167
Southeast Alabama Medical Center	Dothan	98%	594
Baptist Medical Center South	Montgomery	97%	395
Northeast Alabama Regional Medical Center	Anniston	97%	262
Brookwood Medical Center[2]	Birmingham	96%	276
D C H Regional Medical Center[2]	Tuscaloosa	96%	284
Russell Hospital	Alexander City	96%	51
Springhill Medical Center	Mobile	96%	203
Stringfellow Memorial Hospital	Anniston	95%	57
George H. Lanier Memorial Hospital	Valley	94%	35
Decatur Morgan Hospital - Decatur Campus	Decatur	92%	25

Heart Failure Care

ACE Inhibitor or ARB for LVSD

Hospital Name	City	Rate	Cases
Athens - Limestone Hospital	Athens	100%	26
Baptist Medical Center - Princeton	Birmingham	100%	235
Baptist Medical Center East[2]	Montgomery	100%	46
Birmingham VA Medical Center	Birmingham	100%	98
Brookwood Medical Center[2]	Birmingham	100%	111
Coosa Valley Medical Center	Sylacauga	100%	35
Crestwood Medical Center	Huntsville	100%	60
Cullman Regional Medical Center	Cullman	100%	59
East Alabama Medical Center	Opelika	100%	180
Eliza Coffee Memorial Hospital[2]	Florence	100%	78
Flowers Hospital	Dothan	100%	74
George H. Lanier Memorial Hospital	Valley	100%	73
Helen Keller Memorial Hospital	Sheffield	100%	37
Huntsville Hospital[2]	Huntsville	100%	95
Jackson Hospital & Clinic	Montgomery	100%	122
Medical Center Barbour[2]	Eufaula	100%	28
Medical Center Enterprise	Enterprise	100%	27
Medical West	Bessemer	100%	72
Mobile Infirmary[2]	Mobile	100%	93
Riverview Regional Medical Center	Gadsden	100%	46
Saint Vincent's East	Birmingham	100%	120
Shelby Baptist Medical Center	Alabaster	100%	109
South Baldwin Regional Medical Center	Foley	100%	47
Springhill Medical Center	Mobile	100%	149
Trinity Medical Center	Birmingham	100%	103
Univ of S Alabama Med Ctr	Mobile	100%	60
VA Central AL Hlthcare Sys-Montgomery	Montgomery	100%	37
Vaughan Reg Med Ctr Parkway Campus	Selma	100%	122
Walker Baptist Medical Center	Jasper	100%	48
Saint Vincent's Birmingham	Birmingham	99%	127
D C H Regional Medical Center[2]	Tuscaloosa	98%	130
Providence Hospital	Mobile	98%	89
Stringfellow Memorial Hospital	Anniston	98%	59
University of Alabama Hospital[2]	Birmingham	98%	301
Citizens Baptist Medical Center	Talladega	97%	31
Gadsden Regional Medical Center	Gadsden	97%	93
Russell Hospital	Alexander City	97%	33
Thomas Hospital	Fairhope	97%	59
Marshall Medical Center South	Boaz	96%	57
Southeast Alabama Medical Center	Dothan	96%	160
Troy Regional Medical Center	Troy	96%	26
Atmore Community Hospital	Atmore	95%	39
Decatur Morgan Hospital - Decatur Campus	Decatur	95%	103
Northeast Alabama Regional Medical Center	Anniston	95%	116
Baptist Medical Center South[2]	Montgomery	94%	176
L V Stabler Memorial Hospital	Greenville	94%	34
Decatur Morgan Hospital - Parkway Campus	Decatur	79%	28

Discharge Instructions Given

Hospital Name	City	Rate	Cases
Andalusia Regional Hospital[2]	Andalusia	100%	77
Coosa Valley Medical Center	Sylacauga	100%	67
Dekalb Regional Medical Center	Fort Payne	100%	54
Fayette Medical Center	Fayette	100%	40
Lakeland Community Hospital	Haleyville	100%	29
Medical Center Enterprise	Enterprise	100%	69
Riverview Regional Medical Center	Gadsden	100%	138
Russellville Hospital	Russellville	100%	46
Saint Vincent's East	Birmingham	100%	289
South Baldwin Regional Medical Center	Foley	100%	191
Trinity Medical Center	Birmingham	100%	240
Univ of S Alabama Med Ctr	Mobile	100%	103
Vaughan Reg Med Ctr Parkway Campus	Selma	100%	225
Walker Baptist Medical Center	Jasper	100%	132
Wiregrass Medical Center[2]	Geneva	100%	38
Cullman Regional Medical Center	Cullman	98%	223
Dale Medical Center[2]	Ozark	98%	48
Providence Hospital	Mobile	98%	333
Shelby Baptist Medical Center	Alabaster	98%	324
Baptist Medical Center East[2]	Montgomery	97%	193
Birmingham VA Medical Center	Birmingham	97%	199

NOTE: Hospital profiles are in alphabetical order by state, then city, then hospital within the city; Rankings exclude hospitals with less than 25 cases except for patient surveys which excludes hospitals with less than 100 cases; (a) 100-299 cases; (1) The number of cases/patients is too few to report; (2) Data submitted were based on a sample of cases/patients; (3) Results are based on a shorter time period than required; (4) Data suppressed by CMS for one or more quarters; (5) Results are not available for this reporting period; (6) Fewer than 100 patients completed the HCAHPS survey; (7) No cases met the criteria for this measure; (8) The lower limit of the confidence interval cannot be calculated if the number of observed infections equals zero; (9) No data are available from the state/territory for this reporting period; (10) The scores shown reflect fewer than 50 completed surveys; (11) There were discrepancies in the data collection process; (12) This measure does not apply to this hospital for this reporting period; (13) Results cannot be calculated for this reporting period; (14) The results for this state are combined with nearby states to protect confidentiality; Please refer to the User's Guide for a full explanation of data.

Community Hospital	Tallassee	97%	66
Flowers Hospital	Dothan	97%	219
Saint Vincent's Birmingham	Birmingham	97%	360
Saint Vincent's Saint Clair	Pell City	97%	62
Eliza Coffee Memorial Hospital[2]	Florence	96%	216
Jackson Hospital & Clinic	Montgomery	96%	347
Troy Regional Medical Center	Troy	96%	54
University of Alabama Hospital[2]	Birmingham	96%	648
Baptist Medical Center South[2]	Montgomery	95%	437
Brookwood Medical Center[2]	Birmingham	95%	275
East Alabama Medical Center	Opelika	95%	404
Highlands Medical Center	Scottsboro	95%	84
Marshall Medical Center South	Boaz	95%	148
Medical Center Barbour[2]	Eufaula	95%	58
Prattville Baptist Hospital	Prattville	95%	77
Thomas Hospital	Fairhope	95%	182
VA Central AL Hlthcare Sys-Montgomery	Montgomery	95%	60
Baptist Medical Center - Princeton	Birmingham	94%	500
D C H Regional Medical Center[2]	Tuscaloosa	94%	247
L V Stabler Memorial Hospital	Greenville	94%	64
Northwest Medical Center	Winfield	94%	33
Southeast Alabama Medical Center	Dothan	94%	466
Springhill Medical Center	Mobile	94%	424
Citizens Baptist Medical Center	Talladega	92%	102
Medical West	Bessemer	92%	218
D W Mcmillan Memorial Hospital	Brewton	91%	46
Helen Keller Memorial Hospital	Sheffield	91%	152
Russell Hospital	Alexander City	91%	99
Athens - Limestone Hospital	Athens	90%	81
Huntsville Hospital[2]	Huntsville	90%	297
Mobile Infirmary[2]	Mobile	90%	264
Stringfellow Memorial Hospital	Anniston	89%	118
Crestwood Medical Center	Huntsville	87%	190
Monroe County Hospital	Monroeville	87%	31
Gadsden Regional Medical Center	Gadsden	86%	227
North Baldwin Infirmary	Bay Minette	86%	44
Atmore Community Hospital	Atmore	85%	93
Evergreen Medical Center[2]	Evergreen	84%	91
Bryan W Whitfield Memorial Hospital[2]	Demopolis	82%	34
Northeast Alabama Regional Medical Center	Anniston	81%	326
Decatur Morgan Hospital - Decatur Campus	Decatur	72%	289
Decatur Morgan Hospital - Parkway Campus	Decatur	72%	53
George H. Lanier Memorial Hospital	Valley	71%	123
Greene County Hospital[2,3]	Eutaw	69%	26
Mizell Memorial Hospital	Opp	69%	32
Clay County Hospital	Ashland	66%	29
Grove Hill Memorial Hospital[2]	Grove Hill	59%	39
Shoals Hospital	Muscle Shoals	59%	32

Evaluation of LVS Function

Hospital Name	City	Rate	Cases
Andalusia Regional Hospital[2]	Andalusia	100%	84
Athens - Limestone Hospital	Athens	100%	117
Baptist Medical Center - Princeton	Birmingham	100%	585
Baptist Medical Center East[2]	Montgomery	100%	217
Birmingham VA Medical Center	Birmingham	100%	218
Clay County Hospital	Ashland	100%	36
Community Hospital	Tallassee	100%	77
Coosa Valley Medical Center	Sylacauga	100%	97
Crestwood Medical Center	Huntsville	100%	217
Cullman Regional Medical Center	Cullman	100%	291
D C H Regional Medical Center[2]	Tuscaloosa	100%	292
D W Mcmillan Memorial Hospital	Brewton	100%	51
Dale Medical Center[2]	Ozark	100%	62
Dekalb Regional Medical Center	Fort Payne	100%	82
East Alabama Medical Center	Opelika	100%	464
Eliza Coffee Memorial Hospital[2]	Florence	100%	256
Fayette Medical Center	Fayette	100%	47
Flowers Hospital	Dothan	100%	252
Gadsden Regional Medical Center	Gadsden	100%	303
George H. Lanier Memorial Hospital	Valley	100%	146
Helen Keller Memorial Hospital	Sheffield	100%	203
Jackson Hospital & Clinic	Montgomery	100%	426
Lakeland Community Hospital	Haleyville	100%	36
Lawrence Medical Center	Moulton	100%	31
Medical Center Barbour[2]	Eufaula	100%	68
Medical Center Enterprise	Enterprise	100%	79
Medical West	Bessemer	100%	255
Mobile Infirmary[2]	Mobile	100%	308
Pickens County Medical Center[2]	Carrollton	100%	29
Providence Hospital	Mobile	100%	391
Riverview Regional Medical Center	Gadsden	100%	184
Russell Hospital	Alexander City	100%	142
Russellville Hospital	Russellville	100%	66
Saint Vincent's Birmingham	Birmingham	100%	428
Saint Vincent's East	Birmingham	100%	335
Shelby Baptist Medical Center	Alabaster	100%	382
South Baldwin Regional Medical Center	Foley	100%	219
Southeast Alabama Medical Center	Dothan	100%	556
Stringfellow Memorial Hospital	Anniston	100%	133
Thomas Hospital	Fairhope	100%	224
Trinity Medical Center	Birmingham	100%	282
Troy Regional Medical Center	Troy	100%	61
University of Alabama Hospital[2]	Birmingham	100%	702
Univ of S Alabama Med Ctr	Mobile	100%	105
VA Central AL Hlthcare Sys-Montgomery	Montgomery	100%	63
Vaughan Reg Med Ctr Parkway Campus	Selma	100%	270
Walker Baptist Medical Center	Jasper	100%	181
Atmore Community Hospital	Atmore	99%	117
Decatur Morgan Hospital - Decatur Campus	Decatur	99%	353
Huntsville Hospital[2]	Huntsville	99%	368
L V Stabler Memorial Hospital	Greenville	99%	73
Northeast Alabama Regional Medical Center	Anniston	99%	400
Springhill Medical Center	Mobile	99%	495
Baptist Medical Center South[2]	Montgomery	98%	496
Brookwood Medical Center[2]	Birmingham	98%	329
Highlands Medical Center	Scottsboro	98%	103
Mizell Memorial Hospital	Opp	98%	47
Northwest Medical Center	Winfield	98%	43
Citizens Baptist Medical Center	Talladega	97%	118
Prattville Baptist Hospital	Prattville	97%	90
Decatur Morgan Hospital - Parkway Campus	Decatur	96%	70
North Baldwin Infirmary	Bay Minette	96%	48
Shoals Hospital	Muscle Shoals	96%	45
Monroe County Hospital	Monroeville	94%	51
Greene County Hospital[2,3]	Eutaw	93%	30
Saint Vincent's Saint Clair	Pell City	93%	82
Grove Hill Memorial Hospital[2]	Grove Hill	91%	44
Marshall Medical Center South	Boaz	90%	209
Wiregrass Medical Center[2]	Geneva	87%	52
Evergreen Medical Center[2]	Evergreen	86%	99
Bryan W Whitfield Memorial Hospital[2]	Demopolis	41%	37

Medicare Spending

Medicare Spending per Patient (ratio)

Hospital Name	City	Ratio	Cases
Highlands Medical Center	Scottsboro	0.85	-
Marion Regional Medical Center	Hamilton	0.86	-
North Baldwin Infirmary	Bay Minette	0.86	-
Wedowee Hospital	Wedowee	0.86	-
Fayette Medical Center	Fayette	0.87	-
George H. Lanier Memorial Hospital	Valley	0.87	-
Greene County Hospital	Eutaw	0.89	-
Community Hospital	Tallassee	0.90	-
East Alabama Medical Center	Opelika	0.90	-
Lawrence Medical Center	Moulton	0.90	-
Evergreen Medical Center	Evergreen	0.91	-
Medical Center Enterprise	Enterprise	0.92	-
Saint Vincent's Saint Clair	Pell City	0.92	-
Dale Medical Center	Ozark	0.93	-
Atmore Community Hospital	Atmore	0.94	-
Clay County Hospital	Ashland	0.94	-
Cullman Regional Medical Center	Cullman	0.94	-
Jack Hughston Memorial Hospital	Phenix City	0.94	-
Medical West	Bessemer	0.94	-
Univ of S Alabama Med Ctr	Mobile	0.94	-
Wiregrass Medical Center	Geneva	0.94	-
Cherokee Medical Center	Centre	0.95	-
Lakeland Community Hospital	Haleyville	0.95	-
Pickens County Medical Center	Carrollton	0.95	-
Jacksonville Medical Center	Jacksonville	0.96	-
Russell Hospital	Alexander City	0.96	-
University of Alabama Hospital	Birmingham	0.96	-
Bibb Medical Center	Centreville	0.97	-
Crestwood Medical Center	Huntsville	0.97	-
Mobile Infirmary	Mobile	0.97	-
Thomas Hospital	Fairhope	0.97	-
Troy Regional Medical Center	Troy	0.97	-
Walker Baptist Medical Center	Jasper	0.97	-
Athens - Limestone Hospital	Athens	0.98	-
Baptist Medical Center East	Montgomery	0.98	-
D W Mcmillan Memorial Hospital	Brewton	0.98	-
Decatur Morgan Hospital - Decatur Campus	Decatur	0.98	-
Grove Hill Memorial Hospital	Grove Hill	0.98	-
Jackson Medical Center	Jackson	0.98	-
L V Stabler Memorial Hospital	Greenville	0.98	-
Medical Center Barbour	Eufaula	0.98	-
Northeast Alabama Regional Medical Center	Anniston	0.98	-
Providence Hospital	Mobile	0.98	-
Russellville Hospital	Russellville	0.98	-
Saint Vincent's East	Birmingham	0.98	-
Stringfellow Memorial Hospital	Anniston	0.98	-
Andalusia Regional Hospital	Andalusia	0.99	-
Bullock County Hospital	Union Springs	0.99	-
Coosa Valley Medical Center	Sylacauga	0.99	-
Crenshaw Community Hospital	Luverne	0.99	-
Flowers Hospital	Dothan	0.99	-
Prattville Baptist Hospital	Prattville	0.99	-
South Baldwin Regional Medical Center	Foley	0.99	-
Vaughan Reg Med Ctr Parkway Campus	Selma	0.99	-
Baptist Medical Center - Princeton	Birmingham	1.00	-
D C H Regional Medical Center	Tuscaloosa	1.00	-
Dekalb Regional Medical Center	Fort Payne	1.00	-
Eliza Coffee Memorial Hospital	Florence	1.00	-
Georgiana Medical Center	Georgiana	1.00	-
Marshall Medical Center South	Boaz	1.00	-
Mizell Memorial Hospital	Opp	1.00	-
Southeast Alabama Medical Center	Dothan	1.00	-
Citizens Baptist Medical Center	Talladega	1.01	-
Decatur Morgan Hospital - Parkway Campus	Decatur	1.01	-
Huntsville Hospital	Huntsville	1.01	-
Shelby Baptist Medical Center	Alabaster	1.01	-
Springhill Medical Center	Mobile	1.01	-
Trinity Medical Center	Birmingham	1.01	-
Jackson Hospital & Clinic	Montgomery	1.02	-
Northwest Medical Center	Winfield	1.02	-
Bryan W Whitfield Memorial Hospital	Demopolis	1.03	-
Baptist Medical Center South	Montgomery	1.04	-
Brookwood Medical Center	Birmingham	1.04	-
Gadsden Regional Medical Center	Gadsden	1.04	-
Monroe County Hospital	Monroeville	1.04	-
Saint Vincent's Birmingham	Birmingham	1.04	-
Elmore Community Hospital	Wetumpka	1.05	-
Hill Hospital of Sumter County	York	1.05	-
Riverview Regional Medical Center	Gadsden	1.06	-
Shoals Hospital	Muscle Shoals	1.06	-
Helen Keller Memorial Hospital	Sheffield	1.07	-
Hale County Hospital	Greensboro	1.08	-
J Paul Jones Hospital	Camden	1.19	-

Pneumonia Care

Appropriate Initial Antibiotic Given

Hospital Name	City	Rate	Cases
Coosa Valley Medical Center[2]	Sylacauga	100%	56
Crestwood Medical Center	Huntsville	100%	112
Cullman Regional Medical Center[2]	Cullman	100%	58
Eliza Coffee Memorial Hospital[2]	Florence	100%	67
Flowers Hospital	Dothan	100%	138
George H. Lanier Memorial Hospital	Valley	100%	32
Jackson Hospital & Clinic	Montgomery	100%	113
Mobile Infirmary[2]	Mobile	100%	57
Pickens County Medical Center[2]	Carrollton	100%	39
Saint Vincent's Birmingham[2]	Birmingham	100%	106
Saint Vincent's East[2]	Birmingham	100%	81
Trinity Medical Center	Birmingham	100%	63
Baptist Medical Center - Princeton	Birmingham	99%	192
Fayette Medical Center[2]	Fayette	99%	68
Lakeland Community Hospital	Haleyville	99%	82
Northwest Medical Center	Winfield	99%	90
Providence Hospital	Mobile	99%	252
South Baldwin Regional Medical Center	Foley	99%	156
Springhill Medical Center	Mobile	99%	153
Thomas Hospital	Fairhope	99%	75
University of Alabama Hospital[2]	Birmingham	99%	106
Vaughan Reg Med Ctr Parkway Campus	Selma	99%	117
Walker Baptist Medical Center	Jasper	99%	153
D C H Regional Medical Center[2]	Tuscaloosa	98%	185
Decatur Morgan Hospital - Decatur Campus	Decatur	98%	136
Medical Center Enterprise	Enterprise	98%	59
Russellville Hospital	Russellville	98%	83
Shelby Baptist Medical Center	Alabaster	98%	222
Andalusia Regional Hospital	Andalusia	97%	76
Dekalb Regional Medical Center	Fort Payne	97%	60
Medical West	Bessemer	97%	161
Russell Hospital	Alexander City	97%	63
Cherokee Medical Center	Centre	96%	27
Citizens Baptist Medical Center	Talladega	96%	56
East Alabama Medical Center	Opelika	96%	168
Helen Keller Memorial Hospital	Sheffield	96%	173
Huntsville Hospital	Huntsville	96%	366
Shoals Hospital	Muscle Shoals	96%	57
Stringfellow Memorial Hospital	Anniston	96%	93
Baptist Medical Center East[2]	Montgomery	95%	83
Brookwood Medical Center[2]	Birmingham	95%	123
Gadsden Regional Medical Center	Gadsden	95%	237
North Baldwin Infirmary	Bay Minette	95%	40
Prattville Baptist Hospital	Prattville	95%	93
Southeast Alabama Medical Center	Dothan	95%	171
Baptist Medical Center South	Montgomery	94%	96
Birmingham VA Medical Center	Birmingham	94%	48
Marshall Medical Center South	Boaz	94%	160
Lawrence Medical Center	Moulton	93%	56
VA Central AL Hlthcare Sys-Montgomery	Montgomery	93%	41
Atmore Community Hospital	Atmore	92%	50
Decatur Morgan Hospital - Parkway Campus	Decatur	92%	48
Mizell Memorial Hospital	Opp	92%	50
Riverview Regional Medical Center	Gadsden	92%	113
Saint Vincent's Saint Clair	Pell City	92%	181
Troy Regional Medical Center	Troy	92%	39

NOTE: Hospital profiles are in alphabetical order by state, then city, then hospital within the city; Rankings exclude hospitals with less than 25 cases except for patient surveys which excludes hospitals with less than 100 cases; (a) 100-299 cases; (1) The number of cases/patients is too few to report; (2) Data submitted were based on a sample of cases/patients; (3) Results are based on a shorter time period than required; (4) Data suppressed by CMS for one or more quarters; (5) Results are not available for this reporting period; (6) Fewer than 100 patients completed the HCAHPS survey; (7) No cases met the criteria for this measure; (8) The lower limit of the confidence interval cannot be calculated if the number of observed infections equals zero; (9) No data are available from the state/territory for this reporting period; (10) The scores shown reflect fewer than 50 completed surveys; (11) There were discrepancies in the data collection process; (12) This measure does not apply to this hospital for this reporting period; (13) Results cannot be calculated for this reporting period; (14) The results for this state are combined with nearby states to protect confidentiality; Please refer to the User's Guide for a full explanation of data.

Athens - Limestone Hospital	Athens	91%	67
D W Mcmillan Memorial Hospital	Brewton	91%	58
Marion Regional Medical Center	Hamilton	91%	74
Medical Center Barbour[2]	Eufaula	89%	35
Northeast Alabama Regional Medical Center	Anniston	89%	147
Community Hospital	Tallassee	88%	41
Jackson Medical Center	Jackson	88%	26
Wedowee Hospital	Wedowee	88%	42
Clay County Hospital[2]	Ashland	86%	28
Monroe County Hospital	Monroeville	86%	36
Dale Medical Center	Ozark	85%	34
Highlands Medical Center	Scottsboro	83%	143
Evergreen Medical Center[2]	Evergreen	80%	30
Jacksonville Medical Center	Jacksonville	79%	43
Georgiana Medical Center	Georgiana	77%	35
Elmore Community Hospital[2]	Wetumpka	72%	40
Bryan W Whitfield Memorial Hospital[2]	Demopolis	71%	58
Wiregrass Medical Center[2]	Geneva	58%	64

Blood Culture Timing

Hospital Name	City	Rate	Cases
Baptist Medical Center - Princeton	Birmingham	100%	268
Brookwood Medical Center[2]	Birmingham	100%	292
Cherokee Medical Center	Centre	100%	35
Coosa Valley Medical Center[2]	Sylacauga	100%	178
Dale Medical Center	Ozark	100%	56
East Alabama Medical Center	Opelika	100%	214
Flowers Hospital	Dothan	100%	188
Helen Keller Memorial Hospital	Sheffield	100%	244
Jackson Hospital & Clinic	Montgomery	100%	272
Jackson Medical Center	Jackson	100%	25
L V Stabler Memorial Hospital	Greenville	100%	28
Lakeland Community Hospital	Haleyville	100%	67
Monroe County Hospital	Monroeville	100%	45
North Baldwin Infirmary	Bay Minette	100%	53
Providence Hospital	Mobile	100%	212
Russell Hospital	Alexander City	100%	128
Russellville Hospital	Russellville	100%	95
Saint Vincent's Birmingham[2]	Birmingham	100%	153
Saint Vincent's East[2]	Birmingham	100%	133
Shelby Baptist Medical Center	Alabaster	100%	241
South Baldwin Regional Medical Center	Foley	100%	124
Springhill Medical Center	Mobile	100%	192
Thomas Hospital	Fairhope	100%	133
Trinity Medical Center	Birmingham	100%	128
VA Central AL Hlthcare Sys-Montgomery	Montgomery	100%	55
Vaughan Reg Med Ctr Parkway Campus	Selma	100%	151
Walker Baptist Medical Center	Jasper	100%	219
Andalusia Regional Hospital	Andalusia	99%	89
Athens - Limestone Hospital	Athens	99%	144
Citizens Baptist Medical Center	Talladega	99%	95
Decatur Morgan Hospital - Parkway Campus	Decatur	99%	75
Eliza Coffee Memorial Hospital[2]	Florence	99%	99
Gadsden Regional Medical Center	Gadsden	99%	364
Huntsville Hospital	Huntsville	99%	716
Marion Regional Medical Center	Hamilton	99%	85
Marshall Medical Center South	Boaz	99%	360
Medical Center Enterprise	Enterprise	99%	87
Northeast Alabama Regional Medical Center	Anniston	99%	213
Riverview Regional Medical Center	Gadsden	99%	169
Saint Vincent's Saint Clair	Pell City	99%	171
Shoals Hospital	Muscle Shoals	99%	92
Southeast Alabama Medical Center	Dothan	99%	219
Stringfellow Memorial Hospital	Anniston	99%	97
University of Alabama Hospital[2]	Birmingham	99%	258
Univ of S Alabama Med Ctr	Mobile	99%	72
Baptist Medical Center East[2]	Montgomery	98%	127
Cullman Regional Medical Center[2]	Cullman	98%	180
D C H Regional Medical Center[2]	Tuscaloosa	98%	251
Fayette Medical Center[2]	Fayette	98%	95
Medical West	Bessemer	98%	280
Northwest Medical Center	Winfield	98%	98
Pickens County Medical Center[2]	Carrollton	98%	44
Birmingham VA Medical Center	Birmingham	97%	87
Crestwood Medical Center	Huntsville	97%	34
D W Mcmillan Memorial Hospital	Brewton	97%	30
Dekalb Regional Medical Center	Fort Payne	97%	142
Mobile Infirmary[2]	Mobile	97%	75
Prattville Baptist Hospital	Prattville	97%	150
Troy Regional Medical Center	Troy	97%	37
Atmore Community Hospital	Atmore	96%	50
Community Hospital	Tallassee	96%	56
George H. Lanier Memorial Hospital	Valley	96%	55
Highlands Medical Center	Scottsboro	96%	136
Decatur Morgan Hospital - Decatur Campus	Decatur	95%	201
Bibb Medical Center	Centreville	94%	31
Mizell Memorial Hospital	Opp	94%	35
Medical Center Barbour[2]	Eufaula	93%	42
Jacksonville Medical Center	Jacksonville	92%	52
Lawrence Medical Center	Moulton	92%	62
Baptist Medical Center South	Montgomery	91%	111

Wedowee Hospital	Wedowee	91%	47
Lake Martin Community Hospital[2]	Dadeville	80%	25
Wiregrass Medical Center[2]	Geneva	80%	54

Pregnancy and Delivery Care

Newborns whose Deliveries were Scheduled Early

Hospital Name	City	Rate	Cases
Andalusia Regional Hospital[2]	Andalusia	0%	28
Brookwood Medical Center[2]	Birmingham	0%	73
Coosa Valley Medical Center	Sylacauga	0%	139
Flowers Hospital[2]	Dothan	0%	30
South Baldwin Regional Medical Center[2]	Foley	0%	49
Trinity Medical Center[2]	Birmingham	0%	28
University of Alabama Hospital[2]	Birmingham	0%	38
East Alabama Medical Center[2]	Opelika	1%	95
Dekalb Regional Medical Center[2]	Fort Payne	2%	47
Gadsden Regional Medical Center[2]	Gadsden	2%	41
Medical Center Enterprise[2]	Enterprise	2%	41
Crestwood Medical Center[2]	Huntsville	3%	38
Medical West	Bessemer	3%	62
Athens - Limestone Hospital	Athens	4%	57
Baptist Medical Center - Princeton	Birmingham	4%	25
Thomas Hospital	Fairhope	4%	351
Eliza Coffee Memorial Hospital	Florence	5%	84
Shelby Baptist Medical Center[2]	Alabaster	5%	37
Baptist Medical Center East[2]	Montgomery	6%	388
Saint Vincent's Birmingham[2]	Birmingham	6%	54
Walker Baptist Medical Center[2]	Jasper	7%	28
D W Mcmillan Memorial Hospital	Brewton	8%	25
Helen Keller Memorial Hospital[2]	Sheffield	8%	48
George H. Lanier Memorial Hospital	Valley	9%	53
Springhill Medical Center	Mobile	9%	64
Vaughan Reg Med Ctr Parkway Campus[2]	Selma	9%	47
Jackson Hospital & Clinic	Montgomery	10%	133
Providence Hospital	Mobile	10%	201
Northeast Alabama Regional Medical Center[2]	Anniston	12%	48
Russell Hospital[2]	Alexander City	12%	67
D C H Regional Medical Center[2]	Tuscaloosa	13%	54
Highlands Medical Center	Scottsboro	14%	29
Mobile Infirmary[2]	Mobile	14%	56
Baptist Medical Center South	Montgomery	17%	72
Cullman Regional Medical Center	Cullman	19%	63
Decatur Morgan Hospital - Decatur Campus	Decatur	20%	88
Huntsville Hospital[2]	Huntsville	28%	769
Marshall Medical Center South	Boaz	30%	146
Crenshaw Community Hospital[2]	Luverne	74%	27
Bryan W Whitfield Memorial Hospital	Demopolis	96%	55

Preventive Care

Immunization for Influenza

Hospital Name	City	Rate	Cases
Coosa Valley Medical Center[2]	Sylacauga	100%	513
Dekalb Regional Medical Center[2]	Fort Payne	100%	384
Fayette Medical Center[2]	Fayette	100%	293
Flowers Hospital[2]	Dothan	100%	708
L V Stabler Memorial Hospital[2]	Greenville	100%	326
Riverview Regional Medical Center[2]	Gadsden	100%	534
Russellville Hospital[2]	Russellville	100%	298
South Baldwin Regional Medical Center[2]	Foley	100%	626
Trinity Medical Center[2]	Birmingham	100%	642
Vaughan Reg Med Ctr Parkway Campus[2]	Selma	100%	532
Walker Baptist Medical Center[2]	Jasper	100%	536
Athens - Limestone Hospital[2]	Athens	99%	405
Crestwood Medical Center[2]	Huntsville	99%	642
Highlands Medical Center[2]	Scottsboro	99%	423
Medical Center Enterprise[2]	Enterprise	99%	516
Northwest Medical Center[2]	Winfield	99%	297
Providence Hospital[2]	Mobile	99%	539
Univ of S Alabama Med Ctr[2]	Mobile	99%	574
Dale Medical Center[2]	Ozark	98%	354
Eliza Coffee Memorial Hospital[2]	Florence	98%	517
Gadsden Regional Medical Center[2]	Gadsden	98%	673
Jackson Hospital & Clinic[2]	Montgomery	98%	553
Pickens County Medical Center[2]	Carrollton	98%	284
Saint Vincent's Birmingham[2]	Birmingham	98%	500
Stringfellow Memorial Hospital[2]	Anniston	98%	347
Baptist Medical Center - Princeton[2]	Birmingham	97%	596
George H. Lanier Memorial Hospital[2]	Valley	97%	267
Jackson Medical Center	Jackson	97%	175
Saint Vincent's Saint Clair[2]	Pell City	97%	284
Shoals Hospital[2]	Muscle Shoals	97%	312
Troy Regional Medical Center[2]	Troy	97%	300
Bibb Medical Center[2]	Centreville	96%	90
Cullman Regional Medical Center[2]	Cullman	96%	488
Decatur Morgan Hospital - Parkway Campus[2]	Decatur	96%	291
Georgiana Medical Center[2]	Georgiana	96%	220
Helen Keller Memorial Hospital[2]	Sheffield	96%	515
Lakeland Community Hospital[2]	Haleyville	96%	295
Medical Center Barbour[2]	Eufaula	95%	395
Mobile Infirmary[2]	Mobile	95%	602
Springhill Medical Center[2]	Mobile	95%	611
Thomas Hospital[2]	Fairhope	95%	576
Cherokee Medical Center[2]	Centre	94%	301
D C H Regional Medical Center[2]	Tuscaloosa	94%	533
Huntsville Hospital[2]	Huntsville	94%	563
Lawrence Medical Center[2]	Moulton	94%	285
Medical West[2]	Bessemer	94%	577
Red Bay Hospital[2]	Red Bay	94%	52
Andalusia Regional Hospital[2]	Andalusia	93%	340
Clay County Hospital[2]	Ashland	93%	309
Community Hospital[2]	Tallassee	93%	288
D W Mcmillan Memorial Hospital[2]	Brewton	93%	323
Marion Regional Medical Center[2]	Hamilton	93%	305
Southeast Alabama Medical Center[2]	Dothan	93%	558
Atmore Community Hospital[2]	Atmore	92%	264
Brookwood Medical Center[2]	Birmingham	92%	538
Marshall Medical Center South[2]	Boaz	92%	1053
Northeast Alabama Regional Medical Center[2]	Anniston	92%	617
Shelby Baptist Medical Center[2]	Alabaster	92%	561
Baptist Medical Center East[2]	Montgomery	91%	431
Jack Hughston Memorial Hospital[2]	Phenix City	91%	312
Prattville Baptist Hospital[2]	Prattville	91%	339
Russell Hospital[2]	Alexander City	91%	287
Saint Vincent's East[2]	Birmingham	91%	549
Bryan W Whitfield Memorial Hospital[2]	Demopolis	89%	296
Elmore Community Hospital[2]	Wetumpka	88%	319
Baptist Medical Center South[2]	Montgomery	85%	539
Crenshaw Community Hospital[2]	Luverne	85%	283
Citizens Baptist Medical Center[2]	Talladega	82%	286
East Alabama Medical Center[2]	Opelika	82%	750
Grove Hill Memorial Hospital[2]	Grove Hill	82%	320
Decatur Morgan Hospital - Decatur Campus[2]	Decatur	81%	571
University of Alabama Hospital[2]	Birmingham	81%	546
Mizell Memorial Hospital[2]	Opp	80%	334
Monroe County Hospital[2]	Monroeville	74%	259
Jacksonville Medical Center[2]	Jacksonville	67%	244
Wiregrass Medical Center[2]	Geneva	67%	298
North Baldwin Infirmary[2]	Bay Minette	64%	243
Washington County Hospital[2]	Chatom	57%	99
Evergreen Medical Center[2]	Evergreen	56%	295
Bullock County Hospital[2]	Union Springs	55%	298
Hale County Hospital[2]	Greensboro	51%	185
Florala Memorial Hospital[2]	Florala	50%	32
Wedowee Hospital	Wedowee	42%	266
Callahan Eye Hospital	Birmingham	33%	27
Hill Hospital of Sumter County[2]	York	29%	188
Lake Martin Community Hospital[2]	Dadeville	29%	284
Tuscaloosa VA Medical Center[2,3]	Tuscaloosa	24%	131
Greene County Hospital[2]	Eutaw	3%	218
J Paul Jones Hospital	Camden	0%	127

Immunization for Pneumonia

Hospital Name	City	Rate	Cases
Athens - Limestone Hospital[2]	Athens	100%	483
Coosa Valley Medical Center[2]	Sylacauga	100%	652
Crestwood Medical Center[2]	Huntsville	100%	762
Dale Medical Center[2]	Ozark	100%	499
Flowers Hospital[2]	Dothan	100%	777
L V Stabler Memorial Hospital[2]	Greenville	100%	417
Riverview Regional Medical Center[2]	Gadsden	100%	802
Russellville Hospital[2]	Russellville	100%	403
South Baldwin Regional Medical Center[2]	Foley	100%	781
Trinity Medical Center[2]	Birmingham	100%	766
Vaughan Reg Med Ctr Parkway Campus[2]	Selma	100%	644
Walker Baptist Medical Center[2]	Jasper	100%	723
Dekalb Regional Medical Center[2]	Fort Payne	99%	382
Highlands Medical Center[2]	Scottsboro	99%	551
Lawrence Medical Center[2]	Moulton	99%	427
Medical Center Enterprise[2]	Enterprise	99%	516
Providence Hospital[2]	Mobile	99%	683
Stringfellow Memorial Hospital[2]	Anniston	99%	459
Troy Regional Medical Center[2]	Troy	99%	316
Cherokee Medical Center[2]	Centre	98%	430
Cullman Regional Medical Center[2]	Cullman	98%	770
Eliza Coffee Memorial Hospital[2]	Florence	98%	641
Gadsden Regional Medical Center[2]	Gadsden	98%	787
Red Bay Hospital[2]	Red Bay	98%	95
Andalusia Regional Hospital[2]	Andalusia	97%	410
Baptist Medical Center - Princeton[2]	Birmingham	97%	909
D W Mcmillan Memorial Hospital[2]	Brewton	97%	344
Fayette Medical Center[2]	Fayette	97%	471
Georgiana Medical Center[2]	Georgiana	97%	215
Helen Keller Memorial Hospital[2]	Sheffield	97%	579
Lakeland Community Hospital[2]	Haleyville	97%	427
Marshall Medical Center South[2]	Boaz	97%	1271
Medical West[2]	Bessemer	97%	732
Mobile Infirmary[2]	Mobile	97%	768
Saint Vincent's Birmingham[2]	Birmingham	97%	583
Shoals Hospital[2]	Muscle Shoals	97%	479

NOTE: Hospital profiles are in alphabetical order by state, then city, then hospital within the city; Rankings exclude hospitals with less than 25 cases except for patient surveys which excludes hospitals with less than 100 cases; (a) 100-299 cases; (1) The number of cases/patients is too few to report; (2) Data submitted were based on a sample of cases/patients; (3) Results are based on a shorter time period than required; (4) Data suppressed by CMS for one or more quarters; (5) Results are not available for this reporting period; (6) Fewer than 100 patients completed the HCAHPS survey; (7) No cases met the criteria for this measure; (8) The lower limit of the confidence interval cannot be calculated if the number of observed infections equals zero; (9) No data are available from the state/territory for this reporting period; (10) The scores shown reflect fewer than 50 completed surveys; (11) There were discrepancies in the data collection process; (12) This measure does not apply to this hospital for this reporting period; (13) Results cannot be calculated for this reporting period; (14) The results for this state are combined with nearby states to protect confidentiality; Please refer to the User's Guide for a full explanation of data.

Thomas Hospital[2]	Fairhope	97%	731
Univ of S Alabama Med Ctr[2]	Mobile	97%	502
Bryan W Whitfield Memorial Hospital[2]	Demopolis	96%	381
Jackson Hospital & Clinic[2]	Montgomery	96%	737
Northwest Medical Center[2]	Winfield	96%	425
Pickens County Medical Center[2]	Carrollton	96%	424
Saint Vincent's Saint Clair[2]	Pell City	96%	420
George H. Lanier Memorial Hospital[2]	Valley	95%	345
Huntsville Hospital[2]	Huntsville	95%	664
Marion Regional Medical Center[2]	Hamilton	95%	486
Russell Hospital[2]	Alexander City	95%	355
Decatur Morgan Hospital - Decatur Campus[2]	Decatur	94%	683
Jack Hughston Memorial Hospital[2]	Phenix City	94%	397
Jackson Medical Center	Jackson	94%	203
Atmore Community Hospital[2]	Atmore	93%	461
Brookwood Medical Center[2]	Birmingham	93%	507
D C H Regional Medical Center[2]	Tuscaloosa	93%	590
Decatur Morgan Hospital - Parkway Campus[2]	Decatur	93%	433
Elmore Community Hospital[2]	Wetumpka	93%	432
Grove Hill Memorial Hospital[2]	Grove Hill	93%	310
Southeast Alabama Medical Center[2]	Dothan	93%	817
Clay County Hospital[2]	Ashland	92%	257
Medical Center Barbour[2]	Eufaula	91%	526
Baptist Medical Center East[2]	Montgomery	90%	306
Community Hospital[2]	Tallassee	90%	445
Mizell Memorial Hospital[2]	Opp	89%	509
Shelby Baptist Medical Center[2]	Alabaster	89%	737
Saint Vincent's East[2]	Birmingham	88%	700
Springhill Medical Center[2]	Mobile	88%	924
Citizens Baptist Medical Center[2]	Talladega	87%	327
Jacksonville Medical Center[2]	Jacksonville	86%	250
Crenshaw Community Hospital[2]	Luverne	85%	436
Northeast Alabama Regional Medical Center[2]	Anniston	84%	778
University of Alabama Hospital[2]	Birmingham	84%	602
Bullock County Hospital[2]	Union Springs	83%	292
North Baldwin Infirmary[2]	Bay Minette	83%	251
Bibb Medical Center[2]	Centreville	82%	154
Prattville Baptist Hospital[2]	Prattville	82%	493
East Alabama Medical Center[2]	Opelika	80%	771
Monroe County Hospital[2]	Monroeville	80%	277
Baptist Medical Center South[2]	Montgomery	79%	609
Washington County Hospital[2]	Chatom	69%	147
Wiregrass Medical Center[2]	Geneva	63%	445
Evergreen Medical Center[2]	Evergreen	58%	438
Florala Memorial Hospital[2,3]	Florala	57%	54
Wedowee Hospital	Wedowee	50%	373
Hale County Hospital[2]	Greensboro	48%	222
Callahan Eye Hospital	Birmingham	43%	47
Lake Martin Community Hospital[2]	Dadeville	34%	382
Hill Hospital of Sumter County[2]	York	32%	238
Tuscaloosa VA Medical Center[2,3]	Tuscaloosa	32%	156
Greene County Hospital[2]	Eutaw	13%	282
J Paul Jones Hospital[2]	Camden	1%	159

Stroke Care

Anticoagulation Therapy for Atrial Fibrillation

Hospital Name	City	Rate	Cases
Huntsville Hospital	Huntsville	100%	60
Baptist Medical Center South	Montgomery	97%	32
Mobile Infirmary	Mobile	95%	42
Providence Hospital	Mobile	68%	25

Antithrombotic Therapy Timing

Hospital Name	City	Rate	Cases
Coosa Valley Medical Center	Sylacauga	100%	43
Crestwood Medical Center	Huntsville	100%	62
D C H Regional Medical Center[2]	Tuscaloosa	100%	107
East Alabama Medical Center	Opelika	100%	148
Flowers Hospital	Dothan	100%	126
Lakeland Community Hospital	Haleyville	100%	26
Medical Center Enterprise	Enterprise	100%	27
Medical West	Bessemer	100%	81
Russell Hospital	Alexander City	100%	40
Saint Vincent's Birmingham[2]	Birmingham	100%	74
South Baldwin Regional Medical Center	Foley	100%	63
Trinity Medical Center	Birmingham	100%	119
Univ of S Alabama Med Ctr[2]	Mobile	100%	52
Vaughan Reg Med Ctr Parkway Campus[2]	Selma	100%	58
Walker Baptist Medical Center	Jasper	100%	50
Baptist Medical Center - Princeton	Birmingham	99%	219
Brookwood Medical Center[2]	Birmingham	99%	103
Gadsden Regional Medical Center	Gadsden	99%	162
Huntsville Hospital	Huntsville	99%	443
Marshall Medical Center South	Boaz	99%	108
Southeast Alabama Medical Center[2]	Dothan	99%	72
Thomas Hospital[2]	Fairhope	99%	71
Andalusia Regional Hospital	Andalusia	98%	45
Baptist Medical Center South	Montgomery	98%	220
Cullman Regional Medical Center	Cullman	98%	82
Northeast Alabama Regional Medical Center	Anniston	98%	100
Saint Vincent's East[2]	Birmingham	98%	60
Springhill Medical Center	Mobile	98%	100
Eliza Coffee Memorial Hospital	Florence	97%	88
University of Alabama Hospital[2]	Birmingham	97%	67
Citizens Baptist Medical Center	Talladega	96%	48
Highlands Medical Center	Scottsboro	96%	25
Saint Vincent's Saint Clair[2]	Pell City	96%	26
Mobile Infirmary	Mobile	95%	259
Baptist Medical Center East	Montgomery	94%	36
Decatur Morgan Hospital - Decatur Campus	Decatur	94%	89
Helen Keller Memorial Hospital	Sheffield	94%	70
Shelby Baptist Medical Center[2]	Alabaster	94%	105
Athens - Limestone Hospital	Athens	93%	29
Stringfellow Memorial Hospital	Anniston	93%	41
Jackson Hospital & Clinic	Montgomery	92%	111
Prattville Baptist Hospital	Prattville	89%	35
Riverview Regional Medical Center	Gadsden	86%	84
Providence Hospital	Mobile	85%	121
George H. Lanier Memorial Hospital	Valley	83%	29
Evergreen Medical Center	Evergreen	81%	27

Assessed for Rehabilitation

Hospital Name	City	Rate	Cases
Baptist Medical Center East	Montgomery	100%	41
Coosa Valley Medical Center	Sylacauga	100%	36
Cullman Regional Medical Center	Cullman	100%	93
D C H Regional Medical Center[2]	Tuscaloosa	100%	117
Decatur Morgan Hospital - Decatur Campus	Decatur	100%	107
East Alabama Medical Center	Opelika	100%	185
Flowers Hospital	Dothan	100%	148
Huntsville Hospital	Huntsville	100%	543
Medical Center Enterprise	Enterprise	100%	31
Prattville Baptist Hospital	Prattville	100%	39
South Baldwin Regional Medical Center	Foley	100%	82
Trinity Medical Center	Birmingham	100%	169
University of Alabama Hospital[2]	Birmingham	100%	116
Vaughan Reg Med Ctr Parkway Campus[2]	Selma	100%	62
Walker Baptist Medical Center	Jasper	100%	59
Gadsden Regional Medical Center	Gadsden	99%	179
Helen Keller Memorial Hospital	Sheffield	99%	69
Providence Hospital	Mobile	99%	122
Jackson Hospital & Clinic	Montgomery	98%	132
Saint Vincent's Birmingham[2]	Birmingham	98%	91
Saint Vincent's East[2]	Birmingham	98%	65
Univ of S Alabama Med Ctr[2]	Mobile	98%	93
Marshall Medical Center South	Boaz	97%	115
Mobile Infirmary	Mobile	97%	327
Thomas Hospital[2]	Fairhope	97%	72
Baptist Medical Center - Princeton	Birmingham	96%	253
Southeast Alabama Medical Center[2]	Dothan	96%	89
Baptist Medical Center South	Montgomery	95%	285
Crestwood Medical Center	Huntsville	95%	60
Medical West	Bessemer	95%	87
Athens - Limestone Hospital	Athens	94%	33
Andalusia Regional Hospital	Andalusia	93%	55
George H. Lanier Memorial Hospital	Valley	93%	28
Russell Hospital	Alexander City	93%	41
Springhill Medical Center	Mobile	93%	103
Eliza Coffee Memorial Hospital	Florence	92%	100
Evergreen Medical Center	Evergreen	92%	26
Lakeland Community Hospital	Haleyville	92%	26
Shelby Baptist Medical Center[2]	Alabaster	92%	120
Citizens Baptist Medical Center	Talladega	90%	49
Highlands Medical Center	Scottsboro	90%	30
Stringfellow Memorial Hospital	Anniston	87%	46
Decatur Morgan Hospital - Parkway Campus	Decatur	81%	27
Brookwood Medical Center[2]	Birmingham	73%	116
Northeast Alabama Regional Medical Center	Anniston	69%	115
Riverview Regional Medical Center	Gadsden	64%	80

Discharged on Antithrombotic Therapy

Hospital Name	City	Rate	Cases
Baptist Medical Center - Princeton	Birmingham	100%	214
Coosa Valley Medical Center	Sylacauga	100%	34
Crestwood Medical Center	Huntsville	100%	58
Cullman Regional Medical Center	Cullman	100%	87
D C H Regional Medical Center[2]	Tuscaloosa	100%	106
East Alabama Medical Center	Opelika	100%	156
Flowers Hospital	Dothan	100%	139
Gadsden Regional Medical Center	Gadsden	100%	168
George H. Lanier Memorial Hospital	Valley	100%	28
Huntsville Hospital	Huntsville	100%	454
Medical Center Enterprise	Enterprise	100%	31
Northeast Alabama Regional Medical Center	Anniston	100%	109
Russell Hospital	Alexander City	100%	37
Saint Vincent's Birmingham[2]	Birmingham	100%	76
Shelby Baptist Medical Center[2]	Alabaster	100%	113
South Baldwin Regional Medical Center	Foley	100%	78
Trinity Medical Center	Birmingham	100%	122
University of Alabama Hospital[2]	Birmingham	100%	79
Univ of S Alabama Med Ctr[2]	Mobile	100%	61
Vaughan Reg Med Ctr Parkway Campus[2]	Selma	100%	58
Walker Baptist Medical Center	Jasper	100%	59
Baptist Medical Center South	Montgomery	99%	236
Eliza Coffee Memorial Hospital	Florence	99%	89
Jackson Hospital & Clinic	Montgomery	99%	116
Marshall Medical Center South	Boaz	99%	111
Medical West	Bessemer	99%	75
Mobile Infirmary	Mobile	99%	274
Southeast Alabama Medical Center[2]	Dothan	99%	77
Springhill Medical Center	Mobile	99%	96
Helen Keller Memorial Hospital	Sheffield	98%	61
Saint Vincent's East[2]	Birmingham	98%	61
Athens - Limestone Hospital	Athens	97%	30
Baptist Medical Center East	Montgomery	97%	39
Brookwood Medical Center[2]	Birmingham	97%	106
Decatur Morgan Hospital - Decatur Campus	Decatur	97%	100
Thomas Hospital[2]	Fairhope	97%	67
Highlands Medical Center	Scottsboro	96%	28
Providence Hospital	Mobile	96%	106
Stringfellow Memorial Hospital	Anniston	96%	45
Prattville Baptist Hospital	Prattville	95%	38
Andalusia Regional Hospital	Andalusia	93%	46
Citizens Baptist Medical Center	Talladega	92%	48
Riverview Regional Medical Center	Gadsden	91%	80
Decatur Morgan Hospital - Parkway Campus	Decatur	85%	26
Evergreen Medical Center	Evergreen	80%	25

Discharged on Statin Medication

Hospital Name	City	Rate	Cases
Cullman Regional Medical Center	Cullman	100%	68
East Alabama Medical Center	Opelika	100%	138
Flowers Hospital	Dothan	100%	101
South Baldwin Regional Medical Center	Foley	100%	47
Trinity Medical Center	Birmingham	100%	97
University of Alabama Hospital[2]	Birmingham	100%	59
Univ of S Alabama Med Ctr[2]	Mobile	100%	52
Vaughan Reg Med Ctr Parkway Campus[2]	Selma	100%	47
Mobile Infirmary	Mobile	99%	226
Baptist Medical Center South	Montgomery	98%	207
Crestwood Medical Center	Huntsville	98%	44
Helen Keller Memorial Hospital	Sheffield	98%	42
Huntsville Hospital	Huntsville	98%	329
Medical West	Bessemer	97%	62
Gadsden Regional Medical Center	Gadsden	96%	133
Baptist Medical Center - Princeton	Birmingham	95%	186
Prattville Baptist Hospital	Prattville	94%	31
Shelby Baptist Medical Center[2]	Alabaster	94%	82
Decatur Morgan Hospital - Decatur Campus	Decatur	93%	70
Southeast Alabama Medical Center[2]	Dothan	93%	60
Stringfellow Memorial Hospital	Anniston	93%	29
Walker Baptist Medical Center	Jasper	93%	44
Andalusia Regional Hospital	Andalusia	92%	25
Saint Vincent's Birmingham[2]	Birmingham	92%	64
Jackson Hospital & Clinic	Montgomery	91%	101
D C H Regional Medical Center[2]	Tuscaloosa	90%	83
Northeast Alabama Regional Medical Center	Anniston	90%	86
Saint Vincent's East[2]	Birmingham	90%	48
Eliza Coffee Memorial Hospital	Florence	87%	78
Baptist Medical Center East	Montgomery	86%	29
Russell Hospital	Alexander City	82%	34
Marshall Medical Center South	Boaz	81%	93
Springhill Medical Center	Mobile	81%	85
Thomas Hospital[2]	Fairhope	80%	49
Athens - Limestone Hospital	Athens	76%	25
Providence Hospital	Mobile	76%	80
Citizens Baptist Medical Center	Talladega	74%	35
Riverview Regional Medical Center	Gadsden	71%	70
Brookwood Medical Center[2]	Birmingham	62%	90
Highlands Medical Center	Scottsboro	52%	25

Thrombolytic Therapy Timing

Hospital Name	City	Rate	Cases
Baptist Medical Center South	Montgomery	69%	26
Northeast Alabama Regional Medical Center	Anniston	6%	47

Venous Thromboembolism (VTE) Prophylaxis

Hospital Name	City	Rate	Cases
Coosa Valley Medical Center	Sylacauga	100%	43
East Alabama Medical Center	Opelika	100%	181
Lakeland Community Hospital	Haleyville	100%	31
Medical Center Enterprise	Enterprise	100%	25
South Baldwin Regional Medical Center	Foley	100%	72
Trinity Medical Center	Birmingham	100%	188
Univ of S Alabama Med Ctr[2]	Mobile	100%	101
Vaughan Reg Med Ctr Parkway Campus[2]	Selma	100%	69
D C H Regional Medical Center[2]	Tuscaloosa	99%	126
Flowers Hospital	Dothan	99%	154
Huntsville Hospital	Huntsville	99%	554

NOTE: Hospital profiles are in alphabetical order by state, then city, then hospital within the city; Rankings exclude hospitals with less than 25 cases except for patient surveys which excludes hospitals with less than 100 cases; (a) 100-299 cases; (1) The number of cases/patients is too few to report; (2) Data submitted were based on a sample of cases/patients; (3) Results are based on a shorter time period than required; (4) Data suppressed by CMS for one or more quarters; (5) Results are not available for this reporting period; (6) Fewer than 100 patients completed the HCAHPS survey; (7) No cases met the criteria for this measure; (8) The lower limit of the confidence interval cannot be calculated if the number of observed infections equals zero; (9) No data are available from the state/territory for this reporting period; (10) The scores shown reflect fewer than 50 completed surveys; (11) There were discrepancies in the data collection process; (12) This measure does not apply to this hospital for this reporting period; (13) Results cannot be calculated for this reporting period; (14) The results for this state are combined with nearby states to protect confidentiality; Please refer to the User's Guide for a full explanation of data.

Walker Baptist Medical Center	Jasper	98%	60
Baptist Medical Center - Princeton	Birmingham	97%	310
Cullman Regional Medical Center	Cullman	97%	91
Decatur Morgan Hospital - Decatur Campus	Decatur	97%	108
Gadsden Regional Medical Center	Gadsden	97%	176
University of Alabama Hospital[2]	Birmingham	97%	118
Andalusia Regional Hospital	Andalusia	96%	51
Medical West	Bessemer	96%	92
Southeast Alabama Medical Center[2]	Dothan	96%	94
Crestwood Medical Center	Huntsville	95%	65
Citizens Baptist Medical Center	Talladega	92%	48
Mobile Infirmary	Mobile	92%	335
Providence Hospital	Mobile	90%	144
Baptist Medical Center East	Montgomery	89%	35
Shelby Baptist Medical Center[2]	Alabaster	89%	117
Prattville Baptist Hospital	Prattville	88%	40
Helen Keller Memorial Hospital	Sheffield	87%	79
Jackson Hospital & Clinic	Montgomery	87%	140
Baptist Medical Center South	Montgomery	85%	302
Saint Vincent's Birmingham[2]	Birmingham	85%	92
Springhill Medical Center	Mobile	84%	109
Brookwood Medical Center[2]	Birmingham	80%	114
Thomas Hospital[2]	Fairhope	79%	77
Saint Vincent's East[2]	Birmingham	77%	62
Saint Vincent's Saint Clair[2]	Pell City	77%	26
Eliza Coffee Memorial Hospital	Florence	72%	107
Marshall Medical Center South	Boaz	70%	111
Athens - Limestone Hospital	Athens	67%	30
Northeast Alabama Regional Medical Center	Anniston	67%	110
Stringfellow Memorial Hospital	Anniston	66%	44
Russell Hospital	Alexander City	65%	40
George H. Lanier Memorial Hospital	Valley	55%	31
Riverview Regional Medical Center	Gadsden	38%	86
Evergreen Medical Center	Evergreen	28%	29

Written Stroke Educational Materials Given

Hospital Name	City	Rate	Cases
Cullman Regional Medical Center	Cullman	100%	58
Huntsville Hospital	Huntsville	100%	286
South Baldwin Regional Medical Center	Foley	100%	59
Trinity Medical Center	Birmingham	100%	93
Vaughan Reg Med Ctr Parkway Campus[2]	Selma	100%	33
Walker Baptist Medical Center	Jasper	100%	40
Thomas Hospital[2]	Fairhope	98%	49
Andalusia Regional Hospital	Andalusia	97%	29
D C H Regional Medical Center[2]	Tuscaloosa	97%	73
Decatur Morgan Hospital - Decatur Campus	Decatur	97%	61
East Alabama Medical Center	Opelika	96%	102
Providence Hospital	Mobile	95%	61
Crestwood Medical Center	Huntsville	94%	31
Flowers Hospital	Dothan	94%	81
Mobile Infirmary	Mobile	94%	186
Univ of S Alabama Med Ctr[2]	Mobile	94%	69
University of Alabama Hospital[2]	Birmingham	93%	70
Gadsden Regional Medical Center	Gadsden	92%	97
Jackson Hospital & Clinic	Montgomery	92%	62
Shelby Baptist Medical Center[2]	Alabaster	92%	64
Springhill Medical Center	Mobile	91%	64
Stringfellow Memorial Hospital	Anniston	90%	31
Baptist Medical Center - Princeton	Birmingham	88%	155
Baptist Medical Center South	Montgomery	85%	152
Medical West	Bessemer	85%	53
Southeast Alabama Medical Center[2]	Dothan	85%	53
Helen Keller Memorial Hospital	Sheffield	80%	25
Marshall Medical Center South	Boaz	80%	65
Saint Vincent's East[2]	Birmingham	74%	39
Eliza Coffee Memorial Hospital	Florence	71%	49
Saint Vincent's Birmingham[2]	Birmingham	71%	51
Citizens Baptist Medical Center	Talladega	68%	28
Brookwood Medical Center[2]	Birmingham	55%	76
Northeast Alabama Regional Medical Center	Anniston	6%	78
Riverview Regional Medical Center	Gadsden	0%	51

Surgical Care Improvement Project

Appropriate Beta Blocker Usage

Hospital Name	City	Rate	Cases
East Alabama Medical Center	Opelika	100%	415
Flowers Hospital	Dothan	100%	370
Marshall Medical Center South	Boaz	100%	126
Medical Center Enterprise	Enterprise	100%	80
Mobile Infirmary[2]	Mobile	100%	277
Russellville Hospital	Russellville	100%	27
Shelby Baptist Medical Center[2]	Alabaster	100%	253
Trinity Medical Center	Birmingham	100%	390
Vaughan Reg Med Ctr Parkway Campus	Selma	100%	34
Walker Baptist Medical Center	Jasper	100%	128
Baptist Medical Center - Princeton[2]	Birmingham	99%	339
Baptist Medical Center East	Montgomery	99%	75
Crestwood Medical Center	Huntsville	99%	310
Cullman Regional Medical Center[2]	Cullman	99%	97
D C H Regional Medical Center[2]	Tuscaloosa	99%	203
Eliza Coffee Memorial Hospital[2]	Florence	99%	195
Providence Hospital[2]	Mobile	99%	215
Saint Vincent's Birmingham[2]	Birmingham	99%	244
Saint Vincent's East[2]	Birmingham	99%	236
South Baldwin Regional Medical Center	Foley	99%	69
Southeast Alabama Medical Center[2]	Dothan	99%	208
Brookwood Medical Center[2]	Birmingham	98%	378
Coosa Valley Medical Center	Sylacauga	98%	59
Decatur Morgan Hospital - Decatur Campus	Decatur	98%	213
Dekalb Regional Medical Center	Fort Payne	98%	56
Huntsville Hospital[2]	Huntsville	98%	287
Stringfellow Memorial Hospital	Anniston	98%	44
Athens - Limestone Hospital	Athens	97%	63
George H. Lanier Memorial Hospital	Valley	97%	32
Jack Hughston Memorial Hospital[2]	Phenix City	97%	101
Medical West	Bessemer	97%	141
Northeast Alabama Regional Medical Center[2]	Anniston	97%	233
Springhill Medical Center[2]	Mobile	97%	195
Thomas Hospital[2]	Fairhope	97%	142
Helen Keller Memorial Hospital[2]	Sheffield	96%	97
Jackson Hospital & Clinic	Montgomery	96%	384
Riverview Regional Medical Center	Gadsden	96%	151
Univ of S Alabama Med Ctr[2]	Mobile	96%	51
Baptist Medical Center South[2]	Montgomery	95%	342
Andalusia Regional Hospital	Andalusia	94%	32
Birmingham VA Medical Center[2]	Birmingham	94%	127
Gadsden Regional Medical Center	Gadsden	93%	330
University of Alabama Hospital[2]	Birmingham	93%	187
Russell Hospital	Alexander City	92%	64
Shoals Hospital	Muscle Shoals	91%	35
Dale Medical Center	Ozark	53%	30

Appropriate VTP Within 24 Hours

Hospital Name	City	Rate	Cases
Andalusia Regional Hospital	Andalusia	100%	202
Baptist Medical Center - Princeton[2]	Birmingham	100%	439
Baptist Medical Center East	Montgomery	100%	301
Coosa Valley Medical Center	Sylacauga	100%	161
Cullman Regional Medical Center[2]	Cullman	100%	300
D W Mcmillan Memorial Hospital	Brewton	100%	51
Dekalb Regional Medical Center	Fort Payne	100%	126
East Alabama Medical Center	Opelika	100%	1001
Flowers Hospital	Dothan	100%	894
Helen Keller Memorial Hospital[2]	Sheffield	100%	265
Highlands Medical Center	Scottsboro	100%	65
L V Stabler Memorial Hospital	Greenville	100%	68
Medical Center Enterprise	Enterprise	100%	366
Russellville Hospital	Russellville	100%	94
Saint Vincent's Birmingham[2]	Birmingham	100%	384
Shelby Baptist Medical Center[2]	Alabaster	100%	413
South Baldwin Regional Medical Center	Foley	100%	277
Trinity Medical Center	Birmingham	100%	910
Univ of S Alabama Med Ctr[2]	Mobile	100%	201
Walker Baptist Medical Center	Jasper	100%	368
Athens - Limestone Hospital	Athens	99%	193
Birmingham VA Medical Center[2]	Birmingham	99%	204
Crestwood Medical Center	Huntsville	99%	1126
D C H Regional Medical Center[2]	Tuscaloosa	99%	430
Decatur Morgan Hospital - Decatur Campus	Decatur	99%	639
Huntsville Hospital[2]	Huntsville	99%	491
Jackson Hospital & Clinic	Montgomery	99%	674
Mobile Infirmary[2]	Mobile	99%	481
Providence Hospital[2]	Mobile	99%	305
Riverview Regional Medical Center	Gadsden	99%	327
Stringfellow Memorial Hospital	Anniston	99%	136
Vaughan Reg Med Ctr Parkway Campus	Selma	99%	127
Brookwood Medical Center[2]	Birmingham	98%	691
Eliza Coffee Memorial Hospital[2]	Florence	98%	259
Gadsden Regional Medical Center	Gadsden	98%	643
Marshall Medical Center South	Boaz	98%	411
Troy Regional Medical Center	Troy	98%	80
University of Alabama Hospital[2]	Birmingham	98%	414
Dale Medical Center	Ozark	97%	89
George H. Lanier Memorial Hospital	Valley	97%	97
Jack Hughston Memorial Hospital[2]	Phenix City	97%	380
Medical West	Bessemer	97%	383
Springhill Medical Center[2]	Mobile	97%	457
Thomas Hospital[2]	Fairhope	97%	275
Northeast Alabama Regional Medical Center[2]	Anniston	96%	498
Saint Vincent's East[2]	Birmingham	96%	343
Shoals Hospital	Muscle Shoals	96%	114
Southeast Alabama Medical Center[2]	Dothan	96%	295
Prattville Baptist Hospital	Prattville	95%	40
Northwest Medical Center	Winfield	94%	35
Russell Hospital	Alexander City	93%	134
Baptist Medical Center South[2]	Montgomery	91%	627
Citizens Baptist Medical Center	Talladega	91%	44
North Baldwin Infirmary	Bay Minette	88%	43

Controlled Postoperative Blood Glucose

Hospital Name	City	Rate	Cases
Brookwood Medical Center[2]	Birmingham	100%	234
D C H Regional Medical Center[2]	Tuscaloosa	100%	97
Trinity Medical Center	Birmingham	100%	127
East Alabama Medical Center	Opelika	99%	195
Eliza Coffee Memorial Hospital[2]	Florence	99%	87
Huntsville Hospital[2]	Huntsville	99%	161
Mobile Infirmary[2]	Mobile	99%	170
Providence Hospital[2]	Mobile	99%	135
Saint Vincent's Birmingham[2]	Birmingham	99%	132
Thomas Hospital[2]	Fairhope	99%	124
Flowers Hospital	Dothan	98%	132
Baptist Medical Center - Princeton[2]	Birmingham	97%	246
Birmingham VA Medical Center[2]	Birmingham	97%	65
Gadsden Regional Medical Center	Gadsden	97%	172
Shelby Baptist Medical Center[2]	Alabaster	97%	112
Baptist Medical Center South[2]	Montgomery	96%	169
Northeast Alabama Regional Medical Center[2]	Anniston	96%	104
Southeast Alabama Medical Center[2]	Dothan	96%	121
University of Alabama Hospital[2]	Birmingham	96%	137
Jackson Hospital & Clinic	Montgomery	95%	258
Riverview Regional Medical Center	Gadsden	93%	42
Springhill Medical Center[2]	Mobile	92%	96
Saint Vincent's East[2]	Birmingham	89%	116

Perioperative Temperature Management

Hospital Name	City	Rate	Cases
Andalusia Regional Hospital	Andalusia	100%	229
Athens - Limestone Hospital	Athens	100%	220
Baptist Medical Center - Princeton[2]	Birmingham	100%	581
Baptist Medical Center East	Montgomery	100%	392
Baptist Medical Center South[2]	Montgomery	100%	878
Brookwood Medical Center[2]	Birmingham	100%	874
Citizens Baptist Medical Center	Talladega	100%	52
Coosa Valley Medical Center	Sylacauga	100%	203
Crestwood Medical Center	Huntsville	100%	1324
Cullman Regional Medical Center[2]	Cullman	100%	370
D C H Regional Medical Center[2]	Tuscaloosa	100%	574
D W Mcmillan Memorial Hospital	Brewton	100%	106
Dale Medical Center	Ozark	100%	96
Decatur Morgan Hospital - Decatur Campus	Decatur	100%	759
Dekalb Regional Medical Center	Fort Payne	100%	188
East Alabama Medical Center	Opelika	100%	1129
Eliza Coffee Memorial Hospital[2]	Florence	100%	385
Flowers Hospital	Dothan	100%	1159
George H. Lanier Memorial Hospital	Valley	100%	129
Grove Hill Memorial Hospital[2,3]	Grove Hill	100%	28
Helen Keller Memorial Hospital[2]	Sheffield	100%	313
Highlands Medical Center	Scottsboro	100%	94
Jack Hughston Memorial Hospital[2]	Phenix City	100%	412
Jackson Hospital & Clinic	Montgomery	100%	828
L V Stabler Memorial Hospital	Greenville	100%	69
Marshall Medical Center South	Boaz	100%	509
Medical Center Enterprise	Enterprise	100%	404
Medical West	Bessemer	100%	458
Mizell Memorial Hospital	Opp	100%	29
Mobile Infirmary[2]	Mobile	100%	638
Monroe County Hospital[3]	Monroeville	100%	27
Northeast Alabama Regional Medical Center[2]	Anniston	100%	618
Northwest Medical Center	Winfield	100%	85
Providence Hospital[2]	Mobile	100%	407
Riverview Regional Medical Center	Gadsden	100%	386
Russell Hospital	Alexander City	100%	153
Russellville Hospital	Russellville	100%	111
Saint Vincent's Birmingham[2]	Birmingham	100%	507
Saint Vincent's East[2]	Birmingham	100%	405
Shelby Baptist Medical Center[2]	Alabaster	100%	540
Shoals Hospital	Muscle Shoals	100%	126
South Baldwin Regional Medical Center	Foley	100%	330
Southeast Alabama Medical Center[2]	Dothan	100%	365
Springhill Medical Center[2]	Mobile	100%	529
Stringfellow Memorial Hospital	Anniston	100%	156
Thomas Hospital[2]	Fairhope	100%	344
Trinity Medical Center	Birmingham	100%	1107
Troy Regional Medical Center	Troy	100%	87
University of Alabama Hospital[2]	Birmingham	100%	566
Univ of S Alabama Med Ctr[2]	Mobile	100%	254
Vaughan Reg Med Ctr Parkway Campus	Selma	100%	153
Walker Baptist Medical Center	Jasper	100%	400
Birmingham VA Medical Center[2]	Birmingham	99%	298
Gadsden Regional Medical Center	Gadsden	99%	768
Huntsville Hospital[2]	Huntsville	99%	628
Prattville Baptist Hospital	Prattville	98%	44
North Baldwin Infirmary	Bay Minette	94%	54

Prophylactic Antibiotic Selection

Hospital Name	City	Rate	Cases
Baptist Medical Center - Princeton[2]	Birmingham	100%	657

NOTE: Hospital profiles are in alphabetical order by state, then city, then hospital within the city; Rankings exclude hospitals with less than 25 cases except for patient surveys which excludes hospitals with less than 100 cases; (a) 100-299 cases; (1) The number of cases/patients is too few to report; (2) Data submitted were based on a sample of cases/patients; (3) Results are based on a shorter time period than required; (4) Data suppressed by CMS for one or more quarters; (5) Results are not available for this reporting period; (6) Fewer than 100 patients completed the HCAHPS survey; (7) No cases met the criteria for this measure; (8) The lower limit of the confidence interval cannot be calculated if the number of observed infections equals zero; (9) No data are available from the state/territory for this reporting period; (10) The scores shown reflect fewer than 50 completed surveys; (11) There were discrepancies in the data collection process; (12) This measure does not apply to this hospital for this reporting period; (13) Results cannot be calculated for this reporting period; (14) The results for this state are combined with nearby states to protect confidentiality; Please refer to the User's Guide for a full explanation of data.

Hospital Name	City	Rate	Cases
Baptist Medical Center East	Montgomery	100%	217
Birmingham VA Medical Center	Birmingham	100%	207
Crestwood Medical Center	Huntsville	100%	998
Cullman Regional Medical Center[2]	Cullman	100%	272
D W Mcmillan Memorial Hospital	Brewton	100%	66
Dale Medical Center	Ozark	100%	33
East Alabama Medical Center	Opelika	100%	931
Flowers Hospital	Dothan	100%	882
Helen Keller Memorial Hospital[2]	Sheffield	100%	187
Jackson Hospital & Clinic	Montgomery	100%	735
L V Stabler Memorial Hospital	Greenville	100%	48
Marshall Medical Center South	Boaz	100%	378
Medical Center Enterprise	Enterprise	100%	315
Providence Hospital[2]	Mobile	100%	369
Russell Hospital	Alexander City	100%	82
Russellville Hospital	Russellville	100%	71
Shelby Baptist Medical Center[2]	Alabaster	100%	419
Trinity Medical Center	Birmingham	100%	740
Troy Regional Medical Center	Troy	100%	50
University of Alabama Hospital[2]	Birmingham	100%	387
Univ of S Alabama Med Ctr[2]	Mobile	100%	132
Walker Baptist Medical Center	Jasper	100%	284
Andalusia Regional Hospital	Andalusia	99%	181
Athens - Limestone Hospital	Athens	99%	152
Brookwood Medical Center[2]	Birmingham	99%	825
D C H Regional Medical Center[2]	Tuscaloosa	99%	481
Decatur Morgan Hospital - Decatur Campus	Decatur	99%	539
Dekalb Regional Medical Center	Fort Payne	99%	148
Eliza Coffee Memorial Hospital[2]	Florence	99%	334
Gadsden Regional Medical Center	Gadsden	99%	630
George H. Lanier Memorial Hospital	Valley	99%	75
Huntsville Hospital[2]	Huntsville	99%	539
Medical West	Bessemer	99%	215
Mobile Infirmary[2]	Mobile	99%	582
Northeast Alabama Regional Medical Center[2]	Anniston	99%	520
Saint Vincent's Birmingham[2]	Birmingham	99%	482
Saint Vincent's East[2]	Birmingham	99%	363
South Baldwin Regional Medical Center	Foley	99%	188
Southeast Alabama Medical Center[2]	Dothan	99%	329
Springhill Medical Center[2]	Mobile	99%	479
Thomas Hospital[2]	Fairhope	99%	321
Baptist Medical Center South[2]	Montgomery	98%	770
Jack Hughston Memorial Hospital[2]	Phenix City	98%	273
Riverview Regional Medical Center	Gadsden	98%	288
Highlands Medical Center	Scottsboro	97%	79
Shoals Hospital	Muscle Shoals	97%	77
Stringfellow Memorial Hospital	Anniston	97%	99
Coosa Valley Medical Center	Sylacauga	96%	123
Vaughan Reg Med Ctr Parkway Campus	Selma	96%	80

Prophylactic Antibiotic Selection (Outpatient)

Hospital Name	City	Rate	Cases
Andalusia Regional Hospital[3]	Andalusia	100%	26
Crestwood Medical Center	Huntsville	100%	705
Dekalb Regional Medical Center	Fort Payne	100%	75
East Alabama Medical Center	Opelika	100%	848
Flowers Hospital	Dothan	100%	401
Gadsden Regional Medical Center	Gadsden	100%	303
Helen Keller Memorial Hospital	Sheffield	100%	442
Jack Hughston Memorial Hospital	Phenix City	100%	65
Medical Center Enterprise	Enterprise	100%	85
North Baldwin Infirmary	Bay Minette	100%	77
Providence Hospital	Mobile	100%	622
South Baldwin Regional Medical Center	Foley	100%	139
Trinity Medical Center	Birmingham	100%	451
Univ of S Alabama Med Ctr	Mobile	100%	26
Vaughan Reg Med Ctr Parkway Campus	Selma	100%	95
Walker Baptist Medical Center	Jasper	100%	95
Baptist Medical Center East	Montgomery	99%	292
Brookwood Medical Center	Birmingham	99%	941
D C H Regional Medical Center	Tuscaloosa	99%	672
Eliza Coffee Memorial Hospital	Florence	99%	492
George H. Lanier Memorial Hospital	Valley	99%	81
Huntsville Hospital	Huntsville	99%	1031
Jackson Hospital & Clinic	Montgomery	99%	593
Southeast Alabama Medical Center	Dothan	99%	388
Stringfellow Memorial Hospital	Anniston	99%	76
Baptist Medical Center - Princeton	Birmingham	98%	366
Baptist Medical Center South	Montgomery	98%	586
Citizens Baptist Medical Center	Talladega	98%	44
Cullman Regional Medical Center	Cullman	98%	195
Decatur Morgan Hospital - Parkway Campus	Decatur	98%	44
Medical West	Bessemer	98%	145
Saint Vincent's Birmingham	Birmingham	98%	982
Saint Vincent's East	Birmingham	98%	464
Springhill Medical Center	Mobile	98%	216
Jacksonville Medical Center	Jacksonville	97%	96
Mobile Infirmary	Mobile	97%	641
Riverview Regional Medical Center	Gadsden	97%	155
Russell Hospital	Alexander City	97%	307
Thomas Hospital	Fairhope	96%	294
Athens - Limestone Hospital	Athens	95%	128
Decatur Morgan Hospital - Decatur Campus	Decatur	95%	196
Marshall Medical Center South	Boaz	95%	76
Northeast Alabama Regional Medical Center	Anniston	94%	297
Shelby Baptist Medical Center	Alabaster	88%	194
University of Alabama Hospital	Birmingham	85%	609

Prophylactic Antibiotic Stopped

Hospital Name	City	Rate	Cases
Baptist Medical Center - Princeton[2]	Birmingham	100%	630
Birmingham VA Medical Center	Birmingham	100%	205
Flowers Hospital	Dothan	100%	844
Helen Keller Memorial Hospital[2]	Sheffield	100%	176
Marshall Medical Center South	Boaz	100%	376
Medical Center Enterprise	Enterprise	100%	315
South Baldwin Regional Medical Center	Foley	100%	174
Stringfellow Memorial Hospital	Anniston	100%	93
Thomas Hospital[2]	Fairhope	100%	314
Trinity Medical Center	Birmingham	100%	708
Vaughan Reg Med Ctr Parkway Campus	Selma	100%	73
Walker Baptist Medical Center	Jasper	100%	265
Andalusia Regional Hospital	Andalusia	99%	179
Coosa Valley Medical Center	Sylacauga	99%	116
Crestwood Medical Center	Huntsville	99%	978
Cullman Regional Medical Center[2]	Cullman	99%	272
Decatur Morgan Hospital - Decatur Campus	Decatur	99%	533
Dekalb Regional Medical Center	Fort Payne	99%	144
East Alabama Medical Center	Opelika	99%	894
Eliza Coffee Memorial Hospital[2]	Florence	99%	322
Huntsville Hospital[2]	Huntsville	99%	520
Mobile Infirmary[2]	Mobile	99%	539
Russell Hospital	Alexander City	99%	78
Saint Vincent's Birmingham[2]	Birmingham	99%	463
Shelby Baptist Medical Center[2]	Alabaster	99%	380
Springhill Medical Center[2]	Mobile	99%	446
University of Alabama Hospital[2]	Birmingham	99%	378
Brookwood Medical Center[2]	Birmingham	98%	797
D C H Regional Medical Center[2]	Tuscaloosa	98%	459
D W Mcmillan Memorial Hospital	Brewton	98%	65
Jack Hughston Memorial Hospital[2]	Phenix City	98%	269
Jackson Hospital & Clinic	Montgomery	98%	729
L V Stabler Memorial Hospital	Greenville	98%	46
Medical West	Bessemer	98%	211
Northeast Alabama Regional Medical Center[2]	Anniston	98%	507
Providence Hospital[2]	Mobile	98%	341
Saint Vincent's East[2]	Birmingham	98%	345
Russellville Hospital	Russellville	97%	63
Shoals Hospital	Muscle Shoals	97%	73
Baptist Medical Center East	Montgomery	96%	187
Riverview Regional Medical Center	Gadsden	96%	255
Athens - Limestone Hospital	Athens	95%	146
Baptist Medical Center South[2]	Montgomery	95%	761
George H. Lanier Memorial Hospital	Valley	95%	73
Highlands Medical Center	Scottsboro	95%	77
Southeast Alabama Medical Center[2]	Dothan	95%	324
Dale Medical Center	Ozark	94%	32
Gadsden Regional Medical Center	Gadsden	93%	587
Troy Regional Medical Center	Troy	92%	49
Univ of S Alabama Med Ctr[2]	Mobile	90%	122

Prophylactic Antibiotic Timing

Hospital Name	City	Rate	Cases
Andalusia Regional Hospital	Andalusia	100%	182
Baptist Medical Center - Princeton[2]	Birmingham	100%	657
Brookwood Medical Center[2]	Birmingham	100%	825
Coosa Valley Medical Center	Sylacauga	100%	123
Crestwood Medical Center	Huntsville	100%	998
D C H Regional Medical Center[2]	Tuscaloosa	100%	482
Dale Medical Center	Ozark	100%	33
Dekalb Regional Medical Center	Fort Payne	100%	149
East Alabama Medical Center	Opelika	100%	931
Eliza Coffee Memorial Hospital[2]	Florence	100%	334
Flowers Hospital	Dothan	100%	882
Gadsden Regional Medical Center	Gadsden	100%	632
Jackson Hospital & Clinic	Montgomery	100%	736
L V Stabler Memorial Hospital	Greenville	100%	48
Medical Center Enterprise	Enterprise	100%	315
Medical West	Bessemer	100%	215
Providence Hospital[2]	Mobile	100%	372
Russell Hospital	Alexander City	100%	82
Saint Vincent's East[2]	Birmingham	100%	367
Shelby Baptist Medical Center[2]	Alabaster	100%	420
Shoals Hospital	Muscle Shoals	100%	78
South Baldwin Regional Medical Center	Foley	100%	188
Southeast Alabama Medical Center[2]	Dothan	100%	330
Springhill Medical Center[2]	Mobile	100%	481
Trinity Medical Center	Birmingham	100%	743
Troy Regional Medical Center	Troy	100%	50
University of Alabama Hospital[2]	Birmingham	100%	387
Vaughan Reg Med Ctr Parkway Campus	Selma	100%	80
Walker Baptist Medical Center	Jasper	100%	284
Athens - Limestone Hospital	Athens	99%	152
Baptist Medical Center East	Montgomery	99%	217
Cullman Regional Medical Center[2]	Cullman	99%	275
Decatur Morgan Hospital - Decatur Campus	Decatur	99%	539
George H. Lanier Memorial Hospital	Valley	99%	75
Helen Keller Memorial Hospital[2]	Sheffield	99%	188
Huntsville Hospital[2]	Huntsville	99%	540
Marshall Medical Center South	Boaz	99%	380
Mobile Infirmary[2]	Mobile	99%	584
Northeast Alabama Regional Medical Center[2]	Anniston	99%	520
Riverview Regional Medical Center	Gadsden	99%	288
Russellville Hospital	Russellville	99%	71
Saint Vincent's Birmingham[2]	Birmingham	99%	482
Thomas Hospital[2]	Fairhope	99%	321
Univ of S Alabama Med Ctr[2]	Mobile	99%	132
Birmingham VA Medical Center	Birmingham	98%	207
Jack Hughston Memorial Hospital[2]	Phenix City	98%	275
Baptist Medical Center South[2]	Montgomery	97%	778
D W Mcmillan Memorial Hospital	Brewton	97%	67
Stringfellow Memorial Hospital	Anniston	97%	99
Highlands Medical Center	Scottsboro	96%	81

Prophylactic Antibiotic Timing (Outpatient)

Hospital Name	City	Rate	Cases
Andalusia Regional Hospital[3]	Andalusia	100%	26
Baptist Medical Center East	Montgomery	100%	292
Brookwood Medical Center	Birmingham	100%	941
Citizens Baptist Medical Center	Talladega	100%	44
Crestwood Medical Center	Huntsville	100%	705
Cullman Regional Medical Center	Cullman	100%	195
Dekalb Regional Medical Center	Fort Payne	100%	75
East Alabama Medical Center	Opelika	100%	848
Flowers Hospital	Dothan	100%	401
George H. Lanier Memorial Hospital	Valley	100%	81
Providence Hospital	Mobile	100%	622
Russell Hospital	Alexander City	100%	285
South Baldwin Regional Medical Center	Foley	100%	139
Southeast Alabama Medical Center	Dothan	100%	388
Stringfellow Memorial Hospital	Anniston	100%	76
Trinity Medical Center	Birmingham	100%	451
Walker Baptist Medical Center	Jasper	100%	95
Athens - Limestone Hospital	Athens	99%	129
Eliza Coffee Memorial Hospital	Florence	99%	493
Gadsden Regional Medical Center	Gadsden	99%	303
Helen Keller Memorial Hospital	Sheffield	99%	444
Huntsville Hospital	Huntsville	99%	1033
Jackson Hospital & Clinic	Montgomery	99%	596
Medical Center Enterprise	Enterprise	99%	86
Mobile Infirmary	Mobile	99%	645
Saint Vincent's East	Birmingham	99%	465
Springhill Medical Center	Mobile	99%	217
Vaughan Reg Med Ctr Parkway Campus	Selma	99%	93
Baptist Medical Center - Princeton	Birmingham	98%	371
Baptist Medical Center South	Montgomery	98%	592
D C H Regional Medical Center	Tuscaloosa	98%	672
Decatur Morgan Hospital - Decatur Campus	Decatur	98%	200
Jack Hughston Memorial Hospital	Phenix City	98%	65
Saint Vincent's Birmingham	Birmingham	98%	940
Thomas Hospital	Fairhope	98%	296
University of Alabama Hospital	Birmingham	98%	615
Jacksonville Medical Center	Jacksonville	97%	97
North Baldwin Infirmary	Bay Minette	97%	78
Northeast Alabama Regional Medical Center	Anniston	97%	281
Shelby Baptist Medical Center	Alabaster	97%	195
Univ of S Alabama Med Ctr	Mobile	96%	27
Riverview Regional Medical Center	Gadsden	95%	161
Medical West	Bessemer	94%	146
Marshall Medical Center South	Boaz	88%	84
Decatur Morgan Hospital - Parkway Campus	Decatur	84%	37

Urinary Catheter Removal

Hospital Name	City	Rate	Cases
Andalusia Regional Hospital	Andalusia	100%	165
Athens - Limestone Hospital	Athens	100%	151
Coosa Valley Medical Center	Sylacauga	100%	67
Crestwood Medical Center	Huntsville	100%	143
Dale Medical Center	Ozark	100%	79
Dekalb Regional Medical Center	Fort Payne	100%	71
Flowers Hospital	Dothan	100%	667
Helen Keller Memorial Hospital[2]	Sheffield	100%	200
L V Stabler Memorial Hospital	Greenville	100%	59
Medical Center Enterprise	Enterprise	100%	259
Russellville Hospital	Russellville	100%	77
South Baldwin Regional Medical Center	Foley	100%	162
Springhill Medical Center[2]	Mobile	100%	272
Trinity Medical Center	Birmingham	100%	332
Univ of S Alabama Med Ctr[2]	Mobile	100%	131
Birmingham VA Medical Center[2]	Birmingham	99%	154
Brookwood Medical Center[2]	Birmingham	99%	496

NOTE: Hospital profiles are in alphabetical order by state, then city, then hospital within the city; Rankings exclude hospitals with less than 25 cases except for patient surveys which excludes hospitals with less than 100 cases; (a) 100-299 cases; (1) The number of cases/patients is too few to report; (2) Data submitted were based on a sample of cases/patients; (3) Results are based on a shorter time period than required; (4) Data suppressed by CMS for one or more quarters; (5) Results are not available for this reporting period; (6) Fewer than 100 patients completed the HCAHPS survey; (7) No cases met the criteria for this measure; (8) The lower limit of the confidence interval cannot be calculated if the number of observed infections equals zero; (9) No data are available from the state/territory for this reporting period; (10) The scores shown reflect fewer than 50 completed surveys; (11) There were discrepancies in the data collection process; (12) This measure does not apply to this hospital for this reporting period; (13) Results cannot be calculated for this reporting period; (14) The results for this state are combined with nearby states to protect confidentiality; Please refer to the User's Guide for a full explanation of data.

Cullman Regional Medical Center[2]	Cullman	99%	198
D C H Regional Medical Center[2]	Tuscaloosa	99%	367
Decatur Morgan Hospital - Decatur Campus	Decatur	99%	479
East Alabama Medical Center	Opelika	99%	782
Jack Hughston Memorial Hospital[2]	Phenix City	99%	330
Marshall Medical Center South	Boaz	99%	333
Mobile Infirmary[2]	Mobile	99%	465
Providence Hospital[2]	Mobile	99%	341
Riverview Regional Medical Center	Gadsden	99%	288
Saint Vincent's Birmingham[2]	Birmingham	99%	225
Shelby Baptist Medical Center[2]	Alabaster	99%	337
Shoals Hospital	Muscle Shoals	99%	99
Stringfellow Memorial Hospital	Anniston	99%	108
Walker Baptist Medical Center	Jasper	99%	315
Baptist Medical Center - Princeton[2]	Birmingham	98%	336
Huntsville Hospital[2]	Huntsville	98%	322
Saint Vincent's East[2]	Birmingham	98%	339
Jackson Hospital & Clinic	Montgomery	97%	631
Northeast Alabama Regional Medical Center[2]	Anniston	97%	520
Troy Regional Medical Center	Troy	97%	30
University of Alabama Hospital[2]	Birmingham	97%	324
Baptist Medical Center East	Montgomery	96%	91
Eliza Coffee Memorial Hospital[2]	Florence	96%	300
George H. Lanier Memorial Hospital	Valley	96%	70
North Baldwin Infirmary	Bay Minette	96%	28
Thomas Hospital[2]	Fairhope	96%	202
Russell Hospital	Alexander City	95%	94
Medical West	Bessemer	94%	195
Gadsden Regional Medical Center	Gadsden	93%	447
Baptist Medical Center South[2]	Montgomery	91%	454
Southeast Alabama Medical Center[2]	Dothan	91%	312
Highlands Medical Center	Scottsboro	89%	36

Survey of Patients' Hospital Experiences

Area Around Room 'Always' Quiet at Night

Hospital Name	City	Rate	Cases
Marion Regional Medical Center	Hamilton	86%	(a)
Jack Hughston Memorial Hospital	Phenix City	79%	300+
Saint Vincent's Saint Clair	Pell City	78%	300+
Cherokee Medical Center	Centre	77%	(a)
Fayette Medical Center	Fayette	77%	(a)
Mizell Memorial Hospital	Opp	77%	(a)
Northwest Medical Center	Winfield	77%	300+
Russellville Hospital	Russellville	76%	300+
East Alabama Medical Center	Opelika	75%	300+
Elmore Community Hospital	Wetumpka	75%	(a)
Clay County Hospital	Ashland	74%	(a)
Coosa Valley Medical Center	Sylacauga	74%	300+
Monroe County Hospital	Monroeville	74%	(a)
Thomas Hospital	Fairhope	74%	300+
L V Stabler Memorial Hospital	Greenville	73%	(a)
Lake Martin Community Hospital	Dadeville	73%	(a)
Marshall Medical Center South	Boaz	73%	300+
Medical Center Barbour	Eufaula	73%	(a)
North Baldwin Infirmary	Bay Minette	73%	300+
Baptist Medical Center South	Montgomery	72%	300+
Cullman Regional Medical Center	Cullman	72%	300+
Dale Medical Center	Ozark	72%	(a)
Decatur Morgan Hospital - Decatur Campus	Decatur	72%	300+
Evergreen Medical Center	Evergreen	72%	(a)
Georgiana Medical Center	Georgiana	72%	(a)
Prattville Baptist Hospital	Prattville	72%	300+
Russell Hospital	Alexander City	72%	300+
Shoals Hospital	Muscle Shoals	72%	300+
Trinity Medical Center	Birmingham	72%	300+
Crestwood Medical Center	Huntsville	71%	300+
Flowers Hospital	Dothan	71%	300+
Lakeland Community Hospital	Haleyville	71%	300+
Vaughan Reg Med Ctr Parkway Campus	Selma	71%	300+
Andalusia Regional Hospital	Andalusia	70%	300+
Athens - Limestone Hospital	Athens	70%	300+
D W Mcmillan Memorial Hospital	Brewton	70%	(a)
Helen Keller Memorial Hospital	Sheffield	70%	300+
Highlands Medical Center	Scottsboro	70%	(a)
Bryan W Whitfield Memorial Hospital	Demopolis	69%	(a)
Citizens Baptist Medical Center	Talladega	69%	300+
Community Hospital	Tallassee	69%	300+
Huntsville Hospital	Huntsville	69%	300+
South Baldwin Regional Medical Center	Foley	69%	300+
Troy Regional Medical Center	Troy	69%	300+
Jackson Hospital & Clinic	Montgomery	68%	300+
Medical Center Enterprise	Enterprise	68%	300+
Saint Vincent's Birmingham	Birmingham	68%	300+
Southeast Alabama Medical Center	Dothan	68%	300+
University of Alabama Hospital	Birmingham	68%	300+
Wedowee Hospital	Wedowee	68%	(a)
D C H Regional Medical Center	Tuscaloosa	67%	300+
Mobile Infirmary	Mobile	67%	300+
Springhill Medical Center	Mobile	67%	300+
Baptist Medical Center East	Montgomery	66%	300+
Brookwood Medical Center	Birmingham	66%	300+
Dekalb Regional Medical Center	Fort Payne	66%	300+
Gadsden Regional Medical Center	Gadsden	66%	300+
George H. Lanier Memorial Hospital	Valley	66%	300+
Northeast Alabama Regional Medical Center	Anniston	66%	300+
Shelby Baptist Medical Center	Alabaster	66%	300+
Stringfellow Memorial Hospital	Anniston	66%	300+
Atmore Community Hospital	Atmore	65%	(a)
Baptist Medical Center - Princeton	Birmingham	65%	300+
Decatur Morgan Hospital - Parkway Campus	Decatur	65%	(a)
Riverview Regional Medical Center	Gadsden	65%	300+
Univ of S Alabama Med Ctr	Mobile	65%	300+
Crenshaw Community Hospital	Luverne	63%	(a)
Jacksonville Medical Center	Jacksonville	63%	(a)
Medical West	Bessemer	63%	300+
Providence Hospital	Mobile	63%	300+
Walker Baptist Medical Center	Jasper	63%	300+
Lawrence Medical Center	Moulton	62%	(a)
Eliza Coffee Memorial Hospital	Florence	60%	300+
Grove Hill Memorial Hospital	Grove Hill	60%	(a)
Saint Vincent's East	Birmingham	60%	300+
Wiregrass Medical Center	Geneva	59%	(a)

Doctors 'Always' Communicated Well

Hospital Name	City	Rate	Cases
Fayette Medical Center	Fayette	94%	(a)
Crenshaw Community Hospital	Luverne	93%	(a)
Lawrence Medical Center	Moulton	93%	(a)
Monroe County Hospital	Monroeville	92%	(a)
Cherokee Medical Center	Centre	91%	(a)
Marion Regional Medical Center	Hamilton	91%	(a)
Clay County Hospital	Ashland	90%	(a)
Community Hospital	Tallassee	90%	300+
Marshall Medical Center South	Boaz	90%	300+
Mizell Memorial Hospital	Opp	90%	(a)
Saint Vincent's Saint Clair	Pell City	90%	300+
Atmore Community Hospital	Atmore	89%	(a)
Evergreen Medical Center	Evergreen	89%	(a)
Elmore Community Hospital	Wetumpka	88%	(a)
Georgiana Medical Center	Georgiana	88%	(a)
Jack Hughston Memorial Hospital	Phenix City	88%	300+
North Baldwin Infirmary	Bay Minette	88%	300+
Troy Regional Medical Center	Troy	88%	300+
Andalusia Regional Hospital	Andalusia	87%	300+
Bryan W Whitfield Memorial Hospital	Demopolis	87%	(a)
Cullman Regional Medical Center	Cullman	87%	300+
D W Mcmillan Memorial Hospital	Brewton	87%	(a)
Decatur Morgan Hospital - Decatur Campus	Decatur	87%	300+
East Alabama Medical Center	Opelika	87%	300+
L V Stabler Memorial Hospital	Greenville	87%	(a)
Northwest Medical Center	Winfield	87%	300+
Russell Hospital	Alexander City	87%	300+
Russellville Hospital	Russellville	87%	300+
Brookwood Medical Center	Birmingham	86%	300+
Coosa Valley Medical Center	Sylacauga	86%	300+
George H. Lanier Memorial Hospital	Valley	86%	300+
Grove Hill Memorial Hospital	Grove Hill	86%	(a)
Highlands Medical Center	Scottsboro	86%	(a)
South Baldwin Regional Medical Center	Foley	86%	300+
Wiregrass Medical Center	Geneva	86%	(a)
Baptist Medical Center - Princeton	Birmingham	85%	300+
Baptist Medical Center East	Montgomery	85%	300+
Helen Keller Memorial Hospital	Sheffield	85%	300+
Jackson Hospital & Clinic	Montgomery	85%	300+
Jacksonville Medical Center	Jacksonville	85%	(a)
Lake Martin Community Hospital	Dadeville	85%	(a)
Medical Center Enterprise	Enterprise	85%	300+
Saint Vincent's Birmingham	Birmingham	85%	300+
Trinity Medical Center	Birmingham	85%	300+
Medical Center Barbour	Eufaula	84%	(a)
Mobile Infirmary	Mobile	84%	300+
Prattville Baptist Hospital	Prattville	84%	300+
University of Alabama Hospital	Birmingham	84%	300+
Baptist Medical Center South	Montgomery	83%	300+
Citizens Baptist Medical Center	Talladega	83%	300+
Crestwood Medical Center	Huntsville	83%	300+
Dale Medical Center	Ozark	83%	(a)
Flowers Hospital	Dothan	83%	300+
Lakeland Community Hospital	Haleyville	83%	300+
Medical West	Bessemer	83%	300+
Saint Vincent's East	Birmingham	83%	300+
Shoals Hospital	Muscle Shoals	83%	300+
Southeast Alabama Medical Center	Dothan	83%	300+
Springhill Medical Center	Mobile	83%	300+
Thomas Hospital	Fairhope	83%	300+
Athens - Limestone Hospital	Athens	82%	300+
D C H Regional Medical Center	Tuscaloosa	82%	300+
Dekalb Regional Medical Center	Fort Payne	82%	300+
Northeast Alabama Regional Medical Center	Anniston	82%	300+
Univ of S Alabama Med Ctr	Mobile	82%	300+
Vaughan Reg Med Ctr Parkway Campus	Selma	82%	300+
Eliza Coffee Memorial Hospital	Florence	81%	300+
Gadsden Regional Medical Center	Gadsden	81%	300+
Huntsville Hospital	Huntsville	81%	300+
Providence Hospital	Mobile	81%	300+
Shelby Baptist Medical Center	Alabaster	81%	300+
Stringfellow Memorial Hospital	Anniston	81%	300+
Walker Baptist Medical Center	Jasper	81%	300+
Wedowee Hospital	Wedowee	81%	(a)
Riverview Regional Medical Center	Gadsden	77%	300+
Decatur Morgan Hospital - Parkway Campus	Decatur	74%	(a)

Home Recovery Information Given

Hospital Name	City	Rate	Cases
Cherokee Medical Center	Centre	91%	(a)
Fayette Medical Center	Fayette	90%	(a)
South Baldwin Regional Medical Center	Foley	90%	300+
Community Hospital	Tallassee	89%	300+
Jack Hughston Memorial Hospital	Phenix City	89%	300+
Northwest Medical Center	Winfield	89%	300+
Clay County Hospital	Ashland	88%	(a)
Crestwood Medical Center	Huntsville	88%	300+
East Alabama Medical Center	Opelika	88%	300+
Prattville Baptist Hospital	Prattville	88%	300+
Thomas Hospital	Fairhope	88%	300+
Andalusia Regional Hospital	Andalusia	87%	300+
Athens - Limestone Hospital	Athens	87%	300+
Baptist Medical Center East	Montgomery	87%	300+
Decatur Morgan Hospital - Decatur Campus	Decatur	87%	300+
Dekalb Regional Medical Center	Fort Payne	87%	300+
Flowers Hospital	Dothan	87%	300+
Helen Keller Memorial Hospital	Sheffield	87%	300+
Marshall Medical Center South	Boaz	87%	300+
Medical Center Enterprise	Enterprise	87%	300+
Monroe County Hospital	Monroeville	87%	(a)
Saint Vincent's Birmingham	Birmingham	87%	300+
Saint Vincent's Saint Clair	Pell City	87%	300+
Shelby Baptist Medical Center	Alabaster	87%	300+
Evergreen Medical Center	Evergreen	86%	(a)
Georgiana Medical Center	Georgiana	86%	(a)
Huntsville Hospital	Huntsville	86%	300+
Marion Regional Medical Center	Hamilton	86%	(a)
Russell Hospital	Alexander City	86%	300+
Springhill Medical Center	Mobile	86%	300+
Trinity Medical Center	Birmingham	86%	300+
University of Alabama Hospital	Birmingham	86%	300+
Baptist Medical Center - Princeton	Birmingham	85%	300+
Brookwood Medical Center	Birmingham	85%	300+
Gadsden Regional Medical Center	Gadsden	85%	300+
Jackson Hospital & Clinic	Montgomery	85%	300+
Jacksonville Medical Center	Jacksonville	85%	(a)
L V Stabler Memorial Hospital	Greenville	85%	(a)
Lawrence Medical Center	Moulton	85%	(a)
Mobile Infirmary	Mobile	85%	300+
Russellville Hospital	Russellville	85%	300+
Saint Vincent's East	Birmingham	85%	300+
Baptist Medical Center South	Montgomery	84%	300+
Coosa Valley Medical Center	Sylacauga	84%	300+
Cullman Regional Medical Center	Cullman	84%	300+
D C H Regional Medical Center	Tuscaloosa	84%	300+
Highlands Medical Center	Scottsboro	84%	(a)
Medical Center Barbour	Eufaula	84%	(a)
Mizell Memorial Hospital	Opp	84%	(a)
North Baldwin Infirmary	Bay Minette	84%	300+
Northeast Alabama Regional Medical Center	Anniston	84%	300+
Providence Hospital	Mobile	84%	300+
Southeast Alabama Medical Center	Dothan	84%	300+
Atmore Community Hospital	Atmore	83%	(a)
D W Mcmillan Memorial Hospital	Brewton	83%	(a)
Dale Medical Center	Ozark	83%	(a)
Eliza Coffee Memorial Hospital	Florence	83%	300+
George H. Lanier Memorial Hospital	Valley	83%	300+
Lake Martin Community Hospital	Dadeville	83%	(a)
Troy Regional Medical Center	Troy	83%	300+
Univ of S Alabama Med Ctr	Mobile	83%	300+
Walker Baptist Medical Center	Jasper	83%	300+
Wiregrass Medical Center	Geneva	83%	(a)
Lakeland Community Hospital	Haleyville	82%	300+
Citizens Baptist Medical Center	Talladega	81%	300+
Stringfellow Memorial Hospital	Anniston	81%	300+
Crenshaw Community Hospital	Luverne	80%	(a)
Elmore Community Hospital	Wetumpka	80%	(a)
Medical West	Bessemer	80%	300+
Shoals Hospital	Muscle Shoals	80%	300+
Wedowee Hospital	Wedowee	79%	(a)
Grove Hill Memorial Hospital	Grove Hill	78%	(a)
Vaughan Reg Med Ctr Parkway Campus	Selma	77%	300+
Decatur Morgan Hospital - Parkway Campus	Decatur	76%	(a)
Riverview Regional Medical Center	Gadsden	76%	300+
Bryan W Whitfield Memorial Hospital	Demopolis	74%	(a)

NOTE: Hospital profiles are in alphabetical order by state, then city, then hospital within the city; Rankings exclude hospitals with less than 25 cases except for patient surveys which excludes hospitals with less than 100 cases; (a) 100-299 cases; (1) The number of cases/patients is too few to report; (2) Data submitted were based on a sample of cases/patients; (3) Results are based on a shorter time period than required; (4) Data suppressed by CMS for one or more quarters; (5) Results are not available for this reporting period; (6) Fewer than 100 patients completed the HCAHPS survey; (7) No cases met the criteria for this measure; (8) The lower limit of the confidence interval cannot be calculated if the number of observed infections equals zero; (9) No data are available from the state/territory for this reporting period; (10) The scores shown reflect fewer than 50 completed surveys; (11) There were discrepancies in the data collection process; (12) This measure does not apply to this hospital for this reporting period; (13) Results cannot be calculated for this reporting period; (14) The results for this state are combined with nearby states to protect confidentiality; Please refer to the User's Guide for a full explanation of data.

Hospital Given 9 or 10 on 10 Point Scale

Hospital Name	City	Rate	Cases
Fayette Medical Center	Fayette	83%	(a)
University of Alabama Hospital	Birmingham	83%	300+
Marion Regional Medical Center	Hamilton	82%	(a)
Jack Hughston Memorial Hospital	Phenix City	81%	300+
Saint Vincent's Saint Clair	Pell City	81%	300+
Russell Hospital	Alexander City	80%	300+
Trinity Medical Center	Birmingham	79%	300+
Community Hospital	Tallassee	78%	300+
Marshall Medical Center South	Boaz	78%	300+
Saint Vincent's Birmingham	Birmingham	78%	300+
Baptist Medical Center East	Montgomery	77%	300+
Cherokee Medical Center	Centre	77%	(a)
East Alabama Medical Center	Opelika	77%	300+
Flowers Hospital	Dothan	76%	300+
South Baldwin Regional Medical Center	Foley	76%	300+
Thomas Hospital	Fairhope	76%	300+
Baptist Medical Center - Princeton	Birmingham	75%	300+
Crestwood Medical Center	Huntsville	75%	300+
Helen Keller Memorial Hospital	Sheffield	75%	300+
Mobile Infirmary	Mobile	75%	300+
Clay County Hospital	Ashland	74%	(a)
D W Mcmillan Memorial Hospital	Brewton	74%	(a)
Huntsville Hospital	Huntsville	74%	300+
Jackson Hospital & Clinic	Montgomery	74%	300+
North Baldwin Infirmary	Bay Minette	74%	300+
Prattville Baptist Hospital	Prattville	74%	300+
Evergreen Medical Center	Evergreen	73%	(a)
Monroe County Hospital	Monroeville	73%	(a)
Athens - Limestone Hospital	Athens	72%	300+
Cullman Regional Medical Center	Cullman	72%	300+
D C H Regional Medical Center	Tuscaloosa	72%	300+
Highlands Medical Center	Scottsboro	72%	(a)
Medical Center Barbour	Eufaula	72%	(a)
Univ of S Alabama Med Ctr	Mobile	72%	300+
Brookwood Medical Center	Birmingham	71%	300+
Decatur Morgan Hospital - Decatur Campus	Decatur	71%	300+
Gadsden Regional Medical Center	Gadsden	71%	300+
Shoals Hospital	Muscle Shoals	71%	300+
Southeast Alabama Medical Center	Dothan	71%	300+
Coosa Valley Medical Center	Sylacauga	70%	300+
Dekalb Regional Medical Center	Fort Payne	70%	300+
Georgiana Medical Center	Georgiana	70%	(a)
Jacksonville Medical Center	Jacksonville	70%	(a)
L V Stabler Memorial Hospital	Greenville	70%	(a)
Northwest Medical Center	Winfield	70%	300+
Saint Vincent's East	Birmingham	70%	300+
Springhill Medical Center	Mobile	70%	300+
Baptist Medical Center South	Montgomery	69%	300+
Northeast Alabama Regional Medical Center	Anniston	69%	300+
Providence Hospital	Mobile	69%	300+
Walker Baptist Medical Center	Jasper	69%	300+
Elmore Community Hospital	Wetumpka	68%	(a)
Medical Center Enterprise	Enterprise	68%	300+
Shelby Baptist Medical Center	Alabaster	68%	300+
Troy Regional Medical Center	Troy	68%	300+
Bryan W Whitfield Memorial Hospital	Demopolis	67%	(a)
Mizell Memorial Hospital	Opp	67%	(a)
Atmore Community Hospital	Atmore	66%	(a)
Lakeland Community Hospital	Haleyville	66%	300+
Russellville Hospital	Russellville	66%	300+
Andalusia Regional Hospital	Andalusia	65%	300+
Crenshaw Community Hospital	Luverne	65%	(a)
Dale Medical Center	Ozark	65%	(a)
George H. Lanier Memorial Hospital	Valley	65%	300+
Wedowee Hospital	Wedowee	65%	(a)
Lawrence Medical Center	Moulton	64%	(a)
Lake Martin Community Hospital	Dadeville	63%	(a)
Medical West	Bessemer	63%	300+
Stringfellow Memorial Hospital	Anniston	62%	300+
Citizens Baptist Medical Center	Talladega	61%	300+
Riverview Regional Medical Center	Gadsden	61%	300+
Vaughan Reg Med Ctr Parkway Campus	Selma	59%	300+
Decatur Morgan Hospital - Parkway Campus	Decatur	57%	(a)
Wiregrass Medical Center	Geneva	57%	(a)
Eliza Coffee Memorial Hospital	Florence	56%	300+
Grove Hill Memorial Hospital	Grove Hill	54%	(a)

Meds 'Always' Explained Before Given

Hospital Name	City	Rate	Cases
Marion Regional Medical Center	Hamilton	80%	(a)
Georgiana Medical Center	Georgiana	79%	(a)
Fayette Medical Center	Fayette	76%	(a)
Crenshaw Community Hospital	Luverne	75%	(a)
Monroe County Hospital	Monroeville	74%	(a)
D W Mcmillan Memorial Hospital	Brewton	73%	(a)
Cherokee Medical Center	Centre	72%	(a)
Saint Vincent's Saint Clair	Pell City	72%	300+
Coosa Valley Medical Center	Sylacauga	71%	300+
Marshall Medical Center South	Boaz	71%	300+
Russell Hospital	Alexander City	71%	300+
Community Hospital	Tallassee	70%	300+
Flowers Hospital	Dothan	70%	300+
Jack Hughston Memorial Hospital	Phenix City	70%	300+
Mobile Infirmary	Mobile	70%	300+
East Alabama Medical Center	Opelika	69%	300+
L V Stabler Memorial Hospital	Greenville	69%	(a)
Prattville Baptist Hospital	Prattville	69%	300+
Russellville Hospital	Russellville	69%	300+
South Baldwin Regional Medical Center	Foley	69%	300+
University of Alabama Hospital	Birmingham	69%	300+
Huntsville Hospital	Huntsville	68%	300+
Atmore Community Hospital	Atmore	67%	(a)
Dale Medical Center	Ozark	67%	(a)
Mizell Memorial Hospital	Opp	67%	(a)
Thomas Hospital	Fairhope	67%	300+
Trinity Medical Center	Birmingham	67%	300+
Athens - Limestone Hospital	Athens	66%	300+
Baptist Medical Center - Princeton	Birmingham	66%	300+
Crestwood Medical Center	Huntsville	66%	300+
Jackson Hospital & Clinic	Montgomery	66%	300+
Lakeland Community Hospital	Haleyville	66%	300+
Medical Center Barbour	Eufaula	66%	(a)
North Baldwin Infirmary	Bay Minette	66%	300+
Andalusia Regional Hospital	Andalusia	65%	300+
Brookwood Medical Center	Birmingham	65%	300+
D C H Regional Medical Center	Tuscaloosa	65%	300+
Decatur Morgan Hospital - Decatur Campus	Decatur	65%	300+
Highlands Medical Center	Scottsboro	65%	(a)
Lawrence Medical Center	Moulton	65%	(a)
Troy Regional Medical Center	Troy	65%	300+
Univ of S Alabama Med Ctr	Mobile	65%	300+
Wiregrass Medical Center	Geneva	65%	(a)
Baptist Medical Center East	Montgomery	64%	300+
Baptist Medical Center South	Montgomery	64%	300+
Cullman Regional Medical Center	Cullman	64%	300+
Gadsden Regional Medical Center	Gadsden	64%	300+
Helen Keller Memorial Hospital	Sheffield	64%	300+
Medical Center Enterprise	Enterprise	64%	300+
Northwest Medical Center	Winfield	64%	300+
Saint Vincent's Birmingham	Birmingham	64%	300+
Elmore Community Hospital	Wetumpka	63%	(a)
Jacksonville Medical Center	Jacksonville	63%	(a)
Walker Baptist Medical Center	Jasper	63%	300+
Bryan W Whitfield Memorial Hospital	Demopolis	62%	(a)
Clay County Hospital	Ashland	62%	(a)
Providence Hospital	Mobile	62%	300+
Southeast Alabama Medical Center	Dothan	62%	300+
Citizens Baptist Medical Center	Talladega	61%	300+
Dekalb Regional Medical Center	Fort Payne	61%	300+
George H. Lanier Memorial Hospital	Valley	61%	300+
Northeast Alabama Regional Medical Center	Anniston	61%	300+
Saint Vincent's East	Birmingham	61%	300+
Vaughan Reg Med Ctr Parkway Campus	Selma	60%	300+
Evergreen Medical Center	Evergreen	59%	(a)
Lake Martin Community Hospital	Dadeville	59%	(a)
Shelby Baptist Medical Center	Alabaster	59%	300+
Springhill Medical Center	Mobile	59%	300+
Wedowee Hospital	Wedowee	59%	(a)
Eliza Coffee Memorial Hospital	Florence	58%	300+
Grove Hill Memorial Hospital	Grove Hill	57%	(a)
Shoals Hospital	Muscle Shoals	57%	300+
Medical West	Bessemer	56%	300+
Stringfellow Memorial Hospital	Anniston	56%	300+
Riverview Regional Medical Center	Gadsden	55%	300+
Decatur Morgan Hospital - Parkway Campus	Decatur	54%	(a)

Nurses 'Always' Communicated Well

Hospital Name	City	Rate	Cases
Fayette Medical Center	Fayette	90%	(a)
Marion Regional Medical Center	Hamilton	90%	(a)
Community Hospital	Tallassee	88%	300+
Cherokee Medical Center	Centre	87%	(a)
Georgiana Medical Center	Georgiana	85%	(a)
Monroe County Hospital	Monroeville	85%	(a)
Marshall Medical Center South	Boaz	84%	300+
Russell Hospital	Alexander City	84%	300+
Elmore Community Hospital	Wetumpka	83%	(a)
Saint Vincent's Saint Clair	Pell City	83%	300+
South Baldwin Regional Medical Center	Foley	83%	300+
University of Alabama Hospital	Birmingham	83%	300+
Baptist Medical Center East	Montgomery	82%	300+
Jack Hughston Memorial Hospital	Phenix City	82%	300+
Lawrence Medical Center	Moulton	82%	(a)
Prattville Baptist Hospital	Prattville	82%	300+
Thomas Hospital	Fairhope	82%	300+
Trinity Medical Center	Birmingham	82%	300+
Cullman Regional Medical Center	Cullman	81%	300+
D C H Regional Medical Center	Tuscaloosa	81%	300+
D W Mcmillan Memorial Hospital	Brewton	81%	(a)
Dale Medical Center	Ozark	81%	(a)
Decatur Morgan Hospital - Decatur Campus	Decatur	81%	300+
East Alabama Medical Center	Opelika	81%	300+
North Baldwin Infirmary	Bay Minette	81%	300+
Northwest Medical Center	Winfield	81%	300+
Saint Vincent's Birmingham	Birmingham	81%	300+
Athens - Limestone Hospital	Athens	80%	300+
Atmore Community Hospital	Atmore	80%	(a)
Baptist Medical Center - Princeton	Birmingham	80%	300+
Clay County Hospital	Ashland	80%	(a)
Dekalb Regional Medical Center	Fort Payne	80%	300+
Flowers Hospital	Dothan	80%	300+
Gadsden Regional Medical Center	Gadsden	80%	300+
Helen Keller Memorial Hospital	Sheffield	80%	300+
Jacksonville Medical Center	Jacksonville	80%	(a)
Lakeland Community Hospital	Haleyville	80%	300+
Medical Center Barbour	Eufaula	80%	(a)
Medical Center Enterprise	Enterprise	80%	300+
Mobile Infirmary	Mobile	80%	300+
Shoals Hospital	Muscle Shoals	80%	300+
Troy Regional Medical Center	Troy	80%	300+
Coosa Valley Medical Center	Sylacauga	79%	300+
Crestwood Medical Center	Huntsville	79%	300+
Evergreen Medical Center	Evergreen	79%	(a)
Highlands Medical Center	Scottsboro	79%	(a)
Huntsville Hospital	Huntsville	79%	300+
Jackson Hospital & Clinic	Montgomery	79%	300+
Russellville Hospital	Russellville	79%	300+
Wedowee Hospital	Wedowee	79%	(a)
Andalusia Regional Hospital	Andalusia	78%	300+
Baptist Medical Center South	Montgomery	78%	300+
Brookwood Medical Center	Birmingham	78%	300+
L V Stabler Memorial Hospital	Greenville	78%	(a)
Springhill Medical Center	Mobile	78%	300+
Univ of S Alabama Med Ctr	Mobile	78%	300+
Walker Baptist Medical Center	Jasper	78%	300+
Wiregrass Medical Center	Geneva	78%	(a)
Bryan W Whitfield Memorial Hospital	Demopolis	77%	(a)
Eliza Coffee Memorial Hospital	Florence	76%	300+
George H. Lanier Memorial Hospital	Valley	76%	300+
Northeast Alabama Regional Medical Center	Anniston	76%	300+
Saint Vincent's East	Birmingham	76%	300+
Southeast Alabama Medical Center	Dothan	76%	300+
Crenshaw Community Hospital	Luverne	75%	(a)
Lake Martin Community Hospital	Dadeville	75%	(a)
Providence Hospital	Mobile	75%	300+
Grove Hill Memorial Hospital	Grove Hill	74%	(a)
Mizell Memorial Hospital	Opp	74%	(a)
Shelby Baptist Medical Center	Alabaster	74%	300+
Medical West	Bessemer	73%	300+
Citizens Baptist Medical Center	Talladega	72%	300+
Riverview Regional Medical Center	Gadsden	72%	300+
Vaughan Reg Med Ctr Parkway Campus	Selma	72%	300+
Stringfellow Memorial Hospital	Anniston	70%	300+
Decatur Morgan Hospital - Parkway Campus	Decatur	69%	(a)

Pain 'Always' Well Controlled

Hospital Name	City	Rate	Cases
Monroe County Hospital	Monroeville	82%	(a)
Marion Regional Medical Center	Hamilton	81%	(a)
Russell Hospital	Alexander City	79%	300+
Clay County Hospital	Ashland	78%	(a)
Saint Vincent's Saint Clair	Pell City	78%	300+
Baptist Medical Center East	Montgomery	77%	300+
Fayette Medical Center	Fayette	77%	(a)
Marshall Medical Center South	Boaz	77%	300+
South Baldwin Regional Medical Center	Foley	77%	300+
Prattville Baptist Hospital	Prattville	76%	300+
Trinity Medical Center	Birmingham	76%	300+
Coosa Valley Medical Center	Sylacauga	75%	300+
Crenshaw Community Hospital	Luverne	75%	(a)
Cullman Regional Medical Center	Cullman	75%	300+
Thomas Hospital	Fairhope	75%	300+
University of Alabama Hospital	Birmingham	75%	300+
Wedowee Hospital	Wedowee	75%	(a)
East Alabama Medical Center	Opelika	74%	300+
Cherokee Medical Center	Centre	73%	(a)
Community Hospital	Tallassee	73%	300+
Decatur Morgan Hospital - Decatur Campus	Decatur	73%	300+
Elmore Community Hospital	Wetumpka	73%	(a)
Flowers Hospital	Dothan	73%	300+
Jackson Hospital & Clinic	Montgomery	73%	300+
Medical Center Barbour	Eufaula	73%	(a)
Mobile Infirmary	Mobile	73%	300+
North Baldwin Infirmary	Bay Minette	73%	300+
Baptist Medical Center - Princeton	Birmingham	72%	300+
Brookwood Medical Center	Birmingham	72%	300+
Bryan W Whitfield Memorial Hospital	Demopolis	72%	(a)
Crestwood Medical Center	Huntsville	72%	300+
D C H Regional Medical Center	Tuscaloosa	72%	300+
Gadsden Regional Medical Center	Gadsden	72%	300+

NOTE: Hospital profiles are in alphabetical order by state, then city, then hospital within the city; Rankings exclude hospitals with less than 25 cases except for patient surveys which excludes hospitals with less than 100 cases; (a) 100-299 cases; (1) The number of cases/patients is too few to report; (2) Data submitted were based on a sample of cases/patients; (3) Results are based on a shorter time period than required; (4) Data suppressed by CMS for one or more quarters; (5) Results are not available for this reporting period; (6) Fewer than 100 patients completed the HCAHPS survey; (7) No cases met the criteria for this measure; (8) The lower limit of the confidence interval cannot be calculated if the number of observed infections equals zero; (9) No data are available from the state/territory for this reporting period; (10) The scores shown reflect fewer than 50 completed surveys; (11) There were discrepancies in the data collection process; (12) This measure does not apply to this hospital for this reporting period; (13) Results cannot be calculated for this reporting period; (14) The results for this state are combined with nearby states to protect confidentiality; Please refer to the User's Guide for a full explanation of data.

Georgiana Medical Center	Georgiana	72%	(a)
Huntsville Hospital	Huntsville	72%	300+
Jack Hughston Memorial Hospital	Phenix City	72%	300+
Jacksonville Medical Center	Jacksonville	72%	(a)
Northwest Medical Center	Winfield	72%	300+
Russellville Hospital	Russellville	72%	300+
Saint Vincent's Birmingham	Birmingham	72%	300+
Springhill Medical Center	Mobile	72%	300+
Troy Regional Medical Center	Troy	72%	300+
Univ of S Alabama Med Ctr	Mobile	72%	300+
Wiregrass Medical Center	Geneva	72%	(a)
Atmore Community Hospital	Atmore	71%	(a)
D W Mcmillan Memorial Hospital	Brewton	71%	(a)
Evergreen Medical Center	Evergreen	71%	(a)
Highlands Medical Center	Scottsboro	71%	(a)
Lakeland Community Hospital	Haleyville	71%	300+
Medical Center Enterprise	Enterprise	71%	300+
Shoals Hospital	Muscle Shoals	71%	300+
Andalusia Regional Hospital	Andalusia	70%	300+
Athens - Limestone Hospital	Athens	70%	300+
Baptist Medical Center South	Montgomery	70%	300+
Dekalb Regional Medical Center	Fort Payne	70%	300+
Helen Keller Memorial Hospital	Sheffield	70%	300+
Northeast Alabama Regional Medical Center	Anniston	70%	300+
Providence Hospital	Mobile	70%	300+
George H. Lanier Memorial Hospital	Valley	69%	300+
Medical West	Bessemer	69%	300+
Mizell Memorial Hospital	Opp	69%	(a)
Saint Vincent's East	Birmingham	69%	300+
Citizens Baptist Medical Center	Talladega	68%	300+
Dale Medical Center	Ozark	68%	(a)
L V Stabler Memorial Hospital	Greenville	68%	(a)
Shelby Baptist Medical Center	Alabaster	68%	300+
Walker Baptist Medical Center	Jasper	68%	300+
Lawrence Medical Center	Moulton	67%	(a)
Southeast Alabama Medical Center	Dothan	67%	300+
Lake Martin Community Hospital	Dadeville	66%	(a)
Eliza Coffee Memorial Hospital	Florence	65%	300+
Grove Hill Memorial Hospital	Grove Hill	64%	(a)
Vaughan Reg Med Ctr Parkway Campus	Selma	64%	300+
Riverview Regional Medical Center	Gadsden	63%	300+
Stringfellow Memorial Hospital	Anniston	61%	300+
Decatur Morgan Hospital - Parkway Campus	Decatur	60%	(a)

Room and Bathroom 'Always' Clean

Hospital Name	City	Rate	Cases
Marion Regional Medical Center	Hamilton	88%	(a)
Georgiana Medical Center	Georgiana	83%	(a)
Fayette Medical Center	Fayette	82%	(a)
Community Hospital	Tallassee	80%	300+
Monroe County Hospital	Monroeville	78%	(a)
Wedowee Hospital	Wedowee	78%	(a)
Cherokee Medical Center	Centre	76%	(a)
Russell Hospital	Alexander City	76%	300+
South Baldwin Regional Medical Center	Foley	76%	300+
Athens - Limestone Hospital	Athens	75%	300+
Saint Vincent's Saint Clair	Pell City	75%	300+
Lakeland Community Hospital	Haleyville	74%	300+
Lawrence Medical Center	Moulton	74%	(a)
North Baldwin Infirmary	Bay Minette	74%	300+
Crestwood Medical Center	Huntsville	73%	300+
Highlands Medical Center	Scottsboro	73%	(a)
Lake Martin Community Hospital	Dadeville	73%	(a)
University of Alabama Hospital	Birmingham	73%	300+
D W Mcmillan Memorial Hospital	Brewton	72%	(a)
Decatur Morgan Hospital - Parkway Campus	Decatur	72%	(a)
East Alabama Medical Center	Opelika	72%	300+
L V Stabler Memorial Hospital	Greenville	72%	(a)
Medical Center Barbour	Eufaula	72%	(a)
Mizell Memorial Hospital	Opp	72%	(a)
Shoals Hospital	Muscle Shoals	72%	300+
Trinity Medical Center	Birmingham	72%	300+
Wiregrass Medical Center	Geneva	72%	(a)
Bryan W Whitfield Memorial Hospital	Demopolis	71%	(a)
Clay County Hospital	Ashland	71%	(a)
Cullman Regional Medical Center	Cullman	71%	300+
Evergreen Medical Center	Evergreen	71%	(a)
Huntsville Hospital	Huntsville	71%	300+
Jack Hughston Memorial Hospital	Phenix City	71%	300+
Prattville Baptist Hospital	Prattville	71%	300+
Troy Regional Medical Center	Troy	71%	300+
Dale Medical Center	Ozark	70%	(a)
Decatur Morgan Hospital - Decatur Campus	Decatur	70%	300+
Marshall Medical Center South	Boaz	70%	300+
Northwest Medical Center	Winfield	70%	300+
Southeast Alabama Medical Center	Dothan	70%	300+
Andalusia Regional Hospital	Andalusia	69%	300+
Flowers Hospital	Dothan	69%	300+
Helen Keller Memorial Hospital	Sheffield	69%	300+
Jackson Hospital & Clinic	Montgomery	69%	300+
Jacksonville Medical Center	Jacksonville	69%	(a)
Russellville Hospital	Russellville	69%	300+
Vaughan Reg Med Ctr Parkway Campus	Selma	69%	300+
Walker Baptist Medical Center	Jasper	69%	300+
Gadsden Regional Medical Center	Gadsden	68%	300+
Medical Center Enterprise	Enterprise	68%	300+
Thomas Hospital	Fairhope	68%	300+
Baptist Medical Center - Princeton	Birmingham	67%	300+
Baptist Medical Center East	Montgomery	67%	300+
Brookwood Medical Center	Birmingham	67%	300+
Citizens Baptist Medical Center	Talladega	67%	300+
Coosa Valley Medical Center	Sylacauga	67%	300+
D C H Regional Medical Center	Tuscaloosa	67%	300+
Dekalb Regional Medical Center	Fort Payne	67%	300+
Elmore Community Hospital	Wetumpka	67%	(a)
Riverview Regional Medical Center	Gadsden	67%	300+
Univ of S Alabama Med Ctr	Mobile	67%	300+
Atmore Community Hospital	Atmore	66%	(a)
Crenshaw Community Hospital	Luverne	66%	(a)
Providence Hospital	Mobile	66%	300+
Stringfellow Memorial Hospital	Anniston	66%	300+
Baptist Medical Center South	Montgomery	65%	300+
Northeast Alabama Regional Medical Center	Anniston	65%	300+
George H. Lanier Memorial Hospital	Valley	63%	300+
Springhill Medical Center	Mobile	63%	300+
Grove Hill Memorial Hospital	Grove Hill	62%	(a)
Mobile Infirmary	Mobile	62%	300+
Medical West	Bessemer	61%	300+
Saint Vincent's Birmingham	Birmingham	61%	300+
Shelby Baptist Medical Center	Alabaster	61%	300+
Saint Vincent's East	Birmingham	59%	300+
Eliza Coffee Memorial Hospital	Florence	54%	300+

Timely Help 'Always' Received

Hospital Name	City	Rate	Cases
Marion Regional Medical Center	Hamilton	83%	(a)
Elmore Community Hospital	Wetumpka	82%	(a)
Fayette Medical Center	Fayette	81%	(a)
Monroe County Hospital	Monroeville	79%	(a)
Cherokee Medical Center	Centre	78%	(a)
Clay County Hospital	Ashland	78%	(a)
Troy Regional Medical Center	Troy	76%	300+
Community Hospital	Tallassee	75%	300+
Saint Vincent's Saint Clair	Pell City	75%	300+
Georgiana Medical Center	Georgiana	74%	(a)
Marshall Medical Center South	Boaz	74%	300+
Russell Hospital	Alexander City	74%	300+
D W Mcmillan Memorial Hospital	Brewton	73%	(a)
North Baldwin Infirmary	Bay Minette	73%	300+
Wedowee Hospital	Wedowee	73%	(a)
Prattville Baptist Hospital	Prattville	72%	300+
South Baldwin Regional Medical Center	Foley	71%	300+
Thomas Hospital	Fairhope	71%	300+
University of Alabama Hospital	Birmingham	70%	300+
Cullman Regional Medical Center	Cullman	69%	300+
East Alabama Medical Center	Opelika	69%	300+
Helen Keller Memorial Hospital	Sheffield	69%	300+
Jack Hughston Memorial Hospital	Phenix City	69%	300+
Baptist Medical Center East	Montgomery	68%	300+
Lake Martin Community Hospital	Dadeville	68%	(a)
Trinity Medical Center	Birmingham	68%	300+
Andalusia Regional Hospital	Andalusia	67%	300+
Atmore Community Hospital	Atmore	67%	(a)
D C H Regional Medical Center	Tuscaloosa	67%	300+
Decatur Morgan Hospital - Decatur Campus	Decatur	67%	300+
Evergreen Medical Center	Evergreen	67%	(a)
Jacksonville Medical Center	Jacksonville	67%	(a)
L V Stabler Memorial Hospital	Greenville	67%	(a)
Lawrence Medical Center	Moulton	67%	(a)
Russellville Hospital	Russellville	67%	300+
Wiregrass Medical Center	Geneva	67%	(a)
Athens - Limestone Hospital	Athens	66%	300+
Crestwood Medical Center	Huntsville	66%	300+
Dale Medical Center	Ozark	66%	(a)
Dekalb Regional Medical Center	Fort Payne	66%	300+
Highlands Medical Center	Scottsboro	66%	(a)
Huntsville Hospital	Huntsville	66%	300+
Medical Center Enterprise	Enterprise	66%	300+
Saint Vincent's Birmingham	Birmingham	66%	300+
Springhill Medical Center	Mobile	66%	300+
Gadsden Regional Medical Center	Gadsden	65%	300+
Mobile Infirmary	Mobile	65%	300+
Baptist Medical Center - Princeton	Birmingham	64%	300+
Bryan W Whitfield Memorial Hospital	Demopolis	64%	(a)
Crenshaw Community Hospital	Luverne	64%	(a)
Flowers Hospital	Dothan	64%	300+
Jackson Hospital & Clinic	Montgomery	64%	300+
Mizell Memorial Hospital	Opp	64%	(a)
Providence Hospital	Mobile	64%	300+
Shoals Hospital	Muscle Shoals	64%	300+
Univ of S Alabama Med Ctr	Mobile	64%	300+
Walker Baptist Medical Center	Jasper	64%	300+
Brookwood Medical Center	Birmingham	63%	300+
Coosa Valley Medical Center	Sylacauga	63%	300+
Decatur Morgan Hospital - Parkway Campus	Decatur	63%	(a)
Lakeland Community Hospital	Haleyville	63%	300+
Medical Center Barbour	Eufaula	63%	(a)
Northwest Medical Center	Winfield	63%	300+
Baptist Medical Center South	Montgomery	62%	300+
George H. Lanier Memorial Hospital	Valley	62%	300+
Citizens Baptist Medical Center	Talladega	61%	300+
Grove Hill Memorial Hospital	Grove Hill	61%	(a)
Northeast Alabama Regional Medical Center	Anniston	61%	300+
Saint Vincent's East	Birmingham	61%	300+
Shelby Baptist Medical Center	Alabaster	61%	300+
Eliza Coffee Memorial Hospital	Florence	58%	300+
Southeast Alabama Medical Center	Dothan	58%	300+
Vaughan Reg Med Ctr Parkway Campus	Selma	57%	300+
Medical West	Bessemer	56%	300+
Riverview Regional Medical Center	Gadsden	55%	300+
Stringfellow Memorial Hospital	Anniston	51%	300+

Would Definitely Recommend Hospital

Hospital Name	City	Rate	Cases
Jack Hughston Memorial Hospital	Phenix City	85%	300+
University of Alabama Hospital	Birmingham	85%	300+
Fayette Medical Center	Fayette	83%	(a)
Baptist Medical Center East	Montgomery	82%	300+
Saint Vincent's Birmingham	Birmingham	82%	300+
Flowers Hospital	Dothan	80%	300+
Saint Vincent's Saint Clair	Pell City	80%	300+
Thomas Hospital	Fairhope	79%	300+
Trinity Medical Center	Birmingham	79%	300+
Crestwood Medical Center	Huntsville	78%	300+
East Alabama Medical Center	Opelika	78%	300+
Huntsville Hospital	Huntsville	78%	300+
Russell Hospital	Alexander City	78%	300+
Cherokee Medical Center	Centre	77%	(a)
Gadsden Regional Medical Center	Gadsden	76%	300+
Helen Keller Memorial Hospital	Sheffield	76%	300+
Jackson Hospital & Clinic	Montgomery	76%	300+
Marion Regional Medical Center	Hamilton	76%	(a)
Prattville Baptist Hospital	Prattville	76%	300+
Southeast Alabama Medical Center	Dothan	76%	300+
Brookwood Medical Center	Birmingham	75%	300+
Marshall Medical Center South	Boaz	75%	300+
Baptist Medical Center - Princeton	Birmingham	74%	300+
Mobile Infirmary	Mobile	74%	300+
Saint Vincent's East	Birmingham	74%	300+
South Baldwin Regional Medical Center	Foley	74%	300+
Univ of S Alabama Med Ctr	Mobile	74%	300+
Baptist Medical Center South	Montgomery	73%	300+
Decatur Morgan Hospital - Decatur Campus	Decatur	73%	300+
Northeast Alabama Regional Medical Center	Anniston	73%	300+
Providence Hospital	Mobile	73%	300+
Community Hospital	Tallassee	72%	300+
Cullman Regional Medical Center	Cullman	72%	300+
D C H Regional Medical Center	Tuscaloosa	72%	300+
Monroe County Hospital	Monroeville	72%	(a)
Shoals Hospital	Muscle Shoals	72%	300+
Athens - Limestone Hospital	Athens	71%	300+
Shelby Baptist Medical Center	Alabaster	71%	300+
Springhill Medical Center	Mobile	71%	300+
Evergreen Medical Center	Evergreen	70%	(a)
Georgiana Medical Center	Georgiana	70%	(a)
Medical Center Enterprise	Enterprise	70%	300+
North Baldwin Infirmary	Bay Minette	70%	300+
Mizell Memorial Hospital	Opp	69%	(a)
L V Stabler Memorial Hospital	Greenville	68%	(a)
Coosa Valley Medical Center	Sylacauga	67%	300+
D W Mcmillan Memorial Hospital	Brewton	67%	(a)
Medical Center Barbour	Eufaula	67%	(a)
Stringfellow Memorial Hospital	Anniston	67%	300+
Walker Baptist Medical Center	Jasper	67%	300+
Clay County Hospital	Ashland	66%	(a)
Dale Medical Center	Ozark	66%	(a)
Dekalb Regional Medical Center	Fort Payne	65%	300+
Jacksonville Medical Center	Jacksonville	65%	(a)
Northwest Medical Center	Winfield	65%	300+
Andalusia Regional Hospital	Andalusia	64%	300+
Atmore Community Hospital	Atmore	64%	(a)
Highlands Medical Center	Scottsboro	64%	(a)
Russellville Hospital	Russellville	64%	300+
Elmore Community Hospital	Wetumpka	63%	(a)
Lake Martin Community Hospital	Dadeville	63%	(a)
Troy Regional Medical Center	Troy	63%	300+
George H. Lanier Memorial Hospital	Valley	62%	300+
Lawrence Medical Center	Moulton	62%	(a)
Medical West	Bessemer	62%	300+
Wedowee Hospital	Wedowee	60%	(a)
Citizens Baptist Medical Center	Talladega	59%	300+
Riverview Regional Medical Center	Gadsden	59%	300+
Wiregrass Medical Center	Geneva	59%	(a)

NOTE: Hospital profiles are in alphabetical order by state, then city, then hospital within the city; Rankings exclude hospitals with less than 25 cases except for patient surveys which excludes hospitals with less than 100 cases; (a) 100-299 cases; (1) The number of cases/patients is too few to report; (2) Data submitted were based on a sample of cases/patients; (3) Results are based on a shorter time period than required; (4) Data suppressed by CMS for one or more quarters; (5) Results are not available for this reporting period; (6) Fewer than 100 patients completed the HCAHPS survey; (7) No cases met the criteria for this measure; (8) The lower limit of the confidence interval cannot be calculated if the number of observed infections equals zero; (9) No data are available from the state/territory for this reporting period; (10) The scores shown reflect fewer than 50 completed surveys; (11) There were discrepancies in the data collection process; (12) This measure does not apply to this hospital for this reporting period; (13) Results cannot be calculated for this reporting period; (14) The results for this state are combined with nearby states to protect confidentiality; Please refer to the User's Guide for a full explanation of data.

Hospital Name	City	Rate	Cases
Bryan W Whitfield Memorial Hospital	Demopolis	58%	(a)
Decatur Morgan Hospital - Parkway Campus	Decatur	57%	(a)
Lakeland Community Hospital	Haleyville	57%	300+
Grove Hill Memorial Hospital	Grove Hill	56%	(a)
Vaughan Reg Med Ctr Parkway Campus	Selma	56%	300+
Crenshaw Community Hospital	Luverne	53%	(a)
Eliza Coffee Memorial Hospital	Florence	51%	300+

Use of Medical Imaging

Cardiac Imaging Stress Test before OP Surgery

Hospital Name	City	Rate	Cases
L V Stabler Memorial Hospital	Greenville	0.0%	90
Decatur Morgan Hospital - Parkway Campus	Decatur	1.9%	104
Clay County Hospital	Ashland	2.9%	104
Medical Center Barbour	Eufaula	3.0%	202
Walker Baptist Medical Center	Jasper	3.1%	64
Trinity Medical Center	Birmingham	3.2%	63
Shelby Baptist Medical Center	Alabaster	3.6%	112
South Baldwin Regional Medical Center	Foley	3.6%	137
Thomas Hospital	Fairhope	3.7%	54
D W Mcmillan Memorial Hospital	Brewton	4.0%	124
Monroe County Hospital	Monroeville	4.3%	141
Northwest Medical Center	Winfield	4.5%	331
D C H Regional Medical Center	Tuscaloosa	4.6%	700
Dale Medical Center	Ozark	4.8%	166
Eliza Coffee Memorial Hospital	Florence	4.8%	83
Atmore Community Hospital	Atmore	4.9%	223
Coosa Valley Medical Center	Sylacauga	5.0%	338
Northeast Alabama Regional Medical Center	Anniston	5.2%	324
Univ of S Alabama Med Ctr	Mobile	5.2%	96
East Alabama Medical Center	Opelika	5.5%	1428
Lake Martin Community Hospital	Dadeville	5.6%	71
Brookwood Medical Center	Birmingham	5.9%	1364
Dekalb Regional Medical Center	Fort Payne	6.3%	112
Jacksonville Medical Center	Jacksonville	6.3%	79
Saint Vincent's Saint Clair	Pell City	6.3%	79
Gadsden Regional Medical Center	Gadsden	6.6%	91
Mobile Infirmary	Mobile	6.6%	76
Flowers Hospital	Dothan	6.9%	392
Highlands Medical Center	Scottsboro	6.9%	87
Marshall Medical Center South	Boaz	6.9%	590
Citizens Baptist Medical Center	Talladega	7.0%	199
University of Alabama Hospital	Birmingham	7.0%	142
Medical Center Enterprise	Enterprise	7.2%	194
Decatur Morgan Hospital - Decatur Campus	Decatur	7.5%	480
Huntsville Hospital	Huntsville	7.5%	2745
Southeast Alabama Medical Center	Dothan	8.0%	721
Springhill Medical Center	Mobile	8.2%	122
Saint Vincent's Birmingham	Birmingham	8.5%	306
Stringfellow Memorial Hospital	Anniston	8.6%	175
Athens - Limestone Hospital	Athens	10.1%	307
Medical West	Bessemer	10.6%	180
Cullman Regional Medical Center	Cullman	11.3%	71
Troy Regional Medical Center	Troy	12.1%	116

Combination Abdominal CT Scan

Hospital Name	City	Rate	Cases
Hale County Hospital	Greensboro	0.0%	85
Lake Martin Community Hospital	Dadeville	0.0%	62
Bullock County Hospital	Union Springs	1.2%	85
Fayette Medical Center	Fayette	1.7%	354
Cherokee Medical Center	Centre	2.0%	201
D C H Regional Medical Center	Tuscaloosa	2.1%	1846
Jack Hughston Memorial Hospital	Phenix City	2.3%	87
Lawrence Medical Center	Moulton	2.4%	212
Choctaw General Hospital	Butler	2.8%	106
Medical Center Enterprise	Enterprise	3.4%	704
Pickens County Medical Center	Carrollton	3.4%	204
Clay County Hospital	Ashland	3.8%	292
Highlands Medical Center	Scottsboro	3.9%	511
Thomas Hospital	Fairhope	4.0%	748
Decatur Morgan Hospital - Parkway Campus	Decatur	4.2%	264
Southeast Alabama Medical Center	Dothan	4.6%	2158
Saint Vincent's Birmingham	Birmingham	4.8%	1341
Crenshaw Community Hospital	Luverne	5.0%	120
Flowers Hospital	Dothan	5.4%	1713
University of Alabama Hospital	Birmingham	5.4%	782
Crestwood Medical Center	Huntsville	5.5%	676
Saint Vincent's East	Birmingham	6.2%	659
Cullman Regional Medical Center	Cullman	6.6%	815
Vaughan Reg Med Ctr Parkway Campus	Selma	6.8%	676
Medical West	Bessemer	6.9%	656
Riverview Regional Medical Center	Gadsden	7.4%	309
Trinity Medical Center	Birmingham	7.4%	665
Citizens Baptist Medical Center	Talladega	7.5%	320
Russell Hospital	Alexander City	7.7%	1028
Marion Regional Medical Center	Hamilton	7.9%	252
Northwest Medical Center	Winfield	8.0%	389
Georgiana Medical Center	Georgiana	8.5%	71
Coosa Valley Medical Center	Sylacauga	8.6%	717
Wedowee Hospital	Wedowee	8.6%	93
Stringfellow Memorial Hospital	Anniston	8.8%	320
Red Bay Hospital	Red Bay	8.9%	101
Decatur Morgan Hospital - Decatur Campus	Decatur	9.0%	1028
Andalusia Regional Hospital	Andalusia	9.1%	418
Bibb Medical Center	Centreville	9.7%	72
Walker Baptist Medical Center	Jasper	11.1%	593
Monroe County Hospital	Monroeville	11.2%	258
Northeast Alabama Regional Medical Center	Anniston	11.2%	1198
Medical Center Barbour	Eufaula	11.3%	292
Dale Medical Center	Ozark	12.2%	279
Helen Keller Memorial Hospital	Sheffield	12.4%	1048
L V Stabler Memorial Hospital	Greenville	12.4%	185
Marshall Medical Center South	Boaz	12.4%	1598
South Baldwin Regional Medical Center	Foley	12.4%	764
Jackson Hospital & Clinic	Montgomery	12.6%	642
Eliza Coffee Memorial Hospital	Florence	12.8%	1449
Brookwood Medical Center	Birmingham	13.8%	967
Baptist Medical Center - Princeton	Birmingham	14.1%	781
Lakeland Community Hospital	Haleyville	14.2%	155
Dekalb Regional Medical Center	Fort Payne	15.4%	467
Gadsden Regional Medical Center	Gadsden	15.7%	792
Community Hospital	Tallassee	17.9%	112
Russellville Hospital	Russellville	18.1%	227
Washington County Hospital	Chatom	19.1%	68
Saint Vincent's Saint Clair	Pell City	19.4%	407
Bryan W Whitfield Memorial Hospital	Demopolis	19.6%	316
Baptist Medical Center South	Montgomery	20.7%	1712
Troy Regional Medical Center	Troy	21.4%	309
Huntsville Hospital	Huntsville	22.0%	2786
Atmore Community Hospital	Atmore	22.5%	182
J Paul Jones Hospital	Camden	22.5%	89
Elmore Community Hospital	Wetumpka	22.6%	115
Univ of S Alabama Med Ctr	Mobile	22.7%	181
Athens - Limestone Hospital	Athens	24.2%	512
D W Mcmillan Memorial Hospital	Brewton	27.3%	216
North Baldwin Infirmary	Bay Minette	27.7%	184
Shoals Hospital	Muscle Shoals	30.4%	424
Shelby Baptist Medical Center	Alabaster	32.9%	1040
Mizell Memorial Hospital	Opp	34.7%	219
Springhill Medical Center	Mobile	36.7%	708
Grove Hill Memorial Hospital	Grove Hill	36.9%	141
Jackson Medical Center	Jackson	39.1%	110
Jacksonville Medical Center	Jacksonville	39.2%	260
Providence Hospital	Mobile	39.8%	893
Wiregrass Medical Center	Geneva	40.3%	129
Prattville Baptist Hospital	Prattville	46.9%	499
George H. Lanier Memorial Hospital	Valley	48.3%	327
East Alabama Medical Center	Opelika	52.9%	1132
Baptist Medical Center East	Montgomery	54.1%	778
Evergreen Medical Center	Evergreen	66.4%	149
Mobile Infirmary	Mobile	66.9%	1074

Combination Brain/Sinus CT Scan

Hospital Name	City	Rate	Cases
Greene County Hospital	Eutaw	0.0%	64
Hill Hospital of Sumter County	York	0.0%	47
Decatur Morgan Hospital - Decatur Campus	Decatur	0.6%	862
Hale County Hospital	Greensboro	0.7%	147
Wiregrass Medical Center	Geneva	1.1%	185
Springhill Medical Center	Mobile	1.4%	654
Vaughan Reg Med Ctr Parkway Campus	Selma	1.6%	570
Thomas Hospital	Fairhope	1.8%	730
Brookwood Medical Center	Birmingham	2.0%	490
Coosa Valley Medical Center	Sylacauga	2.0%	556
Russell Hospital	Alexander City	2.2%	779
Providence Hospital	Mobile	2.4%	1013
Walker Baptist Medical Center	Jasper	2.4%	552
D C H Regional Medical Center	Tuscaloosa	2.7%	2009
Jackson Hospital & Clinic	Montgomery	2.7%	893
Mobile Infirmary	Mobile	2.9%	790
Saint Vincent's East	Birmingham	2.9%	769
Southeast Alabama Medical Center	Dothan	2.9%	1781
Cullman Regional Medical Center	Cullman	3.1%	1146
South Baldwin Regional Medical Center	Foley	3.1%	687
Shelby Baptist Medical Center	Alabaster	3.2%	654
Flowers Hospital	Dothan	3.4%	987
Eliza Coffee Memorial Hospital	Florence	3.7%	1094
Baptist Medical Center South	Montgomery	3.8%	955
East Alabama Medical Center	Opelika	3.8%	1154
Northeast Alabama Regional Medical Center	Anniston	3.8%	887
Saint Vincent's Birmingham	Birmingham	4.0%	1051
Highlands Medical Center	Scottsboro	4.1%	515
Marshall Medical Center South	Boaz	4.1%	1448
Gadsden Regional Medical Center	Gadsden	4.2%	790
Atmore Community Hospital	Atmore	4.3%	280
Saint Vincent's Saint Clair	Pell City	4.3%	370
University of Alabama Hospital	Birmingham	4.3%	963
Baptist Medical Center - Princeton	Birmingham	4.4%	642
Crestwood Medical Center	Huntsville	4.7%	935
Univ of S Alabama Med Ctr	Mobile	4.8%	227
Huntsville Hospital	Huntsville	5.1%	2947
Medical Center Enterprise	Enterprise	5.1%	644
Trinity Medical Center	Birmingham	5.1%	513
Baptist Medical Center East	Montgomery	5.2%	745
Wedowee Hospital	Wedowee	5.4%	204
Dale Medical Center	Ozark	5.6%	503
Helen Keller Memorial Hospital	Sheffield	5.6%	903
Lawrence Medical Center	Moulton	6.0%	250
L V Stabler Memorial Hospital	Greenville	6.4%	233
Athens - Limestone Hospital	Athens	6.5%	722
Georgiana Medical Center	Georgiana	14.6%	82

Combination Chest CT Scan

Hospital Name	City	Rate	Cases
Athens - Limestone Hospital	Athens	0.0%	288
Brookwood Medical Center	Birmingham	0.0%	539
Choctaw General Hospital	Butler	0.0%	57
Citizens Baptist Medical Center	Talladega	0.0%	115
Crestwood Medical Center	Huntsville	0.0%	267
Decatur Morgan Hospital - Parkway Campus	Decatur	0.0%	194
Highlands Medical Center	Scottsboro	0.0%	167
Jackson Hospital & Clinic	Montgomery	0.0%	333
Lawrence Medical Center	Moulton	0.0%	87
Medical West	Bessemer	0.0%	262
Monroe County Hospital	Monroeville	0.0%	133
Pickens County Medical Center	Carrollton	0.0%	91
Troy Regional Medical Center	Troy	0.0%	116
Wiregrass Medical Center	Geneva	0.0%	62
Saint Vincent's Birmingham	Birmingham	0.1%	721
D C H Regional Medical Center	Tuscaloosa	0.2%	1393
Flowers Hospital	Dothan	0.3%	1196
University of Alabama Hospital	Birmingham	0.3%	290
Mobile Infirmary	Mobile	0.4%	697
Huntsville Hospital	Huntsville	0.5%	1746
Springhill Medical Center	Mobile	0.7%	425
Trinity Medical Center	Birmingham	0.7%	427
East Alabama Medical Center	Opelika	0.8%	729
Helen Keller Memorial Hospital	Sheffield	0.8%	371
Jacksonville Medical Center	Jacksonville	0.9%	114
Northeast Alabama Regional Medical Center	Anniston	0.9%	895
Shelby Baptist Medical Center	Alabaster	1.0%	392
Medical Center Enterprise	Enterprise	1.2%	332
Mizell Memorial Hospital	Opp	1.5%	134
Prattville Baptist Hospital	Prattville	1.5%	271
Fayette Medical Center	Fayette	1.8%	170
Baptist Medical Center South	Montgomery	2.0%	1573
Vaughan Reg Med Ctr Parkway Campus	Selma	2.0%	540
L V Stabler Memorial Hospital	Greenville	2.2%	90
Thomas Hospital	Fairhope	2.3%	488
Southeast Alabama Medical Center	Dothan	2.5%	1371
Baptist Medical Center East	Montgomery	2.6%	267
Northwest Medical Center	Winfield	3.7%	218
Coosa Valley Medical Center	Sylacauga	3.8%	339
Russell Hospital	Alexander City	4.2%	710
D W Mcmillan Memorial Hospital	Brewton	4.5%	244
Marion Regional Medical Center	Hamilton	4.5%	111
Dale Medical Center	Ozark	4.8%	124
Eliza Coffee Memorial Hospital	Florence	5.4%	1051
Clay County Hospital	Ashland	5.5%	127
Decatur Morgan Hospital - Decatur Campus	Decatur	5.6%	789
Cherokee Medical Center	Centre	6.0%	83
Medical Center Barbour	Eufaula	6.0%	167
Baptist Medical Center - Princeton	Birmingham	6.2%	436
South Baldwin Regional Medical Center	Foley	6.8%	427
Bryan W Whitfield Memorial Hospital	Demopolis	8.3%	180
Andalusia Regional Hospital	Andalusia	9.0%	221
Community Hospital	Tallassee	9.1%	77
Riverview Regional Medical Center	Gadsden	9.3%	150
Providence Hospital	Mobile	9.5%	1055
Marshall Medical Center South	Boaz	9.7%	743
Stringfellow Memorial Hospital	Anniston	9.7%	155
Saint Vincent's East	Birmingham	12.9%	139
Cullman Regional Medical Center	Cullman	13.8%	377
North Baldwin Infirmary	Bay Minette	14.1%	71
Univ of S Alabama Med Ctr	Mobile	14.3%	91
Walker Baptist Medical Center	Jasper	14.5%	359
Gadsden Regional Medical Center	Gadsden	15.3%	392
Dekalb Regional Medical Center	Fort Payne	18.9%	180
George H. Lanier Memorial Hospital	Valley	19.1%	215
Shoals Hospital	Muscle Shoals	22.6%	239
Russellville Hospital	Russellville	24.3%	148
Saint Vincent's Saint Clair	Pell City	32.1%	162
Evergreen Medical Center	Evergreen	35.2%	91
Grove Hill Memorial Hospital	Grove Hill	43.8%	73

Follow-up Mammogram/Ultrasound

A follow-up rate near zero may indicate missed cancer; a rate higher than 14% may mean there is unnecessary follow up.

NOTE: Hospital profiles are in alphabetical order by state, then city, then hospital within the city; Rankings exclude hospitals with less than 25 cases except for patient surveys which excludes hospitals with less than 100 cases; (a) 100-299 cases; (1) The number of cases/patients is too few to report; (2) Data submitted were based on a sample of cases/patients; (3) Results are based on a shorter time period than required; (4) Data suppressed by CMS for one or more quarters; (5) Results are not available for this reporting period; (6) Fewer than 100 patients completed the HCAHPS survey; (7) No cases met the criteria for this measure; (8) The lower limit of the confidence interval cannot be calculated if the number of observed infections equals zero; (9) No data are available from the state/territory for this reporting period; (10) The scores shown reflect fewer than 50 completed surveys; (11) There were discrepancies in the data collection process; (12) This measure does not apply to this hospital for this reporting period; (13) Results cannot be calculated for this reporting period; (14) The results for this state are combined with nearby states to protect confidentiality; Please refer to the User's Guide for a full explanation of data.

Hospital Name	City	Rate	Cases
Red Bay Hospital	Red Bay	1.2%	85
Washington County Hospital	Chatom	2.3%	171
Jackson Hospital & Clinic	Montgomery	3.3%	1492
Cherokee Medical Center	Centre	3.4%	234
Marshall Medical Center South	Boaz	3.4%	2262
Helen Keller Memorial Hospital	Sheffield	3.7%	1358
South Baldwin Regional Medical Center	Foley	4.4%	1207
Troy Regional Medical Center	Troy	4.6%	500
Dekalb Regional Medical Center	Fort Payne	5.0%	746
Southeast Alabama Medical Center	Dothan	5.0%	3930
Medical Center Enterprise	Enterprise	5.1%	1089
Walker Baptist Medical Center	Jasper	5.1%	744
Citizens Baptist Medical Center	Talladega	5.4%	572
Grove Hill Memorial Hospital	Grove Hill	5.4%	298
Baptist Medical Center South	Montgomery	5.6%	5937
Flowers Hospital	Dothan	5.8%	3877
Springhill Medical Center	Mobile	5.8%	1633
Atmore Community Hospital	Atmore	6.0%	251
Medical Center Barbour	Eufaula	6.0%	518
Coosa Valley Medical Center	Sylacauga	6.1%	654
Thomas Hospital	Fairhope	6.1%	1977
Andalusia Regional Hospital	Andalusia	6.2%	644
Cullman Regional Medical Center	Cullman	6.2%	738
Baptist Medical Center - Princeton	Birmingham	6.3%	1112
Clay County Hospital	Ashland	6.4%	299
Trinity Medical Center	Birmingham	6.4%	1228
Huntsville Hospital	Huntsville	6.6%	5704
L V Stabler Memorial Hospital	Greenville	6.6%	469
Saint Vincent's Birmingham	Birmingham	6.9%	3645
Dale Medical Center	Ozark	7.0%	469
Gadsden Regional Medical Center	Gadsden	7.0%	688
East Alabama Medical Center	Opelika	7.3%	2066
Crenshaw Community Hospital	Luverne	7.4%	81
Prattville Baptist Hospital	Prattville	7.4%	934
Elmore Community Hospital	Wetumpka	7.7%	207
Saint Vincent's Saint Clair	Pell City	7.8%	257
Vaughan Reg Med Ctr Parkway Campus	Selma	7.8%	1405
Eliza Coffee Memorial Hospital	Florence	8.2%	1484
J Paul Jones Hospital	Camden	8.4%	83
Bryan W Whitfield Memorial Hospital	Demopolis	8.5%	223
Community Hospital	Tallassee	8.9%	271
Crestwood Medical Center	Huntsville	8.9%	1419
Russell Hospital	Alexander City	8.9%	1204
Athens - Limestone Hospital	Athens	9.2%	996
Wiregrass Medical Center	Geneva	9.3%	321
Decatur Morgan Hospital - Decatur Campus	Decatur	9.4%	2344
Northeast Alabama Regional Medical Center	Anniston	9.7%	852
Shelby Baptist Medical Center	Alabaster	9.8%	1222
Evergreen Medical Center	Evergreen	10.1%	247
North Baldwin Infirmary	Bay Minette	10.5%	304
Jackson Medical Center	Jackson	10.6%	189
Shoals Hospital	Muscle Shoals	10.7%	373
Mobile Infirmary	Mobile	10.9%	2802
D W Mcmillan Memorial Hospital	Brewton	11.6%	491
Northwest Medical Center	Winfield	11.6%	748
Bibb Medical Center	Centreville	11.7%	103
Pickens County Medical Center	Carrollton	11.8%	331
Providence Hospital	Mobile	11.9%	1441
Wedowee Hospital	Wedowee	12.0%	108
Russellville Hospital	Russellville	12.1%	339
Lawrence Medical Center	Moulton	12.8%	242
Mizell Memorial Hospital	Opp	12.8%	475
Jacksonville Medical Center	Jacksonville	13.6%	287
Medical West	Bessemer	13.9%	769
George H. Lanier Memorial Hospital	Valley	14.2%	852
Decatur Morgan Hospital - Parkway Campus	Decatur	15.0%	541
D C H Regional Medical Center	Tuscaloosa	15.5%	1884
Lakeland Community Hospital	Haleyville	16.9%	142
Fayette Medical Center	Fayette	18.0%	427
Stringfellow Memorial Hospital	Anniston	19.0%	184
Monroe County Hospital	Monroeville	19.5%	560

Lumbar Spine MRI for Low Back Pain

Hospital Name	City	Rate	Cases
Southeast Alabama Medical Center	Dothan	29.3%	498
University of Alabama Hospital	Birmingham	29.6%	71
Andalusia Regional Hospital	Andalusia	29.9%	134
South Baldwin Regional Medical Center	Foley	31.4%	191
Decatur Morgan Hospital - Parkway Campus	Decatur	32.1%	81
Thomas Hospital	Fairhope	33.2%	235
Highlands Medical Center	Scottsboro	33.3%	51
North Baldwin Infirmary	Bay Minette	33.3%	51
Bryan W Whitfield Memorial Hospital	Demopolis	34.2%	73
Riverview Regional Medical Center	Gadsden	34.8%	46
D W Mcmillan Memorial Hospital	Brewton	35.1%	94
Baptist Medical Center East	Montgomery	35.6%	135
Dekalb Regional Medical Center	Fort Payne	35.9%	64
Baptist Medical Center South	Montgomery	36.4%	214
Flowers Hospital	Dothan	36.6%	134
Huntsville Hospital	Huntsville	37.1%	881
Medical Center Enterprise	Enterprise	37.2%	86
East Alabama Medical Center	Opelika	37.8%	402
Atmore Community Hospital	Atmore	38.0%	50
Mobile Infirmary	Mobile	38.1%	176
Northeast Alabama Regional Medical Center	Anniston	38.2%	259
Trinity Medical Center	Birmingham	38.3%	180
Russell Hospital	Alexander City	38.5%	65
Shelby Baptist Medical Center	Alabaster	38.7%	163
Shoals Hospital	Muscle Shoals	38.7%	199
Vaughan Reg Med Ctr Parkway Campus	Selma	38.8%	134
Decatur Morgan Hospital - Decatur Campus	Decatur	39.0%	141
Walker Baptist Medical Center	Jasper	39.4%	66
Providence Hospital	Mobile	40.0%	185
Helen Keller Memorial Hospital	Sheffield	40.3%	191
Medical West	Bessemer	40.3%	77
Athens - Limestone Hospital	Athens	40.4%	99
Saint Vincent's East	Birmingham	41.4%	116
Prattville Baptist Hospital	Prattville	41.7%	120
Dale Medical Center	Ozark	42.3%	52
Northwest Medical Center	Winfield	42.4%	85
Saint Vincent's Birmingham	Birmingham	42.4%	458
Cullman Regional Medical Center	Cullman	42.6%	54
Fayette Medical Center	Fayette	42.9%	77
Gadsden Regional Medical Center	Gadsden	43.3%	360
Marshall Medical Center South	Boaz	43.5%	490
Crestwood Medical Center	Huntsville	43.7%	199
Eliza Coffee Memorial Hospital	Florence	44.0%	150
Evergreen Medical Center	Evergreen	44.9%	49
Saint Vincent's Saint Clair	Pell City	44.9%	69
Grove Hill Memorial Hospital	Grove Hill	45.7%	35
D C H Regional Medical Center	Tuscaloosa	45.8%	526
Coosa Valley Medical Center	Sylacauga	46.8%	216
Monroe County Hospital	Monroeville	48.6%	37
Jackson Hospital & Clinic	Montgomery	48.9%	182
Stringfellow Memorial Hospital	Anniston	49.6%	119
Russellville Hospital	Russellville	51.6%	62
Marion Regional Medical Center	Hamilton	52.3%	44
Baptist Medical Center - Princeton	Birmingham	53.2%	156
Brookwood Medical Center	Birmingham	53.4%	88
Citizens Baptist Medical Center	Talladega	62.0%	50

NOTE: Hospital profiles are in alphabetical order by state, then city, then hospital within the city; Rankings exclude hospitals with less than 25 cases except for patient surveys which excludes hospitals with less than 100 cases; (a) 100-299 cases; (1) The number of cases/patients is too few to report; (2) Data submitted were based on a sample of cases/patients; (3) Results are based on a shorter time period than required; (4) Data suppressed by CMS for one or more quarters; (5) Results are not available for this reporting period; (6) Fewer than 100 patients completed the HCAHPS survey; (7) No cases met the criteria for this measure; (8) The lower limit of the confidence interval cannot be calculated if the number of observed infections equals zero; (9) No data are available from the state/territory for this reporting period; (10) The scores shown reflect fewer than 50 completed surveys; (11) There were discrepancies in the data collection process; (12) This measure does not apply to this hospital for this reporting period; (13) Results cannot be calculated for this reporting period; (14) The results for this state are combined with nearby states to protect confidentiality; Please refer to the User's Guide for a full explanation of data.

Shelby Baptist Medical Center

1000 First Street North | Phone: 205-620-8100
Alabaster, AL 35007 | Fax: 205-620-7187
E-mail: kay.sertell@bhsala.com
URL: www.baptistmedical.org
Type: Acute Care Hospitals | Emergency Services: Yes
Ownership: Voluntary non-profit - Church | Beds: 210

Key Personnel:
Operating Room. . . . . Carol Adams, RN
Quality Assurance . . . . Judy Blankenship, RN
Chief of Medical Staff. . . . . Elizabeth Ennis, MD
Radiology. . . . . Richard Martin, MD
President/CEO. . . . . Keith Parrott
Emergency Room . . . . Debbie Ritchie, RN

Measure	Cases	This Hosp.	State Avg.	U.S. Avg.
Blood Clot Prevention and Treatment				
Anticoagulation Overlap Therapy[2]	77	95%	91%	93%
ICU Venous Thromboembolism Prophylaxis[2]	123	92%	85%	92%
Incidence of Potentially Preventable VTE[2]	12	8%	18%	10%
UFH with Dosages/Platelet Monitoring[2]	83	100%	95%	97%
Venous Thromboembolism Prophylaxis[2]	318	83%	74%	85%
Warfarin Therapy Discharge Instructions[2]	55	80%	77%	75%
Chest Pain/Possible Heart Attack Care				
Aspirin Given Within 24 Hours of Arrival[1]	-	-	96%	96%
Fibrinolytic Meds Within 30 Min. of Arrival[3,7]	-	-	57%	58%
Average Time to ECG (minutes)[1]	-	-	6	7
Average Time to Transfer (minutes)[3,7]	-	-	61	60
Children's Asthma Care				
Received Home Management Plan of Care	-	-	-	88%
Received Reliever Medication	-	-	-	100%
Received Systemic Corticosteroids	-	-	-	100%
Emergency Department				
Admittance Decision Time (minutes)[2]	736	95	73	98
Head CT Results Within 45 Min. of Arrival[1]	-	-	45%	57%
Patients Who Left ER Before Being Seen	50,185	1%	3%	2%
Time from ER Arrival to Admit. (minutes)[2]	740	303	240	274
Time from ER Arrival to Discharge (minutes)	405	163	126	134
Time in ER Before Being Evaluated (minutes)	421	36	31	26
Time to Pain Meds for Fractures (minutes)	199	65	69	57
Heart Attack Care				
Aspirin Given at Discharge	278	100%	99%	99%
Fibrinolytic Meds Within 30 Min. of Arrival[7]	-	-	77%	54%
PCI Within 90 Minutes of Arrival	52	98%	97%	96%
Statin Prescribed at Discharge	258	99%	98%	98%
Heart Failure Care				
ACE Inhibitor or ARB for LVSD	109	100%	97%	97%
Discharge Instructions Given	324	98%	93%	94%
Evaluation of LVS Function	382	100%	99%	99%
Medicare Spending				
Medicare Spending per Patient (ratio)	-	1.01	0.98	0.98
Pneumonia Care				
Appropriate Initial Antibiotic Given	222	98%	95%	95%
Blood Culture Timing	241	100%	98%	98%
Pregnancy and Delivery Care				
Newborn Deliveries Scheduled Early[2]	37	5%	14%	6%
Preventive Care				
Immunization for Influenza[2]	561	92%	90%	90%
Immunization for Pneumonia[2]	737	89%	91%	92%
Stroke Care				
Anticoagulation Therapy for Atrial Fibrillation[2]	13	100%	92%	95%
Antithrombotic Therapy Timing[2]	105	94%	96%	98%
Assessed for Rehabilitation[2]	120	92%	95%	97%
Discharged on Antithrombotic Therapy[2]	113	100%	98%	99%
Discharged on Statin Medication[2]	82	94%	90%	94%
Thrombolytic Therapy Timing[1,2]	-	-	38%	66%
Venous Thromboembolism Prophylaxis[2]	117	89%	89%	94%
Written Stroke Educational Materials Given[2]	64	92%	85%	88%
Surgical Care Improvement Project				
Appropriate Beta Blocker Usage[2]	253	100%	98%	98%
Appropriate VTP Within 24 Hours[2]	413	100%	98%	98%
Controlled Postoperative Blood Glucose[2]	112	97%	97%	97%
Perioperative Temperature Management[2]	540	100%	100%	100%
Prophylactic Antibiotic Selection[2]	419	100%	99%	99%
Prophylactic Antibiotic Selection (Outpatient)	194	88%	98%	98%
Prophylactic Antibiotic Stopped[2]	380	99%	98%	98%
Prophylactic Antibiotic Timing[2]	420	100%	99%	99%
Prophylactic Antibiotic Timing (Outpatient)	195	97%	99%	98%
Urinary Catheter Removal[2]	337	99%	98%	97%
Survey of Patients' Hospital Experiences				
Area Around Room 'Always' Quiet at Night	300+	66%	71%	61%
Doctors 'Always' Communicated Well	300+	81%	86%	82%
Home Recovery Information Given	300+	87%	84%	85%
Hospital Given 9 or 10 on 10 Point Scale	300+	68%	71%	71%
Meds 'Always' Explained Before Given	300+	59%	66%	64%
Nurses 'Always' Communicated Well	300+	74%	80%	79%
Pain 'Always' Well Controlled	300+	68%	72%	71%
Room and Bathroom 'Always' Clean	300+	61%	71%	73%
Timely Help 'Always' Received	300+	61%	68%	68%
Would Definitely Recommend Hospital	300+	71%	70%	71%
Use of Medical Imaging				
Cardiac Imaging Stress Test before Surgery	112	3.6%	6.5%	5.3%
Combination Abdominal CT Scan	1,040	32.9%	16.5%	10.5%
Combination Brain/Sinus CT Scan	654	3.2%	3.5%	2.7%
Combination Chest CT Scan	392	1.0%	4.2%	2.7%
Follow-up Mammogram/Ultrasound	1,222	9.8%	7.6%	8.8%
Lumbar Spine MRI for Low Back Pain	163	38.7%	40.2%	37.2%

Russell Hospital

3316 Highway 280 | Phone: 256-329-7100
Alexander City, AL 35010 | Fax: 256-329-7186
E-mail: skelley@russellmedcenter.com
URL: www.russellmedcenter.com
Type: Acute Care Hospitals | Emergency Services: Yes
Ownership: Voluntary non-profit - Private | Beds: 75

Key Personnel:
Operating Room. . . . . Scott Cassidy
Intensive Care Unit. . . . . Sharon Davis
Emergency Room . . . . Michelle Goldhagen, MD
CEO/President. . . . . Frank W Harris
Radiology. . . . . Christopher Jah
Quality Assurance . . . . Jan Landers

Measure	Cases	This Hosp.	State Avg.	U.S. Avg.
Blood Clot Prevention and Treatment				
Anticoagulation Overlap Therapy[2]	13	69%	91%	93%
ICU Venous Thromboembolism Prophylaxis[2]	70	89%	85%	92%
Incidence of Potentially Preventable VTE[1,2]	-	-	18%	10%
UFH with Dosages/Platelet Monitoring[1,2]	-	-	95%	97%
Venous Thromboembolism Prophylaxis[2]	209	87%	74%	85%
Warfarin Therapy Discharge Instructions[1,2]	-	-	77%	75%
Chest Pain/Possible Heart Attack Care				
Aspirin Given Within 24 Hours of Arrival[1]	-	-	96%	96%
Fibrinolytic Meds Within 30 Min. of Arrival[3,7]	-	-	57%	58%
Average Time to ECG (minutes)[1]	-	-	6	7
Average Time to Transfer (minutes)[3,7]	-	-	61	60
Children's Asthma Care				
Received Home Management Plan of Care	-	-	-	88%
Received Reliever Medication	-	-	-	100%
Received Systemic Corticosteroids	-	-	-	100%
Emergency Department				
Admittance Decision Time (minutes)[2]	323	98	73	98
Head CT Results Within 45 Min. of Arrival	12	58%	45%	57%
Patients Who Left ER Before Being Seen	24,239	1%	3%	2%
Time from ER Arrival to Admit. (minutes)[2]	368	260	240	274
Time from ER Arrival to Discharge (minutes)	388	108	126	134
Time in ER Before Being Evaluated (minutes)	401	16	31	26
Time to Pain Meds for Fractures (minutes)	78	64	69	57
Heart Attack Care				
Aspirin Given at Discharge	52	100%	99%	99%
Fibrinolytic Meds Within 30 Min. of Arrival[1]	-	-	77%	54%
PCI Within 90 Minutes of Arrival	14	93%	97%	96%
Statin Prescribed at Discharge	51	96%	98%	98%
Heart Failure Care				
ACE Inhibitor or ARB for LVSD	33	97%	97%	97%
Discharge Instructions Given	99	91%	93%	94%
Evaluation of LVS Function	142	100%	99%	99%
Medicare Spending				
Medicare Spending per Patient (ratio)	-	0.96	0.98	0.98
Pneumonia Care				
Appropriate Initial Antibiotic Given	63	97%	95%	95%
Blood Culture Timing	128	100%	98%	98%
Pregnancy and Delivery Care				
Newborn Deliveries Scheduled Early[2]	67	12%	14%	6%
Preventive Care				
Immunization for Influenza[2]	287	91%	90%	90%
Immunization for Pneumonia[2]	355	95%	91%	92%
Stroke Care				
Anticoagulation Therapy for Atrial Fibrillation[1]	-	-	92%	95%
Antithrombotic Therapy Timing	40	100%	96%	98%
Assessed for Rehabilitation	41	93%	95%	97%
Discharged on Antithrombotic Therapy	37	100%	98%	99%
Discharged on Statin Medication	34	82%	90%	94%
Thrombolytic Therapy Timing[1]	-	-	38%	66%
Venous Thromboembolism Prophylaxis	40	65%	89%	94%
Written Stroke Educational Materials Given	22	45%	85%	88%
Surgical Care Improvement Project				
Appropriate Beta Blocker Usage	64	92%	98%	98%
Appropriate VTP Within 24 Hours	134	93%	98%	98%
Controlled Postoperative Blood Glucose[7]	-	-	97%	97%
Perioperative Temperature Management	153	100%	100%	100%
Prophylactic Antibiotic Selection	82	100%	99%	99%
Prophylactic Antibiotic Selection (Outpatient)	307	97%	98%	98%
Prophylactic Antibiotic Stopped	78	99%	98%	98%
Prophylactic Antibiotic Timing	82	100%	99%	99%
Prophylactic Antibiotic Timing (Outpatient)	285	100%	99%	98%
Urinary Catheter Removal	94	95%	98%	97%
Survey of Patients' Hospital Experiences				
Area Around Room 'Always' Quiet at Night	300+	72%	71%	61%
Doctors 'Always' Communicated Well	300+	87%	86%	82%
Home Recovery Information Given	300+	86%	84%	85%
Hospital Given 9 or 10 on 10 Point Scale	300+	80%	71%	71%
Meds 'Always' Explained Before Given	300+	71%	66%	64%
Nurses 'Always' Communicated Well	300+	84%	80%	79%
Pain 'Always' Well Controlled	300+	79%	72%	71%
Room and Bathroom 'Always' Clean	300+	76%	71%	73%
Timely Help 'Always' Received	300+	74%	68%	68%
Would Definitely Recommend Hospital	300+	78%	70%	71%
Use of Medical Imaging				
Cardiac Imaging Stress Test before Surgery[1]	-	-	6.5%	5.3%
Combination Abdominal CT Scan	1,028	7.7%	16.5%	10.5%
Combination Brain/Sinus CT Scan	779	2.2%	3.5%	2.7%
Combination Chest CT Scan	710	4.2%	4.2%	2.7%
Follow-up Mammogram/Ultrasound	1,204	8.9%	7.6%	8.8%
Lumbar Spine MRI for Low Back Pain	65	38.5%	40.2%	37.2%

Andalusia Regional Hospital

849 South Three Notch Street | Phone: 334-222-8466
Andalusia, AL 36420 | Fax: 334-427-0349
URL: www.andalusiaregional.com
Type: Acute Care Hospitals | Emergency Services: Yes
Ownership: Proprietary | Beds: 113

Key Personnel:
CEO/President. . . . . Michael A Callahan
Chief of Medical Staff. . . . . Tim Day, MD
Radiology. . . . . Mary Wilson

Measure	Cases	This Hosp.	State Avg.	U.S. Avg.
Blood Clot Prevention and Treatment				
Anticoagulation Overlap Therapy[2]	15	93%	91%	93%
ICU Venous Thromboembolism Prophylaxis[2]	61	89%	85%	92%
Incidence of Potentially Preventable VTE[2,7]	-	-	18%	10%
UFH with Dosages/Platelet Monitoring[1,2]	-	-	95%	97%
Venous Thromboembolism Prophylaxis[2]	198	93%	74%	85%
Warfarin Therapy Discharge Instructions[1,2]	-	-	77%	75%
Chest Pain/Possible Heart Attack Care				
Aspirin Given Within 24 Hours of Arrival	47	96%	96%	96%
Fibrinolytic Meds Within 30 Min. of Arrival[1]	-	-	57%	58%
Average Time to ECG (minutes)	51	8	6	7
Average Time to Transfer (minutes)[1]	-	-	61	60
Children's Asthma Care				
Received Home Management Plan of Care	-	-	-	88%
Received Reliever Medication	-	-	-	100%
Received Systemic Corticosteroids	-	-	-	100%

NOTE: Hospital profiles are in alphabetical order by state, then city, then hospital within the city; Rankings exclude hospitals with less than 25 cases except for patient surveys which excludes hospitals with less than 100 cases; (a) 100-299 cases; (1) The number of cases/patients is too few to report; (2) Data submitted were based on a sample of cases/patients; (3) Results are based on a shorter time period than required; (4) Data suppressed by CMS for one or more quarters; (5) Results are not available for this reporting period; (6) Fewer than 100 patients completed the HCAHPS survey; (7) No cases met the criteria for this measure; (8) The lower limit of the confidence interval cannot be calculated if the number of observed infections equals zero; (9) No data are available from the state/territory for this reporting period; (10) The scores shown reflect fewer than 50 completed surveys; (11) There were discrepancies in the data collection process; (12) This measure does not apply to this hospital for this reporting period; (13) Results cannot be calculated for this reporting period; (14) The results for this state are combined with nearby states to protect confidentiality; Please refer to the User's Guide for a full explanation of data.

Measure	Cases	This Hosp.	State Avg.	U.S. Avg.
Emergency Department				
Admittance Decision Time (minutes)[2]	385	45	73	98
Head CT Results Within 45 Min. of Arrival[1]	-	-	45%	57%
Patients Who Left ER Before Being Seen	16,364	2%	3%	2%
Time from ER Arrival to Admit. (minutes)[2]	386	184	240	274
Time from ER Arrival to Discharge (minutes)	388	112	126	134
Time in ER Before Being Evaluated (minutes)	404	21	31	26
Time to Pain Meds for Fractures (minutes)	63	46	69	57
Heart Attack Care				
Aspirin Given at Discharge[1]	-	-	99%	99%
Fibrinolytic Meds Within 30 Min. of Arrival[7]	-	-	77%	54%
PCI Within 90 Minutes of Arrival[7]	-	-	97%	96%
Statin Prescribed at Discharge[1]	-	-	98%	98%
Heart Failure Care				
ACE Inhibitor or ARB for LVSD[1,2]	-	-	97%	97%
Discharge Instructions Given[2]	77	100%	93%	94%
Evaluation of LVS Function[2]	84	100%	99%	99%
Medicare Spending				
Medicare Spending per Patient (ratio)	-	0.99	0.98	0.98
Pneumonia Care				
Appropriate Initial Antibiotic Given	76	97%	95%	95%
Blood Culture Timing	89	99%	98%	98%
Pregnancy and Delivery Care				
Newborn Deliveries Scheduled Early[2]	28	0%	14%	6%
Preventive Care				
Immunization for Influenza[2]	340	93%	90%	90%
Immunization for Pneumonia[2]	410	97%	91%	92%
Stroke Care				
Anticoagulation Therapy for Atrial Fibrillation[1]	-	-	92%	95%
Antithrombotic Therapy Timing	45	98%	96%	98%
Assessed for Rehabilitation	55	93%	95%	97%
Discharged on Antithrombotic Therapy	46	93%	98%	99%
Discharged on Statin Medication	25	92%	90%	94%
Thrombolytic Therapy Timing[1]	-	-	38%	66%
Venous Thromboembolism Prophylaxis	51	96%	89%	94%
Written Stroke Educational Materials Given	29	97%	85%	88%
Surgical Care Improvement Project				
Appropriate Beta Blocker Usage	32	94%	98%	98%
Appropriate VTP Within 24 Hours	202	100%	98%	98%
Controlled Postoperative Blood Glucose[7]	-	-	97%	97%
Perioperative Temperature Management	229	100%	100%	100%
Prophylactic Antibiotic Selection	181	99%	99%	99%
Prophylactic Antibiotic Selection (Outpatient)[3]	26	100%	98%	98%
Prophylactic Antibiotic Stopped	179	99%	98%	98%
Prophylactic Antibiotic Timing	182	100%	99%	99%
Prophylactic Antibiotic Timing (Outpatient)[3]	26	100%	99%	98%
Urinary Catheter Removal	165	100%	98%	97%
Survey of Patients' Hospital Experiences				
Area Around Room 'Always' Quiet at Night	300+	70%	71%	61%
Doctors 'Always' Communicated Well	300+	87%	86%	82%
Home Recovery Information Given	300+	87%	84%	85%
Hospital Given 9 or 10 on 10 Point Scale	300+	65%	71%	71%
Meds 'Always' Explained Before Given	300+	65%	66%	64%
Nurses 'Always' Communicated Well	300+	78%	80%	79%
Pain 'Always' Well Controlled	300+	70%	72%	71%
Room and Bathroom 'Always' Clean	300+	69%	71%	73%
Timely Help 'Always' Received	300+	67%	68%	68%
Would Definitely Recommend Hospital	300+	64%	70%	71%
Use of Medical Imaging				
Cardiac Imaging Stress Test before Surgery[7]	-	-	6.5%	5.3%
Combination Abdominal CT Scan	418	9.1%	16.5%	10.5%
Combination Brain/Sinus CT Scan[1]	-	-	3.5%	2.7%
Combination Chest CT Scan	221	9.0%	4.2%	2.7%
Follow-up Mammogram/Ultrasound	644	6.2%	7.6%	8.8%
Lumbar Spine MRI for Low Back Pain	134	29.9%	40.2%	37.2%

Northeast Alabama Regional Medical Center

400 East 10th Street
Anniston, AL 36207
Phone: 256-235-5121
Fax: 256-235-5608
URL: www.rmccares.org
Type: Acute Care Hospitals
Emergency Services: Yes
Ownership: Government - Local
Beds: 336

Key Personnel:

Radiology. . . . . Sheridan Belcher, MD
Coronary Care . . . . Wendy Davidson
Operating Room. . . . . Rochelle Jones
Quality Assurance . . . . Linda McAllister
CEO/President. . . . . J. David McCormack
Infection Control. . . . . Trish Samples
Pediatric In-Patient Care . . . . Mendy Wright, MD
Chief of Medical Staff . . . . David Zinn, MD

Measure	Cases	This Hosp.	State Avg.	U.S. Avg.
Blood Clot Prevention and Treatment				
Anticoagulation Overlap Therapy[2]	85	51%	91%	93%
ICU Venous Thromboembolism Prophylaxis[2]	82	83%	85%	92%
Incidence of Potentially Preventable VTE[2]	39	36%	18%	10%
UFH with Dosages/Platelet Monitoring[2]	58	3%	95%	97%
Venous Thromboembolism Prophylaxis[2]	452	56%	74%	85%
Warfarin Therapy Discharge Instructions[2]	56	20%	77%	75%
Chest Pain/Possible Heart Attack Care				
Aspirin Given Within 24 Hours of Arrival[1]	-	-	96%	96%
Fibrinolytic Meds Within 30 Min. of Arrival[3,7]	-	-	57%	58%
Average Time to ECG (minutes)[1]	-	-	6	7
Average Time to Transfer (minutes)[3,7]	-	-	61	60
Children's Asthma Care				
Received Home Management Plan of Care	-	-	-	88%
Received Reliever Medication	-	-	-	100%
Received Systemic Corticosteroids	-	-	-	100%
Emergency Department				
Admittance Decision Time (minutes)[2]	569	57	73	98
Head CT Results Within 45 Min. of Arrival	23	39%	45%	57%
Patients Who Left ER Before Being Seen	42,018	5%	3%	2%
Time from ER Arrival to Admit. (minutes)[2]	591	224	240	274
Time from ER Arrival to Discharge (minutes)	472	135	126	134
Time in ER Before Being Evaluated (minutes)	504	54	31	26
Time to Pain Meds for Fractures (minutes)	180	90	69	57
Heart Attack Care				
Aspirin Given at Discharge	275	97%	99%	99%
Fibrinolytic Meds Within 30 Min. of Arrival[1]	-	-	77%	54%
PCI Within 90 Minutes of Arrival	37	92%	97%	96%
Statin Prescribed at Discharge	262	97%	98%	98%
Heart Failure Care				
ACE Inhibitor or ARB for LVSD	116	95%	97%	97%
Discharge Instructions Given	326	81%	93%	94%
Evaluation of LVS Function	400	99%	99%	99%
Medicare Spending				
Medicare Spending per Patient (ratio)	-	0.98	0.98	0.98
Pneumonia Care				
Appropriate Initial Antibiotic Given	147	89%	95%	95%
Blood Culture Timing	213	99%	98%	98%
Pregnancy and Delivery Care				
Newborn Deliveries Scheduled Early[2]	48	12%	14%	6%
Preventive Care				
Immunization for Influenza[2]	617	92%	90%	90%
Immunization for Pneumonia[2]	778	84%	91%	92%
Stroke Care				
Anticoagulation Therapy for Atrial Fibrillation	15	67%	92%	95%
Antithrombotic Therapy Timing	100	98%	96%	98%
Assessed for Rehabilitation	115	69%	95%	97%
Discharged on Antithrombotic Therapy	109	100%	98%	99%
Discharged on Statin Medication	86	90%	90%	94%
Thrombolytic Therapy Timing	47	6%	38%	66%
Venous Thromboembolism Prophylaxis	110	67%	89%	94%
Written Stroke Educational Materials Given	78	6%	85%	88%
Surgical Care Improvement Project				
Appropriate Beta Blocker Usage[2]	233	97%	98%	98%
Appropriate VTP Within 24 Hours[2]	498	96%	98%	98%
Controlled Postoperative Blood Glucose[2]	104	96%	97%	97%
Perioperative Temperature Management[2]	618	100%	100%	100%
Prophylactic Antibiotic Selection[2]	520	99%	99%	99%
Prophylactic Antibiotic Selection (Outpatient)	297	94%	98%	98%
Prophylactic Antibiotic Stopped[2]	507	98%	98%	98%
Prophylactic Antibiotic Timing[2]	520	99%	99%	99%
Prophylactic Antibiotic Timing (Outpatient)	281	97%	99%	98%
Urinary Catheter Removal[2]	520	97%	98%	97%
Survey of Patients' Hospital Experiences				
Area Around Room 'Always' Quiet at Night	300+	66%	71%	61%
Doctors 'Always' Communicated Well	300+	82%	86%	82%
Home Recovery Information Given	300+	84%	84%	85%
Hospital Given 9 or 10 on 10 Point Scale	300+	69%	71%	71%
Meds 'Always' Explained Before Given	300+	61%	66%	64%
Nurses 'Always' Communicated Well	300+	76%	80%	79%
Pain 'Always' Well Controlled	300+	70%	72%	71%
Room and Bathroom 'Always' Clean	300+	65%	71%	73%
Timely Help 'Always' Received	300+	61%	68%	68%
Would Definitely Recommend Hospital	300+	73%	70%	71%
Use of Medical Imaging				
Cardiac Imaging Stress Test before Surgery	324	5.2%	6.5%	5.3%
Combination Abdominal CT Scan	1,198	11.2%	16.5%	10.5%
Combination Brain/Sinus CT Scan	887	3.8%	3.5%	2.7%
Combination Chest CT Scan	895	0.9%	4.2%	2.7%
Follow-up Mammogram/Ultrasound	852	9.7%	7.6%	8.8%
Lumbar Spine MRI for Low Back Pain	259	38.2%	40.2%	37.2%

Stringfellow Memorial Hospital

301 East 18th St
Anniston, AL 36201
Phone: 256-235-8900
Fax: 256-235-8751
E-mail: info@stringfellowhealth.com
URL: www.stringfellowhealth.com
Type: Acute Care Hospitals
Emergency Services: Yes
Ownership: Proprietary
Beds: 125

Key Personnel:

Chief of Medical Staff . . . . Igor Bidikov, MD
Operating Room. . . . . Dearl Birdsong
CEO/President. . . . . Linda Burdette
CEO . . . . Jay Hinesley

Measure	Cases	This Hosp.	State Avg.	U.S. Avg.
Blood Clot Prevention and Treatment				
Anticoagulation Overlap Therapy[2]	29	93%	91%	93%
ICU Venous Thromboembolism Prophylaxis[2]	65	88%	85%	92%
Incidence of Potentially Preventable VTE[1,2]	-	-	18%	10%
UFH with Dosages/Platelet Monitoring[1,2]	-	-	95%	97%
Venous Thromboembolism Prophylaxis[2]	305	62%	74%	85%
Warfarin Therapy Discharge Instructions[2]	18	89%	77%	75%
Chest Pain/Possible Heart Attack Care				
Aspirin Given Within 24 Hours of Arrival[1]	-	-	96%	96%
Fibrinolytic Meds Within 30 Min. of Arrival[3,7]	-	-	57%	58%
Average Time to ECG (minutes)[1]	-	-	6	7
Average Time to Transfer (minutes)[3,7]	-	-	61	60
Children's Asthma Care				
Received Home Management Plan of Care	-	-	-	88%
Received Reliever Medication	-	-	-	100%
Received Systemic Corticosteroids	-	-	-	100%
Emergency Department				
Admittance Decision Time (minutes)[2]	487	74	73	98
Head CT Results Within 45 Min. of Arrival[1]	-	-	45%	57%
Patients Who Left ER Before Being Seen	24,793	1%	3%	2%
Time from ER Arrival to Admit. (minutes)[2]	510	198	240	274
Time from ER Arrival to Discharge (minutes)	394	97	126	134
Time in ER Before Being Evaluated (minutes)	406	19	31	26
Time to Pain Meds for Fractures (minutes)	80	62	69	57
Heart Attack Care				
Aspirin Given at Discharge	51	98%	99%	99%
Fibrinolytic Meds Within 30 Min. of Arrival[7]	-	-	77%	54%
PCI Within 90 Minutes of Arrival[1]	-	-	97%	96%
Statin Prescribed at Discharge	57	95%	98%	98%
Heart Failure Care				
ACE Inhibitor or ARB for LVSD	59	98%	97%	97%
Discharge Instructions Given	118	89%	93%	94%
Evaluation of LVS Function	133	100%	99%	99%
Medicare Spending				
Medicare Spending per Patient (ratio)	-	0.98	0.98	0.98
Pneumonia Care				
Appropriate Initial Antibiotic Given	93	96%	95%	95%
Blood Culture Timing	97	99%	98%	98%
Pregnancy and Delivery Care				
Newborn Deliveries Scheduled Early[7]	-	-	14%	6%
Preventive Care				
Immunization for Influenza[2]	347	98%	90%	90%
Immunization for Pneumonia[2]	459	99%	91%	92%
Stroke Care				

NOTE: Hospital profiles are in alphabetical order by state, then city, then hospital within the city; Rankings exclude hospitals with less than 25 cases except for patient surveys which excludes hospitals with less than 100 cases; (a) 100-299 cases; (1) The number of cases/patients is too few to report; (2) Data submitted were based on a sample of cases/patients; (3) Results are based on a shorter time period than required; (4) Data suppressed by CMS for one or more quarters; (5) Results are not available for this reporting period; (6) Fewer than 100 patients completed the HCAHPS survey; (7) No cases met the criteria for this measure; (8) The lower limit of the confidence interval cannot be calculated if the number of observed infections equals zero; (9) No data are available from the state/territory for this reporting period; (10) The scores shown reflect fewer than 50 completed surveys; (11) There were discrepancies in the data collection process; (12) This measure does not apply to this hospital for this reporting period; (13) Results cannot be calculated for this reporting period; (14) The results for this state are combined with nearby states to protect confidentiality; Please refer to the User's Guide for a full explanation of data.

Measure	Cases	This Hosp.	State Avg.	U.S. Avg.
Anticoagulation Therapy for Atrial Fibrillation[1]	-	-	92%	95%
Antithrombotic Therapy Timing	41	93%	96%	98%
Assessed for Rehabilitation	46	87%	95%	97%
Discharged on Antithrombotic Therapy	45	96%	98%	99%
Discharged on Statin Medication	29	93%	90%	94%
Thrombolytic Therapy Timing[7]	-	-	38%	66%
Venous Thromboembolism Prophylaxis	44	66%	89%	94%
Written Stroke Educational Materials Given	31	90%	85%	88%
Surgical Care Improvement Project				
Appropriate Beta Blocker Usage	44	98%	98%	98%
Appropriate VTP Within 24 Hours	136	99%	98%	98%
Controlled Postoperative Blood Glucose[7]	-	-	97%	97%
Perioperative Temperature Management	156	100%	100%	100%
Prophylactic Antibiotic Selection	99	97%	99%	99%
Prophylactic Antibiotic Selection (Outpatient)	76	99%	98%	98%
Prophylactic Antibiotic Stopped	93	100%	98%	98%
Prophylactic Antibiotic Timing	99	97%	99%	99%
Prophylactic Antibiotic Timing (Outpatient)	76	100%	99%	98%
Urinary Catheter Removal	108	99%	98%	97%
Survey of Patients' Hospital Experiences				
Area Around Room 'Always' Quiet at Night	300+	66%	71%	61%
Doctors 'Always' Communicated Well	300+	81%	86%	82%
Home Recovery Information Given	300+	81%	84%	85%
Hospital Given 9 or 10 on 10 Point Scale	300+	62%	71%	71%
Meds 'Always' Explained Before Given	300+	56%	66%	64%
Nurses 'Always' Communicated Well	300+	70%	80%	79%
Pain 'Always' Well Controlled	300+	61%	72%	71%
Room and Bathroom 'Always' Clean	300+	66%	71%	73%
Timely Help 'Always' Received	300+	51%	68%	68%
Would Definitely Recommend Hospital	300+	67%	70%	71%
Use of Medical Imaging				
Cardiac Imaging Stress Test before Surgery	175	8.6%	6.5%	5.3%
Combination Abdominal CT Scan	320	8.8%	16.5%	10.5%
Combination Brain/Sinus CT Scan[1]	-	-	3.5%	2.7%
Combination Chest CT Scan	155	9.7%	4.2%	2.7%
Follow-up Mammogram/Ultrasound	184	19.0%	7.6%	8.8%
Lumbar Spine MRI for Low Back Pain	119	49.6%	40.2%	37.2%

Clay County Hospital

83825 Highway 9
Ashland, AL 36251
Phone: 256-354-2131
Fax: 256-354-1230
E-mail: kjackson@clayhosp.org
URL: www.claycountyhospital.com
Type: Acute Care Hospitals
Emergency Services: Yes
Ownership: Govt - Hospital Dist/Auth
Beds: 53

Key Personnel:

Operating Room. . . . . Julia Carpenter, RN
Quality Assurance . . . . Carolyn Jackson, RN
Infection Control. . . . . Becky Macoy, RN
Emergency Room . . . . Martha Powell, RN
Chief of Medical Staff. . . . . Dwain Rush, MD

Measure	Cases	This Hosp.	State Avg.	U.S. Avg.
Blood Clot Prevention and Treatment				
Anticoagulation Overlap Therapy[1,2]	-	-	91%	93%
ICU Venous Thromboembolism Prophylaxis[2]	75	39%	85%	92%
Incidence of Potentially Preventable VTE[2,7]	-	-	18%	10%
UFH with Dosages/Platelet Monitoring[1,2]	-	-	95%	97%
Venous Thromboembolism Prophylaxis[2]	109	26%	74%	85%
Warfarin Therapy Discharge Instructions[1,2]	-	-	77%	75%
Chest Pain/Possible Heart Attack Care				
Aspirin Given Within 24 Hours of Arrival	69	83%	96%	96%
Fibrinolytic Meds Within 30 Min. of Arrival[1]	-	-	57%	58%
Average Time to ECG (minutes)	75	7	6	7
Average Time to Transfer (minutes)[1]	-	-	61	60
Children's Asthma Care				
Received Home Management Plan of Care	-	-	-	88%
Received Reliever Medication	-	-	-	100%
Received Systemic Corticosteroids	-	-	-	100%
Emergency Department				
Admittance Decision Time (minutes)[2]	131	50	73	98
Head CT Results Within 45 Min. of Arrival[1]	-	-	45%	57%
Patients Who Left ER Before Being Seen	5,158	1%	3%	2%
Time from ER Arrival to Admit. (minutes)[2]	135	200	240	274
Time from ER Arrival to Discharge (minutes)	341	100	126	134
Time in ER Before Being Evaluated (minutes)	397	22	31	26
Time to Pain Meds for Fractures (minutes)	30	50	69	57
Heart Attack Care				
Aspirin Given at Discharge[1,3]	-	-	99%	99%
Fibrinolytic Meds Within 30 Min. of Arrival[3,7]	-	-	77%	54%
PCI Within 90 Minutes of Arrival[3,7]	-	-	97%	96%
Statin Prescribed at Discharge[1,3]	-	-	98%	98%
Heart Failure Care				
ACE Inhibitor or ARB for LVSD	18	50%	97%	97%
Discharge Instructions Given	29	66%	93%	94%
Evaluation of LVS Function	36	100%	99%	99%
Medicare Spending				
Medicare Spending per Patient (ratio)	-	0.94	0.98	0.98
Pneumonia Care				
Appropriate Initial Antibiotic Given[2]	28	86%	95%	95%
Blood Culture Timing[2]	23	100%	98%	98%
Pregnancy and Delivery Care				
Newborn Deliveries Scheduled Early[7]	-	-	14%	6%
Preventive Care				
Immunization for Influenza[2]	309	93%	90%	90%
Immunization for Pneumonia[2]	257	92%	91%	92%
Stroke Care				
Anticoagulation Therapy for Atrial Fibrillation[1]	-	-	92%	95%
Antithrombotic Therapy Timing	11	55%	96%	98%
Assessed for Rehabilitation	12	58%	95%	97%
Discharged on Antithrombotic Therapy	12	58%	98%	99%
Discharged on Statin Medication	12	33%	90%	94%
Thrombolytic Therapy Timing[1]	-	-	38%	66%
Venous Thromboembolism Prophylaxis[1]	-	-	89%	94%
Written Stroke Educational Materials Given[1]	-	-	85%	88%
Surgical Care Improvement Project				
Appropriate Beta Blocker Usage[5]	-	-	98%	98%
Appropriate VTP Within 24 Hours[5]	-	-	98%	98%
Controlled Postoperative Blood Glucose[5]	-	-	97%	97%
Perioperative Temperature Management[5]	-	-	100%	100%
Prophylactic Antibiotic Selection[5]	-	-	99%	99%
Prophylactic Antibiotic Selection (Outpatient)[5]	-	-	98%	98%
Prophylactic Antibiotic Stopped[5]	-	-	98%	98%
Prophylactic Antibiotic Timing[5]	-	-	99%	99%
Prophylactic Antibiotic Timing (Outpatient)[5]	-	-	99%	98%
Urinary Catheter Removal[5]	-	-	98%	97%
Survey of Patients' Hospital Experiences				
Area Around Room 'Always' Quiet at Night	(a)	74%	71%	61%
Doctors 'Always' Communicated Well	(a)	90%	86%	82%
Home Recovery Information Given	(a)	88%	84%	85%
Hospital Given 9 or 10 on 10 Point Scale	(a)	74%	71%	71%
Meds 'Always' Explained Before Given	(a)	62%	66%	64%
Nurses 'Always' Communicated Well	(a)	80%	80%	79%
Pain 'Always' Well Controlled	(a)	78%	72%	71%
Room and Bathroom 'Always' Clean	(a)	71%	71%	73%
Timely Help 'Always' Received	(a)	78%	68%	68%
Would Definitely Recommend Hospital	(a)	66%	70%	71%
Use of Medical Imaging				
Cardiac Imaging Stress Test before Surgery	104	2.9%	6.5%	5.3%
Combination Abdominal CT Scan	292	3.8%	16.5%	10.5%
Combination Brain/Sinus CT Scan[1]	-	-	3.5%	2.7%
Combination Chest CT Scan	127	5.5%	4.2%	2.7%
Follow-up Mammogram/Ultrasound	299	6.4%	7.6%	8.8%
Lumbar Spine MRI for Low Back Pain[7]	-	-	40.2%	37.2%

Athens - Limestone Hospital

700 West Market Street
Athens, AL 35611
Phone: 256-233-9292
Fax: 256-233-9277
E-mail: info@athenslimestonehospital.com
URL: www.athenslimestonehospital.com
Type: Acute Care Hospitals
Emergency Services: Yes
Ownership: Govt - Hospital Dist/Auth
Beds: 101

Key Personnel:

Operating Room. . . . . Nicole Beasley
Radiology. . . . . Paul Jeffrey Fry, PhD
Emergency Room . . . . Doug Moore, RN
Quality Assurance . . . . Patsy Moss, RN JD
Chief of Medical Staff . . . . Paul Edward Noel, MD
President . . . . David Pryor, MSHSA
Infection Control. . . . . Don Stalons, PhD

Measure	Cases	This Hosp.	State Avg.	U.S. Avg.
Blood Clot Prevention and Treatment				
Anticoagulation Overlap Therapy[2]	41	83%	91%	93%
ICU Venous Thromboembolism Prophylaxis[2]	71	86%	85%	92%
Incidence of Potentially Preventable VTE[1,2]	-	-	18%	10%
UFH with Dosages/Platelet Monitoring[2]	23	100%	95%	97%
Venous Thromboembolism Prophylaxis[2]	320	81%	74%	85%
Warfarin Therapy Discharge Instructions[2]	31	94%	77%	75%
Chest Pain/Possible Heart Attack Care				
Aspirin Given Within 24 Hours of Arrival	176	97%	96%	96%
Fibrinolytic Meds Within 30 Min. of Arrival[7]	-	-	57%	58%
Average Time to ECG (minutes)	191	7	6	7
Average Time to Transfer (minutes)[1]	-	-	61	60
Children's Asthma Care				
Received Home Management Plan of Care	-	-	-	88%
Received Reliever Medication	-	-	-	100%
Received Systemic Corticosteroids	-	-	-	100%
Emergency Department				
Admittance Decision Time (minutes)[2]	522	70	73	98
Head CT Results Within 45 Min. of Arrival	21	57%	45%	57%
Patients Who Left ER Before Being Seen	33,762	3%	3%	2%
Time from ER Arrival to Admit. (minutes)[2]	522	248	240	274
Time from ER Arrival to Discharge (minutes)	413	137	126	134
Time in ER Before Being Evaluated (minutes)	448	33	31	26
Time to Pain Meds for Fractures (minutes)	150	72	69	57
Heart Attack Care				
Aspirin Given at Discharge[3,7]	-	-	99%	99%
Fibrinolytic Meds Within 30 Min. of Arrival[3,7]	-	-	77%	54%
PCI Within 90 Minutes of Arrival[3,7]	-	-	97%	96%
Statin Prescribed at Discharge[1,3]	-	-	98%	98%
Heart Failure Care				
ACE Inhibitor or ARB for LVSD	26	100%	97%	97%
Discharge Instructions Given	81	90%	93%	94%
Evaluation of LVS Function	117	100%	99%	99%
Medicare Spending				
Medicare Spending per Patient (ratio)	-	0.98	0.98	0.98
Pneumonia Care				
Appropriate Initial Antibiotic Given	67	91%	95%	95%
Blood Culture Timing	144	99%	98%	98%
Pregnancy and Delivery Care				
Newborn Deliveries Scheduled Early	57	4%	14%	6%
Preventive Care				
Immunization for Influenza[2]	405	99%	90%	90%
Immunization for Pneumonia[2]	483	100%	91%	92%
Stroke Care				
Anticoagulation Therapy for Atrial Fibrillation[1]	-	-	92%	95%
Antithrombotic Therapy Timing	29	93%	96%	98%
Assessed for Rehabilitation	33	94%	95%	97%
Discharged on Antithrombotic Therapy	30	97%	98%	99%
Discharged on Statin Medication	25	76%	90%	94%
Thrombolytic Therapy Timing[1]	-	-	38%	66%
Venous Thromboembolism Prophylaxis	30	67%	89%	94%
Written Stroke Educational Materials Given	15	80%	85%	88%
Surgical Care Improvement Project				
Appropriate Beta Blocker Usage	63	97%	98%	98%
Appropriate VTP Within 24 Hours	193	99%	98%	98%
Controlled Postoperative Blood Glucose[7]	-	-	97%	97%
Perioperative Temperature Management	220	100%	100%	100%
Prophylactic Antibiotic Selection	152	99%	99%	99%
Prophylactic Antibiotic Selection (Outpatient)	128	95%	98%	98%
Prophylactic Antibiotic Stopped	146	95%	98%	98%
Prophylactic Antibiotic Timing	152	99%	99%	99%
Prophylactic Antibiotic Timing (Outpatient)	129	99%	99%	98%
Urinary Catheter Removal	151	100%	98%	97%
Survey of Patients' Hospital Experiences				
Area Around Room 'Always' Quiet at Night	300+	70%	71%	61%
Doctors 'Always' Communicated Well	300+	82%	86%	82%
Home Recovery Information Given	300+	87%	84%	85%
Hospital Given 9 or 10 on 10 Point Scale	300+	72%	71%	71%
Meds 'Always' Explained Before Given	300+	66%	66%	64%
Nurses 'Always' Communicated Well	300+	80%	80%	79%
Pain 'Always' Well Controlled	300+	70%	72%	71%

NOTE: Hospital profiles are in alphabetical order by state, then city, then hospital within the city; Rankings exclude hospitals with less than 25 cases except for patient surveys which excludes hospitals with less than 100 cases; (a) 100-299 cases; (1) The number of cases/patients is too few to report; (2) Data submitted were based on a sample of cases/patients; (3) Results are based on a shorter time period than required; (4) Data suppressed by CMS for one or more quarters; (5) Results are not available for this reporting period; (6) Fewer than 100 patients completed the HCAHPS survey; (7) No cases met the criteria for this measure; (8) The lower limit of the confidence interval cannot be calculated if the number of observed infections equals zero; (9) No data are available from the state/territory for this reporting period; (10) The scores shown reflect fewer than 50 completed surveys; (11) There were discrepancies in the data collection process; (12) This measure does not apply to this hospital for this reporting period; (13) Results cannot be calculated for this reporting period; (14) The results for this state are combined with nearby states to protect confidentiality; Please refer to the User's Guide for a full explanation of data.

Room and Bathroom 'Always' Clean	300+	75%	71%	73%
Timely Help 'Always' Received	300+	66%	68%	68%
Would Definitely Recommend Hospital	300+	71%	70%	71%
Use of Medical Imaging				
Cardiac Imaging Stress Test before Surgery	307	10.1%	6.5%	5.3%
Combination Abdominal CT Scan	512	24.2%	16.5%	10.5%
Combination Brain/Sinus CT Scan	722	6.5%	3.5%	2.7%
Combination Chest CT Scan	288	0.0%	4.2%	2.7%
Follow-up Mammogram/Ultrasound	996	9.2%	7.6%	8.8%
Lumbar Spine MRI for Low Back Pain	99	40.4%	40.2%	37.2%

Atmore Community Hospital

401 Medical Park Drive
Atmore, AL 36502
Phone: 251-368-2500
Fax: 334-368-6362
URL: www.ebaptisthealthcare.org/atmorecommunityhospital
Type: Acute Care Hospitals
Emergency Services: Yes
Ownership: Govt - Hospital Dist/Auth
Beds: 51

Key Personnel:

Radiology. . . . . Larry Arcement
CEO/President. . . . . Mark Faulkner
Chief of Medical Staff. . . . . Michael Oleksyk, MD
Operating Room. . . . . Robert Patacsil
Quality Assurance . . . . Cindi Stephens

Measure	Cases	This Hosp.	State Avg.	U.S. Avg.
Blood Clot Prevention and Treatment				
Anticoagulation Overlap Therapy[2]	17	82%	91%	93%
ICU Venous Thromboembolism Prophylaxis[2]	47	83%	85%	92%
Incidence of Potentially Preventable VTE[1,2]	-	-	18%	10%
UFH with Dosages/Platelet Monitoring[1,2]	-	-	95%	97%
Venous Thromboembolism Prophylaxis[2]	144	79%	74%	85%
Warfarin Therapy Discharge Instructions[2]	15	80%	77%	75%
Chest Pain/Possible Heart Attack Care				
Aspirin Given Within 24 Hours of Arrival	46	91%	96%	96%
Fibrinolytic Meds Within 30 Min. of Arrival[1]	-	-	57%	58%
Average Time to ECG (minutes)	47	9	6	7
Average Time to Transfer (minutes)[1]	-	-	61	60
Children's Asthma Care				
Received Home Management Plan of Care	-	-	-	88%
Received Reliever Medication	-	-	-	100%
Received Systemic Corticosteroids	-	-	-	100%
Emergency Department				
Admittance Decision Time (minutes)[2]	319	60	73	98
Head CT Results Within 45 Min. of Arrival	12	17%	45%	57%
Patients Who Left ER Before Being Seen	10,895	3%	3%	2%
Time from ER Arrival to Admit. (minutes)[2]	319	221	240	274
Time from ER Arrival to Discharge (minutes)	363	128	126	134
Time in ER Before Being Evaluated (minutes)	351	39	31	26
Time to Pain Meds for Fractures (minutes)	21	59	69	57
Heart Attack Care				
Aspirin Given at Discharge[1,3]	-	-	99%	99%
Fibrinolytic Meds Within 30 Min. of Arrival[3,7]	-	-	77%	54%
PCI Within 90 Minutes of Arrival[3,7]	-	-	97%	96%
Statin Prescribed at Discharge[1,3]	-	-	98%	98%
Heart Failure Care				
ACE Inhibitor or ARB for LVSD	39	95%	97%	97%
Discharge Instructions Given	93	85%	93%	94%
Evaluation of LVS Function	117	99%	99%	99%
Medicare Spending				
Medicare Spending per Patient (ratio)	-	0.94	0.98	0.98
Pneumonia Care				
Appropriate Initial Antibiotic Given	50	92%	95%	95%
Blood Culture Timing	50	96%	98%	98%
Pregnancy and Delivery Care				
Newborn Deliveries Scheduled Early[7]	-	-	14%	6%
Preventive Care				
Immunization for Influenza[2]	264	92%	90%	90%
Immunization for Pneumonia[2]	461	93%	91%	92%
Stroke Care				
Anticoagulation Therapy for Atrial Fibrillation[1]	-	-	92%	95%
Antithrombotic Therapy Timing	20	95%	96%	98%
Assessed for Rehabilitation	22	86%	95%	97%
Discharged on Antithrombotic Therapy	19	95%	98%	99%
Discharged on Statin Medication	18	83%	90%	94%
Thrombolytic Therapy Timing[1]	-	-	38%	66%
Venous Thromboembolism Prophylaxis	21	76%	89%	94%
Written Stroke Educational Materials Given	17	29%	85%	88%
Surgical Care Improvement Project				
Appropriate Beta Blocker Usage[1]	-	-	98%	98%
Appropriate VTP Within 24 Hours	12	50%	98%	98%
Controlled Postoperative Blood Glucose[7]	-	-	97%	97%
Perioperative Temperature Management	15	100%	100%	100%
Prophylactic Antibiotic Selection[1]	-	-	99%	99%
Prophylactic Antibiotic Selection (Outpatient)[1]	-	-	98%	98%
Prophylactic Antibiotic Stopped[1]	-	-	98%	98%
Prophylactic Antibiotic Timing[1]	-	-	99%	99%
Prophylactic Antibiotic Timing (Outpatient)[1]	-	-	99%	98%
Urinary Catheter Removal[1]	-	-	98%	97%
Survey of Patients' Hospital Experiences				
Area Around Room 'Always' Quiet at Night	(a)	65%	71%	61%
Doctors 'Always' Communicated Well	(a)	89%	86%	82%
Home Recovery Information Given	(a)	83%	84%	85%
Hospital Given 9 or 10 on 10 Point Scale	(a)	66%	71%	71%
Meds 'Always' Explained Before Given	(a)	67%	66%	64%
Nurses 'Always' Communicated Well	(a)	80%	80%	79%
Pain 'Always' Well Controlled	(a)	71%	72%	71%
Room and Bathroom 'Always' Clean	(a)	66%	71%	73%
Timely Help 'Always' Received	(a)	67%	68%	68%
Would Definitely Recommend Hospital	(a)	64%	70%	71%
Use of Medical Imaging				
Cardiac Imaging Stress Test before Surgery	223	4.9%	6.5%	5.3%
Combination Abdominal CT Scan	182	22.5%	16.5%	10.5%
Combination Brain/Sinus CT Scan	280	4.3%	3.5%	2.7%
Combination Chest CT Scan[1]	-	-	4.2%	2.7%
Follow-up Mammogram/Ultrasound	251	6.0%	7.6%	8.8%
Lumbar Spine MRI for Low Back Pain	50	38.0%	40.2%	37.2%

North Baldwin Infirmary

1815 Hand Avenue
Bay Minette, AL 36507
Phone: 251-937-5521
Fax: 251-937-1657
URL: www.northbaldwinhospital.com
Type: Acute Care Hospitals
Emergency Services: Yes
Ownership: Voluntary non-profit - Private

Key Personnel:

Chief of Medical Staff. . . . . John Crowell
Radiology. . . . . John Doremus, MD
Pediatric Ambulatory Care . . . . . . May Getubig, MD
Pediatric In-Patient Care . . . . May Getubig, MD
Operating Room. . . . . Janet Krettek
Emergency Room . . . . Margaret Roley, RN

Measure	Cases	This Hosp.	State Avg.	U.S. Avg.
Blood Clot Prevention and Treatment				
Anticoagulation Overlap Therapy[1,2]	-	-	91%	93%
ICU Venous Thromboembolism Prophylaxis[2]	28	89%	85%	92%
Incidence of Potentially Preventable VTE[2,7]	-	-	18%	10%
UFH with Dosages/Platelet Monitoring[2,7]	-	-	95%	97%
Venous Thromboembolism Prophylaxis[2]	138	77%	74%	85%
Warfarin Therapy Discharge Instructions[1,2]	-	-	77%	75%
Chest Pain/Possible Heart Attack Care				
Aspirin Given Within 24 Hours of Arrival	44	84%	96%	96%
Fibrinolytic Meds Within 30 Min. of Arrival[7]	-	-	57%	58%
Average Time to ECG (minutes)	45	9	6	7
Average Time to Transfer (minutes)[1]	-	-	61	60
Children's Asthma Care				
Received Home Management Plan of Care	-	-	-	88%
Received Reliever Medication	-	-	-	100%
Received Systemic Corticosteroids	-	-	-	100%
Emergency Department				
Admittance Decision Time (minutes)[2]	288	80	73	98
Head CT Results Within 45 Min. of Arrival[1]	-	-	45%	57%
Patients Who Left ER Before Being Seen	13,927	4%	3%	2%
Time from ER Arrival to Admit. (minutes)[2]	292	275	240	274
Time from ER Arrival to Discharge (minutes)	384	158	126	134
Time in ER Before Being Evaluated (minutes)	404	50	31	26
Time to Pain Meds for Fractures (minutes)	48	74	69	57
Heart Attack Care				
Aspirin Given at Discharge[1]	-	-	99%	99%
Fibrinolytic Meds Within 30 Min. of Arrival[7]	-	-	77%	54%
PCI Within 90 Minutes of Arrival[7]	-	-	97%	96%
Statin Prescribed at Discharge[1]	-	-	98%	98%
Heart Failure Care				
ACE Inhibitor or ARB for LVSD	21	95%	97%	97%
Discharge Instructions Given	44	86%	93%	94%
Evaluation of LVS Function	48	96%	99%	99%
Medicare Spending				
Medicare Spending per Patient (ratio)	-	0.86	0.98	0.98
Pneumonia Care				
Appropriate Initial Antibiotic Given	40	95%	95%	95%
Blood Culture Timing	53	100%	98%	98%
Pregnancy and Delivery Care				
Newborn Deliveries Scheduled Early	22	0%	14%	6%
Preventive Care				
Immunization for Influenza[2]	243	64%	90%	90%
Immunization for Pneumonia[2]	251	83%	91%	92%
Stroke Care				
Anticoagulation Therapy for Atrial Fibrillation[1]	-	-	92%	95%
Antithrombotic Therapy Timing[1]	-	-	96%	98%
Assessed for Rehabilitation[1]	-	-	95%	97%
Discharged on Antithrombotic Therapy[1]	-	-	98%	99%
Discharged on Statin Medication[1]	-	-	90%	94%
Thrombolytic Therapy Timing[7]	-	-	38%	66%
Venous Thromboembolism Prophylaxis	12	83%	89%	94%
Written Stroke Educational Materials Given[1]	-	-	85%	88%
Surgical Care Improvement Project				
Appropriate Beta Blocker Usage[1]	-	-	98%	98%
Appropriate VTP Within 24 Hours	43	88%	98%	98%
Controlled Postoperative Blood Glucose[7]	-	-	97%	97%
Perioperative Temperature Management	54	94%	100%	100%
Prophylactic Antibiotic Selection	20	100%	99%	99%
Prophylactic Antibiotic Selection (Outpatient)	77	100%	98%	98%
Prophylactic Antibiotic Stopped	20	100%	98%	98%
Prophylactic Antibiotic Timing	20	100%	99%	99%
Prophylactic Antibiotic Timing (Outpatient)	78	97%	99%	98%
Urinary Catheter Removal	28	96%	98%	97%
Survey of Patients' Hospital Experiences				
Area Around Room 'Always' Quiet at Night	300+	73%	71%	61%
Doctors 'Always' Communicated Well	300+	88%	86%	82%
Home Recovery Information Given	300+	84%	84%	85%
Hospital Given 9 or 10 on 10 Point Scale	300+	74%	71%	71%
Meds 'Always' Explained Before Given	300+	66%	66%	64%
Nurses 'Always' Communicated Well	300+	81%	80%	79%
Pain 'Always' Well Controlled	300+	73%	72%	71%
Room and Bathroom 'Always' Clean	300+	74%	71%	73%
Timely Help 'Always' Received	300+	73%	68%	68%
Would Definitely Recommend Hospital	300+	70%	70%	71%
Use of Medical Imaging				
Cardiac Imaging Stress Test before Surgery[1]	-	-	6.5%	5.3%
Combination Abdominal CT Scan	184	27.7%	16.5%	10.5%
Combination Brain/Sinus CT Scan[1]	-	-	3.5%	2.7%
Combination Chest CT Scan	71	14.1%	4.2%	2.7%
Follow-up Mammogram/Ultrasound	304	10.5%	7.6%	8.8%
Lumbar Spine MRI for Low Back Pain	51	33.3%	40.2%	37.2%

Medical West

995 9th Avenue Southwest
Bessemer, AL 35021
Phone: 205-481-7000
Fax: 205-481-7994
URL: www.uab.edu
Type: Acute Care Hospitals
Emergency Services: Yes
Ownership: Govt - Hospital Dist/Auth
Beds: 214

Key Personnel:

Operating Room. . . . . Doris Davidson
CEO/President. . . . . David Hoidal
Quality Assurance . . . . Steve Jones

Measure	Cases	This Hosp.	State Avg.	U.S. Avg.
Blood Clot Prevention and Treatment				
Anticoagulation Overlap Therapy[2]	49	88%	91%	93%
ICU Venous Thromboembolism Prophylaxis[2]	103	81%	85%	92%
Incidence of Potentially Preventable VTE[1,2]	-	-	18%	10%
UFH with Dosages/Platelet Monitoring[2]	23	100%	95%	97%
Venous Thromboembolism Prophylaxis[2]	371	75%	74%	85%
Warfarin Therapy Discharge Instructions[2]	28	79%	77%	75%
Chest Pain/Possible Heart Attack Care				

NOTE: Hospital profiles are in alphabetical order by state, then city, then hospital within the city; Rankings exclude hospitals with less than 25 cases except for patient surveys which excludes hospitals with less than 100 cases; (a) 100-299 cases; (1) The number of cases/patients is too few to report; (2) Data submitted were based on a sample of cases/patients; (3) Results are based on a shorter time period than required; (4) Data suppressed by CMS for one or more quarters; (5) Results are not available for this reporting period; (6) Fewer than 100 patients completed the HCAHPS survey; (7) No cases met the criteria for this measure; (8) The lower limit of the confidence interval cannot be calculated if the number of observed infections equals zero; (9) No data are available from the state/territory for this reporting period; (10) The scores shown reflect fewer than 50 completed surveys; (11) There were discrepancies in the data collection process; (12) This measure does not apply to this hospital for this reporting period; (13) Results cannot be calculated for this reporting period; (14) The results for this state are combined with nearby states to protect confidentiality; Please refer to the User's Guide for a full explanation of data.

Measure	Cases	This Hosp.	State Avg.	U.S. Avg.
Aspirin Given Within 24 Hours of Arrival	58	100%	96%	96%
Fibrinolytic Meds Within 30 Min. of Arrival[1]	-	-	57%	58%
Average Time to ECG (minutes)	60	20	6	7
Average Time to Transfer (minutes)	13	108	61	60
Children's Asthma Care				
Received Home Management Plan of Care	-	-	-	88%
Received Reliever Medication	-	-	-	100%
Received Systemic Corticosteroids	-	-	-	100%
Emergency Department				
Admittance Decision Time (minutes)[2]	715	62	73	98
Head CT Results Within 45 Min. of Arrival[1]	-	-	45%	57%
Patients Who Left ER Before Being Seen	44,554	1%	3%	2%
Time from ER Arrival to Admit. (minutes)[2]	744	218	240	274
Time from ER Arrival to Discharge (minutes)	1,331	119	126	134
Time in ER Before Being Evaluated (minutes)	1,481	26	31	26
Time to Pain Meds for Fractures (minutes)	100	72	69	57
Heart Attack Care				
Aspirin Given at Discharge	71	99%	99%	99%
Fibrinolytic Meds Within 30 Min. of Arrival[7]	-	-	77%	54%
PCI Within 90 Minutes of Arrival[7]	-	-	97%	96%
Statin Prescribed at Discharge	64	100%	98%	98%
Heart Failure Care				
ACE Inhibitor or ARB for LVSD	72	100%	97%	97%
Discharge Instructions Given	218	92%	93%	94%
Evaluation of LVS Function	255	100%	99%	99%
Medicare Spending				
Medicare Spending per Patient (ratio)	-	0.94	0.98	0.98
Pneumonia Care				
Appropriate Initial Antibiotic Given	161	97%	95%	95%
Blood Culture Timing	280	98%	98%	98%
Pregnancy and Delivery Care				
Newborn Deliveries Scheduled Early	62	3%	14%	6%
Preventive Care				
Immunization for Influenza[2]	577	94%	90%	90%
Immunization for Pneumonia[2]	732	97%	91%	92%
Stroke Care				
Anticoagulation Therapy for Atrial Fibrillation[1]	-	-	92%	95%
Antithrombotic Therapy Timing	81	100%	96%	98%
Assessed for Rehabilitation	87	95%	95%	97%
Discharged on Antithrombotic Therapy	75	99%	98%	99%
Discharged on Statin Medication	62	97%	90%	94%
Thrombolytic Therapy Timing[1]	-	-	38%	66%
Venous Thromboembolism Prophylaxis	92	96%	89%	94%
Written Stroke Educational Materials Given	53	85%	85%	88%
Surgical Care Improvement Project				
Appropriate Beta Blocker Usage	141	97%	98%	98%
Appropriate VTP Within 24 Hours	383	97%	98%	98%
Controlled Postoperative Blood Glucose[7]	-	-	97%	97%
Perioperative Temperature Management	458	100%	100%	100%
Prophylactic Antibiotic Selection	215	99%	99%	99%
Prophylactic Antibiotic Selection (Outpatient)	145	98%	98%	98%
Prophylactic Antibiotic Stopped	211	98%	98%	98%
Prophylactic Antibiotic Timing	215	100%	99%	99%
Prophylactic Antibiotic Timing (Outpatient)	146	94%	99%	98%
Urinary Catheter Removal	195	94%	98%	97%
Survey of Patients' Hospital Experiences				
Area Around Room 'Always' Quiet at Night	300+	63%	71%	61%
Doctors 'Always' Communicated Well	300+	83%	86%	82%
Home Recovery Information Given	300+	80%	84%	85%
Hospital Given 9 or 10 on 10 Point Scale	300+	63%	71%	71%
Meds 'Always' Explained Before Given	300+	56%	66%	64%
Nurses 'Always' Communicated Well	300+	73%	80%	79%
Pain 'Always' Well Controlled	300+	69%	72%	71%
Room and Bathroom 'Always' Clean	300+	61%	71%	73%
Timely Help 'Always' Received	300+	56%	68%	68%
Would Definitely Recommend Hospital	300+	62%	70%	71%
Use of Medical Imaging				
Cardiac Imaging Stress Test before Surgery	180	10.6%	6.5%	5.3%
Combination Abdominal CT Scan	656	6.9%	16.5%	10.5%
Combination Brain/Sinus CT Scan[1]	-	-	3.5%	2.7%
Combination Chest CT Scan	262	0.0%	4.2%	2.7%
Follow-up Mammogram/Ultrasound	769	13.9%	7.6%	8.8%
Lumbar Spine MRI for Low Back Pain	77	40.3%	40.2%	37.2%

Baptist Medical Center - Princeton

701 Princeton Avenue Southwest
Birmingham, AL 35211
E-mail: info@bhsala.com
URL: www.bhsala.com/princeton
Type: Acute Care Hospitals
Ownership: Voluntary non-profit - Church

Phone: 205-783-3800
Fax: 205-783-7233
Emergency Services: Yes
Beds: 352

Key Personnel:
Infection Control. . . . . Pat Beck
Quality Assurance . . . . Leigh Collier
Chief of Medical Staff. . . . . Elizabeth Ennis, MD
Operating Room. . . . . Jan Howell
Coronary Care . . . . Gary Jones
Radiology. . . . . Terri Lamoas
Cardiac Laboratory. . . . . Leon Pipper
President/CEO. . . . . Betsy Postlethwait

Measure	Cases	This Hosp.	State Avg.	U.S. Avg.
Blood Clot Prevention and Treatment				
Anticoagulation Overlap Therapy[2]	99	97%	91%	93%
ICU Venous Thromboembolism Prophylaxis[2]	151	95%	85%	92%
Incidence of Potentially Preventable VTE[2]	41	0%	18%	10%
UFH with Dosages/Platelet Monitoring[2]	102	100%	95%	97%
Venous Thromboembolism Prophylaxis[2]	280	87%	74%	85%
Warfarin Therapy Discharge Instructions[2]	59	81%	77%	75%
Chest Pain/Possible Heart Attack Care				
Aspirin Given Within 24 Hours of Arrival[1,3]	-	-	96%	96%
Fibrinolytic Meds Within 30 Min. of Arrival[5]	-	-	57%	58%
Average Time to ECG (minutes)[1,3]	-	-	6	7
Average Time to Transfer (minutes)[5]	-	-	61	60
Children's Asthma Care				
Received Home Management Plan of Care	-	-	-	88%
Received Reliever Medication	-	-	-	100%
Received Systemic Corticosteroids	-	-	-	100%
Emergency Department				
Admittance Decision Time (minutes)[2]	582	117	73	98
Head CT Results Within 45 Min. of Arrival[7]	-	-	45%	57%
Patients Who Left ER Before Being Seen	46,891	3%	3%	2%
Time from ER Arrival to Admit. (minutes)[2]	588	308	240	274
Time from ER Arrival to Discharge (minutes)	354	165	126	134
Time in ER Before Being Evaluated (minutes)	409	37	31	26
Time to Pain Meds for Fractures (minutes)	70	74	69	57
Heart Attack Care				
Aspirin Given at Discharge	399	100%	99%	99%
Fibrinolytic Meds Within 30 Min. of Arrival[7]	-	-	77%	54%
PCI Within 90 Minutes of Arrival	56	100%	97%	96%
Statin Prescribed at Discharge	393	100%	98%	98%
Heart Failure Care				
ACE Inhibitor or ARB for LVSD	235	100%	97%	97%
Discharge Instructions Given	500	94%	93%	94%
Evaluation of LVS Function	585	100%	99%	99%
Medicare Spending				
Medicare Spending per Patient (ratio)	-	1.00	0.98	0.98
Pneumonia Care				
Appropriate Initial Antibiotic Given	192	99%	95%	95%
Blood Culture Timing	268	100%	98%	98%
Pregnancy and Delivery Care				
Newborn Deliveries Scheduled Early	25	4%	14%	6%
Preventive Care				
Immunization for Influenza[2]	596	97%	90%	90%
Immunization for Pneumonia[2]	909	97%	91%	92%
Stroke Care				
Anticoagulation Therapy for Atrial Fibrillation	21	95%	92%	95%
Antithrombotic Therapy Timing	219	99%	96%	98%
Assessed for Rehabilitation	253	96%	95%	97%
Discharged on Antithrombotic Therapy	214	100%	98%	99%
Discharged on Statin Medication	186	95%	90%	94%
Thrombolytic Therapy Timing	16	94%	38%	66%
Venous Thromboembolism Prophylaxis	310	97%	89%	94%
Written Stroke Educational Materials Given	155	88%	85%	88%
Surgical Care Improvement Project				
Appropriate Beta Blocker Usage[2]	339	99%	98%	98%
Appropriate VTP Within 24 Hours[2]	439	100%	98%	98%
Controlled Postoperative Blood Glucose[2]	246	97%	97%	97%
Perioperative Temperature Management[2]	581	100%	100%	100%
Prophylactic Antibiotic Selection[2]	657	100%	99%	99%
Prophylactic Antibiotic Selection (Outpatient)	366	98%	98%	98%
Prophylactic Antibiotic Stopped[2]	630	100%	98%	98%
Prophylactic Antibiotic Timing[2]	657	100%	99%	99%
Prophylactic Antibiotic Timing (Outpatient)	371	98%	99%	98%
Urinary Catheter Removal[2]	336	98%	98%	97%
Survey of Patients' Hospital Experiences				
Area Around Room 'Always' Quiet at Night	300+	65%	71%	61%
Doctors 'Always' Communicated Well	300+	85%	86%	82%
Home Recovery Information Given	300+	85%	84%	85%
Hospital Given 9 or 10 on 10 Point Scale	300+	75%	71%	71%
Meds 'Always' Explained Before Given	300+	66%	66%	64%
Nurses 'Always' Communicated Well	300+	80%	80%	79%
Pain 'Always' Well Controlled	300+	72%	72%	71%
Room and Bathroom 'Always' Clean	300+	67%	71%	73%
Timely Help 'Always' Received	300+	64%	68%	68%
Would Definitely Recommend Hospital	300+	74%	70%	71%
Use of Medical Imaging				
Cardiac Imaging Stress Test before Surgery[1]	-	-	6.5%	5.3%
Combination Abdominal CT Scan	781	14.1%	16.5%	10.5%
Combination Brain/Sinus CT Scan	642	4.4%	3.5%	2.7%
Combination Chest CT Scan	436	6.2%	4.2%	2.7%
Follow-up Mammogram/Ultrasound	1,112	6.3%	7.6%	8.8%
Lumbar Spine MRI for Low Back Pain	156	53.2%	40.2%	37.2%

Birmingham VA Medical Center

700 South 19th Street
Birmingham, AL 35233
URL: www.birmingham.va.gov
Type: Acute Care - VA
Ownership: Government Federal

Phone: 205-933-4515
Fax: 205-933-4497
Emergency Services: No
Beds: 314

Key Personnel:
Anesthesiology. . . . . Russell Brockwell, MD
Quality Assurance . . . . Jimmie Davis
Chief of Medical Staff. . . . . John Kennedy, MD
Ambulatory Care . . . . John I Kennedy, MD
Operating Room. . . . . Patricia O'Fallon
CEO/President. . . . . Y C Parris
Infection Control. . . . . Barbara Taylor, RN

Measure	Cases	This Hosp.	State Avg.	U.S. Avg.
Blood Clot Prevention and Treatment				
Anticoagulation Overlap Therapy	-	-	91%	93%
ICU Venous Thromboembolism Prophylaxis	-	-	85%	92%
Incidence of Potentially Preventable VTE	-	-	18%	10%
UFH with Dosages/Platelet Monitoring	-	-	95%	97%
Venous Thromboembolism Prophylaxis	-	-	74%	85%
Warfarin Therapy Discharge Instructions	-	-	77%	75%
Chest Pain/Possible Heart Attack Care				
Aspirin Given Within 24 Hours of Arrival	-	-	96%	96%
Fibrinolytic Meds Within 30 Min. of Arrival	-	-	57%	58%
Average Time to ECG (minutes)	-	-	6	7
Average Time to Transfer (minutes)	-	-	61	60
Children's Asthma Care				
Received Home Management Plan of Care	-	-	-	88%
Received Reliever Medication	-	-	-	100%
Received Systemic Corticosteroids	-	-	-	100%
Emergency Department				
Admittance Decision Time (minutes)	-	-	73	98
Head CT Results Within 45 Min. of Arrival	-	-	45%	57%
Patients Who Left ER Before Being Seen	-	-	3%	2%
Time from ER Arrival to Admit. (minutes)	-	-	240	274
Time from ER Arrival to Discharge (minutes)	-	-	126	134
Time in ER Before Being Evaluated (minutes)	-	-	31	26
Time to Pain Meds for Fractures (minutes)	-	-	69	57
Heart Attack Care				
Aspirin Given at Discharge	54	100%	99%	99%
Fibrinolytic Meds Within 30 Min. of Arrival[5]	-	-	77%	54%
PCI Within 90 Minutes of Arrival[1]	-	-	97%	96%
Statin Prescribed at Discharge	54	100%	98%	98%
Heart Failure Care				
ACE Inhibitor or ARB for LVSD	98	100%	97%	97%
Discharge Instructions Given	199	97%	93%	94%

NOTE: Hospital profiles are in alphabetical order by state, then city, then hospital within the city; Rankings exclude hospitals with less than 25 cases except for patient surveys which excludes hospitals with less than 100 cases; (a) 100-299 cases; (1) The number of cases/patients is too few to report; (2) Data submitted were based on a sample of cases/patients; (3) Results are based on a shorter time period than required; (4) Data suppressed by CMS for one or more quarters; (5) Results are not available for this reporting period; (6) Fewer than 100 patients completed the HCAHPS survey; (7) No cases met the criteria for this measure; (8) The lower limit of the confidence interval cannot be calculated if the number of observed infections equals zero; (9) No data are available from the state/territory for this reporting period; (10) The scores shown reflect fewer than 50 completed surveys; (11) There were discrepancies in the data collection process; (12) This measure does not apply to this hospital for this reporting period; (13) Results cannot be calculated for this reporting period; (14) The results for this state are combined with nearby states to protect confidentiality; Please refer to the User's Guide for a full explanation of data.

Measure	Cases	This Hosp.	State Avg.	U.S. Avg.
Evaluation of LVS Function	218	100%	99%	99%
Medicare Spending				
Medicare Spending per Patient (ratio)	-	-	0.98	0.98
Pneumonia Care				
Appropriate Initial Antibiotic Given	48	94%	95%	95%
Blood Culture Timing	87	97%	98%	98%
Pregnancy and Delivery Care				
Newborn Deliveries Scheduled Early	-	-	14%	6%
Preventive Care				
Immunization for Influenza[5]	-	-	90%	90%
Immunization for Pneumonia[5]	-	-	91%	92%
Stroke Care				
Anticoagulation Therapy for Atrial Fibrillation	-	-	92%	95%
Antithrombotic Therapy Timing	-	-	96%	98%
Assessed for Rehabilitation	-	-	95%	97%
Discharged on Antithrombotic Therapy	-	-	98%	99%
Discharged on Statin Medication	-	-	90%	94%
Thrombolytic Therapy Timing	-	-	38%	66%
Venous Thromboembolism Prophylaxis	-	-	89%	94%
Written Stroke Educational Materials Given	-	-	85%	88%
Surgical Care Improvement Project				
Appropriate Beta Blocker Usage[2]	127	94%	98%	98%
Appropriate VTP Within 24 Hours[2]	204	99%	98%	98%
Controlled Postoperative Blood Glucose[2]	65	97%	97%	97%
Perioperative Temperature Management[2]	298	99%	100%	100%
Prophylactic Antibiotic Selection	207	100%	99%	99%
Prophylactic Antibiotic Selection (Outpatient)	-	-	98%	98%
Prophylactic Antibiotic Stopped	205	100%	98%	98%
Prophylactic Antibiotic Timing	207	98%	99%	99%
Prophylactic Antibiotic Timing (Outpatient)	-	-	99%	98%
Urinary Catheter Removal[2]	154	99%	98%	97%
Survey of Patients' Hospital Experiences				
Area Around Room 'Always' Quiet at Night	-	-	71%	61%
Doctors 'Always' Communicated Well	-	-	86%	82%
Home Recovery Information Given	-	-	84%	85%
Hospital Given 9 or 10 on 10 Point Scale	-	-	71%	71%
Meds 'Always' Explained Before Given	-	-	66%	64%
Nurses 'Always' Communicated Well	-	-	80%	79%
Pain 'Always' Well Controlled	-	-	72%	71%
Room and Bathroom 'Always' Clean	-	-	71%	73%
Timely Help 'Always' Received	-	-	68%	68%
Would Definitely Recommend Hospital	-	-	70%	71%
Use of Medical Imaging				
Cardiac Imaging Stress Test before Surgery	-	-	6.5%	5.3%
Combination Abdominal CT Scan	-	-	16.5%	10.5%
Combination Brain/Sinus CT Scan	-	-	3.5%	2.7%
Combination Chest CT Scan	-	-	4.2%	2.7%
Follow-up Mammogram/Ultrasound	-	-	7.6%	8.8%
Lumbar Spine MRI for Low Back Pain	-	-	40.2%	37.2%

Brookwood Medical Center

2010 Brookwood Medical Center Drive
Birmingham, AL 35209
URL: www.bwmc.com
Phone: 205-877-1000
Fax: 205-871-0534
Type: Acute Care Hospitals
Ownership: Proprietary
Emergency Services: Yes
Beds: 586

Key Personnel:

Chief of Medical Staff.......... Bradley Dennis, MD
Emergency Room .... Jackie Dillard
Quality Assurance .... Sue Esleck
CEO/President............... Garry Gause
Radiology.................... Charlotte Loar
Infection Control.............. Cathy Sanders
Coronary Care................ Linda Suther
Operating Room............... Brenda Traweek

Measure	Cases	This Hosp.	State Avg.	U.S. Avg.
Blood Clot Prevention and Treatment				
Anticoagulation Overlap Therapy[2]	110	96%	91%	93%
ICU Venous Thromboembolism Prophylaxis[2]	108	76%	85%	92%
Incidence of Potentially Preventable VTE[2]	30	13%	18%	10%
UFH with Dosages/Platelet Monitoring[2]	31	100%	95%	97%
Venous Thromboembolism Prophylaxis[2]	270	74%	74%	85%
Warfarin Therapy Discharge Instructions[2]	75	100%	77%	75%
Chest Pain/Possible Heart Attack Care				
Aspirin Given Within 24 Hours of Arrival[3]	20	100%	96%	96%
Fibrinolytic Meds Within 30 Min. of Arrival[5]	-	-	57%	58%
Average Time to ECG (minutes)[3]	22	9	6	7
Average Time to Transfer (minutes)[5]	-	-	61	60
Children's Asthma Care				
Received Home Management Plan of Care	-	-	-	88%
Received Reliever Medication	-	-	-	100%
Received Systemic Corticosteroids	-	-	-	100%
Emergency Department				
Admittance Decision Time (minutes)[2]	437	99	73	98
Head CT Results Within 45 Min. of Arrival[1,3]	-	-	45%	57%
Patients Who Left ER Before Being Seen	42,187	1%	3%	2%
Time from ER Arrival to Admit. (minutes)[2]	439	311	240	274
Time from ER Arrival to Discharge (minutes)	387	195	126	134
Time in ER Before Being Evaluated (minutes)	437	47	31	26
Time to Pain Meds for Fractures (minutes)	143	85	69	57
Heart Attack Care				
Aspirin Given at Discharge[2]	288	99%	99%	99%
Fibrinolytic Meds Within 30 Min. of Arrival[2,7]	-	-	77%	54%
PCI Within 90 Minutes of Arrival[2]	49	98%	97%	96%
Statin Prescribed at Discharge[2]	276	96%	98%	98%
Heart Failure Care				
ACE Inhibitor or ARB for LVSD[2]	111	100%	97%	97%
Discharge Instructions Given[2]	275	95%	93%	94%
Evaluation of LVS Function[2]	329	98%	99%	99%
Medicare Spending				
Medicare Spending per Patient (ratio)	-	1.04	0.98	0.98
Pneumonia Care				
Appropriate Initial Antibiotic Given[2]	123	95%	95%	95%
Blood Culture Timing[2]	292	100%	98%	98%
Pregnancy and Delivery Care				
Newborn Deliveries Scheduled Early[2]	73	0%	14%	6%
Preventive Care				
Immunization for Influenza[2]	538	92%	90%	90%
Immunization for Pneumonia[2]	507	93%	91%	92%
Stroke Care				
Anticoagulation Therapy for Atrial Fibrillation[2]	24	88%	92%	95%
Antithrombotic Therapy Timing[2]	103	99%	96%	98%
Assessed for Rehabilitation[2]	116	73%	95%	97%
Discharged on Antithrombotic Therapy[2]	106	97%	98%	99%
Discharged on Statin Medication[2]	90	62%	90%	94%
Thrombolytic Therapy Timing[1,2]	-	-	38%	66%
Venous Thromboembolism Prophylaxis[2]	114	80%	89%	94%
Written Stroke Educational Materials Given[2]	76	55%	85%	88%
Surgical Care Improvement Project				
Appropriate Beta Blocker Usage[2]	378	98%	98%	98%
Appropriate VTP Within 24 Hours[2]	691	98%	98%	98%
Controlled Postoperative Blood Glucose[2]	234	100%	97%	97%
Perioperative Temperature Management[2]	874	100%	100%	100%
Prophylactic Antibiotic Selection[2]	825	99%	99%	99%
Prophylactic Antibiotic Selection (Outpatient)	941	99%	98%	98%
Prophylactic Antibiotic Stopped[2]	797	98%	98%	98%
Prophylactic Antibiotic Timing[2]	825	100%	99%	99%
Prophylactic Antibiotic Timing (Outpatient)	941	100%	99%	98%
Urinary Catheter Removal[2]	496	99%	98%	97%
Survey of Patients' Hospital Experiences				
Area Around Room 'Always' Quiet at Night	300+	66%	71%	61%
Doctors 'Always' Communicated Well	300+	86%	86%	82%
Home Recovery Information Given	300+	85%	84%	85%
Hospital Given 9 or 10 on 10 Point Scale	300+	71%	71%	71%
Meds 'Always' Explained Before Given	300+	65%	66%	64%
Nurses 'Always' Communicated Well	300+	78%	80%	79%
Pain 'Always' Well Controlled	300+	72%	72%	71%
Room and Bathroom 'Always' Clean	300+	67%	71%	73%
Timely Help 'Always' Received	300+	63%	68%	68%
Would Definitely Recommend Hospital	300+	75%	70%	71%
Use of Medical Imaging				
Cardiac Imaging Stress Test before Surgery	1,364	5.9%	6.5%	5.3%
Combination Abdominal CT Scan	967	13.8%	16.5%	10.5%
Combination Brain/Sinus CT Scan	490	2.0%	3.5%	2.7%
Combination Chest CT Scan	539	0.0%	4.2%	2.7%
Follow-up Mammogram/Ultrasound[7]	-	-	7.6%	8.8%
Lumbar Spine MRI for Low Back Pain	88	53.4%	40.2%	37.2%

Callahan Eye Hospital

1720 University Blvd
Birmingham, AL 35233
URL: www.health.vab.edu/eyes
Phone: 205-325-8100
Fax: 205-325-8547
Type: Acute Care Hospitals
Ownership: Voluntary non-profit - Private
Emergency Services: Yes
Beds: 106

Key Personnel:

Anesthesiology............... Marilyn Allison, CRNA
Patient Relations .... Anne Banks
Radiology................... Polly A Barlow
Quality Assurance .... Karen Burleson
Emergency Room .... Judy Cocheanien, RN
CEO .... Will Ferniany, PhD
Chief of Medical Staff.......... Robert Morris, MD

Measure	Cases	This Hosp.	State Avg.	U.S. Avg.
Blood Clot Prevention and Treatment				
Anticoagulation Overlap Therapy[3,7]	-	-	91%	93%
ICU Venous Thromboembolism Prophylaxis[3,7]	-	-	85%	92%
Incidence of Potentially Preventable VTE[3,7]	-	-	18%	10%
UFH with Dosages/Platelet Monitoring[3,7]	-	-	95%	97%
Venous Thromboembolism Prophylaxis[3]	30	0%	74%	85%
Warfarin Therapy Discharge Instructions[3,7]	-	-	77%	75%
Chest Pain/Possible Heart Attack Care				
Aspirin Given Within 24 Hours of Arrival[5]	-	-	96%	96%
Fibrinolytic Meds Within 30 Min. of Arrival[5]	-	-	57%	58%
Average Time to ECG (minutes)[5]	-	-	6	7
Average Time to Transfer (minutes)[5]	-	-	61	60
Children's Asthma Care				
Received Home Management Plan of Care	-	-	-	88%
Received Reliever Medication	-	-	-	100%
Received Systemic Corticosteroids	-	-	-	100%
Emergency Department				
Admittance Decision Time (minutes)	13	23	73	98
Head CT Results Within 45 Min. of Arrival[5]	-	-	45%	57%
Patients Who Left ER Before Being Seen	5,005	1%	3%	2%
Time from ER Arrival to Admit. (minutes)	14	142	240	274
Time from ER Arrival to Discharge (minutes)	378	100	126	134
Time in ER Before Being Evaluated (minutes)	380	53	31	26
Time to Pain Meds for Fractures (minutes)[5]	-	-	69	57
Heart Attack Care				
Aspirin Given at Discharge[5]	-	-	99%	99%
Fibrinolytic Meds Within 30 Min. of Arrival[5]	-	-	77%	54%
PCI Within 90 Minutes of Arrival[5]	-	-	97%	96%
Statin Prescribed at Discharge[5]	-	-	98%	98%
Heart Failure Care				
ACE Inhibitor or ARB for LVSD[5]	-	-	97%	97%
Discharge Instructions Given[5]	-	-	93%	94%
Evaluation of LVS Function[5]	-	-	99%	99%
Medicare Spending				
Medicare Spending per Patient (ratio)[1]	-	-	0.98	0.98
Pneumonia Care				
Appropriate Initial Antibiotic Given[5]	-	-	95%	95%
Blood Culture Timing[5]	-	-	98%	98%
Pregnancy and Delivery Care				
Newborn Deliveries Scheduled Early[2,7]	-	-	14%	6%
Preventive Care				
Immunization for Influenza	27	33%	90%	90%
Immunization for Pneumonia	47	43%	91%	92%
Stroke Care				
Anticoagulation Therapy for Atrial Fibrillation[5]	-	-	92%	95%
Antithrombotic Therapy Timing[5]	-	-	96%	98%
Assessed for Rehabilitation[5]	-	-	95%	97%
Discharged on Antithrombotic Therapy[5]	-	-	98%	99%
Discharged on Statin Medication[5]	-	-	90%	94%
Thrombolytic Therapy Timing[5]	-	-	38%	66%
Venous Thromboembolism Prophylaxis[5]	-	-	89%	94%
Written Stroke Educational Materials Given[5]	-	-	85%	88%
Surgical Care Improvement Project				
Appropriate Beta Blocker Usage[5]	-	-	98%	98%
Appropriate VTP Within 24 Hours[5]	-	-	98%	98%
Controlled Postoperative Blood Glucose[5]	-	-	97%	97%
Perioperative Temperature Management[5]	-	-	100%	100%

NOTE: Hospital profiles are in alphabetical order by state, then city, then hospital within the city; Rankings exclude hospitals with less than 25 cases except for patient surveys which excludes hospitals with less than 100 cases; (a) 100-299 cases; (1) The number of cases/patients is too few to report; (2) Data submitted were based on a sample of cases/patients; (3) Results are based on a shorter time period than required; (4) Data suppressed by CMS for one or more quarters; (5) Results are not available for this reporting period; (6) Fewer than 100 patients completed the HCAHPS survey; (7) No cases met the criteria for this measure; (8) The lower limit of the confidence interval cannot be calculated if the number of observed infections equals zero; (9) No data are available from the state/territory for this reporting period; (10) The scores shown reflect fewer than 50 completed surveys; (11) There were discrepancies in the data collection process; (12) This measure does not apply to this hospital for this reporting period; (13) Results cannot be calculated for this reporting period; (14) The results for this state are combined with nearby states to protect confidentiality; Please refer to the User's Guide for a full explanation of data.

Measure	Cases	This Hosp.	State Avg.	U.S. Avg.
Prophylactic Antibiotic Selection[5]	-	-	99%	99%
Prophylactic Antibiotic Selection (Outpatient)[5]	-	-	98%	98%
Prophylactic Antibiotic Stopped[5]	-	-	98%	98%
Prophylactic Antibiotic Timing[5]	-	-	99%	99%
Prophylactic Antibiotic Timing (Outpatient)[5]	-	-	99%	98%
Urinary Catheter Removal[5]	-	-	98%	97%
Survey of Patients' Hospital Experiences				
Area Around Room 'Always' Quiet at Night[10]	<100	99%	71%	61%
Doctors 'Always' Communicated Well[10]	<100	94%	86%	82%
Home Recovery Information Given[10]	<100	81%	84%	85%
Hospital Given 9 or 10 on 10 Point Scale[10]	<100	96%	71%	71%
Meds 'Always' Explained Before Given[10]	<100	85%	66%	64%
Nurses 'Always' Communicated Well[10]	<100	100%	80%	79%
Pain 'Always' Well Controlled[10]	<100	90%	72%	71%
Room and Bathroom 'Always' Clean[10]	<100	81%	71%	73%
Timely Help 'Always' Received[10]	<100	100%	68%	68%
Would Definitely Recommend Hospital[10]	<100	97%	70%	71%
Use of Medical Imaging				
Cardiac Imaging Stress Test before Surgery[7]	-	-	6.5%	5.3%
Combination Abdominal CT Scan[7]	-	-	16.5%	10.5%
Combination Brain/Sinus CT Scan[1]	-	-	3.5%	2.7%
Combination Chest CT Scan[7]	-	-	4.2%	2.7%
Follow-up Mammogram/Ultrasound[7]	-	-	7.6%	8.8%
Lumbar Spine MRI for Low Back Pain[7]	-	-	40.2%	37.2%

Saint Vincent's Birmingham

810 Saint Vincent's Drive
Birmingham, AL 35205
Phone: 205-939-7000
Fax: 205-930-2157
URL: www.stv.org
Type: Acute Care Hospitals
Emergency Services: Yes
Ownership: Voluntary non-profit - Private
Beds: 338

Key Personnel:

CEO/President. . . . . Vincent Capone
Quality Assurance . . . . Rebecca Harrison
Radiology. . . . . John Mussleman, MD
Operating Room. . . . . Cheryl Ruttledge, RN
Chief of Medical Staff . . . . Ralph Yarbrough, MD

Measure	Cases	This Hosp.	State Avg.	U.S. Avg.
Blood Clot Prevention and Treatment				
Anticoagulation Overlap Therapy[2]	142	96%	91%	93%
ICU Venous Thromboembolism Prophylaxis[2]	99	76%	85%	92%
Incidence of Potentially Preventable VTE[2]	31	3%	18%	10%
UFH with Dosages/Platelet Monitoring[2]	35	100%	95%	97%
Venous Thromboembolism Prophylaxis[2]	284	64%	74%	85%
Warfarin Therapy Discharge Instructions[2]	103	85%	77%	75%
Chest Pain/Possible Heart Attack Care				
Aspirin Given Within 24 Hours of Arrival[1,3]	-	-	96%	96%
Fibrinolytic Meds Within 30 Min. of Arrival[3,7]	-	-	57%	58%
Average Time to ECG (minutes)[1,3]	-	-	6	7
Average Time to Transfer (minutes)[3,7]	-	-	61	60
Children's Asthma Care				
Received Home Management Plan of Care	-	-	-	88%
Received Reliever Medication	-	-	-	100%
Received Systemic Corticosteroids	-	-	-	100%
Emergency Department				
Admittance Decision Time (minutes)[2]	403	115	73	98
Head CT Results Within 45 Min. of Arrival[1]	-	-	45%	57%
Patients Who Left ER Before Being Seen	49,943	2%	3%	2%
Time from ER Arrival to Admit. (minutes)[2]	405	296	240	274
Time from ER Arrival to Discharge (minutes)	357	195	126	134
Time in ER Before Being Evaluated (minutes)	383	45	31	26
Time to Pain Meds for Fractures (minutes)	174	85	69	57
Heart Attack Care				
Aspirin Given at Discharge	271	100%	99%	99%
Fibrinolytic Meds Within 30 Min. of Arrival[7]	-	-	77%	54%
PCI Within 90 Minutes of Arrival	69	100%	97%	96%
Statin Prescribed at Discharge	265	100%	98%	98%
Heart Failure Care				
ACE Inhibitor or ARB for LVSD	127	99%	97%	97%
Discharge Instructions Given	360	97%	93%	94%
Evaluation of LVS Function	428	100%	99%	99%
Medicare Spending				
Medicare Spending per Patient (ratio)	-	1.04	0.98	0.98
Pneumonia Care				
Appropriate Initial Antibiotic Given[2]	106	100%	95%	95%
Blood Culture Timing[2]	153	100%	98%	98%
Pregnancy and Delivery Care				
Newborn Deliveries Scheduled Early[2]	54	6%	14%	6%
Preventive Care				
Immunization for Influenza[2]	500	98%	90%	90%
Immunization for Pneumonia[2]	583	97%	91%	92%
Stroke Care				
Anticoagulation Therapy for Atrial Fibrillation[2]	11	100%	92%	95%
Antithrombotic Therapy Timing[2]	74	100%	96%	98%
Assessed for Rehabilitation[2]	91	98%	95%	97%
Discharged on Antithrombotic Therapy[2]	76	100%	98%	99%
Discharged on Statin Medication[2]	64	92%	90%	94%
Thrombolytic Therapy Timing[1,2]	-	-	38%	66%
Venous Thromboembolism Prophylaxis[2]	92	85%	89%	94%
Written Stroke Educational Materials Given[2]	51	71%	85%	88%
Surgical Care Improvement Project				
Appropriate Beta Blocker Usage[2]	244	99%	98%	98%
Appropriate VTP Within 24 Hours[2]	384	100%	98%	98%
Controlled Postoperative Blood Glucose[2]	132	99%	97%	97%
Perioperative Temperature Management[2]	507	100%	100%	100%
Prophylactic Antibiotic Selection[2]	482	99%	99%	99%
Prophylactic Antibiotic Selection (Outpatient)	982	98%	98%	98%
Prophylactic Antibiotic Stopped[2]	463	99%	98%	98%
Prophylactic Antibiotic Timing[2]	482	99%	99%	99%
Prophylactic Antibiotic Timing (Outpatient)	940	98%	99%	98%
Urinary Catheter Removal[2]	225	99%	98%	97%
Survey of Patients' Hospital Experiences				
Area Around Room 'Always' Quiet at Night	300+	68%	71%	61%
Doctors 'Always' Communicated Well	300+	85%	86%	82%
Home Recovery Information Given	300+	87%	84%	85%
Hospital Given 9 or 10 on 10 Point Scale	300+	78%	71%	71%
Meds 'Always' Explained Before Given	300+	64%	66%	64%
Nurses 'Always' Communicated Well	300+	81%	80%	79%
Pain 'Always' Well Controlled	300+	72%	72%	71%
Room and Bathroom 'Always' Clean	300+	61%	71%	73%
Timely Help 'Always' Received	300+	66%	68%	68%
Would Definitely Recommend Hospital	300+	82%	70%	71%
Use of Medical Imaging				
Cardiac Imaging Stress Test before Surgery	306	8.5%	6.5%	5.3%
Combination Abdominal CT Scan	1,341	4.8%	16.5%	10.5%
Combination Brain/Sinus CT Scan	1,051	4.0%	3.5%	2.7%
Combination Chest CT Scan	721	0.1%	4.2%	2.7%
Follow-up Mammogram/Ultrasound	3,645	6.9%	7.6%	8.8%
Lumbar Spine MRI for Low Back Pain	458	42.4%	40.2%	37.2%

Saint Vincent's East

50 Medical Park East Drive
Birmingham, AL 35235
Phone: 205-838-3122
Fax: 205-838-5113
E-mail: pmiller@nolandhealth.com
URL: www.nolandhealth.com
Type: Acute Care Hospitals
Emergency Services: Yes
Ownership: Voluntary non-profit - Private
Beds: 45

Key Personnel:

Operating Room. . . . . Denne Cofield
Pediatric In-Patient Care . . . . Rosemarie Faust, MD
President/CEO. . . . . Gary M. Glasscock
Chairman/CEO . . . . Leon C. Hamrick, Sr.
Quality Assurance . . . . Trudie Stricklin
Chief of Medical Staff . . . . Adeeb Thomas, MD

Measure	Cases	This Hosp.	State Avg.	U.S. Avg.
Blood Clot Prevention and Treatment				
Anticoagulation Overlap Therapy[2]	118	100%	91%	93%
ICU Venous Thromboembolism Prophylaxis[2]	100	86%	85%	92%
Incidence of Potentially Preventable VTE[2]	18	0%	18%	10%
UFH with Dosages/Platelet Monitoring[2]	106	100%	95%	97%
Venous Thromboembolism Prophylaxis[2]	263	73%	74%	85%
Warfarin Therapy Discharge Instructions[2]	63	84%	77%	75%
Chest Pain/Possible Heart Attack Care				
Aspirin Given Within 24 Hours of Arrival[5]	-	-	96%	96%
Fibrinolytic Meds Within 30 Min. of Arrival[5]	-	-	57%	58%
Average Time to ECG (minutes)[5]	-	-	6	7
Average Time to Transfer (minutes)[5]	-	-	61	60
Children's Asthma Care				
Received Home Management Plan of Care	-	-	-	88%
Received Reliever Medication	-	-	-	100%
Received Systemic Corticosteroids	-	-	-	100%
Emergency Department				
Admittance Decision Time (minutes)[2]	431	85	73	98
Head CT Results Within 45 Min. of Arrival[1]	-	-	45%	57%
Patients Who Left ER Before Being Seen	52,342	3%	3%	2%
Time from ER Arrival to Admit. (minutes)[2]	451	265	240	274
Time from ER Arrival to Discharge (minutes)	336	146	126	134
Time in ER Before Being Evaluated (minutes)	354	38	31	26
Time to Pain Meds for Fractures (minutes)	201	70	69	57
Heart Attack Care				
Aspirin Given at Discharge	331	100%	99%	99%
Fibrinolytic Meds Within 30 Min. of Arrival[7]	-	-	77%	54%
PCI Within 90 Minutes of Arrival	48	92%	97%	96%
Statin Prescribed at Discharge	327	100%	98%	98%
Heart Failure Care				
ACE Inhibitor or ARB for LVSD	120	100%	97%	97%
Discharge Instructions Given	289	100%	93%	94%
Evaluation of LVS Function	335	100%	99%	99%
Medicare Spending				
Medicare Spending per Patient (ratio)	-	0.98	0.98	0.98
Pneumonia Care				
Appropriate Initial Antibiotic Given[2]	81	100%	95%	95%
Blood Culture Timing[2]	133	100%	98%	98%
Pregnancy and Delivery Care				
Newborn Deliveries Scheduled Early[2]	13	0%	14%	6%
Preventive Care				
Immunization for Influenza[2]	549	91%	90%	90%
Immunization for Pneumonia[2]	700	88%	91%	92%
Stroke Care				
Anticoagulation Therapy for Atrial Fibrillation[2]	13	92%	92%	95%
Antithrombotic Therapy Timing[2]	60	98%	96%	98%
Assessed for Rehabilitation[2]	65	98%	95%	97%
Discharged on Antithrombotic Therapy[2]	61	98%	98%	99%
Discharged on Statin Medication[2]	48	90%	90%	94%
Thrombolytic Therapy Timing[2,7]	-	-	38%	66%
Venous Thromboembolism Prophylaxis[2]	62	77%	89%	94%
Written Stroke Educational Materials Given[2]	39	74%	85%	88%
Surgical Care Improvement Project				
Appropriate Beta Blocker Usage[2]	236	99%	98%	98%
Appropriate VTP Within 24 Hours[2]	343	96%	98%	98%
Controlled Postoperative Blood Glucose[2]	116	89%	97%	97%
Perioperative Temperature Management[2]	405	100%	100%	100%
Prophylactic Antibiotic Selection[2]	363	99%	99%	99%
Prophylactic Antibiotic Selection (Outpatient)	464	98%	98%	98%
Prophylactic Antibiotic Stopped[2]	345	98%	98%	98%
Prophylactic Antibiotic Timing[2]	367	100%	99%	99%
Prophylactic Antibiotic Timing (Outpatient)	465	99%	99%	98%
Urinary Catheter Removal[2]	339	98%	98%	97%
Survey of Patients' Hospital Experiences				
Area Around Room 'Always' Quiet at Night	300+	60%	71%	61%
Doctors 'Always' Communicated Well	300+	83%	86%	82%
Home Recovery Information Given	300+	85%	84%	85%
Hospital Given 9 or 10 on 10 Point Scale	300+	70%	71%	71%
Meds 'Always' Explained Before Given	300+	61%	66%	64%
Nurses 'Always' Communicated Well	300+	76%	80%	79%
Pain 'Always' Well Controlled	300+	69%	72%	71%
Room and Bathroom 'Always' Clean	300+	59%	71%	73%
Timely Help 'Always' Received	300+	61%	68%	68%
Would Definitely Recommend Hospital	300+	74%	70%	71%
Use of Medical Imaging				
Cardiac Imaging Stress Test before Surgery[1]	-	-	6.5%	5.3%
Combination Abdominal CT Scan	659	6.2%	16.5%	10.5%
Combination Brain/Sinus CT Scan	769	2.9%	3.5%	2.7%
Combination Chest CT Scan	139	12.9%	4.2%	2.7%
Follow-up Mammogram/Ultrasound[7]	-	-	7.6%	8.8%
Lumbar Spine MRI for Low Back Pain	116	41.4%	40.2%	37.2%

NOTE: Hospital profiles are in alphabetical order by state, then city, then hospital within the city; Rankings exclude hospitals with less than 25 cases except for patient surveys which excludes hospitals with less than 100 cases; (a) 100-299 cases; (1) The number of cases/patients is too few to report; (2) Data submitted were based on a sample of cases/patients; (3) Results are based on a shorter time period than required; (4) Data suppressed by CMS for one or more quarters; (5) Results are not available for this reporting period; (6) Fewer than 100 patients completed the HCAHPS survey; (7) No cases met the criteria for this measure; (8) The lower limit of the confidence interval cannot be calculated if the number of observed infections equals zero; (9) No data are available from the state/territory for this reporting period; (10) The scores shown reflect fewer than 50 completed surveys; (11) There were discrepancies in the data collection process; (12) This measure does not apply to this hospital for this reporting period; (13) Results cannot be calculated for this reporting period; (14) The results for this state are combined with nearby states to protect confidentiality; Please refer to the User's Guide for a full explanation of data.

Trinity Medical Center

800 Montclair Rd | Phone: 205-592-1000
Birmingham, AL 35213 | Fax: 205-599-4958
E-mail: info@bhsala.com
URL: www.bhsala.com/montclair
Type: Acute Care Hospitals | Emergency Services: Yes
Ownership: Proprietary | Beds: 560

Key Personnel:
CEO/President. . . . . Vicki Briggs
Chief of Medical Staff. . . . . J T Eagan, Jr, MD
Operating Room. . . . . Lynne Hays
Radiology. . . . . Rick Kolaczek
Quality Assurance . . . . Jane Northcutt
Infection Control. . . . . Ginger Smith
Coronary Care . . . . Linda Suther

Measure	Cases	This Hosp.	State Avg.	U.S. Avg.
Blood Clot Prevention and Treatment				
Anticoagulation Overlap Therapy[2]	74	100%	91%	93%
ICU Venous Thromboembolism Prophylaxis[2]	181	100%	85%	92%
Incidence of Potentially Preventable VTE[2]	26	4%	18%	10%
UFH with Dosages/Platelet Monitoring[2]	32	100%	95%	97%
Venous Thromboembolism Prophylaxis[2]	324	98%	74%	85%
Warfarin Therapy Discharge Instructions[2]	54	100%	77%	75%
Chest Pain/Possible Heart Attack Care				
Aspirin Given Within 24 Hours of Arrival[1,3]	-	-	96%	96%
Fibrinolytic Meds Within 30 Min. of Arrival[5]	-	-	57%	58%
Average Time to ECG (minutes)[1,3]	-	-	6	7
Average Time to Transfer (minutes)[5]	-	-	61	60
Children's Asthma Care				
Received Home Management Plan of Care	-	-	-	88%
Received Reliever Medication	-	-	-	100%
Received Systemic Corticosteroids	-	-	-	100%
Emergency Department				
Admittance Decision Time (minutes)[2]	504	55	73	98
Head CT Results Within 45 Min. of Arrival[1]	-	-	45%	57%
Patients Who Left ER Before Being Seen	26,048	1%	3%	2%
Time from ER Arrival to Admit. (minutes)[2]	505	178	240	274
Time from ER Arrival to Discharge (minutes)	393	103	126	134
Time in ER Before Being Evaluated (minutes)	419	17	31	26
Time to Pain Meds for Fractures (minutes)	80	42	69	57
Heart Attack Care				
Aspirin Given at Discharge	269	100%	99%	99%
Fibrinolytic Meds Within 30 Min. of Arrival[7]	-	-	77%	54%
PCI Within 90 Minutes of Arrival	33	97%	97%	96%
Statin Prescribed at Discharge	249	100%	98%	98%
Heart Failure Care				
ACE Inhibitor or ARB for LVSD	103	100%	97%	97%
Discharge Instructions Given	240	100%	93%	94%
Evaluation of LVS Function	282	100%	99%	99%
Medicare Spending				
Medicare Spending per Patient (ratio)	-	1.01	0.98	0.98
Pneumonia Care				
Appropriate Initial Antibiotic Given	63	100%	95%	95%
Blood Culture Timing	128	100%	98%	98%
Pregnancy and Delivery Care				
Newborn Deliveries Scheduled Early[2]	28	0%	14%	6%
Preventive Care				
Immunization for Influenza[2]	642	100%	90%	90%
Immunization for Pneumonia[2]	766	100%	91%	92%
Stroke Care				
Anticoagulation Therapy for Atrial Fibrillation	17	100%	92%	95%
Antithrombotic Therapy Timing	119	100%	96%	98%
Assessed for Rehabilitation	169	100%	95%	97%
Discharged on Antithrombotic Therapy	122	100%	98%	99%
Discharged on Statin Medication	97	100%	90%	94%
Thrombolytic Therapy Timing[1]	-	-	38%	66%
Venous Thromboembolism Prophylaxis	188	100%	89%	94%
Written Stroke Educational Materials Given	93	100%	85%	88%
Surgical Care Improvement Project				
Appropriate Beta Blocker Usage	390	100%	98%	98%
Appropriate VTP Within 24 Hours	910	100%	98%	98%
Controlled Postoperative Blood Glucose	127	100%	97%	97%
Perioperative Temperature Management	1,107	100%	100%	100%
Prophylactic Antibiotic Selection	740	100%	99%	99%
Prophylactic Antibiotic Selection (Outpatient)	451	100%	98%	98%
Prophylactic Antibiotic Stopped	708	100%	98%	98%
Prophylactic Antibiotic Timing	743	100%	99%	99%
Prophylactic Antibiotic Timing (Outpatient)	451	100%	99%	98%
Urinary Catheter Removal	332	100%	98%	97%
Survey of Patients' Hospital Experiences				
Area Around Room 'Always' Quiet at Night	300+	72%	71%	61%
Doctors 'Always' Communicated Well	300+	85%	86%	82%
Home Recovery Information Given	300+	86%	84%	85%
Hospital Given 9 or 10 on 10 Point Scale	300+	79%	71%	71%
Meds 'Always' Explained Before Given	300+	67%	66%	64%
Nurses 'Always' Communicated Well	300+	82%	80%	79%
Pain 'Always' Well Controlled	300+	76%	72%	71%
Room and Bathroom 'Always' Clean	300+	72%	71%	73%
Timely Help 'Always' Received	300+	68%	68%	68%
Would Definitely Recommend Hospital	300+	79%	70%	71%
Use of Medical Imaging				
Cardiac Imaging Stress Test before Surgery	63	3.2%	6.5%	5.3%
Combination Abdominal CT Scan	665	7.4%	16.5%	10.5%
Combination Brain/Sinus CT Scan	513	5.1%	3.5%	2.7%
Combination Chest CT Scan	427	0.7%	4.2%	2.7%
Follow-up Mammogram/Ultrasound	1,228	6.4%	7.6%	8.8%
Lumbar Spine MRI for Low Back Pain	180	38.3%	40.2%	37.2%

University of Alabama Hospital

619 South 19th Street | Phone: 205-934-4011
Birmingham, AL 35233 | Fax: 205-934-1273
URL: www.health.uab.edu
Type: Acute Care Hospitals | Emergency Services: Yes
Ownership: Government - State | Beds: 908

Key Personnel:
Quality Assurance . . . . Arhtur M Boudreaux, MD
Cardiac Laboratory. . . . . Robert C Bourge, MD
Chief of Medical Staff. . . . . Scott Buchalter, MD
Radiology. . . . . Cheri L Canon, MD
Infection Control. . . . . William Dismukes, MD
Operating Room. . . . . Alice Goodwin
Pediatric Ambulatory Care . . . . . . Sergio Stagno, MD
President . . . . Ray L. Watts, MD

Measure	Cases	This Hosp.	State Avg.	U.S. Avg.
Blood Clot Prevention and Treatment				
Anticoagulation Overlap Therapy[2]	226	95%	91%	93%
ICU Venous Thromboembolism Prophylaxis[2]	93	92%	85%	92%
Incidence of Potentially Preventable VTE[2]	124	3%	18%	10%
UFH with Dosages/Platelet Monitoring[2]	110	100%	95%	97%
Venous Thromboembolism Prophylaxis[2]	318	83%	74%	85%
Warfarin Therapy Discharge Instructions[2]	189	83%	77%	75%
Chest Pain/Possible Heart Attack Care				
Aspirin Given Within 24 Hours of Arrival[1,3]	-	-	96%	96%
Fibrinolytic Meds Within 30 Min. of Arrival[5]	-	-	57%	58%
Average Time to ECG (minutes)[1,3]	-	-	6	7
Average Time to Transfer (minutes)[5]	-	-	61	60
Children's Asthma Care				
Received Home Management Plan of Care	-	-	-	88%
Received Reliever Medication	-	-	-	100%
Received Systemic Corticosteroids	-	-	-	100%
Emergency Department				
Admittance Decision Time (minutes)[2]	320	214	73	98
Head CT Results Within 45 Min. of Arrival[7]	-	-	45%	57%
Patients Who Left ER Before Being Seen	86,533	4%	3%	2%
Time from ER Arrival to Admit. (minutes)[2]	523	395	240	274
Time from ER Arrival to Discharge (minutes)	345	190	126	134
Time in ER Before Being Evaluated (minutes)	368	42	31	26
Time to Pain Meds for Fractures (minutes)	151	75	69	57
Heart Attack Care				
Aspirin Given at Discharge	521	99%	99%	99%
Fibrinolytic Meds Within 30 Min. of Arrival[7]	-	-	77%	54%
PCI Within 90 Minutes of Arrival	64	91%	97%	96%
Statin Prescribed at Discharge	503	99%	98%	98%
Heart Failure Care				
ACE Inhibitor or ARB for LVSD[2]	301	98%	97%	97%
Discharge Instructions Given[2]	648	96%	93%	94%
Evaluation of LVS Function[2]	702	100%	99%	99%
Medicare Spending				
Medicare Spending per Patient (ratio)	-	0.96	0.98	0.98
Pneumonia Care				
Appropriate Initial Antibiotic Given[2]	106	99%	95%	95%
Blood Culture Timing[2]	258	99%	98%	98%
Pregnancy and Delivery Care				
Newborn Deliveries Scheduled Early[2]	38	0%	14%	6%
Preventive Care				
Immunization for Influenza[2]	546	81%	90%	90%
Immunization for Pneumonia[2]	602	84%	91%	92%
Stroke Care				
Anticoagulation Therapy for Atrial Fibrillation[1,2]	-	-	92%	95%
Antithrombotic Therapy Timing[2]	67	97%	96%	98%
Assessed for Rehabilitation[2]	116	100%	95%	97%
Discharged on Antithrombotic Therapy[2]	79	100%	98%	99%
Discharged on Statin Medication[2]	59	100%	90%	94%
Thrombolytic Therapy Timing[2]	13	92%	38%	66%
Venous Thromboembolism Prophylaxis[2]	118	97%	89%	94%
Written Stroke Educational Materials Given[2]	70	93%	85%	88%
Surgical Care Improvement Project				
Appropriate Beta Blocker Usage[2]	187	93%	98%	98%
Appropriate VTP Within 24 Hours[2]	414	98%	98%	98%
Controlled Postoperative Blood Glucose[2]	137	96%	97%	97%
Perioperative Temperature Management[2]	566	100%	100%	100%
Prophylactic Antibiotic Selection[2]	387	100%	99%	99%
Prophylactic Antibiotic Selection (Outpatient)	609	85%	98%	98%
Prophylactic Antibiotic Stopped[2]	378	99%	98%	98%
Prophylactic Antibiotic Timing[2]	387	100%	99%	99%
Prophylactic Antibiotic Timing (Outpatient)	615	98%	99%	98%
Urinary Catheter Removal[2]	324	97%	98%	97%
Survey of Patients' Hospital Experiences				
Area Around Room 'Always' Quiet at Night	300+	68%	71%	61%
Doctors 'Always' Communicated Well	300+	84%	86%	82%
Home Recovery Information Given	300+	86%	84%	85%
Hospital Given 9 or 10 on 10 Point Scale	300+	83%	71%	71%
Meds 'Always' Explained Before Given	300+	69%	66%	64%
Nurses 'Always' Communicated Well	300+	83%	80%	79%
Pain 'Always' Well Controlled	300+	75%	72%	71%
Room and Bathroom 'Always' Clean	300+	73%	71%	73%
Timely Help 'Always' Received	300+	70%	68%	68%
Would Definitely Recommend Hospital	300+	85%	70%	71%
Use of Medical Imaging				
Cardiac Imaging Stress Test before Surgery	142	7.0%	6.5%	5.3%
Combination Abdominal CT Scan	782	5.4%	16.5%	10.5%
Combination Brain/Sinus CT Scan	963	4.3%	3.5%	2.7%
Combination Chest CT Scan	290	0.3%	4.2%	2.7%
Follow-up Mammogram/Ultrasound[7]	-	-	7.6%	8.8%
Lumbar Spine MRI for Low Back Pain	71	29.6%	40.2%	37.2%

Marshall Medical Center South

2505 U S Highway 431 North | Phone: 256-593-8310
Boaz, AL 35957 | Fax: 256-840-3636
URL: www.mmcenters.com/mmcsouth.php
Type: Acute Care Hospitals | Emergency Services: Yes
Ownership: Govt - Hospital Dist/Auth | Beds: 150

Key Personnel:
Emergency Room . . . . Ruth Bischoff, RN
CEO . . . . Gary Gore
Administrator . . . . Cheryl Hays
Operating Room. . . . . Cynthia Head, RN
Quality Assurance . . . . Libby McClendon, RN
Intensive Care Unit. . . . . Kerry Quinn, RN
Chief of Medical Staff . . . . Linda Smith
Infection Control. . . . . Ann Thorne

Measure	Cases	This Hosp.	State Avg.	U.S. Avg.
Blood Clot Prevention and Treatment				
Anticoagulation Overlap Therapy[2]	55	95%	91%	93%
ICU Venous Thromboembolism Prophylaxis[2]	85	76%	85%	92%
Incidence of Potentially Preventable VTE[2]	14	29%	18%	10%
UFH with Dosages/Platelet Monitoring[1,2]	-	-	95%	97%
Venous Thromboembolism Prophylaxis[2]	289	55%	74%	85%
Warfarin Therapy Discharge Instructions[2]	40	92%	77%	75%
Chest Pain/Possible Heart Attack Care				
Aspirin Given Within 24 Hours of Arrival	344	98%	96%	96%
Fibrinolytic Meds Within 30 Min. of Arrival[1]	-	-	57%	58%

NOTE: Hospital profiles are in alphabetical order by state, then city, then hospital within the city; Rankings exclude hospitals with less than 25 cases except for patient surveys which excludes hospitals with less than 100 cases; (a) 100-299 cases; (1) The number of cases/patients is too few to report; (2) Data submitted were based on a sample of cases/patients; (3) Results are based on a shorter time period than required; (4) Data suppressed by CMS for one or more quarters; (5) Results are not available for this reporting period; (6) Fewer than 100 patients completed the HCAHPS survey; (7) No cases met the criteria for this measure; (8) The lower limit of the confidence interval cannot be calculated if the number of observed infections equals zero; (9) No data are available from the state/territory for this reporting period; (10) The scores shown reflect fewer than 50 completed surveys; (11) There were discrepancies in the data collection process; (12) This measure does not apply to this hospital for this reporting period; (13) Results cannot be calculated for this reporting period; (14) The results for this state are combined with nearby states to protect confidentiality; Please refer to the User's Guide for a full explanation of data.

Measure	Cases	This Hosp.	State Avg.	U.S. Avg.
Average Time to ECG (minutes)	356	6	6	7
Average Time to Transfer (minutes)	28	56	61	60
Children's Asthma Care				
Received Home Management Plan of Care	-	-	-	88%
Received Reliever Medication	-	-	-	100%
Received Systemic Corticosteroids	-	-	-	100%
Emergency Department				
Admittance Decision Time (minutes)[2]	1,057	65	73	98
Head CT Results Within 45 Min. of Arrival	31	48%	45%	57%
Patients Who Left ER Before Being Seen	75,338	3%	3%	2%
Time from ER Arrival to Admit. (minutes)[2]	1,140	241	240	274
Time from ER Arrival to Discharge (minutes)	1,900	136	126	134
Time in ER Before Being Evaluated (minutes)	1,991	36	31	26
Time to Pain Meds for Fractures (minutes)	310	75	69	57
Heart Attack Care				
Aspirin Given at Discharge	20	100%	99%	99%
Fibrinolytic Meds Within 30 Min. of Arrival[7]	-	-	77%	54%
PCI Within 90 Minutes of Arrival[1]	-	-	97%	96%
Statin Prescribed at Discharge	22	95%	98%	98%
Heart Failure Care				
ACE Inhibitor or ARB for LVSD	57	96%	97%	97%
Discharge Instructions Given	148	95%	93%	94%
Evaluation of LVS Function	209	90%	99%	99%
Medicare Spending				
Medicare Spending per Patient (ratio)	-	1.00	0.98	0.98
Pneumonia Care				
Appropriate Initial Antibiotic Given	160	94%	95%	95%
Blood Culture Timing	360	99%	98%	98%
Pregnancy and Delivery Care				
Newborn Deliveries Scheduled Early	146	30%	14%	6%
Preventive Care				
Immunization for Influenza[2]	1,053	92%	90%	90%
Immunization for Pneumonia[2]	1,271	97%	91%	92%
Stroke Care				
Anticoagulation Therapy for Atrial Fibrillation	14	100%	92%	95%
Antithrombotic Therapy Timing	108	99%	96%	98%
Assessed for Rehabilitation	115	97%	95%	97%
Discharged on Antithrombotic Therapy	111	99%	98%	99%
Discharged on Statin Medication	93	81%	90%	94%
Thrombolytic Therapy Timing	14	0%	38%	66%
Venous Thromboembolism Prophylaxis	111	70%	89%	94%
Written Stroke Educational Materials Given	65	80%	85%	88%
Surgical Care Improvement Project				
Appropriate Beta Blocker Usage	126	100%	98%	98%
Appropriate VTP Within 24 Hours	411	98%	98%	98%
Controlled Postoperative Blood Glucose[7]	-	-	97%	97%
Perioperative Temperature Management	509	100%	100%	100%
Prophylactic Antibiotic Selection	378	100%	99%	99%
Prophylactic Antibiotic Selection (Outpatient)	76	95%	98%	98%
Prophylactic Antibiotic Stopped	376	100%	98%	98%
Prophylactic Antibiotic Timing	380	99%	99%	99%
Prophylactic Antibiotic Timing (Outpatient)	84	88%	99%	98%
Urinary Catheter Removal	333	99%	98%	97%
Survey of Patients' Hospital Experiences				
Area Around Room 'Always' Quiet at Night	300+	73%	71%	61%
Doctors 'Always' Communicated Well	300+	90%	86%	82%
Home Recovery Information Given	300+	87%	84%	85%
Hospital Given 9 or 10 on 10 Point Scale	300+	78%	71%	71%
Meds 'Always' Explained Before Given	300+	71%	66%	64%
Nurses 'Always' Communicated Well	300+	84%	80%	79%
Pain 'Always' Well Controlled	300+	77%	72%	71%
Room and Bathroom 'Always' Clean	300+	70%	71%	73%
Timely Help 'Always' Received	300+	74%	68%	68%
Would Definitely Recommend Hospital	300+	75%	70%	71%
Use of Medical Imaging				
Cardiac Imaging Stress Test before Surgery	590	6.9%	6.5%	5.3%
Combination Abdominal CT Scan	1,598	12.4%	16.5%	10.5%
Combination Brain/Sinus CT Scan	1,448	4.1%	3.5%	2.7%
Combination Chest CT Scan	743	9.7%	4.2%	2.7%
Follow-up Mammogram/Ultrasound	2,262	3.4%	7.6%	8.8%
Lumbar Spine MRI for Low Back Pain	490	43.5%	40.2%	37.2%

D W Mcmillan Memorial Hospital

1301 Belleville Avenue Phone: 251-867-8061
Brewton, AL 36426 Fax: 251-809-8486
URL: www.dwmmh.org
Type: Acute Care Hospitals Emergency Services: Yes
Ownership: Govt - Hospital Dist/Auth Beds: 91

Key Personnel:
CEO/President . . . . Chris Griffin
Quality Assurance . . . . Cindy Lancaster
Surgery . . . . Craig A Peterson

Measure	Cases	This Hosp.	State Avg.	U.S. Avg.
Blood Clot Prevention and Treatment				
Anticoagulation Overlap Therapy[2]	14	86%	91%	93%
ICU Venous Thromboembolism Prophylaxis[2]	83	76%	85%	92%
Incidence of Potentially Preventable VTE[1,2]	-	-	18%	10%
UFH with Dosages/Platelet Monitoring[1,2]	-	-	95%	97%
Venous Thromboembolism Prophylaxis[2]	201	63%	74%	85%
Warfarin Therapy Discharge Instructions[2]	11	100%	77%	75%
Chest Pain/Possible Heart Attack Care				
Aspirin Given Within 24 Hours of Arrival	59	97%	96%	96%
Fibrinolytic Meds Within 30 Min. of Arrival[1]	-	-	57%	58%
Average Time to ECG (minutes)	60	8	6	7
Average Time to Transfer (minutes)[1]	-	-	61	60
Children's Asthma Care				
Received Home Management Plan of Care	-	-	-	88%
Received Reliever Medication	-	-	-	100%
Received Systemic Corticosteroids	-	-	-	100%
Emergency Department				
Admittance Decision Time (minutes)[2]	311	60	73	98
Head CT Results Within 45 Min. of Arrival[1,3]	-	-	45%	57%
Patients Who Left ER Before Being Seen	13,995	2%	3%	2%
Time from ER Arrival to Admit. (minutes)[2]	331	178	240	274
Time from ER Arrival to Discharge (minutes)	559	101	126	134
Time in ER Before Being Evaluated (minutes)	392	28	31	26
Time to Pain Meds for Fractures (minutes)	51	65	69	57
Heart Attack Care				
Aspirin Given at Discharge[1]	-	-	99%	99%
Fibrinolytic Meds Within 30 Min. of Arrival[7]	-	-	77%	54%
PCI Within 90 Minutes of Arrival[7]	-	-	97%	96%
Statin Prescribed at Discharge[1]	-	-	98%	98%
Heart Failure Care				
ACE Inhibitor or ARB for LVSD	16	100%	97%	97%
Discharge Instructions Given	46	91%	93%	94%
Evaluation of LVS Function	51	100%	99%	99%
Medicare Spending				
Medicare Spending per Patient (ratio)	-	0.98	0.98	0.98
Pneumonia Care				
Appropriate Initial Antibiotic Given	58	91%	95%	95%
Blood Culture Timing	30	97%	98%	98%
Pregnancy and Delivery Care				
Newborn Deliveries Scheduled Early	25	8%	14%	6%
Preventive Care				
Immunization for Influenza[2]	323	93%	90%	90%
Immunization for Pneumonia[2]	344	97%	91%	92%
Stroke Care				
Anticoagulation Therapy for Atrial Fibrillation[1]	-	-	92%	95%
Antithrombotic Therapy Timing[1]	-	-	96%	98%
Assessed for Rehabilitation[1]	-	-	95%	97%
Discharged on Antithrombotic Therapy[1]	-	-	98%	99%
Discharged on Statin Medication[1]	-	-	90%	94%
Thrombolytic Therapy Timing[7]	-	-	38%	66%
Venous Thromboembolism Prophylaxis[1]	-	-	89%	94%
Written Stroke Educational Materials Given[1]	-	-	85%	88%
Surgical Care Improvement Project				
Appropriate Beta Blocker Usage	22	91%	98%	98%
Appropriate VTP Within 24 Hours	51	100%	98%	98%
Controlled Postoperative Blood Glucose[7]	-	-	97%	97%
Perioperative Temperature Management	106	100%	100%	100%
Prophylactic Antibiotic Selection	66	100%	99%	99%
Prophylactic Antibiotic Selection (Outpatient)[1]	-	-	98%	98%
Prophylactic Antibiotic Stopped	65	98%	98%	98%
Prophylactic Antibiotic Timing	67	97%	99%	99%
Prophylactic Antibiotic Timing (Outpatient)[1]	-	-	99%	98%
Urinary Catheter Removal	17	94%	98%	97%
Survey of Patients' Hospital Experiences				
Area Around Room 'Always' Quiet at Night	(a)	70%	71%	61%
Doctors 'Always' Communicated Well	(a)	87%	86%	82%
Home Recovery Information Given	(a)	83%	84%	85%
Hospital Given 9 or 10 on 10 Point Scale	(a)	74%	71%	71%
Meds 'Always' Explained Before Given	(a)	73%	66%	64%
Nurses 'Always' Communicated Well	(a)	81%	80%	79%
Pain 'Always' Well Controlled	(a)	71%	72%	71%
Room and Bathroom 'Always' Clean	(a)	72%	71%	73%
Timely Help 'Always' Received	(a)	73%	68%	68%
Would Definitely Recommend Hospital	(a)	67%	70%	71%
Use of Medical Imaging				
Cardiac Imaging Stress Test before Surgery	124	4.0%	6.5%	5.3%
Combination Abdominal CT Scan	216	27.3%	16.5%	10.5%
Combination Brain/Sinus CT Scan[1]	-	-	3.5%	2.7%
Combination Chest CT Scan	244	4.5%	4.2%	2.7%
Follow-up Mammogram/Ultrasound	491	11.6%	7.6%	8.8%
Lumbar Spine MRI for Low Back Pain	94	35.1%	40.2%	37.2%

Choctaw General Hospital

401 Vanity Fair Lane, PO Box 618 Phone: 205-459-9100
Butler, AL 36904
Type: Critical Access Hospitals Emergency Services: Yes
Ownership: Voluntary non-profit - Private

Measure	Cases	This Hosp.	State Avg.	U.S. Avg.
Blood Clot Prevention and Treatment				
Anticoagulation Overlap Therapy[5]	-	-	91%	93%
ICU Venous Thromboembolism Prophylaxis[5]	-	-	85%	92%
Incidence of Potentially Preventable VTE[5]	-	-	18%	10%
UFH with Dosages/Platelet Monitoring[5]	-	-	95%	97%
Venous Thromboembolism Prophylaxis[5]	-	-	74%	85%
Warfarin Therapy Discharge Instructions[5]	-	-	77%	75%
Chest Pain/Possible Heart Attack Care				
Aspirin Given Within 24 Hours of Arrival	11	91%	96%	96%
Fibrinolytic Meds Within 30 Min. of Arrival[7]	-	-	57%	58%
Average Time to ECG (minutes)	11	4	6	7
Average Time to Transfer (minutes)[1]	-	-	61	60
Children's Asthma Care				
Received Home Management Plan of Care	-	-	-	88%
Received Reliever Medication	-	-	-	100%
Received Systemic Corticosteroids	-	-	-	100%
Emergency Department				
Admittance Decision Time (minutes)[5]	-	-	73	98
Head CT Results Within 45 Min. of Arrival[5]	-	-	45%	57%
Patients Who Left ER Before Being Seen	5,445	0%	3%	2%
Time from ER Arrival to Admit. (minutes)[5]	-	-	240	274
Time from ER Arrival to Discharge (minutes)[5]	-	-	126	134
Time in ER Before Being Evaluated (minutes)[5]	-	-	31	26
Time to Pain Meds for Fractures (minutes)[5]	-	-	69	57
Heart Attack Care				
Aspirin Given at Discharge[5]	-	-	99%	99%
Fibrinolytic Meds Within 30 Min. of Arrival[5]	-	-	77%	54%
PCI Within 90 Minutes of Arrival[5]	-	-	97%	96%
Statin Prescribed at Discharge[5]	-	-	98%	98%
Heart Failure Care				
ACE Inhibitor or ARB for LVSD[1,2]	-	-	97%	97%
Discharge Instructions Given[2]	15	93%	93%	94%
Evaluation of LVS Function[2]	16	38%	99%	99%
Medicare Spending				
Medicare Spending per Patient (ratio)	-	-	0.98	0.98
Pneumonia Care				
Appropriate Initial Antibiotic Given[2]	14	86%	95%	95%
Blood Culture Timing[2]	15	100%	98%	98%
Pregnancy and Delivery Care				
Newborn Deliveries Scheduled Early[5]	-	-	14%	6%
Preventive Care				
Immunization for Influenza[5]	-	-	90%	90%
Immunization for Pneumonia[5]	-	-	91%	92%
Stroke Care				
Anticoagulation Therapy for Atrial Fibrillation[5]	-	-	92%	95%
Antithrombotic Therapy Timing[5]	-	-	96%	98%

NOTE: Hospital profiles are in alphabetical order by state, then city, then hospital within the city; Rankings exclude hospitals with less than 25 cases except for patient surveys which excludes hospitals with less than 100 cases; (a) 100-299 cases; (1) The number of cases/patients is too few to report; (2) Data submitted were based on a sample of cases/patients; (3) Results are based on a shorter time period than required; (4) Data suppressed by CMS for one or more quarters; (5) Results are not available for this reporting period; (6) Fewer than 100 patients completed the HCAHPS survey; (7) No cases met the criteria for this measure; (8) The lower limit of the confidence interval cannot be calculated if the number of observed infections equals zero; (9) No data are available from the state/territory for this reporting period; (10) The scores shown reflect fewer than 50 completed surveys; (11) There were discrepancies in the data collection process; (12) This measure does not apply to this hospital for this reporting period; (13) Results cannot be calculated for this reporting period; (14) The results for this state are combined with nearby states to protect confidentiality; Please refer to the User's Guide for a full explanation of data.

Assessed for Rehabilitation[5]	-	-	95%	97%
Discharged on Antithrombotic Therapy[5]	-	-	98%	99%
Discharged on Statin Medication[5]	-	-	90%	94%
Thrombolytic Therapy Timing[5]	-	-	38%	66%
Venous Thromboembolism Prophylaxis[5]	-	-	89%	94%
Written Stroke Educational Materials Given[5]	-	-	85%	88%
Surgical Care Improvement Project				
Appropriate Beta Blocker Usage[5]	-	-	98%	98%
Appropriate VTP Within 24 Hours[5]	-	-	98%	98%
Controlled Postoperative Blood Glucose[5]	-	-	97%	97%
Perioperative Temperature Management[5]	-	-	100%	100%
Prophylactic Antibiotic Selection[5]	-	-	99%	99%
Prophylactic Antibiotic Selection (Outpatient)[5]	-	-	98%	98%
Prophylactic Antibiotic Stopped[5]	-	-	98%	98%
Prophylactic Antibiotic Timing[5]	-	-	99%	99%
Prophylactic Antibiotic Timing (Outpatient)[5]	-	-	99%	98%
Urinary Catheter Removal[5]	-	-	98%	97%
Survey of Patients' Hospital Experiences				
Area Around Room 'Always' Quiet at Night[10]	<100	84%	71%	61%
Doctors 'Always' Communicated Well[10]	<100	90%	86%	82%
Home Recovery Information Given[10]	<100	83%	84%	85%
Hospital Given 9 or 10 on 10 Point Scale[10]	<100	85%	71%	71%
Meds 'Always' Explained Before Given[10]	<100	95%	66%	64%
Nurses 'Always' Communicated Well[10]	<100	92%	80%	79%
Pain 'Always' Well Controlled[10]	<100	75%	72%	71%
Room and Bathroom 'Always' Clean[10]	<100	84%	71%	73%
Timely Help 'Always' Received[10]	<100	88%	68%	68%
Would Definitely Recommend Hospital[10]	<100	86%	70%	71%
Use of Medical Imaging				
Cardiac Imaging Stress Test before Surgery[7]	-	-	6.5%	5.3%
Combination Abdominal CT Scan	106	2.8%	16.5%	10.5%
Combination Brain/Sinus CT Scan[1]	-	-	3.5%	2.7%
Combination Chest CT Scan	57	0.0%	4.2%	2.7%
Follow-up Mammogram/Ultrasound[7]	-	-	7.6%	8.8%
Lumbar Spine MRI for Low Back Pain[1]	-	-	40.2%	37.2%

J Paul Jones Hospital

317 Mcwilliams Avenue
Camden, AL 36726
Phone: 334-682-4131
Fax: 334-682-4131
Type: Acute Care Hospitals
Emergency Services: No
Ownership: Govt - Hospital Dist/Auth
Beds: 32

Key Personnel:
CEO/President. . . . . Libby Kennedy
Infection Control. . . . . Gladys Luker, RN
Emergency Room . . . . Sheila Roe, RN
Quality Assurance . . . . Shirley Short, RN
Chief of Medical Staff. . . . . Willie White, MD

Measure	Cases	This Hosp.	State Avg.	U.S. Avg.
Blood Clot Prevention and Treatment				
Anticoagulation Overlap Therapy[1,2]	-	-	91%	93%
ICU Venous Thromboembolism Prophylaxis[2,7]	-	-	85%	92%
Incidence of Potentially Preventable VTE[2,7]	-	-	18%	10%
UFH with Dosages/Platelet Monitoring[2,7]	-	-	95%	97%
Venous Thromboembolism Prophylaxis[2]	114	11%	74%	85%
Warfarin Therapy Discharge Instructions[1,2]	-	-	77%	75%
Chest Pain/Possible Heart Attack Care				
Aspirin Given Within 24 Hours of Arrival[5]	-	-	96%	96%
Fibrinolytic Meds Within 30 Min. of Arrival[5]	-	-	57%	58%
Average Time to ECG (minutes)[5]	-	-	6	7
Average Time to Transfer (minutes)[5]	-	-	61	60
Children's Asthma Care				
Received Home Management Plan of Care	-	-	-	88%
Received Reliever Medication	-	-	-	100%
Received Systemic Corticosteroids	-	-	-	100%
Emergency Department				
Admittance Decision Time (minutes)	19	0	73	98
Head CT Results Within 45 Min. of Arrival[3,7]	-	-	45%	57%
Patients Who Left ER Before Being Seen	5,276	1%	3%	2%
Time from ER Arrival to Admit. (minutes)	106	178	240	274
Time from ER Arrival to Discharge (minutes)	319	106	126	134
Time in ER Before Being Evaluated (minutes)	211	31	31	26
Time to Pain Meds for Fractures (minutes)[3]	18	64	69	57
Heart Attack Care				
Aspirin Given at Discharge[5]	-	-	99%	99%
Fibrinolytic Meds Within 30 Min. of Arrival[5]	-	-	77%	54%
PCI Within 90 Minutes of Arrival[5]	-	-	97%	96%
Statin Prescribed at Discharge[5]	-	-	98%	98%
Heart Failure Care				
ACE Inhibitor or ARB for LVSD[5]	-	-	97%	97%
Discharge Instructions Given[5]	-	-	93%	94%
Evaluation of LVS Function[5]	-	-	99%	99%
Medicare Spending				
Medicare Spending per Patient (ratio)	-	1.19	0.98	0.98
Pneumonia Care				
Appropriate Initial Antibiotic Given[1,3]	-	-	95%	95%
Blood Culture Timing[1,3]	-	-	98%	98%
Pregnancy and Delivery Care				
Newborn Deliveries Scheduled Early[7]	-	-	14%	6%
Preventive Care				
Immunization for Influenza	127	0%	90%	90%
Immunization for Pneumonia[2]	159	1%	91%	92%
Stroke Care				
Anticoagulation Therapy for Atrial Fibrillation[5]	-	-	92%	95%
Antithrombotic Therapy Timing[5]	-	-	96%	98%
Assessed for Rehabilitation[5]	-	-	95%	97%
Discharged on Antithrombotic Therapy[5]	-	-	98%	99%
Discharged on Statin Medication[5]	-	-	90%	94%
Thrombolytic Therapy Timing[5]	-	-	38%	66%
Venous Thromboembolism Prophylaxis[5]	-	-	89%	94%
Written Stroke Educational Materials Given[5]	-	-	85%	88%
Surgical Care Improvement Project				
Appropriate Beta Blocker Usage[5]	-	-	98%	98%
Appropriate VTP Within 24 Hours[5]	-	-	98%	98%
Controlled Postoperative Blood Glucose[5]	-	-	97%	97%
Perioperative Temperature Management[5]	-	-	100%	100%
Prophylactic Antibiotic Selection[5]	-	-	99%	99%
Prophylactic Antibiotic Selection (Outpatient)[5]	-	-	98%	98%
Prophylactic Antibiotic Stopped[5]	-	-	98%	98%
Prophylactic Antibiotic Timing[5]	-	-	99%	99%
Prophylactic Antibiotic Timing (Outpatient)[5]	-	-	99%	98%
Urinary Catheter Removal[5]	-	-	98%	97%
Survey of Patients' Hospital Experiences				
Area Around Room 'Always' Quiet at Night[10]	<100	86%	71%	61%
Doctors 'Always' Communicated Well[10]	<100	86%	86%	82%
Home Recovery Information Given[10]	<100	91%	84%	85%
Hospital Given 9 or 10 on 10 Point Scale[10]	<100	73%	71%	71%
Meds 'Always' Explained Before Given[10]	<100	60%	66%	64%
Nurses 'Always' Communicated Well[10]	<100	83%	80%	79%
Pain 'Always' Well Controlled[10]	<100	69%	72%	71%
Room and Bathroom 'Always' Clean[10]	<100	71%	71%	73%
Timely Help 'Always' Received[10]	<100	78%	68%	68%
Would Definitely Recommend Hospital[10]	<100	70%	70%	71%
Use of Medical Imaging				
Cardiac Imaging Stress Test before Surgery[7]	-	-	6.5%	5.3%
Combination Abdominal CT Scan	89	22.5%	16.5%	10.5%
Combination Brain/Sinus CT Scan[1]	-	-	3.5%	2.7%
Combination Chest CT Scan[1]	-	-	4.2%	2.7%
Follow-up Mammogram/Ultrasound	83	8.4%	7.6%	8.8%
Lumbar Spine MRI for Low Back Pain[7]	-	-	40.2%	37.2%

Pickens County Medical Center

241 Robert K Wilson Drive
Carrollton, AL 35447
Phone: 205-367-8111
Fax: 205-367-2121
URL: www.dchsystem.com
Type: Acute Care Hospitals
Emergency Services: Yes
Ownership: Govt - Hospital Dist/Auth
Beds: 56

Key Personnel:
Emergency Room . . . . Malika Aryanpure, MD
Radiology. . . . . James Bankston
Operating Room. . . . . Bradley Bilton, RN
Anesthesiology. . . . . Arthur Cheung, CRNA
Quality Assurance . . . . Debbie Elmore, RN
CEO/President. . . . . Wayne McElroy
Chief of Medical Staff. . . . . James L Parker, MD

Measure	Cases	This Hosp.	State Avg.	U.S. Avg.
Blood Clot Prevention and Treatment				
Anticoagulation Overlap Therapy[1,2]	-	-	91%	93%
ICU Venous Thromboembolism Prophylaxis[2]	11	82%	85%	92%
Incidence of Potentially Preventable VTE[1,2]	-	-	18%	10%
UFH with Dosages/Platelet Monitoring[2,7]	-	-	95%	97%
Venous Thromboembolism Prophylaxis[2]	100	64%	74%	85%
Warfarin Therapy Discharge Instructions[1,2]	-	-	77%	75%
Chest Pain/Possible Heart Attack Care				
Aspirin Given Within 24 Hours of Arrival[1,3]	-	-	96%	96%
Fibrinolytic Meds Within 30 Min. of Arrival[3,7]	-	-	57%	58%
Average Time to ECG (minutes)[1,3]	-	-	6	7
Average Time to Transfer (minutes)[3,7]	-	-	61	60
Children's Asthma Care				
Received Home Management Plan of Care	-	-	-	88%
Received Reliever Medication	-	-	-	100%
Received Systemic Corticosteroids	-	-	-	100%
Emergency Department				
Admittance Decision Time (minutes)[2]	343	80	73	98
Head CT Results Within 45 Min. of Arrival[1,3]	-	-	45%	57%
Patients Who Left ER Before Being Seen	11,696	1%	3%	2%
Time from ER Arrival to Admit. (minutes)[2]	347	242	240	274
Time from ER Arrival to Discharge (minutes)	357	124	126	134
Time in ER Before Being Evaluated (minutes)	366	48	31	26
Time to Pain Meds for Fractures (minutes)	26	104	69	57
Heart Attack Care				
Aspirin Given at Discharge[1,2]	-	-	99%	99%
Fibrinolytic Meds Within 30 Min. of Arrival[2,3]	-	-	77%	54%
PCI Within 90 Minutes of Arrival[2,3]	-	-	97%	96%
Statin Prescribed at Discharge[1,2]	-	-	98%	98%
Heart Failure Care				
ACE Inhibitor or ARB for LVSD[1,2]	-	-	97%	97%
Discharge Instructions Given[2]	19	89%	93%	94%
Evaluation of LVS Function[2]	29	100%	99%	99%
Medicare Spending				
Medicare Spending per Patient (ratio)	-	0.95	0.98	0.98
Pneumonia Care				
Appropriate Initial Antibiotic Given[2]	39	100%	95%	95%
Blood Culture Timing[2]	44	98%	98%	98%
Pregnancy and Delivery Care				
Newborn Deliveries Scheduled Early[7]	-	-	14%	6%
Preventive Care				
Immunization for Influenza[2]	284	98%	90%	90%
Immunization for Pneumonia[2]	424	96%	91%	92%
Stroke Care				
Anticoagulation Therapy for Atrial Fibrillation[1]	-	-	92%	95%
Antithrombotic Therapy Timing[1]	-	-	96%	98%
Assessed for Rehabilitation[1]	-	-	95%	97%
Discharged on Antithrombotic Therapy[1]	-	-	98%	99%
Discharged on Statin Medication[1]	-	-	90%	94%
Thrombolytic Therapy Timing[1]	-	-	38%	66%
Venous Thromboembolism Prophylaxis[1]	-	-	89%	94%
Written Stroke Educational Materials Given[1]	-	-	85%	88%
Surgical Care Improvement Project				
Appropriate Beta Blocker Usage[1,3]	-	-	98%	98%
Appropriate VTP Within 24 Hours[1,3]	-	-	98%	98%
Controlled Postoperative Blood Glucose[3,7]	-	-	97%	97%
Perioperative Temperature Management[1,3]	-	-	100%	100%
Prophylactic Antibiotic Selection[1,3]	-	-	99%	99%
Prophylactic Antibiotic Selection (Outpatient)[5]	-	-	98%	98%
Prophylactic Antibiotic Stopped[1,3]	-	-	98%	98%
Prophylactic Antibiotic Timing[1,3]	-	-	99%	99%
Prophylactic Antibiotic Timing (Outpatient)[5]	-	-	99%	98%
Urinary Catheter Removal[1,3]	-	-	98%	97%
Survey of Patients' Hospital Experiences				
Area Around Room 'Always' Quiet at Night[6]	<100	73%	71%	61%
Doctors 'Always' Communicated Well[6]	<100	96%	86%	82%
Home Recovery Information Given[6]	<100	85%	84%	85%
Hospital Given 9 or 10 on 10 Point Scale[6]	<100	76%	71%	71%
Meds 'Always' Explained Before Given[6]	<100	69%	66%	64%
Nurses 'Always' Communicated Well[6]	<100	83%	80%	79%
Pain 'Always' Well Controlled[6]	<100	75%	72%	71%
Room and Bathroom 'Always' Clean[6]	<100	83%	71%	73%
Timely Help 'Always' Received[6]	<100	73%	68%	68%
Would Definitely Recommend Hospital[6]	<100	69%	70%	71%

NOTE: Hospital profiles are in alphabetical order by state, then city, then hospital within the city; Rankings exclude hospitals with less than 25 cases except for patient surveys which excludes hospitals with less than 100 cases; (a) 100-299 cases; (1) The number of cases/patients is too few to report; (2) Data submitted were based on a sample of cases/patients; (3) Results are based on a shorter time period than required; (4) Data suppressed by CMS for one or more quarters; (5) Results are not available for this reporting period; (6) Fewer than 100 patients completed the HCAHPS survey; (7) No cases met the criteria for this measure; (8) The lower limit of the confidence interval cannot be calculated if the number of observed infections equals zero; (9) No data are available from the state/territory for this reporting period; (10) The scores shown reflect fewer than 50 completed surveys; (11) There were discrepancies in the data collection process; (12) This measure does not apply to this hospital for this reporting period; (13) Results cannot be calculated for this reporting period; (14) The results for this state are combined with nearby states to protect confidentiality; Please refer to the User's Guide for a full explanation of data.

Measure	Cases	This Hosp.	State Avg.	U.S. Avg.
Use of Medical Imaging				
Cardiac Imaging Stress Test before Surgery[7]	-	-	6.5%	5.3%
Combination Abdominal CT Scan	204	3.4%	16.5%	10.5%
Combination Brain/Sinus CT Scan[1]	-	-	3.5%	2.7%
Combination Chest CT Scan	91	0.0%	4.2%	2.7%
Follow-up Mammogram/Ultrasound	331	11.8%	7.6%	8.8%
Lumbar Spine MRI for Low Back Pain[1]	-	-	40.2%	37.2%

Cherokee Medical Center

400 Northwood Dr
Centre, AL 35960
Phone: 256-927-5531
Fax: 256-927-1304
URL: www.cherokeemedicalcenter.com
Type: Acute Care Hospitals
Emergency Services: Yes
Ownership: Voluntary non-profit - Private
Beds: 60

Key Personnel:

Radiology. . . . . Teresa Chandler
Operating Room. . . . . Robert Heuermann
Chief of Medical Staff . . . . Thomas Leach
CEO/President. . . . . Jeff Noblin
Quality Assurance . . . . Kay Penland
Emergency Room . . . . Becky Smith, RN

Measure	Cases	This Hosp.	State Avg.	U.S. Avg.
Blood Clot Prevention and Treatment				
Anticoagulation Overlap Therapy[1,2]	-	-	91%	93%
ICU Venous Thromboembolism Prophylaxis[2,7]	-	-	85%	92%
Incidence of Potentially Preventable VTE[1,2]	-	-	18%	10%
UFH with Dosages/Platelet Monitoring[2,7]	-	-	95%	97%
Venous Thromboembolism Prophylaxis[2]	315	88%	74%	85%
Warfarin Therapy Discharge Instructions[1,2]	-	-	77%	75%
Chest Pain/Possible Heart Attack Care				
Aspirin Given Within 24 Hours of Arrival	40	100%	96%	96%
Fibrinolytic Meds Within 30 Min. of Arrival[1]	-	-	57%	58%
Average Time to ECG (minutes)	41	6	6	7
Average Time to Transfer (minutes)[7]	-	-	61	60
Children's Asthma Care				
Received Home Management Plan of Care	-	-	-	88%
Received Reliever Medication	-	-	-	100%
Received Systemic Corticosteroids	-	-	-	100%
Emergency Department				
Admittance Decision Time (minutes)[2]	402	69	73	98
Head CT Results Within 45 Min. of Arrival[1,3]	-	-	45%	57%
Patients Who Left ER Before Being Seen	8,842	1%	3%	2%
Time from ER Arrival to Admit. (minutes)[2]	407	208	240	274
Time from ER Arrival to Discharge (minutes)	384	79	126	134
Time in ER Before Being Evaluated (minutes)	421	12	31	26
Time to Pain Meds for Fractures (minutes)	41	52	69	57
Heart Attack Care				
Aspirin Given at Discharge[3,7]	-	-	99%	99%
Fibrinolytic Meds Within 30 Min. of Arrival[3,7]	-	-	77%	54%
PCI Within 90 Minutes of Arrival[3,7]	-	-	97%	96%
Statin Prescribed at Discharge[3,7]	-	-	98%	98%
Heart Failure Care				
ACE Inhibitor or ARB for LVSD[1]	-	-	97%	97%
Discharge Instructions Given	12	92%	93%	94%
Evaluation of LVS Function	18	94%	99%	99%
Medicare Spending				
Medicare Spending per Patient (ratio)	-	0.95	0.98	0.98
Pneumonia Care				
Appropriate Initial Antibiotic Given	27	96%	95%	95%
Blood Culture Timing	35	100%	98%	98%
Pregnancy and Delivery Care				
Newborn Deliveries Scheduled Early[2,7]	-	-	14%	6%
Preventive Care				
Immunization for Influenza[2]	301	94%	90%	90%
Immunization for Pneumonia[2]	430	98%	91%	92%
Stroke Care				
Anticoagulation Therapy for Atrial Fibrillation[1,3]	-	-	92%	95%
Antithrombotic Therapy Timing[1,3]	-	-	96%	98%
Assessed for Rehabilitation[1,3]	-	-	95%	97%
Discharged on Antithrombotic Therapy[1,3]	-	-	98%	99%
Discharged on Statin Medication[1,3]	-	-	90%	94%
Thrombolytic Therapy Timing[3,7]	-	-	38%	66%
Venous Thromboembolism Prophylaxis[1,3]	-	-	89%	94%
Written Stroke Educational Materials Given[1,3]	-	-	85%	88%
Surgical Care Improvement Project				
Appropriate Beta Blocker Usage[5]	-	-	98%	98%
Appropriate VTP Within 24 Hours[5]	-	-	98%	98%
Controlled Postoperative Blood Glucose[5]	-	-	97%	97%
Perioperative Temperature Management[5]	-	-	100%	100%
Prophylactic Antibiotic Selection[5]	-	-	99%	99%
Prophylactic Antibiotic Selection (Outpatient)[1,3]	-	-	98%	98%
Prophylactic Antibiotic Stopped[5]	-	-	98%	98%
Prophylactic Antibiotic Timing[5]	-	-	99%	99%
Prophylactic Antibiotic Timing (Outpatient)[1,3]	-	-	99%	98%
Urinary Catheter Removal[5]	-	-	98%	97%
Survey of Patients' Hospital Experiences				
Area Around Room 'Always' Quiet at Night	(a)	77%	71%	61%
Doctors 'Always' Communicated Well	(a)	91%	86%	82%
Home Recovery Information Given	(a)	91%	84%	85%
Hospital Given 9 or 10 on 10 Point Scale	(a)	77%	71%	71%
Meds 'Always' Explained Before Given	(a)	72%	66%	64%
Nurses 'Always' Communicated Well	(a)	87%	80%	79%
Pain 'Always' Well Controlled	(a)	73%	72%	71%
Room and Bathroom 'Always' Clean	(a)	76%	71%	73%
Timely Help 'Always' Received	(a)	78%	68%	68%
Would Definitely Recommend Hospital	(a)	77%	70%	71%
Use of Medical Imaging				
Cardiac Imaging Stress Test before Surgery[7]	-	-	6.5%	5.3%
Combination Abdominal CT Scan	201	2.0%	16.5%	10.5%
Combination Brain/Sinus CT Scan[1]	-	-	3.5%	2.7%
Combination Chest CT Scan	83	6.0%	4.2%	2.7%
Follow-up Mammogram/Ultrasound	234	3.4%	7.6%	8.8%
Lumbar Spine MRI for Low Back Pain[1]	-	-	40.2%	37.2%

Bibb Medical Center

208 Pierson Ave
Centreville, AL 35042
Phone: 205-926-4881
Type: Acute Care Hospitals
Emergency Services: Yes
Ownership: Govt - Hospital Dist/Auth

Key Personnel:

Radiology. . . . . Laura McRae
CEO/President. . . . . Terry J Smith

Measure	Cases	This Hosp.	State Avg.	U.S. Avg.
Blood Clot Prevention and Treatment				
Anticoagulation Overlap Therapy[1,2]	-	-	91%	93%
ICU Venous Thromboembolism Prophylaxis[2,7]	-	-	85%	92%
Incidence of Potentially Preventable VTE[1,2]	-	-	18%	10%
UFH with Dosages/Platelet Monitoring[2,7]	-	-	95%	97%
Venous Thromboembolism Prophylaxis[2]	144	44%	74%	85%
Warfarin Therapy Discharge Instructions[1,2]	-	-	77%	75%
Chest Pain/Possible Heart Attack Care				
Aspirin Given Within 24 Hours of Arrival[3]	12	92%	96%	96%
Fibrinolytic Meds Within 30 Min. of Arrival[3,7]	-	-	57%	58%
Average Time to ECG (minutes)[3]	11	5	6	7
Average Time to Transfer (minutes)[1,3]	-	-	61	60
Children's Asthma Care				
Received Home Management Plan of Care	-	-	-	88%
Received Reliever Medication	-	-	-	100%
Received Systemic Corticosteroids	-	-	-	100%
Emergency Department				
Admittance Decision Time (minutes)[2]	64	54	73	98
Head CT Results Within 45 Min. of Arrival[5]	-	-	45%	57%
Patients Who Left ER Before Being Seen	18,244	1%	3%	2%
Time from ER Arrival to Admit. (minutes)[2]	64	192	240	274
Time from ER Arrival to Discharge (minutes)	311	93	126	134
Time in ER Before Being Evaluated (minutes)	387	21	31	26
Time to Pain Meds for Fractures (minutes)	30	90	69	57
Heart Attack Care				
Aspirin Given at Discharge[5]	-	-	99%	99%
Fibrinolytic Meds Within 30 Min. of Arrival[5]	-	-	77%	54%
PCI Within 90 Minutes of Arrival[5]	-	-	97%	96%
Statin Prescribed at Discharge[5]	-	-	98%	98%
Heart Failure Care				
ACE Inhibitor or ARB for LVSD[5]	-	-	97%	97%
Discharge Instructions Given[5]	-	-	93%	94%
Evaluation of LVS Function[5]	-	-	99%	99%
Medicare Spending				
Medicare Spending per Patient (ratio)	-	0.97	0.98	0.98
Pneumonia Care				
Appropriate Initial Antibiotic Given	13	92%	95%	95%
Blood Culture Timing	31	94%	98%	98%
Pregnancy and Delivery Care				
Newborn Deliveries Scheduled Early[7]	-	-	14%	6%
Preventive Care				
Immunization for Influenza[2]	90	96%	90%	90%
Immunization for Pneumonia[2]	154	82%	91%	92%
Stroke Care				
Anticoagulation Therapy for Atrial Fibrillation[3,7]	-	-	92%	95%
Antithrombotic Therapy Timing[1,3]	-	-	96%	98%
Assessed for Rehabilitation[1,3]	-	-	95%	97%
Discharged on Antithrombotic Therapy[1,3]	-	-	98%	99%
Discharged on Statin Medication[1,3]	-	-	90%	94%
Thrombolytic Therapy Timing[3,7]	-	-	38%	66%
Venous Thromboembolism Prophylaxis[1,3]	-	-	89%	94%
Written Stroke Educational Materials Given[3,7]	-	-	85%	88%
Surgical Care Improvement Project				
Appropriate Beta Blocker Usage[5]	-	-	98%	98%
Appropriate VTP Within 24 Hours[5]	-	-	98%	98%
Controlled Postoperative Blood Glucose[5]	-	-	97%	97%
Perioperative Temperature Management[5]	-	-	100%	100%
Prophylactic Antibiotic Selection[5]	-	-	99%	99%
Prophylactic Antibiotic Selection (Outpatient)[5]	-	-	98%	98%
Prophylactic Antibiotic Stopped[5]	-	-	98%	98%
Prophylactic Antibiotic Timing[5]	-	-	99%	99%
Prophylactic Antibiotic Timing (Outpatient)[5]	-	-	99%	98%
Urinary Catheter Removal[5]	-	-	98%	97%
Survey of Patients' Hospital Experiences				
Area Around Room 'Always' Quiet at Night[10]	<100	58%	71%	61%
Doctors 'Always' Communicated Well[10]	<100	78%	86%	82%
Home Recovery Information Given[10]	<100	94%	84%	85%
Hospital Given 9 or 10 on 10 Point Scale[10]	<100	71%	71%	71%
Meds 'Always' Explained Before Given[10]	<100	84%	66%	64%
Nurses 'Always' Communicated Well[10]	<100	81%	80%	79%
Pain 'Always' Well Controlled[10]	<100	65%	72%	71%
Room and Bathroom 'Always' Clean[10]	<100	75%	71%	73%
Timely Help 'Always' Received[10]	<100	48%	68%	68%
Would Definitely Recommend Hospital[10]	<100	70%	70%	71%
Use of Medical Imaging				
Cardiac Imaging Stress Test before Surgery[7]	-	-	6.5%	5.3%
Combination Abdominal CT Scan	72	9.7%	16.5%	10.5%
Combination Brain/Sinus CT Scan[1]	-	-	3.5%	2.7%
Combination Chest CT Scan[1]	-	-	4.2%	2.7%
Follow-up Mammogram/Ultrasound	103	11.7%	7.6%	8.8%
Lumbar Spine MRI for Low Back Pain[7]	-	-	40.2%	37.2%

Washington County Hospital

14600 Saint Stephens Avenue
Chatom, AL 36518
Phone: 251-847-2223
Fax: 251-847-3808
URL: www.wchnh.org
Type: Critical Access Hospitals
Emergency Services: Yes
Ownership: Voluntary non-profit - Other
Beds: 25

Key Personnel:

Chief of Medical Staff . . . . James Hassell
Quality Assurance . . . . Rebecca Johnson
CEO/President. . . . . Douglas Tanner
Infection Control. . . . . Valerie Waddell

Measure	Cases	This Hosp.	State Avg.	U.S. Avg.
Blood Clot Prevention and Treatment				
Anticoagulation Overlap Therapy[2,7]	-	-	91%	93%
ICU Venous Thromboembolism Prophylaxis[2,7]	-	-	85%	92%
Incidence of Potentially Preventable VTE[2,7]	-	-	18%	10%
UFH with Dosages/Platelet Monitoring[2,7]	-	-	95%	97%
Venous Thromboembolism Prophylaxis[2]	111	69%	74%	85%
Warfarin Therapy Discharge Instructions[2,7]	-	-	77%	75%
Chest Pain/Possible Heart Attack Care				
Aspirin Given Within 24 Hours of Arrival	13	92%	96%	96%
Fibrinolytic Meds Within 30 Min. of Arrival[7]	-	-	57%	58%
Average Time to ECG (minutes)	11	8	6	7
Average Time to Transfer (minutes)[1]	-	-	61	60
Children's Asthma Care				

NOTE: Hospital profiles are in alphabetical order by state, then city, then hospital within the city; Rankings exclude hospitals with less than 25 cases except for patient surveys which excludes hospitals with less than 100 cases; (a) 100-299 cases; (1) The number of cases/patients is too few to report; (2) Data submitted were based on a sample of cases/patients; (3) Results are based on a shorter time period than required; (4) Data suppressed by CMS for one or more quarters; (5) Results are not available for this reporting period; (6) Fewer than 100 patients completed the HCAHPS survey; (7) No cases met the criteria for this measure; (8) The lower limit of the confidence interval cannot be calculated if the number of observed infections equals zero; (9) No data are available from the state/territory for this reporting period; (10) The scores shown reflect fewer than 50 completed surveys; (11) There were discrepancies in the data collection process; (12) This measure does not apply to this hospital for this reporting period; (13) Results cannot be calculated for this reporting period; (14) The results for this state are combined with nearby states to protect confidentiality; Please refer to the User's Guide for a full explanation of data.

Measure	Cases	This Hosp.	State Avg.	U.S. Avg.
Received Home Management Plan of Care	-	-	-	88%
Received Reliever Medication	-	-	-	100%
Received Systemic Corticosteroids	-	-	-	100%
Emergency Department				
Admittance Decision Time (minutes)[2]	56	23	73	98
Head CT Results Within 45 Min. of Arrival[1]	-	-	45%	57%
Patients Who Left ER Before Being Seen	3,653	0%	3%	2%
Time from ER Arrival to Admit. (minutes)[2]	84	170	240	274
Time from ER Arrival to Discharge (minutes)	384	100	126	134
Time in ER Before Being Evaluated (minutes)	408	16	31	26
Time to Pain Meds for Fractures (minutes)	20	56	69	57
Heart Attack Care				
Aspirin Given at Discharge[5]	-	-	99%	99%
Fibrinolytic Meds Within 30 Min. of Arrival[5]	-	-	77%	54%
PCI Within 90 Minutes of Arrival[5]	-	-	97%	96%
Statin Prescribed at Discharge[5]	-	-	98%	98%
Heart Failure Care				
ACE Inhibitor or ARB for LVSD[1]	-	-	97%	97%
Discharge Instructions Given[1]	-	-	93%	94%
Evaluation of LVS Function[1]	-	-	99%	99%
Medicare Spending				
Medicare Spending per Patient (ratio)	-	-	0.98	0.98
Pneumonia Care				
Appropriate Initial Antibiotic Given[1,3]	-	-	95%	95%
Blood Culture Timing[1,3]	-	-	98%	98%
Pregnancy and Delivery Care				
Newborn Deliveries Scheduled Early[7]	-	-	14%	6%
Preventive Care				
Immunization for Influenza[2]	99	57%	90%	90%
Immunization for Pneumonia[2]	147	69%	91%	92%
Stroke Care				
Anticoagulation Therapy for Atrial Fibrillation[5]	-	-	92%	95%
Antithrombotic Therapy Timing[5]	-	-	96%	98%
Assessed for Rehabilitation[5]	-	-	95%	97%
Discharged on Antithrombotic Therapy[5]	-	-	98%	99%
Discharged on Statin Medication[5]	-	-	90%	94%
Thrombolytic Therapy Timing[5]	-	-	38%	66%
Venous Thromboembolism Prophylaxis[5]	-	-	89%	94%
Written Stroke Educational Materials Given[5]	-	-	85%	88%
Surgical Care Improvement Project				
Appropriate Beta Blocker Usage[5]	-	-	98%	98%
Appropriate VTP Within 24 Hours[5]	-	-	98%	98%
Controlled Postoperative Blood Glucose[5]	-	-	97%	97%
Perioperative Temperature Management[5]	-	-	100%	100%
Prophylactic Antibiotic Selection[5]	-	-	99%	99%
Prophylactic Antibiotic Selection (Outpatient)[5]	-	-	98%	98%
Prophylactic Antibiotic Stopped[5]	-	-	98%	98%
Prophylactic Antibiotic Timing[5]	-	-	99%	99%
Prophylactic Antibiotic Timing (Outpatient)[5]	-	-	99%	98%
Urinary Catheter Removal[5]	-	-	98%	97%
Survey of Patients' Hospital Experiences				
Area Around Room 'Always' Quiet at Night[10]	<100	77%	71%	61%
Doctors 'Always' Communicated Well[10]	<100	91%	86%	82%
Home Recovery Information Given[10]	<100	81%	84%	85%
Hospital Given 9 or 10 on 10 Point Scale[10]	<100	84%	71%	71%
Meds 'Always' Explained Before Given[10]	<100	87%	66%	64%
Nurses 'Always' Communicated Well[10]	<100	88%	80%	79%
Pain 'Always' Well Controlled[10]	<100	88%	72%	71%
Room and Bathroom 'Always' Clean[10]	<100	77%	71%	73%
Timely Help 'Always' Received[10]	<100	89%	68%	68%
Would Definitely Recommend Hospital[10]	<100	82%	70%	71%
Use of Medical Imaging				
Cardiac Imaging Stress Test before Surgery[7]	-	-	6.5%	5.3%
Combination Abdominal CT Scan	68	19.1%	16.5%	10.5%
Combination Brain/Sinus CT Scan[1]	-	-	3.5%	2.7%
Combination Chest CT Scan[1]	-	-	4.2%	2.7%
Follow-up Mammogram/Ultrasound	171	2.3%	7.6%	8.8%
Lumbar Spine MRI for Low Back Pain[7]	-	-	40.2%	37.2%

Cullman Regional Medical Center

1912 Alabama Highway 157
Cullman, AL 35058
Phone: 256-737-2000
Fax: 256-737-2005
URL: www.crmchospital.com
Type: Acute Care Hospitals
Emergency Services: Yes
Ownership: Govt - Hospital Dist/Auth
Beds: 115

Key Personnel:

CEO . . . . Cheryl Bailey
Ambulatory Care . . . . Susan Copeland
Chief of Medical Staff. . . . . Rick Gober, MD
Chairman/CEO . . . . Todd McLeroy
CEO/President. . . . . Jim Weidner

Measure	Cases	This Hosp.	State Avg.	U.S. Avg.
Blood Clot Prevention and Treatment				
Anticoagulation Overlap Therapy[2]	43	98%	91%	93%
ICU Venous Thromboembolism Prophylaxis[2]	57	96%	85%	92%
Incidence of Potentially Preventable VTE[1,2]	-	-	18%	10%
UFH with Dosages/Platelet Monitoring[2]	17	100%	95%	97%
Venous Thromboembolism Prophylaxis[2]	448	98%	74%	85%
Warfarin Therapy Discharge Instructions[2]	35	100%	77%	75%
Chest Pain/Possible Heart Attack Care				
Aspirin Given Within 24 Hours of Arrival	92	100%	96%	96%
Fibrinolytic Meds Within 30 Min. of Arrival	13	38%	57%	58%
Average Time to ECG (minutes)	94	6	6	7
Average Time to Transfer (minutes)[1]	-	-	61	60
Children's Asthma Care				
Received Home Management Plan of Care	-	-	-	88%
Received Reliever Medication	-	-	-	100%
Received Systemic Corticosteroids	-	-	-	100%
Emergency Department				
Admittance Decision Time (minutes)[2]	650	92	73	98
Head CT Results Within 45 Min. of Arrival	11	82%	45%	57%
Patients Who Left ER Before Being Seen	47,229	1%	3%	2%
Time from ER Arrival to Admit. (minutes)[2]	650	242	240	274
Time from ER Arrival to Discharge (minutes)	546	126	126	134
Time in ER Before Being Evaluated (minutes)	596	26	31	26
Time to Pain Meds for Fractures (minutes)	204	62	69	57
Heart Attack Care				
Aspirin Given at Discharge[2]	70	100%	99%	99%
Fibrinolytic Meds Within 30 Min. of Arrival[1,2]	-	-	77%	54%
PCI Within 90 Minutes of Arrival[2]	11	100%	97%	96%
Statin Prescribed at Discharge[2]	64	98%	98%	98%
Heart Failure Care				
ACE Inhibitor or ARB for LVSD	59	100%	97%	97%
Discharge Instructions Given	223	98%	93%	94%
Evaluation of LVS Function	291	100%	99%	99%
Medicare Spending				
Medicare Spending per Patient (ratio)	-	0.94	0.98	0.98
Pneumonia Care				
Appropriate Initial Antibiotic Given[2]	58	100%	95%	95%
Blood Culture Timing[2]	180	98%	98%	98%
Pregnancy and Delivery Care				
Newborn Deliveries Scheduled Early	63	19%	14%	6%
Preventive Care				
Immunization for Influenza[2]	488	96%	90%	90%
Immunization for Pneumonia[2]	770	98%	91%	92%
Stroke Care				
Anticoagulation Therapy for Atrial Fibrillation[1]	-	-	92%	95%
Antithrombotic Therapy Timing	82	98%	96%	98%
Assessed for Rehabilitation	93	100%	95%	97%
Discharged on Antithrombotic Therapy	87	100%	98%	99%
Discharged on Statin Medication	68	100%	90%	94%
Thrombolytic Therapy Timing	13	54%	38%	66%
Venous Thromboembolism Prophylaxis	91	97%	89%	94%
Written Stroke Educational Materials Given	58	100%	85%	88%
Surgical Care Improvement Project				
Appropriate Beta Blocker Usage[2]	97	99%	98%	98%
Appropriate VTP Within 24 Hours[2]	300	100%	98%	98%
Controlled Postoperative Blood Glucose[2,7]	-	-	97%	97%
Perioperative Temperature Management[2]	370	100%	100%	100%
Prophylactic Antibiotic Selection[2]	272	100%	99%	99%
Prophylactic Antibiotic Selection (Outpatient)	195	98%	98%	98%
Prophylactic Antibiotic Stopped[2]	272	99%	98%	98%
Prophylactic Antibiotic Timing[2]	275	99%	99%	99%
Prophylactic Antibiotic Timing (Outpatient)	195	100%	99%	98%
Urinary Catheter Removal[2]	198	99%	98%	97%
Survey of Patients' Hospital Experiences				
Area Around Room 'Always' Quiet at Night	300+	72%	71%	61%
Doctors 'Always' Communicated Well	300+	87%	86%	82%
Home Recovery Information Given	300+	84%	84%	85%
Hospital Given 9 or 10 on 10 Point Scale	300+	72%	71%	71%
Meds 'Always' Explained Before Given	300+	64%	66%	64%
Nurses 'Always' Communicated Well	300+	81%	80%	79%
Pain 'Always' Well Controlled	300+	75%	72%	71%
Room and Bathroom 'Always' Clean	300+	71%	71%	73%
Timely Help 'Always' Received	300+	69%	68%	68%
Would Definitely Recommend Hospital	300+	72%	70%	71%
Use of Medical Imaging				
Cardiac Imaging Stress Test before Surgery	71	11.3%	6.5%	5.3%
Combination Abdominal CT Scan	815	6.6%	16.5%	10.5%
Combination Brain/Sinus CT Scan	1,146	3.1%	3.5%	2.7%
Combination Chest CT Scan	377	13.8%	4.2%	2.7%
Follow-up Mammogram/Ultrasound	738	6.2%	7.6%	8.8%
Lumbar Spine MRI for Low Back Pain	54	42.6%	40.2%	37.2%

Lake Martin Community Hospital

201 Mariarden Road
Dadeville, AL 36853
Phone: 256-825-7821
Type: Acute Care Hospitals
Emergency Services: Yes
Ownership: Proprietary

Key Personnel:

CEO/President. . . . . Michael Bruce
Radiology. . . . . Joel Partaine

Measure	Cases	This Hosp.	State Avg.	U.S. Avg.
Blood Clot Prevention and Treatment				
Anticoagulation Overlap Therapy[2,7]	-	-	91%	93%
ICU Venous Thromboembolism Prophylaxis[2,7]	-	-	85%	92%
Incidence of Potentially Preventable VTE[2,7]	-	-	18%	10%
UFH with Dosages/Platelet Monitoring[2,7]	-	-	95%	97%
Venous Thromboembolism Prophylaxis[2]	147	33%	74%	85%
Warfarin Therapy Discharge Instructions[2,7]	-	-	77%	75%
Chest Pain/Possible Heart Attack Care				
Aspirin Given Within 24 Hours of Arrival	17	71%	96%	96%
Fibrinolytic Meds Within 30 Min. of Arrival[3,7]	-	-	57%	58%
Average Time to ECG (minutes)	17	12	6	7
Average Time to Transfer (minutes)[1,3]	-	-	61	60
Children's Asthma Care				
Received Home Management Plan of Care	-	-	-	88%
Received Reliever Medication	-	-	-	100%
Received Systemic Corticosteroids	-	-	-	100%
Emergency Department				
Admittance Decision Time (minutes)[2]	479	39	73	98
Head CT Results Within 45 Min. of Arrival[1,3]	-	-	45%	57%
Patients Who Left ER Before Being Seen	5,167	0%	3%	2%
Time from ER Arrival to Admit. (minutes)[2]	532	205	240	274
Time from ER Arrival to Discharge (minutes)	338	106	126	134
Time in ER Before Being Evaluated (minutes)	365	27	31	26
Time to Pain Meds for Fractures (minutes)[3]	20	62	69	57
Heart Attack Care				
Aspirin Given at Discharge[3,7]	-	-	99%	99%
Fibrinolytic Meds Within 30 Min. of Arrival[3,7]	-	-	77%	54%
PCI Within 90 Minutes of Arrival[3,7]	-	-	97%	96%
Statin Prescribed at Discharge[1,3]	-	-	98%	98%
Heart Failure Care				
ACE Inhibitor or ARB for LVSD[1,2]	-	-	97%	97%
Discharge Instructions Given[2]	20	70%	93%	94%
Evaluation of LVS Function[2]	21	67%	99%	99%
Medicare Spending				
Medicare Spending per Patient (ratio)	-	-	0.98	0.98
Pneumonia Care				
Appropriate Initial Antibiotic Given[1,2]	-	-	95%	95%
Blood Culture Timing[2]	25	80%	98%	98%
Pregnancy and Delivery Care				
Newborn Deliveries Scheduled Early[7]	-	-	14%	6%
Preventive Care				
Immunization for Influenza[2]	284	29%	90%	90%

NOTE: Hospital profiles are in alphabetical order by state, then city, then hospital within the city; Rankings exclude hospitals with less than 25 cases except for patient surveys which excludes hospitals with less than 100 cases; (a) 100-299 cases; (1) The number of cases/patients is too few to report; (2) Data submitted were based on a sample of cases/patients; (3) Results are based on a shorter time period than required; (4) Data suppressed by CMS for one or more quarters; (5) Results are not available for this reporting period; (6) Fewer than 100 patients completed the HCAHPS survey; (7) No cases met the criteria for this measure; (8) The lower limit of the confidence interval cannot be calculated if the number of observed infections equals zero; (9) No data are available from the state/territory for this reporting period; (10) The scores shown reflect fewer than 50 completed surveys; (11) There were discrepancies in the data collection process; (12) This measure does not apply to this hospital for this reporting period; (13) Results cannot be calculated for this reporting period; (14) The results for this state are combined with nearby states to protect confidentiality; Please refer to the User's Guide for a full explanation of data.

Measure	Cases	This Hosp.	State Avg.	U.S. Avg.
Immunization for Pneumonia[2]	382	34%	91%	92%
Stroke Care				
Anticoagulation Therapy for Atrial Fibrillation[3,7]	-	-	92%	95%
Antithrombotic Therapy Timing[1,3]	-	-	96%	98%
Assessed for Rehabilitation[1,3]	-	-	95%	97%
Discharged on Antithrombotic Therapy[1,3]	-	-	98%	99%
Discharged on Statin Medication[1,3]	-	-	90%	94%
Thrombolytic Therapy Timing[1,3]	-	-	38%	66%
Venous Thromboembolism Prophylaxis[1,3]	-	-	89%	94%
Written Stroke Educational Materials Given[1,3]	-	-	85%	88%
Surgical Care Improvement Project				
Appropriate Beta Blocker Usage[5]	-	-	98%	98%
Appropriate VTP Within 24 Hours[5]	-	-	98%	98%
Controlled Postoperative Blood Glucose[5]	-	-	97%	97%
Perioperative Temperature Management[5]	-	-	100%	100%
Prophylactic Antibiotic Selection[5]	-	-	99%	99%
Prophylactic Antibiotic Selection (Outpatient)[5]	-	-	98%	98%
Prophylactic Antibiotic Stopped[5]	-	-	98%	98%
Prophylactic Antibiotic Timing[5]	-	-	99%	99%
Prophylactic Antibiotic Timing (Outpatient)[5]	-	-	99%	98%
Urinary Catheter Removal[5]	-	-	98%	97%
Survey of Patients' Hospital Experiences				
Area Around Room 'Always' Quiet at Night	(a)	73%	71%	61%
Doctors 'Always' Communicated Well	(a)	85%	86%	82%
Home Recovery Information Given	(a)	83%	84%	85%
Hospital Given 9 or 10 on 10 Point Scale	(a)	63%	71%	71%
Meds 'Always' Explained Before Given	(a)	59%	66%	64%
Nurses 'Always' Communicated Well	(a)	75%	80%	79%
Pain 'Always' Well Controlled	(a)	66%	72%	71%
Room and Bathroom 'Always' Clean	(a)	73%	71%	73%
Timely Help 'Always' Received	(a)	68%	68%	68%
Would Definitely Recommend Hospital	(a)	63%	70%	71%
Use of Medical Imaging				
Cardiac Imaging Stress Test before Surgery	71	5.6%	6.5%	5.3%
Combination Abdominal CT Scan	62	0.0%	16.5%	10.5%
Combination Brain/Sinus CT Scan[1]	-	-	3.5%	2.7%
Combination Chest CT Scan[1]	-	-	4.2%	2.7%
Follow-up Mammogram/Ultrasound[7]	-	-	7.6%	8.8%
Lumbar Spine MRI for Low Back Pain[1]	-	-	40.2%	37.2%

Decatur Morgan Hospital - Decatur Campus

1201 7th Street Se Phone: 256-341-2000
Decatur, AL 35601 Fax: 256-306-1645
URL: www.decaturgeneral.org
Type: Acute Care Hospitals Emergency Services: Yes
Ownership: Govt - Hospital Dist/Auth Beds: 273

Key Personnel:

Anesthesiology. . . . . Chad Harbin, DO
Pediatrics. . . . . J.W. Hull, MD
Chief of Medical Staff. . . . . Jason Lockette, MD
CEO/President. . . . . Nat Richardson
Surgery . . . . W. Jay Suggs, MD

Measure	Cases	This Hosp.	State Avg.	U.S. Avg.
Blood Clot Prevention and Treatment				
Anticoagulation Overlap Therapy[2]	42	62%	91%	93%
ICU Venous Thromboembolism Prophylaxis[2]	82	71%	85%	92%
Incidence of Potentially Preventable VTE[2]	13	23%	18%	10%
UFH with Dosages/Platelet Monitoring[1,2]	-	-	95%	97%
Venous Thromboembolism Prophylaxis[2]	318	63%	74%	85%
Warfarin Therapy Discharge Instructions[2]	23	48%	77%	75%
Chest Pain/Possible Heart Attack Care				
Aspirin Given Within 24 Hours of Arrival	144	95%	96%	96%
Fibrinolytic Meds Within 30 Min. of Arrival[7]	-	-	57%	58%
Average Time to ECG (minutes)	145	6	6	7
Average Time to Transfer (minutes)[1]	-	-	61	60
Children's Asthma Care				
Received Home Management Plan of Care	-	-	-	88%
Received Reliever Medication	-	-	-	100%
Received Systemic Corticosteroids	-	-	-	100%
Emergency Department				
Admittance Decision Time (minutes)[2]	419	75	73	98
Head CT Results Within 45 Min. of Arrival	24	29%	45%	57%
Patients Who Left ER Before Being Seen	44,362	5%	3%	2%
Time from ER Arrival to Admit. (minutes)[2]	470	286	240	274
Time from ER Arrival to Discharge (minutes)	358	165	126	134
Time in ER Before Being Evaluated (minutes)	368	55	31	26
Time to Pain Meds for Fractures (minutes)	158	80	69	57
Heart Attack Care				
Aspirin Given at Discharge	25	100%	99%	99%
Fibrinolytic Meds Within 30 Min. of Arrival[7]	-	-	77%	54%
PCI Within 90 Minutes of Arrival[7]	-	-	97%	96%
Statin Prescribed at Discharge	25	92%	98%	98%
Heart Failure Care				
ACE Inhibitor or ARB for LVSD	103	95%	97%	97%
Discharge Instructions Given	289	72%	93%	94%
Evaluation of LVS Function	353	99%	99%	99%
Medicare Spending				
Medicare Spending per Patient (ratio)	-	0.98	0.98	0.98
Pneumonia Care				
Appropriate Initial Antibiotic Given	136	98%	95%	95%
Blood Culture Timing	201	95%	98%	98%
Pregnancy and Delivery Care				
Newborn Deliveries Scheduled Early	88	20%	14%	6%
Preventive Care				
Immunization for Influenza[2]	571	81%	90%	90%
Immunization for Pneumonia[2]	683	94%	91%	92%
Stroke Care				
Anticoagulation Therapy for Atrial Fibrillation	13	85%	92%	95%
Antithrombotic Therapy Timing	89	94%	96%	98%
Assessed for Rehabilitation	107	100%	95%	97%
Discharged on Antithrombotic Therapy	100	97%	98%	99%
Discharged on Statin Medication	70	93%	90%	94%
Thrombolytic Therapy Timing	12	58%	38%	66%
Venous Thromboembolism Prophylaxis	108	97%	89%	94%
Written Stroke Educational Materials Given	61	97%	85%	88%
Surgical Care Improvement Project				
Appropriate Beta Blocker Usage	213	98%	98%	98%
Appropriate VTP Within 24 Hours	639	99%	98%	98%
Controlled Postoperative Blood Glucose[7]	-	-	97%	97%
Perioperative Temperature Management	759	100%	100%	100%
Prophylactic Antibiotic Selection	539	99%	99%	99%
Prophylactic Antibiotic Selection (Outpatient)	196	95%	98%	98%
Prophylactic Antibiotic Stopped	533	99%	98%	98%
Prophylactic Antibiotic Timing	539	99%	99%	99%
Prophylactic Antibiotic Timing (Outpatient)	200	98%	99%	98%
Urinary Catheter Removal	479	99%	98%	97%
Survey of Patients' Hospital Experiences				
Area Around Room 'Always' Quiet at Night	300+	72%	71%	61%
Doctors 'Always' Communicated Well	300+	87%	86%	82%
Home Recovery Information Given	300+	87%	84%	85%
Hospital Given 9 or 10 on 10 Point Scale	300+	71%	71%	71%
Meds 'Always' Explained Before Given	300+	65%	66%	64%
Nurses 'Always' Communicated Well	300+	81%	80%	79%
Pain 'Always' Well Controlled	300+	73%	72%	71%
Room and Bathroom 'Always' Clean	300+	70%	71%	73%
Timely Help 'Always' Received	300+	67%	68%	68%
Would Definitely Recommend Hospital	300+	73%	70%	71%
Use of Medical Imaging				
Cardiac Imaging Stress Test before Surgery	480	7.5%	6.5%	5.3%
Combination Abdominal CT Scan	1,028	9.0%	16.5%	10.5%
Combination Brain/Sinus CT Scan	862	0.6%	3.5%	2.7%
Combination Chest CT Scan	789	5.6%	4.2%	2.7%
Follow-up Mammogram/Ultrasound	2,344	9.4%	7.6%	8.8%
Lumbar Spine MRI for Low Back Pain	141	39.0%	40.2%	37.2%

Decatur Morgan Hospital - Parkway Campus

1874 Beltline Rd Sw Phone: 256-350-2211
Decatur, AL 35601 Fax: 256-350-8415
URL: www.parkwaymedicalcenter.com
Type: Acute Care Hospitals Emergency Services: Yes
Ownership: Proprietary Beds: 120

Key Personnel:

Quality Assurance . . . . Deborah Gann
Emergency Room . . . . Ann Harrison
Chief of Medical Staff. . . . . Jason Lockette, MD
CEO/President. . . . . Phillip Mazzuca
Radiology. . . . . Traci Mccormick, MD
Operating Room. . . . . Hugh Comer Nabers, RN
President . . . . Nat Richardson

Measure	Cases	This Hosp.	State Avg.	U.S. Avg.
Blood Clot Prevention and Treatment				
Anticoagulation Overlap Therapy[2]	14	79%	91%	93%
ICU Venous Thromboembolism Prophylaxis[2]	66	83%	85%	92%
Incidence of Potentially Preventable VTE[1,2]	-	-	18%	10%
UFH with Dosages/Platelet Monitoring[1,2]	-	-	95%	97%
Venous Thromboembolism Prophylaxis[2]	125	68%	74%	85%
Warfarin Therapy Discharge Instructions[1,2]	-	-	77%	75%
Chest Pain/Possible Heart Attack Care				
Aspirin Given Within 24 Hours of Arrival	65	94%	96%	96%
Fibrinolytic Meds Within 30 Min. of Arrival[7]	-	-	57%	58%
Average Time to ECG (minutes)	65	4	6	7
Average Time to Transfer (minutes)[1]	-	-	61	60
Children's Asthma Care				
Received Home Management Plan of Care	-	-	-	88%
Received Reliever Medication	-	-	-	100%
Received Systemic Corticosteroids	-	-	-	100%
Emergency Department				
Admittance Decision Time (minutes)[2]	476	73	73	98
Head CT Results Within 45 Min. of Arrival[1,3]	-	-	45%	57%
Patients Who Left ER Before Being Seen	28,693	4%	3%	2%
Time from ER Arrival to Admit. (minutes)[2]	480	235	240	274
Time from ER Arrival to Discharge (minutes)	447	131	126	134
Time in ER Before Being Evaluated (minutes)	469	33	31	26
Time to Pain Meds for Fractures (minutes)	130	76	69	57
Heart Attack Care				
Aspirin Given at Discharge[1]	-	-	99%	99%
Fibrinolytic Meds Within 30 Min. of Arrival[7]	-	-	77%	54%
PCI Within 90 Minutes of Arrival[7]	-	-	97%	96%
Statin Prescribed at Discharge	11	64%	98%	98%
Heart Failure Care				
ACE Inhibitor or ARB for LVSD	28	79%	97%	97%
Discharge Instructions Given	53	72%	93%	94%
Evaluation of LVS Function	70	96%	99%	99%
Medicare Spending				
Medicare Spending per Patient (ratio)	-	1.01	0.98	0.98
Pneumonia Care				
Appropriate Initial Antibiotic Given	48	92%	95%	95%
Blood Culture Timing	75	99%	98%	98%
Pregnancy and Delivery Care				
Newborn Deliveries Scheduled Early[7]	-	-	14%	6%
Preventive Care				
Immunization for Influenza[2]	291	96%	90%	90%
Immunization for Pneumonia[2]	433	93%	91%	92%
Stroke Care				
Anticoagulation Therapy for Atrial Fibrillation[1]	-	-	92%	95%
Antithrombotic Therapy Timing	22	95%	96%	98%
Assessed for Rehabilitation	27	81%	95%	97%
Discharged on Antithrombotic Therapy	26	85%	98%	99%
Discharged on Statin Medication	21	62%	90%	94%
Thrombolytic Therapy Timing[1]	-	-	38%	66%
Venous Thromboembolism Prophylaxis	24	92%	89%	94%
Written Stroke Educational Materials Given	15	7%	85%	88%
Surgical Care Improvement Project				
Appropriate Beta Blocker Usage[1]	-	-	98%	98%
Appropriate VTP Within 24 Hours	15	87%	98%	98%
Controlled Postoperative Blood Glucose[7]	-	-	97%	97%
Perioperative Temperature Management	16	100%	100%	100%
Prophylactic Antibiotic Selection[1]	-	-	99%	99%
Prophylactic Antibiotic Selection (Outpatient)	44	98%	98%	98%
Prophylactic Antibiotic Stopped[1]	-	-	98%	98%
Prophylactic Antibiotic Timing[1]	-	-	99%	99%
Prophylactic Antibiotic Timing (Outpatient)	37	84%	99%	98%
Urinary Catheter Removal	12	50%	98%	97%
Survey of Patients' Hospital Experiences				
Area Around Room 'Always' Quiet at Night	(a)	65%	71%	61%
Doctors 'Always' Communicated Well	(a)	74%	86%	82%
Home Recovery Information Given	(a)	76%	84%	85%
Hospital Given 9 or 10 on 10 Point Scale	(a)	57%	71%	71%
Meds 'Always' Explained Before Given	(a)	54%	66%	64%

NOTE: Hospital profiles are in alphabetical order by state, then city, then hospital within the city; Rankings exclude hospitals with less than 25 cases except for patient surveys which excludes hospitals with less than 100 cases; (a) 100-299 cases; (1) The number of cases/patients is too few to report; (2) Data submitted were based on a sample of cases/patients; (3) Results are based on a shorter time period than required; (4) Data suppressed by CMS for one or more quarters; (5) Results are not available for this reporting period; (6) Fewer than 100 patients completed the HCAHPS survey; (7) No cases met the criteria for this measure; (8) The lower limit of the confidence interval cannot be calculated if the number of observed infections equals zero; (9) No data are available from the state/territory for this reporting period; (10) The scores shown reflect fewer than 50 completed surveys; (11) There were discrepancies in the data collection process; (12) This measure does not apply to this hospital for this reporting period; (13) Results cannot be calculated for this reporting period; (14) The results for this state are combined with nearby states to protect confidentiality; Please refer to the User's Guide for a full explanation of data.

Measure	Cases	This Hosp.	State Avg.	U.S. Avg.
Nurses 'Always' Communicated Well	(a)	69%	80%	79%
Pain 'Always' Well Controlled	(a)	60%	72%	71%
Room and Bathroom 'Always' Clean	(a)	72%	71%	73%
Timely Help 'Always' Received	(a)	63%	68%	68%
Would Definitely Recommend Hospital	(a)	57%	70%	71%
Use of Medical Imaging				
Cardiac Imaging Stress Test before Surgery	104	1.9%	6.5%	5.3%
Combination Abdominal CT Scan	264	4.2%	16.5%	10.5%
Combination Brain/Sinus CT Scan[1]	-	-	3.5%	2.7%
Combination Chest CT Scan	194	0.0%	4.2%	2.7%
Follow-up Mammogram/Ultrasound	541	15.0%	7.6%	8.8%
Lumbar Spine MRI for Low Back Pain	81	32.1%	40.2%	37.2%

Bryan W Whitfield Memorial Hospital

105 Highway 80 East
Demopolis, AL 36732
Phone: 334-289-4000
Fax: 334-287-2594
E-mail: info@bwwmh.com
URL: www.bwwmh.com
Type: Acute Care Hospitals
Emergency Services: Yes
Ownership: Govt - Hospital Dist/Auth
Beds: 99

Key Personnel:

Operating Room. . . . . Fernando Alegria
Chief of Medical Staff. . . . . Ronnie Chu, MD
Intensive Care Unit. . . . . Terry Elmore
Radiology. . . . . Aprile Gibson
Patient Relations . . . . Marcia Lankster
CEO/President. . . . . Mike Marshall
Quality Assurance . . . . Cindy Parten
Hemotology Center . . . . Missy Scarbrough

Measure	Cases	This Hosp.	State Avg.	U.S. Avg.
Blood Clot Prevention and Treatment				
Anticoagulation Overlap Therapy[1,2]	-	-	91%	93%
ICU Venous Thromboembolism Prophylaxis[2]	83	23%	85%	92%
Incidence of Potentially Preventable VTE[2,7]	-	-	18%	10%
UFH with Dosages/Platelet Monitoring[1,2]	-	-	95%	97%
Venous Thromboembolism Prophylaxis[2]	236	7%	74%	85%
Warfarin Therapy Discharge Instructions[1,2]	-	-	77%	75%
Chest Pain/Possible Heart Attack Care				
Aspirin Given Within 24 Hours of Arrival	33	67%	96%	96%
Fibrinolytic Meds Within 30 Min. of Arrival[7]	-	-	57%	58%
Average Time to ECG (minutes)	34	28	6	7
Average Time to Transfer (minutes)[1]	-	-	61	60
Children's Asthma Care				
Received Home Management Plan of Care	-	-	-	88%
Received Reliever Medication	-	-	-	100%
Received Systemic Corticosteroids	-	-	-	100%
Emergency Department				
Admittance Decision Time (minutes)[2]	620	38	73	98
Head CT Results Within 45 Min. of Arrival[1,3]	-	-	45%	57%
Patients Who Left ER Before Being Seen	9,558	2%	3%	2%
Time from ER Arrival to Admit. (minutes)[2]	620	180	240	274
Time from ER Arrival to Discharge (minutes)	341	118	126	134
Time in ER Before Being Evaluated (minutes)	380	35	31	26
Time to Pain Meds for Fractures (minutes)[1,3]	-	-	69	57
Heart Attack Care				
Aspirin Given at Discharge[1]	-	-	99%	99%
Fibrinolytic Meds Within 30 Min. of Arrival[7]	-	-	77%	54%
PCI Within 90 Minutes of Arrival[7]	-	-	97%	96%
Statin Prescribed at Discharge[7]	-	-	98%	98%
Heart Failure Care				
ACE Inhibitor or ARB for LVSD[1,2]	-	-	97%	97%
Discharge Instructions Given[2]	34	82%	93%	94%
Evaluation of LVS Function[2]	37	41%	99%	99%
Medicare Spending				
Medicare Spending per Patient (ratio)	-	1.03	0.98	0.98
Pneumonia Care				
Appropriate Initial Antibiotic Given[2]	58	71%	95%	95%
Blood Culture Timing[2]	21	95%	98%	98%
Pregnancy and Delivery Care				
Newborn Deliveries Scheduled Early	55	96%	14%	6%
Preventive Care				
Immunization for Influenza[2]	296	89%	90%	90%
Immunization for Pneumonia[2]	381	96%	91%	92%
Stroke Care				
Anticoagulation Therapy for Atrial Fibrillation[7]	-	-	92%	95%
Antithrombotic Therapy Timing	11	0%	96%	98%
Assessed for Rehabilitation[1]	-	-	95%	97%
Discharged on Antithrombotic Therapy[1]	-	-	98%	99%
Discharged on Statin Medication[1]	-	-	90%	94%
Thrombolytic Therapy Timing[1]	-	-	38%	66%
Venous Thromboembolism Prophylaxis	11	27%	89%	94%
Written Stroke Educational Materials Given[1]	-	-	85%	88%
Surgical Care Improvement Project				
Appropriate Beta Blocker Usage[1,2]	-	-	98%	98%
Appropriate VTP Within 24 Hours[2]	23	22%	98%	98%
Controlled Postoperative Blood Glucose[2,7]	-	-	97%	97%
Perioperative Temperature Management[2]	24	100%	100%	100%
Prophylactic Antibiotic Selection[2]	22	91%	99%	99%
Prophylactic Antibiotic Selection (Outpatient)[5]	-	-	98%	98%
Prophylactic Antibiotic Stopped[2]	22	14%	98%	98%
Prophylactic Antibiotic Timing[2]	22	73%	99%	99%
Prophylactic Antibiotic Timing (Outpatient)[5]	-	-	99%	98%
Urinary Catheter Removal[1,2]	-	-	98%	97%
Survey of Patients' Hospital Experiences				
Area Around Room 'Always' Quiet at Night	(a)	69%	71%	61%
Doctors 'Always' Communicated Well	(a)	87%	86%	82%
Home Recovery Information Given	(a)	74%	84%	85%
Hospital Given 9 or 10 on 10 Point Scale	(a)	67%	71%	71%
Meds 'Always' Explained Before Given	(a)	62%	66%	64%
Nurses 'Always' Communicated Well	(a)	77%	80%	79%
Pain 'Always' Well Controlled	(a)	72%	72%	71%
Room and Bathroom 'Always' Clean	(a)	71%	71%	73%
Timely Help 'Always' Received	(a)	64%	68%	68%
Would Definitely Recommend Hospital	(a)	58%	70%	71%
Use of Medical Imaging				
Cardiac Imaging Stress Test before Surgery[1]	-	-	6.5%	5.3%
Combination Abdominal CT Scan	316	19.6%	16.5%	10.5%
Combination Brain/Sinus CT Scan[1]	-	-	3.5%	2.7%
Combination Chest CT Scan	180	8.3%	4.2%	2.7%
Follow-up Mammogram/Ultrasound	223	8.5%	7.6%	8.8%
Lumbar Spine MRI for Low Back Pain	73	34.2%	40.2%	37.2%

Flowers Hospital

4370 West Main Street
Dothan, AL 36305
Phone: 334-793-5000
Fax: 334-793-5613
URL: www.flowershospital.com
Type: Acute Care Hospitals
Emergency Services: Yes
Ownership: Proprietary
Beds: 235

Key Personnel:

Radiology. . . . . Christopher R Ahmed
CEO/President. . . . . Keith Granger

Measure	Cases	This Hosp.	State Avg.	U.S. Avg.
Blood Clot Prevention and Treatment				
Anticoagulation Overlap Therapy[2]	52	100%	91%	93%
ICU Venous Thromboembolism Prophylaxis[2]	127	100%	85%	92%
Incidence of Potentially Preventable VTE[1,2]	-	-	18%	10%
UFH with Dosages/Platelet Monitoring[1,2]	-	-	95%	97%
Venous Thromboembolism Prophylaxis[2]	344	100%	74%	85%
Warfarin Therapy Discharge Instructions[2]	41	100%	77%	75%
Chest Pain/Possible Heart Attack Care				
Aspirin Given Within 24 Hours of Arrival[5]	-	-	96%	96%
Fibrinolytic Meds Within 30 Min. of Arrival[5]	-	-	57%	58%
Average Time to ECG (minutes)[5]	-	-	6	7
Average Time to Transfer (minutes)[5]	-	-	61	60
Children's Asthma Care				
Received Home Management Plan of Care	-	-	-	88%
Received Reliever Medication	-	-	-	100%
Received Systemic Corticosteroids	-	-	-	100%
Emergency Department				
Admittance Decision Time (minutes)[2]	566	109	73	98
Head CT Results Within 45 Min. of Arrival[1]	-	-	45%	57%
Patients Who Left ER Before Being Seen	39,118	4%	3%	2%
Time from ER Arrival to Admit. (minutes)[2]	573	278	240	274
Time from ER Arrival to Discharge (minutes)	394	184	126	134
Time in ER Before Being Evaluated (minutes)	395	46	31	26
Time to Pain Meds for Fractures (minutes)	103	76	69	57
Heart Attack Care				
Aspirin Given at Discharge	280	100%	99%	99%
Fibrinolytic Meds Within 30 Min. of Arrival[7]	-	-	77%	54%
PCI Within 90 Minutes of Arrival	35	97%	97%	96%
Statin Prescribed at Discharge	260	100%	98%	98%
Heart Failure Care				
ACE Inhibitor or ARB for LVSD	74	100%	97%	97%
Discharge Instructions Given	219	97%	93%	94%
Evaluation of LVS Function	252	100%	99%	99%
Medicare Spending				
Medicare Spending per Patient (ratio)	-	0.99	0.98	0.98
Pneumonia Care				
Appropriate Initial Antibiotic Given	138	100%	95%	95%
Blood Culture Timing	188	100%	98%	98%
Pregnancy and Delivery Care				
Newborn Deliveries Scheduled Early[2]	30	0%	14%	6%
Preventive Care				
Immunization for Influenza[2]	708	100%	90%	90%
Immunization for Pneumonia[2]	777	100%	91%	92%
Stroke Care				
Anticoagulation Therapy for Atrial Fibrillation	16	100%	92%	95%
Antithrombotic Therapy Timing	126	100%	96%	98%
Assessed for Rehabilitation	148	100%	95%	97%
Discharged on Antithrombotic Therapy	139	100%	98%	99%
Discharged on Statin Medication	101	100%	90%	94%
Thrombolytic Therapy Timing[1]	-	-	38%	66%
Venous Thromboembolism Prophylaxis	154	99%	89%	94%
Written Stroke Educational Materials Given	81	94%	85%	88%
Surgical Care Improvement Project				
Appropriate Beta Blocker Usage	370	100%	98%	98%
Appropriate VTP Within 24 Hours	894	100%	98%	98%
Controlled Postoperative Blood Glucose	132	98%	97%	97%
Perioperative Temperature Management	1,159	100%	100%	100%
Prophylactic Antibiotic Selection	882	100%	99%	99%
Prophylactic Antibiotic Selection (Outpatient)	401	100%	98%	98%
Prophylactic Antibiotic Stopped	844	100%	98%	98%
Prophylactic Antibiotic Timing	882	100%	99%	99%
Prophylactic Antibiotic Timing (Outpatient)	401	100%	99%	98%
Urinary Catheter Removal	667	100%	98%	97%
Survey of Patients' Hospital Experiences				
Area Around Room 'Always' Quiet at Night	300+	71%	71%	61%
Doctors 'Always' Communicated Well	300+	83%	86%	82%
Home Recovery Information Given	300+	87%	84%	85%
Hospital Given 9 or 10 on 10 Point Scale	300+	76%	71%	71%
Meds 'Always' Explained Before Given	300+	70%	66%	64%
Nurses 'Always' Communicated Well	300+	80%	80%	79%
Pain 'Always' Well Controlled	300+	73%	72%	71%
Room and Bathroom 'Always' Clean	300+	69%	71%	73%
Timely Help 'Always' Received	300+	64%	68%	68%
Would Definitely Recommend Hospital	300+	80%	70%	71%
Use of Medical Imaging				
Cardiac Imaging Stress Test before Surgery	392	6.9%	6.5%	5.3%
Combination Abdominal CT Scan	1,713	5.4%	16.5%	10.5%
Combination Brain/Sinus CT Scan	987	3.4%	3.5%	2.7%
Combination Chest CT Scan	1,196	0.3%	4.2%	2.7%
Follow-up Mammogram/Ultrasound	3,877	5.8%	7.6%	8.8%
Lumbar Spine MRI for Low Back Pain	134	36.6%	40.2%	37.2%

Southeast Alabama Medical Center

1108 Ross Clark Circle
Dothan, AL 36301
Phone: 334-793-8701
Fax: 334-793-8751
URL: www.samc.org
Type: Acute Care Hospitals
Emergency Services: Yes
Ownership: Govt - Hospital Dist/Auth
Beds: 400

Key Personnel:

Radiology. . . . . Christopher Ahmed, MD
Quality Assurance . . . . Wanda Fassett
Emergency Room . . . . Jim Jones, DO
Operating Room. . . . . Mike Kay, RN
Chief of Medical Staff. . . . . Guy M. Middleton, MD
CEO/President. . . . . Ronald S Owen
Pediatric Ambulatory Care . . . . . . Lee Scott, MD
Anesthesiology. . . . . James York, MD

Measure	Cases	This Hosp.	State Avg.	U.S. Avg.
Blood Clot Prevention and Treatment				

NOTE: Hospital profiles are in alphabetical order by state, then city, then hospital within the city; Rankings exclude hospitals with less than 25 cases except for patient surveys which excludes hospitals with less than 100 cases; (a) 100-299 cases; (1) The number of cases/patients is too few to report; (2) Data submitted were based on a sample of cases/patients; (3) Results are based on a shorter time period than required; (4) Data suppressed by CMS for one or more quarters; (5) Results are not available for this reporting period; (6) Fewer than 100 patients completed the HCAHPS survey; (7) No cases met the criteria for this measure; (8) The lower limit of the confidence interval cannot be calculated if the number of observed infections equals zero; (9) No data are available from the state/territory for this reporting period; (10) The scores shown reflect fewer than 50 completed surveys; (11) There were discrepancies in the data collection process; (12) This measure does not apply to this hospital for this reporting period; (13) Results cannot be calculated for this reporting period; (14) The results for this state are combined with nearby states to protect confidentiality; Please refer to the User's Guide for a full explanation of data.

Measure	Cases	This Hosp.	State Avg.	U.S. Avg.
Anticoagulation Overlap Therapy[2]	117	85%	91%	93%
ICU Venous Thromboembolism Prophylaxis[2]	85	94%	85%	92%
Incidence of Potentially Preventable VTE[2]	14	7%	18%	10%
UFH with Dosages/Platelet Monitoring[2]	19	89%	95%	97%
Venous Thromboembolism Prophylaxis[2]	337	81%	74%	85%
Warfarin Therapy Discharge Instructions[2]	94	2%	77%	75%
Chest Pain/Possible Heart Attack Care				
Aspirin Given Within 24 Hours of Arrival[1,3]	-	-	96%	96%
Fibrinolytic Meds Within 30 Min. of Arrival[3,7]	-	-	57%	58%
Average Time to ECG (minutes)[1,3]	-	-	6	7
Average Time to Transfer (minutes)[3,7]	-	-	61	60
Children's Asthma Care				
Received Home Management Plan of Care	-	-	-	88%
Received Reliever Medication	-	-	-	100%
Received Systemic Corticosteroids	-	-	-	100%
Emergency Department				
Admittance Decision Time (minutes)[2]	530	66	73	98
Head CT Results Within 45 Min. of Arrival[1]	-	-	45%	57%
Patients Who Left ER Before Being Seen	60,818	4%	3%	2%
Time from ER Arrival to Admit. (minutes)[2]	530	272	240	274
Time from ER Arrival to Discharge (minutes)	361	202	126	134
Time in ER Before Being Evaluated (minutes)	381	62	31	26
Time to Pain Meds for Fractures (minutes)	164	103	69	57
Heart Attack Care				
Aspirin Given at Discharge	601	100%	99%	99%
Fibrinolytic Meds Within 30 Min. of Arrival[7]	-	-	77%	54%
PCI Within 90 Minutes of Arrival	35	91%	97%	96%
Statin Prescribed at Discharge	594	98%	98%	98%
Heart Failure Care				
ACE Inhibitor or ARB for LVSD	160	96%	97%	97%
Discharge Instructions Given	466	94%	93%	94%
Evaluation of LVS Function	556	100%	99%	99%
Medicare Spending				
Medicare Spending per Patient (ratio)	-	1.00	0.98	0.98
Pneumonia Care				
Appropriate Initial Antibiotic Given	171	95%	95%	95%
Blood Culture Timing	219	99%	98%	98%
Pregnancy and Delivery Care				
Newborn Deliveries Scheduled Early[2]	18	0%	14%	6%
Preventive Care				
Immunization for Influenza[2]	558	93%	90%	90%
Immunization for Pneumonia[2]	817	93%	91%	92%
Stroke Care				
Anticoagulation Therapy for Atrial Fibrillation[1,2]	-	-	92%	95%
Antithrombotic Therapy Timing[2]	72	99%	96%	98%
Assessed for Rehabilitation[2]	89	96%	95%	97%
Discharged on Antithrombotic Therapy[2]	77	99%	98%	99%
Discharged on Statin Medication[2]	60	93%	90%	94%
Thrombolytic Therapy Timing[2,7]	-	-	38%	66%
Venous Thromboembolism Prophylaxis[2]	94	96%	89%	94%
Written Stroke Educational Materials Given[2]	53	85%	85%	88%
Surgical Care Improvement Project				
Appropriate Beta Blocker Usage[2]	208	99%	98%	98%
Appropriate VTP Within 24 Hours[2]	295	96%	98%	98%
Controlled Postoperative Blood Glucose[2]	121	96%	97%	97%
Perioperative Temperature Management[2]	365	100%	100%	100%
Prophylactic Antibiotic Selection[2]	329	99%	99%	99%
Prophylactic Antibiotic Selection (Outpatient)	388	99%	98%	98%
Prophylactic Antibiotic Stopped[2]	324	95%	98%	98%
Prophylactic Antibiotic Timing[2]	330	100%	99%	99%
Prophylactic Antibiotic Timing (Outpatient)	388	100%	99%	98%
Urinary Catheter Removal[2]	312	91%	98%	97%
Survey of Patients' Hospital Experiences				
Area Around Room 'Always' Quiet at Night	300+	68%	71%	61%
Doctors 'Always' Communicated Well	300+	83%	86%	82%
Home Recovery Information Given	300+	84%	84%	85%
Hospital Given 9 or 10 on 10 Point Scale	300+	71%	71%	71%
Meds 'Always' Explained Before Given	300+	62%	66%	64%
Nurses 'Always' Communicated Well	300+	76%	80%	79%
Pain 'Always' Well Controlled	300+	67%	72%	71%
Room and Bathroom 'Always' Clean	300+	70%	71%	73%
Timely Help 'Always' Received	300+	58%	68%	68%
Would Definitely Recommend Hospital	300+	76%	70%	71%
Use of Medical Imaging				
Cardiac Imaging Stress Test before Surgery	721	8.0%	6.5%	5.3%
Combination Abdominal CT Scan	2,158	4.6%	16.5%	10.5%
Combination Brain/Sinus CT Scan	1,781	2.9%	3.5%	2.7%
Combination Chest CT Scan	1,371	2.5%	4.2%	2.7%
Follow-up Mammogram/Ultrasound	3,930	5.0%	7.6%	8.8%
Lumbar Spine MRI for Low Back Pain	498	29.3%	40.2%	37.2%

Medical Center Enterprise

400 N Edwards Street　　Phone: 334-347-0584
Enterprise, AL 36330
URL: www.mcehospital.com
Type: Acute Care Hospitals　　Emergency Services: Yes
Ownership: Proprietary　　Beds: 131

Measure	Cases	This Hosp.	State Avg.	U.S. Avg.
Blood Clot Prevention and Treatment				
Anticoagulation Overlap Therapy[2]	14	100%	91%	93%
ICU Venous Thromboembolism Prophylaxis[2]	69	100%	85%	92%
Incidence of Potentially Preventable VTE[2,7]	-	-	18%	10%
UFH with Dosages/Platelet Monitoring[1,2]	-	-	95%	97%
Venous Thromboembolism Prophylaxis[2]	256	98%	74%	85%
Warfarin Therapy Discharge Instructions[2]	14	100%	77%	75%
Chest Pain/Possible Heart Attack Care				
Aspirin Given Within 24 Hours of Arrival	73	99%	96%	96%
Fibrinolytic Meds Within 30 Min. of Arrival[1]	-	-	57%	58%
Average Time to ECG (minutes)	75	7	6	7
Average Time to Transfer (minutes)[7]	-	-	61	60
Children's Asthma Care				
Received Home Management Plan of Care	-	-	-	88%
Received Reliever Medication	-	-	-	100%
Received Systemic Corticosteroids	-	-	-	100%
Emergency Department				
Admittance Decision Time (minutes)[2]	407	63	73	98
Head CT Results Within 45 Min. of Arrival	19	84%	45%	57%
Patients Who Left ER Before Being Seen	29,880	4%	3%	2%
Time from ER Arrival to Admit. (minutes)[2]	410	202	240	274
Time from ER Arrival to Discharge (minutes)	391	119	126	134
Time in ER Before Being Evaluated (minutes)	462	26	31	26
Time to Pain Meds for Fractures (minutes)	162	69	69	57
Heart Attack Care				
Aspirin Given at Discharge[1]	-	-	99%	99%
Fibrinolytic Meds Within 30 Min. of Arrival[7]	-	-	77%	54%
PCI Within 90 Minutes of Arrival[7]	-	-	97%	96%
Statin Prescribed at Discharge[7]	-	-	98%	98%
Heart Failure Care				
ACE Inhibitor or ARB for LVSD	27	100%	97%	97%
Discharge Instructions Given	69	100%	93%	94%
Evaluation of LVS Function	79	100%	99%	99%
Medicare Spending				
Medicare Spending per Patient (ratio)	-	0.92	0.98	0.98
Pneumonia Care				
Appropriate Initial Antibiotic Given	59	98%	95%	95%
Blood Culture Timing	87	99%	98%	98%
Pregnancy and Delivery Care				
Newborn Deliveries Scheduled Early[2]	41	2%	14%	6%
Preventive Care				
Immunization for Influenza[2]	516	99%	90%	90%
Immunization for Pneumonia[2]	516	99%	91%	92%
Stroke Care				
Anticoagulation Therapy for Atrial Fibrillation[1]	-	-	92%	95%
Antithrombotic Therapy Timing	27	100%	96%	98%
Assessed for Rehabilitation	31	100%	95%	97%
Discharged on Antithrombotic Therapy	31	100%	98%	99%
Discharged on Statin Medication	22	95%	90%	94%
Thrombolytic Therapy Timing[7]	-	-	38%	66%
Venous Thromboembolism Prophylaxis	25	100%	89%	94%
Written Stroke Educational Materials Given	18	100%	85%	88%
Surgical Care Improvement Project				
Appropriate Beta Blocker Usage	80	100%	98%	98%
Appropriate VTP Within 24 Hours	366	100%	98%	98%
Controlled Postoperative Blood Glucose[7]	-	-	97%	97%
Perioperative Temperature Management	404	100%	100%	100%
Prophylactic Antibiotic Selection	315	100%	99%	99%
Prophylactic Antibiotic Selection (Outpatient)	85	100%	98%	98%
Prophylactic Antibiotic Stopped	315	100%	98%	98%
Prophylactic Antibiotic Timing	315	100%	99%	99%
Prophylactic Antibiotic Timing (Outpatient)	86	99%	99%	98%
Urinary Catheter Removal	259	100%	98%	97%
Survey of Patients' Hospital Experiences				
Area Around Room 'Always' Quiet at Night	300+	68%	71%	61%
Doctors 'Always' Communicated Well	300+	85%	86%	82%
Home Recovery Information Given	300+	87%	84%	85%
Hospital Given 9 or 10 on 10 Point Scale	300+	68%	71%	71%
Meds 'Always' Explained Before Given	300+	64%	66%	64%
Nurses 'Always' Communicated Well	300+	80%	80%	79%
Pain 'Always' Well Controlled	300+	71%	72%	71%
Room and Bathroom 'Always' Clean	300+	68%	71%	73%
Timely Help 'Always' Received	300+	66%	68%	68%
Would Definitely Recommend Hospital	300+	70%	70%	71%
Use of Medical Imaging				
Cardiac Imaging Stress Test before Surgery	194	7.2%	6.5%	5.3%
Combination Abdominal CT Scan	704	3.4%	16.5%	10.5%
Combination Brain/Sinus CT Scan	644	5.1%	3.5%	2.7%
Combination Chest CT Scan	332	1.2%	4.2%	2.7%
Follow-up Mammogram/Ultrasound	1,089	5.1%	7.6%	8.8%
Lumbar Spine MRI for Low Back Pain	86	37.2%	40.2%	37.2%

Medical Center Barbour

820 W Washington St　　Phone: 334-688-7271
Eufaula, AL 36027　　Fax: 334-687-0028
URL: www.chs.net
Type: Acute Care Hospitals　　Emergency Services: Yes
Ownership: Govt - Hospital Dist/Auth　　Beds: 74

Key Personnel:
Operating Room. . . . . Debbie Homan
CEO/President. . . . . Steve Honeycutt
Chief of Medical Staff . . . . William King, MD

Measure	Cases	This Hosp.	State Avg.	U.S. Avg.
Blood Clot Prevention and Treatment				
Anticoagulation Overlap Therapy[2]	13	100%	91%	93%
ICU Venous Thromboembolism Prophylaxis[2]	173	95%	85%	92%
Incidence of Potentially Preventable VTE[2,7]	-	-	18%	10%
UFH with Dosages/Platelet Monitoring[1,2]	-	-	95%	97%
Venous Thromboembolism Prophylaxis[2]	466	90%	74%	85%
Warfarin Therapy Discharge Instructions[1,2]	-	-	77%	75%
Chest Pain/Possible Heart Attack Care				
Aspirin Given Within 24 Hours of Arrival	54	100%	96%	96%
Fibrinolytic Meds Within 30 Min. of Arrival[1]	-	-	57%	58%
Average Time to ECG (minutes)	59	14	6	7
Average Time to Transfer (minutes)[1]	-	-	61	60
Children's Asthma Care				
Received Home Management Plan of Care	-	-	-	88%
Received Reliever Medication	-	-	-	100%
Received Systemic Corticosteroids	-	-	-	100%
Emergency Department				
Admittance Decision Time (minutes)[2]	667	39	73	98
Head CT Results Within 45 Min. of Arrival	12	8%	45%	57%
Patients Who Left ER Before Being Seen	15,009	2%	3%	2%
Time from ER Arrival to Admit. (minutes)[2]	667	177	240	274
Time from ER Arrival to Discharge (minutes)	318	108	126	134
Time in ER Before Being Evaluated (minutes)	436	21	31	26
Time to Pain Meds for Fractures (minutes)	82	51	69	57
Heart Attack Care				
Aspirin Given at Discharge[1,2]	-	-	99%	99%
Fibrinolytic Meds Within 30 Min. of Arrival[2,7]	-	-	77%	54%
PCI Within 90 Minutes of Arrival[2,7]	-	-	97%	96%
Statin Prescribed at Discharge[1,2]	-	-	98%	98%
Heart Failure Care				
ACE Inhibitor or ARB for LVSD[2]	28	100%	97%	97%
Discharge Instructions Given[2]	58	95%	93%	94%
Evaluation of LVS Function[2]	68	100%	99%	99%
Medicare Spending				
Medicare Spending per Patient (ratio)	-	0.98	0.98	0.98
Pneumonia Care				

NOTE: Hospital profiles are in alphabetical order by state, then city, then hospital within the city; Rankings exclude hospitals with less than 25 cases except for patient surveys which excludes hospitals with less than 100 cases; (a) 100-299 cases; (1) The number of cases/patients is too few to report; (2) Data submitted were based on a sample of cases/patients; (3) Results are based on a shorter time period than required; (4) Data suppressed by CMS for one or more quarters; (5) Results are not available for this reporting period; (6) Fewer than 100 patients completed the HCAHPS survey; (7) No cases met the criteria for this measure; (8) The lower limit of the confidence interval cannot be calculated if the number of observed infections equals zero; (9) No data are available from the state/territory for this reporting period; (10) The scores shown reflect fewer than 50 completed surveys; (11) There were discrepancies in the data collection process; (12) This measure does not apply to this hospital for this reporting period; (13) Results cannot be calculated for this reporting period; (14) The results for this state are combined with nearby states to protect confidentiality; Please refer to the User's Guide for a full explanation of data.

Measure	Cases	This Hosp.	State Avg.	U.S. Avg.
Appropriate Initial Antibiotic Given[2]	35	89%	95%	95%
Blood Culture Timing[2]	42	93%	98%	98%
Pregnancy and Delivery Care				
Newborn Deliveries Scheduled Early[7]	-	-	14%	6%
Preventive Care				
Immunization for Influenza[2]	395	95%	90%	90%
Immunization for Pneumonia[2]	526	91%	91%	92%
Stroke Care				
Anticoagulation Therapy for Atrial Fibrillation[1,2]	-	-	92%	95%
Antithrombotic Therapy Timing[2]	12	100%	96%	98%
Assessed for Rehabilitation[2]	16	88%	95%	97%
Discharged on Antithrombotic Therapy[2]	15	100%	98%	99%
Discharged on Statin Medication[2]	11	82%	90%	94%
Thrombolytic Therapy Timing[1,2]	-	-	38%	66%
Venous Thromboembolism Prophylaxis[2]	17	82%	89%	94%
Written Stroke Educational Materials Given[1,2]	-	-	85%	88%
Surgical Care Improvement Project				
Appropriate Beta Blocker Usage[1,2]	-	-	98%	98%
Appropriate VTP Within 24 Hours[1,2]	-	-	98%	98%
Controlled Postoperative Blood Glucose[2,7]	-	-	97%	97%
Perioperative Temperature Management[2]	21	100%	100%	100%
Prophylactic Antibiotic Selection[1,2]	-	-	99%	99%
Prophylactic Antibiotic Selection (Outpatient)	12	100%	98%	98%
Prophylactic Antibiotic Stopped[1,2]	-	-	98%	98%
Prophylactic Antibiotic Timing[1,2]	-	-	99%	99%
Prophylactic Antibiotic Timing (Outpatient)	14	79%	99%	98%
Urinary Catheter Removal[1,2]	-	-	98%	97%
Survey of Patients' Hospital Experiences				
Area Around Room 'Always' Quiet at Night	(a)	73%	71%	61%
Doctors 'Always' Communicated Well	(a)	84%	86%	82%
Home Recovery Information Given	(a)	84%	84%	85%
Hospital Given 9 or 10 on 10 Point Scale	(a)	72%	71%	71%
Meds 'Always' Explained Before Given	(a)	66%	66%	64%
Nurses 'Always' Communicated Well	(a)	80%	80%	79%
Pain 'Always' Well Controlled	(a)	73%	72%	71%
Room and Bathroom 'Always' Clean	(a)	72%	71%	73%
Timely Help 'Always' Received	(a)	63%	68%	68%
Would Definitely Recommend Hospital	(a)	67%	70%	71%
Use of Medical Imaging				
Cardiac Imaging Stress Test before Surgery	202	3.0%	6.5%	5.3%
Combination Abdominal CT Scan	292	11.3%	16.5%	10.5%
Combination Brain/Sinus CT Scan[1]	-	-	3.5%	2.7%
Combination Chest CT Scan	167	6.0%	4.2%	2.7%
Follow-up Mammogram/Ultrasound	518	6.0%	7.6%	8.8%
Lumbar Spine MRI for Low Back Pain[7]	-	-	40.2%	37.2%

Greene County Hospital

509 Wilson Avenue
Eutaw, AL 35462
Phone: 205-372-3388
Fax: 205-372-2716
Type: Acute Care Hospitals
Ownership: Government - Local
Emergency Services: Yes
Beds: 20

Key Personnel:
CEO/President. . . . . Robert J Coker, Jr
Chief of Medical Staff. . . . . S Faroogai
Emergency Room . . . . Myra Marzette

Measure	Cases	This Hosp.	State Avg.	U.S. Avg.
Blood Clot Prevention and Treatment				
Anticoagulation Overlap Therapy[1,2]	-	-	91%	93%
ICU Venous Thromboembolism Prophylaxis[2,7]	-	-	85%	92%
Incidence of Potentially Preventable VTE[2,7]	-	-	18%	10%
UFH with Dosages/Platelet Monitoring[2,7]	-	-	95%	97%
Venous Thromboembolism Prophylaxis[2]	167	17%	74%	85%
Warfarin Therapy Discharge Instructions[2,7]	-	-	77%	75%
Chest Pain/Possible Heart Attack Care				
Aspirin Given Within 24 Hours of Arrival[5]	-	-	96%	96%
Fibrinolytic Meds Within 30 Min. of Arrival[5]	-	-	57%	58%
Average Time to ECG (minutes)[5]	-	-	6	7
Average Time to Transfer (minutes)[5]	-	-	61	60
Children's Asthma Care				
Received Home Management Plan of Care	-	-	-	88%
Received Reliever Medication	-	-	-	100%
Received Systemic Corticosteroids	-	-	-	100%
Emergency Department				
Admittance Decision Time (minutes)[2]	313	5	73	98
Head CT Results Within 45 Min. of Arrival[5]	-	-	45%	57%
Patients Who Left ER Before Being Seen	5,202	1%	3%	2%
Time from ER Arrival to Admit. (minutes)[2]	321	165	240	274
Time from ER Arrival to Discharge (minutes)	388	137	126	134
Time in ER Before Being Evaluated (minutes)	287	57	31	26
Time to Pain Meds for Fractures (minutes)[1,3]	-	-	69	57
Heart Attack Care				
Aspirin Given at Discharge[5]	-	-	99%	99%
Fibrinolytic Meds Within 30 Min. of Arrival[5]	-	-	77%	54%
PCI Within 90 Minutes of Arrival[5]	-	-	97%	96%
Statin Prescribed at Discharge[5]	-	-	98%	98%
Heart Failure Care				
ACE Inhibitor or ARB for LVSD[2,3]	14	93%	97%	97%
Discharge Instructions Given[2,3]	26	69%	93%	94%
Evaluation of LVS Function[2,3]	30	93%	99%	99%
Medicare Spending				
Medicare Spending per Patient (ratio)	-	0.89	0.98	0.98
Pneumonia Care				
Appropriate Initial Antibiotic Given[2,3]	18	83%	95%	95%
Blood Culture Timing[1,2]	-	-	98%	98%
Pregnancy and Delivery Care				
Newborn Deliveries Scheduled Early[7]	-	-	14%	6%
Preventive Care				
Immunization for Influenza[2]	218	3%	90%	90%
Immunization for Pneumonia[2]	282	13%	91%	92%
Stroke Care				
Anticoagulation Therapy for Atrial Fibrillation[5]	-	-	92%	95%
Antithrombotic Therapy Timing[5]	-	-	96%	98%
Assessed for Rehabilitation[5]	-	-	95%	97%
Discharged on Antithrombotic Therapy[5]	-	-	98%	99%
Discharged on Statin Medication[5]	-	-	90%	94%
Thrombolytic Therapy Timing[5]	-	-	38%	66%
Venous Thromboembolism Prophylaxis[5]	-	-	89%	94%
Written Stroke Educational Materials Given[5]	-	-	85%	88%
Surgical Care Improvement Project				
Appropriate Beta Blocker Usage[5]	-	-	98%	98%
Appropriate VTP Within 24 Hours[5]	-	-	98%	98%
Controlled Postoperative Blood Glucose[5]	-	-	97%	97%
Perioperative Temperature Management[5]	-	-	100%	100%
Prophylactic Antibiotic Selection[5]	-	-	99%	99%
Prophylactic Antibiotic Selection (Outpatient)[5]	-	-	98%	98%
Prophylactic Antibiotic Stopped[5]	-	-	98%	98%
Prophylactic Antibiotic Timing[5]	-	-	99%	99%
Prophylactic Antibiotic Timing (Outpatient)[5]	-	-	99%	98%
Urinary Catheter Removal[5]	-	-	98%	97%
Survey of Patients' Hospital Experiences				
Area Around Room 'Always' Quiet at Night[6]	<100	70%	71%	61%
Doctors 'Always' Communicated Well[6]	<100	92%	86%	82%
Home Recovery Information Given[6]	<100	80%	84%	85%
Hospital Given 9 or 10 on 10 Point Scale[6]	<100	63%	71%	71%
Meds 'Always' Explained Before Given[6]	<100	58%	66%	64%
Nurses 'Always' Communicated Well[6]	<100	79%	80%	79%
Pain 'Always' Well Controlled[6]	<100	66%	72%	71%
Room and Bathroom 'Always' Clean[6]	<100	74%	71%	73%
Timely Help 'Always' Received[6]	<100	67%	68%	68%
Would Definitely Recommend Hospital[6]	<100	71%	70%	71%
Use of Medical Imaging				
Cardiac Imaging Stress Test before Surgery[7]	-	-	6.5%	5.3%
Combination Abdominal CT Scan[1]	-	-	16.5%	10.5%
Combination Brain/Sinus CT Scan	64	0.0%	3.5%	2.7%
Combination Chest CT Scan[1]	-	-	4.2%	2.7%
Follow-up Mammogram/Ultrasound[7]	-	-	7.6%	8.8%
Lumbar Spine MRI for Low Back Pain[7]	-	-	40.2%	37.2%

Evergreen Medical Center

101 Crestview Avenue
Evergreen, AL 36401
Phone: 251-578-2480
URL: www.evergreenmedical.org
Type: Acute Care Hospitals
Ownership: Proprietary
Emergency Services: Yes
Beds: 44

Key Personnel:
Chair/CEO. . . . . Al DeYoung
Administrator . . . . Bob Humphrey
CEO . . . . Robert H. Malte

Measure	Cases	This Hosp.	State Avg.	U.S. Avg.
Blood Clot Prevention and Treatment				
Anticoagulation Overlap Therapy[1,2]	-	-	91%	93%
ICU Venous Thromboembolism Prophylaxis[2,7]	-	-	85%	92%
Incidence of Potentially Preventable VTE[1,2]	-	-	18%	10%
UFH with Dosages/Platelet Monitoring[2,7]	-	-	95%	97%
Venous Thromboembolism Prophylaxis[2]	263	26%	74%	85%
Warfarin Therapy Discharge Instructions[1,2]	-	-	77%	75%
Chest Pain/Possible Heart Attack Care				
Aspirin Given Within 24 Hours of Arrival	11	100%	96%	96%
Fibrinolytic Meds Within 30 Min. of Arrival[3,7]	-	-	57%	58%
Average Time to ECG (minutes)	12	6	6	7
Average Time to Transfer (minutes)[3,7]	-	-	61	60
Children's Asthma Care				
Received Home Management Plan of Care	-	-	-	88%
Received Reliever Medication	-	-	-	100%
Received Systemic Corticosteroids	-	-	-	100%
Emergency Department				
Admittance Decision Time (minutes)[2]	435	60	73	98
Head CT Results Within 45 Min. of Arrival[1]	-	-	45%	57%
Patients Who Left ER Before Being Seen	10,721	1%	3%	2%
Time from ER Arrival to Admit. (minutes)[2]	458	199	240	274
Time from ER Arrival to Discharge (minutes)	520	110	126	134
Time in ER Before Being Evaluated (minutes)	554	40	31	26
Time to Pain Meds for Fractures (minutes)	36	78	69	57
Heart Attack Care				
Aspirin Given at Discharge[1]	-	-	99%	99%
Fibrinolytic Meds Within 30 Min. of Arrival[7]	-	-	77%	54%
PCI Within 90 Minutes of Arrival[7]	-	-	97%	96%
Statin Prescribed at Discharge[1]	-	-	98%	98%
Heart Failure Care				
ACE Inhibitor or ARB for LVSD[2]	18	83%	97%	97%
Discharge Instructions Given[2]	91	84%	93%	94%
Evaluation of LVS Function[2]	99	86%	99%	99%
Medicare Spending				
Medicare Spending per Patient (ratio)	-	0.91	0.98	0.98
Pneumonia Care				
Appropriate Initial Antibiotic Given[2]	30	80%	95%	95%
Blood Culture Timing[2]	23	91%	98%	98%
Pregnancy and Delivery Care				
Newborn Deliveries Scheduled Early[7]	-	-	14%	6%
Preventive Care				
Immunization for Influenza[2]	295	56%	90%	90%
Immunization for Pneumonia[2]	438	58%	91%	92%
Stroke Care				
Anticoagulation Therapy for Atrial Fibrillation[1]	-	-	92%	95%
Antithrombotic Therapy Timing	27	81%	96%	98%
Assessed for Rehabilitation	26	92%	95%	97%
Discharged on Antithrombotic Therapy	25	80%	98%	99%
Discharged on Statin Medication	17	71%	90%	94%
Thrombolytic Therapy Timing	13	0%	38%	66%
Venous Thromboembolism Prophylaxis	29	28%	89%	94%
Written Stroke Educational Materials Given	15	87%	85%	88%
Surgical Care Improvement Project				
Appropriate Beta Blocker Usage[5]	-	-	98%	98%
Appropriate VTP Within 24 Hours[5]	-	-	98%	98%
Controlled Postoperative Blood Glucose[5]	-	-	97%	97%
Perioperative Temperature Management[5]	-	-	100%	100%
Prophylactic Antibiotic Selection[5]	-	-	99%	99%
Prophylactic Antibiotic Selection (Outpatient)[3,7]	-	-	98%	98%
Prophylactic Antibiotic Stopped[5]	-	-	98%	98%
Prophylactic Antibiotic Timing[5]	-	-	99%	99%
Prophylactic Antibiotic Timing (Outpatient)[1,3]	-	-	99%	98%
Urinary Catheter Removal[5]	-	-	98%	97%
Survey of Patients' Hospital Experiences				
Area Around Room 'Always' Quiet at Night	(a)	72%	71%	61%
Doctors 'Always' Communicated Well	(a)	89%	86%	82%
Home Recovery Information Given	(a)	86%	84%	85%
Hospital Given 9 or 10 on 10 Point Scale	(a)	73%	71%	71%
Meds 'Always' Explained Before Given	(a)	59%	66%	64%

NOTE: Hospital profiles are in alphabetical order by state, then city, then hospital within the city; Rankings exclude hospitals with less than 25 cases except for patient surveys which excludes hospitals with less than 100 cases; (a) 100-299 cases; (1) The number of cases/patients is too few to report; (2) Data submitted were based on a sample of cases/patients; (3) Results are based on a shorter time period than required; (4) Data suppressed by CMS for one or more quarters; (5) Results are not available for this reporting period; (6) Fewer than 100 patients completed the HCAHPS survey; (7) No cases met the criteria for this measure; (8) The lower limit of the confidence interval cannot be calculated if the number of observed infections equals zero; (9) No data are available from the state/territory for this reporting period; (10) The scores shown reflect fewer than 50 completed surveys; (11) There were discrepancies in the data collection process; (12) This measure does not apply to this hospital for this reporting period; (13) Results cannot be calculated for this reporting period; (14) The results for this state are combined with nearby states to protect confidentiality; Please refer to the User's Guide for a full explanation of data.

Measure	Cases	This Hosp.	State Avg.	U.S. Avg.
Nurses 'Always' Communicated Well	(a)	79%	80%	79%
Pain 'Always' Well Controlled	(a)	71%	72%	71%
Room and Bathroom 'Always' Clean	(a)	71%	71%	73%
Timely Help 'Always' Received	(a)	67%	68%	68%
Would Definitely Recommend Hospital	(a)	70%	70%	71%
Use of Medical Imaging				
Cardiac Imaging Stress Test before Surgery[7]	-	-	6.5%	5.3%
Combination Abdominal CT Scan	149	66.4%	16.5%	10.5%
Combination Brain/Sinus CT Scan[1]	-	-	3.5%	2.7%
Combination Chest CT Scan	91	35.2%	4.2%	2.7%
Follow-up Mammogram/Ultrasound	247	10.1%	7.6%	8.8%
Lumbar Spine MRI for Low Back Pain	49	44.9%	40.2%	37.2%

Thomas Hospital

750 Morphy Avenue
Fairhope, AL 36532
E-mail: info@thomashospital.com
URL: www.thomashospital.com
Type: Acute Care Hospitals
Ownership: Govt - Hospital Dist/Auth
Phone: 251-928-2375
Fax: 251-928-8028
Emergency Services: Yes
Beds: 150

Key Personnel:
Coronary Care . . . . Kim Devilbiss, RN
Radiology. . . . . Robert Favret, Jr, MD
Operating Room. . . . . Jimmie Gavras, RN
Pediatric In-Patient Care . . . . Sharon Hollingworth, RN
Chief of Medical Staff . . . . Gary W Nelson, MD
CEO/President. . . . . D. Mark Nix
Infection Control . . . . Patti Thames, RN
Quality Assurance . . . . Wanda Winfree

Measure	Cases	This Hosp.	State Avg.	U.S. Avg.
Blood Clot Prevention and Treatment				
Anticoagulation Overlap Therapy[2]	91	87%	91%	93%
ICU Venous Thromboembolism Prophylaxis[2]	78	81%	85%	92%
Incidence of Potentially Preventable VTE[2]	18	11%	18%	10%
UFH with Dosages/Platelet Monitoring[2]	20	100%	95%	97%
Venous Thromboembolism Prophylaxis[2]	293	83%	74%	85%
Warfarin Therapy Discharge Instructions[2]	74	47%	77%	75%
Chest Pain/Possible Heart Attack Care				
Aspirin Given Within 24 Hours of Arrival[3,7]	-	-	96%	96%
Fibrinolytic Meds Within 30 Min. of Arrival[5]	-	-	57%	58%
Average Time to ECG (minutes)[3,7]	-	-	6	7
Average Time to Transfer (minutes)[5]	-	-	61	60
Children's Asthma Care				
Received Home Management Plan of Care	-	-	-	88%
Received Reliever Medication	-	-	-	100%
Received Systemic Corticosteroids	-	-	-	100%
Emergency Department				
Admittance Decision Time (minutes)[2]	494	101	73	98
Head CT Results Within 45 Min. of Arrival	11	9%	45%	57%
Patients Who Left ER Before Being Seen	25,360	2%	3%	2%
Time from ER Arrival to Admit. (minutes)[2]	494	315	240	274
Time from ER Arrival to Discharge (minutes)	378	162	126	134
Time in ER Before Being Evaluated (minutes)	384	35	31	26
Time to Pain Meds for Fractures (minutes)	165	65	69	57
Heart Attack Care				
Aspirin Given at Discharge	271	100%	99%	99%
Fibrinolytic Meds Within 30 Min. of Arrival[7]	-	-	77%	54%
PCI Within 90 Minutes of Arrival	44	100%	97%	96%
Statin Prescribed at Discharge	261	99%	98%	98%
Heart Failure Care				
ACE Inhibitor or ARB for LVSD	59	97%	97%	97%
Discharge Instructions Given	182	95%	93%	94%
Evaluation of LVS Function	224	100%	99%	99%
Medicare Spending				
Medicare Spending per Patient (ratio)	-	0.97	0.98	0.98
Pneumonia Care				
Appropriate Initial Antibiotic Given	75	99%	95%	95%
Blood Culture Timing	133	100%	98%	98%
Pregnancy and Delivery Care				
Newborn Deliveries Scheduled Early	351	4%	14%	6%
Preventive Care				
Immunization for Influenza[2]	576	95%	90%	90%
Immunization for Pneumonia[2]	731	97%	91%	92%
Stroke Care				
Anticoagulation Therapy for Atrial Fibrillation[2]	19	95%	92%	95%
Antithrombotic Therapy Timing[2]	71	99%	96%	98%
Assessed for Rehabilitation[2]	72	97%	95%	97%
Discharged on Antithrombotic Therapy[2]	67	97%	98%	99%
Discharged on Statin Medication[2]	49	80%	90%	94%
Thrombolytic Therapy Timing[1,2]	-	-	38%	66%
Venous Thromboembolism Prophylaxis[2]	77	79%	89%	94%
Written Stroke Educational Materials Given[2]	49	98%	85%	88%
Surgical Care Improvement Project				
Appropriate Beta Blocker Usage[2]	142	97%	98%	98%
Appropriate VTP Within 24 Hours[2]	275	97%	98%	98%
Controlled Postoperative Blood Glucose[2]	124	99%	97%	97%
Perioperative Temperature Management[2]	344	100%	100%	100%
Prophylactic Antibiotic Selection[2]	321	99%	99%	99%
Prophylactic Antibiotic Selection (Outpatient)	294	96%	98%	98%
Prophylactic Antibiotic Stopped[2]	314	100%	98%	98%
Prophylactic Antibiotic Timing[2]	321	99%	99%	99%
Prophylactic Antibiotic Timing (Outpatient)	296	98%	99%	98%
Urinary Catheter Removal[2]	202	96%	98%	97%
Survey of Patients' Hospital Experiences				
Area Around Room 'Always' Quiet at Night	300+	74%	71%	61%
Doctors 'Always' Communicated Well	300+	83%	86%	82%
Home Recovery Information Given	300+	88%	84%	85%
Hospital Given 9 or 10 on 10 Point Scale	300+	76%	71%	71%
Meds 'Always' Explained Before Given	300+	67%	66%	64%
Nurses 'Always' Communicated Well	300+	82%	80%	79%
Pain 'Always' Well Controlled	300+	75%	72%	71%
Room and Bathroom 'Always' Clean	300+	68%	71%	73%
Timely Help 'Always' Received	300+	71%	68%	68%
Would Definitely Recommend Hospital	300+	79%	70%	71%
Use of Medical Imaging				
Cardiac Imaging Stress Test before Surgery	54	3.7%	6.5%	5.3%
Combination Abdominal CT Scan	748	4.0%	16.5%	10.5%
Combination Brain/Sinus CT Scan	730	1.8%	3.5%	2.7%
Combination Chest CT Scan	488	2.3%	4.2%	2.7%
Follow-up Mammogram/Ultrasound	1,977	6.1%	7.6%	8.8%
Lumbar Spine MRI for Low Back Pain	235	33.2%	40.2%	37.2%

Fayette Medical Center

1653 Temple Avenue North
Fayette, AL 35555
URL: www.dchsystem.com
Type: Acute Care Hospitals
Ownership: Voluntary non-profit - Other
Phone: 205-932-5966
Fax: 205-932-1260
Emergency Services: Yes
Beds: 61

Key Personnel:
Chief of Medical Staff . . . . Chelley Kay Alexander
Radiology. . . . . James Bankston
Administrator . . . . Barry S. Cochran
Quality Assurance . . . . Barry Eads

Measure	Cases	This Hosp.	State Avg.	U.S. Avg.
Blood Clot Prevention and Treatment				
Anticoagulation Overlap Therapy[2]	12	100%	91%	93%
ICU Venous Thromboembolism Prophylaxis[2]	23	87%	85%	92%
Incidence of Potentially Preventable VTE[1,2]	-	-	18%	10%
UFH with Dosages/Platelet Monitoring[2,7]	-	-	95%	97%
Venous Thromboembolism Prophylaxis[2]	131	63%	74%	85%
Warfarin Therapy Discharge Instructions[1,2]	-	-	77%	75%
Chest Pain/Possible Heart Attack Care				
Aspirin Given Within 24 Hours of Arrival	101	98%	96%	96%
Fibrinolytic Meds Within 30 Min. of Arrival[1]	-	-	57%	58%
Average Time to ECG (minutes)	106	4	6	7
Average Time to Transfer (minutes)[7]	-	-	61	60
Children's Asthma Care				
Received Home Management Plan of Care	-	-	-	88%
Received Reliever Medication	-	-	-	100%
Received Systemic Corticosteroids	-	-	-	100%
Emergency Department				
Admittance Decision Time (minutes)[2]	433	66	73	98
Head CT Results Within 45 Min. of Arrival[1]	-	-	45%	57%
Patients Who Left ER Before Being Seen	15,025	4%	3%	2%
Time from ER Arrival to Admit. (minutes)[2]	457	208	240	274
Time from ER Arrival to Discharge (minutes)	367	103	126	134
Time in ER Before Being Evaluated (minutes)	393	21	31	26
Time to Pain Meds for Fractures (minutes)	51	40	69	57
Heart Attack Care				
Aspirin Given at Discharge[1]	-	-	99%	99%
Fibrinolytic Meds Within 30 Min. of Arrival[7]	-	-	77%	54%
PCI Within 90 Minutes of Arrival[7]	-	-	97%	96%
Statin Prescribed at Discharge[1]	-	-	98%	98%
Heart Failure Care				
ACE Inhibitor or ARB for LVSD	13	100%	97%	97%
Discharge Instructions Given	40	100%	93%	94%
Evaluation of LVS Function	47	100%	99%	99%
Medicare Spending				
Medicare Spending per Patient (ratio)	-	0.87	0.98	0.98
Pneumonia Care				
Appropriate Initial Antibiotic Given[2]	68	99%	95%	95%
Blood Culture Timing[2]	95	98%	98%	98%
Pregnancy and Delivery Care				
Newborn Deliveries Scheduled Early[7]	-	-	14%	6%
Preventive Care				
Immunization for Influenza[2]	293	100%	90%	90%
Immunization for Pneumonia[2]	471	97%	91%	92%
Stroke Care				
Anticoagulation Therapy for Atrial Fibrillation[1]	-	-	92%	95%
Antithrombotic Therapy Timing	17	94%	96%	98%
Assessed for Rehabilitation	17	88%	95%	97%
Discharged on Antithrombotic Therapy	16	88%	98%	99%
Discharged on Statin Medication	12	83%	90%	94%
Thrombolytic Therapy Timing[1]	-	-	38%	66%
Venous Thromboembolism Prophylaxis	18	94%	89%	94%
Written Stroke Educational Materials Given[1]	-	-	85%	88%
Surgical Care Improvement Project				
Appropriate Beta Blocker Usage[1]	-	-	98%	98%
Appropriate VTP Within 24 Hours	14	100%	98%	98%
Controlled Postoperative Blood Glucose[7]	-	-	97%	97%
Perioperative Temperature Management	17	100%	100%	100%
Prophylactic Antibiotic Selection[1]	-	-	99%	99%
Prophylactic Antibiotic Selection (Outpatient)[1,3]	-	-	98%	98%
Prophylactic Antibiotic Stopped[1]	-	-	98%	98%
Prophylactic Antibiotic Timing[1]	-	-	99%	99%
Prophylactic Antibiotic Timing (Outpatient)[1,3]	-	-	99%	98%
Urinary Catheter Removal	11	100%	98%	97%
Survey of Patients' Hospital Experiences				
Area Around Room 'Always' Quiet at Night	(a)	77%	71%	61%
Doctors 'Always' Communicated Well	(a)	94%	86%	82%
Home Recovery Information Given	(a)	90%	84%	85%
Hospital Given 9 or 10 on 10 Point Scale	(a)	83%	71%	71%
Meds 'Always' Explained Before Given	(a)	76%	66%	64%
Nurses 'Always' Communicated Well	(a)	90%	80%	79%
Pain 'Always' Well Controlled	(a)	77%	72%	71%
Room and Bathroom 'Always' Clean	(a)	82%	71%	73%
Timely Help 'Always' Received	(a)	81%	68%	68%
Would Definitely Recommend Hospital	(a)	83%	70%	71%
Use of Medical Imaging				
Cardiac Imaging Stress Test before Surgery[1]	-	-	6.5%	5.3%
Combination Abdominal CT Scan	354	1.7%	16.5%	10.5%
Combination Brain/Sinus CT Scan[1]	-	-	3.5%	2.7%
Combination Chest CT Scan	170	1.8%	4.2%	2.7%
Follow-up Mammogram/Ultrasound	427	18.0%	7.6%	8.8%
Lumbar Spine MRI for Low Back Pain	77	42.9%	40.2%	37.2%

Florala Memorial Hospital

24273 Fifth Avenue
Florala, AL 36442
Type: Acute Care Hospitals
Ownership: Proprietary
Phone: 334-858-3287
Fax: 334-858-3287
Emergency Services: Yes
Beds: 23

Key Personnel:
Chief of Medical Staff . . . . S Vishwanath, MD

Measure	Cases	This Hosp.	State Avg.	U.S. Avg.
Blood Clot Prevention and Treatment				
Anticoagulation Overlap Therapy[2,3]	-	-	91%	93%
ICU Venous Thromboembolism Prophylaxis[2,3]	-	-	85%	92%
Incidence of Potentially Preventable VTE[2,3]	-	-	18%	10%
UFH with Dosages/Platelet Monitoring[2,3]	-	-	95%	97%

NOTE: Hospital profiles are in alphabetical order by state, then city, then hospital within the city; Rankings exclude hospitals with less than 25 cases except for patient surveys which excludes hospitals with less than 100 cases; (a) 100-299 cases; (1) The number of cases/patients is too few to report; (2) Data submitted were based on a sample of cases/patients; (3) Results are based on a shorter time period than required; (4) Data suppressed by CMS for one or more quarters; (5) Results are not available for this reporting period; (6) Fewer than 100 patients completed the HCAHPS survey; (7) No cases met the criteria for this measure; (8) The lower limit of the confidence interval cannot be calculated if the number of observed infections equals zero; (9) No data are available from the state/territory for this reporting period; (10) The scores shown reflect fewer than 50 completed surveys; (11) There were discrepancies in the data collection process; (12) This measure does not apply to this hospital for this reporting period; (13) Results cannot be calculated for this reporting period; (14) The results for this state are combined with nearby states to protect confidentiality; Please refer to the User's Guide for a full explanation of data.

Measure	Cases	This Hosp.	State Avg.	U.S. Avg.
Venous Thromboembolism Prophylaxis[2,3]	34	6%	74%	85%
Warfarin Therapy Discharge Instructions[2,3]	-	-	77%	75%
Chest Pain/Possible Heart Attack Care				
Aspirin Given Within 24 Hours of Arrival[5]	-	-	96%	96%
Fibrinolytic Meds Within 30 Min. of Arrival[5]	-	-	57%	58%
Average Time to ECG (minutes)[5]	-	-	6	7
Average Time to Transfer (minutes)[5]	-	-	61	60
Children's Asthma Care				
Received Home Management Plan of Care	-	-	-	88%
Received Reliever Medication	-	-	-	100%
Received Systemic Corticosteroids	-	-	-	100%
Emergency Department				
Admittance Decision Time (minutes)[2,3]	46	0	73	98
Head CT Results Within 45 Min. of Arrival[5]	-	-	45%	57%
Patients Who Left ER Before Being Seen	3,211	0%	3%	2%
Time from ER Arrival to Admit. (minutes)[2,3]	46	138	240	274
Time from ER Arrival to Discharge (minutes)	253	78	126	134
Time in ER Before Being Evaluated (minutes)	256	23	31	26
Time to Pain Meds for Fractures (minutes)[1,3]	-	-	69	57
Heart Attack Care				
Aspirin Given at Discharge[1,3]	-	-	99%	99%
Fibrinolytic Meds Within 30 Min. of Arrival[3,7]	-	-	77%	54%
PCI Within 90 Minutes of Arrival[3,7]	-	-	97%	96%
Statin Prescribed at Discharge[1,3]	-	-	98%	98%
Heart Failure Care				
ACE Inhibitor or ARB for LVSD[2,3]	-	-	97%	97%
Discharge Instructions Given[1,2]	-	-	93%	94%
Evaluation of LVS Function[1,2]	-	-	99%	99%
Medicare Spending				
Medicare Spending per Patient (ratio)	-	-	0.98	0.98
Pneumonia Care				
Appropriate Initial Antibiotic Given[2,3]	-	-	95%	95%
Blood Culture Timing[2,3]	-	-	98%	98%
Pregnancy and Delivery Care				
Newborn Deliveries Scheduled Early[2,3]	-	-	14%	6%
Preventive Care				
Immunization for Influenza[2]	32	50%	90%	90%
Immunization for Pneumonia[2,3]	54	57%	91%	92%
Stroke Care				
Anticoagulation Therapy for Atrial Fibrillation[5]	-	-	92%	95%
Antithrombotic Therapy Timing[5]	-	-	96%	98%
Assessed for Rehabilitation[5]	-	-	95%	97%
Discharged on Antithrombotic Therapy[5]	-	-	98%	99%
Discharged on Statin Medication[5]	-	-	90%	94%
Thrombolytic Therapy Timing[5]	-	-	38%	66%
Venous Thromboembolism Prophylaxis[5]	-	-	89%	94%
Written Stroke Educational Materials Given[5]	-	-	85%	88%
Surgical Care Improvement Project				
Appropriate Beta Blocker Usage[5]	-	-	98%	98%
Appropriate VTP Within 24 Hours[5]	-	-	98%	98%
Controlled Postoperative Blood Glucose[5]	-	-	97%	97%
Perioperative Temperature Management[5]	-	-	100%	100%
Prophylactic Antibiotic Selection[5]	-	-	99%	99%
Prophylactic Antibiotic Selection (Outpatient)[5]	-	-	98%	98%
Prophylactic Antibiotic Stopped[5]	-	-	98%	98%
Prophylactic Antibiotic Timing[5]	-	-	99%	99%
Prophylactic Antibiotic Timing (Outpatient)[5]	-	-	99%	98%
Urinary Catheter Removal[5]	-	-	98%	97%
Survey of Patients' Hospital Experiences				
Area Around Room 'Always' Quiet at Night[10]	<100	41%	71%	61%
Doctors 'Always' Communicated Well[10]	<100	94%	86%	82%
Home Recovery Information Given[10]	<100	78%	84%	85%
Hospital Given 9 or 10 on 10 Point Scale[10]	<100	55%	71%	71%
Meds 'Always' Explained Before Given[10]	<100	50%	66%	64%
Nurses 'Always' Communicated Well[10]	<100	80%	80%	79%
Pain 'Always' Well Controlled[10]	<100	85%	72%	71%
Room and Bathroom 'Always' Clean[10]	<100	56%	71%	73%
Timely Help 'Always' Received[10]	<100	68%	68%	68%
Would Definitely Recommend Hospital[10]	<100	52%	70%	71%
Use of Medical Imaging				
Cardiac Imaging Stress Test before Surgery[7]	-	-	6.5%	5.3%
Combination Abdominal CT Scan[1]	-	-	16.5%	10.5%
Combination Brain/Sinus CT Scan[1]	-	-	3.5%	2.7%
Combination Chest CT Scan[1]	-	-	4.2%	2.7%
Follow-up Mammogram/Ultrasound[7]	-	-	7.6%	8.8%
Lumbar Spine MRI for Low Back Pain[7]	-	-	40.2%	37.2%

Eliza Coffee Memorial Hospital

205 Marengo Street
Florence, AL 35631
Phone: 256-768-8400
Fax: 256-768-9420
URL: www.chgroup.org
Type: Acute Care Hospitals
Emergency Services: Yes
Ownership: Govt - Hospital Dist/Auth
Beds: 372

Key Personnel:
CEO/President. . . . . Carl Bailey
Pediatric In-Patient Care . . . . Beth Bevis
Radiology. . . . . Ken Buttone
Coronary Care . . . . Patrice Crosby
Infection Control. . . . . Pam Floyd
Operating Room. . . . . Marty Meadows
Quality Assurance . . . . Karen Ritter
Chief of Medical Staff. . . . . Dan Spangler

Measure	Cases	This Hosp.	State Avg.	U.S. Avg.
Blood Clot Prevention and Treatment				
Anticoagulation Overlap Therapy[2]	71	89%	91%	93%
ICU Venous Thromboembolism Prophylaxis[2]	129	83%	85%	92%
Incidence of Potentially Preventable VTE[1,2]	-	-	18%	10%
UFH with Dosages/Platelet Monitoring[2]	41	98%	95%	97%
Venous Thromboembolism Prophylaxis[2]	284	75%	74%	85%
Warfarin Therapy Discharge Instructions[2]	50	86%	77%	75%
Chest Pain/Possible Heart Attack Care				
Aspirin Given Within 24 Hours of Arrival[1]	-	-	96%	96%
Fibrinolytic Meds Within 30 Min. of Arrival[5]	-	-	57%	58%
Average Time to ECG (minutes)[1]	-	-	6	7
Average Time to Transfer (minutes)[5]	-	-	61	60
Children's Asthma Care				
Received Home Management Plan of Care	-	-	-	88%
Received Reliever Medication	-	-	-	100%
Received Systemic Corticosteroids	-	-	-	100%
Emergency Department				
Admittance Decision Time (minutes)[2]	339	55	73	98
Head CT Results Within 45 Min. of Arrival	11	55%	45%	57%
Patients Who Left ER Before Being Seen	42,353	0%	3%	2%
Time from ER Arrival to Admit. (minutes)[2]	387	214	240	274
Time from ER Arrival to Discharge (minutes)	354	127	126	134
Time in ER Before Being Evaluated (minutes)	379	13	31	26
Time to Pain Meds for Fractures (minutes)	40	64	69	57
Heart Attack Care				
Aspirin Given at Discharge[2]	261	100%	99%	99%
Fibrinolytic Meds Within 30 Min. of Arrival[2,7]	-	-	77%	54%
PCI Within 90 Minutes of Arrival[2]	52	98%	97%	96%
Statin Prescribed at Discharge[2]	254	100%	98%	98%
Heart Failure Care				
ACE Inhibitor or ARB for LVSD[2]	78	100%	97%	97%
Discharge Instructions Given[2]	216	96%	93%	94%
Evaluation of LVS Function[2]	256	100%	99%	99%
Medicare Spending				
Medicare Spending per Patient (ratio)	-	1.00	0.98	0.98
Pneumonia Care				
Appropriate Initial Antibiotic Given[2]	67	100%	95%	95%
Blood Culture Timing[2]	99	99%	98%	98%
Pregnancy and Delivery Care				
Newborn Deliveries Scheduled Early	84	5%	14%	6%
Preventive Care				
Immunization for Influenza[2]	517	98%	90%	90%
Immunization for Pneumonia[2]	641	98%	91%	92%
Stroke Care				
Anticoagulation Therapy for Atrial Fibrillation	17	100%	92%	95%
Antithrombotic Therapy Timing	88	97%	96%	98%
Assessed for Rehabilitation	100	92%	95%	97%
Discharged on Antithrombotic Therapy	89	99%	98%	99%
Discharged on Statin Medication	78	87%	90%	94%
Thrombolytic Therapy Timing[1]	-	-	38%	66%
Venous Thromboembolism Prophylaxis	107	72%	89%	94%
Written Stroke Educational Materials Given	49	71%	85%	88%
Surgical Care Improvement Project				
Appropriate Beta Blocker Usage[2]	195	99%	98%	98%
Appropriate VTP Within 24 Hours[2]	259	98%	98%	98%
Controlled Postoperative Blood Glucose[2]	87	99%	97%	97%
Perioperative Temperature Management[2]	385	100%	100%	100%
Prophylactic Antibiotic Selection[2]	334	99%	99%	99%
Prophylactic Antibiotic Selection (Outpatient)	492	99%	98%	98%
Prophylactic Antibiotic Stopped[2]	322	99%	98%	98%
Prophylactic Antibiotic Timing[2]	334	100%	99%	99%
Prophylactic Antibiotic Timing (Outpatient)	493	99%	99%	98%
Urinary Catheter Removal[2]	300	96%	98%	97%
Survey of Patients' Hospital Experiences				
Area Around Room 'Always' Quiet at Night	300+	60%	71%	61%
Doctors 'Always' Communicated Well	300+	81%	86%	82%
Home Recovery Information Given	300+	83%	84%	85%
Hospital Given 9 or 10 on 10 Point Scale	300+	56%	71%	71%
Meds 'Always' Explained Before Given	300+	58%	66%	64%
Nurses 'Always' Communicated Well	300+	76%	80%	79%
Pain 'Always' Well Controlled	300+	65%	72%	71%
Room and Bathroom 'Always' Clean	300+	54%	71%	73%
Timely Help 'Always' Received	300+	58%	68%	68%
Would Definitely Recommend Hospital	300+	51%	70%	71%
Use of Medical Imaging				
Cardiac Imaging Stress Test before Surgery	83	4.8%	6.5%	5.3%
Combination Abdominal CT Scan	1,449	12.8%	16.5%	10.5%
Combination Brain/Sinus CT Scan	1,094	3.7%	3.5%	2.7%
Combination Chest CT Scan	1,051	5.4%	4.2%	2.7%
Follow-up Mammogram/Ultrasound	1,484	8.2%	7.6%	8.8%
Lumbar Spine MRI for Low Back Pain	150	44.0%	40.2%	37.2%

South Baldwin Regional Medical Center

1613 North Mckenzie Street
Foley, AL 36535
Phone: 251-949-3400
Fax: 251-949-3404
URL: www.southbaldwinrmc.com
Type: Acute Care Hospitals
Emergency Services: Yes
Ownership: Proprietary
Beds: 82

Key Personnel:
Radiology. . . . . John Campbell
Infection Control. . . . . Vicki Coyle
Coronary Care . . . . Sharon Dunkin
Pediatric Ambulatory Care . . . . . . Gary Eberly, MD
Pediatric In-Patient Care . . . . Gary Eberly, MD
Chief of Medical Staff. . . . . Dennis McNulty, DO
Quality Assurance . . . . Linda Mevean
CEO/President. . . . . Stephen Penninoton

Measure	Cases	This Hosp.	State Avg.	U.S. Avg.
Blood Clot Prevention and Treatment				
Anticoagulation Overlap Therapy[2]	110	100%	91%	93%
ICU Venous Thromboembolism Prophylaxis[2]	74	100%	85%	92%
Incidence of Potentially Preventable VTE[2]	13	15%	18%	10%
UFH with Dosages/Platelet Monitoring[2]	11	100%	95%	97%
Venous Thromboembolism Prophylaxis[2]	414	100%	74%	85%
Warfarin Therapy Discharge Instructions[2]	88	100%	77%	75%
Chest Pain/Possible Heart Attack Care				
Aspirin Given Within 24 Hours of Arrival	73	100%	96%	96%
Fibrinolytic Meds Within 30 Min. of Arrival[7]	-	-	57%	58%
Average Time to ECG (minutes)	77	5	6	7
Average Time to Transfer (minutes)	20	28	61	60
Children's Asthma Care				
Received Home Management Plan of Care	-	-	-	88%
Received Reliever Medication	-	-	-	100%
Received Systemic Corticosteroids	-	-	-	100%
Emergency Department				
Admittance Decision Time (minutes)[2]	827	98	73	98
Head CT Results Within 45 Min. of Arrival[1]	-	-	45%	57%
Patients Who Left ER Before Being Seen	28,688	2%	3%	2%
Time from ER Arrival to Admit. (minutes)[2]	838	277	240	274
Time from ER Arrival to Discharge (minutes)	368	153	126	134
Time in ER Before Being Evaluated (minutes)	407	35	31	26
Time to Pain Meds for Fractures (minutes)	182	63	69	57
Heart Attack Care				
Aspirin Given at Discharge	23	100%	99%	99%
Fibrinolytic Meds Within 30 Min. of Arrival[7]	-	-	77%	54%
PCI Within 90 Minutes of Arrival[7]	-	-	97%	96%
Statin Prescribed at Discharge	18	100%	98%	98%

NOTE: Hospital profiles are in alphabetical order by state, then city, then hospital within the city; Rankings exclude hospitals with less than 25 cases except for patient surveys which excludes hospitals with less than 100 cases; (a) 100-299 cases; (1) The number of cases/patients is too few to report; (2) Data submitted were based on a sample of cases/patients; (3) Results are based on a shorter time period than required; (4) Data suppressed by CMS for one or more quarters; (5) Results are not available for this reporting period; (6) Fewer than 100 patients completed the HCAHPS survey; (7) No cases met the criteria for this measure; (8) The lower limit of the confidence interval cannot be calculated if the number of observed infections equals zero; (9) No data are available from the state/territory for this reporting period; (10) The scores shown reflect fewer than 50 completed surveys; (11) There were discrepancies in the data collection process; (12) This measure does not apply to this hospital for this reporting period; (13) Results cannot be calculated for this reporting period; (14) The results for this state are combined with nearby states to protect confidentiality; Please refer to the User's Guide for a full explanation of data.

Measure	Cases	This Hosp.	State Avg.	U.S. Avg.
Heart Failure Care				
ACE Inhibitor or ARB for LVSD	47	100%	97%	97%
Discharge Instructions Given	191	100%	93%	94%
Evaluation of LVS Function	219	100%	99%	99%
Medicare Spending				
Medicare Spending per Patient (ratio)	-	0.99	0.98	0.98
Pneumonia Care				
Appropriate Initial Antibiotic Given	156	99%	95%	95%
Blood Culture Timing	124	100%	98%	98%
Pregnancy and Delivery Care				
Newborn Deliveries Scheduled Early[2]	49	0%	14%	6%
Preventive Care				
Immunization for Influenza[2]	626	100%	90%	90%
Immunization for Pneumonia[2]	781	100%	91%	92%
Stroke Care				
Anticoagulation Therapy for Atrial Fibrillation	13	100%	92%	95%
Antithrombotic Therapy Timing	63	100%	96%	98%
Assessed for Rehabilitation	82	100%	95%	97%
Discharged on Antithrombotic Therapy	78	100%	98%	99%
Discharged on Statin Medication	47	100%	90%	94%
Thrombolytic Therapy Timing[1]	-	-	38%	66%
Venous Thromboembolism Prophylaxis	72	100%	89%	94%
Written Stroke Educational Materials Given	59	100%	85%	88%
Surgical Care Improvement Project				
Appropriate Beta Blocker Usage	69	99%	98%	98%
Appropriate VTP Within 24 Hours	277	100%	98%	98%
Controlled Postoperative Blood Glucose[7]	-	-	97%	97%
Perioperative Temperature Management	330	100%	100%	100%
Prophylactic Antibiotic Selection	188	99%	99%	99%
Prophylactic Antibiotic Selection (Outpatient)	139	100%	98%	98%
Prophylactic Antibiotic Stopped	174	100%	98%	98%
Prophylactic Antibiotic Timing	188	100%	99%	99%
Prophylactic Antibiotic Timing (Outpatient)	139	100%	99%	98%
Urinary Catheter Removal	162	100%	98%	97%
Survey of Patients' Hospital Experiences				
Area Around Room 'Always' Quiet at Night	300+	69%	71%	61%
Doctors 'Always' Communicated Well	300+	86%	86%	82%
Home Recovery Information Given	300+	90%	84%	85%
Hospital Given 9 or 10 on 10 Point Scale	300+	76%	71%	71%
Meds 'Always' Explained Before Given	300+	69%	66%	64%
Nurses 'Always' Communicated Well	300+	83%	80%	79%
Pain 'Always' Well Controlled	300+	77%	72%	71%
Room and Bathroom 'Always' Clean	300+	76%	71%	73%
Timely Help 'Always' Received	300+	71%	68%	68%
Would Definitely Recommend Hospital	300+	74%	70%	71%
Use of Medical Imaging				
Cardiac Imaging Stress Test before Surgery	137	3.6%	6.5%	5.3%
Combination Abdominal CT Scan	764	12.4%	16.5%	10.5%
Combination Brain/Sinus CT Scan	687	3.1%	3.5%	2.7%
Combination Chest CT Scan	427	6.8%	4.2%	2.7%
Follow-up Mammogram/Ultrasound	1,207	4.4%	7.6%	8.8%
Lumbar Spine MRI for Low Back Pain	191	31.4%	40.2%	37.2%

Dekalb Regional Medical Center

200 Medical Center Drive Phone: 256-845-3150
Fort Payne, AL 35968 Fax: 256-997-2512
E-mail: info@bhsala.com
URL: www.baptistmedical.org
Type: Acute Care Hospitals Emergency Services: Yes
Ownership: Proprietary Beds: 134

Key Personnel:
Infection Control. . . . . Patsy Craig, RN
Coronary Care . . . . Cindy Dalton, RN
Emergency Room . . . . Betty Miller, RN
Chief of Medical Staff. . . . . Daniel M Mince, MD
Patient Relations . . . . Alice Parker
CEO/President. . . . . J Peter Selman
Operating Room. . . . . Betty Smith
Quality Assurance . . . . Debra Thomas

Measure	Cases	This Hosp.	State Avg.	U.S. Avg.
Blood Clot Prevention and Treatment				
Anticoagulation Overlap Therapy[2]	18	94%	91%	93%
ICU Venous Thromboembolism Prophylaxis[2]	96	95%	85%	92%
Incidence of Potentially Preventable VTE[1,2]	-	-	18%	10%
UFH with Dosages/Platelet Monitoring[2]	14	100%	95%	97%
Venous Thromboembolism Prophylaxis[2]	209	98%	74%	85%
Warfarin Therapy Discharge Instructions[2]	13	100%	77%	75%
Chest Pain/Possible Heart Attack Care				
Aspirin Given Within 24 Hours of Arrival	37	100%	96%	96%
Fibrinolytic Meds Within 30 Min. of Arrival[1]	-	-	57%	58%
Average Time to ECG (minutes)	39	0	6	7
Average Time to Transfer (minutes)[1]	-	-	61	60
Children's Asthma Care				
Received Home Management Plan of Care	-	-	-	88%
Received Reliever Medication	-	-	-	100%
Received Systemic Corticosteroids	-	-	-	100%
Emergency Department				
Admittance Decision Time (minutes)[2]	491	92	73	98
Head CT Results Within 45 Min. of Arrival	15	80%	45%	57%
Patients Who Left ER Before Being Seen	37,985	1%	3%	2%
Time from ER Arrival to Admit. (minutes)[2]	494	218	240	274
Time from ER Arrival to Discharge (minutes)	398	122	126	134
Time in ER Before Being Evaluated (minutes)	417	18	31	26
Time to Pain Meds for Fractures (minutes)	148	60	69	57
Heart Attack Care				
Aspirin Given at Discharge	58	100%	99%	99%
Fibrinolytic Meds Within 30 Min. of Arrival[7]	-	-	77%	54%
PCI Within 90 Minutes of Arrival[1]	-	-	97%	96%
Statin Prescribed at Discharge	57	100%	98%	98%
Heart Failure Care				
ACE Inhibitor or ARB for LVSD	22	100%	97%	97%
Discharge Instructions Given	54	100%	93%	94%
Evaluation of LVS Function	82	100%	99%	99%
Medicare Spending				
Medicare Spending per Patient (ratio)	-	1.00	0.98	0.98
Pneumonia Care				
Appropriate Initial Antibiotic Given	60	97%	95%	95%
Blood Culture Timing	142	97%	98%	98%
Pregnancy and Delivery Care				
Newborn Deliveries Scheduled Early[2]	47	2%	14%	6%
Preventive Care				
Immunization for Influenza[2]	384	100%	90%	90%
Immunization for Pneumonia[2]	382	99%	91%	92%
Stroke Care				
Anticoagulation Therapy for Atrial Fibrillation[1]	-	-	92%	95%
Antithrombotic Therapy Timing	21	95%	96%	98%
Assessed for Rehabilitation	20	95%	95%	97%
Discharged on Antithrombotic Therapy	18	100%	98%	99%
Discharged on Statin Medication[1]	-	-	90%	94%
Thrombolytic Therapy Timing[7]	-	-	38%	66%
Venous Thromboembolism Prophylaxis	23	100%	89%	94%
Written Stroke Educational Materials Given[1]	-	-	85%	88%
Surgical Care Improvement Project				
Appropriate Beta Blocker Usage	56	98%	98%	98%
Appropriate VTP Within 24 Hours	126	100%	98%	98%
Controlled Postoperative Blood Glucose[7]	-	-	97%	97%
Perioperative Temperature Management	188	100%	100%	100%
Prophylactic Antibiotic Selection	148	99%	99%	99%
Prophylactic Antibiotic Selection (Outpatient)	75	100%	98%	98%
Prophylactic Antibiotic Stopped	144	99%	98%	98%
Prophylactic Antibiotic Timing	149	100%	99%	99%
Prophylactic Antibiotic Timing (Outpatient)	75	100%	99%	98%
Urinary Catheter Removal	71	100%	98%	97%
Survey of Patients' Hospital Experiences				
Area Around Room 'Always' Quiet at Night	300+	66%	71%	61%
Doctors 'Always' Communicated Well	300+	82%	86%	82%
Home Recovery Information Given	300+	87%	84%	85%
Hospital Given 9 or 10 on 10 Point Scale	300+	70%	71%	71%
Meds 'Always' Explained Before Given	300+	61%	66%	64%
Nurses 'Always' Communicated Well	300+	80%	80%	79%
Pain 'Always' Well Controlled	300+	70%	72%	71%
Room and Bathroom 'Always' Clean	300+	67%	71%	73%
Timely Help 'Always' Received	300+	66%	68%	68%
Would Definitely Recommend Hospital	300+	65%	70%	71%
Use of Medical Imaging				
Cardiac Imaging Stress Test before Surgery	112	6.3%	6.5%	5.3%
Combination Abdominal CT Scan	467	15.4%	16.5%	10.5%
Combination Brain/Sinus CT Scan[1]	-	-	3.5%	2.7%
Combination Chest CT Scan	180	18.9%	4.2%	2.7%
Follow-up Mammogram/Ultrasound	746	5.0%	7.6%	8.8%
Lumbar Spine MRI for Low Back Pain	64	35.9%	40.2%	37.2%

Gadsden Regional Medical Center

1007 Goodyear Avenue Phone: 256-494-4000
Gadsden, AL 35903 Fax: 256-494-4474
E-mail: grmcphysicianservices@gadsdenregional.com
URL: www.gadsdenregional.com
Type: Acute Care Hospitals Emergency Services: Yes
Ownership: Proprietary Beds: 346

Key Personnel:
Cardiac Laboratory. . . . . Carol Davis
CEO/President. . . . . Doug DeGraaf
Infection Control. . . . . Teresa Fox, RN
Chief of Medical Staff . . . . Bruce Head, MD
Quality Assurance . . . . Lisa Henderson, RN
Operating Room. . . . . Amy Ragsdale
Radiology. . . . . Bill Ross

Measure	Cases	This Hosp.	State Avg.	U.S. Avg.
Blood Clot Prevention and Treatment				
Anticoagulation Overlap Therapy[2]	80	84%	91%	93%
ICU Venous Thromboembolism Prophylaxis[2]	147	78%	85%	92%
Incidence of Potentially Preventable VTE[2]	23	52%	18%	10%
UFH with Dosages/Platelet Monitoring[2]	66	100%	95%	97%
Venous Thromboembolism Prophylaxis[2]	379	75%	74%	85%
Warfarin Therapy Discharge Instructions[2]	50	94%	77%	75%
Chest Pain/Possible Heart Attack Care				
Aspirin Given Within 24 Hours of Arrival	12	100%	96%	96%
Fibrinolytic Meds Within 30 Min. of Arrival[3,7]	-	-	57%	58%
Average Time to ECG (minutes)	12	0	6	7
Average Time to Transfer (minutes)[3,7]	-	-	61	60
Children's Asthma Care				
Received Home Management Plan of Care	-	-	-	88%
Received Reliever Medication	-	-	-	100%
Received Systemic Corticosteroids	-	-	-	100%
Emergency Department				
Admittance Decision Time (minutes)[2]	592	119	73	98
Head CT Results Within 45 Min. of Arrival[1]	-	-	45%	57%
Patients Who Left ER Before Being Seen	41,653	1%	3%	2%
Time from ER Arrival to Admit. (minutes)[2]	595	365	240	274
Time from ER Arrival to Discharge (minutes)	359	188	126	134
Time in ER Before Being Evaluated (minutes)	410	54	31	26
Time to Pain Meds for Fractures (minutes)	150	73	69	57
Heart Attack Care				
Aspirin Given at Discharge	189	99%	99%	99%
Fibrinolytic Meds Within 30 Min. of Arrival[1]	-	-	77%	54%
PCI Within 90 Minutes of Arrival	36	97%	97%	96%
Statin Prescribed at Discharge	167	98%	98%	98%
Heart Failure Care				
ACE Inhibitor or ARB for LVSD	93	97%	97%	97%
Discharge Instructions Given	227	86%	93%	94%
Evaluation of LVS Function	303	100%	99%	99%
Medicare Spending				
Medicare Spending per Patient (ratio)	-	1.04	0.98	0.98
Pneumonia Care				
Appropriate Initial Antibiotic Given	237	95%	95%	95%
Blood Culture Timing	364	99%	98%	98%
Pregnancy and Delivery Care				
Newborn Deliveries Scheduled Early[2]	41	2%	14%	6%
Preventive Care				
Immunization for Influenza[2]	673	98%	90%	90%
Immunization for Pneumonia[2]	787	98%	91%	92%
Stroke Care				
Anticoagulation Therapy for Atrial Fibrillation	19	100%	92%	95%
Antithrombotic Therapy Timing	162	99%	96%	98%
Assessed for Rehabilitation	179	99%	95%	97%
Discharged on Antithrombotic Therapy	168	100%	98%	99%
Discharged on Statin Medication	133	96%	90%	94%
Thrombolytic Therapy Timing	13	77%	38%	66%
Venous Thromboembolism Prophylaxis	176	97%	89%	94%
Written Stroke Educational Materials Given	97	92%	85%	88%

NOTE: Hospital profiles are in alphabetical order by state, then city, then hospital within the city; Rankings exclude hospitals with less than 25 cases except for patient surveys which excludes hospitals with less than 100 cases; (a) 100-299 cases; (1) The number of cases/patients is too few to report; (2) Data submitted were based on a sample of cases/patients; (3) Results are based on a shorter time period than required; (4) Data suppressed by CMS for one or more quarters; (5) Results are not available for this reporting period; (6) Fewer than 100 patients completed the HCAHPS survey; (7) No cases met the criteria for this measure; (8) The lower limit of the confidence interval cannot be calculated if the number of observed infections equals zero; (9) No data are available from the state/territory for this reporting period; (10) The scores shown reflect fewer than 50 completed surveys; (11) There were discrepancies in the data collection process; (12) This measure does not apply to this hospital for this reporting period; (13) Results cannot be calculated for this reporting period; (14) The results for this state are combined with nearby states to protect confidentiality; Please refer to the User's Guide for a full explanation of data.

Surgical Care Improvement Project				
Appropriate Beta Blocker Usage	330	93%	98%	98%
Appropriate VTP Within 24 Hours	643	98%	98%	98%
Controlled Postoperative Blood Glucose	172	97%	97%	97%
Perioperative Temperature Management	768	99%	100%	100%
Prophylactic Antibiotic Selection	630	99%	99%	99%
Prophylactic Antibiotic Selection (Outpatient)	303	100%	98%	98%
Prophylactic Antibiotic Stopped	587	93%	98%	98%
Prophylactic Antibiotic Timing	632	100%	99%	99%
Prophylactic Antibiotic Timing (Outpatient)	303	99%	99%	98%
Urinary Catheter Removal	447	93%	98%	97%
Survey of Patients' Hospital Experiences				
Area Around Room 'Always' Quiet at Night	300+	66%	71%	61%
Doctors 'Always' Communicated Well	300+	81%	86%	82%
Home Recovery Information Given	300+	85%	84%	85%
Hospital Given 9 or 10 on 10 Point Scale	300+	71%	71%	71%
Meds 'Always' Explained Before Given	300+	64%	66%	64%
Nurses 'Always' Communicated Well	300+	80%	80%	79%
Pain 'Always' Well Controlled	300+	72%	72%	71%
Room and Bathroom 'Always' Clean	300+	68%	71%	73%
Timely Help 'Always' Received	300+	65%	68%	68%
Would Definitely Recommend Hospital	300+	76%	70%	71%
Use of Medical Imaging				
Cardiac Imaging Stress Test before Surgery	91	6.6%	6.5%	5.3%
Combination Abdominal CT Scan	792	15.7%	16.5%	10.5%
Combination Brain/Sinus CT Scan	790	4.2%	3.5%	2.7%
Combination Chest CT Scan	392	15.3%	4.2%	2.7%
Follow-up Mammogram/Ultrasound	688	7.0%	7.6%	8.8%
Lumbar Spine MRI for Low Back Pain	360	43.3%	40.2%	37.2%

Riverview Regional Medical Center

600 South Third Street
Gadsden, AL 35901
Phone: 256-543-5200
Fax: 256-543-5888
E-mail: info@riverviewregional.com
URL: www.riverviewregional.com
Type: Acute Care Hospitals
Emergency Services: Yes
Ownership: Proprietary
Beds: 281

Key Personnel:
Quality Assurance . . . . Paula Day
CEO/President. . . . . Jim Edmondson
Operating Room. . . . . Scott Morris, RN
Infection Control. . . . . Donna Pruin, RN
Pediatric In-Patient Care . . . . Donna Pruitt, RN
Radiology. . . . . Jack Russell
Chief of Medical Staff. . . . . Richael Wells

Measure	Cases	This Hosp.	State Avg.	U.S. Avg.
Blood Clot Prevention and Treatment				
Anticoagulation Overlap Therapy[2]	40	52%	91%	93%
ICU Venous Thromboembolism Prophylaxis[2]	83	51%	85%	92%
Incidence of Potentially Preventable VTE[2]	13	46%	18%	10%
UFH with Dosages/Platelet Monitoring[2]	28	100%	95%	97%
Venous Thromboembolism Prophylaxis[2]	388	28%	74%	85%
Warfarin Therapy Discharge Instructions[2]	28	86%	77%	75%
Chest Pain/Possible Heart Attack Care				
Aspirin Given Within 24 Hours of Arrival[1,3]	-	-	96%	96%
Fibrinolytic Meds Within 30 Min. of Arrival[5]	-	-	57%	58%
Average Time to ECG (minutes)[1,3]	-	-	6	7
Average Time to Transfer (minutes)[5]	-	-	61	60
Children's Asthma Care				
Received Home Management Plan of Care	-	-	-	88%
Received Reliever Medication	-	-	-	100%
Received Systemic Corticosteroids	-	-	-	100%
Emergency Department				
Admittance Decision Time (minutes)[2]	547	125	73	98
Head CT Results Within 45 Min. of Arrival[1]	-	-	45%	57%
Patients Who Left ER Before Being Seen	16,828	0%	3%	2%
Time from ER Arrival to Admit. (minutes)[2]	547	295	240	274
Time from ER Arrival to Discharge (minutes)	888	152	126	134
Time in ER Before Being Evaluated (minutes)	1,038	27	31	26
Time to Pain Meds for Fractures (minutes)	57	73	69	57
Heart Attack Care				
Aspirin Given at Discharge	69	100%	99%	99%
Fibrinolytic Meds Within 30 Min. of Arrival[7]	-	-	77%	54%
PCI Within 90 Minutes of Arrival	12	92%	97%	96%
Statin Prescribed at Discharge	61	100%	98%	98%
Heart Failure Care				
ACE Inhibitor or ARB for LVSD	46	100%	97%	97%
Discharge Instructions Given	138	100%	93%	94%
Evaluation of LVS Function	184	100%	99%	99%
Medicare Spending				
Medicare Spending per Patient (ratio)	-	1.06	0.98	0.98
Pneumonia Care				
Appropriate Initial Antibiotic Given	113	92%	95%	95%
Blood Culture Timing	169	99%	98%	98%
Pregnancy and Delivery Care				
Newborn Deliveries Scheduled Early[7]	-	-	14%	6%
Preventive Care				
Immunization for Influenza[2]	534	100%	90%	90%
Immunization for Pneumonia[2]	802	100%	91%	92%
Stroke Care				
Anticoagulation Therapy for Atrial Fibrillation[1]	-	-	92%	95%
Antithrombotic Therapy Timing	84	86%	96%	98%
Assessed for Rehabilitation	80	64%	95%	97%
Discharged on Antithrombotic Therapy	80	91%	98%	99%
Discharged on Statin Medication	70	71%	90%	94%
Thrombolytic Therapy Timing[1]	-	-	38%	66%
Venous Thromboembolism Prophylaxis	86	38%	89%	94%
Written Stroke Educational Materials Given	51	0%	85%	88%
Surgical Care Improvement Project				
Appropriate Beta Blocker Usage	151	96%	98%	98%
Appropriate VTP Within 24 Hours	327	99%	98%	98%
Controlled Postoperative Blood Glucose	42	93%	97%	97%
Perioperative Temperature Management	386	100%	100%	100%
Prophylactic Antibiotic Selection	288	98%	99%	99%
Prophylactic Antibiotic Selection (Outpatient)	155	97%	98%	98%
Prophylactic Antibiotic Stopped	255	96%	98%	98%
Prophylactic Antibiotic Timing	288	99%	99%	99%
Prophylactic Antibiotic Timing (Outpatient)	161	95%	99%	98%
Urinary Catheter Removal	288	99%	98%	97%
Survey of Patients' Hospital Experiences				
Area Around Room 'Always' Quiet at Night	300+	65%	71%	61%
Doctors 'Always' Communicated Well	300+	77%	86%	82%
Home Recovery Information Given	300+	76%	84%	85%
Hospital Given 9 or 10 on 10 Point Scale	300+	61%	71%	71%
Meds 'Always' Explained Before Given	300+	55%	66%	64%
Nurses 'Always' Communicated Well	300+	72%	80%	79%
Pain 'Always' Well Controlled	300+	63%	72%	71%
Room and Bathroom 'Always' Clean	300+	67%	71%	73%
Timely Help 'Always' Received	300+	55%	68%	68%
Would Definitely Recommend Hospital	300+	59%	70%	71%
Use of Medical Imaging				
Cardiac Imaging Stress Test before Surgery[1]	-	-	6.5%	5.3%
Combination Abdominal CT Scan	309	7.4%	16.5%	10.5%
Combination Brain/Sinus CT Scan[1]	-	-	3.5%	2.7%
Combination Chest CT Scan	150	9.3%	4.2%	2.7%
Follow-up Mammogram/Ultrasound[7]	-	-	7.6%	8.8%
Lumbar Spine MRI for Low Back Pain	46	34.8%	40.2%	37.2%

Wiregrass Medical Center

1200 W Maple Avenue
Geneva, AL 36340
Phone: 334-684-3655
Fax: 334-684-0299
URL: www.wiregrassmedicalcenter.org
Type: Acute Care Hospitals
Emergency Services: Yes
Ownership: Govt - Hospital Dist/Auth
Beds: 83

Key Personnel:
Infection Control. . . . . Judy Brown
Chief of Medical Staff . . . . Christopher S Cosper
CEO/President. . . . . Greg Dykes
Patient Relations . . . . Brenda Fountain
Emergency Room . . . . Jimmy McLeod
Operating Room. . . . . Dale Mitchum
Radiology. . . . . John C Tomberlin
Intensive Care Unit. . . . . Shan Wood

Measure	Cases	This Hosp.	State Avg.	U.S. Avg.
Blood Clot Prevention and Treatment				
Anticoagulation Overlap Therapy[1,2]	-	-	91%	93%
ICU Venous Thromboembolism Prophylaxis[2]	41	20%	85%	92%
Incidence of Potentially Preventable VTE[2,7]	-	-	18%	10%
UFH with Dosages/Platelet Monitoring[2,7]	-	-	95%	97%
Venous Thromboembolism Prophylaxis[2]	146	10%	74%	85%
Warfarin Therapy Discharge Instructions[1,2]	-	-	77%	75%
Chest Pain/Possible Heart Attack Care				
Aspirin Given Within 24 Hours of Arrival	17	88%	96%	96%
Fibrinolytic Meds Within 30 Min. of Arrival[1]	-	-	57%	58%
Average Time to ECG (minutes)	19	9	6	7
Average Time to Transfer (minutes)[1]	-	-	61	60
Children's Asthma Care				
Received Home Management Plan of Care	-	-	-	88%
Received Reliever Medication	-	-	-	100%
Received Systemic Corticosteroids	-	-	-	100%
Emergency Department				
Admittance Decision Time (minutes)[2]	362	50	73	98
Head CT Results Within 45 Min. of Arrival	13	8%	45%	57%
Patients Who Left ER Before Being Seen	11,061	3%	3%	2%
Time from ER Arrival to Admit. (minutes)[2]	394	175	240	274
Time from ER Arrival to Discharge (minutes)	371	113	126	134
Time in ER Before Being Evaluated (minutes)	397	41	31	26
Time to Pain Meds for Fractures (minutes)	42	72	69	57
Heart Attack Care				
Aspirin Given at Discharge[1,2]	-	-	99%	99%
Fibrinolytic Meds Within 30 Min. of Arrival[2,7]	-	-	77%	54%
PCI Within 90 Minutes of Arrival[2,7]	-	-	97%	96%
Statin Prescribed at Discharge[1,2]	-	-	98%	98%
Heart Failure Care				
ACE Inhibitor or ARB for LVSD[2]	16	50%	97%	97%
Discharge Instructions Given[2]	38	100%	93%	94%
Evaluation of LVS Function[2]	52	87%	99%	99%
Medicare Spending				
Medicare Spending per Patient (ratio)	-	0.94	0.98	0.98
Pneumonia Care				
Appropriate Initial Antibiotic Given[2]	64	58%	95%	95%
Blood Culture Timing[2]	54	80%	98%	98%
Pregnancy and Delivery Care				
Newborn Deliveries Scheduled Early[7]	-	-	14%	6%
Preventive Care				
Immunization for Influenza[2]	298	67%	90%	90%
Immunization for Pneumonia[2]	445	63%	91%	92%
Stroke Care				
Anticoagulation Therapy for Atrial Fibrillation[1]	-	-	92%	95%
Antithrombotic Therapy Timing[1]	-	-	96%	98%
Assessed for Rehabilitation[1]	-	-	95%	97%
Discharged on Antithrombotic Therapy[1]	-	-	98%	99%
Discharged on Statin Medication[1]	-	-	90%	94%
Thrombolytic Therapy Timing[1]	-	-	38%	66%
Venous Thromboembolism Prophylaxis[1]	-	-	89%	94%
Written Stroke Educational Materials Given[1]	-	-	85%	88%
Surgical Care Improvement Project				
Appropriate Beta Blocker Usage[1,2]	-	-	98%	98%
Appropriate VTP Within 24 Hours[2]	17	0%	98%	98%
Controlled Postoperative Blood Glucose[2,7]	-	-	97%	97%
Perioperative Temperature Management[2]	16	100%	100%	100%
Prophylactic Antibiotic Selection[2]	11	9%	99%	99%
Prophylactic Antibiotic Selection (Outpatient)[5]	-	-	98%	98%
Prophylactic Antibiotic Stopped[2]	11	9%	98%	98%
Prophylactic Antibiotic Timing[2]	11	27%	99%	99%
Prophylactic Antibiotic Timing (Outpatient)[5]	-	-	99%	98%
Urinary Catheter Removal[1,2]	-	-	98%	97%
Survey of Patients' Hospital Experiences				
Area Around Room 'Always' Quiet at Night	(a)	59%	71%	61%
Doctors 'Always' Communicated Well	(a)	86%	86%	82%
Home Recovery Information Given	(a)	83%	84%	85%
Hospital Given 9 or 10 on 10 Point Scale	(a)	57%	71%	71%
Meds 'Always' Explained Before Given	(a)	65%	66%	64%
Nurses 'Always' Communicated Well	(a)	78%	80%	79%
Pain 'Always' Well Controlled	(a)	72%	72%	71%
Room and Bathroom 'Always' Clean	(a)	72%	71%	73%
Timely Help 'Always' Received	(a)	67%	68%	68%
Would Definitely Recommend Hospital	(a)	59%	70%	71%
Use of Medical Imaging				
Cardiac Imaging Stress Test before Surgery[1]	-	-	6.5%	5.3%

NOTE: Hospital profiles are in alphabetical order by state, then city, then hospital within the city; Rankings exclude hospitals with less than 25 cases except for patient surveys which excludes hospitals with less than 100 cases; (a) 100-299 cases; (1) The number of cases/patients is too few to report; (2) Data submitted were based on a sample of cases/patients; (3) Results are based on a shorter time period than required; (4) Data suppressed by CMS for one or more quarters; (5) Results are not available for this reporting period; (6) Fewer than 100 patients completed the HCAHPS survey; (7) No cases met the criteria for this measure; (8) The lower limit of the confidence interval cannot be calculated if the number of observed infections equals zero; (9) No data are available from the state/territory for this reporting period; (10) The scores shown reflect fewer than 50 completed surveys; (11) There were discrepancies in the data collection process; (12) This measure does not apply to this hospital for this reporting period; (13) Results cannot be calculated for this reporting period; (14) The results for this state are combined with nearby states to protect confidentiality; Please refer to the User's Guide for a full explanation of data.

Measure	Cases	This Hosp.	State Avg.	U.S. Avg.
Combination Abdominal CT Scan	129	40.3%	16.5%	10.5%
Combination Brain/Sinus CT Scan	185	1.1%	3.5%	2.7%
Combination Chest CT Scan	62	0.0%	4.2%	2.7%
Follow-up Mammogram/Ultrasound	321	9.3%	7.6%	8.8%
Lumbar Spine MRI for Low Back Pain[7]	-	-	40.2%	37.2%

Georgiana Medical Center

515 N Miranda Avenue
Georgiana, AL 36033
Type: Acute Care Hospitals
Ownership: Proprietary
Phone: 334-376-2205
Fax: 334-376-9080
Emergency Services: Yes
Beds: 22

Key Personnel:
Emergency Room . . . . Cathy Cates
CEO/President. . . . . Harry Cole
Quality Assurance . . . . Rena McNeet
Chief of Medical Staff . . . . Geoffery Vorts

Measure	Cases	This Hosp.	State Avg.	U.S. Avg.
Blood Clot Prevention and Treatment				
Anticoagulation Overlap Therapy[1,2]	-	-	91%	93%
ICU Venous Thromboembolism Prophylaxis[2,7]	-	-	85%	92%
Incidence of Potentially Preventable VTE[2,7]	-	-	18%	10%
UFH with Dosages/Platelet Monitoring[1,2]	-	-	95%	97%
Venous Thromboembolism Prophylaxis[2]	116	82%	74%	85%
Warfarin Therapy Discharge Instructions[1,2]	-	-	77%	75%
Chest Pain/Possible Heart Attack Care				
Aspirin Given Within 24 Hours of Arrival[1,3]	-	-	96%	96%
Fibrinolytic Meds Within 30 Min. of Arrival[1,3]	-	-	57%	58%
Average Time to ECG (minutes)[1,3]	-	-	6	7
Average Time to Transfer (minutes)[3,7]	-	-	61	60
Children's Asthma Care				
Received Home Management Plan of Care	-	-	-	88%
Received Reliever Medication	-	-	-	100%
Received Systemic Corticosteroids	-	-	-	100%
Emergency Department				
Admittance Decision Time (minutes)[2]	322	40	73	98
Head CT Results Within 45 Min. of Arrival[5]	-	-	45%	57%
Patients Who Left ER Before Being Seen	3,528	0%	3%	2%
Time from ER Arrival to Admit. (minutes)[2]	327	145	240	274
Time from ER Arrival to Discharge (minutes)	388	86	126	134
Time in ER Before Being Evaluated (minutes)	397	45	31	26
Time to Pain Meds for Fractures (minutes)[1]	-	-	69	57
Heart Attack Care				
Aspirin Given at Discharge[1,3]	-	-	99%	99%
Fibrinolytic Meds Within 30 Min. of Arrival[3,7]	-	-	77%	54%
PCI Within 90 Minutes of Arrival[3,7]	-	-	97%	96%
Statin Prescribed at Discharge[1,3]	-	-	98%	98%
Heart Failure Care				
ACE Inhibitor or ARB for LVSD[1]	-	-	97%	97%
Discharge Instructions Given[1]	-	-	93%	94%
Evaluation of LVS Function[1]	-	-	99%	99%
Medicare Spending				
Medicare Spending per Patient (ratio)	-	1.00	0.98	0.98
Pneumonia Care				
Appropriate Initial Antibiotic Given	35	77%	95%	95%
Blood Culture Timing	14	100%	98%	98%
Pregnancy and Delivery Care				
Newborn Deliveries Scheduled Early[7]	-	-	14%	6%
Preventive Care				
Immunization for Influenza[2]	220	96%	90%	90%
Immunization for Pneumonia[2]	215	97%	91%	92%
Stroke Care				
Anticoagulation Therapy for Atrial Fibrillation[1]	-	-	92%	95%
Antithrombotic Therapy Timing[1]	-	-	96%	98%
Assessed for Rehabilitation[1]	-	-	95%	97%
Discharged on Antithrombotic Therapy[1]	-	-	98%	99%
Discharged on Statin Medication[1]	-	-	90%	94%
Thrombolytic Therapy Timing[1]	-	-	38%	66%
Venous Thromboembolism Prophylaxis[1]	-	-	89%	94%
Written Stroke Educational Materials Given[1]	-	-	85%	88%
Surgical Care Improvement Project				
Appropriate Beta Blocker Usage[5]	-	-	98%	98%
Appropriate VTP Within 24 Hours[5]	-	-	98%	98%
Controlled Postoperative Blood Glucose[5]	-	-	97%	97%
Perioperative Temperature Management[5]	-	-	100%	100%
Prophylactic Antibiotic Selection[5]	-	-	99%	99%
Prophylactic Antibiotic Selection (Outpatient)[5]	-	-	98%	98%
Prophylactic Antibiotic Stopped[5]	-	-	98%	98%
Prophylactic Antibiotic Timing[5]	-	-	99%	99%
Prophylactic Antibiotic Timing (Outpatient)[5]	-	-	99%	98%
Urinary Catheter Removal[5]	-	-	98%	97%
Survey of Patients' Hospital Experiences				
Area Around Room 'Always' Quiet at Night	(a)	72%	71%	61%
Doctors 'Always' Communicated Well	(a)	88%	86%	82%
Home Recovery Information Given	(a)	86%	84%	85%
Hospital Given 9 or 10 on 10 Point Scale	(a)	70%	71%	71%
Meds 'Always' Explained Before Given	(a)	79%	66%	64%
Nurses 'Always' Communicated Well	(a)	85%	80%	79%
Pain 'Always' Well Controlled	(a)	72%	72%	71%
Room and Bathroom 'Always' Clean	(a)	83%	71%	73%
Timely Help 'Always' Received	(a)	74%	68%	68%
Would Definitely Recommend Hospital	(a)	70%	70%	71%
Use of Medical Imaging				
Cardiac Imaging Stress Test before Surgery[1]	-	-	6.5%	5.3%
Combination Abdominal CT Scan	71	8.5%	16.5%	10.5%
Combination Brain/Sinus CT Scan	82	14.6%	3.5%	2.7%
Combination Chest CT Scan[1]	-	-	4.2%	2.7%
Follow-up Mammogram/Ultrasound[7]	-	-	7.6%	8.8%
Lumbar Spine MRI for Low Back Pain[7]	-	-	40.2%	37.2%

Hale County Hospital

508 Green Street
Greensboro, AL 36744
Type: Acute Care Hospitals
Ownership: Government - Local
Phone: 334-624-3024
Fax: 334-624-3800
Emergency Services: Yes
Beds: 25

Key Personnel:
Quality Assurance . . . . Melissa Averette
Chief of Medical Staff. . . . . Inkil Hwangpo, MD
CEO/President. . . . . Thomas Lackey

Measure	Cases	This Hosp.	State Avg.	U.S. Avg.
Blood Clot Prevention and Treatment				
Anticoagulation Overlap Therapy[1]	-	-	91%	93%
ICU Venous Thromboembolism Prophylaxis[7]	-	-	85%	92%
Incidence of Potentially Preventable VTE[1]	-	-	18%	10%
UFH with Dosages/Platelet Monitoring[7]	-	-	95%	97%
Venous Thromboembolism Prophylaxis	178	72%	74%	85%
Warfarin Therapy Discharge Instructions[1]	-	-	77%	75%
Chest Pain/Possible Heart Attack Care				
Aspirin Given Within 24 Hours of Arrival	25	80%	96%	96%
Fibrinolytic Meds Within 30 Min. of Arrival[3,7]	-	-	57%	58%
Average Time to ECG (minutes)	27	42	6	7
Average Time to Transfer (minutes)[3,7]	-	-	61	60
Children's Asthma Care				
Received Home Management Plan of Care	-	-	-	88%
Received Reliever Medication	-	-	-	100%
Received Systemic Corticosteroids	-	-	-	100%
Emergency Department				
Admittance Decision Time (minutes)[2]	322	35	73	98
Head CT Results Within 45 Min. of Arrival[1,3]	-	-	45%	57%
Patients Who Left ER Before Being Seen	7,511	2%	3%	2%
Time from ER Arrival to Admit. (minutes)[2]	322	202	240	274
Time from ER Arrival to Discharge (minutes)	345	115	126	134
Time in ER Before Being Evaluated (minutes)	386	32	31	26
Time to Pain Meds for Fractures (minutes)	23	108	69	57
Heart Attack Care				
Aspirin Given at Discharge[1,3]	-	-	99%	99%
Fibrinolytic Meds Within 30 Min. of Arrival[3,7]	-	-	77%	54%
PCI Within 90 Minutes of Arrival[3,7]	-	-	97%	96%
Statin Prescribed at Discharge[1,3]	-	-	98%	98%
Heart Failure Care				
ACE Inhibitor or ARB for LVSD[1]	-	-	97%	97%
Discharge Instructions Given	12	83%	93%	94%
Evaluation of LVS Function	18	94%	99%	99%
Medicare Spending				
Medicare Spending per Patient (ratio)	-	1.08	0.98	0.98
Pneumonia Care				
Appropriate Initial Antibiotic Given	23	65%	95%	95%
Blood Culture Timing	20	75%	98%	98%
Pregnancy and Delivery Care				
Newborn Deliveries Scheduled Early[7]	-	-	14%	6%
Preventive Care				
Immunization for Influenza[2]	185	51%	90%	90%
Immunization for Pneumonia[2]	222	48%	91%	92%
Stroke Care				
Anticoagulation Therapy for Atrial Fibrillation[5]	-	-	92%	95%
Antithrombotic Therapy Timing[5]	-	-	96%	98%
Assessed for Rehabilitation[5]	-	-	95%	97%
Discharged on Antithrombotic Therapy[5]	-	-	98%	99%
Discharged on Statin Medication[5]	-	-	90%	94%
Thrombolytic Therapy Timing[5]	-	-	38%	66%
Venous Thromboembolism Prophylaxis[5]	-	-	89%	94%
Written Stroke Educational Materials Given[5]	-	-	85%	88%
Surgical Care Improvement Project				
Appropriate Beta Blocker Usage[5]	-	-	98%	98%
Appropriate VTP Within 24 Hours[5]	-	-	98%	98%
Controlled Postoperative Blood Glucose[5]	-	-	97%	97%
Perioperative Temperature Management[5]	-	-	100%	100%
Prophylactic Antibiotic Selection[5]	-	-	99%	99%
Prophylactic Antibiotic Selection (Outpatient)[5]	-	-	98%	98%
Prophylactic Antibiotic Stopped[5]	-	-	98%	98%
Prophylactic Antibiotic Timing[5]	-	-	99%	99%
Prophylactic Antibiotic Timing (Outpatient)[5]	-	-	99%	98%
Urinary Catheter Removal[5]	-	-	98%	97%
Survey of Patients' Hospital Experiences				
Area Around Room 'Always' Quiet at Night[6]	<100	80%	71%	61%
Doctors 'Always' Communicated Well[6]	<100	90%	86%	82%
Home Recovery Information Given[6]	<100	87%	84%	85%
Hospital Given 9 or 10 on 10 Point Scale[6]	<100	64%	71%	71%
Meds 'Always' Explained Before Given[6]	<100	61%	66%	64%
Nurses 'Always' Communicated Well[6]	<100	85%	80%	79%
Pain 'Always' Well Controlled[6]	<100	70%	72%	71%
Room and Bathroom 'Always' Clean[6]	<100	81%	71%	73%
Timely Help 'Always' Received[6]	<100	70%	68%	68%
Would Definitely Recommend Hospital[6]	<100	68%	70%	71%
Use of Medical Imaging				
Cardiac Imaging Stress Test before Surgery[7]	-	-	6.5%	5.3%
Combination Abdominal CT Scan	85	0.0%	16.5%	10.5%
Combination Brain/Sinus CT Scan	147	0.7%	3.5%	2.7%
Combination Chest CT Scan[1]	-	-	4.2%	2.7%
Follow-up Mammogram/Ultrasound[7]	-	-	7.6%	8.8%
Lumbar Spine MRI for Low Back Pain[7]	-	-	40.2%	37.2%

L V Stabler Memorial Hospital

29 L V Stabler Drive
Greenville, AL 36037
URL: www.lvstabler.com
Type: Acute Care Hospitals
Ownership: Proprietary
Phone: 334-382-2200
Fax: 334-382-0305
Emergency Services: Yes
Beds: 72

Key Personnel:
Cardiac Laboratory. . . . . Terri Bagents
Operating Room. . . . . Eddie Dunn, RN
CEO/President. . . . . Bobby Ginn
Infection Control. . . . . Chris Killebrew
Chief of Medical Staff . . . . Florencia Sellers
Quality Assurance . . . . Nancy Smith, RN
Coronary Care . . . . Kimberli Weaver
Pediatric In-Patient Care . . . . Kimberli Weaver

Measure	Cases	This Hosp.	State Avg.	U.S. Avg.
Blood Clot Prevention and Treatment				
Anticoagulation Overlap Therapy[1,2]	-	-	91%	93%
ICU Venous Thromboembolism Prophylaxis[2]	138	99%	85%	92%
Incidence of Potentially Preventable VTE[2,7]	-	-	18%	10%
UFH with Dosages/Platelet Monitoring[2,7]	-	-	95%	97%
Venous Thromboembolism Prophylaxis[2]	191	98%	74%	85%
Warfarin Therapy Discharge Instructions[1,2]	-	-	77%	75%
Chest Pain/Possible Heart Attack Care				
Aspirin Given Within 24 Hours of Arrival	24	100%	96%	96%
Fibrinolytic Meds Within 30 Min. of Arrival[1]	-	-	57%	58%
Average Time to ECG (minutes)	27	7	6	7
Average Time to Transfer (minutes)[1]	-	-	61	60
Children's Asthma Care				

NOTE: Hospital profiles are in alphabetical order by state, then city, then hospital within the city; Rankings exclude hospitals with less than 25 cases except for patient surveys which excludes hospitals with less than 100 cases; (a) 100-299 cases; (1) The number of cases/patients is too few to report; (2) Data submitted were based on a sample of cases/patients; (3) Results are based on a shorter time period than required; (4) Data suppressed by CMS for one or more quarters; (5) Results are not available for this reporting period; (6) Fewer than 100 patients completed the HCAHPS survey; (7) No cases met the criteria for this measure; (8) The lower limit of the confidence interval cannot be calculated if the number of observed infections equals zero; (9) No data are available from the state/territory for this reporting period; (10) The scores shown reflect fewer than 50 completed surveys; (11) There were discrepancies in the data collection process; (12) This measure does not apply to this hospital for this reporting period; (13) Results cannot be calculated for this reporting period; (14) The results for this state are combined with nearby states to protect confidentiality; Please refer to the User's Guide for a full explanation of data.

Measure	Cases	This Hosp.	State Avg.	U.S. Avg.
Received Home Management Plan of Care	-	-	-	88%
Received Reliever Medication	-	-	-	100%
Received Systemic Corticosteroids	-	-	-	100%
Emergency Department				
Admittance Decision Time (minutes)[2]	371	56	73	98
Head CT Results Within 45 Min. of Arrival[1]	-	-	45%	57%
Patients Who Left ER Before Being Seen	1,043	1%	3%	2%
Time from ER Arrival to Admit. (minutes)[2]	376	194	240	274
Time from ER Arrival to Discharge (minutes)	393	87	126	134
Time in ER Before Being Evaluated (minutes)	423	25	31	26
Time to Pain Meds for Fractures (minutes)	49	64	69	57
Heart Attack Care				
Aspirin Given at Discharge[1,3]	-	-	99%	99%
Fibrinolytic Meds Within 30 Min. of Arrival[3,7]	-	-	77%	54%
PCI Within 90 Minutes of Arrival[3,7]	-	-	97%	96%
Statin Prescribed at Discharge[1,3]	-	-	98%	98%
Heart Failure Care				
ACE Inhibitor or ARB for LVSD	34	94%	97%	97%
Discharge Instructions Given	64	94%	93%	94%
Evaluation of LVS Function	73	99%	99%	99%
Medicare Spending				
Medicare Spending per Patient (ratio)	-	0.98	0.98	0.98
Pneumonia Care				
Appropriate Initial Antibiotic Given	23	100%	95%	95%
Blood Culture Timing	28	100%	98%	98%
Pregnancy and Delivery Care				
Newborn Deliveries Scheduled Early[2,7]	-	-	14%	6%
Preventive Care				
Immunization for Influenza[2]	326	100%	90%	90%
Immunization for Pneumonia[2]	417	100%	91%	92%
Stroke Care				
Anticoagulation Therapy for Atrial Fibrillation[1]	-	-	92%	95%
Antithrombotic Therapy Timing[1]	-	-	96%	98%
Assessed for Rehabilitation[1]	-	-	95%	97%
Discharged on Antithrombotic Therapy[1]	-	-	98%	99%
Discharged on Statin Medication[1]	-	-	90%	94%
Thrombolytic Therapy Timing[1]	-	-	38%	66%
Venous Thromboembolism Prophylaxis	11	100%	89%	94%
Written Stroke Educational Materials Given[1]	-	-	85%	88%
Surgical Care Improvement Project				
Appropriate Beta Blocker Usage	18	100%	98%	98%
Appropriate VTP Within 24 Hours	68	100%	98%	98%
Controlled Postoperative Blood Glucose[7]	-	-	97%	97%
Perioperative Temperature Management	69	100%	100%	100%
Prophylactic Antibiotic Selection	48	100%	99%	99%
Prophylactic Antibiotic Selection (Outpatient)[1]	-	-	98%	98%
Prophylactic Antibiotic Stopped	46	98%	98%	98%
Prophylactic Antibiotic Timing	48	100%	99%	99%
Prophylactic Antibiotic Timing (Outpatient)[1]	-	-	99%	98%
Urinary Catheter Removal	59	100%	98%	97%
Survey of Patients' Hospital Experiences				
Area Around Room 'Always' Quiet at Night	(a)	73%	71%	61%
Doctors 'Always' Communicated Well	(a)	87%	86%	82%
Home Recovery Information Given	(a)	85%	84%	85%
Hospital Given 9 or 10 on 10 Point Scale	(a)	70%	71%	71%
Meds 'Always' Explained Before Given	(a)	69%	66%	64%
Nurses 'Always' Communicated Well	(a)	78%	80%	79%
Pain 'Always' Well Controlled	(a)	68%	72%	71%
Room and Bathroom 'Always' Clean	(a)	72%	71%	73%
Timely Help 'Always' Received	(a)	67%	68%	68%
Would Definitely Recommend Hospital	(a)	68%	70%	71%
Use of Medical Imaging				
Cardiac Imaging Stress Test before Surgery	90	0.0%	6.5%	5.3%
Combination Abdominal CT Scan	185	12.4%	16.5%	10.5%
Combination Brain/Sinus CT Scan	233	6.4%	3.5%	2.7%
Combination Chest CT Scan	90	2.2%	4.2%	2.7%
Follow-up Mammogram/Ultrasound	469	6.6%	7.6%	8.8%
Lumbar Spine MRI for Low Back Pain[1]	-	-	40.2%	37.2%

Grove Hill Memorial Hospital

295 Jackson Hwy S
Grove Hill, AL 36451
Type: Acute Care Hospitals
Ownership: Government - Local
Phone: 251-275-3191
Fax: 251-275-4281
Emergency Services: Yes
Beds: 50

Key Personnel:
Quality Assurance . . . . Janee Parden
Emergency Room . . . . Dinah Pritchett
CEO/President. . . . . Doug Sewell
Operating Room. . . . . Debbie Stifflemie

Measure	Cases	This Hosp.	State Avg.	U.S. Avg.
Blood Clot Prevention and Treatment				
Anticoagulation Overlap Therapy[1,2]	-	-	91%	93%
ICU Venous Thromboembolism Prophylaxis[2,7]	-	-	85%	92%
Incidence of Potentially Preventable VTE[1,2]	-	-	18%	10%
UFH with Dosages/Platelet Monitoring[1,2]	-	-	95%	97%
Venous Thromboembolism Prophylaxis[2]	157	43%	74%	85%
Warfarin Therapy Discharge Instructions[1,2]	-	-	77%	75%
Chest Pain/Possible Heart Attack Care				
Aspirin Given Within 24 Hours of Arrival[3]	18	89%	96%	96%
Fibrinolytic Meds Within 30 Min. of Arrival[1,3]	-	-	57%	58%
Average Time to ECG (minutes)[3]	17	13	6	7
Average Time to Transfer (minutes)[3,7]	-	-	61	60
Children's Asthma Care				
Received Home Management Plan of Care	-	-	-	88%
Received Reliever Medication	-	-	-	100%
Received Systemic Corticosteroids	-	-	-	100%
Emergency Department				
Admittance Decision Time (minutes)[2]	251	40	73	98
Head CT Results Within 45 Min. of Arrival	11	18%	45%	57%
Patients Who Left ER Before Being Seen	8,837	0%	3%	2%
Time from ER Arrival to Admit. (minutes)[2]	371	188	240	274
Time from ER Arrival to Discharge (minutes)	366	126	126	134
Time in ER Before Being Evaluated (minutes)	361	25	31	26
Time to Pain Meds for Fractures (minutes)	38	52	69	57
Heart Attack Care				
Aspirin Given at Discharge[5]	-	-	99%	99%
Fibrinolytic Meds Within 30 Min. of Arrival[5]	-	-	77%	54%
PCI Within 90 Minutes of Arrival[5]	-	-	97%	96%
Statin Prescribed at Discharge[5]	-	-	98%	98%
Heart Failure Care				
ACE Inhibitor or ARB for LVSD[2]	15	100%	97%	97%
Discharge Instructions Given[2]	39	59%	93%	94%
Evaluation of LVS Function[2]	44	91%	99%	99%
Medicare Spending				
Medicare Spending per Patient (ratio)	-	0.98	0.98	0.98
Pneumonia Care				
Appropriate Initial Antibiotic Given[1,2]	-	-	95%	95%
Blood Culture Timing[2,3]	-	-	98%	98%
Pregnancy and Delivery Care				
Newborn Deliveries Scheduled Early	16	0%	14%	6%
Preventive Care				
Immunization for Influenza[2]	320	82%	90%	90%
Immunization for Pneumonia[2]	310	93%	91%	92%
Stroke Care				
Anticoagulation Therapy for Atrial Fibrillation[3,7]	-	-	92%	95%
Antithrombotic Therapy Timing[3,7]	-	-	96%	98%
Assessed for Rehabilitation[1,3]	-	-	95%	97%
Discharged on Antithrombotic Therapy[1,3]	-	-	98%	99%
Discharged on Statin Medication[1,3]	-	-	90%	94%
Thrombolytic Therapy Timing[1,3]	-	-	38%	66%
Venous Thromboembolism Prophylaxis[1,3]	-	-	89%	94%
Written Stroke Educational Materials Given[1,3]	-	-	85%	88%
Surgical Care Improvement Project				
Appropriate Beta Blocker Usage[1,2]	-	-	98%	98%
Appropriate VTP Within 24 Hours[2,3]	21	95%	98%	98%
Controlled Postoperative Blood Glucose[2,3]	-	-	97%	97%
Perioperative Temperature Management[2,3]	28	100%	100%	100%
Prophylactic Antibiotic Selection[2,3]	18	100%	99%	99%
Prophylactic Antibiotic Selection (Outpatient)[3,7]	-	-	98%	98%
Prophylactic Antibiotic Stopped[2,3]	18	72%	98%	98%
Prophylactic Antibiotic Timing[2,3]	18	94%	99%	99%
Prophylactic Antibiotic Timing (Outpatient)[1,3]	-	-	99%	98%
Urinary Catheter Removal[2,3]	-	-	98%	97%
Survey of Patients' Hospital Experiences				
Area Around Room 'Always' Quiet at Night	(a)	60%	71%	61%
Doctors 'Always' Communicated Well	(a)	86%	86%	82%
Home Recovery Information Given	(a)	78%	84%	85%
Hospital Given 9 or 10 on 10 Point Scale	(a)	54%	71%	71%
Meds 'Always' Explained Before Given	(a)	57%	66%	64%
Nurses 'Always' Communicated Well	(a)	74%	80%	79%
Pain 'Always' Well Controlled	(a)	64%	72%	71%
Room and Bathroom 'Always' Clean	(a)	62%	71%	73%
Timely Help 'Always' Received	(a)	61%	68%	68%
Would Definitely Recommend Hospital	(a)	56%	70%	71%
Use of Medical Imaging				
Cardiac Imaging Stress Test before Surgery[7]	-	-	6.5%	5.3%
Combination Abdominal CT Scan	141	36.9%	16.5%	10.5%
Combination Brain/Sinus CT Scan[1]	-	-	3.5%	2.7%
Combination Chest CT Scan	73	43.8%	4.2%	2.7%
Follow-up Mammogram/Ultrasound	298	5.4%	7.6%	8.8%
Lumbar Spine MRI for Low Back Pain	35	45.7%	40.2%	37.2%

Lakeland Community Hospital

42024 Highway 195 E
Haleyville, AL 35565
URL: www.lifepointhospitals.com
Type: Acute Care Hospitals
Ownership: Voluntary non-profit - Church
Phone: 205-485-7117
Fax: 205-485-7127
Emergency Services: Yes

Key Personnel:
Chief of Medical Staff . . . . Jerry B Harrison, MD
CEO/President. . . . . James P Jeansonne
Infection Control. . . . . Susan Johnson
Radiology. . . . . Regina Mask
Anesthesiology. . . . . Mike Moore
Operating Room. . . . . Bart Seymur
Intensive Care Unit. . . . . Cathleen Valentine

Measure	Cases	This Hosp.	State Avg.	U.S. Avg.
Blood Clot Prevention and Treatment				
Anticoagulation Overlap Therapy[1,2]	-	-	91%	93%
ICU Venous Thromboembolism Prophylaxis[1,2]	-	-	85%	92%
Incidence of Potentially Preventable VTE[1,2]	-	-	18%	10%
UFH with Dosages/Platelet Monitoring[1,2]	-	-	95%	97%
Venous Thromboembolism Prophylaxis[2]	176	91%	74%	85%
Warfarin Therapy Discharge Instructions[1,2]	-	-	77%	75%
Chest Pain/Possible Heart Attack Care				
Aspirin Given Within 24 Hours of Arrival	57	98%	96%	96%
Fibrinolytic Meds Within 30 Min. of Arrival[1]	-	-	57%	58%
Average Time to ECG (minutes)	58	3	6	7
Average Time to Transfer (minutes)[1]	-	-	61	60
Children's Asthma Care				
Received Home Management Plan of Care	-	-	-	88%
Received Reliever Medication	-	-	-	100%
Received Systemic Corticosteroids	-	-	-	100%
Emergency Department				
Admittance Decision Time (minutes)[2]	232	68	73	98
Head CT Results Within 45 Min. of Arrival[1]	-	-	45%	57%
Patients Who Left ER Before Being Seen	8,749	1%	3%	2%
Time from ER Arrival to Admit. (minutes)[2]	233	172	240	274
Time from ER Arrival to Discharge (minutes)	360	70	126	134
Time in ER Before Being Evaluated (minutes)	417	13	31	26
Time to Pain Meds for Fractures (minutes)	30	29	69	57
Heart Attack Care				
Aspirin Given at Discharge[1]	-	-	99%	99%
Fibrinolytic Meds Within 30 Min. of Arrival[7]	-	-	77%	54%
PCI Within 90 Minutes of Arrival[7]	-	-	97%	96%
Statin Prescribed at Discharge[1]	-	-	98%	98%
Heart Failure Care				
ACE Inhibitor or ARB for LVSD[1]	-	-	97%	97%
Discharge Instructions Given	29	100%	93%	94%
Evaluation of LVS Function	36	100%	99%	99%
Medicare Spending				
Medicare Spending per Patient (ratio)	-	0.95	0.98	0.98
Pneumonia Care				
Appropriate Initial Antibiotic Given	82	99%	95%	95%
Blood Culture Timing	67	100%	98%	98%
Pregnancy and Delivery Care				

NOTE: Hospital profiles are in alphabetical order by state, then city, then hospital within the city; Rankings exclude hospitals with less than 25 cases except for patient surveys which excludes hospitals with less than 100 cases; (a) 100-299 cases; (1) The number of cases/patients is too few to report; (2) Data submitted were based on a sample of cases/patients; (3) Results are based on a shorter time period than required; (4) Data suppressed by CMS for one or more quarters; (5) Results are not available for this reporting period; (6) Fewer than 100 patients completed the HCAHPS survey; (7) No cases met the criteria for this measure; (8) The lower limit of the confidence interval cannot be calculated if the number of observed infections equals zero; (9) No data are available from the state/territory for this reporting period; (10) The scores shown reflect fewer than 50 completed surveys; (11) There were discrepancies in the data collection process; (12) This measure does not apply to this hospital for this reporting period; (13) Results cannot be calculated for this reporting period; (14) The results for this state are combined with nearby states to protect confidentiality; Please refer to the User's Guide for a full explanation of data.

Measure	Cases	This Hosp.	State Avg.	U.S. Avg.
Newborn Deliveries Scheduled Early[2,7]	-	-	14%	6%
Preventive Care				
Immunization for Influenza[2]	295	96%	90%	90%
Immunization for Pneumonia[2]	427	97%	91%	92%
Stroke Care				
Anticoagulation Therapy for Atrial Fibrillation[1]	-	-	92%	95%
Antithrombotic Therapy Timing	26	100%	96%	98%
Assessed for Rehabilitation	26	92%	95%	97%
Discharged on Antithrombotic Therapy	22	86%	98%	99%
Discharged on Statin Medication	19	95%	90%	94%
Thrombolytic Therapy Timing[7]	-	-	38%	66%
Venous Thromboembolism Prophylaxis	31	100%	89%	94%
Written Stroke Educational Materials Given	20	80%	85%	88%
Surgical Care Improvement Project				
Appropriate Beta Blocker Usage[1]	-	-	98%	98%
Appropriate VTP Within 24 Hours	12	75%	98%	98%
Controlled Postoperative Blood Glucose[7]	-	-	97%	97%
Perioperative Temperature Management	14	100%	100%	100%
Prophylactic Antibiotic Selection[1]	-	-	99%	99%
Prophylactic Antibiotic Selection (Outpatient)[1]	-	-	98%	98%
Prophylactic Antibiotic Stopped[1]	-	-	98%	98%
Prophylactic Antibiotic Timing[1]	-	-	99%	99%
Prophylactic Antibiotic Timing (Outpatient)[1]	-	-	99%	98%
Urinary Catheter Removal[1]	-	-	98%	97%
Survey of Patients' Hospital Experiences				
Area Around Room 'Always' Quiet at Night	300+	71%	71%	61%
Doctors 'Always' Communicated Well	300+	83%	86%	82%
Home Recovery Information Given	300+	82%	84%	85%
Hospital Given 9 or 10 on 10 Point Scale	300+	66%	71%	71%
Meds 'Always' Explained Before Given	300+	66%	66%	64%
Nurses 'Always' Communicated Well	300+	80%	80%	79%
Pain 'Always' Well Controlled	300+	71%	72%	71%
Room and Bathroom 'Always' Clean	300+	74%	71%	73%
Timely Help 'Always' Received	300+	63%	68%	68%
Would Definitely Recommend Hospital	300+	57%	70%	71%
Use of Medical Imaging				
Cardiac Imaging Stress Test before Surgery[1]	-	-	6.5%	5.3%
Combination Abdominal CT Scan	155	14.2%	16.5%	10.5%
Combination Brain/Sinus CT Scan[1]	-	-	3.5%	2.7%
Combination Chest CT Scan[1]	-	-	4.2%	2.7%
Follow-up Mammogram/Ultrasound	142	16.9%	7.6%	8.8%
Lumbar Spine MRI for Low Back Pain[1]	-	-	40.2%	37.2%

Marion Regional Medical Center

1256 Military Street South
Hamilton, AL 35570
Phone: 205-921-6200
E-mail: mbmc@scnet.net
URL: www.nmhs.net
Type: Acute Care Hospitals
Emergency Services: Yes
Ownership: Voluntary non-profit - Private
Beds: 32

Key Personnel:
Quality Assurance . . . . Holly Cole
CEO/President. . . . . John Heer
Operating Room. . . . . Eric S Young, RN

Measure	Cases	This Hosp.	State Avg.	U.S. Avg.
Blood Clot Prevention and Treatment				
Anticoagulation Overlap Therapy[1,2]	-	-	91%	93%
ICU Venous Thromboembolism Prophylaxis[2]	27	96%	85%	92%
Incidence of Potentially Preventable VTE[2,7]	-	-	18%	10%
UFH with Dosages/Platelet Monitoring[1,2]	-	-	95%	97%
Venous Thromboembolism Prophylaxis[2]	96	92%	74%	85%
Warfarin Therapy Discharge Instructions[1,2]	-	-	77%	75%
Chest Pain/Possible Heart Attack Care				
Aspirin Given Within 24 Hours of Arrival	33	100%	96%	96%
Fibrinolytic Meds Within 30 Min. of Arrival[7]	-	-	57%	58%
Average Time to ECG (minutes)	34	4	6	7
Average Time to Transfer (minutes)[1]	-	-	61	60
Children's Asthma Care				
Received Home Management Plan of Care	-	-	-	88%
Received Reliever Medication	-	-	-	100%
Received Systemic Corticosteroids	-	-	-	100%
Emergency Department				
Admittance Decision Time (minutes)[2]	362	30	73	98
Head CT Results Within 45 Min. of Arrival[7]	-	-	45%	57%
Patients Who Left ER Before Being Seen	9,657	1%	3%	2%
Time from ER Arrival to Admit. (minutes)[2]	409	175	240	274
Time from ER Arrival to Discharge (minutes)	384	101	126	134
Time in ER Before Being Evaluated (minutes)	426	21	31	26
Time to Pain Meds for Fractures (minutes)	28	40	69	57
Heart Attack Care				
Aspirin Given at Discharge[1,3]	-	-	99%	99%
Fibrinolytic Meds Within 30 Min. of Arrival[3,7]	-	-	77%	54%
PCI Within 90 Minutes of Arrival[3,7]	-	-	97%	96%
Statin Prescribed at Discharge[1,3]	-	-	98%	98%
Heart Failure Care				
ACE Inhibitor or ARB for LVSD[1]	-	-	97%	97%
Discharge Instructions Given	23	100%	93%	94%
Evaluation of LVS Function	24	96%	99%	99%
Medicare Spending				
Medicare Spending per Patient (ratio)	-	0.86	0.98	0.98
Pneumonia Care				
Appropriate Initial Antibiotic Given	74	91%	95%	95%
Blood Culture Timing	85	99%	98%	98%
Pregnancy and Delivery Care				
Newborn Deliveries Scheduled Early[7]	-	-	14%	6%
Preventive Care				
Immunization for Influenza[2]	305	93%	90%	90%
Immunization for Pneumonia[2]	486	95%	91%	92%
Stroke Care				
Anticoagulation Therapy for Atrial Fibrillation[1,2]	-	-	92%	95%
Antithrombotic Therapy Timing[2]	17	100%	96%	98%
Assessed for Rehabilitation[2]	12	100%	95%	97%
Discharged on Antithrombotic Therapy[1,2]	-	-	98%	99%
Discharged on Statin Medication[1,2]	-	-	90%	94%
Thrombolytic Therapy Timing[2,7]	-	-	38%	66%
Venous Thromboembolism Prophylaxis[2]	14	100%	89%	94%
Written Stroke Educational Materials Given[1,2]	-	-	85%	88%
Surgical Care Improvement Project				
Appropriate Beta Blocker Usage[1,3]	-	-	98%	98%
Appropriate VTP Within 24 Hours[1,3]	-	-	98%	98%
Controlled Postoperative Blood Glucose[3,7]	-	-	97%	97%
Perioperative Temperature Management[1,3]	-	-	100%	100%
Prophylactic Antibiotic Selection[1,3]	-	-	99%	99%
Prophylactic Antibiotic Selection (Outpatient)[1,3]	-	-	98%	98%
Prophylactic Antibiotic Stopped[1,3]	-	-	98%	98%
Prophylactic Antibiotic Timing[1,3]	-	-	99%	99%
Prophylactic Antibiotic Timing (Outpatient)[1,3]	-	-	99%	98%
Urinary Catheter Removal[1,3]	-	-	98%	97%
Survey of Patients' Hospital Experiences				
Area Around Room 'Always' Quiet at Night	(a)	86%	71%	61%
Doctors 'Always' Communicated Well	(a)	91%	86%	82%
Home Recovery Information Given	(a)	86%	84%	85%
Hospital Given 9 or 10 on 10 Point Scale	(a)	82%	71%	71%
Meds 'Always' Explained Before Given	(a)	80%	66%	64%
Nurses 'Always' Communicated Well	(a)	90%	80%	79%
Pain 'Always' Well Controlled	(a)	81%	72%	71%
Room and Bathroom 'Always' Clean	(a)	88%	71%	73%
Timely Help 'Always' Received	(a)	83%	68%	68%
Would Definitely Recommend Hospital	(a)	76%	70%	71%
Use of Medical Imaging				
Cardiac Imaging Stress Test before Surgery[7]	-	-	6.5%	5.3%
Combination Abdominal CT Scan	252	7.9%	16.5%	10.5%
Combination Brain/Sinus CT Scan[1]	-	-	3.5%	2.7%
Combination Chest CT Scan	111	4.5%	4.2%	2.7%
Follow-up Mammogram/Ultrasound[7]	-	-	7.6%	8.8%
Lumbar Spine MRI for Low Back Pain	44	52.3%	40.2%	37.2%

Crestwood Medical Center

One Hospital Dr Se
Huntsville, AL 35801
Phone: 256-882-3100
Fax: 256-880-4246
URL: www.crestwoodmedcenter.com
Type: Acute Care Hospitals
Emergency Services: Yes
Ownership: Proprietary
Beds: 150

Key Personnel:
Radiology. Robert B Akenhead
Operating Room. . . . . Stephen L Britt
Hemotology Center . . . . Manh Dang, MD
Chief of Medical Staff . . . . James A Flatt, MD
Quality Assurance . . . . Betty Grubb
CEO/President. . . . . Pamela B Hudson
Infection Control. . . . . Mae Mason
Intensive Care Unit. . . . . Lora Porter

Measure	Cases	This Hosp.	State Avg.	U.S. Avg.
Blood Clot Prevention and Treatment				
Anticoagulation Overlap Therapy[2]	54	98%	91%	93%
ICU Venous Thromboembolism Prophylaxis[2]	67	94%	85%	92%
Incidence of Potentially Preventable VTE[1,2]	-	-	18%	10%
UFH with Dosages/Platelet Monitoring[2]	19	100%	95%	97%
Venous Thromboembolism Prophylaxis[2]	356	96%	74%	85%
Warfarin Therapy Discharge Instructions[2]	44	100%	77%	75%
Chest Pain/Possible Heart Attack Care				
Aspirin Given Within 24 Hours of Arrival[1,3]	-	-	96%	96%
Fibrinolytic Meds Within 30 Min. of Arrival[5]	-	-	57%	58%
Average Time to ECG (minutes)[1,3]	-	-	6	7
Average Time to Transfer (minutes)[5]	-	-	61	60
Children's Asthma Care				
Received Home Management Plan of Care	-	-	-	88%
Received Reliever Medication	-	-	-	100%
Received Systemic Corticosteroids	-	-	-	100%
Emergency Department				
Admittance Decision Time (minutes)[2]	579	77	73	98
Head CT Results Within 45 Min. of Arrival[1]	-	-	45%	57%
Patients Who Left ER Before Being Seen	42,713	3%	3%	2%
Time from ER Arrival to Admit. (minutes)[2]	582	243	240	274
Time from ER Arrival to Discharge (minutes)	390	142	126	134
Time in ER Before Being Evaluated (minutes)	419	64	31	26
Time to Pain Meds for Fractures (minutes)	101	81	69	57
Heart Attack Care				
Aspirin Given at Discharge	110	100%	99%	99%
Fibrinolytic Meds Within 30 Min. of Arrival[7]	-	-	77%	54%
PCI Within 90 Minutes of Arrival	16	100%	97%	96%
Statin Prescribed at Discharge	103	100%	98%	98%
Heart Failure Care				
ACE Inhibitor or ARB for LVSD	60	100%	97%	97%
Discharge Instructions Given	190	87%	93%	94%
Evaluation of LVS Function	217	100%	99%	99%
Medicare Spending				
Medicare Spending per Patient (ratio)	-	0.97	0.98	0.98
Pneumonia Care				
Appropriate Initial Antibiotic Given	112	100%	95%	95%
Blood Culture Timing	34	97%	98%	98%
Pregnancy and Delivery Care				
Newborn Deliveries Scheduled Early[2]	38	3%	14%	6%
Preventive Care				
Immunization for Influenza[2]	642	99%	90%	90%
Immunization for Pneumonia[2]	762	100%	91%	92%
Stroke Care				
Anticoagulation Therapy for Atrial Fibrillation	11	100%	92%	95%
Antithrombotic Therapy Timing	62	100%	96%	98%
Assessed for Rehabilitation	60	95%	95%	97%
Discharged on Antithrombotic Therapy	58	100%	98%	99%
Discharged on Statin Medication	44	98%	90%	94%
Thrombolytic Therapy Timing[1]	-	-	38%	66%
Venous Thromboembolism Prophylaxis	65	95%	89%	94%
Written Stroke Educational Materials Given	31	94%	85%	88%
Surgical Care Improvement Project				
Appropriate Beta Blocker Usage	310	99%	98%	98%
Appropriate VTP Within 24 Hours	1,126	99%	98%	98%
Controlled Postoperative Blood Glucose[7]	-	-	97%	97%
Perioperative Temperature Management	1,324	100%	100%	100%
Prophylactic Antibiotic Selection	998	100%	99%	99%
Prophylactic Antibiotic Selection (Outpatient)	705	100%	98%	98%
Prophylactic Antibiotic Stopped	978	99%	98%	98%
Prophylactic Antibiotic Timing	998	100%	99%	99%
Prophylactic Antibiotic Timing (Outpatient)	705	100%	99%	98%
Urinary Catheter Removal	143	100%	98%	97%
Survey of Patients' Hospital Experiences				
Area Around Room 'Always' Quiet at Night	300+	71%	71%	61%
Doctors 'Always' Communicated Well	300+	83%	86%	82%

NOTE: Hospital profiles are in alphabetical order by state, then city, then hospital within the city; Rankings exclude hospitals with less than 25 cases except for patient surveys which excludes hospitals with less than 100 cases; (a) 100-299 cases; (1) The number of cases/patients is too few to report; (2) Data submitted were based on a sample of cases/patients; (3) Results are based on a shorter time period than required; (4) Data suppressed by CMS for one or more quarters; (5) Results are not available for this reporting period; (6) Fewer than 100 patients completed the HCAHPS survey; (7) No cases met the criteria for this measure; (8) The lower limit of the confidence interval cannot be calculated if the number of observed infections equals zero; (9) No data are available from the state/territory for this reporting period; (10) The scores shown reflect fewer than 50 completed surveys; (11) There were discrepancies in the data collection process; (12) This measure does not apply to this hospital for this reporting period; (13) Results cannot be calculated for this reporting period; (14) The results for this state are combined with nearby states to protect confidentiality; Please refer to the User's Guide for a full explanation of data.

Home Recovery Information Given	300+	88%	84%	85%
Hospital Given 9 or 10 on 10 Point Scale	300+	75%	71%	71%
Meds 'Always' Explained Before Given	300+	66%	66%	64%
Nurses 'Always' Communicated Well	300+	79%	80%	79%
Pain 'Always' Well Controlled	300+	72%	72%	71%
Room and Bathroom 'Always' Clean	300+	73%	71%	73%
Timely Help 'Always' Received	300+	66%	68%	68%
Would Definitely Recommend Hospital	300+	78%	70%	71%
Use of Medical Imaging				
Cardiac Imaging Stress Test before Surgery[1]	-	-	6.5%	5.3%
Combination Abdominal CT Scan	676	5.5%	16.5%	10.5%
Combination Brain/Sinus CT Scan	935	4.7%	3.5%	2.7%
Combination Chest CT Scan	267	0.0%	4.2%	2.7%
Follow-up Mammogram/Ultrasound	1,419	8.9%	7.6%	8.8%
Lumbar Spine MRI for Low Back Pain	199	43.7%	40.2%	37.2%

Huntsville Hospital

101 Sivley Rd
Huntsville, AL 35801
Phone: 256-265-1000
Fax: 256-517-8484
URL: www.huntsvillehospital.org
Type: Acute Care Hospitals
Emergency Services: Yes
Ownership: Govt - Hospital Dist/Auth
Beds: 881

Key Personnel:
Chief of Medical Staff . . . . Robert Chappell, MD
Radiology. . . . . Richard J Coleman
Operating Room. . . . . Joseph P Hicks, MD
Pediatric In-Patient Care . . . . Alice McDuffree, MD
Infection Control . . . . Cindy Mize
CEO/President. . . . . David S Spillers
Quality Assurance . . . . Mary Lynne Wright

Measure	Cases	This Hosp.	State Avg.	U.S. Avg.
Blood Clot Prevention and Treatment				
Anticoagulation Overlap Therapy[2]	245	99%	91%	93%
ICU Venous Thromboembolism Prophylaxis[2]	116	91%	85%	92%
Incidence of Potentially Preventable VTE[2]	60	10%	18%	10%
UFH with Dosages/Platelet Monitoring[2]	147	100%	95%	97%
Venous Thromboembolism Prophylaxis[2]	301	79%	74%	85%
Warfarin Therapy Discharge Instructions[2]	183	84%	77%	75%
Chest Pain/Possible Heart Attack Care				
Aspirin Given Within 24 Hours of Arrival[1]	-	-	96%	96%
Fibrinolytic Meds Within 30 Min. of Arrival[3,7]	-	-	57%	58%
Average Time to ECG (minutes)[1]	-	-	6	7
Average Time to Transfer (minutes)[3,7]	-	-	61	60
Children's Asthma Care				
Received Home Management Plan of Care	156	89%	-	88%
Received Reliever Medication	157	100%	-	100%
Received Systemic Corticosteroids	157	100%	-	100%
Emergency Department				
Admittance Decision Time (minutes)[2]	622	99	73	98
Head CT Results Within 45 Min. of Arrival[1]	-	-	45%	57%
Patients Who Left ER Before Being Seen	>100k	4%	3%	2%
Time from ER Arrival to Admit. (minutes)[2]	625	318	240	274
Time from ER Arrival to Discharge (minutes)	369	168	126	134
Time in ER Before Being Evaluated (minutes)	365	52	31	26
Time to Pain Meds for Fractures (minutes)	425	72	69	57
Heart Attack Care				
Aspirin Given at Discharge[2]	377	99%	99%	99%
Fibrinolytic Meds Within 30 Min. of Arrival[2,7]	-	-	77%	54%
PCI Within 90 Minutes of Arrival[2]	45	98%	97%	96%
Statin Prescribed at Discharge[2]	340	99%	98%	98%
Heart Failure Care				
ACE Inhibitor or ARB for LVSD[2]	95	100%	97%	97%
Discharge Instructions Given[2]	297	90%	93%	94%
Evaluation of LVS Function[2]	368	99%	99%	99%
Medicare Spending				
Medicare Spending per Patient (ratio)	-	1.01	0.98	0.98
Pneumonia Care				
Appropriate Initial Antibiotic Given	366	96%	95%	95%
Blood Culture Timing	716	99%	98%	98%
Pregnancy and Delivery Care				
Newborn Deliveries Scheduled Early[2]	769	28%	14%	6%
Preventive Care				
Immunization for Influenza[2]	563	94%	90%	90%
Immunization for Pneumonia[2]	664	95%	91%	92%
Stroke Care				
Anticoagulation Therapy for Atrial Fibrillation	60	100%	92%	95%
Antithrombotic Therapy Timing	443	99%	96%	98%
Assessed for Rehabilitation	543	100%	95%	97%
Discharged on Antithrombotic Therapy	454	100%	98%	99%
Discharged on Statin Medication	329	98%	90%	94%
Thrombolytic Therapy Timing	14	100%	38%	66%
Venous Thromboembolism Prophylaxis	554	99%	89%	94%
Written Stroke Educational Materials Given	286	100%	85%	88%
Surgical Care Improvement Project				
Appropriate Beta Blocker Usage[2]	287	98%	98%	98%
Appropriate VTP Within 24 Hours[2]	491	99%	98%	98%
Controlled Postoperative Blood Glucose[2]	161	99%	97%	97%
Perioperative Temperature Management[2]	628	99%	100%	100%
Prophylactic Antibiotic Selection[2]	539	99%	99%	99%
Prophylactic Antibiotic Selection (Outpatient)	1,031	99%	98%	98%
Prophylactic Antibiotic Stopped[2]	520	99%	98%	98%
Prophylactic Antibiotic Timing[2]	540	99%	99%	99%
Prophylactic Antibiotic Timing (Outpatient)	1,033	99%	99%	98%
Urinary Catheter Removal[2]	322	98%	98%	97%
Survey of Patients' Hospital Experiences				
Area Around Room 'Always' Quiet at Night	300+	69%	71%	61%
Doctors 'Always' Communicated Well	300+	81%	86%	82%
Home Recovery Information Given	300+	86%	84%	85%
Hospital Given 9 or 10 on 10 Point Scale	300+	74%	71%	71%
Meds 'Always' Explained Before Given	300+	68%	66%	64%
Nurses 'Always' Communicated Well	300+	79%	80%	79%
Pain 'Always' Well Controlled	300+	72%	72%	71%
Room and Bathroom 'Always' Clean	300+	71%	71%	73%
Timely Help 'Always' Received	300+	66%	68%	68%
Would Definitely Recommend Hospital	300+	78%	70%	71%
Use of Medical Imaging				
Cardiac Imaging Stress Test before Surgery	2,745	7.5%	6.5%	5.3%
Combination Abdominal CT Scan	2,786	22.0%	16.5%	10.5%
Combination Brain/Sinus CT Scan	2,947	5.1%	3.5%	2.7%
Combination Chest CT Scan	1,746	0.5%	4.2%	2.7%
Follow-up Mammogram/Ultrasound	5,704	6.6%	7.6%	8.8%
Lumbar Spine MRI for Low Back Pain	881	37.1%	40.2%	37.2%

Jackson Medical Center

220 Hospital Drive
Jackson, AL 36545
Phone: 251-246-9021
Fax: 251-246-1108
URL: www.jacksonmedicalcenter.com
Type: Acute Care Hospitals
Emergency Services: Yes
Ownership: Proprietary
Beds: 35

Key Personnel:
Chief of Medical Staff . . . . Jared Ellis, MD
Pediatric Ambulatory Care . . . . . . Lashun Graves, MD
CEO/President. . . . . Teresa F Grimes

Measure	Cases	This Hosp.	State Avg.	U.S. Avg.
Blood Clot Prevention and Treatment				
Anticoagulation Overlap Therapy[2,7]	-	-	91%	93%
ICU Venous Thromboembolism Prophylaxis[2,7]	-	-	85%	92%
Incidence of Potentially Preventable VTE[1,2]	-	-	18%	10%
UFH with Dosages/Platelet Monitoring[2,7]	-	-	95%	97%
Venous Thromboembolism Prophylaxis[2]	155	100%	74%	85%
Warfarin Therapy Discharge Instructions[2,7]	-	-	77%	75%
Chest Pain/Possible Heart Attack Care				
Aspirin Given Within 24 Hours of Arrival	33	97%	96%	96%
Fibrinolytic Meds Within 30 Min. of Arrival[7]	-	-	57%	58%
Average Time to ECG (minutes)	36	9	6	7
Average Time to Transfer (minutes)[1]	-	-	61	60
Children's Asthma Care				
Received Home Management Plan of Care	-	-	-	88%
Received Reliever Medication	-	-	-	100%
Received Systemic Corticosteroids	-	-	-	100%
Emergency Department				
Admittance Decision Time (minutes)	139	52	73	98
Head CT Results Within 45 Min. of Arrival[1]	-	-	45%	57%
Patients Who Left ER Before Being Seen	7,919	3%	3%	2%
Time from ER Arrival to Admit. (minutes)	244	206	240	274
Time from ER Arrival to Discharge (minutes)	368	118	126	134
Time in ER Before Being Evaluated (minutes)	358	41	31	26
Time to Pain Meds for Fractures (minutes)	32	54	69	57
Heart Attack Care				
Aspirin Given at Discharge[3,7]	-	-	99%	99%
Fibrinolytic Meds Within 30 Min. of Arrival[3,7]	-	-	77%	54%
PCI Within 90 Minutes of Arrival[3,7]	-	-	97%	96%
Statin Prescribed at Discharge[3,7]	-	-	98%	98%
Heart Failure Care				
ACE Inhibitor or ARB for LVSD[1]	-	-	97%	97%
Discharge Instructions Given	15	100%	93%	94%
Evaluation of LVS Function	19	100%	99%	99%
Medicare Spending				
Medicare Spending per Patient (ratio)	-	0.98	0.98	0.98
Pneumonia Care				
Appropriate Initial Antibiotic Given	26	88%	95%	95%
Blood Culture Timing	25	100%	98%	98%
Pregnancy and Delivery Care				
Newborn Deliveries Scheduled Early[7]	-	-	14%	6%
Preventive Care				
Immunization for Influenza	175	97%	90%	90%
Immunization for Pneumonia	203	94%	91%	92%
Stroke Care				
Anticoagulation Therapy for Atrial Fibrillation[1]	-	-	92%	95%
Antithrombotic Therapy Timing	13	100%	96%	98%
Assessed for Rehabilitation	11	73%	95%	97%
Discharged on Antithrombotic Therapy	11	82%	98%	99%
Discharged on Statin Medication	11	18%	90%	94%
Thrombolytic Therapy Timing[1]	-	-	38%	66%
Venous Thromboembolism Prophylaxis	14	79%	89%	94%
Written Stroke Educational Materials Given[1]	-	-	85%	88%
Surgical Care Improvement Project				
Appropriate Beta Blocker Usage[5]	-	-	98%	98%
Appropriate VTP Within 24 Hours[5]	-	-	98%	98%
Controlled Postoperative Blood Glucose[5]	-	-	97%	97%
Perioperative Temperature Management[5]	-	-	100%	100%
Prophylactic Antibiotic Selection[5]	-	-	99%	99%
Prophylactic Antibiotic Selection (Outpatient)[5]	-	-	98%	98%
Prophylactic Antibiotic Stopped[5]	-	-	98%	98%
Prophylactic Antibiotic Timing[5]	-	-	99%	99%
Prophylactic Antibiotic Timing (Outpatient)[5]	-	-	99%	98%
Urinary Catheter Removal[5]	-	-	98%	97%
Survey of Patients' Hospital Experiences				
Area Around Room 'Always' Quiet at Night[6]	<100	81%	71%	61%
Doctors 'Always' Communicated Well[6]	<100	89%	86%	82%
Home Recovery Information Given[6]	<100	88%	84%	85%
Hospital Given 9 or 10 on 10 Point Scale[6]	<100	74%	71%	71%
Meds 'Always' Explained Before Given[6]	<100	67%	66%	64%
Nurses 'Always' Communicated Well[6]	<100	85%	80%	79%
Pain 'Always' Well Controlled[6]	<100	74%	72%	71%
Room and Bathroom 'Always' Clean[6]	<100	84%	71%	73%
Timely Help 'Always' Received[6]	<100	86%	68%	68%
Would Definitely Recommend Hospital[6]	<100	75%	70%	71%
Use of Medical Imaging				
Cardiac Imaging Stress Test before Surgery[1]	-	-	6.5%	5.3%
Combination Abdominal CT Scan	110	39.1%	16.5%	10.5%
Combination Brain/Sinus CT Scan[1]	-	-	3.5%	2.7%
Combination Chest CT Scan[1]	-	-	4.2%	2.7%
Follow-up Mammogram/Ultrasound	189	10.6%	7.6%	8.8%
Lumbar Spine MRI for Low Back Pain[1]	-	-	40.2%	37.2%

Jacksonville Medical Center

1701 South Pelham Road
Jacksonville, AL 36265
Phone: 256-782-4538
Fax: 256-435-8116
E-mail: webmaster@jmchealth.com
URL: www.jmchealth.com
Type: Acute Care Hospitals
Emergency Services: Yes
Ownership: Proprietary
Beds: 89

Key Personnel:
Quality Assurance . . . . Cherry Bass
Radiology. . . . . Randy Cortez
Intensive Care Unit. . . . . Mary Ann Crow
Pediatric In-Patient Care . . . . Ebba K Ebba, MD
Operating Room. . . . . Herb Ford
CEO/President. . . . . Russell Ingram
Emergency Room . . . . Rebecca Pierce
Chief of Medical Staff . . . . James Yates

NOTE: Hospital profiles are in alphabetical order by state, then city, then hospital within the city; Rankings exclude hospitals with less than 25 cases except for patient surveys which excludes hospitals with less than 100 cases; (a) 100-299 cases; (1) The number of cases/patients is too few to report; (2) Data submitted were based on a sample of cases/patients; (3) Results are based on a shorter time period than required; (4) Data suppressed by CMS for one or more quarters; (5) Results are not available for this reporting period; (6) Fewer than 100 patients completed the HCAHPS survey; (7) No cases met the criteria for this measure; (8) The lower limit of the confidence interval cannot be calculated if the number of observed infections equals zero; (9) No data are available from the state/territory for this reporting period; (10) The scores shown reflect fewer than 50 completed surveys; (11) There were discrepancies in the data collection process; (12) This measure does not apply to this hospital for this reporting period; (13) Results cannot be calculated for this reporting period; (14) The results for this state are combined with nearby states to protect confidentiality; Please refer to the User's Guide for a full explanation of data.

Measure	Cases	This Hosp.	State Avg.	U.S. Avg.
Blood Clot Prevention and Treatment				
Anticoagulation Overlap Therapy[1,2]	-	-	91%	93%
ICU Venous Thromboembolism Prophylaxis[2]	25	36%	85%	92%
Incidence of Potentially Preventable VTE[1,2]	-	-	18%	10%
UFH with Dosages/Platelet Monitoring[1,2]	-	-	95%	97%
Venous Thromboembolism Prophylaxis[2]	122	39%	74%	85%
Warfarin Therapy Discharge Instructions[1,2]	-	-	77%	75%
Chest Pain/Possible Heart Attack Care				
Aspirin Given Within 24 Hours of Arrival	23	91%	96%	96%
Fibrinolytic Meds Within 30 Min. of Arrival[1]	-	-	57%	58%
Average Time to ECG (minutes)	24	2	6	7
Average Time to Transfer (minutes)[1]	-	-	61	60
Children's Asthma Care				
Received Home Management Plan of Care	-	-	-	88%
Received Reliever Medication	-	-	-	100%
Received Systemic Corticosteroids	-	-	-	100%
Emergency Department				
Admittance Decision Time (minutes)[2]	126	93	73	98
Head CT Results Within 45 Min. of Arrival[1]	-	-	45%	57%
Patients Who Left ER Before Being Seen	14,192	1%	3%	2%
Time from ER Arrival to Admit. (minutes)[2]	180	270	240	274
Time from ER Arrival to Discharge (minutes)	354	128	126	134
Time in ER Before Being Evaluated (minutes)	315	28	31	26
Time to Pain Meds for Fractures (minutes)	58	80	69	57
Heart Attack Care				
Aspirin Given at Discharge[1]	-	-	99%	99%
Fibrinolytic Meds Within 30 Min. of Arrival[7]	-	-	77%	54%
PCI Within 90 Minutes of Arrival[7]	-	-	97%	96%
Statin Prescribed at Discharge[1]	-	-	98%	98%
Heart Failure Care				
ACE Inhibitor or ARB for LVSD[1]	-	-	97%	97%
Discharge Instructions Given	17	53%	93%	94%
Evaluation of LVS Function	22	91%	99%	99%
Medicare Spending				
Medicare Spending per Patient (ratio)	-	0.96	0.98	0.98
Pneumonia Care				
Appropriate Initial Antibiotic Given	43	79%	95%	95%
Blood Culture Timing	52	92%	98%	98%
Pregnancy and Delivery Care				
Newborn Deliveries Scheduled Early[2]	11	45%	14%	6%
Preventive Care				
Immunization for Influenza[2]	244	67%	90%	90%
Immunization for Pneumonia[2]	250	86%	91%	92%
Stroke Care				
Anticoagulation Therapy for Atrial Fibrillation[1]	-	-	92%	95%
Antithrombotic Therapy Timing[1]	-	-	96%	98%
Assessed for Rehabilitation[1]	-	-	95%	97%
Discharged on Antithrombotic Therapy[1]	-	-	98%	99%
Discharged on Statin Medication[1]	-	-	90%	94%
Thrombolytic Therapy Timing[7]	-	-	38%	66%
Venous Thromboembolism Prophylaxis[1]	-	-	89%	94%
Written Stroke Educational Materials Given[1]	-	-	85%	88%
Surgical Care Improvement Project				
Appropriate Beta Blocker Usage[1]	-	-	98%	98%
Appropriate VTP Within 24 Hours[1]	-	-	98%	98%
Controlled Postoperative Blood Glucose[7]	-	-	97%	97%
Perioperative Temperature Management[1]	-	-	100%	100%
Prophylactic Antibiotic Selection[1]	-	-	99%	99%
Prophylactic Antibiotic Selection (Outpatient)	96	97%	98%	98%
Prophylactic Antibiotic Stopped[1]	-	-	98%	98%
Prophylactic Antibiotic Timing[1]	-	-	99%	99%
Prophylactic Antibiotic Timing (Outpatient)	97	97%	99%	98%
Urinary Catheter Removal[1]	-	-	98%	97%
Survey of Patients' Hospital Experiences				
Area Around Room 'Always' Quiet at Night	(a)	63%	71%	61%
Doctors 'Always' Communicated Well	(a)	85%	86%	82%
Home Recovery Information Given	(a)	85%	84%	85%
Hospital Given 9 or 10 on 10 Point Scale	(a)	70%	71%	71%
Meds 'Always' Explained Before Given	(a)	63%	66%	64%
Nurses 'Always' Communicated Well	(a)	80%	80%	79%
Pain 'Always' Well Controlled	(a)	72%	72%	71%
Room and Bathroom 'Always' Clean	(a)	69%	71%	73%
Timely Help 'Always' Received	(a)	67%	68%	68%
Would Definitely Recommend Hospital	(a)	65%	70%	71%
Use of Medical Imaging				
Cardiac Imaging Stress Test before Surgery	79	6.3%	6.5%	5.3%
Combination Abdominal CT Scan	260	39.2%	16.5%	10.5%
Combination Brain/Sinus CT Scan[1]	-	-	3.5%	2.7%
Combination Chest CT Scan	114	0.9%	4.2%	2.7%
Follow-up Mammogram/Ultrasound	287	13.6%	7.6%	8.8%
Lumbar Spine MRI for Low Back Pain[1]	-	-	40.2%	37.2%

Walker Baptist Medical Center

3400 Highway 78 East
Jasper, AL 35502
URL: www.bhsala.com/walker
Phone: 205-387-4000
Fax: 205-387-4011
Type: Acute Care Hospitals
Ownership: Voluntary non-profit - Private
Emergency Services: Yes
Beds: 267

Key Personnel:
Radiology . . . . James Bradley, MD
Quality Assurance . . . . Bob Davenport
Chief of Medical Staff . . . . Elizabeth Ennis, MD
Pediatric Ambulatory Care . . . . . . Patrick Hyland, MD
Pediatric In-Patient Care . . . . Patrick Hyland, MD
CEO/President . . . . Bob Phillips
Operating Room . . . . Kay Weeks

Measure	Cases	This Hosp.	State Avg.	U.S. Avg.
Blood Clot Prevention and Treatment				
Anticoagulation Overlap Therapy[2]	44	95%	91%	93%
ICU Venous Thromboembolism Prophylaxis[2]	106	95%	85%	92%
Incidence of Potentially Preventable VTE[2]	11	0%	18%	10%
UFH with Dosages/Platelet Monitoring[2]	15	100%	95%	97%
Venous Thromboembolism Prophylaxis[2]	306	95%	74%	85%
Warfarin Therapy Discharge Instructions[2]	20	100%	77%	75%
Chest Pain/Possible Heart Attack Care				
Aspirin Given Within 24 Hours of Arrival	95	100%	96%	96%
Fibrinolytic Meds Within 30 Min. of Arrival	14	93%	57%	58%
Average Time to ECG (minutes)	99	0	6	7
Average Time to Transfer (minutes)[7]	-	-	61	60
Children's Asthma Care				
Received Home Management Plan of Care	-	-	-	88%
Received Reliever Medication	-	-	-	100%
Received Systemic Corticosteroids	-	-	-	100%
Emergency Department				
Admittance Decision Time (minutes)[2]	683	74	73	98
Head CT Results Within 45 Min. of Arrival	15	87%	45%	57%
Patients Who Left ER Before Being Seen	37,042	2%	3%	2%
Time from ER Arrival to Admit. (minutes)[2]	683	278	240	274
Time from ER Arrival to Discharge (minutes)	378	140	126	134
Time in ER Before Being Evaluated (minutes)	404	25	31	26
Time to Pain Meds for Fractures (minutes)	162	54	69	57
Heart Attack Care				
Aspirin Given at Discharge	57	100%	99%	99%
Fibrinolytic Meds Within 30 Min. of Arrival[1]	-	-	77%	54%
PCI Within 90 Minutes of Arrival[1]	-	-	97%	96%
Statin Prescribed at Discharge	50	100%	98%	98%
Heart Failure Care				
ACE Inhibitor or ARB for LVSD	48	100%	97%	97%
Discharge Instructions Given	132	100%	93%	94%
Evaluation of LVS Function	181	100%	99%	99%
Medicare Spending				
Medicare Spending per Patient (ratio)	-	0.97	0.98	0.98
Pneumonia Care				
Appropriate Initial Antibiotic Given	153	99%	95%	95%
Blood Culture Timing	219	100%	98%	98%
Pregnancy and Delivery Care				
Newborn Deliveries Scheduled Early[2]	28	7%	14%	6%
Preventive Care				
Immunization for Influenza[2]	536	100%	90%	90%
Immunization for Pneumonia[2]	723	100%	91%	92%
Stroke Care				
Anticoagulation Therapy for Atrial Fibrillation[1]	-	-	92%	95%
Antithrombotic Therapy Timing	50	100%	96%	98%
Assessed for Rehabilitation	59	100%	95%	97%
Discharged on Antithrombotic Therapy	59	100%	98%	99%
Discharged on Statin Medication	44	93%	90%	94%
Thrombolytic Therapy Timing[1]	-	-	38%	66%
Venous Thromboembolism Prophylaxis	60	98%	89%	94%
Written Stroke Educational Materials Given	40	100%	85%	88%
Surgical Care Improvement Project				
Appropriate Beta Blocker Usage	128	100%	98%	98%
Appropriate VTP Within 24 Hours	368	100%	98%	98%
Controlled Postoperative Blood Glucose[7]	-	-	97%	97%
Perioperative Temperature Management	400	100%	100%	100%
Prophylactic Antibiotic Selection	284	100%	99%	99%
Prophylactic Antibiotic Selection (Outpatient)	95	100%	98%	98%
Prophylactic Antibiotic Stopped	265	100%	98%	98%
Prophylactic Antibiotic Timing	284	100%	99%	99%
Prophylactic Antibiotic Timing (Outpatient)	95	100%	99%	98%
Urinary Catheter Removal	315	99%	98%	97%
Survey of Patients' Hospital Experiences				
Area Around Room 'Always' Quiet at Night	300+	63%	71%	61%
Doctors 'Always' Communicated Well	300+	81%	86%	82%
Home Recovery Information Given	300+	83%	84%	85%
Hospital Given 9 or 10 on 10 Point Scale	300+	69%	71%	71%
Meds 'Always' Explained Before Given	300+	63%	66%	64%
Nurses 'Always' Communicated Well	300+	78%	80%	79%
Pain 'Always' Well Controlled	300+	68%	72%	71%
Room and Bathroom 'Always' Clean	300+	69%	71%	73%
Timely Help 'Always' Received	300+	64%	68%	68%
Would Definitely Recommend Hospital	300+	67%	70%	71%
Use of Medical Imaging				
Cardiac Imaging Stress Test before Surgery	64	3.1%	6.5%	5.3%
Combination Abdominal CT Scan	593	11.1%	16.5%	10.5%
Combination Brain/Sinus CT Scan	552	2.4%	3.5%	2.7%
Combination Chest CT Scan	359	14.5%	4.2%	2.7%
Follow-up Mammogram/Ultrasound	744	5.1%	7.6%	8.8%
Lumbar Spine MRI for Low Back Pain	66	39.4%	40.2%	37.2%

Crenshaw Community Hospital

101 Hospital Circle
Luverne, AL 36049
E-mail: mplowden@baptistfirst.org
Phone: 334-335-3374
Fax: 334-335-5636
Type: Acute Care Hospitals
Ownership: Proprietary
Emergency Services: No
Beds: 65

Key Personnel:
Infection Control . . . . Cynthia Butts
Emergency Room . . . . Jeanie Colquitt
Quality Assurance . . . . Deborah Rushing
Operating Room . . . . Patty Rushing, RN
Anesthesiology . . . . Dale Shepherd, CRNA
Ambulatory Care . . . . S Patrick Walker, MD

Measure	Cases	This Hosp.	State Avg.	U.S. Avg.
Blood Clot Prevention and Treatment				
Anticoagulation Overlap Therapy[2,7]	-	-	91%	93%
ICU Venous Thromboembolism Prophylaxis[2,7]	-	-	85%	92%
Incidence of Potentially Preventable VTE[2,7]	-	-	18%	10%
UFH with Dosages/Platelet Monitoring[2,7]	-	-	95%	97%
Venous Thromboembolism Prophylaxis[2]	133	95%	74%	85%
Warfarin Therapy Discharge Instructions[2,7]	-	-	77%	75%
Chest Pain/Possible Heart Attack Care				
Aspirin Given Within 24 Hours of Arrival[1,3]	-	-	96%	96%
Fibrinolytic Meds Within 30 Min. of Arrival[1,3]	-	-	57%	58%
Average Time to ECG (minutes)[1,3]	-	-	6	7
Average Time to Transfer (minutes)[1,3]	-	-	61	60
Children's Asthma Care				
Received Home Management Plan of Care	-	-	-	88%
Received Reliever Medication	-	-	-	100%
Received Systemic Corticosteroids	-	-	-	100%
Emergency Department				
Admittance Decision Time (minutes)[2]	364	50	73	98
Head CT Results Within 45 Min. of Arrival[5]	-	-	45%	57%
Patients Who Left ER Before Being Seen	6,175	1%	3%	2%
Time from ER Arrival to Admit. (minutes)[2]	364	180	240	274
Time from ER Arrival to Discharge (minutes)	375	98	126	134
Time in ER Before Being Evaluated (minutes)	385	29	31	26
Time to Pain Meds for Fractures (minutes)	18	70	69	57
Heart Attack Care				
Aspirin Given at Discharge[5]	-	-	99%	99%

NOTE: Hospital profiles are in alphabetical order by state, then city, then hospital within the city; Rankings exclude hospitals with less than 25 cases except for patient surveys which excludes hospitals with less than 100 cases; (a) 100-299 cases; (1) The number of cases/patients is too few to report; (2) Data submitted were based on a sample of cases/patients; (3) Results are based on a shorter time period than required; (4) Data suppressed by CMS for one or more quarters; (5) Results are not available for this reporting period; (6) Fewer than 100 patients completed the HCAHPS survey; (7) No cases met the criteria for this measure; (8) The lower limit of the confidence interval cannot be calculated if the number of observed infections equals zero; (9) No data are available from the state/territory for this reporting period; (10) The scores shown reflect fewer than 50 completed surveys; (11) There were discrepancies in the data collection process; (12) This measure does not apply to this hospital for this reporting period; (13) Results cannot be calculated for this reporting period; (14) The results for this state are combined with nearby states to protect confidentiality; Please refer to the User's Guide for a full explanation of data.

Fibrinolytic Meds Within 30 Min. of Arrival[5]	-	-	77%	54%
PCI Within 90 Minutes of Arrival[5]	-	-	97%	96%
Statin Prescribed at Discharge[5]	-	-	98%	98%
Heart Failure Care				
ACE Inhibitor or ARB for LVSD[1,3]	-	-	97%	97%
Discharge Instructions Given[3]	17	82%	93%	94%
Evaluation of LVS Function[3]	19	95%	99%	99%
Medicare Spending				
Medicare Spending per Patient (ratio)	-	0.99	0.98	0.98
Pneumonia Care				
Appropriate Initial Antibiotic Given[3]	15	67%	95%	95%
Blood Culture Timing[3]	13	85%	98%	98%
Pregnancy and Delivery Care				
Newborn Deliveries Scheduled Early[2]	27	74%	14%	6%
Preventive Care				
Immunization for Influenza[2]	283	85%	90%	90%
Immunization for Pneumonia[2]	436	85%	91%	92%
Stroke Care				
Anticoagulation Therapy for Atrial Fibrillation[5]	-	-	92%	95%
Antithrombotic Therapy Timing[5]	-	-	96%	98%
Assessed for Rehabilitation[5]	-	-	95%	97%
Discharged on Antithrombotic Therapy[5]	-	-	98%	99%
Discharged on Statin Medication[5]	-	-	90%	94%
Thrombolytic Therapy Timing[5]	-	-	38%	66%
Venous Thromboembolism Prophylaxis[5]	-	-	89%	94%
Written Stroke Educational Materials Given[5]	-	-	85%	88%
Surgical Care Improvement Project				
Appropriate Beta Blocker Usage[5]	-	-	98%	98%
Appropriate VTP Within 24 Hours[5]	-	-	98%	98%
Controlled Postoperative Blood Glucose[5]	-	-	97%	97%
Perioperative Temperature Management[5]	-	-	100%	100%
Prophylactic Antibiotic Selection[5]	-	-	99%	99%
Prophylactic Antibiotic Selection (Outpatient)[5]	-	-	98%	98%
Prophylactic Antibiotic Stopped[5]	-	-	98%	98%
Prophylactic Antibiotic Timing[5]	-	-	99%	99%
Prophylactic Antibiotic Timing (Outpatient)[5]	-	-	99%	98%
Urinary Catheter Removal[5]	-	-	98%	97%
Survey of Patients' Hospital Experiences				
Area Around Room 'Always' Quiet at Night	(a)	63%	71%	61%
Doctors 'Always' Communicated Well	(a)	93%	86%	82%
Home Recovery Information Given	(a)	80%	84%	85%
Hospital Given 9 or 10 on 10 Point Scale	(a)	65%	71%	71%
Meds 'Always' Explained Before Given	(a)	75%	66%	64%
Nurses 'Always' Communicated Well	(a)	75%	80%	79%
Pain 'Always' Well Controlled	(a)	75%	72%	71%
Room and Bathroom 'Always' Clean	(a)	66%	71%	73%
Timely Help 'Always' Received	(a)	64%	68%	68%
Would Definitely Recommend Hospital	(a)	53%	70%	71%
Use of Medical Imaging				
Cardiac Imaging Stress Test before Surgery[7]	-	-	6.5%	5.3%
Combination Abdominal CT Scan	120	5.0%	16.5%	10.5%
Combination Brain/Sinus CT Scan[1]	-	-	3.5%	2.7%
Combination Chest CT Scan[1]	-	-	4.2%	2.7%
Follow-up Mammogram/Ultrasound	81	7.4%	7.6%	8.8%
Lumbar Spine MRI for Low Back Pain[1]	-	-	40.2%	37.2%

Mobile Infirmary

5 Mobile Infirmary Circle
Mobile, AL 36652
Phone: 251-435-4700
Fax: 251-435-3920
E-mail: ihs@infirmaryhealth.org
URL: www.mimc.com
Type: Acute Care Hospitals
Emergency Services: Yes
Ownership: Voluntary non-profit - Private
Beds: 689

Key Personnel:
Emergency Room . . . . William E Admire, Jr
Operating Room. . . . . Sandy Alexander, RN
CEO/President. . . . . E Chandler Bramlett
Intensive Care Unit. . . . . Cindy Buhring, RN
Radiology. . . . . Douglas Hungerford, MD
Pediatric In-Patient Care . . . . . . Dan McCall, III, MD
Quality Assurance . . . . Amy McRae
Chief of Medical Staff . . . . William Schulte, MD

Measure	Cases	This Hosp.	State Avg.	U.S. Avg.
Blood Clot Prevention and Treatment				
Anticoagulation Overlap Therapy[2]	230	92%	91%	93%
ICU Venous Thromboembolism Prophylaxis[2]	97	88%	85%	92%
Incidence of Potentially Preventable VTE[2]	100	15%	18%	10%
UFH with Dosages/Platelet Monitoring[2]	39	100%	95%	97%
Venous Thromboembolism Prophylaxis[2]	354	78%	74%	85%
Warfarin Therapy Discharge Instructions[2]	182	31%	77%	75%
Chest Pain/Possible Heart Attack Care				
Aspirin Given Within 24 Hours of Arrival[3,7]	-	-	96%	96%
Fibrinolytic Meds Within 30 Min. of Arrival[5]	-	-	57%	58%
Average Time to ECG (minutes)[3,7]	-	-	6	7
Average Time to Transfer (minutes)[5]	-	-	61	60
Children's Asthma Care				
Received Home Management Plan of Care	-	-	-	88%
Received Reliever Medication	-	-	-	100%
Received Systemic Corticosteroids	-	-	-	100%
Emergency Department				
Admittance Decision Time (minutes)[2]	612	141	73	98
Head CT Results Within 45 Min. of Arrival[1]	-	-	45%	57%
Patients Who Left ER Before Being Seen	43,352	8%	3%	2%
Time from ER Arrival to Admit. (minutes)[2]	615	384	240	274
Time from ER Arrival to Discharge (minutes)	377	235	126	134
Time in ER Before Being Evaluated (minutes)	417	57	31	26
Time to Pain Meds for Fractures (minutes)	89	98	69	57
Heart Attack Care				
Aspirin Given at Discharge	261	100%	99%	99%
Fibrinolytic Meds Within 30 Min. of Arrival[7]	-	-	77%	54%
PCI Within 90 Minutes of Arrival	29	97%	97%	96%
Statin Prescribed at Discharge	250	100%	98%	98%
Heart Failure Care				
ACE Inhibitor or ARB for LVSD[2]	93	100%	97%	97%
Discharge Instructions Given[2]	264	90%	93%	94%
Evaluation of LVS Function[2]	308	100%	99%	99%
Medicare Spending				
Medicare Spending per Patient (ratio)	-	0.97	0.98	0.98
Pneumonia Care				
Appropriate Initial Antibiotic Given[2]	57	100%	95%	95%
Blood Culture Timing[2]	75	97%	98%	98%
Pregnancy and Delivery Care				
Newborn Deliveries Scheduled Early[2]	56	14%	14%	6%
Preventive Care				
Immunization for Influenza[2]	602	95%	90%	90%
Immunization for Pneumonia[2]	768	97%	91%	92%
Stroke Care				
Anticoagulation Therapy for Atrial Fibrillation	42	95%	92%	95%
Antithrombotic Therapy Timing	259	95%	96%	98%
Assessed for Rehabilitation	327	97%	95%	97%
Discharged on Antithrombotic Therapy	274	99%	98%	99%
Discharged on Statin Medication	226	99%	90%	94%
Thrombolytic Therapy Timing[1]	-	-	38%	66%
Venous Thromboembolism Prophylaxis	335	92%	89%	94%
Written Stroke Educational Materials Given	186	94%	85%	88%
Surgical Care Improvement Project				
Appropriate Beta Blocker Usage[2]	277	100%	98%	98%
Appropriate VTP Within 24 Hours[2]	481	99%	98%	98%
Controlled Postoperative Blood Glucose[2]	170	99%	97%	97%
Perioperative Temperature Management[2]	638	100%	100%	100%
Prophylactic Antibiotic Selection[2]	582	99%	99%	99%
Prophylactic Antibiotic Selection (Outpatient)	641	97%	98%	98%
Prophylactic Antibiotic Stopped[2]	539	99%	98%	98%
Prophylactic Antibiotic Timing[2]	584	99%	99%	99%
Prophylactic Antibiotic Timing (Outpatient)	645	99%	99%	98%
Urinary Catheter Removal[2]	465	99%	98%	97%
Survey of Patients' Hospital Experiences				
Area Around Room 'Always' Quiet at Night	300+	67%	71%	61%
Doctors 'Always' Communicated Well	300+	84%	86%	82%
Home Recovery Information Given	300+	85%	84%	85%
Hospital Given 9 or 10 on 10 Point Scale	300+	75%	71%	71%
Meds 'Always' Explained Before Given	300+	70%	66%	64%
Nurses 'Always' Communicated Well	300+	80%	80%	79%
Pain 'Always' Well Controlled	300+	73%	72%	71%
Room and Bathroom 'Always' Clean	300+	62%	71%	73%
Timely Help 'Always' Received	300+	65%	68%	68%
Would Definitely Recommend Hospital	300+	74%	70%	71%
Use of Medical Imaging				
Cardiac Imaging Stress Test before Surgery	76	6.6%	6.5%	5.3%
Combination Abdominal CT Scan	1,074	66.9%	16.5%	10.5%
Combination Brain/Sinus CT Scan	790	2.9%	3.5%	2.7%
Combination Chest CT Scan	697	0.4%	4.2%	2.7%
Follow-up Mammogram/Ultrasound	2,802	10.9%	7.6%	8.8%
Lumbar Spine MRI for Low Back Pain	176	38.1%	40.2%	37.2%

Providence Hospital

6801 Airport Boulevard
Mobile, AL 36608
Phone: 251-633-1000
Fax: 251-633-1411
URL: www.providencehospital.org
Type: Acute Care Hospitals
Emergency Services: Yes
Ownership: Voluntary non-profit - Church
Beds: 349

Key Personnel:
Coronary Care. . . . . Michael Bolt
Chief of Medical Staff . . . . Carl Brutkiewicz, MD
Operating Room. . . . . Heather Carpenter
CEO/President. . . . . Clark P Christianson
Quality Assurance . . . . Dane Clark
Infection Control. . . . . Ann Doss
Radiology. . . . . Ramona Pickens
Pediatric In-Patient Care . . . . . . Mark Stewart

Measure	Cases	This Hosp.	State Avg.	U.S. Avg.
Blood Clot Prevention and Treatment				
Anticoagulation Overlap Therapy[2]	121	89%	91%	93%
ICU Venous Thromboembolism Prophylaxis[2]	119	86%	85%	92%
Incidence of Potentially Preventable VTE[2]	33	18%	18%	10%
UFH with Dosages/Platelet Monitoring[2]	17	100%	95%	97%
Venous Thromboembolism Prophylaxis[2]	307	74%	74%	85%
Warfarin Therapy Discharge Instructions[2]	89	58%	77%	75%
Chest Pain/Possible Heart Attack Care				
Aspirin Given Within 24 Hours of Arrival[5]	-	-	96%	96%
Fibrinolytic Meds Within 30 Min. of Arrival[5]	-	-	57%	58%
Average Time to ECG (minutes)[5]	-	-	6	7
Average Time to Transfer (minutes)[5]	-	-	61	60
Children's Asthma Care				
Received Home Management Plan of Care	-	-	-	88%
Received Reliever Medication	-	-	-	100%
Received Systemic Corticosteroids	-	-	-	100%
Emergency Department				
Admittance Decision Time (minutes)[2]	416	88	73	98
Head CT Results Within 45 Min. of Arrival[1]	-	-	45%	57%
Patients Who Left ER Before Being Seen	49,564	5%	3%	2%
Time from ER Arrival to Admit. (minutes)[2]	516	286	240	274
Time from ER Arrival to Discharge (minutes)	358	266	126	134
Time in ER Before Being Evaluated (minutes)	384	94	31	26
Time to Pain Meds for Fractures (minutes)	64	97	69	57
Heart Attack Care				
Aspirin Given at Discharge	275	100%	99%	99%
Fibrinolytic Meds Within 30 Min. of Arrival[7]	-	-	77%	54%
PCI Within 90 Minutes of Arrival	65	100%	97%	96%
Statin Prescribed at Discharge	264	100%	98%	98%
Heart Failure Care				
ACE Inhibitor or ARB for LVSD	89	98%	97%	97%
Discharge Instructions Given	333	98%	93%	94%
Evaluation of LVS Function	391	100%	99%	99%
Medicare Spending				
Medicare Spending per Patient (ratio)	-	0.98	0.98	0.98
Pneumonia Care				
Appropriate Initial Antibiotic Given	252	99%	95%	95%
Blood Culture Timing	212	100%	98%	98%
Pregnancy and Delivery Care				
Newborn Deliveries Scheduled Early	201	10%	14%	6%
Preventive Care				
Immunization for Influenza[2]	539	99%	90%	90%
Immunization for Pneumonia[2]	683	99%	91%	92%
Stroke Care				
Anticoagulation Therapy for Atrial Fibrillation	25	68%	92%	95%
Antithrombotic Therapy Timing	121	85%	96%	98%
Assessed for Rehabilitation	122	99%	95%	97%
Discharged on Antithrombotic Therapy	106	96%	98%	99%
Discharged on Statin Medication	80	76%	90%	94%

NOTE: Hospital profiles are in alphabetical order by state, then city, then hospital within the city; Rankings exclude hospitals with less than 25 cases except for patient surveys which excludes hospitals with less than 100 cases; (a) 100-299 cases; (1) The number of cases/patients is too few to report; (2) Data submitted were based on a sample of cases/patients; (3) Results are based on a shorter time period than required; (4) Data suppressed by CMS for one or more quarters; (5) Results are not available for this reporting period; (6) Fewer than 100 patients completed the HCAHPS survey; (7) No cases met the criteria for this measure; (8) The lower limit of the confidence interval cannot be calculated if the number of observed infections equals zero; (9) No data are available from the state/territory for this reporting period; (10) The scores shown reflect fewer than 50 completed surveys; (11) There were discrepancies in the data collection process; (12) This measure does not apply to this hospital for this reporting period; (13) Results cannot be calculated for this reporting period; (14) The results for this state are combined with nearby states to protect confidentiality; Please refer to the User's Guide for a full explanation of data.

Measure	Cases	This Hosp.	State Avg.	U.S. Avg.
Thrombolytic Therapy Timing[1]	-	-	38%	66%
Venous Thromboembolism Prophylaxis	144	90%	89%	94%
Written Stroke Educational Materials Given	61	95%	85%	88%
Surgical Care Improvement Project				
Appropriate Beta Blocker Usage[2]	215	99%	98%	98%
Appropriate VTP Within 24 Hours[2]	305	99%	98%	98%
Controlled Postoperative Blood Glucose[2]	135	99%	97%	97%
Perioperative Temperature Management[2]	407	100%	100%	100%
Prophylactic Antibiotic Selection[2]	369	100%	99%	99%
Prophylactic Antibiotic Selection (Outpatient)	622	100%	98%	98%
Prophylactic Antibiotic Stopped[2]	341	98%	98%	98%
Prophylactic Antibiotic Timing[2]	372	100%	99%	99%
Prophylactic Antibiotic Timing (Outpatient)	622	100%	99%	98%
Urinary Catheter Removal[2]	341	99%	98%	97%
Survey of Patients' Hospital Experiences				
Area Around Room 'Always' Quiet at Night	300+	63%	71%	61%
Doctors 'Always' Communicated Well	300+	81%	86%	82%
Home Recovery Information Given	300+	84%	84%	85%
Hospital Given 9 or 10 on 10 Point Scale	300+	69%	71%	71%
Meds 'Always' Explained Before Given	300+	62%	66%	64%
Nurses 'Always' Communicated Well	300+	75%	80%	79%
Pain 'Always' Well Controlled	300+	70%	72%	71%
Room and Bathroom 'Always' Clean	300+	66%	71%	73%
Timely Help 'Always' Received	300+	64%	68%	68%
Would Definitely Recommend Hospital	300+	73%	70%	71%
Use of Medical Imaging				
Cardiac Imaging Stress Test before Surgery[1]	-	-	6.5%	5.3%
Combination Abdominal CT Scan	893	39.8%	16.5%	10.5%
Combination Brain/Sinus CT Scan	1,013	2.4%	3.5%	2.7%
Combination Chest CT Scan	1,055	9.5%	4.2%	2.7%
Follow-up Mammogram/Ultrasound	1,441	11.9%	7.6%	8.8%
Lumbar Spine MRI for Low Back Pain	185	40.0%	40.2%	37.2%

Springhill Medical Center

3719 Dauphin Street   Phone: 251-344-9630
Mobile, AL 36608   Fax: 251-460-5248
URL: www.springhillmedicalcenter.com
Type: Acute Care Hospitals   Emergency Services: Yes
Ownership: Proprietary   Beds: 252

Key Personnel:
Infection Control. . . . . Beth Beck
Operating Room. . . . . Josie Carter, RN
Quality Assurance . . . . Levita Corbin PhD
Pediatric In-Patient Care . . . . Beth Edwards
Chief of Medical Staff . . . . Alan Shain, MD
President/CEO . . . . Jeffrey M St Clair
Emergency Room . . . . Paul Tomlinson, RN

Measure	Cases	This Hosp.	State Avg.	U.S. Avg.
Blood Clot Prevention and Treatment				
Anticoagulation Overlap Therapy[2]	76	96%	91%	93%
ICU Venous Thromboembolism Prophylaxis[2]	101	89%	85%	92%
Incidence of Potentially Preventable VTE[1,2]	-	-	18%	10%
UFH with Dosages/Platelet Monitoring[2]	11	100%	95%	97%
Venous Thromboembolism Prophylaxis[2]	359	82%	74%	85%
Warfarin Therapy Discharge Instructions[2]	68	100%	77%	75%
Chest Pain/Possible Heart Attack Care				
Aspirin Given Within 24 Hours of Arrival[5]	-	-	96%	96%
Fibrinolytic Meds Within 30 Min. of Arrival[5]	-	-	57%	58%
Average Time to ECG (minutes)[5]	-	-	6	7
Average Time to Transfer (minutes)[5]	-	-	61	60
Children's Asthma Care				
Received Home Management Plan of Care	-	-	-	88%
Received Reliever Medication	-	-	-	100%
Received Systemic Corticosteroids	-	-	-	100%
Emergency Department				
Admittance Decision Time (minutes)[2]	828	92	73	98
Head CT Results Within 45 Min. of Arrival[1]	-	-	45%	57%
Patients Who Left ER Before Being Seen	34,556	5%	3%	2%
Time from ER Arrival to Admit. (minutes)[2]	830	228	240	274
Time from ER Arrival to Discharge (minutes)	379	135	126	134
Time in ER Before Being Evaluated (minutes)	388	38	31	26
Time to Pain Meds for Fractures (minutes)	120	64	69	57
Heart Attack Care				
Aspirin Given at Discharge	206	100%	99%	99%
Fibrinolytic Meds Within 30 Min. of Arrival[7]	-	-	77%	54%
PCI Within 90 Minutes of Arrival	53	98%	97%	96%
Statin Prescribed at Discharge	203	96%	98%	98%
Heart Failure Care				
ACE Inhibitor or ARB for LVSD	149	100%	97%	97%
Discharge Instructions Given	424	94%	93%	94%
Evaluation of LVS Function	495	99%	99%	99%
Medicare Spending				
Medicare Spending per Patient (ratio)	-	1.01	0.98	0.98
Pneumonia Care				
Appropriate Initial Antibiotic Given	153	99%	95%	95%
Blood Culture Timing	192	100%	98%	98%
Pregnancy and Delivery Care				
Newborn Deliveries Scheduled Early	64	9%	14%	6%
Preventive Care				
Immunization for Influenza[2]	611	95%	90%	90%
Immunization for Pneumonia[2]	924	88%	91%	92%
Stroke Care				
Anticoagulation Therapy for Atrial Fibrillation[1]	-	-	92%	95%
Antithrombotic Therapy Timing	100	98%	96%	98%
Assessed for Rehabilitation	103	93%	95%	97%
Discharged on Antithrombotic Therapy	96	99%	98%	99%
Discharged on Statin Medication	85	81%	90%	94%
Thrombolytic Therapy Timing	20	5%	38%	66%
Venous Thromboembolism Prophylaxis	109	84%	89%	94%
Written Stroke Educational Materials Given	64	91%	85%	88%
Surgical Care Improvement Project				
Appropriate Beta Blocker Usage[2]	195	97%	98%	98%
Appropriate VTP Within 24 Hours[2]	457	97%	98%	98%
Controlled Postoperative Blood Glucose[2]	96	92%	97%	97%
Perioperative Temperature Management[2]	529	100%	100%	100%
Prophylactic Antibiotic Selection[2]	479	99%	99%	99%
Prophylactic Antibiotic Selection (Outpatient)	216	98%	98%	98%
Prophylactic Antibiotic Stopped[2]	446	99%	98%	98%
Prophylactic Antibiotic Timing[2]	481	100%	99%	99%
Prophylactic Antibiotic Timing (Outpatient)	217	99%	99%	98%
Urinary Catheter Removal[2]	272	100%	98%	97%
Survey of Patients' Hospital Experiences				
Area Around Room 'Always' Quiet at Night	300+	67%	71%	61%
Doctors 'Always' Communicated Well	300+	83%	86%	82%
Home Recovery Information Given	300+	86%	84%	85%
Hospital Given 9 or 10 on 10 Point Scale	300+	70%	71%	71%
Meds 'Always' Explained Before Given	300+	59%	66%	64%
Nurses 'Always' Communicated Well	300+	78%	80%	79%
Pain 'Always' Well Controlled	300+	72%	72%	71%
Room and Bathroom 'Always' Clean	300+	63%	71%	73%
Timely Help 'Always' Received	300+	66%	68%	68%
Would Definitely Recommend Hospital	300+	71%	70%	71%
Use of Medical Imaging				
Cardiac Imaging Stress Test before Surgery	122	8.2%	6.5%	5.3%
Combination Abdominal CT Scan	708	36.7%	16.5%	10.5%
Combination Brain/Sinus CT Scan	654	1.4%	3.5%	2.7%
Combination Chest CT Scan	425	0.7%	4.2%	2.7%
Follow-up Mammogram/Ultrasound	1,633	5.8%	7.6%	8.8%
Lumbar Spine MRI for Low Back Pain[1]	-	-	40.2%	37.2%

University of South Alabama Children's & Women's Hospital

1700 Center Street   Phone: 251-415-1000
Mobile, AL 36604   Fax: 251-415-1001
URL: www.southalabama.edu/usacwh
Type: Childrens   Emergency Services: Yes
Ownership: Government - State   Beds: 152

Key Personnel:
Operating Room. . . . . Kaye Cooper
Radiology. . . . . Peggy DeArmon
CEO/President. . . . . Stan Hammack
Infection Control. . . . . Amy Hill
Patient Relations . . . . Mary Ellen Laffard
Quality Assurance . . . . Sally Marcinek
Chief of Medical Staff . . . . Richard Teplick, MD
Pediatric In-Patient Care . . . . Terri Wright

Measure	Cases	This Hosp.	State Avg.	U.S. Avg.
Blood Clot Prevention and Treatment				
Anticoagulation Overlap Therapy[5]	-	-	91%	93%
ICU Venous Thromboembolism Prophylaxis[5]	-	-	85%	92%
Incidence of Potentially Preventable VTE[5]	-	-	18%	10%
UFH with Dosages/Platelet Monitoring[5]	-	-	95%	97%
Venous Thromboembolism Prophylaxis[5]	-	-	74%	85%
Warfarin Therapy Discharge Instructions[5]	-	-	77%	75%
Chest Pain/Possible Heart Attack Care				
Aspirin Given Within 24 Hours of Arrival	-	-	96%	96%
Fibrinolytic Meds Within 30 Min. of Arrival	-	-	57%	58%
Average Time to ECG (minutes)	-	-	6	7
Average Time to Transfer (minutes)	-	-	61	60
Children's Asthma Care				
Received Home Management Plan of Care[2]	135	67%	-	88%
Received Reliever Medication[2]	138	100%	-	100%
Received Systemic Corticosteroids[2]	138	99%	-	100%
Emergency Department				
Admittance Decision Time (minutes)[5]	-	-	73	98
Head CT Results Within 45 Min. of Arrival	-	-	45%	57%
Patients Who Left ER Before Being Seen	-	-	3%	2%
Time from ER Arrival to Admit. (minutes)[5]	-	-	240	274
Time from ER Arrival to Discharge (minutes)	-	-	126	134
Time in ER Before Being Evaluated (minutes)	-	-	31	26
Time to Pain Meds for Fractures (minutes)	-	-	69	57
Heart Attack Care				
Aspirin Given at Discharge[5]	-	-	99%	99%
Fibrinolytic Meds Within 30 Min. of Arrival[5]	-	-	77%	54%
PCI Within 90 Minutes of Arrival[5]	-	-	97%	96%
Statin Prescribed at Discharge[5]	-	-	98%	98%
Heart Failure Care				
ACE Inhibitor or ARB for LVSD[5]	-	-	97%	97%
Discharge Instructions Given[5]	-	-	93%	94%
Evaluation of LVS Function[5]	-	-	99%	99%
Medicare Spending				
Medicare Spending per Patient (ratio)	-	-	0.98	0.98
Pneumonia Care				
Appropriate Initial Antibiotic Given[5]	-	-	95%	95%
Blood Culture Timing[5]	-	-	98%	98%
Pregnancy and Delivery Care				
Newborn Deliveries Scheduled Early[5]	-	-	14%	6%
Preventive Care				
Immunization for Influenza[5]	-	-	90%	90%
Immunization for Pneumonia[5]	-	-	91%	92%
Stroke Care				
Anticoagulation Therapy for Atrial Fibrillation[5]	-	-	92%	95%
Antithrombotic Therapy Timing[5]	-	-	96%	98%
Assessed for Rehabilitation[5]	-	-	95%	97%
Discharged on Antithrombotic Therapy[5]	-	-	98%	99%
Discharged on Statin Medication[5]	-	-	90%	94%
Thrombolytic Therapy Timing[5]	-	-	38%	66%
Venous Thromboembolism Prophylaxis[5]	-	-	89%	94%
Written Stroke Educational Materials Given[5]	-	-	85%	88%
Surgical Care Improvement Project				
Appropriate Beta Blocker Usage[5]	-	-	98%	98%
Appropriate VTP Within 24 Hours[5]	-	-	98%	98%
Controlled Postoperative Blood Glucose[5]	-	-	97%	97%
Perioperative Temperature Management[5]	-	-	100%	100%
Prophylactic Antibiotic Selection[5]	-	-	99%	99%
Prophylactic Antibiotic Selection (Outpatient)	-	-	98%	98%
Prophylactic Antibiotic Stopped[5]	-	-	98%	98%
Prophylactic Antibiotic Timing[5]	-	-	99%	99%
Prophylactic Antibiotic Timing (Outpatient)	-	-	99%	98%
Urinary Catheter Removal[5]	-	-	98%	97%
Survey of Patients' Hospital Experiences				
Area Around Room 'Always' Quiet at Night[5]	-	-	71%	61%
Doctors 'Always' Communicated Well[5]	-	-	86%	82%
Home Recovery Information Given[5]	-	-	84%	85%
Hospital Given 9 or 10 on 10 Point Scale[5]	-	-	71%	71%
Meds 'Always' Explained Before Given[5]	-	-	66%	64%
Nurses 'Always' Communicated Well[5]	-	-	80%	79%
Pain 'Always' Well Controlled[5]	-	-	72%	71%
Room and Bathroom 'Always' Clean[5]	-	-	71%	73%
Timely Help 'Always' Received[5]	-	-	68%	68%

NOTE: Hospital profiles are in alphabetical order by state, then city, then hospital within the city; Rankings exclude hospitals with less than 25 cases except for patient surveys which excludes hospitals with less than 100 cases; (a) 100-299 cases; (1) The number of cases/patients is too few to report; (2) Data submitted were based on a sample of cases/patients; (3) Results are based on a shorter time period than required; (4) Data suppressed by CMS for one or more quarters; (5) Results are not available for this reporting period; (6) Fewer than 100 patients completed the HCAHPS survey; (7) No cases met the criteria for this measure; (8) The lower limit of the confidence interval cannot be calculated if the number of observed infections equals zero; (9) No data are available from the state/territory for this reporting period; (10) The scores shown reflect fewer than 50 completed surveys; (11) There were discrepancies in the data collection process; (12) This measure does not apply to this hospital for this reporting period; (13) Results cannot be calculated for this reporting period; (14) The results for this state are combined with nearby states to protect confidentiality; Please refer to the User's Guide for a full explanation of data.

Measure	Cases	This Hosp.	State Avg.	U.S. Avg.
Would Definitely Recommend Hospital[5]	-	-	70%	71%
Use of Medical Imaging				
Cardiac Imaging Stress Test before Surgery	-	-	6.5%	5.3%
Combination Abdominal CT Scan	-	-	16.5%	10.5%
Combination Brain/Sinus CT Scan	-	-	3.5%	2.7%
Combination Chest CT Scan	-	-	4.2%	2.7%
Follow-up Mammogram/Ultrasound	-	-	7.6%	8.8%
Lumbar Spine MRI for Low Back Pain	-	-	40.2%	37.2%

University of South Alabama Medical Center

2451 Fillingim Street Phone: 251-471-7110
Mobile, AL 36617 Fax: 251-470-1672
URL: www.southalabama.edu/usamc
Type: Acute Care Hospitals Emergency Services: Yes
Ownership: Government - State Beds: 406

Key Personnel:
Pediatric Ambulatory Care . . . . . . Robert Boerth, MD
Pediatric In-Patient Care . . . . Robert Boerth, MD
Radiology. . . . . Jeffery C Brandon
Cardiac Laboratory. . . . . Frank Petty John
Quality Assurance . . . . Julie Litzinger
Infection Control. . . . . Keith Ramsey
Chief of Medical Staff. . . . . Richard Teplick, MD

Measure	Cases	This Hosp.	State Avg.	U.S. Avg.
Blood Clot Prevention and Treatment				
Anticoagulation Overlap Therapy[2]	43	98%	91%	93%
ICU Venous Thromboembolism Prophylaxis[2]	85	100%	85%	92%
Incidence of Potentially Preventable VTE[2]	15	0%	18%	10%
UFH with Dosages/Platelet Monitoring[2]	19	100%	95%	97%
Venous Thromboembolism Prophylaxis[2]	298	100%	74%	85%
Warfarin Therapy Discharge Instructions[2]	30	93%	77%	75%
Chest Pain/Possible Heart Attack Care				
Aspirin Given Within 24 Hours of Arrival[5]	-	-	96%	96%
Fibrinolytic Meds Within 30 Min. of Arrival[5]	-	-	57%	58%
Average Time to ECG (minutes)[5]	-	-	6	7
Average Time to Transfer (minutes)[5]	-	-	61	60
Children's Asthma Care				
Received Home Management Plan of Care	-	-	-	88%
Received Reliever Medication	-	-	-	100%
Received Systemic Corticosteroids	-	-	-	100%
Emergency Department				
Admittance Decision Time (minutes)[2]	951	235	73	98
Head CT Results Within 45 Min. of Arrival[1]	-	-	45%	57%
Patients Who Left ER Before Being Seen	29,516	7%	3%	2%
Time from ER Arrival to Admit. (minutes)[2]	952	484	240	274
Time from ER Arrival to Discharge (minutes)	277	285	126	134
Time in ER Before Being Evaluated (minutes)	372	76	31	26
Time to Pain Meds for Fractures (minutes)	113	117	69	57
Heart Attack Care				
Aspirin Given at Discharge	59	100%	99%	99%
Fibrinolytic Meds Within 30 Min. of Arrival[7]	-	-	77%	54%
PCI Within 90 Minutes of Arrival[1]	-	-	97%	96%
Statin Prescribed at Discharge	62	100%	98%	98%
Heart Failure Care				
ACE Inhibitor or ARB for LVSD	60	100%	97%	97%
Discharge Instructions Given	103	100%	93%	94%
Evaluation of LVS Function	105	100%	99%	99%
Medicare Spending				
Medicare Spending per Patient (ratio)	-	0.94	0.98	0.98
Pneumonia Care				
Appropriate Initial Antibiotic Given	20	100%	95%	95%
Blood Culture Timing	72	99%	98%	98%
Pregnancy and Delivery Care				
Newborn Deliveries Scheduled Early[2,7]	-	-	14%	6%
Preventive Care				
Immunization for Influenza[2]	574	99%	90%	90%
Immunization for Pneumonia[2]	502	97%	91%	92%
Stroke Care				
Anticoagulation Therapy for Atrial Fibrillation[1,2]	-	-	92%	95%
Antithrombotic Therapy Timing[2]	52	100%	96%	98%
Assessed for Rehabilitation[2]	93	98%	95%	97%
Discharged on Antithrombotic Therapy[2]	61	100%	98%	99%
Discharged on Statin Medication[2]	52	100%	90%	94%
Thrombolytic Therapy Timing[1,2]	-	-	38%	66%
Venous Thromboembolism Prophylaxis[2]	101	100%	89%	94%
Written Stroke Educational Materials Given[2]	69	94%	85%	88%
Surgical Care Improvement Project				
Appropriate Beta Blocker Usage[2]	51	96%	98%	98%
Appropriate VTP Within 24 Hours[2]	201	100%	98%	98%
Controlled Postoperative Blood Glucose[2]	21	100%	97%	97%
Perioperative Temperature Management[2]	254	100%	100%	100%
Prophylactic Antibiotic Selection[2]	132	100%	99%	99%
Prophylactic Antibiotic Selection (Outpatient)	26	100%	98%	98%
Prophylactic Antibiotic Stopped[2]	122	90%	98%	98%
Prophylactic Antibiotic Timing[2]	132	99%	99%	99%
Prophylactic Antibiotic Timing (Outpatient)	27	96%	99%	98%
Urinary Catheter Removal[2]	131	100%	98%	97%
Survey of Patients' Hospital Experiences				
Area Around Room 'Always' Quiet at Night	300+	65%	71%	61%
Doctors 'Always' Communicated Well	300+	82%	86%	82%
Home Recovery Information Given	300+	83%	84%	85%
Hospital Given 9 or 10 on 10 Point Scale	300+	72%	71%	71%
Meds 'Always' Explained Before Given	300+	65%	66%	64%
Nurses 'Always' Communicated Well	300+	78%	80%	79%
Pain 'Always' Well Controlled	300+	72%	72%	71%
Room and Bathroom 'Always' Clean	300+	67%	71%	73%
Timely Help 'Always' Received	300+	64%	68%	68%
Would Definitely Recommend Hospital	300+	74%	70%	71%
Use of Medical Imaging				
Cardiac Imaging Stress Test before Surgery	96	5.2%	6.5%	5.3%
Combination Abdominal CT Scan	181	22.7%	16.5%	10.5%
Combination Brain/Sinus CT Scan	227	4.8%	3.5%	2.7%
Combination Chest CT Scan	91	14.3%	4.2%	2.7%
Follow-up Mammogram/Ultrasound[7]	-	-	7.6%	8.8%
Lumbar Spine MRI for Low Back Pain[1]	-	-	40.2%	37.2%

Monroe County Hospital

2016 South Alabama Avenue, Box 886 Phone: 251-575-3111
Monroeville, AL 36460
Type: Acute Care Hospitals Emergency Services: Yes
Ownership: Government - Local

Key Personnel:
Emergency Room . . . . Angie Black, RN
Intensive Care Unit. . . . . Kathy Cave, RN
Infection Control. . . . . Leslie Crutchfield
CEO/President. . . . . Vince DiFranco
Radiology. . . . . Amanda Fleming

Measure	Cases	This Hosp.	State Avg.	U.S. Avg.
Blood Clot Prevention and Treatment				
Anticoagulation Overlap Therapy[1,2]	-	-	91%	93%
ICU Venous Thromboembolism Prophylaxis[2]	40	80%	85%	92%
Incidence of Potentially Preventable VTE[2,7]	-	-	18%	10%
UFH with Dosages/Platelet Monitoring[2,7]	-	-	95%	97%
Venous Thromboembolism Prophylaxis[2]	61	69%	74%	85%
Warfarin Therapy Discharge Instructions[1,2]	-	-	77%	75%
Chest Pain/Possible Heart Attack Care				
Aspirin Given Within 24 Hours of Arrival	99	95%	96%	96%
Fibrinolytic Meds Within 30 Min. of Arrival[1]	-	-	57%	58%
Average Time to ECG (minutes)	104	7	6	7
Average Time to Transfer (minutes)[7]	-	-	61	60
Children's Asthma Care				
Received Home Management Plan of Care	-	-	-	88%
Received Reliever Medication	-	-	-	100%
Received Systemic Corticosteroids	-	-	-	100%
Emergency Department				
Admittance Decision Time (minutes)[2]	201	45	73	98
Head CT Results Within 45 Min. of Arrival	12	25%	45%	57%
Patients Who Left ER Before Being Seen	15,319	2%	3%	2%
Time from ER Arrival to Admit. (minutes)[2]	217	220	240	274
Time from ER Arrival to Discharge (minutes)	389	111	126	134
Time in ER Before Being Evaluated (minutes)	349	25	31	26
Time to Pain Meds for Fractures (minutes)	41	55	69	57
Heart Attack Care				
Aspirin Given at Discharge[1]	-	-	99%	99%
Fibrinolytic Meds Within 30 Min. of Arrival[7]	-	-	77%	54%
PCI Within 90 Minutes of Arrival[7]	-	-	97%	96%
Statin Prescribed at Discharge[1]	-	-	98%	98%
Heart Failure Care				
ACE Inhibitor or ARB for LVSD[1]	-	-	97%	97%
Discharge Instructions Given	31	87%	93%	94%
Evaluation of LVS Function	51	94%	99%	99%
Medicare Spending				
Medicare Spending per Patient (ratio)	-	1.04	0.98	0.98
Pneumonia Care				
Appropriate Initial Antibiotic Given	36	86%	95%	95%
Blood Culture Timing	45	100%	98%	98%
Pregnancy and Delivery Care				
Newborn Deliveries Scheduled Early	21	0%	14%	6%
Preventive Care				
Immunization for Influenza[2]	259	74%	90%	90%
Immunization for Pneumonia[2]	277	80%	91%	92%
Stroke Care				
Anticoagulation Therapy for Atrial Fibrillation[1]	-	-	92%	95%
Antithrombotic Therapy Timing	12	100%	96%	98%
Assessed for Rehabilitation	13	77%	95%	97%
Discharged on Antithrombotic Therapy	12	83%	98%	99%
Discharged on Statin Medication	12	67%	90%	94%
Thrombolytic Therapy Timing[1]	-	-	38%	66%
Venous Thromboembolism Prophylaxis	11	91%	89%	94%
Written Stroke Educational Materials Given[1]	-	-	85%	88%
Surgical Care Improvement Project				
Appropriate Beta Blocker Usage[3,7]	-	-	98%	98%
Appropriate VTP Within 24 Hours[3]	23	100%	98%	98%
Controlled Postoperative Blood Glucose[3,7]	-	-	97%	97%
Perioperative Temperature Management[3]	27	100%	100%	100%
Prophylactic Antibiotic Selection[3]	22	95%	99%	99%
Prophylactic Antibiotic Selection (Outpatient)	12	83%	98%	98%
Prophylactic Antibiotic Stopped[3]	22	100%	98%	98%
Prophylactic Antibiotic Timing[3]	22	100%	99%	99%
Prophylactic Antibiotic Timing (Outpatient)	12	100%	99%	98%
Urinary Catheter Removal[1,3]	-	-	98%	97%
Survey of Patients' Hospital Experiences				
Area Around Room 'Always' Quiet at Night	(a)	74%	71%	61%
Doctors 'Always' Communicated Well	(a)	92%	86%	82%
Home Recovery Information Given	(a)	87%	84%	85%
Hospital Given 9 or 10 on 10 Point Scale	(a)	73%	71%	71%
Meds 'Always' Explained Before Given	(a)	74%	66%	64%
Nurses 'Always' Communicated Well	(a)	85%	80%	79%
Pain 'Always' Well Controlled	(a)	82%	72%	71%
Room and Bathroom 'Always' Clean	(a)	78%	71%	73%
Timely Help 'Always' Received	(a)	79%	68%	68%
Would Definitely Recommend Hospital	(a)	72%	70%	71%
Use of Medical Imaging				
Cardiac Imaging Stress Test before Surgery	141	4.3%	6.5%	5.3%
Combination Abdominal CT Scan	258	11.2%	16.5%	10.5%
Combination Brain/Sinus CT Scan[1]	-	-	3.5%	2.7%
Combination Chest CT Scan	133	0.0%	4.2%	2.7%
Follow-up Mammogram/Ultrasound	560	19.5%	7.6%	8.8%
Lumbar Spine MRI for Low Back Pain	37	48.6%	40.2%	37.2%

Baptist Medical Center East

400 Taylor Road Phone: 334-244-8330
Montgomery, AL 36117 Fax: 334-244-8300
URL: www.baptistfirst.org
Type: Acute Care Hospitals Emergency Services: Yes
Ownership: Govt - Hospital Dist/Auth Beds: 150

Key Personnel:
Emergency Room . . . . D Gregory Alexander
Radiology. Joseph M Bailey
Chief of Medical Staff. . . . . Kathy Lindsey
CEO . . . . Peter Selman
CEO/President. . . . . W. Russell Tyner

Measure	Cases	This Hosp.	State Avg.	U.S. Avg.
Blood Clot Prevention and Treatment				
Anticoagulation Overlap Therapy[2]	39	85%	91%	93%
ICU Venous Thromboembolism Prophylaxis[2]	64	61%	85%	92%
Incidence of Potentially Preventable VTE[1,2]	-	-	18%	10%
UFH with Dosages/Platelet Monitoring[1,2]	-	-	95%	97%
Venous Thromboembolism Prophylaxis[2]	356	61%	74%	85%
Warfarin Therapy Discharge Instructions[2]	21	100%	77%	75%
Chest Pain/Possible Heart Attack Care				

NOTE: Hospital profiles are in alphabetical order by state, then city, then hospital within the city; Rankings exclude hospitals with less than 25 cases except for patient surveys which excludes hospitals with less than 100 cases; (a) 100-299 cases; (1) The number of cases/patients is too few to report; (2) Data submitted were based on a sample of cases/patients; (3) Results are based on a shorter time period than required; (4) Data suppressed by CMS for one or more quarters; (5) Results are not available for this reporting period; (6) Fewer than 100 patients completed the HCAHPS survey; (7) No cases met the criteria for this measure; (8) The lower limit of the confidence interval cannot be calculated if the number of observed infections equals zero; (9) No data are available from the state/territory for this reporting period; (10) The scores shown reflect fewer than 50 completed surveys; (11) There were discrepancies in the data collection process; (12) This measure does not apply to this hospital for this reporting period; (13) Results cannot be calculated for this reporting period; (14) The results for this state are combined with nearby states to protect confidentiality; Please refer to the User's Guide for a full explanation of data.

Measure	Cases	This Hosp.	State Avg.	U.S. Avg.
Aspirin Given Within 24 Hours of Arrival	43	98%	96%	96%
Fibrinolytic Meds Within 30 Min. of Arrival[7]	-	-	57%	58%
Average Time to ECG (minutes)	47	7	6	7
Average Time to Transfer (minutes)[1]	-	-	61	60
Children's Asthma Care				
Received Home Management Plan of Care	-	-	-	88%
Received Reliever Medication	-	-	-	100%
Received Systemic Corticosteroids	-	-	-	100%
Emergency Department				
Admittance Decision Time (minutes)[2]	295	122	73	98
Head CT Results Within 45 Min. of Arrival	18	17%	45%	57%
Patients Who Left ER Before Being Seen	43,129	3%	3%	2%
Time from ER Arrival to Admit. (minutes)[2]	307	335	240	274
Time from ER Arrival to Discharge (minutes)	257	198	126	134
Time in ER Before Being Evaluated (minutes)	353	47	31	26
Time to Pain Meds for Fractures (minutes)	130	78	69	57
Heart Attack Care				
Aspirin Given at Discharge	16	100%	99%	99%
Fibrinolytic Meds Within 30 Min. of Arrival[7]	-	-	77%	54%
PCI Within 90 Minutes of Arrival[7]	-	-	97%	96%
Statin Prescribed at Discharge	20	95%	98%	98%
Heart Failure Care				
ACE Inhibitor or ARB for LVSD[2]	46	100%	97%	97%
Discharge Instructions Given[2]	193	97%	93%	94%
Evaluation of LVS Function[2]	217	100%	99%	99%
Medicare Spending				
Medicare Spending per Patient (ratio)	-	0.98	0.98	0.98
Pneumonia Care				
Appropriate Initial Antibiotic Given[2]	83	95%	95%	95%
Blood Culture Timing[2]	127	98%	98%	98%
Pregnancy and Delivery Care				
Newborn Deliveries Scheduled Early[2]	388	6%	14%	6%
Preventive Care				
Immunization for Influenza[2]	431	91%	90%	90%
Immunization for Pneumonia[2]	306	90%	91%	92%
Stroke Care				
Anticoagulation Therapy for Atrial Fibrillation[1]	-	-	92%	95%
Antithrombotic Therapy Timing	36	94%	96%	98%
Assessed for Rehabilitation	41	100%	95%	97%
Discharged on Antithrombotic Therapy	39	97%	98%	99%
Discharged on Statin Medication	29	86%	90%	94%
Thrombolytic Therapy Timing[7]	-	-	38%	66%
Venous Thromboembolism Prophylaxis	35	89%	89%	94%
Written Stroke Educational Materials Given	24	42%	85%	88%
Surgical Care Improvement Project				
Appropriate Beta Blocker Usage	75	99%	98%	98%
Appropriate VTP Within 24 Hours	301	100%	98%	98%
Controlled Postoperative Blood Glucose[7]	-	-	97%	97%
Perioperative Temperature Management	392	100%	100%	100%
Prophylactic Antibiotic Selection	217	100%	99%	99%
Prophylactic Antibiotic Selection (Outpatient)	292	99%	98%	98%
Prophylactic Antibiotic Stopped	187	96%	98%	98%
Prophylactic Antibiotic Timing	217	99%	99%	99%
Prophylactic Antibiotic Timing (Outpatient)	292	100%	99%	98%
Urinary Catheter Removal	91	96%	98%	97%
Survey of Patients' Hospital Experiences				
Area Around Room 'Always' Quiet at Night	300+	66%	71%	61%
Doctors 'Always' Communicated Well	300+	85%	86%	82%
Home Recovery Information Given	300+	87%	84%	85%
Hospital Given 9 or 10 on 10 Point Scale	300+	77%	71%	71%
Meds 'Always' Explained Before Given	300+	64%	66%	64%
Nurses 'Always' Communicated Well	300+	82%	80%	79%
Pain 'Always' Well Controlled	300+	77%	72%	71%
Room and Bathroom 'Always' Clean	300+	67%	71%	73%
Timely Help 'Always' Received	300+	68%	68%	68%
Would Definitely Recommend Hospital	300+	82%	70%	71%
Use of Medical Imaging				
Cardiac Imaging Stress Test before Surgery[1]	-	-	6.5%	5.3%
Combination Abdominal CT Scan	778	54.1%	16.5%	10.5%
Combination Brain/Sinus CT Scan	745	5.2%	3.5%	2.7%
Combination Chest CT Scan	267	2.6%	4.2%	2.7%
Follow-up Mammogram/Ultrasound[7]	-	-	7.6%	8.8%
Lumbar Spine MRI for Low Back Pain	135	35.6%	40.2%	37.2%

Baptist Medical Center South

2105 East South Boulevard
Montgomery, AL 36116
URL: www.baptistfirst.org/south
Type: Acute Care Hospitals
Ownership: Voluntary non-profit - Church
Phone: 334-288-2100
Fax: 334-273-4204
Emergency Services: Yes
Beds: 454

Key Personnel:
Chief of Medical Staff. . . . . C Mason Brown, MD, MBA
Quality Assurance . . . . Kathy Gaston
Radiology. . . . . William McGuffin
Emergency Room . . . . John Moorehouse, MD
Pediatric In-Patient Care . . . . David Morrison
CEO/President. . . . . W Russell Tyner

Measure	Cases	This Hosp.	State Avg.	U.S. Avg.
Blood Clot Prevention and Treatment				
Anticoagulation Overlap Therapy[2]	67	99%	91%	93%
ICU Venous Thromboembolism Prophylaxis[2]	107	68%	85%	92%
Incidence of Potentially Preventable VTE[2]	20	25%	18%	10%
UFH with Dosages/Platelet Monitoring[2]	17	94%	95%	97%
Venous Thromboembolism Prophylaxis[2]	255	78%	74%	85%
Warfarin Therapy Discharge Instructions[2]	45	80%	77%	75%
Chest Pain/Possible Heart Attack Care				
Aspirin Given Within 24 Hours of Arrival[1,3]	-	-	96%	96%
Fibrinolytic Meds Within 30 Min. of Arrival[3,7]	-	-	57%	58%
Average Time to ECG (minutes)[1,3]	-	-	6	7
Average Time to Transfer (minutes)[3,7]	-	-	61	60
Children's Asthma Care				
Received Home Management Plan of Care	-	-	-	88%
Received Reliever Medication	-	-	-	100%
Received Systemic Corticosteroids	-	-	-	100%
Emergency Department				
Admittance Decision Time (minutes)[2]	408	284	73	98
Head CT Results Within 45 Min. of Arrival[1]	-	-	45%	57%
Patients Who Left ER Before Being Seen	62,762	5%	3%	2%
Time from ER Arrival to Admit. (minutes)[2]	415	494	240	274
Time from ER Arrival to Discharge (minutes)	295	200	126	134
Time in ER Before Being Evaluated (minutes)	342	32	31	26
Time to Pain Meds for Fractures (minutes)	125	61	69	57
Heart Attack Care				
Aspirin Given at Discharge	406	98%	99%	99%
Fibrinolytic Meds Within 30 Min. of Arrival[7]	-	-	77%	54%
PCI Within 90 Minutes of Arrival	41	88%	97%	96%
Statin Prescribed at Discharge	395	97%	98%	98%
Heart Failure Care				
ACE Inhibitor or ARB for LVSD[2]	176	94%	97%	97%
Discharge Instructions Given[2]	437	95%	93%	94%
Evaluation of LVS Function[2]	496	98%	99%	99%
Medicare Spending				
Medicare Spending per Patient (ratio)	-	1.04	0.98	0.98
Pneumonia Care				
Appropriate Initial Antibiotic Given	96	94%	95%	95%
Blood Culture Timing	111	91%	98%	98%
Pregnancy and Delivery Care				
Newborn Deliveries Scheduled Early	72	17%	14%	6%
Preventive Care				
Immunization for Influenza[2]	539	85%	90%	90%
Immunization for Pneumonia[2]	609	79%	91%	92%
Stroke Care				
Anticoagulation Therapy for Atrial Fibrillation	32	97%	92%	95%
Antithrombotic Therapy Timing	220	98%	96%	98%
Assessed for Rehabilitation	285	95%	95%	97%
Discharged on Antithrombotic Therapy	236	99%	98%	99%
Discharged on Statin Medication	207	98%	90%	94%
Thrombolytic Therapy Timing	26	69%	38%	66%
Venous Thromboembolism Prophylaxis	302	85%	89%	94%
Written Stroke Educational Materials Given	152	85%	85%	88%
Surgical Care Improvement Project				
Appropriate Beta Blocker Usage[2]	342	95%	98%	98%
Appropriate VTP Within 24 Hours[2]	627	91%	98%	98%
Controlled Postoperative Blood Glucose[2]	169	96%	97%	97%
Perioperative Temperature Management[2]	878	100%	100%	100%
Prophylactic Antibiotic Selection[2]	770	98%	99%	99%
Prophylactic Antibiotic Selection (Outpatient)	586	98%	98%	98%
Prophylactic Antibiotic Stopped[2]	761	95%	98%	98%
Prophylactic Antibiotic Timing[2]	778	97%	99%	99%
Prophylactic Antibiotic Timing (Outpatient)	592	98%	99%	98%
Urinary Catheter Removal[2]	454	91%	98%	97%
Survey of Patients' Hospital Experiences				
Area Around Room 'Always' Quiet at Night	300+	72%	71%	61%
Doctors 'Always' Communicated Well	300+	83%	86%	82%
Home Recovery Information Given	300+	84%	84%	85%
Hospital Given 9 or 10 on 10 Point Scale	300+	69%	71%	71%
Meds 'Always' Explained Before Given	300+	64%	66%	64%
Nurses 'Always' Communicated Well	300+	78%	80%	79%
Pain 'Always' Well Controlled	300+	70%	72%	71%
Room and Bathroom 'Always' Clean	300+	65%	71%	73%
Timely Help 'Always' Received	300+	62%	68%	68%
Would Definitely Recommend Hospital	300+	73%	70%	71%
Use of Medical Imaging				
Cardiac Imaging Stress Test before Surgery[1]	-	-	6.5%	5.3%
Combination Abdominal CT Scan	1,712	20.7%	16.5%	10.5%
Combination Brain/Sinus CT Scan	955	3.8%	3.5%	2.7%
Combination Chest CT Scan	1,573	2.0%	4.2%	2.7%
Follow-up Mammogram/Ultrasound	5,937	5.6%	7.6%	8.8%
Lumbar Spine MRI for Low Back Pain	214	36.4%	40.2%	37.2%

Jackson Hospital & Clinic

1725 Pine Street
Montgomery, AL 36106
URL: www.jackson.org
Type: Acute Care Hospitals
Ownership: Voluntary non-profit - Private
Phone: 334-293-8000
Fax: 334-293-8972
Emergency Services: Yes
Beds: 359

Key Personnel:
Anesthesiology. . . . . Fran Boyette, MD
CEO/President. . . . . Joe B. Riley
Chief of Medical Staff . . . . Patrick Ryan, MD
Infection Control. . . . . Janice Smith
Chairman/CEO . . . . William D. Smith

Measure	Cases	This Hosp.	State Avg.	U.S. Avg.
Blood Clot Prevention and Treatment				
Anticoagulation Overlap Therapy[2]	34	71%	91%	93%
ICU Venous Thromboembolism Prophylaxis[2]	93	78%	85%	92%
Incidence of Potentially Preventable VTE[2]	12	17%	18%	10%
UFH with Dosages/Platelet Monitoring[1,2]	-	-	95%	97%
Venous Thromboembolism Prophylaxis[2]	334	82%	74%	85%
Warfarin Therapy Discharge Instructions[2]	21	76%	77%	75%
Chest Pain/Possible Heart Attack Care				
Aspirin Given Within 24 Hours of Arrival[1,3]	-	-	96%	96%
Fibrinolytic Meds Within 30 Min. of Arrival[5]	-	-	57%	58%
Average Time to ECG (minutes)[1,3]	-	-	6	7
Average Time to Transfer (minutes)[5]	-	-	61	60
Children's Asthma Care				
Received Home Management Plan of Care	-	-	-	88%
Received Reliever Medication	-	-	-	100%
Received Systemic Corticosteroids	-	-	-	100%
Emergency Department				
Admittance Decision Time (minutes)[2]	710	139	73	98
Head CT Results Within 45 Min. of Arrival[1]	-	-	45%	57%
Patients Who Left ER Before Being Seen	44,574	6%	3%	2%
Time from ER Arrival to Admit. (minutes)[2]	710	324	240	274
Time from ER Arrival to Discharge (minutes)	727	186	126	134
Time in ER Before Being Evaluated (minutes)	757	74	31	26
Time to Pain Meds for Fractures (minutes)	36	113	69	57
Heart Attack Care				
Aspirin Given at Discharge	298	99%	99%	99%
Fibrinolytic Meds Within 30 Min. of Arrival[7]	-	-	77%	54%
PCI Within 90 Minutes of Arrival	33	100%	97%	96%
Statin Prescribed at Discharge	243	99%	98%	98%
Heart Failure Care				
ACE Inhibitor or ARB for LVSD	122	100%	97%	97%
Discharge Instructions Given	347	96%	93%	94%
Evaluation of LVS Function	426	100%	99%	99%
Medicare Spending				
Medicare Spending per Patient (ratio)	-	1.02	0.98	0.98
Pneumonia Care				

NOTE: Hospital profiles are in alphabetical order by state, then city, then hospital within the city; Rankings exclude hospitals with less than 25 cases except for patient surveys which excludes hospitals with less than 100 cases; (a) 100-299 cases; (1) The number of cases/patients is too few to report; (2) Data submitted were based on a sample of cases/patients; (3) Results are based on a shorter time period than required; (4) Data suppressed by CMS for one or more quarters; (5) Results are not available for this reporting period; (6) Fewer than 100 patients completed the HCAHPS survey; (7) No cases met the criteria for this measure; (8) The lower limit of the confidence interval cannot be calculated if the number of observed infections equals zero; (9) No data are available from the state/territory for this reporting period; (10) The scores shown reflect fewer than 50 completed surveys; (11) There were discrepancies in the data collection process; (12) This measure does not apply to this hospital for this reporting period; (13) Results cannot be calculated for this reporting period; (14) The results for this state are combined with nearby states to protect confidentiality; Please refer to the User's Guide for a full explanation of data.

Measure	Cases	This Hosp.	State Avg.	U.S. Avg.
Appropriate Initial Antibiotic Given	113	100%	95%	95%
Blood Culture Timing	272	100%	98%	98%
Pregnancy and Delivery Care				
Newborn Deliveries Scheduled Early	133	10%	14%	6%
Preventive Care				
Immunization for Influenza[2]	553	98%	90%	90%
Immunization for Pneumonia[2]	737	96%	91%	92%
Stroke Care				
Anticoagulation Therapy for Atrial Fibrillation	17	100%	92%	95%
Antithrombotic Therapy Timing	111	92%	96%	98%
Assessed for Rehabilitation	132	98%	95%	97%
Discharged on Antithrombotic Therapy	116	99%	98%	99%
Discharged on Statin Medication	101	91%	90%	94%
Thrombolytic Therapy Timing[1]	-	-	38%	66%
Venous Thromboembolism Prophylaxis	140	87%	89%	94%
Written Stroke Educational Materials Given	62	92%	85%	88%
Surgical Care Improvement Project				
Appropriate Beta Blocker Usage	384	96%	98%	98%
Appropriate VTP Within 24 Hours	674	99%	98%	98%
Controlled Postoperative Blood Glucose	258	95%	97%	97%
Perioperative Temperature Management	828	100%	100%	100%
Prophylactic Antibiotic Selection	735	100%	99%	99%
Prophylactic Antibiotic Selection (Outpatient)	593	99%	98%	98%
Prophylactic Antibiotic Stopped	729	98%	98%	98%
Prophylactic Antibiotic Timing	736	100%	99%	99%
Prophylactic Antibiotic Timing (Outpatient)	596	99%	99%	98%
Urinary Catheter Removal	631	97%	98%	97%
Survey of Patients' Hospital Experiences				
Area Around Room 'Always' Quiet at Night	300+	68%	71%	61%
Doctors 'Always' Communicated Well	300+	85%	86%	82%
Home Recovery Information Given	300+	85%	84%	85%
Hospital Given 9 or 10 on 10 Point Scale	300+	74%	71%	71%
Meds 'Always' Explained Before Given	300+	66%	66%	64%
Nurses 'Always' Communicated Well	300+	79%	80%	79%
Pain 'Always' Well Controlled	300+	73%	72%	71%
Room and Bathroom 'Always' Clean	300+	69%	71%	73%
Timely Help 'Always' Received	300+	64%	68%	68%
Would Definitely Recommend Hospital	300+	76%	70%	71%
Use of Medical Imaging				
Cardiac Imaging Stress Test before Surgery[1]	-	-	6.5%	5.3%
Combination Abdominal CT Scan	642	12.6%	16.5%	10.5%
Combination Brain/Sinus CT Scan	893	2.7%	3.5%	2.7%
Combination Chest CT Scan	333	0.0%	4.2%	2.7%
Follow-up Mammogram/Ultrasound	1,492	3.3%	7.6%	8.8%
Lumbar Spine MRI for Low Back Pain	182	48.9%	40.2%	37.2%

VA Central Alabama Healthcare System - Montgomery

215 Perry Hill Road
Montgomery, AL 36109
Phone: 334-260-4100
Fax: 334-260-4143
URL: www.centralalabama.va.gov
Type: Acute Care - VA
Emergency Services: No
Ownership: Government Federal
Beds: 200

Key Personnel:
Chief of Medical Staff . . . . Cliff Robinson, MD
Quality Assurance . . . . Gail Warren, RN

Measure	Cases	This Hosp.	State Avg.	U.S. Avg.
Blood Clot Prevention and Treatment				
Anticoagulation Overlap Therapy	-	-	91%	93%
ICU Venous Thromboembolism Prophylaxis	-	-	85%	92%
Incidence of Potentially Preventable VTE	-	-	18%	10%
UFH with Dosages/Platelet Monitoring	-	-	95%	97%
Venous Thromboembolism Prophylaxis	-	-	74%	85%
Warfarin Therapy Discharge Instructions	-	-	77%	75%
Chest Pain/Possible Heart Attack Care				
Aspirin Given Within 24 Hours of Arrival	-	-	96%	96%
Fibrinolytic Meds Within 30 Min. of Arrival	-	-	57%	58%
Average Time to ECG (minutes)	-	-	6	7
Average Time to Transfer (minutes)	-	-	61	60
Children's Asthma Care				
Received Home Management Plan of Care	-	-	-	88%
Received Reliever Medication	-	-	-	100%
Received Systemic Corticosteroids	-	-	-	100%
Emergency Department				
Admittance Decision Time (minutes)	-	-	73	98
Head CT Results Within 45 Min. of Arrival	-	-	45%	57%
Patients Who Left ER Before Being Seen	-	-	3%	2%
Time from ER Arrival to Admit. (minutes)	-	-	240	274
Time from ER Arrival to Discharge (minutes)	-	-	126	134
Time in ER Before Being Evaluated (minutes)	-	-	31	26
Time to Pain Meds for Fractures (minutes)	-	-	69	57
Heart Attack Care				
Aspirin Given at Discharge[1]	-	-	99%	99%
Fibrinolytic Meds Within 30 Min. of Arrival[5]	-	-	77%	54%
PCI Within 90 Minutes of Arrival[5]	-	-	97%	96%
Statin Prescribed at Discharge[1]	-	-	98%	98%
Heart Failure Care				
ACE Inhibitor or ARB for LVSD	37	100%	97%	97%
Discharge Instructions Given	60	95%	93%	94%
Evaluation of LVS Function	63	100%	99%	99%
Medicare Spending				
Medicare Spending per Patient (ratio)	-	-	0.98	0.98
Pneumonia Care				
Appropriate Initial Antibiotic Given	41	93%	95%	95%
Blood Culture Timing	55	100%	98%	98%
Pregnancy and Delivery Care				
Newborn Deliveries Scheduled Early	-	-	14%	6%
Preventive Care				
Immunization for Influenza[5]	-	-	90%	90%
Immunization for Pneumonia[5]	-	-	91%	92%
Stroke Care				
Anticoagulation Therapy for Atrial Fibrillation	-	-	92%	95%
Antithrombotic Therapy Timing	-	-	96%	98%
Assessed for Rehabilitation	-	-	95%	97%
Discharged on Antithrombotic Therapy	-	-	98%	99%
Discharged on Statin Medication	-	-	90%	94%
Thrombolytic Therapy Timing	-	-	38%	66%
Venous Thromboembolism Prophylaxis	-	-	89%	94%
Written Stroke Educational Materials Given	-	-	85%	88%
Surgical Care Improvement Project				
Appropriate Beta Blocker Usage[5]	-	-	98%	98%
Appropriate VTP Within 24 Hours[5]	-	-	98%	98%
Controlled Postoperative Blood Glucose[5]	-	-	97%	97%
Perioperative Temperature Management[5]	-	-	100%	100%
Prophylactic Antibiotic Selection[5]	-	-	99%	99%
Prophylactic Antibiotic Selection (Outpatient)	-	-	98%	98%
Prophylactic Antibiotic Stopped[5]	-	-	98%	98%
Prophylactic Antibiotic Timing[5]	-	-	99%	99%
Prophylactic Antibiotic Timing (Outpatient)	-	-	99%	98%
Urinary Catheter Removal[5]	-	-	98%	97%
Survey of Patients' Hospital Experiences				
Area Around Room 'Always' Quiet at Night	-	-	71%	61%
Doctors 'Always' Communicated Well	-	-	86%	82%
Home Recovery Information Given	-	-	84%	85%
Hospital Given 9 or 10 on 10 Point Scale	-	-	71%	71%
Meds 'Always' Explained Before Given	-	-	66%	64%
Nurses 'Always' Communicated Well	-	-	80%	79%
Pain 'Always' Well Controlled	-	-	72%	71%
Room and Bathroom 'Always' Clean	-	-	71%	73%
Timely Help 'Always' Received	-	-	68%	68%
Would Definitely Recommend Hospital	-	-	70%	71%
Use of Medical Imaging				
Cardiac Imaging Stress Test before Surgery	-	-	6.5%	5.3%
Combination Abdominal CT Scan	-	-	16.5%	10.5%
Combination Brain/Sinus CT Scan	-	-	3.5%	2.7%
Combination Chest CT Scan	-	-	4.2%	2.7%
Follow-up Mammogram/Ultrasound	-	-	7.6%	8.8%
Lumbar Spine MRI for Low Back Pain	-	-	40.2%	37.2%

Lawrence Medical Center

202 Hospital Street
Moulton, AL 35650
Phone: 256-974-2200
Fax: 256-974-2299
URL: www.lawrencemedicalcenter.com
Type: Acute Care Hospitals
Emergency Services: Yes
Ownership: Govt - Hospital Dist/Auth
Beds: 98

Key Personnel:
Chief of Medical Staff . . . . Charles Coffey
CEO/President . . . . Thomas Dunning
Operating Room . . . . Martha Everly
Infection Control . . . . Melody Farley
Coronary Care . . . . Anita Lacy
Emergency Room . . . . Anita Lacy
Intensive Care Unit . . . . Anita Lacy
Quality Assurance . . . . John Thrasher

Measure	Cases	This Hosp.	State Avg.	U.S. Avg.
Blood Clot Prevention and Treatment				
Anticoagulation Overlap Therapy[1,2]	-	-	91%	93%
ICU Venous Thromboembolism Prophylaxis[2]	25	92%	85%	92%
Incidence of Potentially Preventable VTE[2,7]	-	-	18%	10%
UFH with Dosages/Platelet Monitoring[1,2]	-	-	95%	97%
Venous Thromboembolism Prophylaxis[2]	98	89%	74%	85%
Warfarin Therapy Discharge Instructions[1,2]	-	-	77%	75%
Chest Pain/Possible Heart Attack Care				
Aspirin Given Within 24 Hours of Arrival	39	92%	96%	96%
Fibrinolytic Meds Within 30 Min. of Arrival[1]	-	-	57%	58%
Average Time to ECG (minutes)	41	7	6	7
Average Time to Transfer (minutes)[1]	-	-	61	60
Children's Asthma Care				
Received Home Management Plan of Care	-	-	-	88%
Received Reliever Medication	-	-	-	100%
Received Systemic Corticosteroids	-	-	-	100%
Emergency Department				
Admittance Decision Time (minutes)[2]	297	52	73	98
Head CT Results Within 45 Min. of Arrival[1]	-	-	45%	57%
Patients Who Left ER Before Being Seen	9,273	1%	3%	2%
Time from ER Arrival to Admit. (minutes)[2]	321	191	240	274
Time from ER Arrival to Discharge (minutes)	384	86	126	134
Time in ER Before Being Evaluated (minutes)	405	18	31	26
Time to Pain Meds for Fractures (minutes)	49	40	69	57
Heart Attack Care				
Aspirin Given at Discharge[1]	-	-	99%	99%
Fibrinolytic Meds Within 30 Min. of Arrival[7]	-	-	77%	54%
PCI Within 90 Minutes of Arrival[7]	-	-	97%	96%
Statin Prescribed at Discharge[1]	-	-	98%	98%
Heart Failure Care				
ACE Inhibitor or ARB for LVSD[1]	-	-	97%	97%
Discharge Instructions Given	21	76%	93%	94%
Evaluation of LVS Function	31	100%	99%	99%
Medicare Spending				
Medicare Spending per Patient (ratio)	-	0.90	0.98	0.98
Pneumonia Care				
Appropriate Initial Antibiotic Given	56	93%	95%	95%
Blood Culture Timing	62	92%	98%	98%
Pregnancy and Delivery Care				
Newborn Deliveries Scheduled Early[7]	-	-	14%	6%
Preventive Care				
Immunization for Influenza[2]	285	94%	90%	90%
Immunization for Pneumonia[2]	427	99%	91%	92%
Stroke Care				
Anticoagulation Therapy for Atrial Fibrillation[1]	-	-	92%	95%
Antithrombotic Therapy Timing	16	94%	96%	98%
Assessed for Rehabilitation	13	100%	95%	97%
Discharged on Antithrombotic Therapy	13	100%	98%	99%
Discharged on Statin Medication[1]	-	-	90%	94%
Thrombolytic Therapy Timing[7]	-	-	38%	66%
Venous Thromboembolism Prophylaxis	15	93%	89%	94%
Written Stroke Educational Materials Given[1]	-	-	85%	88%
Surgical Care Improvement Project				
Appropriate Beta Blocker Usage[5]	-	-	98%	98%
Appropriate VTP Within 24 Hours[5]	-	-	98%	98%
Controlled Postoperative Blood Glucose[5]	-	-	97%	97%
Perioperative Temperature Management[5]	-	-	100%	100%
Prophylactic Antibiotic Selection[5]	-	-	99%	99%
Prophylactic Antibiotic Selection (Outpatient)[5]	-	-	98%	98%
Prophylactic Antibiotic Stopped[5]	-	-	98%	98%
Prophylactic Antibiotic Timing[5]	-	-	99%	99%
Prophylactic Antibiotic Timing (Outpatient)[5]	-	-	99%	98%
Urinary Catheter Removal[5]	-	-	98%	97%
Survey of Patients' Hospital Experiences				
Area Around Room 'Always' Quiet at Night	(a)	62%	71%	61%

NOTE: Hospital profiles are in alphabetical order by state, then city, then hospital within the city; Rankings exclude hospitals with less than 25 cases except for patient surveys which excludes hospitals with less than 100 cases; (a) 100-299 cases; (1) The number of cases/patients is too few to report; (2) Data submitted were based on a sample of cases/patients; (3) Results are based on a shorter time period than required; (4) Data suppressed by CMS for one or more quarters; (5) Results are not available for this reporting period; (6) Fewer than 100 patients completed the HCAHPS survey; (7) No cases met the criteria for this measure; (8) The lower limit of the confidence interval cannot be calculated if the number of observed infections equals zero; (9) No data are available from the state/territory for this reporting period; (10) The scores shown reflect fewer than 50 completed surveys; (11) There were discrepancies in the data collection process; (12) This measure does not apply to this hospital for this reporting period; (13) Results cannot be calculated for this reporting period; (14) The results for this state are combined with nearby states to protect confidentiality; Please refer to the User's Guide for a full explanation of data.

Measure	Cases	This Hosp.	State Avg.	U.S. Avg.
Doctors 'Always' Communicated Well	(a)	93%	86%	82%
Home Recovery Information Given	(a)	85%	84%	85%
Hospital Given 9 or 10 on 10 Point Scale	(a)	64%	71%	71%
Meds 'Always' Explained Before Given	(a)	65%	66%	64%
Nurses 'Always' Communicated Well	(a)	82%	80%	79%
Pain 'Always' Well Controlled	(a)	67%	72%	71%
Room and Bathroom 'Always' Clean	(a)	74%	71%	73%
Timely Help 'Always' Received	(a)	67%	68%	68%
Would Definitely Recommend Hospital	(a)	62%	70%	71%
Use of Medical Imaging				
Cardiac Imaging Stress Test before Surgery[7]	-	-	6.5%	5.3%
Combination Abdominal CT Scan	212	2.4%	16.5%	10.5%
Combination Brain/Sinus CT Scan	250	6.0%	3.5%	2.7%
Combination Chest CT Scan	87	0.0%	4.2%	2.7%
Follow-up Mammogram/Ultrasound	242	12.8%	7.6%	8.8%
Lumbar Spine MRI for Low Back Pain[1]	-	-	40.2%	37.2%

Shoals Hospital

201 West Avalon Avenue
Muscle Shoals, AL 35661
URL: www.chgroup.org
Type: Acute Care Hospitals
Ownership: Govt - Hospital Dist/Auth
Phone: 256-386-1601
Fax: 256-386-1115
Emergency Services: Yes
Beds: 144

Key Personnel:
Radiology. . . . . S P Bilyeu
Operating Room. . . . . David Cozart
Emergency Room . . . . Sheila Felton
Intensive Care Unit. . . . . Sheila Felton
Quality Assurance . . . . Kathy Harrison
CEO . . . . Jeff Jennings
Patient Relations . . . . Amanda Mann
Chief of Medical Staff. . . . . Miranda Riley

Measure	Cases	This Hosp.	State Avg.	U.S. Avg.
Blood Clot Prevention and Treatment				
Anticoagulation Overlap Therapy[2]	12	67%	91%	93%
ICU Venous Thromboembolism Prophylaxis[2]	42	79%	85%	92%
Incidence of Potentially Preventable VTE[1,2]	-	-	18%	10%
UFH with Dosages/Platelet Monitoring[2,7]	-	-	95%	97%
Venous Thromboembolism Prophylaxis[2]	142	68%	74%	85%
Warfarin Therapy Discharge Instructions[2]	11	27%	77%	75%
Chest Pain/Possible Heart Attack Care				
Aspirin Given Within 24 Hours of Arrival[1,3]	-	-	96%	96%
Fibrinolytic Meds Within 30 Min. of Arrival[3,7]	-	-	57%	58%
Average Time to ECG (minutes)[1,3]	-	-	6	7
Average Time to Transfer (minutes)[1,3]	-	-	61	60
Children's Asthma Care				
Received Home Management Plan of Care	-	-	-	88%
Received Reliever Medication	-	-	-	100%
Received Systemic Corticosteroids	-	-	-	100%
Emergency Department				
Admittance Decision Time (minutes)[2]	220	52	73	98
Head CT Results Within 45 Min. of Arrival[1]	-	-	45%	57%
Patients Who Left ER Before Being Seen	13,465	4%	3%	2%
Time from ER Arrival to Admit. (minutes)[2]	228	236	240	274
Time from ER Arrival to Discharge (minutes)	442	146	126	134
Time in ER Before Being Evaluated (minutes)	431	23	31	26
Time to Pain Meds for Fractures (minutes)[1]	-	-	69	57
Heart Attack Care				
Aspirin Given at Discharge[1,3]	-	-	99%	99%
Fibrinolytic Meds Within 30 Min. of Arrival[3,7]	-	-	77%	54%
PCI Within 90 Minutes of Arrival[3,7]	-	-	97%	96%
Statin Prescribed at Discharge[1,3]	-	-	98%	98%
Heart Failure Care				
ACE Inhibitor or ARB for LVSD[1]	-	-	97%	97%
Discharge Instructions Given	32	59%	93%	94%
Evaluation of LVS Function	45	96%	99%	99%
Medicare Spending				
Medicare Spending per Patient (ratio)	-	1.06	0.98	0.98
Pneumonia Care				
Appropriate Initial Antibiotic Given	57	96%	95%	95%
Blood Culture Timing	92	99%	98%	98%
Pregnancy and Delivery Care				
Newborn Deliveries Scheduled Early[7]	-	-	14%	6%
Preventive Care				
Immunization for Influenza[2]	312	97%	90%	90%
Immunization for Pneumonia[2]	479	97%	91%	92%
Stroke Care				
Anticoagulation Therapy for Atrial Fibrillation[1]	-	-	92%	95%
Antithrombotic Therapy Timing	19	84%	96%	98%
Assessed for Rehabilitation	18	100%	95%	97%
Discharged on Antithrombotic Therapy	18	89%	98%	99%
Discharged on Statin Medication	15	60%	90%	94%
Thrombolytic Therapy Timing[1]	-	-	38%	66%
Venous Thromboembolism Prophylaxis	20	90%	89%	94%
Written Stroke Educational Materials Given[1]	-	-	85%	88%
Surgical Care Improvement Project				
Appropriate Beta Blocker Usage	35	91%	98%	98%
Appropriate VTP Within 24 Hours	114	96%	98%	98%
Controlled Postoperative Blood Glucose[7]	-	-	97%	97%
Perioperative Temperature Management	126	100%	100%	100%
Prophylactic Antibiotic Selection	77	97%	99%	99%
Prophylactic Antibiotic Selection (Outpatient)[1]	-	-	98%	98%
Prophylactic Antibiotic Stopped	73	97%	98%	98%
Prophylactic Antibiotic Timing	78	100%	99%	99%
Prophylactic Antibiotic Timing (Outpatient)[1]	-	-	99%	98%
Urinary Catheter Removal	99	99%	98%	97%
Survey of Patients' Hospital Experiences				
Area Around Room 'Always' Quiet at Night	300+	72%	71%	61%
Doctors 'Always' Communicated Well	300+	83%	86%	82%
Home Recovery Information Given	300+	80%	84%	85%
Hospital Given 9 or 10 on 10 Point Scale	300+	71%	71%	71%
Meds 'Always' Explained Before Given	300+	57%	66%	64%
Nurses 'Always' Communicated Well	300+	80%	80%	79%
Pain 'Always' Well Controlled	300+	71%	72%	71%
Room and Bathroom 'Always' Clean	300+	72%	71%	73%
Timely Help 'Always' Received	300+	64%	68%	68%
Would Definitely Recommend Hospital	300+	72%	70%	71%
Use of Medical Imaging				
Cardiac Imaging Stress Test before Surgery[1]	-	-	6.5%	5.3%
Combination Abdominal CT Scan	424	30.4%	16.5%	10.5%
Combination Brain/Sinus CT Scan[1]	-	-	3.5%	2.7%
Combination Chest CT Scan	239	22.6%	4.2%	2.7%
Follow-up Mammogram/Ultrasound	373	10.7%	7.6%	8.8%
Lumbar Spine MRI for Low Back Pain	199	38.7%	40.2%	37.2%

East Alabama Medical Center

2000 Pepperell Parkway
Opelika, AL 36801
URL: www.eamc.org
Type: Acute Care Hospitals
Ownership: Govt - Hospital Dist/Auth
Phone: 334-749-3411
Fax: 334-705-1407
Emergency Services: Yes
Beds: 348

Key Personnel:
CEO/President. . . . . Terry Andrus
Quality Assurance . . . . Janice Baker
Emergency Room . . . . Dell Crosby, RN
Radiology. . . . . David Downs, MD
Administrator . . . . Laura D. Grill
Chief of Medical Staff. . . . . Michael Lisenby, MD
Chairman/CEO . . . . Joel Pittard, MD
Operating Room. . . . . Kathy Thomas

Measure	Cases	This Hosp.	State Avg.	U.S. Avg.
Blood Clot Prevention and Treatment				
Anticoagulation Overlap Therapy[2]	87	83%	91%	93%
ICU Venous Thromboembolism Prophylaxis[2]	88	88%	85%	92%
Incidence of Potentially Preventable VTE[2]	15	7%	18%	10%
UFH with Dosages/Platelet Monitoring[2]	13	100%	95%	97%
Venous Thromboembolism Prophylaxis[2]	316	63%	74%	85%
Warfarin Therapy Discharge Instructions[2]	62	87%	77%	75%
Chest Pain/Possible Heart Attack Care				
Aspirin Given Within 24 Hours of Arrival[5]	-	-	96%	96%
Fibrinolytic Meds Within 30 Min. of Arrival[5]	-	-	57%	58%
Average Time to ECG (minutes)[5]	-	-	6	7
Average Time to Transfer (minutes)[5]	-	-	61	60
Children's Asthma Care				
Received Home Management Plan of Care	-	-	-	88%
Received Reliever Medication	-	-	-	100%
Received Systemic Corticosteroids	-	-	-	100%
Emergency Department				
Admittance Decision Time (minutes)[2]	548	45	73	98
Head CT Results Within 45 Min. of Arrival[1]	-	-	45%	57%
Patients Who Left ER Before Being Seen	47,507	3%	3%	2%
Time from ER Arrival to Admit. (minutes)[2]	548	229	240	274
Time from ER Arrival to Discharge (minutes)	446	164	126	134
Time in ER Before Being Evaluated (minutes)	480	53	31	26
Time to Pain Meds for Fractures (minutes)	176	68	69	57
Heart Attack Care				
Aspirin Given at Discharge	241	100%	99%	99%
Fibrinolytic Meds Within 30 Min. of Arrival[7]	-	-	77%	54%
PCI Within 90 Minutes of Arrival	52	98%	97%	96%
Statin Prescribed at Discharge	240	100%	98%	98%
Heart Failure Care				
ACE Inhibitor or ARB for LVSD	180	100%	97%	97%
Discharge Instructions Given	404	95%	93%	94%
Evaluation of LVS Function	464	100%	99%	99%
Medicare Spending				
Medicare Spending per Patient (ratio)	-	0.90	0.98	0.98
Pneumonia Care				
Appropriate Initial Antibiotic Given	168	96%	95%	95%
Blood Culture Timing	214	100%	98%	98%
Pregnancy and Delivery Care				
Newborn Deliveries Scheduled Early[2]	95	1%	14%	6%
Preventive Care				
Immunization for Influenza[2]	750	82%	90%	90%
Immunization for Pneumonia[2]	771	80%	91%	92%
Stroke Care				
Anticoagulation Therapy for Atrial Fibrillation	19	100%	92%	95%
Antithrombotic Therapy Timing	148	100%	96%	98%
Assessed for Rehabilitation	185	100%	95%	97%
Discharged on Antithrombotic Therapy	156	100%	98%	99%
Discharged on Statin Medication	138	100%	90%	94%
Thrombolytic Therapy Timing[1]	-	-	38%	66%
Venous Thromboembolism Prophylaxis	181	100%	89%	94%
Written Stroke Educational Materials Given	102	96%	85%	88%
Surgical Care Improvement Project				
Appropriate Beta Blocker Usage	415	100%	98%	98%
Appropriate VTP Within 24 Hours	1,001	100%	98%	98%
Controlled Postoperative Blood Glucose	195	99%	97%	97%
Perioperative Temperature Management	1,129	100%	100%	100%
Prophylactic Antibiotic Selection	931	100%	99%	99%
Prophylactic Antibiotic Selection (Outpatient)	848	100%	98%	98%
Prophylactic Antibiotic Stopped	894	99%	98%	98%
Prophylactic Antibiotic Timing	931	100%	99%	99%
Prophylactic Antibiotic Timing (Outpatient)	848	100%	99%	98%
Urinary Catheter Removal	782	99%	98%	97%
Survey of Patients' Hospital Experiences				
Area Around Room 'Always' Quiet at Night	300+	75%	71%	61%
Doctors 'Always' Communicated Well	300+	87%	86%	82%
Home Recovery Information Given	300+	88%	84%	85%
Hospital Given 9 or 10 on 10 Point Scale	300+	77%	71%	71%
Meds 'Always' Explained Before Given	300+	69%	66%	64%
Nurses 'Always' Communicated Well	300+	81%	80%	79%
Pain 'Always' Well Controlled	300+	74%	72%	71%
Room and Bathroom 'Always' Clean	300+	72%	71%	73%
Timely Help 'Always' Received	300+	69%	68%	68%
Would Definitely Recommend Hospital	300+	78%	70%	71%
Use of Medical Imaging				
Cardiac Imaging Stress Test before Surgery	1,428	5.5%	6.5%	5.3%
Combination Abdominal CT Scan	1,132	52.9%	16.5%	10.5%
Combination Brain/Sinus CT Scan	1,154	3.8%	3.5%	2.7%
Combination Chest CT Scan	729	0.8%	4.2%	2.7%
Follow-up Mammogram/Ultrasound	2,066	7.3%	7.6%	8.8%
Lumbar Spine MRI for Low Back Pain	402	37.8%	40.2%	37.2%

Mizell Memorial Hospital

702 N Main St
Opp, AL 36467
E-mail: rlemaire@mizellmh.com
URL: www.mizellmh.com
Type: Acute Care Hospitals
Ownership: Voluntary non-profit - Private
Phone: 334-493-3541
Fax: 334-493-9664
Emergency Services: Yes
Beds: 99

Key Personnel:
Pediatric Ambulatory Care . . . . . . Dr Bhagwan Bang

NOTE: Hospital profiles are in alphabetical order by state, then city, then hospital within the city; Rankings exclude hospitals with less than 25 cases except for patient surveys which excludes hospitals with less than 100 cases; (a) 100-299 cases; (1) The number of cases/patients is too few to report; (2) Data submitted were based on a sample of cases/patients; (3) Results are based on a shorter time period than required; (4) Data suppressed by CMS for one or more quarters; (5) Results are not available for this reporting period; (6) Fewer than 100 patients completed the HCAHPS survey; (7) No cases met the criteria for this measure; (8) The lower limit of the confidence interval cannot be calculated if the number of observed infections equals zero; (9) No data are available from the state/territory for this reporting period; (10) The scores shown reflect fewer than 50 completed surveys; (11) There were discrepancies in the data collection process; (12) This measure does not apply to this hospital for this reporting period; (13) Results cannot be calculated for this reporting period; (14) The results for this state are combined with nearby states to protect confidentiality; Please refer to the User's Guide for a full explanation of data.

Emergency Room .... Dr Steve Davis
Operating Room............. Timothy Day
CEO/President.............. Allen Foster
Quality Assurance .... Debbie Franklin
Chief of Medical Staff......... Wheeler A Gunnels, MD
Intensive Care Unit........... Patricia Hill, CRNP
Radiology.................. Vincent E Martin

Measure	Cases	This Hosp.	State Avg.	U.S. Avg.
Blood Clot Prevention and Treatment				
Anticoagulation Overlap Therapy[1,2]	-	-	91%	93%
ICU Venous Thromboembolism Prophylaxis[2]	46	57%	85%	92%
Incidence of Potentially Preventable VTE[2,7]	-	-	18%	10%
UFH with Dosages/Platelet Monitoring[2,7]	-	-	95%	97%
Venous Thromboembolism Prophylaxis[2]	242	62%	74%	85%
Warfarin Therapy Discharge Instructions[1,2]	-	-	77%	75%
Chest Pain/Possible Heart Attack Care				
Aspirin Given Within 24 Hours of Arrival	15	93%	96%	96%
Fibrinolytic Meds Within 30 Min. of Arrival[1]	-	-	57%	58%
Average Time to ECG (minutes)	17	10	6	7
Average Time to Transfer (minutes)[1]	-	-	61	60
Children's Asthma Care				
Received Home Management Plan of Care	-	-	-	88%
Received Reliever Medication	-	-	-	100%
Received Systemic Corticosteroids	-	-	-	100%
Emergency Department				
Admittance Decision Time (minutes)[2]	400	55	73	98
Head CT Results Within 45 Min. of Arrival[1,3]	-	-	45%	57%
Patients Who Left ER Before Being Seen	10,246	3%	3%	2%
Time from ER Arrival to Admit. (minutes)[2]	411	200	240	274
Time from ER Arrival to Discharge (minutes)	278	99	126	134
Time in ER Before Being Evaluated (minutes)	269	28	31	26
Time to Pain Meds for Fractures (minutes)	44	80	69	57
Heart Attack Care				
Aspirin Given at Discharge[1]	-	-	99%	99%
Fibrinolytic Meds Within 30 Min. of Arrival[7]	-	-	77%	54%
PCI Within 90 Minutes of Arrival[7]	-	-	97%	96%
Statin Prescribed at Discharge[1]	-	-	98%	98%
Heart Failure Care				
ACE Inhibitor or ARB for LVSD	12	100%	97%	97%
Discharge Instructions Given	32	69%	93%	94%
Evaluation of LVS Function	47	98%	99%	99%
Medicare Spending				
Medicare Spending per Patient (ratio)	-	1.00	0.98	0.98
Pneumonia Care				
Appropriate Initial Antibiotic Given	50	92%	95%	95%
Blood Culture Timing	35	94%	98%	98%
Pregnancy and Delivery Care				
Newborn Deliveries Scheduled Early[7]	-	-	14%	6%
Preventive Care				
Immunization for Influenza[2]	334	80%	90%	90%
Immunization for Pneumonia[2]	509	89%	91%	92%
Stroke Care				
Anticoagulation Therapy for Atrial Fibrillation[1]	-	-	92%	95%
Antithrombotic Therapy Timing[1]	-	-	96%	98%
Assessed for Rehabilitation[1]	-	-	95%	97%
Discharged on Antithrombotic Therapy[1]	-	-	98%	99%
Discharged on Statin Medication[1]	-	-	90%	94%
Thrombolytic Therapy Timing[7]	-	-	38%	66%
Venous Thromboembolism Prophylaxis[1]	-	-	89%	94%
Written Stroke Educational Materials Given[1]	-	-	85%	88%
Surgical Care Improvement Project				
Appropriate Beta Blocker Usage	11	100%	98%	98%
Appropriate VTP Within 24 Hours	21	95%	98%	98%
Controlled Postoperative Blood Glucose[7]	-	-	97%	97%
Perioperative Temperature Management	29	100%	100%	100%
Prophylactic Antibiotic Selection	16	100%	99%	99%
Prophylactic Antibiotic Selection (Outpatient)[1]	-	-	98%	98%
Prophylactic Antibiotic Stopped	16	94%	98%	98%
Prophylactic Antibiotic Timing	16	100%	99%	99%
Prophylactic Antibiotic Timing (Outpatient)	11	55%	99%	98%
Urinary Catheter Removal	20	95%	98%	97%
Survey of Patients' Hospital Experiences				
Area Around Room 'Always' Quiet at Night	(a)	77%	71%	61%
Doctors 'Always' Communicated Well	(a)	90%	86%	82%
Home Recovery Information Given	(a)	84%	84%	85%
Hospital Given 9 or 10 on 10 Point Scale	(a)	67%	71%	71%
Meds 'Always' Explained Before Given	(a)	67%	66%	64%
Nurses 'Always' Communicated Well	(a)	74%	80%	79%
Pain 'Always' Well Controlled	(a)	69%	72%	71%
Room and Bathroom 'Always' Clean	(a)	72%	71%	73%
Timely Help 'Always' Received	(a)	64%	68%	68%
Would Definitely Recommend Hospital	(a)	69%	70%	71%
Use of Medical Imaging				
Cardiac Imaging Stress Test before Surgery[1]	-	-	6.5%	5.3%
Combination Abdominal CT Scan	219	34.7%	16.5%	10.5%
Combination Brain/Sinus CT Scan[1]	-	-	3.5%	2.7%
Combination Chest CT Scan	134	1.5%	4.2%	2.7%
Follow-up Mammogram/Ultrasound	475	12.8%	7.6%	8.8%
Lumbar Spine MRI for Low Back Pain[1]	-	-	40.2%	37.2%

Dale Medical Center

126 Hospital Ave
Ozark, AL 36360
URL: www.dalemedical.org
Type: Acute Care Hospitals
Ownership: Govt - Hospital Dist/Auth
Phone: 334-774-2601
Fax: 334-774-0258
Emergency Services: Yes
Beds: 89

Key Personnel:
Emergency Room .... Carl W Barlow
Intensive Care Unit........... Lloyd Duncan, RN
Infection Control............. Jan Hamm
CEO/President.............. Vernon Johnson
Pediatric In-Patient Care .... Julie Jones, RN
Radiology.................. Dudley J Terrell

Measure	Cases	This Hosp.	State Avg.	U.S. Avg.
Blood Clot Prevention and Treatment				
Anticoagulation Overlap Therapy[1,2]	-	-	91%	93%
ICU Venous Thromboembolism Prophylaxis[2]	66	100%	85%	92%
Incidence of Potentially Preventable VTE[2,7]	-	-	18%	10%
UFH with Dosages/Platelet Monitoring[2,7]	-	-	95%	97%
Venous Thromboembolism Prophylaxis[2]	221	98%	74%	85%
Warfarin Therapy Discharge Instructions[1,2]	-	-	77%	75%
Chest Pain/Possible Heart Attack Care				
Aspirin Given Within 24 Hours of Arrival	39	95%	96%	96%
Fibrinolytic Meds Within 30 Min. of Arrival[1]	-	-	57%	58%
Average Time to ECG (minutes)	39	6	6	7
Average Time to Transfer (minutes)[7]	-	-	61	60
Children's Asthma Care				
Received Home Management Plan of Care	-	-	-	88%
Received Reliever Medication	-	-	-	100%
Received Systemic Corticosteroids	-	-	-	100%
Emergency Department				
Admittance Decision Time (minutes)[2]	508	50	73	98
Head CT Results Within 45 Min. of Arrival[1,3]	-	-	45%	57%
Patients Who Left ER Before Being Seen	16,986	1%	3%	2%
Time from ER Arrival to Admit. (minutes)[2]	508	164	240	274
Time from ER Arrival to Discharge (minutes)	411	80	126	134
Time in ER Before Being Evaluated (minutes)	521	22	31	26
Time to Pain Meds for Fractures (minutes)	46	46	69	57
Heart Attack Care				
Aspirin Given at Discharge[1,3]	-	-	99%	99%
Fibrinolytic Meds Within 30 Min. of Arrival[3,7]	-	-	77%	54%
PCI Within 90 Minutes of Arrival[3,7]	-	-	97%	96%
Statin Prescribed at Discharge[3,7]	-	-	98%	98%
Heart Failure Care				
ACE Inhibitor or ARB for LVSD[2]	17	94%	97%	97%
Discharge Instructions Given[2]	48	98%	93%	94%
Evaluation of LVS Function[2]	62	100%	99%	99%
Medicare Spending				
Medicare Spending per Patient (ratio)	-	0.93	0.98	0.98
Pneumonia Care				
Appropriate Initial Antibiotic Given	34	85%	95%	95%
Blood Culture Timing	56	100%	98%	98%
Pregnancy and Delivery Care				
Newborn Deliveries Scheduled Early[7]	-	-	14%	6%
Preventive Care				
Immunization for Influenza[2]	354	98%	90%	90%
Immunization for Pneumonia[2]	499	100%	91%	92%
Stroke Care				
Anticoagulation Therapy for Atrial Fibrillation[7]	-	-	92%	95%
Antithrombotic Therapy Timing[1]	-	-	96%	98%
Assessed for Rehabilitation[1]	-	-	95%	97%
Discharged on Antithrombotic Therapy[1]	-	-	98%	99%
Discharged on Statin Medication[1]	-	-	90%	94%
Thrombolytic Therapy Timing[7]	-	-	38%	66%
Venous Thromboembolism Prophylaxis[1]	-	-	89%	94%
Written Stroke Educational Materials Given[1]	-	-	85%	88%
Surgical Care Improvement Project				
Appropriate Beta Blocker Usage	30	53%	98%	98%
Appropriate VTP Within 24 Hours	89	97%	98%	98%
Controlled Postoperative Blood Glucose[7]	-	-	97%	97%
Perioperative Temperature Management	96	100%	100%	100%
Prophylactic Antibiotic Selection	33	100%	99%	99%
Prophylactic Antibiotic Selection (Outpatient)	11	55%	98%	98%
Prophylactic Antibiotic Stopped	32	94%	98%	98%
Prophylactic Antibiotic Timing	33	100%	99%	99%
Prophylactic Antibiotic Timing (Outpatient)	12	83%	99%	98%
Urinary Catheter Removal	79	100%	98%	97%
Survey of Patients' Hospital Experiences				
Area Around Room 'Always' Quiet at Night	(a)	72%	71%	61%
Doctors 'Always' Communicated Well	(a)	83%	86%	82%
Home Recovery Information Given	(a)	83%	84%	85%
Hospital Given 9 or 10 on 10 Point Scale	(a)	65%	71%	71%
Meds 'Always' Explained Before Given	(a)	67%	66%	64%
Nurses 'Always' Communicated Well	(a)	81%	80%	79%
Pain 'Always' Well Controlled	(a)	68%	72%	71%
Room and Bathroom 'Always' Clean	(a)	70%	71%	73%
Timely Help 'Always' Received	(a)	66%	68%	68%
Would Definitely Recommend Hospital	(a)	66%	70%	71%
Use of Medical Imaging				
Cardiac Imaging Stress Test before Surgery	166	4.8%	6.5%	5.3%
Combination Abdominal CT Scan	279	12.2%	16.5%	10.5%
Combination Brain/Sinus CT Scan	503	5.6%	3.5%	2.7%
Combination Chest CT Scan	124	4.8%	4.2%	2.7%
Follow-up Mammogram/Ultrasound	469	7.0%	7.6%	8.8%
Lumbar Spine MRI for Low Back Pain	52	42.3%	40.2%	37.2%

Saint Vincent's Saint Clair

7063 Veterans Parkway
Pell City, AL 35125
URL: www.stclaireregional.com
Type: Acute Care Hospitals
Ownership: Voluntary non-profit - Private
Phone: 205-338-3301
Fax: 205-814-2145
Emergency Services: Yes
Beds: 82

Key Personnel:
CEO/President.............. Douglas H Beverly
Quality Assurance .... Helen Dykes
Radiology.................. Thomas G Loflin
Operating Room............. James West

Measure	Cases	This Hosp.	State Avg.	U.S. Avg.
Blood Clot Prevention and Treatment				
Anticoagulation Overlap Therapy[2]	39	72%	91%	93%
ICU Venous Thromboembolism Prophylaxis[2]	51	65%	85%	92%
Incidence of Potentially Preventable VTE[1,2]	-	-	18%	10%
UFH with Dosages/Platelet Monitoring[2]	26	96%	95%	97%
Venous Thromboembolism Prophylaxis[2]	204	44%	74%	85%
Warfarin Therapy Discharge Instructions[2]	23	91%	77%	75%
Chest Pain/Possible Heart Attack Care				
Aspirin Given Within 24 Hours of Arrival	96	96%	96%	96%
Fibrinolytic Meds Within 30 Min. of Arrival[1]	-	-	57%	58%
Average Time to ECG (minutes)	103	4	6	7
Average Time to Transfer (minutes)[1]	-	-	61	60
Children's Asthma Care				
Received Home Management Plan of Care	-	-	-	88%
Received Reliever Medication	-	-	-	100%
Received Systemic Corticosteroids	-	-	-	100%
Emergency Department				
Admittance Decision Time (minutes)[2]	328	55	73	98
Head CT Results Within 45 Min. of Arrival[1]	-	-	45%	57%
Patients Who Left ER Before Being Seen	25,105	2%	3%	2%
Time from ER Arrival to Admit. (minutes)[2]	330	218	240	274
Time from ER Arrival to Discharge (minutes)	345	107	126	134

NOTE: Hospital profiles are in alphabetical order by state, then city, then hospital within the city; Rankings exclude hospitals with less than 25 cases except for patient surveys which excludes hospitals with less than 100 cases; (a) 100-299 cases; (1) The number of cases/patients is too few to report; (2) Data submitted were based on a sample of cases/patients; (3) Results are based on a shorter time period than required; (4) Data suppressed by CMS for one or more quarters; (5) Results are not available for this reporting period; (6) Fewer than 100 patients completed the HCAHPS survey; (7) No cases met the criteria for this measure; (8) The lower limit of the confidence interval cannot be calculated if the number of observed infections equals zero; (9) No data are available from the state/territory for this reporting period; (10) The scores shown reflect fewer than 50 completed surveys; (11) There were discrepancies in the data collection process; (12) This measure does not apply to this hospital for this reporting period; (13) Results cannot be calculated for this reporting period; (14) The results for this state are combined with nearby states to protect confidentiality; Please refer to the User's Guide for a full explanation of data.

Measure	Cases	This Hosp.	State Avg.	U.S. Avg.
Time in ER Before Being Evaluated (minutes)	356	30	31	26
Time to Pain Meds for Fractures (minutes)	95	68	69	57
Heart Attack Care				
Aspirin Given at Discharge[1]	-	-	99%	99%
Fibrinolytic Meds Within 30 Min. of Arrival[7]	-	-	77%	54%
PCI Within 90 Minutes of Arrival[7]	-	-	97%	96%
Statin Prescribed at Discharge[1]	-	-	98%	98%
Heart Failure Care				
ACE Inhibitor or ARB for LVSD	15	93%	97%	97%
Discharge Instructions Given	62	97%	93%	94%
Evaluation of LVS Function	82	93%	99%	99%
Medicare Spending				
Medicare Spending per Patient (ratio)	-	0.92	0.98	0.98
Pneumonia Care				
Appropriate Initial Antibiotic Given	181	92%	95%	95%
Blood Culture Timing	171	99%	98%	98%
Pregnancy and Delivery Care				
Newborn Deliveries Scheduled Early[7]	-	-	14%	6%
Preventive Care				
Immunization for Influenza[2]	284	97%	90%	90%
Immunization for Pneumonia[2]	420	96%	91%	92%
Stroke Care				
Anticoagulation Therapy for Atrial Fibrillation[1,2]	-	-	92%	95%
Antithrombotic Therapy Timing[2]	26	96%	96%	98%
Assessed for Rehabilitation[2]	23	83%	95%	97%
Discharged on Antithrombotic Therapy[2]	23	96%	98%	99%
Discharged on Statin Medication[2]	21	76%	90%	94%
Thrombolytic Therapy Timing[1,2]	-	-	38%	66%
Venous Thromboembolism Prophylaxis[2]	26	77%	89%	94%
Written Stroke Educational Materials Given[2]	13	92%	85%	88%
Surgical Care Improvement Project				
Appropriate Beta Blocker Usage[1,3]	-	-	98%	98%
Appropriate VTP Within 24 Hours[1,3]	-	-	98%	98%
Controlled Postoperative Blood Glucose[3,7]	-	-	97%	97%
Perioperative Temperature Management[1,3]	-	-	100%	100%
Prophylactic Antibiotic Selection[1,3]	-	-	99%	99%
Prophylactic Antibiotic Selection (Outpatient)[1,3]	-	-	98%	98%
Prophylactic Antibiotic Stopped[1,3]	-	-	98%	98%
Prophylactic Antibiotic Timing[1,3]	-	-	99%	99%
Prophylactic Antibiotic Timing (Outpatient)[1,3]	-	-	99%	98%
Urinary Catheter Removal[1,3]	-	-	98%	97%
Survey of Patients' Hospital Experiences				
Area Around Room 'Always' Quiet at Night	300+	78%	71%	61%
Doctors 'Always' Communicated Well	300+	90%	86%	82%
Home Recovery Information Given	300+	87%	84%	85%
Hospital Given 9 or 10 on 10 Point Scale	300+	81%	71%	71%
Meds 'Always' Explained Before Given	300+	72%	66%	64%
Nurses 'Always' Communicated Well	300+	83%	80%	79%
Pain 'Always' Well Controlled	300+	78%	72%	71%
Room and Bathroom 'Always' Clean	300+	75%	71%	73%
Timely Help 'Always' Received	300+	75%	68%	68%
Would Definitely Recommend Hospital	300+	80%	70%	71%
Use of Medical Imaging				
Cardiac Imaging Stress Test before Surgery	79	6.3%	6.5%	5.3%
Combination Abdominal CT Scan	407	19.4%	16.5%	10.5%
Combination Brain/Sinus CT Scan	370	4.3%	3.5%	2.7%
Combination Chest CT Scan	162	32.1%	4.2%	2.7%
Follow-up Mammogram/Ultrasound	257	7.8%	7.6%	8.8%
Lumbar Spine MRI for Low Back Pain	69	44.9%	40.2%	37.2%

Jack Hughston Memorial Hospital

4401 River Chase Drive | Phone: 334-732-3000
Phenix City, AL 36867
Type: Acute Care Hospitals | Emergency Services: Yes
Ownership: Government - State | Beds: 70

Key Personnel:
CEO . . . . Mark Barker

Measure	Cases	This Hosp.	State Avg.	U.S. Avg.
Blood Clot Prevention and Treatment				
Anticoagulation Overlap Therapy[2]	12	67%	91%	93%
ICU Venous Thromboembolism Prophylaxis[2]	34	79%	85%	92%
Incidence of Potentially Preventable VTE[1,2]	-	-	18%	10%
UFH with Dosages/Platelet Monitoring[1,2]	-	-	95%	97%
Venous Thromboembolism Prophylaxis[2]	118	92%	74%	85%
Warfarin Therapy Discharge Instructions[1,2]	-	-	77%	75%
Chest Pain/Possible Heart Attack Care				
Aspirin Given Within 24 Hours of Arrival[1,3]	-	-	96%	96%
Fibrinolytic Meds Within 30 Min. of Arrival[3,7]	-	-	57%	58%
Average Time to ECG (minutes)[1,3]	-	-	6	7
Average Time to Transfer (minutes)[3,7]	-	-	61	60
Children's Asthma Care				
Received Home Management Plan of Care	-	-	-	88%
Received Reliever Medication	-	-	-	100%
Received Systemic Corticosteroids	-	-	-	100%
Emergency Department				
Admittance Decision Time (minutes)[2]	143	74	73	98
Head CT Results Within 45 Min. of Arrival[1,3]	-	-	45%	57%
Patients Who Left ER Before Being Seen	14,580	1%	3%	2%
Time from ER Arrival to Admit. (minutes)[2]	143	281	240	274
Time from ER Arrival to Discharge (minutes)	425	104	126	134
Time in ER Before Being Evaluated (minutes)	444	48	31	26
Time to Pain Meds for Fractures (minutes)	62	76	69	57
Heart Attack Care				
Aspirin Given at Discharge[1,2]	-	-	99%	99%
Fibrinolytic Meds Within 30 Min. of Arrival[2,3]	-	-	77%	54%
PCI Within 90 Minutes of Arrival[2,3]	-	-	97%	96%
Statin Prescribed at Discharge[1,2]	-	-	98%	98%
Heart Failure Care				
ACE Inhibitor or ARB for LVSD[1,2]	-	-	97%	97%
Discharge Instructions Given[1,2]	-	-	93%	94%
Evaluation of LVS Function[1,2]	-	-	99%	99%
Medicare Spending				
Medicare Spending per Patient (ratio)	-	0.94	0.98	0.98
Pneumonia Care				
Appropriate Initial Antibiotic Given[1,2]	-	-	95%	95%
Blood Culture Timing[2]	12	100%	98%	98%
Pregnancy and Delivery Care				
Newborn Deliveries Scheduled Early[7]	-	-	14%	6%
Preventive Care				
Immunization for Influenza[2]	312	91%	90%	90%
Immunization for Pneumonia[2]	397	94%	91%	92%
Stroke Care				
Anticoagulation Therapy for Atrial Fibrillation[2,3]	-	-	92%	95%
Antithrombotic Therapy Timing[1,2]	-	-	96%	98%
Assessed for Rehabilitation[1,2]	-	-	95%	97%
Discharged on Antithrombotic Therapy[1,2]	-	-	98%	99%
Discharged on Statin Medication[1,2]	-	-	90%	94%
Thrombolytic Therapy Timing[2,3]	-	-	38%	66%
Venous Thromboembolism Prophylaxis[1,2]	-	-	89%	94%
Written Stroke Educational Materials Given[2,3]	-	-	85%	88%
Surgical Care Improvement Project				
Appropriate Beta Blocker Usage[2]	101	97%	98%	98%
Appropriate VTP Within 24 Hours[2]	380	97%	98%	98%
Controlled Postoperative Blood Glucose[2,7]	-	-	97%	97%
Perioperative Temperature Management[2]	412	100%	100%	100%
Prophylactic Antibiotic Selection[2]	273	98%	99%	99%
Prophylactic Antibiotic Selection (Outpatient)	65	100%	98%	98%
Prophylactic Antibiotic Stopped[2]	269	98%	98%	98%
Prophylactic Antibiotic Timing[2]	275	98%	99%	99%
Prophylactic Antibiotic Timing (Outpatient)	65	98%	99%	98%
Urinary Catheter Removal[2]	330	99%	98%	97%
Survey of Patients' Hospital Experiences				
Area Around Room 'Always' Quiet at Night	300+	79%	71%	61%
Doctors 'Always' Communicated Well	300+	88%	86%	82%
Home Recovery Information Given	300+	89%	84%	85%
Hospital Given 9 or 10 on 10 Point Scale	300+	81%	71%	71%
Meds 'Always' Explained Before Given	300+	70%	66%	64%
Nurses 'Always' Communicated Well	300+	82%	80%	79%
Pain 'Always' Well Controlled	300+	72%	72%	71%
Room and Bathroom 'Always' Clean	300+	71%	71%	73%
Timely Help 'Always' Received	300+	69%	68%	68%
Would Definitely Recommend Hospital	300+	85%	70%	71%
Use of Medical Imaging				
Cardiac Imaging Stress Test before Surgery[7]	-	-	6.5%	5.3%
Combination Abdominal CT Scan	87	2.3%	16.5%	10.5%
Combination Brain/Sinus CT Scan[1]	-	-	3.5%	2.7%
Combination Chest CT Scan[1]	-	-	4.2%	2.7%
Follow-up Mammogram/Ultrasound[7]	-	-	7.6%	8.8%
Lumbar Spine MRI for Low Back Pain[1]	-	-	40.2%	37.2%

Prattville Baptist Hospital

124 S Memorial Dr | Phone: 334-361-4267
Prattville, AL 36067 | Fax: 334-361-3131
URL: www.baptistfirst.org/facilities/prattville.htm
Type: Acute Care Hospitals | Emergency Services: Yes
Ownership: Govt - Hospital Dist/Auth | Beds: 85

Key Personnel:
Operating Room. . . . . Deborah Cauthen, RN
Quality Assurance . . . . Doreen Colburn
Chief of Medical Staff . . . . Ed Foxhall
Emergency Room . . . . Danny Perry

Measure	Cases	This Hosp.	State Avg.	U.S. Avg.
Blood Clot Prevention and Treatment				
Anticoagulation Overlap Therapy[2]	16	81%	91%	93%
ICU Venous Thromboembolism Prophylaxis[2]	57	68%	85%	92%
Incidence of Potentially Preventable VTE[1,2]	-	-	18%	10%
UFH with Dosages/Platelet Monitoring[2,7]	-	-	95%	97%
Venous Thromboembolism Prophylaxis[2]	273	70%	74%	85%
Warfarin Therapy Discharge Instructions[2]	12	92%	77%	75%
Chest Pain/Possible Heart Attack Care				
Aspirin Given Within 24 Hours of Arrival	52	98%	96%	96%
Fibrinolytic Meds Within 30 Min. of Arrival[7]	-	-	57%	58%
Average Time to ECG (minutes)	52	12	6	7
Average Time to Transfer (minutes)[1]	-	-	61	60
Children's Asthma Care				
Received Home Management Plan of Care	-	-	-	88%
Received Reliever Medication	-	-	-	100%
Received Systemic Corticosteroids	-	-	-	100%
Emergency Department				
Admittance Decision Time (minutes)[2]	545	248	73	98
Head CT Results Within 45 Min. of Arrival	23	22%	45%	57%
Patients Who Left ER Before Being Seen	31,576	4%	3%	2%
Time from ER Arrival to Admit. (minutes)[2]	550	446	240	274
Time from ER Arrival to Discharge (minutes)	513	161	126	134
Time in ER Before Being Evaluated (minutes)	413	43	31	26
Time to Pain Meds for Fractures (minutes)	118	66	69	57
Heart Attack Care				
Aspirin Given at Discharge[1]	-	-	99%	99%
Fibrinolytic Meds Within 30 Min. of Arrival[7]	-	-	77%	54%
PCI Within 90 Minutes of Arrival[7]	-	-	97%	96%
Statin Prescribed at Discharge[1]	-	-	98%	98%
Heart Failure Care				
ACE Inhibitor or ARB for LVSD	23	96%	97%	97%
Discharge Instructions Given	77	95%	93%	94%
Evaluation of LVS Function	90	97%	99%	99%
Medicare Spending				
Medicare Spending per Patient (ratio)	-	0.99	0.98	0.98
Pneumonia Care				
Appropriate Initial Antibiotic Given	93	95%	95%	95%
Blood Culture Timing	150	97%	98%	98%
Pregnancy and Delivery Care				
Newborn Deliveries Scheduled Early[7]	-	-	14%	6%
Preventive Care				
Immunization for Influenza[2]	339	91%	90%	90%
Immunization for Pneumonia[2]	493	82%	91%	92%
Stroke Care				
Anticoagulation Therapy for Atrial Fibrillation[1]	-	-	92%	95%
Antithrombotic Therapy Timing	35	89%	96%	98%
Assessed for Rehabilitation	39	100%	95%	97%
Discharged on Antithrombotic Therapy	38	95%	98%	99%
Discharged on Statin Medication	31	94%	90%	94%
Thrombolytic Therapy Timing	20	10%	38%	66%
Venous Thromboembolism Prophylaxis	40	88%	89%	94%
Written Stroke Educational Materials Given	24	79%	85%	88%
Surgical Care Improvement Project				
Appropriate Beta Blocker Usage	14	100%	98%	98%
Appropriate VTP Within 24 Hours	40	95%	98%	98%

NOTE: Hospital profiles are in alphabetical order by state, then city, then hospital within the city; Rankings exclude hospitals with less than 25 cases except for patient surveys which excludes hospitals with less than 100 cases; (a) 100-299 cases; (1) The number of cases/patients is too few to report; (2) Data submitted were based on a sample of cases/patients; (3) Results are based on a shorter time period than required; (4) Data suppressed by CMS for one or more quarters; (5) Results are not available for this reporting period; (6) Fewer than 100 patients completed the HCAHPS survey; (7) No cases met the criteria for this measure; (8) The lower limit of the confidence interval cannot be calculated if the number of observed infections equals zero; (9) No data are available from the state/territory for this reporting period; (10) The scores shown reflect fewer than 50 completed surveys; (11) There were discrepancies in the data collection process; (12) This measure does not apply to this hospital for this reporting period; (13) Results cannot be calculated for this reporting period; (14) The results for this state are combined with nearby states to protect confidentiality; Please refer to the User's Guide for a full explanation of data.

Measure	Cases	This Hosp.	State Avg.	U.S. Avg.
Controlled Postoperative Blood Glucose[7]	-	-	97%	97%
Perioperative Temperature Management	44	98%	100%	100%
Prophylactic Antibiotic Selection	12	92%	99%	99%
Prophylactic Antibiotic Selection (Outpatient)[1,3]	-	-	98%	98%
Prophylactic Antibiotic Stopped	11	100%	98%	98%
Prophylactic Antibiotic Timing	12	100%	99%	99%
Prophylactic Antibiotic Timing (Outpatient)[1,3]	-	-	99%	98%
Urinary Catheter Removal[1]	-	-	98%	97%
Survey of Patients' Hospital Experiences				
Area Around Room 'Always' Quiet at Night	300+	72%	71%	61%
Doctors 'Always' Communicated Well	300+	84%	86%	82%
Home Recovery Information Given	300+	88%	84%	85%
Hospital Given 9 or 10 on 10 Point Scale	300+	74%	71%	71%
Meds 'Always' Explained Before Given	300+	69%	66%	64%
Nurses 'Always' Communicated Well	300+	82%	80%	79%
Pain 'Always' Well Controlled	300+	76%	72%	71%
Room and Bathroom 'Always' Clean	300+	71%	71%	73%
Timely Help 'Always' Received	300+	72%	68%	68%
Would Definitely Recommend Hospital	300+	76%	70%	71%
Use of Medical Imaging				
Cardiac Imaging Stress Test before Surgery[1]	-	-	6.5%	5.3%
Combination Abdominal CT Scan	499	46.9%	16.5%	10.5%
Combination Brain/Sinus CT Scan[1]	-	-	3.5%	2.7%
Combination Chest CT Scan	271	1.5%	4.2%	2.7%
Follow-up Mammogram/Ultrasound	934	7.4%	7.6%	8.8%
Lumbar Spine MRI for Low Back Pain	120	41.7%	40.2%	37.2%

Red Bay Hospital

211 Hospital Road
Red Bay, AL 35582
Phone: 256-356-9532
Fax: 256-356-2809
URL: www.redbayhospital.com
Type: Critical Access Hospitals
Emergency Services: Yes
Ownership: Govt - Hospital Dist/Auth
Beds: 33

Key Personnel:
Quality Assurance . . . . Janette Boyd
Operating Room. . . . . Margie Grisson
Infection Control. . . . . K Paten

Measure	Cases	This Hosp.	State Avg.	U.S. Avg.
Blood Clot Prevention and Treatment				
Anticoagulation Overlap Therapy[5]	-	-	91%	93%
ICU Venous Thromboembolism Prophylaxis[5]	-	-	85%	92%
Incidence of Potentially Preventable VTE[5]	-	-	18%	10%
UFH with Dosages/Platelet Monitoring[5]	-	-	95%	97%
Venous Thromboembolism Prophylaxis[5]	-	-	74%	85%
Warfarin Therapy Discharge Instructions[5]	-	-	77%	75%
Chest Pain/Possible Heart Attack Care				
Aspirin Given Within 24 Hours of Arrival	43	100%	96%	96%
Fibrinolytic Meds Within 30 Min. of Arrival[3,7]	-	-	57%	58%
Average Time to ECG (minutes)	45	21	6	7
Average Time to Transfer (minutes)[1,3]	-	-	61	60
Children's Asthma Care				
Received Home Management Plan of Care	-	-	-	88%
Received Reliever Medication	-	-	-	100%
Received Systemic Corticosteroids	-	-	-	100%
Emergency Department				
Admittance Decision Time (minutes)[5]	-	-	73	98
Head CT Results Within 45 Min. of Arrival[5]	-	-	45%	57%
Patients Who Left ER Before Being Seen[5]	-	-	3%	2%
Time from ER Arrival to Admit. (minutes)[5]	-	-	240	274
Time from ER Arrival to Discharge (minutes)[5]	-	-	126	134
Time in ER Before Being Evaluated (minutes)[5]	-	-	31	26
Time to Pain Meds for Fractures (minutes)[5]	-	-	69	57
Heart Attack Care				
Aspirin Given at Discharge[5]	-	-	99%	99%
Fibrinolytic Meds Within 30 Min. of Arrival[5]	-	-	77%	54%
PCI Within 90 Minutes of Arrival[5]	-	-	97%	96%
Statin Prescribed at Discharge[5]	-	-	98%	98%
Heart Failure Care				
ACE Inhibitor or ARB for LVSD[3,7]	-	-	97%	97%
Discharge Instructions Given[1,3]	-	-	93%	94%
Evaluation of LVS Function[1,3]	-	-	99%	99%
Medicare Spending				
Medicare Spending per Patient (ratio)	-	-	0.98	0.98
Pneumonia Care				
Appropriate Initial Antibiotic Given[3]	12	83%	95%	95%
Blood Culture Timing[1,3]	-	-	98%	98%
Pregnancy and Delivery Care				
Newborn Deliveries Scheduled Early[5]	-	-	14%	6%
Preventive Care				
Immunization for Influenza[2]	52	94%	90%	90%
Immunization for Pneumonia[2]	95	98%	91%	92%
Stroke Care				
Anticoagulation Therapy for Atrial Fibrillation[5]	-	-	92%	95%
Antithrombotic Therapy Timing[5]	-	-	96%	98%
Assessed for Rehabilitation[5]	-	-	95%	97%
Discharged on Antithrombotic Therapy[5]	-	-	98%	99%
Discharged on Statin Medication[5]	-	-	90%	94%
Thrombolytic Therapy Timing[5]	-	-	38%	66%
Venous Thromboembolism Prophylaxis[5]	-	-	89%	94%
Written Stroke Educational Materials Given[5]	-	-	85%	88%
Surgical Care Improvement Project				
Appropriate Beta Blocker Usage[5]	-	-	98%	98%
Appropriate VTP Within 24 Hours[5]	-	-	98%	98%
Controlled Postoperative Blood Glucose[5]	-	-	97%	97%
Perioperative Temperature Management[5]	-	-	100%	100%
Prophylactic Antibiotic Selection[5]	-	-	99%	99%
Prophylactic Antibiotic Selection (Outpatient)[5]	-	-	98%	98%
Prophylactic Antibiotic Stopped[5]	-	-	98%	98%
Prophylactic Antibiotic Timing[5]	-	-	99%	99%
Prophylactic Antibiotic Timing (Outpatient)[5]	-	-	99%	98%
Urinary Catheter Removal[5]	-	-	98%	97%
Survey of Patients' Hospital Experiences				
Area Around Room 'Always' Quiet at Night[5]	-	-	71%	61%
Doctors 'Always' Communicated Well[5]	-	-	86%	82%
Home Recovery Information Given[5]	-	-	84%	85%
Hospital Given 9 or 10 on 10 Point Scale[5]	-	-	71%	71%
Meds 'Always' Explained Before Given[5]	-	-	66%	64%
Nurses 'Always' Communicated Well[5]	-	-	80%	79%
Pain 'Always' Well Controlled[5]	-	-	72%	71%
Room and Bathroom 'Always' Clean[5]	-	-	71%	73%
Timely Help 'Always' Received[5]	-	-	68%	68%
Would Definitely Recommend Hospital[5]	-	-	70%	71%
Use of Medical Imaging				
Cardiac Imaging Stress Test before Surgery[7]	-	-	6.5%	5.3%
Combination Abdominal CT Scan	101	8.9%	16.5%	10.5%
Combination Brain/Sinus CT Scan[1]	-	-	3.5%	2.7%
Combination Chest CT Scan[1]	-	-	4.2%	2.7%
Follow-up Mammogram/Ultrasound	85	1.2%	7.6%	8.8%
Lumbar Spine MRI for Low Back Pain[1]	-	-	40.2%	37.2%

Russellville Hospital

15155 Highway 43
Russellville, AL 35653
Phone: 256-332-1611
URL: www.russellvillehospital.com
Type: Acute Care Hospitals
Emergency Services: Yes
Ownership: Proprietary

Key Personnel:
CEO/President. . . . . Christine Stewart

Measure	Cases	This Hosp.	State Avg.	U.S. Avg.
Blood Clot Prevention and Treatment				
Anticoagulation Overlap Therapy[2]	18	100%	91%	93%
ICU Venous Thromboembolism Prophylaxis[2]	57	100%	85%	92%
Incidence of Potentially Preventable VTE[2,7]	-	-	18%	10%
UFH with Dosages/Platelet Monitoring[1,2]	-	-	95%	97%
Venous Thromboembolism Prophylaxis[2]	192	100%	74%	85%
Warfarin Therapy Discharge Instructions[2]	12	100%	77%	75%
Chest Pain/Possible Heart Attack Care				
Aspirin Given Within 24 Hours of Arrival	32	100%	96%	96%
Fibrinolytic Meds Within 30 Min. of Arrival[7]	-	-	57%	58%
Average Time to ECG (minutes)	33	6	6	7
Average Time to Transfer (minutes)[7]	-	-	61	60
Children's Asthma Care				
Received Home Management Plan of Care	-	-	-	88%
Received Reliever Medication	-	-	-	100%
Received Systemic Corticosteroids	-	-	-	100%
Emergency Department				
Admittance Decision Time (minutes)[2]	341	66	73	98
Head CT Results Within 45 Min. of Arrival[1]	-	-	45%	57%
Patients Who Left ER Before Being Seen	11,323	2%	3%	2%
Time from ER Arrival to Admit. (minutes)[2]	341	224	240	274
Time from ER Arrival to Discharge (minutes)	376	98	126	134
Time in ER Before Being Evaluated (minutes)	422	16	31	26
Time to Pain Meds for Fractures (minutes)	58	48	69	57
Heart Attack Care				
Aspirin Given at Discharge	13	100%	99%	99%
Fibrinolytic Meds Within 30 Min. of Arrival[7]	-	-	77%	54%
PCI Within 90 Minutes of Arrival[7]	-	-	97%	96%
Statin Prescribed at Discharge[1]	-	-	98%	98%
Heart Failure Care				
ACE Inhibitor or ARB for LVSD[1]	-	-	97%	97%
Discharge Instructions Given	46	100%	93%	94%
Evaluation of LVS Function	66	100%	99%	99%
Medicare Spending				
Medicare Spending per Patient (ratio)	-	0.98	0.98	0.98
Pneumonia Care				
Appropriate Initial Antibiotic Given	83	98%	95%	95%
Blood Culture Timing	95	100%	98%	98%
Pregnancy and Delivery Care				
Newborn Deliveries Scheduled Early[2,7]	-	-	14%	6%
Preventive Care				
Immunization for Influenza[2]	298	100%	90%	90%
Immunization for Pneumonia[2]	403	100%	91%	92%
Stroke Care				
Anticoagulation Therapy for Atrial Fibrillation[1,2]	-	-	92%	95%
Antithrombotic Therapy Timing[2]	16	100%	96%	98%
Assessed for Rehabilitation[2]	16	100%	95%	97%
Discharged on Antithrombotic Therapy[2]	14	100%	98%	99%
Discharged on Statin Medication[1,2]	-	-	90%	94%
Thrombolytic Therapy Timing[2,7]	-	-	38%	66%
Venous Thromboembolism Prophylaxis[2]	16	100%	89%	94%
Written Stroke Educational Materials Given[2]	12	100%	85%	88%
Surgical Care Improvement Project				
Appropriate Beta Blocker Usage	27	100%	98%	98%
Appropriate VTP Within 24 Hours	94	100%	98%	98%
Controlled Postoperative Blood Glucose[7]	-	-	97%	97%
Perioperative Temperature Management	111	100%	100%	100%
Prophylactic Antibiotic Selection	71	100%	99%	99%
Prophylactic Antibiotic Selection (Outpatient)	18	100%	98%	98%
Prophylactic Antibiotic Stopped	63	97%	98%	98%
Prophylactic Antibiotic Timing	71	99%	99%	99%
Prophylactic Antibiotic Timing (Outpatient)	18	100%	99%	98%
Urinary Catheter Removal	77	100%	98%	97%
Survey of Patients' Hospital Experiences				
Area Around Room 'Always' Quiet at Night	300+	76%	71%	61%
Doctors 'Always' Communicated Well	300+	87%	86%	82%
Home Recovery Information Given	300+	85%	84%	85%
Hospital Given 9 or 10 on 10 Point Scale	300+	66%	71%	71%
Meds 'Always' Explained Before Given	300+	69%	66%	64%
Nurses 'Always' Communicated Well	300+	79%	80%	79%
Pain 'Always' Well Controlled	300+	72%	72%	71%
Room and Bathroom 'Always' Clean	300+	69%	71%	73%
Timely Help 'Always' Received	300+	67%	68%	68%
Would Definitely Recommend Hospital	300+	64%	70%	71%
Use of Medical Imaging				
Cardiac Imaging Stress Test before Surgery[1]	-	-	6.5%	5.3%
Combination Abdominal CT Scan	227	18.1%	16.5%	10.5%
Combination Brain/Sinus CT Scan[1]	-	-	3.5%	2.7%
Combination Chest CT Scan	148	24.3%	4.2%	2.7%
Follow-up Mammogram/Ultrasound	339	12.1%	7.6%	8.8%
Lumbar Spine MRI for Low Back Pain	62	51.6%	40.2%	37.2%

Highlands Medical Center

380 Woods Cove Road
Scottsboro, AL 35768
Phone: 256-259-4444
Fax: 256-218-3656
URL: www.highlandsmedcenter.com
Type: Acute Care Hospitals
Emergency Services: Yes
Ownership: Govt - Hospital Dist/Auth
Beds: 170

Key Personnel:
Chief of Medical Staff . . . . Dr. Lonnie Albin
CEO . . . . Kim Bryant

NOTE: Hospital profiles are in alphabetical order by state, then city, then hospital within the city; Rankings exclude hospitals with less than 25 cases except for patient surveys which excludes hospitals with less than 100 cases; (a) 100-299 cases; (1) The number of cases/patients is too few to report; (2) Data submitted were based on a sample of cases/patients; (3) Results are based on a shorter time period than required; (4) Data suppressed by CMS for one or more quarters; (5) Results are not available for this reporting period; (6) Fewer than 100 patients completed the HCAHPS survey; (7) No cases met the criteria for this measure; (8) The lower limit of the confidence interval cannot be calculated if the number of observed infections equals zero; (9) No data are available from the state/territory for this reporting period; (10) The scores shown reflect fewer than 50 completed surveys; (11) There were discrepancies in the data collection process; (12) This measure does not apply to this hospital for this reporting period; (13) Results cannot be calculated for this reporting period; (14) The results for this state are combined with nearby states to protect confidentiality; Please refer to the User's Guide for a full explanation of data.

Chair/CEO . . . . Chris Gulley
Administrator . . . . Brad Hinton
CEO/President. . . . . Thomas O'Lackey

Measure	Cases	This Hosp.	State Avg.	U.S. Avg.
Blood Clot Prevention and Treatment				
Anticoagulation Overlap Therapy[2]	21	81%	91%	93%
ICU Venous Thromboembolism Prophylaxis[2]	47	72%	85%	92%
Incidence of Potentially Preventable VTE[1,2]	-	-	18%	10%
UFH with Dosages/Platelet Monitoring[1,2]	-	-	95%	97%
Venous Thromboembolism Prophylaxis[2]	318	85%	74%	85%
Warfarin Therapy Discharge Instructions[2]	16	100%	77%	75%
Chest Pain/Possible Heart Attack Care				
Aspirin Given Within 24 Hours of Arrival	88	98%	96%	96%
Fibrinolytic Meds Within 30 Min. of Arrival[7]	-	-	57%	58%
Average Time to ECG (minutes)	92	8	6	7
Average Time to Transfer (minutes)	25	75	61	60
Children's Asthma Care				
Received Home Management Plan of Care	-	-	-	88%
Received Reliever Medication	-	-	-	100%
Received Systemic Corticosteroids	-	-	-	100%
Emergency Department				
Admittance Decision Time (minutes)[2]	311	72	73	98
Head CT Results Within 45 Min. of Arrival[1]	-	-	45%	57%
Patients Who Left ER Before Being Seen	18,334	3%	3%	2%
Time from ER Arrival to Admit. (minutes)[2]	324	254	240	274
Time from ER Arrival to Discharge (minutes)	578	130	126	134
Time in ER Before Being Evaluated (minutes)	594	37	31	26
Time to Pain Meds for Fractures (minutes)	99	77	69	57
Heart Attack Care				
Aspirin Given at Discharge[1]	-	-	99%	99%
Fibrinolytic Meds Within 30 Min. of Arrival[7]	-	-	77%	54%
PCI Within 90 Minutes of Arrival[7]	-	-	97%	96%
Statin Prescribed at Discharge[1]	-	-	98%	98%
Heart Failure Care				
ACE Inhibitor or ARB for LVSD	22	82%	97%	97%
Discharge Instructions Given	84	95%	93%	94%
Evaluation of LVS Function	103	98%	99%	99%
Medicare Spending				
Medicare Spending per Patient (ratio)	-	0.85	0.98	0.98
Pneumonia Care				
Appropriate Initial Antibiotic Given	143	83%	95%	95%
Blood Culture Timing	136	96%	98%	98%
Pregnancy and Delivery Care				
Newborn Deliveries Scheduled Early	29	14%	14%	6%
Preventive Care				
Immunization for Influenza[2]	423	99%	90%	90%
Immunization for Pneumonia[2]	551	99%	91%	92%
Stroke Care				
Anticoagulation Therapy for Atrial Fibrillation[1]	-	-	92%	95%
Antithrombotic Therapy Timing	25	96%	96%	98%
Assessed for Rehabilitation	30	90%	95%	97%
Discharged on Antithrombotic Therapy	28	96%	98%	99%
Discharged on Statin Medication	25	52%	90%	94%
Thrombolytic Therapy Timing[1]	-	-	38%	66%
Venous Thromboembolism Prophylaxis	24	83%	89%	94%
Written Stroke Educational Materials Given	17	100%	85%	88%
Surgical Care Improvement Project				
Appropriate Beta Blocker Usage	21	86%	98%	98%
Appropriate VTP Within 24 Hours	65	100%	98%	98%
Controlled Postoperative Blood Glucose[7]	-	-	97%	97%
Perioperative Temperature Management	94	100%	100%	100%
Prophylactic Antibiotic Selection	79	97%	99%	99%
Prophylactic Antibiotic Selection (Outpatient)[1]	-	-	98%	98%
Prophylactic Antibiotic Stopped	77	95%	98%	98%
Prophylactic Antibiotic Timing	81	96%	99%	99%
Prophylactic Antibiotic Timing (Outpatient)[1]	-	-	99%	98%
Urinary Catheter Removal	36	89%	98%	97%
Survey of Patients' Hospital Experiences				
Area Around Room 'Always' Quiet at Night	(a)	70%	71%	61%
Doctors 'Always' Communicated Well	(a)	86%	86%	82%
Home Recovery Information Given	(a)	84%	84%	85%
Hospital Given 9 or 10 on 10 Point Scale	(a)	72%	71%	71%
Meds 'Always' Explained Before Given	(a)	65%	66%	64%
Nurses 'Always' Communicated Well	(a)	79%	80%	79%
Pain 'Always' Well Controlled	(a)	71%	72%	71%
Room and Bathroom 'Always' Clean	(a)	73%	71%	73%
Timely Help 'Always' Received	(a)	66%	68%	68%
Would Definitely Recommend Hospital	(a)	64%	70%	71%
Use of Medical Imaging				
Cardiac Imaging Stress Test before Surgery	87	6.9%	6.5%	5.3%
Combination Abdominal CT Scan	511	3.9%	16.5%	10.5%
Combination Brain/Sinus CT Scan	515	4.1%	3.5%	2.7%
Combination Chest CT Scan	167	0.0%	4.2%	2.7%
Follow-up Mammogram/Ultrasound[7]	-	-	7.6%	8.8%
Lumbar Spine MRI for Low Back Pain	51	33.3%	40.2%	37.2%

Vaughan Regional Medical Center Parkway Campus

1015 Medical Center Parkway
Selma, AL 36701
Phone: 334-418-4100
Fax: 334-418-3599
URL: www.vaughanregional.com
Type: Acute Care Hospitals
Emergency Services: Yes
Ownership: Proprietary
Beds: 175

Key Personnel:
Pediatric In-Patient Care . . . . Andretta Dallas
Chief of Medical Staff. . . . . Lonnie Felton, MD
Emergency Room . . . . Jason Glass
Cardiac Laboratory. . . . . Jackie Moultrie
Quality Assurance . . . . Susan Painter
CEO/President. . . . . David Sirk
Radiology. . . . . Leland Taylor

Measure	Cases	This Hosp.	State Avg.	U.S. Avg.
Blood Clot Prevention and Treatment				
Anticoagulation Overlap Therapy[2]	65	98%	91%	93%
ICU Venous Thromboembolism Prophylaxis[2]	158	99%	85%	92%
Incidence of Potentially Preventable VTE[1,2]	-	-	18%	10%
UFH with Dosages/Platelet Monitoring[2]	53	100%	95%	97%
Venous Thromboembolism Prophylaxis[2]	293	96%	74%	85%
Warfarin Therapy Discharge Instructions[2]	44	100%	77%	75%
Chest Pain/Possible Heart Attack Care				
Aspirin Given Within 24 Hours of Arrival	21	100%	96%	96%
Fibrinolytic Meds Within 30 Min. of Arrival[1]	-	-	57%	58%
Average Time to ECG (minutes)	25	6	6	7
Average Time to Transfer (minutes)[7]	-	-	61	60
Children's Asthma Care				
Received Home Management Plan of Care	-	-	-	88%
Received Reliever Medication	-	-	-	100%
Received Systemic Corticosteroids	-	-	-	100%
Emergency Department				
Admittance Decision Time (minutes)[2]	670	72	73	98
Head CT Results Within 45 Min. of Arrival[1]	-	-	45%	57%
Patients Who Left ER Before Being Seen	30,759	2%	3%	2%
Time from ER Arrival to Admit. (minutes)[2]	683	243	240	274
Time from ER Arrival to Discharge (minutes)	377	127	126	134
Time in ER Before Being Evaluated (minutes)	445	24	31	26
Time to Pain Meds for Fractures (minutes)	119	69	69	57
Heart Attack Care				
Aspirin Given at Discharge	155	100%	99%	99%
Fibrinolytic Meds Within 30 Min. of Arrival[1]	-	-	77%	54%
PCI Within 90 Minutes of Arrival[1]	-	-	97%	96%
Statin Prescribed at Discharge	147	100%	98%	98%
Heart Failure Care				
ACE Inhibitor or ARB for LVSD	122	100%	97%	97%
Discharge Instructions Given	225	100%	93%	94%
Evaluation of LVS Function	270	100%	99%	99%
Medicare Spending				
Medicare Spending per Patient (ratio)	-	0.99	0.98	0.98
Pneumonia Care				
Appropriate Initial Antibiotic Given	117	99%	95%	95%
Blood Culture Timing	151	100%	98%	98%
Pregnancy and Delivery Care				
Newborn Deliveries Scheduled Early[2]	47	9%	14%	6%
Preventive Care				
Immunization for Influenza[2]	532	100%	90%	90%
Immunization for Pneumonia[2]	644	100%	91%	92%
Stroke Care				
Anticoagulation Therapy for Atrial Fibrillation[1,2]	-	-	92%	95%
Antithrombotic Therapy Timing[2]	58	100%	96%	98%
Assessed for Rehabilitation[2]	62	100%	95%	97%
Discharged on Antithrombotic Therapy[2]	58	100%	98%	99%
Discharged on Statin Medication[2]	47	100%	90%	94%
Thrombolytic Therapy Timing[1,2]	-	-	38%	66%
Venous Thromboembolism Prophylaxis[2]	69	100%	89%	94%
Written Stroke Educational Materials Given[2]	33	100%	85%	88%
Surgical Care Improvement Project				
Appropriate Beta Blocker Usage	34	100%	98%	98%
Appropriate VTP Within 24 Hours	127	99%	98%	98%
Controlled Postoperative Blood Glucose[7]	-	-	97%	97%
Perioperative Temperature Management	153	100%	100%	100%
Prophylactic Antibiotic Selection	80	96%	99%	99%
Prophylactic Antibiotic Selection (Outpatient)	95	100%	98%	98%
Prophylactic Antibiotic Stopped	73	100%	98%	98%
Prophylactic Antibiotic Timing	80	100%	99%	99%
Prophylactic Antibiotic Timing (Outpatient)	93	99%	99%	98%
Urinary Catheter Removal	14	100%	98%	97%
Survey of Patients' Hospital Experiences				
Area Around Room 'Always' Quiet at Night	300+	71%	71%	61%
Doctors 'Always' Communicated Well	300+	82%	86%	82%
Home Recovery Information Given	300+	77%	84%	85%
Hospital Given 9 or 10 on 10 Point Scale	300+	59%	71%	71%
Meds 'Always' Explained Before Given	300+	60%	66%	64%
Nurses 'Always' Communicated Well	300+	72%	80%	79%
Pain 'Always' Well Controlled	300+	64%	72%	71%
Room and Bathroom 'Always' Clean	300+	69%	71%	73%
Timely Help 'Always' Received	300+	57%	68%	68%
Would Definitely Recommend Hospital	300+	56%	70%	71%
Use of Medical Imaging				
Cardiac Imaging Stress Test before Surgery[1]	-	-	6.5%	5.3%
Combination Abdominal CT Scan	676	6.8%	16.5%	10.5%
Combination Brain/Sinus CT Scan	570	1.6%	3.5%	2.7%
Combination Chest CT Scan	540	2.0%	4.2%	2.7%
Follow-up Mammogram/Ultrasound	1,405	7.8%	7.6%	8.8%
Lumbar Spine MRI for Low Back Pain	134	38.8%	40.2%	37.2%

Helen Keller Memorial Hospital

1300 South Montgomery Avenue
Sheffield, AL 35660
Phone: 256-386-4556
Fax: 256-386-4469
E-mail: info@helenkeller.com
URL: www.helenkeller.com
Type: Acute Care Hospitals
Emergency Services: Yes
Ownership: Govt - Hospital Dist/Auth
Beds: 185

Key Personnel:
CEO/President. . . . . William H Anderson, FACHE
Operating Room. . . . . Shelby K Bailey
Quality Assurance . . . . Anna Blair
Chief of Medical Staff. . . . . Richard Deal
Radiology. . . . . Robert F Dunn
Emergency Room . . . . David Gardner
Pediatric Ambulatory Care . . . . . . D Das Kanuru, MD
Pediatric In-Patient Care . . . . D Das Kanuru, MD

Measure	Cases	This Hosp.	State Avg.	U.S. Avg.
Blood Clot Prevention and Treatment				
Anticoagulation Overlap Therapy[2]	32	91%	91%	93%
ICU Venous Thromboembolism Prophylaxis[2]	62	97%	85%	92%
Incidence of Potentially Preventable VTE[1,2]	-	-	18%	10%
UFH with Dosages/Platelet Monitoring[1,2]	-	-	95%	97%
Venous Thromboembolism Prophylaxis[2]	333	83%	74%	85%
Warfarin Therapy Discharge Instructions[2]	19	100%	77%	75%
Chest Pain/Possible Heart Attack Care				
Aspirin Given Within 24 Hours of Arrival	110	99%	96%	96%
Fibrinolytic Meds Within 30 Min. of Arrival[7]	-	-	57%	58%
Average Time to ECG (minutes)	112	6	6	7
Average Time to Transfer (minutes)	20	40	61	60
Children's Asthma Care				
Received Home Management Plan of Care	-	-	-	88%
Received Reliever Medication	-	-	-	100%
Received Systemic Corticosteroids	-	-	-	100%
Emergency Department				
Admittance Decision Time (minutes)[2]	501	66	73	98
Head CT Results Within 45 Min. of Arrival	12	58%	45%	57%
Patients Who Left ER Before Being Seen	37,542	2%	3%	2%

NOTE: Hospital profiles are in alphabetical order by state, then city, then hospital within the city; Rankings exclude hospitals with less than 25 cases except for patient surveys which excludes hospitals with less than 100 cases; (a) 100-299 cases; (1) The number of cases/patients is too few to report; (2) Data submitted were based on a sample of cases/patients; (3) Results are based on a shorter time period than required; (4) Data suppressed by CMS for one or more quarters; (5) Results are not available for this reporting period; (6) Fewer than 100 patients completed the HCAHPS survey; (7) No cases met the criteria for this measure; (8) The lower limit of the confidence interval cannot be calculated if the number of observed infections equals zero; (9) No data are available from the state/territory for this reporting period; (10) The scores shown reflect fewer than 50 completed surveys; (11) There were discrepancies in the data collection process; (12) This measure does not apply to this hospital for this reporting period; (13) Results cannot be calculated for this reporting period; (14) The results for this state are combined with nearby states to protect confidentiality; Please refer to the User's Guide for a full explanation of data.

Measure	Cases	This Hosp.	State Avg.	U.S. Avg.
Time from ER Arrival to Admit. (minutes)[2]	501	195	240	274
Time from ER Arrival to Discharge (minutes)	373	105	126	134
Time in ER Before Being Evaluated (minutes)	383	22	31	26
Time to Pain Meds for Fractures (minutes)	154	60	69	57
Heart Attack Care				
Aspirin Given at Discharge[1]	-	-	99%	99%
Fibrinolytic Meds Within 30 Min. of Arrival[7]	-	-	77%	54%
PCI Within 90 Minutes of Arrival[7]	-	-	97%	96%
Statin Prescribed at Discharge[1]	-	-	98%	98%
Heart Failure Care				
ACE Inhibitor or ARB for LVSD	37	100%	97%	97%
Discharge Instructions Given	152	91%	93%	94%
Evaluation of LVS Function	203	100%	99%	99%
Medicare Spending				
Medicare Spending per Patient (ratio)	-	1.07	0.98	0.98
Pneumonia Care				
Appropriate Initial Antibiotic Given	173	96%	95%	95%
Blood Culture Timing	244	100%	98%	98%
Pregnancy and Delivery Care				
Newborn Deliveries Scheduled Early[2]	48	8%	14%	6%
Preventive Care				
Immunization for Influenza[2]	515	96%	90%	90%
Immunization for Pneumonia[2]	579	97%	91%	92%
Stroke Care				
Anticoagulation Therapy for Atrial Fibrillation[1]	-	-	92%	95%
Antithrombotic Therapy Timing	70	94%	96%	98%
Assessed for Rehabilitation	69	99%	95%	97%
Discharged on Antithrombotic Therapy	61	98%	98%	99%
Discharged on Statin Medication	42	98%	90%	94%
Thrombolytic Therapy Timing[1]	-	-	38%	66%
Venous Thromboembolism Prophylaxis	79	87%	89%	94%
Written Stroke Educational Materials Given	25	80%	85%	88%
Surgical Care Improvement Project				
Appropriate Beta Blocker Usage[2]	97	96%	98%	98%
Appropriate VTP Within 24 Hours[2]	265	100%	98%	98%
Controlled Postoperative Blood Glucose[2,7]	-	-	97%	97%
Perioperative Temperature Management[2]	313	100%	100%	100%
Prophylactic Antibiotic Selection[2]	187	100%	99%	99%
Prophylactic Antibiotic Selection (Outpatient)	442	100%	98%	98%
Prophylactic Antibiotic Stopped[2]	176	100%	98%	98%
Prophylactic Antibiotic Timing[2]	188	99%	99%	99%
Prophylactic Antibiotic Timing (Outpatient)	444	99%	99%	98%
Urinary Catheter Removal[2]	200	100%	98%	97%
Survey of Patients' Hospital Experiences				
Area Around Room 'Always' Quiet at Night	300+	70%	71%	61%
Doctors 'Always' Communicated Well	300+	85%	86%	82%
Home Recovery Information Given	300+	87%	84%	85%
Hospital Given 9 or 10 on 10 Point Scale	300+	75%	71%	71%
Meds 'Always' Explained Before Given	300+	64%	66%	64%
Nurses 'Always' Communicated Well	300+	80%	80%	79%
Pain 'Always' Well Controlled	300+	70%	72%	71%
Room and Bathroom 'Always' Clean	300+	69%	71%	73%
Timely Help 'Always' Received	300+	69%	68%	68%
Would Definitely Recommend Hospital	300+	76%	70%	71%
Use of Medical Imaging				
Cardiac Imaging Stress Test before Surgery[1]	-	-	6.5%	5.3%
Combination Abdominal CT Scan	1,048	12.4%	16.5%	10.5%
Combination Brain/Sinus CT Scan	903	5.6%	3.5%	2.7%
Combination Chest CT Scan	371	0.8%	4.2%	2.7%
Follow-up Mammogram/Ultrasound	1,358	3.7%	7.6%	8.8%
Lumbar Spine MRI for Low Back Pain	191	40.3%	40.2%	37.2%

Coosa Valley Medical Center

315 W Hickory St
Sylacauga, AL 35150
URL: www.cvhealth.net
Phone: 256-249-5000
Fax: 256-249-5622
Type: Acute Care Hospitals
Ownership: Voluntary non-profit - Other
Emergency Services: Yes
Beds: 223

Key Personnel:
Pediatric Ambulatory Care . . . . . . Nader P Bishara, MD
Chief of Medical Staff. . . . . Stephen Bowen, MD
Emergency Room . . . . Tina Brooks, RN
Operating Room. . . . . Juan Campos
Patient Relations . . . . Amy Price
CEO/President. . . . . Glenn C Sisk
Pediatric In-Patient Care . . . . Phillip Smith, MD
Quality Assurance . . . . Carla Taylor

Measure	Cases	This Hosp.	State Avg.	U.S. Avg.
Blood Clot Prevention and Treatment				
Anticoagulation Overlap Therapy[2]	39	97%	91%	93%
ICU Venous Thromboembolism Prophylaxis[2]	101	100%	85%	92%
Incidence of Potentially Preventable VTE[1,2]	-	-	18%	10%
UFH with Dosages/Platelet Monitoring[2]	15	100%	95%	97%
Venous Thromboembolism Prophylaxis[2]	418	99%	74%	85%
Warfarin Therapy Discharge Instructions[2]	20	95%	77%	75%
Chest Pain/Possible Heart Attack Care				
Aspirin Given Within 24 Hours of Arrival	53	100%	96%	96%
Fibrinolytic Meds Within 30 Min. of Arrival[1]	-	-	57%	58%
Average Time to ECG (minutes)	54	3	6	7
Average Time to Transfer (minutes)[7]	-	-	61	60
Children's Asthma Care				
Received Home Management Plan of Care	-	-	-	88%
Received Reliever Medication	-	-	-	100%
Received Systemic Corticosteroids	-	-	-	100%
Emergency Department				
Admittance Decision Time (minutes)[2]	767	76	73	98
Head CT Results Within 45 Min. of Arrival[1]	-	-	45%	57%
Patients Who Left ER Before Being Seen	31,731	0%	3%	2%
Time from ER Arrival to Admit. (minutes)[2]	761	231	240	274
Time from ER Arrival to Discharge (minutes)	381	90	126	134
Time in ER Before Being Evaluated (minutes)	468	18	31	26
Time to Pain Meds for Fractures (minutes)	125	55	69	57
Heart Attack Care				
Aspirin Given at Discharge	15	100%	99%	99%
Fibrinolytic Meds Within 30 Min. of Arrival[7]	-	-	77%	54%
PCI Within 90 Minutes of Arrival[7]	-	-	97%	96%
Statin Prescribed at Discharge	13	100%	98%	98%
Heart Failure Care				
ACE Inhibitor or ARB for LVSD	35	100%	97%	97%
Discharge Instructions Given	67	100%	93%	94%
Evaluation of LVS Function	97	100%	99%	99%
Medicare Spending				
Medicare Spending per Patient (ratio)	-	0.99	0.98	0.98
Pneumonia Care				
Appropriate Initial Antibiotic Given[2]	56	100%	95%	95%
Blood Culture Timing[2]	178	100%	98%	98%
Pregnancy and Delivery Care				
Newborn Deliveries Scheduled Early	139	0%	14%	6%
Preventive Care				
Immunization for Influenza[2]	513	100%	90%	90%
Immunization for Pneumonia[2]	652	100%	91%	92%
Stroke Care				
Anticoagulation Therapy for Atrial Fibrillation[1]	-	-	92%	95%
Antithrombotic Therapy Timing	43	100%	96%	98%
Assessed for Rehabilitation	36	100%	95%	97%
Discharged on Antithrombotic Therapy	34	100%	98%	99%
Discharged on Statin Medication	18	94%	90%	94%
Thrombolytic Therapy Timing[7]	-	-	38%	66%
Venous Thromboembolism Prophylaxis	43	100%	89%	94%
Written Stroke Educational Materials Given	22	86%	85%	88%
Surgical Care Improvement Project				
Appropriate Beta Blocker Usage	59	98%	98%	98%
Appropriate VTP Within 24 Hours	161	100%	98%	98%
Controlled Postoperative Blood Glucose[7]	-	-	97%	97%
Perioperative Temperature Management	203	100%	100%	100%
Prophylactic Antibiotic Selection	123	96%	99%	99%
Prophylactic Antibiotic Selection (Outpatient)	21	95%	98%	98%
Prophylactic Antibiotic Stopped	116	99%	98%	98%
Prophylactic Antibiotic Timing	123	100%	99%	99%
Prophylactic Antibiotic Timing (Outpatient)	21	100%	99%	98%
Urinary Catheter Removal	67	100%	98%	97%
Survey of Patients' Hospital Experiences				
Area Around Room 'Always' Quiet at Night	300+	74%	71%	61%
Doctors 'Always' Communicated Well	300+	86%	86%	82%
Home Recovery Information Given	300+	84%	84%	85%
Hospital Given 9 or 10 on 10 Point Scale	300+	70%	71%	71%
Meds 'Always' Explained Before Given	300+	71%	66%	64%
Nurses 'Always' Communicated Well	300+	79%	80%	79%
Pain 'Always' Well Controlled	300+	75%	72%	71%
Room and Bathroom 'Always' Clean	300+	67%	71%	73%
Timely Help 'Always' Received	300+	63%	68%	68%
Would Definitely Recommend Hospital	300+	67%	70%	71%
Use of Medical Imaging				
Cardiac Imaging Stress Test before Surgery	338	5.0%	6.5%	5.3%
Combination Abdominal CT Scan	717	8.6%	16.5%	10.5%
Combination Brain/Sinus CT Scan	556	2.0%	3.5%	2.7%
Combination Chest CT Scan	339	3.8%	4.2%	2.7%
Follow-up Mammogram/Ultrasound	654	6.1%	7.6%	8.8%
Lumbar Spine MRI for Low Back Pain	216	46.8%	40.2%	37.2%

Citizens Baptist Medical Center

604 Stone Avenue
Talladega, AL 35161
E-mail: info@bhsala.com
URL: www.bhsala.com
Phone: 256-761-4542
Fax: 256-761-4658
Type: Acute Care Hospitals
Ownership: Voluntary non-profit - Private
Emergency Services: Yes
Beds: 122

Key Personnel:
Radiology. . . . . Bryan Edward Billions
Chief of Medical Staff . . . . Elizabeth Ennis, MD
Intensive Care Unit. . . . . Kim Ledbetter
Quality Assurance . . . . Tammy Marshal
CEO/President. . . . . Keith Parrott
Operating Room. . . . . Joyce Pruitt, RN
Emergency Room . . . . Deborah Rutledge
Patient Relations . . . . Danine L Watson, RN

Measure	Cases	This Hosp.	State Avg.	U.S. Avg.
Blood Clot Prevention and Treatment				
Anticoagulation Overlap Therapy[2]	20	95%	91%	93%
ICU Venous Thromboembolism Prophylaxis[2]	69	90%	85%	92%
Incidence of Potentially Preventable VTE[1,2]	-	-	18%	10%
UFH with Dosages/Platelet Monitoring[1,2]	-	-	95%	97%
Venous Thromboembolism Prophylaxis[2]	209	65%	74%	85%
Warfarin Therapy Discharge Instructions[2]	13	46%	77%	75%
Chest Pain/Possible Heart Attack Care				
Aspirin Given Within 24 Hours of Arrival	49	96%	96%	96%
Fibrinolytic Meds Within 30 Min. of Arrival	11	45%	57%	58%
Average Time to ECG (minutes)	51	6	6	7
Average Time to Transfer (minutes)[7]	-	-	61	60
Children's Asthma Care				
Received Home Management Plan of Care	-	-	-	88%
Received Reliever Medication	-	-	-	100%
Received Systemic Corticosteroids	-	-	-	100%
Emergency Department				
Admittance Decision Time (minutes)[2]	357	47	73	98
Head CT Results Within 45 Min. of Arrival[1]	-	-	45%	57%
Patients Who Left ER Before Being Seen	22,590	1%	3%	2%
Time from ER Arrival to Admit. (minutes)[2]	358	188	240	274
Time from ER Arrival to Discharge (minutes)	402	112	126	134
Time in ER Before Being Evaluated (minutes)	422	27	31	26
Time to Pain Meds for Fractures (minutes)	92	61	69	57
Heart Attack Care				
Aspirin Given at Discharge[1]	-	-	99%	99%
Fibrinolytic Meds Within 30 Min. of Arrival[7]	-	-	77%	54%
PCI Within 90 Minutes of Arrival[7]	-	-	97%	96%
Statin Prescribed at Discharge[1]	-	-	98%	98%
Heart Failure Care				
ACE Inhibitor or ARB for LVSD	31	97%	97%	97%
Discharge Instructions Given	102	92%	93%	94%
Evaluation of LVS Function	118	97%	99%	99%
Medicare Spending				
Medicare Spending per Patient (ratio)	-	1.01	0.98	0.98
Pneumonia Care				
Appropriate Initial Antibiotic Given	56	96%	95%	95%
Blood Culture Timing	95	99%	98%	98%
Pregnancy and Delivery Care				
Newborn Deliveries Scheduled Early	20	5%	14%	6%
Preventive Care				
Immunization for Influenza[2]	286	82%	90%	90%
Immunization for Pneumonia[2]	327	87%	91%	92%
Stroke Care				

NOTE: Hospital profiles are in alphabetical order by state, then city, then hospital within the city; Rankings exclude hospitals with less than 25 cases except for patient surveys which excludes hospitals with less than 100 cases; (a) 100-299 cases; (1) The number of cases/patients is too few to report; (2) Data submitted were based on a sample of cases/patients; (3) Results are based on a shorter time period than required; (4) Data suppressed by CMS for one or more quarters; (5) Results are not available for this reporting period; (6) Fewer than 100 patients completed the HCAHPS survey; (7) No cases met the criteria for this measure; (8) The lower limit of the confidence interval cannot be calculated if the number of observed infections equals zero; (9) No data are available from the state/territory for this reporting period; (10) The scores shown reflect fewer than 50 completed surveys; (11) There were discrepancies in the data collection process; (12) This measure does not apply to this hospital for this reporting period; (13) Results cannot be calculated for this reporting period; (14) The results for this state are combined with nearby states to protect confidentiality; Please refer to the User's Guide for a full explanation of data.

Measure	Cases	This Hosp.	State Avg.	U.S. Avg.
Anticoagulation Therapy for Atrial Fibrillation[1]	-	-	92%	95%
Antithrombotic Therapy Timing	48	96%	96%	98%
Assessed for Rehabilitation	49	90%	95%	97%
Discharged on Antithrombotic Therapy	48	92%	98%	99%
Discharged on Statin Medication	35	74%	90%	94%
Thrombolytic Therapy Timing[1]	-	-	38%	66%
Venous Thromboembolism Prophylaxis	48	92%	89%	94%
Written Stroke Educational Materials Given	28	68%	85%	88%
Surgical Care Improvement Project				
Appropriate Beta Blocker Usage[1]	-	-	98%	98%
Appropriate VTP Within 24 Hours	44	91%	98%	98%
Controlled Postoperative Blood Glucose[7]	-	-	97%	97%
Perioperative Temperature Management	52	100%	100%	100%
Prophylactic Antibiotic Selection	24	100%	99%	99%
Prophylactic Antibiotic Selection (Outpatient)	44	98%	98%	98%
Prophylactic Antibiotic Stopped	24	100%	98%	98%
Prophylactic Antibiotic Timing	24	100%	99%	99%
Prophylactic Antibiotic Timing (Outpatient)	44	100%	99%	98%
Urinary Catheter Removal	13	77%	98%	97%
Survey of Patients' Hospital Experiences				
Area Around Room 'Always' Quiet at Night	300+	69%	71%	61%
Doctors 'Always' Communicated Well	300+	83%	86%	82%
Home Recovery Information Given	300+	81%	84%	85%
Hospital Given 9 or 10 on 10 Point Scale	300+	61%	71%	71%
Meds 'Always' Explained Before Given	300+	61%	66%	64%
Nurses 'Always' Communicated Well	300+	72%	80%	79%
Pain 'Always' Well Controlled	300+	68%	72%	71%
Room and Bathroom 'Always' Clean	300+	67%	71%	73%
Timely Help 'Always' Received	300+	61%	68%	68%
Would Definitely Recommend Hospital	300+	59%	70%	71%
Use of Medical Imaging				
Cardiac Imaging Stress Test before Surgery	199	7.0%	6.5%	5.3%
Combination Abdominal CT Scan	320	7.5%	16.5%	10.5%
Combination Brain/Sinus CT Scan[1]	-	-	3.5%	2.7%
Combination Chest CT Scan	115	0.0%	4.2%	2.7%
Follow-up Mammogram/Ultrasound	572	5.4%	7.6%	8.8%
Lumbar Spine MRI for Low Back Pain	50	62.0%	40.2%	37.2%

Community Hospital

805 Friendship Road
Tallassee, AL 36078
Phone: 334-283-6541
Fax: 334-283-3758
E-mail: kmonroe@communityhospitalal.org
URL: www.chal.org
Type: Acute Care Hospitals
Emergency Services: Yes
Ownership: Voluntary non-profit - Private
Beds: 69

Key Personnel:
Radiology. . . . . Jeffrey Adams
Infection Control. . . . . Heather Brawner
Intensive Care Unit. . . . . Gary Corbin
Operating Room. . . . . Faye Kirk
Emergency Room . . . . Kathy Monroe, RN
CEO/President. . . . . Jennie Rhinehart
Quality Assurance . . . . Jennie Rhinehart
Chief of Medical Staff. . . . . Mike Wells

Measure	Cases	This Hosp.	State Avg.	U.S. Avg.
Blood Clot Prevention and Treatment				
Anticoagulation Overlap Therapy[1,2]	-	-	91%	93%
ICU Venous Thromboembolism Prophylaxis[2]	88	77%	85%	92%
Incidence of Potentially Preventable VTE[1,2]	-	-	18%	10%
UFH with Dosages/Platelet Monitoring[1,2]	-	-	95%	97%
Venous Thromboembolism Prophylaxis[2]	231	65%	74%	85%
Warfarin Therapy Discharge Instructions[1,2]	-	-	77%	75%
Chest Pain/Possible Heart Attack Care				
Aspirin Given Within 24 Hours of Arrival	38	100%	96%	96%
Fibrinolytic Meds Within 30 Min. of Arrival[1]	-	-	57%	58%
Average Time to ECG (minutes)	36	14	6	7
Average Time to Transfer (minutes)[1]	-	-	61	60
Children's Asthma Care				
Received Home Management Plan of Care	-	-	-	88%
Received Reliever Medication	-	-	-	100%
Received Systemic Corticosteroids	-	-	-	100%
Emergency Department				
Admittance Decision Time (minutes)[2]	457	67	73	98
Head CT Results Within 45 Min. of Arrival[1]	-	-	45%	57%
Patients Who Left ER Before Being Seen	13,165	2%	3%	2%
Time from ER Arrival to Admit. (minutes)[2]	581	245	240	274
Time from ER Arrival to Discharge (minutes)	548	111	126	134
Time in ER Before Being Evaluated (minutes)	358	34	31	26
Time to Pain Meds for Fractures (minutes)	52	70	69	57
Heart Attack Care				
Aspirin Given at Discharge[1]	-	-	99%	99%
Fibrinolytic Meds Within 30 Min. of Arrival[7]	-	-	77%	54%
PCI Within 90 Minutes of Arrival[7]	-	-	97%	96%
Statin Prescribed at Discharge[1]	-	-	98%	98%
Heart Failure Care				
ACE Inhibitor or ARB for LVSD	18	100%	97%	97%
Discharge Instructions Given	66	97%	93%	94%
Evaluation of LVS Function	77	100%	99%	99%
Medicare Spending				
Medicare Spending per Patient (ratio)	-	0.90	0.98	0.98
Pneumonia Care				
Appropriate Initial Antibiotic Given	41	88%	95%	95%
Blood Culture Timing	56	96%	98%	98%
Pregnancy and Delivery Care				
Newborn Deliveries Scheduled Early[7]	-	-	14%	6%
Preventive Care				
Immunization for Influenza[2]	288	93%	90%	90%
Immunization for Pneumonia[2]	445	90%	91%	92%
Stroke Care				
Anticoagulation Therapy for Atrial Fibrillation[1]	-	-	92%	95%
Antithrombotic Therapy Timing	19	100%	96%	98%
Assessed for Rehabilitation	17	100%	95%	97%
Discharged on Antithrombotic Therapy	17	100%	98%	99%
Discharged on Statin Medication	15	73%	90%	94%
Thrombolytic Therapy Timing[7]	-	-	38%	66%
Venous Thromboembolism Prophylaxis	19	95%	89%	94%
Written Stroke Educational Materials Given[1]	-	-	85%	88%
Surgical Care Improvement Project				
Appropriate Beta Blocker Usage[1]	-	-	98%	98%
Appropriate VTP Within 24 Hours[1]	-	-	98%	98%
Controlled Postoperative Blood Glucose[7]	-	-	97%	97%
Perioperative Temperature Management[1]	-	-	100%	100%
Prophylactic Antibiotic Selection[1]	-	-	99%	99%
Prophylactic Antibiotic Selection (Outpatient)	12	100%	98%	98%
Prophylactic Antibiotic Stopped[1]	-	-	98%	98%
Prophylactic Antibiotic Timing[1]	-	-	99%	99%
Prophylactic Antibiotic Timing (Outpatient)[1]	-	-	99%	98%
Urinary Catheter Removal[1]	-	-	98%	97%
Survey of Patients' Hospital Experiences				
Area Around Room 'Always' Quiet at Night	300+	69%	71%	61%
Doctors 'Always' Communicated Well	300+	90%	86%	82%
Home Recovery Information Given	300+	89%	84%	85%
Hospital Given 9 or 10 on 10 Point Scale	300+	78%	71%	71%
Meds 'Always' Explained Before Given	300+	70%	66%	64%
Nurses 'Always' Communicated Well	300+	88%	80%	79%
Pain 'Always' Well Controlled	300+	73%	72%	71%
Room and Bathroom 'Always' Clean	300+	80%	71%	73%
Timely Help 'Always' Received	300+	75%	68%	68%
Would Definitely Recommend Hospital	300+	72%	70%	71%
Use of Medical Imaging				
Cardiac Imaging Stress Test before Surgery[7]	-	-	6.5%	5.3%
Combination Abdominal CT Scan	112	17.9%	16.5%	10.5%
Combination Brain/Sinus CT Scan[1]	-	-	3.5%	2.7%
Combination Chest CT Scan	77	9.1%	4.2%	2.7%
Follow-up Mammogram/Ultrasound	271	8.9%	7.6%	8.8%
Lumbar Spine MRI for Low Back Pain[1]	-	-	40.2%	37.2%

Troy Regional Medical Center

1330 Highway 231 South
Troy, AL 36081
Phone: 334-670-5000
Fax: 334-566-7490
URL: www.attentushealthcare.com/troyregional
Type: Acute Care Hospitals
Emergency Services: Yes
Ownership: Government - Federal
Beds: 97

Key Personnel:
Pediatric Ambulatory Care . . . . . . Pat Block
Pediatric In-Patient Care . . . . Pat Block
Chief of Medical Staff. . . . . Barkley Davis
CEO/President. . . . . Richard D Gore
Operating Room. . . . . Pamela Hawkins
Quality Assurance . . . . Donna White

Measure	Cases	This Hosp.	State Avg.	U.S. Avg.
Blood Clot Prevention and Treatment				
Anticoagulation Overlap Therapy[1,2]	-	-	91%	93%
ICU Venous Thromboembolism Prophylaxis[2]	41	90%	85%	92%
Incidence of Potentially Preventable VTE[1,2]	-	-	18%	10%
UFH with Dosages/Platelet Monitoring[2,7]	-	-	95%	97%
Venous Thromboembolism Prophylaxis[2]	149	91%	74%	85%
Warfarin Therapy Discharge Instructions[1,2]	-	-	77%	75%
Chest Pain/Possible Heart Attack Care				
Aspirin Given Within 24 Hours of Arrival	42	98%	96%	96%
Fibrinolytic Meds Within 30 Min. of Arrival[1]	-	-	57%	58%
Average Time to ECG (minutes)	44	5	6	7
Average Time to Transfer (minutes)[1]	-	-	61	60
Children's Asthma Care				
Received Home Management Plan of Care	-	-	-	88%
Received Reliever Medication	-	-	-	100%
Received Systemic Corticosteroids	-	-	-	100%
Emergency Department				
Admittance Decision Time (minutes)[2]	435	77	73	98
Head CT Results Within 45 Min. of Arrival[1]	-	-	45%	57%
Patients Who Left ER Before Being Seen	17,415	2%	3%	2%
Time from ER Arrival to Admit. (minutes)[2]	437	203	240	274
Time from ER Arrival to Discharge (minutes)	385	87	126	134
Time in ER Before Being Evaluated (minutes)	404	24	31	26
Time to Pain Meds for Fractures (minutes)	47	39	69	57
Heart Attack Care				
Aspirin Given at Discharge[1]	-	-	99%	99%
Fibrinolytic Meds Within 30 Min. of Arrival[7]	-	-	77%	54%
PCI Within 90 Minutes of Arrival[7]	-	-	97%	96%
Statin Prescribed at Discharge[1]	-	-	98%	98%
Heart Failure Care				
ACE Inhibitor or ARB for LVSD	26	96%	97%	97%
Discharge Instructions Given	54	96%	93%	94%
Evaluation of LVS Function	61	100%	99%	99%
Medicare Spending				
Medicare Spending per Patient (ratio)	-	0.97	0.98	0.98
Pneumonia Care				
Appropriate Initial Antibiotic Given	39	92%	95%	95%
Blood Culture Timing	37	97%	98%	98%
Pregnancy and Delivery Care				
Newborn Deliveries Scheduled Early[7]	-	-	14%	6%
Preventive Care				
Immunization for Influenza[2]	300	97%	90%	90%
Immunization for Pneumonia[2]	316	99%	91%	92%
Stroke Care				
Anticoagulation Therapy for Atrial Fibrillation[7]	-	-	92%	95%
Antithrombotic Therapy Timing	16	94%	96%	98%
Assessed for Rehabilitation	13	100%	95%	97%
Discharged on Antithrombotic Therapy	11	100%	98%	99%
Discharged on Statin Medication[1]	-	-	90%	94%
Thrombolytic Therapy Timing[7]	-	-	38%	66%
Venous Thromboembolism Prophylaxis	16	94%	89%	94%
Written Stroke Educational Materials Given[1]	-	-	85%	88%
Surgical Care Improvement Project				
Appropriate Beta Blocker Usage	13	100%	98%	98%
Appropriate VTP Within 24 Hours	80	98%	98%	98%
Controlled Postoperative Blood Glucose[7]	-	-	97%	97%
Perioperative Temperature Management	87	100%	100%	100%
Prophylactic Antibiotic Selection	50	100%	99%	99%
Prophylactic Antibiotic Selection (Outpatient)[1,3]	-	-	98%	98%
Prophylactic Antibiotic Stopped	49	92%	98%	98%
Prophylactic Antibiotic Timing	50	100%	99%	99%
Prophylactic Antibiotic Timing (Outpatient)[1,3]	-	-	99%	98%
Urinary Catheter Removal	30	97%	98%	97%
Survey of Patients' Hospital Experiences				
Area Around Room 'Always' Quiet at Night	300+	69%	71%	61%
Doctors 'Always' Communicated Well	300+	88%	86%	82%
Home Recovery Information Given	300+	83%	84%	85%
Hospital Given 9 or 10 on 10 Point Scale	300+	68%	71%	71%
Meds 'Always' Explained Before Given	300+	65%	66%	64%

NOTE: Hospital profiles are in alphabetical order by state, then city, then hospital within the city; Rankings exclude hospitals with less than 25 cases except for patient surveys which excludes hospitals with less than 100 cases; (a) 100-299 cases; (1) The number of cases/patients is too few to report; (2) Data submitted were based on a sample of cases/patients; (3) Results are based on a shorter time period than required; (4) Data suppressed by CMS for one or more quarters; (5) Results are not available for this reporting period; (6) Fewer than 100 patients completed the HCAHPS survey; (7) No cases met the criteria for this measure; (8) The lower limit of the confidence interval cannot be calculated if the number of observed infections equals zero; (9) No data are available from the state/territory for this reporting period; (10) The scores shown reflect fewer than 50 completed surveys; (11) There were discrepancies in the data collection process; (12) This measure does not apply to this hospital for this reporting period; (13) Results cannot be calculated for this reporting period; (14) The results for this state are combined with nearby states to protect confidentiality; Please refer to the User's Guide for a full explanation of data.

Nurses 'Always' Communicated Well	300+	80%	80%	79%
Pain 'Always' Well Controlled	300+	72%	72%	71%
Room and Bathroom 'Always' Clean	300+	71%	71%	73%
Timely Help 'Always' Received	300+	76%	68%	68%
Would Definitely Recommend Hospital	300+	63%	70%	71%
Use of Medical Imaging				
Cardiac Imaging Stress Test before Surgery	116	12.1%	6.5%	5.3%
Combination Abdominal CT Scan	309	21.4%	16.5%	10.5%
Combination Brain/Sinus CT Scan[1]	-	-	3.5%	2.7%
Combination Chest CT Scan	116	0.0%	4.2%	2.7%
Follow-up Mammogram/Ultrasound	500	4.6%	7.6%	8.8%
Lumbar Spine MRI for Low Back Pain[1]	-	-	40.2%	37.2%

D C H Regional Medical Center

809 University Boulevard East
Tuscaloosa, AL 35401
Phone: 205-759-7111
Fax: 205-759-6984
URL: www.dchsystem.com
Type: Acute Care Hospitals
Emergency Services: Yes
Ownership: Govt - Hospital Dist/Auth
Beds: 583

Key Personnel:
Intensive Care Unit............ Sheila Bresnahan, RN
Administrator .... Bill Cassels
Emergency Room .... Elvin Crawford, MD
Quality Assurance .... Chris Jones
President/CEO.............. Bryan Kindred
Chief of Medical Staff.......... David Rice, MD
Radiology................... Jim Smith

Measure	Cases	This Hosp.	State Avg.	U.S. Avg.
Blood Clot Prevention and Treatment				
Anticoagulation Overlap Therapy[2]	233	97%	91%	93%
ICU Venous Thromboembolism Prophylaxis[2]	92	92%	85%	92%
Incidence of Potentially Preventable VTE[2]	84	45%	18%	10%
UFH with Dosages/Platelet Monitoring[2]	99	100%	95%	97%
Venous Thromboembolism Prophylaxis[2]	344	94%	74%	85%
Warfarin Therapy Discharge Instructions[2]	165	88%	77%	75%
Chest Pain/Possible Heart Attack Care				
Aspirin Given Within 24 Hours of Arrival[1,3]	-	-	96%	96%
Fibrinolytic Meds Within 30 Min. of Arrival[5]	-	-	57%	58%
Average Time to ECG (minutes)[1,3]	-	-	6	7
Average Time to Transfer (minutes)[5]	-	-	61	60
Children's Asthma Care				
Received Home Management Plan of Care	-	-	-	88%
Received Reliever Medication	-	-	-	100%
Received Systemic Corticosteroids	-	-	-	100%
Emergency Department				
Admittance Decision Time (minutes)[2]	575	86	73	98
Head CT Results Within 45 Min. of Arrival[1]	-	-	45%	57%
Patients Who Left ER Before Being Seen	>100k	4%	3%	2%
Time from ER Arrival to Admit. (minutes)[2]	618	279	240	274
Time from ER Arrival to Discharge (minutes)	416	158	126	134
Time in ER Before Being Evaluated (minutes)	433	45	31	26
Time to Pain Meds for Fractures (minutes)	236	72	69	57
Heart Attack Care				
Aspirin Given at Discharge[2]	294	99%	99%	99%
Fibrinolytic Meds Within 30 Min. of Arrival[2,7]	-	-	77%	54%
PCI Within 90 Minutes of Arrival[2]	34	100%	97%	96%
Statin Prescribed at Discharge[2]	284	96%	98%	98%
Heart Failure Care				
ACE Inhibitor or ARB for LVSD[2]	130	98%	97%	97%
Discharge Instructions Given[2]	247	94%	93%	94%
Evaluation of LVS Function[2]	292	100%	99%	99%
Medicare Spending				
Medicare Spending per Patient (ratio)	-	1.00	0.98	0.98
Pneumonia Care				
Appropriate Initial Antibiotic Given[2]	185	98%	95%	95%
Blood Culture Timing[2]	251	98%	98%	98%
Pregnancy and Delivery Care				
Newborn Deliveries Scheduled Early[2]	54	13%	14%	6%
Preventive Care				
Immunization for Influenza[2]	533	94%	90%	90%
Immunization for Pneumonia[2]	590	93%	91%	92%
Stroke Care				
Anticoagulation Therapy for Atrial Fibrillation[2]	13	100%	92%	95%
Antithrombotic Therapy Timing[2]	107	100%	96%	98%
Assessed for Rehabilitation[2]	117	100%	95%	97%
Discharged on Antithrombotic Therapy[2]	106	100%	98%	99%
Discharged on Statin Medication[2]	83	90%	90%	94%
Thrombolytic Therapy Timing[1,2]	-	-	38%	66%
Venous Thromboembolism Prophylaxis[2]	126	99%	89%	94%
Written Stroke Educational Materials Given[2]	73	97%	85%	88%
Surgical Care Improvement Project				
Appropriate Beta Blocker Usage[2]	203	99%	98%	98%
Appropriate VTP Within 24 Hours[2]	430	99%	98%	98%
Controlled Postoperative Blood Glucose[2]	97	100%	97%	97%
Perioperative Temperature Management[2]	574	100%	100%	100%
Prophylactic Antibiotic Selection[2]	481	99%	99%	99%
Prophylactic Antibiotic Selection (Outpatient)	672	99%	98%	98%
Prophylactic Antibiotic Stopped[2]	459	98%	98%	98%
Prophylactic Antibiotic Timing[2]	482	100%	99%	99%
Prophylactic Antibiotic Timing (Outpatient)	672	98%	99%	98%
Urinary Catheter Removal[2]	367	99%	98%	97%
Survey of Patients' Hospital Experiences				
Area Around Room 'Always' Quiet at Night	300+	67%	71%	61%
Doctors 'Always' Communicated Well	300+	82%	86%	82%
Home Recovery Information Given	300+	84%	84%	85%
Hospital Given 9 or 10 on 10 Point Scale	300+	72%	71%	71%
Meds 'Always' Explained Before Given	300+	65%	66%	64%
Nurses 'Always' Communicated Well	300+	81%	80%	79%
Pain 'Always' Well Controlled	300+	72%	72%	71%
Room and Bathroom 'Always' Clean	300+	67%	71%	73%
Timely Help 'Always' Received	300+	67%	68%	68%
Would Definitely Recommend Hospital	300+	72%	70%	71%
Use of Medical Imaging				
Cardiac Imaging Stress Test before Surgery	700	4.6%	6.5%	5.3%
Combination Abdominal CT Scan	1,846	2.1%	16.5%	10.5%
Combination Brain/Sinus CT Scan	2,009	2.7%	3.5%	2.7%
Combination Chest CT Scan	1,393	0.2%	4.2%	2.7%
Follow-up Mammogram/Ultrasound	1,884	15.5%	7.6%	8.8%
Lumbar Spine MRI for Low Back Pain	526	45.8%	40.2%	37.2%

Tuscaloosa VA Medical Center

3701 Loop Road
Tuscaloosa, AL 35404
Phone: 205-554-2000
Fax: 205-554-2034
URL: www.tuscaloosa.va.gov
Type: Acute Care - VA
Emergency Services: No
Ownership: Government Federal
Beds: 750

Key Personnel:
Infection Control............. Doris Chandler, MSN RNC
Chief of Medical Staff.......... Mark Nissenbaum, MD, MM
Quality Assurance .... Kay Stephens
CEO/President............... Alan J Tyler, MS, MPA

Measure	Cases	This Hosp.	State Avg.	U.S. Avg.
Blood Clot Prevention and Treatment				
Anticoagulation Overlap Therapy	-	-	91%	93%
ICU Venous Thromboembolism Prophylaxis	-	-	85%	92%
Incidence of Potentially Preventable VTE	-	-	18%	10%
UFH with Dosages/Platelet Monitoring	-	-	95%	97%
Venous Thromboembolism Prophylaxis	-	-	74%	85%
Warfarin Therapy Discharge Instructions	-	-	77%	75%
Chest Pain/Possible Heart Attack Care				
Aspirin Given Within 24 Hours of Arrival	-	-	96%	96%
Fibrinolytic Meds Within 30 Min. of Arrival	-	-	57%	58%
Average Time to ECG (minutes)	-	-	6	7
Average Time to Transfer (minutes)	-	-	61	60
Children's Asthma Care				
Received Home Management Plan of Care	-	-	-	88%
Received Reliever Medication	-	-	-	100%
Received Systemic Corticosteroids	-	-	-	100%
Emergency Department				
Admittance Decision Time (minutes)	-	-	73	98
Head CT Results Within 45 Min. of Arrival	-	-	45%	57%
Patients Who Left ER Before Being Seen	-	-	3%	2%
Time from ER Arrival to Admit. (minutes)	-	-	240	274
Time from ER Arrival to Discharge (minutes)	-	-	126	134
Time in ER Before Being Evaluated (minutes)	-	-	31	26
Time to Pain Meds for Fractures (minutes)	-	-	69	57
Heart Attack Care				
Aspirin Given at Discharge[5]	-	-	99%	99%
Fibrinolytic Meds Within 30 Min. of Arrival[5]	-	-	77%	54%
PCI Within 90 Minutes of Arrival[5]	-	-	97%	96%
Statin Prescribed at Discharge[5]	-	-	98%	98%
Heart Failure Care				
ACE Inhibitor or ARB for LVSD[5]	-	-	97%	97%
Discharge Instructions Given[5]	-	-	93%	94%
Evaluation of LVS Function[5]	-	-	99%	99%
Medicare Spending				
Medicare Spending per Patient (ratio)	-	-	0.98	0.98
Pneumonia Care				
Appropriate Initial Antibiotic Given[5]	-	-	95%	95%
Blood Culture Timing[5]	-	-	98%	98%
Pregnancy and Delivery Care				
Newborn Deliveries Scheduled Early	-	-	14%	6%
Preventive Care				
Immunization for Influenza[2,3]	131	24%	90%	90%
Immunization for Pneumonia[2,3]	156	32%	91%	92%
Stroke Care				
Anticoagulation Therapy for Atrial Fibrillation	-	-	92%	95%
Antithrombotic Therapy Timing	-	-	96%	98%
Assessed for Rehabilitation	-	-	95%	97%
Discharged on Antithrombotic Therapy	-	-	98%	99%
Discharged on Statin Medication	-	-	90%	94%
Thrombolytic Therapy Timing	-	-	38%	66%
Venous Thromboembolism Prophylaxis	-	-	89%	94%
Written Stroke Educational Materials Given	-	-	85%	88%
Surgical Care Improvement Project				
Appropriate Beta Blocker Usage[5]	-	-	98%	98%
Appropriate VTP Within 24 Hours[5]	-	-	98%	98%
Controlled Postoperative Blood Glucose[5]	-	-	97%	97%
Perioperative Temperature Management[5]	-	-	100%	100%
Prophylactic Antibiotic Selection[5]	-	-	99%	99%
Prophylactic Antibiotic Selection (Outpatient)	-	-	98%	98%
Prophylactic Antibiotic Stopped[5]	-	-	98%	98%
Prophylactic Antibiotic Timing[5]	-	-	99%	99%
Prophylactic Antibiotic Timing (Outpatient)	-	-	99%	98%
Urinary Catheter Removal[5]	-	-	98%	97%
Survey of Patients' Hospital Experiences				
Area Around Room 'Always' Quiet at Night	-	-	71%	61%
Doctors 'Always' Communicated Well	-	-	86%	82%
Home Recovery Information Given	-	-	84%	85%
Hospital Given 9 or 10 on 10 Point Scale	-	-	71%	71%
Meds 'Always' Explained Before Given	-	-	66%	64%
Nurses 'Always' Communicated Well	-	-	80%	79%
Pain 'Always' Well Controlled	-	-	72%	71%
Room and Bathroom 'Always' Clean	-	-	71%	73%
Timely Help 'Always' Received	-	-	68%	68%
Would Definitely Recommend Hospital	-	-	70%	71%
Use of Medical Imaging				
Cardiac Imaging Stress Test before Surgery	-	-	6.5%	5.3%
Combination Abdominal CT Scan	-	-	16.5%	10.5%
Combination Brain/Sinus CT Scan	-	-	3.5%	2.7%
Combination Chest CT Scan	-	-	4.2%	2.7%
Follow-up Mammogram/Ultrasound	-	-	7.6%	8.8%
Lumbar Spine MRI for Low Back Pain	-	-	40.2%	37.2%

Bullock County Hospital

102 West Conecuh Avenue
Union Springs, AL 36089
Phone: 334-738-2140
Fax: 334-738-2146
E-mail: bullockcountyhospital@hotmail.com
Type: Acute Care Hospitals
Emergency Services: Yes
Ownership: Proprietary
Beds: 30

Key Personnel:
Pediatric Ambulatory Care ...... Maria Bernardo, MD
Pediatric In-Patient Care .... Maria Bernardo
Infection Control............. Concetta Braughton, DON
Emergency Room .... Tahir Siddiq, MD
Chief of Medical Staff.......... Tahir Siddiq, MD

Measure	Cases	This Hosp.	State Avg.	U.S. Avg.
Blood Clot Prevention and Treatment				
Anticoagulation Overlap Therapy[1,2]	-	-	91%	93%
ICU Venous Thromboembolism Prophylaxis[2,7]	-	-	85%	92%

NOTE: Hospital profiles are in alphabetical order by state, then city, then hospital within the city; Rankings exclude hospitals with less than 25 cases except for patient surveys which excludes hospitals with less than 100 cases; (a) 100-299 cases; (1) The number of cases/patients is too few to report; (2) Data submitted were based on a sample of cases/patients; (3) Results are based on a shorter time period than required; (4) Data suppressed by CMS for one or more quarters; (5) Results are not available for this reporting period; (6) Fewer than 100 patients completed the HCAHPS survey; (7) No cases met the criteria for this measure; (8) The lower limit of the confidence interval cannot be calculated if the number of observed infections equals zero; (9) No data are available from the state/territory for this reporting period; (10) The scores shown reflect fewer than 50 completed surveys; (11) There were discrepancies in the data collection process; (12) This measure does not apply to this hospital for this reporting period; (13) Results cannot be calculated for this reporting period; (14) The results for this state are combined with nearby states to protect confidentiality; Please refer to the User's Guide for a full explanation of data.

Incidence of Potentially Preventable VTE[2,7]	-	-	18%	10%
UFH with Dosages/Platelet Monitoring[2,7]	-	-	95%	97%
Venous Thromboembolism Prophylaxis[2]	78	14%	74%	85%
Warfarin Therapy Discharge Instructions[1,2]	-	-	77%	75%
Chest Pain/Possible Heart Attack Care				
Aspirin Given Within 24 Hours of Arrival[5]	-	-	96%	96%
Fibrinolytic Meds Within 30 Min. of Arrival[5]	-	-	57%	58%
Average Time to ECG (minutes)[5]	-	-	6	7
Average Time to Transfer (minutes)[5]	-	-	61	60
Children's Asthma Care				
Received Home Management Plan of Care	-	-	-	88%
Received Reliever Medication	-	-	-	100%
Received Systemic Corticosteroids	-	-	-	100%
Emergency Department				
Admittance Decision Time (minutes)[2]	183	82	73	98
Head CT Results Within 45 Min. of Arrival[5]	-	-	45%	57%
Patients Who Left ER Before Being Seen	5,533	1%	3%	2%
Time from ER Arrival to Admit. (minutes)[2]	191	176	240	274
Time from ER Arrival to Discharge (minutes)	337	90	126	134
Time in ER Before Being Evaluated (minutes)	389	38	31	26
Time to Pain Meds for Fractures (minutes)[5]	-	-	69	57
Heart Attack Care				
Aspirin Given at Discharge[5]	-	-	99%	99%
Fibrinolytic Meds Within 30 Min. of Arrival[5]	-	-	77%	54%
PCI Within 90 Minutes of Arrival[5]	-	-	97%	96%
Statin Prescribed at Discharge[5]	-	-	98%	98%
Heart Failure Care				
ACE Inhibitor or ARB for LVSD[1,3]	-	-	97%	97%
Discharge Instructions Given[3]	14	0%	93%	94%
Evaluation of LVS Function[3]	19	84%	99%	99%
Medicare Spending				
Medicare Spending per Patient (ratio)	-	0.99	0.98	0.98
Pneumonia Care				
Appropriate Initial Antibiotic Given[1,3]	-	-	95%	95%
Blood Culture Timing[1,3]	-	-	98%	98%
Pregnancy and Delivery Care				
Newborn Deliveries Scheduled Early[7]	-	-	14%	6%
Preventive Care				
Immunization for Influenza[2]	298	55%	90%	90%
Immunization for Pneumonia[2]	292	83%	91%	92%
Stroke Care				
Anticoagulation Therapy for Atrial Fibrillation[5]	-	-	92%	95%
Antithrombotic Therapy Timing[5]	-	-	96%	98%
Assessed for Rehabilitation[5]	-	-	95%	97%
Discharged on Antithrombotic Therapy[5]	-	-	98%	99%
Discharged on Statin Medication[5]	-	-	90%	94%
Thrombolytic Therapy Timing[5]	-	-	38%	66%
Venous Thromboembolism Prophylaxis[5]	-	-	89%	94%
Written Stroke Educational Materials Given[5]	-	-	85%	88%
Surgical Care Improvement Project				
Appropriate Beta Blocker Usage[5]	-	-	98%	98%
Appropriate VTP Within 24 Hours[5]	-	-	98%	98%
Controlled Postoperative Blood Glucose[5]	-	-	97%	97%
Perioperative Temperature Management[5]	-	-	100%	100%
Prophylactic Antibiotic Selection[5]	-	-	99%	99%
Prophylactic Antibiotic Selection (Outpatient)[5]	-	-	98%	98%
Prophylactic Antibiotic Stopped[5]	-	-	98%	98%
Prophylactic Antibiotic Timing[5]	-	-	99%	99%
Prophylactic Antibiotic Timing (Outpatient)[5]	-	-	99%	98%
Urinary Catheter Removal[5]	-	-	98%	97%
Survey of Patients' Hospital Experiences				
Area Around Room 'Always' Quiet at Night[6]	<100	84%	71%	61%
Doctors 'Always' Communicated Well[6]	<100	95%	86%	82%
Home Recovery Information Given[6]	<100	82%	84%	85%
Hospital Given 9 or 10 on 10 Point Scale[6]	<100	73%	71%	71%
Meds 'Always' Explained Before Given[6]	<100	81%	66%	64%
Nurses 'Always' Communicated Well[6]	<100	83%	80%	79%
Pain 'Always' Well Controlled[6]	<100	82%	72%	71%
Room and Bathroom 'Always' Clean[6]	<100	88%	71%	73%
Timely Help 'Always' Received[6]	<100	86%	68%	68%
Would Definitely Recommend Hospital[6]	<100	75%	70%	71%
Use of Medical Imaging				
Cardiac Imaging Stress Test before Surgery[7]	-	-	6.5%	5.3%
Combination Abdominal CT Scan	85	1.2%	16.5%	10.5%
Combination Brain/Sinus CT Scan[1]	-	-	3.5%	2.7%
Combination Chest CT Scan[1]	-	-	4.2%	2.7%
Follow-up Mammogram/Ultrasound[1]	-	-	7.6%	8.8%
Lumbar Spine MRI for Low Back Pain[7]	-	-	40.2%	37.2%

George H. Lanier Memorial Hospital

4800 48th St
Valley, AL 36854
Phone: 334-756-1400
Fax: 334-756-6698
URL: www.lanierhospital.com
Type: Acute Care Hospitals
Emergency Services: Yes
Ownership: Voluntary non-profit - Other
Beds: 210

Key Personnel:
Radiology. . . . . J Edward Bass, MD
Chief of Medical Staff . . . . Eric Hemberg
CEO/President. . . . . Robert J Humphrey
Pediatric Ambulatory Care . . . . . . Victor V Pouw, MD
Pediatric In-Patient Care . . . . Victor V Pouw, MD
Emergency Room . . . . Lance Strength, RN
Quality Assurance . . . . Kathy Wilder, RN

Measure	Cases	This Hosp.	State Avg.	U.S. Avg.
Blood Clot Prevention and Treatment				
Anticoagulation Overlap Therapy[1,2]	-	-	91%	93%
ICU Venous Thromboembolism Prophylaxis[2]	32	91%	85%	92%
Incidence of Potentially Preventable VTE[1,2]	-	-	18%	10%
UFH with Dosages/Platelet Monitoring[1,2]	-	-	95%	97%
Venous Thromboembolism Prophylaxis[2]	223	55%	74%	85%
Warfarin Therapy Discharge Instructions[1,2]	-	-	77%	75%
Chest Pain/Possible Heart Attack Care				
Aspirin Given Within 24 Hours of Arrival	11	91%	96%	96%
Fibrinolytic Meds Within 30 Min. of Arrival[3,7]	-	-	57%	58%
Average Time to ECG (minutes)	12	14	6	7
Average Time to Transfer (minutes)[1,3]	-	-	61	60
Children's Asthma Care				
Received Home Management Plan of Care	-	-	-	88%
Received Reliever Medication	-	-	-	100%
Received Systemic Corticosteroids	-	-	-	100%
Emergency Department				
Admittance Decision Time (minutes)[2]	255	76	73	98
Head CT Results Within 45 Min. of Arrival[1]	-	-	45%	57%
Patients Who Left ER Before Being Seen	17,830	1%	3%	2%
Time from ER Arrival to Admit. (minutes)[2]	261	251	240	274
Time from ER Arrival to Discharge (minutes)	348	118	126	134
Time in ER Before Being Evaluated (minutes)	371	24	31	26
Time to Pain Meds for Fractures (minutes)	45	60	69	57
Heart Attack Care				
Aspirin Given at Discharge	36	94%	99%	99%
Fibrinolytic Meds Within 30 Min. of Arrival[7]	-	-	77%	54%
PCI Within 90 Minutes of Arrival[1]	-	-	97%	96%
Statin Prescribed at Discharge	35	94%	98%	98%
Heart Failure Care				
ACE Inhibitor or ARB for LVSD	73	100%	97%	97%
Discharge Instructions Given	123	71%	93%	94%
Evaluation of LVS Function	146	100%	99%	99%
Medicare Spending				
Medicare Spending per Patient (ratio)	-	0.87	0.98	0.98
Pneumonia Care				
Appropriate Initial Antibiotic Given	32	100%	95%	95%
Blood Culture Timing	55	96%	98%	98%
Pregnancy and Delivery Care				
Newborn Deliveries Scheduled Early	53	9%	14%	6%
Preventive Care				
Immunization for Influenza[2]	267	97%	90%	90%
Immunization for Pneumonia[2]	345	95%	91%	92%
Stroke Care				
Anticoagulation Therapy for Atrial Fibrillation[1]	-	-	92%	95%
Antithrombotic Therapy Timing	29	83%	96%	98%
Assessed for Rehabilitation	28	93%	95%	97%
Discharged on Antithrombotic Therapy	28	100%	98%	99%
Discharged on Statin Medication	24	79%	90%	94%
Thrombolytic Therapy Timing[1]	-	-	38%	66%
Venous Thromboembolism Prophylaxis	31	55%	89%	94%
Written Stroke Educational Materials Given	16	69%	85%	88%
Surgical Care Improvement Project				
Appropriate Beta Blocker Usage	32	97%	98%	98%
Appropriate VTP Within 24 Hours	97	97%	98%	98%
Controlled Postoperative Blood Glucose[7]	-	-	97%	97%
Perioperative Temperature Management	129	100%	100%	100%
Prophylactic Antibiotic Selection	75	99%	99%	99%
Prophylactic Antibiotic Selection (Outpatient)	81	99%	98%	98%
Prophylactic Antibiotic Stopped	73	95%	98%	98%
Prophylactic Antibiotic Timing	75	99%	99%	99%
Prophylactic Antibiotic Timing (Outpatient)	81	100%	99%	98%
Urinary Catheter Removal	70	96%	98%	97%
Survey of Patients' Hospital Experiences				
Area Around Room 'Always' Quiet at Night	300+	66%	71%	61%
Doctors 'Always' Communicated Well	300+	86%	86%	82%
Home Recovery Information Given	300+	83%	84%	85%
Hospital Given 9 or 10 on 10 Point Scale	300+	65%	71%	71%
Meds 'Always' Explained Before Given	300+	61%	66%	64%
Nurses 'Always' Communicated Well	300+	76%	80%	79%
Pain 'Always' Well Controlled	300+	69%	72%	71%
Room and Bathroom 'Always' Clean	300+	63%	71%	73%
Timely Help 'Always' Received	300+	62%	68%	68%
Would Definitely Recommend Hospital	300+	62%	70%	71%
Use of Medical Imaging				
Cardiac Imaging Stress Test before Surgery[1]	-	-	6.5%	5.3%
Combination Abdominal CT Scan	327	48.3%	16.5%	10.5%
Combination Brain/Sinus CT Scan[1]	-	-	3.5%	2.7%
Combination Chest CT Scan	215	19.1%	4.2%	2.7%
Follow-up Mammogram/Ultrasound	852	14.2%	7.6%	8.8%
Lumbar Spine MRI for Low Back Pain[1]	-	-	40.2%	37.2%

Wedowee Hospital

209 North Main Street
Wedowee, AL 36278
Phone: 256-357-2111
Fax: 256-357-2165
Type: Acute Care Hospitals
Emergency Services: Yes
Ownership: Government - Local
Beds: 34

Key Personnel:
Administrator . . . . Mike Alexander
Infection Control. . . . . Ruth Bailey
Operating Room. . . . . Ruth Bailey
Quality Assurance . . . . Suzanne Brown
CEO/President. . . . . Ferrel Turner
Radiology. . . . . Tammy Wood

Measure	Cases	This Hosp.	State Avg.	U.S. Avg.
Blood Clot Prevention and Treatment				
Anticoagulation Overlap Therapy[1,2]	-	-	91%	93%
ICU Venous Thromboembolism Prophylaxis[2,7]	-	-	85%	92%
Incidence of Potentially Preventable VTE[2,7]	-	-	18%	10%
UFH with Dosages/Platelet Monitoring[2,7]	-	-	95%	97%
Venous Thromboembolism Prophylaxis[2]	355	55%	74%	85%
Warfarin Therapy Discharge Instructions[1,2]	-	-	77%	75%
Chest Pain/Possible Heart Attack Care				
Aspirin Given Within 24 Hours of Arrival	42	100%	96%	96%
Fibrinolytic Meds Within 30 Min. of Arrival[1]	-	-	57%	58%
Average Time to ECG (minutes)	44	5	6	7
Average Time to Transfer (minutes)[7]	-	-	61	60
Children's Asthma Care				
Received Home Management Plan of Care	-	-	-	88%
Received Reliever Medication	-	-	-	100%
Received Systemic Corticosteroids	-	-	-	100%
Emergency Department				
Admittance Decision Time (minutes)[2]	98	77	73	98
Head CT Results Within 45 Min. of Arrival[3,7]	-	-	45%	57%
Patients Who Left ER Before Being Seen	9,462	0%	3%	2%
Time from ER Arrival to Admit. (minutes)[2]	231	210	240	274
Time from ER Arrival to Discharge (minutes)	270	84	126	134
Time in ER Before Being Evaluated (minutes)	389	20	31	26
Time to Pain Meds for Fractures (minutes)	32	57	69	57
Heart Attack Care				
Aspirin Given at Discharge[1,3]	-	-	99%	99%
Fibrinolytic Meds Within 30 Min. of Arrival[3,7]	-	-	77%	54%
PCI Within 90 Minutes of Arrival[3,7]	-	-	97%	96%
Statin Prescribed at Discharge[1,3]	-	-	98%	98%
Heart Failure Care				

NOTE: Hospital profiles are in alphabetical order by state, then city, then hospital within the city; Rankings exclude hospitals with less than 25 cases except for patient surveys which excludes hospitals with less than 100 cases; (a) 100-299 cases; (1) The number of cases/patients is too few to report; (2) Data submitted were based on a sample of cases/patients; (3) Results are based on a shorter time period than required; (4) Data suppressed by CMS for one or more quarters; (5) Results are not available for this reporting period; (6) Fewer than 100 patients completed the HCAHPS survey; (7) No cases met the criteria for this measure; (8) The lower limit of the confidence interval cannot be calculated if the number of observed infections equals zero; (9) No data are available from the state/territory for this reporting period; (10) The scores shown reflect fewer than 50 completed surveys; (11) There were discrepancies in the data collection process; (12) This measure does not apply to this hospital for this reporting period; (13) Results cannot be calculated for this reporting period; (14) The results for this state are combined with nearby states to protect confidentiality; Please refer to the User's Guide for a full explanation of data.

Measure	Cases	This Hosp.	State Avg.	U.S. Avg.
ACE Inhibitor or ARB for LVSD[1]	-	-	97%	97%
Discharge Instructions Given	17	82%	93%	94%
Evaluation of LVS Function	20	70%	99%	99%
Medicare Spending				
Medicare Spending per Patient (ratio)	-	0.86	0.98	0.98
Pneumonia Care				
Appropriate Initial Antibiotic Given	42	88%	95%	95%
Blood Culture Timing	47	91%	98%	98%
Pregnancy and Delivery Care				
Newborn Deliveries Scheduled Early[7]	-	-	14%	6%
Preventive Care				
Immunization for Influenza	266	42%	90%	90%
Immunization for Pneumonia	373	50%	91%	92%
Stroke Care				
Anticoagulation Therapy for Atrial Fibrillation[7]	-	-	92%	95%
Antithrombotic Therapy Timing[1]	-	-	96%	98%
Assessed for Rehabilitation[1]	-	-	95%	97%
Discharged on Antithrombotic Therapy[1]	-	-	98%	99%
Discharged on Statin Medication[1]	-	-	90%	94%
Thrombolytic Therapy Timing[7]	-	-	38%	66%
Venous Thromboembolism Prophylaxis[1]	-	-	89%	94%
Written Stroke Educational Materials Given[1]	-	-	85%	88%
Surgical Care Improvement Project				
Appropriate Beta Blocker Usage[5]	-	-	98%	98%
Appropriate VTP Within 24 Hours[5]	-	-	98%	98%
Controlled Postoperative Blood Glucose[5]	-	-	97%	97%
Perioperative Temperature Management[5]	-	-	100%	100%
Prophylactic Antibiotic Selection[5]	-	-	99%	99%
Prophylactic Antibiotic Selection (Outpatient)[5]	-	-	98%	98%
Prophylactic Antibiotic Stopped[5]	-	-	98%	98%
Prophylactic Antibiotic Timing[5]	-	-	99%	99%
Prophylactic Antibiotic Timing (Outpatient)[5]	-	-	99%	98%
Urinary Catheter Removal[5]	-	-	98%	97%
Survey of Patients' Hospital Experiences				
Area Around Room 'Always' Quiet at Night	(a)	68%	71%	61%
Doctors 'Always' Communicated Well	(a)	81%	86%	82%
Home Recovery Information Given	(a)	79%	84%	85%
Hospital Given 9 or 10 on 10 Point Scale	(a)	65%	71%	71%
Meds 'Always' Explained Before Given	(a)	59%	66%	64%
Nurses 'Always' Communicated Well	(a)	79%	80%	79%
Pain 'Always' Well Controlled	(a)	75%	72%	71%
Room and Bathroom 'Always' Clean	(a)	78%	71%	73%
Timely Help 'Always' Received	(a)	73%	68%	68%
Would Definitely Recommend Hospital	(a)	60%	70%	71%
Use of Medical Imaging				
Cardiac Imaging Stress Test before Surgery[7]	-	-	6.5%	5.3%
Combination Abdominal CT Scan	93	8.6%	16.5%	10.5%
Combination Brain/Sinus CT Scan	204	5.4%	3.5%	2.7%
Combination Chest CT Scan[1]	-	-	4.2%	2.7%
Follow-up Mammogram/Ultrasound	108	12.0%	7.6%	8.8%
Lumbar Spine MRI for Low Back Pain[7]	-	-	40.2%	37.2%

Elmore Community Hospital

500 Hospital Drive
Wetumpka, AL 36092
Phone: 334-567-4311
Fax: 334-567-5919
Type: Acute Care Hospitals
Emergency Services: Yes
Ownership: Government - State
Beds: 69

Key Personnel:
Chief of Medical Staff . . . . Spencer Coleman, MD
Pediatric Ambulatory Care . . . . . . Spencer Coleman
Pediatric In-Patient Care . . . . Spencer Coleman
Quality Assurance . . . . Anne-Marie Nicholsen
Emergency Room . . . . Becky Turner, RN

Measure	Cases	This Hosp.	State Avg.	U.S. Avg.
Blood Clot Prevention and Treatment				
Anticoagulation Overlap Therapy[2,7]	-	-	91%	93%
ICU Venous Thromboembolism Prophylaxis[2,7]	-	-	85%	92%
Incidence of Potentially Preventable VTE[2,7]	-	-	18%	10%
UFH with Dosages/Platelet Monitoring[2,7]	-	-	95%	97%
Venous Thromboembolism Prophylaxis[2]	204	58%	74%	85%
Warfarin Therapy Discharge Instructions[2,7]	-	-	77%	75%
Chest Pain/Possible Heart Attack Care				
Aspirin Given Within 24 Hours of Arrival[3]	20	90%	96%	96%
Fibrinolytic Meds Within 30 Min. of Arrival[3,7]	-	-	57%	58%
Average Time to ECG (minutes)[3]	21	12	6	7
Average Time to Transfer (minutes)[1,3]	-	-	61	60
Children's Asthma Care				
Received Home Management Plan of Care	-	-	-	88%
Received Reliever Medication	-	-	-	100%
Received Systemic Corticosteroids	-	-	-	100%
Emergency Department				
Admittance Decision Time (minutes)[2]	387	68	73	98
Head CT Results Within 45 Min. of Arrival[1]	-	-	45%	57%
Patients Who Left ER Before Being Seen	12,941	3%	3%	2%
Time from ER Arrival to Admit. (minutes)[2]	421	240	240	274
Time from ER Arrival to Discharge (minutes)	417	105	126	134
Time in ER Before Being Evaluated (minutes)	406	30	31	26
Time to Pain Meds for Fractures (minutes)	34	60	69	57
Heart Attack Care				
Aspirin Given at Discharge[2,3]	-	-	99%	99%
Fibrinolytic Meds Within 30 Min. of Arrival[2,3]	-	-	77%	54%
PCI Within 90 Minutes of Arrival[2,3]	-	-	97%	96%
Statin Prescribed at Discharge[2,3]	-	-	98%	98%
Heart Failure Care				
ACE Inhibitor or ARB for LVSD[1,2]	-	-	97%	97%
Discharge Instructions Given[2]	20	45%	93%	94%
Evaluation of LVS Function[2]	23	74%	99%	99%
Medicare Spending				
Medicare Spending per Patient (ratio)	-	1.05	0.98	0.98
Pneumonia Care				
Appropriate Initial Antibiotic Given[2]	40	72%	95%	95%
Blood Culture Timing[2]	21	86%	98%	98%
Pregnancy and Delivery Care				
Newborn Deliveries Scheduled Early[2,7]	-	-	14%	6%
Preventive Care				
Immunization for Influenza[2]	319	88%	90%	90%
Immunization for Pneumonia[2]	432	93%	91%	92%
Stroke Care				
Anticoagulation Therapy for Atrial Fibrillation[3,7]	-	-	92%	95%
Antithrombotic Therapy Timing[1,3]	-	-	96%	98%
Assessed for Rehabilitation[1,3]	-	-	95%	97%
Discharged on Antithrombotic Therapy[1,3]	-	-	98%	99%
Discharged on Statin Medication[1,3]	-	-	90%	94%
Thrombolytic Therapy Timing[1,3]	-	-	38%	66%
Venous Thromboembolism Prophylaxis[1,3]	-	-	89%	94%
Written Stroke Educational Materials Given[1,3]	-	-	85%	88%
Surgical Care Improvement Project				
Appropriate Beta Blocker Usage[5]	-	-	98%	98%
Appropriate VTP Within 24 Hours[5]	-	-	98%	98%
Controlled Postoperative Blood Glucose[5]	-	-	97%	97%
Perioperative Temperature Management[5]	-	-	100%	100%
Prophylactic Antibiotic Selection[5]	-	-	99%	99%
Prophylactic Antibiotic Selection (Outpatient)[1]	-	-	98%	98%
Prophylactic Antibiotic Stopped[5]	-	-	98%	98%
Prophylactic Antibiotic Timing[5]	-	-	99%	99%
Prophylactic Antibiotic Timing (Outpatient)[1]	-	-	99%	98%
Urinary Catheter Removal[5]	-	-	98%	97%
Survey of Patients' Hospital Experiences				
Area Around Room 'Always' Quiet at Night	(a)	75%	71%	61%
Doctors 'Always' Communicated Well	(a)	88%	86%	82%
Home Recovery Information Given	(a)	80%	84%	85%
Hospital Given 9 or 10 on 10 Point Scale	(a)	68%	71%	71%
Meds 'Always' Explained Before Given	(a)	63%	66%	64%
Nurses 'Always' Communicated Well	(a)	83%	80%	79%
Pain 'Always' Well Controlled	(a)	73%	72%	71%
Room and Bathroom 'Always' Clean	(a)	67%	71%	73%
Timely Help 'Always' Received	(a)	82%	68%	68%
Would Definitely Recommend Hospital	(a)	63%	70%	71%
Use of Medical Imaging				
Cardiac Imaging Stress Test before Surgery[7]	-	-	6.5%	5.3%
Combination Abdominal CT Scan	115	22.6%	16.5%	10.5%
Combination Brain/Sinus CT Scan[1]	-	-	3.5%	2.7%
Combination Chest CT Scan[1]	-	-	4.2%	2.7%
Follow-up Mammogram/Ultrasound	207	7.7%	7.6%	8.8%
Lumbar Spine MRI for Low Back Pain[1]	-	-	40.2%	37.2%

Northwest Medical Center

1530 U S Highway 43
Winfield, AL 35594
Phone: 205-487-7736
Fax: 205-487-7891
URL: www.northwestmedcenter.com
Type: Acute Care Hospitals
Emergency Services: Yes
Ownership: Proprietary
Beds: 71

Key Personnel:
Quality Assurance . . . . Linda Edmond
Chief of Medical Staff . . . . Liz Guyton, MD
Radiology. . . . . Jane Hindman, MD
Operating Room. . . . . Susan Huggins, RN
Radiology. . . . . Steve Martin
Pediatric Ambulatory Care . . . . . . Doug McBride, MD
Pediatric In-Patient Care . . . . Doug McBride, MD
CEO . . . . Chridtine Stewart

Measure	Cases	This Hosp.	State Avg.	U.S. Avg.
Blood Clot Prevention and Treatment				
Anticoagulation Overlap Therapy[2]	14	100%	91%	93%
ICU Venous Thromboembolism Prophylaxis[2]	16	100%	85%	92%
Incidence of Potentially Preventable VTE[1,2]	-	-	18%	10%
UFH with Dosages/Platelet Monitoring[1,2]	-	-	95%	97%
Venous Thromboembolism Prophylaxis[2]	165	96%	74%	85%
Warfarin Therapy Discharge Instructions[1,2]	-	-	77%	75%
Chest Pain/Possible Heart Attack Care				
Aspirin Given Within 24 Hours of Arrival	42	100%	96%	96%
Fibrinolytic Meds Within 30 Min. of Arrival[7]	-	-	57%	58%
Average Time to ECG (minutes)	47	7	6	7
Average Time to Transfer (minutes)[1]	-	-	61	60
Children's Asthma Care				
Received Home Management Plan of Care	-	-	-	88%
Received Reliever Medication	-	-	-	100%
Received Systemic Corticosteroids	-	-	-	100%
Emergency Department				
Admittance Decision Time (minutes)[2]	423	57	73	98
Head CT Results Within 45 Min. of Arrival[1]	-	-	45%	57%
Patients Who Left ER Before Being Seen	12,888	3%	3%	2%
Time from ER Arrival to Admit. (minutes)[2]	428	222	240	274
Time from ER Arrival to Discharge (minutes)	405	113	126	134
Time in ER Before Being Evaluated (minutes)	425	21	31	26
Time to Pain Meds for Fractures (minutes)	47	53	69	57
Heart Attack Care				
Aspirin Given at Discharge[1]	-	-	99%	99%
Fibrinolytic Meds Within 30 Min. of Arrival[7]	-	-	77%	54%
PCI Within 90 Minutes of Arrival[7]	-	-	97%	96%
Statin Prescribed at Discharge[1]	-	-	98%	98%
Heart Failure Care				
ACE Inhibitor or ARB for LVSD	11	91%	97%	97%
Discharge Instructions Given	33	94%	93%	94%
Evaluation of LVS Function	43	98%	99%	99%
Medicare Spending				
Medicare Spending per Patient (ratio)	-	1.02	0.98	0.98
Pneumonia Care				
Appropriate Initial Antibiotic Given	90	99%	95%	95%
Blood Culture Timing	98	98%	98%	98%
Pregnancy and Delivery Care				
Newborn Deliveries Scheduled Early[2,7]	-	-	14%	6%
Preventive Care				
Immunization for Influenza[2]	297	99%	90%	90%
Immunization for Pneumonia[2]	425	96%	91%	92%
Stroke Care				
Anticoagulation Therapy for Atrial Fibrillation[1]	-	-	92%	95%
Antithrombotic Therapy Timing[1]	-	-	96%	98%
Assessed for Rehabilitation	13	100%	95%	97%
Discharged on Antithrombotic Therapy	11	100%	98%	99%
Discharged on Statin Medication[1]	-	-	90%	94%
Thrombolytic Therapy Timing[7]	-	-	38%	66%
Venous Thromboembolism Prophylaxis	15	100%	89%	94%
Written Stroke Educational Materials Given[1]	-	-	85%	88%
Surgical Care Improvement Project				
Appropriate Beta Blocker Usage	17	82%	98%	98%
Appropriate VTP Within 24 Hours	35	94%	98%	98%
Controlled Postoperative Blood Glucose[7]	-	-	97%	97%
Perioperative Temperature Management	85	100%	100%	100%
Prophylactic Antibiotic Selection[1]	-	-	99%	99%

NOTE: Hospital profiles are in alphabetical order by state, then city, then hospital within the city; Rankings exclude hospitals with less than 25 cases except for patient surveys which excludes hospitals with less than 100 cases; (a) 100-299 cases; (1) The number of cases/patients is too few to report; (2) Data submitted were based on a sample of cases/patients; (3) Results are based on a shorter time period than required; (4) Data suppressed by CMS for one or more quarters; (5) Results are not available for this reporting period; (6) Fewer than 100 patients completed the HCAHPS survey; (7) No cases met the criteria for this measure; (8) The lower limit of the confidence interval cannot be calculated if the number of observed infections equals zero; (9) No data are available from the state/territory for this reporting period; (10) The scores shown reflect fewer than 50 completed surveys; (11) There were discrepancies in the data collection process; (12) This measure does not apply to this hospital for this reporting period; (13) Results cannot be calculated for this reporting period; (14) The results for this state are combined with nearby states to protect confidentiality; Please refer to the User's Guide for a full explanation of data.

Measure	Cases	This Hosp.	State Avg.	U.S. Avg.
Prophylactic Antibiotic Selection (Outpatient)	14	100%	98%	98%
Prophylactic Antibiotic Stopped[1]	-	-	98%	98%
Prophylactic Antibiotic Timing[1]	-	-	99%	99%
Prophylactic Antibiotic Timing (Outpatient)	14	100%	99%	98%
Urinary Catheter Removal[1]	-	-	98%	97%
Survey of Patients' Hospital Experiences				
Area Around Room 'Always' Quiet at Night	300+	77%	71%	61%
Doctors 'Always' Communicated Well	300+	87%	86%	82%
Home Recovery Information Given	300+	89%	84%	85%
Hospital Given 9 or 10 on 10 Point Scale	300+	70%	71%	71%
Meds 'Always' Explained Before Given	300+	64%	66%	64%
Nurses 'Always' Communicated Well	300+	81%	80%	79%
Pain 'Always' Well Controlled	300+	72%	72%	71%
Room and Bathroom 'Always' Clean	300+	70%	71%	73%
Timely Help 'Always' Received	300+	63%	68%	68%
Would Definitely Recommend Hospital	300+	65%	70%	71%
Use of Medical Imaging				
Cardiac Imaging Stress Test before Surgery	331	4.5%	6.5%	5.3%
Combination Abdominal CT Scan	389	8.0%	16.5%	10.5%
Combination Brain/Sinus CT Scan[1]	-	-	3.5%	2.7%
Combination Chest CT Scan	218	3.7%	4.2%	2.7%
Follow-up Mammogram/Ultrasound	748	11.6%	7.6%	8.8%
Lumbar Spine MRI for Low Back Pain	85	42.4%	40.2%	37.2%

Hill Hospital of Sumter County

751 Derby Drive
York, AL 36925
Phone: 205-392-5263
Fax: 205-392-9974
E-mail: hillhospital@yahoo.com
URL: www.hillhospitalhomestead.com/hillhospitalhomepage.html

Type: Acute Care Hospitals
Emergency Services: Yes
Ownership: Voluntary non-profit - Other
Beds: 33

Key Personnel:

Infection Control . . . . Cynthia Brown, RN
CEO . . . . Jim Burnett
Patient Relations . . . . Ann Johnson, LPN
Radiology. . . . . Jerry R Luther
Chief of Medical Staff . . . . Gary Walson, DO
Quality Assurance . . . . Donna Wright, RN

Measure	Cases	This Hosp.	State Avg.	U.S. Avg.
Blood Clot Prevention and Treatment				
Anticoagulation Overlap Therapy[2,7]	-	-	91%	93%
ICU Venous Thromboembolism Prophylaxis[2,7]	-	-	85%	92%
Incidence of Potentially Preventable VTE[2,7]	-	-	18%	10%
UFH with Dosages/Platelet Monitoring[2,7]	-	-	95%	97%
Venous Thromboembolism Prophylaxis[2]	110	18%	74%	85%
Warfarin Therapy Discharge Instructions[2,7]	-	-	77%	75%
Chest Pain/Possible Heart Attack Care				
Aspirin Given Within 24 Hours of Arrival[1,3]	-	-	96%	96%
Fibrinolytic Meds Within 30 Min. of Arrival[5]	-	-	57%	58%
Average Time to ECG (minutes)[1,3]	-	-	6	7
Average Time to Transfer (minutes)[5]	-	-	61	60
Children's Asthma Care				
Received Home Management Plan of Care	-	-	-	88%
Received Reliever Medication	-	-	-	100%
Received Systemic Corticosteroids	-	-	-	100%
Emergency Department				
Admittance Decision Time (minutes)	255	60	73	98
Head CT Results Within 45 Min. of Arrival[5]	-	-	45%	57%
Patients Who Left ER Before Being Seen	4,622	1%	3%	2%
Time from ER Arrival to Admit. (minutes)	259	182	240	274
Time from ER Arrival to Discharge (minutes)	353	118	126	134
Time in ER Before Being Evaluated (minutes)	381	42	31	26
Time to Pain Meds for Fractures (minutes)[1,3]	-	-	69	57
Heart Attack Care				
Aspirin Given at Discharge[5]	-	-	99%	99%
Fibrinolytic Meds Within 30 Min. of Arrival[5]	-	-	77%	54%
PCI Within 90 Minutes of Arrival[5]	-	-	97%	96%
Statin Prescribed at Discharge[5]	-	-	98%	98%
Heart Failure Care				
ACE Inhibitor or ARB for LVSD[1]	-	-	97%	97%
Discharge Instructions Given	12	42%	93%	94%
Evaluation of LVS Function	13	46%	99%	99%
Medicare Spending				
Medicare Spending per Patient (ratio)	-	1.05	0.98	0.98
Pneumonia Care				
Appropriate Initial Antibiotic Given[1]	-	-	95%	95%
Blood Culture Timing[1]	-	-	98%	98%
Pregnancy and Delivery Care				
Newborn Deliveries Scheduled Early[7]	-	-	14%	6%
Preventive Care				
Immunization for Influenza[2]	188	29%	90%	90%
Immunization for Pneumonia[2]	238	32%	91%	92%
Stroke Care				
Anticoagulation Therapy for Atrial Fibrillation[3,7]	-	-	92%	95%
Antithrombotic Therapy Timing[1,3]	-	-	96%	98%
Assessed for Rehabilitation[3,7]	-	-	95%	97%
Discharged on Antithrombotic Therapy[3,7]	-	-	98%	99%
Discharged on Statin Medication[3,7]	-	-	90%	94%
Thrombolytic Therapy Timing[1,3]	-	-	38%	66%
Venous Thromboembolism Prophylaxis[1,3]	-	-	89%	94%
Written Stroke Educational Materials Given[3,7]	-	-	85%	88%
Surgical Care Improvement Project				
Appropriate Beta Blocker Usage[5]	-	-	98%	98%
Appropriate VTP Within 24 Hours[5]	-	-	98%	98%
Controlled Postoperative Blood Glucose[5]	-	-	97%	97%
Perioperative Temperature Management[5]	-	-	100%	100%
Prophylactic Antibiotic Selection[5]	-	-	99%	99%
Prophylactic Antibiotic Selection (Outpatient)[5]	-	-	98%	98%
Prophylactic Antibiotic Stopped[5]	-	-	98%	98%
Prophylactic Antibiotic Timing[5]	-	-	99%	99%
Prophylactic Antibiotic Timing (Outpatient)[5]	-	-	99%	98%
Urinary Catheter Removal[5]	-	-	98%	97%
Survey of Patients' Hospital Experiences				
Area Around Room 'Always' Quiet at Night[6]	<100	85%	71%	61%
Doctors 'Always' Communicated Well[6]	<100	93%	86%	82%
Home Recovery Information Given[6]	<100	78%	84%	85%
Hospital Given 9 or 10 on 10 Point Scale[6]	<100	72%	71%	71%
Meds 'Always' Explained Before Given[6]	<100	73%	66%	64%
Nurses 'Always' Communicated Well[6]	<100	87%	80%	79%
Pain 'Always' Well Controlled[6]	<100	70%	72%	71%
Room and Bathroom 'Always' Clean[6]	<100	78%	71%	73%
Timely Help 'Always' Received[6]	<100	74%	68%	68%
Would Definitely Recommend Hospital[6]	<100	72%	70%	71%
Use of Medical Imaging				
Cardiac Imaging Stress Test before Surgery[7]	-	-	6.5%	5.3%
Combination Abdominal CT Scan[1]	-	-	16.5%	10.5%
Combination Brain/Sinus CT Scan	47	0.0%	3.5%	2.7%
Combination Chest CT Scan[1]	-	-	4.2%	2.7%
Follow-up Mammogram/Ultrasound[7]	-	-	7.6%	8.8%
Lumbar Spine MRI for Low Back Pain[7]	-	-	40.2%	37.2%

NOTE: Hospital profiles are in alphabetical order by state, then city, then hospital within the city; Rankings exclude hospitals with less than 25 cases except for patient surveys which excludes hospitals with less than 100 cases; (a) 100-299 cases; (1) The number of cases/patients is too few to report; (2) Data submitted were based on a sample of cases/patients; (3) Results are based on a shorter time period than required; (4) Data suppressed by CMS for one or more quarters; (5) Results are not available for this reporting period; (6) Fewer than 100 patients completed the HCAHPS survey; (7) No cases met the criteria for this measure; (8) The lower limit of the confidence interval cannot be calculated if the number of observed infections equals zero; (9) No data are available from the state/territory for this reporting period; (10) The scores shown reflect fewer than 50 completed surveys; (11) There were discrepancies in the data collection process; (12) This measure does not apply to this hospital for this reporting period; (13) Results cannot be calculated for this reporting period; (14) The results for this state are combined with nearby states to protect confidentiality; Please refer to the User's Guide for a full explanation of data.

Blood Clot Prevention and Treatment

Anticoagulation Overlap Therapy

Hospital Name	City	Rate	Cases
Baptist Health Med Ctr-N Little Rock[2]	North Little Rock	100%	50
Jefferson Regional Medical Center[2]	Pine Bluff	100%	42
Sparks Regional Medical Center[2]	Fort Smith	100%	68
White County Medical Center	Searcy	100%	39
Conway Regional Medical Center[2]	Conway	98%	59
Saint Vincent Infirmary Medical Center[2]	Little Rock	97%	68
UAMS Medical Center[2]	Little Rock	96%	52
Washington Reg Med Ctr at North Hills[2]	Fayetteville	96%	95
Mercy Hospital Northwest Arkansas[2]	Rogers	93%	69
Crittenden Memorial Hospital[2]	West Memphis	92%	25
Saline Memorial Hospital[2]	Benton	91%	34
Baxter Regional Medical Center[2]	Mountain Home	90%	40
NW Arkansas Hospitals[2]	Springdale	89%	74
Saint Edward Mercy Medical Center[2]	Fort Smith	89%	93
Saint Bernards Medical Center[2]	Jonesboro	88%	58
Nea Baptist Memorial Hospital[2]	Jonesboro	86%	28
White River Medical Center[2]	Batesville	81%	37
North Arkansas Regional Medical Center[2]	Harrison	78%	46
Saint Joseph's Mercy Health Center[2]	Hot Springs	78%	59
National Park Medical Center[2]	Hot Springs	76%	29
Saint Marys Regional Medical Center[2]	Russellville	74%	43
Baptist Health Med Ctr-Little Rock[2]	Little Rock	73%	143

ICU Venous Thromboembolism Prophylaxis

Hospital Name	City	Rate	Cases
Crittenden Memorial Hospital[2]	West Memphis	100%	69
Mena Regional Health System[2]	Mena	100%	40
Ouachita County Medical Center[2]	Camden	100%	43
Sparks Regional Medical Center[2]	Fort Smith	100%	66
Washington Reg Med Ctr at North Hills[2]	Fayetteville	100%	93
White County Medical Center	Searcy	100%	438
Arkansas Methodist Medical Center[2]	Paragould	99%	192
Jefferson Regional Medical Center[2]	Pine Bluff	99%	308
NW Arkansas Hospitals[2]	Springdale	99%	81
Saint Joseph's Mercy Health Center[2]	Hot Springs	99%	90
Helena Regional Medical Center[2]	Helena	98%	88
Baptist Health Med Ctr-Hot Springs Co[2]	Malvern	97%	100
Baxter Regional Medical Center[2]	Mountain Home	97%	97
Medical Center South Arkansas[2]	El Dorado	97%	176
Mercy Hospital Northwest Arkansas[2]	Rogers	97%	69
North Arkansas Regional Medical Center[2]	Harrison	97%	88
Johnson Regional Medical Center[2]	Clarksville	96%	212
Saint Bernards Medical Center[2]	Jonesboro	96%	174
Siloam Springs Regional Hospital[2]	Siloam Springs	96%	85
Summit Medical Center[2]	Van Buren	95%	37
Forrest City Medical Center[2]	Forrest City	94%	31
Saint Edward Mercy Medical Center[2]	Fort Smith	94%	84
Saint Marys Regional Medical Center[2]	Russellville	94%	112
Saline Memorial Hospital[2]	Benton	93%	148
Wadley Regional Medical Center at Hope[2]	Hope	93%	74
Harris Hospital[2]	Newport	92%	65
Conway Regional Medical Center[2]	Conway	90%	82
UAMS Medical Center[2]	Little Rock	90%	107
Baptist Health Med Ctr-Little Rock[2]	Little Rock	88%	155
National Park Medical Center[2]	Hot Springs	88%	108
Baptist Health Med Ctr-N Little Rock[2]	North Little Rock	86%	145
White River Medical Center[2]	Batesville	86%	127
Great River Medical Center[2]	Blytheville	85%	53
Nea Baptist Memorial Hospital[2]	Jonesboro	83%	94
Saint Vincent Infirmary Medical Center[2]	Little Rock	82%	115
Magnolia Hospital[2]	Magnolia	79%	28
Saint Vincent Medical Center - North[2]	Sherwood	67%	51
North Metro Medical Center[2]	Jacksonville	64%	25

Incidence of Potentially Preventable VTE

Hospital Name	City	Rate	Cases
UAMS Medical Center[2]	Little Rock	13%	39
Saint Vincent Infirmary Medical Center[2]	Little Rock	15%	27
Baptist Health Med Ctr-Little Rock[2]	Little Rock	22%	46

UFH with Dosages/Platelet Count Monitoring

Hospital Name	City	Rate	Cases
Baptist Health Med Ctr-Little Rock[2]	Little Rock	100%	33
Conway Regional Medical Center[2]	Conway	100%	27
Jefferson Regional Medical Center[2]	Pine Bluff	100%	34
Nea Baptist Memorial Hospital[2]	Jonesboro	100%	30
NW Arkansas Hospitals[2]	Springdale	100%	66
Saint Bernards Medical Center[2]	Jonesboro	100%	39
Saint Edward Mercy Medical Center[2]	Fort Smith	100%	30
UAMS Medical Center[2]	Little Rock	100%	26
Washington Reg Med Ctr at North Hills[2]	Fayetteville	100%	49
Sparks Regional Medical Center[2]	Fort Smith	98%	56

Venous Thromboembolism Prophylaxis

Hospital Name	City	Rate	Cases
Arkansas Heart Hospital[2]	Little Rock	100%	284
Mena Regional Health System[2]	Mena	100%	154
White County Medical Center	Searcy	100%	4364
Five Rivers Medical Center[2]	Pocahontas	99%	94
Arkansas Surgical Hospital[2]	No Little Rock	98%	48
Jefferson Regional Medical Center[2]	Pine Bluff	97%	401
Baptist Health Med Ctr-Hot Springs Co[2]	Malvern	96%	513
North Arkansas Regional Medical Center[2]	Harrison	96%	185
Ouachita County Medical Center[2]	Camden	96%	112
Siloam Springs Regional Hospital[2]	Siloam Springs	96%	201
Helena Regional Medical Center[2]	Helena	95%	279
Medical Center South Arkansas[2]	El Dorado	95%	235
Mercy Hospital Northwest Arkansas[2]	Rogers	95%	284
NW Arkansas Hospitals[2]	Springdale	95%	296
Washington Reg Med Ctr at North Hills[2]	Fayetteville	94%	280
Saint Bernards Medical Center[2]	Jonesboro	93%	224
Saint Marys Regional Medical Center[2]	Russellville	93%	288
Crittenden Memorial Hospital[2]	West Memphis	92%	231
Harris Hospital[2]	Newport	92%	331
Baxter Regional Medical Center[2]	Mountain Home	91%	255
Arkansas Methodist Medical Center[2]	Paragould	90%	559
Chambers Memorial Hospital[2]	Danville	90%	223
Conway Regional Medical Center[2]	Conway	90%	220
Saint Joseph's Mercy Health Center[2]	Hot Springs	90%	336
Baptist Health Med Ctr-Heber Spings[2]	Heber Springs	88%	89
Forrest City Medical Center[2]	Forrest City	88%	151
Saint Edward Mercy Medical Center[2]	Fort Smith	88%	320
UAMS Medical Center[2]	Little Rock	88%	302
Magnolia Hospital[2]	Magnolia	87%	77
Johnson Regional Medical Center[2]	Clarksville	86%	504
Wadley Regional Medical Center at Hope[2]	Hope	86%	111
White River Medical Center[2]	Batesville	86%	355
Great River Medical Center[2]	Blytheville	85%	110
National Park Medical Center[2]	Hot Springs	85%	325
Sparks Regional Medical Center[2]	Fort Smith	85%	385
Saline Memorial Hospital[2]	Benton	84%	214
Nea Baptist Memorial Hospital[2]	Jonesboro	83%	340
Baptist Health Med Ctr-Arkadelphia[2]	Arkadelphia	82%	87
Summit Medical Center[2]	Van Buren	81%	141
Baptist Health Med Ctr-N Little Rock[2]	North Little Rock	78%	232
Saint Vincent Infirmary Medical Center[2]	Little Rock	71%	265
Baptist Health Med Ctr-Little Rock[2]	Little Rock	70%	213
Stone County Medical Center[2,3]	Mountain View	68%	31
Baptist Health Medical Center - Stuttgart[2]	Stuttgart	67%	148
Saint Vincent Medical Center - North[2]	Sherwood	55%	124
Drew Memorial Hospital[2]	Monticello	35%	160

Warfarin Therapy Discharge Instructions

Hospital Name	City	Rate	Cases
Baxter Regional Medical Center[2]	Mountain Home	100%	26
Conway Regional Medical Center[2]	Conway	100%	46
National Park Medical Center[2]	Hot Springs	100%	26
Saline Memorial Hospital[2]	Benton	100%	27
White County Medical Center	Searcy	100%	33
Washington Reg Med Ctr at North Hills[2]	Fayetteville	99%	76
Sparks Regional Medical Center[2]	Fort Smith	98%	53
Baptist Health Med Ctr-N Little Rock[2]	North Little Rock	97%	34
Jefferson Regional Medical Center[2]	Pine Bluff	97%	30
North Arkansas Regional Medical Center[2]	Harrison	97%	39
Saint Bernards Medical Center[2]	Jonesboro	94%	47
NW Arkansas Hospitals[2]	Springdale	83%	46
Saint Vincent Infirmary Medical Center[2]	Little Rock	83%	48
Saint Marys Regional Medical Center[2]	Russellville	76%	33
White River Medical Center[2]	Batesville	73%	26
Baptist Health Med Ctr-Little Rock[2]	Little Rock	66%	95
Mercy Hospital Northwest Arkansas[2]	Rogers	50%	60
Saint Joseph's Mercy Health Center[2]	Hot Springs	49%	45
Saint Edward Mercy Medical Center[2]	Fort Smith	42%	78
UAMS Medical Center[2]	Little Rock	24%	45

Chest Pain/Possible Heart Attack Care

Aspirin Given Within 24 Hours of Arrival

Hospital Name	City	Rate	Cases
Arkansas Methodist Medical Center	Paragould	100%	66
Baptist Health Med Ctr-Heber Spings	Heber Springs	100%	48
Chicot Memorial Medical Center	Lake Village	100%	39
Crossridge Community Hospital	Wynne	100%	27
Five Rivers Medical Center	Pocahontas	100%	38
Helena Regional Medical Center	Helena	100%	57
Mena Regional Health System	Mena	100%	31
Mercy Hospital Berryville	Berryville	100%	26
Siloam Springs Regional Hospital	Siloam Springs	100%	116
Summit Medical Center	Van Buren	100%	50
Johnson Regional Medical Center	Clarksville	99%	102
Ouachita County Medical Center	Camden	99%	113
Ashley County Medical Center	Crossett	98%	43
Howard Memorial Hospital	Nashville	98%	47
Harris Hospital	Newport	97%	31
North Arkansas Regional Medical Center	Harrison	97%	121
Baptist Health Med Ctr-Hot Springs Co	Malvern	96%	73
Baptist Health Medical Center - Stuttgart	Stuttgart	96%	28
Forrest City Medical Center	Forrest City	96%	85
Great River Medical Center	Blytheville	96%	67
Crittenden Memorial Hospital	West Memphis	94%	53
North Metro Medical Center	Jacksonville	93%	28
Baptist Health Med Ctr-Arkadelphia	Arkadelphia	92%	48
Stone County Medical Center	Mountain View	92%	59
Magnolia Hospital	Magnolia	91%	32
Ozark Health	Clinton	91%	53
Drew Memorial Hospital	Monticello	88%	33
Chambers Memorial Hospital	Danville	86%	42

Average Time to ECG (minutes)

Hospital Name	City	Min.	Cases
Helena Regional Medical Center	Helena	1	60
Crossridge Community Hospital	Wynne	2	27
Drew Memorial Hospital	Monticello	2	35
Arkansas Methodist Medical Center	Paragould	4	68
Forrest City Medical Center	Forrest City	4	90
Siloam Springs Regional Hospital	Siloam Springs	4	124
Baptist Health Med Ctr-Hot Springs Co	Malvern	5	86
Johnson Regional Medical Center	Clarksville	5	106
Crittenden Memorial Hospital	West Memphis	6	54
Five Rivers Medical Center	Pocahontas	6	39
Harris Hospital	Newport	6	33
Mena Regional Health System	Mena	6	35
Ozark Health	Clinton	7	55
Howard Memorial Hospital	Nashville	8	48
Magnolia Hospital	Magnolia	8	36
Mercy Hospital Berryville	Berryville	8	26
Ouachita County Medical Center	Camden	8	107
Summit Medical Center	Van Buren	9	57
Baptist Health Med Ctr-Heber Spings	Heber Springs	10	51
Baptist Health Medical Center - Stuttgart	Stuttgart	11	30
Chambers Memorial Hospital	Danville	11	37
Ashley County Medical Center	Crossett	12	43
Great River Medical Center	Blytheville	12	68
North Arkansas Regional Medical Center	Harrison	12	127
Stone County Medical Center	Mountain View	12	64
Chicot Memorial Medical Center	Lake Village	14	41
Baptist Health Med Ctr-Arkadelphia	Arkadelphia	16	48
North Metro Medical Center	Jacksonville	35	27

Children's Asthma Care

Received Home Management Plan of Care

Hospital Name	City	Rate	Cases
Arkansas Children's Hospital	Little Rock	85%	130

Received Reliever Medication

Hospital Name	City	Rate	Cases
Arkansas Children's Hospital	Little Rock	100%	130

Received Systemic Corticosteroids

Hospital Name	City	Rate	Cases
Arkansas Children's Hospital	Little Rock	98%	130

Emergency Department

Admittance Decision Time (minutes)

Hospital Name	City	Min.	Cases
Mercy Hospital Booneville[2]	Booneville	18	108
Ozark Health[2]	Clinton	30	334
Saline Memorial Hospital[2]	Benton	36	119
Baptist Health Med Ctr-Hot Springs Co[2]	Malvern	37	351
Baptist Health Medical Center - Stuttgart[2]	Stuttgart	37	174
Mena Regional Health System[2]	Mena	37	413
Summit Medical Center[2]	Van Buren	43	511
Five Rivers Medical Center[2]	Pocahontas	44	357
Forrest City Medical Center[2]	Forrest City	44	205
Baptist Health Med Ctr-Heber Spings[2]	Heber Springs	45	418
UAMS Medical Center[2]	Little Rock	45	388
Baptist Health Med Ctr-Arkadelphia[2]	Arkadelphia	46	200
Arkansas Heart Hospital[2]	Little Rock	50	253
Howard Memorial Hospital	Nashville	50	256
Magnolia Hospital[2]	Magnolia	50	208
Harris Hospital[2]	Newport	52	516
Jefferson Regional Medical Center[2]	Pine Bluff	52	333
Arkansas Methodist Medical Center[2]	Paragould	55	663
Chambers Memorial Hospital[2]	Danville	55	293
Drew Memorial Hospital[2]	Monticello	55	91
Wadley Regional Medical Center at Hope[2]	Hope	55	370
Baptist Health Med Ctr-N Little Rock[2]	North Little Rock	56	535
Baxter Regional Medical Center[2]	Mountain Home	56	360

NOTE: Hospital profiles are in alphabetical order by state, then city, then hospital within the city; Rankings exclude hospitals with less than 25 cases except for patient surveys which excludes hospitals with less than 100 cases; (a) 100-299 cases; (1) The number of cases/patients is too few to report; (2) Data submitted were based on a sample of cases/patients; (3) Results are based on a shorter time period than required; (4) Data suppressed by CMS for one or more quarters; (5) Results are not available for this reporting period; (6) Fewer than 100 patients completed the HCAHPS survey; (7) No cases met the criteria for this measure; (8) The lower limit of the confidence interval cannot be calculated if the number of observed infections equals zero; (9) No data are available from the state/territory for this reporting period; (10) The scores shown reflect fewer than 50 completed surveys; (11) There were discrepancies in the data collection process; (12) This measure does not apply to this hospital for this reporting period; (13) Results cannot be calculated for this reporting period; (14) The results for this state are combined with nearby states to protect confidentiality; Please refer to the User's Guide for a full explanation of data.

White River Medical Center[2]	Batesville	59	427
Siloam Springs Regional Hospital[2]	Siloam Springs	60	388
Stone County Medical Center[2]	Mountain View	60	196
Baptist Health Med Ctr-Little Rock[2]	Little Rock	61	359
Medical Center South Arkansas[2]	El Dorado	61	505
Great River Medical Center[2]	Blytheville	62	240
Helena Regional Medical Center[2]	Helena	64	476
Saint Joseph's Mercy Health Center[2]	Hot Springs	67	553
Crittenden Memorial Hospital[2]	West Memphis	68	360
Saint Vincent Medical Center - North[2]	Sherwood	68	375
Saint Edward Mercy Medical Center[2]	Fort Smith	70	371
Ouachita County Medical Center[2]	Camden	72	284
National Park Medical Center[2]	Hot Springs	75	541
Saint Marys Regional Medical Center[2]	Russellville	80	458
Saint Vincent Infirmary Medical Center[2]	Little Rock	83	314
Conway Regional Medical Center[2]	Conway	85	497
Nea Baptist Memorial Hospital[2]	Jonesboro	89	397
North Arkansas Regional Medical Center[2]	Harrison	91	325
Mercy Hospital Northwest Arkansas[2]	Rogers	96	392
Johnson Regional Medical Center[2]	Clarksville	99	189
White County Medical Center[2]	Searcy	101	483
Sparks Regional Medical Center[2]	Fort Smith	103	844
NW Arkansas Hospitals[2]	Springdale	112	650
Washington Reg Med Ctr at North Hills[2]	Fayetteville	116	518
Saint Bernards Medical Center[2]	Jonesboro	144	487
North Metro Medical Center[2]	Jacksonville	180	378

Head CT Results Within 45 Minutes of Arrival

Hospital Name	City	Rate	Cases
Baxter Regional Medical Center	Mountain Home	57%	30

Patients Who Left ER Before Being Seen

Hospital Name	City	Rate	Cases
Arkansas Heart Hospital	Little Rock	0%	6152
Arkansas Surgical Hospital	No Little Rock	0%	249
Harris Hospital	Newport	0%	11060
Chicot Memorial Medical Center	Lake Village	1%	6825
Crossridge Community Hospital	Wynne	1%	9012
Drew Memorial Hospital	Monticello	1%	10317
Five Rivers Medical Center	Pocahontas	1%	3597
McGehee Hospital	Mcgehee	1%	4335
Mena Regional Health System	Mena	1%	10222
Physicians' Specialty Hospital	Fayetteville	1%	3540
Arkansas Methodist Medical Center	Paragould	2%	25777
Baptist Health Medical Center - Stuttgart	Stuttgart	2%	10975
Baxter Regional Medical Center	Mountain Home	2%	29300
Chambers Memorial Hospital	Danville	2%	4773
Helena Regional Medical Center	Helena	2%	12209
Howard Memorial Hospital	Nashville	2%	8824
Jefferson Regional Medical Center	Pine Bluff	2%	51896
Medical Center South Arkansas	El Dorado	2%	19175
Mercy Hospital Northwest Arkansas	Rogers	2%	46486
North Arkansas Regional Medical Center	Harrison	2%	23229
NW Arkansas Hospitals	Springdale	2%	75284
Saint Bernards Medical Center	Jonesboro	2%	54865
Siloam Springs Regional Hospital	Siloam Springs	2%	20307
Sparks Regional Medical Center	Fort Smith	2%	66937
Stone County Medical Center	Mountain View	2%	7148
Summit Medical Center	Van Buren	2%	20070
White River Medical Center	Batesville	2%	32757
Baptist Health Med Ctr-Arkadelphia	Arkadelphia	3%	11669
Baptist Health Med Ctr-Heber Spings	Heber Springs	3%	10332
Baptist Health Med Ctr-Little Rock	Little Rock	3%	59054
Crittenden Memorial Hospital	West Memphis	3%	24260
Forrest City Medical Center	Forrest City	3%	17745
Magnolia Hospital	Magnolia	3%	10361
National Park Medical Center	Hot Springs	3%	24377
North Metro Medical Center	Jacksonville	3%	18796
Ozark Health	Clinton	3%	8117
Saint Joseph's Mercy Health Center	Hot Springs	3%	40126
Saint Marys Regional Medical Center	Russellville	3%	26621
Saline Memorial Hospital	Benton	3%	33183
UAMS Medical Center	Little Rock	3%	59065
White County Medical Center	Searcy	3%	50020
Ashley County Medical Center	Crossett	4%	7598
Baptist Health Med Ctr-Hot Springs Co	Malvern	4%	15278
Ouachita County Medical Center	Camden	4%	11429
Saint Vincent Medical Center - North	Sherwood	4%	17785
Conway Regional Medical Center	Conway	5%	40337
Great River Medical Center	Blytheville	5%	12153
Nea Baptist Memorial Hospital	Jonesboro	5%	25199
Washington Reg Med Ctr at North Hills	Fayetteville	5%	51940
Baptist Health Med Ctr-N Little Rock	North Little Rock	6%	49857
Saint Edward Mercy Medical Center	Fort Smith	6%	48125
Saint Vincent Infirmary Medical Center	Little Rock	6%	36214
Wadley Regional Medical Center at Hope	Hope	6%	2660
Johnson Regional Medical Center	Clarksville	7%	15314
River Valley Medical Center	Dardanelle	9%	4943

Time from ER Arrival to Being Admitted (minutes)

Hospital Name	City	Min.	Cases
Baptist Health Med Ctr-Hot Springs Co[2]	Malvern	140	545
Chambers Memorial Hospital[2]	Danville	145	319
Harris Hospital[2]	Newport	155	518
Baptist Health Medical Center - Stuttgart[2]	Stuttgart	159	190
Mercy Hospital Booneville[2]	Booneville	160	142
Baptist Health Med Ctr-Arkadelphia[2]	Arkadelphia	164	210
Summit Medical Center[2]	Van Buren	167	513
Five Rivers Medical Center[2]	Pocahontas	168	378
Forrest City Medical Center[2]	Forrest City	170	213
Saline Memorial Hospital[2]	Benton	170	119
Mena Regional Health System[2]	Mena	176	413
Stone County Medical Center[2]	Mountain View	176	196
Medical Center South Arkansas[2]	El Dorado	177	529
Arkansas Heart Hospital[2]	Little Rock	180	255
Helena Regional Medical Center[2]	Helena	184	477
Arkansas Methodist Medical Center[2]	Paragould	187	665
Drew Memorial Hospital[2]	Monticello	192	89
Great River Medical Center[2]	Blytheville	204	240
Saint Joseph's Mercy Health Center[2]	Hot Springs	204	577
Baxter Regional Medical Center[2]	Mountain Home	205	584
Howard Memorial Hospital	Nashville	208	257
White River Medical Center[2]	Batesville	209	431
Siloam Springs Regional Hospital[2]	Siloam Springs	211	395
Jefferson Regional Medical Center[2]	Pine Bluff	220	562
National Park Medical Center[2]	Hot Springs	221	546
Magnolia Hospital[2]	Magnolia	222	233
Saint Marys Regional Medical Center[2]	Russellville	225	473
Baptist Health Med Ctr-N Little Rock[2]	North Little Rock	226	547
Baptist Health Med Ctr-Heber Spings[2]	Heber Springs	229	458
North Arkansas Regional Medical Center[2]	Harrison	230	329
North Metro Medical Center[2]	Jacksonville	236	387
Mercy Hospital Northwest Arkansas[2]	Rogers	238	415
NW Arkansas Hospitals[2]	Springdale	238	672
Wadley Regional Medical Center at Hope[2]	Hope	238	373
Crittenden Memorial Hospital[2]	West Memphis	240	365
White County Medical Center[2]	Searcy	240	484
Ozark Health[2]	Clinton	242	342
Baptist Health Med Ctr-Little Rock[2]	Little Rock	244	362
Conway Regional Medical Center[2]	Conway	244	497
Saint Vincent Medical Center - North[2]	Sherwood	249	432
Nea Baptist Memorial Hospital[2]	Jonesboro	252	406
Saint Edward Mercy Medical Center[2]	Fort Smith	253	387
Saint Bernards Medical Center[2]	Jonesboro	267	497
Saint Vincent Infirmary Medical Center[2]	Little Rock	268	329
Johnson Regional Medical Center[2]	Clarksville	269	203
Sparks Regional Medical Center[2]	Fort Smith	273	844
Washington Reg Med Ctr at North Hills[2]	Fayetteville	277	531
Ouachita County Medical Center[2]	Camden	285	284
UAMS Medical Center[2]	Little Rock	288	404

Time from ER Arrival to Discharge (minutes)

Hospital Name	City	Min.	Cases
Forrest City Medical Center	Forrest City	86	360
Physicians' Specialty Hospital	Fayetteville	86	352
Harris Hospital	Newport	88	369
Arkansas Surgical Hospital	No Little Rock	91	161
Siloam Springs Regional Hospital	Siloam Springs	94	359
Stone County Medical Center[3]	Mountain View	95	86
Summit Medical Center	Van Buren	95	532
Chambers Memorial Hospital	Danville	97	958
Helena Regional Medical Center	Helena	98	316
Mena Regional Health System	Mena	98	403
Medical Center South Arkansas	El Dorado	99	369
Baptist Health Med Ctr-Arkadelphia	Arkadelphia	100	346
Baptist Health Medical Center - Stuttgart	Stuttgart	100	283
Baptist Health Med Ctr-Hot Springs Co	Malvern	102	346
Five Rivers Medical Center	Pocahontas	102	309
Arkansas Methodist Medical Center	Paragould	104	854
Drew Memorial Hospital	Monticello	105	318
Wadley Regional Medical Center at Hope	Hope	105	456
Saline Memorial Hospital	Benton	107	317
North Metro Medical Center	Jacksonville	112	322
Crittenden Memorial Hospital	West Memphis	115	255
Magnolia Hospital	Magnolia	115	265
Great River Medical Center	Blytheville	122	396
North Arkansas Regional Medical Center	Harrison	123	226
Conway Regional Medical Center	Conway	127	445
White County Medical Center	Searcy	127	473
Johnson Regional Medical Center	Clarksville	128	226
National Park Medical Center	Hot Springs	128	391
Arkansas Heart Hospital	Little Rock	130	299
Baptist Health Med Ctr-Little Rock	Little Rock	130	422
Baxter Regional Medical Center	Mountain Home	130	331
Saint Vincent Medical Center - North	Sherwood	133	339
Baptist Health Med Ctr-Heber Spings	Heber Springs	135	345
Ouachita County Medical Center	Camden	136	216
Jefferson Regional Medical Center	Pine Bluff	141	215
NW Arkansas Hospitals	Springdale	142	366
Nea Baptist Memorial Hospital	Jonesboro	143	365
Sparks Regional Medical Center	Fort Smith	143	401
Saint Marys Regional Medical Center	Russellville	146	427
Saint Bernards Medical Center	Jonesboro	147	427
White River Medical Center	Batesville	148	385
Mercy Hospital Northwest Arkansas	Rogers	154	373
Baptist Health Med Ctr-N Little Rock	North Little Rock	160	396
Saint Vincent Infirmary Medical Center	Little Rock	167	343
UAMS Medical Center	Little Rock	167	357
Saint Joseph's Mercy Health Center	Hot Springs	177	355
Washington Reg Med Ctr at North Hills	Fayetteville	180	359
Saint Edward Mercy Medical Center	Fort Smith	198	374

Time in ER Before Being Evaluated (minutes)

Hospital Name	City	Min.	Cases
Harris Hospital	Newport	9	481
Arkansas Heart Hospital	Little Rock	11	360
Medical Center South Arkansas	El Dorado	13	414
Helena Regional Medical Center	Helena	15	454
Baptist Health Med Ctr-Hot Springs Co	Malvern	18	331
Crittenden Memorial Hospital	West Memphis	18	363
Mena Regional Health System	Mena	18	443
Ouachita County Medical Center	Camden	18	378
Physicians' Specialty Hospital	Fayetteville	18	368
Baxter Regional Medical Center	Mountain Home	19	231
North Arkansas Regional Medical Center	Harrison	19	381
Baptist Health Med Ctr-Arkadelphia	Arkadelphia	20	424
Drew Memorial Hospital	Monticello	20	333
NW Arkansas Hospitals	Springdale	20	368
Saline Memorial Hospital	Benton	20	365
Siloam Springs Regional Hospital	Siloam Springs	20	424
Wadley Regional Medical Center at Hope	Hope	20	428
Arkansas Methodist Medical Center	Paragould	22	954
Five Rivers Medical Center	Pocahontas	22	384
Chambers Memorial Hospital	Danville	24	1046
Forrest City Medical Center	Forrest City	24	408
Stone County Medical Center[3]	Mountain View	24	98
Baptist Health Medical Center - Stuttgart	Stuttgart	25	363
Mercy Hospital Northwest Arkansas	Rogers	28	393
National Park Medical Center	Hot Springs	28	418
Arkansas Surgical Hospital	No Little Rock	30	178
Great River Medical Center	Blytheville	31	570
Magnolia Hospital	Magnolia	31	395
Summit Medical Center	Van Buren	31	591
Baptist Health Med Ctr-Heber Spings	Heber Springs	32	406
Saint Marys Regional Medical Center	Russellville	33	472
UAMS Medical Center	Little Rock	33	352
Johnson Regional Medical Center	Clarksville	34	95
North Metro Medical Center	Jacksonville	34	377
Saint Vincent Medical Center - North	Sherwood	34	330
Saint Edward Mercy Medical Center	Fort Smith	35	393
Baptist Health Med Ctr-N Little Rock	North Little Rock	36	465
Saint Joseph's Mercy Health Center	Hot Springs	38	390
Sparks Regional Medical Center	Fort Smith	38	420
Conway Regional Medical Center	Conway	39	516
Baptist Health Med Ctr-Little Rock	Little Rock	41	452
Nea Baptist Memorial Hospital	Jonesboro	44	388
Saint Bernards Medical Center	Jonesboro	46	391
Saint Vincent Infirmary Medical Center	Little Rock	50	303
White County Medical Center	Searcy	50	545
White River Medical Center	Batesville	50	418
Jefferson Regional Medical Center	Pine Bluff	59	353
Washington Reg Med Ctr at North Hills	Fayetteville	90	323

Time to Pain Meds for Bone Fractures (minutes)

Hospital Name	City	Min.	Cases
Physicians' Specialty Hospital	Fayetteville	30	34
Chicot Memorial Medical Center	Lake Village	40	25
Summit Medical Center	Van Buren	40	27
Helena Regional Medical Center	Helena	42	46
Medical Center South Arkansas	El Dorado	45	78
Stone County Medical Center	Mountain View	46	44
Siloam Springs Regional Hospital	Siloam Springs	47	90
Drew Memorial Hospital	Monticello	49	47
Harris Hospital	Newport	49	37
North Metro Medical Center	Jacksonville	49	62
Magnolia Hospital	Magnolia	50	37
NW Arkansas Hospitals	Springdale	51	171
Baptist Health Med Ctr-Arkadelphia	Arkadelphia	52	52
Five Rivers Medical Center	Pocahontas	52	59
Ouachita County Medical Center	Camden	52	53
White County Medical Center	Searcy	52	184
Saint Vincent Medical Center - North	Sherwood	55	63
Arkansas Methodist Medical Center	Paragould	57	71
Baptist Health Med Ctr-Hot Springs Co	Malvern	57	66
Saint Joseph's Mercy Health Center	Hot Springs	58	102
North Arkansas Regional Medical Center	Harrison	60	86
Saline Memorial Hospital	Benton	63	148
Baptist Health Med Ctr-Little Rock	Little Rock	65	136
Saint Marys Regional Medical Center	Russellville	65	147

NOTE: Hospital profiles are in alphabetical order by state, then city, then hospital within the city; Rankings exclude hospitals with less than 25 cases except for patient surveys which excludes hospitals with less than 100 cases; (a) 100-299 cases; (1) The number of cases/patients is too few to report; (2) Data submitted were based on a sample of cases/patients; (3) Results are based on a shorter time period than required; (4) Data suppressed by CMS for one or more quarters; (5) Results are not available for this reporting period; (6) Fewer than 100 patients completed the HCAHPS survey; (7) No cases met the criteria for this measure; (8) The lower limit of the confidence interval cannot be calculated if the number of observed infections equals zero; (9) No data are available from the state/territory for this reporting period; (10) The scores shown reflect fewer than 50 completed surveys; (11) There were discrepancies in the data collection process; (12) This measure does not apply to this hospital for this reporting period; (13) Results cannot be calculated for this reporting period; (14) The results for this state are combined with nearby states to protect confidentiality; Please refer to the User's Guide for a full explanation of data.

Mercy Hospital Northwest Arkansas	Rogers	67	128
Baxter Regional Medical Center	Mountain Home	69	85
Baptist Health Med Ctr-Heber Spings	Heber Springs	70	62
Crittenden Memorial Hospital	West Memphis	70	85
Johnson Regional Medical Center	Clarksville	70	80
Saint Edward Mercy Medical Center	Fort Smith	70	88
Forrest City Medical Center	Forrest City	71	41
Saint Bernards Medical Center	Jonesboro	72	154
Wadley Regional Medical Center at Hope	Hope	73	28
Baptist Health Medical Center - Stuttgart	Stuttgart	74	37
Conway Regional Medical Center	Conway	74	212
UAMS Medical Center	Little Rock	75	48
Nea Baptist Memorial Hospital	Jonesboro	76	122
Sparks Regional Medical Center	Fort Smith	76	129
National Park Medical Center	Hot Springs	78	87
White River Medical Center	Batesville	78	110
Great River Medical Center	Blytheville	79	41
Chambers Memorial Hospital	Danville	80	25
Saint Vincent Infirmary Medical Center	Little Rock	84	103
Baptist Health Med Ctr-N Little Rock	North Little Rock	85	168
Washington Reg Med Ctr at North Hills	Fayetteville	94	187
Jefferson Regional Medical Center	Pine Bluff	96	146

Heart Attack Care

Aspirin Given at Discharge

Hospital Name	City	Rate	Cases
Arkansas Heart Hospital	Little Rock	100%	368
Arkansas Methodist Medical Center	Paragould	100%	40
Baptist Health Med Ctr-Little Rock[2]	Little Rock	100%	354
Baptist Health Med Ctr-N Little Rock[2]	North Little Rock	100%	252
Medical Center South Arkansas	El Dorado	100%	144
Mercy Hospital Northwest Arkansas	Rogers	100%	229
NW Arkansas Hospitals	Springdale	100%	464
Saint Edward Mercy Medical Center[2]	Fort Smith	100%	253
Saint Joseph's Mercy Health Center	Hot Springs	100%	162
Saint Vincent Infirmary Medical Center	Little Rock	100%	203
Sparks Regional Medical Center[2]	Fort Smith	100%	293
Washington Reg Med Ctr at North Hills[2]	Fayetteville	100%	285
White County Medical Center	Searcy	100%	146
Conway Regional Medical Center	Conway	99%	148
Jefferson Regional Medical Center	Pine Bluff	99%	150
National Park Medical Center	Hot Springs	99%	92
Nea Baptist Memorial Hospital	Jonesboro	99%	166
Saint Bernards Medical Center	Jonesboro	99%	393
Saint Marys Regional Medical Center	Russellville	99%	196
UAMS Medical Center	Little Rock	99%	180
VA Central AR Veterans Healthcare Sys	Little Rock	98%	51
Baxter Regional Medical Center[2]	Mountain Home	97%	212
White River Medical Center	Batesville	96%	189
Saline Memorial Hospital	Benton	89%	102

PCI Within 90 Minutes of Arrival

Hospital Name	City	Rate	Cases
Baptist Health Med Ctr-Little Rock[2]	Little Rock	100%	47
Conway Regional Medical Center	Conway	100%	35
Saint Bernards Medical Center	Jonesboro	100%	29
White County Medical Center	Searcy	100%	29
NW Arkansas Hospitals	Springdale	99%	67
Baptist Health Med Ctr-N Little Rock[2]	North Little Rock	98%	41
Saint Joseph's Mercy Health Center	Hot Springs	98%	56
Washington Reg Med Ctr at North Hills[2]	Fayetteville	98%	47
Saint Vincent Infirmary Medical Center	Little Rock	97%	35
Jefferson Regional Medical Center	Pine Bluff	96%	25
Nea Baptist Memorial Hospital	Jonesboro	96%	27
Baxter Regional Medical Center[2]	Mountain Home	94%	34
Mercy Hospital Northwest Arkansas	Rogers	90%	41
Saint Edward Mercy Medical Center[2]	Fort Smith	89%	36
UAMS Medical Center	Little Rock	87%	31
White River Medical Center	Batesville	86%	36

Statin Prescribed at Discharge

Hospital Name	City	Rate	Cases
Arkansas Heart Hospital	Little Rock	100%	307
Baptist Health Med Ctr-N Little Rock[2]	North Little Rock	100%	241
Medical Center South Arkansas	El Dorado	100%	130
Saint Bernards Medical Center	Jonesboro	100%	380
Saint Joseph's Mercy Health Center	Hot Springs	100%	149
Sparks Regional Medical Center[2]	Fort Smith	100%	299
White County Medical Center	Searcy	100%	139
Baptist Health Med Ctr-Little Rock[2]	Little Rock	99%	350
NW Arkansas Hospitals	Springdale	99%	427
Saint Edward Mercy Medical Center[2]	Fort Smith	99%	247
Mercy Hospital Northwest Arkansas	Rogers	98%	214
Nea Baptist Memorial Hospital	Jonesboro	98%	163
Saint Vincent Infirmary Medical Center	Little Rock	98%	199
Washington Reg Med Ctr at North Hills[2]	Fayetteville	98%	266
Arkansas Methodist Medical Center	Paragould	97%	37
Conway Regional Medical Center	Conway	97%	141
Jefferson Regional Medical Center	Pine Bluff	97%	145
UAMS Medical Center	Little Rock	97%	168
Saint Marys Regional Medical Center	Russellville	96%	190
VA Central AR Veterans Healthcare Sys	Little Rock	94%	49
White River Medical Center	Batesville	94%	179
National Park Medical Center	Hot Springs	91%	82
Baxter Regional Medical Center[2]	Mountain Home	86%	210
Saline Memorial Hospital	Benton	81%	100

Heart Failure Care

ACE Inhibitor or ARB for LVSD

Hospital Name	City	Rate	Cases
Arkansas Heart Hospital	Little Rock	100%	147
Arkansas Methodist Medical Center	Paragould	100%	31
Baptist Health Med Ctr-Little Rock[2]	Little Rock	100%	144
Baptist Health Med Ctr-N Little Rock[2]	North Little Rock	100%	110
Crittenden Memorial Hospital	West Memphis	100%	59
Harris Hospital	Newport	100%	36
Helena Regional Medical Center	Helena	100%	75
Medical Center South Arkansas	El Dorado	100%	47
Sparks Regional Medical Center[2]	Fort Smith	100%	70
UAMS Medical Center	Little Rock	100%	172
White County Medical Center[2]	Searcy	100%	79
Saint Edward Mercy Medical Center[2]	Fort Smith	99%	81
Saint Vincent Infirmary Medical Center	Little Rock	99%	195
Jefferson Regional Medical Center	Pine Bluff	98%	81
Mercy Hospital Northwest Arkansas[2]	Rogers	98%	59
National Park Medical Center	Hot Springs	98%	57
Saint Bernards Medical Center[2]	Jonesboro	98%	200
Forrest City Medical Center	Forrest City	97%	31
Nea Baptist Memorial Hospital	Jonesboro	97%	68
NW Arkansas Hospitals	Springdale	97%	89
Saint Joseph's Mercy Health Center[2]	Hot Springs	97%	95
Saline Memorial Hospital	Benton	95%	42
VA Central AR Veterans Healthcare Sys	Little Rock	95%	168
Washington Reg Med Ctr at North Hills[2]	Fayetteville	94%	105
Fayetteville VA Medical Center	Fayetteville	93%	58
Saint Marys Regional Medical Center	Russellville	90%	29
White River Medical Center	Batesville	90%	100
Conway Regional Medical Center	Conway	89%	28
Great River Medical Center	Blytheville	88%	32
Baxter Regional Medical Center[2]	Mountain Home	86%	83
North Arkansas Regional Medical Center	Harrison	78%	32

Discharge Instructions Given

Hospital Name	City	Rate	Cases
Arkansas Heart Hospital	Little Rock	100%	353
Baptist Health Med Ctr-Little Rock[2]	Little Rock	100%	293
Baptist Health Med Ctr-N Little Rock[2]	North Little Rock	100%	238
Baxter Regional Medical Center[2]	Mountain Home	100%	191
Chambers Memorial Hospital[2]	Danville	100%	37
Crittenden Memorial Hospital	West Memphis	100%	129
Helena Regional Medical Center	Helena	100%	165
Saint Vincent Morrilton	Morrilton	100%	27
Summit Medical Center	Van Buren	100%	30
Baptist Health Medical Center - Stuttgart	Stuttgart	99%	77
Nea Baptist Memorial Hospital	Jonesboro	99%	181
UAMS Medical Center	Little Rock	99%	349
White River Medical Center	Batesville	99%	250
Forrest City Medical Center	Forrest City	98%	59
Medical Center South Arkansas	El Dorado	98%	154
Siloam Springs Regional Hospital	Siloam Springs	98%	45
Washington Reg Med Ctr at North Hills[2]	Fayetteville	98%	201
National Park Medical Center	Hot Springs	97%	170
Sparks Regional Medical Center[2]	Fort Smith	97%	223
White County Medical Center[2]	Searcy	97%	222
Jefferson Regional Medical Center	Pine Bluff	96%	139
Arkansas Methodist Medical Center	Paragould	95%	80
Conway Regional Medical Center	Conway	95%	80
Mercy Hospital Northwest Arkansas[2]	Rogers	95%	170
Saint Joseph's Mercy Health Center[2]	Hot Springs	95%	222
VA Central AR Veterans Healthcare Sys	Little Rock	95%	338
Wadley Regional Medical Center at Hope	Hope	95%	43
Magnolia Hospital	Magnolia	94%	32
NW Arkansas Hospitals	Springdale	94%	252
Saint Edward Mercy Medical Center[2]	Fort Smith	94%	192
Saint Bernards Medical Center[2]	Jonesboro	93%	352
Saint Vincent Infirmary Medical Center	Little Rock	93%	378
Great River Medical Center	Blytheville	92%	77
Ouachita County Medical Center	Camden	92%	52
Baptist Health Med Ctr-Hot Springs Co[2]	Malvern	91%	35
Fayetteville VA Medical Center	Fayetteville	90%	99
South Mississippi County Reg Med Ctr	Osceola	90%	30
Johnson Regional Medical Center	Clarksville	89%	35
North Arkansas Regional Medical Center	Harrison	89%	73
Saint Vincent Medical Center - North	Sherwood	89%	56
Five Rivers Medical Center	Pocahontas	88%	25
Fulton County Hospital	Salem	88%	34
Harris Hospital	Newport	88%	60
Saint Marys Regional Medical Center	Russellville	81%	104
Saline Memorial Hospital	Benton	79%	138

Evaluation of LVS Function

Hospital Name	City	Rate	Cases
Arkansas Heart Hospital	Little Rock	100%	383
Arkansas Methodist Medical Center	Paragould	100%	132
Baptist Health Med Ctr-Heber Spings	Heber Springs	100%	30
Baptist Health Med Ctr-Little Rock[2]	Little Rock	100%	341
Baptist Health Med Ctr-N Little Rock[2]	North Little Rock	100%	298
Crittenden Memorial Hospital	West Memphis	100%	144
Crossridge Community Hospital	Wynne	100%	29
Fayetteville VA Medical Center	Fayetteville	100%	101
Forrest City Medical Center	Forrest City	100%	61
Fulton County Hospital	Salem	100%	52
Helena Regional Medical Center	Helena	100%	185
Jefferson Regional Medical Center	Pine Bluff	100%	168
Magnolia Hospital	Magnolia	100%	54
Medical Center South Arkansas	El Dorado	100%	203
Mena Regional Health System[2]	Mena	100%	37
Mercy Hospital Northwest Arkansas[2]	Rogers	100%	209
National Park Medical Center	Hot Springs	100%	200
Nea Baptist Memorial Hospital	Jonesboro	100%	225
Piggott Community Hospital	Piggott	100%	28
Saint Bernards Medical Center[2]	Jonesboro	100%	423
Saint Edward Mercy Medical Center[2]	Fort Smith	100%	259
Saint Joseph's Mercy Health Center[2]	Hot Springs	100%	269
Saint Vincent Infirmary Medical Center	Little Rock	100%	438
Saint Vincent Medical Center - North	Sherwood	100%	70
Saint Vincent Morrilton	Morrilton	100%	30
Sparks Regional Medical Center[2]	Fort Smith	100%	305
Summit Medical Center	Van Buren	100%	40
UAMS Medical Center	Little Rock	100%	369
VA Central AR Veterans Healthcare Sys	Little Rock	100%	380
Washington Reg Med Ctr at North Hills[2]	Fayetteville	100%	255
White County Medical Center[2]	Searcy	100%	289
White River Medical Center	Batesville	100%	332
Baxter Regional Medical Center[2]	Mountain Home	99%	256
NW Arkansas Hospitals	Springdale	99%	340
Saint Marys Regional Medical Center	Russellville	99%	139
Wadley Regional Medical Center at Hope	Hope	99%	70
Conway Regional Medical Center	Conway	97%	109
Five Rivers Medical Center	Pocahontas	97%	37
Johnson Regional Medical Center	Clarksville	97%	38
Ouachita County Medical Center	Camden	96%	71
Ozark Health	Clinton	96%	28
Siloam Springs Regional Hospital	Siloam Springs	96%	57
Baptist Health Med Ctr-Hot Springs Co[2]	Malvern	95%	44
South Mississippi County Reg Med Ctr	Osceola	95%	39
North Arkansas Regional Medical Center	Harrison	94%	104
Chambers Memorial Hospital[2]	Danville	93%	57
Great River Medical Center	Blytheville	93%	89
Harris Hospital	Newport	93%	73
Baptist Health Medical Center - Stuttgart	Stuttgart	92%	80
Saline Memorial Hospital	Benton	90%	174
Stone County Medical Center	Mountain View	89%	27
Drew Memorial Hospital	Monticello	84%	43
Baptist Health Med Ctr-Arkadelphia	Arkadelphia	79%	38
Ashley County Medical Center[3]	Crossett	62%	26

Medicare Spending

Medicare Spending per Patient (ratio)

Hospital Name	City	Ratio	Cases
Chambers Memorial Hospital	Danville	0.77	-
Helena Regional Medical Center	Helena	0.82	-
Baptist Health Medical Center - Stuttgart	Stuttgart	0.85	-
Forrest City Medical Center	Forrest City	0.88	-
Great River Medical Center	Blytheville	0.89	-
Arkansas Heart Hospital	Little Rock	0.91	-
Arkansas Surgical Hospital	No Little Rock	0.91	-
North Arkansas Regional Medical Center	Harrison	0.91	-
Siloam Springs Regional Hospital	Siloam Springs	0.93	-
Harris Hospital	Newport	0.95	-
Johnson Regional Medical Center	Clarksville	0.95	-
Mercy Hospital Northwest Arkansas	Rogers	0.95	-
Saint Bernards Medical Center	Jonesboro	0.96	-
Saint Joseph's Mercy Health Center	Hot Springs	0.96	-
Saline Memorial Hospital	Benton	0.96	-
Baptist Health Med Ctr-Hot Springs Co	Malvern	0.97	-
Baxter Regional Medical Center	Mountain Home	0.97	-
Saint Vincent Infirmary Medical Center	Little Rock	0.97	-
UAMS Medical Center	Little Rock	0.97	-
Baptist Health Med Ctr-Little Rock	Little Rock	0.98	-
Baptist Health Med Ctr-N Little Rock	North Little Rock	0.98	-
Conway Regional Medical Center	Conway	0.98	-
Saint Marys Regional Medical Center	Russellville	0.98	-
Nea Baptist Memorial Hospital	Jonesboro	0.99	-
NW Arkansas Hospitals	Springdale	0.99	-
White County Medical Center	Searcy	0.99	-

NOTE: Hospital profiles are in alphabetical order by state, then city, then hospital within the city; Rankings exclude hospitals with less than 25 cases except for patient surveys which excludes hospitals with less than 100 cases; (a) 100-299 cases; (1) The number of cases/patients is too few to report; (2) Data submitted were based on a sample of cases/patients; (3) Results are based on a shorter time period than required; (4) Data suppressed by CMS for one or more quarters; (5) Results are not available for this reporting period; (6) Fewer than 100 patients completed the HCAHPS survey; (7) No cases met the criteria for this measure; (8) The lower limit of the confidence interval cannot be calculated if the number of observed infections equals zero; (9) No data are available from the state/territory for this reporting period; (10) The scores shown reflect fewer than 50 completed surveys; (11) There were discrepancies in the data collection process; (12) This measure does not apply to this hospital for this reporting period; (13) Results cannot be calculated for this reporting period; (14) The results for this state are combined with nearby states to protect confidentiality; Please refer to the User's Guide for a full explanation of data.

Hospital Name	City	Rate	Cases
National Park Medical Center	Hot Springs	1.00	-
Saint Edward Mercy Medical Center	Fort Smith	1.00	-
Washington Reg Med Ctr at North Hills	Fayetteville	1.00	-
White River Medical Center	Batesville	1.00	-
Magnolia Hospital	Magnolia	1.01	-
Medical Center South Arkansas	El Dorado	1.01	-
Jefferson Regional Medical Center	Pine Bluff	1.02	-
Mena Regional Health System	Mena	1.03	-
Physicians' Specialty Hospital	Fayetteville	1.03	-
Arkansas Methodist Medical Center	Paragould	1.04	-
Crittenden Memorial Hospital	West Memphis	1.04	-
Sparks Regional Medical Center	Fort Smith	1.04	-
Drew Memorial Hospital	Monticello	1.05	-
Ouachita County Medical Center	Camden	1.05	-
Five Rivers Medical Center	Pocahontas	1.06	-
Summit Medical Center	Van Buren	1.12	-
Saint Vincent Medical Center - North	Sherwood	1.15	-
North Metro Medical Center	Jacksonville	1.26	-

Pneumonia Care

Appropriate Initial Antibiotic Given

Hospital Name	City	Rate	Cases
Forrest City Medical Center	Forrest City	100%	45
Helena Regional Medical Center	Helena	100%	37
Howard Memorial Hospital	Nashville	100%	35
Lawrence Memorial Hospital	Walnut Ridge	100%	30
Mercy Hospital Northwest Arkansas[2]	Rogers	100%	62
Ouachita County Medical Center	Camden	100%	46
Piggott Community Hospital	Piggott	100%	40
Saint Joseph's Mercy Health Center[2]	Hot Springs	100%	56
Sparks Regional Medical Center[2]	Fort Smith	100%	53
Summit Medical Center	Van Buren	100%	49
White County Medical Center[2]	Searcy	100%	83
Arkansas Methodist Medical Center[2]	Paragould	99%	150
Baptist Health Med Ctr-Little Rock[2]	Little Rock	99%	70
Baptist Health Med Ctr-N Little Rock[2]	North Little Rock	99%	88
Crossridge Community Hospital	Wynne	99%	79
Medical Center South Arkansas	El Dorado	99%	71
Ashley County Medical Center	Crossett	98%	40
Baptist Health Med Ctr-Hot Springs Co[2]	Malvern	98%	103
Bradley County Medical Center	Warren	98%	54
Mercy Hospital Berryville[2]	Berryville	98%	66
Nea Baptist Memorial Hospital	Jonesboro	98%	173
Saint Bernards Medical Center[2]	Jonesboro	98%	49
VA Central AR Veterans Healthcare Sys	Little Rock	98%	153
Ozark Health[2]	Clinton	97%	39
Siloam Springs Regional Hospital	Siloam Springs	97%	72
Baxter Regional Medical Center[2]	Mountain Home	96%	91
Chambers Memorial Hospital[2]	Danville	96%	46
National Park Medical Center	Hot Springs	96%	136
Saint Marys Regional Medical Center	Russellville	96%	99
Saline Memorial Hospital[2]	Benton	96%	144
White River Medical Center	Batesville	96%	168
Fayetteville VA Medical Center	Fayetteville	95%	83
Johnson Regional Medical Center	Clarksville	95%	113
NW Arkansas Hospitals	Springdale	95%	167
Washington Reg Med Ctr at North Hills[2]	Fayetteville	95%	87
Baptist Health Med Ctr-Heber Spings	Heber Springs	94%	36
Baptist Health Medical Center - Stuttgart	Stuttgart	94%	47
Crittenden Memorial Hospital[2]	West Memphis	94%	53
Saint Edward Mercy Medical Center[2]	Fort Smith	94%	49
Harris Hospital	Newport	93%	59
Jefferson Regional Medical Center	Pine Bluff	93%	150
Saint Vincent Medical Center - North	Sherwood	92%	71
Five Rivers Medical Center	Pocahontas	91%	47
Ozarks Community Hospital of Gravette[3]	Gravette	91%	33
Saint Vincent Infirmary Medical Center	Little Rock	91%	139
Magnolia Hospital	Magnolia	89%	36
Fulton County Hospital	Salem	88%	33
North Arkansas Regional Medical Center[2]	Harrison	88%	95
St Edward Health Facil-Scott Co	Waldron	88%	34
Great River Medical Center[2]	Blytheville	87%	69
Mena Regional Health System	Mena	86%	43
Wadley Regional Medical Center at Hope	Hope	86%	72
UAMS Medical Center	Little Rock	85%	95
Conway Regional Medical Center[2]	Conway	84%	116
Dallas County Medical Center	Fordyce	84%	31
Drew Memorial Hospital[2]	Monticello	84%	91
Delta Memorial Hospital[2]	Dumas	81%	42
Stone County Medical Center	Mountain View	78%	49

Blood Culture Timing

Hospital Name	City	Rate	Cases
Arkansas Heart Hospital	Little Rock	100%	57
Arkansas Methodist Medical Center[2]	Paragould	100%	201
Baptist Health Med Ctr-Heber Spings	Heber Springs	100%	59
Conway Regional Medical Center[2]	Conway	100%	201
Crossridge Community Hospital	Wynne	100%	34
Five Rivers Medical Center	Pocahontas	100%	63
Helena Regional Medical Center	Helena	100%	42
Howard Memorial Hospital	Nashville	100%	37
Jefferson Regional Medical Center	Pine Bluff	100%	245
Lawrence Memorial Hospital	Walnut Ridge	100%	39
Medical Center South Arkansas	El Dorado	100%	114
Mena Regional Health System	Mena	100%	53
Piggott Community Hospital	Piggott	100%	51
Saint Bernards Medical Center[2]	Jonesboro	100%	84
Saint Joseph's Mercy Health Center[2]	Hot Springs	100%	81
Sparks Regional Medical Center[2]	Fort Smith	100%	120
Summit Medical Center	Van Buren	100%	86
Washington Reg Med Ctr at North Hills[2]	Fayetteville	100%	149
White County Medical Center[2]	Searcy	100%	139
Baptist Health Med Ctr-Little Rock[2]	Little Rock	99%	100
Crittenden Memorial Hospital[2]	West Memphis	99%	127
Fayetteville VA Medical Center	Fayetteville	99%	113
Nea Baptist Memorial Hospital	Jonesboro	99%	269
Saint Marys Regional Medical Center	Russellville	99%	150
Saint Vincent Infirmary Medical Center	Little Rock	99%	188
White River Medical Center	Batesville	99%	239
Baptist Health Med Ctr-Arkadelphia	Arkadelphia	98%	41
Baptist Health Med Ctr-N Little Rock[2]	North Little Rock	98%	163
Forrest City Medical Center	Forrest City	98%	62
Great River Medical Center[2]	Blytheville	98%	123
Magnolia Hospital	Magnolia	98%	48
National Park Medical Center	Hot Springs	98%	148
NW Arkansas Hospitals	Springdale	98%	247
Saint Edward Mercy Medical Center[2]	Fort Smith	98%	102
Saline Memorial Hospital[2]	Benton	98%	268
Siloam Springs Regional Hospital	Siloam Springs	98%	92
Wadley Regional Medical Center at Hope	Hope	98%	54
Mercy Hospital Northwest Arkansas[2]	Rogers	97%	115
VA Central AR Veterans Healthcare Sys	Little Rock	97%	276
Baptist Health Med Ctr-Hot Springs Co[2]	Malvern	96%	100
Baptist Health Medical Center - Stuttgart	Stuttgart	96%	54
Baxter Regional Medical Center[2]	Mountain Home	96%	118
Mercy Hospital Booneville[2]	Booneville	96%	52
South Mississispi County Reg Med Ctr	Osceola	96%	26
Ashley County Medical Center	Crossett	95%	41
Johnson Regional Medical Center	Clarksville	95%	101
Ozark Health[2]	Clinton	95%	55
Saint Vincent Medical Center - North	Sherwood	95%	75
UAMS Medical Center	Little Rock	95%	207
Drew Memorial Hospital[2]	Monticello	94%	81
Ouachita County Medical Center	Camden	94%	33
Fulton County Hospital	Salem	93%	28
Harris Hospital	Newport	93%	85
North Arkansas Regional Medical Center[2]	Harrison	93%	122
Mercy Hospital Berryville[2]	Berryville	91%	78
St Edward Health Facil-Scott Co	Waldron	89%	37
Stone County Medical Center	Mountain View	85%	27
De Queen Medical Center	De Queen	84%	25
Delta Memorial Hospital[2]	Dumas	84%	31

Pregnancy and Delivery Care

Newborns whose Deliveries were Scheduled Early

Hospital Name	City	Rate	Cases
Baptist Health Med Ctr-Little Rock[2]	Little Rock	0%	54
Harris Hospital[2]	Newport	0%	27
Jefferson Regional Medical Center	Pine Bluff	0%	159
Mena Regional Health System[2]	Mena	0%	32
National Park Medical Center[2]	Hot Springs	0%	26
Saint Joseph's Mercy Health Center[2]	Hot Springs	0%	40
Saint Marys Regional Medical Center[2]	Russellville	0%	41
Saint Vincent Infirmary Medical Center[2]	Little Rock	0%	32
Siloam Springs Regional Hospital[2]	Siloam Springs	0%	39
Sparks Regional Medical Center[2]	Fort Smith	0%	26
Baptist Health Med Ctr-Arkadelphia	Arkadelphia	2%	54
Johnson Regional Medical Center[2]	Clarksville	2%	46
Medical Center South Arkansas[2]	El Dorado	4%	50
Ouachita County Medical Center	Camden	4%	25
UAMS Medical Center[2]	Little Rock	4%	26
Washington Reg Med Ctr at North Hills[2]	Fayetteville	4%	50
Crittenden Memorial Hospital[2]	West Memphis	5%	39
Saint Edward Mercy Medical Center[2]	Fort Smith	5%	55
NW Arkansas Hospitals[2]	Springdale	6%	123
Saline Memorial Hospital	Benton	6%	53
Saint Bernards Medical Center[2]	Jonesboro	7%	123
White River Medical Center[2]	Batesville	7%	30
Magnolia Hospital	Magnolia	8%	40
Forrest City Medical Center[2]	Forrest City	9%	46
Baptist Health Med Ctr-N Little Rock[2]	North Little Rock	10%	41
Conway Regional Medical Center[2]	Conway	10%	114
Baxter Regional Medical Center[2]	Mountain Home	14%	28
Arkansas Methodist Medical Center	Paragould	19%	54
Drew Memorial Hospital[2]	Monticello	51%	51

Preventive Care

Immunization for Influenza

Hospital Name	City	Rate	Cases
Helena Regional Medical Center[2]	Helena	100%	415
Medical Center South Arkansas[2]	El Dorado	100%	527
Mercy Hospital Northwest Arkansas[2]	Rogers	100%	541
North Metro Medical Center[2]	Jacksonville	100%	233
Siloam Springs Regional Hospital[2]	Siloam Springs	99%	481
Sparks Regional Medical Center[2]	Fort Smith	99%	628
Summit Medical Center[2]	Van Buren	99%	335
Baptist Health Med Ctr-Hot Springs Co[2]	Malvern	98%	284
National Park Medical Center[2]	Hot Springs	98%	537
NW Arkansas Hospitals[2]	Springdale	98%	700
Ouachita County Medical Center[2]	Camden	98%	270
Saint Marys Regional Medical Center[2]	Russellville	98%	471
Five Rivers Medical Center[2]	Pocahontas	97%	286
Mena Regional Health System[2]	Mena	97%	323
Wadley Regional Medical Center at Hope[2]	Hope	97%	296
Washington Reg Med Ctr at North Hills[2]	Fayetteville	97%	535
White River Medical Center[2]	Batesville	97%	573
Baxter Regional Medical Center[2]	Mountain Home	96%	604
Arkansas Methodist Medical Center[2]	Paragould	95%	566
Jefferson Regional Medical Center[2]	Pine Bluff	95%	880
Nea Baptist Memorial Hospital[2]	Jonesboro	95%	551
Saint Edward Mercy Medical Center[2]	Fort Smith	95%	513
Stone County Medical Center[2]	Mountain View	95%	280
White County Medical Center[2]	Searcy	95%	577
Baptist Health Medical Center - Stuttgart[2]	Stuttgart	94%	252
Harris Hospital[2]	Newport	94%	590
Howard Memorial Hospital	Nashville	94%	208
Johnson Regional Medical Center[2]	Clarksville	94%	222
Saint Bernards Medical Center[2]	Jonesboro	94%	541
Baptist Health Med Ctr-Heber Spings[2]	Heber Springs	93%	279
Forrest City Medical Center[2]	Forrest City	93%	257
Mercy Hospital Berryville[2]	Berryville	93%	290
Saint Vincent Medical Center - North[2]	Sherwood	93%	291
Saline Memorial Hospital[2]	Benton	92%	495
Ozark Health[2]	Clinton	91%	251
Saint Vincent Infirmary Medical Center[2]	Little Rock	90%	548
Saint Joseph's Mercy Health Center[2]	Hot Springs	89%	556
Conway Regional Medical Center[2]	Conway	87%	551
Baptist Health Med Ctr-Arkadelphia[2]	Arkadelphia	86%	244
Chambers Memorial Hospital[2]	Danville	84%	293
North Arkansas Regional Medical Center[2]	Harrison	84%	437
Magnolia Hospital[2]	Magnolia	82%	235
Baptist Health Med Ctr-N Little Rock[2]	North Little Rock	76%	531
Baptist Health Med Ctr-Little Rock[2]	Little Rock	74%	540
Crittenden Memorial Hospital[2]	West Memphis	74%	340
Arkansas Heart Hospital[2]	Little Rock	71%	645
UAMS Medical Center[2]	Little Rock	68%	590
Drew Memorial Hospital[2]	Monticello	56%	244
Mercy Hospital Booneville[2]	Booneville	56%	68
Arkansas Surgical Hospital[2]	No Little Rock	51%	482
Great River Medical Center[2]	Blytheville	51%	236
Physicians' Specialty Hospital[2]	Fayetteville	36%	309

Immunization for Pneumonia

Hospital Name	City	Rate	Cases
Helena Regional Medical Center[2]	Helena	100%	484
Medical Center South Arkansas[2]	El Dorado	100%	604
NW Arkansas Hospitals[2]	Springdale	100%	644
Siloam Springs Regional Hospital[2]	Siloam Springs	100%	420
Sparks Regional Medical Center[2]	Fort Smith	100%	833
Mena Regional Health System[2]	Mena	99%	573
Mercy Hospital Berryville[2]	Berryville	99%	419
Mercy Hospital Northwest Arkansas[2]	Rogers	99%	682
Saint Edward Mercy Medical Center[2]	Fort Smith	99%	617
Baptist Health Med Ctr-Hot Springs Co[2]	Malvern	98%	707
Five Rivers Medical Center[2]	Pocahontas	98%	431
Ouachita County Medical Center[2]	Camden	98%	345
Summit Medical Center[2]	Van Buren	98%	414
Wadley Regional Medical Center at Hope[2]	Hope	98%	449
White River Medical Center[2]	Batesville	98%	722
Harris Hospital[2]	Newport	97%	537
Jefferson Regional Medical Center[2]	Pine Bluff	97%	1268
Johnson Regional Medical Center[2]	Clarksville	97%	234
National Park Medical Center[2]	Hot Springs	97%	702
Baptist Health Med Ctr-Heber Spings[2]	Heber Springs	96%	489
Baxter Regional Medical Center[2]	Mountain Home	96%	875
Forrest City Medical Center[2]	Forrest City	96%	207
Howard Memorial Hospital	Nashville	96%	304
Nea Baptist Memorial Hospital[2]	Jonesboro	96%	723
Stone County Medical Center[2]	Mountain View	96%	447
Arkansas Methodist Medical Center[2]	Paragould	95%	704
Baptist Health Medical Center - Stuttgart[2]	Stuttgart	95%	337
White County Medical Center[2]	Searcy	95%	698
Saint Bernards Medical Center[2]	Jonesboro	93%	689
Washington Reg Med Ctr at North Hills[2]	Fayetteville	93%	682
Saint Joseph's Mercy Health Center[2]	Hot Springs	92%	757

NOTE: Hospital profiles are in alphabetical order by state, then city, then hospital within the city; Rankings exclude hospitals with less than 25 cases except for patient surveys which excludes hospitals with less than 100 cases; (a) 100-299 cases; (1) The number of cases/patients is too few to report; (2) Data submitted were based on a sample of cases/patients; (3) Results are based on a shorter time period than required; (4) Data suppressed by CMS for one or more quarters; (5) Results are not available for this reporting period; (6) Fewer than 100 patients completed the HCAHPS survey; (7) No cases met the criteria for this measure; (8) The lower limit of the confidence interval cannot be calculated if the number of observed infections equals zero; (9) No data are available from the state/territory for this reporting period; (10) The scores shown reflect fewer than 50 completed surveys; (11) There were discrepancies in the data collection process; (12) This measure does not apply to this hospital for this reporting period; (13) Results cannot be calculated for this reporting period; (14) The results for this state are combined with nearby states to protect confidentiality; Please refer to the User's Guide for a full explanation of data.

Hospital Name	City	Rate	Cases
Saint Vincent Medical Center - North[2]	Sherwood	92%	400
Conway Regional Medical Center[2]	Conway	91%	517
Ozark Health[2]	Clinton	91%	433
Saline Memorial Hospital[2]	Benton	91%	597
Crittenden Memorial Hospital[2]	West Memphis	90%	394
Saint Marys Regional Medical Center[2]	Russellville	90%	558
Chambers Memorial Hospital[2]	Danville	89%	331
North Arkansas Regional Medical Center[2]	Harrison	89%	527
Saint Vincent Infirmary Medical Center[2]	Little Rock	88%	684
Magnolia Hospital[2]	Magnolia	86%	281
North Metro Medical Center[2]	Jacksonville	85%	317
Arkansas Heart Hospital[2]	Little Rock	83%	1026
Baptist Health Med Ctr-Arkadelphia[2]	Arkadelphia	82%	228
Baptist Health Med Ctr-N Little Rock[2]	North Little Rock	81%	680
UAMS Medical Center[2]	Little Rock	77%	546
Drew Memorial Hospital[2]	Monticello	73%	176
Baptist Health Med Ctr-Little Rock[2]	Little Rock	71%	599
Great River Medical Center[2]	Blytheville	69%	233
Arkansas Surgical Hospital[2]	No Little Rock	60%	509
Mercy Hospital Booneville[2]	Booneville	55%	120
Physicians' Specialty Hospital[2]	Fayetteville	34%	338

Stroke Care

Anticoagulation Therapy for Atrial Fibrillation

Hospital Name	City	Rate	Cases
Saint Bernards Medical Center	Jonesboro	96%	28

Antithrombotic Therapy Timing

Hospital Name	City	Rate	Cases
Baptist Health Med Ctr-N Little Rock[2]	North Little Rock	100%	76
Mercy Hospital Northwest Arkansas[2]	Rogers	100%	92
NW Arkansas Hospitals	Springdale	100%	94
Saint Marys Regional Medical Center	Russellville	100%	45
Sparks Regional Medical Center[2]	Fort Smith	100%	88
Conway Regional Medical Center	Conway	99%	87
Saint Edward Mercy Medical Center[2]	Fort Smith	99%	67
Washington Reg Med Ctr at North Hills[2]	Fayetteville	98%	66
White County Medical Center	Searcy	98%	99
Arkansas Methodist Medical Center	Paragould	97%	39
Baxter Regional Medical Center[2]	Mountain Home	97%	65
Jefferson Regional Medical Center	Pine Bluff	97%	137
Medical Center South Arkansas	El Dorado	97%	39
Nea Baptist Memorial Hospital[2]	Jonesboro	97%	73
Baptist Health Med Ctr-Little Rock[2]	Little Rock	96%	122
Saint Joseph's Mercy Health Center[2]	Hot Springs	96%	99
Saline Memorial Hospital	Benton	96%	28
UAMS Medical Center[2]	Little Rock	96%	57
Saint Vincent Infirmary Medical Center[2]	Little Rock	95%	43
National Park Medical Center	Hot Springs	91%	55
North Arkansas Regional Medical Center[2]	Harrison	91%	46
Saint Bernards Medical Center	Jonesboro	91%	195
White River Medical Center	Batesville	91%	91

Assessed for Rehabilitation

Hospital Name	City	Rate	Cases
Arkansas Methodist Medical Center	Paragould	100%	38
Medical Center South Arkansas	El Dorado	100%	41
Sparks Regional Medical Center[2]	Fort Smith	100%	107
Baptist Health Med Ctr-Little Rock[2]	Little Rock	99%	161
Jefferson Regional Medical Center	Pine Bluff	99%	144
Saint Bernards Medical Center	Jonesboro	99%	239
Washington Reg Med Ctr at North Hills[2]	Fayetteville	99%	82
White County Medical Center	Searcy	99%	94
UAMS Medical Center[2]	Little Rock	98%	117
Baxter Regional Medical Center[2]	Mountain Home	97%	73
Conway Regional Medical Center	Conway	97%	96
Saline Memorial Hospital	Benton	97%	33
Baptist Health Med Ctr-N Little Rock[2]	North Little Rock	96%	97
NW Arkansas Hospitals	Springdale	96%	103
White River Medical Center	Batesville	95%	82
Mercy Hospital Northwest Arkansas[2]	Rogers	94%	110
Nea Baptist Memorial Hospital[2]	Jonesboro	94%	78
Saint Edward Mercy Medical Center[2]	Fort Smith	94%	77
North Arkansas Regional Medical Center[2]	Harrison	93%	45
National Park Medical Center	Hot Springs	90%	59
Saint Marys Regional Medical Center	Russellville	90%	51
Saint Joseph's Mercy Health Center[2]	Hot Springs	88%	115
Saint Vincent Infirmary Medical Center[2]	Little Rock	80%	85

Discharged on Antithrombotic Therapy

Hospital Name	City	Rate	Cases
Arkansas Methodist Medical Center	Paragould	100%	33
Medical Center South Arkansas	El Dorado	100%	40
NW Arkansas Hospitals	Springdale	100%	90
Saint Edward Mercy Medical Center[2]	Fort Smith	100%	68
Sparks Regional Medical Center[2]	Fort Smith	100%	96
Baptist Health Med Ctr-N Little Rock[2]	North Little Rock	99%	89
Conway Regional Medical Center	Conway	99%	93
Nea Baptist Memorial Hospital[2]	Jonesboro	99%	77
UAMS Medical Center[2]	Little Rock	99%	97
White County Medical Center	Searcy	99%	92
White River Medical Center	Batesville	99%	80
Mercy Hospital Northwest Arkansas[2]	Rogers	98%	106
North Arkansas Regional Medical Center[2]	Harrison	98%	45
Saint Marys Regional Medical Center	Russellville	98%	47
Saint Vincent Infirmary Medical Center[2]	Little Rock	98%	55
Baxter Regional Medical Center[2]	Mountain Home	97%	72
Saint Bernards Medical Center	Jonesboro	97%	203
Saline Memorial Hospital	Benton	97%	31
Washington Reg Med Ctr at North Hills[2]	Fayetteville	97%	63
National Park Medical Center	Hot Springs	96%	57
Jefferson Regional Medical Center	Pine Bluff	94%	126
Saint Joseph's Mercy Health Center[2]	Hot Springs	93%	100
Baptist Health Med Ctr-Little Rock[2]	Little Rock	89%	133

Discharged on Statin Medication

Hospital Name	City	Rate	Cases
Sparks Regional Medical Center[2]	Fort Smith	100%	71
Washington Reg Med Ctr at North Hills[2]	Fayetteville	98%	45
Baptist Health Med Ctr-N Little Rock[2]	North Little Rock	96%	70
Medical Center South Arkansas	El Dorado	96%	25
UAMS Medical Center[2]	Little Rock	95%	75
Saint Bernards Medical Center	Jonesboro	94%	159
Saint Edward Mercy Medical Center[2]	Fort Smith	94%	48
White County Medical Center	Searcy	94%	72
White River Medical Center	Batesville	93%	71
Nea Baptist Memorial Hospital[2]	Jonesboro	92%	59
NW Arkansas Hospitals	Springdale	92%	72
Conway Regional Medical Center	Conway	91%	74
Mercy Hospital Northwest Arkansas[2]	Rogers	91%	90
Saint Marys Regional Medical Center	Russellville	87%	39
Saint Vincent Infirmary Medical Center[2]	Little Rock	87%	45
Jefferson Regional Medical Center	Pine Bluff	85%	94
Baptist Health Med Ctr-Little Rock[2]	Little Rock	81%	98
North Arkansas Regional Medical Center[2]	Harrison	81%	31
National Park Medical Center	Hot Springs	77%	39
Saint Joseph's Mercy Health Center[2]	Hot Springs	76%	93
Baxter Regional Medical Center[2]	Mountain Home	63%	62

Venous Thromboembolism (VTE) Prophylaxis

Hospital Name	City	Rate	Cases
Arkansas Methodist Medical Center	Paragould	100%	42
Sparks Regional Medical Center[2]	Fort Smith	100%	101
Jefferson Regional Medical Center	Pine Bluff	99%	136
Washington Reg Med Ctr at North Hills[2]	Fayetteville	99%	84
White County Medical Center	Searcy	99%	97
North Arkansas Regional Medical Center[2]	Harrison	98%	46
Saint Marys Regional Medical Center	Russellville	98%	48
Saline Memorial Hospital	Benton	97%	36
NW Arkansas Hospitals	Springdale	96%	107
Mercy Hospital Northwest Arkansas[2]	Rogers	94%	97
Saint Bernards Medical Center	Jonesboro	94%	218
Conway Regional Medical Center	Conway	93%	87
Saint Joseph's Mercy Health Center[2]	Hot Springs	93%	123
Saint Edward Mercy Medical Center[2]	Fort Smith	92%	86
UAMS Medical Center[2]	Little Rock	92%	105
National Park Medical Center	Hot Springs	88%	64
Baptist Health Med Ctr-Little Rock[2]	Little Rock	85%	171
Nea Baptist Memorial Hospital[2]	Jonesboro	84%	77
White River Medical Center	Batesville	84%	94
Baxter Regional Medical Center[2]	Mountain Home	81%	64
Medical Center South Arkansas	El Dorado	81%	43
Baptist Health Med Ctr-N Little Rock[2]	North Little Rock	77%	87
Saint Vincent Infirmary Medical Center[2]	Little Rock	77%	93

Written Stroke Educational Materials Given

Hospital Name	City	Rate	Cases
Sparks Regional Medical Center[2]	Fort Smith	100%	57
Conway Regional Medical Center	Conway	98%	55
Jefferson Regional Medical Center	Pine Bluff	97%	70
NW Arkansas Hospitals	Springdale	97%	62
White County Medical Center	Searcy	96%	45
Washington Reg Med Ctr at North Hills[2]	Fayetteville	94%	34
National Park Medical Center	Hot Springs	93%	41
White River Medical Center	Batesville	93%	46
Saint Bernards Medical Center	Jonesboro	92%	119
Baptist Health Med Ctr-N Little Rock[2]	North Little Rock	84%	50
Baxter Regional Medical Center[2]	Mountain Home	84%	38
Baptist Health Med Ctr-Little Rock[2]	Little Rock	82%	66
Saint Edward Mercy Medical Center[2]	Fort Smith	80%	35
UAMS Medical Center[2]	Little Rock	72%	72
Mercy Hospital Northwest Arkansas[2]	Rogers	66%	61
Nea Baptist Memorial Hospital[2]	Jonesboro	62%	42
Saint Joseph's Mercy Health Center[2]	Hot Springs	53%	64
Saint Vincent Infirmary Medical Center[2]	Little Rock	30%	46

Surgical Care Improvement Project

Appropriate Beta Blocker Usage

Hospital Name	City	Rate	Cases
Arkansas Heart Hospital	Little Rock	100%	339
Sparks Regional Medical Center[2]	Fort Smith	100%	189
White County Medical Center[2]	Searcy	100%	131
Baptist Health Med Ctr-N Little Rock[2]	North Little Rock	99%	177
Jefferson Regional Medical Center	Pine Bluff	99%	193
Mercy Hospital Northwest Arkansas[2]	Rogers	99%	153
Saint Edward Mercy Medical Center[2]	Fort Smith	99%	160
White River Medical Center	Batesville	99%	146
Arkansas Surgical Hospital[2]	No Little Rock	98%	119
Baxter Regional Medical Center[2]	Mountain Home	98%	186
Medical Center South Arkansas	El Dorado	98%	132
National Park Medical Center	Hot Springs	98%	119
NW Arkansas Hospitals	Springdale	98%	267
Saint Bernards Medical Center[2]	Jonesboro	98%	280
Saint Joseph's Mercy Health Center[2]	Hot Springs	98%	128
Saline Memorial Hospital	Benton	98%	91
Arkansas Methodist Medical Center	Paragould	97%	31
Conway Regional Medical Center[2]	Conway	97%	107
Nea Baptist Memorial Hospital[2]	Jonesboro	97%	109
UAMS Medical Center[2]	Little Rock	97%	181
VA Central AR Veterans Healthcare Sys[2]	Little Rock	97%	143
Washington Reg Med Ctr at North Hills[2]	Fayetteville	97%	184
Baptist Health Med Ctr-Little Rock[2]	Little Rock	96%	326
Physicians' Specialty Hospital[2]	Fayetteville	96%	25
Saint Vincent Infirmary Medical Center[2]	Little Rock	96%	230
Johnson Regional Medical Center	Clarksville	95%	38
Saint Marys Regional Medical Center	Russellville	95%	58
North Arkansas Regional Medical Center[2]	Harrison	93%	45

Appropriate VTP Within 24 Hours

Hospital Name	City	Rate	Cases
Arkansas Methodist Medical Center	Paragould	100%	101
Baptist Health Med Ctr-N Little Rock[2]	North Little Rock	100%	381
Jefferson Regional Medical Center	Pine Bluff	100%	583
Medical Center South Arkansas	El Dorado	100%	335
Siloam Springs Regional Hospital	Siloam Springs	100%	86
Sparks Regional Medical Center[2]	Fort Smith	100%	260
Stone County Medical Center	Mountain View	100%	68
VA Central AR Veterans Healthcare Sys[2]	Little Rock	100%	301
White County Medical Center[2]	Searcy	100%	282
Arkansas Surgical Hospital[2]	No Little Rock	99%	397
Conway Regional Medical Center[2]	Conway	99%	318
Mercy Hospital Northwest Arkansas[2]	Rogers	99%	321
Saint Edward Mercy Medical Center[2]	Fort Smith	99%	333
Saint Joseph's Mercy Health Center[2]	Hot Springs	99%	343
Saint Marys Regional Medical Center	Russellville	99%	253
Baptist Health Med Ctr-Arkadelphia	Arkadelphia	98%	48
Crittenden Memorial Hospital[2]	West Memphis	98%	101
National Park Medical Center	Hot Springs	98%	321
North Arkansas Regional Medical Center[2]	Harrison	98%	191
NW Arkansas Hospitals	Springdale	98%	433
Physicians' Specialty Hospital[2]	Fayetteville	98%	135
Baptist Health Med Ctr-Little Rock[2]	Little Rock	97%	690
Baxter Regional Medical Center[2]	Mountain Home	97%	273
Saint Vincent Infirmary Medical Center[2]	Little Rock	97%	285
Mena Regional Health System[2]	Mena	96%	28
Ozark Health	Clinton	96%	27
UAMS Medical Center[2]	Little Rock	96%	306
Washington Reg Med Ctr at North Hills[2]	Fayetteville	96%	309
White River Medical Center	Batesville	96%	418
Johnson Regional Medical Center	Clarksville	95%	101
Magnolia Hospital	Magnolia	95%	38
Nea Baptist Memorial Hospital[2]	Jonesboro	95%	296
Saint Bernards Medical Center[2]	Jonesboro	95%	601
Saline Memorial Hospital	Benton	95%	295
Baptist Health Med Ctr-Heber Spings	Heber Springs	94%	54
Ouachita County Medical Center	Camden	94%	49
Summit Medical Center	Van Buren	93%	29
Forrest City Medical Center	Forrest City	91%	35
Saint Vincent Medical Center - North	Sherwood	85%	47

Controlled Postoperative Blood Glucose

Hospital Name	City	Rate	Cases
Arkansas Heart Hospital	Little Rock	100%	685
Jefferson Regional Medical Center	Pine Bluff	100%	63
Mercy Hospital Northwest Arkansas[2]	Rogers	100%	91
National Park Medical Center	Hot Springs	100%	70
NW Arkansas Hospitals	Springdale	100%	216
Saint Edward Mercy Medical Center[2]	Fort Smith	100%	77
Sparks Regional Medical Center[2]	Fort Smith	100%	101
Conway Regional Medical Center[2]	Conway	99%	84
Washington Reg Med Ctr at North Hills[2]	Fayetteville	99%	111
Saint Bernards Medical Center[2]	Jonesboro	98%	178
UAMS Medical Center[2]	Little Rock	98%	128
Baptist Health Med Ctr-Little Rock[2]	Little Rock	97%	240
Baptist Health Med Ctr-N Little Rock[2]	North Little Rock	97%	102

NOTE: Hospital profiles are in alphabetical order by state, then city, then hospital within the city; Rankings exclude hospitals with less than 25 cases except for patient surveys which excludes hospitals with less than 100 cases; (a) 100-299 cases; (1) The number of cases/patients is too few to report; (2) Data submitted were based on a sample of cases/patients; (3) Results are based on a shorter time period than required; (4) Data suppressed by CMS for one or more quarters; (5) Results are not available for this reporting period; (6) Fewer than 100 patients completed the HCAHPS survey; (7) No cases met the criteria for this measure; (8) The lower limit of the confidence interval cannot be calculated if the number of observed infections equals zero; (9) No data are available from the state/territory for this reporting period; (10) The scores shown reflect fewer than 50 completed surveys; (11) There were discrepancies in the data collection process; (12) This measure does not apply to this hospital for this reporting period; (13) Results cannot be calculated for this reporting period; (14) The results for this state are combined with nearby states to protect confidentiality; Please refer to the User's Guide for a full explanation of data.

Baxter Regional Medical Center[2]	Mountain Home	97%	114
Medical Center South Arkansas	El Dorado	97%	65
Nea Baptist Memorial Hospital[2]	Jonesboro	96%	52
Saint Joseph's Mercy Health Center[2]	Hot Springs	96%	74
Saint Vincent Infirmary Medical Center[2]	Little Rock	96%	141

Perioperative Temperature Management

Hospital Name	City	Rate	Cases
Arkansas Heart Hospital	Little Rock	100%	120
Arkansas Methodist Medical Center	Paragould	100%	155
Arkansas Surgical Hospital[2]	No Little Rock	100%	409
Baptist Health Med Ctr-Arkadelphia	Arkadelphia	100%	60
Baptist Health Med Ctr-Heber Spings	Heber Springs	100%	58
Baptist Health Med Ctr-Little Rock[2]	Little Rock	100%	789
Baptist Health Med Ctr-N Little Rock[2]	North Little Rock	100%	449
Baptist Health Medical Center - Stuttgart	Stuttgart	100%	27
Baxter Regional Medical Center[2]	Mountain Home	100%	329
Conway Regional Medical Center[2]	Conway	100%	409
Crittenden Memorial Hospital[2]	West Memphis	100%	120
Forrest City Medical Center	Forrest City	100%	40
Harris Hospital	Newport	100%	42
Jefferson Regional Medical Center	Pine Bluff	100%	681
Johnson Regional Medical Center	Clarksville	100%	119
Magnolia Hospital	Magnolia	100%	42
Medical Center South Arkansas	El Dorado	100%	388
Mena Regional Health System[2]	Mena	100%	38
Mercy Hospital Northwest Arkansas[2]	Rogers	100%	384
National Park Medical Center	Hot Springs	100%	364
North Arkansas Regional Medical Center[2]	Harrison	100%	210
NW Arkansas Hospitals	Springdale	100%	622
Ouachita County Medical Center	Camden	100%	52
Ozark Health	Clinton	100%	28
Saint Bernards Medical Center[2]	Jonesboro	100%	692
Saint Edward Mercy Medical Center[2]	Fort Smith	100%	392
Saint Joseph's Mercy Health Center[2]	Hot Springs	100%	387
Saint Marys Regional Medical Center	Russellville	100%	276
Saint Vincent Medical Center - North	Sherwood	100%	79
Siloam Springs Regional Hospital	Siloam Springs	100%	104
Sparks Regional Medical Center[2]	Fort Smith	100%	371
Stone County Medical Center	Mountain View	100%	73
Summit Medical Center	Van Buren	100%	36
UAMS Medical Center[2]	Little Rock	100%	457
VA Central AR Veterans Healthcare Sys[2]	Little Rock	100%	414
Washington Reg Med Ctr at North Hills[2]	Fayetteville	100%	369
White County Medical Center[2]	Searcy	100%	326
White River Medical Center	Batesville	100%	484
Nea Baptist Memorial Hospital[2]	Jonesboro	99%	368
Physicians' Specialty Hospital[2]	Fayetteville	99%	143
Saint Vincent Infirmary Medical Center[2]	Little Rock	99%	478
Saline Memorial Hospital	Benton	99%	319
Drew Memorial Hospital[2]	Monticello	92%	71

Prophylactic Antibiotic Selection

Hospital Name	City	Rate	Cases
Arkansas Heart Hospital	Little Rock	100%	712
Arkansas Surgical Hospital[2]	No Little Rock	100%	297
Baptist Health Med Ctr-Arkadelphia	Arkadelphia	100%	56
Baptist Health Med Ctr-Heber Spings	Heber Springs	100%	51
Baptist Health Med Ctr-N Little Rock[2]	North Little Rock	100%	397
Harris Hospital	Newport	100%	31
Medical Center South Arkansas	El Dorado	100%	352
Mercy Hospital Northwest Arkansas[2]	Rogers	100%	311
National Park Medical Center	Hot Springs	100%	292
Ouachita County Medical Center	Camden	100%	26
Saint Edward Mercy Medical Center[2]	Fort Smith	100%	323
Saint Vincent Infirmary Medical Center[2]	Little Rock	100%	435
Siloam Springs Regional Hospital	Siloam Springs	100%	63
Sparks Regional Medical Center[2]	Fort Smith	100%	280
Stone County Medical Center	Mountain View	100%	73
White County Medical Center[2]	Searcy	100%	214
Baptist Health Med Ctr-Little Rock[2]	Little Rock	99%	792
Baxter Regional Medical Center[2]	Mountain Home	99%	327
Jefferson Regional Medical Center	Pine Bluff	99%	435
NW Arkansas Hospitals	Springdale	99%	554
Physicians' Specialty Hospital[2]	Fayetteville	99%	105
Saint Bernards Medical Center[2]	Jonesboro	99%	613
Saint Joseph's Mercy Health Center[2]	Hot Springs	99%	318
Saint Marys Regional Medical Center	Russellville	99%	186
UAMS Medical Center[2]	Little Rock	99%	339
VA Central AR Veterans Healthcare Sys	Little Rock	99%	259
Washington Reg Med Ctr at North Hills[2]	Fayetteville	99%	377
White River Medical Center	Batesville	99%	306
Conway Regional Medical Center[2]	Conway	98%	366
North Arkansas Regional Medical Center[2]	Harrison	98%	149
Saline Memorial Hospital	Benton	98%	254
Arkansas Methodist Medical Center	Paragould	97%	70
Nea Baptist Memorial Hospital[2]	Jonesboro	97%	274
Crittenden Memorial Hospital[2]	West Memphis	96%	68
Johnson Regional Medical Center	Clarksville	96%	79
Saint Vincent Medical Center - North	Sherwood	96%	49
Drew Memorial Hospital[2]	Monticello	88%	51

Prophylactic Antibiotic Selection (Outpatient)

Hospital Name	City	Rate	Cases
Arkansas Surgical Hospital	No Little Rock	100%	438
Baptist Health Med Ctr-Arkadelphia	Arkadelphia	100%	63
Ouachita County Medical Center	Camden	100%	26
Sparks Regional Medical Center	Fort Smith	100%	484
Baptist Health Med Ctr-N Little Rock	North Little Rock	99%	547
Jefferson Regional Medical Center	Pine Bluff	99%	423
Medical Center South Arkansas	El Dorado	99%	95
National Park Medical Center	Hot Springs	99%	109
Physicians' Specialty Hospital	Fayetteville	99%	79
Saint Edward Mercy Medical Center	Fort Smith	99%	337
Saint Marys Regional Medical Center	Russellville	99%	74
Saint Vincent Infirmary Medical Center	Little Rock	99%	628
Siloam Springs Regional Hospital	Siloam Springs	99%	74
Baptist Health Med Ctr-Little Rock	Little Rock	98%	1114
Forrest City Medical Center	Forrest City	98%	50
North Arkansas Regional Medical Center	Harrison	98%	172
NW Arkansas Hospitals	Springdale	98%	845
Saint Bernards Medical Center	Jonesboro	98%	776
Saint Joseph's Mercy Health Center	Hot Springs	98%	437
Washington Reg Med Ctr at North Hills	Fayetteville	98%	516
White County Medical Center	Searcy	98%	381
Arkansas Methodist Medical Center	Paragould	97%	75
Johnson Regional Medical Center	Clarksville	97%	60
Mercy Hospital Northwest Arkansas	Rogers	97%	420
Saline Memorial Hospital	Benton	97%	149
Baxter Regional Medical Center	Mountain Home	96%	178
Conway Regional Medical Center	Conway	96%	307
Nea Baptist Memorial Hospital	Jonesboro	96%	414
White River Medical Center	Batesville	96%	166
Crittenden Memorial Hospital	West Memphis	95%	60
UAMS Medical Center	Little Rock	95%	368
Arkansas Heart Hospital	Little Rock	94%	449
Baptist Health Med Ctr-Heber Spings	Heber Springs	94%	32
Saint Vincent Medical Center - North	Sherwood	87%	38

Prophylactic Antibiotic Stopped

Hospital Name	City	Rate	Cases
Arkansas Heart Hospital	Little Rock	100%	706
Arkansas Methodist Medical Center	Paragould	100%	67
Arkansas Surgical Hospital[2]	No Little Rock	100%	295
Jefferson Regional Medical Center	Pine Bluff	100%	417
Medical Center South Arkansas	El Dorado	100%	337
Mercy Hospital Northwest Arkansas[2]	Rogers	100%	299
Ouachita County Medical Center	Camden	100%	26
Saint Marys Regional Medical Center	Russellville	100%	179
Sparks Regional Medical Center[2]	Fort Smith	100%	265
White County Medical Center[2]	Searcy	100%	208
Baptist Health Med Ctr-Little Rock[2]	Little Rock	99%	785
Baptist Health Med Ctr-N Little Rock[2]	North Little Rock	99%	393
National Park Medical Center	Hot Springs	99%	273
Saline Memorial Hospital	Benton	99%	252
Stone County Medical Center	Mountain View	99%	73
Washington Reg Med Ctr at North Hills[2]	Fayetteville	99%	371
Baptist Health Med Ctr-Heber Spings	Heber Springs	98%	50
Drew Memorial Hospital[2]	Monticello	98%	51
NW Arkansas Hospitals	Springdale	98%	539
Saint Bernards Medical Center[2]	Jonesboro	98%	584
Saint Joseph's Mercy Health Center[2]	Hot Springs	98%	298
Saint Vincent Medical Center - North	Sherwood	98%	48
Baxter Regional Medical Center[2]	Mountain Home	97%	306
Nea Baptist Memorial Hospital[2]	Jonesboro	97%	254
Saint Edward Mercy Medical Center[2]	Fort Smith	97%	314
Siloam Springs Regional Hospital	Siloam Springs	97%	59
Conway Regional Medical Center[2]	Conway	96%	356
VA Central AR Veterans Healthcare Sys	Little Rock	96%	246
White River Medical Center	Batesville	96%	302
Saint Vincent Infirmary Medical Center[2]	Little Rock	95%	427
Crittenden Memorial Hospital[2]	West Memphis	94%	67
Harris Hospital	Newport	93%	30
UAMS Medical Center[2]	Little Rock	93%	326
North Arkansas Regional Medical Center[2]	Harrison	92%	144
Johnson Regional Medical Center	Clarksville	91%	77
Physicians' Specialty Hospital[2]	Fayetteville	91%	102
Baptist Health Med Ctr-Arkadelphia	Arkadelphia	89%	55

Prophylactic Antibiotic Timing

Hospital Name	City	Rate	Cases
Arkansas Heart Hospital	Little Rock	100%	712
Arkansas Methodist Medical Center	Paragould	100%	70
Baptist Health Med Ctr-Arkadelphia	Arkadelphia	100%	56
Harris Hospital	Newport	100%	31
Jefferson Regional Medical Center	Pine Bluff	100%	440
Medical Center South Arkansas	El Dorado	100%	352
National Park Medical Center	Hot Springs	100%	292
Saint Edward Mercy Medical Center[2]	Fort Smith	100%	323
Saint Vincent Infirmary Medical Center[2]	Little Rock	100%	435
Siloam Springs Regional Hospital	Siloam Springs	100%	63
Sparks Regional Medical Center[2]	Fort Smith	100%	281
White River Medical Center	Batesville	100%	307
Arkansas Surgical Hospital[2]	No Little Rock	99%	297
Baptist Health Med Ctr-Little Rock[2]	Little Rock	99%	792
Baxter Regional Medical Center[2]	Mountain Home	99%	328
Conway Regional Medical Center[2]	Conway	99%	366
NW Arkansas Hospitals	Springdale	99%	557
Saint Joseph's Mercy Health Center[2]	Hot Springs	99%	318
Saint Marys Regional Medical Center	Russellville	99%	186
Stone County Medical Center	Mountain View	99%	73
VA Central AR Veterans Healthcare Sys	Little Rock	99%	259
White County Medical Center[2]	Searcy	99%	214
Baptist Health Med Ctr-Heber Spings	Heber Springs	98%	51
Baptist Health Med Ctr-N Little Rock[2]	North Little Rock	98%	397
Mercy Hospital Northwest Arkansas[2]	Rogers	98%	311
Nea Baptist Memorial Hospital[2]	Jonesboro	98%	274
Saint Bernards Medical Center[2]	Jonesboro	98%	614
Saline Memorial Hospital	Benton	98%	255
Johnson Regional Medical Center	Clarksville	97%	79
North Arkansas Regional Medical Center[2]	Harrison	97%	149
Physicians' Specialty Hospital[2]	Fayetteville	97%	105
UAMS Medical Center[2]	Little Rock	97%	341
Washington Reg Med Ctr at North Hills[2]	Fayetteville	97%	381
Ouachita County Medical Center	Camden	96%	26
Saint Vincent Medical Center - North	Sherwood	96%	49
Crittenden Memorial Hospital[2]	West Memphis	94%	68
Drew Memorial Hospital[2]	Monticello	65%	66

Prophylactic Antibiotic Timing (Outpatient)

Hospital Name	City	Rate	Cases
Arkansas Heart Hospital	Little Rock	100%	450
Arkansas Surgical Hospital	No Little Rock	100%	439
Baptist Health Med Ctr-N Little Rock	North Little Rock	100%	547
Forrest City Medical Center	Forrest City	100%	50
Jefferson Regional Medical Center	Pine Bluff	100%	423
Ouachita County Medical Center	Camden	100%	26
Physicians' Specialty Hospital	Fayetteville	100%	79
Saline Memorial Hospital	Benton	100%	149
Sparks Regional Medical Center	Fort Smith	100%	484
White County Medical Center	Searcy	100%	376
Mercy Hospital Northwest Arkansas	Rogers	99%	421
NW Arkansas Hospitals	Springdale	99%	847
Saint Bernards Medical Center	Jonesboro	99%	765
Saint Joseph's Mercy Health Center	Hot Springs	99%	439
Saint Vincent Infirmary Medical Center	Little Rock	99%	628
Siloam Springs Regional Hospital	Siloam Springs	99%	74
Baptist Health Med Ctr-Little Rock	Little Rock	98%	1124
Conway Regional Medical Center	Conway	98%	312
Medical Center South Arkansas	El Dorado	98%	96
National Park Medical Center	Hot Springs	98%	111
Nea Baptist Memorial Hospital	Jonesboro	98%	416
Baxter Regional Medical Center	Mountain Home	97%	179
Johnson Regional Medical Center	Clarksville	97%	58
Saint Vincent Medical Center - North	Sherwood	97%	38
Washington Reg Med Ctr at North Hills	Fayetteville	97%	498
Arkansas Methodist Medical Center	Paragould	96%	76
UAMS Medical Center	Little Rock	96%	357
White River Medical Center	Batesville	96%	169
Saint Marys Regional Medical Center	Russellville	95%	76
North Arkansas Regional Medical Center	Harrison	94%	132
Baptist Health Med Ctr-Arkadelphia	Arkadelphia	93%	67
Crittenden Memorial Hospital	West Memphis	93%	61
Saint Edward Mercy Medical Center	Fort Smith	92%	343
Great River Medical Center	Blytheville	77%	26

Urinary Catheter Removal

Hospital Name	City	Rate	Cases
Arkansas Heart Hospital	Little Rock	100%	644
Arkansas Methodist Medical Center	Paragould	100%	53
Baptist Health Med Ctr-N Little Rock[2]	North Little Rock	100%	179
Jefferson Regional Medical Center	Pine Bluff	100%	230
Sparks Regional Medical Center[2]	Fort Smith	100%	200
White County Medical Center[2]	Searcy	100%	225
Arkansas Surgical Hospital[2]	No Little Rock	99%	346
Medical Center South Arkansas	El Dorado	99%	147
NW Arkansas Hospitals	Springdale	99%	373
Saint Marys Regional Medical Center	Russellville	99%	144
Saline Memorial Hospital	Benton	99%	189
White River Medical Center	Batesville	99%	197
Johnson Regional Medical Center	Clarksville	98%	88
Mercy Hospital Northwest Arkansas[2]	Rogers	98%	320
Saint Edward Mercy Medical Center[2]	Fort Smith	98%	248
Saint Joseph's Mercy Health Center[2]	Hot Springs	98%	154
Saint Vincent Infirmary Medical Center[2]	Little Rock	98%	315
Siloam Springs Regional Hospital	Siloam Springs	98%	48
VA Central AR Veterans Healthcare Sys[2]	Little Rock	98%	264
National Park Medical Center	Hot Springs	97%	302
Stone County Medical Center	Mountain View	97%	71
Baptist Health Med Ctr-Little Rock[2]	Little Rock	96%	335

NOTE: Hospital profiles are in alphabetical order by state, then city, then hospital within the city; Rankings exclude hospitals with less than 25 cases except for patient surveys which excludes hospitals with less than 100 cases; (a) 100-299 cases; (1) The number of cases/patients is too few to report; (2) Data submitted were based on a sample of cases/patients; (3) Results are based on a shorter time period than required; (4) Data suppressed by CMS for one or more quarters; (5) Results are not available for this reporting period; (6) Fewer than 100 patients completed the HCAHPS survey; (7) No cases met the criteria for this measure; (8) The lower limit of the confidence interval cannot be calculated if the number of observed infections equals zero; (9) No data are available from the state/territory for this reporting period; (10) The scores shown reflect fewer than 50 completed surveys; (11) There were discrepancies in the data collection process; (12) This measure does not apply to this hospital for this reporting period; (13) Results cannot be calculated for this reporting period; (14) The results for this state are combined with nearby states to protect confidentiality; Please refer to the User's Guide for a full explanation of data.

Nea Baptist Memorial Hospital[2]	Jonesboro	96%	264
Saint Bernards Medical Center[2]	Jonesboro	96%	504
Baxter Regional Medical Center[2]	Mountain Home	95%	288
Conway Regional Medical Center[2]	Conway	94%	184
Washington Reg Med Ctr at North Hills[2]	Fayetteville	94%	196
North Arkansas Regional Medical Center[2]	Harrison	93%	83
UAMS Medical Center[2]	Little Rock	89%	331
Crittenden Memorial Hospital[2]	West Memphis	84%	68
Saint Vincent Medical Center - North	Sherwood	84%	38

Survey of Patients' Hospital Experiences

Area Around Room 'Always' Quiet at Night

Hospital Name	City	Rate	Cases
Arkansas Surgical Hospital	No Little Rock	91%	300+
Physicians' Specialty Hospital	Fayetteville	88%	(a)
Baptist Health Med Ctr-Heber Spings	Heber Springs	79%	(a)
Arkansas Heart Hospital	Little Rock	74%	300+
Chambers Memorial Hospital	Danville	74%	(a)
Magnolia Hospital	Magnolia	72%	(a)
Saint Vincent Medical Center - North	Sherwood	72%	300+
Ashley County Medical Center	Crossett	71%	(a)
Baptist Health Med Ctr-Arkadelphia	Arkadelphia	70%	(a)
Crittenden Memorial Hospital	West Memphis	70%	300+
Forrest City Medical Center	Forrest City	70%	300+
Wadley Regional Medical Center at Hope	Hope	70%	(a)
Conway Regional Medical Center	Conway	69%	300+
Nea Baptist Memorial Hospital	Jonesboro	69%	300+
Ouachita County Medical Center	Camden	69%	300+
Arkansas Methodist Medical Center	Paragould	68%	300+
Baptist Health Med Ctr-Little Rock[11]	Little Rock	68%	300+
Baptist Health Medical Center - Stuttgart	Stuttgart	68%	(a)
Helena Regional Medical Center	Helena	68%	300+
Medical Center South Arkansas	El Dorado	68%	300+
Saint Bernards Medical Center	Jonesboro	68%	300+
Washington Reg Med Ctr at North Hills	Fayetteville	68%	300+
White County Medical Center	Searcy	68%	300+
Saint Vincent Infirmary Medical Center	Little Rock	67%	300+
White River Medical Center	Batesville	67%	300+
North Metro Medical Center[3,11]	Jacksonville	66%	(a)
Saint Vincent Morrilton	Morrilton	66%	(a)
Summit Medical Center	Van Buren	66%	(a)
Baptist Health Med Ctr-Hot Springs Co	Malvern	65%	(a)
Jefferson Regional Medical Center	Pine Bluff	65%	300+
North Arkansas Regional Medical Center	Harrison	65%	300+
UAMS Medical Center	Little Rock	65%	300+
Harris Hospital	Newport	64%	300+
Mena Regional Health System	Mena	64%	(a)
Saline Memorial Hospital	Benton	64%	300+
Five Rivers Medical Center	Pocahontas	63%	(a)
National Park Medical Center	Hot Springs	63%	300+
Baptist Health Med Ctr-N Little Rock	North Little Rock	62%	300+
Siloam Springs Regional Hospital	Siloam Springs	62%	300+
Baxter Regional Medical Center	Mountain Home	61%	300+
Drew Memorial Hospital	Monticello	61%	300+
Great River Medical Center	Blytheville	61%	(a)
NW Arkansas Hospitals	Springdale	61%	300+
Mercy Hospital Northwest Arkansas[11]	Rogers	60%	300+
Johnson Regional Medical Center	Clarksville	59%	300+
Saint Edward Mercy Medical Center[11]	Fort Smith	58%	300+
Saint Joseph's Mercy Health Center[11]	Hot Springs	57%	300+
Sparks Regional Medical Center	Fort Smith	52%	300+
Saint Marys Regional Medical Center	Russellville	51%	300+

Doctors 'Always' Communicated Well

Hospital Name	City	Rate	Cases
Drew Memorial Hospital	Monticello	91%	300+
Physicians' Specialty Hospital	Fayetteville	91%	(a)
Baptist Health Med Ctr-Arkadelphia	Arkadelphia	90%	(a)
Chambers Memorial Hospital	Danville	90%	(a)
Arkansas Surgical Hospital	No Little Rock	89%	300+
Baptist Health Med Ctr-Hot Springs Co	Malvern	88%	(a)
Baptist Health Medical Center - Stuttgart	Stuttgart	88%	(a)
Magnolia Hospital	Magnolia	87%	(a)
Ouachita County Medical Center	Camden	87%	300+
Wadley Regional Medical Center at Hope	Hope	87%	(a)
Baptist Health Med Ctr-Heber Spings	Heber Springs	86%	(a)
Nea Baptist Memorial Hospital	Jonesboro	86%	300+
Arkansas Heart Hospital	Little Rock	85%	300+
Helena Regional Medical Center	Helena	85%	300+
Forrest City Medical Center	Forrest City	84%	300+
Saint Bernards Medical Center	Jonesboro	84%	300+
Saint Vincent Infirmary Medical Center	Little Rock	84%	300+
Saint Vincent Medical Center - North	Sherwood	84%	300+
Saint Vincent Morrilton	Morrilton	84%	(a)
Arkansas Methodist Medical Center	Paragould	83%	300+
Conway Regional Medical Center	Conway	83%	300+
Crittenden Memorial Hospital	West Memphis	83%	300+
Five Rivers Medical Center	Pocahontas	83%	(a)
Saint Edward Mercy Medical Center[11]	Fort Smith	83%	300+
Siloam Springs Regional Hospital	Siloam Springs	83%	300+
White County Medical Center	Searcy	83%	300+
White River Medical Center	Batesville	83%	300+
Jefferson Regional Medical Center	Pine Bluff	82%	300+
Mena Regional Health System	Mena	82%	(a)
Mercy Hospital Northwest Arkansas[11]	Rogers	82%	300+
North Arkansas Regional Medical Center	Harrison	82%	300+
Washington Reg Med Ctr at North Hills	Fayetteville	82%	300+
Baptist Health Med Ctr-Little Rock[11]	Little Rock	81%	300+
Baptist Health Med Ctr-N Little Rock	North Little Rock	81%	300+
Harris Hospital	Newport	81%	300+
Johnson Regional Medical Center	Clarksville	81%	300+
Medical Center South Arkansas	El Dorado	81%	300+
National Park Medical Center	Hot Springs	81%	300+
Summit Medical Center	Van Buren	81%	(a)
Ashley County Medical Center	Crossett	80%	(a)
Baxter Regional Medical Center	Mountain Home	80%	300+
Saint Joseph's Mercy Health Center[11]	Hot Springs	80%	300+
Saline Memorial Hospital	Benton	80%	300+
Saint Marys Regional Medical Center	Russellville	79%	300+
UAMS Medical Center	Little Rock	78%	300+
Great River Medical Center	Blytheville	77%	(a)
North Metro Medical Center[3,11]	Jacksonville	77%	(a)
NW Arkansas Hospitals	Springdale	77%	300+
Sparks Regional Medical Center	Fort Smith	75%	300+

Home Recovery Information Given

Hospital Name	City	Rate	Cases
Physicians' Specialty Hospital	Fayetteville	90%	(a)
Arkansas Surgical Hospital	No Little Rock	89%	300+
Magnolia Hospital	Magnolia	89%	(a)
Siloam Springs Regional Hospital	Siloam Springs	89%	300+
Mercy Hospital Northwest Arkansas[11]	Rogers	88%	300+
Baptist Health Med Ctr-Heber Spings	Heber Springs	87%	(a)
Baxter Regional Medical Center	Mountain Home	87%	300+
Saint Edward Mercy Medical Center[11]	Fort Smith	87%	300+
Washington Reg Med Ctr at North Hills	Fayetteville	87%	300+
Nea Baptist Memorial Hospital	Jonesboro	86%	300+
NW Arkansas Hospitals	Springdale	86%	300+
Arkansas Heart Hospital	Little Rock	85%	300+
Five Rivers Medical Center	Pocahontas	85%	(a)
Harris Hospital	Newport	85%	300+
Jefferson Regional Medical Center	Pine Bluff	85%	300+
Mena Regional Health System	Mena	85%	(a)
Saint Vincent Infirmary Medical Center	Little Rock	85%	300+
White River Medical Center	Batesville	85%	300+
Baptist Health Med Ctr-N Little Rock	North Little Rock	84%	300+
National Park Medical Center	Hot Springs	84%	300+
Saint Vincent Medical Center - North	Sherwood	84%	300+
Saint Vincent Morrilton	Morrilton	84%	(a)
Summit Medical Center	Van Buren	84%	(a)
Wadley Regional Medical Center at Hope	Hope	84%	(a)
Crittenden Memorial Hospital	West Memphis	83%	300+
Saint Bernards Medical Center	Jonesboro	83%	300+
Saint Joseph's Mercy Health Center[11]	Hot Springs	83%	300+
Saline Memorial Hospital	Benton	83%	300+
UAMS Medical Center	Little Rock	83%	300+
Baptist Health Medical Center - Stuttgart	Stuttgart	82%	(a)
Forrest City Medical Center	Forrest City	82%	300+
Saint Marys Regional Medical Center	Russellville	82%	300+
White County Medical Center	Searcy	82%	300+
Baptist Health Med Ctr-Arkadelphia	Arkadelphia	81%	(a)
Baptist Health Med Ctr-Little Rock[11]	Little Rock	81%	300+
Conway Regional Medical Center	Conway	81%	300+
Helena Regional Medical Center	Helena	81%	300+
Medical Center South Arkansas	El Dorado	81%	300+
North Metro Medical Center[3,11]	Jacksonville	81%	(a)
Ouachita County Medical Center	Camden	81%	300+
Arkansas Methodist Medical Center	Paragould	80%	300+
Ashley County Medical Center	Crossett	80%	(a)
Chambers Memorial Hospital	Danville	80%	(a)
Johnson Regional Medical Center	Clarksville	80%	300+
Sparks Regional Medical Center	Fort Smith	80%	300+
North Arkansas Regional Medical Center	Harrison	79%	300+
Baptist Health Med Ctr-Hot Springs Co	Malvern	77%	(a)
Drew Memorial Hospital	Monticello	77%	300+
Great River Medical Center	Blytheville	77%	(a)

Hospital Given 9 or 10 on 10 Point Scale

Hospital Name	City	Rate	Cases
Arkansas Heart Hospital	Little Rock	90%	300+
Arkansas Surgical Hospital	No Little Rock	90%	300+
Physicians' Specialty Hospital	Fayetteville	88%	(a)
Nea Baptist Memorial Hospital	Jonesboro	81%	300+
Baptist Health Med Ctr-Heber Spings	Heber Springs	80%	(a)
Chambers Memorial Hospital	Danville	77%	(a)
Baxter Regional Medical Center	Mountain Home	76%	300+
Baptist Health Med Ctr-N Little Rock	North Little Rock	75%	300+
Mercy Hospital Northwest Arkansas[11]	Rogers	75%	300+
Saint Bernards Medical Center	Jonesboro	75%	300+
UAMS Medical Center	Little Rock	75%	300+
Washington Reg Med Ctr at North Hills	Fayetteville	75%	300+
Baptist Health Med Ctr-Little Rock[11]	Little Rock	74%	300+
Baptist Health Med Ctr-Arkadelphia	Arkadelphia	73%	(a)
Saint Joseph's Mercy Health Center[11]	Hot Springs	73%	300+
Saint Vincent Morrilton	Morrilton	73%	(a)
Conway Regional Medical Center	Conway	72%	300+
National Park Medical Center	Hot Springs	72%	300+
Saint Edward Mercy Medical Center[11]	Fort Smith	72%	300+
White County Medical Center	Searcy	72%	300+
White River Medical Center	Batesville	72%	300+
Saint Vincent Infirmary Medical Center	Little Rock	71%	300+
Saint Vincent Medical Center - North	Sherwood	71%	300+
Saline Memorial Hospital	Benton	71%	300+
Magnolia Hospital	Magnolia	69%	(a)
Ouachita County Medical Center	Camden	69%	300+
Siloam Springs Regional Hospital	Siloam Springs	69%	300+
Wadley Regional Medical Center at Hope	Hope	69%	(a)
Arkansas Methodist Medical Center	Paragould	67%	300+
Mena Regional Health System	Mena	67%	(a)
NW Arkansas Hospitals	Springdale	67%	300+
Baptist Health Med Ctr-Hot Springs Co	Malvern	66%	(a)
Forrest City Medical Center	Forrest City	66%	300+
Helena Regional Medical Center	Helena	66%	300+
Medical Center South Arkansas	El Dorado	66%	300+
Ashley County Medical Center	Crossett	65%	(a)
Crittenden Memorial Hospital	West Memphis	65%	300+
Jefferson Regional Medical Center	Pine Bluff	65%	300+
North Arkansas Regional Medical Center	Harrison	65%	300+
Baptist Health Medical Center - Stuttgart	Stuttgart	64%	(a)
Drew Memorial Hospital	Monticello	64%	300+
Summit Medical Center	Van Buren	64%	(a)
Five Rivers Medical Center	Pocahontas	62%	(a)
Harris Hospital	Newport	61%	300+
North Metro Medical Center[3,11]	Jacksonville	60%	(a)
Johnson Regional Medical Center	Clarksville	59%	300+
Saint Marys Regional Medical Center	Russellville	58%	300+
Sparks Regional Medical Center	Fort Smith	56%	300+
Great River Medical Center	Blytheville	51%	(a)

Meds 'Always' Explained Before Given

Hospital Name	City	Rate	Cases
Physicians' Specialty Hospital	Fayetteville	78%	(a)
Arkansas Surgical Hospital	No Little Rock	77%	300+
Chambers Memorial Hospital	Danville	73%	(a)
Nea Baptist Memorial Hospital	Jonesboro	70%	300+
Baptist Health Med Ctr-Arkadelphia	Arkadelphia	69%	(a)
Baptist Health Med Ctr-Heber Spings	Heber Springs	69%	(a)
Baptist Health Medical Center - Stuttgart	Stuttgart	69%	(a)
Summit Medical Center	Van Buren	68%	(a)
Arkansas Heart Hospital	Little Rock	67%	300+
Harris Hospital	Newport	67%	300+
Washington Reg Med Ctr at North Hills	Fayetteville	67%	300+
Helena Regional Medical Center	Helena	65%	300+
Magnolia Hospital	Magnolia	65%	(a)
Saint Bernards Medical Center	Jonesboro	65%	300+
White County Medical Center	Searcy	65%	300+
White River Medical Center	Batesville	65%	300+
Arkansas Methodist Medical Center	Paragould	64%	300+
Conway Regional Medical Center	Conway	64%	300+
Crittenden Memorial Hospital	West Memphis	64%	300+
Saint Edward Mercy Medical Center[11]	Fort Smith	64%	300+
Saint Vincent Infirmary Medical Center	Little Rock	64%	300+
Saint Vincent Medical Center - North	Sherwood	64%	300+
Ouachita County Medical Center	Camden	63%	300+
Saint Vincent Morrilton	Morrilton	63%	(a)
Saline Memorial Hospital	Benton	63%	300+
Siloam Springs Regional Hospital	Siloam Springs	63%	300+
Baptist Health Med Ctr-N Little Rock	North Little Rock	62%	300+
Baxter Regional Medical Center	Mountain Home	62%	300+
Johnson Regional Medical Center	Clarksville	62%	300+
Wadley Regional Medical Center at Hope	Hope	62%	(a)
Baptist Health Med Ctr-Little Rock[11]	Little Rock	61%	300+
Jefferson Regional Medical Center	Pine Bluff	61%	300+
Medical Center South Arkansas	El Dorado	61%	300+
UAMS Medical Center	Little Rock	61%	300+
Forrest City Medical Center	Forrest City	60%	300+
Mercy Hospital Northwest Arkansas[11]	Rogers	60%	300+
North Arkansas Regional Medical Center	Harrison	60%	300+
Saint Joseph's Mercy Health Center[11]	Hot Springs	60%	300+
Baptist Health Med Ctr-Hot Springs Co	Malvern	59%	(a)
Drew Memorial Hospital	Monticello	59%	300+
NW Arkansas Hospitals	Springdale	59%	300+
Five Rivers Medical Center	Pocahontas	58%	(a)
Mena Regional Health System	Mena	58%	(a)
National Park Medical Center	Hot Springs	58%	300+
Ashley County Medical Center	Crossett	56%	(a)
Great River Medical Center	Blytheville	56%	(a)
North Metro Medical Center[3,11]	Jacksonville	56%	(a)
Saint Marys Regional Medical Center	Russellville	54%	300+
Sparks Regional Medical Center	Fort Smith	49%	300+

NOTE: Hospital profiles are in alphabetical order by state, then city, then hospital within the city; Rankings exclude hospitals with less than 25 cases except for patient surveys which excludes hospitals with less than 100 cases; (a) 100-299 cases; (1) The number of cases/patients is too few to report; (2) Data submitted were based on a sample of cases/patients; (3) Results are based on a shorter time period than required; (4) Data suppressed by CMS for one or more quarters; (5) Results are not available for this reporting period; (6) Fewer than 100 patients completed the HCAHPS survey; (7) No cases met the criteria for this measure; (8) The lower limit of the confidence interval cannot be calculated if the number of observed infections equals zero; (9) No data are available from the state/territory for this reporting period; (10) The scores shown reflect fewer than 50 completed surveys; (11) There were discrepancies in the data collection process; (12) This measure does not apply to this hospital for this reporting period; (13) Results cannot be calculated for this reporting period; (14) The results for this state are combined with nearby states to protect confidentiality; Please refer to the User's Guide for a full explanation of data.

Nurses 'Always' Communicated Well

Hospital Name	City	Rate	Cases
Arkansas Surgical Hospital	No Little Rock	89%	300+
Physicians' Specialty Hospital	Fayetteville	89%	(a)
Arkansas Heart Hospital	Little Rock	87%	300+
Baptist Health Med Ctr-Heber Spings	Heber Springs	87%	(a)
Chambers Memorial Hospital	Danville	85%	(a)
Ouachita County Medical Center	Camden	85%	300+
Nea Baptist Memorial Hospital	Jonesboro	84%	300+
Magnolia Hospital	Magnolia	83%	(a)
Baptist Health Med Ctr-Arkadelphia	Arkadelphia	82%	(a)
Saint Vincent Morrilton	Morrilton	82%	(a)
Wadley Regional Medical Center at Hope	Hope	82%	(a)
Conway Regional Medical Center	Conway	81%	300+
Saint Bernards Medical Center	Jonesboro	81%	300+
Summit Medical Center	Van Buren	81%	(a)
Washington Reg Med Ctr at North Hills	Fayetteville	81%	300+
White River Medical Center	Batesville	81%	300+
Arkansas Methodist Medical Center	Paragould	80%	300+
Saline Memorial Hospital	Benton	80%	300+
Baptist Health Med Ctr-Little Rock[11]	Little Rock	79%	300+
Baptist Health Med Ctr-N Little Rock	North Little Rock	79%	300+
Baxter Regional Medical Center	Mountain Home	79%	300+
Forrest City Medical Center	Forrest City	79%	300+
Helena Regional Medical Center	Helena	79%	300+
Saint Vincent Medical Center - North	Sherwood	79%	300+
Ashley County Medical Center	Crossett	78%	(a)
Baptist Health Medical Center - Stuttgart	Stuttgart	78%	(a)
Crittenden Memorial Hospital	West Memphis	78%	300+
Mercy Hospital Northwest Arkansas[11]	Rogers	78%	300+
White County Medical Center	Searcy	78%	300+
Baptist Health Med Ctr-Hot Springs Co	Malvern	77%	(a)
Mena Regional Health System	Mena	77%	(a)
North Arkansas Regional Medical Center	Harrison	77%	300+
Saint Edward Mercy Medical Center[11]	Fort Smith	77%	300+
Saint Joseph's Mercy Health Center[11]	Hot Springs	77%	300+
Drew Memorial Hospital	Monticello	76%	300+
Saint Vincent Infirmary Medical Center	Little Rock	76%	300+
Siloam Springs Regional Hospital	Siloam Springs	76%	300+
UAMS Medical Center	Little Rock	76%	300+
Five Rivers Medical Center	Pocahontas	75%	(a)
Great River Medical Center	Blytheville	75%	(a)
Harris Hospital	Newport	75%	300+
Jefferson Regional Medical Center	Pine Bluff	75%	300+
Medical Center South Arkansas	El Dorado	75%	300+
National Park Medical Center	Hot Springs	74%	300+
NW Arkansas Hospitals	Springdale	74%	300+
Johnson Regional Medical Center	Clarksville	73%	300+
North Metro Medical Center[3,11]	Jacksonville	71%	(a)
Saint Marys Regional Medical Center	Russellville	71%	300+
Sparks Regional Medical Center	Fort Smith	67%	300+

Pain 'Always' Well Controlled

Hospital Name	City	Rate	Cases
Physicians' Specialty Hospital	Fayetteville	83%	(a)
Arkansas Surgical Hospital	No Little Rock	80%	300+
Chambers Memorial Hospital	Danville	76%	(a)
Nea Baptist Memorial Hospital	Jonesboro	76%	300+
Arkansas Heart Hospital	Little Rock	75%	300+
Baptist Health Med Ctr-Heber Spings	Heber Springs	75%	(a)
Baxter Regional Medical Center	Mountain Home	74%	300+
Five Rivers Medical Center	Pocahontas	74%	(a)
Wadley Regional Medical Center at Hope	Hope	74%	(a)
Washington Reg Med Ctr at North Hills	Fayetteville	74%	300+
Forrest City Medical Center	Forrest City	73%	300+
Ouachita County Medical Center	Camden	73%	300+
Arkansas Methodist Medical Center	Paragould	72%	300+
Baptist Health Med Ctr-Little Rock[11]	Little Rock	72%	300+
Magnolia Hospital	Magnolia	72%	(a)
Saint Bernards Medical Center	Jonesboro	72%	300+
Saline Memorial Hospital	Benton	72%	300+
Summit Medical Center	Van Buren	72%	(a)
White County Medical Center	Searcy	72%	300+
Baptist Health Med Ctr-N Little Rock	North Little Rock	71%	300+
Mercy Hospital Northwest Arkansas[11]	Rogers	71%	300+
Saint Vincent Medical Center - North	Sherwood	71%	300+
Siloam Springs Regional Hospital	Siloam Springs	71%	300+
White River Medical Center	Batesville	71%	300+
Helena Regional Medical Center	Helena	70%	300+
Saint Joseph's Mercy Health Center[11]	Hot Springs	70%	300+
Baptist Health Medical Center - Stuttgart	Stuttgart	69%	(a)
Conway Regional Medical Center	Conway	69%	300+
Crittenden Memorial Hospital	West Memphis	69%	300+
Drew Memorial Hospital	Monticello	69%	300+
Jefferson Regional Medical Center	Pine Bluff	69%	300+
Medical Center South Arkansas	El Dorado	69%	300+
Saint Edward Mercy Medical Center[11]	Fort Smith	69%	300+
Saint Vincent Infirmary Medical Center	Little Rock	69%	300+
UAMS Medical Center	Little Rock	69%	300+
Great River Medical Center	Blytheville	68%	(a)
Harris Hospital	Newport	68%	300+
Johnson Regional Medical Center	Clarksville	68%	300+
National Park Medical Center	Hot Springs	68%	300+
North Arkansas Regional Medical Center	Harrison	68%	300+
Saint Vincent Morrilton	Morrilton	68%	(a)
Ashley County Medical Center	Crossett	67%	(a)
Baptist Health Med Ctr-Arkadelphia	Arkadelphia	67%	(a)
Baptist Health Med Ctr-Hot Springs Co	Malvern	67%	(a)
NW Arkansas Hospitals	Springdale	67%	300+
North Metro Medical Center[3,11]	Jacksonville	66%	(a)
Mena Regional Health System	Mena	65%	(a)
Saint Marys Regional Medical Center	Russellville	65%	300+
Sparks Regional Medical Center	Fort Smith	60%	300+

Room and Bathroom 'Always' Clean

Hospital Name	City	Rate	Cases
Chambers Memorial Hospital	Danville	88%	(a)
Arkansas Heart Hospital	Little Rock	87%	300+
Physicians' Specialty Hospital	Fayetteville	84%	(a)
Arkansas Surgical Hospital	No Little Rock	82%	300+
Baptist Health Med Ctr-Heber Spings	Heber Springs	81%	(a)
Ouachita County Medical Center	Camden	80%	300+
Saint Vincent Morrilton	Morrilton	80%	(a)
Johnson Regional Medical Center	Clarksville	79%	300+
North Arkansas Regional Medical Center	Harrison	79%	300+
Ashley County Medical Center	Crossett	77%	(a)
Baptist Health Med Ctr-Arkadelphia	Arkadelphia	76%	(a)
Arkansas Methodist Medical Center	Paragould	75%	300+
Baptist Health Med Ctr-N Little Rock	North Little Rock	75%	300+
Siloam Springs Regional Hospital	Siloam Springs	75%	300+
Summit Medical Center	Van Buren	75%	(a)
Washington Reg Med Ctr at North Hills	Fayetteville	75%	300+
Baptist Health Med Ctr-Hot Springs Co	Malvern	74%	(a)
Five Rivers Medical Center	Pocahontas	74%	(a)
Saint Bernards Medical Center	Jonesboro	74%	300+
Baptist Health Med Ctr-Little Rock[11]	Little Rock	73%	300+
Conway Regional Medical Center	Conway	73%	300+
Magnolia Hospital	Magnolia	73%	(a)
Mercy Hospital Northwest Arkansas[11]	Rogers	73%	300+
Nea Baptist Memorial Hospital	Jonesboro	72%	300+
Saint Vincent Medical Center - North	Sherwood	72%	300+
Baxter Regional Medical Center	Mountain Home	71%	300+
Helena Regional Medical Center	Helena	71%	300+
UAMS Medical Center	Little Rock	71%	300+
White River Medical Center	Batesville	71%	300+
National Park Medical Center	Hot Springs	70%	300+
NW Arkansas Hospitals	Springdale	70%	300+
Saline Memorial Hospital	Benton	70%	300+
White County Medical Center	Searcy	70%	300+
Forrest City Medical Center	Forrest City	69%	300+
Mena Regional Health System	Mena	69%	(a)
North Metro Medical Center[3,11]	Jacksonville	69%	(a)
Saint Joseph's Mercy Health Center[11]	Hot Springs	69%	300+
Wadley Regional Medical Center at Hope	Hope	68%	(a)
Crittenden Memorial Hospital	West Memphis	66%	300+
Baptist Health Medical Center - Stuttgart	Stuttgart	65%	(a)
Drew Memorial Hospital	Monticello	65%	300+
Saint Edward Mercy Medical Center[11]	Fort Smith	65%	300+
Saint Marys Regional Medical Center	Russellville	65%	300+
Saint Vincent Infirmary Medical Center	Little Rock	65%	300+
Medical Center South Arkansas	El Dorado	64%	300+
Harris Hospital	Newport	63%	300+
Sparks Regional Medical Center	Fort Smith	63%	300+
Jefferson Regional Medical Center	Pine Bluff	62%	300+
Great River Medical Center	Blytheville	60%	(a)

Timely Help 'Always' Received

Hospital Name	City	Rate	Cases
Arkansas Heart Hospital	Little Rock	87%	300+
Physicians' Specialty Hospital	Fayetteville	87%	(a)
Arkansas Surgical Hospital	No Little Rock	79%	300+
Ashley County Medical Center	Crossett	78%	(a)
Ouachita County Medical Center	Camden	78%	300+
Saint Vincent Morrilton	Morrilton	78%	(a)
Baptist Health Med Ctr-Heber Spings	Heber Springs	76%	(a)
Baptist Health Med Ctr-Arkadelphia	Arkadelphia	73%	(a)
Baxter Regional Medical Center	Mountain Home	73%	300+
Chambers Memorial Hospital	Danville	73%	(a)
Nea Baptist Memorial Hospital	Jonesboro	73%	300+
Magnolia Hospital	Magnolia	72%	(a)
Summit Medical Center	Van Buren	72%	(a)
White River Medical Center	Batesville	72%	300+
Baptist Health Medical Center - Stuttgart	Stuttgart	71%	(a)
Harris Hospital	Newport	71%	300+
Saint Vincent Medical Center - North	Sherwood	70%	300+
Wadley Regional Medical Center at Hope	Hope	70%	(a)
Johnson Regional Medical Center	Clarksville	69%	300+
Washington Reg Med Ctr at North Hills	Fayetteville	69%	300+
Arkansas Methodist Medical Center	Paragould	68%	300+
Five Rivers Medical Center	Pocahontas	68%	(a)
Forrest City Medical Center	Forrest City	68%	300+
Baptist Health Med Ctr-N Little Rock	North Little Rock	67%	300+
Medical Center South Arkansas	El Dorado	67%	300+
Saline Memorial Hospital	Benton	67%	300+
Jefferson Regional Medical Center	Pine Bluff	66%	300+
Mena Regional Health System	Mena	66%	(a)
North Arkansas Regional Medical Center	Harrison	66%	300+
Saint Bernards Medical Center	Jonesboro	66%	300+
Siloam Springs Regional Hospital	Siloam Springs	66%	300+
Conway Regional Medical Center	Conway	65%	300+
Crittenden Memorial Hospital	West Memphis	65%	300+
Baptist Health Med Ctr-Little Rock[11]	Little Rock	64%	300+
Helena Regional Medical Center	Helena	64%	300+
North Metro Medical Center[3,11]	Jacksonville	64%	(a)
Baptist Health Med Ctr-Hot Springs Co	Malvern	63%	(a)
Drew Memorial Hospital	Monticello	63%	300+
Mercy Hospital Northwest Arkansas[11]	Rogers	63%	300+
Saint Edward Mercy Medical Center[11]	Fort Smith	63%	300+
Saint Vincent Infirmary Medical Center	Little Rock	63%	300+
White County Medical Center	Searcy	63%	300+
Great River Medical Center	Blytheville	62%	(a)
UAMS Medical Center	Little Rock	62%	300+
Saint Joseph's Mercy Health Center[11]	Hot Springs	61%	300+
National Park Medical Center	Hot Springs	60%	300+
Saint Marys Regional Medical Center	Russellville	60%	300+
NW Arkansas Hospitals	Springdale	57%	300+
Sparks Regional Medical Center	Fort Smith	48%	300+

Would Definitely Recommend Hospital

Hospital Name	City	Rate	Cases
Arkansas Heart Hospital	Little Rock	94%	300+
Arkansas Surgical Hospital	No Little Rock	92%	300+
Physicians' Specialty Hospital	Fayetteville	88%	(a)
Nea Baptist Memorial Hospital	Jonesboro	85%	300+
Mercy Hospital Northwest Arkansas[11]	Rogers	80%	300+
Baptist Health Med Ctr-Heber Spings	Heber Springs	78%	(a)
UAMS Medical Center	Little Rock	78%	300+
Washington Reg Med Ctr at North Hills	Fayetteville	78%	300+
Baptist Health Med Ctr-Little Rock[11]	Little Rock	77%	300+
Baptist Health Med Ctr-N Little Rock	North Little Rock	77%	300+
Saint Vincent Medical Center - North	Sherwood	77%	300+
Baxter Regional Medical Center	Mountain Home	76%	300+
Saint Edward Mercy Medical Center[11]	Fort Smith	76%	300+
National Park Medical Center	Hot Springs	75%	300+
Saint Bernards Medical Center	Jonesboro	75%	300+
Magnolia Hospital	Magnolia	74%	(a)
Saint Joseph's Mercy Health Center[11]	Hot Springs	74%	300+
Saint Vincent Infirmary Medical Center	Little Rock	74%	300+
White County Medical Center	Searcy	72%	300+
Conway Regional Medical Center	Conway	71%	300+
Saline Memorial Hospital	Benton	71%	300+
NW Arkansas Hospitals	Springdale	70%	300+
Ouachita County Medical Center	Camden	69%	300+
Chambers Memorial Hospital	Danville	68%	(a)
Wadley Regional Medical Center at Hope	Hope	68%	(a)
White River Medical Center	Batesville	68%	300+
Summit Medical Center	Van Buren	66%	(a)
Saint Vincent Morrilton	Morrilton	65%	(a)
Siloam Springs Regional Hospital	Siloam Springs	65%	300+
Arkansas Methodist Medical Center	Paragould	64%	300+
Baptist Health Med Ctr-Arkadelphia	Arkadelphia	64%	(a)
Forrest City Medical Center	Forrest City	64%	300+
Drew Memorial Hospital	Monticello	63%	300+
Johnson Regional Medical Center	Clarksville	63%	300+
North Arkansas Regional Medical Center	Harrison	62%	300+
Medical Center South Arkansas	El Dorado	61%	300+
Baptist Health Med Ctr-Hot Springs Co	Malvern	59%	(a)
Crittenden Memorial Hospital	West Memphis	59%	300+
Sparks Regional Medical Center	Fort Smith	59%	300+
Ashley County Medical Center	Crossett	58%	(a)
Five Rivers Medical Center	Pocahontas	58%	(a)
Jefferson Regional Medical Center	Pine Bluff	58%	300+
North Metro Medical Center[3,11]	Jacksonville	57%	(a)
Baptist Health Medical Center - Stuttgart	Stuttgart	56%	(a)
Helena Regional Medical Center	Helena	56%	300+
Saint Marys Regional Medical Center	Russellville	54%	300+
Harris Hospital	Newport	53%	300+
Mena Regional Health System	Mena	53%	(a)
Great River Medical Center	Blytheville	47%	(a)

Use of Medical Imaging

Cardiac Imaging Stress Test before OP Surgery

Hospital Name	City	Rate	Cases
Ashley County Medical Center	Crossett	1.9%	106
White County Medical Center	Searcy	2.2%	413
Jefferson Regional Medical Center	Pine Bluff	2.6%	422
Saline Memorial Hospital	Benton	2.9%	102
Baxter Regional Medical Center	Mountain Home	3.0%	237
Conway Regional Medical Center	Conway	3.1%	128

NOTE: Hospital profiles are in alphabetical order by state, then city, then hospital within the city; Rankings exclude hospitals with less than 25 cases except for patient surveys which excludes hospitals with less than 100 cases; (a) 100-299 cases; (1) The number of cases/patients is too few to report; (2) Data submitted were based on a sample of cases/patients; (3) Results are based on a shorter time period than required; (4) Data suppressed by CMS for one or more quarters; (5) Results are not available for this reporting period; (6) Fewer than 100 patients completed the HCAHPS survey; (7) No cases met the criteria for this measure; (8) The lower limit of the confidence interval cannot be calculated if the number of observed infections equals zero; (9) No data are available from the state/territory for this reporting period; (10) The scores shown reflect fewer than 50 completed surveys; (11) There were discrepancies in the data collection process; (12) This measure does not apply to this hospital for this reporting period; (13) Results cannot be calculated for this reporting period; (14) The results for this state are combined with nearby states to protect confidentiality; Please refer to the User's Guide for a full explanation of data.

Saint Marys Regional Medical Center	Russellville	3.1%	293
Saint Vincent Infirmary Medical Center	Little Rock	3.4%	2759
Medical Center South Arkansas	El Dorado	3.5%	453
Baptist Health Med Ctr-Little Rock	Little Rock	3.8%	993
Washington Reg Med Ctr at North Hills	Fayetteville	3.9%	1138
Mercy Hospital Berryville	Berryville	4.1%	49
Arkansas Heart Hospital	Little Rock	4.2%	2785
Saint Joseph's Mercy Health Center	Hot Springs	4.2%	644
Siloam Springs Regional Hospital	Siloam Springs	4.3%	117
NW Arkansas Hospitals	Springdale	4.4%	546
Baptist Health Med Ctr-N Little Rock	North Little Rock	4.9%	571
Mercy Hospital Northwest Arkansas	Rogers	5.0%	991
Mena Regional Health System	Mena	5.4%	92
Sparks Regional Medical Center	Fort Smith	5.6%	557
Saint Bernards Medical Center	Jonesboro	5.9%	915
Saint Edward Mercy Medical Center	Fort Smith	6.2%	211
White River Medical Center	Batesville	6.3%	348
UAMS Medical Center	Little Rock	6.4%	329
North Arkansas Regional Medical Center	Harrison	6.8%	73
Crittenden Memorial Hospital	West Memphis	7.0%	115
Arkansas Methodist Medical Center	Paragould	11.9%	67

Combination Abdominal CT Scan

Hospital Name	City	Rate	Cases
River Valley Medical Center	Dardanelle	0.0%	132
Mercy Hospital Berryville	Berryville	0.7%	145
Baptist Health Med Ctr-Arkadelphia	Arkadelphia	1.2%	247
Ozark Health	Clinton	1.2%	251
Baptist Health Med Ctr-Little Rock	Little Rock	1.6%	1045
UAMS Medical Center	Little Rock	2.0%	1553
Saint Marys Regional Medical Center	Russellville	3.2%	744
Baptist Health Med Ctr-N Little Rock	North Little Rock	3.4%	1401
Baptist Health Med Ctr-Hot Springs Co	Malvern	4.1%	246
Helena Regional Medical Center	Helena	4.2%	192
Baptist Health Medical Center - Stuttgart	Stuttgart	4.3%	186
Howard Memorial Hospital	Nashville	4.6%	175
Washington Reg Med Ctr at North Hills	Fayetteville	5.2%	917
Chambers Memorial Hospital	Danville	5.4%	129
Mena Regional Health System	Mena	5.5%	293
Medical Center South Arkansas	El Dorado	5.6%	464
Saint Vincent Infirmary Medical Center	Little Rock	5.6%	665
Johnson Regional Medical Center	Clarksville	5.8%	342
McGehee Hospital	Mcgehee	6.5%	77
Baptist Health Med Ctr-Heber Spings	Heber Springs	7.1%	504
Saint Joseph's Mercy Health Center	Hot Springs	7.6%	1518
Conway Regional Medical Center	Conway	7.9%	996
Siloam Springs Regional Hospital	Siloam Springs	8.2%	219
National Park Medical Center	Hot Springs	8.4%	442
Ouachita County Medical Center	Camden	9.4%	319
Saint Vincent Medical Center - North	Sherwood	9.5%	252
Forrest City Medical Center	Forrest City	9.6%	167
Saline Memorial Hospital	Benton	9.7%	638
Magnolia Hospital	Magnolia	11.9%	244
White County Medical Center	Searcy	12.0%	1069
Sparks Regional Medical Center	Fort Smith	12.2%	1421
Baxter Regional Medical Center	Mountain Home	12.6%	676
Mercy Hospital Northwest Arkansas	Rogers	16.2%	902
North Metro Medical Center	Jacksonville	16.3%	202
NW Arkansas Hospitals	Springdale	16.3%	771
Crossridge Community Hospital	Wynne	16.6%	169
Nea Baptist Memorial Hospital	Jonesboro	17.3%	562
Five Rivers Medical Center	Pocahontas	17.6%	159
Crittenden Memorial Hospital	West Memphis	18.3%	366
White River Medical Center	Batesville	20.3%	856
Summit Medical Center	Van Buren	21.4%	187
Ashley County Medical Center	Crossett	21.6%	204
North Arkansas Regional Medical Center	Harrison	21.9%	954
Great River Medical Center	Blytheville	23.7%	224
Jefferson Regional Medical Center	Pine Bluff	24.4%	659
Harris Hospital	Newport	32.5%	166
Arkansas Methodist Medical Center	Paragould	32.6%	399
Wadley Regional Medical Center at Hope	Hope	33.3%	48
Stone County Medical Center	Mountain View	34.4%	285
Drew Memorial Hospital	Monticello	42.1%	299
Saint Bernards Medical Center	Jonesboro	44.7%	2199
Saint Edward Mercy Medical Center	Fort Smith	46.2%	788
Chicot Memorial Medical Center	Lake Village	46.7%	135
Arkansas Heart Hospital	Little Rock	51.2%	84

Combination Brain/Sinus CT Scan

Hospital Name	City	Rate	Cases
Wadley Regional Medical Center at Hope	Hope	0.0%	92
McGehee Hospital	Mcgehee	0.6%	158
Baptist Health Med Ctr-Arkadelphia	Arkadelphia	0.8%	390
North Arkansas Regional Medical Center	Harrison	1.0%	827
Jefferson Regional Medical Center	Pine Bluff	1.1%	965
Mercy Hospital Northwest Arkansas	Rogers	1.1%	880
Saline Memorial Hospital	Benton	1.4%	555
Johnson Regional Medical Center	Clarksville	1.5%	335
Baxter Regional Medical Center	Mountain Home	1.6%	881
Drew Memorial Hospital	Monticello	1.6%	385
Conway Regional Medical Center	Conway	1.9%	903
Medical Center South Arkansas	El Dorado	2.2%	445
Nea Baptist Memorial Hospital	Jonesboro	2.2%	540
UAMS Medical Center	Little Rock	2.2%	597
White County Medical Center	Searcy	2.4%	966
Baptist Health Med Ctr-Little Rock	Little Rock	2.6%	970
Baptist Health Med Ctr-N Little Rock	North Little Rock	2.6%	1044
Sparks Regional Medical Center	Fort Smith	3.0%	1246
Washington Reg Med Ctr at North Hills	Fayetteville	3.1%	980
Saint Joseph's Mercy Health Center	Hot Springs	3.3%	1047
White River Medical Center	Batesville	3.6%	726
Crittenden Memorial Hospital	West Memphis	3.9%	515
Saint Bernards Medical Center	Jonesboro	3.9%	1373
Saint Vincent Infirmary Medical Center	Little Rock	4.1%	834
NW Arkansas Hospitals	Springdale	4.4%	912
Siloam Springs Regional Hospital	Siloam Springs	5.0%	221
Crossridge Community Hospital	Wynne	5.7%	228
North Metro Medical Center	Jacksonville	6.4%	265
Baptist Health Medical Center - Stuttgart	Stuttgart	7.1%	310
Great River Medical Center	Blytheville	7.5%	266
Ouachita County Medical Center	Camden	8.3%	339

Combination Chest CT Scan

Hospital Name	City	Rate	Cases
Arkansas Methodist Medical Center	Paragould	0.0%	262
Chambers Memorial Hospital	Danville	0.0%	69
Mercy Hospital Berryville	Berryville	0.0%	53
Ozark Health	Clinton	0.0%	163
River Valley Medical Center	Dardanelle	0.0%	64
Saint Edward Mercy Medical Center	Fort Smith	0.0%	417
Saline Memorial Hospital	Benton	0.0%	350
White County Medical Center	Searcy	0.0%	605
Baptist Health Med Ctr-N Little Rock	North Little Rock	0.3%	917
Medical Center South Arkansas	El Dorado	0.3%	370
Baptist Health Med Ctr-Hot Springs Co	Malvern	0.6%	176
Saint Vincent Infirmary Medical Center	Little Rock	0.6%	330
Magnolia Hospital	Magnolia	0.8%	125
Baptist Health Med Ctr-Arkadelphia	Arkadelphia	0.9%	108
Ouachita County Medical Center	Camden	0.9%	226
Conway Regional Medical Center	Conway	1.1%	356
Mena Regional Health System	Mena	1.1%	188
Washington Reg Med Ctr at North Hills	Fayetteville	1.1%	281
Saint Bernards Medical Center	Jonesboro	1.2%	1758
UAMS Medical Center	Little Rock	1.2%	1563
Baptist Health Med Ctr-Little Rock	Little Rock	1.3%	523
Forrest City Medical Center	Forrest City	1.3%	77
Siloam Springs Regional Hospital	Siloam Springs	1.4%	73
Five Rivers Medical Center	Pocahontas	1.5%	137
Johnson Regional Medical Center	Clarksville	1.5%	197
Baptist Health Medical Center - Stuttgart	Stuttgart	1.6%	126
Saint Marys Regional Medical Center	Russellville	1.8%	544
Baptist Health Med Ctr-Heber Spings	Heber Springs	2.2%	277
Saint Vincent Medical Center - North	Sherwood	2.2%	92
Baxter Regional Medical Center	Mountain Home	2.3%	476
Saint Joseph's Mercy Health Center	Hot Springs	4.0%	901
Crittenden Memorial Hospital	West Memphis	4.2%	238
Howard Memorial Hospital	Nashville	4.5%	66
North Arkansas Regional Medical Center	Harrison	5.9%	373
NW Arkansas Hospitals	Springdale	7.4%	352
White River Medical Center	Batesville	7.5%	535
North Metro Medical Center	Jacksonville	8.1%	74
Nea Baptist Memorial Hospital	Jonesboro	8.7%	357
Helena Regional Medical Center	Helena	9.5%	84
Sparks Regional Medical Center	Fort Smith	9.6%	806
Mercy Hospital Northwest Arkansas	Rogers	12.5%	574
National Park Medical Center	Hot Springs	13.2%	272
Jefferson Regional Medical Center	Pine Bluff	14.9%	496
Ashley County Medical Center	Crossett	15.3%	131
Crossridge Community Hospital	Wynne	18.7%	107
Harris Hospital	Newport	19.1%	115
Drew Memorial Hospital	Monticello	20.0%	165
Chicot Memorial Medical Center	Lake Village	26.5%	68
Arkansas Heart Hospital	Little Rock	33.8%	130
Great River Medical Center	Blytheville	43.0%	86
Stone County Medical Center	Mountain View	48.8%	125

Follow-up Mammogram/Ultrasound

A follow-up rate near zero may indicate missed cancer; a rate higher than 14% may mean there is unnecessary follow up.

Hospital Name	City	Rate	Cases
Five Rivers Medical Center	Pocahontas	3.4%	175
Crossridge Community Hospital	Wynne	4.5%	179
White River Medical Center	Batesville	4.6%	1426
Arkansas Methodist Medical Center	Paragould	5.0%	598
Medical Center South Arkansas	El Dorado	5.7%	1029
Baptist Health Med Ctr-Heber Spings	Heber Springs	5.8%	642
Ashley County Medical Center	Crossett	5.9%	340
Chicot Memorial Medical Center	Lake Village	5.9%	238
Mercy Hospital Berryville	Berryville	6.1%	278
Saint Edward Mercy Medical Center	Fort Smith	6.2%	1577
Helena Regional Medical Center	Helena	6.5%	199
Sparks Regional Medical Center	Fort Smith	6.6%	2538
Baptist Health Med Ctr-Arkadelphia	Arkadelphia	6.8%	576
Forrest City Medical Center	Forrest City	6.9%	260
Ouachita County Medical Center	Camden	7.8%	232
Great River Medical Center	Blytheville	8.0%	261
Stone County Medical Center	Mountain View	8.0%	137
Baxter Regional Medical Center	Mountain Home	8.3%	2694
North Arkansas Regional Medical Center	Harrison	8.3%	984
Baptist Health Medical Center - Stuttgart	Stuttgart	8.5%	317
Jefferson Regional Medical Center	Pine Bluff	8.5%	1408
Baptist Health Med Ctr-Little Rock	Little Rock	8.8%	4244
Baptist Health Med Ctr-N Little Rock	North Little Rock	9.0%	2021
Ozark Health	Clinton	9.2%	207
Magnolia Hospital	Magnolia	9.5%	497
Mercy Hospital Northwest Arkansas	Rogers	9.8%	2100
Conway Regional Medical Center	Conway	10.3%	2153
Drew Memorial Hospital	Monticello	10.4%	384
UAMS Medical Center	Little Rock	10.7%	1930
Mena Regional Health System	Mena	11.5%	373
Siloam Springs Regional Hospital	Siloam Springs	11.7%	273
Crittenden Memorial Hospital	West Memphis	12.1%	356
Johnson Regional Medical Center	Clarksville	12.1%	363
Saint Bernards Medical Center	Jonesboro	12.7%	2677
Saline Memorial Hospital	Benton	12.9%	752
Washington Reg Med Ctr at North Hills	Fayetteville	13.2%	144
Harris Hospital	Newport	13.5%	156
Saint Vincent Medical Center - North	Sherwood	13.8%	325
Saint Joseph's Mercy Health Center	Hot Springs	14.3%	2786
NW Arkansas Hospitals	Springdale	14.4%	1670
Saint Marys Regional Medical Center	Russellville	15.1%	1083
Summit Medical Center	Van Buren	15.5%	97
Howard Memorial Hospital	Nashville	16.0%	244
National Park Medical Center	Hot Springs	16.3%	710
Baptist Health Med Ctr-Hot Springs Co	Malvern	17.8%	191
North Metro Medical Center	Jacksonville	19.0%	793

Lumbar Spine MRI for Low Back Pain

Hospital Name	City	Rate	Cases
Saint Vincent Medical Center - North	Sherwood	23.8%	84
UAMS Medical Center	Little Rock	30.6%	72
Arkansas Surgical Hospital	No Little Rock	34.7%	294
Saint Joseph's Mercy Health Center	Hot Springs	34.7%	406
Baptist Health Med Ctr-Heber Spings	Heber Springs	35.1%	94
Saint Vincent Infirmary Medical Center	Little Rock	35.3%	173
Baptist Health Med Ctr-Hot Springs Co	Malvern	35.9%	78
National Park Medical Center	Hot Springs	36.5%	104
Mercy Hospital Northwest Arkansas	Rogers	37.3%	236
Baptist Health Med Ctr-N Little Rock	North Little Rock	38.6%	394
Baxter Regional Medical Center	Mountain Home	38.9%	208
Ouachita County Medical Center	Camden	39.3%	56
Physicians' Specialty Hospital	Fayetteville	39.3%	89
Medical Center South Arkansas	El Dorado	39.4%	180
Saint Marys Regional Medical Center	Russellville	39.7%	116
Drew Memorial Hospital	Monticello	39.8%	113
Baptist Health Med Ctr-Arkadelphia	Arkadelphia	41.1%	56
Saint Edward Mercy Medical Center	Fort Smith	41.2%	301
Crittenden Memorial Hospital	West Memphis	41.3%	63
Arkansas Methodist Medical Center	Paragould	41.4%	87
Washington Reg Med Ctr at North Hills	Fayetteville	41.4%	116
White County Medical Center	Searcy	41.7%	216
Saint Bernards Medical Center	Jonesboro	42.9%	469
Conway Regional Medical Center	Conway	43.4%	281
Baptist Health Med Ctr-Little Rock	Little Rock	43.5%	161
NW Arkansas Hospitals	Springdale	44.3%	122
White River Medical Center	Batesville	45.2%	155
Sparks Regional Medical Center	Fort Smith	46.1%	152
Saline Memorial Hospital	Benton	46.2%	130
Ashley County Medical Center	Crossett	47.5%	40
Nea Baptist Memorial Hospital	Jonesboro	47.5%	80
Magnolia Hospital	Magnolia	48.6%	37
Mena Regional Health System	Mena	49.4%	83
North Arkansas Regional Medical Center	Harrison	50.0%	162
Jefferson Regional Medical Center	Pine Bluff	50.5%	200
Ozark Health	Clinton	52.5%	40
North Metro Medical Center	Jacksonville	56.1%	57
Johnson Regional Medical Center	Clarksville	57.7%	52
Forrest City Medical Center	Forrest City	59.1%	44

NOTE: Hospital profiles are in alphabetical order by state, then city, then hospital within the city; Rankings exclude hospitals with less than 25 cases except for patient surveys which excludes hospitals with less than 100 cases; (a) 100-299 cases; (1) The number of cases/patients is too few to report; (2) Data submitted were based on a sample of cases/patients; (3) Results are based on a shorter time period than required; (4) Data suppressed by CMS for one or more quarters; (5) Results are not available for this reporting period; (6) Fewer than 100 patients completed the HCAHPS survey; (7) No cases met the criteria for this measure; (8) The lower limit of the confidence interval cannot be calculated if the number of observed infections equals zero; (9) No data are available from the state/territory for this reporting period; (10) The scores shown reflect fewer than 50 completed surveys; (11) There were discrepancies in the data collection process; (12) This measure does not apply to this hospital for this reporting period; (13) Results cannot be calculated for this reporting period; (14) The results for this state are combined with nearby states to protect confidentiality; Please refer to the User's Guide for a full explanation of data.

Baptist Health Medical Center - Arkadelphia

3050 Twin Rivers Drive Phone: 870-245-2622
Arkadelphia, AR 71923 Fax: 870-245-1198
URL: www.baptist-health.org
Type: Critical Access Hospitals Emergency Services: Yes
Ownership: Voluntary non-profit - Private Beds: 57
Key Personnel:
Quality Assurance . . . . Cathy Abbott, RN
Chief of Medical Staff . . . . Noland Hagood
CEO/President . . . . Russell D Harrington
Emergency Room . . . . McLane Andrew Simpson

Measure	Cases	This Hosp.	State Avg.	U.S. Avg.
Blood Clot Prevention and Treatment				
Anticoagulation Overlap Therapy[2]	14	71%	88%	93%
ICU Venous Thromboembolism Prophylaxis[2]	21	90%	94%	92%
Incidence of Potentially Preventable VTE[1,2]	-	-	12%	10%
UFH with Dosages/Platelet Monitoring[2,7]	-	-	100%	97%
Venous Thromboembolism Prophylaxis[2]	87	82%	91%	85%
Warfarin Therapy Discharge Instructions[2]	12	75%	76%	75%
Chest Pain/Possible Heart Attack Care				
Aspirin Given Within 24 Hours of Arrival	48	92%	96%	96%
Fibrinolytic Meds Within 30 Min. of Arrival[1]	-	-	54%	58%
Average Time to ECG (minutes)	48	16	8	7
Average Time to Transfer (minutes)[1]	-	-	72	60
Children's Asthma Care				
Received Home Management Plan of Care	-	-	-	88%
Received Reliever Medication	-	-	-	100%
Received Systemic Corticosteroids	-	-	-	100%
Emergency Department				
Admittance Decision Time (minutes)[2]	200	46	65	98
Head CT Results Within 45 Min. of Arrival	12	75%	49%	57%
Patients Who Left ER Before Being Seen	11,669	3%	3%	2%
Time from ER Arrival to Admit. (minutes)[2]	210	164	214	274
Time from ER Arrival to Discharge (minutes)	346	100	118	134
Time in ER Before Being Evaluated (minutes)	424	20	26	26
Time to Pain Meds for Fractures (minutes)	52	52	66	57
Heart Attack Care				
Aspirin Given at Discharge[1,3]	-	-	99%	99%
Fibrinolytic Meds Within 30 Min. of Arrival[3,7]	-	-	77%	54%
PCI Within 90 Minutes of Arrival[3,7]	-	-	96%	96%
Statin Prescribed at Discharge[1,3]	-	-	97%	98%
Heart Failure Care				
ACE Inhibitor or ARB for LVSD[1]	-	-	96%	97%
Discharge Instructions Given	23	100%	95%	94%
Evaluation of LVS Function	38	79%	98%	99%
Medicare Spending				
Medicare Spending per Patient (ratio)	-	-	0.98	0.98
Pneumonia Care				
Appropriate Initial Antibiotic Given	20	100%	94%	95%
Blood Culture Timing	41	98%	98%	98%
Pregnancy and Delivery Care				
Newborn Deliveries Scheduled Early	54	2%	6%	6%
Preventive Care				
Immunization for Influenza[2]	244	86%	89%	90%
Immunization for Pneumonia[2]	228	82%	92%	92%
Stroke Care				
Anticoagulation Therapy for Atrial Fibrillation[1]	-	-	90%	95%
Antithrombotic Therapy Timing	14	93%	96%	98%
Assessed for Rehabilitation	14	100%	95%	97%
Discharged on Antithrombotic Therapy	13	92%	96%	99%
Discharged on Statin Medication	11	64%	86%	94%
Thrombolytic Therapy Timing[7]	-	-	35%	66%
Venous Thromboembolism Prophylaxis	17	94%	91%	94%
Written Stroke Educational Materials Given[1]	-	-	81%	88%
Surgical Care Improvement Project				
Appropriate Beta Blocker Usage[1]	-	-	98%	98%
Appropriate VTP Within 24 Hours	48	98%	98%	98%
Controlled Postoperative Blood Glucose[7]	-	-	99%	97%
Perioperative Temperature Management	60	100%	100%	100%
Prophylactic Antibiotic Selection	56	100%	99%	99%
Prophylactic Antibiotic Selection (Outpatient)	63	100%	98%	98%
Prophylactic Antibiotic Stopped	55	89%	98%	98%
Prophylactic Antibiotic Timing	56	100%	99%	99%
Prophylactic Antibiotic Timing (Outpatient)	67	93%	98%	98%
Urinary Catheter Removal[1]	-	-	97%	97%
Survey of Patients' Hospital Experiences				
Area Around Room 'Always' Quiet at Night	(a)	70%	67%	61%
Doctors 'Always' Communicated Well	(a)	90%	83%	82%
Home Recovery Information Given	(a)	81%	83%	85%
Hospital Given 9 or 10 on 10 Point Scale	(a)	73%	70%	71%
Meds 'Always' Explained Before Given	(a)	69%	63%	64%
Nurses 'Always' Communicated Well	(a)	82%	79%	79%
Pain 'Always' Well Controlled	(a)	67%	71%	71%
Room and Bathroom 'Always' Clean	(a)	76%	72%	73%
Timely Help 'Always' Received	(a)	73%	68%	68%
Would Definitely Recommend Hospital	(a)	64%	69%	71%
Use of Medical Imaging				
Cardiac Imaging Stress Test before Surgery[1]	-	-	4.3%	5.3%
Combination Abdominal CT Scan	247	1.2%	15.3%	10.5%
Combination Brain/Sinus CT Scan	390	0.8%	2.9%	2.7%
Combination Chest CT Scan	108	0.9%	5%	2.7%
Follow-up Mammogram/Ultrasound	576	6.8%	9.9%	8.8%
Lumbar Spine MRI for Low Back Pain	56	41.1%	41.6%	37.2%

Little River Memorial Hospital

451 West Locke Street Phone: 870-898-5011
Ashdown, AR 71822
Type: Critical Access Hospitals Emergency Services: Yes
Ownership: Government - Local

Measure	Cases	This Hosp.	State Avg.	U.S. Avg.
Blood Clot Prevention and Treatment				
Anticoagulation Overlap Therapy[5]	-	-	88%	93%
ICU Venous Thromboembolism Prophylaxis[5]	-	-	94%	92%
Incidence of Potentially Preventable VTE[5]	-	-	12%	10%
UFH with Dosages/Platelet Monitoring[5]	-	-	100%	97%
Venous Thromboembolism Prophylaxis[5]	-	-	91%	85%
Warfarin Therapy Discharge Instructions[5]	-	-	76%	75%
Chest Pain/Possible Heart Attack Care				
Aspirin Given Within 24 Hours of Arrival	-	-	96%	96%
Fibrinolytic Meds Within 30 Min. of Arrival	-	-	54%	58%
Average Time to ECG (minutes)	-	-	8	7
Average Time to Transfer (minutes)	-	-	72	60
Children's Asthma Care				
Received Home Management Plan of Care	-	-	-	88%
Received Reliever Medication	-	-	-	100%
Received Systemic Corticosteroids	-	-	-	100%
Emergency Department				
Admittance Decision Time (minutes)[5]	-	-	65	98
Head CT Results Within 45 Min. of Arrival	-	-	49%	57%
Patients Who Left ER Before Being Seen	-	-	3%	2%
Time from ER Arrival to Admit. (minutes)[5]	-	-	214	274
Time from ER Arrival to Discharge (minutes)	-	-	118	134
Time in ER Before Being Evaluated (minutes)	-	-	26	26
Time to Pain Meds for Fractures (minutes)	-	-	66	57
Heart Attack Care				
Aspirin Given at Discharge[5]	-	-	99%	99%
Fibrinolytic Meds Within 30 Min. of Arrival[5]	-	-	77%	54%
PCI Within 90 Minutes of Arrival[5]	-	-	96%	96%
Statin Prescribed at Discharge[5]	-	-	97%	98%
Heart Failure Care				
ACE Inhibitor or ARB for LVSD[1,3]	-	-	96%	97%
Discharge Instructions Given[1,3]	-	-	95%	94%
Evaluation of LVS Function[1,3]	-	-	98%	99%
Medicare Spending				
Medicare Spending per Patient (ratio)	-	-	0.98	0.98
Pneumonia Care				
Appropriate Initial Antibiotic Given	20	80%	94%	95%
Blood Culture Timing	14	86%	98%	98%
Pregnancy and Delivery Care				
Newborn Deliveries Scheduled Early[5]	-	-	6%	6%
Preventive Care				
Immunization for Influenza[5]	-	-	89%	90%
Immunization for Pneumonia[5]	-	-	92%	92%
Stroke Care				
Anticoagulation Therapy for Atrial Fibrillation[5]	-	-	90%	95%
Antithrombotic Therapy Timing[5]	-	-	96%	98%
Assessed for Rehabilitation[5]	-	-	95%	97%
Discharged on Antithrombotic Therapy[5]	-	-	96%	99%
Discharged on Statin Medication[5]	-	-	86%	94%
Thrombolytic Therapy Timing[5]	-	-	35%	66%
Venous Thromboembolism Prophylaxis[5]	-	-	91%	94%
Written Stroke Educational Materials Given[5]	-	-	81%	88%
Surgical Care Improvement Project				
Appropriate Beta Blocker Usage[5]	-	-	98%	98%
Appropriate VTP Within 24 Hours[5]	-	-	98%	98%
Controlled Postoperative Blood Glucose[5]	-	-	99%	97%
Perioperative Temperature Management[5]	-	-	100%	100%
Prophylactic Antibiotic Selection[5]	-	-	99%	99%
Prophylactic Antibiotic Selection (Outpatient)	-	-	98%	98%
Prophylactic Antibiotic Stopped[5]	-	-	98%	98%
Prophylactic Antibiotic Timing[5]	-	-	99%	99%
Prophylactic Antibiotic Timing (Outpatient)	-	-	98%	98%
Urinary Catheter Removal[5]	-	-	97%	97%
Survey of Patients' Hospital Experiences				
Area Around Room 'Always' Quiet at Night[5]	-	-	67%	61%
Doctors 'Always' Communicated Well[5]	-	-	83%	82%
Home Recovery Information Given[5]	-	-	83%	85%
Hospital Given 9 or 10 on 10 Point Scale[5]	-	-	70%	71%
Meds 'Always' Explained Before Given[5]	-	-	63%	64%
Nurses 'Always' Communicated Well[5]	-	-	79%	79%
Pain 'Always' Well Controlled[5]	-	-	71%	71%
Room and Bathroom 'Always' Clean[5]	-	-	72%	73%
Timely Help 'Always' Received[5]	-	-	68%	68%
Would Definitely Recommend Hospital[5]	-	-	69%	71%
Use of Medical Imaging				
Cardiac Imaging Stress Test before Surgery	-	-	4.3%	5.3%
Combination Abdominal CT Scan	-	-	15.3%	10.5%
Combination Brain/Sinus CT Scan	-	-	2.9%	2.7%
Combination Chest CT Scan	-	-	5%	2.7%
Follow-up Mammogram/Ultrasound	-	-	9.9%	8.8%
Lumbar Spine MRI for Low Back Pain	-	-	41.6%	37.2%

White River Medical Center

1710 Harrison Street Phone: 870-262-1200
Batesville, AR 72503 Fax: 870-612-6094
E-mail: smace@mail.wrmc.com
URL: www.wrmc.com
Type: Acute Care Hospitals Emergency Services: Yes
Ownership: Voluntary non-profit - Private Beds: 167
Key Personnel:
CEO . . . . Gary L Bebow
Chief of Medical Staff . . . . Neaville Germ, MD
Quality Assurance . . . . Sandra Jones, RN
Emergency Room . . . . Jeff Mares, RN
Operating Room. . . . . David Posey, RN
President . . . . Charles Schaaf
Cardiac Laboratory. . . . . Robert Wright

Measure	Cases	This Hosp.	State Avg.	U.S. Avg.
Blood Clot Prevention and Treatment				
Anticoagulation Overlap Therapy[2]	37	81%	88%	93%
ICU Venous Thromboembolism Prophylaxis[2]	127	86%	94%	92%
Incidence of Potentially Preventable VTE[1,2]	-	-	12%	10%
UFH with Dosages/Platelet Monitoring[1,2]	-	-	100%	97%
Venous Thromboembolism Prophylaxis[2]	355	86%	91%	85%
Warfarin Therapy Discharge Instructions[2]	26	73%	76%	75%
Chest Pain/Possible Heart Attack Care				
Aspirin Given Within 24 Hours of Arrival[1,3]	-	-	96%	96%
Fibrinolytic Meds Within 30 Min. of Arrival[5]	-	-	54%	58%
Average Time to ECG (minutes)[1,3]	-	-	8	7
Average Time to Transfer (minutes)[5]	-	-	72	60
Children's Asthma Care				
Received Home Management Plan of Care	-	-	-	88%
Received Reliever Medication	-	-	-	100%
Received Systemic Corticosteroids	-	-	-	100%
Emergency Department				
Admittance Decision Time (minutes)[2]	427	59	65	98
Head CT Results Within 45 Min. of Arrival	11	45%	49%	57%
Patients Who Left ER Before Being Seen	32,757	2%	3%	2%
Time from ER Arrival to Admit. (minutes)[2]	431	209	214	274

NOTE: Hospital profiles are in alphabetical order by state, then city, then hospital within the city; Rankings exclude hospitals with less than 25 cases except for patient surveys which excludes hospitals with less than 100 cases; (a) 100-299 cases; (1) The number of cases/patients is too few to report; (2) Data submitted were based on a sample of cases/patients; (3) Results are based on a shorter time period than required; (4) Data suppressed by CMS for one or more quarters; (5) Results are not available for this reporting period; (6) Fewer than 100 patients completed the HCAHPS survey; (7) No cases met the criteria for this measure; (8) The lower limit of the confidence interval cannot be calculated if the number of observed infections equals zero; (9) No data are available from the state/territory for this reporting period; (10) The scores shown reflect fewer than 50 completed surveys; (11) There were discrepancies in the data collection process; (12) This measure does not apply to this hospital for this reporting period; (13) Results cannot be calculated for this reporting period; (14) The results for this state are combined with nearby states to protect confidentiality; Please refer to the User's Guide for a full explanation of data.

Measure	Cases	This Hosp.	State Avg.	U.S. Avg.
Time from ER Arrival to Discharge (minutes)	385	148	118	134
Time in ER Before Being Evaluated (minutes)	418	50	26	26
Time to Pain Meds for Fractures (minutes)	110	78	66	57
Heart Attack Care				
Aspirin Given at Discharge	189	96%	99%	99%
Fibrinolytic Meds Within 30 Min. of Arrival[1]	-	-	77%	54%
PCI Within 90 Minutes of Arrival	36	86%	96%	96%
Statin Prescribed at Discharge	179	94%	97%	98%
Heart Failure Care				
ACE Inhibitor or ARB for LVSD	100	90%	96%	97%
Discharge Instructions Given	250	99%	95%	94%
Evaluation of LVS Function	332	100%	98%	99%
Medicare Spending				
Medicare Spending per Patient (ratio)	-	1.00	0.98	0.98
Pneumonia Care				
Appropriate Initial Antibiotic Given	168	96%	94%	95%
Blood Culture Timing	239	99%	98%	98%
Pregnancy and Delivery Care				
Newborn Deliveries Scheduled Early[2]	30	7%	6%	6%
Preventive Care				
Immunization for Influenza[2]	573	97%	89%	90%
Immunization for Pneumonia[2]	722	98%	92%	92%
Stroke Care				
Anticoagulation Therapy for Atrial Fibrillation[1]	-	-	90%	95%
Antithrombotic Therapy Timing	91	91%	96%	98%
Assessed for Rehabilitation	82	95%	95%	97%
Discharged on Antithrombotic Therapy	80	99%	96%	99%
Discharged on Statin Medication	71	93%	86%	94%
Thrombolytic Therapy Timing[1]	-	-	35%	66%
Venous Thromboembolism Prophylaxis	94	84%	91%	94%
Written Stroke Educational Materials Given	46	93%	81%	88%
Surgical Care Improvement Project				
Appropriate Beta Blocker Usage	146	99%	98%	98%
Appropriate VTP Within 24 Hours	418	96%	98%	98%
Controlled Postoperative Blood Glucose[7]	-	-	99%	97%
Perioperative Temperature Management	484	100%	100%	100%
Prophylactic Antibiotic Selection	306	99%	99%	99%
Prophylactic Antibiotic Selection (Outpatient)	166	96%	98%	98%
Prophylactic Antibiotic Stopped	302	96%	98%	98%
Prophylactic Antibiotic Timing	307	100%	99%	99%
Prophylactic Antibiotic Timing (Outpatient)	169	96%	98%	98%
Urinary Catheter Removal	197	99%	97%	97%
Survey of Patients' Hospital Experiences				
Area Around Room 'Always' Quiet at Night	300+	67%	67%	61%
Doctors 'Always' Communicated Well	300+	83%	83%	82%
Home Recovery Information Given	300+	85%	83%	85%
Hospital Given 9 or 10 on 10 Point Scale	300+	72%	70%	71%
Meds 'Always' Explained Before Given	300+	65%	63%	64%
Nurses 'Always' Communicated Well	300+	81%	79%	79%
Pain 'Always' Well Controlled	300+	71%	71%	71%
Room and Bathroom 'Always' Clean	300+	71%	72%	73%
Timely Help 'Always' Received	300+	72%	68%	68%
Would Definitely Recommend Hospital	300+	68%	69%	71%
Use of Medical Imaging				
Cardiac Imaging Stress Test before Surgery	348	6.3%	4.3%	5.3%
Combination Abdominal CT Scan	856	20.3%	15.3%	10.5%
Combination Brain/Sinus CT Scan	726	3.6%	2.9%	2.7%
Combination Chest CT Scan	535	7.5%	5%	2.7%
Follow-up Mammogram/Ultrasound	1,426	4.6%	9.9%	8.8%
Lumbar Spine MRI for Low Back Pain	155	45.2%	41.6%	37.2%

Saline Memorial Hospital

#1 Medical Park Drive
Benton, AR 72015
Phone: 501-776-6000
Fax: 501-776-6768
E-mail: contactus@salinememorial.org
URL: www.salinememorial.org
Type: Acute Care Hospitals
Emergency Services: Yes
Ownership: Voluntary non-profit - Private
Beds: 153

Key Personnel:
Radiology. . . . . Albert Alexander
Quality Assurance . . . . Kathleen Blackwell
Chief of Medical Staff . . . . Daniel Cartaya
Operating Room. . . . . Jackie Dawson
Emergency Room . . . . Melissa Dockery
CEO/President. . . . . Randy Fortner
Coronary Care . . . . David Gibson
Chairman/CEO . . . . Lance Penfield

Measure	Cases	This Hosp.	State Avg.	U.S. Avg.
Blood Clot Prevention and Treatment				
Anticoagulation Overlap Therapy[2]	34	91%	88%	93%
ICU Venous Thromboembolism Prophylaxis[2]	148	93%	94%	92%
Incidence of Potentially Preventable VTE[2,7]	-	-	12%	10%
UFH with Dosages/Platelet Monitoring[1,2]	-	-	100%	97%
Venous Thromboembolism Prophylaxis[2]	214	84%	91%	85%
Warfarin Therapy Discharge Instructions[2]	27	100%	76%	75%
Chest Pain/Possible Heart Attack Care				
Aspirin Given Within 24 Hours of Arrival	19	95%	96%	96%
Fibrinolytic Meds Within 30 Min. of Arrival[3,7]	-	-	54%	58%
Average Time to ECG (minutes)	20	12	8	7
Average Time to Transfer (minutes)[3,7]	-	-	72	60
Children's Asthma Care				
Received Home Management Plan of Care	-	-	-	88%
Received Reliever Medication	-	-	-	100%
Received Systemic Corticosteroids	-	-	-	100%
Emergency Department				
Admittance Decision Time (minutes)[2]	119	36	65	98
Head CT Results Within 45 Min. of Arrival[1]	-	-	49%	57%
Patients Who Left ER Before Being Seen	33,183	3%	3%	2%
Time from ER Arrival to Admit. (minutes)[2]	119	170	214	274
Time from ER Arrival to Discharge (minutes)	317	107	118	134
Time in ER Before Being Evaluated (minutes)	365	20	26	26
Time to Pain Meds for Fractures (minutes)	148	63	66	57
Heart Attack Care				
Aspirin Given at Discharge	102	89%	99%	99%
Fibrinolytic Meds Within 30 Min. of Arrival[1]	-	-	77%	54%
PCI Within 90 Minutes of Arrival	15	93%	96%	96%
Statin Prescribed at Discharge	100	81%	97%	98%
Heart Failure Care				
ACE Inhibitor or ARB for LVSD	42	95%	96%	97%
Discharge Instructions Given	138	79%	95%	94%
Evaluation of LVS Function	174	90%	98%	99%
Medicare Spending				
Medicare Spending per Patient (ratio)	-	0.96	0.98	0.98
Pneumonia Care				
Appropriate Initial Antibiotic Given[2]	144	96%	94%	95%
Blood Culture Timing[2]	268	98%	98%	98%
Pregnancy and Delivery Care				
Newborn Deliveries Scheduled Early	53	6%	6%	6%
Preventive Care				
Immunization for Influenza[2]	495	92%	89%	90%
Immunization for Pneumonia[2]	597	91%	92%	92%
Stroke Care				
Anticoagulation Therapy for Atrial Fibrillation[1]	-	-	90%	95%
Antithrombotic Therapy Timing	28	96%	96%	98%
Assessed for Rehabilitation	33	97%	95%	97%
Discharged on Antithrombotic Therapy	31	97%	96%	99%
Discharged on Statin Medication	23	74%	86%	94%
Thrombolytic Therapy Timing[1]	-	-	35%	66%
Venous Thromboembolism Prophylaxis	36	97%	91%	94%
Written Stroke Educational Materials Given	21	100%	81%	88%
Surgical Care Improvement Project				
Appropriate Beta Blocker Usage	91	98%	98%	98%
Appropriate VTP Within 24 Hours	295	95%	98%	98%
Controlled Postoperative Blood Glucose[7]	-	-	99%	97%
Perioperative Temperature Management	319	99%	100%	100%
Prophylactic Antibiotic Selection	254	98%	99%	99%
Prophylactic Antibiotic Selection (Outpatient)	149	97%	98%	98%
Prophylactic Antibiotic Stopped	252	99%	98%	98%
Prophylactic Antibiotic Timing	255	98%	99%	99%
Prophylactic Antibiotic Timing (Outpatient)	149	100%	98%	98%
Urinary Catheter Removal	189	99%	97%	97%
Survey of Patients' Hospital Experiences				
Area Around Room 'Always' Quiet at Night	300+	64%	67%	61%
Doctors 'Always' Communicated Well	300+	80%	83%	82%
Home Recovery Information Given	300+	83%	83%	85%
Hospital Given 9 or 10 on 10 Point Scale	300+	71%	70%	71%
Meds 'Always' Explained Before Given	300+	63%	63%	64%
Nurses 'Always' Communicated Well	300+	80%	79%	79%
Pain 'Always' Well Controlled	300+	72%	71%	71%
Room and Bathroom 'Always' Clean	300+	70%	72%	73%
Timely Help 'Always' Received	300+	67%	68%	68%
Would Definitely Recommend Hospital	300+	71%	69%	71%
Use of Medical Imaging				
Cardiac Imaging Stress Test before Surgery	102	2.9%	4.3%	5.3%
Combination Abdominal CT Scan	638	9.7%	15.3%	10.5%
Combination Brain/Sinus CT Scan	555	1.4%	2.9%	2.7%
Combination Chest CT Scan	350	0.0%	5%	2.7%
Follow-up Mammogram/Ultrasound	752	12.9%	9.9%	8.8%
Lumbar Spine MRI for Low Back Pain	130	46.2%	41.6%	37.2%

Mercy Hospital Berryville

214 Carter Street
Berryville, AR 72616
Phone: 870-423-3355
Fax: 870-423-5233
E-mail: info@stjohnsberryville.com
URL: www.carrollregional.com
Type: Critical Access Hospitals
Emergency Services: Yes
Ownership: Voluntary non-profit - Church
Beds: 50

Key Personnel:
CEO/President. . . . . Rudy Darling
Emergency Room . . . . Larry Ginn
Operating Room. . . . . Joyce Pharis, RN
Quality Assurance . . . . Stephanie Rains
Chief of Medical Staff . . . . Richard Taylor, MD

Measure	Cases	This Hosp.	State Avg.	U.S. Avg.
Blood Clot Prevention and Treatment				
Anticoagulation Overlap Therapy[5]	-	-	88%	93%
ICU Venous Thromboembolism Prophylaxis[5]	-	-	94%	92%
Incidence of Potentially Preventable VTE[5]	-	-	12%	10%
UFH with Dosages/Platelet Monitoring[5]	-	-	100%	97%
Venous Thromboembolism Prophylaxis[5]	-	-	91%	85%
Warfarin Therapy Discharge Instructions[5]	-	-	76%	75%
Chest Pain/Possible Heart Attack Care				
Aspirin Given Within 24 Hours of Arrival	26	100%	96%	96%
Fibrinolytic Meds Within 30 Min. of Arrival[7]	-	-	54%	58%
Average Time to ECG (minutes)	26	8	8	7
Average Time to Transfer (minutes)[1]	-	-	72	60
Children's Asthma Care				
Received Home Management Plan of Care	-	-	-	88%
Received Reliever Medication	-	-	-	100%
Received Systemic Corticosteroids	-	-	-	100%
Emergency Department				
Admittance Decision Time (minutes)[5]	-	-	65	98
Head CT Results Within 45 Min. of Arrival[5]	-	-	49%	57%
Patients Who Left ER Before Being Seen[5]	-	-	3%	2%
Time from ER Arrival to Admit. (minutes)[5]	-	-	214	274
Time from ER Arrival to Discharge (minutes)[5]	-	-	118	134
Time in ER Before Being Evaluated (minutes)[5]	-	-	26	26
Time to Pain Meds for Fractures (minutes)[5]	-	-	66	57
Heart Attack Care				
Aspirin Given at Discharge[5]	-	-	99%	99%
Fibrinolytic Meds Within 30 Min. of Arrival[5]	-	-	77%	54%
PCI Within 90 Minutes of Arrival[5]	-	-	96%	96%
Statin Prescribed at Discharge[5]	-	-	97%	98%
Heart Failure Care				
ACE Inhibitor or ARB for LVSD[1]	-	-	96%	97%
Discharge Instructions Given	19	95%	95%	94%
Evaluation of LVS Function	22	95%	98%	99%
Medicare Spending				
Medicare Spending per Patient (ratio)	-	-	0.98	0.98
Pneumonia Care				
Appropriate Initial Antibiotic Given[2]	66	98%	94%	95%
Blood Culture Timing[2]	78	91%	98%	98%
Pregnancy and Delivery Care				
Newborn Deliveries Scheduled Early[5]	-	-	6%	6%
Preventive Care				
Immunization for Influenza[2]	290	93%	89%	90%
Immunization for Pneumonia[2]	419	99%	92%	92%
Stroke Care				
Anticoagulation Therapy for Atrial Fibrillation[5]	-	-	90%	95%
Antithrombotic Therapy Timing[5]	-	-	96%	98%
Assessed for Rehabilitation[5]	-	-	95%	97%

NOTE: Hospital profiles are in alphabetical order by state, then city, then hospital within the city; Rankings exclude hospitals with less than 25 cases except for patient surveys which excludes hospitals with less than 100 cases; (a) 100-299 cases; (1) The number of cases/patients is too few to report; (2) Data submitted were based on a sample of cases/patients; (3) Results are based on a shorter time period than required; (4) Data suppressed by CMS for one or more quarters; (5) Results are not available for this reporting period; (6) Fewer than 100 patients completed the HCAHPS survey; (7) No cases met the criteria for this measure; (8) The lower limit of the confidence interval cannot be calculated if the number of observed infections equals zero; (9) No data are available from the state/territory for this reporting period; (10) The scores shown reflect fewer than 50 completed surveys; (11) There were discrepancies in the data collection process; (12) This measure does not apply to this hospital for this reporting period; (13) Results cannot be calculated for this reporting period; (14) The results for this state are combined with nearby states to protect confidentiality; Please refer to the User's Guide for a full explanation of data.

Measure	Cases	This Hosp.	State Avg.	U.S. Avg.
Discharged on Antithrombotic Therapy[5]	-	-	96%	99%
Discharged on Statin Medication[5]	-	-	86%	94%
Thrombolytic Therapy Timing[5]	-	-	35%	66%
Venous Thromboembolism Prophylaxis[5]	-	-	91%	94%
Written Stroke Educational Materials Given[5]	-	-	81%	88%
Surgical Care Improvement Project				
Appropriate Beta Blocker Usage[1]	-	-	98%	98%
Appropriate VTP Within 24 Hours	13	100%	98%	98%
Controlled Postoperative Blood Glucose[7]	-	-	99%	97%
Perioperative Temperature Management	16	94%	100%	100%
Prophylactic Antibiotic Selection[1]	-	-	99%	99%
Prophylactic Antibiotic Selection (Outpatient)[5]	-	-	98%	98%
Prophylactic Antibiotic Stopped[1]	-	-	98%	98%
Prophylactic Antibiotic Timing[1]	-	-	99%	99%
Prophylactic Antibiotic Timing (Outpatient)[5]	-	-	98%	98%
Urinary Catheter Removal[1]	-	-	97%	97%
Survey of Patients' Hospital Experiences				
Area Around Room 'Always' Quiet at Night[5]	-	-	67%	61%
Doctors 'Always' Communicated Well[5]	-	-	83%	82%
Home Recovery Information Given[5]	-	-	83%	85%
Hospital Given 9 or 10 on 10 Point Scale[5]	-	-	70%	71%
Meds 'Always' Explained Before Given[5]	-	-	63%	64%
Nurses 'Always' Communicated Well[5]	-	-	79%	79%
Pain 'Always' Well Controlled[5]	-	-	71%	71%
Room and Bathroom 'Always' Clean[5]	-	-	72%	73%
Timely Help 'Always' Received[5]	-	-	68%	68%
Would Definitely Recommend Hospital[5]	-	-	69%	71%
Use of Medical Imaging				
Cardiac Imaging Stress Test before Surgery	49	4.1%	4.3%	5.3%
Combination Abdominal CT Scan	145	0.7%	15.3%	10.5%
Combination Brain/Sinus CT Scan[1]	-	-	2.9%	2.7%
Combination Chest CT Scan	53	0.0%	5%	2.7%
Follow-up Mammogram/Ultrasound	278	6.1%	9.9%	8.8%
Lumbar Spine MRI for Low Back Pain[1]	-	-	41.6%	37.2%

Great River Medical Center

1520 N Division Street
Blytheville, AR 72315
Phone: 870-838-7300
Fax: 870-838-7493
E-mail: info@greatrivermc.com
URL: www.greatrivermc.com
Type: Acute Care Hospitals
Emergency Services: Yes
Ownership: Government - Local
Beds: 168

Key Personnel:
Emergency Room . . . . Lisa Alsup
Operating Room. . . . . Gayle Bradford
Radiology. . . . . Dr Dunne
Intensive Care Unit. . . . . Creseana Gist
Chief of Medical Staff . . . . Karen Hester, MD
Hemotology Center . . . . Mike Viar
Infection Control. . . . . Willa Warren

Measure	Cases	This Hosp.	State Avg.	U.S. Avg.
Blood Clot Prevention and Treatment				
Anticoagulation Overlap Therapy[1,2]	-	-	88%	93%
ICU Venous Thromboembolism Prophylaxis[2]	53	85%	94%	92%
Incidence of Potentially Preventable VTE[1,2]	-	-	12%	10%
UFH with Dosages/Platelet Monitoring[1,2]	-	-	100%	97%
Venous Thromboembolism Prophylaxis[2]	110	85%	91%	85%
Warfarin Therapy Discharge Instructions[1,2]	-	-	76%	75%
Chest Pain/Possible Heart Attack Care				
Aspirin Given Within 24 Hours of Arrival	67	96%	96%	96%
Fibrinolytic Meds Within 30 Min. of Arrival[1]	-	-	54%	58%
Average Time to ECG (minutes)	68	12	8	7
Average Time to Transfer (minutes)	11	69	72	60
Children's Asthma Care				
Received Home Management Plan of Care	-	-	-	88%
Received Reliever Medication	-	-	-	100%
Received Systemic Corticosteroids	-	-	-	100%
Emergency Department				
Admittance Decision Time (minutes)[2]	240	62	65	98
Head CT Results Within 45 Min. of Arrival[1]	-	-	49%	57%
Patients Who Left ER Before Being Seen	12,153	5%	3%	2%
Time from ER Arrival to Admit. (minutes)[2]	240	204	214	274
Time from ER Arrival to Discharge (minutes)	396	122	118	134
Time in ER Before Being Evaluated (minutes)	570	31	26	26
Time to Pain Meds for Fractures (minutes)	41	79	66	57
Heart Attack Care				
Aspirin Given at Discharge[1]	-	-	99%	99%
Fibrinolytic Meds Within 30 Min. of Arrival[7]	-	-	77%	54%
PCI Within 90 Minutes of Arrival[7]	-	-	96%	96%
Statin Prescribed at Discharge[1]	-	-	97%	98%
Heart Failure Care				
ACE Inhibitor or ARB for LVSD	32	88%	96%	97%
Discharge Instructions Given	77	92%	95%	94%
Evaluation of LVS Function	89	93%	98%	99%
Medicare Spending				
Medicare Spending per Patient (ratio)	-	0.89	0.98	0.98
Pneumonia Care				
Appropriate Initial Antibiotic Given[2]	69	87%	94%	95%
Blood Culture Timing[2]	123	98%	98%	98%
Pregnancy and Delivery Care				
Newborn Deliveries Scheduled Early[1,2]	-	-	6%	6%
Preventive Care				
Immunization for Influenza[2]	236	51%	89%	90%
Immunization for Pneumonia[2]	233	69%	92%	92%
Stroke Care				
Anticoagulation Therapy for Atrial Fibrillation[7]	-	-	90%	95%
Antithrombotic Therapy Timing[1]	-	-	96%	98%
Assessed for Rehabilitation[1]	-	-	95%	97%
Discharged on Antithrombotic Therapy[1]	-	-	96%	99%
Discharged on Statin Medication[1]	-	-	86%	94%
Thrombolytic Therapy Timing[1]	-	-	35%	66%
Venous Thromboembolism Prophylaxis[1]	-	-	91%	94%
Written Stroke Educational Materials Given[1]	-	-	81%	88%
Surgical Care Improvement Project				
Appropriate Beta Blocker Usage[7]	-	-	98%	98%
Appropriate VTP Within 24 Hours	11	100%	98%	98%
Controlled Postoperative Blood Glucose[7]	-	-	99%	97%
Perioperative Temperature Management	13	100%	100%	100%
Prophylactic Antibiotic Selection	11	82%	99%	99%
Prophylactic Antibiotic Selection (Outpatient)	20	80%	98%	98%
Prophylactic Antibiotic Stopped	11	91%	98%	98%
Prophylactic Antibiotic Timing	11	100%	99%	99%
Prophylactic Antibiotic Timing (Outpatient)	26	77%	98%	98%
Urinary Catheter Removal[1]	-	-	97%	97%
Survey of Patients' Hospital Experiences				
Area Around Room 'Always' Quiet at Night	(a)	61%	67%	61%
Doctors 'Always' Communicated Well	(a)	77%	83%	82%
Home Recovery Information Given	(a)	77%	83%	85%
Hospital Given 9 or 10 on 10 Point Scale	(a)	51%	70%	71%
Meds 'Always' Explained Before Given	(a)	56%	63%	64%
Nurses 'Always' Communicated Well	(a)	75%	79%	79%
Pain 'Always' Well Controlled	(a)	68%	71%	71%
Room and Bathroom 'Always' Clean	(a)	60%	72%	73%
Timely Help 'Always' Received	(a)	62%	68%	68%
Would Definitely Recommend Hospital	(a)	47%	69%	71%
Use of Medical Imaging				
Cardiac Imaging Stress Test before Surgery[1]	-	-	4.3%	5.3%
Combination Abdominal CT Scan	224	23.7%	15.3%	10.5%
Combination Brain/Sinus CT Scan	266	7.5%	2.9%	2.7%
Combination Chest CT Scan	86	43.0%	5%	2.7%
Follow-up Mammogram/Ultrasound	261	8.0%	9.9%	8.8%
Lumbar Spine MRI for Low Back Pain[1]	-	-	41.6%	37.2%

Mercy Hospital Booneville

880 West Main
Booneville, AR 72927
Phone: 479-675-2800
Fax: 479-675-4842
E-mail: gldelforge@hotmail.com
URL: www.boonevillehospital.com
Type: Critical Access Hospitals
Emergency Services: Yes
Ownership: Voluntary non-profit - Private
Beds: 25

Key Personnel:
Emergency Room . . . . LeAnn Box
Quality Assurance . . . . Lucia Brasher
Chief of Medical Staff. . . . . William Daniel, MD
CEO/President. . . . . Gary DelForge
Pediatric Ambulatory Care . . . . . . Samina Nadvi, MD
Pediatric In-Patient Care . . . . Samina Nadvi, MD
Infection Control. . . . . Nikki Parker
Operating Room. . . . . Barbara Templeman, RN

Measure	Cases	This Hosp.	State Avg.	U.S. Avg.
Blood Clot Prevention and Treatment				
Anticoagulation Overlap Therapy[5]	-	-	88%	93%
ICU Venous Thromboembolism Prophylaxis[5]	-	-	94%	92%
Incidence of Potentially Preventable VTE[5]	-	-	12%	10%
UFH with Dosages/Platelet Monitoring[5]	-	-	100%	97%
Venous Thromboembolism Prophylaxis[5]	-	-	91%	85%
Warfarin Therapy Discharge Instructions[5]	-	-	76%	75%
Chest Pain/Possible Heart Attack Care				
Aspirin Given Within 24 Hours of Arrival	-	-	96%	96%
Fibrinolytic Meds Within 30 Min. of Arrival	-	-	54%	58%
Average Time to ECG (minutes)	-	-	8	7
Average Time to Transfer (minutes)	-	-	72	60
Children's Asthma Care				
Received Home Management Plan of Care	-	-	-	88%
Received Reliever Medication	-	-	-	100%
Received Systemic Corticosteroids	-	-	-	100%
Emergency Department				
Admittance Decision Time (minutes)[2]	108	18	65	98
Head CT Results Within 45 Min. of Arrival	-	-	49%	57%
Patients Who Left ER Before Being Seen	-	-	3%	2%
Time from ER Arrival to Admit. (minutes)[2]	142	160	214	274
Time from ER Arrival to Discharge (minutes)	-	-	118	134
Time in ER Before Being Evaluated (minutes)	-	-	26	26
Time to Pain Meds for Fractures (minutes)	-	-	66	57
Heart Attack Care				
Aspirin Given at Discharge[1,3]	-	-	99%	99%
Fibrinolytic Meds Within 30 Min. of Arrival[3,7]	-	-	77%	54%
PCI Within 90 Minutes of Arrival[3,7]	-	-	96%	96%
Statin Prescribed at Discharge[1,3]	-	-	97%	98%
Heart Failure Care				
ACE Inhibitor or ARB for LVSD[1,2]	-	-	96%	97%
Discharge Instructions Given[1,2]	-	-	95%	94%
Evaluation of LVS Function[2]	12	75%	98%	99%
Medicare Spending				
Medicare Spending per Patient (ratio)	-	-	0.98	0.98
Pneumonia Care				
Appropriate Initial Antibiotic Given[2]	22	77%	94%	95%
Blood Culture Timing[2]	52	96%	98%	98%
Pregnancy and Delivery Care				
Newborn Deliveries Scheduled Early[5]	-	-	6%	6%
Preventive Care				
Immunization for Influenza[2]	68	56%	89%	90%
Immunization for Pneumonia[2]	120	55%	92%	92%
Stroke Care				
Anticoagulation Therapy for Atrial Fibrillation[2,3]	-	-	90%	95%
Antithrombotic Therapy Timing[1,2]	-	-	96%	98%
Assessed for Rehabilitation[1,2]	-	-	95%	97%
Discharged on Antithrombotic Therapy[1,2]	-	-	96%	99%
Discharged on Statin Medication[1,2]	-	-	86%	94%
Thrombolytic Therapy Timing[2,3]	-	-	35%	66%
Venous Thromboembolism Prophylaxis[1,2]	-	-	91%	94%
Written Stroke Educational Materials Given[2,3]	-	-	81%	88%
Surgical Care Improvement Project				
Appropriate Beta Blocker Usage[5]	-	-	98%	98%
Appropriate VTP Within 24 Hours[5]	-	-	98%	98%
Controlled Postoperative Blood Glucose[5]	-	-	99%	97%
Perioperative Temperature Management[5]	-	-	100%	100%
Prophylactic Antibiotic Selection[5]	-	-	99%	99%
Prophylactic Antibiotic Selection (Outpatient)	-	-	98%	98%
Prophylactic Antibiotic Stopped[5]	-	-	98%	98%
Prophylactic Antibiotic Timing[5]	-	-	99%	99%
Prophylactic Antibiotic Timing (Outpatient)	-	-	98%	98%
Urinary Catheter Removal[5]	-	-	97%	97%
Survey of Patients' Hospital Experiences				
Area Around Room 'Always' Quiet at Night[5]	-	-	67%	61%
Doctors 'Always' Communicated Well[5]	-	-	83%	82%
Home Recovery Information Given[5]	-	-	83%	85%
Hospital Given 9 or 10 on 10 Point Scale[5]	-	-	70%	71%
Meds 'Always' Explained Before Given[5]	-	-	63%	64%
Nurses 'Always' Communicated Well[5]	-	-	79%	79%
Pain 'Always' Well Controlled[5]	-	-	71%	71%

NOTE: Hospital profiles are in alphabetical order by state, then city, then hospital within the city; Rankings exclude hospitals with less than 25 cases except for patient surveys which excludes hospitals with less than 100 cases; (a) 100-299 cases; (1) The number of cases/patients is too few to report; (2) Data submitted were based on a sample of cases/patients; (3) Results are based on a shorter time period than required; (4) Data suppressed by CMS for one or more quarters; (5) Results are not available for this reporting period; (6) Fewer than 100 patients completed the HCAHPS survey; (7) No cases met the criteria for this measure; (8) The lower limit of the confidence interval cannot be calculated if the number of observed infections equals zero; (9) No data are available from the state/territory for this reporting period; (10) The scores shown reflect fewer than 50 completed surveys; (11) There were discrepancies in the data collection process; (12) This measure does not apply to this hospital for this reporting period; (13) Results cannot be calculated for this reporting period; (14) The results for this state are combined with nearby states to protect confidentiality; Please refer to the User's Guide for a full explanation of data.

Measure	Cases	This Hosp.	State Avg.	U.S. Avg.
Room and Bathroom 'Always' Clean[5]	-	-	72%	73%
Timely Help 'Always' Received[5]	-	-	68%	68%
Would Definitely Recommend Hospital[5]	-	-	69%	71%
Use of Medical Imaging				
Cardiac Imaging Stress Test before Surgery	-	-	4.3%	5.3%
Combination Abdominal CT Scan	-	-	15.3%	10.5%
Combination Brain/Sinus CT Scan	-	-	2.9%	2.7%
Combination Chest CT Scan	-	-	5%	2.7%
Follow-up Mammogram/Ultrasound	-	-	9.9%	8.8%
Lumbar Spine MRI for Low Back Pain	-	-	41.6%	37.2%

Community Medical Center Izard County

103 Grasse Street
Calico Rock, AR 72519
Phone: 870-297-3726
Type: Critical Access Hospitals
Emergency Services: No
Ownership: Voluntary non-profit - Private

Measure	Cases	This Hosp.	State Avg.	U.S. Avg.
Blood Clot Prevention and Treatment				
Anticoagulation Overlap Therapy[5]	-	-	88%	93%
ICU Venous Thromboembolism Prophylaxis[5]	-	-	94%	92%
Incidence of Potentially Preventable VTE[5]	-	-	12%	10%
UFH with Dosages/Platelet Monitoring[5]	-	-	100%	97%
Venous Thromboembolism Prophylaxis[5]	-	-	91%	85%
Warfarin Therapy Discharge Instructions[5]	-	-	76%	75%
Chest Pain/Possible Heart Attack Care				
Aspirin Given Within 24 Hours of Arrival	-	-	96%	96%
Fibrinolytic Meds Within 30 Min. of Arrival	-	-	54%	58%
Average Time to ECG (minutes)	-	-	8	7
Average Time to Transfer (minutes)	-	-	72	60
Children's Asthma Care				
Received Home Management Plan of Care	-	-	-	88%
Received Reliever Medication	-	-	-	100%
Received Systemic Corticosteroids	-	-	-	100%
Emergency Department				
Admittance Decision Time (minutes)[5]	-	-	65	98
Head CT Results Within 45 Min. of Arrival	-	-	49%	57%
Patients Who Left ER Before Being Seen	-	-	3%	2%
Time from ER Arrival to Admit. (minutes)[5]	-	-	214	274
Time from ER Arrival to Discharge (minutes)	-	-	118	134
Time in ER Before Being Evaluated (minutes)	-	-	26	26
Time to Pain Meds for Fractures (minutes)	-	-	66	57
Heart Attack Care				
Aspirin Given at Discharge[5]	-	-	99%	99%
Fibrinolytic Meds Within 30 Min. of Arrival[5]	-	-	77%	54%
PCI Within 90 Minutes of Arrival[5]	-	-	96%	96%
Statin Prescribed at Discharge[5]	-	-	97%	98%
Heart Failure Care				
ACE Inhibitor or ARB for LVSD[1,2]	-	-	96%	97%
Discharge Instructions Given[2]	16	56%	95%	94%
Evaluation of LVS Function[2]	14	79%	98%	99%
Medicare Spending				
Medicare Spending per Patient (ratio)	-	-	0.98	0.98
Pneumonia Care				
Appropriate Initial Antibiotic Given[1,2]	-	-	94%	95%
Blood Culture Timing[1,2]	-	-	98%	98%
Pregnancy and Delivery Care				
Newborn Deliveries Scheduled Early[5]	-	-	6%	6%
Preventive Care				
Immunization for Influenza[5]	-	-	89%	90%
Immunization for Pneumonia[5]	-	-	92%	92%
Stroke Care				
Anticoagulation Therapy for Atrial Fibrillation[5]	-	-	90%	95%
Antithrombotic Therapy Timing[5]	-	-	96%	98%
Assessed for Rehabilitation[5]	-	-	95%	97%
Discharged on Antithrombotic Therapy[5]	-	-	96%	99%
Discharged on Statin Medication[5]	-	-	86%	94%
Thrombolytic Therapy Timing[5]	-	-	35%	66%
Venous Thromboembolism Prophylaxis[5]	-	-	91%	94%
Written Stroke Educational Materials Given[5]	-	-	81%	88%
Surgical Care Improvement Project				
Appropriate Beta Blocker Usage[5]	-	-	98%	98%
Appropriate VTP Within 24 Hours[5]	-	-	98%	98%
Controlled Postoperative Blood Glucose[5]	-	-	99%	97%
Perioperative Temperature Management[5]	-	-	100%	100%
Prophylactic Antibiotic Selection[5]	-	-	99%	99%
Prophylactic Antibiotic Selection (Outpatient)	-	-	98%	98%
Prophylactic Antibiotic Stopped[5]	-	-	98%	98%
Prophylactic Antibiotic Timing[5]	-	-	99%	99%
Prophylactic Antibiotic Timing (Outpatient)	-	-	98%	98%
Urinary Catheter Removal[5]	-	-	97%	97%
Survey of Patients' Hospital Experiences				
Area Around Room 'Always' Quiet at Night[5]	-	-	67%	61%
Doctors 'Always' Communicated Well[5]	-	-	83%	82%
Home Recovery Information Given[5]	-	-	83%	85%
Hospital Given 9 or 10 on 10 Point Scale[5]	-	-	70%	71%
Meds 'Always' Explained Before Given[5]	-	-	63%	64%
Nurses 'Always' Communicated Well[5]	-	-	79%	79%
Pain 'Always' Well Controlled[5]	-	-	71%	71%
Room and Bathroom 'Always' Clean[5]	-	-	72%	73%
Timely Help 'Always' Received[5]	-	-	68%	68%
Would Definitely Recommend Hospital[5]	-	-	69%	71%
Use of Medical Imaging				
Cardiac Imaging Stress Test before Surgery	-	-	4.3%	5.3%
Combination Abdominal CT Scan	-	-	15.3%	10.5%
Combination Brain/Sinus CT Scan	-	-	2.9%	2.7%
Combination Chest CT Scan	-	-	5%	2.7%
Follow-up Mammogram/Ultrasound	-	-	9.9%	8.8%
Lumbar Spine MRI for Low Back Pain	-	-	41.6%	37.2%

Ouachita County Medical Center

638 California Avenue
Camden, AR 71701
Phone: 870-836-1000
Fax: 870-836-1358
E-mail: ocmc@ipa.net
URL: www.ouachitamedcenter.com
Type: Acute Care Hospitals
Emergency Services: Yes
Ownership: Voluntary non-profit - Private
Beds: 98

Key Personnel:
Chief of Medical Staff. . . . . Dr Gale Allen McFarland
CEO/President. . . . . David Cicero
Quality Assurance . . . . Connie Davis
Operating Room. . . . . Melodee Sanders

Measure	Cases	This Hosp.	State Avg.	U.S. Avg.
Blood Clot Prevention and Treatment				
Anticoagulation Overlap Therapy[2]	16	81%	88%	93%
ICU Venous Thromboembolism Prophylaxis[2]	43	100%	94%	92%
Incidence of Potentially Preventable VTE[1,2]	-	-	12%	10%
UFH with Dosages/Platelet Monitoring[2,7]	-	-	100%	97%
Venous Thromboembolism Prophylaxis[2]	112	96%	91%	85%
Warfarin Therapy Discharge Instructions[2]	11	91%	76%	75%
Chest Pain/Possible Heart Attack Care				
Aspirin Given Within 24 Hours of Arrival	113	99%	96%	96%
Fibrinolytic Meds Within 30 Min. of Arrival	11	64%	54%	58%
Average Time to ECG (minutes)	107	8	8	7
Average Time to Transfer (minutes)[1]	-	-	72	60
Children's Asthma Care				
Received Home Management Plan of Care	-	-	-	88%
Received Reliever Medication	-	-	-	100%
Received Systemic Corticosteroids	-	-	-	100%
Emergency Department				
Admittance Decision Time (minutes)[2]	284	72	65	98
Head CT Results Within 45 Min. of Arrival[1]	-	-	49%	57%
Patients Who Left ER Before Being Seen	11,429	4%	3%	2%
Time from ER Arrival to Admit. (minutes)[2]	284	285	214	274
Time from ER Arrival to Discharge (minutes)	216	136	118	134
Time in ER Before Being Evaluated (minutes)	378	18	26	26
Time to Pain Meds for Fractures (minutes)	53	52	66	57
Heart Attack Care				
Aspirin Given at Discharge[7]	-	-	99%	99%
Fibrinolytic Meds Within 30 Min. of Arrival[7]	-	-	77%	54%
PCI Within 90 Minutes of Arrival[7]	-	-	96%	96%
Statin Prescribed at Discharge[7]	-	-	97%	98%
Heart Failure Care				
ACE Inhibitor or ARB for LVSD	13	85%	96%	97%
Discharge Instructions Given	52	92%	95%	94%
Evaluation of LVS Function	71	96%	98%	99%
Medicare Spending				
Medicare Spending per Patient (ratio)	-	1.05	0.98	0.98
Pneumonia Care				
Appropriate Initial Antibiotic Given	46	100%	94%	95%
Blood Culture Timing	33	94%	98%	98%
Pregnancy and Delivery Care				
Newborn Deliveries Scheduled Early	25	4%	6%	6%
Preventive Care				
Immunization for Influenza[2]	270	98%	89%	90%
Immunization for Pneumonia[2]	345	98%	92%	92%
Stroke Care				
Anticoagulation Therapy for Atrial Fibrillation[1]	-	-	90%	95%
Antithrombotic Therapy Timing	22	82%	96%	98%
Assessed for Rehabilitation	22	100%	95%	97%
Discharged on Antithrombotic Therapy	21	81%	96%	99%
Discharged on Statin Medication	19	63%	86%	94%
Thrombolytic Therapy Timing[7]	-	-	35%	66%
Venous Thromboembolism Prophylaxis	22	95%	91%	94%
Written Stroke Educational Materials Given[1]	-	-	81%	88%
Surgical Care Improvement Project				
Appropriate Beta Blocker Usage[7]	-	-	98%	98%
Appropriate VTP Within 24 Hours	49	94%	98%	98%
Controlled Postoperative Blood Glucose[7]	-	-	99%	97%
Perioperative Temperature Management	52	100%	100%	100%
Prophylactic Antibiotic Selection	26	100%	99%	99%
Prophylactic Antibiotic Selection (Outpatient)	26	100%	98%	98%
Prophylactic Antibiotic Stopped	26	100%	98%	98%
Prophylactic Antibiotic Timing	26	96%	99%	99%
Prophylactic Antibiotic Timing (Outpatient)	26	100%	98%	98%
Urinary Catheter Removal[1]	-	-	97%	97%
Survey of Patients' Hospital Experiences				
Area Around Room 'Always' Quiet at Night	300+	69%	67%	61%
Doctors 'Always' Communicated Well	300+	87%	83%	82%
Home Recovery Information Given	300+	81%	83%	85%
Hospital Given 9 or 10 on 10 Point Scale	300+	69%	70%	71%
Meds 'Always' Explained Before Given	300+	63%	63%	64%
Nurses 'Always' Communicated Well	300+	85%	79%	79%
Pain 'Always' Well Controlled	300+	73%	71%	71%
Room and Bathroom 'Always' Clean	300+	80%	72%	73%
Timely Help 'Always' Received	300+	78%	68%	68%
Would Definitely Recommend Hospital	300+	69%	69%	71%
Use of Medical Imaging				
Cardiac Imaging Stress Test before Surgery[1]	-	-	4.3%	5.3%
Combination Abdominal CT Scan	319	9.4%	15.3%	10.5%
Combination Brain/Sinus CT Scan	339	8.3%	2.9%	2.7%
Combination Chest CT Scan	226	0.9%	5%	2.7%
Follow-up Mammogram/Ultrasound	232	7.8%	9.9%	8.8%
Lumbar Spine MRI for Low Back Pain	56	39.3%	41.6%	37.2%

Johnson Regional Medical Center

1100 East Poplar Street
Clarksville, AR 72830
Phone: 479-754-5454
Fax: 501-754-4019
URL: www.jrmc.com
Type: Acute Care Hospitals
Emergency Services: Yes
Ownership: Voluntary non-profit - Private
Beds: 68

Key Personnel:
Quality Assurance . . . . Maribel Baker
Intensive Care Unit. . . . . Lisa Carlton
Chief of Medical Staff . . . . Joe Dunanon
Radiology. . . . . Jeffrey Hale
CEO/President. . . . . Larry Morse
Patient Relations . . . . Terri Shumbaugh
Infection Control. . . . . Renay Storms
Operating Room. . . . . Lynn Yarbrough

Measure	Cases	This Hosp.	State Avg.	U.S. Avg.
Blood Clot Prevention and Treatment				
Anticoagulation Overlap Therapy[2]	13	38%	88%	93%
ICU Venous Thromboembolism Prophylaxis[2]	212	96%	94%	92%
Incidence of Potentially Preventable VTE[2,7]	-	-	12%	10%
UFH with Dosages/Platelet Monitoring[2,7]	-	-	100%	97%
Venous Thromboembolism Prophylaxis[2]	504	86%	91%	85%
Warfarin Therapy Discharge Instructions[1,2]	-	-	76%	75%
Chest Pain/Possible Heart Attack Care				
Aspirin Given Within 24 Hours of Arrival	102	99%	96%	96%

NOTE: Hospital profiles are in alphabetical order by state, then city, then hospital within the city; Rankings exclude hospitals with less than 25 cases except for patient surveys which excludes hospitals with less than 100 cases; (a) 100-299 cases; (1) The number of cases/patients is too few to report; (2) Data submitted were based on a sample of cases/patients; (3) Results are based on a shorter time period than required; (4) Data suppressed by CMS for one or more quarters; (5) Results are not available for this reporting period; (6) Fewer than 100 patients completed the HCAHPS survey; (7) No cases met the criteria for this measure; (8) The lower limit of the confidence interval cannot be calculated if the number of observed infections equals zero; (9) No data are available from the state/territory for this reporting period; (10) The scores shown reflect fewer than 50 completed surveys; (11) There were discrepancies in the data collection process; (12) This measure does not apply to this hospital for this reporting period; (13) Results cannot be calculated for this reporting period; (14) The results for this state are combined with nearby states to protect confidentiality; Please refer to the User's Guide for a full explanation of data.

Measure	Cases	This Hosp.	State Avg.	U.S. Avg.
Fibrinolytic Meds Within 30 Min. of Arrival[1]	-	-	54%	58%
Average Time to ECG (minutes)	106	5	8	7
Average Time to Transfer (minutes)[1]	-	-	72	60
Children's Asthma Care				
Received Home Management Plan of Care	-	-	-	88%
Received Reliever Medication	-	-	-	100%
Received Systemic Corticosteroids	-	-	-	100%
Emergency Department				
Admittance Decision Time (minutes)[2]	189	99	65	98
Head CT Results Within 45 Min. of Arrival[1]	-	-	49%	57%
Patients Who Left ER Before Being Seen	15,314	7%	3%	2%
Time from ER Arrival to Admit. (minutes)[2]	203	269	214	274
Time from ER Arrival to Discharge (minutes)	226	128	118	134
Time in ER Before Being Evaluated (minutes)	95	34	26	26
Time to Pain Meds for Fractures (minutes)	80	70	66	57
Heart Attack Care				
Aspirin Given at Discharge[1]	-	-	99%	99%
Fibrinolytic Meds Within 30 Min. of Arrival[7]	-	-	77%	54%
PCI Within 90 Minutes of Arrival[7]	-	-	96%	96%
Statin Prescribed at Discharge[1]	-	-	97%	98%
Heart Failure Care				
ACE Inhibitor or ARB for LVSD	11	82%	96%	97%
Discharge Instructions Given	35	89%	95%	94%
Evaluation of LVS Function	38	97%	98%	99%
Medicare Spending				
Medicare Spending per Patient (ratio)	-	0.95	0.98	0.98
Pneumonia Care				
Appropriate Initial Antibiotic Given	113	95%	94%	95%
Blood Culture Timing	101	95%	98%	98%
Pregnancy and Delivery Care				
Newborn Deliveries Scheduled Early[2]	46	2%	6%	6%
Preventive Care				
Immunization for Influenza[2]	222	94%	89%	90%
Immunization for Pneumonia[2]	234	97%	92%	92%
Stroke Care				
Anticoagulation Therapy for Atrial Fibrillation[1]	-	-	90%	95%
Antithrombotic Therapy Timing	19	84%	96%	98%
Assessed for Rehabilitation	17	88%	95%	97%
Discharged on Antithrombotic Therapy	16	88%	96%	99%
Discharged on Statin Medication	15	87%	86%	94%
Thrombolytic Therapy Timing[7]	-	-	35%	66%
Venous Thromboembolism Prophylaxis	19	89%	91%	94%
Written Stroke Educational Materials Given[1]	-	-	81%	88%
Surgical Care Improvement Project				
Appropriate Beta Blocker Usage	38	95%	98%	98%
Appropriate VTP Within 24 Hours	101	95%	98%	98%
Controlled Postoperative Blood Glucose[7]	-	-	99%	97%
Perioperative Temperature Management	119	100%	100%	100%
Prophylactic Antibiotic Selection	79	96%	99%	99%
Prophylactic Antibiotic Selection (Outpatient)	60	97%	98%	98%
Prophylactic Antibiotic Stopped	77	91%	98%	98%
Prophylactic Antibiotic Timing	79	97%	99%	99%
Prophylactic Antibiotic Timing (Outpatient)	58	97%	98%	98%
Urinary Catheter Removal	88	98%	97%	97%
Survey of Patients' Hospital Experiences				
Area Around Room 'Always' Quiet at Night	300+	59%	67%	61%
Doctors 'Always' Communicated Well	300+	81%	83%	82%
Home Recovery Information Given	300+	80%	83%	85%
Hospital Given 9 or 10 on 10 Point Scale	300+	59%	70%	71%
Meds 'Always' Explained Before Given	300+	62%	63%	64%
Nurses 'Always' Communicated Well	300+	73%	79%	79%
Pain 'Always' Well Controlled	300+	68%	71%	71%
Room and Bathroom 'Always' Clean	300+	79%	72%	73%
Timely Help 'Always' Received	300+	69%	68%	68%
Would Definitely Recommend Hospital	300+	63%	69%	71%
Use of Medical Imaging				
Cardiac Imaging Stress Test before Surgery[1]	-	-	4.3%	5.3%
Combination Abdominal CT Scan	342	5.8%	15.3%	10.5%
Combination Brain/Sinus CT Scan	335	1.5%	2.9%	2.7%
Combination Chest CT Scan	197	1.5%	5%	2.7%
Follow-up Mammogram/Ultrasound	363	12.1%	9.9%	8.8%
Lumbar Spine MRI for Low Back Pain	52	57.7%	41.6%	37.2%

Ozark Health

2500 Highway 65 South
Clinton, AR 72031
Phone: 501-745-7004
Fax: 501-745-2472
E-mail: ozark@artelco.com
Type: Critical Access Hospitals
Emergency Services: Yes
Ownership: Voluntary non-profit - Private
Beds: 25

Key Personnel:

Pediatrics. . . . . Keith Coward
CEO . . . . David Deaton
Emergency Room . . . . Harriet Guglielmo
Quality Assurance . . . . Sandy Presley
Operating Room. . . . . Steve Schoettle, RN
Surgery . . . . Steve Schoettle
Chief of Medical Staff . . . . Harry Starnes

Measure	Cases	This Hosp.	State Avg.	U.S. Avg.
Blood Clot Prevention and Treatment				
Anticoagulation Overlap Therapy[5]	-	-	88%	93%
ICU Venous Thromboembolism Prophylaxis[5]	-	-	94%	92%
Incidence of Potentially Preventable VTE[5]	-	-	12%	10%
UFH with Dosages/Platelet Monitoring[5]	-	-	100%	97%
Venous Thromboembolism Prophylaxis[5]	-	-	91%	85%
Warfarin Therapy Discharge Instructions[5]	-	-	76%	75%
Chest Pain/Possible Heart Attack Care				
Aspirin Given Within 24 Hours of Arrival	53	91%	96%	96%
Fibrinolytic Meds Within 30 Min. of Arrival[1]	-	-	54%	58%
Average Time to ECG (minutes)	55	7	8	7
Average Time to Transfer (minutes)[7]	-	-	72	60
Children's Asthma Care				
Received Home Management Plan of Care	-	-	-	88%
Received Reliever Medication	-	-	-	100%
Received Systemic Corticosteroids	-	-	-	100%
Emergency Department				
Admittance Decision Time (minutes)[2]	334	30	65	98
Head CT Results Within 45 Min. of Arrival[3]	14	36%	49%	57%
Patients Who Left ER Before Being Seen	8,117	3%	3%	2%
Time from ER Arrival to Admit. (minutes)[2]	342	242	214	274
Time from ER Arrival to Discharge (minutes)[5]	-	-	118	134
Time in ER Before Being Evaluated (minutes)[5]	-	-	26	26
Time to Pain Meds for Fractures (minutes)[5]	-	-	66	57
Heart Attack Care				
Aspirin Given at Discharge[1,3]	-	-	99%	99%
Fibrinolytic Meds Within 30 Min. of Arrival[3,7]	-	-	77%	54%
PCI Within 90 Minutes of Arrival[3,7]	-	-	96%	96%
Statin Prescribed at Discharge[1,3]	-	-	97%	98%
Heart Failure Care				
ACE Inhibitor or ARB for LVSD[1]	-	-	96%	97%
Discharge Instructions Given	16	75%	95%	94%
Evaluation of LVS Function	28	96%	98%	99%
Medicare Spending				
Medicare Spending per Patient (ratio)	-	-	0.98	0.98
Pneumonia Care				
Appropriate Initial Antibiotic Given[2]	39	97%	94%	95%
Blood Culture Timing[2]	55	95%	98%	98%
Pregnancy and Delivery Care				
Newborn Deliveries Scheduled Early[3,7]	-	-	6%	6%
Preventive Care				
Immunization for Influenza[2]	251	91%	89%	90%
Immunization for Pneumonia[2]	433	91%	92%	92%
Stroke Care				
Anticoagulation Therapy for Atrial Fibrillation[1]	-	-	90%	95%
Antithrombotic Therapy Timing	13	100%	96%	98%
Assessed for Rehabilitation	12	100%	95%	97%
Discharged on Antithrombotic Therapy	12	100%	96%	99%
Discharged on Statin Medication[1]	-	-	86%	94%
Thrombolytic Therapy Timing[7]	-	-	35%	66%
Venous Thromboembolism Prophylaxis	14	100%	91%	94%
Written Stroke Educational Materials Given[1]	-	-	81%	88%
Surgical Care Improvement Project				
Appropriate Beta Blocker Usage[1]	-	-	98%	98%
Appropriate VTP Within 24 Hours	27	96%	98%	98%
Controlled Postoperative Blood Glucose[7]	-	-	99%	97%
Perioperative Temperature Management	28	100%	100%	100%
Prophylactic Antibiotic Selection	22	100%	99%	99%
Prophylactic Antibiotic Selection (Outpatient)[1,3]	-	-	98%	98%
Prophylactic Antibiotic Stopped	22	100%	98%	98%
Prophylactic Antibiotic Timing	22	100%	99%	99%
Prophylactic Antibiotic Timing (Outpatient)[1,3]	-	-	98%	98%
Urinary Catheter Removal	23	100%	97%	97%
Survey of Patients' Hospital Experiences				
Area Around Room 'Always' Quiet at Night[5]	-	-	67%	61%
Doctors 'Always' Communicated Well[5]	-	-	83%	82%
Home Recovery Information Given[5]	-	-	83%	85%
Hospital Given 9 or 10 on 10 Point Scale[5]	-	-	70%	71%
Meds 'Always' Explained Before Given[5]	-	-	63%	64%
Nurses 'Always' Communicated Well[5]	-	-	79%	79%
Pain 'Always' Well Controlled[5]	-	-	71%	71%
Room and Bathroom 'Always' Clean[5]	-	-	72%	73%
Timely Help 'Always' Received[5]	-	-	68%	68%
Would Definitely Recommend Hospital[5]	-	-	69%	71%
Use of Medical Imaging				
Cardiac Imaging Stress Test before Surgery[1]	-	-	4.3%	5.3%
Combination Abdominal CT Scan	251	1.2%	15.3%	10.5%
Combination Brain/Sinus CT Scan[1]	-	-	2.9%	2.7%
Combination Chest CT Scan	163	0.0%	5%	2.7%
Follow-up Mammogram/Ultrasound	207	9.2%	9.9%	8.8%
Lumbar Spine MRI for Low Back Pain	40	52.5%	41.6%	37.2%

Conway Regional Medical Center

2302 College Avenue
Conway, AR 72034
Phone: 501-329-3831
Fax: 501-450-2283
E-mail: info@conwayregional.org
URL: www.conwayregional.org
Type: Acute Care Hospitals
Emergency Services: Yes
Ownership: Voluntary non-profit - Private
Beds: 146

Key Personnel:

Radiology. . . . . Keith Bell
Chair/CEO . . . . Charlie DeBoard
Quality Assurance . . . . Tanya Gierke
CEO/President. . . . . Jim Lambert
Chief of Medical Staff . . . . Don Steely
Operating Room. . . . . Stephanie Strickland, RN

Measure	Cases	This Hosp.	State Avg.	U.S. Avg.
Blood Clot Prevention and Treatment				
Anticoagulation Overlap Therapy[2]	59	98%	88%	93%
ICU Venous Thromboembolism Prophylaxis[2]	82	90%	94%	92%
Incidence of Potentially Preventable VTE[1,2]	-	-	12%	10%
UFH with Dosages/Platelet Monitoring[2]	27	100%	100%	97%
Venous Thromboembolism Prophylaxis[2]	220	90%	91%	85%
Warfarin Therapy Discharge Instructions[2]	46	100%	76%	75%
Chest Pain/Possible Heart Attack Care				
Aspirin Given Within 24 Hours of Arrival[1,3]	-	-	96%	96%
Fibrinolytic Meds Within 30 Min. of Arrival[5]	-	-	54%	58%
Average Time to ECG (minutes)[1,3]	-	-	8	7
Average Time to Transfer (minutes)[5]	-	-	72	60
Children's Asthma Care				
Received Home Management Plan of Care	-	-	-	88%
Received Reliever Medication	-	-	-	100%
Received Systemic Corticosteroids	-	-	-	100%
Emergency Department				
Admittance Decision Time (minutes)[2]	497	85	65	98
Head CT Results Within 45 Min. of Arrival	14	100%	49%	57%
Patients Who Left ER Before Being Seen	40,337	5%	3%	2%
Time from ER Arrival to Admit. (minutes)[2]	497	244	214	274
Time from ER Arrival to Discharge (minutes)	445	127	118	134
Time in ER Before Being Evaluated (minutes)	516	39	26	26
Time to Pain Meds for Fractures (minutes)	212	74	66	57
Heart Attack Care				
Aspirin Given at Discharge	148	99%	99%	99%
Fibrinolytic Meds Within 30 Min. of Arrival[7]	-	-	77%	54%
PCI Within 90 Minutes of Arrival	35	100%	96%	96%
Statin Prescribed at Discharge	141	97%	97%	98%
Heart Failure Care				
ACE Inhibitor or ARB for LVSD	28	89%	96%	97%
Discharge Instructions Given	80	95%	95%	94%
Evaluation of LVS Function	109	97%	98%	99%
Medicare Spending				
Medicare Spending per Patient (ratio)	-	0.98	0.98	0.98
Pneumonia Care				

NOTE: Hospital profiles are in alphabetical order by state, then city, then hospital within the city; Rankings exclude hospitals with less than 25 cases except for patient surveys which excludes hospitals with less than 100 cases; (a) 100-299 cases; (1) The number of cases/patients is too few to report; (2) Data submitted were based on a sample of cases/patients; (3) Results are based on a shorter time period than required; (4) Data suppressed by CMS for one or more quarters; (5) Results are not available for this reporting period; (6) Fewer than 100 patients completed the HCAHPS survey; (7) No cases met the criteria for this measure; (8) The lower limit of the confidence interval cannot be calculated if the number of observed infections equals zero; (9) No data are available from the state/territory for this reporting period; (10) The scores shown reflect fewer than 50 completed surveys; (11) There were discrepancies in the data collection process; (12) This measure does not apply to this hospital for this reporting period; (13) Results cannot be calculated for this reporting period; (14) The results for this state are combined with nearby states to protect confidentiality; Please refer to the User's Guide for a full explanation of data.

Appropriate Initial Antibiotic Given[2]	116	84%	94%	95%
Blood Culture Timing[2]	201	100%	98%	98%
Pregnancy and Delivery Care				
Newborn Deliveries Scheduled Early[2]	114	10%	6%	6%
Preventive Care				
Immunization for Influenza[2]	551	87%	89%	90%
Immunization for Pneumonia[2]	517	91%	92%	92%
Stroke Care				
Anticoagulation Therapy for Atrial Fibrillation	16	100%	90%	95%
Antithrombotic Therapy Timing	87	99%	96%	98%
Assessed for Rehabilitation	96	97%	95%	97%
Discharged on Antithrombotic Therapy	93	99%	96%	99%
Discharged on Statin Medication	74	91%	86%	94%
Thrombolytic Therapy Timing[1]	-	-	35%	66%
Venous Thromboembolism Prophylaxis	87	93%	91%	94%
Written Stroke Educational Materials Given	55	98%	81%	88%
Surgical Care Improvement Project				
Appropriate Beta Blocker Usage[2]	107	97%	98%	98%
Appropriate VTP Within 24 Hours[2]	318	99%	98%	98%
Controlled Postoperative Blood Glucose[2]	84	99%	99%	97%
Perioperative Temperature Management[2]	409	100%	100%	100%
Prophylactic Antibiotic Selection[2]	366	98%	99%	99%
Prophylactic Antibiotic Selection (Outpatient)	307	96%	98%	98%
Prophylactic Antibiotic Stopped[2]	356	96%	98%	98%
Prophylactic Antibiotic Timing[2]	366	99%	99%	99%
Prophylactic Antibiotic Timing (Outpatient)	312	98%	98%	98%
Urinary Catheter Removal[2]	184	94%	97%	97%
Survey of Patients' Hospital Experiences				
Area Around Room 'Always' Quiet at Night	300+	69%	67%	61%
Doctors 'Always' Communicated Well	300+	83%	83%	82%
Home Recovery Information Given	300+	81%	83%	85%
Hospital Given 9 or 10 on 10 Point Scale	300+	72%	70%	71%
Meds 'Always' Explained Before Given	300+	64%	63%	64%
Nurses 'Always' Communicated Well	300+	81%	79%	79%
Pain 'Always' Well Controlled	300+	69%	71%	71%
Room and Bathroom 'Always' Clean	300+	73%	72%	73%
Timely Help 'Always' Received	300+	65%	68%	68%
Would Definitely Recommend Hospital	300+	71%	69%	71%
Use of Medical Imaging				
Cardiac Imaging Stress Test before Surgery	128	3.1%	4.3%	5.3%
Combination Abdominal CT Scan	996	7.9%	15.3%	10.5%
Combination Brain/Sinus CT Scan	903	1.9%	2.9%	2.7%
Combination Chest CT Scan	356	1.1%	5%	2.7%
Follow-up Mammogram/Ultrasound	2,153	10.3%	9.9%	8.8%
Lumbar Spine MRI for Low Back Pain	281	43.4%	41.6%	37.2%

Ashley County Medical Center

1015 Unity Road
Crossett, AR 71635
URL: www.acmonline.org
Phone: 870-364-4111
Fax: 870-364-1245
Type: Critical Access Hospitals
Emergency Services: Yes
Ownership: Voluntary non-profit - Private
Beds: 46

Key Personnel:
Infection Control. . . . . Myrna Bryan
Anesthesiology. . . . . Warren Gouner
Emergency Room . . . . William Lynn, MD
Intensive Care Unit. . . . . Nicki Miller
Operating Room. . . . . Margaret Pope, RN
Chief of Medical Staff . . . . Phillip Rindt, MD
CEO/President. . . . . Russ D Sword
Quality Assurance . . . . Donna White, RN

Measure	Cases	This Hosp.	State Avg.	U.S. Avg.
Blood Clot Prevention and Treatment				
Anticoagulation Overlap Therapy[5]	-	-	88%	93%
ICU Venous Thromboembolism Prophylaxis[5]	-	-	94%	92%
Incidence of Potentially Preventable VTE[5]	-	-	12%	10%
UFH with Dosages/Platelet Monitoring[5]	-	-	100%	97%
Venous Thromboembolism Prophylaxis[5]	-	-	91%	85%
Warfarin Therapy Discharge Instructions[5]	-	-	76%	75%
Chest Pain/Possible Heart Attack Care				
Aspirin Given Within 24 Hours of Arrival	43	98%	96%	96%
Fibrinolytic Meds Within 30 Min. of Arrival[1]	-	-	54%	58%
Average Time to ECG (minutes)	43	12	8	7
Average Time to Transfer (minutes)[7]	-	-	72	60
Children's Asthma Care				
Received Home Management Plan of Care	-	-	-	88%
Received Reliever Medication	-	-	-	100%
Received Systemic Corticosteroids	-	-	-	100%
Emergency Department				
Admittance Decision Time (minutes)[5]	-	-	65	98
Head CT Results Within 45 Min. of Arrival[5]	-	-	49%	57%
Patients Who Left ER Before Being Seen	7,598	4%	3%	2%
Time from ER Arrival to Admit. (minutes)[5]	-	-	214	274
Time from ER Arrival to Discharge (minutes)[5]	-	-	118	134
Time in ER Before Being Evaluated (minutes)[5]	-	-	26	26
Time to Pain Meds for Fractures (minutes)[5]	-	-	66	57
Heart Attack Care				
Aspirin Given at Discharge[5]	-	-	99%	99%
Fibrinolytic Meds Within 30 Min. of Arrival[5]	-	-	77%	54%
PCI Within 90 Minutes of Arrival[5]	-	-	96%	96%
Statin Prescribed at Discharge[5]	-	-	97%	98%
Heart Failure Care				
ACE Inhibitor or ARB for LVSD[1,3]	-	-	96%	97%
Discharge Instructions Given[3]	21	57%	95%	94%
Evaluation of LVS Function[3]	26	62%	98%	99%
Medicare Spending				
Medicare Spending per Patient (ratio)	-	-	0.98	0.98
Pneumonia Care				
Appropriate Initial Antibiotic Given	40	98%	94%	95%
Blood Culture Timing	41	95%	98%	98%
Pregnancy and Delivery Care				
Newborn Deliveries Scheduled Early[5]	-	-	6%	6%
Preventive Care				
Immunization for Influenza[5]	-	-	89%	90%
Immunization for Pneumonia[5]	-	-	92%	92%
Stroke Care				
Anticoagulation Therapy for Atrial Fibrillation[5]	-	-	90%	95%
Antithrombotic Therapy Timing[5]	-	-	96%	98%
Assessed for Rehabilitation[5]	-	-	95%	97%
Discharged on Antithrombotic Therapy[5]	-	-	96%	99%
Discharged on Statin Medication[5]	-	-	86%	94%
Thrombolytic Therapy Timing[5]	-	-	35%	66%
Venous Thromboembolism Prophylaxis[5]	-	-	91%	94%
Written Stroke Educational Materials Given[5]	-	-	81%	88%
Surgical Care Improvement Project				
Appropriate Beta Blocker Usage[5]	-	-	98%	98%
Appropriate VTP Within 24 Hours[5]	-	-	98%	98%
Controlled Postoperative Blood Glucose[5]	-	-	99%	97%
Perioperative Temperature Management[5]	-	-	100%	100%
Prophylactic Antibiotic Selection[5]	-	-	99%	99%
Prophylactic Antibiotic Selection (Outpatient)[1,3]	-	-	98%	98%
Prophylactic Antibiotic Stopped[5]	-	-	98%	98%
Prophylactic Antibiotic Timing[5]	-	-	99%	99%
Prophylactic Antibiotic Timing (Outpatient)[1,3]	-	-	98%	98%
Urinary Catheter Removal[5]	-	-	97%	97%
Survey of Patients' Hospital Experiences				
Area Around Room 'Always' Quiet at Night	(a)	71%	67%	61%
Doctors 'Always' Communicated Well	(a)	80%	83%	82%
Home Recovery Information Given	(a)	80%	83%	85%
Hospital Given 9 or 10 on 10 Point Scale	(a)	65%	70%	71%
Meds 'Always' Explained Before Given	(a)	56%	63%	64%
Nurses 'Always' Communicated Well	(a)	78%	79%	79%
Pain 'Always' Well Controlled	(a)	67%	71%	71%
Room and Bathroom 'Always' Clean	(a)	77%	72%	73%
Timely Help 'Always' Received	(a)	78%	68%	68%
Would Definitely Recommend Hospital	(a)	58%	69%	71%
Use of Medical Imaging				
Cardiac Imaging Stress Test before Surgery	106	1.9%	4.3%	5.3%
Combination Abdominal CT Scan	204	21.6%	15.3%	10.5%
Combination Brain/Sinus CT Scan[1]	-	-	2.9%	2.7%
Combination Chest CT Scan	131	15.3%	5%	2.7%
Follow-up Mammogram/Ultrasound	340	5.9%	9.9%	8.8%
Lumbar Spine MRI for Low Back Pain	40	47.5%	41.6%	37.2%

Chambers Memorial Hospital

719 Detroit Street
Danville, AR 72833
URL: www.chambershospital.com
Phone: 479-495-2241
Fax: 479-495-6290
Type: Acute Care Hospitals
Emergency Services: Yes
Ownership: Voluntary non-profit - Private
Beds: 41

Key Personnel:
Operating Room. . . . . Pat Briley
Quality Assurance . . . . Mary Anne Daves
CEO/President. . . . . Scott Peek
Radiology. . . . . Don Riley
Chief of Medical Staff . . . . Philip Tippin, MD

Measure	Cases	This Hosp.	State Avg.	U.S. Avg.
Blood Clot Prevention and Treatment				
Anticoagulation Overlap Therapy[1,2]	-	-	88%	93%
ICU Venous Thromboembolism Prophylaxis[1,2]	-	-	94%	92%
Incidence of Potentially Preventable VTE[2,7]	-	-	12%	10%
UFH with Dosages/Platelet Monitoring[2,7]	-	-	100%	97%
Venous Thromboembolism Prophylaxis[2]	223	90%	91%	85%
Warfarin Therapy Discharge Instructions[2,7]	-	-	76%	75%
Chest Pain/Possible Heart Attack Care				
Aspirin Given Within 24 Hours of Arrival	42	86%	96%	96%
Fibrinolytic Meds Within 30 Min. of Arrival[1,3]	-	-	54%	58%
Average Time to ECG (minutes)	37	11	8	7
Average Time to Transfer (minutes)[3,7]	-	-	72	60
Children's Asthma Care				
Received Home Management Plan of Care	-	-	-	88%
Received Reliever Medication	-	-	-	100%
Received Systemic Corticosteroids	-	-	-	100%
Emergency Department				
Admittance Decision Time (minutes)[2]	293	55	65	98
Head CT Results Within 45 Min. of Arrival[1]	-	-	49%	57%
Patients Who Left ER Before Being Seen	4,773	2%	3%	2%
Time from ER Arrival to Admit. (minutes)[2]	319	145	214	274
Time from ER Arrival to Discharge (minutes)	958	97	118	134
Time in ER Before Being Evaluated (minutes)	1,046	24	26	26
Time to Pain Meds for Fractures (minutes)	25	80	66	57
Heart Attack Care				
Aspirin Given at Discharge[1,3]	-	-	99%	99%
Fibrinolytic Meds Within 30 Min. of Arrival[3,7]	-	-	77%	54%
PCI Within 90 Minutes of Arrival[3,7]	-	-	96%	96%
Statin Prescribed at Discharge[3,7]	-	-	97%	98%
Heart Failure Care				
ACE Inhibitor or ARB for LVSD[1,2]	-	-	96%	97%
Discharge Instructions Given[2]	37	100%	95%	94%
Evaluation of LVS Function[2]	57	93%	98%	99%
Medicare Spending				
Medicare Spending per Patient (ratio)	-	0.77	0.98	0.98
Pneumonia Care				
Appropriate Initial Antibiotic Given[2]	46	96%	94%	95%
Blood Culture Timing[1,2]	-	-	98%	98%
Pregnancy and Delivery Care				
Newborn Deliveries Scheduled Early[7]	-	-	6%	6%
Preventive Care				
Immunization for Influenza[2]	293	84%	89%	90%
Immunization for Pneumonia[2]	331	89%	92%	92%
Stroke Care				
Anticoagulation Therapy for Atrial Fibrillation[1,2]	-	-	90%	95%
Antithrombotic Therapy Timing[2]	14	79%	96%	98%
Assessed for Rehabilitation[2]	20	75%	95%	97%
Discharged on Antithrombotic Therapy[2]	13	85%	96%	99%
Discharged on Statin Medication[1,2]	-	-	86%	94%
Thrombolytic Therapy Timing[2,7]	-	-	35%	66%
Venous Thromboembolism Prophylaxis[2]	18	78%	91%	94%
Written Stroke Educational Materials Given[1,2]	-	-	81%	88%
Surgical Care Improvement Project				
Appropriate Beta Blocker Usage[5]	-	-	98%	98%
Appropriate VTP Within 24 Hours[5]	-	-	98%	98%
Controlled Postoperative Blood Glucose[5]	-	-	99%	97%
Perioperative Temperature Management[5]	-	-	100%	100%
Prophylactic Antibiotic Selection[5]	-	-	99%	99%
Prophylactic Antibiotic Selection (Outpatient)[3,7]	-	-	98%	98%
Prophylactic Antibiotic Stopped[5]	-	-	98%	98%

NOTE: Hospital profiles are in alphabetical order by state, then city, then hospital within the city; Rankings exclude hospitals with less than 25 cases except for patient surveys which excludes hospitals with less than 100 cases; (a) 100-299 cases; (1) The number of cases/patients is too few to report; (2) Data submitted were based on a sample of cases/patients; (3) Results are based on a shorter time period than required; (4) Data suppressed by CMS for one or more quarters; (5) Results are not available for this reporting period; (6) Fewer than 100 patients completed the HCAHPS survey; (7) No cases met the criteria for this measure; (8) The lower limit of the confidence interval cannot be calculated if the number of observed infections equals zero; (9) No data are available from the state/territory for this reporting period; (10) The scores shown reflect fewer than 50 completed surveys; (11) There were discrepancies in the data collection process; (12) This measure does not apply to this hospital for this reporting period; (13) Results cannot be calculated for this reporting period; (14) The results for this state are combined with nearby states to protect confidentiality; Please refer to the User's Guide for a full explanation of data.

Measure	Cases	This Hosp.	State Avg.	U.S. Avg.
Prophylactic Antibiotic Timing[5]	-	-	99%	99%
Prophylactic Antibiotic Timing (Outpatient)[1,3]	-	-	98%	98%
Urinary Catheter Removal[5]	-	-	97%	97%
Survey of Patients' Hospital Experiences				
Area Around Room 'Always' Quiet at Night	(a)	74%	67%	61%
Doctors 'Always' Communicated Well	(a)	90%	83%	82%
Home Recovery Information Given	(a)	80%	83%	85%
Hospital Given 9 or 10 on 10 Point Scale	(a)	77%	70%	71%
Meds 'Always' Explained Before Given	(a)	73%	63%	64%
Nurses 'Always' Communicated Well	(a)	85%	79%	79%
Pain 'Always' Well Controlled	(a)	76%	71%	71%
Room and Bathroom 'Always' Clean	(a)	88%	72%	73%
Timely Help 'Always' Received	(a)	73%	68%	68%
Would Definitely Recommend Hospital	(a)	68%	69%	71%
Use of Medical Imaging				
Cardiac Imaging Stress Test before Surgery[7]	-	-	4.3%	5.3%
Combination Abdominal CT Scan	129	5.4%	15.3%	10.5%
Combination Brain/Sinus CT Scan[1]	-	-	2.9%	2.7%
Combination Chest CT Scan	69	0.0%	5%	2.7%
Follow-up Mammogram/Ultrasound[7]	-	-	9.9%	8.8%
Lumbar Spine MRI for Low Back Pain[1]	-	-	41.6%	37.2%

River Valley Medical Center

200 North Third Street
Dardanelle, AR 72834
Phone: 479-229-4677
Fax: 479-229-2738
Type: Critical Access Hospitals
Emergency Services: Yes
Ownership: Proprietary
Beds: 85

Key Personnel:
CEO/President. . . . . Sandra Wear

Measure	Cases	This Hosp.	State Avg.	U.S. Avg.
Blood Clot Prevention and Treatment				
Anticoagulation Overlap Therapy[5]	-	-	88%	93%
ICU Venous Thromboembolism Prophylaxis[5]	-	-	94%	92%
Incidence of Potentially Preventable VTE[5]	-	-	12%	10%
UFH with Dosages/Platelet Monitoring[5]	-	-	100%	97%
Venous Thromboembolism Prophylaxis[5]	-	-	91%	85%
Warfarin Therapy Discharge Instructions[5]	-	-	76%	75%
Chest Pain/Possible Heart Attack Care				
Aspirin Given Within 24 Hours of Arrival	17	82%	96%	96%
Fibrinolytic Meds Within 30 Min. of Arrival[1,3]	-	-	54%	58%
Average Time to ECG (minutes)	18	6	8	7
Average Time to Transfer (minutes)[1,3]	-	-	72	60
Children's Asthma Care				
Received Home Management Plan of Care	-	-	-	88%
Received Reliever Medication	-	-	-	100%
Received Systemic Corticosteroids	-	-	-	100%
Emergency Department				
Admittance Decision Time (minutes)[5]	-	-	65	98
Head CT Results Within 45 Min. of Arrival[5]	-	-	49%	57%
Patients Who Left ER Before Being Seen	4,943	9%	3%	2%
Time from ER Arrival to Admit. (minutes)[5]	-	-	214	274
Time from ER Arrival to Discharge (minutes)[5]	-	-	118	134
Time in ER Before Being Evaluated (minutes)[5]	-	-	26	26
Time to Pain Meds for Fractures (minutes)[1,3]	-	-	66	57
Heart Attack Care				
Aspirin Given at Discharge[5]	-	-	99%	99%
Fibrinolytic Meds Within 30 Min. of Arrival[5]	-	-	77%	54%
PCI Within 90 Minutes of Arrival[5]	-	-	96%	96%
Statin Prescribed at Discharge[5]	-	-	97%	98%
Heart Failure Care				
ACE Inhibitor or ARB for LVSD[1]	-	-	96%	97%
Discharge Instructions Given[1]	-	-	95%	94%
Evaluation of LVS Function	19	63%	98%	99%
Medicare Spending				
Medicare Spending per Patient (ratio)	-	-	0.98	0.98
Pneumonia Care				
Appropriate Initial Antibiotic Given	12	100%	94%	95%
Blood Culture Timing	16	88%	98%	98%
Pregnancy and Delivery Care				
Newborn Deliveries Scheduled Early[5]	-	-	6%	6%
Preventive Care				
Immunization for Influenza[5]	-	-	89%	90%
Immunization for Pneumonia[5]	-	-	92%	92%
Stroke Care				
Anticoagulation Therapy for Atrial Fibrillation[5]	-	-	90%	95%
Antithrombotic Therapy Timing[5]	-	-	96%	98%
Assessed for Rehabilitation[5]	-	-	95%	97%
Discharged on Antithrombotic Therapy[5]	-	-	96%	99%
Discharged on Statin Medication[5]	-	-	86%	94%
Thrombolytic Therapy Timing[5]	-	-	35%	66%
Venous Thromboembolism Prophylaxis[5]	-	-	91%	94%
Written Stroke Educational Materials Given[5]	-	-	81%	88%
Surgical Care Improvement Project				
Appropriate Beta Blocker Usage[5]	-	-	98%	98%
Appropriate VTP Within 24 Hours[5]	-	-	98%	98%
Controlled Postoperative Blood Glucose[5]	-	-	99%	97%
Perioperative Temperature Management[5]	-	-	100%	100%
Prophylactic Antibiotic Selection[5]	-	-	99%	99%
Prophylactic Antibiotic Selection (Outpatient)[1,3]	-	-	98%	98%
Prophylactic Antibiotic Stopped[5]	-	-	98%	98%
Prophylactic Antibiotic Timing[5]	-	-	99%	99%
Prophylactic Antibiotic Timing (Outpatient)[1,3]	-	-	98%	98%
Urinary Catheter Removal[5]	-	-	97%	97%
Survey of Patients' Hospital Experiences				
Area Around Room 'Always' Quiet at Night[5]	-	-	67%	61%
Doctors 'Always' Communicated Well[5]	-	-	83%	82%
Home Recovery Information Given[5]	-	-	83%	85%
Hospital Given 9 or 10 on 10 Point Scale[5]	-	-	70%	71%
Meds 'Always' Explained Before Given[5]	-	-	63%	64%
Nurses 'Always' Communicated Well[5]	-	-	79%	79%
Pain 'Always' Well Controlled[5]	-	-	71%	71%
Room and Bathroom 'Always' Clean[5]	-	-	72%	73%
Timely Help 'Always' Received[5]	-	-	68%	68%
Would Definitely Recommend Hospital[5]	-	-	69%	71%
Use of Medical Imaging				
Cardiac Imaging Stress Test before Surgery[7]	-	-	4.3%	5.3%
Combination Abdominal CT Scan	132	0.0%	15.3%	10.5%
Combination Brain/Sinus CT Scan[1]	-	-	2.9%	2.7%
Combination Chest CT Scan	64	0.0%	5%	2.7%
Follow-up Mammogram/Ultrasound[7]	-	-	9.9%	8.8%
Lumbar Spine MRI for Low Back Pain[7]	-	-	41.6%	37.2%

De Queen Medical Center

1306 West Collin Raye Drive
De Queen, AR 71832
Phone: 870-584-4111
Fax: 870-584-4100
URL: www.dequeenmedicalcenter.com
Type: Critical Access Hospitals
Emergency Services: Yes
Ownership: Voluntary non-profit - Other
Beds: 35

Key Personnel:
Pediatric Ambulatory Care . . . . . . Susan Couture, MD
Chief of Medical Staff. . . . . Cheryl Vogan, MD
CEO/President. . . . . Layne Webb

Measure	Cases	This Hosp.	State Avg.	U.S. Avg.
Blood Clot Prevention and Treatment				
Anticoagulation Overlap Therapy[5]	-	-	88%	93%
ICU Venous Thromboembolism Prophylaxis[5]	-	-	94%	92%
Incidence of Potentially Preventable VTE[5]	-	-	12%	10%
UFH with Dosages/Platelet Monitoring[5]	-	-	100%	97%
Venous Thromboembolism Prophylaxis[5]	-	-	91%	85%
Warfarin Therapy Discharge Instructions[5]	-	-	76%	75%
Chest Pain/Possible Heart Attack Care				
Aspirin Given Within 24 Hours of Arrival	-	-	96%	96%
Fibrinolytic Meds Within 30 Min. of Arrival	-	-	54%	58%
Average Time to ECG (minutes)	-	-	8	7
Average Time to Transfer (minutes)	-	-	72	60
Children's Asthma Care				
Received Home Management Plan of Care	-	-	-	88%
Received Reliever Medication	-	-	-	100%
Received Systemic Corticosteroids	-	-	-	100%
Emergency Department				
Admittance Decision Time (minutes)[5]	-	-	65	98
Head CT Results Within 45 Min. of Arrival	-	-	49%	57%
Patients Who Left ER Before Being Seen	-	-	3%	2%
Time from ER Arrival to Admit. (minutes)[5]	-	-	214	274
Time from ER Arrival to Discharge (minutes)	-	-	118	134
Time in ER Before Being Evaluated (minutes)	-	-	26	26
Time to Pain Meds for Fractures (minutes)	-	-	66	57
Heart Attack Care				
Aspirin Given at Discharge[5]	-	-	99%	99%
Fibrinolytic Meds Within 30 Min. of Arrival[5]	-	-	77%	54%
PCI Within 90 Minutes of Arrival[5]	-	-	96%	96%
Statin Prescribed at Discharge[5]	-	-	97%	98%
Heart Failure Care				
ACE Inhibitor or ARB for LVSD[1]	-	-	96%	97%
Discharge Instructions Given[1]	-	-	95%	94%
Evaluation of LVS Function[1]	-	-	98%	99%
Medicare Spending				
Medicare Spending per Patient (ratio)	-	-	0.98	0.98
Pneumonia Care				
Appropriate Initial Antibiotic Given	19	53%	94%	95%
Blood Culture Timing	25	84%	98%	98%
Pregnancy and Delivery Care				
Newborn Deliveries Scheduled Early[5]	-	-	6%	6%
Preventive Care				
Immunization for Influenza[5]	-	-	89%	90%
Immunization for Pneumonia[5]	-	-	92%	92%
Stroke Care				
Anticoagulation Therapy for Atrial Fibrillation[5]	-	-	90%	95%
Antithrombotic Therapy Timing[5]	-	-	96%	98%
Assessed for Rehabilitation[5]	-	-	95%	97%
Discharged on Antithrombotic Therapy[5]	-	-	96%	99%
Discharged on Statin Medication[5]	-	-	86%	94%
Thrombolytic Therapy Timing[5]	-	-	35%	66%
Venous Thromboembolism Prophylaxis[5]	-	-	91%	94%
Written Stroke Educational Materials Given[5]	-	-	81%	88%
Surgical Care Improvement Project				
Appropriate Beta Blocker Usage[5]	-	-	98%	98%
Appropriate VTP Within 24 Hours[5]	-	-	98%	98%
Controlled Postoperative Blood Glucose[5]	-	-	99%	97%
Perioperative Temperature Management[5]	-	-	100%	100%
Prophylactic Antibiotic Selection[5]	-	-	99%	99%
Prophylactic Antibiotic Selection (Outpatient)	-	-	98%	98%
Prophylactic Antibiotic Stopped[5]	-	-	98%	98%
Prophylactic Antibiotic Timing[5]	-	-	99%	99%
Prophylactic Antibiotic Timing (Outpatient)	-	-	98%	98%
Urinary Catheter Removal[5]	-	-	97%	97%
Survey of Patients' Hospital Experiences				
Area Around Room 'Always' Quiet at Night[5]	-	-	67%	61%
Doctors 'Always' Communicated Well[5]	-	-	83%	82%
Home Recovery Information Given[5]	-	-	83%	85%
Hospital Given 9 or 10 on 10 Point Scale[5]	-	-	70%	71%
Meds 'Always' Explained Before Given[5]	-	-	63%	64%
Nurses 'Always' Communicated Well[5]	-	-	79%	79%
Pain 'Always' Well Controlled[5]	-	-	71%	71%
Room and Bathroom 'Always' Clean[5]	-	-	72%	73%
Timely Help 'Always' Received[5]	-	-	68%	68%
Would Definitely Recommend Hospital[5]	-	-	69%	71%
Use of Medical Imaging				
Cardiac Imaging Stress Test before Surgery	-	-	4.3%	5.3%
Combination Abdominal CT Scan	-	-	15.3%	10.5%
Combination Brain/Sinus CT Scan	-	-	2.9%	2.7%
Combination Chest CT Scan	-	-	5%	2.7%
Follow-up Mammogram/Ultrasound	-	-	9.9%	8.8%
Lumbar Spine MRI for Low Back Pain	-	-	41.6%	37.2%

Dewitt Hospital & Nursing Home

1641 Whitehead Drive
De Witt, AR 72042
Phone: 870-946-3571
Fax: 870-946-4377
Type: Critical Access Hospitals
Emergency Services: Yes
Ownership: Voluntary non-profit - Private
Beds: 25

Key Personnel:
CEO/President. . . . . Darren Caldwell
Quality Assurance . . . . Darren Caldwell
Emergency Room . . . . Karen Campbell, RN
Chief of Medical Staff. . . . . Stan Purleson

Measure	Cases	This Hosp.	State Avg.	U.S. Avg.
Blood Clot Prevention and Treatment				
Anticoagulation Overlap Therapy[5]	-	-	88%	93%
ICU Venous Thromboembolism Prophylaxis[5]	-	-	94%	92%

NOTE: Hospital profiles are in alphabetical order by state, then city, then hospital within the city; Rankings exclude hospitals with less than 25 cases except for patient surveys which excludes hospitals with less than 100 cases; (a) 100-299 cases; (1) The number of cases/patients is too few to report; (2) Data submitted were based on a sample of cases/patients; (3) Results are based on a shorter time period than required; (4) Data suppressed by CMS for one or more quarters; (5) Results are not available for this reporting period; (6) Fewer than 100 patients completed the HCAHPS survey; (7) No cases met the criteria for this measure; (8) The lower limit of the confidence interval cannot be calculated if the number of observed infections equals zero; (9) No data are available from the state/territory for this reporting period; (10) The scores shown reflect fewer than 50 completed surveys; (11) There were discrepancies in the data collection process; (12) This measure does not apply to this hospital for this reporting period; (13) Results cannot be calculated for this reporting period; (14) The results for this state are combined with nearby states to protect confidentiality; Please refer to the User's Guide for a full explanation of data.

Measure	Cases	This Hosp.	State Avg.	U.S. Avg.
Incidence of Potentially Preventable VTE[5]	-	-	12%	10%
UFH with Dosages/Platelet Monitoring[5]	-	-	100%	97%
Venous Thromboembolism Prophylaxis[5]	-	-	91%	85%
Warfarin Therapy Discharge Instructions[5]	-	-	76%	75%
Chest Pain/Possible Heart Attack Care				
Aspirin Given Within 24 Hours of Arrival	-	-	96%	96%
Fibrinolytic Meds Within 30 Min. of Arrival	-	-	54%	58%
Average Time to ECG (minutes)	-	-	8	7
Average Time to Transfer (minutes)	-	-	72	60
Children's Asthma Care				
Received Home Management Plan of Care	-	-	-	88%
Received Reliever Medication	-	-	-	100%
Received Systemic Corticosteroids	-	-	-	100%
Emergency Department				
Admittance Decision Time (minutes)[5]	-	-	65	98
Head CT Results Within 45 Min. of Arrival	-	-	49%	57%
Patients Who Left ER Before Being Seen	-	-	3%	2%
Time from ER Arrival to Admit. (minutes)[5]	-	-	214	274
Time from ER Arrival to Discharge (minutes)	-	-	118	134
Time in ER Before Being Evaluated (minutes)	-	-	26	26
Time to Pain Meds for Fractures (minutes)	-	-	66	57
Heart Attack Care				
Aspirin Given at Discharge[5]	-	-	99%	99%
Fibrinolytic Meds Within 30 Min. of Arrival[5]	-	-	77%	54%
PCI Within 90 Minutes of Arrival[5]	-	-	96%	96%
Statin Prescribed at Discharge[5]	-	-	97%	98%
Heart Failure Care				
ACE Inhibitor or ARB for LVSD[1]	-	-	96%	97%
Discharge Instructions Given	19	100%	95%	94%
Evaluation of LVS Function	20	40%	98%	99%
Medicare Spending				
Medicare Spending per Patient (ratio)	-	-	0.98	0.98
Pneumonia Care				
Appropriate Initial Antibiotic Given	12	92%	94%	95%
Blood Culture Timing[1]	-	-	98%	98%
Pregnancy and Delivery Care				
Newborn Deliveries Scheduled Early[5]	-	-	6%	6%
Preventive Care				
Immunization for Influenza[5]	-	-	89%	90%
Immunization for Pneumonia[5]	-	-	92%	92%
Stroke Care				
Anticoagulation Therapy for Atrial Fibrillation[5]	-	-	90%	95%
Antithrombotic Therapy Timing[5]	-	-	96%	98%
Assessed for Rehabilitation[5]	-	-	95%	97%
Discharged on Antithrombotic Therapy[5]	-	-	96%	99%
Discharged on Statin Medication[5]	-	-	86%	94%
Thrombolytic Therapy Timing[5]	-	-	35%	66%
Venous Thromboembolism Prophylaxis[5]	-	-	91%	94%
Written Stroke Educational Materials Given[5]	-	-	81%	88%
Surgical Care Improvement Project				
Appropriate Beta Blocker Usage[5]	-	-	98%	98%
Appropriate VTP Within 24 Hours[5]	-	-	98%	98%
Controlled Postoperative Blood Glucose[5]	-	-	99%	97%
Perioperative Temperature Management[5]	-	-	100%	100%
Prophylactic Antibiotic Selection[5]	-	-	99%	99%
Prophylactic Antibiotic Selection (Outpatient)	-	-	98%	98%
Prophylactic Antibiotic Stopped[5]	-	-	98%	98%
Prophylactic Antibiotic Timing[5]	-	-	99%	99%
Prophylactic Antibiotic Timing (Outpatient)	-	-	98%	98%
Urinary Catheter Removal[5]	-	-	97%	97%
Survey of Patients' Hospital Experiences				
Area Around Room 'Always' Quiet at Night[5]	-	-	67%	61%
Doctors 'Always' Communicated Well[5]	-	-	83%	82%
Home Recovery Information Given[5]	-	-	83%	85%
Hospital Given 9 or 10 on 10 Point Scale[5]	-	-	70%	71%
Meds 'Always' Explained Before Given[5]	-	-	63%	64%
Nurses 'Always' Communicated Well[5]	-	-	79%	79%
Pain 'Always' Well Controlled[5]	-	-	71%	71%
Room and Bathroom 'Always' Clean[5]	-	-	72%	73%
Timely Help 'Always' Received[5]	-	-	68%	68%
Would Definitely Recommend Hospital[5]	-	-	69%	71%
Use of Medical Imaging				
Cardiac Imaging Stress Test before Surgery	-	-	4.3%	5.3%
Combination Abdominal CT Scan	-	-	15.3%	10.5%
Combination Brain/Sinus CT Scan	-	-	2.9%	2.7%
Combination Chest CT Scan	-	-	5%	2.7%
Follow-up Mammogram/Ultrasound	-	-	9.9%	8.8%
Lumbar Spine MRI for Low Back Pain	-	-	41.6%	37.2%

Delta Memorial Hospital

300 East Pickens
Dumas, AR 71639
Phone: 870-382-4303
Fax: 870-382-6555
E-mail: xray@deltamem.org
URL: www.dumasar.org
Type: Critical Access Hospitals
Emergency Services: Yes
Ownership: Voluntary non-profit - Private
Beds: 50

Key Personnel:
Chief of Medical Staff.......... David Chambers
Quality Assurance .... Jania Karr
Chairman/CEO .... David A. Lane
Pediatric Ambulatory Care ...... Hemal Mehta
Pediatric In-Patient Care .... Hemal Mehta
CEO/President............... Craig Ortego

Measure	Cases	This Hosp.	State Avg.	U.S. Avg.
Blood Clot Prevention and Treatment				
Anticoagulation Overlap Therapy[5]	-	-	88%	93%
ICU Venous Thromboembolism Prophylaxis[5]	-	-	94%	92%
Incidence of Potentially Preventable VTE[5]	-	-	12%	10%
UFH with Dosages/Platelet Monitoring[5]	-	-	100%	97%
Venous Thromboembolism Prophylaxis[5]	-	-	91%	85%
Warfarin Therapy Discharge Instructions[5]	-	-	76%	75%
Chest Pain/Possible Heart Attack Care				
Aspirin Given Within 24 Hours of Arrival	-	-	96%	96%
Fibrinolytic Meds Within 30 Min. of Arrival	-	-	54%	58%
Average Time to ECG (minutes)	-	-	8	7
Average Time to Transfer (minutes)	-	-	72	60
Children's Asthma Care				
Received Home Management Plan of Care	-	-	-	88%
Received Reliever Medication	-	-	-	100%
Received Systemic Corticosteroids	-	-	-	100%
Emergency Department				
Admittance Decision Time (minutes)[5]	-	-	65	98
Head CT Results Within 45 Min. of Arrival	-	-	49%	57%
Patients Who Left ER Before Being Seen	-	-	3%	2%
Time from ER Arrival to Admit. (minutes)[5]	-	-	214	274
Time from ER Arrival to Discharge (minutes)	-	-	118	134
Time in ER Before Being Evaluated (minutes)	-	-	26	26
Time to Pain Meds for Fractures (minutes)	-	-	66	57
Heart Attack Care				
Aspirin Given at Discharge[2,3]	-	-	99%	99%
Fibrinolytic Meds Within 30 Min. of Arrival[2,3]	-	-	77%	54%
PCI Within 90 Minutes of Arrival[2,3]	-	-	96%	96%
Statin Prescribed at Discharge[2,3]	-	-	97%	98%
Heart Failure Care				
ACE Inhibitor or ARB for LVSD[1,2]	-	-	96%	97%
Discharge Instructions Given[2]	17	53%	95%	94%
Evaluation of LVS Function[2]	17	82%	98%	99%
Medicare Spending				
Medicare Spending per Patient (ratio)	-	-	0.98	0.98
Pneumonia Care				
Appropriate Initial Antibiotic Given[2]	42	81%	94%	95%
Blood Culture Timing[2]	31	84%	98%	98%
Pregnancy and Delivery Care				
Newborn Deliveries Scheduled Early[5]	-	-	6%	6%
Preventive Care				
Immunization for Influenza[5]	-	-	89%	90%
Immunization for Pneumonia[5]	-	-	92%	92%
Stroke Care				
Anticoagulation Therapy for Atrial Fibrillation[5]	-	-	90%	95%
Antithrombotic Therapy Timing[5]	-	-	96%	98%
Assessed for Rehabilitation[5]	-	-	95%	97%
Discharged on Antithrombotic Therapy[5]	-	-	96%	99%
Discharged on Statin Medication[5]	-	-	86%	94%
Thrombolytic Therapy Timing[5]	-	-	35%	66%
Venous Thromboembolism Prophylaxis[5]	-	-	91%	94%
Written Stroke Educational Materials Given[5]	-	-	81%	88%
Surgical Care Improvement Project				
Appropriate Beta Blocker Usage[2,7]	-	-	98%	98%
Appropriate VTP Within 24 Hours[1,2]	-	-	98%	98%
Controlled Postoperative Blood Glucose[2,7]	-	-	99%	97%
Perioperative Temperature Management[1,2]	-	-	100%	100%
Prophylactic Antibiotic Selection[1,2]	-	-	99%	99%
Prophylactic Antibiotic Selection (Outpatient)	-	-	98%	98%
Prophylactic Antibiotic Stopped[1,2]	-	-	98%	98%
Prophylactic Antibiotic Timing[1,2]	-	-	99%	99%
Prophylactic Antibiotic Timing (Outpatient)	-	-	98%	98%
Urinary Catheter Removal[2,7]	-	-	97%	97%
Survey of Patients' Hospital Experiences				
Area Around Room 'Always' Quiet at Night[5]	-	-	67%	61%
Doctors 'Always' Communicated Well[5]	-	-	83%	82%
Home Recovery Information Given[5]	-	-	83%	85%
Hospital Given 9 or 10 on 10 Point Scale[5]	-	-	70%	71%
Meds 'Always' Explained Before Given[5]	-	-	63%	64%
Nurses 'Always' Communicated Well[5]	-	-	79%	79%
Pain 'Always' Well Controlled[5]	-	-	71%	71%
Room and Bathroom 'Always' Clean[5]	-	-	72%	73%
Timely Help 'Always' Received[5]	-	-	68%	68%
Would Definitely Recommend Hospital[5]	-	-	69%	71%
Use of Medical Imaging				
Cardiac Imaging Stress Test before Surgery	-	-	4.3%	5.3%
Combination Abdominal CT Scan	-	-	15.3%	10.5%
Combination Brain/Sinus CT Scan	-	-	2.9%	2.7%
Combination Chest CT Scan	-	-	5%	2.7%
Follow-up Mammogram/Ultrasound	-	-	9.9%	8.8%
Lumbar Spine MRI for Low Back Pain	-	-	41.6%	37.2%

Medical Center South Arkansas

700 West Grove Street
El Dorado, AR 71731
Phone: 870-863-2000
Fax: 870-863-2500
E-mail: mary.dumas@triadhospitals.com
URL: www.themedcenter.net
Type: Acute Care Hospitals
Emergency Services: Yes
Ownership: Proprietary
Beds: 360

Key Personnel:
Chief of Medical Staff.......... Cheryl Barenberg
Quality Assurance .... Cheryl Barenberg
Infection Control............. Bob Cook, RN
Radiology.................. Robert B Forward
CEO/President.............. Luther J Lewis
Emergency Room .... Marie Owens
Intensive Care Unit........... Becky Parnell
Operating Room............. Margaret Wilson, RN

Measure	Cases	This Hosp.	State Avg.	U.S. Avg.
Blood Clot Prevention and Treatment				
Anticoagulation Overlap Therapy[2]	23	96%	88%	93%
ICU Venous Thromboembolism Prophylaxis[2]	176	97%	94%	92%
Incidence of Potentially Preventable VTE[1,2]	-	-	12%	10%
UFH with Dosages/Platelet Monitoring[1,2]	-	-	100%	97%
Venous Thromboembolism Prophylaxis[2]	235	95%	91%	85%
Warfarin Therapy Discharge Instructions[2]	18	89%	76%	75%
Chest Pain/Possible Heart Attack Care				
Aspirin Given Within 24 Hours of Arrival[1]	-	-	96%	96%
Fibrinolytic Meds Within 30 Min. of Arrival[5]	-	-	54%	58%
Average Time to ECG (minutes)[1]	-	-	8	7
Average Time to Transfer (minutes)[5]	-	-	72	60
Children's Asthma Care				
Received Home Management Plan of Care	-	-	-	88%
Received Reliever Medication	-	-	-	100%
Received Systemic Corticosteroids	-	-	-	100%
Emergency Department				
Admittance Decision Time (minutes)[2]	505	61	65	98
Head CT Results Within 45 Min. of Arrival	11	55%	49%	57%
Patients Who Left ER Before Being Seen	19,175	2%	3%	2%
Time from ER Arrival to Admit. (minutes)[2]	529	177	214	274
Time from ER Arrival to Discharge (minutes)	369	99	118	134
Time in ER Before Being Evaluated (minutes)	414	13	26	26
Time to Pain Meds for Fractures (minutes)	78	45	66	57
Heart Attack Care				
Aspirin Given at Discharge	144	100%	99%	99%
Fibrinolytic Meds Within 30 Min. of Arrival[7]	-	-	77%	54%

NOTE: Hospital profiles are in alphabetical order by state, then city, then hospital within the city; Rankings exclude hospitals with less than 25 cases except for patient surveys which excludes hospitals with less than 100 cases; (a) 100-299 cases; (1) The number of cases/patients is too few to report; (2) Data submitted were based on a sample of cases/patients; (3) Results are based on a shorter time period than required; (4) Data suppressed by CMS for one or more quarters; (5) Results are not available for this reporting period; (6) Fewer than 100 patients completed the HCAHPS survey; (7) No cases met the criteria for this measure; (8) The lower limit of the confidence interval cannot be calculated if the number of observed infections equals zero; (9) No data are available from the state/territory for this reporting period; (10) The scores shown reflect fewer than 50 completed surveys; (11) There were discrepancies in the data collection process; (12) This measure does not apply to this hospital for this reporting period; (13) Results cannot be calculated for this reporting period; (14) The results for this state are combined with nearby states to protect confidentiality; Please refer to the User's Guide for a full explanation of data.

Measure	Cases	This Hosp.	State Avg.	U.S. Avg.
PCI Within 90 Minutes of Arrival	22	100%	96%	96%
Statin Prescribed at Discharge	130	100%	97%	98%
Heart Failure Care				
ACE Inhibitor or ARB for LVSD	47	100%	96%	97%
Discharge Instructions Given	154	98%	95%	94%
Evaluation of LVS Function	203	100%	98%	99%
Medicare Spending				
Medicare Spending per Patient (ratio)	-	1.01	0.98	0.98
Pneumonia Care				
Appropriate Initial Antibiotic Given	71	99%	94%	95%
Blood Culture Timing	114	100%	98%	98%
Pregnancy and Delivery Care				
Newborn Deliveries Scheduled Early[2]	50	4%	6%	6%
Preventive Care				
Immunization for Influenza[2]	527	100%	89%	90%
Immunization for Pneumonia[2]	604	100%	92%	92%
Stroke Care				
Anticoagulation Therapy for Atrial Fibrillation[1]	-	-	90%	95%
Antithrombotic Therapy Timing	39	97%	96%	98%
Assessed for Rehabilitation	41	100%	95%	97%
Discharged on Antithrombotic Therapy	40	100%	96%	99%
Discharged on Statin Medication	25	96%	86%	94%
Thrombolytic Therapy Timing[7]	-	-	35%	66%
Venous Thromboembolism Prophylaxis	43	81%	91%	94%
Written Stroke Educational Materials Given	21	95%	81%	88%
Surgical Care Improvement Project				
Appropriate Beta Blocker Usage	132	98%	98%	98%
Appropriate VTP Within 24 Hours	335	100%	98%	98%
Controlled Postoperative Blood Glucose	65	97%	99%	97%
Perioperative Temperature Management	388	100%	100%	100%
Prophylactic Antibiotic Selection	352	100%	99%	99%
Prophylactic Antibiotic Selection (Outpatient)	95	99%	98%	98%
Prophylactic Antibiotic Stopped	337	100%	98%	98%
Prophylactic Antibiotic Timing	352	100%	99%	99%
Prophylactic Antibiotic Timing (Outpatient)	96	98%	98%	98%
Urinary Catheter Removal	147	99%	97%	97%
Survey of Patients' Hospital Experiences				
Area Around Room 'Always' Quiet at Night	300+	68%	67%	61%
Doctors 'Always' Communicated Well	300+	81%	83%	82%
Home Recovery Information Given	300+	81%	83%	85%
Hospital Given 9 or 10 on 10 Point Scale	300+	66%	70%	71%
Meds 'Always' Explained Before Given	300+	61%	63%	64%
Nurses 'Always' Communicated Well	300+	75%	79%	79%
Pain 'Always' Well Controlled	300+	69%	71%	71%
Room and Bathroom 'Always' Clean	300+	64%	72%	73%
Timely Help 'Always' Received	300+	67%	68%	68%
Would Definitely Recommend Hospital	300+	61%	69%	71%
Use of Medical Imaging				
Cardiac Imaging Stress Test before Surgery	453	3.5%	4.3%	5.3%
Combination Abdominal CT Scan	464	5.6%	15.3%	10.5%
Combination Brain/Sinus CT Scan	445	2.2%	2.9%	2.7%
Combination Chest CT Scan	370	0.3%	5%	2.7%
Follow-up Mammogram/Ultrasound	1,029	5.7%	9.9%	8.8%
Lumbar Spine MRI for Low Back Pain	180	39.4%	41.6%	37.2%

Eureka Springs Hospital

24 Norris Street
Eureka Springs, AR 72632
Phone: 479-253-7400
Type: Critical Access Hospitals
Emergency Services: Yes
Ownership: Proprietary

Measure	Cases	This Hosp.	State Avg.	U.S. Avg.
Blood Clot Prevention and Treatment				
Anticoagulation Overlap Therapy[5]	-	-	88%	93%
ICU Venous Thromboembolism Prophylaxis[5]	-	-	94%	92%
Incidence of Potentially Preventable VTE[5]	-	-	12%	10%
UFH with Dosages/Platelet Monitoring[5]	-	-	100%	97%
Venous Thromboembolism Prophylaxis[5]	-	-	91%	85%
Warfarin Therapy Discharge Instructions[5]	-	-	76%	75%
Chest Pain/Possible Heart Attack Care				
Aspirin Given Within 24 Hours of Arrival	-	-	96%	96%
Fibrinolytic Meds Within 30 Min. of Arrival	-	-	54%	58%
Average Time to ECG (minutes)	-	-	8	7
Average Time to Transfer (minutes)	-	-	72	60
Children's Asthma Care				
Received Home Management Plan of Care	-	-	-	88%
Received Reliever Medication	-	-	-	100%
Received Systemic Corticosteroids	-	-	-	100%
Emergency Department				
Admittance Decision Time (minutes)[5]	-	-	65	98
Head CT Results Within 45 Min. of Arrival	-	-	49%	57%
Patients Who Left ER Before Being Seen	-	-	3%	2%
Time from ER Arrival to Admit. (minutes)[5]	-	-	214	274
Time from ER Arrival to Discharge (minutes)	-	-	118	134
Time in ER Before Being Evaluated (minutes)	-	-	26	26
Time to Pain Meds for Fractures (minutes)	-	-	66	57
Heart Attack Care				
Aspirin Given at Discharge[5]	-	-	99%	99%
Fibrinolytic Meds Within 30 Min. of Arrival[5]	-	-	77%	54%
PCI Within 90 Minutes of Arrival[5]	-	-	96%	96%
Statin Prescribed at Discharge[5]	-	-	97%	98%
Heart Failure Care				
ACE Inhibitor or ARB for LVSD[2,3]	-	-	96%	97%
Discharge Instructions Given[1,2]	-	-	95%	94%
Evaluation of LVS Function[1,2]	-	-	98%	99%
Medicare Spending				
Medicare Spending per Patient (ratio)	-	-	0.98	0.98
Pneumonia Care				
Appropriate Initial Antibiotic Given[1,2]	-	-	94%	95%
Blood Culture Timing[1,2]	-	-	98%	98%
Pregnancy and Delivery Care				
Newborn Deliveries Scheduled Early[5]	-	-	6%	6%
Preventive Care				
Immunization for Influenza[5]	-	-	89%	90%
Immunization for Pneumonia[5]	-	-	92%	92%
Stroke Care				
Anticoagulation Therapy for Atrial Fibrillation[5]	-	-	90%	95%
Antithrombotic Therapy Timing[5]	-	-	96%	98%
Assessed for Rehabilitation[5]	-	-	95%	97%
Discharged on Antithrombotic Therapy[5]	-	-	96%	99%
Discharged on Statin Medication[5]	-	-	86%	94%
Thrombolytic Therapy Timing[5]	-	-	35%	66%
Venous Thromboembolism Prophylaxis[5]	-	-	91%	94%
Written Stroke Educational Materials Given[5]	-	-	81%	88%
Surgical Care Improvement Project				
Appropriate Beta Blocker Usage[5]	-	-	98%	98%
Appropriate VTP Within 24 Hours[5]	-	-	98%	98%
Controlled Postoperative Blood Glucose[5]	-	-	99%	97%
Perioperative Temperature Management[5]	-	-	100%	100%
Prophylactic Antibiotic Selection[5]	-	-	99%	99%
Prophylactic Antibiotic Selection (Outpatient)	-	-	98%	98%
Prophylactic Antibiotic Stopped[5]	-	-	98%	98%
Prophylactic Antibiotic Timing[5]	-	-	99%	99%
Prophylactic Antibiotic Timing (Outpatient)	-	-	98%	98%
Urinary Catheter Removal[5]	-	-	97%	97%
Survey of Patients' Hospital Experiences				
Area Around Room 'Always' Quiet at Night[5]	-	-	67%	61%
Doctors 'Always' Communicated Well[5]	-	-	83%	82%
Home Recovery Information Given[5]	-	-	83%	85%
Hospital Given 9 or 10 on 10 Point Scale[5]	-	-	70%	71%
Meds 'Always' Explained Before Given[5]	-	-	63%	64%
Nurses 'Always' Communicated Well[5]	-	-	79%	79%
Pain 'Always' Well Controlled[5]	-	-	71%	71%
Room and Bathroom 'Always' Clean[5]	-	-	72%	73%
Timely Help 'Always' Received[5]	-	-	68%	68%
Would Definitely Recommend Hospital[5]	-	-	69%	71%
Use of Medical Imaging				
Cardiac Imaging Stress Test before Surgery	-	-	4.3%	5.3%
Combination Abdominal CT Scan	-	-	15.3%	10.5%
Combination Brain/Sinus CT Scan	-	-	2.9%	2.7%
Combination Chest CT Scan	-	-	5%	2.7%
Follow-up Mammogram/Ultrasound	-	-	9.9%	8.8%
Lumbar Spine MRI for Low Back Pain	-	-	41.6%	37.2%

Fayetteville VA Medical Center

1100 N. College Avenue
Fayetteville, AR 72703
Phone: 479-444-5058
Fax: 501-444-5062
URL: www.va.gov/sta/guide/home.asp
Type: Acute Care - VA
Emergency Services: No
Ownership: Government Federal
Beds: 53

Key Personnel:

Chief of Medical Staff. . . . . Gregory A Antoine, MD
Operating Room. . . . . Kay Collins, RN
Quality Assurance . . . . Jeri Elizandro
Infection Control. . . . . Mary Ann Harris, RN
Radiology. . . . . Mary Jo Henry, MD
Intensive Care Unit. . . . . Theresa Jones, RN

Measure	Cases	This Hosp.	State Avg.	U.S. Avg.
Blood Clot Prevention and Treatment				
Anticoagulation Overlap Therapy	-	-	88%	93%
ICU Venous Thromboembolism Prophylaxis	-	-	94%	92%
Incidence of Potentially Preventable VTE	-	-	12%	10%
UFH with Dosages/Platelet Monitoring	-	-	100%	97%
Venous Thromboembolism Prophylaxis	-	-	91%	85%
Warfarin Therapy Discharge Instructions	-	-	76%	75%
Chest Pain/Possible Heart Attack Care				
Aspirin Given Within 24 Hours of Arrival	-	-	96%	96%
Fibrinolytic Meds Within 30 Min. of Arrival	-	-	54%	58%
Average Time to ECG (minutes)	-	-	8	7
Average Time to Transfer (minutes)	-	-	72	60
Children's Asthma Care				
Received Home Management Plan of Care	-	-	-	88%
Received Reliever Medication	-	-	-	100%
Received Systemic Corticosteroids	-	-	-	100%
Emergency Department				
Admittance Decision Time (minutes)	-	-	65	98
Head CT Results Within 45 Min. of Arrival	-	-	49%	57%
Patients Who Left ER Before Being Seen	-	-	3%	2%
Time from ER Arrival to Admit. (minutes)	-	-	214	274
Time from ER Arrival to Discharge (minutes)	-	-	118	134
Time in ER Before Being Evaluated (minutes)	-	-	26	26
Time to Pain Meds for Fractures (minutes)	-	-	66	57
Heart Attack Care				
Aspirin Given at Discharge[5]	-	-	99%	99%
Fibrinolytic Meds Within 30 Min. of Arrival[5]	-	-	77%	54%
PCI Within 90 Minutes of Arrival[5]	-	-	96%	96%
Statin Prescribed at Discharge[5]	-	-	97%	98%
Heart Failure Care				
ACE Inhibitor or ARB for LVSD	58	93%	96%	97%
Discharge Instructions Given	99	90%	95%	94%
Evaluation of LVS Function	101	100%	98%	99%
Medicare Spending				
Medicare Spending per Patient (ratio)	-	-	0.98	0.98
Pneumonia Care				
Appropriate Initial Antibiotic Given	83	95%	94%	95%
Blood Culture Timing	113	99%	98%	98%
Pregnancy and Delivery Care				
Newborn Deliveries Scheduled Early	-	-	6%	6%
Preventive Care				
Immunization for Influenza[5]	-	-	89%	90%
Immunization for Pneumonia[5]	-	-	92%	92%
Stroke Care				
Anticoagulation Therapy for Atrial Fibrillation	-	-	90%	95%
Antithrombotic Therapy Timing	-	-	96%	98%
Assessed for Rehabilitation	-	-	95%	97%
Discharged on Antithrombotic Therapy	-	-	96%	99%
Discharged on Statin Medication	-	-	86%	94%
Thrombolytic Therapy Timing	-	-	35%	66%
Venous Thromboembolism Prophylaxis	-	-	91%	94%
Written Stroke Educational Materials Given	-	-	81%	88%
Surgical Care Improvement Project				
Appropriate Beta Blocker Usage[1,2]	-	-	98%	98%
Appropriate VTP Within 24 Hours[1,2]	11	100%	98%	98%
Controlled Postoperative Blood Glucose[5]	-	-	99%	97%
Perioperative Temperature Management[1,2]	11	100%	100%	100%
Prophylactic Antibiotic Selection[1]	-	-	99%	99%
Prophylactic Antibiotic Selection (Outpatient)	-	-	98%	98%
Prophylactic Antibiotic Stopped[1]	-	-	98%	98%

NOTE: Hospital profiles are in alphabetical order by state, then city, then hospital within the city; Rankings exclude hospitals with less than 25 cases except for patient surveys which excludes hospitals with less than 100 cases; (a) 100-299 cases; (1) The number of cases/patients is too few to report; (2) Data submitted were based on a sample of cases/patients; (3) Results are based on a shorter time period than required; (4) Data suppressed by CMS for one or more quarters; (5) Results are not available for this reporting period; (6) Fewer than 100 patients completed the HCAHPS survey; (7) No cases met the criteria for this measure; (8) The lower limit of the confidence interval cannot be calculated if the number of observed infections equals zero; (9) No data are available from the state/territory for this reporting period; (10) The scores shown reflect fewer than 50 completed surveys; (11) There were discrepancies in the data collection process; (12) This measure does not apply to this hospital for this reporting period; (13) Results cannot be calculated for this reporting period; (14) The results for this state are combined with nearby states to protect confidentiality; Please refer to the User's Guide for a full explanation of data.

Measure	Cases	This Hosp.	State Avg.	U.S. Avg.
Prophylactic Antibiotic Timing[1]	-	-	99%	99%
Prophylactic Antibiotic Timing (Outpatient)	-	-	98%	98%
Urinary Catheter Removal[1,2]	-	-	97%	97%
Survey of Patients' Hospital Experiences				
Area Around Room 'Always' Quiet at Night	-	-	67%	61%
Doctors 'Always' Communicated Well	-	-	83%	82%
Home Recovery Information Given	-	-	83%	85%
Hospital Given 9 or 10 on 10 Point Scale	-	-	70%	71%
Meds 'Always' Explained Before Given	-	-	63%	64%
Nurses 'Always' Communicated Well	-	-	79%	79%
Pain 'Always' Well Controlled	-	-	71%	71%
Room and Bathroom 'Always' Clean	-	-	72%	73%
Timely Help 'Always' Received	-	-	68%	68%
Would Definitely Recommend Hospital	-	-	69%	71%
Use of Medical Imaging				
Cardiac Imaging Stress Test before Surgery	-	-	4.3%	5.3%
Combination Abdominal CT Scan	-	-	15.3%	10.5%
Combination Brain/Sinus CT Scan	-	-	2.9%	2.7%
Combination Chest CT Scan	-	-	5%	2.7%
Follow-up Mammogram/Ultrasound	-	-	9.9%	8.8%
Lumbar Spine MRI for Low Back Pain	-	-	41.6%	37.2%

Physicians' Specialty Hospital

3873 North Parkview Drive Phone: 479-571-7002
Fayetteville, AR 72703
URL: www.pshfay.com
Type: Acute Care Hospitals Emergency Services: Yes
Ownership: Physician
Key Personnel:
CEO . . . . D Greene
Anesthesiology. . . . . William Murry, MD
Pediatrics. . . . . Martha Sharkey, MD

Measure	Cases	This Hosp.	State Avg.	U.S. Avg.
Blood Clot Prevention and Treatment				
Anticoagulation Overlap Therapy[2,7]	-	-	88%	93%
ICU Venous Thromboembolism Prophylaxis[2,7]	-	-	94%	92%
Incidence of Potentially Preventable VTE[2,7]	-	-	12%	10%
UFH with Dosages/Platelet Monitoring[2,7]	-	-	100%	97%
Venous Thromboembolism Prophylaxis[1,2]	-	-	91%	85%
Warfarin Therapy Discharge Instructions[2,7]	-	-	76%	75%
Chest Pain/Possible Heart Attack Care				
Aspirin Given Within 24 Hours of Arrival[1,3]	-	-	96%	96%
Fibrinolytic Meds Within 30 Min. of Arrival[5]	-	-	54%	58%
Average Time to ECG (minutes)[1,3]	-	-	8	7
Average Time to Transfer (minutes)[5]	-	-	72	60
Children's Asthma Care				
Received Home Management Plan of Care	-	-	-	88%
Received Reliever Medication	-	-	-	100%
Received Systemic Corticosteroids	-	-	-	100%
Emergency Department				
Admittance Decision Time (minutes)[1,2]	-	-	65	98
Head CT Results Within 45 Min. of Arrival[1,3]	-	-	49%	57%
Patients Who Left ER Before Being Seen	3,540	1%	3%	2%
Time from ER Arrival to Admit. (minutes)[1,2]	-	-	214	274
Time from ER Arrival to Discharge (minutes)	352	86	118	134
Time in ER Before Being Evaluated (minutes)	368	18	26	26
Time to Pain Meds for Fractures (minutes)	34	30	66	57
Heart Attack Care				
Aspirin Given at Discharge[5]	-	-	99%	99%
Fibrinolytic Meds Within 30 Min. of Arrival[5]	-	-	77%	54%
PCI Within 90 Minutes of Arrival[5]	-	-	96%	96%
Statin Prescribed at Discharge[5]	-	-	97%	98%
Heart Failure Care				
ACE Inhibitor or ARB for LVSD[5]	-	-	96%	97%
Discharge Instructions Given[5]	-	-	95%	94%
Evaluation of LVS Function[5]	-	-	98%	99%
Medicare Spending				
Medicare Spending per Patient (ratio)	-	1.03	0.98	0.98
Pneumonia Care				
Appropriate Initial Antibiotic Given[5]	-	-	94%	95%
Blood Culture Timing[5]	-	-	98%	98%
Pregnancy and Delivery Care				
Newborn Deliveries Scheduled Early[2,7]	-	-	6%	6%
Preventive Care				
Immunization for Influenza[2]	309	36%	89%	90%
Immunization for Pneumonia[2]	338	34%	92%	92%
Stroke Care				
Anticoagulation Therapy for Atrial Fibrillation[5]	-	-	90%	95%
Antithrombotic Therapy Timing[5]	-	-	96%	98%
Assessed for Rehabilitation[5]	-	-	95%	97%
Discharged on Antithrombotic Therapy[5]	-	-	96%	99%
Discharged on Statin Medication[5]	-	-	86%	94%
Thrombolytic Therapy Timing[5]	-	-	35%	66%
Venous Thromboembolism Prophylaxis[5]	-	-	91%	94%
Written Stroke Educational Materials Given[5]	-	-	81%	88%
Surgical Care Improvement Project				
Appropriate Beta Blocker Usage[2]	25	96%	98%	98%
Appropriate VTP Within 24 Hours[2]	135	98%	98%	98%
Controlled Postoperative Blood Glucose[2,7]	-	-	99%	97%
Perioperative Temperature Management[2]	143	99%	100%	100%
Prophylactic Antibiotic Selection[2]	105	99%	99%	99%
Prophylactic Antibiotic Selection (Outpatient)	79	99%	98%	98%
Prophylactic Antibiotic Stopped[2]	102	91%	98%	98%
Prophylactic Antibiotic Timing[2]	105	97%	99%	99%
Prophylactic Antibiotic Timing (Outpatient)	79	100%	98%	98%
Urinary Catheter Removal[2]	11	73%	97%	97%
Survey of Patients' Hospital Experiences				
Area Around Room 'Always' Quiet at Night	(a)	88%	67%	61%
Doctors 'Always' Communicated Well	(a)	91%	83%	82%
Home Recovery Information Given	(a)	90%	83%	85%
Hospital Given 9 or 10 on 10 Point Scale	(a)	88%	70%	71%
Meds 'Always' Explained Before Given	(a)	78%	63%	64%
Nurses 'Always' Communicated Well	(a)	89%	79%	79%
Pain 'Always' Well Controlled	(a)	83%	71%	71%
Room and Bathroom 'Always' Clean	(a)	84%	72%	73%
Timely Help 'Always' Received	(a)	87%	68%	68%
Would Definitely Recommend Hospital	(a)	88%	69%	71%
Use of Medical Imaging				
Cardiac Imaging Stress Test before Surgery[7]	-	-	4.3%	5.3%
Combination Abdominal CT Scan[1]	-	-	15.3%	10.5%
Combination Brain/Sinus CT Scan[1]	-	-	2.9%	2.7%
Combination Chest CT Scan[1]	-	-	5%	2.7%
Follow-up Mammogram/Ultrasound[7]	-	-	9.9%	8.8%
Lumbar Spine MRI for Low Back Pain	89	39.3%	41.6%	37.2%

Washington Regional Medical Center at North Hills

3215 N North Hills Blvd Phone: 479-463-5113
Fayetteville, AR 72703 Fax: 479-713-1296
URL: www.wregional.com
Type: Acute Care Hospitals Emergency Services: Yes
Ownership: Government - Local Beds: 366
Key Personnel:
CEO/President. . . . . Bill Bradley
Quality Assurance . . . . Susan Michie
Pediatric Ambulatory Care . . . . . . Terry Payton, MD
Pediatric In-Patient Care . . . . Terry Payton, MD
Radiology. . . . . Kevin Pope, MD
Chief of Medical Staff. . . . . David Ratcliffee
Cardiac Laboratory. . . . . Dixie Sharp
Operating Room. . . . . Evelyn Wheeler, RN

Measure	Cases	This Hosp.	State Avg.	U.S. Avg.
Blood Clot Prevention and Treatment				
Anticoagulation Overlap Therapy[2]	95	96%	88%	93%
ICU Venous Thromboembolism Prophylaxis[2]	93	100%	94%	92%
Incidence of Potentially Preventable VTE[2]	18	0%	12%	10%
UFH with Dosages/Platelet Monitoring[2]	49	100%	100%	97%
Venous Thromboembolism Prophylaxis[2]	280	94%	91%	85%
Warfarin Therapy Discharge Instructions[2]	76	99%	76%	75%
Chest Pain/Possible Heart Attack Care				
Aspirin Given Within 24 Hours of Arrival[5]	-	-	96%	96%
Fibrinolytic Meds Within 30 Min. of Arrival[5]	-	-	54%	58%
Average Time to ECG (minutes)[5]	-	-	8	7
Average Time to Transfer (minutes)[5]	-	-	72	60
Children's Asthma Care				
Received Home Management Plan of Care	-	-	-	88%
Received Reliever Medication	-	-	-	100%
Received Systemic Corticosteroids	-	-	-	100%
Emergency Department				
Admittance Decision Time (minutes)[2]	518	116	65	98
Head CT Results Within 45 Min. of Arrival[1]	-	-	49%	57%
Patients Who Left ER Before Being Seen	51,940	5%	3%	2%
Time from ER Arrival to Admit. (minutes)[2]	531	277	214	274
Time from ER Arrival to Discharge (minutes)	359	180	118	134
Time in ER Before Being Evaluated (minutes)	323	90	26	26
Time to Pain Meds for Fractures (minutes)	187	94	66	57
Heart Attack Care				
Aspirin Given at Discharge[2]	285	100%	99%	99%
Fibrinolytic Meds Within 30 Min. of Arrival[2,7]	-	-	77%	54%
PCI Within 90 Minutes of Arrival[2]	47	98%	96%	96%
Statin Prescribed at Discharge[2]	266	98%	97%	98%
Heart Failure Care				
ACE Inhibitor or ARB for LVSD[2]	105	94%	96%	97%
Discharge Instructions Given[2]	201	98%	95%	94%
Evaluation of LVS Function[2]	255	100%	98%	99%
Medicare Spending				
Medicare Spending per Patient (ratio)	-	1.00	0.98	0.98
Pneumonia Care				
Appropriate Initial Antibiotic Given[2]	87	95%	94%	95%
Blood Culture Timing[2]	149	100%	98%	98%
Pregnancy and Delivery Care				
Newborn Deliveries Scheduled Early[2]	50	4%	6%	6%
Preventive Care				
Immunization for Influenza[2]	535	97%	89%	90%
Immunization for Pneumonia[2]	682	93%	92%	92%
Stroke Care				
Anticoagulation Therapy for Atrial Fibrillation[1,2]	-	-	90%	95%
Antithrombotic Therapy Timing[2]	66	98%	96%	98%
Assessed for Rehabilitation[2]	82	99%	95%	97%
Discharged on Antithrombotic Therapy[2]	63	97%	96%	99%
Discharged on Statin Medication[2]	45	98%	86%	94%
Thrombolytic Therapy Timing[1,2]	-	-	35%	66%
Venous Thromboembolism Prophylaxis[2]	84	99%	91%	94%
Written Stroke Educational Materials Given[2]	34	94%	81%	88%
Surgical Care Improvement Project				
Appropriate Beta Blocker Usage[2]	184	97%	98%	98%
Appropriate VTP Within 24 Hours[2]	309	96%	98%	98%
Controlled Postoperative Blood Glucose[2]	111	99%	99%	97%
Perioperative Temperature Management[2]	369	100%	100%	100%
Prophylactic Antibiotic Selection[2]	377	99%	99%	99%
Prophylactic Antibiotic Selection (Outpatient)	516	98%	98%	98%
Prophylactic Antibiotic Stopped[2]	371	99%	98%	98%
Prophylactic Antibiotic Timing[2]	381	97%	99%	99%
Prophylactic Antibiotic Timing (Outpatient)	498	97%	98%	98%
Urinary Catheter Removal[2]	196	94%	97%	97%
Survey of Patients' Hospital Experiences				
Area Around Room 'Always' Quiet at Night	300+	68%	67%	61%
Doctors 'Always' Communicated Well	300+	82%	83%	82%
Home Recovery Information Given	300+	87%	83%	85%
Hospital Given 9 or 10 on 10 Point Scale	300+	75%	70%	71%
Meds 'Always' Explained Before Given	300+	67%	63%	64%
Nurses 'Always' Communicated Well	300+	81%	79%	79%
Pain 'Always' Well Controlled	300+	74%	71%	71%
Room and Bathroom 'Always' Clean	300+	75%	72%	73%
Timely Help 'Always' Received	300+	69%	68%	68%
Would Definitely Recommend Hospital	300+	78%	69%	71%
Use of Medical Imaging				
Cardiac Imaging Stress Test before Surgery	1,138	3.9%	4.3%	5.3%
Combination Abdominal CT Scan	917	5.2%	15.3%	10.5%
Combination Brain/Sinus CT Scan	980	3.1%	2.9%	2.7%
Combination Chest CT Scan	281	1.1%	5%	2.7%
Follow-up Mammogram/Ultrasound	144	13.2%	9.9%	8.8%
Lumbar Spine MRI for Low Back Pain	116	41.4%	41.6%	37.2%

Dallas County Medical Center

201 Clifton Street Phone: 870-352-6300
Fordyce, AR 71742 Fax: 870-352-6391
URL: www.dallascountymedicalcenter.com
Type: Critical Access Hospitals Emergency Services: Yes
Ownership: Government - Local Beds: 25
Key Personnel:
Quality Assurance . . . . Scott Manes, RN

NOTE: Hospital profiles are in alphabetical order by state, then city, then hospital within the city; Rankings exclude hospitals with less than 25 cases except for patient surveys which excludes hospitals with less than 100 cases; (a) 100-299 cases; (1) The number of cases/patients is too few to report; (2) Data submitted were based on a sample of cases/patients; (3) Results are based on a shorter time period than required; (4) Data suppressed by CMS for one or more quarters; (5) Results are not available for this reporting period; (6) Fewer than 100 patients completed the HCAHPS survey; (7) No cases met the criteria for this measure; (8) The lower limit of the confidence interval cannot be calculated if the number of observed infections equals zero; (9) No data are available from the state/territory for this reporting period; (10) The scores shown reflect fewer than 50 completed surveys; (11) There were discrepancies in the data collection process; (12) This measure does not apply to this hospital for this reporting period; (13) Results cannot be calculated for this reporting period; (14) The results for this state are combined with nearby states to protect confidentiality; Please refer to the User's Guide for a full explanation of data.

Chief of Medical Staff.......... Michael D Payne, MD
CEO .... Matt Wille
Emergency Room .... Shelley Young, RN
Infection Control.............. Shelley Young, RN

Measure	Cases	This Hosp.	State Avg.	U.S. Avg.
Blood Clot Prevention and Treatment				
Anticoagulation Overlap Therapy[5]	-	-	88%	93%
ICU Venous Thromboembolism Prophylaxis[5]	-	-	94%	92%
Incidence of Potentially Preventable VTE[5]	-	-	12%	10%
UFH with Dosages/Platelet Monitoring[5]	-	-	100%	97%
Venous Thromboembolism Prophylaxis[5]	-	-	91%	85%
Warfarin Therapy Discharge Instructions[5]	-	-	76%	75%
Chest Pain/Possible Heart Attack Care				
Aspirin Given Within 24 Hours of Arrival	-	-	96%	96%
Fibrinolytic Meds Within 30 Min. of Arrival	-	-	54%	58%
Average Time to ECG (minutes)	-	-	8	7
Average Time to Transfer (minutes)	-	-	72	60
Children's Asthma Care				
Received Home Management Plan of Care	-	-	-	88%
Received Reliever Medication	-	-	-	100%
Received Systemic Corticosteroids	-	-	-	100%
Emergency Department				
Admittance Decision Time (minutes)[5]	-	-	65	98
Head CT Results Within 45 Min. of Arrival	-	-	49%	57%
Patients Who Left ER Before Being Seen	-	-	3%	2%
Time from ER Arrival to Admit. (minutes)[5]	-	-	214	274
Time from ER Arrival to Discharge (minutes)	-	-	118	134
Time in ER Before Being Evaluated (minutes)	-	-	26	26
Time to Pain Meds for Fractures (minutes)	-	-	66	57
Heart Attack Care				
Aspirin Given at Discharge[5]	-	-	99%	99%
Fibrinolytic Meds Within 30 Min. of Arrival[5]	-	-	77%	54%
PCI Within 90 Minutes of Arrival[5]	-	-	96%	96%
Statin Prescribed at Discharge[5]	-	-	97%	98%
Heart Failure Care				
ACE Inhibitor or ARB for LVSD[1,3]	-	-	96%	97%
Discharge Instructions Given[1,3]	-	-	95%	94%
Evaluation of LVS Function[1,3]	-	-	98%	99%
Medicare Spending				
Medicare Spending per Patient (ratio)	-	-	0.98	0.98
Pneumonia Care				
Appropriate Initial Antibiotic Given	31	84%	94%	95%
Blood Culture Timing	12	67%	98%	98%
Pregnancy and Delivery Care				
Newborn Deliveries Scheduled Early[5]	-	-	6%	6%
Preventive Care				
Immunization for Influenza[5]	-	-	89%	90%
Immunization for Pneumonia[5]	-	-	92%	92%
Stroke Care				
Anticoagulation Therapy for Atrial Fibrillation[5]	-	-	90%	95%
Antithrombotic Therapy Timing[5]	-	-	96%	98%
Assessed for Rehabilitation[5]	-	-	95%	97%
Discharged on Antithrombotic Therapy[5]	-	-	96%	99%
Discharged on Statin Medication[5]	-	-	86%	94%
Thrombolytic Therapy Timing[5]	-	-	35%	66%
Venous Thromboembolism Prophylaxis[5]	-	-	91%	94%
Written Stroke Educational Materials Given[5]	-	-	81%	88%
Surgical Care Improvement Project				
Appropriate Beta Blocker Usage[5]	-	-	98%	98%
Appropriate VTP Within 24 Hours[5]	-	-	98%	98%
Controlled Postoperative Blood Glucose[5]	-	-	99%	97%
Perioperative Temperature Management[5]	-	-	100%	100%
Prophylactic Antibiotic Selection[5]	-	-	99%	99%
Prophylactic Antibiotic Selection (Outpatient)	-	-	98%	98%
Prophylactic Antibiotic Stopped[5]	-	-	98%	98%
Prophylactic Antibiotic Timing[5]	-	-	99%	99%
Prophylactic Antibiotic Timing (Outpatient)	-	-	98%	98%
Urinary Catheter Removal[5]	-	-	97%	97%
Survey of Patients' Hospital Experiences				
Area Around Room 'Always' Quiet at Night[5]	-	-	67%	61%
Doctors 'Always' Communicated Well[5]	-	-	83%	82%
Home Recovery Information Given[5]	-	-	83%	85%
Hospital Given 9 or 10 on 10 Point Scale[5]	-	-	70%	71%
Meds 'Always' Explained Before Given[5]	-	-	63%	64%
Nurses 'Always' Communicated Well[5]	-	-	79%	79%
Pain 'Always' Well Controlled[5]	-	-	71%	71%
Room and Bathroom 'Always' Clean[5]	-	-	72%	73%
Timely Help 'Always' Received[5]	-	-	68%	68%
Would Definitely Recommend Hospital[5]	-	-	69%	71%
Use of Medical Imaging				
Cardiac Imaging Stress Test before Surgery	-	-	4.3%	5.3%
Combination Abdominal CT Scan	-	-	15.3%	10.5%
Combination Brain/Sinus CT Scan	-	-	2.9%	2.7%
Combination Chest CT Scan	-	-	5%	2.7%
Follow-up Mammogram/Ultrasound	-	-	9.9%	8.8%
Lumbar Spine MRI for Low Back Pain	-	-	41.6%	37.2%

Forrest City Medical Center

1601 Newcastle Road
Forrest City, AR 72335
Phone: 870-261-0000
Fax: 970-277-3516
URL: www.bmhcc.org
Type: Acute Care Hospitals
Emergency Services: Yes
Ownership: Proprietary
Beds: 118

Key Personnel:

Intensive Care Unit............ Mary Baker, RN
Infection Control.............. Jerre Fisher, RN
Quality Assurance .... Pat Hamilton, RN
Emergency Room .... Barbara McGill, RN
Pediatric Ambulatory Care ...... Ganapathy Rama, MD
Pediatric In-Patient Care .... Ganapathy Rama, MD
Chief of Medical Staff.......... Frank Schwartz, MD
Operating Room.............. Kenny Worley, RN

Measure	Cases	This Hosp.	State Avg.	U.S. Avg.
Blood Clot Prevention and Treatment				
Anticoagulation Overlap Therapy[1,2]	-	-	88%	93%
ICU Venous Thromboembolism Prophylaxis[2]	31	94%	94%	92%
Incidence of Potentially Preventable VTE[1,2]	-	-	12%	10%
UFH with Dosages/Platelet Monitoring[1,2]	-	-	100%	97%
Venous Thromboembolism Prophylaxis[2]	151	88%	91%	85%
Warfarin Therapy Discharge Instructions[1,2]	-	-	76%	75%
Chest Pain/Possible Heart Attack Care				
Aspirin Given Within 24 Hours of Arrival	85	96%	96%	96%
Fibrinolytic Meds Within 30 Min. of Arrival[7]	-	-	54%	58%
Average Time to ECG (minutes)	90	4	8	7
Average Time to Transfer (minutes)[1]	-	-	72	60
Children's Asthma Care				
Received Home Management Plan of Care	-	-	-	88%
Received Reliever Medication	-	-	-	100%
Received Systemic Corticosteroids	-	-	-	100%
Emergency Department				
Admittance Decision Time (minutes)[2]	205	44	65	98
Head CT Results Within 45 Min. of Arrival[1]	-	-	49%	57%
Patients Who Left ER Before Being Seen	17,745	3%	3%	2%
Time from ER Arrival to Admit. (minutes)[2]	213	170	214	274
Time from ER Arrival to Discharge (minutes)	360	86	118	134
Time in ER Before Being Evaluated (minutes)	408	24	26	26
Time to Pain Meds for Fractures (minutes)	41	71	66	57
Heart Attack Care				
Aspirin Given at Discharge[1]	-	-	99%	99%
Fibrinolytic Meds Within 30 Min. of Arrival[7]	-	-	77%	54%
PCI Within 90 Minutes of Arrival[7]	-	-	96%	96%
Statin Prescribed at Discharge[1]	-	-	97%	98%
Heart Failure Care				
ACE Inhibitor or ARB for LVSD	31	97%	96%	97%
Discharge Instructions Given	59	98%	95%	94%
Evaluation of LVS Function	61	100%	98%	99%
Medicare Spending				
Medicare Spending per Patient (ratio)	-	0.88	0.98	0.98
Pneumonia Care				
Appropriate Initial Antibiotic Given	45	100%	94%	95%
Blood Culture Timing	62	98%	98%	98%
Pregnancy and Delivery Care				
Newborn Deliveries Scheduled Early[2]	46	9%	6%	6%
Preventive Care				
Immunization for Influenza[2]	257	93%	89%	90%
Immunization for Pneumonia[2]	207	96%	92%	92%
Stroke Care				
Anticoagulation Therapy for Atrial Fibrillation[1]	-	-	90%	95%
Antithrombotic Therapy Timing	21	95%	96%	98%
Assessed for Rehabilitation	19	89%	95%	97%
Discharged on Antithrombotic Therapy	19	95%	96%	99%
Discharged on Statin Medication	17	65%	86%	94%
Thrombolytic Therapy Timing[7]	-	-	35%	66%
Venous Thromboembolism Prophylaxis	18	89%	91%	94%
Written Stroke Educational Materials Given	14	43%	81%	88%
Surgical Care Improvement Project				
Appropriate Beta Blocker Usage[1]	-	-	98%	98%
Appropriate VTP Within 24 Hours	35	91%	98%	98%
Controlled Postoperative Blood Glucose[7]	-	-	99%	97%
Perioperative Temperature Management	40	100%	100%	100%
Prophylactic Antibiotic Selection	20	100%	99%	99%
Prophylactic Antibiotic Selection (Outpatient)	50	98%	98%	98%
Prophylactic Antibiotic Stopped	19	100%	98%	98%
Prophylactic Antibiotic Timing	20	100%	99%	99%
Prophylactic Antibiotic Timing (Outpatient)	50	100%	98%	98%
Urinary Catheter Removal[1]	-	-	97%	97%
Survey of Patients' Hospital Experiences				
Area Around Room 'Always' Quiet at Night	300+	70%	67%	61%
Doctors 'Always' Communicated Well	300+	84%	83%	82%
Home Recovery Information Given	300+	82%	83%	85%
Hospital Given 9 or 10 on 10 Point Scale	300+	66%	70%	71%
Meds 'Always' Explained Before Given	300+	60%	63%	64%
Nurses 'Always' Communicated Well	300+	79%	79%	79%
Pain 'Always' Well Controlled	300+	73%	71%	71%
Room and Bathroom 'Always' Clean	300+	69%	72%	73%
Timely Help 'Always' Received	300+	68%	68%	68%
Would Definitely Recommend Hospital	300+	64%	69%	71%
Use of Medical Imaging				
Cardiac Imaging Stress Test before Surgery[7]	-	-	4.3%	5.3%
Combination Abdominal CT Scan	187	9.6%	15.3%	10.5%
Combination Brain/Sinus CT Scan[1]	-	-	2.9%	2.7%
Combination Chest CT Scan	77	1.3%	5%	2.7%
Follow-up Mammogram/Ultrasound	260	6.9%	9.9%	8.8%
Lumbar Spine MRI for Low Back Pain	44	59.1%	41.6%	37.2%

Saint Edward Mercy Medical Center

7301 Rogers Ave
Fort Smith, AR 72917
Phone: 479-314-6000
Fax: 479-314-1770
URL: www.stedwardmercy.com
Type: Acute Care Hospitals
Emergency Services: Yes
Ownership: Voluntary non-profit - Private
Beds: 336

Key Personnel:

Radiology.................. Kenneth Gardner, MD
CEO/President............... Ryan Gehrig
Quality Assurance .... Eileen Kradel
Operating Room.............. Deena Lee
Chief of Medical Staff.......... Chrisca Van Asche, MD
Cardiac Laboratory............ Timothy Waack
Emergency Room .... Jackie Wallace, RN

Measure	Cases	This Hosp.	State Avg.	U.S. Avg.
Blood Clot Prevention and Treatment				
Anticoagulation Overlap Therapy[2]	93	89%	88%	93%
ICU Venous Thromboembolism Prophylaxis[2]	84	94%	94%	92%
Incidence of Potentially Preventable VTE[2]	15	13%	12%	10%
UFH with Dosages/Platelet Monitoring[2]	30	100%	100%	97%
Venous Thromboembolism Prophylaxis[2]	320	88%	91%	85%
Warfarin Therapy Discharge Instructions[2]	78	42%	76%	75%
Chest Pain/Possible Heart Attack Care				
Aspirin Given Within 24 Hours of Arrival[1,3]	-	-	96%	96%
Fibrinolytic Meds Within 30 Min. of Arrival[5]	-	-	54%	58%
Average Time to ECG (minutes)[1,3]	-	-	8	7
Average Time to Transfer (minutes)[5]	-	-	72	60
Children's Asthma Care				
Received Home Management Plan of Care	-	-	-	88%
Received Reliever Medication	-	-	-	100%
Received Systemic Corticosteroids	-	-	-	100%
Emergency Department				
Admittance Decision Time (minutes)[2]	371	70	65	98
Head CT Results Within 45 Min. of Arrival[1]	-	-	49%	57%
Patients Who Left ER Before Being Seen	48,125	6%	3%	2%

NOTE: Hospital profiles are in alphabetical order by state, then city, then hospital within the city; Rankings exclude hospitals with less than 25 cases except for patient surveys which excludes hospitals with less than 100 cases; (a) 100-299 cases; (1) The number of cases/patients is too few to report; (2) Data submitted were based on a sample of cases/patients; (3) Results are based on a shorter time period than required; (4) Data suppressed by CMS for one or more quarters; (5) Results are not available for this reporting period; (6) Fewer than 100 patients completed the HCAHPS survey; (7) No cases met the criteria for this measure; (8) The lower limit of the confidence interval cannot be calculated if the number of observed infections equals zero; (9) No data are available from the state/territory for this reporting period; (10) The scores shown reflect fewer than 50 completed surveys; (11) There were discrepancies in the data collection process; (12) This measure does not apply to this hospital for this reporting period; (13) Results cannot be calculated for this reporting period; (14) The results for this state are combined with nearby states to protect confidentiality; Please refer to the User's Guide for a full explanation of data.

Measure	Cases	This Hosp.	State Avg.	U.S. Avg.
Time from ER Arrival to Admit. (minutes)[2]	387	253	214	274
Time from ER Arrival to Discharge (minutes)	374	198	118	134
Time in ER Before Being Evaluated (minutes)	393	35	26	26
Time to Pain Meds for Fractures (minutes)	88	70	66	57
Heart Attack Care				
Aspirin Given at Discharge[2]	253	100%	99%	99%
Fibrinolytic Meds Within 30 Min. of Arrival[1,2]	-	-	77%	54%
PCI Within 90 Minutes of Arrival[2]	36	89%	96%	96%
Statin Prescribed at Discharge[2]	247	99%	97%	98%
Heart Failure Care				
ACE Inhibitor or ARB for LVSD[2]	81	99%	96%	97%
Discharge Instructions Given[2]	192	94%	95%	94%
Evaluation of LVS Function[2]	259	100%	98%	99%
Medicare Spending				
Medicare Spending per Patient (ratio)	-	1.00	0.98	0.98
Pneumonia Care				
Appropriate Initial Antibiotic Given[2]	49	94%	94%	95%
Blood Culture Timing[2]	102	98%	98%	98%
Pregnancy and Delivery Care				
Newborn Deliveries Scheduled Early[2]	55	5%	6%	6%
Preventive Care				
Immunization for Influenza[2]	513	95%	89%	90%
Immunization for Pneumonia[2]	617	99%	92%	92%
Stroke Care				
Anticoagulation Therapy for Atrial Fibrillation[2]	15	87%	90%	95%
Antithrombotic Therapy Timing[2]	67	99%	96%	98%
Assessed for Rehabilitation[2]	77	94%	95%	97%
Discharged on Antithrombotic Therapy[2]	68	100%	96%	99%
Discharged on Statin Medication[2]	48	94%	86%	94%
Thrombolytic Therapy Timing[1,2]	-	-	35%	66%
Venous Thromboembolism Prophylaxis[2]	86	92%	91%	94%
Written Stroke Educational Materials Given[2]	35	80%	81%	88%
Surgical Care Improvement Project				
Appropriate Beta Blocker Usage[2]	160	99%	98%	98%
Appropriate VTP Within 24 Hours[2]	333	99%	98%	98%
Controlled Postoperative Blood Glucose[2]	77	100%	99%	97%
Perioperative Temperature Management[2]	392	100%	100%	100%
Prophylactic Antibiotic Selection[2]	323	100%	99%	99%
Prophylactic Antibiotic Selection (Outpatient)	337	99%	98%	98%
Prophylactic Antibiotic Stopped[2]	314	97%	98%	98%
Prophylactic Antibiotic Timing[2]	323	100%	99%	99%
Prophylactic Antibiotic Timing (Outpatient)	343	92%	98%	98%
Urinary Catheter Removal[2]	248	98%	97%	97%
Survey of Patients' Hospital Experiences				
Area Around Room 'Always' Quiet at Night[11]	300+	58%	67%	61%
Doctors 'Always' Communicated Well[11]	300+	83%	83%	82%
Home Recovery Information Given[11]	300+	87%	83%	85%
Hospital Given 9 or 10 on 10 Point Scale[11]	300+	72%	70%	71%
Meds 'Always' Explained Before Given[11]	300+	64%	63%	64%
Nurses 'Always' Communicated Well[11]	300+	77%	79%	79%
Pain 'Always' Well Controlled[11]	300+	69%	71%	71%
Room and Bathroom 'Always' Clean[11]	300+	65%	72%	73%
Timely Help 'Always' Received[11]	300+	63%	68%	68%
Would Definitely Recommend Hospital[11]	300+	76%	69%	71%
Use of Medical Imaging				
Cardiac Imaging Stress Test before Surgery	211	6.2%	4.3%	5.3%
Combination Abdominal CT Scan	788	46.2%	15.3%	10.5%
Combination Brain/Sinus CT Scan[1]	-	-	2.9%	2.7%
Combination Chest CT Scan	417	0.0%	5%	2.7%
Follow-up Mammogram/Ultrasound	1,577	6.2%	9.9%	8.8%
Lumbar Spine MRI for Low Back Pain	301	41.2%	41.6%	37.2%

Sparks Regional Medical Center

1001 Towson Avenue | Phone: 501-441-4000
Fort Smith, AR 72902 | Fax: 479-441-5462
URL: www.sparks.org
Type: Acute Care Hospitals | Emergency Services: Yes
Ownership: Proprietary | Beds: 510

Key Personnel:
Quality Assurance . . . . Jane Ball
Operating Room. . . . . Janina Bonwich
Emergency Room . . . . Kelly Hill
Chief of Medical Staff. . . . . Katherine Irish Clardy, MD
CEO/President. . . . . Dan McKay
Surgery . . . . Lori Sallee
Coronary Care . . . . Rebecca Vonderheide

Measure	Cases	This Hosp.	State Avg.	U.S. Avg.
Blood Clot Prevention and Treatment				
Anticoagulation Overlap Therapy[2]	68	100%	88%	93%
ICU Venous Thromboembolism Prophylaxis[2]	66	100%	94%	92%
Incidence of Potentially Preventable VTE[2]	13	8%	12%	10%
UFH with Dosages/Platelet Monitoring[2]	56	98%	100%	97%
Venous Thromboembolism Prophylaxis[2]	385	85%	91%	85%
Warfarin Therapy Discharge Instructions[2]	53	98%	76%	75%
Chest Pain/Possible Heart Attack Care				
Aspirin Given Within 24 Hours of Arrival[1,3]	-	-	96%	96%
Fibrinolytic Meds Within 30 Min. of Arrival[5]	-	-	54%	58%
Average Time to ECG (minutes)[1,3]	-	-	8	7
Average Time to Transfer (minutes)[5]	-	-	72	60
Children's Asthma Care				
Received Home Management Plan of Care	-	-	-	88%
Received Reliever Medication	-	-	-	100%
Received Systemic Corticosteroids	-	-	-	100%
Emergency Department				
Admittance Decision Time (minutes)[2]	844	103	65	98
Head CT Results Within 45 Min. of Arrival[1]	-	-	49%	57%
Patients Who Left ER Before Being Seen	66,937	2%	3%	2%
Time from ER Arrival to Admit. (minutes)[2]	844	273	214	274
Time from ER Arrival to Discharge (minutes)	401	143	118	134
Time in ER Before Being Evaluated (minutes)	420	38	26	26
Time to Pain Meds for Fractures (minutes)	129	76	66	57
Heart Attack Care				
Aspirin Given at Discharge[2]	293	100%	99%	99%
Fibrinolytic Meds Within 30 Min. of Arrival[2,7]	-	-	77%	54%
PCI Within 90 Minutes of Arrival[2]	21	100%	96%	96%
Statin Prescribed at Discharge[2]	299	100%	97%	98%
Heart Failure Care				
ACE Inhibitor or ARB for LVSD[2]	70	100%	96%	97%
Discharge Instructions Given[2]	223	97%	95%	94%
Evaluation of LVS Function[2]	305	100%	98%	99%
Medicare Spending				
Medicare Spending per Patient (ratio)	-	1.04	0.98	0.98
Pneumonia Care				
Appropriate Initial Antibiotic Given[2]	53	100%	94%	95%
Blood Culture Timing[2]	120	100%	98%	98%
Pregnancy and Delivery Care				
Newborn Deliveries Scheduled Early[2]	26	0%	6%	6%
Preventive Care				
Immunization for Influenza[2]	628	99%	89%	90%
Immunization for Pneumonia[2]	833	100%	92%	92%
Stroke Care				
Anticoagulation Therapy for Atrial Fibrillation[2]	17	100%	90%	95%
Antithrombotic Therapy Timing[2]	88	100%	96%	98%
Assessed for Rehabilitation[2]	107	100%	95%	97%
Discharged on Antithrombotic Therapy[2]	96	100%	96%	99%
Discharged on Statin Medication[2]	71	100%	86%	94%
Thrombolytic Therapy Timing[1,2]	-	-	35%	66%
Venous Thromboembolism Prophylaxis[2]	101	100%	91%	94%
Written Stroke Educational Materials Given[2]	57	100%	81%	88%
Surgical Care Improvement Project				
Appropriate Beta Blocker Usage[2]	189	100%	98%	98%
Appropriate VTP Within 24 Hours[2]	260	100%	98%	98%
Controlled Postoperative Blood Glucose[2]	101	100%	99%	97%
Perioperative Temperature Management[2]	371	100%	100%	100%
Prophylactic Antibiotic Selection[2]	280	100%	99%	99%
Prophylactic Antibiotic Selection (Outpatient)	484	100%	98%	98%
Prophylactic Antibiotic Stopped[2]	265	100%	98%	98%
Prophylactic Antibiotic Timing[2]	281	100%	99%	99%
Prophylactic Antibiotic Timing (Outpatient)	484	100%	98%	98%
Urinary Catheter Removal[2]	200	100%	97%	97%
Survey of Patients' Hospital Experiences				
Area Around Room 'Always' Quiet at Night	300+	52%	67%	61%
Doctors 'Always' Communicated Well	300+	75%	83%	82%
Home Recovery Information Given	300+	80%	83%	85%
Hospital Given 9 or 10 on 10 Point Scale	300+	56%	70%	71%
Meds 'Always' Explained Before Given	300+	49%	63%	64%
Nurses 'Always' Communicated Well	300+	67%	79%	79%
Pain 'Always' Well Controlled	300+	60%	71%	71%
Room and Bathroom 'Always' Clean	300+	63%	72%	73%
Timely Help 'Always' Received	300+	48%	68%	68%
Would Definitely Recommend Hospital	300+	59%	69%	71%
Use of Medical Imaging				
Cardiac Imaging Stress Test before Surgery	557	5.6%	4.3%	5.3%
Combination Abdominal CT Scan	1,421	12.2%	15.3%	10.5%
Combination Brain/Sinus CT Scan	1,246	3.0%	2.9%	2.7%
Combination Chest CT Scan	806	9.6%	5%	2.7%
Follow-up Mammogram/Ultrasound	2,538	6.6%	9.9%	8.8%
Lumbar Spine MRI for Low Back Pain	152	46.1%	41.6%	37.2%

Ozarks Community Hospital of Gravette

1101 Jackson Street Sw | Phone: 479-787-5291
Gravette, AR 72736
URL: www.ochonline.com
Type: Critical Access Hospitals | Emergency Services: Yes
Ownership: Proprietary

Measure	Cases	This Hosp.	State Avg.	U.S. Avg.
Blood Clot Prevention and Treatment				
Anticoagulation Overlap Therapy[5]	-	-	88%	93%
ICU Venous Thromboembolism Prophylaxis[5]	-	-	94%	92%
Incidence of Potentially Preventable VTE[5]	-	-	12%	10%
UFH with Dosages/Platelet Monitoring[5]	-	-	100%	97%
Venous Thromboembolism Prophylaxis[5]	-	-	91%	85%
Warfarin Therapy Discharge Instructions[5]	-	-	76%	75%
Chest Pain/Possible Heart Attack Care				
Aspirin Given Within 24 Hours of Arrival[5]	-	-	96%	96%
Fibrinolytic Meds Within 30 Min. of Arrival[5]	-	-	54%	58%
Average Time to ECG (minutes)[5]	-	-	8	7
Average Time to Transfer (minutes)[5]	-	-	72	60
Children's Asthma Care				
Received Home Management Plan of Care	-	-	-	88%
Received Reliever Medication	-	-	-	100%
Received Systemic Corticosteroids	-	-	-	100%
Emergency Department				
Admittance Decision Time (minutes)[5]	-	-	65	98
Head CT Results Within 45 Min. of Arrival[5]	-	-	49%	57%
Patients Who Left ER Before Being Seen[5]	-	-	3%	2%
Time from ER Arrival to Admit. (minutes)[5]	-	-	214	274
Time from ER Arrival to Discharge (minutes)[5]	-	-	118	134
Time in ER Before Being Evaluated (minutes)[5]	-	-	26	26
Time to Pain Meds for Fractures (minutes)[5]	-	-	66	57
Heart Attack Care				
Aspirin Given at Discharge[3,7]	-	-	99%	99%
Fibrinolytic Meds Within 30 Min. of Arrival[3,7]	-	-	77%	54%
PCI Within 90 Minutes of Arrival[3,7]	-	-	96%	96%
Statin Prescribed at Discharge[3,7]	-	-	97%	98%
Heart Failure Care				
ACE Inhibitor or ARB for LVSD[1,3]	-	-	96%	97%
Discharge Instructions Given[3]	12	33%	95%	94%
Evaluation of LVS Function[3]	17	53%	98%	99%
Medicare Spending				
Medicare Spending per Patient (ratio)	-	-	0.98	0.98
Pneumonia Care				
Appropriate Initial Antibiotic Given[3]	33	91%	94%	95%
Blood Culture Timing[1,3]	-	-	98%	98%
Pregnancy and Delivery Care				
Newborn Deliveries Scheduled Early[5]	-	-	6%	6%
Preventive Care				
Immunization for Influenza[5]	-	-	89%	90%
Immunization for Pneumonia[5]	-	-	92%	92%
Stroke Care				
Anticoagulation Therapy for Atrial Fibrillation[5]	-	-	90%	95%
Antithrombotic Therapy Timing[5]	-	-	96%	98%
Assessed for Rehabilitation[5]	-	-	95%	97%
Discharged on Antithrombotic Therapy[5]	-	-	96%	99%
Discharged on Statin Medication[5]	-	-	86%	94%
Thrombolytic Therapy Timing[5]	-	-	35%	66%
Venous Thromboembolism Prophylaxis[5]	-	-	91%	94%
Written Stroke Educational Materials Given[5]	-	-	81%	88%

NOTE: Hospital profiles are in alphabetical order by state, then city, then hospital within the city; Rankings exclude hospitals with less than 25 cases except for patient surveys which excludes hospitals with less than 100 cases; (a) 100-299 cases; (1) The number of cases/patients is too few to report; (2) Data submitted were based on a sample of cases/patients; (3) Results are based on a shorter time period than required; (4) Data suppressed by CMS for one or more quarters; (5) Results are not available for this reporting period; (6) Fewer than 100 patients completed the HCAHPS survey; (7) No cases met the criteria for this measure; (8) The lower limit of the confidence interval cannot be calculated if the number of observed infections equals zero; (9) No data are available from the state/territory for this reporting period; (10) The scores shown reflect fewer than 50 completed surveys; (11) There were discrepancies in the data collection process; (12) This measure does not apply to this hospital for this reporting period; (13) Results cannot be calculated for this reporting period; (14) The results for this state are combined with nearby states to protect confidentiality; Please refer to the User's Guide for a full explanation of data.

Measure	Cases	This Hosp.	State Avg.	U.S. Avg.
Surgical Care Improvement Project				
Appropriate Beta Blocker Usage[5]	-	-	98%	98%
Appropriate VTP Within 24 Hours[5]	-	-	98%	98%
Controlled Postoperative Blood Glucose[5]	-	-	99%	97%
Perioperative Temperature Management[5]	-	-	100%	100%
Prophylactic Antibiotic Selection[5]	-	-	99%	99%
Prophylactic Antibiotic Selection (Outpatient)[5]	-	-	98%	98%
Prophylactic Antibiotic Stopped[5]	-	-	98%	98%
Prophylactic Antibiotic Timing[5]	-	-	99%	99%
Prophylactic Antibiotic Timing (Outpatient)[5]	-	-	98%	98%
Urinary Catheter Removal[5]	-	-	97%	97%
Survey of Patients' Hospital Experiences				
Area Around Room 'Always' Quiet at Night[5]	-	-	67%	61%
Doctors 'Always' Communicated Well[5]	-	-	83%	82%
Home Recovery Information Given[5]	-	-	83%	85%
Hospital Given 9 or 10 on 10 Point Scale[5]	-	-	70%	71%
Meds 'Always' Explained Before Given[5]	-	-	63%	64%
Nurses 'Always' Communicated Well[5]	-	-	79%	79%
Pain 'Always' Well Controlled[5]	-	-	71%	71%
Room and Bathroom 'Always' Clean[5]	-	-	72%	73%
Timely Help 'Always' Received[5]	-	-	68%	68%
Would Definitely Recommend Hospital[5]	-	-	69%	71%
Use of Medical Imaging				
Cardiac Imaging Stress Test before Surgery[7]	-	-	4.3%	5.3%
Combination Abdominal CT Scan[1]	-	-	15.3%	10.5%
Combination Brain/Sinus CT Scan[1]	-	-	2.9%	2.7%
Combination Chest CT Scan[1]	-	-	5%	2.7%
Follow-up Mammogram/Ultrasound[7]	-	-	9.9%	8.8%
Lumbar Spine MRI for Low Back Pain[1]	-	-	41.6%	37.2%

North Arkansas Regional Medical Center

620 North Main Street — Phone: 870-414-4000
Harrison, AR 72601 — Fax: 870-365-2430
URL: www.narmc.com
Type: Acute Care Hospitals — Emergency Services: Yes
Ownership: Voluntary non-profit - Private — Beds: 174

Key Personnel:
Chief of Medical Staff.......... Brad Allen
Quality Assurance .... Sharon Bates
Operating Room............... Thomas Bell
Radiology.................... Chris Bennett, MD
Pediatric Ambulatory Care ...... Asish Ghosh, MD
CEO/President............... Timothy E Hill
Anesthesiology............... James D. Waters
Infection Control............. Kalen Youngs

Measure	Cases	This Hosp.	State Avg.	U.S. Avg.
Blood Clot Prevention and Treatment				
Anticoagulation Overlap Therapy[2]	46	78%	88%	93%
ICU Venous Thromboembolism Prophylaxis[2]	88	97%	94%	92%
Incidence of Potentially Preventable VTE[1,2]	-	-	12%	10%
UFH with Dosages/Platelet Monitoring[1,2]	-	-	100%	97%
Venous Thromboembolism Prophylaxis[2]	185	96%	91%	85%
Warfarin Therapy Discharge Instructions[2]	39	97%	76%	75%
Chest Pain/Possible Heart Attack Care				
Aspirin Given Within 24 Hours of Arrival	121	97%	96%	96%
Fibrinolytic Meds Within 30 Min. of Arrival[7]	-	-	54%	58%
Average Time to ECG (minutes)	127	12	8	7
Average Time to Transfer (minutes)[1]	-	-	72	60
Children's Asthma Care				
Received Home Management Plan of Care	-	-	-	88%
Received Reliever Medication	-	-	-	100%
Received Systemic Corticosteroids	-	-	-	100%
Emergency Department				
Admittance Decision Time (minutes)[2]	325	91	65	98
Head CT Results Within 45 Min. of Arrival[1]	-	-	49%	57%
Patients Who Left ER Before Being Seen	23,229	2%	3%	2%
Time from ER Arrival to Admit. (minutes)[2]	329	230	214	274
Time from ER Arrival to Discharge (minutes)	226	123	118	134
Time in ER Before Being Evaluated (minutes)	381	19	26	26
Time to Pain Meds for Fractures (minutes)	86	60	66	57
Heart Attack Care				
Aspirin Given at Discharge[1]	-	-	99%	99%
Fibrinolytic Meds Within 30 Min. of Arrival[7]	-	-	77%	54%
PCI Within 90 Minutes of Arrival[7]	-	-	96%	96%
Statin Prescribed at Discharge[1]	-	-	97%	98%
Heart Failure Care				
ACE Inhibitor or ARB for LVSD	32	78%	96%	97%
Discharge Instructions Given	72	89%	95%	94%
Evaluation of LVS Function	104	94%	98%	99%
Medicare Spending				
Medicare Spending per Patient (ratio)	-	0.91	0.98	0.98
Pneumonia Care				
Appropriate Initial Antibiotic Given[2]	95	88%	94%	95%
Blood Culture Timing[2]	122	93%	98%	98%
Pregnancy and Delivery Care				
Newborn Deliveries Scheduled Early[2]	21	14%	6%	6%
Preventive Care				
Immunization for Influenza[2]	437	84%	89%	90%
Immunization for Pneumonia[2]	527	89%	92%	92%
Stroke Care				
Anticoagulation Therapy for Atrial Fibrillation[1,2]	-	-	90%	95%
Antithrombotic Therapy Timing[2]	46	91%	96%	98%
Assessed for Rehabilitation[2]	45	93%	95%	97%
Discharged on Antithrombotic Therapy[2]	45	98%	96%	99%
Discharged on Statin Medication[2]	31	81%	86%	94%
Thrombolytic Therapy Timing[1,2]	-	-	35%	66%
Venous Thromboembolism Prophylaxis[2]	46	98%	91%	94%
Written Stroke Educational Materials Given[2]	23	78%	81%	88%
Surgical Care Improvement Project				
Appropriate Beta Blocker Usage[2]	45	93%	98%	98%
Appropriate VTP Within 24 Hours[2]	191	98%	98%	98%
Controlled Postoperative Blood Glucose[2,7]	-	-	99%	97%
Perioperative Temperature Management[2]	210	100%	100%	100%
Prophylactic Antibiotic Selection[2]	149	98%	99%	99%
Prophylactic Antibiotic Selection (Outpatient)	172	98%	98%	98%
Prophylactic Antibiotic Stopped[2]	144	92%	98%	98%
Prophylactic Antibiotic Timing[2]	149	97%	99%	99%
Prophylactic Antibiotic Timing (Outpatient)	132	94%	98%	98%
Urinary Catheter Removal[2]	83	93%	97%	97%
Survey of Patients' Hospital Experiences				
Area Around Room 'Always' Quiet at Night	300+	65%	67%	61%
Doctors 'Always' Communicated Well	300+	82%	83%	82%
Home Recovery Information Given	300+	79%	83%	85%
Hospital Given 9 or 10 on 10 Point Scale	300+	65%	70%	71%
Meds 'Always' Explained Before Given	300+	60%	63%	64%
Nurses 'Always' Communicated Well	300+	77%	79%	79%
Pain 'Always' Well Controlled	300+	68%	71%	71%
Room and Bathroom 'Always' Clean	300+	79%	72%	73%
Timely Help 'Always' Received	300+	66%	68%	68%
Would Definitely Recommend Hospital	300+	62%	69%	71%
Use of Medical Imaging				
Cardiac Imaging Stress Test before Surgery	73	6.8%	4.3%	5.3%
Combination Abdominal CT Scan	954	21.9%	15.3%	10.5%
Combination Brain/Sinus CT Scan	827	1.0%	2.9%	2.7%
Combination Chest CT Scan	373	5.9%	5%	2.7%
Follow-up Mammogram/Ultrasound	984	8.3%	9.9%	8.8%
Lumbar Spine MRI for Low Back Pain	162	50.0%	41.6%	37.2%

Baptist Health Medical Center - Heber Spings

1800 Bypass Road — Phone: 501-887-3000
Heber Springs, AR 72543 — Fax: 501-206-3390
URL: www.baptist-health.org
Type: Critical Access Hospitals — Emergency Services: Yes
Ownership: Voluntary non-profit - Private — Beds: 49

Key Personnel:
Operating Room............. Rhonda Clark
Emergency Room .... Kari M Kramer Kajitani, RN
CEO/President.............. Edward Lacy
Chief of Medical Staff.......... Tonya Little, MD
Quality Assurance .... Crystal Muirhead
Infection Control............ Tamara Wright

Measure	Cases	This Hosp.	State Avg.	U.S. Avg.
Blood Clot Prevention and Treatment				
Anticoagulation Overlap Therapy[1,2]	-	-	88%	93%
ICU Venous Thromboembolism Prophylaxis[1,2]	-	-	94%	92%
Incidence of Potentially Preventable VTE[2,7]	-	-	12%	10%
UFH with Dosages/Platelet Monitoring[2,7]	-	-	100%	97%
Venous Thromboembolism Prophylaxis[2]	89	88%	91%	85%
Warfarin Therapy Discharge Instructions[1,2]	-	-	76%	75%
Chest Pain/Possible Heart Attack Care				
Aspirin Given Within 24 Hours of Arrival	48	100%	96%	96%
Fibrinolytic Meds Within 30 Min. of Arrival[1]	-	-	54%	58%
Average Time to ECG (minutes)	51	10	8	7
Average Time to Transfer (minutes)[1]	-	-	72	60
Children's Asthma Care				
Received Home Management Plan of Care	-	-	-	88%
Received Reliever Medication	-	-	-	100%
Received Systemic Corticosteroids	-	-	-	100%
Emergency Department				
Admittance Decision Time (minutes)[2]	418	45	65	98
Head CT Results Within 45 Min. of Arrival[1]	-	-	49%	57%
Patients Who Left ER Before Being Seen	10,332	3%	3%	2%
Time from ER Arrival to Admit. (minutes)[2]	458	229	214	274
Time from ER Arrival to Discharge (minutes)	345	135	118	134
Time in ER Before Being Evaluated (minutes)	406	32	26	26
Time to Pain Meds for Fractures (minutes)	62	70	66	57
Heart Attack Care				
Aspirin Given at Discharge[1,3]	-	-	99%	99%
Fibrinolytic Meds Within 30 Min. of Arrival[3,7]	-	-	77%	54%
PCI Within 90 Minutes of Arrival[3,7]	-	-	96%	96%
Statin Prescribed at Discharge[1,3]	-	-	97%	98%
Heart Failure Care				
ACE Inhibitor or ARB for LVSD[1]	-	-	96%	97%
Discharge Instructions Given	22	100%	95%	94%
Evaluation of LVS Function	30	100%	98%	99%
Medicare Spending				
Medicare Spending per Patient (ratio)	-	-	0.98	0.98
Pneumonia Care				
Appropriate Initial Antibiotic Given	36	94%	94%	95%
Blood Culture Timing	59	100%	98%	98%
Pregnancy and Delivery Care				
Newborn Deliveries Scheduled Early[7]	-	-	6%	6%
Preventive Care				
Immunization for Influenza[2]	279	93%	89%	90%
Immunization for Pneumonia[2]	489	96%	92%	92%
Stroke Care				
Anticoagulation Therapy for Atrial Fibrillation[1]	-	-	90%	95%
Antithrombotic Therapy Timing[1]	-	-	96%	98%
Assessed for Rehabilitation[1]	-	-	95%	97%
Discharged on Antithrombotic Therapy[1]	-	-	96%	99%
Discharged on Statin Medication[1]	-	-	86%	94%
Thrombolytic Therapy Timing[7]	-	-	35%	66%
Venous Thromboembolism Prophylaxis[1]	-	-	91%	94%
Written Stroke Educational Materials Given[1]	-	-	81%	88%
Surgical Care Improvement Project				
Appropriate Beta Blocker Usage	19	100%	98%	98%
Appropriate VTP Within 24 Hours	54	94%	98%	98%
Controlled Postoperative Blood Glucose[7]	-	-	99%	97%
Perioperative Temperature Management	58	100%	100%	100%
Prophylactic Antibiotic Selection	51	100%	99%	99%
Prophylactic Antibiotic Selection (Outpatient)	32	94%	98%	98%
Prophylactic Antibiotic Stopped	50	98%	98%	98%
Prophylactic Antibiotic Timing	51	98%	99%	99%
Prophylactic Antibiotic Timing (Outpatient)[1]	-	-	98%	98%
Urinary Catheter Removal	17	82%	97%	97%
Survey of Patients' Hospital Experiences				
Area Around Room 'Always' Quiet at Night	(a)	79%	67%	61%
Doctors 'Always' Communicated Well	(a)	86%	83%	82%
Home Recovery Information Given	(a)	87%	83%	85%
Hospital Given 9 or 10 on 10 Point Scale	(a)	80%	70%	71%
Meds 'Always' Explained Before Given	(a)	69%	63%	64%
Nurses 'Always' Communicated Well	(a)	87%	79%	79%
Pain 'Always' Well Controlled	(a)	75%	71%	71%
Room and Bathroom 'Always' Clean	(a)	81%	72%	73%
Timely Help 'Always' Received	(a)	76%	68%	68%
Would Definitely Recommend Hospital	(a)	78%	69%	71%
Use of Medical Imaging				
Cardiac Imaging Stress Test before Surgery[7]	-	-	4.3%	5.3%
Combination Abdominal CT Scan	504	7.1%	15.3%	10.5%
Combination Brain/Sinus CT Scan[1]	-	-	2.9%	2.7%

NOTE: Hospital profiles are in alphabetical order by state, then city, then hospital within the city; Rankings exclude hospitals with less than 25 cases except for patient surveys which excludes hospitals with less than 100 cases; (a) 100-299 cases; (1) The number of cases/patients is too few to report; (2) Data submitted were based on a sample of cases/patients; (3) Results are based on a shorter time period than required; (4) Data suppressed by CMS for one or more quarters; (5) Results are not available for this reporting period; (6) Fewer than 100 patients completed the HCAHPS survey; (7) No cases met the criteria for this measure; (8) The lower limit of the confidence interval cannot be calculated if the number of observed infections equals zero; (9) No data are available from the state/territory for this reporting period; (10) The scores shown reflect fewer than 50 completed surveys; (11) There were discrepancies in the data collection process; (12) This measure does not apply to this hospital for this reporting period; (13) Results cannot be calculated for this reporting period; (14) The results for this state are combined with nearby states to protect confidentiality; Please refer to the User's Guide for a full explanation of data.

Measure	Cases	This Hosp.	State Avg.	U.S. Avg.
Combination Chest CT Scan	277	2.2%	5%	2.7%
Follow-up Mammogram/Ultrasound	642	5.8%	9.9%	8.8%
Lumbar Spine MRI for Low Back Pain	94	35.1%	41.6%	37.2%

Helena Regional Medical Center

1801 Martin Luther King Drive Phone: 870-338-5800
Helena, AR 72342 Fax: 870-816-3944
URL: www.helenaregionalmedicalcenter.com
Type: Acute Care Hospitals Emergency Services: Yes
Ownership: Proprietary Beds: 155

Key Personnel:
Chief of Medical Staff.......... Thomas Bailey
Emergency Room .... Don Ball
Radiology.................. John Chang
Operating Room.............. Courtney Dillard
Quality Assurance .... Joanne Hardin
Intensive Care Unit............ Mattie Littlejohn, MD
Infection Control.............. Jamie Pryor
CEO/President............... Tom Sewell

Measure	Cases	This Hosp.	State Avg.	U.S. Avg.
Blood Clot Prevention and Treatment				
Anticoagulation Overlap Therapy[1,2]	-	-	88%	93%
ICU Venous Thromboembolism Prophylaxis[2]	88	98%	94%	92%
Incidence of Potentially Preventable VTE[1,2]	-	-	12%	10%
UFH with Dosages/Platelet Monitoring[1,2]	-	-	100%	97%
Venous Thromboembolism Prophylaxis[2]	279	95%	91%	85%
Warfarin Therapy Discharge Instructions[1,2]	-	-	76%	75%
Chest Pain/Possible Heart Attack Care				
Aspirin Given Within 24 Hours of Arrival	57	100%	96%	96%
Fibrinolytic Meds Within 30 Min. of Arrival[1]	-	-	54%	58%
Average Time to ECG (minutes)	60	1	8	7
Average Time to Transfer (minutes)[7]	-	-	72	60
Children's Asthma Care				
Received Home Management Plan of Care	-	-	-	88%
Received Reliever Medication	-	-	-	100%
Received Systemic Corticosteroids	-	-	-	100%
Emergency Department				
Admittance Decision Time (minutes)[2]	476	64	65	98
Head CT Results Within 45 Min. of Arrival[1]	-	-	49%	57%
Patients Who Left ER Before Being Seen	12,209	2%	3%	2%
Time from ER Arrival to Admit. (minutes)[2]	477	184	214	274
Time from ER Arrival to Discharge (minutes)	316	98	118	134
Time in ER Before Being Evaluated (minutes)	454	15	26	26
Time to Pain Meds for Fractures (minutes)	46	42	66	57
Heart Attack Care				
Aspirin Given at Discharge[1]	-	-	99%	99%
Fibrinolytic Meds Within 30 Min. of Arrival[7]	-	-	77%	54%
PCI Within 90 Minutes of Arrival[7]	-	-	96%	96%
Statin Prescribed at Discharge[1]	-	-	97%	98%
Heart Failure Care				
ACE Inhibitor or ARB for LVSD	75	100%	96%	97%
Discharge Instructions Given	165	100%	95%	94%
Evaluation of LVS Function	185	100%	98%	99%
Medicare Spending				
Medicare Spending per Patient (ratio)	-	0.82	0.98	0.98
Pneumonia Care				
Appropriate Initial Antibiotic Given	37	100%	94%	95%
Blood Culture Timing	42	100%	98%	98%
Pregnancy and Delivery Care				
Newborn Deliveries Scheduled Early[2]	19	0%	6%	6%
Preventive Care				
Immunization for Influenza[2]	415	100%	89%	90%
Immunization for Pneumonia[2]	484	100%	92%	92%
Stroke Care				
Anticoagulation Therapy for Atrial Fibrillation[1]	-	-	90%	95%
Antithrombotic Therapy Timing	17	100%	96%	98%
Assessed for Rehabilitation	16	94%	95%	97%
Discharged on Antithrombotic Therapy	15	87%	96%	99%
Discharged on Statin Medication	12	75%	86%	94%
Thrombolytic Therapy Timing[7]	-	-	35%	66%
Venous Thromboembolism Prophylaxis	16	100%	91%	94%
Written Stroke Educational Materials Given[1]	-	-	81%	88%
Surgical Care Improvement Project				
Appropriate Beta Blocker Usage[1]	-	-	98%	98%
Appropriate VTP Within 24 Hours	11	100%	98%	98%
Controlled Postoperative Blood Glucose[7]	-	-	99%	97%
Perioperative Temperature Management	12	100%	100%	100%
Prophylactic Antibiotic Selection[1]	-	-	99%	99%
Prophylactic Antibiotic Selection (Outpatient)[1,3]	-	-	98%	98%
Prophylactic Antibiotic Stopped[1]	-	-	98%	98%
Prophylactic Antibiotic Timing[1]	-	-	99%	99%
Prophylactic Antibiotic Timing (Outpatient)[1,3]	-	-	98%	98%
Urinary Catheter Removal[1]	-	-	97%	97%
Survey of Patients' Hospital Experiences				
Area Around Room 'Always' Quiet at Night	300+	68%	67%	61%
Doctors 'Always' Communicated Well	300+	85%	83%	82%
Home Recovery Information Given	300+	81%	83%	85%
Hospital Given 9 or 10 on 10 Point Scale	300+	66%	70%	71%
Meds 'Always' Explained Before Given	300+	65%	63%	64%
Nurses 'Always' Communicated Well	300+	79%	79%	79%
Pain 'Always' Well Controlled	300+	70%	71%	71%
Room and Bathroom 'Always' Clean	300+	71%	72%	73%
Timely Help 'Always' Received	300+	64%	68%	68%
Would Definitely Recommend Hospital	300+	56%	69%	71%
Use of Medical Imaging				
Cardiac Imaging Stress Test before Surgery[7]	-	-	4.3%	5.3%
Combination Abdominal CT Scan	192	4.2%	15.3%	10.5%
Combination Brain/Sinus CT Scan[1]	-	-	2.9%	2.7%
Combination Chest CT Scan	84	9.5%	5%	2.7%
Follow-up Mammogram/Ultrasound	199	6.5%	9.9%	8.8%
Lumbar Spine MRI for Low Back Pain[1]	-	-	41.6%	37.2%

Wadley Regional Medical Center at Hope

2001 South Main Phone: 870-777-2323
Hope, AR 71801
Type: Acute Care Hospitals Emergency Services: Yes
Ownership: Proprietary

Measure	Cases	This Hosp.	State Avg.	U.S. Avg.
Blood Clot Prevention and Treatment				
Anticoagulation Overlap Therapy[1,2]	-	-	88%	93%
ICU Venous Thromboembolism Prophylaxis[2]	74	93%	94%	92%
Incidence of Potentially Preventable VTE[2,7]	-	-	12%	10%
UFH with Dosages/Platelet Monitoring[2,7]	-	-	100%	97%
Venous Thromboembolism Prophylaxis[2]	111	86%	91%	85%
Warfarin Therapy Discharge Instructions[1,2]	-	-	76%	75%
Chest Pain/Possible Heart Attack Care				
Aspirin Given Within 24 Hours of Arrival[1,3]	-	-	96%	96%
Fibrinolytic Meds Within 30 Min. of Arrival[3,7]	-	-	54%	58%
Average Time to ECG (minutes)[1,3]	-	-	8	7
Average Time to Transfer (minutes)[3,7]	-	-	72	60
Children's Asthma Care				
Received Home Management Plan of Care	-	-	-	88%
Received Reliever Medication	-	-	-	100%
Received Systemic Corticosteroids	-	-	-	100%
Emergency Department				
Admittance Decision Time (minutes)[2]	370	55	65	98
Head CT Results Within 45 Min. of Arrival[1]	-	-	49%	57%
Patients Who Left ER Before Being Seen	2,660	6%	3%	2%
Time from ER Arrival to Admit. (minutes)[2]	373	238	214	274
Time from ER Arrival to Discharge (minutes)	456	105	118	134
Time in ER Before Being Evaluated (minutes)	428	20	26	26
Time to Pain Meds for Fractures (minutes)	28	73	66	57
Heart Attack Care				
Aspirin Given at Discharge[1,3]	-	-	99%	99%
Fibrinolytic Meds Within 30 Min. of Arrival[3,7]	-	-	77%	54%
PCI Within 90 Minutes of Arrival[3,7]	-	-	96%	96%
Statin Prescribed at Discharge[1,3]	-	-	97%	98%
Heart Failure Care				
ACE Inhibitor or ARB for LVSD	11	82%	96%	97%
Discharge Instructions Given	43	95%	95%	94%
Evaluation of LVS Function	70	99%	98%	99%
Medicare Spending				
Medicare Spending per Patient (ratio)	-	-	0.98	0.98
Pneumonia Care				
Appropriate Initial Antibiotic Given	72	86%	94%	95%
Blood Culture Timing	54	98%	98%	98%
Pregnancy and Delivery Care				
Newborn Deliveries Scheduled Early[7]	-	-	6%	6%
Preventive Care				
Immunization for Influenza[2]	296	97%	89%	90%
Immunization for Pneumonia[2]	449	98%	92%	92%
Stroke Care				
Anticoagulation Therapy for Atrial Fibrillation[7]	-	-	90%	95%
Antithrombotic Therapy Timing[1]	-	-	96%	98%
Assessed for Rehabilitation[1]	-	-	95%	97%
Discharged on Antithrombotic Therapy[1]	-	-	96%	99%
Discharged on Statin Medication[1]	-	-	86%	94%
Thrombolytic Therapy Timing[7]	-	-	35%	66%
Venous Thromboembolism Prophylaxis[1]	-	-	91%	94%
Written Stroke Educational Materials Given[1]	-	-	81%	88%
Surgical Care Improvement Project				
Appropriate Beta Blocker Usage[5]	-	-	98%	98%
Appropriate VTP Within 24 Hours[5]	-	-	98%	98%
Controlled Postoperative Blood Glucose[5]	-	-	99%	97%
Perioperative Temperature Management[5]	-	-	100%	100%
Prophylactic Antibiotic Selection[5]	-	-	99%	99%
Prophylactic Antibiotic Selection (Outpatient)[5]	-	-	98%	98%
Prophylactic Antibiotic Stopped[5]	-	-	98%	98%
Prophylactic Antibiotic Timing[5]	-	-	99%	99%
Prophylactic Antibiotic Timing (Outpatient)[5]	-	-	98%	98%
Urinary Catheter Removal[5]	-	-	97%	97%
Survey of Patients' Hospital Experiences				
Area Around Room 'Always' Quiet at Night	(a)	70%	67%	61%
Doctors 'Always' Communicated Well	(a)	87%	83%	82%
Home Recovery Information Given	(a)	84%	83%	85%
Hospital Given 9 or 10 on 10 Point Scale	(a)	69%	70%	71%
Meds 'Always' Explained Before Given	(a)	62%	63%	64%
Nurses 'Always' Communicated Well	(a)	82%	79%	79%
Pain 'Always' Well Controlled	(a)	74%	71%	71%
Room and Bathroom 'Always' Clean	(a)	68%	72%	73%
Timely Help 'Always' Received	(a)	70%	68%	68%
Would Definitely Recommend Hospital	(a)	68%	69%	71%
Use of Medical Imaging				
Cardiac Imaging Stress Test before Surgery[1]	-	-	4.3%	5.3%
Combination Abdominal CT Scan	48	33.3%	15.3%	10.5%
Combination Brain/Sinus CT Scan	92	0.0%	2.9%	2.7%
Combination Chest CT Scan[1]	-	-	5%	2.7%
Follow-up Mammogram/Ultrasound[1]	-	-	9.9%	8.8%
Lumbar Spine MRI for Low Back Pain[1]	-	-	41.6%	37.2%

Leo N Levi National Arthritis Hospital

300 Prospect Ave Phone: 501-624-1281
Hot Springs, AR 71901 Fax: 501-622-3500
E-mail: bholsomback@levihospital.com
URL: www.levihospital.com
Type: Acute Care Hospitals Emergency Services: Yes
Ownership: Voluntary non-profit - Private Beds: 89

Key Personnel:
Pediatric Ambulatory Care ...... Laura Dunn, MD
Pediatric In-Patient Care .... Laura Dunn, MD
Chief of Medical Staff.......... Michael Goldman
Quality Assurance .... Beverley Jackson
CEO/President............... Patrick G McCabe Jr, Jr

Measure	Cases	This Hosp.	State Avg.	U.S. Avg.
Blood Clot Prevention and Treatment				
Anticoagulation Overlap Therapy[5]	-	-	88%	93%
ICU Venous Thromboembolism Prophylaxis[5]	-	-	94%	92%
Incidence of Potentially Preventable VTE[5]	-	-	12%	10%
UFH with Dosages/Platelet Monitoring[5]	-	-	100%	97%
Venous Thromboembolism Prophylaxis[5]	-	-	91%	85%
Warfarin Therapy Discharge Instructions[5]	-	-	76%	75%
Chest Pain/Possible Heart Attack Care				
Aspirin Given Within 24 Hours of Arrival[5]	-	-	96%	96%
Fibrinolytic Meds Within 30 Min. of Arrival[5]	-	-	54%	58%
Average Time to ECG (minutes)[5]	-	-	8	7
Average Time to Transfer (minutes)[5]	-	-	72	60
Children's Asthma Care				
Received Home Management Plan of Care	-	-	-	88%
Received Reliever Medication	-	-	-	100%
Received Systemic Corticosteroids	-	-	-	100%

NOTE: Hospital profiles are in alphabetical order by state, then city, then hospital within the city; Rankings exclude hospitals with less than 25 cases except for patient surveys which excludes hospitals with less than 100 cases; (a) 100-299 cases; (1) The number of cases/patients is too few to report; (2) Data submitted were based on a sample of cases/patients; (3) Results are based on a shorter time period than required; (4) Data suppressed by CMS for one or more quarters; (5) Results are not available for this reporting period; (6) Fewer than 100 patients completed the HCAHPS survey; (7) No cases met the criteria for this measure; (8) The lower limit of the confidence interval cannot be calculated if the number of observed infections equals zero; (9) No data are available from the state/territory for this reporting period; (10) The scores shown reflect fewer than 50 completed surveys; (11) There were discrepancies in the data collection process; (12) This measure does not apply to this hospital for this reporting period; (13) Results cannot be calculated for this reporting period; (14) The results for this state are combined with nearby states to protect confidentiality; Please refer to the User's Guide for a full explanation of data.

Measure	Cases	This Hosp.	State Avg.	U.S. Avg.
Emergency Department				
Admittance Decision Time (minutes)[5]	-	-	65	98
Head CT Results Within 45 Min. of Arrival[5]	-	-	49%	57%
Patients Who Left ER Before Being Seen[5]	-	-	3%	2%
Time from ER Arrival to Admit. (minutes)[5]	-	-	214	274
Time from ER Arrival to Discharge (minutes)[5]	-	-	118	134
Time in ER Before Being Evaluated (minutes)[5]	-	-	26	26
Time to Pain Meds for Fractures (minutes)[5]	-	-	66	57
Heart Attack Care				
Aspirin Given at Discharge[5]	-	-	99%	99%
Fibrinolytic Meds Within 30 Min. of Arrival[5]	-	-	77%	54%
PCI Within 90 Minutes of Arrival[5]	-	-	96%	96%
Statin Prescribed at Discharge[5]	-	-	97%	98%
Heart Failure Care				
ACE Inhibitor or ARB for LVSD[5]	-	-	96%	97%
Discharge Instructions Given[5]	-	-	95%	94%
Evaluation of LVS Function[5]	-	-	98%	99%
Medicare Spending				
Medicare Spending per Patient (ratio)	-	-	0.98	0.98
Pneumonia Care				
Appropriate Initial Antibiotic Given[5]	-	-	94%	95%
Blood Culture Timing[5]	-	-	98%	98%
Pregnancy and Delivery Care				
Newborn Deliveries Scheduled Early[7]	-	-	6%	6%
Preventive Care				
Immunization for Influenza[5]	-	-	89%	90%
Immunization for Pneumonia[5]	-	-	92%	92%
Stroke Care				
Anticoagulation Therapy for Atrial Fibrillation[5]	-	-	90%	95%
Antithrombotic Therapy Timing[5]	-	-	96%	98%
Assessed for Rehabilitation[5]	-	-	95%	97%
Discharged on Antithrombotic Therapy[5]	-	-	96%	99%
Discharged on Statin Medication[5]	-	-	86%	94%
Thrombolytic Therapy Timing[5]	-	-	35%	66%
Venous Thromboembolism Prophylaxis[5]	-	-	91%	94%
Written Stroke Educational Materials Given[5]	-	-	81%	88%
Surgical Care Improvement Project				
Appropriate Beta Blocker Usage[5]	-	-	98%	98%
Appropriate VTP Within 24 Hours[5]	-	-	98%	98%
Controlled Postoperative Blood Glucose[5]	-	-	99%	97%
Perioperative Temperature Management[5]	-	-	100%	100%
Prophylactic Antibiotic Selection[5]	-	-	99%	99%
Prophylactic Antibiotic Selection (Outpatient)[5]	-	-	98%	98%
Prophylactic Antibiotic Stopped[5]	-	-	98%	98%
Prophylactic Antibiotic Timing[5]	-	-	99%	99%
Prophylactic Antibiotic Timing (Outpatient)[5]	-	-	98%	98%
Urinary Catheter Removal[5]	-	-	97%	97%
Survey of Patients' Hospital Experiences				
Area Around Room 'Always' Quiet at Night[1]	-	-	67%	61%
Doctors 'Always' Communicated Well[1]	-	-	83%	82%
Home Recovery Information Given[1]	-	-	83%	85%
Hospital Given 9 or 10 on 10 Point Scale[1]	-	-	70%	71%
Meds 'Always' Explained Before Given[1]	-	-	63%	64%
Nurses 'Always' Communicated Well[1]	-	-	79%	79%
Pain 'Always' Well Controlled[1]	-	-	71%	71%
Room and Bathroom 'Always' Clean[1]	-	-	72%	73%
Timely Help 'Always' Received[1]	-	-	68%	68%
Would Definitely Recommend Hospital[1]	-	-	69%	71%
Use of Medical Imaging				
Cardiac Imaging Stress Test before Surgery[7]	-	-	4.3%	5.3%
Combination Abdominal CT Scan[7]	-	-	15.3%	10.5%
Combination Brain/Sinus CT Scan[7]	-	-	2.9%	2.7%
Combination Chest CT Scan[7]	-	-	5%	2.7%
Follow-up Mammogram/Ultrasound[7]	-	-	9.9%	8.8%
Lumbar Spine MRI for Low Back Pain[7]	-	-	41.6%	37.2%

National Park Medical Center

1910 Malvern Avenue Phone: 501-321-1000
Hot Springs, AR 71901 Fax: 501-321-2922
URL: www.nationalparkmedical.com
Type: Acute Care Hospitals Emergency Services: Yes
Ownership: Proprietary Beds: 166

Key Personnel:

Chief of Medical Staff.......... Scott Anderson
Radiology.................. Cecil W Cupp, III
CEO .... Jerry D Mabry

Measure	Cases	This Hosp.	State Avg.	U.S. Avg.
Blood Clot Prevention and Treatment				
Anticoagulation Overlap Therapy[2]	29	76%	88%	93%
ICU Venous Thromboembolism Prophylaxis[2]	108	88%	94%	92%
Incidence of Potentially Preventable VTE[1,2]	-	-	12%	10%
UFH with Dosages/Platelet Monitoring[1,2]	-	-	100%	97%
Venous Thromboembolism Prophylaxis[2]	325	85%	91%	85%
Warfarin Therapy Discharge Instructions[2]	26	100%	76%	75%
Chest Pain/Possible Heart Attack Care				
Aspirin Given Within 24 Hours of Arrival[1]	-	-	96%	96%
Fibrinolytic Meds Within 30 Min. of Arrival[5]	-	-	54%	58%
Average Time to ECG (minutes)[1]	-	-	8	7
Average Time to Transfer (minutes)[5]	-	-	72	60
Children's Asthma Care				
Received Home Management Plan of Care	-	-	-	88%
Received Reliever Medication	-	-	-	100%
Received Systemic Corticosteroids	-	-	-	100%
Emergency Department				
Admittance Decision Time (minutes)[2]	541	75	65	98
Head CT Results Within 45 Min. of Arrival[1]	-	-	49%	57%
Patients Who Left ER Before Being Seen	24,377	3%	3%	2%
Time from ER Arrival to Admit. (minutes)[2]	546	221	214	274
Time from ER Arrival to Discharge (minutes)	391	128	118	134
Time in ER Before Being Evaluated (minutes)	418	28	26	26
Time to Pain Meds for Fractures (minutes)	87	78	66	57
Heart Attack Care				
Aspirin Given at Discharge	92	99%	99%	99%
Fibrinolytic Meds Within 30 Min. of Arrival[1]	-	-	77%	54%
PCI Within 90 Minutes of Arrival[1]	-	-	96%	96%
Statin Prescribed at Discharge	82	91%	97%	98%
Heart Failure Care				
ACE Inhibitor or ARB for LVSD	57	98%	96%	97%
Discharge Instructions Given	170	97%	95%	94%
Evaluation of LVS Function	200	100%	98%	99%
Medicare Spending				
Medicare Spending per Patient (ratio)	-	1.00	0.98	0.98
Pneumonia Care				
Appropriate Initial Antibiotic Given	136	96%	94%	95%
Blood Culture Timing	148	98%	98%	98%
Pregnancy and Delivery Care				
Newborn Deliveries Scheduled Early[2]	26	0%	6%	6%
Preventive Care				
Immunization for Influenza[2]	537	98%	89%	90%
Immunization for Pneumonia[2]	702	97%	92%	92%
Stroke Care				
Anticoagulation Therapy for Atrial Fibrillation	14	86%	90%	95%
Antithrombotic Therapy Timing	55	91%	96%	98%
Assessed for Rehabilitation	59	90%	95%	97%
Discharged on Antithrombotic Therapy	57	96%	96%	99%
Discharged on Statin Medication	39	77%	86%	94%
Thrombolytic Therapy Timing[1]	-	-	35%	66%
Venous Thromboembolism Prophylaxis	64	88%	91%	94%
Written Stroke Educational Materials Given	41	93%	81%	88%
Surgical Care Improvement Project				
Appropriate Beta Blocker Usage	119	98%	98%	98%
Appropriate VTP Within 24 Hours	321	98%	98%	98%
Controlled Postoperative Blood Glucose	70	100%	99%	97%
Perioperative Temperature Management	364	100%	100%	100%
Prophylactic Antibiotic Selection	292	100%	99%	99%
Prophylactic Antibiotic Selection (Outpatient)	109	99%	98%	98%
Prophylactic Antibiotic Stopped	273	99%	98%	98%
Prophylactic Antibiotic Timing	292	100%	99%	99%
Prophylactic Antibiotic Timing (Outpatient)	111	98%	98%	98%
Urinary Catheter Removal	302	97%	97%	97%
Survey of Patients' Hospital Experiences				
Area Around Room 'Always' Quiet at Night	300+	63%	67%	61%
Doctors 'Always' Communicated Well	300+	81%	83%	82%
Home Recovery Information Given	300+	84%	83%	85%
Hospital Given 9 or 10 on 10 Point Scale	300+	72%	70%	71%
Meds 'Always' Explained Before Given	300+	58%	63%	64%
Nurses 'Always' Communicated Well	300+	74%	79%	79%
Pain 'Always' Well Controlled	300+	68%	71%	71%
Room and Bathroom 'Always' Clean	300+	70%	72%	73%
Timely Help 'Always' Received	300+	60%	68%	68%
Would Definitely Recommend Hospital	300+	75%	69%	71%
Use of Medical Imaging				
Cardiac Imaging Stress Test before Surgery[1]	-	-	4.3%	5.3%
Combination Abdominal CT Scan	442	8.4%	15.3%	10.5%
Combination Brain/Sinus CT Scan[1]	-	-	2.9%	2.7%
Combination Chest CT Scan	272	13.2%	5%	2.7%
Follow-up Mammogram/Ultrasound	710	16.3%	9.9%	8.8%
Lumbar Spine MRI for Low Back Pain	104	36.5%	41.6%	37.2%

Saint Joseph's Mercy Health Center

300 Werner Street Phone: 501-622-1000
Hot Springs, AR 71903 Fax: 501-622-1199
URL: www.saintjosephs.com
Type: Acute Care Hospitals Emergency Services: Yes
Ownership: Voluntary non-profit - Church Beds: 317

Key Personnel:

CEO/President............... Randy Fale
Intensive Care Unit............ Steve Henson
Chief of Medical Staff.......... Mark Larey, DO
Radiology.................. Chuck Miles

Measure	Cases	This Hosp.	State Avg.	U.S. Avg.
Blood Clot Prevention and Treatment				
Anticoagulation Overlap Therapy[2]	59	78%	88%	93%
ICU Venous Thromboembolism Prophylaxis[2]	90	99%	94%	92%
Incidence of Potentially Preventable VTE[1,2]	-	-	12%	10%
UFH with Dosages/Platelet Monitoring[2]	18	100%	100%	97%
Venous Thromboembolism Prophylaxis[2]	336	90%	91%	85%
Warfarin Therapy Discharge Instructions[2]	45	49%	76%	75%
Chest Pain/Possible Heart Attack Care				
Aspirin Given Within 24 Hours of Arrival[1]	-	-	96%	96%
Fibrinolytic Meds Within 30 Min. of Arrival[3,7]	-	-	54%	58%
Average Time to ECG (minutes)[1]	-	-	8	7
Average Time to Transfer (minutes)[3,7]	-	-	72	60
Children's Asthma Care				
Received Home Management Plan of Care	-	-	-	88%
Received Reliever Medication	-	-	-	100%
Received Systemic Corticosteroids	-	-	-	100%
Emergency Department				
Admittance Decision Time (minutes)[2]	553	67	65	98
Head CT Results Within 45 Min. of Arrival[1]	-	-	49%	57%
Patients Who Left ER Before Being Seen	40,126	3%	3%	2%
Time from ER Arrival to Admit. (minutes)[2]	577	204	214	274
Time from ER Arrival to Discharge (minutes)	355	177	118	134
Time in ER Before Being Evaluated (minutes)	390	38	26	26
Time to Pain Meds for Fractures (minutes)	102	58	66	57
Heart Attack Care				
Aspirin Given at Discharge	162	100%	99%	99%
Fibrinolytic Meds Within 30 Min. of Arrival[1]	-	-	77%	54%
PCI Within 90 Minutes of Arrival	56	98%	96%	96%
Statin Prescribed at Discharge	149	100%	97%	98%
Heart Failure Care				
ACE Inhibitor or ARB for LVSD[2]	95	97%	96%	97%
Discharge Instructions Given[2]	222	95%	95%	94%
Evaluation of LVS Function[2]	269	100%	98%	99%
Medicare Spending				
Medicare Spending per Patient (ratio)	-	0.96	0.98	0.98
Pneumonia Care				
Appropriate Initial Antibiotic Given[2]	56	100%	94%	95%
Blood Culture Timing[2]	81	100%	98%	98%
Pregnancy and Delivery Care				
Newborn Deliveries Scheduled Early[2]	40	0%	6%	6%
Preventive Care				
Immunization for Influenza[2]	556	89%	89%	90%
Immunization for Pneumonia[2]	757	92%	92%	92%
Stroke Care				
Anticoagulation Therapy for Atrial Fibrillation[2]	22	73%	90%	95%
Antithrombotic Therapy Timing[2]	99	96%	96%	98%
Assessed for Rehabilitation[2]	115	88%	95%	97%
Discharged on Antithrombotic Therapy[2]	100	93%	96%	99%

NOTE: Hospital profiles are in alphabetical order by state, then city, then hospital within the city; Rankings exclude hospitals with less than 25 cases except for patient surveys which excludes hospitals with less than 100 cases; (a) 100-299 cases; (1) The number of cases/patients is too few to report; (2) Data submitted were based on a sample of cases/patients; (3) Results are based on a shorter time period than required; (4) Data suppressed by CMS for one or more quarters; (5) Results are not available for this reporting period; (6) Fewer than 100 patients completed the HCAHPS survey; (7) No cases met the criteria for this measure; (8) The lower limit of the confidence interval cannot be calculated if the number of observed infections equals zero; (9) No data are available from the state/territory for this reporting period; (10) The scores shown reflect fewer than 50 completed surveys; (11) There were discrepancies in the data collection process; (12) This measure does not apply to this hospital for this reporting period; (13) Results cannot be calculated for this reporting period; (14) The results for this state are combined with nearby states to protect confidentiality; Please refer to the User's Guide for a full explanation of data.

Measure	Cases	This Hosp.	State Avg.	U.S. Avg.
Discharged on Statin Medication[2]	93	76%	86%	94%
Thrombolytic Therapy Timing[2]	16	38%	35%	66%
Venous Thromboembolism Prophylaxis[2]	123	93%	91%	94%
Written Stroke Educational Materials Given[2]	64	53%	81%	88%
Surgical Care Improvement Project				
Appropriate Beta Blocker Usage[2]	128	98%	98%	98%
Appropriate VTP Within 24 Hours[2]	343	99%	98%	98%
Controlled Postoperative Blood Glucose[2]	74	96%	99%	97%
Perioperative Temperature Management[2]	387	100%	100%	100%
Prophylactic Antibiotic Selection[2]	318	99%	99%	99%
Prophylactic Antibiotic Selection (Outpatient)	437	98%	98%	98%
Prophylactic Antibiotic Stopped[2]	298	98%	98%	98%
Prophylactic Antibiotic Timing[2]	318	99%	99%	99%
Prophylactic Antibiotic Timing (Outpatient)	439	99%	98%	98%
Urinary Catheter Removal[2]	154	98%	97%	97%
Survey of Patients' Hospital Experiences				
Area Around Room 'Always' Quiet at Night[11]	300+	57%	67%	61%
Doctors 'Always' Communicated Well[11]	300+	80%	83%	82%
Home Recovery Information Given[11]	300+	83%	83%	85%
Hospital Given 9 or 10 on 10 Point Scale[11]	300+	73%	70%	71%
Meds 'Always' Explained Before Given[11]	300+	60%	63%	64%
Nurses 'Always' Communicated Well[11]	300+	77%	79%	79%
Pain 'Always' Well Controlled[11]	300+	70%	71%	71%
Room and Bathroom 'Always' Clean[11]	300+	69%	72%	73%
Timely Help 'Always' Received[11]	300+	61%	68%	68%
Would Definitely Recommend Hospital[11]	300+	74%	69%	71%
Use of Medical Imaging				
Cardiac Imaging Stress Test before Surgery	644	4.2%	4.3%	5.3%
Combination Abdominal CT Scan	1,518	7.6%	15.3%	10.5%
Combination Brain/Sinus CT Scan	1,047	3.3%	2.9%	2.7%
Combination Chest CT Scan	901	4.0%	5%	2.7%
Follow-up Mammogram/Ultrasound	2,786	14.3%	9.9%	8.8%
Lumbar Spine MRI for Low Back Pain	406	34.7%	41.6%	37.2%

North Metro Medical Center

1400 Braden Street
Jacksonville, AR 72076
Type: Acute Care Hospitals
Ownership: Voluntary non-profit - Private
Phone: 501-985-7000
Fax: 501-982-3055
Emergency Services: Yes
Beds: 113

Key Personnel:
Radiology. . . . . Albert Alexande
President/CEO. . . . . Rock Bordelon
Quality Assurance . . . . Margaret Corbett
Operating Room. . . . . Susie Hickman, RN
CEO . . . . Cindy Stafford

Measure	Cases	This Hosp.	State Avg.	U.S. Avg.
Blood Clot Prevention and Treatment				
Anticoagulation Overlap Therapy[1,2]	-	-	88%	93%
ICU Venous Thromboembolism Prophylaxis[2]	25	64%	94%	92%
Incidence of Potentially Preventable VTE[2,7]	-	-	12%	10%
UFH with Dosages/Platelet Monitoring[1,2]	-	-	100%	97%
Venous Thromboembolism Prophylaxis[2]	24	83%	91%	85%
Warfarin Therapy Discharge Instructions[2]	15	67%	76%	75%
Chest Pain/Possible Heart Attack Care				
Aspirin Given Within 24 Hours of Arrival	28	93%	96%	96%
Fibrinolytic Meds Within 30 Min. of Arrival[1]	-	-	54%	58%
Average Time to ECG (minutes)	27	35	8	7
Average Time to Transfer (minutes)[1]	-	-	72	60
Children's Asthma Care				
Received Home Management Plan of Care	-	-	-	88%
Received Reliever Medication	-	-	-	100%
Received Systemic Corticosteroids	-	-	-	100%
Emergency Department				
Admittance Decision Time (minutes)[2]	378	180	65	98
Head CT Results Within 45 Min. of Arrival[1]	-	-	49%	57%
Patients Who Left ER Before Being Seen	18,796	3%	3%	2%
Time from ER Arrival to Admit. (minutes)[2]	387	236	214	274
Time from ER Arrival to Discharge (minutes)	322	112	118	134
Time in ER Before Being Evaluated (minutes)	377	34	26	26
Time to Pain Meds for Fractures (minutes)	62	49	66	57
Heart Attack Care				
Aspirin Given at Discharge[1]	-	-	99%	99%
Fibrinolytic Meds Within 30 Min. of Arrival[1]	-	-	77%	54%
PCI Within 90 Minutes of Arrival[7]	-	-	96%	96%
Statin Prescribed at Discharge[1]	-	-	97%	98%
Heart Failure Care				
ACE Inhibitor or ARB for LVSD[1]	-	-	96%	97%
Discharge Instructions Given[1]	-	-	95%	94%
Evaluation of LVS Function[1]	-	-	98%	99%
Medicare Spending				
Medicare Spending per Patient (ratio)	-	1.26	0.98	0.98
Pneumonia Care				
Appropriate Initial Antibiotic Given	11	91%	94%	95%
Blood Culture Timing	19	74%	98%	98%
Pregnancy and Delivery Care				
Newborn Deliveries Scheduled Early[7]	-	-	6%	6%
Preventive Care				
Immunization for Influenza[2]	233	100%	89%	90%
Immunization for Pneumonia[2]	317	85%	92%	92%
Stroke Care				
Anticoagulation Therapy for Atrial Fibrillation[7]	-	-	90%	95%
Antithrombotic Therapy Timing[1]	-	-	96%	98%
Assessed for Rehabilitation[1]	-	-	95%	97%
Discharged on Antithrombotic Therapy[7]	-	-	96%	99%
Discharged on Statin Medication[7]	-	-	86%	94%
Thrombolytic Therapy Timing[1]	-	-	35%	66%
Venous Thromboembolism Prophylaxis[1]	-	-	91%	94%
Written Stroke Educational Materials Given[1]	-	-	81%	88%
Surgical Care Improvement Project				
Appropriate Beta Blocker Usage[1]	-	-	98%	98%
Appropriate VTP Within 24 Hours[1]	-	-	98%	98%
Controlled Postoperative Blood Glucose[7]	-	-	99%	97%
Perioperative Temperature Management[1]	-	-	100%	100%
Prophylactic Antibiotic Selection[7]	-	-	99%	99%
Prophylactic Antibiotic Selection (Outpatient)[3]	12	50%	98%	98%
Prophylactic Antibiotic Stopped[7]	-	-	98%	98%
Prophylactic Antibiotic Timing[1]	-	-	99%	99%
Prophylactic Antibiotic Timing (Outpatient)[3]	12	92%	98%	98%
Urinary Catheter Removal[1]	-	-	97%	97%
Survey of Patients' Hospital Experiences				
Area Around Room 'Always' Quiet at Night[3,11]	(a)	66%	67%	61%
Doctors 'Always' Communicated Well[3,11]	(a)	77%	83%	82%
Home Recovery Information Given[3,11]	(a)	81%	83%	85%
Hospital Given 9 or 10 on 10 Point Scale[3,11]	(a)	60%	70%	71%
Meds 'Always' Explained Before Given[3,11]	(a)	56%	63%	64%
Nurses 'Always' Communicated Well[3,11]	(a)	71%	79%	79%
Pain 'Always' Well Controlled[3,11]	(a)	66%	71%	71%
Room and Bathroom 'Always' Clean[3,11]	(a)	69%	72%	73%
Timely Help 'Always' Received[3,11]	(a)	64%	68%	68%
Would Definitely Recommend Hospital[3,11]	(a)	57%	69%	71%
Use of Medical Imaging				
Cardiac Imaging Stress Test before Surgery[1]	-	-	4.3%	5.3%
Combination Abdominal CT Scan	202	16.3%	15.3%	10.5%
Combination Brain/Sinus CT Scan	265	6.4%	2.9%	2.7%
Combination Chest CT Scan	74	8.1%	5%	2.7%
Follow-up Mammogram/Ultrasound	793	19.0%	9.9%	8.8%
Lumbar Spine MRI for Low Back Pain	57	56.1%	41.6%	37.2%

Nea Baptist Memorial Hospital

3024 Stadium Boulevard
Jonesboro, AR 72401
URL: www.baptistonline.com
Type: Acute Care Hospitals
Ownership: Voluntary non-profit - Private
Phone: 870-972-7000
Emergency Services: Yes
Beds: 100

Key Personnel:
Administrator . . . . Brad Parsons
CEO . . . . Brad Parsons

Measure	Cases	This Hosp.	State Avg.	U.S. Avg.
Blood Clot Prevention and Treatment				
Anticoagulation Overlap Therapy[2]	28	86%	88%	93%
ICU Venous Thromboembolism Prophylaxis[2]	94	83%	94%	92%
Incidence of Potentially Preventable VTE[1,2]	-	-	12%	10%
UFH with Dosages/Platelet Monitoring[2]	30	100%	100%	97%
Venous Thromboembolism Prophylaxis[2]	340	83%	91%	85%
Warfarin Therapy Discharge Instructions[2]	24	46%	76%	75%
Chest Pain/Possible Heart Attack Care				
Aspirin Given Within 24 Hours of Arrival[1,3]	-	-	96%	96%
Fibrinolytic Meds Within 30 Min. of Arrival[3,7]	-	-	54%	58%
Average Time to ECG (minutes)[1,3]	-	-	8	7
Average Time to Transfer (minutes)[3,7]	-	-	72	60
Children's Asthma Care				
Received Home Management Plan of Care	-	-	-	88%
Received Reliever Medication	-	-	-	100%
Received Systemic Corticosteroids	-	-	-	100%
Emergency Department				
Admittance Decision Time (minutes)[2]	397	89	65	98
Head CT Results Within 45 Min. of Arrival	13	23%	49%	57%
Patients Who Left ER Before Being Seen	25,199	5%	3%	2%
Time from ER Arrival to Admit. (minutes)[2]	406	252	214	274
Time from ER Arrival to Discharge (minutes)	365	143	118	134
Time in ER Before Being Evaluated (minutes)	388	44	26	26
Time to Pain Meds for Fractures (minutes)	122	76	66	57
Heart Attack Care				
Aspirin Given at Discharge	166	99%	99%	99%
Fibrinolytic Meds Within 30 Min. of Arrival[7]	-	-	77%	54%
PCI Within 90 Minutes of Arrival	27	96%	96%	96%
Statin Prescribed at Discharge	163	98%	97%	98%
Heart Failure Care				
ACE Inhibitor or ARB for LVSD	68	97%	96%	97%
Discharge Instructions Given	181	99%	95%	94%
Evaluation of LVS Function	225	100%	98%	99%
Medicare Spending				
Medicare Spending per Patient (ratio)	-	0.99	0.98	0.98
Pneumonia Care				
Appropriate Initial Antibiotic Given	173	98%	94%	95%
Blood Culture Timing	269	99%	98%	98%
Pregnancy and Delivery Care				
Newborn Deliveries Scheduled Early[2]	18	0%	6%	6%
Preventive Care				
Immunization for Influenza[2]	551	95%	89%	90%
Immunization for Pneumonia[2]	723	96%	92%	92%
Stroke Care				
Anticoagulation Therapy for Atrial Fibrillation[2]	15	87%	90%	95%
Antithrombotic Therapy Timing[2]	73	97%	96%	98%
Assessed for Rehabilitation[2]	78	94%	95%	97%
Discharged on Antithrombotic Therapy[2]	77	99%	96%	99%
Discharged on Statin Medication[2]	59	92%	86%	94%
Thrombolytic Therapy Timing[2]	18	0%	35%	66%
Venous Thromboembolism Prophylaxis[2]	77	84%	91%	94%
Written Stroke Educational Materials Given[2]	42	62%	81%	88%
Surgical Care Improvement Project				
Appropriate Beta Blocker Usage[2]	109	97%	98%	98%
Appropriate VTP Within 24 Hours[2]	296	95%	98%	98%
Controlled Postoperative Blood Glucose[2]	52	96%	99%	97%
Perioperative Temperature Management[2]	368	99%	100%	100%
Prophylactic Antibiotic Selection[2]	274	97%	99%	99%
Prophylactic Antibiotic Selection (Outpatient)	414	96%	98%	98%
Prophylactic Antibiotic Stopped[2]	254	97%	98%	98%
Prophylactic Antibiotic Timing[2]	274	98%	99%	99%
Prophylactic Antibiotic Timing (Outpatient)	416	98%	98%	98%
Urinary Catheter Removal[2]	264	96%	97%	97%
Survey of Patients' Hospital Experiences				
Area Around Room 'Always' Quiet at Night	300+	69%	67%	61%
Doctors 'Always' Communicated Well	300+	86%	83%	82%
Home Recovery Information Given	300+	86%	83%	85%
Hospital Given 9 or 10 on 10 Point Scale	300+	81%	70%	71%
Meds 'Always' Explained Before Given	300+	70%	63%	64%
Nurses 'Always' Communicated Well	300+	84%	79%	79%
Pain 'Always' Well Controlled	300+	76%	71%	71%
Room and Bathroom 'Always' Clean	300+	72%	72%	73%
Timely Help 'Always' Received	300+	73%	68%	68%
Would Definitely Recommend Hospital	300+	85%	69%	71%
Use of Medical Imaging				
Cardiac Imaging Stress Test before Surgery[1]	-	-	4.3%	5.3%
Combination Abdominal CT Scan	562	17.3%	15.3%	10.5%
Combination Brain/Sinus CT Scan	540	2.2%	2.9%	2.7%
Combination Chest CT Scan	357	8.7%	5%	2.7%
Follow-up Mammogram/Ultrasound[7]	-	-	9.9%	8.8%

NOTE: Hospital profiles are in alphabetical order by state, then city, then hospital within the city; Rankings exclude hospitals with less than 25 cases except for patient surveys which excludes hospitals with less than 100 cases; (a) 100-299 cases; (1) The number of cases/patients is too few to report; (2) Data submitted were based on a sample of cases/patients; (3) Results are based on a shorter time period than required; (4) Data suppressed by CMS for one or more quarters; (5) Results are not available for this reporting period; (6) Fewer than 100 patients completed the HCAHPS survey; (7) No cases met the criteria for this measure; (8) The lower limit of the confidence interval cannot be calculated if the number of observed infections equals zero; (9) No data are available from the state/territory for this reporting period; (10) The scores shown reflect fewer than 50 completed surveys; (11) There were discrepancies in the data collection process; (12) This measure does not apply to this hospital for this reporting period; (13) Results cannot be calculated for this reporting period; (14) The results for this state are combined with nearby states to protect confidentiality; Please refer to the User's Guide for a full explanation of data.

Measure	Cases	This Hosp.	State Avg.	U.S. Avg.
Lumbar Spine MRI for Low Back Pain	80	47.5%	41.6%	37.2%

Saint Bernards Medical Center

225 E Jackson Phone: 870-972-4100
Jonesboro, AR 72401 Fax: 870-974-5112
URL: www.sbrmc.com
Type: Acute Care Hospitals Emergency Services: Yes
Ownership: Voluntary non-profit - Private Beds: 375

Key Personnel:

CEO/President. . . . . Chris Barber
Emergency Room . . . . Katheryn Blackman
Operating Room. . . . . Dorothy Byford, RN
Chief of Medical Staff. . . . . BJ Cranfill, MD
Radiology. . . . . Kevin Hawley
Infection Control. . . . . Debbi Ledbetter, RN
Patient Relations . . . . Brenda Million
Cardiac Laboratory. . . . . Jo Yawn

Measure	Cases	This Hosp.	State Avg.	U.S. Avg.
Blood Clot Prevention and Treatment				
Anticoagulation Overlap Therapy[2]	58	88%	88%	93%
ICU Venous Thromboembolism Prophylaxis[2]	174	96%	94%	92%
Incidence of Potentially Preventable VTE[2]	15	13%	12%	10%
UFH with Dosages/Platelet Monitoring[2]	39	100%	100%	97%
Venous Thromboembolism Prophylaxis[2]	224	93%	91%	85%
Warfarin Therapy Discharge Instructions[2]	47	94%	76%	75%
Chest Pain/Possible Heart Attack Care				
Aspirin Given Within 24 Hours of Arrival[1,3]	-	-	96%	96%
Fibrinolytic Meds Within 30 Min. of Arrival[5]	-	-	54%	58%
Average Time to ECG (minutes)[3,7]	-	-	8	7
Average Time to Transfer (minutes)[5]	-	-	72	60
Children's Asthma Care				
Received Home Management Plan of Care	22	91%	-	88%
Received Reliever Medication	23	100%	-	100%
Received Systemic Corticosteroids	23	100%	-	100%
Emergency Department				
Admittance Decision Time (minutes)[2]	487	144	65	98
Head CT Results Within 45 Min. of Arrival[1]	-	-	49%	57%
Patients Who Left ER Before Being Seen	54,865	2%	3%	2%
Time from ER Arrival to Admit. (minutes)[2]	497	267	214	274
Time from ER Arrival to Discharge (minutes)	427	147	118	134
Time in ER Before Being Evaluated (minutes)	391	46	26	26
Time to Pain Meds for Fractures (minutes)	154	72	66	57
Heart Attack Care				
Aspirin Given at Discharge	393	99%	99%	99%
Fibrinolytic Meds Within 30 Min. of Arrival[7]	-	-	77%	54%
PCI Within 90 Minutes of Arrival	29	100%	96%	96%
Statin Prescribed at Discharge	380	100%	97%	98%
Heart Failure Care				
ACE Inhibitor or ARB for LVSD[2]	200	98%	96%	97%
Discharge Instructions Given[2]	352	93%	95%	94%
Evaluation of LVS Function[2]	423	100%	98%	99%
Medicare Spending				
Medicare Spending per Patient (ratio)	-	0.96	0.98	0.98
Pneumonia Care				
Appropriate Initial Antibiotic Given[2]	49	98%	94%	95%
Blood Culture Timing[2]	84	100%	98%	98%
Pregnancy and Delivery Care				
Newborn Deliveries Scheduled Early[2]	123	7%	6%	6%
Preventive Care				
Immunization for Influenza[2]	541	94%	89%	90%
Immunization for Pneumonia[2]	689	93%	92%	92%
Stroke Care				
Anticoagulation Therapy for Atrial Fibrillation	28	96%	90%	95%
Antithrombotic Therapy Timing	195	91%	96%	98%
Assessed for Rehabilitation	239	99%	95%	97%
Discharged on Antithrombotic Therapy	203	97%	96%	99%
Discharged on Statin Medication	159	94%	86%	94%
Thrombolytic Therapy Timing[1]	-	-	35%	66%
Venous Thromboembolism Prophylaxis	218	94%	91%	94%
Written Stroke Educational Materials Given	119	92%	81%	88%
Surgical Care Improvement Project				
Appropriate Beta Blocker Usage[2]	280	98%	98%	98%
Appropriate VTP Within 24 Hours[2]	601	95%	98%	98%
Controlled Postoperative Blood Glucose[2]	178	98%	99%	97%
Perioperative Temperature Management[2]	692	100%	100%	100%
Prophylactic Antibiotic Selection[2]	613	99%	99%	99%
Prophylactic Antibiotic Selection (Outpatient)	776	98%	98%	98%
Prophylactic Antibiotic Stopped[2]	584	98%	98%	98%
Prophylactic Antibiotic Timing[2]	614	98%	99%	99%
Prophylactic Antibiotic Timing (Outpatient)	765	99%	98%	98%
Urinary Catheter Removal[2]	504	96%	97%	97%
Survey of Patients' Hospital Experiences				
Area Around Room 'Always' Quiet at Night	300+	68%	67%	61%
Doctors 'Always' Communicated Well	300+	84%	83%	82%
Home Recovery Information Given	300+	83%	83%	85%
Hospital Given 9 or 10 on 10 Point Scale	300+	75%	70%	71%
Meds 'Always' Explained Before Given	300+	65%	63%	64%
Nurses 'Always' Communicated Well	300+	81%	79%	79%
Pain 'Always' Well Controlled	300+	72%	71%	71%
Room and Bathroom 'Always' Clean	300+	74%	72%	73%
Timely Help 'Always' Received	300+	66%	68%	68%
Would Definitely Recommend Hospital	300+	75%	69%	71%
Use of Medical Imaging				
Cardiac Imaging Stress Test before Surgery	915	5.9%	4.3%	5.3%
Combination Abdominal CT Scan	2,199	44.7%	15.3%	10.5%
Combination Brain/Sinus CT Scan	1,373	3.9%	2.9%	2.7%
Combination Chest CT Scan	1,758	1.2%	5%	2.7%
Follow-up Mammogram/Ultrasound	2,677	12.7%	9.9%	8.8%
Lumbar Spine MRI for Low Back Pain	469	42.9%	41.6%	37.2%

Chicot Memorial Medical Center

2729 South Highway 65 & 82 Phone: 870-265-5351
Lake Village, AR 71653 Fax: 870-265-2091
URL: www.chicotmemorial.com
Type: Critical Access Hospitals Emergency Services: Yes
Ownership: Voluntary non-profit - Private Beds: 25

Key Personnel:

CEO/President. . . . . David A Chumley
Chief of Medical Staff. . . . . Joann Gregory, MD
Quality Assurance . . . . Holda Laukon, RN
Emergency Room . . . . Tara Olivi, RN
Radiology. . . . . R Smithsith, MD

Measure	Cases	This Hosp.	State Avg.	U.S. Avg.
Blood Clot Prevention and Treatment				
Anticoagulation Overlap Therapy[5]	-	-	88%	93%
ICU Venous Thromboembolism Prophylaxis[5]	-	-	94%	92%
Incidence of Potentially Preventable VTE[5]	-	-	12%	10%
UFH with Dosages/Platelet Monitoring[5]	-	-	100%	97%
Venous Thromboembolism Prophylaxis[5]	-	-	91%	85%
Warfarin Therapy Discharge Instructions[5]	-	-	76%	75%
Chest Pain/Possible Heart Attack Care				
Aspirin Given Within 24 Hours of Arrival	39	100%	96%	96%
Fibrinolytic Meds Within 30 Min. of Arrival[1]	-	-	54%	58%
Average Time to ECG (minutes)	41	14	8	7
Average Time to Transfer (minutes)[7]	-	-	72	60
Children's Asthma Care				
Received Home Management Plan of Care	-	-	-	88%
Received Reliever Medication	-	-	-	100%
Received Systemic Corticosteroids	-	-	-	100%
Emergency Department				
Admittance Decision Time (minutes)[5]	-	-	65	98
Head CT Results Within 45 Min. of Arrival[1]	-	-	49%	57%
Patients Who Left ER Before Being Seen	6,825	1%	3%	2%
Time from ER Arrival to Admit. (minutes)[5]	-	-	214	274
Time from ER Arrival to Discharge (minutes)[5]	-	-	118	134
Time in ER Before Being Evaluated (minutes)[5]	-	-	26	26
Time to Pain Meds for Fractures (minutes)	25	40	66	57
Heart Attack Care				
Aspirin Given at Discharge[1,3]	-	-	99%	99%
Fibrinolytic Meds Within 30 Min. of Arrival[3,7]	-	-	77%	54%
PCI Within 90 Minutes of Arrival[3,7]	-	-	96%	96%
Statin Prescribed at Discharge[1,3]	-	-	97%	98%
Heart Failure Care				
ACE Inhibitor or ARB for LVSD[1]	-	-	96%	97%
Discharge Instructions Given	18	100%	95%	94%
Evaluation of LVS Function	24	92%	98%	99%
Medicare Spending				
Medicare Spending per Patient (ratio)	-	-	0.98	0.98
Pneumonia Care				
Appropriate Initial Antibiotic Given	12	100%	94%	95%
Blood Culture Timing[1]	-	-	98%	98%
Pregnancy and Delivery Care				
Newborn Deliveries Scheduled Early[5]	-	-	6%	6%
Preventive Care				
Immunization for Influenza[5]	-	-	89%	90%
Immunization for Pneumonia[5]	-	-	92%	92%
Stroke Care				
Anticoagulation Therapy for Atrial Fibrillation[5]	-	-	90%	95%
Antithrombotic Therapy Timing[5]	-	-	96%	98%
Assessed for Rehabilitation[5]	-	-	95%	97%
Discharged on Antithrombotic Therapy[5]	-	-	96%	99%
Discharged on Statin Medication[5]	-	-	86%	94%
Thrombolytic Therapy Timing[5]	-	-	35%	66%
Venous Thromboembolism Prophylaxis[5]	-	-	91%	94%
Written Stroke Educational Materials Given[5]	-	-	81%	88%
Surgical Care Improvement Project				
Appropriate Beta Blocker Usage[1]	-	-	98%	98%
Appropriate VTP Within 24 Hours	13	100%	98%	98%
Controlled Postoperative Blood Glucose[7]	-	-	99%	97%
Perioperative Temperature Management	17	100%	100%	100%
Prophylactic Antibiotic Selection[1]	-	-	99%	99%
Prophylactic Antibiotic Selection (Outpatient)[1,3]	-	-	98%	98%
Prophylactic Antibiotic Stopped[1]	-	-	98%	98%
Prophylactic Antibiotic Timing[1]	-	-	99%	99%
Prophylactic Antibiotic Timing (Outpatient)[1,3]	-	-	98%	98%
Urinary Catheter Removal[1]	-	-	97%	97%
Survey of Patients' Hospital Experiences				
Area Around Room 'Always' Quiet at Night[5]	-	-	67%	61%
Doctors 'Always' Communicated Well[5]	-	-	83%	82%
Home Recovery Information Given[5]	-	-	83%	85%
Hospital Given 9 or 10 on 10 Point Scale[5]	-	-	70%	71%
Meds 'Always' Explained Before Given[5]	-	-	63%	64%
Nurses 'Always' Communicated Well[5]	-	-	79%	79%
Pain 'Always' Well Controlled[5]	-	-	71%	71%
Room and Bathroom 'Always' Clean[5]	-	-	72%	73%
Timely Help 'Always' Received[5]	-	-	68%	68%
Would Definitely Recommend Hospital[5]	-	-	69%	71%
Use of Medical Imaging				
Cardiac Imaging Stress Test before Surgery[7]	-	-	4.3%	5.3%
Combination Abdominal CT Scan	135	46.7%	15.3%	10.5%
Combination Brain/Sinus CT Scan[1]	-	-	2.9%	2.7%
Combination Chest CT Scan	68	26.5%	5%	2.7%
Follow-up Mammogram/Ultrasound	238	5.9%	9.9%	8.8%
Lumbar Spine MRI for Low Back Pain[1]	-	-	41.6%	37.2%

Arkansas Children's Hospital

800 Marshall Street Slot 301 Phone: 501-364-1100
Little Rock, AR 72202 Fax: 501-364-2806
URL: www.archildrens.org
Type: Childrens Emergency Services: Yes
Ownership: Voluntary non-profit - Private Beds: 370

Key Personnel:

CEO/President. . . . . Jonathan Bates
Pediatric Ambulatory Care . . . . . . Debra Fiser, MD
Pediatric In-Patient Care . . . . Debra Fiser, MD
Quality Assurance . . . . Patricia Higginbotham
Emergency Room . . . . Jacqueline Jardine
Operating Room. . . . . Kathy Lindstrom
Radiology. . . . . Joanna Seibert, MD
Chief of Medical Staff. . . . . Bonnie Taylor

Measure	Cases	This Hosp.	State Avg.	U.S. Avg.
Blood Clot Prevention and Treatment				
Anticoagulation Overlap Therapy[5]	-	-	88%	93%
ICU Venous Thromboembolism Prophylaxis[5]	-	-	94%	92%
Incidence of Potentially Preventable VTE[5]	-	-	12%	10%
UFH with Dosages/Platelet Monitoring[5]	-	-	100%	97%
Venous Thromboembolism Prophylaxis[5]	-	-	91%	85%
Warfarin Therapy Discharge Instructions[5]	-	-	76%	75%
Chest Pain/Possible Heart Attack Care				
Aspirin Given Within 24 Hours of Arrival	-	-	96%	96%
Fibrinolytic Meds Within 30 Min. of Arrival	-	-	54%	58%

NOTE: Hospital profiles are in alphabetical order by state, then city, then hospital within the city; Rankings exclude hospitals with less than 25 cases except for patient surveys which excludes hospitals with less than 100 cases; (a) 100-299 cases; (1) The number of cases/patients is too few to report; (2) Data submitted were based on a sample of cases/patients; (3) Results are based on a shorter time period than required; (4) Data suppressed by CMS for one or more quarters; (5) Results are not available for this reporting period; (6) Fewer than 100 patients completed the HCAHPS survey; (7) No cases met the criteria for this measure; (8) The lower limit of the confidence interval cannot be calculated if the number of observed infections equals zero; (9) No data are available from the state/territory for this reporting period; (10) The scores shown reflect fewer than 50 completed surveys; (11) There were discrepancies in the data collection process; (12) This measure does not apply to this hospital for this reporting period; (13) Results cannot be calculated for this reporting period; (14) The results for this state are combined with nearby states to protect confidentiality; Please refer to the User's Guide for a full explanation of data.

Measure	Cases	This Hosp.	State Avg.	U.S. Avg.
Average Time to ECG (minutes)	-	-	8	7
Average Time to Transfer (minutes)	-	-	72	60
Children's Asthma Care				
Received Home Management Plan of Care	130	85%	-	88%
Received Reliever Medication	130	100%	-	100%
Received Systemic Corticosteroids	130	98%	-	100%
Emergency Department				
Admittance Decision Time (minutes)[5]	-	-	65	98
Head CT Results Within 45 Min. of Arrival	-	-	49%	57%
Patients Who Left ER Before Being Seen	-	-	3%	2%
Time from ER Arrival to Admit. (minutes)[5]	-	-	214	274
Time from ER Arrival to Discharge (minutes)	-	-	118	134
Time in ER Before Being Evaluated (minutes)	-	-	26	26
Time to Pain Meds for Fractures (minutes)	-	-	66	57
Heart Attack Care				
Aspirin Given at Discharge[5]	-	-	99%	99%
Fibrinolytic Meds Within 30 Min. of Arrival[5]	-	-	77%	54%
PCI Within 90 Minutes of Arrival[5]	-	-	96%	96%
Statin Prescribed at Discharge[5]	-	-	97%	98%
Heart Failure Care				
ACE Inhibitor or ARB for LVSD[5]	-	-	96%	97%
Discharge Instructions Given[5]	-	-	95%	94%
Evaluation of LVS Function[5]	-	-	98%	99%
Medicare Spending				
Medicare Spending per Patient (ratio)	-	-	0.98	0.98
Pneumonia Care				
Appropriate Initial Antibiotic Given[5]	-	-	94%	95%
Blood Culture Timing[5]	-	-	98%	98%
Pregnancy and Delivery Care				
Newborn Deliveries Scheduled Early[5]	-	-	6%	6%
Preventive Care				
Immunization for Influenza[5]	-	-	89%	90%
Immunization for Pneumonia[5]	-	-	92%	92%
Stroke Care				
Anticoagulation Therapy for Atrial Fibrillation[5]	-	-	90%	95%
Antithrombotic Therapy Timing[5]	-	-	96%	98%
Assessed for Rehabilitation[5]	-	-	95%	97%
Discharged on Antithrombotic Therapy[5]	-	-	96%	99%
Discharged on Statin Medication[5]	-	-	86%	94%
Thrombolytic Therapy Timing[5]	-	-	35%	66%
Venous Thromboembolism Prophylaxis[5]	-	-	91%	94%
Written Stroke Educational Materials Given[5]	-	-	81%	88%
Surgical Care Improvement Project				
Appropriate Beta Blocker Usage[5]	-	-	98%	98%
Appropriate VTP Within 24 Hours[5]	-	-	98%	98%
Controlled Postoperative Blood Glucose[5]	-	-	99%	97%
Perioperative Temperature Management[5]	-	-	100%	100%
Prophylactic Antibiotic Selection[5]	-	-	99%	99%
Prophylactic Antibiotic Selection (Outpatient)	-	-	98%	98%
Prophylactic Antibiotic Stopped[5]	-	-	98%	98%
Prophylactic Antibiotic Timing[5]	-	-	99%	99%
Prophylactic Antibiotic Timing (Outpatient)	-	-	98%	98%
Urinary Catheter Removal[5]	-	-	97%	97%
Survey of Patients' Hospital Experiences				
Area Around Room 'Always' Quiet at Night[5]	-	-	67%	61%
Doctors 'Always' Communicated Well[5]	-	-	83%	82%
Home Recovery Information Given[5]	-	-	83%	85%
Hospital Given 9 or 10 on 10 Point Scale[5]	-	-	70%	71%
Meds 'Always' Explained Before Given[5]	-	-	63%	64%
Nurses 'Always' Communicated Well[5]	-	-	79%	79%
Pain 'Always' Well Controlled[5]	-	-	71%	71%
Room and Bathroom 'Always' Clean[5]	-	-	72%	73%
Timely Help 'Always' Received[5]	-	-	68%	68%
Would Definitely Recommend Hospital[5]	-	-	69%	71%
Use of Medical Imaging				
Cardiac Imaging Stress Test before Surgery	-	-	4.3%	5.3%
Combination Abdominal CT Scan	-	-	15.3%	10.5%
Combination Brain/Sinus CT Scan	-	-	2.9%	2.7%
Combination Chest CT Scan	-	-	5%	2.7%
Follow-up Mammogram/Ultrasound	-	-	9.9%	8.8%
Lumbar Spine MRI for Low Back Pain	-	-	41.6%	37.2%

Arkansas Heart Hospital

1701 S Shackleford Road
Little Rock, AR 72211
URL: www.arheart.com
Type: Acute Care Hospitals
Ownership: Proprietary
Phone: 501-219-7000
Fax: 501-219-7402
Emergency Services: Yes
Beds: 84

Key Personnel:
Chief of Medical Staff.......... Bruce Murphy
CEO/President.............. Charlie Smith
Operating Room.............. C O Williams

Measure	Cases	This Hosp.	State Avg.	U.S. Avg.
Blood Clot Prevention and Treatment				
Anticoagulation Overlap Therapy[2]	24	96%	88%	93%
ICU Venous Thromboembolism Prophylaxis[2,7]	-	-	94%	92%
Incidence of Potentially Preventable VTE[1,2]	-	-	12%	10%
UFH with Dosages/Platelet Monitoring[2]	11	100%	100%	97%
Venous Thromboembolism Prophylaxis[2]	284	100%	91%	85%
Warfarin Therapy Discharge Instructions[2]	21	100%	76%	75%
Chest Pain/Possible Heart Attack Care				
Aspirin Given Within 24 Hours of Arrival[5]	-	-	96%	96%
Fibrinolytic Meds Within 30 Min. of Arrival[5]	-	-	54%	58%
Average Time to ECG (minutes)[5]	-	-	8	7
Average Time to Transfer (minutes)[5]	-	-	72	60
Children's Asthma Care				
Received Home Management Plan of Care	-	-	-	88%
Received Reliever Medication	-	-	-	100%
Received Systemic Corticosteroids	-	-	-	100%
Emergency Department				
Admittance Decision Time (minutes)[2]	253	50	65	98
Head CT Results Within 45 Min. of Arrival[1]	-	-	49%	57%
Patients Who Left ER Before Being Seen	6,152	0%	3%	2%
Time from ER Arrival to Admit. (minutes)[2]	255	180	214	274
Time from ER Arrival to Discharge (minutes)	299	130	118	134
Time in ER Before Being Evaluated (minutes)	360	11	26	26
Time to Pain Meds for Fractures (minutes)[3,7]	-	-	66	57
Heart Attack Care				
Aspirin Given at Discharge	368	100%	99%	99%
Fibrinolytic Meds Within 30 Min. of Arrival[7]	-	-	77%	54%
PCI Within 90 Minutes of Arrival	12	100%	96%	96%
Statin Prescribed at Discharge	307	100%	97%	98%
Heart Failure Care				
ACE Inhibitor or ARB for LVSD	147	100%	96%	97%
Discharge Instructions Given	353	100%	95%	94%
Evaluation of LVS Function	383	100%	98%	99%
Medicare Spending				
Medicare Spending per Patient (ratio)	-	0.91	0.98	0.98
Pneumonia Care				
Appropriate Initial Antibiotic Given	17	100%	94%	95%
Blood Culture Timing	57	100%	98%	98%
Pregnancy and Delivery Care				
Newborn Deliveries Scheduled Early[7]	-	-	6%	6%
Preventive Care				
Immunization for Influenza[2]	645	71%	89%	90%
Immunization for Pneumonia[2]	1,026	83%	92%	92%
Stroke Care				
Anticoagulation Therapy for Atrial Fibrillation[1]	-	-	90%	95%
Antithrombotic Therapy Timing	13	100%	96%	98%
Assessed for Rehabilitation	19	79%	95%	97%
Discharged on Antithrombotic Therapy	17	100%	96%	99%
Discharged on Statin Medication	17	94%	86%	94%
Thrombolytic Therapy Timing[1]	-	-	35%	66%
Venous Thromboembolism Prophylaxis	16	88%	91%	94%
Written Stroke Educational Materials Given	14	100%	81%	88%
Surgical Care Improvement Project				
Appropriate Beta Blocker Usage	339	100%	98%	98%
Appropriate VTP Within 24 Hours[1]	-	-	98%	98%
Controlled Postoperative Blood Glucose	685	100%	99%	97%
Perioperative Temperature Management	120	100%	100%	100%
Prophylactic Antibiotic Selection	712	100%	99%	99%
Prophylactic Antibiotic Selection (Outpatient)	449	94%	98%	98%
Prophylactic Antibiotic Stopped	706	100%	98%	98%
Prophylactic Antibiotic Timing	712	100%	99%	99%
Prophylactic Antibiotic Timing (Outpatient)	450	100%	98%	98%
Urinary Catheter Removal	644	100%	97%	97%
Survey of Patients' Hospital Experiences				
Area Around Room 'Always' Quiet at Night	300+	74%	67%	61%
Doctors 'Always' Communicated Well	300+	85%	83%	82%
Home Recovery Information Given	300+	85%	83%	85%
Hospital Given 9 or 10 on 10 Point Scale	300+	90%	70%	71%
Meds 'Always' Explained Before Given	300+	67%	63%	64%
Nurses 'Always' Communicated Well	300+	87%	79%	79%
Pain 'Always' Well Controlled	300+	75%	71%	71%
Room and Bathroom 'Always' Clean	300+	87%	72%	73%
Timely Help 'Always' Received	300+	87%	68%	68%
Would Definitely Recommend Hospital	300+	94%	69%	71%
Use of Medical Imaging				
Cardiac Imaging Stress Test before Surgery	2,785	4.2%	4.3%	5.3%
Combination Abdominal CT Scan	84	51.2%	15.3%	10.5%
Combination Brain/Sinus CT Scan[1]	-	-	2.9%	2.7%
Combination Chest CT Scan	130	33.8%	5%	2.7%
Follow-up Mammogram/Ultrasound[7]	-	-	9.9%	8.8%
Lumbar Spine MRI for Low Back Pain[1]	-	-	41.6%	37.2%

Baptist Health Medical Center - Little Rock

9601 Interstate 630, Exit 7
Little Rock, AR 72205
URL: www.baptist-health.com
Type: Acute Care Hospitals
Ownership: Voluntary non-profit - Private
Phone: 501-202-2000
Fax: 501-202-1280
Emergency Services: Yes
Beds: 724

Key Personnel:
Chief of Medical Staff.......... Neal Beaton, MD
Pediatric In-Patient Care .... Jerry Byrum, MD
Intensive Care Unit........... Donnie Floyd
CEO/President.............. Russel D Harrington Jr
Quality Assurance .... Sue Hylton
Emergency Room .... Marvin Leibovich, MD
Infection Control............. John Schultz, MD
Radiology.................. Cecile Shoptan, MD

Measure	Cases	This Hosp.	State Avg.	U.S. Avg.
Blood Clot Prevention and Treatment				
Anticoagulation Overlap Therapy[2]	143	73%	88%	93%
ICU Venous Thromboembolism Prophylaxis[2]	155	88%	94%	92%
Incidence of Potentially Preventable VTE[2]	46	22%	12%	10%
UFH with Dosages/Platelet Monitoring[2]	33	100%	100%	97%
Venous Thromboembolism Prophylaxis[2]	213	70%	91%	85%
Warfarin Therapy Discharge Instructions[2]	95	66%	76%	75%
Chest Pain/Possible Heart Attack Care				
Aspirin Given Within 24 Hours of Arrival[5]	-	-	96%	96%
Fibrinolytic Meds Within 30 Min. of Arrival[5]	-	-	54%	58%
Average Time to ECG (minutes)[5]	-	-	8	7
Average Time to Transfer (minutes)[5]	-	-	72	60
Children's Asthma Care				
Received Home Management Plan of Care	-	-	-	88%
Received Reliever Medication	-	-	-	100%
Received Systemic Corticosteroids	-	-	-	100%
Emergency Department				
Admittance Decision Time (minutes)[2]	359	61	65	98
Head CT Results Within 45 Min. of Arrival[1]	-	-	49%	57%
Patients Who Left ER Before Being Seen	59,054	3%	3%	2%
Time from ER Arrival to Admit. (minutes)[2]	362	244	214	274
Time from ER Arrival to Discharge (minutes)	422	130	118	134
Time in ER Before Being Evaluated (minutes)	452	41	26	26
Time to Pain Meds for Fractures (minutes)	136	65	66	57
Heart Attack Care				
Aspirin Given at Discharge[2]	354	100%	99%	99%
Fibrinolytic Meds Within 30 Min. of Arrival[2,7]	-	-	77%	54%
PCI Within 90 Minutes of Arrival[2]	47	100%	96%	96%
Statin Prescribed at Discharge[2]	350	99%	97%	98%
Heart Failure Care				
ACE Inhibitor or ARB for LVSD[2]	144	100%	96%	97%
Discharge Instructions Given[2]	293	100%	95%	94%
Evaluation of LVS Function[2]	341	100%	98%	99%
Medicare Spending				
Medicare Spending per Patient (ratio)	-	0.98	0.98	0.98
Pneumonia Care				
Appropriate Initial Antibiotic Given[2]	70	99%	94%	95%
Blood Culture Timing[2]	100	99%	98%	98%

NOTE: Hospital profiles are in alphabetical order by state, then city, then hospital within the city; Rankings exclude hospitals with less than 25 cases except for patient surveys which excludes hospitals with less than 100 cases; (a) 100-299 cases; (1) The number of cases/patients is too few to report; (2) Data submitted were based on a sample of cases/patients; (3) Results are based on a shorter time period than required; (4) Data suppressed by CMS for one or more quarters; (5) Results are not available for this reporting period; (6) Fewer than 100 patients completed the HCAHPS survey; (7) No cases met the criteria for this measure; (8) The lower limit of the confidence interval cannot be calculated if the number of observed infections equals zero; (9) No data are available from the state/territory for this reporting period; (10) The scores shown reflect fewer than 50 completed surveys; (11) There were discrepancies in the data collection process; (12) This measure does not apply to this hospital for this reporting period; (13) Results cannot be calculated for this reporting period; (14) The results for this state are combined with nearby states to protect confidentiality; Please refer to the User's Guide for a full explanation of data.

Measure	Cases	This Hosp.	State Avg.	U.S. Avg.
Pregnancy and Delivery Care				
Newborn Deliveries Scheduled Early[2]	54	0%	6%	6%
Preventive Care				
Immunization for Influenza[2]	540	74%	89%	90%
Immunization for Pneumonia[2]	599	71%	92%	92%
Stroke Care				
Anticoagulation Therapy for Atrial Fibrillation[2]	24	92%	90%	95%
Antithrombotic Therapy Timing[2]	122	96%	96%	98%
Assessed for Rehabilitation[2]	161	99%	95%	97%
Discharged on Antithrombotic Therapy[2]	133	89%	96%	99%
Discharged on Statin Medication[2]	98	81%	86%	94%
Thrombolytic Therapy Timing[1,2]	-	-	35%	66%
Venous Thromboembolism Prophylaxis[2]	171	85%	91%	94%
Written Stroke Educational Materials Given[2]	66	82%	81%	88%
Surgical Care Improvement Project				
Appropriate Beta Blocker Usage[2]	326	96%	98%	98%
Appropriate VTP Within 24 Hours[2]	690	97%	98%	98%
Controlled Postoperative Blood Glucose[2]	240	97%	99%	97%
Perioperative Temperature Management[2]	789	100%	100%	100%
Prophylactic Antibiotic Selection[2]	792	99%	99%	99%
Prophylactic Antibiotic Selection (Outpatient)	1,114	98%	98%	98%
Prophylactic Antibiotic Stopped[2]	785	99%	98%	98%
Prophylactic Antibiotic Timing[2]	792	99%	99%	99%
Prophylactic Antibiotic Timing (Outpatient)	1,124	98%	98%	98%
Urinary Catheter Removal[2]	335	96%	97%	97%
Survey of Patients' Hospital Experiences				
Area Around Room 'Always' Quiet at Night[11]	300+	68%	67%	61%
Doctors 'Always' Communicated Well[11]	300+	81%	83%	82%
Home Recovery Information Given[11]	300+	81%	83%	85%
Hospital Given 9 or 10 on 10 Point Scale[11]	300+	74%	70%	71%
Meds 'Always' Explained Before Given[11]	300+	61%	63%	64%
Nurses 'Always' Communicated Well[11]	300+	79%	79%	79%
Pain 'Always' Well Controlled[11]	300+	72%	71%	71%
Room and Bathroom 'Always' Clean[11]	300+	73%	72%	73%
Timely Help 'Always' Received[11]	300+	64%	68%	68%
Would Definitely Recommend Hospital[11]	300+	77%	69%	71%
Use of Medical Imaging				
Cardiac Imaging Stress Test before Surgery	993	3.8%	4.3%	5.3%
Combination Abdominal CT Scan	1,045	1.6%	15.3%	10.5%
Combination Brain/Sinus CT Scan	970	2.6%	2.9%	2.7%
Combination Chest CT Scan	523	1.3%	5%	2.7%
Follow-up Mammogram/Ultrasound	4,244	8.8%	9.9%	8.8%
Lumbar Spine MRI for Low Back Pain	161	43.5%	41.6%	37.2%

Saint Vincent Infirmary Medical Center

Two Saint Vincent Circle Phone: 501-552-3000
Little Rock, AR 72205 Fax: 501-552-4510
URL: www.stvincenthealth.org
Type: Acute Care Hospitals Emergency Services: Yes
Ownership: Voluntary non-profit - Private Beds: 611

Key Personnel:
CEO/President. . . . . Diana T Hueter
Pediatric Ambulatory Care . . . . . . Sue Keathley, MD
Pediatric In-Patient Care . . . . Sue Keathley, MD
Infection Control. . . . . Kenny Kemp
Chief of Medical Staff. . . . . Gail A McCracken, MD
Emergency Room . . . . Leslie H Sessions, MD
Radiology. . . . . David Tamas, MD
Quality Assurance . . . . Rebecca Tutton

Measure	Cases	This Hosp.	State Avg.	U.S. Avg.
Blood Clot Prevention and Treatment				
Anticoagulation Overlap Therapy[2]	68	97%	88%	93%
ICU Venous Thromboembolism Prophylaxis[2]	115	82%	94%	92%
Incidence of Potentially Preventable VTE[2]	27	15%	12%	10%
UFH with Dosages/Platelet Monitoring[2]	19	100%	100%	97%
Venous Thromboembolism Prophylaxis[2]	265	71%	91%	85%
Warfarin Therapy Discharge Instructions[2]	48	83%	76%	75%
Chest Pain/Possible Heart Attack Care				
Aspirin Given Within 24 Hours of Arrival[3,7]	-	-	96%	96%
Fibrinolytic Meds Within 30 Min. of Arrival[5]	-	-	54%	58%
Average Time to ECG (minutes)[3,7]	-	-	8	7
Average Time to Transfer (minutes)[5]	-	-	72	60
Children's Asthma Care				
Received Home Management Plan of Care	-	-	-	88%
Received Reliever Medication	-	-	-	100%
Received Systemic Corticosteroids	-	-	-	100%
Emergency Department				
Admittance Decision Time (minutes)[2]	314	83	65	98
Head CT Results Within 45 Min. of Arrival[7]	-	-	49%	57%
Patients Who Left ER Before Being Seen	36,214	6%	3%	2%
Time from ER Arrival to Admit. (minutes)[2]	329	268	214	274
Time from ER Arrival to Discharge (minutes)	343	167	118	134
Time in ER Before Being Evaluated (minutes)	303	50	26	26
Time to Pain Meds for Fractures (minutes)	103	84	66	57
Heart Attack Care				
Aspirin Given at Discharge	203	100%	99%	99%
Fibrinolytic Meds Within 30 Min. of Arrival[7]	-	-	77%	54%
PCI Within 90 Minutes of Arrival	35	97%	96%	96%
Statin Prescribed at Discharge	199	98%	97%	98%
Heart Failure Care				
ACE Inhibitor or ARB for LVSD	195	99%	96%	97%
Discharge Instructions Given	378	93%	95%	94%
Evaluation of LVS Function	438	100%	98%	99%
Medicare Spending				
Medicare Spending per Patient (ratio)	-	0.97	0.98	0.98
Pneumonia Care				
Appropriate Initial Antibiotic Given	139	91%	94%	95%
Blood Culture Timing	188	99%	98%	98%
Pregnancy and Delivery Care				
Newborn Deliveries Scheduled Early[2]	32	0%	6%	6%
Preventive Care				
Immunization for Influenza[2]	548	90%	89%	90%
Immunization for Pneumonia[2]	684	88%	92%	92%
Stroke Care				
Anticoagulation Therapy for Atrial Fibrillation[1,2]	-	-	90%	95%
Antithrombotic Therapy Timing[2]	43	95%	96%	98%
Assessed for Rehabilitation[2]	85	80%	95%	97%
Discharged on Antithrombotic Therapy[2]	55	98%	96%	99%
Discharged on Statin Medication[2]	45	87%	86%	94%
Thrombolytic Therapy Timing[1,2]	-	-	35%	66%
Venous Thromboembolism Prophylaxis[2]	93	77%	91%	94%
Written Stroke Educational Materials Given[2]	46	30%	81%	88%
Surgical Care Improvement Project				
Appropriate Beta Blocker Usage[2]	230	96%	98%	98%
Appropriate VTP Within 24 Hours[2]	285	97%	98%	98%
Controlled Postoperative Blood Glucose[2]	141	96%	99%	97%
Perioperative Temperature Management[2]	478	99%	100%	100%
Prophylactic Antibiotic Selection[2]	435	100%	99%	99%
Prophylactic Antibiotic Selection (Outpatient)	628	99%	98%	98%
Prophylactic Antibiotic Stopped[2]	427	95%	98%	98%
Prophylactic Antibiotic Timing[2]	435	100%	99%	99%
Prophylactic Antibiotic Timing (Outpatient)	628	99%	98%	98%
Urinary Catheter Removal[2]	315	98%	97%	97%
Survey of Patients' Hospital Experiences				
Area Around Room 'Always' Quiet at Night	300+	67%	67%	61%
Doctors 'Always' Communicated Well	300+	84%	83%	82%
Home Recovery Information Given	300+	85%	83%	85%
Hospital Given 9 or 10 on 10 Point Scale	300+	71%	70%	71%
Meds 'Always' Explained Before Given	300+	64%	63%	64%
Nurses 'Always' Communicated Well	300+	76%	79%	79%
Pain 'Always' Well Controlled	300+	69%	71%	71%
Room and Bathroom 'Always' Clean	300+	65%	72%	73%
Timely Help 'Always' Received	300+	63%	68%	68%
Would Definitely Recommend Hospital	300+	74%	69%	71%
Use of Medical Imaging				
Cardiac Imaging Stress Test before Surgery	2,759	3.4%	4.3%	5.3%
Combination Abdominal CT Scan	665	5.6%	15.3%	10.5%
Combination Brain/Sinus CT Scan	834	4.1%	2.9%	2.7%
Combination Chest CT Scan	330	0.6%	5%	2.7%
Follow-up Mammogram/Ultrasound[7]	-	-	9.9%	8.8%
Lumbar Spine MRI for Low Back Pain	173	35.3%	41.6%	37.2%

UAMS Medical Center

4301 West Markham Street Mail Slot 612 Phone: 501-686-5000
Little Rock, AR 72205 Fax: 501-661-7968
URL: www.uams.edu/medcenter
Type: Acute Care Hospitals Emergency Services: Yes
Ownership: Government - State Beds: 400

Key Personnel:
Infection Control. . . . . Robert W Bradsher, MD
Chief of Medical Staff . . . . Christina L. Clark, B.A.
Radiology. . . . . Ernest Ferris, MD
Operating Room. . . . . Betty Piatt, RN
Quality Assurance . . . . Richard L Smith
CEO/President. . . . . Roxane A. Townsend, MD
Pediatric Ambulatory Care . . . . . Terry Yamauchi, MD
Pediatric In-Patient Care . . . . . . Terry Yamauchi, MD

Measure	Cases	This Hosp.	State Avg.	U.S. Avg.
Blood Clot Prevention and Treatment				
Anticoagulation Overlap Therapy[2]	52	96%	88%	93%
ICU Venous Thromboembolism Prophylaxis[2]	107	90%	94%	92%
Incidence of Potentially Preventable VTE[2]	39	13%	12%	10%
UFH with Dosages/Platelet Monitoring[2]	26	100%	100%	97%
Venous Thromboembolism Prophylaxis[2]	302	88%	91%	85%
Warfarin Therapy Discharge Instructions[2]	45	24%	76%	75%
Chest Pain/Possible Heart Attack Care				
Aspirin Given Within 24 Hours of Arrival[5]	-	-	96%	96%
Fibrinolytic Meds Within 30 Min. of Arrival[5]	-	-	54%	58%
Average Time to ECG (minutes)[5]	-	-	8	7
Average Time to Transfer (minutes)[5]	-	-	72	60
Children's Asthma Care				
Received Home Management Plan of Care	-	-	-	88%
Received Reliever Medication	-	-	-	100%
Received Systemic Corticosteroids	-	-	-	100%
Emergency Department				
Admittance Decision Time (minutes)[2]	388	45	65	98
Head CT Results Within 45 Min. of Arrival[1,3]	-	-	49%	57%
Patients Who Left ER Before Being Seen	59,065	3%	3%	2%
Time from ER Arrival to Admit. (minutes)[2]	404	288	214	274
Time from ER Arrival to Discharge (minutes)	357	167	118	134
Time in ER Before Being Evaluated (minutes)	352	33	26	26
Time to Pain Meds for Fractures (minutes)	48	75	66	57
Heart Attack Care				
Aspirin Given at Discharge	180	99%	99%	99%
Fibrinolytic Meds Within 30 Min. of Arrival[7]	-	-	77%	54%
PCI Within 90 Minutes of Arrival	31	87%	96%	96%
Statin Prescribed at Discharge	168	97%	97%	98%
Heart Failure Care				
ACE Inhibitor or ARB for LVSD	172	100%	96%	97%
Discharge Instructions Given	349	99%	95%	94%
Evaluation of LVS Function	369	100%	98%	99%
Medicare Spending				
Medicare Spending per Patient (ratio)	-	0.97	0.98	0.98
Pneumonia Care				
Appropriate Initial Antibiotic Given	95	85%	94%	95%
Blood Culture Timing	207	95%	98%	98%
Pregnancy and Delivery Care				
Newborn Deliveries Scheduled Early[2]	26	4%	6%	6%
Preventive Care				
Immunization for Influenza[2]	590	68%	89%	90%
Immunization for Pneumonia[2]	546	77%	92%	92%
Stroke Care				
Anticoagulation Therapy for Atrial Fibrillation[2]	11	100%	90%	95%
Antithrombotic Therapy Timing[2]	57	96%	96%	98%
Assessed for Rehabilitation[2]	117	98%	95%	97%
Discharged on Antithrombotic Therapy[2]	97	99%	96%	99%
Discharged on Statin Medication[2]	75	95%	86%	94%
Thrombolytic Therapy Timing[1,2]	-	-	35%	66%
Venous Thromboembolism Prophylaxis[2]	105	92%	91%	94%
Written Stroke Educational Materials Given[2]	72	72%	81%	88%
Surgical Care Improvement Project				
Appropriate Beta Blocker Usage[2]	181	97%	98%	98%
Appropriate VTP Within 24 Hours[2]	306	96%	98%	98%
Controlled Postoperative Blood Glucose[2]	128	98%	99%	97%
Perioperative Temperature Management[2]	457	100%	100%	100%
Prophylactic Antibiotic Selection[2]	339	99%	99%	99%

NOTE: Hospital profiles are in alphabetical order by state, then city, then hospital within the city; Rankings exclude hospitals with less than 25 cases except for patient surveys which excludes hospitals with less than 100 cases; (a) 100-299 cases; (1) The number of cases/patients is too few to report; (2) Data submitted were based on a sample of cases/patients; (3) Results are based on a shorter time period than required; (4) Data suppressed by CMS for one or more quarters; (5) Results are not available for this reporting period; (6) Fewer than 100 patients completed the HCAHPS survey; (7) No cases met the criteria for this measure; (8) The lower limit of the confidence interval cannot be calculated if the number of observed infections equals zero; (9) No data are available from the state/territory for this reporting period; (10) The scores shown reflect fewer than 50 completed surveys; (11) There were discrepancies in the data collection process; (12) This measure does not apply to this hospital for this reporting period; (13) Results cannot be calculated for this reporting period; (14) The results for this state are combined with nearby states to protect confidentiality; Please refer to the User's Guide for a full explanation of data.

Measure	Cases	This Hosp.	State Avg.	U.S. Avg.
Prophylactic Antibiotic Selection (Outpatient)	368	95%	98%	98%
Prophylactic Antibiotic Stopped[2]	326	93%	98%	98%
Prophylactic Antibiotic Timing[2]	341	97%	99%	99%
Prophylactic Antibiotic Timing (Outpatient)	357	96%	98%	98%
Urinary Catheter Removal[2]	331	89%	97%	97%
Survey of Patients' Hospital Experiences				
Area Around Room 'Always' Quiet at Night	300+	65%	67%	61%
Doctors 'Always' Communicated Well	300+	78%	83%	82%
Home Recovery Information Given	300+	83%	83%	85%
Hospital Given 9 or 10 on 10 Point Scale	300+	75%	70%	71%
Meds 'Always' Explained Before Given	300+	61%	63%	64%
Nurses 'Always' Communicated Well	300+	76%	79%	79%
Pain 'Always' Well Controlled	300+	69%	71%	71%
Room and Bathroom 'Always' Clean	300+	71%	72%	73%
Timely Help 'Always' Received	300+	62%	68%	68%
Would Definitely Recommend Hospital	300+	78%	69%	71%
Use of Medical Imaging				
Cardiac Imaging Stress Test before Surgery	329	6.4%	4.3%	5.3%
Combination Abdominal CT Scan	1,553	2.0%	15.3%	10.5%
Combination Brain/Sinus CT Scan	597	2.2%	2.9%	2.7%
Combination Chest CT Scan	1,563	1.2%	5%	2.7%
Follow-up Mammogram/Ultrasound	1,930	10.7%	9.9%	8.8%
Lumbar Spine MRI for Low Back Pain	72	30.6%	41.6%	37.2%

VA Central Arkansas Veterans Healthcare System

4300 West Seventh Street — Phone: 501-257-1000
Little Rock, AR 72205 — Fax: 401-257-5404
URL: www.visn16.med.va.gov
Type: Acute Care - VA — Emergency Services: No
Ownership: Government Federal — Beds: 664

Key Personnel:
CEO/President . . . . George H Gray Jr
Emergency Room . . . . Tim Holcomb, MD
Chief of Medical Staff . . . . Michael R. Winn

Measure	Cases	This Hosp.	State Avg.	U.S. Avg.
Blood Clot Prevention and Treatment				
Anticoagulation Overlap Therapy	-	-	88%	93%
ICU Venous Thromboembolism Prophylaxis	-	-	94%	92%
Incidence of Potentially Preventable VTE	-	-	12%	10%
UFH with Dosages/Platelet Monitoring	-	-	100%	97%
Venous Thromboembolism Prophylaxis	-	-	91%	85%
Warfarin Therapy Discharge Instructions	-	-	76%	75%
Chest Pain/Possible Heart Attack Care				
Aspirin Given Within 24 Hours of Arrival	-	-	96%	96%
Fibrinolytic Meds Within 30 Min. of Arrival	-	-	54%	58%
Average Time to ECG (minutes)	-	-	8	7
Average Time to Transfer (minutes)	-	-	72	60
Children's Asthma Care				
Received Home Management Plan of Care	-	-	-	88%
Received Reliever Medication	-	-	-	100%
Received Systemic Corticosteroids	-	-	-	100%
Emergency Department				
Admittance Decision Time (minutes)	-	-	65	98
Head CT Results Within 45 Min. of Arrival	-	-	49%	57%
Patients Who Left ER Before Being Seen	-	-	3%	2%
Time from ER Arrival to Admit. (minutes)	-	-	214	274
Time from ER Arrival to Discharge (minutes)	-	-	118	134
Time in ER Before Being Evaluated (minutes)	-	-	26	26
Time to Pain Meds for Fractures (minutes)	-	-	66	57
Heart Attack Care				
Aspirin Given at Discharge	51	98%	99%	99%
Fibrinolytic Meds Within 30 Min. of Arrival[5]	-	-	77%	54%
PCI Within 90 Minutes of Arrival[1]	17	65%	96%	96%
Statin Prescribed at Discharge	49	94%	97%	98%
Heart Failure Care				
ACE Inhibitor or ARB for LVSD	168	95%	96%	97%
Discharge Instructions Given	338	95%	95%	94%
Evaluation of LVS Function	380	100%	98%	99%
Medicare Spending				
Medicare Spending per Patient (ratio)	-	-	0.98	0.98
Pneumonia Care				
Appropriate Initial Antibiotic Given	153	98%	94%	95%
Blood Culture Timing	276	97%	98%	98%
Pregnancy and Delivery Care				
Newborn Deliveries Scheduled Early	-	-	6%	6%
Preventive Care				
Immunization for Influenza[5]	-	-	89%	90%
Immunization for Pneumonia[5]	-	-	92%	92%
Stroke Care				
Anticoagulation Therapy for Atrial Fibrillation	-	-	90%	95%
Antithrombotic Therapy Timing	-	-	96%	98%
Assessed for Rehabilitation	-	-	95%	97%
Discharged on Antithrombotic Therapy	-	-	96%	99%
Discharged on Statin Medication	-	-	86%	94%
Thrombolytic Therapy Timing	-	-	35%	66%
Venous Thromboembolism Prophylaxis	-	-	91%	94%
Written Stroke Educational Materials Given	-	-	81%	88%
Surgical Care Improvement Project				
Appropriate Beta Blocker Usage[2]	143	97%	98%	98%
Appropriate VTP Within 24 Hours[2]	301	100%	98%	98%
Controlled Postoperative Blood Glucose[5]	-	-	99%	97%
Perioperative Temperature Management[2]	414	100%	100%	100%
Prophylactic Antibiotic Selection	259	99%	99%	99%
Prophylactic Antibiotic Selection (Outpatient)	-	-	98%	98%
Prophylactic Antibiotic Stopped	246	96%	98%	98%
Prophylactic Antibiotic Timing	259	99%	99%	99%
Prophylactic Antibiotic Timing (Outpatient)	-	-	98%	98%
Urinary Catheter Removal[2]	264	98%	97%	97%
Survey of Patients' Hospital Experiences				
Area Around Room 'Always' Quiet at Night	-	-	67%	61%
Doctors 'Always' Communicated Well	-	-	83%	82%
Home Recovery Information Given	-	-	83%	85%
Hospital Given 9 or 10 on 10 Point Scale	-	-	70%	71%
Meds 'Always' Explained Before Given	-	-	63%	64%
Nurses 'Always' Communicated Well	-	-	79%	79%
Pain 'Always' Well Controlled	-	-	71%	71%
Room and Bathroom 'Always' Clean	-	-	72%	73%
Timely Help 'Always' Received	-	-	68%	68%
Would Definitely Recommend Hospital	-	-	69%	71%
Use of Medical Imaging				
Cardiac Imaging Stress Test before Surgery	-	-	4.3%	5.3%
Combination Abdominal CT Scan	-	-	15.3%	10.5%
Combination Brain/Sinus CT Scan	-	-	2.9%	2.7%
Combination Chest CT Scan	-	-	5%	2.7%
Follow-up Mammogram/Ultrasound	-	-	9.9%	8.8%
Lumbar Spine MRI for Low Back Pain	-	-	41.6%	37.2%

Magnolia Hospital

101 Hospital Drive — Phone: 870-235-3000
Magnolia, AR 71754
URL: www.magnoliahospital.org
Type: Acute Care Hospitals — Emergency Services: Yes
Ownership: Government - Local — Beds: 70

Key Personnel:
Radiology . . . . Jamie Rayburn
Chief of Medical Staff . . . . Karen Weido

Measure	Cases	This Hosp.	State Avg.	U.S. Avg.
Blood Clot Prevention and Treatment				
Anticoagulation Overlap Therapy[1,2]	-	-	88%	93%
ICU Venous Thromboembolism Prophylaxis[2]	28	79%	94%	92%
Incidence of Potentially Preventable VTE[1,2]	-	-	12%	10%
UFH with Dosages/Platelet Monitoring[2,7]	-	-	100%	97%
Venous Thromboembolism Prophylaxis[2]	77	87%	91%	85%
Warfarin Therapy Discharge Instructions[1,2]	-	-	76%	75%
Chest Pain/Possible Heart Attack Care				
Aspirin Given Within 24 Hours of Arrival	32	91%	96%	96%
Fibrinolytic Meds Within 30 Min. of Arrival[1]	-	-	54%	58%
Average Time to ECG (minutes)	36	8	8	7
Average Time to Transfer (minutes)[7]	-	-	72	60
Children's Asthma Care				
Received Home Management Plan of Care	-	-	-	88%
Received Reliever Medication	-	-	-	100%
Received Systemic Corticosteroids	-	-	-	100%
Emergency Department				
Admittance Decision Time (minutes)[2]	208	50	65	98
Head CT Results Within 45 Min. of Arrival	12	8%	49%	57%
Patients Who Left ER Before Being Seen	10,361	3%	3%	2%
Time from ER Arrival to Admit. (minutes)[2]	233	222	214	274
Time from ER Arrival to Discharge (minutes)	265	115	118	134
Time in ER Before Being Evaluated (minutes)	395	31	26	26
Time to Pain Meds for Fractures (minutes)	37	50	66	57
Heart Attack Care				
Aspirin Given at Discharge[1]	-	-	99%	99%
Fibrinolytic Meds Within 30 Min. of Arrival[7]	-	-	77%	54%
PCI Within 90 Minutes of Arrival[7]	-	-	96%	96%
Statin Prescribed at Discharge[1]	-	-	97%	98%
Heart Failure Care				
ACE Inhibitor or ARB for LVSD	17	88%	96%	97%
Discharge Instructions Given	32	94%	95%	94%
Evaluation of LVS Function	54	100%	98%	99%
Medicare Spending				
Medicare Spending per Patient (ratio)	-	1.01	0.98	0.98
Pneumonia Care				
Appropriate Initial Antibiotic Given	36	89%	94%	95%
Blood Culture Timing	48	98%	98%	98%
Pregnancy and Delivery Care				
Newborn Deliveries Scheduled Early	40	8%	6%	6%
Preventive Care				
Immunization for Influenza[2]	235	82%	89%	90%
Immunization for Pneumonia[2]	281	86%	92%	92%
Stroke Care				
Anticoagulation Therapy for Atrial Fibrillation[1]	-	-	90%	95%
Antithrombotic Therapy Timing	14	79%	96%	98%
Assessed for Rehabilitation	14	93%	95%	97%
Discharged on Antithrombotic Therapy	14	86%	96%	99%
Discharged on Statin Medication	14	43%	86%	94%
Thrombolytic Therapy Timing[1]	-	-	35%	66%
Venous Thromboembolism Prophylaxis	14	36%	91%	94%
Written Stroke Educational Materials Given[1]	-	-	81%	88%
Surgical Care Improvement Project				
Appropriate Beta Blocker Usage[1]	-	-	98%	98%
Appropriate VTP Within 24 Hours	38	95%	98%	98%
Controlled Postoperative Blood Glucose[7]	-	-	99%	97%
Perioperative Temperature Management	42	100%	100%	100%
Prophylactic Antibiotic Selection	18	100%	99%	99%
Prophylactic Antibiotic Selection (Outpatient)[1,3]	-	-	98%	98%
Prophylactic Antibiotic Stopped	18	100%	98%	98%
Prophylactic Antibiotic Timing	18	94%	99%	99%
Prophylactic Antibiotic Timing (Outpatient)[1,3]	-	-	98%	98%
Urinary Catheter Removal[1]	-	-	97%	97%
Survey of Patients' Hospital Experiences				
Area Around Room 'Always' Quiet at Night	(a)	72%	67%	61%
Doctors 'Always' Communicated Well	(a)	87%	83%	82%
Home Recovery Information Given	(a)	89%	83%	85%
Hospital Given 9 or 10 on 10 Point Scale	(a)	69%	70%	71%
Meds 'Always' Explained Before Given	(a)	65%	63%	64%
Nurses 'Always' Communicated Well	(a)	83%	79%	79%
Pain 'Always' Well Controlled	(a)	72%	71%	71%
Room and Bathroom 'Always' Clean	(a)	73%	72%	73%
Timely Help 'Always' Received	(a)	72%	68%	68%
Would Definitely Recommend Hospital	(a)	74%	69%	71%
Use of Medical Imaging				
Cardiac Imaging Stress Test before Surgery[7]	-	-	4.3%	5.3%
Combination Abdominal CT Scan	244	11.9%	15.3%	10.5%
Combination Brain/Sinus CT Scan[1]	-	-	2.9%	2.7%
Combination Chest CT Scan	125	0.8%	5%	2.7%
Follow-up Mammogram/Ultrasound	497	9.5%	9.9%	8.8%
Lumbar Spine MRI for Low Back Pain	37	48.6%	41.6%	37.2%

Baptist Health Medical Center - Hot Springs County

1001 Schneider Drive — Phone: 501-337-4911
Malvern, AR 72104 — Fax: 501-332-7395
E-mail: info@hscmc.org
URL: www.hscmc.org
Type: Acute Care Hospitals — Emergency Services: Yes
Ownership: Voluntary non-profit - Private — Beds: 92

Key Personnel:
Chief of Medical Staff . . . . Larry Brashears, MD
Radiology . . . . George Brenner
Emergency Room . . . . Robert Brown
Coronary Care . . . . Charles Clogston

NOTE: Hospital profiles are in alphabetical order by state, then city, then hospital within the city; Rankings exclude hospitals with less than 25 cases except for patient surveys which excludes hospitals with less than 100 cases; (a) 100-299 cases; (1) The number of cases/patients is too few to report; (2) Data submitted were based on a sample of cases/patients; (3) Results are based on a shorter time period than required; (4) Data suppressed by CMS for one or more quarters; (5) Results are not available for this reporting period; (6) Fewer than 100 patients completed the HCAHPS survey; (7) No cases met the criteria for this measure; (8) The lower limit of the confidence interval cannot be calculated if the number of observed infections equals zero; (9) No data are available from the state/territory for this reporting period; (10) The scores shown reflect fewer than 50 completed surveys; (11) There were discrepancies in the data collection process; (12) This measure does not apply to this hospital for this reporting period; (13) Results cannot be calculated for this reporting period; (14) The results for this state are combined with nearby states to protect confidentiality; Please refer to the User's Guide for a full explanation of data.

CEO/President. . . . . Sheila Williams

Measure	Cases	This Hosp.	State Avg.	U.S. Avg.
Blood Clot Prevention and Treatment				
Anticoagulation Overlap Therapy[1,2]	-	-	88%	93%
ICU Venous Thromboembolism Prophylaxis[2]	100	97%	94%	92%
Incidence of Potentially Preventable VTE[1,2]	-	-	12%	10%
UFH with Dosages/Platelet Monitoring[1,2]	-	-	100%	97%
Venous Thromboembolism Prophylaxis[2]	513	96%	91%	85%
Warfarin Therapy Discharge Instructions[1,2]	-	-	76%	75%
Chest Pain/Possible Heart Attack Care				
Aspirin Given Within 24 Hours of Arrival	73	96%	96%	96%
Fibrinolytic Meds Within 30 Min. of Arrival[1]	-	-	54%	58%
Average Time to ECG (minutes)	86	5	8	7
Average Time to Transfer (minutes)[1]	-	-	72	60
Children's Asthma Care				
Received Home Management Plan of Care	-	-	-	88%
Received Reliever Medication	-	-	-	100%
Received Systemic Corticosteroids	-	-	-	100%
Emergency Department				
Admittance Decision Time (minutes)[2]	351	37	65	98
Head CT Results Within 45 Min. of Arrival[1]	-	-	49%	57%
Patients Who Left ER Before Being Seen	15,278	4%	3%	2%
Time from ER Arrival to Admit. (minutes)[2]	545	140	214	274
Time from ER Arrival to Discharge (minutes)	346	102	118	134
Time in ER Before Being Evaluated (minutes)	331	18	26	26
Time to Pain Meds for Fractures (minutes)	66	57	66	57
Heart Attack Care				
Aspirin Given at Discharge[1,3]	-	-	99%	99%
Fibrinolytic Meds Within 30 Min. of Arrival[3,7]	-	-	77%	54%
PCI Within 90 Minutes of Arrival[3,7]	-	-	96%	96%
Statin Prescribed at Discharge[1,3]	-	-	97%	98%
Heart Failure Care				
ACE Inhibitor or ARB for LVSD[2]	11	55%	96%	97%
Discharge Instructions Given[2]	35	91%	95%	94%
Evaluation of LVS Function[2]	44	95%	98%	99%
Medicare Spending				
Medicare Spending per Patient (ratio)	-	0.97	0.98	0.98
Pneumonia Care				
Appropriate Initial Antibiotic Given[2]	103	98%	94%	95%
Blood Culture Timing[2]	100	96%	98%	98%
Pregnancy and Delivery Care				
Newborn Deliveries Scheduled Early[7]	-	-	6%	6%
Preventive Care				
Immunization for Influenza[2]	284	98%	89%	90%
Immunization for Pneumonia[2]	707	98%	92%	92%
Stroke Care				
Anticoagulation Therapy for Atrial Fibrillation[1]	-	-	90%	95%
Antithrombotic Therapy Timing	12	100%	96%	98%
Assessed for Rehabilitation	13	100%	95%	97%
Discharged on Antithrombotic Therapy	11	91%	96%	99%
Discharged on Statin Medication[1]	-	-	86%	94%
Thrombolytic Therapy Timing[1]	-	-	35%	66%
Venous Thromboembolism Prophylaxis	18	94%	91%	94%
Written Stroke Educational Materials Given[1]	-	-	81%	88%
Surgical Care Improvement Project				
Appropriate Beta Blocker Usage[1,3]	-	-	98%	98%
Appropriate VTP Within 24 Hours[1,3]	-	-	98%	98%
Controlled Postoperative Blood Glucose[3,7]	-	-	99%	97%
Perioperative Temperature Management[3]	11	100%	100%	100%
Prophylactic Antibiotic Selection[1,3]	-	-	99%	99%
Prophylactic Antibiotic Selection (Outpatient)[1]	-	-	98%	98%
Prophylactic Antibiotic Stopped[1,3]	-	-	98%	98%
Prophylactic Antibiotic Timing[1,3]	-	-	99%	99%
Prophylactic Antibiotic Timing (Outpatient)[1]	-	-	98%	98%
Urinary Catheter Removal[1,3]	-	-	97%	97%
Survey of Patients' Hospital Experiences				
Area Around Room 'Always' Quiet at Night	(a)	65%	67%	61%
Doctors 'Always' Communicated Well	(a)	88%	83%	82%
Home Recovery Information Given	(a)	77%	83%	85%
Hospital Given 9 or 10 on 10 Point Scale	(a)	66%	70%	71%
Meds 'Always' Explained Before Given	(a)	59%	63%	64%
Nurses 'Always' Communicated Well	(a)	77%	79%	79%
Pain 'Always' Well Controlled	(a)	67%	71%	71%
Room and Bathroom 'Always' Clean	(a)	74%	72%	73%
Timely Help 'Always' Received	(a)	63%	68%	68%
Would Definitely Recommend Hospital	(a)	59%	69%	71%
Use of Medical Imaging				
Cardiac Imaging Stress Test before Surgery[7]	-	-	4.3%	5.3%
Combination Abdominal CT Scan	246	4.1%	15.3%	10.5%
Combination Brain/Sinus CT Scan[1]	-	-	2.9%	2.7%
Combination Chest CT Scan	176	0.6%	5%	2.7%
Follow-up Mammogram/Ultrasound	191	17.8%	9.9%	8.8%
Lumbar Spine MRI for Low Back Pain	78	35.9%	41.6%	37.2%

McGehee Hospital

900 South Third Street
Mcgehee, AR 71654
Phone: 870-222-5600
Fax: 870-222-4253
Type: Critical Access Hospitals
Emergency Services: Yes
Ownership: Voluntary non-profit - Private
Beds: 34

Key Personnel:

Infection Control. . . . . Sarah Calvert
CEO/President. . . . . John Heard
Quality Assurance . . . . Cynthia Smith

Measure	Cases	This Hosp.	State Avg.	U.S. Avg.
Blood Clot Prevention and Treatment				
Anticoagulation Overlap Therapy[5]	-	-	88%	93%
ICU Venous Thromboembolism Prophylaxis[5]	-	-	94%	92%
Incidence of Potentially Preventable VTE[5]	-	-	12%	10%
UFH with Dosages/Platelet Monitoring[5]	-	-	100%	97%
Venous Thromboembolism Prophylaxis[5]	-	-	91%	85%
Warfarin Therapy Discharge Instructions[5]	-	-	76%	75%
Chest Pain/Possible Heart Attack Care				
Aspirin Given Within 24 Hours of Arrival	18	78%	96%	96%
Fibrinolytic Meds Within 30 Min. of Arrival[1]	-	-	54%	58%
Average Time to ECG (minutes)	21	10	8	7
Average Time to Transfer (minutes)[7]	-	-	72	60
Children's Asthma Care				
Received Home Management Plan of Care	-	-	-	88%
Received Reliever Medication	-	-	-	100%
Received Systemic Corticosteroids	-	-	-	100%
Emergency Department				
Admittance Decision Time (minutes)[5]	-	-	65	98
Head CT Results Within 45 Min. of Arrival[3,7]	-	-	49%	57%
Patients Who Left ER Before Being Seen	4,335	1%	3%	2%
Time from ER Arrival to Admit. (minutes)[5]	-	-	214	274
Time from ER Arrival to Discharge (minutes)[5]	-	-	118	134
Time in ER Before Being Evaluated (minutes)[5]	-	-	26	26
Time to Pain Meds for Fractures (minutes)[1,3]	-	-	66	57
Heart Attack Care				
Aspirin Given at Discharge[3,7]	-	-	99%	99%
Fibrinolytic Meds Within 30 Min. of Arrival[3,7]	-	-	77%	54%
PCI Within 90 Minutes of Arrival[5]	-	-	96%	96%
Statin Prescribed at Discharge[3,7]	-	-	97%	98%
Heart Failure Care				
ACE Inhibitor or ARB for LVSD	15	100%	96%	97%
Discharge Instructions Given	22	95%	95%	94%
Evaluation of LVS Function	24	92%	98%	99%
Medicare Spending				
Medicare Spending per Patient (ratio)	-	-	0.98	0.98
Pneumonia Care				
Appropriate Initial Antibiotic Given	11	82%	94%	95%
Blood Culture Timing	12	83%	98%	98%
Pregnancy and Delivery Care				
Newborn Deliveries Scheduled Early[5]	-	-	6%	6%
Preventive Care				
Immunization for Influenza[5]	-	-	89%	90%
Immunization for Pneumonia[5]	-	-	92%	92%
Stroke Care				
Anticoagulation Therapy for Atrial Fibrillation[5]	-	-	90%	95%
Antithrombotic Therapy Timing[5]	-	-	96%	98%
Assessed for Rehabilitation[5]	-	-	95%	97%
Discharged on Antithrombotic Therapy[5]	-	-	96%	99%
Discharged on Statin Medication[5]	-	-	86%	94%
Thrombolytic Therapy Timing[5]	-	-	35%	66%
Venous Thromboembolism Prophylaxis[5]	-	-	91%	94%
Written Stroke Educational Materials Given[5]	-	-	81%	88%
Surgical Care Improvement Project				
Appropriate Beta Blocker Usage[5]	-	-	98%	98%
Appropriate VTP Within 24 Hours[5]	-	-	98%	98%
Controlled Postoperative Blood Glucose[5]	-	-	99%	97%
Perioperative Temperature Management[5]	-	-	100%	100%
Prophylactic Antibiotic Selection[5]	-	-	99%	99%
Prophylactic Antibiotic Selection (Outpatient)[5]	-	-	98%	98%
Prophylactic Antibiotic Stopped[5]	-	-	98%	98%
Prophylactic Antibiotic Timing[5]	-	-	99%	99%
Prophylactic Antibiotic Timing (Outpatient)[5]	-	-	98%	98%
Urinary Catheter Removal[5]	-	-	97%	97%
Survey of Patients' Hospital Experiences				
Area Around Room 'Always' Quiet at Night[5]	-	-	67%	61%
Doctors 'Always' Communicated Well[5]	-	-	83%	82%
Home Recovery Information Given[5]	-	-	83%	85%
Hospital Given 9 or 10 on 10 Point Scale[5]	-	-	70%	71%
Meds 'Always' Explained Before Given[5]	-	-	63%	64%
Nurses 'Always' Communicated Well[5]	-	-	79%	79%
Pain 'Always' Well Controlled[5]	-	-	71%	71%
Room and Bathroom 'Always' Clean[5]	-	-	72%	73%
Timely Help 'Always' Received[5]	-	-	68%	68%
Would Definitely Recommend Hospital[5]	-	-	69%	71%
Use of Medical Imaging				
Cardiac Imaging Stress Test before Surgery[7]	-	-	4.3%	5.3%
Combination Abdominal CT Scan	77	6.5%	15.3%	10.5%
Combination Brain/Sinus CT Scan	158	0.6%	2.9%	2.7%
Combination Chest CT Scan[1]	-	-	5%	2.7%
Follow-up Mammogram/Ultrasound[7]	-	-	9.9%	8.8%
Lumbar Spine MRI for Low Back Pain[1]	-	-	41.6%	37.2%

Mena Regional Health System

311 North Morrow Street
Mena, AR 71953
Phone: 479-394-6100
Fax: 501-394-4577
Type: Acute Care Hospitals
Emergency Services: Yes
Ownership: Government - Local
Beds: 65

Key Personnel:

CEO/President. . . . . Tim Bowen
Intensive Care Unit. . . . . Darlene Hesterlee
Infection Control. . . . . Pam Posey, RN
Chief of Medical Staff . . . . Melinda Richardson
Operating Room. . . . . Thomas Tinnesz, RN
Radiology. . . . . Jonathan C Welsh

Measure	Cases	This Hosp.	State Avg.	U.S. Avg.
Blood Clot Prevention and Treatment				
Anticoagulation Overlap Therapy[2]	11	82%	88%	93%
ICU Venous Thromboembolism Prophylaxis[2]	40	100%	94%	92%
Incidence of Potentially Preventable VTE[2,7]	-	-	12%	10%
UFH with Dosages/Platelet Monitoring[2,7]	-	-	100%	97%
Venous Thromboembolism Prophylaxis[2]	154	100%	91%	85%
Warfarin Therapy Discharge Instructions[1,2]	-	-	76%	75%
Chest Pain/Possible Heart Attack Care				
Aspirin Given Within 24 Hours of Arrival	31	100%	96%	96%
Fibrinolytic Meds Within 30 Min. of Arrival[1,3]	-	-	54%	58%
Average Time to ECG (minutes)	35	6	8	7
Average Time to Transfer (minutes)[1,3]	-	-	72	60
Children's Asthma Care				
Received Home Management Plan of Care	-	-	-	88%
Received Reliever Medication	-	-	-	100%
Received Systemic Corticosteroids	-	-	-	100%
Emergency Department				
Admittance Decision Time (minutes)[2]	413	37	65	98
Head CT Results Within 45 Min. of Arrival[1,3]	-	-	49%	57%
Patients Who Left ER Before Being Seen	10,222	1%	3%	2%
Time from ER Arrival to Admit. (minutes)[2]	413	176	214	274
Time from ER Arrival to Discharge (minutes)	403	98	118	134
Time in ER Before Being Evaluated (minutes)	443	18	26	26
Time to Pain Meds for Fractures (minutes)	21	80	66	57
Heart Attack Care				
Aspirin Given at Discharge[1]	-	-	99%	99%
Fibrinolytic Meds Within 30 Min. of Arrival[7]	-	-	77%	54%
PCI Within 90 Minutes of Arrival[7]	-	-	96%	96%

NOTE: Hospital profiles are in alphabetical order by state, then city, then hospital within the city; Rankings exclude hospitals with less than 25 cases except for patient surveys which excludes hospitals with less than 100 cases; (a) 100-299 cases; (1) The number of cases/patients is too few to report; (2) Data submitted were based on a sample of cases/patients; (3) Results are based on a shorter time period than required; (4) Data suppressed by CMS for one or more quarters; (5) Results are not available for this reporting period; (6) Fewer than 100 patients completed the HCAHPS survey; (7) No cases met the criteria for this measure; (8) The lower limit of the confidence interval cannot be calculated if the number of observed infections equals zero; (9) No data are available from the state/territory for this reporting period; (10) The scores shown reflect fewer than 50 completed surveys; (11) There were discrepancies in the data collection process; (12) This measure does not apply to this hospital for this reporting period; (13) Results cannot be calculated for this reporting period; (14) The results for this state are combined with nearby states to protect confidentiality; Please refer to the User's Guide for a full explanation of data.

Measure	Cases	This Hosp.	State Avg.	U.S. Avg.
Statin Prescribed at Discharge[1]	-	-	97%	98%
Heart Failure Care				
ACE Inhibitor or ARB for LVSD[1,2]	-	-	96%	97%
Discharge Instructions Given[2]	22	100%	95%	94%
Evaluation of LVS Function[2]	37	100%	98%	99%
Medicare Spending				
Medicare Spending per Patient (ratio)	-	1.03	0.98	0.98
Pneumonia Care				
Appropriate Initial Antibiotic Given	43	86%	94%	95%
Blood Culture Timing	53	100%	98%	98%
Pregnancy and Delivery Care				
Newborn Deliveries Scheduled Early[2]	32	0%	6%	6%
Preventive Care				
Immunization for Influenza[2]	323	97%	89%	90%
Immunization for Pneumonia[2]	573	99%	92%	92%
Stroke Care				
Anticoagulation Therapy for Atrial Fibrillation[1]	-	-	90%	95%
Antithrombotic Therapy Timing	12	100%	96%	98%
Assessed for Rehabilitation	14	100%	95%	97%
Discharged on Antithrombotic Therapy	14	93%	96%	99%
Discharged on Statin Medication	13	69%	86%	94%
Thrombolytic Therapy Timing[7]	-	-	35%	66%
Venous Thromboembolism Prophylaxis	14	100%	91%	94%
Written Stroke Educational Materials Given[1]	-	-	81%	88%
Surgical Care Improvement Project				
Appropriate Beta Blocker Usage[1,2]	-	-	98%	98%
Appropriate VTP Within 24 Hours[2]	28	96%	98%	98%
Controlled Postoperative Blood Glucose[2,7]	-	-	99%	97%
Perioperative Temperature Management[2]	38	100%	100%	100%
Prophylactic Antibiotic Selection[2]	24	100%	99%	99%
Prophylactic Antibiotic Selection (Outpatient)[1,3]	-	-	98%	98%
Prophylactic Antibiotic Stopped[2]	23	100%	98%	98%
Prophylactic Antibiotic Timing[2]	24	100%	99%	99%
Prophylactic Antibiotic Timing (Outpatient)[1,3]	-	-	98%	98%
Urinary Catheter Removal[1,2]	-	-	97%	97%
Survey of Patients' Hospital Experiences				
Area Around Room 'Always' Quiet at Night	(a)	64%	67%	61%
Doctors 'Always' Communicated Well	(a)	82%	83%	82%
Home Recovery Information Given	(a)	85%	83%	85%
Hospital Given 9 or 10 on 10 Point Scale	(a)	67%	70%	71%
Meds 'Always' Explained Before Given	(a)	58%	63%	64%
Nurses 'Always' Communicated Well	(a)	77%	79%	79%
Pain 'Always' Well Controlled	(a)	65%	71%	71%
Room and Bathroom 'Always' Clean	(a)	69%	72%	73%
Timely Help 'Always' Received	(a)	66%	68%	68%
Would Definitely Recommend Hospital	(a)	53%	69%	71%
Use of Medical Imaging				
Cardiac Imaging Stress Test before Surgery	92	5.4%	4.3%	5.3%
Combination Abdominal CT Scan	293	5.5%	15.3%	10.5%
Combination Brain/Sinus CT Scan[1]	-	-	2.9%	2.7%
Combination Chest CT Scan	188	1.1%	5%	2.7%
Follow-up Mammogram/Ultrasound	373	11.5%	9.9%	8.8%
Lumbar Spine MRI for Low Back Pain	83	49.4%	41.6%	37.2%

Drew Memorial Hospital

778 Scogin Drive — Phone: 870-367-2411
Monticello, AR 71655 — Fax: 870-460-3562
E-mail: sweast@drewmemorial.org
URL: www.drewmemorial.org
Type: Acute Care Hospitals — Emergency Services: Yes
Ownership: Voluntary non-profit - Other — Beds: 50

Key Personnel:

Infection Control. . . . . Barbara Barnes, RN
CEO . . . . Scott Barrilleaux
Quality Assurance . . . . Karen Donaldson
Radiology. . . . . David Gossman, BSRT
Operating Room. . . . . Ginger Jeffers, RN
CEO/President. . . . . Bart Millstead, MA
Coronary Care . . . . Zelda Pryor, RN
Chief of Medical Staff. . . . . Tim Simon, MD

Measure	Cases	This Hosp.	State Avg.	U.S. Avg.
Blood Clot Prevention and Treatment				
Anticoagulation Overlap Therapy[2]	13	46%	88%	93%
ICU Venous Thromboembolism Prophylaxis[2]	23	61%	94%	92%
Incidence of Potentially Preventable VTE[1,2]	-	-	12%	10%
UFH with Dosages/Platelet Monitoring[2,7]	-	-	100%	97%
Venous Thromboembolism Prophylaxis[2]	160	35%	91%	85%
Warfarin Therapy Discharge Instructions[1,2]	-	-	76%	75%
Chest Pain/Possible Heart Attack Care				
Aspirin Given Within 24 Hours of Arrival	33	88%	96%	96%
Fibrinolytic Meds Within 30 Min. of Arrival[1]	-	-	54%	58%
Average Time to ECG (minutes)	35	2	8	7
Average Time to Transfer (minutes)[1]	-	-	72	60
Children's Asthma Care				
Received Home Management Plan of Care	-	-	-	88%
Received Reliever Medication	-	-	-	100%
Received Systemic Corticosteroids	-	-	-	100%
Emergency Department				
Admittance Decision Time (minutes)[2]	91	55	65	98
Head CT Results Within 45 Min. of Arrival[1]	-	-	49%	57%
Patients Who Left ER Before Being Seen	10,317	1%	3%	2%
Time from ER Arrival to Admit. (minutes)[2]	89	192	214	274
Time from ER Arrival to Discharge (minutes)	318	105	118	134
Time in ER Before Being Evaluated (minutes)	333	20	26	26
Time to Pain Meds for Fractures (minutes)	47	49	66	57
Heart Attack Care				
Aspirin Given at Discharge[1,2]	-	-	99%	99%
Fibrinolytic Meds Within 30 Min. of Arrival[2,7]	-	-	77%	54%
PCI Within 90 Minutes of Arrival[2,7]	-	-	96%	96%
Statin Prescribed at Discharge[1,2]	-	-	97%	98%
Heart Failure Care				
ACE Inhibitor or ARB for LVSD	14	50%	96%	97%
Discharge Instructions Given	22	82%	95%	94%
Evaluation of LVS Function	43	84%	98%	99%
Medicare Spending				
Medicare Spending per Patient (ratio)	-	1.05	0.98	0.98
Pneumonia Care				
Appropriate Initial Antibiotic Given[2]	91	84%	94%	95%
Blood Culture Timing[2]	81	94%	98%	98%
Pregnancy and Delivery Care				
Newborn Deliveries Scheduled Early[2]	51	51%	6%	6%
Preventive Care				
Immunization for Influenza[2]	244	56%	89%	90%
Immunization for Pneumonia[2]	176	73%	92%	92%
Stroke Care				
Anticoagulation Therapy for Atrial Fibrillation[1,2]	-	-	90%	95%
Antithrombotic Therapy Timing[2]	13	100%	96%	98%
Assessed for Rehabilitation[2]	12	92%	95%	97%
Discharged on Antithrombotic Therapy[2]	12	92%	96%	99%
Discharged on Statin Medication[1,2]	-	-	86%	94%
Thrombolytic Therapy Timing[1,2]	-	-	35%	66%
Venous Thromboembolism Prophylaxis[2]	12	100%	91%	94%
Written Stroke Educational Materials Given[1,2]	-	-	81%	88%
Surgical Care Improvement Project				
Appropriate Beta Blocker Usage[1,2]	-	-	98%	98%
Appropriate VTP Within 24 Hours[2]	20	100%	98%	98%
Controlled Postoperative Blood Glucose[2,7]	-	-	99%	97%
Perioperative Temperature Management[2]	71	92%	100%	100%
Prophylactic Antibiotic Selection[2]	51	88%	99%	99%
Prophylactic Antibiotic Selection (Outpatient)[1]	-	-	98%	98%
Prophylactic Antibiotic Stopped[2]	51	98%	98%	98%
Prophylactic Antibiotic Timing[2]	66	65%	99%	99%
Prophylactic Antibiotic Timing (Outpatient)	11	45%	98%	98%
Urinary Catheter Removal[2,7]	-	-	97%	97%
Survey of Patients' Hospital Experiences				
Area Around Room 'Always' Quiet at Night	300+	61%	67%	61%
Doctors 'Always' Communicated Well	300+	91%	83%	82%
Home Recovery Information Given	300+	77%	83%	85%
Hospital Given 9 or 10 on 10 Point Scale	300+	64%	70%	71%
Meds 'Always' Explained Before Given	300+	59%	63%	64%
Nurses 'Always' Communicated Well	300+	76%	79%	79%
Pain 'Always' Well Controlled	300+	69%	71%	71%
Room and Bathroom 'Always' Clean	300+	65%	72%	73%
Timely Help 'Always' Received	300+	63%	68%	68%
Would Definitely Recommend Hospital	300+	63%	69%	71%
Use of Medical Imaging				
Cardiac Imaging Stress Test before Surgery[7]	-	-	4.3%	5.3%
Combination Abdominal CT Scan	299	42.1%	15.3%	10.5%
Combination Brain/Sinus CT Scan	385	1.6%	2.9%	2.7%
Combination Chest CT Scan	165	20.0%	5%	2.7%
Follow-up Mammogram/Ultrasound	384	10.4%	9.9%	8.8%
Lumbar Spine MRI for Low Back Pain	113	39.8%	41.6%	37.2%

Saint Vincent Morrilton

#4 Hospital Drive — Phone: 501-977-2300
Morrilton, AR 72110 — Fax: 501-977-2400
URL: www.stvincenthealth.com
Type: Critical Access Hospitals — Emergency Services: Yes
Ownership: Voluntary non-profit - Church — Beds: 84

Key Personnel:

Emergency Room . . . . Daphne Brown
Infection Control. . . . . Holly Campbell
Quality Assurance . . . . Holly Campbell
CEO/President. . . . . Jonathan Davis
Intensive Care Unit. . . . . Gwyned Hill
Chief of Medical Staff. . . . . Jack Lyon, MD
Operating Room. . . . . Jeanie Stracner
Cardiac Laboratory. . . . . A Westerfield

Measure	Cases	This Hosp.	State Avg.	U.S. Avg.
Blood Clot Prevention and Treatment				
Anticoagulation Overlap Therapy[5]	-	-	88%	93%
ICU Venous Thromboembolism Prophylaxis[5]	-	-	94%	92%
Incidence of Potentially Preventable VTE[5]	-	-	12%	10%
UFH with Dosages/Platelet Monitoring[5]	-	-	100%	97%
Venous Thromboembolism Prophylaxis[5]	-	-	91%	85%
Warfarin Therapy Discharge Instructions[5]	-	-	76%	75%
Chest Pain/Possible Heart Attack Care				
Aspirin Given Within 24 Hours of Arrival	-	-	96%	96%
Fibrinolytic Meds Within 30 Min. of Arrival	-	-	54%	58%
Average Time to ECG (minutes)	-	-	8	7
Average Time to Transfer (minutes)	-	-	72	60
Children's Asthma Care				
Received Home Management Plan of Care	-	-	-	88%
Received Reliever Medication	-	-	-	100%
Received Systemic Corticosteroids	-	-	-	100%
Emergency Department				
Admittance Decision Time (minutes)[5]	-	-	65	98
Head CT Results Within 45 Min. of Arrival	-	-	49%	57%
Patients Who Left ER Before Being Seen	-	-	3%	2%
Time from ER Arrival to Admit. (minutes)[5]	-	-	214	274
Time from ER Arrival to Discharge (minutes)	-	-	118	134
Time in ER Before Being Evaluated (minutes)	-	-	26	26
Time to Pain Meds for Fractures (minutes)	-	-	66	57
Heart Attack Care				
Aspirin Given at Discharge[3,7]	-	-	99%	99%
Fibrinolytic Meds Within 30 Min. of Arrival[3,7]	-	-	77%	54%
PCI Within 90 Minutes of Arrival[3,7]	-	-	96%	96%
Statin Prescribed at Discharge[3,7]	-	-	97%	98%
Heart Failure Care				
ACE Inhibitor or ARB for LVSD	18	100%	96%	97%
Discharge Instructions Given	27	100%	95%	94%
Evaluation of LVS Function	30	100%	98%	99%
Medicare Spending				
Medicare Spending per Patient (ratio)	-	-	0.98	0.98
Pneumonia Care				
Appropriate Initial Antibiotic Given	24	92%	94%	95%
Blood Culture Timing	23	96%	98%	98%
Pregnancy and Delivery Care				
Newborn Deliveries Scheduled Early[5]	-	-	6%	6%
Preventive Care				
Immunization for Influenza[5]	-	-	89%	90%
Immunization for Pneumonia[5]	-	-	92%	92%
Stroke Care				
Anticoagulation Therapy for Atrial Fibrillation[5]	-	-	90%	95%
Antithrombotic Therapy Timing[5]	-	-	96%	98%
Assessed for Rehabilitation[5]	-	-	95%	97%
Discharged on Antithrombotic Therapy[5]	-	-	96%	99%
Discharged on Statin Medication[5]	-	-	86%	94%
Thrombolytic Therapy Timing[5]	-	-	35%	66%
Venous Thromboembolism Prophylaxis[5]	-	-	91%	94%

NOTE: Hospital profiles are in alphabetical order by state, then city, then hospital within the city; Rankings exclude hospitals with less than 25 cases except for patient surveys which excludes hospitals with less than 100 cases; (a) 100-299 cases; (1) The number of cases/patients is too few to report; (2) Data submitted were based on a sample of cases/patients; (3) Results are based on a shorter time period than required; (4) Data suppressed by CMS for one or more quarters; (5) Results are not available for this reporting period; (6) Fewer than 100 patients completed the HCAHPS survey; (7) No cases met the criteria for this measure; (8) The lower limit of the confidence interval cannot be calculated if the number of observed infections equals zero; (9) No data are available from the state/territory for this reporting period; (10) The scores shown reflect fewer than 50 completed surveys; (11) There were discrepancies in the data collection process; (12) This measure does not apply to this hospital for this reporting period; (13) Results cannot be calculated for this reporting period; (14) The results for this state are combined with nearby states to protect confidentiality; Please refer to the User's Guide for a full explanation of data.

Measure	Cases	This Hosp.	State Avg.	U.S. Avg.
Written Stroke Educational Materials Given[5]	-	-	81%	88%
Surgical Care Improvement Project				
Appropriate Beta Blocker Usage[1]	-	-	98%	98%
Appropriate VTP Within 24 Hours	17	100%	98%	98%
Controlled Postoperative Blood Glucose[7]	-	-	99%	97%
Perioperative Temperature Management	20	100%	100%	100%
Prophylactic Antibiotic Selection[1]	-	-	99%	99%
Prophylactic Antibiotic Selection (Outpatient)	-	-	98%	98%
Prophylactic Antibiotic Stopped[1]	-	-	98%	98%
Prophylactic Antibiotic Timing[1]	-	-	99%	99%
Prophylactic Antibiotic Timing (Outpatient)	-	-	98%	98%
Urinary Catheter Removal[1]	-	-	97%	97%
Survey of Patients' Hospital Experiences				
Area Around Room 'Always' Quiet at Night	(a)	66%	67%	61%
Doctors 'Always' Communicated Well	(a)	84%	83%	82%
Home Recovery Information Given	(a)	84%	83%	85%
Hospital Given 9 or 10 on 10 Point Scale	(a)	73%	70%	71%
Meds 'Always' Explained Before Given	(a)	63%	63%	64%
Nurses 'Always' Communicated Well	(a)	82%	79%	79%
Pain 'Always' Well Controlled	(a)	68%	71%	71%
Room and Bathroom 'Always' Clean	(a)	80%	72%	73%
Timely Help 'Always' Received	(a)	78%	68%	68%
Would Definitely Recommend Hospital	(a)	65%	69%	71%
Use of Medical Imaging				
Cardiac Imaging Stress Test before Surgery	-	-	4.3%	5.3%
Combination Abdominal CT Scan	-	-	15.3%	10.5%
Combination Brain/Sinus CT Scan	-	-	2.9%	2.7%
Combination Chest CT Scan	-	-	5%	2.7%
Follow-up Mammogram/Ultrasound	-	-	9.9%	8.8%
Lumbar Spine MRI for Low Back Pain	-	-	41.6%	37.2%

Baxter Regional Medical Center

624 Hospital Drive — Phone: 870-508-1000
Mountain Home, AR 72653 — Fax: 870-424-1650
URL: www.baxterregional.org
Type: Acute Care Hospitals — Emergency Services: Yes
Ownership: Voluntary non-profit - Private — Beds: 268

Key Personnel:

Pediatric Ambulatory Care . . . . . . Yoland Condery, MD
Quality Assurance . . . . Carla Day
Radiology. Randy Gontens, MD
Infection Control. . . . . Sherry McGoldrick
CEO/President. . . . . Ron Peterson
Operating Room. . . . . Carol Piakowski
Pediatric In-Patient Care . . . . Jessica Snodgrass
Chief of Medical Staff. . . . . Ed White, MD

Measure	Cases	This Hosp.	State Avg.	U.S. Avg.
Blood Clot Prevention and Treatment				
Anticoagulation Overlap Therapy[2]	40	90%	88%	93%
ICU Venous Thromboembolism Prophylaxis[2]	97	97%	94%	92%
Incidence of Potentially Preventable VTE[1,2]	-	-	12%	10%
UFH with Dosages/Platelet Monitoring[1,2]	-	-	100%	97%
Venous Thromboembolism Prophylaxis[2]	255	91%	91%	85%
Warfarin Therapy Discharge Instructions[2]	26	100%	76%	75%
Chest Pain/Possible Heart Attack Care				
Aspirin Given Within 24 Hours of Arrival[1]	-	-	96%	96%
Fibrinolytic Meds Within 30 Min. of Arrival[3,7]	-	-	54%	58%
Average Time to ECG (minutes)[1]	-	-	8	7
Average Time to Transfer (minutes)[3,7]	-	-	72	60
Children's Asthma Care				
Received Home Management Plan of Care	-	-	-	88%
Received Reliever Medication	-	-	-	100%
Received Systemic Corticosteroids	-	-	-	100%
Emergency Department				
Admittance Decision Time (minutes)[2]	360	56	65	98
Head CT Results Within 45 Min. of Arrival	30	57%	49%	57%
Patients Who Left ER Before Being Seen	29,300	2%	3%	2%
Time from ER Arrival to Admit. (minutes)[2]	584	205	214	274
Time from ER Arrival to Discharge (minutes)	331	130	118	134
Time in ER Before Being Evaluated (minutes)	231	19	26	26
Time to Pain Meds for Fractures (minutes)	85	69	66	57
Heart Attack Care				
Aspirin Given at Discharge[2]	212	97%	99%	99%
Fibrinolytic Meds Within 30 Min. of Arrival[2,7]	-	-	77%	54%
PCI Within 90 Minutes of Arrival[2]	34	94%	96%	96%
Statin Prescribed at Discharge[2]	210	86%	97%	98%
Heart Failure Care				
ACE Inhibitor or ARB for LVSD[2]	83	86%	96%	97%
Discharge Instructions Given[2]	191	100%	95%	94%
Evaluation of LVS Function[2]	256	99%	98%	99%
Medicare Spending				
Medicare Spending per Patient (ratio)	-	0.97	0.98	0.98
Pneumonia Care				
Appropriate Initial Antibiotic Given[2]	91	96%	94%	95%
Blood Culture Timing[2]	118	96%	98%	98%
Pregnancy and Delivery Care				
Newborn Deliveries Scheduled Early[2]	28	14%	6%	6%
Preventive Care				
Immunization for Influenza[2]	604	96%	89%	90%
Immunization for Pneumonia[2]	875	96%	92%	92%
Stroke Care				
Anticoagulation Therapy for Atrial Fibrillation[1,2]	-	-	90%	95%
Antithrombotic Therapy Timing[2]	65	97%	96%	98%
Assessed for Rehabilitation[2]	73	97%	95%	97%
Discharged on Antithrombotic Therapy[2]	72	97%	96%	99%
Discharged on Statin Medication[2]	62	63%	86%	94%
Thrombolytic Therapy Timing[1,2]	-	-	35%	66%
Venous Thromboembolism Prophylaxis[2]	64	81%	91%	94%
Written Stroke Educational Materials Given[2]	38	84%	81%	88%
Surgical Care Improvement Project				
Appropriate Beta Blocker Usage[2]	186	98%	98%	98%
Appropriate VTP Within 24 Hours[2]	273	97%	98%	98%
Controlled Postoperative Blood Glucose[2]	114	97%	99%	97%
Perioperative Temperature Management[2]	329	100%	100%	100%
Prophylactic Antibiotic Selection[2]	327	99%	99%	99%
Prophylactic Antibiotic Selection (Outpatient)	178	96%	98%	98%
Prophylactic Antibiotic Stopped[2]	306	97%	98%	98%
Prophylactic Antibiotic Timing[2]	328	99%	99%	99%
Prophylactic Antibiotic Timing (Outpatient)	179	97%	98%	98%
Urinary Catheter Removal[2]	288	95%	97%	97%
Survey of Patients' Hospital Experiences				
Area Around Room 'Always' Quiet at Night	300+	61%	67%	61%
Doctors 'Always' Communicated Well	300+	80%	83%	82%
Home Recovery Information Given	300+	87%	83%	85%
Hospital Given 9 or 10 on 10 Point Scale	300+	76%	70%	71%
Meds 'Always' Explained Before Given	300+	62%	63%	64%
Nurses 'Always' Communicated Well	300+	79%	79%	79%
Pain 'Always' Well Controlled	300+	74%	71%	71%
Room and Bathroom 'Always' Clean	300+	71%	72%	73%
Timely Help 'Always' Received	300+	73%	68%	68%
Would Definitely Recommend Hospital	300+	76%	69%	71%
Use of Medical Imaging				
Cardiac Imaging Stress Test before Surgery	237	3.0%	4.3%	5.3%
Combination Abdominal CT Scan	676	12.6%	15.3%	10.5%
Combination Brain/Sinus CT Scan	881	1.6%	2.9%	2.7%
Combination Chest CT Scan	476	2.3%	5%	2.7%
Follow-up Mammogram/Ultrasound	2,694	8.3%	9.9%	8.8%
Lumbar Spine MRI for Low Back Pain	208	38.9%	41.6%	37.2%

Stone County Medical Center

Highway 14 East — Phone: 870-269-4361
Mountain View, AR 72560 — Fax: 870-269-6593
Type: Critical Access Hospitals — Emergency Services: Yes
Ownership: Voluntary non-profit - Private — Beds: 25

Key Personnel:

Operating Room. . . . . Pat Bracken, RN

Measure	Cases	This Hosp.	State Avg.	U.S. Avg.
Blood Clot Prevention and Treatment				
Anticoagulation Overlap Therapy[1,2]	-	-	88%	93%
ICU Venous Thromboembolism Prophylaxis[1,2]	-	-	94%	92%
Incidence of Potentially Preventable VTE[2,3]	-	-	12%	10%
UFH with Dosages/Platelet Monitoring[2,3]	-	-	100%	97%
Venous Thromboembolism Prophylaxis[2,3]	31	68%	91%	85%
Warfarin Therapy Discharge Instructions[1,2]	-	-	76%	75%
Chest Pain/Possible Heart Attack Care				
Aspirin Given Within 24 Hours of Arrival	59	92%	96%	96%
Fibrinolytic Meds Within 30 Min. of Arrival[1]	-	-	54%	58%
Average Time to ECG (minutes)	64	12	8	7
Average Time to Transfer (minutes)[1]	-	-	72	60
Children's Asthma Care				
Received Home Management Plan of Care	-	-	-	88%
Received Reliever Medication	-	-	-	100%
Received Systemic Corticosteroids	-	-	-	100%
Emergency Department				
Admittance Decision Time (minutes)[2]	196	60	65	98
Head CT Results Within 45 Min. of Arrival	12	17%	49%	57%
Patients Who Left ER Before Being Seen	7,148	2%	3%	2%
Time from ER Arrival to Admit. (minutes)[2]	196	176	214	274
Time from ER Arrival to Discharge (minutes)[3]	86	95	118	134
Time in ER Before Being Evaluated (minutes)[3]	98	24	26	26
Time to Pain Meds for Fractures (minutes)	44	46	66	57
Heart Attack Care				
Aspirin Given at Discharge[1,3]	-	-	99%	99%
Fibrinolytic Meds Within 30 Min. of Arrival[3,7]	-	-	77%	54%
PCI Within 90 Minutes of Arrival[3,7]	-	-	96%	96%
Statin Prescribed at Discharge[1,3]	-	-	97%	98%
Heart Failure Care				
ACE Inhibitor or ARB for LVSD[1]	-	-	96%	97%
Discharge Instructions Given	19	100%	95%	94%
Evaluation of LVS Function	27	89%	98%	99%
Medicare Spending				
Medicare Spending per Patient (ratio)	-	-	0.98	0.98
Pneumonia Care				
Appropriate Initial Antibiotic Given	49	78%	94%	95%
Blood Culture Timing	27	85%	98%	98%
Pregnancy and Delivery Care				
Newborn Deliveries Scheduled Early[3,7]	-	-	6%	6%
Preventive Care				
Immunization for Influenza[2]	280	95%	89%	90%
Immunization for Pneumonia[2]	447	96%	92%	92%
Stroke Care				
Anticoagulation Therapy for Atrial Fibrillation[1,3]	-	-	90%	95%
Antithrombotic Therapy Timing[1,3]	-	-	96%	98%
Assessed for Rehabilitation[1,3]	-	-	95%	97%
Discharged on Antithrombotic Therapy[1,3]	-	-	96%	99%
Discharged on Statin Medication[1,3]	-	-	86%	94%
Thrombolytic Therapy Timing[1,3]	-	-	35%	66%
Venous Thromboembolism Prophylaxis[1,3]	-	-	91%	94%
Written Stroke Educational Materials Given[1,3]	-	-	81%	88%
Surgical Care Improvement Project				
Appropriate Beta Blocker Usage	17	100%	98%	98%
Appropriate VTP Within 24 Hours	68	100%	98%	98%
Controlled Postoperative Blood Glucose[7]	-	-	99%	97%
Perioperative Temperature Management	73	100%	100%	100%
Prophylactic Antibiotic Selection	73	100%	99%	99%
Prophylactic Antibiotic Selection (Outpatient)[5]	-	-	98%	98%
Prophylactic Antibiotic Stopped	73	99%	98%	98%
Prophylactic Antibiotic Timing	73	99%	99%	99%
Prophylactic Antibiotic Timing (Outpatient)[5]	-	-	98%	98%
Urinary Catheter Removal	71	97%	97%	97%
Survey of Patients' Hospital Experiences				
Area Around Room 'Always' Quiet at Night[5]	-	-	67%	61%
Doctors 'Always' Communicated Well[5]	-	-	83%	82%
Home Recovery Information Given[5]	-	-	83%	85%
Hospital Given 9 or 10 on 10 Point Scale[5]	-	-	70%	71%
Meds 'Always' Explained Before Given[5]	-	-	63%	64%
Nurses 'Always' Communicated Well[5]	-	-	79%	79%
Pain 'Always' Well Controlled[5]	-	-	71%	71%
Room and Bathroom 'Always' Clean[5]	-	-	72%	73%
Timely Help 'Always' Received[5]	-	-	68%	68%
Would Definitely Recommend Hospital[5]	-	-	69%	71%
Use of Medical Imaging				
Cardiac Imaging Stress Test before Surgery[7]	-	-	4.3%	5.3%
Combination Abdominal CT Scan	285	34.4%	15.3%	10.5%
Combination Brain/Sinus CT Scan[1]	-	-	2.9%	2.7%
Combination Chest CT Scan	125	48.8%	5%	2.7%
Follow-up Mammogram/Ultrasound	137	8.0%	9.9%	8.8%
Lumbar Spine MRI for Low Back Pain[1]	-	-	41.6%	37.2%

NOTE: Hospital profiles are in alphabetical order by state, then city, then hospital within the city; Rankings exclude hospitals with less than 25 cases except for patient surveys which excludes hospitals with less than 100 cases; (a) 100-299 cases; (1) The number of cases/patients is too few to report; (2) Data submitted were based on a sample of cases/patients; (3) Results are based on a shorter time period than required; (4) Data suppressed by CMS for one or more quarters; (5) Results are not available for this reporting period; (6) Fewer than 100 patients completed the HCAHPS survey; (7) No cases met the criteria for this measure; (8) The lower limit of the confidence interval cannot be calculated if the number of observed infections equals zero; (9) No data are available from the state/territory for this reporting period; (10) The scores shown reflect fewer than 50 completed surveys; (11) There were discrepancies in the data collection process; (12) This measure does not apply to this hospital for this reporting period; (13) Results cannot be calculated for this reporting period; (14) The results for this state are combined with nearby states to protect confidentiality; Please refer to the User's Guide for a full explanation of data.

Howard Memorial Hospital

130 Medical Circle Phone: 870-845-4400
Nashville, AR 71852 Fax: 870-845-4178
E-mail: hmh@cswnet.com
URL: www.howardmemorial.com
Type: Critical Access Hospitals Emergency Services: Yes
Ownership: Voluntary non-profit - Private Beds: 25

Key Personnel:
Radiology. . . . . Gayla Beaird
Operating Room. . . . . Sibbie Burrow
Intensive Care Unit. . . . . Rae Dowda, RN
Quality Assurance . . . . Angelia Hanson, RN
CEO . . . . Debra J. Wright, MS
Chief of Medical Staff . . . . Hasmukh Patel
Emergency Room . . . . Sam Peebles, MD
Infection Control. . . . . Conley Venable, RN

Measure	Cases	This Hosp.	State Avg.	U.S. Avg.
Blood Clot Prevention and Treatment				
Anticoagulation Overlap Therapy[5]	-	-	88%	93%
ICU Venous Thromboembolism Prophylaxis[5]	-	-	94%	92%
Incidence of Potentially Preventable VTE[5]	-	-	12%	10%
UFH with Dosages/Platelet Monitoring[5]	-	-	100%	97%
Venous Thromboembolism Prophylaxis[5]	-	-	91%	85%
Warfarin Therapy Discharge Instructions[5]	-	-	76%	75%
Chest Pain/Possible Heart Attack Care				
Aspirin Given Within 24 Hours of Arrival	47	98%	96%	96%
Fibrinolytic Meds Within 30 Min. of Arrival[1]	-	-	54%	58%
Average Time to ECG (minutes)	48	8	8	7
Average Time to Transfer (minutes)[7]	-	-	72	60
Children's Asthma Care				
Received Home Management Plan of Care	-	-	-	88%
Received Reliever Medication	-	-	-	100%
Received Systemic Corticosteroids	-	-	-	100%
Emergency Department				
Admittance Decision Time (minutes)	256	50	65	98
Head CT Results Within 45 Min. of Arrival[5]	-	-	49%	57%
Patients Who Left ER Before Being Seen	8,824	2%	3%	2%
Time from ER Arrival to Admit. (minutes)	257	208	214	274
Time from ER Arrival to Discharge (minutes)[5]	-	-	118	134
Time in ER Before Being Evaluated (minutes)[5]	-	-	26	26
Time to Pain Meds for Fractures (minutes)[5]	-	-	66	57
Heart Attack Care				
Aspirin Given at Discharge[3,7]	-	-	99%	99%
Fibrinolytic Meds Within 30 Min. of Arrival[3,7]	-	-	77%	54%
PCI Within 90 Minutes of Arrival[3,7]	-	-	96%	96%
Statin Prescribed at Discharge[3,7]	-	-	97%	98%
Heart Failure Care				
ACE Inhibitor or ARB for LVSD[1,3]	-	-	96%	97%
Discharge Instructions Given[1,3]	-	-	95%	94%
Evaluation of LVS Function[1,3]	-	-	98%	99%
Medicare Spending				
Medicare Spending per Patient (ratio)	-	-	0.98	0.98
Pneumonia Care				
Appropriate Initial Antibiotic Given	35	100%	94%	95%
Blood Culture Timing	37	100%	98%	98%
Pregnancy and Delivery Care				
Newborn Deliveries Scheduled Early[5]	-	-	6%	6%
Preventive Care				
Immunization for Influenza	208	94%	89%	90%
Immunization for Pneumonia	304	96%	92%	92%
Stroke Care				
Anticoagulation Therapy for Atrial Fibrillation[5]	-	-	90%	95%
Antithrombotic Therapy Timing[5]	-	-	96%	98%
Assessed for Rehabilitation[5]	-	-	95%	97%
Discharged on Antithrombotic Therapy[5]	-	-	96%	99%
Discharged on Statin Medication[5]	-	-	86%	94%
Thrombolytic Therapy Timing[5]	-	-	35%	66%
Venous Thromboembolism Prophylaxis[5]	-	-	91%	94%
Written Stroke Educational Materials Given[5]	-	-	81%	88%
Surgical Care Improvement Project				
Appropriate Beta Blocker Usage[3,7]	-	-	98%	98%
Appropriate VTP Within 24 Hours[3,7]	-	-	98%	98%
Controlled Postoperative Blood Glucose[3,7]	-	-	99%	97%
Perioperative Temperature Management[1,3]	-	-	100%	100%
Prophylactic Antibiotic Selection[3,7]	-	-	99%	99%
Prophylactic Antibiotic Selection (Outpatient)[5]	-	-	98%	98%
Prophylactic Antibiotic Stopped[3,7]	-	-	98%	98%
Prophylactic Antibiotic Timing[3,7]	-	-	99%	99%
Prophylactic Antibiotic Timing (Outpatient)[5]	-	-	98%	98%
Urinary Catheter Removal[3,7]	-	-	97%	97%
Survey of Patients' Hospital Experiences				
Area Around Room 'Always' Quiet at Night[6]	<100	79%	67%	61%
Doctors 'Always' Communicated Well[6]	<100	85%	83%	82%
Home Recovery Information Given[6]	<100	75%	83%	85%
Hospital Given 9 or 10 on 10 Point Scale[6]	<100	81%	70%	71%
Meds 'Always' Explained Before Given[6]	<100	75%	63%	64%
Nurses 'Always' Communicated Well[6]	<100	83%	79%	79%
Pain 'Always' Well Controlled[6]	<100	80%	71%	71%
Room and Bathroom 'Always' Clean[6]	<100	84%	72%	73%
Timely Help 'Always' Received[6]	<100	82%	68%	68%
Would Definitely Recommend Hospital[6]	<100	81%	69%	71%
Use of Medical Imaging				
Cardiac Imaging Stress Test before Surgery[7]	-	-	4.3%	5.3%
Combination Abdominal CT Scan	175	4.6%	15.3%	10.5%
Combination Brain/Sinus CT Scan[1]	-	-	2.9%	2.7%
Combination Chest CT Scan	66	4.5%	5%	2.7%
Follow-up Mammogram/Ultrasound	244	16.0%	9.9%	8.8%
Lumbar Spine MRI for Low Back Pain[1]	-	-	41.6%	37.2%

Harris Hospital

1205 Mclain Street Phone: 870-523-8911
Newport, AR 72112 Fax: 870-523-0225
URL: www.harrishospital.com
Type: Acute Care Hospitals Emergency Services: Yes
Ownership: Proprietary Beds: 132

Key Personnel:
Emergency Room . . . . Mohammed Ahmed
Radiology. . . . . Melissa Bloch-Mensch
CEO/President. . . . . Claude Camp
Chief of Medical Staff . . . . Mufiz Chauhan, MD
Pediatric Ambulatory Care . . . . . . Mohamed Hasan, MD
Operating Room. . . . . Hon Poon
Quality Assurance . . . . Ana Stapleton

Measure	Cases	This Hosp.	State Avg.	U.S. Avg.
Blood Clot Prevention and Treatment				
Anticoagulation Overlap Therapy[2]	12	100%	88%	93%
ICU Venous Thromboembolism Prophylaxis[2]	65	92%	94%	92%
Incidence of Potentially Preventable VTE[1,2]	-	-	12%	10%
UFH with Dosages/Platelet Monitoring[2,7]	-	-	100%	97%
Venous Thromboembolism Prophylaxis[2]	331	92%	91%	85%
Warfarin Therapy Discharge Instructions[1,2]	-	-	76%	75%
Chest Pain/Possible Heart Attack Care				
Aspirin Given Within 24 Hours of Arrival	31	97%	96%	96%
Fibrinolytic Meds Within 30 Min. of Arrival[1]	-	-	54%	58%
Average Time to ECG (minutes)	33	6	8	7
Average Time to Transfer (minutes)[1]	-	-	72	60
Children's Asthma Care				
Received Home Management Plan of Care	-	-	-	88%
Received Reliever Medication	-	-	-	100%
Received Systemic Corticosteroids	-	-	-	100%
Emergency Department				
Admittance Decision Time (minutes)[2]	516	52	65	98
Head CT Results Within 45 Min. of Arrival[1]	-	-	49%	57%
Patients Who Left ER Before Being Seen	11,060	0%	3%	2%
Time from ER Arrival to Admit. (minutes)[2]	518	155	214	274
Time from ER Arrival to Discharge (minutes)	369	88	118	134
Time in ER Before Being Evaluated (minutes)	481	9	26	26
Time to Pain Meds for Fractures (minutes)	37	49	66	57
Heart Attack Care				
Aspirin Given at Discharge[1,3]	-	-	99%	99%
Fibrinolytic Meds Within 30 Min. of Arrival[3,7]	-	-	77%	54%
PCI Within 90 Minutes of Arrival[3,7]	-	-	96%	96%
Statin Prescribed at Discharge[1,3]	-	-	97%	98%
Heart Failure Care				
ACE Inhibitor or ARB for LVSD	36	100%	96%	97%
Discharge Instructions Given	60	88%	95%	94%
Evaluation of LVS Function	73	93%	98%	99%
Medicare Spending				
Medicare Spending per Patient (ratio)	-	0.95	0.98	0.98
Pneumonia Care				
Appropriate Initial Antibiotic Given	59	93%	94%	95%
Blood Culture Timing	85	93%	98%	98%
Pregnancy and Delivery Care				
Newborn Deliveries Scheduled Early[2]	27	0%	6%	6%
Preventive Care				
Immunization for Influenza[2]	590	94%	89%	90%
Immunization for Pneumonia[2]	537	97%	92%	92%
Stroke Care				
Anticoagulation Therapy for Atrial Fibrillation[1]	-	-	90%	95%
Antithrombotic Therapy Timing[1]	-	-	96%	98%
Assessed for Rehabilitation[1]	-	-	95%	97%
Discharged on Antithrombotic Therapy[1]	-	-	96%	99%
Discharged on Statin Medication[1]	-	-	86%	94%
Thrombolytic Therapy Timing[1]	-	-	35%	66%
Venous Thromboembolism Prophylaxis[1]	-	-	91%	94%
Written Stroke Educational Materials Given[1]	-	-	81%	88%
Surgical Care Improvement Project				
Appropriate Beta Blocker Usage[1]	-	-	98%	98%
Appropriate VTP Within 24 Hours	24	100%	98%	98%
Controlled Postoperative Blood Glucose[7]	-	-	99%	97%
Perioperative Temperature Management	42	100%	100%	100%
Prophylactic Antibiotic Selection	31	100%	99%	99%
Prophylactic Antibiotic Selection (Outpatient)	16	94%	98%	98%
Prophylactic Antibiotic Stopped	30	93%	98%	98%
Prophylactic Antibiotic Timing	31	100%	99%	99%
Prophylactic Antibiotic Timing (Outpatient)	16	100%	98%	98%
Urinary Catheter Removal[1]	-	-	97%	97%
Survey of Patients' Hospital Experiences				
Area Around Room 'Always' Quiet at Night	300+	64%	67%	61%
Doctors 'Always' Communicated Well	300+	81%	83%	82%
Home Recovery Information Given	300+	85%	83%	85%
Hospital Given 9 or 10 on 10 Point Scale	300+	61%	70%	71%
Meds 'Always' Explained Before Given	300+	67%	63%	64%
Nurses 'Always' Communicated Well	300+	75%	79%	79%
Pain 'Always' Well Controlled	300+	68%	71%	71%
Room and Bathroom 'Always' Clean	300+	63%	72%	73%
Timely Help 'Always' Received	300+	71%	68%	68%
Would Definitely Recommend Hospital	300+	53%	69%	71%
Use of Medical Imaging				
Cardiac Imaging Stress Test before Surgery[1]	-	-	4.3%	5.3%
Combination Abdominal CT Scan	166	32.5%	15.3%	10.5%
Combination Brain/Sinus CT Scan[1]	-	-	2.9%	2.7%
Combination Chest CT Scan	115	19.1%	5%	2.7%
Follow-up Mammogram/Ultrasound	156	13.5%	9.9%	8.8%
Lumbar Spine MRI for Low Back Pain[1]	-	-	41.6%	37.2%

Arkansas Surgical Hospital

5201 North Shore Drive Phone: 501-748-8000
No Little Rock, AR 72118
E-mail: questions@asksurgicalhospital.com
URL: www.arksurgicalhospital.com
Type: Acute Care Hospitals Emergency Services: Yes
Ownership: Physician Beds: 20

Measure	Cases	This Hosp.	State Avg.	U.S. Avg.
Blood Clot Prevention and Treatment				
Anticoagulation Overlap Therapy[2,7]	-	-	88%	93%
ICU Venous Thromboembolism Prophylaxis[2,7]	-	-	94%	92%
Incidence of Potentially Preventable VTE[1,2]	-	-	12%	10%
UFH with Dosages/Platelet Monitoring[2,7]	-	-	100%	97%
Venous Thromboembolism Prophylaxis[2]	48	98%	91%	85%
Warfarin Therapy Discharge Instructions[2,7]	-	-	76%	75%
Chest Pain/Possible Heart Attack Care				
Aspirin Given Within 24 Hours of Arrival[5]	-	-	96%	96%
Fibrinolytic Meds Within 30 Min. of Arrival[5]	-	-	54%	58%
Average Time to ECG (minutes)[5]	-	-	8	7
Average Time to Transfer (minutes)[5]	-	-	72	60
Children's Asthma Care				
Received Home Management Plan of Care	-	-	-	88%
Received Reliever Medication	-	-	-	100%
Received Systemic Corticosteroids	-	-	-	100%

NOTE: Hospital profiles are in alphabetical order by state, then city, then hospital within the city; Rankings exclude hospitals with less than 25 cases except for patient surveys which excludes hospitals with less than 100 cases; (a) 100-299 cases; (1) The number of cases/patients is too few to report; (2) Data submitted were based on a sample of cases/patients; (3) Results are based on a shorter time period than required; (4) Data suppressed by CMS for one or more quarters; (5) Results are not available for this reporting period; (6) Fewer than 100 patients completed the HCAHPS survey; (7) No cases met the criteria for this measure; (8) The lower limit of the confidence interval cannot be calculated if the number of observed infections equals zero; (9) No data are available from the state/territory for this reporting period; (10) The scores shown reflect fewer than 50 completed surveys; (11) There were discrepancies in the data collection process; (12) This measure does not apply to this hospital for this reporting period; (13) Results cannot be calculated for this reporting period; (14) The results for this state are combined with nearby states to protect confidentiality; Please refer to the User's Guide for a full explanation of data.

Measure	Cases	This Hosp.	State Avg.	U.S. Avg.
Emergency Department				
Admittance Decision Time (minutes)[2,7]	-	-	65	98
Head CT Results Within 45 Min. of Arrival[1,3]	-	-	49%	57%
Patients Who Left ER Before Being Seen	249	0%	3%	2%
Time from ER Arrival to Admit. (minutes)[2,7]	-	-	214	274
Time from ER Arrival to Discharge (minutes)	161	91	118	134
Time in ER Before Being Evaluated (minutes)	178	30	26	26
Time to Pain Meds for Fractures (minutes)[1,3]	-	-	66	57
Heart Attack Care				
Aspirin Given at Discharge[5]	-	-	99%	99%
Fibrinolytic Meds Within 30 Min. of Arrival[5]	-	-	77%	54%
PCI Within 90 Minutes of Arrival[5]	-	-	96%	96%
Statin Prescribed at Discharge[5]	-	-	97%	98%
Heart Failure Care				
ACE Inhibitor or ARB for LVSD[5]	-	-	96%	97%
Discharge Instructions Given[5]	-	-	95%	94%
Evaluation of LVS Function[5]	-	-	98%	99%
Medicare Spending				
Medicare Spending per Patient (ratio)	-	0.91	0.98	0.98
Pneumonia Care				
Appropriate Initial Antibiotic Given[5]	-	-	94%	95%
Blood Culture Timing[5]	-	-	98%	98%
Pregnancy and Delivery Care				
Newborn Deliveries Scheduled Early[7]	-	-	6%	6%
Preventive Care				
Immunization for Influenza[2]	482	51%	89%	90%
Immunization for Pneumonia[2]	509	60%	92%	92%
Stroke Care				
Anticoagulation Therapy for Atrial Fibrillation[5]	-	-	90%	95%
Antithrombotic Therapy Timing[5]	-	-	96%	98%
Assessed for Rehabilitation[5]	-	-	95%	97%
Discharged on Antithrombotic Therapy[5]	-	-	96%	99%
Discharged on Statin Medication[5]	-	-	86%	94%
Thrombolytic Therapy Timing[5]	-	-	35%	66%
Venous Thromboembolism Prophylaxis[5]	-	-	91%	94%
Written Stroke Educational Materials Given[5]	-	-	81%	88%
Surgical Care Improvement Project				
Appropriate Beta Blocker Usage[2]	119	98%	98%	98%
Appropriate VTP Within 24 Hours[2]	397	99%	98%	98%
Controlled Postoperative Blood Glucose[2,7]	-	-	99%	97%
Perioperative Temperature Management[2]	409	100%	100%	100%
Prophylactic Antibiotic Selection[2]	297	100%	99%	99%
Prophylactic Antibiotic Selection (Outpatient)	438	100%	98%	98%
Prophylactic Antibiotic Stopped[2]	295	100%	98%	98%
Prophylactic Antibiotic Timing[2]	297	99%	99%	99%
Prophylactic Antibiotic Timing (Outpatient)	439	100%	98%	98%
Urinary Catheter Removal[2]	346	99%	97%	97%
Survey of Patients' Hospital Experiences				
Area Around Room 'Always' Quiet at Night	300+	91%	67%	61%
Doctors 'Always' Communicated Well	300+	89%	83%	82%
Home Recovery Information Given	300+	89%	83%	85%
Hospital Given 9 or 10 on 10 Point Scale	300+	90%	70%	71%
Meds 'Always' Explained Before Given	300+	77%	63%	64%
Nurses 'Always' Communicated Well	300+	89%	79%	79%
Pain 'Always' Well Controlled	300+	80%	71%	71%
Room and Bathroom 'Always' Clean	300+	82%	72%	73%
Timely Help 'Always' Received	300+	79%	68%	68%
Would Definitely Recommend Hospital	300+	92%	69%	71%
Use of Medical Imaging				
Cardiac Imaging Stress Test before Surgery[7]	-	-	4.3%	5.3%
Combination Abdominal CT Scan[1]	-	-	15.3%	10.5%
Combination Brain/Sinus CT Scan[1]	-	-	2.9%	2.7%
Combination Chest CT Scan[1]	-	-	5%	2.7%
Follow-up Mammogram/Ultrasound[7]	-	-	9.9%	8.8%
Lumbar Spine MRI for Low Back Pain	294	34.7%	41.6%	37.2%

Baptist Health Medical Center - North Little Rock

3333 Springhill Drive Phone: 501-202-3000
North Little Rock, AR 72117 Fax: 501-202-3813
E-mail: roxannel@baptist-health.org
URL: www.baptist-health.org
Type: Acute Care Hospitals Emergency Services: Yes
Ownership: Voluntary non-profit - Other Beds: 248

Key Personnel:

Operating Room. . . . . David W Bevans, III
Quality Assurance . . . . Donna Gershner
CEO/President. . . . . Russell D Harrington
Infection Control. . . . . Becky Hawley
Radiology. . . . . David C Kolb
Chief of Medical Staff . . . . Valerie McNee
Coronary Care . . . . Faye Nipps
Pediatric In-Patient Care . . . . Naomi Wallis

Measure	Cases	This Hosp.	State Avg.	U.S. Avg.
Blood Clot Prevention and Treatment				
Anticoagulation Overlap Therapy[2]	50	100%	88%	93%
ICU Venous Thromboembolism Prophylaxis[2]	145	86%	94%	92%
Incidence of Potentially Preventable VTE[1,2]	-	-	12%	10%
UFH with Dosages/Platelet Monitoring[2]	14	100%	100%	97%
Venous Thromboembolism Prophylaxis[2]	232	78%	91%	85%
Warfarin Therapy Discharge Instructions[2]	34	97%	76%	75%
Chest Pain/Possible Heart Attack Care				
Aspirin Given Within 24 Hours of Arrival[5]	-	-	96%	96%
Fibrinolytic Meds Within 30 Min. of Arrival[5]	-	-	54%	58%
Average Time to ECG (minutes)[5]	-	-	8	7
Average Time to Transfer (minutes)[5]	-	-	72	60
Children's Asthma Care				
Received Home Management Plan of Care	-	-	-	88%
Received Reliever Medication	-	-	-	100%
Received Systemic Corticosteroids	-	-	-	100%
Emergency Department				
Admittance Decision Time (minutes)[2]	535	56	65	98
Head CT Results Within 45 Min. of Arrival	24	29%	49%	57%
Patients Who Left ER Before Being Seen	49,857	6%	3%	2%
Time from ER Arrival to Admit. (minutes)[2]	547	226	214	274
Time from ER Arrival to Discharge (minutes)	396	160	118	134
Time in ER Before Being Evaluated (minutes)	465	36	26	26
Time to Pain Meds for Fractures (minutes)	168	85	66	57
Heart Attack Care				
Aspirin Given at Discharge[2]	252	100%	99%	99%
Fibrinolytic Meds Within 30 Min. of Arrival[2,7]	-	-	77%	54%
PCI Within 90 Minutes of Arrival[2]	41	98%	96%	96%
Statin Prescribed at Discharge[2]	241	100%	97%	98%
Heart Failure Care				
ACE Inhibitor or ARB for LVSD[2]	110	100%	96%	97%
Discharge Instructions Given[2]	238	100%	95%	94%
Evaluation of LVS Function[2]	298	100%	98%	99%
Medicare Spending				
Medicare Spending per Patient (ratio)	-	0.98	0.98	0.98
Pneumonia Care				
Appropriate Initial Antibiotic Given[2]	88	99%	94%	95%
Blood Culture Timing[2]	163	98%	98%	98%
Pregnancy and Delivery Care				
Newborn Deliveries Scheduled Early[2]	41	10%	6%	6%
Preventive Care				
Immunization for Influenza[2]	531	76%	89%	90%
Immunization for Pneumonia[2]	680	81%	92%	92%
Stroke Care				
Anticoagulation Therapy for Atrial Fibrillation[2]	15	100%	90%	95%
Antithrombotic Therapy Timing[2]	76	100%	96%	98%
Assessed for Rehabilitation[2]	97	96%	95%	97%
Discharged on Antithrombotic Therapy[2]	89	99%	96%	99%
Discharged on Statin Medication[2]	70	96%	86%	94%
Thrombolytic Therapy Timing[1,2]	-	-	35%	66%
Venous Thromboembolism Prophylaxis[2]	87	77%	91%	94%
Written Stroke Educational Materials Given[2]	50	84%	81%	88%
Surgical Care Improvement Project				
Appropriate Beta Blocker Usage[2]	177	99%	98%	98%
Appropriate VTP Within 24 Hours[2]	381	100%	98%	98%
Controlled Postoperative Blood Glucose[2]	102	97%	99%	97%
Perioperative Temperature Management[2]	449	100%	100%	100%
Prophylactic Antibiotic Selection[2]	397	100%	99%	99%
Prophylactic Antibiotic Selection (Outpatient)	547	99%	98%	98%
Prophylactic Antibiotic Stopped[2]	393	99%	98%	98%
Prophylactic Antibiotic Timing[2]	397	98%	99%	99%
Prophylactic Antibiotic Timing (Outpatient)	547	100%	98%	98%
Urinary Catheter Removal[2]	179	100%	97%	97%
Survey of Patients' Hospital Experiences				
Area Around Room 'Always' Quiet at Night	300+	62%	67%	61%
Doctors 'Always' Communicated Well	300+	81%	83%	82%
Home Recovery Information Given	300+	84%	83%	85%
Hospital Given 9 or 10 on 10 Point Scale	300+	75%	70%	71%
Meds 'Always' Explained Before Given	300+	62%	63%	64%
Nurses 'Always' Communicated Well	300+	79%	79%	79%
Pain 'Always' Well Controlled	300+	71%	71%	71%
Room and Bathroom 'Always' Clean	300+	75%	72%	73%
Timely Help 'Always' Received	300+	67%	68%	68%
Would Definitely Recommend Hospital	300+	77%	69%	71%
Use of Medical Imaging				
Cardiac Imaging Stress Test before Surgery	571	4.9%	4.3%	5.3%
Combination Abdominal CT Scan	1,401	3.4%	15.3%	10.5%
Combination Brain/Sinus CT Scan	1,044	2.6%	2.9%	2.7%
Combination Chest CT Scan	917	0.3%	5%	2.7%
Follow-up Mammogram/Ultrasound	2,021	9.0%	9.9%	8.8%
Lumbar Spine MRI for Low Back Pain	394	38.6%	41.6%	37.2%

South Mississippi County Regional Medical Center

611 West Lee Avenue Phone: 870-563-7000
Osceola, AR 72370 Fax: 615-327-0898
Type: Critical Access Hospitals Emergency Services: Yes
Ownership: Government - Local Beds: 25

Key Personnel:

CEO/President. . . . . Keith Broach
Intensive Care Unit. . . . . Renee Debald
Coronary Care . . . . Tammy Fleming
Quality Assurance . . . . Joanne Hardin
Chief of Medical Staff . . . . James Hudson, MD
Patient Relations . . . . Scott Husted
Operating Room. . . . . Jerrilyn Talley
Infection Control. . . . . Willa Warren

Measure	Cases	This Hosp.	State Avg.	U.S. Avg.
Blood Clot Prevention and Treatment				
Anticoagulation Overlap Therapy[5]	-	-	88%	93%
ICU Venous Thromboembolism Prophylaxis[5]	-	-	94%	92%
Incidence of Potentially Preventable VTE[5]	-	-	12%	10%
UFH with Dosages/Platelet Monitoring[5]	-	-	100%	97%
Venous Thromboembolism Prophylaxis[5]	-	-	91%	85%
Warfarin Therapy Discharge Instructions[5]	-	-	76%	75%
Chest Pain/Possible Heart Attack Care				
Aspirin Given Within 24 Hours of Arrival	-	-	96%	96%
Fibrinolytic Meds Within 30 Min. of Arrival	-	-	54%	58%
Average Time to ECG (minutes)	-	-	8	7
Average Time to Transfer (minutes)	-	-	72	60
Children's Asthma Care				
Received Home Management Plan of Care	-	-	-	88%
Received Reliever Medication	-	-	-	100%
Received Systemic Corticosteroids	-	-	-	100%
Emergency Department				
Admittance Decision Time (minutes)[5]	-	-	65	98
Head CT Results Within 45 Min. of Arrival	-	-	49%	57%
Patients Who Left ER Before Being Seen	-	-	3%	2%
Time from ER Arrival to Admit. (minutes)[5]	-	-	214	274
Time from ER Arrival to Discharge (minutes)	-	-	118	134
Time in ER Before Being Evaluated (minutes)	-	-	26	26
Time to Pain Meds for Fractures (minutes)	-	-	66	57
Heart Attack Care				
Aspirin Given at Discharge[1,3]	-	-	99%	99%
Fibrinolytic Meds Within 30 Min. of Arrival[3,7]	-	-	77%	54%
PCI Within 90 Minutes of Arrival[3,7]	-	-	96%	96%
Statin Prescribed at Discharge[1,3]	-	-	97%	98%
Heart Failure Care				
ACE Inhibitor or ARB for LVSD	13	77%	96%	97%
Discharge Instructions Given	30	90%	95%	94%
Evaluation of LVS Function	39	95%	98%	99%
Medicare Spending				

NOTE: Hospital profiles are in alphabetical order by state, then city, then hospital within the city; Rankings exclude hospitals with less than 25 cases except for patient surveys which excludes hospitals with less than 100 cases; (a) 100-299 cases; (1) The number of cases/patients is too few to report; (2) Data submitted were based on a sample of cases/patients; (3) Results are based on a shorter time period than required; (4) Data suppressed by CMS for one or more quarters; (5) Results are not available for this reporting period; (6) Fewer than 100 patients completed the HCAHPS survey; (7) No cases met the criteria for this measure; (8) The lower limit of the confidence interval cannot be calculated if the number of observed infections equals zero; (9) No data are available from the state/territory for this reporting period; (10) The scores shown reflect fewer than 50 completed surveys; (11) There were discrepancies in the data collection process; (12) This measure does not apply to this hospital for this reporting period; (13) Results cannot be calculated for this reporting period; (14) The results for this state are combined with nearby states to protect confidentiality; Please refer to the User's Guide for a full explanation of data.

Measure	Cases	This Hosp.	State Avg.	U.S. Avg.
Medicare Spending per Patient (ratio)	-	-	0.98	0.98
Pneumonia Care				
Appropriate Initial Antibiotic Given	22	95%	94%	95%
Blood Culture Timing	26	96%	98%	98%
Pregnancy and Delivery Care				
Newborn Deliveries Scheduled Early[3,7]	-	-	6%	6%
Preventive Care				
Immunization for Influenza[5]	-	-	89%	90%
Immunization for Pneumonia[5]	-	-	92%	92%
Stroke Care				
Anticoagulation Therapy for Atrial Fibrillation[5]	-	-	90%	95%
Antithrombotic Therapy Timing[5]	-	-	96%	98%
Assessed for Rehabilitation[5]	-	-	95%	97%
Discharged on Antithrombotic Therapy[5]	-	-	96%	99%
Discharged on Statin Medication[5]	-	-	86%	94%
Thrombolytic Therapy Timing[5]	-	-	35%	66%
Venous Thromboembolism Prophylaxis[5]	-	-	91%	94%
Written Stroke Educational Materials Given[5]	-	-	81%	88%
Surgical Care Improvement Project				
Appropriate Beta Blocker Usage[5]	-	-	98%	98%
Appropriate VTP Within 24 Hours[5]	-	-	98%	98%
Controlled Postoperative Blood Glucose[5]	-	-	99%	97%
Perioperative Temperature Management[5]	-	-	100%	100%
Prophylactic Antibiotic Selection[5]	-	-	99%	99%
Prophylactic Antibiotic Selection (Outpatient)	-	-	98%	98%
Prophylactic Antibiotic Stopped[5]	-	-	98%	98%
Prophylactic Antibiotic Timing[5]	-	-	99%	99%
Prophylactic Antibiotic Timing (Outpatient)	-	-	98%	98%
Urinary Catheter Removal[5]	-	-	97%	97%
Survey of Patients' Hospital Experiences				
Area Around Room 'Always' Quiet at Night[5]	-	-	67%	61%
Doctors 'Always' Communicated Well[5]	-	-	83%	82%
Home Recovery Information Given[5]	-	-	83%	85%
Hospital Given 9 or 10 on 10 Point Scale[5]	-	-	70%	71%
Meds 'Always' Explained Before Given[5]	-	-	63%	64%
Nurses 'Always' Communicated Well[5]	-	-	79%	79%
Pain 'Always' Well Controlled[5]	-	-	71%	71%
Room and Bathroom 'Always' Clean[5]	-	-	72%	73%
Timely Help 'Always' Received[5]	-	-	68%	68%
Would Definitely Recommend Hospital[5]	-	-	69%	71%
Use of Medical Imaging				
Cardiac Imaging Stress Test before Surgery	-	-	4.3%	5.3%
Combination Abdominal CT Scan	-	-	15.3%	10.5%
Combination Brain/Sinus CT Scan	-	-	2.9%	2.7%
Combination Chest CT Scan	-	-	5%	2.7%
Follow-up Mammogram/Ultrasound	-	-	9.9%	8.8%
Lumbar Spine MRI for Low Back Pain	-	-	41.6%	37.2%

Mercy Hospital Turner Memorial

801 West River Street
Ozark, AR 72949
Phone: 479-667-4138
Fax: 479-667-4751
Type: Critical Access Hospitals
Emergency Services: Yes
Ownership: Government - Local
Beds: 39

Key Personnel:
Chief of Medical Staff . . . . Garth Carrick, MD
Quality Assurance . . . . Randall Dickerson
Operating Room. . . . . Mary Foster, RN
CEO/President. . . . . Jim Maddox

Measure	Cases	This Hosp.	State Avg.	U.S. Avg.
Blood Clot Prevention and Treatment				
Anticoagulation Overlap Therapy[5]	-	-	88%	93%
ICU Venous Thromboembolism Prophylaxis[5]	-	-	94%	92%
Incidence of Potentially Preventable VTE[5]	-	-	12%	10%
UFH with Dosages/Platelet Monitoring[5]	-	-	100%	97%
Venous Thromboembolism Prophylaxis[5]	-	-	91%	85%
Warfarin Therapy Discharge Instructions[5]	-	-	76%	75%
Chest Pain/Possible Heart Attack Care				
Aspirin Given Within 24 Hours of Arrival	-	-	96%	96%
Fibrinolytic Meds Within 30 Min. of Arrival	-	-	54%	58%
Average Time to ECG (minutes)	-	-	8	7
Average Time to Transfer (minutes)	-	-	72	60
Children's Asthma Care				
Received Home Management Plan of Care	-	-	-	88%
Received Reliever Medication	-	-	-	100%
Received Systemic Corticosteroids	-	-	-	100%
Emergency Department				
Admittance Decision Time (minutes)[5]	-	-	65	98
Head CT Results Within 45 Min. of Arrival	-	-	49%	57%
Patients Who Left ER Before Being Seen	-	-	3%	2%
Time from ER Arrival to Admit. (minutes)[5]	-	-	214	274
Time from ER Arrival to Discharge (minutes)	-	-	118	134
Time in ER Before Being Evaluated (minutes)	-	-	26	26
Time to Pain Meds for Fractures (minutes)	-	-	66	57
Heart Attack Care				
Aspirin Given at Discharge[5]	-	-	99%	99%
Fibrinolytic Meds Within 30 Min. of Arrival[5]	-	-	77%	54%
PCI Within 90 Minutes of Arrival[5]	-	-	96%	96%
Statin Prescribed at Discharge[5]	-	-	97%	98%
Heart Failure Care				
ACE Inhibitor or ARB for LVSD[1]	-	-	96%	97%
Discharge Instructions Given	21	90%	95%	94%
Evaluation of LVS Function	18	67%	98%	99%
Medicare Spending				
Medicare Spending per Patient (ratio)	-	-	0.98	0.98
Pneumonia Care				
Appropriate Initial Antibiotic Given[1]	-	-	94%	95%
Blood Culture Timing	17	100%	98%	98%
Pregnancy and Delivery Care				
Newborn Deliveries Scheduled Early[3,7]	-	-	6%	6%
Preventive Care				
Immunization for Influenza[5]	-	-	89%	90%
Immunization for Pneumonia[5]	-	-	92%	92%
Stroke Care				
Anticoagulation Therapy for Atrial Fibrillation[5]	-	-	90%	95%
Antithrombotic Therapy Timing[5]	-	-	96%	98%
Assessed for Rehabilitation[5]	-	-	95%	97%
Discharged on Antithrombotic Therapy[5]	-	-	96%	99%
Discharged on Statin Medication[5]	-	-	86%	94%
Thrombolytic Therapy Timing[5]	-	-	35%	66%
Venous Thromboembolism Prophylaxis[5]	-	-	91%	94%
Written Stroke Educational Materials Given[5]	-	-	81%	88%
Surgical Care Improvement Project				
Appropriate Beta Blocker Usage[3,7]	-	-	98%	98%
Appropriate VTP Within 24 Hours[1,3]	-	-	98%	98%
Controlled Postoperative Blood Glucose[3,7]	-	-	99%	97%
Perioperative Temperature Management[1,3]	-	-	100%	100%
Prophylactic Antibiotic Selection[3,7]	-	-	99%	99%
Prophylactic Antibiotic Selection (Outpatient)	-	-	98%	98%
Prophylactic Antibiotic Stopped[3,7]	-	-	98%	98%
Prophylactic Antibiotic Timing[3,7]	-	-	99%	99%
Prophylactic Antibiotic Timing (Outpatient)	-	-	98%	98%
Urinary Catheter Removal[3,7]	-	-	97%	97%
Survey of Patients' Hospital Experiences				
Area Around Room 'Always' Quiet at Night[5]	-	-	67%	61%
Doctors 'Always' Communicated Well[5]	-	-	83%	82%
Home Recovery Information Given[5]	-	-	83%	85%
Hospital Given 9 or 10 on 10 Point Scale[5]	-	-	70%	71%
Meds 'Always' Explained Before Given[5]	-	-	63%	64%
Nurses 'Always' Communicated Well[5]	-	-	79%	79%
Pain 'Always' Well Controlled[5]	-	-	71%	71%
Room and Bathroom 'Always' Clean[5]	-	-	72%	73%
Timely Help 'Always' Received[5]	-	-	68%	68%
Would Definitely Recommend Hospital[5]	-	-	69%	71%
Use of Medical Imaging				
Cardiac Imaging Stress Test before Surgery	-	-	4.3%	5.3%
Combination Abdominal CT Scan	-	-	15.3%	10.5%
Combination Brain/Sinus CT Scan	-	-	2.9%	2.7%
Combination Chest CT Scan	-	-	5%	2.7%
Follow-up Mammogram/Ultrasound	-	-	9.9%	8.8%
Lumbar Spine MRI for Low Back Pain	-	-	41.6%	37.2%

Arkansas Methodist Medical Center

900 West Kingshighway
Paragould, AR 72450
Phone: 870-239-7000
Fax: 870-239-7400
URL: www.arkansasmethodist.org
Type: Acute Care Hospitals
Emergency Services: Yes
Ownership: Voluntary non-profit - Private
Beds: 129

Key Personnel:
Radiology. . . . . John Collier, MD
CEO/President. . . . . Barry Davis, FACHE
Chairman/CEO . . . . Rhonda Davis
Emergency Room . . . . Christi Foust, RN
Operating Room. . . . . Adel Hassan, RN
Chief of Medical Staff. . . . . Norman Smith
Quality Assurance . . . . Lana Williams

Measure	Cases	This Hosp.	State Avg.	U.S. Avg.
Blood Clot Prevention and Treatment				
Anticoagulation Overlap Therapy[2]	16	100%	88%	93%
ICU Venous Thromboembolism Prophylaxis[2]	192	99%	94%	92%
Incidence of Potentially Preventable VTE[1,2]	-	-	12%	10%
UFH with Dosages/Platelet Monitoring[2]	14	100%	100%	97%
Venous Thromboembolism Prophylaxis[2]	559	90%	91%	85%
Warfarin Therapy Discharge Instructions[1,2]	-	-	76%	75%
Chest Pain/Possible Heart Attack Care				
Aspirin Given Within 24 Hours of Arrival	66	100%	96%	96%
Fibrinolytic Meds Within 30 Min. of Arrival[7]	-	-	54%	58%
Average Time to ECG (minutes)	68	4	8	7
Average Time to Transfer (minutes)[1]	-	-	72	60
Children's Asthma Care				
Received Home Management Plan of Care	-	-	-	88%
Received Reliever Medication	-	-	-	100%
Received Systemic Corticosteroids	-	-	-	100%
Emergency Department				
Admittance Decision Time (minutes)[2]	663	55	65	98
Head CT Results Within 45 Min. of Arrival[1]	-	-	49%	57%
Patients Who Left ER Before Being Seen	25,777	2%	3%	2%
Time from ER Arrival to Admit. (minutes)[2]	665	187	214	274
Time from ER Arrival to Discharge (minutes)	854	104	118	134
Time in ER Before Being Evaluated (minutes)	954	22	26	26
Time to Pain Meds for Fractures (minutes)	71	57	66	57
Heart Attack Care				
Aspirin Given at Discharge	40	100%	99%	99%
Fibrinolytic Meds Within 30 Min. of Arrival[7]	-	-	77%	54%
PCI Within 90 Minutes of Arrival[1]	-	-	96%	96%
Statin Prescribed at Discharge	37	97%	97%	98%
Heart Failure Care				
ACE Inhibitor or ARB for LVSD	31	100%	96%	97%
Discharge Instructions Given	93	95%	95%	94%
Evaluation of LVS Function	132	100%	98%	99%
Medicare Spending				
Medicare Spending per Patient (ratio)	-	1.04	0.98	0.98
Pneumonia Care				
Appropriate Initial Antibiotic Given[2]	150	99%	94%	95%
Blood Culture Timing[2]	201	100%	98%	98%
Pregnancy and Delivery Care				
Newborn Deliveries Scheduled Early	54	19%	6%	6%
Preventive Care				
Immunization for Influenza[2]	566	95%	89%	90%
Immunization for Pneumonia[2]	704	95%	92%	92%
Stroke Care				
Anticoagulation Therapy for Atrial Fibrillation[1]	-	-	90%	95%
Antithrombotic Therapy Timing	39	97%	96%	98%
Assessed for Rehabilitation	38	100%	95%	97%
Discharged on Antithrombotic Therapy	33	100%	96%	99%
Discharged on Statin Medication	23	96%	86%	94%
Thrombolytic Therapy Timing[7]	-	-	35%	66%
Venous Thromboembolism Prophylaxis	42	100%	91%	94%
Written Stroke Educational Materials Given	12	75%	81%	88%
Surgical Care Improvement Project				
Appropriate Beta Blocker Usage	31	97%	98%	98%
Appropriate VTP Within 24 Hours	101	100%	98%	98%
Controlled Postoperative Blood Glucose[7]	-	-	99%	97%
Perioperative Temperature Management	155	100%	100%	100%
Prophylactic Antibiotic Selection	70	97%	99%	99%
Prophylactic Antibiotic Selection (Outpatient)	75	97%	98%	98%

NOTE: Hospital profiles are in alphabetical order by state, then city, then hospital within the city; Rankings exclude hospitals with less than 25 cases except for patient surveys which excludes hospitals with less than 100 cases; (a) 100-299 cases; (1) The number of cases/patients is too few to report; (2) Data submitted were based on a sample of cases/patients; (3) Results are based on a shorter time period than required; (4) Data suppressed by CMS for one or more quarters; (5) Results are not available for this reporting period; (6) Fewer than 100 patients completed the HCAHPS survey; (7) No cases met the criteria for this measure; (8) The lower limit of the confidence interval cannot be calculated if the number of observed infections equals zero; (9) No data are available from the state/territory for this reporting period; (10) The scores shown reflect fewer than 50 completed surveys; (11) There were discrepancies in the data collection process; (12) This measure does not apply to this hospital for this reporting period; (13) Results cannot be calculated for this reporting period; (14) The results for this state are combined with nearby states to protect confidentiality; Please refer to the User's Guide for a full explanation of data.

Measure	Cases	This Hosp.	State Avg.	U.S. Avg.
Prophylactic Antibiotic Stopped	67	100%	98%	98%
Prophylactic Antibiotic Timing	70	100%	99%	99%
Prophylactic Antibiotic Timing (Outpatient)	76	96%	98%	98%
Urinary Catheter Removal	53	100%	97%	97%
Survey of Patients' Hospital Experiences				
Area Around Room 'Always' Quiet at Night	300+	68%	67%	61%
Doctors 'Always' Communicated Well	300+	83%	83%	82%
Home Recovery Information Given	300+	80%	83%	85%
Hospital Given 9 or 10 on 10 Point Scale	300+	67%	70%	71%
Meds 'Always' Explained Before Given	300+	64%	63%	64%
Nurses 'Always' Communicated Well	300+	80%	79%	79%
Pain 'Always' Well Controlled	300+	72%	71%	71%
Room and Bathroom 'Always' Clean	300+	75%	72%	73%
Timely Help 'Always' Received	300+	68%	68%	68%
Would Definitely Recommend Hospital	300+	64%	69%	71%
Use of Medical Imaging				
Cardiac Imaging Stress Test before Surgery	67	11.9%	4.3%	5.3%
Combination Abdominal CT Scan	399	32.6%	15.3%	10.5%
Combination Brain/Sinus CT Scan[1]	-	-	2.9%	2.7%
Combination Chest CT Scan	262	0.0%	5%	2.7%
Follow-up Mammogram/Ultrasound	598	5.0%	9.9%	8.8%
Lumbar Spine MRI for Low Back Pain	87	41.4%	41.6%	37.2%

North Logan Mercy Hospital

500 East Academy
Paris, AR 72855
Phone: 479-963-6101
Fax: 501-963-6155
Type: Critical Access Hospitals
Emergency Services: Yes
Ownership: Voluntary non-profit - Private
Beds: 16

Key Personnel:
Chief of Medical Staff. . . . . WP Enns, MD
Operating Room. . . . . Peggy Kleiss, RN
CEO/President. . . . . Michael Morgan

Measure	Cases	This Hosp.	State Avg.	U.S. Avg.
Blood Clot Prevention and Treatment				
Anticoagulation Overlap Therapy[5]	-	-	88%	93%
ICU Venous Thromboembolism Prophylaxis[5]	-	-	94%	92%
Incidence of Potentially Preventable VTE[5]	-	-	12%	10%
UFH with Dosages/Platelet Monitoring[5]	-	-	100%	97%
Venous Thromboembolism Prophylaxis[5]	-	-	91%	85%
Warfarin Therapy Discharge Instructions[5]	-	-	76%	75%
Chest Pain/Possible Heart Attack Care				
Aspirin Given Within 24 Hours of Arrival	-	-	96%	96%
Fibrinolytic Meds Within 30 Min. of Arrival	-	-	54%	58%
Average Time to ECG (minutes)	-	-	8	7
Average Time to Transfer (minutes)	-	-	72	60
Children's Asthma Care				
Received Home Management Plan of Care	-	-	-	88%
Received Reliever Medication	-	-	-	100%
Received Systemic Corticosteroids	-	-	-	100%
Emergency Department				
Admittance Decision Time (minutes)[5]	-	-	65	98
Head CT Results Within 45 Min. of Arrival	-	-	49%	57%
Patients Who Left ER Before Being Seen	-	-	3%	2%
Time from ER Arrival to Admit. (minutes)[5]	-	-	214	274
Time from ER Arrival to Discharge (minutes)	-	-	118	134
Time in ER Before Being Evaluated (minutes)	-	-	26	26
Time to Pain Meds for Fractures (minutes)	-	-	66	57
Heart Attack Care				
Aspirin Given at Discharge[3,7]	-	-	99%	99%
Fibrinolytic Meds Within 30 Min. of Arrival[3,7]	-	-	77%	54%
PCI Within 90 Minutes of Arrival[3,7]	-	-	96%	96%
Statin Prescribed at Discharge[3,7]	-	-	97%	98%
Heart Failure Care				
ACE Inhibitor or ARB for LVSD[1,3]	-	-	96%	97%
Discharge Instructions Given[1,3]	-	-	95%	94%
Evaluation of LVS Function[1,3]	-	-	98%	99%
Medicare Spending				
Medicare Spending per Patient (ratio)	-	-	0.98	0.98
Pneumonia Care				
Appropriate Initial Antibiotic Given[1]	-	-	94%	95%
Blood Culture Timing[1]	-	-	98%	98%
Pregnancy and Delivery Care				
Newborn Deliveries Scheduled Early[3,7]	-	-	6%	6%
Preventive Care				
Immunization for Influenza[5]	-	-	89%	90%
Immunization for Pneumonia[5]	-	-	92%	92%
Stroke Care				
Anticoagulation Therapy for Atrial Fibrillation[5]	-	-	90%	95%
Antithrombotic Therapy Timing[5]	-	-	96%	98%
Assessed for Rehabilitation[5]	-	-	95%	97%
Discharged on Antithrombotic Therapy[5]	-	-	96%	99%
Discharged on Statin Medication[5]	-	-	86%	94%
Thrombolytic Therapy Timing[5]	-	-	35%	66%
Venous Thromboembolism Prophylaxis[5]	-	-	91%	94%
Written Stroke Educational Materials Given[5]	-	-	81%	88%
Surgical Care Improvement Project				
Appropriate Beta Blocker Usage[5]	-	-	98%	98%
Appropriate VTP Within 24 Hours[5]	-	-	98%	98%
Controlled Postoperative Blood Glucose[5]	-	-	99%	97%
Perioperative Temperature Management[5]	-	-	100%	100%
Prophylactic Antibiotic Selection[5]	-	-	99%	99%
Prophylactic Antibiotic Selection (Outpatient)	-	-	98%	98%
Prophylactic Antibiotic Stopped[5]	-	-	98%	98%
Prophylactic Antibiotic Timing[5]	-	-	99%	99%
Prophylactic Antibiotic Timing (Outpatient)	-	-	98%	98%
Urinary Catheter Removal[5]	-	-	97%	97%
Survey of Patients' Hospital Experiences				
Area Around Room 'Always' Quiet at Night[5]	-	-	67%	61%
Doctors 'Always' Communicated Well[5]	-	-	83%	82%
Home Recovery Information Given[5]	-	-	83%	85%
Hospital Given 9 or 10 on 10 Point Scale[5]	-	-	70%	71%
Meds 'Always' Explained Before Given[5]	-	-	63%	64%
Nurses 'Always' Communicated Well[5]	-	-	79%	79%
Pain 'Always' Well Controlled[5]	-	-	71%	71%
Room and Bathroom 'Always' Clean[5]	-	-	72%	73%
Timely Help 'Always' Received[5]	-	-	68%	68%
Would Definitely Recommend Hospital[5]	-	-	69%	71%
Use of Medical Imaging				
Cardiac Imaging Stress Test before Surgery	-	-	4.3%	5.3%
Combination Abdominal CT Scan	-	-	15.3%	10.5%
Combination Brain/Sinus CT Scan	-	-	2.9%	2.7%
Combination Chest CT Scan	-	-	5%	2.7%
Follow-up Mammogram/Ultrasound	-	-	9.9%	8.8%
Lumbar Spine MRI for Low Back Pain	-	-	41.6%	37.2%

Piggott Community Hospital

1206 Gordon Duckworth Drive
Piggott, AR 72454
Phone: 870-598-3881
Fax: 870-598-2437
E-mail: info@piggottcommunityhospital.com
URL: www.piggottcommunityhospital.com
Type: Critical Access Hospitals
Emergency Services: Yes
Ownership: Government - Local
Beds: 35

Key Personnel:
Radiology. . . . . Suzie Countzler Daffron, RT
Emergency Room . . . . Tammye Hendrix, RN
Infection Control. . . . . Judy Nettles, RN
Chief of Medical Staff. . . . . David Owens

Measure	Cases	This Hosp.	State Avg.	U.S. Avg.
Blood Clot Prevention and Treatment				
Anticoagulation Overlap Therapy[5]	-	-	88%	93%
ICU Venous Thromboembolism Prophylaxis[5]	-	-	94%	92%
Incidence of Potentially Preventable VTE[5]	-	-	12%	10%
UFH with Dosages/Platelet Monitoring[5]	-	-	100%	97%
Venous Thromboembolism Prophylaxis[5]	-	-	91%	85%
Warfarin Therapy Discharge Instructions[5]	-	-	76%	75%
Chest Pain/Possible Heart Attack Care				
Aspirin Given Within 24 Hours of Arrival	-	-	96%	96%
Fibrinolytic Meds Within 30 Min. of Arrival	-	-	54%	58%
Average Time to ECG (minutes)	-	-	8	7
Average Time to Transfer (minutes)	-	-	72	60
Children's Asthma Care				
Received Home Management Plan of Care	-	-	-	88%
Received Reliever Medication	-	-	-	100%
Received Systemic Corticosteroids	-	-	-	100%
Emergency Department				
Admittance Decision Time (minutes)[5]	-	-	65	98
Head CT Results Within 45 Min. of Arrival	-	-	49%	57%
Patients Who Left ER Before Being Seen	-	-	3%	2%
Time from ER Arrival to Admit. (minutes)[5]	-	-	214	274
Time from ER Arrival to Discharge (minutes)	-	-	118	134
Time in ER Before Being Evaluated (minutes)	-	-	26	26
Time to Pain Meds for Fractures (minutes)	-	-	66	57
Heart Attack Care				
Aspirin Given at Discharge[3,7]	-	-	99%	99%
Fibrinolytic Meds Within 30 Min. of Arrival[3,7]	-	-	77%	54%
PCI Within 90 Minutes of Arrival[3,7]	-	-	96%	96%
Statin Prescribed at Discharge[3,7]	-	-	97%	98%
Heart Failure Care				
ACE Inhibitor or ARB for LVSD[1]	-	-	96%	97%
Discharge Instructions Given	18	100%	95%	94%
Evaluation of LVS Function	28	100%	98%	99%
Medicare Spending				
Medicare Spending per Patient (ratio)	-	-	0.98	0.98
Pneumonia Care				
Appropriate Initial Antibiotic Given	40	100%	94%	95%
Blood Culture Timing	51	100%	98%	98%
Pregnancy and Delivery Care				
Newborn Deliveries Scheduled Early[5]	-	-	6%	6%
Preventive Care				
Immunization for Influenza[5]	-	-	89%	90%
Immunization for Pneumonia[5]	-	-	92%	92%
Stroke Care				
Anticoagulation Therapy for Atrial Fibrillation[5]	-	-	90%	95%
Antithrombotic Therapy Timing[5]	-	-	96%	98%
Assessed for Rehabilitation[5]	-	-	95%	97%
Discharged on Antithrombotic Therapy[5]	-	-	96%	99%
Discharged on Statin Medication[5]	-	-	86%	94%
Thrombolytic Therapy Timing[5]	-	-	35%	66%
Venous Thromboembolism Prophylaxis[5]	-	-	91%	94%
Written Stroke Educational Materials Given[5]	-	-	81%	88%
Surgical Care Improvement Project				
Appropriate Beta Blocker Usage[5]	-	-	98%	98%
Appropriate VTP Within 24 Hours[5]	-	-	98%	98%
Controlled Postoperative Blood Glucose[5]	-	-	99%	97%
Perioperative Temperature Management[5]	-	-	100%	100%
Prophylactic Antibiotic Selection[5]	-	-	99%	99%
Prophylactic Antibiotic Selection (Outpatient)	-	-	98%	98%
Prophylactic Antibiotic Stopped[5]	-	-	98%	98%
Prophylactic Antibiotic Timing[5]	-	-	99%	99%
Prophylactic Antibiotic Timing (Outpatient)	-	-	98%	98%
Urinary Catheter Removal[5]	-	-	97%	97%
Survey of Patients' Hospital Experiences				
Area Around Room 'Always' Quiet at Night[5]	-	-	67%	61%
Doctors 'Always' Communicated Well[5]	-	-	83%	82%
Home Recovery Information Given[5]	-	-	83%	85%
Hospital Given 9 or 10 on 10 Point Scale[5]	-	-	70%	71%
Meds 'Always' Explained Before Given[5]	-	-	63%	64%
Nurses 'Always' Communicated Well[5]	-	-	79%	79%
Pain 'Always' Well Controlled[5]	-	-	71%	71%
Room and Bathroom 'Always' Clean[5]	-	-	72%	73%
Timely Help 'Always' Received[5]	-	-	68%	68%
Would Definitely Recommend Hospital[5]	-	-	69%	71%
Use of Medical Imaging				
Cardiac Imaging Stress Test before Surgery	-	-	4.3%	5.3%
Combination Abdominal CT Scan	-	-	15.3%	10.5%
Combination Brain/Sinus CT Scan	-	-	2.9%	2.7%
Combination Chest CT Scan	-	-	5%	2.7%
Follow-up Mammogram/Ultrasound	-	-	9.9%	8.8%
Lumbar Spine MRI for Low Back Pain	-	-	41.6%	37.2%

Jefferson Regional Medical Center

1600 West 40th Avenue
Pine Bluff, AR 71603
Phone: 870-541-7100
Fax: 870-541-7204
URL: www.jrmc.org
Type: Acute Care Hospitals
Emergency Services: Yes
Ownership: Voluntary non-profit - Private
Beds: 471

Key Personnel:
Pediatric Ambulatory Care . . . . . . Lloyene Bruce-Roid, MD
Pediatric In-Patient Care . . . . Lloyene Bruce-Roid, MD
CEO/President. . . . . Walter Johnson

NOTE: Hospital profiles are in alphabetical order by state, then city, then hospital within the city; Rankings exclude hospitals with less than 25 cases except for patient surveys which excludes hospitals with less than 100 cases; (a) 100-299 cases; (1) The number of cases/patients is too few to report; (2) Data submitted were based on a sample of cases/patients; (3) Results are based on a shorter time period than required; (4) Data suppressed by CMS for one or more quarters; (5) Results are not available for this reporting period; (6) Fewer than 100 patients completed the HCAHPS survey; (7) No cases met the criteria for this measure; (8) The lower limit of the confidence interval cannot be calculated if the number of observed infections equals zero; (9) No data are available from the state/territory for this reporting period; (10) The scores shown reflect fewer than 50 completed surveys; (11) There were discrepancies in the data collection process; (12) This measure does not apply to this hospital for this reporting period; (13) Results cannot be calculated for this reporting period; (14) The results for this state are combined with nearby states to protect confidentiality; Please refer to the User's Guide for a full explanation of data.

Radiology . . . . Joyce Linzy
Chief of Medical Staff . . . . Reid Pierce, MD
Infection Control . . . . Michaelle Roberts
Quality Assurance . . . . Connie Rodgers
Operating Room . . . . Ruth Rogers

Measure	Cases	This Hosp.	State Avg.	U.S. Avg.
Blood Clot Prevention and Treatment				
Anticoagulation Overlap Therapy[2]	42	100%	88%	93%
ICU Venous Thromboembolism Prophylaxis[2]	308	99%	94%	92%
Incidence of Potentially Preventable VTE[2]	17	18%	12%	10%
UFH with Dosages/Platelet Monitoring[2]	34	100%	100%	97%
Venous Thromboembolism Prophylaxis[2]	401	97%	91%	85%
Warfarin Therapy Discharge Instructions[2]	30	97%	76%	75%
Chest Pain/Possible Heart Attack Care				
Aspirin Given Within 24 Hours of Arrival[1]	-	-	96%	96%
Fibrinolytic Meds Within 30 Min. of Arrival[3,7]	-	-	54%	58%
Average Time to ECG (minutes)[1]	-	-	8	7
Average Time to Transfer (minutes)[3,7]	-	-	72	60
Children's Asthma Care				
Received Home Management Plan of Care	-	-	-	88%
Received Reliever Medication	-	-	-	100%
Received Systemic Corticosteroids	-	-	-	100%
Emergency Department				
Admittance Decision Time (minutes)[2]	333	52	65	98
Head CT Results Within 45 Min. of Arrival	12	67%	49%	57%
Patients Who Left ER Before Being Seen	51,896	2%	3%	2%
Time from ER Arrival to Admit. (minutes)[2]	562	220	214	274
Time from ER Arrival to Discharge (minutes)	215	141	118	134
Time in ER Before Being Evaluated (minutes)	353	59	26	26
Time to Pain Meds for Fractures (minutes)	146	96	66	57
Heart Attack Care				
Aspirin Given at Discharge	150	99%	99%	99%
Fibrinolytic Meds Within 30 Min. of Arrival[1]	-	-	77%	54%
PCI Within 90 Minutes of Arrival	25	96%	96%	96%
Statin Prescribed at Discharge	145	97%	97%	98%
Heart Failure Care				
ACE Inhibitor or ARB for LVSD	81	98%	96%	97%
Discharge Instructions Given	139	96%	95%	94%
Evaluation of LVS Function	168	100%	98%	99%
Medicare Spending				
Medicare Spending per Patient (ratio)	-	1.02	0.98	0.98
Pneumonia Care				
Appropriate Initial Antibiotic Given	150	93%	94%	95%
Blood Culture Timing	245	100%	98%	98%
Pregnancy and Delivery Care				
Newborn Deliveries Scheduled Early	159	0%	6%	6%
Preventive Care				
Immunization for Influenza[2]	880	95%	89%	90%
Immunization for Pneumonia[2]	1,268	97%	92%	92%
Stroke Care				
Anticoagulation Therapy for Atrial Fibrillation	15	80%	90%	95%
Antithrombotic Therapy Timing	137	97%	96%	98%
Assessed for Rehabilitation	144	99%	95%	97%
Discharged on Antithrombotic Therapy	126	94%	96%	99%
Discharged on Statin Medication	94	85%	86%	94%
Thrombolytic Therapy Timing[1]	-	-	35%	66%
Venous Thromboembolism Prophylaxis	136	99%	91%	94%
Written Stroke Educational Materials Given	70	97%	81%	88%
Surgical Care Improvement Project				
Appropriate Beta Blocker Usage	193	99%	98%	98%
Appropriate VTP Within 24 Hours	583	100%	98%	98%
Controlled Postoperative Blood Glucose	63	100%	99%	97%
Perioperative Temperature Management	681	100%	100%	100%
Prophylactic Antibiotic Selection	435	99%	99%	99%
Prophylactic Antibiotic Selection (Outpatient)	423	99%	98%	98%
Prophylactic Antibiotic Stopped	417	100%	98%	98%
Prophylactic Antibiotic Timing	440	100%	99%	99%
Prophylactic Antibiotic Timing (Outpatient)	423	100%	98%	98%
Urinary Catheter Removal	230	100%	97%	97%
Survey of Patients' Hospital Experiences				
Area Around Room 'Always' Quiet at Night	300+	65%	67%	61%
Doctors 'Always' Communicated Well	300+	82%	83%	82%
Home Recovery Information Given	300+	85%	83%	85%
Hospital Given 9 or 10 on 10 Point Scale	300+	65%	70%	71%
Meds 'Always' Explained Before Given	300+	61%	63%	64%
Nurses 'Always' Communicated Well	300+	75%	79%	79%
Pain 'Always' Well Controlled	300+	69%	71%	71%
Room and Bathroom 'Always' Clean	300+	62%	72%	73%
Timely Help 'Always' Received	300+	66%	68%	68%
Would Definitely Recommend Hospital	300+	58%	69%	71%
Use of Medical Imaging				
Cardiac Imaging Stress Test before Surgery	422	2.6%	4.3%	5.3%
Combination Abdominal CT Scan	659	24.4%	15.3%	10.5%
Combination Brain/Sinus CT Scan	965	1.1%	2.9%	2.7%
Combination Chest CT Scan	496	14.9%	5%	2.7%
Follow-up Mammogram/Ultrasound	1,408	8.5%	9.9%	8.8%
Lumbar Spine MRI for Low Back Pain	200	50.5%	41.6%	37.2%

Five Rivers Medical Center

2801 Medical Center Drive
Pocahontas, AR 72455
Type: Acute Care Hospitals
Ownership: Government - Local
Phone: 870-892-6000
Fax: 870-892-8100
Emergency Services: Yes
Beds: 50

Key Personnel:
Quality Assurance . . . . Jody Ayers, RN
Radiology . . . . Becky Brown
Infection Control . . . . Judy Downs, RN
Emergency Room . . . . Danna Guntharp, RN
Intensive Care Unit . . . . Linda Leach, RN
Hemotology Center . . . . Rose Throesch, RN
CEO/President . . . . John Tucker
Operating Room . . . . Sharrie Weissenbach, RN

Measure	Cases	This Hosp.	State Avg.	U.S. Avg.
Blood Clot Prevention and Treatment				
Anticoagulation Overlap Therapy[1,2]	-	-	88%	93%
ICU Venous Thromboembolism Prophylaxis[1,2]	-	-	94%	92%
Incidence of Potentially Preventable VTE[2,7]	-	-	12%	10%
UFH with Dosages/Platelet Monitoring[2,7]	-	-	100%	97%
Venous Thromboembolism Prophylaxis[2]	94	99%	91%	85%
Warfarin Therapy Discharge Instructions[1,2]	-	-	76%	75%
Chest Pain/Possible Heart Attack Care				
Aspirin Given Within 24 Hours of Arrival	38	100%	96%	96%
Fibrinolytic Meds Within 30 Min. of Arrival[7]	-	-	54%	58%
Average Time to ECG (minutes)	39	6	8	7
Average Time to Transfer (minutes)[1]	-	-	72	60
Children's Asthma Care				
Received Home Management Plan of Care	-	-	-	88%
Received Reliever Medication	-	-	-	100%
Received Systemic Corticosteroids	-	-	-	100%
Emergency Department				
Admittance Decision Time (minutes)[2]	357	44	65	98
Head CT Results Within 45 Min. of Arrival[1,3]	-	-	49%	57%
Patients Who Left ER Before Being Seen	3,597	1%	3%	2%
Time from ER Arrival to Admit. (minutes)[2]	378	168	214	274
Time from ER Arrival to Discharge (minutes)	309	102	118	134
Time in ER Before Being Evaluated (minutes)	384	22	26	26
Time to Pain Meds for Fractures (minutes)	59	52	66	57
Heart Attack Care				
Aspirin Given at Discharge[5]	-	-	99%	99%
Fibrinolytic Meds Within 30 Min. of Arrival[5]	-	-	77%	54%
PCI Within 90 Minutes of Arrival[5]	-	-	96%	96%
Statin Prescribed at Discharge[5]	-	-	97%	98%
Heart Failure Care				
ACE Inhibitor or ARB for LVSD[1]	-	-	96%	97%
Discharge Instructions Given	25	88%	95%	94%
Evaluation of LVS Function	37	97%	98%	99%
Medicare Spending				
Medicare Spending per Patient (ratio)	-	1.06	0.98	0.98
Pneumonia Care				
Appropriate Initial Antibiotic Given	47	91%	94%	95%
Blood Culture Timing	63	100%	98%	98%
Pregnancy and Delivery Care				
Newborn Deliveries Scheduled Early[7]	-	-	6%	6%
Preventive Care				
Immunization for Influenza[2]	286	97%	89%	90%
Immunization for Pneumonia[2]	431	98%	92%	92%
Stroke Care				
Anticoagulation Therapy for Atrial Fibrillation[1,3]	-	-	90%	95%
Antithrombotic Therapy Timing[1,3]	-	-	96%	98%
Assessed for Rehabilitation[3]	12	100%	95%	97%
Discharged on Antithrombotic Therapy[3]	11	100%	96%	99%
Discharged on Statin Medication[1,3]	-	-	86%	94%
Thrombolytic Therapy Timing[1,3]	-	-	35%	66%
Venous Thromboembolism Prophylaxis[1,3]	-	-	91%	94%
Written Stroke Educational Materials Given[1,3]	-	-	81%	88%
Surgical Care Improvement Project				
Appropriate Beta Blocker Usage[1,3]	-	-	98%	98%
Appropriate VTP Within 24 Hours[1,3]	-	-	98%	98%
Controlled Postoperative Blood Glucose[3,7]	-	-	99%	97%
Perioperative Temperature Management[1,3]	-	-	100%	100%
Prophylactic Antibiotic Selection[1,3]	-	-	99%	99%
Prophylactic Antibiotic Selection (Outpatient)[3,7]	-	-	98%	98%
Prophylactic Antibiotic Stopped[1,3]	-	-	98%	98%
Prophylactic Antibiotic Timing[1,3]	-	-	99%	99%
Prophylactic Antibiotic Timing (Outpatient)[3,7]	-	-	98%	98%
Urinary Catheter Removal[1,3]	-	-	97%	97%
Survey of Patients' Hospital Experiences				
Area Around Room 'Always' Quiet at Night	(a)	63%	67%	61%
Doctors 'Always' Communicated Well	(a)	83%	83%	82%
Home Recovery Information Given	(a)	85%	83%	85%
Hospital Given 9 or 10 on 10 Point Scale	(a)	62%	70%	71%
Meds 'Always' Explained Before Given	(a)	58%	63%	64%
Nurses 'Always' Communicated Well	(a)	75%	79%	79%
Pain 'Always' Well Controlled	(a)	74%	71%	71%
Room and Bathroom 'Always' Clean	(a)	74%	72%	73%
Timely Help 'Always' Received	(a)	68%	68%	68%
Would Definitely Recommend Hospital	(a)	58%	69%	71%
Use of Medical Imaging				
Cardiac Imaging Stress Test before Surgery[1]	-	-	4.3%	5.3%
Combination Abdominal CT Scan	159	17.6%	15.3%	10.5%
Combination Brain/Sinus CT Scan[1]	-	-	2.9%	2.7%
Combination Chest CT Scan	137	1.5%	5%	2.7%
Follow-up Mammogram/Ultrasound	175	3.4%	9.9%	8.8%
Lumbar Spine MRI for Low Back Pain[1]	-	-	41.6%	37.2%

Mercy Hospital Northwest Arkansas

2710 Rife Medical Lane
Rogers, AR 72758
URL: www.mercy4u.com
Type: Acute Care Hospitals
Ownership: Voluntary non-profit - Church
Phone: 479-338-8000
Emergency Services: Yes

Key Personnel:
CEO/President . . . . Lynn Britton
Emergency . . . . Brad Johnson, MD

Measure	Cases	This Hosp.	State Avg.	U.S. Avg.
Blood Clot Prevention and Treatment				
Anticoagulation Overlap Therapy[2]	69	93%	88%	93%
ICU Venous Thromboembolism Prophylaxis[2]	69	97%	94%	92%
Incidence of Potentially Preventable VTE[2]	11	9%	12%	10%
UFH with Dosages/Platelet Monitoring[2]	22	100%	100%	97%
Venous Thromboembolism Prophylaxis[2]	284	95%	91%	85%
Warfarin Therapy Discharge Instructions[2]	60	50%	76%	75%
Chest Pain/Possible Heart Attack Care				
Aspirin Given Within 24 Hours of Arrival[1,3]	-	-	96%	96%
Fibrinolytic Meds Within 30 Min. of Arrival[5]	-	-	54%	58%
Average Time to ECG (minutes)[1,3]	-	-	8	7
Average Time to Transfer (minutes)[5]	-	-	72	60
Children's Asthma Care				
Received Home Management Plan of Care	-	-	-	88%
Received Reliever Medication	-	-	-	100%
Received Systemic Corticosteroids	-	-	-	100%
Emergency Department				
Admittance Decision Time (minutes)[2]	392	96	65	98
Head CT Results Within 45 Min. of Arrival[1,3]	-	-	49%	57%
Patients Who Left ER Before Being Seen	46,486	2%	3%	2%
Time from ER Arrival to Admit. (minutes)[2]	415	238	214	274
Time from ER Arrival to Discharge (minutes)	373	154	118	134
Time in ER Before Being Evaluated (minutes)	393	28	26	26
Time to Pain Meds for Fractures (minutes)	128	67	66	57

NOTE: Hospital profiles are in alphabetical order by state, then city, then hospital within the city; Rankings exclude hospitals with less than 25 cases except for patient surveys which excludes hospitals with less than 100 cases; (a) 100-299 cases; (1) The number of cases/patients is too few to report; (2) Data submitted were based on a sample of cases/patients; (3) Results are based on a shorter time period than required; (4) Data suppressed by CMS for one or more quarters; (5) Results are not available for this reporting period; (6) Fewer than 100 patients completed the HCAHPS survey; (7) No cases met the criteria for this measure; (8) The lower limit of the confidence interval cannot be calculated if the number of observed infections equals zero; (9) No data are available from the state/territory for this reporting period; (10) The scores shown reflect fewer than 50 completed surveys; (11) There were discrepancies in the data collection process; (12) This measure does not apply to this hospital for this reporting period; (13) Results cannot be calculated for this reporting period; (14) The results for this state are combined with nearby states to protect confidentiality; Please refer to the User's Guide for a full explanation of data.

Measure	Cases	This Hosp.	State Avg.	U.S. Avg.
Heart Attack Care				
Aspirin Given at Discharge	229	100%	99%	99%
Fibrinolytic Meds Within 30 Min. of Arrival[7]	-	-	77%	54%
PCI Within 90 Minutes of Arrival	41	90%	96%	96%
Statin Prescribed at Discharge	214	98%	97%	98%
Heart Failure Care				
ACE Inhibitor or ARB for LVSD[2]	59	98%	96%	97%
Discharge Instructions Given[2]	170	95%	95%	94%
Evaluation of LVS Function[2]	209	100%	98%	99%
Medicare Spending				
Medicare Spending per Patient (ratio)	-	0.95	0.98	0.98
Pneumonia Care				
Appropriate Initial Antibiotic Given[2]	62	100%	94%	95%
Blood Culture Timing[2]	115	97%	98%	98%
Pregnancy and Delivery Care				
Newborn Deliveries Scheduled Early[2]	22	5%	6%	6%
Preventive Care				
Immunization for Influenza[2]	541	100%	89%	90%
Immunization for Pneumonia[2]	682	99%	92%	92%
Stroke Care				
Anticoagulation Therapy for Atrial Fibrillation[2]	17	71%	90%	95%
Antithrombotic Therapy Timing[2]	92	100%	96%	98%
Assessed for Rehabilitation[2]	110	94%	95%	97%
Discharged on Antithrombotic Therapy[2]	106	98%	96%	99%
Discharged on Statin Medication[2]	90	91%	86%	94%
Thrombolytic Therapy Timing[2]	20	55%	35%	66%
Venous Thromboembolism Prophylaxis[2]	97	94%	91%	94%
Written Stroke Educational Materials Given[2]	61	66%	81%	88%
Surgical Care Improvement Project				
Appropriate Beta Blocker Usage[2]	153	99%	98%	98%
Appropriate VTP Within 24 Hours[2]	321	99%	98%	98%
Controlled Postoperative Blood Glucose[2]	91	100%	99%	97%
Perioperative Temperature Management[2]	384	100%	100%	100%
Prophylactic Antibiotic Selection[2]	311	100%	99%	99%
Prophylactic Antibiotic Selection (Outpatient)	420	97%	98%	98%
Prophylactic Antibiotic Stopped[2]	299	100%	98%	98%
Prophylactic Antibiotic Timing[2]	311	98%	99%	99%
Prophylactic Antibiotic Timing (Outpatient)	421	99%	98%	98%
Urinary Catheter Removal[2]	320	98%	97%	97%
Survey of Patients' Hospital Experiences				
Area Around Room 'Always' Quiet at Night[11]	300+	60%	67%	61%
Doctors 'Always' Communicated Well[11]	300+	82%	83%	82%
Home Recovery Information Given[11]	300+	88%	83%	85%
Hospital Given 9 or 10 on 10 Point Scale[11]	300+	75%	70%	71%
Meds 'Always' Explained Before Given[11]	300+	60%	63%	64%
Nurses 'Always' Communicated Well[11]	300+	78%	79%	79%
Pain 'Always' Well Controlled[11]	300+	71%	71%	71%
Room and Bathroom 'Always' Clean[11]	300+	73%	72%	73%
Timely Help 'Always' Received[11]	300+	63%	68%	68%
Would Definitely Recommend Hospital[11]	300+	80%	69%	71%
Use of Medical Imaging				
Cardiac Imaging Stress Test before Surgery	991	5.0%	4.3%	5.3%
Combination Abdominal CT Scan	902	16.2%	15.3%	10.5%
Combination Brain/Sinus CT Scan	880	1.1%	2.9%	2.7%
Combination Chest CT Scan	574	12.5%	5%	2.7%
Follow-up Mammogram/Ultrasound	2,100	9.8%	9.9%	8.8%
Lumbar Spine MRI for Low Back Pain	236	37.3%	41.6%	37.2%

Saint Marys Regional Medical Center

1808 West Main Street
Russellville, AR 72801
Phone: 479-968-2841
Fax: 479-964-9287
URL: www.saintmarysregional.com
Type: Acute Care Hospitals
Emergency Services: Yes
Ownership: Proprietary
Beds: 170

Key Personnel:
Radiology. Ashley Burnham
Emergency Room . . . . Todd Carter, MD
CEO/President. . . . . Lee Myles
Chief of Medical Staff. . . . . Ira Shapiro, MD

Measure	Cases	This Hosp.	State Avg.	U.S. Avg.
Blood Clot Prevention and Treatment				
Anticoagulation Overlap Therapy[2]	43	74%	88%	93%
ICU Venous Thromboembolism Prophylaxis[2]	112	94%	94%	92%
Incidence of Potentially Preventable VTE[1,2]	-	-	12%	10%
UFH with Dosages/Platelet Monitoring[1,2]	-	-	100%	97%
Venous Thromboembolism Prophylaxis[2]	288	93%	91%	85%
Warfarin Therapy Discharge Instructions[2]	33	76%	76%	75%
Chest Pain/Possible Heart Attack Care				
Aspirin Given Within 24 Hours of Arrival	23	100%	96%	96%
Fibrinolytic Meds Within 30 Min. of Arrival[3,7]	-	-	54%	58%
Average Time to ECG (minutes)	23	2	8	7
Average Time to Transfer (minutes)[3,7]	-	-	72	60
Children's Asthma Care				
Received Home Management Plan of Care	-	-	-	88%
Received Reliever Medication	-	-	-	100%
Received Systemic Corticosteroids	-	-	-	100%
Emergency Department				
Admittance Decision Time (minutes)[2]	458	80	65	98
Head CT Results Within 45 Min. of Arrival	21	24%	49%	57%
Patients Who Left ER Before Being Seen	26,621	3%	3%	2%
Time from ER Arrival to Admit. (minutes)[2]	473	225	214	274
Time from ER Arrival to Discharge (minutes)	427	146	118	134
Time in ER Before Being Evaluated (minutes)	472	33	26	26
Time to Pain Meds for Fractures (minutes)	147	65	66	57
Heart Attack Care				
Aspirin Given at Discharge	196	99%	99%	99%
Fibrinolytic Meds Within 30 Min. of Arrival[7]	-	-	77%	54%
PCI Within 90 Minutes of Arrival	21	86%	96%	96%
Statin Prescribed at Discharge	190	96%	97%	98%
Heart Failure Care				
ACE Inhibitor or ARB for LVSD	29	90%	96%	97%
Discharge Instructions Given	104	81%	95%	94%
Evaluation of LVS Function	139	99%	98%	99%
Medicare Spending				
Medicare Spending per Patient (ratio)	-	0.98	0.98	0.98
Pneumonia Care				
Appropriate Initial Antibiotic Given	99	96%	94%	95%
Blood Culture Timing	150	99%	98%	98%
Pregnancy and Delivery Care				
Newborn Deliveries Scheduled Early[2]	41	0%	6%	6%
Preventive Care				
Immunization for Influenza[2]	471	98%	89%	90%
Immunization for Pneumonia[2]	558	90%	92%	92%
Stroke Care				
Anticoagulation Therapy for Atrial Fibrillation[1]	-	-	90%	95%
Antithrombotic Therapy Timing	45	100%	96%	98%
Assessed for Rehabilitation	51	90%	95%	97%
Discharged on Antithrombotic Therapy	47	98%	96%	99%
Discharged on Statin Medication	39	87%	86%	94%
Thrombolytic Therapy Timing[1]	-	-	35%	66%
Venous Thromboembolism Prophylaxis	48	98%	91%	94%
Written Stroke Educational Materials Given	23	78%	81%	88%
Surgical Care Improvement Project				
Appropriate Beta Blocker Usage	58	95%	98%	98%
Appropriate VTP Within 24 Hours	253	99%	98%	98%
Controlled Postoperative Blood Glucose[7]	-	-	99%	97%
Perioperative Temperature Management	276	100%	100%	100%
Prophylactic Antibiotic Selection	186	99%	99%	99%
Prophylactic Antibiotic Selection (Outpatient)	74	99%	98%	98%
Prophylactic Antibiotic Stopped	179	100%	98%	98%
Prophylactic Antibiotic Timing	186	99%	99%	99%
Prophylactic Antibiotic Timing (Outpatient)	76	95%	98%	98%
Urinary Catheter Removal	144	99%	97%	97%
Survey of Patients' Hospital Experiences				
Area Around Room 'Always' Quiet at Night	300+	51%	67%	61%
Doctors 'Always' Communicated Well	300+	79%	83%	82%
Home Recovery Information Given	300+	82%	83%	85%
Hospital Given 9 or 10 on 10 Point Scale	300+	58%	70%	71%
Meds 'Always' Explained Before Given	300+	54%	63%	64%
Nurses 'Always' Communicated Well	300+	71%	79%	79%
Pain 'Always' Well Controlled	300+	65%	71%	71%
Room and Bathroom 'Always' Clean	300+	65%	72%	73%
Timely Help 'Always' Received	300+	60%	68%	68%
Would Definitely Recommend Hospital	300+	54%	69%	71%
Use of Medical Imaging				
Cardiac Imaging Stress Test before Surgery	293	3.1%	4.3%	5.3%
Combination Abdominal CT Scan	744	3.2%	15.3%	10.5%
Combination Brain/Sinus CT Scan[1]	-	-	2.9%	2.7%
Combination Chest CT Scan	544	1.8%	5%	2.7%
Follow-up Mammogram/Ultrasound	1,083	15.1%	9.9%	8.8%
Lumbar Spine MRI for Low Back Pain	116	39.7%	41.6%	37.2%

Fulton County Hospital

679 North Main Street
Phone: 870-895-2691
Salem, AR 72576
URL: www.fultoncountyhospital.org
Type: Critical Access Hospitals
Emergency Services: Yes
Ownership: Government - Local

Measure	Cases	This Hosp.	State Avg.	U.S. Avg.
Blood Clot Prevention and Treatment				
Anticoagulation Overlap Therapy[5]	-	-	88%	93%
ICU Venous Thromboembolism Prophylaxis[5]	-	-	94%	92%
Incidence of Potentially Preventable VTE[5]	-	-	12%	10%
UFH with Dosages/Platelet Monitoring[5]	-	-	100%	97%
Venous Thromboembolism Prophylaxis[5]	-	-	91%	85%
Warfarin Therapy Discharge Instructions[5]	-	-	76%	75%
Chest Pain/Possible Heart Attack Care				
Aspirin Given Within 24 Hours of Arrival	-	-	96%	96%
Fibrinolytic Meds Within 30 Min. of Arrival	-	-	54%	58%
Average Time to ECG (minutes)	-	-	8	7
Average Time to Transfer (minutes)	-	-	72	60
Children's Asthma Care				
Received Home Management Plan of Care	-	-	-	88%
Received Reliever Medication	-	-	-	100%
Received Systemic Corticosteroids	-	-	-	100%
Emergency Department				
Admittance Decision Time (minutes)[5]	-	-	65	98
Head CT Results Within 45 Min. of Arrival	-	-	49%	57%
Patients Who Left ER Before Being Seen	-	-	3%	2%
Time from ER Arrival to Admit. (minutes)[5]	-	-	214	274
Time from ER Arrival to Discharge (minutes)	-	-	118	134
Time in ER Before Being Evaluated (minutes)	-	-	26	26
Time to Pain Meds for Fractures (minutes)	-	-	66	57
Heart Attack Care				
Aspirin Given at Discharge[3,7]	-	-	99%	99%
Fibrinolytic Meds Within 30 Min. of Arrival[3,7]	-	-	77%	54%
PCI Within 90 Minutes of Arrival[3,7]	-	-	96%	96%
Statin Prescribed at Discharge[3,7]	-	-	97%	98%
Heart Failure Care				
ACE Inhibitor or ARB for LVSD[1]	-	-	96%	97%
Discharge Instructions Given	34	88%	95%	94%
Evaluation of LVS Function	52	100%	98%	99%
Medicare Spending				
Medicare Spending per Patient (ratio)	-	-	0.98	0.98
Pneumonia Care				
Appropriate Initial Antibiotic Given	33	88%	94%	95%
Blood Culture Timing	28	93%	98%	98%
Pregnancy and Delivery Care				
Newborn Deliveries Scheduled Early[5]	-	-	6%	6%
Preventive Care				
Immunization for Influenza[5]	-	-	89%	90%
Immunization for Pneumonia[5]	-	-	92%	92%
Stroke Care				
Anticoagulation Therapy for Atrial Fibrillation[5]	-	-	90%	95%
Antithrombotic Therapy Timing[5]	-	-	96%	98%
Assessed for Rehabilitation[5]	-	-	95%	97%
Discharged on Antithrombotic Therapy[5]	-	-	96%	99%
Discharged on Statin Medication[5]	-	-	86%	94%
Thrombolytic Therapy Timing[5]	-	-	35%	66%
Venous Thromboembolism Prophylaxis[5]	-	-	91%	94%
Written Stroke Educational Materials Given[5]	-	-	81%	88%
Surgical Care Improvement Project				
Appropriate Beta Blocker Usage[5]	-	-	98%	98%
Appropriate VTP Within 24 Hours[5]	-	-	98%	98%
Controlled Postoperative Blood Glucose[5]	-	-	99%	97%
Perioperative Temperature Management[5]	-	-	100%	100%
Prophylactic Antibiotic Selection[5]	-	-	99%	99%

NOTE: Hospital profiles are in alphabetical order by state, then city, then hospital within the city; Rankings exclude hospitals with less than 25 cases except for patient surveys which excludes hospitals with less than 100 cases; (a) 100-299 cases; (1) The number of cases/patients is too few to report; (2) Data submitted were based on a sample of cases/patients; (3) Results are based on a shorter time period than required; (4) Data suppressed by CMS for one or more quarters; (5) Results are not available for this reporting period; (6) Fewer than 100 patients completed the HCAHPS survey; (7) No cases met the criteria for this measure; (8) The lower limit of the confidence interval cannot be calculated if the number of observed infections equals zero; (9) No data are available from the state/territory for this reporting period; (10) The scores shown reflect fewer than 50 completed surveys; (11) There were discrepancies in the data collection process; (12) This measure does not apply to this hospital for this reporting period; (13) Results cannot be calculated for this reporting period; (14) The results for this state are combined with nearby states to protect confidentiality; Please refer to the User's Guide for a full explanation of data.

Measure	Cases	This Hosp.	State Avg.	U.S. Avg.
Prophylactic Antibiotic Selection (Outpatient)	-	-	98%	98%
Prophylactic Antibiotic Stopped[5]	-	-	98%	98%
Prophylactic Antibiotic Timing[5]	-	-	99%	99%
Prophylactic Antibiotic Timing (Outpatient)	-	-	98%	98%
Urinary Catheter Removal[5]	-	-	97%	97%
Survey of Patients' Hospital Experiences				
Area Around Room 'Always' Quiet at Night[5]	-	-	67%	61%
Doctors 'Always' Communicated Well[5]	-	-	83%	82%
Home Recovery Information Given[5]	-	-	83%	85%
Hospital Given 9 or 10 on 10 Point Scale[5]	-	-	70%	71%
Meds 'Always' Explained Before Given[5]	-	-	63%	64%
Nurses 'Always' Communicated Well[5]	-	-	79%	79%
Pain 'Always' Well Controlled[5]	-	-	71%	71%
Room and Bathroom 'Always' Clean[5]	-	-	72%	73%
Timely Help 'Always' Received[5]	-	-	68%	68%
Would Definitely Recommend Hospital[5]	-	-	69%	71%
Use of Medical Imaging				
Cardiac Imaging Stress Test before Surgery	-	-	4.3%	5.3%
Combination Abdominal CT Scan	-	-	15.3%	10.5%
Combination Brain/Sinus CT Scan	-	-	2.9%	2.7%
Combination Chest CT Scan	-	-	5%	2.7%
Follow-up Mammogram/Ultrasound	-	-	9.9%	8.8%
Lumbar Spine MRI for Low Back Pain	-	-	41.6%	37.2%

White County Medical Center

3214 East Race Avenue — Phone: 501-278-3100
Searcy, AR 72143 — Fax: 501-278-3344
URL: www.centralarkhospital.com
Type: Acute Care Hospitals — Emergency Services: Yes
Ownership: Voluntary non-profit - Private — Beds: 193

Key Personnel:
President/CEO. . . . . Joan Coffman
Radiology. . . . . Cody Haines, MD
Emergency Room . . . . Keri Larough
Pediatric Ambulatory Care . . . . . . J Lewis, MD
Pediatric In-Patient Care . . . . J Lewis, MD
Operating Room. . . . . Nora Osbourne
Chief of Medical Staff . . . . Shelly Tobey

Measure	Cases	This Hosp.	State Avg.	U.S. Avg.
Blood Clot Prevention and Treatment				
Anticoagulation Overlap Therapy	39	100%	88%	93%
ICU Venous Thromboembolism Prophylaxis	438	100%	94%	92%
Incidence of Potentially Preventable VTE[1]	-	-	12%	10%
UFH with Dosages/Platelet Monitoring[7]	-	-	100%	97%
Venous Thromboembolism Prophylaxis	4,364	100%	91%	85%
Warfarin Therapy Discharge Instructions	33	100%	76%	75%
Chest Pain/Possible Heart Attack Care				
Aspirin Given Within 24 Hours of Arrival	17	100%	96%	96%
Fibrinolytic Meds Within 30 Min. of Arrival[3,7]	-	-	54%	58%
Average Time to ECG (minutes)	18	3	8	7
Average Time to Transfer (minutes)[3,7]	-	-	72	60
Children's Asthma Care				
Received Home Management Plan of Care	-	-	-	88%
Received Reliever Medication	-	-	-	100%
Received Systemic Corticosteroids	-	-	-	100%
Emergency Department				
Admittance Decision Time (minutes)[2]	483	101	65	98
Head CT Results Within 45 Min. of Arrival	24	67%	49%	57%
Patients Who Left ER Before Being Seen	50,020	3%	3%	2%
Time from ER Arrival to Admit. (minutes)[2]	484	240	214	274
Time from ER Arrival to Discharge (minutes)	473	127	118	134
Time in ER Before Being Evaluated (minutes)	545	50	26	26
Time to Pain Meds for Fractures (minutes)	184	52	66	57
Heart Attack Care				
Aspirin Given at Discharge	146	100%	99%	99%
Fibrinolytic Meds Within 30 Min. of Arrival[7]	-	-	77%	54%
PCI Within 90 Minutes of Arrival	29	100%	96%	96%
Statin Prescribed at Discharge	139	100%	97%	98%
Heart Failure Care				
ACE Inhibitor or ARB for LVSD[2]	79	100%	96%	97%
Discharge Instructions Given[2]	222	97%	95%	94%
Evaluation of LVS Function[2]	289	100%	98%	99%
Medicare Spending				
Medicare Spending per Patient (ratio)	-	0.99	0.98	0.98
Pneumonia Care				
Appropriate Initial Antibiotic Given[2]	83	100%	94%	95%
Blood Culture Timing[2]	139	100%	98%	98%
Pregnancy and Delivery Care				
Newborn Deliveries Scheduled Early[2]	21	0%	6%	6%
Preventive Care				
Immunization for Influenza[2]	577	95%	89%	90%
Immunization for Pneumonia[2]	698	95%	92%	92%
Stroke Care				
Anticoagulation Therapy for Atrial Fibrillation	13	100%	90%	95%
Antithrombotic Therapy Timing	99	98%	96%	98%
Assessed for Rehabilitation	94	99%	95%	97%
Discharged on Antithrombotic Therapy	92	99%	96%	99%
Discharged on Statin Medication	72	94%	86%	94%
Thrombolytic Therapy Timing[1]	-	-	35%	66%
Venous Thromboembolism Prophylaxis	97	99%	91%	94%
Written Stroke Educational Materials Given	45	96%	81%	88%
Surgical Care Improvement Project				
Appropriate Beta Blocker Usage[2]	131	100%	98%	98%
Appropriate VTP Within 24 Hours[2]	282	100%	98%	98%
Controlled Postoperative Blood Glucose[2,7]	-	-	99%	97%
Perioperative Temperature Management[2]	326	100%	100%	100%
Prophylactic Antibiotic Selection[2]	214	100%	99%	99%
Prophylactic Antibiotic Selection (Outpatient)	381	98%	98%	98%
Prophylactic Antibiotic Stopped[2]	208	100%	98%	98%
Prophylactic Antibiotic Timing[2]	214	99%	99%	99%
Prophylactic Antibiotic Timing (Outpatient)	376	100%	98%	98%
Urinary Catheter Removal[2]	225	100%	97%	97%
Survey of Patients' Hospital Experiences				
Area Around Room 'Always' Quiet at Night	300+	68%	67%	61%
Doctors 'Always' Communicated Well	300+	83%	83%	82%
Home Recovery Information Given	300+	82%	83%	85%
Hospital Given 9 or 10 on 10 Point Scale	300+	72%	70%	71%
Meds 'Always' Explained Before Given	300+	65%	63%	64%
Nurses 'Always' Communicated Well	300+	78%	79%	79%
Pain 'Always' Well Controlled	300+	72%	71%	71%
Room and Bathroom 'Always' Clean	300+	70%	72%	73%
Timely Help 'Always' Received	300+	63%	68%	68%
Would Definitely Recommend Hospital	300+	72%	69%	71%
Use of Medical Imaging				
Cardiac Imaging Stress Test before Surgery	413	2.2%	4.3%	5.3%
Combination Abdominal CT Scan	1,069	12.0%	15.3%	10.5%
Combination Brain/Sinus CT Scan	966	2.4%	2.9%	2.7%
Combination Chest CT Scan	605	0.0%	5%	2.7%
Follow-up Mammogram/Ultrasound[7]	-	-	9.9%	8.8%
Lumbar Spine MRI for Low Back Pain	216	41.7%	41.6%	37.2%

Saint Vincent Medical Center - North

2215 Wildwood Avenue — Phone: 501-552-7100
Sherwood, AR 72120
Type: Acute Care Hospitals — Emergency Services: Yes
Ownership: Voluntary non-profit - Private — Beds: 50

Key Personnel:
CEO/President. . . . . Peter D. Banko
Chief of Medical Staff . . . . Tom Cummins, MD
President . . . . David Foster

Measure	Cases	This Hosp.	State Avg.	U.S. Avg.
Blood Clot Prevention and Treatment				
Anticoagulation Overlap Therapy[2]	15	100%	88%	93%
ICU Venous Thromboembolism Prophylaxis[2]	51	67%	94%	92%
Incidence of Potentially Preventable VTE[1,2]	-	-	12%	10%
UFH with Dosages/Platelet Monitoring[1,2]	-	-	100%	97%
Venous Thromboembolism Prophylaxis[2]	124	55%	91%	85%
Warfarin Therapy Discharge Instructions[1,2]	-	-	76%	75%
Chest Pain/Possible Heart Attack Care				
Aspirin Given Within 24 Hours of Arrival[1]	-	-	96%	96%
Fibrinolytic Meds Within 30 Min. of Arrival[3,7]	-	-	54%	58%
Average Time to ECG (minutes)[1]	-	-	8	7
Average Time to Transfer (minutes)[1,3]	-	-	72	60
Children's Asthma Care				
Received Home Management Plan of Care	-	-	-	88%
Received Reliever Medication	-	-	-	100%
Received Systemic Corticosteroids	-	-	-	100%
Emergency Department				
Admittance Decision Time (minutes)[2]	375	68	65	98
Head CT Results Within 45 Min. of Arrival	13	62%	49%	57%
Patients Who Left ER Before Being Seen	17,785	4%	3%	2%
Time from ER Arrival to Admit. (minutes)[2]	432	249	214	274
Time from ER Arrival to Discharge (minutes)	339	133	118	134
Time in ER Before Being Evaluated (minutes)	330	34	26	26
Time to Pain Meds for Fractures (minutes)	63	55	66	57
Heart Attack Care				
Aspirin Given at Discharge	13	100%	99%	99%
Fibrinolytic Meds Within 30 Min. of Arrival[7]	-	-	77%	54%
PCI Within 90 Minutes of Arrival[7]	-	-	96%	96%
Statin Prescribed at Discharge	13	77%	97%	98%
Heart Failure Care				
ACE Inhibitor or ARB for LVSD	24	92%	96%	97%
Discharge Instructions Given	56	89%	95%	94%
Evaluation of LVS Function	70	100%	98%	99%
Medicare Spending				
Medicare Spending per Patient (ratio)	-	1.15	0.98	0.98
Pneumonia Care				
Appropriate Initial Antibiotic Given	71	92%	94%	95%
Blood Culture Timing	75	95%	98%	98%
Pregnancy and Delivery Care				
Newborn Deliveries Scheduled Early[7]	-	-	6%	6%
Preventive Care				
Immunization for Influenza[2]	291	93%	89%	90%
Immunization for Pneumonia[2]	400	92%	92%	92%
Stroke Care				
Anticoagulation Therapy for Atrial Fibrillation[2,7]	-	-	90%	95%
Antithrombotic Therapy Timing[2]	13	92%	96%	98%
Assessed for Rehabilitation[2]	14	93%	95%	97%
Discharged on Antithrombotic Therapy[2]	13	92%	96%	99%
Discharged on Statin Medication[2]	12	33%	86%	94%
Thrombolytic Therapy Timing[1,2]	-	-	35%	66%
Venous Thromboembolism Prophylaxis[2]	16	75%	91%	94%
Written Stroke Educational Materials Given[1,2]	-	-	81%	88%
Surgical Care Improvement Project				
Appropriate Beta Blocker Usage	16	88%	98%	98%
Appropriate VTP Within 24 Hours	47	85%	98%	98%
Controlled Postoperative Blood Glucose[7]	-	-	99%	97%
Perioperative Temperature Management	79	100%	100%	100%
Prophylactic Antibiotic Selection	49	96%	99%	99%
Prophylactic Antibiotic Selection (Outpatient)	38	87%	98%	98%
Prophylactic Antibiotic Stopped	48	98%	98%	98%
Prophylactic Antibiotic Timing	49	96%	99%	99%
Prophylactic Antibiotic Timing (Outpatient)	38	97%	98%	98%
Urinary Catheter Removal	38	84%	97%	97%
Survey of Patients' Hospital Experiences				
Area Around Room 'Always' Quiet at Night	300+	72%	67%	61%
Doctors 'Always' Communicated Well	300+	84%	83%	82%
Home Recovery Information Given	300+	84%	83%	85%
Hospital Given 9 or 10 on 10 Point Scale	300+	71%	70%	71%
Meds 'Always' Explained Before Given	300+	64%	63%	64%
Nurses 'Always' Communicated Well	300+	79%	79%	79%
Pain 'Always' Well Controlled	300+	71%	71%	71%
Room and Bathroom 'Always' Clean	300+	72%	72%	73%
Timely Help 'Always' Received	300+	70%	68%	68%
Would Definitely Recommend Hospital	300+	77%	69%	71%
Use of Medical Imaging				
Cardiac Imaging Stress Test before Surgery[1]	-	-	4.3%	5.3%
Combination Abdominal CT Scan	252	9.5%	15.3%	10.5%
Combination Brain/Sinus CT Scan[1]	-	-	2.9%	2.7%
Combination Chest CT Scan	92	2.2%	5%	2.7%
Follow-up Mammogram/Ultrasound	325	13.8%	9.9%	8.8%
Lumbar Spine MRI for Low Back Pain	84	23.8%	41.6%	37.2%

Siloam Springs Regional Hospital

603 North Progress Avenue — Phone: 479-524-4141
Siloam Springs, AR 72761 — Fax: 501-549-2486
Type: Acute Care Hospitals — Emergency Services: Yes
Ownership: Proprietary — Beds: 73

Key Personnel:
Quality Assurance . . . . Scott Harris
Emergency Room . . . . Robin McAlister

NOTE: Hospital profiles are in alphabetical order by state, then city, then hospital within the city; Rankings exclude hospitals with less than 25 cases except for patient surveys which excludes hospitals with less than 100 cases; (a) 100-299 cases; (1) The number of cases/patients is too few to report; (2) Data submitted were based on a sample of cases/patients; (3) Results are based on a shorter time period than required; (4) Data suppressed by CMS for one or more quarters; (5) Results are not available for this reporting period; (6) Fewer than 100 patients completed the HCAHPS survey; (7) No cases met the criteria for this measure; (8) The lower limit of the confidence interval cannot be calculated if the number of observed infections equals zero; (9) No data are available from the state/territory for this reporting period; (10) The scores shown reflect fewer than 50 completed surveys; (11) There were discrepancies in the data collection process; (12) This measure does not apply to this hospital for this reporting period; (13) Results cannot be calculated for this reporting period; (14) The results for this state are combined with nearby states to protect confidentiality; Please refer to the User's Guide for a full explanation of data.

CEO/President. . . . . Tinny Mclean
Operating Room. . . . . Leah Oman, RN
Chief of Medical Staff. . . . . Angela Sanmeier

Measure	Cases	This Hosp.	State Avg.	U.S. Avg.
Blood Clot Prevention and Treatment				
Anticoagulation Overlap Therapy[1,2]	-	-	88%	93%
ICU Venous Thromboembolism Prophylaxis[2]	85	96%	94%	92%
Incidence of Potentially Preventable VTE[2,7]	-	-	12%	10%
UFH with Dosages/Platelet Monitoring[1,2]	-	-	100%	97%
Venous Thromboembolism Prophylaxis[2]	201	96%	91%	85%
Warfarin Therapy Discharge Instructions[1,2]	-	-	76%	75%
Chest Pain/Possible Heart Attack Care				
Aspirin Given Within 24 Hours of Arrival	116	100%	96%	96%
Fibrinolytic Meds Within 30 Min. of Arrival[1]	-	-	54%	58%
Average Time to ECG (minutes)	124	4	8	7
Average Time to Transfer (minutes)[1]	-	-	72	60
Children's Asthma Care				
Received Home Management Plan of Care	-	-	-	88%
Received Reliever Medication	-	-	-	100%
Received Systemic Corticosteroids	-	-	-	100%
Emergency Department				
Admittance Decision Time (minutes)[2]	388	60	65	98
Head CT Results Within 45 Min. of Arrival[1]	-	-	49%	57%
Patients Who Left ER Before Being Seen	20,307	2%	3%	2%
Time from ER Arrival to Admit. (minutes)[2]	395	211	214	274
Time from ER Arrival to Discharge (minutes)	359	94	118	134
Time in ER Before Being Evaluated (minutes)	424	20	26	26
Time to Pain Meds for Fractures (minutes)	90	47	66	57
Heart Attack Care				
Aspirin Given at Discharge[1]	-	-	99%	99%
Fibrinolytic Meds Within 30 Min. of Arrival[7]	-	-	77%	54%
PCI Within 90 Minutes of Arrival[7]	-	-	96%	96%
Statin Prescribed at Discharge[1]	-	-	97%	98%
Heart Failure Care				
ACE Inhibitor or ARB for LVSD	12	100%	96%	97%
Discharge Instructions Given	45	98%	95%	94%
Evaluation of LVS Function	57	96%	98%	99%
Medicare Spending				
Medicare Spending per Patient (ratio)	-	0.93	0.98	0.98
Pneumonia Care				
Appropriate Initial Antibiotic Given	72	97%	94%	95%
Blood Culture Timing	92	98%	98%	98%
Pregnancy and Delivery Care				
Newborn Deliveries Scheduled Early[2]	39	0%	6%	6%
Preventive Care				
Immunization for Influenza[2]	481	99%	89%	90%
Immunization for Pneumonia[2]	420	100%	92%	92%
Stroke Care				
Anticoagulation Therapy for Atrial Fibrillation[1]	-	-	90%	95%
Antithrombotic Therapy Timing	16	100%	96%	98%
Assessed for Rehabilitation	17	100%	95%	97%
Discharged on Antithrombotic Therapy	17	100%	96%	99%
Discharged on Statin Medication	16	100%	86%	94%
Thrombolytic Therapy Timing[1]	-	-	35%	66%
Venous Thromboembolism Prophylaxis	20	100%	91%	94%
Written Stroke Educational Materials Given[1]	-	-	81%	88%
Surgical Care Improvement Project				
Appropriate Beta Blocker Usage	19	95%	98%	98%
Appropriate VTP Within 24 Hours	86	100%	98%	98%
Controlled Postoperative Blood Glucose[7]	-	-	99%	97%
Perioperative Temperature Management	104	100%	100%	100%
Prophylactic Antibiotic Selection	63	100%	99%	99%
Prophylactic Antibiotic Selection (Outpatient)	74	99%	98%	98%
Prophylactic Antibiotic Stopped	59	97%	98%	98%
Prophylactic Antibiotic Timing	63	100%	99%	99%
Prophylactic Antibiotic Timing (Outpatient)	74	99%	98%	98%
Urinary Catheter Removal	48	98%	97%	97%
Survey of Patients' Hospital Experiences				
Area Around Room 'Always' Quiet at Night	300+	62%	67%	61%
Doctors 'Always' Communicated Well	300+	83%	83%	82%
Home Recovery Information Given	300+	89%	83%	85%
Hospital Given 9 or 10 on 10 Point Scale	300+	69%	70%	71%
Meds 'Always' Explained Before Given	300+	63%	63%	64%
Nurses 'Always' Communicated Well	300+	76%	79%	79%
Pain 'Always' Well Controlled	300+	71%	71%	71%
Room and Bathroom 'Always' Clean	300+	75%	72%	73%
Timely Help 'Always' Received	300+	66%	68%	68%
Would Definitely Recommend Hospital	300+	65%	69%	71%
Use of Medical Imaging				
Cardiac Imaging Stress Test before Surgery	117	4.3%	4.3%	5.3%
Combination Abdominal CT Scan	219	8.2%	15.3%	10.5%
Combination Brain/Sinus CT Scan	221	5.0%	2.9%	2.7%
Combination Chest CT Scan	73	1.4%	5%	2.7%
Follow-up Mammogram/Ultrasound	273	11.7%	9.9%	8.8%
Lumbar Spine MRI for Low Back Pain[1]	-	-	41.6%	37.2%

NW Arkansas Hospitals

609 West Maple Avenue — Phone: 479-751-5711
Springdale, AR 72764 — Fax: 479-757-2928
URL: www.northwesthealth.org
Type: Acute Care Hospitals — Emergency Services: Yes
Ownership: Proprietary — Beds: 222

Key Personnel:
Emergency Room . . . . Dana Bell, MD
Quality Assurance . . . . Amy Forest
Pediatric Ambulatory Care . . . . . . Elizabeth Froman, MD
Pediatric In-Patient Care . . . . Elizabeth Froman, MD
Infection Control. . . . . Sharon Jorde
President . . . . Nichole Maher, MPH
Chief of Medical Staff. . . . . Sanjay Patel, MD
Intensive Care Unit. . . . . Carol Tulobaski

Measure	Cases	This Hosp.	State Avg.	U.S. Avg.
Blood Clot Prevention and Treatment				
Anticoagulation Overlap Therapy[2]	74	89%	88%	93%
ICU Venous Thromboembolism Prophylaxis[2]	81	99%	94%	92%
Incidence of Potentially Preventable VTE[2]	18	0%	12%	10%
UFH with Dosages/Platelet Monitoring[2]	66	100%	100%	97%
Venous Thromboembolism Prophylaxis[2]	296	95%	91%	85%
Warfarin Therapy Discharge Instructions[2]	46	83%	76%	75%
Chest Pain/Possible Heart Attack Care				
Aspirin Given Within 24 Hours of Arrival[3,7]	-	-	96%	96%
Fibrinolytic Meds Within 30 Min. of Arrival[5]	-	-	54%	58%
Average Time to ECG (minutes)[3,7]	-	-	8	7
Average Time to Transfer (minutes)[5]	-	-	72	60
Children's Asthma Care				
Received Home Management Plan of Care	-	-	-	88%
Received Reliever Medication	-	-	-	100%
Received Systemic Corticosteroids	-	-	-	100%
Emergency Department				
Admittance Decision Time (minutes)[2]	650	112	65	98
Head CT Results Within 45 Min. of Arrival	17	94%	49%	57%
Patients Who Left ER Before Being Seen	75,284	2%	3%	2%
Time from ER Arrival to Admit. (minutes)[2]	672	238	214	274
Time from ER Arrival to Discharge (minutes)	366	142	118	134
Time in ER Before Being Evaluated (minutes)	368	20	26	26
Time to Pain Meds for Fractures (minutes)	171	51	66	57
Heart Attack Care				
Aspirin Given at Discharge	464	100%	99%	99%
Fibrinolytic Meds Within 30 Min. of Arrival[7]	-	-	77%	54%
PCI Within 90 Minutes of Arrival	67	99%	96%	96%
Statin Prescribed at Discharge	427	99%	97%	98%
Heart Failure Care				
ACE Inhibitor or ARB for LVSD	89	97%	96%	97%
Discharge Instructions Given	252	94%	95%	94%
Evaluation of LVS Function	340	99%	98%	99%
Medicare Spending				
Medicare Spending per Patient (ratio)	-	0.99	0.98	0.98
Pneumonia Care				
Appropriate Initial Antibiotic Given	167	95%	94%	95%
Blood Culture Timing	247	98%	98%	98%
Pregnancy and Delivery Care				
Newborn Deliveries Scheduled Early[2]	123	6%	6%	6%
Preventive Care				
Immunization for Influenza[2]	700	98%	89%	90%
Immunization for Pneumonia[2]	644	100%	92%	92%
Stroke Care				
Anticoagulation Therapy for Atrial Fibrillation[1]	-	-	90%	95%
Antithrombotic Therapy Timing	94	100%	96%	98%
Assessed for Rehabilitation	103	96%	95%	97%
Discharged on Antithrombotic Therapy	90	100%	96%	99%
Discharged on Statin Medication	72	92%	86%	94%
Thrombolytic Therapy Timing[1]	-	-	35%	66%
Venous Thromboembolism Prophylaxis	107	96%	91%	94%
Written Stroke Educational Materials Given	62	97%	81%	88%
Surgical Care Improvement Project				
Appropriate Beta Blocker Usage	267	98%	98%	98%
Appropriate VTP Within 24 Hours	433	98%	98%	98%
Controlled Postoperative Blood Glucose	216	100%	99%	97%
Perioperative Temperature Management	622	100%	100%	100%
Prophylactic Antibiotic Selection	554	99%	99%	99%
Prophylactic Antibiotic Selection (Outpatient)	845	98%	98%	98%
Prophylactic Antibiotic Stopped	539	98%	98%	98%
Prophylactic Antibiotic Timing	557	99%	99%	99%
Prophylactic Antibiotic Timing (Outpatient)	847	99%	98%	98%
Urinary Catheter Removal	373	99%	97%	97%
Survey of Patients' Hospital Experiences				
Area Around Room 'Always' Quiet at Night	300+	61%	67%	61%
Doctors 'Always' Communicated Well	300+	77%	83%	82%
Home Recovery Information Given	300+	86%	83%	85%
Hospital Given 9 or 10 on 10 Point Scale	300+	67%	70%	71%
Meds 'Always' Explained Before Given	300+	59%	63%	64%
Nurses 'Always' Communicated Well	300+	74%	79%	79%
Pain 'Always' Well Controlled	300+	67%	71%	71%
Room and Bathroom 'Always' Clean	300+	70%	72%	73%
Timely Help 'Always' Received	300+	57%	68%	68%
Would Definitely Recommend Hospital	300+	70%	69%	71%
Use of Medical Imaging				
Cardiac Imaging Stress Test before Surgery	546	4.4%	4.3%	5.3%
Combination Abdominal CT Scan	771	16.3%	15.3%	10.5%
Combination Brain/Sinus CT Scan	912	4.4%	2.9%	2.7%
Combination Chest CT Scan	352	7.4%	5%	2.7%
Follow-up Mammogram/Ultrasound	1,670	14.4%	9.9%	8.8%
Lumbar Spine MRI for Low Back Pain	122	44.3%	41.6%	37.2%

Baptist Health Medical Center - Stuttgart

1703 North Buerkle Road — Phone: 870-673-3511
Stuttgart, AR 72160 — Fax: 870-672-6869
E-mail: aholstead@stuttgart-medical.org
URL: www.stuttgart-medical.org
Type: Acute Care Hospitals — Emergency Services: Yes
Ownership: Proprietary — Beds: 49

Key Personnel:
Operating Room. . . . . Dr Gilbert, RN
Chief of Medical Staff. . . . . Dr Hord, MD
Infection Control. . . . . Rachelle McCarthy, RN
Quality Assurance . . . . Joy Neighbors
CEO/President. . . . . Bob Phillips
Coronary Care . . . . Janice York

Measure	Cases	This Hosp.	State Avg.	U.S. Avg.
Blood Clot Prevention and Treatment				
Anticoagulation Overlap Therapy[1,2]	-	-	88%	93%
ICU Venous Thromboembolism Prophylaxis[2]	14	57%	94%	92%
Incidence of Potentially Preventable VTE[2,7]	-	-	12%	10%
UFH with Dosages/Platelet Monitoring[1,2]	-	-	100%	97%
Venous Thromboembolism Prophylaxis[2]	148	67%	91%	85%
Warfarin Therapy Discharge Instructions[1,2]	-	-	76%	75%
Chest Pain/Possible Heart Attack Care				
Aspirin Given Within 24 Hours of Arrival	28	96%	96%	96%
Fibrinolytic Meds Within 30 Min. of Arrival[1]	-	-	54%	58%
Average Time to ECG (minutes)	30	11	8	7
Average Time to Transfer (minutes)[1]	-	-	72	60
Children's Asthma Care				
Received Home Management Plan of Care	-	-	-	88%
Received Reliever Medication	-	-	-	100%
Received Systemic Corticosteroids	-	-	-	100%
Emergency Department				
Admittance Decision Time (minutes)[2]	174	37	65	98
Head CT Results Within 45 Min. of Arrival[1]	-	-	49%	57%
Patients Who Left ER Before Being Seen	10,975	2%	3%	2%
Time from ER Arrival to Admit. (minutes)[2]	190	159	214	274

NOTE: Hospital profiles are in alphabetical order by state, then city, then hospital within the city; Rankings exclude hospitals with less than 25 cases except for patient surveys which excludes hospitals with less than 100 cases; (a) 100-299 cases; (1) The number of cases/patients is too few to report; (2) Data submitted were based on a sample of cases/patients; (3) Results are based on a shorter time period than required; (4) Data suppressed by CMS for one or more quarters; (5) Results are not available for this reporting period; (6) Fewer than 100 patients completed the HCAHPS survey; (7) No cases met the criteria for this measure; (8) The lower limit of the confidence interval cannot be calculated if the number of observed infections equals zero; (9) No data are available from the state/territory for this reporting period; (10) The scores shown reflect fewer than 50 completed surveys; (11) There were discrepancies in the data collection process; (12) This measure does not apply to this hospital for this reporting period; (13) Results cannot be calculated for this reporting period; (14) The results for this state are combined with nearby states to protect confidentiality; Please refer to the User's Guide for a full explanation of data.

Measure	Cases	This Hosp.	State Avg.	U.S. Avg.
Time from ER Arrival to Discharge (minutes)	283	100	118	134
Time in ER Before Being Evaluated (minutes)	363	25	26	26
Time to Pain Meds for Fractures (minutes)	37	74	66	57
Heart Attack Care				
Aspirin Given at Discharge[1]	-	-	99%	99%
Fibrinolytic Meds Within 30 Min. of Arrival[7]	-	-	77%	54%
PCI Within 90 Minutes of Arrival[7]	-	-	96%	96%
Statin Prescribed at Discharge[1]	-	-	97%	98%
Heart Failure Care				
ACE Inhibitor or ARB for LVSD	20	100%	96%	97%
Discharge Instructions Given	77	99%	95%	94%
Evaluation of LVS Function	80	92%	98%	99%
Medicare Spending				
Medicare Spending per Patient (ratio)	-	0.85	0.98	0.98
Pneumonia Care				
Appropriate Initial Antibiotic Given	47	94%	94%	95%
Blood Culture Timing	54	96%	98%	98%
Pregnancy and Delivery Care				
Newborn Deliveries Scheduled Early	24	12%	6%	6%
Preventive Care				
Immunization for Influenza[2]	252	94%	89%	90%
Immunization for Pneumonia[2]	337	95%	92%	92%
Stroke Care				
Anticoagulation Therapy for Atrial Fibrillation[1]	-	-	90%	95%
Antithrombotic Therapy Timing	13	85%	96%	98%
Assessed for Rehabilitation	14	71%	95%	97%
Discharged on Antithrombotic Therapy	12	83%	96%	99%
Discharged on Statin Medication	13	46%	86%	94%
Thrombolytic Therapy Timing[7]	-	-	35%	66%
Venous Thromboembolism Prophylaxis	16	75%	91%	94%
Written Stroke Educational Materials Given	11	55%	81%	88%
Surgical Care Improvement Project				
Appropriate Beta Blocker Usage[7]	-	-	98%	98%
Appropriate VTP Within 24 Hours	24	100%	98%	98%
Controlled Postoperative Blood Glucose[7]	-	-	99%	97%
Perioperative Temperature Management	27	100%	100%	100%
Prophylactic Antibiotic Selection	22	91%	99%	99%
Prophylactic Antibiotic Selection (Outpatient)	24	100%	98%	98%
Prophylactic Antibiotic Stopped	22	100%	98%	98%
Prophylactic Antibiotic Timing	22	95%	99%	99%
Prophylactic Antibiotic Timing (Outpatient)	24	96%	98%	98%
Urinary Catheter Removal[7]	-	-	97%	97%
Survey of Patients' Hospital Experiences				
Area Around Room 'Always' Quiet at Night	(a)	68%	67%	61%
Doctors 'Always' Communicated Well	(a)	88%	83%	82%
Home Recovery Information Given	(a)	82%	83%	85%
Hospital Given 9 or 10 on 10 Point Scale	(a)	64%	70%	71%
Meds 'Always' Explained Before Given	(a)	69%	63%	64%
Nurses 'Always' Communicated Well	(a)	78%	79%	79%
Pain 'Always' Well Controlled	(a)	69%	71%	71%
Room and Bathroom 'Always' Clean	(a)	65%	72%	73%
Timely Help 'Always' Received	(a)	71%	68%	68%
Would Definitely Recommend Hospital	(a)	56%	69%	71%
Use of Medical Imaging				
Cardiac Imaging Stress Test before Surgery[1]	-	-	4.3%	5.3%
Combination Abdominal CT Scan	186	4.3%	15.3%	10.5%
Combination Brain/Sinus CT Scan	310	7.1%	2.9%	2.7%
Combination Chest CT Scan	126	1.6%	5%	2.7%
Follow-up Mammogram/Ultrasound	317	8.5%	9.9%	8.8%
Lumbar Spine MRI for Low Back Pain[1]	-	-	41.6%	37.2%

Summit Medical Center

East Main & South 20th Street
Van Buren, AR 72956
URL: www.summitmc.net
Phone: 479-471-4300
Fax: 501-474-4458
Type: Acute Care Hospitals
Emergency Services: Yes
Ownership: Proprietary
Beds: 103

Key Personnel:

Quality Assurance . . . . Mary Jo Brinkman
Operating Room. . . . . Larry Edwards, RN
Intensive Care Unit. . . . . Landon Horton, RN
Radiology. . . . . Shawn Imhoof
Infection Control. . . . . Beth Puckett, RN
Emergency Room . . . . Perryes Stilwell, RN
CEO/President. . . . . Pam Tahan
Chief of Medical Staff. . . . . Brett Whatcott, DO

Measure	Cases	This Hosp.	State Avg.	U.S. Avg.
Blood Clot Prevention and Treatment				
Anticoagulation Overlap Therapy[1,2]	-	-	88%	93%
ICU Venous Thromboembolism Prophylaxis[2]	37	95%	94%	92%
Incidence of Potentially Preventable VTE[2,7]	-	-	12%	10%
UFH with Dosages/Platelet Monitoring[1,2]	-	-	100%	97%
Venous Thromboembolism Prophylaxis[2]	141	81%	91%	85%
Warfarin Therapy Discharge Instructions[1,2]	-	-	76%	75%
Chest Pain/Possible Heart Attack Care				
Aspirin Given Within 24 Hours of Arrival	50	100%	96%	96%
Fibrinolytic Meds Within 30 Min. of Arrival[1]	-	-	54%	58%
Average Time to ECG (minutes)	57	9	8	7
Average Time to Transfer (minutes)[1]	-	-	72	60
Children's Asthma Care				
Received Home Management Plan of Care	-	-	-	88%
Received Reliever Medication	-	-	-	100%
Received Systemic Corticosteroids	-	-	-	100%
Emergency Department				
Admittance Decision Time (minutes)[2]	511	43	65	98
Head CT Results Within 45 Min. of Arrival[1,3]	-	-	49%	57%
Patients Who Left ER Before Being Seen	20,070	2%	3%	2%
Time from ER Arrival to Admit. (minutes)[2]	513	167	214	274
Time from ER Arrival to Discharge (minutes)	532	95	118	134
Time in ER Before Being Evaluated (minutes)	591	31	26	26
Time to Pain Meds for Fractures (minutes)	27	40	66	57
Heart Attack Care				
Aspirin Given at Discharge[1]	-	-	99%	99%
Fibrinolytic Meds Within 30 Min. of Arrival[7]	-	-	77%	54%
PCI Within 90 Minutes of Arrival[7]	-	-	96%	96%
Statin Prescribed at Discharge[1]	-	-	97%	98%
Heart Failure Care				
ACE Inhibitor or ARB for LVSD	17	100%	96%	97%
Discharge Instructions Given	30	100%	95%	94%
Evaluation of LVS Function	40	100%	98%	99%
Medicare Spending				
Medicare Spending per Patient (ratio)	-	1.12	0.98	0.98
Pneumonia Care				
Appropriate Initial Antibiotic Given	49	100%	94%	95%
Blood Culture Timing	86	100%	98%	98%
Pregnancy and Delivery Care				
Newborn Deliveries Scheduled Early[7]	-	-	6%	6%
Preventive Care				
Immunization for Influenza[2]	335	99%	89%	90%
Immunization for Pneumonia[2]	414	98%	92%	92%
Stroke Care				
Anticoagulation Therapy for Atrial Fibrillation[1]	-	-	90%	95%
Antithrombotic Therapy Timing[1]	-	-	96%	98%
Assessed for Rehabilitation[1]	-	-	95%	97%
Discharged on Antithrombotic Therapy[1]	-	-	96%	99%
Discharged on Statin Medication[1]	-	-	86%	94%
Thrombolytic Therapy Timing[1]	-	-	35%	66%
Venous Thromboembolism Prophylaxis	11	73%	91%	94%
Written Stroke Educational Materials Given[1]	-	-	81%	88%
Surgical Care Improvement Project				
Appropriate Beta Blocker Usage[1]	-	-	98%	98%
Appropriate VTP Within 24 Hours	29	93%	98%	98%
Controlled Postoperative Blood Glucose[7]	-	-	99%	97%
Perioperative Temperature Management	36	100%	100%	100%
Prophylactic Antibiotic Selection	17	100%	99%	99%
Prophylactic Antibiotic Selection (Outpatient)	20	95%	98%	98%
Prophylactic Antibiotic Stopped	17	100%	98%	98%
Prophylactic Antibiotic Timing	17	100%	99%	99%
Prophylactic Antibiotic Timing (Outpatient)	20	100%	98%	98%
Urinary Catheter Removal	14	93%	97%	97%
Survey of Patients' Hospital Experiences				
Area Around Room 'Always' Quiet at Night	(a)	66%	67%	61%
Doctors 'Always' Communicated Well	(a)	81%	83%	82%
Home Recovery Information Given	(a)	84%	83%	85%
Hospital Given 9 or 10 on 10 Point Scale	(a)	64%	70%	71%
Meds 'Always' Explained Before Given	(a)	68%	63%	64%
Nurses 'Always' Communicated Well	(a)	81%	79%	79%
Pain 'Always' Well Controlled	(a)	72%	71%	71%
Room and Bathroom 'Always' Clean	(a)	75%	72%	73%
Timely Help 'Always' Received	(a)	72%	68%	68%
Would Definitely Recommend Hospital	(a)	66%	69%	71%
Use of Medical Imaging				
Cardiac Imaging Stress Test before Surgery[1]	-	-	4.3%	5.3%
Combination Abdominal CT Scan	187	21.4%	15.3%	10.5%
Combination Brain/Sinus CT Scan[1]	-	-	2.9%	2.7%
Combination Chest CT Scan[1]	-	-	5%	2.7%
Follow-up Mammogram/Ultrasound	97	15.5%	9.9%	8.8%
Lumbar Spine MRI for Low Back Pain[1]	-	-	41.6%	37.2%

Saint Edward Health Facilities of Scott County

1341 West Sixth Street
Waldron, AR 72958
Phone: 479-637-4135
Fax: 501-637-3523
Type: Critical Access Hospitals
Emergency Services: Yes
Ownership: Voluntary non-profit - Private
Beds: 24

Key Personnel:

Chief of Medical Staff. . . . . Nathan Bennett, DO
Operating Room. . . . . Bonnie Gray
CEO/President. . . . . Dorothy O'Bar, RN
Emergency Room . . . . Dorothy O'Bar, RN
Quality Assurance . . . . Dorothy O'Bar, RN

Measure	Cases	This Hosp.	State Avg.	U.S. Avg.
Blood Clot Prevention and Treatment				
Anticoagulation Overlap Therapy[5]	-	-	88%	93%
ICU Venous Thromboembolism Prophylaxis[5]	-	-	94%	92%
Incidence of Potentially Preventable VTE[5]	-	-	12%	10%
UFH with Dosages/Platelet Monitoring[5]	-	-	100%	97%
Venous Thromboembolism Prophylaxis[5]	-	-	91%	85%
Warfarin Therapy Discharge Instructions[5]	-	-	76%	75%
Chest Pain/Possible Heart Attack Care				
Aspirin Given Within 24 Hours of Arrival	-	-	96%	96%
Fibrinolytic Meds Within 30 Min. of Arrival	-	-	54%	58%
Average Time to ECG (minutes)	-	-	8	7
Average Time to Transfer (minutes)	-	-	72	60
Children's Asthma Care				
Received Home Management Plan of Care	-	-	-	88%
Received Reliever Medication	-	-	-	100%
Received Systemic Corticosteroids	-	-	-	100%
Emergency Department				
Admittance Decision Time (minutes)[5]	-	-	65	98
Head CT Results Within 45 Min. of Arrival	-	-	49%	57%
Patients Who Left ER Before Being Seen	-	-	3%	2%
Time from ER Arrival to Admit. (minutes)[5]	-	-	214	274
Time from ER Arrival to Discharge (minutes)	-	-	118	134
Time in ER Before Being Evaluated (minutes)	-	-	26	26
Time to Pain Meds for Fractures (minutes)	-	-	66	57
Heart Attack Care				
Aspirin Given at Discharge[1,3]	-	-	99%	99%
Fibrinolytic Meds Within 30 Min. of Arrival[3,7]	-	-	77%	54%
PCI Within 90 Minutes of Arrival[3,7]	-	-	96%	96%
Statin Prescribed at Discharge[1,3]	-	-	97%	98%
Heart Failure Care				
ACE Inhibitor or ARB for LVSD[1]	-	-	96%	97%
Discharge Instructions Given	20	95%	95%	94%
Evaluation of LVS Function	23	74%	98%	99%
Medicare Spending				
Medicare Spending per Patient (ratio)	-	-	0.98	0.98
Pneumonia Care				
Appropriate Initial Antibiotic Given	34	88%	94%	95%
Blood Culture Timing	37	89%	98%	98%
Pregnancy and Delivery Care				
Newborn Deliveries Scheduled Early[3,7]	-	-	6%	6%
Preventive Care				
Immunization for Influenza[5]	-	-	89%	90%
Immunization for Pneumonia[5]	-	-	92%	92%
Stroke Care				
Anticoagulation Therapy for Atrial Fibrillation[5]	-	-	90%	95%
Antithrombotic Therapy Timing[5]	-	-	96%	98%
Assessed for Rehabilitation[5]	-	-	95%	97%
Discharged on Antithrombotic Therapy[5]	-	-	96%	99%

NOTE: Hospital profiles are in alphabetical order by state, then city, then hospital within the city; Rankings exclude hospitals with less than 25 cases except for patient surveys which excludes hospitals with less than 100 cases; (a) 100-299 cases; (1) The number of cases/patients is too few to report; (2) Data submitted were based on a sample of cases/patients; (3) Results are based on a shorter time period than required; (4) Data suppressed by CMS for one or more quarters; (5) Results are not available for this reporting period; (6) Fewer than 100 patients completed the HCAHPS survey; (7) No cases met the criteria for this measure; (8) The lower limit of the confidence interval cannot be calculated if the number of observed infections equals zero; (9) No data are available from the state/territory for this reporting period; (10) The scores shown reflect fewer than 50 completed surveys; (11) There were discrepancies in the data collection process; (12) This measure does not apply to this hospital for this reporting period; (13) Results cannot be calculated for this reporting period; (14) The results for this state are combined with nearby states to protect confidentiality; Please refer to the User's Guide for a full explanation of data.

Measure	Cases	This Hosp.	State Avg.	U.S. Avg.
Discharged on Statin Medication[5]	-	-	86%	94%
Thrombolytic Therapy Timing[5]	-	-	35%	66%
Venous Thromboembolism Prophylaxis[5]	-	-	91%	94%
Written Stroke Educational Materials Given[5]	-	-	81%	88%
Surgical Care Improvement Project				
Appropriate Beta Blocker Usage[5]	-	-	98%	98%
Appropriate VTP Within 24 Hours[5]	-	-	98%	98%
Controlled Postoperative Blood Glucose[5]	-	-	99%	97%
Perioperative Temperature Management[5]	-	-	100%	100%
Prophylactic Antibiotic Selection[5]	-	-	99%	99%
Prophylactic Antibiotic Selection (Outpatient)	-	-	98%	98%
Prophylactic Antibiotic Stopped[5]	-	-	98%	98%
Prophylactic Antibiotic Timing[5]	-	-	99%	99%
Prophylactic Antibiotic Timing (Outpatient)	-	-	98%	98%
Urinary Catheter Removal[5]	-	-	97%	97%
Survey of Patients' Hospital Experiences				
Area Around Room 'Always' Quiet at Night[5]	-	-	67%	61%
Doctors 'Always' Communicated Well[5]	-	-	83%	82%
Home Recovery Information Given[5]	-	-	83%	85%
Hospital Given 9 or 10 on 10 Point Scale[5]	-	-	70%	71%
Meds 'Always' Explained Before Given[5]	-	-	63%	64%
Nurses 'Always' Communicated Well[5]	-	-	79%	79%
Pain 'Always' Well Controlled[5]	-	-	71%	71%
Room and Bathroom 'Always' Clean[5]	-	-	72%	73%
Timely Help 'Always' Received[5]	-	-	68%	68%
Would Definitely Recommend Hospital[5]	-	-	69%	71%
Use of Medical Imaging				
Cardiac Imaging Stress Test before Surgery	-	-	4.3%	5.3%
Combination Abdominal CT Scan	-	-	15.3%	10.5%
Combination Brain/Sinus CT Scan	-	-	2.9%	2.7%
Combination Chest CT Scan	-	-	5%	2.7%
Follow-up Mammogram/Ultrasound	-	-	9.9%	8.8%
Lumbar Spine MRI for Low Back Pain	-	-	41.6%	37.2%

Lawrence Memorial Hospital

1309 West Main
Walnut Ridge, AR 72476
Phone: 870-886-1200
Fax: 870-886-5340
E-mail: beagan@lawrencehealth.net
URL: www.lawrencehealth.net
Type: Critical Access Hospitals
Emergency Services: Yes
Ownership: Government - Local
Beds: 195

Key Personnel:
Quality Assurance .... Junior Briner
Emergency Room .... Dennise Chadwick
Intensive Care Unit............ D Cousins
President .... George Fray
Infection Control............. Teresa Milam
Radiology.................. Bill Rex
Operating Room.............. Susan Simmons
Chief of Medical Staff.......... Paul Vellozo

Measure	Cases	This Hosp.	State Avg.	U.S. Avg.
Blood Clot Prevention and Treatment				
Anticoagulation Overlap Therapy[5]	-	-	88%	93%
ICU Venous Thromboembolism Prophylaxis[5]	-	-	94%	92%
Incidence of Potentially Preventable VTE[5]	-	-	12%	10%
UFH with Dosages/Platelet Monitoring[5]	-	-	100%	97%
Venous Thromboembolism Prophylaxis[5]	-	-	91%	85%
Warfarin Therapy Discharge Instructions[5]	-	-	76%	75%
Chest Pain/Possible Heart Attack Care				
Aspirin Given Within 24 Hours of Arrival	-	-	96%	96%
Fibrinolytic Meds Within 30 Min. of Arrival	-	-	54%	58%
Average Time to ECG (minutes)	-	-	8	7
Average Time to Transfer (minutes)	-	-	72	60
Children's Asthma Care				
Received Home Management Plan of Care	-	-	-	88%
Received Reliever Medication	-	-	-	100%
Received Systemic Corticosteroids	-	-	-	100%
Emergency Department				
Admittance Decision Time (minutes)[5]	-	-	65	98
Head CT Results Within 45 Min. of Arrival	-	-	49%	57%
Patients Who Left ER Before Being Seen	-	-	3%	2%
Time from ER Arrival to Admit. (minutes)[5]	-	-	214	274
Time from ER Arrival to Discharge (minutes)	-	-	118	134
Time in ER Before Being Evaluated (minutes)	-	-	26	26
Time to Pain Meds for Fractures (minutes)	-	-	66	57
Heart Attack Care				
Aspirin Given at Discharge[5]	-	-	99%	99%
Fibrinolytic Meds Within 30 Min. of Arrival[5]	-	-	77%	54%
PCI Within 90 Minutes of Arrival[5]	-	-	96%	96%
Statin Prescribed at Discharge[5]	-	-	97%	98%
Heart Failure Care				
ACE Inhibitor or ARB for LVSD[1]	-	-	96%	97%
Discharge Instructions Given[1]	-	-	95%	94%
Evaluation of LVS Function	18	100%	98%	99%
Medicare Spending				
Medicare Spending per Patient (ratio)	-	-	0.98	0.98
Pneumonia Care				
Appropriate Initial Antibiotic Given	30	100%	94%	95%
Blood Culture Timing	39	100%	98%	98%
Pregnancy and Delivery Care				
Newborn Deliveries Scheduled Early[5]	-	-	6%	6%
Preventive Care				
Immunization for Influenza[5]	-	-	89%	90%
Immunization for Pneumonia[5]	-	-	92%	92%
Stroke Care				
Anticoagulation Therapy for Atrial Fibrillation[5]	-	-	90%	95%
Antithrombotic Therapy Timing[5]	-	-	96%	98%
Assessed for Rehabilitation[5]	-	-	95%	97%
Discharged on Antithrombotic Therapy[5]	-	-	96%	99%
Discharged on Statin Medication[5]	-	-	86%	94%
Thrombolytic Therapy Timing[5]	-	-	35%	66%
Venous Thromboembolism Prophylaxis[5]	-	-	91%	94%
Written Stroke Educational Materials Given[5]	-	-	81%	88%
Surgical Care Improvement Project				
Appropriate Beta Blocker Usage[5]	-	-	98%	98%
Appropriate VTP Within 24 Hours[5]	-	-	98%	98%
Controlled Postoperative Blood Glucose[5]	-	-	99%	97%
Perioperative Temperature Management[5]	-	-	100%	100%
Prophylactic Antibiotic Selection[5]	-	-	99%	99%
Prophylactic Antibiotic Selection (Outpatient)	-	-	98%	98%
Prophylactic Antibiotic Stopped[5]	-	-	98%	98%
Prophylactic Antibiotic Timing[5]	-	-	99%	99%
Prophylactic Antibiotic Timing (Outpatient)	-	-	98%	98%
Urinary Catheter Removal[5]	-	-	97%	97%
Survey of Patients' Hospital Experiences				
Area Around Room 'Always' Quiet at Night[5]	-	-	67%	61%
Doctors 'Always' Communicated Well[5]	-	-	83%	82%
Home Recovery Information Given[5]	-	-	83%	85%
Hospital Given 9 or 10 on 10 Point Scale[5]	-	-	70%	71%
Meds 'Always' Explained Before Given[5]	-	-	63%	64%
Nurses 'Always' Communicated Well[5]	-	-	79%	79%
Pain 'Always' Well Controlled[5]	-	-	71%	71%
Room and Bathroom 'Always' Clean[5]	-	-	72%	73%
Timely Help 'Always' Received[5]	-	-	68%	68%
Would Definitely Recommend Hospital[5]	-	-	69%	71%
Use of Medical Imaging				
Cardiac Imaging Stress Test before Surgery	-	-	4.3%	5.3%
Combination Abdominal CT Scan	-	-	15.3%	10.5%
Combination Brain/Sinus CT Scan	-	-	2.9%	2.7%
Combination Chest CT Scan	-	-	5%	2.7%
Follow-up Mammogram/Ultrasound	-	-	9.9%	8.8%
Lumbar Spine MRI for Low Back Pain	-	-	41.6%	37.2%

Bradley County Medical Center

404 South Bradley Street
Warren, AR 71671
Phone: 870-226-3731
Fax: 870-226-7049
URL: www.bradleycountymedicalcenter.com
Type: Critical Access Hospitals
Emergency Services: Yes
Ownership: Voluntary non-profit - Private
Beds: 49

Key Personnel:
Operating Room.............. Kathy Hall, RN
CEO .... Rex Jones
Radiology.................. Charlotte Laster
Chief of Medical Staff.......... James W Marsh, MD
CEO/President............... Harold Mitchell
Chairman/CEO .... Freddie Mobley
Quality Assurance .... Lucille Shank
Emergency Room .... Page Stell, RN

Measure	Cases	This Hosp.	State Avg.	U.S. Avg.
Blood Clot Prevention and Treatment				
Anticoagulation Overlap Therapy[5]	-	-	88%	93%
ICU Venous Thromboembolism Prophylaxis[5]	-	-	94%	92%
Incidence of Potentially Preventable VTE[5]	-	-	12%	10%
UFH with Dosages/Platelet Monitoring[5]	-	-	100%	97%
Venous Thromboembolism Prophylaxis[5]	-	-	91%	85%
Warfarin Therapy Discharge Instructions[5]	-	-	76%	75%
Chest Pain/Possible Heart Attack Care				
Aspirin Given Within 24 Hours of Arrival	-	-	96%	96%
Fibrinolytic Meds Within 30 Min. of Arrival	-	-	54%	58%
Average Time to ECG (minutes)	-	-	8	7
Average Time to Transfer (minutes)	-	-	72	60
Children's Asthma Care				
Received Home Management Plan of Care	-	-	-	88%
Received Reliever Medication	-	-	-	100%
Received Systemic Corticosteroids	-	-	-	100%
Emergency Department				
Admittance Decision Time (minutes)[5]	-	-	65	98
Head CT Results Within 45 Min. of Arrival	-	-	49%	57%
Patients Who Left ER Before Being Seen	-	-	3%	2%
Time from ER Arrival to Admit. (minutes)[5]	-	-	214	274
Time from ER Arrival to Discharge (minutes)	-	-	118	134
Time in ER Before Being Evaluated (minutes)	-	-	26	26
Time to Pain Meds for Fractures (minutes)	-	-	66	57
Heart Attack Care				
Aspirin Given at Discharge[5]	-	-	99%	99%
Fibrinolytic Meds Within 30 Min. of Arrival[5]	-	-	77%	54%
PCI Within 90 Minutes of Arrival[5]	-	-	96%	96%
Statin Prescribed at Discharge[5]	-	-	97%	98%
Heart Failure Care				
ACE Inhibitor or ARB for LVSD[1]	-	-	96%	97%
Discharge Instructions Given	11	91%	95%	94%
Evaluation of LVS Function	20	60%	98%	99%
Medicare Spending				
Medicare Spending per Patient (ratio)	-	-	0.98	0.98
Pneumonia Care				
Appropriate Initial Antibiotic Given	54	98%	94%	95%
Blood Culture Timing	22	95%	98%	98%
Pregnancy and Delivery Care				
Newborn Deliveries Scheduled Early[5]	-	-	6%	6%
Preventive Care				
Immunization for Influenza[5]	-	-	89%	90%
Immunization for Pneumonia[5]	-	-	92%	92%
Stroke Care				
Anticoagulation Therapy for Atrial Fibrillation[5]	-	-	90%	95%
Antithrombotic Therapy Timing[5]	-	-	96%	98%
Assessed for Rehabilitation[5]	-	-	95%	97%
Discharged on Antithrombotic Therapy[5]	-	-	96%	99%
Discharged on Statin Medication[5]	-	-	86%	94%
Thrombolytic Therapy Timing[5]	-	-	35%	66%
Venous Thromboembolism Prophylaxis[5]	-	-	91%	94%
Written Stroke Educational Materials Given[5]	-	-	81%	88%
Surgical Care Improvement Project				
Appropriate Beta Blocker Usage[5]	-	-	98%	98%
Appropriate VTP Within 24 Hours[5]	-	-	98%	98%
Controlled Postoperative Blood Glucose[5]	-	-	99%	97%
Perioperative Temperature Management[5]	-	-	100%	100%
Prophylactic Antibiotic Selection[5]	-	-	99%	99%
Prophylactic Antibiotic Selection (Outpatient)	-	-	98%	98%
Prophylactic Antibiotic Stopped[5]	-	-	98%	98%
Prophylactic Antibiotic Timing[5]	-	-	99%	99%
Prophylactic Antibiotic Timing (Outpatient)	-	-	98%	98%
Urinary Catheter Removal[5]	-	-	97%	97%
Survey of Patients' Hospital Experiences				
Area Around Room 'Always' Quiet at Night[5]	-	-	67%	61%
Doctors 'Always' Communicated Well[5]	-	-	83%	82%
Home Recovery Information Given[5]	-	-	83%	85%
Hospital Given 9 or 10 on 10 Point Scale[5]	-	-	70%	71%
Meds 'Always' Explained Before Given[5]	-	-	63%	64%
Nurses 'Always' Communicated Well[5]	-	-	79%	79%
Pain 'Always' Well Controlled[5]	-	-	71%	71%

NOTE: Hospital profiles are in alphabetical order by state, then city, then hospital within the city; Rankings exclude hospitals with less than 25 cases except for patient surveys which excludes hospitals with less than 100 cases; (a) 100-299 cases; (1) The number of cases/patients is too few to report; (2) Data submitted were based on a sample of cases/patients; (3) Results are based on a shorter time period than required; (4) Data suppressed by CMS for one or more quarters; (5) Results are not available for this reporting period; (6) Fewer than 100 patients completed the HCAHPS survey; (7) No cases met the criteria for this measure; (8) The lower limit of the confidence interval cannot be calculated if the number of observed infections equals zero; (9) No data are available from the state/territory for this reporting period; (10) The scores shown reflect fewer than 50 completed surveys; (11) There were discrepancies in the data collection process; (12) This measure does not apply to this hospital for this reporting period; (13) Results cannot be calculated for this reporting period; (14) The results for this state are combined with nearby states to protect confidentiality; Please refer to the User's Guide for a full explanation of data.

Measure	Cases	This Hosp.	State Avg.	U.S. Avg.
Room and Bathroom 'Always' Clean[5]	-	-	72%	73%
Timely Help 'Always' Received[5]	-	-	68%	68%
Would Definitely Recommend Hospital[5]	-	-	69%	71%
Use of Medical Imaging				
Cardiac Imaging Stress Test before Surgery	-	-	4.3%	5.3%
Combination Abdominal CT Scan	-	-	15.3%	10.5%
Combination Brain/Sinus CT Scan	-	-	2.9%	2.7%
Combination Chest CT Scan	-	-	5%	2.7%
Follow-up Mammogram/Ultrasound	-	-	9.9%	8.8%
Lumbar Spine MRI for Low Back Pain	-	-	41.6%	37.2%

Crittenden Memorial Hospital

200 Tyler
West Memphis, AR 72301
Phone: 870-735-1500
Fax: 870-732-7710
URL: www.crittendenmemorial.org
Type: Acute Care Hospitals
Emergency Services: Yes
Ownership: Voluntary non-profit - Private
Beds: 152

Key Personnel:

CEO .... Gene Cashman
Emergency Room .... Lance Herrell
CEO/President............... Ross Hooper
Chief of Medical Staff.......... Paul J Huffstutter, MD
Quality Assurance .... Nancy Hunter
Intensive Care Unit.......... Donna Lanier
Cardiac Laboratory............ Frank Martin, MD
Infection Control.............. Laura Staveley

Measure	Cases	This Hosp.	State Avg.	U.S. Avg.
Blood Clot Prevention and Treatment				
Anticoagulation Overlap Therapy[2]	25	92%	88%	93%
ICU Venous Thromboembolism Prophylaxis[2]	69	100%	94%	92%
Incidence of Potentially Preventable VTE[1,2]	-	-	12%	10%
UFH with Dosages/Platelet Monitoring[2]	19	100%	100%	97%
Venous Thromboembolism Prophylaxis[2]	231	92%	91%	85%
Warfarin Therapy Discharge Instructions[2]	15	27%	76%	75%
Chest Pain/Possible Heart Attack Care				
Aspirin Given Within 24 Hours of Arrival	53	94%	96%	96%
Fibrinolytic Meds Within 30 Min. of Arrival[7]	-	-	54%	58%
Average Time to ECG (minutes)	54	6	8	7
Average Time to Transfer (minutes)[1]	-	-	72	60
Children's Asthma Care				
Received Home Management Plan of Care	-	-	-	88%
Received Reliever Medication	-	-	-	100%
Received Systemic Corticosteroids	-	-	-	100%
Emergency Department				
Admittance Decision Time (minutes)[2]	360	68	65	98
Head CT Results Within 45 Min. of Arrival	16	12%	49%	57%
Patients Who Left ER Before Being Seen	24,260	3%	3%	2%
Time from ER Arrival to Admit. (minutes)[2]	365	240	214	274
Time from ER Arrival to Discharge (minutes)	255	115	118	134
Time in ER Before Being Evaluated (minutes)	363	18	26	26
Time to Pain Meds for Fractures (minutes)	85	70	66	57
Heart Attack Care				
Aspirin Given at Discharge	13	85%	99%	99%
Fibrinolytic Meds Within 30 Min. of Arrival[7]	-	-	77%	54%
PCI Within 90 Minutes of Arrival[7]	-	-	96%	96%
Statin Prescribed at Discharge	13	100%	97%	98%
Heart Failure Care				
ACE Inhibitor or ARB for LVSD	59	100%	96%	97%
Discharge Instructions Given	129	100%	95%	94%
Evaluation of LVS Function	144	100%	98%	99%
Medicare Spending				
Medicare Spending per Patient (ratio)	-	1.04	0.98	0.98
Pneumonia Care				
Appropriate Initial Antibiotic Given[2]	53	94%	94%	95%
Blood Culture Timing[2]	127	99%	98%	98%
Pregnancy and Delivery Care				
Newborn Deliveries Scheduled Early[2]	39	5%	6%	6%
Preventive Care				
Immunization for Influenza[2]	340	74%	89%	90%
Immunization for Pneumonia[2]	394	90%	92%	92%
Stroke Care				
Anticoagulation Therapy for Atrial Fibrillation[1]	-	-	90%	95%
Antithrombotic Therapy Timing	21	90%	96%	98%
Assessed for Rehabilitation	22	91%	95%	97%
Discharged on Antithrombotic Therapy	22	100%	96%	99%
Discharged on Statin Medication	20	85%	86%	94%
Thrombolytic Therapy Timing[1]	-	-	35%	66%
Venous Thromboembolism Prophylaxis	20	90%	91%	94%
Written Stroke Educational Materials Given	14	0%	81%	88%
Surgical Care Improvement Project				
Appropriate Beta Blocker Usage[2]	21	95%	98%	98%
Appropriate VTP Within 24 Hours[2]	101	98%	98%	98%
Controlled Postoperative Blood Glucose[2,7]	-	-	99%	97%
Perioperative Temperature Management[2]	120	100%	100%	100%
Prophylactic Antibiotic Selection[2]	68	96%	99%	99%
Prophylactic Antibiotic Selection (Outpatient)	60	95%	98%	98%
Prophylactic Antibiotic Stopped[2]	67	94%	98%	98%
Prophylactic Antibiotic Timing[2]	68	94%	99%	99%
Prophylactic Antibiotic Timing (Outpatient)	61	93%	98%	98%
Urinary Catheter Removal[2]	68	84%	97%	97%
Survey of Patients' Hospital Experiences				
Area Around Room 'Always' Quiet at Night	300+	70%	67%	61%
Doctors 'Always' Communicated Well	300+	83%	83%	82%
Home Recovery Information Given	300+	83%	83%	85%
Hospital Given 9 or 10 on 10 Point Scale	300+	65%	70%	71%
Meds 'Always' Explained Before Given	300+	64%	63%	64%
Nurses 'Always' Communicated Well	300+	78%	79%	79%
Pain 'Always' Well Controlled	300+	69%	71%	71%
Room and Bathroom 'Always' Clean	300+	66%	72%	73%
Timely Help 'Always' Received	300+	65%	68%	68%
Would Definitely Recommend Hospital	300+	59%	69%	71%
Use of Medical Imaging				
Cardiac Imaging Stress Test before Surgery	115	7.0%	4.3%	5.3%
Combination Abdominal CT Scan	366	18.3%	15.3%	10.5%
Combination Brain/Sinus CT Scan	515	3.9%	2.9%	2.7%
Combination Chest CT Scan	238	4.2%	5%	2.7%
Follow-up Mammogram/Ultrasound	356	12.1%	9.9%	8.8%
Lumbar Spine MRI for Low Back Pain	63	41.3%	41.6%	37.2%

Crossridge Community Hospital

310 South Falls Boulevard
Wynne, AR 72396
Phone: 870-238-3300
Fax: 870-238-7432
Type: Critical Access Hospitals
Emergency Services: Yes
Ownership: Voluntary non-profit - Private
Beds: 25

Key Personnel:

Radiology.................... Adam Cabell
Quality Assurance .... Pat Hamilton

Measure	Cases	This Hosp.	State Avg.	U.S. Avg.
Blood Clot Prevention and Treatment				
Anticoagulation Overlap Therapy[5]	-	-	88%	93%
ICU Venous Thromboembolism Prophylaxis[5]	-	-	94%	92%
Incidence of Potentially Preventable VTE[5]	-	-	12%	10%
UFH with Dosages/Platelet Monitoring[5]	-	-	100%	97%
Venous Thromboembolism Prophylaxis[5]	-	-	91%	85%
Warfarin Therapy Discharge Instructions[5]	-	-	76%	75%
Chest Pain/Possible Heart Attack Care				
Aspirin Given Within 24 Hours of Arrival	27	100%	96%	96%
Fibrinolytic Meds Within 30 Min. of Arrival[1]	-	-	54%	58%
Average Time to ECG (minutes)	27	2	8	7
Average Time to Transfer (minutes)	12	61	72	60
Children's Asthma Care				
Received Home Management Plan of Care	-	-	-	88%
Received Reliever Medication	-	-	-	100%
Received Systemic Corticosteroids	-	-	-	100%
Emergency Department				
Admittance Decision Time (minutes)[5]	-	-	65	98
Head CT Results Within 45 Min. of Arrival[5]	-	-	49%	57%
Patients Who Left ER Before Being Seen	9,012	1%	3%	2%
Time from ER Arrival to Admit. (minutes)[5]	-	-	214	274
Time from ER Arrival to Discharge (minutes)[5]	-	-	118	134
Time in ER Before Being Evaluated (minutes)[5]	-	-	26	26
Time to Pain Meds for Fractures (minutes)[5]	-	-	66	57
Heart Attack Care				
Aspirin Given at Discharge[5]	-	-	99%	99%
Fibrinolytic Meds Within 30 Min. of Arrival[5]	-	-	77%	54%
PCI Within 90 Minutes of Arrival[5]	-	-	96%	96%
Statin Prescribed at Discharge[5]	-	-	97%	98%
Heart Failure Care				
ACE Inhibitor or ARB for LVSD[1]	-	-	96%	97%
Discharge Instructions Given	19	100%	95%	94%
Evaluation of LVS Function	29	100%	98%	99%
Medicare Spending				
Medicare Spending per Patient (ratio)	-	-	0.98	0.98
Pneumonia Care				
Appropriate Initial Antibiotic Given	79	99%	94%	95%
Blood Culture Timing	34	100%	98%	98%
Pregnancy and Delivery Care				
Newborn Deliveries Scheduled Early[5]	-	-	6%	6%
Preventive Care				
Immunization for Influenza[5]	-	-	89%	90%
Immunization for Pneumonia[5]	-	-	92%	92%
Stroke Care				
Anticoagulation Therapy for Atrial Fibrillation[5]	-	-	90%	95%
Antithrombotic Therapy Timing[5]	-	-	96%	98%
Assessed for Rehabilitation[5]	-	-	95%	97%
Discharged on Antithrombotic Therapy[5]	-	-	96%	99%
Discharged on Statin Medication[5]	-	-	86%	94%
Thrombolytic Therapy Timing[5]	-	-	35%	66%
Venous Thromboembolism Prophylaxis[5]	-	-	91%	94%
Written Stroke Educational Materials Given[5]	-	-	81%	88%
Surgical Care Improvement Project				
Appropriate Beta Blocker Usage[5]	-	-	98%	98%
Appropriate VTP Within 24 Hours[5]	-	-	98%	98%
Controlled Postoperative Blood Glucose[5]	-	-	99%	97%
Perioperative Temperature Management[5]	-	-	100%	100%
Prophylactic Antibiotic Selection[5]	-	-	99%	99%
Prophylactic Antibiotic Selection (Outpatient)[5]	-	-	98%	98%
Prophylactic Antibiotic Stopped[5]	-	-	98%	98%
Prophylactic Antibiotic Timing[5]	-	-	99%	99%
Prophylactic Antibiotic Timing (Outpatient)[5]	-	-	98%	98%
Urinary Catheter Removal[5]	-	-	97%	97%
Survey of Patients' Hospital Experiences				
Area Around Room 'Always' Quiet at Night[5]	-	-	67%	61%
Doctors 'Always' Communicated Well[5]	-	-	83%	82%
Home Recovery Information Given[5]	-	-	83%	85%
Hospital Given 9 or 10 on 10 Point Scale[5]	-	-	70%	71%
Meds 'Always' Explained Before Given[5]	-	-	63%	64%
Nurses 'Always' Communicated Well[5]	-	-	79%	79%
Pain 'Always' Well Controlled[5]	-	-	71%	71%
Room and Bathroom 'Always' Clean[5]	-	-	72%	73%
Timely Help 'Always' Received[5]	-	-	68%	68%
Would Definitely Recommend Hospital[5]	-	-	69%	71%
Use of Medical Imaging				
Cardiac Imaging Stress Test before Surgery[7]	-	-	4.3%	5.3%
Combination Abdominal CT Scan	169	16.6%	15.3%	10.5%
Combination Brain/Sinus CT Scan	228	5.7%	2.9%	2.7%
Combination Chest CT Scan	107	18.7%	5%	2.7%
Follow-up Mammogram/Ultrasound	179	4.5%	9.9%	8.8%
Lumbar Spine MRI for Low Back Pain[1]	-	-	41.6%	37.2%

NOTE: Hospital profiles are in alphabetical order by state, then city, then hospital within the city; Rankings exclude hospitals with less than 25 cases except for patient surveys which excludes hospitals with less than 100 cases; (a) 100-299 cases; (1) The number of cases/patients is too few to report; (2) Data submitted were based on a sample of cases/patients; (3) Results are based on a shorter time period than required; (4) Data suppressed by CMS for one or more quarters; (5) Results are not available for this reporting period; (6) Fewer than 100 patients completed the HCAHPS survey; (7) No cases met the criteria for this measure; (8) The lower limit of the confidence interval cannot be calculated if the number of observed infections equals zero; (9) No data are available from the state/territory for this reporting period; (10) The scores shown reflect fewer than 50 completed surveys; (11) There were discrepancies in the data collection process; (12) This measure does not apply to this hospital for this reporting period; (13) Results cannot be calculated for this reporting period; (14) The results for this state are combined with nearby states to protect confidentiality; Please refer to the User's Guide for a full explanation of data.

Blood Clot Prevention and Treatment

Anticoagulation Overlap Therapy

Hospital Name	City	Rate	Cases
Baptist Hospital of Miami[2]	Miami	100%	87
Boca Raton Regional Hospital[2]	Boca Raton	100%	129
Broward Health Coral Springs[2]	Coral Springs	100%	66
Capital Regional Medical Center[2]	Tallahassee	100%	75
Central Florida Regional Hospital[2]	Sanford	100%	70
Delray Medical Center[2]	Delray Beach	100%	114
Edward White Hospital[2]	St Petersburg	100%	26
Fawcett Memorial Hospital[2]	Port Charlotte	100%	134
Florida Hospital Flagler[2]	Palm Coast	100%	71
Florida Hospital North Pinellas[2]	Tarpon Springs	100%	28
Florida Hospital Waterman[2]	Tavares	100%	115
Fort Walton Beach Medical Center[2]	Fort Walton Bch	100%	43
Health Central[2]	Ocoee	100%	86
Holmes Regional Medical Center[2]	Melbourne	100%	218
Homestead Hospital[2]	Homestead	100%	53
Jupiter Medical Center[2]	Jupiter	100%	125
Lake City Medical Center[2]	Lake City	100%	27
Lake Wales Medical Center[2]	Lake Wales	100%	47
Lower Keys Medical Center[2]	Key West	100%	30
Memorial Hospital Pembroke[2]	Pembroke Pines	100%	57
Memorial Hospital West[2]	Pembroke Pines	100%	132
Memorial Regional Hospital[2]	Hollywood	100%	159
North Florida Regional Medical Center[2]	Gainesville	100%	115
Orange Park Medical Center[2]	Orange Park	100%	113
Palmetto General Hospital[2]	Hialeah	100%	53
Raulerson Hospital[2]	Okeechobee	100%	32
Regional Medical Center Bayonet Point[2]	Hudson	100%	83
Sacred Heart Hosp-Emerald Coast[2]	Miramar Beach	100%	31
Saint Lucie Medical Center[2]	Port Saint Lucie	100%	125
Saint Mary's Medical Center[2]	W Palm Beach	100%	45
Sebastian River Medical Center[2]	Sebastian	100%	39
South Miami Hospital[2]	South Miami	100%	63
Town & Country Hospital[2]	Tampa	100%	26
Venice Reg Med Ctr-Bayfront Health[2]	Venice	100%	115
Viera Hospital[2]	Melbourne	100%	48
Wellington Regional Medical Center[2]	Wellington	100%	52
West Boca Medical Center[2]	Boca Raton	100%	46
West Kendall Baptist Hospital[2]	Miami	100%	31
Brandon Regional Hospital[2]	Brandon	99%	199
Florida Hospital Heartland Medical Center[2]	Sebring	99%	69
Good Samaritan Medical Center[2]	W Palm Beach	99%	72
Kendall Regional Medical Center[2]	Miami	99%	77
Lakeland Regional Medical Center[2]	Lakeland	99%	303
Lawnwood Reg Med Ctr & Heart Inst[2]	Fort Pierce	99%	107
Oak Hill Hospital[2]	Brooksville	99%	132
Sacred Heart Hospital[2]	Pensacola	99%	95
Saint Vincent's Medical Center[2]	Jacksonville	99%	139
Sarasota Memorial Hospital[2]	Sarasota	99%	126
South Bay Hospital[2]	Sun City Center	99%	73
Cleveland Clinic Hospital[2]	Weston	98%	41
Doctors Hospital of Sarasota[2]	Sarasota	98%	61
Flagler Hospital[2]	St Augustine	98%	88
Gulf Coast Regional Medical Center[2]	Panama City	98%	62
Holy Cross Hospital[2]	Fort Lauderdale	98%	45
Largo Medical Center[2]	Largo	98%	123
Saint Petersburg General Hospital[2]	St Petersburg	98%	51
Aventura Hospital & Medical Center[2]	Aventura	97%	154
Bay Med Ctr Sacred Heart Health Sys[2]	Panama City	97%	79
Blake Medical Center[2]	Bradenton	97%	126
Florida Hospital Tampa[2]	Tampa	97%	107
Florida Hospital Zephyrhills[2]	Zephyrhills	97%	32
JFK Medical Center[2]	Atlantis	97%	196
Medical Center of Trinity[2]	Trinity	97%	67
Northside Hospital[2]	St Petersburg	97%	58
Ocala Regional Medical Center[2]	Ocala	97%	158
Palm Bay Hospital[2]	Palm Bay	97%	75
Physicians Reg Med Ctr-Pine Ridge[2]	Naples	97%	104
Plantation General Hospital[2]	Plantation	97%	92
Saint Vincent's Medical Center Southside[2]	Jacksonville	97%	78
University Hospital & Medical Center[2]	Tamarac	97%	34
Florida Hospital[2]	Orlando	96%	476
Florida Hospital Memorial Medical Center[2]	Daytona Bch	96%	103
Manatee Memorial Hospital[2]	Bradenton	96%	106
Martin Medical Center[2]	Stuart	96%	152
Orlando Health[2]	Orlando	96%	324
Parrish Medical Center[2]	Titusville	96%	48
UF Health Shands Hospital[2]	Gainesville	96%	188
Westside Regional Medical Center[2]	Plantation	96%	76
Winter Haven Hospital[2]	Winter Haven	96%	134
Baptist Medical Center Beaches[2]	Jcksnvl Bch	95%	63
Bayfront Health Brooksville[2]	Brooksville	95%	75
Bethesda Hospital East[2]	Boynton Beach	95%	127
Cape Canaveral Hospital[2]	Cocoa Beach	95%	59
Englewood Community Hospital[2]	Englewood	95%	39
Palms West Hospital[2]	Loxahatchee	95%	62
Broward Health Imperial Point[2]	Fort Lauderdale	94%	48
Florida Hospital Carrollwood[2]	Tampa	94%	54
Memorial Hospital Miramar[2]	Miramar	94%	68
Santa Rosa Medical Center[2]	Milton	94%	32
University of Miami Hospital[2]	Miami	94%	63
The Villages Regional Hospital[2]	The Villages	94%	178
West Palm Hospital[2]	W Palm Beach	94%	32
Doctors Hospital[2]	Coral Gables	93%	27
Hialeah Hospital[2]	Hialeah	93%	45
Mease Countryside Hospital[2]	Safety Harbor	93%	106
Osceola Regional Medical Center[2]	Kissimmee	93%	141
UF Health Jacksonville[2]	Jacksonville	93%	128
Bayfront Health Port Charlotte[2]	Port Charlotte	92%	76
Florida Hospital Deland[2]	Deland	92%	88
Florida Hospital Fish Memorial[2]	Orange City	92%	66
Halifax Health Medical Center[2]	Daytona Bch	92%	127
Leesburg Regional Medical Center[2]	Leesburg	92%	107
Naples Community Hospital[2]	Naples	92%	248
Saint Joseph's Hospital[2]	Tampa	92%	232
Broward Health Medical Center[2]	Fort Lauderdale	91%	94
Bartow Regional Medical Center[2]	Bartow	90%	48
Bayfront Health - Saint Petersburg[2]	St Petersburg	90%	79
Heart of Florida Regional Medical Center[2]	Davenport	90%	63
Mayo Clinic[2]	Jacksonville	90%	118
Memorial Hospital of Tampa[2]	Tampa	90%	48
Northwest Medical Center[2]	Margate	90%	71
Palm Beach Gardens Medical Center[2]	Palm Bch Grdns	90%	89
Tampa General Hospital[2]	Tampa	90%	327
West Florida Hospital[2]	Pensacola	90%	71
Bert Fish Medical Center[2]	New Smyrn Bch	89%	66
Wuesthoff Medical Center Rockledge[2]	Rockledge	89%	70
Citrus Memorial Hospital[2]	Inverness	87%	173
Jackson Memorial Hospital[2]	Miami	87%	269
Morton Plant Hospital[2]	Clearwater	87%	157
Morton Plant North Bay Hospital[2]	New Port Richey	87%	45
South Lake Hospital[2]	Clermont	86%	87
Broward Health North[2]	Pompano Bch	85%	81
Lehigh Regional Medical Center[2]	Lehigh Acres	85%	27
Gulf Coast Med Ctr Lee Mem Health Sys[2]	Fort Myers	84%	216
Memorial Hospital Jacksonville[2]	Jacksonville	84%	146
North Shore Medical Center[2]	Miami	84%	92
Munroe Regional Medical Center[2]	Ocala	82%	182
South Florida Baptist Hospital[2]	Plant City	82%	51
Tallahassee Memorial Hospital[2]	Tallahassee	82%	83
Baptist Medical Center[2]	Jacksonville	81%	276
Cape Coral Hospital[2]	Cape Coral	81%	128
Indian River Medical Center[2]	Vero Beach	81%	119
Lee Memorial Hospital[2]	Fort Myers	81%	212
Mease Hospital Dunedin[2]	Dunedin	81%	37
Gulf Breeze Hospital[2]	Gulf Breeze	78%	32
Putnam Community Medical Center[2]	Palatka	78%	45
Seven Rivers Regional Medical Center[2]	Crystal River	78%	32
Lakewood Ranch Medical Center[2]	Bradenton	77%	31
Baptist Medical Center - Nassau[2]	Fernandina Bch	74%	27
Mount Sinai Medical Center[2]	Miami Beach	74%	98
Saint Anthony's Hospital[2]	St Petersburg	72%	141
Wuesthoff Medical Center - Melbourne[2]	Melbourne	72%	46
Saint Cloud Regional Medical Center[2]	Saint Cloud	70%	27
Baptist Hospital[2]	Pensacola	64%	81
Highlands Regional Medical Center[2]	Sebring	40%	42

ICU Venous Thromboembolism Prophylaxis

Hospital Name	City	Rate	Cases
Baptist Hospital of Miami[2]	Miami	100%	54
Boca Raton Regional Hospital[2]	Boca Raton	100%	79
Brandon Regional Hospital[2]	Brandon	100%	96
Cape Canaveral Hospital[2]	Cocoa Beach	100%	60
Capital Regional Medical Center[2]	Tallahassee	100%	57
Central Florida Regional Hospital[2]	Sanford	100%	118
Cleveland Clinic Hospital[2]	Weston	100%	54
Delray Medical Center[2]	Delray Beach	100%	105
Doctors Hospital[2]	Coral Gables	100%	46
Doctors Hospital of Sarasota[2]	Sarasota	100%	75
Edward White Hospital[2]	St Petersburg	100%	88
Englewood Community Hospital[2]	Englewood	100%	73
Florida Hospital Wesley Chapel[2,3]	Wesley Chapel	100%	26
Gulf Coast Regional Medical Center[2]	Panama City	100%	69
Health Central[2]	Ocoee	100%	38
Holy Cross Hospital[2]	Fort Lauderdale	100%	35
Homestead Hospital[2]	Homestead	100%	60
JFK Medical Center[2]	Atlantis	100%	87
Kendall Regional Medical Center[2]	Miami	100%	82
Lake Wales Medical Center[2]	Lake Wales	100%	73
Lawnwood Reg Med Ctr & Heart Inst[2]	Fort Pierce	100%	124
Medical Center of Trinity[2]	Trinity	100%	80
Memorial Hospital Miramar[2]	Miramar	100%	58
Memorial Hospital Pembroke[2]	Pembroke Pines	100%	71
Memorial Regional Hospital[2]	Hollywood	100%	80
Oak Hill Hospital[2]	Brooksville	100%	55
Ocala Regional Medical Center[2]	Ocala	100%	95
Orange Park Medical Center[2]	Orange Park	100%	63
Osceola Regional Medical Center[2]	Kissimmee	100%	72
Raulerson Hospital[2]	Okeechobee	100%	88
Regional Medical Center Bayonet Point[2]	Hudson	100%	143
Saint Lucie Medical Center[2]	Port Saint Lucie	100%	61
Saint Mary's Medical Center[2]	W Palm Beach	100%	71
Saint Vincent's Medical Center Southside[2]	Jacksonville	100%	43
Santa Rosa Medical Center[2]	Milton	100%	101
South Bay Hospital[2]	Sun City Center	100%	60
South Miami Hospital[2]	South Miami	100%	117
Twin Cities Hospital[2]	Niceville	100%	82
Venice Reg Med Ctr-Bayfront Health[2]	Venice	100%	31
Viera Hospital[2]	Melbourne	100%	43
West Kendall Baptist Hospital[2]	Miami	100%	91
Baptist Medical Center - Nassau[2]	Fernandina Bch	99%	75
Blake Medical Center[2]	Bradenton	99%	100
Coral Gables Hospital[2]	Coral Gables	99%	78
Lakewood Ranch Medical Center[2]	Bradenton	99%	76
North Florida Regional Medical Center[2]	Gainesville	99%	77
Orlando Health[2]	Orlando	99%	96
Palm Bay Hospital[2]	Palm Bay	99%	77
Physicians Reg Med Ctr-Pine Ridge[2]	Naples	99%	76
Plantation General Hospital[2]	Plantation	99%	73
Saint Joseph's Hospital[2]	Tampa	99%	94
South Lake Hospital[2]	Clermont	99%	254
West Boca Medical Center[2]	Boca Raton	99%	93
West Palm Hospital[2]	W Palm Beach	99%	79
Westside Regional Medical Center[2]	Plantation	99%	98
Aventura Hospital & Medical Center[2]	Aventura	98%	110
Bethesda Hospital East[2]	Boynton Beach	98%	63
Florida Hospital North Pinellas[2]	Tarpon Springs	98%	62
Florida Hospital Tampa[2]	Tampa	98%	66
Lake City Medical Center[2]	Lake City	98%	96
Lakeside Medical Center[2]	Belle Glade	98%	64
Largo Medical Center[2]	Largo	98%	123
Lehigh Regional Medical Center[2]	Lehigh Acres	98%	55
Mease Countryside Hospital[2]	Safety Harbor	98%	82
Mease Hospital Dunedin[2]	Dunedin	98%	103
Memorial Hospital West[2]	Pembroke Pines	98%	62
Mount Sinai Medical Center[2]	Miami Beach	98%	55
Wuesthoff Medical Center Rockledge[2]	Rockledge	98%	65
Fawcett Memorial Hospital[2]	Port Charlotte	97%	76
Flagler Hospital[2]	St Augustine	97%	90
Florida Hospital[2]	Orlando	97%	137
Florida Hospital Carrollwood[2]	Tampa	97%	37
Florida Hospital Flagler[2]	Palm Coast	97%	91
Good Samaritan Medical Center[2]	W Palm Beach	97%	64
Holmes Regional Medical Center[2]	Melbourne	97%	93
Lower Keys Medical Center[2]	Key West	97%	58
Mayo Clinic[2]	Jacksonville	97%	86
Morton Plant North Bay Hospital[2]	New Port Richey	97%	68
North Okaloosa Medical Center[2]	Crestview	97%	101
Northwest Medical Center[2]	Margate	97%	76
Palms of Pasadena Hospital[2]	St Petersburg	97%	104
Parrish Medical Center[2]	Titusville	97%	69
Saint Petersburg General Hospital[2]	St Petersburg	97%	103
Sarasota Memorial Hospital[2]	Sarasota	97%	70
Tallahassee Memorial Hospital[2]	Tallahassee	97%	134
Bartow Regional Medical Center[2]	Bartow	96%	52
Broward Health Medical Center[2]	Fort Lauderdale	96%	57
Florida Hospital Memorial Medical Center[2]	Daytona Bch	96%	82
Jupiter Medical Center[2]	Jupiter	96%	51
Larkin Community Hospital[2]	South Miami	96%	48
Northside Hospital[2]	St Petersburg	96%	121
UF Health Jacksonville[2]	Jacksonville	96%	112
University Hospital & Medical Center[2]	Tamarac	96%	76
Wellington Regional Medical Center[2]	Wellington	96%	53
Baptist Medical Center[2]	Jacksonville	95%	95
Florida Hospital Fish Memorial[2]	Orange City	95%	93
Florida Hospital Waterman[2]	Tavares	95%	55
Hialeah Hospital[2]	Hialeah	95%	107
Lakeland Regional Medical Center[2]	Lakeland	95%	91
Martin Medical Center[2]	Stuart	95%	60
Memorial Hospital Jacksonville[2]	Jacksonville	95%	87
Broward Health North[2]	Pompano Bch	94%	70
Florida Hospital Zephyrhills[2]	Zephyrhills	94%	69
Fort Walton Beach Medical Center[2]	Fort Walton Bch	94%	125
Morton Plant Hospital[2]	Clearwater	94%	99
North Shore Medical Center[2]	Miami	94%	214
UF Health Shands Hospital[2]	Gainesville	94%	101
West Florida Hospital[2]	Pensacola	94%	139
Winter Haven Hospital[2]	Winter Haven	94%	98
Bayfront Health Punta Gorda[2]	Punta Gorda	93%	55
Highlands Regional Medical Center[2]	Sebring	93%	117
Munroe Regional Medical Center[2]	Ocala	93%	42
Palm Beach Gardens Medical Center[2]	Palm Bch Grdns	93%	149
Palmetto General Hospital[2]	Hialeah	93%	92
University of Miami Hospital[2]	Miami	93%	113
Baptist Medical Center Beaches[2]	Jcksnvl Bch	92%	101
Bay Med Ctr Sacred Heart Health Sys[2]	Panama City	92%	263
Halifax Health Medical Center[2]	Daytona Bch	92%	75
Naples Community Hospital[2]	Naples	92%	38
Palms West Hospital[2]	Loxahatchee	92%	61

NOTE: Hospital profiles are in alphabetical order by state, then city, then hospital within the city; Rankings exclude hospitals with less than 25 cases except for patient surveys which excludes hospitals with less than 100 cases; (a) 100-299 cases; (1) The number of cases/patients is too few to report; (2) Data submitted were based on a sample of cases/patients; (3) Results are based on a shorter time period than required; (4) Data suppressed by CMS for one or more quarters; (5) Results are not available for this reporting period; (6) Fewer than 100 patients completed the HCAHPS survey; (7) No cases met the criteria for this measure; (8) The lower limit of the confidence interval cannot be calculated if the number of observed infections equals zero; (9) No data are available from the state/territory for this reporting period; (10) The scores shown reflect fewer than 50 completed surveys; (11) There were discrepancies in the data collection process; (12) This measure does not apply to this hospital for this reporting period; (13) Results cannot be calculated for this reporting period; (14) The results for this state are combined with nearby states to protect confidentiality; Please refer to the User's Guide for a full explanation of data.

Hospital Name	City	Rate	Cases
Sacred Heart Hospital[2]	Pensacola	92%	76
Saint Anthony's Hospital[2]	St Petersburg	92%	88
Saint Vincent's Medical Center[2]	Jacksonville	92%	63
Bayfront Health Brooksville[2]	Brooksville	91%	94
Bayfront Health Port Charlotte[2]	Port Charlotte	91%	64
Palm Springs General Hospital[2]	Hialeah	91%	100
Baptist Hospital[2]	Pensacola	90%	69
Bayfront Health - Saint Petersburg[2]	St Petersburg	90%	145
Cape Coral Hospital[2]	Cape Coral	90%	59
Desoto Memorial Hospital[2]	Arcadia	90%	79
Florida Hospital Heartland Medical Center[2]	Sebring	90%	147
Leesburg Regional Medical Center[2]	Leesburg	90%	60
Broward Health Coral Springs[2]	Coral Springs	89%	55
South Florida Baptist Hospital[2]	Plant City	89%	81
Jackson Memorial Hospital[2]	Miami	88%	216
Sacred Heart Hosp-Emerald Coast[2]	Miramar Beach	88%	52
Town & Country Hospital[2]	Tampa	88%	52
Indian River Medical Center[2]	Vero Beach	86%	70
Seven Rivers Regional Medical Center[2]	Crystal River	86%	74
Tampa General Hospital[2]	Tampa	86%	116
Wuesthoff Medical Center - Melbourne[2]	Melbourne	86%	57
Bayfront Health Dade City[2]	Dade City	85%	100
Florida Hospital Deland[2]	Deland	84%	114
Manatee Memorial Hospital[2]	Bradenton	84%	82
Putnam Community Medical Center[2]	Palatka	84%	69
The Villages Regional Hospital[2]	The Villages	84%	25
Bert Fish Medical Center[2]	New Smyrn Bch	83%	90
Broward Health Imperial Point[2]	Fort Lauderdale	83%	47
Gulf Breeze Hospital[2]	Gulf Breeze	83%	48
Lee Memorial Hospital[2]	Fort Myers	83%	71
Metropolitan Hospital of Miami[2]	Miami	83%	30
Memorial Hospital of Tampa[2]	Tampa	82%	77
Gulf Coast Med Ctr Lee Mem Health Sys[2]	Fort Myers	77%	52
Westchester General Hospital[2]	Miami	77%	96
Jackson Hospital[2]	Marianna	76%	42
Doctor's Memorial Hospital[2]	Perry	71%	38
Saint Cloud Regional Medical Center[2]	Saint Cloud	71%	59
Citrus Memorial Hospital[2]	Inverness	70%	82
Heart of Florida Regional Medical Center[2]	Davenport	68%	47
Shands Lake Shore Regional Medical Center[2]	Lake City	57%	136
Healthmark Regional Medical Center[2]	Defuniak Spgs	34%	56

Incidence of Potentially Preventable VTE

Hospital Name	City	Rate	Cases
Boca Raton Regional Hospital[2]	Boca Raton	0%	58
Brandon Regional Hospital[2]	Brandon	0%	29
Broward Health North[2]	Pompano Bch	0%	26
Fawcett Memorial Hospital[2]	Port Charlotte	0%	30
Florida Hospital Waterman[2]	Tavares	0%	27
Memorial Hospital West[2]	Pembroke Pines	0%	43
Memorial Regional Hospital[2]	Hollywood	0%	53
Morton Plant Hospital[2]	Clearwater	0%	27
Baptist Hospital of Miami[2]	Miami	2%	52
Orlando Health[2]	Orlando	2%	63
Mayo Clinic[2]	Jacksonville	3%	86
Naples Community Hospital[2]	Naples	3%	63
UF Health Shands Hospital[2]	Gainesville	4%	80
Holmes Regional Medical Center[2]	Melbourne	5%	40
Aventura Hospital & Medical Center[2]	Aventura	6%	33
Bethesda Hospital East[2]	Boynton Beach	6%	31
Mount Sinai Medical Center[2]	Miami Beach	6%	48
Saint Joseph's Hospital[2]	Tampa	6%	47
Florida Hospital[2]	Orlando	7%	113
UF Health Jacksonville[2]	Jacksonville	7%	28
Blake Medical Center[2]	Bradenton	8%	25
Florida Hospital Tampa[2]	Tampa	8%	49
JFK Medical Center[2]	Atlantis	8%	36
Broward Health Medical Center[2]	Fort Lauderdale	10%	40
Tampa General Hospital[2]	Tampa	10%	103
Jackson Memorial Hospital[2]	Miami	11%	120
Memorial Hospital Jacksonville[2]	Jacksonville	11%	35
Sacred Heart Hospital[2]	Pensacola	11%	28
Lee Memorial Hospital[2]	Fort Myers	13%	54
Baptist Medical Center[2]	Jacksonville	15%	47
Bayfront Health - Saint Petersburg[2]	St Petersburg	15%	27
Gulf Coast Med Ctr Lee Mem Health Sys[2]	Fort Myers	15%	73
University of Miami Hospital[2]	Miami	18%	33
Lakeland Regional Medical Center[2]	Lakeland	19%	53
Saint Anthony's Hospital[2]	St Petersburg	24%	42
Cape Coral Hospital[2]	Cape Coral	28%	29
Halifax Health Medical Center[2]	Daytona Bch	38%	26

UFH with Dosages/Platelet Count Monitoring

Hospital Name	City	Rate	Cases
Baptist Hospital of Miami[2]	Miami	100%	145
Baptist Medical Center[2]	Jacksonville	100%	228
Baptist Medical Center Beaches[2]	Jcksnvll Bch	100%	47
Bartow Regional Medical Center[2]	Bartow	100%	30
Bay Med Ctr Sacred Heart Health Sys[2]	Panama City	100%	94
Bayfront Health Brooksville[2]	Brooksville	100%	50
Bayfront Health Port Charlotte[2]	Port Charlotte	100%	70
Bert Fish Medical Center[2]	New Smyrn Bch	100%	38
Bethesda Hospital East[2]	Boynton Beach	100%	107
Blake Medical Center[2]	Bradenton	100%	41
Boca Raton Regional Hospital[2]	Boca Raton	100%	117
Brandon Regional Hospital[2]	Brandon	100%	74
Broward Health North[2]	Pompano Bch	100%	28
Cape Canaveral Hospital[2]	Cocoa Beach	100%	39
Cape Coral Hospital[2]	Cape Coral	100%	115
Capital Regional Medical Center[2]	Tallahassee	100%	62
Citrus Memorial Hospital[2]	Inverness	100%	88
Cleveland Clinic Hospital[2]	Weston	100%	45
Delray Medical Center[2]	Delray Beach	100%	108
Doctors Hospital[2]	Coral Gables	100%	37
Fawcett Memorial Hospital[2]	Port Charlotte	100%	113
Flagler Hospital[2]	St Augustine	100%	89
Florida Hospital[2]	Orlando	100%	218
Florida Hospital Deland[2]	Deland	100%	32
Florida Hospital Fish Memorial[2]	Orange City	100%	43
Florida Hospital Flagler[2]	Palm Coast	100%	35
Florida Hospital Heartland Medical Center[2]	Sebring	100%	37
Florida Hospital Memorial Medical Center[2]	Daytona Bch	100%	31
Florida Hospital Tampa[2]	Tampa	100%	42
Florida Hospital Waterman[2]	Tavares	100%	38
Good Samaritan Medical Center[2]	W Palm Beach	100%	36
Gulf Coast Regional Medical Center[2]	Panama City	100%	57
Halifax Health Medical Center[2]	Daytona Bch	100%	77
Heart of Florida Regional Medical Center[2]	Davenport	100%	28
Highlands Regional Medical Center[2]	Sebring	100%	35
Holmes Regional Medical Center[2]	Melbourne	100%	228
JFK Medical Center[2]	Atlantis	100%	209
Jupiter Medical Center[2]	Jupiter	100%	130
Kendall Regional Medical Center[2]	Miami	100%	55
Lakeland Regional Medical Center[2]	Lakeland	100%	248
Largo Medical Center[2]	Largo	100%	40
Lawnwood Reg Med Ctr & Heart Inst[2]	Fort Pierce	100%	97
Lee Memorial Hospital[2]	Fort Myers	100%	79
Mayo Clinic[2]	Jacksonville	100%	93
Medical Center of Trinity[2]	Trinity	100%	27
Memorial Hospital Pembroke[2]	Pembroke Pines	100%	35
Memorial Hospital West[2]	Pembroke Pines	100%	38
Memorial Regional Hospital[2]	Hollywood	100%	56
Morton Plant Hospital[2]	Clearwater	100%	39
Morton Plant North Bay Hospital[2]	New Port Richey	100%	37
Munroe Regional Medical Center[2]	Ocala	100%	204
Naples Community Hospital[2]	Naples	100%	241
North Florida Regional Medical Center[2]	Gainesville	100%	78
Northside Hospital[2]	St Petersburg	100%	30
Oak Hill Hospital[2]	Brooksville	100%	63
Ocala Regional Medical Center[2]	Ocala	100%	179
Orange Park Medical Center[2]	Orange Park	100%	84
Orlando Health[2]	Orlando	100%	106
Osceola Regional Medical Center[2]	Kissimmee	100%	36
Palm Bay Hospital[2]	Palm Bay	100%	74
Palm Beach Gardens Medical Center[2]	Palm Bch Grdns	100%	80
Palms West Hospital[2]	Loxahatchee	100%	55
Physicians Reg Med Ctr-Pine Ridge[2]	Naples	100%	98
Putnam Community Medical Center[2]	Palatka	100%	36
Regional Medical Center Bayonet Point[2]	Hudson	100%	45
Saint Anthony's Hospital[2]	St Petersburg	100%	50
Saint Joseph's Hospital[2]	Tampa	100%	62
Saint Lucie Medical Center[2]	Port Saint Lucie	100%	74
Saint Mary's Medical Center[2]	W Palm Beach	100%	31
Saint Vincent's Medical Center[2]	Jacksonville	100%	88
Saint Vincent's Medical Center Southside[2]	Jacksonville	100%	64
Santa Rosa Medical Center[2]	Milton	100%	34
Sarasota Memorial Hospital[2]	Sarasota	100%	41
Sebastian River Medical Center[2]	Sebastian	100%	41
South Lake Hospital[2]	Clermont	100%	63
South Miami Hospital[2]	South Miami	100%	45
Tallahassee Memorial Hospital[2]	Tallahassee	100%	84
UF Health Jacksonville[2]	Jacksonville	100%	70
UF Health Shands Hospital[2]	Gainesville	100%	238
University of Miami Hospital[2]	Miami	100%	64
Venice Reg Med Ctr-Bayfront Health[2]	Venice	100%	110
Wellington Regional Medical Center[2]	Wellington	100%	35
West Boca Medical Center[2]	Boca Raton	100%	30
West Kendall Baptist Hospital[2]	Miami	100%	34
West Palm Hospital[2]	W Palm Beach	100%	29
Winter Haven Hospital[2]	Winter Haven	100%	78
Wuesthoff Medical Center Rockledge[2]	Rockledge	100%	59
Gulf Coast Med Ctr Lee Mem Health Sys[2]	Fort Myers	99%	194
Memorial Hospital Jacksonville[2]	Jacksonville	99%	151
The Villages Regional Hospital[2]	The Villages	99%	185
Aventura Hospital & Medical Center[2]	Aventura	98%	62
Central Florida Regional Hospital[2]	Sanford	98%	58
Indian River Medical Center[2]	Vero Beach	98%	85
Jackson Memorial Hospital[2]	Miami	98%	212
Leesburg Regional Medical Center[2]	Leesburg	98%	104
Mease Countryside Hospital[2]	Safety Harbor	98%	56
Parrish Medical Center[2]	Titusville	98%	40
Plantation General Hospital[2]	Plantation	98%	44
Tampa General Hospital[2]	Tampa	98%	257
Wuesthoff Medical Center - Melbourne[2]	Melbourne	98%	41
Manatee Memorial Hospital[2]	Bradenton	97%	61
Viera Hospital[2]	Melbourne	97%	34
Martin Medical Center[2]	Stuart	96%	72
North Shore Medical Center[2]	Miami	93%	30

Venous Thromboembolism Prophylaxis

Hospital Name	City	Rate	Cases
Boca Raton Regional Hospital[2]	Boca Raton	100%	337
Delray Medical Center[2]	Delray Beach	100%	347
Doctors Hospital[2]	Coral Gables	100%	351
Doctors Hospital of Sarasota[2]	Sarasota	100%	297
Edward White Hospital[2]	St Petersburg	100%	217
Florida Hospital Wesley Chapel[2,3]	Wesley Chapel	100%	151
Memorial Regional Hospital[2]	Hollywood	100%	491
Oak Hill Hospital[2]	Brooksville	100%	383
Regional Medical Center Bayonet Point[2]	Hudson	100%	360
Saint Vincent's Medical Center Southside[2]	Jacksonville	100%	304
Sebastian River Medical Center[2]	Sebastian	100%	364
Shands Starke Regional Medical Center[2]	Starke	100%	233
Twin Cities Hospital[2]	Niceville	100%	139
West Kendall Baptist Hospital[2]	Miami	100%	484
Baptist Hospital of Miami[2]	Miami	99%	396
Englewood Community Hospital[2]	Englewood	99%	311
Florida Hospital North Pinellas[2]	Tarpon Springs	99%	317
Florida Hospital Wauchula[2]	Wauchula	99%	142
Health Central[2]	Ocoee	99%	549
Holy Cross Hospital[2]	Fort Lauderdale	99%	386
Lawnwood Reg Med Ctr & Heart Inst[2]	Fort Pierce	99%	340
Medical Center of Trinity[2]	Trinity	99%	393
Memorial Hospital Miramar[2]	Miramar	99%	342
North Okaloosa Medical Center[2]	Crestview	99%	426
South Miami Hospital[2]	South Miami	99%	418
Blake Medical Center[2]	Bradenton	98%	383
Brandon Regional Hospital[2]	Brandon	98%	350
Capital Regional Medical Center[2]	Tallahassee	98%	422
Kendall Regional Medical Center[2]	Miami	98%	362
Lake Wales Medical Center[2]	Lake Wales	98%	448
Lakeside Medical Center[2]	Belle Glade	98%	324
Mease Hospital Dunedin[2]	Dunedin	98%	354
Memorial Hospital Pembroke[2]	Pembroke Pines	98%	308
Orange Park Medical Center[2]	Orange Park	98%	408
Raulerson Hospital[2]	Okeechobee	98%	365
Saint Lucie Medical Center[2]	Port Saint Lucie	98%	383
Saint Mary's Medical Center[2]	W Palm Beach	98%	347
Saint Vincent's Medical Center[2]	Jacksonville	98%	336
Viera Hospital[2]	Melbourne	98%	306
Central Florida Regional Hospital[2]	Sanford	97%	330
Florida Hospital Memorial Medical Center[2]	Daytona Bch	97%	365
Florida Hospital Waterman[2]	Tavares	97%	388
Gulf Coast Regional Medical Center[2]	Panama City	97%	371
Homestead Hospital[2]	Homestead	97%	332
Mease Countryside Hospital[2]	Safety Harbor	97%	385
Memorial Hospital West[2]	Pembroke Pines	97%	365
Saint Petersburg General Hospital[2]	St Petersburg	97%	307
South Bay Hospital[2]	Sun City Center	97%	385
Venice Reg Med Ctr-Bayfront Health[2]	Venice	97%	338
Cape Canaveral Hospital[2]	Cocoa Beach	96%	344
Lake City Medical Center[2]	Lake City	96%	364
Lehigh Regional Medical Center[2]	Lehigh Acres	96%	241
North Florida Regional Medical Center[2]	Gainesville	96%	393
Ocala Regional Medical Center[2]	Ocala	96%	356
Orlando Health[2]	Orlando	96%	606
Santa Rosa Medical Center[2]	Milton	96%	274
Aventura Hospital & Medical Center[2]	Aventura	95%	372
Broward Health Coral Springs[2]	Coral Springs	95%	347
Cleveland Clinic Hospital[2]	Weston	95%	311
Coral Gables Hospital[2]	Coral Gables	95%	332
Florida Hospital[2]	Orlando	95%	1114
Good Samaritan Medical Center[2]	W Palm Beach	95%	357
Jupiter Medical Center[2]	Jupiter	95%	377
Mariners Hospital	Tavernier	95%	297
Plantation General Hospital[2]	Plantation	95%	375
West Palm Hospital[2]	W Palm Beach	95%	275
Bethesda Hospital East[2]	Boynton Beach	94%	350
Florida Hospital Flagler[2]	Palm Coast	94%	327
Morton Plant North Bay Hospital[2]	New Port Richey	94%	260
Osceola Regional Medical Center[2]	Kissimmee	94%	399
South Lake Hospital[2]	Clermont	94%	2477
West Boca Medical Center[2]	Boca Raton	94%	332
Fawcett Memorial Hospital[2]	Port Charlotte	93%	382
JFK Medical Center[2]	Atlantis	93%	381
Palm Bay Hospital[2]	Palm Bay	93%	353
Putnam Community Medical Center[2]	Palatka	93%	392
UF Health Jacksonville[2]	Jacksonville	93%	246
Broward Health North[2]	Pompano Bch	92%	337
Hialeah Hospital[2]	Hialeah	92%	367
Mayo Clinic[2]	Jacksonville	92%	312
Northside Hospital[2]	St Petersburg	92%	324

NOTE: Hospital profiles are in alphabetical order by state, then city, then hospital within the city; Rankings exclude hospitals with less than 25 cases except for patient surveys which excludes hospitals with less than 100 cases; (a) 100-299 cases; (1) The number of cases/patients is too few to report; (2) Data submitted were based on a sample of cases/patients; (3) Results are based on a shorter time period than required; (4) Data suppressed by CMS for one or more quarters; (5) Results are not available for this reporting period; (6) Fewer than 100 patients completed the HCAHPS survey; (7) No cases met the criteria for this measure; (8) The lower limit of the confidence interval cannot be calculated if the number of observed infections equals zero; (9) No data are available from the state/territory for this reporting period; (10) The scores shown reflect fewer than 50 completed surveys; (11) There were discrepancies in the data collection process; (12) This measure does not apply to this hospital for this reporting period; (13) Results cannot be calculated for this reporting period; (14) The results for this state are combined with nearby states to protect confidentiality; Please refer to the User's Guide for a full explanation of data.

Hospital Name	City	Rate	Cases
Flagler Hospital[2]	St Augustine	91%	328
Fort Walton Beach Medical Center[2]	Fort Walton Bch	91%	296
Palms of Pasadena Hospital[2]	St Petersburg	91%	366
Saint Joseph's Hospital[2]	Tampa	91%	311
Holmes Regional Medical Center[2]	Melbourne	90%	377
Lower Keys Medical Center[2]	Key West	90%	255
Physicians Reg Med Ctr-Pine Ridge[2]	Naples	90%	355
Florida Hospital Heartland Medical Center[2]	Sebring	89%	511
Florida Hospital Zephyrhills[2]	Zephyrhills	89%	332
Morton Plant Hospital[2]	Clearwater	89%	367
Palm Beach Gardens Medical Center[2]	Palm Bch Grdns	89%	314
Sacred Heart Hospital on the Gulf	Port Saint Joe	89%	224
Sarasota Memorial Hospital[2]	Sarasota	89%	334
University of Miami Hospital[2]	Miami	89%	282
Baptist Medical Center[2]	Jacksonville	88%	342
Baptist Medical Center Beaches[2]	Jcksnvl Bch	88%	301
Shands Live Oak Regional Medical Center[2]	Live Oak	88%	132
Tallahassee Memorial Hospital[2]	Tallahassee	88%	504
Westside Regional Medical Center[2]	Plantation	88%	337
Florida Hospital Deland[2]	Deland	87%	286
Florida Hospital Fish Memorial[2]	Orange City	87%	356
Lakewood Ranch Medical Center[2]	Bradenton	87%	278
Memorial Hospital Jacksonville[2]	Jacksonville	87%	403
Sacred Heart Hosp-Emerald Coast[2]	Miramar Beach	87%	303
UF Health Shands Hospital[2]	Gainesville	87%	321
Wuesthoff Medical Center - Melbourne[2]	Melbourne	87%	369
Desoto Memorial Hospital[2]	Arcadia	86%	115
Florida Hospital Tampa[2]	Tampa	86%	333
Largo Medical Center[2]	Largo	86%	343
Northwest Medical Center[2]	Margate	86%	369
Jay Hospital[2]	Jay	85%	146
Parrish Medical Center[2]	Titusville	85%	390
Florida Hospital Carrollwood[2]	Tampa	84%	327
Highlands Regional Medical Center[2]	Sebring	84%	300
Martin Medical Center[2]	Stuart	84%	348
Palmetto General Hospital[2]	Hialeah	84%	256
Saint Anthony's Hospital[2]	St Petersburg	84%	335
Cape Coral Hospital[2]	Cape Coral	83%	356
Gulf Breeze Hospital[2]	Gulf Breeze	83%	346
Palm Springs General Hospital[2]	Hialeah	83%	358
Larkin Community Hospital[2]	South Miami	82%	229
Lee Memorial Hospital[2]	Fort Myers	82%	314
Town & Country Hospital[2]	Tampa	82%	279
University Hospital & Medical Center[2]	Tamarac	82%	377
West Florida Hospital[2]	Pensacola	82%	285
Gulf Coast Med Ctr Lee Mem Health Sys[2]	Fort Myers	81%	341
Naples Community Hospital[2]	Naples	81%	365
North Shore Medical Center[2]	Miami	81%	529
The Villages Regional Hospital[2]	The Villages	81%	381
Wellington Regional Medical Center[2]	Wellington	81%	374
Bert Fish Medical Center[2]	New Smyrn Bch	80%	320
Broward Health Medical Center[2]	Fort Lauderdale	80%	314
Mount Sinai Medical Center[2]	Miami Beach	80%	332
Sacred Heart Hospital[2]	Pensacola	80%	342
Palms West Hospital[2]	Loxahatchee	79%	369
Bartow Regional Medical Center[2]	Bartow	78%	318
Jackson Memorial Hospital[2]	Miami	78%	931
Wuesthoff Medical Center Rockledge[2]	Rockledge	78%	345
Baptist Medical Center - Nassau[2]	Fernandina Bch	76%	259
Bay Med Ctr Sacred Heart Health Sys[2]	Panama City	76%	703
Bayfront Health Port Charlotte[2]	Port Charlotte	76%	383
Halifax Health Medical Center[2]	Daytona Bch	76%	280
Jackson Hospital[2]	Marianna	76%	313
Leesburg Regional Medical Center[2]	Leesburg	76%	372
Memorial Hospital of Tampa[2]	Tampa	76%	398
Winter Haven Hospital[2]	Winter Haven	76%	279
Tampa General Hospital[2]	Tampa	75%	311
Baptist Hospital[2]	Pensacola	74%	337
Bayfront Health Punta Gorda[2]	Punta Gorda	73%	342
Lakeland Regional Medical Center[2]	Lakeland	73%	332
South Florida Baptist Hospital[2]	Plant City	73%	339
Bayfront Health - Saint Petersburg[2]	St Petersburg	71%	331
Indian River Medical Center[2]	Vero Beach	71%	347
Broward Health Imperial Point[2]	Fort Lauderdale	68%	242
Doctor's Memorial Hospital[2]	Perry	67%	98
Munroe Regional Medical Center[2]	Ocala	67%	354
Westchester General Hospital[2]	Miami	65%	422
Bayfront Health Brooksville[2]	Brooksville	64%	365
Saint Cloud Regional Medical Center[2]	Saint Cloud	64%	386
Bayfront Health Dade City[2]	Dade City	63%	186
Manatee Memorial Hospital[2]	Bradenton	60%	347
Citrus Memorial Hospital[2]	Inverness	58%	440
Metropolitan Hospital of Miami[2]	Miami	56%	380
Seven Rivers Regional Medical Center[2]	Crystal River	51%	318
Heart of Florida Regional Medical Center[2]	Davenport	46%	312
Douglas Gardens Hospital[2]	Miami	42%	156
Shands Lake Shore Regional Medical Center[2]	Lake City	41%	250
Healthmark Regional Medical Center[2]	Defuniak Spgs	17%	100
Anne Bates Leach Eye Hospital	Miami	0%	29

Warfarin Therapy Discharge Instructions

Hospital Name	City	Rate	Cases
Baptist Hospital of Miami[2]	Miami	100%	66
Boca Raton Regional Hospital[2]	Boca Raton	100%	93
Brandon Regional Hospital[2]	Brandon	100%	149
Broward Health Coral Springs[2]	Coral Springs	100%	47
Broward Health Imperial Point[2]	Fort Lauderdale	100%	40
Broward Health Medical Center[2]	Fort Lauderdale	100%	66
Broward Health North[2]	Pompano Bch	100%	51
Capital Regional Medical Center[2]	Tallahassee	100%	53
Delray Medical Center[2]	Delray Beach	100%	67
Florida Hospital Waterman[2]	Tavares	100%	93
Fort Walton Beach Medical Center[2]	Fort Walton Bch	100%	32
Good Samaritan Medical Center[2]	W Palm Beach	100%	39
Highlands Regional Medical Center[2]	Sebring	100%	27
Holy Cross Hospital[2]	Fort Lauderdale	100%	28
Homestead Hospital[2]	Homestead	100%	37
JFK Medical Center[2]	Atlantis	100%	131
Lake Wales Medical Center[2]	Lake Wales	100%	39
Memorial Hospital Jacksonville[2]	Jacksonville	100%	99
Memorial Hospital Miramar[2]	Miramar	100%	59
Memorial Hospital Pembroke[2]	Pembroke Pines	100%	49
Memorial Hospital West[2]	Pembroke Pines	100%	101
Memorial Regional Hospital[2]	Hollywood	100%	116
North Florida Regional Medical Center[2]	Gainesville	100%	85
Northside Hospital[2]	St Petersburg	100%	39
Northwest Medical Center[2]	Margate	100%	55
Oak Hill Hospital[2]	Brooksville	100%	106
Ocala Regional Medical Center[2]	Ocala	100%	120
Orange Park Medical Center[2]	Orange Park	100%	71
Palmetto General Hospital[2]	Hialeah	100%	35
Palms West Hospital[2]	Loxahatchee	100%	33
Raulerson Hospital[2]	Okeechobee	100%	25
Regional Medical Center Bayonet Point[2]	Hudson	100%	69
Saint Lucie Medical Center[2]	Port Saint Lucie	100%	86
Saint Mary's Medical Center[2]	W Palm Beach	100%	29
Sarasota Memorial Hospital[2]	Sarasota	100%	95
Sebastian River Medical Center[2]	Sebastian	100%	35
South Bay Hospital[2]	Sun City Center	100%	43
South Miami Hospital[2]	South Miami	100%	38
Venice Reg Med Ctr-Bayfront Health[2]	Venice	100%	86
West Boca Medical Center[2]	Boca Raton	100%	35
West Florida Hospital[2]	Pensacola	100%	51
West Palm Hospital[2]	W Palm Beach	100%	25
Westside Regional Medical Center[2]	Plantation	100%	47
Fawcett Memorial Hospital[2]	Port Charlotte	99%	96
Osceola Regional Medical Center[2]	Kissimmee	99%	116
Physicians Reg Med Ctr-Pine Ridge[2]	Naples	99%	86
Aventura Hospital & Medical Center[2]	Aventura	98%	108
Cape Canaveral Hospital[2]	Cocoa Beach	98%	53
Halifax Health Medical Center[2]	Daytona Bch	98%	84
Health Central[2]	Ocoee	98%	66
Jupiter Medical Center[2]	Jupiter	98%	91
Kendall Regional Medical Center[2]	Miami	98%	52
Saint Vincent's Medical Center Southside[2]	Jacksonville	98%	49
The Villages Regional Hospital[2]	The Villages	98%	144
Central Florida Regional Hospital[2]	Sanford	97%	64
Gulf Coast Regional Medical Center[2]	Panama City	97%	38
Hialeah Hospital[2]	Hialeah	97%	36
Lakeland Regional Medical Center[2]	Lakeland	97%	243
Memorial Hospital of Tampa[2]	Tampa	97%	32
Plantation General Hospital[2]	Plantation	97%	64
Viera Hospital[2]	Melbourne	97%	35
Blake Medical Center[2]	Bradenton	96%	93
Englewood Community Hospital[2]	Englewood	96%	25
Leesburg Regional Medical Center[2]	Leesburg	96%	75
Morton Plant North Bay Hospital[2]	New Port Richey	96%	25
Manatee Memorial Hospital[2]	Bradenton	95%	65
Saint Anthony's Hospital[2]	St Petersburg	95%	95
University of Miami Hospital[2]	Miami	95%	41
Bartow Regional Medical Center[2]	Bartow	94%	35
Florida Hospital Deland[2]	Deland	94%	62
Lee Memorial Hospital[2]	Fort Myers	94%	160
Bay Med Ctr Sacred Heart Health Sys[2]	Panama City	93%	60
Bethesda Hospital East[2]	Boynton Beach	93%	92
Doctors Hospital of Sarasota[2]	Sarasota	93%	41
Largo Medical Center[2]	Largo	93%	85
Lawnwood Reg Med Ctr & Heart Inst[2]	Fort Pierce	93%	84
Mease Countryside Hospital[2]	Safety Harbor	93%	70
Medical Center of Trinity[2]	Trinity	93%	41
Baptist Medical Center Beaches[2]	Jcksnvl Bch	92%	50
Cape Coral Hospital[2]	Cape Coral	92%	95
Gulf Coast Med Ctr Lee Mem Health Sys[2]	Fort Myers	92%	154
Morton Plant Hospital[2]	Clearwater	92%	114
Saint Vincent's Medical Center[2]	Jacksonville	92%	93
Florida Hospital Memorial Medical Center[2]	Daytona Bch	91%	76
Palm Beach Gardens Medical Center[2]	Palm Bch Grdns	91%	65
Wellington Regional Medical Center[2]	Wellington	91%	35
North Shore Medical Center[2]	Miami	90%	63
Mayo Clinic[2]	Jacksonville	89%	87
Flagler Hospital[2]	St Augustine	88%	59
Florida Hospital Heartland Medical Center[2]	Sebring	88%	42
Wuesthoff Medical Center - Melbourne[2]	Melbourne	88%	32
Florida Hospital Tampa[2]	Tampa	87%	70
Martin Medical Center[2]	Stuart	87%	112
Wuesthoff Medical Center Rockledge[2]	Rockledge	87%	39
Putnam Community Medical Center[2]	Palatka	86%	36
Saint Petersburg General Hospital[2]	St Petersburg	86%	36
Florida Hospital Fish Memorial[2]	Orange City	85%	41
Holmes Regional Medical Center[2]	Melbourne	85%	132
Saint Joseph's Hospital[2]	Tampa	85%	185
South Florida Baptist Hospital[2]	Plant City	84%	43
Florida Hospital[2]	Orlando	83%	349
South Lake Hospital[2]	Clermont	83%	64
UF Health Shands Hospital[2]	Gainesville	83%	135
Tallahassee Memorial Hospital[2]	Tallahassee	81%	53
Florida Hospital Flagler[2]	Palm Coast	80%	49
Parrish Medical Center[2]	Titusville	79%	38
Bayfront Health Brooksville[2]	Brooksville	76%	54
Winter Haven Hospital[2]	Winter Haven	76%	87
Naples Community Hospital[2]	Naples	72%	199
Indian River Medical Center[2]	Vero Beach	71%	86
Santa Rosa Medical Center[2]	Milton	70%	27
Bert Fish Medical Center[2]	New Smyrn Bch	69%	45
Palm Bay Hospital[2]	Palm Bay	69%	52
Bayfront Health - Saint Petersburg[2]	St Petersburg	67%	52
Mount Sinai Medical Center[2]	Miami Beach	66%	44
Citrus Memorial Hospital[2]	Inverness	65%	120
Baptist Medical Center[2]	Jacksonville	64%	225
Jackson Memorial Hospital[2]	Miami	63%	197
Florida Hospital Carrollwood[2]	Tampa	62%	40
Heart of Florida Regional Medical Center[2]	Davenport	53%	43
Tampa General Hospital[2]	Tampa	53%	241
Orlando Health[2]	Orlando	51%	254
Cleveland Clinic Hospital[2]	Weston	41%	27
Sacred Heart Hospital[2]	Pensacola	26%	73
Bayfront Health Port Charlotte[2]	Port Charlotte	25%	55
UF Health Jacksonville[2]	Jacksonville	24%	92
Baptist Hospital[2]	Pensacola	4%	56
Munroe Regional Medical Center[2]	Ocala	0%	146

Chest Pain/Possible Heart Attack Care

Aspirin Given Within 24 Hours of Arrival

Hospital Name	City	Rate	Cases
Bayfront Health Dade City[3]	Dade City	100%	27
Bayfront Health Punta Gorda	Punta Gorda	100%	37
Broward Health Imperial Point	Fort Lauderdale	100%	36
Desoto Memorial Hospital	Arcadia	100%	52
Florida Hospital Carrollwood	Tampa	100%	45
Hialeah Hospital	Hialeah	100%	57
Homestead Hospital	Homestead	100%	57
Jupiter Medical Center	Jupiter	100%	66
Mariners Hospital	Tavernier	100%	81
Mease Hospital Dunedin	Dunedin	100%	40
Memorial Hospital Miramar	Miramar	100%	42
Plantation General Hospital	Plantation	100%	27
Raulerson Hospital	Okeechobee	100%	58
Saint Cloud Regional Medical Center	Saint Cloud	100%	35
Saint Lucie Medical Center	Port Saint Lucie	100%	64
Saint Petersburg General Hospital	St Petersburg	100%	32
Seven Rivers Regional Medical Center	Crystal River	100%	29
South Florida Baptist Hospital	Plant City	100%	36
University Hospital & Medical Center	Tamarac	100%	38
Viera Hospital	Melbourne	100%	62
West Boca Medical Center	Boca Raton	100%	40
West Kendall Baptist Hospital	Miami	100%	85
Gulf Breeze Hospital	Gulf Breeze	99%	69
Memorial Hospital Pembroke	Pembroke Pines	99%	78
Doctor's Memorial Hospital	Perry	98%	89
Englewood Community Hospital	Englewood	98%	64
Lake City Medical Center	Lake City	98%	132
Lehigh Regional Medical Center	Lehigh Acres	98%	55
Palm Bay Hospital	Palm Bay	98%	47
Shands Live Oak Regional Medical Center	Live Oak	98%	172
Baptist Medical Center Beaches	Jcksnvl Bch	97%	76
Broward Health Coral Springs	Coral Springs	97%	109
Cape Coral Hospital	Cape Coral	97%	67
Sacred Heart Hospital on the Gulf	Port Saint Joe	97%	36
Twin Cities Hospital	Niceville	97%	34
Baptist Medical Center - Nassau	Fernandina Bch	96%	95
Jackson Hospital	Marianna	95%	59
Martin Medical Center	Stuart	95%	38
Florida Hospital Wauchula	Wauchula	94%	51
Lakeside Medical Center	Belle Glade	94%	34
North Shore Medical Center	Miami	93%	42
Santa Rosa Medical Center	Milton	93%	72
Florida Hospital Fish Memorial	Orange City	92%	49
Baptist Medical Center	Jacksonville	91%	33
Shands Lake Shore Regional Medical Center	Lake City	91%	91

NOTE: Hospital profiles are in alphabetical order by state, then city, then hospital within the city; Rankings exclude hospitals with less than 25 cases except for patient surveys which excludes hospitals with less than 100 cases; (a) 100-299 cases; (1) The number of cases/patients is too few to report; (2) Data submitted were based on a sample of cases/patients; (3) Results are based on a shorter time period than required; (4) Data suppressed by CMS for one or more quarters; (5) Results are not available for this reporting period; (6) Fewer than 100 patients completed the HCAHPS survey; (7) No cases met the criteria for this measure; (8) The lower limit of the confidence interval cannot be calculated if the number of observed infections equals zero; (9) No data are available from the state/territory for this reporting period; (10) The scores shown reflect fewer than 50 completed surveys; (11) There were discrepancies in the data collection process; (12) This measure does not apply to this hospital for this reporting period; (13) Results cannot be calculated for this reporting period; (14) The results for this state are combined with nearby states to protect confidentiality; Please refer to the User's Guide for a full explanation of data.

Average Time to ECG (minutes)

Hospital Name	City	Min.	Cases
Bayfront Health Dade City[3]	Dade City	0	27
Bayfront Health Punta Gorda	Punta Gorda	0	38
Homestead Hospital	Homestead	0	58
Saint Lucie Medical Center	Port Saint Lucie	0	67
Englewood Community Hospital	Englewood	1	65
West Kendall Baptist Hospital	Miami	1	90
Desoto Memorial Hospital	Arcadia	2	54
Lehigh Regional Medical Center	Lehigh Acres	2	57
Mariners Hospital	Tavernier	2	81
Palm Bay Hospital	Palm Bay	2	48
Cape Coral Hospital	Cape Coral	5	67
Florida Hospital Carrollwood	Tampa	5	46
Jupiter Medical Center	Jupiter	5	69
Martin Medical Center	Stuart	5	41
Memorial Hospital Miramar	Miramar	5	45
Saint Cloud Regional Medical Center	Saint Cloud	5	40
Florida Hospital Wauchula	Wauchula	6	54
Santa Rosa Medical Center	Milton	6	75
Twin Cities Hospital	Niceville	6	34
Viera Hospital	Melbourne	6	62
Bayfront Health Brooksville	Brooksville	7	25
Florida Hospital Fish Memorial	Orange City	7	44
Memorial Hospital Pembroke	Pembroke Pines	7	80
Raulerson Hospital	Okeechobee	7	61
Saint Petersburg General Hospital	St Petersburg	7	35
Seven Rivers Regional Medical Center	Crystal River	7	29
Shands Lake Shore Regional Medical Center	Lake City	7	93
South Florida Baptist Hospital	Plant City	7	36
Baptist Medical Center	Jacksonville	8	30
Baptist Medical Center - Nassau	Fernandina Bch	8	99
Broward Health Coral Springs	Coral Springs	8	113
Doctor's Memorial Hospital	Perry	8	92
Gulf Breeze Hospital	Gulf Breeze	8	71
Jackson Hospital	Marianna	8	61
Lakeside Medical Center	Belle Glade	8	34
Mease Hospital Dunedin	Dunedin	8	40
Shands Live Oak Regional Medical Center	Live Oak	8	179
West Boca Medical Center	Boca Raton	8	41
Baptist Medical Center Beaches	Jcksnvll Bch	9	80
Broward Health Imperial Point	Fort Lauderdale	10	37
Sacred Heart Hospital on the Gulf	Port Saint Joe	12	36
North Shore Medical Center	Miami	13	41
Lake City Medical Center	Lake City	14	143
Hialeah Hospital	Hialeah	15	58
Plantation General Hospital	Plantation	16	27
University Hospital & Medical Center	Tamarac	21	39

Average Time to Transfer (minutes)

Hospital Name	City	Min.	Cases
Baptist Medical Center Beaches	Jcksnvll Bch	35	25
Saint Lucie Medical Center	Port Saint Lucie	36	30
Gulf Breeze Hospital	Gulf Breeze	43	25

Children's Asthma Care

Received Home Management Plan of Care

Hospital Name	City	Rate	Cases
Lawnwood Reg Med Ctr & Heart Inst	Fort Pierce	100%	76
Memorial Regional Hospital	Hollywood	100%	262
Orlando Health	Orlando	94%	371
Baptist Medical Center	Jacksonville	91%	491

Received Reliever Medication

Hospital Name	City	Rate	Cases
Baptist Medical Center	Jacksonville	100%	493
Lawnwood Reg Med Ctr & Heart Inst	Fort Pierce	100%	77
Memorial Regional Hospital	Hollywood	100%	262
Orlando Health	Orlando	100%	371

Received Systemic Corticosteroids

Hospital Name	City	Rate	Cases
Baptist Medical Center	Jacksonville	100%	491
Lawnwood Reg Med Ctr & Heart Inst	Fort Pierce	100%	77
Memorial Regional Hospital	Hollywood	100%	262
Orlando Health	Orlando	100%	371

Emergency Department

Admittance Decision Time (minutes)

Hospital Name	City	Min.	Cases
Healthmark Regional Medical Center[2]	Defuniak Spgs	0	414
Lakeland Regional Medical Center[2]	Lakeland	27	632
Edward White Hospital[2]	St Petersburg	34	439
Fawcett Memorial Hospital[2]	Port Charlotte	37	847
Oak Hill Hospital[2]	Brooksville	49	865
Blake Medical Center[2]	Bradenton	51	964
Jay Hospital[2]	Jay	52	480
Doctors Hospital of Sarasota[2]	Sarasota	56	757
Florida Hospital North Pinellas[2]	Tarpon Springs	56	585
Lower Keys Medical Center[2]	Key West	58	563
Northside Hospital[2]	St Petersburg	59	996
Baptist Medical Center Beaches[2]	Jcksnvll Bch	61	576
Kendall Regional Medical Center[2]	Miami	62	1086
Bartow Regional Medical Center[2]	Bartow	63	531
Regional Medical Center Bayonet Point[2]	Hudson	64	1078
Shands Live Oak Regional Medical Center[2]	Live Oak	67	569
Twin Cities Hospital[2]	Niceville	69	353
Doctor's Memorial Hospital[2]	Perry	70	569
Gulf Coast Regional Medical Center[2]	Panama City	71	663
Plantation General Hospital[2]	Plantation	71	778
Raulerson Hospital[2]	Okeechobee	71	888
Saint Joseph's Hospital[2]	Tampa	71	578
Shands Starke Regional Medical Center[2]	Starke	71	797
Fort Walton Beach Medical Center[2]	Fort Walton Bch	72	789
Englewood Community Hospital[2]	Englewood	73	666
Bayfront Health - Saint Petersburg[2]	St Petersburg	74	500
Westside Regional Medical Center[2]	Plantation	75	1038
Shands Lake Shore Regional Medical Center[2]	Lake City	76	443
Westchester General Hospital[2]	Miami	76	974
Florida Hospital Wauchula[2]	Wauchula	77	178
Medical Center of Trinity[2]	Trinity	77	858
Saint Petersburg General Hospital[2]	St Petersburg	79	720
Florida Hospital Wesley Chapel[2,3]	Wesley Chapel	80	142
Florida Hospital Memorial Medical Center[2]	Daytona Bch	81	642
Largo Medical Center[2]	Largo	81	761
Town & Country Hospital[2]	Tampa	81	395
West Palm Hospital[2]	W Palm Beach	81	895
Central Florida Regional Hospital[2]	Sanford	82	860
South Lake Hospital[2]	Clermont	82	1263
Saint Vincent's Medical Center Southside[2]	Jacksonville	83	465
Palms West Hospital[2]	Loxahatchee	84	842
Mariners Hospital[2]	Tavernier	85	422
Sacred Heart Hospital on the Gulf[2]	Port Saint Joe	85	105
Saint Cloud Regional Medical Center[2]	Saint Cloud	85	896
Naples Community Hospital[2]	Naples	86	737
Santa Rosa Medical Center[2]	Milton	86	537
Viera Hospital[2]	Melbourne	86	495
West Florida Hospital[2]	Pensacola	86	796
Florida Hospital Waterman[2]	Tavares	88	825
Gulf Breeze Hospital[2]	Gulf Breeze	88	483
Morton Plant Hospital[2]	Clearwater	89	443
Lakewood Ranch Medical Center[2]	Bradenton	90	380
Highlands Regional Medical Center[2]	Sebring	91	649
South Bay Hospital[2]	Sun City Center	91	1022
Florida Hospital Zephyrhills[2]	Zephyrhills	93	713
Jackson Hospital[2]	Marianna	93	316
Lake Wales Medical Center[2]	Lake Wales	94	835
Lakeside Medical Center[2]	Belle Glade	95	430
Florida Hospital Carrollwood[2]	Tampa	96	508
Memorial Hospital of Tampa[2]	Tampa	96	664
Orlando Health[2]	Orlando	96	456
Sacred Heart Hospital[2]	Pensacola	96	366
Saint Lucie Medical Center[2]	Port Saint Lucie	96	882
University Hospital & Medical Center[2]	Tamarac	96	964
Cape Canaveral Hospital[2]	Cocoa Beach	97	777
Sebastian River Medical Center[2]	Sebastian	97	647
Bayfront Health Brooksville[2]	Brooksville	98	783
Desoto Memorial Hospital[2]	Arcadia	99	189
Boca Raton Regional Hospital[2]	Boca Raton	100	613
South Florida Baptist Hospital[2]	Plant City	100	407
JFK Medical Center[2]	Atlantis	102	920
Brandon Regional Hospital[2]	Brandon	103	821
Aventura Hospital & Medical Center[2]	Aventura	104	1131
Lawnwood Reg Med Ctr & Heart Inst[2]	Fort Pierce	104	835
Mayo Clinic[2]	Jacksonville	104	521
Palm Bay Hospital[2]	Palm Bay	104	950
Seven Rivers Regional Medical Center[2]	Crystal River	104	796
Bayfront Health Dade City[2]	Dade City	106	436
Saint Anthony's Hospital[2]	St Petersburg	106	778
Florida Hospital Heartland Medical Center[2]	Sebring	107	1142
Health Central[2]	Ocoee	107	990
Mease Hospital Dunedin[2]	Dunedin	108	733
Palms of Pasadena Hospital[2]	St Petersburg	108	739
Morton Plant North Bay Hospital[2]	New Port Richey	109	442
Florida Hospital Deland[2]	Deland	111	819
Venice Reg Med Ctr-Bayfront Health[2]	Venice	111	759
Putnam Community Medical Center[2]	Palatka	113	701
Tallahassee Memorial Hospital[2]	Tallahassee	113	460
Citrus Memorial Hospital[2]	Inverness	114	325
North Okaloosa Medical Center[2]	Crestview	114	901
Sacred Heart Hosp-Emerald Coast[2]	Miramar Beach	114	420
Ocala Regional Medical Center[2]	Ocala	116	995
Osceola Regional Medical Center[2]	Kissimmee	116	920
South Miami Hospital[2]	South Miami	116	525
Holmes Regional Medical Center[2]	Melbourne	117	646
North Florida Regional Medical Center[2]	Gainesville	117	966
Sarasota Memorial Hospital[2]	Sarasota	117	449
Memorial Hospital Jacksonville[2]	Jacksonville	118	851
Coral Gables Hospital[2]	Coral Gables	119	1121
Bert Fish Medical Center[2]	New Smyrn Bch	120	499
Capital Regional Medical Center[2]	Tallahassee	120	956
Holy Cross Hospital[2]	Fort Lauderdale	121	655
Baptist Medical Center - Nassau[2]	Fernandina Bch	122	271
Florida Hospital[2]	Orlando	122	754
Parrish Medical Center[2]	Titusville	122	819
Bayfront Health Punta Gorda[2]	Punta Gorda	123	618
Wuesthoff Medical Center - Melbourne[2]	Melbourne	123	484
Lake City Medical Center[2]	Lake City	125	574
Larkin Community Hospital[2]	South Miami	125	379
Mease Countryside Hospital[2]	Safety Harbor	125	721
Baptist Medical Center[2]	Jacksonville	127	487
Florida Hospital Tampa[2]	Tampa	128	624
Manatee Memorial Hospital[2]	Bradenton	129	427
Homestead Hospital[2]	Homestead	131	667
Lehigh Regional Medical Center[2]	Lehigh Acres	131	503
Baptist Hospital[2]	Pensacola	132	631
Broward Health North[2]	Pompano Bch	133	947
West Boca Medical Center[2]	Boca Raton	133	744
Delray Medical Center[2]	Delray Beach	136	1059
Northwest Medical Center[2]	Margate	136	811
Florida Hospital Flagler[2]	Palm Coast	139	698
Jupiter Medical Center[2]	Jupiter	140	790
The Villages Regional Hospital[2]	The Villages	141	693
Palm Beach Gardens Medical Center[2]	Palm Bch Grdns	142	1036
Bethesda Hospital East[2]	Boynton Beach	143	459
Florida Hospital Fish Memorial[2]	Orange City	143	566
Physicians Reg Med Ctr-Pine Ridge[2]	Naples	143	876
Palm Springs General Hospital[2]	Hialeah	145	752
Wuesthoff Medical Center Rockledge[2]	Rockledge	146	688
Saint Mary's Medical Center[2]	W Palm Beach	147	626
Heart of Florida Regional Medical Center[2]	Davenport	150	806
Flagler Hospital[2]	St Augustine	152	620
Gulf Coast Med Ctr Lee Mem Health Sys[2]	Fort Myers	152	762
Memorial Regional Hospital[2]	Hollywood	154	502
Broward Health Imperial Point[2]	Fort Lauderdale	157	635
Lee Memorial Hospital[2]	Fort Myers	157	661
Halifax Health Medical Center[2]	Daytona Bch	162	590
Bay Med Ctr Sacred Heart Health Sys[2]	Panama City	164	822
Winter Haven Hospital[2]	Winter Haven	164	684
Indian River Medical Center[2]	Vero Beach	165	679
Bayfront Health Port Charlotte[2]	Port Charlotte	166	565
West Kendall Baptist Hospital[2]	Miami	166	858
Memorial Hospital Miramar[2]	Miramar	171	465
Munroe Regional Medical Center[2]	Ocala	172	639
Tampa General Hospital[2]	Tampa	172	536
North Shore Medical Center[2]	Miami	174	1431
Martin Medical Center[2]	Stuart	176	532
University of Miami Hospital[2]	Miami	177	475
Good Samaritan Medical Center[2]	W Palm Beach	178	766
Memorial Hospital West[2]	Pembroke Pines	178	478
Metropolitan Hospital of Miami[2]	Miami	182	771
Wellington Regional Medical Center[2]	Wellington	184	719
Memorial Hospital Pembroke[2]	Pembroke Pines	185	705
UF Health Shands Hospital[2]	Gainesville	191	441
Broward Health Medical Center[2]	Fort Lauderdale	194	622
Leesburg Regional Medical Center[2]	Leesburg	194	497
Cape Coral Hospital[2]	Cape Coral	195	842
Orange Park Medical Center[2]	Orange Park	198	881
Baptist Hospital of Miami[2]	Miami	201	622
Broward Health Coral Springs[2]	Coral Springs	204	584
Saint Vincent's Medical Center[2]	Jacksonville	210	501
Cleveland Clinic Hospital[2]	Weston	214	559
Doctors Hospital[2]	Coral Gables	224	678
Mount Sinai Medical Center[2]	Miami Beach	233	583
UF Health Jacksonville[2]	Jacksonville	292	595
Jackson Memorial Hospital[2]	Miami	316	1685
Hialeah Hospital[2]	Hialeah	324	840
Palmetto General Hospital[2]	Hialeah	335	785

Head CT Results Within 45 Minutes of Arrival

Hospital Name	City	Rate	Cases
Englewood Community Hospital	Englewood	96%	28
Health Central	Ocoee	84%	25
The Villages Regional Hospital	The Villages	65%	26
Shands Live Oak Regional Medical Center	Live Oak	28%	25

Patients Who Left ER Before Being Seen

Hospital Name	City	Rate	Cases
Anne Bates Leach Eye Hospital	Miami	0%	17234
Aventura Hospital & Medical Center	Aventura	0%	65029
Broward Health Medical Center	Fort Lauderdale	0%	102335
Cape Coral Hospital	Cape Coral	0%	28928
Cleveland Clinic Hospital	Weston	0%	33380
Doctors Hospital of Sarasota	Sarasota	0%	23085
Englewood Community Hospital	Englewood	0%	15527
Florida Hospital Wauchula	Wauchula	0%	13900
Gulf Coast Med Ctr Lee Mem Health Sys	Fort Myers	0%	29554

NOTE: Hospital profiles are in alphabetical order by state, then city, then hospital within the city; Rankings exclude hospitals with less than 25 cases except for patient surveys which excludes hospitals with less than 100 cases; (a) 100-299 cases; (1) The number of cases/patients is too few to report; (2) Data submitted were based on a sample of cases/patients; (3) Results are based on a shorter time period than required; (4) Data suppressed by CMS for one or more quarters; (5) Results are not available for this reporting period; (6) Fewer than 100 patients completed the HCAHPS survey; (7) No cases met the criteria for this measure; (8) The lower limit of the confidence interval cannot be calculated if the number of observed infections equals zero; (9) No data are available from the state/territory for this reporting period; (10) The scores shown reflect fewer than 50 completed surveys; (11) There were discrepancies in the data collection process; (12) This measure does not apply to this hospital for this reporting period; (13) Results cannot be calculated for this reporting period; (14) The results for this state are combined with nearby states to protect confidentiality; Please refer to the User's Guide for a full explanation of data.

Holy Cross Hospital	Fort Lauderdale	0%	51075
Kendall Regional Medical Center	Miami	0%	73287
Largo Medical Center	Largo	0%	43020
Lawnwood Reg Med Ctr & Heart Inst	Fort Pierce	0%	55333
Lee Memorial Hospital	Fort Myers	0%	70513
Mease Hospital Dunedin	Dunedin	0%	24605
Mount Sinai Medical Center	Miami Beach	0%	63203
North Florida Regional Medical Center	Gainesville	0%	66691
Northside Hospital	St Petersburg	0%	31437
Palm Beach Gardens Medical Center	Palm Bch Grdns	0%	30258
Raulerson Hospital	Okeechobee	0%	25018
Sacred Heart Hospital on the Gulf	Port Saint Joe	0%	8791
Saint Lucie Medical Center	Port Saint Lucie	0%	44560
Westside Regional Medical Center	Plantation	0%	44675
Baptist Hospital of Miami	Miami	1%	112785
Bartow Regional Medical Center	Bartow	1%	29929
Bayfront Health - Saint Petersburg	St Petersburg	1%	49049
Bayfront Health Brooksville	Brooksville	1%	54863
Bayfront Health Dade City	Dade City	1%	23362
Bethesda Hospital East	Boynton Beach	1%	62580
Blake Medical Center	Bradenton	1%	37485
Boca Raton Regional Hospital	Boca Raton	1%	43414
Brandon Regional Hospital	Brandon	1%	103150
Capital Regional Medical Center	Tallahassee	1%	87494
Central Florida Regional Hospital	Sanford	1%	45492
Coral Gables Hospital	Coral Gables	1%	15973
Delray Medical Center	Delray Beach	1%	46311
Doctors Hospital	Coral Gables	1%	18500
Edward White Hospital	St Petersburg	1%	11542
Florida Hospital Flagler	Palm Coast	1%	39984
Florida Hospital Memorial Medical Center	Daytona Bch	1%	46637
Florida Hospital North Pinellas	Tarpon Springs	1%	19378
Fort Walton Beach Medical Center	Fort Walton Bch	1%	63370
Gulf Coast Regional Medical Center	Panama City	1%	55320
Health Central	Ocoee	1%	63021
Heart of Florida Regional Medical Center	Davenport	1%	50878
Hialeah Hospital	Hialeah	1%	32086
Highlands Regional Medical Center	Sebring	1%	18960
Holmes Regional Medical Center	Melbourne	1%	67599
Homestead Hospital	Homestead	1%	90752
Jackson Hospital	Marianna	1%	26319
Jay Hospital	Jay	1%	9972
JFK Medical Center	Atlantis	1%	78098
Jupiter Medical Center	Jupiter	1%	30831
Lakeland Regional Medical Center	Lakeland	1%	172449
Lakeside Medical Center	Belle Glade	1%	22710
Lehigh Regional Medical Center	Lehigh Acres	1%	35503
Lower Keys Medical Center	Key West	1%	24879
Martin Medical Center	Stuart	1%	83241
Mayo Clinic	Jacksonville	1%	26995
Mease Countryside Hospital	Safety Harbor	1%	53117
Medical Center of Trinity	Trinity	1%	43159
Memorial Hospital Jacksonville	Jacksonville	1%	90556
Memorial Hospital Miramar	Miramar	1%	59764
Memorial Hospital of Tampa	Tampa	1%	16074
Memorial Hospital Pembroke	Pembroke Pines	1%	91152
Memorial Regional Hospital	Hollywood	1%	176592
North Okaloosa Medical Center	Crestview	1%	31085
Oak Hill Hospital	Brooksville	1%	38228
Ocala Regional Medical Center	Ocala	1%	75969
Orange Park Medical Center	Orange Park	1%	88906
Osceola Regional Medical Center	Kissimmee	1%	87813
Palmetto General Hospital	Hialeah	1%	63004
Palms of Pasadena Hospital	St Petersburg	1%	14533
Palms West Hospital	Loxahatchee	1%	45364
Physicians Reg Med Ctr-Pine Ridge	Naples	1%	49549
Plantation General Hospital	Plantation	1%	52315
Regional Medical Center Bayonet Point	Hudson	1%	40919
Sacred Heart Hosp-Emerald Coast	Miramar Beach	1%	27979
Saint Petersburg General Hospital	St Petersburg	1%	31914
Saint Vincent's Medical Center Southside	Jacksonville	1%	35682
Sarasota Memorial Hospital	Sarasota	1%	134712
Sebastian River Medical Center	Sebastian	1%	19243
Seven Rivers Regional Medical Center	Crystal River	1%	22310
Shands Live Oak Regional Medical Center	Live Oak	1%	22926
South Bay Hospital	Sun City Center	1%	27709
South Miami Hospital	South Miami	1%	30826
University Hospital & Medical Center	Tamarac	1%	33142
University of Miami Hospital	Miami	1%	33036
Venice Reg Med Ctr-Bayfront Health	Venice	1%	33164
Viera Hospital	Melbourne	1%	16594
Wellington Regional Medical Center	Wellington	1%	21741
West Boca Medical Center	Boca Raton	1%	35504
West Florida Hospital	Pensacola	1%	50551
West Kendall Baptist Hospital	Miami	1%	45135
West Palm Hospital	W Palm Beach	1%	25606
Westchester General Hospital	Miami	1%	10642
Wuesthoff Medical Center Rockledge	Rockledge	1%	36758
Baptist Medical Center Beaches	Jcksnvll Bch	2%	37249
Bay Med Ctr Sacred Heart Health Sys	Panama City	2%	58249
Bayfront Health Punta Gorda	Punta Gorda	2%	18040
Bert Fish Medical Center	New Smyrn Bch	2%	31295
Broward Health Imperial Point	Fort Lauderdale	2%	33984
Broward Health North	Pompano Bch	2%	61284
Fawcett Memorial Hospital	Port Charlotte	2%	24704
Flagler Hospital	St Augustine	2%	53515
Florida Hospital	Orlando	2%	446576
Florida Hospital Heartland Medical Center	Sebring	2%	27389
Florida Hospital Waterman	Tavares	2%	53598
Gulf Breeze Hospital	Gulf Breeze	2%	28182
Halifax Health Medical Center	Daytona Bch	2%	116800
Healthmark Regional Medical Center	Defuniak Spgs	2%	11734
Indian River Medical Center	Vero Beach	2%	57166
Lake City Medical Center	Lake City	2%	28047
Leesburg Regional Medical Center	Leesburg	2%	47702
Manatee Memorial Hospital	Bradenton	2%	66066
Mariners Hospital	Tavernier	2%	11830
Memorial Hospital West	Pembroke Pines	2%	93015
Naples Community Hospital	Naples	2%	89925
Northwest Medical Center	Margate	2%	45369
Orlando Health	Orlando	2%	282258
Palm Bay Hospital	Palm Bay	2%	40194
Palm Springs General Hospital	Hialeah	2%	5473
Parrish Medical Center	Titusville	2%	41852
Saint Anthony's Hospital	St Petersburg	2%	42523
Saint Cloud Regional Medical Center	Saint Cloud	2%	25684
Saint Joseph's Hospital	Tampa	2%	186053
Santa Rosa Medical Center	Milton	2%	32263
Shands Lake Shore Regional Medical Center	Lake City	2%	28715
South Florida Baptist Hospital	Plant City	2%	42151
South Lake Hospital	Clermont	2%	47763
Town & Country Hospital	Tampa	2%	22411
Twin Cities Hospital	Niceville	2%	15173
Wuesthoff Medical Center - Melbourne	Melbourne	2%	18510
Baptist Medical Center - Nassau	Fernandina Bch	3%	25949
Bayfront Health Port Charlotte	Port Charlotte	3%	26844
Cape Canaveral Hospital	Cocoa Beach	3%	27399
Desoto Memorial Hospital	Arcadia	3%	16448
Florida Hospital Carrollwood	Tampa	3%	22915
Florida Hospital Deland	Deland	3%	50588
Florida Hospital Fish Memorial	Orange City	3%	49712
Lakewood Ranch Medical Center	Bradenton	3%	2298
Larkin Community Hospital	South Miami	3%	7440
Morton Plant Hospital	Clearwater	3%	77818
North Shore Medical Center	Miami	3%	71850
Sacred Heart Hospital	Pensacola	3%	89018
Saint Vincent's Medical Center	Jacksonville	3%	72403
Baptist Hospital	Pensacola	4%	51366
Baptist Medical Center	Jacksonville	4%	183384
Broward Health Coral Springs	Coral Springs	4%	56693
Florida Hospital Zephyrhills	Zephyrhills	4%	34813
Good Samaritan Medical Center	W Palm Beach	4%	30808
Lake Wales Medical Center	Lake Wales	4%	5306
Putnam Community Medical Center	Palatka	4%	29472
Tampa General Hospital	Tampa	4%	84754
UF Health Shands Hospital	Gainesville	4%	87842
The Villages Regional Hospital	The Villages	4%	42673
Winter Haven Hospital	Winter Haven	4%	64685
Doctor's Memorial Hospital	Perry	5%	14523
Munroe Regional Medical Center	Ocala	5%	104099
Saint Mary's Medical Center	W Palm Beach	5%	61273
Citrus Memorial Hospital	Inverness	6%	42018
Florida Hospital Tampa	Tampa	6%	51700
Jackson Memorial Hospital	Miami	6%	195889
Morton Plant North Bay Hospital	New Port Richey	6%	35364
Tallahassee Memorial Hospital	Tallahassee	6%	74082
UF Health Jacksonville	Jacksonville	8%	89453

Time from ER Arrival to Being Admitted (minutes)

Hospital Name	City	Min.	Cases
Lakeland Regional Medical Center[2]	Lakeland	168	761
Florida Hospital North Pinellas[2]	Tarpon Springs	175	585
Edward White Hospital[2]	St Petersburg	180	439
Sacred Heart Hospital on the Gulf[2]	Port Saint Joe	182	191
Englewood Community Hospital[2]	Englewood	183	666
Healthmark Regional Medical Center[2]	Defuniak Spgs	188	426
Fawcett Memorial Hospital[2]	Port Charlotte	196	847
Doctors Hospital of Sarasota[2]	Sarasota	201	757
Palms West Hospital[2]	Loxahatchee	205	851
JFK Medical Center[2]	Atlantis	207	920
Blake Medical Center[2]	Bradenton	211	968
Northside Hospital[2]	St Petersburg	214	996
Aventura Hospital & Medical Center[2]	Aventura	217	1131
Raulerson Hospital[2]	Okeechobee	217	888
Jackson Hospital[2]	Marianna	219	316
Jay Hospital[2]	Jay	220	481
Plantation General Hospital[2]	Plantation	221	778
Santa Rosa Medical Center[2]	Milton	221	536
Bayfront Health Dade City[2]	Dade City	223	436
West Palm Hospital[2]	W Palm Beach	223	895
Florida Hospital Wesley Chapel[2,3]	Wesley Chapel	224	142
Saint Petersburg General Hospital[2]	St Petersburg	224	721
Florida Hospital Wauchula[2]	Wauchula	226	252
Saint Joseph's Hospital[2]	Tampa	227	594
Saint Vincent's Medical Center Southside[2]	Jacksonville	228	467
Twin Cities Hospital[2]	Niceville	228	353
University Hospital & Medical Center[2]	Tamarac	228	964
Largo Medical Center[2]	Largo	232	766
Bartow Regional Medical Center[2]	Bartow	233	531
Highlands Regional Medical Center[2]	Sebring	233	649
Medical Center of Trinity[2]	Trinity	234	858
Regional Medical Center Bayonet Point[2]	Hudson	234	1078
Gulf Coast Regional Medical Center[2]	Panama City	237	663
Kendall Regional Medical Center[2]	Miami	237	1086
Fort Walton Beach Medical Center[2]	Fort Walton Bch	239	789
Oak Hill Hospital[2]	Brooksville	240	865
North Okaloosa Medical Center[2]	Crestview	241	902
West Florida Hospital[2]	Pensacola	241	796
Boca Raton Regional Hospital[2]	Boca Raton	242	618
Viera Hospital[2]	Melbourne	242	495
Baptist Medical Center Beaches[2]	Jcksnvll Bch	246	578
Shands Starke Regional Medical Center[2]	Starke	246	797
Lakeside Medical Center[2]	Belle Glade	247	431
Sebastian River Medical Center[2]	Sebastian	248	650
Florida Hospital Carrollwood[2]	Tampa	249	541
Naples Community Hospital[2]	Naples	249	756
Bayfront Health - Saint Petersburg[2]	St Petersburg	251	522
Westside Regional Medical Center[2]	Plantation	251	1038
South Bay Hospital[2]	Sun City Center	252	1022
Saint Lucie Medical Center[2]	Port Saint Lucie	254	882
Saint Cloud Regional Medical Center[2]	Saint Cloud	255	898
Lake Wales Medical Center[2]	Lake Wales	256	835
Lawnwood Reg Med Ctr & Heart Inst[2]	Fort Pierce	256	835
Lower Keys Medical Center[2]	Key West	256	566
Venice Reg Med Ctr-Bayfront Health[2]	Venice	257	783
Palm Beach Gardens Medical Center[2]	Palm Bch Grdns	258	1036
Palms of Pasadena Hospital[2]	St Petersburg	262	745
Sacred Heart Hosp-Emerald Coast[2]	Miramar Beach	262	467
Northwest Medical Center[2]	Margate	263	835
Capital Regional Medical Center[2]	Tallahassee	264	956
Holmes Regional Medical Center[2]	Melbourne	264	649
Wuesthoff Medical Center - Melbourne[2]	Melbourne	264	518
Central Florida Regional Hospital[2]	Sanford	265	860
Bayfront Health Punta Gorda[2]	Punta Gorda	266	620
Palm Bay Hospital[2]	Palm Bay	266	950
Mariners Hospital[2]	Tavernier	267	437
Cape Canaveral Hospital[2]	Cocoa Beach	268	777
Shands Lake Shore Regional Medical Center[2]	Lake City	268	444
Florida Hospital Waterman[2]	Tavares	270	832
South Florida Baptist Hospital[2]	Plant City	271	409
Gulf Breeze Hospital[2]	Gulf Breeze	273	491
Mayo Clinic[2]	Jacksonville	274	522
Florida Hospital Memorial Medical Center[2]	Daytona Bch	275	659
Mease Hospital Dunedin[2]	Dunedin	275	735
Putnam Community Medical Center[2]	Palatka	275	720
Florida Hospital Heartland Medical Center[2]	Sebring	276	1241
North Florida Regional Medical Center[2]	Gainesville	276	966
Memorial Hospital of Tampa[2]	Tampa	277	664
Bayfront Health Brooksville[2]	Brooksville	280	783
Shands Live Oak Regional Medical Center[2]	Live Oak	280	570
Wuesthoff Medical Center Rockledge[2]	Rockledge	281	727
Doctor's Memorial Hospital[2]	Perry	284	652
Memorial Hospital Jacksonville[2]	Jacksonville	284	852
Parrish Medical Center[2]	Titusville	286	822
Physicians Reg Med Ctr-Pine Ridge[2]	Naples	288	876
Bethesda Hospital East[2]	Boynton Beach	290	483
Brandon Regional Hospital[2]	Brandon	290	826
Osceola Regional Medical Center[2]	Kissimmee	290	920
Florida Hospital Zephyrhills[2]	Zephyrhills	292	719
Lakewood Ranch Medical Center[2]	Bradenton	294	382
Saint Anthony's Hospital[2]	St Petersburg	296	789
Seven Rivers Regional Medical Center[2]	Crystal River	296	797
Ocala Regional Medical Center[2]	Ocala	299	995
Lehigh Regional Medical Center[2]	Lehigh Acres	300	505
Morton Plant Hospital[2]	Clearwater	300	447
Baptist Medical Center - Nassau[2]	Fernandina Bch	302	272
Town & Country Hospital[2]	Tampa	302	429
Bert Fish Medical Center[2]	New Smyrn Bch	305	517
Mease Countryside Hospital[2]	Safety Harbor	305	733
Jupiter Medical Center[2]	Jupiter	306	793
Sacred Heart Hospital[2]	Pensacola	310	400
Baptist Hospital[2]	Pensacola	311	665
Morton Plant North Bay Hospital[2]	New Port Richey	311	458
Westchester General Hospital[2]	Miami	312	974
South Lake Hospital[2]	Clermont	313	1731
Florida Hospital Deland[2]	Deland	316	856
Florida Hospital Tampa[2]	Tampa	316	626
Sarasota Memorial Hospital[2]	Sarasota	317	453
Desoto Memorial Hospital[2]	Arcadia	318	232
Lake City Medical Center[2]	Lake City	318	574
Memorial Regional Hospital[2]	Hollywood	318	505
Holy Cross Hospital[2]	Fort Lauderdale	320	656
Delray Medical Center[2]	Delray Beach	322	1059

NOTE: Hospital profiles are in alphabetical order by state, then city, then hospital within the city; Rankings exclude hospitals with less than 25 cases except for patient surveys which excludes hospitals with less than 100 cases; (a) 100-299 cases; (1) The number of cases/patients is too few to report; (2) Data submitted were based on a sample of cases/patients; (3) Results are based on a shorter time period than required; (4) Data suppressed by CMS for one or more quarters; (5) Results are not available for this reporting period; (6) Fewer than 100 patients completed the HCAHPS survey; (7) No cases met the criteria for this measure; (8) The lower limit of the confidence interval cannot be calculated if the number of observed infections equals zero; (9) No data are available from the state/territory for this reporting period; (10) The scores shown reflect fewer than 50 completed surveys; (11) There were discrepancies in the data collection process; (12) This measure does not apply to this hospital for this reporting period; (13) Results cannot be calculated for this reporting period; (14) The results for this state are combined with nearby states to protect confidentiality; Please refer to the User's Guide for a full explanation of data.

Bayfront Health Port Charlotte[2]	Port Charlotte	326	607
Coral Gables Hospital[2]	Coral Gables	326	1121
Florida Hospital[2]	Orlando	328	768
Lee Memorial Hospital[2]	Fort Myers	329	669
Baptist Medical Center[2]	Jacksonville	330	498
Larkin Community Hospital[2]	South Miami	330	380
Citrus Memorial Hospital[2]	Inverness	334	335
Orlando Health[2]	Orlando	335	541
West Boca Medical Center[2]	Boca Raton	335	744
Broward Health Imperial Point[2]	Fort Lauderdale	337	659
Halifax Health Medical Center[2]	Daytona Bch	337	590
Memorial Hospital Pembroke[2]	Pembroke Pines	339	726
Good Samaritan Medical Center[2]	W Palm Beach	340	766
Gulf Coast Med Ctr Lee Mem Health Sys[2]	Fort Myers	340	766
Saint Mary's Medical Center[2]	W Palm Beach	340	626
Doctors Hospital[2]	Coral Gables	343	814
Memorial Hospital West[2]	Pembroke Pines	343	478
Indian River Medical Center[2]	Vero Beach	346	691
Broward Health North[2]	Pompano Bch	350	949
Bay Med Ctr Sacred Heart Health Sys[2]	Panama City	351	829
Broward Health Medical Center[2]	Fort Lauderdale	351	624
Memorial Hospital Miramar[2]	Miramar	353	468
Cleveland Clinic Hospital[2]	Weston	355	562
Orange Park Medical Center[2]	Orange Park	355	881
Cape Coral Hospital[2]	Cape Coral	356	842
Heart of Florida Regional Medical Center[2]	Davenport	356	808
Florida Hospital Flagler[2]	Palm Coast	359	884
Martin Medical Center[2]	Stuart	360	534
North Shore Medical Center[2]	Miami	362	1434
Flagler Hospital[2]	St Augustine	364	620
University of Miami Hospital[2]	Miami	366	478
South Miami Hospital[2]	South Miami	367	529
Health Central[2]	Ocoee	373	990
Manatee Memorial Hospital[2]	Bradenton	380	429
Homestead Hospital[2]	Homestead	382	677
Wellington Regional Medical Center[2]	Wellington	383	725
Saint Vincent's Medical Center[2]	Jacksonville	386	513
Tallahassee Memorial Hospital[2]	Tallahassee	386	490
Palm Springs General Hospital[2]	Hialeah	390	752
West Kendall Baptist Hospital[2]	Miami	394	858
Winter Haven Hospital[2]	Winter Haven	394	695
Mount Sinai Medical Center[2]	Miami Beach	399	586
The Villages Regional Hospital[2]	The Villages	399	739
Munroe Regional Medical Center[2]	Ocala	413	643
UF Health Shands Hospital[2]	Gainesville	414	442
Broward Health Coral Springs[2]	Coral Springs	415	584
Florida Hospital Fish Memorial[2]	Orange City	416	568
Metropolitan Hospital of Miami[2]	Miami	416	771
Tampa General Hospital[2]	Tampa	418	540
Baptist Hospital of Miami[2]	Miami	432	746
Leesburg Regional Medical Center[2]	Leesburg	434	548
Hialeah Hospital[2]	Hialeah	518	842
Palmetto General Hospital[2]	Hialeah	535	785
UF Health Jacksonville[2]	Jacksonville	626	629
Jackson Memorial Hospital[2]	Miami	692	1702

Time from ER Arrival to Discharge (minutes)

Hospital Name	City	Min.	Cases
Sacred Heart Hospital on the Gulf	Port Saint Joe	74	349
Lehigh Regional Medical Center	Lehigh Acres	89	381
Florida Hospital Wauchula	Wauchula	90	390
Heart of Florida Regional Medical Center	Davenport	95	723
Lake Wales Medical Center	Lake Wales	97	392
Florida Hospital Memorial Medical Center	Daytona Bch	99	712
Bartow Regional Medical Center	Bartow	100	588
Edward White Hospital	St Petersburg	100	391
Healthmark Regional Medical Center	Defuniak Spgs	100	321
Jackson Hospital	Marianna	101	1156
Englewood Community Hospital	Englewood	102	370
Santa Rosa Medical Center	Milton	103	351
Mariners Hospital	Tavernier	104	339
Jay Hospital	Jay	105	449
Bayfront Health Dade City	Dade City	108	971
Fort Walton Beach Medical Center	Fort Walton Bch	108	486
Putnam Community Medical Center	Palatka	109	440
Shands Live Oak Regional Medical Center	Live Oak	111	889
Lakeland Regional Medical Center	Lakeland	112	445
Physicians Reg Med Ctr-Pine Ridge	Naples	113	683
Saint Petersburg General Hospital	St Petersburg	114	450
Sebastian River Medical Center	Sebastian	114	367
Florida Hospital North Pinellas	Tarpon Springs	115	381
Capital Regional Medical Center	Tallahassee	116	491
Lakeside Medical Center	Belle Glade	116	448
Lower Keys Medical Center	Key West	116	1130
Twin Cities Hospital	Niceville	116	388
West Palm Hospital	W Palm Beach	116	398
Wuesthoff Medical Center - Melbourne	Melbourne	116	362
Memorial Hospital Pembroke	Pembroke Pines	121	353
Doctors Hospital of Sarasota	Sarasota	122	416
Kendall Regional Medical Center	Miami	122	470
Raulerson Hospital	Okeechobee	122	449
South Florida Baptist Hospital	Plant City	122	357
Bert Fish Medical Center	New Smyrn Bch	123	477
Memorial Regional Hospital	Hollywood	123	684
Saint Lucie Medical Center	Port Saint Lucie	124	448
Shands Lake Shore Regional Medical Center	Lake City	124	1053
Memorial Hospital Jacksonville	Jacksonville	125	508
Munroe Regional Medical Center	Ocala	125	341
Palms West Hospital	Loxahatchee	125	441
Westside Regional Medical Center	Plantation	125	430
Wuesthoff Medical Center Rockledge	Rockledge	125	361
Bayfront Health Punta Gorda	Punta Gorda	126	389
Lake City Medical Center	Lake City	126	376
Northside Hospital	St Petersburg	126	436
Fawcett Memorial Hospital	Port Charlotte	127	410
Baptist Medical Center - Nassau	Fernandina Bch	128	408
Bayfront Health Brooksville	Brooksville	128	1136
Gulf Coast Regional Medical Center	Panama City	128	511
North Okaloosa Medical Center	Crestview	129	393
Orange Park Medical Center	Orange Park	129	502
University Hospital & Medical Center	Tamarac	129	383
Cleveland Clinic Hospital	Weston	130	386
Saint Cloud Regional Medical Center	Saint Cloud	130	678
Seven Rivers Regional Medical Center	Crystal River	130	446
Blake Medical Center	Bradenton	131	444
Florida Hospital Deland	Deland	131	357
Town & Country Hospital	Tampa	131	1091
Highlands Regional Medical Center	Sebring	132	413
Good Samaritan Medical Center	W Palm Beach	133	387
Saint Mary's Medical Center	W Palm Beach	133	471
Florida Hospital Carrollwood	Tampa	134	344
Halifax Health Medical Center	Daytona Bch	134	391
Naples Community Hospital	Naples	134	395
Plantation General Hospital	Plantation	134	468
JFK Medical Center	Atlantis	135	402
Hendry Regional Medical Center[3]	Clewiston	136	279
Lawnwood Reg Med Ctr & Heart Inst	Fort Pierce	136	459
Regional Medical Center Bayonet Point	Hudson	136	404
Northwest Medical Center	Margate	137	409
Martin Medical Center	Stuart	138	380
Palms of Pasadena Hospital	St Petersburg	139	487
Gulf Breeze Hospital	Gulf Breeze	140	458
Florida Hospital Wesley Chapel[3]	Wesley Chapel	141	93
Palm Beach Gardens Medical Center	Palm Bch Grdns	141	357
Sacred Heart Hosp-Emerald Coast	Miramar Beach	141	389
Manatee Memorial Hospital	Bradenton	142	382
Aventura Hospital & Medical Center	Aventura	143	436
Boca Raton Regional Hospital	Boca Raton	143	325
Doctor's Memorial Hospital	Perry	143	371
Palm Bay Hospital	Palm Bay	143	380
Mease Hospital Dunedin	Dunedin	144	358
Medical Center of Trinity	Trinity	144	454
Wellington Regional Medical Center	Wellington	144	408
Bethesda Hospital East	Boynton Beach	145	355
Florida Hospital Heartland Medical Center	Sebring	145	776
Lakewood Ranch Medical Center	Bradenton	145	385
South Bay Hospital	Sun City Center	145	421
Viera Hospital	Melbourne	145	383
Anne Bates Leach Eye Hospital	Miami	147	407
Central Florida Regional Hospital	Sanford	147	455
Desoto Memorial Hospital	Arcadia	147	365
Brandon Regional Hospital	Brandon	148	497
Florida Hospital Waterman	Tavares	149	335
Baptist Medical Center Beaches	Jcksnvll Bch	150	400
Memorial Hospital West	Pembroke Pines	151	335
Florida Hospital Zephyrhills	Zephyrhills	152	298
Holy Cross Hospital	Fort Lauderdale	152	389
Memorial Hospital of Tampa	Tampa	152	371
Largo Medical Center	Largo	153	407
Osceola Regional Medical Center	Kissimmee	154	443
Saint Joseph's Hospital	Tampa	154	352
Florida Hospital Flagler	Palm Coast	155	342
Flagler Hospital	St Augustine	156	370
Jupiter Medical Center	Jupiter	156	374
Oak Hill Hospital	Brooksville	156	444
Saint Vincent's Medical Center Southside	Jacksonville	156	375
Indian River Medical Center	Vero Beach	157	364
Venice Reg Med Ctr-Bayfront Health	Venice	157	363
West Boca Medical Center	Boca Raton	158	418
Broward Health North	Pompano Bch	159	375
Ocala Regional Medical Center	Ocala	159	445
Holmes Regional Medical Center	Melbourne	160	412
Baptist Hospital	Pensacola	162	432
Citrus Memorial Hospital	Inverness	162	522
Mount Sinai Medical Center	Miami Beach	162	364
Parrish Medical Center	Titusville	162	420
Bayfront Health - Saint Petersburg	St Petersburg	163	433
Broward Health Medical Center	Fort Lauderdale	163	384
Delray Medical Center	Delray Beach	163	382
Bay Med Ctr Sacred Heart Health Sys	Panama City	164	416
Mayo Clinic	Jacksonville	164	385
Memorial Hospital Miramar	Miramar	164	362
Baptist Medical Center	Jacksonville	165	401
Broward Health Imperial Point	Fort Lauderdale	165	367
Sarasota Memorial Hospital	Sarasota	165	396
Bayfront Health Port Charlotte	Port Charlotte	166	394
Florida Hospital	Orlando	168	1396
Florida Hospital Fish Memorial	Orange City	170	337
Morton Plant Hospital	Clearwater	170	368
Morton Plant North Bay Hospital	New Port Richey	170	321
West Florida Hospital	Pensacola	170	450
Lee Memorial Hospital	Fort Myers	172	369
South Lake Hospital	Clermont	172	2276
Cape Canaveral Hospital	Cocoa Beach	174	367
Florida Hospital Tampa	Tampa	174	326
Homestead Hospital	Homestead	174	729
Westchester General Hospital	Miami	174	1115
Orlando Health	Orlando	176	1587
North Shore Medical Center	Miami	177	877
Sacred Heart Hospital	Pensacola	179	309
Mease Countryside Hospital	Safety Harbor	180	364
Broward Health Coral Springs	Coral Springs	183	370
Coral Gables Hospital	Coral Gables	186	405
North Florida Regional Medical Center	Gainesville	188	460
Health Central	Ocoee	196	4741
Leesburg Regional Medical Center	Leesburg	197	325
Palmetto General Hospital	Hialeah	198	342
Saint Vincent's Medical Center	Jacksonville	198	335
University of Miami Hospital	Miami	202	455
Cape Coral Hospital	Cape Coral	203	359
Saint Anthony's Hospital	St Petersburg	206	548
Gulf Coast Med Ctr Lee Mem Health Sys	Fort Myers	208	368
Hialeah Hospital	Hialeah	208	453
Doctors Hospital	Coral Gables	209	360
West Kendall Baptist Hospital	Miami	216	1196
Baptist Hospital of Miami	Miami	223	363
Palm Springs General Hospital	Hialeah	224	308
The Villages Regional Hospital	The Villages	232	293
Winter Haven Hospital	Winter Haven	236	407
UF Health Jacksonville	Jacksonville	237	337
Tallahassee Memorial Hospital	Tallahassee	241	327
UF Health Shands Hospital	Gainesville	242	308
South Miami Hospital	South Miami	261	381
Larkin Community Hospital	South Miami	262	191
Jackson Memorial Hospital	Miami	281	954
Tampa General Hospital	Tampa	330	316

Time in ER Before Being Evaluated (minutes)

Hospital Name	City	Min.	Cases
Bayfront Health Dade City	Dade City	4	1056
Hialeah Hospital	Hialeah	4	500
West Palm Hospital	W Palm Beach	4	453
Kendall Regional Medical Center	Miami	5	505
Edward White Hospital	St Petersburg	7	442
West Florida Hospital	Pensacola	7	512
Brandon Regional Hospital	Brandon	8	542
Englewood Community Hospital	Englewood	8	433
Lake City Medical Center	Lake City	8	452
Raulerson Hospital	Okeechobee	8	501
Fawcett Memorial Hospital	Port Charlotte	9	431
Fort Walton Beach Medical Center	Fort Walton Bch	9	518
Northwest Medical Center	Margate	9	495
Palms West Hospital	Loxahatchee	9	453
Aventura Hospital & Medical Center	Aventura	10	471
Saint Petersburg General Hospital	St Petersburg	10	500
Northside Hospital	St Petersburg	11	498
Palm Beach Gardens Medical Center	Palm Bch Grdns	11	384
Saint Lucie Medical Center	Port Saint Lucie	11	499
University Hospital & Medical Center	Tamarac	11	476
Westside Regional Medical Center	Plantation	11	461
Good Samaritan Medical Center	W Palm Beach	12	454
South Bay Hospital	Sun City Center	12	467
Gulf Coast Regional Medical Center	Panama City	13	535
Lawnwood Reg Med Ctr & Heart Inst	Fort Pierce	13	520
Osceola Regional Medical Center	Kissimmee	13	521
Plantation General Hospital	Plantation	13	536
Shands Live Oak Regional Medical Center	Live Oak	13	991
Cleveland Clinic Hospital	Weston	14	415
Desoto Memorial Hospital	Arcadia	14	407
Doctors Hospital of Sarasota	Sarasota	14	441
JFK Medical Center	Atlantis	14	533
Bartow Regional Medical Center	Bartow	15	626
Central Florida Regional Hospital	Sanford	15	499
Doctors Hospital	Coral Gables	15	394
Florida Hospital Memorial Medical Center	Daytona Bch	15	669
Highlands Regional Medical Center	Sebring	15	433
Largo Medical Center	Largo	15	463
Capital Regional Medical Center	Tallahassee	16	531
Homestead Hospital	Homestead	16	805
Medical Center of Trinity	Trinity	16	469
Oak Hill Hospital	Brooksville	16	496
Sacred Heart Hospital on the Gulf	Port Saint Joe	16	355
Wuesthoff Medical Center Rockledge	Rockledge	16	416

NOTE: Hospital profiles are in alphabetical order by state, then city, then hospital within the city; Rankings exclude hospitals with less than 25 cases except for patient surveys which excludes hospitals with less than 100 cases; (a) 100-299 cases; (1) The number of cases/patients is too few to report; (2) Data submitted were based on a sample of cases/patients; (3) Results are based on a shorter time period than required; (4) Data suppressed by CMS for one or more quarters; (5) Results are not available for this reporting period; (6) Fewer than 100 patients completed the HCAHPS survey; (7) No cases met the criteria for this measure; (8) The lower limit of the confidence interval cannot be calculated if the number of observed infections equals zero; (9) No data are available from the state/territory for this reporting period; (10) The scores shown reflect fewer than 50 completed surveys; (11) There were discrepancies in the data collection process; (12) This measure does not apply to this hospital for this reporting period; (13) Results cannot be calculated for this reporting period; (14) The results for this state are combined with nearby states to protect confidentiality; Please refer to the User's Guide for a full explanation of data.

Coral Gables Hospital	Coral Gables	17	477
Heart of Florida Regional Medical Center	Davenport	17	767
Lakeland Regional Medical Center	Lakeland	17	461
Twin Cities Hospital	Niceville	17	429
Bethesda Hospital East	Boynton Beach	18	402
Holy Cross Hospital	Fort Lauderdale	18	421
Memorial Hospital Jacksonville	Jacksonville	18	544
Physicians Reg Med Ctr-Pine Ridge	Naples	18	736
Regional Medical Center Bayonet Point	Hudson	18	439
Shands Lake Shore Regional Medical Center	Lake City	18	1148
Broward Health Medical Center	Fort Lauderdale	19	408
Florida Hospital North Pinellas	Tarpon Springs	19	430
Lakeside Medical Center	Belle Glade	19	469
Larkin Community Hospital	South Miami	19	285
Martin Medical Center	Stuart	19	399
Bayfront Health Punta Gorda	Punta Gorda	20	417
Blake Medical Center	Bradenton	20	478
North Florida Regional Medical Center	Gainesville	20	509
Ocala Regional Medical Center	Ocala	20	532
Bayfront Health Brooksville	Brooksville	21	1240
Delray Medical Center	Delray Beach	21	423
Lake Wales Medical Center	Lake Wales	21	419
Lakewood Ranch Medical Center	Bradenton	21	365
Mease Hospital Dunedin	Dunedin	21	381
Seven Rivers Regional Medical Center	Crystal River	21	469
Wellington Regional Medical Center	Wellington	21	378
Broward Health Coral Springs	Coral Springs	22	433
Florida Hospital Wauchula	Wauchula	22	327
Orange Park Medical Center	Orange Park	22	528
Palm Bay Hospital	Palm Bay	22	405
Wuesthoff Medical Center - Melbourne	Melbourne	22	411
Viera Hospital	Melbourne	23	374
Florida Hospital Wesley Chapel[3]	Wesley Chapel	24	102
Jupiter Medical Center	Jupiter	24	415
Lehigh Regional Medical Center	Lehigh Acres	24	388
Memorial Regional Hospital	Hollywood	24	752
North Okaloosa Medical Center	Crestview	24	416
Bert Fish Medical Center	New Smyrn Bch	26	518
Florida Hospital Carrollwood	Tampa	26	373
Putnam Community Medical Center	Palatka	26	486
Town & Country Hospital	Tampa	26	1151
West Boca Medical Center	Boca Raton	26	447
Holmes Regional Medical Center	Melbourne	27	443
Mariners Hospital	Tavernier	27	379
Palms of Pasadena Hospital	St Petersburg	27	555
Broward Health North	Pompano Bch	28	406
Flagler Hospital	St Augustine	28	415
Santa Rosa Medical Center	Milton	28	384
South Florida Baptist Hospital	Plant City	28	406
Florida Hospital Zephyrhills	Zephyrhills	29	367
Jackson Hospital	Marianna	30	1195
Mount Sinai Medical Center	Miami Beach	30	332
Saint Mary's Medical Center	W Palm Beach	30	497
Baptist Medical Center Beaches	Jcksnvl Bch	31	501
Bayfront Health - Saint Petersburg	St Petersburg	31	246
Bayfront Health Port Charlotte	Port Charlotte	31	405
Healthmark Regional Medical Center	Defuniak Spgs	31	289
Lower Keys Medical Center	Key West	32	1244
Mayo Clinic	Jacksonville	32	373
Memorial Hospital Miramar	Miramar	33	359
Saint Vincent's Medical Center Southside	Jacksonville	33	395
Baptist Medical Center - Nassau	Fernandina Bch	34	501
Cape Canaveral Hospital	Cocoa Beach	34	377
Florida Hospital Heartland Medical Center	Sebring	34	821
Cape Coral Hospital	Cape Coral	35	371
Halifax Health Medical Center	Daytona Bch	35	409
Memorial Hospital of Tampa	Tampa	35	403
Palmetto General Hospital	Hialeah	35	381
Sacred Heart Hosp-Emerald Coast	Miramar Beach	36	356
Sebastian River Medical Center	Sebastian	36	405
Bay Med Ctr Sacred Heart Health Sys	Panama City	37	441
Hendry Regional Medical Center[3]	Clewiston	37	300
Broward Health Imperial Point	Fort Lauderdale	38	417
Florida Hospital Waterman	Tavares	38	369
Memorial Hospital West	Pembroke Pines	38	382
Naples Community Hospital	Naples	38	317
Saint Joseph's Hospital	Tampa	38	344
Westchester General Hospital	Miami	38	1214
Morton Plant Hospital	Clearwater	39	431
Venice Reg Med Ctr-Bayfront Health	Venice	39	396
Manatee Memorial Hospital	Bradenton	40	420
Munroe Regional Medical Center	Ocala	40	369
Saint Anthony's Hospital	St Petersburg	40	626
Sarasota Memorial Hospital	Sarasota	40	430
Doctor's Memorial Hospital	Perry	41	405
Florida Hospital	Orlando	41	1526
Gulf Coast Med Ctr Lee Mem Health Sys	Fort Myers	41	371
Palm Springs General Hospital	Hialeah	41	405
Saint Cloud Regional Medical Center	Saint Cloud	41	698
Gulf Breeze Hospital	Gulf Breeze	42	471
Memorial Hospital Pembroke	Pembroke Pines	43	378
West Kendall Baptist Hospital	Miami	43	1301
Florida Hospital Deland	Deland	44	357
UF Health Shands Hospital	Gainesville	44	358
Baptist Medical Center	Jacksonville	45	494
Parrish Medical Center	Titusville	46	448
Florida Hospital Flagler	Palm Coast	47	358
Lee Memorial Hospital	Fort Myers	47	354
Mease Countryside Hospital	Safety Harbor	47	440
Florida Hospital Tampa	Tampa	48	362
The Villages Regional Hospital	The Villages	48	366
Boca Raton Regional Hospital	Boca Raton	51	383
South Lake Hospital	Clermont	51	1855
Baptist Hospital	Pensacola	52	421
Jay Hospital	Jay	52	469
Baptist Hospital of Miami	Miami	53	414
Indian River Medical Center	Vero Beach	53	395
Morton Plant North Bay Hospital	New Port Richey	53	382
South Miami Hospital	South Miami	55	435
Saint Vincent's Medical Center	Jacksonville	57	399
Florida Hospital Fish Memorial	Orange City	58	358
Leesburg Regional Medical Center	Leesburg	58	358
North Shore Medical Center	Miami	58	943
Sacred Heart Hospital	Pensacola	60	255
Citrus Memorial Hospital	Inverness	70	486
Tallahassee Memorial Hospital	Tallahassee	70	324
Tampa General Hospital	Tampa	70	369
UF Health Jacksonville	Jacksonville	76	92
Jackson Memorial Hospital	Miami	81	996
Health Central	Ocoee	83	5077
University of Miami Hospital	Miami	91	297
Orlando Health	Orlando	95	356
Winter Haven Hospital	Winter Haven	102	390
Anne Bates Leach Eye Hospital	Miami	118	280

Time to Pain Meds for Bone Fractures (minutes)

Hospital Name	City	Min.	Cases
Bartow Regional Medical Center	Bartow	31	112
Florida Hospital Wauchula	Wauchula	33	65
Lakeland Regional Medical Center	Lakeland	35	403
Memorial Hospital West	Pembroke Pines	35	368
Broward Health Medical Center	Fort Lauderdale	36	198
Heart of Florida Regional Medical Center	Davenport	37	74
Lehigh Regional Medical Center	Lehigh Acres	37	80
Saint Petersburg General Hospital	St Petersburg	37	65
Medical Center of Trinity	Trinity	38	104
Cleveland Clinic Hospital	Weston	39	90
Northwest Medical Center	Margate	39	113
Doctor's Memorial Hospital	Perry	40	64
Doctors Hospital of Sarasota	Sarasota	40	67
Englewood Community Hospital	Englewood	40	58
Kendall Regional Medical Center	Miami	40	174
Mease Hospital Dunedin	Dunedin	40	46
Baptist Medical Center - Nassau	Fernandina Bch	41	69
Memorial Regional Hospital	Hollywood	41	480
Palm Beach Gardens Medical Center	Palm Bch Grdns	41	142
West Kendall Baptist Hospital	Miami	41	143
Gulf Coast Regional Medical Center	Panama City	42	173
Northside Hospital	St Petersburg	42	55
Plantation General Hospital	Plantation	42	186
Baptist Hospital of Miami	Miami	43	184
Bayfront Health Port Charlotte	Port Charlotte	43	57
Florida Hospital North Pinellas	Tarpon Springs	43	75
Wuesthoff Medical Center - Melbourne	Melbourne	43	58
Bayfront Health Dade City	Dade City	44	78
Good Samaritan Medical Center	W Palm Beach	44	32
Santa Rosa Medical Center	Milton	45	99
Aventura Hospital & Medical Center	Aventura	46	179
Bayfront Health Brooksville	Brooksville	46	158
Highlands Regional Medical Center	Sebring	46	58
Lower Keys Medical Center	Key West	46	123
Town & Country Hospital	Tampa	46	56
South Bay Hospital	Sun City Center	47	73
Westside Regional Medical Center	Plantation	47	109
Regional Medical Center Bayonet Point	Hudson	48	109
Sebastian River Medical Center	Sebastian	48	92
JFK Medical Center	Atlantis	50	77
Largo Medical Center	Largo	50	66
Memorial Hospital Miramar	Miramar	50	286
Palms of Pasadena Hospital	St Petersburg	50	78
Putnam Community Medical Center	Palatka	50	82
Raulerson Hospital	Okeechobee	50	93
University Hospital & Medical Center	Tamarac	50	129
West Palm Hospital	W Palm Beach	50	36
Bethesda Hospital East	Boynton Beach	51	181
Capital Regional Medical Center	Tallahassee	51	145
Lakeside Medical Center	Belle Glade	52	77
Naples Community Hospital	Naples	52	212
Oak Hill Hospital	Brooksville	52	120
Saint Cloud Regional Medical Center	Saint Cloud	52	70
Viera Hospital	Melbourne	52	68
Mease Countryside Hospital	Safety Harbor	53	122
Saint Lucie Medical Center	Port Saint Lucie	53	88
Blake Medical Center	Bradenton	54	141
Desoto Memorial Hospital	Arcadia	54	39
Holmes Regional Medical Center	Melbourne	54	274
Jackson Hospital	Marianna	54	115
Lake Wales Medical Center	Lake Wales	54	76
Osceola Regional Medical Center	Kissimmee	54	212
Venice Reg Med Ctr-Bayfront Health	Venice	54	74
Wuesthoff Medical Center Rockledge	Rockledge	54	71
Mariners Hospital	Tavernier	55	42
Bayfront Health Punta Gorda	Punta Gorda	56	56
Hialeah Hospital	Hialeah	56	46
Homestead Hospital	Homestead	56	244
Lakewood Ranch Medical Center	Bradenton	56	121
Ocala Regional Medical Center	Ocala	56	117
Florida Hospital Zephyrhills	Zephyrhills	57	46
Fort Walton Beach Medical Center	Fort Walton Bch	57	121
Palms West Hospital	Loxahatchee	57	160
Physicians Reg Med Ctr-Pine Ridge	Naples	57	156
Bayfront Health - Saint Petersburg	St Petersburg	58	36
Broward Health North	Pompano Bch	58	237
Coral Gables Hospital	Coral Gables	58	41
Florida Hospital Carrollwood	Tampa	58	53
Saint Mary's Medical Center	W Palm Beach	58	148
South Lake Hospital	Clermont	58	164
Mount Sinai Medical Center	Miami Beach	59	121
South Florida Baptist Hospital	Plant City	59	81
Brandon Regional Hospital	Brandon	60	253
Fawcett Memorial Hospital	Port Charlotte	60	57
Flagler Hospital	St Augustine	60	131
Florida Hospital Flagler	Palm Coast	60	126
Morton Plant Hospital	Clearwater	60	128
Palm Bay Hospital	Palm Bay	60	162
Saint Joseph's Hospital	Tampa	60	293
Palm Springs General Hospital	Hialeah	61	37
Broward Health Coral Springs	Coral Springs	62	186
Central Florida Regional Hospital	Sanford	62	97
Jupiter Medical Center	Jupiter	62	129
Lawnwood Reg Med Ctr & Heart Inst	Fort Pierce	62	134
Mayo Clinic	Jacksonville	62	59
Twin Cities Hospital	Niceville	63	50
Bert Fish Medical Center	New Smyrn Bch	64	74
Boca Raton Regional Hospital	Boca Raton	64	197
Doctors Hospital	Coral Gables	64	44
Lake City Medical Center	Lake City	64	71
Morton Plant North Bay Hospital	New Port Richey	64	98
Shands Live Oak Regional Medical Center	Live Oak	64	61
Baptist Medical Center Beaches	Jcksnvl Bch	65	139
Shands Lake Shore Regional Medical Center	Lake City	65	55
West Boca Medical Center	Boca Raton	65	205
Delray Medical Center	Delray Beach	66	188
Florida Hospital Memorial Medical Center	Daytona Bch	66	140
Manatee Memorial Hospital	Bradenton	66	270
Munroe Regional Medical Center	Ocala	66	257
Florida Hospital Heartland Medical Center	Sebring	68	189
Gulf Coast Med Ctr Lee Mem Health Sys	Fort Myers	68	88
Holy Cross Hospital	Fort Lauderdale	68	208
Indian River Medical Center	Vero Beach	68	134
Lee Memorial Hospital	Fort Myers	68	264
Memorial Hospital Jacksonville	Jacksonville	68	141
North Okaloosa Medical Center	Crestview	68	130
North Shore Medical Center	Miami	68	115
North Florida Regional Medical Center	Gainesville	69	86
UF Health Shands Hospital	Gainesville	69	321
Florida Hospital Tampa	Tampa	70	132
Sacred Heart Hospital	Pensacola	71	225
Wellington Regional Medical Center	Wellington	71	102
Bay Med Ctr Sacred Heart Health Sys	Panama City	72	130
Palmetto General Hospital	Hialeah	72	189
Seven Rivers Regional Medical Center	Crystal River	72	56
Florida Hospital Waterman	Tavares	73	109
Halifax Health Medical Center	Daytona Bch	73	291
Martin Medical Center	Stuart	73	183
Saint Vincent's Medical Center Southside	Jacksonville	73	25
Tallahassee Memorial Hospital	Tallahassee	74	197
Cape Coral Hospital	Cape Coral	75	89
Memorial Hospital Pembroke	Pembroke Pines	75	102
Orange Park Medical Center	Orange Park	75	287
Saint Anthony's Hospital	St Petersburg	75	45
South Miami Hospital	South Miami	75	40
University of Miami Hospital	Miami	75	38
West Florida Hospital	Pensacola	75	117
Gulf Breeze Hospital	Gulf Breeze	76	102
Sacred Heart Hosp-Emerald Coast	Miramar Beach	76	211
Cape Canaveral Hospital	Cocoa Beach	79	114
Parrish Medical Center	Titusville	80	173
Saint Vincent's Medical Center	Jacksonville	80	61
Sarasota Memorial Hospital	Sarasota	80	184
Florida Hospital Deland	Deland	81	130
Florida Hospital	Orlando	86	435
Memorial Hospital of Tampa	Tampa	86	44

NOTE: Hospital profiles are in alphabetical order by state, then city, then hospital within the city; Rankings exclude hospitals with less than 25 cases except for patient surveys which excludes hospitals with less than 100 cases; (a) 100-299 cases; (1) The number of cases/patients is too few to report; (2) Data submitted were based on a sample of cases/patients; (3) Results are based on a shorter time period than required; (4) Data suppressed by CMS for one or more quarters; (5) Results are not available for this reporting period; (6) Fewer than 100 patients completed the HCAHPS survey; (7) No cases met the criteria for this measure; (8) The lower limit of the confidence interval cannot be calculated if the number of observed infections equals zero; (9) No data are available from the state/territory for this reporting period; (10) The scores shown reflect fewer than 50 completed surveys; (11) There were discrepancies in the data collection process; (12) This measure does not apply to this hospital for this reporting period; (13) Results cannot be calculated for this reporting period; (14) The results for this state are combined with nearby states to protect confidentiality; Please refer to the User's Guide for a full explanation of data.

Hospital Name	City	Rate	Cases
UF Health Jacksonville	Jacksonville	86	206
Baptist Medical Center	Jacksonville	87	528
Orlando Health	Orlando	87	568
Florida Hospital Fish Memorial	Orange City	91	133
Baptist Hospital	Pensacola	92	54
Health Central	Ocoee	93	237
Tampa General Hospital	Tampa	93	200
Citrus Memorial Hospital	Inverness	100	136
Leesburg Regional Medical Center	Leesburg	100	55
Winter Haven Hospital	Winter Haven	100	191
Jackson Memorial Hospital	Miami	101	425
The Villages Regional Hospital	The Villages	122	61

Heart Attack Care

Aspirin Given at Discharge

Hospital Name	City	Rate	Cases
Aventura Hospital & Medical Center[2]	Aventura	100%	265
Baptist Hospital[2]	Pensacola	100%	260
Baptist Hospital of Miami[2]	Miami	100%	279
Bay Med Ctr Sacred Heart Health Sys	Panama City	100%	366
Bay Pines VA Medical Center	Bay Pines	100%	57
Bethesda Hospital East[2]	Boynton Beach	100%	231
Boca Raton Regional Hospital	Boca Raton	100%	197
Brandon Regional Hospital[2]	Brandon	100%	272
Broward Health Medical Center[2]	Fort Lauderdale	100%	290
Broward Health North	Pompano Bch	100%	142
Capital Regional Medical Center	Tallahassee	100%	187
Central Florida Regional Hospital	Sanford	100%	255
Cleveland Clinic Hospital	Weston	100%	122
Delray Medical Center	Delray Beach	100%	268
Doctors Hospital of Sarasota	Sarasota	100%	94
Fawcett Memorial Hospital[2]	Port Charlotte	100%	202
Florida Hospital[2]	Orlando	100%	1069
Florida Hospital Fish Memorial	Orange City	100%	53
Florida Hospital Flagler	Palm Coast	100%	140
Florida Hospital Heartland Medical Center	Sebring	100%	277
Florida Hospital Memorial Medical Center	Daytona Bch	100%	209
Florida Hospital North Pinellas	Tarpon Springs	100%	90
Florida Hospital Zephyrhills	Zephyrhills	100%	177
Fort Walton Beach Medical Center	Fort Walton Bch	100%	237
Good Samaritan Medical Center	W Palm Beach	100%	53
Gulf Coast Regional Medical Center[2]	Panama City	100%	122
Halifax Health Medical Center[2]	Daytona Bch	100%	305
Health Central	Ocoee	100%	145
Hialeah Hospital	Hialeah	100%	98
Highlands Regional Medical Center	Sebring	100%	107
Holy Cross Hospital	Fort Lauderdale	100%	309
Homestead Hospital	Homestead	100%	42
JFK Medical Center	Atlantis	100%	546
Kendall Regional Medical Center	Miami	100%	430
Lake Wales Medical Center	Lake Wales	100%	28
Largo Medical Center	Largo	100%	330
Lawnwood Reg Med Ctr & Heart Inst	Fort Pierce	100%	577
Lower Keys Medical Center	Key West	100%	35
Manatee Memorial Hospital[2]	Bradenton	100%	272
Martin Medical Center[2]	Stuart	100%	256
Mayo Clinic	Jacksonville	100%	102
Mease Countryside Hospital	Safety Harbor	100%	381
Medical Center of Trinity	Trinity	100%	214
Memorial Hospital Jacksonville	Jacksonville	100%	332
Memorial Hospital West	Pembroke Pines	100%	331
Memorial Regional Hospital	Hollywood	100%	450
Metropolitan Hospital of Miami	Miami	100%	52
Morton Plant Hospital	Clearwater	100%	548
Morton Plant North Bay Hospital	New Port Richey	100%	185
North Florida Regional Medical Center	Gainesville	100%	481
North Okaloosa Medical Center	Crestview	100%	80
North Shore Medical Center	Miami	100%	216
Northside Hospital[2]	St Petersburg	100%	282
Northwest Medical Center	Margate	100%	336
Oak Hill Hospital[2]	Brooksville	100%	259
Ocala Regional Medical Center	Ocala	100%	298
Orange Park Medical Center	Orange Park	100%	272
Osceola Regional Medical Center[2]	Kissimmee	100%	430
Palm Beach Gardens Medical Center	Palm Bch Grdns	100%	426
Palmetto General Hospital[2]	Hialeah	100%	379
Palms West Hospital	Loxahatchee	100%	154
Parrish Medical Center	Titusville	100%	104
Plantation General Hospital[2]	Plantation	100%	237
Raulerson Hospital	Okeechobee	100%	32
Saint Anthony's Hospital	St Petersburg	100%	202
Saint Lucie Medical Center	Port Saint Lucie	100%	95
Saint Vincent's Medical Center Southside[2]	Jacksonville	100%	79
Sarasota Memorial Hospital	Sarasota	100%	491
Sebastian River Medical Center	Sebastian	100%	103
Seven Rivers Regional Medical Center	Crystal River	100%	73
South Florida Baptist Hospital	Plant City	100%	58
South Miami Hospital	South Miami	100%	223
Tallahassee Memorial Hospital	Tallahassee	100%	457
University Hospital & Medical Center	Tamarac	100%	38
University of Miami Hospital	Miami	100%	221
VA N Florida/S Georgia Healthcare Sys	Gainesville	100%	117
Venice Reg Med Ctr-Bayfront Health[2]	Venice	100%	269
The Villages Regional Hospital[2]	The Villages	100%	297
Wellington Regional Medical Center	Wellington	100%	91
West Florida Hospital	Pensacola	100%	208
Baptist Medical Center[2]	Jacksonville	99%	339
Bayfront Health Dade City	Dade City	99%	69
Blake Medical Center[2]	Bradenton	99%	243
Cape Canaveral Hospital	Cocoa Beach	99%	122
Florida Hospital Waterman[2]	Tavares	99%	183
Gulf Coast Med Ctr Lee Mem Health Sys[2]	Fort Myers	99%	270
Holmes Regional Medical Center	Melbourne	99%	527
Indian River Medical Center[2]	Vero Beach	99%	265
Jackson Memorial Hospital[2]	Miami	99%	497
Lakeland Regional Medical Center[2]	Lakeland	99%	291
Leesburg Regional Medical Center[2]	Leesburg	99%	278
Mount Sinai Medical Center	Miami Beach	99%	473
Munroe Regional Medical Center	Ocala	99%	559
Orlando Health	Orlando	99%	724
Physicians Reg Med Ctr-Pine Ridge	Naples	99%	152
Putnam Community Medical Center	Palatka	99%	113
Regional Medical Center Bayonet Point[2]	Hudson	99%	272
Sacred Heart Hosp-Emerald Coast	Miramar Beach	99%	87
Saint Joseph's Hospital	Tampa	99%	583
Saint Vincent's Medical Center[2]	Jacksonville	99%	308
Tampa VA Medical Center	Tampa	99%	146
UF Health Jacksonville[2]	Jacksonville	99%	276
UF Health Shands Hospital	Gainesville	99%	265
Westside Regional Medical Center[2]	Plantation	99%	283
Bayfront Health - Saint Petersburg[2]	St Petersburg	98%	178
Bayfront Health Port Charlotte	Port Charlotte	98%	221
Bert Fish Medical Center	New Smyrn Bch	98%	182
Flagler Hospital[2]	St Augustine	98%	225
Florida Hospital Deland	Deland	98%	178
Florida Hospital Tampa	Tampa	98%	295
Lee Memorial Hospital[2]	Fort Myers	98%	297
Naples Community Hospital	Naples	98%	494
Palm Springs General Hospital	Hialeah	98%	54
Sacred Heart Hospital[2]	Pensacola	98%	311
Wuesthoff Medical Center Rockledge	Rockledge	98%	175
Citrus Memorial Hospital	Inverness	97%	289
Miami VA Medical Center	Miami	97%	29
Tampa General Hospital	Tampa	97%	295
Winter Haven Hospital	Winter Haven	97%	355
Bayfront Health Brooksville	Brooksville	96%	134
Cape Coral Hospital	Cape Coral	96%	56
Mease Hospital Dunedin	Dunedin	96%	25
South Lake Hospital	Clermont	96%	168
Wuesthoff Medical Center - Melbourne	Melbourne	96%	50
Baptist Medical Center Beaches[2]	Jcksnvll Bch	95%	41
Lakewood Ranch Medical Center	Bradenton	95%	104
Heart of Florida Regional Medical Center	Davenport	92%	128

PCI Within 90 Minutes of Arrival

Hospital Name	City	Rate	Cases
Aventura Hospital & Medical Center[2]	Aventura	100%	40
Baptist Hospital of Miami[2]	Miami	100%	46
Boca Raton Regional Hospital	Boca Raton	100%	46
Capital Regional Medical Center	Tallahassee	100%	42
Delray Medical Center	Delray Beach	100%	35
Florida Hospital[2]	Orlando	100%	135
Florida Hospital North Pinellas	Tarpon Springs	100%	28
Florida Hospital Zephyrhills	Zephyrhills	100%	43
Fort Walton Beach Medical Center	Fort Walton Bch	100%	34
Halifax Health Medical Center[2]	Daytona Bch	100%	44
Health Central	Ocoee	100%	32
Holmes Regional Medical Center	Melbourne	100%	58
JFK Medical Center	Atlantis	100%	85
Kendall Regional Medical Center	Miami	100%	107
Largo Medical Center	Largo	100%	66
Lawnwood Reg Med Ctr & Heart Inst	Fort Pierce	100%	32
Leesburg Regional Medical Center[2]	Leesburg	100%	36
Manatee Memorial Hospital[2]	Bradenton	100%	32
Medical Center of Trinity	Trinity	100%	33
Memorial Regional Hospital	Hollywood	100%	55
Mount Sinai Medical Center	Miami Beach	100%	47
North Florida Regional Medical Center	Gainesville	100%	64
North Okaloosa Medical Center	Crestview	100%	27
North Shore Medical Center	Miami	100%	31
Northside Hospital[2]	St Petersburg	100%	43
Orange Park Medical Center	Orange Park	100%	39
Osceola Regional Medical Center[2]	Kissimmee	100%	55
Palm Beach Gardens Medical Center	Palm Bch Grdns	100%	78
Palmetto General Hospital[2]	Hialeah	100%	84
Parrish Medical Center	Titusville	100%	36
Regional Medical Center Bayonet Point[2]	Hudson	100%	44
Tallahassee Memorial Hospital	Tallahassee	100%	58
UF Health Shands Hospital	Gainesville	100%	52
Venice Reg Med Ctr-Bayfront Health[2]	Venice	100%	53
Wellington Regional Medical Center	Wellington	100%	33
West Florida Hospital	Pensacola	100%	50
Westside Regional Medical Center[2]	Plantation	100%	43
Wuesthoff Medical Center Rockledge	Rockledge	100%	33
Florida Hospital Tampa	Tampa	99%	78
Bay Med Ctr Sacred Heart Health Sys	Panama City	98%	40
Brandon Regional Hospital[2]	Brandon	98%	54
Broward Health Medical Center[2]	Fort Lauderdale	98%	42
Central Florida Regional Hospital	Sanford	98%	40
Florida Hospital Waterman[2]	Tavares	98%	58
Holy Cross Hospital	Fort Lauderdale	98%	43
Indian River Medical Center[2]	Vero Beach	98%	50
Lakeland Regional Medical Center[2]	Lakeland	98%	57
Memorial Hospital West	Pembroke Pines	98%	65
Morton Plant Hospital	Clearwater	98%	49
Baptist Hospital[2]	Pensacola	97%	66
Florida Hospital Memorial Medical Center	Daytona Bch	97%	37
Heart of Florida Regional Medical Center	Davenport	97%	32
Physicians Reg Med Ctr-Pine Ridge	Naples	97%	35
Sacred Heart Hosp-Emerald Coast	Miramar Beach	97%	30
Saint Anthony's Hospital	St Petersburg	97%	32
South Miami Hospital	South Miami	97%	36
The Villages Regional Hospital[2]	The Villages	97%	34
Blake Medical Center[2]	Bradenton	96%	27
Cape Canaveral Hospital	Cocoa Beach	96%	26
Doctors Hospital of Sarasota	Sarasota	96%	27
Fawcett Memorial Hospital[2]	Port Charlotte	96%	28
Jackson Memorial Hospital[2]	Miami	96%	129
Baptist Medical Center[2]	Jacksonville	95%	38
Florida Hospital Heartland Medical Center	Sebring	95%	38
Highlands Regional Medical Center	Sebring	95%	43
Mease Countryside Hospital	Safety Harbor	95%	79
Naples Community Hospital	Naples	95%	42
Oak Hill Hospital[2]	Brooksville	95%	40
Sacred Heart Hospital[2]	Pensacola	95%	37
Saint Joseph's Hospital	Tampa	95%	86
Saint Vincent's Medical Center[2]	Jacksonville	95%	43
UF Health Jacksonville[2]	Jacksonville	95%	42
Bayfront Health - Saint Petersburg[2]	St Petersburg	94%	49
Bethesda Hospital East[2]	Boynton Beach	93%	41
Florida Hospital Flagler	Palm Coast	93%	29
Martin Medical Center[2]	Stuart	93%	41
Orlando Health	Orlando	93%	89
Plantation General Hospital[2]	Plantation	93%	29
Winter Haven Hospital	Winter Haven	93%	55
Tampa General Hospital	Tampa	92%	40
Munroe Regional Medical Center	Ocala	91%	58
South Lake Hospital	Clermont	91%	32
Gulf Coast Med Ctr Lee Mem Health Sys[2]	Fort Myers	90%	60
Citrus Memorial Hospital	Inverness	87%	91
Florida Hospital Deland	Deland	87%	30
Putnam Community Medical Center	Palatka	87%	31
Sarasota Memorial Hospital	Sarasota	87%	63
Bert Fish Medical Center	New Smyrn Bch	85%	33
Flagler Hospital[2]	St Augustine	82%	34
Lee Memorial Hospital[2]	Fort Myers	82%	33
Bayfront Health Port Charlotte	Port Charlotte	80%	35

Statin Prescribed at Discharge

Hospital Name	City	Rate	Cases
Aventura Hospital & Medical Center[2]	Aventura	100%	274
Baptist Hospital[2]	Pensacola	100%	251
Baptist Hospital of Miami[2]	Miami	100%	283
Bay Med Ctr Sacred Heart Health Sys	Panama City	100%	332
Bay Pines VA Medical Center	Bay Pines	100%	56
Boca Raton Regional Hospital	Boca Raton	100%	188
Brandon Regional Hospital[2]	Brandon	100%	257
Broward Health Medical Center[2]	Fort Lauderdale	100%	285
Broward Health North	Pompano Bch	100%	138
Central Florida Regional Hospital	Sanford	100%	225
Cleveland Clinic Hospital	Weston	100%	118
Delray Medical Center	Delray Beach	100%	250
Fawcett Memorial Hospital[2]	Port Charlotte	100%	174
Florida Hospital[2]	Orlando	100%	1034
Florida Hospital Fish Memorial	Orange City	100%	49
Florida Hospital Flagler	Palm Coast	100%	125
Florida Hospital Memorial Medical Center	Daytona Bch	100%	198
Florida Hospital North Pinellas	Tarpon Springs	100%	84
Fort Walton Beach Medical Center	Fort Walton Bch	100%	217
Good Samaritan Medical Center	W Palm Beach	100%	54
Health Central	Ocoee	100%	138
Hialeah Hospital	Hialeah	100%	111
Highlands Regional Medical Center	Sebring	100%	99
Holy Cross Hospital	Fort Lauderdale	100%	315
Homestead Hospital	Homestead	100%	42
JFK Medical Center	Atlantis	100%	527
Kendall Regional Medical Center	Miami	100%	437
Lakeland Regional Medical Center[2]	Lakeland	100%	290
Lawnwood Reg Med Ctr & Heart Inst	Fort Pierce	100%	570
Manatee Memorial Hospital[2]	Bradenton	100%	258
Martin Medical Center[2]	Stuart	100%	250

NOTE: Hospital profiles are in alphabetical order by state, then city, then hospital within the city; Rankings exclude hospitals with less than 25 cases except for patient surveys which excludes hospitals with less than 100 cases; (a) 100-299 cases; (1) The number of cases/patients is too few to report; (2) Data submitted were based on a sample of cases/patients; (3) Results are based on a shorter time period than required; (4) Data suppressed by CMS for one or more quarters; (5) Results are not available for this reporting period; (6) Fewer than 100 patients completed the HCAHPS survey; (7) No cases met the criteria for this measure; (8) The lower limit of the confidence interval cannot be calculated if the number of observed infections equals zero; (9) No data are available from the state/territory for this reporting period; (10) The scores shown reflect fewer than 50 completed surveys; (11) There were discrepancies in the data collection process; (12) This measure does not apply to this hospital for this reporting period; (13) Results cannot be calculated for this reporting period; (14) The results for this state are combined with nearby states to protect confidentiality; Please refer to the User's Guide for a full explanation of data.

Mayo Clinic	Jacksonville	100%	103
Medical Center of Trinity	Trinity	100%	211
Memorial Hospital West	Pembroke Pines	100%	325
Memorial Regional Hospital	Hollywood	100%	439
Metropolitan Hospital of Miami	Miami	100%	52
Miami VA Medical Center	Miami	100%	32
Morton Plant Hospital	Clearwater	100%	520
Morton Plant North Bay Hospital	New Port Richey	100%	180
North Florida Regional Medical Center	Gainesville	100%	436
North Okaloosa Medical Center	Crestview	100%	72
North Shore Medical Center	Miami	100%	217
Northwest Medical Center	Margate	100%	320
Oak Hill Hospital[2]	Brooksville	100%	237
Ocala Regional Medical Center	Ocala	100%	289
Orange Park Medical Center	Orange Park	100%	260
Osceola Regional Medical Center[2]	Kissimmee	100%	427
Palm Beach Gardens Medical Center	Palm Bch Grdns	100%	397
Palms West Hospital	Loxahatchee	100%	152
Parrish Medical Center	Titusville	100%	98
Raulerson Hospital	Okeechobee	100%	30
Regional Medical Center Bayonet Point[2]	Hudson	100%	250
Saint Lucie Medical Center	Port Saint Lucie	100%	91
Sarasota Memorial Hospital	Sarasota	100%	491
Sebastian River Medical Center	Sebastian	100%	105
South Bay Hospital	Sun City Center	100%	28
South Florida Baptist Hospital	Plant City	100%	54
South Miami Hospital	South Miami	100%	227
University of Miami Hospital	Miami	100%	217
Venice Reg Med Ctr-Bayfront Health[2]	Venice	100%	264
Wellington Regional Medical Center	Wellington	100%	93
West Florida Hospital	Pensacola	100%	203
Baptist Medical Center[2]	Jacksonville	99%	319
Blake Medical Center[2]	Bradenton	99%	221
Capital Regional Medical Center	Tallahassee	99%	179
Doctors Hospital of Sarasota	Sarasota	99%	91
Florida Hospital Deland	Deland	99%	173
Florida Hospital Waterman[2]	Tavares	99%	166
Florida Hospital Zephyrhills	Zephyrhills	99%	171
Halifax Health Medical Center[2]	Daytona Bch	99%	281
Indian River Medical Center[2]	Vero Beach	99%	242
Lakewood Ranch Medical Center	Bradenton	99%	90
Largo Medical Center	Largo	99%	317
Mease Countryside Hospital	Safety Harbor	99%	363
Memorial Hospital Jacksonville	Jacksonville	99%	325
Mount Sinai Medical Center	Miami Beach	99%	473
Northside Hospital[2]	St Petersburg	99%	266
Orlando Health	Orlando	99%	720
Palmetto General Hospital[2]	Hialeah	99%	381
Physicians Reg Med Ctr-Pine Ridge	Naples	99%	134
Plantation General Hospital[2]	Plantation	99%	236
Sacred Heart Hosp-Emerald Coast	Miramar Beach	99%	85
Saint Anthony's Hospital	St Petersburg	99%	204
Saint Joseph's Hospital	Tampa	99%	577
Saint Vincent's Medical Center Southside[2]	Jacksonville	99%	77
Seven Rivers Regional Medical Center	Crystal River	99%	68
Tallahassee Memorial Hospital	Tallahassee	99%	446
UF Health Jacksonville[2]	Jacksonville	99%	273
UF Health Shands Hospital	Gainesville	99%	259
VA N Florida/S Georgia Healthcare Sys	Gainesville	99%	114
Westside Regional Medical Center[2]	Plantation	99%	281
Wuesthoff Medical Center Rockledge	Rockledge	99%	154
Bayfront Health Brooksville	Brooksville	98%	115
Cape Canaveral Hospital	Cocoa Beach	98%	114
Cape Coral Hospital	Cape Coral	98%	47
Florida Hospital Heartland Medical Center	Sebring	98%	274
Florida Hospital Tampa	Tampa	98%	288
Gulf Coast Med Ctr Lee Mem Health Sys[2]	Fort Myers	98%	257
Gulf Coast Regional Medical Center[2]	Panama City	98%	107
Holmes Regional Medical Center	Melbourne	98%	507
Jackson Memorial Hospital[2]	Miami	98%	505
Naples Community Hospital	Naples	98%	476
Sacred Heart Hospital[2]	Pensacola	98%	293
Saint Vincent's Medical Center[2]	Jacksonville	98%	285
Bayfront Health - Saint Petersburg[2]	St Petersburg	97%	161
Bayfront Health Dade City	Dade City	97%	65
Bert Fish Medical Center	New Smyrn Bch	97%	176
Bethesda Hospital East[2]	Boynton Beach	97%	228
Flagler Hospital[2]	St Augustine	97%	212
Lee Memorial Hospital[2]	Fort Myers	97%	283
Lower Keys Medical Center	Key West	97%	33
Tampa VA Medical Center	Tampa	97%	138
University Hospital & Medical Center	Tamarac	97%	29
Bayfront Health Port Charlotte	Port Charlotte	96%	206
Lake Wales Medical Center	Lake Wales	96%	25
The Villages Regional Hospital[2]	The Villages	96%	277
Baptist Medical Center Beaches[2]	Jcksnvl Bch	95%	37
Winter Haven Hospital	Winter Haven	95%	348
Heart of Florida Regional Medical Center	Davenport	94%	124
Putnam Community Medical Center	Palatka	94%	110
South Lake Hospital	Clermont	94%	161
Wuesthoff Medical Center - Melbourne	Melbourne	94%	48
Citrus Memorial Hospital	Inverness	93%	277
Leesburg Regional Medical Center[2]	Leesburg	92%	259
Tampa General Hospital	Tampa	92%	290
Munroe Regional Medical Center	Ocala	91%	545
Jackson Hospital	Marianna	84%	25
Palm Springs General Hospital	Hialeah	81%	54

Heart Failure Care

ACE Inhibitor or ARB for LVSD

Hospital Name	City	Rate	Cases
Baptist Hospital[2]	Pensacola	100%	130
Baptist Hospital of Miami[2]	Miami	100%	76
Bartow Regional Medical Center	Bartow	100%	32
Bayfront Health Brooksville	Brooksville	100%	60
Bayfront Health Dade City	Dade City	100%	28
Boca Raton Regional Hospital[2]	Boca Raton	100%	55
Brandon Regional Hospital[2]	Brandon	100%	132
Broward Health Coral Springs	Coral Springs	100%	60
Broward Health Imperial Point	Fort Lauderdale	100%	62
Broward Health Medical Center[2]	Fort Lauderdale	100%	164
Broward Health North[2]	Pompano Bch	100%	121
Cape Canaveral Hospital	Cocoa Beach	100%	58
Capital Regional Medical Center	Tallahassee	100%	163
Central Florida Regional Hospital	Sanford	100%	113
Coral Gables Hospital	Coral Gables	100%	68
Delray Medical Center[2]	Delray Beach	100%	70
Doctors Hospital	Coral Gables	100%	36
Doctors Hospital of Sarasota	Sarasota	100%	57
Englewood Community Hospital	Englewood	100%	37
Fawcett Memorial Hospital[2]	Port Charlotte	100%	58
Florida Hospital Carrollwood[2]	Tampa	100%	27
Florida Hospital Flagler	Palm Coast	100%	80
Florida Hospital Heartland Medical Center	Sebring	100%	127
Florida Hospital North Pinellas	Tarpon Springs	100%	36
Florida Hospital Waterman[2]	Tavares	100%	93
Fort Walton Beach Medical Center	Fort Walton Bch	100%	94
Good Samaritan Medical Center	W Palm Beach	100%	55
Gulf Breeze Hospital	Gulf Breeze	100%	25
Gulf Coast Regional Medical Center[2]	Panama City	100%	58
Halifax Health Medical Center[2]	Daytona Bch	100%	142
Health Central	Ocoee	100%	90
Highlands Regional Medical Center	Sebring	100%	34
Holy Cross Hospital	Fort Lauderdale	100%	144
Homestead Hospital	Homestead	100%	52
Jackson Hospital	Marianna	100%	28
JFK Medical Center	Atlantis	100%	266
Kendall Regional Medical Center	Miami	100%	231
Lake City Medical Center[2]	Lake City	100%	53
Lakeside Medical Center	Belle Glade	100%	32
Largo Medical Center	Largo	100%	106
Lawnwood Reg Med Ctr & Heart Inst	Fort Pierce	100%	217
Leesburg Regional Medical Center[2]	Leesburg	100%	96
Manatee Memorial Hospital[2]	Bradenton	100%	85
Medical Center of Trinity	Trinity	100%	94
Memorial Hospital Jacksonville[2]	Jacksonville	100%	71
Memorial Hospital Miramar	Miramar	100%	29
Memorial Hospital of Tampa	Tampa	100%	30
Memorial Hospital Pembroke	Pembroke Pines	100%	54
Memorial Hospital West	Pembroke Pines	100%	184
Memorial Regional Hospital	Hollywood	100%	281
Metropolitan Hospital of Miami	Miami	100%	46
Miami VA Medical Center	Miami	100%	88
Mount Sinai Medical Center	Miami Beach	100%	185
North Florida Regional Medical Center[2]	Gainesville	100%	72
North Okaloosa Medical Center	Crestview	100%	73
Northwest Medical Center	Margate	100%	143
Oak Hill Hospital[2]	Brooksville	100%	75
Ocala Regional Medical Center[2]	Ocala	100%	108
Orange Park Medical Center	Orange Park	100%	100
Palm Beach Gardens Medical Center	Palm Bch Grdns	100%	144
Palm Springs General Hospital	Hialeah	100%	57
Palms of Pasadena Hospital	St Petersburg	100%	25
Palms West Hospital	Loxahatchee	100%	53
Parrish Medical Center	Titusville	100%	58
Physicians Reg Med Ctr-Pine Ridge	Naples	100%	71
Raulerson Hospital	Okeechobee	100%	76
Sacred Heart Hospital[2]	Pensacola	100%	110
Saint Cloud Regional Medical Center	Saint Cloud	100%	41
Saint Joseph's Hospital	Tampa	100%	303
Saint Lucie Medical Center	Port Saint Lucie	100%	102
Saint Petersburg General Hospital	St Petersburg	100%	27
Saint Vincent's Medical Center[2]	Jacksonville	100%	121
Saint Vincent's Medical Center Southside[2]	Jacksonville	100%	64
Sebastian River Medical Center	Sebastian	100%	90
Seven Rivers Regional Medical Center	Crystal River	100%	78
South Bay Hospital	Sun City Center	100%	84
South Florida Baptist Hospital	Plant City	100%	55
South Miami Hospital	South Miami	100%	112
UF Health Shands Hospital[2]	Gainesville	100%	138
Venice Reg Med Ctr-Bayfront Health[2]	Venice	100%	62
The Villages Regional Hospital[2]	The Villages	100%	92
Wellington Regional Medical Center[2]	Wellington	100%	54
West Boca Medical Center	Boca Raton	100%	60
West Florida Hospital	Pensacola	100%	111
West Kendall Baptist Hospital	Miami	100%	65
Aventura Hospital & Medical Center[2]	Aventura	99%	143
Bay Med Ctr Sacred Heart Health Sys[2]	Panama City	99%	144
Bay Pines VA Medical Center	Bay Pines	99%	85
Florida Hospital[2]	Orlando	99%	696
Florida Hospital Deland	Deland	99%	115
Florida Hospital Fish Memorial	Orange City	99%	142
Florida Hospital Memorial Medical Center	Daytona Bch	99%	149
Florida Hospital Zephyrhills	Zephyrhills	99%	95
Lakeland Regional Medical Center[2]	Lakeland	99%	118
Mease Countryside Hospital	Safety Harbor	99%	110
Morton Plant North Bay Hospital	New Port Richey	99%	70
North Shore Medical Center[2]	Miami	99%	285
Northside Hospital[2]	St Petersburg	99%	88
Orlando Health	Orlando	99%	402
Osceola Regional Medical Center[2]	Kissimmee	99%	116
Palm Bay Hospital	Palm Bay	99%	70
Palmetto General Hospital[2]	Hialeah	99%	145
Plantation General Hospital[2]	Plantation	99%	127
Regional Medical Center Bayonet Point[2]	Hudson	99%	80
Saint Anthony's Hospital	St Petersburg	99%	112
UF Health Jacksonville[2]	Jacksonville	99%	154
W Palm Beach VA Medical Center	W Palm Beach	99%	78
Baptist Medical Center Beaches[2]	Jcksnvl Bch	98%	47
Blake Medical Center[2]	Bradenton	98%	66
Hialeah Hospital[2]	Hialeah	98%	81
Holmes Regional Medical Center	Melbourne	98%	332
Indian River Medical Center[2]	Vero Beach	98%	82
Jackson Memorial Hospital[2]	Miami	98%	405
Jupiter Medical Center	Jupiter	98%	48
Lehigh Regional Medical Center	Lehigh Acres	98%	41
Mease Hospital Dunedin	Dunedin	98%	45
Morton Plant Hospital	Clearwater	98%	165
Saint Mary's Medical Center	W Palm Beach	98%	51
Tallahassee Memorial Hospital	Tallahassee	98%	253
Baptist Medical Center - Nassau[2]	Fernandina Bch	97%	38
Bayfront Health Port Charlotte	Port Charlotte	97%	97
Cleveland Clinic Hospital	Weston	97%	78
Flagler Hospital[2]	St Augustine	97%	94
Heart of Florida Regional Medical Center	Davenport	97%	130
Sacred Heart Hosp-Emerald Coast	Miramar Beach	97%	37
Sarasota Memorial Hospital[2]	Sarasota	97%	108
Shands Lake Shore Regional Medical Center	Lake City	97%	33
University Hospital & Medical Center	Tamarac	97%	35
Westside Regional Medical Center[2]	Plantation	97%	146
Baptist Medical Center[2]	Jacksonville	96%	85
Bayfront Health - Saint Petersburg[2]	St Petersburg	96%	73
Florida Hospital Tampa	Tampa	96%	155
Martin Medical Center[2]	Stuart	96%	82
Mayo Clinic	Jacksonville	96%	68
Tampa VA Medical Center	Tampa	96%	162
Wuesthoff Medical Center Rockledge	Rockledge	96%	91
Bethesda Hospital East[2]	Boynton Beach	95%	83
University of Miami Hospital	Miami	95%	304
Wuesthoff Medical Center - Melbourne	Melbourne	95%	41
Lakewood Ranch Medical Center	Bradenton	94%	47
VA N Florida/S Georgia Healthcare Sys	Gainesville	94%	219
Bert Fish Medical Center	New Smyrn Bch	93%	29
Lake Wales Medical Center	Lake Wales	93%	71
Naples Community Hospital[2]	Naples	93%	86
Citrus Memorial Hospital	Inverness	92%	132
Tampa General Hospital[2]	Tampa	92%	111
Lee Memorial Hospital[2]	Fort Myers	91%	120
Putnam Community Medical Center	Palatka	91%	76
Winter Haven Hospital[2]	Winter Haven	91%	141
Bayfront Health Punta Gorda	Punta Gorda	90%	41
Cape Coral Hospital[2]	Cape Coral	90%	81
Desoto Memorial Hospital	Arcadia	89%	35
Lower Keys Medical Center	Key West	89%	27
Munroe Regional Medical Center[2]	Ocala	89%	87
South Lake Hospital	Clermont	89%	66
Gulf Coast Med Ctr Lee Mem Health Sys[2]	Fort Myers	87%	91
Larkin Community Hospital	South Miami	85%	27

Discharge Instructions Given

Hospital Name	City	Rate	Cases
Baptist Hospital of Miami[2]	Miami	100%	265
Boca Raton Regional Hospital[2]	Boca Raton	100%	237
Broward Health Medical Center[2]	Fort Lauderdale	100%	313
Broward Health North[2]	Pompano Bch	100%	256
Capital Regional Medical Center	Tallahassee	100%	362
Coral Gables Hospital	Coral Gables	100%	197
Delray Medical Center[2]	Delray Beach	100%	280
Doctor's Memorial Hospital	Perry	100%	32
Doctors Memorial Hospital	Bonifay	100%	57
Englewood Community Hospital	Englewood	100%	139

NOTE: Hospital profiles are in alphabetical order by state, then city, then hospital within the city; Rankings exclude hospitals with less than 25 cases except for patient surveys which excludes hospitals with less than 100 cases; (a) 100-299 cases; (1) The number of cases/patients is too few to report; (2) Data submitted were based on a sample of cases/patients; (3) Results are based on a shorter time period than required; (4) Data suppressed by CMS for one or more quarters; (5) Results are not available for this reporting period; (6) Fewer than 100 patients completed the HCAHPS survey; (7) No cases met the criteria for this measure; (8) The lower limit of the confidence interval cannot be calculated if the number of observed infections equals zero; (9) No data are available from the state/territory for this reporting period; (10) The scores shown reflect fewer than 50 completed surveys; (11) There were discrepancies in the data collection process; (12) This measure does not apply to this hospital for this reporting period; (13) Results cannot be calculated for this reporting period; (14) The results for this state are combined with nearby states to protect confidentiality; Please refer to the User's Guide for a full explanation of data.

Fawcett Memorial Hospital[2]	Port Charlotte	100%	201
Florida Hospital[2]	Orlando	100%	2142
Florida Hospital North Pinellas	Tarpon Springs	100%	96
Florida Hospital Waterman[2]	Tavares	100%	224
Health Central	Ocoee	100%	261
Hendry Regional Medical Center	Clewiston	100%	47
Highlands Regional Medical Center	Sebring	100%	108
Holy Cross Hospital	Fort Lauderdale	100%	428
Homestead Hospital	Homestead	100%	240
Jay Hospital	Jay	100%	40
JFK Medical Center	Atlantis	100%	764
Lake City Medical Center[2]	Lake City	100%	197
Larkin Community Hospital	South Miami	100%	31
Lawnwood Reg Med Ctr & Heart Inst	Fort Pierce	100%	463
Manatee Memorial Hospital[2]	Bradenton	100%	237
Mariners Hospital	Tavernier	100%	25
Medical Center of Trinity	Trinity	100%	250
Memorial Hospital Miramar	Miramar	100%	116
Memorial Hospital Pembroke	Pembroke Pines	100%	157
Memorial Hospital West	Pembroke Pines	100%	519
Memorial Regional Hospital	Hollywood	100%	581
Metropolitan Hospital of Miami	Miami	100%	110
Mount Sinai Medical Center	Miami Beach	100%	405
North Florida Regional Medical Center[2]	Gainesville	100%	278
North Okaloosa Medical Center	Crestview	100%	204
Northside Hospital[2]	St Petersburg	100%	233
Oak Hill Hospital[2]	Brooksville	100%	241
Ocala Regional Medical Center[2]	Ocala	100%	235
Orange Park Medical Center	Orange Park	100%	383
Osceola Regional Medical Center[2]	Kissimmee	100%	250
Palmetto General Hospital[2]	Hialeah	100%	322
Palms West Hospital	Loxahatchee	100%	188
Raulerson Hospital	Okeechobee	100%	201
Regional Medical Center Bayonet Point[2]	Hudson	100%	234
Saint Lucie Medical Center	Port Saint Lucie	100%	315
Saint Mary's Medical Center	W Palm Beach	100%	105
Saint Vincent's Medical Center Southside[2]	Jacksonville	100%	158
Sebastian River Medical Center	Sebastian	100%	167
Seven Rivers Regional Medical Center	Crystal River	100%	116
Shands Starke Regional Medical Center	Starke	100%	58
South Bay Hospital	Sun City Center	100%	203
Twin Cities Hospital	Niceville	100%	49
University Hospital & Medical Center	Tamarac	100%	155
Venice Reg Med Ctr-Bayfront Health[2]	Venice	100%	186
West Boca Medical Center	Boca Raton	100%	196
West Florida Hospital	Pensacola	100%	306
West Kendall Baptist Hospital	Miami	100%	171
West Palm Hospital	W Palm Beach	100%	98
Westside Regional Medical Center[2]	Plantation	100%	312
Baptist Medical Center Beaches[2]	Jcksnvll Bch	99%	151
Bay Pines VA Medical Center	Bay Pines	99%	204
Cleveland Clinic Hospital	Weston	99%	256
Doctors Hospital	Coral Gables	99%	154
Florida Hospital Deland	Deland	99%	278
Good Samaritan Medical Center	W Palm Beach	99%	160
Halifax Health Medical Center[2]	Daytona Bch	99%	336
Hialeah Hospital[2]	Hialeah	99%	204
Holmes Regional Medical Center	Melbourne	99%	633
Jupiter Medical Center	Jupiter	99%	166
Kendall Regional Medical Center	Miami	99%	577
Lakewood Ranch Medical Center	Bradenton	99%	104
Plantation General Hospital[2]	Plantation	99%	268
Saint Joseph's Hospital	Tampa	99%	608
South Florida Baptist Hospital	Plant City	99%	171
South Lake Hospital	Clermont	99%	229
South Miami Hospital	South Miami	99%	299
VA N Florida/S Georgia Healthcare Sys	Gainesville	99%	486
Wellington Regional Medical Center[2]	Wellington	99%	155
Bayfront Health Dade City	Dade City	98%	85
Brandon Regional Hospital[2]	Brandon	98%	328
Doctors Hospital of Sarasota	Sarasota	98%	165
Florida Hospital Fish Memorial	Orange City	98%	352
Florida Hospital Tampa	Tampa	98%	370
Florida Hospital Zephyrhills	Zephyrhills	98%	232
Fort Walton Beach Medical Center	Fort Walton Bch	98%	236
Lakeland Regional Medical Center[2]	Lakeland	98%	262
Mease Hospital Dunedin	Dunedin	98%	105
Memorial Hospital Jacksonville[2]	Jacksonville	98%	252
Northwest Medical Center	Margate	98%	427
Palm Bay Hospital	Palm Bay	98%	157
Parrish Medical Center	Titusville	98%	143
Sarasota Memorial Hospital[2]	Sarasota	98%	285
Viera Hospital	Melbourne	98%	48
Aventura Hospital & Medical Center[2]	Aventura	97%	256
Cape Canaveral Hospital	Cocoa Beach	97%	134
Gulf Coast Regional Medical Center[2]	Panama City	97%	156
Mayo Clinic	Jacksonville	97%	219
Miami VA Medical Center	Miami	97%	149
Morton Plant Hospital	Clearwater	97%	461
Morton Plant North Bay Hospital	New Port Richey	97%	232
Palm Beach Gardens Medical Center	Palm Bch Grdns	97%	373
Saint Vincent's Medical Center[2]	Jacksonville	97%	260
Bethesda Hospital East[2]	Boynton Beach	96%	216
Blake Medical Center[2]	Bradenton	96%	213
Central Florida Regional Hospital	Sanford	96%	350
Florida Hospital Memorial Medical Center	Daytona Bch	96%	362
Indian River Medical Center[2]	Vero Beach	96%	257
Tampa General Hospital[2]	Tampa	96%	227
The Villages Regional Hospital[2]	The Villages	96%	249
Baptist Hospital[2]	Pensacola	95%	290
Baptist Medical Center - Nassau[2]	Fernandina Bch	95%	74
Bayfront Health Brooksville	Brooksville	95%	229
Edward White Hospital	St Petersburg	95%	39
Florida Hospital Flagler	Palm Coast	95%	224
Florida Hospital Heartland Medical Center	Sebring	95%	326
Largo Medical Center	Largo	95%	309
Lower Keys Medical Center	Key West	95%	58
Mease Countryside Hospital	Safety Harbor	95%	335
Palms of Pasadena Hospital	St Petersburg	95%	88
W Palm Beach VA Medical Center	W Palm Beach	95%	222
Heart of Florida Regional Medical Center	Davenport	94%	294
Lake Wales Medical Center	Lake Wales	94%	220
Sacred Heart Hospital[2]	Pensacola	94%	250
Sacred Heart Hosp-Emerald Coast	Miramar Beach	94%	84
Tampa VA Medical Center	Tampa	94%	328
Town & Country Hospital	Tampa	94%	49
UF Health Jacksonville[2]	Jacksonville	94%	256
Bartow Regional Medical Center	Bartow	93%	109
Bayfront Health Punta Gorda	Punta Gorda	93%	107
Broward Health Coral Springs	Coral Springs	93%	138
Broward Health Imperial Point	Fort Lauderdale	93%	134
Gulf Breeze Hospital	Gulf Breeze	93%	94
Martin Medical Center[2]	Stuart	93%	232
UF Health Shands Hospital[2]	Gainesville	93%	243
Baptist Medical Center[2]	Jacksonville	92%	274
Flagler Hospital[2]	St Augustine	92%	263
Jackson Memorial Hospital[2]	Miami	92%	768
North Shore Medical Center[2]	Miami	92%	653
Saint Anthony's Hospital	St Petersburg	92%	284
Saint Petersburg General Hospital	St Petersburg	92%	88
Tallahassee Memorial Hospital	Tallahassee	92%	493
Bay Med Ctr Sacred Heart Health Sys[2]	Panama City	91%	388
Lehigh Regional Medical Center	Lehigh Acres	91%	93
Orlando Health	Orlando	91%	926
Citrus Memorial Hospital	Inverness	90%	305
Naples Community Hospital[2]	Naples	90%	255
Shands Lake Shore Regional Medical Center	Lake City	90%	132
Desoto Memorial Hospital	Arcadia	89%	61
Gulf Coast Med Ctr Lee Mem Health Sys[2]	Fort Myers	89%	252
Putnam Community Medical Center	Palatka	89%	180
Santa Rosa Medical Center	Milton	89%	87
Cape Coral Hospital[2]	Cape Coral	88%	249
Palm Springs General Hospital	Hialeah	88%	147
Bert Fish Medical Center	New Smyrn Bch	87%	87
Leesburg Regional Medical Center[2]	Leesburg	87%	306
Wuesthoff Medical Center Rockledge	Rockledge	87%	272
Jackson Hospital	Marianna	86%	95
Lakeside Medical Center	Belle Glade	86%	98
Munroe Regional Medical Center[2]	Ocala	86%	222
Bayfront Health - Saint Petersburg[2]	St Petersburg	85%	224
University of Miami Hospital	Miami	85%	589
Bayfront Health Port Charlotte	Port Charlotte	84%	262
Florida Hospital Carrollwood[2]	Tampa	84%	75
Winter Haven Hospital[2]	Winter Haven	83%	235
Lee Memorial Hospital[2]	Fort Myers	82%	257
Physicians Reg Med Ctr-Pine Ridge	Naples	77%	209
Shands Live Oak Regional Medical Center	Live Oak	71%	45
Wuesthoff Medical Center - Melbourne	Melbourne	70%	63
Memorial Hospital of Tampa	Tampa	67%	79
Saint Cloud Regional Medical Center	Saint Cloud	65%	89
Westchester General Hospital[2]	Miami	62%	26
Healthmark Regional Medical Center[2]	Defuniak Spgs	43%	35

Evaluation of LVS Function

Hospital Name	City	Rate	Cases
Aventura Hospital & Medical Center[2]	Aventura	100%	320
Baptist Hospital[2]	Pensacola	100%	330
Baptist Hospital of Miami[2]	Miami	100%	311
Baptist Medical Center[2]	Jacksonville	100%	349
Baptist Medical Center - Nassau[2]	Fernandina Bch	100%	91
Baptist Medical Center Beaches[2]	Jcksnvll Bch	100%	192
Bartow Regional Medical Center	Bartow	100%	123
Bay Med Ctr Sacred Heart Health Sys[2]	Panama City	100%	483
Bay Pines VA Medical Center	Bay Pines	100%	233
Bayfront Health - Saint Petersburg[2]	St Petersburg	100%	276
Bayfront Health Dade City	Dade City	100%	98
Bayfront Health Port Charlotte	Port Charlotte	100%	308
Bayfront Health Punta Gorda	Punta Gorda	100%	136
Blake Medical Center[2]	Bradenton	100%	290
Boca Raton Regional Hospital[2]	Boca Raton	100%	313
Brandon Regional Hospital[2]	Brandon	100%	400
Broward Health Coral Springs	Coral Springs	100%	166
Broward Health Medical Center[2]	Fort Lauderdale	100%	334
Broward Health North[2]	Pompano Bch	100%	292
Cape Canaveral Hospital	Cocoa Beach	100%	164
Capital Regional Medical Center	Tallahassee	100%	428
Central Florida Regional Hospital	Sanford	100%	414
Cleveland Clinic Hospital	Weston	100%	297
Coral Gables Hospital	Coral Gables	100%	202
Delray Medical Center[2]	Delray Beach	100%	374
Desoto Memorial Hospital	Arcadia	100%	70
Doctor's Memorial Hospital	Perry	100%	36
Doctors Hospital	Coral Gables	100%	179
Doctors Hospital of Sarasota	Sarasota	100%	235
Edward White Hospital	St Petersburg	100%	63
Englewood Community Hospital	Englewood	100%	170
Fawcett Memorial Hospital[2]	Port Charlotte	100%	264
Florida Hospital[2]	Orlando	100%	2544
Florida Hospital Carrollwood[2]	Tampa	100%	89
Florida Hospital Deland	Deland	100%	357
Florida Hospital Fish Memorial	Orange City	100%	466
Florida Hospital Flagler	Palm Coast	100%	283
Florida Hospital Memorial Medical Center	Daytona Bch	100%	459
Florida Hospital North Pinellas	Tarpon Springs	100%	127
Florida Hospital Waterman[2]	Tavares	100%	276
Florida Hospital Zephyrhills	Zephyrhills	100%	285
Fort Walton Beach Medical Center	Fort Walton Bch	100%	293
Good Samaritan Medical Center	W Palm Beach	100%	198
Gulf Breeze Hospital	Gulf Breeze	100%	118
Gulf Coast Regional Medical Center[2]	Panama City	100%	200
Halifax Health Medical Center[2]	Daytona Bch	100%	434
Health Central	Ocoee	100%	317
Hendry Regional Medical Center	Clewiston	100%	47
Hialeah Hospital[2]	Hialeah	100%	258
Highlands Regional Medical Center	Sebring	100%	136
Holmes Regional Medical Center	Melbourne	100%	787
Holy Cross Hospital	Fort Lauderdale	100%	506
Homestead Hospital	Homestead	100%	264
Indian River Medical Center[2]	Vero Beach	100%	326
Jackson Memorial Hospital[2]	Miami	100%	868
Jay Hospital	Jay	100%	52
JFK Medical Center	Atlantis	100%	988
Jupiter Medical Center	Jupiter	100%	200
Kendall Regional Medical Center	Miami	100%	635
Lake City Medical Center[2]	Lake City	100%	254
Lake Wales Medical Center	Lake Wales	100%	272
Lakeland Regional Medical Center[2]	Lakeland	100%	318
Lakeside Medical Center	Belle Glade	100%	103
Largo Medical Center	Largo	100%	439
Larkin Community Hospital	South Miami	100%	41
Lawnwood Reg Med Ctr & Heart Inst	Fort Pierce	100%	532
Lee Memorial Hospital[2]	Fort Myers	100%	297
Lehigh Regional Medical Center	Lehigh Acres	100%	110
Lower Keys Medical Center	Key West	100%	67
Manatee Memorial Hospital[2]	Bradenton	100%	304
Mariners Hospital	Tavernier	100%	29
Martin Medical Center[2]	Stuart	100%	282
Mease Countryside Hospital	Safety Harbor	100%	445
Mease Hospital Dunedin	Dunedin	100%	142
Medical Center of Trinity	Trinity	100%	336
Memorial Hospital Jacksonville[2]	Jacksonville	100%	325
Memorial Hospital Miramar	Miramar	100%	137
Memorial Hospital of Tampa	Tampa	100%	103
Memorial Hospital Pembroke	Pembroke Pines	100%	176
Memorial Hospital West	Pembroke Pines	100%	596
Memorial Regional Hospital	Hollywood	100%	677
Metropolitan Hospital of Miami	Miami	100%	107
Miami VA Medical Center	Miami	100%	156
Morton Plant Hospital	Clearwater	100%	595
Morton Plant North Bay Hospital	New Port Richey	100%	302
Mount Sinai Medical Center	Miami Beach	100%	517
Munroe Regional Medical Center[2]	Ocala	100%	269
North Florida Regional Medical Center[2]	Gainesville	100%	329
North Okaloosa Medical Center	Crestview	100%	240
North Shore Medical Center[2]	Miami	100%	814
Northside Hospital[2]	St Petersburg	100%	293
Northwest Medical Center	Margate	100%	533
Oak Hill Hospital[2]	Brooksville	100%	283
Ocala Regional Medical Center[2]	Ocala	100%	274
Orange Park Medical Center	Orange Park	100%	528
Orlando Health	Orlando	100%	1054
Osceola Regional Medical Center[2]	Kissimmee	100%	300
Palm Beach Gardens Medical Center	Palm Bch Grdns	100%	439
Palmetto General Hospital[2]	Hialeah	100%	391
Palms West Hospital	Loxahatchee	100%	225
Parrish Medical Center	Titusville	100%	176
Physicians Reg Med Ctr-Pine Ridge	Naples	100%	231
Plantation General Hospital[2]	Plantation	100%	301
Raulerson Hospital	Okeechobee	100%	235
Regional Medical Center Bayonet Point[2]	Hudson	100%	287
Sacred Heart Hospital[2]	Pensacola	100%	310
Sacred Heart Hosp-Emerald Coast	Miramar Beach	100%	97
Saint Anthony's Hospital	St Petersburg	100%	375

NOTE: Hospital profiles are in alphabetical order by state, then city, then hospital within the city; Rankings exclude hospitals with less than 25 cases except for patient surveys which excludes hospitals with less than 100 cases; (a) 100-299 cases; (1) The number of cases/patients is too few to report; (2) Data submitted were based on a sample of cases/patients; (3) Results are based on a shorter time period than required; (4) Data suppressed by CMS for one or more quarters; (5) Results are not available for this reporting period; (6) Fewer than 100 patients completed the HCAHPS survey; (7) No cases met the criteria for this measure; (8) The lower limit of the confidence interval cannot be calculated if the number of observed infections equals zero; (9) No data are available from the state/territory for this reporting period; (10) The scores shown reflect fewer than 50 completed surveys; (11) There were discrepancies in the data collection process; (12) This measure does not apply to this hospital for this reporting period; (13) Results cannot be calculated for this reporting period; (14) The results for this state are combined with nearby states to protect confidentiality; Please refer to the User's Guide for a full explanation of data.

Hospital Name	City	Rate	Cases
Saint Cloud Regional Medical Center	Saint Cloud	100%	119
Saint Joseph's Hospital	Tampa	100%	734
Saint Lucie Medical Center	Port Saint Lucie	100%	414
Saint Mary's Medical Center	W Palm Beach	100%	125
Saint Petersburg General Hospital	St Petersburg	100%	110
Saint Vincent's Medical Center[2]	Jacksonville	100%	301
Saint Vincent's Medical Center Southside[2]	Jacksonville	100%	200
Santa Rosa Medical Center	Milton	100%	102
Sarasota Memorial Hospital[2]	Sarasota	100%	409
Sebastian River Medical Center	Sebastian	100%	188
Seven Rivers Regional Medical Center	Crystal River	100%	150
Shands Live Oak Regional Medical Center	Live Oak	100%	73
South Bay Hospital	Sun City Center	100%	293
South Florida Baptist Hospital	Plant City	100%	199
South Miami Hospital	South Miami	100%	358
Tallahassee Memorial Hospital	Tallahassee	100%	588
Tampa VA Medical Center	Tampa	100%	361
Town & Country Hospital	Tampa	100%	60
Twin Cities Hospital	Niceville	100%	66
UF Health Jacksonville[2]	Jacksonville	100%	287
UF Health Shands Hospital[2]	Gainesville	100%	274
University Hospital & Medical Center	Tamarac	100%	198
University of Miami Hospital	Miami	100%	699
VA N Florida/S Georgia Healthcare Sys	Gainesville	100%	527
Venice Reg Med Ctr-Bayfront Health[2]	Venice	100%	259
Viera Hospital	Melbourne	100%	63
The Villages Regional Hospital[2]	The Villages	100%	328
W Palm Beach VA Medical Center	W Palm Beach	100%	250
Wellington Regional Medical Center[2]	Wellington	100%	208
West Boca Medical Center	Boca Raton	100%	253
West Florida Hospital	Pensacola	100%	369
West Kendall Baptist Hospital	Miami	100%	200
West Palm Hospital	W Palm Beach	100%	135
Westside Regional Medical Center[2]	Plantation	100%	391
Winter Haven Hospital[2]	Winter Haven	100%	330
Wuesthoff Medical Center - Melbourne	Melbourne	100%	90
Wuesthoff Medical Center Rockledge	Rockledge	100%	341
Bayfront Health Brooksville	Brooksville	99%	270
Bethesda Hospital East[2]	Boynton Beach	99%	301
Broward Health Imperial Point	Fort Lauderdale	99%	162
Cape Coral Hospital[2]	Cape Coral	99%	285
Flagler Hospital[2]	St Augustine	99%	324
Florida Hospital Heartland Medical Center	Sebring	99%	400
Florida Hospital Tampa	Tampa	99%	464
Gulf Coast Med Ctr Lee Mem Health Sys[2]	Fort Myers	99%	298
Heart of Florida Regional Medical Center	Davenport	99%	340
Jackson Hospital	Marianna	99%	106
Lakewood Ranch Medical Center	Bradenton	99%	133
Mayo Clinic	Jacksonville	99%	251
Naples Community Hospital[2]	Naples	99%	295
Palm Bay Hospital	Palm Bay	99%	199
Shands Lake Shore Regional Medical Center	Lake City	99%	160
Shands Starke Regional Medical Center	Starke	99%	69
South Lake Hospital	Clermont	99%	249
Tampa General Hospital[2]	Tampa	99%	257
Leesburg Regional Medical Center[2]	Leesburg	98%	385
Palm Springs General Hospital	Hialeah	98%	195
Palms of Pasadena Hospital	St Petersburg	98%	124
Citrus Memorial Hospital	Inverness	97%	393
Putnam Community Medical Center	Palatka	97%	234
Bert Fish Medical Center	New Smyrn Bch	95%	103
Westchester General Hospital[2]	Miami	93%	41
Doctors Memorial Hospital	Bonifay	17%	64
Healthmark Regional Medical Center[2]	Defuniak Spgs	15%	47

Medicare Spending

Medicare Spending per Patient (ratio)

Hospital Name	City	Ratio	Cases
Jay Hospital	Jay	0.86	-
Douglas Gardens Hospital	Miami	0.90	-
Lower Keys Medical Center	Key West	0.93	-
Desoto Memorial Hospital	Arcadia	0.95	-
Twin Cities Hospital	Niceville	0.95	-
Englewood Community Hospital	Englewood	0.96	-
Florida Hospital Zephyrhills	Zephyrhills	0.96	-
Lakeside Medical Center	Belle Glade	0.96	-
Raulerson Hospital	Okeechobee	0.96	-
Bert Fish Medical Center	New Smyrn Bch	0.97	-
Florida Hospital Wesley Chapel	Wesley Chapel	0.97	-
Gulf Breeze Hospital	Gulf Breeze	0.97	-
Memorial Hospital Pembroke	Pembroke Pines	0.97	-
Fort Walton Beach Medical Center	Fort Walton Bch	0.98	-
Mayo Clinic	Jacksonville	0.98	-
North Florida Regional Medical Center	Gainesville	0.99	-
North Okaloosa Medical Center	Crestview	0.99	-
Sacred Heart Hosp-Emerald Coast	Miramar Beach	0.99	-
Sacred Heart Hospital on the Gulf	Port Saint Joe	0.99	-
Baptist Medical Center - Nassau	Fernandina Bch	1.00	-
Bayfront Health Punta Gorda	Punta Gorda	1.00	-
Physicians Reg Med Ctr-Pine Ridge	Naples	1.00	-
Tampa General Hospital	Tampa	1.00	-
UF Health Jacksonville	Jacksonville	1.00	-
UF Health Shands Hospital	Gainesville	1.00	-
West Florida Hospital	Pensacola	1.00	-
Cleveland Clinic Hospital	Weston	1.01	-
Healthmark Regional Medical Center	Defuniak Spgs	1.01	-
Jackson Hospital	Marianna	1.01	-
Jupiter Medical Center	Jupiter	1.01	-
Lake Wales Medical Center	Lake Wales	1.01	-
Lee Memorial Hospital	Fort Myers	1.01	-
Ocala Regional Medical Center	Ocala	1.01	-
Santa Rosa Medical Center	Milton	1.01	-
Sebastian River Medical Center	Sebastian	1.01	-
The Villages Regional Hospital	The Villages	1.01	-
Baptist Hospital	Pensacola	1.02	-
Baptist Hospital of Miami	Miami	1.02	-
Bartow Regional Medical Center	Bartow	1.02	-
Cape Coral Hospital	Cape Coral	1.02	-
Central Florida Regional Hospital	Sanford	1.02	-
Florida Hospital Deland	Deland	1.02	-
Gulf Coast Med Ctr Lee Mem Health Sys	Fort Myers	1.02	-
Leesburg Regional Medical Center	Leesburg	1.02	-
Lehigh Regional Medical Center	Lehigh Acres	1.02	-
Memorial Hospital Miramar	Miramar	1.02	-
Orlando Health	Orlando	1.02	-
Osceola Regional Medical Center	Kissimmee	1.02	-
Sacred Heart Hospital	Pensacola	1.02	-
South Florida Baptist Hospital	Plant City	1.02	-
South Lake Hospital	Clermont	1.02	-
South Miami Hospital	South Miami	1.02	-
Bayfront Health Port Charlotte	Port Charlotte	1.03	-
Brandon Regional Hospital	Brandon	1.03	-
Doctor's Memorial Hospital	Perry	1.03	-
Flagler Hospital	St Augustine	1.03	-
Florida Hospital Memorial Medical Center	Daytona Bch	1.03	-
Florida Hospital Waterman	Tavares	1.03	-
Highlands Regional Medical Center	Sebring	1.03	-
Kendall Regional Medical Center	Miami	1.03	-
Lake City Medical Center	Lake City	1.03	-
Lakeland Regional Medical Center	Lakeland	1.03	-
Naples Community Hospital	Naples	1.03	-
Parrish Medical Center	Titusville	1.03	-
Regional Medical Center Bayonet Point	Hudson	1.03	-
Saint Vincent's Medical Center	Jacksonville	1.03	-
Saint Vincent's Medical Center Southside	Jacksonville	1.03	-
Seven Rivers Regional Medical Center	Crystal River	1.03	-
Shands Lake Shore Regional Medical Center	Lake City	1.03	-
Town & Country Hospital	Tampa	1.03	-
Bayfront Health Brooksville	Brooksville	1.04	-
Broward Health Medical Center	Fort Lauderdale	1.04	-
Cape Canaveral Hospital	Cocoa Beach	1.04	-
Florida Hospital	Orlando	1.04	-
Florida Hospital Fish Memorial	Orange City	1.04	-
Florida Hospital Heartland Medical Center	Sebring	1.04	-
Heart of Florida Regional Medical Center	Davenport	1.04	-
Indian River Medical Center	Vero Beach	1.04	-
Jackson Memorial Hospital	Miami	1.04	-
Martin Medical Center	Stuart	1.04	-
Memorial Hospital of Tampa	Tampa	1.04	-
Memorial Hospital West	Pembroke Pines	1.04	-
Metropolitan Hospital of Miami	Miami	1.04	-
Munroe Regional Medical Center	Ocala	1.04	-
Saint Cloud Regional Medical Center	Saint Cloud	1.04	-
Venice Reg Med Ctr-Bayfront Health	Venice	1.04	-
Viera Hospital	Melbourne	1.04	-
Bay Med Ctr Sacred Heart Health Sys	Panama City	1.05	-
Bayfront Health Dade City	Dade City	1.05	-
Boca Raton Regional Hospital	Boca Raton	1.05	-
Broward Health Imperial Point	Fort Lauderdale	1.05	-
Citrus Memorial Hospital	Inverness	1.05	-
Doctors Hospital	Coral Gables	1.05	-
Florida Hospital Flagler	Palm Coast	1.05	-
Halifax Health Medical Center	Daytona Bch	1.05	-
Memorial Regional Hospital	Hollywood	1.05	-
Morton Plant Hospital	Clearwater	1.05	-
Oak Hill Hospital	Brooksville	1.05	-
Putnam Community Medical Center	Palatka	1.05	-
Saint Anthony's Hospital	St Petersburg	1.05	-
Saint Lucie Medical Center	Port Saint Lucie	1.05	-
Tallahassee Memorial Hospital	Tallahassee	1.05	-
Edward White Hospital	St Petersburg	1.06	-
Fawcett Memorial Hospital	Port Charlotte	1.06	-
Florida Hospital Carrollwood	Tampa	1.06	-
Florida Hospital North Pinellas	Tarpon Springs	1.06	-
Health Central	Ocoee	1.06	-
Holy Cross Hospital	Fort Lauderdale	1.06	-
Larkin Community Hospital	South Miami	1.06	-
Lawnwood Reg Med Ctr & Heart Inst	Fort Pierce	1.06	-
Plantation General Hospital	Plantation	1.06	-
Saint Joseph's Hospital	Tampa	1.06	-
Blake Medical Center	Bradenton	1.07	-
Broward Health North	Pompano Bch	1.07	-
Good Samaritan Medical Center	W Palm Beach	1.07	-
Homestead Hospital	Homestead	1.07	-
JFK Medical Center	Atlantis	1.07	-
Manatee Memorial Hospital	Bradenton	1.07	-
Mease Countryside Hospital	Safety Harbor	1.07	-
Palm Beach Gardens Medical Center	Palm Bch Grdns	1.07	-
Palms West Hospital	Loxahatchee	1.07	-
University of Miami Hospital	Miami	1.07	-
Baptist Medical Center Beaches	Jcksnvl Bch	1.08	-
Broward Health Coral Springs	Coral Springs	1.08	-
Capital Regional Medical Center	Tallahassee	1.08	-
Doctors Hospital of Sarasota	Sarasota	1.08	-
Gulf Coast Regional Medical Center	Panama City	1.08	-
Mount Sinai Medical Center	Miami Beach	1.08	-
Saint Mary's Medical Center	W Palm Beach	1.08	-
Saint Petersburg General Hospital	St Petersburg	1.08	-
West Palm Hospital	W Palm Beach	1.08	-
Westchester General Hospital	Miami	1.08	-
Wuesthoff Medical Center Rockledge	Rockledge	1.08	-
Florida Hospital Tampa	Tampa	1.09	-
Holmes Regional Medical Center	Melbourne	1.09	-
Medical Center of Trinity	Trinity	1.09	-
Northside Hospital	St Petersburg	1.09	-
Northwest Medical Center	Margate	1.09	-
Palm Bay Hospital	Palm Bay	1.09	-
Sarasota Memorial Hospital	Sarasota	1.09	-
South Bay Hospital	Sun City Center	1.09	-
Aventura Hospital & Medical Center	Aventura	1.10	-
Baptist Medical Center	Jacksonville	1.10	-
Bayfront Health - Saint Petersburg	St Petersburg	1.10	-
Delray Medical Center	Delray Beach	1.10	-
Palm Springs General Hospital	Hialeah	1.10	-
West Kendall Baptist Hospital	Miami	1.10	-
Bethesda Hospital East	Boynton Beach	1.11	-
Coral Gables Hospital	Coral Gables	1.11	-
Lakewood Ranch Medical Center	Bradenton	1.11	-
Largo Medical Center	Largo	1.11	-
Orange Park Medical Center	Orange Park	1.11	-
University Hospital & Medical Center	Tamarac	1.11	-
Wellington Regional Medical Center	Wellington	1.11	-
Westside Regional Medical Center	Plantation	1.11	-
Winter Haven Hospital	Winter Haven	1.11	-
Morton Plant North Bay Hospital	New Port Richey	1.12	-
West Boca Medical Center	Boca Raton	1.12	-
Hialeah Hospital	Hialeah	1.13	-
Memorial Hospital Jacksonville	Jacksonville	1.13	-
Palmetto General Hospital	Hialeah	1.13	-
Mease Hospital Dunedin	Dunedin	1.14	-
North Shore Medical Center	Miami	1.14	-
Palms of Pasadena Hospital	St Petersburg	1.14	-
Wuesthoff Medical Center - Melbourne	Melbourne	1.15	-

Pneumonia Care

Appropriate Initial Antibiotic Given

Hospital Name	City	Rate	Cases
Aventura Hospital & Medical Center[2]	Aventura	100%	78
Baptist Hospital of Miami[2]	Miami	100%	78
Broward Health Medical Center[2]	Fort Lauderdale	100%	146
Broward Health North[2]	Pompano Bch	100%	71
Coral Gables Hospital	Coral Gables	100%	74
Delray Medical Center[2]	Delray Beach	100%	132
Englewood Community Hospital	Englewood	100%	54
Fawcett Memorial Hospital[2]	Port Charlotte	100%	45
Fishermen's Hospital	Marathon	100%	31
Florida Hospital North Pinellas	Tarpon Springs	100%	84
Gulf Breeze Hospital[2]	Gulf Breeze	100%	119
Health Central	Ocoee	100%	148
Holy Cross Hospital	Fort Lauderdale	100%	115
Jay Hospital	Jay	100%	26
JFK Medical Center	Atlantis	100%	208
Kendall Regional Medical Center	Miami	100%	192
Lake City Medical Center[2]	Lake City	100%	84
Lake Wales Medical Center	Lake Wales	100%	63
Lakeside Medical Center	Belle Glade	100%	59
Largo Medical Center	Largo	100%	131
Lawnwood Reg Med Ctr & Heart Inst	Fort Pierce	100%	143
Leesburg Regional Medical Center[2]	Leesburg	100%	117
Lehigh Regional Medical Center	Lehigh Acres	100%	72
Lower Keys Medical Center	Key West	100%	42
Manatee Memorial Hospital[2]	Bradenton	100%	89
Martin Medical Center[2]	Stuart	100%	76
Mease Hospital Dunedin	Dunedin	100%	81
Medical Center of Trinity[2]	Trinity	100%	75
Memorial Hospital Miramar	Miramar	100%	114
Memorial Hospital Pembroke	Pembroke Pines	100%	152
Memorial Hospital West	Pembroke Pines	100%	270
Memorial Regional Hospital	Hollywood	100%	238

NOTE: Hospital profiles are in alphabetical order by state, then city, then hospital within the city; Rankings exclude hospitals with less than 25 cases except for patient surveys which excludes hospitals with less than 100 cases; (a) 100-299 cases; (1) The number of cases/patients is too few to report; (2) Data submitted were based on a sample of cases/patients; (3) Results are based on a shorter time period than required; (4) Data suppressed by CMS for one or more quarters; (5) Results are not available for this reporting period; (6) Fewer than 100 patients completed the HCAHPS survey; (7) No cases met the criteria for this measure; (8) The lower limit of the confidence interval cannot be calculated if the number of observed infections equals zero; (9) No data are available from the state/territory for this reporting period; (10) The scores shown reflect fewer than 50 completed surveys; (11) There were discrepancies in the data collection process; (12) This measure does not apply to this hospital for this reporting period; (13) Results cannot be calculated for this reporting period; (14) The results for this state are combined with nearby states to protect confidentiality; Please refer to the User's Guide for a full explanation of data.

North Florida Regional Medical Center	Gainesville	100%	291
North Shore Medical Center[2]	Miami	100%	206
Northside Hospital[2]	St Petersburg	100%	66
Oak Hill Hospital	Brooksville	100%	158
Ocala Regional Medical Center[2]	Ocala	100%	102
Orange Park Medical Center[2]	Orange Park	100%	65
Palm Bay Hospital	Palm Bay	100%	132
Raulerson Hospital	Okeechobee	100%	57
Regional Medical Center Bayonet Point[2]	Hudson	100%	63
Sacred Heart Hosp-Emerald Coast	Miramar Beach	100%	91
Saint Lucie Medical Center	Port Saint Lucie	100%	150
Saint Mary's Medical Center	W Palm Beach	100%	53
Saint Vincent's Medical Center[2]	Jacksonville	100%	81
Saint Vincent's Medical Center Southside[2]	Jacksonville	100%	66
Santa Rosa Medical Center	Milton	100%	58
Sebastian River Medical Center	Sebastian	100%	144
Shands Lake Shore Regional Medical Center	Lake City	100%	54
South Miami Hospital	South Miami	100%	88
Twin Cities Hospital	Niceville	100%	41
University of Miami Hospital	Miami	100%	67
Venice Reg Med Ctr-Bayfront Health[2]	Venice	100%	109
Viera Hospital	Melbourne	100%	68
W Palm Beach VA Medical Center	W Palm Beach	100%	101
Wellington Regional Medical Center[2]	Wellington	100%	109
West Kendall Baptist Hospital	Miami	100%	100
West Palm Hospital	W Palm Beach	100%	47
Westchester General Hospital[2]	Miami	100%	48
Westside Regional Medical Center	Plantation	100%	108
Baptist Hospital[2]	Pensacola	99%	106
Bethesda Hospital East[2]	Boynton Beach	99%	92
Blake Medical Center	Bradenton	99%	111
Boca Raton Regional Hospital[2]	Boca Raton	99%	106
Brandon Regional Hospital[2]	Brandon	99%	180
Broward Health Coral Springs[2]	Coral Springs	99%	144
Broward Health Imperial Point	Fort Lauderdale	99%	69
Central Florida Regional Hospital	Sanford	99%	155
Cleveland Clinic Hospital	Weston	99%	88
Doctors Hospital	Coral Gables	99%	70
Florida Hospital[2]	Orlando	99%	1121
Florida Hospital Heartland Medical Center	Sebring	99%	135
Florida Hospital Waterman[2]	Tavares	99%	94
Hialeah Hospital[2]	Hialeah	99%	155
Highlands Regional Medical Center	Sebring	99%	71
Holmes Regional Medical Center	Melbourne	99%	298
Homestead Hospital	Homestead	99%	127
Jackson Hospital	Marianna	99%	99
Jupiter Medical Center[2]	Jupiter	99%	90
Lakeland Regional Medical Center[2]	Lakeland	99%	105
Mease Countryside Hospital	Safety Harbor	99%	178
North Okaloosa Medical Center	Crestview	99%	74
Northwest Medical Center	Margate	99%	137
Palm Beach Gardens Medical Center	Palm Bch Grdns	99%	87
Palmetto General Hospital[2]	Hialeah	99%	123
Palms of Pasadena Hospital	St Petersburg	99%	104
Palms West Hospital	Loxahatchee	99%	110
Parrish Medical Center	Titusville	99%	108
Physicians Reg Med Ctr-Pine Ridge	Naples	99%	159
Saint Cloud Regional Medical Center	Saint Cloud	99%	70
Sarasota Memorial Hospital[2]	Sarasota	99%	100
Shands Starke Regional Medical Center	Starke	99%	92
South Bay Hospital	Sun City Center	99%	151
University Hospital & Medical Center	Tamarac	99%	76
West Florida Hospital[2]	Pensacola	99%	71
Bartow Regional Medical Center	Bartow	98%	94
Bayfront Health Port Charlotte	Port Charlotte	98%	145
Capital Regional Medical Center	Tallahassee	98%	114
Doctors Hospital of Sarasota	Sarasota	98%	104
Edward White Hospital[2]	St Petersburg	98%	56
Florida Hospital Fish Memorial	Orange City	98%	175
Florida Hospital Flagler	Palm Coast	98%	156
Fort Walton Beach Medical Center	Fort Walton Bch	98%	118
Good Samaritan Medical Center	W Palm Beach	98%	122
Indian River Medical Center[2]	Vero Beach	98%	127
Mayo Clinic	Jacksonville	98%	56
Memorial Hospital Jacksonville[2]	Jacksonville	98%	59
Memorial Hospital of Tampa	Tampa	98%	103
Morton Plant Hospital	Clearwater	98%	140
Mount Sinai Medical Center	Miami Beach	98%	192
Osceola Regional Medical Center[2]	Kissimmee	98%	262
Plantation General Hospital[2]	Plantation	98%	105
Saint Joseph's Hospital	Tampa	98%	349
South Florida Baptist Hospital	Plant City	98%	116
Town & Country Hospital	Tampa	98%	47
The Villages Regional Hospital[2]	The Villages	98%	96
West Boca Medical Center	Boca Raton	98%	98
Baptist Medical Center - Nassau[2]	Fernandina Bch	97%	121
Bay Med Ctr Sacred Heart Health Sys[2]	Panama City	97%	151
Bay Pines VA Medical Center	Bay Pines	97%	74
Bayfront Health Punta Gorda[2]	Punta Gorda	97%	90
Bert Fish Medical Center	New Smyrn Bch	97%	59
Cape Canaveral Hospital	Cocoa Beach	97%	145
Cape Coral Hospital[2]	Cape Coral	97%	94
Florida Hospital Carrollwood[2]	Tampa	97%	75
Florida Hospital Deland	Deland	97%	142
Florida Hospital Memorial Medical Center	Daytona Bch	97%	182
Gulf Coast Regional Medical Center[2]	Panama City	97%	72
Halifax Health Medical Center[2]	Daytona Bch	97%	209
Jackson Memorial Hospital[2]	Miami	97%	185
Naples Community Hospital[2]	Naples	97%	143
Putnam Community Medical Center	Palatka	97%	73
Saint Anthony's Hospital	St Petersburg	97%	150
Baptist Medical Center Beaches[2]	Jcksnvll Bch	96%	156
Bayfront Health Brooksville	Brooksville	96%	157
Citrus Memorial Hospital	Inverness	96%	190
Florida Hospital Zephyrhills	Zephyrhills	96%	102
Lakewood Ranch Medical Center[2]	Bradenton	96%	55
Larkin Community Hospital	South Miami	96%	57
Metropolitan Hospital of Miami	Miami	96%	67
Munroe Regional Medical Center[2]	Ocala	96%	96
Palm Springs General Hospital	Hialeah	96%	163
Sacred Heart Hospital[2]	Pensacola	96%	89
South Lake Hospital	Clermont	96%	96
Tallahassee Memorial Hospital	Tallahassee	96%	147
Bayfront Health Dade City	Dade City	95%	40
Florida Hospital Tampa	Tampa	95%	199
Gulf Coast Med Ctr Lee Mem Health Sys[2]	Fort Myers	95%	83
Morton Plant North Bay Hospital	New Port Richey	95%	100
Saint Petersburg General Hospital[2]	St Petersburg	95%	62
Tampa VA Medical Center	Tampa	95%	120
Baptist Medical Center[2]	Jacksonville	94%	116
Bayfront Health - Saint Petersburg[2]	St Petersburg	94%	64
Flagler Hospital[2]	St Augustine	94%	66
Lee Memorial Hospital[2]	Fort Myers	94%	102
Orlando Health[2]	Orlando	94%	291
VA N Florida/S Georgia Healthcare Sys	Gainesville	94%	119
Wuesthoff Medical Center Rockledge	Rockledge	94%	137
Desoto Memorial Hospital	Arcadia	93%	61
Seven Rivers Regional Medical Center	Crystal River	93%	61
Shands Live Oak Regional Medical Center	Live Oak	93%	57
UF Health Jacksonville[2]	Jacksonville	93%	43
Wuesthoff Medical Center - Melbourne	Melbourne	93%	71
Heart of Florida Regional Medical Center	Davenport	92%	92
Tampa General Hospital[2]	Tampa	91%	35
Winter Haven Hospital[2]	Winter Haven	89%	80
Doctor's Memorial Hospital	Perry	81%	37
Healthmark Regional Medical Center[2]	Defuniak Spgs	50%	40
Doctors Memorial Hospital	Bonifay	44%	70

Blood Culture Timing

Hospital Name	City	Rate	Cases
Aventura Hospital & Medical Center[2]	Aventura	100%	167
Baptist Hospital of Miami[2]	Miami	100%	123
Bayfront Health Brooksville	Brooksville	100%	224
Blake Medical Center	Bradenton	100%	177
Boca Raton Regional Hospital[2]	Boca Raton	100%	140
Broward Health North[2]	Pompano Bch	100%	142
Cape Canaveral Hospital	Cocoa Beach	100%	210
Capital Regional Medical Center	Tallahassee	100%	198
Cleveland Clinic Hospital	Weston	100%	191
Coral Gables Hospital	Coral Gables	100%	105
Delray Medical Center[2]	Delray Beach	100%	219
Doctor's Memorial Hospital	Perry	100%	50
Doctors Hospital	Coral Gables	100%	148
Doctors Hospital of Sarasota	Sarasota	100%	162
Englewood Community Hospital	Englewood	100%	92
Fawcett Memorial Hospital[2]	Port Charlotte	100%	90
Flagler Hospital[2]	St Augustine	100%	123
Florida Hospital Deland	Deland	100%	299
Florida Hospital North Pinellas	Tarpon Springs	100%	124
Florida Hospital Waterman[2]	Tavares	100%	110
Fort Walton Beach Medical Center	Fort Walton Bch	100%	203
Highlands Regional Medical Center	Sebring	100%	109
Homestead Hospital	Homestead	100%	225
Jay Hospital	Jay	100%	26
JFK Medical Center	Atlantis	100%	357
Kendall Regional Medical Center	Miami	100%	371
Lake City Medical Center[2]	Lake City	100%	136
Lake Wales Medical Center	Lake Wales	100%	113
Lakeland Regional Medical Center[2]	Lakeland	100%	131
Largo Medical Center	Largo	100%	219
Lawnwood Reg Med Ctr & Heart Inst	Fort Pierce	100%	337
Lehigh Regional Medical Center	Lehigh Acres	100%	99
Mariners Hospital	Tavernier	100%	32
Mayo Clinic	Jacksonville	100%	161
Mease Hospital Dunedin	Dunedin	100%	182
Medical Center of Trinity[2]	Trinity	100%	104
Memorial Hospital Jacksonville[2]	Jacksonville	100%	92
Memorial Hospital Pembroke	Pembroke Pines	100%	228
Memorial Hospital West	Pembroke Pines	100%	434
Memorial Regional Hospital	Hollywood	100%	477
Morton Plant Hospital	Clearwater	100%	415
North Florida Regional Medical Center	Gainesville	100%	562
North Shore Medical Center[2]	Miami	100%	414
Northside Hospital[2]	St Petersburg	100%	127
Northwest Medical Center	Margate	100%	230
Oak Hill Hospital	Brooksville	100%	222
Orange Park Medical Center[2]	Orange Park	100%	71
Palm Bay Hospital	Palm Bay	100%	218
Palm Beach Gardens Medical Center	Palm Bch Grdns	100%	145
Physicians Reg Med Ctr-Pine Ridge	Naples	100%	227
Raulerson Hospital	Okeechobee	100%	115
Sacred Heart Hospital on the Gulf	Port Saint Joe	100%	25
Saint Lucie Medical Center	Port Saint Lucie	100%	377
Saint Vincent's Medical Center Southside[2]	Jacksonville	100%	142
Sebastian River Medical Center	Sebastian	100%	179
Shands Lake Shore Regional Medical Center	Lake City	100%	67
Shands Starke Regional Medical Center	Starke	100%	101
South Bay Hospital	Sun City Center	100%	243
South Florida Baptist Hospital	Plant City	100%	228
South Miami Hospital	South Miami	100%	198
Twin Cities Hospital	Niceville	100%	79
University Hospital & Medical Center	Tamarac	100%	144
University of Miami Hospital	Miami	100%	173
Venice Reg Med Ctr-Bayfront Health[2]	Venice	100%	160
Viera Hospital	Melbourne	100%	95
West Florida Hospital[2]	Pensacola	100%	148
West Palm Hospital	W Palm Beach	100%	109
Wuesthoff Medical Center - Melbourne	Melbourne	100%	132
Baptist Hospital[2]	Pensacola	99%	170
Baptist Medical Center Beaches[2]	Jcksnvll Bch	99%	232
Bayfront Health - Saint Petersburg[2]	St Petersburg	99%	170
Bayfront Health Punta Gorda[2]	Punta Gorda	99%	132
Brandon Regional Hospital[2]	Brandon	99%	214
Broward Health Coral Springs[2]	Coral Springs	99%	141
Broward Health Imperial Point	Fort Lauderdale	99%	114
Broward Health Medical Center[2]	Fort Lauderdale	99%	272
Desoto Memorial Hospital	Arcadia	99%	83
Edward White Hospital[2]	St Petersburg	99%	69
Florida Hospital[2]	Orlando	99%	863
Florida Hospital Memorial Medical Center	Daytona Bch	99%	304
Florida Hospital Tampa	Tampa	99%	475
Florida Hospital Zephyrhills	Zephyrhills	99%	178
Gulf Breeze Hospital[2]	Gulf Breeze	99%	145
Gulf Coast Regional Medical Center[2]	Panama City	99%	139
Health Central	Ocoee	99%	215
Heart of Florida Regional Medical Center	Davenport	99%	170
Holmes Regional Medical Center	Melbourne	99%	617
Jupiter Medical Center[2]	Jupiter	99%	154
Lakewood Ranch Medical Center[2]	Bradenton	99%	80
Larkin Community Hospital	South Miami	99%	99
Mease Countryside Hospital	Safety Harbor	99%	367
Memorial Hospital Miramar	Miramar	99%	197
Miami VA Medical Center	Miami	99%	89
Morton Plant North Bay Hospital	New Port Richey	99%	183
Mount Sinai Medical Center	Miami Beach	99%	378
Ocala Regional Medical Center[2]	Ocala	99%	203
Osceola Regional Medical Center[2]	Kissimmee	99%	249
Palm Springs General Hospital	Hialeah	99%	335
Palms West Hospital	Loxahatchee	99%	191
Plantation General Hospital[2]	Plantation	99%	185
Sacred Heart Hosp-Emerald Coast	Miramar Beach	99%	163
Saint Anthony's Hospital	St Petersburg	99%	325
Saint Petersburg General Hospital[2]	St Petersburg	99%	126
Santa Rosa Medical Center	Milton	99%	90
Tampa VA Medical Center	Tampa	99%	242
UF Health Shands Hospital[2]	Gainesville	99%	107
W Palm Beach VA Medical Center	W Palm Beach	99%	143
West Boca Medical Center	Boca Raton	99%	145
Westchester General Hospital[2]	Miami	99%	86
Westside Regional Medical Center	Plantation	99%	193
Baptist Medical Center - Nassau[2]	Fernandina Bch	98%	183
Bartow Regional Medical Center	Bartow	98%	130
Bayfront Health Port Charlotte	Port Charlotte	98%	242
Bethesda Hospital East[2]	Boynton Beach	98%	124
Central Florida Regional Hospital	Sanford	98%	193
Florida Hospital Carrollwood[2]	Tampa	98%	122
Florida Hospital Flagler	Palm Coast	98%	317
Florida Hospital Heartland Medical Center	Sebring	98%	282
Good Samaritan Medical Center	W Palm Beach	98%	199
Gulf Coast Med Ctr Lee Mem Health Sys[2]	Fort Myers	98%	171
Hialeah Hospital[2]	Hialeah	98%	162
Holy Cross Hospital	Fort Lauderdale	98%	275
Indian River Medical Center[2]	Vero Beach	98%	179
Lower Keys Medical Center	Key West	98%	60
Memorial Hospital of Tampa	Tampa	98%	130
Palmetto General Hospital[2]	Hialeah	98%	184
Regional Medical Center Bayonet Point[2]	Hudson	98%	47
Sacred Heart Hospital[2]	Pensacola	98%	174
Saint Cloud Regional Medical Center	Saint Cloud	98%	108
Saint Joseph's Hospital	Tampa	98%	579
West Kendall Baptist Hospital	Miami	98%	196
Wuesthoff Medical Center Rockledge	Rockledge	98%	266
Baptist Medical Center[2]	Jacksonville	97%	221

NOTE: Hospital profiles are in alphabetical order by state, then city, then hospital within the city; Rankings exclude hospitals with less than 25 cases except for patient surveys which excludes hospitals with less than 100 cases; (a) 100-299 cases; (1) The number of cases/patients is too few to report; (2) Data submitted were based on a sample of cases/patients; (3) Results are based on a shorter time period than required; (4) Data suppressed by CMS for one or more quarters; (5) Results are not available for this reporting period; (6) Fewer than 100 patients completed the HCAHPS survey; (7) No cases met the criteria for this measure; (8) The lower limit of the confidence interval cannot be calculated if the number of observed infections equals zero; (9) No data are available from the state/territory for this reporting period; (10) The scores shown reflect fewer than 50 completed surveys; (11) There were discrepancies in the data collection process; (12) This measure does not apply to this hospital for this reporting period; (13) Results cannot be calculated for this reporting period; (14) The results for this state are combined with nearby states to protect confidentiality; Please refer to the User's Guide for a full explanation of data.

Hospital Name	City	Rate	Cases
Bay Med Ctr Sacred Heart Health Sys[2]	Panama City	97%	218
Bay Pines VA Medical Center	Bay Pines	97%	131
Bayfront Health Dade City	Dade City	97%	58
Bert Fish Medical Center	New Smyrn Bch	97%	124
Florida Hospital Fish Memorial	Orange City	97%	339
Halifax Health Medical Center[2]	Daytona Bch	97%	363
Manatee Memorial Hospital[2]	Bradenton	97%	157
Martin Medical Center[2]	Stuart	97%	152
Naples Community Hospital[2]	Naples	97%	213
Saint Mary's Medical Center	W Palm Beach	97%	102
Saint Vincent's Medical Center[2]	Jacksonville	97%	73
Shands Live Oak Regional Medical Center	Live Oak	97%	91
Tallahassee Memorial Hospital	Tallahassee	97%	196
Town & Country Hospital	Tampa	97%	65
The Villages Regional Hospital[2]	The Villages	97%	74
Wellington Regional Medical Center[2]	Wellington	97%	190
Winter Haven Hospital[2]	Winter Haven	97%	153
Lee Memorial Hospital[2]	Fort Myers	96%	163
Leesburg Regional Medical Center[2]	Leesburg	96%	105
Munroe Regional Medical Center[2]	Ocala	96%	150
Sarasota Memorial Hospital[2]	Sarasota	96%	165
Cape Coral Hospital[2]	Cape Coral	95%	155
Citrus Memorial Hospital	Inverness	95%	262
Jackson Hospital	Marianna	95%	167
Lakeside Medical Center	Belle Glade	95%	108
Palms of Pasadena Hospital	St Petersburg	95%	129
Parrish Medical Center	Titusville	95%	163
Jackson Memorial Hospital[2]	Miami	94%	358
Orlando Health[2]	Orlando	94%	534
South Lake Hospital	Clermont	94%	160
VA N Florida/S Georgia Healthcare Sys	Gainesville	94%	232
Fishermen's Hospital	Marathon	93%	41
Seven Rivers Regional Medical Center	Crystal River	90%	94
Putnam Community Medical Center	Palatka	89%	106
Tampa General Hospital[2]	Tampa	89%	70
UF Health Jacksonville[2]	Jacksonville	89%	89

Pregnancy and Delivery Care

Newborns whose Deliveries were Scheduled Early

Hospital Name	City	Rate	Cases
Baptist Hospital of Miami[2]	Miami	0%	71
Baptist Medical Center[2]	Jacksonville	0%	65
Baptist Medical Center Beaches[2]	Jcksnvll Bch	0%	30
Bay Med Ctr Sacred Heart Health Sys	Panama City	0%	35
Broward Health Coral Springs[2]	Coral Springs	0%	47
Broward Health Medical Center[2]	Fort Lauderdale	0%	93
Capital Regional Medical Center[2]	Tallahassee	0%	30
Central Florida Regional Hospital[2]	Sanford	0%	34
Desoto Memorial Hospital[2]	Arcadia	0%	28
Flagler Hospital	St Augustine	0%	104
Florida Hospital Deland[2]	Deland	0%	39
Fort Walton Beach Medical Center[2]	Fort Walton Bch	0%	27
Hialeah Hospital[2]	Hialeah	0%	44
Leesburg Regional Medical Center[2]	Leesburg	0%	34
Medical Center of Trinity[2]	Trinity	0%	34
Memorial Hospital Jacksonville[2]	Jacksonville	0%	36
Memorial Hospital West[2]	Pembroke Pines	0%	77
Memorial Regional Hospital[2]	Hollywood	0%	77
North Shore Medical Center[2]	Miami	0%	54
Northwest Medical Center[2]	Margate	0%	40
Orange Park Medical Center[2]	Orange Park	0%	66
Osceola Regional Medical Center[2]	Kissimmee	0%	46
Palms West Hospital[2]	Loxahatchee	0%	47
Parrish Medical Center	Titusville	0%	53
Putnam Community Medical Center[2]	Palatka	0%	37
Saint Petersburg General Hospital[2]	St Petersburg	0%	38
Saint Vincent's Medical Center Southside[2]	Jacksonville	0%	34
South Lake Hospital	Clermont	0%	40
UF Health Jacksonville[2]	Jacksonville	0%	46
West Kendall Baptist Hospital	Miami	0%	80
Brandon Regional Hospital[2]	Brandon	1%	71
Florida Hospital Memorial Medical Center[2]	Daytona Bch	1%	140
Lawnwood Reg Med Ctr & Heart Inst	Fort Pierce	1%	138
Shands Lake Shore Regional Medical Center	Lake City	1%	120
Lakeland Regional Medical Center	Lakeland	2%	264
Palmetto General Hospital[2]	Hialeah	2%	42
Saint Mary's Medical Center[2]	W Palm Beach	2%	58
Bayfront Health - Saint Petersburg[2]	St Petersburg	3%	62
Bayfront Health Brooksville	Brooksville	3%	147
Cape Coral Hospital[2]	Cape Coral	3%	33
Citrus Memorial Hospital[2]	Inverness	3%	37
Florida Hospital[2]	Orlando	3%	177
Good Samaritan Medical Center[2]	W Palm Beach	3%	35
Holy Cross Hospital	Fort Lauderdale	3%	98
Lower Keys Medical Center	Key West	3%	32
North Florida Regional Medical Center[2]	Gainesville	3%	38
Sacred Heart Hosp-Emerald Coast[2]	Miramar Beach	3%	34
Saint Lucie Medical Center[2]	Port Saint Lucie	3%	34
Winter Haven Hospital[2]	Winter Haven	3%	32
Florida Hospital Zephyrhills	Zephyrhills	4%	28
Gulf Coast Regional Medical Center[2]	Panama City	4%	56
Highlands Regional Medical Center	Sebring	4%	25
Homestead Hospital[2]	Homestead	4%	178
Jupiter Medical Center	Jupiter	4%	160
Kendall Regional Medical Center[2]	Miami	4%	28
Lakewood Ranch Medical Center[2]	Bradenton	4%	26
Mount Sinai Medical Center[2]	Miami Beach	4%	55
Orlando Health[2]	Orlando	4%	208
Sacred Heart Hospital[2]	Pensacola	4%	69
Tampa General Hospital[2]	Tampa	4%	45
West Florida Hospital[2]	Pensacola	4%	45
Bethesda Hospital East[2]	Boynton Beach	5%	80
Florida Hospital Heartland Medical Center[2]	Sebring	5%	38
Plantation General Hospital[2]	Plantation	5%	111
Wellington Regional Medical Center[2]	Wellington	5%	43
Cape Canaveral Hospital[2]	Cocoa Beach	6%	34
Lee Memorial Hospital[2]	Fort Myers	6%	67
Martin Medical Center	Stuart	6%	138
South Florida Baptist Hospital[2]	Plant City	6%	36
Wuesthoff Medical Center Rockledge	Rockledge	6%	47
Jackson Memorial Hospital[2]	Miami	7%	146
Tallahassee Memorial Hospital[2]	Tallahassee	7%	227
UF Health Shands Hospital[2]	Gainesville	7%	30
West Boca Medical Center[2]	Boca Raton	7%	42
Gulf Coast Med Ctr Lee Mem Health Sys[2]	Fort Myers	8%	49
Holmes Regional Medical Center[2]	Melbourne	8%	36
Jackson Hospital	Marianna	8%	40
Manatee Memorial Hospital[2]	Bradenton	8%	60
Sarasota Memorial Hospital[2]	Sarasota	8%	48
Halifax Health Medical Center[2]	Daytona Bch	9%	89
Memorial Hospital Miramar[2]	Miramar	9%	55
Health Central	Ocoee	10%	73
South Miami Hospital[2]	South Miami	10%	89
Baptist Medical Center - Nassau[2]	Fernandina Bch	11%	56
Saint Joseph's Hospital[2]	Tampa	14%	137
Naples Community Hospital[2]	Naples	17%	59
Bayfront Health Port Charlotte[2]	Port Charlotte	18%	38
Physicians Reg Med Ctr-Pine Ridge	Naples	18%	28
Munroe Regional Medical Center	Ocala	19%	318
Boca Raton Regional Hospital[2]	Boca Raton	20%	44
Heart of Florida Regional Medical Center	Davenport	29%	101
Wuesthoff Medical Center - Melbourne	Melbourne	31%	32
Baptist Hospital[2]	Pensacola	32%	47
Morton Plant Hospital[2]	Clearwater	34%	50
Santa Rosa Medical Center	Milton	41%	39
Mease Countryside Hospital[2]	Safety Harbor	54%	70

Preventive Care

Immunization for Influenza

Hospital Name	City	Rate	Cases
Baptist Hospital of Miami[2]	Miami	100%	527
Broward Health North[2]	Pompano Bch	100%	585
Coral Gables Hospital[2]	Coral Gables	100%	611
Delray Medical Center[2]	Delray Beach	100%	652
Doctors Hospital of Sarasota[2]	Sarasota	100%	602
Highlands Regional Medical Center[2]	Sebring	100%	437
Jay Hospital[2]	Jay	100%	259
JFK Medical Center[2]	Atlantis	100%	723
Largo Medical Center[2]	Largo	100%	649
Lawnwood Reg Med Ctr & Heart Inst[2]	Fort Pierce	100%	598
Lehigh Regional Medical Center[2]	Lehigh Acres	100%	306
Lower Keys Medical Center[2]	Key West	100%	402
Memorial Hospital Pembroke[2]	Pembroke Pines	100%	557
Memorial Hospital West[2]	Pembroke Pines	100%	518
North Okaloosa Medical Center[2]	Crestview	100%	612
Northside Hospital[2]	St Petersburg	100%	613
Ocala Regional Medical Center[2]	Ocala	100%	697
Orange Park Medical Center[2]	Orange Park	100%	548
Palm Springs General Hospital[2]	Hialeah	100%	409
Raulerson Hospital[2]	Okeechobee	100%	509
Regional Medical Center Bayonet Point[2]	Hudson	100%	684
Sebastian River Medical Center[2]	Sebastian	100%	470
South Bay Hospital[2]	Sun City Center	100%	585
Twin Cities Hospital[2]	Niceville	100%	289
Venice Reg Med Ctr-Bayfront Health[2]	Venice	100%	607
West Kendall Baptist Hospital[2]	Miami	100%	501
West Palm Hospital[2]	W Palm Beach	100%	594
Westside Regional Medical Center[2]	Plantation	100%	627
Aventura Hospital & Medical Center[2]	Aventura	99%	686
Boca Raton Regional Hospital[2]	Boca Raton	99%	494
Cape Canaveral Hospital[2]	Cocoa Beach	99%	581
Capital Regional Medical Center[2]	Tallahassee	99%	611
Edward White Hospital[2]	St Petersburg	99%	356
Flagler Hospital[2]	St Augustine	99%	597
Lake Wales Medical Center[2]	Lake Wales	99%	567
Mariners Hospital[2]	Tavernier	99%	301
Mease Hospital Dunedin[2]	Dunedin	99%	477
Memorial Hospital Jacksonville[2]	Jacksonville	99%	639
Memorial Regional Hospital[2]	Hollywood	99%	812
North Florida Regional Medical Center[2]	Gainesville	99%	654
Oak Hill Hospital[2]	Brooksville	99%	657
Osceola Regional Medical Center[2]	Kissimmee	99%	595
Plantation General Hospital[2]	Plantation	99%	604
Saint Vincent's Medical Center Southside[2]	Jacksonville	99%	567
Santa Rosa Medical Center[2]	Milton	99%	371
Shands Live Oak Regional Medical Center[2]	Live Oak	99%	275
Viera Hospital[2]	Melbourne	99%	366
Bayfront Health Punta Gorda[2]	Punta Gorda	98%	441
Bethesda Hospital East[2]	Boynton Beach	98%	515
Blake Medical Center[2]	Bradenton	98%	666
Central Florida Regional Hospital[2]	Sanford	98%	570
Englewood Community Hospital[2]	Englewood	98%	370
Fawcett Memorial Hospital[2]	Port Charlotte	98%	642
Fort Walton Beach Medical Center[2]	Fort Walton Bch	98%	565
Kendall Regional Medical Center[2]	Miami	98%	645
Lake City Medical Center[2]	Lake City	98%	455
Medical Center of Trinity[2]	Trinity	98%	652
Northwest Medical Center[2]	Margate	98%	588
Palms West Hospital[2]	Loxahatchee	98%	562
Putnam Community Medical Center[2]	Palatka	98%	517
Sacred Heart Hospital on the Gulf[2]	Port Saint Joe	98%	217
Saint Lucie Medical Center[2]	Port Saint Lucie	98%	600
Shands Lake Shore Regional Medical Center[2]	Lake City	98%	433
University Hospital & Medical Center[2]	Tamarac	98%	616
West Florida Hospital[2]	Pensacola	98%	641
Bartow Regional Medical Center[2]	Bartow	97%	405
Brandon Regional Hospital[2]	Brandon	97%	619
Broward Health Coral Springs[2]	Coral Springs	97%	538
Broward Health Medical Center[2]	Fort Lauderdale	97%	503
Doctors Hospital[2]	Coral Gables	97%	596
Florida Hospital North Pinellas[2]	Tarpon Springs	97%	508
Florida Hospital Wauchula[2]	Wauchula	97%	139
Gulf Coast Regional Medical Center[2]	Panama City	97%	537
Hialeah Hospital[2]	Hialeah	97%	541
Jupiter Medical Center[2]	Jupiter	97%	597
Martin Medical Center[2]	Stuart	97%	554
Memorial Hospital of Tampa[2]	Tampa	97%	443
Palm Beach Gardens Medical Center[2]	Palm Bch Grdns	97%	648
Palms of Pasadena Hospital[2]	St Petersburg	97%	440
Saint Petersburg General Hospital[2]	St Petersburg	97%	553
Shands Starke Regional Medical Center[2]	Starke	97%	515
South Florida Baptist Hospital[2]	Plant City	97%	565
South Miami Hospital[2]	South Miami	97%	635
Tallahassee Memorial Hospital[2]	Tallahassee	97%	491
Town & Country Hospital[2]	Tampa	97%	353
Westchester General Hospital[2]	Miami	97%	512
Baptist Medical Center Beaches[2]	Jcksnvll Bch	96%	536
Bay Med Ctr Sacred Heart Health Sys[2]	Panama City	96%	568
Bayfront Health Port Charlotte[2]	Port Charlotte	96%	588
Cleveland Clinic Hospital[2]	Weston	96%	620
Lakeland Regional Medical Center[2]	Lakeland	96%	553
Lakewood Ranch Medical Center[2]	Bradenton	96%	512
Mease Countryside Hospital[2]	Safety Harbor	96%	602
Memorial Hospital Miramar[2]	Miramar	96%	476
Morton Plant Hospital[2]	Clearwater	96%	530
Morton Plant North Bay Hospital[2]	New Port Richey	96%	604
Saint Mary's Medical Center[2]	W Palm Beach	96%	507
Seven Rivers Regional Medical Center[2]	Crystal River	96%	598
South Lake Hospital[2]	Clermont	96%	1743
Bayfront Health Brooksville[2]	Brooksville	95%	527
Florida Hospital Carrollwood[2]	Tampa	95%	481
Homestead Hospital[2]	Homestead	95%	553
Jackson Hospital[2]	Marianna	95%	364
Physicians Reg Med Ctr-Pine Ridge[2]	Naples	95%	680
Sacred Heart Hosp-Emerald Coast[2]	Miramar Beach	95%	503
Saint Anthony's Hospital[2]	St Petersburg	95%	693
Sarasota Memorial Hospital[2]	Sarasota	95%	559
The Villages Regional Hospital[2]	The Villages	95%	588
Broward Health Imperial Point[2]	Fort Lauderdale	94%	608
Florida Hospital Flagler[2]	Palm Coast	94%	589
Gulf Breeze Hospital[2]	Gulf Breeze	94%	451
Saint Cloud Regional Medical Center[2]	Saint Cloud	94%	615
Saint Vincent's Medical Center[2]	Jacksonville	94%	599
West Boca Medical Center[2]	Boca Raton	94%	522
Wuesthoff Medical Center Rockledge[2]	Rockledge	94%	598
Baptist Medical Center[2]	Jacksonville	93%	544
Florida Hospital Waterman[2]	Tavares	93%	569
Lakeside Medical Center[2]	Belle Glade	93%	299
Munroe Regional Medical Center[2]	Ocala	93%	528
Orlando Health[2]	Orlando	93%	629
Parrish Medical Center[2]	Titusville	93%	539
Desoto Memorial Hospital[2]	Arcadia	92%	237
Florida Hospital Zephyrhills[2]	Zephyrhills	92%	570
Health Central[2]	Ocoee	92%	613
Heart of Florida Regional Medical Center[2]	Davenport	92%	563
Palmetto General Hospital[2]	Hialeah	92%	573
Saint Joseph's Hospital[2]	Tampa	92%	509
UF Health Jacksonville[2]	Jacksonville	92%	520
UF Health Shands Hospital[2]	Gainesville	92%	532

NOTE: Hospital profiles are in alphabetical order by state, then city, then hospital within the city; Rankings exclude hospitals with less than 25 cases except for patient surveys which excludes hospitals with less than 100 cases; (a) 100-299 cases; (1) The number of cases/patients is too few to report; (2) Data submitted were based on a sample of cases/patients; (3) Results are based on a shorter time period than required; (4) Data suppressed by CMS for one or more quarters; (5) Results are not available for this reporting period; (6) Fewer than 100 patients completed the HCAHPS survey; (7) No cases met the criteria for this measure; (8) The lower limit of the confidence interval cannot be calculated if the number of observed infections equals zero; (9) No data are available from the state/territory for this reporting period; (10) The scores shown reflect fewer than 50 completed surveys; (11) There were discrepancies in the data collection process; (12) This measure does not apply to this hospital for this reporting period; (13) Results cannot be calculated for this reporting period; (14) The results for this state are combined with nearby states to protect confidentiality; Please refer to the User's Guide for a full explanation of data.

Hospital Name	City	Rate	Cases
Bayfront Health Dade City[2]	Dade City	91%	325
Florida Hospital Memorial Medical Center[2]	Daytona Bch	91%	555
Good Samaritan Medical Center[2]	W Palm Beach	91%	598
Manatee Memorial Hospital[2]	Bradenton	91%	537
Naples Community Hospital[2]	Naples	91%	621
Sacred Heart Hospital[2]	Pensacola	91%	524
Florida Hospital Heartland Medical Center[2]	Sebring	90%	886
Indian River Medical Center[2]	Vero Beach	90%	582
Baptist Hospital[2]	Pensacola	89%	605
Bert Fish Medical Center[2]	New Smyrn Bch	89%	378
Holmes Regional Medical Center[2]	Melbourne	89%	559
Leesburg Regional Medical Center[2]	Leesburg	89%	594
Florida Hospital[2]	Orlando	88%	563
Florida Hospital Tampa[2]	Tampa	88%	551
Holy Cross Hospital[2]	Fort Lauderdale	88%	580
Winter Haven Hospital[2]	Winter Haven	88%	574
Mount Sinai Medical Center[2]	Miami Beach	87%	536
Palm Bay Hospital[2]	Palm Bay	87%	564
Wuesthoff Medical Center - Melbourne[2]	Melbourne	87%	482
Baptist Medical Center - Nassau[2]	Fernandina Bch	86%	302
Citrus Memorial Hospital[2]	Inverness	86%	666
North Shore Medical Center[2]	Miami	85%	1201
Florida Hospital Fish Memorial[2]	Orange City	84%	587
University of Miami Hospital[2]	Miami	84%	609
Wellington Regional Medical Center[2]	Wellington	84%	502
Gulf Coast Med Ctr Lee Mem Health Sys[2]	Fort Myers	83%	585
Doctor's Memorial Hospital[2]	Perry	82%	326
Jackson Memorial Hospital[2]	Miami	82%	1583
Larkin Community Hospital[2]	South Miami	80%	369
Cape Coral Hospital[2]	Cape Coral	79%	558
Florida Hospital Deland[2]	Deland	79%	531
Mayo Clinic[2]	Jacksonville	79%	612
Tampa General Hospital[2]	Tampa	78%	542
Bayfront Health - Saint Petersburg[2]	St Petersburg	77%	461
Halifax Health Medical Center[2]	Daytona Bch	76%	579
Lee Memorial Hospital[2]	Fort Myers	75%	556
Metropolitan Hospital of Miami[2]	Miami	75%	419
Douglas Gardens Hospital[2]	Miami	73%	164
Healthmark Regional Medical Center[2]	Defuniak Spgs	54%	294

Immunization for Pneumonia

Hospital Name	City	Rate	Cases
Aventura Hospital & Medical Center[2]	Aventura	100%	1002
Baptist Hospital of Miami[2]	Miami	100%	566
Broward Health North[2]	Pompano Bch	100%	797
Cape Canaveral Hospital[2]	Cocoa Beach	100%	799
Coral Gables Hospital[2]	Coral Gables	100%	891
Delray Medical Center[2]	Delray Beach	100%	1057
Highlands Regional Medical Center[2]	Sebring	100%	571
JFK Medical Center[2]	Atlantis	100%	1054
Kendall Regional Medical Center[2]	Miami	100%	791
Lake Wales Medical Center[2]	Lake Wales	100%	834
Lawnwood Reg Med Ctr & Heart Inst[2]	Fort Pierce	100%	682
Lehigh Regional Medical Center[2]	Lehigh Acres	100%	417
Memorial Hospital Pembroke[2]	Pembroke Pines	100%	737
Memorial Hospital West[2]	Pembroke Pines	100%	524
North Florida Regional Medical Center[2]	Gainesville	100%	921
Northwest Medical Center[2]	Margate	100%	713
Ocala Regional Medical Center[2]	Ocala	100%	1065
Orange Park Medical Center[2]	Orange Park	100%	688
Palm Springs General Hospital[2]	Hialeah	100%	752
Plantation General Hospital[2]	Plantation	100%	634
Raulerson Hospital[2]	Okeechobee	100%	802
Regional Medical Center Bayonet Point[2]	Hudson	100%	1019
Sacred Heart Hospital on the Gulf[2]	Port Saint Joe	100%	333
Saint Lucie Medical Center[2]	Port Saint Lucie	100%	885
Sebastian River Medical Center[2]	Sebastian	100%	700
South Bay Hospital[2]	Sun City Center	100%	1016
Twin Cities Hospital[2]	Niceville	100%	434
Viera Hospital[2]	Melbourne	100%	518
West Kendall Baptist Hospital[2]	Miami	100%	666
West Palm Hospital[2]	W Palm Beach	100%	744
Westside Regional Medical Center[2]	Plantation	100%	899
Bethesda Hospital East[2]	Boynton Beach	99%	623
Boca Raton Regional Hospital[2]	Boca Raton	99%	728
Capital Regional Medical Center[2]	Tallahassee	99%	751
Central Florida Regional Hospital[2]	Sanford	99%	777
Doctors Hospital of Sarasota[2]	Sarasota	99%	1018
Edward White Hospital[2]	St Petersburg	99%	495
Florida Hospital North Pinellas[2]	Tarpon Springs	99%	652
Florida Hospital Wauchula[2]	Wauchula	99%	229
Gulf Coast Regional Medical Center[2]	Panama City	99%	597
Hialeah Hospital[2]	Hialeah	99%	676
Jupiter Medical Center[2]	Jupiter	99%	769
Largo Medical Center[2]	Largo	99%	1016
Lower Keys Medical Center[2]	Key West	99%	386
Mariners Hospital[2]	Tavernier	99%	362
Mease Countryside Hospital[2]	Safety Harbor	99%	767
Medical Center of Trinity[2]	Trinity	99%	899
Memorial Regional Hospital[2]	Hollywood	99%	882
North Okaloosa Medical Center[2]	Crestview	99%	848
Northside Hospital[2]	St Petersburg	99%	945
Palms of Pasadena Hospital[2]	St Petersburg	99%	744
Palms West Hospital[2]	Loxahatchee	99%	500
Saint Vincent's Medical Center Southside[2]	Jacksonville	99%	614
Shands Live Oak Regional Medical Center[2]	Live Oak	99%	432
Shands Starke Regional Medical Center[2]	Starke	99%	722
South Miami Hospital[2]	South Miami	99%	597
University Hospital & Medical Center[2]	Tamarac	99%	932
Venice Reg Med Ctr-Bayfront Health[2]	Venice	99%	1049
Westchester General Hospital[2]	Miami	99%	769
Bartow Regional Medical Center[2]	Bartow	98%	554
Bay Med Ctr Sacred Heart Health Sys[2]	Panama City	98%	832
Bayfront Health Brooksville[2]	Brooksville	98%	705
Desoto Memorial Hospital[2]	Arcadia	98%	291
Englewood Community Hospital[2]	Englewood	98%	602
Heart of Florida Regional Medical Center[2]	Davenport	98%	725
Homestead Hospital[2]	Homestead	98%	544
Lake City Medical Center[2]	Lake City	98%	748
Lakewood Ranch Medical Center[2]	Bradenton	98%	596
Martin Medical Center[2]	Stuart	98%	747
Mease Hospital Dunedin[2]	Dunedin	98%	712
Memorial Hospital Jacksonville[2]	Jacksonville	98%	850
Memorial Hospital Miramar[2]	Miramar	98%	351
Oak Hill Hospital[2]	Brooksville	98%	1036
Osceola Regional Medical Center[2]	Kissimmee	98%	801
Putnam Community Medical Center[2]	Palatka	98%	761
Saint Vincent's Medical Center[2]	Jacksonville	98%	856
Santa Rosa Medical Center[2]	Milton	98%	459
Wuesthoff Medical Center Rockledge[2]	Rockledge	98%	800
Bayfront Health Port Charlotte[2]	Port Charlotte	97%	769
Bayfront Health Punta Gorda[2]	Punta Gorda	97%	633
Blake Medical Center[2]	Bradenton	97%	986
Broward Health Coral Springs[2]	Coral Springs	97%	478
Broward Health Medical Center[2]	Fort Lauderdale	97%	455
Doctors Hospital[2]	Coral Gables	97%	863
Flagler Hospital[2]	St Augustine	97%	773
Florida Hospital Waterman[2]	Tavares	97%	841
Fort Walton Beach Medical Center[2]	Fort Walton Bch	97%	739
Jay Hospital[2]	Jay	97%	385
Lakeland Regional Medical Center[2]	Lakeland	97%	706
Memorial Hospital of Tampa[2]	Tampa	97%	593
Palm Beach Gardens Medical Center[2]	Palm Bch Grdns	97%	1015
Palmetto General Hospital[2]	Hialeah	97%	635
Parrish Medical Center[2]	Titusville	97%	773
Saint Mary's Medical Center[2]	W Palm Beach	97%	260
Saint Petersburg General Hospital[2]	St Petersburg	97%	618
Town & Country Hospital[2]	Tampa	97%	432
The Villages Regional Hospital[2]	The Villages	97%	1043
West Florida Hospital[2]	Pensacola	97%	931
Baptist Medical Center Beaches[2]	Jcksnvll Bch	96%	574
Holmes Regional Medical Center[2]	Melbourne	96%	765
Jackson Hospital[2]	Marianna	96%	434
Leesburg Regional Medical Center[2]	Leesburg	96%	872
Physicians Reg Med Ctr-Pine Ridge[2]	Naples	96%	975
Saint Cloud Regional Medical Center[2]	Saint Cloud	96%	717
Seven Rivers Regional Medical Center[2]	Crystal River	96%	875
Shands Lake Shore Regional Medical Center[2]	Lake City	96%	444
South Lake Hospital[2]	Clermont	96%	2371
West Boca Medical Center[2]	Boca Raton	96%	479
Brandon Regional Hospital[2]	Brandon	95%	638
Broward Health Imperial Point[2]	Fort Lauderdale	95%	685
Cleveland Clinic Hospital[2]	Weston	95%	763
Fawcett Memorial Hospital[2]	Port Charlotte	95%	1061
Florida Hospital Memorial Medical Center[2]	Daytona Bch	95%	782
Florida Hospital Tampa[2]	Tampa	95%	664
Florida Hospital Zephyrhills[2]	Zephyrhills	95%	829
Good Samaritan Medical Center[2]	W Palm Beach	95%	743
Health Central[2]	Ocoee	95%	763
Lakeside Medical Center[2]	Belle Glade	95%	241
Morton Plant North Bay Hospital[2]	New Port Richey	95%	646
Naples Community Hospital[2]	Naples	95%	794
Palm Bay Hospital[2]	Palm Bay	95%	867
Sacred Heart Hosp-Emerald Coast[2]	Miramar Beach	95%	593
Sarasota Memorial Hospital[2]	Sarasota	95%	752
Baptist Hospital[2]	Pensacola	94%	790
Florida Hospital[2]	Orlando	94%	654
Florida Hospital Carrollwood[2]	Tampa	94%	584
Florida Hospital Flagler[2]	Palm Coast	94%	929
Florida Hospital Heartland Medical Center[2]	Sebring	94%	1409
Manatee Memorial Hospital[2]	Bradenton	94%	683
Mount Sinai Medical Center[2]	Miami Beach	94%	635
North Shore Medical Center[2]	Miami	94%	1410
UF Health Jacksonville[2]	Jacksonville	94%	528
Anne Bates Leach Eye Hospital	Miami	93%	28
Indian River Medical Center[2]	Vero Beach	93%	817
Morton Plant Hospital[2]	Clearwater	93%	692
UF Health Shands Hospital[2]	Gainesville	93%	513
Wellington Regional Medical Center[2]	Wellington	93%	534
Florida Hospital Wesley Chapel[2,3]	Wesley Chapel	92%	92
Halifax Health Medical Center[2]	Daytona Bch	92%	609
Munroe Regional Medical Center[2]	Ocala	92%	783
Tallahassee Memorial Hospital[2]	Tallahassee	92%	539
Winter Haven Hospital[2]	Winter Haven	92%	735
Baptist Medical Center[2]	Jacksonville	91%	539
Baptist Medical Center - Nassau[2]	Fernandina Bch	91%	312
Florida Hospital Deland[2]	Deland	91%	740
Gulf Breeze Hospital[2]	Gulf Breeze	91%	622
Sacred Heart Hospital[2]	Pensacola	91%	506
Saint Joseph's Hospital[2]	Tampa	91%	460
Wuesthoff Medical Center - Melbourne[2]	Melbourne	91%	569
Bayfront Health Dade City[2]	Dade City	90%	418
Jackson Memorial Hospital[2]	Miami	90%	1506
Bert Fish Medical Center[2]	New Smyrn Bch	89%	599
South Florida Baptist Hospital[2]	Plant City	89%	733
Citrus Memorial Hospital[2]	Inverness	88%	988
Florida Hospital Fish Memorial[2]	Orange City	88%	887
Holy Cross Hospital[2]	Fort Lauderdale	87%	765
Saint Anthony's Hospital[2]	St Petersburg	86%	1000
Doctor's Memorial Hospital[2]	Perry	85%	438
Gulf Coast Med Ctr Lee Mem Health Sys[2]	Fort Myers	84%	820
Bayfront Health - Saint Petersburg[2]	St Petersburg	83%	524
Larkin Community Hospital[2]	South Miami	83%	571
Mayo Clinic[2]	Jacksonville	83%	790
Orlando Health[2]	Orlando	83%	559
University of Miami Hospital[2]	Miami	82%	799
Cape Coral Hospital[2]	Cape Coral	81%	770
Douglas Gardens Hospital[2]	Miami	77%	314
Lee Memorial Hospital[2]	Fort Myers	77%	641
Tampa General Hospital[2]	Tampa	76%	562
Metropolitan Hospital of Miami[2]	Miami	69%	658
Healthmark Regional Medical Center[2]	Defuniak Spgs	66%	444

Stroke Care

Anticoagulation Therapy for Atrial Fibrillation

Hospital Name	City	Rate	Cases
Baptist Hospital of Miami[2]	Miami	100%	29
Boca Raton Regional Hospital	Boca Raton	100%	35
Broward Health North[2]	Pompano Bch	100%	27
Delray Medical Center	Delray Beach	100%	41
Flagler Hospital	St Augustine	100%	30
Florida Hospital Memorial Medical Center	Daytona Bch	100%	33
Florida Hospital Tampa	Tampa	100%	33
Holmes Regional Medical Center	Melbourne	100%	34
Holy Cross Hospital	Fort Lauderdale	100%	35
Largo Medical Center[2]	Largo	100%	25
Lawnwood Reg Med Ctr & Heart Inst	Fort Pierce	100%	32
Lee Memorial Hospital[2]	Fort Myers	100%	29
Memorial Hospital West	Pembroke Pines	100%	29
Memorial Regional Hospital	Hollywood	100%	27
Mount Sinai Medical Center	Miami Beach	100%	26
Physicians Reg Med Ctr-Pine Ridge	Naples	100%	34
Sarasota Memorial Hospital	Sarasota	100%	51
Mease Countryside Hospital	Safety Harbor	98%	44
Saint Joseph's Hospital	Tampa	98%	51
Florida Hospital	Orlando	97%	143
Orlando Health	Orlando	97%	36
Tallahassee Memorial Hospital	Tallahassee	97%	33
Blake Medical Center	Bradenton	96%	27
Brandon Regional Hospital	Brandon	96%	27
Morton Plant Hospital	Clearwater	95%	37
Munroe Regional Medical Center[2]	Ocala	93%	28
Morton Plant North Bay Hospital	New Port Richey	88%	25
Bay Med Ctr Sacred Heart Health Sys	Panama City	79%	34

Antithrombotic Therapy Timing

Hospital Name	City	Rate	Cases
Baptist Hospital of Miami[2]	Miami	100%	121
Baptist Medical Center Beaches[2]	Jcksnvll Bch	100%	50
Bethesda Hospital East[2]	Boynton Beach	100%	80
Boca Raton Regional Hospital	Boca Raton	100%	148
Broward Health Coral Springs	Coral Springs	100%	49
Broward Health North[2]	Pompano Bch	100%	147
Cape Coral Hospital[2]	Cape Coral	100%	99
Capital Regional Medical Center[2]	Tallahassee	100%	125
Cleveland Clinic Hospital	Weston	100%	47
Coral Gables Hospital	Coral Gables	100%	39
Delray Medical Center	Delray Beach	100%	169
Doctors Hospital	Coral Gables	100%	37
Doctors Hospital of Sarasota[2]	Sarasota	100%	63
Fawcett Memorial Hospital[2]	Port Charlotte	100%	69
Flagler Hospital	St Augustine	100%	146
Florida Hospital Carrollwood[2]	Tampa	100%	28
Florida Hospital Heartland Medical Center	Sebring	100%	97
Florida Hospital North Pinellas[2]	Tarpon Springs	100%	31
Florida Hospital Waterman[2]	Tavares	100%	85
Florida Hospital Zephyrhills	Zephyrhills	100%	93
Fort Walton Beach Medical Center[2]	Fort Walton Bch	100%	89
Good Samaritan Medical Center	W Palm Beach	100%	52
Gulf Breeze Hospital	Gulf Breeze	100%	43
Gulf Coast Regional Medical Center	Panama City	100%	75

NOTE: Hospital profiles are in alphabetical order by state, then city, then hospital within the city; Rankings exclude hospitals with less than 25 cases except for patient surveys which excludes hospitals with less than 100 cases; (a) 100-299 cases; (1) The number of cases/patients is too few to report; (2) Data submitted were based on a sample of cases/patients; (3) Results are based on a shorter time period than required; (4) Data suppressed by CMS for one or more quarters; (5) Results are not available for this reporting period; (6) Fewer than 100 patients completed the HCAHPS survey; (7) No cases met the criteria for this measure; (8) The lower limit of the confidence interval cannot be calculated if the number of observed infections equals zero; (9) No data are available from the state/territory for this reporting period; (10) The scores shown reflect fewer than 50 completed surveys; (11) There were discrepancies in the data collection process; (12) This measure does not apply to this hospital for this reporting period; (13) Results cannot be calculated for this reporting period; (14) The results for this state are combined with nearby states to protect confidentiality; Please refer to the User's Guide for a full explanation of data.

Health Central	Ocoee	100%	72
Highlands Regional Medical Center	Sebring	100%	30
Holmes Regional Medical Center	Melbourne	100%	237
Homestead Hospital	Homestead	100%	80
Jackson Hospital	Marianna	100%	51
JFK Medical Center[2]	Atlantis	100%	93
Jupiter Medical Center	Jupiter	100%	74
Lake City Medical Center[2]	Lake City	100%	48
Lakewood Ranch Medical Center	Bradenton	100%	60
Lawnwood Reg Med Ctr & Heart Inst	Fort Pierce	100%	324
Medical Center of Trinity[2]	Trinity	100%	95
Memorial Hospital Pembroke	Pembroke Pines	100%	54
Memorial Hospital West	Pembroke Pines	100%	206
Memorial Regional Hospital	Hollywood	100%	246
Morton Plant Hospital	Clearwater	100%	183
North Okaloosa Medical Center	Crestview	100%	37
Northside Hospital[2]	St Petersburg	100%	84
Oak Hill Hospital[2]	Brooksville	100%	90
Orange Park Medical Center[2]	Orange Park	100%	115
Osceola Regional Medical Center[2]	Kissimmee	100%	98
Palm Bay Hospital	Palm Bay	100%	56
Palm Beach Gardens Medical Center	Palm Bch Grdns	100%	89
Palmetto General Hospital	Hialeah	100%	209
Palms of Pasadena Hospital	St Petersburg	100%	61
Plantation General Hospital[2]	Plantation	100%	82
Putnam Community Medical Center	Palatka	100%	61
Raulerson Hospital[2]	Okeechobee	100%	46
Sacred Heart Hosp-Emerald Coast	Miramar Beach	100%	37
Saint Mary's Medical Center[2]	W Palm Beach	100%	119
Saint Petersburg General Hospital	St Petersburg	100%	42
Santa Rosa Medical Center	Milton	100%	28
Sarasota Memorial Hospital	Sarasota	100%	212
Sebastian River Medical Center	Sebastian	100%	62
Seven Rivers Regional Medical Center	Crystal River	100%	58
South Bay Hospital[2]	Sun City Center	100%	84
South Lake Hospital	Clermont	100%	58
South Miami Hospital	South Miami	100%	86
Tallahassee Memorial Hospital	Tallahassee	100%	251
UF Health Jacksonville[2]	Jacksonville	100%	71
University Hospital & Medical Center	Tamarac	100%	64
West Florida Hospital[2]	Pensacola	100%	110
West Kendall Baptist Hospital	Miami	100%	44
West Palm Hospital[2]	W Palm Beach	100%	32
Wuesthoff Medical Center - Melbourne	Melbourne	100%	27
Aventura Hospital & Medical Center[2]	Aventura	99%	92
Blake Medical Center	Bradenton	99%	112
Brandon Regional Hospital	Brandon	99%	180
Broward Health Medical Center	Fort Lauderdale	99%	138
Cape Canaveral Hospital	Cocoa Beach	99%	80
Citrus Memorial Hospital	Inverness	99%	142
Florida Hospital	Orlando	99%	969
Florida Hospital Tampa	Tampa	99%	156
Indian River Medical Center[2]	Vero Beach	99%	81
Kendall Regional Medical Center[2]	Miami	99%	110
Lakeland Regional Medical Center[2]	Lakeland	99%	104
Martin Medical Center[2]	Stuart	99%	84
Memorial Hospital Jacksonville[2]	Jacksonville	99%	88
Mount Sinai Medical Center	Miami Beach	99%	119
North Florida Regional Medical Center	Gainesville	99%	220
Ocala Regional Medical Center[2]	Ocala	99%	99
Parrish Medical Center	Titusville	99%	105
Regional Medical Center Bayonet Point[2]	Hudson	99%	73
Saint Vincent's Medical Center[2]	Jacksonville	99%	81
Venice Reg Med Ctr-Bayfront Health[2]	Venice	99%	83
Westside Regional Medical Center[2]	Plantation	99%	94
Baptist Medical Center[2]	Jacksonville	98%	110
Florida Hospital Flagler	Palm Coast	98%	122
Florida Hospital Memorial Medical Center	Daytona Bch	98%	151
Gulf Coast Med Ctr Lee Mem Health Sys[2]	Fort Myers	98%	111
Halifax Health Medical Center[2]	Daytona Bch	98%	161
Largo Medical Center[2]	Largo	98%	132
Mayo Clinic[2]	Jacksonville	98%	45
Mease Countryside Hospital	Safety Harbor	98%	178
Mease Hospital Dunedin	Dunedin	98%	63
Naples Community Hospital[2]	Naples	98%	90
Orlando Health	Orlando	98%	398
Physicians Reg Med Ctr-Pine Ridge	Naples	98%	132
Saint Vincent's Medical Center Southside[2]	Jacksonville	98%	56
Tampa General Hospital[2]	Tampa	98%	57
UF Health Shands Hospital[2]	Gainesville	98%	44
West Boca Medical Center	Boca Raton	98%	85
Bartow Regional Medical Center	Bartow	97%	39
Bay Med Ctr Sacred Heart Health Sys	Panama City	97%	206
Bayfront Health Dade City	Dade City	97%	39
Florida Hospital Fish Memorial[2]	Orange City	97%	101
Lake Wales Medical Center	Lake Wales	97%	61
North Shore Medical Center	Miami	97%	216
Northwest Medical Center	Margate	97%	137
Saint Lucie Medical Center[2]	Port Saint Lucie	97%	75
Wellington Regional Medical Center	Wellington	97%	78
Bayfront Health Brooksville	Brooksville	96%	95
Bert Fish Medical Center	New Smyrn Bch	96%	55
Central Florida Regional Hospital[2]	Sanford	96%	102
Edward White Hospital	St Petersburg	96%	25
Florida Hospital Deland[2]	Deland	96%	84
Leesburg Regional Medical Center[2]	Leesburg	96%	74
Lower Keys Medical Center	Key West	96%	27
Manatee Memorial Hospital[2]	Bradenton	96%	67
Morton Plant North Bay Hospital	New Port Richey	96%	94
Sacred Heart Hospital[2]	Pensacola	96%	57
Saint Joseph's Hospital	Tampa	96%	392
Viera Hospital	Melbourne	96%	28
Wuesthoff Medical Center Rockledge	Rockledge	96%	116
Hialeah Hospital	Hialeah	95%	98
Munroe Regional Medical Center[2]	Ocala	95%	119
Saint Anthony's Hospital	St Petersburg	95%	138
The Villages Regional Hospital[2]	The Villages	95%	95
Baptist Hospital	Pensacola	94%	143
Bayfront Health - Saint Petersburg[2]	St Petersburg	94%	89
Bayfront Health Punta Gorda	Punta Gorda	94%	53
South Florida Baptist Hospital	Plant City	94%	49
Holy Cross Hospital	Fort Lauderdale	93%	165
Lee Memorial Hospital[2]	Fort Myers	93%	153
Palms West Hospital	Loxahatchee	93%	107
Bayfront Health Port Charlotte	Port Charlotte	92%	83
Jackson Memorial Hospital[2]	Miami	92%	213
Memorial Hospital Miramar	Miramar	92%	48
Winter Haven Hospital	Winter Haven	92%	142
University of Miami Hospital	Miami	91%	75
Heart of Florida Regional Medical Center[2]	Davenport	85%	79
Saint Cloud Regional Medical Center	Saint Cloud	85%	26
Larkin Community Hospital	South Miami	84%	25

Assessed for Rehabilitation

Hospital Name	City	Rate	Cases
Baptist Hospital	Pensacola	100%	173
Baptist Hospital of Miami[2]	Miami	100%	154
Bartow Regional Medical Center	Bartow	100%	43
Bert Fish Medical Center	New Smyrn Bch	100%	63
Boca Raton Regional Hospital	Boca Raton	100%	185
Broward Health Coral Springs	Coral Springs	100%	57
Broward Health North[2]	Pompano Bch	100%	201
Cleveland Clinic Hospital	Weston	100%	78
Delray Medical Center	Delray Beach	100%	249
Doctors Hospital	Coral Gables	100%	45
Fawcett Memorial Hospital[2]	Port Charlotte	100%	79
Florida Hospital Deland[2]	Deland	100%	93
Florida Hospital Flagler	Palm Coast	100%	138
Florida Hospital Tampa	Tampa	100%	201
Florida Hospital Waterman[2]	Tavares	100%	88
Fort Walton Beach Medical Center[2]	Fort Walton Bch	100%	118
Gulf Coast Regional Medical Center	Panama City	100%	89
Health Central	Ocoee	100%	79
Holmes Regional Medical Center	Melbourne	100%	286
Holy Cross Hospital	Fort Lauderdale	100%	202
Homestead Hospital	Homestead	100%	82
Jackson Hospital	Marianna	100%	56
Jupiter Medical Center	Jupiter	100%	79
Lake City Medical Center[2]	Lake City	100%	48
Largo Medical Center[2]	Largo	100%	149
Lawnwood Reg Med Ctr & Heart Inst	Fort Pierce	100%	378
Mayo Clinic[2]	Jacksonville	100%	113
Mease Hospital Dunedin	Dunedin	100%	62
Medical Center of Trinity[2]	Trinity	100%	94
Memorial Hospital Jacksonville[2]	Jacksonville	100%	97
Memorial Hospital Pembroke	Pembroke Pines	100%	56
Memorial Hospital West	Pembroke Pines	100%	228
Memorial Regional Hospital	Hollywood	100%	349
North Okaloosa Medical Center	Crestview	100%	38
North Shore Medical Center	Miami	100%	257
Northside Hospital[2]	St Petersburg	100%	111
Oak Hill Hospital[2]	Brooksville	100%	98
Palms of Pasadena Hospital	St Petersburg	100%	69
Raulerson Hospital[2]	Okeechobee	100%	48
Saint Vincent's Medical Center Southside[2]	Jacksonville	100%	63
Sebastian River Medical Center	Sebastian	100%	66
South Bay Hospital[2]	Sun City Center	100%	84
South Miami Hospital	South Miami	100%	103
Tallahassee Memorial Hospital	Tallahassee	100%	299
Venice Reg Med Ctr-Bayfront Health[2]	Venice	100%	101
Viera Hospital	Melbourne	100%	28
West Florida Hospital[2]	Pensacola	100%	109
West Kendall Baptist Hospital	Miami	100%	35
Westside Regional Medical Center[2]	Plantation	100%	111
Aventura Hospital & Medical Center[2]	Aventura	99%	119
Blake Medical Center	Bradenton	99%	143
Broward Health Medical Center	Fort Lauderdale	99%	175
Cape Canaveral Hospital	Cocoa Beach	99%	86
Capital Regional Medical Center[2]	Tallahassee	99%	135
Central Florida Regional Hospital[2]	Sanford	99%	110
Doctors Hospital of Sarasota[2]	Sarasota	99%	77
Flagler Hospital	St Augustine	99%	174
Florida Hospital Heartland Medical Center	Sebring	99%	127
Florida Hospital Memorial Medical Center	Daytona Bch	99%	189
Florida Hospital Zephyrhills	Zephyrhills	99%	113
Gulf Coast Med Ctr Lee Mem Health Sys[2]	Fort Myers	99%	147
Halifax Health Medical Center[2]	Daytona Bch	99%	192
Hialeah Hospital	Hialeah	99%	112
Indian River Medical Center[2]	Vero Beach	99%	92
JFK Medical Center[2]	Atlantis	99%	116
Lakewood Ranch Medical Center	Bradenton	99%	69
Martin Medical Center[2]	Stuart	99%	97
Morton Plant North Bay Hospital	New Port Richey	99%	92
Mount Sinai Medical Center	Miami Beach	99%	166
Munroe Regional Medical Center[2]	Ocala	99%	132
Osceola Regional Medical Center[2]	Kissimmee	99%	122
Palm Beach Gardens Medical Center	Palm Bch Grdns	99%	95
Physicians Reg Med Ctr-Pine Ridge	Naples	99%	213
Plantation General Hospital[2]	Plantation	99%	95
Regional Medical Center Bayonet Point[2]	Hudson	99%	86
Sacred Heart Hospital[2]	Pensacola	99%	101
Saint Mary's Medical Center[2]	W Palm Beach	99%	188
Saint Vincent's Medical Center[2]	Jacksonville	99%	86
Baptist Medical Center Beaches[2]	Jcksnvl Bch	98%	47
Bayfront Health - Saint Petersburg[2]	St Petersburg	98%	125
Good Samaritan Medical Center	W Palm Beach	98%	50
Gulf Breeze Hospital	Gulf Breeze	98%	49
Lake Wales Medical Center	Lake Wales	98%	59
Memorial Hospital Miramar	Miramar	98%	47
Morton Plant Hospital	Clearwater	98%	259
North Florida Regional Medical Center	Gainesville	98%	225
Ocala Regional Medical Center[2]	Ocala	98%	99
Orange Park Medical Center[2]	Orange Park	98%	115
Orlando Health	Orlando	98%	499
Palm Bay Hospital	Palm Bay	98%	54
Palmetto General Hospital	Hialeah	98%	257
South Florida Baptist Hospital	Plant City	98%	51
Wellington Regional Medical Center	Wellington	98%	91
West Boca Medical Center	Boca Raton	98%	96
Winter Haven Hospital	Winter Haven	98%	159
Cape Coral Hospital[2]	Cape Coral	97%	114
Florida Hospital Carrollwood[2]	Tampa	97%	29
Lakeland Regional Medical Center[2]	Lakeland	97%	130
Leesburg Regional Medical Center[2]	Leesburg	97%	91
Manatee Memorial Hospital[2]	Bradenton	97%	92
Mease Countryside Hospital	Safety Harbor	97%	178
Saint Anthony's Hospital	St Petersburg	97%	166
Saint Joseph's Hospital	Tampa	97%	483
Saint Petersburg General Hospital	St Petersburg	97%	38
UF Health Jacksonville[2]	Jacksonville	97%	96
University Hospital & Medical Center	Tamarac	97%	68
Wuesthoff Medical Center - Melbourne	Melbourne	97%	30
Brandon Regional Hospital	Brandon	96%	224
Florida Hospital	Orlando	96%	1251
Lee Memorial Hospital[2]	Fort Myers	96%	195
Northwest Medical Center	Margate	96%	161
Palms West Hospital	Loxahatchee	96%	118
Parrish Medical Center	Titusville	96%	120
Saint Lucie Medical Center[2]	Port Saint Lucie	96%	74
Santa Rosa Medical Center	Milton	96%	27
UF Health Shands Hospital[2]	Gainesville	96%	117
Wuesthoff Medical Center Rockledge	Rockledge	96%	126
Bayfront Health Brooksville	Brooksville	95%	92
Bethesda Hospital East[2]	Boynton Beach	95%	102
Coral Gables Hospital	Coral Gables	95%	37
Florida Hospital Fish Memorial[2]	Orange City	95%	102
Sarasota Memorial Hospital	Sarasota	95%	298
The Villages Regional Hospital[2]	The Villages	95%	110
Baptist Medical Center[2]	Jacksonville	94%	118
Florida Hospital North Pinellas[2]	Tarpon Springs	94%	33
Naples Community Hospital[2]	Naples	94%	106
South Lake Hospital	Clermont	94%	62
University of Miami Hospital	Miami	94%	97
West Palm Hospital[2]	W Palm Beach	94%	33
Bayfront Health Punta Gorda	Punta Gorda	93%	59
Broward Health Imperial Point	Fort Lauderdale	93%	29
Jackson Memorial Hospital[2]	Miami	93%	279
Kendall Regional Medical Center[2]	Miami	93%	126
Tampa General Hospital[2]	Tampa	93%	110
Bayfront Health Port Charlotte	Port Charlotte	92%	91
Citrus Memorial Hospital	Inverness	90%	135
Seven Rivers Regional Medical Center	Crystal River	90%	50
Bayfront Health Dade City	Dade City	89%	37
Highlands Regional Medical Center	Sebring	89%	28
Memorial Hospital of Tampa	Tampa	88%	25
Putnam Community Medical Center	Palatka	84%	61
Bay Med Ctr Sacred Heart Health Sys	Panama City	83%	235
Heart of Florida Regional Medical Center[2]	Davenport	83%	87
Sacred Heart Hosp-Emerald Coast	Miramar Beach	83%	47
Saint Cloud Regional Medical Center	Saint Cloud	82%	28
Lower Keys Medical Center	Key West	81%	27

NOTE: Hospital profiles are in alphabetical order by state, then city, then hospital within the city; Rankings exclude hospitals with less than 25 cases except for patient surveys which excludes hospitals with less than 100 cases; (a) 100-299 cases; (1) The number of cases/patients is too few to report; (2) Data submitted were based on a sample of cases/patients; (3) Results are based on a shorter time period than required; (4) Data suppressed by CMS for one or more quarters; (5) Results are not available for this reporting period; (6) Fewer than 100 patients completed the HCAHPS survey; (7) No cases met the criteria for this measure; (8) The lower limit of the confidence interval cannot be calculated if the number of observed infections equals zero; (9) No data are available from the state/territory for this reporting period; (10) The scores shown reflect fewer than 50 completed surveys; (11) There were discrepancies in the data collection process; (12) This measure does not apply to this hospital for this reporting period; (13) Results cannot be calculated for this reporting period; (14) The results for this state are combined with nearby states to protect confidentiality; Please refer to the User's Guide for a full explanation of data.

Discharged on Antithrombotic Therapy

Hospital Name	City	Rate	Cases
Aventura Hospital & Medical Center[2]	Aventura	100%	96
Baptist Hospital of Miami[2]	Miami	100%	130
Bartow Regional Medical Center	Bartow	100%	42
Bay Med Ctr Sacred Heart Health Sys	Panama City	100%	207
Bayfront Health - Saint Petersburg[2]	St Petersburg	100%	90
Bayfront Health Dade City	Dade City	100%	37
Bayfront Health Punta Gorda	Punta Gorda	100%	50
Bethesda Hospital East[2]	Boynton Beach	100%	84
Boca Raton Regional Hospital	Boca Raton	100%	155
Brandon Regional Hospital	Brandon	100%	199
Broward Health Coral Springs	Coral Springs	100%	55
Broward Health Imperial Point	Fort Lauderdale	100%	27
Broward Health Medical Center	Fort Lauderdale	100%	148
Cape Canaveral Hospital	Cocoa Beach	100%	78
Cape Coral Hospital[2]	Cape Coral	100%	100
Capital Regional Medical Center[2]	Tallahassee	100%	127
Cleveland Clinic Hospital	Weston	100%	68
Coral Gables Hospital	Coral Gables	100%	33
Delray Medical Center	Delray Beach	100%	204
Doctors Hospital	Coral Gables	100%	37
Doctors Hospital of Sarasota[2]	Sarasota	100%	71
Fawcett Memorial Hospital[2]	Port Charlotte	100%	73
Flagler Hospital	St Augustine	100%	144
Florida Hospital Deland[2]	Deland	100%	88
Florida Hospital Fish Memorial[2]	Orange City	100%	101
Florida Hospital Waterman[2]	Tavares	100%	81
Florida Hospital Zephyrhills	Zephyrhills	100%	95
Fort Walton Beach Medical Center[2]	Fort Walton Bch	100%	108
Gulf Breeze Hospital	Gulf Breeze	100%	47
Gulf Coast Med Ctr Lee Mem Health Sys[2]	Fort Myers	100%	132
Gulf Coast Regional Medical Center	Panama City	100%	84
Halifax Health Medical Center[2]	Daytona Bch	100%	153
Health Central	Ocoee	100%	69
Holmes Regional Medical Center	Melbourne	100%	235
Homestead Hospital	Homestead	100%	79
Jackson Hospital	Marianna	100%	53
Jupiter Medical Center	Jupiter	100%	75
Kendall Regional Medical Center[2]	Miami	100%	117
Lake City Medical Center[2]	Lake City	100%	48
Lake Wales Medical Center	Lake Wales	100%	58
Largo Medical Center[2]	Largo	100%	127
Lawnwood Reg Med Ctr & Heart Inst	Fort Pierce	100%	325
Leesburg Regional Medical Center[2]	Leesburg	100%	75
Lower Keys Medical Center	Key West	100%	27
Mease Countryside Hospital	Safety Harbor	100%	173
Mease Hospital Dunedin	Dunedin	100%	58
Memorial Hospital Jacksonville[2]	Jacksonville	100%	85
Memorial Hospital Pembroke	Pembroke Pines	100%	53
Memorial Hospital West	Pembroke Pines	100%	206
Memorial Regional Hospital	Hollywood	100%	250
Morton Plant North Bay Hospital	New Port Richey	100%	91
North Florida Regional Medical Center	Gainesville	100%	216
Northside Hospital[2]	St Petersburg	100%	84
Oak Hill Hospital[2]	Brooksville	100%	98
Orange Park Medical Center[2]	Orange Park	100%	100
Orlando Health	Orlando	100%	410
Palmetto General Hospital	Hialeah	100%	214
Palms of Pasadena Hospital	St Petersburg	100%	63
Parrish Medical Center	Titusville	100%	110
Putnam Community Medical Center	Palatka	100%	60
Regional Medical Center Bayonet Point[2]	Hudson	100%	64
Sacred Heart Hospital[2]	Pensacola	100%	82
Sacred Heart Hosp-Emerald Coast	Miramar Beach	100%	39
Saint Anthony's Hospital	St Petersburg	100%	149
Saint Mary's Medical Center[2]	W Palm Beach	100%	132
Saint Petersburg General Hospital	St Petersburg	100%	36
Saint Vincent's Medical Center[2]	Jacksonville	100%	76
Saint Vincent's Medical Center Southside[2]	Jacksonville	100%	56
Santa Rosa Medical Center	Milton	100%	25
Sarasota Memorial Hospital	Sarasota	100%	256
Sebastian River Medical Center	Sebastian	100%	61
Seven Rivers Regional Medical Center	Crystal River	100%	48
South Bay Hospital[2]	Sun City Center	100%	79
South Miami Hospital	South Miami	100%	92
Tallahassee Memorial Hospital	Tallahassee	100%	241
UF Health Shands Hospital[2]	Gainesville	100%	69
University Hospital & Medical Center	Tamarac	100%	63
Venice Reg Med Ctr-Bayfront Health[2]	Venice	100%	93
Viera Hospital	Melbourne	100%	27
The Villages Regional Hospital[2]	The Villages	100%	92
Wellington Regional Medical Center	Wellington	100%	84
West Boca Medical Center	Boca Raton	100%	87
West Florida Hospital[2]	Pensacola	100%	108
West Kendall Baptist Hospital	Miami	100%	30
West Palm Hospital[2]	W Palm Beach	100%	31
Westside Regional Medical Center[2]	Plantation	100%	88
Wuesthoff Medical Center - Melbourne	Melbourne	100%	28
Baptist Hospital	Pensacola	99%	151
Blake Medical Center	Bradenton	99%	121
Broward Health North[2]	Pompano Bch	99%	154
Florida Hospital	Orlando	99%	1037
Florida Hospital Flagler	Palm Coast	99%	129
Florida Hospital Heartland Medical Center	Sebring	99%	118
Florida Hospital Memorial Medical Center	Daytona Bch	99%	157
Florida Hospital Tampa	Tampa	99%	172
Hialeah Hospital	Hialeah	99%	93
Holy Cross Hospital	Fort Lauderdale	99%	167
Indian River Medical Center[2]	Vero Beach	99%	82
JFK Medical Center[2]	Atlantis	99%	94
Lakeland Regional Medical Center[2]	Lakeland	99%	106
Lee Memorial Hospital[2]	Fort Myers	99%	174
Manatee Memorial Hospital[2]	Bradenton	99%	78
Martin Medical Center[2]	Stuart	99%	92
Ocala Regional Medical Center[2]	Ocala	99%	95
Osceola Regional Medical Center[2]	Kissimmee	99%	100
Palms West Hospital	Loxahatchee	99%	100
Physicians Reg Med Ctr-Pine Ridge	Naples	99%	152
Plantation General Hospital[2]	Plantation	99%	80
Saint Joseph's Hospital	Tampa	99%	395
Saint Lucie Medical Center[2]	Port Saint Lucie	99%	72
Baptist Medical Center Beaches[2]	Jcksnvl Bch	98%	47
Bayfront Health Port Charlotte	Port Charlotte	98%	81
Bert Fish Medical Center	New Smyrn Bch	98%	61
Central Florida Regional Hospital[2]	Sanford	98%	103
Citrus Memorial Hospital	Inverness	98%	131
Good Samaritan Medical Center	W Palm Beach	98%	46
Lakewood Ranch Medical Center	Bradenton	98%	63
Morton Plant Hospital	Clearwater	98%	200
Mount Sinai Medical Center	Miami Beach	98%	128
Munroe Regional Medical Center[2]	Ocala	98%	124
Naples Community Hospital[2]	Naples	98%	94
North Shore Medical Center	Miami	98%	226
Palm Bay Hospital	Palm Bay	98%	54
Palm Beach Gardens Medical Center	Palm Bch Grdns	98%	91
Raulerson Hospital[2]	Okeechobee	98%	44
South Florida Baptist Hospital	Plant City	98%	51
Winter Haven Hospital	Winter Haven	98%	155
Wuesthoff Medical Center Rockledge	Rockledge	98%	115
Bayfront Health Brooksville	Brooksville	97%	92
Florida Hospital Carrollwood[2]	Tampa	97%	29
Florida Hospital North Pinellas[2]	Tarpon Springs	97%	32
Jackson Memorial Hospital[2]	Miami	97%	229
Mayo Clinic[2]	Jacksonville	97%	75
Medical Center of Trinity[2]	Trinity	97%	89
North Okaloosa Medical Center	Crestview	97%	37
Northwest Medical Center	Margate	97%	149
South Lake Hospital	Clermont	97%	60
Baptist Medical Center[2]	Jacksonville	96%	104
Highlands Regional Medical Center	Sebring	96%	27
Tampa General Hospital[2]	Tampa	95%	64
UF Health Jacksonville[2]	Jacksonville	95%	85
Heart of Florida Regional Medical Center[2]	Davenport	94%	83
University of Miami Hospital	Miami	94%	88
Saint Cloud Regional Medical Center	Saint Cloud	92%	25
Memorial Hospital Miramar	Miramar	83%	46

Discharged on Statin Medication

Hospital Name	City	Rate	Cases
Bert Fish Medical Center	New Smyrn Bch	100%	54
Boca Raton Regional Hospital	Boca Raton	100%	124
Broward Health Coral Springs	Coral Springs	100%	45
Capital Regional Medical Center[2]	Tallahassee	100%	101
Cleveland Clinic Hospital	Weston	100%	54
Delray Medical Center	Delray Beach	100%	165
Doctors Hospital	Coral Gables	100%	28
Doctors Hospital of Sarasota[2]	Sarasota	100%	58
Fawcett Memorial Hospital[2]	Port Charlotte	100%	52
Florida Hospital North Pinellas[2]	Tarpon Springs	100%	25
Fort Walton Beach Medical Center[2]	Fort Walton Bch	100%	91
Lawnwood Reg Med Ctr & Heart Inst	Fort Pierce	100%	255
Memorial Hospital Pembroke	Pembroke Pines	100%	39
Memorial Hospital West	Pembroke Pines	100%	148
Oak Hill Hospital[2]	Brooksville	100%	74
Palmetto General Hospital	Hialeah	100%	174
Saint Petersburg General Hospital	St Petersburg	100%	25
Saint Vincent's Medical Center[2]	Jacksonville	100%	60
Saint Vincent's Medical Center Southside[2]	Jacksonville	100%	44
Sebastian River Medical Center	Sebastian	100%	60
South Bay Hospital[2]	Sun City Center	100%	55
South Miami Hospital	South Miami	100%	68
Tallahassee Memorial Hospital	Tallahassee	100%	205
West Boca Medical Center	Boca Raton	100%	69
West Palm Hospital[2]	W Palm Beach	100%	26
Aventura Hospital & Medical Center[2]	Aventura	99%	79
Baptist Hospital of Miami[2]	Miami	99%	102
Broward Health Medical Center	Fort Lauderdale	99%	117
Central Florida Regional Hospital[2]	Sanford	99%	74
Florida Hospital Heartland Medical Center	Sebring	99%	96
Florida Hospital Zephyrhills	Zephyrhills	99%	80
Memorial Regional Hospital	Hollywood	99%	205
North Florida Regional Medical Center	Gainesville	99%	170
Orange Park Medical Center[2]	Orange Park	99%	76
Osceola Regional Medical Center[2]	Kissimmee	99%	84
Palms West Hospital	Loxahatchee	99%	77
Saint Mary's Medical Center[2]	W Palm Beach	99%	98
Sarasota Memorial Hospital	Sarasota	99%	181
West Florida Hospital[2]	Pensacola	99%	82
Brandon Regional Hospital	Brandon	98%	164
Broward Health North[2]	Pompano Bch	98%	123
Cape Canaveral Hospital	Cocoa Beach	98%	61
Florida Hospital	Orlando	98%	836
Florida Hospital Deland[2]	Deland	98%	61
Florida Hospital Waterman[2]	Tavares	98%	62
Holmes Regional Medical Center	Melbourne	98%	175
Homestead Hospital	Homestead	98%	62
Jupiter Medical Center	Jupiter	98%	60
Lake City Medical Center[2]	Lake City	98%	41
Lakewood Ranch Medical Center	Bradenton	98%	41
North Shore Medical Center	Miami	98%	164
Northside Hospital[2]	St Petersburg	98%	66
Orlando Health	Orlando	98%	326
Palms of Pasadena Hospital	St Petersburg	98%	42
UF Health Shands Hospital[2]	Gainesville	98%	49
Venice Reg Med Ctr-Bayfront Health[2]	Venice	98%	66
Bayfront Health Dade City	Dade City	97%	35
Blake Medical Center	Bradenton	97%	92
Coral Gables Hospital	Coral Gables	97%	29
Good Samaritan Medical Center	W Palm Beach	97%	36
Gulf Coast Med Ctr Lee Mem Health Sys[2]	Fort Myers	97%	104
JFK Medical Center[2]	Atlantis	97%	70
Kendall Regional Medical Center[2]	Miami	97%	88
Mount Sinai Medical Center	Miami Beach	97%	122
Ocala Regional Medical Center[2]	Ocala	97%	75
Palm Beach Gardens Medical Center	Palm Bch Grdns	97%	69
Plantation General Hospital[2]	Plantation	97%	59
Raulerson Hospital[2]	Okeechobee	97%	32
Sacred Heart Hospital[2]	Pensacola	97%	64
Saint Anthony's Hospital	St Petersburg	97%	129
Westside Regional Medical Center[2]	Plantation	97%	59
Baptist Hospital	Pensacola	96%	105
Bayfront Health - Saint Petersburg[2]	St Petersburg	96%	70
Flagler Hospital	St Augustine	96%	109
Florida Hospital Memorial Medical Center	Daytona Bch	96%	124
Halifax Health Medical Center[2]	Daytona Bch	96%	111
Health Central	Ocoee	96%	57
Hialeah Hospital	Hialeah	96%	83
Holy Cross Hospital	Fort Lauderdale	96%	130
Manatee Memorial Hospital[2]	Bradenton	96%	57
Mease Countryside Hospital	Safety Harbor	96%	143
Memorial Hospital Jacksonville[2]	Jacksonville	96%	70
Morton Plant North Bay Hospital	New Port Richey	96%	70
Parrish Medical Center	Titusville	96%	78
Regional Medical Center Bayonet Point[2]	Hudson	96%	49
Wellington Regional Medical Center	Wellington	96%	73
Wuesthoff Medical Center Rockledge	Rockledge	96%	91
Cape Coral Hospital[2]	Cape Coral	95%	75
Gulf Breeze Hospital	Gulf Breeze	95%	41
Gulf Coast Regional Medical Center	Panama City	95%	63
Indian River Medical Center[2]	Vero Beach	95%	58
Lakeland Regional Medical Center[2]	Lakeland	95%	88
Martin Medical Center[2]	Stuart	95%	65
Mease Hospital Dunedin	Dunedin	95%	44
Morton Plant Hospital	Clearwater	95%	147
Palm Bay Hospital	Palm Bay	95%	38
UF Health Jacksonville[2]	Jacksonville	95%	66
Bethesda Hospital East[2]	Boynton Beach	94%	68
Florida Hospital Flagler	Palm Coast	94%	98
Largo Medical Center[2]	Largo	94%	99
Mayo Clinic[2]	Jacksonville	94%	53
Saint Joseph's Hospital	Tampa	94%	319
University Hospital & Medical Center	Tamarac	94%	48
Bartow Regional Medical Center	Bartow	93%	29
Jackson Memorial Hospital[2]	Miami	93%	195
Lee Memorial Hospital[2]	Fort Myers	93%	141
University of Miami Hospital	Miami	93%	70
Winter Haven Hospital	Winter Haven	93%	107
Baptist Medical Center Beaches[2]	Jcksnvl Bch	92%	37
Florida Hospital Fish Memorial[2]	Orange City	92%	83
Florida Hospital Tampa	Tampa	92%	132
Leesburg Regional Medical Center[2]	Leesburg	92%	65
Medical Center of Trinity[2]	Trinity	92%	73
Putnam Community Medical Center	Palatka	92%	48
Sacred Heart Hosp-Emerald Coast	Miramar Beach	92%	39
Saint Lucie Medical Center[2]	Port Saint Lucie	92%	50
Northwest Medical Center	Margate	91%	129
The Villages Regional Hospital[2]	The Villages	91%	85
Baptist Medical Center[2]	Jacksonville	90%	72
Bay Med Ctr Sacred Heart Health Sys	Panama City	89%	169
Citrus Memorial Hospital	Inverness	89%	114
South Florida Baptist Hospital	Plant City	89%	37

NOTE: Hospital profiles are in alphabetical order by state, then city, then hospital within the city; Rankings exclude hospitals with less than 25 cases except for patient surveys which excludes hospitals with less than 100 cases; (a) 100-299 cases; (1) The number of cases/patients is too few to report; (2) Data submitted were based on a sample of cases/patients; (3) Results are based on a shorter time period than required; (4) Data suppressed by CMS for one or more quarters; (5) Results are not available for this reporting period; (6) Fewer than 100 patients completed the HCAHPS survey; (7) No cases met the criteria for this measure; (8) The lower limit of the confidence interval cannot be calculated if the number of observed infections equals zero; (9) No data are available from the state/territory for this reporting period; (10) The scores shown reflect fewer than 50 completed surveys; (11) There were discrepancies in the data collection process; (12) This measure does not apply to this hospital for this reporting period; (13) Results cannot be calculated for this reporting period; (14) The results for this state are combined with nearby states to protect confidentiality; Please refer to the User's Guide for a full explanation of data.

South Lake Hospital	Clermont	89%	46
Tampa General Hospital[2]	Tampa	89%	46
Bayfront Health Punta Gorda	Punta Gorda	88%	42
Naples Community Hospital[2]	Naples	88%	68
Munroe Regional Medical Center[2]	Ocala	87%	87
North Okaloosa Medical Center	Crestview	87%	31
Seven Rivers Regional Medical Center	Crystal River	85%	40
Lake Wales Medical Center	Lake Wales	84%	43
Bayfront Health Port Charlotte	Port Charlotte	83%	66
Memorial Hospital Miramar	Miramar	82%	40
Heart of Florida Regional Medical Center[2]	Davenport	81%	69
Bayfront Health Brooksville	Brooksville	77%	66
Jackson Hospital	Marianna	77%	47
Physicians Reg Med Ctr-Pine Ridge	Naples	75%	126
Saint Cloud Regional Medical Center	Saint Cloud	68%	25

Thrombolytic Therapy Timing

Hospital Name	City	Rate	Cases
Delray Medical Center	Delray Beach	100%	29
Gulf Coast Med Ctr Lee Mem Health Sys[2]	Fort Myers	100%	27
Palmetto General Hospital	Hialeah	100%	33
Florida Hospital	Orlando	88%	90
Lee Memorial Hospital[2]	Fort Myers	87%	30
North Shore Medical Center	Miami	82%	28
Jackson Memorial Hospital[2]	Miami	59%	29
Physicians Reg Med Ctr-Pine Ridge	Naples	51%	45
Bay Med Ctr Sacred Heart Health Sys	Panama City	43%	37
UF Health Jacksonville[2]	Jacksonville	33%	30

Venous Thromboembolism (VTE) Prophylaxis

Hospital Name	City	Rate	Cases
Baptist Hospital of Miami[2]	Miami	100%	148
Broward Health North[2]	Pompano Bch	100%	218
Cape Canaveral Hospital	Cocoa Beach	100%	85
Central Florida Regional Hospital[2]	Sanford	100%	115
Cleveland Clinic Hospital	Weston	100%	65
Delray Medical Center	Delray Beach	100%	262
Doctors Hospital	Coral Gables	100%	46
Florida Hospital North Pinellas[2]	Tarpon Springs	100%	38
Gulf Coast Regional Medical Center	Panama City	100%	88
Homestead Hospital	Homestead	100%	75
Lawnwood Reg Med Ctr & Heart Inst	Fort Pierce	100%	407
Mease Hospital Dunedin	Dunedin	100%	68
Memorial Hospital Pembroke	Pembroke Pines	100%	56
Memorial Hospital West	Pembroke Pines	100%	232
Northside Hospital[2]	St Petersburg	100%	125
Oak Hill Hospital[2]	Brooksville	100%	100
Palms of Pasadena Hospital	St Petersburg	100%	73
Saint Lucie Medical Center[2]	Port Saint Lucie	100%	84
Saint Mary's Medical Center[2]	W Palm Beach	100%	243
Saint Petersburg General Hospital	St Petersburg	100%	45
Saint Vincent's Medical Center Southside[2]	Jacksonville	100%	67
Santa Rosa Medical Center	Milton	100%	29
Sebastian River Medical Center	Sebastian	100%	68
South Bay Hospital[2]	Sun City Center	100%	92
South Miami Hospital	South Miami	100%	110
Tallahassee Memorial Hospital	Tallahassee	100%	343
Viera Hospital	Melbourne	100%	25
West Boca Medical Center	Boca Raton	100%	94
West Kendall Baptist Hospital	Miami	100%	46
Boca Raton Regional Hospital	Boca Raton	99%	195
Brandon Regional Hospital	Brandon	99%	221
Broward Health Medical Center	Fort Lauderdale	99%	190
Capital Regional Medical Center[2]	Tallahassee	99%	135
Florida Hospital	Orlando	99%	1335
Florida Hospital Waterman[2]	Tavares	99%	100
Holmes Regional Medical Center	Melbourne	99%	306
JFK Medical Center[2]	Atlantis	99%	120
Martin Medical Center[2]	Stuart	99%	95
Memorial Regional Hospital	Hollywood	99%	389
Morton Plant Hospital	Clearwater	99%	275
Morton Plant North Bay Hospital	New Port Richey	99%	96
North Florida Regional Medical Center	Gainesville	99%	225
Orange Park Medical Center[2]	Orange Park	99%	129
Orlando Health	Orlando	99%	515
Venice Reg Med Ctr-Bayfront Health[2]	Venice	99%	106
West Florida Hospital[2]	Pensacola	99%	109
Aventura Hospital & Medical Center[2]	Aventura	98%	124
Bert Fish Medical Center	New Smyrn Bch	98%	51
Blake Medical Center	Bradenton	98%	150
Coral Gables Hospital	Coral Gables	98%	43
Fawcett Memorial Hospital[2]	Port Charlotte	98%	88
Flagler Hospital	St Augustine	98%	173
Florida Hospital Zephyrhills	Zephyrhills	98%	121
Fort Walton Beach Medical Center[2]	Fort Walton Bch	98%	117
Good Samaritan Medical Center	W Palm Beach	98%	54
Jupiter Medical Center	Jupiter	98%	93
Lakeland Regional Medical Center[2]	Lakeland	98%	136
Lakewood Ranch Medical Center	Bradenton	98%	64
Largo Medical Center[2]	Largo	98%	174
Mayo Clinic[2]	Jacksonville	98%	108
Mease Countryside Hospital	Safety Harbor	98%	186
Osceola Regional Medical Center[2]	Kissimmee	98%	132
Raulerson Hospital[2]	Okeechobee	98%	48
Saint Anthony's Hospital	St Petersburg	98%	168
Saint Joseph's Hospital	Tampa	98%	510
Saint Vincent's Medical Center[2]	Jacksonville	98%	95
UF Health Shands Hospital[2]	Gainesville	98%	130
Bartow Regional Medical Center	Bartow	97%	39
Bayfront Health - Saint Petersburg[2]	St Petersburg	97%	138
Doctors Hospital of Sarasota[2]	Sarasota	97%	75
Gulf Coast Med Ctr Lee Mem Health Sys[2]	Fort Myers	97%	158
Memorial Hospital Jacksonville[2]	Jacksonville	97%	111
Mount Sinai Medical Center	Miami Beach	97%	181
North Okaloosa Medical Center	Crestview	97%	38
Ocala Regional Medical Center[2]	Ocala	97%	112
Plantation General Hospital[2]	Plantation	97%	96
Regional Medical Center Bayonet Point[2]	Hudson	97%	105
Sarasota Memorial Hospital	Sarasota	97%	278
South Lake Hospital	Clermont	97%	59
West Palm Hospital[2]	W Palm Beach	97%	33
Winter Haven Hospital	Winter Haven	97%	158
Edward White Hospital	St Petersburg	96%	26
Florida Hospital Heartland Medical Center	Sebring	96%	123
Florida Hospital Memorial Medical Center	Daytona Bch	96%	199
Gulf Breeze Hospital	Gulf Breeze	96%	48
Halifax Health Medical Center[2]	Daytona Bch	96%	213
Health Central	Ocoee	96%	85
Indian River Medical Center[2]	Vero Beach	96%	98
Kendall Regional Medical Center[2]	Miami	96%	135
North Shore Medical Center	Miami	96%	277
Palm Beach Gardens Medical Center	Palm Bch Grdns	96%	103
Parrish Medical Center	Titusville	96%	128
Baptist Medical Center[2]	Jacksonville	95%	119
Bethesda Hospital East[2]	Boynton Beach	95%	103
Florida Hospital Tampa	Tampa	95%	211
Holy Cross Hospital	Fort Lauderdale	95%	226
Palmetto General Hospital	Hialeah	95%	282
UF Health Jacksonville[2]	Jacksonville	95%	99
Westside Regional Medical Center[2]	Plantation	95%	133
Baptist Hospital	Pensacola	94%	191
Bayfront Health Port Charlotte	Port Charlotte	94%	93
Florida Hospital Flagler	Palm Coast	94%	132
Hialeah Hospital	Hialeah	94%	127
Lee Memorial Hospital[2]	Fort Myers	94%	211
Memorial Hospital Miramar	Miramar	94%	47
Sacred Heart Hospital[2]	Pensacola	94%	99
Munroe Regional Medical Center[2]	Ocala	93%	130
Wuesthoff Medical Center Rockledge	Rockledge	93%	137
Broward Health Coral Springs	Coral Springs	92%	59
Florida Hospital Deland[2]	Deland	92%	91
Florida Hospital Fish Memorial[2]	Orange City	92%	103
Northwest Medical Center	Margate	92%	154
Putnam Community Medical Center	Palatka	92%	62
University Hospital & Medical Center	Tamarac	92%	77
Physicians Reg Med Ctr-Pine Ridge	Naples	91%	232
Wellington Regional Medical Center	Wellington	91%	101
Cape Coral Hospital[2]	Cape Coral	90%	125
Jackson Hospital	Marianna	90%	52
Larkin Community Hospital	South Miami	90%	29
Medical Center of Trinity[2]	Trinity	90%	103
Naples Community Hospital[2]	Naples	90%	109
Wuesthoff Medical Center - Melbourne	Melbourne	90%	31
Bayfront Health Punta Gorda	Punta Gorda	89%	64
Lake City Medical Center[2]	Lake City	89%	47
Manatee Memorial Hospital[2]	Bradenton	89%	99
Tampa General Hospital[2]	Tampa	89%	108
Memorial Hospital of Tampa	Tampa	88%	25
Palms West Hospital	Loxahatchee	88%	129
Baptist Medical Center Beaches[2]	Jcksnvl Bch	87%	47
Highlands Regional Medical Center	Sebring	87%	30
Palm Bay Hospital	Palm Bay	87%	54
Jackson Memorial Hospital[2]	Miami	86%	300
Sacred Heart Hosp-Emerald Coast	Miramar Beach	86%	36
Florida Hospital Carrollwood[2]	Tampa	85%	26
Leesburg Regional Medical Center[2]	Leesburg	85%	101
Lower Keys Medical Center	Key West	85%	26
Bay Med Ctr Sacred Heart Health Sys	Panama City	84%	251
The Villages Regional Hospital[2]	The Villages	81%	108
Bayfront Health Dade City	Dade City	78%	37
University of Miami Hospital	Miami	75%	105
Lake Wales Medical Center	Lake Wales	74%	69
South Florida Baptist Hospital	Plant City	69%	51
Broward Health Imperial Point	Fort Lauderdale	68%	28
Metropolitan Hospital of Miami	Miami	68%	31
Saint Cloud Regional Medical Center	Saint Cloud	68%	28
Citrus Memorial Hospital	Inverness	67%	156
Seven Rivers Regional Medical Center	Crystal River	66%	65
Bayfront Health Brooksville	Brooksville	65%	103
Heart of Florida Regional Medical Center[2]	Davenport	33%	90

Written Stroke Educational Materials Given

Hospital Name	City	Rate	Cases
Aventura Hospital & Medical Center[2]	Aventura	100%	69
Baptist Hospital of Miami[2]	Miami	100%	86
Bartow Regional Medical Center	Bartow	100%	29
Bayfront Health Punta Gorda	Punta Gorda	100%	29
Bethesda Hospital East[2]	Boynton Beach	100%	57
Boca Raton Regional Hospital	Boca Raton	100%	103
Broward Health Coral Springs	Coral Springs	100%	44
Cape Coral Hospital[2]	Cape Coral	100%	89
Capital Regional Medical Center[2]	Tallahassee	100%	76
Delray Medical Center	Delray Beach	100%	123
Fawcett Memorial Hospital[2]	Port Charlotte	100%	40
Florida Hospital Waterman[2]	Tavares	100%	60
Fort Walton Beach Medical Center[2]	Fort Walton Bch	100%	67
Good Samaritan Medical Center	W Palm Beach	100%	25
Gulf Coast Med Ctr Lee Mem Health Sys[2]	Fort Myers	100%	71
Health Central	Ocoee	100%	56
Homestead Hospital	Homestead	100%	53
Jackson Hospital	Marianna	100%	36
JFK Medical Center[2]	Atlantis	100%	70
Jupiter Medical Center	Jupiter	100%	47
Lake City Medical Center[2]	Lake City	100%	38
Lakeland Regional Medical Center[2]	Lakeland	100%	83
Lawnwood Reg Med Ctr & Heart Inst	Fort Pierce	100%	234
Lee Memorial Hospital[2]	Fort Myers	100%	127
Martin Medical Center[2]	Stuart	100%	53
Mease Hospital Dunedin	Dunedin	100%	38
Memorial Hospital Jacksonville[2]	Jacksonville	100%	51
Memorial Hospital Miramar	Miramar	100%	29
Memorial Hospital Pembroke	Pembroke Pines	100%	40
North Florida Regional Medical Center	Gainesville	100%	151
Northside Hospital[2]	St Petersburg	100%	56
Oak Hill Hospital[2]	Brooksville	100%	62
Ocala Regional Medical Center[2]	Ocala	100%	69
Orange Park Medical Center[2]	Orange Park	100%	74
Osceola Regional Medical Center[2]	Kissimmee	100%	80
Palms of Pasadena Hospital	St Petersburg	100%	35
Parrish Medical Center	Titusville	100%	72
Plantation General Hospital[2]	Plantation	100%	59
Raulerson Hospital[2]	Okeechobee	100%	39
Regional Medical Center Bayonet Point[2]	Hudson	100%	38
Saint Lucie Medical Center[2]	Port Saint Lucie	100%	45
Sebastian River Medical Center	Sebastian	100%	37
South Bay Hospital[2]	Sun City Center	100%	45
South Miami Hospital	South Miami	100%	57
University Hospital & Medical Center	Tamarac	100%	33
Wellington Regional Medical Center	Wellington	100%	50
West Florida Hospital[2]	Pensacola	100%	60
Westside Regional Medical Center[2]	Plantation	100%	56
Broward Health Medical Center	Fort Lauderdale	99%	118
Citrus Memorial Hospital	Inverness	99%	79
Florida Hospital Flagler	Palm Coast	99%	80
Florida Hospital Zephyrhills	Zephyrhills	99%	68
Memorial Hospital West	Pembroke Pines	99%	151
Saint Mary's Medical Center[2]	W Palm Beach	99%	105
Blake Medical Center	Bradenton	98%	58
Cape Canaveral Hospital	Cocoa Beach	98%	54
Cleveland Clinic Hospital	Weston	98%	61
Doctors Hospital of Sarasota[2]	Sarasota	98%	41
Florida Hospital Heartland Medical Center	Sebring	98%	83
Gulf Coast Regional Medical Center	Panama City	98%	49
Halifax Health Medical Center[2]	Daytona Bch	98%	115
Kendall Regional Medical Center[2]	Miami	98%	87
Lakewood Ranch Medical Center	Bradenton	98%	43
Memorial Regional Hospital	Hollywood	98%	174
Northwest Medical Center	Margate	98%	93
Palmetto General Hospital	Hialeah	98%	157
Palms West Hospital	Loxahatchee	98%	88
Saint Anthony's Hospital	St Petersburg	98%	93
Tallahassee Memorial Hospital	Tallahassee	98%	162
West Boca Medical Center	Boca Raton	98%	59
Winter Haven Hospital	Winter Haven	98%	88
Baptist Hospital	Pensacola	97%	88
Brandon Regional Hospital	Brandon	97%	149
Doctors Hospital	Coral Gables	97%	32
Florida Hospital	Orlando	97%	779
Florida Hospital Memorial Medical Center	Daytona Bch	97%	93
Holmes Regional Medical Center	Melbourne	97%	150
Largo Medical Center[2]	Largo	97%	59
Mount Sinai Medical Center	Miami Beach	97%	73
University of Miami Hospital	Miami	97%	60
Holy Cross Hospital	Fort Lauderdale	96%	117
Indian River Medical Center[2]	Vero Beach	96%	49
Morton Plant North Bay Hospital	New Port Richey	96%	52
North Okaloosa Medical Center	Crestview	96%	28
Saint Vincent's Medical Center[2]	Jacksonville	96%	46
Broward Health North[2]	Pompano Bch	95%	110
Florida Hospital Deland[2]	Deland	95%	44
Venice Reg Med Ctr-Bayfront Health[2]	Venice	95%	57

NOTE: Hospital profiles are in alphabetical order by state, then city, then hospital within the city; Rankings exclude hospitals with less than 25 cases except for patient surveys which excludes hospitals with less than 100 cases; (a) 100-299 cases; (1) The number of cases/patients is too few to report; (2) Data submitted were based on a sample of cases/patients; (3) Results are based on a shorter time period than required; (4) Data suppressed by CMS for one or more quarters; (5) Results are not available for this reporting period; (6) Fewer than 100 patients completed the HCAHPS survey; (7) No cases met the criteria for this measure; (8) The lower limit of the confidence interval cannot be calculated if the number of observed infections equals zero; (9) No data are available from the state/territory for this reporting period; (10) The scores shown reflect fewer than 50 completed surveys; (11) There were discrepancies in the data collection process; (12) This measure does not apply to this hospital for this reporting period; (13) Results cannot be calculated for this reporting period; (14) The results for this state are combined with nearby states to protect confidentiality; Please refer to the User's Guide for a full explanation of data.

Hospital Name	City	Rate	Cases
Bert Fish Medical Center	New Smyrn Bch	94%	35
Florida Hospital Tampa	Tampa	94%	116
Mayo Clinic[2]	Jacksonville	94%	69
Medical Center of Trinity[2]	Trinity	94%	67
Sarasota Memorial Hospital	Sarasota	94%	126
South Florida Baptist Hospital	Plant City	94%	35
Hialeah Hospital	Hialeah	93%	71
Palm Beach Gardens Medical Center	Palm Bch Grdns	93%	56
Saint Joseph's Hospital	Tampa	93%	292
Bayfront Health Dade City	Dade City	92%	25
Central Florida Regional Hospital[2]	Sanford	92%	76
Flagler Hospital	St Augustine	92%	108
Manatee Memorial Hospital[2]	Bradenton	92%	53
Morton Plant Hospital	Clearwater	92%	131
Munroe Regional Medical Center[2]	Ocala	92%	91
North Shore Medical Center	Miami	92%	142
South Lake Hospital	Clermont	92%	50
Baptist Medical Center Beaches[2]	Jcksnvl Bch	91%	32
Bayfront Health - Saint Petersburg[2]	St Petersburg	91%	69
Mease Countryside Hospital	Safety Harbor	91%	98
Palm Bay Hospital	Palm Bay	91%	34
Saint Vincent's Medical Center Southside[2]	Jacksonville	91%	45
Orlando Health	Orlando	90%	319
Baptist Medical Center[2]	Jacksonville	89%	79
Leesburg Regional Medical Center[2]	Leesburg	88%	58
Bayfront Health Port Charlotte	Port Charlotte	85%	48
Lake Wales Medical Center	Lake Wales	85%	34
Bayfront Health Brooksville	Brooksville	84%	50
UF Health Jacksonville[2]	Jacksonville	82%	49
The Villages Regional Hospital[2]	The Villages	81%	57
Tampa General Hospital[2]	Tampa	80%	66
Florida Hospital Fish Memorial[2]	Orange City	79%	58
Putnam Community Medical Center	Palatka	79%	33
Wuesthoff Medical Center Rockledge	Rockledge	78%	60
Gulf Breeze Hospital	Gulf Breeze	77%	35
Sacred Heart Hospital[2]	Pensacola	77%	64
UF Health Shands Hospital[2]	Gainesville	76%	55
Bay Med Ctr Sacred Heart Health Sys	Panama City	75%	137
Jackson Memorial Hospital[2]	Miami	75%	183
Physicians Reg Med Ctr-Pine Ridge	Naples	63%	123
Seven Rivers Regional Medical Center	Crystal River	61%	33
Sacred Heart Hosp-Emerald Coast	Miramar Beach	58%	33
Naples Community Hospital[2]	Naples	51%	70
Heart of Florida Regional Medical Center[2]	Davenport	48%	56

Surgical Care Improvement Project

Appropriate Beta Blocker Usage

Hospital Name	City	Rate	Cases
Bay Med Ctr Sacred Heart Health Sys[2]	Panama City	100%	337
Blake Medical Center[2]	Bradenton	100%	279
Broward Health Coral Springs[2]	Coral Springs	100%	125
Broward Health Imperial Point	Fort Lauderdale	100%	99
Broward Health Medical Center[2]	Fort Lauderdale	100%	206
Broward Health North[2]	Pompano Bch	100%	99
Capital Regional Medical Center	Tallahassee	100%	98
Central Florida Regional Hospital[2]	Sanford	100%	203
Coral Gables Hospital[2]	Coral Gables	100%	97
Delray Medical Center[2]	Delray Beach	100%	422
Doctors Hospital	Coral Gables	100%	154
Doctors Hospital of Sarasota[2]	Sarasota	100%	138
Edward White Hospital	St Petersburg	100%	59
Englewood Community Hospital	Englewood	100%	37
Florida Hospital Deland	Deland	100%	177
Florida Hospital Flagler	Palm Coast	100%	124
Florida Hospital Memorial Medical Center[2]	Daytona Bch	100%	381
Florida Hospital North Pinellas[2]	Tarpon Springs	100%	76
Florida Hospital Waterman[2]	Tavares	100%	132
Florida Hospital Zephyrhills	Zephyrhills	100%	207
Gulf Breeze Hospital[2]	Gulf Breeze	100%	105
Hialeah Hospital[2]	Hialeah	100%	74
Highlands Regional Medical Center[2]	Sebring	100%	67
Holy Cross Hospital[2]	Fort Lauderdale	100%	215
Homestead Hospital	Homestead	100%	56
JFK Medical Center[2]	Atlantis	100%	309
Jupiter Medical Center[2]	Jupiter	100%	145
Lake City Medical Center[2]	Lake City	100%	50
Largo Medical Center[2]	Largo	100%	228
Lawnwood Reg Med Ctr & Heart Inst	Fort Pierce	100%	296
Memorial Hospital Jacksonville[2]	Jacksonville	100%	290
Memorial Hospital Pembroke[2]	Pembroke Pines	100%	96
Memorial Hospital West[2]	Pembroke Pines	100%	121
Memorial Regional Hospital[2]	Hollywood	100%	317
North Florida Regional Medical Center[2]	Gainesville	100%	269
North Okaloosa Medical Center	Crestview	100%	54
Northside Hospital[2]	St Petersburg	100%	191
Northwest Medical Center[2]	Margate	100%	170
Oak Hill Hospital[2]	Brooksville	100%	280
Orange Park Medical Center[2]	Orange Park	100%	187
Palm Bay Hospital	Palm Bay	100%	117
Palm Beach Gardens Medical Center	Palm Bch Grdns	100%	324
Palms of Pasadena Hospital	St Petersburg	100%	150
Palms West Hospital[2]	Loxahatchee	100%	84
Parrish Medical Center	Titusville	100%	120
Physicians Reg Med Ctr-Pine Ridge	Naples	100%	346
Plantation General Hospital[2]	Plantation	100%	245
Raulerson Hospital	Okeechobee	100%	48
Regional Medical Center Bayonet Point[2]	Hudson	100%	235
Sacred Heart Hosp-Emerald Coast[2]	Miramar Beach	100%	117
Saint Lucie Medical Center[2]	Port Saint Lucie	100%	148
Sebastian River Medical Center	Sebastian	100%	178
South Miami Hospital[2]	South Miami	100%	177
Tallahassee Memorial Hospital[2]	Tallahassee	100%	527
Twin Cities Hospital	Niceville	100%	58
Venice Reg Med Ctr-Bayfront Health[2]	Venice	100%	299
Viera Hospital	Melbourne	100%	154
W Palm Beach VA Medical Center[2]	W Palm Beach	100%	54
West Florida Hospital[2]	Pensacola	100%	223
West Kendall Baptist Hospital	Miami	100%	41
West Palm Hospital	W Palm Beach	100%	66
Westside Regional Medical Center[2]	Plantation	100%	202
Aventura Hospital & Medical Center[2]	Aventura	99%	235
Baptist Hospital[2]	Pensacola	99%	309
Baptist Hospital of Miami[2]	Miami	99%	216
Bay Pines VA Medical Center[2]	Bay Pines	99%	143
Bayfront Health Brooksville	Brooksville	99%	160
Bayfront Health Punta Gorda[2]	Punta Gorda	99%	106
Boca Raton Regional Hospital[2]	Boca Raton	99%	189
Brandon Regional Hospital[2]	Brandon	99%	218
Cape Canaveral Hospital[2]	Cocoa Beach	99%	115
Cape Coral Hospital[2]	Cape Coral	99%	162
Fawcett Memorial Hospital[2]	Port Charlotte	99%	155
Flagler Hospital[2]	St Augustine	99%	179
Florida Hospital[2]	Orlando	99%	2121
Florida Hospital Heartland Medical Center	Sebring	99%	196
Florida Hospital Tampa[2]	Tampa	99%	154
Fort Walton Beach Medical Center[2]	Fort Walton Bch	99%	154
Gulf Coast Med Ctr Lee Mem Health Sys[2]	Fort Myers	99%	237
Gulf Coast Regional Medical Center[2]	Panama City	99%	184
Halifax Health Medical Center[2]	Daytona Bch	99%	274
Holmes Regional Medical Center[2]	Melbourne	99%	597
Mayo Clinic[2]	Jacksonville	99%	317
Medical Center of Trinity[2]	Trinity	99%	178
Morton Plant Hospital[2]	Clearwater	99%	659
Munroe Regional Medical Center[2]	Ocala	99%	265
Ocala Regional Medical Center[2]	Ocala	99%	227
Palmetto General Hospital[2]	Hialeah	99%	303
Saint Petersburg General Hospital[2]	St Petersburg	99%	81
Saint Vincent's Medical Center[2]	Jacksonville	99%	247
Saint Vincent's Medical Center Southside[2]	Jacksonville	99%	109
Tampa General Hospital[2]	Tampa	99%	540
UF Health Jacksonville[2]	Jacksonville	99%	165
Wellington Regional Medical Center[2]	Wellington	99%	107
Winter Haven Hospital[2]	Winter Haven	99%	260
Baptist Medical Center Beaches[2]	Jcksnvl Bch	98%	139
Bayfront Health Port Charlotte[2]	Port Charlotte	98%	297
Florida Hospital Fish Memorial	Orange City	98%	112
Good Samaritan Medical Center[2]	W Palm Beach	98%	137
Health Central	Ocoee	98%	197
Kendall Regional Medical Center[2]	Miami	98%	278
Lakeland Regional Medical Center[2]	Lakeland	98%	291
Lee Memorial Hospital[2]	Fort Myers	98%	369
Lower Keys Medical Center[2]	Key West	98%	65
Manatee Memorial Hospital[2]	Bradenton	98%	249
Mease Hospital Dunedin[2]	Dunedin	98%	63
Mount Sinai Medical Center[2]	Miami Beach	98%	533
Naples Community Hospital[2]	Naples	98%	346
Saint Anthony's Hospital[2]	St Petersburg	98%	230
Saint Joseph's Hospital[2]	Tampa	98%	380
Saint Mary's Medical Center[2]	W Palm Beach	98%	62
Santa Rosa Medical Center	Milton	98%	59
South Bay Hospital[2]	Sun City Center	98%	125
UF Health Shands Hospital[2]	Gainesville	98%	216
University of Miami Hospital	Miami	98%	432
Baptist Medical Center[2]	Jacksonville	97%	329
Bartow Regional Medical Center	Bartow	97%	58
Bayfront Health - Saint Petersburg[2]	St Petersburg	97%	157
Bert Fish Medical Center	New Smyrn Bch	97%	97
Cleveland Clinic Hospital[2]	Weston	97%	172
Jackson Memorial Hospital[2]	Miami	97%	233
Leesburg Regional Medical Center[2]	Leesburg	97%	417
Lehigh Regional Medical Center	Lehigh Acres	97%	63
Memorial Hospital of Tampa	Tampa	97%	78
Morton Plant North Bay Hospital[2]	New Port Richey	97%	70
Orlando Health[2]	Orlando	97%	1103
Osceola Regional Medical Center[2]	Kissimmee	97%	193
Sarasota Memorial Hospital[2]	Sarasota	97%	306
Tampa VA Medical Center[2]	Tampa	97%	188
University Hospital & Medical Center[2]	Tamarac	97%	112
Wuesthoff Medical Center - Melbourne[2]	Melbourne	97%	125
Wuesthoff Medical Center Rockledge[2]	Rockledge	97%	215
Bayfront Health Dade City	Dade City	96%	54
Citrus Memorial Hospital	Inverness	96%	279
Heart of Florida Regional Medical Center	Davenport	96%	238
Jackson Hospital	Marianna	96%	54
Martin Medical Center[2]	Stuart	96%	171
Mease Countryside Hospital[2]	Safety Harbor	96%	174
Sacred Heart Hospital[2]	Pensacola	96%	215
South Florida Baptist Hospital	Plant City	96%	108
Town & Country Hospital	Tampa	96%	50
VA N Florida/S Georgia Healthcare Sys[2]	Gainesville	96%	275
The Villages Regional Hospital	The Villages	96%	218
Indian River Medical Center[2]	Vero Beach	95%	271
Lake Wales Medical Center	Lake Wales	95%	44
Seven Rivers Regional Medical Center	Crystal River	95%	246
South Lake Hospital	Clermont	95%	182
Bethesda Hospital East[2]	Boynton Beach	94%	215
North Shore Medical Center	Miami	94%	168
Florida Hospital Carrollwood[2]	Tampa	93%	88
Miami VA Medical Center[2]	Miami	92%	115
Lakewood Ranch Medical Center[2]	Bradenton	90%	105
West Boca Medical Center[2]	Boca Raton	90%	63
Palm Springs General Hospital	Hialeah	81%	36

Appropriate VTP Within 24 Hours

Hospital Name	City	Rate	Cases
Baptist Hospital of Miami[2]	Miami	100%	440
Blake Medical Center[2]	Bradenton	100%	425
Boca Raton Regional Hospital[2]	Boca Raton	100%	337
Broward Health Coral Springs[2]	Coral Springs	100%	443
Broward Health Medical Center[2]	Fort Lauderdale	100%	508
Broward Health North[2]	Pompano Bch	100%	364
Coral Gables Hospital[2]	Coral Gables	100%	303
Delray Medical Center[2]	Delray Beach	100%	689
Doctor's Memorial Hospital	Perry	100%	69
Doctors Hospital	Coral Gables	100%	515
Englewood Community Hospital	Englewood	100%	134
Fawcett Memorial Hospital[2]	Port Charlotte	100%	388
Fishermen's Hospital	Marathon	100%	44
Florida Hospital Flagler	Palm Coast	100%	451
Florida Hospital Memorial Medical Center[2]	Daytona Bch	100%	667
Florida Hospital North Pinellas[2]	Tarpon Springs	100%	218
Florida Hospital Waterman[2]	Tavares	100%	275
Florida Hospital Wesley Chapel[3]	Wesley Chapel	100%	29
Gulf Coast Regional Medical Center[2]	Panama City	100%	393
Health Central	Ocoee	100%	570
Highlands Regional Medical Center[2]	Sebring	100%	153
Holy Cross Hospital[2]	Fort Lauderdale	100%	518
Homestead Hospital	Homestead	100%	222
JFK Medical Center[2]	Atlantis	100%	472
Jupiter Medical Center[2]	Jupiter	100%	483
Kendall Regional Medical Center[2]	Miami	100%	488
Lake City Medical Center[2]	Lake City	100%	143
Largo Medical Center[2]	Largo	100%	424
Lawnwood Reg Med Ctr & Heart Inst	Fort Pierce	100%	434
Mariners Hospital	Tavernier	100%	39
Medical Center of Trinity[2]	Trinity	100%	414
Memorial Hospital Jacksonville[2]	Jacksonville	100%	533
Memorial Hospital Pembroke[2]	Pembroke Pines	100%	282
Memorial Hospital West[2]	Pembroke Pines	100%	383
Memorial Regional Hospital[2]	Hollywood	100%	432
Metropolitan Hospital of Miami	Miami	100%	106
Miami VA Medical Center[2]	Miami	100%	242
Northside Hospital[2]	St Petersburg	100%	185
Northwest Medical Center[2]	Margate	100%	294
Ocala Regional Medical Center[2]	Ocala	100%	521
Orange Park Medical Center[2]	Orange Park	100%	357
Osceola Regional Medical Center[2]	Kissimmee	100%	445
Palms of Pasadena Hospital	St Petersburg	100%	506
Raulerson Hospital	Okeechobee	100%	125
Saint Lucie Medical Center[2]	Port Saint Lucie	100%	440
Saint Petersburg General Hospital[2]	St Petersburg	100%	260
Saint Vincent's Medical Center[2]	Jacksonville	100%	350
Saint Vincent's Medical Center Southside[2]	Jacksonville	100%	318
Sebastian River Medical Center	Sebastian	100%	415
South Bay Hospital[2]	Sun City Center	100%	304
South Miami Hospital[2]	South Miami	100%	360
University Hospital & Medical Center[2]	Tamarac	100%	300
Venice Reg Med Ctr-Bayfront Health[2]	Venice	100%	434
W Palm Beach VA Medical Center[2]	W Palm Beach	100%	156
West Florida Hospital[2]	Pensacola	100%	442
West Kendall Baptist Hospital	Miami	100%	177
Aventura Hospital & Medical Center[2]	Aventura	99%	421
Baptist Medical Center[2]	Jacksonville	99%	599
Baptist Medical Center Beaches[2]	Jcksnvl Bch	99%	416
Bartow Regional Medical Center	Bartow	99%	166
Bayfront Health Dade City	Dade City	99%	143
Bert Fish Medical Center	New Smyrn Bch	99%	267
Brandon Regional Hospital[2]	Brandon	99%	482
Broward Health Imperial Point	Fort Lauderdale	99%	368
Cape Canaveral Hospital[2]	Cocoa Beach	99%	360
Capital Regional Medical Center	Tallahassee	99%	458

NOTE: Hospital profiles are in alphabetical order by state, then city, then hospital within the city; Rankings exclude hospitals with less than 25 cases except for patient surveys which excludes hospitals with less than 100 cases; (a) 100-299 cases; (1) The number of cases/patients is too few to report; (2) Data submitted were based on a sample of cases/patients; (3) Results are based on a shorter time period than required; (4) Data suppressed by CMS for one or more quarters; (5) Results are not available for this reporting period; (6) Fewer than 100 patients completed the HCAHPS survey; (7) No cases met the criteria for this measure; (8) The lower limit of the confidence interval cannot be calculated if the number of observed infections equals zero; (9) No data are available from the state/territory for this reporting period; (10) The scores shown reflect fewer than 50 completed surveys; (11) There were discrepancies in the data collection process; (12) This measure does not apply to this hospital for this reporting period; (13) Results cannot be calculated for this reporting period; (14) The results for this state are combined with nearby states to protect confidentiality; Please refer to the User's Guide for a full explanation of data.

Hospital Name	City	Rate	Cases
Central Florida Regional Hospital[2]	Sanford	99%	351
Cleveland Clinic Hospital[2]	Weston	99%	322
Doctors Hospital of Sarasota[2]	Sarasota	99%	399
Edward White Hospital	St Petersburg	99%	197
Florida Hospital[2]	Orlando	99%	5531
Florida Hospital Deland	Deland	99%	528
Florida Hospital Fish Memorial	Orange City	99%	353
Florida Hospital Heartland Medical Center	Sebring	99%	424
Fort Walton Beach Medical Center[2]	Fort Walton Bch	99%	359
Holmes Regional Medical Center[2]	Melbourne	99%	892
Lakewood Ranch Medical Center[2]	Bradenton	99%	363
Memorial Hospital Miramar[2]	Miramar	99%	214
Morton Plant Hospital[2]	Clearwater	99%	1225
North Florida Regional Medical Center[2]	Gainesville	99%	530
Oak Hill Hospital[2]	Brooksville	99%	380
Palm Bay Hospital	Palm Bay	99%	321
Palmetto General Hospital[2]	Hialeah	99%	450
Palms West Hospital[2]	Loxahatchee	99%	344
Parrish Medical Center	Titusville	99%	383
Plantation General Hospital[2]	Plantation	99%	513
Regional Medical Center Bayonet Point[2]	Hudson	99%	353
Saint Anthony's Hospital[2]	St Petersburg	99%	590
Saint Cloud Regional Medical Center	Saint Cloud	99%	80
Saint Joseph's Hospital[2]	Tampa	99%	799
Saint Mary's Medical Center[2]	W Palm Beach	99%	248
Santa Rosa Medical Center	Milton	99%	155
South Florida Baptist Hospital	Plant City	99%	398
Tallahassee Memorial Hospital[2]	Tallahassee	99%	1110
Twin Cities Hospital	Niceville	99%	156
UF Health Jacksonville[2]	Jacksonville	99%	294
UF Health Shands Hospital[2]	Gainesville	99%	437
Viera Hospital	Melbourne	99%	539
Wellington Regional Medical Center[2]	Wellington	99%	401
West Boca Medical Center[2]	Boca Raton	99%	233
West Palm Hospital	W Palm Beach	99%	183
Westside Regional Medical Center[2]	Plantation	99%	439
Baptist Hospital[2]	Pensacola	98%	461
Baptist Medical Center - Nassau[2]	Fernandina Bch	98%	122
Bayfront Health - Saint Petersburg[2]	St Petersburg	98%	303
Bayfront Health Brooksville	Brooksville	98%	452
Bayfront Health Port Charlotte[2]	Port Charlotte	98%	440
Bayfront Health Punta Gorda[2]	Punta Gorda	98%	235
Flagler Hospital[2]	St Augustine	98%	318
Florida Hospital Carrollwood[2]	Tampa	98%	296
Florida Hospital Zephyrhills	Zephyrhills	98%	313
Gulf Breeze Hospital[2]	Gulf Breeze	98%	295
Halifax Health Medical Center[2]	Daytona Bch	98%	720
Hialeah Hospital[2]	Hialeah	98%	291
Jackson Hospital	Marianna	98%	146
Jackson Memorial Hospital[2]	Miami	98%	762
Lakeland Regional Medical Center[2]	Lakeland	98%	492
Lakeside Medical Center	Belle Glade	98%	42
Lehigh Regional Medical Center	Lehigh Acres	98%	170
Mayo Clinic[2]	Jacksonville	98%	450
Mease Countryside Hospital[2]	Safety Harbor	98%	462
Mease Hospital Dunedin[2]	Dunedin	98%	235
Morton Plant North Bay Hospital[2]	New Port Richey	98%	155
Mount Sinai Medical Center[2]	Miami Beach	98%	526
Naples Community Hospital[2]	Naples	98%	517
North Okaloosa Medical Center	Crestview	98%	159
North Shore Medical Center	Miami	98%	355
Orlando Health[2]	Orlando	98%	2587
Sacred Heart Hosp-Emerald Coast[2]	Miramar Beach	98%	330
Sarasota Memorial Hospital[2]	Sarasota	98%	461
South Lake Hospital	Clermont	98%	520
Tampa General Hospital[2]	Tampa	98%	926
Town & Country Hospital	Tampa	98%	168
VA N Florida/S Georgia Healthcare Sys[2]	Gainesville	98%	411
Winter Haven Hospital[2]	Winter Haven	98%	340
Bay Pines VA Medical Center[2]	Bay Pines	97%	272
Gulf Coast Med Ctr Lee Mem Health Sys[2]	Fort Myers	97%	420
Indian River Medical Center[2]	Vero Beach	97%	408
Leesburg Regional Medical Center[2]	Leesburg	97%	521
Manatee Memorial Hospital[2]	Bradenton	97%	420
Martin Medical Center[2]	Stuart	97%	387
Memorial Hospital of Tampa	Tampa	97%	196
Sacred Heart Hospital[2]	Pensacola	97%	481
Tampa VA Medical Center[2]	Tampa	97%	239
University of Miami Hospital	Miami	97%	1126
Westchester General Hospital[2]	Miami	97%	31
Wuesthoff Medical Center Rockledge[2]	Rockledge	97%	346
Bethesda Hospital East[2]	Boynton Beach	96%	396
Lee Memorial Hospital[2]	Fort Myers	96%	504
Palm Beach Gardens Medical Center	Palm Bch Grdns	96%	233
Putnam Community Medical Center	Palatka	96%	164
Seven Rivers Regional Medical Center	Crystal River	96%	675
Wuesthoff Medical Center - Melbourne[2]	Melbourne	96%	341
Bay Med Ctr Sacred Heart Health Sys[2]	Panama City	95%	381
Good Samaritan Medical Center[2]	W Palm Beach	95%	444
Heart of Florida Regional Medical Center	Davenport	95%	803
Lower Keys Medical Center[2]	Key West	95%	184
Munroe Regional Medical Center[2]	Ocala	95%	292
Physicians Reg Med Ctr-Pine Ridge	Naples	95%	1090
Cape Coral Hospital[2]	Cape Coral	94%	429
Desoto Memorial Hospital	Arcadia	94%	34
Lake Wales Medical Center	Lake Wales	94%	106
Shands Lake Shore Regional Medical Center	Lake City	94%	68
Citrus Memorial Hospital	Inverness	93%	550
Florida Hospital Tampa[2]	Tampa	93%	252
Palm Springs General Hospital	Hialeah	93%	122
The Villages Regional Hospital	The Villages	93%	532
Larkin Community Hospital	South Miami	85%	33

Controlled Postoperative Blood Glucose

Hospital Name	City	Rate	Cases
Broward Health Medical Center[2]	Fort Lauderdale	100%	166
Citrus Memorial Hospital	Inverness	100%	144
Florida Hospital Memorial Medical Center[2]	Daytona Bch	100%	237
Florida Hospital Tampa[2]	Tampa	100%	120
Florida Hospital Waterman[2]	Tavares	100%	60
Florida Hospital Zephyrhills	Zephyrhills	100%	96
Fort Walton Beach Medical Center[2]	Fort Walton Bch	100%	95
JFK Medical Center[2]	Atlantis	100%	182
Lawnwood Reg Med Ctr & Heart Inst	Fort Pierce	100%	213
Memorial Regional Hospital[2]	Hollywood	100%	235
North Florida Regional Medical Center[2]	Gainesville	100%	143
Orange Park Medical Center[2]	Orange Park	100%	71
Palm Beach Gardens Medical Center	Palm Bch Grdns	100%	256
Regional Medical Center Bayonet Point[2]	Hudson	100%	145
Venice Reg Med Ctr-Bayfront Health[2]	Venice	100%	135
West Florida Hospital[2]	Pensacola	100%	102
Westside Regional Medical Center[2]	Plantation	100%	91
Bayfront Health Port Charlotte[2]	Port Charlotte	99%	148
Blake Medical Center[2]	Bradenton	99%	144
Boca Raton Regional Hospital[2]	Boca Raton	99%	118
Central Florida Regional Hospital[2]	Sanford	99%	114
Halifax Health Medical Center[2]	Daytona Bch	99%	125
Kendall Regional Medical Center[2]	Miami	99%	79
Largo Medical Center[2]	Largo	99%	94
Morton Plant Hospital[2]	Clearwater	99%	295
Northside Hospital[2]	St Petersburg	99%	139
Northwest Medical Center[2]	Margate	99%	106
Osceola Regional Medical Center[2]	Kissimmee	99%	75
Palmetto General Hospital[2]	Hialeah	99%	151
Saint Joseph's Hospital[2]	Tampa	99%	282
Saint Vincent's Medical Center[2]	Jacksonville	99%	144
Tallahassee Memorial Hospital[2]	Tallahassee	99%	315
Aventura Hospital & Medical Center[2]	Aventura	98%	112
Baptist Medical Center[2]	Jacksonville	98%	244
Bayfront Health - Saint Petersburg[2]	St Petersburg	98%	82
Brandon Regional Hospital[2]	Brandon	98%	126
Florida Hospital[2]	Orlando	98%	929
Gulf Coast Med Ctr Lee Mem Health Sys[2]	Fort Myers	98%	57
Holy Cross Hospital[2]	Fort Lauderdale	98%	212
Memorial Hospital Jacksonville[2]	Jacksonville	98%	136
Mount Sinai Medical Center[2]	Miami Beach	98%	690
Oak Hill Hospital[2]	Brooksville	98%	106
Ocala Regional Medical Center[2]	Ocala	98%	89
South Miami Hospital[2]	South Miami	98%	66
UF Health Jacksonville[2]	Jacksonville	98%	95
Winter Haven Hospital[2]	Winter Haven	98%	180
Baptist Hospital[2]	Pensacola	97%	178
Baptist Hospital of Miami[2]	Miami	97%	151
Holmes Regional Medical Center[2]	Melbourne	97%	323
Indian River Medical Center[2]	Vero Beach	97%	174
Lakeland Regional Medical Center[2]	Lakeland	97%	181
Lee Memorial Hospital[2]	Fort Myers	97%	192
Manatee Memorial Hospital[2]	Bradenton	97%	165
Munroe Regional Medical Center[2]	Ocala	97%	136
Naples Community Hospital[2]	Naples	97%	204
Orlando Health[2]	Orlando	97%	265
Sarasota Memorial Hospital[2]	Sarasota	97%	178
VA N Florida/S Georgia Healthcare Sys[2]	Gainesville	97%	130
Wuesthoff Medical Center Rockledge[2]	Rockledge	97%	104
Bethesda Hospital East[2]	Boynton Beach	96%	121
Delray Medical Center[2]	Delray Beach	96%	171
Leesburg Regional Medical Center[2]	Leesburg	96%	343
Martin Medical Center[2]	Stuart	96%	93
UF Health Shands Hospital[2]	Gainesville	96%	112
Bay Med Ctr Sacred Heart Health Sys[2]	Panama City	95%	282
Cleveland Clinic Hospital[2]	Weston	95%	133
Jackson Memorial Hospital[2]	Miami	95%	94
Mayo Clinic[2]	Jacksonville	95%	184
Plantation General Hospital[2]	Plantation	95%	87
Tampa VA Medical Center[2]	Tampa	95%	76
North Shore Medical Center	Miami	94%	87
Tampa General Hospital[2]	Tampa	94%	252
Capital Regional Medical Center	Tallahassee	93%	46
University of Miami Hospital	Miami	92%	126
Sacred Heart Hospital[2]	Pensacola	91%	103
Flagler Hospital[2]	St Augustine	90%	101

Perioperative Temperature Management

Hospital Name	City	Rate	Cases
Aventura Hospital & Medical Center[2]	Aventura	100%	512
Baptist Hospital[2]	Pensacola	100%	628
Baptist Hospital of Miami[2]	Miami	100%	519
Baptist Medical Center[2]	Jacksonville	100%	806
Baptist Medical Center - Nassau[2]	Fernandina Bch	100%	129
Baptist Medical Center Beaches[2]	Jcksnvl Bch	100%	462
Bartow Regional Medical Center	Bartow	100%	202
Bay Med Ctr Sacred Heart Health Sys[2]	Panama City	100%	546
Bay Pines VA Medical Center[2]	Bay Pines	100%	352
Bayfront Health - Saint Petersburg[2]	St Petersburg	100%	372
Bayfront Health Brooksville	Brooksville	100%	460
Bayfront Health Dade City	Dade City	100%	187
Bayfront Health Port Charlotte[2]	Port Charlotte	100%	529
Bayfront Health Punta Gorda[2]	Punta Gorda	100%	266
Bert Fish Medical Center	New Smyrn Bch	100%	303
Bethesda Hospital East[2]	Boynton Beach	100%	481
Blake Medical Center[2]	Bradenton	100%	482
Boca Raton Regional Hospital[2]	Boca Raton	100%	525
Brandon Regional Hospital[2]	Brandon	100%	594
Broward Health Coral Springs[2]	Coral Springs	100%	468
Broward Health Imperial Point	Fort Lauderdale	100%	397
Broward Health Medical Center[2]	Fort Lauderdale	100%	637
Broward Health North[2]	Pompano Bch	100%	411
Cape Canaveral Hospital[2]	Cocoa Beach	100%	395
Cape Coral Hospital[2]	Cape Coral	100%	510
Capital Regional Medical Center	Tallahassee	100%	559
Central Florida Regional Hospital[2]	Sanford	100%	403
Citrus Memorial Hospital	Inverness	100%	672
Cleveland Clinic Hospital[2]	Weston	100%	404
Coral Gables Hospital[2]	Coral Gables	100%	349
Delray Medical Center[2]	Delray Beach	100%	810
Desoto Memorial Hospital	Arcadia	100%	34
Doctor's Memorial Hospital	Perry	100%	76
Doctors Hospital	Coral Gables	100%	594
Doctors Hospital of Sarasota[2]	Sarasota	100%	466
Edward White Hospital	St Petersburg	100%	214
Englewood Community Hospital	Englewood	100%	145
Fawcett Memorial Hospital[2]	Port Charlotte	100%	462
Fishermen's Hospital	Marathon	100%	51
Flagler Hospital[2]	St Augustine	100%	415
Florida Hospital[2]	Orlando	100%	7658
Florida Hospital Deland	Deland	100%	551
Florida Hospital Fish Memorial	Orange City	100%	399
Florida Hospital Flagler	Palm Coast	100%	496
Florida Hospital Heartland Medical Center	Sebring	100%	500
Florida Hospital Memorial Medical Center[2]	Daytona Bch	100%	777
Florida Hospital North Pinellas[2]	Tarpon Springs	100%	250
Florida Hospital Tampa[2]	Tampa	100%	426
Florida Hospital Waterman[2]	Tavares	100%	367
Florida Hospital Wesley Chapel[3]	Wesley Chapel	100%	29
Florida Hospital Zephyrhills	Zephyrhills	100%	404
Fort Walton Beach Medical Center[2]	Fort Walton Bch	100%	494
Good Samaritan Medical Center[2]	W Palm Beach	100%	509
Gulf Breeze Hospital[2]	Gulf Breeze	100%	355
Gulf Coast Med Ctr Lee Mem Health Sys[2]	Fort Myers	100%	570
Gulf Coast Regional Medical Center[2]	Panama City	100%	529
Halifax Health Medical Center[2]	Daytona Bch	100%	831
Health Central	Ocoee	100%	655
Heart of Florida Regional Medical Center	Davenport	100%	852
Hialeah Hospital[2]	Hialeah	100%	345
Highlands Regional Medical Center[2]	Sebring	100%	188
Holmes Regional Medical Center[2]	Melbourne	100%	1126
Holy Cross Hospital[2]	Fort Lauderdale	100%	628
Homestead Hospital	Homestead	100%	241
Jackson Hospital	Marianna	100%	157
Jackson Memorial Hospital[2]	Miami	100%	1092
JFK Medical Center[2]	Atlantis	100%	591
Jupiter Medical Center[2]	Jupiter	100%	530
Kendall Regional Medical Center[2]	Miami	100%	577
Lake City Medical Center[2]	Lake City	100%	150
Lakeland Regional Medical Center[2]	Lakeland	100%	645
Lakeside Medical Center	Belle Glade	100%	51
Lakewood Ranch Medical Center[2]	Bradenton	100%	446
Largo Medical Center[2]	Largo	100%	509
Lawnwood Reg Med Ctr & Heart Inst	Fort Pierce	100%	544
Leesburg Regional Medical Center[2]	Leesburg	100%	646
Lehigh Regional Medical Center	Lehigh Acres	100%	205
Lower Keys Medical Center[2]	Key West	100%	218
Manatee Memorial Hospital[2]	Bradenton	100%	475
Mariners Hospital	Tavernier	100%	42
Mayo Clinic[2]	Jacksonville	100%	538
Mease Countryside Hospital[2]	Safety Harbor	100%	568
Mease Hospital Dunedin[2]	Dunedin	100%	251
Medical Center of Trinity[2]	Trinity	100%	483
Memorial Hospital Jacksonville[2]	Jacksonville	100%	646
Memorial Hospital Miramar[2]	Miramar	100%	261
Memorial Hospital of Tampa	Tampa	100%	228
Memorial Hospital Pembroke[2]	Pembroke Pines	100%	338

NOTE: Hospital profiles are in alphabetical order by state, then city, then hospital within the city; Rankings exclude hospitals with less than 25 cases except for patient surveys which excludes hospitals with less than 100 cases; (a) 100-299 cases; (1) The number of cases/patients is too few to report; (2) Data submitted were based on a sample of cases/patients; (3) Results are based on a shorter time period than required; (4) Data suppressed by CMS for one or more quarters; (5) Results are not available for this reporting period; (6) Fewer than 100 patients completed the HCAHPS survey; (7) No cases met the criteria for this measure; (8) The lower limit of the confidence interval cannot be calculated if the number of observed infections equals zero; (9) No data are available from the state/territory for this reporting period; (10) The scores shown reflect fewer than 50 completed surveys; (11) There were discrepancies in the data collection process; (12) This measure does not apply to this hospital for this reporting period; (13) Results cannot be calculated for this reporting period; (14) The results for this state are combined with nearby states to protect confidentiality; Please refer to the User's Guide for a full explanation of data.

Hospital Name	City	Rate	Cases
Memorial Hospital West[2]	Pembroke Pines	100%	429
Memorial Regional Hospital[2]	Hollywood	100%	527
Metropolitan Hospital of Miami	Miami	100%	162
Morton Plant Hospital[2]	Clearwater	100%	1522
Morton Plant North Bay Hospital[2]	New Port Richey	100%	189
Mount Sinai Medical Center[2]	Miami Beach	100%	652
Naples Community Hospital[2]	Naples	100%	662
North Florida Regional Medical Center[2]	Gainesville	100%	675
North Okaloosa Medical Center	Crestview	100%	216
Northside Hospital[2]	St Petersburg	100%	240
Northwest Medical Center[2]	Margate	100%	340
Oak Hill Hospital[2]	Brooksville	100%	471
Ocala Regional Medical Center[2]	Ocala	100%	640
Orange Park Medical Center[2]	Orange Park	100%	435
Orlando Health[2]	Orlando	100%	3220
Osceola Regional Medical Center[2]	Kissimmee	100%	518
Palm Bay Hospital	Palm Bay	100%	344
Palm Beach Gardens Medical Center	Palm Bch Grdns	100%	450
Palm Springs General Hospital	Hialeah	100%	143
Palmetto General Hospital[2]	Hialeah	100%	529
Palms of Pasadena Hospital	St Petersburg	100%	545
Palms West Hospital[2]	Loxahatchee	100%	384
Parrish Medical Center	Titusville	100%	421
Physicians Reg Med Ctr-Pine Ridge	Naples	100%	1317
Plantation General Hospital[2]	Plantation	100%	668
Putnam Community Medical Center	Palatka	100%	228
Raulerson Hospital	Okeechobee	100%	141
Regional Medical Center Bayonet Point[2]	Hudson	100%	411
Sacred Heart Hospital[2]	Pensacola	100%	676
Sacred Heart Hosp-Emerald Coast[2]	Miramar Beach	100%	391
Saint Anthony's Hospital[2]	St Petersburg	100%	692
Saint Cloud Regional Medical Center	Saint Cloud	100%	82
Saint Joseph's Hospital[2]	Tampa	100%	1119
Saint Lucie Medical Center[2]	Port Saint Lucie	100%	510
Saint Mary's Medical Center[2]	W Palm Beach	100%	302
Saint Petersburg General Hospital[2]	St Petersburg	100%	296
Saint Vincent's Medical Center[2]	Jacksonville	100%	522
Saint Vincent's Medical Center Southside[2]	Jacksonville	100%	361
Santa Rosa Medical Center	Milton	100%	197
Sarasota Memorial Hospital[2]	Sarasota	100%	644
Sebastian River Medical Center	Sebastian	100%	524
Seven Rivers Regional Medical Center	Crystal River	100%	795
Shands Lake Shore Regional Medical Center	Lake City	100%	82
Shands Starke Regional Medical Center	Starke	100%	30
South Bay Hospital[2]	Sun City Center	100%	344
South Florida Baptist Hospital	Plant City	100%	444
South Lake Hospital	Clermont	100%	575
South Miami Hospital[2]	South Miami	100%	474
Tallahassee Memorial Hospital[2]	Tallahassee	100%	1355
Tampa General Hospital[2]	Tampa	100%	1268
Town & Country Hospital	Tampa	100%	204
Twin Cities Hospital	Niceville	100%	178
UF Health Jacksonville[2]	Jacksonville	100%	401
UF Health Shands Hospital[2]	Gainesville	100%	556
University Hospital & Medical Center[2]	Tamarac	100%	319
University of Miami Hospital	Miami	100%	1253
Venice Reg Med Ctr-Bayfront Health[2]	Venice	100%	502
Viera Hospital	Melbourne	100%	577
W Palm Beach VA Medical Center[2]	W Palm Beach	100%	170
Wellington Regional Medical Center[2]	Wellington	100%	434
West Boca Medical Center[2]	Boca Raton	100%	276
West Florida Hospital[2]	Pensacola	100%	537
West Kendall Baptist Hospital	Miami	100%	179
West Palm Hospital	W Palm Beach	100%	208
Westchester General Hospital[2]	Miami	100%	35
Westside Regional Medical Center[2]	Plantation	100%	483
Winter Haven Hospital[2]	Winter Haven	100%	417
Wuesthoff Medical Center - Melbourne[2]	Melbourne	100%	390
Wuesthoff Medical Center Rockledge[2]	Rockledge	100%	425
Florida Hospital Carrollwood[2]	Tampa	99%	324
Indian River Medical Center[2]	Vero Beach	99%	521
Lake Wales Medical Center	Lake Wales	99%	137
Lee Memorial Hospital[2]	Fort Myers	99%	657
Martin Medical Center[2]	Stuart	99%	488
Miami VA Medical Center[2]	Miami	99%	303
Munroe Regional Medical Center[2]	Ocala	99%	422
North Shore Medical Center	Miami	99%	392
VA N Florida/S Georgia Healthcare Sys[2]	Gainesville	99%	499
The Villages Regional Hospital	The Villages	99%	625
Larkin Community Hospital	South Miami	98%	44
Tampa VA Medical Center[2]	Tampa	96%	312

Prophylactic Antibiotic Selection

Hospital Name	City	Rate	Cases
Aventura Hospital & Medical Center[2]	Aventura	100%	381
Baptist Hospital[2]	Pensacola	100%	524
Baptist Hospital of Miami[2]	Miami	100%	455
Baptist Medical Center Beaches[2]	Jcksnvll Bch	100%	302
Bethesda Hospital East[2]	Boynton Beach	100%	390
Boca Raton Regional Hospital[2]	Boca Raton	100%	452
Brandon Regional Hospital[2]	Brandon	100%	459
Broward Health Coral Springs[2]	Coral Springs	100%	289
Broward Health Imperial Point	Fort Lauderdale	100%	268
Broward Health Medical Center[2]	Fort Lauderdale	100%	559
Capital Regional Medical Center	Tallahassee	100%	372
Central Florida Regional Hospital[2]	Sanford	100%	339
Cleveland Clinic Hospital[2]	Weston	100%	329
Delray Medical Center[2]	Delray Beach	100%	693
Doctor's Memorial Hospital	Perry	100%	48
Doctors Hospital	Coral Gables	100%	358
Doctors Hospital of Sarasota[2]	Sarasota	100%	276
Edward White Hospital	St Petersburg	100%	132
Fishermen's Hospital	Marathon	100%	32
Florida Hospital Deland	Deland	100%	419
Florida Hospital Fish Memorial	Orange City	100%	202
Florida Hospital Memorial Medical Center[2]	Daytona Bch	100%	771
Florida Hospital Waterman[2]	Tavares	100%	240
Florida Hospital Zephyrhills	Zephyrhills	100%	287
Fort Walton Beach Medical Center[2]	Fort Walton Bch	100%	346
Gulf Breeze Hospital[2]	Gulf Breeze	100%	229
Hialeah Hospital[2]	Hialeah	100%	170
Highlands Regional Medical Center[2]	Sebring	100%	107
Holmes Regional Medical Center[2]	Melbourne	100%	1137
Homestead Hospital	Homestead	100%	89
JFK Medical Center[2]	Atlantis	100%	505
Jupiter Medical Center[2]	Jupiter	100%	342
Kendall Regional Medical Center[2]	Miami	100%	409
Lake City Medical Center[2]	Lake City	100%	98
Largo Medical Center[2]	Largo	100%	371
Lawnwood Reg Med Ctr & Heart Inst	Fort Pierce	100%	394
Leesburg Regional Medical Center[2]	Leesburg	100%	802
Lehigh Regional Medical Center	Lehigh Acres	100%	118
Lower Keys Medical Center[2]	Key West	100%	110
Mariners Hospital	Tavernier	100%	29
Mease Countryside Hospital[2]	Safety Harbor	100%	437
Mease Hospital Dunedin[2]	Dunedin	100%	189
Medical Center of Trinity[2]	Trinity	100%	284
Memorial Hospital Pembroke[2]	Pembroke Pines	100%	200
Memorial Hospital West[2]	Pembroke Pines	100%	300
Memorial Regional Hospital[2]	Hollywood	100%	530
Morton Plant Hospital[2]	Clearwater	100%	1450
North Florida Regional Medical Center[2]	Gainesville	100%	573
North Okaloosa Medical Center	Crestview	100%	149
Northside Hospital[2]	St Petersburg	100%	222
Oak Hill Hospital[2]	Brooksville	100%	352
Ocala Regional Medical Center[2]	Ocala	100%	476
Orange Park Medical Center[2]	Orange Park	100%	286
Palm Bay Hospital	Palm Bay	100%	264
Palms of Pasadena Hospital	St Petersburg	100%	284
Palms West Hospital[2]	Loxahatchee	100%	215
Parrish Medical Center	Titusville	100%	238
Raulerson Hospital	Okeechobee	100%	59
Regional Medical Center Bayonet Point[2]	Hudson	100%	349
Sacred Heart Hosp-Emerald Coast[2]	Miramar Beach	100%	297
Saint Cloud Regional Medical Center	Saint Cloud	100%	28
Saint Lucie Medical Center[2]	Port Saint Lucie	100%	324
Saint Vincent's Medical Center[2]	Jacksonville	100%	473
Saint Vincent's Medical Center Southside[2]	Jacksonville	100%	216
Santa Rosa Medical Center	Milton	100%	110
Sarasota Memorial Hospital[2]	Sarasota	100%	567
Sebastian River Medical Center	Sebastian	100%	279
South Bay Hospital[2]	Sun City Center	100%	193
South Florida Baptist Hospital	Plant City	100%	281
South Lake Hospital	Clermont	100%	408
Tallahassee Memorial Hospital[2]	Tallahassee	100%	1189
Town & Country Hospital	Tampa	100%	91
Twin Cities Hospital	Niceville	100%	121
UF Health Jacksonville[2]	Jacksonville	100%	367
UF Health Shands Hospital[2]	Gainesville	100%	383
University Hospital & Medical Center[2]	Tamarac	100%	195
Venice Reg Med Ctr-Bayfront Health[2]	Venice	100%	476
Viera Hospital	Melbourne	100%	385
West Florida Hospital[2]	Pensacola	100%	388
West Kendall Baptist Hospital	Miami	100%	81
West Palm Hospital	W Palm Beach	100%	117
Winter Haven Hospital[2]	Winter Haven	100%	384
Wuesthoff Medical Center - Melbourne[2]	Melbourne	100%	275
Baptist Medical Center[2]	Jacksonville	99%	747
Bay Med Ctr Sacred Heart Health Sys[2]	Panama City	99%	630
Bay Pines VA Medical Center	Bay Pines	99%	230
Bayfront Health Brooksville	Brooksville	99%	309
Bayfront Health Port Charlotte[2]	Port Charlotte	99%	469
Bert Fish Medical Center	New Smyrn Bch	99%	192
Broward Health North[2]	Pompano Bch	99%	258
Cape Canaveral Hospital[2]	Cocoa Beach	99%	258
Coral Gables Hospital[2]	Coral Gables	99%	263
Englewood Community Hospital	Englewood	99%	106
Fawcett Memorial Hospital[2]	Port Charlotte	99%	290
Flagler Hospital[2]	St Augustine	99%	347
Florida Hospital[2]	Orlando	99%	4027
Florida Hospital Carrollwood[2]	Tampa	99%	202
Florida Hospital Flagler	Palm Coast	99%	308
Florida Hospital Heartland Medical Center	Sebring	99%	306
Gulf Coast Regional Medical Center[2]	Panama City	99%	318
Halifax Health Medical Center[2]	Daytona Bch	99%	741
Health Central	Ocoee	99%	493
Holy Cross Hospital[2]	Fort Lauderdale	99%	544
Jackson Memorial Hospital[2]	Miami	99%	540
Lakewood Ranch Medical Center[2]	Bradenton	99%	338
Manatee Memorial Hospital[2]	Bradenton	99%	447
Mayo Clinic[2]	Jacksonville	99%	460
Memorial Hospital Jacksonville[2]	Jacksonville	99%	537
Memorial Hospital Miramar[2]	Miramar	99%	138
Miami VA Medical Center	Miami	99%	172
Morton Plant North Bay Hospital[2]	New Port Richey	99%	85
Mount Sinai Medical Center[2]	Miami Beach	99%	1122
North Shore Medical Center	Miami	99%	263
Northwest Medical Center[2]	Margate	99%	238
Osceola Regional Medical Center[2]	Kissimmee	99%	389
Palm Beach Gardens Medical Center	Palm Bch Grdns	99%	431
Palm Springs General Hospital	Hialeah	99%	77
Putnam Community Medical Center	Palatka	99%	160
Sacred Heart Hospital[2]	Pensacola	99%	483
Saint Anthony's Hospital[2]	St Petersburg	99%	513
Saint Joseph's Hospital[2]	Tampa	99%	889
Saint Petersburg General Hospital[2]	St Petersburg	99%	172
Seven Rivers Regional Medical Center	Crystal River	99%	613
South Miami Hospital[2]	South Miami	99%	342
Tampa VA Medical Center	Tampa	99%	256
VA N Florida/S Georgia Healthcare Sys	Gainesville	99%	473
West Boca Medical Center[2]	Boca Raton	99%	173
Westside Regional Medical Center[2]	Plantation	99%	358
Wuesthoff Medical Center Rockledge[2]	Rockledge	99%	364
Bayfront Health - Saint Petersburg[2]	St Petersburg	98%	321
Blake Medical Center[2]	Bradenton	98%	415
Florida Hospital North Pinellas[2]	Tarpon Springs	98%	162
Florida Hospital Tampa[2]	Tampa	98%	277
Good Samaritan Medical Center[2]	W Palm Beach	98%	278
Gulf Coast Med Ctr Lee Mem Health Sys[2]	Fort Myers	98%	424
Indian River Medical Center[2]	Vero Beach	98%	468
Lakeland Regional Medical Center[2]	Lakeland	98%	554
Martin Medical Center[2]	Stuart	98%	388
Munroe Regional Medical Center[2]	Ocala	98%	386
Naples Community Hospital[2]	Naples	98%	629
Orlando Health[2]	Orlando	98%	2012
Palmetto General Hospital[2]	Hialeah	98%	533
Plantation General Hospital[2]	Plantation	98%	494
Tampa General Hospital[2]	Tampa	98%	817
University of Miami Hospital	Miami	98%	490
The Villages Regional Hospital	The Villages	98%	337
W Palm Beach VA Medical Center	W Palm Beach	98%	90
Bayfront Health Punta Gorda[2]	Punta Gorda	97%	170
Citrus Memorial Hospital	Inverness	97%	549
Jackson Hospital	Marianna	97%	118
Lake Wales Medical Center	Lake Wales	97%	58
Lee Memorial Hospital[2]	Fort Myers	97%	583
Wellington Regional Medical Center[2]	Wellington	97%	251
Bartow Regional Medical Center	Bartow	96%	114
Heart of Florida Regional Medical Center	Davenport	96%	618
Memorial Hospital of Tampa	Tampa	96%	139
Saint Mary's Medical Center[2]	W Palm Beach	96%	196
Cape Coral Hospital[2]	Cape Coral	95%	289
Bayfront Health Dade City	Dade City	94%	89
Metropolitan Hospital of Miami	Miami	93%	123
Shands Lake Shore Regional Medical Center	Lake City	93%	46
Physicians Reg Med Ctr-Pine Ridge	Naples	92%	816
Baptist Medical Center - Nassau[2]	Fernandina Bch	91%	55

Prophylactic Antibiotic Selection (Outpatient)

Hospital Name	City	Rate	Cases
Baptist Hospital of Miami	Miami	100%	682
Boca Raton Regional Hospital	Boca Raton	100%	534
Cape Canaveral Hospital	Cocoa Beach	100%	95
Edward White Hospital	St Petersburg	100%	45
Englewood Community Hospital	Englewood	100%	42
Florida Hospital Wesley Chapel[3]	Wesley Chapel	100%	25
Fort Walton Beach Medical Center	Fort Walton Bch	100%	167
Hialeah Hospital	Hialeah	100%	65
JFK Medical Center	Atlantis	100%	516
Lake City Medical Center	Lake City	100%	40
Lawnwood Reg Med Ctr & Heart Inst	Fort Pierce	100%	273
Lower Keys Medical Center	Key West	100%	49
Mease Hospital Dunedin	Dunedin	100%	71
Memorial Hospital Miramar	Miramar	100%	353
Memorial Hospital West	Pembroke Pines	100%	370
Memorial Regional Hospital	Hollywood	100%	314
North Florida Regional Medical Center	Gainesville	100%	741
Northside Hospital	St Petersburg	100%	203
Ocala Regional Medical Center	Ocala	100%	324
Palm Beach Gardens Medical Center	Palm Bch Grdns	100%	375
Putnam Community Medical Center	Palatka	100%	87
Raulerson Hospital	Okeechobee	100%	100
Regional Medical Center Bayonet Point	Hudson	100%	303

NOTE: Hospital profiles are in alphabetical order by state, then city, then hospital within the city; Rankings exclude hospitals with less than 25 cases except for patient surveys which excludes hospitals with less than 100 cases; (a) 100-299 cases; (1) The number of cases/patients is too few to report; (2) Data submitted were based on a sample of cases/patients; (3) Results are based on a shorter time period than required; (4) Data suppressed by CMS for one or more quarters; (5) Results are not available for this reporting period; (6) Fewer than 100 patients completed the HCAHPS survey; (7) No cases met the criteria for this measure; (8) The lower limit of the confidence interval cannot be calculated if the number of observed infections equals zero; (9) No data are available from the state/territory for this reporting period; (10) The scores shown reflect fewer than 50 completed surveys; (11) There were discrepancies in the data collection process; (12) This measure does not apply to this hospital for this reporting period; (13) Results cannot be calculated for this reporting period; (14) The results for this state are combined with nearby states to protect confidentiality; Please refer to the User's Guide for a full explanation of data.

Hospital Name	City	Rate	Cases
Saint Lucie Medical Center	Port Saint Lucie	100%	80
Santa Rosa Medical Center	Milton	100%	151
Sebastian River Medical Center	Sebastian	100%	138
South Miami Hospital	South Miami	100%	732
Twin Cities Hospital	Niceville	100%	25
Venice Reg Med Ctr-Bayfront Health	Venice	100%	460
West Boca Medical Center	Boca Raton	100%	287
West Kendall Baptist Hospital	Miami	100%	25
West Palm Hospital	W Palm Beach	100%	51
Westside Regional Medical Center	Plantation	100%	209
Bayfront Health - Saint Petersburg	St Petersburg	99%	303
Bert Fish Medical Center	New Smyrn Bch	99%	67
Blake Medical Center	Bradenton	99%	292
Brandon Regional Hospital	Brandon	99%	482
Broward Health Coral Springs	Coral Springs	99%	132
Broward Health Imperial Point	Fort Lauderdale	99%	184
Capital Regional Medical Center	Tallahassee	99%	320
Coral Gables Hospital	Coral Gables	99%	399
Delray Medical Center	Delray Beach	99%	564
Doctors Hospital	Coral Gables	99%	359
Doctors Hospital of Sarasota	Sarasota	99%	350
Fawcett Memorial Hospital	Port Charlotte	99%	321
Flagler Hospital	St Augustine	99%	233
Florida Hospital Deland	Deland	99%	73
Florida Hospital North Pinellas	Tarpon Springs	99%	76
Florida Hospital Waterman	Tavares	99%	306
Gulf Coast Regional Medical Center	Panama City	99%	378
Holy Cross Hospital	Fort Lauderdale	99%	474
Kendall Regional Medical Center	Miami	99%	154
Largo Medical Center	Largo	99%	564
Memorial Hospital Jacksonville	Jacksonville	99%	451
Memorial Hospital Pembroke	Pembroke Pines	99%	134
North Okaloosa Medical Center	Crestview	99%	114
Northwest Medical Center	Margate	99%	303
Oak Hill Hospital	Brooksville	99%	167
Orange Park Medical Center	Orange Park	99%	486
Orlando Health	Orlando	99%	982
Osceola Regional Medical Center	Kissimmee	99%	295
Parrish Medical Center	Titusville	99%	144
Physicians Reg Med Ctr-Pine Ridge	Naples	99%	534
Sacred Heart Hosp-Emerald Coast	Miramar Beach	99%	195
Saint Petersburg General Hospital	St Petersburg	99%	239
Saint Vincent's Medical Center Southside	Jacksonville	99%	424
Tallahassee Memorial Hospital	Tallahassee	99%	1211
UF Health Jacksonville	Jacksonville	99%	272
UF Health Shands Hospital	Gainesville	99%	423
West Florida Hospital	Pensacola	99%	378
Winter Haven Hospital	Winter Haven	99%	550
Aventura Hospital & Medical Center	Aventura	98%	247
Baptist Hospital	Pensacola	98%	571
Baptist Medical Center	Jacksonville	98%	946
Bay Med Ctr Sacred Heart Health Sys	Panama City	98%	424
Bayfront Health Punta Gorda	Punta Gorda	98%	105
Broward Health Medical Center	Fort Lauderdale	98%	341
Central Florida Regional Hospital	Sanford	98%	198
Citrus Memorial Hospital	Inverness	98%	296
Florida Hospital Carrollwood	Tampa	98%	129
Florida Hospital Fish Memorial	Orange City	98%	133
Gulf Breeze Hospital	Gulf Breeze	98%	143
Health Central	Ocoee	98%	196
Holmes Regional Medical Center	Melbourne	98%	699
Jupiter Medical Center	Jupiter	98%	366
Lakewood Ranch Medical Center	Bradenton	98%	116
Lee Memorial Hospital	Fort Myers	98%	702
Mease Countryside Hospital	Safety Harbor	98%	358
Medical Center of Trinity	Trinity	98%	161
Morton Plant Hospital	Clearwater	98%	645
Mount Sinai Medical Center	Miami Beach	98%	696
North Shore Medical Center	Miami	98%	156
Palmetto General Hospital	Hialeah	98%	455
Saint Cloud Regional Medical Center	Saint Cloud	98%	48
Saint Joseph's Hospital	Tampa	98%	414
Saint Vincent's Medical Center	Jacksonville	98%	725
Sarasota Memorial Hospital	Sarasota	98%	881
Bayfront Health Brooksville	Brooksville	97%	185
Bayfront Health Port Charlotte	Port Charlotte	97%	401
Cape Coral Hospital	Cape Coral	97%	361
Cleveland Clinic Hospital	Weston	97%	761
Florida Hospital Heartland Medical Center	Sebring	97%	102
Florida Hospital Zephyrhills	Zephyrhills	97%	257
Gulf Coast Med Ctr Lee Mem Health Sys	Fort Myers	97%	417
Halifax Health Medical Center	Daytona Bch	97%	663
Indian River Medical Center	Vero Beach	97%	224
Naples Community Hospital	Naples	97%	592
Palm Springs General Hospital	Hialeah	97%	167
Palms West Hospital	Loxahatchee	97%	197
Plantation General Hospital	Plantation	97%	361
Sacred Heart Hospital	Pensacola	97%	444
South Bay Hospital	Sun City Center	97%	78
South Lake Hospital	Clermont	97%	109
University Hospital & Medical Center	Tamarac	97%	29
Wuesthoff Medical Center Rockledge	Rockledge	97%	342
Bartow Regional Medical Center	Bartow	96%	81
Florida Hospital	Orlando	96%	2257
Florida Hospital Memorial Medical Center	Daytona Bch	96%	715
Highlands Regional Medical Center	Sebring	96%	138
Lake Wales Medical Center	Lake Wales	96%	54
Lakeland Regional Medical Center	Lakeland	96%	533
Leesburg Regional Medical Center	Leesburg	96%	397
Martin Medical Center	Stuart	96%	573
Munroe Regional Medical Center	Ocala	96%	545
Saint Anthony's Hospital	St Petersburg	96%	293
Viera Hospital	Melbourne	96%	69
The Villages Regional Hospital	The Villages	96%	515
Wellington Regional Medical Center	Wellington	96%	98
Bayfront Health Dade City	Dade City	95%	141
Broward Health North	Pompano Bch	95%	199
Heart of Florida Regional Medical Center	Davenport	95%	245
Jackson Memorial Hospital	Miami	95%	432
Manatee Memorial Hospital	Bradenton	95%	351
Bethesda Hospital East	Boynton Beach	94%	342
Town & Country Hospital	Tampa	94%	51
University of Miami Hospital	Miami	94%	327
Morton Plant North Bay Hospital	New Port Richey	93%	55
Seven Rivers Regional Medical Center	Crystal River	93%	103
Baptist Medical Center Beaches	Jcksnvl Bch	92%	91
Florida Hospital Flagler	Palm Coast	92%	101
Florida Hospital Tampa	Tampa	92%	421
Good Samaritan Medical Center	W Palm Beach	92%	286
South Florida Baptist Hospital	Plant City	89%	76
Wuesthoff Medical Center - Melbourne	Melbourne	88%	235
Mayo Clinic	Jacksonville	87%	515
Tampa General Hospital	Tampa	86%	592
Baptist Medical Center - Nassau	Fernandina Bch	78%	27
Palm Bay Hospital	Palm Bay	68%	25

Prophylactic Antibiotic Stopped

Hospital Name	City	Rate	Cases
Baptist Hospital[2]	Pensacola	100%	515
Baptist Hospital of Miami[2]	Miami	100%	445
Bartow Regional Medical Center	Bartow	100%	107
Blake Medical Center[2]	Bradenton	100%	397
Boca Raton Regional Hospital[2]	Boca Raton	100%	305
Broward Health Imperial Point	Fort Lauderdale	100%	256
Broward Health Medical Center[2]	Fort Lauderdale	100%	535
Broward Health North[2]	Pompano Bch	100%	250
Capital Regional Medical Center	Tallahassee	100%	362
Coral Gables Hospital[2]	Coral Gables	100%	252
Englewood Community Hospital	Englewood	100%	103
Fawcett Memorial Hospital[2]	Port Charlotte	100%	266
Florida Hospital Flagler	Palm Coast	100%	296
Gulf Breeze Hospital[2]	Gulf Breeze	100%	224
JFK Medical Center[2]	Atlantis	100%	470
Jupiter Medical Center[2]	Jupiter	100%	337
Lake City Medical Center[2]	Lake City	100%	95
Lawnwood Reg Med Ctr & Heart Inst	Fort Pierce	100%	362
Lehigh Regional Medical Center	Lehigh Acres	100%	114
Medical Center of Trinity[2]	Trinity	100%	266
Memorial Hospital Miramar[2]	Miramar	100%	136
Memorial Hospital Pembroke[2]	Pembroke Pines	100%	186
Memorial Hospital West[2]	Pembroke Pines	100%	291
Metropolitan Hospital of Miami	Miami	100%	123
Morton Plant Hospital[2]	Clearwater	100%	1412
North Florida Regional Medical Center[2]	Gainesville	100%	565
Northwest Medical Center[2]	Margate	100%	227
Oak Hill Hospital[2]	Brooksville	100%	341
Ocala Regional Medical Center[2]	Ocala	100%	445
Orange Park Medical Center[2]	Orange Park	100%	275
Osceola Regional Medical Center[2]	Kissimmee	100%	379
Parrish Medical Center	Titusville	100%	238
Raulerson Hospital	Okeechobee	100%	49
Saint Cloud Regional Medical Center	Saint Cloud	100%	26
Saint Lucie Medical Center[2]	Port Saint Lucie	100%	276
Saint Vincent's Medical Center Southside[2]	Jacksonville	100%	213
Santa Rosa Medical Center	Milton	100%	105
Sebastian River Medical Center	Sebastian	100%	279
Shands Lake Shore Regional Medical Center	Lake City	100%	46
South Miami Hospital[2]	South Miami	100%	321
Tallahassee Memorial Hospital[2]	Tallahassee	100%	1173
Venice Reg Med Ctr-Bayfront Health[2]	Venice	100%	446
Wellington Regional Medical Center[2]	Wellington	100%	242
West Boca Medical Center[2]	Boca Raton	100%	170
West Florida Hospital[2]	Pensacola	100%	359
West Kendall Baptist Hospital	Miami	100%	76
West Palm Hospital	W Palm Beach	100%	107
Aventura Hospital & Medical Center[2]	Aventura	99%	357
Bay Med Ctr Sacred Heart Health Sys[2]	Panama City	99%	619
Bayfront Health - Saint Petersburg[2]	St Petersburg	99%	311
Bayfront Health Punta Gorda[2]	Punta Gorda	99%	166
Brandon Regional Hospital[2]	Brandon	99%	440
Broward Health Coral Springs[2]	Coral Springs	99%	278
Cape Canaveral Hospital[2]	Cocoa Beach	99%	257
Central Florida Regional Hospital[2]	Sanford	99%	323
Cleveland Clinic Hospital[2]	Weston	99%	320
Delray Medical Center[2]	Delray Beach	99%	675
Doctors Hospital	Coral Gables	99%	340
Flagler Hospital[2]	St Augustine	99%	336
Florida Hospital[2]	Orlando	99%	3817
Florida Hospital Carrollwood[2]	Tampa	99%	191
Florida Hospital Deland	Deland	99%	407
Florida Hospital Memorial Medical Center[2]	Daytona Bch	99%	746
Florida Hospital Waterman[2]	Tavares	99%	222
Florida Hospital Zephyrhills	Zephyrhills	99%	273
Fort Walton Beach Medical Center[2]	Fort Walton Bch	99%	327
Gulf Coast Regional Medical Center[2]	Panama City	99%	195
Halifax Health Medical Center[2]	Daytona Bch	99%	719
Health Central	Ocoee	99%	475
Highlands Regional Medical Center[2]	Sebring	99%	97
Holmes Regional Medical Center[2]	Melbourne	99%	1111
Holy Cross Hospital[2]	Fort Lauderdale	99%	537
Homestead Hospital	Homestead	99%	87
Kendall Regional Medical Center[2]	Miami	99%	390
Largo Medical Center[2]	Largo	99%	353
Lower Keys Medical Center[2]	Key West	99%	108
Mease Countryside Hospital[2]	Safety Harbor	99%	430
Memorial Hospital Jacksonville[2]	Jacksonville	99%	483
Memorial Hospital of Tampa	Tampa	99%	130
Memorial Regional Hospital[2]	Hollywood	99%	502
Morton Plant North Bay Hospital[2]	New Port Richey	99%	83
Palm Bay Hospital	Palm Bay	99%	261
Palm Beach Gardens Medical Center	Palm Bch Grdns	99%	394
Palmetto General Hospital[2]	Hialeah	99%	511
Palms of Pasadena Hospital	St Petersburg	99%	283
Palms West Hospital[2]	Loxahatchee	99%	183
Plantation General Hospital[2]	Plantation	99%	479
Saint Mary's Medical Center[2]	W Palm Beach	99%	183
Saint Petersburg General Hospital[2]	St Petersburg	99%	165
Saint Vincent's Medical Center[2]	Jacksonville	99%	457
Sarasota Memorial Hospital[2]	Sarasota	99%	544
Seven Rivers Regional Medical Center	Crystal River	99%	610
South Bay Hospital[2]	Sun City Center	99%	188
South Florida Baptist Hospital	Plant City	99%	268
Town & Country Hospital	Tampa	99%	88
Twin Cities Hospital	Niceville	99%	120
UF Health Jacksonville[2]	Jacksonville	99%	357
University Hospital & Medical Center[2]	Tamarac	99%	192
Viera Hospital	Melbourne	99%	382
Westside Regional Medical Center[2]	Plantation	99%	347
Baptist Medical Center[2]	Jacksonville	98%	731
Baptist Medical Center Beaches[2]	Jcksnvl Bch	98%	294
Doctor's Memorial Hospital	Perry	98%	48
Doctors Hospital of Sarasota[2]	Sarasota	98%	275
Edward White Hospital	St Petersburg	98%	126
Florida Hospital Fish Memorial	Orange City	98%	194
Florida Hospital North Pinellas[2]	Tarpon Springs	98%	160
Florida Hospital Tampa[2]	Tampa	98%	273
Jackson Hospital	Marianna	98%	116
Lakewood Ranch Medical Center[2]	Bradenton	98%	334
Leesburg Regional Medical Center[2]	Leesburg	98%	794
Manatee Memorial Hospital[2]	Bradenton	98%	424
Mease Hospital Dunedin[2]	Dunedin	98%	183
Mount Sinai Medical Center[2]	Miami Beach	98%	1107
Northside Hospital[2]	St Petersburg	98%	211
Orlando Health[2]	Orlando	98%	1956
Putnam Community Medical Center	Palatka	98%	159
Regional Medical Center Bayonet Point[2]	Hudson	98%	330
Saint Anthony's Hospital[2]	St Petersburg	98%	496
Saint Joseph's Hospital[2]	Tampa	98%	853
South Lake Hospital	Clermont	98%	393
UF Health Shands Hospital[2]	Gainesville	98%	365
The Villages Regional Hospital	The Villages	98%	326
Winter Haven Hospital[2]	Winter Haven	98%	376
Bay Pines VA Medical Center	Bay Pines	97%	222
Bayfront Health Brooksville	Brooksville	97%	291
Bayfront Health Dade City	Dade City	97%	74
Florida Hospital Heartland Medical Center	Sebring	97%	302
Jackson Memorial Hospital[2]	Miami	97%	520
Lakeland Regional Medical Center[2]	Lakeland	97%	527
Martin Medical Center[2]	Stuart	97%	370
Mayo Clinic[2]	Jacksonville	97%	428
North Okaloosa Medical Center	Crestview	97%	136
North Shore Medical Center	Miami	97%	245
Sacred Heart Hospital[2]	Pensacola	97%	462
Sacred Heart Hosp-Emerald Coast[2]	Miramar Beach	97%	293
Tampa General Hospital[2]	Tampa	97%	786
W Palm Beach VA Medical Center	W Palm Beach	97%	88
Bayfront Health Port Charlotte[2]	Port Charlotte	96%	439
Bethesda Hospital East[2]	Boynton Beach	96%	383
Citrus Memorial Hospital	Inverness	96%	541
Good Samaritan Medical Center[2]	W Palm Beach	96%	252
Indian River Medical Center[2]	Vero Beach	96%	452
Lake Wales Medical Center	Lake Wales	96%	56
Mariners Hospital	Tavernier	96%	26

NOTE: Hospital profiles are in alphabetical order by state, then city, then hospital within the city; Rankings exclude hospitals with less than 25 cases except for patient surveys which excludes hospitals with less than 100 cases; (a) 100-299 cases; (1) The number of cases/patients is too few to report; (2) Data submitted were based on a sample of cases/patients; (3) Results are based on a shorter time period than required; (4) Data suppressed by CMS for one or more quarters; (5) Results are not available for this reporting period; (6) Fewer than 100 patients completed the HCAHPS survey; (7) No cases met the criteria for this measure; (8) The lower limit of the confidence interval cannot be calculated if the number of observed infections equals zero; (9) No data are available from the state/territory for this reporting period; (10) The scores shown reflect fewer than 50 completed surveys; (11) There were discrepancies in the data collection process; (12) This measure does not apply to this hospital for this reporting period; (13) Results cannot be calculated for this reporting period; (14) The results for this state are combined with nearby states to protect confidentiality; Please refer to the User's Guide for a full explanation of data.

Hospital Name	City	Rate	Cases
VA N Florida/S Georgia Healthcare Sys	Gainesville	96%	457
Gulf Coast Med Ctr Lee Mem Health Sys[2]	Fort Myers	95%	403
Naples Community Hospital[2]	Naples	95%	608
Tampa VA Medical Center	Tampa	95%	252
Wuesthoff Medical Center Rockledge[2]	Rockledge	95%	350
Bert Fish Medical Center	New Smyrn Bch	94%	189
Fishermen's Hospital	Marathon	94%	31
Munroe Regional Medical Center[2]	Ocala	94%	373
University of Miami Hospital	Miami	94%	478
Lee Memorial Hospital[2]	Fort Myers	93%	562
Heart of Florida Regional Medical Center	Davenport	92%	573
Miami VA Medical Center	Miami	91%	169
Physicians Reg Med Ctr-Pine Ridge	Naples	91%	787
Cape Coral Hospital[2]	Cape Coral	90%	275
Hialeah Hospital[2]	Hialeah	90%	163
Baptist Medical Center - Nassau[2]	Fernandina Bch	89%	53
Wuesthoff Medical Center - Melbourne[2]	Melbourne	89%	268
Palm Springs General Hospital	Hialeah	88%	77

Prophylactic Antibiotic Timing

Hospital Name	City	Rate	Cases
Baptist Hospital[2]	Pensacola	100%	526
Baptist Hospital of Miami[2]	Miami	100%	456
Bay Med Ctr Sacred Heart Health Sys[2]	Panama City	100%	631
Bayfront Health Punta Gorda[2]	Punta Gorda	100%	170
Blake Medical Center[2]	Bradenton	100%	415
Boca Raton Regional Hospital[2]	Boca Raton	100%	310
Brandon Regional Hospital[2]	Brandon	100%	454
Broward Health Coral Springs[2]	Coral Springs	100%	292
Broward Health Imperial Point	Fort Lauderdale	100%	268
Broward Health Medical Center[2]	Fort Lauderdale	100%	559
Broward Health North[2]	Pompano Bch	100%	258
Cape Canaveral Hospital[2]	Cocoa Beach	100%	258
Capital Regional Medical Center	Tallahassee	100%	372
Coral Gables Hospital[2]	Coral Gables	100%	263
Delray Medical Center[2]	Delray Beach	100%	694
Doctor's Memorial Hospital	Perry	100%	48
Doctors Hospital	Coral Gables	100%	358
Doctors Hospital of Sarasota[2]	Sarasota	100%	277
Edward White Hospital	St Petersburg	100%	132
Englewood Community Hospital	Englewood	100%	106
Fawcett Memorial Hospital[2]	Port Charlotte	100%	290
Fishermen's Hospital	Marathon	100%	32
Florida Hospital[2]	Orlando	100%	4036
Florida Hospital Deland	Deland	100%	419
Florida Hospital Fish Memorial	Orange City	100%	202
Florida Hospital Flagler	Palm Coast	100%	308
Florida Hospital Memorial Medical Center[2]	Daytona Bch	100%	772
Florida Hospital Tampa[2]	Tampa	100%	279
Florida Hospital Waterman[2]	Tavares	100%	240
Florida Hospital Zephyrhills	Zephyrhills	100%	289
Fort Walton Beach Medical Center[2]	Fort Walton Bch	100%	348
Gulf Breeze Hospital[2]	Gulf Breeze	100%	229
Gulf Coast Regional Medical Center[2]	Panama City	100%	318
Halifax Health Medical Center[2]	Daytona Bch	100%	745
Health Central	Ocoee	100%	493
Highlands Regional Medical Center[2]	Sebring	100%	107
Holy Cross Hospital[2]	Fort Lauderdale	100%	545
Homestead Hospital	Homestead	100%	89
Jackson Memorial Hospital[2]	Miami	100%	540
JFK Medical Center[2]	Atlantis	100%	507
Jupiter Medical Center[2]	Jupiter	100%	343
Kendall Regional Medical Center[2]	Miami	100%	409
Lake City Medical Center[2]	Lake City	100%	98
Lake Wales Medical Center	Lake Wales	100%	58
Lawnwood Reg Med Ctr & Heart Inst	Fort Pierce	100%	395
Lehigh Regional Medical Center	Lehigh Acres	100%	118
Lower Keys Medical Center[2]	Key West	100%	110
Mariners Hospital	Tavernier	100%	31
Mease Hospital Dunedin[2]	Dunedin	100%	189
Medical Center of Trinity[2]	Trinity	100%	283
Memorial Hospital Jacksonville[2]	Jacksonville	100%	537
Memorial Hospital Miramar[2]	Miramar	100%	138
Memorial Hospital West[2]	Pembroke Pines	100%	301
Memorial Regional Hospital[2]	Hollywood	100%	531
Mount Sinai Medical Center[2]	Miami Beach	100%	1122
North Florida Regional Medical Center[2]	Gainesville	100%	574
North Shore Medical Center	Miami	100%	263
Northside Hospital[2]	St Petersburg	100%	222
Northwest Medical Center[2]	Margate	100%	240
Oak Hill Hospital[2]	Brooksville	100%	352
Ocala Regional Medical Center[2]	Ocala	100%	477
Orange Park Medical Center[2]	Orange Park	100%	286
Palm Beach Gardens Medical Center	Palm Bch Grdns	100%	431
Palm Springs General Hospital	Hialeah	100%	77
Palms of Pasadena Hospital	St Petersburg	100%	284
Palms West Hospital[2]	Loxahatchee	100%	215
Plantation General Hospital[2]	Plantation	100%	494
Putnam Community Medical Center	Palatka	100%	160
Raulerson Hospital	Okeechobee	100%	59
Sacred Heart Hosp-Emerald Coast[2]	Miramar Beach	100%	297
Saint Anthony's Hospital[2]	St Petersburg	100%	514
Saint Cloud Regional Medical Center	Saint Cloud	100%	28
Saint Lucie Medical Center[2]	Port Saint Lucie	100%	324
Saint Petersburg General Hospital[2]	St Petersburg	100%	172
Saint Vincent's Medical Center[2]	Jacksonville	100%	477
Saint Vincent's Medical Center Southside[2]	Jacksonville	100%	216
Santa Rosa Medical Center	Milton	100%	110
Sarasota Memorial Hospital[2]	Sarasota	100%	570
Sebastian River Medical Center	Sebastian	100%	280
South Lake Hospital	Clermont	100%	408
South Miami Hospital[2]	South Miami	100%	344
Tallahassee Memorial Hospital[2]	Tallahassee	100%	1194
Town & Country Hospital	Tampa	100%	91
Twin Cities Hospital	Niceville	100%	121
UF Health Shands Hospital[2]	Gainesville	100%	387
University Hospital & Medical Center[2]	Tamarac	100%	195
Venice Reg Med Ctr-Bayfront Health[2]	Venice	100%	476
Viera Hospital	Melbourne	100%	385
Wellington Regional Medical Center[2]	Wellington	100%	251
West Boca Medical Center[2]	Boca Raton	100%	173
West Florida Hospital[2]	Pensacola	100%	389
West Kendall Baptist Hospital	Miami	100%	81
West Palm Hospital	W Palm Beach	100%	117
Westside Regional Medical Center[2]	Plantation	100%	359
Aventura Hospital & Medical Center[2]	Aventura	99%	382
Bay Pines VA Medical Center	Bay Pines	99%	230
Bayfront Health - Saint Petersburg[2]	St Petersburg	99%	321
Bayfront Health Brooksville	Brooksville	99%	310
Bayfront Health Port Charlotte[2]	Port Charlotte	99%	470
Bethesda Hospital East[2]	Boynton Beach	99%	390
Cape Coral Hospital[2]	Cape Coral	99%	289
Central Florida Regional Hospital[2]	Sanford	99%	340
Cleveland Clinic Hospital[2]	Weston	99%	330
Florida Hospital Carrollwood[2]	Tampa	99%	203
Florida Hospital North Pinellas[2]	Tarpon Springs	99%	162
Good Samaritan Medical Center[2]	W Palm Beach	99%	279
Gulf Coast Med Ctr Lee Mem Health Sys[2]	Fort Myers	99%	425
Holmes Regional Medical Center[2]	Melbourne	99%	1137
Jackson Hospital	Marianna	99%	118
Lakeland Regional Medical Center[2]	Lakeland	99%	555
Largo Medical Center[2]	Largo	99%	371
Mayo Clinic[2]	Jacksonville	99%	460
Memorial Hospital Pembroke[2]	Pembroke Pines	99%	200
Metropolitan Hospital of Miami	Miami	99%	123
Miami VA Medical Center	Miami	99%	172
Morton Plant Hospital[2]	Clearwater	99%	1459
Morton Plant North Bay Hospital[2]	New Port Richey	99%	85
Naples Community Hospital[2]	Naples	99%	632
North Okaloosa Medical Center	Crestview	99%	150
Orlando Health[2]	Orlando	99%	2015
Osceola Regional Medical Center[2]	Kissimmee	99%	389
Palm Bay Hospital	Palm Bay	99%	264
Palmetto General Hospital[2]	Hialeah	99%	537
Parrish Medical Center	Titusville	99%	244
Physicians Reg Med Ctr-Pine Ridge	Naples	99%	816
Regional Medical Center Bayonet Point[2]	Hudson	99%	351
Sacred Heart Hospital[2]	Pensacola	99%	483
Saint Joseph's Hospital[2]	Tampa	99%	893
South Bay Hospital[2]	Sun City Center	99%	193
South Florida Baptist Hospital	Plant City	99%	281
UF Health Jacksonville[2]	Jacksonville	99%	367
University of Miami Hospital	Miami	99%	492
VA N Florida/S Georgia Healthcare Sys	Gainesville	99%	474
W Palm Beach VA Medical Center	W Palm Beach	99%	90
Wuesthoff Medical Center Rockledge[2]	Rockledge	99%	364
Baptist Medical Center[2]	Jacksonville	98%	749
Baptist Medical Center - Nassau[2]	Fernandina Bch	98%	55
Baptist Medical Center Beaches[2]	Jcksnvl Bch	98%	302
Bayfront Health Dade City	Dade City	98%	89
Citrus Memorial Hospital	Inverness	98%	550
Flagler Hospital[2]	St Augustine	98%	347
Florida Hospital Heartland Medical Center	Sebring	98%	307
Heart of Florida Regional Medical Center	Davenport	98%	620
Hialeah Hospital[2]	Hialeah	98%	170
Indian River Medical Center[2]	Vero Beach	98%	468
Lee Memorial Hospital[2]	Fort Myers	98%	584
Saint Mary's Medical Center[2]	W Palm Beach	98%	196
The Villages Regional Hospital	The Villages	98%	339
Winter Haven Hospital[2]	Winter Haven	98%	385
Wuesthoff Medical Center - Melbourne[2]	Melbourne	98%	277
Bartow Regional Medical Center	Bartow	97%	115
Bert Fish Medical Center	New Smyrn Bch	97%	192
Lakewood Ranch Medical Center[2]	Bradenton	97%	338
Leesburg Regional Medical Center[2]	Leesburg	97%	802
Manatee Memorial Hospital[2]	Bradenton	97%	450
Martin Medical Center[2]	Stuart	97%	391
Mease Countryside Hospital[2]	Safety Harbor	97%	438
Memorial Hospital of Tampa	Tampa	97%	140
Tampa VA Medical Center	Tampa	97%	258
Munroe Regional Medical Center[2]	Ocala	96%	387
Seven Rivers Regional Medical Center	Crystal River	96%	615
Tampa General Hospital[2]	Tampa	96%	822
Shands Lake Shore Regional Medical Center	Lake City	91%	46

Prophylactic Antibiotic Timing (Outpatient)

Hospital Name	City	Rate	Cases
Baptist Hospital of Miami	Miami	100%	677
Bay Med Ctr Sacred Heart Health Sys	Panama City	100%	425
Boca Raton Regional Hospital	Boca Raton	100%	534
Broward Health Coral Springs	Coral Springs	100%	132
Broward Health Imperial Point	Fort Lauderdale	100%	184
Central Florida Regional Hospital	Sanford	100%	198
Cleveland Clinic Hospital	Weston	100%	762
Delray Medical Center	Delray Beach	100%	564
Doctors Hospital of Sarasota	Sarasota	100%	350
Edward White Hospital	St Petersburg	100%	45
Englewood Community Hospital	Englewood	100%	42
Fawcett Memorial Hospital	Port Charlotte	100%	322
Florida Hospital Flagler	Palm Coast	100%	70
Florida Hospital Wesley Chapel[3]	Wesley Chapel	100%	25
Fort Walton Beach Medical Center	Fort Walton Bch	100%	167
Gulf Coast Regional Medical Center	Panama City	100%	378
Hialeah Hospital	Hialeah	100%	60
Highlands Regional Medical Center	Sebring	100%	138
Holy Cross Hospital	Fort Lauderdale	100%	474
JFK Medical Center	Atlantis	100%	517
Jupiter Medical Center	Jupiter	100%	365
Kendall Regional Medical Center	Miami	100%	154
Lake City Medical Center	Lake City	100%	40
Lake Wales Medical Center	Lake Wales	100%	54
Lakeland Regional Medical Center	Lakeland	100%	440
Largo Medical Center	Largo	100%	564
Lawnwood Reg Med Ctr & Heart Inst	Fort Pierce	100%	273
Mease Hospital Dunedin	Dunedin	100%	71
Medical Center of Trinity	Trinity	100%	161
Memorial Hospital Jacksonville	Jacksonville	100%	451
Memorial Hospital Miramar	Miramar	100%	353
Memorial Hospital Pembroke	Pembroke Pines	100%	134
Memorial Hospital West	Pembroke Pines	100%	370
North Florida Regional Medical Center	Gainesville	100%	741
Northwest Medical Center	Margate	100%	303
Oak Hill Hospital	Brooksville	100%	167
Ocala Regional Medical Center	Ocala	100%	324
Orange Park Medical Center	Orange Park	100%	486
Osceola Regional Medical Center	Kissimmee	100%	295
Palm Bay Hospital	Palm Bay	100%	25
Palm Beach Gardens Medical Center	Palm Bch Grdns	100%	375
Palmetto General Hospital	Hialeah	100%	455
Palms West Hospital	Loxahatchee	100%	197
Raulerson Hospital	Okeechobee	100%	100
Sacred Heart Hospital	Pensacola	100%	445
Saint Cloud Regional Medical Center	Saint Cloud	100%	48
Saint Lucie Medical Center	Port Saint Lucie	100%	80
Saint Petersburg General Hospital	St Petersburg	100%	239
Saint Vincent's Medical Center Southside	Jacksonville	100%	425
Santa Rosa Medical Center	Milton	100%	151
Sebastian River Medical Center	Sebastian	100%	138
South Miami Hospital	South Miami	100%	733
Twin Cities Hospital	Niceville	100%	25
University Hospital & Medical Center	Tamarac	100%	29
Venice Reg Med Ctr-Bayfront Health	Venice	100%	460
West Boca Medical Center	Boca Raton	100%	287
West Kendall Baptist Hospital	Miami	100%	25
West Palm Hospital	W Palm Beach	100%	51
Westside Regional Medical Center	Plantation	100%	209
Bayfront Health - Saint Petersburg	St Petersburg	99%	302
Bayfront Health Brooksville	Brooksville	99%	185
Bayfront Health Dade City	Dade City	99%	142
Bayfront Health Punta Gorda	Punta Gorda	99%	105
Blake Medical Center	Bradenton	99%	293
Brandon Regional Hospital	Brandon	99%	482
Broward Health Medical Center	Fort Lauderdale	99%	325
Capital Regional Medical Center	Tallahassee	99%	320
Coral Gables Hospital	Coral Gables	99%	401
Doctors Hospital	Coral Gables	99%	360
Florida Hospital	Orlando	99%	2266
Florida Hospital Deland	Deland	99%	74
Florida Hospital Tampa	Tampa	99%	423
Florida Hospital Waterman	Tavares	99%	306
Florida Hospital Zephyrhills	Zephyrhills	99%	257
Gulf Breeze Hospital	Gulf Breeze	99%	143
Halifax Health Medical Center	Daytona Bch	99%	666
Health Central	Ocoee	99%	197
Holmes Regional Medical Center	Melbourne	99%	702
Leesburg Regional Medical Center	Leesburg	99%	399
Martin Medical Center	Stuart	99%	575
Mease Countryside Hospital	Safety Harbor	99%	358
Memorial Regional Hospital	Hollywood	99%	314
Mount Sinai Medical Center	Miami Beach	99%	695
North Shore Medical Center	Miami	99%	157
Northside Hospital	St Petersburg	99%	203
Orlando Health	Orlando	99%	982

NOTE: Hospital profiles are in alphabetical order by state, then city, then hospital within the city; Rankings exclude hospitals with less than 25 cases except for patient surveys which excludes hospitals with less than 100 cases; (a) 100-299 cases; (1) The number of cases/patients is too few to report; (2) Data submitted were based on a sample of cases/patients; (3) Results are based on a shorter time period than required; (4) Data suppressed by CMS for one or more quarters; (5) Results are not available for this reporting period; (6) Fewer than 100 patients completed the HCAHPS survey; (7) No cases met the criteria for this measure; (8) The lower limit of the confidence interval cannot be calculated if the number of observed infections equals zero; (9) No data are available from the state/territory for this reporting period; (10) The scores shown reflect fewer than 50 completed surveys; (11) There were discrepancies in the data collection process; (12) This measure does not apply to this hospital for this reporting period; (13) Results cannot be calculated for this reporting period; (14) The results for this state are combined with nearby states to protect confidentiality; Please refer to the User's Guide for a full explanation of data.

Parrish Medical Center	Titusville	99%	145
Physicians Reg Med Ctr-Pine Ridge	Naples	99%	535
Plantation General Hospital	Plantation	99%	362
Putnam Community Medical Center	Palatka	99%	88
Regional Medical Center Bayonet Point	Hudson	99%	303
Saint Vincent's Medical Center	Jacksonville	99%	726
Sarasota Memorial Hospital	Sarasota	99%	883
South Bay Hospital	Sun City Center	99%	78
Tallahassee Memorial Hospital	Tallahassee	99%	1216
UF Health Jacksonville	Jacksonville	99%	274
Viera Hospital	Melbourne	99%	70
The Villages Regional Hospital	The Villages	99%	516
Wellington Regional Medical Center	Wellington	99%	99
West Florida Hospital	Pensacola	99%	378
Wuesthoff Medical Center Rockledge	Rockledge	99%	343
Aventura Hospital & Medical Center	Aventura	98%	248
Bayfront Health Port Charlotte	Port Charlotte	98%	406
Cape Canaveral Hospital	Cocoa Beach	98%	96
Florida Hospital Fish Memorial	Orange City	98%	135
Florida Hospital Heartland Medical Center	Sebring	98%	102
Good Samaritan Medical Center	W Palm Beach	98%	289
Lower Keys Medical Center	Key West	98%	50
Morton Plant Hospital	Clearwater	98%	647
Morton Plant North Bay Hospital	New Port Richey	98%	55
Naples Community Hospital	Naples	98%	597
North Okaloosa Medical Center	Crestview	98%	115
Palm Springs General Hospital	Hialeah	98%	171
Saint Joseph's Hospital	Tampa	98%	417
South Lake Hospital	Clermont	98%	108
UF Health Shands Hospital	Gainesville	98%	423
Winter Haven Hospital	Winter Haven	98%	549
Baptist Hospital	Pensacola	97%	578
Cape Coral Hospital	Cape Coral	97%	363
Citrus Memorial Hospital	Inverness	97%	296
Florida Hospital Memorial Medical Center	Daytona Bch	97%	731
Florida Hospital North Pinellas	Tarpon Springs	97%	78
Gulf Coast Med Ctr Lee Mem Health Sys	Fort Myers	97%	419
Heart of Florida Regional Medical Center	Davenport	97%	244
Jackson Memorial Hospital	Miami	97%	264
Mayo Clinic	Jacksonville	97%	519
Sacred Heart Hosp-Emerald Coast	Miramar Beach	97%	198
Seven Rivers Regional Medical Center	Crystal River	97%	102
University of Miami Hospital	Miami	97%	328
Baptist Medical Center	Jacksonville	96%	963
Baptist Medical Center - Nassau	Fernandina Bch	96%	28
Baptist Medical Center Beaches	Jcksnvll Bch	96%	92
Bartow Regional Medical Center	Bartow	96%	81
Flagler Hospital	St Augustine	96%	235
Florida Hospital Carrollwood	Tampa	96%	130
Indian River Medical Center	Vero Beach	96%	228
Manatee Memorial Hospital	Bradenton	96%	361
Saint Anthony's Hospital	St Petersburg	96%	296
Wuesthoff Medical Center - Melbourne	Melbourne	95%	237
Tampa General Hospital	Tampa	94%	598
Bethesda Hospital East	Boynton Beach	93%	344
Broward Health North	Pompano Bch	93%	201
Lee Memorial Hospital	Fort Myers	93%	709
Munroe Regional Medical Center	Ocala	93%	559
Lakewood Ranch Medical Center	Bradenton	92%	121
Town & Country Hospital	Tampa	92%	52
South Florida Baptist Hospital	Plant City	91%	79
Bert Fish Medical Center	New Smyrn Bch	85%	75

Urinary Catheter Removal

Hospital Name	City	Rate	Cases
Aventura Hospital & Medical Center[2]	Aventura	100%	264
Baptist Hospital of Miami[2]	Miami	100%	416
Bayfront Health Dade City	Dade City	100%	112
Boca Raton Regional Hospital[2]	Boca Raton	100%	255
Brandon Regional Hospital[2]	Brandon	100%	387
Broward Health Coral Springs[2]	Coral Springs	100%	272
Broward Health Imperial Point	Fort Lauderdale	100%	110
Broward Health Medical Center[2]	Fort Lauderdale	100%	351
Broward Health North[2]	Pompano Bch	100%	270
Cape Canaveral Hospital[2]	Cocoa Beach	100%	263
Capital Regional Medical Center	Tallahassee	100%	346
Central Florida Regional Hospital[2]	Sanford	100%	276
Coral Gables Hospital[2]	Coral Gables	100%	203
Delray Medical Center[2]	Delray Beach	100%	425
Doctor's Memorial Hospital	Perry	100%	55
Doctors Hospital	Coral Gables	100%	263
Fawcett Memorial Hospital[2]	Port Charlotte	100%	341
Florida Hospital[2]	Orlando	100%	4316
Florida Hospital Fish Memorial	Orange City	100%	224
Fort Walton Beach Medical Center[2]	Fort Walton Bch	100%	279
Gulf Breeze Hospital[2]	Gulf Breeze	100%	222
Gulf Coast Regional Medical Center[2]	Panama City	100%	327
Health Central	Ocoee	100%	452
Highlands Regional Medical Center[2]	Sebring	100%	98
Holy Cross Hospital[2]	Fort Lauderdale	100%	558
Homestead Hospital	Homestead	100%	125
JFK Medical Center[2]	Atlantis	100%	354
Jupiter Medical Center[2]	Jupiter	100%	329
Lake City Medical Center[2]	Lake City	100%	112
Lawnwood Reg Med Ctr & Heart Inst	Fort Pierce	100%	365
Mariners Hospital	Tavernier	100%	39
Medical Center of Trinity[2]	Trinity	100%	207
Memorial Hospital Pembroke[2]	Pembroke Pines	100%	147
Memorial Hospital West[2]	Pembroke Pines	100%	213
Memorial Regional Hospital[2]	Hollywood	100%	369
Metropolitan Hospital of Miami	Miami	100%	67
Morton Plant Hospital[2]	Clearwater	100%	1326
North Florida Regional Medical Center[2]	Gainesville	100%	518
Northwest Medical Center[2]	Margate	100%	201
Oak Hill Hospital[2]	Brooksville	100%	377
Ocala Regional Medical Center[2]	Ocala	100%	483
Orange Park Medical Center[2]	Orange Park	100%	176
Palm Bay Hospital	Palm Bay	100%	235
Palmetto General Hospital[2]	Hialeah	100%	252
Palms West Hospital[2]	Loxahatchee	100%	159
Parrish Medical Center	Titusville	100%	270
Plantation General Hospital[2]	Plantation	100%	399
Raulerson Hospital	Okeechobee	100%	52
Saint Cloud Regional Medical Center	Saint Cloud	100%	44
Saint Joseph's Hospital[2]	Tampa	100%	805
Saint Lucie Medical Center[2]	Port Saint Lucie	100%	210
Saint Vincent's Medical Center Southside[2]	Jacksonville	100%	93
Sebastian River Medical Center	Sebastian	100%	381
South Bay Hospital[2]	Sun City Center	100%	273
South Miami Hospital[2]	South Miami	100%	232
Twin Cities Hospital	Niceville	100%	126
UF Health Jacksonville[2]	Jacksonville	100%	266
University Hospital & Medical Center[2]	Tamarac	100%	240
Venice Reg Med Ctr-Bayfront Health[2]	Venice	100%	379
Viera Hospital	Melbourne	100%	521
W Palm Beach VA Medical Center[2]	W Palm Beach	100%	86
West Florida Hospital[2]	Pensacola	100%	256
West Kendall Baptist Hospital	Miami	100%	91
West Palm Hospital	W Palm Beach	100%	99
Baptist Hospital[2]	Pensacola	99%	418
Bay Pines VA Medical Center[2]	Bay Pines	99%	291
Blake Medical Center[2]	Bradenton	99%	333
Doctors Hospital of Sarasota[2]	Sarasota	99%	281
Edward White Hospital	St Petersburg	99%	139
Englewood Community Hospital	Englewood	99%	84
Florida Hospital Carrollwood[2]	Tampa	99%	280
Florida Hospital Deland	Deland	99%	461
Florida Hospital Flagler	Palm Coast	99%	366
Florida Hospital Heartland Medical Center	Sebring	99%	354
Florida Hospital Memorial Medical Center[2]	Daytona Bch	99%	638
Florida Hospital North Pinellas[2]	Tarpon Springs	99%	165
Florida Hospital Zephyrhills	Zephyrhills	99%	231
Holmes Regional Medical Center[2]	Melbourne	99%	1021
Kendall Regional Medical Center[2]	Miami	99%	232
Mease Hospital Dunedin[2]	Dunedin	99%	219
Memorial Hospital Jacksonville[2]	Jacksonville	99%	302
Memorial Hospital Miramar[2]	Miramar	99%	117
Palms of Pasadena Hospital	St Petersburg	99%	288
Physicians Reg Med Ctr-Pine Ridge	Naples	99%	404
Regional Medical Center Bayonet Point[2]	Hudson	99%	370
Sacred Heart Hosp-Emerald Coast[2]	Miramar Beach	99%	280
Saint Mary's Medical Center[2]	W Palm Beach	99%	181
Saint Petersburg General Hospital[2]	St Petersburg	99%	158
Sarasota Memorial Hospital[2]	Sarasota	99%	407
South Florida Baptist Hospital	Plant City	99%	112
Tallahassee Memorial Hospital[2]	Tallahassee	99%	1118
Wellington Regional Medical Center[2]	Wellington	99%	291
Westside Regional Medical Center[2]	Plantation	99%	206
Bayfront Health - Saint Petersburg[2]	St Petersburg	98%	262
Bayfront Health Port Charlotte[2]	Port Charlotte	98%	493
Florida Hospital Waterman[2]	Tavares	98%	267
Good Samaritan Medical Center[2]	W Palm Beach	98%	256
Halifax Health Medical Center[2]	Daytona Bch	98%	651
Lakewood Ranch Medical Center[2]	Bradenton	98%	279
Largo Medical Center[2]	Largo	98%	315
Mayo Clinic[2]	Jacksonville	98%	498
Mease Countryside Hospital[2]	Safety Harbor	98%	438
Memorial Hospital of Tampa	Tampa	98%	145
Morton Plant North Bay Hospital[2]	New Port Richey	98%	134
Northside Hospital[2]	St Petersburg	98%	255
Palm Beach Gardens Medical Center	Palm Bch Grdns	98%	270
Saint Anthony's Hospital[2]	St Petersburg	98%	489
Santa Rosa Medical Center	Milton	98%	101
Tampa General Hospital[2]	Tampa	98%	866
Tampa VA Medical Center[2]	Tampa	98%	263
UF Health Shands Hospital[2]	Gainesville	98%	345
University of Miami Hospital	Miami	98%	570
Bartow Regional Medical Center	Bartow	97%	97
Bayfront Health Brooksville	Brooksville	97%	308
Cleveland Clinic Hospital[2]	Weston	97%	331
Flagler Hospital[2]	St Augustine	97%	237
Florida Hospital Tampa[2]	Tampa	97%	264
Hialeah Hospital[2]	Hialeah	97%	107
Manatee Memorial Hospital[2]	Bradenton	97%	357
Mount Sinai Medical Center[2]	Miami Beach	97%	927
Orlando Health[2]	Orlando	97%	2083
Osceola Regional Medical Center[2]	Kissimmee	97%	366
Putnam Community Medical Center	Palatka	97%	90
Saint Vincent's Medical Center[2]	Jacksonville	97%	118
South Lake Hospital	Clermont	97%	147
VA N Florida/S Georgia Healthcare Sys[2]	Gainesville	97%	475
Winter Haven Hospital[2]	Winter Haven	97%	372
Wuesthoff Medical Center - Melbourne[2]	Melbourne	97%	272
Baptist Medical Center Beaches[2]	Jcksnvll Bch	96%	138
Bay Med Ctr Sacred Heart Health Sys[2]	Panama City	96%	592
Bayfront Health Punta Gorda[2]	Punta Gorda	96%	162
Jackson Hospital	Marianna	96%	73
Jackson Memorial Hospital[2]	Miami	96%	517
Lakeland Regional Medical Center[2]	Lakeland	96%	373
Miami VA Medical Center[2]	Miami	96%	174
Seven Rivers Regional Medical Center	Crystal River	96%	668
Wuesthoff Medical Center Rockledge[2]	Rockledge	96%	355
Baptist Medical Center[2]	Jacksonville	95%	400
Bert Fish Medical Center	New Smyrn Bch	95%	212
Bethesda Hospital East[2]	Boynton Beach	95%	247
Lake Wales Medical Center	Lake Wales	95%	94
Lower Keys Medical Center[2]	Key West	95%	130
North Shore Medical Center	Miami	95%	202
West Boca Medical Center[2]	Boca Raton	95%	131
Gulf Coast Med Ctr Lee Mem Health Sys[2]	Fort Myers	94%	217
Martin Medical Center[2]	Stuart	94%	277
Palm Springs General Hospital	Hialeah	94%	64
Leesburg Regional Medical Center[2]	Leesburg	93%	483
Naples Community Hospital[2]	Naples	93%	643
North Okaloosa Medical Center	Crestview	92%	60
Town & Country Hospital	Tampa	92%	80
Indian River Medical Center[2]	Vero Beach	91%	465
The Villages Regional Hospital	The Villages	91%	408
Citrus Memorial Hospital	Inverness	90%	480
Munroe Regional Medical Center[2]	Ocala	90%	381
Sacred Heart Hospital[2]	Pensacola	90%	438
Heart of Florida Regional Medical Center	Davenport	89%	236
Lehigh Regional Medical Center	Lehigh Acres	89%	28
Cape Coral Hospital[2]	Cape Coral	87%	152
Baptist Medical Center - Nassau[2]	Fernandina Bch	82%	45
Lee Memorial Hospital[2]	Fort Myers	79%	202

Survey of Patients' Hospital Experiences

Area Around Room 'Always' Quiet at Night

Hospital Name	City	Rate	Cases
Sacred Heart Hospital on the Gulf	Port Saint Joe	86%	(a)
Healthmark Regional Medical Center	Defuniak Spgs	80%	(a)
West Kendall Baptist Hospital	Miami	77%	300+
Homestead Hospital	Homestead	76%	300+
Jay Hospital	Jay	76%	(a)
Hendry Regional Medical Center	Clewiston	73%	(a)
Florida Hospital Memorial Medical Center[11]	Daytona Bch	72%	300+
Gulf Breeze Hospital	Gulf Breeze	71%	300+
Capital Regional Medical Center	Tallahassee	70%	300+
Doctor's Memorial Hospital	Perry	70%	(a)
Jackson Hospital	Marianna	70%	300+
Mariners Hospital	Tavernier	70%	(a)
Palm Bay Hospital	Palm Bay	70%	300+
Lakeside Medical Center	Belle Glade	69%	300+
Mayo Clinic[11]	Jacksonville	69%	300+
Memorial Hospital Miramar	Miramar	69%	300+
Viera Hospital	Melbourne	69%	300+
Baptist Medical Center - Nassau	Fernandina Bch	68%	300+
Cleveland Clinic Hospital	Weston	68%	300+
Medical Center of Trinity	Trinity	68%	300+
Fishermen's Hospital	Marathon	66%	(a)
Florida Hospital	Orlando	66%	300+
Memorial Hospital West	Pembroke Pines	66%	300+
Sacred Heart Hosp-Emerald Coast	Miramar Beach	66%	300+
Saint Vincent's Medical Center Southside	Jacksonville	66%	300+
Aventura Hospital & Medical Center	Aventura	65%	300+
Baptist Hospital	Pensacola	65%	300+
Fort Walton Beach Medical Center	Fort Walton Bch	65%	300+
Halifax Health Medical Center	Daytona Bch	65%	300+
Town & Country Hospital	Tampa	65%	300+
West Palm Hospital	W Palm Beach	65%	300+
Baptist Medical Center Beaches	Jcksnvll Bch	64%	300+
Health Central	Ocoee	64%	300+
Memorial Hospital Pembroke	Pembroke Pines	64%	300+
Parrish Medical Center	Titusville	64%	300+
Saint Joseph's Hospital	Tampa	64%	300+
South Miami Hospital	South Miami	64%	300+
Broward Health North	Pompano Bch	63%	300+
Doctors Hospital	Coral Gables	63%	300+
Good Samaritan Medical Center	W Palm Beach	63%	300+
Memorial Regional Hospital	Hollywood	63%	300+

NOTE: Hospital profiles are in alphabetical order by state, then city, then hospital within the city; Rankings exclude hospitals with less than 25 cases except for patient surveys which excludes hospitals with less than 100 cases; (a) 100-299 cases; (1) The number of cases/patients is too few to report; (2) Data submitted were based on a sample of cases/patients; (3) Results are based on a shorter time period than required; (4) Data suppressed by CMS for one or more quarters; (5) Results are not available for this reporting period; (6) Fewer than 100 patients completed the HCAHPS survey; (7) No cases met the criteria for this measure; (8) The lower limit of the confidence interval cannot be calculated if the number of observed infections equals zero; (9) No data are available from the state/territory for this reporting period; (10) The scores shown reflect fewer than 50 completed surveys; (11) There were discrepancies in the data collection process; (12) This measure does not apply to this hospital for this reporting period; (13) Results cannot be calculated for this reporting period; (14) The results for this state are combined with nearby states to protect confidentiality; Please refer to the User's Guide for a full explanation of data.

Orlando Health	Orlando	63%	300+
Plantation General Hospital	Plantation	63%	300+
University of Miami Hospital	Miami	63%	300+
West Florida Hospital	Pensacola	63%	300+
Memorial Hospital Jacksonville	Jacksonville	62%	300+
Memorial Hospital of Tampa	Tampa	62%	300+
Baptist Hospital of Miami	Miami	61%	300+
Bert Fish Medical Center	New Smyrn Bch	61%	300+
Broward Health Imperial Point	Fort Lauderdale	61%	300+
Florida Hospital Carrollwood[11]	Tampa	61%	300+
Lake Wales Medical Center	Lake Wales	61%	300+
Lakewood Ranch Medical Center	Bradenton	61%	300+
North Okaloosa Medical Center	Crestview	61%	300+
Physicians Reg Med Ctr-Pine Ridge	Naples	61%	300+
Saint Petersburg General Hospital	St Petersburg	61%	300+
Baptist Medical Center	Jacksonville	60%	300+
Bay Med Ctr Sacred Heart Health Sys	Panama City	60%	300+
Brandon Regional Hospital	Brandon	60%	300+
Cape Canaveral Hospital	Cocoa Beach	60%	300+
Coral Gables Hospital	Coral Gables	60%	300+
Edward White Hospital	St Petersburg	60%	300+
Florida Hospital Heartland Medical Center[11]	Sebring	60%	300+
Hialeah Hospital	Hialeah	60%	300+
Raulerson Hospital	Okeechobee	60%	300+
South Florida Baptist Hospital[11]	Plant City	60%	300+
Twin Cities Hospital	Niceville	60%	300+
Palmetto General Hospital	Hialeah	59%	300+
Sacred Heart Hospital	Pensacola	59%	300+
Saint Vincent's Medical Center	Jacksonville	59%	(a)
South Lake Hospital	Clermont	59%	300+
UF Health Jacksonville	Jacksonville	59%	300+
Jupiter Medical Center	Jupiter	58%	300+
Kendall Regional Medical Center	Miami	58%	300+
Lee Memorial Hospital	Fort Myers	58%	300+
Ocala Regional Medical Center	Ocala	58%	300+
Palms of Pasadena Hospital	St Petersburg	58%	300+
Saint Lucie Medical Center	Port Saint Lucie	58%	300+
Tallahassee Memorial Hospital	Tallahassee	58%	300+
University Hospital & Medical Center	Tamarac	58%	300+
Wellington Regional Medical Center	Wellington	58%	300+
Englewood Community Hospital	Englewood	57%	300+
Florida Hospital Fish Memorial[11]	Orange City	57%	300+
Florida Hospital Tampa[11]	Tampa	57%	300+
Florida Hospital Waterman[11]	Tavares	57%	300+
Lake City Medical Center	Lake City	57%	300+
Mease Hospital Dunedin[11]	Dunedin	57%	300+
Osceola Regional Medical Center	Kissimmee	57%	300+
Palm Beach Gardens Medical Center	Palm Bch Grdns	57%	300+
UF Health Shands Hospital	Gainesville	57%	300+
Bethesda Hospital East	Boynton Beach	56%	300+
Central Florida Regional Hospital	Sanford	56%	300+
Desoto Memorial Hospital	Arcadia	56%	300+
Doctors Hospital of Sarasota	Sarasota	56%	300+
Flagler Hospital	St Augustine	56%	300+
Lakeland Regional Medical Center	Lakeland	56%	300+
Larkin Community Hospital	South Miami	56%	(a)
Oak Hill Hospital	Brooksville	56%	300+
Palm Springs General Hospital	Hialeah	56%	300+
Saint Anthony's Hospital	St Petersburg	56%	300+
Sarasota Memorial Hospital	Sarasota	56%	300+
Tampa General Hospital	Tampa	56%	300+
Cape Coral Hospital	Cape Coral	55%	300+
Florida Hospital North Pinellas[11]	Tarpon Springs	55%	300+
Jackson Memorial Hospital	Miami	55%	300+
North Florida Regional Medical Center	Gainesville	55%	300+
Orange Park Medical Center	Orange Park	55%	300+
Saint Mary's Medical Center	W Palm Beach	55%	300+
Sebastian River Medical Center	Sebastian	55%	300+
Bayfront Health - Saint Petersburg	St Petersburg	54%	300+
Broward Health Coral Springs	Coral Springs	54%	300+
Broward Health Medical Center	Fort Lauderdale	54%	300+
Florida Hospital Flagler[11]	Palm Coast	54%	300+
Gulf Coast Med Ctr Lee Mem Health Sys	Fort Myers	54%	300+
Holmes Regional Medical Center	Melbourne	54%	300+
Munroe Regional Medical Center	Ocala	54%	300+
Naples Community Hospital	Naples	54%	300+
North Shore Medical Center	Miami	54%	300+
Northwest Medical Center	Margate	54%	300+
Palms West Hospital	Loxahatchee	54%	300+
Winter Haven Hospital	Winter Haven	54%	300+
Florida Hospital Zephyrhills[11]	Zephyrhills	53%	300+
Holy Cross Hospital	Fort Lauderdale	53%	300+
Manatee Memorial Hospital	Bradenton	53%	300+
Santa Rosa Medical Center	Milton	53%	300+
Westchester General Hospital	Miami	53%	300+
Bartow Regional Medical Center	Bartow	52%	300+
Blake Medical Center	Bradenton	52%	300+
Gulf Coast Regional Medical Center	Panama City	52%	300+
Largo Medical Center	Largo	52%	300+
Morton Plant North Bay Hospital[11]	New Port Richey	52%	300+
Putnam Community Medical Center	Palatka	52%	300+
Wuesthoff Medical Center - Melbourne	Melbourne	52%	300+
JFK Medical Center	Atlantis	51%	300+
Lehigh Regional Medical Center	Lehigh Acres	51%	300+
Mount Sinai Medical Center	Miami Beach	51%	300+
Northside Hospital	St Petersburg	51%	300+
Bayfront Health Punta Gorda	Punta Gorda	50%	300+
Florida Hospital Deland[11]	Deland	50%	300+
Lawnwood Reg Med Ctr & Heart Inst	Fort Pierce	50%	300+
Morton Plant Hospital[11]	Clearwater	50%	300+
South Bay Hospital	Sun City Center	50%	300+
Heart of Florida Regional Medical Center	Davenport	49%	300+
Regional Medical Center Bayonet Point	Hudson	49%	300+
Saint Cloud Regional Medical Center	Saint Cloud	49%	300+
Shands Lake Shore Regional Medical Center	Lake City	49%	300+
Westside Regional Medical Center	Plantation	49%	300+
Wuesthoff Medical Center Rockledge	Rockledge	49%	300+
Boca Raton Regional Hospital	Boca Raton	48%	300+
Highlands Regional Medical Center	Sebring	48%	300+
Leesburg Regional Medical Center	Leesburg	48%	300+
Lower Keys Medical Center	Key West	48%	300+
Martin Medical Center	Stuart	48%	300+
The Villages Regional Hospital	The Villages	47%	300+
Bayfront Health Dade City	Dade City	46%	300+
Bayfront Health Port Charlotte	Port Charlotte	46%	300+
Mease Countryside Hospital[11]	Safety Harbor	46%	300+
Venice Reg Med Ctr-Bayfront Health	Venice	46%	300+
Delray Medical Center	Delray Beach	45%	300+
Fawcett Memorial Hospital	Port Charlotte	45%	300+
Indian River Medical Center	Vero Beach	45%	300+
West Boca Medical Center	Boca Raton	45%	300+
Bayfront Health Brooksville	Brooksville	43%	300+
Citrus Memorial Hospital	Inverness	43%	300+
Seven Rivers Regional Medical Center	Crystal River	43%	300+

Doctors 'Always' Communicated Well

Hospital Name	City	Rate	Cases
Healthmark Regional Medical Center	Defuniak Spgs	94%	(a)
Sacred Heart Hospital on the Gulf	Port Saint Joe	92%	(a)
Jackson Hospital	Marianna	89%	300+
Jay Hospital	Jay	89%	(a)
Twin Cities Hospital	Niceville	88%	300+
Doctors Hospital	Coral Gables	87%	300+
Mariners Hospital	Tavernier	87%	(a)
West Kendall Baptist Hospital	Miami	87%	300+
Mayo Clinic[11]	Jacksonville	86%	300+
South Miami Hospital	South Miami	85%	300+
Baptist Medical Center - Nassau	Fernandina Bch	84%	300+
Coral Gables Hospital	Coral Gables	84%	300+
Gulf Breeze Hospital	Gulf Breeze	84%	300+
Sacred Heart Hosp-Emerald Coast	Miramar Beach	84%	300+
Baptist Hospital	Pensacola	83%	300+
Baptist Hospital of Miami	Miami	83%	300+
Hendry Regional Medical Center	Clewiston	83%	(a)
Lakeside Medical Center	Belle Glade	83%	300+
Palm Beach Gardens Medical Center	Palm Bch Grdns	83%	300+
Palms of Pasadena Hospital	St Petersburg	83%	300+
Bert Fish Medical Center	New Smyrn Bch	82%	300+
Cleveland Clinic Hospital	Weston	82%	300+
Good Samaritan Medical Center	W Palm Beach	82%	300+
Homestead Hospital	Homestead	82%	300+
Memorial Hospital Miramar	Miramar	82%	300+
Palm Springs General Hospital	Hialeah	82%	300+
Palmetto General Hospital	Hialeah	82%	300+
Sacred Heart Hospital	Pensacola	82%	300+
Sarasota Memorial Hospital	Sarasota	82%	300+
Viera Hospital	Melbourne	82%	300+
Baptist Medical Center Beaches	Jcksnvll Bch	81%	300+
Boca Raton Regional Hospital	Boca Raton	81%	300+
Doctor's Memorial Hospital	Perry	81%	(a)
Lake City Medical Center	Lake City	81%	300+
Memorial Hospital West	Pembroke Pines	81%	300+
Parrish Medical Center	Titusville	81%	300+
Tallahassee Memorial Hospital	Tallahassee	81%	300+
University of Miami Hospital	Miami	81%	300+
Westchester General Hospital	Miami	81%	300+
Capital Regional Medical Center	Tallahassee	80%	300+
Hialeah Hospital	Hialeah	80%	300+
Holy Cross Hospital	Fort Lauderdale	80%	300+
Lower Keys Medical Center	Key West	80%	300+
Memorial Regional Hospital	Hollywood	80%	300+
Plantation General Hospital	Plantation	80%	300+
Saint Vincent's Medical Center Southside	Jacksonville	80%	300+
Town & Country Hospital	Tampa	80%	300+
UF Health Shands Hospital	Gainesville	80%	300+
Fishermen's Hospital	Marathon	79%	(a)
Florida Hospital Memorial Medical Center[11]	Daytona Bch	79%	300+
Florida Hospital North Pinellas[11]	Tarpon Springs	79%	300+
North Okaloosa Medical Center	Crestview	79%	300+
Saint Joseph's Hospital	Tampa	79%	300+
Saint Vincent's Medical Center	Jacksonville	79%	(a)
Santa Rosa Medical Center	Milton	79%	300+
UF Health Jacksonville	Jacksonville	79%	300+
Cape Canaveral Hospital	Cocoa Beach	78%	300+
Desoto Memorial Hospital	Arcadia	78%	300+
Doctors Hospital of Sarasota	Sarasota	78%	300+
Florida Hospital	Orlando	78%	300+
Florida Hospital Carrollwood[11]	Tampa	78%	300+
Florida Hospital Flagler[11]	Palm Coast	78%	300+
Fort Walton Beach Medical Center	Fort Walton Bch	78%	300+
Jackson Memorial Hospital	Miami	78%	300+
Jupiter Medical Center	Jupiter	78%	300+
Kendall Regional Medical Center	Miami	78%	300+
Morton Plant Hospital[11]	Clearwater	78%	300+
Mount Sinai Medical Center	Miami Beach	78%	300+
North Florida Regional Medical Center	Gainesville	78%	300+
North Shore Medical Center	Miami	78%	300+
Putnam Community Medical Center	Palatka	78%	300+
Sebastian River Medical Center	Sebastian	78%	300+
South Florida Baptist Hospital[11]	Plant City	78%	300+
West Florida Hospital	Pensacola	78%	300+
Aventura Hospital & Medical Center	Aventura	77%	300+
Baptist Medical Center	Jacksonville	77%	300+
Englewood Community Hospital	Englewood	77%	300+
Florida Hospital Tampa[11]	Tampa	77%	300+
Gulf Coast Regional Medical Center	Panama City	77%	300+
Halifax Health Medical Center	Daytona Bch	77%	300+
Lakeland Regional Medical Center	Lakeland	77%	300+
Lakewood Ranch Medical Center	Bradenton	77%	300+
Memorial Hospital of Tampa	Tampa	77%	300+
Naples Community Hospital	Naples	77%	300+
Orlando Health	Orlando	77%	300+
Physicians Reg Med Ctr-Pine Ridge	Naples	77%	300+
Raulerson Hospital	Okeechobee	77%	300+
Tampa General Hospital	Tampa	77%	300+
West Palm Hospital	W Palm Beach	77%	300+
Bay Med Ctr Sacred Heart Health Sys	Panama City	76%	300+
Bayfront Health - Saint Petersburg	St Petersburg	76%	300+
Broward Health North	Pompano Bch	76%	300+
Central Florida Regional Hospital	Sanford	76%	300+
Edward White Hospital	St Petersburg	76%	300+
Flagler Hospital	St Augustine	76%	300+
Florida Hospital Heartland Medical Center[11]	Sebring	76%	300+
Florida Hospital Zephyrhills[11]	Zephyrhills	76%	300+
Health Central	Ocoee	76%	300+
Indian River Medical Center	Vero Beach	76%	300+
Manatee Memorial Hospital	Bradenton	76%	300+
Mease Countryside Hospital[11]	Safety Harbor	76%	300+
Medical Center of Trinity	Trinity	76%	300+
Memorial Hospital Pembroke	Pembroke Pines	76%	300+
Saint Mary's Medical Center	W Palm Beach	76%	300+
Saint Petersburg General Hospital	St Petersburg	76%	300+
Venice Reg Med Ctr-Bayfront Health	Venice	76%	300+
West Boca Medical Center	Boca Raton	76%	300+
Bartow Regional Medical Center	Bartow	75%	300+
Blake Medical Center	Bradenton	75%	300+
Broward Health Imperial Point	Fort Lauderdale	75%	300+
Holmes Regional Medical Center	Melbourne	75%	300+
Lake Wales Medical Center	Lake Wales	75%	300+
Larkin Community Hospital	South Miami	75%	(a)
Lee Memorial Hospital	Fort Myers	75%	300+
Memorial Hospital Jacksonville	Jacksonville	75%	300+
Orange Park Medical Center	Orange Park	75%	300+
Osceola Regional Medical Center	Kissimmee	75%	300+
Palm Bay Hospital	Palm Bay	75%	300+
Saint Lucie Medical Center	Port Saint Lucie	75%	300+
University Hospital & Medical Center	Tamarac	75%	300+
Westside Regional Medical Center	Plantation	75%	300+
Bayfront Health Punta Gorda	Punta Gorda	74%	300+
Fawcett Memorial Hospital	Port Charlotte	74%	300+
Florida Hospital Deland[11]	Deland	74%	300+
Florida Hospital Fish Memorial[11]	Orange City	74%	300+
Northside Hospital	St Petersburg	74%	300+
Oak Hill Hospital	Brooksville	74%	300+
Ocala Regional Medical Center	Ocala	74%	300+
Saint Anthony's Hospital	St Petersburg	74%	300+
Winter Haven Hospital	Winter Haven	74%	300+
Bayfront Health Dade City	Dade City	73%	300+
Brandon Regional Hospital	Brandon	73%	300+
Broward Health Coral Springs	Coral Springs	73%	300+
Citrus Memorial Hospital	Inverness	73%	300+
Delray Medical Center	Delray Beach	73%	300+
Florida Hospital Waterman[11]	Tavares	73%	300+
Highlands Regional Medical Center	Sebring	73%	300+
Largo Medical Center	Largo	73%	300+
Lawnwood Reg Med Ctr & Heart Inst	Fort Pierce	73%	300+
Martin Medical Center	Stuart	73%	300+
Mease Hospital Dunedin[11]	Dunedin	73%	300+
Shands Lake Shore Regional Medical Center	Lake City	73%	300+
Broward Health Medical Center	Fort Lauderdale	72%	300+
Cape Coral Hospital	Cape Coral	72%	300+
JFK Medical Center	Atlantis	72%	300+
Munroe Regional Medical Center	Ocala	72%	300+

NOTE: Hospital profiles are in alphabetical order by state, then city, then hospital within the city; Rankings exclude hospitals with less than 25 cases except for patient surveys which excludes hospitals with less than 100 cases; (a) 100-299 cases; (1) The number of cases/patients is too few to report; (2) Data submitted were based on a sample of cases/patients; (3) Results are based on a shorter time period than required; (4) Data suppressed by CMS for one or more quarters; (5) Results are not available for this reporting period; (6) Fewer than 100 patients completed the HCAHPS survey; (7) No cases met the criteria for this measure; (8) The lower limit of the confidence interval cannot be calculated if the number of observed infections equals zero; (9) No data are available from the state/territory for this reporting period; (10) The scores shown reflect fewer than 50 completed surveys; (11) There were discrepancies in the data collection process; (12) This measure does not apply to this hospital for this reporting period; (13) Results cannot be calculated for this reporting period; (14) The results for this state are combined with nearby states to protect confidentiality; Please refer to the User's Guide for a full explanation of data.

Hospital Name	City	Rate	Cases
Palms West Hospital	Loxahatchee	72%	300+
Saint Cloud Regional Medical Center	Saint Cloud	72%	300+
Seven Rivers Regional Medical Center	Crystal River	72%	300+
Wuesthoff Medical Center Rockledge	Rockledge	72%	300+
Lehigh Regional Medical Center	Lehigh Acres	71%	300+
Morton Plant North Bay Hospital[11]	New Port Richey	71%	300+
Northwest Medical Center	Margate	71%	300+
Regional Medical Center Bayonet Point	Hudson	71%	300+
South Bay Hospital	Sun City Center	71%	300+
South Lake Hospital	Clermont	71%	300+
Wellington Regional Medical Center	Wellington	71%	300+
Bayfront Health Port Charlotte	Port Charlotte	70%	300+
Gulf Coast Med Ctr Lee Mem Health Sys	Fort Myers	70%	300+
Bayfront Health Brooksville	Brooksville	69%	300+
Bethesda Hospital East	Boynton Beach	69%	300+
Heart of Florida Regional Medical Center	Davenport	69%	300+
The Villages Regional Hospital	The Villages	68%	300+
Leesburg Regional Medical Center	Leesburg	66%	300+
Wuesthoff Medical Center - Melbourne	Melbourne	65%	300+

Home Recovery Information Given

Hospital Name	City	Rate	Cases
Sacred Heart Hospital on the Gulf	Port Saint Joe	95%	(a)
Twin Cities Hospital	Niceville	93%	300+
Healthmark Regional Medical Center	Defuniak Spgs	92%	(a)
Mariners Hospital	Tavernier	91%	(a)
Mayo Clinic[11]	Jacksonville	90%	300+
Jackson Hospital	Marianna	89%	300+
Sacred Heart Hosp-Emerald Coast	Miramar Beach	89%	300+
Saint Vincent's Medical Center Southside	Jacksonville	89%	300+
UF Health Shands Hospital	Gainesville	89%	300+
Gulf Breeze Hospital	Gulf Breeze	88%	300+
Mease Hospital Dunedin[11]	Dunedin	88%	300+
South Florida Baptist Hospital[11]	Plant City	88%	300+
Baptist Hospital	Pensacola	87%	300+
Baptist Medical Center Beaches	Jcksnvl Bch	87%	300+
Doctors Hospital of Sarasota	Sarasota	87%	300+
Fawcett Memorial Hospital	Port Charlotte	87%	300+
Florida Hospital	Orlando	87%	300+
Florida Hospital Heartland Medical Center[11]	Sebring	87%	300+
Florida Hospital Memorial Medical Center[11]	Daytona Bch	87%	300+
Gulf Coast Regional Medical Center	Panama City	87%	300+
Jupiter Medical Center	Jupiter	87%	300+
Lakewood Ranch Medical Center	Bradenton	87%	300+
Morton Plant Hospital[11]	Clearwater	87%	300+
Sacred Heart Hospital	Pensacola	87%	300+
Sarasota Memorial Hospital	Sarasota	87%	300+
Viera Hospital	Melbourne	87%	300+
Bert Fish Medical Center	New Smyrn Bch	86%	300+
Broward Health North	Pompano Bch	86%	300+
Doctors Hospital	Coral Gables	86%	300+
Edward White Hospital	St Petersburg	86%	300+
Florida Hospital Carrollwood[11]	Tampa	86%	300+
Florida Hospital Deland[11]	Deland	86%	300+
Highlands Regional Medical Center	Sebring	86%	300+
Lake City Medical Center	Lake City	86%	300+
Manatee Memorial Hospital	Bradenton	86%	300+
Memorial Hospital Miramar	Miramar	86%	300+
Oak Hill Hospital	Brooksville	86%	300+
Orange Park Medical Center	Orange Park	86%	300+
West Florida Hospital	Pensacola	86%	300+
West Kendall Baptist Hospital	Miami	86%	300+
Cape Canaveral Hospital	Cocoa Beach	85%	300+
Florida Hospital Waterman[11]	Tavares	85%	300+
Fort Walton Beach Medical Center	Fort Walton Bch	85%	300+
Hendry Regional Medical Center	Clewiston	85%	(a)
Lee Memorial Hospital	Fort Myers	85%	300+
Mease Countryside Hospital[11]	Safety Harbor	85%	300+
Memorial Regional Hospital	Hollywood	85%	300+
Morton Plant North Bay Hospital[11]	New Port Richey	85%	300+
Ocala Regional Medical Center	Ocala	85%	300+
Parrish Medical Center	Titusville	85%	300+
Saint Joseph's Hospital	Tampa	85%	300+
Saint Lucie Medical Center	Port Saint Lucie	85%	300+
Saint Petersburg General Hospital	St Petersburg	85%	300+
Tampa General Hospital	Tampa	85%	300+
UF Health Jacksonville	Jacksonville	85%	300+
Baptist Hospital of Miami	Miami	84%	300+
Baptist Medical Center	Jacksonville	84%	300+
Bay Med Ctr Sacred Heart Health Sys	Panama City	84%	300+
Blake Medical Center	Bradenton	84%	300+
Broward Health Imperial Point	Fort Lauderdale	84%	300+
Cape Coral Hospital	Cape Coral	84%	300+
Capital Regional Medical Center	Tallahassee	84%	300+
Central Florida Regional Hospital	Sanford	84%	300+
Florida Hospital Flagler[11]	Palm Coast	84%	300+
Florida Hospital Tampa[11]	Tampa	84%	300+
Gulf Coast Med Ctr Lee Mem Health Sys	Fort Myers	84%	300+
Halifax Health Medical Center	Daytona Bch	84%	300+
Homestead Hospital	Homestead	84%	300+
Lake Wales Medical Center	Lake Wales	84%	300+
Martin Medical Center	Stuart	84%	300+
Palm Bay Hospital	Palm Bay	84%	300+
Raulerson Hospital	Okeechobee	84%	300+
Saint Vincent's Medical Center	Jacksonville	84%	(a)
South Lake Hospital	Clermont	84%	300+
Tallahassee Memorial Hospital	Tallahassee	84%	300+
Winter Haven Hospital	Winter Haven	84%	300+
Baptist Medical Center - Nassau	Fernandina Bch	83%	300+
Brandon Regional Hospital	Brandon	83%	300+
Citrus Memorial Hospital	Inverness	83%	300+
Cleveland Clinic Hospital	Weston	83%	300+
Doctor's Memorial Hospital	Perry	83%	(a)
Englewood Community Hospital	Englewood	83%	300+
Flagler Hospital	St Augustine	83%	300+
Florida Hospital Fish Memorial[11]	Orange City	83%	300+
Florida Hospital Zephyrhills[11]	Zephyrhills	83%	300+
Holmes Regional Medical Center	Melbourne	83%	300+
Indian River Medical Center	Vero Beach	83%	300+
Jay Hospital	Jay	83%	(a)
Lakeside Medical Center	Belle Glade	83%	300+
Larkin Community Hospital	South Miami	83%	(a)
Memorial Hospital Jacksonville	Jacksonville	83%	300+
Memorial Hospital Pembroke	Pembroke Pines	83%	300+
North Florida Regional Medical Center	Gainesville	83%	300+
North Okaloosa Medical Center	Crestview	83%	300+
Palms of Pasadena Hospital	St Petersburg	83%	300+
Regional Medical Center Bayonet Point	Hudson	83%	300+
Santa Rosa Medical Center	Milton	83%	300+
South Miami Hospital	South Miami	83%	300+
Town & Country Hospital	Tampa	83%	300+
Desoto Memorial Hospital	Arcadia	82%	300+
Fishermen's Hospital	Marathon	82%	(a)
Florida Hospital North Pinellas[11]	Tarpon Springs	82%	300+
Lakeland Regional Medical Center	Lakeland	82%	300+
Lawnwood Reg Med Ctr & Heart Inst	Fort Pierce	82%	300+
Medical Center of Trinity	Trinity	82%	300+
Munroe Regional Medical Center	Ocala	82%	300+
Northside Hospital	St Petersburg	82%	300+
Palm Beach Gardens Medical Center	Palm Bch Grdns	82%	300+
Physicians Reg Med Ctr-Pine Ridge	Naples	82%	300+
Saint Anthony's Hospital	St Petersburg	82%	300+
Venice Reg Med Ctr-Bayfront Health	Venice	82%	300+
West Palm Hospital	W Palm Beach	82%	300+
Bayfront Health - Saint Petersburg	St Petersburg	81%	300+
Delray Medical Center	Delray Beach	81%	300+
Holy Cross Hospital	Fort Lauderdale	81%	300+
Largo Medical Center	Largo	81%	300+
Lower Keys Medical Center	Key West	81%	300+
Mount Sinai Medical Center	Miami Beach	81%	300+
Orlando Health	Orlando	81%	300+
Osceola Regional Medical Center	Kissimmee	81%	300+
South Bay Hospital	Sun City Center	81%	300+
Bayfront Health Punta Gorda	Punta Gorda	80%	300+
Good Samaritan Medical Center	W Palm Beach	80%	300+
Kendall Regional Medical Center	Miami	80%	300+
Memorial Hospital of Tampa	Tampa	80%	300+
Memorial Hospital West	Pembroke Pines	80%	300+
Palms West Hospital	Loxahatchee	80%	300+
Plantation General Hospital	Plantation	80%	300+
Putnam Community Medical Center	Palatka	80%	300+
Saint Mary's Medical Center	W Palm Beach	80%	300+
Seven Rivers Regional Medical Center	Crystal River	80%	300+
University Hospital & Medical Center	Tamarac	80%	300+
University of Miami Hospital	Miami	80%	300+
Bartow Regional Medical Center	Bartow	79%	300+
Bayfront Health Brooksville	Brooksville	79%	300+
Bayfront Health Port Charlotte	Port Charlotte	79%	300+
Broward Health Coral Springs	Coral Springs	79%	300+
Broward Health Medical Center	Fort Lauderdale	79%	300+
Naples Community Hospital	Naples	79%	300+
Northwest Medical Center	Margate	79%	300+
Wellington Regional Medical Center	Wellington	79%	300+
Westchester General Hospital	Miami	79%	300+
Wuesthoff Medical Center Rockledge	Rockledge	79%	300+
Aventura Hospital & Medical Center	Aventura	78%	300+
Boca Raton Regional Hospital	Boca Raton	78%	300+
Heart of Florida Regional Medical Center	Davenport	78%	300+
Hialeah Hospital	Hialeah	78%	300+
North Shore Medical Center	Miami	78%	300+
Saint Cloud Regional Medical Center	Saint Cloud	78%	300+
Sebastian River Medical Center	Sebastian	78%	300+
Westside Regional Medical Center	Plantation	78%	300+
Bayfront Health Dade City	Dade City	77%	300+
Bethesda Hospital East	Boynton Beach	77%	300+
Coral Gables Hospital	Coral Gables	77%	300+
JFK Medical Center	Atlantis	77%	300+
Leesburg Regional Medical Center	Leesburg	77%	300+
Lehigh Regional Medical Center	Lehigh Acres	77%	300+
West Boca Medical Center	Boca Raton	77%	300+
Wuesthoff Medical Center - Melbourne	Melbourne	77%	300+
Health Central	Ocoee	76%	300+
Jackson Memorial Hospital	Miami	75%	300+
Palm Springs General Hospital	Hialeah	75%	300+
Palmetto General Hospital	Hialeah	75%	300+
The Villages Regional Hospital	The Villages	75%	300+
Shands Lake Shore Regional Medical Center	Lake City	73%	300+

Hospital Given 9 or 10 on 10 Point Scale

Hospital Name	City	Rate	Cases
Sacred Heart Hospital on the Gulf	Port Saint Joe	90%	(a)
Mayo Clinic[11]	Jacksonville	89%	300+
West Kendall Baptist Hospital	Miami	84%	300+
Healthmark Regional Medical Center	Defuniak Spgs	83%	(a)
Mariners Hospital	Tavernier	83%	(a)
Memorial Hospital Miramar	Miramar	83%	300+
Sacred Heart Hosp-Emerald Coast	Miramar Beach	82%	300+
Viera Hospital	Melbourne	82%	300+
Florida Hospital Memorial Medical Center[11]	Daytona Bch	81%	300+
Gulf Breeze Hospital	Gulf Breeze	81%	300+
South Miami Hospital	South Miami	81%	300+
Cleveland Clinic Hospital	Weston	80%	300+
Baptist Hospital of Miami	Miami	78%	300+
Doctors Hospital	Coral Gables	78%	300+
Homestead Hospital	Homestead	77%	300+
Memorial Regional Hospital	Hollywood	77%	300+
Morton Plant Hospital[11]	Clearwater	77%	300+
Saint Joseph's Hospital	Tampa	77%	300+
UF Health Shands Hospital	Gainesville	77%	300+
Baptist Hospital	Pensacola	76%	300+
Baptist Medical Center - Nassau	Fernandina Bch	76%	300+
Florida Hospital	Orlando	76%	300+
Mease Hospital Dunedin[11]	Dunedin	76%	300+
Sarasota Memorial Hospital	Sarasota	76%	300+
Twin Cities Hospital	Niceville	76%	300+
Baptist Medical Center Beaches	Jcksnvl Bch	75%	300+
Jackson Hospital	Marianna	75%	300+
Jay Hospital	Jay	75%	(a)
Palm Bay Hospital	Palm Bay	75%	300+
Tampa General Hospital	Tampa	75%	300+
Jupiter Medical Center	Jupiter	74%	300+
Memorial Hospital West	Pembroke Pines	74%	300+
West Florida Hospital	Pensacola	74%	300+
Baptist Medical Center	Jacksonville	73%	300+
Broward Health North	Pompano Bch	73%	300+
Cape Canaveral Hospital	Cocoa Beach	73%	300+
Doctors Hospital of Sarasota	Sarasota	73%	300+
Mease Countryside Hospital[11]	Safety Harbor	73%	300+
Memorial Hospital Pembroke	Pembroke Pines	73%	300+
Orlando Health	Orlando	73%	300+
South Florida Baptist Hospital[11]	Plant City	73%	300+
Broward Health Imperial Point	Fort Lauderdale	72%	300+
Doctor's Memorial Hospital	Perry	72%	(a)
Lakewood Ranch Medical Center	Bradenton	72%	300+
Parrish Medical Center	Titusville	72%	300+
Sacred Heart Hospital	Pensacola	72%	300+
Saint Anthony's Hospital	St Petersburg	72%	300+
Bert Fish Medical Center	New Smyrn Bch	71%	300+
Boca Raton Regional Hospital	Boca Raton	71%	300+
Fishermen's Hospital	Marathon	71%	(a)
Lake City Medical Center	Lake City	71%	300+
Morton Plant North Bay Hospital[11]	New Port Richey	71%	300+
Palms of Pasadena Hospital	St Petersburg	71%	300+
Bayfront Health - Saint Petersburg	St Petersburg	70%	300+
Holy Cross Hospital	Fort Lauderdale	70%	300+
Martin Medical Center	Stuart	70%	300+
Bay Med Ctr Sacred Heart Health Sys	Panama City	69%	300+
Florida Hospital North Pinellas[11]	Tarpon Springs	69%	300+
Lakeland Regional Medical Center	Lakeland	69%	300+
Medical Center of Trinity	Trinity	69%	300+
Oak Hill Hospital	Brooksville	69%	300+
Palm Beach Gardens Medical Center	Palm Bch Grdns	69%	300+
Saint Petersburg General Hospital	St Petersburg	69%	300+
Saint Vincent's Medical Center Southside	Jacksonville	69%	300+
University of Miami Hospital	Miami	69%	300+
Capital Regional Medical Center	Tallahassee	68%	300+
Flagler Hospital	St Augustine	68%	300+
Florida Hospital Carrollwood[11]	Tampa	68%	300+
Health Central	Ocoee	68%	300+
Lake Wales Medical Center	Lake Wales	68%	300+
Lee Memorial Hospital	Fort Myers	68%	300+
Saint Vincent's Medical Center	Jacksonville	68%	(a)
Winter Haven Hospital	Winter Haven	68%	300+
Bethesda Hospital East	Boynton Beach	67%	300+
Desoto Memorial Hospital	Arcadia	67%	300+
Florida Hospital Heartland Medical Center[11]	Sebring	67%	300+
Halifax Health Medical Center	Daytona Bch	67%	300+
Raulerson Hospital	Okeechobee	67%	300+
South Lake Hospital	Clermont	67%	300+
Tallahassee Memorial Hospital	Tallahassee	67%	300+
West Palm Hospital	W Palm Beach	67%	300+
Edward White Hospital	St Petersburg	66%	300+
Florida Hospital Waterman[11]	Tavares	66%	300+

NOTE: Hospital profiles are in alphabetical order by state, then city, then hospital within the city; Rankings exclude hospitals with less than 25 cases except for patient surveys which excludes hospitals with less than 100 cases; (a) 100-299 cases; (1) The number of cases/patients is too few to report; (2) Data submitted were based on a sample of cases/patients; (3) Results are based on a shorter time period than required; (4) Data suppressed by CMS for one or more quarters; (5) Results are not available for this reporting period; (6) Fewer than 100 patients completed the HCAHPS survey; (7) No cases met the criteria for this measure; (8) The lower limit of the confidence interval cannot be calculated if the number of observed infections equals zero; (9) No data are available from the state/territory for this reporting period; (10) The scores shown reflect fewer than 50 completed surveys; (11) There were discrepancies in the data collection process; (12) This measure does not apply to this hospital for this reporting period; (13) Results cannot be calculated for this reporting period; (14) The results for this state are combined with nearby states to protect confidentiality; Please refer to the User's Guide for a full explanation of data.

Hospital Name	City	Rate	Cases
Florida Hospital Zephyrhills[11]	Zephyrhills	66%	300+
Gulf Coast Regional Medical Center	Panama City	66%	300+
Hendry Regional Medical Center	Clewiston	66%	(a)
Holmes Regional Medical Center	Melbourne	66%	300+
Memorial Hospital of Tampa	Tampa	66%	300+
Munroe Regional Medical Center	Ocala	66%	300+
Naples Community Hospital	Naples	66%	300+
North Florida Regional Medical Center	Gainesville	66%	300+
North Okaloosa Medical Center	Crestview	66%	300+
UF Health Jacksonville	Jacksonville	66%	300+
Good Samaritan Medical Center	W Palm Beach	65%	300+
Manatee Memorial Hospital	Bradenton	65%	300+
Mount Sinai Medical Center	Miami Beach	65%	300+
Plantation General Hospital	Plantation	65%	300+
Saint Mary's Medical Center	W Palm Beach	65%	300+
Florida Hospital Flagler[11]	Palm Coast	64%	300+
Gulf Coast Med Ctr Lee Mem Health Sys	Fort Myers	64%	300+
Ocala Regional Medical Center	Ocala	64%	300+
Orange Park Medical Center	Orange Park	64%	300+
Physicians Reg Med Ctr-Pine Ridge	Naples	64%	300+
Saint Lucie Medical Center	Port Saint Lucie	64%	300+
Aventura Hospital & Medical Center	Aventura	63%	300+
Blake Medical Center	Bradenton	63%	300+
Broward Health Medical Center	Fort Lauderdale	63%	300+
Central Florida Regional Hospital	Sanford	63%	300+
Englewood Community Hospital	Englewood	63%	300+
Fawcett Memorial Hospital	Port Charlotte	63%	300+
Florida Hospital Deland[11]	Deland	63%	300+
Florida Hospital Fish Memorial[11]	Orange City	63%	300+
Indian River Medical Center	Vero Beach	63%	300+
Memorial Hospital Jacksonville	Jacksonville	63%	300+
Town & Country Hospital	Tampa	63%	300+
Cape Coral Hospital	Cape Coral	62%	300+
Fort Walton Beach Medical Center	Fort Walton Bch	62%	300+
Hialeah Hospital	Hialeah	62%	300+
Northside Hospital	St Petersburg	62%	300+
Coral Gables Hospital	Coral Gables	61%	300+
Florida Hospital Tampa[11]	Tampa	61%	300+
Jackson Memorial Hospital	Miami	61%	300+
Kendall Regional Medical Center	Miami	61%	300+
Lakeside Medical Center	Belle Glade	61%	300+
Palm Springs General Hospital	Hialeah	61%	300+
Palmetto General Hospital	Hialeah	61%	300+
Citrus Memorial Hospital	Inverness	60%	300+
Larkin Community Hospital	South Miami	60%	(a)
Palms West Hospital	Loxahatchee	60%	300+
Regional Medical Center Bayonet Point	Hudson	60%	300+
Westchester General Hospital	Miami	60%	300+
Bayfront Health Punta Gorda	Punta Gorda	59%	300+
Broward Health Coral Springs	Coral Springs	59%	300+
Largo Medical Center	Largo	59%	300+
Lawnwood Reg Med Ctr & Heart Inst	Fort Pierce	59%	300+
Osceola Regional Medical Center	Kissimmee	59%	300+
JFK Medical Center	Atlantis	58%	300+
Putnam Community Medical Center	Palatka	58%	300+
Sebastian River Medical Center	Sebastian	58%	300+
South Bay Hospital	Sun City Center	58%	300+
Wellington Regional Medical Center	Wellington	58%	300+
Brandon Regional Hospital	Brandon	57%	300+
North Shore Medical Center	Miami	57%	300+
Santa Rosa Medical Center	Milton	57%	300+
Venice Reg Med Ctr-Bayfront Health	Venice	57%	300+
West Boca Medical Center	Boca Raton	57%	300+
Westside Regional Medical Center	Plantation	57%	300+
Delray Medical Center	Delray Beach	56%	300+
Seven Rivers Regional Medical Center	Crystal River	56%	300+
The Villages Regional Hospital	The Villages	56%	300+
Bartow Regional Medical Center	Bartow	55%	300+
Leesburg Regional Medical Center	Leesburg	55%	300+
Northwest Medical Center	Margate	55%	300+
University Hospital & Medical Center	Tamarac	55%	300+
Wuesthoff Medical Center - Melbourne	Melbourne	55%	300+
Highlands Regional Medical Center	Sebring	54%	300+
Bayfront Health Dade City	Dade City	52%	300+
Bayfront Health Port Charlotte	Port Charlotte	51%	300+
Heart of Florida Regional Medical Center	Davenport	50%	300+
Saint Cloud Regional Medical Center	Saint Cloud	50%	300+
Shands Lake Shore Regional Medical Center	Lake City	50%	300+
Lower Keys Medical Center	Key West	49%	300+
Wuesthoff Medical Center Rockledge	Rockledge	48%	300+
Bayfront Health Brooksville	Brooksville	45%	300+
Lehigh Regional Medical Center	Lehigh Acres	45%	300+

Meds 'Always' Explained Before Given

Hospital Name	City	Rate	Cases
Sacred Heart Hospital on the Gulf	Port Saint Joe	84%	(a)
Mariners Hospital	Tavernier	76%	(a)
Jay Hospital	Jay	73%	(a)
Fishermen's Hospital	Marathon	71%	(a)
Viera Hospital	Melbourne	71%	300+
Twin Cities Hospital	Niceville	70%	300+
West Kendall Baptist Hospital	Miami	70%	300+
Cape Canaveral Hospital	Cocoa Beach	69%	300+
Cleveland Clinic Hospital	Weston	69%	300+
Homestead Hospital	Homestead	69%	300+
Jackson Hospital	Marianna	69%	300+
Sacred Heart Hosp-Emerald Coast	Miramar Beach	69%	300+
Florida Hospital	Orlando	68%	300+
Baptist Hospital	Pensacola	67%	300+
Broward Health North	Pompano Bch	67%	300+
Gulf Breeze Hospital	Gulf Breeze	67%	300+
Memorial Hospital Miramar	Miramar	67%	300+
Baptist Hospital of Miami	Miami	66%	300+
Doctor's Memorial Hospital	Perry	66%	(a)
Doctors Hospital	Coral Gables	66%	300+
Larkin Community Hospital	South Miami	66%	(a)
Mayo Clinic[11]	Jacksonville	66%	300+
Memorial Regional Hospital	Hollywood	66%	300+
Sarasota Memorial Hospital	Sarasota	66%	300+
Tallahassee Memorial Hospital	Tallahassee	66%	300+
Broward Health Imperial Point	Fort Lauderdale	65%	300+
Florida Hospital Memorial Medical Center[11]	Daytona Bch	65%	300+
Saint Vincent's Medical Center Southside	Jacksonville	65%	300+
South Miami Hospital	South Miami	65%	300+
Coral Gables Hospital	Coral Gables	64%	300+
Memorial Hospital Pembroke	Pembroke Pines	64%	300+
Palm Bay Hospital	Palm Bay	64%	300+
Raulerson Hospital	Okeechobee	64%	300+
Tampa General Hospital	Tampa	64%	300+
UF Health Jacksonville	Jacksonville	64%	300+
Baptist Medical Center - Nassau	Fernandina Bch	63%	300+
Baptist Medical Center Beaches	Jcksnvll Bch	63%	300+
Florida Hospital Carrollwood[11]	Tampa	63%	300+
Health Central	Ocoee	63%	300+
Lake City Medical Center	Lake City	63%	300+
Morton Plant Hospital[11]	Clearwater	63%	300+
Parrish Medical Center	Titusville	63%	300+
South Florida Baptist Hospital[11]	Plant City	63%	300+
UF Health Shands Hospital	Gainesville	63%	300+
Lake Wales Medical Center	Lake Wales	62%	300+
Lakeland Regional Medical Center	Lakeland	62%	300+
Lee Memorial Hospital	Fort Myers	62%	300+
Mease Countryside Hospital[11]	Safety Harbor	62%	300+
Memorial Hospital West	Pembroke Pines	62%	300+
Sacred Heart Hospital	Pensacola	62%	300+
Saint Joseph's Hospital	Tampa	62%	300+
University of Miami Hospital	Miami	62%	300+
West Florida Hospital	Pensacola	62%	300+
West Palm Hospital	W Palm Beach	62%	300+
Bert Fish Medical Center	New Smyrn Bch	61%	300+
Broward Health Coral Springs	Coral Springs	61%	300+
Central Florida Regional Hospital	Sanford	61%	300+
Edward White Hospital	St Petersburg	61%	300+
Florida Hospital Fish Memorial[11]	Orange City	61%	300+
Florida Hospital North Pinellas[11]	Tarpon Springs	61%	300+
Fort Walton Beach Medical Center	Fort Walton Bch	61%	300+
Holmes Regional Medical Center	Melbourne	61%	300+
Mease Hospital Dunedin[11]	Dunedin	61%	300+
North Okaloosa Medical Center	Crestview	61%	300+
Palm Springs General Hospital	Hialeah	61%	300+
Plantation General Hospital	Plantation	61%	300+
Saint Anthony's Hospital	St Petersburg	61%	300+
Saint Petersburg General Hospital	St Petersburg	61%	300+
Saint Vincent's Medical Center	Jacksonville	61%	(a)
Westchester General Hospital	Miami	61%	300+
Aventura Hospital & Medical Center	Aventura	60%	300+
Bay Med Ctr Sacred Heart Health Sys	Panama City	60%	300+
Cape Coral Hospital	Cape Coral	60%	300+
Capital Regional Medical Center	Tallahassee	60%	300+
Florida Hospital Deland[11]	Deland	60%	300+
Florida Hospital Flagler[11]	Palm Coast	60%	300+
Florida Hospital Heartland Medical Center[11]	Sebring	60%	300+
Hendry Regional Medical Center	Clewiston	60%	(a)
Hialeah Hospital	Hialeah	60%	300+
Holy Cross Hospital	Fort Lauderdale	60%	300+
Jupiter Medical Center	Jupiter	60%	300+
Lakewood Ranch Medical Center	Bradenton	60%	300+
Mount Sinai Medical Center	Miami Beach	60%	300+
Orange Park Medical Center	Orange Park	60%	300+
Palm Beach Gardens Medical Center	Palm Bch Grdns	60%	300+
Palms of Pasadena Hospital	St Petersburg	60%	300+
Putnam Community Medical Center	Palatka	60%	300+
Saint Lucie Medical Center	Port Saint Lucie	60%	300+
Saint Mary's Medical Center	W Palm Beach	60%	300+
Town & Country Hospital	Tampa	60%	300+
Florida Hospital Tampa[11]	Tampa	59%	300+
Florida Hospital Zephyrhills[11]	Zephyrhills	59%	300+
Kendall Regional Medical Center	Miami	59%	300+
Morton Plant North Bay Hospital[11]	New Port Richey	59%	300+
Oak Hill Hospital	Brooksville	59%	300+
Orlando Health	Orlando	59%	300+
Baptist Medical Center	Jacksonville	58%	300+
Bethesda Hospital East	Boynton Beach	58%	300+
Boca Raton Regional Hospital	Boca Raton	58%	300+
Desoto Memorial Hospital	Arcadia	58%	300+
Doctors Hospital of Sarasota	Sarasota	58%	300+
Florida Hospital Waterman[11]	Tavares	58%	300+
Gulf Coast Med Ctr Lee Mem Health Sys	Fort Myers	58%	300+
Indian River Medical Center	Vero Beach	58%	300+
JFK Medical Center	Atlantis	58%	300+
Lower Keys Medical Center	Key West	58%	300+
North Florida Regional Medical Center	Gainesville	58%	300+
Palmetto General Hospital	Hialeah	58%	300+
Santa Rosa Medical Center	Milton	58%	300+
Bayfront Health - Saint Petersburg	St Petersburg	57%	300+
Englewood Community Hospital	Englewood	57%	300+
Flagler Hospital	St Augustine	57%	300+
Gulf Coast Regional Medical Center	Panama City	57%	300+
Lakeside Medical Center	Belle Glade	57%	300+
Lawnwood Reg Med Ctr & Heart Inst	Fort Pierce	57%	300+
Martin Medical Center	Stuart	57%	300+
Medical Center of Trinity	Trinity	57%	300+
Memorial Hospital of Tampa	Tampa	57%	300+
Naples Community Hospital	Naples	57%	300+
Osceola Regional Medical Center	Kissimmee	57%	300+
Physicians Reg Med Ctr-Pine Ridge	Naples	57%	300+
South Lake Hospital	Clermont	57%	300+
Winter Haven Hospital	Winter Haven	57%	300+
Fawcett Memorial Hospital	Port Charlotte	56%	300+
Halifax Health Medical Center	Daytona Bch	56%	300+
Healthmark Regional Medical Center	Defuniak Spgs	56%	(a)
Largo Medical Center	Largo	56%	300+
North Shore Medical Center	Miami	56%	300+
Ocala Regional Medical Center	Ocala	56%	300+
University Hospital & Medical Center	Tamarac	56%	300+
Bayfront Health Punta Gorda	Punta Gorda	55%	300+
Blake Medical Center	Bradenton	55%	300+
Broward Health Medical Center	Fort Lauderdale	55%	300+
Good Samaritan Medical Center	W Palm Beach	55%	300+
Memorial Hospital Jacksonville	Jacksonville	55%	300+
Munroe Regional Medical Center	Ocala	55%	300+
Palms West Hospital	Loxahatchee	55%	300+
Regional Medical Center Bayonet Point	Hudson	55%	300+
South Bay Hospital	Sun City Center	55%	300+
Delray Medical Center	Delray Beach	54%	300+
Leesburg Regional Medical Center	Leesburg	54%	300+
Northside Hospital	St Petersburg	54%	300+
Sebastian River Medical Center	Sebastian	54%	300+
Seven Rivers Regional Medical Center	Crystal River	54%	300+
Shands Lake Shore Regional Medical Center	Lake City	54%	300+
West Boca Medical Center	Boca Raton	54%	300+
Wuesthoff Medical Center Rockledge	Rockledge	54%	300+
Citrus Memorial Hospital	Inverness	53%	300+
Manatee Memorial Hospital	Bradenton	53%	300+
Northwest Medical Center	Margate	53%	300+
Wuesthoff Medical Center - Melbourne	Melbourne	53%	300+
Brandon Regional Hospital	Brandon	52%	300+
Highlands Regional Medical Center	Sebring	52%	300+
Jackson Memorial Hospital	Miami	52%	300+
Venice Reg Med Ctr-Bayfront Health	Venice	52%	300+
Wellington Regional Medical Center	Wellington	52%	300+
Westside Regional Medical Center	Plantation	52%	300+
Bartow Regional Medical Center	Bartow	51%	300+
Bayfront Health Dade City	Dade City	50%	300+
Heart of Florida Regional Medical Center	Davenport	50%	300+
The Villages Regional Hospital	The Villages	50%	300+
Bayfront Health Brooksville	Brooksville	48%	300+
Bayfront Health Port Charlotte	Port Charlotte	48%	300+
Saint Cloud Regional Medical Center	Saint Cloud	46%	300+
Lehigh Regional Medical Center	Lehigh Acres	45%	300+

Nurses 'Always' Communicated Well

Hospital Name	City	Rate	Cases
Sacred Heart Hospital on the Gulf	Port Saint Joe	91%	(a)
Mariners Hospital	Tavernier	89%	(a)
Jay Hospital	Jay	86%	(a)
Gulf Breeze Hospital	Gulf Breeze	84%	300+
Memorial Hospital Miramar	Miramar	84%	300+
Viera Hospital	Melbourne	84%	300+
West Kendall Baptist Hospital	Miami	84%	300+
Fishermen's Hospital	Marathon	83%	(a)
Mayo Clinic[11]	Jacksonville	83%	300+
Sacred Heart Hosp-Emerald Coast	Miramar Beach	83%	300+
South Miami Hospital	South Miami	83%	300+
Cape Canaveral Hospital	Cocoa Beach	82%	300+
Doctors Hospital	Coral Gables	82%	300+
Healthmark Regional Medical Center	Defuniak Spgs	82%	(a)
Hendry Regional Medical Center	Clewiston	82%	(a)
Baptist Hospital	Pensacola	81%	300+
Baptist Hospital of Miami	Miami	81%	300+
Baptist Medical Center - Nassau	Fernandina Bch	81%	300+
Doctor's Memorial Hospital	Perry	81%	(a)
Florida Hospital	Orlando	81%	300+

NOTE: Hospital profiles are in alphabetical order by state, then city, then hospital within the city; Rankings exclude hospitals with less than 25 cases except for patient surveys which excludes hospitals with less than 100 cases; (a) 100-299 cases; (1) The number of cases/patients is too few to report; (2) Data submitted were based on a sample of cases/patients; (3) Results are based on a shorter time period than required; (4) Data suppressed by CMS for one or more quarters; (5) Results are not available for this reporting period; (6) Fewer than 100 patients completed the HCAHPS survey; (7) No cases met the criteria for this measure; (8) The lower limit of the confidence interval cannot be calculated if the number of observed infections equals zero; (9) No data are available from the state/territory for this reporting period; (10) The scores shown reflect fewer than 50 completed surveys; (11) There were discrepancies in the data collection process; (12) This measure does not apply to this hospital for this reporting period; (13) Results cannot be calculated for this reporting period; (14) The results for this state are combined with nearby states to protect confidentiality; Please refer to the User's Guide for a full explanation of data.

Homestead Hospital	Homestead	81%	300+
Jackson Hospital	Marianna	81%	300+
Palm Bay Hospital	Palm Bay	81%	300+
Sarasota Memorial Hospital	Sarasota	81%	300+
Twin Cities Hospital	Niceville	81%	300+
Baptist Medical Center Beaches	Jcksnvl Bch	80%	300+
Memorial Hospital Pembroke	Pembroke Pines	80%	300+
Memorial Regional Hospital	Hollywood	80%	300+
Parrish Medical Center	Titusville	80%	300+
Sacred Heart Hospital	Pensacola	80%	300+
Bert Fish Medical Center	New Smyrn Bch	79%	300+
Cleveland Clinic Hospital	Weston	79%	300+
Florida Hospital Memorial Medical Center[11]	Daytona Bch	79%	300+
Health Central	Ocoee	79%	300+
Saint Joseph's Hospital	Tampa	79%	300+
Saint Vincent's Medical Center Southside	Jacksonville	79%	300+
UF Health Shands Hospital	Gainesville	79%	300+
Broward Health North	Pompano Bch	78%	300+
Florida Hospital Heartland Medical Center[11]	Sebring	78%	300+
Florida Hospital North Pinellas[11]	Tarpon Springs	78%	300+
Lee Memorial Hospital	Fort Myers	78%	300+
Mease Countryside Hospital[11]	Safety Harbor	78%	300+
Memorial Hospital West	Pembroke Pines	78%	300+
Morton Plant Hospital[11]	Clearwater	78%	300+
North Okaloosa Medical Center	Crestview	78%	300+
Raulerson Hospital	Okeechobee	78%	300+
South Florida Baptist Hospital[11]	Plant City	78%	300+
West Florida Hospital	Pensacola	78%	300+
Florida Hospital Carrollwood[11]	Tampa	77%	300+
Florida Hospital Deland[11]	Deland	77%	300+
Florida Hospital Zephyrhills[11]	Zephyrhills	77%	300+
Holmes Regional Medical Center	Melbourne	77%	300+
Lake City Medical Center	Lake City	77%	300+
Lakeland Regional Medical Center	Lakeland	77%	300+
Morton Plant North Bay Hospital[11]	New Port Richey	77%	300+
Oak Hill Hospital	Brooksville	77%	300+
Palms of Pasadena Hospital	St Petersburg	77%	300+
Saint Vincent's Medical Center	Jacksonville	77%	(a)
Tampa General Hospital	Tampa	77%	300+
UF Health Jacksonville	Jacksonville	77%	300+
Winter Haven Hospital	Winter Haven	77%	300+
Baptist Medical Center	Jacksonville	76%	300+
Bay Med Ctr Sacred Heart Health Sys	Panama City	76%	300+
Boca Raton Regional Hospital	Boca Raton	76%	300+
Cape Coral Hospital	Cape Coral	76%	300+
Doctors Hospital of Sarasota	Sarasota	76%	300+
Florida Hospital Tampa[11]	Tampa	76%	300+
Gulf Coast Regional Medical Center	Panama City	76%	300+
Jupiter Medical Center	Jupiter	76%	300+
Lake Wales Medical Center	Lake Wales	76%	300+
Lakewood Ranch Medical Center	Bradenton	76%	300+
Mease Hospital Dunedin[11]	Dunedin	76%	300+
Palm Springs General Hospital	Hialeah	76%	300+
Saint Anthony's Hospital	St Petersburg	76%	300+
Saint Petersburg General Hospital	St Petersburg	76%	300+
Tallahassee Memorial Hospital	Tallahassee	76%	300+
University of Miami Hospital	Miami	76%	300+
Bayfront Health - Saint Petersburg	St Petersburg	75%	300+
Capital Regional Medical Center	Tallahassee	75%	300+
Central Florida Regional Hospital	Sanford	75%	300+
Coral Gables Hospital	Coral Gables	75%	300+
Desoto Memorial Hospital	Arcadia	75%	300+
Florida Hospital Fish Memorial[11]	Orange City	75%	300+
Florida Hospital Flagler[11]	Palm Coast	75%	300+
Gulf Coast Med Ctr Lee Mem Health Sys	Fort Myers	75%	300+
Orlando Health	Orlando	75%	300+
Palm Beach Gardens Medical Center	Palm Bch Grdns	75%	300+
Saint Lucie Medical Center	Port Saint Lucie	75%	300+
Westchester General Hospital	Miami	75%	300+
Broward Health Imperial Point	Fort Lauderdale	74%	300+
Englewood Community Hospital	Englewood	74%	300+
Halifax Health Medical Center	Daytona Bch	74%	300+
Hialeah Hospital	Hialeah	74%	300+
Holy Cross Hospital	Fort Lauderdale	74%	300+
Kendall Regional Medical Center	Miami	74%	300+
Martin Medical Center	Stuart	74%	300+
Medical Center of Trinity	Trinity	74%	300+
Town & Country Hospital	Tampa	74%	300+
West Palm Hospital	W Palm Beach	74%	300+
Fawcett Memorial Hospital	Port Charlotte	73%	300+
Flagler Hospital	St Augustine	73%	300+
Florida Hospital Waterman[11]	Tavares	73%	300+
Fort Walton Beach Medical Center	Fort Walton Bch	73%	300+
Indian River Medical Center	Vero Beach	73%	300+
Lower Keys Medical Center	Key West	73%	300+
Manatee Memorial Hospital	Bradenton	73%	300+
Memorial Hospital Jacksonville	Jacksonville	73%	300+
Memorial Hospital of Tampa	Tampa	73%	300+
Mount Sinai Medical Center	Miami Beach	73%	300+
Munroe Regional Medical Center	Ocala	73%	300+
Naples Community Hospital	Naples	73%	300+
North Florida Regional Medical Center	Gainesville	73%	300+
Orange Park Medical Center	Orange Park	73%	300+
Palmetto General Hospital	Hialeah	73%	300+
Plantation General Hospital	Plantation	73%	300+
Putnam Community Medical Center	Palatka	73%	300+
Saint Mary's Medical Center	W Palm Beach	73%	300+
Santa Rosa Medical Center	Milton	73%	300+
Aventura Hospital & Medical Center	Aventura	72%	300+
Good Samaritan Medical Center	W Palm Beach	72%	300+
South Bay Hospital	Sun City Center	72%	300+
South Lake Hospital	Clermont	72%	300+
Bayfront Health Punta Gorda	Punta Gorda	71%	300+
Broward Health Coral Springs	Coral Springs	71%	300+
Citrus Memorial Hospital	Inverness	71%	300+
Edward White Hospital	St Petersburg	71%	300+
Lakeside Medical Center	Belle Glade	71%	300+
Larkin Community Hospital	South Miami	71%	(a)
Lawnwood Reg Med Ctr & Heart Inst	Fort Pierce	71%	300+
North Shore Medical Center	Miami	71%	300+
Northside Hospital	St Petersburg	71%	300+
Ocala Regional Medical Center	Ocala	71%	300+
Osceola Regional Medical Center	Kissimmee	71%	300+
Seven Rivers Regional Medical Center	Crystal River	71%	300+
Venice Reg Med Ctr-Bayfront Health	Venice	71%	300+
The Villages Regional Hospital	The Villages	71%	300+
Blake Medical Center	Bradenton	70%	300+
Broward Health Medical Center	Fort Lauderdale	70%	300+
Delray Medical Center	Delray Beach	70%	300+
Largo Medical Center	Largo	70%	300+
Physicians Reg Med Ctr-Pine Ridge	Naples	70%	300+
Regional Medical Center Bayonet Point	Hudson	70%	300+
West Boca Medical Center	Boca Raton	70%	300+
Bartow Regional Medical Center	Bartow	69%	300+
Bethesda Hospital East	Boynton Beach	69%	300+
Highlands Regional Medical Center	Sebring	69%	300+
Leesburg Regional Medical Center	Leesburg	69%	300+
Palms West Hospital	Loxahatchee	69%	300+
Shands Lake Shore Regional Medical Center	Lake City	69%	300+
Brandon Regional Hospital	Brandon	68%	300+
Jackson Memorial Hospital	Miami	68%	300+
JFK Medical Center	Atlantis	68%	300+
Sebastian River Medical Center	Sebastian	68%	300+
University Hospital & Medical Center	Tamarac	68%	300+
Wellington Regional Medical Center	Wellington	68%	300+
Westside Regional Medical Center	Plantation	68%	300+
Wuesthoff Medical Center - Melbourne	Melbourne	68%	300+
Northwest Medical Center	Margate	67%	300+
Wuesthoff Medical Center Rockledge	Rockledge	66%	300+
Bayfront Health Brooksville	Brooksville	64%	300+
Bayfront Health Port Charlotte	Port Charlotte	64%	300+
Bayfront Health Dade City	Dade City	63%	300+
Lehigh Regional Medical Center	Lehigh Acres	63%	300+
Heart of Florida Regional Medical Center	Davenport	62%	300+
Saint Cloud Regional Medical Center	Saint Cloud	62%	300+

Pain 'Always' Well Controlled

Hospital Name	City	Rate	Cases
Sacred Heart Hospital on the Gulf	Port Saint Joe	90%	(a)
Mariners Hospital	Tavernier	80%	(a)
Healthmark Regional Medical Center	Defuniak Spgs	79%	(a)
West Kendall Baptist Hospital	Miami	78%	300+
Memorial Hospital Miramar	Miramar	77%	300+
Doctor's Memorial Hospital	Perry	76%	(a)
Doctors Hospital	Coral Gables	76%	300+
Viera Hospital	Melbourne	76%	300+
Baptist Hospital of Miami	Miami	75%	300+
Fishermen's Hospital	Marathon	75%	(a)
Gulf Breeze Hospital	Gulf Breeze	75%	300+
Sacred Heart Hosp-Emerald Coast	Miramar Beach	75%	300+
Twin Cities Hospital	Niceville	75%	300+
Cape Canaveral Hospital	Cocoa Beach	74%	300+
Homestead Hospital	Homestead	74%	300+
Jay Hospital	Jay	74%	(a)
Mayo Clinic[11]	Jacksonville	74%	300+
South Miami Hospital	South Miami	74%	300+
UF Health Shands Hospital	Gainesville	74%	300+
Baptist Hospital	Pensacola	73%	300+
Baptist Medical Center Beaches	Jcksnvl Bch	73%	300+
Broward Health North	Pompano Bch	73%	300+
Jackson Hospital	Marianna	73%	300+
Palm Bay Hospital	Palm Bay	73%	300+
Sarasota Memorial Hospital	Sarasota	73%	300+
Bert Fish Medical Center	New Smyrn Bch	72%	300+
Cleveland Clinic Hospital	Weston	72%	300+
Desoto Memorial Hospital	Arcadia	72%	300+
Florida Hospital	Orlando	72%	300+
Memorial Regional Hospital	Hollywood	72%	300+
Parrish Medical Center	Titusville	72%	300+
Sacred Heart Hospital	Pensacola	72%	300+
Westchester General Hospital	Miami	72%	300+
Bayfront Health - Saint Petersburg	St Petersburg	71%	300+
Florida Hospital Memorial Medical Center[11]	Daytona Bch	71%	300+
Lake City Medical Center	Lake City	71%	300+
Lakewood Ranch Medical Center	Bradenton	71%	300+
Memorial Hospital West	Pembroke Pines	71%	300+
Oak Hill Hospital	Brooksville	71%	300+
Saint Joseph's Hospital	Tampa	71%	300+
Saint Vincent's Medical Center Southside	Jacksonville	71%	300+
Winter Haven Hospital	Winter Haven	71%	300+
Baptist Medical Center	Jacksonville	70%	300+
Baptist Medical Center - Nassau	Fernandina Bch	70%	300+
Boca Raton Regional Hospital	Boca Raton	70%	300+
Hendry Regional Medical Center	Clewiston	70%	(a)
Hialeah Hospital	Hialeah	70%	300+
Kendall Regional Medical Center	Miami	70%	300+
Lee Memorial Hospital	Fort Myers	70%	300+
Memorial Hospital Pembroke	Pembroke Pines	70%	300+
Morton Plant Hospital[11]	Clearwater	70%	300+
Palm Beach Gardens Medical Center	Palm Bch Grdns	70%	300+
Palms of Pasadena Hospital	St Petersburg	70%	300+
South Florida Baptist Hospital[11]	Plant City	70%	300+
Tallahassee Memorial Hospital	Tallahassee	70%	300+
Town & Country Hospital	Tampa	70%	300+
University of Miami Hospital	Miami	70%	300+
Broward Health Coral Springs	Coral Springs	69%	300+
Broward Health Imperial Point	Fort Lauderdale	69%	300+
Florida Hospital Flagler[11]	Palm Coast	69%	300+
Florida Hospital Zephyrhills[11]	Zephyrhills	69%	300+
Fort Walton Beach Medical Center	Fort Walton Bch	69%	300+
Gulf Coast Regional Medical Center	Panama City	69%	300+
Health Central	Ocoee	69%	300+
Jupiter Medical Center	Jupiter	69%	300+
Lake Wales Medical Center	Lake Wales	69%	300+
North Okaloosa Medical Center	Crestview	69%	300+
Palmetto General Hospital	Hialeah	69%	300+
Raulerson Hospital	Okeechobee	69%	300+
Saint Lucie Medical Center	Port Saint Lucie	69%	300+
Tampa General Hospital	Tampa	69%	300+
West Florida Hospital	Pensacola	69%	300+
West Palm Hospital	W Palm Beach	69%	300+
Bay Med Ctr Sacred Heart Health Sys	Panama City	68%	300+
Cape Coral Hospital	Cape Coral	68%	300+
Coral Gables Hospital	Coral Gables	68%	300+
Englewood Community Hospital	Englewood	68%	300+
Florida Hospital Heartland Medical Center[11]	Sebring	68%	300+
Florida Hospital North Pinellas[11]	Tarpon Springs	68%	300+
Gulf Coast Med Ctr Lee Mem Health Sys	Fort Myers	68%	300+
Lakeland Regional Medical Center	Lakeland	68%	300+
Lower Keys Medical Center	Key West	68%	300+
Martin Medical Center	Stuart	68%	300+
Saint Anthony's Hospital	St Petersburg	68%	300+
Saint Mary's Medical Center	W Palm Beach	68%	300+
UF Health Jacksonville	Jacksonville	68%	300+
Capital Regional Medical Center	Tallahassee	67%	300+
Central Florida Regional Hospital	Sanford	67%	300+
Doctors Hospital of Sarasota	Sarasota	67%	300+
Fawcett Memorial Hospital	Port Charlotte	67%	300+
Flagler Hospital	St Augustine	67%	300+
Florida Hospital Carrollwood[11]	Tampa	67%	300+
Florida Hospital Deland[11]	Deland	67%	300+
Florida Hospital Fish Memorial[11]	Orange City	67%	300+
Florida Hospital Tampa[11]	Tampa	67%	300+
Florida Hospital Waterman[11]	Tavares	67%	300+
Holmes Regional Medical Center	Melbourne	67%	300+
Holy Cross Hospital	Fort Lauderdale	67%	300+
Indian River Medical Center	Vero Beach	67%	300+
Mease Countryside Hospital[11]	Safety Harbor	67%	300+
Mease Hospital Dunedin[11]	Dunedin	67%	300+
Medical Center of Trinity	Trinity	67%	300+
Morton Plant North Bay Hospital[11]	New Port Richey	67%	300+
Mount Sinai Medical Center	Miami Beach	67%	300+
Munroe Regional Medical Center	Ocala	67%	300+
North Florida Regional Medical Center	Gainesville	67%	300+
Orange Park Medical Center	Orange Park	67%	300+
Orlando Health	Orlando	67%	300+
Plantation General Hospital	Plantation	67%	300+
Saint Petersburg General Hospital	St Petersburg	67%	300+
Aventura Hospital & Medical Center	Aventura	66%	300+
Edward White Hospital	St Petersburg	66%	300+
Good Samaritan Medical Center	W Palm Beach	66%	300+
Halifax Health Medical Center	Daytona Bch	66%	300+
Lawnwood Reg Med Ctr & Heart Inst	Fort Pierce	66%	300+
Manatee Memorial Hospital	Bradenton	66%	300+
Memorial Hospital Jacksonville	Jacksonville	66%	300+
Memorial Hospital of Tampa	Tampa	66%	300+
Naples Community Hospital	Naples	66%	300+
Osceola Regional Medical Center	Kissimmee	66%	300+
Palm Springs General Hospital	Hialeah	66%	300+
Saint Vincent's Medical Center	Jacksonville	66%	(a)
South Lake Hospital	Clermont	66%	300+
Bayfront Health Punta Gorda	Punta Gorda	65%	300+
Jackson Memorial Hospital	Miami	65%	300+

NOTE: Hospital profiles are in alphabetical order by state, then city, then hospital within the city; Rankings exclude hospitals with less than 25 cases except for patient surveys which excludes hospitals with less than 100 cases; (a) 100-299 cases; (1) The number of cases/patients is too few to report; (2) Data submitted were based on a sample of cases/patients; (3) Results are based on a shorter time period than required; (4) Data suppressed by CMS for one or more quarters; (5) Results are not available for this reporting period; (6) Fewer than 100 patients completed the HCAHPS survey; (7) No cases met the criteria for this measure; (8) The lower limit of the confidence interval cannot be calculated if the number of observed infections equals zero; (9) No data are available from the state/territory for this reporting period; (10) The scores shown reflect fewer than 50 completed surveys; (11) There were discrepancies in the data collection process; (12) This measure does not apply to this hospital for this reporting period; (13) Results cannot be calculated for this reporting period; (14) The results for this state are combined with nearby states to protect confidentiality; Please refer to the User's Guide for a full explanation of data.

Putnam Community Medical Center	Palatka	65%	300+
Santa Rosa Medical Center	Milton	65%	300+
Shands Lake Shore Regional Medical Center	Lake City	65%	300+
West Boca Medical Center	Boca Raton	65%	300+
Blake Medical Center	Bradenton	64%	300+
North Shore Medical Center	Miami	64%	300+
Ocala Regional Medical Center	Ocala	64%	300+
Palms West Hospital	Loxahatchee	64%	300+
Physicians Reg Med Ctr-Pine Ridge	Naples	64%	300+
Sebastian River Medical Center	Sebastian	64%	300+
Wuesthoff Medical Center - Melbourne	Melbourne	64%	300+
Bayfront Health Port Charlotte	Port Charlotte	63%	300+
Brandon Regional Hospital	Brandon	63%	300+
Broward Health Medical Center	Fort Lauderdale	63%	300+
Citrus Memorial Hospital	Inverness	63%	300+
Largo Medical Center	Largo	63%	300+
Leesburg Regional Medical Center	Leesburg	63%	300+
South Bay Hospital	Sun City Center	63%	300+
University Hospital & Medical Center	Tamarac	63%	300+
Westside Regional Medical Center	Plantation	63%	300+
Bethesda Hospital East	Boynton Beach	62%	300+
Northwest Medical Center	Margate	62%	300+
Regional Medical Center Bayonet Point	Hudson	62%	300+
Venice Reg Med Ctr-Bayfront Health	Venice	62%	300+
Delray Medical Center	Delray Beach	61%	300+
Lakeside Medical Center	Belle Glade	61%	300+
Saint Cloud Regional Medical Center	Saint Cloud	61%	300+
Seven Rivers Regional Medical Center	Crystal River	61%	300+
The Villages Regional Hospital	The Villages	61%	300+
Wellington Regional Medical Center	Wellington	61%	300+
Bartow Regional Medical Center	Bartow	60%	300+
Highlands Regional Medical Center	Sebring	60%	300+
JFK Medical Center	Atlantis	60%	300+
Northside Hospital	St Petersburg	60%	300+
Wuesthoff Medical Center Rockledge	Rockledge	60%	300+
Bayfront Health Brooksville	Brooksville	58%	300+
Bayfront Health Dade City	Dade City	58%	300+
Larkin Community Hospital	South Miami	58%	(a)
Heart of Florida Regional Medical Center	Davenport	57%	300+
Lehigh Regional Medical Center	Lehigh Acres	53%	300+

Room and Bathroom 'Always' Clean

Hospital Name	City	Rate	Cases
Mariners Hospital	Tavernier	89%	(a)
Sacred Heart Hospital on the Gulf	Port Saint Joe	89%	(a)
West Kendall Baptist Hospital	Miami	87%	300+
Doctor's Memorial Hospital	Perry	85%	(a)
Memorial Hospital Miramar	Miramar	83%	300+
Palm Bay Hospital	Palm Bay	81%	300+
Cape Canaveral Hospital	Cocoa Beach	80%	300+
Healthmark Regional Medical Center	Defuniak Spgs	80%	(a)
Lakeside Medical Center	Belle Glade	79%	300+
Larkin Community Hospital	South Miami	79%	(a)
Mayo Clinic[11]	Jacksonville	79%	300+
Viera Hospital	Melbourne	79%	300+
Palm Springs General Hospital	Hialeah	78%	300+
South Florida Baptist Hospital[11]	Plant City	78%	300+
Florida Hospital	Orlando	77%	300+
Homestead Hospital	Homestead	77%	300+
Jay Hospital	Jay	77%	(a)
Memorial Hospital West	Pembroke Pines	77%	300+
Saint Joseph's Hospital	Tampa	77%	300+
Doctors Hospital	Coral Gables	76%	300+
Health Central	Ocoee	76%	300+
Memorial Regional Hospital	Hollywood	76%	300+
Palmetto General Hospital	Hialeah	76%	300+
Florida Hospital Heartland Medical Center[11]	Sebring	75%	300+
Florida Hospital Memorial Medical Center[11]	Daytona Bch	75%	300+
Florida Hospital North Pinellas[11]	Tarpon Springs	75%	300+
Mease Hospital Dunedin[11]	Dunedin	75%	300+
Memorial Hospital Pembroke	Pembroke Pines	75%	300+
South Miami Hospital	South Miami	75%	300+
Tallahassee Memorial Hospital	Tallahassee	75%	300+
Baptist Hospital	Pensacola	74%	300+
Coral Gables Hospital	Coral Gables	74%	300+
Gulf Breeze Hospital	Gulf Breeze	74%	300+
Mease Countryside Hospital[11]	Safety Harbor	74%	300+
Morton Plant Hospital[11]	Clearwater	74%	300+
Parrish Medical Center	Titusville	74%	300+
Baptist Hospital of Miami	Miami	73%	300+
Baptist Medical Center Beaches	Jcksnvll Bch	73%	300+
Florida Hospital Waterman[11]	Tavares	73%	300+
Jackson Hospital	Marianna	73%	300+
Lake Wales Medical Center	Lake Wales	73%	300+
Sacred Heart Hosp-Emerald Coast	Miramar Beach	73%	300+
Saint Petersburg General Hospital	St Petersburg	73%	300+
Westchester General Hospital	Miami	73%	300+
Cleveland Clinic Hospital	Weston	72%	300+
Fishermen's Hospital	Marathon	72%	(a)
Flagler Hospital	St Augustine	72%	300+
Florida Hospital Flagler[11]	Palm Coast	72%	300+
Kendall Regional Medical Center	Miami	72%	300+
Medical Center of Trinity	Trinity	72%	300+
Santa Rosa Medical Center	Milton	72%	300+
Winter Haven Hospital	Winter Haven	72%	300+
Baptist Medical Center	Jacksonville	71%	300+
Broward Health North	Pompano Bch	71%	300+
Doctors Hospital of Sarasota	Sarasota	71%	300+
Florida Hospital Carrollwood[11]	Tampa	71%	300+
Hialeah Hospital	Hialeah	71%	300+
Saint Vincent's Medical Center Southside	Jacksonville	71%	300+
Sarasota Memorial Hospital	Sarasota	71%	300+
University of Miami Hospital	Miami	71%	300+
Bert Fish Medical Center	New Smyrn Bch	70%	300+
Broward Health Imperial Point	Fort Lauderdale	70%	300+
Capital Regional Medical Center	Tallahassee	70%	300+
Edward White Hospital	St Petersburg	70%	300+
Holmes Regional Medical Center	Melbourne	70%	300+
Lake City Medical Center	Lake City	70%	300+
Morton Plant North Bay Hospital[11]	New Port Richey	70%	300+
Northside Hospital	St Petersburg	70%	300+
Orange Park Medical Center	Orange Park	70%	300+
Palms of Pasadena Hospital	St Petersburg	70%	300+
Physicians Reg Med Ctr-Pine Ridge	Naples	70%	300+
Raulerson Hospital	Okeechobee	70%	300+
Saint Anthony's Hospital	St Petersburg	70%	300+
South Lake Hospital	Clermont	70%	300+
Twin Cities Hospital	Niceville	70%	300+
Baptist Medical Center - Nassau	Fernandina Bch	69%	300+
Bayfront Health - Saint Petersburg	St Petersburg	69%	300+
Cape Coral Hospital	Cape Coral	69%	300+
Florida Hospital Fish Memorial[11]	Orange City	69%	300+
Memorial Hospital of Tampa	Tampa	69%	300+
Orlando Health	Orlando	69%	300+
Plantation General Hospital	Plantation	69%	300+
West Palm Hospital	W Palm Beach	69%	300+
Bartow Regional Medical Center	Bartow	68%	300+
Halifax Health Medical Center	Daytona Bch	68%	300+
Lakewood Ranch Medical Center	Bradenton	68%	300+
Lee Memorial Hospital	Fort Myers	68%	300+
Mount Sinai Medical Center	Miami Beach	68%	300+
North Okaloosa Medical Center	Crestview	68%	300+
Saint Lucie Medical Center	Port Saint Lucie	68%	300+
Town & Country Hospital	Tampa	68%	300+
Aventura Hospital & Medical Center	Aventura	67%	300+
Desoto Memorial Hospital	Arcadia	67%	300+
Florida Hospital Tampa[11]	Tampa	67%	300+
Florida Hospital Zephyrhills[11]	Zephyrhills	67%	300+
Highlands Regional Medical Center	Sebring	67%	300+
Holy Cross Hospital	Fort Lauderdale	67%	300+
Jupiter Medical Center	Jupiter	67%	300+
Leesburg Regional Medical Center	Leesburg	67%	300+
Naples Community Hospital	Naples	67%	300+
Wuesthoff Medical Center - Melbourne	Melbourne	67%	300+
Bayfront Health Brooksville	Brooksville	66%	300+
Bayfront Health Punta Gorda	Punta Gorda	66%	300+
Broward Health Coral Springs	Coral Springs	66%	300+
Central Florida Regional Hospital	Sanford	66%	300+
Florida Hospital Deland[11]	Deland	66%	300+
Gulf Coast Regional Medical Center	Panama City	66%	300+
Lehigh Regional Medical Center	Lehigh Acres	66%	300+
Manatee Memorial Hospital	Bradenton	66%	300+
Martin Medical Center	Stuart	66%	300+
Oak Hill Hospital	Brooksville	66%	300+
Ocala Regional Medical Center	Ocala	66%	300+
Putnam Community Medical Center	Palatka	66%	300+
Sebastian River Medical Center	Sebastian	66%	300+
Shands Lake Shore Regional Medical Center	Lake City	66%	300+
South Bay Hospital	Sun City Center	66%	300+
UF Health Shands Hospital	Gainesville	66%	300+
The Villages Regional Hospital	The Villages	66%	300+
Wellington Regional Medical Center	Wellington	66%	300+
West Florida Hospital	Pensacola	66%	300+
Bayfront Health Dade City	Dade City	65%	300+
Bethesda Hospital East	Boynton Beach	65%	300+
Boca Raton Regional Hospital	Boca Raton	65%	300+
Broward Health Medical Center	Fort Lauderdale	65%	300+
Citrus Memorial Hospital	Inverness	65%	300+
Munroe Regional Medical Center	Ocala	65%	300+
Osceola Regional Medical Center	Kissimmee	65%	300+
Sacred Heart Hospital	Pensacola	65%	300+
Tampa General Hospital	Tampa	65%	300+
UF Health Jacksonville	Jacksonville	65%	300+
Bay Med Ctr Sacred Heart Health Sys	Panama City	64%	300+
Blake Medical Center	Bradenton	64%	300+
Brandon Regional Hospital	Brandon	64%	300+
Englewood Community Hospital	Englewood	64%	300+
Fort Walton Beach Medical Center	Fort Walton Bch	64%	300+
Gulf Coast Med Ctr Lee Mem Health Sys	Fort Myers	64%	300+
Heart of Florida Regional Medical Center	Davenport	64%	300+
Indian River Medical Center	Vero Beach	64%	300+
Lakeland Regional Medical Center	Lakeland	64%	300+
Largo Medical Center	Largo	64%	300+
Memorial Hospital Jacksonville	Jacksonville	64%	300+
North Shore Medical Center	Miami	64%	300+
Regional Medical Center Bayonet Point	Hudson	64%	300+
Saint Cloud Regional Medical Center	Saint Cloud	64%	300+
University Hospital & Medical Center	Tamarac	64%	300+
Bayfront Health Port Charlotte	Port Charlotte	63%	300+
Hendry Regional Medical Center	Clewiston	63%	(a)
Lawnwood Reg Med Ctr & Heart Inst	Fort Pierce	63%	300+
Palm Beach Gardens Medical Center	Palm Bch Grdns	63%	300+
Saint Mary's Medical Center	W Palm Beach	63%	300+
Saint Vincent's Medical Center	Jacksonville	63%	(a)
Westside Regional Medical Center	Plantation	63%	300+
North Florida Regional Medical Center	Gainesville	62%	300+
Palms West Hospital	Loxahatchee	62%	300+
Venice Reg Med Ctr-Bayfront Health	Venice	62%	300+
Jackson Memorial Hospital	Miami	61%	300+
Lower Keys Medical Center	Key West	61%	300+
Northwest Medical Center	Margate	61%	300+
Fawcett Memorial Hospital	Port Charlotte	60%	300+
Good Samaritan Medical Center	W Palm Beach	60%	300+
JFK Medical Center	Atlantis	60%	300+
Wuesthoff Medical Center Rockledge	Rockledge	60%	300+
Seven Rivers Regional Medical Center	Crystal River	59%	300+
West Boca Medical Center	Boca Raton	56%	300+
Delray Medical Center	Delray Beach	55%	300+

Timely Help 'Always' Received

Hospital Name	City	Rate	Cases
Mariners Hospital	Tavernier	89%	(a)
Sacred Heart Hospital on the Gulf	Port Saint Joe	88%	(a)
Jay Hospital	Jay	80%	(a)
Healthmark Regional Medical Center	Defuniak Spgs	75%	(a)
Hendry Regional Medical Center	Clewiston	75%	(a)
Doctor's Memorial Hospital	Perry	74%	(a)
Gulf Breeze Hospital	Gulf Breeze	74%	300+
Viera Hospital	Melbourne	73%	300+
Fishermen's Hospital	Marathon	72%	(a)
Sacred Heart Hosp-Emerald Coast	Miramar Beach	72%	300+
Twin Cities Hospital	Niceville	72%	300+
Memorial Hospital Pembroke	Pembroke Pines	71%	300+
Parrish Medical Center	Titusville	71%	300+
Mayo Clinic[11]	Jacksonville	70%	300+
Memorial Hospital Miramar	Miramar	70%	300+
South Florida Baptist Hospital[11]	Plant City	70%	300+
West Kendall Baptist Hospital	Miami	70%	300+
Baptist Hospital	Pensacola	69%	300+
Doctors Hospital	Coral Gables	69%	300+
Lake City Medical Center	Lake City	69%	300+
Cape Canaveral Hospital	Cocoa Beach	68%	300+
Florida Hospital Memorial Medical Center[11]	Daytona Bch	68%	300+
Jackson Hospital	Marianna	68%	300+
Lower Keys Medical Center	Key West	68%	300+
Palm Bay Hospital	Palm Bay	68%	300+
Baptist Medical Center - Nassau	Fernandina Bch	67%	300+
Florida Hospital	Orlando	67%	300+
Memorial Regional Hospital	Hollywood	67%	300+
Morton Plant Hospital[11]	Clearwater	67%	300+
North Okaloosa Medical Center	Crestview	67%	300+
Palm Beach Gardens Medical Center	Palm Bch Grdns	67%	300+
Raulerson Hospital	Okeechobee	67%	300+
Winter Haven Hospital	Winter Haven	67%	300+
Cleveland Clinic Hospital	Weston	66%	300+
Palms of Pasadena Hospital	St Petersburg	66%	300+
Saint Vincent's Medical Center Southside	Jacksonville	66%	300+
Sarasota Memorial Hospital	Sarasota	66%	300+
South Miami Hospital	South Miami	66%	300+
Florida Hospital Zephyrhills[11]	Zephyrhills	65%	300+
Homestead Hospital	Homestead	65%	300+
Mease Hospital Dunedin[11]	Dunedin	65%	300+
Sacred Heart Hospital	Pensacola	65%	300+
Baptist Hospital of Miami	Miami	64%	300+
Baptist Medical Center	Jacksonville	64%	300+
Baptist Medical Center Beaches	Jcksnvll Bch	64%	300+
Bert Fish Medical Center	New Smyrn Bch	64%	300+
Broward Health North	Pompano Bch	64%	300+
Florida Hospital Deland[11]	Deland	64%	300+
Florida Hospital Heartland Medical Center[11]	Sebring	64%	300+
Florida Hospital Waterman[11]	Tavares	64%	300+
Health Central	Ocoee	64%	300+
Jupiter Medical Center	Jupiter	64%	300+
Lee Memorial Hospital	Fort Myers	64%	300+
Saint Joseph's Hospital	Tampa	64%	300+
Tampa General Hospital	Tampa	64%	300+
West Florida Hospital	Pensacola	64%	300+
Desoto Memorial Hospital	Arcadia	63%	300+
Flagler Hospital	St Augustine	63%	300+
Florida Hospital Carrollwood[11]	Tampa	63%	300+
Florida Hospital Fish Memorial[11]	Orange City	63%	300+
Florida Hospital North Pinellas[11]	Tarpon Springs	63%	300+
Halifax Health Medical Center	Daytona Bch	63%	300+

NOTE: Hospital profiles are in alphabetical order by state, then city, then hospital within the city; Rankings exclude hospitals with less than 25 cases except for patient surveys which excludes hospitals with less than 100 cases; (a) 100-299 cases; (1) The number of cases/patients is too few to report; (2) Data submitted were based on a sample of cases/patients; (3) Results are based on a shorter time period than required; (4) Data suppressed by CMS for one or more quarters; (5) Results are not available for this reporting period; (6) Fewer than 100 patients completed the HCAHPS survey; (7) No cases met the criteria for this measure; (8) The lower limit of the confidence interval cannot be calculated if the number of observed infections equals zero; (9) No data are available from the state/territory for this reporting period; (10) The scores shown reflect fewer than 50 completed surveys; (11) There were discrepancies in the data collection process; (12) This measure does not apply to this hospital for this reporting period; (13) Results cannot be calculated for this reporting period; (14) The results for this state are combined with nearby states to protect confidentiality; Please refer to the User's Guide for a full explanation of data.

Hospital Name	City	Rate	Cases
Medical Center of Trinity	Trinity	63%	300+
Memorial Hospital West	Pembroke Pines	63%	300+
Palmetto General Hospital	Hialeah	63%	300+
Saint Petersburg General Hospital	St Petersburg	63%	300+
Santa Rosa Medical Center	Milton	63%	300+
West Palm Hospital	W Palm Beach	63%	300+
Coral Gables Hospital	Coral Gables	62%	300+
Gulf Coast Med Ctr Lee Mem Health Sys	Fort Myers	62%	300+
Kendall Regional Medical Center	Miami	62%	300+
Lakeland Regional Medical Center	Lakeland	62%	300+
Mease Countryside Hospital[11]	Safety Harbor	62%	300+
Oak Hill Hospital	Brooksville	62%	300+
Orlando Health	Orlando	62%	300+
Saint Anthony's Hospital	St Petersburg	62%	300+
South Lake Hospital	Clermont	62%	300+
UF Health Shands Hospital	Gainesville	62%	300+
Aventura Hospital & Medical Center	Aventura	61%	300+
Bay Med Ctr Sacred Heart Health Sys	Panama City	61%	300+
Bayfront Health Punta Gorda	Punta Gorda	61%	300+
Broward Health Imperial Point	Fort Lauderdale	61%	300+
Englewood Community Hospital	Englewood	61%	300+
Florida Hospital Flagler[11]	Palm Coast	61%	300+
Florida Hospital Tampa[11]	Tampa	61%	300+
Hialeah Hospital	Hialeah	61%	300+
Holmes Regional Medical Center	Melbourne	61%	300+
Martin Medical Center	Stuart	61%	300+
Morton Plant North Bay Hospital[11]	New Port Richey	61%	300+
Palm Springs General Hospital	Hialeah	61%	300+
Saint Lucie Medical Center	Port Saint Lucie	61%	300+
Tallahassee Memorial Hospital	Tallahassee	61%	300+
Bayfront Health - Saint Petersburg	St Petersburg	60%	300+
Central Florida Regional Hospital	Sanford	60%	300+
Fort Walton Beach Medical Center	Fort Walton Bch	60%	300+
Lake Wales Medical Center	Lake Wales	60%	300+
Lakewood Ranch Medical Center	Bradenton	60%	300+
Largo Medical Center	Largo	60%	300+
Osceola Regional Medical Center	Kissimmee	60%	300+
Saint Vincent's Medical Center	Jacksonville	60%	(a)
UF Health Jacksonville	Jacksonville	60%	300+
Boca Raton Regional Hospital	Boca Raton	59%	300+
Capital Regional Medical Center	Tallahassee	59%	300+
Doctors Hospital of Sarasota	Sarasota	59%	300+
Gulf Coast Regional Medical Center	Panama City	59%	300+
Memorial Hospital of Tampa	Tampa	59%	300+
Mount Sinai Medical Center	Miami Beach	59%	300+
Naples Community Hospital	Naples	59%	300+
Shands Lake Shore Regional Medical Center	Lake City	59%	300+
South Bay Hospital	Sun City Center	59%	300+
University of Miami Hospital	Miami	59%	300+
Bartow Regional Medical Center	Bartow	58%	300+
Cape Coral Hospital	Cape Coral	58%	300+
Edward White Hospital	St Petersburg	58%	300+
Lakeside Medical Center	Belle Glade	58%	300+
Northside Hospital	St Petersburg	58%	300+
Plantation General Hospital	Plantation	58%	300+
Saint Mary's Medical Center	W Palm Beach	58%	300+
Westchester General Hospital	Miami	58%	300+
Holy Cross Hospital	Fort Lauderdale	57%	300+
Leesburg Regional Medical Center	Leesburg	57%	300+
North Florida Regional Medical Center	Gainesville	57%	300+
Seven Rivers Regional Medical Center	Crystal River	57%	300+
Town & Country Hospital	Tampa	57%	300+
Venice Reg Med Ctr-Bayfront Health	Venice	57%	300+
West Boca Medical Center	Boca Raton	57%	300+
Blake Medical Center	Bradenton	56%	300+
Highlands Regional Medical Center	Sebring	56%	300+
Indian River Medical Center	Vero Beach	56%	300+
Jackson Memorial Hospital	Miami	56%	300+
Larkin Community Hospital	South Miami	56%	(a)
Manatee Memorial Hospital	Bradenton	56%	300+
Orange Park Medical Center	Orange Park	56%	300+
Putnam Community Medical Center	Palatka	56%	300+
The Villages Regional Hospital	The Villages	56%	300+
Good Samaritan Medical Center	W Palm Beach	55%	300+
Lawnwood Reg Med Ctr & Heart Inst	Fort Pierce	55%	300+
Memorial Hospital Jacksonville	Jacksonville	55%	300+
Munroe Regional Medical Center	Ocala	55%	300+
Ocala Regional Medical Center	Ocala	55%	300+
Palms West Hospital	Loxahatchee	55%	300+
Sebastian River Medical Center	Sebastian	55%	300+
Westside Regional Medical Center	Plantation	55%	300+
Bayfront Health Dade City	Dade City	54%	300+
Bayfront Health Port Charlotte	Port Charlotte	54%	300+
Brandon Regional Hospital	Brandon	54%	300+
Citrus Memorial Hospital	Inverness	54%	300+
Fawcett Memorial Hospital	Port Charlotte	54%	300+
JFK Medical Center	Atlantis	54%	300+
Regional Medical Center Bayonet Point	Hudson	54%	300+
University Hospital & Medical Center	Tamarac	54%	300+
Delray Medical Center	Delray Beach	53%	300+
North Shore Medical Center	Miami	53%	300+
Physicians Reg Med Ctr-Pine Ridge	Naples	53%	300+
Bethesda Hospital East	Boynton Beach	52%	300+
Broward Health Coral Springs	Coral Springs	52%	300+
Wuesthoff Medical Center Rockledge	Rockledge	52%	300+
Northwest Medical Center	Margate	51%	300+
Wuesthoff Medical Center - Melbourne	Melbourne	51%	300+
Broward Health Medical Center	Fort Lauderdale	50%	300+
Heart of Florida Regional Medical Center	Davenport	50%	300+
Saint Cloud Regional Medical Center	Saint Cloud	50%	300+
Wellington Regional Medical Center	Wellington	49%	300+
Lehigh Regional Medical Center	Lehigh Acres	48%	300+
Bayfront Health Brooksville	Brooksville	46%	300+

Would Definitely Recommend Hospital

Hospital Name	City	Rate	Cases
Mayo Clinic[11]	Jacksonville	92%	300+
Sacred Heart Hospital on the Gulf	Port Saint Joe	90%	(a)
Viera Hospital	Melbourne	88%	300+
West Kendall Baptist Hospital	Miami	86%	300+
Gulf Breeze Hospital	Gulf Breeze	85%	300+
Memorial Hospital Miramar	Miramar	85%	300+
Sacred Heart Hosp-Emerald Coast	Miramar Beach	85%	300+
Cleveland Clinic Hospital	Weston	84%	300+
Florida Hospital Memorial Medical Center[11]	Daytona Bch	84%	300+
Doctors Hospital	Coral Gables	83%	300+
Sarasota Memorial Hospital	Sarasota	83%	300+
Mariners Hospital	Tavernier	82%	(a)
Morton Plant Hospital[11]	Clearwater	81%	300+
South Miami Hospital	South Miami	81%	300+
UF Health Shands Hospital	Gainesville	81%	300+
Baptist Hospital of Miami	Miami	80%	300+
Memorial Regional Hospital	Hollywood	80%	300+
Saint Joseph's Hospital	Tampa	80%	300+
Twin Cities Hospital	Niceville	80%	300+
Baptist Medical Center - Nassau	Fernandina Bch	79%	300+
Baptist Medical Center Beaches	Jcksnvll Bch	79%	300+
Homestead Hospital	Homestead	79%	300+
Jupiter Medical Center	Jupiter	79%	300+
Memorial Hospital West	Pembroke Pines	79%	300+
Tampa General Hospital	Tampa	79%	300+
Baptist Medical Center	Jacksonville	78%	300+
Boca Raton Regional Hospital	Boca Raton	78%	300+
Cape Canaveral Hospital	Cocoa Beach	78%	300+
Florida Hospital	Orlando	78%	300+
Baptist Hospital	Pensacola	77%	300+
Mease Countryside Hospital[11]	Safety Harbor	77%	300+
Saint Anthony's Hospital	St Petersburg	77%	300+
Broward Health Imperial Point	Fort Lauderdale	76%	300+
Doctors Hospital of Sarasota	Sarasota	76%	300+
Holy Cross Hospital	Fort Lauderdale	76%	300+
Lake City Medical Center	Lake City	76%	300+
Mease Hospital Dunedin[11]	Dunedin	76%	300+
Memorial Hospital Pembroke	Pembroke Pines	76%	300+
Palm Bay Hospital	Palm Bay	76%	300+
Sacred Heart Hospital	Pensacola	76%	300+
West Florida Hospital	Pensacola	76%	300+
Lakewood Ranch Medical Center	Bradenton	75%	300+
Lee Memorial Hospital	Fort Myers	75%	300+
Morton Plant North Bay Hospital[11]	New Port Richey	75%	300+
Saint Vincent's Medical Center Southside	Jacksonville	75%	300+
Broward Health North	Pompano Bch	74%	300+
Capital Regional Medical Center	Tallahassee	74%	300+
Jay Hospital	Jay	74%	(a)
Martin Medical Center	Stuart	74%	300+
Orlando Health	Orlando	74%	300+
Parrish Medical Center	Titusville	74%	300+
Tallahassee Memorial Hospital	Tallahassee	74%	300+
Lakeland Regional Medical Center	Lakeland	73%	300+
Naples Community Hospital	Naples	73%	300+
North Florida Regional Medical Center	Gainesville	73%	300+
Palm Beach Gardens Medical Center	Palm Bch Grdns	73%	300+
South Florida Baptist Hospital[11]	Plant City	73%	300+
University of Miami Hospital	Miami	73%	300+
Winter Haven Hospital	Winter Haven	73%	300+
Bay Med Ctr Sacred Heart Health Sys	Panama City	72%	300+
Bert Fish Medical Center	New Smyrn Bch	72%	300+
Gulf Coast Regional Medical Center	Panama City	72%	300+
Holmes Regional Medical Center	Melbourne	72%	300+
Jackson Hospital	Marianna	72%	300+
Oak Hill Hospital	Brooksville	72%	300+
Flagler Hospital	St Augustine	71%	300+
Florida Hospital Heartland Medical Center[11]	Sebring	71%	300+
Medical Center of Trinity	Trinity	71%	300+
Munroe Regional Medical Center	Ocala	71%	300+
Saint Vincent's Medical Center	Jacksonville	71%	(a)
Florida Hospital North Pinellas[11]	Tarpon Springs	70%	300+
Good Samaritan Medical Center	W Palm Beach	70%	300+
Gulf Coast Med Ctr Lee Mem Health Sys	Fort Myers	70%	300+
Mount Sinai Medical Center	Miami Beach	70%	300+
Palms of Pasadena Hospital	St Petersburg	70%	300+
Broward Health Medical Center	Fort Lauderdale	69%	300+
Edward White Hospital	St Petersburg	69%	300+
Fishermen's Hospital	Marathon	69%	(a)
Florida Hospital Carrollwood[11]	Tampa	69%	300+
Halifax Health Medical Center	Daytona Bch	69%	300+
Health Central	Ocoee	69%	300+
West Palm Hospital	W Palm Beach	69%	300+
Bethesda Hospital East	Boynton Beach	68%	300+
Doctor's Memorial Hospital	Perry	68%	(a)
Fawcett Memorial Hospital	Port Charlotte	68%	300+
Indian River Medical Center	Vero Beach	68%	300+
Ocala Regional Medical Center	Ocala	68%	300+
Physicians Reg Med Ctr-Pine Ridge	Naples	68%	300+
Saint Mary's Medical Center	W Palm Beach	68%	300+
Saint Petersburg General Hospital	St Petersburg	68%	300+
Bayfront Health - Saint Petersburg	St Petersburg	67%	300+
Blake Medical Center	Bradenton	67%	300+
Florida Hospital Waterman[11]	Tavares	67%	300+
Manatee Memorial Hospital	Bradenton	67%	300+
South Lake Hospital	Clermont	67%	300+
Aventura Hospital & Medical Center	Aventura	66%	300+
Florida Hospital Zephyrhills[11]	Zephyrhills	66%	300+
Memorial Hospital of Tampa	Tampa	66%	300+
Plantation General Hospital	Plantation	66%	300+
Cape Coral Hospital	Cape Coral	65%	300+
Central Florida Regional Hospital	Sanford	65%	300+
Coral Gables Hospital	Coral Gables	65%	300+
Florida Hospital Flagler[11]	Palm Coast	65%	300+
Florida Hospital Tampa[11]	Tampa	65%	300+
Healthmark Regional Medical Center	Defuniak Spgs	65%	(a)
Jackson Memorial Hospital	Miami	65%	300+
Lake Wales Medical Center	Lake Wales	65%	300+
North Okaloosa Medical Center	Crestview	65%	300+
Palms West Hospital	Loxahatchee	65%	300+
Saint Lucie Medical Center	Port Saint Lucie	65%	300+
UF Health Jacksonville	Jacksonville	65%	300+
Memorial Hospital Jacksonville	Jacksonville	64%	300+
Northside Hospital	St Petersburg	64%	300+
Raulerson Hospital	Okeechobee	64%	300+
Sebastian River Medical Center	Sebastian	64%	300+
Venice Reg Med Ctr-Bayfront Health	Venice	64%	300+
Citrus Memorial Hospital	Inverness	63%	300+
Delray Medical Center	Delray Beach	63%	300+
Florida Hospital Deland[11]	Deland	63%	300+
Fort Walton Beach Medical Center	Fort Walton Bch	63%	300+
Hialeah Hospital	Hialeah	63%	300+
JFK Medical Center	Atlantis	63%	300+
Largo Medical Center	Largo	63%	300+
Orange Park Medical Center	Orange Park	63%	300+
Town & Country Hospital	Tampa	63%	300+
Bayfront Health Punta Gorda	Punta Gorda	62%	300+
Kendall Regional Medical Center	Miami	62%	300+
Lakeside Medical Center	Belle Glade	62%	300+
Palm Springs General Hospital	Hialeah	62%	300+
Palmetto General Hospital	Hialeah	62%	300+
Regional Medical Center Bayonet Point	Hudson	62%	300+
Wellington Regional Medical Center	Wellington	62%	300+
West Boca Medical Center	Boca Raton	62%	300+
Bartow Regional Medical Center	Bartow	61%	300+
Broward Health Coral Springs	Coral Springs	61%	300+
Desoto Memorial Hospital	Arcadia	61%	300+
Florida Hospital Fish Memorial[11]	Orange City	61%	300+
Lawnwood Reg Med Ctr & Heart Inst	Fort Pierce	61%	300+
Osceola Regional Medical Center	Kissimmee	61%	300+
Seven Rivers Regional Medical Center	Crystal River	61%	300+
Westside Regional Medical Center	Plantation	61%	300+
Englewood Community Hospital	Englewood	60%	300+
Hendry Regional Medical Center	Clewiston	60%	(a)
Northwest Medical Center	Margate	60%	300+
Leesburg Regional Medical Center	Leesburg	59%	300+
South Bay Hospital	Sun City Center	59%	300+
University Hospital & Medical Center	Tamarac	59%	300+
North Shore Medical Center	Miami	58%	300+
The Villages Regional Hospital	The Villages	58%	300+
Westchester General Hospital	Miami	58%	300+
Wuesthoff Medical Center - Melbourne	Melbourne	58%	300+
Highlands Regional Medical Center	Sebring	57%	300+
Larkin Community Hospital	South Miami	57%	(a)
Bayfront Health Dade City	Dade City	56%	300+
Brandon Regional Hospital	Brandon	56%	300+
Santa Rosa Medical Center	Milton	55%	300+
Bayfront Health Port Charlotte	Port Charlotte	54%	300+
Lower Keys Medical Center	Key West	53%	300+
Saint Cloud Regional Medical Center	Saint Cloud	52%	300+
Shands Lake Shore Regional Medical Center	Lake City	52%	300+
Putnam Community Medical Center	Palatka	51%	300+
Heart of Florida Regional Medical Center	Davenport	50%	300+
Bayfront Health Brooksville	Brooksville	49%	300+
Wuesthoff Medical Center Rockledge	Rockledge	48%	300+
Lehigh Regional Medical Center	Lehigh Acres	45%	300+

NOTE: Hospital profiles are in alphabetical order by state, then city, then hospital within the city; Rankings exclude hospitals with less than 25 cases except for patient surveys which excludes hospitals with less than 100 cases; (a) 100-299 cases; (1) The number of cases/patients is too few to report; (2) Data submitted were based on a sample of cases/patients; (3) Results are based on a shorter time period than required; (4) Data suppressed by CMS for one or more quarters; (5) Results are not available for this reporting period; (6) Fewer than 100 patients completed the HCAHPS survey; (7) No cases met the criteria for this measure; (8) The lower limit of the confidence interval cannot be calculated if the number of observed infections equals zero; (9) No data are available from the state/territory for this reporting period; (10) The scores shown reflect fewer than 50 completed surveys; (11) There were discrepancies in the data collection process; (12) This measure does not apply to this hospital for this reporting period; (13) Results cannot be calculated for this reporting period; (14) The results for this state are combined with nearby states to protect confidentiality; Please refer to the User's Guide for a full explanation of data.

Use of Medical Imaging

Cardiac Imaging Stress Test before OP Surgery

Hospital Name	City	Rate	Cases
Homestead Hospital	Homestead	1.2%	82
Palm Bay Hospital	Palm Bay	2.2%	178
Lakewood Ranch Medical Center	Bradenton	2.7%	74
Tallahassee Memorial Hospital	Tallahassee	2.8%	325
Gulf Coast Regional Medical Center	Panama City	3.0%	67
Lower Keys Medical Center	Key West	3.1%	288
Capital Regional Medical Center	Tallahassee	3.2%	186
Heart of Florida Regional Medical Center	Davenport	3.3%	90
Mease Countryside Hospital	Safety Harbor	3.3%	61
Ocala Regional Medical Center	Ocala	3.3%	273
UF Health Jacksonville	Jacksonville	3.3%	521
Florida Hospital Tampa	Tampa	3.4%	146
Gulf Breeze Hospital	Gulf Breeze	3.4%	471
North Okaloosa Medical Center	Crestview	3.6%	110
South Miami Hospital	South Miami	3.6%	140
Plantation General Hospital	Plantation	3.7%	136
Jackson Hospital	Marianna	3.8%	131
Lake Wales Medical Center	Lake Wales	3.8%	78
Saint Cloud Regional Medical Center	Saint Cloud	3.8%	79
Broward Health Imperial Point	Fort Lauderdale	4.0%	75
Gulf Coast Med Ctr Lee Mem Health Sys	Fort Myers	4.0%	227
Shands Live Oak Regional Medical Center	Live Oak	4.0%	75
Florida Hospital Waterman	Tavares	4.1%	266
Broward Health Medical Center	Fort Lauderdale	4.3%	210
Cleveland Clinic Hospital	Weston	4.3%	46
North Florida Regional Medical Center	Gainesville	4.4%	617
Winter Haven Hospital	Winter Haven	4.4%	204
Florida Hospital Deland	Deland	4.5%	110
Leesburg Regional Medical Center	Leesburg	4.5%	313
Florida Hospital Heartland Medical Center	Sebring	4.6%	591
Halifax Health Medical Center	Daytona Bch	4.6%	173
Sacred Heart Hosp-Emerald Coast	Miramar Beach	4.7%	446
South Bay Hospital	Sun City Center	4.8%	62
Saint Vincent's Medical Center	Jacksonville	4.9%	2572
Venice Reg Med Ctr-Bayfront Health	Venice	4.9%	182
Holmes Regional Medical Center	Melbourne	5.0%	542
Central Florida Regional Hospital	Sanford	5.1%	59
Town & Country Hospital	Tampa	5.1%	79
Baptist Hospital	Pensacola	5.2%	1415
Memorial Hospital of Tampa	Tampa	5.2%	96
UF Health Shands Hospital	Gainesville	5.3%	339
Florida Hospital Memorial Medical Center	Daytona Bch	5.5%	110
Lake City Medical Center	Lake City	5.5%	145
Florida Hospital	Orlando	5.6%	817
Munroe Regional Medical Center	Ocala	5.6%	576
Parrish Medical Center	Titusville	5.6%	287
Sacred Heart Hospital	Pensacola	5.6%	771
Fort Walton Beach Medical Center	Fort Walton Bch	5.7%	210
Health Central	Ocoee	5.7%	192
Putnam Community Medical Center	Palatka	5.7%	192
Bayfront Health - Saint Petersburg	St Petersburg	5.8%	138
Jackson Memorial Hospital	Miami	5.8%	275
Baptist Medical Center Beaches	Jcksnvl Bch	5.9%	1219
Lee Memorial Hospital	Fort Myers	5.9%	2080
Wuesthoff Medical Center Rockledge	Rockledge	5.9%	409
Cape Canaveral Hospital	Cocoa Beach	6.0%	434
Baptist Hospital of Miami	Miami	6.1%	295
Bert Fish Medical Center	New Smyrn Bch	6.1%	261
Holy Cross Hospital	Fort Lauderdale	6.1%	2376
Indian River Medical Center	Vero Beach	6.2%	1278
West Florida Hospital	Pensacola	6.2%	762
Baptist Medical Center - Nassau	Fernandina Bch	6.3%	473
Fishermen's Hospital	Marathon	6.3%	95
Bayfront Health Brooksville	Brooksville	6.4%	204
Physicians Reg Med Ctr-Pine Ridge	Naples	6.4%	453
Wuesthoff Medical Center - Melbourne	Melbourne	6.4%	109
Lawnwood Reg Med Ctr & Heart Inst	Fort Pierce	6.5%	62
Cape Coral Hospital	Cape Coral	6.6%	229
Florida Hospital Flagler	Palm Coast	6.6%	213
JFK Medical Center	Atlantis	6.6%	196
Osceola Regional Medical Center	Kissimmee	6.7%	254
South Florida Baptist Hospital	Plant City	6.7%	90
Viera Hospital	Melbourne	6.7%	90
Saint Vincent's Medical Center Southside	Jacksonville	6.8%	585
Tampa General Hospital	Tampa	6.9%	475
Naples Community Hospital	Naples	7.1%	2459
Orange Park Medical Center	Orange Park	7.1%	410
Saint Joseph's Hospital	Tampa	7.2%	456
Bethesda Hospital East	Boynton Beach	7.3%	151
Manatee Memorial Hospital	Bradenton	7.3%	729
Orlando Health	Orlando	7.3%	2677
Oak Hill Hospital	Brooksville	7.4%	136
Sarasota Memorial Hospital	Sarasota	7.4%	326
South Lake Hospital	Clermont	7.5%	241
Baptist Medical Center	Jacksonville	7.6%	2500
Memorial Hospital Jacksonville	Jacksonville	7.6%	118
Mariners Hospital	Tavernier	7.7%	143
Brandon Regional Hospital	Brandon	7.8%	219
The Villages Regional Hospital	The Villages	7.8%	383
Citrus Memorial Hospital	Inverness	8.0%	175
Lehigh Regional Medical Center	Lehigh Acres	8.0%	87
Sebastian River Medical Center	Sebastian	8.0%	100
University of Miami Hospital	Miami	8.0%	539
Mount Sinai Medical Center	Miami Beach	8.2%	256
Twin Cities Hospital	Niceville	8.2%	98
Florida Hospital Fish Memorial	Orange City	8.4%	119
Saint Anthony's Hospital	St Petersburg	8.5%	117
Good Samaritan Medical Center	W Palm Beach	8.6%	210
Santa Rosa Medical Center	Milton	8.8%	171
Seven Rivers Regional Medical Center	Crystal River	8.9%	135
Lakeland Regional Medical Center	Lakeland	9.2%	501
Martin Medical Center	Stuart	9.2%	304
Broward Health North	Pompano Bch	9.3%	108
Flagler Hospital	St Augustine	9.3%	611
Bay Med Ctr Sacred Heart Health Sys	Panama City	10.0%	210
Shands Lake Shore Regional Medical Center	Lake City	10.1%	89
Morton Plant Hospital	Clearwater	10.7%	122
Boca Raton Regional Hospital	Boca Raton	10.9%	375
Mayo Clinic	Jacksonville	10.9%	751
Morton Plant North Bay Hospital	New Port Richey	11.1%	72
Delray Medical Center	Delray Beach	11.3%	265
Florida Hospital Zephyrhills	Zephyrhills	14.9%	67

Combination Abdominal CT Scan

Hospital Name	City	Rate	Cases
Halifax Health Medical Center	Daytona Bch	0.3%	632
Palms West Hospital	Loxahatchee	0.5%	198
North Florida Regional Medical Center	Gainesville	0.8%	1159
Delray Medical Center	Delray Beach	1.0%	824
Jackson Memorial Hospital	Miami	1.0%	780
Bethesda Hospital East	Boynton Beach	1.2%	736
Naples Community Hospital	Naples	1.2%	1352
Hialeah Hospital	Hialeah	1.3%	397
West Kendall Baptist Hospital	Miami	1.3%	541
Saint Joseph's Hospital	Tampa	1.4%	1252
Capital Regional Medical Center	Tallahassee	1.5%	537
Brandon Regional Hospital	Brandon	1.6%	643
Kendall Regional Medical Center	Miami	1.6%	618
Mayo Clinic	Jacksonville	1.6%	490
Homestead Hospital	Homestead	1.7%	605
Aventura Hospital & Medical Center	Aventura	1.8%	794
Baptist Hospital of Miami	Miami	1.8%	1458
Lake City Medical Center	Lake City	1.8%	488
West Palm Hospital	W Palm Beach	1.9%	156
Ocala Regional Medical Center	Ocala	2.0%	1150
Baptist Medical Center - Nassau	Fernandina Bch	2.2%	650
Palm Springs General Hospital	Hialeah	2.2%	417
Lawnwood Reg Med Ctr & Heart Inst	Fort Pierce	2.4%	541
Munroe Regional Medical Center	Ocala	2.4%	1239
Saint Mary's Medical Center	W Palm Beach	2.4%	168
Doctors Hospital	Coral Gables	2.5%	322
Regional Medical Center Bayonet Point	Hudson	2.5%	356
South Lake Hospital	Clermont	2.5%	966
Doctors Hospital of Sarasota	Sarasota	2.6%	302
South Bay Hospital	Sun City Center	2.6%	545
Manatee Memorial Hospital	Bradenton	2.7%	547
Morton Plant Hospital	Clearwater	2.8%	815
Tallahassee Memorial Hospital	Tallahassee	2.8%	503
South Miami Hospital	South Miami	2.9%	547
Lakeland Regional Medical Center	Lakeland	3.1%	1217
Health Central	Ocoee	3.2%	532
Florida Hospital Carrollwood	Tampa	3.3%	181
Edward White Hospital	St Petersburg	3.4%	118
Fawcett Memorial Hospital	Port Charlotte	3.4%	557
Lehigh Regional Medical Center	Lehigh Acres	3.4%	204
JFK Medical Center	Atlantis	3.5%	1074
Bert Fish Medical Center	New Smyrn Bch	3.7%	651
Saint Cloud Regional Medical Center	Saint Cloud	3.7%	323
Coral Gables Hospital	Coral Gables	3.8%	312
Martin Medical Center	Stuart	3.8%	1598
Memorial Hospital Miramar	Miramar	3.8%	420
Wellington Regional Medical Center	Wellington	3.8%	366
Morton Plant North Bay Hospital	New Port Richey	3.9%	306
Saint Vincent's Medical Center	Jacksonville	3.9%	1219
Bartow Regional Medical Center	Bartow	4.0%	199
Holy Cross Hospital	Fort Lauderdale	4.1%	1542
Shands Live Oak Regional Medical Center	Live Oak	4.1%	488
Viera Hospital	Melbourne	4.1%	339
Florida Hospital Memorial Medical Center	Daytona Bch	4.2%	873
Lower Keys Medical Center	Key West	4.2%	261
Mariners Hospital	Tavernier	4.2%	384
Orange Park Medical Center	Orange Park	4.4%	804
Palm Beach Gardens Medical Center	Palm Bch Grdns	4.4%	455
West Florida Hospital	Pensacola	4.5%	938
Fishermen's Hospital	Marathon	4.6%	260
Medical Center of Trinity	Trinity	4.7%	365
Orlando Health	Orlando	4.9%	2656
South Florida Baptist Hospital	Plant City	4.9%	408
Memorial Hospital West	Pembroke Pines	5.0%	862
Osceola Regional Medical Center	Kissimmee	5.1%	572
Plantation General Hospital	Plantation	5.1%	778
Lakewood Ranch Medical Center	Bradenton	5.2%	405
Memorial Regional Hospital	Hollywood	5.2%	985
Saint Vincent's Medical Center Southside	Jacksonville	5.3%	341
Broward Health North	Pompano Bch	5.4%	392
Memorial Hospital Pembroke	Pembroke Pines	5.4%	390
Palmetto General Hospital	Hialeah	5.4%	706
Saint Lucie Medical Center	Port Saint Lucie	5.4%	719
Leesburg Regional Medical Center	Leesburg	5.5%	456
Westside Regional Medical Center	Plantation	5.5%	458
Broward Health Imperial Point	Fort Lauderdale	5.7%	332
Doctor's Memorial Hospital	Perry	5.8%	259
West Boca Medical Center	Boca Raton	5.9%	340
Bayfront Health - Saint Petersburg	St Petersburg	6.0%	315
Broward Health Coral Springs	Coral Springs	6.0%	536
Shands Lake Shore Regional Medical Center	Lake City	6.0%	417
Sacred Heart Hospital on the Gulf	Port Saint Joe	6.1%	132
Jackson Hospital	Marianna	6.2%	482
Memorial Hospital Jacksonville	Jacksonville	6.2%	793
Baptist Medical Center	Jacksonville	6.3%	2304
Central Florida Regional Hospital	Sanford	6.3%	366
Putnam Community Medical Center	Palatka	6.4%	534
Florida Hospital Deland	Deland	6.6%	632
Florida Hospital Fish Memorial	Orange City	6.7%	705
Bayfront Health Punta Gorda	Punta Gorda	6.9%	406
University of Miami Hospital	Miami	7.1%	701
Northwest Medical Center	Margate	7.2%	568
Parrish Medical Center	Titusville	7.2%	971
Venice Reg Med Ctr-Bayfront Health	Venice	7.2%	1377
Saint Petersburg General Hospital	St Petersburg	7.3%	177
The Villages Regional Hospital	The Villages	7.3%	951
North Shore Medical Center	Miami	7.6%	607
Saint Anthony's Hospital	St Petersburg	7.9%	860
Florida Hospital Flagler	Palm Coast	8.0%	1032
Holmes Regional Medical Center	Melbourne	8.0%	736
Boca Raton Regional Hospital	Boca Raton	8.1%	3891
Bayfront Health Brooksville	Brooksville	8.7%	681
Florida Hospital Wesley Chapel	Wesley Chapel	8.8%	148
Flagler Hospital	St Augustine	8.9%	1509
George E Weems Memorial Hospital	Apalachicola	9.0%	67
Raulerson Hospital	Okeechobee	9.0%	434
Northside Hospital	St Petersburg	9.3%	237
Sacred Heart Hosp-Emerald Coast	Miramar Beach	9.3%	849
Winter Haven Hospital	Winter Haven	9.4%	896
Seven Rivers Regional Medical Center	Crystal River	9.7%	413
Mease Hospital Dunedin	Dunedin	9.9%	374
Santa Rosa Medical Center	Milton	9.9%	487
Largo Medical Center	Largo	10.2%	401
Sacred Heart Hospital	Pensacola	10.4%	1616
Florida Hospital Waterman	Tavares	10.5%	1906
Gulf Coast Regional Medical Center	Panama City	10.5%	1013
University Hospital & Medical Center	Tamarac	10.5%	361
Bayfront Health Port Charlotte	Port Charlotte	10.7%	428
Florida Hospital Tampa	Tampa	10.7%	477
Mease Countryside Hospital	Safety Harbor	10.8%	1153
Blake Medical Center	Bradenton	10.9%	495
Baptist Medical Center Beaches	Jcksnvl Bch	11.6%	868
Hendry Regional Medical Center	Clewiston	11.7%	265
Broward Health Medical Center	Fort Lauderdale	11.8%	617
Englewood Community Hospital	Englewood	12.0%	308
Physicians Reg Med Ctr-Pine Ridge	Naples	12.6%	1634
Gulf Breeze Hospital	Gulf Breeze	12.9%	587
Palm Bay Hospital	Palm Bay	12.9%	404
Bayfront Health Dade City	Dade City	13.0%	138
Citrus Memorial Hospital	Inverness	13.0%	1124
Mount Sinai Medical Center	Miami Beach	13.3%	1649
Bay Med Ctr Sacred Heart Health Sys	Panama City	13.6%	1342
Indian River Medical Center	Vero Beach	13.7%	940
Town & Country Hospital	Tampa	13.8%	239
Wuesthoff Medical Center - Melbourne	Melbourne	14.0%	429
Cape Canaveral Hospital	Cocoa Beach	14.1%	799
Sarasota Memorial Hospital	Sarasota	14.2%	2760
Good Samaritan Medical Center	W Palm Beach	14.5%	1195
Highlands Regional Medical Center	Sebring	14.7%	632
Heart of Florida Regional Medical Center	Davenport	14.8%	520
Florida Hospital North Pinellas	Tarpon Springs	15.0%	253
Westchester General Hospital	Miami	15.3%	137
Healthmark Regional Medical Center	Defuniak Spgs	15.7%	134
Jupiter Medical Center	Jupiter	15.9%	1620
UF Health Shands Hospital	Gainesville	16.6%	2513
Lakeside Medical Center	Belle Glade	16.7%	120
Fort Walton Beach Medical Center	Fort Walton Bch	17.2%	548
Palms of Pasadena Hospital	St Petersburg	17.4%	558
North Okaloosa Medical Center	Crestview	17.6%	632
Desoto Memorial Hospital	Arcadia	18.7%	418
Lake Wales Medical Center	Lake Wales	20.7%	275
Tampa General Hospital	Tampa	20.8%	662
Twin Cities Hospital	Niceville	22.4%	335
Baptist Hospital	Pensacola	23.0%	880

NOTE: Hospital profiles are in alphabetical order by state, then city, then hospital within the city; Rankings exclude hospitals with less than 25 cases except for patient surveys which excludes hospitals with less than 100 cases; (a) 100-299 cases; (1) The number of cases/patients is too few to report; (2) Data submitted were based on a sample of cases/patients; (3) Results are based on a shorter time period than required; (4) Data suppressed by CMS for one or more quarters; (5) Results are not available for this reporting period; (6) Fewer than 100 patients completed the HCAHPS survey; (7) No cases met the criteria for this measure; (8) The lower limit of the confidence interval cannot be calculated if the number of observed infections equals zero; (9) No data are available from the state/territory for this reporting period; (10) The scores shown reflect fewer than 50 completed surveys; (11) There were discrepancies in the data collection process; (12) This measure does not apply to this hospital for this reporting period; (13) Results cannot be calculated for this reporting period; (14) The results for this state are combined with nearby states to protect confidentiality; Please refer to the User's Guide for a full explanation of data.

Hospital Name	City	Rate	Cases
Florida Hospital Zephyrhills	Zephyrhills	25.4%	504
Cleveland Clinic Hospital	Weston	26.6%	1161
Larkin Community Hospital	South Miami	26.6%	128
Florida Hospital	Orlando	28.5%	5975
Jay Hospital	Jay	33.3%	99
UF Health Jacksonville	Jacksonville	33.5%	744
Sebastian River Medical Center	Sebastian	36.2%	663
Oak Hill Hospital	Brooksville	40.4%	708
Florida Hospital Wauchula	Wauchula	41.9%	203
Wuesthoff Medical Center Rockledge	Rockledge	45.5%	881
Gulf Coast Med Ctr Lee Mem Health Sys	Fort Myers	51.2%	555
Florida Hospital Heartland Medical Center	Sebring	51.9%	1386
Cape Coral Hospital	Cape Coral	58.1%	742
Lee Memorial Hospital	Fort Myers	58.2%	1480
Memorial Hospital of Tampa	Tampa	60.9%	353

Combination Brain/Sinus CT Scan

Hospital Name	City	Rate	Cases
Jay Hospital	Jay	0.0%	93
Holmes Regional Medical Center	Melbourne	0.6%	1405
Parrish Medical Center	Titusville	0.6%	967
Cleveland Clinic Hospital	Weston	0.9%	540
Jackson Hospital	Marianna	1.0%	508
Palm Bay Hospital	Palm Bay	1.2%	502
Holy Cross Hospital	Fort Lauderdale	1.3%	949
Shands Live Oak Regional Medical Center	Live Oak	1.3%	595
West Boca Medical Center	Boca Raton	1.3%	458
Memorial Hospital Pembroke	Pembroke Pines	1.4%	359
Memorial Hospital West	Pembroke Pines	1.6%	701
Palm Beach Gardens Medical Center	Palm Bch Grdns	1.6%	749
Florida Hospital Memorial Medical Center	Daytona Bch	1.8%	975
Putnam Community Medical Center	Palatka	1.9%	681
Mayo Clinic	Jacksonville	2.0%	1035
Saint Lucie Medical Center	Port Saint Lucie	2.0%	1318
South Lake Hospital	Clermont	2.0%	762
Winter Haven Hospital	Winter Haven	2.0%	1174
North Shore Medical Center	Miami	2.1%	775
Wellington Regional Medical Center	Wellington	2.1%	435
Bay Med Ctr Sacred Heart Health Sys	Panama City	2.2%	1321
Bert Fish Medical Center	New Smyrn Bch	2.2%	677
Boca Raton Regional Hospital	Boca Raton	2.2%	2596
Florida Hospital Heartland Medical Center	Sebring	2.2%	1334
Martin Medical Center	Stuart	2.2%	2089
Munroe Regional Medical Center	Ocala	2.2%	1899
Baptist Hospital of Miami	Miami	2.3%	1394
North Florida Regional Medical Center	Gainesville	2.3%	1643
University Hospital & Medical Center	Tamarac	2.3%	619
Flagler Hospital	St Augustine	2.4%	1400
Good Samaritan Medical Center	W Palm Beach	2.4%	891
West Kendall Baptist Hospital	Miami	2.4%	548
JFK Medical Center	Atlantis	2.5%	1247
Palmetto General Hospital	Hialeah	2.5%	602
Saint Anthony's Hospital	St Petersburg	2.5%	970
Tallahassee Memorial Hospital	Tallahassee	2.5%	904
West Florida Hospital	Pensacola	2.5%	1163
Cape Coral Hospital	Cape Coral	2.6%	838
Blake Medical Center	Bradenton	2.7%	848
Florida Hospital Flagler	Palm Coast	2.7%	927
Plantation General Hospital	Plantation	2.7%	752
Delray Medical Center	Delray Beach	2.8%	1262
Florida Hospital Deland	Deland	2.8%	773
Kendall Regional Medical Center	Miami	2.8%	712
Memorial Regional Hospital	Hollywood	2.8%	1124
Aventura Hospital & Medical Center	Aventura	2.9%	816
Palms of Pasadena Hospital	St Petersburg	2.9%	660
Sacred Heart Hospital	Pensacola	2.9%	1327
Sacred Heart Hosp-Emerald Coast	Miramar Beach	2.9%	631
Physicians Reg Med Ctr-Pine Ridge	Naples	3.0%	1439
Saint Vincent's Medical Center	Jacksonville	3.0%	1406
Venice Reg Med Ctr-Bayfront Health	Venice	3.0%	1613
Mount Sinai Medical Center	Miami Beach	3.1%	1010
UF Health Shands Hospital	Gainesville	3.1%	1013
Baptist Hospital	Pensacola	3.2%	948
Baptist Medical Center - Nassau	Fernandina Bch	3.2%	812
Florida Hospital Fish Memorial	Orange City	3.2%	660
Bayfront Health Brooksville	Brooksville	3.3%	857
Florida Hospital	Orlando	3.4%	4115
Largo Medical Center	Largo	3.4%	789
Memorial Hospital Jacksonville	Jacksonville	3.4%	730
Baptist Medical Center	Jacksonville	3.5%	2639
Citrus Memorial Hospital	Inverness	3.5%	1559
Lake City Medical Center	Lake City	3.5%	773
Orlando Health	Orlando	3.5%	2120
UF Health Jacksonville	Jacksonville	3.5%	767
Fort Walton Beach Medical Center	Fort Walton Bch	3.7%	803
Indian River Medical Center	Vero Beach	3.7%	1167
Jackson Memorial Hospital	Miami	3.7%	947
Morton Plant Hospital	Clearwater	3.7%	1664
Orange Park Medical Center	Orange Park	3.7%	928
Central Florida Regional Hospital	Sanford	3.8%	598
Fawcett Memorial Hospital	Port Charlotte	3.8%	825
Gulf Coast Regional Medical Center	Panama City	3.8%	847
Halifax Health Medical Center	Daytona Bch	3.8%	1360
Ocala Regional Medical Center	Ocala	3.8%	1384
Sarasota Memorial Hospital	Sarasota	3.8%	3137
Sebastian River Medical Center	Sebastian	3.8%	601
Desoto Memorial Hospital	Arcadia	3.9%	407
Florida Hospital Tampa	Tampa	3.9%	947
Gulf Coast Med Ctr Lee Mem Health Sys	Fort Myers	4.0%	991
Jupiter Medical Center	Jupiter	4.0%	1408
Northside Hospital	St Petersburg	4.0%	422
Saint Joseph's Hospital	Tampa	4.0%	1816
The Villages Regional Hospital	The Villages	4.0%	1638
Westside Regional Medical Center	Plantation	4.0%	544
Capital Regional Medical Center	Tallahassee	4.1%	749
Gulf Breeze Hospital	Gulf Breeze	4.1%	665
Mease Hospital Dunedin	Dunedin	4.1%	631
Broward Health Coral Springs	Coral Springs	4.2%	430
Florida Hospital Waterman	Tavares	4.2%	1570
Naples Community Hospital	Naples	4.2%	2042
Lee Memorial Hospital	Fort Myers	4.3%	1635
South Florida Baptist Hospital	Plant City	4.3%	445
Tampa General Hospital	Tampa	4.3%	604
Bayfront Health Port Charlotte	Port Charlotte	4.4%	570
Lawnwood Reg Med Ctr & Heart Inst	Fort Pierce	4.4%	726
Morton Plant North Bay Hospital	New Port Richey	4.4%	618
Osceola Regional Medical Center	Kissimmee	4.4%	632
Baptist Medical Center Beaches	Jcksnvl Bch	4.5%	1069
Lakeland Regional Medical Center	Lakeland	4.5%	1849
Twin Cities Hospital	Niceville	4.5%	441
Bethesda Hospital East	Boynton Beach	4.6%	1538
Homestead Hospital	Homestead	4.6%	703
Manatee Memorial Hospital	Bradenton	4.6%	717
Wuesthoff Medical Center Rockledge	Rockledge	4.6%	702
Saint Cloud Regional Medical Center	Saint Cloud	4.7%	344
Seven Rivers Regional Medical Center	Crystal River	4.7%	572
Palm Springs General Hospital	Hialeah	4.8%	567
Mease Countryside Hospital	Safety Harbor	4.9%	1806
Memorial Hospital of Tampa	Tampa	4.9%	246
Bayfront Health Punta Gorda	Punta Gorda	5.0%	581
Lakewood Ranch Medical Center	Bradenton	5.0%	519
Wuesthoff Medical Center - Melbourne	Melbourne	5.0%	362
Englewood Community Hospital	Englewood	5.1%	605
Northwest Medical Center	Margate	5.1%	591
South Miami Hospital	South Miami	5.1%	720
Brandon Regional Hospital	Brandon	5.3%	879
Broward Health Imperial Point	Fort Lauderdale	5.4%	408
Cape Canaveral Hospital	Cocoa Beach	5.4%	690
Florida Hospital Wesley Chapel	Wesley Chapel	5.4%	184
Health Central	Ocoee	5.6%	734
Leesburg Regional Medical Center	Leesburg	5.6%	942
Santa Rosa Medical Center	Milton	5.6%	468
Palms West Hospital	Loxahatchee	5.7%	261
Oak Hill Hospital	Brooksville	5.8%	138
Regional Medical Center Bayonet Point	Hudson	6.0%	569
Broward Health North	Pompano Bch	6.2%	731
South Bay Hospital	Sun City Center	6.2%	940
Medical Center of Trinity	Trinity	6.6%	575
Bayfront Health - Saint Petersburg	St Petersburg	6.9%	462
Broward Health Medical Center	Fort Lauderdale	7.3%	753
Fishermen's Hospital	Marathon	7.4%	272
Coral Gables Hospital	Coral Gables	7.5%	295

Combination Chest CT Scan

Hospital Name	City	Rate	Cases
Aventura Hospital & Medical Center	Aventura	0.0%	520
Baptist Medical Center - Nassau	Fernandina Bch	0.0%	447
Bayfront Health - Saint Petersburg	St Petersburg	0.0%	164
Cape Coral Hospital	Cape Coral	0.0%	324
Capital Regional Medical Center	Tallahassee	0.0%	128
Doctors Hospital	Coral Gables	0.0%	148
Englewood Community Hospital	Englewood	0.0%	53
Fishermen's Hospital	Marathon	0.0%	108
Florida Hospital Deland	Deland	0.0%	576
Hialeah Hospital	Hialeah	0.0%	94
Holy Cross Hospital	Fort Lauderdale	0.0%	1359
Kendall Regional Medical Center	Miami	0.0%	200
Lake City Medical Center	Lake City	0.0%	107
Medical Center of Trinity	Trinity	0.0%	105
Memorial Hospital Miramar	Miramar	0.0%	222
Morton Plant Hospital	Clearwater	0.0%	118
North Florida Regional Medical Center	Gainesville	0.0%	122
North Okaloosa Medical Center	Crestview	0.0%	270
Northside Hospital	St Petersburg	0.0%	71
Oak Hill Hospital	Brooksville	0.0%	215
Palms of Pasadena Hospital	St Petersburg	0.0%	346
Palms West Hospital	Loxahatchee	0.0%	50
Regional Medical Center Bayonet Point	Hudson	0.0%	71
Twin Cities Hospital	Niceville	0.0%	134
Venice Reg Med Ctr-Bayfront Health	Venice	0.0%	793
The Villages Regional Hospital	The Villages	0.0%	213
West Kendall Baptist Hospital	Miami	0.0%	234
Westside Regional Medical Center	Plantation	0.0%	223
Boca Raton Regional Hospital	Boca Raton	0.1%	4222
Lee Memorial Hospital	Fort Myers	0.1%	783
Mease Countryside Hospital	Safety Harbor	0.1%	740
Orange Park Medical Center	Orange Park	0.1%	962
Florida Hospital Fish Memorial	Orange City	0.2%	553
South Lake Hospital	Clermont	0.2%	413
UF Health Shands Hospital	Gainesville	0.2%	2474
Cape Canaveral Hospital	Cocoa Beach	0.3%	643
Florida Hospital	Orlando	0.3%	3604
Homestead Hospital	Homestead	0.3%	313
Lakeland Regional Medical Center	Lakeland	0.3%	305
Palmetto General Hospital	Hialeah	0.3%	335
Saint Vincent's Medical Center	Jacksonville	0.3%	1034
Baptist Hospital of Miami	Miami	0.4%	476
Parrish Medical Center	Titusville	0.4%	511
South Bay Hospital	Sun City Center	0.4%	252
Viera Hospital	Melbourne	0.4%	264
Bert Fish Medical Center	New Smyrn Bch	0.5%	406
West Boca Medical Center	Boca Raton	0.5%	191
Florida Hospital Heartland Medical Center	Sebring	0.6%	844
Mease Hospital Dunedin	Dunedin	0.6%	179
Naples Community Hospital	Naples	0.6%	344
Osceola Regional Medical Center	Kissimmee	0.6%	166
Saint Anthony's Hospital	St Petersburg	0.6%	477
South Florida Baptist Hospital	Plant City	0.6%	164
Florida Hospital Waterman	Tavares	0.7%	1346
Plantation General Hospital	Plantation	0.7%	303
Saint Lucie Medical Center	Port Saint Lucie	0.7%	138
South Miami Hospital	South Miami	0.7%	437
Bethesda Hospital East	Boynton Beach	0.8%	126
Cleveland Clinic Hospital	Weston	0.8%	1147
Delray Medical Center	Delray Beach	0.8%	132
Gulf Coast Med Ctr Lee Mem Health Sys	Fort Myers	0.8%	132
Tallahassee Memorial Hospital	Tallahassee	0.8%	132
Baptist Medical Center Beaches	Jcksnvl Bch	0.9%	579
Manatee Memorial Hospital	Bradenton	1.0%	194
Orlando Health	Orlando	1.0%	2418
University of Miami Hospital	Miami	1.0%	397
Central Florida Regional Hospital	Sanford	1.1%	181
Good Samaritan Medical Center	W Palm Beach	1.1%	760
Holmes Regional Medical Center	Melbourne	1.1%	714
Memorial Hospital Jacksonville	Jacksonville	1.2%	489
West Florida Hospital	Pensacola	1.2%	481
Bay Med Ctr Sacred Heart Health Sys	Panama City	1.3%	1196
Jackson Memorial Hospital	Miami	1.3%	462
Ocala Regional Medical Center	Ocala	1.3%	240
Palm Bay Hospital	Palm Bay	1.3%	389
Sacred Heart Hospital	Pensacola	1.3%	1065
Saint Cloud Regional Medical Center	Saint Cloud	1.3%	150
Tampa General Hospital	Tampa	1.3%	305
Doctors Hospital of Sarasota	Sarasota	1.4%	73
Florida Hospital Memorial Medical Center	Daytona Bch	1.4%	920
Gulf Breeze Hospital	Gulf Breeze	1.4%	222
Halifax Health Medical Center	Daytona Bch	1.4%	72
Baptist Medical Center	Jacksonville	1.5%	1619
Memorial Regional Hospital	Hollywood	1.5%	895
Saint Joseph's Hospital	Tampa	1.5%	205
Wellington Regional Medical Center	Wellington	1.6%	127
Blake Medical Center	Bradenton	1.7%	117
Morton Plant North Bay Hospital	New Port Richey	1.7%	60
Broward Health Imperial Point	Fort Lauderdale	1.9%	212
Broward Health Coral Springs	Coral Springs	2.0%	200
Lawnwood Reg Med Ctr & Heart Inst	Fort Pierce	2.0%	247
Mariners Hospital	Tavernier	2.0%	199
North Shore Medical Center	Miami	2.0%	354
Palm Beach Gardens Medical Center	Palm Bch Grdns	2.0%	249
Leesburg Regional Medical Center	Leesburg	2.1%	95
Munroe Regional Medical Center	Ocala	2.1%	327
George E Weems Memorial Hospital	Apalachicola	2.2%	46
Martin Medical Center	Stuart	2.2%	914
Memorial Hospital West	Pembroke Pines	2.3%	823
Physicians Reg Med Ctr-Pine Ridge	Naples	2.3%	569
Wuesthoff Medical Center - Melbourne	Melbourne	2.4%	169
Flagler Hospital	St Augustine	2.7%	1380
Florida Hospital Flagler	Palm Coast	2.9%	834
Saint Vincent's Medical Center Southside	Jacksonville	2.9%	137
Sebastian River Medical Center	Sebastian	2.9%	491
Lakewood Ranch Medical Center	Bradenton	3.2%	124
Shands Live Oak Regional Medical Center	Live Oak	3.3%	362
Lehigh Regional Medical Center	Lehigh Acres	3.5%	57
Broward Health North	Pompano Bch	3.6%	279
University Hospital & Medical Center	Tamarac	3.7%	242
Lower Keys Medical Center	Key West	3.8%	159
Saint Petersburg General Hospital	St Petersburg	3.8%	53
Fawcett Memorial Hospital	Port Charlotte	4.0%	150
Sacred Heart Hosp-Emerald Coast	Miramar Beach	4.1%	556
Saint Mary's Medical Center	W Palm Beach	4.1%	49
Mayo Clinic	Jacksonville	4.3%	46
Northwest Medical Center	Margate	4.5%	266
Palm Springs General Hospital	Hialeah	4.5%	155

NOTE: Hospital profiles are in alphabetical order by state, then city, then hospital within the city; Rankings exclude hospitals with less than 25 cases except for patient surveys which excludes hospitals with less than 100 cases; (a) 100-299 cases; (1) The number of cases/patients is too few to report; (2) Data submitted were based on a sample of cases/patients; (3) Results are based on a shorter time period than required; (4) Data suppressed by CMS for one or more quarters; (5) Results are not available for this reporting period; (6) Fewer than 100 patients completed the HCAHPS survey; (7) No cases met the criteria for this measure; (8) The lower limit of the confidence interval cannot be calculated if the number of observed infections equals zero; (9) No data are available from the state/territory for this reporting period; (10) The scores shown reflect fewer than 50 completed surveys; (11) There were discrepancies in the data collection process; (12) This measure does not apply to this hospital for this reporting period; (13) Results cannot be calculated for this reporting period; (14) The results for this state are combined with nearby states to protect confidentiality; Please refer to the User's Guide for a full explanation of data.

Hospital Name	City	Rate	Cases
Florida Hospital Zephyrhills	Zephyrhills	4.6%	153
Broward Health Medical Center	Fort Lauderdale	4.7%	365
Florida Hospital Wauchula	Wauchula	4.8%	104
Putnam Community Medical Center	Palatka	5.0%	201
Doctor's Memorial Hospital	Perry	5.5%	109
Sarasota Memorial Hospital	Sarasota	5.6%	1816
Sacred Heart Hospital on the Gulf	Port Saint Joe	5.8%	69
Florida Hospital North Pinellas	Tarpon Springs	6.0%	100
Citrus Memorial Hospital	Inverness	6.3%	668
Jackson Hospital	Marianna	6.3%	160
Shands Lake Shore Regional Medical Center	Lake City	6.4%	171
Bayfront Health Port Charlotte	Port Charlotte	6.5%	154
Gulf Coast Regional Medical Center	Panama City	6.8%	717
Wuesthoff Medical Center Rockledge	Rockledge	6.8%	453
Bayfront Health Brooksville	Brooksville	7.1%	395
Brandon Regional Hospital	Brandon	7.8%	116
Baptist Hospital	Pensacola	8.0%	465
Memorial Hospital Pembroke	Pembroke Pines	8.3%	228
Raulerson Hospital	Okeechobee	8.3%	144
Seven Rivers Regional Medical Center	Crystal River	8.5%	106
Indian River Medical Center	Vero Beach	8.6%	327
JFK Medical Center	Atlantis	9.1%	309
Jupiter Medical Center	Jupiter	9.7%	1529
Mount Sinai Medical Center	Miami Beach	9.7%	1280
Winter Haven Hospital	Winter Haven	11.0%	273
Fort Walton Beach Medical Center	Fort Walton Bch	12.2%	221
Health Central	Ocoee	12.2%	246
Highlands Regional Medical Center	Sebring	13.4%	298
Bayfront Health Punta Gorda	Punta Gorda	14.3%	119
Florida Hospital Tampa	Tampa	15.5%	200
Largo Medical Center	Largo	15.7%	102
Desoto Memorial Hospital	Arcadia	16.2%	154
Heart of Florida Regional Medical Center	Davenport	16.2%	167
UF Health Jacksonville	Jacksonville	16.8%	606
Hendry Regional Medical Center	Clewiston	19.2%	104
Santa Rosa Medical Center	Milton	23.0%	100
Memorial Hospital of Tampa	Tampa	29.6%	199
Town & Country Hospital	Tampa	32.0%	97
Lake Wales Medical Center	Lake Wales	37.3%	118

Follow-up Mammogram/Ultrasound

A follow-up rate near zero may indicate missed cancer; a rate higher than 14% may mean there is unnecessary follow up.

Hospital Name	City	Rate	Cases
Seven Rivers Regional Medical Center	Crystal River	2.7%	930
Palms of Pasadena Hospital	St Petersburg	3.1%	701
Palms West Hospital	Loxahatchee	4.2%	331
Lakewood Ranch Medical Center	Bradenton	4.5%	531
Parrish Medical Center	Titusville	4.5%	1728
Largo Medical Center	Largo	4.7%	423
Lake Wales Medical Center	Lake Wales	4.9%	493
Raulerson Hospital	Okeechobee	4.9%	629
Coral Gables Hospital	Coral Gables	5.1%	117
Sarasota Memorial Hospital	Sarasota	5.2%	8687
Mease Hospital Dunedin	Dunedin	5.4%	913
Doctors Hospital of Sarasota	Sarasota	5.5%	778
Florida Hospital	Orlando	5.7%	5930
Venice Reg Med Ctr-Bayfront Health	Venice	5.7%	2367
Central Florida Regional Hospital	Sanford	5.8%	310
Aventura Hospital & Medical Center	Aventura	5.9%	929
Englewood Community Hospital	Englewood	5.9%	373
Tampa General Hospital	Tampa	5.9%	324
Manatee Memorial Hospital	Bradenton	6.0%	486
Orange Park Medical Center	Orange Park	6.0%	1170
Physicians Reg Med Ctr-Pine Ridge	Naples	6.4%	1824
University Hospital & Medical Center	Tamarac	6.5%	294
North Florida Regional Medical Center	Gainesville	6.8%	222
Gulf Breeze Hospital	Gulf Breeze	6.9%	1028
Saint Petersburg General Hospital	St Petersburg	6.9%	568
Health Central	Ocoee	7.0%	790
Lee Memorial Hospital	Fort Myers	7.0%	3309
Putnam Community Medical Center	Palatka	7.1%	1020
Bayfront Health Port Charlotte	Port Charlotte	7.5%	1096
Cape Coral Hospital	Cape Coral	7.6%	1422
Mease Countryside Hospital	Safety Harbor	7.7%	2776
South Bay Hospital	Sun City Center	7.7%	1127
Town & Country Hospital	Tampa	7.7%	248
Holmes Regional Medical Center	Melbourne	7.8%	1632
Orlando Health	Orlando	7.8%	1717
Saint Anthony's Hospital	St Petersburg	7.8%	1344
Lakeside Medical Center	Belle Glade	7.9%	203
Baptist Medical Center - Nassau	Fernandina Bch	8.0%	1427
Jay Hospital	Jay	8.0%	138
Sacred Heart Hospital on the Gulf	Port Saint Joe	8.0%	174
North Okaloosa Medical Center	Crestview	8.1%	1242
UF Health Shands Hospital	Gainesville	8.2%	1818
Wellington Regional Medical Center	Wellington	8.3%	599
Florida Hospital Tampa	Tampa	8.4%	371
Saint Joseph's Hospital	Tampa	8.4%	1185
South Lake Hospital	Clermont	8.4%	1222
Florida Hospital Heartland Medical Center	Sebring	8.5%	1690
Jackson Memorial Hospital	Miami	8.5%	575
University of Miami Hospital	Miami	8.5%	117
Baptist Medical Center	Jacksonville	8.6%	3594
Blake Medical Center	Bradenton	8.6%	1072
Fishermen's Hospital	Marathon	8.9%	157
Florida Hospital Waterman	Tavares	9.1%	2832
Saint Lucie Medical Center	Port Saint Lucie	9.1%	747
Baptist Medical Center Beaches	Jcksnvl Bch	9.2%	1953
Jackson Hospital	Marianna	9.2%	917
Shands Live Oak Regional Medical Center	Live Oak	9.2%	459
Florida Hospital Memorial Medical Center	Daytona Bch	9.3%	1216
Oak Hill Hospital	Brooksville	9.5%	1006
Palmetto General Hospital	Hialeah	9.5%	548
Sacred Heart Hosp-Emerald Coast	Miramar Beach	9.5%	1005
South Florida Baptist Hospital	Plant City	9.5%	724
Cape Canaveral Hospital	Cocoa Beach	9.6%	1687
Heart of Florida Regional Medical Center	Davenport	9.6%	438
UF Health Jacksonville	Jacksonville	9.6%	1851
Plantation General Hospital	Plantation	10.0%	958
Winter Haven Hospital	Winter Haven	10.0%	962
South Miami Hospital	South Miami	10.1%	426
Boca Raton Regional Hospital	Boca Raton	10.2%	9526
Palm Bay Hospital	Palm Bay	10.3%	789
Gulf Coast Regional Medical Center	Panama City	10.4%	616
Florida Hospital Zephyrhills	Zephyrhills	10.6%	529
Leesburg Regional Medical Center	Leesburg	10.8%	148
Memorial Hospital Jacksonville	Jacksonville	10.8%	1770
Doctor's Memorial Hospital	Perry	10.9%	331
Flagler Hospital	St Augustine	10.9%	2507
Florida Hospital North Pinellas	Tarpon Springs	10.9%	303
Memorial Hospital of Tampa	Tampa	10.9%	395
Bayfront Health - Saint Petersburg	St Petersburg	11.1%	433
Homestead Hospital	Homestead	11.1%	395
Sacred Heart Hospital	Pensacola	11.1%	2845
Santa Rosa Medical Center	Milton	11.1%	451
Viera Hospital	Melbourne	11.1%	235
Bartow Regional Medical Center	Bartow	11.2%	258
Broward Health North	Pompano Bch	11.4%	317
Desoto Memorial Hospital	Arcadia	11.4%	420
Baptist Hospital	Pensacola	11.5%	1797
Fawcett Memorial Hospital	Port Charlotte	11.5%	365
Broward Health Coral Springs	Coral Springs	11.6%	605
Wuesthoff Medical Center Rockledge	Rockledge	11.6%	1233
Bert Fish Medical Center	New Smyrn Bch	11.7%	1053
Northwest Medical Center	Margate	11.8%	279
Saint Mary's Medical Center	W Palm Beach	12.0%	133
Broward Health Medical Center	Fort Lauderdale	12.1%	643
Osceola Regional Medical Center	Kissimmee	12.2%	526
Martin Medical Center	Stuart	12.3%	721
Saint Vincent's Medical Center	Jacksonville	12.4%	3837
Kendall Regional Medical Center	Miami	12.7%	212
West Florida Hospital	Pensacola	12.9%	2240
Florida Hospital Fish Memorial	Orange City	13.0%	928
West Boca Medical Center	Boca Raton	13.0%	601
Bay Med Ctr Sacred Heart Health Sys	Panama City	13.1%	703
Citrus Memorial Hospital	Inverness	13.4%	2637
Memorial Hospital Miramar	Miramar	13.5%	356
Memorial Hospital West	Pembroke Pines	13.8%	1286
Lower Keys Medical Center	Key West	14.0%	559
Hialeah Hospital	Hialeah	14.1%	220
Florida Hospital Deland	Deland	14.2%	1384
Good Samaritan Medical Center	W Palm Beach	14.4%	2020
Saint Cloud Regional Medical Center	Saint Cloud	14.9%	484
Tallahassee Memorial Hospital	Tallahassee	14.9%	161
Broward Health Imperial Point	Fort Lauderdale	15.5%	502
Palm Beach Gardens Medical Center	Palm Bch Grdns	15.5%	187
Saint Vincent's Medical Center Southside	Jacksonville	16.0%	194
Fort Walton Beach Medical Center	Fort Walton Bch	16.1%	347
Mount Sinai Medical Center	Miami Beach	16.5%	1519
Capital Regional Medical Center	Tallahassee	16.7%	444
Holy Cross Hospital	Fort Lauderdale	16.9%	2200
North Shore Medical Center	Miami	17.1%	387
Shands Lake Shore Regional Medical Center	Lake City	17.2%	425
Twin Cities Hospital	Niceville	17.4%	385
Sebastian River Medical Center	Sebastian	17.9%	988
Memorial Regional Hospital	Hollywood	18.0%	1286
Bayfront Health Dade City	Dade City	18.3%	82
Wuesthoff Medical Center - Melbourne	Melbourne	18.6%	236
Cleveland Clinic Hospital	Weston	19.1%	1127
JFK Medical Center	Atlantis	19.1%	742
Mariners Hospital	Tavernier	19.1%	346
Highlands Regional Medical Center	Sebring	19.6%	97
Hendry Regional Medical Center	Clewiston	20.1%	194
Bayfront Health Brooksville	Brooksville	20.2%	564
Florida Hospital Flagler	Palm Coast	20.2%	1041
Jupiter Medical Center	Jupiter	21.0%	2161
Westside Regional Medical Center	Plantation	22.8%	372
West Palm Hospital	W Palm Beach	23.5%	68
Bayfront Health Punta Gorda	Punta Gorda	27.5%	69

Lumbar Spine MRI for Low Back Pain

Hospital Name	City	Rate	Cases
Jupiter Medical Center	Jupiter	22.1%	149
Boca Raton Regional Hospital	Boca Raton	25.0%	535
Santa Rosa Medical Center	Milton	26.3%	57
Sebastian River Medical Center	Sebastian	26.3%	76
Plantation General Hospital	Plantation	27.4%	73
Cape Canaveral Hospital	Cocoa Beach	27.8%	54
Palmetto General Hospital	Hialeah	28.1%	57
Baptist Medical Center Beaches	Jcksnvl Bch	28.6%	119
Mariners Hospital	Tavernier	28.8%	59
Mease Countryside Hospital	Safety Harbor	30.1%	133
Baptist Medical Center	Jacksonville	31.2%	503
Florida Hospital Flagler	Palm Coast	31.5%	73
Sacred Heart Hosp-Emerald Coast	Miramar Beach	31.8%	129
Citrus Memorial Hospital	Inverness	31.9%	91
Flagler Hospital	St Augustine	31.9%	141
Palms of Pasadena Hospital	St Petersburg	32.0%	50
University of Miami Hospital	Miami	32.0%	50
Holy Cross Hospital	Fort Lauderdale	32.3%	155
Baptist Hospital	Pensacola	32.5%	243
Lee Memorial Hospital	Fort Myers	32.6%	291
North Okaloosa Medical Center	Crestview	32.7%	52
Sarasota Memorial Hospital	Sarasota	33.1%	284
Health Central	Ocoee	33.3%	51
Parrish Medical Center	Titusville	33.3%	183
Saint Vincent's Medical Center Southside	Jacksonville	33.3%	63
Florida Hospital Deland	Deland	34.4%	96
Florida Hospital Heartland Medical Center	Sebring	34.4%	180
Bay Med Ctr Sacred Heart Health Sys	Panama City	34.5%	119
Shands Lake Shore Regional Medical Center	Lake City	34.6%	52
Gulf Breeze Hospital	Gulf Breeze	34.9%	166
West Florida Hospital	Pensacola	34.9%	83
Orlando Health	Orlando	35.3%	116
Florida Hospital	Orlando	36.3%	460
Physicians Reg Med Ctr-Pine Ridge	Naples	36.3%	179
South Lake Hospital	Clermont	36.5%	52
Cape Coral Hospital	Cape Coral	36.7%	98
Florida Hospital Memorial Medical Center	Daytona Bch	36.7%	60
UF Health Shands Hospital	Gainesville	36.9%	149
Orange Park Medical Center	Orange Park	37.1%	97
Saint Vincent's Medical Center	Jacksonville	37.2%	164
Putnam Community Medical Center	Palatka	37.3%	59
Memorial Hospital Jacksonville	Jacksonville	37.5%	96
Cleveland Clinic Hospital	Weston	37.6%	157
Good Samaritan Medical Center	W Palm Beach	37.6%	242
UF Health Jacksonville	Jacksonville	37.7%	138
Florida Hospital Waterman	Tavares	37.8%	164
Sacred Heart Hospital	Pensacola	37.8%	262
Memorial Regional Hospital	Hollywood	37.9%	58
North Shore Medical Center	Miami	38.7%	62
Venice Reg Med Ctr-Bayfront Health	Venice	39.5%	76
Broward Health Medical Center	Fort Lauderdale	40.5%	42
South Miami Hospital	South Miami	40.5%	74
Baptist Medical Center - Nassau	Fernandina Bch	40.8%	76
South Bay Hospital	Sun City Center	40.9%	44
Mease Hospital Dunedin	Dunedin	42.2%	45
Mount Sinai Medical Center	Miami Beach	42.8%	180
Winter Haven Hospital	Winter Haven	43.2%	37
Bert Fish Medical Center	New Smyrn Bch	43.3%	60
Fort Walton Beach Medical Center	Fort Walton Bch	43.8%	48
Memorial Hospital West	Pembroke Pines	43.9%	66
Memorial Hospital Miramar	Miramar	44.0%	50
Florida Hospital Fish Memorial	Orange City	44.4%	63
Gulf Coast Regional Medical Center	Panama City	44.4%	45
Saint Anthony's Hospital	St Petersburg	44.4%	72
Baptist Hospital of Miami	Miami	45.5%	110
Homestead Hospital	Homestead	47.3%	55
Florida Hospital Zephyrhills	Zephyrhills	47.4%	38
Fishermen's Hospital	Marathon	47.7%	44
West Kendall Baptist Hospital	Miami	50.9%	53
Hialeah Hospital	Hialeah	63.0%	46

NOTE: Hospital profiles are in alphabetical order by state, then city, then hospital within the city; Rankings exclude hospitals with less than 25 cases except for patient surveys which excludes hospitals with less than 100 cases; (a) 100-299 cases; (1) The number of cases/patients is too few to report; (2) Data submitted were based on a sample of cases/patients; (3) Results are based on a shorter time period than required; (4) Data suppressed by CMS for one or more quarters; (5) Results are not available for this reporting period; (6) Fewer than 100 patients completed the HCAHPS survey; (7) No cases met the criteria for this measure; (8) The lower limit of the confidence interval cannot be calculated if the number of observed infections equals zero; (9) No data are available from the state/territory for this reporting period; (10) The scores shown reflect fewer than 50 completed surveys; (11) There were discrepancies in the data collection process; (12) This measure does not apply to this hospital for this reporting period; (13) Results cannot be calculated for this reporting period; (14) The results for this state are combined with nearby states to protect confidentiality; Please refer to the User's Guide for a full explanation of data.

George E Weems Memorial Hospital

135 Ave G Phone: 850-653-8853
Apalachicola, FL 32320
Type: Critical Access Hospitals Emergency Services: Yes
Ownership: Government - Local

Measure	Cases	This Hosp.	State Avg.	U.S. Avg.
Blood Clot Prevention and Treatment				
Anticoagulation Overlap Therapy[5]	-	-	93%	93%
ICU Venous Thromboembolism Prophylaxis[5]	-	-	94%	92%
Incidence of Potentially Preventable VTE[5]	-	-	10%	10%
UFH with Dosages/Platelet Monitoring[5]	-	-	100%	97%
Venous Thromboembolism Prophylaxis[5]	-	-	88%	85%
Warfarin Therapy Discharge Instructions[5]	-	-	85%	75%
Chest Pain/Possible Heart Attack Care				
Aspirin Given Within 24 Hours of Arrival[5]	-	-	98%	96%
Fibrinolytic Meds Within 30 Min. of Arrival[5]	-	-	81%	58%
Average Time to ECG (minutes)[5]	-	-	7	7
Average Time to Transfer (minutes)[5]	-	-	53	60
Children's Asthma Care				
Received Home Management Plan of Care	-	-	-	88%
Received Reliever Medication	-	-	-	100%
Received Systemic Corticosteroids	-	-	-	100%
Emergency Department				
Admittance Decision Time (minutes)[5]	-	-	111	98
Head CT Results Within 45 Min. of Arrival[5]	-	-	64%	57%
Patients Who Left ER Before Being Seen[5]	-	-	2%	2%
Time from ER Arrival to Admit. (minutes)[5]	-	-	289	274
Time from ER Arrival to Discharge (minutes)[5]	-	-	147	134
Time in ER Before Being Evaluated (minutes)[5]	-	-	26	26
Time to Pain Meds for Fractures (minutes)[5]	-	-	60	57
Heart Attack Care				
Aspirin Given at Discharge[5]	-	-	99%	99%
Fibrinolytic Meds Within 30 Min. of Arrival[5]	-	-	50%	54%
PCI Within 90 Minutes of Arrival[5]	-	-	96%	96%
Statin Prescribed at Discharge[5]	-	-	99%	98%
Heart Failure Care				
ACE Inhibitor or ARB for LVSD[3,7]	-	-	98%	97%
Discharge Instructions Given[1,3]	-	-	96%	94%
Evaluation of LVS Function[1,3]	-	-	100%	99%
Medicare Spending				
Medicare Spending per Patient (ratio)	-	-	1.04	0.98
Pneumonia Care				
Appropriate Initial Antibiotic Given[3,7]	-	-	98%	95%
Blood Culture Timing[3,7]	-	-	99%	98%
Pregnancy and Delivery Care				
Newborn Deliveries Scheduled Early[5]	-	-	6%	6%
Preventive Care				
Immunization for Influenza[5]	-	-	94%	90%
Immunization for Pneumonia[5]	-	-	96%	92%
Stroke Care				
Anticoagulation Therapy for Atrial Fibrillation[5]	-	-	97%	95%
Antithrombotic Therapy Timing[5]	-	-	98%	98%
Assessed for Rehabilitation[5]	-	-	97%	97%
Discharged on Antithrombotic Therapy[5]	-	-	99%	99%
Discharged on Statin Medication[5]	-	-	96%	94%
Thrombolytic Therapy Timing[5]	-	-	76%	66%
Venous Thromboembolism Prophylaxis[5]	-	-	95%	94%
Written Stroke Educational Materials Given[5]	-	-	94%	88%
Surgical Care Improvement Project				
Appropriate Beta Blocker Usage[5]	-	-	99%	98%
Appropriate VTP Within 24 Hours[5]	-	-	99%	98%
Controlled Postoperative Blood Glucose[5]	-	-	98%	97%
Perioperative Temperature Management[5]	-	-	100%	100%
Prophylactic Antibiotic Selection[5]	-	-	99%	99%
Prophylactic Antibiotic Selection (Outpatient)[5]	-	-	98%	98%
Prophylactic Antibiotic Stopped[5]	-	-	98%	98%
Prophylactic Antibiotic Timing[5]	-	-	99%	99%
Prophylactic Antibiotic Timing (Outpatient)[5]	-	-	98%	98%
Urinary Catheter Removal[5]	-	-	98%	97%
Survey of Patients' Hospital Experiences				
Area Around Room 'Always' Quiet at Night[5]	-	-	58%	61%
Doctors 'Always' Communicated Well[5]	-	-	77%	82%
Home Recovery Information Given[5]	-	-	83%	85%
Hospital Given 9 or 10 on 10 Point Scale[5]	-	-	67%	71%
Meds 'Always' Explained Before Given[5]	-	-	60%	64%
Nurses 'Always' Communicated Well[5]	-	-	75%	79%
Pain 'Always' Well Controlled[5]	-	-	68%	71%
Room and Bathroom 'Always' Clean[5]	-	-	69%	73%
Timely Help 'Always' Received[5]	-	-	62%	68%
Would Definitely Recommend Hospital[5]	-	-	69%	71%
Use of Medical Imaging				
Cardiac Imaging Stress Test before Surgery[7]	-	-	6.4%	5.3%
Combination Abdominal CT Scan	67	9.0%	11.8%	10.5%
Combination Brain/Sinus CT Scan[1]	-	-	3.4%	2.7%
Combination Chest CT Scan	46	2.2%	2.4%	2.7%
Follow-up Mammogram/Ultrasound[1]	-	-	10.2%	8.8%
Lumbar Spine MRI for Low Back Pain[7]	-	-	35.2%	37.2%

Desoto Memorial Hospital

900 N Robert Ave Phone: 863-494-3535
Arcadia, FL 34265 Fax: 863-494-8400
E-mail: hr@dmh.org
URL: www.dmh.org
Type: Acute Care Hospitals Emergency Services: Yes
Ownership: Voluntary non-profit - Private Beds: 49

Key Personnel:
Chief of Medical Staff. . . . . Wael Alokeh
Operating Room. . . . . Tammy Ford
Infection Control. . . . . Yvonne Hunt
Emergency Room . . . . Steven Mishkind
President . . . . Steven Mishkind
Intensive Care Unit. . . . . Lori Prescott
Quality Assurance . . . . Audrey Proudfit
CEO/President. . . . . Vince Sica

Measure	Cases	This Hosp.	State Avg.	U.S. Avg.
Blood Clot Prevention and Treatment				
Anticoagulation Overlap Therapy[1,2]	-	-	93%	93%
ICU Venous Thromboembolism Prophylaxis[2]	79	90%	94%	92%
Incidence of Potentially Preventable VTE[2,7]	-	-	10%	10%
UFH with Dosages/Platelet Monitoring[1,2]	-	-	100%	97%
Venous Thromboembolism Prophylaxis[2]	115	86%	88%	85%
Warfarin Therapy Discharge Instructions[1,2]	-	-	85%	75%
Chest Pain/Possible Heart Attack Care				
Aspirin Given Within 24 Hours of Arrival	52	100%	98%	96%
Fibrinolytic Meds Within 30 Min. of Arrival[1]	-	-	81%	58%
Average Time to ECG (minutes)	54	2	7	7
Average Time to Transfer (minutes)[1]	-	-	53	60
Children's Asthma Care				
Received Home Management Plan of Care	-	-	-	88%
Received Reliever Medication	-	-	-	100%
Received Systemic Corticosteroids	-	-	-	100%
Emergency Department				
Admittance Decision Time (minutes)[2]	189	99	111	98
Head CT Results Within 45 Min. of Arrival[1]	-	-	64%	57%
Patients Who Left ER Before Being Seen	16,448	3%	2%	2%
Time from ER Arrival to Admit. (minutes)[2]	232	318	289	274
Time from ER Arrival to Discharge (minutes)	365	147	147	134
Time in ER Before Being Evaluated (minutes)	407	14	26	26
Time to Pain Meds for Fractures (minutes)	39	54	60	57
Heart Attack Care				
Aspirin Given at Discharge[1]	-	-	99%	99%
Fibrinolytic Meds Within 30 Min. of Arrival[7]	-	-	50%	54%
PCI Within 90 Minutes of Arrival[7]	-	-	96%	96%
Statin Prescribed at Discharge[1]	-	-	99%	98%
Heart Failure Care				
ACE Inhibitor or ARB for LVSD	35	89%	98%	97%
Discharge Instructions Given	61	89%	96%	94%
Evaluation of LVS Function	70	100%	100%	99%
Medicare Spending				
Medicare Spending per Patient (ratio)	-	0.95	1.04	0.98
Pneumonia Care				
Appropriate Initial Antibiotic Given	61	93%	98%	95%
Blood Culture Timing	83	99%	99%	98%
Pregnancy and Delivery Care				
Newborn Deliveries Scheduled Early[2]	28	0%	6%	6%
Preventive Care				
Immunization for Influenza[2]	237	92%	94%	90%
Immunization for Pneumonia[2]	291	98%	96%	92%
Stroke Care				
Anticoagulation Therapy for Atrial Fibrillation[1]	-	-	97%	95%
Antithrombotic Therapy Timing	19	95%	98%	98%
Assessed for Rehabilitation	17	94%	97%	97%
Discharged on Antithrombotic Therapy	17	100%	99%	99%
Discharged on Statin Medication	15	73%	96%	94%
Thrombolytic Therapy Timing[7]	-	-	76%	66%
Venous Thromboembolism Prophylaxis	17	65%	95%	94%
Written Stroke Educational Materials Given	11	0%	94%	88%
Surgical Care Improvement Project				
Appropriate Beta Blocker Usage[1]	-	-	99%	98%
Appropriate VTP Within 24 Hours	34	94%	99%	98%
Controlled Postoperative Blood Glucose[7]	-	-	98%	97%
Perioperative Temperature Management	34	100%	100%	100%
Prophylactic Antibiotic Selection	19	89%	99%	99%
Prophylactic Antibiotic Selection (Outpatient)	18	100%	98%	98%
Prophylactic Antibiotic Stopped	17	71%	98%	98%
Prophylactic Antibiotic Timing	19	100%	99%	99%
Prophylactic Antibiotic Timing (Outpatient)[1]	-	-	98%	98%
Urinary Catheter Removal	20	85%	98%	97%
Survey of Patients' Hospital Experiences				
Area Around Room 'Always' Quiet at Night	300+	56%	58%	61%
Doctors 'Always' Communicated Well	300+	78%	77%	82%
Home Recovery Information Given	300+	82%	83%	85%
Hospital Given 9 or 10 on 10 Point Scale	300+	67%	67%	71%
Meds 'Always' Explained Before Given	300+	58%	60%	64%
Nurses 'Always' Communicated Well	300+	75%	75%	79%
Pain 'Always' Well Controlled	300+	72%	68%	71%
Room and Bathroom 'Always' Clean	300+	67%	69%	73%
Timely Help 'Always' Received	300+	63%	62%	68%
Would Definitely Recommend Hospital	300+	61%	69%	71%
Use of Medical Imaging				
Cardiac Imaging Stress Test before Surgery[1]	-	-	6.4%	5.3%
Combination Abdominal CT Scan	418	18.7%	11.8%	10.5%
Combination Brain/Sinus CT Scan	407	3.9%	3.4%	2.7%
Combination Chest CT Scan	154	16.2%	2.4%	2.7%
Follow-up Mammogram/Ultrasound	420	11.4%	10.2%	8.8%
Lumbar Spine MRI for Low Back Pain[1]	-	-	35.2%	37.2%

JFK Medical Center

5301 S Congress Ave Phone: 561-965-7300
Atlantis, FL 33462 Fax: 561-642-3684
E-mail: nicole.baxter@hcahealthcare.com
URL: www.jfkmc.com
Type: Acute Care Hospitals Emergency Services: Yes
Ownership: Proprietary Beds: 424

Key Personnel:
Chief of Medical Staff. . . . . Jose F Arrascue, MD
Anesthesiology. . . . . Gary Dellerson, MD
CEO/President. . . . . Gina Melby
Infection Control. . . . . Ellen Minden
Quality Assurance . . . . Carole Morgan
Radiology. . . . . Ann Regueiro
Operating Room. . . . . Cindy Schuetz
Emergency Room . . . . Randall Wolff, MD

Measure	Cases	This Hosp.	State Avg.	U.S. Avg.
Blood Clot Prevention and Treatment				
Anticoagulation Overlap Therapy[2]	196	97%	93%	93%
ICU Venous Thromboembolism Prophylaxis[2]	87	100%	94%	92%
Incidence of Potentially Preventable VTE[2]	36	8%	10%	10%
UFH with Dosages/Platelet Monitoring[2]	209	100%	100%	97%
Venous Thromboembolism Prophylaxis[2]	381	93%	88%	85%
Warfarin Therapy Discharge Instructions[2]	131	100%	85%	75%
Chest Pain/Possible Heart Attack Care				
Aspirin Given Within 24 Hours of Arrival	15	100%	98%	96%
Fibrinolytic Meds Within 30 Min. of Arrival[3,7]	-	-	81%	58%
Average Time to ECG (minutes)	15	5	7	7
Average Time to Transfer (minutes)[3,7]	-	-	53	60
Children's Asthma Care				
Received Home Management Plan of Care	-	-	-	88%
Received Reliever Medication	-	-	-	100%
Received Systemic Corticosteroids	-	-	-	100%

NOTE: Hospital profiles are in alphabetical order by state, then city, then hospital within the city; Rankings exclude hospitals with less than 25 cases except for patient surveys which excludes hospitals with less than 100 cases; (a) 100-299 cases; (1) The number of cases/patients is too few to report; (2) Data submitted were based on a sample of cases/patients; (3) Results are based on a shorter time period than required; (4) Data suppressed by CMS for one or more quarters; (5) Results are not available for this reporting period; (6) Fewer than 100 patients completed the HCAHPS survey; (7) No cases met the criteria for this measure; (8) The lower limit of the confidence interval cannot be calculated if the number of observed infections equals zero; (9) No data are available from the state/territory for this reporting period; (10) The scores shown reflect fewer than 50 completed surveys; (11) There were discrepancies in the data collection process; (12) This measure does not apply to this hospital for this reporting period; (13) Results cannot be calculated for this reporting period; (14) The results for this state are combined with nearby states to protect confidentiality; Please refer to the User's Guide for a full explanation of data.

Emergency Department				
Admittance Decision Time (minutes)[2]	920	102	111	98
Head CT Results Within 45 Min. of Arrival[1]	-	-	64%	57%
Patients Who Left ER Before Being Seen	78,098	1%	2%	2%
Time from ER Arrival to Admit. (minutes)[2]	920	207	289	274
Time from ER Arrival to Discharge (minutes)	402	135	147	134
Time in ER Before Being Evaluated (minutes)	533	14	26	26
Time to Pain Meds for Fractures (minutes)	77	50	60	57
Heart Attack Care				
Aspirin Given at Discharge	546	100%	99%	99%
Fibrinolytic Meds Within 30 Min. of Arrival[7]	-	-	50%	54%
PCI Within 90 Minutes of Arrival	85	100%	96%	96%
Statin Prescribed at Discharge	527	100%	99%	98%
Heart Failure Care				
ACE Inhibitor or ARB for LVSD	266	100%	98%	97%
Discharge Instructions Given	764	100%	96%	94%
Evaluation of LVS Function	988	100%	100%	99%
Medicare Spending				
Medicare Spending per Patient (ratio)	-	1.07	1.04	0.98
Pneumonia Care				
Appropriate Initial Antibiotic Given	208	100%	98%	95%
Blood Culture Timing	357	100%	99%	98%
Pregnancy and Delivery Care				
Newborn Deliveries Scheduled Early[2,7]	-	-	6%	6%
Preventive Care				
Immunization for Influenza[2]	723	100%	94%	90%
Immunization for Pneumonia[2]	1,054	100%	96%	92%
Stroke Care				
Anticoagulation Therapy for Atrial Fibrillation[2]	15	100%	97%	95%
Antithrombotic Therapy Timing[2]	93	100%	98%	98%
Assessed for Rehabilitation[2]	116	99%	97%	97%
Discharged on Antithrombotic Therapy[2]	94	99%	99%	99%
Discharged on Statin Medication[2]	70	97%	96%	94%
Thrombolytic Therapy Timing[1,2]	-	-	76%	66%
Venous Thromboembolism Prophylaxis[2]	120	99%	95%	94%
Written Stroke Educational Materials Given[2]	70	100%	94%	88%
Surgical Care Improvement Project				
Appropriate Beta Blocker Usage[2]	309	100%	99%	98%
Appropriate VTP Within 24 Hours[2]	472	100%	99%	98%
Controlled Postoperative Blood Glucose[2]	182	100%	98%	97%
Perioperative Temperature Management[2]	591	100%	100%	100%
Prophylactic Antibiotic Selection[2]	505	100%	99%	99%
Prophylactic Antibiotic Selection (Outpatient)	516	100%	98%	98%
Prophylactic Antibiotic Stopped[2]	470	100%	98%	98%
Prophylactic Antibiotic Timing[2]	507	100%	99%	99%
Prophylactic Antibiotic Timing (Outpatient)	517	100%	98%	98%
Urinary Catheter Removal[2]	354	100%	98%	97%
Survey of Patients' Hospital Experiences				
Area Around Room 'Always' Quiet at Night	300+	51%	58%	61%
Doctors 'Always' Communicated Well	300+	72%	77%	82%
Home Recovery Information Given	300+	77%	83%	85%
Hospital Given 9 or 10 on 10 Point Scale	300+	58%	67%	71%
Meds 'Always' Explained Before Given	300+	58%	60%	64%
Nurses 'Always' Communicated Well	300+	68%	75%	79%
Pain 'Always' Well Controlled	300+	60%	68%	71%
Room and Bathroom 'Always' Clean	300+	60%	69%	73%
Timely Help 'Always' Received	300+	54%	62%	68%
Would Definitely Recommend Hospital	300+	63%	69%	71%
Use of Medical Imaging				
Cardiac Imaging Stress Test before Surgery	196	6.6%	6.4%	5.3%
Combination Abdominal CT Scan	1,074	3.5%	11.8%	10.5%
Combination Brain/Sinus CT Scan	1,247	2.5%	3.4%	2.7%
Combination Chest CT Scan	309	9.1%	2.4%	2.7%
Follow-up Mammogram/Ultrasound	742	19.1%	10.2%	8.8%
Lumbar Spine MRI for Low Back Pain[1]	-	-	35.2%	37.2%

Aventura Hospital & Medical Center

20900 Biscayne Blvd Phone: 305-682-7000
Aventura, FL 33180 Fax: 305-682-7105
URL: www.aventurahospital.com
Type: Acute Care Hospitals Emergency Services: Yes
Ownership: Voluntary non-profit - Private Beds: 407

Key Personnel:

Pediatric Ambulatory Care . . . . . . Charles Azan, MD
Chief of Medical Staff . . . . Mark Firestone, MD
Operating Room. . . . . Allen Kantrowitz, MD
Infection Control. . . . . Linda Kusek
Radiology. . . . . Shlomo Leibowich, MD
Quality Assurance . . . . Kathleen Morris
CEO/President. . . . . Heather J Rohan

Measure	Cases	This Hosp.	State Avg.	U.S. Avg.
Blood Clot Prevention and Treatment				
Anticoagulation Overlap Therapy[2]	154	97%	93%	93%
ICU Venous Thromboembolism Prophylaxis[2]	110	98%	94%	92%
Incidence of Potentially Preventable VTE[2]	33	6%	10%	10%
UFH with Dosages/Platelet Monitoring[2]	62	98%	100%	97%
Venous Thromboembolism Prophylaxis[2]	372	95%	88%	85%
Warfarin Therapy Discharge Instructions[2]	108	98%	85%	75%
Chest Pain/Possible Heart Attack Care				
Aspirin Given Within 24 Hours of Arrival[5]	-	-	98%	96%
Fibrinolytic Meds Within 30 Min. of Arrival[5]	-	-	81%	58%
Average Time to ECG (minutes)[5]	-	-	7	7
Average Time to Transfer (minutes)[5]	-	-	53	60
Children's Asthma Care				
Received Home Management Plan of Care	-	-	-	88%
Received Reliever Medication	-	-	-	100%
Received Systemic Corticosteroids	-	-	-	100%
Emergency Department				
Admittance Decision Time (minutes)[2]	1,131	104	111	98
Head CT Results Within 45 Min. of Arrival[1,3]	-	-	64%	57%
Patients Who Left ER Before Being Seen	65,029	0%	2%	2%
Time from ER Arrival to Admit. (minutes)[2]	1,131	217	289	274
Time from ER Arrival to Discharge (minutes)	436	143	147	134
Time in ER Before Being Evaluated (minutes)	471	10	26	26
Time to Pain Meds for Fractures (minutes)	179	46	60	57
Heart Attack Care				
Aspirin Given at Discharge[2]	265	100%	99%	99%
Fibrinolytic Meds Within 30 Min. of Arrival[2,7]	-	-	50%	54%
PCI Within 90 Minutes of Arrival[2]	40	100%	96%	96%
Statin Prescribed at Discharge[2]	274	100%	99%	98%
Heart Failure Care				
ACE Inhibitor or ARB for LVSD[2]	143	99%	98%	97%
Discharge Instructions Given[2]	256	97%	96%	94%
Evaluation of LVS Function[2]	320	100%	100%	99%
Medicare Spending				
Medicare Spending per Patient (ratio)	-	1.10	1.04	0.98
Pneumonia Care				
Appropriate Initial Antibiotic Given[2]	78	100%	98%	95%
Blood Culture Timing[2]	167	100%	99%	98%
Pregnancy and Delivery Care				
Newborn Deliveries Scheduled Early[2,7]	-	-	6%	6%
Preventive Care				
Immunization for Influenza[2]	686	99%	94%	90%
Immunization for Pneumonia[2]	1,002	100%	96%	92%
Stroke Care				
Anticoagulation Therapy for Atrial Fibrillation[2]	13	100%	97%	95%
Antithrombotic Therapy Timing[2]	92	99%	98%	98%
Assessed for Rehabilitation[2]	119	99%	97%	97%
Discharged on Antithrombotic Therapy[2]	96	100%	99%	99%
Discharged on Statin Medication[2]	79	99%	96%	94%
Thrombolytic Therapy Timing[1,2]	-	-	76%	66%
Venous Thromboembolism Prophylaxis[2]	124	98%	95%	94%
Written Stroke Educational Materials Given[2]	69	100%	94%	88%
Surgical Care Improvement Project				
Appropriate Beta Blocker Usage[2]	235	99%	99%	98%
Appropriate VTP Within 24 Hours[2]	421	99%	99%	98%
Controlled Postoperative Blood Glucose[2]	112	98%	98%	97%
Perioperative Temperature Management[2]	512	100%	100%	100%
Prophylactic Antibiotic Selection[2]	381	100%	99%	99%
Prophylactic Antibiotic Selection (Outpatient)	247	98%	98%	98%
Prophylactic Antibiotic Stopped[2]	357	99%	98%	98%
Prophylactic Antibiotic Timing[2]	382	99%	99%	99%
Prophylactic Antibiotic Timing (Outpatient)	248	98%	98%	98%
Urinary Catheter Removal[2]	264	100%	98%	97%
Survey of Patients' Hospital Experiences				
Area Around Room 'Always' Quiet at Night	300+	65%	58%	61%
Doctors 'Always' Communicated Well	300+	77%	77%	82%
Home Recovery Information Given	300+	78%	83%	85%
Hospital Given 9 or 10 on 10 Point Scale	300+	63%	67%	71%
Meds 'Always' Explained Before Given	300+	60%	60%	64%
Nurses 'Always' Communicated Well	300+	72%	75%	79%
Pain 'Always' Well Controlled	300+	66%	68%	71%
Room and Bathroom 'Always' Clean	300+	67%	69%	73%
Timely Help 'Always' Received	300+	61%	62%	68%
Would Definitely Recommend Hospital	300+	66%	69%	71%
Use of Medical Imaging				
Cardiac Imaging Stress Test before Surgery[1]	-	-	6.4%	5.3%
Combination Abdominal CT Scan	794	1.8%	11.8%	10.5%
Combination Brain/Sinus CT Scan	816	2.9%	3.4%	2.7%
Combination Chest CT Scan	520	0.0%	2.4%	2.7%
Follow-up Mammogram/Ultrasound	929	5.9%	10.2%	8.8%
Lumbar Spine MRI for Low Back Pain[1]	-	-	35.2%	37.2%

Bartow Regional Medical Center

2200 Osprey Blvd Phone: 863-533-8111
Bartow, FL 33831 Fax: 863-519-1420
URL: www.bartowregional.com
Type: Acute Care Hospitals Emergency Services: Yes
Ownership: Proprietary Beds: 72

Key Personnel:

Radiology. Darren M Buono, MD
Emergency Room . . . . Catherine Crichlow, RN
Chief of Medical Staff . . . . Terrance Delikat, DO
Pediatric Ambulatory Care . . . . . . Luis Favilli, MD
Pediatric In-Patient Care . . . . Luis Favilli, MD
CEO/President. . . . . Phil Minden
Surgery . . . . Stuart D Patterson, MD
Quality Assurance . . . . George Wenner, RN

Measure	Cases	This Hosp.	State Avg.	U.S. Avg.
Blood Clot Prevention and Treatment				
Anticoagulation Overlap Therapy[2]	48	90%	93%	93%
ICU Venous Thromboembolism Prophylaxis[2]	52	96%	94%	92%
Incidence of Potentially Preventable VTE[1,2]	-	-	10%	10%
UFH with Dosages/Platelet Monitoring[2]	30	100%	100%	97%
Venous Thromboembolism Prophylaxis[2]	318	78%	88%	85%
Warfarin Therapy Discharge Instructions[2]	35	94%	85%	75%
Chest Pain/Possible Heart Attack Care				
Aspirin Given Within 24 Hours of Arrival	15	93%	98%	96%
Fibrinolytic Meds Within 30 Min. of Arrival[1,3]	-	-	81%	58%
Average Time to ECG (minutes)	17	6	7	7
Average Time to Transfer (minutes)[1,3]	-	-	53	60
Children's Asthma Care				
Received Home Management Plan of Care	-	-	-	88%
Received Reliever Medication	-	-	-	100%
Received Systemic Corticosteroids	-	-	-	100%
Emergency Department				
Admittance Decision Time (minutes)[2]	531	63	111	98
Head CT Results Within 45 Min. of Arrival[1]	-	-	64%	57%
Patients Who Left ER Before Being Seen	29,929	1%	2%	2%
Time from ER Arrival to Admit. (minutes)[2]	531	233	289	274
Time from ER Arrival to Discharge (minutes)	588	100	147	134
Time in ER Before Being Evaluated (minutes)	626	15	26	26
Time to Pain Meds for Fractures (minutes)	112	31	60	57
Heart Attack Care				
Aspirin Given at Discharge	14	100%	99%	99%
Fibrinolytic Meds Within 30 Min. of Arrival[7]	-	-	50%	54%
PCI Within 90 Minutes of Arrival[7]	-	-	96%	96%
Statin Prescribed at Discharge	11	100%	99%	98%
Heart Failure Care				
ACE Inhibitor or ARB for LVSD	32	100%	98%	97%
Discharge Instructions Given	109	93%	96%	94%
Evaluation of LVS Function	123	100%	100%	99%
Medicare Spending				
Medicare Spending per Patient (ratio)	-	1.02	1.04	0.98
Pneumonia Care				
Appropriate Initial Antibiotic Given	94	98%	98%	95%
Blood Culture Timing	130	98%	99%	98%
Pregnancy and Delivery Care				
Newborn Deliveries Scheduled Early[7]	-	-	6%	6%
Preventive Care				
Immunization for Influenza[2]	405	97%	94%	90%

NOTE: Hospital profiles are in alphabetical order by state, then city, then hospital within the city; Rankings exclude hospitals with less than 25 cases except for patient surveys which excludes hospitals with less than 100 cases; (a) 100-299 cases; (1) The number of cases/patients is too few to report; (2) Data submitted were based on a sample of cases/patients; (3) Results are based on a shorter time period than required; (4) Data suppressed by CMS for one or more quarters; (5) Results are not available for this reporting period; (6) Fewer than 100 patients completed the HCAHPS survey; (7) No cases met the criteria for this measure; (8) The lower limit of the confidence interval cannot be calculated if the number of observed infections equals zero; (9) No data are available from the state/territory for this reporting period; (10) The scores shown reflect fewer than 50 completed surveys; (11) There were discrepancies in the data collection process; (12) This measure does not apply to this hospital for this reporting period; (13) Results cannot be calculated for this reporting period; (14) The results for this state are combined with nearby states to protect confidentiality; Please refer to the User's Guide for a full explanation of data.

Measure	Cases	This Hosp.	State Avg.	U.S. Avg.
Immunization for Pneumonia[2]	554	98%	96%	92%
Stroke Care				
Anticoagulation Therapy for Atrial Fibrillation[1]	-	-	97%	95%
Antithrombotic Therapy Timing	39	97%	98%	98%
Assessed for Rehabilitation	43	100%	97%	97%
Discharged on Antithrombotic Therapy	42	100%	99%	99%
Discharged on Statin Medication	29	93%	96%	94%
Thrombolytic Therapy Timing[1]	-	-	76%	66%
Venous Thromboembolism Prophylaxis	39	97%	95%	94%
Written Stroke Educational Materials Given	29	100%	94%	88%
Surgical Care Improvement Project				
Appropriate Beta Blocker Usage	58	97%	99%	98%
Appropriate VTP Within 24 Hours	166	99%	99%	98%
Controlled Postoperative Blood Glucose[7]	-	-	98%	97%
Perioperative Temperature Management	202	100%	100%	100%
Prophylactic Antibiotic Selection	114	96%	99%	99%
Prophylactic Antibiotic Selection (Outpatient)	81	96%	98%	98%
Prophylactic Antibiotic Stopped	107	100%	98%	98%
Prophylactic Antibiotic Timing	115	97%	99%	99%
Prophylactic Antibiotic Timing (Outpatient)	81	96%	98%	98%
Urinary Catheter Removal	97	97%	98%	97%
Survey of Patients' Hospital Experiences				
Area Around Room 'Always' Quiet at Night	300+	52%	58%	61%
Doctors 'Always' Communicated Well	300+	75%	77%	82%
Home Recovery Information Given	300+	79%	83%	85%
Hospital Given 9 or 10 on 10 Point Scale	300+	55%	67%	71%
Meds 'Always' Explained Before Given	300+	51%	60%	64%
Nurses 'Always' Communicated Well	300+	69%	75%	79%
Pain 'Always' Well Controlled	300+	60%	68%	71%
Room and Bathroom 'Always' Clean	300+	68%	69%	73%
Timely Help 'Always' Received	300+	58%	62%	68%
Would Definitely Recommend Hospital	300+	61%	69%	71%
Use of Medical Imaging				
Cardiac Imaging Stress Test before Surgery[1]	-	-	6.4%	5.3%
Combination Abdominal CT Scan	199	4.0%	11.8%	10.5%
Combination Brain/Sinus CT Scan[1]	-	-	3.4%	2.7%
Combination Chest CT Scan[1]	-	-	2.4%	2.7%
Follow-up Mammogram/Ultrasound	258	11.2%	10.2%	8.8%
Lumbar Spine MRI for Low Back Pain[1]	-	-	35.2%	37.2%

Bay Pines VA Medical Center

10000 Bay Pines Blvd. Phone: 727-398-6661
Bay Pines, FL 33708 Fax: 727-398-9442
URL: www.baypines.va.gov
Type: Acute Care - VA Emergency Services: No
Ownership: Government Federal Beds: 469

Key Personnel:
Emergency Room . . . . Jeffery Abraham, MD
Patient Relations . . . . Patti DeFalco
Quality Assurance . . . . JoAnne Elkins, RN
CEO/President. . . . . Wallace M Hopkins, FACHE
Infection Control. . . . . David Johnson, MD
Radiology. . . . . Bruce Kudryk, MD
Intensive Care Unit. . . . . Janie McGrew, RN
Chief of Medical Staff. . . . . George Van Buskirk

Measure	Cases	This Hosp.	State Avg.	U.S. Avg.
Blood Clot Prevention and Treatment				
Anticoagulation Overlap Therapy	-	-	93%	93%
ICU Venous Thromboembolism Prophylaxis	-	-	94%	92%
Incidence of Potentially Preventable VTE	-	-	10%	10%
UFH with Dosages/Platelet Monitoring	-	-	100%	97%
Venous Thromboembolism Prophylaxis	-	-	88%	85%
Warfarin Therapy Discharge Instructions	-	-	85%	75%
Chest Pain/Possible Heart Attack Care				
Aspirin Given Within 24 Hours of Arrival	-	-	98%	96%
Fibrinolytic Meds Within 30 Min. of Arrival	-	-	81%	58%
Average Time to ECG (minutes)	-	-	7	7
Average Time to Transfer (minutes)	-	-	53	60
Children's Asthma Care				
Received Home Management Plan of Care	-	-	-	88%
Received Reliever Medication	-	-	-	100%
Received Systemic Corticosteroids	-	-	-	100%
Emergency Department				
Admittance Decision Time (minutes)	-	-	111	98
Head CT Results Within 45 Min. of Arrival	-	-	64%	57%
Patients Who Left ER Before Being Seen	-	-	2%	2%
Time from ER Arrival to Admit. (minutes)	-	-	289	274
Time from ER Arrival to Discharge (minutes)	-	-	147	134
Time in ER Before Being Evaluated (minutes)	-	-	26	26
Time to Pain Meds for Fractures (minutes)	-	-	60	57
Heart Attack Care				
Aspirin Given at Discharge	57	100%	99%	99%
Fibrinolytic Meds Within 30 Min. of Arrival[5]	-	-	50%	54%
PCI Within 90 Minutes of Arrival[1]	-	-	96%	96%
Statin Prescribed at Discharge	56	100%	99%	98%
Heart Failure Care				
ACE Inhibitor or ARB for LVSD	85	99%	98%	97%
Discharge Instructions Given	204	99%	96%	94%
Evaluation of LVS Function	233	100%	100%	99%
Medicare Spending				
Medicare Spending per Patient (ratio)	-	-	1.04	0.98
Pneumonia Care				
Appropriate Initial Antibiotic Given	74	97%	98%	95%
Blood Culture Timing	131	97%	99%	98%
Pregnancy and Delivery Care				
Newborn Deliveries Scheduled Early	-	-	6%	6%
Preventive Care				
Immunization for Influenza[5]	-	-	94%	90%
Immunization for Pneumonia[5]	-	-	96%	92%
Stroke Care				
Anticoagulation Therapy for Atrial Fibrillation	-	-	97%	95%
Antithrombotic Therapy Timing	-	-	98%	98%
Assessed for Rehabilitation	-	-	97%	97%
Discharged on Antithrombotic Therapy	-	-	99%	99%
Discharged on Statin Medication	-	-	96%	94%
Thrombolytic Therapy Timing	-	-	76%	66%
Venous Thromboembolism Prophylaxis	-	-	95%	94%
Written Stroke Educational Materials Given	-	-	94%	88%
Surgical Care Improvement Project				
Appropriate Beta Blocker Usage[2]	143	99%	99%	98%
Appropriate VTP Within 24 Hours[2]	272	97%	99%	98%
Controlled Postoperative Blood Glucose[5]	-	-	98%	97%
Perioperative Temperature Management[2]	352	100%	100%	100%
Prophylactic Antibiotic Selection	230	99%	99%	99%
Prophylactic Antibiotic Selection (Outpatient)	-	-	98%	98%
Prophylactic Antibiotic Stopped	222	97%	98%	98%
Prophylactic Antibiotic Timing	230	99%	99%	99%
Prophylactic Antibiotic Timing (Outpatient)	-	-	98%	98%
Urinary Catheter Removal[2]	291	99%	98%	97%
Survey of Patients' Hospital Experiences				
Area Around Room 'Always' Quiet at Night	-	-	58%	61%
Doctors 'Always' Communicated Well	-	-	77%	82%
Home Recovery Information Given	-	-	83%	85%
Hospital Given 9 or 10 on 10 Point Scale	-	-	67%	71%
Meds 'Always' Explained Before Given	-	-	60%	64%
Nurses 'Always' Communicated Well	-	-	75%	79%
Pain 'Always' Well Controlled	-	-	68%	71%
Room and Bathroom 'Always' Clean	-	-	69%	73%
Timely Help 'Always' Received	-	-	62%	68%
Would Definitely Recommend Hospital	-	-	69%	71%
Use of Medical Imaging				
Cardiac Imaging Stress Test before Surgery	-	-	6.4%	5.3%
Combination Abdominal CT Scan	-	-	11.8%	10.5%
Combination Brain/Sinus CT Scan	-	-	3.4%	2.7%
Combination Chest CT Scan	-	-	2.4%	2.7%
Follow-up Mammogram/Ultrasound	-	-	10.2%	8.8%
Lumbar Spine MRI for Low Back Pain	-	-	35.2%	37.2%

Lakeside Medical Center

39200 Hooker Hwy Phone: 561-996-6571
Belle Glade, FL 33430 Fax: 561-996-2898
URL: www.gladesgeneral.org
Type: Acute Care Hospitals Emergency Services: Yes
Ownership: Govt - Hospital Dist/Auth Beds: 73

Key Personnel:
Patient Relations . . . . Terry Calsetto
Emergency Room . . . . Sharon Jones
CEO/President. . . . . Ruth McDaniel
Chief of Medical Staff . . . . Antonio Mendez, MD
Infection Control. . . . . Nancy O'Neal
Quality Assurance . . . . Nancy O'Neal
Operating Room. . . . . Kimberley Sample

Measure	Cases	This Hosp.	State Avg.	U.S. Avg.
Blood Clot Prevention and Treatment				
Anticoagulation Overlap Therapy[2]	20	100%	93%	93%
ICU Venous Thromboembolism Prophylaxis[2]	64	98%	94%	92%
Incidence of Potentially Preventable VTE[1,2]	-	-	10%	10%
UFH with Dosages/Platelet Monitoring[1,2]	-	-	100%	97%
Venous Thromboembolism Prophylaxis[2]	324	98%	88%	85%
Warfarin Therapy Discharge Instructions[2]	16	94%	85%	75%
Chest Pain/Possible Heart Attack Care				
Aspirin Given Within 24 Hours of Arrival	34	94%	98%	96%
Fibrinolytic Meds Within 30 Min. of Arrival[3,7]	-	-	81%	58%
Average Time to ECG (minutes)	34	8	7	7
Average Time to Transfer (minutes)[1,3]	-	-	53	60
Children's Asthma Care				
Received Home Management Plan of Care	-	-	-	88%
Received Reliever Medication	-	-	-	100%
Received Systemic Corticosteroids	-	-	-	100%
Emergency Department				
Admittance Decision Time (minutes)[2]	430	95	111	98
Head CT Results Within 45 Min. of Arrival[1]	-	-	64%	57%
Patients Who Left ER Before Being Seen	22,710	1%	2%	2%
Time from ER Arrival to Admit. (minutes)[2]	431	247	289	274
Time from ER Arrival to Discharge (minutes)	448	116	147	134
Time in ER Before Being Evaluated (minutes)	469	19	26	26
Time to Pain Meds for Fractures (minutes)	77	52	60	57
Heart Attack Care				
Aspirin Given at Discharge	23	91%	99%	99%
Fibrinolytic Meds Within 30 Min. of Arrival[7]	-	-	50%	54%
PCI Within 90 Minutes of Arrival[7]	-	-	96%	96%
Statin Prescribed at Discharge	23	96%	99%	98%
Heart Failure Care				
ACE Inhibitor or ARB for LVSD	32	100%	98%	97%
Discharge Instructions Given	98	86%	96%	94%
Evaluation of LVS Function	103	100%	100%	99%
Medicare Spending				
Medicare Spending per Patient (ratio)	-	0.96	1.04	0.98
Pneumonia Care				
Appropriate Initial Antibiotic Given	59	100%	98%	95%
Blood Culture Timing	108	95%	99%	98%
Pregnancy and Delivery Care				
Newborn Deliveries Scheduled Early[2]	19	0%	6%	6%
Preventive Care				
Immunization for Influenza[2]	299	93%	94%	90%
Immunization for Pneumonia[2]	241	95%	96%	92%
Stroke Care				
Anticoagulation Therapy for Atrial Fibrillation[5]	-	-	97%	95%
Antithrombotic Therapy Timing[5]	-	-	98%	98%
Assessed for Rehabilitation[5]	-	-	97%	97%
Discharged on Antithrombotic Therapy[5]	-	-	99%	99%
Discharged on Statin Medication[5]	-	-	96%	94%
Thrombolytic Therapy Timing[5]	-	-	76%	66%
Venous Thromboembolism Prophylaxis[5]	-	-	95%	94%
Written Stroke Educational Materials Given[5]	-	-	94%	88%
Surgical Care Improvement Project				
Appropriate Beta Blocker Usage[1]	-	-	99%	98%
Appropriate VTP Within 24 Hours	42	98%	99%	98%
Controlled Postoperative Blood Glucose[7]	-	-	98%	97%
Perioperative Temperature Management	51	100%	100%	100%
Prophylactic Antibiotic Selection	17	100%	99%	99%
Prophylactic Antibiotic Selection (Outpatient)[5]	-	-	98%	98%
Prophylactic Antibiotic Stopped	17	100%	98%	98%
Prophylactic Antibiotic Timing	17	100%	99%	99%
Prophylactic Antibiotic Timing (Outpatient)[5]	-	-	98%	98%
Urinary Catheter Removal	14	93%	98%	97%
Survey of Patients' Hospital Experiences				
Area Around Room 'Always' Quiet at Night	300+	69%	58%	61%
Doctors 'Always' Communicated Well	300+	83%	77%	82%
Home Recovery Information Given	300+	83%	83%	85%

NOTE: Hospital profiles are in alphabetical order by state, then city, then hospital within the city; Rankings exclude hospitals with less than 25 cases except for patient surveys which excludes hospitals with less than 100 cases; (a) 100-299 cases; (1) The number of cases/patients is too few to report; (2) Data submitted were based on a sample of cases/patients; (3) Results are based on a shorter time period than required; (4) Data suppressed by CMS for one or more quarters; (5) Results are not available for this reporting period; (6) Fewer than 100 patients completed the HCAHPS survey; (7) No cases met the criteria for this measure; (8) The lower limit of the confidence interval cannot be calculated if the number of observed infections equals zero; (9) No data are available from the state/territory for this reporting period; (10) The scores shown reflect fewer than 50 completed surveys; (11) There were discrepancies in the data collection process; (12) This measure does not apply to this hospital for this reporting period; (13) Results cannot be calculated for this reporting period; (14) The results for this state are combined with nearby states to protect confidentiality; Please refer to the User's Guide for a full explanation of data.

Hospital Given 9 or 10 on 10 Point Scale	300+	61%	67%	71%
Meds 'Always' Explained Before Given	300+	57%	60%	64%
Nurses 'Always' Communicated Well	300+	71%	75%	79%
Pain 'Always' Well Controlled	300+	61%	68%	71%
Room and Bathroom 'Always' Clean	300+	79%	69%	73%
Timely Help 'Always' Received	300+	58%	62%	68%
Would Definitely Recommend Hospital	300+	62%	69%	71%
Use of Medical Imaging				
Cardiac Imaging Stress Test before Surgery[7]	-	-	6.4%	5.3%
Combination Abdominal CT Scan	120	16.7%	11.8%	10.5%
Combination Brain/Sinus CT Scan[1]	-	-	3.4%	2.7%
Combination Chest CT Scan[1]	-	-	2.4%	2.7%
Follow-up Mammogram/Ultrasound	203	7.9%	10.2%	8.8%
Lumbar Spine MRI for Low Back Pain[1]	-	-	35.2%	37.2%

Calhoun - Liberty Hospital

20370 Ne Burns Ave Phone: 850-674-3493
Blountstown, FL 32424
Type: Critical Access Hospitals Emergency Services: Yes
Ownership: Voluntary non-profit - Private

Measure	Cases	This Hosp.	State Avg.	U.S. Avg.
Blood Clot Prevention and Treatment				
Anticoagulation Overlap Therapy[5]	-	-	93%	93%
ICU Venous Thromboembolism Prophylaxis[5]	-	-	94%	92%
Incidence of Potentially Preventable VTE[5]	-	-	10%	10%
UFH with Dosages/Platelet Monitoring[5]	-	-	100%	97%
Venous Thromboembolism Prophylaxis[5]	-	-	88%	85%
Warfarin Therapy Discharge Instructions[5]	-	-	85%	75%
Chest Pain/Possible Heart Attack Care				
Aspirin Given Within 24 Hours of Arrival	-	-	98%	96%
Fibrinolytic Meds Within 30 Min. of Arrival	-	-	81%	58%
Average Time to ECG (minutes)	-	-	7	7
Average Time to Transfer (minutes)	-	-	53	60
Children's Asthma Care				
Received Home Management Plan of Care	-	-	-	88%
Received Reliever Medication	-	-	-	100%
Received Systemic Corticosteroids	-	-	-	100%
Emergency Department				
Admittance Decision Time (minutes)[5]	-	-	111	98
Head CT Results Within 45 Min. of Arrival	-	-	64%	57%
Patients Who Left ER Before Being Seen	-	-	2%	2%
Time from ER Arrival to Admit. (minutes)[5]	-	-	289	274
Time from ER Arrival to Discharge (minutes)	-	-	147	134
Time in ER Before Being Evaluated (minutes)	-	-	26	26
Time to Pain Meds for Fractures (minutes)	-	-	60	57
Heart Attack Care				
Aspirin Given at Discharge[5]	-	-	99%	99%
Fibrinolytic Meds Within 30 Min. of Arrival[5]	-	-	50%	54%
PCI Within 90 Minutes of Arrival[5]	-	-	96%	96%
Statin Prescribed at Discharge[5]	-	-	99%	98%
Heart Failure Care				
ACE Inhibitor or ARB for LVSD[5]	-	-	98%	97%
Discharge Instructions Given[5]	-	-	96%	94%
Evaluation of LVS Function[5]	-	-	100%	99%
Medicare Spending				
Medicare Spending per Patient (ratio)	-	-	1.04	0.98
Pneumonia Care				
Appropriate Initial Antibiotic Given[5]	-	-	98%	95%
Blood Culture Timing[5]	-	-	99%	98%
Pregnancy and Delivery Care				
Newborn Deliveries Scheduled Early[5]	-	-	6%	6%
Preventive Care				
Immunization for Influenza[5]	-	-	94%	90%
Immunization for Pneumonia[5]	-	-	96%	92%
Stroke Care				
Anticoagulation Therapy for Atrial Fibrillation[5]	-	-	97%	95%
Antithrombotic Therapy Timing[5]	-	-	98%	98%
Assessed for Rehabilitation[5]	-	-	97%	97%
Discharged on Antithrombotic Therapy[5]	-	-	99%	99%
Discharged on Statin Medication[5]	-	-	96%	94%
Thrombolytic Therapy Timing[5]	-	-	76%	66%
Venous Thromboembolism Prophylaxis[5]	-	-	95%	94%
Written Stroke Educational Materials Given[5]	-	-	94%	88%
Surgical Care Improvement Project				
Appropriate Beta Blocker Usage[5]	-	-	99%	98%
Appropriate VTP Within 24 Hours[5]	-	-	99%	98%
Controlled Postoperative Blood Glucose[5]	-	-	98%	97%
Perioperative Temperature Management[5]	-	-	100%	100%
Prophylactic Antibiotic Selection[5]	-	-	99%	99%
Prophylactic Antibiotic Selection (Outpatient)	-	-	98%	98%
Prophylactic Antibiotic Stopped[5]	-	-	98%	98%
Prophylactic Antibiotic Timing[5]	-	-	99%	99%
Prophylactic Antibiotic Timing (Outpatient)	-	-	98%	98%
Urinary Catheter Removal[5]	-	-	98%	97%
Survey of Patients' Hospital Experiences				
Area Around Room 'Always' Quiet at Night[5]	-	-	58%	61%
Doctors 'Always' Communicated Well[5]	-	-	77%	82%
Home Recovery Information Given[5]	-	-	83%	85%
Hospital Given 9 or 10 on 10 Point Scale[5]	-	-	67%	71%
Meds 'Always' Explained Before Given[5]	-	-	60%	64%
Nurses 'Always' Communicated Well[5]	-	-	75%	79%
Pain 'Always' Well Controlled[5]	-	-	68%	71%
Room and Bathroom 'Always' Clean[5]	-	-	69%	73%
Timely Help 'Always' Received[5]	-	-	62%	68%
Would Definitely Recommend Hospital[5]	-	-	69%	71%
Use of Medical Imaging				
Cardiac Imaging Stress Test before Surgery	-	-	6.4%	5.3%
Combination Abdominal CT Scan	-	-	11.8%	10.5%
Combination Brain/Sinus CT Scan	-	-	3.4%	2.7%
Combination Chest CT Scan	-	-	2.4%	2.7%
Follow-up Mammogram/Ultrasound	-	-	10.2%	8.8%
Lumbar Spine MRI for Low Back Pain	-	-	35.2%	37.2%

Boca Raton Regional Hospital

800 Meadows Rd Phone: 561-362-5002
Boca Raton, FL 33486
URL: www.brrh.com
Type: Acute Care Hospitals Emergency Services: Yes
Ownership: Voluntary non-profit - Private Beds: 400
Key Personnel:
CEO/President. . . . . Jerry J Fedele
Chief of Medical Staff . . . . Charles Posternack, MD, FACP, FRCPC

Measure	Cases	This Hosp.	State Avg.	U.S. Avg.
Blood Clot Prevention and Treatment				
Anticoagulation Overlap Therapy[2]	129	100%	93%	93%
ICU Venous Thromboembolism Prophylaxis[2]	79	100%	94%	92%
Incidence of Potentially Preventable VTE[2]	58	0%	10%	10%
UFH with Dosages/Platelet Monitoring[2]	117	100%	100%	97%
Venous Thromboembolism Prophylaxis[2]	337	100%	88%	85%
Warfarin Therapy Discharge Instructions[2]	93	100%	85%	75%
Chest Pain/Possible Heart Attack Care				
Aspirin Given Within 24 Hours of Arrival[1,3]	-	-	98%	96%
Fibrinolytic Meds Within 30 Min. of Arrival[5]	-	-	81%	58%
Average Time to ECG (minutes)[1,3]	-	-	7	7
Average Time to Transfer (minutes)[5]	-	-	53	60
Children's Asthma Care				
Received Home Management Plan of Care	-	-	-	88%
Received Reliever Medication	-	-	-	100%
Received Systemic Corticosteroids	-	-	-	100%
Emergency Department				
Admittance Decision Time (minutes)[2]	613	100	111	98
Head CT Results Within 45 Min. of Arrival[1]	-	-	64%	57%
Patients Who Left ER Before Being Seen	43,414	1%	2%	2%
Time from ER Arrival to Admit. (minutes)[2]	618	242	289	274
Time from ER Arrival to Discharge (minutes)	325	143	147	134
Time in ER Before Being Evaluated (minutes)	383	51	26	26
Time to Pain Meds for Fractures (minutes)	197	64	60	57
Heart Attack Care				
Aspirin Given at Discharge	197	100%	99%	99%
Fibrinolytic Meds Within 30 Min. of Arrival[7]	-	-	50%	54%
PCI Within 90 Minutes of Arrival	46	100%	96%	96%
Statin Prescribed at Discharge	188	100%	99%	98%
Heart Failure Care				
ACE Inhibitor or ARB for LVSD[2]	55	100%	98%	97%
Discharge Instructions Given[2]	237	100%	96%	94%
Evaluation of LVS Function[2]	313	100%	100%	99%
Medicare Spending				
Medicare Spending per Patient (ratio)	-	1.05	1.04	0.98
Pneumonia Care				
Appropriate Initial Antibiotic Given[2]	106	99%	98%	95%
Blood Culture Timing[2]	140	100%	99%	98%
Pregnancy and Delivery Care				
Newborn Deliveries Scheduled Early[2]	44	20%	6%	6%
Preventive Care				
Immunization for Influenza[2]	494	99%	94%	90%
Immunization for Pneumonia[2]	728	99%	96%	92%
Stroke Care				
Anticoagulation Therapy for Atrial Fibrillation	35	100%	97%	95%
Antithrombotic Therapy Timing	148	100%	98%	98%
Assessed for Rehabilitation	185	100%	97%	97%
Discharged on Antithrombotic Therapy	155	100%	99%	99%
Discharged on Statin Medication	124	100%	96%	94%
Thrombolytic Therapy Timing[1]	-	-	76%	66%
Venous Thromboembolism Prophylaxis	195	99%	95%	94%
Written Stroke Educational Materials Given	103	100%	94%	88%
Surgical Care Improvement Project				
Appropriate Beta Blocker Usage[2]	189	99%	99%	98%
Appropriate VTP Within 24 Hours[2]	337	100%	99%	98%
Controlled Postoperative Blood Glucose[2]	118	99%	98%	97%
Perioperative Temperature Management[2]	525	100%	100%	100%
Prophylactic Antibiotic Selection[2]	309	100%	99%	99%
Prophylactic Antibiotic Selection (Outpatient)	534	100%	98%	98%
Prophylactic Antibiotic Stopped[2]	305	100%	98%	98%
Prophylactic Antibiotic Timing[2]	310	100%	99%	99%
Prophylactic Antibiotic Timing (Outpatient)	534	100%	98%	98%
Urinary Catheter Removal[2]	255	100%	98%	97%
Survey of Patients' Hospital Experiences				
Area Around Room 'Always' Quiet at Night	300+	48%	58%	61%
Doctors 'Always' Communicated Well	300+	81%	77%	82%
Home Recovery Information Given	300+	78%	83%	85%
Hospital Given 9 or 10 on 10 Point Scale	300+	71%	67%	71%
Meds 'Always' Explained Before Given	300+	58%	60%	64%
Nurses 'Always' Communicated Well	300+	76%	75%	79%
Pain 'Always' Well Controlled	300+	70%	68%	71%
Room and Bathroom 'Always' Clean	300+	65%	69%	73%
Timely Help 'Always' Received	300+	59%	62%	68%
Would Definitely Recommend Hospital	300+	78%	69%	71%
Use of Medical Imaging				
Cardiac Imaging Stress Test before Surgery	375	10.9%	6.4%	5.3%
Combination Abdominal CT Scan	3,891	8.1%	11.8%	10.5%
Combination Brain/Sinus CT Scan	2,596	2.2%	3.4%	2.7%
Combination Chest CT Scan	4,222	0.1%	2.4%	2.7%
Follow-up Mammogram/Ultrasound	9,526	10.2%	10.2%	8.8%
Lumbar Spine MRI for Low Back Pain	535	25.0%	35.2%	37.2%

West Boca Medical Center

21644 State Rd 7 Phone: 561-488-8000
Boca Raton, FL 33428 Fax: 561-488-8105
URL: www.westbocamedctr.com
Type: Acute Care Hospitals Emergency Services: Yes
Ownership: Proprietary Beds: 185
Key Personnel:
Chief of Medical Staff . . . . Dr Jennifer Daley
CEO . . . . Mitch Feldman
Quality Assurance . . . . Sandra Henbest
Pediatric Ambulatory Care . . . . . . S Randel, MD
Pediatric In-Patient Care . . . . S Randel, MD
Operating Room. . . . . Roger Royal
Radiology. . . . . Mintra Sukal, MD

Measure	Cases	This Hosp.	State Avg.	U.S. Avg.
Blood Clot Prevention and Treatment				
Anticoagulation Overlap Therapy[2]	46	100%	93%	93%
ICU Venous Thromboembolism Prophylaxis[2]	93	99%	94%	92%
Incidence of Potentially Preventable VTE[1,2]	-	-	10%	10%
UFH with Dosages/Platelet Monitoring[2]	30	100%	100%	97%
Venous Thromboembolism Prophylaxis[2]	332	94%	88%	85%
Warfarin Therapy Discharge Instructions[2]	35	100%	85%	75%
Chest Pain/Possible Heart Attack Care				

NOTE: Hospital profiles are in alphabetical order by state, then city, then hospital within the city; Rankings exclude hospitals with less than 25 cases except for patient surveys which excludes hospitals with less than 100 cases; (a) 100-299 cases; (1) The number of cases/patients is too few to report; (2) Data submitted were based on a sample of cases/patients; (3) Results are based on a shorter time period than required; (4) Data suppressed by CMS for one or more quarters; (5) Results are not available for this reporting period; (6) Fewer than 100 patients completed the HCAHPS survey; (7) No cases met the criteria for this measure; (8) The lower limit of the confidence interval cannot be calculated if the number of observed infections equals zero; (9) No data are available from the state/territory for this reporting period; (10) The scores shown reflect fewer than 50 completed surveys; (11) There were discrepancies in the data collection process; (12) This measure does not apply to this hospital for this reporting period; (13) Results cannot be calculated for this reporting period; (14) The results for this state are combined with nearby states to protect confidentiality; Please refer to the User's Guide for a full explanation of data.

Measure	Cases	This Hosp.	State Avg.	U.S. Avg.
Aspirin Given Within 24 Hours of Arrival	40	100%	98%	96%
Fibrinolytic Meds Within 30 Min. of Arrival[7]	-	-	81%	58%
Average Time to ECG (minutes)	41	8	7	7
Average Time to Transfer (minutes)[1]	-	-	53	60
Children's Asthma Care				
Received Home Management Plan of Care	-	-	-	88%
Received Reliever Medication	-	-	-	100%
Received Systemic Corticosteroids	-	-	-	100%
Emergency Department				
Admittance Decision Time (minutes)[2]	744	133	111	98
Head CT Results Within 45 Min. of Arrival[1]	-	-	64%	57%
Patients Who Left ER Before Being Seen	35,504	1%	2%	2%
Time from ER Arrival to Admit. (minutes)[2]	744	335	289	274
Time from ER Arrival to Discharge (minutes)	418	158	147	134
Time in ER Before Being Evaluated (minutes)	447	26	26	26
Time to Pain Meds for Fractures (minutes)	205	65	60	57
Heart Attack Care				
Aspirin Given at Discharge	21	90%	99%	99%
Fibrinolytic Meds Within 30 Min. of Arrival[7]	-	-	50%	54%
PCI Within 90 Minutes of Arrival[7]	-	-	96%	96%
Statin Prescribed at Discharge	23	100%	99%	98%
Heart Failure Care				
ACE Inhibitor or ARB for LVSD	60	100%	98%	97%
Discharge Instructions Given	196	100%	96%	94%
Evaluation of LVS Function	253	100%	100%	99%
Medicare Spending				
Medicare Spending per Patient (ratio)	-	1.12	1.04	0.98
Pneumonia Care				
Appropriate Initial Antibiotic Given	98	98%	98%	95%
Blood Culture Timing	145	99%	99%	98%
Pregnancy and Delivery Care				
Newborn Deliveries Scheduled Early[2]	42	7%	6%	6%
Preventive Care				
Immunization for Influenza[2]	522	94%	94%	90%
Immunization for Pneumonia[2]	479	96%	96%	92%
Stroke Care				
Anticoagulation Therapy for Atrial Fibrillation	11	100%	97%	95%
Antithrombotic Therapy Timing	85	98%	98%	98%
Assessed for Rehabilitation	96	98%	97%	97%
Discharged on Antithrombotic Therapy	87	100%	99%	99%
Discharged on Statin Medication	69	100%	96%	94%
Thrombolytic Therapy Timing[1]	-	-	76%	66%
Venous Thromboembolism Prophylaxis	94	100%	95%	94%
Written Stroke Educational Materials Given	59	98%	94%	88%
Surgical Care Improvement Project				
Appropriate Beta Blocker Usage[2]	63	90%	99%	98%
Appropriate VTP Within 24 Hours[2]	233	99%	99%	98%
Controlled Postoperative Blood Glucose[2,7]	-	-	98%	97%
Perioperative Temperature Management[2]	276	100%	100%	100%
Prophylactic Antibiotic Selection[2]	173	99%	99%	99%
Prophylactic Antibiotic Selection (Outpatient)	287	100%	98%	98%
Prophylactic Antibiotic Stopped[2]	170	100%	98%	98%
Prophylactic Antibiotic Timing[2]	173	100%	99%	99%
Prophylactic Antibiotic Timing (Outpatient)	287	100%	98%	98%
Urinary Catheter Removal[2]	131	95%	98%	97%
Survey of Patients' Hospital Experiences				
Area Around Room 'Always' Quiet at Night	300+	45%	58%	61%
Doctors 'Always' Communicated Well	300+	76%	77%	82%
Home Recovery Information Given	300+	77%	83%	85%
Hospital Given 9 or 10 on 10 Point Scale	300+	57%	67%	71%
Meds 'Always' Explained Before Given	300+	54%	60%	64%
Nurses 'Always' Communicated Well	300+	70%	75%	79%
Pain 'Always' Well Controlled	300+	65%	68%	71%
Room and Bathroom 'Always' Clean	300+	56%	69%	73%
Timely Help 'Always' Received	300+	57%	62%	68%
Would Definitely Recommend Hospital	300+	62%	69%	71%
Use of Medical Imaging				
Cardiac Imaging Stress Test before Surgery[1]	-	-	6.4%	5.3%
Combination Abdominal CT Scan	340	5.9%	11.8%	10.5%
Combination Brain/Sinus CT Scan	458	1.3%	3.4%	2.7%
Combination Chest CT Scan	191	0.5%	2.4%	2.7%
Follow-up Mammogram/Ultrasound	601	13.0%	10.2%	8.8%
Lumbar Spine MRI for Low Back Pain[1]	-	-	35.2%	37.2%

Doctors Memorial Hospital

2600 Hospital Dr
Bonifay, FL 32425
Phone: 850-547-1120
Fax: 850-547-8006
URL: www.pahn.org/dmh.cfm
Type: Critical Access Hospitals
Emergency Services: Yes
Ownership: Govt - Hospital Dist/Auth
Beds: 20

Key Personnel:
Radiology. . . . . Rohan Anderson
Chief of Medical Staff . . . . Leisa Bailey
CEO/President. . . . . Joann Baker
Patient Relations . . . . Brenda Blitch
Quality Assurance . . . . Christy Booth
Operating Room. . . . . Kathy Ramsey
Infection Control. . . . . Renny Sanders

Measure	Cases	This Hosp.	State Avg.	U.S. Avg.
Blood Clot Prevention and Treatment				
Anticoagulation Overlap Therapy[5]	-	-	93%	93%
ICU Venous Thromboembolism Prophylaxis[5]	-	-	94%	92%
Incidence of Potentially Preventable VTE[5]	-	-	10%	10%
UFH with Dosages/Platelet Monitoring[5]	-	-	100%	97%
Venous Thromboembolism Prophylaxis[5]	-	-	88%	85%
Warfarin Therapy Discharge Instructions[5]	-	-	85%	75%
Chest Pain/Possible Heart Attack Care				
Aspirin Given Within 24 Hours of Arrival	-	-	98%	96%
Fibrinolytic Meds Within 30 Min. of Arrival	-	-	81%	58%
Average Time to ECG (minutes)	-	-	7	7
Average Time to Transfer (minutes)	-	-	53	60
Children's Asthma Care				
Received Home Management Plan of Care	-	-	-	88%
Received Reliever Medication	-	-	-	100%
Received Systemic Corticosteroids	-	-	-	100%
Emergency Department				
Admittance Decision Time (minutes)[5]	-	-	111	98
Head CT Results Within 45 Min. of Arrival	-	-	64%	57%
Patients Who Left ER Before Being Seen	-	-	2%	2%
Time from ER Arrival to Admit. (minutes)[5]	-	-	289	274
Time from ER Arrival to Discharge (minutes)	-	-	147	134
Time in ER Before Being Evaluated (minutes)	-	-	26	26
Time to Pain Meds for Fractures (minutes)	-	-	60	57
Heart Attack Care				
Aspirin Given at Discharge[5]	-	-	99%	99%
Fibrinolytic Meds Within 30 Min. of Arrival[5]	-	-	50%	54%
PCI Within 90 Minutes of Arrival[5]	-	-	96%	96%
Statin Prescribed at Discharge[5]	-	-	99%	98%
Heart Failure Care				
ACE Inhibitor or ARB for LVSD[1]	-	-	98%	97%
Discharge Instructions Given	57	100%	96%	94%
Evaluation of LVS Function	64	17%	100%	99%
Medicare Spending				
Medicare Spending per Patient (ratio)	-	-	1.04	0.98
Pneumonia Care				
Appropriate Initial Antibiotic Given	70	44%	98%	95%
Blood Culture Timing[1]	-	-	99%	98%
Pregnancy and Delivery Care				
Newborn Deliveries Scheduled Early[5]	-	-	6%	6%
Preventive Care				
Immunization for Influenza[5]	-	-	94%	90%
Immunization for Pneumonia[5]	-	-	96%	92%
Stroke Care				
Anticoagulation Therapy for Atrial Fibrillation[5]	-	-	97%	95%
Antithrombotic Therapy Timing[5]	-	-	98%	98%
Assessed for Rehabilitation[5]	-	-	97%	97%
Discharged on Antithrombotic Therapy[5]	-	-	99%	99%
Discharged on Statin Medication[5]	-	-	96%	94%
Thrombolytic Therapy Timing[5]	-	-	76%	66%
Venous Thromboembolism Prophylaxis[5]	-	-	95%	94%
Written Stroke Educational Materials Given[5]	-	-	94%	88%
Surgical Care Improvement Project				
Appropriate Beta Blocker Usage[5]	-	-	99%	98%
Appropriate VTP Within 24 Hours[5]	-	-	99%	98%
Controlled Postoperative Blood Glucose[5]	-	-	98%	97%
Perioperative Temperature Management[5]	-	-	100%	100%
Prophylactic Antibiotic Selection[5]	-	-	99%	99%
Prophylactic Antibiotic Selection (Outpatient)	-	-	98%	98%
Prophylactic Antibiotic Stopped[5]	-	-	98%	98%
Prophylactic Antibiotic Timing[5]	-	-	99%	99%
Prophylactic Antibiotic Timing (Outpatient)	-	-	98%	98%
Urinary Catheter Removal[5]	-	-	98%	97%
Survey of Patients' Hospital Experiences				
Area Around Room 'Always' Quiet at Night[5]	-	-	58%	61%
Doctors 'Always' Communicated Well[5]	-	-	77%	82%
Home Recovery Information Given[5]	-	-	83%	85%
Hospital Given 9 or 10 on 10 Point Scale[5]	-	-	67%	71%
Meds 'Always' Explained Before Given[5]	-	-	60%	64%
Nurses 'Always' Communicated Well[5]	-	-	75%	79%
Pain 'Always' Well Controlled[5]	-	-	68%	71%
Room and Bathroom 'Always' Clean[5]	-	-	69%	73%
Timely Help 'Always' Received[5]	-	-	62%	68%
Would Definitely Recommend Hospital[5]	-	-	69%	71%
Use of Medical Imaging				
Cardiac Imaging Stress Test before Surgery	-	-	6.4%	5.3%
Combination Abdominal CT Scan	-	-	11.8%	10.5%
Combination Brain/Sinus CT Scan	-	-	3.4%	2.7%
Combination Chest CT Scan	-	-	2.4%	2.7%
Follow-up Mammogram/Ultrasound	-	-	10.2%	8.8%
Lumbar Spine MRI for Low Back Pain	-	-	35.2%	37.2%

Bethesda Hospital East

2815 S Seacrest Blvd
Boynton Beach, FL 33435
Phone: 561-737-7733
Fax: 561-737-4534
URL: www.bethesdahealthcare.com
Type: Acute Care Hospitals
Emergency Services: Yes
Ownership: Voluntary non-profit - Private
Beds: 390

Key Personnel:
Chief of Medical Staff . . . . James Byrnes, MD
CEO/President. . . . . Roger L. Kirk, FACHE
Quality Assurance . . . . Gary Ritson
Emergency Room . . . . Christopher Schirmer, MD
Patient Relations . . . . Ernestine Ziacik

Measure	Cases	This Hosp.	State Avg.	U.S. Avg.
Blood Clot Prevention and Treatment				
Anticoagulation Overlap Therapy[2]	127	95%	93%	93%
ICU Venous Thromboembolism Prophylaxis[2]	63	98%	94%	92%
Incidence of Potentially Preventable VTE[2]	31	6%	10%	10%
UFH with Dosages/Platelet Monitoring[2]	107	100%	100%	97%
Venous Thromboembolism Prophylaxis[2]	350	94%	88%	85%
Warfarin Therapy Discharge Instructions[2]	92	93%	85%	75%
Chest Pain/Possible Heart Attack Care				
Aspirin Given Within 24 Hours of Arrival[1,3]	-	-	98%	96%
Fibrinolytic Meds Within 30 Min. of Arrival[5]	-	-	81%	58%
Average Time to ECG (minutes)[1,3]	-	-	7	7
Average Time to Transfer (minutes)[5]	-	-	53	60
Children's Asthma Care				
Received Home Management Plan of Care	-	-	-	88%
Received Reliever Medication	-	-	-	100%
Received Systemic Corticosteroids	-	-	-	100%
Emergency Department				
Admittance Decision Time (minutes)[2]	459	143	111	98
Head CT Results Within 45 Min. of Arrival	14	64%	64%	57%
Patients Who Left ER Before Being Seen	62,580	1%	2%	2%
Time from ER Arrival to Admit. (minutes)[2]	483	290	289	274
Time from ER Arrival to Discharge (minutes)	355	145	147	134
Time in ER Before Being Evaluated (minutes)	402	18	26	26
Time to Pain Meds for Fractures (minutes)	181	51	60	57
Heart Attack Care				
Aspirin Given at Discharge[2]	231	100%	99%	99%
Fibrinolytic Meds Within 30 Min. of Arrival[2,7]	-	-	50%	54%
PCI Within 90 Minutes of Arrival[2]	41	93%	96%	96%
Statin Prescribed at Discharge[2]	228	97%	99%	98%
Heart Failure Care				
ACE Inhibitor or ARB for LVSD[2]	83	95%	98%	97%
Discharge Instructions Given[2]	216	96%	96%	94%
Evaluation of LVS Function[2]	301	99%	100%	99%
Medicare Spending				
Medicare Spending per Patient (ratio)	-	1.11	1.04	0.98

NOTE: Hospital profiles are in alphabetical order by state, then city, then hospital within the city; Rankings exclude hospitals with less than 25 cases except for patient surveys which excludes hospitals with less than 100 cases; (a) 100-299 cases; (1) The number of cases/patients is too few to report; (2) Data submitted were based on a sample of cases/patients; (3) Results are based on a shorter time period than required; (4) Data suppressed by CMS for one or more quarters; (5) Results are not available for this reporting period; (6) Fewer than 100 patients completed the HCAHPS survey; (7) No cases met the criteria for this measure; (8) The lower limit of the confidence interval cannot be calculated if the number of observed infections equals zero; (9) No data are available from the state/territory for this reporting period; (10) The scores shown reflect fewer than 50 completed surveys; (11) There were discrepancies in the data collection process; (12) This measure does not apply to this hospital for this reporting period; (13) Results cannot be calculated for this reporting period; (14) The results for this state are combined with nearby states to protect confidentiality; Please refer to the User's Guide for a full explanation of data.

Measure	Cases	This Hosp.	State Avg.	U.S. Avg.
Pneumonia Care				
Appropriate Initial Antibiotic Given[2]	92	99%	98%	95%
Blood Culture Timing[2]	124	98%	99%	98%
Pregnancy and Delivery Care				
Newborn Deliveries Scheduled Early[2]	80	5%	6%	6%
Preventive Care				
Immunization for Influenza[2]	515	98%	94%	90%
Immunization for Pneumonia[2]	623	99%	96%	92%
Stroke Care				
Anticoagulation Therapy for Atrial Fibrillation[2]	21	100%	97%	95%
Antithrombotic Therapy Timing[2]	80	100%	98%	98%
Assessed for Rehabilitation[2]	102	95%	97%	97%
Discharged on Antithrombotic Therapy[2]	84	100%	99%	99%
Discharged on Statin Medication[2]	68	94%	96%	94%
Thrombolytic Therapy Timing[2]	14	86%	76%	66%
Venous Thromboembolism Prophylaxis[2]	103	95%	95%	94%
Written Stroke Educational Materials Given[2]	57	100%	94%	88%
Surgical Care Improvement Project				
Appropriate Beta Blocker Usage[2]	215	94%	99%	98%
Appropriate VTP Within 24 Hours[2]	396	96%	99%	98%
Controlled Postoperative Blood Glucose[2]	121	96%	98%	97%
Perioperative Temperature Management[2]	481	100%	100%	100%
Prophylactic Antibiotic Selection[2]	390	100%	99%	99%
Prophylactic Antibiotic Selection (Outpatient)	342	94%	98%	98%
Prophylactic Antibiotic Stopped[2]	383	96%	98%	98%
Prophylactic Antibiotic Timing[2]	390	99%	99%	99%
Prophylactic Antibiotic Timing (Outpatient)	344	93%	98%	98%
Urinary Catheter Removal[2]	247	95%	98%	97%
Survey of Patients' Hospital Experiences				
Area Around Room 'Always' Quiet at Night	300+	56%	58%	61%
Doctors 'Always' Communicated Well	300+	69%	77%	82%
Home Recovery Information Given	300+	77%	83%	85%
Hospital Given 9 or 10 on 10 Point Scale	300+	67%	67%	71%
Meds 'Always' Explained Before Given	300+	58%	60%	64%
Nurses 'Always' Communicated Well	300+	69%	75%	79%
Pain 'Always' Well Controlled	300+	62%	68%	71%
Room and Bathroom 'Always' Clean	300+	65%	69%	73%
Timely Help 'Always' Received	300+	52%	62%	68%
Would Definitely Recommend Hospital	300+	68%	69%	71%
Use of Medical Imaging				
Cardiac Imaging Stress Test before Surgery	151	7.3%	6.4%	5.3%
Combination Abdominal CT Scan	736	1.2%	11.8%	10.5%
Combination Brain/Sinus CT Scan	1,538	4.6%	3.4%	2.7%
Combination Chest CT Scan	126	0.8%	2.4%	2.7%
Follow-up Mammogram/Ultrasound[7]	-	-	10.2%	8.8%
Lumbar Spine MRI for Low Back Pain[1]	-	-	35.2%	37.2%

Blake Medical Center

2020 59th Saint W
Bradenton, FL 34209
Phone: 941-792-6611
URL: www.blakemedicalcenter.com
Type: Acute Care Hospitals
Emergency Services: Yes
Ownership: Proprietary
Beds: 383

Key Personnel:

Radiology. Osarugue A Aideyan
CEO/President. . . . . Daniel J Friedrich III
Chief of Medical Staff . . . . Janine Mylett, MD

Measure	Cases	This Hosp.	State Avg.	U.S. Avg.
Blood Clot Prevention and Treatment				
Anticoagulation Overlap Therapy[2]	126	97%	93%	93%
ICU Venous Thromboembolism Prophylaxis[2]	100	99%	94%	92%
Incidence of Potentially Preventable VTE[2]	25	8%	10%	10%
UFH with Dosages/Platelet Monitoring[2]	41	100%	100%	97%
Venous Thromboembolism Prophylaxis[2]	383	98%	88%	85%
Warfarin Therapy Discharge Instructions[2]	93	96%	85%	75%
Chest Pain/Possible Heart Attack Care				
Aspirin Given Within 24 Hours of Arrival[5]	-	-	98%	96%
Fibrinolytic Meds Within 30 Min. of Arrival[5]	-	-	81%	58%
Average Time to ECG (minutes)[5]	-	-	7	7
Average Time to Transfer (minutes)[5]	-	-	53	60
Children's Asthma Care				
Received Home Management Plan of Care	-	-	-	88%
Received Reliever Medication	-	-	-	100%
Received Systemic Corticosteroids	-	-	-	100%
Emergency Department				
Admittance Decision Time (minutes)[2]	964	51	111	98
Head CT Results Within 45 Min. of Arrival[1,3]	-	-	64%	57%
Patients Who Left ER Before Being Seen	37,485	1%	2%	2%
Time from ER Arrival to Admit. (minutes)[2]	968	211	289	274
Time from ER Arrival to Discharge (minutes)	444	131	147	134
Time in ER Before Being Evaluated (minutes)	478	20	26	26
Time to Pain Meds for Fractures (minutes)	141	54	60	57
Heart Attack Care				
Aspirin Given at Discharge[2]	243	99%	99%	99%
Fibrinolytic Meds Within 30 Min. of Arrival[2,7]	-	-	50%	54%
PCI Within 90 Minutes of Arrival[2]	27	96%	96%	96%
Statin Prescribed at Discharge[2]	221	99%	99%	98%
Heart Failure Care				
ACE Inhibitor or ARB for LVSD[2]	66	98%	98%	97%
Discharge Instructions Given[2]	213	96%	96%	94%
Evaluation of LVS Function[2]	290	100%	100%	99%
Medicare Spending				
Medicare Spending per Patient (ratio)	-	1.07	1.04	0.98
Pneumonia Care				
Appropriate Initial Antibiotic Given	111	99%	98%	95%
Blood Culture Timing	177	100%	99%	98%
Pregnancy and Delivery Care				
Newborn Deliveries Scheduled Early[2,7]	-	-	6%	6%
Preventive Care				
Immunization for Influenza[2]	666	98%	94%	90%
Immunization for Pneumonia[2]	986	97%	96%	92%
Stroke Care				
Anticoagulation Therapy for Atrial Fibrillation	27	96%	97%	95%
Antithrombotic Therapy Timing	112	99%	98%	98%
Assessed for Rehabilitation	143	99%	97%	97%
Discharged on Antithrombotic Therapy	121	99%	99%	99%
Discharged on Statin Medication	92	97%	96%	94%
Thrombolytic Therapy Timing	16	94%	76%	66%
Venous Thromboembolism Prophylaxis	150	98%	95%	94%
Written Stroke Educational Materials Given	58	98%	94%	88%
Surgical Care Improvement Project				
Appropriate Beta Blocker Usage[2]	279	100%	99%	98%
Appropriate VTP Within 24 Hours[2]	425	100%	99%	98%
Controlled Postoperative Blood Glucose[2]	144	99%	98%	97%
Perioperative Temperature Management[2]	482	100%	100%	100%
Prophylactic Antibiotic Selection[2]	415	98%	99%	99%
Prophylactic Antibiotic Selection (Outpatient)	292	99%	98%	98%
Prophylactic Antibiotic Stopped[2]	397	100%	98%	98%
Prophylactic Antibiotic Timing[2]	415	100%	99%	99%
Prophylactic Antibiotic Timing (Outpatient)	293	99%	98%	98%
Urinary Catheter Removal[2]	333	99%	98%	97%
Survey of Patients' Hospital Experiences				
Area Around Room 'Always' Quiet at Night	300+	52%	58%	61%
Doctors 'Always' Communicated Well	300+	75%	77%	82%
Home Recovery Information Given	300+	84%	83%	85%
Hospital Given 9 or 10 on 10 Point Scale	300+	63%	67%	71%
Meds 'Always' Explained Before Given	300+	55%	60%	64%
Nurses 'Always' Communicated Well	300+	70%	75%	79%
Pain 'Always' Well Controlled	300+	64%	68%	71%
Room and Bathroom 'Always' Clean	300+	64%	69%	73%
Timely Help 'Always' Received	300+	56%	62%	68%
Would Definitely Recommend Hospital	300+	67%	69%	71%
Use of Medical Imaging				
Cardiac Imaging Stress Test before Surgery[1]	-	-	6.4%	5.3%
Combination Abdominal CT Scan	495	10.9%	11.8%	10.5%
Combination Brain/Sinus CT Scan	848	2.7%	3.4%	2.7%
Combination Chest CT Scan	117	1.7%	2.4%	2.7%
Follow-up Mammogram/Ultrasound	1,072	8.6%	10.2%	8.8%
Lumbar Spine MRI for Low Back Pain[1]	-	-	35.2%	37.2%

Lakewood Ranch Medical Center

8330 Lakewood Ranch Boulevard
Bradenton, FL 34202
Phone: 941-782-2100
Fax: 941-782-2575
URL: www.lakewoodranchmedicalcenter.com
Type: Acute Care Hospitals
Emergency Services: Yes
Ownership: Proprietary
Beds: 120

Key Personnel:

Chief of Medical Staff . . . . Richard Aranibar
Radiology. Alebert Berje
CEO . . . . Richard Fletcher
Chairman/CEO . . . . Robert Hillstrom, MD
Operating Room. . . . . Alan Miller
Chief of Medical Staff . . . . Aaron Sudbury, MD
CEO/President. . . . . Jim Wilson

Measure	Cases	This Hosp.	State Avg.	U.S. Avg.
Blood Clot Prevention and Treatment				
Anticoagulation Overlap Therapy[2]	31	77%	93%	93%
ICU Venous Thromboembolism Prophylaxis[2]	76	99%	94%	92%
Incidence of Potentially Preventable VTE[1,2]	-	-	10%	10%
UFH with Dosages/Platelet Monitoring[2]	13	100%	100%	97%
Venous Thromboembolism Prophylaxis[2]	278	87%	88%	85%
Warfarin Therapy Discharge Instructions[2]	21	95%	85%	75%
Chest Pain/Possible Heart Attack Care				
Aspirin Given Within 24 Hours of Arrival[1,3]	-	-	98%	96%
Fibrinolytic Meds Within 30 Min. of Arrival[3,7]	-	-	81%	58%
Average Time to ECG (minutes)[1,3]	-	-	7	7
Average Time to Transfer (minutes)[3,7]	-	-	53	60
Children's Asthma Care				
Received Home Management Plan of Care	-	-	-	88%
Received Reliever Medication	-	-	-	100%
Received Systemic Corticosteroids	-	-	-	100%
Emergency Department				
Admittance Decision Time (minutes)[2]	380	90	111	98
Head CT Results Within 45 Min. of Arrival[1]	-	-	64%	57%
Patients Who Left ER Before Being Seen	2,298	3%	2%	2%
Time from ER Arrival to Admit. (minutes)[2]	382	294	289	274
Time from ER Arrival to Discharge (minutes)	385	145	147	134
Time in ER Before Being Evaluated (minutes)	365	21	26	26
Time to Pain Meds for Fractures (minutes)	121	56	60	57
Heart Attack Care				
Aspirin Given at Discharge	104	95%	99%	99%
Fibrinolytic Meds Within 30 Min. of Arrival[7]	-	-	50%	54%
PCI Within 90 Minutes of Arrival	21	81%	96%	96%
Statin Prescribed at Discharge	90	99%	99%	98%
Heart Failure Care				
ACE Inhibitor or ARB for LVSD	47	94%	98%	97%
Discharge Instructions Given	104	99%	96%	94%
Evaluation of LVS Function	133	99%	100%	99%
Medicare Spending				
Medicare Spending per Patient (ratio)	-	1.11	1.04	0.98
Pneumonia Care				
Appropriate Initial Antibiotic Given[2]	55	96%	98%	95%
Blood Culture Timing[2]	80	99%	99%	98%
Pregnancy and Delivery Care				
Newborn Deliveries Scheduled Early[2]	26	4%	6%	6%
Preventive Care				
Immunization for Influenza[2]	512	96%	94%	90%
Immunization for Pneumonia[2]	596	98%	96%	92%
Stroke Care				
Anticoagulation Therapy for Atrial Fibrillation[1]	-	-	97%	95%
Antithrombotic Therapy Timing	60	100%	98%	98%
Assessed for Rehabilitation	69	99%	97%	97%
Discharged on Antithrombotic Therapy	63	98%	99%	99%
Discharged on Statin Medication	41	98%	96%	94%
Thrombolytic Therapy Timing[1]	-	-	76%	66%
Venous Thromboembolism Prophylaxis	64	98%	95%	94%
Written Stroke Educational Materials Given	43	98%	94%	88%
Surgical Care Improvement Project				
Appropriate Beta Blocker Usage[2]	105	90%	99%	98%
Appropriate VTP Within 24 Hours[2]	363	99%	99%	98%
Controlled Postoperative Blood Glucose[2,7]	-	-	98%	97%
Perioperative Temperature Management[2]	446	100%	100%	100%
Prophylactic Antibiotic Selection[2]	338	99%	99%	99%
Prophylactic Antibiotic Selection (Outpatient)	116	98%	98%	98%

NOTE: Hospital profiles are in alphabetical order by state, then city, then hospital within the city; Rankings exclude hospitals with less than 25 cases except for patient surveys which excludes hospitals with less than 100 cases; (a) 100-299 cases; (1) The number of cases/patients is too few to report; (2) Data submitted were based on a sample of cases/patients; (3) Results are based on a shorter time period than required; (4) Data suppressed by CMS for one or more quarters; (5) Results are not available for this reporting period; (6) Fewer than 100 patients completed the HCAHPS survey; (7) No cases met the criteria for this measure; (8) The lower limit of the confidence interval cannot be calculated if the number of observed infections equals zero; (9) No data are available from the state/territory for this reporting period; (10) The scores shown reflect fewer than 50 completed surveys; (11) There were discrepancies in the data collection process; (12) This measure does not apply to this hospital for this reporting period; (13) Results cannot be calculated for this reporting period; (14) The results for this state are combined with nearby states to protect confidentiality; Please refer to the User's Guide for a full explanation of data.

Prophylactic Antibiotic Stopped[2]	334	98%	98%	98%
Prophylactic Antibiotic Timing[2]	338	97%	99%	99%
Prophylactic Antibiotic Timing (Outpatient)	121	92%	98%	98%
Urinary Catheter Removal[2]	279	98%	98%	97%
Survey of Patients' Hospital Experiences				
Area Around Room 'Always' Quiet at Night	300+	61%	58%	61%
Doctors 'Always' Communicated Well	300+	77%	77%	82%
Home Recovery Information Given	300+	87%	83%	85%
Hospital Given 9 or 10 on 10 Point Scale	300+	72%	67%	71%
Meds 'Always' Explained Before Given	300+	60%	60%	64%
Nurses 'Always' Communicated Well	300+	76%	75%	79%
Pain 'Always' Well Controlled	300+	71%	68%	71%
Room and Bathroom 'Always' Clean	300+	68%	69%	73%
Timely Help 'Always' Received	300+	60%	62%	68%
Would Definitely Recommend Hospital	300+	75%	69%	71%
Use of Medical Imaging				
Cardiac Imaging Stress Test before Surgery	74	2.7%	6.4%	5.3%
Combination Abdominal CT Scan	405	5.2%	11.8%	10.5%
Combination Brain/Sinus CT Scan	519	5.0%	3.4%	2.7%
Combination Chest CT Scan	124	3.2%	2.4%	2.7%
Follow-up Mammogram/Ultrasound	531	4.5%	10.2%	8.8%
Lumbar Spine MRI for Low Back Pain[1]	-	-	35.2%	37.2%

Manatee Memorial Hospital

206 2nd Saint E
Bradenton, FL 34208
Phone: 941-746-5111
Fax: 941-745-6826
E-mail: betty.chambliss@mmhhs.com
URL: www.manateememorial.com
Type: Acute Care Hospitals
Emergency Services: Yes
Ownership: Proprietary
Beds: 319

Key Personnel:
Emergency Room . . . . Linda Antes
Quality Assurance . . . . Tina Buchanan
Chief of Medical Staff . . . . Linda Christmann, MD
CEO/President . . . . Kevin Dilallo
Radiology . . . . Paula Jefferson
Operating Room . . . . Dan Magnusson
Infection Control . . . . Cassie Molina
Anesthesiology . . . . Barry Severs, MD

Measure	Cases	This Hosp.	State Avg.	U.S. Avg.
Blood Clot Prevention and Treatment				
Anticoagulation Overlap Therapy[2]	106	96%	93%	93%
ICU Venous Thromboembolism Prophylaxis[2]	82	84%	94%	92%
Incidence of Potentially Preventable VTE[2]	21	14%	10%	10%
UFH with Dosages/Platelet Monitoring[2]	61	97%	100%	97%
Venous Thromboembolism Prophylaxis[2]	347	60%	88%	85%
Warfarin Therapy Discharge Instructions[2]	65	95%	85%	75%
Chest Pain/Possible Heart Attack Care				
Aspirin Given Within 24 Hours of Arrival[1,3]	-	-	98%	96%
Fibrinolytic Meds Within 30 Min. of Arrival[5]	-	-	81%	58%
Average Time to ECG (minutes)[1,3]	-	-	7	7
Average Time to Transfer (minutes)[5]	-	-	53	60
Children's Asthma Care				
Received Home Management Plan of Care	-	-	-	88%
Received Reliever Medication	-	-	-	100%
Received Systemic Corticosteroids	-	-	-	100%
Emergency Department				
Admittance Decision Time (minutes)[2]	427	129	111	98
Head CT Results Within 45 Min. of Arrival[1]	-	-	64%	57%
Patients Who Left ER Before Being Seen	66,066	2%	2%	2%
Time from ER Arrival to Admit. (minutes)[2]	429	380	289	274
Time from ER Arrival to Discharge (minutes)	382	142	147	134
Time in ER Before Being Evaluated (minutes)	420	40	26	26
Time to Pain Meds for Fractures (minutes)	270	66	60	57
Heart Attack Care				
Aspirin Given at Discharge[2]	272	100%	99%	99%
Fibrinolytic Meds Within 30 Min. of Arrival[2,7]	-	-	50%	54%
PCI Within 90 Minutes of Arrival[2]	32	100%	96%	96%
Statin Prescribed at Discharge[2]	258	100%	99%	98%
Heart Failure Care				
ACE Inhibitor or ARB for LVSD[2]	85	100%	98%	97%
Discharge Instructions Given[2]	237	100%	96%	94%
Evaluation of LVS Function[2]	304	100%	100%	99%
Medicare Spending				
Medicare Spending per Patient (ratio)	-	1.07	1.04	0.98
Pneumonia Care				
Appropriate Initial Antibiotic Given[2]	89	100%	98%	95%
Blood Culture Timing[2]	157	97%	99%	98%
Pregnancy and Delivery Care				
Newborn Deliveries Scheduled Early[2]	60	8%	6%	6%
Preventive Care				
Immunization for Influenza[2]	537	91%	94%	90%
Immunization for Pneumonia[2]	683	94%	96%	92%
Stroke Care				
Anticoagulation Therapy for Atrial Fibrillation[2]	13	77%	97%	95%
Antithrombotic Therapy Timing[2]	67	96%	98%	98%
Assessed for Rehabilitation[2]	92	97%	97%	97%
Discharged on Antithrombotic Therapy[2]	78	99%	99%	99%
Discharged on Statin Medication[2]	57	96%	96%	94%
Thrombolytic Therapy Timing[2]	16	81%	76%	66%
Venous Thromboembolism Prophylaxis[2]	99	89%	95%	94%
Written Stroke Educational Materials Given[2]	53	92%	94%	88%
Surgical Care Improvement Project				
Appropriate Beta Blocker Usage[2]	249	98%	99%	98%
Appropriate VTP Within 24 Hours[2]	420	97%	99%	98%
Controlled Postoperative Blood Glucose[2]	165	97%	98%	97%
Perioperative Temperature Management[2]	475	100%	100%	100%
Prophylactic Antibiotic Selection[2]	447	99%	99%	99%
Prophylactic Antibiotic Selection (Outpatient)	351	95%	98%	98%
Prophylactic Antibiotic Stopped[2]	424	98%	98%	98%
Prophylactic Antibiotic Timing[2]	450	97%	99%	99%
Prophylactic Antibiotic Timing (Outpatient)	361	96%	98%	98%
Urinary Catheter Removal[2]	357	97%	98%	97%
Survey of Patients' Hospital Experiences				
Area Around Room 'Always' Quiet at Night	300+	53%	58%	61%
Doctors 'Always' Communicated Well	300+	76%	77%	82%
Home Recovery Information Given	300+	86%	83%	85%
Hospital Given 9 or 10 on 10 Point Scale	300+	65%	67%	71%
Meds 'Always' Explained Before Given	300+	53%	60%	64%
Nurses 'Always' Communicated Well	300+	73%	75%	79%
Pain 'Always' Well Controlled	300+	66%	68%	71%
Room and Bathroom 'Always' Clean	300+	66%	69%	73%
Timely Help 'Always' Received	300+	56%	62%	68%
Would Definitely Recommend Hospital	300+	67%	69%	71%
Use of Medical Imaging				
Cardiac Imaging Stress Test before Surgery	729	7.3%	6.4%	5.3%
Combination Abdominal CT Scan	547	2.7%	11.8%	10.5%
Combination Brain/Sinus CT Scan	717	4.6%	3.4%	2.7%
Combination Chest CT Scan	194	1.0%	2.4%	2.7%
Follow-up Mammogram/Ultrasound	486	6.0%	10.2%	8.8%
Lumbar Spine MRI for Low Back Pain[1]	-	-	35.2%	37.2%

Brandon Regional Hospital

119 Oakfield Dr
Brandon, FL 33511
Phone: 813-681-5551
Fax: 813-654-7203
URL: www.brandonregionalhospital.com
Type: Acute Care Hospitals
Emergency Services: Yes
Ownership: Proprietary
Beds: 407

Key Personnel:
Cardiac Laboratory . . . . Jill Benford
Emergency Room . . . . Roderick Bennett
Chief of Medical Staff . . . . Dr. Joe Corcoran, MD
CEO/President . . . . Blang Eng
Quality Assurance . . . . Roger Fournier
Pediatric In-Patient Care . . . . Hamid Latif, MD
Radiology . . . . Gary Litvin
Operating Room . . . . Nancy Pickens

Measure	Cases	This Hosp.	State Avg.	U.S. Avg.
Blood Clot Prevention and Treatment				
Anticoagulation Overlap Therapy[2]	199	99%	93%	93%
ICU Venous Thromboembolism Prophylaxis[2]	96	100%	94%	92%
Incidence of Potentially Preventable VTE[2]	29	0%	10%	10%
UFH with Dosages/Platelet Monitoring[2]	74	100%	100%	97%
Venous Thromboembolism Prophylaxis[2]	350	98%	88%	85%
Warfarin Therapy Discharge Instructions[2]	149	100%	85%	75%
Chest Pain/Possible Heart Attack Care				
Aspirin Given Within 24 Hours of Arrival[1,3]	-	-	98%	96%
Fibrinolytic Meds Within 30 Min. of Arrival[5]	-	-	81%	58%
Average Time to ECG (minutes)[1,3]	-	-	7	7
Average Time to Transfer (minutes)[5]	-	-	53	60
Children's Asthma Care				
Received Home Management Plan of Care	-	-	-	88%
Received Reliever Medication	-	-	-	100%
Received Systemic Corticosteroids	-	-	-	100%
Emergency Department				
Admittance Decision Time (minutes)[2]	821	103	111	98
Head CT Results Within 45 Min. of Arrival[1]	-	-	64%	57%
Patients Who Left ER Before Being Seen	>100k	1%	2%	2%
Time from ER Arrival to Admit. (minutes)[2]	826	290	289	274
Time from ER Arrival to Discharge (minutes)	497	148	147	134
Time in ER Before Being Evaluated (minutes)	542	8	26	26
Time to Pain Meds for Fractures (minutes)	253	60	60	57
Heart Attack Care				
Aspirin Given at Discharge[2]	272	100%	99%	99%
Fibrinolytic Meds Within 30 Min. of Arrival[2,7]	-	-	50%	54%
PCI Within 90 Minutes of Arrival[2]	54	98%	96%	96%
Statin Prescribed at Discharge[2]	257	100%	99%	98%
Heart Failure Care				
ACE Inhibitor or ARB for LVSD[2]	132	100%	98%	97%
Discharge Instructions Given[2]	328	98%	96%	94%
Evaluation of LVS Function[2]	400	100%	100%	99%
Medicare Spending				
Medicare Spending per Patient (ratio)	-	1.03	1.04	0.98
Pneumonia Care				
Appropriate Initial Antibiotic Given[2]	180	99%	98%	95%
Blood Culture Timing[2]	214	99%	99%	98%
Pregnancy and Delivery Care				
Newborn Deliveries Scheduled Early[2]	71	1%	6%	6%
Preventive Care				
Immunization for Influenza[2]	619	97%	94%	90%
Immunization for Pneumonia[2]	638	95%	96%	92%
Stroke Care				
Anticoagulation Therapy for Atrial Fibrillation	27	96%	97%	95%
Antithrombotic Therapy Timing	180	99%	98%	98%
Assessed for Rehabilitation	224	96%	97%	97%
Discharged on Antithrombotic Therapy	199	100%	99%	99%
Discharged on Statin Medication	164	98%	96%	94%
Thrombolytic Therapy Timing	16	81%	76%	66%
Venous Thromboembolism Prophylaxis	221	99%	95%	94%
Written Stroke Educational Materials Given	149	97%	94%	88%
Surgical Care Improvement Project				
Appropriate Beta Blocker Usage[2]	218	99%	99%	98%
Appropriate VTP Within 24 Hours[2]	482	99%	99%	98%
Controlled Postoperative Blood Glucose[2]	126	98%	98%	97%
Perioperative Temperature Management[2]	594	100%	100%	100%
Prophylactic Antibiotic Selection[2]	452	100%	99%	99%
Prophylactic Antibiotic Selection (Outpatient)	482	99%	98%	98%
Prophylactic Antibiotic Stopped[2]	440	99%	98%	98%
Prophylactic Antibiotic Timing[2]	454	100%	99%	99%
Prophylactic Antibiotic Timing (Outpatient)	482	99%	98%	98%
Urinary Catheter Removal[2]	387	100%	98%	97%
Survey of Patients' Hospital Experiences				
Area Around Room 'Always' Quiet at Night	300+	60%	58%	61%
Doctors 'Always' Communicated Well	300+	73%	77%	82%
Home Recovery Information Given	300+	83%	83%	85%
Hospital Given 9 or 10 on 10 Point Scale	300+	57%	67%	71%
Meds 'Always' Explained Before Given	300+	52%	60%	64%
Nurses 'Always' Communicated Well	300+	68%	75%	79%
Pain 'Always' Well Controlled	300+	63%	68%	71%
Room and Bathroom 'Always' Clean	300+	64%	69%	73%
Timely Help 'Always' Received	300+	54%	62%	68%
Would Definitely Recommend Hospital	300+	56%	69%	71%
Use of Medical Imaging				
Cardiac Imaging Stress Test before Surgery	219	7.8%	6.4%	5.3%
Combination Abdominal CT Scan	643	1.6%	11.8%	10.5%
Combination Brain/Sinus CT Scan	879	5.3%	3.4%	2.7%
Combination Chest CT Scan	116	7.8%	2.4%	2.7%
Follow-up Mammogram/Ultrasound[7]	-	-	10.2%	8.8%
Lumbar Spine MRI for Low Back Pain[1]	-	-	35.2%	37.2%

NOTE: Hospital profiles are in alphabetical order by state, then city, then hospital within the city; Rankings exclude hospitals with less than 25 cases except for patient surveys which excludes hospitals with less than 100 cases; (a) 100-299 cases; (1) The number of cases/patients is too few to report; (2) Data submitted were based on a sample of cases/patients; (3) Results are based on a shorter time period than required; (4) Data suppressed by CMS for one or more quarters; (5) Results are not available for this reporting period; (6) Fewer than 100 patients completed the HCAHPS survey; (7) No cases met the criteria for this measure; (8) The lower limit of the confidence interval cannot be calculated if the number of observed infections equals zero; (9) No data are available from the state/territory for this reporting period; (10) The scores shown reflect fewer than 50 completed surveys; (11) There were discrepancies in the data collection process; (12) This measure does not apply to this hospital for this reporting period; (13) Results cannot be calculated for this reporting period; (14) The results for this state are combined with nearby states to protect confidentiality; Please refer to the User's Guide for a full explanation of data.

Bayfront Health Brooksville

17240 Cortez Blvd
Brooksville, FL 34601
Phone: 352-796-5111
Fax: 352-544-5711
E-mail: elaine.rothen@brh.hma-corp.com
URL: www.brooksvilleregionalhospital.org
Type: Acute Care Hospitals
Emergency Services: Yes
Ownership: Voluntary non-profit - Church
Beds: 120

Key Personnel:
Chief of Medical Staff. . . . . Mahmood Akel, MD
Emergency Room . . . . Ralph Brown, RN
CEO/President. . . . . Kathy Burke
Radiology. . . . . Sanford Davis
Quality Assurance . . . . Cheryl Love
Operating Room. . . . . Shauna McKinnon
Infection Control. . . . . Susan Napoleon
Intensive Care Unit. . . . . Gina Swaggerty, RN

Measure	Cases	This Hosp.	State Avg.	U.S. Avg.
Blood Clot Prevention and Treatment				
Anticoagulation Overlap Therapy[2]	75	95%	93%	93%
ICU Venous Thromboembolism Prophylaxis[2]	94	91%	94%	92%
Incidence of Potentially Preventable VTE[2]	12	25%	10%	10%
UFH with Dosages/Platelet Monitoring[2]	50	100%	100%	97%
Venous Thromboembolism Prophylaxis[2]	365	64%	88%	85%
Warfarin Therapy Discharge Instructions[2]	54	76%	85%	75%
Chest Pain/Possible Heart Attack Care				
Aspirin Given Within 24 Hours of Arrival	24	100%	98%	96%
Fibrinolytic Meds Within 30 Min. of Arrival[7]	-	-	81%	58%
Average Time to ECG (minutes)	25	7	7	7
Average Time to Transfer (minutes)[1]	-	-	53	60
Children's Asthma Care				
Received Home Management Plan of Care	-	-	-	88%
Received Reliever Medication	-	-	-	100%
Received Systemic Corticosteroids	-	-	-	100%
Emergency Department				
Admittance Decision Time (minutes)[2]	783	98	111	98
Head CT Results Within 45 Min. of Arrival[1]	-	-	64%	57%
Patients Who Left ER Before Being Seen	54,863	1%	2%	2%
Time from ER Arrival to Admit. (minutes)[2]	783	280	289	274
Time from ER Arrival to Discharge (minutes)	1,136	128	147	134
Time in ER Before Being Evaluated (minutes)	1,240	21	26	26
Time to Pain Meds for Fractures (minutes)	158	46	60	57
Heart Attack Care				
Aspirin Given at Discharge	134	96%	99%	99%
Fibrinolytic Meds Within 30 Min. of Arrival[7]	-	-	50%	54%
PCI Within 90 Minutes of Arrival	20	95%	96%	96%
Statin Prescribed at Discharge	115	98%	99%	98%
Heart Failure Care				
ACE Inhibitor or ARB for LVSD	60	100%	98%	97%
Discharge Instructions Given	229	95%	96%	94%
Evaluation of LVS Function	270	99%	100%	99%
Medicare Spending				
Medicare Spending per Patient (ratio)	-	1.04	1.04	0.98
Pneumonia Care				
Appropriate Initial Antibiotic Given	157	96%	98%	95%
Blood Culture Timing	224	100%	99%	98%
Pregnancy and Delivery Care				
Newborn Deliveries Scheduled Early	147	3%	6%	6%
Preventive Care				
Immunization for Influenza[2]	527	95%	94%	90%
Immunization for Pneumonia[2]	705	98%	96%	92%
Stroke Care				
Anticoagulation Therapy for Atrial Fibrillation	14	100%	97%	95%
Antithrombotic Therapy Timing	95	96%	98%	98%
Assessed for Rehabilitation	92	95%	97%	97%
Discharged on Antithrombotic Therapy	92	97%	99%	99%
Discharged on Statin Medication	66	77%	96%	94%
Thrombolytic Therapy Timing[1]	-	-	76%	66%
Venous Thromboembolism Prophylaxis	103	65%	95%	94%
Written Stroke Educational Materials Given	50	84%	94%	88%
Surgical Care Improvement Project				
Appropriate Beta Blocker Usage	160	99%	99%	98%
Appropriate VTP Within 24 Hours	452	98%	99%	98%
Controlled Postoperative Blood Glucose[7]	-	-	98%	97%
Perioperative Temperature Management	460	100%	100%	100%
Prophylactic Antibiotic Selection	309	99%	99%	99%
Prophylactic Antibiotic Selection (Outpatient)	185	97%	98%	98%
Prophylactic Antibiotic Stopped	291	97%	98%	98%
Prophylactic Antibiotic Timing	310	99%	99%	99%
Prophylactic Antibiotic Timing (Outpatient)	185	99%	98%	98%
Urinary Catheter Removal	308	97%	98%	97%
Survey of Patients' Hospital Experiences				
Area Around Room 'Always' Quiet at Night	300+	43%	58%	61%
Doctors 'Always' Communicated Well	300+	69%	77%	82%
Home Recovery Information Given	300+	79%	83%	85%
Hospital Given 9 or 10 on 10 Point Scale	300+	45%	67%	71%
Meds 'Always' Explained Before Given	300+	48%	60%	64%
Nurses 'Always' Communicated Well	300+	64%	75%	79%
Pain 'Always' Well Controlled	300+	58%	68%	71%
Room and Bathroom 'Always' Clean	300+	66%	69%	73%
Timely Help 'Always' Received	300+	46%	62%	68%
Would Definitely Recommend Hospital	300+	49%	69%	71%
Use of Medical Imaging				
Cardiac Imaging Stress Test before Surgery	204	6.4%	6.4%	5.3%
Combination Abdominal CT Scan	681	8.7%	11.8%	10.5%
Combination Brain/Sinus CT Scan	857	3.3%	3.4%	2.7%
Combination Chest CT Scan	395	7.1%	2.4%	2.7%
Follow-up Mammogram/Ultrasound	564	20.2%	10.2%	8.8%
Lumbar Spine MRI for Low Back Pain[1]	-	-	35.2%	37.2%

Oak Hill Hospital

11375 Cortez Blvd
Brooksville, FL 34613
Phone: 352-596-6632
Fax: 352-597-3024
URL: www.oakhillhospital.com
Type: Acute Care Hospitals
Emergency Services: Yes
Ownership: Voluntary non-profit - Other
Beds: 204

Key Personnel:
Chief of Medical Staff. . . . . Mahmoud Nimer, MD
Quality Assurance . . . . Bertha O'Leary
CEO . . . . Mickey Smith

Measure	Cases	This Hosp.	State Avg.	U.S. Avg.
Blood Clot Prevention and Treatment				
Anticoagulation Overlap Therapy[2]	132	99%	93%	93%
ICU Venous Thromboembolism Prophylaxis[2]	55	100%	94%	92%
Incidence of Potentially Preventable VTE[2]	16	0%	10%	10%
UFH with Dosages/Platelet Monitoring[2]	63	100%	100%	97%
Venous Thromboembolism Prophylaxis[2]	383	100%	88%	85%
Warfarin Therapy Discharge Instructions[2]	106	100%	85%	75%
Chest Pain/Possible Heart Attack Care				
Aspirin Given Within 24 Hours of Arrival[1,3]	-	-	98%	96%
Fibrinolytic Meds Within 30 Min. of Arrival[5]	-	-	81%	58%
Average Time to ECG (minutes)[3,7]	-	-	7	7
Average Time to Transfer (minutes)[5]	-	-	53	60
Children's Asthma Care				
Received Home Management Plan of Care	-	-	-	88%
Received Reliever Medication	-	-	-	100%
Received Systemic Corticosteroids	-	-	-	100%
Emergency Department				
Admittance Decision Time (minutes)[2]	865	49	111	98
Head CT Results Within 45 Min. of Arrival	14	86%	64%	57%
Patients Who Left ER Before Being Seen	38,228	1%	2%	2%
Time from ER Arrival to Admit. (minutes)[2]	865	240	289	274
Time from ER Arrival to Discharge (minutes)	444	156	147	134
Time in ER Before Being Evaluated (minutes)	496	16	26	26
Time to Pain Meds for Fractures (minutes)	120	52	60	57
Heart Attack Care				
Aspirin Given at Discharge[2]	259	100%	99%	99%
Fibrinolytic Meds Within 30 Min. of Arrival[2,7]	-	-	50%	54%
PCI Within 90 Minutes of Arrival[2]	40	95%	96%	96%
Statin Prescribed at Discharge[2]	237	100%	99%	98%
Heart Failure Care				
ACE Inhibitor or ARB for LVSD[2]	75	100%	98%	97%
Discharge Instructions Given[2]	241	100%	96%	94%
Evaluation of LVS Function[2]	283	100%	100%	99%
Medicare Spending				
Medicare Spending per Patient (ratio)	-	1.05	1.04	0.98
Pneumonia Care				
Appropriate Initial Antibiotic Given	158	100%	98%	95%
Blood Culture Timing	222	100%	99%	98%
Pregnancy and Delivery Care				
Newborn Deliveries Scheduled Early[2,7]	-	-	6%	6%
Preventive Care				
Immunization for Influenza[2]	657	99%	94%	90%
Immunization for Pneumonia[2]	1,036	98%	96%	92%
Stroke Care				
Anticoagulation Therapy for Atrial Fibrillation[2]	19	100%	97%	95%
Antithrombotic Therapy Timing[2]	90	100%	98%	98%
Assessed for Rehabilitation[2]	98	100%	97%	97%
Discharged on Antithrombotic Therapy[2]	98	100%	99%	99%
Discharged on Statin Medication[2]	74	100%	96%	94%
Thrombolytic Therapy Timing[1,2]	-	-	76%	66%
Venous Thromboembolism Prophylaxis[2]	100	100%	95%	94%
Written Stroke Educational Materials Given[2]	62	100%	94%	88%
Surgical Care Improvement Project				
Appropriate Beta Blocker Usage[2]	280	100%	99%	98%
Appropriate VTP Within 24 Hours[2]	380	99%	99%	98%
Controlled Postoperative Blood Glucose[2]	106	98%	98%	97%
Perioperative Temperature Management[2]	471	100%	100%	100%
Prophylactic Antibiotic Selection[2]	352	100%	99%	99%
Prophylactic Antibiotic Selection (Outpatient)	167	99%	98%	98%
Prophylactic Antibiotic Stopped[2]	341	100%	98%	98%
Prophylactic Antibiotic Timing[2]	352	100%	99%	99%
Prophylactic Antibiotic Timing (Outpatient)	167	100%	98%	98%
Urinary Catheter Removal[2]	377	100%	98%	97%
Survey of Patients' Hospital Experiences				
Area Around Room 'Always' Quiet at Night	300+	56%	58%	61%
Doctors 'Always' Communicated Well	300+	74%	77%	82%
Home Recovery Information Given	300+	86%	83%	85%
Hospital Given 9 or 10 on 10 Point Scale	300+	69%	67%	71%
Meds 'Always' Explained Before Given	300+	59%	60%	64%
Nurses 'Always' Communicated Well	300+	77%	75%	79%
Pain 'Always' Well Controlled	300+	71%	68%	71%
Room and Bathroom 'Always' Clean	300+	66%	69%	73%
Timely Help 'Always' Received	300+	62%	62%	68%
Would Definitely Recommend Hospital	300+	72%	69%	71%
Use of Medical Imaging				
Cardiac Imaging Stress Test before Surgery	136	7.4%	6.4%	5.3%
Combination Abdominal CT Scan	708	40.4%	11.8%	10.5%
Combination Brain/Sinus CT Scan	138	5.8%	3.4%	2.7%
Combination Chest CT Scan	215	0.0%	2.4%	2.7%
Follow-up Mammogram/Ultrasound	1,006	9.5%	10.2%	8.8%
Lumbar Spine MRI for Low Back Pain[1]	-	-	35.2%	37.2%

Cape Coral Hospital

636 Del Prado Blvd
Cape Coral, FL 33990
Phone: 239-574-2323
URL: www.leememorial.org
Type: Acute Care Hospitals
Emergency Services: Yes
Ownership: Govt - Hospital Dist/Auth

Key Personnel:
CEO/President. . . . . James Nathan

Measure	Cases	This Hosp.	State Avg.	U.S. Avg.
Blood Clot Prevention and Treatment				
Anticoagulation Overlap Therapy[2]	128	81%	93%	93%
ICU Venous Thromboembolism Prophylaxis[2]	59	90%	94%	92%
Incidence of Potentially Preventable VTE[2]	29	28%	10%	10%
UFH with Dosages/Platelet Monitoring[2]	115	100%	100%	97%
Venous Thromboembolism Prophylaxis[2]	356	83%	88%	85%
Warfarin Therapy Discharge Instructions[2]	95	92%	85%	75%
Chest Pain/Possible Heart Attack Care				
Aspirin Given Within 24 Hours of Arrival	67	97%	98%	96%
Fibrinolytic Meds Within 30 Min. of Arrival[7]	-	-	81%	58%
Average Time to ECG (minutes)	67	5	7	7
Average Time to Transfer (minutes)	17	29	53	60
Children's Asthma Care				
Received Home Management Plan of Care	-	-	-	88%
Received Reliever Medication	-	-	-	100%
Received Systemic Corticosteroids	-	-	-	100%
Emergency Department				
Admittance Decision Time (minutes)[2]	842	195	111	98
Head CT Results Within 45 Min. of Arrival[7]	-	-	64%	57%

NOTE: Hospital profiles are in alphabetical order by state, then city, then hospital within the city; Rankings exclude hospitals with less than 25 cases except for patient surveys which excludes hospitals with less than 100 cases; (a) 100-299 cases; (1) The number of cases/patients is too few to report; (2) Data submitted were based on a sample of cases/patients; (3) Results are based on a shorter time period than required; (4) Data suppressed by CMS for one or more quarters; (5) Results are not available for this reporting period; (6) Fewer than 100 patients completed the HCAHPS survey; (7) No cases met the criteria for this measure; (8) The lower limit of the confidence interval cannot be calculated if the number of observed infections equals zero; (9) No data are available from the state/territory for this reporting period; (10) The scores shown reflect fewer than 50 completed surveys; (11) There were discrepancies in the data collection process; (12) This measure does not apply to this hospital for this reporting period; (13) Results cannot be calculated for this reporting period; (14) The results for this state are combined with nearby states to protect confidentiality; Please refer to the User's Guide for a full explanation of data.

Measure	Cases	This Hosp.	State Avg.	U.S. Avg.
Patients Who Left ER Before Being Seen	28,928	0%	2%	2%
Time from ER Arrival to Admit. (minutes)[2]	842	356	289	274
Time from ER Arrival to Discharge (minutes)	359	203	147	134
Time in ER Before Being Evaluated (minutes)	371	35	26	26
Time to Pain Meds for Fractures (minutes)	89	75	60	57
Heart Attack Care				
Aspirin Given at Discharge	56	96%	99%	99%
Fibrinolytic Meds Within 30 Min. of Arrival[7]	-	-	50%	54%
PCI Within 90 Minutes of Arrival[7]	-	-	96%	96%
Statin Prescribed at Discharge	47	98%	99%	98%
Heart Failure Care				
ACE Inhibitor or ARB for LVSD[2]	81	90%	98%	97%
Discharge Instructions Given[2]	249	88%	96%	94%
Evaluation of LVS Function[2]	285	99%	100%	99%
Medicare Spending				
Medicare Spending per Patient (ratio)	-	1.02	1.04	0.98
Pneumonia Care				
Appropriate Initial Antibiotic Given[2]	94	97%	98%	95%
Blood Culture Timing[2]	155	95%	99%	98%
Pregnancy and Delivery Care				
Newborn Deliveries Scheduled Early[2]	33	3%	6%	6%
Preventive Care				
Immunization for Influenza[2]	558	79%	94%	90%
Immunization for Pneumonia[2]	770	81%	96%	92%
Stroke Care				
Anticoagulation Therapy for Atrial Fibrillation[2]	19	95%	97%	95%
Antithrombotic Therapy Timing[2]	99	100%	98%	98%
Assessed for Rehabilitation[2]	114	97%	97%	97%
Discharged on Antithrombotic Therapy[2]	100	100%	99%	99%
Discharged on Statin Medication[2]	75	95%	96%	94%
Thrombolytic Therapy Timing[1,2]	-	-	76%	66%
Venous Thromboembolism Prophylaxis[2]	125	90%	95%	94%
Written Stroke Educational Materials Given[2]	89	100%	94%	88%
Surgical Care Improvement Project				
Appropriate Beta Blocker Usage[2]	162	99%	99%	98%
Appropriate VTP Within 24 Hours[2]	429	94%	99%	98%
Controlled Postoperative Blood Glucose[2,7]	-	-	98%	97%
Perioperative Temperature Management[2]	510	100%	100%	100%
Prophylactic Antibiotic Selection[2]	289	95%	99%	99%
Prophylactic Antibiotic Selection (Outpatient)	361	97%	98%	98%
Prophylactic Antibiotic Stopped[2]	275	90%	98%	98%
Prophylactic Antibiotic Timing[2]	289	99%	99%	99%
Prophylactic Antibiotic Timing (Outpatient)	363	97%	98%	98%
Urinary Catheter Removal[2]	152	87%	98%	97%
Survey of Patients' Hospital Experiences				
Area Around Room 'Always' Quiet at Night	300+	55%	58%	61%
Doctors 'Always' Communicated Well	300+	72%	77%	82%
Home Recovery Information Given	300+	84%	83%	85%
Hospital Given 9 or 10 on 10 Point Scale	300+	62%	67%	71%
Meds 'Always' Explained Before Given	300+	60%	60%	64%
Nurses 'Always' Communicated Well	300+	76%	75%	79%
Pain 'Always' Well Controlled	300+	68%	68%	71%
Room and Bathroom 'Always' Clean	300+	69%	69%	73%
Timely Help 'Always' Received	300+	58%	62%	68%
Would Definitely Recommend Hospital	300+	65%	69%	71%
Use of Medical Imaging				
Cardiac Imaging Stress Test before Surgery	229	6.6%	6.4%	5.3%
Combination Abdominal CT Scan	742	58.1%	11.8%	10.5%
Combination Brain/Sinus CT Scan	838	2.6%	3.4%	2.7%
Combination Chest CT Scan	324	0.0%	2.4%	2.7%
Follow-up Mammogram/Ultrasound	1,422	7.6%	10.2%	8.8%
Lumbar Spine MRI for Low Back Pain	98	36.7%	35.2%	37.2%

Northwest Florida Community Hospital

1360 Brickyard Rd
Chipley, FL 32428
Phone: 850-638-1610
Fax: 850-638-6106
E-mail: marketing@nfch.org
URL: www.nfch.org
Type: Critical Access Hospitals
Emergency Services: Yes
Ownership: Voluntary non-profit - Private
Beds: 59

Key Personnel:
Quality Assurance . . . . John E Allen
Anesthesiology. . . . . Gabriel E Berry, MD
Operating Room. . . . . Terry Dasinger, RN
Intensive Care Unit. . . . . Anita Dowd, RN
Infection Control. . . . . Michelle W Fuller, RN
Emergency Room . . . . Patricia Pickron, RN
CEO/President. . . . . Patrick A Schlenker
Chief of Medical Staff. . . . . Samuel E. Ward, MD

Measure	Cases	This Hosp.	State Avg.	U.S. Avg.
Blood Clot Prevention and Treatment				
Anticoagulation Overlap Therapy[5]	-	-	93%	93%
ICU Venous Thromboembolism Prophylaxis[5]	-	-	94%	92%
Incidence of Potentially Preventable VTE[5]	-	-	10%	10%
UFH with Dosages/Platelet Monitoring[5]	-	-	100%	97%
Venous Thromboembolism Prophylaxis[5]	-	-	88%	85%
Warfarin Therapy Discharge Instructions[5]	-	-	85%	75%
Chest Pain/Possible Heart Attack Care				
Aspirin Given Within 24 Hours of Arrival	-	-	98%	96%
Fibrinolytic Meds Within 30 Min. of Arrival	-	-	81%	58%
Average Time to ECG (minutes)	-	-	7	7
Average Time to Transfer (minutes)	-	-	53	60
Children's Asthma Care				
Received Home Management Plan of Care	-	-	-	88%
Received Reliever Medication	-	-	-	100%
Received Systemic Corticosteroids	-	-	-	100%
Emergency Department				
Admittance Decision Time (minutes)[5]	-	-	111	98
Head CT Results Within 45 Min. of Arrival	-	-	64%	57%
Patients Who Left ER Before Being Seen	-	-	2%	2%
Time from ER Arrival to Admit. (minutes)[5]	-	-	289	274
Time from ER Arrival to Discharge (minutes)	-	-	147	134
Time in ER Before Being Evaluated (minutes)	-	-	26	26
Time to Pain Meds for Fractures (minutes)	-	-	60	57
Heart Attack Care				
Aspirin Given at Discharge[5]	-	-	99%	99%
Fibrinolytic Meds Within 30 Min. of Arrival[5]	-	-	50%	54%
PCI Within 90 Minutes of Arrival[5]	-	-	96%	96%
Statin Prescribed at Discharge[5]	-	-	99%	98%
Heart Failure Care				
ACE Inhibitor or ARB for LVSD[3,7]	-	-	98%	97%
Discharge Instructions Given[1,3]	-	-	96%	94%
Evaluation of LVS Function[1,3]	-	-	100%	99%
Medicare Spending				
Medicare Spending per Patient (ratio)	-	-	1.04	0.98
Pneumonia Care				
Appropriate Initial Antibiotic Given[3,7]	-	-	98%	95%
Blood Culture Timing[3,7]	-	-	99%	98%
Pregnancy and Delivery Care				
Newborn Deliveries Scheduled Early[5]	-	-	6%	6%
Preventive Care				
Immunization for Influenza[5]	-	-	94%	90%
Immunization for Pneumonia[5]	-	-	96%	92%
Stroke Care				
Anticoagulation Therapy for Atrial Fibrillation[5]	-	-	97%	95%
Antithrombotic Therapy Timing[5]	-	-	98%	98%
Assessed for Rehabilitation[5]	-	-	97%	97%
Discharged on Antithrombotic Therapy[5]	-	-	99%	99%
Discharged on Statin Medication[5]	-	-	96%	94%
Thrombolytic Therapy Timing[5]	-	-	76%	66%
Venous Thromboembolism Prophylaxis[5]	-	-	95%	94%
Written Stroke Educational Materials Given[5]	-	-	94%	88%
Surgical Care Improvement Project				
Appropriate Beta Blocker Usage[5]	-	-	99%	98%
Appropriate VTP Within 24 Hours[5]	-	-	99%	98%
Controlled Postoperative Blood Glucose[5]	-	-	98%	97%
Perioperative Temperature Management[5]	-	-	100%	100%
Prophylactic Antibiotic Selection[5]	-	-	99%	99%
Prophylactic Antibiotic Selection (Outpatient)	-	-	98%	98%
Prophylactic Antibiotic Stopped[5]	-	-	98%	98%
Prophylactic Antibiotic Timing[5]	-	-	99%	99%
Prophylactic Antibiotic Timing (Outpatient)	-	-	98%	98%
Urinary Catheter Removal[5]	-	-	98%	97%
Survey of Patients' Hospital Experiences				
Area Around Room 'Always' Quiet at Night[5]	-	-	58%	61%
Doctors 'Always' Communicated Well[5]	-	-	77%	82%
Home Recovery Information Given[5]	-	-	83%	85%
Hospital Given 9 or 10 on 10 Point Scale[5]	-	-	67%	71%
Meds 'Always' Explained Before Given[5]	-	-	60%	64%
Nurses 'Always' Communicated Well[5]	-	-	75%	79%
Pain 'Always' Well Controlled[5]	-	-	68%	71%
Room and Bathroom 'Always' Clean[5]	-	-	69%	73%
Timely Help 'Always' Received[5]	-	-	62%	68%
Would Definitely Recommend Hospital[5]	-	-	69%	71%
Use of Medical Imaging				
Cardiac Imaging Stress Test before Surgery	-	-	6.4%	5.3%
Combination Abdominal CT Scan	-	-	11.8%	10.5%
Combination Brain/Sinus CT Scan	-	-	3.4%	2.7%
Combination Chest CT Scan	-	-	2.4%	2.7%
Follow-up Mammogram/Ultrasound	-	-	10.2%	8.8%
Lumbar Spine MRI for Low Back Pain	-	-	35.2%	37.2%

Morton Plant Hospital

300 Pinellas St
Clearwater, FL 33756
Phone: 727-462-7000
Fax: 727-461-8101
URL: www.measehospitals.com
Type: Acute Care Hospitals
Emergency Services: Yes
Ownership: Voluntary non-profit - Private
Beds: 687

Key Personnel:
Radiology. . . . . Paul Amberg
Chief of Medical Staff . . . . John Babka, MD
CEO/President. . . . . Philip K Beauchamp, FACHE
Infection Control. . . . . Rebecca Carlson
Quality Assurance . . . . June Delapp
Pediatric In-Patient Care . . . . Greg Savel, MD
Operating Room. . . . . Cheryl Young, RN

Measure	Cases	This Hosp.	State Avg.	U.S. Avg.
Blood Clot Prevention and Treatment				
Anticoagulation Overlap Therapy[2]	157	87%	93%	93%
ICU Venous Thromboembolism Prophylaxis[2]	99	94%	94%	92%
Incidence of Potentially Preventable VTE[2]	27	0%	10%	10%
UFH with Dosages/Platelet Monitoring[2]	39	100%	100%	97%
Venous Thromboembolism Prophylaxis[2]	367	89%	88%	85%
Warfarin Therapy Discharge Instructions[2]	114	92%	85%	75%
Chest Pain/Possible Heart Attack Care				
Aspirin Given Within 24 Hours of Arrival[1,3]	-	-	98%	96%
Fibrinolytic Meds Within 30 Min. of Arrival[5]	-	-	81%	58%
Average Time to ECG (minutes)[1,3]	-	-	7	7
Average Time to Transfer (minutes)[5]	-	-	53	60
Children's Asthma Care				
Received Home Management Plan of Care	-	-	-	88%
Received Reliever Medication	-	-	-	100%
Received Systemic Corticosteroids	-	-	-	100%
Emergency Department				
Admittance Decision Time (minutes)[2]	443	89	111	98
Head CT Results Within 45 Min. of Arrival[1]	-	-	64%	57%
Patients Who Left ER Before Being Seen	77,818	3%	2%	2%
Time from ER Arrival to Admit. (minutes)[2]	447	300	289	274
Time from ER Arrival to Discharge (minutes)	368	170	147	134
Time in ER Before Being Evaluated (minutes)	431	39	26	26
Time to Pain Meds for Fractures (minutes)	128	60	60	57
Heart Attack Care				
Aspirin Given at Discharge	548	100%	99%	99%
Fibrinolytic Meds Within 30 Min. of Arrival[7]	-	-	50%	54%
PCI Within 90 Minutes of Arrival	49	98%	96%	96%
Statin Prescribed at Discharge	520	100%	99%	98%
Heart Failure Care				
ACE Inhibitor or ARB for LVSD	165	98%	98%	97%
Discharge Instructions Given	461	97%	96%	94%
Evaluation of LVS Function	595	100%	100%	99%
Medicare Spending				
Medicare Spending per Patient (ratio)	-	1.05	1.04	0.98
Pneumonia Care				
Appropriate Initial Antibiotic Given	140	98%	98%	95%
Blood Culture Timing	415	100%	99%	98%
Pregnancy and Delivery Care				
Newborn Deliveries Scheduled Early[2]	50	34%	6%	6%
Preventive Care				
Immunization for Influenza[2]	530	96%	94%	90%
Immunization for Pneumonia[2]	692	93%	96%	92%
Stroke Care				

NOTE: Hospital profiles are in alphabetical order by state, then city, then hospital within the city; Rankings exclude hospitals with less than 25 cases except for patient surveys which excludes hospitals with less than 100 cases; (a) 100-299 cases; (1) The number of cases/patients is too few to report; (2) Data submitted were based on a sample of cases/patients; (3) Results are based on a shorter time period than required; (4) Data suppressed by CMS for one or more quarters; (5) Results are not available for this reporting period; (6) Fewer than 100 patients completed the HCAHPS survey; (7) No cases met the criteria for this measure; (8) The lower limit of the confidence interval cannot be calculated if the number of observed infections equals zero; (9) No data are available from the state/territory for this reporting period; (10) The scores shown reflect fewer than 50 completed surveys; (11) There were discrepancies in the data collection process; (12) This measure does not apply to this hospital for this reporting period; (13) Results cannot be calculated for this reporting period; (14) The results for this state are combined with nearby states to protect confidentiality; Please refer to the User's Guide for a full explanation of data.

Anticoagulation Therapy for Atrial Fibrillation	37	95%	97%	95%
Antithrombotic Therapy Timing	183	100%	98%	98%
Assessed for Rehabilitation	259	98%	97%	97%
Discharged on Antithrombotic Therapy	200	98%	99%	99%
Discharged on Statin Medication	147	95%	96%	94%
Thrombolytic Therapy Timing	18	89%	76%	66%
Venous Thromboembolism Prophylaxis	275	99%	95%	94%
Written Stroke Educational Materials Given	131	92%	94%	88%
Surgical Care Improvement Project				
Appropriate Beta Blocker Usage[2]	659	99%	99%	98%
Appropriate VTP Within 24 Hours[2]	1,225	99%	99%	98%
Controlled Postoperative Blood Glucose[2]	295	99%	98%	97%
Perioperative Temperature Management[2]	1,522	100%	100%	100%
Prophylactic Antibiotic Selection[2]	1,450	100%	99%	99%
Prophylactic Antibiotic Selection (Outpatient)	645	98%	98%	98%
Prophylactic Antibiotic Stopped[2]	1,412	100%	98%	98%
Prophylactic Antibiotic Timing[2]	1,459	99%	99%	99%
Prophylactic Antibiotic Timing (Outpatient)	647	98%	98%	98%
Urinary Catheter Removal[2]	1,326	100%	98%	97%
Survey of Patients' Hospital Experiences				
Area Around Room 'Always' Quiet at Night[11]	300+	50%	58%	61%
Doctors 'Always' Communicated Well[11]	300+	78%	77%	82%
Home Recovery Information Given[11]	300+	87%	83%	85%
Hospital Given 9 or 10 on 10 Point Scale[11]	300+	77%	67%	71%
Meds 'Always' Explained Before Given[11]	300+	63%	60%	64%
Nurses 'Always' Communicated Well[11]	300+	78%	75%	79%
Pain 'Always' Well Controlled[11]	300+	70%	68%	71%
Room and Bathroom 'Always' Clean[11]	300+	74%	69%	73%
Timely Help 'Always' Received[11]	300+	67%	62%	68%
Would Definitely Recommend Hospital[11]	300+	81%	69%	71%
Use of Medical Imaging				
Cardiac Imaging Stress Test before Surgery	122	10.7%	6.4%	5.3%
Combination Abdominal CT Scan	815	2.8%	11.8%	10.5%
Combination Brain/Sinus CT Scan	1,664	3.7%	3.4%	2.7%
Combination Chest CT Scan	118	0.0%	2.4%	2.7%
Follow-up Mammogram/Ultrasound[7]	-	-	10.2%	8.8%
Lumbar Spine MRI for Low Back Pain[1]	-	-	35.2%	37.2%

South Lake Hospital

1900 Don Wickham Dr
Clermont, FL 34711
Phone: 352-394-4071
Fax: 352-394-7179
URL: www.southlakehospital.com
Type: Acute Care Hospitals
Emergency Services: Yes
Ownership: Govt - Hospital Dist/Auth
Beds: 104

Key Personnel:
Radiology. . . . . Robert Anderson
Chief of Medical Staff. . . . . Eric Carter
CEO/President. . . . . Leslie Longacre

Measure	Cases	This Hosp.	State Avg.	U.S. Avg.
Blood Clot Prevention and Treatment				
Anticoagulation Overlap Therapy[2]	87	86%	93%	93%
ICU Venous Thromboembolism Prophylaxis[2]	254	99%	94%	92%
Incidence of Potentially Preventable VTE[2]	13	15%	10%	10%
UFH with Dosages/Platelet Monitoring[2]	63	100%	100%	97%
Venous Thromboembolism Prophylaxis[2]	2,477	94%	88%	85%
Warfarin Therapy Discharge Instructions[2]	64	83%	85%	75%
Chest Pain/Possible Heart Attack Care				
Aspirin Given Within 24 Hours of Arrival[1]	-	-	98%	96%
Fibrinolytic Meds Within 30 Min. of Arrival[7]	-	-	81%	58%
Average Time to ECG (minutes)[1]	-	-	7	7
Average Time to Transfer (minutes)[1]	-	-	53	60
Children's Asthma Care				
Received Home Management Plan of Care	-	-	-	88%
Received Reliever Medication	-	-	-	100%
Received Systemic Corticosteroids	-	-	-	100%
Emergency Department				
Admittance Decision Time (minutes)[2]	1,263	82	111	98
Head CT Results Within 45 Min. of Arrival[1]	-	-	64%	57%
Patients Who Left ER Before Being Seen	47,763	2%	2%	2%
Time from ER Arrival to Admit. (minutes)[2]	1,731	313	289	274
Time from ER Arrival to Discharge (minutes)	2,276	172	147	134
Time in ER Before Being Evaluated (minutes)	1,855	51	26	26
Time to Pain Meds for Fractures (minutes)	164	58	60	57
Heart Attack Care				
Aspirin Given at Discharge	168	96%	99%	99%
Fibrinolytic Meds Within 30 Min. of Arrival[7]	-	-	50%	54%
PCI Within 90 Minutes of Arrival	32	91%	96%	96%
Statin Prescribed at Discharge	161	94%	99%	98%
Heart Failure Care				
ACE Inhibitor or ARB for LVSD	66	89%	98%	97%
Discharge Instructions Given	229	99%	96%	94%
Evaluation of LVS Function	249	99%	100%	99%
Medicare Spending				
Medicare Spending per Patient (ratio)	-	1.02	1.04	0.98
Pneumonia Care				
Appropriate Initial Antibiotic Given	96	96%	98%	95%
Blood Culture Timing	160	94%	99%	98%
Pregnancy and Delivery Care				
Newborn Deliveries Scheduled Early	40	0%	6%	6%
Preventive Care				
Immunization for Influenza[2]	1,743	96%	94%	90%
Immunization for Pneumonia[2]	2,371	96%	96%	92%
Stroke Care				
Anticoagulation Therapy for Atrial Fibrillation[1]	-	-	97%	95%
Antithrombotic Therapy Timing	58	100%	98%	98%
Assessed for Rehabilitation	62	94%	97%	97%
Discharged on Antithrombotic Therapy	60	97%	99%	99%
Discharged on Statin Medication	46	89%	96%	94%
Thrombolytic Therapy Timing[1]	-	-	76%	66%
Venous Thromboembolism Prophylaxis	59	97%	95%	94%
Written Stroke Educational Materials Given	50	92%	94%	88%
Surgical Care Improvement Project				
Appropriate Beta Blocker Usage	182	95%	99%	98%
Appropriate VTP Within 24 Hours	520	98%	99%	98%
Controlled Postoperative Blood Glucose[7]	-	-	98%	97%
Perioperative Temperature Management	575	100%	100%	100%
Prophylactic Antibiotic Selection	408	100%	99%	99%
Prophylactic Antibiotic Selection (Outpatient)	109	97%	98%	98%
Prophylactic Antibiotic Stopped	393	98%	98%	98%
Prophylactic Antibiotic Timing	408	100%	99%	99%
Prophylactic Antibiotic Timing (Outpatient)	108	98%	98%	98%
Urinary Catheter Removal	147	97%	98%	97%
Survey of Patients' Hospital Experiences				
Area Around Room 'Always' Quiet at Night	300+	59%	58%	61%
Doctors 'Always' Communicated Well	300+	71%	77%	82%
Home Recovery Information Given	300+	84%	83%	85%
Hospital Given 9 or 10 on 10 Point Scale	300+	67%	67%	71%
Meds 'Always' Explained Before Given	300+	57%	60%	64%
Nurses 'Always' Communicated Well	300+	72%	75%	79%
Pain 'Always' Well Controlled	300+	66%	68%	71%
Room and Bathroom 'Always' Clean	300+	70%	69%	73%
Timely Help 'Always' Received	300+	62%	62%	68%
Would Definitely Recommend Hospital	300+	67%	69%	71%
Use of Medical Imaging				
Cardiac Imaging Stress Test before Surgery	241	7.5%	6.4%	5.3%
Combination Abdominal CT Scan	966	2.5%	11.8%	10.5%
Combination Brain/Sinus CT Scan	762	2.0%	3.4%	2.7%
Combination Chest CT Scan	413	0.2%	2.4%	2.7%
Follow-up Mammogram/Ultrasound	1,222	8.4%	10.2%	8.8%
Lumbar Spine MRI for Low Back Pain	52	36.5%	35.2%	37.2%

Hendry Regional Medical Center

524 W Sagamore Ave
Clewiston, FL 33440
Phone: 863-902-3033
Fax: 863-983-0805
URL: www.hendryregional.org
Type: Critical Access Hospitals
Emergency Services: Yes
Ownership: Voluntary non-profit - Other
Beds: 66

Key Personnel:
Pediatric Ambulatory Care . . . . . . Charles Azan, MD
Radiology. . . . . Hardman Corman
CEO . . . . Raymond Draper
Chief of Medical Staff. . . . . Adrian Fedele, MD
Quality Assurance . . . . Chris Hamilton, RN
Infection Control. . . . . Linda Reecer, RN
Operating Room. . . . . Linda Reecer, RN

Measure	Cases	This Hosp.	State Avg.	U.S. Avg.
Blood Clot Prevention and Treatment				
Anticoagulation Overlap Therapy[5]	-	-	93%	93%
ICU Venous Thromboembolism Prophylaxis[5]	-	-	94%	92%
Incidence of Potentially Preventable VTE[5]	-	-	10%	10%
UFH with Dosages/Platelet Monitoring[5]	-	-	100%	97%
Venous Thromboembolism Prophylaxis[5]	-	-	88%	85%
Warfarin Therapy Discharge Instructions[5]	-	-	85%	75%
Chest Pain/Possible Heart Attack Care				
Aspirin Given Within 24 Hours of Arrival[5]	-	-	98%	96%
Fibrinolytic Meds Within 30 Min. of Arrival[5]	-	-	81%	58%
Average Time to ECG (minutes)[5]	-	-	7	7
Average Time to Transfer (minutes)[5]	-	-	53	60
Children's Asthma Care				
Received Home Management Plan of Care	-	-	-	88%
Received Reliever Medication	-	-	-	100%
Received Systemic Corticosteroids	-	-	-	100%
Emergency Department				
Admittance Decision Time (minutes)[5]	-	-	111	98
Head CT Results Within 45 Min. of Arrival[5]	-	-	64%	57%
Patients Who Left ER Before Being Seen[5]	-	-	2%	2%
Time from ER Arrival to Admit. (minutes)[5]	-	-	289	274
Time from ER Arrival to Discharge (minutes)[3]	279	136	147	134
Time in ER Before Being Evaluated (minutes)[3]	300	37	26	26
Time to Pain Meds for Fractures (minutes)[5]	-	-	60	57
Heart Attack Care				
Aspirin Given at Discharge[1]	-	-	99%	99%
Fibrinolytic Meds Within 30 Min. of Arrival[7]	-	-	50%	54%
PCI Within 90 Minutes of Arrival[7]	-	-	96%	96%
Statin Prescribed at Discharge[7]	-	-	99%	98%
Heart Failure Care				
ACE Inhibitor or ARB for LVSD	11	100%	98%	97%
Discharge Instructions Given	47	100%	96%	94%
Evaluation of LVS Function	47	100%	100%	99%
Medicare Spending				
Medicare Spending per Patient (ratio)	-	-	1.04	0.98
Pneumonia Care				
Appropriate Initial Antibiotic Given[1]	-	-	98%	95%
Blood Culture Timing	13	100%	99%	98%
Pregnancy and Delivery Care				
Newborn Deliveries Scheduled Early[5]	-	-	6%	6%
Preventive Care				
Immunization for Influenza[5]	-	-	94%	90%
Immunization for Pneumonia[5]	-	-	96%	92%
Stroke Care				
Anticoagulation Therapy for Atrial Fibrillation[5]	-	-	97%	95%
Antithrombotic Therapy Timing[5]	-	-	98%	98%
Assessed for Rehabilitation[5]	-	-	97%	97%
Discharged on Antithrombotic Therapy[5]	-	-	99%	99%
Discharged on Statin Medication[5]	-	-	96%	94%
Thrombolytic Therapy Timing[5]	-	-	76%	66%
Venous Thromboembolism Prophylaxis[5]	-	-	95%	94%
Written Stroke Educational Materials Given[5]	-	-	94%	88%
Surgical Care Improvement Project				
Appropriate Beta Blocker Usage[1]	-	-	99%	98%
Appropriate VTP Within 24 Hours[1]	-	-	99%	98%
Controlled Postoperative Blood Glucose[7]	-	-	98%	97%
Perioperative Temperature Management[1]	-	-	100%	100%
Prophylactic Antibiotic Selection[1]	-	-	99%	99%
Prophylactic Antibiotic Selection (Outpatient)[5]	-	-	98%	98%
Prophylactic Antibiotic Stopped[1]	-	-	98%	98%
Prophylactic Antibiotic Timing[1]	-	-	99%	99%
Prophylactic Antibiotic Timing (Outpatient)[5]	-	-	98%	98%
Urinary Catheter Removal[1]	-	-	98%	97%
Survey of Patients' Hospital Experiences				
Area Around Room 'Always' Quiet at Night	(a)	73%	58%	61%
Doctors 'Always' Communicated Well	(a)	83%	77%	82%
Home Recovery Information Given	(a)	85%	83%	85%
Hospital Given 9 or 10 on 10 Point Scale	(a)	66%	67%	71%
Meds 'Always' Explained Before Given	(a)	60%	60%	64%
Nurses 'Always' Communicated Well	(a)	82%	75%	79%
Pain 'Always' Well Controlled	(a)	70%	68%	71%
Room and Bathroom 'Always' Clean	(a)	63%	69%	73%
Timely Help 'Always' Received	(a)	75%	62%	68%

NOTE: Hospital profiles are in alphabetical order by state, then city, then hospital within the city; Rankings exclude hospitals with less than 25 cases except for patient surveys which excludes hospitals with less than 100 cases; (a) 100-299 cases; (1) The number of cases/patients is too few to report; (2) Data submitted were based on a sample of cases/patients; (3) Results are based on a shorter time period than required; (4) Data suppressed by CMS for one or more quarters; (5) Results are not available for this reporting period; (6) Fewer than 100 patients completed the HCAHPS survey; (7) No cases met the criteria for this measure; (8) The lower limit of the confidence interval cannot be calculated if the number of observed infections equals zero; (9) No data are available from the state/territory for this reporting period; (10) The scores shown reflect fewer than 50 completed surveys; (11) There were discrepancies in the data collection process; (12) This measure does not apply to this hospital for this reporting period; (13) Results cannot be calculated for this reporting period; (14) The results for this state are combined with nearby states to protect confidentiality; Please refer to the User's Guide for a full explanation of data.

Would Definitely Recommend Hospital	(a)	60%	69%	71%
Use of Medical Imaging				
Cardiac Imaging Stress Test before Surgery[1]	-	-	6.4%	5.3%
Combination Abdominal CT Scan	265	11.7%	11.8%	10.5%
Combination Brain/Sinus CT Scan[1]	-	-	3.4%	2.7%
Combination Chest CT Scan	104	19.2%	2.4%	2.7%
Follow-up Mammogram/Ultrasound	194	20.1%	10.2%	8.8%
Lumbar Spine MRI for Low Back Pain[1]	-	-	35.2%	37.2%

Cape Canaveral Hospital

701 W Cocoa Beach Causeway
Cocoa Beach, FL 32932
Phone: 321-799-7111
URL: www.health-first.org
Type: Acute Care Hospitals
Emergency Services: Yes
Ownership: Voluntary non-profit - Private
Beds: 150

Key Personnel:
Radiology. . . . . Bradley Barnes
Intensive Care Unit. . . . . Jane Curts, RN
Operating Room. . . . . Candace Dukes
Chief of Medical Staff . . . . Scott Gettings, MD
CEO/President. . . . . Steven P. Johnson
Quality Assurance . . . . Joy Presser
Infection Control. . . . . Joan Scabarozi

Measure	Cases	This Hosp.	State Avg.	U.S. Avg.
Blood Clot Prevention and Treatment				
Anticoagulation Overlap Therapy[2]	59	95%	93%	93%
ICU Venous Thromboembolism Prophylaxis[2]	60	100%	94%	92%
Incidence of Potentially Preventable VTE[1,2]	-	-	10%	10%
UFH with Dosages/Platelet Monitoring[2]	39	100%	100%	97%
Venous Thromboembolism Prophylaxis[2]	344	96%	88%	85%
Warfarin Therapy Discharge Instructions[2]	53	98%	85%	75%
Chest Pain/Possible Heart Attack Care				
Aspirin Given Within 24 Hours of Arrival[1]	-	-	98%	96%
Fibrinolytic Meds Within 30 Min. of Arrival[3,7]	-	-	81%	58%
Average Time to ECG (minutes)[1]	-	-	7	7
Average Time to Transfer (minutes)[1,3]	-	-	53	60
Children's Asthma Care				
Received Home Management Plan of Care	-	-	-	88%
Received Reliever Medication	-	-	-	100%
Received Systemic Corticosteroids	-	-	-	100%
Emergency Department				
Admittance Decision Time (minutes)[2]	777	97	111	98
Head CT Results Within 45 Min. of Arrival[1]	-	-	64%	57%
Patients Who Left ER Before Being Seen	27,399	3%	2%	2%
Time from ER Arrival to Admit. (minutes)[2]	777	268	289	274
Time from ER Arrival to Discharge (minutes)	367	174	147	134
Time in ER Before Being Evaluated (minutes)	377	34	26	26
Time to Pain Meds for Fractures (minutes)	114	79	60	57
Heart Attack Care				
Aspirin Given at Discharge	122	99%	99%	99%
Fibrinolytic Meds Within 30 Min. of Arrival[7]	-	-	50%	54%
PCI Within 90 Minutes of Arrival	26	96%	96%	96%
Statin Prescribed at Discharge	114	98%	99%	98%
Heart Failure Care				
ACE Inhibitor or ARB for LVSD	58	100%	98%	97%
Discharge Instructions Given	134	97%	96%	94%
Evaluation of LVS Function	164	100%	100%	99%
Medicare Spending				
Medicare Spending per Patient (ratio)	-	1.04	1.04	0.98
Pneumonia Care				
Appropriate Initial Antibiotic Given	145	97%	98%	95%
Blood Culture Timing	210	100%	99%	98%
Pregnancy and Delivery Care				
Newborn Deliveries Scheduled Early[2]	34	6%	6%	6%
Preventive Care				
Immunization for Influenza[2]	581	99%	94%	90%
Immunization for Pneumonia[2]	799	100%	96%	92%
Stroke Care				
Anticoagulation Therapy for Atrial Fibrillation	12	92%	97%	95%
Antithrombotic Therapy Timing	80	99%	98%	98%
Assessed for Rehabilitation	86	99%	97%	97%
Discharged on Antithrombotic Therapy	78	100%	99%	99%
Discharged on Statin Medication	61	98%	96%	94%
Thrombolytic Therapy Timing[1]	-	-	76%	66%
Venous Thromboembolism Prophylaxis	85	100%	95%	94%
Written Stroke Educational Materials Given	54	98%	94%	88%
Surgical Care Improvement Project				
Appropriate Beta Blocker Usage[2]	115	99%	99%	98%
Appropriate VTP Within 24 Hours[2]	360	99%	99%	98%
Controlled Postoperative Blood Glucose[2,7]	-	-	98%	97%
Perioperative Temperature Management[2]	395	100%	100%	100%
Prophylactic Antibiotic Selection[2]	258	99%	99%	99%
Prophylactic Antibiotic Selection (Outpatient)	95	100%	98%	98%
Prophylactic Antibiotic Stopped[2]	257	99%	98%	98%
Prophylactic Antibiotic Timing[2]	258	100%	99%	99%
Prophylactic Antibiotic Timing (Outpatient)	96	98%	98%	98%
Urinary Catheter Removal[2]	263	100%	98%	97%
Survey of Patients' Hospital Experiences				
Area Around Room 'Always' Quiet at Night	300+	60%	58%	61%
Doctors 'Always' Communicated Well	300+	78%	77%	82%
Home Recovery Information Given	300+	85%	83%	85%
Hospital Given 9 or 10 on 10 Point Scale	300+	73%	67%	71%
Meds 'Always' Explained Before Given	300+	69%	60%	64%
Nurses 'Always' Communicated Well	300+	82%	75%	79%
Pain 'Always' Well Controlled	300+	74%	68%	71%
Room and Bathroom 'Always' Clean	300+	80%	69%	73%
Timely Help 'Always' Received	300+	68%	62%	68%
Would Definitely Recommend Hospital	300+	78%	69%	71%
Use of Medical Imaging				
Cardiac Imaging Stress Test before Surgery	434	6.0%	6.4%	5.3%
Combination Abdominal CT Scan	799	14.1%	11.8%	10.5%
Combination Brain/Sinus CT Scan	690	5.4%	3.4%	2.7%
Combination Chest CT Scan	643	0.3%	2.4%	2.7%
Follow-up Mammogram/Ultrasound	1,687	9.6%	10.2%	8.8%
Lumbar Spine MRI for Low Back Pain	54	27.8%	35.2%	37.2%

Coral Gables Hospital

3100 Douglas Rd
Coral Gables, FL 33134
Phone: 305-445-8461
Fax: 305-441-6879
URL: www.coralgableshospital.com
Type: Acute Care Hospitals
Emergency Services: Yes
Ownership: Proprietary
Beds: 256

Key Personnel:
Quality Assurance . . . . Jan Bennett
Radiology. . . . . Morton Blumberg, MD
Emergency Room . . . . Donna Stevens, RN
CEO . . . . Jeffrey M Welch

Measure	Cases	This Hosp.	State Avg.	U.S. Avg.
Blood Clot Prevention and Treatment				
Anticoagulation Overlap Therapy[2]	16	100%	93%	93%
ICU Venous Thromboembolism Prophylaxis[2]	78	99%	94%	92%
Incidence of Potentially Preventable VTE[1,2]	-	-	10%	10%
UFH with Dosages/Platelet Monitoring[1,2]	-	-	100%	97%
Venous Thromboembolism Prophylaxis[2]	332	95%	88%	85%
Warfarin Therapy Discharge Instructions[2]	11	100%	85%	75%
Chest Pain/Possible Heart Attack Care				
Aspirin Given Within 24 Hours of Arrival	18	100%	98%	96%
Fibrinolytic Meds Within 30 Min. of Arrival[7]	-	-	81%	58%
Average Time to ECG (minutes)	20	4	7	7
Average Time to Transfer (minutes)[1]	-	-	53	60
Children's Asthma Care				
Received Home Management Plan of Care	-	-	-	88%
Received Reliever Medication	-	-	-	100%
Received Systemic Corticosteroids	-	-	-	100%
Emergency Department				
Admittance Decision Time (minutes)[2]	1,121	119	111	98
Head CT Results Within 45 Min. of Arrival[1,3]	-	-	64%	57%
Patients Who Left ER Before Being Seen	15,973	1%	2%	2%
Time from ER Arrival to Admit. (minutes)[2]	1,121	326	289	274
Time from ER Arrival to Discharge (minutes)	405	186	147	134
Time in ER Before Being Evaluated (minutes)	477	17	26	26
Time to Pain Meds for Fractures (minutes)	41	58	60	57
Heart Attack Care				
Aspirin Given at Discharge	12	100%	99%	99%
Fibrinolytic Meds Within 30 Min. of Arrival[7]	-	-	50%	54%
PCI Within 90 Minutes of Arrival[7]	-	-	96%	96%
Statin Prescribed at Discharge	11	100%	99%	98%
Heart Failure Care				
ACE Inhibitor or ARB for LVSD	68	100%	98%	97%
Discharge Instructions Given	197	100%	96%	94%
Evaluation of LVS Function	202	100%	100%	99%
Medicare Spending				
Medicare Spending per Patient (ratio)	-	1.11	1.04	0.98
Pneumonia Care				
Appropriate Initial Antibiotic Given	74	100%	98%	95%
Blood Culture Timing	105	100%	99%	98%
Pregnancy and Delivery Care				
Newborn Deliveries Scheduled Early[7]	-	-	6%	6%
Preventive Care				
Immunization for Influenza[2]	611	100%	94%	90%
Immunization for Pneumonia[2]	891	100%	96%	92%
Stroke Care				
Anticoagulation Therapy for Atrial Fibrillation[1]	-	-	97%	95%
Antithrombotic Therapy Timing	39	100%	98%	98%
Assessed for Rehabilitation	37	95%	97%	97%
Discharged on Antithrombotic Therapy	33	100%	99%	99%
Discharged on Statin Medication	29	97%	96%	94%
Thrombolytic Therapy Timing[1]	-	-	76%	66%
Venous Thromboembolism Prophylaxis	43	98%	95%	94%
Written Stroke Educational Materials Given	21	100%	94%	88%
Surgical Care Improvement Project				
Appropriate Beta Blocker Usage[2]	97	100%	99%	98%
Appropriate VTP Within 24 Hours[2]	303	100%	99%	98%
Controlled Postoperative Blood Glucose[2,7]	-	-	98%	97%
Perioperative Temperature Management[2]	349	100%	100%	100%
Prophylactic Antibiotic Selection[2]	263	99%	99%	99%
Prophylactic Antibiotic Selection (Outpatient)	399	99%	98%	98%
Prophylactic Antibiotic Stopped[2]	252	100%	98%	98%
Prophylactic Antibiotic Timing[2]	263	100%	99%	99%
Prophylactic Antibiotic Timing (Outpatient)	401	99%	98%	98%
Urinary Catheter Removal[2]	203	100%	98%	97%
Survey of Patients' Hospital Experiences				
Area Around Room 'Always' Quiet at Night	300+	60%	58%	61%
Doctors 'Always' Communicated Well	300+	84%	77%	82%
Home Recovery Information Given	300+	77%	83%	85%
Hospital Given 9 or 10 on 10 Point Scale	300+	61%	67%	71%
Meds 'Always' Explained Before Given	300+	64%	60%	64%
Nurses 'Always' Communicated Well	300+	75%	75%	79%
Pain 'Always' Well Controlled	300+	68%	68%	71%
Room and Bathroom 'Always' Clean	300+	74%	69%	73%
Timely Help 'Always' Received	300+	62%	62%	68%
Would Definitely Recommend Hospital	300+	65%	69%	71%
Use of Medical Imaging				
Cardiac Imaging Stress Test before Surgery[1]	-	-	6.4%	5.3%
Combination Abdominal CT Scan	312	3.8%	11.8%	10.5%
Combination Brain/Sinus CT Scan	295	7.5%	3.4%	2.7%
Combination Chest CT Scan[1]	-	-	2.4%	2.7%
Follow-up Mammogram/Ultrasound	117	5.1%	10.2%	8.8%
Lumbar Spine MRI for Low Back Pain[1]	-	-	35.2%	37.2%

Doctors Hospital

5000 University Dr
Coral Gables, FL 33146
Phone: 305-666-2111
Fax: 786-308-3201
URL: www.baptisthealth.net
Type: Acute Care Hospitals
Emergency Services: Yes
Ownership: Voluntary non-profit - Other
Beds: 281

Key Personnel:
CEO/President. . . . . Brian E Keeley
Chief of Medical Staff . . . . Richard Whittington, MD

Measure	Cases	This Hosp.	State Avg.	U.S. Avg.
Blood Clot Prevention and Treatment				
Anticoagulation Overlap Therapy[2]	27	93%	93%	93%
ICU Venous Thromboembolism Prophylaxis[2]	46	100%	94%	92%
Incidence of Potentially Preventable VTE[1,2]	-	-	10%	10%
UFH with Dosages/Platelet Monitoring[2]	37	100%	100%	97%
Venous Thromboembolism Prophylaxis[2]	351	100%	88%	85%
Warfarin Therapy Discharge Instructions[2]	22	100%	85%	75%
Chest Pain/Possible Heart Attack Care				
Aspirin Given Within 24 Hours of Arrival	22	100%	98%	96%
Fibrinolytic Meds Within 30 Min. of Arrival[7]	-	-	81%	58%

NOTE: Hospital profiles are in alphabetical order by state, then city, then hospital within the city; Rankings exclude hospitals with less than 25 cases except for patient surveys which excludes hospitals with less than 100 cases; (a) 100-299 cases; (1) The number of cases/patients is too few to report; (2) Data submitted were based on a sample of cases/patients; (3) Results are based on a shorter time period than required; (4) Data suppressed by CMS for one or more quarters; (5) Results are not available for this reporting period; (6) Fewer than 100 patients completed the HCAHPS survey; (7) No cases met the criteria for this measure; (8) The lower limit of the confidence interval cannot be calculated if the number of observed infections equals zero; (9) No data are available from the state/territory for this reporting period; (10) The scores shown reflect fewer than 50 completed surveys; (11) There were discrepancies in the data collection process; (12) This measure does not apply to this hospital for this reporting period; (13) Results cannot be calculated for this reporting period; (14) The results for this state are combined with nearby states to protect confidentiality; Please refer to the User's Guide for a full explanation of data.

Measure	Cases	This Hosp.	State Avg.	U.S. Avg.
Average Time to ECG (minutes)	24	2	7	7
Average Time to Transfer (minutes)[1]	-	-	53	60
Children's Asthma Care				
Received Home Management Plan of Care	-	-	-	88%
Received Reliever Medication	-	-	-	100%
Received Systemic Corticosteroids	-	-	-	100%
Emergency Department				
Admittance Decision Time (minutes)[2]	678	224	111	98
Head CT Results Within 45 Min. of Arrival[1]	-	-	64%	57%
Patients Who Left ER Before Being Seen	18,500	1%	2%	2%
Time from ER Arrival to Admit. (minutes)[2]	814	343	289	274
Time from ER Arrival to Discharge (minutes)	360	209	147	134
Time in ER Before Being Evaluated (minutes)	394	15	26	26
Time to Pain Meds for Fractures (minutes)	44	64	60	57
Heart Attack Care				
Aspirin Given at Discharge[1]	-	-	99%	99%
Fibrinolytic Meds Within 30 Min. of Arrival[7]	-	-	50%	54%
PCI Within 90 Minutes of Arrival[7]	-	-	96%	96%
Statin Prescribed at Discharge[1]	-	-	99%	98%
Heart Failure Care				
ACE Inhibitor or ARB for LVSD	36	100%	98%	97%
Discharge Instructions Given	154	99%	96%	94%
Evaluation of LVS Function	179	100%	100%	99%
Medicare Spending				
Medicare Spending per Patient (ratio)	-	1.05	1.04	0.98
Pneumonia Care				
Appropriate Initial Antibiotic Given	70	99%	98%	95%
Blood Culture Timing	148	100%	99%	98%
Pregnancy and Delivery Care				
Newborn Deliveries Scheduled Early[7]	-	-	6%	6%
Preventive Care				
Immunization for Influenza[2]	596	97%	94%	90%
Immunization for Pneumonia[2]	863	97%	96%	92%
Stroke Care				
Anticoagulation Therapy for Atrial Fibrillation[1]	-	-	97%	95%
Antithrombotic Therapy Timing	37	100%	98%	98%
Assessed for Rehabilitation	45	100%	97%	97%
Discharged on Antithrombotic Therapy	37	100%	99%	99%
Discharged on Statin Medication	28	100%	96%	94%
Thrombolytic Therapy Timing[7]	-	-	76%	66%
Venous Thromboembolism Prophylaxis	46	100%	95%	94%
Written Stroke Educational Materials Given	32	97%	94%	88%
Surgical Care Improvement Project				
Appropriate Beta Blocker Usage	154	100%	99%	98%
Appropriate VTP Within 24 Hours	515	100%	99%	98%
Controlled Postoperative Blood Glucose[7]	-	-	98%	97%
Perioperative Temperature Management	594	100%	100%	100%
Prophylactic Antibiotic Selection	358	100%	99%	99%
Prophylactic Antibiotic Selection (Outpatient)	359	99%	98%	98%
Prophylactic Antibiotic Stopped	340	99%	98%	98%
Prophylactic Antibiotic Timing	358	100%	99%	99%
Prophylactic Antibiotic Timing (Outpatient)	360	99%	98%	98%
Urinary Catheter Removal	263	100%	98%	97%
Survey of Patients' Hospital Experiences				
Area Around Room 'Always' Quiet at Night	300+	63%	58%	61%
Doctors 'Always' Communicated Well	300+	87%	77%	82%
Home Recovery Information Given	300+	86%	83%	85%
Hospital Given 9 or 10 on 10 Point Scale	300+	78%	67%	71%
Meds 'Always' Explained Before Given	300+	66%	60%	64%
Nurses 'Always' Communicated Well	300+	82%	75%	79%
Pain 'Always' Well Controlled	300+	76%	68%	71%
Room and Bathroom 'Always' Clean	300+	76%	69%	73%
Timely Help 'Always' Received	300+	69%	62%	68%
Would Definitely Recommend Hospital	300+	83%	69%	71%
Use of Medical Imaging				
Cardiac Imaging Stress Test before Surgery[1]	-	-	6.4%	5.3%
Combination Abdominal CT Scan	322	2.5%	11.8%	10.5%
Combination Brain/Sinus CT Scan[1]	-	-	3.4%	2.7%
Combination Chest CT Scan	148	0.0%	2.4%	2.7%
Follow-up Mammogram/Ultrasound[7]	-	-	10.2%	8.8%
Lumbar Spine MRI for Low Back Pain[1]	-	-	35.2%	37.2%

Broward Health Coral Springs

3000 Coral Hills Dr
Coral Springs, FL 33065
URL: www.coralspringsmedicalcenter.org
Type: Acute Care Hospitals
Ownership: Govt - Hospital Dist/Auth
Phone: 954-344-3000
Fax: 954-344-3146
Emergency Services: Yes
Beds: 200

Key Personnel:
Infection Control. . . . . Ava Dobin
Operating Room. . . . . Sue Florentini
Chief of Medical Staff. . . . . Thomas Goldschmidt
CEO/President. . . . . Deborah Mulvihill, RN, MSN
Quality Assurance . . . . Barry Rosen
Emergency Room . . . . Rachelle Zahniser

Measure	Cases	This Hosp.	State Avg.	U.S. Avg.
Blood Clot Prevention and Treatment				
Anticoagulation Overlap Therapy[2]	66	100%	93%	93%
ICU Venous Thromboembolism Prophylaxis[2]	55	89%	94%	92%
Incidence of Potentially Preventable VTE[1,2]	-	-	10%	10%
UFH with Dosages/Platelet Monitoring[1,2]	-	-	100%	97%
Venous Thromboembolism Prophylaxis[2]	347	95%	88%	85%
Warfarin Therapy Discharge Instructions[2]	47	100%	85%	75%
Chest Pain/Possible Heart Attack Care				
Aspirin Given Within 24 Hours of Arrival	109	97%	98%	96%
Fibrinolytic Meds Within 30 Min. of Arrival[7]	-	-	81%	58%
Average Time to ECG (minutes)	113	8	7	7
Average Time to Transfer (minutes)	15	49	53	60
Children's Asthma Care				
Received Home Management Plan of Care	-	-	-	88%
Received Reliever Medication	-	-	-	100%
Received Systemic Corticosteroids	-	-	-	100%
Emergency Department				
Admittance Decision Time (minutes)[2]	584	204	111	98
Head CT Results Within 45 Min. of Arrival[1]	-	-	64%	57%
Patients Who Left ER Before Being Seen	56,693	4%	2%	2%
Time from ER Arrival to Admit. (minutes)[2]	584	415	289	274
Time from ER Arrival to Discharge (minutes)	370	183	147	134
Time in ER Before Being Evaluated (minutes)	433	22	26	26
Time to Pain Meds for Fractures (minutes)	186	62	60	57
Heart Attack Care				
Aspirin Given at Discharge	13	100%	99%	99%
Fibrinolytic Meds Within 30 Min. of Arrival[7]	-	-	50%	54%
PCI Within 90 Minutes of Arrival[7]	-	-	96%	96%
Statin Prescribed at Discharge[1]	-	-	99%	98%
Heart Failure Care				
ACE Inhibitor or ARB for LVSD	60	100%	98%	97%
Discharge Instructions Given	138	93%	96%	94%
Evaluation of LVS Function	166	100%	100%	99%
Medicare Spending				
Medicare Spending per Patient (ratio)	-	1.08	1.04	0.98
Pneumonia Care				
Appropriate Initial Antibiotic Given[2]	144	99%	98%	95%
Blood Culture Timing[2]	141	99%	99%	98%
Pregnancy and Delivery Care				
Newborn Deliveries Scheduled Early[2]	47	0%	6%	6%
Preventive Care				
Immunization for Influenza[2]	538	97%	94%	90%
Immunization for Pneumonia[2]	478	97%	96%	92%
Stroke Care				
Anticoagulation Therapy for Atrial Fibrillation[1]	-	-	97%	95%
Antithrombotic Therapy Timing	49	100%	98%	98%
Assessed for Rehabilitation	57	100%	97%	97%
Discharged on Antithrombotic Therapy	55	100%	99%	99%
Discharged on Statin Medication	45	100%	96%	94%
Thrombolytic Therapy Timing[1]	-	-	76%	66%
Venous Thromboembolism Prophylaxis	59	92%	95%	94%
Written Stroke Educational Materials Given	44	100%	94%	88%
Surgical Care Improvement Project				
Appropriate Beta Blocker Usage[2]	125	100%	99%	98%
Appropriate VTP Within 24 Hours[2]	443	100%	99%	98%
Controlled Postoperative Blood Glucose[2,7]	-	-	98%	97%
Perioperative Temperature Management[2]	468	100%	100%	100%
Prophylactic Antibiotic Selection[2]	289	100%	99%	99%
Prophylactic Antibiotic Selection (Outpatient)	132	99%	98%	98%
Prophylactic Antibiotic Stopped[2]	278	99%	98%	98%
Prophylactic Antibiotic Timing[2]	292	100%	99%	99%
Prophylactic Antibiotic Timing (Outpatient)	132	100%	98%	98%
Urinary Catheter Removal[2]	272	100%	98%	97%
Survey of Patients' Hospital Experiences				
Area Around Room 'Always' Quiet at Night	300+	54%	58%	61%
Doctors 'Always' Communicated Well	300+	73%	77%	82%
Home Recovery Information Given	300+	79%	83%	85%
Hospital Given 9 or 10 on 10 Point Scale	300+	59%	67%	71%
Meds 'Always' Explained Before Given	300+	61%	60%	64%
Nurses 'Always' Communicated Well	300+	71%	75%	79%
Pain 'Always' Well Controlled	300+	69%	68%	71%
Room and Bathroom 'Always' Clean	300+	66%	69%	73%
Timely Help 'Always' Received	300+	52%	62%	68%
Would Definitely Recommend Hospital	300+	61%	69%	71%
Use of Medical Imaging				
Cardiac Imaging Stress Test before Surgery[1]	-	-	6.4%	5.3%
Combination Abdominal CT Scan	536	6.0%	11.8%	10.5%
Combination Brain/Sinus CT Scan	430	4.2%	3.4%	2.7%
Combination Chest CT Scan	200	2.0%	2.4%	2.7%
Follow-up Mammogram/Ultrasound	605	11.6%	10.2%	8.8%
Lumbar Spine MRI for Low Back Pain[1]	-	-	35.2%	37.2%

North Okaloosa Medical Center

151 Redstone Ave Se
Crestview, FL 32539
URL: www.northokaloosa.com
Type: Acute Care Hospitals
Ownership: Voluntary non-profit - Private
Phone: 850-689-8100
Fax: 850-689-8484
Emergency Services: Yes
Beds: 110

Key Personnel:
CEO/President. . . . . Brad Goodson
Emergency Room . . . . Russall Lewis
Cardiac Laboratory. . . . . Perry Thomas

Measure	Cases	This Hosp.	State Avg.	U.S. Avg.
Blood Clot Prevention and Treatment				
Anticoagulation Overlap Therapy[2]	13	92%	93%	93%
ICU Venous Thromboembolism Prophylaxis[2]	101	97%	94%	92%
Incidence of Potentially Preventable VTE[1,2]	-	-	10%	10%
UFH with Dosages/Platelet Monitoring[1,2]	-	-	100%	97%
Venous Thromboembolism Prophylaxis[2]	426	99%	88%	85%
Warfarin Therapy Discharge Instructions[1,2]	-	-	85%	75%
Chest Pain/Possible Heart Attack Care				
Aspirin Given Within 24 Hours of Arrival[1]	-	-	98%	96%
Fibrinolytic Meds Within 30 Min. of Arrival[3,7]	-	-	81%	58%
Average Time to ECG (minutes)[1]	-	-	7	7
Average Time to Transfer (minutes)[1,3]	-	-	53	60
Children's Asthma Care				
Received Home Management Plan of Care	-	-	-	88%
Received Reliever Medication	-	-	-	100%
Received Systemic Corticosteroids	-	-	-	100%
Emergency Department				
Admittance Decision Time (minutes)[2]	901	114	111	98
Head CT Results Within 45 Min. of Arrival	14	93%	64%	57%
Patients Who Left ER Before Being Seen	31,085	1%	2%	2%
Time from ER Arrival to Admit. (minutes)[2]	902	241	289	274
Time from ER Arrival to Discharge (minutes)	393	129	147	134
Time in ER Before Being Evaluated (minutes)	416	24	26	26
Time to Pain Meds for Fractures (minutes)	130	68	60	57
Heart Attack Care				
Aspirin Given at Discharge	80	100%	99%	99%
Fibrinolytic Meds Within 30 Min. of Arrival[7]	-	-	50%	54%
PCI Within 90 Minutes of Arrival	27	100%	96%	96%
Statin Prescribed at Discharge	72	100%	99%	98%
Heart Failure Care				
ACE Inhibitor or ARB for LVSD	73	100%	98%	97%
Discharge Instructions Given	204	100%	96%	94%
Evaluation of LVS Function	240	100%	100%	99%
Medicare Spending				
Medicare Spending per Patient (ratio)	-	0.99	1.04	0.98
Pneumonia Care				
Appropriate Initial Antibiotic Given	74	99%	98%	95%
Blood Culture Timing[1]	-	-	99%	98%
Pregnancy and Delivery Care				
Newborn Deliveries Scheduled Early[2]	24	0%	6%	6%

NOTE: Hospital profiles are in alphabetical order by state, then city, then hospital within the city; Rankings exclude hospitals with less than 25 cases except for patient surveys which excludes hospitals with less than 100 cases; (a) 100-299 cases; (1) The number of cases/patients is too few to report; (2) Data submitted were based on a sample of cases/patients; (3) Results are based on a shorter time period than required; (4) Data suppressed by CMS for one or more quarters; (5) Results are not available for this reporting period; (6) Fewer than 100 patients completed the HCAHPS survey; (7) No cases met the criteria for this measure; (8) The lower limit of the confidence interval cannot be calculated if the number of observed infections equals zero; (9) No data are available from the state/territory for this reporting period; (10) The scores shown reflect fewer than 50 completed surveys; (11) There were discrepancies in the data collection process; (12) This measure does not apply to this hospital for this reporting period; (13) Results cannot be calculated for this reporting period; (14) The results for this state are combined with nearby states to protect confidentiality; Please refer to the User's Guide for a full explanation of data.

Preventive Care				
Immunization for Influenza[2]	612	100%	94%	90%
Immunization for Pneumonia[2]	848	99%	96%	92%
Stroke Care				
Anticoagulation Therapy for Atrial Fibrillation[1]	-	-	97%	95%
Antithrombotic Therapy Timing	37	100%	98%	98%
Assessed for Rehabilitation	38	100%	97%	97%
Discharged on Antithrombotic Therapy	37	97%	99%	99%
Discharged on Statin Medication	31	87%	96%	94%
Thrombolytic Therapy Timing[7]	-	-	76%	66%
Venous Thromboembolism Prophylaxis	38	97%	95%	94%
Written Stroke Educational Materials Given	28	96%	94%	88%
Surgical Care Improvement Project				
Appropriate Beta Blocker Usage	54	100%	99%	98%
Appropriate VTP Within 24 Hours	159	98%	99%	98%
Controlled Postoperative Blood Glucose[7]	-	-	98%	97%
Perioperative Temperature Management	216	100%	100%	100%
Prophylactic Antibiotic Selection	149	100%	99%	99%
Prophylactic Antibiotic Selection (Outpatient)	114	99%	98%	98%
Prophylactic Antibiotic Stopped	136	97%	98%	98%
Prophylactic Antibiotic Timing	150	99%	99%	99%
Prophylactic Antibiotic Timing (Outpatient)	115	98%	98%	98%
Urinary Catheter Removal	60	92%	98%	97%
Survey of Patients' Hospital Experiences				
Area Around Room 'Always' Quiet at Night	300+	61%	58%	61%
Doctors 'Always' Communicated Well	300+	79%	77%	82%
Home Recovery Information Given	300+	83%	83%	85%
Hospital Given 9 or 10 on 10 Point Scale	300+	66%	67%	71%
Meds 'Always' Explained Before Given	300+	61%	60%	64%
Nurses 'Always' Communicated Well	300+	78%	75%	79%
Pain 'Always' Well Controlled	300+	69%	68%	71%
Room and Bathroom 'Always' Clean	300+	68%	69%	73%
Timely Help 'Always' Received	300+	67%	62%	68%
Would Definitely Recommend Hospital	300+	65%	69%	71%
Use of Medical Imaging				
Cardiac Imaging Stress Test before Surgery	110	3.6%	6.4%	5.3%
Combination Abdominal CT Scan	632	17.6%	11.8%	10.5%
Combination Brain/Sinus CT Scan[1]	-	-	3.4%	2.7%
Combination Chest CT Scan	270	0.0%	2.4%	2.7%
Follow-up Mammogram/Ultrasound	1,242	8.1%	10.2%	8.8%
Lumbar Spine MRI for Low Back Pain	52	32.7%	35.2%	37.2%

Seven Rivers Regional Medical Center

6201 N Suncoast Blvd
Crystal River, FL 34428
E-mail: info@srrmc.hma-corp.com
URL: www.srrmc.com
Type: Acute Care Hospitals
Ownership: Proprietary
Phone: 352-795-6560
Fax: 352-795-8369
Emergency Services: Yes
Beds: 128

Key Personnel:
Coronary Care . . . . Deanna Beverly, RN
Intensive Care Unit. . . . . Deanna Beverly, RN
CEO/President. . . . . Joyce Brancato
Operating Room. . . . . Anne Gilley
Quality Assurance . . . . Ann Grant
Emergency Room . . . . Mary Martin
Chief of Medical Staff. . . . . Grigor Varlakov
Infection Control. . . . . Teresa Wright, RN

Measure	Cases	This Hosp.	State Avg.	U.S. Avg.
Blood Clot Prevention and Treatment				
Anticoagulation Overlap Therapy[2]	32	78%	93%	93%
ICU Venous Thromboembolism Prophylaxis[2]	74	86%	94%	92%
Incidence of Potentially Preventable VTE[1,2]	-	-	10%	10%
UFH with Dosages/Platelet Monitoring[2]	18	100%	100%	97%
Venous Thromboembolism Prophylaxis[2]	318	51%	88%	85%
Warfarin Therapy Discharge Instructions[2]	23	65%	85%	75%
Chest Pain/Possible Heart Attack Care				
Aspirin Given Within 24 Hours of Arrival	29	100%	98%	96%
Fibrinolytic Meds Within 30 Min. of Arrival[7]	-	-	81%	58%
Average Time to ECG (minutes)	29	7	7	7
Average Time to Transfer (minutes)[1]	-	-	53	60
Children's Asthma Care				
Received Home Management Plan of Care	-	-	-	88%
Received Reliever Medication	-	-	-	100%
Received Systemic Corticosteroids	-	-	-	100%
Emergency Department				
Admittance Decision Time (minutes)[2]	796	104	111	98
Head CT Results Within 45 Min. of Arrival	12	67%	64%	57%
Patients Who Left ER Before Being Seen	22,310	1%	2%	2%
Time from ER Arrival to Admit. (minutes)[2]	797	296	289	274
Time from ER Arrival to Discharge (minutes)	446	130	147	134
Time in ER Before Being Evaluated (minutes)	469	21	26	26
Time to Pain Meds for Fractures (minutes)	56	72	60	57
Heart Attack Care				
Aspirin Given at Discharge	73	100%	99%	99%
Fibrinolytic Meds Within 30 Min. of Arrival[7]	-	-	50%	54%
PCI Within 90 Minutes of Arrival[1]	-	-	96%	96%
Statin Prescribed at Discharge	68	99%	99%	98%
Heart Failure Care				
ACE Inhibitor or ARB for LVSD	78	100%	98%	97%
Discharge Instructions Given	116	100%	96%	94%
Evaluation of LVS Function	150	100%	100%	99%
Medicare Spending				
Medicare Spending per Patient (ratio)	-	1.03	1.04	0.98
Pneumonia Care				
Appropriate Initial Antibiotic Given	61	93%	98%	95%
Blood Culture Timing	94	90%	99%	98%
Pregnancy and Delivery Care				
Newborn Deliveries Scheduled Early	16	0%	6%	6%
Preventive Care				
Immunization for Influenza[2]	598	96%	94%	90%
Immunization for Pneumonia[2]	875	96%	96%	92%
Stroke Care				
Anticoagulation Therapy for Atrial Fibrillation[1]	-	-	97%	95%
Antithrombotic Therapy Timing	58	100%	98%	98%
Assessed for Rehabilitation	50	90%	97%	97%
Discharged on Antithrombotic Therapy	48	100%	99%	99%
Discharged on Statin Medication	40	85%	96%	94%
Thrombolytic Therapy Timing[1]	-	-	76%	66%
Venous Thromboembolism Prophylaxis	65	66%	95%	94%
Written Stroke Educational Materials Given	33	61%	94%	88%
Surgical Care Improvement Project				
Appropriate Beta Blocker Usage	246	95%	99%	98%
Appropriate VTP Within 24 Hours	675	96%	99%	98%
Controlled Postoperative Blood Glucose[7]	-	-	98%	97%
Perioperative Temperature Management	795	100%	100%	100%
Prophylactic Antibiotic Selection	613	99%	99%	99%
Prophylactic Antibiotic Selection (Outpatient)	103	93%	98%	98%
Prophylactic Antibiotic Stopped	610	99%	98%	98%
Prophylactic Antibiotic Timing	615	96%	99%	99%
Prophylactic Antibiotic Timing (Outpatient)	102	97%	98%	98%
Urinary Catheter Removal	668	96%	98%	97%
Survey of Patients' Hospital Experiences				
Area Around Room 'Always' Quiet at Night	300+	43%	58%	61%
Doctors 'Always' Communicated Well	300+	72%	77%	82%
Home Recovery Information Given	300+	80%	83%	85%
Hospital Given 9 or 10 on 10 Point Scale	300+	56%	67%	71%
Meds 'Always' Explained Before Given	300+	54%	60%	64%
Nurses 'Always' Communicated Well	300+	71%	75%	79%
Pain 'Always' Well Controlled	300+	61%	68%	71%
Room and Bathroom 'Always' Clean	300+	59%	69%	73%
Timely Help 'Always' Received	300+	57%	62%	68%
Would Definitely Recommend Hospital	300+	61%	69%	71%
Use of Medical Imaging				
Cardiac Imaging Stress Test before Surgery	135	8.9%	6.4%	5.3%
Combination Abdominal CT Scan	413	9.7%	11.8%	10.5%
Combination Brain/Sinus CT Scan	572	4.7%	3.4%	2.7%
Combination Chest CT Scan	106	8.5%	2.4%	2.7%
Follow-up Mammogram/Ultrasound	930	2.7%	10.2%	8.8%
Lumbar Spine MRI for Low Back Pain[1]	-	-	35.2%	37.2%

Bayfront Health Dade City

13100 Ft King Road
Dade City, FL 33525
URL: www.pascoregionalmc.com
Type: Acute Care Hospitals
Ownership: Proprietary
Phone: 352-568-3174
Fax: 352-521-1196
Emergency Services: Yes
Beds: 120

Key Personnel:
Emergency Room . . . . Thomas Carpenter
Infection Control. . . . . Rita Clark
Radiology. . . . . Pedro J Duarte
CEO/President. . . . . Stan Holm
Chief of Medical Staff. . . . . Elizabeth John, MD
Operating Room. . . . . Pandurangan Krishnar
Intensive Care Unit. . . . . Tina Nelson
Quality Assurance . . . . Carolyn Newton

Measure	Cases	This Hosp.	State Avg.	U.S. Avg.
Blood Clot Prevention and Treatment				
Anticoagulation Overlap Therapy[2]	15	53%	93%	93%
ICU Venous Thromboembolism Prophylaxis[2]	100	85%	94%	92%
Incidence of Potentially Preventable VTE[1,2]	-	-	10%	10%
UFH with Dosages/Platelet Monitoring[1,2]	-	-	100%	97%
Venous Thromboembolism Prophylaxis[2]	186	63%	88%	85%
Warfarin Therapy Discharge Instructions[1,2]	-	-	85%	75%
Chest Pain/Possible Heart Attack Care				
Aspirin Given Within 24 Hours of Arrival[3]	27	100%	98%	96%
Fibrinolytic Meds Within 30 Min. of Arrival[5]	-	-	81%	58%
Average Time to ECG (minutes)[3]	27	0	7	7
Average Time to Transfer (minutes)[5]	-	-	53	60
Children's Asthma Care				
Received Home Management Plan of Care	-	-	-	88%
Received Reliever Medication	-	-	-	100%
Received Systemic Corticosteroids	-	-	-	100%
Emergency Department				
Admittance Decision Time (minutes)[2]	436	106	111	98
Head CT Results Within 45 Min. of Arrival[1]	-	-	64%	57%
Patients Who Left ER Before Being Seen	23,362	1%	2%	2%
Time from ER Arrival to Admit. (minutes)[2]	436	223	289	274
Time from ER Arrival to Discharge (minutes)	971	108	147	134
Time in ER Before Being Evaluated (minutes)	1,056	4	26	26
Time to Pain Meds for Fractures (minutes)	78	44	60	57
Heart Attack Care				
Aspirin Given at Discharge	69	99%	99%	99%
Fibrinolytic Meds Within 30 Min. of Arrival[7]	-	-	50%	54%
PCI Within 90 Minutes of Arrival	12	100%	96%	96%
Statin Prescribed at Discharge	65	97%	99%	98%
Heart Failure Care				
ACE Inhibitor or ARB for LVSD	28	100%	98%	97%
Discharge Instructions Given	85	98%	96%	94%
Evaluation of LVS Function	98	100%	100%	99%
Medicare Spending				
Medicare Spending per Patient (ratio)	-	1.05	1.04	0.98
Pneumonia Care				
Appropriate Initial Antibiotic Given	40	95%	98%	95%
Blood Culture Timing	58	97%	99%	98%
Pregnancy and Delivery Care				
Newborn Deliveries Scheduled Early	19	11%	6%	6%
Preventive Care				
Immunization for Influenza[2]	325	91%	94%	90%
Immunization for Pneumonia[2]	418	90%	96%	92%
Stroke Care				
Anticoagulation Therapy for Atrial Fibrillation[7]	-	-	97%	95%
Antithrombotic Therapy Timing	39	97%	98%	98%
Assessed for Rehabilitation	37	89%	97%	97%
Discharged on Antithrombotic Therapy	37	100%	99%	99%
Discharged on Statin Medication	35	97%	96%	94%
Thrombolytic Therapy Timing[1]	-	-	76%	66%
Venous Thromboembolism Prophylaxis	37	78%	95%	94%
Written Stroke Educational Materials Given	25	92%	94%	88%
Surgical Care Improvement Project				
Appropriate Beta Blocker Usage	54	96%	99%	98%
Appropriate VTP Within 24 Hours	143	99%	99%	98%
Controlled Postoperative Blood Glucose[7]	-	-	98%	97%
Perioperative Temperature Management	187	100%	100%	100%
Prophylactic Antibiotic Selection	89	94%	99%	99%

NOTE: Hospital profiles are in alphabetical order by state, then city, then hospital within the city; Rankings exclude hospitals with less than 25 cases except for patient surveys which excludes hospitals with less than 100 cases; (a) 100-299 cases; (1) The number of cases/patients is too few to report; (2) Data submitted were based on a sample of cases/patients; (3) Results are based on a shorter time period than required; (4) Data suppressed by CMS for one or more quarters; (5) Results are not available for this reporting period; (6) Fewer than 100 patients completed the HCAHPS survey; (7) No cases met the criteria for this measure; (8) The lower limit of the confidence interval cannot be calculated if the number of observed infections equals zero; (9) No data are available from the state/territory for this reporting period; (10) The scores shown reflect fewer than 50 completed surveys; (11) There were discrepancies in the data collection process; (12) This measure does not apply to this hospital for this reporting period; (13) Results cannot be calculated for this reporting period; (14) The results for this state are combined with nearby states to protect confidentiality; Please refer to the User's Guide for a full explanation of data.

Prophylactic Antibiotic Selection (Outpatient)	141	95%	98%	98%
Prophylactic Antibiotic Stopped	74	97%	98%	98%
Prophylactic Antibiotic Timing	89	98%	99%	99%
Prophylactic Antibiotic Timing (Outpatient)	142	99%	98%	98%
Urinary Catheter Removal	112	100%	98%	97%
Survey of Patients' Hospital Experiences				
Area Around Room 'Always' Quiet at Night	300+	46%	58%	61%
Doctors 'Always' Communicated Well	300+	73%	77%	82%
Home Recovery Information Given	300+	77%	83%	85%
Hospital Given 9 or 10 on 10 Point Scale	300+	52%	67%	71%
Meds 'Always' Explained Before Given	300+	50%	60%	64%
Nurses 'Always' Communicated Well	300+	63%	75%	79%
Pain 'Always' Well Controlled	300+	58%	68%	71%
Room and Bathroom 'Always' Clean	300+	65%	69%	73%
Timely Help 'Always' Received	300+	54%	62%	68%
Would Definitely Recommend Hospital	300+	56%	69%	71%
Use of Medical Imaging				
Cardiac Imaging Stress Test before Surgery[1]	-	-	6.4%	5.3%
Combination Abdominal CT Scan	138	13.0%	11.8%	10.5%
Combination Brain/Sinus CT Scan[1]	-	-	3.4%	2.7%
Combination Chest CT Scan[1]	-	-	2.4%	2.7%
Follow-up Mammogram/Ultrasound	82	18.3%	10.2%	8.8%
Lumbar Spine MRI for Low Back Pain[1]	-	-	35.2%	37.2%

Heart of Florida Regional Medical Center

40100 Us Hwy 27 N Phone: 863-422-4971
Davenport, FL 33837 Fax: 863-419-2465
E-mail: hofrmc@gte.net
URL: www.heartofflorida.com
Type: Acute Care Hospitals Emergency Services: Yes
Ownership: Proprietary Beds: 142

Key Personnel:
Radiology.................. Adel Abdulla
CEO .... Ann Barnhart
Operating Room.............. John Bateman, RN
Infection Control.............. Nancy Draves
Quality Assurance .... Ken Emmitt
Chief of Medical Staff.......... Devendra Kahlon, MD
Intensive Care Unit............ Lee Mead
Pediatric In-Patient Care .... Beth Schneider

Measure	Cases	This Hosp.	State Avg.	U.S. Avg.
Blood Clot Prevention and Treatment				
Anticoagulation Overlap Therapy[2]	63	90%	93%	93%
ICU Venous Thromboembolism Prophylaxis[2]	47	68%	94%	92%
Incidence of Potentially Preventable VTE[2]	16	62%	10%	10%
UFH with Dosages/Platelet Monitoring[2]	28	100%	100%	97%
Venous Thromboembolism Prophylaxis[2]	312	46%	88%	85%
Warfarin Therapy Discharge Instructions[2]	43	53%	85%	75%
Chest Pain/Possible Heart Attack Care				
Aspirin Given Within 24 Hours of Arrival[1]	-	-	98%	96%
Fibrinolytic Meds Within 30 Min. of Arrival[5]	-	-	81%	58%
Average Time to ECG (minutes)[1]	-	-	7	7
Average Time to Transfer (minutes)[5]	-	-	53	60
Children's Asthma Care				
Received Home Management Plan of Care	-	-	-	88%
Received Reliever Medication	-	-	-	100%
Received Systemic Corticosteroids	-	-	-	100%
Emergency Department				
Admittance Decision Time (minutes)[2]	806	150	111	98
Head CT Results Within 45 Min. of Arrival[1]	-	-	64%	57%
Patients Who Left ER Before Being Seen	50,878	1%	2%	2%
Time from ER Arrival to Admit. (minutes)[2]	808	356	289	274
Time from ER Arrival to Discharge (minutes)	723	95	147	134
Time in ER Before Being Evaluated (minutes)	767	17	26	26
Time to Pain Meds for Fractures (minutes)	74	37	60	57
Heart Attack Care				
Aspirin Given at Discharge	128	92%	99%	99%
Fibrinolytic Meds Within 30 Min. of Arrival[7]	-	-	50%	54%
PCI Within 90 Minutes of Arrival	32	97%	96%	96%
Statin Prescribed at Discharge	124	94%	99%	98%
Heart Failure Care				
ACE Inhibitor or ARB for LVSD	130	97%	98%	97%
Discharge Instructions Given	294	94%	96%	94%
Evaluation of LVS Function	340	99%	100%	99%
Medicare Spending				
Medicare Spending per Patient (ratio)	-	1.04	1.04	0.98
Pneumonia Care				
Appropriate Initial Antibiotic Given	92	92%	98%	95%
Blood Culture Timing	170	99%	99%	98%
Pregnancy and Delivery Care				
Newborn Deliveries Scheduled Early	101	29%	6%	6%
Preventive Care				
Immunization for Influenza[2]	563	92%	94%	90%
Immunization for Pneumonia[2]	725	98%	96%	92%
Stroke Care				
Anticoagulation Therapy for Atrial Fibrillation[1,2]	-	-	97%	95%
Antithrombotic Therapy Timing[2]	79	85%	98%	98%
Assessed for Rehabilitation[2]	87	83%	97%	97%
Discharged on Antithrombotic Therapy[2]	83	94%	99%	99%
Discharged on Statin Medication[2]	69	81%	96%	94%
Thrombolytic Therapy Timing[1,2]	-	-	76%	66%
Venous Thromboembolism Prophylaxis[2]	90	33%	95%	94%
Written Stroke Educational Materials Given[2]	56	48%	94%	88%
Surgical Care Improvement Project				
Appropriate Beta Blocker Usage	238	96%	99%	98%
Appropriate VTP Within 24 Hours	803	95%	99%	98%
Controlled Postoperative Blood Glucose[7]	-	-	98%	97%
Perioperative Temperature Management	852	100%	100%	100%
Prophylactic Antibiotic Selection	618	96%	99%	99%
Prophylactic Antibiotic Selection (Outpatient)	245	95%	98%	98%
Prophylactic Antibiotic Stopped	573	92%	98%	98%
Prophylactic Antibiotic Timing	620	98%	99%	99%
Prophylactic Antibiotic Timing (Outpatient)	244	97%	98%	98%
Urinary Catheter Removal	236	89%	98%	97%
Survey of Patients' Hospital Experiences				
Area Around Room 'Always' Quiet at Night	300+	49%	58%	61%
Doctors 'Always' Communicated Well	300+	69%	77%	82%
Home Recovery Information Given	300+	78%	83%	85%
Hospital Given 9 or 10 on 10 Point Scale	300+	50%	67%	71%
Meds 'Always' Explained Before Given	300+	50%	60%	64%
Nurses 'Always' Communicated Well	300+	62%	75%	79%
Pain 'Always' Well Controlled	300+	57%	68%	71%
Room and Bathroom 'Always' Clean	300+	64%	69%	73%
Timely Help 'Always' Received	300+	50%	62%	68%
Would Definitely Recommend Hospital	300+	50%	69%	71%
Use of Medical Imaging				
Cardiac Imaging Stress Test before Surgery	90	3.3%	6.4%	5.3%
Combination Abdominal CT Scan	520	14.8%	11.8%	10.5%
Combination Brain/Sinus CT Scan[1]	-	-	3.4%	2.7%
Combination Chest CT Scan	167	16.2%	2.4%	2.7%
Follow-up Mammogram/Ultrasound	438	9.6%	10.2%	8.8%
Lumbar Spine MRI for Low Back Pain[1]	-	-	35.2%	37.2%

Florida Hospital Memorial Medical Center

301 Memorial Medical Parkway Phone: 386-676-6000
Daytona Beach, FL 32117 Fax: 386-671-5099
URL: www.fhmd.com
Type: Acute Care Hospitals Emergency Services: Yes
Ownership: Voluntary non-profit - Church Beds: 400

Measure	Cases	This Hosp.	State Avg.	U.S. Avg.
Blood Clot Prevention and Treatment				
Anticoagulation Overlap Therapy[2]	103	96%	93%	93%
ICU Venous Thromboembolism Prophylaxis[2]	82	96%	94%	92%
Incidence of Potentially Preventable VTE[1,2]	-	-	10%	10%
UFH with Dosages/Platelet Monitoring[2]	31	100%	100%	97%
Venous Thromboembolism Prophylaxis[2]	365	97%	88%	85%
Warfarin Therapy Discharge Instructions[2]	76	91%	85%	75%
Chest Pain/Possible Heart Attack Care				
Aspirin Given Within 24 Hours of Arrival	18	94%	98%	96%
Fibrinolytic Meds Within 30 Min. of Arrival[3,7]	-	-	81%	58%
Average Time to ECG (minutes)	18	5	7	7
Average Time to Transfer (minutes)[1,3]	-	-	53	60
Children's Asthma Care				
Received Home Management Plan of Care	-	-	-	88%
Received Reliever Medication	-	-	-	100%
Received Systemic Corticosteroids	-	-	-	100%
Emergency Department				
Admittance Decision Time (minutes)[2]	642	81	111	98
Head CT Results Within 45 Min. of Arrival[1]	-	-	64%	57%
Patients Who Left ER Before Being Seen	46,637	1%	2%	2%
Time from ER Arrival to Admit. (minutes)[2]	659	275	289	274
Time from ER Arrival to Discharge (minutes)	712	99	147	134
Time in ER Before Being Evaluated (minutes)	669	15	26	26
Time to Pain Meds for Fractures (minutes)	140	66	60	57
Heart Attack Care				
Aspirin Given at Discharge	209	100%	99%	99%
Fibrinolytic Meds Within 30 Min. of Arrival[7]	-	-	50%	54%
PCI Within 90 Minutes of Arrival	37	97%	96%	96%
Statin Prescribed at Discharge	198	100%	99%	98%
Heart Failure Care				
ACE Inhibitor or ARB for LVSD	149	99%	98%	97%
Discharge Instructions Given	362	96%	96%	94%
Evaluation of LVS Function	459	100%	100%	99%
Medicare Spending				
Medicare Spending per Patient (ratio)	-	1.03	1.04	0.98
Pneumonia Care				
Appropriate Initial Antibiotic Given	182	97%	98%	95%
Blood Culture Timing	304	99%	99%	98%
Pregnancy and Delivery Care				
Newborn Deliveries Scheduled Early[2]	140	1%	6%	6%
Preventive Care				
Immunization for Influenza[2]	555	91%	94%	90%
Immunization for Pneumonia[2]	782	95%	96%	92%
Stroke Care				
Anticoagulation Therapy for Atrial Fibrillation	33	100%	97%	95%
Antithrombotic Therapy Timing	151	98%	98%	98%
Assessed for Rehabilitation	189	99%	97%	97%
Discharged on Antithrombotic Therapy	157	99%	99%	99%
Discharged on Statin Medication	124	96%	96%	94%
Thrombolytic Therapy Timing	14	100%	76%	66%
Venous Thromboembolism Prophylaxis	199	96%	95%	94%
Written Stroke Educational Materials Given	93	97%	94%	88%
Surgical Care Improvement Project				
Appropriate Beta Blocker Usage[2]	381	100%	99%	98%
Appropriate VTP Within 24 Hours[2]	667	100%	99%	98%
Controlled Postoperative Blood Glucose[2]	237	100%	98%	97%
Perioperative Temperature Management[2]	777	100%	100%	100%
Prophylactic Antibiotic Selection[2]	771	100%	99%	99%
Prophylactic Antibiotic Selection (Outpatient)	715	96%	98%	98%
Prophylactic Antibiotic Stopped[2]	746	99%	98%	98%
Prophylactic Antibiotic Timing[2]	772	100%	99%	99%
Prophylactic Antibiotic Timing (Outpatient)	731	97%	98%	98%
Urinary Catheter Removal[2]	638	99%	98%	97%
Survey of Patients' Hospital Experiences				
Area Around Room 'Always' Quiet at Night[11]	300+	72%	58%	61%
Doctors 'Always' Communicated Well[11]	300+	79%	77%	82%
Home Recovery Information Given[11]	300+	87%	83%	85%
Hospital Given 9 or 10 on 10 Point Scale[11]	300+	81%	67%	71%
Meds 'Always' Explained Before Given[11]	300+	65%	60%	64%
Nurses 'Always' Communicated Well[11]	300+	79%	75%	79%
Pain 'Always' Well Controlled[11]	300+	71%	68%	71%
Room and Bathroom 'Always' Clean[11]	300+	75%	69%	73%
Timely Help 'Always' Received[11]	300+	68%	62%	68%
Would Definitely Recommend Hospital[11]	300+	84%	69%	71%
Use of Medical Imaging				
Cardiac Imaging Stress Test before Surgery	110	5.5%	6.4%	5.3%
Combination Abdominal CT Scan	873	4.2%	11.8%	10.5%
Combination Brain/Sinus CT Scan	975	1.8%	3.4%	2.7%
Combination Chest CT Scan	920	1.4%	2.4%	2.7%
Follow-up Mammogram/Ultrasound	1,216	9.3%	10.2%	8.8%
Lumbar Spine MRI for Low Back Pain	60	36.7%	35.2%	37.2%

Halifax Health Medical Center

303 N Clyde Morris Blvd Phone: 386-254-4000
Daytona Beach, FL 32114 Fax: 386-258-4860
URL: www.halifax.org
Type: Acute Care Hospitals Emergency Services: Yes
Ownership: Govt - Hospital Dist/Auth Beds: 764

Key Personnel:
Infection Control.............. Richard Duma, MD

NOTE: Hospital profiles are in alphabetical order by state, then city, then hospital within the city; Rankings exclude hospitals with less than 25 cases except for patient surveys which excludes hospitals with less than 100 cases; (a) 100-299 cases; (1) The number of cases/patients is too few to report; (2) Data submitted were based on a sample of cases/patients; (3) Results are based on a shorter time period than required; (4) Data suppressed by CMS for one or more quarters; (5) Results are not available for this reporting period; (6) Fewer than 100 patients completed the HCAHPS survey; (7) No cases met the criteria for this measure; (8) The lower limit of the confidence interval cannot be calculated if the number of observed infections equals zero; (9) No data are available from the state/territory for this reporting period; (10) The scores shown reflect fewer than 50 completed surveys; (11) There were discrepancies in the data collection process; (12) This measure does not apply to this hospital for this reporting period; (13) Results cannot be calculated for this reporting period; (14) The results for this state are combined with nearby states to protect confidentiality; Please refer to the User's Guide for a full explanation of data.

CEO/President. . . . . Jeff Feasel
Quality Assurance . . . . Pat Llamas
Coronary Care. . . . . Lori Myers, RN
Pediatric In-Patient Care . . . . Catherine Privett, RN
Chief of Medical Staff . . . . Don Stoner, MD
Radiology. . . . . Alberto Tineo, MD
Operating Room. . . . . Linda Vossler

Measure	Cases	This Hosp.	State Avg.	U.S. Avg.
Blood Clot Prevention and Treatment				
Anticoagulation Overlap Therapy[2]	127	92%	93%	93%
ICU Venous Thromboembolism Prophylaxis[2]	75	92%	94%	92%
Incidence of Potentially Preventable VTE[2]	26	38%	10%	10%
UFH with Dosages/Platelet Monitoring[2]	77	100%	100%	97%
Venous Thromboembolism Prophylaxis[2]	280	76%	88%	85%
Warfarin Therapy Discharge Instructions[2]	84	98%	85%	75%
Chest Pain/Possible Heart Attack Care				
Aspirin Given Within 24 Hours of Arrival[5]	-	-	98%	96%
Fibrinolytic Meds Within 30 Min. of Arrival[5]	-	-	81%	58%
Average Time to ECG (minutes)[5]	-	-	7	7
Average Time to Transfer (minutes)[5]	-	-	53	60
Children's Asthma Care				
Received Home Management Plan of Care	-	-	-	88%
Received Reliever Medication	-	-	-	100%
Received Systemic Corticosteroids	-	-	-	100%
Emergency Department				
Admittance Decision Time (minutes)[2]	590	162	111	98
Head CT Results Within 45 Min. of Arrival[1]	-	-	64%	57%
Patients Who Left ER Before Being Seen	>100k	2%	2%	2%
Time from ER Arrival to Admit. (minutes)[2]	590	337	289	274
Time from ER Arrival to Discharge (minutes)	391	134	147	134
Time in ER Before Being Evaluated (minutes)	409	35	26	26
Time to Pain Meds for Fractures (minutes)	291	73	60	57
Heart Attack Care				
Aspirin Given at Discharge[2]	305	100%	99%	99%
Fibrinolytic Meds Within 30 Min. of Arrival[2,7]	-	-	50%	54%
PCI Within 90 Minutes of Arrival[2]	44	100%	96%	96%
Statin Prescribed at Discharge[2]	281	99%	99%	98%
Heart Failure Care				
ACE Inhibitor or ARB for LVSD[2]	142	100%	98%	97%
Discharge Instructions Given[2]	336	99%	96%	94%
Evaluation of LVS Function[2]	434	100%	100%	99%
Medicare Spending				
Medicare Spending per Patient (ratio)	-	1.05	1.04	0.98
Pneumonia Care				
Appropriate Initial Antibiotic Given[2]	209	97%	98%	95%
Blood Culture Timing[2]	363	97%	99%	98%
Pregnancy and Delivery Care				
Newborn Deliveries Scheduled Early[2]	89	9%	6%	6%
Preventive Care				
Immunization for Influenza[2]	579	76%	94%	90%
Immunization for Pneumonia[2]	609	92%	96%	92%
Stroke Care				
Anticoagulation Therapy for Atrial Fibrillation[2]	24	100%	97%	95%
Antithrombotic Therapy Timing[2]	161	98%	98%	98%
Assessed for Rehabilitation[2]	192	99%	97%	97%
Discharged on Antithrombotic Therapy[2]	153	100%	99%	99%
Discharged on Statin Medication[2]	111	96%	96%	94%
Thrombolytic Therapy Timing[2]	12	92%	76%	66%
Venous Thromboembolism Prophylaxis[2]	213	96%	95%	94%
Written Stroke Educational Materials Given[2]	115	98%	94%	88%
Surgical Care Improvement Project				
Appropriate Beta Blocker Usage[2]	274	99%	99%	98%
Appropriate VTP Within 24 Hours[2]	720	98%	99%	98%
Controlled Postoperative Blood Glucose[2]	125	99%	98%	97%
Perioperative Temperature Management[2]	831	100%	100%	100%
Prophylactic Antibiotic Selection[2]	741	99%	99%	99%
Prophylactic Antibiotic Selection (Outpatient)	663	97%	98%	98%
Prophylactic Antibiotic Stopped[2]	719	99%	98%	98%
Prophylactic Antibiotic Timing[2]	745	100%	99%	99%
Prophylactic Antibiotic Timing (Outpatient)	666	99%	98%	98%
Urinary Catheter Removal[2]	651	98%	98%	97%
Survey of Patients' Hospital Experiences				
Area Around Room 'Always' Quiet at Night	300+	65%	58%	61%
Doctors 'Always' Communicated Well	300+	77%	77%	82%
Home Recovery Information Given	300+	84%	83%	85%
Hospital Given 9 or 10 on 10 Point Scale	300+	67%	67%	71%
Meds 'Always' Explained Before Given	300+	56%	60%	64%
Nurses 'Always' Communicated Well	300+	74%	75%	79%
Pain 'Always' Well Controlled	300+	66%	68%	71%
Room and Bathroom 'Always' Clean	300+	68%	69%	73%
Timely Help 'Always' Received	300+	63%	62%	68%
Would Definitely Recommend Hospital	300+	69%	69%	71%
Use of Medical Imaging				
Cardiac Imaging Stress Test before Surgery	173	4.6%	6.4%	5.3%
Combination Abdominal CT Scan	632	0.3%	11.8%	10.5%
Combination Brain/Sinus CT Scan	1,360	3.8%	3.4%	2.7%
Combination Chest CT Scan	72	1.4%	2.4%	2.7%
Follow-up Mammogram/Ultrasound[7]	-	-	10.2%	8.8%
Lumbar Spine MRI for Low Back Pain[1]	-	-	35.2%	37.2%

Healthmark Regional Medical Center

4413 Us Hwy 331 S Phone: 850-951-4500
Defuniak Springs, FL 32435
URL: www.healthmarkregional.com
Type: Acute Care Hospitals Emergency Services: Yes
Ownership: Government - State
Key Personnel:
Anesthesiology. . . . . Scott Haufe, M.D.
Quality Assurance . . . . Violet Kennison RN DON
Cardiology . . . . Paul Tamburro, M.D.
CEO/President. . . . . James Thompson PhD
Radiology. . . . . John Tomberlin, M.D.

Measure	Cases	This Hosp.	State Avg.	U.S. Avg.
Blood Clot Prevention and Treatment				
Anticoagulation Overlap Therapy[1,2]	-	-	93%	93%
ICU Venous Thromboembolism Prophylaxis[2]	56	34%	94%	92%
Incidence of Potentially Preventable VTE[2,7]	-	-	10%	10%
UFH with Dosages/Platelet Monitoring[2,7]	-	-	100%	97%
Venous Thromboembolism Prophylaxis[2]	100	17%	88%	85%
Warfarin Therapy Discharge Instructions[1,2]	-	-	85%	75%
Chest Pain/Possible Heart Attack Care				
Aspirin Given Within 24 Hours of Arrival	20	95%	98%	96%
Fibrinolytic Meds Within 30 Min. of Arrival[7]	-	-	81%	58%
Average Time to ECG (minutes)	20	27	7	7
Average Time to Transfer (minutes)[1]	-	-	53	60
Children's Asthma Care				
Received Home Management Plan of Care	-	-	-	88%
Received Reliever Medication	-	-	-	100%
Received Systemic Corticosteroids	-	-	-	100%
Emergency Department				
Admittance Decision Time (minutes)[2]	414	0	111	98
Head CT Results Within 45 Min. of Arrival[5]	-	-	64%	57%
Patients Who Left ER Before Being Seen	11,734	2%	2%	2%
Time from ER Arrival to Admit. (minutes)[2]	426	188	289	274
Time from ER Arrival to Discharge (minutes)	321	100	147	134
Time in ER Before Being Evaluated (minutes)	289	31	26	26
Time to Pain Meds for Fractures (minutes)	17	64	60	57
Heart Attack Care				
Aspirin Given at Discharge[1,2]	-	-	99%	99%
Fibrinolytic Meds Within 30 Min. of Arrival[2,7]	-	-	50%	54%
PCI Within 90 Minutes of Arrival[2,7]	-	-	96%	96%
Statin Prescribed at Discharge[1,2]	-	-	99%	98%
Heart Failure Care				
ACE Inhibitor or ARB for LVSD[1,2]	-	-	98%	97%
Discharge Instructions Given[2]	35	43%	96%	94%
Evaluation of LVS Function[2]	47	15%	100%	99%
Medicare Spending				
Medicare Spending per Patient (ratio)	-	1.01	1.04	0.98
Pneumonia Care				
Appropriate Initial Antibiotic Given[2]	40	50%	98%	95%
Blood Culture Timing[2]	22	91%	99%	98%
Pregnancy and Delivery Care				
Newborn Deliveries Scheduled Early[7]	-	-	6%	6%
Preventive Care				
Immunization for Influenza[2]	294	54%	94%	90%
Immunization for Pneumonia[2]	444	66%	96%	92%
Stroke Care				
Anticoagulation Therapy for Atrial Fibrillation[1,2]	-	-	97%	95%
Antithrombotic Therapy Timing[1,2]	-	-	98%	98%
Assessed for Rehabilitation[1,2]	-	-	97%	97%
Discharged on Antithrombotic Therapy[1,2]	-	-	99%	99%
Discharged on Statin Medication[1,2]	-	-	96%	94%
Thrombolytic Therapy Timing[1,2]	-	-	76%	66%
Venous Thromboembolism Prophylaxis[1,2]	-	-	95%	94%
Written Stroke Educational Materials Given[1,2]	-	-	94%	88%
Surgical Care Improvement Project				
Appropriate Beta Blocker Usage[1,2]	-	-	99%	98%
Appropriate VTP Within 24 Hours[1,2]	-	-	99%	98%
Controlled Postoperative Blood Glucose[2,7]	-	-	98%	97%
Perioperative Temperature Management[2]	14	100%	100%	100%
Prophylactic Antibiotic Selection[1,2]	-	-	99%	99%
Prophylactic Antibiotic Selection (Outpatient)[3,7]	-	-	98%	98%
Prophylactic Antibiotic Stopped[1,2]	-	-	98%	98%
Prophylactic Antibiotic Timing[1,2]	-	-	99%	99%
Prophylactic Antibiotic Timing (Outpatient)[1,3]	-	-	98%	98%
Urinary Catheter Removal[1,2]	-	-	98%	97%
Survey of Patients' Hospital Experiences				
Area Around Room 'Always' Quiet at Night	(a)	80%	58%	61%
Doctors 'Always' Communicated Well	(a)	94%	77%	82%
Home Recovery Information Given	(a)	92%	83%	85%
Hospital Given 9 or 10 on 10 Point Scale	(a)	83%	67%	71%
Meds 'Always' Explained Before Given	(a)	56%	60%	64%
Nurses 'Always' Communicated Well	(a)	82%	75%	79%
Pain 'Always' Well Controlled	(a)	79%	68%	71%
Room and Bathroom 'Always' Clean	(a)	80%	69%	73%
Timely Help 'Always' Received	(a)	75%	62%	68%
Would Definitely Recommend Hospital	(a)	65%	69%	71%
Use of Medical Imaging				
Cardiac Imaging Stress Test before Surgery[1]	-	-	6.4%	5.3%
Combination Abdominal CT Scan	134	15.7%	11.8%	10.5%
Combination Brain/Sinus CT Scan[1]	-	-	3.4%	2.7%
Combination Chest CT Scan[1]	-	-	2.4%	2.7%
Follow-up Mammogram/Ultrasound[7]	-	-	10.2%	8.8%
Lumbar Spine MRI for Low Back Pain[1]	-	-	35.2%	37.2%

Florida Hospital Deland

701 W Plymouth Ave Phone: 386-943-4772
Deland, FL 32720 Fax: 386-943-3674
URL: www.fhdeland.org
Type: Acute Care Hospitals Emergency Services: Yes
Ownership: Voluntary non-profit - Church Beds: 156
Key Personnel:
Infection Control. . . . . Maria Cuccinello
Chief of Medical Staff . . . . Mark Hollmann
Emergency Room . . . . Beth Hooks
Quality Assurance . . . . Leanna Nichols
Operating Room. . . . . Jim Stoll
CEO/President. . . . . Daryl Tol
Intensive Care Unit. . . . . Elisha Voigt

Measure	Cases	This Hosp.	State Avg.	U.S. Avg.
Blood Clot Prevention and Treatment				
Anticoagulation Overlap Therapy[2]	88	92%	93%	93%
ICU Venous Thromboembolism Prophylaxis[2]	114	84%	94%	92%
Incidence of Potentially Preventable VTE[1,2]	-	-	10%	10%
UFH with Dosages/Platelet Monitoring[2]	32	100%	100%	97%
Venous Thromboembolism Prophylaxis[2]	286	87%	88%	85%
Warfarin Therapy Discharge Instructions[2]	62	94%	85%	75%
Chest Pain/Possible Heart Attack Care				
Aspirin Given Within 24 Hours of Arrival[1,3]	-	-	98%	96%
Fibrinolytic Meds Within 30 Min. of Arrival[3,7]	-	-	81%	58%
Average Time to ECG (minutes)[1,3]	-	-	7	7
Average Time to Transfer (minutes)[1,3]	-	-	53	60
Children's Asthma Care				
Received Home Management Plan of Care	-	-	-	88%
Received Reliever Medication	-	-	-	100%
Received Systemic Corticosteroids	-	-	-	100%
Emergency Department				
Admittance Decision Time (minutes)[2]	819	111	111	98
Head CT Results Within 45 Min. of Arrival[1]	-	-	64%	57%
Patients Who Left ER Before Being Seen	50,588	3%	2%	2%
Time from ER Arrival to Admit. (minutes)[2]	856	316	289	274

NOTE: Hospital profiles are in alphabetical order by state, then city, then hospital within the city; Rankings exclude hospitals with less than 25 cases except for patient surveys which excludes hospitals with less than 100 cases; (a) 100-299 cases; (1) The number of cases/patients is too few to report; (2) Data submitted were based on a sample of cases/patients; (3) Results are based on a shorter time period than required; (4) Data suppressed by CMS for one or more quarters; (5) Results are not available for this reporting period; (6) Fewer than 100 patients completed the HCAHPS survey; (7) No cases met the criteria for this measure; (8) The lower limit of the confidence interval cannot be calculated if the number of observed infections equals zero; (9) No data are available from the state/territory for this reporting period; (10) The scores shown reflect fewer than 50 completed surveys; (11) There were discrepancies in the data collection process; (12) This measure does not apply to this hospital for this reporting period; (13) Results cannot be calculated for this reporting period; (14) The results for this state are combined with nearby states to protect confidentiality; Please refer to the User's Guide for a full explanation of data.

Measure	Cases	This Hosp.	State Avg.	U.S. Avg.
Time from ER Arrival to Discharge (minutes)	357	131	147	134
Time in ER Before Being Evaluated (minutes)	357	44	26	26
Time to Pain Meds for Fractures (minutes)	130	81	60	57
Heart Attack Care				
Aspirin Given at Discharge	178	98%	99%	99%
Fibrinolytic Meds Within 30 Min. of Arrival[7]	-	-	50%	54%
PCI Within 90 Minutes of Arrival	30	87%	96%	96%
Statin Prescribed at Discharge	173	99%	99%	98%
Heart Failure Care				
ACE Inhibitor or ARB for LVSD	115	99%	98%	97%
Discharge Instructions Given	278	99%	96%	94%
Evaluation of LVS Function	357	100%	100%	99%
Medicare Spending				
Medicare Spending per Patient (ratio)	-	1.02	1.04	0.98
Pneumonia Care				
Appropriate Initial Antibiotic Given	142	97%	98%	95%
Blood Culture Timing	299	100%	99%	98%
Pregnancy and Delivery Care				
Newborn Deliveries Scheduled Early[2]	39	0%	6%	6%
Preventive Care				
Immunization for Influenza[2]	531	79%	94%	90%
Immunization for Pneumonia[2]	740	91%	96%	92%
Stroke Care				
Anticoagulation Therapy for Atrial Fibrillation[1,2]	-	-	97%	95%
Antithrombotic Therapy Timing[2]	84	96%	98%	98%
Assessed for Rehabilitation[2]	93	100%	97%	97%
Discharged on Antithrombotic Therapy[2]	88	100%	99%	99%
Discharged on Statin Medication[2]	61	98%	96%	94%
Thrombolytic Therapy Timing[1,2]	-	-	76%	66%
Venous Thromboembolism Prophylaxis[2]	91	92%	95%	94%
Written Stroke Educational Materials Given[2]	44	95%	94%	88%
Surgical Care Improvement Project				
Appropriate Beta Blocker Usage	177	100%	99%	98%
Appropriate VTP Within 24 Hours	528	99%	99%	98%
Controlled Postoperative Blood Glucose[7]	-	-	98%	97%
Perioperative Temperature Management	551	100%	100%	100%
Prophylactic Antibiotic Selection	419	100%	99%	99%
Prophylactic Antibiotic Selection (Outpatient)	73	99%	98%	98%
Prophylactic Antibiotic Stopped	407	99%	98%	98%
Prophylactic Antibiotic Timing	419	100%	99%	99%
Prophylactic Antibiotic Timing (Outpatient)	74	99%	98%	98%
Urinary Catheter Removal	461	99%	98%	97%
Survey of Patients' Hospital Experiences				
Area Around Room 'Always' Quiet at Night[11]	300+	50%	58%	61%
Doctors 'Always' Communicated Well[11]	300+	74%	77%	82%
Home Recovery Information Given[11]	300+	86%	83%	85%
Hospital Given 9 or 10 on 10 Point Scale[11]	300+	63%	67%	71%
Meds 'Always' Explained Before Given[11]	300+	60%	60%	64%
Nurses 'Always' Communicated Well[11]	300+	77%	75%	79%
Pain 'Always' Well Controlled[11]	300+	67%	68%	71%
Room and Bathroom 'Always' Clean[11]	300+	66%	69%	73%
Timely Help 'Always' Received[11]	300+	64%	62%	68%
Would Definitely Recommend Hospital[11]	300+	63%	69%	71%
Use of Medical Imaging				
Cardiac Imaging Stress Test before Surgery	110	4.5%	6.4%	5.3%
Combination Abdominal CT Scan	632	6.6%	11.8%	10.5%
Combination Brain/Sinus CT Scan	773	2.8%	3.4%	2.7%
Combination Chest CT Scan	576	0.0%	2.4%	2.7%
Follow-up Mammogram/Ultrasound	1,384	14.2%	10.2%	8.8%
Lumbar Spine MRI for Low Back Pain	96	34.4%	35.2%	37.2%

Delray Medical Center

5352 Linton Blvd
Delray Beach, FL 33484
URL: www.delraymedicalctr.com
Phone: 561-498-4440
Fax: 561-495-3103
Type: Acute Care Hospitals
Ownership: Proprietary
Emergency Services: Yes
Beds: 343

Key Personnel:
Chief of Medical Staff . . . . Bruce Barton, MD
Quality Assurance . . . . Richard Bluni
CEO . . . . Mark Bryan
CEO/President . . . . Mitch Feldman
Emergency Room . . . . Audrey Gregory
Radiology . . . . Theresa Griffith

Measure	Cases	This Hosp.	State Avg.	U.S. Avg.
Blood Clot Prevention and Treatment				
Anticoagulation Overlap Therapy[2]	114	100%	93%	93%
ICU Venous Thromboembolism Prophylaxis[2]	105	100%	94%	92%
Incidence of Potentially Preventable VTE[2]	16	0%	10%	10%
UFH with Dosages/Platelet Monitoring[2]	108	100%	100%	97%
Venous Thromboembolism Prophylaxis[2]	347	100%	88%	85%
Warfarin Therapy Discharge Instructions[2]	67	100%	85%	75%
Chest Pain/Possible Heart Attack Care				
Aspirin Given Within 24 Hours of Arrival[1,3]	-	-	98%	96%
Fibrinolytic Meds Within 30 Min. of Arrival[3,7]	-	-	81%	58%
Average Time to ECG (minutes)[1,3]	-	-	7	7
Average Time to Transfer (minutes)[3,7]	-	-	53	60
Children's Asthma Care				
Received Home Management Plan of Care	-	-	-	88%
Received Reliever Medication	-	-	-	100%
Received Systemic Corticosteroids	-	-	-	100%
Emergency Department				
Admittance Decision Time (minutes)[2]	1,059	136	111	98
Head CT Results Within 45 Min. of Arrival[1]	-	-	64%	57%
Patients Who Left ER Before Being Seen	46,311	1%	2%	2%
Time from ER Arrival to Admit. (minutes)[2]	1,059	322	289	274
Time from ER Arrival to Discharge (minutes)	382	163	147	134
Time in ER Before Being Evaluated (minutes)	423	21	26	26
Time to Pain Meds for Fractures (minutes)	188	66	60	57
Heart Attack Care				
Aspirin Given at Discharge	268	100%	99%	99%
Fibrinolytic Meds Within 30 Min. of Arrival[7]	-	-	50%	54%
PCI Within 90 Minutes of Arrival	35	100%	96%	96%
Statin Prescribed at Discharge	250	100%	99%	98%
Heart Failure Care				
ACE Inhibitor or ARB for LVSD[2]	70	100%	98%	97%
Discharge Instructions Given[2]	280	100%	96%	94%
Evaluation of LVS Function[2]	374	100%	100%	99%
Medicare Spending				
Medicare Spending per Patient (ratio)	-	1.10	1.04	0.98
Pneumonia Care				
Appropriate Initial Antibiotic Given[2]	132	100%	98%	95%
Blood Culture Timing[2]	219	100%	99%	98%
Pregnancy and Delivery Care				
Newborn Deliveries Scheduled Early[7]	-	-	6%	6%
Preventive Care				
Immunization for Influenza[2]	652	100%	94%	90%
Immunization for Pneumonia[2]	1,057	100%	96%	92%
Stroke Care				
Anticoagulation Therapy for Atrial Fibrillation	41	100%	97%	95%
Antithrombotic Therapy Timing	169	100%	98%	98%
Assessed for Rehabilitation	249	100%	97%	97%
Discharged on Antithrombotic Therapy	204	100%	99%	99%
Discharged on Statin Medication	165	100%	96%	94%
Thrombolytic Therapy Timing	29	100%	76%	66%
Venous Thromboembolism Prophylaxis	262	100%	95%	94%
Written Stroke Educational Materials Given	123	100%	94%	88%
Surgical Care Improvement Project				
Appropriate Beta Blocker Usage[2]	422	100%	99%	98%
Appropriate VTP Within 24 Hours[2]	689	100%	99%	98%
Controlled Postoperative Blood Glucose[2]	171	96%	98%	97%
Perioperative Temperature Management[2]	810	100%	100%	100%
Prophylactic Antibiotic Selection[2]	693	100%	99%	99%
Prophylactic Antibiotic Selection (Outpatient)	564	99%	98%	98%
Prophylactic Antibiotic Stopped[2]	675	99%	98%	98%
Prophylactic Antibiotic Timing[2]	694	100%	99%	99%
Prophylactic Antibiotic Timing (Outpatient)	564	100%	98%	98%
Urinary Catheter Removal[2]	425	100%	98%	97%
Survey of Patients' Hospital Experiences				
Area Around Room 'Always' Quiet at Night	300+	45%	58%	61%
Doctors 'Always' Communicated Well	300+	73%	77%	82%
Home Recovery Information Given	300+	81%	83%	85%
Hospital Given 9 or 10 on 10 Point Scale	300+	56%	67%	71%
Meds 'Always' Explained Before Given	300+	54%	60%	64%
Nurses 'Always' Communicated Well	300+	70%	75%	79%
Pain 'Always' Well Controlled	300+	61%	68%	71%
Room and Bathroom 'Always' Clean	300+	55%	69%	73%
Timely Help 'Always' Received	300+	53%	62%	68%
Would Definitely Recommend Hospital	300+	63%	69%	71%
Use of Medical Imaging				
Cardiac Imaging Stress Test before Surgery	265	11.3%	6.4%	5.3%
Combination Abdominal CT Scan	824	1.0%	11.8%	10.5%
Combination Brain/Sinus CT Scan	1,262	2.8%	3.4%	2.7%
Combination Chest CT Scan	132	0.8%	2.4%	2.7%
Follow-up Mammogram/Ultrasound[7]	-	-	10.2%	8.8%
Lumbar Spine MRI for Low Back Pain[1]	-	-	35.2%	37.2%

Mease Hospital Dunedin

601 Main Street
Dunedin, FL 34698
URL: www.measehospitals.com
Phone: 727-733-1111
Type: Acute Care Hospitals
Ownership: Voluntary non-profit - Private
Emergency Services: Yes
Beds: 143

Measure	Cases	This Hosp.	State Avg.	U.S. Avg.
Blood Clot Prevention and Treatment				
Anticoagulation Overlap Therapy[2]	37	81%	93%	93%
ICU Venous Thromboembolism Prophylaxis[2]	103	98%	94%	92%
Incidence of Potentially Preventable VTE[1,2]	-	-	10%	10%
UFH with Dosages/Platelet Monitoring[2]	12	100%	100%	97%
Venous Thromboembolism Prophylaxis[2]	354	98%	88%	85%
Warfarin Therapy Discharge Instructions[2]	20	95%	85%	75%
Chest Pain/Possible Heart Attack Care				
Aspirin Given Within 24 Hours of Arrival	40	100%	98%	96%
Fibrinolytic Meds Within 30 Min. of Arrival[7]	-	-	81%	58%
Average Time to ECG (minutes)	40	8	7	7
Average Time to Transfer (minutes)[1]	-	-	53	60
Children's Asthma Care				
Received Home Management Plan of Care	-	-	-	88%
Received Reliever Medication	-	-	-	100%
Received Systemic Corticosteroids	-	-	-	100%
Emergency Department				
Admittance Decision Time (minutes)[2]	733	108	111	98
Head CT Results Within 45 Min. of Arrival[1]	-	-	64%	57%
Patients Who Left ER Before Being Seen	24,605	0%	2%	2%
Time from ER Arrival to Admit. (minutes)[2]	735	275	289	274
Time from ER Arrival to Discharge (minutes)	358	144	147	134
Time in ER Before Being Evaluated (minutes)	381	21	26	26
Time to Pain Meds for Fractures (minutes)	46	40	60	57
Heart Attack Care				
Aspirin Given at Discharge	25	96%	99%	99%
Fibrinolytic Meds Within 30 Min. of Arrival[7]	-	-	50%	54%
PCI Within 90 Minutes of Arrival[7]	-	-	96%	96%
Statin Prescribed at Discharge	20	95%	99%	98%
Heart Failure Care				
ACE Inhibitor or ARB for LVSD	45	98%	98%	97%
Discharge Instructions Given	105	98%	96%	94%
Evaluation of LVS Function	142	100%	100%	99%
Medicare Spending				
Medicare Spending per Patient (ratio)	-	1.14	1.04	0.98
Pneumonia Care				
Appropriate Initial Antibiotic Given	81	100%	98%	95%
Blood Culture Timing	182	100%	99%	98%
Pregnancy and Delivery Care				
Newborn Deliveries Scheduled Early[7]	-	-	6%	6%
Preventive Care				
Immunization for Influenza[2]	477	99%	94%	90%
Immunization for Pneumonia[2]	712	98%	96%	92%
Stroke Care				
Anticoagulation Therapy for Atrial Fibrillation	12	92%	97%	95%
Antithrombotic Therapy Timing	63	98%	98%	98%
Assessed for Rehabilitation	62	100%	97%	97%
Discharged on Antithrombotic Therapy	58	100%	99%	99%
Discharged on Statin Medication	44	95%	96%	94%
Thrombolytic Therapy Timing[1]	-	-	76%	66%
Venous Thromboembolism Prophylaxis	68	100%	95%	94%
Written Stroke Educational Materials Given	38	100%	94%	88%
Surgical Care Improvement Project				
Appropriate Beta Blocker Usage[2]	63	98%	99%	98%

NOTE: Hospital profiles are in alphabetical order by state, then city, then hospital within the city; Rankings exclude hospitals with less than 25 cases except for patient surveys which excludes hospitals with less than 100 cases; (a) 100-299 cases; (1) The number of cases/patients is too few to report; (2) Data submitted were based on a sample of cases/patients; (3) Results are based on a shorter time period than required; (4) Data suppressed by CMS for one or more quarters; (5) Results are not available for this reporting period; (6) Fewer than 100 patients completed the HCAHPS survey; (7) No cases met the criteria for this measure; (8) The lower limit of the confidence interval cannot be calculated if the number of observed infections equals zero; (9) No data are available from the state/territory for this reporting period; (10) The scores shown reflect fewer than 50 completed surveys; (11) There were discrepancies in the data collection process; (12) This measure does not apply to this hospital for this reporting period; (13) Results cannot be calculated for this reporting period; (14) The results for this state are combined with nearby states to protect confidentiality; Please refer to the User's Guide for a full explanation of data.

Appropriate VTP Within 24 Hours[2]	235	98%	99%	98%
Controlled Postoperative Blood Glucose[2,7]	-	-	98%	97%
Perioperative Temperature Management[2]	251	100%	100%	100%
Prophylactic Antibiotic Selection[2]	189	100%	99%	99%
Prophylactic Antibiotic Selection (Outpatient)	71	100%	98%	98%
Prophylactic Antibiotic Stopped[2]	183	98%	98%	98%
Prophylactic Antibiotic Timing[2]	189	100%	99%	99%
Prophylactic Antibiotic Timing (Outpatient)	71	100%	98%	98%
Urinary Catheter Removal[2]	219	99%	98%	97%
Survey of Patients' Hospital Experiences				
Area Around Room 'Always' Quiet at Night[11]	300+	57%	58%	61%
Doctors 'Always' Communicated Well[11]	300+	73%	77%	82%
Home Recovery Information Given[11]	300+	88%	83%	85%
Hospital Given 9 or 10 on 10 Point Scale[11]	300+	76%	67%	71%
Meds 'Always' Explained Before Given[11]	300+	61%	60%	64%
Nurses 'Always' Communicated Well[11]	300+	76%	75%	79%
Pain 'Always' Well Controlled[11]	300+	67%	68%	71%
Room and Bathroom 'Always' Clean[11]	300+	75%	69%	73%
Timely Help 'Always' Received[11]	300+	65%	62%	68%
Would Definitely Recommend Hospital[11]	300+	76%	69%	71%
Use of Medical Imaging				
Cardiac Imaging Stress Test before Surgery[1]	-	-	6.4%	5.3%
Combination Abdominal CT Scan	374	9.9%	11.8%	10.5%
Combination Brain/Sinus CT Scan	631	4.1%	3.4%	2.7%
Combination Chest CT Scan	179	0.6%	2.4%	2.7%
Follow-up Mammogram/Ultrasound	913	5.4%	10.2%	8.8%
Lumbar Spine MRI for Low Back Pain	45	42.2%	35.2%	37.2%

Englewood Community Hospital

700 Medical Blvd
Englewood, FL 34223
Phone: 941-475-6571
Fax: 941-473-7259
URL: www.englewoodcommunityhospital.com
Type: Acute Care Hospitals
Emergency Services: Yes
Ownership: Proprietary
Beds: 100

Key Personnel:
CEO . . . . Dale Alward
Chief of Medical Staff. . . . . Raul Verde, MD

Measure	Cases	This Hosp.	State Avg.	U.S. Avg.
Blood Clot Prevention and Treatment				
Anticoagulation Overlap Therapy[2]	39	95%	93%	93%
ICU Venous Thromboembolism Prophylaxis[2]	73	100%	94%	92%
Incidence of Potentially Preventable VTE[1,2]	-	-	10%	10%
UFH with Dosages/Platelet Monitoring[2]	19	100%	100%	97%
Venous Thromboembolism Prophylaxis[2]	311	99%	88%	85%
Warfarin Therapy Discharge Instructions[2]	25	96%	85%	75%
Chest Pain/Possible Heart Attack Care				
Aspirin Given Within 24 Hours of Arrival	64	98%	98%	96%
Fibrinolytic Meds Within 30 Min. of Arrival[7]	-	-	81%	58%
Average Time to ECG (minutes)	65	1	7	7
Average Time to Transfer (minutes)	17	52	53	60
Children's Asthma Care				
Received Home Management Plan of Care	-	-	-	88%
Received Reliever Medication	-	-	-	100%
Received Systemic Corticosteroids	-	-	-	100%
Emergency Department				
Admittance Decision Time (minutes)[2]	666	73	111	98
Head CT Results Within 45 Min. of Arrival	28	96%	64%	57%
Patients Who Left ER Before Being Seen	15,527	0%	2%	2%
Time from ER Arrival to Admit. (minutes)[2]	666	183	289	274
Time from ER Arrival to Discharge (minutes)	370	102	147	134
Time in ER Before Being Evaluated (minutes)	433	8	26	26
Time to Pain Meds for Fractures (minutes)	58	40	60	57
Heart Attack Care				
Aspirin Given at Discharge	11	100%	99%	99%
Fibrinolytic Meds Within 30 Min. of Arrival[7]	-	-	50%	54%
PCI Within 90 Minutes of Arrival[7]	-	-	96%	96%
Statin Prescribed at Discharge[1]	-	-	99%	98%
Heart Failure Care				
ACE Inhibitor or ARB for LVSD	37	100%	98%	97%
Discharge Instructions Given	139	100%	96%	94%
Evaluation of LVS Function	170	100%	100%	99%
Medicare Spending				
Medicare Spending per Patient (ratio)	-	0.96	1.04	0.98
Pneumonia Care				
Appropriate Initial Antibiotic Given	54	100%	98%	95%
Blood Culture Timing	92	100%	99%	98%
Pregnancy and Delivery Care				
Newborn Deliveries Scheduled Early[7]	-	-	6%	6%
Preventive Care				
Immunization for Influenza[2]	370	98%	94%	90%
Immunization for Pneumonia[2]	602	98%	96%	92%
Stroke Care				
Anticoagulation Therapy for Atrial Fibrillation[1,2]	-	-	97%	95%
Antithrombotic Therapy Timing[1,2]	-	-	98%	98%
Assessed for Rehabilitation[1,2]	-	-	97%	97%
Discharged on Antithrombotic Therapy[1,2]	-	-	99%	99%
Discharged on Statin Medication[1,2]	-	-	96%	94%
Thrombolytic Therapy Timing[2,7]	-	-	76%	66%
Venous Thromboembolism Prophylaxis[1,2]	-	-	95%	94%
Written Stroke Educational Materials Given[1,2]	-	-	94%	88%
Surgical Care Improvement Project				
Appropriate Beta Blocker Usage	37	100%	99%	98%
Appropriate VTP Within 24 Hours	134	100%	99%	98%
Controlled Postoperative Blood Glucose[7]	-	-	98%	97%
Perioperative Temperature Management	145	100%	100%	100%
Prophylactic Antibiotic Selection	106	99%	99%	99%
Prophylactic Antibiotic Selection (Outpatient)	42	100%	98%	98%
Prophylactic Antibiotic Stopped	103	100%	98%	98%
Prophylactic Antibiotic Timing	106	100%	99%	99%
Prophylactic Antibiotic Timing (Outpatient)	42	100%	98%	98%
Urinary Catheter Removal	84	99%	98%	97%
Survey of Patients' Hospital Experiences				
Area Around Room 'Always' Quiet at Night	300+	57%	58%	61%
Doctors 'Always' Communicated Well	300+	77%	77%	82%
Home Recovery Information Given	300+	83%	83%	85%
Hospital Given 9 or 10 on 10 Point Scale	300+	63%	67%	71%
Meds 'Always' Explained Before Given	300+	57%	60%	64%
Nurses 'Always' Communicated Well	300+	74%	75%	79%
Pain 'Always' Well Controlled	300+	68%	68%	71%
Room and Bathroom 'Always' Clean	300+	64%	69%	73%
Timely Help 'Always' Received	300+	61%	62%	68%
Would Definitely Recommend Hospital	300+	60%	69%	71%
Use of Medical Imaging				
Cardiac Imaging Stress Test before Surgery[1]	-	-	6.4%	5.3%
Combination Abdominal CT Scan	308	12.0%	11.8%	10.5%
Combination Brain/Sinus CT Scan	605	5.1%	3.4%	2.7%
Combination Chest CT Scan	53	0.0%	2.4%	2.7%
Follow-up Mammogram/Ultrasound	373	5.9%	10.2%	8.8%
Lumbar Spine MRI for Low Back Pain[1]	-	-	35.2%	37.2%

Baptist Medical Center - Nassau

1250 S 18th St
Fernandina Beach, FL 32034
Phone: 904-321-3500
Fax: 904-321-3511
URL: www.e-baptisthealth.com
Type: Acute Care Hospitals
Emergency Services: Yes
Ownership: Government - Local
Beds: 54

Key Personnel:
Radiology. Mary Alderman, MD
Coronary Care . . . . Debbie Dunman
Infection Control. . . . . Ted Jones, RN
Operating Room. . . . . Joan Knerr, RN
CEO/President. . . . . Stephen Lee, FACHE, EdD
Chief of Medical Staff . . . . David Murray, MD
Pediatric Ambulatory Care . . . . . . Tae Rho, MD
Pediatric In-Patient Care . . . . Tae Rho, MD

Measure	Cases	This Hosp.	State Avg.	U.S. Avg.
Blood Clot Prevention and Treatment				
Anticoagulation Overlap Therapy[2]	27	74%	93%	93%
ICU Venous Thromboembolism Prophylaxis[2]	75	99%	94%	92%
Incidence of Potentially Preventable VTE[2,7]	-	-	10%	10%
UFH with Dosages/Platelet Monitoring[1,2]	-	-	100%	97%
Venous Thromboembolism Prophylaxis[2]	259	76%	88%	85%
Warfarin Therapy Discharge Instructions[2]	23	83%	85%	75%
Chest Pain/Possible Heart Attack Care				
Aspirin Given Within 24 Hours of Arrival	95	96%	98%	96%
Fibrinolytic Meds Within 30 Min. of Arrival[7]	-	-	81%	58%
Average Time to ECG (minutes)	99	8	7	7
Average Time to Transfer (minutes)[1]	-	-	53	60
Children's Asthma Care				
Received Home Management Plan of Care	-	-	-	88%
Received Reliever Medication	-	-	-	100%
Received Systemic Corticosteroids	-	-	-	100%
Emergency Department				
Admittance Decision Time (minutes)[2]	271	122	111	98
Head CT Results Within 45 Min. of Arrival	12	83%	64%	57%
Patients Who Left ER Before Being Seen	25,949	3%	2%	2%
Time from ER Arrival to Admit. (minutes)[2]	272	302	289	274
Time from ER Arrival to Discharge (minutes)	408	128	147	134
Time in ER Before Being Evaluated (minutes)	501	34	26	26
Time to Pain Meds for Fractures (minutes)	69	41	60	57
Heart Attack Care				
Aspirin Given at Discharge[1,2]	-	-	99%	99%
Fibrinolytic Meds Within 30 Min. of Arrival[2,7]	-	-	50%	54%
PCI Within 90 Minutes of Arrival[2,7]	-	-	96%	96%
Statin Prescribed at Discharge[2]	11	64%	99%	98%
Heart Failure Care				
ACE Inhibitor or ARB for LVSD[2]	38	97%	98%	97%
Discharge Instructions Given[2]	74	95%	96%	94%
Evaluation of LVS Function[2]	91	100%	100%	99%
Medicare Spending				
Medicare Spending per Patient (ratio)	-	1.00	1.04	0.98
Pneumonia Care				
Appropriate Initial Antibiotic Given[2]	121	97%	98%	95%
Blood Culture Timing[2]	183	98%	99%	98%
Pregnancy and Delivery Care				
Newborn Deliveries Scheduled Early[2]	56	11%	6%	6%
Preventive Care				
Immunization for Influenza[2]	302	86%	94%	90%
Immunization for Pneumonia[2]	312	91%	96%	92%
Stroke Care				
Anticoagulation Therapy for Atrial Fibrillation[1,2]	-	-	97%	95%
Antithrombotic Therapy Timing[2]	19	100%	98%	98%
Assessed for Rehabilitation[2]	22	100%	97%	97%
Discharged on Antithrombotic Therapy[2]	22	100%	99%	99%
Discharged on Statin Medication[2]	16	100%	96%	94%
Thrombolytic Therapy Timing[2,7]	-	-	76%	66%
Venous Thromboembolism Prophylaxis[2]	19	89%	95%	94%
Written Stroke Educational Materials Given[2]	16	94%	94%	88%
Surgical Care Improvement Project				
Appropriate Beta Blocker Usage[2]	20	100%	99%	98%
Appropriate VTP Within 24 Hours[2]	122	98%	99%	98%
Controlled Postoperative Blood Glucose[2,7]	-	-	98%	97%
Perioperative Temperature Management[2]	129	100%	100%	100%
Prophylactic Antibiotic Selection[2]	55	91%	99%	99%
Prophylactic Antibiotic Selection (Outpatient)	27	78%	98%	98%
Prophylactic Antibiotic Stopped[2]	53	89%	98%	98%
Prophylactic Antibiotic Timing[2]	55	98%	99%	99%
Prophylactic Antibiotic Timing (Outpatient)	28	96%	98%	98%
Urinary Catheter Removal[2]	45	82%	98%	97%
Survey of Patients' Hospital Experiences				
Area Around Room 'Always' Quiet at Night	300+	68%	58%	61%
Doctors 'Always' Communicated Well	300+	84%	77%	82%
Home Recovery Information Given	300+	83%	83%	85%
Hospital Given 9 or 10 on 10 Point Scale	300+	76%	67%	71%
Meds 'Always' Explained Before Given	300+	63%	60%	64%
Nurses 'Always' Communicated Well	300+	81%	75%	79%
Pain 'Always' Well Controlled	300+	70%	68%	71%
Room and Bathroom 'Always' Clean	300+	69%	69%	73%
Timely Help 'Always' Received	300+	67%	62%	68%
Would Definitely Recommend Hospital	300+	79%	69%	71%
Use of Medical Imaging				
Cardiac Imaging Stress Test before Surgery	473	6.3%	6.4%	5.3%
Combination Abdominal CT Scan	650	2.2%	11.8%	10.5%
Combination Brain/Sinus CT Scan	812	3.2%	3.4%	2.7%
Combination Chest CT Scan	447	0.0%	2.4%	2.7%
Follow-up Mammogram/Ultrasound	1,427	8.0%	10.2%	8.8%
Lumbar Spine MRI for Low Back Pain	76	40.8%	35.2%	37.2%

NOTE: Hospital profiles are in alphabetical order by state, then city, then hospital within the city; Rankings exclude hospitals with less than 25 cases except for patient surveys which excludes hospitals with less than 100 cases; (a) 100-299 cases; (1) The number of cases/patients is too few to report; (2) Data submitted were based on a sample of cases/patients; (3) Results are based on a shorter time period than required; (4) Data suppressed by CMS for one or more quarters; (5) Results are not available for this reporting period; (6) Fewer than 100 patients completed the HCAHPS survey; (7) No cases met the criteria for this measure; (8) The lower limit of the confidence interval cannot be calculated if the number of observed infections equals zero; (9) No data are available from the state/territory for this reporting period; (10) The scores shown reflect fewer than 50 completed surveys; (11) There were discrepancies in the data collection process; (12) This measure does not apply to this hospital for this reporting period; (13) Results cannot be calculated for this reporting period; (14) The results for this state are combined with nearby states to protect confidentiality; Please refer to the User's Guide for a full explanation of data.

Broward Health Imperial Point

6401 N Federal Hwy
Fort Lauderdale, FL 33308
URL: www.nbhd.org
Type: Acute Care Hospitals
Ownership: Govt - Hospital Dist/Auth
Phone: 954-776-8500
Fax: 954-776-8520
Emergency Services: Yes
Beds: 204

Key Personnel:
Radiology. . . . . Carlos Duran
CEO/President. . . . . Calvin Glidewell
Operating Room. . . . . Cassandra Jackson
Chief of Medical Staff . . . . William Jensen
Infection Control. . . . . Ruthie Moncilovich
Quality Assurance . . . . Ruthie Moncilovich

Measure	Cases	This Hosp.	State Avg.	U.S. Avg.
Blood Clot Prevention and Treatment				
Anticoagulation Overlap Therapy[2]	48	94%	93%	93%
ICU Venous Thromboembolism Prophylaxis[2]	47	83%	94%	92%
Incidence of Potentially Preventable VTE[1,2]	-	-	10%	10%
UFH with Dosages/Platelet Monitoring[1,2]	-	-	100%	97%
Venous Thromboembolism Prophylaxis[2]	242	68%	88%	85%
Warfarin Therapy Discharge Instructions[2]	40	100%	85%	75%
Chest Pain/Possible Heart Attack Care				
Aspirin Given Within 24 Hours of Arrival	36	100%	98%	96%
Fibrinolytic Meds Within 30 Min. of Arrival[7]	-	-	81%	58%
Average Time to ECG (minutes)	37	10	7	7
Average Time to Transfer (minutes)[1]	-	-	53	60
Children's Asthma Care				
Received Home Management Plan of Care	-	-	-	88%
Received Reliever Medication	-	-	-	100%
Received Systemic Corticosteroids	-	-	-	100%
Emergency Department				
Admittance Decision Time (minutes)[2]	635	157	111	98
Head CT Results Within 45 Min. of Arrival[7]	-	-	64%	57%
Patients Who Left ER Before Being Seen	33,984	2%	2%	2%
Time from ER Arrival to Admit. (minutes)[2]	659	337	289	274
Time from ER Arrival to Discharge (minutes)	367	165	147	134
Time in ER Before Being Evaluated (minutes)	417	38	26	26
Time to Pain Meds for Fractures (minutes)	23	70	60	57
Heart Attack Care				
Aspirin Given at Discharge	13	100%	99%	99%
Fibrinolytic Meds Within 30 Min. of Arrival[7]	-	-	50%	54%
PCI Within 90 Minutes of Arrival[7]	-	-	96%	96%
Statin Prescribed at Discharge[1]	-	-	99%	98%
Heart Failure Care				
ACE Inhibitor or ARB for LVSD	62	100%	98%	97%
Discharge Instructions Given	134	93%	96%	94%
Evaluation of LVS Function	162	99%	100%	99%
Medicare Spending				
Medicare Spending per Patient (ratio)	-	1.05	1.04	0.98
Pneumonia Care				
Appropriate Initial Antibiotic Given	69	99%	98%	95%
Blood Culture Timing	114	99%	99%	98%
Pregnancy and Delivery Care				
Newborn Deliveries Scheduled Early[7]	-	-	6%	6%
Preventive Care				
Immunization for Influenza[2]	608	94%	94%	90%
Immunization for Pneumonia[2]	685	95%	96%	92%
Stroke Care				
Anticoagulation Therapy for Atrial Fibrillation[1]	-	-	97%	95%
Antithrombotic Therapy Timing	22	100%	98%	98%
Assessed for Rehabilitation	29	93%	97%	97%
Discharged on Antithrombotic Therapy	27	100%	99%	99%
Discharged on Statin Medication	23	100%	96%	94%
Thrombolytic Therapy Timing[1]	-	-	76%	66%
Venous Thromboembolism Prophylaxis	28	68%	95%	94%
Written Stroke Educational Materials Given	17	100%	94%	88%
Surgical Care Improvement Project				
Appropriate Beta Blocker Usage	99	100%	99%	98%
Appropriate VTP Within 24 Hours	368	99%	99%	98%
Controlled Postoperative Blood Glucose[7]	-	-	98%	97%
Perioperative Temperature Management	397	100%	100%	100%
Prophylactic Antibiotic Selection	268	100%	99%	99%
Prophylactic Antibiotic Selection (Outpatient)	184	99%	98%	98%
Prophylactic Antibiotic Stopped	256	100%	98%	98%
Prophylactic Antibiotic Timing	268	100%	99%	99%
Prophylactic Antibiotic Timing (Outpatient)	184	100%	98%	98%
Urinary Catheter Removal	110	100%	98%	97%
Survey of Patients' Hospital Experiences				
Area Around Room 'Always' Quiet at Night	300+	61%	58%	61%
Doctors 'Always' Communicated Well	300+	75%	77%	82%
Home Recovery Information Given	300+	84%	83%	85%
Hospital Given 9 or 10 on 10 Point Scale	300+	72%	67%	71%
Meds 'Always' Explained Before Given	300+	65%	60%	64%
Nurses 'Always' Communicated Well	300+	74%	75%	79%
Pain 'Always' Well Controlled	300+	69%	68%	71%
Room and Bathroom 'Always' Clean	300+	70%	69%	73%
Timely Help 'Always' Received	300+	61%	62%	68%
Would Definitely Recommend Hospital	300+	76%	69%	71%
Use of Medical Imaging				
Cardiac Imaging Stress Test before Surgery	75	4.0%	6.4%	5.3%
Combination Abdominal CT Scan	332	5.7%	11.8%	10.5%
Combination Brain/Sinus CT Scan	408	5.4%	3.4%	2.7%
Combination Chest CT Scan	212	1.9%	2.4%	2.7%
Follow-up Mammogram/Ultrasound	502	15.5%	10.2%	8.8%
Lumbar Spine MRI for Low Back Pain[1]	-	-	35.2%	37.2%

Broward Health Medical Center

1600 S Andrews Ave
Fort Lauderdale, FL 33316
URL: www.browardhealth.org
Type: Acute Care Hospitals
Ownership: Govt - Hospital Dist/Auth
Phone: 954-355-4400
Fax: 954-468-8046
Emergency Services: Yes
Beds: 592

Key Personnel:
Pediatric In-Patient Care . . . . Carol Bhim
Chief of Medical Staff . . . . Dr. Georges Boutlin, MD
Coronary Care . . . . Julie Gabriel
Radiology. . . . . Stuart Glassberg
Pediatric Ambulatory Care . . . . . . Corinne Hall
Quality Assurance . . . . Ela Lena
CEO/President. . . . . Frank Nash
Infection Control. . . . . Shirley Ochipa

Measure	Cases	This Hosp.	State Avg.	U.S. Avg.
Blood Clot Prevention and Treatment				
Anticoagulation Overlap Therapy[2]	94	91%	93%	93%
ICU Venous Thromboembolism Prophylaxis[2]	57	96%	94%	92%
Incidence of Potentially Preventable VTE[2]	40	10%	10%	10%
UFH with Dosages/Platelet Monitoring[2]	14	100%	100%	97%
Venous Thromboembolism Prophylaxis[2]	314	80%	88%	85%
Warfarin Therapy Discharge Instructions[2]	66	100%	85%	75%
Chest Pain/Possible Heart Attack Care				
Aspirin Given Within 24 Hours of Arrival[1,3]	-	-	98%	96%
Fibrinolytic Meds Within 30 Min. of Arrival[3,7]	-	-	81%	58%
Average Time to ECG (minutes)[1,3]	-	-	7	7
Average Time to Transfer (minutes)[3,7]	-	-	53	60
Children's Asthma Care				
Received Home Management Plan of Care	-	-	-	88%
Received Reliever Medication	-	-	-	100%
Received Systemic Corticosteroids	-	-	-	100%
Emergency Department				
Admittance Decision Time (minutes)[2]	622	194	111	98
Head CT Results Within 45 Min. of Arrival[1]	-	-	64%	57%
Patients Who Left ER Before Being Seen	>100k	0%	2%	2%
Time from ER Arrival to Admit. (minutes)[2]	624	351	289	274
Time from ER Arrival to Discharge (minutes)	384	163	147	134
Time in ER Before Being Evaluated (minutes)	408	19	26	26
Time to Pain Meds for Fractures (minutes)	198	36	60	57
Heart Attack Care				
Aspirin Given at Discharge[2]	290	100%	99%	99%
Fibrinolytic Meds Within 30 Min. of Arrival[2,7]	-	-	50%	54%
PCI Within 90 Minutes of Arrival[2]	42	98%	96%	96%
Statin Prescribed at Discharge[2]	285	100%	99%	98%
Heart Failure Care				
ACE Inhibitor or ARB for LVSD[2]	164	100%	98%	97%
Discharge Instructions Given[2]	313	100%	96%	94%
Evaluation of LVS Function[2]	334	100%	100%	99%
Medicare Spending				
Medicare Spending per Patient (ratio)	-	1.04	1.04	0.98
Pneumonia Care				
Appropriate Initial Antibiotic Given[2]	146	100%	98%	95%
Blood Culture Timing[2]	272	99%	99%	98%
Pregnancy and Delivery Care				
Newborn Deliveries Scheduled Early[2]	93	0%	6%	6%
Preventive Care				
Immunization for Influenza[2]	503	97%	94%	90%
Immunization for Pneumonia[2]	455	97%	96%	92%
Stroke Care				
Anticoagulation Therapy for Atrial Fibrillation	17	100%	97%	95%
Antithrombotic Therapy Timing	138	99%	98%	98%
Assessed for Rehabilitation	175	99%	97%	97%
Discharged on Antithrombotic Therapy	148	100%	99%	99%
Discharged on Statin Medication	117	99%	96%	94%
Thrombolytic Therapy Timing[1]	-	-	76%	66%
Venous Thromboembolism Prophylaxis	190	99%	95%	94%
Written Stroke Educational Materials Given	118	99%	94%	88%
Surgical Care Improvement Project				
Appropriate Beta Blocker Usage[2]	206	100%	99%	98%
Appropriate VTP Within 24 Hours[2]	508	100%	99%	98%
Controlled Postoperative Blood Glucose[2]	166	100%	98%	97%
Perioperative Temperature Management[2]	637	100%	100%	100%
Prophylactic Antibiotic Selection[2]	559	100%	99%	99%
Prophylactic Antibiotic Selection (Outpatient)	341	98%	98%	98%
Prophylactic Antibiotic Stopped[2]	535	100%	98%	98%
Prophylactic Antibiotic Timing[2]	559	100%	99%	99%
Prophylactic Antibiotic Timing (Outpatient)	325	99%	98%	98%
Urinary Catheter Removal[2]	351	100%	98%	97%
Survey of Patients' Hospital Experiences				
Area Around Room 'Always' Quiet at Night	300+	54%	58%	61%
Doctors 'Always' Communicated Well	300+	72%	77%	82%
Home Recovery Information Given	300+	79%	83%	85%
Hospital Given 9 or 10 on 10 Point Scale	300+	63%	67%	71%
Meds 'Always' Explained Before Given	300+	55%	60%	64%
Nurses 'Always' Communicated Well	300+	70%	75%	79%
Pain 'Always' Well Controlled	300+	63%	68%	71%
Room and Bathroom 'Always' Clean	300+	65%	69%	73%
Timely Help 'Always' Received	300+	50%	62%	68%
Would Definitely Recommend Hospital	300+	69%	69%	71%
Use of Medical Imaging				
Cardiac Imaging Stress Test before Surgery	210	4.3%	6.4%	5.3%
Combination Abdominal CT Scan	617	11.8%	11.8%	10.5%
Combination Brain/Sinus CT Scan	753	7.3%	3.4%	2.7%
Combination Chest CT Scan	365	4.7%	2.4%	2.7%
Follow-up Mammogram/Ultrasound	643	12.1%	10.2%	8.8%
Lumbar Spine MRI for Low Back Pain	42	40.5%	35.2%	37.2%

Holy Cross Hospital

4725 N Federal Hwy
Fort Lauderdale, FL 33308
E-mail: luisa.gutman@holy-cross.com
URL: www.holy-cross.com
Type: Acute Care Hospitals
Ownership: Voluntary non-profit - Church
Phone: 954-771-8000
Fax: 954-267-6896
Emergency Services: Yes
Beds: 581

Key Personnel:
Radiology. . . . . Carlos Duran
Patient Relations . . . . Amy Emmel
Infection Control. . . . . Elisa Fabian
Quality Assurance . . . . Sherri Gilbert
Chief of Medical Staff . . . . Kenneth Homer, MD
Pediatric Ambulatory Care . . . . . . Joanne MacLean
Hemotology Center . . . . Maureen Mann
CEO/President. . . . . Patrick Taylor, MD, MBA

Measure	Cases	This Hosp.	State Avg.	U.S. Avg.
Blood Clot Prevention and Treatment				
Anticoagulation Overlap Therapy[2]	45	98%	93%	93%
ICU Venous Thromboembolism Prophylaxis[2]	35	100%	94%	92%
Incidence of Potentially Preventable VTE[1,2]	-	-	10%	10%
UFH with Dosages/Platelet Monitoring[2]	11	100%	100%	97%
Venous Thromboembolism Prophylaxis[2]	386	99%	88%	85%
Warfarin Therapy Discharge Instructions[2]	28	100%	85%	75%
Chest Pain/Possible Heart Attack Care				
Aspirin Given Within 24 Hours of Arrival[5]	-	-	98%	96%
Fibrinolytic Meds Within 30 Min. of Arrival[5]	-	-	81%	58%
Average Time to ECG (minutes)[5]	-	-	7	7

NOTE: Hospital profiles are in alphabetical order by state, then city, then hospital within the city; Rankings exclude hospitals with less than 25 cases except for patient surveys which excludes hospitals with less than 100 cases; (a) 100-299 cases; (1) The number of cases/patients is too few to report; (2) Data submitted were based on a sample of cases/patients; (3) Results are based on a shorter time period than required; (4) Data suppressed by CMS for one or more quarters; (5) Results are not available for this reporting period; (6) Fewer than 100 patients completed the HCAHPS survey; (7) No cases met the criteria for this measure; (8) The lower limit of the confidence interval cannot be calculated if the number of observed infections equals zero; (9) No data are available from the state/territory for this reporting period; (10) The scores shown reflect fewer than 50 completed surveys; (11) There were discrepancies in the data collection process; (12) This measure does not apply to this hospital for this reporting period; (13) Results cannot be calculated for this reporting period; (14) The results for this state are combined with nearby states to protect confidentiality; Please refer to the User's Guide for a full explanation of data.

Measure	Cases	This Hosp.	State Avg.	U.S. Avg.
Average Time to Transfer (minutes)[5]	-	-	53	60
Children's Asthma Care				
Received Home Management Plan of Care	-	-	-	88%
Received Reliever Medication	-	-	-	100%
Received Systemic Corticosteroids	-	-	-	100%
Emergency Department				
Admittance Decision Time (minutes)[2]	655	121	111	98
Head CT Results Within 45 Min. of Arrival	11	55%	64%	57%
Patients Who Left ER Before Being Seen	51,075	0%	2%	2%
Time from ER Arrival to Admit. (minutes)[2]	656	320	289	274
Time from ER Arrival to Discharge (minutes)	389	152	147	134
Time in ER Before Being Evaluated (minutes)	421	18	26	26
Time to Pain Meds for Fractures (minutes)	208	68	60	57
Heart Attack Care				
Aspirin Given at Discharge	309	100%	99%	99%
Fibrinolytic Meds Within 30 Min. of Arrival[7]	-	-	50%	54%
PCI Within 90 Minutes of Arrival	43	98%	96%	96%
Statin Prescribed at Discharge	315	100%	99%	98%
Heart Failure Care				
ACE Inhibitor or ARB for LVSD	144	100%	98%	97%
Discharge Instructions Given	428	100%	96%	94%
Evaluation of LVS Function	506	100%	100%	99%
Medicare Spending				
Medicare Spending per Patient (ratio)	-	1.06	1.04	0.98
Pneumonia Care				
Appropriate Initial Antibiotic Given	115	100%	98%	95%
Blood Culture Timing	275	98%	99%	98%
Pregnancy and Delivery Care				
Newborn Deliveries Scheduled Early	98	3%	6%	6%
Preventive Care				
Immunization for Influenza[2]	580	88%	94%	90%
Immunization for Pneumonia[2]	765	87%	96%	92%
Stroke Care				
Anticoagulation Therapy for Atrial Fibrillation	35	100%	97%	95%
Antithrombotic Therapy Timing	165	93%	98%	98%
Assessed for Rehabilitation	202	100%	97%	97%
Discharged on Antithrombotic Therapy	167	99%	99%	99%
Discharged on Statin Medication	130	96%	96%	94%
Thrombolytic Therapy Timing	18	72%	76%	66%
Venous Thromboembolism Prophylaxis	226	95%	95%	94%
Written Stroke Educational Materials Given	117	96%	94%	88%
Surgical Care Improvement Project				
Appropriate Beta Blocker Usage[2]	215	100%	99%	98%
Appropriate VTP Within 24 Hours[2]	518	100%	99%	98%
Controlled Postoperative Blood Glucose[2]	212	98%	98%	97%
Perioperative Temperature Management[2]	628	100%	100%	100%
Prophylactic Antibiotic Selection[2]	544	99%	99%	99%
Prophylactic Antibiotic Selection (Outpatient)	474	99%	98%	98%
Prophylactic Antibiotic Stopped[2]	537	99%	98%	98%
Prophylactic Antibiotic Timing[2]	545	100%	99%	99%
Prophylactic Antibiotic Timing (Outpatient)	474	100%	98%	98%
Urinary Catheter Removal[2]	558	100%	98%	97%
Survey of Patients' Hospital Experiences				
Area Around Room 'Always' Quiet at Night	300+	53%	58%	61%
Doctors 'Always' Communicated Well	300+	80%	77%	82%
Home Recovery Information Given	300+	81%	83%	85%
Hospital Given 9 or 10 on 10 Point Scale	300+	70%	67%	71%
Meds 'Always' Explained Before Given	300+	60%	60%	64%
Nurses 'Always' Communicated Well	300+	74%	75%	79%
Pain 'Always' Well Controlled	300+	67%	68%	71%
Room and Bathroom 'Always' Clean	300+	67%	69%	73%
Timely Help 'Always' Received	300+	57%	62%	68%
Would Definitely Recommend Hospital	300+	76%	69%	71%
Use of Medical Imaging				
Cardiac Imaging Stress Test before Surgery	2,376	6.1%	6.4%	5.3%
Combination Abdominal CT Scan	1,542	4.1%	11.8%	10.5%
Combination Brain/Sinus CT Scan	949	1.3%	3.4%	2.7%
Combination Chest CT Scan	1,359	0.0%	2.4%	2.7%
Follow-up Mammogram/Ultrasound	2,200	16.9%	10.2%	8.8%
Lumbar Spine MRI for Low Back Pain	155	32.3%	35.2%	37.2%

Gulf Coast Medical Center Lee Memorial Health System

13681 Doctor's Way
Fort Myers, FL 33912
URL: www.leememorial.org
Phone: 239-768-5000
Fax: 239-768-8379
Type: Acute Care Hospitals
Ownership: Govt - Hospital Dist/Auth
Emergency Services: Yes
Beds: 120

Key Personnel:
Emergency Room . . . . Myrian Alea
Chairman/CEO . . . . Sanford Cohen, MD
Chief of Medical Staff . . . . Gary J Correnti
Patient Relations . . . . Donna Giannuzzi
CEO/President . . . . James R Nathan

Measure	Cases	This Hosp.	State Avg.	U.S. Avg.
Blood Clot Prevention and Treatment				
Anticoagulation Overlap Therapy[2]	216	84%	93%	93%
ICU Venous Thromboembolism Prophylaxis[2]	52	77%	94%	92%
Incidence of Potentially Preventable VTE[2]	73	15%	10%	10%
UFH with Dosages/Platelet Monitoring[2]	194	99%	100%	97%
Venous Thromboembolism Prophylaxis[2]	341	81%	88%	85%
Warfarin Therapy Discharge Instructions[2]	154	92%	85%	75%
Chest Pain/Possible Heart Attack Care				
Aspirin Given Within 24 Hours of Arrival[1]	-	-	98%	96%
Fibrinolytic Meds Within 30 Min. of Arrival[5]	-	-	81%	58%
Average Time to ECG (minutes)[1]	-	-	7	7
Average Time to Transfer (minutes)[5]	-	-	53	60
Children's Asthma Care				
Received Home Management Plan of Care	-	-	-	88%
Received Reliever Medication	-	-	-	100%
Received Systemic Corticosteroids	-	-	-	100%
Emergency Department				
Admittance Decision Time (minutes)[2]	762	152	111	98
Head CT Results Within 45 Min. of Arrival[1]	-	-	64%	57%
Patients Who Left ER Before Being Seen	29,554	0%	2%	2%
Time from ER Arrival to Admit. (minutes)[2]	766	340	289	274
Time from ER Arrival to Discharge (minutes)	368	208	147	134
Time in ER Before Being Evaluated (minutes)	371	41	26	26
Time to Pain Meds for Fractures (minutes)	88	68	60	57
Heart Attack Care				
Aspirin Given at Discharge[2]	270	99%	99%	99%
Fibrinolytic Meds Within 30 Min. of Arrival[2,7]	-	-	50%	54%
PCI Within 90 Minutes of Arrival[2]	60	90%	96%	96%
Statin Prescribed at Discharge[2]	257	98%	99%	98%
Heart Failure Care				
ACE Inhibitor or ARB for LVSD[2]	91	87%	98%	97%
Discharge Instructions Given[2]	252	89%	96%	94%
Evaluation of LVS Function[2]	298	99%	100%	99%
Medicare Spending				
Medicare Spending per Patient (ratio)	-	1.02	1.04	0.98
Pneumonia Care				
Appropriate Initial Antibiotic Given[2]	83	95%	98%	95%
Blood Culture Timing[2]	171	98%	99%	98%
Pregnancy and Delivery Care				
Newborn Deliveries Scheduled Early[2]	49	8%	6%	6%
Preventive Care				
Immunization for Influenza[2]	585	83%	94%	90%
Immunization for Pneumonia[2]	820	84%	96%	92%
Stroke Care				
Anticoagulation Therapy for Atrial Fibrillation[2]	22	100%	97%	95%
Antithrombotic Therapy Timing[2]	111	98%	98%	98%
Assessed for Rehabilitation[2]	147	99%	97%	97%
Discharged on Antithrombotic Therapy[2]	132	100%	99%	99%
Discharged on Statin Medication[2]	104	97%	96%	94%
Thrombolytic Therapy Timing[2]	27	100%	76%	66%
Venous Thromboembolism Prophylaxis[2]	158	97%	95%	94%
Written Stroke Educational Materials Given[2]	71	100%	94%	88%
Surgical Care Improvement Project				
Appropriate Beta Blocker Usage[2]	237	99%	99%	98%
Appropriate VTP Within 24 Hours[2]	420	97%	99%	98%
Controlled Postoperative Blood Glucose[2]	57	98%	98%	97%
Perioperative Temperature Management[2]	570	100%	100%	100%
Prophylactic Antibiotic Selection[2]	424	98%	99%	99%
Prophylactic Antibiotic Selection (Outpatient)	417	97%	98%	98%
Prophylactic Antibiotic Stopped[2]	403	95%	98%	98%
Prophylactic Antibiotic Timing[2]	425	99%	99%	99%
Prophylactic Antibiotic Timing (Outpatient)	419	97%	98%	98%
Urinary Catheter Removal[2]	217	94%	98%	97%
Survey of Patients' Hospital Experiences				
Area Around Room 'Always' Quiet at Night	300+	54%	58%	61%
Doctors 'Always' Communicated Well	300+	70%	77%	82%
Home Recovery Information Given	300+	84%	83%	85%
Hospital Given 9 or 10 on 10 Point Scale	300+	64%	67%	71%
Meds 'Always' Explained Before Given	300+	58%	60%	64%
Nurses 'Always' Communicated Well	300+	75%	75%	79%
Pain 'Always' Well Controlled	300+	68%	68%	71%
Room and Bathroom 'Always' Clean	300+	64%	69%	73%
Timely Help 'Always' Received	300+	62%	62%	68%
Would Definitely Recommend Hospital	300+	70%	69%	71%
Use of Medical Imaging				
Cardiac Imaging Stress Test before Surgery	227	4.0%	6.4%	5.3%
Combination Abdominal CT Scan	555	51.2%	11.8%	10.5%
Combination Brain/Sinus CT Scan	991	4.0%	3.4%	2.7%
Combination Chest CT Scan	132	0.8%	2.4%	2.7%
Follow-up Mammogram/Ultrasound[7]	-	-	10.2%	8.8%
Lumbar Spine MRI for Low Back Pain[1]	-	-	35.2%	37.2%

Lee Memorial Hospital

2776 Cleveland Ave
Fort Myers, FL 33901
URL: www.leememorial.org
Phone: 239-332-1111
Fax: 239-772-6565
Type: Acute Care Hospitals
Ownership: Govt - Hospital Dist/Auth
Emergency Services: Yes
Beds: 367

Key Personnel:
Chairman/CEO . . . . Sanford Cohen, MD
Patient Relations . . . . Donna Giannuzzi
Chief of Medical Staff . . . . Chuck Krivenko, MD
CEO/President . . . . James R Nathan

Measure	Cases	This Hosp.	State Avg.	U.S. Avg.
Blood Clot Prevention and Treatment				
Anticoagulation Overlap Therapy[2]	212	81%	93%	93%
ICU Venous Thromboembolism Prophylaxis[2]	71	83%	94%	92%
Incidence of Potentially Preventable VTE[2]	54	13%	10%	10%
UFH with Dosages/Platelet Monitoring[2]	79	100%	100%	97%
Venous Thromboembolism Prophylaxis[2]	314	82%	88%	85%
Warfarin Therapy Discharge Instructions[2]	160	94%	85%	75%
Chest Pain/Possible Heart Attack Care				
Aspirin Given Within 24 Hours of Arrival	15	100%	98%	96%
Fibrinolytic Meds Within 30 Min. of Arrival[3,7]	-	-	81%	58%
Average Time to ECG (minutes)	15	9	7	7
Average Time to Transfer (minutes)[3,7]	-	-	53	60
Children's Asthma Care				
Received Home Management Plan of Care	-	-	-	88%
Received Reliever Medication	-	-	-	100%
Received Systemic Corticosteroids	-	-	-	100%
Emergency Department				
Admittance Decision Time (minutes)[2]	661	157	111	98
Head CT Results Within 45 Min. of Arrival[1]	-	-	64%	57%
Patients Who Left ER Before Being Seen	70,513	0%	2%	2%
Time from ER Arrival to Admit. (minutes)[2]	669	329	289	274
Time from ER Arrival to Discharge (minutes)	369	172	147	134
Time in ER Before Being Evaluated (minutes)	354	47	26	26
Time to Pain Meds for Fractures (minutes)	264	68	60	57
Heart Attack Care				
Aspirin Given at Discharge[2]	297	98%	99%	99%
Fibrinolytic Meds Within 30 Min. of Arrival[2,7]	-	-	50%	54%
PCI Within 90 Minutes of Arrival[2]	33	82%	96%	96%
Statin Prescribed at Discharge[2]	283	97%	99%	98%
Heart Failure Care				
ACE Inhibitor or ARB for LVSD[2]	120	91%	98%	97%
Discharge Instructions Given[2]	257	82%	96%	94%
Evaluation of LVS Function[2]	297	100%	100%	99%
Medicare Spending				
Medicare Spending per Patient (ratio)	-	1.01	1.04	0.98
Pneumonia Care				
Appropriate Initial Antibiotic Given[2]	102	94%	98%	95%
Blood Culture Timing[2]	163	96%	99%	98%
Pregnancy and Delivery Care				

NOTE: Hospital profiles are in alphabetical order by state, then city, then hospital within the city; Rankings exclude hospitals with less than 25 cases except for patient surveys which excludes hospitals with less than 100 cases; (a) 100-299 cases; (1) The number of cases/patients is too few to report; (2) Data submitted were based on a sample of cases/patients; (3) Results are based on a shorter time period than required; (4) Data suppressed by CMS for one or more quarters; (5) Results are not available for this reporting period; (6) Fewer than 100 patients completed the HCAHPS survey; (7) No cases met the criteria for this measure; (8) The lower limit of the confidence interval cannot be calculated if the number of observed infections equals zero; (9) No data are available from the state/territory for this reporting period; (10) The scores shown reflect fewer than 50 completed surveys; (11) There were discrepancies in the data collection process; (12) This measure does not apply to this hospital for this reporting period; (13) Results cannot be calculated for this reporting period; (14) The results for this state are combined with nearby states to protect confidentiality; Please refer to the User's Guide for a full explanation of data.

Measure	Cases	This Hosp.	State Avg.	U.S. Avg.
Newborn Deliveries Scheduled Early[2]	67	6%	6%	6%
Preventive Care				
Immunization for Influenza[2]	556	75%	94%	90%
Immunization for Pneumonia[2]	641	77%	96%	92%
Stroke Care				
Anticoagulation Therapy for Atrial Fibrillation[2]	29	100%	97%	95%
Antithrombotic Therapy Timing[2]	153	93%	98%	98%
Assessed for Rehabilitation[2]	195	96%	97%	97%
Discharged on Antithrombotic Therapy[2]	174	99%	99%	99%
Discharged on Statin Medication[2]	141	93%	96%	94%
Thrombolytic Therapy Timing[2]	30	87%	76%	66%
Venous Thromboembolism Prophylaxis[2]	211	94%	95%	94%
Written Stroke Educational Materials Given[2]	127	100%	94%	88%
Surgical Care Improvement Project				
Appropriate Beta Blocker Usage[2]	369	98%	99%	98%
Appropriate VTP Within 24 Hours[2]	504	96%	99%	98%
Controlled Postoperative Blood Glucose[2]	192	97%	98%	97%
Perioperative Temperature Management[2]	657	99%	100%	100%
Prophylactic Antibiotic Selection[2]	583	97%	99%	99%
Prophylactic Antibiotic Selection (Outpatient)	702	98%	98%	98%
Prophylactic Antibiotic Stopped[2]	562	93%	98%	98%
Prophylactic Antibiotic Timing[2]	584	98%	99%	99%
Prophylactic Antibiotic Timing (Outpatient)	709	93%	98%	98%
Urinary Catheter Removal[2]	202	79%	98%	97%
Survey of Patients' Hospital Experiences				
Area Around Room 'Always' Quiet at Night	300+	58%	58%	61%
Doctors 'Always' Communicated Well	300+	75%	77%	82%
Home Recovery Information Given	300+	85%	83%	85%
Hospital Given 9 or 10 on 10 Point Scale	300+	68%	67%	71%
Meds 'Always' Explained Before Given	300+	62%	60%	64%
Nurses 'Always' Communicated Well	300+	78%	75%	79%
Pain 'Always' Well Controlled	300+	70%	68%	71%
Room and Bathroom 'Always' Clean	300+	68%	69%	73%
Timely Help 'Always' Received	300+	64%	62%	68%
Would Definitely Recommend Hospital	300+	75%	69%	71%
Use of Medical Imaging				
Cardiac Imaging Stress Test before Surgery	2,080	5.9%	6.4%	5.3%
Combination Abdominal CT Scan	1,480	58.2%	11.8%	10.5%
Combination Brain/Sinus CT Scan	1,635	4.3%	3.4%	2.7%
Combination Chest CT Scan	783	0.1%	2.4%	2.7%
Follow-up Mammogram/Ultrasound	3,309	7.0%	10.2%	8.8%
Lumbar Spine MRI for Low Back Pain	291	32.6%	35.2%	37.2%

Lawnwood Regional Medical Center & Heart Institute

1700 S 23rd St
Fort Pierce, FL 34950
URL: www.lawnwoodmed.com
Type: Acute Care Hospitals
Ownership: Proprietary
Phone: 772-461-4000
Fax: 877-567-8583
Emergency Services: Yes
Beds: 36

Measure	Cases	This Hosp.	State Avg.	U.S. Avg.
Blood Clot Prevention and Treatment				
Anticoagulation Overlap Therapy[2]	107	99%	93%	93%
ICU Venous Thromboembolism Prophylaxis[2]	124	100%	94%	92%
Incidence of Potentially Preventable VTE[2]	19	0%	10%	10%
UFH with Dosages/Platelet Monitoring[2]	97	100%	100%	97%
Venous Thromboembolism Prophylaxis[2]	340	99%	88%	85%
Warfarin Therapy Discharge Instructions[2]	84	93%	85%	75%
Chest Pain/Possible Heart Attack Care				
Aspirin Given Within 24 Hours of Arrival[5]	-	-	98%	96%
Fibrinolytic Meds Within 30 Min. of Arrival[5]	-	-	81%	58%
Average Time to ECG (minutes)[5]	-	-	7	7
Average Time to Transfer (minutes)[5]	-	-	53	60
Children's Asthma Care				
Received Home Management Plan of Care	76	100%	-	88%
Received Reliever Medication	77	100%	-	100%
Received Systemic Corticosteroids	77	100%	-	100%
Emergency Department				
Admittance Decision Time (minutes)[2]	835	104	111	98
Head CT Results Within 45 Min. of Arrival[1]	-	-	64%	57%
Patients Who Left ER Before Being Seen	55,333	0%	2%	2%
Time from ER Arrival to Admit. (minutes)[2]	835	256	289	274
Time from ER Arrival to Discharge (minutes)	459	136	147	134
Time in ER Before Being Evaluated (minutes)	520	13	26	26
Time to Pain Meds for Fractures (minutes)	134	62	60	57
Heart Attack Care				
Aspirin Given at Discharge	577	100%	99%	99%
Fibrinolytic Meds Within 30 Min. of Arrival[7]	-	-	50%	54%
PCI Within 90 Minutes of Arrival	32	100%	96%	96%
Statin Prescribed at Discharge	570	100%	99%	98%
Heart Failure Care				
ACE Inhibitor or ARB for LVSD	217	100%	98%	97%
Discharge Instructions Given	463	100%	96%	94%
Evaluation of LVS Function	532	100%	100%	99%
Medicare Spending				
Medicare Spending per Patient (ratio)	-	1.06	1.04	0.98
Pneumonia Care				
Appropriate Initial Antibiotic Given	143	100%	98%	95%
Blood Culture Timing	337	100%	99%	98%
Pregnancy and Delivery Care				
Newborn Deliveries Scheduled Early	138	1%	6%	6%
Preventive Care				
Immunization for Influenza[2]	598	100%	94%	90%
Immunization for Pneumonia[2]	682	100%	96%	92%
Stroke Care				
Anticoagulation Therapy for Atrial Fibrillation	32	100%	97%	95%
Antithrombotic Therapy Timing	324	100%	98%	98%
Assessed for Rehabilitation	378	100%	97%	97%
Discharged on Antithrombotic Therapy	325	100%	99%	99%
Discharged on Statin Medication	255	100%	96%	94%
Thrombolytic Therapy Timing[1]	-	-	76%	66%
Venous Thromboembolism Prophylaxis	407	100%	95%	94%
Written Stroke Educational Materials Given	234	100%	94%	88%
Surgical Care Improvement Project				
Appropriate Beta Blocker Usage	296	100%	99%	98%
Appropriate VTP Within 24 Hours	434	100%	99%	98%
Controlled Postoperative Blood Glucose	213	100%	98%	97%
Perioperative Temperature Management	544	100%	100%	100%
Prophylactic Antibiotic Selection	394	100%	99%	99%
Prophylactic Antibiotic Selection (Outpatient)	273	100%	98%	98%
Prophylactic Antibiotic Stopped	362	100%	98%	98%
Prophylactic Antibiotic Timing	395	100%	99%	99%
Prophylactic Antibiotic Timing (Outpatient)	273	100%	98%	98%
Urinary Catheter Removal	365	100%	98%	97%
Survey of Patients' Hospital Experiences				
Area Around Room 'Always' Quiet at Night	300+	50%	58%	61%
Doctors 'Always' Communicated Well	300+	73%	77%	82%
Home Recovery Information Given	300+	82%	83%	85%
Hospital Given 9 or 10 on 10 Point Scale	300+	59%	67%	71%
Meds 'Always' Explained Before Given	300+	57%	60%	64%
Nurses 'Always' Communicated Well	300+	71%	75%	79%
Pain 'Always' Well Controlled	300+	66%	68%	71%
Room and Bathroom 'Always' Clean	300+	63%	69%	73%
Timely Help 'Always' Received	300+	55%	62%	68%
Would Definitely Recommend Hospital	300+	61%	69%	71%
Use of Medical Imaging				
Cardiac Imaging Stress Test before Surgery	62	6.5%	6.4%	5.3%
Combination Abdominal CT Scan	541	2.4%	11.8%	10.5%
Combination Brain/Sinus CT Scan	726	4.4%	3.4%	2.7%
Combination Chest CT Scan	247	2.0%	2.4%	2.7%
Follow-up Mammogram/Ultrasound[7]	-	-	10.2%	8.8%
Lumbar Spine MRI for Low Back Pain[1]	-	-	35.2%	37.2%

Fort Walton Beach Medical Center

1000 Mar - Walt Dr
Fort Walton Beach, FL 32547
URL: www.fwbmedicalcenter.com
Type: Acute Care Hospitals
Ownership: Proprietary
Phone: 850-862-1111
Fax: 850-862-9149
Emergency Services: Yes
Beds: 247

Key Personnel:
Operating Room. . . . . David W Burkland
Cardiac Laboratory. . . . . Stan Clark
Intensive Care Unit. . . . . Linda Davis
Chief of Medical Staff. . . . . Thomas Holt
Emergency Room . . . . Cathy McIntyre
CEO . . . . Mitch Mongell, FACHE
Quality Assurance . . . . Evelyn Ross

Measure	Cases	This Hosp.	State Avg.	U.S. Avg.
Blood Clot Prevention and Treatment				
Anticoagulation Overlap Therapy[2]	43	100%	93%	93%
ICU Venous Thromboembolism Prophylaxis[2]	125	94%	94%	92%
Incidence of Potentially Preventable VTE[1,2]	-	-	10%	10%
UFH with Dosages/Platelet Monitoring[1,2]	-	-	100%	97%
Venous Thromboembolism Prophylaxis[2]	296	91%	88%	85%
Warfarin Therapy Discharge Instructions[2]	32	100%	85%	75%
Chest Pain/Possible Heart Attack Care				
Aspirin Given Within 24 Hours of Arrival[1,3]	-	-	98%	96%
Fibrinolytic Meds Within 30 Min. of Arrival[5]	-	-	81%	58%
Average Time to ECG (minutes)[1,3]	-	-	7	7
Average Time to Transfer (minutes)[5]	-	-	53	60
Children's Asthma Care				
Received Home Management Plan of Care	-	-	-	88%
Received Reliever Medication	-	-	-	100%
Received Systemic Corticosteroids	-	-	-	100%
Emergency Department				
Admittance Decision Time (minutes)[2]	789	72	111	98
Head CT Results Within 45 Min. of Arrival[3,7]	-	-	64%	57%
Patients Who Left ER Before Being Seen	63,370	1%	2%	2%
Time from ER Arrival to Admit. (minutes)[2]	789	239	289	274
Time from ER Arrival to Discharge (minutes)	486	108	147	134
Time in ER Before Being Evaluated (minutes)	518	9	26	26
Time to Pain Meds for Fractures (minutes)	121	57	60	57
Heart Attack Care				
Aspirin Given at Discharge	237	100%	99%	99%
Fibrinolytic Meds Within 30 Min. of Arrival[7]	-	-	50%	54%
PCI Within 90 Minutes of Arrival	34	100%	96%	96%
Statin Prescribed at Discharge	217	100%	99%	98%
Heart Failure Care				
ACE Inhibitor or ARB for LVSD	94	100%	98%	97%
Discharge Instructions Given	236	98%	96%	94%
Evaluation of LVS Function	293	100%	100%	99%
Medicare Spending				
Medicare Spending per Patient (ratio)	-	0.98	1.04	0.98
Pneumonia Care				
Appropriate Initial Antibiotic Given	118	98%	98%	95%
Blood Culture Timing	203	100%	99%	98%
Pregnancy and Delivery Care				
Newborn Deliveries Scheduled Early[2]	27	0%	6%	6%
Preventive Care				
Immunization for Influenza[2]	565	98%	94%	90%
Immunization for Pneumonia[2]	739	97%	96%	92%
Stroke Care				
Anticoagulation Therapy for Atrial Fibrillation[2]	13	100%	97%	95%
Antithrombotic Therapy Timing[2]	89	100%	98%	98%
Assessed for Rehabilitation[2]	118	100%	97%	97%
Discharged on Antithrombotic Therapy[2]	108	100%	99%	99%
Discharged on Statin Medication[2]	91	100%	96%	94%
Thrombolytic Therapy Timing[2]	12	83%	76%	66%
Venous Thromboembolism Prophylaxis[2]	117	98%	95%	94%
Written Stroke Educational Materials Given[2]	67	100%	94%	88%
Surgical Care Improvement Project				
Appropriate Beta Blocker Usage[2]	154	99%	99%	98%
Appropriate VTP Within 24 Hours[2]	359	99%	99%	98%
Controlled Postoperative Blood Glucose[2]	95	100%	98%	97%
Perioperative Temperature Management[2]	494	100%	100%	100%
Prophylactic Antibiotic Selection[2]	346	100%	99%	99%
Prophylactic Antibiotic Selection (Outpatient)	167	100%	98%	98%
Prophylactic Antibiotic Stopped[2]	327	99%	98%	98%
Prophylactic Antibiotic Timing[2]	348	100%	99%	99%
Prophylactic Antibiotic Timing (Outpatient)	167	100%	98%	98%
Urinary Catheter Removal[2]	279	100%	98%	97%
Survey of Patients' Hospital Experiences				
Area Around Room 'Always' Quiet at Night	300+	65%	58%	61%
Doctors 'Always' Communicated Well	300+	78%	77%	82%
Home Recovery Information Given	300+	85%	83%	85%
Hospital Given 9 or 10 on 10 Point Scale	300+	62%	67%	71%
Meds 'Always' Explained Before Given	300+	61%	60%	64%
Nurses 'Always' Communicated Well	300+	73%	75%	79%
Pain 'Always' Well Controlled	300+	69%	68%	71%

NOTE: Hospital profiles are in alphabetical order by state, then city, then hospital within the city; Rankings exclude hospitals with less than 25 cases except for patient surveys which excludes hospitals with less than 100 cases; (a) 100-299 cases; (1) The number of cases/patients is too few to report; (2) Data submitted were based on a sample of cases/patients; (3) Results are based on a shorter time period than required; (4) Data suppressed by CMS for one or more quarters; (5) Results are not available for this reporting period; (6) Fewer than 100 patients completed the HCAHPS survey; (7) No cases met the criteria for this measure; (8) The lower limit of the confidence interval cannot be calculated if the number of observed infections equals zero; (9) No data are available from the state/territory for this reporting period; (10) The scores shown reflect fewer than 50 completed surveys; (11) There were discrepancies in the data collection process; (12) This measure does not apply to this hospital for this reporting period; (13) Results cannot be calculated for this reporting period; (14) The results for this state are combined with nearby states to protect confidentiality; Please refer to the User's Guide for a full explanation of data.

Room and Bathroom 'Always' Clean	300+	64%	69%	73%
Timely Help 'Always' Received	300+	60%	62%	68%
Would Definitely Recommend Hospital	300+	63%	69%	71%
Use of Medical Imaging				
Cardiac Imaging Stress Test before Surgery	210	5.7%	6.4%	5.3%
Combination Abdominal CT Scan	548	17.2%	11.8%	10.5%
Combination Brain/Sinus CT Scan	803	3.7%	3.4%	2.7%
Combination Chest CT Scan	221	12.2%	2.4%	2.7%
Follow-up Mammogram/Ultrasound	347	16.1%	10.2%	8.8%
Lumbar Spine MRI for Low Back Pain	48	43.8%	35.2%	37.2%

North Florida Regional Medical Center

6500 Newberry Rd Phone: 352-333-4100
Gainesville, FL 32605 Fax: 352-333-4800
URL: www.nfrmc.com
Type: Acute Care Hospitals Emergency Services: Yes
Ownership: Proprietary Beds: 353
Key Personnel:
CEO/President. . . . . Wardn Boston III
Quality Assurance . . . . Jane Patterson
Radiology. . . . . Robert Stouffer

Measure	Cases	This Hosp.	State Avg.	U.S. Avg.
Blood Clot Prevention and Treatment				
Anticoagulation Overlap Therapy[2]	115	100%	93%	93%
ICU Venous Thromboembolism Prophylaxis[2]	77	99%	94%	92%
Incidence of Potentially Preventable VTE[2]	20	0%	10%	10%
UFH with Dosages/Platelet Monitoring[2]	78	100%	100%	97%
Venous Thromboembolism Prophylaxis[2]	393	96%	88%	85%
Warfarin Therapy Discharge Instructions[2]	85	100%	85%	75%
Chest Pain/Possible Heart Attack Care				
Aspirin Given Within 24 Hours of Arrival[5]	-	-	98%	96%
Fibrinolytic Meds Within 30 Min. of Arrival[5]	-	-	81%	58%
Average Time to ECG (minutes)[5]	-	-	7	7
Average Time to Transfer (minutes)[5]	-	-	53	60
Children's Asthma Care				
Received Home Management Plan of Care	-	-	-	88%
Received Reliever Medication	-	-	-	100%
Received Systemic Corticosteroids	-	-	-	100%
Emergency Department				
Admittance Decision Time (minutes)[2]	966	117	111	98
Head CT Results Within 45 Min. of Arrival	16	81%	64%	57%
Patients Who Left ER Before Being Seen	66,691	0%	2%	2%
Time from ER Arrival to Admit. (minutes)[2]	966	276	289	274
Time from ER Arrival to Discharge (minutes)	460	188	147	134
Time in ER Before Being Evaluated (minutes)	509	20	26	26
Time to Pain Meds for Fractures (minutes)	86	69	60	57
Heart Attack Care				
Aspirin Given at Discharge	481	100%	99%	99%
Fibrinolytic Meds Within 30 Min. of Arrival[7]	-	-	50%	54%
PCI Within 90 Minutes of Arrival	64	100%	96%	96%
Statin Prescribed at Discharge	436	100%	99%	98%
Heart Failure Care				
ACE Inhibitor or ARB for LVSD[2]	72	100%	98%	97%
Discharge Instructions Given[2]	278	100%	96%	94%
Evaluation of LVS Function[2]	329	100%	100%	99%
Medicare Spending				
Medicare Spending per Patient (ratio)	-	0.99	1.04	0.98
Pneumonia Care				
Appropriate Initial Antibiotic Given	291	100%	98%	95%
Blood Culture Timing	562	100%	99%	98%
Pregnancy and Delivery Care				
Newborn Deliveries Scheduled Early[2]	38	3%	6%	6%
Preventive Care				
Immunization for Influenza[2]	654	99%	94%	90%
Immunization for Pneumonia[2]	921	100%	96%	92%
Stroke Care				
Anticoagulation Therapy for Atrial Fibrillation	23	100%	97%	95%
Antithrombotic Therapy Timing	220	99%	98%	98%
Assessed for Rehabilitation	225	98%	97%	97%
Discharged on Antithrombotic Therapy	216	100%	99%	99%
Discharged on Statin Medication	170	99%	96%	94%
Thrombolytic Therapy Timing	12	92%	76%	66%
Venous Thromboembolism Prophylaxis	225	99%	95%	94%
Written Stroke Educational Materials Given	151	100%	94%	88%
Surgical Care Improvement Project				
Appropriate Beta Blocker Usage[2]	269	100%	99%	98%
Appropriate VTP Within 24 Hours[2]	530	99%	99%	98%
Controlled Postoperative Blood Glucose[2]	143	100%	98%	97%
Perioperative Temperature Management[2]	675	100%	100%	100%
Prophylactic Antibiotic Selection[2]	573	100%	99%	99%
Prophylactic Antibiotic Selection (Outpatient)	741	100%	98%	98%
Prophylactic Antibiotic Stopped[2]	565	100%	98%	98%
Prophylactic Antibiotic Timing[2]	574	100%	99%	99%
Prophylactic Antibiotic Timing (Outpatient)	741	100%	98%	98%
Urinary Catheter Removal[2]	518	100%	98%	97%
Survey of Patients' Hospital Experiences				
Area Around Room 'Always' Quiet at Night	300+	55%	58%	61%
Doctors 'Always' Communicated Well	300+	78%	77%	82%
Home Recovery Information Given	300+	83%	83%	85%
Hospital Given 9 or 10 on 10 Point Scale	300+	66%	67%	71%
Meds 'Always' Explained Before Given	300+	58%	60%	64%
Nurses 'Always' Communicated Well	300+	73%	75%	79%
Pain 'Always' Well Controlled	300+	67%	68%	71%
Room and Bathroom 'Always' Clean	300+	62%	69%	73%
Timely Help 'Always' Received	300+	57%	62%	68%
Would Definitely Recommend Hospital	300+	73%	69%	71%
Use of Medical Imaging				
Cardiac Imaging Stress Test before Surgery	617	4.4%	6.4%	5.3%
Combination Abdominal CT Scan	1,159	0.8%	11.8%	10.5%
Combination Brain/Sinus CT Scan	1,643	2.3%	3.4%	2.7%
Combination Chest CT Scan	122	0.0%	2.4%	2.7%
Follow-up Mammogram/Ultrasound	222	6.8%	10.2%	8.8%
Lumbar Spine MRI for Low Back Pain[1]	-	-	35.2%	37.2%

UF Health Shands Hospital

1600 Sw Archer Rd Phone: 352-265-8000
Gainesville, FL 32610 Fax: 352-265-7948
E-mail: consult@shands.ufl.edu
URL: www.shands.org
Type: Acute Care Hospitals Emergency Services: Yes
Ownership: Government - Federal Beds: 2,000
Key Personnel:
Radiology. . . . . Steven Blumberg
Administrator . . . . Marina Cecchini, M.B.A.
Pediatric In-Patient Care . . . . Terrance R Flotte, MD
Chief of Medical Staff. . . . . Timothy Flynn, M.D., F.A.C.S.
President. . . . . David S. Guzick, M.D., Ph.D.
Quality Assurance . . . . Randy Harmatz, M.B.A

Measure	Cases	This Hosp.	State Avg.	U.S. Avg.
Blood Clot Prevention and Treatment				
Anticoagulation Overlap Therapy[2]	188	96%	93%	93%
ICU Venous Thromboembolism Prophylaxis[2]	101	94%	94%	92%
Incidence of Potentially Preventable VTE[2]	80	4%	10%	10%
UFH with Dosages/Platelet Monitoring[2]	238	100%	100%	97%
Venous Thromboembolism Prophylaxis[2]	321	87%	88%	85%
Warfarin Therapy Discharge Instructions[2]	135	83%	85%	75%
Chest Pain/Possible Heart Attack Care				
Aspirin Given Within 24 Hours of Arrival[1,3]	-	-	98%	96%
Fibrinolytic Meds Within 30 Min. of Arrival[5]	-	-	81%	58%
Average Time to ECG (minutes)[1,3]	-	-	7	7
Average Time to Transfer (minutes)[5]	-	-	53	60
Children's Asthma Care				
Received Home Management Plan of Care	-	-	-	88%
Received Reliever Medication	-	-	-	100%
Received Systemic Corticosteroids	-	-	-	100%
Emergency Department				
Admittance Decision Time (minutes)[2]	441	191	111	98
Head CT Results Within 45 Min. of Arrival[1]	-	-	64%	57%
Patients Who Left ER Before Being Seen	87,842	4%	2%	2%
Time from ER Arrival to Admit. (minutes)[2]	442	414	289	274
Time from ER Arrival to Discharge (minutes)	308	242	147	134
Time in ER Before Being Evaluated (minutes)	358	44	26	26
Time to Pain Meds for Fractures (minutes)	321	69	60	57
Heart Attack Care				
Aspirin Given at Discharge	265	99%	99%	99%
Fibrinolytic Meds Within 30 Min. of Arrival[7]	-	-	50%	54%
PCI Within 90 Minutes of Arrival	52	100%	96%	96%
Statin Prescribed at Discharge	259	99%	99%	98%
Heart Failure Care				
ACE Inhibitor or ARB for LVSD[2]	138	100%	98%	97%
Discharge Instructions Given[2]	243	93%	96%	94%
Evaluation of LVS Function[2]	274	100%	100%	99%
Medicare Spending				
Medicare Spending per Patient (ratio)	-	1.00	1.04	0.98
Pneumonia Care				
Appropriate Initial Antibiotic Given[2]	22	95%	98%	95%
Blood Culture Timing[2]	107	99%	99%	98%
Pregnancy and Delivery Care				
Newborn Deliveries Scheduled Early[2]	30	7%	6%	6%
Preventive Care				
Immunization for Influenza[2]	532	92%	94%	90%
Immunization for Pneumonia[2]	513	93%	96%	92%
Stroke Care				
Anticoagulation Therapy for Atrial Fibrillation[2]	11	100%	97%	95%
Antithrombotic Therapy Timing[2]	44	98%	98%	98%
Assessed for Rehabilitation[2]	117	96%	97%	97%
Discharged on Antithrombotic Therapy[2]	69	100%	99%	99%
Discharged on Statin Medication[2]	49	98%	96%	94%
Thrombolytic Therapy Timing[2]	11	100%	76%	66%
Venous Thromboembolism Prophylaxis[2]	130	98%	95%	94%
Written Stroke Educational Materials Given[2]	55	76%	94%	88%
Surgical Care Improvement Project				
Appropriate Beta Blocker Usage[2]	216	98%	99%	98%
Appropriate VTP Within 24 Hours[2]	437	99%	99%	98%
Controlled Postoperative Blood Glucose[2]	112	96%	98%	97%
Perioperative Temperature Management[2]	556	100%	100%	100%
Prophylactic Antibiotic Selection[2]	383	100%	99%	99%
Prophylactic Antibiotic Selection (Outpatient)	423	99%	98%	98%
Prophylactic Antibiotic Stopped[2]	365	98%	98%	98%
Prophylactic Antibiotic Timing[2]	387	100%	99%	99%
Prophylactic Antibiotic Timing (Outpatient)	423	98%	98%	98%
Urinary Catheter Removal[2]	345	98%	98%	97%
Survey of Patients' Hospital Experiences				
Area Around Room 'Always' Quiet at Night	300+	57%	58%	61%
Doctors 'Always' Communicated Well	300+	80%	77%	82%
Home Recovery Information Given	300+	89%	83%	85%
Hospital Given 9 or 10 on 10 Point Scale	300+	77%	67%	71%
Meds 'Always' Explained Before Given	300+	63%	60%	64%
Nurses 'Always' Communicated Well	300+	79%	75%	79%
Pain 'Always' Well Controlled	300+	74%	68%	71%
Room and Bathroom 'Always' Clean	300+	66%	69%	73%
Timely Help 'Always' Received	300+	62%	62%	68%
Would Definitely Recommend Hospital	300+	81%	69%	71%
Use of Medical Imaging				
Cardiac Imaging Stress Test before Surgery	339	5.3%	6.4%	5.3%
Combination Abdominal CT Scan	2,513	16.6%	11.8%	10.5%
Combination Brain/Sinus CT Scan	1,013	3.1%	3.4%	2.7%
Combination Chest CT Scan	2,474	0.2%	2.4%	2.7%
Follow-up Mammogram/Ultrasound	1,818	8.2%	10.2%	8.8%
Lumbar Spine MRI for Low Back Pain	149	36.9%	35.2%	37.2%

VA North Florida/South Georgia Healthcare System

1601 S W Archer Road Phone: 352-376-1611
Gainesville, FL 32608 Fax: 352-374-6113
URL: www.northflorida.va.gov
Type: Acute Care - VA Emergency Services: No
Ownership: Government Federal Beds: 323
Key Personnel:
Emergency Room . . . . Mary Allen, MD
Chief of Medical Staff . . . . Bradley S. Bender, MD
CEO/President. . . . . Elwood Headley, MD

Measure	Cases	This Hosp.	State Avg.	U.S. Avg.
Blood Clot Prevention and Treatment				
Anticoagulation Overlap Therapy	-	-	93%	93%
ICU Venous Thromboembolism Prophylaxis	-	-	94%	92%
Incidence of Potentially Preventable VTE	-	-	10%	10%
UFH with Dosages/Platelet Monitoring	-	-	100%	97%
Venous Thromboembolism Prophylaxis	-	-	88%	85%
Warfarin Therapy Discharge Instructions	-	-	85%	75%
Chest Pain/Possible Heart Attack Care				

NOTE: Hospital profiles are in alphabetical order by state, then city, then hospital within the city; Rankings exclude hospitals with less than 25 cases except for patient surveys which excludes hospitals with less than 100 cases; (a) 100-299 cases; (1) The number of cases/patients is too few to report; (2) Data submitted were based on a sample of cases/patients; (3) Results are based on a shorter time period than required; (4) Data suppressed by CMS for one or more quarters; (5) Results are not available for this reporting period; (6) Fewer than 100 patients completed the HCAHPS survey; (7) No cases met the criteria for this measure; (8) The lower limit of the confidence interval cannot be calculated if the number of observed infections equals zero; (9) No data are available from the state/territory for this reporting period; (10) The scores shown reflect fewer than 50 completed surveys; (11) There were discrepancies in the data collection process; (12) This measure does not apply to this hospital for this reporting period; (13) Results cannot be calculated for this reporting period; (14) The results for this state are combined with nearby states to protect confidentiality; Please refer to the User's Guide for a full explanation of data.

Aspirin Given Within 24 Hours of Arrival	-	-	98%	96%
Fibrinolytic Meds Within 30 Min. of Arrival	-	-	81%	58%
Average Time to ECG (minutes)	-	-	7	7
Average Time to Transfer (minutes)	-	-	53	60
Children's Asthma Care				
Received Home Management Plan of Care	-	-	-	88%
Received Reliever Medication	-	-	-	100%
Received Systemic Corticosteroids	-	-	-	100%
Emergency Department				
Admittance Decision Time (minutes)	-	-	111	98
Head CT Results Within 45 Min. of Arrival	-	-	64%	57%
Patients Who Left ER Before Being Seen	-	-	2%	2%
Time from ER Arrival to Admit. (minutes)	-	-	289	274
Time from ER Arrival to Discharge (minutes)	-	-	147	134
Time in ER Before Being Evaluated (minutes)	-	-	26	26
Time to Pain Meds for Fractures (minutes)	-	-	60	57
Heart Attack Care				
Aspirin Given at Discharge	117	100%	99%	99%
Fibrinolytic Meds Within 30 Min. of Arrival[5]	-	-	50%	54%
PCI Within 90 Minutes of Arrival[1]	-	-	96%	96%
Statin Prescribed at Discharge	114	99%	99%	98%
Heart Failure Care				
ACE Inhibitor or ARB for LVSD	219	94%	98%	97%
Discharge Instructions Given	486	99%	96%	94%
Evaluation of LVS Function	527	100%	100%	99%
Medicare Spending				
Medicare Spending per Patient (ratio)	-	-	1.04	0.98
Pneumonia Care				
Appropriate Initial Antibiotic Given	119	94%	98%	95%
Blood Culture Timing	232	94%	99%	98%
Pregnancy and Delivery Care				
Newborn Deliveries Scheduled Early	-	-	6%	6%
Preventive Care				
Immunization for Influenza[5]	-	-	94%	90%
Immunization for Pneumonia[5]	-	-	96%	92%
Stroke Care				
Anticoagulation Therapy for Atrial Fibrillation	-	-	97%	95%
Antithrombotic Therapy Timing	-	-	98%	98%
Assessed for Rehabilitation	-	-	97%	97%
Discharged on Antithrombotic Therapy	-	-	99%	99%
Discharged on Statin Medication	-	-	96%	94%
Thrombolytic Therapy Timing	-	-	76%	66%
Venous Thromboembolism Prophylaxis	-	-	95%	94%
Written Stroke Educational Materials Given	-	-	94%	88%
Surgical Care Improvement Project				
Appropriate Beta Blocker Usage[2]	275	96%	99%	98%
Appropriate VTP Within 24 Hours[2]	411	98%	99%	98%
Controlled Postoperative Blood Glucose[2]	130	97%	98%	97%
Perioperative Temperature Management[2]	499	99%	100%	100%
Prophylactic Antibiotic Selection	473	99%	99%	99%
Prophylactic Antibiotic Selection (Outpatient)	-	-	98%	98%
Prophylactic Antibiotic Stopped	457	96%	98%	98%
Prophylactic Antibiotic Timing	474	99%	99%	99%
Prophylactic Antibiotic Timing (Outpatient)	-	-	98%	98%
Urinary Catheter Removal[2]	475	97%	98%	97%
Survey of Patients' Hospital Experiences				
Area Around Room 'Always' Quiet at Night	-	-	58%	61%
Doctors 'Always' Communicated Well	-	-	77%	82%
Home Recovery Information Given	-	-	83%	85%
Hospital Given 9 or 10 on 10 Point Scale	-	-	67%	71%
Meds 'Always' Explained Before Given	-	-	60%	64%
Nurses 'Always' Communicated Well	-	-	75%	79%
Pain 'Always' Well Controlled	-	-	68%	71%
Room and Bathroom 'Always' Clean	-	-	69%	73%
Timely Help 'Always' Received	-	-	62%	68%
Would Definitely Recommend Hospital	-	-	69%	71%
Use of Medical Imaging				
Cardiac Imaging Stress Test before Surgery	-	-	6.4%	5.3%
Combination Abdominal CT Scan	-	-	11.8%	10.5%
Combination Brain/Sinus CT Scan	-	-	3.4%	2.7%
Combination Chest CT Scan	-	-	2.4%	2.7%
Follow-up Mammogram/Ultrasound	-	-	10.2%	8.8%
Lumbar Spine MRI for Low Back Pain	-	-	35.2%	37.2%

Campbellton Graceville Hospital

5429 College Drive
Graceville, FL 32440
Phone: 850-263-7201
Type: Critical Access Hospitals
Emergency Services: Yes
Ownership: Government - State

Key Personnel:
CEO . . . . H.D. Cannington
Radiology. . . . . John Carey Tomberlin, M.D.
Cardiology . . . . Ray Marling

Measure	Cases	This Hosp.	State Avg.	U.S. Avg.
Blood Clot Prevention and Treatment				
Anticoagulation Overlap Therapy[5]	-	-	93%	93%
ICU Venous Thromboembolism Prophylaxis[5]	-	-	94%	92%
Incidence of Potentially Preventable VTE[5]	-	-	10%	10%
UFH with Dosages/Platelet Monitoring[5]	-	-	100%	97%
Venous Thromboembolism Prophylaxis[5]	-	-	88%	85%
Warfarin Therapy Discharge Instructions[5]	-	-	85%	75%
Chest Pain/Possible Heart Attack Care				
Aspirin Given Within 24 Hours of Arrival	-	-	98%	96%
Fibrinolytic Meds Within 30 Min. of Arrival	-	-	81%	58%
Average Time to ECG (minutes)	-	-	7	7
Average Time to Transfer (minutes)	-	-	53	60
Children's Asthma Care				
Received Home Management Plan of Care	-	-	-	88%
Received Reliever Medication	-	-	-	100%
Received Systemic Corticosteroids	-	-	-	100%
Emergency Department				
Admittance Decision Time (minutes)[5]	-	-	111	98
Head CT Results Within 45 Min. of Arrival	-	-	64%	57%
Patients Who Left ER Before Being Seen	-	-	2%	2%
Time from ER Arrival to Admit. (minutes)[5]	-	-	289	274
Time from ER Arrival to Discharge (minutes)	-	-	147	134
Time in ER Before Being Evaluated (minutes)	-	-	26	26
Time to Pain Meds for Fractures (minutes)	-	-	60	57
Heart Attack Care				
Aspirin Given at Discharge[3,7]	-	-	99%	99%
Fibrinolytic Meds Within 30 Min. of Arrival[3,7]	-	-	50%	54%
PCI Within 90 Minutes of Arrival[3,7]	-	-	96%	96%
Statin Prescribed at Discharge[3,7]	-	-	99%	98%
Heart Failure Care				
ACE Inhibitor or ARB for LVSD[1]	-	-	98%	97%
Discharge Instructions Given[1]	-	-	96%	94%
Evaluation of LVS Function	19	89%	100%	99%
Medicare Spending				
Medicare Spending per Patient (ratio)	-	-	1.04	0.98
Pneumonia Care				
Appropriate Initial Antibiotic Given[7]	-	-	98%	95%
Blood Culture Timing[1]	-	-	99%	98%
Pregnancy and Delivery Care				
Newborn Deliveries Scheduled Early[5]	-	-	6%	6%
Preventive Care				
Immunization for Influenza[5]	-	-	94%	90%
Immunization for Pneumonia[5]	-	-	96%	92%
Stroke Care				
Anticoagulation Therapy for Atrial Fibrillation[5]	-	-	97%	95%
Antithrombotic Therapy Timing[5]	-	-	98%	98%
Assessed for Rehabilitation[5]	-	-	97%	97%
Discharged on Antithrombotic Therapy[5]	-	-	99%	99%
Discharged on Statin Medication[5]	-	-	96%	94%
Thrombolytic Therapy Timing[5]	-	-	76%	66%
Venous Thromboembolism Prophylaxis[5]	-	-	95%	94%
Written Stroke Educational Materials Given[5]	-	-	94%	88%
Surgical Care Improvement Project				
Appropriate Beta Blocker Usage[5]	-	-	99%	98%
Appropriate VTP Within 24 Hours[5]	-	-	99%	98%
Controlled Postoperative Blood Glucose[5]	-	-	98%	97%
Perioperative Temperature Management[5]	-	-	100%	100%
Prophylactic Antibiotic Selection[5]	-	-	99%	99%
Prophylactic Antibiotic Selection (Outpatient)	-	-	98%	98%
Prophylactic Antibiotic Stopped[5]	-	-	98%	98%
Prophylactic Antibiotic Timing[5]	-	-	99%	99%
Prophylactic Antibiotic Timing (Outpatient)	-	-	98%	98%
Urinary Catheter Removal[5]	-	-	98%	97%
Survey of Patients' Hospital Experiences				
Area Around Room 'Always' Quiet at Night[5]	-	-	58%	61%
Doctors 'Always' Communicated Well[5]	-	-	77%	82%
Home Recovery Information Given[5]	-	-	83%	85%
Hospital Given 9 or 10 on 10 Point Scale[5]	-	-	67%	71%
Meds 'Always' Explained Before Given[5]	-	-	60%	64%
Nurses 'Always' Communicated Well[5]	-	-	75%	79%
Pain 'Always' Well Controlled[5]	-	-	68%	71%
Room and Bathroom 'Always' Clean[5]	-	-	69%	73%
Timely Help 'Always' Received[5]	-	-	62%	68%
Would Definitely Recommend Hospital[5]	-	-	69%	71%
Use of Medical Imaging				
Cardiac Imaging Stress Test before Surgery	-	-	6.4%	5.3%
Combination Abdominal CT Scan	-	-	11.8%	10.5%
Combination Brain/Sinus CT Scan	-	-	3.4%	2.7%
Combination Chest CT Scan	-	-	2.4%	2.7%
Follow-up Mammogram/Ultrasound	-	-	10.2%	8.8%
Lumbar Spine MRI for Low Back Pain	-	-	35.2%	37.2%

Gulf Breeze Hospital

1110 Gulf Breeze Pkwy
Gulf Breeze, FL 32561
Phone: 850-934-2000
Fax: 850-934-2069
URL: www.ebaptisthealthcare.org
Type: Acute Care Hospitals
Emergency Services: Yes
Ownership: Voluntary non-profit - Other
Beds: 77

Key Personnel:
Operating Room. . . . . Terry Evans
Infection Control. . . . . Mark Faulkner

Measure	Cases	This Hosp.	State Avg.	U.S. Avg.
Blood Clot Prevention and Treatment				
Anticoagulation Overlap Therapy[2]	32	78%	93%	93%
ICU Venous Thromboembolism Prophylaxis[2]	48	83%	94%	92%
Incidence of Potentially Preventable VTE[1,2]	-	-	10%	10%
UFH with Dosages/Platelet Monitoring[1,2]	-	-	100%	97%
Venous Thromboembolism Prophylaxis[2]	346	83%	88%	85%
Warfarin Therapy Discharge Instructions[2]	24	17%	85%	75%
Chest Pain/Possible Heart Attack Care				
Aspirin Given Within 24 Hours of Arrival	69	99%	98%	96%
Fibrinolytic Meds Within 30 Min. of Arrival[7]	-	-	81%	58%
Average Time to ECG (minutes)	71	8	7	7
Average Time to Transfer (minutes)	25	43	53	60
Children's Asthma Care				
Received Home Management Plan of Care	-	-	-	88%
Received Reliever Medication	-	-	-	100%
Received Systemic Corticosteroids	-	-	-	100%
Emergency Department				
Admittance Decision Time (minutes)[2]	483	88	111	98
Head CT Results Within 45 Min. of Arrival[1]	-	-	64%	57%
Patients Who Left ER Before Being Seen	28,182	2%	2%	2%
Time from ER Arrival to Admit. (minutes)[2]	491	273	289	274
Time from ER Arrival to Discharge (minutes)	458	140	147	134
Time in ER Before Being Evaluated (minutes)	471	42	26	26
Time to Pain Meds for Fractures (minutes)	102	76	60	57
Heart Attack Care				
Aspirin Given at Discharge[1]	-	-	99%	99%
Fibrinolytic Meds Within 30 Min. of Arrival[7]	-	-	50%	54%
PCI Within 90 Minutes of Arrival[7]	-	-	96%	96%
Statin Prescribed at Discharge[1]	-	-	99%	98%
Heart Failure Care				
ACE Inhibitor or ARB for LVSD	25	100%	98%	97%
Discharge Instructions Given	94	93%	96%	94%
Evaluation of LVS Function	118	100%	100%	99%
Medicare Spending				
Medicare Spending per Patient (ratio)	-	0.97	1.04	0.98
Pneumonia Care				
Appropriate Initial Antibiotic Given[2]	119	100%	98%	95%
Blood Culture Timing[2]	145	99%	99%	98%
Pregnancy and Delivery Care				
Newborn Deliveries Scheduled Early[7]	-	-	6%	6%
Preventive Care				
Immunization for Influenza[2]	451	94%	94%	90%

NOTE: Hospital profiles are in alphabetical order by state, then city, then hospital within the city; Rankings exclude hospitals with less than 25 cases except for patient surveys which excludes hospitals with less than 100 cases; (a) 100-299 cases; (1) The number of cases/patients is too few to report; (2) Data submitted were based on a sample of cases/patients; (3) Results are based on a shorter time period than required; (4) Data suppressed by CMS for one or more quarters; (5) Results are not available for this reporting period; (6) Fewer than 100 patients completed the HCAHPS survey; (7) No cases met the criteria for this measure; (8) The lower limit of the confidence interval cannot be calculated if the number of observed infections equals zero; (9) No data are available from the state/territory for this reporting period; (10) The scores shown reflect fewer than 50 completed surveys; (11) There were discrepancies in the data collection process; (12) This measure does not apply to this hospital for this reporting period; (13) Results cannot be calculated for this reporting period; (14) The results for this state are combined with nearby states to protect confidentiality; Please refer to the User's Guide for a full explanation of data.

Measure	Cases	This Hosp.	State Avg.	U.S. Avg.
Immunization for Pneumonia[2]	622	91%	96%	92%
Stroke Care				
Anticoagulation Therapy for Atrial Fibrillation[1]	-	-	97%	95%
Antithrombotic Therapy Timing	43	100%	98%	98%
Assessed for Rehabilitation	49	98%	97%	97%
Discharged on Antithrombotic Therapy	47	100%	99%	99%
Discharged on Statin Medication	41	95%	96%	94%
Thrombolytic Therapy Timing[1]	-	-	76%	66%
Venous Thromboembolism Prophylaxis	48	96%	95%	94%
Written Stroke Educational Materials Given	35	77%	94%	88%
Surgical Care Improvement Project				
Appropriate Beta Blocker Usage[2]	105	100%	99%	98%
Appropriate VTP Within 24 Hours[2]	295	98%	99%	98%
Controlled Postoperative Blood Glucose[2,7]	-	-	98%	97%
Perioperative Temperature Management[2]	355	100%	100%	100%
Prophylactic Antibiotic Selection[2]	229	100%	99%	99%
Prophylactic Antibiotic Selection (Outpatient)	143	98%	98%	98%
Prophylactic Antibiotic Stopped[2]	224	100%	98%	98%
Prophylactic Antibiotic Timing[2]	229	100%	99%	99%
Prophylactic Antibiotic Timing (Outpatient)	143	99%	98%	98%
Urinary Catheter Removal[2]	222	100%	98%	97%
Survey of Patients' Hospital Experiences				
Area Around Room 'Always' Quiet at Night	300+	71%	58%	61%
Doctors 'Always' Communicated Well	300+	84%	77%	82%
Home Recovery Information Given	300+	88%	83%	85%
Hospital Given 9 or 10 on 10 Point Scale	300+	81%	67%	71%
Meds 'Always' Explained Before Given	300+	67%	60%	64%
Nurses 'Always' Communicated Well	300+	84%	75%	79%
Pain 'Always' Well Controlled	300+	75%	68%	71%
Room and Bathroom 'Always' Clean	300+	74%	69%	73%
Timely Help 'Always' Received	300+	74%	62%	68%
Would Definitely Recommend Hospital	300+	85%	69%	71%
Use of Medical Imaging				
Cardiac Imaging Stress Test before Surgery	471	3.4%	6.4%	5.3%
Combination Abdominal CT Scan	587	12.9%	11.8%	10.5%
Combination Brain/Sinus CT Scan	665	4.1%	3.4%	2.7%
Combination Chest CT Scan	222	1.4%	2.4%	2.7%
Follow-up Mammogram/Ultrasound	1,028	6.9%	10.2%	8.8%
Lumbar Spine MRI for Low Back Pain	166	34.9%	35.2%	37.2%

Hialeah Hospital

651 E 25th St
Hialeah, FL 33013
Phone: 305-693-6100
Fax: 305-835-4252
URL: www.hialeahhosp.com
Type: Acute Care Hospitals
Emergency Services: Yes
Ownership: Proprietary
Beds: 378

Key Personnel:
Operating Room. . . . . Barbara Blanco, RN
Pediatric In-Patient Care . . . . Jorge Cabrera, MD
Radiology. . . . . Mark Fasbinder, MD
Infection Control. . . . . Maggie Kane
Chief of Medical Staff. . . . . Jose Nunez, MD
CEO/President. . . . . Ben A. Rodriguez
Quality Assurance . . . . Karin Williamson

Measure	Cases	This Hosp.	State Avg.	U.S. Avg.
Blood Clot Prevention and Treatment				
Anticoagulation Overlap Therapy[2]	45	93%	93%	93%
ICU Venous Thromboembolism Prophylaxis[2]	107	95%	94%	92%
Incidence of Potentially Preventable VTE[1,2]	-	-	10%	10%
UFH with Dosages/Platelet Monitoring[2]	20	100%	100%	97%
Venous Thromboembolism Prophylaxis[2]	367	92%	88%	85%
Warfarin Therapy Discharge Instructions[2]	36	97%	85%	75%
Chest Pain/Possible Heart Attack Care				
Aspirin Given Within 24 Hours of Arrival	57	100%	98%	96%
Fibrinolytic Meds Within 30 Min. of Arrival[7]	-	-	81%	58%
Average Time to ECG (minutes)	58	15	7	7
Average Time to Transfer (minutes)	20	83	53	60
Children's Asthma Care				
Received Home Management Plan of Care	-	-	-	88%
Received Reliever Medication	-	-	-	100%
Received Systemic Corticosteroids	-	-	-	100%
Emergency Department				
Admittance Decision Time (minutes)[2]	840	324	111	98
Head CT Results Within 45 Min. of Arrival	11	73%	64%	57%
Patients Who Left ER Before Being Seen	32,086	1%	2%	2%
Time from ER Arrival to Admit. (minutes)[2]	842	518	289	274
Time from ER Arrival to Discharge (minutes)	453	208	147	134
Time in ER Before Being Evaluated (minutes)	500	4	26	26
Time to Pain Meds for Fractures (minutes)	46	56	60	57
Heart Attack Care				
Aspirin Given at Discharge	98	100%	99%	99%
Fibrinolytic Meds Within 30 Min. of Arrival[7]	-	-	50%	54%
PCI Within 90 Minutes of Arrival[7]	-	-	96%	96%
Statin Prescribed at Discharge	111	100%	99%	98%
Heart Failure Care				
ACE Inhibitor or ARB for LVSD[2]	81	98%	98%	97%
Discharge Instructions Given[2]	204	99%	96%	94%
Evaluation of LVS Function[2]	258	100%	100%	99%
Medicare Spending				
Medicare Spending per Patient (ratio)	-	1.13	1.04	0.98
Pneumonia Care				
Appropriate Initial Antibiotic Given[2]	155	99%	98%	95%
Blood Culture Timing[2]	162	98%	99%	98%
Pregnancy and Delivery Care				
Newborn Deliveries Scheduled Early[2]	44	0%	6%	6%
Preventive Care				
Immunization for Influenza[2]	541	97%	94%	90%
Immunization for Pneumonia[2]	676	99%	96%	92%
Stroke Care				
Anticoagulation Therapy for Atrial Fibrillation[1]	-	-	97%	95%
Antithrombotic Therapy Timing	98	95%	98%	98%
Assessed for Rehabilitation	112	99%	97%	97%
Discharged on Antithrombotic Therapy	93	99%	99%	99%
Discharged on Statin Medication	83	96%	96%	94%
Thrombolytic Therapy Timing[1]	-	-	76%	66%
Venous Thromboembolism Prophylaxis	127	94%	95%	94%
Written Stroke Educational Materials Given	71	93%	94%	88%
Surgical Care Improvement Project				
Appropriate Beta Blocker Usage[2]	74	100%	99%	98%
Appropriate VTP Within 24 Hours[2]	291	98%	99%	98%
Controlled Postoperative Blood Glucose[2,7]	-	-	98%	97%
Perioperative Temperature Management[2]	345	100%	100%	100%
Prophylactic Antibiotic Selection[2]	170	100%	99%	99%
Prophylactic Antibiotic Selection (Outpatient)	65	100%	98%	98%
Prophylactic Antibiotic Stopped[2]	163	90%	98%	98%
Prophylactic Antibiotic Timing[2]	170	98%	99%	99%
Prophylactic Antibiotic Timing (Outpatient)	60	100%	98%	98%
Urinary Catheter Removal[2]	107	97%	98%	97%
Survey of Patients' Hospital Experiences				
Area Around Room 'Always' Quiet at Night	300+	60%	58%	61%
Doctors 'Always' Communicated Well	300+	80%	77%	82%
Home Recovery Information Given	300+	78%	83%	85%
Hospital Given 9 or 10 on 10 Point Scale	300+	62%	67%	71%
Meds 'Always' Explained Before Given	300+	60%	60%	64%
Nurses 'Always' Communicated Well	300+	74%	75%	79%
Pain 'Always' Well Controlled	300+	70%	68%	71%
Room and Bathroom 'Always' Clean	300+	71%	69%	73%
Timely Help 'Always' Received	300+	61%	62%	68%
Would Definitely Recommend Hospital	300+	63%	69%	71%
Use of Medical Imaging				
Cardiac Imaging Stress Test before Surgery[7]	-	-	6.4%	5.3%
Combination Abdominal CT Scan	397	1.3%	11.8%	10.5%
Combination Brain/Sinus CT Scan[1]	-	-	3.4%	2.7%
Combination Chest CT Scan	94	0.0%	2.4%	2.7%
Follow-up Mammogram/Ultrasound	220	14.1%	10.2%	8.8%
Lumbar Spine MRI for Low Back Pain	46	63.0%	35.2%	37.2%

Palm Springs General Hospital

1475 W 49th St
Hialeah, FL 33012
Phone: 305-558-2500
Fax: 305-558-8679
URL: www.psghosp.com
Type: Acute Care Hospitals
Emergency Services: Yes
Ownership: Voluntary non-profit - Private
Beds: 247

Key Personnel:
Emergency Room . . . . Theresa Bernanrd, RN
Operating Room. . . . . Jackie Esbaugh, RN
Chief of Medical Staff. . . . . Roberto Fernandez, MD
CEO/President. . . . . Carlos Milanes

Measure	Cases	This Hosp.	State Avg.	U.S. Avg.
Blood Clot Prevention and Treatment				
Anticoagulation Overlap Therapy[2]	20	80%	93%	93%
ICU Venous Thromboembolism Prophylaxis[2]	100	91%	94%	92%
Incidence of Potentially Preventable VTE[2,7]	-	-	10%	10%
UFH with Dosages/Platelet Monitoring[1,2]	-	-	100%	97%
Venous Thromboembolism Prophylaxis[2]	358	83%	88%	85%
Warfarin Therapy Discharge Instructions[2]	15	93%	85%	75%
Chest Pain/Possible Heart Attack Care				
Aspirin Given Within 24 Hours of Arrival	21	100%	98%	96%
Fibrinolytic Meds Within 30 Min. of Arrival[3,7]	-	-	81%	58%
Average Time to ECG (minutes)	21	12	7	7
Average Time to Transfer (minutes)[3,7]	-	-	53	60
Children's Asthma Care				
Received Home Management Plan of Care	-	-	-	88%
Received Reliever Medication	-	-	-	100%
Received Systemic Corticosteroids	-	-	-	100%
Emergency Department				
Admittance Decision Time (minutes)[2]	752	145	111	98
Head CT Results Within 45 Min. of Arrival[1]	-	-	64%	57%
Patients Who Left ER Before Being Seen	5,473	2%	2%	2%
Time from ER Arrival to Admit. (minutes)[2]	752	390	289	274
Time from ER Arrival to Discharge (minutes)	308	224	147	134
Time in ER Before Being Evaluated (minutes)	405	41	26	26
Time to Pain Meds for Fractures (minutes)	37	61	60	57
Heart Attack Care				
Aspirin Given at Discharge	54	98%	99%	99%
Fibrinolytic Meds Within 30 Min. of Arrival[7]	-	-	50%	54%
PCI Within 90 Minutes of Arrival[7]	-	-	96%	96%
Statin Prescribed at Discharge	54	81%	99%	98%
Heart Failure Care				
ACE Inhibitor or ARB for LVSD	57	100%	98%	97%
Discharge Instructions Given	147	88%	96%	94%
Evaluation of LVS Function	195	98%	100%	99%
Medicare Spending				
Medicare Spending per Patient (ratio)	-	1.10	1.04	0.98
Pneumonia Care				
Appropriate Initial Antibiotic Given	163	96%	98%	95%
Blood Culture Timing	335	99%	99%	98%
Pregnancy and Delivery Care				
Newborn Deliveries Scheduled Early[7]	-	-	6%	6%
Preventive Care				
Immunization for Influenza[2]	409	100%	94%	90%
Immunization for Pneumonia[2]	752	100%	96%	92%
Stroke Care				
Anticoagulation Therapy for Atrial Fibrillation[1]	-	-	97%	95%
Antithrombotic Therapy Timing	20	95%	98%	98%
Assessed for Rehabilitation	22	73%	97%	97%
Discharged on Antithrombotic Therapy	22	100%	99%	99%
Discharged on Statin Medication	19	79%	96%	94%
Thrombolytic Therapy Timing[7]	-	-	76%	66%
Venous Thromboembolism Prophylaxis	22	64%	95%	94%
Written Stroke Educational Materials Given	18	22%	94%	88%
Surgical Care Improvement Project				
Appropriate Beta Blocker Usage	36	81%	99%	98%
Appropriate VTP Within 24 Hours	122	93%	99%	98%
Controlled Postoperative Blood Glucose[7]	-	-	98%	97%
Perioperative Temperature Management	143	100%	100%	100%
Prophylactic Antibiotic Selection	77	99%	99%	99%
Prophylactic Antibiotic Selection (Outpatient)	167	97%	98%	98%
Prophylactic Antibiotic Stopped	77	88%	98%	98%
Prophylactic Antibiotic Timing	77	100%	99%	99%
Prophylactic Antibiotic Timing (Outpatient)	171	98%	98%	98%
Urinary Catheter Removal	64	94%	98%	97%
Survey of Patients' Hospital Experiences				
Area Around Room 'Always' Quiet at Night	300+	56%	58%	61%
Doctors 'Always' Communicated Well	300+	82%	77%	82%
Home Recovery Information Given	300+	75%	83%	85%
Hospital Given 9 or 10 on 10 Point Scale	300+	61%	67%	71%
Meds 'Always' Explained Before Given	300+	61%	60%	64%
Nurses 'Always' Communicated Well	300+	76%	75%	79%
Pain 'Always' Well Controlled	300+	66%	68%	71%

NOTE: Hospital profiles are in alphabetical order by state, then city, then hospital within the city; Rankings exclude hospitals with less than 25 cases except for patient surveys which excludes hospitals with less than 100 cases; (a) 100-299 cases; (1) The number of cases/patients is too few to report; (2) Data submitted were based on a sample of cases/patients; (3) Results are based on a shorter time period than required; (4) Data suppressed by CMS for one or more quarters; (5) Results are not available for this reporting period; (6) Fewer than 100 patients completed the HCAHPS survey; (7) No cases met the criteria for this measure; (8) The lower limit of the confidence interval cannot be calculated if the number of observed infections equals zero; (9) No data are available from the state/territory for this reporting period; (10) The scores shown reflect fewer than 50 completed surveys; (11) There were discrepancies in the data collection process; (12) This measure does not apply to this hospital for this reporting period; (13) Results cannot be calculated for this reporting period; (14) The results for this state are combined with nearby states to protect confidentiality; Please refer to the User's Guide for a full explanation of data.

Measure	Cases	This Hosp.	State Avg.	U.S. Avg.
Room and Bathroom 'Always' Clean	300+	78%	69%	73%
Timely Help 'Always' Received	300+	61%	62%	68%
Would Definitely Recommend Hospital	300+	62%	69%	71%
Use of Medical Imaging				
Cardiac Imaging Stress Test before Surgery[1]	-	-	6.4%	5.3%
Combination Abdominal CT Scan	417	2.2%	11.8%	10.5%
Combination Brain/Sinus CT Scan	567	4.8%	3.4%	2.7%
Combination Chest CT Scan	155	4.5%	2.4%	2.7%
Follow-up Mammogram/Ultrasound[1]	-	-	10.2%	8.8%
Lumbar Spine MRI for Low Back Pain[1]	-	-	35.2%	37.2%

Palmetto General Hospital

2001 W 68th St Phone: 305-823-5000
Hialeah, FL 33016 Fax: 305-364-2173
URL: www.palmettogeneral.com
Type: Acute Care Hospitals Emergency Services: Yes
Ownership: Proprietary Beds: 360

Key Personnel:
Radiology.................... Simi Anidjar
Cardiac Laboratory............ Gonzalo Arcentales
Operating Room............... Edgardo Ariza
Quality Assurance .... Ruben De La Vega
Chief of Medical Staff.......... Jose Gamez, MD
Coronary Care .... Judy Martin
CEO/President................ Ana Mederos, MBA
Infection Control.............. Jose Luis Ruiz

Measure	Cases	This Hosp.	State Avg.	U.S. Avg.
Blood Clot Prevention and Treatment				
Anticoagulation Overlap Therapy[2]	53	100%	93%	93%
ICU Venous Thromboembolism Prophylaxis[2]	92	93%	94%	92%
Incidence of Potentially Preventable VTE[2]	14	21%	10%	10%
UFH with Dosages/Platelet Monitoring[2]	24	100%	100%	97%
Venous Thromboembolism Prophylaxis[2]	256	84%	88%	85%
Warfarin Therapy Discharge Instructions[2]	35	100%	85%	75%
Chest Pain/Possible Heart Attack Care				
Aspirin Given Within 24 Hours of Arrival[3,7]	-	-	98%	96%
Fibrinolytic Meds Within 30 Min. of Arrival[3,7]	-	-	81%	58%
Average Time to ECG (minutes)[1,3]	-	-	7	7
Average Time to Transfer (minutes)[3,7]	-	-	53	60
Children's Asthma Care				
Received Home Management Plan of Care	-	-	-	88%
Received Reliever Medication	-	-	-	100%
Received Systemic Corticosteroids	-	-	-	100%
Emergency Department				
Admittance Decision Time (minutes)[2]	785	335	111	98
Head CT Results Within 45 Min. of Arrival	13	77%	64%	57%
Patients Who Left ER Before Being Seen	63,004	1%	2%	2%
Time from ER Arrival to Admit. (minutes)[2]	785	535	289	274
Time from ER Arrival to Discharge (minutes)	342	198	147	134
Time in ER Before Being Evaluated (minutes)	381	35	26	26
Time to Pain Meds for Fractures (minutes)	189	72	60	57
Heart Attack Care				
Aspirin Given at Discharge[2]	379	100%	99%	99%
Fibrinolytic Meds Within 30 Min. of Arrival[2,7]	-	-	50%	54%
PCI Within 90 Minutes of Arrival[2]	84	100%	96%	96%
Statin Prescribed at Discharge[2]	381	99%	99%	98%
Heart Failure Care				
ACE Inhibitor or ARB for LVSD[2]	145	99%	98%	97%
Discharge Instructions Given[2]	322	100%	96%	94%
Evaluation of LVS Function[2]	391	100%	100%	99%
Medicare Spending				
Medicare Spending per Patient (ratio)	-	1.13	1.04	0.98
Pneumonia Care				
Appropriate Initial Antibiotic Given[2]	123	99%	98%	95%
Blood Culture Timing[2]	184	98%	99%	98%
Pregnancy and Delivery Care				
Newborn Deliveries Scheduled Early[2]	42	2%	6%	6%
Preventive Care				
Immunization for Influenza[2]	573	92%	94%	90%
Immunization for Pneumonia[2]	635	97%	96%	92%
Stroke Care				
Anticoagulation Therapy for Atrial Fibrillation	16	100%	97%	95%
Antithrombotic Therapy Timing	209	100%	98%	98%
Assessed for Rehabilitation	257	98%	97%	97%
Discharged on Antithrombotic Therapy	214	100%	99%	99%
Discharged on Statin Medication	174	100%	96%	94%
Thrombolytic Therapy Timing	33	100%	76%	66%
Venous Thromboembolism Prophylaxis	282	95%	95%	94%
Written Stroke Educational Materials Given	157	98%	94%	88%
Surgical Care Improvement Project				
Appropriate Beta Blocker Usage[2]	303	99%	99%	98%
Appropriate VTP Within 24 Hours[2]	450	99%	99%	98%
Controlled Postoperative Blood Glucose[2]	151	99%	98%	97%
Perioperative Temperature Management[2]	529	100%	100%	100%
Prophylactic Antibiotic Selection[2]	533	98%	99%	99%
Prophylactic Antibiotic Selection (Outpatient)	455	98%	98%	98%
Prophylactic Antibiotic Stopped[2]	511	99%	98%	98%
Prophylactic Antibiotic Timing[2]	537	99%	99%	99%
Prophylactic Antibiotic Timing (Outpatient)	455	100%	98%	98%
Urinary Catheter Removal[2]	252	100%	98%	97%
Survey of Patients' Hospital Experiences				
Area Around Room 'Always' Quiet at Night	300+	59%	58%	61%
Doctors 'Always' Communicated Well	300+	82%	77%	82%
Home Recovery Information Given	300+	75%	83%	85%
Hospital Given 9 or 10 on 10 Point Scale	300+	61%	67%	71%
Meds 'Always' Explained Before Given	300+	58%	60%	64%
Nurses 'Always' Communicated Well	300+	73%	75%	79%
Pain 'Always' Well Controlled	300+	69%	68%	71%
Room and Bathroom 'Always' Clean	300+	76%	69%	73%
Timely Help 'Always' Received	300+	63%	62%	68%
Would Definitely Recommend Hospital	300+	62%	69%	71%
Use of Medical Imaging				
Cardiac Imaging Stress Test before Surgery[1]	-	-	6.4%	5.3%
Combination Abdominal CT Scan	706	5.4%	11.8%	10.5%
Combination Brain/Sinus CT Scan	602	2.5%	3.4%	2.7%
Combination Chest CT Scan	335	0.3%	2.4%	2.7%
Follow-up Mammogram/Ultrasound	548	9.5%	10.2%	8.8%
Lumbar Spine MRI for Low Back Pain	57	28.1%	35.2%	37.2%

Memorial Regional Hospital

3501 Johnson St Phone: 954-987-2000
Hollywood, FL 33021 Fax: 954-985-3453
URL: www.memorialregional.com
Type: Acute Care Hospitals Emergency Services: Yes
Ownership: Govt - Hospital Dist/Auth Beds: 690

Key Personnel:
Operating Room.............. Mary Ann Crawford
Radiology.................... Benjamin Freedman, MD
Chief of Medical Staff.......... Kenneth Gelman, MD
Hemotology Center .... Atif Hussein, MD
Quality Assurance .... Patricia Jackson
Emergency Room .... Randy Katz, DO
Cardiology.................. Ralph Levy, MD
Anesthesiology............... Joseph Loskove, MD

Measure	Cases	This Hosp.	State Avg.	U.S. Avg.
Blood Clot Prevention and Treatment				
Anticoagulation Overlap Therapy[2]	159	100%	93%	93%
ICU Venous Thromboembolism Prophylaxis[2]	80	100%	94%	92%
Incidence of Potentially Preventable VTE[2]	53	0%	10%	10%
UFH with Dosages/Platelet Monitoring[2]	56	100%	100%	97%
Venous Thromboembolism Prophylaxis[2]	491	100%	88%	85%
Warfarin Therapy Discharge Instructions[2]	116	100%	85%	75%
Chest Pain/Possible Heart Attack Care				
Aspirin Given Within 24 Hours of Arrival[1,3]	-	-	98%	96%
Fibrinolytic Meds Within 30 Min. of Arrival[3,7]	-	-	81%	58%
Average Time to ECG (minutes)[1,3]	-	-	7	7
Average Time to Transfer (minutes)[3,7]	-	-	53	60
Children's Asthma Care				
Received Home Management Plan of Care	262	100%	-	88%
Received Reliever Medication	262	100%	-	100%
Received Systemic Corticosteroids	262	100%	-	100%
Emergency Department				
Admittance Decision Time (minutes)[2]	502	154	111	98
Head CT Results Within 45 Min. of Arrival[1]	-	-	64%	57%
Patients Who Left ER Before Being Seen	>100k	1%	2%	2%
Time from ER Arrival to Admit. (minutes)[2]	505	318	289	274
Time from ER Arrival to Discharge (minutes)	684	123	147	134
Time in ER Before Being Evaluated (minutes)	752	24	26	26
Time to Pain Meds for Fractures (minutes)	480	41	60	57
Heart Attack Care				
Aspirin Given at Discharge	450	100%	99%	99%
Fibrinolytic Meds Within 30 Min. of Arrival[7]	-	-	50%	54%
PCI Within 90 Minutes of Arrival	55	100%	96%	96%
Statin Prescribed at Discharge	439	100%	99%	98%
Heart Failure Care				
ACE Inhibitor or ARB for LVSD	281	100%	98%	97%
Discharge Instructions Given	581	100%	96%	94%
Evaluation of LVS Function	677	100%	100%	99%
Medicare Spending				
Medicare Spending per Patient (ratio)	-	1.05	1.04	0.98
Pneumonia Care				
Appropriate Initial Antibiotic Given	238	100%	98%	95%
Blood Culture Timing	477	100%	99%	98%
Pregnancy and Delivery Care				
Newborn Deliveries Scheduled Early[2]	77	0%	6%	6%
Preventive Care				
Immunization for Influenza[2]	812	99%	94%	90%
Immunization for Pneumonia[2]	882	99%	96%	92%
Stroke Care				
Anticoagulation Therapy for Atrial Fibrillation	27	100%	97%	95%
Antithrombotic Therapy Timing	246	100%	98%	98%
Assessed for Rehabilitation	349	100%	97%	97%
Discharged on Antithrombotic Therapy	250	100%	99%	99%
Discharged on Statin Medication	205	99%	96%	94%
Thrombolytic Therapy Timing	20	95%	76%	66%
Venous Thromboembolism Prophylaxis	389	99%	95%	94%
Written Stroke Educational Materials Given	174	98%	94%	88%
Surgical Care Improvement Project				
Appropriate Beta Blocker Usage[2]	317	100%	99%	98%
Appropriate VTP Within 24 Hours[2]	432	100%	99%	98%
Controlled Postoperative Blood Glucose[2]	235	100%	98%	97%
Perioperative Temperature Management[2]	527	100%	100%	100%
Prophylactic Antibiotic Selection[2]	530	100%	99%	99%
Prophylactic Antibiotic Selection (Outpatient)	314	100%	98%	98%
Prophylactic Antibiotic Stopped[2]	502	99%	98%	98%
Prophylactic Antibiotic Timing[2]	531	100%	99%	99%
Prophylactic Antibiotic Timing (Outpatient)	314	99%	98%	98%
Urinary Catheter Removal[2]	369	100%	98%	97%
Survey of Patients' Hospital Experiences				
Area Around Room 'Always' Quiet at Night	300+	63%	58%	61%
Doctors 'Always' Communicated Well	300+	80%	77%	82%
Home Recovery Information Given	300+	85%	83%	85%
Hospital Given 9 or 10 on 10 Point Scale	300+	77%	67%	71%
Meds 'Always' Explained Before Given	300+	66%	60%	64%
Nurses 'Always' Communicated Well	300+	80%	75%	79%
Pain 'Always' Well Controlled	300+	72%	68%	71%
Room and Bathroom 'Always' Clean	300+	76%	69%	73%
Timely Help 'Always' Received	300+	67%	62%	68%
Would Definitely Recommend Hospital	300+	80%	69%	71%
Use of Medical Imaging				
Cardiac Imaging Stress Test before Surgery[1]	-	-	6.4%	5.3%
Combination Abdominal CT Scan	985	5.2%	11.8%	10.5%
Combination Brain/Sinus CT Scan	1,124	2.8%	3.4%	2.7%
Combination Chest CT Scan	895	1.5%	2.4%	2.7%
Follow-up Mammogram/Ultrasound	1,286	18.0%	10.2%	8.8%
Lumbar Spine MRI for Low Back Pain	58	37.9%	35.2%	37.2%

Homestead Hospital

975 Baptist Way Phone: 786-243-8000
Homestead, FL 33033 Fax: 305-242-3557
URL: www.baptisthealth.net
Type: Acute Care Hospitals Emergency Services: Yes
Ownership: Voluntary non-profit - Private Beds: 120

Key Personnel:
CEO/President................ Bo Boulenger
Chief of Medical Staff........... J Rudolph Gossman Jr, DMD
Anesthesiology............... Samir Kulkarni, MD
Emergency Room .... Lloyd Tucker
Quality Assurance .... Jill White

Measure	Cases	This Hosp.	State Avg.	U.S. Avg.
Blood Clot Prevention and Treatment				
Anticoagulation Overlap Therapy[2]	53	100%	93%	93%

NOTE: Hospital profiles are in alphabetical order by state, then city, then hospital within the city; Rankings exclude hospitals with less than 25 cases except for patient surveys which excludes hospitals with less than 100 cases; (a) 100-299 cases; (1) The number of cases/patients is too few to report; (2) Data submitted were based on a sample of cases/patients; (3) Results are based on a shorter time period than required; (4) Data suppressed by CMS for one or more quarters; (5) Results are not available for this reporting period; (6) Fewer than 100 patients completed the HCAHPS survey; (7) No cases met the criteria for this measure; (8) The lower limit of the confidence interval cannot be calculated if the number of observed infections equals zero; (9) No data are available from the state/territory for this reporting period; (10) The scores shown reflect fewer than 50 completed surveys; (11) There were discrepancies in the data collection process; (12) This measure does not apply to this hospital for this reporting period; (13) Results cannot be calculated for this reporting period; (14) The results for this state are combined with nearby states to protect confidentiality; Please refer to the User's Guide for a full explanation of data.

Measure	Cases	This Hosp.	State Avg.	U.S. Avg.
ICU Venous Thromboembolism Prophylaxis[2]	60	100%	94%	92%
Incidence of Potentially Preventable VTE[1,2]	-	-	10%	10%
UFH with Dosages/Platelet Monitoring[2]	20	100%	100%	97%
Venous Thromboembolism Prophylaxis[2]	332	97%	88%	85%
Warfarin Therapy Discharge Instructions[2]	37	100%	85%	75%
Chest Pain/Possible Heart Attack Care				
Aspirin Given Within 24 Hours of Arrival	57	100%	98%	96%
Fibrinolytic Meds Within 30 Min. of Arrival[7]	-	-	81%	58%
Average Time to ECG (minutes)	58	0	7	7
Average Time to Transfer (minutes)[1]	-	-	53	60
Children's Asthma Care				
Received Home Management Plan of Care	-	-	-	88%
Received Reliever Medication	-	-	-	100%
Received Systemic Corticosteroids	-	-	-	100%
Emergency Department				
Admittance Decision Time (minutes)[2]	667	131	111	98
Head CT Results Within 45 Min. of Arrival	11	27%	64%	57%
Patients Who Left ER Before Being Seen	90,752	1%	2%	2%
Time from ER Arrival to Admit. (minutes)[2]	677	382	289	274
Time from ER Arrival to Discharge (minutes)	729	174	147	134
Time in ER Before Being Evaluated (minutes)	805	16	26	26
Time to Pain Meds for Fractures (minutes)	244	56	60	57
Heart Attack Care				
Aspirin Given at Discharge	42	100%	99%	99%
Fibrinolytic Meds Within 30 Min. of Arrival[7]	-	-	50%	54%
PCI Within 90 Minutes of Arrival[7]	-	-	96%	96%
Statin Prescribed at Discharge	42	100%	99%	98%
Heart Failure Care				
ACE Inhibitor or ARB for LVSD	52	100%	98%	97%
Discharge Instructions Given	240	100%	96%	94%
Evaluation of LVS Function	264	100%	100%	99%
Medicare Spending				
Medicare Spending per Patient (ratio)	-	1.07	1.04	0.98
Pneumonia Care				
Appropriate Initial Antibiotic Given	127	99%	98%	95%
Blood Culture Timing	225	100%	99%	98%
Pregnancy and Delivery Care				
Newborn Deliveries Scheduled Early[2]	178	4%	6%	6%
Preventive Care				
Immunization for Influenza[2]	553	95%	94%	90%
Immunization for Pneumonia[2]	544	98%	96%	92%
Stroke Care				
Anticoagulation Therapy for Atrial Fibrillation[1]	-	-	97%	95%
Antithrombotic Therapy Timing	80	100%	98%	98%
Assessed for Rehabilitation	82	100%	97%	97%
Discharged on Antithrombotic Therapy	79	100%	99%	99%
Discharged on Statin Medication	62	98%	96%	94%
Thrombolytic Therapy Timing[7]	-	-	76%	66%
Venous Thromboembolism Prophylaxis	75	100%	95%	94%
Written Stroke Educational Materials Given	53	100%	94%	88%
Surgical Care Improvement Project				
Appropriate Beta Blocker Usage	56	100%	99%	98%
Appropriate VTP Within 24 Hours	222	100%	99%	98%
Controlled Postoperative Blood Glucose[7]	-	-	98%	97%
Perioperative Temperature Management	241	100%	100%	100%
Prophylactic Antibiotic Selection	89	100%	99%	99%
Prophylactic Antibiotic Selection (Outpatient)	14	100%	98%	98%
Prophylactic Antibiotic Stopped	87	99%	98%	98%
Prophylactic Antibiotic Timing	89	100%	99%	99%
Prophylactic Antibiotic Timing (Outpatient)	14	93%	98%	98%
Urinary Catheter Removal	125	100%	98%	97%
Survey of Patients' Hospital Experiences				
Area Around Room 'Always' Quiet at Night	300+	76%	58%	61%
Doctors 'Always' Communicated Well	300+	82%	77%	82%
Home Recovery Information Given	300+	84%	83%	85%
Hospital Given 9 or 10 on 10 Point Scale	300+	77%	67%	71%
Meds 'Always' Explained Before Given	300+	69%	60%	64%
Nurses 'Always' Communicated Well	300+	81%	75%	79%
Pain 'Always' Well Controlled	300+	74%	68%	71%
Room and Bathroom 'Always' Clean	300+	77%	69%	73%
Timely Help 'Always' Received	300+	65%	62%	68%
Would Definitely Recommend Hospital	300+	79%	69%	71%
Use of Medical Imaging				
Cardiac Imaging Stress Test before Surgery	82	1.2%	6.4%	5.3%
Combination Abdominal CT Scan	605	1.7%	11.8%	10.5%
Combination Brain/Sinus CT Scan	703	4.6%	3.4%	2.7%
Combination Chest CT Scan	313	0.3%	2.4%	2.7%
Follow-up Mammogram/Ultrasound	395	11.1%	10.2%	8.8%
Lumbar Spine MRI for Low Back Pain	55	47.3%	35.2%	37.2%

Regional Medical Center Bayonet Point

14000 Fivay Road
Hudson, FL 34667
Phone: 727-819-2929
Fax: 727-868-6431
URL: www.mchealth.comorwww.heartoftampa.com
Type: Acute Care Hospitals
Emergency Services: Yes
Ownership: Proprietary
Beds: 290

Key Personnel:

Quality Assurance . . . . Ken Emmitt
Radiology. . . . . Alexander Fernandez, MD
Intensive Care Unit. . . . . Cavoy Foelders
CEO/President. . . . . Shayne George, MBA, MHA, FACHE
Infection Control. . . . . Barbara Haner
Chief of Medical Staff. . . . . Joseph Pino, M.D., MBA, FAAF
Emergency Room . . . . Kenneth Steinberg, DO
Operating Room. . . . . Laura Tischler

Measure	Cases	This Hosp.	State Avg.	U.S. Avg.
Blood Clot Prevention and Treatment				
Anticoagulation Overlap Therapy[2]	83	100%	93%	93%
ICU Venous Thromboembolism Prophylaxis[2]	143	100%	94%	92%
Incidence of Potentially Preventable VTE[1,2]	-	-	10%	10%
UFH with Dosages/Platelet Monitoring[2]	45	100%	100%	97%
Venous Thromboembolism Prophylaxis[2]	360	100%	88%	85%
Warfarin Therapy Discharge Instructions[2]	69	100%	85%	75%
Chest Pain/Possible Heart Attack Care				
Aspirin Given Within 24 Hours of Arrival[5]	-	-	98%	96%
Fibrinolytic Meds Within 30 Min. of Arrival[5]	-	-	81%	58%
Average Time to ECG (minutes)[5]	-	-	7	7
Average Time to Transfer (minutes)[5]	-	-	53	60
Children's Asthma Care				
Received Home Management Plan of Care	-	-	-	88%
Received Reliever Medication	-	-	-	100%
Received Systemic Corticosteroids	-	-	-	100%
Emergency Department				
Admittance Decision Time (minutes)[2]	1,078	64	111	98
Head CT Results Within 45 Min. of Arrival[1]	-	-	64%	57%
Patients Who Left ER Before Being Seen	40,919	1%	2%	2%
Time from ER Arrival to Admit. (minutes)[2]	1,078	234	289	274
Time from ER Arrival to Discharge (minutes)	404	136	147	134
Time in ER Before Being Evaluated (minutes)	439	18	26	26
Time to Pain Meds for Fractures (minutes)	109	48	60	57
Heart Attack Care				
Aspirin Given at Discharge[2]	272	99%	99%	99%
Fibrinolytic Meds Within 30 Min. of Arrival[2,7]	-	-	50%	54%
PCI Within 90 Minutes of Arrival[2]	44	100%	96%	96%
Statin Prescribed at Discharge[2]	250	100%	99%	98%
Heart Failure Care				
ACE Inhibitor or ARB for LVSD[2]	80	99%	98%	97%
Discharge Instructions Given[2]	234	100%	96%	94%
Evaluation of LVS Function[2]	287	100%	100%	99%
Medicare Spending				
Medicare Spending per Patient (ratio)	-	1.03	1.04	0.98
Pneumonia Care				
Appropriate Initial Antibiotic Given[2]	63	100%	98%	95%
Blood Culture Timing[2]	47	98%	99%	98%
Pregnancy and Delivery Care				
Newborn Deliveries Scheduled Early[2,7]	-	-	6%	6%
Preventive Care				
Immunization for Influenza[2]	684	100%	94%	90%
Immunization for Pneumonia[2]	1,019	100%	96%	92%
Stroke Care				
Anticoagulation Therapy for Atrial Fibrillation[2]	13	100%	97%	95%
Antithrombotic Therapy Timing[2]	73	99%	98%	98%
Assessed for Rehabilitation[2]	86	99%	97%	97%
Discharged on Antithrombotic Therapy[2]	64	100%	99%	99%
Discharged on Statin Medication[2]	49	96%	96%	94%
Thrombolytic Therapy Timing[1,2]	-	-	76%	66%
Venous Thromboembolism Prophylaxis[2]	105	97%	95%	94%
Written Stroke Educational Materials Given[2]	38	100%	94%	88%
Surgical Care Improvement Project				
Appropriate Beta Blocker Usage[2]	235	100%	99%	98%
Appropriate VTP Within 24 Hours[2]	353	99%	99%	98%
Controlled Postoperative Blood Glucose[2]	145	100%	98%	97%
Perioperative Temperature Management[2]	411	100%	100%	100%
Prophylactic Antibiotic Selection[2]	349	100%	99%	99%
Prophylactic Antibiotic Selection (Outpatient)	303	100%	98%	98%
Prophylactic Antibiotic Stopped[2]	330	98%	98%	98%
Prophylactic Antibiotic Timing[2]	351	99%	99%	99%
Prophylactic Antibiotic Timing (Outpatient)	303	99%	98%	98%
Urinary Catheter Removal[2]	370	99%	98%	97%
Survey of Patients' Hospital Experiences				
Area Around Room 'Always' Quiet at Night	300+	49%	58%	61%
Doctors 'Always' Communicated Well	300+	71%	77%	82%
Home Recovery Information Given	300+	83%	83%	85%
Hospital Given 9 or 10 on 10 Point Scale	300+	60%	67%	71%
Meds 'Always' Explained Before Given	300+	55%	60%	64%
Nurses 'Always' Communicated Well	300+	70%	75%	79%
Pain 'Always' Well Controlled	300+	62%	68%	71%
Room and Bathroom 'Always' Clean	300+	64%	69%	73%
Timely Help 'Always' Received	300+	54%	62%	68%
Would Definitely Recommend Hospital	300+	62%	69%	71%
Use of Medical Imaging				
Cardiac Imaging Stress Test before Surgery[1]	-	-	6.4%	5.3%
Combination Abdominal CT Scan	356	2.5%	11.8%	10.5%
Combination Brain/Sinus CT Scan	569	6.0%	3.4%	2.7%
Combination Chest CT Scan	71	0.0%	2.4%	2.7%
Follow-up Mammogram/Ultrasound[7]	-	-	10.2%	8.8%
Lumbar Spine MRI for Low Back Pain[1]	-	-	35.2%	37.2%

Citrus Memorial Hospital

502 W Highland Blvd
Inverness, FL 34452
Phone: 352-726-1551
Fax: 352-341-0136
E-mail: lringquist@citrusmh.org
URL: www.citrusmh.com
Type: Acute Care Hospitals
Emergency Services: Yes
Ownership: Govt - Hospital Dist/Auth
Beds: 171

Key Personnel:

Infection Control. . . . . Rosemary Barker
CEO/President. . . . . Ryan Beaty
Radiology. . . . . Michael Berlow
Coronary Care . . . . Maggie Brest, RN
Operating Room. . . . . Thomas Hendrick, ADON
Quality Assurance . . . . Pat Leach
Chief of Medical Staff. . . . . Rama Nathan
Pediatric Ambulatory Care . . . . . . Sheila Stone, ADON

Measure	Cases	This Hosp.	State Avg.	U.S. Avg.
Blood Clot Prevention and Treatment				
Anticoagulation Overlap Therapy[2]	173	87%	93%	93%
ICU Venous Thromboembolism Prophylaxis[2]	82	70%	94%	92%
Incidence of Potentially Preventable VTE[2]	24	12%	10%	10%
UFH with Dosages/Platelet Monitoring[2]	88	100%	100%	97%
Venous Thromboembolism Prophylaxis[2]	440	58%	88%	85%
Warfarin Therapy Discharge Instructions[2]	120	65%	85%	75%
Chest Pain/Possible Heart Attack Care				
Aspirin Given Within 24 Hours of Arrival[1,3]	-	-	98%	96%
Fibrinolytic Meds Within 30 Min. of Arrival[5]	-	-	81%	58%
Average Time to ECG (minutes)[1,3]	-	-	7	7
Average Time to Transfer (minutes)[5]	-	-	53	60
Children's Asthma Care				
Received Home Management Plan of Care	-	-	-	88%
Received Reliever Medication	-	-	-	100%
Received Systemic Corticosteroids	-	-	-	100%
Emergency Department				
Admittance Decision Time (minutes)[2]	325	114	111	98
Head CT Results Within 45 Min. of Arrival[1]	-	-	64%	57%
Patients Who Left ER Before Being Seen	42,018	6%	2%	2%
Time from ER Arrival to Admit. (minutes)[2]	335	334	289	274
Time from ER Arrival to Discharge (minutes)	522	162	147	134
Time in ER Before Being Evaluated (minutes)	486	70	26	26
Time to Pain Meds for Fractures (minutes)	136	100	60	57

NOTE: Hospital profiles are in alphabetical order by state, then city, then hospital within the city; Rankings exclude hospitals with less than 25 cases except for patient surveys which excludes hospitals with less than 100 cases; (a) 100-299 cases; (1) The number of cases/patients is too few to report; (2) Data submitted were based on a sample of cases/patients; (3) Results are based on a shorter time period than required; (4) Data suppressed by CMS for one or more quarters; (5) Results are not available for this reporting period; (6) Fewer than 100 patients completed the HCAHPS survey; (7) No cases met the criteria for this measure; (8) The lower limit of the confidence interval cannot be calculated if the number of observed infections equals zero; (9) No data are available from the state/territory for this reporting period; (10) The scores shown reflect fewer than 50 completed surveys; (11) There were discrepancies in the data collection process; (12) This measure does not apply to this hospital for this reporting period; (13) Results cannot be calculated for this reporting period; (14) The results for this state are combined with nearby states to protect confidentiality; Please refer to the User's Guide for a full explanation of data.

Measure	Cases	This Hosp.	State Avg.	U.S. Avg.
Heart Attack Care				
Aspirin Given at Discharge	289	97%	99%	99%
Fibrinolytic Meds Within 30 Min. of Arrival[7]	-	-	50%	54%
PCI Within 90 Minutes of Arrival	91	87%	96%	96%
Statin Prescribed at Discharge	277	93%	99%	98%
Heart Failure Care				
ACE Inhibitor or ARB for LVSD	132	92%	98%	97%
Discharge Instructions Given	305	90%	96%	94%
Evaluation of LVS Function	393	97%	100%	99%
Medicare Spending				
Medicare Spending per Patient (ratio)	-	1.05	1.04	0.98
Pneumonia Care				
Appropriate Initial Antibiotic Given	190	96%	98%	95%
Blood Culture Timing	262	95%	99%	98%
Pregnancy and Delivery Care				
Newborn Deliveries Scheduled Early[2]	37	3%	6%	6%
Preventive Care				
Immunization for Influenza[2]	666	86%	94%	90%
Immunization for Pneumonia[2]	988	88%	96%	92%
Stroke Care				
Anticoagulation Therapy for Atrial Fibrillation	23	100%	97%	95%
Antithrombotic Therapy Timing	142	99%	98%	98%
Assessed for Rehabilitation	135	90%	97%	97%
Discharged on Antithrombotic Therapy	131	98%	99%	99%
Discharged on Statin Medication	114	89%	96%	94%
Thrombolytic Therapy Timing	19	47%	76%	66%
Venous Thromboembolism Prophylaxis	156	67%	95%	94%
Written Stroke Educational Materials Given	79	99%	94%	88%
Surgical Care Improvement Project				
Appropriate Beta Blocker Usage	279	96%	99%	98%
Appropriate VTP Within 24 Hours	550	93%	99%	98%
Controlled Postoperative Blood Glucose	144	100%	98%	97%
Perioperative Temperature Management	672	100%	100%	100%
Prophylactic Antibiotic Selection	549	97%	99%	99%
Prophylactic Antibiotic Selection (Outpatient)	296	98%	98%	98%
Prophylactic Antibiotic Stopped	541	96%	98%	98%
Prophylactic Antibiotic Timing	550	98%	99%	99%
Prophylactic Antibiotic Timing (Outpatient)	296	97%	98%	98%
Urinary Catheter Removal	480	90%	98%	97%
Survey of Patients' Hospital Experiences				
Area Around Room 'Always' Quiet at Night	300+	43%	58%	61%
Doctors 'Always' Communicated Well	300+	73%	77%	82%
Home Recovery Information Given	300+	83%	83%	85%
Hospital Given 9 or 10 on 10 Point Scale	300+	60%	67%	71%
Meds 'Always' Explained Before Given	300+	53%	60%	64%
Nurses 'Always' Communicated Well	300+	71%	75%	79%
Pain 'Always' Well Controlled	300+	63%	68%	71%
Room and Bathroom 'Always' Clean	300+	65%	69%	73%
Timely Help 'Always' Received	300+	54%	62%	68%
Would Definitely Recommend Hospital	300+	63%	69%	71%
Use of Medical Imaging				
Cardiac Imaging Stress Test before Surgery	175	8.0%	6.4%	5.3%
Combination Abdominal CT Scan	1,124	13.0%	11.8%	10.5%
Combination Brain/Sinus CT Scan	1,559	3.5%	3.4%	2.7%
Combination Chest CT Scan	668	6.3%	2.4%	2.7%
Follow-up Mammogram/Ultrasound	2,637	13.4%	10.2%	8.8%
Lumbar Spine MRI for Low Back Pain	91	31.9%	35.2%	37.2%

Baptist Medical Center

800 Prudential Dr
Jacksonville, FL 32207
Phone: 904-202-2000
Fax: 904-202-4920
URL: www.ebaptisthealth.com
Type: Acute Care Hospitals
Emergency Services: Yes
Ownership: Voluntary non-profit - Private
Beds: 579

Key Personnel:

Pediatric In-Patient Care .... Terry Bridgham, MD
Operating Room............. Ed Hubel
Infection Control............. Edna Javis
CEO/President.............. Michael Mayo, FACHE
Quality Assurance .... Cory Meyers
Chief of Medical Staff.......... Keith Stein, MD, FCCM, FCCP
Emergency Room .... Richard Stomberg, MD

Measure	Cases	This Hosp.	State Avg.	U.S. Avg.
Blood Clot Prevention and Treatment				
Anticoagulation Overlap Therapy[2]	276	81%	93%	93%
ICU Venous Thromboembolism Prophylaxis[2]	95	95%	94%	92%
Incidence of Potentially Preventable VTE[2]	47	15%	10%	10%
UFH with Dosages/Platelet Monitoring[2]	228	100%	100%	97%
Venous Thromboembolism Prophylaxis[2]	342	88%	88%	85%
Warfarin Therapy Discharge Instructions[2]	225	64%	85%	75%
Chest Pain/Possible Heart Attack Care				
Aspirin Given Within 24 Hours of Arrival	33	91%	98%	96%
Fibrinolytic Meds Within 30 Min. of Arrival[7]	-	-	81%	58%
Average Time to ECG (minutes)	30	8	7	7
Average Time to Transfer (minutes)[1]	-	-	53	60
Children's Asthma Care				
Received Home Management Plan of Care	491	91%	-	88%
Received Reliever Medication	493	100%	-	100%
Received Systemic Corticosteroids	491	100%	-	100%
Emergency Department				
Admittance Decision Time (minutes)[2]	487	127	111	98
Head CT Results Within 45 Min. of Arrival	21	57%	64%	57%
Patients Who Left ER Before Being Seen	>100k	4%	2%	2%
Time from ER Arrival to Admit. (minutes)[2]	498	330	289	274
Time from ER Arrival to Discharge (minutes)	401	165	147	134
Time in ER Before Being Evaluated (minutes)	494	45	26	26
Time to Pain Meds for Fractures (minutes)	528	87	60	57
Heart Attack Care				
Aspirin Given at Discharge[2]	339	99%	99%	99%
Fibrinolytic Meds Within 30 Min. of Arrival[2,7]	-	-	50%	54%
PCI Within 90 Minutes of Arrival[2]	38	95%	96%	96%
Statin Prescribed at Discharge[2]	319	99%	99%	98%
Heart Failure Care				
ACE Inhibitor or ARB for LVSD[2]	85	96%	98%	97%
Discharge Instructions Given[2]	274	92%	96%	94%
Evaluation of LVS Function[2]	349	100%	100%	99%
Medicare Spending				
Medicare Spending per Patient (ratio)	-	1.10	1.04	0.98
Pneumonia Care				
Appropriate Initial Antibiotic Given[2]	116	94%	98%	95%
Blood Culture Timing[2]	221	97%	99%	98%
Pregnancy and Delivery Care				
Newborn Deliveries Scheduled Early[2]	65	0%	6%	6%
Preventive Care				
Immunization for Influenza[2]	544	93%	94%	90%
Immunization for Pneumonia[2]	539	91%	96%	92%
Stroke Care				
Anticoagulation Therapy for Atrial Fibrillation[2]	13	100%	97%	95%
Antithrombotic Therapy Timing[2]	110	98%	98%	98%
Assessed for Rehabilitation[2]	118	94%	97%	97%
Discharged on Antithrombotic Therapy[2]	104	96%	99%	99%
Discharged on Statin Medication[2]	72	90%	96%	94%
Thrombolytic Therapy Timing[1,2]	-	-	76%	66%
Venous Thromboembolism Prophylaxis[2]	119	95%	95%	94%
Written Stroke Educational Materials Given[2]	79	89%	94%	88%
Surgical Care Improvement Project				
Appropriate Beta Blocker Usage[2]	329	97%	99%	98%
Appropriate VTP Within 24 Hours[2]	599	99%	99%	98%
Controlled Postoperative Blood Glucose[2]	244	98%	98%	97%
Perioperative Temperature Management[2]	806	100%	100%	100%
Prophylactic Antibiotic Selection[2]	747	99%	99%	99%
Prophylactic Antibiotic Selection (Outpatient)	946	98%	98%	98%
Prophylactic Antibiotic Stopped[2]	731	98%	98%	98%
Prophylactic Antibiotic Timing[2]	749	98%	99%	99%
Prophylactic Antibiotic Timing (Outpatient)	963	96%	98%	98%
Urinary Catheter Removal[2]	400	95%	98%	97%
Survey of Patients' Hospital Experiences				
Area Around Room 'Always' Quiet at Night	300+	60%	58%	61%
Doctors 'Always' Communicated Well	300+	77%	77%	82%
Home Recovery Information Given	300+	84%	83%	85%
Hospital Given 9 or 10 on 10 Point Scale	300+	73%	67%	71%
Meds 'Always' Explained Before Given	300+	58%	60%	64%
Nurses 'Always' Communicated Well	300+	76%	75%	79%
Pain 'Always' Well Controlled	300+	70%	68%	71%
Room and Bathroom 'Always' Clean	300+	71%	69%	73%
Timely Help 'Always' Received	300+	64%	62%	68%
Would Definitely Recommend Hospital	300+	78%	69%	71%
Use of Medical Imaging				
Cardiac Imaging Stress Test before Surgery	2,500	7.6%	6.4%	5.3%
Combination Abdominal CT Scan	2,304	6.3%	11.8%	10.5%
Combination Brain/Sinus CT Scan	2,639	3.5%	3.4%	2.7%
Combination Chest CT Scan	1,619	1.5%	2.4%	2.7%
Follow-up Mammogram/Ultrasound	3,594	8.6%	10.2%	8.8%
Lumbar Spine MRI for Low Back Pain	503	31.2%	35.2%	37.2%

Mayo Clinic

4500 San Pablo Rd
Jacksonville, FL 32224
Phone: 904-953-2000
Fax: 904-953-0430
URL: www.mayoclinic.org/jacksonville
Type: Acute Care Hospitals
Emergency Services: Yes
Ownership: Voluntary non-profit - Private

Key Personnel:

Radiology.................. Anthony Adelson
CEO/President.............. Denis A Cortese, MD

Measure	Cases	This Hosp.	State Avg.	U.S. Avg.
Blood Clot Prevention and Treatment				
Anticoagulation Overlap Therapy[2]	118	90%	93%	93%
ICU Venous Thromboembolism Prophylaxis[2]	86	97%	94%	92%
Incidence of Potentially Preventable VTE[2]	86	3%	10%	10%
UFH with Dosages/Platelet Monitoring[2]	93	100%	100%	97%
Venous Thromboembolism Prophylaxis[2]	312	92%	88%	85%
Warfarin Therapy Discharge Instructions[2]	87	89%	85%	75%
Chest Pain/Possible Heart Attack Care				
Aspirin Given Within 24 Hours of Arrival[5]	-	-	98%	96%
Fibrinolytic Meds Within 30 Min. of Arrival[5]	-	-	81%	58%
Average Time to ECG (minutes)[5]	-	-	7	7
Average Time to Transfer (minutes)[5]	-	-	53	60
Children's Asthma Care				
Received Home Management Plan of Care	-	-	-	88%
Received Reliever Medication	-	-	-	100%
Received Systemic Corticosteroids	-	-	-	100%
Emergency Department				
Admittance Decision Time (minutes)[2]	521	104	111	98
Head CT Results Within 45 Min. of Arrival[1]	-	-	64%	57%
Patients Who Left ER Before Being Seen	26,995	1%	2%	2%
Time from ER Arrival to Admit. (minutes)[2]	522	274	289	274
Time from ER Arrival to Discharge (minutes)	385	164	147	134
Time in ER Before Being Evaluated (minutes)	373	32	26	26
Time to Pain Meds for Fractures (minutes)	59	62	60	57
Heart Attack Care				
Aspirin Given at Discharge	102	100%	99%	99%
Fibrinolytic Meds Within 30 Min. of Arrival[7]	-	-	50%	54%
PCI Within 90 Minutes of Arrival	20	100%	96%	96%
Statin Prescribed at Discharge	103	100%	99%	98%
Heart Failure Care				
ACE Inhibitor or ARB for LVSD	68	96%	98%	97%
Discharge Instructions Given	219	97%	96%	94%
Evaluation of LVS Function	251	99%	100%	99%
Medicare Spending				
Medicare Spending per Patient (ratio)	-	0.98	1.04	0.98
Pneumonia Care				
Appropriate Initial Antibiotic Given	56	98%	98%	95%
Blood Culture Timing	161	100%	99%	98%
Pregnancy and Delivery Care				
Newborn Deliveries Scheduled Early[7]	-	-	6%	6%
Preventive Care				
Immunization for Influenza[2]	612	79%	94%	90%
Immunization for Pneumonia[2]	790	83%	96%	92%
Stroke Care				
Anticoagulation Therapy for Atrial Fibrillation[1,2]	-	-	97%	95%
Antithrombotic Therapy Timing[2]	45	98%	98%	98%
Assessed for Rehabilitation[2]	113	100%	97%	97%
Discharged on Antithrombotic Therapy[2]	75	97%	99%	99%
Discharged on Statin Medication[2]	53	94%	96%	94%
Thrombolytic Therapy Timing[2]	11	64%	76%	66%
Venous Thromboembolism Prophylaxis[2]	108	98%	95%	94%
Written Stroke Educational Materials Given[2]	69	94%	94%	88%
Surgical Care Improvement Project				
Appropriate Beta Blocker Usage[2]	317	99%	99%	98%

NOTE: Hospital profiles are in alphabetical order by state, then city, then hospital within the city; Rankings exclude hospitals with less than 25 cases except for patient surveys which excludes hospitals with less than 100 cases; (a) 100-299 cases; (1) The number of cases/patients is too few to report; (2) Data submitted were based on a sample of cases/patients; (3) Results are based on a shorter time period than required; (4) Data suppressed by CMS for one or more quarters; (5) Results are not available for this reporting period; (6) Fewer than 100 patients completed the HCAHPS survey; (7) No cases met the criteria for this measure; (8) The lower limit of the confidence interval cannot be calculated if the number of observed infections equals zero; (9) No data are available from the state/territory for this reporting period; (10) The scores shown reflect fewer than 50 completed surveys; (11) There were discrepancies in the data collection process; (12) This measure does not apply to this hospital for this reporting period; (13) Results cannot be calculated for this reporting period; (14) The results for this state are combined with nearby states to protect confidentiality; Please refer to the User's Guide for a full explanation of data.

Measure	Cases	This Hosp.	State Avg.	U.S. Avg.
Appropriate VTP Within 24 Hours[2]	450	98%	99%	98%
Controlled Postoperative Blood Glucose[2]	184	95%	98%	97%
Perioperative Temperature Management[2]	538	100%	100%	100%
Prophylactic Antibiotic Selection[2]	460	99%	99%	99%
Prophylactic Antibiotic Selection (Outpatient)	515	87%	98%	98%
Prophylactic Antibiotic Stopped[2]	428	97%	98%	98%
Prophylactic Antibiotic Timing[2]	460	99%	99%	99%
Prophylactic Antibiotic Timing (Outpatient)	519	97%	98%	98%
Urinary Catheter Removal[2]	498	98%	98%	97%
Survey of Patients' Hospital Experiences				
Area Around Room 'Always' Quiet at Night[11]	300+	69%	58%	61%
Doctors 'Always' Communicated Well[11]	300+	86%	77%	82%
Home Recovery Information Given[11]	300+	90%	83%	85%
Hospital Given 9 or 10 on 10 Point Scale[11]	300+	89%	67%	71%
Meds 'Always' Explained Before Given[11]	300+	66%	60%	64%
Nurses 'Always' Communicated Well[11]	300+	83%	75%	79%
Pain 'Always' Well Controlled[11]	300+	74%	68%	71%
Room and Bathroom 'Always' Clean[11]	300+	79%	69%	73%
Timely Help 'Always' Received[11]	300+	70%	62%	68%
Would Definitely Recommend Hospital[11]	300+	92%	69%	71%
Use of Medical Imaging				
Cardiac Imaging Stress Test before Surgery	751	10.9%	6.4%	5.3%
Combination Abdominal CT Scan	490	1.6%	11.8%	10.5%
Combination Brain/Sinus CT Scan	1,035	2.0%	3.4%	2.7%
Combination Chest CT Scan	46	4.3%	2.4%	2.7%
Follow-up Mammogram/Ultrasound[7]	-	-	10.2%	8.8%
Lumbar Spine MRI for Low Back Pain[1]	-	-	35.2%	37.2%

Memorial Hospital Jacksonville

3625 University Blvd S
Jacksonville, FL 32216
Phone: 904-399-6111
Fax: 904-399-6817
URL: www.memorialhospitaljax.com
Type: Acute Care Hospitals
Emergency Services: Yes
Ownership: Proprietary
Beds: 418

Key Personnel:
Chief of Medical Staff. . . . . Osvaldo Contarini, MD
Cardiac Laboratory. . . . . Rob Grant, RN
Radiology. . . . . Rafael Irizarry, MD
Operating Room. . . . . Gail Luther, RN
Quality Assurance . . . . Kelly Mullee
CEO/President. . . . . Jim O'Loughlin
Pediatric In-Patient Care . . . . Rudolfo Pena-Ariet, MD
Infection Control. . . . . Jennifer Sackett, RN

Measure	Cases	This Hosp.	State Avg.	U.S. Avg.
Blood Clot Prevention and Treatment				
Anticoagulation Overlap Therapy[2]	146	84%	93%	93%
ICU Venous Thromboembolism Prophylaxis[2]	87	95%	94%	92%
Incidence of Potentially Preventable VTE[2]	35	11%	10%	10%
UFH with Dosages/Platelet Monitoring[2]	151	99%	100%	97%
Venous Thromboembolism Prophylaxis[2]	403	87%	88%	85%
Warfarin Therapy Discharge Instructions[2]	99	100%	85%	75%
Chest Pain/Possible Heart Attack Care				
Aspirin Given Within 24 Hours of Arrival[5]	-	-	98%	96%
Fibrinolytic Meds Within 30 Min. of Arrival[5]	-	-	81%	58%
Average Time to ECG (minutes)[1]	-	-	7	7
Average Time to Transfer (minutes)[5]	-	-	53	60
Children's Asthma Care				
Received Home Management Plan of Care	-	-	-	88%
Received Reliever Medication	-	-	-	100%
Received Systemic Corticosteroids	-	-	-	100%
Emergency Department				
Admittance Decision Time (minutes)[2]	851	118	111	98
Head CT Results Within 45 Min. of Arrival[1]	-	-	64%	57%
Patients Who Left ER Before Being Seen	90,556	1%	2%	2%
Time from ER Arrival to Admit. (minutes)[2]	852	284	289	274
Time from ER Arrival to Discharge (minutes)	508	125	147	134
Time in ER Before Being Evaluated (minutes)	544	18	26	26
Time to Pain Meds for Fractures (minutes)	141	68	60	57
Heart Attack Care				
Aspirin Given at Discharge	332	100%	99%	99%
Fibrinolytic Meds Within 30 Min. of Arrival[7]	-	-	50%	54%
PCI Within 90 Minutes of Arrival	19	100%	96%	96%
Statin Prescribed at Discharge	325	99%	99%	98%
Heart Failure Care				
ACE Inhibitor or ARB for LVSD[2]	71	100%	98%	97%
Discharge Instructions Given[2]	252	98%	96%	94%
Evaluation of LVS Function[2]	325	100%	100%	99%
Medicare Spending				
Medicare Spending per Patient (ratio)	-	1.13	1.04	0.98
Pneumonia Care				
Appropriate Initial Antibiotic Given[2]	59	98%	98%	95%
Blood Culture Timing[2]	92	100%	99%	98%
Pregnancy and Delivery Care				
Newborn Deliveries Scheduled Early[2]	36	0%	6%	6%
Preventive Care				
Immunization for Influenza[2]	639	99%	94%	90%
Immunization for Pneumonia[2]	850	98%	96%	92%
Stroke Care				
Anticoagulation Therapy for Atrial Fibrillation[1,2]	-	-	97%	95%
Antithrombotic Therapy Timing[2]	88	99%	98%	98%
Assessed for Rehabilitation[2]	97	100%	97%	97%
Discharged on Antithrombotic Therapy[2]	85	100%	99%	99%
Discharged on Statin Medication[2]	70	96%	96%	94%
Thrombolytic Therapy Timing[1,2]	-	-	76%	66%
Venous Thromboembolism Prophylaxis[2]	111	97%	95%	94%
Written Stroke Educational Materials Given[2]	51	100%	94%	88%
Surgical Care Improvement Project				
Appropriate Beta Blocker Usage[2]	290	100%	99%	98%
Appropriate VTP Within 24 Hours[2]	533	100%	99%	98%
Controlled Postoperative Blood Glucose[2]	136	98%	98%	97%
Perioperative Temperature Management[2]	646	100%	100%	100%
Prophylactic Antibiotic Selection[2]	537	99%	99%	99%
Prophylactic Antibiotic Selection (Outpatient)	451	99%	98%	98%
Prophylactic Antibiotic Stopped[2]	483	99%	98%	98%
Prophylactic Antibiotic Timing[2]	537	100%	99%	99%
Prophylactic Antibiotic Timing (Outpatient)	451	100%	98%	98%
Urinary Catheter Removal[2]	302	99%	98%	97%
Survey of Patients' Hospital Experiences				
Area Around Room 'Always' Quiet at Night	300+	62%	58%	61%
Doctors 'Always' Communicated Well	300+	75%	77%	82%
Home Recovery Information Given	300+	83%	83%	85%
Hospital Given 9 or 10 on 10 Point Scale	300+	63%	67%	71%
Meds 'Always' Explained Before Given	300+	55%	60%	64%
Nurses 'Always' Communicated Well	300+	73%	75%	79%
Pain 'Always' Well Controlled	300+	66%	68%	71%
Room and Bathroom 'Always' Clean	300+	64%	69%	73%
Timely Help 'Always' Received	300+	55%	62%	68%
Would Definitely Recommend Hospital	300+	64%	69%	71%
Use of Medical Imaging				
Cardiac Imaging Stress Test before Surgery	118	7.6%	6.4%	5.3%
Combination Abdominal CT Scan	793	6.2%	11.8%	10.5%
Combination Brain/Sinus CT Scan	730	3.4%	3.4%	2.7%
Combination Chest CT Scan	489	1.2%	2.4%	2.7%
Follow-up Mammogram/Ultrasound	1,770	10.8%	10.2%	8.8%
Lumbar Spine MRI for Low Back Pain	96	37.5%	35.2%	37.2%

Saint Vincent's Medical Center

1 Shircliff Way
Jacksonville, FL 32204
Phone: 904-308-7300
Fax: 904-308-7941
URL: www.jaxhealth.com
Type: Acute Care Hospitals
Emergency Services: Yes
Ownership: Voluntary non-profit - Church
Beds: 528

Key Personnel:
Operating Room. . . . . Sohrab E Afshari, RN
Radiology. . . . . Peter R Bream
CEO/President. . . . . Moody Chisholm
Coronary Care . . . . Lorraine Keith, RN
Quality Assurance . . . . Tracy Mondel
Chief of Medical Staff. . . . . David E Pirrung, MD
Cardiac Laboratory. . . . . Patti Stephenson
Infection Control. . . . . Bonnie Viergutz

Measure	Cases	This Hosp.	State Avg.	U.S. Avg.
Blood Clot Prevention and Treatment				
Anticoagulation Overlap Therapy[2]	139	99%	93%	93%
ICU Venous Thromboembolism Prophylaxis[2]	63	92%	94%	92%
Incidence of Potentially Preventable VTE[2]	21	0%	10%	10%
UFH with Dosages/Platelet Monitoring[2]	88	100%	100%	97%
Venous Thromboembolism Prophylaxis[2]	336	98%	88%	85%
Warfarin Therapy Discharge Instructions[2]	93	92%	85%	75%
Chest Pain/Possible Heart Attack Care				
Aspirin Given Within 24 Hours of Arrival[5]	-	-	98%	96%
Fibrinolytic Meds Within 30 Min. of Arrival[5]	-	-	81%	58%
Average Time to ECG (minutes)[5]	-	-	7	7
Average Time to Transfer (minutes)[5]	-	-	53	60
Children's Asthma Care				
Received Home Management Plan of Care	-	-	-	88%
Received Reliever Medication	-	-	-	100%
Received Systemic Corticosteroids	-	-	-	100%
Emergency Department				
Admittance Decision Time (minutes)[2]	501	210	111	98
Head CT Results Within 45 Min. of Arrival[1]	-	-	64%	57%
Patients Who Left ER Before Being Seen	72,403	3%	2%	2%
Time from ER Arrival to Admit. (minutes)[2]	513	386	289	274
Time from ER Arrival to Discharge (minutes)	335	198	147	134
Time in ER Before Being Evaluated (minutes)	399	57	26	26
Time to Pain Meds for Fractures (minutes)	61	80	60	57
Heart Attack Care				
Aspirin Given at Discharge[2]	308	99%	99%	99%
Fibrinolytic Meds Within 30 Min. of Arrival[2,7]	-	-	50%	54%
PCI Within 90 Minutes of Arrival[2]	43	95%	96%	96%
Statin Prescribed at Discharge[2]	285	98%	99%	98%
Heart Failure Care				
ACE Inhibitor or ARB for LVSD[2]	121	100%	98%	97%
Discharge Instructions Given[2]	260	97%	96%	94%
Evaluation of LVS Function[2]	301	100%	100%	99%
Medicare Spending				
Medicare Spending per Patient (ratio)	-	1.03	1.04	0.98
Pneumonia Care				
Appropriate Initial Antibiotic Given[2]	81	100%	98%	95%
Blood Culture Timing[2]	73	97%	99%	98%
Pregnancy and Delivery Care				
Newborn Deliveries Scheduled Early[2]	24	12%	6%	6%
Preventive Care				
Immunization for Influenza[2]	599	94%	94%	90%
Immunization for Pneumonia[2]	856	98%	96%	92%
Stroke Care				
Anticoagulation Therapy for Atrial Fibrillation[1,2]	-	-	97%	95%
Antithrombotic Therapy Timing[2]	81	99%	98%	98%
Assessed for Rehabilitation[2]	86	99%	97%	97%
Discharged on Antithrombotic Therapy[2]	76	100%	99%	99%
Discharged on Statin Medication[2]	60	100%	96%	94%
Thrombolytic Therapy Timing[1,2]	-	-	76%	66%
Venous Thromboembolism Prophylaxis[2]	95	98%	95%	94%
Written Stroke Educational Materials Given[2]	46	96%	94%	88%
Surgical Care Improvement Project				
Appropriate Beta Blocker Usage[2]	247	99%	99%	98%
Appropriate VTP Within 24 Hours[2]	350	100%	99%	98%
Controlled Postoperative Blood Glucose[2]	144	99%	98%	97%
Perioperative Temperature Management[2]	522	100%	100%	100%
Prophylactic Antibiotic Selection[2]	473	100%	99%	99%
Prophylactic Antibiotic Selection (Outpatient)	725	98%	98%	98%
Prophylactic Antibiotic Stopped[2]	457	99%	98%	98%
Prophylactic Antibiotic Timing[2]	477	100%	99%	99%
Prophylactic Antibiotic Timing (Outpatient)	726	99%	98%	98%
Urinary Catheter Removal[2]	118	97%	98%	97%
Survey of Patients' Hospital Experiences				
Area Around Room 'Always' Quiet at Night	(a)	59%	58%	61%
Doctors 'Always' Communicated Well	(a)	79%	77%	82%
Home Recovery Information Given	(a)	84%	83%	85%
Hospital Given 9 or 10 on 10 Point Scale	(a)	68%	67%	71%
Meds 'Always' Explained Before Given	(a)	61%	60%	64%
Nurses 'Always' Communicated Well	(a)	77%	75%	79%
Pain 'Always' Well Controlled	(a)	66%	68%	71%
Room and Bathroom 'Always' Clean	(a)	63%	69%	73%
Timely Help 'Always' Received	(a)	60%	62%	68%
Would Definitely Recommend Hospital	(a)	71%	69%	71%
Use of Medical Imaging				
Cardiac Imaging Stress Test before Surgery	2,572	4.9%	6.4%	5.3%
Combination Abdominal CT Scan	1,219	3.9%	11.8%	10.5%
Combination Brain/Sinus CT Scan	1,406	3.0%	3.4%	2.7%

NOTE: Hospital profiles are in alphabetical order by state, then city, then hospital within the city; Rankings exclude hospitals with less than 25 cases except for patient surveys which excludes hospitals with less than 100 cases; (a) 100-299 cases; (1) The number of cases/patients is too few to report; (2) Data submitted were based on a sample of cases/patients; (3) Results are based on a shorter time period than required; (4) Data suppressed by CMS for one or more quarters; (5) Results are not available for this reporting period; (6) Fewer than 100 patients completed the HCAHPS survey; (7) No cases met the criteria for this measure; (8) The lower limit of the confidence interval cannot be calculated if the number of observed infections equals zero; (9) No data are available from the state/territory for this reporting period; (10) The scores shown reflect fewer than 50 completed surveys; (11) There were discrepancies in the data collection process; (12) This measure does not apply to this hospital for this reporting period; (13) Results cannot be calculated for this reporting period; (14) The results for this state are combined with nearby states to protect confidentiality; Please refer to the User's Guide for a full explanation of data.

Measure	Cases	This Hosp.	State Avg.	U.S. Avg.
Combination Chest CT Scan	1,034	0.3%	2.4%	2.7%
Follow-up Mammogram/Ultrasound	3,837	12.4%	10.2%	8.8%
Lumbar Spine MRI for Low Back Pain	164	37.2%	35.2%	37.2%

Saint Vincent's Medical Center Southside

4201 Belfort Rd Phone: 904-296-3700
Jacksonville, FL 32216 Fax: 904-296-7941
URL: www.jaxhealth.com
Type: Acute Care Hospitals Emergency Services: Yes
Ownership: Voluntary non-profit - Private Beds: 313

Key Personnel:
Operating Room. . . . . Scott Carpenter
Emergency Room . . . . Kathy Coley, RN
Chief of Medical Staff. . . . . Steven Nauman, MD
Quality Assurance . . . . Diane Rabideau-Wise
CEO/President. . . . . Kyle Sanders
Radiology. . . . . Neal Wilson

Measure	Cases	This Hosp.	State Avg.	U.S. Avg.
Blood Clot Prevention and Treatment				
Anticoagulation Overlap Therapy[2]	78	97%	93%	93%
ICU Venous Thromboembolism Prophylaxis[2]	43	100%	94%	92%
Incidence of Potentially Preventable VTE[2]	14	0%	10%	10%
UFH with Dosages/Platelet Monitoring[2]	64	100%	100%	97%
Venous Thromboembolism Prophylaxis[2]	304	100%	88%	85%
Warfarin Therapy Discharge Instructions[2]	49	98%	85%	75%
Chest Pain/Possible Heart Attack Care				
Aspirin Given Within 24 Hours of Arrival[1,3]	-	-	98%	96%
Fibrinolytic Meds Within 30 Min. of Arrival[3,7]	-	-	81%	58%
Average Time to ECG (minutes)[1,3]	-	-	7	7
Average Time to Transfer (minutes)[3,7]	-	-	53	60
Children's Asthma Care				
Received Home Management Plan of Care	-	-	-	88%
Received Reliever Medication	-	-	-	100%
Received Systemic Corticosteroids	-	-	-	100%
Emergency Department				
Admittance Decision Time (minutes)[2]	465	83	111	98
Head CT Results Within 45 Min. of Arrival[5]	-	-	64%	57%
Patients Who Left ER Before Being Seen	35,682	1%	2%	2%
Time from ER Arrival to Admit. (minutes)[2]	467	228	289	274
Time from ER Arrival to Discharge (minutes)	375	156	147	134
Time in ER Before Being Evaluated (minutes)	395	33	26	26
Time to Pain Meds for Fractures (minutes)	25	73	60	57
Heart Attack Care				
Aspirin Given at Discharge[2]	79	100%	99%	99%
Fibrinolytic Meds Within 30 Min. of Arrival[2,7]	-	-	50%	54%
PCI Within 90 Minutes of Arrival[2]	11	100%	96%	96%
Statin Prescribed at Discharge[2]	77	99%	99%	98%
Heart Failure Care				
ACE Inhibitor or ARB for LVSD[2]	64	100%	98%	97%
Discharge Instructions Given[2]	158	100%	96%	94%
Evaluation of LVS Function[2]	200	100%	100%	99%
Medicare Spending				
Medicare Spending per Patient (ratio)	-	1.03	1.04	0.98
Pneumonia Care				
Appropriate Initial Antibiotic Given[2]	66	100%	98%	95%
Blood Culture Timing[2]	142	100%	99%	98%
Pregnancy and Delivery Care				
Newborn Deliveries Scheduled Early[2]	34	0%	6%	6%
Preventive Care				
Immunization for Influenza[2]	567	99%	94%	90%
Immunization for Pneumonia[2]	614	99%	96%	92%
Stroke Care				
Anticoagulation Therapy for Atrial Fibrillation[1,2]	-	-	97%	95%
Antithrombotic Therapy Timing[2]	56	98%	98%	98%
Assessed for Rehabilitation[2]	63	100%	97%	97%
Discharged on Antithrombotic Therapy[2]	56	100%	99%	99%
Discharged on Statin Medication[2]	44	100%	96%	94%
Thrombolytic Therapy Timing[1,2]	-	-	76%	66%
Venous Thromboembolism Prophylaxis[2]	67	100%	95%	94%
Written Stroke Educational Materials Given[2]	45	91%	94%	88%
Surgical Care Improvement Project				
Appropriate Beta Blocker Usage[2]	109	99%	99%	98%
Appropriate VTP Within 24 Hours[2]	318	100%	99%	98%
Controlled Postoperative Blood Glucose[2,7]	-	-	98%	97%
Perioperative Temperature Management[2]	361	100%	100%	100%
Prophylactic Antibiotic Selection[2]	216	100%	99%	99%
Prophylactic Antibiotic Selection (Outpatient)	424	99%	98%	98%
Prophylactic Antibiotic Stopped[2]	213	100%	98%	98%
Prophylactic Antibiotic Timing[2]	216	100%	99%	99%
Prophylactic Antibiotic Timing (Outpatient)	425	100%	98%	98%
Urinary Catheter Removal[2]	93	100%	98%	97%
Survey of Patients' Hospital Experiences				
Area Around Room 'Always' Quiet at Night	300+	66%	58%	61%
Doctors 'Always' Communicated Well	300+	80%	77%	82%
Home Recovery Information Given	300+	89%	83%	85%
Hospital Given 9 or 10 on 10 Point Scale	300+	69%	67%	71%
Meds 'Always' Explained Before Given	300+	65%	60%	64%
Nurses 'Always' Communicated Well	300+	79%	75%	79%
Pain 'Always' Well Controlled	300+	71%	68%	71%
Room and Bathroom 'Always' Clean	300+	71%	69%	73%
Timely Help 'Always' Received	300+	66%	62%	68%
Would Definitely Recommend Hospital	300+	75%	69%	71%
Use of Medical Imaging				
Cardiac Imaging Stress Test before Surgery	585	6.8%	6.4%	5.3%
Combination Abdominal CT Scan	341	5.3%	11.8%	10.5%
Combination Brain/Sinus CT Scan[1]	-	-	3.4%	2.7%
Combination Chest CT Scan	137	2.9%	2.4%	2.7%
Follow-up Mammogram/Ultrasound	194	16.0%	10.2%	8.8%
Lumbar Spine MRI for Low Back Pain	63	33.3%	35.2%	37.2%

UF Health Jacksonville

655 W 8th St Phone: 904-244-0411
Jacksonville, FL 32209 Fax: 904-244-9668
URL: www.shandsjacksonville.org
Type: Acute Care Hospitals Emergency Services: Yes
Ownership: Voluntary non-profit - Private Beds: 695

Key Personnel:
CEO . . . . Russell E. Armistead, MBA
Coronary Care . . . . Ginger Campbell, CNO
Radiology. . . . . Kevin Cuda
CEO/President. . . . . David S. Guzick, MD, PhD
Pediatric Ambulatory Care . . . . . . Rita James
Pediatric In-Patient Care . . . . Sandy McDonald, RN
Infection Control. . . . . Becky Saltford, RN
Chief of Medical Staff. . . . . David Vukich, MD

Measure	Cases	This Hosp.	State Avg.	U.S. Avg.
Blood Clot Prevention and Treatment				
Anticoagulation Overlap Therapy[2]	128	93%	93%	93%
ICU Venous Thromboembolism Prophylaxis[2]	112	96%	94%	92%
Incidence of Potentially Preventable VTE[2]	28	7%	10%	10%
UFH with Dosages/Platelet Monitoring[2]	70	100%	100%	97%
Venous Thromboembolism Prophylaxis[2]	246	93%	88%	85%
Warfarin Therapy Discharge Instructions[2]	92	24%	85%	75%
Chest Pain/Possible Heart Attack Care				
Aspirin Given Within 24 Hours of Arrival[5]	-	-	98%	96%
Fibrinolytic Meds Within 30 Min. of Arrival[5]	-	-	81%	58%
Average Time to ECG (minutes)[5]	-	-	7	7
Average Time to Transfer (minutes)[5]	-	-	53	60
Children's Asthma Care				
Received Home Management Plan of Care	-	-	-	88%
Received Reliever Medication	-	-	-	100%
Received Systemic Corticosteroids	-	-	-	100%
Emergency Department				
Admittance Decision Time (minutes)[2]	595	292	111	98
Head CT Results Within 45 Min. of Arrival[1]	-	-	64%	57%
Patients Who Left ER Before Being Seen	89,453	8%	2%	2%
Time from ER Arrival to Admit. (minutes)[2]	629	626	289	274
Time from ER Arrival to Discharge (minutes)	337	237	147	134
Time in ER Before Being Evaluated (minutes)	92	76	26	26
Time to Pain Meds for Fractures (minutes)	206	86	60	57
Heart Attack Care				
Aspirin Given at Discharge[2]	276	99%	99%	99%
Fibrinolytic Meds Within 30 Min. of Arrival[2,7]	-	-	50%	54%
PCI Within 90 Minutes of Arrival[2]	42	95%	96%	96%
Statin Prescribed at Discharge[2]	273	99%	99%	98%
Heart Failure Care				
ACE Inhibitor or ARB for LVSD[2]	154	99%	98%	97%
Discharge Instructions Given[2]	256	94%	96%	94%
Evaluation of LVS Function[2]	287	100%	100%	99%
Medicare Spending				
Medicare Spending per Patient (ratio)	-	1.00	1.04	0.98
Pneumonia Care				
Appropriate Initial Antibiotic Given[2]	43	93%	98%	95%
Blood Culture Timing[2]	89	89%	99%	98%
Pregnancy and Delivery Care				
Newborn Deliveries Scheduled Early[2]	46	0%	6%	6%
Preventive Care				
Immunization for Influenza[2]	520	92%	94%	90%
Immunization for Pneumonia[2]	528	94%	96%	92%
Stroke Care				
Anticoagulation Therapy for Atrial Fibrillation[1,2]	-	-	97%	95%
Antithrombotic Therapy Timing[2]	71	100%	98%	98%
Assessed for Rehabilitation[2]	96	97%	97%	97%
Discharged on Antithrombotic Therapy[2]	85	95%	99%	99%
Discharged on Statin Medication[2]	66	95%	96%	94%
Thrombolytic Therapy Timing[2]	30	33%	76%	66%
Venous Thromboembolism Prophylaxis[2]	99	95%	95%	94%
Written Stroke Educational Materials Given[2]	49	82%	94%	88%
Surgical Care Improvement Project				
Appropriate Beta Blocker Usage[2]	165	99%	99%	98%
Appropriate VTP Within 24 Hours[2]	294	99%	99%	98%
Controlled Postoperative Blood Glucose[2]	95	98%	98%	97%
Perioperative Temperature Management[2]	401	100%	100%	100%
Prophylactic Antibiotic Selection[2]	367	100%	99%	99%
Prophylactic Antibiotic Selection (Outpatient)	272	99%	98%	98%
Prophylactic Antibiotic Stopped[2]	357	99%	98%	98%
Prophylactic Antibiotic Timing[2]	367	99%	99%	99%
Prophylactic Antibiotic Timing (Outpatient)	274	99%	98%	98%
Urinary Catheter Removal[2]	266	100%	98%	97%
Survey of Patients' Hospital Experiences				
Area Around Room 'Always' Quiet at Night	300+	59%	58%	61%
Doctors 'Always' Communicated Well	300+	79%	77%	82%
Home Recovery Information Given	300+	85%	83%	85%
Hospital Given 9 or 10 on 10 Point Scale	300+	66%	67%	71%
Meds 'Always' Explained Before Given	300+	64%	60%	64%
Nurses 'Always' Communicated Well	300+	77%	75%	79%
Pain 'Always' Well Controlled	300+	68%	68%	71%
Room and Bathroom 'Always' Clean	300+	65%	69%	73%
Timely Help 'Always' Received	300+	60%	62%	68%
Would Definitely Recommend Hospital	300+	65%	69%	71%
Use of Medical Imaging				
Cardiac Imaging Stress Test before Surgery	521	3.3%	6.4%	5.3%
Combination Abdominal CT Scan	744	33.5%	11.8%	10.5%
Combination Brain/Sinus CT Scan	767	3.5%	3.4%	2.7%
Combination Chest CT Scan	606	16.8%	2.4%	2.7%
Follow-up Mammogram/Ultrasound	1,851	9.6%	10.2%	8.8%
Lumbar Spine MRI for Low Back Pain	138	37.7%	35.2%	37.2%

Baptist Medical Center Beaches

1350 13th Ave S Phone: 904-247-2900
Jacksonville Beach, FL 32250 Fax: 904-627-2975
URL: www.e-baptisthealth.com/about_us/hospitals/beaches.html
Type: Acute Care Hospitals Emergency Services: Yes
Ownership: Voluntary non-profit - Private Beds: 146

Key Personnel:
Radiology. . . . . Dana Beighley
Operating Room. . . . . Donna Bowen
Quality Assurance . . . . Debra Dilibero
CEO/President. . . . . A. Hugh Greene, FACHE
Patient Relations . . . . Janice Kiernan
President . . . . Joseph Mitrick, FACHE
Chief of Medical Staff. . . . . Pamela Rama, MD

Measure	Cases	This Hosp.	State Avg.	U.S. Avg.
Blood Clot Prevention and Treatment				
Anticoagulation Overlap Therapy[2]	63	95%	93%	93%
ICU Venous Thromboembolism Prophylaxis[2]	101	92%	94%	92%
Incidence of Potentially Preventable VTE[1,2]	-	-	10%	10%
UFH with Dosages/Platelet Monitoring[2]	47	100%	100%	97%
Venous Thromboembolism Prophylaxis[2]	301	88%	88%	85%
Warfarin Therapy Discharge Instructions[2]	50	92%	85%	75%
Chest Pain/Possible Heart Attack Care				
Aspirin Given Within 24 Hours of Arrival	76	97%	98%	96%

NOTE: Hospital profiles are in alphabetical order by state, then city, then hospital within the city; Rankings exclude hospitals with less than 25 cases except for patient surveys which excludes hospitals with less than 100 cases; (a) 100-299 cases; (1) The number of cases/patients is too few to report; (2) Data submitted were based on a sample of cases/patients; (3) Results are based on a shorter time period than required; (4) Data suppressed by CMS for one or more quarters; (5) Results are not available for this reporting period; (6) Fewer than 100 patients completed the HCAHPS survey; (7) No cases met the criteria for this measure; (8) The lower limit of the confidence interval cannot be calculated if the number of observed infections equals zero; (9) No data are available from the state/territory for this reporting period; (10) The scores shown reflect fewer than 50 completed surveys; (11) There were discrepancies in the data collection process; (12) This measure does not apply to this hospital for this reporting period; (13) Results cannot be calculated for this reporting period; (14) The results for this state are combined with nearby states to protect confidentiality; Please refer to the User's Guide for a full explanation of data.

Measure	Cases	This Hosp.	State Avg.	U.S. Avg.
Fibrinolytic Meds Within 30 Min. of Arrival[1]	-	-	81%	58%
Average Time to ECG (minutes)	80	9	7	7
Average Time to Transfer (minutes)	25	35	53	60
Children's Asthma Care				
Received Home Management Plan of Care	-	-	-	88%
Received Reliever Medication	-	-	-	100%
Received Systemic Corticosteroids	-	-	-	100%
Emergency Department				
Admittance Decision Time (minutes)[2]	576	61	111	98
Head CT Results Within 45 Min. of Arrival[1]	-	-	64%	57%
Patients Who Left ER Before Being Seen	37,249	2%	2%	2%
Time from ER Arrival to Admit. (minutes)[2]	578	246	289	274
Time from ER Arrival to Discharge (minutes)	400	150	147	134
Time in ER Before Being Evaluated (minutes)	501	31	26	26
Time to Pain Meds for Fractures (minutes)	139	65	60	57
Heart Attack Care				
Aspirin Given at Discharge[2]	41	95%	99%	99%
Fibrinolytic Meds Within 30 Min. of Arrival[2,7]	-	-	50%	54%
PCI Within 90 Minutes of Arrival[2,7]	-	-	96%	96%
Statin Prescribed at Discharge[2]	37	95%	99%	98%
Heart Failure Care				
ACE Inhibitor or ARB for LVSD[2]	47	98%	98%	97%
Discharge Instructions Given[2]	151	99%	96%	94%
Evaluation of LVS Function[2]	192	100%	100%	99%
Medicare Spending				
Medicare Spending per Patient (ratio)	-	1.08	1.04	0.98
Pneumonia Care				
Appropriate Initial Antibiotic Given[2]	156	96%	98%	95%
Blood Culture Timing[2]	232	99%	99%	98%
Pregnancy and Delivery Care				
Newborn Deliveries Scheduled Early[2]	30	0%	6%	6%
Preventive Care				
Immunization for Influenza[2]	536	96%	94%	90%
Immunization for Pneumonia[2]	574	96%	96%	92%
Stroke Care				
Anticoagulation Therapy for Atrial Fibrillation[1,2]	-	-	97%	95%
Antithrombotic Therapy Timing[2]	50	100%	98%	98%
Assessed for Rehabilitation[2]	47	98%	97%	97%
Discharged on Antithrombotic Therapy[2]	47	98%	99%	99%
Discharged on Statin Medication[2]	37	92%	96%	94%
Thrombolytic Therapy Timing[1,2]	-	-	76%	66%
Venous Thromboembolism Prophylaxis[2]	47	87%	95%	94%
Written Stroke Educational Materials Given[2]	32	91%	94%	88%
Surgical Care Improvement Project				
Appropriate Beta Blocker Usage[2]	139	98%	99%	98%
Appropriate VTP Within 24 Hours[2]	416	99%	99%	98%
Controlled Postoperative Blood Glucose[2,7]	-	-	98%	97%
Perioperative Temperature Management[2]	462	100%	100%	100%
Prophylactic Antibiotic Selection[2]	302	100%	99%	99%
Prophylactic Antibiotic Selection (Outpatient)	91	92%	98%	98%
Prophylactic Antibiotic Stopped[2]	294	98%	98%	98%
Prophylactic Antibiotic Timing[2]	302	98%	99%	99%
Prophylactic Antibiotic Timing (Outpatient)	92	96%	98%	98%
Urinary Catheter Removal[2]	138	96%	98%	97%
Survey of Patients' Hospital Experiences				
Area Around Room 'Always' Quiet at Night	300+	64%	58%	61%
Doctors 'Always' Communicated Well	300+	81%	77%	82%
Home Recovery Information Given	300+	87%	83%	85%
Hospital Given 9 or 10 on 10 Point Scale	300+	75%	67%	71%
Meds 'Always' Explained Before Given	300+	63%	60%	64%
Nurses 'Always' Communicated Well	300+	80%	75%	79%
Pain 'Always' Well Controlled	300+	73%	68%	71%
Room and Bathroom 'Always' Clean	300+	73%	69%	73%
Timely Help 'Always' Received	300+	64%	62%	68%
Would Definitely Recommend Hospital	300+	79%	69%	71%
Use of Medical Imaging				
Cardiac Imaging Stress Test before Surgery	1,219	5.9%	6.4%	5.3%
Combination Abdominal CT Scan	868	11.6%	11.8%	10.5%
Combination Brain/Sinus CT Scan	1,069	4.5%	3.4%	2.7%
Combination Chest CT Scan	579	0.9%	2.4%	2.7%
Follow-up Mammogram/Ultrasound	1,953	9.2%	10.2%	8.8%
Lumbar Spine MRI for Low Back Pain	119	28.6%	35.2%	37.2%

Jay Hospital

14114 Alabama St
Jay, FL 32565
Phone: 850-675-4532
Fax: 850-675-8070
URL: www.bhcpns.org
Type: Acute Care Hospitals
Emergency Services: Yes
Ownership: Voluntary non-profit - Private
Beds: 55

Key Personnel:

Cardiology . . . . Luther Carter, M.D., F.A.C.C.,
CEO/President. . . . . Mark Faulkner
Emergency Room . . . . Kaprena Kelley, RN
Quality Assurance . . . . Robert Lindenborn
Surgery . . . . George Rees, MD
Pediatrics. . . . . Marian Stewart, MD

Measure	Cases	This Hosp.	State Avg.	U.S. Avg.
Blood Clot Prevention and Treatment				
Anticoagulation Overlap Therapy[1,2]	-	-	93%	93%
ICU Venous Thromboembolism Prophylaxis[2,7]	-	-	94%	92%
Incidence of Potentially Preventable VTE[2,7]	-	-	10%	10%
UFH with Dosages/Platelet Monitoring[2,7]	-	-	100%	97%
Venous Thromboembolism Prophylaxis[2]	146	85%	88%	85%
Warfarin Therapy Discharge Instructions[1,2]	-	-	85%	75%
Chest Pain/Possible Heart Attack Care				
Aspirin Given Within 24 Hours of Arrival	11	100%	98%	96%
Fibrinolytic Meds Within 30 Min. of Arrival[3,7]	-	-	81%	58%
Average Time to ECG (minutes)	14	10	7	7
Average Time to Transfer (minutes)[3,7]	-	-	53	60
Children's Asthma Care				
Received Home Management Plan of Care	-	-	-	88%
Received Reliever Medication	-	-	-	100%
Received Systemic Corticosteroids	-	-	-	100%
Emergency Department				
Admittance Decision Time (minutes)[2]	480	52	111	98
Head CT Results Within 45 Min. of Arrival[1]	-	-	64%	57%
Patients Who Left ER Before Being Seen	9,972	1%	2%	2%
Time from ER Arrival to Admit. (minutes)[2]	481	220	289	274
Time from ER Arrival to Discharge (minutes)	449	105	147	134
Time in ER Before Being Evaluated (minutes)	469	52	26	26
Time to Pain Meds for Fractures (minutes)	20	61	60	57
Heart Attack Care				
Aspirin Given at Discharge[1,3]	-	-	99%	99%
Fibrinolytic Meds Within 30 Min. of Arrival[3,7]	-	-	50%	54%
PCI Within 90 Minutes of Arrival[3,7]	-	-	96%	96%
Statin Prescribed at Discharge[1,3]	-	-	99%	98%
Heart Failure Care				
ACE Inhibitor or ARB for LVSD	12	100%	98%	97%
Discharge Instructions Given	40	100%	96%	94%
Evaluation of LVS Function	52	100%	100%	99%
Medicare Spending				
Medicare Spending per Patient (ratio)	-	0.86	1.04	0.98
Pneumonia Care				
Appropriate Initial Antibiotic Given	26	100%	98%	95%
Blood Culture Timing	26	100%	99%	98%
Pregnancy and Delivery Care				
Newborn Deliveries Scheduled Early[7]	-	-	6%	6%
Preventive Care				
Immunization for Influenza[2]	259	100%	94%	90%
Immunization for Pneumonia[2]	385	97%	96%	92%
Stroke Care				
Anticoagulation Therapy for Atrial Fibrillation[7]	-	-	97%	95%
Antithrombotic Therapy Timing[1]	-	-	98%	98%
Assessed for Rehabilitation[1]	-	-	97%	97%
Discharged on Antithrombotic Therapy[1]	-	-	99%	99%
Discharged on Statin Medication[1]	-	-	96%	94%
Thrombolytic Therapy Timing[1]	-	-	76%	66%
Venous Thromboembolism Prophylaxis[1]	-	-	95%	94%
Written Stroke Educational Materials Given[1]	-	-	94%	88%
Surgical Care Improvement Project				
Appropriate Beta Blocker Usage[5]	-	-	99%	98%
Appropriate VTP Within 24 Hours[5]	-	-	99%	98%
Controlled Postoperative Blood Glucose[5]	-	-	98%	97%
Perioperative Temperature Management[5]	-	-	100%	100%
Prophylactic Antibiotic Selection[5]	-	-	99%	99%
Prophylactic Antibiotic Selection (Outpatient)[5]	-	-	98%	98%
Prophylactic Antibiotic Stopped[5]	-	-	98%	98%
Prophylactic Antibiotic Timing[5]	-	-	99%	99%
Prophylactic Antibiotic Timing (Outpatient)[5]	-	-	98%	98%
Urinary Catheter Removal[5]	-	-	98%	97%
Survey of Patients' Hospital Experiences				
Area Around Room 'Always' Quiet at Night	(a)	76%	58%	61%
Doctors 'Always' Communicated Well	(a)	89%	77%	82%
Home Recovery Information Given	(a)	83%	83%	85%
Hospital Given 9 or 10 on 10 Point Scale	(a)	75%	67%	71%
Meds 'Always' Explained Before Given	(a)	73%	60%	64%
Nurses 'Always' Communicated Well	(a)	86%	75%	79%
Pain 'Always' Well Controlled	(a)	74%	68%	71%
Room and Bathroom 'Always' Clean	(a)	77%	69%	73%
Timely Help 'Always' Received	(a)	80%	62%	68%
Would Definitely Recommend Hospital	(a)	74%	69%	71%
Use of Medical Imaging				
Cardiac Imaging Stress Test before Surgery[1]	-	-	6.4%	5.3%
Combination Abdominal CT Scan	99	33.3%	11.8%	10.5%
Combination Brain/Sinus CT Scan	93	0.0%	3.4%	2.7%
Combination Chest CT Scan[1]	-	-	2.4%	2.7%
Follow-up Mammogram/Ultrasound	138	8.0%	10.2%	8.8%
Lumbar Spine MRI for Low Back Pain[1]	-	-	35.2%	37.2%

Jupiter Medical Center

1210 S Old Dixie Hwy
Jupiter, FL 33458
Phone: 561-747-2234
Fax: 561-743-5042
E-mail: ljones@jupitermed.com
URL: www.jupitermed.com
Type: Acute Care Hospitals
Emergency Services: Yes
Ownership: Voluntary non-profit - Private
Beds: 156

Key Personnel:

Emergency Room . . . . Michael Collins, MD
CEO/President. . . . . John D. Couris
Quality Assurance . . . . Terri Freeman
Chief of Medical Staff . . . . Thomas Rowe, MD
Operating Room. . . . . Beth Suriano
Ambulatory Care . . . . Terri Wentz

Measure	Cases	This Hosp.	State Avg.	U.S. Avg.
Blood Clot Prevention and Treatment				
Anticoagulation Overlap Therapy[2]	125	100%	93%	93%
ICU Venous Thromboembolism Prophylaxis[2]	51	96%	94%	92%
Incidence of Potentially Preventable VTE[2]	17	0%	10%	10%
UFH with Dosages/Platelet Monitoring[2]	130	100%	100%	97%
Venous Thromboembolism Prophylaxis[2]	377	95%	88%	85%
Warfarin Therapy Discharge Instructions[2]	91	98%	85%	75%
Chest Pain/Possible Heart Attack Care				
Aspirin Given Within 24 Hours of Arrival	66	100%	98%	96%
Fibrinolytic Meds Within 30 Min. of Arrival[7]	-	-	81%	58%
Average Time to ECG (minutes)	69	5	7	7
Average Time to Transfer (minutes)	16	62	53	60
Children's Asthma Care				
Received Home Management Plan of Care	-	-	-	88%
Received Reliever Medication	-	-	-	100%
Received Systemic Corticosteroids	-	-	-	100%
Emergency Department				
Admittance Decision Time (minutes)[2]	790	140	111	98
Head CT Results Within 45 Min. of Arrival	23	74%	64%	57%
Patients Who Left ER Before Being Seen	30,831	1%	2%	2%
Time from ER Arrival to Admit. (minutes)[2]	793	306	289	274
Time from ER Arrival to Discharge (minutes)	374	156	147	134
Time in ER Before Being Evaluated (minutes)	415	24	26	26
Time to Pain Meds for Fractures (minutes)	129	62	60	57
Heart Attack Care				
Aspirin Given at Discharge	13	100%	99%	99%
Fibrinolytic Meds Within 30 Min. of Arrival[7]	-	-	50%	54%
PCI Within 90 Minutes of Arrival[7]	-	-	96%	96%
Statin Prescribed at Discharge	13	100%	99%	98%
Heart Failure Care				
ACE Inhibitor or ARB for LVSD	48	98%	98%	97%
Discharge Instructions Given	166	99%	96%	94%
Evaluation of LVS Function	200	100%	100%	99%
Medicare Spending				
Medicare Spending per Patient (ratio)	-	1.01	1.04	0.98
Pneumonia Care				
Appropriate Initial Antibiotic Given[2]	90	99%	98%	95%

NOTE: Hospital profiles are in alphabetical order by state, then city, then hospital within the city; Rankings exclude hospitals with less than 25 cases except for patient surveys which excludes hospitals with less than 100 cases; (a) 100-299 cases; (1) The number of cases/patients is too few to report; (2) Data submitted were based on a sample of cases/patients; (3) Results are based on a shorter time period than required; (4) Data suppressed by CMS for one or more quarters; (5) Results are not available for this reporting period; (6) Fewer than 100 patients completed the HCAHPS survey; (7) No cases met the criteria for this measure; (8) The lower limit of the confidence interval cannot be calculated if the number of observed infections equals zero; (9) No data are available from the state/territory for this reporting period; (10) The scores shown reflect fewer than 50 completed surveys; (11) There were discrepancies in the data collection process; (12) This measure does not apply to this hospital for this reporting period; (13) Results cannot be calculated for this reporting period; (14) The results for this state are combined with nearby states to protect confidentiality; Please refer to the User's Guide for a full explanation of data.

Blood Culture Timing[2]	154	99%	99%	98%
Pregnancy and Delivery Care				
Newborn Deliveries Scheduled Early	160	4%	6%	6%
Preventive Care				
Immunization for Influenza[2]	597	97%	94%	90%
Immunization for Pneumonia[2]	769	99%	96%	92%
Stroke Care				
Anticoagulation Therapy for Atrial Fibrillation	17	100%	97%	95%
Antithrombotic Therapy Timing	74	100%	98%	98%
Assessed for Rehabilitation	79	100%	97%	97%
Discharged on Antithrombotic Therapy	75	100%	99%	99%
Discharged on Statin Medication	60	98%	96%	94%
Thrombolytic Therapy Timing[1]	-	-	76%	66%
Venous Thromboembolism Prophylaxis	93	98%	95%	94%
Written Stroke Educational Materials Given	47	100%	94%	88%
Surgical Care Improvement Project				
Appropriate Beta Blocker Usage[2]	145	100%	99%	98%
Appropriate VTP Within 24 Hours[2]	483	100%	99%	98%
Controlled Postoperative Blood Glucose[2,7]	-	-	98%	97%
Perioperative Temperature Management[2]	530	100%	100%	100%
Prophylactic Antibiotic Selection[2]	342	100%	99%	99%
Prophylactic Antibiotic Selection (Outpatient)	366	98%	98%	98%
Prophylactic Antibiotic Stopped[2]	337	100%	98%	98%
Prophylactic Antibiotic Timing[2]	343	100%	99%	99%
Prophylactic Antibiotic Timing (Outpatient)	365	100%	98%	98%
Urinary Catheter Removal[2]	329	100%	98%	97%
Survey of Patients' Hospital Experiences				
Area Around Room 'Always' Quiet at Night	300+	58%	58%	61%
Doctors 'Always' Communicated Well	300+	78%	77%	82%
Home Recovery Information Given	300+	87%	83%	85%
Hospital Given 9 or 10 on 10 Point Scale	300+	74%	67%	71%
Meds 'Always' Explained Before Given	300+	60%	60%	64%
Nurses 'Always' Communicated Well	300+	76%	75%	79%
Pain 'Always' Well Controlled	300+	69%	68%	71%
Room and Bathroom 'Always' Clean	300+	67%	69%	73%
Timely Help 'Always' Received	300+	64%	62%	68%
Would Definitely Recommend Hospital	300+	79%	69%	71%
Use of Medical Imaging				
Cardiac Imaging Stress Test before Surgery[1]	-	-	6.4%	5.3%
Combination Abdominal CT Scan	1,620	15.9%	11.8%	10.5%
Combination Brain/Sinus CT Scan	1,408	4.0%	3.4%	2.7%
Combination Chest CT Scan	1,529	9.7%	2.4%	2.7%
Follow-up Mammogram/Ultrasound	2,161	21.0%	10.2%	8.8%
Lumbar Spine MRI for Low Back Pain	149	22.1%	35.2%	37.2%

Lower Keys Medical Center

5900 College Road
Key West, FL 33040
URL: www.lkmc.com
Phone: 305-294-5531
Fax: 305-296-2520
Type: Acute Care Hospitals
Ownership: Proprietary
Emergency Services: Yes
Beds: 169

Key Personnel:

Infection Control . . . . Alice Brady
Cardiac Laboratory. . . . . Dan Courtney
Chief of Medical Staff . . . . Jerome Covington, MD
Emergency Room . . . . Sheila Duncan
Radiology. . . . . Jose Hernandez
Quality Assurance . . . . Barbara Southwell
Operating Room. . . . . Phllis Stout
CEO/President. . . . . Nicki Will

Measure	Cases	This Hosp.	State Avg.	U.S. Avg.
Blood Clot Prevention and Treatment				
Anticoagulation Overlap Therapy[2]	30	100%	93%	93%
ICU Venous Thromboembolism Prophylaxis[2]	58	97%	94%	92%
Incidence of Potentially Preventable VTE[1,2]	-	-	10%	10%
UFH with Dosages/Platelet Monitoring[2]	20	100%	100%	97%
Venous Thromboembolism Prophylaxis[2]	255	90%	88%	85%
Warfarin Therapy Discharge Instructions[2]	24	100%	85%	75%
Chest Pain/Possible Heart Attack Care				
Aspirin Given Within 24 Hours of Arrival	23	96%	98%	96%
Fibrinolytic Meds Within 30 Min. of Arrival[3,7]	-	-	81%	58%
Average Time to ECG (minutes)	23	2	7	7
Average Time to Transfer (minutes)[1,3]	-	-	53	60
Children's Asthma Care				
Received Home Management Plan of Care	-	-	-	88%
Received Reliever Medication	-	-	-	100%
Received Systemic Corticosteroids	-	-	-	100%
Emergency Department				
Admittance Decision Time (minutes)[2]	563	58	111	98
Head CT Results Within 45 Min. of Arrival[1]	-	-	64%	57%
Patients Who Left ER Before Being Seen	24,879	1%	2%	2%
Time from ER Arrival to Admit. (minutes)[2]	566	256	289	274
Time from ER Arrival to Discharge (minutes)	1,130	116	147	134
Time in ER Before Being Evaluated (minutes)	1,244	32	26	26
Time to Pain Meds for Fractures (minutes)	123	46	60	57
Heart Attack Care				
Aspirin Given at Discharge	35	100%	99%	99%
Fibrinolytic Meds Within 30 Min. of Arrival[7]	-	-	50%	54%
PCI Within 90 Minutes of Arrival[1]	-	-	96%	96%
Statin Prescribed at Discharge	33	97%	99%	98%
Heart Failure Care				
ACE Inhibitor or ARB for LVSD	27	89%	98%	97%
Discharge Instructions Given	58	95%	96%	94%
Evaluation of LVS Function	67	100%	100%	99%
Medicare Spending				
Medicare Spending per Patient (ratio)	-	0.93	1.04	0.98
Pneumonia Care				
Appropriate Initial Antibiotic Given	42	100%	98%	95%
Blood Culture Timing	60	98%	99%	98%
Pregnancy and Delivery Care				
Newborn Deliveries Scheduled Early	32	3%	6%	6%
Preventive Care				
Immunization for Influenza[2]	402	100%	94%	90%
Immunization for Pneumonia[2]	386	99%	96%	92%
Stroke Care				
Anticoagulation Therapy for Atrial Fibrillation[1]	-	-	97%	95%
Antithrombotic Therapy Timing	27	96%	98%	98%
Assessed for Rehabilitation	27	81%	97%	97%
Discharged on Antithrombotic Therapy	27	100%	99%	99%
Discharged on Statin Medication	23	96%	96%	94%
Thrombolytic Therapy Timing[1]	-	-	76%	66%
Venous Thromboembolism Prophylaxis	26	85%	95%	94%
Written Stroke Educational Materials Given	21	100%	94%	88%
Surgical Care Improvement Project				
Appropriate Beta Blocker Usage[2]	65	98%	99%	98%
Appropriate VTP Within 24 Hours[2]	184	95%	99%	98%
Controlled Postoperative Blood Glucose[2,7]	-	-	98%	97%
Perioperative Temperature Management[2]	218	100%	100%	100%
Prophylactic Antibiotic Selection[2]	110	100%	99%	99%
Prophylactic Antibiotic Selection (Outpatient)	49	100%	98%	98%
Prophylactic Antibiotic Stopped[2]	108	99%	98%	98%
Prophylactic Antibiotic Timing[2]	110	100%	99%	99%
Prophylactic Antibiotic Timing (Outpatient)	50	98%	98%	98%
Urinary Catheter Removal[2]	130	95%	98%	97%
Survey of Patients' Hospital Experiences				
Area Around Room 'Always' Quiet at Night	300+	48%	58%	61%
Doctors 'Always' Communicated Well	300+	80%	77%	82%
Home Recovery Information Given	300+	81%	83%	85%
Hospital Given 9 or 10 on 10 Point Scale	300+	49%	67%	71%
Meds 'Always' Explained Before Given	300+	58%	60%	64%
Nurses 'Always' Communicated Well	300+	73%	75%	79%
Pain 'Always' Well Controlled	300+	68%	68%	71%
Room and Bathroom 'Always' Clean	300+	61%	69%	73%
Timely Help 'Always' Received	300+	68%	62%	68%
Would Definitely Recommend Hospital	300+	53%	69%	71%
Use of Medical Imaging				
Cardiac Imaging Stress Test before Surgery	288	3.1%	6.4%	5.3%
Combination Abdominal CT Scan	261	4.2%	11.8%	10.5%
Combination Brain/Sinus CT Scan[1]	-	-	3.4%	2.7%
Combination Chest CT Scan	159	3.8%	2.4%	2.7%
Follow-up Mammogram/Ultrasound	559	14.0%	10.2%	8.8%
Lumbar Spine MRI for Low Back Pain[1]	-	-	35.2%	37.2%

Osceola Regional Medical Center

700 West Oak Street
Kissimmee, FL 34741
URL: www.osceolaregional.com
Phone: 407-846-2266
Fax: 407-518-3616
Type: Acute Care Hospitals
Ownership: Proprietary
Emergency Services: Yes
Beds: 231

Key Personnel:

Emergency Room . . . . Anthony Alatriste
Radiology. . . . . Stewart Bakst, MD
Ambulatory Care . . . . Louis Caputo
Operating Room. . . . . Napoleon N Estrada
Chief of Medical Staff . . . . Aida Sanchez Jimenez, MD
CEO . . . . Robert Krieger
Quality Assurance . . . . Linda Lemon-Steiner
Intensive Care Unit. . . . . Richard Puerce

Measure	Cases	This Hosp.	State Avg.	U.S. Avg.
Blood Clot Prevention and Treatment				
Anticoagulation Overlap Therapy[2]	141	93%	93%	93%
ICU Venous Thromboembolism Prophylaxis[2]	72	100%	94%	92%
Incidence of Potentially Preventable VTE[2]	16	6%	10%	10%
UFH with Dosages/Platelet Monitoring[2]	36	100%	100%	97%
Venous Thromboembolism Prophylaxis[2]	399	94%	88%	85%
Warfarin Therapy Discharge Instructions[2]	116	99%	85%	75%
Chest Pain/Possible Heart Attack Care				
Aspirin Given Within 24 Hours of Arrival[5]	-	-	98%	96%
Fibrinolytic Meds Within 30 Min. of Arrival[5]	-	-	81%	58%
Average Time to ECG (minutes)[5]	-	-	7	7
Average Time to Transfer (minutes)[5]	-	-	53	60
Children's Asthma Care				
Received Home Management Plan of Care	-	-	-	88%
Received Reliever Medication	-	-	-	100%
Received Systemic Corticosteroids	-	-	-	100%
Emergency Department				
Admittance Decision Time (minutes)[2]	920	116	111	98
Head CT Results Within 45 Min. of Arrival	22	77%	64%	57%
Patients Who Left ER Before Being Seen	87,813	1%	2%	2%
Time from ER Arrival to Admit. (minutes)[2]	920	290	289	274
Time from ER Arrival to Discharge (minutes)	443	154	147	134
Time in ER Before Being Evaluated (minutes)	521	13	26	26
Time to Pain Meds for Fractures (minutes)	212	54	60	57
Heart Attack Care				
Aspirin Given at Discharge[2]	430	100%	99%	99%
Fibrinolytic Meds Within 30 Min. of Arrival[2,7]	-	-	50%	54%
PCI Within 90 Minutes of Arrival[2]	55	100%	96%	96%
Statin Prescribed at Discharge[2]	427	100%	99%	98%
Heart Failure Care				
ACE Inhibitor or ARB for LVSD[2]	116	99%	98%	97%
Discharge Instructions Given[2]	250	100%	96%	94%
Evaluation of LVS Function[2]	300	100%	100%	99%
Medicare Spending				
Medicare Spending per Patient (ratio)	-	1.02	1.04	0.98
Pneumonia Care				
Appropriate Initial Antibiotic Given[2]	262	98%	98%	95%
Blood Culture Timing[2]	249	99%	99%	98%
Pregnancy and Delivery Care				
Newborn Deliveries Scheduled Early[2]	46	0%	6%	6%
Preventive Care				
Immunization for Influenza[2]	595	99%	94%	90%
Immunization for Pneumonia[2]	801	98%	96%	92%
Stroke Care				
Anticoagulation Therapy for Atrial Fibrillation[2]	11	91%	97%	95%
Antithrombotic Therapy Timing[2]	98	100%	98%	98%
Assessed for Rehabilitation[2]	122	99%	97%	97%
Discharged on Antithrombotic Therapy[2]	100	99%	99%	99%
Discharged on Statin Medication[2]	84	99%	96%	94%
Thrombolytic Therapy Timing[1,2]	-	-	76%	66%
Venous Thromboembolism Prophylaxis[2]	132	98%	95%	94%
Written Stroke Educational Materials Given[2]	80	100%	94%	88%
Surgical Care Improvement Project				
Appropriate Beta Blocker Usage[2]	193	97%	99%	98%
Appropriate VTP Within 24 Hours[2]	445	100%	99%	98%
Controlled Postoperative Blood Glucose[2]	75	99%	98%	97%
Perioperative Temperature Management[2]	518	100%	100%	100%
Prophylactic Antibiotic Selection[2]	389	99%	99%	99%

NOTE: Hospital profiles are in alphabetical order by state, then city, then hospital within the city; Rankings exclude hospitals with less than 25 cases except for patient surveys which excludes hospitals with less than 100 cases; (a) 100-299 cases; (1) The number of cases/patients is too few to report; (2) Data submitted were based on a sample of cases/patients; (3) Results are based on a shorter time period than required; (4) Data suppressed by CMS for one or more quarters; (5) Results are not available for this reporting period; (6) Fewer than 100 patients completed the HCAHPS survey; (7) No cases met the criteria for this measure; (8) The lower limit of the confidence interval cannot be calculated if the number of observed infections equals zero; (9) No data are available from the state/territory for this reporting period; (10) The scores shown reflect fewer than 50 completed surveys; (11) There were discrepancies in the data collection process; (12) This measure does not apply to this hospital for this reporting period; (13) Results cannot be calculated for this reporting period; (14) The results for this state are combined with nearby states to protect confidentiality; Please refer to the User's Guide for a full explanation of data.

Measure	Cases	This Hosp.	State Avg.	U.S. Avg.
Prophylactic Antibiotic Selection (Outpatient)	295	99%	98%	98%
Prophylactic Antibiotic Stopped[2]	379	100%	98%	98%
Prophylactic Antibiotic Timing[2]	389	99%	99%	99%
Prophylactic Antibiotic Timing (Outpatient)	295	100%	98%	98%
Urinary Catheter Removal[2]	366	97%	98%	97%
Survey of Patients' Hospital Experiences				
Area Around Room 'Always' Quiet at Night	300+	57%	58%	61%
Doctors 'Always' Communicated Well	300+	75%	77%	82%
Home Recovery Information Given	300+	81%	83%	85%
Hospital Given 9 or 10 on 10 Point Scale	300+	59%	67%	71%
Meds 'Always' Explained Before Given	300+	57%	60%	64%
Nurses 'Always' Communicated Well	300+	71%	75%	79%
Pain 'Always' Well Controlled	300+	66%	68%	71%
Room and Bathroom 'Always' Clean	300+	65%	69%	73%
Timely Help 'Always' Received	300+	60%	62%	68%
Would Definitely Recommend Hospital	300+	61%	69%	71%
Use of Medical Imaging				
Cardiac Imaging Stress Test before Surgery	254	6.7%	6.4%	5.3%
Combination Abdominal CT Scan	572	5.1%	11.8%	10.5%
Combination Brain/Sinus CT Scan	632	4.4%	3.4%	2.7%
Combination Chest CT Scan	166	0.6%	2.4%	2.7%
Follow-up Mammogram/Ultrasound	526	12.2%	10.2%	8.8%
Lumbar Spine MRI for Low Back Pain[1]	-	-	35.2%	37.2%

Lake Butler Hospital Hand Surgery Center

850 E Main St Phone: 386-496-2323
Lake Butler, FL 32054
Type: Critical Access Hospitals Emergency Services: Yes
Ownership: Voluntary non-profit - Private

Measure	Cases	This Hosp.	State Avg.	U.S. Avg.
Blood Clot Prevention and Treatment				
Anticoagulation Overlap Therapy[5]	-	-	93%	93%
ICU Venous Thromboembolism Prophylaxis[5]	-	-	94%	92%
Incidence of Potentially Preventable VTE[5]	-	-	10%	10%
UFH with Dosages/Platelet Monitoring[5]	-	-	100%	97%
Venous Thromboembolism Prophylaxis[5]	-	-	88%	85%
Warfarin Therapy Discharge Instructions[5]	-	-	85%	75%
Chest Pain/Possible Heart Attack Care				
Aspirin Given Within 24 Hours of Arrival	-	-	98%	96%
Fibrinolytic Meds Within 30 Min. of Arrival	-	-	81%	58%
Average Time to ECG (minutes)	-	-	7	7
Average Time to Transfer (minutes)	-	-	53	60
Children's Asthma Care				
Received Home Management Plan of Care	-	-	-	88%
Received Reliever Medication	-	-	-	100%
Received Systemic Corticosteroids	-	-	-	100%
Emergency Department				
Admittance Decision Time (minutes)[5]	-	-	111	98
Head CT Results Within 45 Min. of Arrival	-	-	64%	57%
Patients Who Left ER Before Being Seen	-	-	2%	2%
Time from ER Arrival to Admit. (minutes)[5]	-	-	289	274
Time from ER Arrival to Discharge (minutes)	-	-	147	134
Time in ER Before Being Evaluated (minutes)	-	-	26	26
Time to Pain Meds for Fractures (minutes)	-	-	60	57
Heart Attack Care				
Aspirin Given at Discharge[5]	-	-	99%	99%
Fibrinolytic Meds Within 30 Min. of Arrival[5]	-	-	50%	54%
PCI Within 90 Minutes of Arrival[5]	-	-	96%	96%
Statin Prescribed at Discharge[5]	-	-	99%	98%
Heart Failure Care				
ACE Inhibitor or ARB for LVSD[3,7]	-	-	98%	97%
Discharge Instructions Given[3,7]	-	-	96%	94%
Evaluation of LVS Function[1,3]	-	-	100%	99%
Medicare Spending				
Medicare Spending per Patient (ratio)	-	-	1.04	0.98
Pneumonia Care				
Appropriate Initial Antibiotic Given[1]	-	-	98%	95%
Blood Culture Timing[7]	-	-	99%	98%
Pregnancy and Delivery Care				
Newborn Deliveries Scheduled Early[5]	-	-	6%	6%
Preventive Care				
Immunization for Influenza[5]	-	-	94%	90%
Immunization for Pneumonia[5]	-	-	96%	92%
Stroke Care				
Anticoagulation Therapy for Atrial Fibrillation[5]	-	-	97%	95%
Antithrombotic Therapy Timing[5]	-	-	98%	98%
Assessed for Rehabilitation[5]	-	-	97%	97%
Discharged on Antithrombotic Therapy[5]	-	-	99%	99%
Discharged on Statin Medication[5]	-	-	96%	94%
Thrombolytic Therapy Timing[5]	-	-	76%	66%
Venous Thromboembolism Prophylaxis[5]	-	-	95%	94%
Written Stroke Educational Materials Given[5]	-	-	94%	88%
Surgical Care Improvement Project				
Appropriate Beta Blocker Usage[5]	-	-	99%	98%
Appropriate VTP Within 24 Hours[5]	-	-	99%	98%
Controlled Postoperative Blood Glucose[5]	-	-	98%	97%
Perioperative Temperature Management[5]	-	-	100%	100%
Prophylactic Antibiotic Selection[5]	-	-	99%	99%
Prophylactic Antibiotic Selection (Outpatient)	-	-	98%	98%
Prophylactic Antibiotic Stopped[5]	-	-	98%	98%
Prophylactic Antibiotic Timing[5]	-	-	99%	99%
Prophylactic Antibiotic Timing (Outpatient)	-	-	98%	98%
Urinary Catheter Removal[5]	-	-	98%	97%
Survey of Patients' Hospital Experiences				
Area Around Room 'Always' Quiet at Night[5]	-	-	58%	61%
Doctors 'Always' Communicated Well[5]	-	-	77%	82%
Home Recovery Information Given[5]	-	-	83%	85%
Hospital Given 9 or 10 on 10 Point Scale[5]	-	-	67%	71%
Meds 'Always' Explained Before Given[5]	-	-	60%	64%
Nurses 'Always' Communicated Well[5]	-	-	75%	79%
Pain 'Always' Well Controlled[5]	-	-	68%	71%
Room and Bathroom 'Always' Clean[5]	-	-	69%	73%
Timely Help 'Always' Received[5]	-	-	62%	68%
Would Definitely Recommend Hospital[5]	-	-	69%	71%
Use of Medical Imaging				
Cardiac Imaging Stress Test before Surgery	-	-	6.4%	5.3%
Combination Abdominal CT Scan	-	-	11.8%	10.5%
Combination Brain/Sinus CT Scan	-	-	3.4%	2.7%
Combination Chest CT Scan	-	-	2.4%	2.7%
Follow-up Mammogram/Ultrasound	-	-	10.2%	8.8%
Lumbar Spine MRI for Low Back Pain	-	-	35.2%	37.2%

Lake City Medical Center

340 Nw Commerce Dr Phone: 386-719-9000
Lake City, FL 32055 Fax: 386-719-7787
URL: www.lakecitymedical.com
Type: Acute Care Hospitals Emergency Services: Yes
Ownership: Voluntary non-profit - Private Beds: 75

Key Personnel:
Radiology. . . . . Andres R Acosla
Emergency Room . . . . Mark A Dobbertien, RN
Intensive Care Unit. . . . . Mark Fontaine
Infection Control. . . . . Mary Fuller
Quality Assurance . . . . Louise McKernan
Operating Room. . . . . Debby Moore, RN
Chief of Medical Staff . . . . Eric Ordinario, DO
CEO . . . . Mark Robinson

Measure	Cases	This Hosp.	State Avg.	U.S. Avg.
Blood Clot Prevention and Treatment				
Anticoagulation Overlap Therapy[2]	27	100%	93%	93%
ICU Venous Thromboembolism Prophylaxis[2]	96	98%	94%	92%
Incidence of Potentially Preventable VTE[1,2]	-	-	10%	10%
UFH with Dosages/Platelet Monitoring[2]	18	100%	100%	97%
Venous Thromboembolism Prophylaxis[2]	364	96%	88%	85%
Warfarin Therapy Discharge Instructions[2]	20	100%	85%	75%
Chest Pain/Possible Heart Attack Care				
Aspirin Given Within 24 Hours of Arrival	132	98%	98%	96%
Fibrinolytic Meds Within 30 Min. of Arrival[7]	-	-	81%	58%
Average Time to ECG (minutes)	143	14	7	7
Average Time to Transfer (minutes)	15	84	53	60
Children's Asthma Care				
Received Home Management Plan of Care	-	-	-	88%
Received Reliever Medication	-	-	-	100%
Received Systemic Corticosteroids	-	-	-	100%
Emergency Department				
Admittance Decision Time (minutes)[2]	574	125	111	98
Head CT Results Within 45 Min. of Arrival[1]	-	-	64%	57%
Patients Who Left ER Before Being Seen	28,047	2%	2%	2%
Time from ER Arrival to Admit. (minutes)[2]	574	318	289	274
Time from ER Arrival to Discharge (minutes)	376	126	147	134
Time in ER Before Being Evaluated (minutes)	452	8	26	26
Time to Pain Meds for Fractures (minutes)	71	64	60	57
Heart Attack Care				
Aspirin Given at Discharge[2]	18	100%	99%	99%
Fibrinolytic Meds Within 30 Min. of Arrival[2,7]	-	-	50%	54%
PCI Within 90 Minutes of Arrival[2,7]	-	-	96%	96%
Statin Prescribed at Discharge[2]	14	100%	99%	98%
Heart Failure Care				
ACE Inhibitor or ARB for LVSD[2]	53	100%	98%	97%
Discharge Instructions Given[2]	197	100%	96%	94%
Evaluation of LVS Function[2]	254	100%	100%	99%
Medicare Spending				
Medicare Spending per Patient (ratio)	-	1.03	1.04	0.98
Pneumonia Care				
Appropriate Initial Antibiotic Given[2]	84	100%	98%	95%
Blood Culture Timing[2]	136	100%	99%	98%
Pregnancy and Delivery Care				
Newborn Deliveries Scheduled Early[2,7]	-	-	6%	6%
Preventive Care				
Immunization for Influenza[2]	455	98%	94%	90%
Immunization for Pneumonia[2]	748	98%	96%	92%
Stroke Care				
Anticoagulation Therapy for Atrial Fibrillation[1,2]	-	-	97%	95%
Antithrombotic Therapy Timing[2]	48	100%	98%	98%
Assessed for Rehabilitation[2]	48	100%	97%	97%
Discharged on Antithrombotic Therapy[2]	48	100%	99%	99%
Discharged on Statin Medication[2]	41	98%	96%	94%
Thrombolytic Therapy Timing[2,7]	-	-	76%	66%
Venous Thromboembolism Prophylaxis[2]	47	89%	95%	94%
Written Stroke Educational Materials Given[2]	38	100%	94%	88%
Surgical Care Improvement Project				
Appropriate Beta Blocker Usage[2]	50	100%	99%	98%
Appropriate VTP Within 24 Hours[2]	143	100%	99%	98%
Controlled Postoperative Blood Glucose[2,7]	-	-	98%	97%
Perioperative Temperature Management[2]	150	100%	100%	100%
Prophylactic Antibiotic Selection[2]	98	100%	99%	99%
Prophylactic Antibiotic Selection (Outpatient)	40	100%	98%	98%
Prophylactic Antibiotic Stopped[2]	95	100%	98%	98%
Prophylactic Antibiotic Timing[2]	98	100%	99%	99%
Prophylactic Antibiotic Timing (Outpatient)	40	100%	98%	98%
Urinary Catheter Removal[2]	112	100%	98%	97%
Survey of Patients' Hospital Experiences				
Area Around Room 'Always' Quiet at Night	300+	57%	58%	61%
Doctors 'Always' Communicated Well	300+	81%	77%	82%
Home Recovery Information Given	300+	86%	83%	85%
Hospital Given 9 or 10 on 10 Point Scale	300+	71%	67%	71%
Meds 'Always' Explained Before Given	300+	63%	60%	64%
Nurses 'Always' Communicated Well	300+	77%	75%	79%
Pain 'Always' Well Controlled	300+	71%	68%	71%
Room and Bathroom 'Always' Clean	300+	70%	69%	73%
Timely Help 'Always' Received	300+	69%	62%	68%
Would Definitely Recommend Hospital	300+	76%	69%	71%
Use of Medical Imaging				
Cardiac Imaging Stress Test before Surgery	145	5.5%	6.4%	5.3%
Combination Abdominal CT Scan	488	1.8%	11.8%	10.5%
Combination Brain/Sinus CT Scan	773	3.5%	3.4%	2.7%
Combination Chest CT Scan	107	0.0%	2.4%	2.7%
Follow-up Mammogram/Ultrasound[7]	-	-	10.2%	8.8%
Lumbar Spine MRI for Low Back Pain[1]	-	-	35.2%	37.2%

Shands Lake Shore Regional Medical Center

368 Ne Franklin St Phone: 386-292-8000
Lake City, FL 32055 Fax: 386-754-8121
URL: www.shands.org
Type: Acute Care Hospitals Emergency Services: Yes
Ownership: Voluntary non-profit - Private Beds: 99

Key Personnel:
Radiology. . . . . Jeffrey Bennet
Chief of Medical Staff . . . . Jerry J Berger
Emergency Room . . . . Noel Braseth

NOTE: Hospital profiles are in alphabetical order by state, then city, then hospital within the city; Rankings exclude hospitals with less than 25 cases except for patient surveys which excludes hospitals with less than 100 cases; (a) 100-299 cases; (1) The number of cases/patients is too few to report; (2) Data submitted were based on a sample of cases/patients; (3) Results are based on a shorter time period than required; (4) Data suppressed by CMS for one or more quarters; (5) Results are not available for this reporting period; (6) Fewer than 100 patients completed the HCAHPS survey; (7) No cases met the criteria for this measure; (8) The lower limit of the confidence interval cannot be calculated if the number of observed infections equals zero; (9) No data are available from the state/territory for this reporting period; (10) The scores shown reflect fewer than 50 completed surveys; (11) There were discrepancies in the data collection process; (12) This measure does not apply to this hospital for this reporting period; (13) Results cannot be calculated for this reporting period; (14) The results for this state are combined with nearby states to protect confidentiality; Please refer to the User's Guide for a full explanation of data.

Pediatric Ambulatory Care . . . . . . Kelly Carmen
CEO/President. . . . . Tim Goldfarb
Operating Room. . . . . Dee McRae
Intensive Care Unit. . . . . Donna Reagan
Quality Assurance . . . . Janice Watson

Measure	Cases	This Hosp.	State Avg.	U.S. Avg.
Blood Clot Prevention and Treatment				
Anticoagulation Overlap Therapy[2]	22	45%	93%	93%
ICU Venous Thromboembolism Prophylaxis[2]	136	57%	94%	92%
Incidence of Potentially Preventable VTE[1,2]	-	-	10%	10%
UFH with Dosages/Platelet Monitoring[1,2]	-	-	100%	97%
Venous Thromboembolism Prophylaxis[2]	250	41%	88%	85%
Warfarin Therapy Discharge Instructions[2]	15	47%	85%	75%
Chest Pain/Possible Heart Attack Care				
Aspirin Given Within 24 Hours of Arrival	91	91%	98%	96%
Fibrinolytic Meds Within 30 Min. of Arrival[7]	-	-	81%	58%
Average Time to ECG (minutes)	93	7	7	7
Average Time to Transfer (minutes)[1]	-	-	53	60
Children's Asthma Care				
Received Home Management Plan of Care	-	-	-	88%
Received Reliever Medication	-	-	-	100%
Received Systemic Corticosteroids	-	-	-	100%
Emergency Department				
Admittance Decision Time (minutes)[2]	443	76	111	98
Head CT Results Within 45 Min. of Arrival[1]	-	-	64%	57%
Patients Who Left ER Before Being Seen	28,715	2%	2%	2%
Time from ER Arrival to Admit. (minutes)[2]	444	268	289	274
Time from ER Arrival to Discharge (minutes)	1,053	124	147	134
Time in ER Before Being Evaluated (minutes)	1,148	18	26	26
Time to Pain Meds for Fractures (minutes)	55	65	60	57
Heart Attack Care				
Aspirin Given at Discharge	19	74%	99%	99%
Fibrinolytic Meds Within 30 Min. of Arrival[7]	-	-	50%	54%
PCI Within 90 Minutes of Arrival[7]	-	-	96%	96%
Statin Prescribed at Discharge	16	94%	99%	98%
Heart Failure Care				
ACE Inhibitor or ARB for LVSD	33	97%	98%	97%
Discharge Instructions Given	132	90%	96%	94%
Evaluation of LVS Function	160	99%	100%	99%
Medicare Spending				
Medicare Spending per Patient (ratio)	-	1.03	1.04	0.98
Pneumonia Care				
Appropriate Initial Antibiotic Given	54	100%	98%	95%
Blood Culture Timing	67	100%	99%	98%
Pregnancy and Delivery Care				
Newborn Deliveries Scheduled Early	120	1%	6%	6%
Preventive Care				
Immunization for Influenza[2]	433	98%	94%	90%
Immunization for Pneumonia[2]	444	96%	96%	92%
Stroke Care				
Anticoagulation Therapy for Atrial Fibrillation[7]	-	-	97%	95%
Antithrombotic Therapy Timing[1]	-	-	98%	98%
Assessed for Rehabilitation[1]	-	-	97%	97%
Discharged on Antithrombotic Therapy[1]	-	-	99%	99%
Discharged on Statin Medication[1]	-	-	96%	94%
Thrombolytic Therapy Timing[7]	-	-	76%	66%
Venous Thromboembolism Prophylaxis[1]	-	-	95%	94%
Written Stroke Educational Materials Given[1]	-	-	94%	88%
Surgical Care Improvement Project				
Appropriate Beta Blocker Usage[1]	-	-	99%	98%
Appropriate VTP Within 24 Hours	68	94%	99%	98%
Controlled Postoperative Blood Glucose[7]	-	-	98%	97%
Perioperative Temperature Management	82	100%	100%	100%
Prophylactic Antibiotic Selection	46	93%	99%	99%
Prophylactic Antibiotic Selection (Outpatient)[1]	-	-	98%	98%
Prophylactic Antibiotic Stopped	46	100%	98%	98%
Prophylactic Antibiotic Timing	46	91%	99%	99%
Prophylactic Antibiotic Timing (Outpatient)	11	73%	98%	98%
Urinary Catheter Removal	23	100%	98%	97%
Survey of Patients' Hospital Experiences				
Area Around Room 'Always' Quiet at Night	300+	49%	58%	61%
Doctors 'Always' Communicated Well	300+	73%	77%	82%
Home Recovery Information Given	300+	73%	83%	85%
Hospital Given 9 or 10 on 10 Point Scale	300+	50%	67%	71%
Meds 'Always' Explained Before Given	300+	54%	60%	64%
Nurses 'Always' Communicated Well	300+	69%	75%	79%
Pain 'Always' Well Controlled	300+	65%	68%	71%
Room and Bathroom 'Always' Clean	300+	66%	69%	73%
Timely Help 'Always' Received	300+	59%	62%	68%
Would Definitely Recommend Hospital	300+	52%	69%	71%
Use of Medical Imaging				
Cardiac Imaging Stress Test before Surgery	89	10.1%	6.4%	5.3%
Combination Abdominal CT Scan	417	6.0%	11.8%	10.5%
Combination Brain/Sinus CT Scan[1]	-	-	3.4%	2.7%
Combination Chest CT Scan	171	6.4%	2.4%	2.7%
Follow-up Mammogram/Ultrasound	425	17.2%	10.2%	8.8%
Lumbar Spine MRI for Low Back Pain	52	34.6%	35.2%	37.2%

Lake Wales Medical Center

410 S 11th St
Lake Wales, FL 33853
Phone: 863-676-1433
Fax: 863-676-9323
URL: www.lakewalesmedicalcenter.com
Type: Acute Care Hospitals
Emergency Services: Yes
Ownership: Proprietary
Beds: 154

Key Personnel:
Anesthesiology. . . . . Thomas G Bouwkamp, MD
Emergency Room . . . . Michael Boyer
Chief of Medical Staff. . . . . Caroline Honculada, MD
Infection Control. . . . . Marvette Isom, RN
Quality Assurance . . . . Rafael Pabor, RN
Intensive Care Unit. . . . . Flora Wilson, RN
CEO/President. . . . . Michael J Yungmann

Measure	Cases	This Hosp.	State Avg.	U.S. Avg.
Blood Clot Prevention and Treatment				
Anticoagulation Overlap Therapy[2]	47	100%	93%	93%
ICU Venous Thromboembolism Prophylaxis[2]	73	100%	94%	92%
Incidence of Potentially Preventable VTE[1,2]	-	-	10%	10%
UFH with Dosages/Platelet Monitoring[2]	22	100%	100%	97%
Venous Thromboembolism Prophylaxis[2]	448	98%	88%	85%
Warfarin Therapy Discharge Instructions[2]	39	100%	85%	75%
Chest Pain/Possible Heart Attack Care				
Aspirin Given Within 24 Hours of Arrival	21	100%	98%	96%
Fibrinolytic Meds Within 30 Min. of Arrival[3,7]	-	-	81%	58%
Average Time to ECG (minutes)	24	6	7	7
Average Time to Transfer (minutes)[1,3]	-	-	53	60
Children's Asthma Care				
Received Home Management Plan of Care	-	-	-	88%
Received Reliever Medication	-	-	-	100%
Received Systemic Corticosteroids	-	-	-	100%
Emergency Department				
Admittance Decision Time (minutes)[2]	835	94	111	98
Head CT Results Within 45 Min. of Arrival[1]	-	-	64%	57%
Patients Who Left ER Before Being Seen	5,306	4%	2%	2%
Time from ER Arrival to Admit. (minutes)[2]	835	256	289	274
Time from ER Arrival to Discharge (minutes)	392	97	147	134
Time in ER Before Being Evaluated (minutes)	419	21	26	26
Time to Pain Meds for Fractures (minutes)	76	54	60	57
Heart Attack Care				
Aspirin Given at Discharge	28	100%	99%	99%
Fibrinolytic Meds Within 30 Min. of Arrival[7]	-	-	50%	54%
PCI Within 90 Minutes of Arrival[7]	-	-	96%	96%
Statin Prescribed at Discharge	25	96%	99%	98%
Heart Failure Care				
ACE Inhibitor or ARB for LVSD	71	93%	98%	97%
Discharge Instructions Given	220	94%	96%	94%
Evaluation of LVS Function	272	100%	100%	99%
Medicare Spending				
Medicare Spending per Patient (ratio)	-	1.01	1.04	0.98
Pneumonia Care				
Appropriate Initial Antibiotic Given	63	100%	98%	95%
Blood Culture Timing	113	100%	99%	98%
Pregnancy and Delivery Care				
Newborn Deliveries Scheduled Early[2,7]	-	-	6%	6%
Preventive Care				
Immunization for Influenza[2]	567	99%	94%	90%
Immunization for Pneumonia[2]	834	100%	96%	92%
Stroke Care				
Anticoagulation Therapy for Atrial Fibrillation[1]	-	-	97%	95%
Antithrombotic Therapy Timing	61	97%	98%	98%
Assessed for Rehabilitation	59	98%	97%	97%
Discharged on Antithrombotic Therapy	58	100%	99%	99%
Discharged on Statin Medication	43	84%	96%	94%
Thrombolytic Therapy Timing[1]	-	-	76%	66%
Venous Thromboembolism Prophylaxis	69	74%	95%	94%
Written Stroke Educational Materials Given	34	85%	94%	88%
Surgical Care Improvement Project				
Appropriate Beta Blocker Usage	44	95%	99%	98%
Appropriate VTP Within 24 Hours	106	94%	99%	98%
Controlled Postoperative Blood Glucose[7]	-	-	98%	97%
Perioperative Temperature Management	137	99%	100%	100%
Prophylactic Antibiotic Selection	58	97%	99%	99%
Prophylactic Antibiotic Selection (Outpatient)	54	96%	98%	98%
Prophylactic Antibiotic Stopped	56	96%	98%	98%
Prophylactic Antibiotic Timing	58	100%	99%	99%
Prophylactic Antibiotic Timing (Outpatient)	54	100%	98%	98%
Urinary Catheter Removal	94	95%	98%	97%
Survey of Patients' Hospital Experiences				
Area Around Room 'Always' Quiet at Night	300+	61%	58%	61%
Doctors 'Always' Communicated Well	300+	75%	77%	82%
Home Recovery Information Given	300+	84%	83%	85%
Hospital Given 9 or 10 on 10 Point Scale	300+	68%	67%	71%
Meds 'Always' Explained Before Given	300+	62%	60%	64%
Nurses 'Always' Communicated Well	300+	76%	75%	79%
Pain 'Always' Well Controlled	300+	69%	68%	71%
Room and Bathroom 'Always' Clean	300+	73%	69%	73%
Timely Help 'Always' Received	300+	60%	62%	68%
Would Definitely Recommend Hospital	300+	65%	69%	71%
Use of Medical Imaging				
Cardiac Imaging Stress Test before Surgery	78	3.8%	6.4%	5.3%
Combination Abdominal CT Scan	275	20.7%	11.8%	10.5%
Combination Brain/Sinus CT Scan[1]	-	-	3.4%	2.7%
Combination Chest CT Scan	118	37.3%	2.4%	2.7%
Follow-up Mammogram/Ultrasound	493	4.9%	10.2%	8.8%
Lumbar Spine MRI for Low Back Pain[1]	-	-	35.2%	37.2%

Lakeland Regional Medical Center

1324 Lakeland Hills Blvd
Lakeland, FL 33805
Phone: 863-687-1100
Fax: 863-284-1979
E-mail: info@lrmc.com
URL: www.lrmc.com
Type: Acute Care Hospitals
Emergency Services: Yes
Ownership: Voluntary non-profit - Private
Beds: 851

Key Personnel:
Quality Assurance . . . . Gloria Cason
Emergency Room . . . . Marge Keck
Intensive Care Unit. . . . . Carrie Ogilvie
Infection Control. . . . . Theresa Ohrmund
Radiology. . . . . Kim Pyles
Chief of Medical Staff. . . . . Edwin Sammer, MD
CEO/President. . . . . Jack T Stephens
Anesthesiology. . . . . Margie Voyles

Measure	Cases	This Hosp.	State Avg.	U.S. Avg.
Blood Clot Prevention and Treatment				
Anticoagulation Overlap Therapy[2]	303	99%	93%	93%
ICU Venous Thromboembolism Prophylaxis[2]	91	95%	94%	92%
Incidence of Potentially Preventable VTE[2]	53	19%	10%	10%
UFH with Dosages/Platelet Monitoring[2]	248	100%	100%	97%
Venous Thromboembolism Prophylaxis[2]	332	73%	88%	85%
Warfarin Therapy Discharge Instructions[2]	243	97%	85%	75%
Chest Pain/Possible Heart Attack Care				
Aspirin Given Within 24 Hours of Arrival[1,3]	-	-	98%	96%
Fibrinolytic Meds Within 30 Min. of Arrival[5]	-	-	81%	58%
Average Time to ECG (minutes)[1,3]	-	-	7	7
Average Time to Transfer (minutes)[5]	-	-	53	60
Children's Asthma Care				
Received Home Management Plan of Care	-	-	-	88%
Received Reliever Medication	-	-	-	100%
Received Systemic Corticosteroids	-	-	-	100%
Emergency Department				
Admittance Decision Time (minutes)[2]	632	27	111	98

NOTE: Hospital profiles are in alphabetical order by state, then city, then hospital within the city; Rankings exclude hospitals with less than 25 cases except for patient surveys which excludes hospitals with less than 100 cases; (a) 100-299 cases; (1) The number of cases/patients is too few to report; (2) Data submitted were based on a sample of cases/patients; (3) Results are based on a shorter time period than required; (4) Data suppressed by CMS for one or more quarters; (5) Results are not available for this reporting period; (6) Fewer than 100 patients completed the HCAHPS survey; (7) No cases met the criteria for this measure; (8) The lower limit of the confidence interval cannot be calculated if the number of observed infections equals zero; (9) No data are available from the state/territory for this reporting period; (10) The scores shown reflect fewer than 50 completed surveys; (11) There were discrepancies in the data collection process; (12) This measure does not apply to this hospital for this reporting period; (13) Results cannot be calculated for this reporting period; (14) The results for this state are combined with nearby states to protect confidentiality; Please refer to the User's Guide for a full explanation of data.

Measure	Cases	This Hosp.	State Avg.	U.S. Avg.
Head CT Results Within 45 Min. of Arrival[1]	-	-	64%	57%
Patients Who Left ER Before Being Seen	>100k	1%	2%	2%
Time from ER Arrival to Admit. (minutes)[2]	761	168	289	274
Time from ER Arrival to Discharge (minutes)	445	112	147	134
Time in ER Before Being Evaluated (minutes)	461	17	26	26
Time to Pain Meds for Fractures (minutes)	403	35	60	57
Heart Attack Care				
Aspirin Given at Discharge[2]	291	99%	99%	99%
Fibrinolytic Meds Within 30 Min. of Arrival[2,7]	-	-	50%	54%
PCI Within 90 Minutes of Arrival[2]	57	98%	96%	96%
Statin Prescribed at Discharge[2]	290	100%	99%	98%
Heart Failure Care				
ACE Inhibitor or ARB for LVSD[2]	118	99%	98%	97%
Discharge Instructions Given[2]	262	98%	96%	94%
Evaluation of LVS Function[2]	318	100%	100%	99%
Medicare Spending				
Medicare Spending per Patient (ratio)	-	1.03	1.04	0.98
Pneumonia Care				
Appropriate Initial Antibiotic Given[2]	105	99%	98%	95%
Blood Culture Timing[2]	131	100%	99%	98%
Pregnancy and Delivery Care				
Newborn Deliveries Scheduled Early	264	2%	6%	6%
Preventive Care				
Immunization for Influenza[2]	553	96%	94%	90%
Immunization for Pneumonia[2]	706	97%	96%	92%
Stroke Care				
Anticoagulation Therapy for Atrial Fibrillation[2]	16	88%	97%	95%
Antithrombotic Therapy Timing[2]	104	99%	98%	98%
Assessed for Rehabilitation[2]	130	97%	97%	97%
Discharged on Antithrombotic Therapy[2]	106	99%	99%	99%
Discharged on Statin Medication[2]	88	95%	96%	94%
Thrombolytic Therapy Timing[1,2]	-	-	76%	66%
Venous Thromboembolism Prophylaxis[2]	136	98%	95%	94%
Written Stroke Educational Materials Given[2]	83	100%	94%	88%
Surgical Care Improvement Project				
Appropriate Beta Blocker Usage[2]	291	98%	99%	98%
Appropriate VTP Within 24 Hours[2]	492	98%	99%	98%
Controlled Postoperative Blood Glucose[2]	181	97%	98%	97%
Perioperative Temperature Management[2]	645	100%	100%	100%
Prophylactic Antibiotic Selection[2]	554	98%	99%	99%
Prophylactic Antibiotic Selection (Outpatient)	533	96%	98%	98%
Prophylactic Antibiotic Stopped[2]	527	97%	98%	98%
Prophylactic Antibiotic Timing[2]	555	99%	99%	99%
Prophylactic Antibiotic Timing (Outpatient)	440	100%	98%	98%
Urinary Catheter Removal[2]	373	96%	98%	97%
Survey of Patients' Hospital Experiences				
Area Around Room 'Always' Quiet at Night	300+	56%	58%	61%
Doctors 'Always' Communicated Well	300+	77%	77%	82%
Home Recovery Information Given	300+	82%	83%	85%
Hospital Given 9 or 10 on 10 Point Scale	300+	69%	67%	71%
Meds 'Always' Explained Before Given	300+	62%	60%	64%
Nurses 'Always' Communicated Well	300+	77%	75%	79%
Pain 'Always' Well Controlled	300+	68%	68%	71%
Room and Bathroom 'Always' Clean	300+	64%	69%	73%
Timely Help 'Always' Received	300+	62%	62%	68%
Would Definitely Recommend Hospital	300+	73%	69%	71%
Use of Medical Imaging				
Cardiac Imaging Stress Test before Surgery	501	9.2%	6.4%	5.3%
Combination Abdominal CT Scan	1,217	3.1%	11.8%	10.5%
Combination Brain/Sinus CT Scan	1,849	4.5%	3.4%	2.7%
Combination Chest CT Scan	305	0.3%	2.4%	2.7%
Follow-up Mammogram/Ultrasound[7]	-	-	10.2%	8.8%
Lumbar Spine MRI for Low Back Pain[1]	-	-	35.2%	37.2%

Largo Medical Center

201 14th Saint Sw
Largo, FL 33770
Phone: 727-588-5200
Fax: 727-588-5907
URL: www.largomedical.com
Type: Acute Care Hospitals
Emergency Services: Yes
Ownership: Proprietary
Beds: 256

Key Personnel:

Infection Control. . . . . Paula Bates
CEO . . . . Anthony Degina
Intensive Care Unit. . . . . Susan Finch
Quality Assurance . . . . Karen Meno
Operating Room. . . . . Ricardo Requena, DO
Surgery . . . . Richard Requena, D.O.
Chief of Medical Staff. . . . . Rakesh K Sharma, MD
Radiology. . . . . Harvey Wiener, D.O.

Measure	Cases	This Hosp.	State Avg.	U.S. Avg.
Blood Clot Prevention and Treatment				
Anticoagulation Overlap Therapy[2]	123	98%	93%	93%
ICU Venous Thromboembolism Prophylaxis[2]	123	98%	94%	92%
Incidence of Potentially Preventable VTE[2]	24	8%	10%	10%
UFH with Dosages/Platelet Monitoring[2]	40	100%	100%	97%
Venous Thromboembolism Prophylaxis[2]	343	86%	88%	85%
Warfarin Therapy Discharge Instructions[2]	85	93%	85%	75%
Chest Pain/Possible Heart Attack Care				
Aspirin Given Within 24 Hours of Arrival[1,3]	-	-	98%	96%
Fibrinolytic Meds Within 30 Min. of Arrival[5]	-	-	81%	58%
Average Time to ECG (minutes)[1,3]	-	-	7	7
Average Time to Transfer (minutes)[5]	-	-	53	60
Children's Asthma Care				
Received Home Management Plan of Care	-	-	-	88%
Received Reliever Medication	-	-	-	100%
Received Systemic Corticosteroids	-	-	-	100%
Emergency Department				
Admittance Decision Time (minutes)[2]	761	81	111	98
Head CT Results Within 45 Min. of Arrival[1]	-	-	64%	57%
Patients Who Left ER Before Being Seen	43,020	0%	2%	2%
Time from ER Arrival to Admit. (minutes)[2]	766	232	289	274
Time from ER Arrival to Discharge (minutes)	407	153	147	134
Time in ER Before Being Evaluated (minutes)	463	15	26	26
Time to Pain Meds for Fractures (minutes)	66	50	60	57
Heart Attack Care				
Aspirin Given at Discharge	330	100%	99%	99%
Fibrinolytic Meds Within 30 Min. of Arrival[7]	-	-	50%	54%
PCI Within 90 Minutes of Arrival	66	100%	96%	96%
Statin Prescribed at Discharge	317	99%	99%	98%
Heart Failure Care				
ACE Inhibitor or ARB for LVSD	106	100%	98%	97%
Discharge Instructions Given	309	95%	96%	94%
Evaluation of LVS Function	439	100%	100%	99%
Medicare Spending				
Medicare Spending per Patient (ratio)	-	1.11	1.04	0.98
Pneumonia Care				
Appropriate Initial Antibiotic Given	131	100%	98%	95%
Blood Culture Timing	219	100%	99%	98%
Pregnancy and Delivery Care				
Newborn Deliveries Scheduled Early[2,7]	-	-	6%	6%
Preventive Care				
Immunization for Influenza[2]	649	100%	94%	90%
Immunization for Pneumonia[2]	1,016	99%	96%	92%
Stroke Care				
Anticoagulation Therapy for Atrial Fibrillation[2]	25	100%	97%	95%
Antithrombotic Therapy Timing[2]	132	98%	98%	98%
Assessed for Rehabilitation[2]	149	100%	97%	97%
Discharged on Antithrombotic Therapy[2]	127	100%	99%	99%
Discharged on Statin Medication[2]	99	94%	96%	94%
Thrombolytic Therapy Timing[1,2]	-	-	76%	66%
Venous Thromboembolism Prophylaxis[2]	174	98%	95%	94%
Written Stroke Educational Materials Given[2]	59	97%	94%	88%
Surgical Care Improvement Project				
Appropriate Beta Blocker Usage[2]	228	100%	99%	98%
Appropriate VTP Within 24 Hours[2]	424	100%	99%	98%
Controlled Postoperative Blood Glucose[2]	94	99%	98%	97%
Perioperative Temperature Management[2]	509	100%	100%	100%
Prophylactic Antibiotic Selection[2]	371	100%	99%	99%
Prophylactic Antibiotic Selection (Outpatient)	564	99%	98%	98%
Prophylactic Antibiotic Stopped[2]	353	99%	98%	98%
Prophylactic Antibiotic Timing[2]	371	99%	99%	99%
Prophylactic Antibiotic Timing (Outpatient)	564	100%	98%	98%
Urinary Catheter Removal[2]	315	98%	98%	97%
Survey of Patients' Hospital Experiences				
Area Around Room 'Always' Quiet at Night	300+	52%	58%	61%
Doctors 'Always' Communicated Well	300+	73%	77%	82%
Home Recovery Information Given	300+	81%	83%	85%
Hospital Given 9 or 10 on 10 Point Scale	300+	59%	67%	71%
Meds 'Always' Explained Before Given	300+	56%	60%	64%
Nurses 'Always' Communicated Well	300+	70%	75%	79%
Pain 'Always' Well Controlled	300+	63%	68%	71%
Room and Bathroom 'Always' Clean	300+	64%	69%	73%
Timely Help 'Always' Received	300+	60%	62%	68%
Would Definitely Recommend Hospital	300+	63%	69%	71%
Use of Medical Imaging				
Cardiac Imaging Stress Test before Surgery[1]	-	-	6.4%	5.3%
Combination Abdominal CT Scan	401	10.2%	11.8%	10.5%
Combination Brain/Sinus CT Scan	789	3.4%	3.4%	2.7%
Combination Chest CT Scan	102	15.7%	2.4%	2.7%
Follow-up Mammogram/Ultrasound	423	4.7%	10.2%	8.8%
Lumbar Spine MRI for Low Back Pain[1]	-	-	35.2%	37.2%

Leesburg Regional Medical Center

600 E Dixie Ave
Leesburg, FL 34748
Phone: 352-323-5762
Fax: 352-323-5009
URL: www.leesburgregional.org
Type: Acute Care Hospitals
Emergency Services: Yes
Ownership: Voluntary non-profit - Private
Beds: 322

Key Personnel:

Emergency Room . . . . Sharon Garbaravage
Chairman/CEO . . . . Don V. Hahnfeldt
Radiology. . . . . Steve Smith
CEO/President. . . . . Ted Williams, CFRE, CFRM

Measure	Cases	This Hosp.	State Avg.	U.S. Avg.
Blood Clot Prevention and Treatment				
Anticoagulation Overlap Therapy[2]	107	92%	93%	93%
ICU Venous Thromboembolism Prophylaxis[2]	60	90%	94%	92%
Incidence of Potentially Preventable VTE[2]	14	36%	10%	10%
UFH with Dosages/Platelet Monitoring[2]	104	98%	100%	97%
Venous Thromboembolism Prophylaxis[2]	372	76%	88%	85%
Warfarin Therapy Discharge Instructions[2]	75	96%	85%	75%
Chest Pain/Possible Heart Attack Care				
Aspirin Given Within 24 Hours of Arrival[1,3]	-	-	98%	96%
Fibrinolytic Meds Within 30 Min. of Arrival[5]	-	-	81%	58%
Average Time to ECG (minutes)[1,3]	-	-	7	7
Average Time to Transfer (minutes)[5]	-	-	53	60
Children's Asthma Care				
Received Home Management Plan of Care	-	-	-	88%
Received Reliever Medication	-	-	-	100%
Received Systemic Corticosteroids	-	-	-	100%
Emergency Department				
Admittance Decision Time (minutes)[2]	497	194	111	98
Head CT Results Within 45 Min. of Arrival[1]	-	-	64%	57%
Patients Who Left ER Before Being Seen	47,702	2%	2%	2%
Time from ER Arrival to Admit. (minutes)[2]	548	434	289	274
Time from ER Arrival to Discharge (minutes)	325	197	147	134
Time in ER Before Being Evaluated (minutes)	358	58	26	26
Time to Pain Meds for Fractures (minutes)	55	100	60	57
Heart Attack Care				
Aspirin Given at Discharge[2]	278	99%	99%	99%
Fibrinolytic Meds Within 30 Min. of Arrival[2,7]	-	-	50%	54%
PCI Within 90 Minutes of Arrival[2]	36	100%	96%	96%
Statin Prescribed at Discharge[2]	259	92%	99%	98%
Heart Failure Care				
ACE Inhibitor or ARB for LVSD[2]	96	100%	98%	97%
Discharge Instructions Given[2]	306	87%	96%	94%
Evaluation of LVS Function[2]	385	98%	100%	99%
Medicare Spending				
Medicare Spending per Patient (ratio)	-	1.02	1.04	0.98
Pneumonia Care				
Appropriate Initial Antibiotic Given[2]	117	100%	98%	95%
Blood Culture Timing[2]	105	96%	99%	98%
Pregnancy and Delivery Care				
Newborn Deliveries Scheduled Early[2]	34	0%	6%	6%
Preventive Care				
Immunization for Influenza[2]	594	89%	94%	90%
Immunization for Pneumonia[2]	872	96%	96%	92%
Stroke Care				
Anticoagulation Therapy for Atrial Fibrillation[2]	11	100%	97%	95%

NOTE: Hospital profiles are in alphabetical order by state, then city, then hospital within the city; Rankings exclude hospitals with less than 25 cases except for patient surveys which excludes hospitals with less than 100 cases; (a) 100-299 cases; (1) The number of cases/patients is too few to report; (2) Data submitted were based on a sample of cases/patients; (3) Results are based on a shorter time period than required; (4) Data suppressed by CMS for one or more quarters; (5) Results are not available for this reporting period; (6) Fewer than 100 patients completed the HCAHPS survey; (7) No cases met the criteria for this measure; (8) The lower limit of the confidence interval cannot be calculated if the number of observed infections equals zero; (9) No data are available from the state/territory for this reporting period; (10) The scores shown reflect fewer than 50 completed surveys; (11) There were discrepancies in the data collection process; (12) This measure does not apply to this hospital for this reporting period; (13) Results cannot be calculated for this reporting period; (14) The results for this state are combined with nearby states to protect confidentiality; Please refer to the User's Guide for a full explanation of data.

Measure	Cases	This Hosp.	State Avg.	U.S. Avg.
Antithrombotic Therapy Timing[2]	74	96%	98%	98%
Assessed for Rehabilitation[2]	91	97%	97%	97%
Discharged on Antithrombotic Therapy[2]	75	100%	99%	99%
Discharged on Statin Medication[2]	65	92%	96%	94%
Thrombolytic Therapy Timing[1,2]	-	-	76%	66%
Venous Thromboembolism Prophylaxis[2]	101	85%	95%	94%
Written Stroke Educational Materials Given[2]	58	88%	94%	88%
Surgical Care Improvement Project				
Appropriate Beta Blocker Usage[2]	417	97%	99%	98%
Appropriate VTP Within 24 Hours[2]	521	97%	99%	98%
Controlled Postoperative Blood Glucose[2]	343	96%	98%	97%
Perioperative Temperature Management[2]	646	100%	100%	100%
Prophylactic Antibiotic Selection[2]	802	100%	99%	99%
Prophylactic Antibiotic Selection (Outpatient)	397	96%	98%	98%
Prophylactic Antibiotic Stopped[2]	794	98%	98%	98%
Prophylactic Antibiotic Timing[2]	802	97%	99%	99%
Prophylactic Antibiotic Timing (Outpatient)	399	99%	98%	98%
Urinary Catheter Removal[2]	483	93%	98%	97%
Survey of Patients' Hospital Experiences				
Area Around Room 'Always' Quiet at Night	300+	48%	58%	61%
Doctors 'Always' Communicated Well	300+	66%	77%	82%
Home Recovery Information Given	300+	77%	83%	85%
Hospital Given 9 or 10 on 10 Point Scale	300+	55%	67%	71%
Meds 'Always' Explained Before Given	300+	54%	60%	64%
Nurses 'Always' Communicated Well	300+	69%	75%	79%
Pain 'Always' Well Controlled	300+	63%	68%	71%
Room and Bathroom 'Always' Clean	300+	67%	69%	73%
Timely Help 'Always' Received	300+	57%	62%	68%
Would Definitely Recommend Hospital	300+	59%	69%	71%
Use of Medical Imaging				
Cardiac Imaging Stress Test before Surgery	313	4.5%	6.4%	5.3%
Combination Abdominal CT Scan	456	5.5%	11.8%	10.5%
Combination Brain/Sinus CT Scan	942	5.6%	3.4%	2.7%
Combination Chest CT Scan	95	2.1%	2.4%	2.7%
Follow-up Mammogram/Ultrasound	148	10.8%	10.2%	8.8%
Lumbar Spine MRI for Low Back Pain[1]	-	-	35.2%	37.2%

Lehigh Regional Medical Center

1500 Lee Blvd
Lehigh Acres, FL 33936
Phone: 239-369-2101
Fax: 239-368-4510
URL: www.lehighregional.com
Type: Acute Care Hospitals
Emergency Services: Yes
Ownership: Voluntary non-profit - Private
Beds: 88

Key Personnel:
Pediatric Ambulatory Care . . . . . . Jose Arroyo, MD
Pediatric In-Patient Care . . . . Jose Arroyo, MD
Chief of Medical Staff . . . . Barry K Butler
Operating Room. . . . . Beth Gratkowski
CEO/President. . . . . Jos_ F Morillo
Radiology. . . . . Margo H Roca
Quality Assurance . . . . Shirley Spicer

Measure	Cases	This Hosp.	State Avg.	U.S. Avg.
Blood Clot Prevention and Treatment				
Anticoagulation Overlap Therapy[2]	27	85%	93%	93%
ICU Venous Thromboembolism Prophylaxis[2]	55	98%	94%	92%
Incidence of Potentially Preventable VTE[2,7]	-	-	10%	10%
UFH with Dosages/Platelet Monitoring[2]	24	100%	100%	97%
Venous Thromboembolism Prophylaxis[2]	241	96%	88%	85%
Warfarin Therapy Discharge Instructions[2]	21	100%	85%	75%
Chest Pain/Possible Heart Attack Care				
Aspirin Given Within 24 Hours of Arrival	55	98%	98%	96%
Fibrinolytic Meds Within 30 Min. of Arrival[7]	-	-	81%	58%
Average Time to ECG (minutes)	57	2	7	7
Average Time to Transfer (minutes)[1]	-	-	53	60
Children's Asthma Care				
Received Home Management Plan of Care	-	-	-	88%
Received Reliever Medication	-	-	-	100%
Received Systemic Corticosteroids	-	-	-	100%
Emergency Department				
Admittance Decision Time (minutes)[2]	503	131	111	98
Head CT Results Within 45 Min. of Arrival[1]	-	-	64%	57%
Patients Who Left ER Before Being Seen	35,503	1%	2%	2%
Time from ER Arrival to Admit. (minutes)[2]	505	300	289	274
Time from ER Arrival to Discharge (minutes)	381	89	147	134
Time in ER Before Being Evaluated (minutes)	388	24	26	26
Time to Pain Meds for Fractures (minutes)	80	37	60	57
Heart Attack Care				
Aspirin Given at Discharge	18	100%	99%	99%
Fibrinolytic Meds Within 30 Min. of Arrival[7]	-	-	50%	54%
PCI Within 90 Minutes of Arrival[7]	-	-	96%	96%
Statin Prescribed at Discharge	14	100%	99%	98%
Heart Failure Care				
ACE Inhibitor or ARB for LVSD	41	98%	98%	97%
Discharge Instructions Given	93	91%	96%	94%
Evaluation of LVS Function	110	100%	100%	99%
Medicare Spending				
Medicare Spending per Patient (ratio)	-	1.02	1.04	0.98
Pneumonia Care				
Appropriate Initial Antibiotic Given	72	100%	98%	95%
Blood Culture Timing	99	100%	99%	98%
Pregnancy and Delivery Care				
Newborn Deliveries Scheduled Early[7]	-	-	6%	6%
Preventive Care				
Immunization for Influenza[2]	306	100%	94%	90%
Immunization for Pneumonia[2]	417	100%	96%	92%
Stroke Care				
Anticoagulation Therapy for Atrial Fibrillation[7]	-	-	97%	95%
Antithrombotic Therapy Timing	20	90%	98%	98%
Assessed for Rehabilitation	19	100%	97%	97%
Discharged on Antithrombotic Therapy	19	100%	99%	99%
Discharged on Statin Medication	16	94%	96%	94%
Thrombolytic Therapy Timing[7]	-	-	76%	66%
Venous Thromboembolism Prophylaxis	19	95%	95%	94%
Written Stroke Educational Materials Given	13	100%	94%	88%
Surgical Care Improvement Project				
Appropriate Beta Blocker Usage	63	97%	99%	98%
Appropriate VTP Within 24 Hours	170	98%	99%	98%
Controlled Postoperative Blood Glucose[7]	-	-	98%	97%
Perioperative Temperature Management	205	100%	100%	100%
Prophylactic Antibiotic Selection	118	100%	99%	99%
Prophylactic Antibiotic Selection (Outpatient)	16	100%	98%	98%
Prophylactic Antibiotic Stopped	114	100%	98%	98%
Prophylactic Antibiotic Timing	118	100%	99%	99%
Prophylactic Antibiotic Timing (Outpatient)	16	100%	98%	98%
Urinary Catheter Removal	28	89%	98%	97%
Survey of Patients' Hospital Experiences				
Area Around Room 'Always' Quiet at Night	300+	51%	58%	61%
Doctors 'Always' Communicated Well	300+	71%	77%	82%
Home Recovery Information Given	300+	77%	83%	85%
Hospital Given 9 or 10 on 10 Point Scale	300+	45%	67%	71%
Meds 'Always' Explained Before Given	300+	45%	60%	64%
Nurses 'Always' Communicated Well	300+	63%	75%	79%
Pain 'Always' Well Controlled	300+	53%	68%	71%
Room and Bathroom 'Always' Clean	300+	66%	69%	73%
Timely Help 'Always' Received	300+	48%	62%	68%
Would Definitely Recommend Hospital	300+	45%	69%	71%
Use of Medical Imaging				
Cardiac Imaging Stress Test before Surgery	87	8.0%	6.4%	5.3%
Combination Abdominal CT Scan	204	3.4%	11.8%	10.5%
Combination Brain/Sinus CT Scan[1]	-	-	3.4%	2.7%
Combination Chest CT Scan	57	3.5%	2.4%	2.7%
Follow-up Mammogram/Ultrasound[7]	-	-	10.2%	8.8%
Lumbar Spine MRI for Low Back Pain[1]	-	-	35.2%	37.2%

Shands Live Oak Regional Medical Center

1100 Sw 11th St
Live Oak, FL 32060
Phone: 904-362-1413
Fax: 386-362-0841
URL: www.shands.org
Type: Critical Access Hospitals
Emergency Services: Yes
Ownership: Proprietary
Beds: 30

Key Personnel:
Chief of Medical Staff . . . . Andrew Baff, MD
Emergency Room . . . . Robert Ftindell
Operating Room. . . . . Bunny Motes

Measure	Cases	This Hosp.	State Avg.	U.S. Avg.
Blood Clot Prevention and Treatment				
Anticoagulation Overlap Therapy[1,2]	-	-	93%	93%
ICU Venous Thromboembolism Prophylaxis[2,7]	-	-	94%	92%
Incidence of Potentially Preventable VTE[2,7]	-	-	10%	10%
UFH with Dosages/Platelet Monitoring[1,2]	-	-	100%	97%
Venous Thromboembolism Prophylaxis[2]	132	88%	88%	85%
Warfarin Therapy Discharge Instructions[1,2]	-	-	85%	75%
Chest Pain/Possible Heart Attack Care				
Aspirin Given Within 24 Hours of Arrival	172	98%	98%	96%
Fibrinolytic Meds Within 30 Min. of Arrival[7]	-	-	81%	58%
Average Time to ECG (minutes)	179	8	7	7
Average Time to Transfer (minutes)[1]	-	-	53	60
Children's Asthma Care				
Received Home Management Plan of Care	-	-	-	88%
Received Reliever Medication	-	-	-	100%
Received Systemic Corticosteroids	-	-	-	100%
Emergency Department				
Admittance Decision Time (minutes)[2]	569	67	111	98
Head CT Results Within 45 Min. of Arrival	25	28%	64%	57%
Patients Who Left ER Before Being Seen	22,926	1%	2%	2%
Time from ER Arrival to Admit. (minutes)[2]	570	280	289	274
Time from ER Arrival to Discharge (minutes)	889	111	147	134
Time in ER Before Being Evaluated (minutes)	991	13	26	26
Time to Pain Meds for Fractures (minutes)	61	64	60	57
Heart Attack Care				
Aspirin Given at Discharge[1]	-	-	99%	99%
Fibrinolytic Meds Within 30 Min. of Arrival[7]	-	-	50%	54%
PCI Within 90 Minutes of Arrival[7]	-	-	96%	96%
Statin Prescribed at Discharge[1]	-	-	99%	98%
Heart Failure Care				
ACE Inhibitor or ARB for LVSD	16	100%	98%	97%
Discharge Instructions Given	45	71%	96%	94%
Evaluation of LVS Function	73	100%	100%	99%
Medicare Spending				
Medicare Spending per Patient (ratio)	-	-	1.04	0.98
Pneumonia Care				
Appropriate Initial Antibiotic Given	57	93%	98%	95%
Blood Culture Timing	91	97%	99%	98%
Pregnancy and Delivery Care				
Newborn Deliveries Scheduled Early[7]	-	-	6%	6%
Preventive Care				
Immunization for Influenza[2]	275	99%	94%	90%
Immunization for Pneumonia[2]	432	99%	96%	92%
Stroke Care				
Anticoagulation Therapy for Atrial Fibrillation[3,7]	-	-	97%	95%
Antithrombotic Therapy Timing[1,3]	-	-	98%	98%
Assessed for Rehabilitation[1,3]	-	-	97%	97%
Discharged on Antithrombotic Therapy[1,3]	-	-	99%	99%
Discharged on Statin Medication[1,3]	-	-	96%	94%
Thrombolytic Therapy Timing[1,3]	-	-	76%	66%
Venous Thromboembolism Prophylaxis[1,3]	-	-	95%	94%
Written Stroke Educational Materials Given[1,3]	-	-	94%	88%
Surgical Care Improvement Project				
Appropriate Beta Blocker Usage[5]	-	-	99%	98%
Appropriate VTP Within 24 Hours[5]	-	-	99%	98%
Controlled Postoperative Blood Glucose[5]	-	-	98%	97%
Perioperative Temperature Management[5]	-	-	100%	100%
Prophylactic Antibiotic Selection[5]	-	-	99%	99%
Prophylactic Antibiotic Selection (Outpatient)[5]	-	-	98%	98%
Prophylactic Antibiotic Stopped[5]	-	-	98%	98%
Prophylactic Antibiotic Timing[5]	-	-	99%	99%
Prophylactic Antibiotic Timing (Outpatient)[5]	-	-	98%	98%
Urinary Catheter Removal[5]	-	-	98%	97%
Survey of Patients' Hospital Experiences				
Area Around Room 'Always' Quiet at Night[5]	-	-	58%	61%
Doctors 'Always' Communicated Well[5]	-	-	77%	82%
Home Recovery Information Given[5]	-	-	83%	85%
Hospital Given 9 or 10 on 10 Point Scale[5]	-	-	67%	71%
Meds 'Always' Explained Before Given[5]	-	-	60%	64%
Nurses 'Always' Communicated Well[5]	-	-	75%	79%
Pain 'Always' Well Controlled[5]	-	-	68%	71%
Room and Bathroom 'Always' Clean[5]	-	-	69%	73%
Timely Help 'Always' Received[5]	-	-	62%	68%
Would Definitely Recommend Hospital[5]	-	-	69%	71%

NOTE: Hospital profiles are in alphabetical order by state, then city, then hospital within the city; Rankings exclude hospitals with less than 25 cases except for patient surveys which excludes hospitals with less than 100 cases; (a) 100-299 cases; (1) The number of cases/patients is too few to report; (2) Data submitted were based on a sample of cases/patients; (3) Results are based on a shorter time period than required; (4) Data suppressed by CMS for one or more quarters; (5) Results are not available for this reporting period; (6) Fewer than 100 patients completed the HCAHPS survey; (7) No cases met the criteria for this measure; (8) The lower limit of the confidence interval cannot be calculated if the number of observed infections equals zero; (9) No data are available from the state/territory for this reporting period; (10) The scores shown reflect fewer than 50 completed surveys; (11) There were discrepancies in the data collection process; (12) This measure does not apply to this hospital for this reporting period; (13) Results cannot be calculated for this reporting period; (14) The results for this state are combined with nearby states to protect confidentiality; Please refer to the User's Guide for a full explanation of data.

Use of Medical Imaging				
Cardiac Imaging Stress Test before Surgery	75	4.0%	6.4%	5.3%
Combination Abdominal CT Scan	488	4.1%	11.8%	10.5%
Combination Brain/Sinus CT Scan	595	1.3%	3.4%	2.7%
Combination Chest CT Scan	362	3.3%	2.4%	2.7%
Follow-up Mammogram/Ultrasound	459	9.2%	10.2%	8.8%
Lumbar Spine MRI for Low Back Pain[1]	-	-	35.2%	37.2%

Palms West Hospital

13001 Southern Blvd
Loxahatchee, FL 33470
Phone: 561-753-4245
Fax: 561-791-8108
URL: www.palmswesthospital.com
Type: Acute Care Hospitals
Emergency Services: Yes
Ownership: Proprietary
Beds: 175

Key Personnel:
Pediatric Ambulatory Care .... Juan Abellon, MD
Pediatric In-Patient Care .... Juan Abellon, MD
Quality Assurance .... Debbie Adkins
Emergency Room .... Judy Charriez, RN
CEO .... Eric Goldman
Operating Room.............. June Shipp, RN

Measure	Cases	This Hosp.	State Avg.	U.S. Avg.
Blood Clot Prevention and Treatment				
Anticoagulation Overlap Therapy[2]	62	95%	93%	93%
ICU Venous Thromboembolism Prophylaxis[2]	61	92%	94%	92%
Incidence of Potentially Preventable VTE[1,2]	-	-	10%	10%
UFH with Dosages/Platelet Monitoring[2]	55	100%	100%	97%
Venous Thromboembolism Prophylaxis[2]	369	79%	88%	85%
Warfarin Therapy Discharge Instructions[2]	33	100%	85%	75%
Chest Pain/Possible Heart Attack Care				
Aspirin Given Within 24 Hours of Arrival[1]	-	-	98%	96%
Fibrinolytic Meds Within 30 Min. of Arrival[3,7]	-	-	81%	58%
Average Time to ECG (minutes)[1]	-	-	7	7
Average Time to Transfer (minutes)[3,7]	-	-	53	60
Children's Asthma Care				
Received Home Management Plan of Care	-	-	-	88%
Received Reliever Medication	-	-	-	100%
Received Systemic Corticosteroids	-	-	-	100%
Emergency Department				
Admittance Decision Time (minutes)[2]	842	84	111	98
Head CT Results Within 45 Min. of Arrival[1]	-	-	64%	57%
Patients Who Left ER Before Being Seen	45,364	1%	2%	2%
Time from ER Arrival to Admit. (minutes)[2]	851	205	289	274
Time from ER Arrival to Discharge (minutes)	441	125	147	134
Time in ER Before Being Evaluated (minutes)	453	9	26	26
Time to Pain Meds for Fractures (minutes)	160	57	60	57
Heart Attack Care				
Aspirin Given at Discharge	154	100%	99%	99%
Fibrinolytic Meds Within 30 Min. of Arrival[7]	-	-	50%	54%
PCI Within 90 Minutes of Arrival	17	100%	96%	96%
Statin Prescribed at Discharge	152	100%	99%	98%
Heart Failure Care				
ACE Inhibitor or ARB for LVSD	53	100%	98%	97%
Discharge Instructions Given	188	100%	96%	94%
Evaluation of LVS Function	225	100%	100%	99%
Medicare Spending				
Medicare Spending per Patient (ratio)	-	1.07	1.04	0.98
Pneumonia Care				
Appropriate Initial Antibiotic Given	110	99%	98%	95%
Blood Culture Timing	191	99%	99%	98%
Pregnancy and Delivery Care				
Newborn Deliveries Scheduled Early[2]	47	0%	6%	6%
Preventive Care				
Immunization for Influenza[2]	562	98%	94%	90%
Immunization for Pneumonia[2]	500	99%	96%	92%
Stroke Care				
Anticoagulation Therapy for Atrial Fibrillation[1]	-	-	97%	95%
Antithrombotic Therapy Timing	107	93%	98%	98%
Assessed for Rehabilitation	118	96%	97%	97%
Discharged on Antithrombotic Therapy	100	99%	99%	99%
Discharged on Statin Medication	77	99%	96%	94%
Thrombolytic Therapy Timing[1]	-	-	76%	66%
Venous Thromboembolism Prophylaxis	129	88%	95%	94%
Written Stroke Educational Materials Given	88	98%	94%	88%
Surgical Care Improvement Project				
Appropriate Beta Blocker Usage[2]	84	100%	99%	98%
Appropriate VTP Within 24 Hours[2]	344	99%	99%	98%
Controlled Postoperative Blood Glucose[2,7]	-	-	98%	97%
Perioperative Temperature Management[2]	384	100%	100%	100%
Prophylactic Antibiotic Selection[2]	215	100%	99%	99%
Prophylactic Antibiotic Selection (Outpatient)	197	97%	98%	98%
Prophylactic Antibiotic Stopped[2]	183	99%	98%	98%
Prophylactic Antibiotic Timing[2]	215	100%	99%	99%
Prophylactic Antibiotic Timing (Outpatient)	197	100%	98%	98%
Urinary Catheter Removal[2]	159	100%	98%	97%
Survey of Patients' Hospital Experiences				
Area Around Room 'Always' Quiet at Night	300+	54%	58%	61%
Doctors 'Always' Communicated Well	300+	72%	77%	82%
Home Recovery Information Given	300+	80%	83%	85%
Hospital Given 9 or 10 on 10 Point Scale	300+	60%	67%	71%
Meds 'Always' Explained Before Given	300+	55%	60%	64%
Nurses 'Always' Communicated Well	300+	69%	75%	79%
Pain 'Always' Well Controlled	300+	64%	68%	71%
Room and Bathroom 'Always' Clean	300+	62%	69%	73%
Timely Help 'Always' Received	300+	55%	62%	68%
Would Definitely Recommend Hospital	300+	65%	69%	71%
Use of Medical Imaging				
Cardiac Imaging Stress Test before Surgery[1]	-	-	6.4%	5.3%
Combination Abdominal CT Scan	198	0.5%	11.8%	10.5%
Combination Brain/Sinus CT Scan	261	5.7%	3.4%	2.7%
Combination Chest CT Scan	50	0.0%	2.4%	2.7%
Follow-up Mammogram/Ultrasound	331	4.2%	10.2%	8.8%
Lumbar Spine MRI for Low Back Pain[1]	-	-	35.2%	37.2%

Madison County Memorial Hospital

309 Ne Marion St
Madison, FL 32340
Phone: 850-973-2271
Type: Critical Access Hospitals
Emergency Services: Yes
Ownership: Govt - Hospital Dist/Auth

Measure	Cases	This Hosp.	State Avg.	U.S. Avg.
Blood Clot Prevention and Treatment				
Anticoagulation Overlap Therapy[5]	-	-	93%	93%
ICU Venous Thromboembolism Prophylaxis[5]	-	-	94%	92%
Incidence of Potentially Preventable VTE[5]	-	-	10%	10%
UFH with Dosages/Platelet Monitoring[5]	-	-	100%	97%
Venous Thromboembolism Prophylaxis[5]	-	-	88%	85%
Warfarin Therapy Discharge Instructions[5]	-	-	85%	75%
Chest Pain/Possible Heart Attack Care				
Aspirin Given Within 24 Hours of Arrival	-	-	98%	96%
Fibrinolytic Meds Within 30 Min. of Arrival	-	-	81%	58%
Average Time to ECG (minutes)	-	-	7	7
Average Time to Transfer (minutes)	-	-	53	60
Children's Asthma Care				
Received Home Management Plan of Care	-	-	-	88%
Received Reliever Medication	-	-	-	100%
Received Systemic Corticosteroids	-	-	-	100%
Emergency Department				
Admittance Decision Time (minutes)[5]	-	-	111	98
Head CT Results Within 45 Min. of Arrival	-	-	64%	57%
Patients Who Left ER Before Being Seen	-	-	2%	2%
Time from ER Arrival to Admit. (minutes)[5]	-	-	289	274
Time from ER Arrival to Discharge (minutes)	-	-	147	134
Time in ER Before Being Evaluated (minutes)	-	-	26	26
Time to Pain Meds for Fractures (minutes)	-	-	60	57
Heart Attack Care				
Aspirin Given at Discharge[5]	-	-	99%	99%
Fibrinolytic Meds Within 30 Min. of Arrival[5]	-	-	50%	54%
PCI Within 90 Minutes of Arrival[5]	-	-	96%	96%
Statin Prescribed at Discharge[5]	-	-	99%	98%
Heart Failure Care				
ACE Inhibitor or ARB for LVSD[1,2]	-	-	98%	97%
Discharge Instructions Given[2]	12	92%	96%	94%
Evaluation of LVS Function[2]	22	27%	100%	99%
Medicare Spending				
Medicare Spending per Patient (ratio)	-	-	1.04	0.98
Pneumonia Care				
Appropriate Initial Antibiotic Given[2]	20	40%	98%	95%
Blood Culture Timing[2]	22	86%	99%	98%
Pregnancy and Delivery Care				
Newborn Deliveries Scheduled Early[3,7]	-	-	6%	6%
Preventive Care				
Immunization for Influenza[5]	-	-	94%	90%
Immunization for Pneumonia[5]	-	-	96%	92%
Stroke Care				
Anticoagulation Therapy for Atrial Fibrillation[2,3]	-	-	97%	95%
Antithrombotic Therapy Timing[1,2]	-	-	98%	98%
Assessed for Rehabilitation[1,2]	-	-	97%	97%
Discharged on Antithrombotic Therapy[1,2]	-	-	99%	99%
Discharged on Statin Medication[1,2]	-	-	96%	94%
Thrombolytic Therapy Timing[2,3]	-	-	76%	66%
Venous Thromboembolism Prophylaxis[1,2]	-	-	95%	94%
Written Stroke Educational Materials Given[2,3]	-	-	94%	88%
Surgical Care Improvement Project				
Appropriate Beta Blocker Usage[5]	-	-	99%	98%
Appropriate VTP Within 24 Hours[5]	-	-	99%	98%
Controlled Postoperative Blood Glucose[5]	-	-	98%	97%
Perioperative Temperature Management[5]	-	-	100%	100%
Prophylactic Antibiotic Selection[5]	-	-	99%	99%
Prophylactic Antibiotic Selection (Outpatient)	-	-	98%	98%
Prophylactic Antibiotic Stopped[5]	-	-	98%	98%
Prophylactic Antibiotic Timing[5]	-	-	99%	99%
Prophylactic Antibiotic Timing (Outpatient)	-	-	98%	98%
Urinary Catheter Removal[5]	-	-	98%	97%
Survey of Patients' Hospital Experiences				
Area Around Room 'Always' Quiet at Night[5]	-	-	58%	61%
Doctors 'Always' Communicated Well[5]	-	-	77%	82%
Home Recovery Information Given[5]	-	-	83%	85%
Hospital Given 9 or 10 on 10 Point Scale[5]	-	-	67%	71%
Meds 'Always' Explained Before Given[5]	-	-	60%	64%
Nurses 'Always' Communicated Well[5]	-	-	75%	79%
Pain 'Always' Well Controlled[5]	-	-	68%	71%
Room and Bathroom 'Always' Clean[5]	-	-	69%	73%
Timely Help 'Always' Received[5]	-	-	62%	68%
Would Definitely Recommend Hospital[5]	-	-	69%	71%
Use of Medical Imaging				
Cardiac Imaging Stress Test before Surgery	-	-	6.4%	5.3%
Combination Abdominal CT Scan	-	-	11.8%	10.5%
Combination Brain/Sinus CT Scan	-	-	3.4%	2.7%
Combination Chest CT Scan	-	-	2.4%	2.7%
Follow-up Mammogram/Ultrasound	-	-	10.2%	8.8%
Lumbar Spine MRI for Low Back Pain	-	-	35.2%	37.2%

Fishermen's Hospital

3301 Overseas Hwy
Marathon, FL 33050
Phone: 305-743-5533
Fax: 305-743-3962
URL: www.fishermenshospital.com
Type: Critical Access Hospitals
Emergency Services: Yes
Ownership: Proprietary
Beds: 25

Key Personnel:
CEO/President.............. Kim Bassett
Radiology.................. Hugo Diaz
Quality Assurance .... Kelly Reid
Emergency Room .... Jerilyn Town, RN

Measure	Cases	This Hosp.	State Avg.	U.S. Avg.
Blood Clot Prevention and Treatment				
Anticoagulation Overlap Therapy[5]	-	-	93%	93%
ICU Venous Thromboembolism Prophylaxis[5]	-	-	94%	92%
Incidence of Potentially Preventable VTE[5]	-	-	10%	10%
UFH with Dosages/Platelet Monitoring[5]	-	-	100%	97%
Venous Thromboembolism Prophylaxis[5]	-	-	88%	85%
Warfarin Therapy Discharge Instructions[5]	-	-	85%	75%
Chest Pain/Possible Heart Attack Care				
Aspirin Given Within 24 Hours of Arrival[5]	-	-	98%	96%
Fibrinolytic Meds Within 30 Min. of Arrival[5]	-	-	81%	58%
Average Time to ECG (minutes)[5]	-	-	7	7
Average Time to Transfer (minutes)[5]	-	-	53	60
Children's Asthma Care				
Received Home Management Plan of Care	-	-	-	88%
Received Reliever Medication	-	-	-	100%

NOTE: Hospital profiles are in alphabetical order by state, then city, then hospital within the city; Rankings exclude hospitals with less than 25 cases except for patient surveys which excludes hospitals with less than 100 cases; (a) 100-299 cases; (1) The number of cases/patients is too few to report; (2) Data submitted were based on a sample of cases/patients; (3) Results are based on a shorter time period than required; (4) Data suppressed by CMS for one or more quarters; (5) Results are not available for this reporting period; (6) Fewer than 100 patients completed the HCAHPS survey; (7) No cases met the criteria for this measure; (8) The lower limit of the confidence interval cannot be calculated if the number of observed infections equals zero; (9) No data are available from the state/territory for this reporting period; (10) The scores shown reflect fewer than 50 completed surveys; (11) There were discrepancies in the data collection process; (12) This measure does not apply to this hospital for this reporting period; (13) Results cannot be calculated for this reporting period; (14) The results for this state are combined with nearby states to protect confidentiality; Please refer to the User's Guide for a full explanation of data.

Received Systemic Corticosteroids	-	-	-	100%
Emergency Department				
Admittance Decision Time (minutes)[5]	-	-	111	98
Head CT Results Within 45 Min. of Arrival[5]	-	-	64%	57%
Patients Who Left ER Before Being Seen[5]	-	-	2%	2%
Time from ER Arrival to Admit. (minutes)[5]	-	-	289	274
Time from ER Arrival to Discharge (minutes)[5]	-	-	147	134
Time in ER Before Being Evaluated (minutes)[5]	-	-	26	26
Time to Pain Meds for Fractures (minutes)[5]	-	-	60	57
Heart Attack Care				
Aspirin Given at Discharge[3,7]	-	-	99%	99%
Fibrinolytic Meds Within 30 Min. of Arrival[3,7]	-	-	50%	54%
PCI Within 90 Minutes of Arrival[3,7]	-	-	96%	96%
Statin Prescribed at Discharge[3,7]	-	-	99%	98%
Heart Failure Care				
ACE Inhibitor or ARB for LVSD[1]	-	-	98%	97%
Discharge Instructions Given	20	100%	96%	94%
Evaluation of LVS Function	21	100%	100%	99%
Medicare Spending				
Medicare Spending per Patient (ratio)	-	-	1.04	0.98
Pneumonia Care				
Appropriate Initial Antibiotic Given	31	100%	98%	95%
Blood Culture Timing	41	93%	99%	98%
Pregnancy and Delivery Care				
Newborn Deliveries Scheduled Early[3,7]	-	-	6%	6%
Preventive Care				
Immunization for Influenza[5]	-	-	94%	90%
Immunization for Pneumonia[5]	-	-	96%	92%
Stroke Care				
Anticoagulation Therapy for Atrial Fibrillation[5]	-	-	97%	95%
Antithrombotic Therapy Timing[5]	-	-	98%	98%
Assessed for Rehabilitation[5]	-	-	97%	97%
Discharged on Antithrombotic Therapy[5]	-	-	99%	99%
Discharged on Statin Medication[5]	-	-	96%	94%
Thrombolytic Therapy Timing[5]	-	-	76%	66%
Venous Thromboembolism Prophylaxis[5]	-	-	95%	94%
Written Stroke Educational Materials Given[5]	-	-	94%	88%
Surgical Care Improvement Project				
Appropriate Beta Blocker Usage	16	100%	99%	98%
Appropriate VTP Within 24 Hours	44	100%	99%	98%
Controlled Postoperative Blood Glucose[7]	-	-	98%	97%
Perioperative Temperature Management	51	100%	100%	100%
Prophylactic Antibiotic Selection	32	100%	99%	99%
Prophylactic Antibiotic Selection (Outpatient)[5]	-	-	98%	98%
Prophylactic Antibiotic Stopped	31	94%	98%	98%
Prophylactic Antibiotic Timing	32	100%	99%	99%
Prophylactic Antibiotic Timing (Outpatient)[5]	-	-	98%	98%
Urinary Catheter Removal	13	100%	98%	97%
Survey of Patients' Hospital Experiences				
Area Around Room 'Always' Quiet at Night	(a)	66%	58%	61%
Doctors 'Always' Communicated Well	(a)	79%	77%	82%
Home Recovery Information Given	(a)	82%	83%	85%
Hospital Given 9 or 10 on 10 Point Scale	(a)	71%	67%	71%
Meds 'Always' Explained Before Given	(a)	71%	60%	64%
Nurses 'Always' Communicated Well	(a)	83%	75%	79%
Pain 'Always' Well Controlled	(a)	75%	68%	71%
Room and Bathroom 'Always' Clean	(a)	72%	69%	73%
Timely Help 'Always' Received	(a)	72%	62%	68%
Would Definitely Recommend Hospital	(a)	69%	69%	71%
Use of Medical Imaging				
Cardiac Imaging Stress Test before Surgery	95	6.3%	6.4%	5.3%
Combination Abdominal CT Scan	260	4.6%	11.8%	10.5%
Combination Brain/Sinus CT Scan	272	7.4%	3.4%	2.7%
Combination Chest CT Scan	108	0.0%	2.4%	2.7%
Follow-up Mammogram/Ultrasound	157	8.9%	10.2%	8.8%
Lumbar Spine MRI for Low Back Pain	44	47.7%	35.2%	37.2%

Northwest Medical Center

2801 N State Rd 7
Margate, FL 33063
Phone: 954-974-0400
Fax: 954-978-4183
URL: www.northwestmed.com
Type: Acute Care Hospitals
Emergency Services: Yes
Ownership: Proprietary
Beds: 215

Key Personnel:
Quality Assurance . . . . Diane Batten, RN
Infection Control. . . . . Jeannette Callaway
Chief of Medical Staff. . . . . Steve Foster, MD
Emergency Room . . . . Nadiney Giudice, RN
Operating Room. . . . . Lisa Havaas, RN
CEO . . . . Mark Rader, FACHE
Intensive Care Unit. . . . . Carol Rhorstad, RN
Radiology. . . . . Todd Schwartz

Measure	Cases	This Hosp.	State Avg.	U.S. Avg.
Blood Clot Prevention and Treatment				
Anticoagulation Overlap Therapy[2]	71	90%	93%	93%
ICU Venous Thromboembolism Prophylaxis[2]	76	97%	94%	92%
Incidence of Potentially Preventable VTE[1,2]	-	-	10%	10%
UFH with Dosages/Platelet Monitoring[1,2]	-	-	100%	97%
Venous Thromboembolism Prophylaxis[2]	369	86%	88%	85%
Warfarin Therapy Discharge Instructions[2]	55	100%	85%	75%
Chest Pain/Possible Heart Attack Care				
Aspirin Given Within 24 Hours of Arrival[5]	-	-	98%	96%
Fibrinolytic Meds Within 30 Min. of Arrival[5]	-	-	81%	58%
Average Time to ECG (minutes)[5]	-	-	7	7
Average Time to Transfer (minutes)[5]	-	-	53	60
Children's Asthma Care				
Received Home Management Plan of Care	-	-	-	88%
Received Reliever Medication	-	-	-	100%
Received Systemic Corticosteroids	-	-	-	100%
Emergency Department				
Admittance Decision Time (minutes)[2]	811	136	111	98
Head CT Results Within 45 Min. of Arrival[1]	-	-	64%	57%
Patients Who Left ER Before Being Seen	45,369	2%	2%	2%
Time from ER Arrival to Admit. (minutes)[2]	835	263	289	274
Time from ER Arrival to Discharge (minutes)	409	137	147	134
Time in ER Before Being Evaluated (minutes)	495	9	26	26
Time to Pain Meds for Fractures (minutes)	113	39	60	57
Heart Attack Care				
Aspirin Given at Discharge	336	100%	99%	99%
Fibrinolytic Meds Within 30 Min. of Arrival[7]	-	-	50%	54%
PCI Within 90 Minutes of Arrival	24	100%	96%	96%
Statin Prescribed at Discharge	320	100%	99%	98%
Heart Failure Care				
ACE Inhibitor or ARB for LVSD	143	100%	98%	97%
Discharge Instructions Given	427	98%	96%	94%
Evaluation of LVS Function	533	100%	100%	99%
Medicare Spending				
Medicare Spending per Patient (ratio)	-	1.09	1.04	0.98
Pneumonia Care				
Appropriate Initial Antibiotic Given	137	99%	98%	95%
Blood Culture Timing	230	100%	99%	98%
Pregnancy and Delivery Care				
Newborn Deliveries Scheduled Early[2]	40	0%	6%	6%
Preventive Care				
Immunization for Influenza[2]	588	98%	94%	90%
Immunization for Pneumonia[2]	713	100%	96%	92%
Stroke Care				
Anticoagulation Therapy for Atrial Fibrillation	20	95%	97%	95%
Antithrombotic Therapy Timing	137	97%	98%	98%
Assessed for Rehabilitation	161	96%	97%	97%
Discharged on Antithrombotic Therapy	149	97%	99%	99%
Discharged on Statin Medication	129	91%	96%	94%
Thrombolytic Therapy Timing	12	58%	76%	66%
Venous Thromboembolism Prophylaxis	154	92%	95%	94%
Written Stroke Educational Materials Given	93	98%	94%	88%
Surgical Care Improvement Project				
Appropriate Beta Blocker Usage[2]	170	100%	99%	98%
Appropriate VTP Within 24 Hours[2]	294	100%	99%	98%
Controlled Postoperative Blood Glucose[2]	106	99%	98%	97%
Perioperative Temperature Management[2]	340	100%	100%	100%
Prophylactic Antibiotic Selection[2]	238	99%	99%	99%
Prophylactic Antibiotic Selection (Outpatient)	303	99%	98%	98%
Prophylactic Antibiotic Stopped[2]	227	100%	98%	98%
Prophylactic Antibiotic Timing[2]	240	100%	99%	99%
Prophylactic Antibiotic Timing (Outpatient)	303	100%	98%	98%
Urinary Catheter Removal[2]	201	100%	98%	97%
Survey of Patients' Hospital Experiences				
Area Around Room 'Always' Quiet at Night	300+	54%	58%	61%
Doctors 'Always' Communicated Well	300+	71%	77%	82%
Home Recovery Information Given	300+	79%	83%	85%
Hospital Given 9 or 10 on 10 Point Scale	300+	55%	67%	71%
Meds 'Always' Explained Before Given	300+	53%	60%	64%
Nurses 'Always' Communicated Well	300+	67%	75%	79%
Pain 'Always' Well Controlled	300+	62%	68%	71%
Room and Bathroom 'Always' Clean	300+	61%	69%	73%
Timely Help 'Always' Received	300+	51%	62%	68%
Would Definitely Recommend Hospital	300+	60%	69%	71%
Use of Medical Imaging				
Cardiac Imaging Stress Test before Surgery[1]	-	-	6.4%	5.3%
Combination Abdominal CT Scan	568	7.2%	11.8%	10.5%
Combination Brain/Sinus CT Scan	591	5.1%	3.4%	2.7%
Combination Chest CT Scan	266	4.5%	2.4%	2.7%
Follow-up Mammogram/Ultrasound	279	11.8%	10.2%	8.8%
Lumbar Spine MRI for Low Back Pain[1]	-	-	35.2%	37.2%

Jackson Hospital

4250 Hospital Dr
Marianna, FL 32446
Phone: 850-718-2620
Fax: 850-482-6374
E-mail: webmaster@jacksonhosp.com
URL: www.jacksonhosp.com
Type: Acute Care Hospitals
Emergency Services: Yes
Ownership: Govt - Hospital Dist/Auth
Beds: 100

Key Personnel:
Operating Room. . . . . Nikorn Arunakul
Radiology. . . . . Glenn Clark
Quality Assurance . . . . Brooke Donaldson
Chief of Medical Staff . . . . Gonzalo Oria, MD
CEO/President. . . . . John West

Measure	Cases	This Hosp.	State Avg.	U.S. Avg.
Blood Clot Prevention and Treatment				
Anticoagulation Overlap Therapy[1,2]	-	-	93%	93%
ICU Venous Thromboembolism Prophylaxis[2]	42	76%	94%	92%
Incidence of Potentially Preventable VTE[2,7]	-	-	10%	10%
UFH with Dosages/Platelet Monitoring[2,7]	-	-	100%	97%
Venous Thromboembolism Prophylaxis[2]	313	76%	88%	85%
Warfarin Therapy Discharge Instructions[1,2]	-	-	85%	75%
Chest Pain/Possible Heart Attack Care				
Aspirin Given Within 24 Hours of Arrival	59	95%	98%	96%
Fibrinolytic Meds Within 30 Min. of Arrival[1]	-	-	81%	58%
Average Time to ECG (minutes)	61	8	7	7
Average Time to Transfer (minutes)	19	141	53	60
Children's Asthma Care				
Received Home Management Plan of Care	-	-	-	88%
Received Reliever Medication	-	-	-	100%
Received Systemic Corticosteroids	-	-	-	100%
Emergency Department				
Admittance Decision Time (minutes)[2]	316	93	111	98
Head CT Results Within 45 Min. of Arrival[1]	-	-	64%	57%
Patients Who Left ER Before Being Seen	26,319	1%	2%	2%
Time from ER Arrival to Admit. (minutes)[2]	316	219	289	274
Time from ER Arrival to Discharge (minutes)	1,156	101	147	134
Time in ER Before Being Evaluated (minutes)	1,195	30	26	26
Time to Pain Meds for Fractures (minutes)	115	54	60	57
Heart Attack Care				
Aspirin Given at Discharge	24	100%	99%	99%
Fibrinolytic Meds Within 30 Min. of Arrival[7]	-	-	50%	54%
PCI Within 90 Minutes of Arrival[7]	-	-	96%	96%
Statin Prescribed at Discharge	25	84%	99%	98%
Heart Failure Care				
ACE Inhibitor or ARB for LVSD	28	100%	98%	97%
Discharge Instructions Given	95	86%	96%	94%
Evaluation of LVS Function	106	99%	100%	99%
Medicare Spending				
Medicare Spending per Patient (ratio)	-	1.01	1.04	0.98
Pneumonia Care				

NOTE: Hospital profiles are in alphabetical order by state, then city, then hospital within the city; Rankings exclude hospitals with less than 25 cases except for patient surveys which excludes hospitals with less than 100 cases; (a) 100-299 cases; (1) The number of cases/patients is too few to report; (2) Data submitted were based on a sample of cases/patients; (3) Results are based on a shorter time period than required; (4) Data suppressed by CMS for one or more quarters; (5) Results are not available for this reporting period; (6) Fewer than 100 patients completed the HCAHPS survey; (7) No cases met the criteria for this measure; (8) The lower limit of the confidence interval cannot be calculated if the number of observed infections equals zero; (9) No data are available from the state/territory for this reporting period; (10) The scores shown reflect fewer than 50 completed surveys; (11) There were discrepancies in the data collection process; (12) This measure does not apply to this hospital for this reporting period; (13) Results cannot be calculated for this reporting period; (14) The results for this state are combined with nearby states to protect confidentiality; Please refer to the User's Guide for a full explanation of data.

Measure	Cases	This Hosp.	State Avg.	U.S. Avg.
Appropriate Initial Antibiotic Given	99	99%	98%	95%
Blood Culture Timing	167	95%	99%	98%
Pregnancy and Delivery Care				
Newborn Deliveries Scheduled Early	40	8%	6%	6%
Preventive Care				
Immunization for Influenza[2]	364	95%	94%	90%
Immunization for Pneumonia[2]	434	96%	96%	92%
Stroke Care				
Anticoagulation Therapy for Atrial Fibrillation[1]	-	-	97%	95%
Antithrombotic Therapy Timing	51	100%	98%	98%
Assessed for Rehabilitation	56	100%	97%	97%
Discharged on Antithrombotic Therapy	53	100%	99%	99%
Discharged on Statin Medication	47	77%	96%	94%
Thrombolytic Therapy Timing[1]	-	-	76%	66%
Venous Thromboembolism Prophylaxis	52	90%	95%	94%
Written Stroke Educational Materials Given	36	100%	94%	88%
Surgical Care Improvement Project				
Appropriate Beta Blocker Usage	54	96%	99%	98%
Appropriate VTP Within 24 Hours	146	98%	99%	98%
Controlled Postoperative Blood Glucose[7]	-	-	98%	97%
Perioperative Temperature Management	157	100%	100%	100%
Prophylactic Antibiotic Selection	118	97%	99%	99%
Prophylactic Antibiotic Selection (Outpatient)	21	100%	98%	98%
Prophylactic Antibiotic Stopped	116	98%	98%	98%
Prophylactic Antibiotic Timing	118	99%	99%	99%
Prophylactic Antibiotic Timing (Outpatient)	20	85%	98%	98%
Urinary Catheter Removal	73	96%	98%	97%
Survey of Patients' Hospital Experiences				
Area Around Room 'Always' Quiet at Night	300+	70%	58%	61%
Doctors 'Always' Communicated Well	300+	89%	77%	82%
Home Recovery Information Given	300+	89%	83%	85%
Hospital Given 9 or 10 on 10 Point Scale	300+	75%	67%	71%
Meds 'Always' Explained Before Given	300+	69%	60%	64%
Nurses 'Always' Communicated Well	300+	81%	75%	79%
Pain 'Always' Well Controlled	300+	73%	68%	71%
Room and Bathroom 'Always' Clean	300+	73%	69%	73%
Timely Help 'Always' Received	300+	68%	62%	68%
Would Definitely Recommend Hospital	300+	72%	69%	71%
Use of Medical Imaging				
Cardiac Imaging Stress Test before Surgery	131	3.8%	6.4%	5.3%
Combination Abdominal CT Scan	482	6.2%	11.8%	10.5%
Combination Brain/Sinus CT Scan	508	1.0%	3.4%	2.7%
Combination Chest CT Scan	160	6.3%	2.4%	2.7%
Follow-up Mammogram/Ultrasound	917	9.2%	10.2%	8.8%
Lumbar Spine MRI for Low Back Pain[1]	-	-	35.2%	37.2%

Holmes Regional Medical Center

1350 S Hickory St — Phone: 321-434-7000
Melbourne, FL 32901 — Fax: 321-434-8587
URL: www.healthfirst.org
Type: Acute Care Hospitals — Emergency Services: Yes
Ownership: Voluntary non-profit - Private — Beds: 515

Key Personnel:

Operating Room. . . . . Judy Bourne
Emergency Room . . . . Scott Gettings, MD
CEO/President. . . . . Stephen P. Johnson, PhD
Intensive Care Unit. . . . . Rose Mazanec-Freeman, RN
Quality Assurance . . . . James V Palermo, MD
Pediatric In-Patient Care . . . . Mahesh Soni, MD
Radiology. . . . . Martin Stern, MD
Infection Control. . . . . Stacy Westphal

Measure	Cases	This Hosp.	State Avg.	U.S. Avg.
Blood Clot Prevention and Treatment				
Anticoagulation Overlap Therapy[2]	218	100%	93%	93%
ICU Venous Thromboembolism Prophylaxis[2]	93	97%	94%	92%
Incidence of Potentially Preventable VTE[2]	40	5%	10%	10%
UFH with Dosages/Platelet Monitoring[2]	228	100%	100%	97%
Venous Thromboembolism Prophylaxis[2]	377	90%	88%	85%
Warfarin Therapy Discharge Instructions[2]	132	85%	85%	75%
Chest Pain/Possible Heart Attack Care				
Aspirin Given Within 24 Hours of Arrival[1,3]	-	-	98%	96%
Fibrinolytic Meds Within 30 Min. of Arrival[5]	-	-	81%	58%
Average Time to ECG (minutes)[1,3]	-	-	7	7
Average Time to Transfer (minutes)[5]	-	-	53	60
Children's Asthma Care				
Received Home Management Plan of Care	-	-	-	88%
Received Reliever Medication	-	-	-	100%
Received Systemic Corticosteroids	-	-	-	100%
Emergency Department				
Admittance Decision Time (minutes)[2]	646	117	111	98
Head CT Results Within 45 Min. of Arrival[1]	-	-	64%	57%
Patients Who Left ER Before Being Seen	67,599	1%	2%	2%
Time from ER Arrival to Admit. (minutes)[2]	649	264	289	274
Time from ER Arrival to Discharge (minutes)	412	160	147	134
Time in ER Before Being Evaluated (minutes)	443	27	26	26
Time to Pain Meds for Fractures (minutes)	274	54	60	57
Heart Attack Care				
Aspirin Given at Discharge	527	99%	99%	99%
Fibrinolytic Meds Within 30 Min. of Arrival[7]	-	-	50%	54%
PCI Within 90 Minutes of Arrival	58	100%	96%	96%
Statin Prescribed at Discharge	507	98%	99%	98%
Heart Failure Care				
ACE Inhibitor or ARB for LVSD	332	98%	98%	97%
Discharge Instructions Given	633	99%	96%	94%
Evaluation of LVS Function	787	100%	100%	99%
Medicare Spending				
Medicare Spending per Patient (ratio)	-	1.09	1.04	0.98
Pneumonia Care				
Appropriate Initial Antibiotic Given	298	99%	98%	95%
Blood Culture Timing	617	99%	99%	98%
Pregnancy and Delivery Care				
Newborn Deliveries Scheduled Early[2]	36	8%	6%	6%
Preventive Care				
Immunization for Influenza[2]	559	89%	94%	90%
Immunization for Pneumonia[2]	765	96%	96%	92%
Stroke Care				
Anticoagulation Therapy for Atrial Fibrillation	34	100%	97%	95%
Antithrombotic Therapy Timing	237	100%	98%	98%
Assessed for Rehabilitation	286	100%	97%	97%
Discharged on Antithrombotic Therapy	235	100%	99%	99%
Discharged on Statin Medication	175	98%	96%	94%
Thrombolytic Therapy Timing	14	100%	76%	66%
Venous Thromboembolism Prophylaxis	306	99%	95%	94%
Written Stroke Educational Materials Given	150	97%	94%	88%
Surgical Care Improvement Project				
Appropriate Beta Blocker Usage[2]	597	99%	99%	98%
Appropriate VTP Within 24 Hours[2]	892	99%	99%	98%
Controlled Postoperative Blood Glucose[2]	323	97%	98%	97%
Perioperative Temperature Management[2]	1,126	100%	100%	100%
Prophylactic Antibiotic Selection[2]	1,137	100%	99%	99%
Prophylactic Antibiotic Selection (Outpatient)	699	98%	98%	98%
Prophylactic Antibiotic Stopped[2]	1,111	99%	98%	98%
Prophylactic Antibiotic Timing[2]	1,137	99%	99%	99%
Prophylactic Antibiotic Timing (Outpatient)	702	99%	98%	98%
Urinary Catheter Removal[2]	1,021	99%	98%	97%
Survey of Patients' Hospital Experiences				
Area Around Room 'Always' Quiet at Night	300+	54%	58%	61%
Doctors 'Always' Communicated Well	300+	75%	77%	82%
Home Recovery Information Given	300+	83%	83%	85%
Hospital Given 9 or 10 on 10 Point Scale	300+	66%	67%	71%
Meds 'Always' Explained Before Given	300+	61%	60%	64%
Nurses 'Always' Communicated Well	300+	77%	75%	79%
Pain 'Always' Well Controlled	300+	67%	68%	71%
Room and Bathroom 'Always' Clean	300+	70%	69%	73%
Timely Help 'Always' Received	300+	61%	62%	68%
Would Definitely Recommend Hospital	300+	72%	69%	71%
Use of Medical Imaging				
Cardiac Imaging Stress Test before Surgery	542	5.0%	6.4%	5.3%
Combination Abdominal CT Scan	736	8.0%	11.8%	10.5%
Combination Brain/Sinus CT Scan	1,405	0.6%	3.4%	2.7%
Combination Chest CT Scan	714	1.1%	2.4%	2.7%
Follow-up Mammogram/Ultrasound	1,632	7.8%	10.2%	8.8%
Lumbar Spine MRI for Low Back Pain[1]	-	-	35.2%	37.2%

Viera Hospital

8745 N Wickham Rd — Phone: 321-434-9000
Melbourne, FL 32940
URL: www.health-first.org
Type: Acute Care Hospitals — Emergency Services: Yes
Ownership: Voluntary non-profit - Private

Measure	Cases	This Hosp.	State Avg.	U.S. Avg.
Blood Clot Prevention and Treatment				
Anticoagulation Overlap Therapy[2]	48	100%	93%	93%
ICU Venous Thromboembolism Prophylaxis[2]	43	100%	94%	92%
Incidence of Potentially Preventable VTE[2]	11	0%	10%	10%
UFH with Dosages/Platelet Monitoring[2]	34	97%	100%	97%
Venous Thromboembolism Prophylaxis[2]	306	98%	88%	85%
Warfarin Therapy Discharge Instructions[2]	35	97%	85%	75%
Chest Pain/Possible Heart Attack Care				
Aspirin Given Within 24 Hours of Arrival	62	100%	98%	96%
Fibrinolytic Meds Within 30 Min. of Arrival[7]	-	-	81%	58%
Average Time to ECG (minutes)	62	6	7	7
Average Time to Transfer (minutes)[1]	-	-	53	60
Children's Asthma Care				
Received Home Management Plan of Care	-	-	-	88%
Received Reliever Medication	-	-	-	100%
Received Systemic Corticosteroids	-	-	-	100%
Emergency Department				
Admittance Decision Time (minutes)[2]	495	86	111	98
Head CT Results Within 45 Min. of Arrival[7]	-	-	64%	57%
Patients Who Left ER Before Being Seen	16,594	1%	2%	2%
Time from ER Arrival to Admit. (minutes)[2]	495	242	289	274
Time from ER Arrival to Discharge (minutes)	383	145	147	134
Time in ER Before Being Evaluated (minutes)	374	23	26	26
Time to Pain Meds for Fractures (minutes)	68	52	60	57
Heart Attack Care				
Aspirin Given at Discharge[1]	-	-	99%	99%
Fibrinolytic Meds Within 30 Min. of Arrival[7]	-	-	50%	54%
PCI Within 90 Minutes of Arrival[7]	-	-	96%	96%
Statin Prescribed at Discharge[1]	-	-	99%	98%
Heart Failure Care				
ACE Inhibitor or ARB for LVSD	19	100%	98%	97%
Discharge Instructions Given	48	98%	96%	94%
Evaluation of LVS Function	63	100%	100%	99%
Medicare Spending				
Medicare Spending per Patient (ratio)	-	1.04	1.04	0.98
Pneumonia Care				
Appropriate Initial Antibiotic Given	68	100%	98%	95%
Blood Culture Timing	95	100%	99%	98%
Pregnancy and Delivery Care				
Newborn Deliveries Scheduled Early[7]	-	-	6%	6%
Preventive Care				
Immunization for Influenza[2]	366	99%	94%	90%
Immunization for Pneumonia[2]	518	100%	96%	92%
Stroke Care				
Anticoagulation Therapy for Atrial Fibrillation[1]	-	-	97%	95%
Antithrombotic Therapy Timing	28	96%	98%	98%
Assessed for Rehabilitation	28	100%	97%	97%
Discharged on Antithrombotic Therapy	27	100%	99%	99%
Discharged on Statin Medication	19	100%	96%	94%
Thrombolytic Therapy Timing[1]	-	-	76%	66%
Venous Thromboembolism Prophylaxis	25	100%	95%	94%
Written Stroke Educational Materials Given	23	100%	94%	88%
Surgical Care Improvement Project				
Appropriate Beta Blocker Usage	154	100%	99%	98%
Appropriate VTP Within 24 Hours	539	99%	99%	98%
Controlled Postoperative Blood Glucose[7]	-	-	98%	97%
Perioperative Temperature Management	577	100%	100%	100%
Prophylactic Antibiotic Selection	385	100%	99%	99%
Prophylactic Antibiotic Selection (Outpatient)	69	96%	98%	98%
Prophylactic Antibiotic Stopped	382	99%	98%	98%
Prophylactic Antibiotic Timing	385	100%	99%	99%
Prophylactic Antibiotic Timing (Outpatient)	70	99%	98%	98%
Urinary Catheter Removal	521	100%	98%	97%
Survey of Patients' Hospital Experiences				
Area Around Room 'Always' Quiet at Night	300+	69%	58%	61%

NOTE: Hospital profiles are in alphabetical order by state, then city, then hospital within the city; Rankings exclude hospitals with less than 25 cases except for patient surveys which excludes hospitals with less than 100 cases; (a) 100-299 cases; (1) The number of cases/patients is too few to report; (2) Data submitted were based on a sample of cases/patients; (3) Results are based on a shorter time period than required; (4) Data suppressed by CMS for one or more quarters; (5) Results are not available for this reporting period; (6) Fewer than 100 patients completed the HCAHPS survey; (7) No cases met the criteria for this measure; (8) The lower limit of the confidence interval cannot be calculated if the number of observed infections equals zero; (9) No data are available from the state/territory for this reporting period; (10) The scores shown reflect fewer than 50 completed surveys; (11) There were discrepancies in the data collection process; (12) This measure does not apply to this hospital for this reporting period; (13) Results cannot be calculated for this reporting period; (14) The results for this state are combined with nearby states to protect confidentiality; Please refer to the User's Guide for a full explanation of data.

Doctors 'Always' Communicated Well	300+	82%	77%	82%
Home Recovery Information Given	300+	87%	83%	85%
Hospital Given 9 or 10 on 10 Point Scale	300+	82%	67%	71%
Meds 'Always' Explained Before Given	300+	71%	60%	64%
Nurses 'Always' Communicated Well	300+	84%	75%	79%
Pain 'Always' Well Controlled	300+	76%	68%	71%
Room and Bathroom 'Always' Clean	300+	79%	69%	73%
Timely Help 'Always' Received	300+	73%	62%	68%
Would Definitely Recommend Hospital	300+	88%	69%	71%
Use of Medical Imaging				
Cardiac Imaging Stress Test before Surgery	90	6.7%	6.4%	5.3%
Combination Abdominal CT Scan	339	4.1%	11.8%	10.5%
Combination Brain/Sinus CT Scan[1]	-	-	3.4%	2.7%
Combination Chest CT Scan	264	0.4%	2.4%	2.7%
Follow-up Mammogram/Ultrasound	235	11.1%	10.2%	8.8%
Lumbar Spine MRI for Low Back Pain[1]	-	-	35.2%	37.2%

Wuesthoff Medical Center - Melbourne

250 North Wickham Road
Melbourne, FL 32935
Phone: 321-752-1200
Fax: 321-752-1698
URL: www.wuesthoff.org
Type: Acute Care Hospitals
Emergency Services: Yes
Ownership: Voluntary non-profit - Private
Beds: 65

Key Personnel:
CEO/President. . . . . Richard Frank
Chief of Medical Staff . . . . Kent N Leifer

Measure	Cases	This Hosp.	State Avg.	U.S. Avg.
Blood Clot Prevention and Treatment				
Anticoagulation Overlap Therapy[2]	46	72%	93%	93%
ICU Venous Thromboembolism Prophylaxis[2]	57	86%	94%	92%
Incidence of Potentially Preventable VTE[1,2]	-	-	10%	10%
UFH with Dosages/Platelet Monitoring[2]	41	98%	100%	97%
Venous Thromboembolism Prophylaxis[2]	369	87%	88%	85%
Warfarin Therapy Discharge Instructions[2]	32	88%	85%	75%
Chest Pain/Possible Heart Attack Care				
Aspirin Given Within 24 Hours of Arrival[1,3]	-	-	98%	96%
Fibrinolytic Meds Within 30 Min. of Arrival[3,7]	-	-	81%	58%
Average Time to ECG (minutes)[1,3]	-	-	7	7
Average Time to Transfer (minutes)[3,7]	-	-	53	60
Children's Asthma Care				
Received Home Management Plan of Care	-	-	-	88%
Received Reliever Medication	-	-	-	100%
Received Systemic Corticosteroids	-	-	-	100%
Emergency Department				
Admittance Decision Time (minutes)[2]	484	123	111	98
Head CT Results Within 45 Min. of Arrival[1]	-	-	64%	57%
Patients Who Left ER Before Being Seen	18,510	2%	2%	2%
Time from ER Arrival to Admit. (minutes)[2]	518	264	289	274
Time from ER Arrival to Discharge (minutes)	362	116	147	134
Time in ER Before Being Evaluated (minutes)	411	22	26	26
Time to Pain Meds for Fractures (minutes)	58	43	60	57
Heart Attack Care				
Aspirin Given at Discharge	50	96%	99%	99%
Fibrinolytic Meds Within 30 Min. of Arrival[7]	-	-	50%	54%
PCI Within 90 Minutes of Arrival	11	82%	96%	96%
Statin Prescribed at Discharge	48	94%	99%	98%
Heart Failure Care				
ACE Inhibitor or ARB for LVSD	41	95%	98%	97%
Discharge Instructions Given	63	70%	96%	94%
Evaluation of LVS Function	90	100%	100%	99%
Medicare Spending				
Medicare Spending per Patient (ratio)	-	1.15	1.04	0.98
Pneumonia Care				
Appropriate Initial Antibiotic Given	71	93%	98%	95%
Blood Culture Timing	132	100%	99%	98%
Pregnancy and Delivery Care				
Newborn Deliveries Scheduled Early	32	31%	6%	6%
Preventive Care				
Immunization for Influenza[2]	482	87%	94%	90%
Immunization for Pneumonia[2]	569	91%	96%	92%
Stroke Care				
Anticoagulation Therapy for Atrial Fibrillation[1]	-	-	97%	95%
Antithrombotic Therapy Timing	27	100%	98%	98%
Assessed for Rehabilitation	30	97%	97%	97%
Discharged on Antithrombotic Therapy	28	100%	99%	99%
Discharged on Statin Medication	17	100%	96%	94%
Thrombolytic Therapy Timing[1]	-	-	76%	66%
Venous Thromboembolism Prophylaxis	31	90%	95%	94%
Written Stroke Educational Materials Given	17	59%	94%	88%
Surgical Care Improvement Project				
Appropriate Beta Blocker Usage[2]	125	97%	99%	98%
Appropriate VTP Within 24 Hours[2]	341	96%	99%	98%
Controlled Postoperative Blood Glucose[2,7]	-	-	98%	97%
Perioperative Temperature Management[2]	390	100%	100%	100%
Prophylactic Antibiotic Selection[2]	275	100%	99%	99%
Prophylactic Antibiotic Selection (Outpatient)	235	88%	98%	98%
Prophylactic Antibiotic Stopped[2]	268	89%	98%	98%
Prophylactic Antibiotic Timing[2]	277	98%	99%	99%
Prophylactic Antibiotic Timing (Outpatient)	237	95%	98%	98%
Urinary Catheter Removal[2]	272	97%	98%	97%
Survey of Patients' Hospital Experiences				
Area Around Room 'Always' Quiet at Night	300+	52%	58%	61%
Doctors 'Always' Communicated Well	300+	65%	77%	82%
Home Recovery Information Given	300+	77%	83%	85%
Hospital Given 9 or 10 on 10 Point Scale	300+	55%	67%	71%
Meds 'Always' Explained Before Given	300+	53%	60%	64%
Nurses 'Always' Communicated Well	300+	68%	75%	79%
Pain 'Always' Well Controlled	300+	64%	68%	71%
Room and Bathroom 'Always' Clean	300+	67%	69%	73%
Timely Help 'Always' Received	300+	51%	62%	68%
Would Definitely Recommend Hospital	300+	58%	69%	71%
Use of Medical Imaging				
Cardiac Imaging Stress Test before Surgery	109	6.4%	6.4%	5.3%
Combination Abdominal CT Scan	429	14.0%	11.8%	10.5%
Combination Brain/Sinus CT Scan	362	5.0%	3.4%	2.7%
Combination Chest CT Scan	169	2.4%	2.4%	2.7%
Follow-up Mammogram/Ultrasound	236	18.6%	10.2%	8.8%
Lumbar Spine MRI for Low Back Pain[1]	-	-	35.2%	37.2%

Anne Bates Leach Eye Hospital

900 Nw 17th St
Miami, FL 33136
Phone: 305-326-6000
Fax: 305-326-6311
URL: www.bascompalmer.org
Type: Acute Care Hospitals
Emergency Services: Yes
Ownership: Voluntary non-profit - Other
Beds: 100

Key Personnel:
CEO/President. . . . . Eduardo C Alfonso
Chief of Medical Staff . . . . Byron L Lam

Measure	Cases	This Hosp.	State Avg.	U.S. Avg.
Blood Clot Prevention and Treatment				
Anticoagulation Overlap Therapy[7]	-	-	93%	93%
ICU Venous Thromboembolism Prophylaxis[7]	-	-	94%	92%
Incidence of Potentially Preventable VTE[7]	-	-	10%	10%
UFH with Dosages/Platelet Monitoring[7]	-	-	100%	97%
Venous Thromboembolism Prophylaxis	29	0%	88%	85%
Warfarin Therapy Discharge Instructions[7]	-	-	85%	75%
Chest Pain/Possible Heart Attack Care				
Aspirin Given Within 24 Hours of Arrival[5]	-	-	98%	96%
Fibrinolytic Meds Within 30 Min. of Arrival[5]	-	-	81%	58%
Average Time to ECG (minutes)[5]	-	-	7	7
Average Time to Transfer (minutes)[5]	-	-	53	60
Children's Asthma Care				
Received Home Management Plan of Care	-	-	-	88%
Received Reliever Medication	-	-	-	100%
Received Systemic Corticosteroids	-	-	-	100%
Emergency Department				
Admittance Decision Time (minutes)	13	57	111	98
Head CT Results Within 45 Min. of Arrival[5]	-	-	64%	57%
Patients Who Left ER Before Being Seen	17,234	0%	2%	2%
Time from ER Arrival to Admit. (minutes)	13	391	289	274
Time from ER Arrival to Discharge (minutes)	407	147	147	134
Time in ER Before Being Evaluated (minutes)	280	118	26	26
Time to Pain Meds for Fractures (minutes)[5]	-	-	60	57
Heart Attack Care				
Aspirin Given at Discharge[5]	-	-	99%	99%
Fibrinolytic Meds Within 30 Min. of Arrival[5]	-	-	50%	54%
PCI Within 90 Minutes of Arrival[5]	-	-	96%	96%
Statin Prescribed at Discharge[5]	-	-	99%	98%
Heart Failure Care				
ACE Inhibitor or ARB for LVSD[5]	-	-	98%	97%
Discharge Instructions Given[5]	-	-	96%	94%
Evaluation of LVS Function[5]	-	-	100%	99%
Medicare Spending				
Medicare Spending per Patient (ratio)[1]	-	-	1.04	0.98
Pneumonia Care				
Appropriate Initial Antibiotic Given[5]	-	-	98%	95%
Blood Culture Timing[5]	-	-	99%	98%
Pregnancy and Delivery Care				
Newborn Deliveries Scheduled Early[7]	-	-	6%	6%
Preventive Care				
Immunization for Influenza	20	75%	94%	90%
Immunization for Pneumonia	28	93%	96%	92%
Stroke Care				
Anticoagulation Therapy for Atrial Fibrillation[5]	-	-	97%	95%
Antithrombotic Therapy Timing[5]	-	-	98%	98%
Assessed for Rehabilitation[5]	-	-	97%	97%
Discharged on Antithrombotic Therapy[5]	-	-	99%	99%
Discharged on Statin Medication[5]	-	-	96%	94%
Thrombolytic Therapy Timing[5]	-	-	76%	66%
Venous Thromboembolism Prophylaxis[5]	-	-	95%	94%
Written Stroke Educational Materials Given[5]	-	-	94%	88%
Surgical Care Improvement Project				
Appropriate Beta Blocker Usage[5]	-	-	99%	98%
Appropriate VTP Within 24 Hours[5]	-	-	99%	98%
Controlled Postoperative Blood Glucose[5]	-	-	98%	97%
Perioperative Temperature Management[5]	-	-	100%	100%
Prophylactic Antibiotic Selection[5]	-	-	99%	99%
Prophylactic Antibiotic Selection (Outpatient)[5]	-	-	98%	98%
Prophylactic Antibiotic Stopped[5]	-	-	98%	98%
Prophylactic Antibiotic Timing[5]	-	-	99%	99%
Prophylactic Antibiotic Timing (Outpatient)[5]	-	-	98%	98%
Urinary Catheter Removal[5]	-	-	98%	97%
Survey of Patients' Hospital Experiences				
Area Around Room 'Always' Quiet at Night[10]	<100	67%	58%	61%
Doctors 'Always' Communicated Well[10]	<100	97%	77%	82%
Home Recovery Information Given[10]	<100	78%	83%	85%
Hospital Given 9 or 10 on 10 Point Scale[10]	<100	91%	67%	71%
Meds 'Always' Explained Before Given[10]	<100	59%	60%	64%
Nurses 'Always' Communicated Well[10]	<100	96%	75%	79%
Pain 'Always' Well Controlled[10]	<100	85%	68%	71%
Room and Bathroom 'Always' Clean[10]	<100	72%	69%	73%
Timely Help 'Always' Received[10]	<100	87%	62%	68%
Would Definitely Recommend Hospital[10]	<100	89%	69%	71%
Use of Medical Imaging				
Cardiac Imaging Stress Test before Surgery[7]	-	-	6.4%	5.3%
Combination Abdominal CT Scan[7]	-	-	11.8%	10.5%
Combination Brain/Sinus CT Scan[7]	-	-	3.4%	2.7%
Combination Chest CT Scan[7]	-	-	2.4%	2.7%
Follow-up Mammogram/Ultrasound[7]	-	-	10.2%	8.8%
Lumbar Spine MRI for Low Back Pain[1]	-	-	35.2%	37.2%

Baptist Hospital of Miami

8900 N Kendall Dr
Miami, FL 33176
Phone: 786-596-1960
Fax: 786-596-2428
URL: www.baptisthealth.net
Type: Acute Care Hospitals
Emergency Services: Yes
Ownership: Voluntary non-profit - Private
Beds: 513

Key Personnel:
Chief of Medical Staff . . . . Eugene Eisher, MD
Pediatric Ambulatory Care . . . . . . Denise Harris, RN
CEO/President. . . . . Brian E. Keeley
Radiology. . . . . Neil Messinger, MD
Infection Control. . . . . Barbara Russell, RN
Operating Room. . . . . Michelle Ryder
Quality Assurance . . . . Lynne Thompson

Measure	Cases	This Hosp.	State Avg.	U.S. Avg.
Blood Clot Prevention and Treatment				
Anticoagulation Overlap Therapy[2]	87	100%	93%	93%
ICU Venous Thromboembolism Prophylaxis[2]	54	100%	94%	92%
Incidence of Potentially Preventable VTE[2]	52	2%	10%	10%

NOTE: Hospital profiles are in alphabetical order by state, then city, then hospital within the city; Rankings exclude hospitals with less than 25 cases except for patient surveys which excludes hospitals with less than 100 cases; (a) 100-299 cases; (1) The number of cases/patients is too few to report; (2) Data submitted were based on a sample of cases/patients; (3) Results are based on a shorter time period than required; (4) Data suppressed by CMS for one or more quarters; (5) Results are not available for this reporting period; (6) Fewer than 100 patients completed the HCAHPS survey; (7) No cases met the criteria for this measure; (8) The lower limit of the confidence interval cannot be calculated if the number of observed infections equals zero; (9) No data are available from the state/territory for this reporting period; (10) The scores shown reflect fewer than 50 completed surveys; (11) There were discrepancies in the data collection process; (12) This measure does not apply to this hospital for this reporting period; (13) Results cannot be calculated for this reporting period; (14) The results for this state are combined with nearby states to protect confidentiality; Please refer to the User's Guide for a full explanation of data.

Measure	Cases	This Hosp.	State Avg.	U.S. Avg.
UFH with Dosages/Platelet Monitoring[2]	145	100%	100%	97%
Venous Thromboembolism Prophylaxis[2]	396	99%	88%	85%
Warfarin Therapy Discharge Instructions[2]	66	100%	85%	75%
Chest Pain/Possible Heart Attack Care				
Aspirin Given Within 24 Hours of Arrival[1,3]	-	-	98%	96%
Fibrinolytic Meds Within 30 Min. of Arrival[5]	-	-	81%	58%
Average Time to ECG (minutes)[1,3]	-	-	7	7
Average Time to Transfer (minutes)[5]	-	-	53	60
Children's Asthma Care				
Received Home Management Plan of Care	-	-	-	88%
Received Reliever Medication	-	-	-	100%
Received Systemic Corticosteroids	-	-	-	100%
Emergency Department				
Admittance Decision Time (minutes)[2]	622	201	111	98
Head CT Results Within 45 Min. of Arrival[1]	-	-	64%	57%
Patients Who Left ER Before Being Seen	>100k	1%	2%	2%
Time from ER Arrival to Admit. (minutes)[2]	746	432	289	274
Time from ER Arrival to Discharge (minutes)	363	223	147	134
Time in ER Before Being Evaluated (minutes)	414	53	26	26
Time to Pain Meds for Fractures (minutes)	184	43	60	57
Heart Attack Care				
Aspirin Given at Discharge[2]	279	100%	99%	99%
Fibrinolytic Meds Within 30 Min. of Arrival[1,2]	-	-	50%	54%
PCI Within 90 Minutes of Arrival[2]	46	100%	96%	96%
Statin Prescribed at Discharge[2]	283	100%	99%	98%
Heart Failure Care				
ACE Inhibitor or ARB for LVSD[2]	76	100%	98%	97%
Discharge Instructions Given[2]	265	100%	96%	94%
Evaluation of LVS Function[2]	311	100%	100%	99%
Medicare Spending				
Medicare Spending per Patient (ratio)	-	1.02	1.04	0.98
Pneumonia Care				
Appropriate Initial Antibiotic Given[2]	78	100%	98%	95%
Blood Culture Timing[2]	123	100%	99%	98%
Pregnancy and Delivery Care				
Newborn Deliveries Scheduled Early[2]	71	0%	6%	6%
Preventive Care				
Immunization for Influenza[2]	527	100%	94%	90%
Immunization for Pneumonia[2]	566	100%	96%	92%
Stroke Care				
Anticoagulation Therapy for Atrial Fibrillation[2]	29	100%	97%	95%
Antithrombotic Therapy Timing[2]	121	100%	98%	98%
Assessed for Rehabilitation[2]	154	100%	97%	97%
Discharged on Antithrombotic Therapy[2]	130	100%	99%	99%
Discharged on Statin Medication[2]	102	99%	96%	94%
Thrombolytic Therapy Timing[1,2]	-	-	76%	66%
Venous Thromboembolism Prophylaxis[2]	148	100%	95%	94%
Written Stroke Educational Materials Given[2]	86	100%	94%	88%
Surgical Care Improvement Project				
Appropriate Beta Blocker Usage[2]	216	99%	99%	98%
Appropriate VTP Within 24 Hours[2]	440	100%	99%	98%
Controlled Postoperative Blood Glucose[2]	151	97%	98%	97%
Perioperative Temperature Management[2]	519	100%	100%	100%
Prophylactic Antibiotic Selection[2]	455	100%	99%	99%
Prophylactic Antibiotic Selection (Outpatient)	682	100%	98%	98%
Prophylactic Antibiotic Stopped[2]	445	100%	98%	98%
Prophylactic Antibiotic Timing[2]	456	100%	99%	99%
Prophylactic Antibiotic Timing (Outpatient)	677	100%	98%	98%
Urinary Catheter Removal[2]	416	100%	98%	97%
Survey of Patients' Hospital Experiences				
Area Around Room 'Always' Quiet at Night	300+	61%	58%	61%
Doctors 'Always' Communicated Well	300+	83%	77%	82%
Home Recovery Information Given	300+	84%	83%	85%
Hospital Given 9 or 10 on 10 Point Scale	300+	78%	67%	71%
Meds 'Always' Explained Before Given	300+	66%	60%	64%
Nurses 'Always' Communicated Well	300+	81%	75%	79%
Pain 'Always' Well Controlled	300+	75%	68%	71%
Room and Bathroom 'Always' Clean	300+	73%	69%	73%
Timely Help 'Always' Received	300+	64%	62%	68%
Would Definitely Recommend Hospital	300+	80%	69%	71%
Use of Medical Imaging				
Cardiac Imaging Stress Test before Surgery	295	6.1%	6.4%	5.3%
Combination Abdominal CT Scan	1,458	1.8%	11.8%	10.5%
Combination Brain/Sinus CT Scan	1,394	2.3%	3.4%	2.7%
Combination Chest CT Scan	476	0.4%	2.4%	2.7%
Follow-up Mammogram/Ultrasound[7]	-	-	10.2%	8.8%
Lumbar Spine MRI for Low Back Pain	110	45.5%	35.2%	37.2%

Douglas Gardens Hospital

5200 Ne 2nd Ave
Miami, FL 33137
E-mail: info@mjhha.org
URL: www.mjhha.org
Phone: 305-751-8626
Fax: 305-754-4530
Type: Acute Care Hospitals
Emergency Services: No
Ownership: Voluntary non-profit - Private
Beds: 494

Key Personnel:
CEO/President. . . . . Jeffrey P Freimark
Quality Assurance . . . . Lelani Kicklighter
Chief of Medical Staff. . . . . Brian J. Kiedrowski, MD
Ambulatory Care . . . . Mindy Tucker
Infection Control. . . . . Erna Zemel

Measure	Cases	This Hosp.	State Avg.	U.S. Avg.
Blood Clot Prevention and Treatment				
Anticoagulation Overlap Therapy[2,7]	-	-	93%	93%
ICU Venous Thromboembolism Prophylaxis[2,7]	-	-	94%	92%
Incidence of Potentially Preventable VTE[2,7]	-	-	10%	10%
UFH with Dosages/Platelet Monitoring[2,7]	-	-	100%	97%
Venous Thromboembolism Prophylaxis[2]	156	42%	88%	85%
Warfarin Therapy Discharge Instructions[2,7]	-	-	85%	75%
Chest Pain/Possible Heart Attack Care				
Aspirin Given Within 24 Hours of Arrival	-	-	98%	96%
Fibrinolytic Meds Within 30 Min. of Arrival	-	-	81%	58%
Average Time to ECG (minutes)	-	-	7	7
Average Time to Transfer (minutes)	-	-	53	60
Children's Asthma Care				
Received Home Management Plan of Care	-	-	-	88%
Received Reliever Medication	-	-	-	100%
Received Systemic Corticosteroids	-	-	-	100%
Emergency Department				
Admittance Decision Time (minutes)[2,7]	-	-	111	98
Head CT Results Within 45 Min. of Arrival	-	-	64%	57%
Patients Who Left ER Before Being Seen	-	-	2%	2%
Time from ER Arrival to Admit. (minutes)[2,7]	-	-	289	274
Time from ER Arrival to Discharge (minutes)	-	-	147	134
Time in ER Before Being Evaluated (minutes)	-	-	26	26
Time to Pain Meds for Fractures (minutes)	-	-	60	57
Heart Attack Care				
Aspirin Given at Discharge[5]	-	-	99%	99%
Fibrinolytic Meds Within 30 Min. of Arrival[5]	-	-	50%	54%
PCI Within 90 Minutes of Arrival[5]	-	-	96%	96%
Statin Prescribed at Discharge[5]	-	-	99%	98%
Heart Failure Care				
ACE Inhibitor or ARB for LVSD[1,2]	-	-	98%	97%
Discharge Instructions Given[1,2]	-	-	96%	94%
Evaluation of LVS Function[1,2]	-	-	100%	99%
Medicare Spending				
Medicare Spending per Patient (ratio)	-	0.90	1.04	0.98
Pneumonia Care				
Appropriate Initial Antibiotic Given[1,2]	-	-	98%	95%
Blood Culture Timing[2,7]	-	-	99%	98%
Pregnancy and Delivery Care				
Newborn Deliveries Scheduled Early[7]	-	-	6%	6%
Preventive Care				
Immunization for Influenza[2]	164	73%	94%	90%
Immunization for Pneumonia[2]	314	77%	96%	92%
Stroke Care				
Anticoagulation Therapy for Atrial Fibrillation[5]	-	-	97%	95%
Antithrombotic Therapy Timing[5]	-	-	98%	98%
Assessed for Rehabilitation[5]	-	-	97%	97%
Discharged on Antithrombotic Therapy[5]	-	-	99%	99%
Discharged on Statin Medication[5]	-	-	96%	94%
Thrombolytic Therapy Timing[5]	-	-	76%	66%
Venous Thromboembolism Prophylaxis[5]	-	-	95%	94%
Written Stroke Educational Materials Given[5]	-	-	94%	88%
Surgical Care Improvement Project				
Appropriate Beta Blocker Usage[5]	-	-	99%	98%
Appropriate VTP Within 24 Hours[5]	-	-	99%	98%
Controlled Postoperative Blood Glucose[5]	-	-	98%	97%
Perioperative Temperature Management[5]	-	-	100%	100%
Prophylactic Antibiotic Selection[5]	-	-	99%	99%
Prophylactic Antibiotic Selection (Outpatient)	-	-	98%	98%
Prophylactic Antibiotic Stopped[5]	-	-	98%	98%
Prophylactic Antibiotic Timing[5]	-	-	99%	99%
Prophylactic Antibiotic Timing (Outpatient)	-	-	98%	98%
Urinary Catheter Removal[5]	-	-	98%	97%
Survey of Patients' Hospital Experiences				
Area Around Room 'Always' Quiet at Night[10]	<100	69%	58%	61%
Doctors 'Always' Communicated Well[10]	<100	80%	77%	82%
Home Recovery Information Given[10]	<100	87%	83%	85%
Hospital Given 9 or 10 on 10 Point Scale[10]	<100	59%	67%	71%
Meds 'Always' Explained Before Given[10]	<100	62%	60%	64%
Nurses 'Always' Communicated Well[10]	<100	90%	75%	79%
Pain 'Always' Well Controlled[10]	<100	61%	68%	71%
Room and Bathroom 'Always' Clean[10]	<100	80%	69%	73%
Timely Help 'Always' Received[10]	<100	81%	62%	68%
Would Definitely Recommend Hospital[10]	<100	56%	69%	71%
Use of Medical Imaging				
Cardiac Imaging Stress Test before Surgery	-	-	6.4%	5.3%
Combination Abdominal CT Scan	-	-	11.8%	10.5%
Combination Brain/Sinus CT Scan	-	-	3.4%	2.7%
Combination Chest CT Scan	-	-	2.4%	2.7%
Follow-up Mammogram/Ultrasound	-	-	10.2%	8.8%
Lumbar Spine MRI for Low Back Pain	-	-	35.2%	37.2%

Jackson Memorial Hospital

1611 Nw 12th Ave
Miami, FL 33136
URL: www.jhsmiami.org
Phone: 305-585-1111
Fax: 305-326-8630
Type: Acute Care Hospitals
Emergency Services: Yes
Ownership: Govt - Hospital Dist/Auth
Beds: 1,558

Key Personnel:
Chief of Medical Staff. . . . . Gerard A Kaiser, MD
Quality Assurance . . . . Ted Lucas
CEO/President. . . . . Carlos A. Migoya

Measure	Cases	This Hosp.	State Avg.	U.S. Avg.
Blood Clot Prevention and Treatment				
Anticoagulation Overlap Therapy[2]	269	87%	93%	93%
ICU Venous Thromboembolism Prophylaxis[2]	216	88%	94%	92%
Incidence of Potentially Preventable VTE[2]	120	11%	10%	10%
UFH with Dosages/Platelet Monitoring[2]	212	98%	100%	97%
Venous Thromboembolism Prophylaxis[2]	931	78%	88%	85%
Warfarin Therapy Discharge Instructions[2]	197	63%	85%	75%
Chest Pain/Possible Heart Attack Care				
Aspirin Given Within 24 Hours of Arrival[1,3]	-	-	98%	96%
Fibrinolytic Meds Within 30 Min. of Arrival[3,7]	-	-	81%	58%
Average Time to ECG (minutes)[1,3]	-	-	7	7
Average Time to Transfer (minutes)[1,3]	-	-	53	60
Children's Asthma Care				
Received Home Management Plan of Care	-	-	-	88%
Received Reliever Medication	-	-	-	100%
Received Systemic Corticosteroids	-	-	-	100%
Emergency Department				
Admittance Decision Time (minutes)[2]	1,685	316	111	98
Head CT Results Within 45 Min. of Arrival	17	24%	64%	57%
Patients Who Left ER Before Being Seen	>100k	6%	2%	2%
Time from ER Arrival to Admit. (minutes)[2]	1,702	692	289	274
Time from ER Arrival to Discharge (minutes)	954	281	147	134
Time in ER Before Being Evaluated (minutes)	996	81	26	26
Time to Pain Meds for Fractures (minutes)	425	101	60	57
Heart Attack Care				
Aspirin Given at Discharge[2]	497	99%	99%	99%
Fibrinolytic Meds Within 30 Min. of Arrival[2,7]	-	-	50%	54%
PCI Within 90 Minutes of Arrival[2]	129	96%	96%	96%
Statin Prescribed at Discharge[2]	505	98%	99%	98%
Heart Failure Care				
ACE Inhibitor or ARB for LVSD[2]	405	98%	98%	97%
Discharge Instructions Given[2]	768	92%	96%	94%
Evaluation of LVS Function[2]	868	100%	100%	99%
Medicare Spending				

NOTE: Hospital profiles are in alphabetical order by state, then city, then hospital within the city; Rankings exclude hospitals with less than 25 cases except for patient surveys which excludes hospitals with less than 100 cases; (a) 100-299 cases; (1) The number of cases/patients is too few to report; (2) Data submitted were based on a sample of cases/patients; (3) Results are based on a shorter time period than required; (4) Data suppressed by CMS for one or more quarters; (5) Results are not available for this reporting period; (6) Fewer than 100 patients completed the HCAHPS survey; (7) No cases met the criteria for this measure; (8) The lower limit of the confidence interval cannot be calculated if the number of observed infections equals zero; (9) No data are available from the state/territory for this reporting period; (10) The scores shown reflect fewer than 50 completed surveys; (11) There were discrepancies in the data collection process; (12) This measure does not apply to this hospital for this reporting period; (13) Results cannot be calculated for this reporting period; (14) The results for this state are combined with nearby states to protect confidentiality; Please refer to the User's Guide for a full explanation of data.

Medicare Spending per Patient (ratio)	-	1.04	1.04	0.98
Pneumonia Care				
Appropriate Initial Antibiotic Given[2]	185	97%	98%	95%
Blood Culture Timing[2]	358	94%	99%	98%
Pregnancy and Delivery Care				
Newborn Deliveries Scheduled Early[2]	146	7%	6%	6%
Preventive Care				
Immunization for Influenza[2]	1,583	82%	94%	90%
Immunization for Pneumonia[2]	1,506	90%	96%	92%
Stroke Care				
Anticoagulation Therapy for Atrial Fibrillation[2]	23	100%	97%	95%
Antithrombotic Therapy Timing[2]	213	92%	98%	98%
Assessed for Rehabilitation[2]	279	93%	97%	97%
Discharged on Antithrombotic Therapy[2]	229	97%	99%	99%
Discharged on Statin Medication[2]	195	93%	96%	94%
Thrombolytic Therapy Timing[2]	29	59%	76%	66%
Venous Thromboembolism Prophylaxis[2]	300	86%	95%	94%
Written Stroke Educational Materials Given[2]	183	75%	94%	88%
Surgical Care Improvement Project				
Appropriate Beta Blocker Usage[2]	233	97%	99%	98%
Appropriate VTP Within 24 Hours[2]	762	98%	99%	98%
Controlled Postoperative Blood Glucose[2]	94	95%	98%	97%
Perioperative Temperature Management[2]	1,092	100%	100%	100%
Prophylactic Antibiotic Selection[2]	540	99%	99%	99%
Prophylactic Antibiotic Selection (Outpatient)	432	95%	98%	98%
Prophylactic Antibiotic Stopped[2]	520	97%	98%	98%
Prophylactic Antibiotic Timing[2]	540	100%	99%	99%
Prophylactic Antibiotic Timing (Outpatient)	264	97%	98%	98%
Urinary Catheter Removal[2]	517	96%	98%	97%
Survey of Patients' Hospital Experiences				
Area Around Room 'Always' Quiet at Night	300+	55%	58%	61%
Doctors 'Always' Communicated Well	300+	78%	77%	82%
Home Recovery Information Given	300+	75%	83%	85%
Hospital Given 9 or 10 on 10 Point Scale	300+	61%	67%	71%
Meds 'Always' Explained Before Given	300+	52%	60%	64%
Nurses 'Always' Communicated Well	300+	68%	75%	79%
Pain 'Always' Well Controlled	300+	65%	68%	71%
Room and Bathroom 'Always' Clean	300+	61%	69%	73%
Timely Help 'Always' Received	300+	56%	62%	68%
Would Definitely Recommend Hospital	300+	65%	69%	71%
Use of Medical Imaging				
Cardiac Imaging Stress Test before Surgery	275	5.8%	6.4%	5.3%
Combination Abdominal CT Scan	780	1.0%	11.8%	10.5%
Combination Brain/Sinus CT Scan	947	3.7%	3.4%	2.7%
Combination Chest CT Scan	462	1.3%	2.4%	2.7%
Follow-up Mammogram/Ultrasound	575	8.5%	10.2%	8.8%
Lumbar Spine MRI for Low Back Pain[1]	-	-	35.2%	37.2%

Kendall Regional Medical Center

11750 Bird Rd
Miami, FL 33175
Phone: 305-223-3000
Fax: 305-227-5503
URL: www.kendallmed.com
Type: Acute Care Hospitals
Emergency Services: Yes
Ownership: Proprietary
Beds: 412

Key Personnel:
Infection Control. . . . . Alberto Alea, MD
Intensive Care Unit. . . . . Vangie Bustos, RN
Radiology. . . . . Roberto Calderon, MD
CEO/President. . . . . Scott A. Cihak
Quality Assurance . . . . Shirley Minier, RN
Patient Relations . . . . JoAnne Plumlee
Operating Room. . . . . Joann Plumlee, RN
Emergency Room . . . . Juan J Remos, MD

Measure	Cases	This Hosp.	State Avg.	U.S. Avg.
Blood Clot Prevention and Treatment				
Anticoagulation Overlap Therapy[2]	77	99%	93%	93%
ICU Venous Thromboembolism Prophylaxis[2]	82	100%	94%	92%
Incidence of Potentially Preventable VTE[2]	21	0%	10%	10%
UFH with Dosages/Platelet Monitoring[2]	55	100%	100%	97%
Venous Thromboembolism Prophylaxis[2]	362	98%	88%	85%
Warfarin Therapy Discharge Instructions[2]	52	98%	85%	75%
Chest Pain/Possible Heart Attack Care				
Aspirin Given Within 24 Hours of Arrival[1,3]	-	-	98%	96%
Fibrinolytic Meds Within 30 Min. of Arrival[5]	-	-	81%	58%
Average Time to ECG (minutes)[1,3]	-	-	7	7
Average Time to Transfer (minutes)[5]	-	-	53	60
Children's Asthma Care				
Received Home Management Plan of Care	-	-	-	88%
Received Reliever Medication	-	-	-	100%
Received Systemic Corticosteroids	-	-	-	100%
Emergency Department				
Admittance Decision Time (minutes)[2]	1,086	62	111	98
Head CT Results Within 45 Min. of Arrival[1]	-	-	64%	57%
Patients Who Left ER Before Being Seen	73,287	0%	2%	2%
Time from ER Arrival to Admit. (minutes)[2]	1,086	237	289	274
Time from ER Arrival to Discharge (minutes)	470	122	147	134
Time in ER Before Being Evaluated (minutes)	505	5	26	26
Time to Pain Meds for Fractures (minutes)	174	40	60	57
Heart Attack Care				
Aspirin Given at Discharge	430	100%	99%	99%
Fibrinolytic Meds Within 30 Min. of Arrival[1]	-	-	50%	54%
PCI Within 90 Minutes of Arrival	107	100%	96%	96%
Statin Prescribed at Discharge	437	100%	99%	98%
Heart Failure Care				
ACE Inhibitor or ARB for LVSD	231	100%	98%	97%
Discharge Instructions Given	577	99%	96%	94%
Evaluation of LVS Function	635	100%	100%	99%
Medicare Spending				
Medicare Spending per Patient (ratio)	-	1.03	1.04	0.98
Pneumonia Care				
Appropriate Initial Antibiotic Given	192	100%	98%	95%
Blood Culture Timing	371	100%	99%	98%
Pregnancy and Delivery Care				
Newborn Deliveries Scheduled Early[2]	28	4%	6%	6%
Preventive Care				
Immunization for Influenza[2]	645	98%	94%	90%
Immunization for Pneumonia[2]	791	100%	96%	92%
Stroke Care				
Anticoagulation Therapy for Atrial Fibrillation[2]	17	100%	97%	95%
Antithrombotic Therapy Timing[2]	110	99%	98%	98%
Assessed for Rehabilitation[2]	126	93%	97%	97%
Discharged on Antithrombotic Therapy[2]	117	100%	99%	99%
Discharged on Statin Medication[2]	88	97%	96%	94%
Thrombolytic Therapy Timing[1,2]	-	-	76%	66%
Venous Thromboembolism Prophylaxis[2]	135	96%	95%	94%
Written Stroke Educational Materials Given[2]	87	98%	94%	88%
Surgical Care Improvement Project				
Appropriate Beta Blocker Usage[2]	278	98%	99%	98%
Appropriate VTP Within 24 Hours[2]	488	100%	99%	98%
Controlled Postoperative Blood Glucose[2]	79	99%	98%	97%
Perioperative Temperature Management[2]	577	100%	100%	100%
Prophylactic Antibiotic Selection[2]	409	100%	99%	99%
Prophylactic Antibiotic Selection (Outpatient)	154	99%	98%	98%
Prophylactic Antibiotic Stopped[2]	390	99%	98%	98%
Prophylactic Antibiotic Timing[2]	409	100%	99%	99%
Prophylactic Antibiotic Timing (Outpatient)	154	100%	98%	98%
Urinary Catheter Removal[2]	232	99%	98%	97%
Survey of Patients' Hospital Experiences				
Area Around Room 'Always' Quiet at Night	300+	58%	58%	61%
Doctors 'Always' Communicated Well	300+	78%	77%	82%
Home Recovery Information Given	300+	80%	83%	85%
Hospital Given 9 or 10 on 10 Point Scale	300+	61%	67%	71%
Meds 'Always' Explained Before Given	300+	59%	60%	64%
Nurses 'Always' Communicated Well	300+	74%	75%	79%
Pain 'Always' Well Controlled	300+	70%	68%	71%
Room and Bathroom 'Always' Clean	300+	72%	69%	73%
Timely Help 'Always' Received	300+	62%	62%	68%
Would Definitely Recommend Hospital	300+	62%	69%	71%
Use of Medical Imaging				
Cardiac Imaging Stress Test before Surgery[1]	-	-	6.4%	5.3%
Combination Abdominal CT Scan	618	1.6%	11.8%	10.5%
Combination Brain/Sinus CT Scan	712	2.8%	3.4%	2.7%
Combination Chest CT Scan	200	0.0%	2.4%	2.7%
Follow-up Mammogram/Ultrasound	212	12.7%	10.2%	8.8%
Lumbar Spine MRI for Low Back Pain[1]	-	-	35.2%	37.2%

Metropolitan Hospital of Miami

5959 Nw 7th St
Miami, FL 33126
Phone: 305-264-1000
Fax: 305-265-6504
E-mail: hospital@pahnet.org
URL: www.pahnet.org
Type: Acute Care Hospitals
Emergency Services: Yes
Ownership: Proprietary
Beds: 146

Measure	Cases	This Hosp.	State Avg.	U.S. Avg.
Blood Clot Prevention and Treatment				
Anticoagulation Overlap Therapy[1,2]	-	-	93%	93%
ICU Venous Thromboembolism Prophylaxis[2]	30	83%	94%	92%
Incidence of Potentially Preventable VTE[2,7]	-	-	10%	10%
UFH with Dosages/Platelet Monitoring[1,2]	-	-	100%	97%
Venous Thromboembolism Prophylaxis[2]	380	56%	88%	85%
Warfarin Therapy Discharge Instructions[1,2]	-	-	85%	75%
Chest Pain/Possible Heart Attack Care				
Aspirin Given Within 24 Hours of Arrival[5]	-	-	98%	96%
Fibrinolytic Meds Within 30 Min. of Arrival[5]	-	-	81%	58%
Average Time to ECG (minutes)[5]	-	-	7	7
Average Time to Transfer (minutes)[5]	-	-	53	60
Children's Asthma Care				
Received Home Management Plan of Care	-	-	-	88%
Received Reliever Medication	-	-	-	100%
Received Systemic Corticosteroids	-	-	-	100%
Emergency Department				
Admittance Decision Time (minutes)[2]	771	182	111	98
Head CT Results Within 45 Min. of Arrival[5]	-	-	64%	57%
Patients Who Left ER Before Being Seen[5]	-	-	2%	2%
Time from ER Arrival to Admit. (minutes)[2]	771	416	289	274
Time from ER Arrival to Discharge (minutes)[5]	-	-	147	134
Time in ER Before Being Evaluated (minutes)[5]	-	-	26	26
Time to Pain Meds for Fractures (minutes)[5]	-	-	60	57
Heart Attack Care				
Aspirin Given at Discharge	52	100%	99%	99%
Fibrinolytic Meds Within 30 Min. of Arrival[7]	-	-	50%	54%
PCI Within 90 Minutes of Arrival[7]	-	-	96%	96%
Statin Prescribed at Discharge	52	100%	99%	98%
Heart Failure Care				
ACE Inhibitor or ARB for LVSD	46	100%	98%	97%
Discharge Instructions Given	110	100%	96%	94%
Evaluation of LVS Function	107	100%	100%	99%
Medicare Spending				
Medicare Spending per Patient (ratio)	-	1.04	1.04	0.98
Pneumonia Care				
Appropriate Initial Antibiotic Given	67	96%	98%	95%
Blood Culture Timing[1]	-	-	99%	98%
Pregnancy and Delivery Care				
Newborn Deliveries Scheduled Early[7]	-	-	6%	6%
Preventive Care				
Immunization for Influenza[2]	419	75%	94%	90%
Immunization for Pneumonia[2]	658	69%	96%	92%
Stroke Care				
Anticoagulation Therapy for Atrial Fibrillation	13	100%	97%	95%
Antithrombotic Therapy Timing	11	18%	98%	98%
Assessed for Rehabilitation	24	92%	97%	97%
Discharged on Antithrombotic Therapy	19	63%	99%	99%
Discharged on Statin Medication	21	100%	96%	94%
Thrombolytic Therapy Timing[7]	-	-	76%	66%
Venous Thromboembolism Prophylaxis	31	68%	95%	94%
Written Stroke Educational Materials Given	15	100%	94%	88%
Surgical Care Improvement Project				
Appropriate Beta Blocker Usage[1]	-	-	99%	98%
Appropriate VTP Within 24 Hours	106	100%	99%	98%
Controlled Postoperative Blood Glucose[7]	-	-	98%	97%
Perioperative Temperature Management	162	100%	100%	100%
Prophylactic Antibiotic Selection	123	93%	99%	99%
Prophylactic Antibiotic Selection (Outpatient)[5]	-	-	98%	98%
Prophylactic Antibiotic Stopped	123	100%	98%	98%
Prophylactic Antibiotic Timing	123	99%	99%	99%
Prophylactic Antibiotic Timing (Outpatient)[5]	-	-	98%	98%
Urinary Catheter Removal	67	100%	98%	97%
Survey of Patients' Hospital Experiences				

NOTE: Hospital profiles are in alphabetical order by state, then city, then hospital within the city; Rankings exclude hospitals with less than 25 cases except for patient surveys which excludes hospitals with less than 100 cases; (a) 100-299 cases; (1) The number of cases/patients is too few to report; (2) Data submitted were based on a sample of cases/patients; (3) Results are based on a shorter time period than required; (4) Data suppressed by CMS for one or more quarters; (5) Results are not available for this reporting period; (6) Fewer than 100 patients completed the HCAHPS survey; (7) No cases met the criteria for this measure; (8) The lower limit of the confidence interval cannot be calculated if the number of observed infections equals zero; (9) No data are available from the state/territory for this reporting period; (10) The scores shown reflect fewer than 50 completed surveys; (11) There were discrepancies in the data collection process; (12) This measure does not apply to this hospital for this reporting period; (13) Results cannot be calculated for this reporting period; (14) The results for this state are combined with nearby states to protect confidentiality; Please refer to the User's Guide for a full explanation of data.

Measure	Cases	This Hosp.	State Avg.	U.S. Avg.
Area Around Room 'Always' Quiet at Night[5]	-	-	58%	61%
Doctors 'Always' Communicated Well[5]	-	-	77%	82%
Home Recovery Information Given[5]	-	-	83%	85%
Hospital Given 9 or 10 on 10 Point Scale[5]	-	-	67%	71%
Meds 'Always' Explained Before Given[5]	-	-	60%	64%
Nurses 'Always' Communicated Well[5]	-	-	75%	79%
Pain 'Always' Well Controlled[5]	-	-	68%	71%
Room and Bathroom 'Always' Clean[5]	-	-	69%	73%
Timely Help 'Always' Received[5]	-	-	62%	68%
Would Definitely Recommend Hospital[5]	-	-	69%	71%
Use of Medical Imaging				
Cardiac Imaging Stress Test before Surgery[5]	-	-	6.4%	5.3%
Combination Abdominal CT Scan[5]	-	-	11.8%	10.5%
Combination Brain/Sinus CT Scan[5]	-	-	3.4%	2.7%
Combination Chest CT Scan[5]	-	-	2.4%	2.7%
Follow-up Mammogram/Ultrasound[5]	-	-	10.2%	8.8%
Lumbar Spine MRI for Low Back Pain[5]	-	-	35.2%	37.2%

Miami VA Medical Center

1201 N W 16th Street
Miami, FL 33125
Phone: 305-324-4455
Fax: 305-575-3266
URL: www1.va.gov/visn8/miami/facilities/miami.asp
Type: Acute Care - VA
Emergency Services: No
Ownership: Government Federal
Beds: 415

Key Personnel:
Quality Assurance .... Kathleen Coniglio, RN
Chief of Medical Staff .... Vincent DeGennaro, MD
Anesthesiology............... EA DeLisser, MD
Infection Control.............. Richard Greenman, MD
Emergency Room .... Jack Yaffa, MD

Measure	Cases	This Hosp.	State Avg.	U.S. Avg.
Blood Clot Prevention and Treatment				
Anticoagulation Overlap Therapy	-	-	93%	93%
ICU Venous Thromboembolism Prophylaxis	-	-	94%	92%
Incidence of Potentially Preventable VTE	-	-	10%	10%
UFH with Dosages/Platelet Monitoring	-	-	100%	97%
Venous Thromboembolism Prophylaxis	-	-	88%	85%
Warfarin Therapy Discharge Instructions	-	-	85%	75%
Chest Pain/Possible Heart Attack Care				
Aspirin Given Within 24 Hours of Arrival	-	-	98%	96%
Fibrinolytic Meds Within 30 Min. of Arrival	-	-	81%	58%
Average Time to ECG (minutes)	-	-	7	7
Average Time to Transfer (minutes)	-	-	53	60
Children's Asthma Care				
Received Home Management Plan of Care	-	-	-	88%
Received Reliever Medication	-	-	-	100%
Received Systemic Corticosteroids	-	-	-	100%
Emergency Department				
Admittance Decision Time (minutes)	-	-	111	98
Head CT Results Within 45 Min. of Arrival	-	-	64%	57%
Patients Who Left ER Before Being Seen	-	-	2%	2%
Time from ER Arrival to Admit. (minutes)	-	-	289	274
Time from ER Arrival to Discharge (minutes)	-	-	147	134
Time in ER Before Being Evaluated (minutes)	-	-	26	26
Time to Pain Meds for Fractures (minutes)	-	-	60	57
Heart Attack Care				
Aspirin Given at Discharge	29	97%	99%	99%
Fibrinolytic Meds Within 30 Min. of Arrival[5]	-	-	50%	54%
PCI Within 90 Minutes of Arrival[1]	-	-	96%	96%
Statin Prescribed at Discharge	32	100%	99%	98%
Heart Failure Care				
ACE Inhibitor or ARB for LVSD	88	100%	98%	97%
Discharge Instructions Given	149	97%	96%	94%
Evaluation of LVS Function	156	100%	100%	99%
Medicare Spending				
Medicare Spending per Patient (ratio)	-	-	1.04	0.98
Pneumonia Care				
Appropriate Initial Antibiotic Given[1]	24	96%	98%	95%
Blood Culture Timing	89	99%	99%	98%
Pregnancy and Delivery Care				
Newborn Deliveries Scheduled Early	-	-	6%	6%
Preventive Care				
Immunization for Influenza[5]	-	-	94%	90%
Immunization for Pneumonia[5]	-	-	96%	92%
Stroke Care				
Anticoagulation Therapy for Atrial Fibrillation	-	-	97%	95%
Antithrombotic Therapy Timing	-	-	98%	98%
Assessed for Rehabilitation	-	-	97%	97%
Discharged on Antithrombotic Therapy	-	-	99%	99%
Discharged on Statin Medication	-	-	96%	94%
Thrombolytic Therapy Timing	-	-	76%	66%
Venous Thromboembolism Prophylaxis	-	-	95%	94%
Written Stroke Educational Materials Given	-	-	94%	88%
Surgical Care Improvement Project				
Appropriate Beta Blocker Usage[2]	115	92%	99%	98%
Appropriate VTP Within 24 Hours[2]	242	100%	99%	98%
Controlled Postoperative Blood Glucose[5]	-	-	98%	97%
Perioperative Temperature Management[2]	303	99%	100%	100%
Prophylactic Antibiotic Selection	172	99%	99%	99%
Prophylactic Antibiotic Selection (Outpatient)	-	-	98%	98%
Prophylactic Antibiotic Stopped	169	91%	98%	98%
Prophylactic Antibiotic Timing	172	99%	99%	99%
Prophylactic Antibiotic Timing (Outpatient)	-	-	98%	98%
Urinary Catheter Removal[2]	174	96%	98%	97%
Survey of Patients' Hospital Experiences				
Area Around Room 'Always' Quiet at Night	-	-	58%	61%
Doctors 'Always' Communicated Well	-	-	77%	82%
Home Recovery Information Given	-	-	83%	85%
Hospital Given 9 or 10 on 10 Point Scale	-	-	67%	71%
Meds 'Always' Explained Before Given	-	-	60%	64%
Nurses 'Always' Communicated Well	-	-	75%	79%
Pain 'Always' Well Controlled	-	-	68%	71%
Room and Bathroom 'Always' Clean	-	-	69%	73%
Timely Help 'Always' Received	-	-	62%	68%
Would Definitely Recommend Hospital	-	-	69%	71%
Use of Medical Imaging				
Cardiac Imaging Stress Test before Surgery	-	-	6.4%	5.3%
Combination Abdominal CT Scan	-	-	11.8%	10.5%
Combination Brain/Sinus CT Scan	-	-	3.4%	2.7%
Combination Chest CT Scan	-	-	2.4%	2.7%
Follow-up Mammogram/Ultrasound	-	-	10.2%	8.8%
Lumbar Spine MRI for Low Back Pain	-	-	35.2%	37.2%

North Shore Medical Center

1100 Nw 95th St
Miami, FL 33150
Phone: 305-835-6000
Fax: 305-835-6163
URL: www.northshoremedical.com
Type: Acute Care Hospitals
Emergency Services: Yes
Ownership: Proprietary
Beds: 357

Key Personnel:
Anesthesiology............... David Acosta, MD
Emergency Room .... Vera Burke
Intensive Care Unit............ Edwina Crum, RN
Hemotology Center .... Carolyn Gilleand
Chief of Medical Staff.......... Constantine Kitsos, MD
CEO/President............... Manny Linares
Cardiac Laboratory............ Dennis Reese
Infection Control.............. Veronica Torres

Measure	Cases	This Hosp.	State Avg.	U.S. Avg.
Blood Clot Prevention and Treatment				
Anticoagulation Overlap Therapy[2]	92	84%	93%	93%
ICU Venous Thromboembolism Prophylaxis[2]	214	94%	94%	92%
Incidence of Potentially Preventable VTE[2]	14	29%	10%	10%
UFH with Dosages/Platelet Monitoring[2]	30	93%	100%	97%
Venous Thromboembolism Prophylaxis[2]	529	81%	88%	85%
Warfarin Therapy Discharge Instructions[2]	63	90%	85%	75%
Chest Pain/Possible Heart Attack Care				
Aspirin Given Within 24 Hours of Arrival	42	93%	98%	96%
Fibrinolytic Meds Within 30 Min. of Arrival[7]	-	-	81%	58%
Average Time to ECG (minutes)	41	13	7	7
Average Time to Transfer (minutes)	18	76	53	60
Children's Asthma Care				
Received Home Management Plan of Care	-	-	-	88%
Received Reliever Medication	-	-	-	100%
Received Systemic Corticosteroids	-	-	-	100%
Emergency Department				
Admittance Decision Time (minutes)[2]	1,431	174	111	98
Head CT Results Within 45 Min. of Arrival[1]	-	-	64%	57%
Patients Who Left ER Before Being Seen	71,850	3%	2%	2%
Time from ER Arrival to Admit. (minutes)[2]	1,434	362	289	274
Time from ER Arrival to Discharge (minutes)	877	177	147	134
Time in ER Before Being Evaluated (minutes)	943	58	26	26
Time to Pain Meds for Fractures (minutes)	115	68	60	57
Heart Attack Care				
Aspirin Given at Discharge	216	100%	99%	99%
Fibrinolytic Meds Within 30 Min. of Arrival[7]	-	-	50%	54%
PCI Within 90 Minutes of Arrival	31	100%	96%	96%
Statin Prescribed at Discharge	217	100%	99%	98%
Heart Failure Care				
ACE Inhibitor or ARB for LVSD[2]	285	99%	98%	97%
Discharge Instructions Given[2]	653	92%	96%	94%
Evaluation of LVS Function[2]	814	100%	100%	99%
Medicare Spending				
Medicare Spending per Patient (ratio)	-	1.14	1.04	0.98
Pneumonia Care				
Appropriate Initial Antibiotic Given[2]	206	100%	98%	95%
Blood Culture Timing[2]	414	100%	99%	98%
Pregnancy and Delivery Care				
Newborn Deliveries Scheduled Early[2]	54	0%	6%	6%
Preventive Care				
Immunization for Influenza[2]	1,201	85%	94%	90%
Immunization for Pneumonia[2]	1,410	94%	96%	92%
Stroke Care				
Anticoagulation Therapy for Atrial Fibrillation	16	100%	97%	95%
Antithrombotic Therapy Timing	216	97%	98%	98%
Assessed for Rehabilitation	257	100%	97%	97%
Discharged on Antithrombotic Therapy	226	98%	99%	99%
Discharged on Statin Medication	164	98%	96%	94%
Thrombolytic Therapy Timing	28	82%	76%	66%
Venous Thromboembolism Prophylaxis	277	96%	95%	94%
Written Stroke Educational Materials Given	142	92%	94%	88%
Surgical Care Improvement Project				
Appropriate Beta Blocker Usage	168	94%	99%	98%
Appropriate VTP Within 24 Hours	355	98%	99%	98%
Controlled Postoperative Blood Glucose	87	94%	98%	97%
Perioperative Temperature Management	392	99%	100%	100%
Prophylactic Antibiotic Selection	263	99%	99%	99%
Prophylactic Antibiotic Selection (Outpatient)	156	98%	98%	98%
Prophylactic Antibiotic Stopped	245	97%	98%	98%
Prophylactic Antibiotic Timing	263	100%	99%	99%
Prophylactic Antibiotic Timing (Outpatient)	157	99%	98%	98%
Urinary Catheter Removal	202	95%	98%	97%
Survey of Patients' Hospital Experiences				
Area Around Room 'Always' Quiet at Night	300+	54%	58%	61%
Doctors 'Always' Communicated Well	300+	78%	77%	82%
Home Recovery Information Given	300+	78%	83%	85%
Hospital Given 9 or 10 on 10 Point Scale	300+	57%	67%	71%
Meds 'Always' Explained Before Given	300+	56%	60%	64%
Nurses 'Always' Communicated Well	300+	71%	75%	79%
Pain 'Always' Well Controlled	300+	64%	68%	71%
Room and Bathroom 'Always' Clean	300+	64%	69%	73%
Timely Help 'Always' Received	300+	53%	62%	68%
Would Definitely Recommend Hospital	300+	58%	69%	71%
Use of Medical Imaging				
Cardiac Imaging Stress Test before Surgery[1]	-	-	6.4%	5.3%
Combination Abdominal CT Scan	607	7.6%	11.8%	10.5%
Combination Brain/Sinus CT Scan	775	2.1%	3.4%	2.7%
Combination Chest CT Scan	354	2.0%	2.4%	2.7%
Follow-up Mammogram/Ultrasound	387	17.1%	10.2%	8.8%
Lumbar Spine MRI for Low Back Pain	62	38.7%	35.2%	37.2%

University of Miami Hospital

1400 Nw 12th Ave
Miami, FL 33136
Phone: 305-325-5511
Fax: 305-325-4673
URL: www.cedarsmedicalcenter.com
Type: Acute Care Hospitals
Emergency Services: Yes
Ownership: Voluntary non-profit - Private
Beds: 560

Key Personnel:
Operating Room............. Leonidas Ahumada
Radiology.................... Robert E Beasley
Cardiac Laboratory............ Anne Lee, RN
Infection Control............. Anexis Lopez
Quality Assurance .... Cathy J McClellan

NOTE: Hospital profiles are in alphabetical order by state, then city, then hospital within the city; Rankings exclude hospitals with less than 25 cases except for patient surveys which excludes hospitals with less than 100 cases; (a) 100-299 cases; (1) The number of cases/patients is too few to report; (2) Data submitted were based on a sample of cases/patients; (3) Results are based on a shorter time period than required; (4) Data suppressed by CMS for one or more quarters; (5) Results are not available for this reporting period; (6) Fewer than 100 patients completed the HCAHPS survey; (7) No cases met the criteria for this measure; (8) The lower limit of the confidence interval cannot be calculated if the number of observed infections equals zero; (9) No data are available from the state/territory for this reporting period; (10) The scores shown reflect fewer than 50 completed surveys; (11) There were discrepancies in the data collection process; (12) This measure does not apply to this hospital for this reporting period; (13) Results cannot be calculated for this reporting period; (14) The results for this state are combined with nearby states to protect confidentiality; Please refer to the User's Guide for a full explanation of data.

Chief of Medical Staff . . . . Jolly Varki, MD
CEO/President . . . . David Zambrana, D.N.P., M.B.A.,

Measure	Cases	This Hosp.	State Avg.	U.S. Avg.
Blood Clot Prevention and Treatment				
Anticoagulation Overlap Therapy[2]	63	94%	93%	93%
ICU Venous Thromboembolism Prophylaxis[2]	113	93%	94%	92%
Incidence of Potentially Preventable VTE[2]	33	18%	10%	10%
UFH with Dosages/Platelet Monitoring[2]	64	100%	100%	97%
Venous Thromboembolism Prophylaxis[2]	282	89%	88%	85%
Warfarin Therapy Discharge Instructions[2]	41	95%	85%	75%
Chest Pain/Possible Heart Attack Care				
Aspirin Given Within 24 Hours of Arrival[1,3]	-	-	98%	96%
Fibrinolytic Meds Within 30 Min. of Arrival[5]	-	-	81%	58%
Average Time to ECG (minutes)[1,3]	-	-	7	7
Average Time to Transfer (minutes)[5]	-	-	53	60
Children's Asthma Care				
Received Home Management Plan of Care	-	-	-	88%
Received Reliever Medication	-	-	-	100%
Received Systemic Corticosteroids	-	-	-	100%
Emergency Department				
Admittance Decision Time (minutes)[2]	475	177	111	98
Head CT Results Within 45 Min. of Arrival[1]	-	-	64%	57%
Patients Who Left ER Before Being Seen	33,036	1%	2%	2%
Time from ER Arrival to Admit. (minutes)[2]	478	366	289	274
Time from ER Arrival to Discharge (minutes)	455	202	147	134
Time in ER Before Being Evaluated (minutes)	297	91	26	26
Time to Pain Meds for Fractures (minutes)	38	75	60	57
Heart Attack Care				
Aspirin Given at Discharge	221	100%	99%	99%
Fibrinolytic Meds Within 30 Min. of Arrival[7]	-	-	50%	54%
PCI Within 90 Minutes of Arrival	23	78%	96%	96%
Statin Prescribed at Discharge	217	100%	99%	98%
Heart Failure Care				
ACE Inhibitor or ARB for LVSD	304	95%	98%	97%
Discharge Instructions Given	589	85%	96%	94%
Evaluation of LVS Function	699	100%	100%	99%
Medicare Spending				
Medicare Spending per Patient (ratio)	-	1.07	1.04	0.98
Pneumonia Care				
Appropriate Initial Antibiotic Given	67	100%	98%	95%
Blood Culture Timing	173	100%	99%	98%
Pregnancy and Delivery Care				
Newborn Deliveries Scheduled Early[7]	-	-	6%	6%
Preventive Care				
Immunization for Influenza[2]	609	84%	94%	90%
Immunization for Pneumonia[2]	799	82%	96%	92%
Stroke Care				
Anticoagulation Therapy for Atrial Fibrillation	17	88%	97%	95%
Antithrombotic Therapy Timing	75	91%	98%	98%
Assessed for Rehabilitation	97	94%	97%	97%
Discharged on Antithrombotic Therapy	88	94%	99%	99%
Discharged on Statin Medication	70	93%	96%	94%
Thrombolytic Therapy Timing	13	46%	76%	66%
Venous Thromboembolism Prophylaxis	105	75%	95%	94%
Written Stroke Educational Materials Given	60	97%	94%	88%
Surgical Care Improvement Project				
Appropriate Beta Blocker Usage	432	98%	99%	98%
Appropriate VTP Within 24 Hours	1,126	97%	99%	98%
Controlled Postoperative Blood Glucose	126	92%	98%	97%
Perioperative Temperature Management	1,253	100%	100%	100%
Prophylactic Antibiotic Selection	490	98%	99%	99%
Prophylactic Antibiotic Selection (Outpatient)	327	94%	98%	98%
Prophylactic Antibiotic Stopped	478	94%	98%	98%
Prophylactic Antibiotic Timing	492	99%	99%	99%
Prophylactic Antibiotic Timing (Outpatient)	328	97%	98%	98%
Urinary Catheter Removal	570	98%	98%	97%
Survey of Patients' Hospital Experiences				
Area Around Room 'Always' Quiet at Night	300+	63%	58%	61%
Doctors 'Always' Communicated Well	300+	81%	77%	82%
Home Recovery Information Given	300+	80%	83%	85%
Hospital Given 9 or 10 on 10 Point Scale	300+	69%	67%	71%
Meds 'Always' Explained Before Given	300+	62%	60%	64%
Nurses 'Always' Communicated Well	300+	76%	75%	79%
Pain 'Always' Well Controlled	300+	70%	68%	71%
Room and Bathroom 'Always' Clean	300+	71%	69%	73%
Timely Help 'Always' Received	300+	59%	62%	68%
Would Definitely Recommend Hospital	300+	73%	69%	71%
Use of Medical Imaging				
Cardiac Imaging Stress Test before Surgery	539	8.0%	6.4%	5.3%
Combination Abdominal CT Scan	701	7.1%	11.8%	10.5%
Combination Brain/Sinus CT Scan[1]	-	-	3.4%	2.7%
Combination Chest CT Scan	397	1.0%	2.4%	2.7%
Follow-up Mammogram/Ultrasound	117	8.5%	10.2%	8.8%
Lumbar Spine MRI for Low Back Pain	50	32.0%	35.2%	37.2%

West Kendall Baptist Hospital

9555 Sw 162 Ave
Miami, FL 33196
Phone: 786-467-2011
URL: www.baptisthealth.net
Type: Acute Care Hospitals
Emergency Services: Yes
Ownership: Voluntary non-profit - Private

Measure	Cases	This Hosp.	State Avg.	U.S. Avg.
Blood Clot Prevention and Treatment				
Anticoagulation Overlap Therapy[2]	31	100%	93%	93%
ICU Venous Thromboembolism Prophylaxis[2]	91	100%	94%	92%
Incidence of Potentially Preventable VTE[1,2]	-	-	10%	10%
UFH with Dosages/Platelet Monitoring[2]	34	100%	100%	97%
Venous Thromboembolism Prophylaxis[2]	484	100%	88%	85%
Warfarin Therapy Discharge Instructions[2]	19	100%	85%	75%
Chest Pain/Possible Heart Attack Care				
Aspirin Given Within 24 Hours of Arrival	85	100%	98%	96%
Fibrinolytic Meds Within 30 Min. of Arrival[7]	-	-	81%	58%
Average Time to ECG (minutes)	90	1	7	7
Average Time to Transfer (minutes)	12	30	53	60
Children's Asthma Care				
Received Home Management Plan of Care	-	-	-	88%
Received Reliever Medication	-	-	-	100%
Received Systemic Corticosteroids	-	-	-	100%
Emergency Department				
Admittance Decision Time (minutes)[2]	858	166	111	98
Head CT Results Within 45 Min. of Arrival[1]	-	-	64%	57%
Patients Who Left ER Before Being Seen	45,135	1%	2%	2%
Time from ER Arrival to Admit. (minutes)[2]	858	394	289	274
Time from ER Arrival to Discharge (minutes)	1,196	216	147	134
Time in ER Before Being Evaluated (minutes)	1,301	43	26	26
Time to Pain Meds for Fractures (minutes)	143	41	60	57
Heart Attack Care				
Aspirin Given at Discharge	17	100%	99%	99%
Fibrinolytic Meds Within 30 Min. of Arrival[7]	-	-	50%	54%
PCI Within 90 Minutes of Arrival[7]	-	-	96%	96%
Statin Prescribed at Discharge	18	100%	99%	98%
Heart Failure Care				
ACE Inhibitor or ARB for LVSD	65	100%	98%	97%
Discharge Instructions Given	171	100%	96%	94%
Evaluation of LVS Function	200	100%	100%	99%
Medicare Spending				
Medicare Spending per Patient (ratio)	-	1.10	1.04	0.98
Pneumonia Care				
Appropriate Initial Antibiotic Given	100	100%	98%	95%
Blood Culture Timing	196	98%	99%	98%
Pregnancy and Delivery Care				
Newborn Deliveries Scheduled Early	80	0%	6%	6%
Preventive Care				
Immunization for Influenza[2]	501	100%	94%	90%
Immunization for Pneumonia[2]	666	100%	96%	92%
Stroke Care				
Anticoagulation Therapy for Atrial Fibrillation[1]	-	-	97%	95%
Antithrombotic Therapy Timing	44	100%	98%	98%
Assessed for Rehabilitation	35	100%	97%	97%
Discharged on Antithrombotic Therapy	30	100%	99%	99%
Discharged on Statin Medication	24	100%	96%	94%
Thrombolytic Therapy Timing[7]	-	-	76%	66%
Venous Thromboembolism Prophylaxis	46	100%	95%	94%
Written Stroke Educational Materials Given	22	100%	94%	88%
Surgical Care Improvement Project				
Appropriate Beta Blocker Usage	41	100%	99%	98%
Appropriate VTP Within 24 Hours	177	100%	99%	98%
Controlled Postoperative Blood Glucose[7]	-	-	98%	97%
Perioperative Temperature Management	179	100%	100%	100%
Prophylactic Antibiotic Selection	81	100%	99%	99%
Prophylactic Antibiotic Selection (Outpatient)	25	100%	98%	98%
Prophylactic Antibiotic Stopped	76	100%	98%	98%
Prophylactic Antibiotic Timing	81	100%	99%	99%
Prophylactic Antibiotic Timing (Outpatient)	25	100%	98%	98%
Urinary Catheter Removal	91	100%	98%	97%
Survey of Patients' Hospital Experiences				
Area Around Room 'Always' Quiet at Night	300+	77%	58%	61%
Doctors 'Always' Communicated Well	300+	87%	77%	82%
Home Recovery Information Given	300+	86%	83%	85%
Hospital Given 9 or 10 on 10 Point Scale	300+	84%	67%	71%
Meds 'Always' Explained Before Given	300+	70%	60%	64%
Nurses 'Always' Communicated Well	300+	84%	75%	79%
Pain 'Always' Well Controlled	300+	78%	68%	71%
Room and Bathroom 'Always' Clean	300+	87%	69%	73%
Timely Help 'Always' Received	300+	70%	62%	68%
Would Definitely Recommend Hospital	300+	86%	69%	71%
Use of Medical Imaging				
Cardiac Imaging Stress Test before Surgery[1]	-	-	6.4%	5.3%
Combination Abdominal CT Scan	541	1.3%	11.8%	10.5%
Combination Brain/Sinus CT Scan	548	2.4%	3.4%	2.7%
Combination Chest CT Scan	234	0.0%	2.4%	2.7%
Follow-up Mammogram/Ultrasound[7]	-	-	10.2%	8.8%
Lumbar Spine MRI for Low Back Pain	53	50.9%	35.2%	37.2%

Westchester General Hospital

2500 Sw 75th Ave
Miami, FL 33155
Phone: 305-263-9270
Fax: 305-267-6920
URL: www.westchestergeneralhospital.com
Type: Acute Care Hospitals
Emergency Services: Yes
Ownership: Proprietary
Beds: 160

Key Personnel:
CEO . . . . Gilda Baldwin
Administrator . . . . Loretta Grossman, RN,BSN
Emergency Room . . . . Torres Pelayo
Quality Assurance . . . . Marlene Rabinovich
Chief of Medical Staff . . . . Rogelio Zaldivar, MD

Measure	Cases	This Hosp.	State Avg.	U.S. Avg.
Blood Clot Prevention and Treatment				
Anticoagulation Overlap Therapy[1,2]	-	-	93%	93%
ICU Venous Thromboembolism Prophylaxis[2]	96	77%	94%	92%
Incidence of Potentially Preventable VTE[2]	22	95%	10%	10%
UFH with Dosages/Platelet Monitoring[1,2]	-	-	100%	97%
Venous Thromboembolism Prophylaxis[2]	422	65%	88%	85%
Warfarin Therapy Discharge Instructions[1,2]	-	-	85%	75%
Chest Pain/Possible Heart Attack Care				
Aspirin Given Within 24 Hours of Arrival[1,3]	-	-	98%	96%
Fibrinolytic Meds Within 30 Min. of Arrival[3,7]	-	-	81%	58%
Average Time to ECG (minutes)[1,3]	-	-	7	7
Average Time to Transfer (minutes)[3,7]	-	-	53	60
Children's Asthma Care				
Received Home Management Plan of Care	-	-	-	88%
Received Reliever Medication	-	-	-	100%
Received Systemic Corticosteroids	-	-	-	100%
Emergency Department				
Admittance Decision Time (minutes)[2]	974	76	111	98
Head CT Results Within 45 Min. of Arrival[3,7]	-	-	64%	57%
Patients Who Left ER Before Being Seen	10,642	1%	2%	2%
Time from ER Arrival to Admit. (minutes)[2]	974	312	289	274
Time from ER Arrival to Discharge (minutes)	1,115	174	147	134
Time in ER Before Being Evaluated (minutes)	1,214	38	26	26
Time to Pain Meds for Fractures (minutes)[1]	-	-	60	57
Heart Attack Care				
Aspirin Given at Discharge[1,2]	-	-	99%	99%
Fibrinolytic Meds Within 30 Min. of Arrival[1,2]	-	-	50%	54%
PCI Within 90 Minutes of Arrival[2,7]	-	-	96%	96%
Statin Prescribed at Discharge[1,2]	-	-	99%	98%
Heart Failure Care				

NOTE: *Hospital profiles are in alphabetical order by state, then city, then hospital within the city; Rankings exclude hospitals with less than 25 cases except for patient surveys which excludes hospitals with less than 100 cases; (a) 100-299 cases; (1) The number of cases/patients is too few to report; (2) Data submitted were based on a sample of cases/patients; (3) Results are based on a shorter time period than required; (4) Data suppressed by CMS for one or more quarters; (5) Results are not available for this reporting period; (6) Fewer than 100 patients completed the HCAHPS survey; (7) No cases met the criteria for this measure; (8) The lower limit of the confidence interval cannot be calculated if the number of observed infections equals zero; (9) No data are available from the state/territory for this reporting period; (10) The scores shown reflect fewer than 50 completed surveys; (11) There were discrepancies in the data collection process; (12) This measure does not apply to this hospital for this reporting period; (13) Results cannot be calculated for this reporting period; (14) The results for this state are combined with nearby states to protect confidentiality; Please refer to the User's Guide for a full explanation of data.*

Measure	Cases	This Hosp.	State Avg.	U.S. Avg.
ACE Inhibitor or ARB for LVSD[1,2]	-	-	98%	97%
Discharge Instructions Given[2]	26	62%	96%	94%
Evaluation of LVS Function[2]	41	93%	100%	99%
Medicare Spending				
Medicare Spending per Patient (ratio)	-	1.08	1.04	0.98
Pneumonia Care				
Appropriate Initial Antibiotic Given[2]	48	100%	98%	95%
Blood Culture Timing[2]	86	99%	99%	98%
Pregnancy and Delivery Care				
Newborn Deliveries Scheduled Early[7]	-	-	6%	6%
Preventive Care				
Immunization for Influenza[2]	512	97%	94%	90%
Immunization for Pneumonia[2]	769	99%	96%	92%
Stroke Care				
Anticoagulation Therapy for Atrial Fibrillation[1,2]	-	-	97%	95%
Antithrombotic Therapy Timing[1,2]	-	-	98%	98%
Assessed for Rehabilitation[1,2]	-	-	97%	97%
Discharged on Antithrombotic Therapy[1,2]	-	-	99%	99%
Discharged on Statin Medication[1,2]	-	-	96%	94%
Thrombolytic Therapy Timing[1,2]	-	-	76%	66%
Venous Thromboembolism Prophylaxis[1,2]	-	-	95%	94%
Written Stroke Educational Materials Given[1,2]	-	-	94%	88%
Surgical Care Improvement Project				
Appropriate Beta Blocker Usage[1,2]	-	-	99%	98%
Appropriate VTP Within 24 Hours[2]	31	97%	99%	98%
Controlled Postoperative Blood Glucose[2,7]	-	-	98%	97%
Perioperative Temperature Management[2]	35	100%	100%	100%
Prophylactic Antibiotic Selection[2]	13	92%	99%	99%
Prophylactic Antibiotic Selection (Outpatient)	11	91%	98%	98%
Prophylactic Antibiotic Stopped[2]	12	100%	98%	98%
Prophylactic Antibiotic Timing[2]	13	100%	99%	99%
Prophylactic Antibiotic Timing (Outpatient)	19	58%	98%	98%
Urinary Catheter Removal[1,2]	-	-	98%	97%
Survey of Patients' Hospital Experiences				
Area Around Room 'Always' Quiet at Night	300+	53%	58%	61%
Doctors 'Always' Communicated Well	300+	81%	77%	82%
Home Recovery Information Given	300+	79%	83%	85%
Hospital Given 9 or 10 on 10 Point Scale	300+	60%	67%	71%
Meds 'Always' Explained Before Given	300+	61%	60%	64%
Nurses 'Always' Communicated Well	300+	75%	75%	79%
Pain 'Always' Well Controlled	300+	72%	68%	71%
Room and Bathroom 'Always' Clean	300+	73%	69%	73%
Timely Help 'Always' Received	300+	58%	62%	68%
Would Definitely Recommend Hospital	300+	58%	69%	71%
Use of Medical Imaging				
Cardiac Imaging Stress Test before Surgery[1]	-	-	6.4%	5.3%
Combination Abdominal CT Scan	137	15.3%	11.8%	10.5%
Combination Brain/Sinus CT Scan[1]	-	-	3.4%	2.7%
Combination Chest CT Scan[1]	-	-	2.4%	2.7%
Follow-up Mammogram/Ultrasound[1]	-	-	10.2%	8.8%
Lumbar Spine MRI for Low Back Pain[7]	-	-	35.2%	37.2%

Mount Sinai Medical Center

4300 Alton Rd
Miami Beach, FL 33140
E-mail: webmaster@msmc.com
URL: www.msmc.com
Type: Acute Care Hospitals
Ownership: Proprietary
Phone: 305-674-2121
Fax: 305-674-2334
Emergency Services: Yes
Beds: 672

Key Personnel:
Emergency Room . . . . Art Diskin, MD
Quality Assurance . . . . Ellen Heines
Cardiac Laboratory. . . . . Gervasio Lamas, MD
Hemotology Center . . . . Jose Lutzky, MD
Radiology. . . . . Jeffrey D Neitlich, MD
Chief of Medical Staff . . . . Peter H Segall, MD
CEO/President. . . . . Steven D Sonenreich
Anesthesiology. . . . . S Howard Wittels, MD

Measure	Cases	This Hosp.	State Avg.	U.S. Avg.
Blood Clot Prevention and Treatment				
Anticoagulation Overlap Therapy[2]	98	74%	93%	93%
ICU Venous Thromboembolism Prophylaxis[2]	55	98%	94%	92%
Incidence of Potentially Preventable VTE[2]	48	6%	10%	10%
UFH with Dosages/Platelet Monitoring[2]	17	100%	100%	97%
Venous Thromboembolism Prophylaxis[2]	332	80%	88%	85%
Warfarin Therapy Discharge Instructions[2]	44	66%	85%	75%
Chest Pain/Possible Heart Attack Care				
Aspirin Given Within 24 Hours of Arrival[1]	-	-	98%	96%
Fibrinolytic Meds Within 30 Min. of Arrival[5]	-	-	81%	58%
Average Time to ECG (minutes)[1]	-	-	7	7
Average Time to Transfer (minutes)[5]	-	-	53	60
Children's Asthma Care				
Received Home Management Plan of Care	-	-	-	88%
Received Reliever Medication	-	-	-	100%
Received Systemic Corticosteroids	-	-	-	100%
Emergency Department				
Admittance Decision Time (minutes)[2]	583	233	111	98
Head CT Results Within 45 Min. of Arrival[3,7]	-	-	64%	57%
Patients Who Left ER Before Being Seen	63,203	0%	2%	2%
Time from ER Arrival to Admit. (minutes)[2]	586	399	289	274
Time from ER Arrival to Discharge (minutes)	364	162	147	134
Time in ER Before Being Evaluated (minutes)	332	30	26	26
Time to Pain Meds for Fractures (minutes)	121	59	60	57
Heart Attack Care				
Aspirin Given at Discharge	473	99%	99%	99%
Fibrinolytic Meds Within 30 Min. of Arrival[7]	-	-	50%	54%
PCI Within 90 Minutes of Arrival	47	100%	96%	96%
Statin Prescribed at Discharge	473	99%	99%	98%
Heart Failure Care				
ACE Inhibitor or ARB for LVSD	185	100%	98%	97%
Discharge Instructions Given	405	100%	96%	94%
Evaluation of LVS Function	517	100%	100%	99%
Medicare Spending				
Medicare Spending per Patient (ratio)	-	1.08	1.04	0.98
Pneumonia Care				
Appropriate Initial Antibiotic Given	192	98%	98%	95%
Blood Culture Timing	378	99%	99%	98%
Pregnancy and Delivery Care				
Newborn Deliveries Scheduled Early[2]	55	4%	6%	6%
Preventive Care				
Immunization for Influenza[2]	536	87%	94%	90%
Immunization for Pneumonia[2]	635	94%	96%	92%
Stroke Care				
Anticoagulation Therapy for Atrial Fibrillation	26	100%	97%	95%
Antithrombotic Therapy Timing	119	99%	98%	98%
Assessed for Rehabilitation	166	99%	97%	97%
Discharged on Antithrombotic Therapy	128	98%	99%	99%
Discharged on Statin Medication	122	97%	96%	94%
Thrombolytic Therapy Timing[1]	-	-	76%	66%
Venous Thromboembolism Prophylaxis	181	97%	95%	94%
Written Stroke Educational Materials Given	73	97%	94%	88%
Surgical Care Improvement Project				
Appropriate Beta Blocker Usage[2]	533	98%	99%	98%
Appropriate VTP Within 24 Hours[2]	526	98%	99%	98%
Controlled Postoperative Blood Glucose[2]	690	98%	98%	97%
Perioperative Temperature Management[2]	652	100%	100%	100%
Prophylactic Antibiotic Selection[2]	1,122	99%	99%	99%
Prophylactic Antibiotic Selection (Outpatient)	696	98%	98%	98%
Prophylactic Antibiotic Stopped[2]	1,107	98%	98%	98%
Prophylactic Antibiotic Timing[2]	1,122	100%	99%	99%
Prophylactic Antibiotic Timing (Outpatient)	695	99%	98%	98%
Urinary Catheter Removal[2]	927	97%	98%	97%
Survey of Patients' Hospital Experiences				
Area Around Room 'Always' Quiet at Night	300+	51%	58%	61%
Doctors 'Always' Communicated Well	300+	78%	77%	82%
Home Recovery Information Given	300+	81%	83%	85%
Hospital Given 9 or 10 on 10 Point Scale	300+	65%	67%	71%
Meds 'Always' Explained Before Given	300+	60%	60%	64%
Nurses 'Always' Communicated Well	300+	73%	75%	79%
Pain 'Always' Well Controlled	300+	67%	68%	71%
Room and Bathroom 'Always' Clean	300+	68%	69%	73%
Timely Help 'Always' Received	300+	59%	62%	68%
Would Definitely Recommend Hospital	300+	70%	69%	71%
Use of Medical Imaging				
Cardiac Imaging Stress Test before Surgery	256	8.2%	6.4%	5.3%
Combination Abdominal CT Scan	1,649	13.3%	11.8%	10.5%
Combination Brain/Sinus CT Scan	1,010	3.1%	3.4%	2.7%
Combination Chest CT Scan	1,280	9.7%	2.4%	2.7%
Follow-up Mammogram/Ultrasound	1,519	16.5%	10.2%	8.8%
Lumbar Spine MRI for Low Back Pain	180	42.8%	35.2%	37.2%

Santa Rosa Medical Center

6002 Berryhill Rd
Milton, FL 32570
Type: Acute Care Hospitals
Ownership: Proprietary
Phone: 850-626-7762
Fax: 850-623-5083
Emergency Services: Yes
Beds: 129

Key Personnel:
Operating Room. . . . . Robert A Althar
Radiology. . . . . Thomas Ballard
CEO/President. . . . . Pete Gandy
Quality Assurance . . . . Mike Howatt
Emergency Room . . . . Kathy Rowe
Infection Control. . . . . Judy Wolfe
Intensive Care Unit. . . . . Cecilia Wood
CEO . . . . Phillip Wright, FACHE

Measure	Cases	This Hosp.	State Avg.	U.S. Avg.
Blood Clot Prevention and Treatment				
Anticoagulation Overlap Therapy[2]	32	94%	93%	93%
ICU Venous Thromboembolism Prophylaxis[2]	101	100%	94%	92%
Incidence of Potentially Preventable VTE[1,2]	-	-	10%	10%
UFH with Dosages/Platelet Monitoring[2]	34	100%	100%	97%
Venous Thromboembolism Prophylaxis[2]	274	96%	88%	85%
Warfarin Therapy Discharge Instructions[2]	27	70%	85%	75%
Chest Pain/Possible Heart Attack Care				
Aspirin Given Within 24 Hours of Arrival	72	93%	98%	96%
Fibrinolytic Meds Within 30 Min. of Arrival[7]	-	-	81%	58%
Average Time to ECG (minutes)	75	6	7	7
Average Time to Transfer (minutes)[1]	-	-	53	60
Children's Asthma Care				
Received Home Management Plan of Care	-	-	-	88%
Received Reliever Medication	-	-	-	100%
Received Systemic Corticosteroids	-	-	-	100%
Emergency Department				
Admittance Decision Time (minutes)[2]	537	86	111	98
Head CT Results Within 45 Min. of Arrival[1]	-	-	64%	57%
Patients Who Left ER Before Being Seen	32,263	2%	2%	2%
Time from ER Arrival to Admit. (minutes)[2]	536	221	289	274
Time from ER Arrival to Discharge (minutes)	351	103	147	134
Time in ER Before Being Evaluated (minutes)	384	28	26	26
Time to Pain Meds for Fractures (minutes)	99	45	60	57
Heart Attack Care				
Aspirin Given at Discharge	11	100%	99%	99%
Fibrinolytic Meds Within 30 Min. of Arrival[7]	-	-	50%	54%
PCI Within 90 Minutes of Arrival[7]	-	-	96%	96%
Statin Prescribed at Discharge	11	91%	99%	98%
Heart Failure Care				
ACE Inhibitor or ARB for LVSD	17	100%	98%	97%
Discharge Instructions Given	87	89%	96%	94%
Evaluation of LVS Function	102	100%	100%	99%
Medicare Spending				
Medicare Spending per Patient (ratio)	-	1.01	1.04	0.98
Pneumonia Care				
Appropriate Initial Antibiotic Given	58	100%	98%	95%
Blood Culture Timing	90	99%	99%	98%
Pregnancy and Delivery Care				
Newborn Deliveries Scheduled Early	39	41%	6%	6%
Preventive Care				
Immunization for Influenza[2]	371	99%	94%	90%
Immunization for Pneumonia[2]	459	98%	96%	92%
Stroke Care				
Anticoagulation Therapy for Atrial Fibrillation[1]	-	-	97%	95%
Antithrombotic Therapy Timing	28	100%	98%	98%
Assessed for Rehabilitation	27	96%	97%	97%
Discharged on Antithrombotic Therapy	25	100%	99%	99%
Discharged on Statin Medication	17	100%	96%	94%
Thrombolytic Therapy Timing[7]	-	-	76%	66%
Venous Thromboembolism Prophylaxis	29	100%	95%	94%
Written Stroke Educational Materials Given	24	100%	94%	88%
Surgical Care Improvement Project				
Appropriate Beta Blocker Usage	59	98%	99%	98%

NOTE: Hospital profiles are in alphabetical order by state, then city, then hospital within the city; Rankings exclude hospitals with less than 25 cases except for patient surveys which excludes hospitals with less than 100 cases; (a) 100-299 cases; (1) The number of cases/patients is too few to report; (2) Data submitted were based on a sample of cases/patients; (3) Results are based on a shorter time period than required; (4) Data suppressed by CMS for one or more quarters; (5) Results are not available for this reporting period; (6) Fewer than 100 patients completed the HCAHPS survey; (7) No cases met the criteria for this measure; (8) The lower limit of the confidence interval cannot be calculated if the number of observed infections equals zero; (9) No data are available from the state/territory for this reporting period; (10) The scores shown reflect fewer than 50 completed surveys; (11) There were discrepancies in the data collection process; (12) This measure does not apply to this hospital for this reporting period; (13) Results cannot be calculated for this reporting period; (14) The results for this state are combined with nearby states to protect confidentiality; Please refer to the User's Guide for a full explanation of data.

Appropriate VTP Within 24 Hours	155	99%	99%	98%
Controlled Postoperative Blood Glucose[7]	-	-	98%	97%
Perioperative Temperature Management	197	100%	100%	100%
Prophylactic Antibiotic Selection	110	100%	99%	99%
Prophylactic Antibiotic Selection (Outpatient)	151	100%	98%	98%
Prophylactic Antibiotic Stopped	105	100%	98%	98%
Prophylactic Antibiotic Timing	110	100%	99%	99%
Prophylactic Antibiotic Timing (Outpatient)	151	100%	98%	98%
Urinary Catheter Removal	101	98%	98%	97%
Survey of Patients' Hospital Experiences				
Area Around Room 'Always' Quiet at Night	300+	53%	58%	61%
Doctors 'Always' Communicated Well	300+	79%	77%	82%
Home Recovery Information Given	300+	83%	83%	85%
Hospital Given 9 or 10 on 10 Point Scale	300+	57%	67%	71%
Meds 'Always' Explained Before Given	300+	58%	60%	64%
Nurses 'Always' Communicated Well	300+	73%	75%	79%
Pain 'Always' Well Controlled	300+	65%	68%	71%
Room and Bathroom 'Always' Clean	300+	72%	69%	73%
Timely Help 'Always' Received	300+	63%	62%	68%
Would Definitely Recommend Hospital	300+	55%	69%	71%
Use of Medical Imaging				
Cardiac Imaging Stress Test before Surgery	171	8.8%	6.4%	5.3%
Combination Abdominal CT Scan	487	9.9%	11.8%	10.5%
Combination Brain/Sinus CT Scan	468	5.6%	3.4%	2.7%
Combination Chest CT Scan	100	23.0%	2.4%	2.7%
Follow-up Mammogram/Ultrasound	451	11.1%	10.2%	8.8%
Lumbar Spine MRI for Low Back Pain	57	26.3%	35.2%	37.2%

Memorial Hospital Miramar

1901 Sw 172nd Ave Phone: 954-538-4810
Miramar, FL 33029
Type: Acute Care Hospitals Emergency Services: Yes
Ownership: Voluntary non-profit - Other
Key Personnel:
Operating Room. . . . . Anel Alvarado, MD
CEO . . . . Leah A. Carpenter
Chief of Medical Staff. . . . . Jay B. Fine, MD
Anesthesiology. . . . . Gary Gomez, MD
Pediatrics. . . . . Ana Roig-Cantisano, MD
Pediatric In-Patient Care . . . . Ben-Emir Sanchez, MD

Measure	Cases	This Hosp.	State Avg.	U.S. Avg.
Blood Clot Prevention and Treatment				
Anticoagulation Overlap Therapy[2]	68	94%	93%	93%
ICU Venous Thromboembolism Prophylaxis[2]	58	100%	94%	92%
Incidence of Potentially Preventable VTE[1,2]	-	-	10%	10%
UFH with Dosages/Platelet Monitoring[2]	14	100%	100%	97%
Venous Thromboembolism Prophylaxis[2]	342	99%	88%	85%
Warfarin Therapy Discharge Instructions[2]	59	100%	85%	75%
Chest Pain/Possible Heart Attack Care				
Aspirin Given Within 24 Hours of Arrival	42	100%	98%	96%
Fibrinolytic Meds Within 30 Min. of Arrival[7]	-	-	81%	58%
Average Time to ECG (minutes)	45	5	7	7
Average Time to Transfer (minutes)[1]	-	-	53	60
Children's Asthma Care				
Received Home Management Plan of Care	-	-	-	88%
Received Reliever Medication	-	-	-	100%
Received Systemic Corticosteroids	-	-	-	100%
Emergency Department				
Admittance Decision Time (minutes)[2]	465	171	111	98
Head CT Results Within 45 Min. of Arrival[1]	-	-	64%	57%
Patients Who Left ER Before Being Seen	59,764	1%	2%	2%
Time from ER Arrival to Admit. (minutes)[2]	468	353	289	274
Time from ER Arrival to Discharge (minutes)	362	164	147	134
Time in ER Before Being Evaluated (minutes)	359	33	26	26
Time to Pain Meds for Fractures (minutes)	286	50	60	57
Heart Attack Care				
Aspirin Given at Discharge	11	100%	99%	99%
Fibrinolytic Meds Within 30 Min. of Arrival[7]	-	-	50%	54%
PCI Within 90 Minutes of Arrival[7]	-	-	96%	96%
Statin Prescribed at Discharge[1]	-	-	99%	98%
Heart Failure Care				
ACE Inhibitor or ARB for LVSD	29	100%	98%	97%
Discharge Instructions Given	116	100%	96%	94%
Evaluation of LVS Function	137	100%	100%	99%
Medicare Spending				
Medicare Spending per Patient (ratio)	-	1.02	1.04	0.98
Pneumonia Care				
Appropriate Initial Antibiotic Given	114	100%	98%	95%
Blood Culture Timing	197	99%	99%	98%
Pregnancy and Delivery Care				
Newborn Deliveries Scheduled Early[2]	55	9%	6%	6%
Preventive Care				
Immunization for Influenza[2]	476	96%	94%	90%
Immunization for Pneumonia[2]	351	98%	96%	92%
Stroke Care				
Anticoagulation Therapy for Atrial Fibrillation[1]	-	-	97%	95%
Antithrombotic Therapy Timing	48	92%	98%	98%
Assessed for Rehabilitation	47	98%	97%	97%
Discharged on Antithrombotic Therapy	46	83%	99%	99%
Discharged on Statin Medication	40	82%	96%	94%
Thrombolytic Therapy Timing[1]	-	-	76%	66%
Venous Thromboembolism Prophylaxis	47	94%	95%	94%
Written Stroke Educational Materials Given	29	100%	94%	88%
Surgical Care Improvement Project				
Appropriate Beta Blocker Usage[2]	16	100%	99%	98%
Appropriate VTP Within 24 Hours[2]	214	99%	99%	98%
Controlled Postoperative Blood Glucose[2,7]	-	-	98%	97%
Perioperative Temperature Management[2]	261	100%	100%	100%
Prophylactic Antibiotic Selection[2]	138	99%	99%	99%
Prophylactic Antibiotic Selection (Outpatient)	353	100%	98%	98%
Prophylactic Antibiotic Stopped[2]	136	100%	98%	98%
Prophylactic Antibiotic Timing[2]	138	100%	99%	99%
Prophylactic Antibiotic Timing (Outpatient)	353	100%	98%	98%
Urinary Catheter Removal[2]	117	99%	98%	97%
Survey of Patients' Hospital Experiences				
Area Around Room 'Always' Quiet at Night	300+	69%	58%	61%
Doctors 'Always' Communicated Well	300+	82%	77%	82%
Home Recovery Information Given	300+	86%	83%	85%
Hospital Given 9 or 10 on 10 Point Scale	300+	83%	67%	71%
Meds 'Always' Explained Before Given	300+	67%	60%	64%
Nurses 'Always' Communicated Well	300+	84%	75%	79%
Pain 'Always' Well Controlled	300+	77%	68%	71%
Room and Bathroom 'Always' Clean	300+	83%	69%	73%
Timely Help 'Always' Received	300+	70%	62%	68%
Would Definitely Recommend Hospital	300+	85%	69%	71%
Use of Medical Imaging				
Cardiac Imaging Stress Test before Surgery[7]	-	-	6.4%	5.3%
Combination Abdominal CT Scan	420	3.8%	11.8%	10.5%
Combination Brain/Sinus CT Scan[1]	-	-	3.4%	2.7%
Combination Chest CT Scan	222	0.0%	2.4%	2.7%
Follow-up Mammogram/Ultrasound	356	13.5%	10.2%	8.8%
Lumbar Spine MRI for Low Back Pain	50	44.0%	35.2%	37.2%

Sacred Heart Hospital on the Emerald Coast

7800 Us Hwy 98 W Phone: 850-278-3600
Miramar Beach, FL 32550 Fax: 850-278-3010
URL: www.sacredheartemerald.org
Type: Acute Care Hospitals Emergency Services: Yes
Ownership: Voluntary non-profit - Other
Key Personnel:
Radiology. . . . . Franklin D Abbot
Chief of Medical Staff. . . . . Calvin L Blount Jr
CEO/President. . . . . Roger Hall

Measure	Cases	This Hosp.	State Avg.	U.S. Avg.
Blood Clot Prevention and Treatment				
Anticoagulation Overlap Therapy[2]	31	100%	93%	93%
ICU Venous Thromboembolism Prophylaxis[2]	52	88%	94%	92%
Incidence of Potentially Preventable VTE[1,2]	-	-	10%	10%
UFH with Dosages/Platelet Monitoring[1,2]	-	-	100%	97%
Venous Thromboembolism Prophylaxis[2]	303	87%	88%	85%
Warfarin Therapy Discharge Instructions[2]	23	100%	85%	75%
Chest Pain/Possible Heart Attack Care				
Aspirin Given Within 24 Hours of Arrival[1]	-	-	98%	96%
Fibrinolytic Meds Within 30 Min. of Arrival[3,7]	-	-	81%	58%
Average Time to ECG (minutes)[1]	-	-	7	7
Average Time to Transfer (minutes)[3,7]	-	-	53	60
Children's Asthma Care				
Received Home Management Plan of Care	-	-	-	88%
Received Reliever Medication	-	-	-	100%
Received Systemic Corticosteroids	-	-	-	100%
Emergency Department				
Admittance Decision Time (minutes)[2]	420	114	111	98
Head CT Results Within 45 Min. of Arrival	18	44%	64%	57%
Patients Who Left ER Before Being Seen	27,979	1%	2%	2%
Time from ER Arrival to Admit. (minutes)[2]	467	262	289	274
Time from ER Arrival to Discharge (minutes)	389	141	147	134
Time in ER Before Being Evaluated (minutes)	356	36	26	26
Time to Pain Meds for Fractures (minutes)	211	76	60	57
Heart Attack Care				
Aspirin Given at Discharge	87	99%	99%	99%
Fibrinolytic Meds Within 30 Min. of Arrival[7]	-	-	50%	54%
PCI Within 90 Minutes of Arrival	30	97%	96%	96%
Statin Prescribed at Discharge	85	99%	99%	98%
Heart Failure Care				
ACE Inhibitor or ARB for LVSD	37	97%	98%	97%
Discharge Instructions Given	84	94%	96%	94%
Evaluation of LVS Function	97	100%	100%	99%
Medicare Spending				
Medicare Spending per Patient (ratio)	-	0.99	1.04	0.98
Pneumonia Care				
Appropriate Initial Antibiotic Given	91	100%	98%	95%
Blood Culture Timing	163	99%	99%	98%
Pregnancy and Delivery Care				
Newborn Deliveries Scheduled Early[2]	34	3%	6%	6%
Preventive Care				
Immunization for Influenza[2]	503	95%	94%	90%
Immunization for Pneumonia[2]	593	95%	96%	92%
Stroke Care				
Anticoagulation Therapy for Atrial Fibrillation[1]	-	-	97%	95%
Antithrombotic Therapy Timing	37	100%	98%	98%
Assessed for Rehabilitation	47	83%	97%	97%
Discharged on Antithrombotic Therapy	39	100%	99%	99%
Discharged on Statin Medication	39	92%	96%	94%
Thrombolytic Therapy Timing[1]	-	-	76%	66%
Venous Thromboembolism Prophylaxis	36	86%	95%	94%
Written Stroke Educational Materials Given	33	58%	94%	88%
Surgical Care Improvement Project				
Appropriate Beta Blocker Usage[2]	117	100%	99%	98%
Appropriate VTP Within 24 Hours[2]	330	98%	99%	98%
Controlled Postoperative Blood Glucose[2,7]	-	-	98%	97%
Perioperative Temperature Management[2]	391	100%	100%	100%
Prophylactic Antibiotic Selection[2]	297	100%	99%	99%
Prophylactic Antibiotic Selection (Outpatient)	195	99%	98%	98%
Prophylactic Antibiotic Stopped[2]	293	97%	98%	98%
Prophylactic Antibiotic Timing[2]	297	100%	99%	99%
Prophylactic Antibiotic Timing (Outpatient)	198	97%	98%	98%
Urinary Catheter Removal[2]	280	99%	98%	97%
Survey of Patients' Hospital Experiences				
Area Around Room 'Always' Quiet at Night	300+	66%	58%	61%
Doctors 'Always' Communicated Well	300+	84%	77%	82%
Home Recovery Information Given	300+	89%	83%	85%
Hospital Given 9 or 10 on 10 Point Scale	300+	82%	67%	71%
Meds 'Always' Explained Before Given	300+	69%	60%	64%
Nurses 'Always' Communicated Well	300+	83%	75%	79%
Pain 'Always' Well Controlled	300+	75%	68%	71%
Room and Bathroom 'Always' Clean	300+	73%	69%	73%
Timely Help 'Always' Received	300+	72%	62%	68%
Would Definitely Recommend Hospital	300+	85%	69%	71%
Use of Medical Imaging				
Cardiac Imaging Stress Test before Surgery	446	4.7%	6.4%	5.3%
Combination Abdominal CT Scan	849	9.3%	11.8%	10.5%
Combination Brain/Sinus CT Scan	631	2.9%	3.4%	2.7%
Combination Chest CT Scan	556	4.1%	2.4%	2.7%
Follow-up Mammogram/Ultrasound	1,005	9.5%	10.2%	8.8%
Lumbar Spine MRI for Low Back Pain	129	31.8%	35.2%	37.2%

NOTE: Hospital profiles are in alphabetical order by state, then city, then hospital within the city; Rankings exclude hospitals with less than 25 cases except for patient surveys which excludes hospitals with less than 100 cases; (a) 100-299 cases; (1) The number of cases/patients is too few to report; (2) Data submitted were based on a sample of cases/patients; (3) Results are based on a shorter time period than required; (4) Data suppressed by CMS for one or more quarters; (5) Results are not available for this reporting period; (6) Fewer than 100 patients completed the HCAHPS survey; (7) No cases met the criteria for this measure; (8) The lower limit of the confidence interval cannot be calculated if the number of observed infections equals zero; (9) No data are available from the state/territory for this reporting period; (10) The scores shown reflect fewer than 50 completed surveys; (11) There were discrepancies in the data collection process; (12) This measure does not apply to this hospital for this reporting period; (13) Results cannot be calculated for this reporting period; (14) The results for this state are combined with nearby states to protect confidentiality; Please refer to the User's Guide for a full explanation of data.

Naples Community Hospital

350 7th Saint N | Phone: 239-436-5000
Naples, FL 34102 | Fax: 239-436-5048
URL: www.nchmd.org
Type: Acute Care Hospitals | Emergency Services: Yes
Ownership: Voluntary non-profit - Private | Beds: 390

Key Personnel:
Anesthesiology. . . . . Lee Anderson, MD
Quality Assurance . . . . Barbara Cain
Chief of Medical Staff. . . . . Kevin D Cooper
Operating Room. . . . . Bill Diamond
Pediatric Ambulatory Care . . . . . . Debra Shepard, MD
Emergency Room . . . . Andrew C Shuter, DO
Radiology. . . . . Michael Theobald, MD
CEO/President. . . . . Allen S Weiss, MD

Measure	Cases	This Hosp.	State Avg.	U.S. Avg.
Blood Clot Prevention and Treatment				
Anticoagulation Overlap Therapy[2]	248	92%	93%	93%
ICU Venous Thromboembolism Prophylaxis[2]	38	92%	94%	92%
Incidence of Potentially Preventable VTE[2]	63	3%	10%	10%
UFH with Dosages/Platelet Monitoring[2]	241	100%	100%	97%
Venous Thromboembolism Prophylaxis[2]	365	81%	88%	85%
Warfarin Therapy Discharge Instructions[2]	199	72%	85%	75%
Chest Pain/Possible Heart Attack Care				
Aspirin Given Within 24 Hours of Arrival[1,3]	-	-	98%	96%
Fibrinolytic Meds Within 30 Min. of Arrival[3,7]	-	-	81%	58%
Average Time to ECG (minutes)[1,3]	-	-	7	7
Average Time to Transfer (minutes)[3,7]	-	-	53	60
Children's Asthma Care				
Received Home Management Plan of Care	-	-	-	88%
Received Reliever Medication	-	-	-	100%
Received Systemic Corticosteroids	-	-	-	100%
Emergency Department				
Admittance Decision Time (minutes)[2]	737	86	111	98
Head CT Results Within 45 Min. of Arrival	11	64%	64%	57%
Patients Who Left ER Before Being Seen	89,925	2%	2%	2%
Time from ER Arrival to Admit. (minutes)[2]	756	249	289	274
Time from ER Arrival to Discharge (minutes)	395	134	147	134
Time in ER Before Being Evaluated (minutes)	317	38	26	26
Time to Pain Meds for Fractures (minutes)	212	52	60	57
Heart Attack Care				
Aspirin Given at Discharge	494	98%	99%	99%
Fibrinolytic Meds Within 30 Min. of Arrival[7]	-	-	50%	54%
PCI Within 90 Minutes of Arrival	42	95%	96%	96%
Statin Prescribed at Discharge	476	98%	99%	98%
Heart Failure Care				
ACE Inhibitor or ARB for LVSD[2]	86	93%	98%	97%
Discharge Instructions Given[2]	255	90%	96%	94%
Evaluation of LVS Function[2]	295	99%	100%	99%
Medicare Spending				
Medicare Spending per Patient (ratio)	-	1.03	1.04	0.98
Pneumonia Care				
Appropriate Initial Antibiotic Given[2]	143	97%	98%	95%
Blood Culture Timing[2]	213	97%	99%	98%
Pregnancy and Delivery Care				
Newborn Deliveries Scheduled Early[2]	59	17%	6%	6%
Preventive Care				
Immunization for Influenza[2]	621	91%	94%	90%
Immunization for Pneumonia[2]	794	95%	96%	92%
Stroke Care				
Anticoagulation Therapy for Atrial Fibrillation[2]	20	100%	97%	95%
Antithrombotic Therapy Timing[2]	90	98%	98%	98%
Assessed for Rehabilitation[2]	106	94%	97%	97%
Discharged on Antithrombotic Therapy[2]	94	98%	99%	99%
Discharged on Statin Medication[2]	68	88%	96%	94%
Thrombolytic Therapy Timing[1,2]	-	-	76%	66%
Venous Thromboembolism Prophylaxis[2]	109	90%	95%	94%
Written Stroke Educational Materials Given[2]	70	51%	94%	88%
Surgical Care Improvement Project				
Appropriate Beta Blocker Usage[2]	346	98%	99%	98%
Appropriate VTP Within 24 Hours[2]	517	98%	99%	98%
Controlled Postoperative Blood Glucose[2]	204	97%	98%	97%
Perioperative Temperature Management[2]	662	100%	100%	100%
Prophylactic Antibiotic Selection[2]	629	98%	99%	99%
Prophylactic Antibiotic Selection (Outpatient)	592	97%	98%	98%
Prophylactic Antibiotic Stopped[2]	608	95%	98%	98%
Prophylactic Antibiotic Timing[2]	632	99%	99%	99%
Prophylactic Antibiotic Timing (Outpatient)	597	98%	98%	98%
Urinary Catheter Removal[2]	643	93%	98%	97%
Survey of Patients' Hospital Experiences				
Area Around Room 'Always' Quiet at Night	300+	54%	58%	61%
Doctors 'Always' Communicated Well	300+	77%	77%	82%
Home Recovery Information Given	300+	79%	83%	85%
Hospital Given 9 or 10 on 10 Point Scale	300+	66%	67%	71%
Meds 'Always' Explained Before Given	300+	57%	60%	64%
Nurses 'Always' Communicated Well	300+	73%	75%	79%
Pain 'Always' Well Controlled	300+	66%	68%	71%
Room and Bathroom 'Always' Clean	300+	67%	69%	73%
Timely Help 'Always' Received	300+	59%	62%	68%
Would Definitely Recommend Hospital	300+	73%	69%	71%
Use of Medical Imaging				
Cardiac Imaging Stress Test before Surgery	2,459	7.1%	6.4%	5.3%
Combination Abdominal CT Scan	1,352	1.2%	11.8%	10.5%
Combination Brain/Sinus CT Scan	2,042	4.2%	3.4%	2.7%
Combination Chest CT Scan	344	0.6%	2.4%	2.7%
Follow-up Mammogram/Ultrasound[7]	-	-	10.2%	8.8%
Lumbar Spine MRI for Low Back Pain[1]	-	-	35.2%	37.2%

Physicians Regional Medical Center - Pine Ridge

6101 Pine Ridge Road | Phone: 239-348-4000
Naples, FL 34119 | Fax: 239-348-4140
URL: www.physiciansregional.com
Type: Acute Care Hospitals | Emergency Services: Yes
Ownership: Proprietary | Beds: 83

Key Personnel:
Chief of Medical Staff. . . . . Lawrence H Albert
Radiology. . . . . Michael F DAngelo
Infection Control. . . . . Nicholas J Lekas, MD/FACP
CEO/President. . . . . Geoffrey D Moebius, MD

Measure	Cases	This Hosp.	State Avg.	U.S. Avg.
Blood Clot Prevention and Treatment				
Anticoagulation Overlap Therapy[2]	104	97%	93%	93%
ICU Venous Thromboembolism Prophylaxis[2]	76	99%	94%	92%
Incidence of Potentially Preventable VTE[2]	24	0%	10%	10%
UFH with Dosages/Platelet Monitoring[2]	98	100%	100%	97%
Venous Thromboembolism Prophylaxis[2]	355	90%	88%	85%
Warfarin Therapy Discharge Instructions[2]	86	99%	85%	75%
Chest Pain/Possible Heart Attack Care				
Aspirin Given Within 24 Hours of Arrival	18	100%	98%	96%
Fibrinolytic Meds Within 30 Min. of Arrival[3,7]	-	-	81%	58%
Average Time to ECG (minutes)	19	15	7	7
Average Time to Transfer (minutes)[3,7]	-	-	53	60
Children's Asthma Care				
Received Home Management Plan of Care	-	-	-	88%
Received Reliever Medication	-	-	-	100%
Received Systemic Corticosteroids	-	-	-	100%
Emergency Department				
Admittance Decision Time (minutes)[2]	876	143	111	98
Head CT Results Within 45 Min. of Arrival	19	0%	64%	57%
Patients Who Left ER Before Being Seen	49,549	1%	2%	2%
Time from ER Arrival to Admit. (minutes)[2]	876	288	289	274
Time from ER Arrival to Discharge (minutes)	683	113	147	134
Time in ER Before Being Evaluated (minutes)	736	18	26	26
Time to Pain Meds for Fractures (minutes)	156	57	60	57
Heart Attack Care				
Aspirin Given at Discharge	152	99%	99%	99%
Fibrinolytic Meds Within 30 Min. of Arrival[7]	-	-	50%	54%
PCI Within 90 Minutes of Arrival	35	97%	96%	96%
Statin Prescribed at Discharge	134	99%	99%	98%
Heart Failure Care				
ACE Inhibitor or ARB for LVSD	71	100%	98%	97%
Discharge Instructions Given	209	77%	96%	94%
Evaluation of LVS Function	231	100%	100%	99%
Medicare Spending				
Medicare Spending per Patient (ratio)	-	1.00	1.04	0.98
Pneumonia Care				
Appropriate Initial Antibiotic Given	159	99%	98%	95%
Blood Culture Timing	227	100%	99%	98%
Pregnancy and Delivery Care				
Newborn Deliveries Scheduled Early	28	18%	6%	6%
Preventive Care				
Immunization for Influenza[2]	680	95%	94%	90%
Immunization for Pneumonia[2]	975	96%	96%	92%
Stroke Care				
Anticoagulation Therapy for Atrial Fibrillation	34	100%	97%	95%
Antithrombotic Therapy Timing	132	98%	98%	98%
Assessed for Rehabilitation	213	99%	97%	97%
Discharged on Antithrombotic Therapy	152	99%	99%	99%
Discharged on Statin Medication	126	75%	96%	94%
Thrombolytic Therapy Timing	45	51%	76%	66%
Venous Thromboembolism Prophylaxis	232	91%	95%	94%
Written Stroke Educational Materials Given	123	63%	94%	88%
Surgical Care Improvement Project				
Appropriate Beta Blocker Usage	346	100%	99%	98%
Appropriate VTP Within 24 Hours	1,090	95%	99%	98%
Controlled Postoperative Blood Glucose[7]	-	-	98%	97%
Perioperative Temperature Management	1,317	100%	100%	100%
Prophylactic Antibiotic Selection	816	92%	99%	99%
Prophylactic Antibiotic Selection (Outpatient)	534	99%	98%	98%
Prophylactic Antibiotic Stopped	787	91%	98%	98%
Prophylactic Antibiotic Timing	816	99%	99%	99%
Prophylactic Antibiotic Timing (Outpatient)	535	99%	98%	98%
Urinary Catheter Removal	404	99%	98%	97%
Survey of Patients' Hospital Experiences				
Area Around Room 'Always' Quiet at Night	300+	61%	58%	61%
Doctors 'Always' Communicated Well	300+	77%	77%	82%
Home Recovery Information Given	300+	82%	83%	85%
Hospital Given 9 or 10 on 10 Point Scale	300+	64%	67%	71%
Meds 'Always' Explained Before Given	300+	57%	60%	64%
Nurses 'Always' Communicated Well	300+	70%	75%	79%
Pain 'Always' Well Controlled	300+	64%	68%	71%
Room and Bathroom 'Always' Clean	300+	70%	69%	73%
Timely Help 'Always' Received	300+	53%	62%	68%
Would Definitely Recommend Hospital	300+	68%	69%	71%
Use of Medical Imaging				
Cardiac Imaging Stress Test before Surgery	453	6.4%	6.4%	5.3%
Combination Abdominal CT Scan	1,634	12.6%	11.8%	10.5%
Combination Brain/Sinus CT Scan	1,439	3.0%	3.4%	2.7%
Combination Chest CT Scan	569	2.3%	2.4%	2.7%
Follow-up Mammogram/Ultrasound	1,824	6.4%	10.2%	8.8%
Lumbar Spine MRI for Low Back Pain	179	36.3%	35.2%	37.2%

Morton Plant North Bay Hospital

6600 Madison Street | Phone: 727-842-8468
New Port Richey, FL 34652 | Fax: 727-848-8762
URL: www.mortonplant.com
Type: Acute Care Hospitals | Emergency Services: Yes
Ownership: Voluntary non-profit - Private | Beds: 122

Key Personnel:
Quality Assurance . . . . Sandy Karsersas
Operating Room. . . . . Neal Roeper

Measure	Cases	This Hosp.	State Avg.	U.S. Avg.
Blood Clot Prevention and Treatment				
Anticoagulation Overlap Therapy[2]	45	87%	93%	93%
ICU Venous Thromboembolism Prophylaxis[2]	68	97%	94%	92%
Incidence of Potentially Preventable VTE[1,2]	-	-	10%	10%
UFH with Dosages/Platelet Monitoring[2]	37	100%	100%	97%
Venous Thromboembolism Prophylaxis[2]	260	94%	88%	85%
Warfarin Therapy Discharge Instructions[2]	25	96%	85%	75%
Chest Pain/Possible Heart Attack Care				
Aspirin Given Within 24 Hours of Arrival[1,3]	-	-	98%	96%
Fibrinolytic Meds Within 30 Min. of Arrival[3,7]	-	-	81%	58%
Average Time to ECG (minutes)[1,3]	-	-	7	7
Average Time to Transfer (minutes)[3,7]	-	-	53	60
Children's Asthma Care				
Received Home Management Plan of Care	-	-	-	88%
Received Reliever Medication	-	-	-	100%
Received Systemic Corticosteroids	-	-	-	100%
Emergency Department				
Admittance Decision Time (minutes)[2]	442	109	111	98

NOTE: Hospital profiles are in alphabetical order by state, then city, then hospital within the city; Rankings exclude hospitals with less than 25 cases except for patient surveys which excludes hospitals with less than 100 cases; (a) 100-299 cases; (1) The number of cases/patients is too few to report; (2) Data submitted were based on a sample of cases/patients; (3) Results are based on a shorter time period than required; (4) Data suppressed by CMS for one or more quarters; (5) Results are not available for this reporting period; (6) Fewer than 100 patients completed the HCAHPS survey; (7) No cases met the criteria for this measure; (8) The lower limit of the confidence interval cannot be calculated if the number of observed infections equals zero; (9) No data are available from the state/territory for this reporting period; (10) The scores shown reflect fewer than 50 completed surveys; (11) There were discrepancies in the data collection process; (12) This measure does not apply to this hospital for this reporting period; (13) Results cannot be calculated for this reporting period; (14) The results for this state are combined with nearby states to protect confidentiality; Please refer to the User's Guide for a full explanation of data.

Measure	Cases	This Hosp.	State Avg.	U.S. Avg.
Head CT Results Within 45 Min. of Arrival[1]	-	-	64%	57%
Patients Who Left ER Before Being Seen	35,364	6%	2%	2%
Time from ER Arrival to Admit. (minutes)[2]	458	311	289	274
Time from ER Arrival to Discharge (minutes)	321	170	147	134
Time in ER Before Being Evaluated (minutes)	382	53	26	26
Time to Pain Meds for Fractures (minutes)	98	64	60	57
Heart Attack Care				
Aspirin Given at Discharge	185	100%	99%	99%
Fibrinolytic Meds Within 30 Min. of Arrival[7]	-	-	50%	54%
PCI Within 90 Minutes of Arrival	19	100%	96%	96%
Statin Prescribed at Discharge	180	100%	99%	98%
Heart Failure Care				
ACE Inhibitor or ARB for LVSD	70	99%	98%	97%
Discharge Instructions Given	232	97%	96%	94%
Evaluation of LVS Function	302	100%	100%	99%
Medicare Spending				
Medicare Spending per Patient (ratio)	-	1.12	1.04	0.98
Pneumonia Care				
Appropriate Initial Antibiotic Given	100	95%	98%	95%
Blood Culture Timing	183	99%	99%	98%
Pregnancy and Delivery Care				
Newborn Deliveries Scheduled Early[7]	-	-	6%	6%
Preventive Care				
Immunization for Influenza[2]	604	96%	94%	90%
Immunization for Pneumonia[2]	646	95%	96%	92%
Stroke Care				
Anticoagulation Therapy for Atrial Fibrillation	25	88%	97%	95%
Antithrombotic Therapy Timing	94	96%	98%	98%
Assessed for Rehabilitation	92	99%	97%	97%
Discharged on Antithrombotic Therapy	91	100%	99%	99%
Discharged on Statin Medication	70	96%	96%	94%
Thrombolytic Therapy Timing[1]	-	-	76%	66%
Venous Thromboembolism Prophylaxis	96	99%	95%	94%
Written Stroke Educational Materials Given	52	96%	94%	88%
Surgical Care Improvement Project				
Appropriate Beta Blocker Usage[2]	70	97%	99%	98%
Appropriate VTP Within 24 Hours[2]	155	98%	99%	98%
Controlled Postoperative Blood Glucose[2,7]	-	-	98%	97%
Perioperative Temperature Management[2]	189	100%	100%	100%
Prophylactic Antibiotic Selection[2]	85	99%	99%	99%
Prophylactic Antibiotic Selection (Outpatient)	55	93%	98%	98%
Prophylactic Antibiotic Stopped[2]	83	99%	98%	98%
Prophylactic Antibiotic Timing[2]	85	99%	99%	99%
Prophylactic Antibiotic Timing (Outpatient)	55	98%	98%	98%
Urinary Catheter Removal[2]	134	98%	98%	97%
Survey of Patients' Hospital Experiences				
Area Around Room 'Always' Quiet at Night[11]	300+	52%	58%	61%
Doctors 'Always' Communicated Well[11]	300+	71%	77%	82%
Home Recovery Information Given[11]	300+	85%	83%	85%
Hospital Given 9 or 10 on 10 Point Scale[11]	300+	71%	67%	71%
Meds 'Always' Explained Before Given[11]	300+	59%	60%	64%
Nurses 'Always' Communicated Well[11]	300+	77%	75%	79%
Pain 'Always' Well Controlled[11]	300+	67%	68%	71%
Room and Bathroom 'Always' Clean[11]	300+	70%	69%	73%
Timely Help 'Always' Received[11]	300+	61%	62%	68%
Would Definitely Recommend Hospital[11]	300+	75%	69%	71%
Use of Medical Imaging				
Cardiac Imaging Stress Test before Surgery	72	11.1%	6.4%	5.3%
Combination Abdominal CT Scan	306	3.9%	11.8%	10.5%
Combination Brain/Sinus CT Scan	618	4.4%	3.4%	2.7%
Combination Chest CT Scan	60	1.7%	2.4%	2.7%
Follow-up Mammogram/Ultrasound[7]	-	-	10.2%	8.8%
Lumbar Spine MRI for Low Back Pain[1]	-	-	35.2%	37.2%

Bert Fish Medical Center

401 Palmetto St — Phone: 386-424-5000
New Smyrna Beach, FL 32170
URL: www.bertfish.com
Type: Acute Care Hospitals — Emergency Services: Yes
Ownership: Voluntary non-profit - Private — Beds: 116

Key Personnel:
Chief of Medical Staff. . . . . Jean L Ackerman
Radiology. . . . . Bradley Barnes, MD
Cardiac Laboratory. . . . . Ashraf S Elsakr, MD
CEO . . . . Steve Harrell
Infection Control. . . . . Reba Kiran Isaac Ailani, MD
Operating Room. . . . . Heather M Metchick, MD FACOG
Quality Assurance . . . . Wayne Pearson
CEO/President. . . . . Bob Williams

Measure	Cases	This Hosp.	State Avg.	U.S. Avg.
Blood Clot Prevention and Treatment				
Anticoagulation Overlap Therapy[2]	66	89%	93%	93%
ICU Venous Thromboembolism Prophylaxis[2]	90	83%	94%	92%
Incidence of Potentially Preventable VTE[2]	13	23%	10%	10%
UFH with Dosages/Platelet Monitoring[2]	38	100%	100%	97%
Venous Thromboembolism Prophylaxis[2]	320	80%	88%	85%
Warfarin Therapy Discharge Instructions[2]	45	69%	85%	75%
Chest Pain/Possible Heart Attack Care				
Aspirin Given Within 24 Hours of Arrival[1,3]	-	-	98%	96%
Fibrinolytic Meds Within 30 Min. of Arrival[5]	-	-	81%	58%
Average Time to ECG (minutes)[1,3]	-	-	7	7
Average Time to Transfer (minutes)[5]	-	-	53	60
Children's Asthma Care				
Received Home Management Plan of Care	-	-	-	88%
Received Reliever Medication	-	-	-	100%
Received Systemic Corticosteroids	-	-	-	100%
Emergency Department				
Admittance Decision Time (minutes)[2]	499	120	111	98
Head CT Results Within 45 Min. of Arrival	13	62%	64%	57%
Patients Who Left ER Before Being Seen	31,295	2%	2%	2%
Time from ER Arrival to Admit. (minutes)[2]	517	305	289	274
Time from ER Arrival to Discharge (minutes)	477	123	147	134
Time in ER Before Being Evaluated (minutes)	518	26	26	26
Time to Pain Meds for Fractures (minutes)	74	64	60	57
Heart Attack Care				
Aspirin Given at Discharge	182	98%	99%	99%
Fibrinolytic Meds Within 30 Min. of Arrival[7]	-	-	50%	54%
PCI Within 90 Minutes of Arrival	33	85%	96%	96%
Statin Prescribed at Discharge	176	97%	99%	98%
Heart Failure Care				
ACE Inhibitor or ARB for LVSD	29	93%	98%	97%
Discharge Instructions Given	87	87%	96%	94%
Evaluation of LVS Function	103	95%	100%	99%
Medicare Spending				
Medicare Spending per Patient (ratio)	-	0.97	1.04	0.98
Pneumonia Care				
Appropriate Initial Antibiotic Given	59	97%	98%	95%
Blood Culture Timing	124	97%	99%	98%
Pregnancy and Delivery Care				
Newborn Deliveries Scheduled Early[7]	-	-	6%	6%
Preventive Care				
Immunization for Influenza[2]	378	89%	94%	90%
Immunization for Pneumonia[2]	599	89%	96%	92%
Stroke Care				
Anticoagulation Therapy for Atrial Fibrillation	19	95%	97%	95%
Antithrombotic Therapy Timing	55	96%	98%	98%
Assessed for Rehabilitation	63	100%	97%	97%
Discharged on Antithrombotic Therapy	61	98%	99%	99%
Discharged on Statin Medication	54	100%	96%	94%
Thrombolytic Therapy Timing[1]	-	-	76%	66%
Venous Thromboembolism Prophylaxis	51	98%	95%	94%
Written Stroke Educational Materials Given	35	94%	94%	88%
Surgical Care Improvement Project				
Appropriate Beta Blocker Usage	97	97%	99%	98%
Appropriate VTP Within 24 Hours	267	99%	99%	98%
Controlled Postoperative Blood Glucose[7]	-	-	98%	97%
Perioperative Temperature Management	303	100%	100%	100%
Prophylactic Antibiotic Selection	192	99%	99%	99%
Prophylactic Antibiotic Selection (Outpatient)	67	99%	98%	98%
Prophylactic Antibiotic Stopped	189	94%	98%	98%
Prophylactic Antibiotic Timing	192	97%	99%	99%
Prophylactic Antibiotic Timing (Outpatient)	75	85%	98%	98%
Urinary Catheter Removal	212	95%	98%	97%
Survey of Patients' Hospital Experiences				
Area Around Room 'Always' Quiet at Night	300+	61%	58%	61%
Doctors 'Always' Communicated Well	300+	82%	77%	82%
Home Recovery Information Given	300+	86%	83%	85%
Hospital Given 9 or 10 on 10 Point Scale	300+	71%	67%	71%
Meds 'Always' Explained Before Given	300+	61%	60%	64%
Nurses 'Always' Communicated Well	300+	79%	75%	79%
Pain 'Always' Well Controlled	300+	72%	68%	71%
Room and Bathroom 'Always' Clean	300+	70%	69%	73%
Timely Help 'Always' Received	300+	64%	62%	68%
Would Definitely Recommend Hospital	300+	72%	69%	71%
Use of Medical Imaging				
Cardiac Imaging Stress Test before Surgery	261	6.1%	6.4%	5.3%
Combination Abdominal CT Scan	651	3.7%	11.8%	10.5%
Combination Brain/Sinus CT Scan	677	2.2%	3.4%	2.7%
Combination Chest CT Scan	406	0.5%	2.4%	2.7%
Follow-up Mammogram/Ultrasound	1,053	11.7%	10.2%	8.8%
Lumbar Spine MRI for Low Back Pain	60	43.3%	35.2%	37.2%

Twin Cities Hospital

2190 Hwy 85 N — Phone: 850-678-4131
Niceville, FL 32578 — Fax: 850-729-9473
URL: www.tchealthcare.com
Type: Acute Care Hospitals — Emergency Services: Yes
Ownership: Proprietary — Beds: 65

Key Personnel:
Chief of Medical Staff. . . . . William Abernathy, MD
Radiology. . . . . Thomas Ballard
Operating Room. . . . . Belinda Richardson, RN
Quality Assurance . . . . Evelyn Ross
CEO/President. . . . . David A Whalen

Measure	Cases	This Hosp.	State Avg.	U.S. Avg.
Blood Clot Prevention and Treatment				
Anticoagulation Overlap Therapy[2]	12	100%	93%	93%
ICU Venous Thromboembolism Prophylaxis[2]	82	100%	94%	92%
Incidence of Potentially Preventable VTE[2,7]	-	-	10%	10%
UFH with Dosages/Platelet Monitoring[1,2]	-	-	100%	97%
Venous Thromboembolism Prophylaxis[2]	139	100%	88%	85%
Warfarin Therapy Discharge Instructions[2]	11	100%	85%	75%
Chest Pain/Possible Heart Attack Care				
Aspirin Given Within 24 Hours of Arrival	34	97%	98%	96%
Fibrinolytic Meds Within 30 Min. of Arrival[7]	-	-	81%	58%
Average Time to ECG (minutes)	34	6	7	7
Average Time to Transfer (minutes)[1]	-	-	53	60
Children's Asthma Care				
Received Home Management Plan of Care	-	-	-	88%
Received Reliever Medication	-	-	-	100%
Received Systemic Corticosteroids	-	-	-	100%
Emergency Department				
Admittance Decision Time (minutes)[2]	353	69	111	98
Head CT Results Within 45 Min. of Arrival[1]	-	-	64%	57%
Patients Who Left ER Before Being Seen	15,173	2%	2%	2%
Time from ER Arrival to Admit. (minutes)[2]	353	228	289	274
Time from ER Arrival to Discharge (minutes)	388	116	147	134
Time in ER Before Being Evaluated (minutes)	429	17	26	26
Time to Pain Meds for Fractures (minutes)	50	63	60	57
Heart Attack Care				
Aspirin Given at Discharge[1]	-	-	99%	99%
Fibrinolytic Meds Within 30 Min. of Arrival[7]	-	-	50%	54%
PCI Within 90 Minutes of Arrival[7]	-	-	96%	96%
Statin Prescribed at Discharge[1]	-	-	99%	98%
Heart Failure Care				
ACE Inhibitor or ARB for LVSD	15	100%	98%	97%
Discharge Instructions Given	49	100%	96%	94%
Evaluation of LVS Function	66	100%	100%	99%
Medicare Spending				
Medicare Spending per Patient (ratio)	-	0.95	1.04	0.98
Pneumonia Care				
Appropriate Initial Antibiotic Given	41	100%	98%	95%
Blood Culture Timing	79	100%	99%	98%
Pregnancy and Delivery Care				
Newborn Deliveries Scheduled Early[2,7]	-	-	6%	6%
Preventive Care				
Immunization for Influenza[2]	289	100%	94%	90%
Immunization for Pneumonia[2]	434	100%	96%	92%
Stroke Care				
Anticoagulation Therapy for Atrial Fibrillation[2,3]	-	-	97%	95%

NOTE: Hospital profiles are in alphabetical order by state, then city, then hospital within the city; Rankings exclude hospitals with less than 25 cases except for patient surveys which excludes hospitals with less than 100 cases; (a) 100-299 cases; (1) The number of cases/patients is too few to report; (2) Data submitted were based on a sample of cases/patients; (3) Results are based on a shorter time period than required; (4) Data suppressed by CMS for one or more quarters; (5) Results are not available for this reporting period; (6) Fewer than 100 patients completed the HCAHPS survey; (7) No cases met the criteria for this measure; (8) The lower limit of the confidence interval cannot be calculated if the number of observed infections equals zero; (9) No data are available from the state/territory for this reporting period; (10) The scores shown reflect fewer than 50 completed surveys; (11) There were discrepancies in the data collection process; (12) This measure does not apply to this hospital for this reporting period; (13) Results cannot be calculated for this reporting period; (14) The results for this state are combined with nearby states to protect confidentiality; Please refer to the User's Guide for a full explanation of data.

Measure	Cases	This Hosp.	State Avg.	U.S. Avg.
Antithrombotic Therapy Timing[1,2]	-	-	98%	98%
Assessed for Rehabilitation[1,2]	-	-	97%	97%
Discharged on Antithrombotic Therapy[1,2]	-	-	99%	99%
Discharged on Statin Medication[1,2]	-	-	96%	94%
Thrombolytic Therapy Timing[2,3]	-	-	76%	66%
Venous Thromboembolism Prophylaxis[1,2]	-	-	95%	94%
Written Stroke Educational Materials Given[1,2]	-	-	94%	88%
Surgical Care Improvement Project				
Appropriate Beta Blocker Usage	58	100%	99%	98%
Appropriate VTP Within 24 Hours	156	99%	99%	98%
Controlled Postoperative Blood Glucose[7]	-	-	98%	97%
Perioperative Temperature Management	178	100%	100%	100%
Prophylactic Antibiotic Selection	121	100%	99%	99%
Prophylactic Antibiotic Selection (Outpatient)	25	100%	98%	98%
Prophylactic Antibiotic Stopped	120	99%	98%	98%
Prophylactic Antibiotic Timing	121	100%	99%	99%
Prophylactic Antibiotic Timing (Outpatient)	25	100%	98%	98%
Urinary Catheter Removal	126	100%	98%	97%
Survey of Patients' Hospital Experiences				
Area Around Room 'Always' Quiet at Night	300+	60%	58%	61%
Doctors 'Always' Communicated Well	300+	88%	77%	82%
Home Recovery Information Given	300+	93%	83%	85%
Hospital Given 9 or 10 on 10 Point Scale	300+	76%	67%	71%
Meds 'Always' Explained Before Given	300+	70%	60%	64%
Nurses 'Always' Communicated Well	300+	81%	75%	79%
Pain 'Always' Well Controlled	300+	75%	68%	71%
Room and Bathroom 'Always' Clean	300+	70%	69%	73%
Timely Help 'Always' Received	300+	72%	62%	68%
Would Definitely Recommend Hospital	300+	80%	69%	71%
Use of Medical Imaging				
Cardiac Imaging Stress Test before Surgery	98	8.2%	6.4%	5.3%
Combination Abdominal CT Scan	335	22.4%	11.8%	10.5%
Combination Brain/Sinus CT Scan	441	4.5%	3.4%	2.7%
Combination Chest CT Scan	134	0.0%	2.4%	2.7%
Follow-up Mammogram/Ultrasound	385	17.4%	10.2%	8.8%
Lumbar Spine MRI for Low Back Pain[1]	-	-	35.2%	37.2%

Munroe Regional Medical Center

1500 Sw 1st Ave
Ocala, FL 34474
Phone: 352-351-7200
Fax: 352-351-7201
URL: www.munroeregional.com
Type: Acute Care Hospitals
Emergency Services: Yes
Ownership: Govt - Hospital Dist/Auth
Beds: 421

Key Personnel:

Chief of Medical Staff. . . . . Perin Alfred, MD
Radiology. . . . . Karn Lappi
CEO/President. . . . . Richard D. Mutarelli, CPA, MBA
Emergency Room . . . . Vicky Nelson
Quality Assurance . . . . Cynthia Prewitt
Pediatric In-Patient Care . . . . Humerea Qamar

Measure	Cases	This Hosp.	State Avg.	U.S. Avg.
Blood Clot Prevention and Treatment				
Anticoagulation Overlap Therapy[2]	182	82%	93%	93%
ICU Venous Thromboembolism Prophylaxis[2]	42	93%	94%	92%
Incidence of Potentially Preventable VTE[2]	15	27%	10%	10%
UFH with Dosages/Platelet Monitoring[2]	204	100%	100%	97%
Venous Thromboembolism Prophylaxis[2]	354	67%	88%	85%
Warfarin Therapy Discharge Instructions[2]	146	0%	85%	75%
Chest Pain/Possible Heart Attack Care				
Aspirin Given Within 24 Hours of Arrival[1,3]	-	-	98%	96%
Fibrinolytic Meds Within 30 Min. of Arrival[5]	-	-	81%	58%
Average Time to ECG (minutes)[1,3]	-	-	7	7
Average Time to Transfer (minutes)[5]	-	-	53	60
Children's Asthma Care				
Received Home Management Plan of Care	-	-	-	88%
Received Reliever Medication	-	-	-	100%
Received Systemic Corticosteroids	-	-	-	100%
Emergency Department				
Admittance Decision Time (minutes)[2]	639	172	111	98
Head CT Results Within 45 Min. of Arrival[1]	-	-	64%	57%
Patients Who Left ER Before Being Seen	>100k	5%	2%	2%
Time from ER Arrival to Admit. (minutes)[2]	643	413	289	274
Time from ER Arrival to Discharge (minutes)	341	125	147	134
Time in ER Before Being Evaluated (minutes)	369	40	26	26
Time to Pain Meds for Fractures (minutes)	257	66	60	57
Heart Attack Care				
Aspirin Given at Discharge	559	99%	99%	99%
Fibrinolytic Meds Within 30 Min. of Arrival[7]	-	-	50%	54%
PCI Within 90 Minutes of Arrival	58	91%	96%	96%
Statin Prescribed at Discharge	545	91%	99%	98%
Heart Failure Care				
ACE Inhibitor or ARB for LVSD[2]	87	89%	98%	97%
Discharge Instructions Given[2]	222	86%	96%	94%
Evaluation of LVS Function[2]	269	100%	100%	99%
Medicare Spending				
Medicare Spending per Patient (ratio)	-	1.04	1.04	0.98
Pneumonia Care				
Appropriate Initial Antibiotic Given[2]	96	96%	98%	95%
Blood Culture Timing[2]	150	96%	99%	98%
Pregnancy and Delivery Care				
Newborn Deliveries Scheduled Early	318	19%	6%	6%
Preventive Care				
Immunization for Influenza[2]	528	93%	94%	90%
Immunization for Pneumonia[2]	783	92%	96%	92%
Stroke Care				
Anticoagulation Therapy for Atrial Fibrillation[2]	28	93%	97%	95%
Antithrombotic Therapy Timing[2]	119	95%	98%	98%
Assessed for Rehabilitation[2]	132	99%	97%	97%
Discharged on Antithrombotic Therapy[2]	124	98%	99%	99%
Discharged on Statin Medication[2]	87	87%	96%	94%
Thrombolytic Therapy Timing[1,2]	-	-	76%	66%
Venous Thromboembolism Prophylaxis[2]	130	93%	95%	94%
Written Stroke Educational Materials Given[2]	91	92%	94%	88%
Surgical Care Improvement Project				
Appropriate Beta Blocker Usage[2]	265	99%	99%	98%
Appropriate VTP Within 24 Hours[2]	292	95%	99%	98%
Controlled Postoperative Blood Glucose[2]	136	97%	98%	97%
Perioperative Temperature Management[2]	422	99%	100%	100%
Prophylactic Antibiotic Selection[2]	386	98%	99%	99%
Prophylactic Antibiotic Selection (Outpatient)	545	96%	98%	98%
Prophylactic Antibiotic Stopped[2]	373	94%	98%	98%
Prophylactic Antibiotic Timing[2]	387	96%	99%	99%
Prophylactic Antibiotic Timing (Outpatient)	559	93%	98%	98%
Urinary Catheter Removal[2]	381	90%	98%	97%
Survey of Patients' Hospital Experiences				
Area Around Room 'Always' Quiet at Night	300+	54%	58%	61%
Doctors 'Always' Communicated Well	300+	72%	77%	82%
Home Recovery Information Given	300+	82%	83%	85%
Hospital Given 9 or 10 on 10 Point Scale	300+	66%	67%	71%
Meds 'Always' Explained Before Given	300+	55%	60%	64%
Nurses 'Always' Communicated Well	300+	73%	75%	79%
Pain 'Always' Well Controlled	300+	67%	68%	71%
Room and Bathroom 'Always' Clean	300+	65%	69%	73%
Timely Help 'Always' Received	300+	55%	62%	68%
Would Definitely Recommend Hospital	300+	71%	69%	71%
Use of Medical Imaging				
Cardiac Imaging Stress Test before Surgery	576	5.6%	6.4%	5.3%
Combination Abdominal CT Scan	1,239	2.4%	11.8%	10.5%
Combination Brain/Sinus CT Scan	1,899	2.2%	3.4%	2.7%
Combination Chest CT Scan	327	2.1%	2.4%	2.7%
Follow-up Mammogram/Ultrasound[7]	-	-	10.2%	8.8%
Lumbar Spine MRI for Low Back Pain[1]	-	-	35.2%	37.2%

Ocala Regional Medical Center

1431 Sw 1st Ave
Ocala, FL 34478
Phone: 352-401-1000
Fax: 352-401-1198
URL: www.ocalaregional.com
Type: Acute Care Hospitals
Emergency Services: Yes
Ownership: Proprietary
Beds: 200

Key Personnel:

Radiology. . . . . Dana Mark Allen
Emergency Room . . . . Susan Atkin
Hemotology Center . . . . Linda Dolhay
Operating Room. . . . . Rochelle Jones
President . . . . Michael Joyce
Quality Assurance . . . . Carol Marlin
Cardiac Laboratory. . . . . Gloria Nolan
Chief of Medical Staff . . . . Larry Popeil

Measure	Cases	This Hosp.	State Avg.	U.S. Avg.
Blood Clot Prevention and Treatment				
Anticoagulation Overlap Therapy[2]	158	97%	93%	93%
ICU Venous Thromboembolism Prophylaxis[2]	95	100%	94%	92%
Incidence of Potentially Preventable VTE[2]	21	0%	10%	10%
UFH with Dosages/Platelet Monitoring[2]	179	100%	100%	97%
Venous Thromboembolism Prophylaxis[2]	356	96%	88%	85%
Warfarin Therapy Discharge Instructions[2]	120	100%	85%	75%
Chest Pain/Possible Heart Attack Care				
Aspirin Given Within 24 Hours of Arrival[1,3]	-	-	98%	96%
Fibrinolytic Meds Within 30 Min. of Arrival[5]	-	-	81%	58%
Average Time to ECG (minutes)[1,3]	-	-	7	7
Average Time to Transfer (minutes)[5]	-	-	53	60
Children's Asthma Care				
Received Home Management Plan of Care	-	-	-	88%
Received Reliever Medication	-	-	-	100%
Received Systemic Corticosteroids	-	-	-	100%
Emergency Department				
Admittance Decision Time (minutes)[2]	995	116	111	98
Head CT Results Within 45 Min. of Arrival[1]	-	-	64%	57%
Patients Who Left ER Before Being Seen	75,969	1%	2%	2%
Time from ER Arrival to Admit. (minutes)[2]	995	299	289	274
Time from ER Arrival to Discharge (minutes)	445	159	147	134
Time in ER Before Being Evaluated (minutes)	532	20	26	26
Time to Pain Meds for Fractures (minutes)	117	56	60	57
Heart Attack Care				
Aspirin Given at Discharge	298	100%	99%	99%
Fibrinolytic Meds Within 30 Min. of Arrival[7]	-	-	50%	54%
PCI Within 90 Minutes of Arrival	18	89%	96%	96%
Statin Prescribed at Discharge	289	100%	99%	98%
Heart Failure Care				
ACE Inhibitor or ARB for LVSD[2]	108	100%	98%	97%
Discharge Instructions Given[2]	235	100%	96%	94%
Evaluation of LVS Function[2]	274	100%	100%	99%
Medicare Spending				
Medicare Spending per Patient (ratio)	-	1.01	1.04	0.98
Pneumonia Care				
Appropriate Initial Antibiotic Given[2]	102	100%	98%	95%
Blood Culture Timing[2]	203	99%	99%	98%
Pregnancy and Delivery Care				
Newborn Deliveries Scheduled Early[2,7]	-	-	6%	6%
Preventive Care				
Immunization for Influenza[2]	697	100%	94%	90%
Immunization for Pneumonia[2]	1,065	100%	96%	92%
Stroke Care				
Anticoagulation Therapy for Atrial Fibrillation[1,2]	-	-	97%	95%
Antithrombotic Therapy Timing[2]	99	99%	98%	98%
Assessed for Rehabilitation[2]	99	98%	97%	97%
Discharged on Antithrombotic Therapy[2]	95	99%	99%	99%
Discharged on Statin Medication[2]	75	97%	96%	94%
Thrombolytic Therapy Timing[1,2]	-	-	76%	66%
Venous Thromboembolism Prophylaxis[2]	112	97%	95%	94%
Written Stroke Educational Materials Given[2]	69	100%	94%	88%
Surgical Care Improvement Project				
Appropriate Beta Blocker Usage[2]	227	99%	99%	98%
Appropriate VTP Within 24 Hours[2]	521	100%	99%	98%
Controlled Postoperative Blood Glucose[2]	89	98%	98%	97%
Perioperative Temperature Management[2]	640	100%	100%	100%
Prophylactic Antibiotic Selection[2]	476	100%	99%	99%
Prophylactic Antibiotic Selection (Outpatient)	324	100%	98%	98%
Prophylactic Antibiotic Stopped[2]	445	100%	98%	98%
Prophylactic Antibiotic Timing[2]	477	100%	99%	99%
Prophylactic Antibiotic Timing (Outpatient)	324	100%	98%	98%
Urinary Catheter Removal[2]	483	100%	98%	97%
Survey of Patients' Hospital Experiences				
Area Around Room 'Always' Quiet at Night	300+	58%	58%	61%
Doctors 'Always' Communicated Well	300+	74%	77%	82%
Home Recovery Information Given	300+	85%	83%	85%
Hospital Given 9 or 10 on 10 Point Scale	300+	64%	67%	71%
Meds 'Always' Explained Before Given	300+	56%	60%	64%
Nurses 'Always' Communicated Well	300+	71%	75%	79%
Pain 'Always' Well Controlled	300+	64%	68%	71%

NOTE: Hospital profiles are in alphabetical order by state, then city, then hospital within the city; Rankings exclude hospitals with less than 25 cases except for patient surveys which excludes hospitals with less than 100 cases; (a) 100-299 cases; (1) The number of cases/patients is too few to report; (2) Data submitted were based on a sample of cases/patients; (3) Results are based on a shorter time period than required; (4) Data suppressed by CMS for one or more quarters; (5) Results are not available for this reporting period; (6) Fewer than 100 patients completed the HCAHPS survey; (7) No cases met the criteria for this measure; (8) The lower limit of the confidence interval cannot be calculated if the number of observed infections equals zero; (9) No data are available from the state/territory for this reporting period; (10) The scores shown reflect fewer than 50 completed surveys; (11) There were discrepancies in the data collection process; (12) This measure does not apply to this hospital for this reporting period; (13) Results cannot be calculated for this reporting period; (14) The results for this state are combined with nearby states to protect confidentiality; Please refer to the User's Guide for a full explanation of data.

Measure	Cases	This Hosp.	State Avg.	U.S. Avg.
Room and Bathroom 'Always' Clean	300+	66%	69%	73%
Timely Help 'Always' Received	300+	55%	62%	68%
Would Definitely Recommend Hospital	300+	68%	69%	71%
Use of Medical Imaging				
Cardiac Imaging Stress Test before Surgery	273	3.3%	6.4%	5.3%
Combination Abdominal CT Scan	1,150	2.0%	11.8%	10.5%
Combination Brain/Sinus CT Scan	1,384	3.8%	3.4%	2.7%
Combination Chest CT Scan	240	1.3%	2.4%	2.7%
Follow-up Mammogram/Ultrasound[7]	-	-	10.2%	8.8%
Lumbar Spine MRI for Low Back Pain[1]	-	-	35.2%	37.2%

Health Central

10000 W Colonial Dr
Ocoee, FL 34761
Phone: 407-296-1820
Fax: 407-290-2118
E-mail: darlenel@health-central.org
URL: www.health-central.org
Type: Acute Care Hospitals
Emergency Services: Yes
Ownership: Government - State
Beds: 171

Key Personnel:

Radiology. . . . . Neil W Baron, MD
Operating Room. . . . . Matthew D Hurbanis, MD
CEO/President. . . . . Richard M Irwin, Jr
Chief of Medical Staff . . . . Pran M Kar, MD
Emergency Room . . . . Terry Kemp
Quality Assurance . . . . Bart Rodier, MD
Pediatric Ambulatory Care . . . . . . Lewis Wasserman, MD
Pediatric In-Patient Care . . . . Lewis Wasserman, MD

Measure	Cases	This Hosp.	State Avg.	U.S. Avg.
Blood Clot Prevention and Treatment				
Anticoagulation Overlap Therapy[2]	86	100%	93%	93%
ICU Venous Thromboembolism Prophylaxis[2]	38	100%	94%	92%
Incidence of Potentially Preventable VTE[1,2]	-	-	10%	10%
UFH with Dosages/Platelet Monitoring[2]	23	100%	100%	97%
Venous Thromboembolism Prophylaxis[2]	549	99%	88%	85%
Warfarin Therapy Discharge Instructions[2]	66	98%	85%	75%
Chest Pain/Possible Heart Attack Care				
Aspirin Given Within 24 Hours of Arrival[1,3]	-	-	98%	96%
Fibrinolytic Meds Within 30 Min. of Arrival[3,7]	-	-	81%	58%
Average Time to ECG (minutes)[1,3]	-	-	7	7
Average Time to Transfer (minutes)[3,7]	-	-	53	60
Children's Asthma Care				
Received Home Management Plan of Care	-	-	-	88%
Received Reliever Medication	-	-	-	100%
Received Systemic Corticosteroids	-	-	-	100%
Emergency Department				
Admittance Decision Time (minutes)[2]	990	107	111	98
Head CT Results Within 45 Min. of Arrival	25	84%	64%	57%
Patients Who Left ER Before Being Seen	63,021	1%	2%	2%
Time from ER Arrival to Admit. (minutes)[2]	990	373	289	274
Time from ER Arrival to Discharge (minutes)	4,741	196	147	134
Time in ER Before Being Evaluated (minutes)	5,077	83	26	26
Time to Pain Meds for Fractures (minutes)	237	93	60	57
Heart Attack Care				
Aspirin Given at Discharge	145	100%	99%	99%
Fibrinolytic Meds Within 30 Min. of Arrival[7]	-	-	50%	54%
PCI Within 90 Minutes of Arrival	32	100%	96%	96%
Statin Prescribed at Discharge	138	100%	99%	98%
Heart Failure Care				
ACE Inhibitor or ARB for LVSD	90	100%	98%	97%
Discharge Instructions Given	261	100%	96%	94%
Evaluation of LVS Function	317	100%	100%	99%
Medicare Spending				
Medicare Spending per Patient (ratio)	-	1.06	1.04	0.98
Pneumonia Care				
Appropriate Initial Antibiotic Given	148	100%	98%	95%
Blood Culture Timing	215	99%	99%	98%
Pregnancy and Delivery Care				
Newborn Deliveries Scheduled Early	73	10%	6%	6%
Preventive Care				
Immunization for Influenza[2]	613	92%	94%	90%
Immunization for Pneumonia[2]	763	95%	96%	92%
Stroke Care				
Anticoagulation Therapy for Atrial Fibrillation[1]	-	-	97%	95%
Antithrombotic Therapy Timing	72	100%	98%	98%
Assessed for Rehabilitation	79	100%	97%	97%
Discharged on Antithrombotic Therapy	69	100%	99%	99%
Discharged on Statin Medication	57	96%	96%	94%
Thrombolytic Therapy Timing[7]	-	-	76%	66%
Venous Thromboembolism Prophylaxis	85	96%	95%	94%
Written Stroke Educational Materials Given	56	100%	94%	88%
Surgical Care Improvement Project				
Appropriate Beta Blocker Usage	197	98%	99%	98%
Appropriate VTP Within 24 Hours	570	100%	99%	98%
Controlled Postoperative Blood Glucose[7]	-	-	98%	97%
Perioperative Temperature Management	655	100%	100%	100%
Prophylactic Antibiotic Selection	493	99%	99%	99%
Prophylactic Antibiotic Selection (Outpatient)	196	98%	98%	98%
Prophylactic Antibiotic Stopped	475	99%	98%	98%
Prophylactic Antibiotic Timing	493	100%	99%	99%
Prophylactic Antibiotic Timing (Outpatient)	197	99%	98%	98%
Urinary Catheter Removal	452	100%	98%	97%
Survey of Patients' Hospital Experiences				
Area Around Room 'Always' Quiet at Night	300+	64%	58%	61%
Doctors 'Always' Communicated Well	300+	76%	77%	82%
Home Recovery Information Given	300+	76%	83%	85%
Hospital Given 9 or 10 on 10 Point Scale	300+	68%	67%	71%
Meds 'Always' Explained Before Given	300+	63%	60%	64%
Nurses 'Always' Communicated Well	300+	79%	75%	79%
Pain 'Always' Well Controlled	300+	69%	68%	71%
Room and Bathroom 'Always' Clean	300+	76%	69%	73%
Timely Help 'Always' Received	300+	64%	62%	68%
Would Definitely Recommend Hospital	300+	69%	69%	71%
Use of Medical Imaging				
Cardiac Imaging Stress Test before Surgery	192	5.7%	6.4%	5.3%
Combination Abdominal CT Scan	532	3.2%	11.8%	10.5%
Combination Brain/Sinus CT Scan	734	5.6%	3.4%	2.7%
Combination Chest CT Scan	246	12.2%	2.4%	2.7%
Follow-up Mammogram/Ultrasound	790	7.0%	10.2%	8.8%
Lumbar Spine MRI for Low Back Pain	51	33.3%	35.2%	37.2%

Raulerson Hospital

1796 Hwy 441 North
Okeechobee, FL 34972
Phone: 863-763-2151
Fax: 863-824-2991
URL: www.raulersonhospital.com
Type: Acute Care Hospitals
Emergency Services: Yes
Ownership: Proprietary
Beds: 101

Key Personnel:

Chief of Medical Staff. . . . . Iqbal Ahmed
CEO/President. . . . . Robert Lee

Measure	Cases	This Hosp.	State Avg.	U.S. Avg.
Blood Clot Prevention and Treatment				
Anticoagulation Overlap Therapy[2]	32	100%	93%	93%
ICU Venous Thromboembolism Prophylaxis[2]	88	100%	94%	92%
Incidence of Potentially Preventable VTE[1,2]	-	-	10%	10%
UFH with Dosages/Platelet Monitoring[2]	11	100%	100%	97%
Venous Thromboembolism Prophylaxis[2]	365	98%	88%	85%
Warfarin Therapy Discharge Instructions[2]	25	100%	85%	75%
Chest Pain/Possible Heart Attack Care				
Aspirin Given Within 24 Hours of Arrival	58	100%	98%	96%
Fibrinolytic Meds Within 30 Min. of Arrival[1]	-	-	81%	58%
Average Time to ECG (minutes)	61	7	7	7
Average Time to Transfer (minutes)[1]	-	-	53	60
Children's Asthma Care				
Received Home Management Plan of Care	-	-	-	88%
Received Reliever Medication	-	-	-	100%
Received Systemic Corticosteroids	-	-	-	100%
Emergency Department				
Admittance Decision Time (minutes)[2]	888	71	111	98
Head CT Results Within 45 Min. of Arrival[1]	-	-	64%	57%
Patients Who Left ER Before Being Seen	25,018	0%	2%	2%
Time from ER Arrival to Admit. (minutes)[2]	888	217	289	274
Time from ER Arrival to Discharge (minutes)	449	122	147	134
Time in ER Before Being Evaluated (minutes)	501	8	26	26
Time to Pain Meds for Fractures (minutes)	93	50	60	57
Heart Attack Care				
Aspirin Given at Discharge	32	100%	99%	99%
Fibrinolytic Meds Within 30 Min. of Arrival[7]	-	-	50%	54%
PCI Within 90 Minutes of Arrival[7]	-	-	96%	96%
Statin Prescribed at Discharge	30	100%	99%	98%
Heart Failure Care				
ACE Inhibitor or ARB for LVSD	76	100%	98%	97%
Discharge Instructions Given	201	100%	96%	94%
Evaluation of LVS Function	235	100%	100%	99%
Medicare Spending				
Medicare Spending per Patient (ratio)	-	0.96	1.04	0.98
Pneumonia Care				
Appropriate Initial Antibiotic Given	57	100%	98%	95%
Blood Culture Timing	115	100%	99%	98%
Pregnancy and Delivery Care				
Newborn Deliveries Scheduled Early[2,7]	-	-	6%	6%
Preventive Care				
Immunization for Influenza[2]	509	100%	94%	90%
Immunization for Pneumonia[2]	802	100%	96%	92%
Stroke Care				
Anticoagulation Therapy for Atrial Fibrillation[1,2]	-	-	97%	95%
Antithrombotic Therapy Timing[2]	46	100%	98%	98%
Assessed for Rehabilitation[2]	48	100%	97%	97%
Discharged on Antithrombotic Therapy[2]	44	98%	99%	99%
Discharged on Statin Medication[2]	32	97%	96%	94%
Thrombolytic Therapy Timing[1,2]	-	-	76%	66%
Venous Thromboembolism Prophylaxis[2]	48	98%	95%	94%
Written Stroke Educational Materials Given[2]	39	100%	94%	88%
Surgical Care Improvement Project				
Appropriate Beta Blocker Usage	48	100%	99%	98%
Appropriate VTP Within 24 Hours	125	100%	99%	98%
Controlled Postoperative Blood Glucose[7]	-	-	98%	97%
Perioperative Temperature Management	141	100%	100%	100%
Prophylactic Antibiotic Selection	59	100%	99%	99%
Prophylactic Antibiotic Selection (Outpatient)	100	100%	98%	98%
Prophylactic Antibiotic Stopped	49	100%	98%	98%
Prophylactic Antibiotic Timing	59	100%	99%	99%
Prophylactic Antibiotic Timing (Outpatient)	100	100%	98%	98%
Urinary Catheter Removal	52	100%	98%	97%
Survey of Patients' Hospital Experiences				
Area Around Room 'Always' Quiet at Night	300+	60%	58%	61%
Doctors 'Always' Communicated Well	300+	77%	77%	82%
Home Recovery Information Given	300+	84%	83%	85%
Hospital Given 9 or 10 on 10 Point Scale	300+	67%	67%	71%
Meds 'Always' Explained Before Given	300+	64%	60%	64%
Nurses 'Always' Communicated Well	300+	78%	75%	79%
Pain 'Always' Well Controlled	300+	69%	68%	71%
Room and Bathroom 'Always' Clean	300+	70%	69%	73%
Timely Help 'Always' Received	300+	67%	62%	68%
Would Definitely Recommend Hospital	300+	64%	69%	71%
Use of Medical Imaging				
Cardiac Imaging Stress Test before Surgery[1]	-	-	6.4%	5.3%
Combination Abdominal CT Scan	434	9.0%	11.8%	10.5%
Combination Brain/Sinus CT Scan[1]	-	-	3.4%	2.7%
Combination Chest CT Scan	144	8.3%	2.4%	2.7%
Follow-up Mammogram/Ultrasound	629	4.9%	10.2%	8.8%
Lumbar Spine MRI for Low Back Pain[1]	-	-	35.2%	37.2%

Florida Hospital Fish Memorial

1055 Saxon Blvd
Orange City, FL 32763
Phone: 386-917-5000
Fax: 386-917-5425
URL: www.fhfishmemorial.org
Type: Acute Care Hospitals
Emergency Services: Yes
Ownership: Voluntary non-profit - Church
Beds: 139

Key Personnel:

Infection Control. . . . . Jackie Adkins
Operating Room. . . . . Rene A Capulong
CEO/President. . . . . Joe Johnson
Intensive Care Unit. . . . . Evelyn Lopez
Quality Assurance . . . . Jill Pace
Emergency Room . . . . Deborah Palmer
Radiology. . . . . Mike Wilmore

Measure	Cases	This Hosp.	State Avg.	U.S. Avg.
Blood Clot Prevention and Treatment				
Anticoagulation Overlap Therapy[2]	66	92%	93%	93%
ICU Venous Thromboembolism Prophylaxis[2]	93	95%	94%	92%
Incidence of Potentially Preventable VTE[2]	16	19%	10%	10%

NOTE: Hospital profiles are in alphabetical order by state, then city, then hospital within the city; Rankings exclude hospitals with less than 25 cases except for patient surveys which excludes hospitals with less than 100 cases; (a) 100-299 cases; (1) The number of cases/patients is too few to report; (2) Data submitted were based on a sample of cases/patients; (3) Results are based on a shorter time period than required; (4) Data suppressed by CMS for one or more quarters; (5) Results are not available for this reporting period; (6) Fewer than 100 patients completed the HCAHPS survey; (7) No cases met the criteria for this measure; (8) The lower limit of the confidence interval cannot be calculated if the number of observed infections equals zero; (9) No data are available from the state/territory for this reporting period; (10) The scores shown reflect fewer than 50 completed surveys; (11) There were discrepancies in the data collection process; (12) This measure does not apply to this hospital for this reporting period; (13) Results cannot be calculated for this reporting period; (14) The results for this state are combined with nearby states to protect confidentiality; Please refer to the User's Guide for a full explanation of data.

UFH with Dosages/Platelet Monitoring[2]	43	100%	100%	97%
Venous Thromboembolism Prophylaxis[2]	356	87%	88%	85%
Warfarin Therapy Discharge Instructions[2]	41	85%	85%	75%
Chest Pain/Possible Heart Attack Care				
Aspirin Given Within 24 Hours of Arrival	49	92%	98%	96%
Fibrinolytic Meds Within 30 Min. of Arrival[7]	-	-	81%	58%
Average Time to ECG (minutes)	44	7	7	7
Average Time to Transfer (minutes)	21	57	53	60
Children's Asthma Care				
Received Home Management Plan of Care	-	-	-	88%
Received Reliever Medication	-	-	-	100%
Received Systemic Corticosteroids	-	-	-	100%
Emergency Department				
Admittance Decision Time (minutes)[2]	566	143	111	98
Head CT Results Within 45 Min. of Arrival	15	40%	64%	57%
Patients Who Left ER Before Being Seen	49,712	3%	2%	2%
Time from ER Arrival to Admit. (minutes)[2]	568	416	289	274
Time from ER Arrival to Discharge (minutes)	337	170	147	134
Time in ER Before Being Evaluated (minutes)	358	58	26	26
Time to Pain Meds for Fractures (minutes)	133	91	60	57
Heart Attack Care				
Aspirin Given at Discharge	53	100%	99%	99%
Fibrinolytic Meds Within 30 Min. of Arrival[7]	-	-	50%	54%
PCI Within 90 Minutes of Arrival[7]	-	-	96%	96%
Statin Prescribed at Discharge	49	100%	99%	98%
Heart Failure Care				
ACE Inhibitor or ARB for LVSD	142	99%	98%	97%
Discharge Instructions Given	352	98%	96%	94%
Evaluation of LVS Function	466	100%	100%	99%
Medicare Spending				
Medicare Spending per Patient (ratio)	-	1.04	1.04	0.98
Pneumonia Care				
Appropriate Initial Antibiotic Given	175	98%	98%	95%
Blood Culture Timing	339	97%	99%	98%
Pregnancy and Delivery Care				
Newborn Deliveries Scheduled Early[7]	-	-	6%	6%
Preventive Care				
Immunization for Influenza[2]	587	84%	94%	90%
Immunization for Pneumonia[2]	887	88%	96%	92%
Stroke Care				
Anticoagulation Therapy for Atrial Fibrillation[2]	22	100%	97%	95%
Antithrombotic Therapy Timing[2]	101	97%	98%	98%
Assessed for Rehabilitation[2]	102	95%	97%	97%
Discharged on Antithrombotic Therapy[2]	101	100%	99%	99%
Discharged on Statin Medication[2]	83	92%	96%	94%
Thrombolytic Therapy Timing[1,2]	-	-	76%	66%
Venous Thromboembolism Prophylaxis[2]	103	92%	95%	94%
Written Stroke Educational Materials Given[2]	58	79%	94%	88%
Surgical Care Improvement Project				
Appropriate Beta Blocker Usage	112	98%	99%	98%
Appropriate VTP Within 24 Hours	353	99%	99%	98%
Controlled Postoperative Blood Glucose[7]	-	-	98%	97%
Perioperative Temperature Management	399	100%	100%	100%
Prophylactic Antibiotic Selection	202	100%	99%	99%
Prophylactic Antibiotic Selection (Outpatient)	133	98%	98%	98%
Prophylactic Antibiotic Stopped	194	98%	98%	98%
Prophylactic Antibiotic Timing	202	100%	99%	99%
Prophylactic Antibiotic Timing (Outpatient)	135	98%	98%	98%
Urinary Catheter Removal	224	100%	98%	97%
Survey of Patients' Hospital Experiences				
Area Around Room 'Always' Quiet at Night[11]	300+	57%	58%	61%
Doctors 'Always' Communicated Well[11]	300+	74%	77%	82%
Home Recovery Information Given[11]	300+	83%	83%	85%
Hospital Given 9 or 10 on 10 Point Scale[11]	300+	63%	67%	71%
Meds 'Always' Explained Before Given[11]	300+	61%	60%	64%
Nurses 'Always' Communicated Well[11]	300+	75%	75%	79%
Pain 'Always' Well Controlled[11]	300+	67%	68%	71%
Room and Bathroom 'Always' Clean[11]	300+	69%	69%	73%
Timely Help 'Always' Received[11]	300+	63%	62%	68%
Would Definitely Recommend Hospital[11]	300+	61%	69%	71%
Use of Medical Imaging				
Cardiac Imaging Stress Test before Surgery	119	8.4%	6.4%	5.3%
Combination Abdominal CT Scan	705	6.7%	11.8%	10.5%
Combination Brain/Sinus CT Scan	660	3.2%	3.4%	2.7%
Combination Chest CT Scan	553	0.2%	2.4%	2.7%
Follow-up Mammogram/Ultrasound	928	13.0%	10.2%	8.8%
Lumbar Spine MRI for Low Back Pain	63	44.4%	35.2%	37.2%

Orange Park Medical Center

2001 Kingsley Ave
Orange Park, FL 32073
URL: www.opmedical.com
Type: Acute Care Hospitals
Ownership: Voluntary non-profit - Other
Phone: 904-276-8500
Fax: 904-276-8703
Emergency Services: Yes
Beds: 224

Key Personnel:
Emergency Room . . . . John Cole
CEO/President. . . . . Robert Krieger
Quality Assurance . . . . Sandra Oliver
Chief of Medical Staff . . . . Tony Tullot, MD

Measure	Cases	This Hosp.	State Avg.	U.S. Avg.
Blood Clot Prevention and Treatment				
Anticoagulation Overlap Therapy[2]	113	100%	93%	93%
ICU Venous Thromboembolism Prophylaxis[2]	63	100%	94%	92%
Incidence of Potentially Preventable VTE[2]	24	0%	10%	10%
UFH with Dosages/Platelet Monitoring[2]	84	100%	100%	97%
Venous Thromboembolism Prophylaxis[2]	408	98%	88%	85%
Warfarin Therapy Discharge Instructions[2]	71	100%	85%	75%
Chest Pain/Possible Heart Attack Care				
Aspirin Given Within 24 Hours of Arrival[1,3]	-	-	98%	96%
Fibrinolytic Meds Within 30 Min. of Arrival[3,7]	-	-	81%	58%
Average Time to ECG (minutes)[1,3]	-	-	7	7
Average Time to Transfer (minutes)[3,7]	-	-	53	60
Children's Asthma Care				
Received Home Management Plan of Care	-	-	-	88%
Received Reliever Medication	-	-	-	100%
Received Systemic Corticosteroids	-	-	-	100%
Emergency Department				
Admittance Decision Time (minutes)[2]	881	198	111	98
Head CT Results Within 45 Min. of Arrival[1]	-	-	64%	57%
Patients Who Left ER Before Being Seen	88,906	1%	2%	2%
Time from ER Arrival to Admit. (minutes)[2]	881	355	289	274
Time from ER Arrival to Discharge (minutes)	502	129	147	134
Time in ER Before Being Evaluated (minutes)	528	22	26	26
Time to Pain Meds for Fractures (minutes)	287	75	60	57
Heart Attack Care				
Aspirin Given at Discharge	272	100%	99%	99%
Fibrinolytic Meds Within 30 Min. of Arrival[7]	-	-	50%	54%
PCI Within 90 Minutes of Arrival	39	100%	96%	96%
Statin Prescribed at Discharge	260	100%	99%	98%
Heart Failure Care				
ACE Inhibitor or ARB for LVSD	100	100%	98%	97%
Discharge Instructions Given	383	100%	96%	94%
Evaluation of LVS Function	528	100%	100%	99%
Medicare Spending				
Medicare Spending per Patient (ratio)	-	1.11	1.04	0.98
Pneumonia Care				
Appropriate Initial Antibiotic Given[2]	65	100%	98%	95%
Blood Culture Timing[2]	71	100%	99%	98%
Pregnancy and Delivery Care				
Newborn Deliveries Scheduled Early[2]	66	0%	6%	6%
Preventive Care				
Immunization for Influenza[2]	548	100%	94%	90%
Immunization for Pneumonia[2]	688	100%	96%	92%
Stroke Care				
Anticoagulation Therapy for Atrial Fibrillation[1,2]	-	-	97%	95%
Antithrombotic Therapy Timing[2]	115	100%	98%	98%
Assessed for Rehabilitation[2]	115	98%	97%	97%
Discharged on Antithrombotic Therapy[2]	100	100%	99%	99%
Discharged on Statin Medication[2]	76	99%	96%	94%
Thrombolytic Therapy Timing[1,2]	-	-	76%	66%
Venous Thromboembolism Prophylaxis[2]	129	99%	95%	94%
Written Stroke Educational Materials Given[2]	74	100%	94%	88%
Surgical Care Improvement Project				
Appropriate Beta Blocker Usage[2]	187	100%	99%	98%
Appropriate VTP Within 24 Hours[2]	357	100%	99%	98%
Controlled Postoperative Blood Glucose[2]	71	100%	98%	97%
Perioperative Temperature Management[2]	435	100%	100%	100%
Prophylactic Antibiotic Selection[2]	286	100%	99%	99%
Prophylactic Antibiotic Selection (Outpatient)	486	99%	98%	98%
Prophylactic Antibiotic Stopped[2]	275	100%	98%	98%
Prophylactic Antibiotic Timing[2]	286	100%	99%	99%
Prophylactic Antibiotic Timing (Outpatient)	486	100%	98%	98%
Urinary Catheter Removal[2]	176	100%	98%	97%
Survey of Patients' Hospital Experiences				
Area Around Room 'Always' Quiet at Night	300+	55%	58%	61%
Doctors 'Always' Communicated Well	300+	75%	77%	82%
Home Recovery Information Given	300+	86%	83%	85%
Hospital Given 9 or 10 on 10 Point Scale	300+	64%	67%	71%
Meds 'Always' Explained Before Given	300+	60%	60%	64%
Nurses 'Always' Communicated Well	300+	73%	75%	79%
Pain 'Always' Well Controlled	300+	67%	68%	71%
Room and Bathroom 'Always' Clean	300+	70%	69%	73%
Timely Help 'Always' Received	300+	56%	62%	68%
Would Definitely Recommend Hospital	300+	63%	69%	71%
Use of Medical Imaging				
Cardiac Imaging Stress Test before Surgery	410	7.1%	6.4%	5.3%
Combination Abdominal CT Scan	804	4.4%	11.8%	10.5%
Combination Brain/Sinus CT Scan	928	3.7%	3.4%	2.7%
Combination Chest CT Scan	962	0.1%	2.4%	2.7%
Follow-up Mammogram/Ultrasound	1,170	6.0%	10.2%	8.8%
Lumbar Spine MRI for Low Back Pain	97	37.1%	35.2%	37.2%

Florida Hospital

601 E Rollins St
Orlando, FL 32803
URL: www.floridahospital.com
Type: Acute Care Hospitals
Ownership: Voluntary non-profit - Private
Phone: 407-303-1976
Fax: 407-200-4938
Emergency Services: Yes
Beds: 2,188

Key Personnel:
CEO/President. . . . . Don Jernigan
Chief of Medical Staff . . . . Robert Reynolds, MD

Measure	Cases	This Hosp.	State Avg.	U.S. Avg.
Blood Clot Prevention and Treatment				
Anticoagulation Overlap Therapy[2]	476	96%	93%	93%
ICU Venous Thromboembolism Prophylaxis[2]	137	97%	94%	92%
Incidence of Potentially Preventable VTE[2]	113	7%	10%	10%
UFH with Dosages/Platelet Monitoring[2]	218	100%	100%	97%
Venous Thromboembolism Prophylaxis[2]	1,114	95%	88%	85%
Warfarin Therapy Discharge Instructions[2]	349	83%	85%	75%
Chest Pain/Possible Heart Attack Care				
Aspirin Given Within 24 Hours of Arrival[1,3]	-	-	98%	96%
Fibrinolytic Meds Within 30 Min. of Arrival[3,7]	-	-	81%	58%
Average Time to ECG (minutes)[1,3]	-	-	7	7
Average Time to Transfer (minutes)[1,3]	-	-	53	60
Children's Asthma Care				
Received Home Management Plan of Care	-	-	-	88%
Received Reliever Medication	-	-	-	100%
Received Systemic Corticosteroids	-	-	-	100%
Emergency Department				
Admittance Decision Time (minutes)[2]	754	122	111	98
Head CT Results Within 45 Min. of Arrival[1]	-	-	64%	57%
Patients Who Left ER Before Being Seen	>100k	2%	2%	2%
Time from ER Arrival to Admit. (minutes)[2]	768	328	289	274
Time from ER Arrival to Discharge (minutes)	1,396	168	147	134
Time in ER Before Being Evaluated (minutes)	1,526	41	26	26
Time to Pain Meds for Fractures (minutes)	435	86	60	57
Heart Attack Care				
Aspirin Given at Discharge[2]	1,069	100%	99%	99%
Fibrinolytic Meds Within 30 Min. of Arrival[2,7]	-	-	50%	54%
PCI Within 90 Minutes of Arrival[2]	135	100%	96%	96%
Statin Prescribed at Discharge[2]	1,034	100%	99%	98%
Heart Failure Care				
ACE Inhibitor or ARB for LVSD[2]	696	99%	98%	97%
Discharge Instructions Given[2]	2,142	100%	96%	94%
Evaluation of LVS Function[2]	2,544	100%	100%	99%
Medicare Spending				
Medicare Spending per Patient (ratio)	-	1.04	1.04	0.98
Pneumonia Care				

NOTE: Hospital profiles are in alphabetical order by state, then city, then hospital within the city; Rankings exclude hospitals with less than 25 cases except for patient surveys which excludes hospitals with less than 100 cases; (a) 100-299 cases; (1) The number of cases/patients is too few to report; (2) Data submitted were based on a sample of cases/patients; (3) Results are based on a shorter time period than required; (4) Data suppressed by CMS for one or more quarters; (5) Results are not available for this reporting period; (6) Fewer than 100 patients completed the HCAHPS survey; (7) No cases met the criteria for this measure; (8) The lower limit of the confidence interval cannot be calculated if the number of observed infections equals zero; (9) No data are available from the state/territory for this reporting period; (10) The scores shown reflect fewer than 50 completed surveys; (11) There were discrepancies in the data collection process; (12) This measure does not apply to this hospital for this reporting period; (13) Results cannot be calculated for this reporting period; (14) The results for this state are combined with nearby states to protect confidentiality; Please refer to the User's Guide for a full explanation of data.

Appropriate Initial Antibiotic Given[2]	1,121	99%	98%	95%
Blood Culture Timing[2]	863	99%	99%	98%
Pregnancy and Delivery Care				
Newborn Deliveries Scheduled Early[2]	177	3%	6%	6%
Preventive Care				
Immunization for Influenza[2]	563	88%	94%	90%
Immunization for Pneumonia[2]	654	94%	96%	92%
Stroke Care				
Anticoagulation Therapy for Atrial Fibrillation	143	97%	97%	95%
Antithrombotic Therapy Timing	969	99%	98%	98%
Assessed for Rehabilitation	1,251	96%	97%	97%
Discharged on Antithrombotic Therapy	1,037	99%	99%	99%
Discharged on Statin Medication	836	98%	96%	94%
Thrombolytic Therapy Timing	90	88%	76%	66%
Venous Thromboembolism Prophylaxis	1,335	99%	95%	94%
Written Stroke Educational Materials Given	779	97%	94%	88%
Surgical Care Improvement Project				
Appropriate Beta Blocker Usage[2]	2,121	99%	99%	98%
Appropriate VTP Within 24 Hours[2]	5,531	99%	99%	98%
Controlled Postoperative Blood Glucose[2]	929	98%	98%	97%
Perioperative Temperature Management[2]	7,658	100%	100%	100%
Prophylactic Antibiotic Selection[2]	4,027	99%	99%	99%
Prophylactic Antibiotic Selection (Outpatient)	2,257	96%	98%	98%
Prophylactic Antibiotic Stopped[2]	3,817	99%	98%	98%
Prophylactic Antibiotic Timing[2]	4,036	100%	99%	99%
Prophylactic Antibiotic Timing (Outpatient)	2,266	99%	98%	98%
Urinary Catheter Removal[2]	4,316	100%	98%	97%
Survey of Patients' Hospital Experiences				
Area Around Room 'Always' Quiet at Night	300+	66%	58%	61%
Doctors 'Always' Communicated Well	300+	78%	77%	82%
Home Recovery Information Given	300+	87%	83%	85%
Hospital Given 9 or 10 on 10 Point Scale	300+	76%	67%	71%
Meds 'Always' Explained Before Given	300+	68%	60%	64%
Nurses 'Always' Communicated Well	300+	81%	75%	79%
Pain 'Always' Well Controlled	300+	72%	68%	71%
Room and Bathroom 'Always' Clean	300+	77%	69%	73%
Timely Help 'Always' Received	300+	67%	62%	68%
Would Definitely Recommend Hospital	300+	78%	69%	71%
Use of Medical Imaging				
Cardiac Imaging Stress Test before Surgery	817	5.6%	6.4%	5.3%
Combination Abdominal CT Scan	5,975	28.5%	11.8%	10.5%
Combination Brain/Sinus CT Scan	4,115	3.4%	3.4%	2.7%
Combination Chest CT Scan	3,604	0.3%	2.4%	2.7%
Follow-up Mammogram/Ultrasound	5,930	5.7%	10.2%	8.8%
Lumbar Spine MRI for Low Back Pain	460	36.3%	35.2%	37.2%

Orlando Health

1414 S Kuhl Ave
Orlando, FL 32806
Phone: 321-841-5111
Fax: 407-237-6374
URL: www.orlandoregionalmedicalcenter.org
Type: Acute Care Hospitals
Emergency Services: Yes
Ownership: Voluntary non-profit - Private
Beds: 581

Key Personnel:

Pediatric In-Patient Care .... Raymond Caron, MD
Chief of Medical Staff........... Arnold Lazar, MD
Radiology.................. Mark Mahan, MD
Operating Room.............. Deb Monroe, RN
CEO/President.............. Sherrie Sitarik
Emergency Room .... Lisa Smith

Measure	Cases	This Hosp.	State Avg.	U.S. Avg.
Blood Clot Prevention and Treatment				
Anticoagulation Overlap Therapy[2]	324	96%	93%	93%
ICU Venous Thromboembolism Prophylaxis[2]	96	99%	94%	92%
Incidence of Potentially Preventable VTE[2]	63	2%	10%	10%
UFH with Dosages/Platelet Monitoring[2]	106	100%	100%	97%
Venous Thromboembolism Prophylaxis[2]	606	96%	88%	85%
Warfarin Therapy Discharge Instructions[2]	254	51%	85%	75%
Chest Pain/Possible Heart Attack Care				
Aspirin Given Within 24 Hours of Arrival[1]	-	-	98%	96%
Fibrinolytic Meds Within 30 Min. of Arrival[3,7]	-	-	81%	58%
Average Time to ECG (minutes)[1]	-	-	7	7
Average Time to Transfer (minutes)[3,7]	-	-	53	60
Children's Asthma Care				
Received Home Management Plan of Care	371	94%	-	88%
Received Reliever Medication	371	100%	-	100%
Received Systemic Corticosteroids	371	100%	-	100%
Emergency Department				
Admittance Decision Time (minutes)[2]	456	96	111	98
Head CT Results Within 45 Min. of Arrival[1]	-	-	64%	57%
Patients Who Left ER Before Being Seen	>100k	2%	2%	2%
Time from ER Arrival to Admit. (minutes)[2]	541	335	289	274
Time from ER Arrival to Discharge (minutes)	1,587	176	147	134
Time in ER Before Being Evaluated (minutes)	356	95	26	26
Time to Pain Meds for Fractures (minutes)	568	87	60	57
Heart Attack Care				
Aspirin Given at Discharge	724	99%	99%	99%
Fibrinolytic Meds Within 30 Min. of Arrival[7]	-	-	50%	54%
PCI Within 90 Minutes of Arrival	89	93%	96%	96%
Statin Prescribed at Discharge	720	99%	99%	98%
Heart Failure Care				
ACE Inhibitor or ARB for LVSD	402	99%	98%	97%
Discharge Instructions Given	926	91%	96%	94%
Evaluation of LVS Function	1,054	100%	100%	99%
Medicare Spending				
Medicare Spending per Patient (ratio)	-	1.02	1.04	0.98
Pneumonia Care				
Appropriate Initial Antibiotic Given[2]	291	94%	98%	95%
Blood Culture Timing[2]	534	94%	99%	98%
Pregnancy and Delivery Care				
Newborn Deliveries Scheduled Early[2]	208	4%	6%	6%
Preventive Care				
Immunization for Influenza[2]	629	93%	94%	90%
Immunization for Pneumonia[2]	559	83%	96%	92%
Stroke Care				
Anticoagulation Therapy for Atrial Fibrillation	36	97%	97%	95%
Antithrombotic Therapy Timing	398	98%	98%	98%
Assessed for Rehabilitation	499	98%	97%	97%
Discharged on Antithrombotic Therapy	410	100%	99%	99%
Discharged on Statin Medication	326	98%	96%	94%
Thrombolytic Therapy Timing	24	71%	76%	66%
Venous Thromboembolism Prophylaxis	515	99%	95%	94%
Written Stroke Educational Materials Given	319	90%	94%	88%
Surgical Care Improvement Project				
Appropriate Beta Blocker Usage[2]	1,103	97%	99%	98%
Appropriate VTP Within 24 Hours[2]	2,587	98%	99%	98%
Controlled Postoperative Blood Glucose[2]	265	97%	98%	97%
Perioperative Temperature Management[2]	3,220	100%	100%	100%
Prophylactic Antibiotic Selection[2]	2,012	98%	99%	99%
Prophylactic Antibiotic Selection (Outpatient)	982	99%	98%	98%
Prophylactic Antibiotic Stopped[2]	1,956	98%	98%	98%
Prophylactic Antibiotic Timing[2]	2,015	99%	99%	99%
Prophylactic Antibiotic Timing (Outpatient)	982	99%	98%	98%
Urinary Catheter Removal[2]	2,083	97%	98%	97%
Survey of Patients' Hospital Experiences				
Area Around Room 'Always' Quiet at Night	300+	63%	58%	61%
Doctors 'Always' Communicated Well	300+	77%	77%	82%
Home Recovery Information Given	300+	81%	83%	85%
Hospital Given 9 or 10 on 10 Point Scale	300+	73%	67%	71%
Meds 'Always' Explained Before Given	300+	59%	60%	64%
Nurses 'Always' Communicated Well	300+	75%	75%	79%
Pain 'Always' Well Controlled	300+	67%	68%	71%
Room and Bathroom 'Always' Clean	300+	69%	69%	73%
Timely Help 'Always' Received	300+	62%	62%	68%
Would Definitely Recommend Hospital	300+	74%	69%	71%
Use of Medical Imaging				
Cardiac Imaging Stress Test before Surgery	2,677	7.3%	6.4%	5.3%
Combination Abdominal CT Scan	2,656	4.9%	11.8%	10.5%
Combination Brain/Sinus CT Scan	2,120	3.5%	3.4%	2.7%
Combination Chest CT Scan	2,418	1.0%	2.4%	2.7%
Follow-up Mammogram/Ultrasound	1,717	7.8%	10.2%	8.8%
Lumbar Spine MRI for Low Back Pain	116	35.3%	35.2%	37.2%

Putnam Community Medical Center

611 Zeagler Dr
Palatka, FL 32177
Phone: 386-326-8500
Fax: 386-325-8178
URL: www.pcmcfl.com
Type: Acute Care Hospitals
Emergency Services: Yes
Ownership: Proprietary
Beds: 141

Key Personnel:

CEO/President.............. Bruce A Baldwin
Chief of Medical Staff.......... David W Burkland, MD
Emergency Room .... Charles Donaldson
Quality Assurance .... Bobbie Long
Radiology.................. Gray Mason

Measure	Cases	This Hosp.	State Avg.	U.S. Avg.
Blood Clot Prevention and Treatment				
Anticoagulation Overlap Therapy[2]	45	78%	93%	93%
ICU Venous Thromboembolism Prophylaxis[2]	69	84%	94%	92%
Incidence of Potentially Preventable VTE[1,2]	-	-	10%	10%
UFH with Dosages/Platelet Monitoring[2]	36	100%	100%	97%
Venous Thromboembolism Prophylaxis[2]	392	93%	88%	85%
Warfarin Therapy Discharge Instructions[2]	36	86%	85%	75%
Chest Pain/Possible Heart Attack Care				
Aspirin Given Within 24 Hours of Arrival[1,3]	-	-	98%	96%
Fibrinolytic Meds Within 30 Min. of Arrival[5]	-	-	81%	58%
Average Time to ECG (minutes)[1,3]	-	-	7	7
Average Time to Transfer (minutes)[5]	-	-	53	60
Children's Asthma Care				
Received Home Management Plan of Care	-	-	-	88%
Received Reliever Medication	-	-	-	100%
Received Systemic Corticosteroids	-	-	-	100%
Emergency Department				
Admittance Decision Time (minutes)[2]	701	113	111	98
Head CT Results Within 45 Min. of Arrival[1]	-	-	64%	57%
Patients Who Left ER Before Being Seen	29,472	4%	2%	2%
Time from ER Arrival to Admit. (minutes)[2]	720	275	289	274
Time from ER Arrival to Discharge (minutes)	440	109	147	134
Time in ER Before Being Evaluated (minutes)	486	26	26	26
Time to Pain Meds for Fractures (minutes)	82	50	60	57
Heart Attack Care				
Aspirin Given at Discharge	113	99%	99%	99%
Fibrinolytic Meds Within 30 Min. of Arrival[1]	-	-	50%	54%
PCI Within 90 Minutes of Arrival	31	87%	96%	96%
Statin Prescribed at Discharge	110	94%	99%	98%
Heart Failure Care				
ACE Inhibitor or ARB for LVSD	76	91%	98%	97%
Discharge Instructions Given	180	89%	96%	94%
Evaluation of LVS Function	234	97%	100%	99%
Medicare Spending				
Medicare Spending per Patient (ratio)	-	1.05	1.04	0.98
Pneumonia Care				
Appropriate Initial Antibiotic Given	73	97%	98%	95%
Blood Culture Timing	106	89%	99%	98%
Pregnancy and Delivery Care				
Newborn Deliveries Scheduled Early[2]	37	0%	6%	6%
Preventive Care				
Immunization for Influenza[2]	517	98%	94%	90%
Immunization for Pneumonia[2]	761	98%	96%	92%
Stroke Care				
Anticoagulation Therapy for Atrial Fibrillation[1]	-	-	97%	95%
Antithrombotic Therapy Timing	61	100%	98%	98%
Assessed for Rehabilitation	61	84%	97%	97%
Discharged on Antithrombotic Therapy	60	100%	99%	99%
Discharged on Statin Medication	48	92%	96%	94%
Thrombolytic Therapy Timing[1]	-	-	76%	66%
Venous Thromboembolism Prophylaxis	62	92%	95%	94%
Written Stroke Educational Materials Given	33	79%	94%	88%
Surgical Care Improvement Project				
Appropriate Beta Blocker Usage	20	95%	99%	98%
Appropriate VTP Within 24 Hours	164	96%	99%	98%
Controlled Postoperative Blood Glucose[7]	-	-	98%	97%
Perioperative Temperature Management	228	100%	100%	100%
Prophylactic Antibiotic Selection	160	99%	99%	99%
Prophylactic Antibiotic Selection (Outpatient)	87	100%	98%	98%
Prophylactic Antibiotic Stopped	159	98%	98%	98%

NOTE: Hospital profiles are in alphabetical order by state, then city, then hospital within the city; Rankings exclude hospitals with less than 25 cases except for patient surveys which excludes hospitals with less than 100 cases; (a) 100-299 cases; (1) The number of cases/patients is too few to report; (2) Data submitted were based on a sample of cases/patients; (3) Results are based on a shorter time period than required; (4) Data suppressed by CMS for one or more quarters; (5) Results are not available for this reporting period; (6) Fewer than 100 patients completed the HCAHPS survey; (7) No cases met the criteria for this measure; (8) The lower limit of the confidence interval cannot be calculated if the number of observed infections equals zero; (9) No data are available from the state/territory for this reporting period; (10) The scores shown reflect fewer than 50 completed surveys; (11) There were discrepancies in the data collection process; (12) This measure does not apply to this hospital for this reporting period; (13) Results cannot be calculated for this reporting period; (14) The results for this state are combined with nearby states to protect confidentiality; Please refer to the User's Guide for a full explanation of data.

Measure	Cases	This Hosp.	State Avg.	U.S. Avg.
Prophylactic Antibiotic Timing	160	100%	99%	99%
Prophylactic Antibiotic Timing (Outpatient)	88	99%	98%	98%
Urinary Catheter Removal	90	97%	98%	97%
Survey of Patients' Hospital Experiences				
Area Around Room 'Always' Quiet at Night	300+	52%	58%	61%
Doctors 'Always' Communicated Well	300+	78%	77%	82%
Home Recovery Information Given	300+	80%	83%	85%
Hospital Given 9 or 10 on 10 Point Scale	300+	58%	67%	71%
Meds 'Always' Explained Before Given	300+	60%	60%	64%
Nurses 'Always' Communicated Well	300+	73%	75%	79%
Pain 'Always' Well Controlled	300+	65%	68%	71%
Room and Bathroom 'Always' Clean	300+	66%	69%	73%
Timely Help 'Always' Received	300+	56%	62%	68%
Would Definitely Recommend Hospital	300+	51%	69%	71%
Use of Medical Imaging				
Cardiac Imaging Stress Test before Surgery	192	5.7%	6.4%	5.3%
Combination Abdominal CT Scan	534	6.4%	11.8%	10.5%
Combination Brain/Sinus CT Scan	681	1.9%	3.4%	2.7%
Combination Chest CT Scan	201	5.0%	2.4%	2.7%
Follow-up Mammogram/Ultrasound	1,020	7.1%	10.2%	8.8%
Lumbar Spine MRI for Low Back Pain	59	37.3%	35.2%	37.2%

Palm Bay Hospital

1425 Malabar Rd, Ne
Palm Bay, FL 32907
Phone: 321-434-8000
URL: www.health-first.org
Type: Acute Care Hospitals
Emergency Services: Yes
Ownership: Proprietary

Measure	Cases	This Hosp.	State Avg.	U.S. Avg.
Blood Clot Prevention and Treatment				
Anticoagulation Overlap Therapy[2]	75	97%	93%	93%
ICU Venous Thromboembolism Prophylaxis[2]	77	99%	94%	92%
Incidence of Potentially Preventable VTE[1,2]	-	-	10%	10%
UFH with Dosages/Platelet Monitoring[2]	74	100%	100%	97%
Venous Thromboembolism Prophylaxis[2]	353	93%	88%	85%
Warfarin Therapy Discharge Instructions[2]	52	69%	85%	75%
Chest Pain/Possible Heart Attack Care				
Aspirin Given Within 24 Hours of Arrival	47	98%	98%	96%
Fibrinolytic Meds Within 30 Min. of Arrival[7]	-	-	81%	58%
Average Time to ECG (minutes)	48	2	7	7
Average Time to Transfer (minutes)	11	59	53	60
Children's Asthma Care				
Received Home Management Plan of Care	-	-	-	88%
Received Reliever Medication	-	-	-	100%
Received Systemic Corticosteroids	-	-	-	100%
Emergency Department				
Admittance Decision Time (minutes)[2]	950	104	111	98
Head CT Results Within 45 Min. of Arrival[1]	-	-	64%	57%
Patients Who Left ER Before Being Seen	40,194	2%	2%	2%
Time from ER Arrival to Admit. (minutes)[2]	950	266	289	274
Time from ER Arrival to Discharge (minutes)	380	143	147	134
Time in ER Before Being Evaluated (minutes)	405	22	26	26
Time to Pain Meds for Fractures (minutes)	162	60	60	57
Heart Attack Care				
Aspirin Given at Discharge	20	95%	99%	99%
Fibrinolytic Meds Within 30 Min. of Arrival[7]	-	-	50%	54%
PCI Within 90 Minutes of Arrival[7]	-	-	96%	96%
Statin Prescribed at Discharge	21	95%	99%	98%
Heart Failure Care				
ACE Inhibitor or ARB for LVSD	70	99%	98%	97%
Discharge Instructions Given	157	98%	96%	94%
Evaluation of LVS Function	199	99%	100%	99%
Medicare Spending				
Medicare Spending per Patient (ratio)	-	1.09	1.04	0.98
Pneumonia Care				
Appropriate Initial Antibiotic Given	132	100%	98%	95%
Blood Culture Timing	218	100%	99%	98%
Pregnancy and Delivery Care				
Newborn Deliveries Scheduled Early[7]	-	-	6%	6%
Preventive Care				
Immunization for Influenza[2]	564	87%	94%	90%
Immunization for Pneumonia[2]	867	95%	96%	92%
Stroke Care				
Anticoagulation Therapy for Atrial Fibrillation[1]	-	-	97%	95%
Antithrombotic Therapy Timing	56	100%	98%	98%
Assessed for Rehabilitation	54	98%	97%	97%
Discharged on Antithrombotic Therapy	54	98%	99%	99%
Discharged on Statin Medication	38	95%	96%	94%
Thrombolytic Therapy Timing[7]	-	-	76%	66%
Venous Thromboembolism Prophylaxis	54	87%	95%	94%
Written Stroke Educational Materials Given	34	91%	94%	88%
Surgical Care Improvement Project				
Appropriate Beta Blocker Usage	117	100%	99%	98%
Appropriate VTP Within 24 Hours	321	99%	99%	98%
Controlled Postoperative Blood Glucose[7]	-	-	98%	97%
Perioperative Temperature Management	344	100%	100%	100%
Prophylactic Antibiotic Selection	264	100%	99%	99%
Prophylactic Antibiotic Selection (Outpatient)	25	68%	98%	98%
Prophylactic Antibiotic Stopped	261	99%	98%	98%
Prophylactic Antibiotic Timing	264	99%	99%	99%
Prophylactic Antibiotic Timing (Outpatient)	25	100%	98%	98%
Urinary Catheter Removal	235	100%	98%	97%
Survey of Patients' Hospital Experiences				
Area Around Room 'Always' Quiet at Night	300+	70%	58%	61%
Doctors 'Always' Communicated Well	300+	75%	77%	82%
Home Recovery Information Given	300+	84%	83%	85%
Hospital Given 9 or 10 on 10 Point Scale	300+	75%	67%	71%
Meds 'Always' Explained Before Given	300+	64%	60%	64%
Nurses 'Always' Communicated Well	300+	81%	75%	79%
Pain 'Always' Well Controlled	300+	73%	68%	71%
Room and Bathroom 'Always' Clean	300+	81%	69%	73%
Timely Help 'Always' Received	300+	68%	62%	68%
Would Definitely Recommend Hospital	300+	76%	69%	71%
Use of Medical Imaging				
Cardiac Imaging Stress Test before Surgery	178	2.2%	6.4%	5.3%
Combination Abdominal CT Scan	404	12.9%	11.8%	10.5%
Combination Brain/Sinus CT Scan	502	1.2%	3.4%	2.7%
Combination Chest CT Scan	389	1.3%	2.4%	2.7%
Follow-up Mammogram/Ultrasound	789	10.3%	10.2%	8.8%
Lumbar Spine MRI for Low Back Pain[1]	-	-	35.2%	37.2%

Palm Beach Gardens Medical Center

3360 Burns Rd
Palm Beach Gardens, FL 33410
Phone: 561-622-1411
Fax: 561-694-7160
URL: www.pbgmc.com
Type: Acute Care Hospitals
Emergency Services: Yes
Ownership: Proprietary
Beds: 199

Key Personnel:
Cardiac Laboratory. . . . . Melanie Giles
Quality Assurance . . . . Rita Mack
Operating Room. . . . . Stephen Martyak
CEO/President. . . . . David A Pettit
Pediatric In-Patient Care . . . . . . Luis Pineiro, MD
Chief of Medical Staff. . . . . Richard Pomerantz, MD
Emergency Room . . . . Neil Stern
Radiology. . . . . Brian Young

Measure	Cases	This Hosp.	State Avg.	U.S. Avg.
Blood Clot Prevention and Treatment				
Anticoagulation Overlap Therapy[2]	89	90%	93%	93%
ICU Venous Thromboembolism Prophylaxis[2]	149	93%	94%	92%
Incidence of Potentially Preventable VTE[2]	12	0%	10%	10%
UFH with Dosages/Platelet Monitoring[2]	80	100%	100%	97%
Venous Thromboembolism Prophylaxis[2]	314	89%	88%	85%
Warfarin Therapy Discharge Instructions[2]	65	91%	85%	75%
Chest Pain/Possible Heart Attack Care				
Aspirin Given Within 24 Hours of Arrival[1,3]	-	-	98%	96%
Fibrinolytic Meds Within 30 Min. of Arrival[3,7]	-	-	81%	58%
Average Time to ECG (minutes)[1,3]	-	-	7	7
Average Time to Transfer (minutes)[3,7]	-	-	53	60
Children's Asthma Care				
Received Home Management Plan of Care	-	-	-	88%
Received Reliever Medication	-	-	-	100%
Received Systemic Corticosteroids	-	-	-	100%
Emergency Department				
Admittance Decision Time (minutes)[2]	1,036	142	111	98
Head CT Results Within 45 Min. of Arrival[1]	-	-	64%	57%
Patients Who Left ER Before Being Seen	30,258	0%	2%	2%
Time from ER Arrival to Admit. (minutes)[2]	1,036	258	289	274
Time from ER Arrival to Discharge (minutes)	357	141	147	134
Time in ER Before Being Evaluated (minutes)	384	11	26	26
Time to Pain Meds for Fractures (minutes)	142	41	60	57
Heart Attack Care				
Aspirin Given at Discharge	426	100%	99%	99%
Fibrinolytic Meds Within 30 Min. of Arrival[7]	-	-	50%	54%
PCI Within 90 Minutes of Arrival	78	100%	96%	96%
Statin Prescribed at Discharge	397	100%	99%	98%
Heart Failure Care				
ACE Inhibitor or ARB for LVSD	144	100%	98%	97%
Discharge Instructions Given	373	97%	96%	94%
Evaluation of LVS Function	439	100%	100%	99%
Medicare Spending				
Medicare Spending per Patient (ratio)	-	1.07	1.04	0.98
Pneumonia Care				
Appropriate Initial Antibiotic Given	87	99%	98%	95%
Blood Culture Timing	145	100%	99%	98%
Pregnancy and Delivery Care				
Newborn Deliveries Scheduled Early[7]	-	-	6%	6%
Preventive Care				
Immunization for Influenza[2]	648	97%	94%	90%
Immunization for Pneumonia[2]	1,015	97%	96%	92%
Stroke Care				
Anticoagulation Therapy for Atrial Fibrillation	21	100%	97%	95%
Antithrombotic Therapy Timing	89	100%	98%	98%
Assessed for Rehabilitation	95	99%	97%	97%
Discharged on Antithrombotic Therapy	91	98%	99%	99%
Discharged on Statin Medication	69	97%	96%	94%
Thrombolytic Therapy Timing	13	100%	76%	66%
Venous Thromboembolism Prophylaxis	103	96%	95%	94%
Written Stroke Educational Materials Given	56	93%	94%	88%
Surgical Care Improvement Project				
Appropriate Beta Blocker Usage	324	100%	99%	98%
Appropriate VTP Within 24 Hours	233	96%	99%	98%
Controlled Postoperative Blood Glucose	256	100%	98%	97%
Perioperative Temperature Management	450	100%	100%	100%
Prophylactic Antibiotic Selection	431	99%	99%	99%
Prophylactic Antibiotic Selection (Outpatient)	375	100%	98%	98%
Prophylactic Antibiotic Stopped	394	99%	98%	98%
Prophylactic Antibiotic Timing	431	100%	99%	99%
Prophylactic Antibiotic Timing (Outpatient)	375	100%	98%	98%
Urinary Catheter Removal	270	98%	98%	97%
Survey of Patients' Hospital Experiences				
Area Around Room 'Always' Quiet at Night	300+	57%	58%	61%
Doctors 'Always' Communicated Well	300+	83%	77%	82%
Home Recovery Information Given	300+	82%	83%	85%
Hospital Given 9 or 10 on 10 Point Scale	300+	69%	67%	71%
Meds 'Always' Explained Before Given	300+	60%	60%	64%
Nurses 'Always' Communicated Well	300+	75%	75%	79%
Pain 'Always' Well Controlled	300+	70%	68%	71%
Room and Bathroom 'Always' Clean	300+	63%	69%	73%
Timely Help 'Always' Received	300+	67%	62%	68%
Would Definitely Recommend Hospital	300+	73%	69%	71%
Use of Medical Imaging				
Cardiac Imaging Stress Test before Surgery[1]	-	-	6.4%	5.3%
Combination Abdominal CT Scan	455	4.4%	11.8%	10.5%
Combination Brain/Sinus CT Scan	749	1.6%	3.4%	2.7%
Combination Chest CT Scan	249	2.0%	2.4%	2.7%
Follow-up Mammogram/Ultrasound	187	15.5%	10.2%	8.8%
Lumbar Spine MRI for Low Back Pain[1]	-	-	35.2%	37.2%

Florida Hospital Flagler

60 Memorial Medical Pkwy
Palm Coast, FL 32164
Phone: 386-586-2000
Fax: 386-586-4620
Type: Acute Care Hospitals
Emergency Services: Yes
Ownership: Voluntary non-profit - Church
Beds: 81

Key Personnel:
Operating Room. . . . . Alfred L Alson
Quality Assurance . . . . Connie Amatucci
Radiology. . . . . Josiah W Bancroft
Chief of Medical Staff . . . . Robert Bianco, MD
CEO/President. . . . . Richard Lind
Emergency Room . . . . Maureen Sabella

NOTE: Hospital profiles are in alphabetical order by state, then city, then hospital within the city; Rankings exclude hospitals with less than 25 cases except for patient surveys which excludes hospitals with less than 100 cases; (a) 100-299 cases; (1) The number of cases/patients is too few to report; (2) Data submitted were based on a sample of cases/patients; (3) Results are based on a shorter time period than required; (4) Data suppressed by CMS for one or more quarters; (5) Results are not available for this reporting period; (6) Fewer than 100 patients completed the HCAHPS survey; (7) No cases met the criteria for this measure; (8) The lower limit of the confidence interval cannot be calculated if the number of observed infections equals zero; (9) No data are available from the state/territory for this reporting period; (10) The scores shown reflect fewer than 50 completed surveys; (11) There were discrepancies in the data collection process; (12) This measure does not apply to this hospital for this reporting period; (13) Results cannot be calculated for this reporting period; (14) The results for this state are combined with nearby states to protect confidentiality; Please refer to the User's Guide for a full explanation of data.

Measure	Cases	This Hosp.	State Avg.	U.S. Avg.
Blood Clot Prevention and Treatment				
Anticoagulation Overlap Therapy[2]	71	100%	93%	93%
ICU Venous Thromboembolism Prophylaxis[2]	91	97%	94%	92%
Incidence of Potentially Preventable VTE[2]	16	0%	10%	10%
UFH with Dosages/Platelet Monitoring[2]	35	100%	100%	97%
Venous Thromboembolism Prophylaxis[2]	327	94%	88%	85%
Warfarin Therapy Discharge Instructions[2]	49	80%	85%	75%
Chest Pain/Possible Heart Attack Care				
Aspirin Given Within 24 Hours of Arrival[1,3]	-	-	98%	96%
Fibrinolytic Meds Within 30 Min. of Arrival[3,7]	-	-	81%	58%
Average Time to ECG (minutes)[1,3]	-	-	7	7
Average Time to Transfer (minutes)[3,7]	-	-	53	60
Children's Asthma Care				
Received Home Management Plan of Care	-	-	-	88%
Received Reliever Medication	-	-	-	100%
Received Systemic Corticosteroids	-	-	-	100%
Emergency Department				
Admittance Decision Time (minutes)[2]	698	139	111	98
Head CT Results Within 45 Min. of Arrival	12	67%	64%	57%
Patients Who Left ER Before Being Seen	39,984	1%	2%	2%
Time from ER Arrival to Admit. (minutes)[2]	884	359	289	274
Time from ER Arrival to Discharge (minutes)	342	155	147	134
Time in ER Before Being Evaluated (minutes)	358	47	26	26
Time to Pain Meds for Fractures (minutes)	126	60	60	57
Heart Attack Care				
Aspirin Given at Discharge	140	100%	99%	99%
Fibrinolytic Meds Within 30 Min. of Arrival[7]	-	-	50%	54%
PCI Within 90 Minutes of Arrival	29	93%	96%	96%
Statin Prescribed at Discharge	125	100%	99%	98%
Heart Failure Care				
ACE Inhibitor or ARB for LVSD	80	100%	98%	97%
Discharge Instructions Given	224	95%	96%	94%
Evaluation of LVS Function	283	100%	100%	99%
Medicare Spending				
Medicare Spending per Patient (ratio)	-	1.05	1.04	0.98
Pneumonia Care				
Appropriate Initial Antibiotic Given	156	98%	98%	95%
Blood Culture Timing	317	98%	99%	98%
Pregnancy and Delivery Care				
Newborn Deliveries Scheduled Early[7]	-	-	6%	6%
Preventive Care				
Immunization for Influenza[2]	589	94%	94%	90%
Immunization for Pneumonia[2]	929	94%	96%	92%
Stroke Care				
Anticoagulation Therapy for Atrial Fibrillation	12	100%	97%	95%
Antithrombotic Therapy Timing	122	98%	98%	98%
Assessed for Rehabilitation	138	100%	97%	97%
Discharged on Antithrombotic Therapy	129	99%	99%	99%
Discharged on Statin Medication	98	94%	96%	94%
Thrombolytic Therapy Timing	11	73%	76%	66%
Venous Thromboembolism Prophylaxis	132	94%	95%	94%
Written Stroke Educational Materials Given	80	99%	94%	88%
Surgical Care Improvement Project				
Appropriate Beta Blocker Usage	124	100%	99%	98%
Appropriate VTP Within 24 Hours	451	100%	99%	98%
Controlled Postoperative Blood Glucose[7]	-	-	98%	97%
Perioperative Temperature Management	496	100%	100%	100%
Prophylactic Antibiotic Selection	308	99%	99%	99%
Prophylactic Antibiotic Selection (Outpatient)	101	92%	98%	98%
Prophylactic Antibiotic Stopped	296	100%	98%	98%
Prophylactic Antibiotic Timing	308	100%	99%	99%
Prophylactic Antibiotic Timing (Outpatient)	70	100%	98%	98%
Urinary Catheter Removal	366	99%	98%	97%
Survey of Patients' Hospital Experiences				
Area Around Room 'Always' Quiet at Night[11]	300+	54%	58%	61%
Doctors 'Always' Communicated Well[11]	300+	78%	77%	82%
Home Recovery Information Given[11]	300+	84%	83%	85%
Hospital Given 9 or 10 on 10 Point Scale[11]	300+	64%	67%	71%
Meds 'Always' Explained Before Given[11]	300+	60%	60%	64%
Nurses 'Always' Communicated Well[11]	300+	75%	75%	79%
Pain 'Always' Well Controlled[11]	300+	69%	68%	71%
Room and Bathroom 'Always' Clean[11]	300+	72%	69%	73%
Timely Help 'Always' Received[11]	300+	61%	62%	68%
Would Definitely Recommend Hospital[11]	300+	65%	69%	71%
Use of Medical Imaging				
Cardiac Imaging Stress Test before Surgery	213	6.6%	6.4%	5.3%
Combination Abdominal CT Scan	1,032	8.0%	11.8%	10.5%
Combination Brain/Sinus CT Scan	927	2.7%	3.4%	2.7%
Combination Chest CT Scan	834	2.9%	2.4%	2.7%
Follow-up Mammogram/Ultrasound	1,041	20.2%	10.2%	8.8%
Lumbar Spine MRI for Low Back Pain	73	31.5%	35.2%	37.2%

Bay Medical Center Sacred Heart Health System

615 N Bonita Ave
Panama City, FL 32401
URL: www.baymedical.org
Phone: 850-769-1511
Fax: 850-747-6443
Type: Acute Care Hospitals
Ownership: Govt - Hospital Dist/Auth
Emergency Services: Yes
Beds: 413

Key Personnel:
Anesthesiology. . . . . John Gooding, DO
Emergency Room . . . . Kevin Groves, MD
CEO/President. . . . . Barry Keel
Operating Room. . . . . Brenda Kingdon
Chief of Medical Staff . . . . Todd Minga, MD
Infection Control. . . . . Nina O'Flaherty
Pediatric Ambulatory Care . . . . . . Ingrid Rachesky, MD
Radiology. . . . . Martin Sheline, MD

Measure	Cases	This Hosp.	State Avg.	U.S. Avg.
Blood Clot Prevention and Treatment				
Anticoagulation Overlap Therapy[2]	79	97%	93%	93%
ICU Venous Thromboembolism Prophylaxis[2]	263	92%	94%	92%
Incidence of Potentially Preventable VTE[1,2]	-	-	10%	10%
UFH with Dosages/Platelet Monitoring[2]	94	100%	100%	97%
Venous Thromboembolism Prophylaxis[2]	703	76%	88%	85%
Warfarin Therapy Discharge Instructions[2]	60	93%	85%	75%
Chest Pain/Possible Heart Attack Care				
Aspirin Given Within 24 Hours of Arrival[1,3]	-	-	98%	96%
Fibrinolytic Meds Within 30 Min. of Arrival[5]	-	-	81%	58%
Average Time to ECG (minutes)[1,3]	-	-	7	7
Average Time to Transfer (minutes)[5]	-	-	53	60
Children's Asthma Care				
Received Home Management Plan of Care	-	-	-	88%
Received Reliever Medication	-	-	-	100%
Received Systemic Corticosteroids	-	-	-	100%
Emergency Department				
Admittance Decision Time (minutes)[2]	822	164	111	98
Head CT Results Within 45 Min. of Arrival	12	50%	64%	57%
Patients Who Left ER Before Being Seen	58,249	2%	2%	2%
Time from ER Arrival to Admit. (minutes)[2]	829	351	289	274
Time from ER Arrival to Discharge (minutes)	416	164	147	134
Time in ER Before Being Evaluated (minutes)	441	37	26	26
Time to Pain Meds for Fractures (minutes)	130	72	60	57
Heart Attack Care				
Aspirin Given at Discharge	366	100%	99%	99%
Fibrinolytic Meds Within 30 Min. of Arrival[7]	-	-	50%	54%
PCI Within 90 Minutes of Arrival	40	98%	96%	96%
Statin Prescribed at Discharge	332	100%	99%	98%
Heart Failure Care				
ACE Inhibitor or ARB for LVSD[2]	144	99%	98%	97%
Discharge Instructions Given[2]	388	91%	96%	94%
Evaluation of LVS Function[2]	483	100%	100%	99%
Medicare Spending				
Medicare Spending per Patient (ratio)	-	1.05	1.04	0.98
Pneumonia Care				
Appropriate Initial Antibiotic Given[2]	151	97%	98%	95%
Blood Culture Timing[2]	218	97%	99%	98%
Pregnancy and Delivery Care				
Newborn Deliveries Scheduled Early	35	0%	6%	6%
Preventive Care				
Immunization for Influenza[2]	568	96%	94%	90%
Immunization for Pneumonia[2]	832	98%	96%	92%
Stroke Care				
Anticoagulation Therapy for Atrial Fibrillation	34	79%	97%	95%
Antithrombotic Therapy Timing	206	97%	98%	98%
Assessed for Rehabilitation	235	83%	97%	97%
Discharged on Antithrombotic Therapy	207	100%	99%	99%
Discharged on Statin Medication	169	89%	96%	94%
Thrombolytic Therapy Timing	37	43%	76%	66%
Venous Thromboembolism Prophylaxis	251	84%	95%	94%
Written Stroke Educational Materials Given	137	75%	94%	88%
Surgical Care Improvement Project				
Appropriate Beta Blocker Usage[2]	337	100%	99%	98%
Appropriate VTP Within 24 Hours[2]	381	95%	99%	98%
Controlled Postoperative Blood Glucose[2]	282	95%	98%	97%
Perioperative Temperature Management[2]	546	100%	100%	100%
Prophylactic Antibiotic Selection[2]	630	99%	99%	99%
Prophylactic Antibiotic Selection (Outpatient)	424	98%	98%	98%
Prophylactic Antibiotic Stopped[2]	619	99%	98%	98%
Prophylactic Antibiotic Timing[2]	631	100%	99%	99%
Prophylactic Antibiotic Timing (Outpatient)	425	100%	98%	98%
Urinary Catheter Removal[2]	592	96%	98%	97%
Survey of Patients' Hospital Experiences				
Area Around Room 'Always' Quiet at Night	300+	60%	58%	61%
Doctors 'Always' Communicated Well	300+	76%	77%	82%
Home Recovery Information Given	300+	84%	83%	85%
Hospital Given 9 or 10 on 10 Point Scale	300+	69%	67%	71%
Meds 'Always' Explained Before Given	300+	60%	60%	64%
Nurses 'Always' Communicated Well	300+	76%	75%	79%
Pain 'Always' Well Controlled	300+	68%	68%	71%
Room and Bathroom 'Always' Clean	300+	64%	69%	73%
Timely Help 'Always' Received	300+	61%	62%	68%
Would Definitely Recommend Hospital	300+	72%	69%	71%
Use of Medical Imaging				
Cardiac Imaging Stress Test before Surgery	210	10.0%	6.4%	5.3%
Combination Abdominal CT Scan	1,342	13.6%	11.8%	10.5%
Combination Brain/Sinus CT Scan	1,321	2.2%	3.4%	2.7%
Combination Chest CT Scan	1,196	1.3%	2.4%	2.7%
Follow-up Mammogram/Ultrasound	703	13.1%	10.2%	8.8%
Lumbar Spine MRI for Low Back Pain	119	34.5%	35.2%	37.2%

Gulf Coast Regional Medical Center

449 W 23rd St
Panama City, FL 32405
URL: www.egulfcoastmedical.com
Phone: 850-747-7926
Fax: 850-747-7907
Type: Acute Care Hospitals
Ownership: Proprietary
Emergency Services: Yes
Beds: 176

Key Personnel:
Infection Control. . . . . William Bone, MD
Patient Relations . . . . Nueva Cowart
Radiology. . . . . Wendy W. Kriegel, MD
Quality Assurance . . . . Laura Meese
Intensive Care Unit. . . . . Victor Ortega, MD
CEO . . . . Carlton Ulmer
Chief of Medical Staff. . . . . Richard B. Wilson, MD
Operating Room. . . . . Sharon Wolfrom

Measure	Cases	This Hosp.	State Avg.	U.S. Avg.
Blood Clot Prevention and Treatment				
Anticoagulation Overlap Therapy[2]	62	98%	93%	93%
ICU Venous Thromboembolism Prophylaxis[2]	69	100%	94%	92%
Incidence of Potentially Preventable VTE[1,2]	-	-	10%	10%
UFH with Dosages/Platelet Monitoring[2]	57	100%	100%	97%
Venous Thromboembolism Prophylaxis[2]	371	97%	88%	85%
Warfarin Therapy Discharge Instructions[2]	38	97%	85%	75%
Chest Pain/Possible Heart Attack Care				
Aspirin Given Within 24 Hours of Arrival[5]	-	-	98%	96%
Fibrinolytic Meds Within 30 Min. of Arrival[5]	-	-	81%	58%
Average Time to ECG (minutes)[5]	-	-	7	7
Average Time to Transfer (minutes)[5]	-	-	53	60
Children's Asthma Care				
Received Home Management Plan of Care	-	-	-	88%
Received Reliever Medication	-	-	-	100%
Received Systemic Corticosteroids	-	-	-	100%
Emergency Department				
Admittance Decision Time (minutes)[2]	663	71	111	98
Head CT Results Within 45 Min. of Arrival[1]	-	-	64%	57%
Patients Who Left ER Before Being Seen	55,320	1%	2%	2%
Time from ER Arrival to Admit. (minutes)[2]	663	237	289	274
Time from ER Arrival to Discharge (minutes)	511	128	147	134
Time in ER Before Being Evaluated (minutes)	535	13	26	26

NOTE: Hospital profiles are in alphabetical order by state, then city, then hospital within the city; Rankings exclude hospitals with less than 25 cases except for patient surveys which excludes hospitals with less than 100 cases; (a) 100-299 cases; (1) The number of cases/patients is too few to report; (2) Data submitted were based on a sample of cases/patients; (3) Results are based on a shorter time period than required; (4) Data suppressed by CMS for one or more quarters; (5) Results are not available for this reporting period; (6) Fewer than 100 patients completed the HCAHPS survey; (7) No cases met the criteria for this measure; (8) The lower limit of the confidence interval cannot be calculated if the number of observed infections equals zero; (9) No data are available from the state/territory for this reporting period; (10) The scores shown reflect fewer than 50 completed surveys; (11) There were discrepancies in the data collection process; (12) This measure does not apply to this hospital for this reporting period; (13) Results cannot be calculated for this reporting period; (14) The results for this state are combined with nearby states to protect confidentiality; Please refer to the User's Guide for a full explanation of data.

Measure	Cases	This Hosp.	State Avg.	U.S. Avg.
Time to Pain Meds for Fractures (minutes)	173	42	60	57
Heart Attack Care				
Aspirin Given at Discharge[2]	122	100%	99%	99%
Fibrinolytic Meds Within 30 Min. of Arrival[2,7]	-	-	50%	54%
PCI Within 90 Minutes of Arrival[2]	15	93%	96%	96%
Statin Prescribed at Discharge[2]	107	98%	99%	98%
Heart Failure Care				
ACE Inhibitor or ARB for LVSD[2]	58	100%	98%	97%
Discharge Instructions Given[2]	156	97%	96%	94%
Evaluation of LVS Function[2]	200	100%	100%	99%
Medicare Spending				
Medicare Spending per Patient (ratio)	-	1.08	1.04	0.98
Pneumonia Care				
Appropriate Initial Antibiotic Given[2]	72	97%	98%	95%
Blood Culture Timing[2]	139	99%	99%	98%
Pregnancy and Delivery Care				
Newborn Deliveries Scheduled Early[2]	56	4%	6%	6%
Preventive Care				
Immunization for Influenza[2]	537	97%	94%	90%
Immunization for Pneumonia[2]	597	99%	96%	92%
Stroke Care				
Anticoagulation Therapy for Atrial Fibrillation	16	94%	97%	95%
Antithrombotic Therapy Timing	75	100%	98%	98%
Assessed for Rehabilitation	89	100%	97%	97%
Discharged on Antithrombotic Therapy	84	100%	99%	99%
Discharged on Statin Medication	63	95%	96%	94%
Thrombolytic Therapy Timing[1]	-	-	76%	66%
Venous Thromboembolism Prophylaxis	88	100%	95%	94%
Written Stroke Educational Materials Given	49	98%	94%	88%
Surgical Care Improvement Project				
Appropriate Beta Blocker Usage[2]	184	99%	99%	98%
Appropriate VTP Within 24 Hours[2]	393	100%	99%	98%
Controlled Postoperative Blood Glucose[2,7]	-	-	98%	97%
Perioperative Temperature Management[2]	529	100%	100%	100%
Prophylactic Antibiotic Selection[2]	318	99%	99%	99%
Prophylactic Antibiotic Selection (Outpatient)	378	99%	98%	98%
Prophylactic Antibiotic Stopped[2]	195	99%	98%	98%
Prophylactic Antibiotic Timing[2]	318	100%	99%	99%
Prophylactic Antibiotic Timing (Outpatient)	378	100%	98%	98%
Urinary Catheter Removal[2]	327	100%	98%	97%
Survey of Patients' Hospital Experiences				
Area Around Room 'Always' Quiet at Night	300+	52%	58%	61%
Doctors 'Always' Communicated Well	300+	77%	77%	82%
Home Recovery Information Given	300+	87%	83%	85%
Hospital Given 9 or 10 on 10 Point Scale	300+	66%	67%	71%
Meds 'Always' Explained Before Given	300+	57%	60%	64%
Nurses 'Always' Communicated Well	300+	76%	75%	79%
Pain 'Always' Well Controlled	300+	69%	68%	71%
Room and Bathroom 'Always' Clean	300+	66%	69%	73%
Timely Help 'Always' Received	300+	59%	62%	68%
Would Definitely Recommend Hospital	300+	72%	69%	71%
Use of Medical Imaging				
Cardiac Imaging Stress Test before Surgery	67	3.0%	6.4%	5.3%
Combination Abdominal CT Scan	1,013	10.5%	11.8%	10.5%
Combination Brain/Sinus CT Scan	847	3.8%	3.4%	2.7%
Combination Chest CT Scan	717	6.8%	2.4%	2.7%
Follow-up Mammogram/Ultrasound	616	10.4%	10.2%	8.8%
Lumbar Spine MRI for Low Back Pain	45	44.4%	35.2%	37.2%

Memorial Hospital Pembroke

7800 Sheridan St
Pembroke Pines, FL 33024
Phone: 954-962-9650
Fax: 954-963-8471
E-mail: info@mhs.net
URL: www.memorialpembroke.com\
Type: Acute Care Hospitals
Emergency Services: Yes
Ownership: Govt - Hospital Dist/Auth
Beds: 149

Key Personnel:
Emergency Room .... Inemesit Abia
Operating Room.............. Anel Alvarado
Anesthesiology............... Kenneth Kirzner, MD
Chief of Medical Staff.......... Jorge Luna, DO
Patient Relations .... Sandra Sanchez-Perez
Radiology..................... Trevor Swerdlow, MD

Measure	Cases	This Hosp.	State Avg.	U.S. Avg.
Blood Clot Prevention and Treatment				
Anticoagulation Overlap Therapy[2]	57	100%	93%	93%
ICU Venous Thromboembolism Prophylaxis[2]	71	100%	94%	92%
Incidence of Potentially Preventable VTE[1,2]	-	-	10%	10%
UFH with Dosages/Platelet Monitoring[2]	35	100%	100%	97%
Venous Thromboembolism Prophylaxis[2]	308	98%	88%	85%
Warfarin Therapy Discharge Instructions[2]	49	100%	85%	75%
Chest Pain/Possible Heart Attack Care				
Aspirin Given Within 24 Hours of Arrival	78	99%	98%	96%
Fibrinolytic Meds Within 30 Min. of Arrival[7]	-	-	81%	58%
Average Time to ECG (minutes)	80	7	7	7
Average Time to Transfer (minutes)	15	41	53	60
Children's Asthma Care				
Received Home Management Plan of Care	-	-	-	88%
Received Reliever Medication	-	-	-	100%
Received Systemic Corticosteroids	-	-	-	100%
Emergency Department				
Admittance Decision Time (minutes)[2]	705	185	111	98
Head CT Results Within 45 Min. of Arrival[1]	-	-	64%	57%
Patients Who Left ER Before Being Seen	91,152	1%	2%	2%
Time from ER Arrival to Admit. (minutes)[2]	726	339	289	274
Time from ER Arrival to Discharge (minutes)	353	121	147	134
Time in ER Before Being Evaluated (minutes)	378	43	26	26
Time to Pain Meds for Fractures (minutes)	102	75	60	57
Heart Attack Care				
Aspirin Given at Discharge	11	100%	99%	99%
Fibrinolytic Meds Within 30 Min. of Arrival[7]	-	-	50%	54%
PCI Within 90 Minutes of Arrival[7]	-	-	96%	96%
Statin Prescribed at Discharge[1]	-	-	99%	98%
Heart Failure Care				
ACE Inhibitor or ARB for LVSD	54	100%	98%	97%
Discharge Instructions Given	157	100%	96%	94%
Evaluation of LVS Function	176	100%	100%	99%
Medicare Spending				
Medicare Spending per Patient (ratio)	-	0.97	1.04	0.98
Pneumonia Care				
Appropriate Initial Antibiotic Given	152	100%	98%	95%
Blood Culture Timing	228	100%	99%	98%
Pregnancy and Delivery Care				
Newborn Deliveries Scheduled Early[7]	-	-	6%	6%
Preventive Care				
Immunization for Influenza[2]	557	100%	94%	90%
Immunization for Pneumonia[2]	737	100%	96%	92%
Stroke Care				
Anticoagulation Therapy for Atrial Fibrillation[1]	-	-	97%	95%
Antithrombotic Therapy Timing	54	100%	98%	98%
Assessed for Rehabilitation	56	100%	97%	97%
Discharged on Antithrombotic Therapy	53	100%	99%	99%
Discharged on Statin Medication	39	100%	96%	94%
Thrombolytic Therapy Timing[1]	-	-	76%	66%
Venous Thromboembolism Prophylaxis	56	100%	95%	94%
Written Stroke Educational Materials Given	40	100%	94%	88%
Surgical Care Improvement Project				
Appropriate Beta Blocker Usage[2]	96	100%	99%	98%
Appropriate VTP Within 24 Hours[2]	282	100%	99%	98%
Controlled Postoperative Blood Glucose[2,7]	-	-	98%	97%
Perioperative Temperature Management[2]	338	100%	100%	100%
Prophylactic Antibiotic Selection[2]	200	100%	99%	99%
Prophylactic Antibiotic Selection (Outpatient)	134	99%	98%	98%
Prophylactic Antibiotic Stopped[2]	186	100%	98%	98%
Prophylactic Antibiotic Timing[2]	200	99%	99%	99%
Prophylactic Antibiotic Timing (Outpatient)	134	100%	98%	98%
Urinary Catheter Removal[2]	147	100%	98%	97%
Survey of Patients' Hospital Experiences				
Area Around Room 'Always' Quiet at Night	300+	64%	58%	61%
Doctors 'Always' Communicated Well	300+	76%	77%	82%
Home Recovery Information Given	300+	83%	83%	85%
Hospital Given 9 or 10 on 10 Point Scale	300+	73%	67%	71%
Meds 'Always' Explained Before Given	300+	64%	60%	64%
Nurses 'Always' Communicated Well	300+	80%	75%	79%
Pain 'Always' Well Controlled	300+	70%	68%	71%
Room and Bathroom 'Always' Clean	300+	75%	69%	73%
Timely Help 'Always' Received	300+	71%	62%	68%
Would Definitely Recommend Hospital	300+	76%	69%	71%
Use of Medical Imaging				
Cardiac Imaging Stress Test before Surgery[7]	-	-	6.4%	5.3%
Combination Abdominal CT Scan	390	5.4%	11.8%	10.5%
Combination Brain/Sinus CT Scan	359	1.4%	3.4%	2.7%
Combination Chest CT Scan	228	8.3%	2.4%	2.7%
Follow-up Mammogram/Ultrasound[1]	-	-	10.2%	8.8%
Lumbar Spine MRI for Low Back Pain[1]	-	-	35.2%	37.2%

Memorial Hospital West

703 N Flamingo Rd
Pembroke Pines, FL 33028
Phone: 954-436-5000
Fax: 954-433-7155
URL: www.memorialwest.com
Type: Acute Care Hospitals
Emergency Services: Yes
Ownership: Govt - Hospital Dist/Auth
Beds: 220

Key Personnel:
Radiology.......................... Lester Goldberg, MD
Chief of Medical Staff.......... Beverly Greenberg, DO
Pediatric Ambulatory Care ...... Sue Kleet
Pediatric In-Patient Care .... Sue Kleet
Infection Control................. Kim Mahon
Operating Room.................. Phyllis Neimark
Coronary Care.................... Lisa Quintero
Quality Assurance .... Beatrix Thom

Measure	Cases	This Hosp.	State Avg.	U.S. Avg.
Blood Clot Prevention and Treatment				
Anticoagulation Overlap Therapy[2]	132	100%	93%	93%
ICU Venous Thromboembolism Prophylaxis[2]	62	98%	94%	92%
Incidence of Potentially Preventable VTE[2]	43	0%	10%	10%
UFH with Dosages/Platelet Monitoring[2]	38	100%	100%	97%
Venous Thromboembolism Prophylaxis[2]	365	97%	88%	85%
Warfarin Therapy Discharge Instructions[2]	101	100%	85%	75%
Chest Pain/Possible Heart Attack Care				
Aspirin Given Within 24 Hours of Arrival[1,3]	-	-	98%	96%
Fibrinolytic Meds Within 30 Min. of Arrival[5]	-	-	81%	58%
Average Time to ECG (minutes)[1,3]	-	-	7	7
Average Time to Transfer (minutes)[5]	-	-	53	60
Children's Asthma Care				
Received Home Management Plan of Care	-	-	-	88%
Received Reliever Medication	-	-	-	100%
Received Systemic Corticosteroids	-	-	-	100%
Emergency Department				
Admittance Decision Time (minutes)[2]	478	178	111	98
Head CT Results Within 45 Min. of Arrival	19	89%	64%	57%
Patients Who Left ER Before Being Seen	93,015	2%	2%	2%
Time from ER Arrival to Admit. (minutes)[2]	478	343	289	274
Time from ER Arrival to Discharge (minutes)	335	151	147	134
Time in ER Before Being Evaluated (minutes)	382	38	26	26
Time to Pain Meds for Fractures (minutes)	368	35	60	57
Heart Attack Care				
Aspirin Given at Discharge	331	100%	99%	99%
Fibrinolytic Meds Within 30 Min. of Arrival[7]	-	-	50%	54%
PCI Within 90 Minutes of Arrival	65	98%	96%	96%
Statin Prescribed at Discharge	325	100%	99%	98%
Heart Failure Care				
ACE Inhibitor or ARB for LVSD	184	100%	98%	97%
Discharge Instructions Given	519	100%	96%	94%
Evaluation of LVS Function	596	100%	100%	99%
Medicare Spending				
Medicare Spending per Patient (ratio)	-	1.04	1.04	0.98
Pneumonia Care				
Appropriate Initial Antibiotic Given	270	100%	98%	95%
Blood Culture Timing	434	100%	99%	98%
Pregnancy and Delivery Care				
Newborn Deliveries Scheduled Early[2]	77	0%	6%	6%
Preventive Care				
Immunization for Influenza[2]	518	100%	94%	90%
Immunization for Pneumonia[2]	524	100%	96%	92%
Stroke Care				
Anticoagulation Therapy for Atrial Fibrillation	29	100%	97%	95%
Antithrombotic Therapy Timing	206	100%	98%	98%
Assessed for Rehabilitation	228	100%	97%	97%
Discharged on Antithrombotic Therapy	206	100%	99%	99%

NOTE: Hospital profiles are in alphabetical order by state, then city, then hospital within the city; Rankings exclude hospitals with less than 25 cases except for patient surveys which excludes hospitals with less than 100 cases; (a) 100-299 cases; (1) The number of cases/patients is too few to report; (2) Data submitted were based on a sample of cases/patients; (3) Results are based on a shorter time period than required; (4) Data suppressed by CMS for one or more quarters; (5) Results are not available for this reporting period; (6) Fewer than 100 patients completed the HCAHPS survey; (7) No cases met the criteria for this measure; (8) The lower limit of the confidence interval cannot be calculated if the number of observed infections equals zero; (9) No data are available from the state/territory for this reporting period; (10) The scores shown reflect fewer than 50 completed surveys; (11) There were discrepancies in the data collection process; (12) This measure does not apply to this hospital for this reporting period; (13) Results cannot be calculated for this reporting period; (14) The results for this state are combined with nearby states to protect confidentiality; Please refer to the User's Guide for a full explanation of data.

Measure	Cases	This Hosp.	State Avg.	U.S. Avg.
Discharged on Statin Medication	148	100%	96%	94%
Thrombolytic Therapy Timing[1]	-	-	76%	66%
Venous Thromboembolism Prophylaxis	232	100%	95%	94%
Written Stroke Educational Materials Given	151	99%	94%	88%
Surgical Care Improvement Project				
Appropriate Beta Blocker Usage[2]	121	100%	99%	98%
Appropriate VTP Within 24 Hours[2]	383	100%	99%	98%
Controlled Postoperative Blood Glucose[2,7]	-	-	98%	97%
Perioperative Temperature Management[2]	429	100%	100%	100%
Prophylactic Antibiotic Selection[2]	300	100%	99%	99%
Prophylactic Antibiotic Selection (Outpatient)	370	100%	98%	98%
Prophylactic Antibiotic Stopped[2]	291	100%	98%	98%
Prophylactic Antibiotic Timing[2]	301	100%	99%	99%
Prophylactic Antibiotic Timing (Outpatient)	370	100%	98%	98%
Urinary Catheter Removal[2]	213	100%	98%	97%
Survey of Patients' Hospital Experiences				
Area Around Room 'Always' Quiet at Night	300+	66%	58%	61%
Doctors 'Always' Communicated Well	300+	81%	77%	82%
Home Recovery Information Given	300+	80%	83%	85%
Hospital Given 9 or 10 on 10 Point Scale	300+	74%	67%	71%
Meds 'Always' Explained Before Given	300+	62%	60%	64%
Nurses 'Always' Communicated Well	300+	78%	75%	79%
Pain 'Always' Well Controlled	300+	71%	68%	71%
Room and Bathroom 'Always' Clean	300+	77%	69%	73%
Timely Help 'Always' Received	300+	63%	62%	68%
Would Definitely Recommend Hospital	300+	79%	69%	71%
Use of Medical Imaging				
Cardiac Imaging Stress Test before Surgery[1]	-	-	6.4%	5.3%
Combination Abdominal CT Scan	862	5.0%	11.8%	10.5%
Combination Brain/Sinus CT Scan	701	1.6%	3.4%	2.7%
Combination Chest CT Scan	823	2.3%	2.4%	2.7%
Follow-up Mammogram/Ultrasound	1,286	13.8%	10.2%	8.8%
Lumbar Spine MRI for Low Back Pain	66	43.9%	35.2%	37.2%

Baptist Hospital

1000 W Moreno St
Pensacola, FL 32501
Phone: 850-434-4011
Fax: 850-469-2307
URL: www.ebaptisthealthcare.org
Type: Acute Care Hospitals
Emergency Services: Yes
Ownership: Voluntary non-profit - Private
Beds: 492

Key Personnel:

Hemotology Center . . . . Donna Campbell
CEO/President. . . . . Mark Faulkner
Infection Control. . . . . Tammy Jernigan
Chief of Medical Staff. . . . . Michael Oleksyk, MD
Radiology. . . . . Carolyn Schuster
Quality Assurance . . . . Alicia Snyder
Intensive Care Unit. . . . . Terrie Wood

Measure	Cases	This Hosp.	State Avg.	U.S. Avg.
Blood Clot Prevention and Treatment				
Anticoagulation Overlap Therapy[2]	81	64%	93%	93%
ICU Venous Thromboembolism Prophylaxis[2]	69	90%	94%	92%
Incidence of Potentially Preventable VTE[2]	24	21%	10%	10%
UFH with Dosages/Platelet Monitoring[2]	19	79%	100%	97%
Venous Thromboembolism Prophylaxis[2]	337	74%	88%	85%
Warfarin Therapy Discharge Instructions[2]	56	4%	85%	75%
Chest Pain/Possible Heart Attack Care				
Aspirin Given Within 24 Hours of Arrival[5]	-	-	98%	96%
Fibrinolytic Meds Within 30 Min. of Arrival[5]	-	-	81%	58%
Average Time to ECG (minutes)[5]	-	-	7	7
Average Time to Transfer (minutes)[5]	-	-	53	60
Children's Asthma Care				
Received Home Management Plan of Care	-	-	-	88%
Received Reliever Medication	-	-	-	100%
Received Systemic Corticosteroids	-	-	-	100%
Emergency Department				
Admittance Decision Time (minutes)[2]	631	132	111	98
Head CT Results Within 45 Min. of Arrival[1]	-	-	64%	57%
Patients Who Left ER Before Being Seen	51,366	4%	2%	2%
Time from ER Arrival to Admit. (minutes)[2]	665	311	289	274
Time from ER Arrival to Discharge (minutes)	432	162	147	134
Time in ER Before Being Evaluated (minutes)	421	52	26	26
Time to Pain Meds for Fractures (minutes)	54	92	60	57
Heart Attack Care				
Aspirin Given at Discharge[2]	260	100%	99%	99%
Fibrinolytic Meds Within 30 Min. of Arrival[2,7]	-	-	50%	54%
PCI Within 90 Minutes of Arrival[2]	66	97%	96%	96%
Statin Prescribed at Discharge[2]	251	100%	99%	98%
Heart Failure Care				
ACE Inhibitor or ARB for LVSD[2]	130	100%	98%	97%
Discharge Instructions Given[2]	290	95%	96%	94%
Evaluation of LVS Function[2]	330	100%	100%	99%
Medicare Spending				
Medicare Spending per Patient (ratio)	-	1.02	1.04	0.98
Pneumonia Care				
Appropriate Initial Antibiotic Given[2]	106	99%	98%	95%
Blood Culture Timing[2]	170	99%	99%	98%
Pregnancy and Delivery Care				
Newborn Deliveries Scheduled Early[2]	47	32%	6%	6%
Preventive Care				
Immunization for Influenza[2]	605	89%	94%	90%
Immunization for Pneumonia[2]	790	94%	96%	92%
Stroke Care				
Anticoagulation Therapy for Atrial Fibrillation	24	88%	97%	95%
Antithrombotic Therapy Timing	143	94%	98%	98%
Assessed for Rehabilitation	173	100%	97%	97%
Discharged on Antithrombotic Therapy	151	99%	99%	99%
Discharged on Statin Medication	105	96%	96%	94%
Thrombolytic Therapy Timing	17	88%	76%	66%
Venous Thromboembolism Prophylaxis	191	94%	95%	94%
Written Stroke Educational Materials Given	88	97%	94%	88%
Surgical Care Improvement Project				
Appropriate Beta Blocker Usage[2]	309	99%	99%	98%
Appropriate VTP Within 24 Hours[2]	461	98%	99%	98%
Controlled Postoperative Blood Glucose[2]	178	97%	98%	97%
Perioperative Temperature Management[2]	628	100%	100%	100%
Prophylactic Antibiotic Selection[2]	524	100%	99%	99%
Prophylactic Antibiotic Selection (Outpatient)	571	98%	98%	98%
Prophylactic Antibiotic Stopped[2]	515	100%	98%	98%
Prophylactic Antibiotic Timing[2]	526	100%	99%	99%
Prophylactic Antibiotic Timing (Outpatient)	578	97%	98%	98%
Urinary Catheter Removal[2]	418	99%	98%	97%
Survey of Patients' Hospital Experiences				
Area Around Room 'Always' Quiet at Night	300+	65%	58%	61%
Doctors 'Always' Communicated Well	300+	83%	77%	82%
Home Recovery Information Given	300+	87%	83%	85%
Hospital Given 9 or 10 on 10 Point Scale	300+	76%	67%	71%
Meds 'Always' Explained Before Given	300+	67%	60%	64%
Nurses 'Always' Communicated Well	300+	81%	75%	79%
Pain 'Always' Well Controlled	300+	73%	68%	71%
Room and Bathroom 'Always' Clean	300+	74%	69%	73%
Timely Help 'Always' Received	300+	69%	62%	68%
Would Definitely Recommend Hospital	300+	77%	69%	71%
Use of Medical Imaging				
Cardiac Imaging Stress Test before Surgery	1,415	5.2%	6.4%	5.3%
Combination Abdominal CT Scan	880	23.0%	11.8%	10.5%
Combination Brain/Sinus CT Scan	948	3.2%	3.4%	2.7%
Combination Chest CT Scan	465	8.0%	2.4%	2.7%
Follow-up Mammogram/Ultrasound	1,797	11.5%	10.2%	8.8%
Lumbar Spine MRI for Low Back Pain	243	32.5%	35.2%	37.2%

Sacred Heart Hospital

5151 N 9th Ave
Pensacola, FL 32504
Phone: 850-416-7000
Fax: 850-416-6740
URL: www.sacred-heart.org
Type: Acute Care Hospitals
Emergency Services: Yes
Ownership: Voluntary non-profit - Other
Beds: 449

Key Personnel:

Chief of Medical Staff . . . . Stephanie Duggan, MD
Quality Assurance . . . . Debra Foshee
CEO/President. . . . . Henry Stovall
Radiology. . . . . Ron Thompson
Infection Control. . . . . Barbara Wade, MD
Pediatric Ambulatory Care . . . . . . Cynthia Worrell-White
Pediatric In-Patient Care . . . . Cynthia Worrell-White

Measure	Cases	This Hosp.	State Avg.	U.S. Avg.
Blood Clot Prevention and Treatment				
Anticoagulation Overlap Therapy[2]	95	99%	93%	93%
ICU Venous Thromboembolism Prophylaxis[2]	76	92%	94%	92%
Incidence of Potentially Preventable VTE[2]	28	11%	10%	10%
UFH with Dosages/Platelet Monitoring[2]	17	100%	100%	97%
Venous Thromboembolism Prophylaxis[2]	342	80%	88%	85%
Warfarin Therapy Discharge Instructions[2]	73	26%	85%	75%
Chest Pain/Possible Heart Attack Care				
Aspirin Given Within 24 Hours of Arrival[5]	-	-	98%	96%
Fibrinolytic Meds Within 30 Min. of Arrival[5]	-	-	81%	58%
Average Time to ECG (minutes)[5]	-	-	7	7
Average Time to Transfer (minutes)[5]	-	-	53	60
Children's Asthma Care				
Received Home Management Plan of Care	-	-	-	88%
Received Reliever Medication	-	-	-	100%
Received Systemic Corticosteroids	-	-	-	100%
Emergency Department				
Admittance Decision Time (minutes)[2]	366	96	111	98
Head CT Results Within 45 Min. of Arrival[1]	-	-	64%	57%
Patients Who Left ER Before Being Seen	89,018	3%	2%	2%
Time from ER Arrival to Admit. (minutes)[2]	400	310	289	274
Time from ER Arrival to Discharge (minutes)	309	179	147	134
Time in ER Before Being Evaluated (minutes)	255	60	26	26
Time to Pain Meds for Fractures (minutes)	225	71	60	57
Heart Attack Care				
Aspirin Given at Discharge[2]	311	98%	99%	99%
Fibrinolytic Meds Within 30 Min. of Arrival[1,2]	-	-	50%	54%
PCI Within 90 Minutes of Arrival[2]	37	95%	96%	96%
Statin Prescribed at Discharge[2]	293	98%	99%	98%
Heart Failure Care				
ACE Inhibitor or ARB for LVSD[2]	110	100%	98%	97%
Discharge Instructions Given[2]	250	94%	96%	94%
Evaluation of LVS Function[2]	310	100%	100%	99%
Medicare Spending				
Medicare Spending per Patient (ratio)	-	1.02	1.04	0.98
Pneumonia Care				
Appropriate Initial Antibiotic Given[2]	89	96%	98%	95%
Blood Culture Timing[2]	174	98%	99%	98%
Pregnancy and Delivery Care				
Newborn Deliveries Scheduled Early[2]	69	4%	6%	6%
Preventive Care				
Immunization for Influenza[2]	524	91%	94%	90%
Immunization for Pneumonia[2]	506	91%	96%	92%
Stroke Care				
Anticoagulation Therapy for Atrial Fibrillation[2]	12	100%	97%	95%
Antithrombotic Therapy Timing[2]	57	96%	98%	98%
Assessed for Rehabilitation[2]	101	99%	97%	97%
Discharged on Antithrombotic Therapy[2]	82	100%	99%	99%
Discharged on Statin Medication[2]	64	97%	96%	94%
Thrombolytic Therapy Timing[2]	18	11%	76%	66%
Venous Thromboembolism Prophylaxis[2]	99	94%	95%	94%
Written Stroke Educational Materials Given[2]	64	77%	94%	88%
Surgical Care Improvement Project				
Appropriate Beta Blocker Usage[2]	215	96%	99%	98%
Appropriate VTP Within 24 Hours[2]	481	97%	99%	98%
Controlled Postoperative Blood Glucose[2]	103	91%	98%	97%
Perioperative Temperature Management[2]	676	100%	100%	100%
Prophylactic Antibiotic Selection[2]	483	99%	99%	99%
Prophylactic Antibiotic Selection (Outpatient)	444	97%	98%	98%
Prophylactic Antibiotic Stopped[2]	462	97%	98%	98%
Prophylactic Antibiotic Timing[2]	483	99%	99%	99%
Prophylactic Antibiotic Timing (Outpatient)	445	100%	98%	98%
Urinary Catheter Removal[2]	438	90%	98%	97%
Survey of Patients' Hospital Experiences				
Area Around Room 'Always' Quiet at Night	300+	59%	58%	61%
Doctors 'Always' Communicated Well	300+	82%	77%	82%
Home Recovery Information Given	300+	87%	83%	85%
Hospital Given 9 or 10 on 10 Point Scale	300+	72%	67%	71%
Meds 'Always' Explained Before Given	300+	62%	60%	64%
Nurses 'Always' Communicated Well	300+	80%	75%	79%
Pain 'Always' Well Controlled	300+	72%	68%	71%
Room and Bathroom 'Always' Clean	300+	65%	69%	73%
Timely Help 'Always' Received	300+	65%	62%	68%
Would Definitely Recommend Hospital	300+	76%	69%	71%

NOTE: Hospital profiles are in alphabetical order by state, then city, then hospital within the city; Rankings exclude hospitals with less than 25 cases except for patient surveys which excludes hospitals with less than 100 cases; (a) 100-299 cases; (1) The number of cases/patients is too few to report; (2) Data submitted were based on a sample of cases/patients; (3) Results are based on a shorter time period than required; (4) Data suppressed by CMS for one or more quarters; (5) Results are not available for this reporting period; (6) Fewer than 100 patients completed the HCAHPS survey; (7) No cases met the criteria for this measure; (8) The lower limit of the confidence interval cannot be calculated if the number of observed infections equals zero; (9) No data are available from the state/territory for this reporting period; (10) The scores shown reflect fewer than 50 completed surveys; (11) There were discrepancies in the data collection process; (12) This measure does not apply to this hospital for this reporting period; (13) Results cannot be calculated for this reporting period; (14) The results for this state are combined with nearby states to protect confidentiality; Please refer to the User's Guide for a full explanation of data.

Use of Medical Imaging				
Cardiac Imaging Stress Test before Surgery	771	5.6%	6.4%	5.3%
Combination Abdominal CT Scan	1,616	10.4%	11.8%	10.5%
Combination Brain/Sinus CT Scan	1,327	2.9%	3.4%	2.7%
Combination Chest CT Scan	1,065	1.3%	2.4%	2.7%
Follow-up Mammogram/Ultrasound	2,845	11.1%	10.2%	8.8%
Lumbar Spine MRI for Low Back Pain	262	37.8%	35.2%	37.2%

West Florida Hospital

8383 N Davis Hwy
Pensacola, FL 32514
URL: www.westfloridahospital.com
Type: Acute Care Hospitals
Ownership: Proprietary
Phone: 850-494-4000
Fax: 850-494-5216
Emergency Services: Yes
Beds: 531

Key Personnel:
Radiology. . . . . Lisa Harrison
Emergency Room . . . . Margie Hobbs
Operating Room. . . . . Pam Parker
Coronary Care . . . . Jacque Posey
Intensive Care Unit. . . . . Jacque Posey
Infection Control. . . . . Lorraine Price
Quality Assurance . . . . Sharon Smith
CEO/President. . . . . Dennis A Taylor

Measure	Cases	This Hosp.	State Avg.	U.S. Avg.
Blood Clot Prevention and Treatment				
Anticoagulation Overlap Therapy[2]	71	90%	93%	93%
ICU Venous Thromboembolism Prophylaxis[2]	139	94%	94%	92%
Incidence of Potentially Preventable VTE[1,2]	-	-	10%	10%
UFH with Dosages/Platelet Monitoring[2]	18	100%	100%	97%
Venous Thromboembolism Prophylaxis[2]	285	82%	88%	85%
Warfarin Therapy Discharge Instructions[2]	51	100%	85%	75%
Chest Pain/Possible Heart Attack Care				
Aspirin Given Within 24 Hours of Arrival[3,7]	-	-	98%	96%
Fibrinolytic Meds Within 30 Min. of Arrival[5]	-	-	81%	58%
Average Time to ECG (minutes)[3,7]	-	-	7	7
Average Time to Transfer (minutes)[5]	-	-	53	60
Children's Asthma Care				
Received Home Management Plan of Care	-	-	-	88%
Received Reliever Medication	-	-	-	100%
Received Systemic Corticosteroids	-	-	-	100%
Emergency Department				
Admittance Decision Time (minutes)[2]	796	86	111	98
Head CT Results Within 45 Min. of Arrival	18	56%	64%	57%
Patients Who Left ER Before Being Seen	50,551	1%	2%	2%
Time from ER Arrival to Admit. (minutes)[2]	796	241	289	274
Time from ER Arrival to Discharge (minutes)	450	170	147	134
Time in ER Before Being Evaluated (minutes)	512	7	26	26
Time to Pain Meds for Fractures (minutes)	117	75	60	57
Heart Attack Care				
Aspirin Given at Discharge	208	100%	99%	99%
Fibrinolytic Meds Within 30 Min. of Arrival[7]	-	-	50%	54%
PCI Within 90 Minutes of Arrival	50	100%	96%	96%
Statin Prescribed at Discharge	203	100%	99%	98%
Heart Failure Care				
ACE Inhibitor or ARB for LVSD	111	100%	98%	97%
Discharge Instructions Given	306	100%	96%	94%
Evaluation of LVS Function	369	100%	100%	99%
Medicare Spending				
Medicare Spending per Patient (ratio)	-	1.00	1.04	0.98
Pneumonia Care				
Appropriate Initial Antibiotic Given[2]	71	99%	98%	95%
Blood Culture Timing[2]	148	100%	99%	98%
Pregnancy and Delivery Care				
Newborn Deliveries Scheduled Early[2]	45	4%	6%	6%
Preventive Care				
Immunization for Influenza[2]	641	98%	94%	90%
Immunization for Pneumonia[2]	931	97%	96%	92%
Stroke Care				
Anticoagulation Therapy for Atrial Fibrillation[2]	13	100%	97%	95%
Antithrombotic Therapy Timing[2]	110	100%	98%	98%
Assessed for Rehabilitation[2]	109	100%	97%	97%
Discharged on Antithrombotic Therapy[2]	108	100%	99%	99%
Discharged on Statin Medication[2]	82	99%	96%	94%
Thrombolytic Therapy Timing[1,2]	-	-	76%	66%
Venous Thromboembolism Prophylaxis[2]	109	99%	95%	94%
Written Stroke Educational Materials Given[2]	60	100%	94%	88%
Surgical Care Improvement Project				
Appropriate Beta Blocker Usage[2]	223	100%	99%	98%
Appropriate VTP Within 24 Hours[2]	442	100%	99%	98%
Controlled Postoperative Blood Glucose[2]	102	100%	98%	97%
Perioperative Temperature Management[2]	537	100%	100%	100%
Prophylactic Antibiotic Selection[2]	388	100%	99%	99%
Prophylactic Antibiotic Selection (Outpatient)	378	99%	98%	98%
Prophylactic Antibiotic Stopped[2]	359	100%	98%	98%
Prophylactic Antibiotic Timing[2]	389	100%	99%	99%
Prophylactic Antibiotic Timing (Outpatient)	378	99%	98%	98%
Urinary Catheter Removal[2]	256	100%	98%	97%
Survey of Patients' Hospital Experiences				
Area Around Room 'Always' Quiet at Night	300+	63%	58%	61%
Doctors 'Always' Communicated Well	300+	78%	77%	82%
Home Recovery Information Given	300+	86%	83%	85%
Hospital Given 9 or 10 on 10 Point Scale	300+	74%	67%	71%
Meds 'Always' Explained Before Given	300+	62%	60%	64%
Nurses 'Always' Communicated Well	300+	78%	75%	79%
Pain 'Always' Well Controlled	300+	69%	68%	71%
Room and Bathroom 'Always' Clean	300+	66%	69%	73%
Timely Help 'Always' Received	300+	64%	62%	68%
Would Definitely Recommend Hospital	300+	76%	69%	71%
Use of Medical Imaging				
Cardiac Imaging Stress Test before Surgery	762	6.2%	6.4%	5.3%
Combination Abdominal CT Scan	938	4.5%	11.8%	10.5%
Combination Brain/Sinus CT Scan	1,163	2.5%	3.4%	2.7%
Combination Chest CT Scan	481	1.2%	2.4%	2.7%
Follow-up Mammogram/Ultrasound	2,240	12.9%	10.2%	8.8%
Lumbar Spine MRI for Low Back Pain	83	34.9%	35.2%	37.2%

Doctor's Memorial Hospital

333 N Byron Butler Pkwy
Perry, FL 32348
E-mail: adnun@doctorsmemorial.com
URL: www.doctorsmemorial.com
Type: Acute Care Hospitals
Ownership: Voluntary non-profit - Private
Phone: 850-584-0800
Fax: 850-584-2524
Emergency Services: Yes
Beds: 48

Key Personnel:
Emergency Room . . . . Deborah Dorman, RN
Quality Assurance . . . . Ann Gray, RN
CEO/President. . . . . Richard Huth
Operating Room. . . . . Lisa Noles
Radiology. . . . . Lyn Odom
Intensive Care Unit. . . . . Lisa Story, RN
Cardiac Laboratory. . . . . Tulio Sulbaran
Infection Control. . . . . Delores Weldon, RN

Measure	Cases	This Hosp.	State Avg.	U.S. Avg.
Blood Clot Prevention and Treatment				
Anticoagulation Overlap Therapy[1,2]	-	-	93%	93%
ICU Venous Thromboembolism Prophylaxis[2]	38	71%	94%	92%
Incidence of Potentially Preventable VTE[2,7]	-	-	10%	10%
UFH with Dosages/Platelet Monitoring[1,2]	-	-	100%	97%
Venous Thromboembolism Prophylaxis[2]	98	67%	88%	85%
Warfarin Therapy Discharge Instructions[1,2]	-	-	85%	75%
Chest Pain/Possible Heart Attack Care				
Aspirin Given Within 24 Hours of Arrival	89	98%	98%	96%
Fibrinolytic Meds Within 30 Min. of Arrival[1]	-	-	81%	58%
Average Time to ECG (minutes)	92	8	7	7
Average Time to Transfer (minutes)[1]	-	-	53	60
Children's Asthma Care				
Received Home Management Plan of Care	-	-	-	88%
Received Reliever Medication	-	-	-	100%
Received Systemic Corticosteroids	-	-	-	100%
Emergency Department				
Admittance Decision Time (minutes)[2]	569	70	111	98
Head CT Results Within 45 Min. of Arrival[1]	-	-	64%	57%
Patients Who Left ER Before Being Seen	14,523	5%	2%	2%
Time from ER Arrival to Admit. (minutes)[2]	652	284	289	274
Time from ER Arrival to Discharge (minutes)	371	143	147	134
Time in ER Before Being Evaluated (minutes)	405	41	26	26
Time to Pain Meds for Fractures (minutes)	64	40	60	57
Heart Attack Care				
Aspirin Given at Discharge[1,3]	-	-	99%	99%
Fibrinolytic Meds Within 30 Min. of Arrival[3,7]	-	-	50%	54%
PCI Within 90 Minutes of Arrival[3,7]	-	-	96%	96%
Statin Prescribed at Discharge[3,7]	-	-	99%	98%
Heart Failure Care				
ACE Inhibitor or ARB for LVSD	20	90%	98%	97%
Discharge Instructions Given	32	100%	96%	94%
Evaluation of LVS Function	36	100%	100%	99%
Medicare Spending				
Medicare Spending per Patient (ratio)	-	1.03	1.04	0.98
Pneumonia Care				
Appropriate Initial Antibiotic Given	37	81%	98%	95%
Blood Culture Timing	50	100%	99%	98%
Pregnancy and Delivery Care				
Newborn Deliveries Scheduled Early[7]	-	-	6%	6%
Preventive Care				
Immunization for Influenza[2]	326	82%	94%	90%
Immunization for Pneumonia[2]	438	85%	96%	92%
Stroke Care				
Anticoagulation Therapy for Atrial Fibrillation[7]	-	-	97%	95%
Antithrombotic Therapy Timing[1]	-	-	98%	98%
Assessed for Rehabilitation[1]	-	-	97%	97%
Discharged on Antithrombotic Therapy[1]	-	-	99%	99%
Discharged on Statin Medication[1]	-	-	96%	94%
Thrombolytic Therapy Timing[7]	-	-	76%	66%
Venous Thromboembolism Prophylaxis[1]	-	-	95%	94%
Written Stroke Educational Materials Given[1]	-	-	94%	88%
Surgical Care Improvement Project				
Appropriate Beta Blocker Usage	14	100%	99%	98%
Appropriate VTP Within 24 Hours	69	100%	99%	98%
Controlled Postoperative Blood Glucose[7]	-	-	98%	97%
Perioperative Temperature Management	76	100%	100%	100%
Prophylactic Antibiotic Selection	48	100%	99%	99%
Prophylactic Antibiotic Selection (Outpatient)[1,3]	-	-	98%	98%
Prophylactic Antibiotic Stopped	48	98%	98%	98%
Prophylactic Antibiotic Timing	48	100%	99%	99%
Prophylactic Antibiotic Timing (Outpatient)[1,3]	-	-	98%	98%
Urinary Catheter Removal	55	100%	98%	97%
Survey of Patients' Hospital Experiences				
Area Around Room 'Always' Quiet at Night	(a)	70%	58%	61%
Doctors 'Always' Communicated Well	(a)	81%	77%	82%
Home Recovery Information Given	(a)	83%	83%	85%
Hospital Given 9 or 10 on 10 Point Scale	(a)	72%	67%	71%
Meds 'Always' Explained Before Given	(a)	66%	60%	64%
Nurses 'Always' Communicated Well	(a)	81%	75%	79%
Pain 'Always' Well Controlled	(a)	76%	68%	71%
Room and Bathroom 'Always' Clean	(a)	85%	69%	73%
Timely Help 'Always' Received	(a)	74%	62%	68%
Would Definitely Recommend Hospital	(a)	68%	69%	71%
Use of Medical Imaging				
Cardiac Imaging Stress Test before Surgery[1]	-	-	6.4%	5.3%
Combination Abdominal CT Scan	259	5.8%	11.8%	10.5%
Combination Brain/Sinus CT Scan[1]	-	-	3.4%	2.7%
Combination Chest CT Scan	109	5.5%	2.4%	2.7%
Follow-up Mammogram/Ultrasound	331	10.9%	10.2%	8.8%
Lumbar Spine MRI for Low Back Pain[1]	-	-	35.2%	37.2%

South Florida Baptist Hospital

301 N Alexander St
Plant City, FL 33563
URL: www.sjbhealth.org
Type: Acute Care Hospitals
Ownership: Voluntary non-profit - Private
Phone: 813-757-1200
Fax: 813-757-1255
Emergency Services: Yes
Beds: 147

Key Personnel:
Radiology. . . . . Axel Frank Campbell, MD
CEO/President. . . . . Issac Mallah
Emergency Room . . . . Natalie Rivera, RN
Pediatric Ambulatory Care . . . . . . Michael Salvato, MD
Pediatric In-Patient Care . . . . Michael Salvato, MD
Chief of Medical Staff. . . . . Steve Smith, MD

Measure	Cases	This Hosp.	State Avg.	U.S. Avg.
Blood Clot Prevention and Treatment				
Anticoagulation Overlap Therapy[2]	51	82%	93%	93%
ICU Venous Thromboembolism Prophylaxis[2]	81	89%	94%	92%

NOTE: Hospital profiles are in alphabetical order by state, then city, then hospital within the city; Rankings exclude hospitals with less than 25 cases except for patient surveys which excludes hospitals with less than 100 cases; (a) 100-299 cases; (1) The number of cases/patients is too few to report; (2) Data submitted were based on a sample of cases/patients; (3) Results are based on a shorter time period than required; (4) Data suppressed by CMS for one or more quarters; (5) Results are not available for this reporting period; (6) Fewer than 100 patients completed the HCAHPS survey; (7) No cases met the criteria for this measure; (8) The lower limit of the confidence interval cannot be calculated if the number of observed infections equals zero; (9) No data are available from the state/territory for this reporting period; (10) The scores shown reflect fewer than 50 completed surveys; (11) There were discrepancies in the data collection process; (12) This measure does not apply to this hospital for this reporting period; (13) Results cannot be calculated for this reporting period; (14) The results for this state are combined with nearby states to protect confidentiality; Please refer to the User's Guide for a full explanation of data.

Measure	Cases	This Hosp.	State Avg.	U.S. Avg.
Incidence of Potentially Preventable VTE[1,2]	-	-	10%	10%
UFH with Dosages/Platelet Monitoring[2]	15	100%	100%	97%
Venous Thromboembolism Prophylaxis[2]	339	73%	88%	85%
Warfarin Therapy Discharge Instructions[2]	43	84%	85%	75%
Chest Pain/Possible Heart Attack Care				
Aspirin Given Within 24 Hours of Arrival	36	100%	98%	96%
Fibrinolytic Meds Within 30 Min. of Arrival[1]	-	-	81%	58%
Average Time to ECG (minutes)	36	7	7	7
Average Time to Transfer (minutes)[1]	-	-	53	60
Children's Asthma Care				
Received Home Management Plan of Care	-	-	-	88%
Received Reliever Medication	-	-	-	100%
Received Systemic Corticosteroids	-	-	-	100%
Emergency Department				
Admittance Decision Time (minutes)[2]	407	100	111	98
Head CT Results Within 45 Min. of Arrival[1]	-	-	64%	57%
Patients Who Left ER Before Being Seen	42,151	2%	2%	2%
Time from ER Arrival to Admit. (minutes)[2]	409	271	289	274
Time from ER Arrival to Discharge (minutes)	357	122	147	134
Time in ER Before Being Evaluated (minutes)	406	28	26	26
Time to Pain Meds for Fractures (minutes)	81	59	60	57
Heart Attack Care				
Aspirin Given at Discharge	58	100%	99%	99%
Fibrinolytic Meds Within 30 Min. of Arrival[7]	-	-	50%	54%
PCI Within 90 Minutes of Arrival[7]	-	-	96%	96%
Statin Prescribed at Discharge	54	100%	99%	98%
Heart Failure Care				
ACE Inhibitor or ARB for LVSD	55	100%	98%	97%
Discharge Instructions Given	171	99%	96%	94%
Evaluation of LVS Function	199	100%	100%	99%
Medicare Spending				
Medicare Spending per Patient (ratio)	-	1.02	1.04	0.98
Pneumonia Care				
Appropriate Initial Antibiotic Given	116	98%	98%	95%
Blood Culture Timing	228	100%	99%	98%
Pregnancy and Delivery Care				
Newborn Deliveries Scheduled Early[2]	36	6%	6%	6%
Preventive Care				
Immunization for Influenza[2]	565	97%	94%	90%
Immunization for Pneumonia[2]	733	89%	96%	92%
Stroke Care				
Anticoagulation Therapy for Atrial Fibrillation[1]	-	-	97%	95%
Antithrombotic Therapy Timing	49	94%	98%	98%
Assessed for Rehabilitation	51	98%	97%	97%
Discharged on Antithrombotic Therapy	51	98%	99%	99%
Discharged on Statin Medication	37	89%	96%	94%
Thrombolytic Therapy Timing[1]	-	-	76%	66%
Venous Thromboembolism Prophylaxis	51	69%	95%	94%
Written Stroke Educational Materials Given	35	94%	94%	88%
Surgical Care Improvement Project				
Appropriate Beta Blocker Usage	108	96%	99%	98%
Appropriate VTP Within 24 Hours	398	99%	99%	98%
Controlled Postoperative Blood Glucose[7]	-	-	98%	97%
Perioperative Temperature Management	444	100%	100%	100%
Prophylactic Antibiotic Selection	281	100%	99%	99%
Prophylactic Antibiotic Selection (Outpatient)	76	89%	98%	98%
Prophylactic Antibiotic Stopped	268	99%	98%	98%
Prophylactic Antibiotic Timing	281	99%	99%	99%
Prophylactic Antibiotic Timing (Outpatient)	79	91%	98%	98%
Urinary Catheter Removal	112	99%	98%	97%
Survey of Patients' Hospital Experiences				
Area Around Room 'Always' Quiet at Night[11]	300+	60%	58%	61%
Doctors 'Always' Communicated Well[11]	300+	78%	77%	82%
Home Recovery Information Given[11]	300+	88%	83%	85%
Hospital Given 9 or 10 on 10 Point Scale[11]	300+	73%	67%	71%
Meds 'Always' Explained Before Given[11]	300+	63%	60%	64%
Nurses 'Always' Communicated Well[11]	300+	78%	75%	79%
Pain 'Always' Well Controlled[11]	300+	70%	68%	71%
Room and Bathroom 'Always' Clean[11]	300+	78%	69%	73%
Timely Help 'Always' Received[11]	300+	70%	62%	68%
Would Definitely Recommend Hospital[11]	300+	73%	69%	71%
Use of Medical Imaging				
Cardiac Imaging Stress Test before Surgery	90	6.7%	6.4%	5.3%
Combination Abdominal CT Scan	408	4.9%	11.8%	10.5%
Combination Brain/Sinus CT Scan	445	4.3%	3.4%	2.7%
Combination Chest CT Scan	164	0.6%	2.4%	2.7%
Follow-up Mammogram/Ultrasound	724	9.5%	10.2%	8.8%
Lumbar Spine MRI for Low Back Pain[1]	-	-	35.2%	37.2%

Plantation General Hospital

401 Nw 42nd Ave
Plantation, FL 33317
URL: www.plantationgeneral.com
Type: Acute Care Hospitals
Ownership: Proprietary
Phone: 954-587-5010
Fax: 954-587-3220
Emergency Services: Yes
Beds: 264

Key Personnel:
Radiology. . . . . Jocelyn Bowman
CEO/President. . . . . Randy Gross
Chairman/CEO . . . . Joel M. Jancko, MD
Operating Room. . . . . Ruth Nash
Quality Assurance . . . . Cindy Rogers

Measure	Cases	This Hosp.	State Avg.	U.S. Avg.
Blood Clot Prevention and Treatment				
Anticoagulation Overlap Therapy[2]	92	97%	93%	93%
ICU Venous Thromboembolism Prophylaxis[2]	73	99%	94%	92%
Incidence of Potentially Preventable VTE[2]	18	6%	10%	10%
UFH with Dosages/Platelet Monitoring[2]	44	98%	100%	97%
Venous Thromboembolism Prophylaxis[2]	375	95%	88%	85%
Warfarin Therapy Discharge Instructions[2]	64	97%	85%	75%
Chest Pain/Possible Heart Attack Care				
Aspirin Given Within 24 Hours of Arrival	27	100%	98%	96%
Fibrinolytic Meds Within 30 Min. of Arrival[7]	-	-	81%	58%
Average Time to ECG (minutes)	27	16	7	7
Average Time to Transfer (minutes)[1]	-	-	53	60
Children's Asthma Care				
Received Home Management Plan of Care	-	-	-	88%
Received Reliever Medication	-	-	-	100%
Received Systemic Corticosteroids	-	-	-	100%
Emergency Department				
Admittance Decision Time (minutes)[2]	778	71	111	98
Head CT Results Within 45 Min. of Arrival[1]	-	-	64%	57%
Patients Who Left ER Before Being Seen	52,315	1%	2%	2%
Time from ER Arrival to Admit. (minutes)[2]	778	221	289	274
Time from ER Arrival to Discharge (minutes)	468	134	147	134
Time in ER Before Being Evaluated (minutes)	536	13	26	26
Time to Pain Meds for Fractures (minutes)	186	42	60	57
Heart Attack Care				
Aspirin Given at Discharge[2]	237	100%	99%	99%
Fibrinolytic Meds Within 30 Min. of Arrival[2,7]	-	-	50%	54%
PCI Within 90 Minutes of Arrival[2]	29	93%	96%	96%
Statin Prescribed at Discharge[2]	236	99%	99%	98%
Heart Failure Care				
ACE Inhibitor or ARB for LVSD[2]	127	99%	98%	97%
Discharge Instructions Given[2]	268	99%	96%	94%
Evaluation of LVS Function[2]	301	100%	100%	99%
Medicare Spending				
Medicare Spending per Patient (ratio)	-	1.06	1.04	0.98
Pneumonia Care				
Appropriate Initial Antibiotic Given[2]	105	98%	98%	95%
Blood Culture Timing[2]	185	99%	99%	98%
Pregnancy and Delivery Care				
Newborn Deliveries Scheduled Early[2]	111	5%	6%	6%
Preventive Care				
Immunization for Influenza[2]	604	99%	94%	90%
Immunization for Pneumonia[2]	634	100%	96%	92%
Stroke Care				
Anticoagulation Therapy for Atrial Fibrillation[2]	14	100%	97%	95%
Antithrombotic Therapy Timing[2]	82	100%	98%	98%
Assessed for Rehabilitation[2]	95	99%	97%	97%
Discharged on Antithrombotic Therapy[2]	80	99%	99%	99%
Discharged on Statin Medication[2]	59	97%	96%	94%
Thrombolytic Therapy Timing[2,7]	-	-	76%	66%
Venous Thromboembolism Prophylaxis[2]	96	97%	95%	94%
Written Stroke Educational Materials Given[2]	59	100%	94%	88%
Surgical Care Improvement Project				
Appropriate Beta Blocker Usage[2]	245	100%	99%	98%
Appropriate VTP Within 24 Hours[2]	513	99%	99%	98%
Controlled Postoperative Blood Glucose[2]	87	95%	98%	97%
Perioperative Temperature Management[2]	668	100%	100%	100%
Prophylactic Antibiotic Selection[2]	494	98%	99%	99%
Prophylactic Antibiotic Selection (Outpatient)	361	97%	98%	98%
Prophylactic Antibiotic Stopped[2]	479	99%	98%	98%
Prophylactic Antibiotic Timing[2]	494	100%	99%	99%
Prophylactic Antibiotic Timing (Outpatient)	362	99%	98%	98%
Urinary Catheter Removal[2]	399	100%	98%	97%
Survey of Patients' Hospital Experiences				
Area Around Room 'Always' Quiet at Night	300+	63%	58%	61%
Doctors 'Always' Communicated Well	300+	80%	77%	82%
Home Recovery Information Given	300+	80%	83%	85%
Hospital Given 9 or 10 on 10 Point Scale	300+	65%	67%	71%
Meds 'Always' Explained Before Given	300+	61%	60%	64%
Nurses 'Always' Communicated Well	300+	73%	75%	79%
Pain 'Always' Well Controlled	300+	67%	68%	71%
Room and Bathroom 'Always' Clean	300+	69%	69%	73%
Timely Help 'Always' Received	300+	58%	62%	68%
Would Definitely Recommend Hospital	300+	66%	69%	71%
Use of Medical Imaging				
Cardiac Imaging Stress Test before Surgery	136	3.7%	6.4%	5.3%
Combination Abdominal CT Scan	778	5.1%	11.8%	10.5%
Combination Brain/Sinus CT Scan	752	2.7%	3.4%	2.7%
Combination Chest CT Scan	303	0.7%	2.4%	2.7%
Follow-up Mammogram/Ultrasound	958	10.0%	10.2%	8.8%
Lumbar Spine MRI for Low Back Pain	73	27.4%	35.2%	37.2%

Westside Regional Medical Center

8201 W Broward Blvd
Plantation, FL 33324
URL: www.westsidehospital.com
Type: Acute Care Hospitals
Ownership: Proprietary
Phone: 954-473-6600
Fax: 954-452-2133
Emergency Services: Yes
Beds: 224

Key Personnel:
Radiology. . . . . Andrew Akerman, MD
Chief of Medical Staff . . . . Paul Bates, MD
Operating Room. . . . . Fernando Bayron-Vele
Quality Assurance . . . . Debi Brindley
CEO . . . . Lee Chaykin, FACHE
Pediatric In-Patient Care . . . . Lawrence Pearson
Emergency Room . . . . Susan West

Measure	Cases	This Hosp.	State Avg.	U.S. Avg.
Blood Clot Prevention and Treatment				
Anticoagulation Overlap Therapy[2]	76	96%	93%	93%
ICU Venous Thromboembolism Prophylaxis[2]	98	99%	94%	92%
Incidence of Potentially Preventable VTE[2]	12	0%	10%	10%
UFH with Dosages/Platelet Monitoring[2]	13	100%	100%	97%
Venous Thromboembolism Prophylaxis[2]	337	88%	88%	85%
Warfarin Therapy Discharge Instructions[2]	47	100%	85%	75%
Chest Pain/Possible Heart Attack Care				
Aspirin Given Within 24 Hours of Arrival[1,3]	-	-	98%	96%
Fibrinolytic Meds Within 30 Min. of Arrival[5]	-	-	81%	58%
Average Time to ECG (minutes)[1,3]	-	-	7	7
Average Time to Transfer (minutes)[5]	-	-	53	60
Children's Asthma Care				
Received Home Management Plan of Care	-	-	-	88%
Received Reliever Medication	-	-	-	100%
Received Systemic Corticosteroids	-	-	-	100%
Emergency Department				
Admittance Decision Time (minutes)[2]	1,038	75	111	98
Head CT Results Within 45 Min. of Arrival[1]	-	-	64%	57%
Patients Who Left ER Before Being Seen	44,675	0%	2%	2%
Time from ER Arrival to Admit. (minutes)[2]	1,038	251	289	274
Time from ER Arrival to Discharge (minutes)	430	125	147	134
Time in ER Before Being Evaluated (minutes)	461	11	26	26
Time to Pain Meds for Fractures (minutes)	109	47	60	57
Heart Attack Care				
Aspirin Given at Discharge[2]	283	99%	99%	99%
Fibrinolytic Meds Within 30 Min. of Arrival[2,7]	-	-	50%	54%
PCI Within 90 Minutes of Arrival[2]	43	100%	96%	96%
Statin Prescribed at Discharge[2]	281	99%	99%	98%
Heart Failure Care				
ACE Inhibitor or ARB for LVSD[2]	146	97%	98%	97%

NOTE: Hospital profiles are in alphabetical order by state, then city, then hospital within the city; Rankings exclude hospitals with less than 25 cases except for patient surveys which excludes hospitals with less than 100 cases; (a) 100-299 cases; (1) The number of cases/patients is too few to report; (2) Data submitted were based on a sample of cases/patients; (3) Results are based on a shorter time period than required; (4) Data suppressed by CMS for one or more quarters; (5) Results are not available for this reporting period; (6) Fewer than 100 patients completed the HCAHPS survey; (7) No cases met the criteria for this measure; (8) The lower limit of the confidence interval cannot be calculated if the number of observed infections equals zero; (9) No data are available from the state/territory for this reporting period; (10) The scores shown reflect fewer than 50 completed surveys; (11) There were discrepancies in the data collection process; (12) This measure does not apply to this hospital for this reporting period; (13) Results cannot be calculated for this reporting period; (14) The results for this state are combined with nearby states to protect confidentiality; Please refer to the User's Guide for a full explanation of data.

Discharge Instructions Given[2]	312	100%	96%	94%
Evaluation of LVS Function[2]	391	100%	100%	99%
Medicare Spending				
Medicare Spending per Patient (ratio)	-	1.11	1.04	0.98
Pneumonia Care				
Appropriate Initial Antibiotic Given	108	100%	98%	95%
Blood Culture Timing	193	99%	99%	98%
Pregnancy and Delivery Care				
Newborn Deliveries Scheduled Early[2,7]	-	-	6%	6%
Preventive Care				
Immunization for Influenza[2]	627	100%	94%	90%
Immunization for Pneumonia[2]	899	100%	96%	92%
Stroke Care				
Anticoagulation Therapy for Atrial Fibrillation[2]	21	90%	97%	95%
Antithrombotic Therapy Timing[2]	94	99%	98%	98%
Assessed for Rehabilitation[2]	111	100%	97%	97%
Discharged on Antithrombotic Therapy[2]	88	100%	99%	99%
Discharged on Statin Medication[2]	59	97%	96%	94%
Thrombolytic Therapy Timing[1,2]	-	-	76%	66%
Venous Thromboembolism Prophylaxis[2]	133	95%	95%	94%
Written Stroke Educational Materials Given[2]	56	100%	94%	88%
Surgical Care Improvement Project				
Appropriate Beta Blocker Usage[2]	202	100%	99%	98%
Appropriate VTP Within 24 Hours[2]	439	99%	99%	98%
Controlled Postoperative Blood Glucose[2]	91	100%	98%	97%
Perioperative Temperature Management[2]	483	100%	100%	100%
Prophylactic Antibiotic Selection[2]	358	99%	99%	99%
Prophylactic Antibiotic Selection (Outpatient)	209	100%	98%	98%
Prophylactic Antibiotic Stopped[2]	347	99%	98%	98%
Prophylactic Antibiotic Timing[2]	359	100%	99%	99%
Prophylactic Antibiotic Timing (Outpatient)	209	100%	98%	98%
Urinary Catheter Removal[2]	206	99%	98%	97%
Survey of Patients' Hospital Experiences				
Area Around Room 'Always' Quiet at Night	300+	49%	58%	61%
Doctors 'Always' Communicated Well	300+	75%	77%	82%
Home Recovery Information Given	300+	78%	83%	85%
Hospital Given 9 or 10 on 10 Point Scale	300+	57%	67%	71%
Meds 'Always' Explained Before Given	300+	52%	60%	64%
Nurses 'Always' Communicated Well	300+	68%	75%	79%
Pain 'Always' Well Controlled	300+	63%	68%	71%
Room and Bathroom 'Always' Clean	300+	63%	69%	73%
Timely Help 'Always' Received	300+	55%	62%	68%
Would Definitely Recommend Hospital	300+	61%	69%	71%
Use of Medical Imaging				
Cardiac Imaging Stress Test before Surgery[1]	-	-	6.4%	5.3%
Combination Abdominal CT Scan	458	5.5%	11.8%	10.5%
Combination Brain/Sinus CT Scan	544	4.0%	3.4%	2.7%
Combination Chest CT Scan	223	0.0%	2.4%	2.7%
Follow-up Mammogram/Ultrasound	372	22.8%	10.2%	8.8%
Lumbar Spine MRI for Low Back Pain[1]	-	-	35.2%	37.2%

Broward Health North

201 E Sample Rd
Pompano Beach, FL 33064
URL: www.browardhealth.org
Type: Acute Care Hospitals
Ownership: Govt - Hospital Dist/Auth
Phone: 954-786-6950
Fax: 954-781-4224
Emergency Services: Yes
Beds: 419

Key Personnel:

Pediatric Ambulatory Care . . . . . . Navinbai Ali, MD
Hemotology Center . . . . Dennis Grady
Infection Control. . . . . Mel Koham, MD
Radiology. . . . . Dan Lowdher
CEO/President. . . . . Patrick Maloney
Intensive Care Unit. . . . . Eileen Maniste
Chief of Medical Staff . . . . Steven Shapiro, MD
Operating Room. . . . . Cassandra Whitney

Measure	Cases	This Hosp.	State Avg.	U.S. Avg.
Blood Clot Prevention and Treatment				
Anticoagulation Overlap Therapy[2]	81	85%	93%	93%
ICU Venous Thromboembolism Prophylaxis[2]	70	94%	94%	92%
Incidence of Potentially Preventable VTE[2]	26	0%	10%	10%
UFH with Dosages/Platelet Monitoring[2]	28	100%	100%	97%
Venous Thromboembolism Prophylaxis[2]	337	92%	88%	85%
Warfarin Therapy Discharge Instructions[2]	51	100%	85%	75%
Chest Pain/Possible Heart Attack Care				
Aspirin Given Within 24 Hours of Arrival	11	100%	98%	96%
Fibrinolytic Meds Within 30 Min. of Arrival[3,7]	-	-	81%	58%
Average Time to ECG (minutes)[1]	-	-	7	7
Average Time to Transfer (minutes)[3,7]	-	-	53	60
Children's Asthma Care				
Received Home Management Plan of Care	-	-	-	88%
Received Reliever Medication	-	-	-	100%
Received Systemic Corticosteroids	-	-	-	100%
Emergency Department				
Admittance Decision Time (minutes)[2]	947	133	111	98
Head CT Results Within 45 Min. of Arrival[1]	-	-	64%	57%
Patients Who Left ER Before Being Seen	61,284	2%	2%	2%
Time from ER Arrival to Admit. (minutes)[2]	949	350	289	274
Time from ER Arrival to Discharge (minutes)	375	159	147	134
Time in ER Before Being Evaluated (minutes)	406	28	26	26
Time to Pain Meds for Fractures (minutes)	237	58	60	57
Heart Attack Care				
Aspirin Given at Discharge	142	100%	99%	99%
Fibrinolytic Meds Within 30 Min. of Arrival[7]	-	-	50%	54%
PCI Within 90 Minutes of Arrival	21	90%	96%	96%
Statin Prescribed at Discharge	138	100%	99%	98%
Heart Failure Care				
ACE Inhibitor or ARB for LVSD[2]	121	100%	98%	97%
Discharge Instructions Given[2]	256	100%	96%	94%
Evaluation of LVS Function[2]	292	100%	100%	99%
Medicare Spending				
Medicare Spending per Patient (ratio)	-	1.07	1.04	0.98
Pneumonia Care				
Appropriate Initial Antibiotic Given[2]	71	100%	98%	95%
Blood Culture Timing[2]	142	100%	99%	98%
Pregnancy and Delivery Care				
Newborn Deliveries Scheduled Early[7]	-	-	6%	6%
Preventive Care				
Immunization for Influenza[2]	585	100%	94%	90%
Immunization for Pneumonia[2]	797	100%	96%	92%
Stroke Care				
Anticoagulation Therapy for Atrial Fibrillation[2]	27	100%	97%	95%
Antithrombotic Therapy Timing[2]	147	100%	98%	98%
Assessed for Rehabilitation[2]	201	100%	97%	97%
Discharged on Antithrombotic Therapy[2]	154	99%	99%	99%
Discharged on Statin Medication[2]	123	98%	96%	94%
Thrombolytic Therapy Timing[2]	13	92%	76%	66%
Venous Thromboembolism Prophylaxis[2]	218	100%	95%	94%
Written Stroke Educational Materials Given[2]	110	95%	94%	88%
Surgical Care Improvement Project				
Appropriate Beta Blocker Usage[2]	99	100%	99%	98%
Appropriate VTP Within 24 Hours[2]	364	100%	99%	98%
Controlled Postoperative Blood Glucose[2,7]	-	-	98%	97%
Perioperative Temperature Management[2]	411	100%	100%	100%
Prophylactic Antibiotic Selection[2]	258	99%	99%	99%
Prophylactic Antibiotic Selection (Outpatient)	199	95%	98%	98%
Prophylactic Antibiotic Stopped[2]	250	100%	98%	98%
Prophylactic Antibiotic Timing[2]	258	100%	99%	99%
Prophylactic Antibiotic Timing (Outpatient)	201	93%	98%	98%
Urinary Catheter Removal[2]	270	100%	98%	97%
Survey of Patients' Hospital Experiences				
Area Around Room 'Always' Quiet at Night	300+	63%	58%	61%
Doctors 'Always' Communicated Well	300+	76%	77%	82%
Home Recovery Information Given	300+	86%	83%	85%
Hospital Given 9 or 10 on 10 Point Scale	300+	73%	67%	71%
Meds 'Always' Explained Before Given	300+	67%	60%	64%
Nurses 'Always' Communicated Well	300+	78%	75%	79%
Pain 'Always' Well Controlled	300+	73%	68%	71%
Room and Bathroom 'Always' Clean	300+	71%	69%	73%
Timely Help 'Always' Received	300+	64%	62%	68%
Would Definitely Recommend Hospital	300+	74%	69%	71%
Use of Medical Imaging				
Cardiac Imaging Stress Test before Surgery	108	9.3%	6.4%	5.3%
Combination Abdominal CT Scan	392	5.4%	11.8%	10.5%
Combination Brain/Sinus CT Scan	731	6.2%	3.4%	2.7%
Combination Chest CT Scan	279	3.6%	2.4%	2.7%
Follow-up Mammogram/Ultrasound	317	11.4%	10.2%	8.8%
Lumbar Spine MRI for Low Back Pain[1]	-	-	35.2%	37.2%

Bayfront Health Port Charlotte

2500 Harbor Blvd
Port Charlotte, FL 33952
Type: Acute Care Hospitals
Ownership: Proprietary
Phone: 941-766-4122
Fax: 941-766-4140
Emergency Services: Yes
Beds: 212

Key Personnel:

Radiology. . . . . Harold Ackerstei
Operating Room. . . . . Casey DeVries
Infection Control. . . . . Joyce Dulmage
Chief of Medical Staff . . . . David McAtee, DO
CEO/President. . . . . J David McCormack
Quality Assurance . . . . Gary Miles

Measure	Cases	This Hosp.	State Avg.	U.S. Avg.
Blood Clot Prevention and Treatment				
Anticoagulation Overlap Therapy[2]	76	92%	93%	93%
ICU Venous Thromboembolism Prophylaxis[2]	64	91%	94%	92%
Incidence of Potentially Preventable VTE[2]	17	0%	10%	10%
UFH with Dosages/Platelet Monitoring[2]	70	100%	100%	97%
Venous Thromboembolism Prophylaxis[2]	383	76%	88%	85%
Warfarin Therapy Discharge Instructions[2]	55	25%	85%	75%
Chest Pain/Possible Heart Attack Care				
Aspirin Given Within 24 Hours of Arrival[5]	-	-	98%	96%
Fibrinolytic Meds Within 30 Min. of Arrival[5]	-	-	81%	58%
Average Time to ECG (minutes)[5]	-	-	7	7
Average Time to Transfer (minutes)[5]	-	-	53	60
Children's Asthma Care				
Received Home Management Plan of Care	-	-	-	88%
Received Reliever Medication	-	-	-	100%
Received Systemic Corticosteroids	-	-	-	100%
Emergency Department				
Admittance Decision Time (minutes)[2]	565	166	111	98
Head CT Results Within 45 Min. of Arrival[1]	-	-	64%	57%
Patients Who Left ER Before Being Seen	26,844	3%	2%	2%
Time from ER Arrival to Admit. (minutes)[2]	607	326	289	274
Time from ER Arrival to Discharge (minutes)	394	166	147	134
Time in ER Before Being Evaluated (minutes)	405	31	26	26
Time to Pain Meds for Fractures (minutes)	57	43	60	57
Heart Attack Care				
Aspirin Given at Discharge	221	98%	99%	99%
Fibrinolytic Meds Within 30 Min. of Arrival[7]	-	-	50%	54%
PCI Within 90 Minutes of Arrival	35	80%	96%	96%
Statin Prescribed at Discharge	206	96%	99%	98%
Heart Failure Care				
ACE Inhibitor or ARB for LVSD	97	97%	98%	97%
Discharge Instructions Given	262	84%	96%	94%
Evaluation of LVS Function	308	100%	100%	99%
Medicare Spending				
Medicare Spending per Patient (ratio)	-	1.03	1.04	0.98
Pneumonia Care				
Appropriate Initial Antibiotic Given	145	98%	98%	95%
Blood Culture Timing	242	98%	99%	98%
Pregnancy and Delivery Care				
Newborn Deliveries Scheduled Early[2]	38	18%	6%	6%
Preventive Care				
Immunization for Influenza[2]	588	96%	94%	90%
Immunization for Pneumonia[2]	769	97%	96%	92%
Stroke Care				
Anticoagulation Therapy for Atrial Fibrillation	16	100%	97%	95%
Antithrombotic Therapy Timing	83	92%	98%	98%
Assessed for Rehabilitation	91	92%	97%	97%
Discharged on Antithrombotic Therapy	81	98%	99%	99%
Discharged on Statin Medication	66	83%	96%	94%
Thrombolytic Therapy Timing[1]	-	-	76%	66%
Venous Thromboembolism Prophylaxis	93	94%	95%	94%
Written Stroke Educational Materials Given	48	85%	94%	88%
Surgical Care Improvement Project				
Appropriate Beta Blocker Usage[2]	297	98%	99%	98%
Appropriate VTP Within 24 Hours[2]	440	98%	99%	98%
Controlled Postoperative Blood Glucose[2]	148	99%	98%	97%
Perioperative Temperature Management[2]	529	100%	100%	100%
Prophylactic Antibiotic Selection[2]	469	99%	99%	99%

NOTE: Hospital profiles are in alphabetical order by state, then city, then hospital within the city; Rankings exclude hospitals with less than 25 cases except for patient surveys which excludes hospitals with less than 100 cases; (a) 100-299 cases; (1) The number of cases/patients is too few to report; (2) Data submitted were based on a sample of cases/patients; (3) Results are based on a shorter time period than required; (4) Data suppressed by CMS for one or more quarters; (5) Results are not available for this reporting period; (6) Fewer than 100 patients completed the HCAHPS survey; (7) No cases met the criteria for this measure; (8) The lower limit of the confidence interval cannot be calculated if the number of observed infections equals zero; (9) No data are available from the state/territory for this reporting period; (10) The scores shown reflect fewer than 50 completed surveys; (11) There were discrepancies in the data collection process; (12) This measure does not apply to this hospital for this reporting period; (13) Results cannot be calculated for this reporting period; (14) The results for this state are combined with nearby states to protect confidentiality; Please refer to the User's Guide for a full explanation of data.

Measure	Cases	This Hosp.	State Avg.	U.S. Avg.
Prophylactic Antibiotic Selection (Outpatient)	401	97%	98%	98%
Prophylactic Antibiotic Stopped[2]	439	96%	98%	98%
Prophylactic Antibiotic Timing[2]	470	99%	99%	99%
Prophylactic Antibiotic Timing (Outpatient)	406	98%	98%	98%
Urinary Catheter Removal[2]	493	98%	98%	97%
Survey of Patients' Hospital Experiences				
Area Around Room 'Always' Quiet at Night	300+	46%	58%	61%
Doctors 'Always' Communicated Well	300+	70%	77%	82%
Home Recovery Information Given	300+	79%	83%	85%
Hospital Given 9 or 10 on 10 Point Scale	300+	51%	67%	71%
Meds 'Always' Explained Before Given	300+	48%	60%	64%
Nurses 'Always' Communicated Well	300+	64%	75%	79%
Pain 'Always' Well Controlled	300+	63%	68%	71%
Room and Bathroom 'Always' Clean	300+	63%	69%	73%
Timely Help 'Always' Received	300+	54%	62%	68%
Would Definitely Recommend Hospital	300+	54%	69%	71%
Use of Medical Imaging				
Cardiac Imaging Stress Test before Surgery[1]	-	-	6.4%	5.3%
Combination Abdominal CT Scan	428	10.7%	11.8%	10.5%
Combination Brain/Sinus CT Scan	570	4.4%	3.4%	2.7%
Combination Chest CT Scan	154	6.5%	2.4%	2.7%
Follow-up Mammogram/Ultrasound	1,096	7.5%	10.2%	8.8%
Lumbar Spine MRI for Low Back Pain[1]	-	-	35.2%	37.2%

Fawcett Memorial Hospital

21298 Olean Blvd
Port Charlotte, FL 33952
Phone: 941-629-1181
Fax: 941-627-6142
URL: www.fawcetthospital.com
Type: Acute Care Hospitals
Emergency Services: Yes
Ownership: Proprietary
Beds: 238

Key Personnel:
Operating Room. . . . . Alvaro Bada
Radiology. . . . . Bruce Bielfelt
Chief of Medical Staff. . . . . Nasir Khalidi, MD
Infection Control. . . . . Vicki Pellenz
CEO/President. . . . . Thomas J Rice
Cardiac Laboratory. . . . . Dennis Valera
Quality Assurance . . . . Nancy Whaley

Measure	Cases	This Hosp.	State Avg.	U.S. Avg.
Blood Clot Prevention and Treatment				
Anticoagulation Overlap Therapy[2]	134	100%	93%	93%
ICU Venous Thromboembolism Prophylaxis[2]	76	97%	94%	92%
Incidence of Potentially Preventable VTE[2]	30	0%	10%	10%
UFH with Dosages/Platelet Monitoring[2]	113	100%	100%	97%
Venous Thromboembolism Prophylaxis[2]	382	93%	88%	85%
Warfarin Therapy Discharge Instructions[2]	96	99%	85%	75%
Chest Pain/Possible Heart Attack Care				
Aspirin Given Within 24 Hours of Arrival[1,3]	-	-	98%	96%
Fibrinolytic Meds Within 30 Min. of Arrival[5]	-	-	81%	58%
Average Time to ECG (minutes)[1,3]	-	-	7	7
Average Time to Transfer (minutes)[5]	-	-	53	60
Children's Asthma Care				
Received Home Management Plan of Care	-	-	-	88%
Received Reliever Medication	-	-	-	100%
Received Systemic Corticosteroids	-	-	-	100%
Emergency Department				
Admittance Decision Time (minutes)[2]	847	47	111	98
Head CT Results Within 45 Min. of Arrival[3,7]	-	-	64%	57%
Patients Who Left ER Before Being Seen	24,704	2%	2%	2%
Time from ER Arrival to Admit. (minutes)[2]	847	196	289	274
Time from ER Arrival to Discharge (minutes)	410	127	147	134
Time in ER Before Being Evaluated (minutes)	431	9	26	26
Time to Pain Meds for Fractures (minutes)	57	60	60	57
Heart Attack Care				
Aspirin Given at Discharge[2]	202	100%	99%	99%
Fibrinolytic Meds Within 30 Min. of Arrival[2,7]	-	-	50%	54%
PCI Within 90 Minutes of Arrival[2]	28	96%	96%	96%
Statin Prescribed at Discharge[2]	174	100%	99%	98%
Heart Failure Care				
ACE Inhibitor or ARB for LVSD[2]	58	100%	98%	97%
Discharge Instructions Given[2]	201	100%	96%	94%
Evaluation of LVS Function[2]	264	100%	100%	99%
Medicare Spending				
Medicare Spending per Patient (ratio)	-	1.06	1.04	0.98
Pneumonia Care				
Appropriate Initial Antibiotic Given[2]	45	100%	98%	95%
Blood Culture Timing[2]	90	100%	99%	98%
Pregnancy and Delivery Care				
Newborn Deliveries Scheduled Early[2,7]	-	-	6%	6%
Preventive Care				
Immunization for Influenza[2]	642	98%	94%	90%
Immunization for Pneumonia[2]	1,061	95%	96%	92%
Stroke Care				
Anticoagulation Therapy for Atrial Fibrillation[1,2]	-	-	97%	95%
Antithrombotic Therapy Timing[2]	69	100%	98%	98%
Assessed for Rehabilitation[2]	79	100%	97%	97%
Discharged on Antithrombotic Therapy[2]	73	100%	99%	99%
Discharged on Statin Medication[2]	52	100%	96%	94%
Thrombolytic Therapy Timing[1,2]	-	-	76%	66%
Venous Thromboembolism Prophylaxis[2]	88	98%	95%	94%
Written Stroke Educational Materials Given[2]	40	100%	94%	88%
Surgical Care Improvement Project				
Appropriate Beta Blocker Usage[2]	155	99%	99%	98%
Appropriate VTP Within 24 Hours[2]	388	100%	99%	98%
Controlled Postoperative Blood Glucose[1,2]	-	-	98%	97%
Perioperative Temperature Management[2]	462	100%	100%	100%
Prophylactic Antibiotic Selection[2]	290	99%	99%	99%
Prophylactic Antibiotic Selection (Outpatient)	321	99%	98%	98%
Prophylactic Antibiotic Stopped[2]	266	100%	98%	98%
Prophylactic Antibiotic Timing[2]	290	100%	99%	99%
Prophylactic Antibiotic Timing (Outpatient)	322	100%	98%	98%
Urinary Catheter Removal[2]	341	100%	98%	97%
Survey of Patients' Hospital Experiences				
Area Around Room 'Always' Quiet at Night	300+	45%	58%	61%
Doctors 'Always' Communicated Well	300+	74%	77%	82%
Home Recovery Information Given	300+	87%	83%	85%
Hospital Given 9 or 10 on 10 Point Scale	300+	63%	67%	71%
Meds 'Always' Explained Before Given	300+	56%	60%	64%
Nurses 'Always' Communicated Well	300+	73%	75%	79%
Pain 'Always' Well Controlled	300+	67%	68%	71%
Room and Bathroom 'Always' Clean	300+	60%	69%	73%
Timely Help 'Always' Received	300+	54%	62%	68%
Would Definitely Recommend Hospital	300+	68%	69%	71%
Use of Medical Imaging				
Cardiac Imaging Stress Test before Surgery[1]	-	-	6.4%	5.3%
Combination Abdominal CT Scan	557	3.4%	11.8%	10.5%
Combination Brain/Sinus CT Scan	825	3.8%	3.4%	2.7%
Combination Chest CT Scan	150	4.0%	2.4%	2.7%
Follow-up Mammogram/Ultrasound	365	11.5%	10.2%	8.8%
Lumbar Spine MRI for Low Back Pain[1]	-	-	35.2%	37.2%

Sacred Heart Hospital on the Gulf

3801 E Hwy 98
Port Saint Joe, FL 32456
Phone: 850-229-5600
URL: www.sacred-heart.org/gulf
Type: Acute Care Hospitals
Emergency Services: Yes
Ownership: Voluntary non-profit - Private
Beds: 25

Key Personnel:
President . . . . Roger Hall

Measure	Cases	This Hosp.	State Avg.	U.S. Avg.
Blood Clot Prevention and Treatment				
Anticoagulation Overlap Therapy	11	100%	93%	93%
ICU Venous Thromboembolism Prophylaxis[7]	-	-	94%	92%
Incidence of Potentially Preventable VTE[7]	-	-	10%	10%
UFH with Dosages/Platelet Monitoring[7]	-	-	100%	97%
Venous Thromboembolism Prophylaxis	224	89%	88%	85%
Warfarin Therapy Discharge Instructions[1]	-	-	85%	75%
Chest Pain/Possible Heart Attack Care				
Aspirin Given Within 24 Hours of Arrival	36	97%	98%	96%
Fibrinolytic Meds Within 30 Min. of Arrival[7]	-	-	81%	58%
Average Time to ECG (minutes)	36	12	7	7
Average Time to Transfer (minutes)[1]	-	-	53	60
Children's Asthma Care				
Received Home Management Plan of Care	-	-	-	88%
Received Reliever Medication	-	-	-	100%
Received Systemic Corticosteroids	-	-	-	100%
Emergency Department				
Admittance Decision Time (minutes)[2]	105	85	111	98
Head CT Results Within 45 Min. of Arrival[1]	-	-	64%	57%
Patients Who Left ER Before Being Seen	8,791	0%	2%	2%
Time from ER Arrival to Admit. (minutes)[2]	191	182	289	274
Time from ER Arrival to Discharge (minutes)	349	74	147	134
Time in ER Before Being Evaluated (minutes)	355	16	26	26
Time to Pain Meds for Fractures (minutes)	24	50	60	57
Heart Attack Care				
Aspirin Given at Discharge[1,3]	-	-	99%	99%
Fibrinolytic Meds Within 30 Min. of Arrival[3,7]	-	-	50%	54%
PCI Within 90 Minutes of Arrival[3,7]	-	-	96%	96%
Statin Prescribed at Discharge[1,3]	-	-	99%	98%
Heart Failure Care				
ACE Inhibitor or ARB for LVSD[1]	-	-	98%	97%
Discharge Instructions Given	16	100%	96%	94%
Evaluation of LVS Function	16	100%	100%	99%
Medicare Spending				
Medicare Spending per Patient (ratio)	-	0.99	1.04	0.98
Pneumonia Care				
Appropriate Initial Antibiotic Given	17	100%	98%	95%
Blood Culture Timing	25	100%	99%	98%
Pregnancy and Delivery Care				
Newborn Deliveries Scheduled Early[7]	-	-	6%	6%
Preventive Care				
Immunization for Influenza[2]	217	98%	94%	90%
Immunization for Pneumonia[2]	333	100%	96%	92%
Stroke Care				
Anticoagulation Therapy for Atrial Fibrillation[3,7]	-	-	97%	95%
Antithrombotic Therapy Timing[1,3]	-	-	98%	98%
Assessed for Rehabilitation[1,3]	-	-	97%	97%
Discharged on Antithrombotic Therapy[1,3]	-	-	99%	99%
Discharged on Statin Medication[1,3]	-	-	96%	94%
Thrombolytic Therapy Timing[3,7]	-	-	76%	66%
Venous Thromboembolism Prophylaxis[1,3]	-	-	95%	94%
Written Stroke Educational Materials Given[1,3]	-	-	94%	88%
Surgical Care Improvement Project				
Appropriate Beta Blocker Usage[1,2]	-	-	99%	98%
Appropriate VTP Within 24 Hours[1,2]	-	-	99%	98%
Controlled Postoperative Blood Glucose[2,7]	-	-	98%	97%
Perioperative Temperature Management[1,2]	-	-	100%	100%
Prophylactic Antibiotic Selection[1,2]	-	-	99%	99%
Prophylactic Antibiotic Selection (Outpatient)[1,3]	-	-	98%	98%
Prophylactic Antibiotic Stopped[1,2]	-	-	98%	98%
Prophylactic Antibiotic Timing[1,2]	-	-	99%	99%
Prophylactic Antibiotic Timing (Outpatient)[1,3]	-	-	98%	98%
Urinary Catheter Removal[1,2]	-	-	98%	97%
Survey of Patients' Hospital Experiences				
Area Around Room 'Always' Quiet at Night	(a)	86%	58%	61%
Doctors 'Always' Communicated Well	(a)	92%	77%	82%
Home Recovery Information Given	(a)	95%	83%	85%
Hospital Given 9 or 10 on 10 Point Scale	(a)	90%	67%	71%
Meds 'Always' Explained Before Given	(a)	84%	60%	64%
Nurses 'Always' Communicated Well	(a)	91%	75%	79%
Pain 'Always' Well Controlled	(a)	90%	68%	71%
Room and Bathroom 'Always' Clean	(a)	89%	69%	73%
Timely Help 'Always' Received	(a)	88%	62%	68%
Would Definitely Recommend Hospital	(a)	90%	69%	71%
Use of Medical Imaging				
Cardiac Imaging Stress Test before Surgery[1]	-	-	6.4%	5.3%
Combination Abdominal CT Scan	132	6.1%	11.8%	10.5%
Combination Brain/Sinus CT Scan[1]	-	-	3.4%	2.7%
Combination Chest CT Scan	69	5.8%	2.4%	2.7%
Follow-up Mammogram/Ultrasound	174	8.0%	10.2%	8.8%
Lumbar Spine MRI for Low Back Pain[1]	-	-	35.2%	37.2%

Saint Lucie Medical Center

1800 Se Tiffany Ave
Port Saint Lucie, FL 34952
Phone: 772-335-4000
Fax: 772-398-3742
URL: www.stluciemed.com
Type: Acute Care Hospitals
Emergency Services: Yes
Ownership: Proprietary
Beds: 194

Key Personnel:
Operating Room. . . . . Terri Benedict
CEO . . . . Jay Finnegan

NOTE: Hospital profiles are in alphabetical order by state, then city, then hospital within the city; Rankings exclude hospitals with less than 25 cases except for patient surveys which excludes hospitals with less than 100 cases; (a) 100-299 cases; (1) The number of cases/patients is too few to report; (2) Data submitted were based on a sample of cases/patients; (3) Results are based on a shorter time period than required; (4) Data suppressed by CMS for one or more quarters; (5) Results are not available for this reporting period; (6) Fewer than 100 patients completed the HCAHPS survey; (7) No cases met the criteria for this measure; (8) The lower limit of the confidence interval cannot be calculated if the number of observed infections equals zero; (9) No data are available from the state/territory for this reporting period; (10) The scores shown reflect fewer than 50 completed surveys; (11) There were discrepancies in the data collection process; (12) This measure does not apply to this hospital for this reporting period; (13) Results cannot be calculated for this reporting period; (14) The results for this state are combined with nearby states to protect confidentiality; Please refer to the User's Guide for a full explanation of data.

Radiology. . . . . William Merrell
Chief of Medical Staff. . . . . Michael Paul, MD
Infection Control. . . . . Suzane Perry, RN
Cardiac Laboratory. . . . . Shawn Poland
Quality Assurance . . . . Diana Stobete

Measure	Cases	This Hosp.	State Avg.	U.S. Avg.
Blood Clot Prevention and Treatment				
Anticoagulation Overlap Therapy[2]	125	100%	93%	93%
ICU Venous Thromboembolism Prophylaxis[2]	61	100%	94%	92%
Incidence of Potentially Preventable VTE[2]	23	4%	10%	10%
UFH with Dosages/Platelet Monitoring[2]	74	100%	100%	97%
Venous Thromboembolism Prophylaxis[2]	383	98%	88%	85%
Warfarin Therapy Discharge Instructions[2]	86	100%	85%	75%
Chest Pain/Possible Heart Attack Care				
Aspirin Given Within 24 Hours of Arrival	64	100%	98%	96%
Fibrinolytic Meds Within 30 Min. of Arrival[7]	-	-	81%	58%
Average Time to ECG (minutes)	67	0	7	7
Average Time to Transfer (minutes)	30	36	53	60
Children's Asthma Care				
Received Home Management Plan of Care	-	-	-	88%
Received Reliever Medication	-	-	-	100%
Received Systemic Corticosteroids	-	-	-	100%
Emergency Department				
Admittance Decision Time (minutes)[2]	882	96	111	98
Head CT Results Within 45 Min. of Arrival	21	86%	64%	57%
Patients Who Left ER Before Being Seen	44,560	0%	2%	2%
Time from ER Arrival to Admit. (minutes)[2]	882	254	289	274
Time from ER Arrival to Discharge (minutes)	448	124	147	134
Time in ER Before Being Evaluated (minutes)	499	11	26	26
Time to Pain Meds for Fractures (minutes)	88	53	60	57
Heart Attack Care				
Aspirin Given at Discharge	95	100%	99%	99%
Fibrinolytic Meds Within 30 Min. of Arrival[7]	-	-	50%	54%
PCI Within 90 Minutes of Arrival[7]	-	-	96%	96%
Statin Prescribed at Discharge	91	100%	99%	98%
Heart Failure Care				
ACE Inhibitor or ARB for LVSD	102	100%	98%	97%
Discharge Instructions Given	315	100%	96%	94%
Evaluation of LVS Function	414	100%	100%	99%
Medicare Spending				
Medicare Spending per Patient (ratio)	-	1.05	1.04	0.98
Pneumonia Care				
Appropriate Initial Antibiotic Given	150	100%	98%	95%
Blood Culture Timing	377	100%	99%	98%
Pregnancy and Delivery Care				
Newborn Deliveries Scheduled Early[2]	34	3%	6%	6%
Preventive Care				
Immunization for Influenza[2]	600	98%	94%	90%
Immunization for Pneumonia[2]	885	100%	96%	92%
Stroke Care				
Anticoagulation Therapy for Atrial Fibrillation[2]	12	100%	97%	95%
Antithrombotic Therapy Timing[2]	75	97%	98%	98%
Assessed for Rehabilitation[2]	74	96%	97%	97%
Discharged on Antithrombotic Therapy[2]	72	99%	99%	99%
Discharged on Statin Medication[2]	50	92%	96%	94%
Thrombolytic Therapy Timing[1,2]	-	-	76%	66%
Venous Thromboembolism Prophylaxis[2]	84	100%	95%	94%
Written Stroke Educational Materials Given[2]	45	100%	94%	88%
Surgical Care Improvement Project				
Appropriate Beta Blocker Usage[2]	148	100%	99%	98%
Appropriate VTP Within 24 Hours[2]	440	100%	99%	98%
Controlled Postoperative Blood Glucose[2,7]	-	-	98%	97%
Perioperative Temperature Management[2]	510	100%	100%	100%
Prophylactic Antibiotic Selection[2]	324	100%	99%	99%
Prophylactic Antibiotic Selection (Outpatient)	80	100%	98%	98%
Prophylactic Antibiotic Stopped[2]	276	100%	98%	98%
Prophylactic Antibiotic Timing[2]	324	100%	99%	99%
Prophylactic Antibiotic Timing (Outpatient)	80	100%	98%	98%
Urinary Catheter Removal[2]	210	100%	98%	97%
Survey of Patients' Hospital Experiences				
Area Around Room 'Always' Quiet at Night	300+	58%	58%	61%
Doctors 'Always' Communicated Well	300+	75%	77%	82%
Home Recovery Information Given	300+	85%	83%	85%
Hospital Given 9 or 10 on 10 Point Scale	300+	64%	67%	71%
Meds 'Always' Explained Before Given	300+	60%	60%	64%
Nurses 'Always' Communicated Well	300+	75%	75%	79%
Pain 'Always' Well Controlled	300+	69%	68%	71%
Room and Bathroom 'Always' Clean	300+	68%	69%	73%
Timely Help 'Always' Received	300+	61%	62%	68%
Would Definitely Recommend Hospital	300+	65%	69%	71%
Use of Medical Imaging				
Cardiac Imaging Stress Test before Surgery[1]	-	-	6.4%	5.3%
Combination Abdominal CT Scan	719	5.4%	11.8%	10.5%
Combination Brain/Sinus CT Scan	1,318	2.0%	3.4%	2.7%
Combination Chest CT Scan	138	0.7%	2.4%	2.7%
Follow-up Mammogram/Ultrasound	747	9.1%	10.2%	8.8%
Lumbar Spine MRI for Low Back Pain[1]	-	-	35.2%	37.2%

Bayfront Health Punta Gorda

809 E Marion Ave Phone: 941-639-3131
Punta Gorda, FL 33950 Fax: 941-637-2454
URL: www.charlotteregional.com
Type: Acute Care Hospitals Emergency Services: Yes
Ownership: Proprietary Beds: 208

Key Personnel:

Emergency Room . . . . Larry R Bachle
Quality Assurance . . . . Denise Barnett
CEO . . . . Brandon W. Downey
Chief of Medical Staff . . . . Thomas Noone, MD
President . . . . Andre Williams, D.P.M.

Measure	Cases	This Hosp.	State Avg.	U.S. Avg.
Blood Clot Prevention and Treatment				
Anticoagulation Overlap Therapy[2]	24	88%	93%	93%
ICU Venous Thromboembolism Prophylaxis[2]	55	93%	94%	92%
Incidence of Potentially Preventable VTE[1,2]	-	-	10%	10%
UFH with Dosages/Platelet Monitoring[2]	13	100%	100%	97%
Venous Thromboembolism Prophylaxis[2]	342	73%	88%	85%
Warfarin Therapy Discharge Instructions[2]	15	73%	85%	75%
Chest Pain/Possible Heart Attack Care				
Aspirin Given Within 24 Hours of Arrival	37	100%	98%	96%
Fibrinolytic Meds Within 30 Min. of Arrival[7]	-	-	81%	58%
Average Time to ECG (minutes)	38	0	7	7
Average Time to Transfer (minutes)[1]	-	-	53	60
Children's Asthma Care				
Received Home Management Plan of Care	-	-	-	88%
Received Reliever Medication	-	-	-	100%
Received Systemic Corticosteroids	-	-	-	100%
Emergency Department				
Admittance Decision Time (minutes)[2]	618	123	111	98
Head CT Results Within 45 Min. of Arrival[1]	-	-	64%	57%
Patients Who Left ER Before Being Seen	18,040	2%	2%	2%
Time from ER Arrival to Admit. (minutes)[2]	620	266	289	274
Time from ER Arrival to Discharge (minutes)	389	126	147	134
Time in ER Before Being Evaluated (minutes)	417	20	26	26
Time to Pain Meds for Fractures (minutes)	56	56	60	57
Heart Attack Care				
Aspirin Given at Discharge[1]	-	-	99%	99%
Fibrinolytic Meds Within 30 Min. of Arrival[7]	-	-	50%	54%
PCI Within 90 Minutes of Arrival[7]	-	-	96%	96%
Statin Prescribed at Discharge[1]	-	-	99%	98%
Heart Failure Care				
ACE Inhibitor or ARB for LVSD	41	90%	98%	97%
Discharge Instructions Given	107	93%	96%	94%
Evaluation of LVS Function	136	100%	100%	99%
Medicare Spending				
Medicare Spending per Patient (ratio)	-	1.00	1.04	0.98
Pneumonia Care				
Appropriate Initial Antibiotic Given[2]	90	97%	98%	95%
Blood Culture Timing[2]	132	99%	99%	98%
Pregnancy and Delivery Care				
Newborn Deliveries Scheduled Early[7]	-	-	6%	6%
Preventive Care				
Immunization for Influenza[2]	441	98%	94%	90%
Immunization for Pneumonia[2]	633	97%	96%	92%
Stroke Care				
Anticoagulation Therapy for Atrial Fibrillation[1]	-	-	97%	95%
Antithrombotic Therapy Timing	53	94%	98%	98%
Assessed for Rehabilitation	59	93%	97%	97%
Discharged on Antithrombotic Therapy	50	100%	99%	99%
Discharged on Statin Medication	42	88%	96%	94%
Thrombolytic Therapy Timing[1]	-	-	76%	66%
Venous Thromboembolism Prophylaxis	64	89%	95%	94%
Written Stroke Educational Materials Given	29	100%	94%	88%
Surgical Care Improvement Project				
Appropriate Beta Blocker Usage[2]	106	99%	99%	98%
Appropriate VTP Within 24 Hours[2]	235	98%	99%	98%
Controlled Postoperative Blood Glucose[2,7]	-	-	98%	97%
Perioperative Temperature Management[2]	266	100%	100%	100%
Prophylactic Antibiotic Selection[2]	170	97%	99%	99%
Prophylactic Antibiotic Selection (Outpatient)	105	98%	98%	98%
Prophylactic Antibiotic Stopped[2]	166	99%	98%	98%
Prophylactic Antibiotic Timing[2]	170	100%	99%	99%
Prophylactic Antibiotic Timing (Outpatient)	105	99%	98%	98%
Urinary Catheter Removal[2]	162	96%	98%	97%
Survey of Patients' Hospital Experiences				
Area Around Room 'Always' Quiet at Night	300+	50%	58%	61%
Doctors 'Always' Communicated Well	300+	74%	77%	82%
Home Recovery Information Given	300+	80%	83%	85%
Hospital Given 9 or 10 on 10 Point Scale	300+	59%	67%	71%
Meds 'Always' Explained Before Given	300+	55%	60%	64%
Nurses 'Always' Communicated Well	300+	71%	75%	79%
Pain 'Always' Well Controlled	300+	65%	68%	71%
Room and Bathroom 'Always' Clean	300+	66%	69%	73%
Timely Help 'Always' Received	300+	61%	62%	68%
Would Definitely Recommend Hospital	300+	62%	69%	71%
Use of Medical Imaging				
Cardiac Imaging Stress Test before Surgery[1]	-	-	6.4%	5.3%
Combination Abdominal CT Scan	406	6.9%	11.8%	10.5%
Combination Brain/Sinus CT Scan	581	5.0%	3.4%	2.7%
Combination Chest CT Scan	119	14.3%	2.4%	2.7%
Follow-up Mammogram/Ultrasound	69	27.5%	10.2%	8.8%
Lumbar Spine MRI for Low Back Pain[1]	-	-	35.2%	37.2%

Wuesthoff Medical Center Rockledge

110 Longwood Ave Phone: 321-637-2603
Rockledge, FL 32955 Fax: 321-690-6617
URL: www.wuesthoff.org
Type: Acute Care Hospitals Emergency Services: Yes
Ownership: Voluntary non-profit - Private Beds: 298

Key Personnel:

CEO . . . . Tim Cerullo
Pediatric Ambulatory Care . . . . . . Javier Diaz, MD
Infection Control. . . . . Mukul Garg, MD
Quality Assurance . . . . Damon Newton
Radiology. . . . . Robert Page, MD
Chief of Medical Staff. . . . . Duff Sprawls, MD
Operating Room. . . . . Linda Taylor

Measure	Cases	This Hosp.	State Avg.	U.S. Avg.
Blood Clot Prevention and Treatment				
Anticoagulation Overlap Therapy[2]	70	89%	93%	93%
ICU Venous Thromboembolism Prophylaxis[2]	65	98%	94%	92%
Incidence of Potentially Preventable VTE[1,2]	-	-	10%	10%
UFH with Dosages/Platelet Monitoring[2]	59	100%	100%	97%
Venous Thromboembolism Prophylaxis[2]	345	78%	88%	85%
Warfarin Therapy Discharge Instructions[2]	39	87%	85%	75%
Chest Pain/Possible Heart Attack Care				
Aspirin Given Within 24 Hours of Arrival[1,3]	-	-	98%	96%
Fibrinolytic Meds Within 30 Min. of Arrival[5]	-	-	81%	58%
Average Time to ECG (minutes)[1,3]	-	-	7	7
Average Time to Transfer (minutes)[5]	-	-	53	60
Children's Asthma Care				
Received Home Management Plan of Care	-	-	-	88%
Received Reliever Medication	-	-	-	100%
Received Systemic Corticosteroids	-	-	-	100%
Emergency Department				
Admittance Decision Time (minutes)[2]	688	146	111	98
Head CT Results Within 45 Min. of Arrival[1]	-	-	64%	57%
Patients Who Left ER Before Being Seen	36,758	1%	2%	2%
Time from ER Arrival to Admit. (minutes)[2]	727	281	289	274
Time from ER Arrival to Discharge (minutes)	361	125	147	134

NOTE: Hospital profiles are in alphabetical order by state, then city, then hospital within the city; Rankings exclude hospitals with less than 25 cases except for patient surveys which excludes hospitals with less than 100 cases; (a) 100-299 cases; (1) The number of cases/patients is too few to report; (2) Data submitted were based on a sample of cases/patients; (3) Results are based on a shorter time period than required; (4) Data suppressed by CMS for one or more quarters; (5) Results are not available for this reporting period; (6) Fewer than 100 patients completed the HCAHPS survey; (7) No cases met the criteria for this measure; (8) The lower limit of the confidence interval cannot be calculated if the number of observed infections equals zero; (9) No data are available from the state/territory for this reporting period; (10) The scores shown reflect fewer than 50 completed surveys; (11) There were discrepancies in the data collection process; (12) This measure does not apply to this hospital for this reporting period; (13) Results cannot be calculated for this reporting period; (14) The results for this state are combined with nearby states to protect confidentiality; Please refer to the User's Guide for a full explanation of data.

Measure	Cases	This Hosp.	State Avg.	U.S. Avg.
Time in ER Before Being Evaluated (minutes)	416	16	26	26
Time to Pain Meds for Fractures (minutes)	71	54	60	57
Heart Attack Care				
Aspirin Given at Discharge	175	98%	99%	99%
Fibrinolytic Meds Within 30 Min. of Arrival[7]	-	-	50%	54%
PCI Within 90 Minutes of Arrival	33	100%	96%	96%
Statin Prescribed at Discharge	154	99%	99%	98%
Heart Failure Care				
ACE Inhibitor or ARB for LVSD	91	96%	98%	97%
Discharge Instructions Given	272	87%	96%	94%
Evaluation of LVS Function	341	100%	100%	99%
Medicare Spending				
Medicare Spending per Patient (ratio)	-	1.08	1.04	0.98
Pneumonia Care				
Appropriate Initial Antibiotic Given	137	94%	98%	95%
Blood Culture Timing	266	98%	99%	98%
Pregnancy and Delivery Care				
Newborn Deliveries Scheduled Early	47	6%	6%	6%
Preventive Care				
Immunization for Influenza[2]	598	94%	94%	90%
Immunization for Pneumonia[2]	800	98%	96%	92%
Stroke Care				
Anticoagulation Therapy for Atrial Fibrillation	20	85%	97%	95%
Antithrombotic Therapy Timing	116	96%	98%	98%
Assessed for Rehabilitation	126	96%	97%	97%
Discharged on Antithrombotic Therapy	115	98%	99%	99%
Discharged on Statin Medication	91	96%	96%	94%
Thrombolytic Therapy Timing[1]	-	-	76%	66%
Venous Thromboembolism Prophylaxis	137	93%	95%	94%
Written Stroke Educational Materials Given	60	78%	94%	88%
Surgical Care Improvement Project				
Appropriate Beta Blocker Usage[2]	215	97%	99%	98%
Appropriate VTP Within 24 Hours[2]	346	97%	99%	98%
Controlled Postoperative Blood Glucose[2]	104	97%	98%	97%
Perioperative Temperature Management[2]	425	100%	100%	100%
Prophylactic Antibiotic Selection[2]	364	99%	99%	99%
Prophylactic Antibiotic Selection (Outpatient)	342	97%	98%	98%
Prophylactic Antibiotic Stopped[2]	350	95%	98%	98%
Prophylactic Antibiotic Timing[2]	364	99%	99%	99%
Prophylactic Antibiotic Timing (Outpatient)	343	99%	98%	98%
Urinary Catheter Removal[2]	355	96%	98%	97%
Survey of Patients' Hospital Experiences				
Area Around Room 'Always' Quiet at Night	300+	49%	58%	61%
Doctors 'Always' Communicated Well	300+	72%	77%	82%
Home Recovery Information Given	300+	79%	83%	85%
Hospital Given 9 or 10 on 10 Point Scale	300+	48%	67%	71%
Meds 'Always' Explained Before Given	300+	54%	60%	64%
Nurses 'Always' Communicated Well	300+	66%	75%	79%
Pain 'Always' Well Controlled	300+	60%	68%	71%
Room and Bathroom 'Always' Clean	300+	60%	69%	73%
Timely Help 'Always' Received	300+	52%	62%	68%
Would Definitely Recommend Hospital	300+	48%	69%	71%
Use of Medical Imaging				
Cardiac Imaging Stress Test before Surgery	409	5.9%	6.4%	5.3%
Combination Abdominal CT Scan	881	45.5%	11.8%	10.5%
Combination Brain/Sinus CT Scan	702	4.6%	3.4%	2.7%
Combination Chest CT Scan	453	6.8%	2.4%	2.7%
Follow-up Mammogram/Ultrasound	1,233	11.6%	10.2%	8.8%
Lumbar Spine MRI for Low Back Pain[1]	-	-	35.2%	37.2%

Mease Countryside Hospital

3231 Mcmullen Booth Rd
Safety Harbor, FL 34695
Phone: 727-734-6950
Fax: 727-725-6181
URL: www.measehospitals.com
Type: Acute Care Hospitals
Emergency Services: Yes
Ownership: Voluntary non-profit - Private
Beds: 205

Key Personnel:

Pediatric Ambulatory Care . . . . . . Janet Allen, MD
Radiology. . . . . Brian L Anderson
President . . . . Lou Galdieri, MHA, BSN
President . . . . Kristopher Hoce
Quality Assurance . . . . Stuart Jonap
Ambulatory Care . . . . Jerome Ladous
Operating Room. . . . . Celia Larimore
Emergency Room . . . . Kelly Triolo, RN

Measure	Cases	This Hosp.	State Avg.	U.S. Avg.
Blood Clot Prevention and Treatment				
Anticoagulation Overlap Therapy[2]	106	93%	93%	93%
ICU Venous Thromboembolism Prophylaxis[2]	82	98%	94%	92%
Incidence of Potentially Preventable VTE[2]	14	0%	10%	10%
UFH with Dosages/Platelet Monitoring[2]	56	98%	100%	97%
Venous Thromboembolism Prophylaxis[2]	385	97%	88%	85%
Warfarin Therapy Discharge Instructions[2]	70	93%	85%	75%
Chest Pain/Possible Heart Attack Care				
Aspirin Given Within 24 Hours of Arrival[1]	-	-	98%	96%
Fibrinolytic Meds Within 30 Min. of Arrival[3,7]	-	-	81%	58%
Average Time to ECG (minutes)[1]	-	-	7	7
Average Time to Transfer (minutes)[3,7]	-	-	53	60
Children's Asthma Care				
Received Home Management Plan of Care	-	-	-	88%
Received Reliever Medication	-	-	-	100%
Received Systemic Corticosteroids	-	-	-	100%
Emergency Department				
Admittance Decision Time (minutes)[2]	721	125	111	98
Head CT Results Within 45 Min. of Arrival	21	81%	64%	57%
Patients Who Left ER Before Being Seen	53,117	1%	2%	2%
Time from ER Arrival to Admit. (minutes)[2]	733	305	289	274
Time from ER Arrival to Discharge (minutes)	364	180	147	134
Time in ER Before Being Evaluated (minutes)	440	47	26	26
Time to Pain Meds for Fractures (minutes)	122	53	60	57
Heart Attack Care				
Aspirin Given at Discharge	381	100%	99%	99%
Fibrinolytic Meds Within 30 Min. of Arrival[1]	-	-	50%	54%
PCI Within 90 Minutes of Arrival	79	95%	96%	96%
Statin Prescribed at Discharge	363	99%	99%	98%
Heart Failure Care				
ACE Inhibitor or ARB for LVSD	110	99%	98%	97%
Discharge Instructions Given	335	95%	96%	94%
Evaluation of LVS Function	445	100%	100%	99%
Medicare Spending				
Medicare Spending per Patient (ratio)	-	1.07	1.04	0.98
Pneumonia Care				
Appropriate Initial Antibiotic Given	178	99%	98%	95%
Blood Culture Timing	367	99%	99%	98%
Pregnancy and Delivery Care				
Newborn Deliveries Scheduled Early[2]	70	54%	6%	6%
Preventive Care				
Immunization for Influenza[2]	602	96%	94%	90%
Immunization for Pneumonia[2]	767	99%	96%	92%
Stroke Care				
Anticoagulation Therapy for Atrial Fibrillation	44	98%	97%	95%
Antithrombotic Therapy Timing	178	98%	98%	98%
Assessed for Rehabilitation	178	97%	97%	97%
Discharged on Antithrombotic Therapy	173	100%	99%	99%
Discharged on Statin Medication	143	96%	96%	94%
Thrombolytic Therapy Timing[1]	-	-	76%	66%
Venous Thromboembolism Prophylaxis	186	98%	95%	94%
Written Stroke Educational Materials Given	98	91%	94%	88%
Surgical Care Improvement Project				
Appropriate Beta Blocker Usage[2]	174	96%	99%	98%
Appropriate VTP Within 24 Hours[2]	462	98%	99%	98%
Controlled Postoperative Blood Glucose[2,7]	-	-	98%	97%
Perioperative Temperature Management[2]	568	100%	100%	100%
Prophylactic Antibiotic Selection[2]	437	100%	99%	99%
Prophylactic Antibiotic Selection (Outpatient)	358	98%	98%	98%
Prophylactic Antibiotic Stopped[2]	430	99%	98%	98%
Prophylactic Antibiotic Timing[2]	438	97%	99%	99%
Prophylactic Antibiotic Timing (Outpatient)	358	99%	98%	98%
Urinary Catheter Removal[2]	438	98%	98%	97%
Survey of Patients' Hospital Experiences				
Area Around Room 'Always' Quiet at Night[11]	300+	46%	58%	61%
Doctors 'Always' Communicated Well[11]	300+	76%	77%	82%
Home Recovery Information Given[11]	300+	85%	83%	85%
Hospital Given 9 or 10 on 10 Point Scale[11]	300+	73%	67%	71%
Meds 'Always' Explained Before Given[11]	300+	62%	60%	64%
Nurses 'Always' Communicated Well[11]	300+	78%	75%	79%
Pain 'Always' Well Controlled[11]	300+	67%	68%	71%
Room and Bathroom 'Always' Clean[11]	300+	74%	69%	73%
Timely Help 'Always' Received[11]	300+	62%	62%	68%
Would Definitely Recommend Hospital[11]	300+	77%	69%	71%
Use of Medical Imaging				
Cardiac Imaging Stress Test before Surgery	61	3.3%	6.4%	5.3%
Combination Abdominal CT Scan	1,153	10.8%	11.8%	10.5%
Combination Brain/Sinus CT Scan	1,806	4.9%	3.4%	2.7%
Combination Chest CT Scan	740	0.1%	2.4%	2.7%
Follow-up Mammogram/Ultrasound	2,776	7.7%	10.2%	8.8%
Lumbar Spine MRI for Low Back Pain	133	30.1%	35.2%	37.2%

Flagler Hospital

400 Health Park Blvd
Saint Augustine, FL 32086
Phone: 904-819-4426
Fax: 904-819-4472
URL: www.flaglerhospital.com
Type: Acute Care Hospitals
Emergency Services: Yes
Ownership: Voluntary non-profit - Private
Beds: 321

Key Personnel:

Quality Assurance . . . . Michael Dibella
CEO/President. . . . . Joseph Gordy
Operating Room. . . . . Sandi Raburn
Chairman/CEO . . . . Len Tucker

Measure	Cases	This Hosp.	State Avg.	U.S. Avg.
Blood Clot Prevention and Treatment				
Anticoagulation Overlap Therapy[2]	88	98%	93%	93%
ICU Venous Thromboembolism Prophylaxis[2]	90	97%	94%	92%
Incidence of Potentially Preventable VTE[2]	20	0%	10%	10%
UFH with Dosages/Platelet Monitoring[2]	89	100%	100%	97%
Venous Thromboembolism Prophylaxis[2]	328	91%	88%	85%
Warfarin Therapy Discharge Instructions[2]	59	88%	85%	75%
Chest Pain/Possible Heart Attack Care				
Aspirin Given Within 24 Hours of Arrival[1,3]	-	-	98%	96%
Fibrinolytic Meds Within 30 Min. of Arrival[5]	-	-	81%	58%
Average Time to ECG (minutes)[1,3]	-	-	7	7
Average Time to Transfer (minutes)[5]	-	-	53	60
Children's Asthma Care				
Received Home Management Plan of Care	-	-	-	88%
Received Reliever Medication	-	-	-	100%
Received Systemic Corticosteroids	-	-	-	100%
Emergency Department				
Admittance Decision Time (minutes)[2]	620	152	111	98
Head CT Results Within 45 Min. of Arrival[1]	-	-	64%	57%
Patients Who Left ER Before Being Seen	53,515	2%	2%	2%
Time from ER Arrival to Admit. (minutes)[2]	620	364	289	274
Time from ER Arrival to Discharge (minutes)	370	156	147	134
Time in ER Before Being Evaluated (minutes)	415	28	26	26
Time to Pain Meds for Fractures (minutes)	131	60	60	57
Heart Attack Care				
Aspirin Given at Discharge[2]	225	98%	99%	99%
Fibrinolytic Meds Within 30 Min. of Arrival[2,7]	-	-	50%	54%
PCI Within 90 Minutes of Arrival[2]	34	82%	96%	96%
Statin Prescribed at Discharge[2]	212	97%	99%	98%
Heart Failure Care				
ACE Inhibitor or ARB for LVSD[2]	94	97%	98%	97%
Discharge Instructions Given[2]	263	92%	96%	94%
Evaluation of LVS Function[2]	324	99%	100%	99%
Medicare Spending				
Medicare Spending per Patient (ratio)	-	1.03	1.04	0.98
Pneumonia Care				
Appropriate Initial Antibiotic Given[2]	66	94%	98%	95%
Blood Culture Timing[2]	123	100%	99%	98%
Pregnancy and Delivery Care				
Newborn Deliveries Scheduled Early	104	0%	6%	6%
Preventive Care				
Immunization for Influenza[2]	597	99%	94%	90%
Immunization for Pneumonia[2]	773	97%	96%	92%
Stroke Care				
Anticoagulation Therapy for Atrial Fibrillation	30	100%	97%	95%
Antithrombotic Therapy Timing	146	100%	98%	98%
Assessed for Rehabilitation	174	99%	97%	97%
Discharged on Antithrombotic Therapy	144	100%	99%	99%
Discharged on Statin Medication	109	96%	96%	94%
Thrombolytic Therapy Timing[1]	-	-	76%	66%

NOTE: Hospital profiles are in alphabetical order by state, then city, then hospital within the city; Rankings exclude hospitals with less than 25 cases except for patient surveys which excludes hospitals with less than 100 cases; (a) 100-299 cases; (1) The number of cases/patients is too few to report; (2) Data submitted were based on a sample of cases/patients; (3) Results are based on a shorter time period than required; (4) Data suppressed by CMS for one or more quarters; (5) Results are not available for this reporting period; (6) Fewer than 100 patients completed the HCAHPS survey; (7) No cases met the criteria for this measure; (8) The lower limit of the confidence interval cannot be calculated if the number of observed infections equals zero; (9) No data are available from the state/territory for this reporting period; (10) The scores shown reflect fewer than 50 completed surveys; (11) There were discrepancies in the data collection process; (12) This measure does not apply to this hospital for this reporting period; (13) Results cannot be calculated for this reporting period; (14) The results for this state are combined with nearby states to protect confidentiality; Please refer to the User's Guide for a full explanation of data.

Venous Thromboembolism Prophylaxis	173	98%	95%	94%
Written Stroke Educational Materials Given	108	92%	94%	88%
Surgical Care Improvement Project				
Appropriate Beta Blocker Usage[2]	179	99%	99%	98%
Appropriate VTP Within 24 Hours[2]	318	98%	99%	98%
Controlled Postoperative Blood Glucose[2]	101	90%	98%	97%
Perioperative Temperature Management[2]	415	100%	100%	100%
Prophylactic Antibiotic Selection[2]	347	99%	99%	99%
Prophylactic Antibiotic Selection (Outpatient)	233	99%	98%	98%
Prophylactic Antibiotic Stopped[2]	336	99%	98%	98%
Prophylactic Antibiotic Timing[2]	347	98%	99%	99%
Prophylactic Antibiotic Timing (Outpatient)	235	96%	98%	98%
Urinary Catheter Removal[2]	237	97%	98%	97%
Survey of Patients' Hospital Experiences				
Area Around Room 'Always' Quiet at Night	300+	56%	58%	61%
Doctors 'Always' Communicated Well	300+	76%	77%	82%
Home Recovery Information Given	300+	83%	83%	85%
Hospital Given 9 or 10 on 10 Point Scale	300+	68%	67%	71%
Meds 'Always' Explained Before Given	300+	57%	60%	64%
Nurses 'Always' Communicated Well	300+	73%	75%	79%
Pain 'Always' Well Controlled	300+	67%	68%	71%
Room and Bathroom 'Always' Clean	300+	72%	69%	73%
Timely Help 'Always' Received	300+	63%	62%	68%
Would Definitely Recommend Hospital	300+	71%	69%	71%
Use of Medical Imaging				
Cardiac Imaging Stress Test before Surgery	611	9.3%	6.4%	5.3%
Combination Abdominal CT Scan	1,509	8.9%	11.8%	10.5%
Combination Brain/Sinus CT Scan	1,400	2.4%	3.4%	2.7%
Combination Chest CT Scan	1,380	2.7%	2.4%	2.7%
Follow-up Mammogram/Ultrasound	2,507	10.9%	10.2%	8.8%
Lumbar Spine MRI for Low Back Pain	141	31.9%	35.2%	37.2%

Saint Cloud Regional Medical Center

2906 17th Street Phone: 407-498-3432
Saint Cloud, FL 34769 Fax: 407-892-4835
URL: www.stcloudregional.com
Type: Acute Care Hospitals Emergency Services: Yes
Ownership: Proprietary Beds: 84

Key Personnel:
Hemotology Center . . . . Alka Arora
CEO/President. . . . . Ronald Beer
Anesthesiology. . . . . Nipa Gandhi
Pediatrics. . . . . Vasanthy Raghavan
Pediatrics. . . . . Rosela Rich
Pediatrics. . . . . Archana Watane

Measure	Cases	This Hosp.	State Avg.	U.S. Avg.
Blood Clot Prevention and Treatment				
Anticoagulation Overlap Therapy[2]	27	70%	93%	93%
ICU Venous Thromboembolism Prophylaxis[2]	59	71%	94%	92%
Incidence of Potentially Preventable VTE[1,2]	-	-	10%	10%
UFH with Dosages/Platelet Monitoring[1,2]	-	-	100%	97%
Venous Thromboembolism Prophylaxis[2]	386	64%	88%	85%
Warfarin Therapy Discharge Instructions[2]	23	87%	85%	75%
Chest Pain/Possible Heart Attack Care				
Aspirin Given Within 24 Hours of Arrival	35	100%	98%	96%
Fibrinolytic Meds Within 30 Min. of Arrival[7]	-	-	81%	58%
Average Time to ECG (minutes)	40	5	7	7
Average Time to Transfer (minutes)[1]	-	-	53	60
Children's Asthma Care				
Received Home Management Plan of Care	-	-	-	88%
Received Reliever Medication	-	-	-	100%
Received Systemic Corticosteroids	-	-	-	100%
Emergency Department				
Admittance Decision Time (minutes)[2]	896	85	111	98
Head CT Results Within 45 Min. of Arrival[1,3]	-	-	64%	57%
Patients Who Left ER Before Being Seen	25,684	2%	2%	2%
Time from ER Arrival to Admit. (minutes)[2]	898	255	289	274
Time from ER Arrival to Discharge (minutes)	678	130	147	134
Time in ER Before Being Evaluated (minutes)	698	41	26	26
Time to Pain Meds for Fractures (minutes)	70	52	60	57
Heart Attack Care				
Aspirin Given at Discharge	11	100%	99%	99%
Fibrinolytic Meds Within 30 Min. of Arrival[7]	-	-	50%	54%
PCI Within 90 Minutes of Arrival[7]	-	-	96%	96%
Statin Prescribed at Discharge	12	100%	99%	98%
Heart Failure Care				
ACE Inhibitor or ARB for LVSD	41	100%	98%	97%
Discharge Instructions Given	89	65%	96%	94%
Evaluation of LVS Function	119	100%	100%	99%
Medicare Spending				
Medicare Spending per Patient (ratio)	-	1.04	1.04	0.98
Pneumonia Care				
Appropriate Initial Antibiotic Given	70	99%	98%	95%
Blood Culture Timing	108	98%	99%	98%
Pregnancy and Delivery Care				
Newborn Deliveries Scheduled Early[2,7]	-	-	6%	6%
Preventive Care				
Immunization for Influenza[2]	615	94%	94%	90%
Immunization for Pneumonia[2]	717	96%	96%	92%
Stroke Care				
Anticoagulation Therapy for Atrial Fibrillation[1]	-	-	97%	95%
Antithrombotic Therapy Timing	26	85%	98%	98%
Assessed for Rehabilitation	28	82%	97%	97%
Discharged on Antithrombotic Therapy	25	92%	99%	99%
Discharged on Statin Medication	25	68%	96%	94%
Thrombolytic Therapy Timing[1]	-	-	76%	66%
Venous Thromboembolism Prophylaxis	28	68%	95%	94%
Written Stroke Educational Materials Given	19	74%	94%	88%
Surgical Care Improvement Project				
Appropriate Beta Blocker Usage	20	90%	99%	98%
Appropriate VTP Within 24 Hours	80	99%	99%	98%
Controlled Postoperative Blood Glucose[7]	-	-	98%	97%
Perioperative Temperature Management	82	100%	100%	100%
Prophylactic Antibiotic Selection	28	100%	99%	99%
Prophylactic Antibiotic Selection (Outpatient)	48	98%	98%	98%
Prophylactic Antibiotic Stopped	26	100%	98%	98%
Prophylactic Antibiotic Timing	28	100%	99%	99%
Prophylactic Antibiotic Timing (Outpatient)	48	100%	98%	98%
Urinary Catheter Removal	44	100%	98%	97%
Survey of Patients' Hospital Experiences				
Area Around Room 'Always' Quiet at Night	300+	49%	58%	61%
Doctors 'Always' Communicated Well	300+	72%	77%	82%
Home Recovery Information Given	300+	78%	83%	85%
Hospital Given 9 or 10 on 10 Point Scale	300+	50%	67%	71%
Meds 'Always' Explained Before Given	300+	46%	60%	64%
Nurses 'Always' Communicated Well	300+	62%	75%	79%
Pain 'Always' Well Controlled	300+	61%	68%	71%
Room and Bathroom 'Always' Clean	300+	64%	69%	73%
Timely Help 'Always' Received	300+	50%	62%	68%
Would Definitely Recommend Hospital	300+	52%	69%	71%
Use of Medical Imaging				
Cardiac Imaging Stress Test before Surgery	79	3.8%	6.4%	5.3%
Combination Abdominal CT Scan	323	3.7%	11.8%	10.5%
Combination Brain/Sinus CT Scan	344	4.7%	3.4%	2.7%
Combination Chest CT Scan	150	1.3%	2.4%	2.7%
Follow-up Mammogram/Ultrasound	484	14.9%	10.2%	8.8%
Lumbar Spine MRI for Low Back Pain[1]	-	-	35.2%	37.2%

Bayfront Health - Saint Petersburg

701 6th Saint S Phone: 727-823-1234
Saint Petersburg, FL 33701 Fax: 727-893-6962
URL: www.bayfront.org
Type: Acute Care Hospitals Emergency Services: Yes
Ownership: Voluntary non-profit - Private Beds: 502

Key Personnel:
CEO/President. . . . . Kathryn Gillette
Chief of Medical Staff. . . . . Arnold Ramirez

Measure	Cases	This Hosp.	State Avg.	U.S. Avg.
Blood Clot Prevention and Treatment				
Anticoagulation Overlap Therapy[2]	79	90%	93%	93%
ICU Venous Thromboembolism Prophylaxis[2]	145	90%	94%	92%
Incidence of Potentially Preventable VTE[2]	27	15%	10%	10%
UFH with Dosages/Platelet Monitoring[2]	24	96%	100%	97%
Venous Thromboembolism Prophylaxis[2]	331	71%	88%	85%
Warfarin Therapy Discharge Instructions[2]	52	67%	85%	75%
Chest Pain/Possible Heart Attack Care				
Aspirin Given Within 24 Hours of Arrival[3,7]	-	-	98%	96%
Fibrinolytic Meds Within 30 Min. of Arrival[5]	-	-	81%	58%
Average Time to ECG (minutes)[3,7]	-	-	7	7
Average Time to Transfer (minutes)[5]	-	-	53	60
Children's Asthma Care				
Received Home Management Plan of Care	-	-	-	88%
Received Reliever Medication	-	-	-	100%
Received Systemic Corticosteroids	-	-	-	100%
Emergency Department				
Admittance Decision Time (minutes)[2]	500	74	111	98
Head CT Results Within 45 Min. of Arrival[7]	-	-	64%	57%
Patients Who Left ER Before Being Seen	49,049	1%	2%	2%
Time from ER Arrival to Admit. (minutes)[2]	522	251	289	274
Time from ER Arrival to Discharge (minutes)	433	163	147	134
Time in ER Before Being Evaluated (minutes)	246	31	26	26
Time to Pain Meds for Fractures (minutes)	36	58	60	57
Heart Attack Care				
Aspirin Given at Discharge[2]	178	98%	99%	99%
Fibrinolytic Meds Within 30 Min. of Arrival[2,7]	-	-	50%	54%
PCI Within 90 Minutes of Arrival[2]	49	94%	96%	96%
Statin Prescribed at Discharge[2]	161	97%	99%	98%
Heart Failure Care				
ACE Inhibitor or ARB for LVSD[2]	73	96%	98%	97%
Discharge Instructions Given[2]	224	85%	96%	94%
Evaluation of LVS Function[2]	276	100%	100%	99%
Medicare Spending				
Medicare Spending per Patient (ratio)	-	1.10	1.04	0.98
Pneumonia Care				
Appropriate Initial Antibiotic Given[2]	64	94%	98%	95%
Blood Culture Timing[2]	170	99%	99%	98%
Pregnancy and Delivery Care				
Newborn Deliveries Scheduled Early[2]	62	3%	6%	6%
Preventive Care				
Immunization for Influenza[2]	461	77%	94%	90%
Immunization for Pneumonia[2]	524	83%	96%	92%
Stroke Care				
Anticoagulation Therapy for Atrial Fibrillation[2]	19	95%	97%	95%
Antithrombotic Therapy Timing[2]	89	94%	98%	98%
Assessed for Rehabilitation[2]	125	98%	97%	97%
Discharged on Antithrombotic Therapy[2]	90	100%	99%	99%
Discharged on Statin Medication[2]	70	96%	96%	94%
Thrombolytic Therapy Timing[1,2]	-	-	76%	66%
Venous Thromboembolism Prophylaxis[2]	138	97%	95%	94%
Written Stroke Educational Materials Given[2]	69	91%	94%	88%
Surgical Care Improvement Project				
Appropriate Beta Blocker Usage[2]	157	97%	99%	98%
Appropriate VTP Within 24 Hours[2]	303	98%	99%	98%
Controlled Postoperative Blood Glucose[2]	82	98%	98%	97%
Perioperative Temperature Management[2]	372	100%	100%	100%
Prophylactic Antibiotic Selection[2]	321	98%	99%	99%
Prophylactic Antibiotic Selection (Outpatient)	303	99%	98%	98%
Prophylactic Antibiotic Stopped[2]	311	99%	98%	98%
Prophylactic Antibiotic Timing[2]	321	99%	99%	99%
Prophylactic Antibiotic Timing (Outpatient)	302	99%	98%	98%
Urinary Catheter Removal[2]	262	98%	98%	97%
Survey of Patients' Hospital Experiences				
Area Around Room 'Always' Quiet at Night	300+	54%	58%	61%
Doctors 'Always' Communicated Well	300+	76%	77%	82%
Home Recovery Information Given	300+	81%	83%	85%
Hospital Given 9 or 10 on 10 Point Scale	300+	70%	67%	71%
Meds 'Always' Explained Before Given	300+	57%	60%	64%
Nurses 'Always' Communicated Well	300+	75%	75%	79%
Pain 'Always' Well Controlled	300+	71%	68%	71%
Room and Bathroom 'Always' Clean	300+	69%	69%	73%
Timely Help 'Always' Received	300+	60%	62%	68%
Would Definitely Recommend Hospital	300+	67%	69%	71%
Use of Medical Imaging				
Cardiac Imaging Stress Test before Surgery	138	5.8%	6.4%	5.3%
Combination Abdominal CT Scan	315	6.0%	11.8%	10.5%
Combination Brain/Sinus CT Scan	462	6.9%	3.4%	2.7%
Combination Chest CT Scan	164	0.0%	2.4%	2.7%
Follow-up Mammogram/Ultrasound	433	11.1%	10.2%	8.8%
Lumbar Spine MRI for Low Back Pain[1]	-	-	35.2%	37.2%

NOTE: Hospital profiles are in alphabetical order by state, then city, then hospital within the city; Rankings exclude hospitals with less than 25 cases except for patient surveys which excludes hospitals with less than 100 cases; (a) 100-299 cases; (1) The number of cases/patients is too few to report; (2) Data submitted were based on a sample of cases/patients; (3) Results are based on a shorter time period than required; (4) Data suppressed by CMS for one or more quarters; (5) Results are not available for this reporting period; (6) Fewer than 100 patients completed the HCAHPS survey; (7) No cases met the criteria for this measure; (8) The lower limit of the confidence interval cannot be calculated if the number of observed infections equals zero; (9) No data are available from the state/territory for this reporting period; (10) The scores shown reflect fewer than 50 completed surveys; (11) There were discrepancies in the data collection process; (12) This measure does not apply to this hospital for this reporting period; (13) Results cannot be calculated for this reporting period; (14) The results for this state are combined with nearby states to protect confidentiality; Please refer to the User's Guide for a full explanation of data.

Edward White Hospital

2323 9th Ave N
Saint Petersburg, FL 33713
Phone: 727-323-1111
Fax: 727-328-6135
URL: www.edwhitehospital.com
Type: Acute Care Hospitals
Emergency Services: Yes
Ownership: Proprietary
Beds: 167

Key Personnel:

Radiology. . . . . Chester Babat
Chief of Medical Staff. . . . . Clinton Davis, MD
Emergency Room . . . . Nagy Farag, MD
CEO/President. . . . . Peggy Gatliff
Infection Control. . . . . Michelle Haynes
Intensive Care Unit. . . . . Claudia Leon
Quality Assurance . . . . Lura Nelms
Operating Room. . . . . Gayle Wheelter

Measure	Cases	This Hosp.	State Avg.	U.S. Avg.
Blood Clot Prevention and Treatment				
Anticoagulation Overlap Therapy[2]	26	100%	93%	93%
ICU Venous Thromboembolism Prophylaxis[2]	88	100%	94%	92%
Incidence of Potentially Preventable VTE[1,2]	-	-	10%	10%
UFH with Dosages/Platelet Monitoring[1,2]	-	-	100%	97%
Venous Thromboembolism Prophylaxis[2]	217	100%	88%	85%
Warfarin Therapy Discharge Instructions[2]	13	77%	85%	75%
Chest Pain/Possible Heart Attack Care				
Aspirin Given Within 24 Hours of Arrival[1]	-	-	98%	96%
Fibrinolytic Meds Within 30 Min. of Arrival[3,7]	-	-	81%	58%
Average Time to ECG (minutes)[1]	-	-	7	7
Average Time to Transfer (minutes)[1,3]	-	-	53	60
Children's Asthma Care				
Received Home Management Plan of Care	-	-	-	88%
Received Reliever Medication	-	-	-	100%
Received Systemic Corticosteroids	-	-	-	100%
Emergency Department				
Admittance Decision Time (minutes)[2]	439	34	111	98
Head CT Results Within 45 Min. of Arrival[1,3]	-	-	64%	57%
Patients Who Left ER Before Being Seen	11,542	1%	2%	2%
Time from ER Arrival to Admit. (minutes)[2]	439	180	289	274
Time from ER Arrival to Discharge (minutes)	391	100	147	134
Time in ER Before Being Evaluated (minutes)	442	7	26	26
Time to Pain Meds for Fractures (minutes)	13	51	60	57
Heart Attack Care				
Aspirin Given at Discharge[1]	-	-	99%	99%
Fibrinolytic Meds Within 30 Min. of Arrival[7]	-	-	50%	54%
PCI Within 90 Minutes of Arrival[7]	-	-	96%	96%
Statin Prescribed at Discharge[1]	-	-	99%	98%
Heart Failure Care				
ACE Inhibitor or ARB for LVSD	12	100%	98%	97%
Discharge Instructions Given	39	95%	96%	94%
Evaluation of LVS Function	63	100%	100%	99%
Medicare Spending				
Medicare Spending per Patient (ratio)	-	1.06	1.04	0.98
Pneumonia Care				
Appropriate Initial Antibiotic Given[2]	56	98%	98%	95%
Blood Culture Timing[2]	69	99%	99%	98%
Pregnancy and Delivery Care				
Newborn Deliveries Scheduled Early[2,7]	-	-	6%	6%
Preventive Care				
Immunization for Influenza[2]	356	99%	94%	90%
Immunization for Pneumonia[2]	495	99%	96%	92%
Stroke Care				
Anticoagulation Therapy for Atrial Fibrillation[1]	-	-	97%	95%
Antithrombotic Therapy Timing	25	96%	98%	98%
Assessed for Rehabilitation	23	100%	97%	97%
Discharged on Antithrombotic Therapy	22	100%	99%	99%
Discharged on Statin Medication	14	100%	96%	94%
Thrombolytic Therapy Timing[1]	-	-	76%	66%
Venous Thromboembolism Prophylaxis	26	96%	95%	94%
Written Stroke Educational Materials Given[1]	-	-	94%	88%
Surgical Care Improvement Project				
Appropriate Beta Blocker Usage	59	100%	99%	98%
Appropriate VTP Within 24 Hours	197	99%	99%	98%
Controlled Postoperative Blood Glucose[7]	-	-	98%	97%
Perioperative Temperature Management	214	100%	100%	100%
Prophylactic Antibiotic Selection	132	100%	99%	99%
Prophylactic Antibiotic Selection (Outpatient)	45	100%	98%	98%
Prophylactic Antibiotic Stopped	126	98%	98%	98%
Prophylactic Antibiotic Timing	132	100%	99%	99%
Prophylactic Antibiotic Timing (Outpatient)	45	100%	98%	98%
Urinary Catheter Removal	139	99%	98%	97%
Survey of Patients' Hospital Experiences				
Area Around Room 'Always' Quiet at Night	300+	60%	58%	61%
Doctors 'Always' Communicated Well	300+	76%	77%	82%
Home Recovery Information Given	300+	86%	83%	85%
Hospital Given 9 or 10 on 10 Point Scale	300+	66%	67%	71%
Meds 'Always' Explained Before Given	300+	61%	60%	64%
Nurses 'Always' Communicated Well	300+	71%	75%	79%
Pain 'Always' Well Controlled	300+	66%	68%	71%
Room and Bathroom 'Always' Clean	300+	70%	69%	73%
Timely Help 'Always' Received	300+	58%	62%	68%
Would Definitely Recommend Hospital	300+	69%	69%	71%
Use of Medical Imaging				
Cardiac Imaging Stress Test before Surgery[1]	-	-	6.4%	5.3%
Combination Abdominal CT Scan	118	3.4%	11.8%	10.5%
Combination Brain/Sinus CT Scan[1]	-	-	3.4%	2.7%
Combination Chest CT Scan[1]	-	-	2.4%	2.7%
Follow-up Mammogram/Ultrasound[7]	-	-	10.2%	8.8%
Lumbar Spine MRI for Low Back Pain[1]	-	-	35.2%	37.2%

Northside Hospital

6000 49th Street N
Saint Petersburg, FL 33709
Phone: 813-521-5000
Fax: 727-521-5007
URL: www.northsidehospital.com
Type: Acute Care Hospitals
Emergency Services: Yes
Ownership: Proprietary
Beds: 288

Key Personnel:

Chief of Medical Staff. . . . . Syed H Abid
Operating Room. . . . . William M Blackshear, RN
Chairman/CEO . . . . Dominic J. Connelly
Intensive Care Unit. . . . . Mary Ellen Jackson, RN
CEO/President. . . . . Dia Nichols
Radiology. . . . . Dennis J Pevarski

Measure	Cases	This Hosp.	State Avg.	U.S. Avg.
Blood Clot Prevention and Treatment				
Anticoagulation Overlap Therapy[2]	58	97%	93%	93%
ICU Venous Thromboembolism Prophylaxis[2]	121	96%	94%	92%
Incidence of Potentially Preventable VTE[2]	20	20%	10%	10%
UFH with Dosages/Platelet Monitoring[2]	30	100%	100%	97%
Venous Thromboembolism Prophylaxis[2]	324	92%	88%	85%
Warfarin Therapy Discharge Instructions[2]	39	100%	85%	75%
Chest Pain/Possible Heart Attack Care				
Aspirin Given Within 24 Hours of Arrival[1,3]	-	-	98%	96%
Fibrinolytic Meds Within 30 Min. of Arrival[5]	-	-	81%	58%
Average Time to ECG (minutes)[1,3]	-	-	7	7
Average Time to Transfer (minutes)[5]	-	-	53	60
Children's Asthma Care				
Received Home Management Plan of Care	-	-	-	88%
Received Reliever Medication	-	-	-	100%
Received Systemic Corticosteroids	-	-	-	100%
Emergency Department				
Admittance Decision Time (minutes)[2]	996	59	111	98
Head CT Results Within 45 Min. of Arrival[7]	-	-	64%	57%
Patients Who Left ER Before Being Seen	31,437	0%	2%	2%
Time from ER Arrival to Admit. (minutes)[2]	996	214	289	274
Time from ER Arrival to Discharge (minutes)	436	126	147	134
Time in ER Before Being Evaluated (minutes)	498	11	26	26
Time to Pain Meds for Fractures (minutes)	55	42	60	57
Heart Attack Care				
Aspirin Given at Discharge[2]	282	100%	99%	99%
Fibrinolytic Meds Within 30 Min. of Arrival[2,7]	-	-	50%	54%
PCI Within 90 Minutes of Arrival[2]	43	100%	96%	96%
Statin Prescribed at Discharge[2]	266	99%	99%	98%
Heart Failure Care				
ACE Inhibitor or ARB for LVSD[2]	88	99%	98%	97%
Discharge Instructions Given[2]	233	100%	96%	94%
Evaluation of LVS Function[2]	293	100%	100%	99%
Medicare Spending				
Medicare Spending per Patient (ratio)	-	1.09	1.04	0.98
Pneumonia Care				
Appropriate Initial Antibiotic Given[2]	66	100%	98%	95%
Blood Culture Timing[2]	127	100%	99%	98%
Pregnancy and Delivery Care				
Newborn Deliveries Scheduled Early[2,7]	-	-	6%	6%
Preventive Care				
Immunization for Influenza[2]	613	100%	94%	90%
Immunization for Pneumonia[2]	945	99%	96%	92%
Stroke Care				
Anticoagulation Therapy for Atrial Fibrillation[2]	18	100%	97%	95%
Antithrombotic Therapy Timing[2]	84	100%	98%	98%
Assessed for Rehabilitation[2]	111	100%	97%	97%
Discharged on Antithrombotic Therapy[2]	84	100%	99%	99%
Discharged on Statin Medication[2]	66	98%	96%	94%
Thrombolytic Therapy Timing[1,2]	-	-	76%	66%
Venous Thromboembolism Prophylaxis[2]	125	100%	95%	94%
Written Stroke Educational Materials Given[2]	56	100%	94%	88%
Surgical Care Improvement Project				
Appropriate Beta Blocker Usage[2]	191	100%	99%	98%
Appropriate VTP Within 24 Hours[2]	185	100%	99%	98%
Controlled Postoperative Blood Glucose[2]	139	99%	98%	97%
Perioperative Temperature Management[2]	240	100%	100%	100%
Prophylactic Antibiotic Selection[2]	222	100%	99%	99%
Prophylactic Antibiotic Selection (Outpatient)	203	100%	98%	98%
Prophylactic Antibiotic Stopped[2]	211	98%	98%	98%
Prophylactic Antibiotic Timing[2]	222	100%	99%	99%
Prophylactic Antibiotic Timing (Outpatient)	203	99%	98%	98%
Urinary Catheter Removal[2]	255	98%	98%	97%
Survey of Patients' Hospital Experiences				
Area Around Room 'Always' Quiet at Night	300+	51%	58%	61%
Doctors 'Always' Communicated Well	300+	74%	77%	82%
Home Recovery Information Given	300+	82%	83%	85%
Hospital Given 9 or 10 on 10 Point Scale	300+	62%	67%	71%
Meds 'Always' Explained Before Given	300+	54%	60%	64%
Nurses 'Always' Communicated Well	300+	71%	75%	79%
Pain 'Always' Well Controlled	300+	60%	68%	71%
Room and Bathroom 'Always' Clean	300+	70%	69%	73%
Timely Help 'Always' Received	300+	58%	62%	68%
Would Definitely Recommend Hospital	300+	64%	69%	71%
Use of Medical Imaging				
Cardiac Imaging Stress Test before Surgery[1]	-	-	6.4%	5.3%
Combination Abdominal CT Scan	237	9.3%	11.8%	10.5%
Combination Brain/Sinus CT Scan	422	4.0%	3.4%	2.7%
Combination Chest CT Scan	71	0.0%	2.4%	2.7%
Follow-up Mammogram/Ultrasound[7]	-	-	10.2%	8.8%
Lumbar Spine MRI for Low Back Pain[1]	-	-	35.2%	37.2%

Palms of Pasadena Hospital

1501 Pasadena Ave South
Saint Petersburg, FL 33707
Phone: 727-381-1000
Fax: 727-341-7009
E-mail: palms@palmspasadena.com
URL: www.palmspasadena.com
Type: Acute Care Hospitals
Emergency Services: Yes
Ownership: Proprietary
Beds: 307

Key Personnel:

Infection Control. . . . . Phyllis Elliott
CEO/President. . . . . Sharon Hayes, RN, BSN, MBA
Quality Assurance . . . . Sharon Milbourn
Radiology. . . . . Stephanie Poveromo
Operating Room. . . . . Judy Stewart
Cardiac Laboratory. . . . . Lynn Stilwell
Chief of Medical Staff. . . . . Robert Wharton, MD

Measure	Cases	This Hosp.	State Avg.	U.S. Avg.
Blood Clot Prevention and Treatment				
Anticoagulation Overlap Therapy[2]	21	100%	93%	93%
ICU Venous Thromboembolism Prophylaxis[2]	104	97%	94%	92%
Incidence of Potentially Preventable VTE[2,7]	-	-	10%	10%
UFH with Dosages/Platelet Monitoring[1,2]	-	-	100%	97%
Venous Thromboembolism Prophylaxis[2]	366	91%	88%	85%
Warfarin Therapy Discharge Instructions[2]	14	86%	85%	75%
Chest Pain/Possible Heart Attack Care				
Aspirin Given Within 24 Hours of Arrival[1,3]	-	-	98%	96%
Fibrinolytic Meds Within 30 Min. of Arrival[1,3]	-	-	81%	58%
Average Time to ECG (minutes)[3]	12	2	7	7
Average Time to Transfer (minutes)[1,3]	-	-	53	60

NOTE: Hospital profiles are in alphabetical order by state, then city, then hospital within the city; Rankings exclude hospitals with less than 25 cases except for patient surveys which excludes hospitals with less than 100 cases; (a) 100-299 cases; (1) The number of cases/patients is too few to report; (2) Data submitted were based on a sample of cases/patients; (3) Results are based on a shorter time period than required; (4) Data suppressed by CMS for one or more quarters; (5) Results are not available for this reporting period; (6) Fewer than 100 patients completed the HCAHPS survey; (7) No cases met the criteria for this measure; (8) The lower limit of the confidence interval cannot be calculated if the number of observed infections equals zero; (9) No data are available from the state/territory for this reporting period; (10) The scores shown reflect fewer than 50 completed surveys; (11) There were discrepancies in the data collection process; (12) This measure does not apply to this hospital for this reporting period; (13) Results cannot be calculated for this reporting period; (14) The results for this state are combined with nearby states to protect confidentiality; Please refer to the User's Guide for a full explanation of data.

Children's Asthma Care				
Received Home Management Plan of Care	-	-	-	88%
Received Reliever Medication	-	-	-	100%
Received Systemic Corticosteroids	-	-	-	100%
Emergency Department				
Admittance Decision Time (minutes)[2]	739	108	111	98
Head CT Results Within 45 Min. of Arrival[3,7]	-	-	64%	57%
Patients Who Left ER Before Being Seen	14,533	1%	2%	2%
Time from ER Arrival to Admit. (minutes)[2]	745	262	289	274
Time from ER Arrival to Discharge (minutes)	487	139	147	134
Time in ER Before Being Evaluated (minutes)	555	27	26	26
Time to Pain Meds for Fractures (minutes)	78	50	60	57
Heart Attack Care				
Aspirin Given at Discharge	14	100%	99%	99%
Fibrinolytic Meds Within 30 Min. of Arrival[7]	-	-	50%	54%
PCI Within 90 Minutes of Arrival[7]	-	-	96%	96%
Statin Prescribed at Discharge	13	85%	99%	98%
Heart Failure Care				
ACE Inhibitor or ARB for LVSD	25	100%	98%	97%
Discharge Instructions Given	88	95%	96%	94%
Evaluation of LVS Function	124	98%	100%	99%
Medicare Spending				
Medicare Spending per Patient (ratio)	-	1.14	1.04	0.98
Pneumonia Care				
Appropriate Initial Antibiotic Given	104	99%	98%	95%
Blood Culture Timing	129	95%	99%	98%
Pregnancy and Delivery Care				
Newborn Deliveries Scheduled Early[7]	-	-	6%	6%
Preventive Care				
Immunization for Influenza[2]	440	97%	94%	90%
Immunization for Pneumonia[2]	744	99%	96%	92%
Stroke Care				
Anticoagulation Therapy for Atrial Fibrillation	18	100%	97%	95%
Antithrombotic Therapy Timing	61	100%	98%	98%
Assessed for Rehabilitation	69	100%	97%	97%
Discharged on Antithrombotic Therapy	63	100%	99%	99%
Discharged on Statin Medication	42	98%	96%	94%
Thrombolytic Therapy Timing[1]	-	-	76%	66%
Venous Thromboembolism Prophylaxis	73	100%	95%	94%
Written Stroke Educational Materials Given	35	100%	94%	88%
Surgical Care Improvement Project				
Appropriate Beta Blocker Usage	150	100%	99%	98%
Appropriate VTP Within 24 Hours	506	100%	99%	98%
Controlled Postoperative Blood Glucose[7]	-	-	98%	97%
Perioperative Temperature Management	545	100%	100%	100%
Prophylactic Antibiotic Selection	284	100%	99%	99%
Prophylactic Antibiotic Selection (Outpatient)	14	100%	98%	98%
Prophylactic Antibiotic Stopped	283	99%	98%	98%
Prophylactic Antibiotic Timing	284	100%	99%	99%
Prophylactic Antibiotic Timing (Outpatient)	14	100%	98%	98%
Urinary Catheter Removal	288	99%	98%	97%
Survey of Patients' Hospital Experiences				
Area Around Room 'Always' Quiet at Night	300+	58%	58%	61%
Doctors 'Always' Communicated Well	300+	83%	77%	82%
Home Recovery Information Given	300+	83%	83%	85%
Hospital Given 9 or 10 on 10 Point Scale	300+	71%	67%	71%
Meds 'Always' Explained Before Given	300+	60%	60%	64%
Nurses 'Always' Communicated Well	300+	77%	75%	79%
Pain 'Always' Well Controlled	300+	70%	68%	71%
Room and Bathroom 'Always' Clean	300+	70%	69%	73%
Timely Help 'Always' Received	300+	66%	62%	68%
Would Definitely Recommend Hospital	300+	70%	69%	71%
Use of Medical Imaging				
Cardiac Imaging Stress Test before Surgery[1]	-	-	6.4%	5.3%
Combination Abdominal CT Scan	558	17.4%	11.8%	10.5%
Combination Brain/Sinus CT Scan	660	2.9%	3.4%	2.7%
Combination Chest CT Scan	346	0.0%	2.4%	2.7%
Follow-up Mammogram/Ultrasound	701	3.1%	10.2%	8.8%
Lumbar Spine MRI for Low Back Pain	50	32.0%	35.2%	37.2%

Saint Anthony's Hospital

1200 7th Avenue North
Saint Petersburg, FL 33705
URL: www.stanthonys.com
Type: Acute Care Hospitals
Ownership: Voluntary non-profit - Church
Phone: 727-825-1100
Fax: 727-825-1302
Emergency Services: Yes
Beds: 405

Key Personnel:

Radiology. Glen Alan Call
Anesthesiology. . . . . Thomas Conroy, MD
Chief of Medical Staff. . . . . James McClintic, MD
Emergency Room . . . . R Michael Smith, MD
CEO/President. . . . . William Ulbricht

Measure	Cases	This Hosp.	State Avg.	U.S. Avg.
Blood Clot Prevention and Treatment				
Anticoagulation Overlap Therapy[2]	141	72%	93%	93%
ICU Venous Thromboembolism Prophylaxis[2]	88	92%	94%	92%
Incidence of Potentially Preventable VTE[2]	42	24%	10%	10%
UFH with Dosages/Platelet Monitoring[2]	50	100%	100%	97%
Venous Thromboembolism Prophylaxis[2]	335	84%	88%	85%
Warfarin Therapy Discharge Instructions[2]	95	95%	85%	75%
Chest Pain/Possible Heart Attack Care				
Aspirin Given Within 24 Hours of Arrival[5]	-	-	98%	96%
Fibrinolytic Meds Within 30 Min. of Arrival[5]	-	-	81%	58%
Average Time to ECG (minutes)[5]	-	-	7	7
Average Time to Transfer (minutes)[5]	-	-	53	60
Children's Asthma Care				
Received Home Management Plan of Care	-	-	-	88%
Received Reliever Medication	-	-	-	100%
Received Systemic Corticosteroids	-	-	-	100%
Emergency Department				
Admittance Decision Time (minutes)[2]	778	106	111	98
Head CT Results Within 45 Min. of Arrival[1]	-	-	64%	57%
Patients Who Left ER Before Being Seen	42,523	2%	2%	2%
Time from ER Arrival to Admit. (minutes)[2]	789	296	289	274
Time from ER Arrival to Discharge (minutes)	548	206	147	134
Time in ER Before Being Evaluated (minutes)	626	40	26	26
Time to Pain Meds for Fractures (minutes)	45	75	60	57
Heart Attack Care				
Aspirin Given at Discharge	202	100%	99%	99%
Fibrinolytic Meds Within 30 Min. of Arrival[7]	-	-	50%	54%
PCI Within 90 Minutes of Arrival	32	97%	96%	96%
Statin Prescribed at Discharge	204	99%	99%	98%
Heart Failure Care				
ACE Inhibitor or ARB for LVSD	112	99%	98%	97%
Discharge Instructions Given	284	92%	96%	94%
Evaluation of LVS Function	375	100%	100%	99%
Medicare Spending				
Medicare Spending per Patient (ratio)	-	1.05	1.04	0.98
Pneumonia Care				
Appropriate Initial Antibiotic Given	150	97%	98%	95%
Blood Culture Timing	325	99%	99%	98%
Pregnancy and Delivery Care				
Newborn Deliveries Scheduled Early[7]	-	-	6%	6%
Preventive Care				
Immunization for Influenza[2]	693	95%	94%	90%
Immunization for Pneumonia[2]	1,000	86%	96%	92%
Stroke Care				
Anticoagulation Therapy for Atrial Fibrillation[1]	-	-	97%	95%
Antithrombotic Therapy Timing	138	95%	98%	98%
Assessed for Rehabilitation	166	97%	97%	97%
Discharged on Antithrombotic Therapy	149	100%	99%	99%
Discharged on Statin Medication	129	97%	96%	94%
Thrombolytic Therapy Timing[1]	-	-	76%	66%
Venous Thromboembolism Prophylaxis	168	98%	95%	94%
Written Stroke Educational Materials Given	93	98%	94%	88%
Surgical Care Improvement Project				
Appropriate Beta Blocker Usage[2]	230	98%	99%	98%
Appropriate VTP Within 24 Hours[2]	590	99%	99%	98%
Controlled Postoperative Blood Glucose[2,7]	-	-	98%	97%
Perioperative Temperature Management[2]	692	100%	100%	100%
Prophylactic Antibiotic Selection[2]	513	99%	99%	99%
Prophylactic Antibiotic Selection (Outpatient)	293	96%	98%	98%
Prophylactic Antibiotic Stopped[2]	496	98%	98%	98%
Prophylactic Antibiotic Timing[2]	514	100%	99%	99%
Prophylactic Antibiotic Timing (Outpatient)	296	96%	98%	98%
Urinary Catheter Removal[2]	489	98%	98%	97%
Survey of Patients' Hospital Experiences				
Area Around Room 'Always' Quiet at Night	300+	56%	58%	61%
Doctors 'Always' Communicated Well	300+	74%	77%	82%
Home Recovery Information Given	300+	82%	83%	85%
Hospital Given 9 or 10 on 10 Point Scale	300+	72%	67%	71%
Meds 'Always' Explained Before Given	300+	61%	60%	64%
Nurses 'Always' Communicated Well	300+	76%	75%	79%
Pain 'Always' Well Controlled	300+	68%	68%	71%
Room and Bathroom 'Always' Clean	300+	70%	69%	73%
Timely Help 'Always' Received	300+	62%	62%	68%
Would Definitely Recommend Hospital	300+	77%	69%	71%
Use of Medical Imaging				
Cardiac Imaging Stress Test before Surgery	117	8.5%	6.4%	5.3%
Combination Abdominal CT Scan	860	7.9%	11.8%	10.5%
Combination Brain/Sinus CT Scan	970	2.5%	3.4%	2.7%
Combination Chest CT Scan	477	0.6%	2.4%	2.7%
Follow-up Mammogram/Ultrasound	1,344	7.8%	10.2%	8.8%
Lumbar Spine MRI for Low Back Pain	72	44.4%	35.2%	37.2%

Saint Petersburg General Hospital

6500 38th Ave N
Saint Petersburg, FL 33710
URL: www.stpetegeneralhospital.com
Type: Acute Care Hospitals
Ownership: Proprietary
Phone: 727-384-1414
Fax: 727-341-4889
Emergency Services: Yes
Beds: 219

Key Personnel:

Chief of Medical Staff. . . . . Romeo Acosta, MD
Radiology. Chester Babat
Emergency Room . . . . Andrew Basile
Quality Assurance . . . . Rosemary Bloomfield
CEO . . . . Robert Conroy, Jr
Intensive Care Unit. . . . . Debby Garreck
President/CEO. . . . . Peter A. Marmerstein

Measure	Cases	This Hosp.	State Avg.	U.S. Avg.
Blood Clot Prevention and Treatment				
Anticoagulation Overlap Therapy[2]	51	98%	93%	93%
ICU Venous Thromboembolism Prophylaxis[2]	103	97%	94%	92%
Incidence of Potentially Preventable VTE[1,2]	-	-	10%	10%
UFH with Dosages/Platelet Monitoring[2]	17	100%	100%	97%
Venous Thromboembolism Prophylaxis[2]	307	97%	88%	85%
Warfarin Therapy Discharge Instructions[2]	36	86%	85%	75%
Chest Pain/Possible Heart Attack Care				
Aspirin Given Within 24 Hours of Arrival	32	100%	98%	96%
Fibrinolytic Meds Within 30 Min. of Arrival[7]	-	-	81%	58%
Average Time to ECG (minutes)	35	7	7	7
Average Time to Transfer (minutes)	17	55	53	60
Children's Asthma Care				
Received Home Management Plan of Care	-	-	-	88%
Received Reliever Medication	-	-	-	100%
Received Systemic Corticosteroids	-	-	-	100%
Emergency Department				
Admittance Decision Time (minutes)[2]	720	79	111	98
Head CT Results Within 45 Min. of Arrival[1]	-	-	64%	57%
Patients Who Left ER Before Being Seen	31,914	1%	2%	2%
Time from ER Arrival to Admit. (minutes)[2]	721	224	289	274
Time from ER Arrival to Discharge (minutes)	450	114	147	134
Time in ER Before Being Evaluated (minutes)	500	10	26	26
Time to Pain Meds for Fractures (minutes)	65	37	60	57
Heart Attack Care				
Aspirin Given at Discharge[1]	-	-	99%	99%
Fibrinolytic Meds Within 30 Min. of Arrival[7]	-	-	50%	54%
PCI Within 90 Minutes of Arrival[7]	-	-	96%	96%
Statin Prescribed at Discharge[1]	-	-	99%	98%
Heart Failure Care				
ACE Inhibitor or ARB for LVSD	27	100%	98%	97%
Discharge Instructions Given	88	92%	96%	94%
Evaluation of LVS Function	110	100%	100%	99%
Medicare Spending				
Medicare Spending per Patient (ratio)	-	1.08	1.04	0.98
Pneumonia Care				
Appropriate Initial Antibiotic Given[2]	62	95%	98%	95%

NOTE: Hospital profiles are in alphabetical order by state, then city, then hospital within the city; Rankings exclude hospitals with less than 25 cases except for patient surveys which excludes hospitals with less than 100 cases; (a) 100-299 cases; (1) The number of cases/patients is too few to report; (2) Data submitted were based on a sample of cases/patients; (3) Results are based on a shorter time period than required; (4) Data suppressed by CMS for one or more quarters; (5) Results are not available for this reporting period; (6) Fewer than 100 patients completed the HCAHPS survey; (7) No cases met the criteria for this measure; (8) The lower limit of the confidence interval cannot be calculated if the number of observed infections equals zero; (9) No data are available from the state/territory for this reporting period; (10) The scores shown reflect fewer than 50 completed surveys; (11) There were discrepancies in the data collection process; (12) This measure does not apply to this hospital for this reporting period; (13) Results cannot be calculated for this reporting period; (14) The results for this state are combined with nearby states to protect confidentiality; Please refer to the User's Guide for a full explanation of data.

Measure	Cases	This Hosp.	State Avg.	U.S. Avg.
Blood Culture Timing[2]	126	99%	99%	98%
Pregnancy and Delivery Care				
Newborn Deliveries Scheduled Early[2]	38	0%	6%	6%
Preventive Care				
Immunization for Influenza[2]	553	97%	94%	90%
Immunization for Pneumonia[2]	618	97%	96%	92%
Stroke Care				
Anticoagulation Therapy for Atrial Fibrillation[1]	-	-	97%	95%
Antithrombotic Therapy Timing	42	100%	98%	98%
Assessed for Rehabilitation	38	97%	97%	97%
Discharged on Antithrombotic Therapy	36	100%	99%	99%
Discharged on Statin Medication	25	100%	96%	94%
Thrombolytic Therapy Timing[1]	-	-	76%	66%
Venous Thromboembolism Prophylaxis	45	100%	95%	94%
Written Stroke Educational Materials Given	21	100%	94%	88%
Surgical Care Improvement Project				
Appropriate Beta Blocker Usage[2]	81	99%	99%	98%
Appropriate VTP Within 24 Hours[2]	260	100%	99%	98%
Controlled Postoperative Blood Glucose[2,7]	-	-	98%	97%
Perioperative Temperature Management[2]	296	100%	100%	100%
Prophylactic Antibiotic Selection[2]	172	99%	99%	99%
Prophylactic Antibiotic Selection (Outpatient)	239	99%	98%	98%
Prophylactic Antibiotic Stopped[2]	165	99%	98%	98%
Prophylactic Antibiotic Timing[2]	172	100%	99%	99%
Prophylactic Antibiotic Timing (Outpatient)	239	100%	98%	98%
Urinary Catheter Removal[2]	158	99%	98%	97%
Survey of Patients' Hospital Experiences				
Area Around Room 'Always' Quiet at Night	300+	61%	58%	61%
Doctors 'Always' Communicated Well	300+	76%	77%	82%
Home Recovery Information Given	300+	85%	83%	85%
Hospital Given 9 or 10 on 10 Point Scale	300+	69%	67%	71%
Meds 'Always' Explained Before Given	300+	61%	60%	64%
Nurses 'Always' Communicated Well	300+	76%	75%	79%
Pain 'Always' Well Controlled	300+	67%	68%	71%
Room and Bathroom 'Always' Clean	300+	73%	69%	73%
Timely Help 'Always' Received	300+	63%	62%	68%
Would Definitely Recommend Hospital	300+	68%	69%	71%
Use of Medical Imaging				
Cardiac Imaging Stress Test before Surgery[1]	-	-	6.4%	5.3%
Combination Abdominal CT Scan	177	7.3%	11.8%	10.5%
Combination Brain/Sinus CT Scan[1]	-	-	3.4%	2.7%
Combination Chest CT Scan	53	3.8%	2.4%	2.7%
Follow-up Mammogram/Ultrasound	568	6.9%	10.2%	8.8%
Lumbar Spine MRI for Low Back Pain[7]	-	-	35.2%	37.2%

Central Florida Regional Hospital

1401 W Seminole Blvd
Sanford, FL 32771
Phone: 407-321-4500
Fax: 407-302-7310
URL: www.centralfloridaregional.com
Type: Acute Care Hospitals
Ownership: Proprietary
Emergency Services: Yes
Beds: 226

Key Personnel:

Quality Assurance . . . . Debbie Arruda
CEO/President. . . . . Wendy H Brandon
Emergency Room . . . . Linda Breum
Operating Room. . . . . Franklin D Clontz
Chief of Medical Staff. . . . . Meureen Daniel
Radiology. . . . . Juan A Lopez

Measure	Cases	This Hosp.	State Avg.	U.S. Avg.
Blood Clot Prevention and Treatment				
Anticoagulation Overlap Therapy[2]	70	100%	93%	93%
ICU Venous Thromboembolism Prophylaxis[2]	118	100%	94%	92%
Incidence of Potentially Preventable VTE[1,2]	-	-	10%	10%
UFH with Dosages/Platelet Monitoring[2]	58	98%	100%	97%
Venous Thromboembolism Prophylaxis[2]	330	97%	88%	85%
Warfarin Therapy Discharge Instructions[2]	64	97%	85%	75%
Chest Pain/Possible Heart Attack Care				
Aspirin Given Within 24 Hours of Arrival[3,7]	-	-	98%	96%
Fibrinolytic Meds Within 30 Min. of Arrival[5]	-	-	81%	58%
Average Time to ECG (minutes)[3,7]	-	-	7	7
Average Time to Transfer (minutes)[5]	-	-	53	60
Children's Asthma Care				
Received Home Management Plan of Care	-	-	-	88%
Received Reliever Medication	-	-	-	100%
Received Systemic Corticosteroids	-	-	-	100%
Emergency Department				
Admittance Decision Time (minutes)[2]	860	82	111	98
Head CT Results Within 45 Min. of Arrival	14	71%	64%	57%
Patients Who Left ER Before Being Seen	45,492	1%	2%	2%
Time from ER Arrival to Admit. (minutes)[2]	860	265	289	274
Time from ER Arrival to Discharge (minutes)	455	147	147	134
Time in ER Before Being Evaluated (minutes)	499	15	26	26
Time to Pain Meds for Fractures (minutes)	97	62	60	57
Heart Attack Care				
Aspirin Given at Discharge	255	100%	99%	99%
Fibrinolytic Meds Within 30 Min. of Arrival[7]	-	-	50%	54%
PCI Within 90 Minutes of Arrival	40	98%	96%	96%
Statin Prescribed at Discharge	225	100%	99%	98%
Heart Failure Care				
ACE Inhibitor or ARB for LVSD	113	100%	98%	97%
Discharge Instructions Given	350	96%	96%	94%
Evaluation of LVS Function	414	100%	100%	99%
Medicare Spending				
Medicare Spending per Patient (ratio)	-	1.02	1.04	0.98
Pneumonia Care				
Appropriate Initial Antibiotic Given	155	99%	98%	95%
Blood Culture Timing	193	98%	99%	98%
Pregnancy and Delivery Care				
Newborn Deliveries Scheduled Early[2]	34	0%	6%	6%
Preventive Care				
Immunization for Influenza[2]	570	98%	94%	90%
Immunization for Pneumonia[2]	777	99%	96%	92%
Stroke Care				
Anticoagulation Therapy for Atrial Fibrillation[2]	17	100%	97%	95%
Antithrombotic Therapy Timing[2]	102	96%	98%	98%
Assessed for Rehabilitation[2]	110	99%	97%	97%
Discharged on Antithrombotic Therapy[2]	103	98%	99%	99%
Discharged on Statin Medication[2]	74	99%	96%	94%
Thrombolytic Therapy Timing[1,2]	-	-	76%	66%
Venous Thromboembolism Prophylaxis[2]	115	100%	95%	94%
Written Stroke Educational Materials Given[2]	76	92%	94%	88%
Surgical Care Improvement Project				
Appropriate Beta Blocker Usage[2]	203	100%	99%	98%
Appropriate VTP Within 24 Hours[2]	351	99%	99%	98%
Controlled Postoperative Blood Glucose[2]	114	99%	98%	97%
Perioperative Temperature Management[2]	403	100%	100%	100%
Prophylactic Antibiotic Selection[2]	339	100%	99%	99%
Prophylactic Antibiotic Selection (Outpatient)	198	98%	98%	98%
Prophylactic Antibiotic Stopped[2]	323	99%	98%	98%
Prophylactic Antibiotic Timing[2]	340	99%	99%	99%
Prophylactic Antibiotic Timing (Outpatient)	198	100%	98%	98%
Urinary Catheter Removal[2]	276	100%	98%	97%
Survey of Patients' Hospital Experiences				
Area Around Room 'Always' Quiet at Night	300+	56%	58%	61%
Doctors 'Always' Communicated Well	300+	76%	77%	82%
Home Recovery Information Given	300+	84%	83%	85%
Hospital Given 9 or 10 on 10 Point Scale	300+	63%	67%	71%
Meds 'Always' Explained Before Given	300+	61%	60%	64%
Nurses 'Always' Communicated Well	300+	75%	75%	79%
Pain 'Always' Well Controlled	300+	67%	68%	71%
Room and Bathroom 'Always' Clean	300+	66%	69%	73%
Timely Help 'Always' Received	300+	60%	62%	68%
Would Definitely Recommend Hospital	300+	65%	69%	71%
Use of Medical Imaging				
Cardiac Imaging Stress Test before Surgery	59	5.1%	6.4%	5.3%
Combination Abdominal CT Scan	366	6.3%	11.8%	10.5%
Combination Brain/Sinus CT Scan	598	3.8%	3.4%	2.7%
Combination Chest CT Scan	181	1.1%	2.4%	2.7%
Follow-up Mammogram/Ultrasound	310	5.8%	10.2%	8.8%
Lumbar Spine MRI for Low Back Pain[1]	-	-	35.2%	37.2%

Doctors Hospital of Sarasota

5731 Bee Ridge Rd
Sarasota, FL 34233
Phone: 941-342-1100
Fax: 941-377-7127
URL: www.doctorsofsarasota.com
Type: Acute Care Hospitals
Ownership: Proprietary
Emergency Services: Yes
Beds: 168

Key Personnel:

Chief of Medical Staff. . . . . Michael Barron, MD
Anesthesiology. . . . . Christopher Brukoff, MD
Operating Room. . . . . Richard Golub, MD
CEO . . . . Robert Meade
CEO/President. . . . . Lindell F Orn

Measure	Cases	This Hosp.	State Avg.	U.S. Avg.
Blood Clot Prevention and Treatment				
Anticoagulation Overlap Therapy[2]	61	98%	93%	93%
ICU Venous Thromboembolism Prophylaxis[2]	75	100%	94%	92%
Incidence of Potentially Preventable VTE[1,2]	-	-	10%	10%
UFH with Dosages/Platelet Monitoring[2]	15	100%	100%	97%
Venous Thromboembolism Prophylaxis[2]	297	100%	88%	85%
Warfarin Therapy Discharge Instructions[2]	41	93%	85%	75%
Chest Pain/Possible Heart Attack Care				
Aspirin Given Within 24 Hours of Arrival[1,3]	-	-	98%	96%
Fibrinolytic Meds Within 30 Min. of Arrival[3,7]	-	-	81%	58%
Average Time to ECG (minutes)[1,3]	-	-	7	7
Average Time to Transfer (minutes)[3,7]	-	-	53	60
Children's Asthma Care				
Received Home Management Plan of Care	-	-	-	88%
Received Reliever Medication	-	-	-	100%
Received Systemic Corticosteroids	-	-	-	100%
Emergency Department				
Admittance Decision Time (minutes)[2]	757	56	111	98
Head CT Results Within 45 Min. of Arrival[1]	-	-	64%	57%
Patients Who Left ER Before Being Seen	23,085	0%	2%	2%
Time from ER Arrival to Admit. (minutes)[2]	757	201	289	274
Time from ER Arrival to Discharge (minutes)	416	122	147	134
Time in ER Before Being Evaluated (minutes)	441	14	26	26
Time to Pain Meds for Fractures (minutes)	67	40	60	57
Heart Attack Care				
Aspirin Given at Discharge	94	100%	99%	99%
Fibrinolytic Meds Within 30 Min. of Arrival[7]	-	-	50%	54%
PCI Within 90 Minutes of Arrival	27	96%	96%	96%
Statin Prescribed at Discharge	91	99%	99%	98%
Heart Failure Care				
ACE Inhibitor or ARB for LVSD	57	100%	98%	97%
Discharge Instructions Given	165	98%	96%	94%
Evaluation of LVS Function	235	100%	100%	99%
Medicare Spending				
Medicare Spending per Patient (ratio)	-	1.08	1.04	0.98
Pneumonia Care				
Appropriate Initial Antibiotic Given	104	98%	98%	95%
Blood Culture Timing	162	100%	99%	98%
Pregnancy and Delivery Care				
Newborn Deliveries Scheduled Early[2,7]	-	-	6%	6%
Preventive Care				
Immunization for Influenza[2]	602	100%	94%	90%
Immunization for Pneumonia[2]	1,018	99%	96%	92%
Stroke Care				
Anticoagulation Therapy for Atrial Fibrillation[2]	15	100%	97%	95%
Antithrombotic Therapy Timing[2]	63	100%	98%	98%
Assessed for Rehabilitation[2]	77	99%	97%	97%
Discharged on Antithrombotic Therapy[2]	71	100%	99%	99%
Discharged on Statin Medication[2]	58	100%	96%	94%
Thrombolytic Therapy Timing[1,2]	-	-	76%	66%
Venous Thromboembolism Prophylaxis[2]	75	97%	95%	94%
Written Stroke Educational Materials Given[2]	41	98%	94%	88%
Surgical Care Improvement Project				
Appropriate Beta Blocker Usage[2]	138	100%	99%	98%
Appropriate VTP Within 24 Hours[2]	399	99%	99%	98%
Controlled Postoperative Blood Glucose[2,7]	-	-	98%	97%
Perioperative Temperature Management[2]	466	100%	100%	100%
Prophylactic Antibiotic Selection[2]	276	100%	99%	99%
Prophylactic Antibiotic Selection (Outpatient)	350	99%	98%	98%
Prophylactic Antibiotic Stopped[2]	275	98%	98%	98%

NOTE: Hospital profiles are in alphabetical order by state, then city, then hospital within the city; Rankings exclude hospitals with less than 25 cases except for patient surveys which excludes hospitals with less than 100 cases; (a) 100-299 cases; (1) The number of cases/patients is too few to report; (2) Data submitted were based on a sample of cases/patients; (3) Results are based on a shorter time period than required; (4) Data suppressed by CMS for one or more quarters; (5) Results are not available for this reporting period; (6) Fewer than 100 patients completed the HCAHPS survey; (7) No cases met the criteria for this measure; (8) The lower limit of the confidence interval cannot be calculated if the number of observed infections equals zero; (9) No data are available from the state/territory for this reporting period; (10) The scores shown reflect fewer than 50 completed surveys; (11) There were discrepancies in the data collection process; (12) This measure does not apply to this hospital for this reporting period; (13) Results cannot be calculated for this reporting period; (14) The results for this state are combined with nearby states to protect confidentiality; Please refer to the User's Guide for a full explanation of data.

Measure	Cases	This Hosp.	State Avg.	U.S. Avg.
Prophylactic Antibiotic Timing[2]	277	100%	99%	99%
Prophylactic Antibiotic Timing (Outpatient)	350	100%	98%	98%
Urinary Catheter Removal[2]	281	99%	98%	97%
Survey of Patients' Hospital Experiences				
Area Around Room 'Always' Quiet at Night	300+	56%	58%	61%
Doctors 'Always' Communicated Well	300+	78%	77%	82%
Home Recovery Information Given	300+	87%	83%	85%
Hospital Given 9 or 10 on 10 Point Scale	300+	73%	67%	71%
Meds 'Always' Explained Before Given	300+	58%	60%	64%
Nurses 'Always' Communicated Well	300+	76%	75%	79%
Pain 'Always' Well Controlled	300+	67%	68%	71%
Room and Bathroom 'Always' Clean	300+	71%	69%	73%
Timely Help 'Always' Received	300+	59%	62%	68%
Would Definitely Recommend Hospital	300+	76%	69%	71%
Use of Medical Imaging				
Cardiac Imaging Stress Test before Surgery[1]	-	-	6.4%	5.3%
Combination Abdominal CT Scan	302	2.6%	11.8%	10.5%
Combination Brain/Sinus CT Scan[1]	-	-	3.4%	2.7%
Combination Chest CT Scan	73	1.4%	2.4%	2.7%
Follow-up Mammogram/Ultrasound	778	5.5%	10.2%	8.8%
Lumbar Spine MRI for Low Back Pain[1]	-	-	35.2%	37.2%

Sarasota Memorial Hospital

1700 S Tamiami Trl
Sarasota, FL 34239
Phone: 941-917-9000
Fax: 941-917-1930
E-mail: webcoordinator@smh.com
URL: www.smh.com
Type: Acute Care Hospitals
Emergency Services: Yes
Ownership: Govt - Hospital Dist/Auth
Beds: 845

Key Personnel:

Coronary Care . . . . Marie Barth
Operating Room. . . . . Bert A Bowers
Pediatric In-Patient Care . . . . Gerry Connors, RN
Infection Control. . . . . Susan Gray, RN
Radiology. . . . . Karen M Gross
Chair/CEO . . . . Marguerite G. Malone, Ed.D.
Chief of Medical Staff. . . . . R. Stephen Taylor, MD, MBA
CEO/President. . . . . David Verinder

Measure	Cases	This Hosp.	State Avg.	U.S. Avg.
Blood Clot Prevention and Treatment				
Anticoagulation Overlap Therapy[2]	126	99%	93%	93%
ICU Venous Thromboembolism Prophylaxis[2]	70	97%	94%	92%
Incidence of Potentially Preventable VTE[1,2]	-	-	10%	10%
UFH with Dosages/Platelet Monitoring[2]	41	100%	100%	97%
Venous Thromboembolism Prophylaxis[2]	334	89%	88%	85%
Warfarin Therapy Discharge Instructions[2]	95	100%	85%	75%
Chest Pain/Possible Heart Attack Care				
Aspirin Given Within 24 Hours of Arrival	16	94%	98%	96%
Fibrinolytic Meds Within 30 Min. of Arrival[3,7]	-	-	81%	58%
Average Time to ECG (minutes)	16	2	7	7
Average Time to Transfer (minutes)[3,7]	-	-	53	60
Children's Asthma Care				
Received Home Management Plan of Care	-	-	-	88%
Received Reliever Medication	-	-	-	100%
Received Systemic Corticosteroids	-	-	-	100%
Emergency Department				
Admittance Decision Time (minutes)[2]	449	117	111	98
Head CT Results Within 45 Min. of Arrival[1]	-	-	64%	57%
Patients Who Left ER Before Being Seen	>100k	1%	2%	2%
Time from ER Arrival to Admit. (minutes)[2]	453	317	289	274
Time from ER Arrival to Discharge (minutes)	396	165	147	134
Time in ER Before Being Evaluated (minutes)	430	40	26	26
Time to Pain Meds for Fractures (minutes)	184	80	60	57
Heart Attack Care				
Aspirin Given at Discharge	491	100%	99%	99%
Fibrinolytic Meds Within 30 Min. of Arrival[7]	-	-	50%	54%
PCI Within 90 Minutes of Arrival	63	87%	96%	96%
Statin Prescribed at Discharge	491	100%	99%	98%
Heart Failure Care				
ACE Inhibitor or ARB for LVSD[2]	108	97%	98%	97%
Discharge Instructions Given[2]	285	98%	96%	94%
Evaluation of LVS Function[2]	409	100%	100%	99%
Medicare Spending				
Medicare Spending per Patient (ratio)	-	1.09	1.04	0.98
Pneumonia Care				
Appropriate Initial Antibiotic Given[2]	100	99%	98%	95%
Blood Culture Timing[2]	165	96%	99%	98%
Pregnancy and Delivery Care				
Newborn Deliveries Scheduled Early[2]	48	8%	6%	6%
Preventive Care				
Immunization for Influenza[2]	559	95%	94%	90%
Immunization for Pneumonia[2]	752	95%	96%	92%
Stroke Care				
Anticoagulation Therapy for Atrial Fibrillation	51	100%	97%	95%
Antithrombotic Therapy Timing	212	100%	98%	98%
Assessed for Rehabilitation	298	95%	97%	97%
Discharged on Antithrombotic Therapy	256	100%	99%	99%
Discharged on Statin Medication	181	99%	96%	94%
Thrombolytic Therapy Timing	19	100%	76%	66%
Venous Thromboembolism Prophylaxis	278	97%	95%	94%
Written Stroke Educational Materials Given	126	94%	94%	88%
Surgical Care Improvement Project				
Appropriate Beta Blocker Usage[2]	306	97%	99%	98%
Appropriate VTP Within 24 Hours[2]	461	98%	99%	98%
Controlled Postoperative Blood Glucose[2]	178	97%	98%	97%
Perioperative Temperature Management[2]	644	100%	100%	100%
Prophylactic Antibiotic Selection[2]	567	100%	99%	99%
Prophylactic Antibiotic Selection (Outpatient)	881	98%	98%	98%
Prophylactic Antibiotic Stopped[2]	544	99%	98%	98%
Prophylactic Antibiotic Timing[2]	570	100%	99%	99%
Prophylactic Antibiotic Timing (Outpatient)	883	99%	98%	98%
Urinary Catheter Removal[2]	407	99%	98%	97%
Survey of Patients' Hospital Experiences				
Area Around Room 'Always' Quiet at Night	300+	56%	58%	61%
Doctors 'Always' Communicated Well	300+	82%	77%	82%
Home Recovery Information Given	300+	87%	83%	85%
Hospital Given 9 or 10 on 10 Point Scale	300+	76%	67%	71%
Meds 'Always' Explained Before Given	300+	66%	60%	64%
Nurses 'Always' Communicated Well	300+	81%	75%	79%
Pain 'Always' Well Controlled	300+	73%	68%	71%
Room and Bathroom 'Always' Clean	300+	71%	69%	73%
Timely Help 'Always' Received	300+	66%	62%	68%
Would Definitely Recommend Hospital	300+	83%	69%	71%
Use of Medical Imaging				
Cardiac Imaging Stress Test before Surgery	326	7.4%	6.4%	5.3%
Combination Abdominal CT Scan	2,760	14.2%	11.8%	10.5%
Combination Brain/Sinus CT Scan	3,137	3.8%	3.4%	2.7%
Combination Chest CT Scan	1,816	5.6%	2.4%	2.7%
Follow-up Mammogram/Ultrasound	8,687	5.2%	10.2%	8.8%
Lumbar Spine MRI for Low Back Pain	284	33.1%	35.2%	37.2%

Sebastian River Medical Center

13695 Us Hwy 1
Sebastian, FL 32978
Phone: 772-589-3187
Fax: 772-388-3689
E-mail: info@srmc.hma-corp.com
URL: www.srmcenter.com
Type: Acute Care Hospitals
Emergency Services: Yes
Ownership: Proprietary
Beds: 129

Key Personnel:

Quality Assurance . . . . Coleen Bailey
Radiology. . . . . Robert Bisset
Chief of Medical Staff. . . . . Ralph Geiger, MD
CEO/President. . . . . Emily Holliman
Operating Room. . . . . Hadi Shalhoub
Infection Control. . . . . Denise Stidham, RN

Measure	Cases	This Hosp.	State Avg.	U.S. Avg.
Blood Clot Prevention and Treatment				
Anticoagulation Overlap Therapy[2]	39	100%	93%	93%
ICU Venous Thromboembolism Prophylaxis[2]	20	100%	94%	92%
Incidence of Potentially Preventable VTE[1,2]	-	-	10%	10%
UFH with Dosages/Platelet Monitoring[2]	41	100%	100%	97%
Venous Thromboembolism Prophylaxis[2]	364	100%	88%	85%
Warfarin Therapy Discharge Instructions[2]	35	100%	85%	75%
Chest Pain/Possible Heart Attack Care				
Aspirin Given Within 24 Hours of Arrival[1,3]	-	-	98%	96%
Fibrinolytic Meds Within 30 Min. of Arrival[3,7]	-	-	81%	58%
Average Time to ECG (minutes)[1,3]	-	-	7	7
Average Time to Transfer (minutes)[3,7]	-	-	53	60
Children's Asthma Care				
Received Home Management Plan of Care	-	-	-	88%
Received Reliever Medication	-	-	-	100%
Received Systemic Corticosteroids	-	-	-	100%
Emergency Department				
Admittance Decision Time (minutes)[2]	647	97	111	98
Head CT Results Within 45 Min. of Arrival[1]	-	-	64%	57%
Patients Who Left ER Before Being Seen	19,243	1%	2%	2%
Time from ER Arrival to Admit. (minutes)[2]	650	248	289	274
Time from ER Arrival to Discharge (minutes)	367	114	147	134
Time in ER Before Being Evaluated (minutes)	405	36	26	26
Time to Pain Meds for Fractures (minutes)	92	48	60	57
Heart Attack Care				
Aspirin Given at Discharge	103	100%	99%	99%
Fibrinolytic Meds Within 30 Min. of Arrival[7]	-	-	50%	54%
PCI Within 90 Minutes of Arrival[1]	-	-	96%	96%
Statin Prescribed at Discharge	105	100%	99%	98%
Heart Failure Care				
ACE Inhibitor or ARB for LVSD	90	100%	98%	97%
Discharge Instructions Given	167	100%	96%	94%
Evaluation of LVS Function	188	100%	100%	99%
Medicare Spending				
Medicare Spending per Patient (ratio)	-	1.01	1.04	0.98
Pneumonia Care				
Appropriate Initial Antibiotic Given	144	100%	98%	95%
Blood Culture Timing	179	100%	99%	98%
Pregnancy and Delivery Care				
Newborn Deliveries Scheduled Early[7]	-	-	6%	6%
Preventive Care				
Immunization for Influenza[2]	470	100%	94%	90%
Immunization for Pneumonia[2]	700	100%	96%	92%
Stroke Care				
Anticoagulation Therapy for Atrial Fibrillation[1]	-	-	97%	95%
Antithrombotic Therapy Timing	62	100%	98%	98%
Assessed for Rehabilitation	66	100%	97%	97%
Discharged on Antithrombotic Therapy	61	100%	99%	99%
Discharged on Statin Medication	60	100%	96%	94%
Thrombolytic Therapy Timing[1]	-	-	76%	66%
Venous Thromboembolism Prophylaxis	68	100%	95%	94%
Written Stroke Educational Materials Given	37	100%	94%	88%
Surgical Care Improvement Project				
Appropriate Beta Blocker Usage	178	100%	99%	98%
Appropriate VTP Within 24 Hours	415	100%	99%	98%
Controlled Postoperative Blood Glucose[7]	-	-	98%	97%
Perioperative Temperature Management	524	100%	100%	100%
Prophylactic Antibiotic Selection	279	100%	99%	99%
Prophylactic Antibiotic Selection (Outpatient)	138	100%	98%	98%
Prophylactic Antibiotic Stopped	279	100%	98%	98%
Prophylactic Antibiotic Timing	280	100%	99%	99%
Prophylactic Antibiotic Timing (Outpatient)	138	100%	98%	98%
Urinary Catheter Removal	381	100%	98%	97%
Survey of Patients' Hospital Experiences				
Area Around Room 'Always' Quiet at Night	300+	55%	58%	61%
Doctors 'Always' Communicated Well	300+	78%	77%	82%
Home Recovery Information Given	300+	78%	83%	85%
Hospital Given 9 or 10 on 10 Point Scale	300+	58%	67%	71%
Meds 'Always' Explained Before Given	300+	54%	60%	64%
Nurses 'Always' Communicated Well	300+	68%	75%	79%
Pain 'Always' Well Controlled	300+	64%	68%	71%
Room and Bathroom 'Always' Clean	300+	66%	69%	73%
Timely Help 'Always' Received	300+	55%	62%	68%
Would Definitely Recommend Hospital	300+	64%	69%	71%
Use of Medical Imaging				
Cardiac Imaging Stress Test before Surgery	100	8.0%	6.4%	5.3%
Combination Abdominal CT Scan	663	36.2%	11.8%	10.5%
Combination Brain/Sinus CT Scan	601	3.8%	3.4%	2.7%
Combination Chest CT Scan	491	2.9%	2.4%	2.7%
Follow-up Mammogram/Ultrasound	988	17.9%	10.2%	8.8%
Lumbar Spine MRI for Low Back Pain	76	26.3%	35.2%	37.2%

NOTE: Hospital profiles are in alphabetical order by state, then city, then hospital within the city; Rankings exclude hospitals with less than 25 cases except for patient surveys which excludes hospitals with less than 100 cases; (a) 100-299 cases; (1) The number of cases/patients is too few to report; (2) Data submitted were based on a sample of cases/patients; (3) Results are based on a shorter time period than required; (4) Data suppressed by CMS for one or more quarters; (5) Results are not available for this reporting period; (6) Fewer than 100 patients completed the HCAHPS survey; (7) No cases met the criteria for this measure; (8) The lower limit of the confidence interval cannot be calculated if the number of observed infections equals zero; (9) No data are available from the state/territory for this reporting period; (10) The scores shown reflect fewer than 50 completed surveys; (11) There were discrepancies in the data collection process; (12) This measure does not apply to this hospital for this reporting period; (13) Results cannot be calculated for this reporting period; (14) The results for this state are combined with nearby states to protect confidentiality; Please refer to the User's Guide for a full explanation of data.

Florida Hospital Heartland Medical Center

4200 Sun N' Lake Blvd Phone: 863-314-4466
Sebring, FL 33871 Fax: 863-402-3415
URL: www.fhhd.org
Type: Acute Care Hospitals Emergency Services: Yes
Ownership: Voluntary non-profit - Church Beds: 111

Key Personnel:
Radiology.................... James B Ball
Chief of Medical Staff.......... Hanford G Brace
Emergency Room .... William Crankshaw
CEO/President............... John Harding
Hemotology Center .... A I Shah

Measure	Cases	This Hosp.	State Avg.	U.S. Avg.
Blood Clot Prevention and Treatment				
Anticoagulation Overlap Therapy[2]	69	99%	93%	93%
ICU Venous Thromboembolism Prophylaxis[2]	147	90%	94%	92%
Incidence of Potentially Preventable VTE[1,2]	-	-	10%	10%
UFH with Dosages/Platelet Monitoring[2]	37	100%	100%	97%
Venous Thromboembolism Prophylaxis[2]	511	89%	88%	85%
Warfarin Therapy Discharge Instructions[2]	42	88%	85%	75%
Chest Pain/Possible Heart Attack Care				
Aspirin Given Within 24 Hours of Arrival[1,3]	-	-	98%	96%
Fibrinolytic Meds Within 30 Min. of Arrival[3,7]	-	-	81%	58%
Average Time to ECG (minutes)[1,3]	-	-	7	7
Average Time to Transfer (minutes)[1,3]	-	-	53	60
Children's Asthma Care				
Received Home Management Plan of Care	-	-	-	88%
Received Reliever Medication	-	-	-	100%
Received Systemic Corticosteroids	-	-	-	100%
Emergency Department				
Admittance Decision Time (minutes)[2]	1,142	107	111	98
Head CT Results Within 45 Min. of Arrival	16	44%	64%	57%
Patients Who Left ER Before Being Seen	27,389	2%	2%	2%
Time from ER Arrival to Admit. (minutes)[2]	1,241	276	289	274
Time from ER Arrival to Discharge (minutes)	776	145	147	134
Time in ER Before Being Evaluated (minutes)	821	34	26	26
Time to Pain Meds for Fractures (minutes)	189	68	60	57
Heart Attack Care				
Aspirin Given at Discharge	277	100%	99%	99%
Fibrinolytic Meds Within 30 Min. of Arrival[7]	-	-	50%	54%
PCI Within 90 Minutes of Arrival	38	95%	96%	96%
Statin Prescribed at Discharge	274	98%	99%	98%
Heart Failure Care				
ACE Inhibitor or ARB for LVSD	127	100%	98%	97%
Discharge Instructions Given	326	95%	96%	94%
Evaluation of LVS Function	400	99%	100%	99%
Medicare Spending				
Medicare Spending per Patient (ratio)	-	1.04	1.04	0.98
Pneumonia Care				
Appropriate Initial Antibiotic Given	135	99%	98%	95%
Blood Culture Timing	282	98%	99%	98%
Pregnancy and Delivery Care				
Newborn Deliveries Scheduled Early[2]	38	5%	6%	6%
Preventive Care				
Immunization for Influenza[2]	886	90%	94%	90%
Immunization for Pneumonia[2]	1,409	94%	96%	92%
Stroke Care				
Anticoagulation Therapy for Atrial Fibrillation	13	92%	97%	95%
Antithrombotic Therapy Timing	97	100%	98%	98%
Assessed for Rehabilitation	127	99%	97%	97%
Discharged on Antithrombotic Therapy	118	99%	99%	99%
Discharged on Statin Medication	96	99%	96%	94%
Thrombolytic Therapy Timing	13	100%	76%	66%
Venous Thromboembolism Prophylaxis	123	96%	95%	94%
Written Stroke Educational Materials Given	83	98%	94%	88%
Surgical Care Improvement Project				
Appropriate Beta Blocker Usage	196	99%	99%	98%
Appropriate VTP Within 24 Hours	424	99%	99%	98%
Controlled Postoperative Blood Glucose[7]	-	-	98%	97%
Perioperative Temperature Management	500	100%	100%	100%
Prophylactic Antibiotic Selection	306	99%	99%	99%
Prophylactic Antibiotic Selection (Outpatient)	102	97%	98%	98%
Prophylactic Antibiotic Stopped	302	97%	98%	98%
Prophylactic Antibiotic Timing	307	98%	99%	99%
Prophylactic Antibiotic Timing (Outpatient)	102	98%	98%	98%
Urinary Catheter Removal	354	99%	98%	97%
Survey of Patients' Hospital Experiences				
Area Around Room 'Always' Quiet at Night[11]	300+	60%	58%	61%
Doctors 'Always' Communicated Well[11]	300+	76%	77%	82%
Home Recovery Information Given[11]	300+	87%	83%	85%
Hospital Given 9 or 10 on 10 Point Scale[11]	300+	67%	67%	71%
Meds 'Always' Explained Before Given[11]	300+	60%	60%	64%
Nurses 'Always' Communicated Well[11]	300+	78%	75%	79%
Pain 'Always' Well Controlled[11]	300+	68%	68%	71%
Room and Bathroom 'Always' Clean[11]	300+	75%	69%	73%
Timely Help 'Always' Received[11]	300+	64%	62%	68%
Would Definitely Recommend Hospital[11]	300+	71%	69%	71%
Use of Medical Imaging				
Cardiac Imaging Stress Test before Surgery	591	4.6%	6.4%	5.3%
Combination Abdominal CT Scan	1,386	51.9%	11.8%	10.5%
Combination Brain/Sinus CT Scan	1,334	2.2%	3.4%	2.7%
Combination Chest CT Scan	844	0.6%	2.4%	2.7%
Follow-up Mammogram/Ultrasound	1,690	8.5%	10.2%	8.8%
Lumbar Spine MRI for Low Back Pain	180	34.4%	35.2%	37.2%

Highlands Regional Medical Center

3600 S Highlands Ave Phone: 863-385-6101
Sebring, FL 33870 Fax: 863-385-3489
URL: www.highlandsregional.com
Type: Acute Care Hospitals Emergency Services: Yes
Ownership: Proprietary Beds: 126

Key Personnel:
CEO .... Joseph Bernard
Chief of Medical Staff.......... P Chockalingam
Operating Room.............. Daphne DuVall, RN
CEO/President............... Robert G Mahaffey
Quality Assurance .... Denise Pietri
Emergency Room .... Dorothy Reed, RN

Measure	Cases	This Hosp.	State Avg.	U.S. Avg.
Blood Clot Prevention and Treatment				
Anticoagulation Overlap Therapy[2]	42	40%	93%	93%
ICU Venous Thromboembolism Prophylaxis[2]	117	93%	94%	92%
Incidence of Potentially Preventable VTE[1,2]	-	-	10%	10%
UFH with Dosages/Platelet Monitoring[2]	35	100%	100%	97%
Venous Thromboembolism Prophylaxis[2]	300	84%	88%	85%
Warfarin Therapy Discharge Instructions[2]	27	100%	85%	75%
Chest Pain/Possible Heart Attack Care				
Aspirin Given Within 24 Hours of Arrival	16	100%	98%	96%
Fibrinolytic Meds Within 30 Min. of Arrival[7]	-	-	81%	58%
Average Time to ECG (minutes)	16	5	7	7
Average Time to Transfer (minutes)[1]	-	-	53	60
Children's Asthma Care				
Received Home Management Plan of Care	-	-	-	88%
Received Reliever Medication	-	-	-	100%
Received Systemic Corticosteroids	-	-	-	100%
Emergency Department				
Admittance Decision Time (minutes)[2]	649	91	111	98
Head CT Results Within 45 Min. of Arrival[1]	-	-	64%	57%
Patients Who Left ER Before Being Seen	18,960	1%	2%	2%
Time from ER Arrival to Admit. (minutes)[2]	649	233	289	274
Time from ER Arrival to Discharge (minutes)	413	132	147	134
Time in ER Before Being Evaluated (minutes)	433	15	26	26
Time to Pain Meds for Fractures (minutes)	58	46	60	57
Heart Attack Care				
Aspirin Given at Discharge	107	100%	99%	99%
Fibrinolytic Meds Within 30 Min. of Arrival[7]	-	-	50%	54%
PCI Within 90 Minutes of Arrival	43	95%	96%	96%
Statin Prescribed at Discharge	99	100%	99%	98%
Heart Failure Care				
ACE Inhibitor or ARB for LVSD	34	100%	98%	97%
Discharge Instructions Given	108	100%	96%	94%
Evaluation of LVS Function	136	100%	100%	99%
Medicare Spending				
Medicare Spending per Patient (ratio)	-	1.03	1.04	0.98
Pneumonia Care				
Appropriate Initial Antibiotic Given	71	99%	98%	95%
Blood Culture Timing	109	100%	99%	98%
Pregnancy and Delivery Care				
Newborn Deliveries Scheduled Early	25	4%	6%	6%
Preventive Care				
Immunization for Influenza[2]	437	100%	94%	90%
Immunization for Pneumonia[2]	571	100%	96%	92%
Stroke Care				
Anticoagulation Therapy for Atrial Fibrillation[1]	-	-	97%	95%
Antithrombotic Therapy Timing	30	100%	98%	98%
Assessed for Rehabilitation	28	89%	97%	97%
Discharged on Antithrombotic Therapy	27	96%	99%	99%
Discharged on Statin Medication	20	65%	96%	94%
Thrombolytic Therapy Timing[1]	-	-	76%	66%
Venous Thromboembolism Prophylaxis	30	87%	95%	94%
Written Stroke Educational Materials Given	16	100%	94%	88%
Surgical Care Improvement Project				
Appropriate Beta Blocker Usage[2]	67	100%	99%	98%
Appropriate VTP Within 24 Hours[2]	153	100%	99%	98%
Controlled Postoperative Blood Glucose[2,7]	-	-	98%	97%
Perioperative Temperature Management[2]	188	100%	100%	100%
Prophylactic Antibiotic Selection[2]	107	100%	99%	99%
Prophylactic Antibiotic Selection (Outpatient)	138	96%	98%	98%
Prophylactic Antibiotic Stopped[2]	97	99%	98%	98%
Prophylactic Antibiotic Timing[2]	107	100%	99%	99%
Prophylactic Antibiotic Timing (Outpatient)	138	100%	98%	98%
Urinary Catheter Removal[2]	98	100%	98%	97%
Survey of Patients' Hospital Experiences				
Area Around Room 'Always' Quiet at Night	300+	48%	58%	61%
Doctors 'Always' Communicated Well	300+	73%	77%	82%
Home Recovery Information Given	300+	86%	83%	85%
Hospital Given 9 or 10 on 10 Point Scale	300+	54%	67%	71%
Meds 'Always' Explained Before Given	300+	52%	60%	64%
Nurses 'Always' Communicated Well	300+	69%	75%	79%
Pain 'Always' Well Controlled	300+	60%	68%	71%
Room and Bathroom 'Always' Clean	300+	67%	69%	73%
Timely Help 'Always' Received	300+	56%	62%	68%
Would Definitely Recommend Hospital	300+	57%	69%	71%
Use of Medical Imaging				
Cardiac Imaging Stress Test before Surgery[1]	-	-	6.4%	5.3%
Combination Abdominal CT Scan	632	14.7%	11.8%	10.5%
Combination Brain/Sinus CT Scan[1]	-	-	3.4%	2.7%
Combination Chest CT Scan	298	13.4%	2.4%	2.7%
Follow-up Mammogram/Ultrasound	97	19.6%	10.2%	8.8%
Lumbar Spine MRI for Low Back Pain[1]	-	-	35.2%	37.2%

Larkin Community Hospital

7031 Sw 62nd Ave Phone: 305-284-7500
South Miami, FL 33143 Fax: 305-284-7545
E-mail: sgonzalez@larkinhospital.com
URL: www.larkinhospital.com
Type: Acute Care Hospitals Emergency Services: Yes
Ownership: Proprietary Beds: 112

Key Personnel:
Quality Assurance .... Lourdes Arcos
Chief of Medical Staff.......... Gustavo Leon
Operating Room.............. Paulien Radix
Emergency Room .... Pauline Radix
Intensive Care Unit............ Pauline Radix
Patient Relations .... Carlota Solorzano
CEO .... Sandy Sosa-Guerrero
Infection Control.............. Marcia Trader

Measure	Cases	This Hosp.	State Avg.	U.S. Avg.
Blood Clot Prevention and Treatment				
Anticoagulation Overlap Therapy[2]	12	67%	93%	93%
ICU Venous Thromboembolism Prophylaxis[2]	48	96%	94%	92%
Incidence of Potentially Preventable VTE[1,2]	-	-	10%	10%
UFH with Dosages/Platelet Monitoring[1,2]	-	-	100%	97%
Venous Thromboembolism Prophylaxis[2]	229	82%	88%	85%
Warfarin Therapy Discharge Instructions[1,2]	-	-	85%	75%
Chest Pain/Possible Heart Attack Care				
Aspirin Given Within 24 Hours of Arrival[3,7]	-	-	98%	96%
Fibrinolytic Meds Within 30 Min. of Arrival[5]	-	-	81%	58%
Average Time to ECG (minutes)[3,7]	-	-	7	7
Average Time to Transfer (minutes)[5]	-	-	53	60
Children's Asthma Care				

NOTE: Hospital profiles are in alphabetical order by state, then city, then hospital within the city; Rankings exclude hospitals with less than 25 cases except for patient surveys which excludes hospitals with less than 100 cases; (a) 100-299 cases; (1) The number of cases/patients is too few to report; (2) Data submitted were based on a sample of cases/patients; (3) Results are based on a shorter time period than required; (4) Data suppressed by CMS for one or more quarters; (5) Results are not available for this reporting period; (6) Fewer than 100 patients completed the HCAHPS survey; (7) No cases met the criteria for this measure; (8) The lower limit of the confidence interval cannot be calculated if the number of observed infections equals zero; (9) No data are available from the state/territory for this reporting period; (10) The scores shown reflect fewer than 50 completed surveys; (11) There were discrepancies in the data collection process; (12) This measure does not apply to this hospital for this reporting period; (13) Results cannot be calculated for this reporting period; (14) The results for this state are combined with nearby states to protect confidentiality; Please refer to the User's Guide for a full explanation of data.

Measure	Cases	This Hosp.	State Avg.	U.S. Avg.
Received Home Management Plan of Care	-	-	-	88%
Received Reliever Medication	-	-	-	100%
Received Systemic Corticosteroids	-	-	-	100%
Emergency Department				
Admittance Decision Time (minutes)[2]	379	125	111	98
Head CT Results Within 45 Min. of Arrival[3,7]	-	-	64%	57%
Patients Who Left ER Before Being Seen	7,440	3%	2%	2%
Time from ER Arrival to Admit. (minutes)[2]	380	330	289	274
Time from ER Arrival to Discharge (minutes)	191	262	147	134
Time in ER Before Being Evaluated (minutes)	285	19	26	26
Time to Pain Meds for Fractures (minutes)	11	116	60	57
Heart Attack Care				
Aspirin Given at Discharge[1,3]	-	-	99%	99%
Fibrinolytic Meds Within 30 Min. of Arrival[3,7]	-	-	50%	54%
PCI Within 90 Minutes of Arrival[3,7]	-	-	96%	96%
Statin Prescribed at Discharge[1,3]	-	-	99%	98%
Heart Failure Care				
ACE Inhibitor or ARB for LVSD	27	85%	98%	97%
Discharge Instructions Given	31	100%	96%	94%
Evaluation of LVS Function	41	100%	100%	99%
Medicare Spending				
Medicare Spending per Patient (ratio)	-	1.06	1.04	0.98
Pneumonia Care				
Appropriate Initial Antibiotic Given	57	96%	98%	95%
Blood Culture Timing	99	99%	99%	98%
Pregnancy and Delivery Care				
Newborn Deliveries Scheduled Early[7]	-	-	6%	6%
Preventive Care				
Immunization for Influenza[2]	369	80%	94%	90%
Immunization for Pneumonia[2]	571	83%	96%	92%
Stroke Care				
Anticoagulation Therapy for Atrial Fibrillation[7]	-	-	97%	95%
Antithrombotic Therapy Timing	25	84%	98%	98%
Assessed for Rehabilitation	24	71%	97%	97%
Discharged on Antithrombotic Therapy	22	68%	99%	99%
Discharged on Statin Medication	16	62%	96%	94%
Thrombolytic Therapy Timing[1]	-	-	76%	66%
Venous Thromboembolism Prophylaxis	29	90%	95%	94%
Written Stroke Educational Materials Given	14	86%	94%	88%
Surgical Care Improvement Project				
Appropriate Beta Blocker Usage	15	93%	99%	98%
Appropriate VTP Within 24 Hours	33	85%	99%	98%
Controlled Postoperative Blood Glucose[7]	-	-	98%	97%
Perioperative Temperature Management	44	98%	100%	100%
Prophylactic Antibiotic Selection	20	100%	99%	99%
Prophylactic Antibiotic Selection (Outpatient)	12	92%	98%	98%
Prophylactic Antibiotic Stopped	20	100%	98%	98%
Prophylactic Antibiotic Timing	20	95%	99%	99%
Prophylactic Antibiotic Timing (Outpatient)	12	100%	98%	98%
Urinary Catheter Removal	11	82%	98%	97%
Survey of Patients' Hospital Experiences				
Area Around Room 'Always' Quiet at Night	(a)	56%	58%	61%
Doctors 'Always' Communicated Well	(a)	75%	77%	82%
Home Recovery Information Given	(a)	83%	83%	85%
Hospital Given 9 or 10 on 10 Point Scale	(a)	60%	67%	71%
Meds 'Always' Explained Before Given	(a)	66%	60%	64%
Nurses 'Always' Communicated Well	(a)	71%	75%	79%
Pain 'Always' Well Controlled	(a)	58%	68%	71%
Room and Bathroom 'Always' Clean	(a)	79%	69%	73%
Timely Help 'Always' Received	(a)	56%	62%	68%
Would Definitely Recommend Hospital	(a)	57%	69%	71%
Use of Medical Imaging				
Cardiac Imaging Stress Test before Surgery[7]	-	-	6.4%	5.3%
Combination Abdominal CT Scan	128	26.6%	11.8%	10.5%
Combination Brain/Sinus CT Scan[1]	-	-	3.4%	2.7%
Combination Chest CT Scan[1]	-	-	2.4%	2.7%
Follow-up Mammogram/Ultrasound[7]	-	-	10.2%	8.8%
Lumbar Spine MRI for Low Back Pain[1]	-	-	35.2%	37.2%

South Miami Hospital

6200 Sw 73rd St
South Miami, FL 33143
Phone: 786-662-4000
Fax: 305-662-2759
E-mail: corporatepr@baptisthealth.net
URL: www.baptisthealth.net
Type: Acute Care Hospitals
Emergency Services: Yes
Ownership: Voluntary non-profit - Private
Beds: 452

Key Personnel:

Infection Control. . . . . Vicki Heitzer
CEO/President. . . . . Brian E. Keeley
Chief of Medical Staff . . . . Juan Mella, MD
Radiology. . . . . Steven Olfzewski, MD
Quality Assurance . . . . Kathryn Townsend
Pediatric Ambulatory Care . . . . . . Ernesta Valdes, MD
Pediatric In-Patient Care . . . . Ernesta Valdes, MD
Operating Room. . . . . Denise Woods

Measure	Cases	This Hosp.	State Avg.	U.S. Avg.
Blood Clot Prevention and Treatment				
Anticoagulation Overlap Therapy[2]	63	100%	93%	93%
ICU Venous Thromboembolism Prophylaxis[2]	117	100%	94%	92%
Incidence of Potentially Preventable VTE[2]	24	0%	10%	10%
UFH with Dosages/Platelet Monitoring[2]	45	100%	100%	97%
Venous Thromboembolism Prophylaxis[2]	418	99%	88%	85%
Warfarin Therapy Discharge Instructions[2]	38	100%	85%	75%
Chest Pain/Possible Heart Attack Care				
Aspirin Given Within 24 Hours of Arrival[1,3]	-	-	98%	96%
Fibrinolytic Meds Within 30 Min. of Arrival[5]	-	-	81%	58%
Average Time to ECG (minutes)[1,3]	-	-	7	7
Average Time to Transfer (minutes)[5]	-	-	53	60
Children's Asthma Care				
Received Home Management Plan of Care	-	-	-	88%
Received Reliever Medication	-	-	-	100%
Received Systemic Corticosteroids	-	-	-	100%
Emergency Department				
Admittance Decision Time (minutes)[2]	525	116	111	98
Head CT Results Within 45 Min. of Arrival	11	73%	64%	57%
Patients Who Left ER Before Being Seen	30,826	1%	2%	2%
Time from ER Arrival to Admit. (minutes)[2]	529	367	289	274
Time from ER Arrival to Discharge (minutes)	381	261	147	134
Time in ER Before Being Evaluated (minutes)	435	55	26	26
Time to Pain Meds for Fractures (minutes)	40	75	60	57
Heart Attack Care				
Aspirin Given at Discharge	223	100%	99%	99%
Fibrinolytic Meds Within 30 Min. of Arrival[7]	-	-	50%	54%
PCI Within 90 Minutes of Arrival	36	97%	96%	96%
Statin Prescribed at Discharge	227	100%	99%	98%
Heart Failure Care				
ACE Inhibitor or ARB for LVSD	112	100%	98%	97%
Discharge Instructions Given	299	99%	96%	94%
Evaluation of LVS Function	358	100%	100%	99%
Medicare Spending				
Medicare Spending per Patient (ratio)	-	1.02	1.04	0.98
Pneumonia Care				
Appropriate Initial Antibiotic Given	88	100%	98%	95%
Blood Culture Timing	198	100%	99%	98%
Pregnancy and Delivery Care				
Newborn Deliveries Scheduled Early[2]	89	10%	6%	6%
Preventive Care				
Immunization for Influenza[2]	635	97%	94%	90%
Immunization for Pneumonia[2]	597	99%	96%	92%
Stroke Care				
Anticoagulation Therapy for Atrial Fibrillation	19	100%	97%	95%
Antithrombotic Therapy Timing	86	100%	98%	98%
Assessed for Rehabilitation	103	100%	97%	97%
Discharged on Antithrombotic Therapy	92	100%	99%	99%
Discharged on Statin Medication	68	100%	96%	94%
Thrombolytic Therapy Timing[1]	-	-	76%	66%
Venous Thromboembolism Prophylaxis	110	100%	95%	94%
Written Stroke Educational Materials Given	57	100%	94%	88%
Surgical Care Improvement Project				
Appropriate Beta Blocker Usage[2]	177	100%	99%	98%
Appropriate VTP Within 24 Hours[2]	360	100%	99%	98%
Controlled Postoperative Blood Glucose[2]	66	98%	98%	97%
Perioperative Temperature Management[2]	474	100%	100%	100%
Prophylactic Antibiotic Selection[2]	342	99%	99%	99%
Prophylactic Antibiotic Selection (Outpatient)	732	100%	98%	98%
Prophylactic Antibiotic Stopped[2]	321	100%	98%	98%
Prophylactic Antibiotic Timing[2]	344	100%	99%	99%
Prophylactic Antibiotic Timing (Outpatient)	733	100%	98%	98%
Urinary Catheter Removal[2]	232	100%	98%	97%
Survey of Patients' Hospital Experiences				
Area Around Room 'Always' Quiet at Night	300+	64%	58%	61%
Doctors 'Always' Communicated Well	300+	85%	77%	82%
Home Recovery Information Given	300+	83%	83%	85%
Hospital Given 9 or 10 on 10 Point Scale	300+	81%	67%	71%
Meds 'Always' Explained Before Given	300+	65%	60%	64%
Nurses 'Always' Communicated Well	300+	83%	75%	79%
Pain 'Always' Well Controlled	300+	74%	68%	71%
Room and Bathroom 'Always' Clean	300+	75%	69%	73%
Timely Help 'Always' Received	300+	66%	62%	68%
Would Definitely Recommend Hospital	300+	81%	69%	71%
Use of Medical Imaging				
Cardiac Imaging Stress Test before Surgery	140	3.6%	6.4%	5.3%
Combination Abdominal CT Scan	547	2.9%	11.8%	10.5%
Combination Brain/Sinus CT Scan	720	5.1%	3.4%	2.7%
Combination Chest CT Scan	437	0.7%	2.4%	2.7%
Follow-up Mammogram/Ultrasound	426	10.1%	10.2%	8.8%
Lumbar Spine MRI for Low Back Pain	74	40.5%	35.2%	37.2%

Shands Starke Regional Medical Center

922 E Call St
Starke, FL 32091
Phone: 904-368-2300
Fax: 904-368-2306
URL: www.shands.com
Type: Critical Access Hospitals
Emergency Services: Yes
Ownership: Proprietary
Beds: 49

Key Personnel:

CEO/President. . . . . Jeannie Baker
Chief of Medical Staff . . . . Carl Eison
Quality Assurance . . . . Martha Epps
Emergency Room . . . . Dann Mann
Operating Room. . . . . Lynda Pepe, RN

Measure	Cases	This Hosp.	State Avg.	U.S. Avg.
Blood Clot Prevention and Treatment				
Anticoagulation Overlap Therapy[1,2]	-	-	93%	93%
ICU Venous Thromboembolism Prophylaxis[2,7]	-	-	94%	92%
Incidence of Potentially Preventable VTE[2,7]	-	-	10%	10%
UFH with Dosages/Platelet Monitoring[1,2]	-	-	100%	97%
Venous Thromboembolism Prophylaxis[2]	233	100%	88%	85%
Warfarin Therapy Discharge Instructions[1,2]	-	-	85%	75%
Chest Pain/Possible Heart Attack Care				
Aspirin Given Within 24 Hours of Arrival	-	-	98%	96%
Fibrinolytic Meds Within 30 Min. of Arrival	-	-	81%	58%
Average Time to ECG (minutes)	-	-	7	7
Average Time to Transfer (minutes)	-	-	53	60
Children's Asthma Care				
Received Home Management Plan of Care	-	-	-	88%
Received Reliever Medication	-	-	-	100%
Received Systemic Corticosteroids	-	-	-	100%
Emergency Department				
Admittance Decision Time (minutes)[2]	797	71	111	98
Head CT Results Within 45 Min. of Arrival	-	-	64%	57%
Patients Who Left ER Before Being Seen	-	-	2%	2%
Time from ER Arrival to Admit. (minutes)[2]	797	246	289	274
Time from ER Arrival to Discharge (minutes)	-	-	147	134
Time in ER Before Being Evaluated (minutes)	-	-	26	26
Time to Pain Meds for Fractures (minutes)	-	-	60	57
Heart Attack Care				
Aspirin Given at Discharge[1]	-	-	99%	99%
Fibrinolytic Meds Within 30 Min. of Arrival[7]	-	-	50%	54%
PCI Within 90 Minutes of Arrival[7]	-	-	96%	96%
Statin Prescribed at Discharge[1]	-	-	99%	98%
Heart Failure Care				
ACE Inhibitor or ARB for LVSD	13	100%	98%	97%
Discharge Instructions Given	58	100%	96%	94%
Evaluation of LVS Function	69	99%	100%	99%
Medicare Spending				
Medicare Spending per Patient (ratio)	-	-	1.04	0.98

NOTE: Hospital profiles are in alphabetical order by state, then city, then hospital within the city; Rankings exclude hospitals with less than 25 cases except for patient surveys which excludes hospitals with less than 100 cases; (a) 100-299 cases; (1) The number of cases/patients is too few to report; (2) Data submitted were based on a sample of cases/patients; (3) Results are based on a shorter time period than required; (4) Data suppressed by CMS for one or more quarters; (5) Results are not available for this reporting period; (6) Fewer than 100 patients completed the HCAHPS survey; (7) No cases met the criteria for this measure; (8) The lower limit of the confidence interval cannot be calculated if the number of observed infections equals zero; (9) No data are available from the state/territory for this reporting period; (10) The scores shown reflect fewer than 50 completed surveys; (11) There were discrepancies in the data collection process; (12) This measure does not apply to this hospital for this reporting period; (13) Results cannot be calculated for this reporting period; (14) The results for this state are combined with nearby states to protect confidentiality; Please refer to the User's Guide for a full explanation of data.

Measure	Cases	This Hosp.	State Avg.	U.S. Avg.
Pneumonia Care				
Appropriate Initial Antibiotic Given	92	99%	98%	95%
Blood Culture Timing	101	100%	99%	98%
Pregnancy and Delivery Care				
Newborn Deliveries Scheduled Early[7]	-	-	6%	6%
Preventive Care				
Immunization for Influenza[2]	515	97%	94%	90%
Immunization for Pneumonia[2]	722	99%	96%	92%
Stroke Care				
Anticoagulation Therapy for Atrial Fibrillation[1]	-	-	97%	95%
Antithrombotic Therapy Timing[1]	-	-	98%	98%
Assessed for Rehabilitation[1]	-	-	97%	97%
Discharged on Antithrombotic Therapy[1]	-	-	99%	99%
Discharged on Statin Medication[1]	-	-	96%	94%
Thrombolytic Therapy Timing[7]	-	-	76%	66%
Venous Thromboembolism Prophylaxis[1]	-	-	95%	94%
Written Stroke Educational Materials Given[1]	-	-	94%	88%
Surgical Care Improvement Project				
Appropriate Beta Blocker Usage	11	100%	99%	98%
Appropriate VTP Within 24 Hours	14	100%	99%	98%
Controlled Postoperative Blood Glucose[7]	-	-	98%	97%
Perioperative Temperature Management	30	100%	100%	100%
Prophylactic Antibiotic Selection[1]	-	-	99%	99%
Prophylactic Antibiotic Selection (Outpatient)	-	-	98%	98%
Prophylactic Antibiotic Stopped[1]	-	-	98%	98%
Prophylactic Antibiotic Timing[1]	-	-	99%	99%
Prophylactic Antibiotic Timing (Outpatient)	-	-	98%	98%
Urinary Catheter Removal	24	100%	98%	97%
Survey of Patients' Hospital Experiences				
Area Around Room 'Always' Quiet at Night[5]	-	-	58%	61%
Doctors 'Always' Communicated Well[5]	-	-	77%	82%
Home Recovery Information Given[5]	-	-	83%	85%
Hospital Given 9 or 10 on 10 Point Scale[5]	-	-	67%	71%
Meds 'Always' Explained Before Given[5]	-	-	60%	64%
Nurses 'Always' Communicated Well[5]	-	-	75%	79%
Pain 'Always' Well Controlled[5]	-	-	68%	71%
Room and Bathroom 'Always' Clean[5]	-	-	69%	73%
Timely Help 'Always' Received[5]	-	-	62%	68%
Would Definitely Recommend Hospital[5]	-	-	69%	71%
Use of Medical Imaging				
Cardiac Imaging Stress Test before Surgery	-	-	6.4%	5.3%
Combination Abdominal CT Scan	-	-	11.8%	10.5%
Combination Brain/Sinus CT Scan	-	-	3.4%	2.7%
Combination Chest CT Scan	-	-	2.4%	2.7%
Follow-up Mammogram/Ultrasound	-	-	10.2%	8.8%
Lumbar Spine MRI for Low Back Pain	-	-	35.2%	37.2%

Martin Medical Center

200 Se Hospital Ave Phone: 772-287-5200
Stuart, FL 34995 Fax: 772-223-2801
URL: www.mmhs.com
Type: Acute Care Hospitals Emergency Services: Yes
Ownership: Voluntary non-profit - Private Beds: 244

Key Personnel:
Quality Assurance . . . . Christine Friedman
Chief of Medical Staff. . . . . Howard M Robbins, MD
CEO/President. . . . . Mark E Robitaille
Infection Control. . . . . Lynn Sullivan
Operating Room. . . . . Heather Wood
Radiology. . . . . Ralph Young

Measure	Cases	This Hosp.	State Avg.	U.S. Avg.
Blood Clot Prevention and Treatment				
Anticoagulation Overlap Therapy[2]	152	96%	93%	93%
ICU Venous Thromboembolism Prophylaxis[2]	60	95%	94%	92%
Incidence of Potentially Preventable VTE[2]	12	17%	10%	10%
UFH with Dosages/Platelet Monitoring[2]	72	96%	100%	97%
Venous Thromboembolism Prophylaxis[2]	348	84%	88%	85%
Warfarin Therapy Discharge Instructions[2]	112	87%	85%	75%
Chest Pain/Possible Heart Attack Care				
Aspirin Given Within 24 Hours of Arrival	38	95%	98%	96%
Fibrinolytic Meds Within 30 Min. of Arrival[3,7]	-	-	81%	58%
Average Time to ECG (minutes)	41	5	7	7
Average Time to Transfer (minutes)[3,7]	-	-	53	60
Children's Asthma Care				
Received Home Management Plan of Care	-	-	-	88%
Received Reliever Medication	-	-	-	100%
Received Systemic Corticosteroids	-	-	-	100%
Emergency Department				
Admittance Decision Time (minutes)[2]	532	176	111	98
Head CT Results Within 45 Min. of Arrival	13	62%	64%	57%
Patients Who Left ER Before Being Seen	83,241	1%	2%	2%
Time from ER Arrival to Admit. (minutes)[2]	534	360	289	274
Time from ER Arrival to Discharge (minutes)	380	138	147	134
Time in ER Before Being Evaluated (minutes)	399	19	26	26
Time to Pain Meds for Fractures (minutes)	183	73	60	57
Heart Attack Care				
Aspirin Given at Discharge[2]	256	100%	99%	99%
Fibrinolytic Meds Within 30 Min. of Arrival[2,7]	-	-	50%	54%
PCI Within 90 Minutes of Arrival[2]	41	93%	96%	96%
Statin Prescribed at Discharge[2]	250	100%	99%	98%
Heart Failure Care				
ACE Inhibitor or ARB for LVSD[2]	82	96%	98%	97%
Discharge Instructions Given[2]	232	93%	96%	94%
Evaluation of LVS Function[2]	282	100%	100%	99%
Medicare Spending				
Medicare Spending per Patient (ratio)	-	1.04	1.04	0.98
Pneumonia Care				
Appropriate Initial Antibiotic Given[2]	76	100%	98%	95%
Blood Culture Timing[2]	152	97%	99%	98%
Pregnancy and Delivery Care				
Newborn Deliveries Scheduled Early	138	6%	6%	6%
Preventive Care				
Immunization for Influenza[2]	554	97%	94%	90%
Immunization for Pneumonia[2]	747	98%	96%	92%
Stroke Care				
Anticoagulation Therapy for Atrial Fibrillation[2]	16	94%	97%	95%
Antithrombotic Therapy Timing[2]	84	99%	98%	98%
Assessed for Rehabilitation[2]	97	99%	97%	97%
Discharged on Antithrombotic Therapy[2]	92	99%	99%	99%
Discharged on Statin Medication[2]	65	95%	96%	94%
Thrombolytic Therapy Timing[1,2]	-	-	76%	66%
Venous Thromboembolism Prophylaxis[2]	95	99%	95%	94%
Written Stroke Educational Materials Given[2]	53	100%	94%	88%
Surgical Care Improvement Project				
Appropriate Beta Blocker Usage[2]	171	96%	99%	98%
Appropriate VTP Within 24 Hours[2]	387	97%	99%	98%
Controlled Postoperative Blood Glucose[2]	93	96%	98%	97%
Perioperative Temperature Management[2]	488	99%	100%	100%
Prophylactic Antibiotic Selection[2]	388	98%	99%	99%
Prophylactic Antibiotic Selection (Outpatient)	573	96%	98%	98%
Prophylactic Antibiotic Stopped[2]	370	97%	98%	98%
Prophylactic Antibiotic Timing[2]	391	97%	99%	99%
Prophylactic Antibiotic Timing (Outpatient)	575	99%	98%	98%
Urinary Catheter Removal[2]	277	94%	98%	97%
Survey of Patients' Hospital Experiences				
Area Around Room 'Always' Quiet at Night	300+	48%	58%	61%
Doctors 'Always' Communicated Well	300+	73%	77%	82%
Home Recovery Information Given	300+	84%	83%	85%
Hospital Given 9 or 10 on 10 Point Scale	300+	70%	67%	71%
Meds 'Always' Explained Before Given	300+	57%	60%	64%
Nurses 'Always' Communicated Well	300+	74%	75%	79%
Pain 'Always' Well Controlled	300+	68%	68%	71%
Room and Bathroom 'Always' Clean	300+	66%	69%	73%
Timely Help 'Always' Received	300+	61%	62%	68%
Would Definitely Recommend Hospital	300+	74%	69%	71%
Use of Medical Imaging				
Cardiac Imaging Stress Test before Surgery	304	9.2%	6.4%	5.3%
Combination Abdominal CT Scan	1,598	3.8%	11.8%	10.5%
Combination Brain/Sinus CT Scan	2,089	2.2%	3.4%	2.7%
Combination Chest CT Scan	914	2.2%	2.4%	2.7%
Follow-up Mammogram/Ultrasound	721	12.3%	10.2%	8.8%
Lumbar Spine MRI for Low Back Pain[1]	-	-	35.2%	37.2%

South Bay Hospital

4016 Sun City Center Blvd Phone: 813-634-3301
Sun City Center, FL 33573 Fax: 813-634-0466
URL: www.southbayhospital.com
Type: Acute Care Hospitals Emergency Services: Yes
Ownership: Proprietary Beds: 112

Key Personnel:
Radiology. . . . . Jose Arjona
Surgery . . . . Angelo Paola, MD
Chief of Medical Staff . . . . Shahul Riazudeen, MD
CEO . . . . Sharon Roush

Measure	Cases	This Hosp.	State Avg.	U.S. Avg.
Blood Clot Prevention and Treatment				
Anticoagulation Overlap Therapy[2]	73	99%	93%	93%
ICU Venous Thromboembolism Prophylaxis[2]	60	100%	94%	92%
Incidence of Potentially Preventable VTE[2]	12	0%	10%	10%
UFH with Dosages/Platelet Monitoring[2]	20	100%	100%	97%
Venous Thromboembolism Prophylaxis[2]	385	97%	88%	85%
Warfarin Therapy Discharge Instructions[2]	43	100%	85%	75%
Chest Pain/Possible Heart Attack Care				
Aspirin Given Within 24 Hours of Arrival	14	100%	98%	96%
Fibrinolytic Meds Within 30 Min. of Arrival[3,7]	-	-	81%	58%
Average Time to ECG (minutes)	15	7	7	7
Average Time to Transfer (minutes)[3,7]	-	-	53	60
Children's Asthma Care				
Received Home Management Plan of Care	-	-	-	88%
Received Reliever Medication	-	-	-	100%
Received Systemic Corticosteroids	-	-	-	100%
Emergency Department				
Admittance Decision Time (minutes)[2]	1,022	91	111	98
Head CT Results Within 45 Min. of Arrival	17	35%	64%	57%
Patients Who Left ER Before Being Seen	27,709	1%	2%	2%
Time from ER Arrival to Admit. (minutes)[2]	1,022	252	289	274
Time from ER Arrival to Discharge (minutes)	421	145	147	134
Time in ER Before Being Evaluated (minutes)	467	12	26	26
Time to Pain Meds for Fractures (minutes)	73	47	60	57
Heart Attack Care				
Aspirin Given at Discharge	24	100%	99%	99%
Fibrinolytic Meds Within 30 Min. of Arrival[7]	-	-	50%	54%
PCI Within 90 Minutes of Arrival[7]	-	-	96%	96%
Statin Prescribed at Discharge	28	100%	99%	98%
Heart Failure Care				
ACE Inhibitor or ARB for LVSD	84	100%	98%	97%
Discharge Instructions Given	203	100%	96%	94%
Evaluation of LVS Function	293	100%	100%	99%
Medicare Spending				
Medicare Spending per Patient (ratio)	-	1.09	1.04	0.98
Pneumonia Care				
Appropriate Initial Antibiotic Given	151	99%	98%	95%
Blood Culture Timing	243	100%	99%	98%
Pregnancy and Delivery Care				
Newborn Deliveries Scheduled Early[2,7]	-	-	6%	6%
Preventive Care				
Immunization for Influenza[2]	585	100%	94%	90%
Immunization for Pneumonia[2]	1,016	100%	96%	92%
Stroke Care				
Anticoagulation Therapy for Atrial Fibrillation[1,2]	-	-	97%	95%
Antithrombotic Therapy Timing[2]	84	100%	98%	98%
Assessed for Rehabilitation[2]	84	100%	97%	97%
Discharged on Antithrombotic Therapy[2]	79	100%	99%	99%
Discharged on Statin Medication[2]	55	100%	96%	94%
Thrombolytic Therapy Timing[1,2]	-	-	76%	66%
Venous Thromboembolism Prophylaxis[2]	92	100%	95%	94%
Written Stroke Educational Materials Given[2]	45	100%	94%	88%
Surgical Care Improvement Project				
Appropriate Beta Blocker Usage[2]	125	98%	99%	98%
Appropriate VTP Within 24 Hours[2]	304	100%	99%	98%
Controlled Postoperative Blood Glucose[2,7]	-	-	98%	97%
Perioperative Temperature Management[2]	344	100%	100%	100%
Prophylactic Antibiotic Selection[2]	193	100%	99%	99%
Prophylactic Antibiotic Selection (Outpatient)	78	97%	98%	98%
Prophylactic Antibiotic Stopped[2]	188	99%	98%	98%
Prophylactic Antibiotic Timing[2]	193	99%	99%	99%

NOTE: Hospital profiles are in alphabetical order by state, then city, then hospital within the city; Rankings exclude hospitals with less than 25 cases except for patient surveys which excludes hospitals with less than 100 cases; (a) 100-299 cases; (1) The number of cases/patients is too few to report; (2) Data submitted were based on a sample of cases/patients; (3) Results are based on a shorter time period than required; (4) Data suppressed by CMS for one or more quarters; (5) Results are not available for this reporting period; (6) Fewer than 100 patients completed the HCAHPS survey; (7) No cases met the criteria for this measure; (8) The lower limit of the confidence interval cannot be calculated if the number of observed infections equals zero; (9) No data are available from the state/territory for this reporting period; (10) The scores shown reflect fewer than 50 completed surveys; (11) There were discrepancies in the data collection process; (12) This measure does not apply to this hospital for this reporting period; (13) Results cannot be calculated for this reporting period; (14) The results for this state are combined with nearby states to protect confidentiality; Please refer to the User's Guide for a full explanation of data.

Measure	Cases	This Hosp.	State Avg.	U.S. Avg.
Prophylactic Antibiotic Timing (Outpatient)	78	99%	98%	98%
Urinary Catheter Removal[2]	273	100%	98%	97%
Survey of Patients' Hospital Experiences				
Area Around Room 'Always' Quiet at Night	300+	50%	58%	61%
Doctors 'Always' Communicated Well	300+	71%	77%	82%
Home Recovery Information Given	300+	81%	83%	85%
Hospital Given 9 or 10 on 10 Point Scale	300+	58%	67%	71%
Meds 'Always' Explained Before Given	300+	55%	60%	64%
Nurses 'Always' Communicated Well	300+	72%	75%	79%
Pain 'Always' Well Controlled	300+	63%	68%	71%
Room and Bathroom 'Always' Clean	300+	66%	69%	73%
Timely Help 'Always' Received	300+	59%	62%	68%
Would Definitely Recommend Hospital	300+	59%	69%	71%
Use of Medical Imaging				
Cardiac Imaging Stress Test before Surgery	62	4.8%	6.4%	5.3%
Combination Abdominal CT Scan	545	2.6%	11.8%	10.5%
Combination Brain/Sinus CT Scan	940	6.2%	3.4%	2.7%
Combination Chest CT Scan	252	0.4%	2.4%	2.7%
Follow-up Mammogram/Ultrasound	1,127	7.7%	10.2%	8.8%
Lumbar Spine MRI for Low Back Pain	44	40.9%	35.2%	37.2%

Capital Regional Medical Center

2626 Capital Medical Blvd
Tallahassee, FL 32308
Phone: 850-656-5000
Fax: 850-656-5198
URL: www.capitalregionalmedicalcenter.com
Type: Acute Care Hospitals
Emergency Services: Yes
Ownership: Proprietary
Beds: 198

Key Personnel:
Radiology. . . . . Gregory Albrigh, RT
CEO . . . . Brain T. Cook
Quality Assurance . . . . Linda Deeb
Infection Control. . . . . Carol Frank, RN
Cardiac Laboratory. . . . . Barry Hamp
Chief of Medical Staff . . . . John Thoebes, MD
Operating Room. . . . . Linda Thombs, RN
Emergency Room . . . . Susie West

Measure	Cases	This Hosp.	State Avg.	U.S. Avg.
Blood Clot Prevention and Treatment				
Anticoagulation Overlap Therapy[2]	75	100%	93%	93%
ICU Venous Thromboembolism Prophylaxis[2]	57	100%	94%	92%
Incidence of Potentially Preventable VTE[1,2]	-	-	10%	10%
UFH with Dosages/Platelet Monitoring[2]	62	100%	100%	97%
Venous Thromboembolism Prophylaxis[2]	422	98%	88%	85%
Warfarin Therapy Discharge Instructions[2]	53	100%	85%	75%
Chest Pain/Possible Heart Attack Care				
Aspirin Given Within 24 Hours of Arrival[1]	-	-	98%	96%
Fibrinolytic Meds Within 30 Min. of Arrival[7]	-	-	81%	58%
Average Time to ECG (minutes)[1]	-	-	7	7
Average Time to Transfer (minutes)[7]	-	-	53	60
Children's Asthma Care				
Received Home Management Plan of Care	-	-	-	88%
Received Reliever Medication	-	-	-	100%
Received Systemic Corticosteroids	-	-	-	100%
Emergency Department				
Admittance Decision Time (minutes)[2]	956	120	111	98
Head CT Results Within 45 Min. of Arrival[1]	-	-	64%	57%
Patients Who Left ER Before Being Seen	87,494	1%	2%	2%
Time from ER Arrival to Admit. (minutes)[2]	956	264	289	274
Time from ER Arrival to Discharge (minutes)	491	116	147	134
Time in ER Before Being Evaluated (minutes)	531	16	26	26
Time to Pain Meds for Fractures (minutes)	145	51	60	57
Heart Attack Care				
Aspirin Given at Discharge	187	100%	99%	99%
Fibrinolytic Meds Within 30 Min. of Arrival[7]	-	-	50%	54%
PCI Within 90 Minutes of Arrival	42	100%	96%	96%
Statin Prescribed at Discharge	179	99%	99%	98%
Heart Failure Care				
ACE Inhibitor or ARB for LVSD	163	100%	98%	97%
Discharge Instructions Given	362	100%	96%	94%
Evaluation of LVS Function	428	100%	100%	99%
Medicare Spending				
Medicare Spending per Patient (ratio)	-	1.08	1.04	0.98
Pneumonia Care				
Appropriate Initial Antibiotic Given	114	98%	98%	95%
Blood Culture Timing	198	100%	99%	98%
Pregnancy and Delivery Care				
Newborn Deliveries Scheduled Early[2]	30	0%	6%	6%
Preventive Care				
Immunization for Influenza[2]	611	99%	94%	90%
Immunization for Pneumonia[2]	751	99%	96%	92%
Stroke Care				
Anticoagulation Therapy for Atrial Fibrillation[2]	11	100%	97%	95%
Antithrombotic Therapy Timing[2]	125	100%	98%	98%
Assessed for Rehabilitation[2]	135	99%	97%	97%
Discharged on Antithrombotic Therapy[2]	127	100%	99%	99%
Discharged on Statin Medication[2]	101	100%	96%	94%
Thrombolytic Therapy Timing[1,2]	-	-	76%	66%
Venous Thromboembolism Prophylaxis[2]	135	99%	95%	94%
Written Stroke Educational Materials Given[2]	76	100%	94%	88%
Surgical Care Improvement Project				
Appropriate Beta Blocker Usage	98	100%	99%	98%
Appropriate VTP Within 24 Hours	458	99%	99%	98%
Controlled Postoperative Blood Glucose	46	93%	98%	97%
Perioperative Temperature Management	559	100%	100%	100%
Prophylactic Antibiotic Selection	372	100%	99%	99%
Prophylactic Antibiotic Selection (Outpatient)	320	99%	98%	98%
Prophylactic Antibiotic Stopped	362	100%	98%	98%
Prophylactic Antibiotic Timing	372	100%	99%	99%
Prophylactic Antibiotic Timing (Outpatient)	320	99%	98%	98%
Urinary Catheter Removal	346	100%	98%	97%
Survey of Patients' Hospital Experiences				
Area Around Room 'Always' Quiet at Night	300+	70%	58%	61%
Doctors 'Always' Communicated Well	300+	80%	77%	82%
Home Recovery Information Given	300+	84%	83%	85%
Hospital Given 9 or 10 on 10 Point Scale	300+	68%	67%	71%
Meds 'Always' Explained Before Given	300+	60%	60%	64%
Nurses 'Always' Communicated Well	300+	75%	75%	79%
Pain 'Always' Well Controlled	300+	67%	68%	71%
Room and Bathroom 'Always' Clean	300+	70%	69%	73%
Timely Help 'Always' Received	300+	59%	62%	68%
Would Definitely Recommend Hospital	300+	74%	69%	71%
Use of Medical Imaging				
Cardiac Imaging Stress Test before Surgery	186	3.2%	6.4%	5.3%
Combination Abdominal CT Scan	537	1.5%	11.8%	10.5%
Combination Brain/Sinus CT Scan	749	4.1%	3.4%	2.7%
Combination Chest CT Scan	128	0.0%	2.4%	2.7%
Follow-up Mammogram/Ultrasound	444	16.7%	10.2%	8.8%
Lumbar Spine MRI for Low Back Pain[1]	-	-	35.2%	37.2%

Tallahassee Memorial Hospital

1300 Miccosukee Rd
Tallahassee, FL 32308
Phone: 850-431-1155
Fax: 850-431-6489
URL: www.tmh.org
Type: Acute Care Hospitals
Emergency Services: Yes
Ownership: Voluntary non-profit - Private
Beds: 770

Key Personnel:
Radiology. . . . . Gregory R Albright, MD
Operating Room. . . . . Shelby L Blank
Quality Assurance . . . . Judy Davis
Infection Control. . . . . Martha DeCastro, RN
Pediatric Ambulatory Care . . . . . . David Guttman, MD
Cardiac Laboratory. . . . . Lisa Mullee
CEO/President. . . . . G Mark O'Bryant
Chief of Medical Staff . . . . Dean Watson, MD

Measure	Cases	This Hosp.	State Avg.	U.S. Avg.
Blood Clot Prevention and Treatment				
Anticoagulation Overlap Therapy[2]	83	82%	93%	93%
ICU Venous Thromboembolism Prophylaxis[2]	134	97%	94%	92%
Incidence of Potentially Preventable VTE[2]	11	0%	10%	10%
UFH with Dosages/Platelet Monitoring[2]	84	100%	100%	97%
Venous Thromboembolism Prophylaxis[2]	504	88%	88%	85%
Warfarin Therapy Discharge Instructions[2]	53	81%	85%	75%
Chest Pain/Possible Heart Attack Care				
Aspirin Given Within 24 Hours of Arrival[1,3]	-	-	98%	96%
Fibrinolytic Meds Within 30 Min. of Arrival[5]	-	-	81%	58%
Average Time to ECG (minutes)[1,3]	-	-	7	7
Average Time to Transfer (minutes)[5]	-	-	53	60
Children's Asthma Care				
Received Home Management Plan of Care	-	-	-	88%
Received Reliever Medication	-	-	-	100%
Received Systemic Corticosteroids	-	-	-	100%
Emergency Department				
Admittance Decision Time (minutes)[2]	460	113	111	98
Head CT Results Within 45 Min. of Arrival[1]	-	-	64%	57%
Patients Who Left ER Before Being Seen	74,082	6%	2%	2%
Time from ER Arrival to Admit. (minutes)[2]	490	386	289	274
Time from ER Arrival to Discharge (minutes)	327	241	147	134
Time in ER Before Being Evaluated (minutes)	324	70	26	26
Time to Pain Meds for Fractures (minutes)	197	74	60	57
Heart Attack Care				
Aspirin Given at Discharge	457	100%	99%	99%
Fibrinolytic Meds Within 30 Min. of Arrival[7]	-	-	50%	54%
PCI Within 90 Minutes of Arrival	58	100%	96%	96%
Statin Prescribed at Discharge	446	99%	99%	98%
Heart Failure Care				
ACE Inhibitor or ARB for LVSD	253	98%	98%	97%
Discharge Instructions Given	493	92%	96%	94%
Evaluation of LVS Function	588	100%	100%	99%
Medicare Spending				
Medicare Spending per Patient (ratio)	-	1.05	1.04	0.98
Pneumonia Care				
Appropriate Initial Antibiotic Given	147	96%	98%	95%
Blood Culture Timing	196	97%	99%	98%
Pregnancy and Delivery Care				
Newborn Deliveries Scheduled Early[2]	227	7%	6%	6%
Preventive Care				
Immunization for Influenza[2]	491	97%	94%	90%
Immunization for Pneumonia[2]	539	92%	96%	92%
Stroke Care				
Anticoagulation Therapy for Atrial Fibrillation	33	97%	97%	95%
Antithrombotic Therapy Timing	251	100%	98%	98%
Assessed for Rehabilitation	299	100%	97%	97%
Discharged on Antithrombotic Therapy	241	100%	99%	99%
Discharged on Statin Medication	205	100%	96%	94%
Thrombolytic Therapy Timing	13	92%	76%	66%
Venous Thromboembolism Prophylaxis	343	100%	95%	94%
Written Stroke Educational Materials Given	162	98%	94%	88%
Surgical Care Improvement Project				
Appropriate Beta Blocker Usage[2]	527	100%	99%	98%
Appropriate VTP Within 24 Hours[2]	1,110	99%	99%	98%
Controlled Postoperative Blood Glucose[2]	315	99%	98%	97%
Perioperative Temperature Management[2]	1,355	100%	100%	100%
Prophylactic Antibiotic Selection[2]	1,189	100%	99%	99%
Prophylactic Antibiotic Selection (Outpatient)	1,211	99%	98%	98%
Prophylactic Antibiotic Stopped[2]	1,173	100%	98%	98%
Prophylactic Antibiotic Timing[2]	1,194	100%	99%	99%
Prophylactic Antibiotic Timing (Outpatient)	1,216	99%	98%	98%
Urinary Catheter Removal[2]	1,118	99%	98%	97%
Survey of Patients' Hospital Experiences				
Area Around Room 'Always' Quiet at Night	300+	58%	58%	61%
Doctors 'Always' Communicated Well	300+	81%	77%	82%
Home Recovery Information Given	300+	84%	83%	85%
Hospital Given 9 or 10 on 10 Point Scale	300+	67%	67%	71%
Meds 'Always' Explained Before Given	300+	66%	60%	64%
Nurses 'Always' Communicated Well	300+	76%	75%	79%
Pain 'Always' Well Controlled	300+	70%	68%	71%
Room and Bathroom 'Always' Clean	300+	75%	69%	73%
Timely Help 'Always' Received	300+	61%	62%	68%
Would Definitely Recommend Hospital	300+	74%	69%	71%
Use of Medical Imaging				
Cardiac Imaging Stress Test before Surgery	325	2.8%	6.4%	5.3%
Combination Abdominal CT Scan	503	2.8%	11.8%	10.5%
Combination Brain/Sinus CT Scan	904	2.5%	3.4%	2.7%
Combination Chest CT Scan	132	0.8%	2.4%	2.7%
Follow-up Mammogram/Ultrasound	161	14.9%	10.2%	8.8%
Lumbar Spine MRI for Low Back Pain[1]	-	-	35.2%	37.2%

NOTE: Hospital profiles are in alphabetical order by state, then city, then hospital within the city; Rankings exclude hospitals with less than 25 cases except for patient surveys which excludes hospitals with less than 100 cases; (a) 100-299 cases; (1) The number of cases/patients is too few to report; (2) Data submitted were based on a sample of cases/patients; (3) Results are based on a shorter time period than required; (4) Data suppressed by CMS for one or more quarters; (5) Results are not available for this reporting period; (6) Fewer than 100 patients completed the HCAHPS survey; (7) No cases met the criteria for this measure; (8) The lower limit of the confidence interval cannot be calculated if the number of observed infections equals zero; (9) No data are available from the state/territory for this reporting period; (10) The scores shown reflect fewer than 50 completed surveys; (11) There were discrepancies in the data collection process; (12) This measure does not apply to this hospital for this reporting period; (13) Results cannot be calculated for this reporting period; (14) The results for this state are combined with nearby states to protect confidentiality; Please refer to the User's Guide for a full explanation of data.

University Hospital & Medical Center

7201 N University Dr — Phone: 954-721-2200
Tamarac, FL 33321 — Fax: 954-724-6666
URL: www.uhmchealth.com
Type: Acute Care Hospitals — Emergency Services: Yes
Ownership: Proprietary — Beds: 317

Key Personnel:
Emergency Room . . . . Denise Eichenblat, RN
CEO/President. . . . . Michael G Joseph
Chief of Medical Staff . . . . Nichols Katz, MD
Radiology. . . . . Gaston Mendez, MD
Operating Room. . . . . Yvonne Slaughter, RN

Measure	Cases	This Hosp.	State Avg.	U.S. Avg.
Blood Clot Prevention and Treatment				
Anticoagulation Overlap Therapy[2]	34	97%	93%	93%
ICU Venous Thromboembolism Prophylaxis[2]	76	96%	94%	92%
Incidence of Potentially Preventable VTE[1,2]	-	-	10%	10%
UFH with Dosages/Platelet Monitoring[1,2]	-	-	100%	97%
Venous Thromboembolism Prophylaxis[2]	377	82%	88%	85%
Warfarin Therapy Discharge Instructions[2]	21	100%	85%	75%
Chest Pain/Possible Heart Attack Care				
Aspirin Given Within 24 Hours of Arrival	38	100%	98%	96%
Fibrinolytic Meds Within 30 Min. of Arrival[7]	-	-	81%	58%
Average Time to ECG (minutes)	39	21	7	7
Average Time to Transfer (minutes)	17	67	53	60
Children's Asthma Care				
Received Home Management Plan of Care	-	-	-	88%
Received Reliever Medication	-	-	-	100%
Received Systemic Corticosteroids	-	-	-	100%
Emergency Department				
Admittance Decision Time (minutes)[2]	964	96	111	98
Head CT Results Within 45 Min. of Arrival	11	73%	64%	57%
Patients Who Left ER Before Being Seen	33,142	1%	2%	2%
Time from ER Arrival to Admit. (minutes)[2]	964	228	289	274
Time from ER Arrival to Discharge (minutes)	383	129	147	134
Time in ER Before Being Evaluated (minutes)	476	11	26	26
Time to Pain Meds for Fractures (minutes)	129	50	60	57
Heart Attack Care				
Aspirin Given at Discharge	38	100%	99%	99%
Fibrinolytic Meds Within 30 Min. of Arrival[7]	-	-	50%	54%
PCI Within 90 Minutes of Arrival[7]	-	-	96%	96%
Statin Prescribed at Discharge	29	97%	99%	98%
Heart Failure Care				
ACE Inhibitor or ARB for LVSD	35	97%	98%	97%
Discharge Instructions Given	155	100%	96%	94%
Evaluation of LVS Function	198	100%	100%	99%
Medicare Spending				
Medicare Spending per Patient (ratio)	-	1.11	1.04	0.98
Pneumonia Care				
Appropriate Initial Antibiotic Given	76	99%	98%	95%
Blood Culture Timing	144	100%	99%	98%
Pregnancy and Delivery Care				
Newborn Deliveries Scheduled Early[2,7]	-	-	6%	6%
Preventive Care				
Immunization for Influenza[2]	616	98%	94%	90%
Immunization for Pneumonia[2]	932	99%	96%	92%
Stroke Care				
Anticoagulation Therapy for Atrial Fibrillation[1]	-	-	97%	95%
Antithrombotic Therapy Timing	64	100%	98%	98%
Assessed for Rehabilitation	68	97%	97%	97%
Discharged on Antithrombotic Therapy	63	100%	99%	99%
Discharged on Statin Medication	48	94%	96%	94%
Thrombolytic Therapy Timing[1]	-	-	76%	66%
Venous Thromboembolism Prophylaxis	77	92%	95%	94%
Written Stroke Educational Materials Given	33	100%	94%	88%
Surgical Care Improvement Project				
Appropriate Beta Blocker Usage[2]	112	97%	99%	98%
Appropriate VTP Within 24 Hours[2]	300	100%	99%	98%
Controlled Postoperative Blood Glucose[2,7]	-	-	98%	97%
Perioperative Temperature Management[2]	319	100%	100%	100%
Prophylactic Antibiotic Selection[2]	195	100%	99%	99%
Prophylactic Antibiotic Selection (Outpatient)	29	97%	98%	98%
Prophylactic Antibiotic Stopped[2]	192	99%	98%	98%
Prophylactic Antibiotic Timing[2]	195	100%	99%	99%
Prophylactic Antibiotic Timing (Outpatient)	29	100%	98%	98%
Urinary Catheter Removal[2]	240	100%	98%	97%
Survey of Patients' Hospital Experiences				
Area Around Room 'Always' Quiet at Night	300+	58%	58%	61%
Doctors 'Always' Communicated Well	300+	75%	77%	82%
Home Recovery Information Given	300+	80%	83%	85%
Hospital Given 9 or 10 on 10 Point Scale	300+	55%	67%	71%
Meds 'Always' Explained Before Given	300+	56%	60%	64%
Nurses 'Always' Communicated Well	300+	68%	75%	79%
Pain 'Always' Well Controlled	300+	63%	68%	71%
Room and Bathroom 'Always' Clean	300+	64%	69%	73%
Timely Help 'Always' Received	300+	54%	62%	68%
Would Definitely Recommend Hospital	300+	59%	69%	71%
Use of Medical Imaging				
Cardiac Imaging Stress Test before Surgery[1]	-	-	6.4%	5.3%
Combination Abdominal CT Scan	361	10.5%	11.8%	10.5%
Combination Brain/Sinus CT Scan	619	2.3%	3.4%	2.7%
Combination Chest CT Scan	242	3.7%	2.4%	2.7%
Follow-up Mammogram/Ultrasound	294	6.5%	10.2%	8.8%
Lumbar Spine MRI for Low Back Pain[1]	-	-	35.2%	37.2%

Florida Hospital Carrollwood

7171 North Dale Mabry — Phone: 813-932-2222
Tampa, FL 33614 — Fax: 813-558-8011
URL: www.uchcarrollwood.com
Type: Acute Care Hospitals — Emergency Services: Yes
Ownership: Voluntary non-profit - Church — Beds: 120

Key Personnel:
Chief of Medical Staff . . . . Scott Bronleewe
CEO/President. . . . . Donald Evans
Quality Assurance . . . . George Foley
Operating Room. . . . . Susan March, RN
Emergency Room . . . . Brenda McCartney

Measure	Cases	This Hosp.	State Avg.	U.S. Avg.
Blood Clot Prevention and Treatment				
Anticoagulation Overlap Therapy[2]	54	94%	93%	93%
ICU Venous Thromboembolism Prophylaxis[2]	37	97%	94%	92%
Incidence of Potentially Preventable VTE[2]	11	45%	10%	10%
UFH with Dosages/Platelet Monitoring[1,2]	-	-	100%	97%
Venous Thromboembolism Prophylaxis[2]	327	84%	88%	85%
Warfarin Therapy Discharge Instructions[2]	40	62%	85%	75%
Chest Pain/Possible Heart Attack Care				
Aspirin Given Within 24 Hours of Arrival	45	100%	98%	96%
Fibrinolytic Meds Within 30 Min. of Arrival[7]	-	-	81%	58%
Average Time to ECG (minutes)	46	5	7	7
Average Time to Transfer (minutes)[1]	-	-	53	60
Children's Asthma Care				
Received Home Management Plan of Care	-	-	-	88%
Received Reliever Medication	-	-	-	100%
Received Systemic Corticosteroids	-	-	-	100%
Emergency Department				
Admittance Decision Time (minutes)[2]	508	96	111	98
Head CT Results Within 45 Min. of Arrival[1]	-	-	64%	57%
Patients Who Left ER Before Being Seen	22,915	3%	2%	2%
Time from ER Arrival to Admit. (minutes)[2]	541	249	289	274
Time from ER Arrival to Discharge (minutes)	344	134	147	134
Time in ER Before Being Evaluated (minutes)	373	26	26	26
Time to Pain Meds for Fractures (minutes)	53	58	60	57
Heart Attack Care				
Aspirin Given at Discharge[1,2]	-	-	99%	99%
Fibrinolytic Meds Within 30 Min. of Arrival[2,7]	-	-	50%	54%
PCI Within 90 Minutes of Arrival[2,7]	-	-	96%	96%
Statin Prescribed at Discharge[1,2]	-	-	99%	98%
Heart Failure Care				
ACE Inhibitor or ARB for LVSD[2]	27	100%	98%	97%
Discharge Instructions Given[2]	75	84%	96%	94%
Evaluation of LVS Function[2]	89	100%	100%	99%
Medicare Spending				
Medicare Spending per Patient (ratio)	-	1.06	1.04	0.98
Pneumonia Care				
Appropriate Initial Antibiotic Given[2]	75	97%	98%	95%
Blood Culture Timing[2]	122	98%	99%	98%
Pregnancy and Delivery Care				
Newborn Deliveries Scheduled Early[2,7]	-	-	6%	6%
Preventive Care				
Immunization for Influenza[2]	481	95%	94%	90%
Immunization for Pneumonia[2]	584	94%	96%	92%
Stroke Care				
Anticoagulation Therapy for Atrial Fibrillation[1,2]	-	-	97%	95%
Antithrombotic Therapy Timing[2]	28	100%	98%	98%
Assessed for Rehabilitation[2]	29	97%	97%	97%
Discharged on Antithrombotic Therapy[2]	29	97%	99%	99%
Discharged on Statin Medication[2]	23	91%	96%	94%
Thrombolytic Therapy Timing[2,7]	-	-	76%	66%
Venous Thromboembolism Prophylaxis[2]	26	85%	95%	94%
Written Stroke Educational Materials Given[2]	20	75%	94%	88%
Surgical Care Improvement Project				
Appropriate Beta Blocker Usage[2]	88	93%	99%	98%
Appropriate VTP Within 24 Hours[2]	296	98%	99%	98%
Controlled Postoperative Blood Glucose[2,7]	-	-	98%	97%
Perioperative Temperature Management[2]	324	99%	100%	100%
Prophylactic Antibiotic Selection[2]	202	99%	99%	99%
Prophylactic Antibiotic Selection (Outpatient)	129	98%	98%	98%
Prophylactic Antibiotic Stopped[2]	191	99%	98%	98%
Prophylactic Antibiotic Timing[2]	203	99%	99%	99%
Prophylactic Antibiotic Timing (Outpatient)	130	96%	98%	98%
Urinary Catheter Removal[2]	280	99%	98%	97%
Survey of Patients' Hospital Experiences				
Area Around Room 'Always' Quiet at Night[11]	300+	61%	58%	61%
Doctors 'Always' Communicated Well[11]	300+	78%	77%	82%
Home Recovery Information Given[11]	300+	86%	83%	85%
Hospital Given 9 or 10 on 10 Point Scale[11]	300+	68%	67%	71%
Meds 'Always' Explained Before Given[11]	300+	63%	60%	64%
Nurses 'Always' Communicated Well[11]	300+	77%	75%	79%
Pain 'Always' Well Controlled[11]	300+	67%	68%	71%
Room and Bathroom 'Always' Clean[11]	300+	71%	69%	73%
Timely Help 'Always' Received[11]	300+	63%	62%	68%
Would Definitely Recommend Hospital[11]	300+	69%	69%	71%
Use of Medical Imaging				
Cardiac Imaging Stress Test before Surgery[1]	-	-	6.4%	5.3%
Combination Abdominal CT Scan	181	3.3%	11.8%	10.5%
Combination Brain/Sinus CT Scan[1]	-	-	3.4%	2.7%
Combination Chest CT Scan[1]	-	-	2.4%	2.7%
Follow-up Mammogram/Ultrasound[1]	-	-	10.2%	8.8%
Lumbar Spine MRI for Low Back Pain[1]	-	-	35.2%	37.2%

Florida Hospital Tampa

3100 E Fletcher Ave — Phone: 813-615-7200
Tampa, FL 33613 — Fax: 813-615-7313
URL: www.uch.org
Type: Acute Care Hospitals — Emergency Services: Yes
Ownership: Voluntary non-profit - Private — Beds: 2,247

Key Personnel:
CEO/President. . . . . Calvin Glidwell
Pediatric In-Patient Care . . . . Rosemary Jarvis, RN
Quality Assurance . . . . Barry Jeff
Chief of Medical Staff . . . . Kurt Stonesifer, MD
Radiology. . . . . Habib Tannir
Operating Room. . . . . Laura Tischler, RN
Infection Control. . . . . Jackie Whittaker

Measure	Cases	This Hosp.	State Avg.	U.S. Avg.
Blood Clot Prevention and Treatment				
Anticoagulation Overlap Therapy[2]	107	97%	93%	93%
ICU Venous Thromboembolism Prophylaxis[2]	66	98%	94%	92%
Incidence of Potentially Preventable VTE[2]	49	8%	10%	10%
UFH with Dosages/Platelet Monitoring[2]	42	100%	100%	97%
Venous Thromboembolism Prophylaxis[2]	333	86%	88%	85%
Warfarin Therapy Discharge Instructions[2]	70	87%	85%	75%
Chest Pain/Possible Heart Attack Care				
Aspirin Given Within 24 Hours of Arrival[1,3]	-	-	98%	96%
Fibrinolytic Meds Within 30 Min. of Arrival[5]	-	-	81%	58%
Average Time to ECG (minutes)[1,3]	-	-	7	7
Average Time to Transfer (minutes)[5]	-	-	53	60
Children's Asthma Care				
Received Home Management Plan of Care	-	-	-	88%
Received Reliever Medication	-	-	-	100%
Received Systemic Corticosteroids	-	-	-	100%

NOTE: Hospital profiles are in alphabetical order by state, then city, then hospital within the city; Rankings exclude hospitals with less than 25 cases except for patient surveys which excludes hospitals with less than 100 cases; (a) 100-299 cases; (1) The number of cases/patients is too few to report; (2) Data submitted were based on a sample of cases/patients; (3) Results are based on a shorter time period than required; (4) Data suppressed by CMS for one or more quarters; (5) Results are not available for this reporting period; (6) Fewer than 100 patients completed the HCAHPS survey; (7) No cases met the criteria for this measure; (8) The lower limit of the confidence interval cannot be calculated if the number of observed infections equals zero; (9) No data are available from the state/territory for this reporting period; (10) The scores shown reflect fewer than 50 completed surveys; (11) There were discrepancies in the data collection process; (12) This measure does not apply to this hospital for this reporting period; (13) Results cannot be calculated for this reporting period; (14) The results for this state are combined with nearby states to protect confidentiality; Please refer to the User's Guide for a full explanation of data.

Measure	Cases	This Hosp.	State Avg.	U.S. Avg.
Emergency Department				
Admittance Decision Time (minutes)[2]	624	128	111	98
Head CT Results Within 45 Min. of Arrival[1]	-	-	64%	57%
Patients Who Left ER Before Being Seen	51,700	6%	2%	2%
Time from ER Arrival to Admit. (minutes)[2]	626	316	289	274
Time from ER Arrival to Discharge (minutes)	326	174	147	134
Time in ER Before Being Evaluated (minutes)	362	48	26	26
Time to Pain Meds for Fractures (minutes)	132	70	60	57
Heart Attack Care				
Aspirin Given at Discharge	295	98%	99%	99%
Fibrinolytic Meds Within 30 Min. of Arrival[7]	-	-	50%	54%
PCI Within 90 Minutes of Arrival	78	99%	96%	96%
Statin Prescribed at Discharge	288	98%	99%	98%
Heart Failure Care				
ACE Inhibitor or ARB for LVSD	155	96%	98%	97%
Discharge Instructions Given	370	98%	96%	94%
Evaluation of LVS Function	464	99%	100%	99%
Medicare Spending				
Medicare Spending per Patient (ratio)	-	1.09	1.04	0.98
Pneumonia Care				
Appropriate Initial Antibiotic Given	199	95%	98%	95%
Blood Culture Timing	475	99%	99%	98%
Pregnancy and Delivery Care				
Newborn Deliveries Scheduled Early[2]	23	13%	6%	6%
Preventive Care				
Immunization for Influenza[2]	551	88%	94%	90%
Immunization for Pneumonia[2]	664	95%	96%	92%
Stroke Care				
Anticoagulation Therapy for Atrial Fibrillation	33	100%	97%	95%
Antithrombotic Therapy Timing	156	99%	98%	98%
Assessed for Rehabilitation	201	100%	97%	97%
Discharged on Antithrombotic Therapy	172	99%	99%	99%
Discharged on Statin Medication	132	92%	96%	94%
Thrombolytic Therapy Timing	11	91%	76%	66%
Venous Thromboembolism Prophylaxis	211	95%	95%	94%
Written Stroke Educational Materials Given	116	94%	94%	88%
Surgical Care Improvement Project				
Appropriate Beta Blocker Usage[2]	154	99%	99%	98%
Appropriate VTP Within 24 Hours[2]	252	93%	99%	98%
Controlled Postoperative Blood Glucose[2]	120	100%	98%	97%
Perioperative Temperature Management[2]	426	100%	100%	100%
Prophylactic Antibiotic Selection[2]	277	98%	99%	99%
Prophylactic Antibiotic Selection (Outpatient)	421	92%	98%	98%
Prophylactic Antibiotic Stopped[2]	273	98%	98%	98%
Prophylactic Antibiotic Timing[2]	279	100%	99%	99%
Prophylactic Antibiotic Timing (Outpatient)	423	99%	98%	98%
Urinary Catheter Removal[2]	264	97%	98%	97%
Survey of Patients' Hospital Experiences				
Area Around Room 'Always' Quiet at Night[11]	300+	57%	58%	61%
Doctors 'Always' Communicated Well[11]	300+	77%	77%	82%
Home Recovery Information Given[11]	300+	84%	83%	85%
Hospital Given 9 or 10 on 10 Point Scale[11]	300+	61%	67%	71%
Meds 'Always' Explained Before Given[11]	300+	59%	60%	64%
Nurses 'Always' Communicated Well[11]	300+	76%	75%	79%
Pain 'Always' Well Controlled[11]	300+	67%	68%	71%
Room and Bathroom 'Always' Clean[11]	300+	67%	69%	73%
Timely Help 'Always' Received[11]	300+	61%	62%	68%
Would Definitely Recommend Hospital[11]	300+	65%	69%	71%
Use of Medical Imaging				
Cardiac Imaging Stress Test before Surgery	146	3.4%	6.4%	5.3%
Combination Abdominal CT Scan	477	10.7%	11.8%	10.5%
Combination Brain/Sinus CT Scan	947	3.9%	3.4%	2.7%
Combination Chest CT Scan	200	15.5%	2.4%	2.7%
Follow-up Mammogram/Ultrasound	371	8.4%	10.2%	8.8%
Lumbar Spine MRI for Low Back Pain[1]	-	-	35.2%	37.2%

Memorial Hospital of Tampa

2901 Swann Ave
Tampa, FL 33609
Phone: 813-873-6400
Fax: 813-874-8685
E-mail: info@memorialhospitaltampa.com
URL: www.memorialhospitaltampa.com

Type: Acute Care Hospitals
Emergency Services: Yes
Ownership: Proprietary
Beds: 180

Key Personnel:

Operating Room. . . . . Susan Caldwell
Patient Relations . . . . Starlin Favors
Infection Control. . . . . Dennis Gonzales
Chief of Medical Staff . . . . James Hankerson
CEO . . . . John Mainieri
Emergency Room . . . . Sue Neil
Quality Assurance . . . . Linda Weisweaver

Measure	Cases	This Hosp.	State Avg.	U.S. Avg.
Blood Clot Prevention and Treatment				
Anticoagulation Overlap Therapy[2]	48	90%	93%	93%
ICU Venous Thromboembolism Prophylaxis[2]	77	82%	94%	92%
Incidence of Potentially Preventable VTE[1,2]	-	-	10%	10%
UFH with Dosages/Platelet Monitoring[1,2]	-	-	100%	97%
Venous Thromboembolism Prophylaxis[2]	398	76%	88%	85%
Warfarin Therapy Discharge Instructions[2]	32	97%	85%	75%
Chest Pain/Possible Heart Attack Care				
Aspirin Given Within 24 Hours of Arrival[1,3]	-	-	98%	96%
Fibrinolytic Meds Within 30 Min. of Arrival[3,7]	-	-	81%	58%
Average Time to ECG (minutes)[1,3]	-	-	7	7
Average Time to Transfer (minutes)[1,3]	-	-	53	60
Children's Asthma Care				
Received Home Management Plan of Care	-	-	-	88%
Received Reliever Medication	-	-	-	100%
Received Systemic Corticosteroids	-	-	-	100%
Emergency Department				
Admittance Decision Time (minutes)[2]	664	96	111	98
Head CT Results Within 45 Min. of Arrival[3,7]	-	-	64%	57%
Patients Who Left ER Before Being Seen	16,074	1%	2%	2%
Time from ER Arrival to Admit. (minutes)[2]	664	277	289	274
Time from ER Arrival to Discharge (minutes)	371	152	147	134
Time in ER Before Being Evaluated (minutes)	403	35	26	26
Time to Pain Meds for Fractures (minutes)	44	86	60	57
Heart Attack Care				
Aspirin Given at Discharge[1]	-	-	99%	99%
Fibrinolytic Meds Within 30 Min. of Arrival[7]	-	-	50%	54%
PCI Within 90 Minutes of Arrival[7]	-	-	96%	96%
Statin Prescribed at Discharge[1]	-	-	99%	98%
Heart Failure Care				
ACE Inhibitor or ARB for LVSD	30	100%	98%	97%
Discharge Instructions Given	79	67%	96%	94%
Evaluation of LVS Function	103	100%	100%	99%
Medicare Spending				
Medicare Spending per Patient (ratio)	-	1.04	1.04	0.98
Pneumonia Care				
Appropriate Initial Antibiotic Given	103	98%	98%	95%
Blood Culture Timing	130	98%	99%	98%
Pregnancy and Delivery Care				
Newborn Deliveries Scheduled Early[7]	-	-	6%	6%
Preventive Care				
Immunization for Influenza[2]	443	97%	94%	90%
Immunization for Pneumonia[2]	593	97%	96%	92%
Stroke Care				
Anticoagulation Therapy for Atrial Fibrillation[1]	-	-	97%	95%
Antithrombotic Therapy Timing	24	100%	98%	98%
Assessed for Rehabilitation	25	88%	97%	97%
Discharged on Antithrombotic Therapy	24	100%	99%	99%
Discharged on Statin Medication	21	86%	96%	94%
Thrombolytic Therapy Timing[1]	-	-	76%	66%
Venous Thromboembolism Prophylaxis	25	88%	95%	94%
Written Stroke Educational Materials Given	18	78%	94%	88%
Surgical Care Improvement Project				
Appropriate Beta Blocker Usage	78	97%	99%	98%
Appropriate VTP Within 24 Hours	196	97%	99%	98%
Controlled Postoperative Blood Glucose[7]	-	-	98%	97%
Perioperative Temperature Management	228	100%	100%	100%
Prophylactic Antibiotic Selection	139	96%	99%	99%
Prophylactic Antibiotic Selection (Outpatient)	20	85%	98%	98%
Prophylactic Antibiotic Stopped	130	99%	98%	98%
Prophylactic Antibiotic Timing	140	97%	99%	99%
Prophylactic Antibiotic Timing (Outpatient)	20	100%	98%	98%
Urinary Catheter Removal	145	98%	98%	97%
Survey of Patients' Hospital Experiences				
Area Around Room 'Always' Quiet at Night	300+	62%	58%	61%
Doctors 'Always' Communicated Well	300+	77%	77%	82%
Home Recovery Information Given	300+	80%	83%	85%
Hospital Given 9 or 10 on 10 Point Scale	300+	66%	67%	71%
Meds 'Always' Explained Before Given	300+	57%	60%	64%
Nurses 'Always' Communicated Well	300+	73%	75%	79%
Pain 'Always' Well Controlled	300+	66%	68%	71%
Room and Bathroom 'Always' Clean	300+	69%	69%	73%
Timely Help 'Always' Received	300+	59%	62%	68%
Would Definitely Recommend Hospital	300+	66%	69%	71%
Use of Medical Imaging				
Cardiac Imaging Stress Test before Surgery	96	5.2%	6.4%	5.3%
Combination Abdominal CT Scan	353	60.9%	11.8%	10.5%
Combination Brain/Sinus CT Scan	246	4.9%	3.4%	2.7%
Combination Chest CT Scan	199	29.6%	2.4%	2.7%
Follow-up Mammogram/Ultrasound	395	10.9%	10.2%	8.8%
Lumbar Spine MRI for Low Back Pain[1]	-	-	35.2%	37.2%

Saint Joseph's Hospital

3001 W Martin Luther King Jr Blvd
Tampa, FL 33677
Phone: 813-870-4398
Fax: 813-870-4639
URL: www.stjosephstampa.org

Type: Acute Care Hospitals
Emergency Services: Yes
Ownership: Voluntary non-profit - Church
Beds: 521

Key Personnel:

Operating Room. . . . . Dennis Anthony Alfonso
Radiology. . . . . David R Babin
CEO/President. . . . . Lorraine Lutton
Pediatric Ambulatory Care . . . . . . Ovidio Mendez
Pediatric In-Patient Care . . . . Ovidio Mendez
Infection Control. . . . . Cathy Ricchezza
Quality Assurance . . . . Glenn Simpson
Chief of Medical Staff . . . . Mark D Vaaler, MD

Measure	Cases	This Hosp.	State Avg.	U.S. Avg.
Blood Clot Prevention and Treatment				
Anticoagulation Overlap Therapy[2]	232	92%	93%	93%
ICU Venous Thromboembolism Prophylaxis[2]	94	99%	94%	92%
Incidence of Potentially Preventable VTE[2]	47	6%	10%	10%
UFH with Dosages/Platelet Monitoring[2]	62	100%	100%	97%
Venous Thromboembolism Prophylaxis[2]	311	91%	88%	85%
Warfarin Therapy Discharge Instructions[2]	185	85%	85%	75%
Chest Pain/Possible Heart Attack Care				
Aspirin Given Within 24 Hours of Arrival[1,3]	-	-	98%	96%
Fibrinolytic Meds Within 30 Min. of Arrival[5]	-	-	81%	58%
Average Time to ECG (minutes)[1,3]	-	-	7	7
Average Time to Transfer (minutes)[5]	-	-	53	60
Children's Asthma Care				
Received Home Management Plan of Care	-	-	-	88%
Received Reliever Medication	-	-	-	100%
Received Systemic Corticosteroids	-	-	-	100%
Emergency Department				
Admittance Decision Time (minutes)[2]	578	71	111	98
Head CT Results Within 45 Min. of Arrival[1]	-	-	64%	57%
Patients Who Left ER Before Being Seen	>100k	2%	2%	2%
Time from ER Arrival to Admit. (minutes)[2]	594	227	289	274
Time from ER Arrival to Discharge (minutes)	352	154	147	134
Time in ER Before Being Evaluated (minutes)	344	38	26	26
Time to Pain Meds for Fractures (minutes)	293	60	60	57
Heart Attack Care				
Aspirin Given at Discharge	583	99%	99%	99%
Fibrinolytic Meds Within 30 Min. of Arrival[7]	-	-	50%	54%
PCI Within 90 Minutes of Arrival	86	95%	96%	96%
Statin Prescribed at Discharge	577	99%	99%	98%
Heart Failure Care				
ACE Inhibitor or ARB for LVSD	303	100%	98%	97%
Discharge Instructions Given	608	99%	96%	94%
Evaluation of LVS Function	734	100%	100%	99%
Medicare Spending				

NOTE: Hospital profiles are in alphabetical order by state, then city, then hospital within the city; Rankings exclude hospitals with less than 25 cases except for patient surveys which excludes hospitals with less than 100 cases; (a) 100-299 cases; (1) The number of cases/patients is too few to report; (2) Data submitted were based on a sample of cases/patients; (3) Results are based on a shorter time period than required; (4) Data suppressed by CMS for one or more quarters; (5) Results are not available for this reporting period; (6) Fewer than 100 patients completed the HCAHPS survey; (7) No cases met the criteria for this measure; (8) The lower limit of the confidence interval cannot be calculated if the number of observed infections equals zero; (9) No data are available from the state/territory for this reporting period; (10) The scores shown reflect fewer than 50 completed surveys; (11) There were discrepancies in the data collection process; (12) This measure does not apply to this hospital for this reporting period; (13) Results cannot be calculated for this reporting period; (14) The results for this state are combined with nearby states to protect confidentiality; Please refer to the User's Guide for a full explanation of data.

Measure	Cases	This Hosp.	State Avg.	U.S. Avg.
Medicare Spending per Patient (ratio)	-	1.06	1.04	0.98
Pneumonia Care				
Appropriate Initial Antibiotic Given	349	98%	98%	95%
Blood Culture Timing	579	98%	99%	98%
Pregnancy and Delivery Care				
Newborn Deliveries Scheduled Early[2]	137	14%	6%	6%
Preventive Care				
Immunization for Influenza[2]	509	92%	94%	90%
Immunization for Pneumonia[2]	460	91%	96%	92%
Stroke Care				
Anticoagulation Therapy for Atrial Fibrillation	51	98%	97%	95%
Antithrombotic Therapy Timing	392	96%	98%	98%
Assessed for Rehabilitation	483	97%	97%	97%
Discharged on Antithrombotic Therapy	395	99%	99%	99%
Discharged on Statin Medication	319	94%	96%	94%
Thrombolytic Therapy Timing[1]	-	-	76%	66%
Venous Thromboembolism Prophylaxis	510	98%	95%	94%
Written Stroke Educational Materials Given	292	93%	94%	88%
Surgical Care Improvement Project				
Appropriate Beta Blocker Usage[2]	380	98%	99%	98%
Appropriate VTP Within 24 Hours[2]	799	99%	99%	98%
Controlled Postoperative Blood Glucose[2]	282	99%	98%	97%
Perioperative Temperature Management[2]	1,119	100%	100%	100%
Prophylactic Antibiotic Selection[2]	889	99%	99%	99%
Prophylactic Antibiotic Selection (Outpatient)	414	98%	98%	98%
Prophylactic Antibiotic Stopped[2]	853	98%	98%	98%
Prophylactic Antibiotic Timing[2]	893	99%	99%	99%
Prophylactic Antibiotic Timing (Outpatient)	417	98%	98%	98%
Urinary Catheter Removal[2]	805	100%	98%	97%
Survey of Patients' Hospital Experiences				
Area Around Room 'Always' Quiet at Night	300+	64%	58%	61%
Doctors 'Always' Communicated Well	300+	79%	77%	82%
Home Recovery Information Given	300+	85%	83%	85%
Hospital Given 9 or 10 on 10 Point Scale	300+	77%	67%	71%
Meds 'Always' Explained Before Given	300+	62%	60%	64%
Nurses 'Always' Communicated Well	300+	79%	75%	79%
Pain 'Always' Well Controlled	300+	71%	68%	71%
Room and Bathroom 'Always' Clean	300+	77%	69%	73%
Timely Help 'Always' Received	300+	64%	62%	68%
Would Definitely Recommend Hospital	300+	80%	69%	71%
Use of Medical Imaging				
Cardiac Imaging Stress Test before Surgery	456	7.2%	6.4%	5.3%
Combination Abdominal CT Scan	1,252	1.4%	11.8%	10.5%
Combination Brain/Sinus CT Scan	1,816	4.0%	3.4%	2.7%
Combination Chest CT Scan	205	1.5%	2.4%	2.7%
Follow-up Mammogram/Ultrasound	1,185	8.4%	10.2%	8.8%
Lumbar Spine MRI for Low Back Pain[1]	-	-	35.2%	37.2%

Tampa General Hospital

1 Tampa General Circle
Tampa, FL 33606
Phone: 813-844-7000
Fax: 813-844-4057
E-mail: jstone@tgh.org
URL: www.tgh.org
Type: Acute Care Hospitals
Emergency Services: Yes
Ownership: Voluntary non-profit - Private
Beds: 988

Key Personnel:

Pediatric Ambulatory Care . . . . . . John Curran, MD
Pediatric In-Patient Care . . . . John Curran, MD
Emergency Room . . . . James V Hillman
CEO/President. . . . . Ronald A Hytoff
Chief of Medical Staff. . . . . Devanand Mangar, MD
Radiology. . . . . Carlos Martinez
Infection Control. . . . . John Sinnott, MD
Quality Assurance . . . . Frank Testa

Measure	Cases	This Hosp.	State Avg.	U.S. Avg.
Blood Clot Prevention and Treatment				
Anticoagulation Overlap Therapy[2]	327	90%	93%	93%
ICU Venous Thromboembolism Prophylaxis[2]	116	86%	94%	92%
Incidence of Potentially Preventable VTE[2]	103	10%	10%	10%
UFH with Dosages/Platelet Monitoring[2]	257	98%	100%	97%
Venous Thromboembolism Prophylaxis[2]	311	75%	88%	85%
Warfarin Therapy Discharge Instructions[2]	241	53%	85%	75%
Chest Pain/Possible Heart Attack Care				
Aspirin Given Within 24 Hours of Arrival[5]	-	-	98%	96%
Fibrinolytic Meds Within 30 Min. of Arrival[5]	-	-	81%	58%
Average Time to ECG (minutes)[5]	-	-	7	7
Average Time to Transfer (minutes)[5]	-	-	53	60
Children's Asthma Care				
Received Home Management Plan of Care	-	-	-	88%
Received Reliever Medication	-	-	-	100%
Received Systemic Corticosteroids	-	-	-	100%
Emergency Department				
Admittance Decision Time (minutes)[2]	536	172	111	98
Head CT Results Within 45 Min. of Arrival[1]	-	-	64%	57%
Patients Who Left ER Before Being Seen	84,754	4%	2%	2%
Time from ER Arrival to Admit. (minutes)[2]	540	418	289	274
Time from ER Arrival to Discharge (minutes)	316	330	147	134
Time in ER Before Being Evaluated (minutes)	369	70	26	26
Time to Pain Meds for Fractures (minutes)	200	93	60	57
Heart Attack Care				
Aspirin Given at Discharge	295	97%	99%	99%
Fibrinolytic Meds Within 30 Min. of Arrival[7]	-	-	50%	54%
PCI Within 90 Minutes of Arrival	40	92%	96%	96%
Statin Prescribed at Discharge	290	92%	99%	98%
Heart Failure Care				
ACE Inhibitor or ARB for LVSD[2]	111	92%	98%	97%
Discharge Instructions Given[2]	227	96%	96%	94%
Evaluation of LVS Function[2]	257	99%	100%	99%
Medicare Spending				
Medicare Spending per Patient (ratio)	-	1.00	1.04	0.98
Pneumonia Care				
Appropriate Initial Antibiotic Given[2]	35	91%	98%	95%
Blood Culture Timing[2]	70	89%	99%	98%
Pregnancy and Delivery Care				
Newborn Deliveries Scheduled Early[2]	45	4%	6%	6%
Preventive Care				
Immunization for Influenza[2]	542	78%	94%	90%
Immunization for Pneumonia[2]	562	76%	96%	92%
Stroke Care				
Anticoagulation Therapy for Atrial Fibrillation[1,2]	-	-	97%	95%
Antithrombotic Therapy Timing[2]	57	98%	98%	98%
Assessed for Rehabilitation[2]	110	93%	97%	97%
Discharged on Antithrombotic Therapy[2]	64	95%	99%	99%
Discharged on Statin Medication[2]	46	89%	96%	94%
Thrombolytic Therapy Timing[1,2]	-	-	76%	66%
Venous Thromboembolism Prophylaxis[2]	108	89%	95%	94%
Written Stroke Educational Materials Given[2]	66	80%	94%	88%
Surgical Care Improvement Project				
Appropriate Beta Blocker Usage[2]	540	99%	99%	98%
Appropriate VTP Within 24 Hours[2]	926	98%	99%	98%
Controlled Postoperative Blood Glucose[2]	252	94%	98%	97%
Perioperative Temperature Management[2]	1,268	100%	100%	100%
Prophylactic Antibiotic Selection[2]	817	98%	99%	99%
Prophylactic Antibiotic Selection (Outpatient)	592	86%	98%	98%
Prophylactic Antibiotic Stopped[2]	786	97%	98%	98%
Prophylactic Antibiotic Timing[2]	822	96%	99%	99%
Prophylactic Antibiotic Timing (Outpatient)	598	94%	98%	98%
Urinary Catheter Removal[2]	866	98%	98%	97%
Survey of Patients' Hospital Experiences				
Area Around Room 'Always' Quiet at Night	300+	56%	58%	61%
Doctors 'Always' Communicated Well	300+	77%	77%	82%
Home Recovery Information Given	300+	85%	83%	85%
Hospital Given 9 or 10 on 10 Point Scale	300+	75%	67%	71%
Meds 'Always' Explained Before Given	300+	64%	60%	64%
Nurses 'Always' Communicated Well	300+	77%	75%	79%
Pain 'Always' Well Controlled	300+	69%	68%	71%
Room and Bathroom 'Always' Clean	300+	65%	69%	73%
Timely Help 'Always' Received	300+	64%	62%	68%
Would Definitely Recommend Hospital	300+	79%	69%	71%
Use of Medical Imaging				
Cardiac Imaging Stress Test before Surgery	475	6.9%	6.4%	5.3%
Combination Abdominal CT Scan	662	20.8%	11.8%	10.5%
Combination Brain/Sinus CT Scan	604	4.3%	3.4%	2.7%
Combination Chest CT Scan	305	1.3%	2.4%	2.7%
Follow-up Mammogram/Ultrasound	324	5.9%	10.2%	8.8%
Lumbar Spine MRI for Low Back Pain[1]	-	-	35.2%	37.2%

Tampa VA Medical Center

13000 Bruce B Downs Blvd.
Tampa, FL 33612
Phone: 813-972-2000
Fax: 813-978-5922
URL: www.tampa.va.gov
Type: Acute Care - VA
Emergency Services: No
Ownership: Government Federal
Beds: 581

Key Personnel:

Intensive Care Unit. . . . . Susan George, RN
Chief of Medical Staff. . . . . Willard Harris, MD
Operating Room. . . . . Sandra Jansen, RN
Emergency Room . . . . James V Snapp, MD
Infection Control. . . . . John Toney, MD
Radiology. . . . . Michael Vermes, MD
Quality Assurance . . . . Jan Webb

Measure	Cases	This Hosp.	State Avg.	U.S. Avg.
Blood Clot Prevention and Treatment				
Anticoagulation Overlap Therapy	-	-	93%	93%
ICU Venous Thromboembolism Prophylaxis	-	-	94%	92%
Incidence of Potentially Preventable VTE	-	-	10%	10%
UFH with Dosages/Platelet Monitoring	-	-	100%	97%
Venous Thromboembolism Prophylaxis	-	-	88%	85%
Warfarin Therapy Discharge Instructions	-	-	85%	75%
Chest Pain/Possible Heart Attack Care				
Aspirin Given Within 24 Hours of Arrival	-	-	98%	96%
Fibrinolytic Meds Within 30 Min. of Arrival	-	-	81%	58%
Average Time to ECG (minutes)	-	-	7	7
Average Time to Transfer (minutes)	-	-	53	60
Children's Asthma Care				
Received Home Management Plan of Care	-	-	-	88%
Received Reliever Medication	-	-	-	100%
Received Systemic Corticosteroids	-	-	-	100%
Emergency Department				
Admittance Decision Time (minutes)	-	-	111	98
Head CT Results Within 45 Min. of Arrival	-	-	64%	57%
Patients Who Left ER Before Being Seen	-	-	2%	2%
Time from ER Arrival to Admit. (minutes)	-	-	289	274
Time from ER Arrival to Discharge (minutes)	-	-	147	134
Time in ER Before Being Evaluated (minutes)	-	-	26	26
Time to Pain Meds for Fractures (minutes)	-	-	60	57
Heart Attack Care				
Aspirin Given at Discharge	146	99%	99%	99%
Fibrinolytic Meds Within 30 Min. of Arrival[5]	-	-	50%	54%
PCI Within 90 Minutes of Arrival[1]	-	-	96%	96%
Statin Prescribed at Discharge	138	97%	99%	98%
Heart Failure Care				
ACE Inhibitor or ARB for LVSD	162	96%	98%	97%
Discharge Instructions Given	328	94%	96%	94%
Evaluation of LVS Function	361	100%	100%	99%
Medicare Spending				
Medicare Spending per Patient (ratio)	-	-	1.04	0.98
Pneumonia Care				
Appropriate Initial Antibiotic Given	120	95%	98%	95%
Blood Culture Timing	242	99%	99%	98%
Pregnancy and Delivery Care				
Newborn Deliveries Scheduled Early	-	-	6%	6%
Preventive Care				
Immunization for Influenza[5]	-	-	94%	90%
Immunization for Pneumonia[5]	-	-	96%	92%
Stroke Care				
Anticoagulation Therapy for Atrial Fibrillation	-	-	97%	95%
Antithrombotic Therapy Timing	-	-	98%	98%
Assessed for Rehabilitation	-	-	97%	97%
Discharged on Antithrombotic Therapy	-	-	99%	99%
Discharged on Statin Medication	-	-	96%	94%
Thrombolytic Therapy Timing	-	-	76%	66%
Venous Thromboembolism Prophylaxis	-	-	95%	94%
Written Stroke Educational Materials Given	-	-	94%	88%
Surgical Care Improvement Project				
Appropriate Beta Blocker Usage[2]	188	97%	99%	98%
Appropriate VTP Within 24 Hours[2]	239	97%	99%	98%
Controlled Postoperative Blood Glucose[2]	76	95%	98%	97%
Perioperative Temperature Management[2]	312	96%	100%	100%
Prophylactic Antibiotic Selection	256	99%	99%	99%
Prophylactic Antibiotic Selection (Outpatient)	-	-	98%	98%

NOTE: Hospital profiles are in alphabetical order by state, then city, then hospital within the city; Rankings exclude hospitals with less than 25 cases except for patient surveys which excludes hospitals with less than 100 cases; (a) 100-299 cases; (1) The number of cases/patients is too few to report; (2) Data submitted were based on a sample of cases/patients; (3) Results are based on a shorter time period than required; (4) Data suppressed by CMS for one or more quarters; (5) Results are not available for this reporting period; (6) Fewer than 100 patients completed the HCAHPS survey; (7) No cases met the criteria for this measure; (8) The lower limit of the confidence interval cannot be calculated if the number of observed infections equals zero; (9) No data are available from the state/territory for this reporting period; (10) The scores shown reflect fewer than 50 completed surveys; (11) There were discrepancies in the data collection process; (12) This measure does not apply to this hospital for this reporting period; (13) Results cannot be calculated for this reporting period; (14) The results for this state are combined with nearby states to protect confidentiality; Please refer to the User's Guide for a full explanation of data.

Measure	Cases	This Hosp.	State Avg.	U.S. Avg.
Prophylactic Antibiotic Stopped	252	95%	98%	98%
Prophylactic Antibiotic Timing	258	97%	99%	99%
Prophylactic Antibiotic Timing (Outpatient)	-	-	98%	98%
Urinary Catheter Removal[2]	263	98%	98%	97%
Survey of Patients' Hospital Experiences				
Area Around Room 'Always' Quiet at Night	-	-	58%	61%
Doctors 'Always' Communicated Well	-	-	77%	82%
Home Recovery Information Given	-	-	83%	85%
Hospital Given 9 or 10 on 10 Point Scale	-	-	67%	71%
Meds 'Always' Explained Before Given	-	-	60%	64%
Nurses 'Always' Communicated Well	-	-	75%	79%
Pain 'Always' Well Controlled	-	-	68%	71%
Room and Bathroom 'Always' Clean	-	-	69%	73%
Timely Help 'Always' Received	-	-	62%	68%
Would Definitely Recommend Hospital	-	-	69%	71%
Use of Medical Imaging				
Cardiac Imaging Stress Test before Surgery	-	-	6.4%	5.3%
Combination Abdominal CT Scan	-	-	11.8%	10.5%
Combination Brain/Sinus CT Scan	-	-	3.4%	2.7%
Combination Chest CT Scan	-	-	2.4%	2.7%
Follow-up Mammogram/Ultrasound	-	-	10.2%	8.8%
Lumbar Spine MRI for Low Back Pain	-	-	35.2%	37.2%

Town & Country Hospital

6001 Webb Rd
Tampa, FL 33615
Phone: 813-882-7159
Fax: 813-887-5112
E-mail: townandcountry@iasishealthcare.com
URL: www.townandcountryhospital.com
Type: Acute Care Hospitals
Emergency Services: Yes
Ownership: Proprietary
Beds: 201

Key Personnel:
Cardiac Laboratory. . . . . William Capo
CEO . . . . Jake Fisher
Chief of Medical Staff. . . . . Patrick D Horan, MD
Radiology. . . . . David Jermain
Coronary Care. . . . . Wilma Marshall
Emergency Room . . . . Andrea Platt, MD
Quality Assurance . . . . Ciindy Price
Intensive Care Unit. . . . . Patty Wall

Measure	Cases	This Hosp.	State Avg.	U.S. Avg.
Blood Clot Prevention and Treatment				
Anticoagulation Overlap Therapy[2]	26	100%	93%	93%
ICU Venous Thromboembolism Prophylaxis[2]	52	88%	94%	92%
Incidence of Potentially Preventable VTE[1,2]	-	-	10%	10%
UFH with Dosages/Platelet Monitoring[2]	15	100%	100%	97%
Venous Thromboembolism Prophylaxis[2]	279	82%	88%	85%
Warfarin Therapy Discharge Instructions[2]	18	94%	85%	75%
Chest Pain/Possible Heart Attack Care				
Aspirin Given Within 24 Hours of Arrival[1,3]	-	-	98%	96%
Fibrinolytic Meds Within 30 Min. of Arrival[3,7]	-	-	81%	58%
Average Time to ECG (minutes)[1,3]	-	-	7	7
Average Time to Transfer (minutes)[3,7]	-	-	53	60
Children's Asthma Care				
Received Home Management Plan of Care	-	-	-	88%
Received Reliever Medication	-	-	-	100%
Received Systemic Corticosteroids	-	-	-	100%
Emergency Department				
Admittance Decision Time (minutes)[2]	395	81	111	98
Head CT Results Within 45 Min. of Arrival[1]	-	-	64%	57%
Patients Who Left ER Before Being Seen	22,411	2%	2%	2%
Time from ER Arrival to Admit. (minutes)[2]	429	302	289	274
Time from ER Arrival to Discharge (minutes)	1,091	131	147	134
Time in ER Before Being Evaluated (minutes)	1,151	26	26	26
Time to Pain Meds for Fractures (minutes)	56	46	60	57
Heart Attack Care				
Aspirin Given at Discharge	11	100%	99%	99%
Fibrinolytic Meds Within 30 Min. of Arrival[7]	-	-	50%	54%
PCI Within 90 Minutes of Arrival[7]	-	-	96%	96%
Statin Prescribed at Discharge[1]	-	-	99%	98%
Heart Failure Care				
ACE Inhibitor or ARB for LVSD	20	100%	98%	97%
Discharge Instructions Given	49	94%	96%	94%
Evaluation of LVS Function	60	100%	100%	99%
Medicare Spending				
Medicare Spending per Patient (ratio)	-	1.03	1.04	0.98
Pneumonia Care				
Appropriate Initial Antibiotic Given	47	98%	98%	95%
Blood Culture Timing	65	97%	99%	98%
Pregnancy and Delivery Care				
Newborn Deliveries Scheduled Early[7]	-	-	6%	6%
Preventive Care				
Immunization for Influenza[2]	353	97%	94%	90%
Immunization for Pneumonia[2]	432	97%	96%	92%
Stroke Care				
Anticoagulation Therapy for Atrial Fibrillation[1]	-	-	97%	95%
Antithrombotic Therapy Timing	19	95%	98%	98%
Assessed for Rehabilitation	17	100%	97%	97%
Discharged on Antithrombotic Therapy	16	100%	99%	99%
Discharged on Statin Medication	13	92%	96%	94%
Thrombolytic Therapy Timing[1]	-	-	76%	66%
Venous Thromboembolism Prophylaxis	19	89%	95%	94%
Written Stroke Educational Materials Given	14	100%	94%	88%
Surgical Care Improvement Project				
Appropriate Beta Blocker Usage	50	96%	99%	98%
Appropriate VTP Within 24 Hours	168	98%	99%	98%
Controlled Postoperative Blood Glucose[7]	-	-	98%	97%
Perioperative Temperature Management	204	100%	100%	100%
Prophylactic Antibiotic Selection	91	100%	99%	99%
Prophylactic Antibiotic Selection (Outpatient)	51	94%	98%	98%
Prophylactic Antibiotic Stopped	88	99%	98%	98%
Prophylactic Antibiotic Timing	91	100%	99%	99%
Prophylactic Antibiotic Timing (Outpatient)	52	92%	98%	98%
Urinary Catheter Removal	80	92%	98%	97%
Survey of Patients' Hospital Experiences				
Area Around Room 'Always' Quiet at Night	300+	65%	58%	61%
Doctors 'Always' Communicated Well	300+	80%	77%	82%
Home Recovery Information Given	300+	83%	83%	85%
Hospital Given 9 or 10 on 10 Point Scale	300+	63%	67%	71%
Meds 'Always' Explained Before Given	300+	60%	60%	64%
Nurses 'Always' Communicated Well	300+	74%	75%	79%
Pain 'Always' Well Controlled	300+	70%	68%	71%
Room and Bathroom 'Always' Clean	300+	68%	69%	73%
Timely Help 'Always' Received	300+	57%	62%	68%
Would Definitely Recommend Hospital	300+	63%	69%	71%
Use of Medical Imaging				
Cardiac Imaging Stress Test before Surgery	79	5.1%	6.4%	5.3%
Combination Abdominal CT Scan	239	13.8%	11.8%	10.5%
Combination Brain/Sinus CT Scan[1]	-	-	3.4%	2.7%
Combination Chest CT Scan	97	32.0%	2.4%	2.7%
Follow-up Mammogram/Ultrasound	248	7.7%	10.2%	8.8%
Lumbar Spine MRI for Low Back Pain[1]	-	-	35.2%	37.2%

Florida Hospital North Pinellas

1395 S Pinellas Ave
Tarpon Springs, FL 34689
Phone: 727-942-5000
Fax: 727-942-5161
E-mail: heinfo@mail.uch.org
URL: www.hemh.com
Type: Acute Care Hospitals
Emergency Services: Yes
Ownership: Voluntary non-profit - Other
Beds: 168

Key Personnel:
Radiology. . . . . Anjali Agrawal
Intensive Care Unit. . . . . Beth Carter
Chief of Medical Staff. . . . . John Dallman, MD
Infection Control. . . . . Paula Hartzel, RN
CEO/President. . . . . Steve MacLauchlan
Quality Assurance . . . . John McPherson
Operating Room. . . . . Lois Petrosky
Cardiac Laboratory. . . . . Cheryl Sotrop

Measure	Cases	This Hosp.	State Avg.	U.S. Avg.
Blood Clot Prevention and Treatment				
Anticoagulation Overlap Therapy[2]	28	100%	93%	93%
ICU Venous Thromboembolism Prophylaxis[2]	62	98%	94%	92%
Incidence of Potentially Preventable VTE[1,2]	-	-	10%	10%
UFH with Dosages/Platelet Monitoring[1,2]	-	-	100%	97%
Venous Thromboembolism Prophylaxis[2]	317	99%	88%	85%
Warfarin Therapy Discharge Instructions[2]	21	100%	85%	75%
Chest Pain/Possible Heart Attack Care				
Aspirin Given Within 24 Hours of Arrival[5]	-	-	98%	96%
Fibrinolytic Meds Within 30 Min. of Arrival[5]	-	-	81%	58%
Average Time to ECG (minutes)[5]	-	-	7	7
Average Time to Transfer (minutes)[5]	-	-	53	60
Children's Asthma Care				
Received Home Management Plan of Care	-	-	-	88%
Received Reliever Medication	-	-	-	100%
Received Systemic Corticosteroids	-	-	-	100%
Emergency Department				
Admittance Decision Time (minutes)[2]	585	56	111	98
Head CT Results Within 45 Min. of Arrival[1]	-	-	64%	57%
Patients Who Left ER Before Being Seen	19,378	1%	2%	2%
Time from ER Arrival to Admit. (minutes)[2]	585	175	289	274
Time from ER Arrival to Discharge (minutes)	381	115	147	134
Time in ER Before Being Evaluated (minutes)	430	19	26	26
Time to Pain Meds for Fractures (minutes)	75	43	60	57
Heart Attack Care				
Aspirin Given at Discharge	90	100%	99%	99%
Fibrinolytic Meds Within 30 Min. of Arrival[7]	-	-	50%	54%
PCI Within 90 Minutes of Arrival	28	100%	96%	96%
Statin Prescribed at Discharge	84	100%	99%	98%
Heart Failure Care				
ACE Inhibitor or ARB for LVSD	36	100%	98%	97%
Discharge Instructions Given	96	100%	96%	94%
Evaluation of LVS Function	127	100%	100%	99%
Medicare Spending				
Medicare Spending per Patient (ratio)	-	1.06	1.04	0.98
Pneumonia Care				
Appropriate Initial Antibiotic Given	84	100%	98%	95%
Blood Culture Timing	124	100%	99%	98%
Pregnancy and Delivery Care				
Newborn Deliveries Scheduled Early[2]	12	0%	6%	6%
Preventive Care				
Immunization for Influenza[2]	508	97%	94%	90%
Immunization for Pneumonia[2]	652	99%	96%	92%
Stroke Care				
Anticoagulation Therapy for Atrial Fibrillation[1,2]	-	-	97%	95%
Antithrombotic Therapy Timing[2]	31	100%	98%	98%
Assessed for Rehabilitation[2]	33	94%	97%	97%
Discharged on Antithrombotic Therapy[2]	32	97%	99%	99%
Discharged on Statin Medication[2]	25	100%	96%	94%
Thrombolytic Therapy Timing[1,2]	-	-	76%	66%
Venous Thromboembolism Prophylaxis[2]	38	100%	95%	94%
Written Stroke Educational Materials Given[2]	19	95%	94%	88%
Surgical Care Improvement Project				
Appropriate Beta Blocker Usage[2]	76	100%	99%	98%
Appropriate VTP Within 24 Hours[2]	218	100%	99%	98%
Controlled Postoperative Blood Glucose[2,7]	-	-	98%	97%
Perioperative Temperature Management[2]	250	100%	100%	100%
Prophylactic Antibiotic Selection[2]	162	98%	99%	99%
Prophylactic Antibiotic Selection (Outpatient)	76	99%	98%	98%
Prophylactic Antibiotic Stopped[2]	160	98%	98%	98%
Prophylactic Antibiotic Timing[2]	162	99%	99%	99%
Prophylactic Antibiotic Timing (Outpatient)	78	97%	98%	98%
Urinary Catheter Removal[2]	165	99%	98%	97%
Survey of Patients' Hospital Experiences				
Area Around Room 'Always' Quiet at Night[11]	300+	55%	58%	61%
Doctors 'Always' Communicated Well[11]	300+	79%	77%	82%
Home Recovery Information Given[11]	300+	82%	83%	85%
Hospital Given 9 or 10 on 10 Point Scale[11]	300+	69%	67%	71%
Meds 'Always' Explained Before Given[11]	300+	61%	60%	64%
Nurses 'Always' Communicated Well[11]	300+	78%	75%	79%
Pain 'Always' Well Controlled[11]	300+	68%	68%	71%
Room and Bathroom 'Always' Clean[11]	300+	75%	69%	73%
Timely Help 'Always' Received[11]	300+	63%	62%	68%
Would Definitely Recommend Hospital[11]	300+	70%	69%	71%
Use of Medical Imaging				
Cardiac Imaging Stress Test before Surgery[1]	-	-	6.4%	5.3%
Combination Abdominal CT Scan	253	15.0%	11.8%	10.5%
Combination Brain/Sinus CT Scan[1]	-	-	3.4%	2.7%
Combination Chest CT Scan	100	6.0%	2.4%	2.7%
Follow-up Mammogram/Ultrasound	303	10.9%	10.2%	8.8%
Lumbar Spine MRI for Low Back Pain[1]	-	-	35.2%	37.2%

NOTE: Hospital profiles are in alphabetical order by state, then city, then hospital within the city; Rankings exclude hospitals with less than 25 cases except for patient surveys which excludes hospitals with less than 100 cases; (a) 100-299 cases; (1) The number of cases/patients is too few to report; (2) Data submitted were based on a sample of cases/patients; (3) Results are based on a shorter time period than required; (4) Data suppressed by CMS for one or more quarters; (5) Results are not available for this reporting period; (6) Fewer than 100 patients completed the HCAHPS survey; (7) No cases met the criteria for this measure; (8) The lower limit of the confidence interval cannot be calculated if the number of observed infections equals zero; (9) No data are available from the state/territory for this reporting period; (10) The scores shown reflect fewer than 50 completed surveys; (11) There were discrepancies in the data collection process; (12) This measure does not apply to this hospital for this reporting period; (13) Results cannot be calculated for this reporting period; (14) The results for this state are combined with nearby states to protect confidentiality; Please refer to the User's Guide for a full explanation of data.

Florida Hospital Waterman

1000 Waterman Way
Tavares, FL 32778
Phone: 352-253-3300
Fax: 352-253-3927
E-mail: cindi.harrod@ahss.org
URL: www.fhwat.org
Type: Acute Care Hospitals
Emergency Services: Yes
Ownership: Voluntary non-profit - Church
Beds: 204

Key Personnel:
Emergency Room . . . . Annie Akkara
Cardiac Laboratory. . . . . Eric Blamick
Chief of Medical Staff . . . . Rosemary Cirelli, MD
Quality Assurance . . . . Carol Jeffes
Radiology. . . . . Robert Kittyle
Hemotology Center . . . . Pamela Marrero
CEO/President. . . . . Kenneth R Mattison
Operating Room. . . . . Heather Wood

Measure	Cases	This Hosp.	State Avg.	U.S. Avg.
Blood Clot Prevention and Treatment				
Anticoagulation Overlap Therapy[2]	115	100%	93%	93%
ICU Venous Thromboembolism Prophylaxis[2]	55	95%	94%	92%
Incidence of Potentially Preventable VTE[2]	27	0%	10%	10%
UFH with Dosages/Platelet Monitoring[2]	38	100%	100%	97%
Venous Thromboembolism Prophylaxis[2]	388	97%	88%	85%
Warfarin Therapy Discharge Instructions[2]	93	100%	85%	75%
Chest Pain/Possible Heart Attack Care				
Aspirin Given Within 24 Hours of Arrival[1,3]	-	-	98%	96%
Fibrinolytic Meds Within 30 Min. of Arrival[3,7]	-	-	81%	58%
Average Time to ECG (minutes)[1,3]	-	-	7	7
Average Time to Transfer (minutes)[3,7]	-	-	53	60
Children's Asthma Care				
Received Home Management Plan of Care	-	-	-	88%
Received Reliever Medication	-	-	-	100%
Received Systemic Corticosteroids	-	-	-	100%
Emergency Department				
Admittance Decision Time (minutes)[2]	825	88	111	98
Head CT Results Within 45 Min. of Arrival	16	38%	64%	57%
Patients Who Left ER Before Being Seen	53,598	2%	2%	2%
Time from ER Arrival to Admit. (minutes)[2]	832	270	289	274
Time from ER Arrival to Discharge (minutes)	335	149	147	134
Time in ER Before Being Evaluated (minutes)	369	38	26	26
Time to Pain Meds for Fractures (minutes)	109	73	60	57
Heart Attack Care				
Aspirin Given at Discharge[2]	183	99%	99%	99%
Fibrinolytic Meds Within 30 Min. of Arrival[2,7]	-	-	50%	54%
PCI Within 90 Minutes of Arrival[2]	58	98%	96%	96%
Statin Prescribed at Discharge[2]	166	99%	99%	98%
Heart Failure Care				
ACE Inhibitor or ARB for LVSD[2]	93	100%	98%	97%
Discharge Instructions Given[2]	224	100%	96%	94%
Evaluation of LVS Function[2]	276	100%	100%	99%
Medicare Spending				
Medicare Spending per Patient (ratio)	-	1.03	1.04	0.98
Pneumonia Care				
Appropriate Initial Antibiotic Given[2]	94	99%	98%	95%
Blood Culture Timing[2]	110	100%	99%	98%
Pregnancy and Delivery Care				
Newborn Deliveries Scheduled Early[2]	20	10%	6%	6%
Preventive Care				
Immunization for Influenza[2]	569	93%	94%	90%
Immunization for Pneumonia[2]	841	97%	96%	92%
Stroke Care				
Anticoagulation Therapy for Atrial Fibrillation[1,2]	-	-	97%	95%
Antithrombotic Therapy Timing[2]	85	100%	98%	98%
Assessed for Rehabilitation[2]	88	100%	97%	97%
Discharged on Antithrombotic Therapy[2]	81	100%	99%	99%
Discharged on Statin Medication[2]	62	98%	96%	94%
Thrombolytic Therapy Timing[1,2]	-	-	76%	66%
Venous Thromboembolism Prophylaxis[2]	100	99%	95%	94%
Written Stroke Educational Materials Given[2]	60	100%	94%	88%
Surgical Care Improvement Project				
Appropriate Beta Blocker Usage[2]	132	100%	99%	98%
Appropriate VTP Within 24 Hours[2]	275	100%	99%	98%
Controlled Postoperative Blood Glucose[2]	60	100%	98%	97%
Perioperative Temperature Management[2]	367	100%	100%	100%
Prophylactic Antibiotic Selection[2]	240	100%	99%	99%
Prophylactic Antibiotic Selection (Outpatient)	306	99%	98%	98%
Prophylactic Antibiotic Stopped[2]	222	99%	98%	98%
Prophylactic Antibiotic Timing[2]	240	100%	99%	99%
Prophylactic Antibiotic Timing (Outpatient)	306	99%	98%	98%
Urinary Catheter Removal[2]	267	98%	98%	97%
Survey of Patients' Hospital Experiences				
Area Around Room 'Always' Quiet at Night[11]	300+	57%	58%	61%
Doctors 'Always' Communicated Well[11]	300+	73%	77%	82%
Home Recovery Information Given[11]	300+	85%	83%	85%
Hospital Given 9 or 10 on 10 Point Scale[11]	300+	66%	67%	71%
Meds 'Always' Explained Before Given[11]	300+	58%	60%	64%
Nurses 'Always' Communicated Well[11]	300+	73%	75%	79%
Pain 'Always' Well Controlled[11]	300+	67%	68%	71%
Room and Bathroom 'Always' Clean[11]	300+	73%	69%	73%
Timely Help 'Always' Received[11]	300+	64%	62%	68%
Would Definitely Recommend Hospital[11]	300+	67%	69%	71%
Use of Medical Imaging				
Cardiac Imaging Stress Test before Surgery	266	4.1%	6.4%	5.3%
Combination Abdominal CT Scan	1,906	10.5%	11.8%	10.5%
Combination Brain/Sinus CT Scan	1,570	4.2%	3.4%	2.7%
Combination Chest CT Scan	1,346	0.7%	2.4%	2.7%
Follow-up Mammogram/Ultrasound	2,832	9.1%	10.2%	8.8%
Lumbar Spine MRI for Low Back Pain	164	37.8%	35.2%	37.2%

Mariners Hospital

91500 Overseas Highway
Tavernier, FL 33070
Phone: 305-434-3000
Fax: 305-853-1581
E-mail: corporatepr@baptisthealth.net
URL: www.baptisthealth.net
Type: Critical Access Hospitals
Emergency Services: Yes
Ownership: Voluntary non-profit - Private
Beds: 25

Key Personnel:
Intensive Care Unit. . . . . Roberta Fismer, RN
CEO/President. . . . . Brian E. Keeley
Infection Control. . . . . Gisele Monson
Operating Room. . . . . Orlando Morej_n, RN
Emergency Room . . . . Tracy Murrell
Quality Assurance . . . . John Sohn

Measure	Cases	This Hosp.	State Avg.	U.S. Avg.
Blood Clot Prevention and Treatment				
Anticoagulation Overlap Therapy[1]	-	-	93%	93%
ICU Venous Thromboembolism Prophylaxis[1]	-	-	94%	92%
Incidence of Potentially Preventable VTE[7]	-	-	10%	10%
UFH with Dosages/Platelet Monitoring[1]	-	-	100%	97%
Venous Thromboembolism Prophylaxis	297	95%	88%	85%
Warfarin Therapy Discharge Instructions[1]	-	-	85%	75%
Chest Pain/Possible Heart Attack Care				
Aspirin Given Within 24 Hours of Arrival	81	100%	98%	96%
Fibrinolytic Meds Within 30 Min. of Arrival[1]	-	-	81%	58%
Average Time to ECG (minutes)	81	2	7	7
Average Time to Transfer (minutes)[7]	-	-	53	60
Children's Asthma Care				
Received Home Management Plan of Care	-	-	-	88%
Received Reliever Medication	-	-	-	100%
Received Systemic Corticosteroids	-	-	-	100%
Emergency Department				
Admittance Decision Time (minutes)[2]	422	85	111	98
Head CT Results Within 45 Min. of Arrival	12	67%	64%	57%
Patients Who Left ER Before Being Seen	11,830	2%	2%	2%
Time from ER Arrival to Admit. (minutes)[2]	437	267	289	274
Time from ER Arrival to Discharge (minutes)	339	104	147	134
Time in ER Before Being Evaluated (minutes)	379	27	26	26
Time to Pain Meds for Fractures (minutes)	42	55	60	57
Heart Attack Care				
Aspirin Given at Discharge[5]	-	-	99%	99%
Fibrinolytic Meds Within 30 Min. of Arrival[5]	-	-	50%	54%
PCI Within 90 Minutes of Arrival[5]	-	-	96%	96%
Statin Prescribed at Discharge[5]	-	-	99%	98%
Heart Failure Care				
ACE Inhibitor or ARB for LVSD	11	100%	98%	97%
Discharge Instructions Given	25	100%	96%	94%
Evaluation of LVS Function	29	100%	100%	99%
Medicare Spending				
Medicare Spending per Patient (ratio)	-	-	1.04	0.98
Pneumonia Care				
Appropriate Initial Antibiotic Given	19	100%	98%	95%
Blood Culture Timing	32	100%	99%	98%
Pregnancy and Delivery Care				
Newborn Deliveries Scheduled Early[5]	-	-	6%	6%
Preventive Care				
Immunization for Influenza[2]	301	99%	94%	90%
Immunization for Pneumonia[2]	362	99%	96%	92%
Stroke Care				
Anticoagulation Therapy for Atrial Fibrillation[3,7]	-	-	97%	95%
Antithrombotic Therapy Timing[1,3]	-	-	98%	98%
Assessed for Rehabilitation[1,3]	-	-	97%	97%
Discharged on Antithrombotic Therapy[1,3]	-	-	99%	99%
Discharged on Statin Medication[3,7]	-	-	96%	94%
Thrombolytic Therapy Timing[3,7]	-	-	76%	66%
Venous Thromboembolism Prophylaxis[1,3]	-	-	95%	94%
Written Stroke Educational Materials Given[1,3]	-	-	94%	88%
Surgical Care Improvement Project				
Appropriate Beta Blocker Usage[1]	-	-	99%	98%
Appropriate VTP Within 24 Hours	39	100%	99%	98%
Controlled Postoperative Blood Glucose[7]	-	-	98%	97%
Perioperative Temperature Management	42	100%	100%	100%
Prophylactic Antibiotic Selection	29	100%	99%	99%
Prophylactic Antibiotic Selection (Outpatient)[1,3]	-	-	98%	98%
Prophylactic Antibiotic Stopped	26	96%	98%	98%
Prophylactic Antibiotic Timing	31	100%	99%	99%
Prophylactic Antibiotic Timing (Outpatient)[1,3]	-	-	98%	98%
Urinary Catheter Removal	39	100%	98%	97%
Survey of Patients' Hospital Experiences				
Area Around Room 'Always' Quiet at Night	(a)	70%	58%	61%
Doctors 'Always' Communicated Well	(a)	87%	77%	82%
Home Recovery Information Given	(a)	91%	83%	85%
Hospital Given 9 or 10 on 10 Point Scale	(a)	83%	67%	71%
Meds 'Always' Explained Before Given	(a)	76%	60%	64%
Nurses 'Always' Communicated Well	(a)	89%	75%	79%
Pain 'Always' Well Controlled	(a)	80%	68%	71%
Room and Bathroom 'Always' Clean	(a)	89%	69%	73%
Timely Help 'Always' Received	(a)	89%	62%	68%
Would Definitely Recommend Hospital	(a)	82%	69%	71%
Use of Medical Imaging				
Cardiac Imaging Stress Test before Surgery	143	7.7%	6.4%	5.3%
Combination Abdominal CT Scan	384	4.2%	11.8%	10.5%
Combination Brain/Sinus CT Scan[1]	-	-	3.4%	2.7%
Combination Chest CT Scan	199	2.0%	2.4%	2.7%
Follow-up Mammogram/Ultrasound	346	19.1%	10.2%	8.8%
Lumbar Spine MRI for Low Back Pain	59	28.8%	35.2%	37.2%

The Villages Regional Hospital

1451 El Camino Real
The Villages, FL 32159
Phone: 352-751-8000
Fax: 352-751-8975
URL: www.tvrh.org
Type: Acute Care Hospitals
Emergency Services: Yes
Ownership: Voluntary non-profit - Private
Beds: 66

Key Personnel:
Chief of Medical Staff . . . . Dr Dan Carlson
CEO/President. . . . . Don Henderson, FACHE

Measure	Cases	This Hosp.	State Avg.	U.S. Avg.
Blood Clot Prevention and Treatment				
Anticoagulation Overlap Therapy[2]	178	94%	93%	93%
ICU Venous Thromboembolism Prophylaxis[2]	25	84%	94%	92%
Incidence of Potentially Preventable VTE[2]	16	31%	10%	10%
UFH with Dosages/Platelet Monitoring[2]	185	99%	100%	97%
Venous Thromboembolism Prophylaxis[2]	381	81%	88%	85%
Warfarin Therapy Discharge Instructions[2]	144	98%	85%	75%
Chest Pain/Possible Heart Attack Care				
Aspirin Given Within 24 Hours of Arrival[1]	-	-	98%	96%
Fibrinolytic Meds Within 30 Min. of Arrival[3,7]	-	-	81%	58%
Average Time to ECG (minutes)[1]	-	-	7	7
Average Time to Transfer (minutes)[3,7]	-	-	53	60
Children's Asthma Care				
Received Home Management Plan of Care	-	-	-	88%
Received Reliever Medication	-	-	-	100%

NOTE: Hospital profiles are in alphabetical order by state, then city, then hospital within the city; Rankings exclude hospitals with less than 25 cases except for patient surveys which excludes hospitals with less than 100 cases; (a) 100-299 cases; (1) The number of cases/patients is too few to report; (2) Data submitted were based on a sample of cases/patients; (3) Results are based on a shorter time period than required; (4) Data suppressed by CMS for one or more quarters; (5) Results are not available for this reporting period; (6) Fewer than 100 patients completed the HCAHPS survey; (7) No cases met the criteria for this measure; (8) The lower limit of the confidence interval cannot be calculated if the number of observed infections equals zero; (9) No data are available from the state/territory for this reporting period; (10) The scores shown reflect fewer than 50 completed surveys; (11) There were discrepancies in the data collection process; (12) This measure does not apply to this hospital for this reporting period; (13) Results cannot be calculated for this reporting period; (14) The results for this state are combined with nearby states to protect confidentiality; Please refer to the User's Guide for a full explanation of data.

Measure	Cases	This Hosp.	State Avg.	U.S. Avg.
Received Systemic Corticosteroids	-	-	-	100%
Emergency Department				
Admittance Decision Time (minutes)[2]	693	141	111	98
Head CT Results Within 45 Min. of Arrival	26	65%	64%	57%
Patients Who Left ER Before Being Seen	42,673	4%	2%	2%
Time from ER Arrival to Admit. (minutes)[2]	739	399	289	274
Time from ER Arrival to Discharge (minutes)	293	232	147	134
Time in ER Before Being Evaluated (minutes)	366	48	26	26
Time to Pain Meds for Fractures (minutes)	61	122	60	57
Heart Attack Care				
Aspirin Given at Discharge[2]	297	100%	99%	99%
Fibrinolytic Meds Within 30 Min. of Arrival[2,7]	-	-	50%	54%
PCI Within 90 Minutes of Arrival[2]	34	97%	96%	96%
Statin Prescribed at Discharge[2]	277	96%	99%	98%
Heart Failure Care				
ACE Inhibitor or ARB for LVSD[2]	92	100%	98%	97%
Discharge Instructions Given[2]	249	96%	96%	94%
Evaluation of LVS Function[2]	328	100%	100%	99%
Medicare Spending				
Medicare Spending per Patient (ratio)	-	1.01	1.04	0.98
Pneumonia Care				
Appropriate Initial Antibiotic Given[2]	96	98%	98%	95%
Blood Culture Timing[2]	74	97%	99%	98%
Pregnancy and Delivery Care				
Newborn Deliveries Scheduled Early[7]	-	-	6%	6%
Preventive Care				
Immunization for Influenza[2]	588	95%	94%	90%
Immunization for Pneumonia[2]	1,043	97%	96%	92%
Stroke Care				
Anticoagulation Therapy for Atrial Fibrillation[2]	13	100%	97%	95%
Antithrombotic Therapy Timing[2]	95	95%	98%	98%
Assessed for Rehabilitation[2]	110	95%	97%	97%
Discharged on Antithrombotic Therapy[2]	92	100%	99%	99%
Discharged on Statin Medication[2]	85	91%	96%	94%
Thrombolytic Therapy Timing[1,2]	-	-	76%	66%
Venous Thromboembolism Prophylaxis[2]	108	81%	95%	94%
Written Stroke Educational Materials Given[2]	57	81%	94%	88%
Surgical Care Improvement Project				
Appropriate Beta Blocker Usage	218	96%	99%	98%
Appropriate VTP Within 24 Hours	532	93%	99%	98%
Controlled Postoperative Blood Glucose[7]	-	-	98%	97%
Perioperative Temperature Management	625	99%	100%	100%
Prophylactic Antibiotic Selection	337	98%	99%	99%
Prophylactic Antibiotic Selection (Outpatient)	515	96%	98%	98%
Prophylactic Antibiotic Stopped	326	98%	98%	98%
Prophylactic Antibiotic Timing	339	98%	99%	99%
Prophylactic Antibiotic Timing (Outpatient)	516	99%	98%	98%
Urinary Catheter Removal	408	91%	98%	97%
Survey of Patients' Hospital Experiences				
Area Around Room 'Always' Quiet at Night	300+	47%	58%	61%
Doctors 'Always' Communicated Well	300+	68%	77%	82%
Home Recovery Information Given	300+	75%	83%	85%
Hospital Given 9 or 10 on 10 Point Scale	300+	56%	67%	71%
Meds 'Always' Explained Before Given	300+	50%	60%	64%
Nurses 'Always' Communicated Well	300+	71%	75%	79%
Pain 'Always' Well Controlled	300+	61%	68%	71%
Room and Bathroom 'Always' Clean	300+	66%	69%	73%
Timely Help 'Always' Received	300+	56%	62%	68%
Would Definitely Recommend Hospital	300+	58%	69%	71%
Use of Medical Imaging				
Cardiac Imaging Stress Test before Surgery	383	7.8%	6.4%	5.3%
Combination Abdominal CT Scan	951	7.3%	11.8%	10.5%
Combination Brain/Sinus CT Scan	1,638	4.0%	3.4%	2.7%
Combination Chest CT Scan	213	0.0%	2.4%	2.7%
Follow-up Mammogram/Ultrasound[7]	-	-	10.2%	8.8%
Lumbar Spine MRI for Low Back Pain[1]	-	-	35.2%	37.2%

Parrish Medical Center

951 N Washington Ave
Titusville, FL 32796
Phone: 321-268-6111
Fax: 321-268-6231
URL: www.parrishmed.com
Type: Acute Care Hospitals
Emergency Services: Yes
Ownership: Govt - Hospital Dist/Auth
Beds: 210

Key Personnel:
Pediatric In-Patient Care . . . . Angel Acevedo, MD
Chief of Medical Staff. . . . . Lisa Alexander, MD
Radiology. . . . . Wasfi A Makar
President/CEO. . . . . George Mikitarian
Quality Assurance . . . . Sheryl O'Connor, RN
Operating Room. . . . . Ramesh P Patel, RN

Measure	Cases	This Hosp.	State Avg.	U.S. Avg.
Blood Clot Prevention and Treatment				
Anticoagulation Overlap Therapy[2]	48	96%	93%	93%
ICU Venous Thromboembolism Prophylaxis[2]	69	97%	94%	92%
Incidence of Potentially Preventable VTE[1,2]	-	-	10%	10%
UFH with Dosages/Platelet Monitoring[2]	40	98%	100%	97%
Venous Thromboembolism Prophylaxis[2]	390	85%	88%	85%
Warfarin Therapy Discharge Instructions[2]	38	79%	85%	75%
Chest Pain/Possible Heart Attack Care				
Aspirin Given Within 24 Hours of Arrival[1]	-	-	98%	96%
Fibrinolytic Meds Within 30 Min. of Arrival[5]	-	-	81%	58%
Average Time to ECG (minutes)[1]	-	-	7	7
Average Time to Transfer (minutes)[5]	-	-	53	60
Children's Asthma Care				
Received Home Management Plan of Care	-	-	-	88%
Received Reliever Medication	-	-	-	100%
Received Systemic Corticosteroids	-	-	-	100%
Emergency Department				
Admittance Decision Time (minutes)[2]	819	122	111	98
Head CT Results Within 45 Min. of Arrival	16	62%	64%	57%
Patients Who Left ER Before Being Seen	41,852	2%	2%	2%
Time from ER Arrival to Admit. (minutes)[2]	822	286	289	274
Time from ER Arrival to Discharge (minutes)	420	162	147	134
Time in ER Before Being Evaluated (minutes)	448	46	26	26
Time to Pain Meds for Fractures (minutes)	173	80	60	57
Heart Attack Care				
Aspirin Given at Discharge	104	100%	99%	99%
Fibrinolytic Meds Within 30 Min. of Arrival[7]	-	-	50%	54%
PCI Within 90 Minutes of Arrival	36	100%	96%	96%
Statin Prescribed at Discharge	98	100%	99%	98%
Heart Failure Care				
ACE Inhibitor or ARB for LVSD	58	100%	98%	97%
Discharge Instructions Given	143	98%	96%	94%
Evaluation of LVS Function	176	100%	100%	99%
Medicare Spending				
Medicare Spending per Patient (ratio)	-	1.03	1.04	0.98
Pneumonia Care				
Appropriate Initial Antibiotic Given	108	99%	98%	95%
Blood Culture Timing	163	95%	99%	98%
Pregnancy and Delivery Care				
Newborn Deliveries Scheduled Early	53	0%	6%	6%
Preventive Care				
Immunization for Influenza[2]	539	93%	94%	90%
Immunization for Pneumonia[2]	773	97%	96%	92%
Stroke Care				
Anticoagulation Therapy for Atrial Fibrillation	19	100%	97%	95%
Antithrombotic Therapy Timing	105	99%	98%	98%
Assessed for Rehabilitation	120	96%	97%	97%
Discharged on Antithrombotic Therapy	110	100%	99%	99%
Discharged on Statin Medication	78	96%	96%	94%
Thrombolytic Therapy Timing	19	84%	76%	66%
Venous Thromboembolism Prophylaxis	128	96%	95%	94%
Written Stroke Educational Materials Given	72	100%	94%	88%
Surgical Care Improvement Project				
Appropriate Beta Blocker Usage	120	100%	99%	98%
Appropriate VTP Within 24 Hours	383	99%	99%	98%
Controlled Postoperative Blood Glucose[7]	-	-	98%	97%
Perioperative Temperature Management	421	100%	100%	100%
Prophylactic Antibiotic Selection	238	100%	99%	99%
Prophylactic Antibiotic Selection (Outpatient)	144	99%	98%	98%
Prophylactic Antibiotic Stopped	238	100%	98%	98%
Prophylactic Antibiotic Timing	244	99%	99%	99%
Prophylactic Antibiotic Timing (Outpatient)	145	99%	98%	98%
Urinary Catheter Removal	270	100%	98%	97%
Survey of Patients' Hospital Experiences				
Area Around Room 'Always' Quiet at Night	300+	64%	58%	61%
Doctors 'Always' Communicated Well	300+	81%	77%	82%
Home Recovery Information Given	300+	85%	83%	85%
Hospital Given 9 or 10 on 10 Point Scale	300+	72%	67%	71%
Meds 'Always' Explained Before Given	300+	63%	60%	64%
Nurses 'Always' Communicated Well	300+	80%	75%	79%
Pain 'Always' Well Controlled	300+	72%	68%	71%
Room and Bathroom 'Always' Clean	300+	74%	69%	73%
Timely Help 'Always' Received	300+	71%	62%	68%
Would Definitely Recommend Hospital	300+	74%	69%	71%
Use of Medical Imaging				
Cardiac Imaging Stress Test before Surgery	287	5.6%	6.4%	5.3%
Combination Abdominal CT Scan	971	7.2%	11.8%	10.5%
Combination Brain/Sinus CT Scan	967	0.6%	3.4%	2.7%
Combination Chest CT Scan	511	0.4%	2.4%	2.7%
Follow-up Mammogram/Ultrasound	1,728	4.5%	10.2%	8.8%
Lumbar Spine MRI for Low Back Pain	183	33.3%	35.2%	37.2%

Medical Center of Trinity

9330 Sr 54
Trinity, FL 34655
Phone: 727-848-1733
Fax: 727-845-9167
URL: www.communityhospitalnpr.com
Type: Acute Care Hospitals
Emergency Services: Yes
Ownership: Proprietary
Beds: 389

Key Personnel:
Chief of Medical Staff. . . . . Peter Candelora, MD
Operating Room. . . . . Peter Candelora, MD
Infection Control. . . . . Michelle DeWatt
CEO/President. . . . . Kathryn Gillette
Quality Assurance . . . . Peggy Green, RN
Emergency Room . . . . Terry Meadows, MD
Chairman/CEO . . . . Richard A. Miller, DO
Anesthesiology. . . . . Christor J Pitarys, MD

Measure	Cases	This Hosp.	State Avg.	U.S. Avg.
Blood Clot Prevention and Treatment				
Anticoagulation Overlap Therapy[2]	67	97%	93%	93%
ICU Venous Thromboembolism Prophylaxis[2]	80	100%	94%	92%
Incidence of Potentially Preventable VTE[2]	21	5%	10%	10%
UFH with Dosages/Platelet Monitoring[2]	27	100%	100%	97%
Venous Thromboembolism Prophylaxis[2]	393	99%	88%	85%
Warfarin Therapy Discharge Instructions[2]	41	93%	85%	75%
Chest Pain/Possible Heart Attack Care				
Aspirin Given Within 24 Hours of Arrival[5]	-	-	98%	96%
Fibrinolytic Meds Within 30 Min. of Arrival[5]	-	-	81%	58%
Average Time to ECG (minutes)[5]	-	-	7	7
Average Time to Transfer (minutes)[5]	-	-	53	60
Children's Asthma Care				
Received Home Management Plan of Care	-	-	-	88%
Received Reliever Medication	-	-	-	100%
Received Systemic Corticosteroids	-	-	-	100%
Emergency Department				
Admittance Decision Time (minutes)[2]	858	77	111	98
Head CT Results Within 45 Min. of Arrival[1]	-	-	64%	57%
Patients Who Left ER Before Being Seen	43,159	1%	2%	2%
Time from ER Arrival to Admit. (minutes)[2]	858	234	289	274
Time from ER Arrival to Discharge (minutes)	454	144	147	134
Time in ER Before Being Evaluated (minutes)	469	16	26	26
Time to Pain Meds for Fractures (minutes)	104	38	60	57
Heart Attack Care				
Aspirin Given at Discharge	214	100%	99%	99%
Fibrinolytic Meds Within 30 Min. of Arrival[7]	-	-	50%	54%
PCI Within 90 Minutes of Arrival	33	100%	96%	96%
Statin Prescribed at Discharge	211	100%	99%	98%
Heart Failure Care				
ACE Inhibitor or ARB for LVSD	94	100%	98%	97%
Discharge Instructions Given	250	100%	96%	94%
Evaluation of LVS Function	336	100%	100%	99%
Medicare Spending				
Medicare Spending per Patient (ratio)	-	1.09	1.04	0.98
Pneumonia Care				

NOTE: Hospital profiles are in alphabetical order by state, then city, then hospital within the city; Rankings exclude hospitals with less than 25 cases except for patient surveys which excludes hospitals with less than 100 cases; (a) 100-299 cases; (1) The number of cases/patients is too few to report; (2) Data submitted were based on a sample of cases/patients; (3) Results are based on a shorter time period than required; (4) Data suppressed by CMS for one or more quarters; (5) Results are not available for this reporting period; (6) Fewer than 100 patients completed the HCAHPS survey; (7) No cases met the criteria for this measure; (8) The lower limit of the confidence interval cannot be calculated if the number of observed infections equals zero; (9) No data are available from the state/territory for this reporting period; (10) The scores shown reflect fewer than 50 completed surveys; (11) There were discrepancies in the data collection process; (12) This measure does not apply to this hospital for this reporting period; (13) Results cannot be calculated for this reporting period; (14) The results for this state are combined with nearby states to protect confidentiality; Please refer to the User's Guide for a full explanation of data.

Measure	Cases	This Hosp.	State Avg.	U.S. Avg.
Appropriate Initial Antibiotic Given[2]	75	100%	98%	95%
Blood Culture Timing[2]	104	100%	99%	98%
Pregnancy and Delivery Care				
Newborn Deliveries Scheduled Early[2]	34	0%	6%	6%
Preventive Care				
Immunization for Influenza[2]	652	98%	94%	90%
Immunization for Pneumonia[2]	899	99%	96%	92%
Stroke Care				
Anticoagulation Therapy for Atrial Fibrillation[2]	15	93%	97%	95%
Antithrombotic Therapy Timing[2]	95	100%	98%	98%
Assessed for Rehabilitation[2]	94	100%	97%	97%
Discharged on Antithrombotic Therapy[2]	89	97%	99%	99%
Discharged on Statin Medication[2]	73	92%	96%	94%
Thrombolytic Therapy Timing[1,2]	-	-	76%	66%
Venous Thromboembolism Prophylaxis[2]	103	90%	95%	94%
Written Stroke Educational Materials Given[2]	67	94%	94%	88%
Surgical Care Improvement Project				
Appropriate Beta Blocker Usage[2]	178	99%	99%	98%
Appropriate VTP Within 24 Hours[2]	414	100%	99%	98%
Controlled Postoperative Blood Glucose[2,7]	-	-	98%	97%
Perioperative Temperature Management[2]	483	100%	100%	100%
Prophylactic Antibiotic Selection[2]	284	100%	99%	99%
Prophylactic Antibiotic Selection (Outpatient)	161	98%	98%	98%
Prophylactic Antibiotic Stopped[2]	266	100%	98%	98%
Prophylactic Antibiotic Timing[2]	283	100%	99%	99%
Prophylactic Antibiotic Timing (Outpatient)	161	100%	98%	98%
Urinary Catheter Removal[2]	207	100%	98%	97%
Survey of Patients' Hospital Experiences				
Area Around Room 'Always' Quiet at Night	300+	68%	58%	61%
Doctors 'Always' Communicated Well	300+	76%	77%	82%
Home Recovery Information Given	300+	82%	83%	85%
Hospital Given 9 or 10 on 10 Point Scale	300+	69%	67%	71%
Meds 'Always' Explained Before Given	300+	57%	60%	64%
Nurses 'Always' Communicated Well	300+	74%	75%	79%
Pain 'Always' Well Controlled	300+	67%	68%	71%
Room and Bathroom 'Always' Clean	300+	72%	69%	73%
Timely Help 'Always' Received	300+	63%	62%	68%
Would Definitely Recommend Hospital	300+	71%	69%	71%
Use of Medical Imaging				
Cardiac Imaging Stress Test before Surgery[1]	-	-	6.4%	5.3%
Combination Abdominal CT Scan	365	4.7%	11.8%	10.5%
Combination Brain/Sinus CT Scan	575	6.6%	3.4%	2.7%
Combination Chest CT Scan	105	0.0%	2.4%	2.7%
Follow-up Mammogram/Ultrasound[1]	-	-	10.2%	8.8%
Lumbar Spine MRI for Low Back Pain[1]	-	-	35.2%	37.2%

Venice Regional Medical Center - Bayfront Health

540 the Rialto
Venice, FL 34285
Phone: 941-485-7711
Fax: 941-483-7621
URL: www.veniceregional.com
Type: Acute Care Hospitals
Emergency Services: Yes
Ownership: Proprietary
Beds: 312

Key Personnel:

Emergency Room .... Linda Caissie
Quality Assurance .... Diane Petty
Operating Room.............. Michelle Walker
CEO/President................ Peter Wozniak

Measure	Cases	This Hosp.	State Avg.	U.S. Avg.
Blood Clot Prevention and Treatment				
Anticoagulation Overlap Therapy[2]	115	100%	93%	93%
ICU Venous Thromboembolism Prophylaxis[2]	31	100%	94%	92%
Incidence of Potentially Preventable VTE[2]	13	0%	10%	10%
UFH with Dosages/Platelet Monitoring[2]	110	100%	100%	97%
Venous Thromboembolism Prophylaxis[2]	338	97%	88%	85%
Warfarin Therapy Discharge Instructions[2]	86	100%	85%	75%
Chest Pain/Possible Heart Attack Care				
Aspirin Given Within 24 Hours of Arrival[5]	-	-	98%	96%
Fibrinolytic Meds Within 30 Min. of Arrival[5]	-	-	81%	58%
Average Time to ECG (minutes)[5]	-	-	7	7
Average Time to Transfer (minutes)[5]	-	-	53	60
Children's Asthma Care				
Received Home Management Plan of Care	-	-	-	88%
Received Reliever Medication	-	-	-	100%
Received Systemic Corticosteroids	-	-	-	100%
Emergency Department				
Admittance Decision Time (minutes)[2]	759	111	111	98
Head CT Results Within 45 Min. of Arrival[3,7]	-	-	64%	57%
Patients Who Left ER Before Being Seen	33,164	1%	2%	2%
Time from ER Arrival to Admit. (minutes)[2]	783	257	289	274
Time from ER Arrival to Discharge (minutes)	363	157	147	134
Time in ER Before Being Evaluated (minutes)	396	39	26	26
Time to Pain Meds for Fractures (minutes)	74	54	60	57
Heart Attack Care				
Aspirin Given at Discharge[2]	269	100%	99%	99%
Fibrinolytic Meds Within 30 Min. of Arrival[2,7]	-	-	50%	54%
PCI Within 90 Minutes of Arrival[2]	53	100%	96%	96%
Statin Prescribed at Discharge[2]	264	100%	99%	98%
Heart Failure Care				
ACE Inhibitor or ARB for LVSD[2]	62	100%	98%	97%
Discharge Instructions Given[2]	186	100%	96%	94%
Evaluation of LVS Function[2]	259	100%	100%	99%
Medicare Spending				
Medicare Spending per Patient (ratio)	-	1.04	1.04	0.98
Pneumonia Care				
Appropriate Initial Antibiotic Given[2]	109	100%	98%	95%
Blood Culture Timing[2]	160	100%	99%	98%
Pregnancy and Delivery Care				
Newborn Deliveries Scheduled Early[7]	-	-	6%	6%
Preventive Care				
Immunization for Influenza[2]	607	100%	94%	90%
Immunization for Pneumonia[2]	1,049	99%	96%	92%
Stroke Care				
Anticoagulation Therapy for Atrial Fibrillation[2]	21	100%	97%	95%
Antithrombotic Therapy Timing[2]	83	99%	98%	98%
Assessed for Rehabilitation[2]	101	100%	97%	97%
Discharged on Antithrombotic Therapy[2]	93	100%	99%	99%
Discharged on Statin Medication[2]	66	98%	96%	94%
Thrombolytic Therapy Timing[1,2]	-	-	76%	66%
Venous Thromboembolism Prophylaxis[2]	106	99%	95%	94%
Written Stroke Educational Materials Given[2]	57	95%	94%	88%
Surgical Care Improvement Project				
Appropriate Beta Blocker Usage[2]	299	100%	99%	98%
Appropriate VTP Within 24 Hours[2]	434	100%	99%	98%
Controlled Postoperative Blood Glucose[2]	135	100%	98%	97%
Perioperative Temperature Management[2]	502	100%	100%	100%
Prophylactic Antibiotic Selection[2]	476	100%	99%	99%
Prophylactic Antibiotic Selection (Outpatient)	460	100%	98%	98%
Prophylactic Antibiotic Stopped[2]	446	100%	98%	98%
Prophylactic Antibiotic Timing[2]	476	100%	99%	99%
Prophylactic Antibiotic Timing (Outpatient)	460	100%	98%	98%
Urinary Catheter Removal[2]	379	100%	98%	97%
Survey of Patients' Hospital Experiences				
Area Around Room 'Always' Quiet at Night	300+	46%	58%	61%
Doctors 'Always' Communicated Well	300+	76%	77%	82%
Home Recovery Information Given	300+	82%	83%	85%
Hospital Given 9 or 10 on 10 Point Scale	300+	57%	67%	71%
Meds 'Always' Explained Before Given	300+	52%	60%	64%
Nurses 'Always' Communicated Well	300+	71%	75%	79%
Pain 'Always' Well Controlled	300+	62%	68%	71%
Room and Bathroom 'Always' Clean	300+	62%	69%	73%
Timely Help 'Always' Received	300+	57%	62%	68%
Would Definitely Recommend Hospital	300+	64%	69%	71%
Use of Medical Imaging				
Cardiac Imaging Stress Test before Surgery	182	4.9%	6.4%	5.3%
Combination Abdominal CT Scan	1,377	7.2%	11.8%	10.5%
Combination Brain/Sinus CT Scan	1,613	3.0%	3.4%	2.7%
Combination Chest CT Scan	793	0.0%	2.4%	2.7%
Follow-up Mammogram/Ultrasound	2,367	5.7%	10.2%	8.8%
Lumbar Spine MRI for Low Back Pain	76	39.5%	35.2%	37.2%

Indian River Medical Center

1000 36th St
Vero Beach, FL 32960
Phone: 772-567-4311
Fax: 772-562-5628
URL: www.irmh.com
Type: Acute Care Hospitals
Emergency Services: Yes
Ownership: Govt - Hospital Dist/Auth
Beds: 335

Key Personnel:

Quality Assurance .... Annette Barton-Riley
Radiology.................... Jay Colella, MD
Emergency Room .... Brad Damiani, MD
Cardiac Laboratory............ Robert Hendley, MD
Chief of Medical Staff.......... Charles Mackett III, MD
Pediatric In-Patient Care .... Marc McCain, MD
Operating Room............... Theodore Perry, MD
CEO/President................ Jeffrey L Susi, FACHE

Measure	Cases	This Hosp.	State Avg.	U.S. Avg.
Blood Clot Prevention and Treatment				
Anticoagulation Overlap Therapy[2]	119	81%	93%	93%
ICU Venous Thromboembolism Prophylaxis[2]	70	86%	94%	92%
Incidence of Potentially Preventable VTE[2]	14	21%	10%	10%
UFH with Dosages/Platelet Monitoring[2]	85	98%	100%	97%
Venous Thromboembolism Prophylaxis[2]	347	71%	88%	85%
Warfarin Therapy Discharge Instructions[2]	86	71%	85%	75%
Chest Pain/Possible Heart Attack Care				
Aspirin Given Within 24 Hours of Arrival[5]	-	-	98%	96%
Fibrinolytic Meds Within 30 Min. of Arrival[5]	-	-	81%	58%
Average Time to ECG (minutes)[5]	-	-	7	7
Average Time to Transfer (minutes)[5]	-	-	53	60
Children's Asthma Care				
Received Home Management Plan of Care	-	-	-	88%
Received Reliever Medication	-	-	-	100%
Received Systemic Corticosteroids	-	-	-	100%
Emergency Department				
Admittance Decision Time (minutes)[2]	679	165	111	98
Head CT Results Within 45 Min. of Arrival[1]	-	-	64%	57%
Patients Who Left ER Before Being Seen	57,166	2%	2%	2%
Time from ER Arrival to Admit. (minutes)[2]	691	346	289	274
Time from ER Arrival to Discharge (minutes)	364	157	147	134
Time in ER Before Being Evaluated (minutes)	395	53	26	26
Time to Pain Meds for Fractures (minutes)	134	68	60	57
Heart Attack Care				
Aspirin Given at Discharge[2]	265	99%	99%	99%
Fibrinolytic Meds Within 30 Min. of Arrival[2,7]	-	-	50%	54%
PCI Within 90 Minutes of Arrival[2]	50	98%	96%	96%
Statin Prescribed at Discharge[2]	242	99%	99%	98%
Heart Failure Care				
ACE Inhibitor or ARB for LVSD[2]	82	98%	98%	97%
Discharge Instructions Given[2]	257	96%	96%	94%
Evaluation of LVS Function[2]	326	100%	100%	99%
Medicare Spending				
Medicare Spending per Patient (ratio)	-	1.04	1.04	0.98
Pneumonia Care				
Appropriate Initial Antibiotic Given[2]	127	98%	98%	95%
Blood Culture Timing[2]	179	98%	99%	98%
Pregnancy and Delivery Care				
Newborn Deliveries Scheduled Early[2]	21	0%	6%	6%
Preventive Care				
Immunization for Influenza[2]	582	90%	94%	90%
Immunization for Pneumonia[2]	817	93%	96%	92%
Stroke Care				
Anticoagulation Therapy for Atrial Fibrillation[2]	15	100%	97%	95%
Antithrombotic Therapy Timing[2]	81	99%	98%	98%
Assessed for Rehabilitation[2]	92	99%	97%	97%
Discharged on Antithrombotic Therapy[2]	82	99%	99%	99%
Discharged on Statin Medication[2]	58	95%	96%	94%
Thrombolytic Therapy Timing[1,2]	-	-	76%	66%
Venous Thromboembolism Prophylaxis[2]	98	96%	95%	94%
Written Stroke Educational Materials Given[2]	49	96%	94%	88%
Surgical Care Improvement Project				
Appropriate Beta Blocker Usage[2]	271	95%	99%	98%
Appropriate VTP Within 24 Hours[2]	408	97%	99%	98%
Controlled Postoperative Blood Glucose[2]	174	97%	98%	97%
Perioperative Temperature Management[2]	521	99%	100%	100%
Prophylactic Antibiotic Selection[2]	468	98%	99%	99%

NOTE: Hospital profiles are in alphabetical order by state, then city, then hospital within the city; Rankings exclude hospitals with less than 25 cases except for patient surveys which excludes hospitals with less than 100 cases; (a) 100-299 cases; (1) The number of cases/patients is too few to report; (2) Data submitted were based on a sample of cases/patients; (3) Results are based on a shorter time period than required; (4) Data suppressed by CMS for one or more quarters; (5) Results are not available for this reporting period; (6) Fewer than 100 patients completed the HCAHPS survey; (7) No cases met the criteria for this measure; (8) The lower limit of the confidence interval cannot be calculated if the number of observed infections equals zero; (9) No data are available from the state/territory for this reporting period; (10) The scores shown reflect fewer than 50 completed surveys; (11) There were discrepancies in the data collection process; (12) This measure does not apply to this hospital for this reporting period; (13) Results cannot be calculated for this reporting period; (14) The results for this state are combined with nearby states to protect confidentiality; Please refer to the User's Guide for a full explanation of data.

Prophylactic Antibiotic Selection (Outpatient)	224	97%	98%	98%
Prophylactic Antibiotic Stopped[2]	452	96%	98%	98%
Prophylactic Antibiotic Timing[2]	468	98%	99%	99%
Prophylactic Antibiotic Timing (Outpatient)	228	96%	98%	98%
Urinary Catheter Removal[2]	465	91%	98%	97%
Survey of Patients' Hospital Experiences				
Area Around Room 'Always' Quiet at Night	300+	45%	58%	61%
Doctors 'Always' Communicated Well	300+	76%	77%	82%
Home Recovery Information Given	300+	83%	83%	85%
Hospital Given 9 or 10 on 10 Point Scale	300+	63%	67%	71%
Meds 'Always' Explained Before Given	300+	58%	60%	64%
Nurses 'Always' Communicated Well	300+	73%	75%	79%
Pain 'Always' Well Controlled	300+	67%	68%	71%
Room and Bathroom 'Always' Clean	300+	64%	69%	73%
Timely Help 'Always' Received	300+	56%	62%	68%
Would Definitely Recommend Hospital	300+	68%	69%	71%
Use of Medical Imaging				
Cardiac Imaging Stress Test before Surgery	1,278	6.2%	6.4%	5.3%
Combination Abdominal CT Scan	940	13.7%	11.8%	10.5%
Combination Brain/Sinus CT Scan	1,167	3.7%	3.4%	2.7%
Combination Chest CT Scan	327	8.6%	2.4%	2.7%
Follow-up Mammogram/Ultrasound[7]	-	-	10.2%	8.8%
Lumbar Spine MRI for Low Back Pain[1]	-	-	35.2%	37.2%

Florida Hospital Wauchula

533 Carlton St Phone: 863-773-3101
Wauchula, FL 33873 Fax: 863-773-0126
Type: Critical Access Hospitals Emergency Services: Yes
Ownership: Voluntary non-profit - Church Beds: 25

Key Personnel:
Radiology. . . . . James B Ball
CEO/President. . . . . John Harding

Measure	Cases	This Hosp.	State Avg.	U.S. Avg.
Blood Clot Prevention and Treatment				
Anticoagulation Overlap Therapy[1,2]	-	-	93%	93%
ICU Venous Thromboembolism Prophylaxis[2,7]	-	-	94%	92%
Incidence of Potentially Preventable VTE[2,7]	-	-	10%	10%
UFH with Dosages/Platelet Monitoring[2,7]	-	-	100%	97%
Venous Thromboembolism Prophylaxis[2]	142	99%	88%	85%
Warfarin Therapy Discharge Instructions[1,2]	-	-	85%	75%
Chest Pain/Possible Heart Attack Care				
Aspirin Given Within 24 Hours of Arrival	51	94%	98%	96%
Fibrinolytic Meds Within 30 Min. of Arrival[1]	-	-	81%	58%
Average Time to ECG (minutes)	54	6	7	7
Average Time to Transfer (minutes)	12	44	53	60
Children's Asthma Care				
Received Home Management Plan of Care	-	-	-	88%
Received Reliever Medication	-	-	-	100%
Received Systemic Corticosteroids	-	-	-	100%
Emergency Department				
Admittance Decision Time (minutes)[2]	178	77	111	98
Head CT Results Within 45 Min. of Arrival[1]	-	-	64%	57%
Patients Who Left ER Before Being Seen	13,900	0%	2%	2%
Time from ER Arrival to Admit. (minutes)[2]	252	226	289	274
Time from ER Arrival to Discharge (minutes)	390	90	147	134
Time in ER Before Being Evaluated (minutes)	327	22	26	26
Time to Pain Meds for Fractures (minutes)	65	33	60	57
Heart Attack Care				
Aspirin Given at Discharge[1,3]	-	-	99%	99%
Fibrinolytic Meds Within 30 Min. of Arrival[5]	-	-	50%	54%
PCI Within 90 Minutes of Arrival[5]	-	-	96%	96%
Statin Prescribed at Discharge[1,3]	-	-	99%	98%
Heart Failure Care				
ACE Inhibitor or ARB for LVSD[1]	-	-	98%	97%
Discharge Instructions Given	12	92%	96%	94%
Evaluation of LVS Function	18	100%	100%	99%
Medicare Spending				
Medicare Spending per Patient (ratio)	-	-	1.04	0.98
Pneumonia Care				
Appropriate Initial Antibiotic Given	11	91%	98%	95%
Blood Culture Timing	20	100%	99%	98%
Pregnancy and Delivery Care				
Newborn Deliveries Scheduled Early[5]	-	-	6%	6%
Preventive Care				
Immunization for Influenza[2]	139	97%	94%	90%
Immunization for Pneumonia[2]	229	99%	96%	92%
Stroke Care				
Anticoagulation Therapy for Atrial Fibrillation[3,7]	-	-	97%	95%
Antithrombotic Therapy Timing[1,3]	-	-	98%	98%
Assessed for Rehabilitation[1,3]	-	-	97%	97%
Discharged on Antithrombotic Therapy[1,3]	-	-	99%	99%
Discharged on Statin Medication[3,7]	-	-	96%	94%
Thrombolytic Therapy Timing[3,7]	-	-	76%	66%
Venous Thromboembolism Prophylaxis[1,3]	-	-	95%	94%
Written Stroke Educational Materials Given[1,3]	-	-	94%	88%
Surgical Care Improvement Project				
Appropriate Beta Blocker Usage[5]	-	-	99%	98%
Appropriate VTP Within 24 Hours[5]	-	-	99%	98%
Controlled Postoperative Blood Glucose[5]	-	-	98%	97%
Perioperative Temperature Management[5]	-	-	100%	100%
Prophylactic Antibiotic Selection[5]	-	-	99%	99%
Prophylactic Antibiotic Selection (Outpatient)[5]	-	-	98%	98%
Prophylactic Antibiotic Stopped[5]	-	-	98%	98%
Prophylactic Antibiotic Timing[5]	-	-	99%	99%
Prophylactic Antibiotic Timing (Outpatient)[5]	-	-	98%	98%
Urinary Catheter Removal[5]	-	-	98%	97%
Survey of Patients' Hospital Experiences				
Area Around Room 'Always' Quiet at Night[10,11]	<100	68%	58%	61%
Doctors 'Always' Communicated Well[10,11]	<100	80%	77%	82%
Home Recovery Information Given[10,11]	<100	92%	83%	85%
Hospital Given 9 or 10 on 10 Point Scale[10,11]	<100	71%	67%	71%
Meds 'Always' Explained Before Given[10,11]	<100	75%	60%	64%
Nurses 'Always' Communicated Well[10,11]	<100	85%	75%	79%
Pain 'Always' Well Controlled[10,11]	<100	83%	68%	71%
Room and Bathroom 'Always' Clean[10,11]	<100	75%	69%	73%
Timely Help 'Always' Received[10,11]	<100	71%	62%	68%
Would Definitely Recommend Hospital[10,11]	<100	71%	69%	71%
Use of Medical Imaging				
Cardiac Imaging Stress Test before Surgery[7]	-	-	6.4%	5.3%
Combination Abdominal CT Scan	203	41.9%	11.8%	10.5%
Combination Brain/Sinus CT Scan[1]	-	-	3.4%	2.7%
Combination Chest CT Scan	104	4.8%	2.4%	2.7%
Follow-up Mammogram/Ultrasound[7]	-	-	10.2%	8.8%
Lumbar Spine MRI for Low Back Pain[1]	-	-	35.2%	37.2%

Wellington Regional Medical Center

10101 Forest Hill Blvd Phone: 561-798-8500
Wellington, FL 33414 Fax: 561-753-2619
URL: www.wellingtonregional.com
Type: Acute Care Hospitals Emergency Services: Yes
Ownership: Proprietary Beds: 143

Key Personnel:
CEO/President. . . . . Kevin DiLallo

Measure	Cases	This Hosp.	State Avg.	U.S. Avg.
Blood Clot Prevention and Treatment				
Anticoagulation Overlap Therapy[2]	52	100%	93%	93%
ICU Venous Thromboembolism Prophylaxis[2]	53	96%	94%	92%
Incidence of Potentially Preventable VTE[2]	19	11%	10%	10%
UFH with Dosages/Platelet Monitoring[2]	35	100%	100%	97%
Venous Thromboembolism Prophylaxis[2]	374	81%	88%	85%
Warfarin Therapy Discharge Instructions[2]	35	91%	85%	75%
Chest Pain/Possible Heart Attack Care				
Aspirin Given Within 24 Hours of Arrival[1,3]	-	-	98%	96%
Fibrinolytic Meds Within 30 Min. of Arrival[3,7]	-	-	81%	58%
Average Time to ECG (minutes)[1,3]	-	-	7	7
Average Time to Transfer (minutes)[3,7]	-	-	53	60
Children's Asthma Care				
Received Home Management Plan of Care	-	-	-	88%
Received Reliever Medication	-	-	-	100%
Received Systemic Corticosteroids	-	-	-	100%
Emergency Department				
Admittance Decision Time (minutes)[2]	719	184	111	98
Head CT Results Within 45 Min. of Arrival[1]	-	-	64%	57%
Patients Who Left ER Before Being Seen	21,741	1%	2%	2%
Time from ER Arrival to Admit. (minutes)[2]	725	383	289	274
Time from ER Arrival to Discharge (minutes)	408	144	147	134
Time in ER Before Being Evaluated (minutes)	378	21	26	26
Time to Pain Meds for Fractures (minutes)	102	71	60	57
Heart Attack Care				
Aspirin Given at Discharge	91	100%	99%	99%
Fibrinolytic Meds Within 30 Min. of Arrival[7]	-	-	50%	54%
PCI Within 90 Minutes of Arrival	33	100%	96%	96%
Statin Prescribed at Discharge	93	100%	99%	98%
Heart Failure Care				
ACE Inhibitor or ARB for LVSD[2]	54	100%	98%	97%
Discharge Instructions Given[2]	155	99%	96%	94%
Evaluation of LVS Function[2]	208	100%	100%	99%
Medicare Spending				
Medicare Spending per Patient (ratio)	-	1.11	1.04	0.98
Pneumonia Care				
Appropriate Initial Antibiotic Given[2]	109	100%	98%	95%
Blood Culture Timing[2]	190	97%	99%	98%
Pregnancy and Delivery Care				
Newborn Deliveries Scheduled Early[2]	43	5%	6%	6%
Preventive Care				
Immunization for Influenza[2]	502	84%	94%	90%
Immunization for Pneumonia[2]	534	93%	96%	92%
Stroke Care				
Anticoagulation Therapy for Atrial Fibrillation	11	100%	97%	95%
Antithrombotic Therapy Timing	78	97%	98%	98%
Assessed for Rehabilitation	91	98%	97%	97%
Discharged on Antithrombotic Therapy	84	100%	99%	99%
Discharged on Statin Medication	73	96%	96%	94%
Thrombolytic Therapy Timing[1]	-	-	76%	66%
Venous Thromboembolism Prophylaxis	101	91%	95%	94%
Written Stroke Educational Materials Given	50	100%	94%	88%
Surgical Care Improvement Project				
Appropriate Beta Blocker Usage[2]	107	99%	99%	98%
Appropriate VTP Within 24 Hours[2]	401	99%	99%	98%
Controlled Postoperative Blood Glucose[2,7]	-	-	98%	97%
Perioperative Temperature Management[2]	434	100%	100%	100%
Prophylactic Antibiotic Selection[2]	251	97%	99%	99%
Prophylactic Antibiotic Selection (Outpatient)	98	96%	98%	98%
Prophylactic Antibiotic Stopped[2]	242	100%	98%	98%
Prophylactic Antibiotic Timing[2]	251	100%	99%	99%
Prophylactic Antibiotic Timing (Outpatient)	99	99%	98%	98%
Urinary Catheter Removal[2]	291	99%	98%	97%
Survey of Patients' Hospital Experiences				
Area Around Room 'Always' Quiet at Night	300+	58%	58%	61%
Doctors 'Always' Communicated Well	300+	71%	77%	82%
Home Recovery Information Given	300+	79%	83%	85%
Hospital Given 9 or 10 on 10 Point Scale	300+	58%	67%	71%
Meds 'Always' Explained Before Given	300+	52%	60%	64%
Nurses 'Always' Communicated Well	300+	68%	75%	79%
Pain 'Always' Well Controlled	300+	61%	68%	71%
Room and Bathroom 'Always' Clean	300+	66%	69%	73%
Timely Help 'Always' Received	300+	49%	62%	68%
Would Definitely Recommend Hospital	300+	62%	69%	71%
Use of Medical Imaging				
Cardiac Imaging Stress Test before Surgery[1]	-	-	6.4%	5.3%
Combination Abdominal CT Scan	366	3.8%	11.8%	10.5%
Combination Brain/Sinus CT Scan	435	2.1%	3.4%	2.7%
Combination Chest CT Scan	127	1.6%	2.4%	2.7%
Follow-up Mammogram/Ultrasound	599	8.3%	10.2%	8.8%
Lumbar Spine MRI for Low Back Pain[1]	-	-	35.2%	37.2%

Florida Hospital Wesley Chapel

2600 Bruce B Downs Blvd Phone: 813-929-5490
Wesley Chapel, FL 33544
Type: Acute Care Hospitals Emergency Services: Yes
Ownership: Voluntary non-profit - Private

Measure	Cases	This Hosp.	State Avg.	U.S. Avg.
Blood Clot Prevention and Treatment				
Anticoagulation Overlap Therapy[2,3]	11	100%	93%	93%
ICU Venous Thromboembolism Prophylaxis[2,3]	26	100%	94%	92%
Incidence of Potentially Preventable VTE[1,2]	-	-	10%	10%
UFH with Dosages/Platelet Monitoring[1,2]	-	-	100%	97%
Venous Thromboembolism Prophylaxis[2,3]	151	100%	88%	85%

NOTE: Hospital profiles are in alphabetical order by state, then city, then hospital within the city; Rankings exclude hospitals with less than 25 cases except for patient surveys which excludes hospitals with less than 100 cases; (a) 100-299 cases; (1) The number of cases/patients is too few to report; (2) Data submitted were based on a sample of cases/patients; (3) Results are based on a shorter time period than required; (4) Data suppressed by CMS for one or more quarters; (5) Results are not available for this reporting period; (6) Fewer than 100 patients completed the HCAHPS survey; (7) No cases met the criteria for this measure; (8) The lower limit of the confidence interval cannot be calculated if the number of observed infections equals zero; (9) No data are available from the state/territory for this reporting period; (10) The scores shown reflect fewer than 50 completed surveys; (11) There were discrepancies in the data collection process; (12) This measure does not apply to this hospital for this reporting period; (13) Results cannot be calculated for this reporting period; (14) The results for this state are combined with nearby states to protect confidentiality; Please refer to the User's Guide for a full explanation of data.

Measure	Cases	This Hosp.	State Avg.	U.S. Avg.
Warfarin Therapy Discharge Instructions[1,2]	-	-	85%	75%
Chest Pain/Possible Heart Attack Care				
Aspirin Given Within 24 Hours of Arrival[1,3]	-	-	98%	96%
Fibrinolytic Meds Within 30 Min. of Arrival[3,7]	-	-	81%	58%
Average Time to ECG (minutes)[1,3]	-	-	7	7
Average Time to Transfer (minutes)[1,3]	-	-	53	60
Children's Asthma Care				
Received Home Management Plan of Care	-	-	-	88%
Received Reliever Medication	-	-	-	100%
Received Systemic Corticosteroids	-	-	-	100%
Emergency Department				
Admittance Decision Time (minutes)[2,3]	142	80	111	98
Head CT Results Within 45 Min. of Arrival[1,3]	-	-	64%	57%
Patients Who Left ER Before Being Seen[5]	-	-	2%	2%
Time from ER Arrival to Admit. (minutes)[2,3]	142	224	289	274
Time from ER Arrival to Discharge (minutes)[3]	93	141	147	134
Time in ER Before Being Evaluated (minutes)[3]	102	24	26	26
Time to Pain Meds for Fractures (minutes)[3]	21	44	60	57
Heart Attack Care				
Aspirin Given at Discharge[1,3]	-	-	99%	99%
Fibrinolytic Meds Within 30 Min. of Arrival[3,7]	-	-	50%	54%
PCI Within 90 Minutes of Arrival[3,7]	-	-	96%	96%
Statin Prescribed at Discharge[1,3]	-	-	99%	98%
Heart Failure Care				
ACE Inhibitor or ARB for LVSD[3]	11	100%	98%	97%
Discharge Instructions Given[3]	16	100%	96%	94%
Evaluation of LVS Function[3]	18	100%	100%	99%
Medicare Spending				
Medicare Spending per Patient (ratio)	-	0.97	1.04	0.98
Pneumonia Care				
Appropriate Initial Antibiotic Given[3]	12	100%	98%	95%
Blood Culture Timing[3]	22	100%	99%	98%
Pregnancy and Delivery Care				
Newborn Deliveries Scheduled Early[3]	13	15%	6%	6%
Preventive Care				
Immunization for Influenza[5]	-	-	94%	90%
Immunization for Pneumonia[2,3]	92	92%	96%	92%
Stroke Care				
Anticoagulation Therapy for Atrial Fibrillation[1,3]	-	-	97%	95%
Antithrombotic Therapy Timing[1,3]	-	-	98%	98%
Assessed for Rehabilitation[3]	13	100%	97%	97%
Discharged on Antithrombotic Therapy[3]	12	100%	99%	99%
Discharged on Statin Medication[1,3]	-	-	96%	94%
Thrombolytic Therapy Timing[1,3]	-	-	76%	66%
Venous Thromboembolism Prophylaxis[3]	13	100%	95%	94%
Written Stroke Educational Materials Given[1,3]	-	-	94%	88%
Surgical Care Improvement Project				
Appropriate Beta Blocker Usage[1,3]	-	-	99%	98%
Appropriate VTP Within 24 Hours[3]	29	100%	99%	98%
Controlled Postoperative Blood Glucose[3,7]	-	-	98%	97%
Perioperative Temperature Management[3]	29	100%	100%	100%
Prophylactic Antibiotic Selection[3]	17	94%	99%	99%
Prophylactic Antibiotic Selection (Outpatient)[3]	25	100%	98%	98%
Prophylactic Antibiotic Stopped[3]	15	100%	98%	98%
Prophylactic Antibiotic Timing[3]	17	100%	99%	99%
Prophylactic Antibiotic Timing (Outpatient)[3]	25	100%	98%	98%
Urinary Catheter Removal[3]	16	100%	98%	97%
Survey of Patients' Hospital Experiences				
Area Around Room 'Always' Quiet at Night[5]	-	-	58%	61%
Doctors 'Always' Communicated Well[5]	-	-	77%	82%
Home Recovery Information Given[5]	-	-	83%	85%
Hospital Given 9 or 10 on 10 Point Scale[5]	-	-	67%	71%
Meds 'Always' Explained Before Given[5]	-	-	60%	64%
Nurses 'Always' Communicated Well[5]	-	-	75%	79%
Pain 'Always' Well Controlled[5]	-	-	68%	71%
Room and Bathroom 'Always' Clean[5]	-	-	69%	73%
Timely Help 'Always' Received[5]	-	-	62%	68%
Would Definitely Recommend Hospital[5]	-	-	69%	71%
Use of Medical Imaging				
Cardiac Imaging Stress Test before Surgery[1]	-	-	6.4%	5.3%
Combination Abdominal CT Scan	148	8.8%	11.8%	10.5%
Combination Brain/Sinus CT Scan	184	5.4%	3.4%	2.7%
Combination Chest CT Scan[1]	-	-	2.4%	2.7%
Follow-up Mammogram/Ultrasound[1]	-	-	10.2%	8.8%
Lumbar Spine MRI for Low Back Pain[1]	-	-	35.2%	37.2%

Good Samaritan Medical Center

1309 N Flagler Dr
West Palm Beach, FL 33401
Phone: 561-655-5511
Fax: 561-650-6127
URL: www.goodsamaritanmc.com
Type: Acute Care Hospitals
Emergency Services: Yes
Ownership: Proprietary
Beds: 341

Key Personnel:
Quality Assurance . . . . Peter Bleswas
Radiology. . . . . David Herold, MD
Chief of Medical Staff . . . . Daniel R Higgins, MD
Infection Control. . . . . Arlene Merrill
CEO/President . . . . Mark Nosacka
Pediatric Ambulatory Care . . . . . . Ronald A Romear, MD
Pediatric In-Patient Care . . . . Ronald A Romear, MD

Measure	Cases	This Hosp.	State Avg.	U.S. Avg.
Blood Clot Prevention and Treatment				
Anticoagulation Overlap Therapy[2]	72	99%	93%	93%
ICU Venous Thromboembolism Prophylaxis[2]	64	97%	94%	92%
Incidence of Potentially Preventable VTE[1,2]	-	-	10%	10%
UFH with Dosages/Platelet Monitoring[2]	36	100%	100%	97%
Venous Thromboembolism Prophylaxis[2]	357	95%	88%	85%
Warfarin Therapy Discharge Instructions[2]	39	100%	85%	75%
Chest Pain/Possible Heart Attack Care				
Aspirin Given Within 24 Hours of Arrival[1,3]	-	-	98%	96%
Fibrinolytic Meds Within 30 Min. of Arrival[5]	-	-	81%	58%
Average Time to ECG (minutes)[1,3]	-	-	7	7
Average Time to Transfer (minutes)[5]	-	-	53	60
Children's Asthma Care				
Received Home Management Plan of Care	-	-	-	88%
Received Reliever Medication	-	-	-	100%
Received Systemic Corticosteroids	-	-	-	100%
Emergency Department				
Admittance Decision Time (minutes)[2]	766	178	111	98
Head CT Results Within 45 Min. of Arrival	13	85%	64%	57%
Patients Who Left ER Before Being Seen	30,808	4%	2%	2%
Time from ER Arrival to Admit. (minutes)[2]	766	340	289	274
Time from ER Arrival to Discharge (minutes)	387	133	147	134
Time in ER Before Being Evaluated (minutes)	454	12	26	26
Time to Pain Meds for Fractures (minutes)	32	44	60	57
Heart Attack Care				
Aspirin Given at Discharge	53	100%	99%	99%
Fibrinolytic Meds Within 30 Min. of Arrival[7]	-	-	50%	54%
PCI Within 90 Minutes of Arrival	22	100%	96%	96%
Statin Prescribed at Discharge	54	100%	99%	98%
Heart Failure Care				
ACE Inhibitor or ARB for LVSD	55	100%	98%	97%
Discharge Instructions Given	160	99%	96%	94%
Evaluation of LVS Function	198	100%	100%	99%
Medicare Spending				
Medicare Spending per Patient (ratio)	-	1.07	1.04	0.98
Pneumonia Care				
Appropriate Initial Antibiotic Given	122	98%	98%	95%
Blood Culture Timing	199	98%	99%	98%
Pregnancy and Delivery Care				
Newborn Deliveries Scheduled Early[2]	35	3%	6%	6%
Preventive Care				
Immunization for Influenza[2]	598	91%	94%	90%
Immunization for Pneumonia[2]	743	95%	96%	92%
Stroke Care				
Anticoagulation Therapy for Atrial Fibrillation[1]	-	-	97%	95%
Antithrombotic Therapy Timing	52	100%	98%	98%
Assessed for Rehabilitation	50	98%	97%	97%
Discharged on Antithrombotic Therapy	46	98%	99%	99%
Discharged on Statin Medication	36	97%	96%	94%
Thrombolytic Therapy Timing[1]	-	-	76%	66%
Venous Thromboembolism Prophylaxis	54	98%	95%	94%
Written Stroke Educational Materials Given	25	100%	94%	88%
Surgical Care Improvement Project				
Appropriate Beta Blocker Usage[2]	137	98%	99%	98%
Appropriate VTP Within 24 Hours[2]	444	95%	99%	98%
Controlled Postoperative Blood Glucose[2,7]	-	-	98%	97%
Perioperative Temperature Management[2]	509	100%	100%	100%
Prophylactic Antibiotic Selection[2]	278	98%	99%	99%
Prophylactic Antibiotic Selection (Outpatient)	286	92%	98%	98%
Prophylactic Antibiotic Stopped[2]	252	96%	98%	98%
Prophylactic Antibiotic Timing[2]	279	99%	99%	99%
Prophylactic Antibiotic Timing (Outpatient)	289	98%	98%	98%
Urinary Catheter Removal[2]	256	98%	98%	97%
Survey of Patients' Hospital Experiences				
Area Around Room 'Always' Quiet at Night	300+	63%	58%	61%
Doctors 'Always' Communicated Well	300+	82%	77%	82%
Home Recovery Information Given	300+	80%	83%	85%
Hospital Given 9 or 10 on 10 Point Scale	300+	65%	67%	71%
Meds 'Always' Explained Before Given	300+	55%	60%	64%
Nurses 'Always' Communicated Well	300+	72%	75%	79%
Pain 'Always' Well Controlled	300+	66%	68%	71%
Room and Bathroom 'Always' Clean	300+	60%	69%	73%
Timely Help 'Always' Received	300+	55%	62%	68%
Would Definitely Recommend Hospital	300+	70%	69%	71%
Use of Medical Imaging				
Cardiac Imaging Stress Test before Surgery	210	8.6%	6.4%	5.3%
Combination Abdominal CT Scan	1,195	14.5%	11.8%	10.5%
Combination Brain/Sinus CT Scan	891	2.4%	3.4%	2.7%
Combination Chest CT Scan	760	1.1%	2.4%	2.7%
Follow-up Mammogram/Ultrasound	2,020	14.4%	10.2%	8.8%
Lumbar Spine MRI for Low Back Pain	242	37.6%	35.2%	37.2%

Saint Mary's Medical Center

901 45th St
West Palm Beach, FL 33407
Phone: 561-840-6202
Fax: 561-882-1025
URL: www.stmarysmc.com
Type: Acute Care Hospitals
Emergency Services: Yes
Ownership: Proprietary
Beds: 460

Key Personnel:
Infection Control. . . . . G Alexander Carden, MD
Emergency Room . . . . Patricia Connor, RN
Chief of Medical Staff . . . . David Dodson, MD
Intensive Care Unit. . . . . Connie Rigg, RN
Radiology. . . . . Nicholas Rojo, MD
Pediatric In-Patient Care . . . . Tommy Schechtman, MD
Anesthesiology. . . . . Mitchell Untracht, MD

Measure	Cases	This Hosp.	State Avg.	U.S. Avg.
Blood Clot Prevention and Treatment				
Anticoagulation Overlap Therapy[2]	45	100%	93%	93%
ICU Venous Thromboembolism Prophylaxis[2]	71	100%	94%	92%
Incidence of Potentially Preventable VTE[2]	20	0%	10%	10%
UFH with Dosages/Platelet Monitoring[2]	31	100%	100%	97%
Venous Thromboembolism Prophylaxis[2]	347	98%	88%	85%
Warfarin Therapy Discharge Instructions[2]	29	100%	85%	75%
Chest Pain/Possible Heart Attack Care				
Aspirin Given Within 24 Hours of Arrival	15	93%	98%	96%
Fibrinolytic Meds Within 30 Min. of Arrival[7]	-	-	81%	58%
Average Time to ECG (minutes)	15	12	7	7
Average Time to Transfer (minutes)[1]	-	-	53	60
Children's Asthma Care				
Received Home Management Plan of Care	-	-	-	88%
Received Reliever Medication	-	-	-	100%
Received Systemic Corticosteroids	-	-	-	100%
Emergency Department				
Admittance Decision Time (minutes)[2]	626	147	111	98
Head CT Results Within 45 Min. of Arrival[1]	-	-	64%	57%
Patients Who Left ER Before Being Seen	61,273	5%	2%	2%
Time from ER Arrival to Admit. (minutes)[2]	626	340	289	274
Time from ER Arrival to Discharge (minutes)	471	133	147	134
Time in ER Before Being Evaluated (minutes)	497	30	26	26
Time to Pain Meds for Fractures (minutes)	148	58	60	57
Heart Attack Care				
Aspirin Given at Discharge	11	100%	99%	99%
Fibrinolytic Meds Within 30 Min. of Arrival[7]	-	-	50%	54%
PCI Within 90 Minutes of Arrival[7]	-	-	96%	96%
Statin Prescribed at Discharge	12	100%	99%	98%
Heart Failure Care				
ACE Inhibitor or ARB for LVSD	51	98%	98%	97%
Discharge Instructions Given	105	100%	96%	94%

NOTE: Hospital profiles are in alphabetical order by state, then city, then hospital within the city; Rankings exclude hospitals with less than 25 cases except for patient surveys which excludes hospitals with less than 100 cases; (a) 100-299 cases; (1) The number of cases/patients is too few to report; (2) Data submitted were based on a sample of cases/patients; (3) Results are based on a shorter time period than required; (4) Data suppressed by CMS for one or more quarters; (5) Results are not available for this reporting period; (6) Fewer than 100 patients completed the HCAHPS survey; (7) No cases met the criteria for this measure; (8) The lower limit of the confidence interval cannot be calculated if the number of observed infections equals zero; (9) No data are available from the state/territory for this reporting period; (10) The scores shown reflect fewer than 50 completed surveys; (11) There were discrepancies in the data collection process; (12) This measure does not apply to this hospital for this reporting period; (13) Results cannot be calculated for this reporting period; (14) The results for this state are combined with nearby states to protect confidentiality; Please refer to the User's Guide for a full explanation of data.

Measure	Cases	This Hosp.	State Avg.	U.S. Avg.
Evaluation of LVS Function	125	100%	100%	99%
Medicare Spending				
Medicare Spending per Patient (ratio)	-	1.08	1.04	0.98
Pneumonia Care				
Appropriate Initial Antibiotic Given	53	100%	98%	95%
Blood Culture Timing	102	97%	99%	98%
Pregnancy and Delivery Care				
Newborn Deliveries Scheduled Early[2]	58	2%	6%	6%
Preventive Care				
Immunization for Influenza[2]	507	96%	94%	90%
Immunization for Pneumonia[2]	260	97%	96%	92%
Stroke Care				
Anticoagulation Therapy for Atrial Fibrillation[2]	11	91%	97%	95%
Antithrombotic Therapy Timing[2]	119	100%	98%	98%
Assessed for Rehabilitation[2]	188	99%	97%	97%
Discharged on Antithrombotic Therapy[2]	132	100%	99%	99%
Discharged on Statin Medication[2]	98	99%	96%	94%
Thrombolytic Therapy Timing[2]	21	95%	76%	66%
Venous Thromboembolism Prophylaxis[2]	243	100%	95%	94%
Written Stroke Educational Materials Given[2]	105	99%	94%	88%
Surgical Care Improvement Project				
Appropriate Beta Blocker Usage[2]	62	98%	99%	98%
Appropriate VTP Within 24 Hours[2]	248	99%	99%	98%
Controlled Postoperative Blood Glucose[1,2]	-	-	98%	97%
Perioperative Temperature Management[2]	302	100%	100%	100%
Prophylactic Antibiotic Selection[2]	196	96%	99%	99%
Prophylactic Antibiotic Selection (Outpatient)	18	89%	98%	98%
Prophylactic Antibiotic Stopped[2]	183	99%	98%	98%
Prophylactic Antibiotic Timing[2]	196	98%	99%	99%
Prophylactic Antibiotic Timing (Outpatient)	20	90%	98%	98%
Urinary Catheter Removal[2]	181	99%	98%	97%
Survey of Patients' Hospital Experiences				
Area Around Room 'Always' Quiet at Night	300+	55%	58%	61%
Doctors 'Always' Communicated Well	300+	76%	77%	82%
Home Recovery Information Given	300+	80%	83%	85%
Hospital Given 9 or 10 on 10 Point Scale	300+	65%	67%	71%
Meds 'Always' Explained Before Given	300+	60%	60%	64%
Nurses 'Always' Communicated Well	300+	73%	75%	79%
Pain 'Always' Well Controlled	300+	68%	68%	71%
Room and Bathroom 'Always' Clean	300+	63%	69%	73%
Timely Help 'Always' Received	300+	58%	62%	68%
Would Definitely Recommend Hospital	300+	68%	69%	71%
Use of Medical Imaging				
Cardiac Imaging Stress Test before Surgery[1]	-	-	6.4%	5.3%
Combination Abdominal CT Scan	168	2.4%	11.8%	10.5%
Combination Brain/Sinus CT Scan[1]	-	-	3.4%	2.7%
Combination Chest CT Scan	49	4.1%	2.4%	2.7%
Follow-up Mammogram/Ultrasound	133	12.0%	10.2%	8.8%
Lumbar Spine MRI for Low Back Pain[1]	-	-	35.2%	37.2%

W Palm Beach VA Medical Center

7305 N. Military Trail
West Palm Beach, FL 33410
Phone: 561-422-8600
Fax: 561-422-7706
URL: www.va.gov
Type: Acute Care - VA
Emergency Services: No
Ownership: Government Federal
Beds: 270
Key Personnel:
Chief of Medical Staff .... Deepak Mandi, MD

Measure	Cases	This Hosp.	State Avg.	U.S. Avg.
Blood Clot Prevention and Treatment				
Anticoagulation Overlap Therapy	-	-	93%	93%
ICU Venous Thromboembolism Prophylaxis	-	-	94%	92%
Incidence of Potentially Preventable VTE	-	-	10%	10%
UFH with Dosages/Platelet Monitoring	-	-	100%	97%
Venous Thromboembolism Prophylaxis	-	-	88%	85%
Warfarin Therapy Discharge Instructions	-	-	85%	75%
Chest Pain/Possible Heart Attack Care				
Aspirin Given Within 24 Hours of Arrival	-	-	98%	96%
Fibrinolytic Meds Within 30 Min. of Arrival	-	-	81%	58%
Average Time to ECG (minutes)	-	-	7	7
Average Time to Transfer (minutes)	-	-	53	60
Children's Asthma Care				
Received Home Management Plan of Care	-	-	-	88%
Received Reliever Medication	-	-	-	100%
Received Systemic Corticosteroids	-	-	-	100%
Emergency Department				
Admittance Decision Time (minutes)	-	-	111	98
Head CT Results Within 45 Min. of Arrival	-	-	64%	57%
Patients Who Left ER Before Being Seen	-	-	2%	2%
Time from ER Arrival to Admit. (minutes)	-	-	289	274
Time from ER Arrival to Discharge (minutes)	-	-	147	134
Time in ER Before Being Evaluated (minutes)	-	-	26	26
Time to Pain Meds for Fractures (minutes)	-	-	60	57
Heart Attack Care				
Aspirin Given at Discharge[1]	13	100%	99%	99%
Fibrinolytic Meds Within 30 Min. of Arrival[5]	-	-	50%	54%
PCI Within 90 Minutes of Arrival[5]	-	-	96%	96%
Statin Prescribed at Discharge[1]	15	93%	99%	98%
Heart Failure Care				
ACE Inhibitor or ARB for LVSD	78	99%	98%	97%
Discharge Instructions Given	222	95%	96%	94%
Evaluation of LVS Function	250	100%	100%	99%
Medicare Spending				
Medicare Spending per Patient (ratio)	-	-	1.04	0.98
Pneumonia Care				
Appropriate Initial Antibiotic Given	101	100%	98%	95%
Blood Culture Timing	143	99%	99%	98%
Pregnancy and Delivery Care				
Newborn Deliveries Scheduled Early	-	-	6%	6%
Preventive Care				
Immunization for Influenza[5]	-	-	94%	90%
Immunization for Pneumonia[5]	-	-	96%	92%
Stroke Care				
Anticoagulation Therapy for Atrial Fibrillation	-	-	97%	95%
Antithrombotic Therapy Timing	-	-	98%	98%
Assessed for Rehabilitation	-	-	97%	97%
Discharged on Antithrombotic Therapy	-	-	99%	99%
Discharged on Statin Medication	-	-	96%	94%
Thrombolytic Therapy Timing	-	-	76%	66%
Venous Thromboembolism Prophylaxis	-	-	95%	94%
Written Stroke Educational Materials Given	-	-	94%	88%
Surgical Care Improvement Project				
Appropriate Beta Blocker Usage[2]	54	100%	99%	98%
Appropriate VTP Within 24 Hours[2]	156	100%	99%	98%
Controlled Postoperative Blood Glucose[5]	-	-	98%	97%
Perioperative Temperature Management[2]	170	100%	100%	100%
Prophylactic Antibiotic Selection	90	98%	99%	99%
Prophylactic Antibiotic Selection (Outpatient)	-	-	98%	98%
Prophylactic Antibiotic Stopped	88	97%	98%	98%
Prophylactic Antibiotic Timing	90	99%	99%	99%
Prophylactic Antibiotic Timing (Outpatient)	-	-	98%	98%
Urinary Catheter Removal[2]	86	100%	98%	97%
Survey of Patients' Hospital Experiences				
Area Around Room 'Always' Quiet at Night	-	-	58%	61%
Doctors 'Always' Communicated Well	-	-	77%	82%
Home Recovery Information Given	-	-	83%	85%
Hospital Given 9 or 10 on 10 Point Scale	-	-	67%	71%
Meds 'Always' Explained Before Given	-	-	60%	64%
Nurses 'Always' Communicated Well	-	-	75%	79%
Pain 'Always' Well Controlled	-	-	68%	71%
Room and Bathroom 'Always' Clean	-	-	69%	73%
Timely Help 'Always' Received	-	-	62%	68%
Would Definitely Recommend Hospital	-	-	69%	71%
Use of Medical Imaging				
Cardiac Imaging Stress Test before Surgery	-	-	6.4%	5.3%
Combination Abdominal CT Scan	-	-	11.8%	10.5%
Combination Brain/Sinus CT Scan	-	-	3.4%	2.7%
Combination Chest CT Scan	-	-	2.4%	2.7%
Follow-up Mammogram/Ultrasound	-	-	10.2%	8.8%
Lumbar Spine MRI for Low Back Pain	-	-	35.2%	37.2%

West Palm Hospital

2201 45th St
West Palm Beach, FL 33407
Phone: 561-844-6141
Fax: 561-844-8955
URL: www.columbiahospital.com
Type: Acute Care Hospitals
Emergency Services: Yes
Ownership: Proprietary
Beds: 250
Key Personnel:
Quality Assurance .... Mary Kelly
Emergency Room .... Dennis Keown
Radiology.................. Kim Mullin
CEO .... Dana C. Oaks
Operating Room.............. Gary Reardon
Patient Relations .... Simone Scime

Measure	Cases	This Hosp.	State Avg.	U.S. Avg.
Blood Clot Prevention and Treatment				
Anticoagulation Overlap Therapy[2]	32	94%	93%	93%
ICU Venous Thromboembolism Prophylaxis[2]	79	99%	94%	92%
Incidence of Potentially Preventable VTE[1,2]	-	-	10%	10%
UFH with Dosages/Platelet Monitoring[2]	29	100%	100%	97%
Venous Thromboembolism Prophylaxis[2]	275	95%	88%	85%
Warfarin Therapy Discharge Instructions[2]	25	100%	85%	75%
Chest Pain/Possible Heart Attack Care				
Aspirin Given Within 24 Hours of Arrival	20	100%	98%	96%
Fibrinolytic Meds Within 30 Min. of Arrival[7]	-	-	81%	58%
Average Time to ECG (minutes)	20	10	7	7
Average Time to Transfer (minutes)[1]	-	-	53	60
Children's Asthma Care				
Received Home Management Plan of Care	-	-	-	88%
Received Reliever Medication	-	-	-	100%
Received Systemic Corticosteroids	-	-	-	100%
Emergency Department				
Admittance Decision Time (minutes)[2]	895	81	111	98
Head CT Results Within 45 Min. of Arrival[1]	-	-	64%	57%
Patients Who Left ER Before Being Seen	25,606	1%	2%	2%
Time from ER Arrival to Admit. (minutes)[2]	895	223	289	274
Time from ER Arrival to Discharge (minutes)	398	116	147	134
Time in ER Before Being Evaluated (minutes)	453	4	26	26
Time to Pain Meds for Fractures (minutes)	36	50	60	57
Heart Attack Care				
Aspirin Given at Discharge	16	100%	99%	99%
Fibrinolytic Meds Within 30 Min. of Arrival[7]	-	-	50%	54%
PCI Within 90 Minutes of Arrival[7]	-	-	96%	96%
Statin Prescribed at Discharge	17	100%	99%	98%
Heart Failure Care				
ACE Inhibitor or ARB for LVSD	19	100%	98%	97%
Discharge Instructions Given	98	100%	96%	94%
Evaluation of LVS Function	135	100%	100%	99%
Medicare Spending				
Medicare Spending per Patient (ratio)	-	1.08	1.04	0.98
Pneumonia Care				
Appropriate Initial Antibiotic Given	47	100%	98%	95%
Blood Culture Timing	109	100%	99%	98%
Pregnancy and Delivery Care				
Newborn Deliveries Scheduled Early[2,7]	-	-	6%	6%
Preventive Care				
Immunization for Influenza[2]	594	100%	94%	90%
Immunization for Pneumonia[2]	744	100%	96%	92%
Stroke Care				
Anticoagulation Therapy for Atrial Fibrillation[1,2]	-	-	97%	95%
Antithrombotic Therapy Timing[2]	32	100%	98%	98%
Assessed for Rehabilitation[2]	33	94%	97%	97%
Discharged on Antithrombotic Therapy[2]	31	100%	99%	99%
Discharged on Statin Medication[2]	26	100%	96%	94%
Thrombolytic Therapy Timing[1,2]	-	-	76%	66%
Venous Thromboembolism Prophylaxis[2]	33	97%	95%	94%
Written Stroke Educational Materials Given[2]	18	100%	94%	88%
Surgical Care Improvement Project				
Appropriate Beta Blocker Usage	66	100%	99%	98%
Appropriate VTP Within 24 Hours	183	99%	99%	98%
Controlled Postoperative Blood Glucose[7]	-	-	98%	97%
Perioperative Temperature Management	208	100%	100%	100%
Prophylactic Antibiotic Selection	117	100%	99%	99%
Prophylactic Antibiotic Selection (Outpatient)	51	100%	98%	98%
Prophylactic Antibiotic Stopped	107	100%	98%	98%

NOTE: Hospital profiles are in alphabetical order by state, then city, then hospital within the city; Rankings exclude hospitals with less than 25 cases except for patient surveys which excludes hospitals with less than 100 cases; (a) 100-299 cases; (1) The number of cases/patients is too few to report; (2) Data submitted were based on a sample of cases/patients; (3) Results are based on a shorter time period than required; (4) Data suppressed by CMS for one or more quarters; (5) Results are not available for this reporting period; (6) Fewer than 100 patients completed the HCAHPS survey; (7) No cases met the criteria for this measure; (8) The lower limit of the confidence interval cannot be calculated if the number of observed infections equals zero; (9) No data are available from the state/territory for this reporting period; (10) The scores shown reflect fewer than 50 completed surveys; (11) There were discrepancies in the data collection process; (12) This measure does not apply to this hospital for this reporting period; (13) Results cannot be calculated for this reporting period; (14) The results for this state are combined with nearby states to protect confidentiality; Please refer to the User's Guide for a full explanation of data.

Prophylactic Antibiotic Timing	117	100%	99%	99%
Prophylactic Antibiotic Timing (Outpatient)	51	100%	98%	98%
Urinary Catheter Removal	99	100%	98%	97%
Survey of Patients' Hospital Experiences				
Area Around Room 'Always' Quiet at Night	300+	65%	58%	61%
Doctors 'Always' Communicated Well	300+	77%	77%	82%
Home Recovery Information Given	300+	82%	83%	85%
Hospital Given 9 or 10 on 10 Point Scale	300+	67%	67%	71%
Meds 'Always' Explained Before Given	300+	62%	60%	64%
Nurses 'Always' Communicated Well	300+	74%	75%	79%
Pain 'Always' Well Controlled	300+	69%	68%	71%
Room and Bathroom 'Always' Clean	300+	69%	69%	73%
Timely Help 'Always' Received	300+	63%	62%	68%
Would Definitely Recommend Hospital	300+	69%	69%	71%
Use of Medical Imaging				
Cardiac Imaging Stress Test before Surgery[1]	-	-	6.4%	5.3%
Combination Abdominal CT Scan	156	1.9%	11.8%	10.5%
Combination Brain/Sinus CT Scan[1]	-	-	3.4%	2.7%
Combination Chest CT Scan[1]	-	-	2.4%	2.7%
Follow-up Mammogram/Ultrasound	68	23.5%	10.2%	8.8%
Lumbar Spine MRI for Low Back Pain[1]	-	-	35.2%	37.2%

Cleveland Clinic Hospital

3100 Weston Rd
Weston, FL 33331
Phone: 954-689-5000
Fax: 954-689-5058
URL: www.clevelandclinic.org
Type: Acute Care Hospitals
Emergency Services: Yes
Ownership: Proprietary
Beds: 150

Key Personnel:
Radiology. . . . . Manzoor Ahmed
CEO/President. . . . . Bernardo Fernandez
Infection Control. . . . . Margaret Govensele, MD
Operating Room. . . . . Juan Noqueras
Chief of Medical Staff. . . . . Eduardo Oliviera
Pediatric Ambulatory Care . . . . . . Rudolph R Roskos, MD
Pediatric In-Patient Care . . . . Rudolph R Roskos, MD
Quality Assurance . . . . Georgia Ruf, RN

Measure	Cases	This Hosp.	State Avg.	U.S. Avg.
Blood Clot Prevention and Treatment				
Anticoagulation Overlap Therapy[2]	41	98%	93%	93%
ICU Venous Thromboembolism Prophylaxis[2]	54	100%	94%	92%
Incidence of Potentially Preventable VTE[2]	21	10%	10%	10%
UFH with Dosages/Platelet Monitoring[2]	45	100%	100%	97%
Venous Thromboembolism Prophylaxis[2]	311	95%	88%	85%
Warfarin Therapy Discharge Instructions[2]	27	41%	85%	75%
Chest Pain/Possible Heart Attack Care				
Aspirin Given Within 24 Hours of Arrival[1,3]	-	-	98%	96%
Fibrinolytic Meds Within 30 Min. of Arrival[5]	-	-	81%	58%
Average Time to ECG (minutes)[1,3]	-	-	7	7
Average Time to Transfer (minutes)[5]	-	-	53	60
Children's Asthma Care				
Received Home Management Plan of Care	-	-	-	88%
Received Reliever Medication	-	-	-	100%
Received Systemic Corticosteroids	-	-	-	100%
Emergency Department				
Admittance Decision Time (minutes)[2]	559	214	111	98
Head CT Results Within 45 Min. of Arrival[1]	-	-	64%	57%
Patients Who Left ER Before Being Seen	33,380	0%	2%	2%
Time from ER Arrival to Admit. (minutes)[2]	562	355	289	274
Time from ER Arrival to Discharge (minutes)	386	130	147	134
Time in ER Before Being Evaluated (minutes)	415	14	26	26
Time to Pain Meds for Fractures (minutes)	90	39	60	57
Heart Attack Care				
Aspirin Given at Discharge	122	100%	99%	99%
Fibrinolytic Meds Within 30 Min. of Arrival[7]	-	-	50%	54%
PCI Within 90 Minutes of Arrival	22	91%	96%	96%
Statin Prescribed at Discharge	118	100%	99%	98%
Heart Failure Care				
ACE Inhibitor or ARB for LVSD	78	97%	98%	97%
Discharge Instructions Given	256	99%	96%	94%
Evaluation of LVS Function	297	100%	100%	99%
Medicare Spending				
Medicare Spending per Patient (ratio)	-	1.01	1.04	0.98
Pneumonia Care				
Appropriate Initial Antibiotic Given	88	99%	98%	95%
Blood Culture Timing	191	100%	99%	98%
Pregnancy and Delivery Care				
Newborn Deliveries Scheduled Early[2,7]	-	-	6%	6%
Preventive Care				
Immunization for Influenza[2]	620	96%	94%	90%
Immunization for Pneumonia[2]	763	95%	96%	92%
Stroke Care				
Anticoagulation Therapy for Atrial Fibrillation[1]	-	-	97%	95%
Antithrombotic Therapy Timing	47	100%	98%	98%
Assessed for Rehabilitation	78	100%	97%	97%
Discharged on Antithrombotic Therapy	68	100%	99%	99%
Discharged on Statin Medication	54	100%	96%	94%
Thrombolytic Therapy Timing[1]	-	-	76%	66%
Venous Thromboembolism Prophylaxis	65	100%	95%	94%
Written Stroke Educational Materials Given	61	98%	94%	88%
Surgical Care Improvement Project				
Appropriate Beta Blocker Usage[2]	172	97%	99%	98%
Appropriate VTP Within 24 Hours[2]	322	99%	99%	98%
Controlled Postoperative Blood Glucose[2]	133	95%	98%	97%
Perioperative Temperature Management[2]	404	100%	100%	100%
Prophylactic Antibiotic Selection[2]	329	100%	99%	99%
Prophylactic Antibiotic Selection (Outpatient)	761	97%	98%	98%
Prophylactic Antibiotic Stopped[2]	320	99%	98%	98%
Prophylactic Antibiotic Timing[2]	330	99%	99%	99%
Prophylactic Antibiotic Timing (Outpatient)	762	100%	98%	98%
Urinary Catheter Removal[2]	331	97%	98%	97%
Survey of Patients' Hospital Experiences				
Area Around Room 'Always' Quiet at Night	300+	68%	58%	61%
Doctors 'Always' Communicated Well	300+	82%	77%	82%
Home Recovery Information Given	300+	83%	83%	85%
Hospital Given 9 or 10 on 10 Point Scale	300+	80%	67%	71%
Meds 'Always' Explained Before Given	300+	69%	60%	64%
Nurses 'Always' Communicated Well	300+	79%	75%	79%
Pain 'Always' Well Controlled	300+	72%	68%	71%
Room and Bathroom 'Always' Clean	300+	72%	69%	73%
Timely Help 'Always' Received	300+	66%	62%	68%
Would Definitely Recommend Hospital	300+	84%	69%	71%
Use of Medical Imaging				
Cardiac Imaging Stress Test before Surgery	46	4.3%	6.4%	5.3%
Combination Abdominal CT Scan	1,161	26.6%	11.8%	10.5%
Combination Brain/Sinus CT Scan	540	0.9%	3.4%	2.7%
Combination Chest CT Scan	1,147	0.8%	2.4%	2.7%
Follow-up Mammogram/Ultrasound	1,127	19.1%	10.2%	8.8%
Lumbar Spine MRI for Low Back Pain	157	37.6%	35.2%	37.2%

Winter Haven Hospital

200 Ave F Ne
Winter Haven, FL 33881
Phone: 863-293-1121
Fax: 863-291-6028
URL: www.winterhavenhospital.com
Type: Acute Care Hospitals
Emergency Services: Yes
Ownership: Voluntary non-profit - Private
Beds: 604

Key Personnel:
CEO/President. . . . . Lance Anastasio
Quality Assurance . . . . Merle Libby
Operating Room. . . . . Delores Miley, RN
Radiology. . . . . Tony Patrick
Pediatric Ambulatory Care . . . . . . George Pilapil, MD
Pediatric In-Patient Care . . . . George Pilapil, MD
Infection Control. . . . . Larry Vargo
Chief of Medical Staff. . . . . Peter Verril, MD

Measure	Cases	This Hosp.	State Avg.	U.S. Avg.
Blood Clot Prevention and Treatment				
Anticoagulation Overlap Therapy[2]	134	96%	93%	93%
ICU Venous Thromboembolism Prophylaxis[2]	98	94%	94%	92%
Incidence of Potentially Preventable VTE[2]	13	23%	10%	10%
UFH with Dosages/Platelet Monitoring[2]	78	100%	100%	97%
Venous Thromboembolism Prophylaxis[2]	279	76%	88%	85%
Warfarin Therapy Discharge Instructions[2]	87	76%	85%	75%
Chest Pain/Possible Heart Attack Care				
Aspirin Given Within 24 Hours of Arrival[1]	-	-	98%	96%
Fibrinolytic Meds Within 30 Min. of Arrival[3,7]	-	-	81%	58%
Average Time to ECG (minutes)[1]	-	-	7	7
Average Time to Transfer (minutes)[3,7]	-	-	53	60
Children's Asthma Care				
Received Home Management Plan of Care	-	-	-	88%
Received Reliever Medication	-	-	-	100%
Received Systemic Corticosteroids	-	-	-	100%
Emergency Department				
Admittance Decision Time (minutes)[2]	684	164	111	98
Head CT Results Within 45 Min. of Arrival	20	70%	64%	57%
Patients Who Left ER Before Being Seen	64,685	4%	2%	2%
Time from ER Arrival to Admit. (minutes)[2]	695	394	289	274
Time from ER Arrival to Discharge (minutes)	407	236	147	134
Time in ER Before Being Evaluated (minutes)	390	102	26	26
Time to Pain Meds for Fractures (minutes)	191	100	60	57
Heart Attack Care				
Aspirin Given at Discharge	355	97%	99%	99%
Fibrinolytic Meds Within 30 Min. of Arrival[7]	-	-	50%	54%
PCI Within 90 Minutes of Arrival	55	93%	96%	96%
Statin Prescribed at Discharge	348	95%	99%	98%
Heart Failure Care				
ACE Inhibitor or ARB for LVSD[2]	141	91%	98%	97%
Discharge Instructions Given[2]	235	83%	96%	94%
Evaluation of LVS Function[2]	330	100%	100%	99%
Medicare Spending				
Medicare Spending per Patient (ratio)	-	1.11	1.04	0.98
Pneumonia Care				
Appropriate Initial Antibiotic Given[2]	80	89%	98%	95%
Blood Culture Timing[2]	153	97%	99%	98%
Pregnancy and Delivery Care				
Newborn Deliveries Scheduled Early[2]	32	3%	6%	6%
Preventive Care				
Immunization for Influenza[2]	574	88%	94%	90%
Immunization for Pneumonia[2]	735	92%	96%	92%
Stroke Care				
Anticoagulation Therapy for Atrial Fibrillation	20	95%	97%	95%
Antithrombotic Therapy Timing	142	92%	98%	98%
Assessed for Rehabilitation	159	98%	97%	97%
Discharged on Antithrombotic Therapy	155	98%	99%	99%
Discharged on Statin Medication	107	93%	96%	94%
Thrombolytic Therapy Timing	14	79%	76%	66%
Venous Thromboembolism Prophylaxis	158	97%	95%	94%
Written Stroke Educational Materials Given	88	98%	94%	88%
Surgical Care Improvement Project				
Appropriate Beta Blocker Usage[2]	260	99%	99%	98%
Appropriate VTP Within 24 Hours[2]	340	98%	99%	98%
Controlled Postoperative Blood Glucose[2]	180	98%	98%	97%
Perioperative Temperature Management[2]	417	100%	100%	100%
Prophylactic Antibiotic Selection[2]	384	100%	99%	99%
Prophylactic Antibiotic Selection (Outpatient)	550	99%	98%	98%
Prophylactic Antibiotic Stopped[2]	376	98%	98%	98%
Prophylactic Antibiotic Timing[2]	385	98%	99%	99%
Prophylactic Antibiotic Timing (Outpatient)	549	98%	98%	98%
Urinary Catheter Removal[2]	372	97%	98%	97%
Survey of Patients' Hospital Experiences				
Area Around Room 'Always' Quiet at Night	300+	54%	58%	61%
Doctors 'Always' Communicated Well	300+	74%	77%	82%
Home Recovery Information Given	300+	84%	83%	85%
Hospital Given 9 or 10 on 10 Point Scale	300+	68%	67%	71%
Meds 'Always' Explained Before Given	300+	57%	60%	64%
Nurses 'Always' Communicated Well	300+	77%	75%	79%
Pain 'Always' Well Controlled	300+	71%	68%	71%
Room and Bathroom 'Always' Clean	300+	72%	69%	73%
Timely Help 'Always' Received	300+	67%	62%	68%
Would Definitely Recommend Hospital	300+	73%	69%	71%
Use of Medical Imaging				
Cardiac Imaging Stress Test before Surgery	204	4.4%	6.4%	5.3%
Combination Abdominal CT Scan	896	9.4%	11.8%	10.5%
Combination Brain/Sinus CT Scan	1,174	2.0%	3.4%	2.7%
Combination Chest CT Scan	273	11.0%	2.4%	2.7%
Follow-up Mammogram/Ultrasound	962	10.0%	10.2%	8.8%
Lumbar Spine MRI for Low Back Pain	37	43.2%	35.2%	37.2%

NOTE: Hospital profiles are in alphabetical order by state, then city, then hospital within the city; Rankings exclude hospitals with less than 25 cases except for patient surveys which excludes hospitals with less than 100 cases; (a) 100-299 cases; (1) The number of cases/patients is too few to report; (2) Data submitted were based on a sample of cases/patients; (3) Results are based on a shorter time period than required; (4) Data suppressed by CMS for one or more quarters; (5) Results are not available for this reporting period; (6) Fewer than 100 patients completed the HCAHPS survey; (7) No cases met the criteria for this measure; (8) The lower limit of the confidence interval cannot be calculated if the number of observed infections equals zero; (9) No data are available from the state/territory for this reporting period; (10) The scores shown reflect fewer than 50 completed surveys; (11) There were discrepancies in the data collection process; (12) This measure does not apply to this hospital for this reporting period; (13) Results cannot be calculated for this reporting period; (14) The results for this state are combined with nearby states to protect confidentiality; Please refer to the User's Guide for a full explanation of data.

Florida Hospital Zephyrhills

7050 Gall Blvd
Zephyrhills, FL 33541
Phone: 813-788-0411
Fax: 813-783-6196
URL: www.epmc.org
Type: Acute Care Hospitals
Emergency Services: Yes
Ownership: Voluntary non-profit - Church
Beds: 154

Key Personnel:

Chief of Medical Staff.......... Paul Citrin, MD
Infection Control.............. Xiomara Hewitt-Jeffrey
Emergency Room .... Barbara Neal
CEO/President................ Paul Norman
Quality Assurance .... Robert Ruchti
Operating Room............... Caroline Whitis

Measure	Cases	This Hosp.	State Avg.	U.S. Avg.
Blood Clot Prevention and Treatment				
Anticoagulation Overlap Therapy[2]	32	97%	93%	93%
ICU Venous Thromboembolism Prophylaxis[2]	69	94%	94%	92%
Incidence of Potentially Preventable VTE[1,2]	-	-	10%	10%
UFH with Dosages/Platelet Monitoring[1,2]	-	-	100%	97%
Venous Thromboembolism Prophylaxis[2]	332	89%	88%	85%
Warfarin Therapy Discharge Instructions[2]	24	92%	85%	75%
Chest Pain/Possible Heart Attack Care				
Aspirin Given Within 24 Hours of Arrival[3,7]	-	-	98%	96%
Fibrinolytic Meds Within 30 Min. of Arrival[5]	-	-	81%	58%
Average Time to ECG (minutes)[3,7]	-	-	7	7
Average Time to Transfer (minutes)[5]	-	-	53	60
Children's Asthma Care				
Received Home Management Plan of Care	-	-	-	88%
Received Reliever Medication	-	-	-	100%
Received Systemic Corticosteroids	-	-	-	100%
Emergency Department				
Admittance Decision Time (minutes)[2]	713	93	111	98
Head CT Results Within 45 Min. of Arrival[1]	-	-	64%	57%
Patients Who Left ER Before Being Seen	34,813	4%	2%	2%
Time from ER Arrival to Admit. (minutes)[2]	719	292	289	274
Time from ER Arrival to Discharge (minutes)	298	152	147	134
Time in ER Before Being Evaluated (minutes)	367	29	26	26
Time to Pain Meds for Fractures (minutes)	46	57	60	57
Heart Attack Care				
Aspirin Given at Discharge	177	100%	99%	99%
Fibrinolytic Meds Within 30 Min. of Arrival[7]	-	-	50%	54%
PCI Within 90 Minutes of Arrival	43	100%	96%	96%
Statin Prescribed at Discharge	171	99%	99%	98%
Heart Failure Care				
ACE Inhibitor or ARB for LVSD	95	99%	98%	97%
Discharge Instructions Given	232	98%	96%	94%
Evaluation of LVS Function	285	100%	100%	99%
Medicare Spending				
Medicare Spending per Patient (ratio)	-	0.96	1.04	0.98
Pneumonia Care				
Appropriate Initial Antibiotic Given	102	96%	98%	95%
Blood Culture Timing	178	99%	99%	98%
Pregnancy and Delivery Care				
Newborn Deliveries Scheduled Early	28	4%	6%	6%
Preventive Care				
Immunization for Influenza[2]	570	92%	94%	90%
Immunization for Pneumonia[2]	829	95%	96%	92%
Stroke Care				
Anticoagulation Therapy for Atrial Fibrillation[1]	-	-	97%	95%
Antithrombotic Therapy Timing	93	100%	98%	98%
Assessed for Rehabilitation	113	99%	97%	97%
Discharged on Antithrombotic Therapy	95	100%	99%	99%
Discharged on Statin Medication	80	99%	96%	94%
Thrombolytic Therapy Timing[1]	-	-	76%	66%
Venous Thromboembolism Prophylaxis	121	98%	95%	94%
Written Stroke Educational Materials Given	68	99%	94%	88%
Surgical Care Improvement Project				
Appropriate Beta Blocker Usage	207	100%	99%	98%
Appropriate VTP Within 24 Hours	313	98%	99%	98%
Controlled Postoperative Blood Glucose	96	100%	98%	97%
Perioperative Temperature Management	404	100%	100%	100%
Prophylactic Antibiotic Selection	287	100%	99%	99%
Prophylactic Antibiotic Selection (Outpatient)	257	97%	98%	98%
Prophylactic Antibiotic Stopped	273	99%	98%	98%
Prophylactic Antibiotic Timing	289	100%	99%	99%
Prophylactic Antibiotic Timing (Outpatient)	257	99%	98%	98%
Urinary Catheter Removal	231	99%	98%	97%
Survey of Patients' Hospital Experiences				
Area Around Room 'Always' Quiet at Night[11]	300+	53%	58%	61%
Doctors 'Always' Communicated Well[11]	300+	76%	77%	82%
Home Recovery Information Given[11]	300+	83%	83%	85%
Hospital Given 9 or 10 on 10 Point Scale[11]	300+	66%	67%	71%
Meds 'Always' Explained Before Given[11]	300+	59%	60%	64%
Nurses 'Always' Communicated Well[11]	300+	77%	75%	79%
Pain 'Always' Well Controlled[11]	300+	69%	68%	71%
Room and Bathroom 'Always' Clean[11]	300+	67%	69%	73%
Timely Help 'Always' Received[11]	300+	65%	62%	68%
Would Definitely Recommend Hospital[11]	300+	66%	69%	71%
Use of Medical Imaging				
Cardiac Imaging Stress Test before Surgery	67	14.9%	6.4%	5.3%
Combination Abdominal CT Scan	504	25.4%	11.8%	10.5%
Combination Brain/Sinus CT Scan[1]	-	-	3.4%	2.7%
Combination Chest CT Scan	153	4.6%	2.4%	2.7%
Follow-up Mammogram/Ultrasound	529	10.6%	10.2%	8.8%
Lumbar Spine MRI for Low Back Pain	38	47.4%	35.2%	37.2%

NOTE: Hospital profiles are in alphabetical order by state, then city, then hospital within the city; Rankings exclude hospitals with less than 25 cases except for patient surveys which excludes hospitals with less than 100 cases; (a) 100-299 cases; (1) The number of cases/patients is too few to report; (2) Data submitted were based on a sample of cases/patients; (3) Results are based on a shorter time period than required; (4) Data suppressed by CMS for one or more quarters; (5) Results are not available for this reporting period; (6) Fewer than 100 patients completed the HCAHPS survey; (7) No cases met the criteria for this measure; (8) The lower limit of the confidence interval cannot be calculated if the number of observed infections equals zero; (9) No data are available from the state/territory for this reporting period; (10) The scores shown reflect fewer than 50 completed surveys; (11) There were discrepancies in the data collection process; (12) This measure does not apply to this hospital for this reporting period; (13) Results cannot be calculated for this reporting period; (14) The results for this state are combined with nearby states to protect confidentiality; Please refer to the User's Guide for a full explanation of data.

Blood Clot Prevention and Treatment

Anticoagulation Overlap Therapy

Hospital Name	City	Rate	Cases
Cartersville Medical Center[2]	Cartersville	100%	46
Doctors Hospital[2]	Augusta	100%	51
Emory - Adventist Hospital[2]	Smyrna	100%	25
Northside Hospital[2]	Atlanta	100%	136
Northside Hospital Cherokee[2]	Canton	100%	59
Northside Hospital Forsyth[2]	Cumming	100%	66
Rockdale Medical Center[2]	Conyers	100%	92
West Georgia Medical Center[2]	Lagrange	100%	75
Athens Regional Medical Center[2]	Athens	99%	140
John D Archbold Memorial Hospital[2]	Thomasville	99%	76
Eastside Medical Center[2]	Snellville	98%	92
Grady Memorial Hospital[2]	Atlanta	98%	196
Hamilton Medical Center[2]	Dalton	98%	58
Med College of Georgia Hosps[2]	Augusta	98%	82
Piedmont Fayette Hospital[2]	Fayetteville	98%	109
Wellstar Douglas Hospital[2]	Douglasville	98%	65
Wellstar Kennestone Hospital[2]	Marietta	98%	229
Coffee Regional Medical Center[2]	Douglas	97%	35
Dekalb Medical Center at Hillandale[2]	Lithonia	97%	92
Saint Joseph's Hospital of Atlanta[2]	Atlanta	97%	104
Barrow Regional Medical Center[2]	Winder	96%	28
Candler Hospital[2]	Savannah	96%	95
Emory University Hospital Midtown[2]	Atlanta	96%	196
Gwinnett Medical Center[2]	Lawrenceville	96%	263
Piedmont Henry Hospital[2]	Stockbridge	96%	132
Saint Joseph's Hospital - Savannah[2]	Savannah	96%	138
Saint Mary's Hospital[2]	Athens	96%	54
Spalding Regional Hospital[2]	Griffin	96%	78
Crisp Regional Hospital[2]	Cordele	95%	40
Emory Johns Creek Hospital[2]	Johns Creek	95%	39
Redmond Regional Medical Center[2]	Rome	94%	97
Wellstar Cobb Hospital[2]	Austell	94%	127
Dekalb Medical Center[2]	Decatur	93%	196
Piedmont Hospital[2]	Atlanta	93%	198
SE Georgia Health Sys-Brunswick[2]	Brunswick	93%	72
Phoebe Putney Memorial Hospital[2]	Albany	92%	160
Piedmont Newnan Hospital[2]	Newnan	92%	50
Emory University Hospital[2]	Atlanta	91%	164
Fairview Park Hospital[2]	Dublin	91%	45
Floyd Medical Center[2]	Rome	91%	78
Midtown Medical Center[2]	Columbus	91%	77
Northeast Georgia Medical Center[2]	Gainesville	91%	192
Southern Regional Medical Center[2]	Riverdale	90%	120
Memorial Health Univ Medical Center[2]	Savannah	89%	155
Newton Medical Center[2]	Covington	89%	45
Saint Francis Hospital[2]	Columbus	89%	119
Atlanta Medical Center[2]	Atlanta	87%	91
Colquitt Regional Medical Center[2]	Moultrie	86%	28
Tanner Medical Center Villa Rica[2]	Villa Rica	85%	27
Tift Regional Medical Center[2]	Tifton	85%	75
Meadows Regional Medical Center[2]	Vidalia	84%	38
Gordon Hospital[2]	Calhoun	82%	28
North Fulton Hospital[2]	Roswell	81%	42
University Hospital[2]	Augusta	81%	176
Tanner Medical Center - Carrollton[2]	Carrollton	80%	75
East Georgia Regional Medical Center[2]	Statesboro	79%	81
Mayo Clinic Health System - Waycross[2]	Waycross	79%	75
Coliseum Medical Center[2]	Macon	77%	71
Houston Medical Center[2]	Warner Robins	69%	113
Oconee Regional Medical Center[2]	Milledgeville	68%	41
Medical Center of Central Georgia[2]	Macon	64%	188
South Georgia Medical Center[2]	Valdosta	61%	103

ICU Venous Thromboembolism Prophylaxis

Hospital Name	City	Rate	Cases
Cartersville Medical Center[2]	Cartersville	100%	111
Coliseum Northside Hospital[2]	Macon	100%	55
Emory - Adventist Hospital[2]	Smyrna	100%	32
Fannin Regional Hospital[2]	Blue Ridge	100%	34
Gordon Hospital[2]	Calhoun	100%	142
Northside Hospital[2]	Atlanta	100%	44
Northside Hospital Cherokee[2]	Canton	100%	88
Northside Medical Center[2]	Columbus	100%	50
Rockdale Medical Center[2]	Conyers	100%	86
Tift Regional Medical Center[2]	Tifton	100%	62
Trinity Hospital of Augusta[2]	Augusta	100%	55
Union General Hospital[2]	Blairsville	100%	38
Emory University Hospital Midtown[2]	Atlanta	99%	130
Northside Hospital Forsyth[2]	Cumming	99%	88
Piedmont Henry Hospital[2]	Stockbridge	99%	82
Eastside Medical Center[2]	Snellville	98%	91
Fairview Park Hospital[2]	Dublin	98%	185
Medical Center of Central Georgia[2]	Macon	98%	87
Newton Medical Center[2]	Covington	98%	94
Wellstar Cobb Hospital[2]	Austell	98%	88
Wellstar Kennestone Hospital[2]	Marietta	98%	97
West Georgia Medical Center[2]	Lagrange	98%	120
Dekalb Medical Center[2]	Decatur	97%	87
Doctors Hospital[2]	Augusta	97%	78
Gwinnett Medical Center[2]	Lawrenceville	97%	59
Med College of Georgia Hosps[2]	Augusta	97%	124
University Hospital[2]	Augusta	97%	58
Barrow Regional Medical Center[2]	Winder	96%	77
Coliseum Medical Center[2]	Macon	96%	108
Emory Johns Creek Hospital[2]	Johns Creek	96%	91
Floyd Medical Center[2]	Rome	96%	71
North Fulton Hospital[2]	Roswell	96%	125
Tanner Medical Center - Carrollton[2]	Carrollton	96%	83
Tanner Medical Center Villa Rica[2]	Villa Rica	96%	51
Grady Memorial Hospital[2]	Atlanta	95%	93
John D Archbold Memorial Hospital[2]	Thomasville	95%	63
Phoebe Sumter Medical Center[2]	Americus	95%	93
Wellstar Douglas Hospital[2]	Douglasville	95%	80
Doctors Specialty Hospital[2]	Columbus	94%	48
Emory University Hospital[2]	Atlanta	94%	78
Piedmont Fayette Hospital[2]	Fayetteville	94%	54
SE Georgia Health Sys-Brunswick[2]	Brunswick	94%	98
Spalding Regional Hospital[2]	Griffin	94%	116
Hamilton Medical Center[2]	Dalton	93%	81
Midtown Medical Center[2]	Columbus	93%	56
Piedmont Hospital[2]	Atlanta	93%	86
Saint Mary's Hospital[2]	Athens	93%	73
Taylor Regional Hospital[2]	Hawkinsville	93%	60
Wayne Memorial Hospital[2]	Jesup	93%	120
Candler Hospital[2]	Savannah	92%	60
Memorial Health Univ Medical Center[2]	Savannah	92%	66
Wellstar Paulding Hospital[2]	Hiram	92%	25
Dekalb Medical Center at Hillandale[2]	Lithonia	91%	68
Clearview Regional Medical Center[2]	Monroe	90%	83
Oconee Regional Medical Center[2]	Milledgeville	90%	122
Redmond Regional Medical Center[2]	Rome	90%	122
Atlanta Medical Center[2]	Atlanta	89%	149
Piedmont Newnan Hospital[2]	Newnan	89%	80
Southern Regional Medical Center[2]	Riverdale	89%	120
Chestatee Regional Hospital[2]	Dahlonega	88%	25
Hutcheson Medical Center[2]	Fort Oglethorpe	88%	133
Piedmont Mountainside Hospital[2]	Jasper	88%	50
Dorminy Medical Center[2]	Fitzgerald	86%	44
Mayo Clinic Health System - Waycross[2]	Waycross	85%	95
Athens Regional Medical Center[2]	Athens	84%	92
Colquitt Regional Medical Center[2]	Moultrie	84%	77
East Georgia Regional Medical Center[2]	Statesboro	84%	81
Habersham County Medical Center[2]	Demorest	83%	58
Northeast Georgia Medical Center[2]	Gainesville	83%	155
Saint Joseph's Hospital - Savannah[2]	Savannah	83%	108
Stephens County Hospital[2]	Toccoa	83%	29
Saint Joseph's Hospital of Atlanta[2]	Atlanta	82%	112
Memorial Hospital & Manor[2]	Bainbridge	81%	67
Meadows Regional Medical Center[2]	Vidalia	80%	96
Phoebe Putney Memorial Hospital[2]	Albany	79%	97
Saint Francis Hospital[2]	Columbus	77%	87
SE Georgia Health Sys-Camden Campus[2]	Saint Marys	76%	37
Coffee Regional Medical Center[2]	Douglas	74%	93
Crisp Regional Hospital[2]	Cordele	74%	135
Dodge County Hospital[2]	Eastman	73%	41
Houston Medical Center[2]	Warner Robins	72%	25
Upson Regional Medical Center[2]	Thomaston	71%	48
South Georgia Medical Center[2]	Valdosta	69%	192
Washington County Regional Medical Center[2]	Sandersville	68%	44
Elbert Memorial Hospital[2]	Elberton	66%	32
Ty Cobb Regional Medical Center[2]	Lavonia	56%	34
Appling Hospital[2]	Baxley	52%	40
Emanuel County Hospital Authority[2]	Swainsboro	48%	40
North Georgia Medical Center[2]	Ellijay	27%	66

Incidence of Potentially Preventable VTE

Hospital Name	City	Rate	Cases
Dekalb Medical Center[2]	Decatur	0%	26
Gwinnett Medical Center[2]	Lawrenceville	0%	32
Northside Hospital[2]	Atlanta	0%	48
Atlanta Medical Center[2]	Atlanta	3%	29
Med College of Georgia Hosps[2]	Augusta	3%	67
Medical Center of Central Georgia[2]	Macon	6%	51
Emory University Hospital[2]	Atlanta	7%	71
Memorial Health Univ Medical Center[2]	Savannah	7%	45
Doctors Hospital[2]	Augusta	9%	35
Saint Joseph's Hospital - Savannah[2]	Savannah	9%	35
Emory University Hospital Midtown[2]	Atlanta	10%	69
Piedmont Hospital[2]	Atlanta	10%	62
Wellstar Kennestone Hospital[2]	Marietta	15%	67
Grady Memorial Hospital[2]	Atlanta	16%	64
Phoebe Putney Memorial Hospital[2]	Albany	21%	34
Northeast Georgia Medical Center[2]	Gainesville	22%	37
University Hospital[2]	Augusta	23%	39

UFH with Dosages/Platelet Count Monitoring

Hospital Name	City	Rate	Cases
Athens Regional Medical Center[2]	Athens	100%	115
Barrow Regional Medical Center[2]	Winder	100%	25
Cartersville Medical Center[2]	Cartersville	100%	57
Coffee Regional Medical Center[2]	Douglas	100%	25
Coliseum Medical Center[2]	Macon	100%	80
Dekalb Medical Center[2]	Decatur	100%	165
Dekalb Medical Center at Hillandale[2]	Lithonia	100%	72
East Georgia Regional Medical Center[2]	Statesboro	100%	28
Eastside Medical Center[2]	Snellville	100%	41
Emory University Hospital[2]	Atlanta	100%	157
Emory University Hospital Midtown[2]	Atlanta	100%	207
Fairview Park Hospital[2]	Dublin	100%	45
Floyd Medical Center[2]	Rome	100%	31
Grady Memorial Hospital[2]	Atlanta	100%	177
Gwinnett Medical Center[2]	Lawrenceville	100%	173
Hamilton Medical Center[2]	Dalton	100%	47
John D Archbold Memorial Hospital[2]	Thomasville	100%	63
Mayo Clinic Health System - Waycross[2]	Waycross	100%	43
Memorial Health Univ Medical Center[2]	Savannah	100%	30
Midtown Medical Center[2]	Columbus	100%	38
North Fulton Hospital[2]	Roswell	100%	43
Northeast Georgia Medical Center[2]	Gainesville	100%	191
Northside Hospital[2]	Atlanta	100%	121
Northside Hospital Cherokee[2]	Canton	100%	38
Northside Hospital Forsyth[2]	Cumming	100%	80
Oconee Regional Medical Center[2]	Milledgeville	100%	29
Piedmont Fayette Hospital[2]	Fayetteville	100%	104
Piedmont Henry Hospital[2]	Stockbridge	100%	92
Piedmont Newnan Hospital[2]	Newnan	100%	46
Redmond Regional Medical Center[2]	Rome	100%	39
Rockdale Medical Center[2]	Conyers	100%	25
Saint Francis Hospital[2]	Columbus	100%	41
Saint Joseph's Hospital - Savannah[2]	Savannah	100%	46
Saint Joseph's Hospital of Atlanta[2]	Atlanta	100%	108
Saint Mary's Hospital[2]	Athens	100%	39
SE Georgia Health Sys-Brunswick[2]	Brunswick	100%	52
Southern Regional Medical Center[2]	Riverdale	100%	79
Spalding Regional Hospital[2]	Griffin	100%	57
Tift Regional Medical Center[2]	Tifton	100%	38
Wellstar Cobb Hospital[2]	Austell	100%	129
Wellstar Douglas Hospital[2]	Douglasville	100%	35
Wellstar Kennestone Hospital[2]	Marietta	100%	199
West Georgia Medical Center[2]	Lagrange	100%	68
Medical Center of Central Georgia[2]	Macon	99%	199
Med College of Georgia Hosps[2]	Augusta	99%	73
Tanner Medical Center - Carrollton[2]	Carrollton	99%	69
University Hospital[2]	Augusta	99%	81
Atlanta Medical Center[2]	Atlanta	97%	66
Phoebe Putney Memorial Hospital[2]	Albany	97%	70
Tanner Medical Center Villa Rica[2]	Villa Rica	97%	29
Piedmont Hospital[2]	Atlanta	95%	213
Houston Medical Center[2]	Warner Robins	94%	49
South Georgia Medical Center[2]	Valdosta	67%	30

Venous Thromboembolism Prophylaxis

Hospital Name	City	Rate	Cases
Chatuge Regional Hospital[2]	Hiawassee	100%	79
Trinity Hospital of Augusta[2]	Augusta	100%	272
Emory - Adventist Hospital[2]	Smyrna	99%	159
Fannin Regional Hospital[2]	Blue Ridge	99%	146
Northside Hospital Cherokee[2]	Canton	99%	370
Northside Hospital Forsyth[2]	Cumming	99%	377
Doctors Hospital[2]	Augusta	98%	330
Eastside Medical Center[2]	Snellville	98%	359
Fairview Park Hospital[2]	Dublin	98%	286
Gordon Hospital[2]	Calhoun	98%	388
Northside Medical Center[2]	Columbus	98%	110
West Georgia Medical Center[2]	Lagrange	98%	292
Hamilton Medical Center[2]	Dalton	97%	302
Northside Hospital[2]	Atlanta	97%	413
Rockdale Medical Center[2]	Conyers	97%	356
Southeastern Regional Medical Center[2]	Newnan	97%	89
Cartersville Medical Center[2]	Cartersville	96%	307
Northridge Medical Center[2]	Commerce	96%	112
Emory Johns Creek Hospital[2]	Johns Creek	95%	326
Higgins General Hospital[2]	Bremen	95%	138
Piedmont Henry Hospital[2]	Stockbridge	95%	347
Floyd Medical Center[2]	Rome	94%	319
John D Archbold Memorial Hospital[2]	Thomasville	94%	326
Tanner Medical Center - Carrollton[2]	Carrollton	94%	326
Union General Hospital[2]	Blairsville	94%	178
Dekalb Medical Center[2]	Decatur	93%	321
Dekalb Medical Center at Hillandale[2]	Lithonia	93%	398
Emory University Hospital[2]	Atlanta	93%	309
Emory University Hospital Midtown[2]	Atlanta	93%	351
Tanner Medical Center Villa Rica[2]	Villa Rica	93%	137
Coliseum Northside Hospital[2]	Macon	92%	204
Barrow Regional Medical Center[2]	Winder	91%	225

NOTE: Hospital profiles are in alphabetical order by state, then city, then hospital within the city; Rankings exclude hospitals with less than 25 cases except for patient surveys which excludes hospitals with less than 100 cases; (a) 100-299 cases; (1) The number of cases/patients is too few to report; (2) Data submitted were based on a sample of cases/patients; (3) Results are based on a shorter time period than required; (4) Data suppressed by CMS for one or more quarters; (5) Results are not available for this reporting period; (6) Fewer than 100 patients completed the HCAHPS survey; (7) No cases met the criteria for this measure; (8) The lower limit of the confidence interval cannot be calculated if the number of observed infections equals zero; (9) No data are available from the state/territory for this reporting period; (10) The scores shown reflect fewer than 50 completed surveys; (11) There were discrepancies in the data collection process; (12) This measure does not apply to this hospital for this reporting period; (13) Results cannot be calculated for this reporting period; (14) The results for this state are combined with nearby states to protect confidentiality; Please refer to the User's Guide for a full explanation of data.

Midtown Medical Center[2]	Columbus	91%	377
Spalding Regional Hospital[2]	Griffin	91%	350
Wayne Memorial Hospital[2]	Jesup	91%	314
Gwinnett Medical Center[2]	Lawrenceville	90%	378
Tift Regional Medical Center[2]	Tifton	90%	336
Grady Memorial Hospital[2]	Atlanta	89%	334
Saint Mary's Hospital[2]	Athens	89%	248
Putnam General Hospital[2,3]	Eatonton	88%	34
Redmond Regional Medical Center[2]	Rome	88%	339
University Hospital[2]	Augusta	88%	372
Wellstar Paulding Hospital[2]	Hiram	88%	184
North Fulton Hospital[2]	Roswell	87%	279
Piedmont Fayette Hospital[2]	Fayetteville	87%	389
Coliseum Medical Center[2]	Macon	86%	333
Med College of Georgia Hosps[2]	Augusta	86%	269
Piedmont Newnan Hospital[2]	Newnan	86%	389
Doctors Specialty Hospital[2]	Columbus	85%	348
Newton Medical Center[2]	Covington	85%	350
Phoebe Sumter Medical Center[2]	Americus	85%	213
Piedmont Mountainside Hospital[2]	Jasper	85%	246
Clearview Regional Medical Center[2]	Monroe	84%	247
Liberty Regional Medical Center[2,3]	Hinesville	83%	89
Wellstar Kennestone Hospital[2]	Marietta	83%	332
SE Georgia Health Sys-Brunswick[2]	Brunswick	82%	338
Wellstar Cobb Hospital[2]	Austell	82%	350
Medical Center of Central Georgia[2]	Macon	81%	312
Oconee Regional Medical Center[2]	Milledgeville	81%	384
Saint Joseph's Hospital of Atlanta[2]	Atlanta	81%	318
Memorial Health Univ Medical Center[2]	Savannah	80%	307
Candler Hospital[2]	Savannah	79%	396
Memorial Hospital & Manor[2]	Bainbridge	79%	208
East Georgia Regional Medical Center[2]	Statesboro	78%	389
SE Georgia Health Sys-Camden Campus[2]	Saint Marys	78%	130
Athens Regional Medical Center[2]	Athens	77%	316
Chestatee Regional Hospital[2]	Dahlonega	77%	123
Habersham County Medical Center[2]	Demorest	77%	238
Piedmont Hospital[2]	Atlanta	77%	372
Wellstar Douglas Hospital[2]	Douglasville	77%	379
Grady General Hospital[2]	Cairo	76%	123
Hutcheson Medical Center[2]	Fort Oglethorpe	76%	324
Saint Francis Hospital[2]	Columbus	76%	338
Saint Joseph's Hospital - Savannah[2]	Savannah	76%	310
Atlanta Medical Center[2]	Atlanta	75%	280
Mayo Clinic Health System - Waycross[2]	Waycross	74%	382
Phoebe Putney Memorial Hospital[2]	Albany	74%	316
Washington County Regional Medical Center[2]	Sandersville	73%	282
Northeast Georgia Medical Center[2]	Gainesville	72%	296
South Georgia Medical Center[2]	Valdosta	72%	438
Colquitt Regional Medical Center[2]	Moultrie	71%	326
Southern Regional Medical Center[2]	Riverdale	71%	382
Crisp Regional Hospital[2]	Cordele	70%	184
Dorminy Medical Center[2]	Fitzgerald	70%	126
Taylor Regional Hospital[2]	Hawkinsville	69%	128
Dodge County Hospital[2]	Eastman	68%	159
Stephens County Hospital[2]	Toccoa	68%	202
Meadows Regional Medical Center[2]	Vidalia	66%	345
Perry Hospital[2]	Perry	64%	153
Polk Medical Center[2]	Cedartown	63%	71
Mountain Lakes Medical Center[2]	Clayton	61%	173
Appling Hospital[2]	Baxley	56%	232
Elbert Memorial Hospital[2]	Elberton	56%	140
Coffee Regional Medical Center[2]	Douglas	54%	377
Houston Medical Center[2]	Warner Robins	52%	381
Upson Regional Medical Center[2]	Thomaston	49%	339
Cook Medical Center[2]	Adel	47%	118
Murray Medical Center[2]	Chatsworth	46%	128
Ty Cobb Regional Medical Center[2]	Lavonia	44%	108
Jefferson Hospital[2]	Louisville	40%	126
Burke Medical Center[2]	Waynesboro	38%	114
Effingham County Hospital	Springfield	38%	60
Univ McDuffie Co Reg Med Ctr[2]	Thomson	34%	145
Donalsonville Hospital[2]	Donalsonville	31%	336
North Georgia Medical Center[2]	Ellijay	30%	126
Emanuel County Hospital Authority[2]	Swainsboro	26%	118
Flint River Hospital[2]	Montezuma	19%	68
Evans Memorial Hospital[2]	Claxton	18%	222
Irwin County Hospital[2]	Ocilla	5%	126

Warfarin Therapy Discharge Instructions

Hospital Name	City	Rate	Cases
Coliseum Medical Center[2]	Macon	100%	57
Crisp Regional Hospital[2]	Cordele	100%	25
Doctors Hospital[2]	Augusta	100%	42
Eastside Medical Center[2]	Snellville	100%	68
Fairview Park Hospital[2]	Dublin	100%	36
Northeast Georgia Medical Center[2]	Gainesville	100%	149
Northside Hospital[2]	Atlanta	100%	105
Northside Hospital Cherokee[2]	Canton	100%	44
Northside Hospital Forsyth[2]	Cumming	100%	50
Spalding Regional Hospital[2]	Griffin	100%	56
West Georgia Medical Center[2]	Lagrange	100%	61
Midtown Medical Center[2]	Columbus	98%	61
Rockdale Medical Center[2]	Conyers	98%	80
Wellstar Douglas Hospital[2]	Douglasville	98%	55
John D Archbold Memorial Hospital[2]	Thomasville	97%	67
North Fulton Hospital[2]	Roswell	97%	30
Redmond Regional Medical Center[2]	Rome	97%	75
Gordon Hospital[2]	Calhoun	96%	25
Candler Hospital[2]	Savannah	95%	65
Piedmont Henry Hospital[2]	Stockbridge	95%	106
SE Georgia Health Sys-Brunswick[2]	Brunswick	94%	54
Mayo Clinic Health System - Waycross[2]	Waycross	93%	58
Dekalb Medical Center at Hillandale[2]	Lithonia	92%	80
Piedmont Newnan Hospital[2]	Newnan	91%	43
Cartersville Medical Center[2]	Cartersville	90%	41
Grady Memorial Hospital[2]	Atlanta	90%	160
Piedmont Hospital[2]	Atlanta	90%	135
Floyd Medical Center[2]	Rome	89%	65
Gwinnett Medical Center[2]	Lawrenceville	88%	203
Saint Joseph's Hospital - Savannah[2]	Savannah	87%	118
Piedmont Fayette Hospital[2]	Fayetteville	85%	89
Dekalb Medical Center[2]	Decatur	84%	143
Hamilton Medical Center[2]	Dalton	84%	45
Wellstar Kennestone Hospital[2]	Marietta	84%	154
Coffee Regional Medical Center[2]	Douglas	83%	30
Tanner Medical Center Villa Rica[2]	Villa Rica	81%	27
Wellstar Cobb Hospital[2]	Austell	80%	90
Saint Francis Hospital[2]	Columbus	78%	97
South Georgia Medical Center[2]	Valdosta	74%	82
Newton Medical Center[2]	Covington	72%	43
University Hospital[2]	Augusta	72%	134
Memorial Health Univ Medical Center[2]	Savannah	70%	96
East Georgia Regional Medical Center[2]	Statesboro	67%	70
Saint Mary's Hospital[2]	Athens	65%	37
Southern Regional Medical Center[2]	Riverdale	65%	99
Emory University Hospital[2]	Atlanta	61%	121
Medical Center of Central Georgia[2]	Macon	61%	148
Saint Joseph's Hospital of Atlanta[2]	Atlanta	60%	77
Med College of Georgia Hosps[2]	Augusta	58%	48
Emory University Hospital Midtown[2]	Atlanta	56%	156
Atlanta Medical Center[2]	Atlanta	55%	67
Tanner Medical Center - Carrollton[2]	Carrollton	53%	60
Oconee Regional Medical Center[2]	Milledgeville	50%	30
Emory Johns Creek Hospital[2]	Johns Creek	48%	27
Houston Medical Center[2]	Warner Robins	34%	88
Phoebe Putney Memorial Hospital[2]	Albany	30%	130
Meadows Regional Medical Center[2]	Vidalia	26%	27
Athens Regional Medical Center[2]	Athens	9%	111
Tift Regional Medical Center[2]	Tifton	6%	63

Chest Pain/Possible Heart Attack Care

Aspirin Given Within 24 Hours of Arrival

Hospital Name	City	Rate	Cases
Colquitt Regional Medical Center	Moultrie	100%	54
Crisp Regional Hospital	Cordele	100%	62
East Georgia Regional Medical Center[3]	Statesboro	100%	47
Evans Memorial Hospital	Claxton	100%	27
Gordon Hospital	Calhoun	100%	51
Habersham County Medical Center	Demorest	100%	101
North Fulton Hospital	Roswell	100%	88
Northside Hospital Forsyth	Cumming	100%	25
Oconee Regional Medical Center	Milledgeville	100%	105
Piedmont Fayette Hospital	Fayetteville	100%	37
SE Georgia Health Sys-Camden Campus	Saint Marys	100%	64
Stephens County Hospital	Toccoa	100%	70
Tanner Medical Center Villa Rica	Villa Rica	100%	52
Candler Hospital	Savannah	98%	42
Dekalb Medical Center at Hillandale	Lithonia	98%	51
Piedmont Newnan Hospital	Newnan	98%	41
Rockdale Medical Center	Conyers	98%	49
Clearview Regional Medical Center	Monroe	97%	36
Dorminy Medical Center	Fitzgerald	97%	35
Fannin Regional Hospital	Blue Ridge	97%	34
Higgins General Hospital	Bremen	97%	60
Hutcheson Medical Center	Fort Oglethorpe	97%	36
Newton Medical Center	Covington	97%	74
Northside Hospital Cherokee	Canton	97%	31
Coffee Regional Medical Center	Douglas	96%	57
Houston Medical Center	Warner Robins	96%	28
Barrow Regional Medical Center	Winder	95%	43
Chatuge Regional Hospital	Hiawassee	95%	37
Putnam General Hospital	Eatonton	95%	78
Chestatee Regional Hospital	Dahlonega	94%	31
Coliseum Northside Hospital	Macon	94%	33
Liberty Regional Medical Center	Hinesville	94%	52
Mayo Clinic Health System - Waycross	Waycross	94%	34
Phoebe Sumter Medical Center	Americus	94%	52
Taylor Regional Hospital	Hawkinsville	94%	32
Wayne Memorial Hospital	Jesup	94%	50
Wellstar Paulding Hospital	Hiram	94%	150
Wellstar Douglas Hospital	Douglasville	93%	29
Emanuel County Hospital Authority[3]	Swainsboro	92%	25
Polk Medical Center	Cedartown	92%	171
Ty Cobb Regional Medical Center	Lavonia	92%	52
Union General Hospital	Blairsville	92%	100
Jefferson Hospital	Louisville	91%	45
Memorial Hospital & Manor	Bainbridge	89%	27
Wellstar Kennestone Hospital	Marietta	89%	37
Upson Regional Medical Center	Thomaston	88%	97
Piedmont Mountainside Hospital	Jasper	87%	75
Univ McDuffie Co Reg Med Ctr	Thomson	87%	60
Washington County Regional Medical Center	Sandersville	85%	55
Wellstar Cobb Hospital	Austell	85%	33
Dodge County Hospital	Eastman	81%	37
North Georgia Medical Center	Ellijay	63%	27

Average Time to ECG (minutes)

Hospital Name	City	Min.	Cases
Houston Medical Center	Warner Robins	0	28
Northside Hospital Forsyth	Cumming	0	27
Wellstar Kennestone Hospital	Marietta	0	38
Wellstar Paulding Hospital	Hiram	0	152
Northside Hospital Cherokee	Canton	2	33
Piedmont Newnan Hospital	Newnan	2	42
Piedmont Fayette Hospital	Fayetteville	3	39
Tanner Medical Center Villa Rica	Villa Rica	3	54
Wellstar Douglas Hospital	Douglasville	3	31
Clearview Regional Medical Center	Monroe	4	39
Coffee Regional Medical Center	Douglas	4	58
Wellstar Cobb Hospital	Austell	4	34
Fannin Regional Hospital	Blue Ridge	5	37
Newton Medical Center	Covington	5	79
Taylor Regional Hospital	Hawkinsville	5	30
Gordon Hospital	Calhoun	6	50
Union General Hospital	Blairsville	6	100
Liberty Regional Medical Center	Hinesville	7	25
North Fulton Hospital	Roswell	7	88
Piedmont Mountainside Hospital	Jasper	7	73
Stephens County Hospital	Toccoa	7	70
Crisp Regional Hospital	Cordele	8	64
Higgins General Hospital	Bremen	8	62
Hutcheson Medical Center	Fort Oglethorpe	8	36
Oconee Regional Medical Center	Milledgeville	8	107
Polk Medical Center	Cedartown	8	171
Rockdale Medical Center	Conyers	8	49
Upson Regional Medical Center	Thomaston	8	102
Habersham County Medical Center	Demorest	9	101
Jefferson Hospital	Louisville	9	44
Mayo Clinic Health System - Waycross	Waycross	9	37
Putnam General Hospital	Eatonton	9	81
Washington County Regional Medical Center	Sandersville	9	59
Barrow Regional Medical Center	Winder	10	46
Dekalb Medical Center at Hillandale	Lithonia	10	52
Dodge County Hospital	Eastman	10	42
Phoebe Sumter Medical Center	Americus	10	53
East Georgia Regional Medical Center[3]	Statesboro	11	50
Coliseum Northside Hospital	Macon	12	33
Wayne Memorial Hospital	Jesup	12	53
Ty Cobb Regional Medical Center	Lavonia	13	48
Dorminy Medical Center	Fitzgerald	14	38
North Georgia Medical Center	Ellijay	14	26
Bacon County Hospital	Alma	17	26
Univ McDuffie Co Reg Med Ctr	Thomson	17	61
Candler Hospital	Savannah	18	42
Colquitt Regional Medical Center	Moultrie	18	60
Chestatee Regional Hospital	Dahlonega	19	31
SE Georgia Health Sys-Camden Campus	Saint Marys	20	67
Chatuge Regional Hospital	Hiawassee	21	38
Evans Memorial Hospital	Claxton	22	30

Average Time to Transfer (minutes)

Hospital Name	City	Min.	Cases
North Fulton Hospital	Roswell	77	25

Children's Asthma Care

Received Home Management Plan of Care

Hospital Name	City	Rate	Cases
Med College of Georgia Hosps[2]	Augusta	88%	167
Tift Regional Medical Center	Tifton	78%	27

Received Reliever Medication

Hospital Name	City	Rate	Cases
Med College of Georgia Hosps[2]	Augusta	100%	167
Tift Regional Medical Center	Tifton	100%	28

NOTE: Hospital profiles are in alphabetical order by state, then city, then hospital within the city; Rankings exclude hospitals with less than 25 cases except for patient surveys which excludes hospitals with less than 100 cases; (a) 100-299 cases; (1) The number of cases/patients is too few to report; (2) Data submitted were based on a sample of cases/patients; (3) Results are based on a shorter time period than required; (4) Data suppressed by CMS for one or more quarters; (5) Results are not available for this reporting period; (6) Fewer than 100 patients completed the HCAHPS survey; (7) No cases met the criteria for this measure; (8) The lower limit of the confidence interval cannot be calculated if the number of observed infections equals zero; (9) No data are available from the state/territory for this reporting period; (10) The scores shown reflect fewer than 50 completed surveys; (11) There were discrepancies in the data collection process; (12) This measure does not apply to this hospital for this reporting period; (13) Results cannot be calculated for this reporting period; (14) The results for this state are combined with nearby states to protect confidentiality; Please refer to the User's Guide for a full explanation of data.

Received Systemic Corticosteroids

Hospital Name	City	Rate	Cases
Med College of Georgia Hosps[2]	Augusta	100%	167
Tift Regional Medical Center	Tifton	100%	27

Emergency Department

Admittance Decision Time (minutes)

Hospital Name	City	Min.	Cases
Polk Medical Center[2]	Cedartown	25	31
Stephens County Hospital[2]	Toccoa	34	510
Donalsonville Hospital[2]	Donalsonville	40	79
Elbert Memorial Hospital[2]	Elberton	40	410
Wills Memorial Hospital[2]	Washington	40	286
Evans Memorial Hospital[2]	Claxton	42	362
Memorial Hospital & Manor[2]	Bainbridge	44	271
Washington County Regional Medical Center[2]	Sandersville	44	302
Dorminy Medical Center[2]	Fitzgerald	48	508
Tanner Medical Center - Carrollton[2]	Carrollton	48	391
Bacon County Hospital[2]	Alma	49	235
Murray Medical Center	Chatsworth	50	130
Ty Cobb Regional Medical Center[2]	Lavonia	50	291
Tanner Medical Center Villa Rica[2]	Villa Rica	52	246
Cook Medical Center[2]	Adel	53	203
Coffee Regional Medical Center[2]	Douglas	55	427
Emory - Adventist Hospital[2]	Smyrna	55	463
Jasper Memorial Hospital	Monticello	55	37
Wellstar Paulding Hospital[2]	Hiram	55	388
Flint River Hospital[2]	Montezuma	56	160
Jeff Davis Hospital[2]	Hazlehurst	56	78
Morgan Memorial Hospital	Madison	56	86
Union General Hospital[2]	Blairsville	56	256
Doctors Hospital[2]	Augusta	57	553
Wayne Memorial Hospital[2]	Jesup	59	403
Dodge County Hospital[2]	Eastman	60	280
Grady General Hospital[2]	Cairo	60	281
North Georgia Medical Center[2]	Ellijay	61	469
Coliseum Northside Hospital[2]	Macon	62	410
Mountain Lakes Medical Center[2]	Clayton	62	225
Newton Medical Center[2]	Covington	62	897
Hutcheson Medical Center[2]	Fort Oglethorpe	64	461
Jefferson Hospital[2]	Louisville	65	263
Northridge Medical Center[2]	Commerce	65	429
Putnam General Hospital[2]	Eatonton	65	295
Higgins General Hospital[2]	Bremen	67	339
Chatuge Regional Hospital	Hiawassee	68	51
Effingham County Hospital	Springfield	68	91
Trinity Hospital of Augusta[2]	Augusta	68	368
Upson Regional Medical Center[2]	Thomaston	68	400
Chestatee Regional Hospital[2]	Dahlonega	70	364
Colquitt Regional Medical Center[2]	Moultrie	70	545
Saint Mary's Good Samaritan Hospital[2,3]	Greensboro	70	47
Liberty Regional Medical Center[2]	Hinesville	72	125
Univ McDuffie Co Reg Med Ctr[2]	Thomson	73	168
Taylor Regional Hospital[2]	Hawkinsville	75	298
Coliseum Medical Center[2]	Macon	78	641
Appling Hospital[2]	Baxley	79	233
Habersham County Medical Center[2]	Demorest	79	479
Gordon Hospital[2]	Calhoun	81	1122
Crisp Regional Hospital[2]	Cordele	82	563
Mayo Clinic Health System - Waycross[2]	Waycross	82	993
Burke Medical Center[2]	Waynesboro	83	95
SE Georgia Health Sys-Camden Campus[2]	Saint Marys	83	164
Floyd Medical Center[2]	Rome	84	450
Perry Hospital[2]	Perry	85	353
West Georgia Medical Center[2]	Lagrange	88	625
Emanuel County Hospital Authority[2]	Swainsboro	90	489
Fairview Park Hospital[2]	Dublin	90	713
Fannin Regional Hospital[2]	Blue Ridge	92	244
Northside Hospital Forsyth[2]	Cumming	92	517
Meadows Regional Medical Center[2]	Vidalia	93	465
Northside Hospital Cherokee[2]	Canton	98	361
Redmond Regional Medical Center[2]	Rome	98	678
Wellstar Douglas Hospital[2]	Douglasville	98	354
Cartersville Medical Center[2]	Cartersville	100	599
Hamilton Medical Center[2]	Dalton	100	406
SE Georgia Health Sys-Brunswick[2]	Brunswick	103	519
Clearview Regional Medical Center[2]	Monroe	106	512
Northside Hospital[2]	Atlanta	106	146
Spalding Regional Hospital[2]	Griffin	106	530
North Fulton Hospital[2]	Roswell	110	681
Wellstar Cobb Hospital[2]	Austell	110	333
Northeast Georgia Medical Center[2]	Gainesville	113	541
Athens Regional Medical Center[2]	Athens	115	478
Rockdale Medical Center[2]	Conyers	116	665
University Hospital[2]	Augusta	116	494
Saint Mary's Hospital[2]	Athens	118	452
Emory Johns Creek Hospital[2]	Johns Creek	119	683
Saint Joseph's Hospital - Savannah[2]	Savannah	122	516
Phoebe Sumter Medical Center[2]	Americus	125	510
Wellstar Kennestone Hospital[2]	Marietta	125	540
Piedmont Newnan Hospital[2]	Newnan	126	706
Emory University Hospital Midtown[2]	Atlanta	128	396
East Georgia Regional Medical Center[2]	Statesboro	129	563
Houston Medical Center[2]	Warner Robins	130	627
Oconee Regional Medical Center[2]	Milledgeville	130	690
Saint Joseph's Hospital of Atlanta[2]	Atlanta	135	503
Grady Memorial Hospital[2]	Atlanta	136	381
Phoebe Putney Memorial Hospital[2]	Albany	138	550
Tift Regional Medical Center[2]	Tifton	146	624
South Georgia Medical Center[2]	Valdosta	150	636
Emory University Hospital[2]	Atlanta	152	364
Piedmont Hospital[2]	Atlanta	159	446
Barrow Regional Medical Center[2]	Winder	161	548
Dekalb Medical Center[2]	Decatur	162	503
John D Archbold Memorial Hospital[2]	Thomasville	163	622
Southern Regional Medical Center[2]	Riverdale	175	669
Piedmont Henry Hospital[2]	Stockbridge	177	671
Gwinnett Medical Center[2]	Lawrenceville	181	884
Piedmont Fayette Hospital[2]	Fayetteville	188	624
Med College of Georgia Hosps[2]	Augusta	192	530
Saint Francis Hospital[2]	Columbus	195	1004
Eastside Medical Center[2]	Snellville	197	577
Atlanta Medical Center[2]	Atlanta	207	568
Medical Center of Central Georgia[2]	Macon	218	528
Dekalb Medical Center at Hillandale[2]	Lithonia	227	1060
Candler Hospital[2]	Savannah	230	340
Memorial Health Univ Medical Center[2]	Savannah	277	562
Midtown Medical Center[2]	Columbus	315	350

Head CT Results Within 45 Minutes of Arrival

Hospital Name	City	Rate	Cases
Spalding Regional Hospital	Griffin	92%	25
Gwinnett Medical Center	Lawrenceville	72%	39
Wellstar Kennestone Hospital	Marietta	55%	31

Patients Who Left ER Before Being Seen

Hospital Name	City	Rate	Cases
Chatuge Regional Hospital	Hiawassee	0%	5491
Clinch Memorial Hospital	Homerville	0%	5902
Fairview Park Hospital	Dublin	0%	37598
Miller County Hospital	Colquitt	0%	4731
Union General Hospital	Blairsville	0%	19268
Wayne Memorial Hospital	Jesup	0%	29320
Wills Memorial Hospital	Washington	0%	5521
Appling Hospital	Baxley	1%	8987
Bacon County Hospital	Alma	1%	7994
Bleckley Memorial Hospital	Cochran	1%	4946
Burke Medical Center	Waynesboro	1%	8729
Coliseum Medical Center	Macon	1%	41650
Coliseum Northside Hospital	Macon	1%	23478
Cook Medical Center	Adel	1%	9999
Doctors Hospital	Augusta	1%	48685
Eastside Medical Center	Snellville	1%	61866
Effingham County Hospital	Springfield	1%	13410
Emory Johns Creek Hospital	Johns Creek	1%	24292
Evans Memorial Hospital	Claxton	1%	9773
Grady General Hospital	Cairo	1%	11215
Habersham County Medical Center	Demorest	1%	13503
Jasper Memorial Hospital	Monticello	1%	4842
Liberty Regional Medical Center	Hinesville	1%	23987
Meadows Regional Medical Center	Vidalia	1%	30298
Memorial Health Univ Medical Center	Savannah	1%	101509
Memorial Hospital & Manor	Bainbridge	1%	18000
Morgan Memorial Hospital	Madison	1%	7375
Northeast Georgia Medical Center	Gainesville	1%	106621
Northside Hospital	Atlanta	1%	26545
Northside Hospital Cherokee	Canton	1%	18896
Northside Hospital Forsyth	Cumming	1%	27752
Redmond Regional Medical Center	Rome	1%	39685
Saint Joseph's Hospital of Atlanta	Atlanta	1%	33790
Saint Mary's Good Samaritan Hospital	Greensboro	1%	8698
Stephens County Hospital	Toccoa	1%	21444
Taylor Regional Hospital	Hawkinsville	1%	10099
Trinity Hospital of Augusta	Augusta	1%	18138
Upson Regional Medical Center	Thomaston	1%	33329
Wellstar Cobb Hospital	Austell	1%	106913
West Georgia Medical Center	Lagrange	1%	66895
Athens Regional Medical Center	Athens	2%	78426
Candler Hospital	Savannah	2%	54486
Cartersville Medical Center	Cartersville	2%	49298
Chestatee Regional Hospital	Dahlonega	2%	11636
Dekalb Medical Center	Decatur	2%	66193
Dekalb Medical Center at Hillandale	Lithonia	2%	60407
Dorminy Medical Center	Fitzgerald	2%	11111
Elbert Memorial Hospital	Elberton	2%	8356
Emory - Adventist Hospital	Smyrna	2%	28429
Emory University Hospital	Atlanta	2%	37754
Fannin Regional Hospital	Blue Ridge	2%	10945
Floyd Medical Center	Rome	2%	79941
Gordon Hospital	Calhoun	2%	39036
Hutcheson Medical Center	Fort Oglethorpe	2%	34410
Irwin County Hospital	Ocilla	2%	4661
Jefferson Hospital	Louisville	2%	4983
Monroe County Hospital	Forsyth	2%	8726
North Fulton Hospital	Roswell	2%	40016
Northridge Medical Center	Commerce	2%	12699
Oconee Regional Medical Center	Milledgeville	2%	31175
Perry Hospital	Perry	2%	15116
Phoebe Sumter Medical Center	Americus	2%	23329
Piedmont Fayette Hospital	Fayetteville	2%	63594
Piedmont Hospital	Atlanta	2%	50506
Putnam General Hospital	Eatonton	2%	11507
Rockdale Medical Center	Conyers	2%	49002
Saint Joseph's Hospital - Savannah	Savannah	2%	36124
Saint Mary's Hospital	Athens	2%	40033
Southwest Georgia Regional Medical Center	Cuthbert	2%	5560
Spalding Regional Hospital	Griffin	2%	54365
Tanner Medical Center - Carrollton	Carrollton	2%	48291
Tift Regional Medical Center	Tifton	2%	55045
Ty Cobb Regional Medical Center	Lavonia	2%	17186
Washington County Regional Medical Center	Sandersville	2%	12095
Atlanta Medical Center	Atlanta	3%	58630
Barrow Regional Medical Center	Winder	3%	23213
Clearview Regional Medical Center	Monroe	3%	32076
Coffee Regional Medical Center	Douglas	3%	33332
Colquitt Regional Medical Center	Moultrie	3%	27825
Dodge County Hospital	Eastman	3%	13602
Donalsonville Hospital	Donalsonville	3%	6784
Emanuel County Hospital Authority	Swainsboro	3%	12922
Gwinnett Medical Center	Lawrenceville	3%	140830
Mayo Clinic Health System - Waycross	Waycross	3%	48775
The Medical Center of Peach County	Byron	3%	12970
North Georgia Medical Center	Ellijay	3%	10647
Phoebe Putney Memorial Hospital	Albany	3%	76537
Piedmont Newnan Hospital	Newnan	3%	47951
Tanner Medical Center Villa Rica	Villa Rica	3%	39689
Univ McDuffie Co Reg Med Ctr	Thomson	3%	13649
Wellstar Douglas Hospital	Douglasville	3%	64011
Wellstar Kennestone Hospital	Marietta	3%	129651
Wellstar Paulding Hospital	Hiram	3%	42324
Crisp Regional Hospital	Cordele	4%	18499
East Georgia Regional Medical Center	Statesboro	4%	41075
Hamilton Medical Center	Dalton	4%	65492
Med College of Georgia Hosps	Augusta	4%	88653
Piedmont Henry Hospital	Stockbridge	4%	79978
Piedmont Mountainside Hospital	Jasper	4%	22131
Polk Medical Center	Cedartown	4%	23258
South Georgia Medical Center	Valdosta	4%	74751
Emory University Hospital Midtown	Atlanta	5%	59922
Higgins General Hospital	Bremen	5%	23880
Medical Center of Central Georgia	Macon	5%	66546
Murray Medical Center	Chatsworth	5%	18076
Newton Medical Center	Covington	5%	50687
Saint Francis Hospital	Columbus	5%	58011
SE Georgia Health Sys-Camden Campus	Saint Marys	5%	30511
University Hospital	Augusta	5%	80877
Doctors Specialty Hospital	Columbus	6%	9577
Jeff Davis Hospital	Hazlehurst	6%	8794
SE Georgia Health Sys-Brunswick	Brunswick	6%	55965
Southern Regional Medical Center	Riverdale	6%	85352
John D Archbold Memorial Hospital	Thomasville	7%	32335
Midtown Medical Center	Columbus	9%	66781
Grady Memorial Hospital	Atlanta	10%	110403
Houston Medical Center	Warner Robins	10%	26978

Time from ER Arrival to Being Admitted (minutes)

Hospital Name	City	Min.	Cases
Polk Medical Center[2]	Cedartown	131	33
Wills Memorial Hospital[2]	Washington	150	286
Cook Medical Center[2]	Adel	172	233
Grady General Hospital[2]	Cairo	180	281
Stephens County Hospital[2]	Toccoa	181	510
Evans Memorial Hospital[2]	Claxton	183	362
Jeff Davis Hospital[2]	Hazlehurst	198	78
Elbert Memorial Hospital[2]	Elberton	200	414
Redmond Regional Medical Center[2]	Rome	201	680
Coffee Regional Medical Center[2]	Douglas	203	437
Doctors Hospital[2]	Augusta	203	553
Donalsonville Hospital[2]	Donalsonville	205	79
Putnam General Hospital[2]	Eatonton	206	388
Bacon County Hospital[2]	Alma	208	257
Fannin Regional Hospital[2]	Blue Ridge	212	298
West Georgia Medical Center[2]	Lagrange	212	626
Emory - Adventist Hospital[2]	Smyrna	214	506
Memorial Hospital & Manor[2]	Bainbridge	214	276
Jefferson Hospital[2]	Louisville	215	283
Wayne Memorial Hospital[2]	Jesup	215	405
Morgan Memorial Hospital	Madison	216	91
Dorminy Medical Center[2]	Fitzgerald	218	514
Taylor Regional Hospital[2]	Hawkinsville	222	318

NOTE: Hospital profiles are in alphabetical order by state, then city, then hospital within the city; Rankings exclude hospitals with less than 25 cases except for patient surveys which excludes hospitals with less than 100 cases; (a) 100-299 cases; (1) The number of cases/patients is too few to report; (2) Data submitted were based on a sample of cases/patients; (3) Results are based on a shorter time period than required; (4) Data suppressed by CMS for one or more quarters; (5) Results are not available for this reporting period; (6) Fewer than 100 patients completed the HCAHPS survey; (7) No cases met the criteria for this measure; (8) The lower limit of the confidence interval cannot be calculated if the number of observed infections equals zero; (9) No data are available from the state/territory for this reporting period; (10) The scores shown reflect fewer than 50 completed surveys; (11) There were discrepancies in the data collection process; (12) This measure does not apply to this hospital for this reporting period; (13) Results cannot be calculated for this reporting period; (14) The results for this state are combined with nearby states to protect confidentiality; Please refer to the User's Guide for a full explanation of data.

Hospital Name	City	Min.	Cases
Coliseum Northside Hospital[2]	Macon	224	410
Northridge Medical Center[2]	Commerce	225	429
Hutcheson Medical Center[2]	Fort Oglethorpe	226	496
Tanner Medical Center - Carrollton[2]	Carrollton	226	474
North Georgia Medical Center[2]	Ellijay	227	518
Habersham County Medical Center[2]	Demorest	228	482
Washington County Regional Medical Center[2]	Sandersville	228	302
Ty Cobb Regional Medical Center[2]	Lavonia	229	393
Jasper Memorial Hospital	Monticello	232	46
Union General Hospital[2]	Blairsville	232	300
Burke Medical Center[2]	Waynesboro	234	108
Tanner Medical Center Villa Rica[2]	Villa Rica	235	257
Floyd Medical Center[2]	Rome	238	509
Northside Hospital Forsyth[2]	Cumming	238	517
Coliseum Medical Center[2]	Macon	239	641
Gordon Hospital[2]	Calhoun	239	1129
Trinity Hospital of Augusta[2]	Augusta	240	392
Chestatee Regional Hospital[2]	Dahlonega	244	366
Mayo Clinic Health System - Waycross[2]	Waycross	244	995
Murray Medical Center	Chatsworth	246	136
Mountain Lakes Medical Center[2]	Clayton	248	226
Saint Mary's Good Samaritan Hospital[2,3]	Greensboro	248	48
Dodge County Hospital[2]	Eastman	250	291
Saint Mary's Hospital[2]	Athens	254	463
Appling Hospital[2]	Baxley	255	249
Chatuge Regional Hospital	Hiawassee	255	52
Fairview Park Hospital[2]	Dublin	255	713
Northside Hospital[2]	Atlanta	256	151
Univ McDuffie Co Reg Med Ctr[2]	Thomson	256	172
Wellstar Paulding Hospital[2]	Hiram	257	412
Upson Regional Medical Center[2]	Thomaston	258	423
Effingham County Hospital	Springfield	259	91
Newton Medical Center[2]	Covington	260	962
Higgins General Hospital[2]	Bremen	264	339
Colquitt Regional Medical Center[2]	Moultrie	265	562
Emanuel County Hospital Authority[2]	Swainsboro	268	493
Athens Regional Medical Center[2]	Athens	270	482
Flint River Hospital[2]	Montezuma	274	174
Liberty Regional Medical Center[2]	Hinesville	274	125
North Fulton Hospital[2]	Roswell	274	682
Meadows Regional Medical Center[2]	Vidalia	277	485
Northeast Georgia Medical Center[2]	Gainesville	281	549
Cartersville Medical Center[2]	Cartersville	284	600
SE Georgia Health Sys-Camden Campus[2]	Saint Marys	284	165
Hamilton Medical Center[2]	Dalton	286	440
Spalding Regional Hospital[2]	Griffin	286	598
SE Georgia Health Sys-Brunswick[2]	Brunswick	294	533
Crisp Regional Hospital[2]	Cordele	297	614
Perry Hospital[2]	Perry	298	354
Phoebe Sumter Medical Center[2]	Americus	298	516
Clearview Regional Medical Center[2]	Monroe	303	515
Rockdale Medical Center[2]	Conyers	304	666
Northside Hospital Cherokee[2]	Canton	306	375
Saint Joseph's Hospital of Atlanta[2]	Atlanta	311	535
Wellstar Kennestone Hospital[2]	Marietta	312	570
Barrow Regional Medical Center[2]	Winder	316	550
University Hospital[2]	Augusta	318	498
Emory Johns Creek Hospital[2]	Johns Creek	322	683
Wellstar Douglas Hospital[2]	Douglasville	323	396
Tift Regional Medical Center[2]	Tifton	326	626
East Georgia Regional Medical Center[2]	Statesboro	328	563
Piedmont Newnan Hospital[2]	Newnan	335	714
Wellstar Cobb Hospital[2]	Austell	335	372
Eastside Medical Center[2]	Snellville	340	607
Phoebe Putney Memorial Hospital[2]	Albany	340	574
John D Archbold Memorial Hospital[2]	Thomasville	356	622
Saint Joseph's Hospital - Savannah[2]	Savannah	356	516
South Georgia Medical Center[2]	Valdosta	366	650
Emory University Hospital Midtown[2]	Atlanta	374	407
Med College of Georgia Hosps[2]	Augusta	374	534
Gwinnett Medical Center[2]	Lawrenceville	378	922
Houston Medical Center[2]	Warner Robins	380	640
Oconee Regional Medical Center[2]	Milledgeville	385	690
Piedmont Hospital[2]	Atlanta	398	456
Piedmont Henry Hospital[2]	Stockbridge	402	671
Dekalb Medical Center[2]	Decatur	405	505
Emory University Hospital[2]	Atlanta	408	378
Piedmont Fayette Hospital[2]	Fayetteville	414	630
Southern Regional Medical Center[2]	Riverdale	415	850
Atlanta Medical Center[2]	Atlanta	417	573
Saint Francis Hospital[2]	Columbus	430	1004
Dekalb Medical Center at Hillandale[2]	Lithonia	465	1061
Medical Center of Central Georgia[2]	Macon	482	530
Grady Memorial Hospital[2]	Atlanta	511	403
Memorial Health Univ Medical Center[2]	Savannah	521	575
Candler Hospital[2]	Savannah	538	341
Midtown Medical Center[2]	Columbus	602	376

Time from ER Arrival to Discharge (minutes)

Hospital Name	City	Min.	Cases
Polk Medical Center	Cedartown	72	396
Morgan Memorial Hospital	Madison	79	363
Burke Medical Center[11]	Waynesboro	89	407
Evans Memorial Hospital	Claxton	90	295
Saint Mary's Good Samaritan Hospital[3]	Greensboro	90	209
Cook Medical Center[11]	Adel	94	414
Stephens County Hospital	Toccoa	95	371
Fannin Regional Hospital	Blue Ridge	96	362
Grady General Hospital	Cairo	97	451
Coffee Regional Medical Center	Douglas	102	444
Taylor Regional Hospital	Hawkinsville	104	391
Chatuge Regional Hospital[11]	Hiawassee	105	395
Irwin County Hospital	Ocilla	105	396
Doctors Hospital	Augusta	106	486
Effingham County Hospital	Springfield	106	426
West Georgia Medical Center	Lagrange	106	357
Chestatee Regional Hospital	Dahlonega	107	412
Washington County Regional Medical Center	Sandersville	107	379
Gordon Hospital	Calhoun	108	454
Liberty Regional Medical Center	Hinesville	110	214
Bacon County Hospital	Alma	112	411
Elbert Memorial Hospital	Elberton	112	443
Coliseum Northside Hospital	Macon	114	453
Hutcheson Medical Center	Fort Oglethorpe	114	431
Appling Hospital	Baxley	115	240
Northridge Medical Center	Commerce	115	426
Higgins General Hospital	Bremen	116	369
Univ McDuffie Co Reg Med Ctr[11]	Thomson	116	412
Dorminy Medical Center	Fitzgerald	117	419
Wayne Memorial Hospital	Jesup	117	429
Ty Cobb Regional Medical Center	Lavonia	118	417
Donalsonville Hospital	Donalsonville	119	433
Barrow Regional Medical Center	Winder	120	437
Emory - Adventist Hospital	Smyrna	120	350
Habersham County Medical Center	Demorest	121	469
Trinity Hospital of Augusta	Augusta	122	400
Jefferson Hospital	Louisville	125	338
Clearview Regional Medical Center	Monroe	128	529
Tanner Medical Center - Carrollton	Carrollton	128	390
Hamilton Medical Center	Dalton	129	351
Memorial Health Univ Medical Center	Savannah	130	334
Wellstar Paulding Hospital	Hiram	132	402
Dodge County Hospital	Eastman	133	414
North Georgia Medical Center[11]	Ellijay	133	383
Saint Mary's Hospital	Athens	134	407
Murray Medical Center	Chatsworth	135	341
North Fulton Hospital	Roswell	135	346
Wellstar Cobb Hospital	Austell	135	400
Colquitt Regional Medical Center	Moultrie	136	341
Mayo Clinic Health System - Waycross	Waycross	136	443
Perry Hospital	Perry	137	401
Upson Regional Medical Center	Thomaston	137	372
Tanner Medical Center Villa Rica	Villa Rica	139	385
Fairview Park Hospital	Dublin	140	426
Redmond Regional Medical Center	Rome	140	458
Meadows Regional Medical Center	Vidalia	142	396
Northside Hospital Forsyth	Cumming	144	406
Emanuel County Hospital Authority	Swainsboro	145	561
Memorial Hospital & Manor[3]	Bainbridge	145	311
Northside Hospital	Atlanta	145	402
Piedmont Mountainside Hospital	Jasper	145	393
Floyd Medical Center	Rome	146	338
Union General Hospital	Blairsville	146	410
Atlanta Medical Center	Atlanta	147	458
SE Georgia Health Sys-Camden Campus[11]	Saint Marys	147	437
Phoebe Sumter Medical Center	Americus	148	419
Flint River Hospital	Montezuma	150	188
Northeast Georgia Medical Center	Gainesville	150	395
Phoebe Putney Memorial Hospital	Albany	150	827
Wellstar Douglas Hospital	Douglasville	150	399
East Georgia Regional Medical Center	Statesboro	151	665
Newton Medical Center[11]	Covington	151	420
Candler Hospital	Savannah	154	370
Saint Joseph's Hospital - Savannah	Savannah	157	367
Tift Regional Medical Center	Tifton	160	454
Athens Regional Medical Center	Athens	161	305
Northside Hospital Cherokee	Canton	161	420
Coliseum Medical Center	Macon	162	455
Dekalb Medical Center at Hillandale	Lithonia	162	398
Spalding Regional Hospital	Griffin	162	446
South Georgia Medical Center	Valdosta	164	432
SE Georgia Health Sys-Brunswick[11]	Brunswick	166	445
John D Archbold Memorial Hospital[11]	Thomasville	167	452
Midtown Medical Center	Columbus	169	507
University Hospital	Augusta	170	400
Emory Johns Creek Hospital	Johns Creek	172	380
Cartersville Medical Center	Cartersville	173	430
Gwinnett Medical Center	Lawrenceville	177	811
Rockdale Medical Center	Conyers	180	470
Med College of Georgia Hosps	Augusta	181	335
Southern Regional Medical Center	Riverdale	186	1010
Piedmont Fayette Hospital	Fayetteville	188	411
Crisp Regional Hospital	Cordele	190	434
Piedmont Henry Hospital	Stockbridge	192	413
Eastside Medical Center	Snellville	195	491
Saint Francis Hospital	Columbus	196	408
Saint Joseph's Hospital of Atlanta	Atlanta	197	395
Oconee Regional Medical Center	Milledgeville	198	404
Wellstar Kennestone Hospital	Marietta	201	384
Piedmont Newnan Hospital	Newnan	203	470
Houston Medical Center	Warner Robins	206	380
Dekalb Medical Center	Decatur	209	357
Piedmont Hospital	Atlanta	219	401
Medical Center of Central Georgia	Macon	243	359
Emory University Hospital Midtown	Atlanta	302	355
Emory University Hospital	Atlanta	324	347
Grady Memorial Hospital	Atlanta	477	299

Time in ER Before Being Evaluated (minutes)

Hospital Name	City	Min.	Cases
Cartersville Medical Center	Cartersville	7	510
Appling Hospital	Baxley	8	249
Coliseum Northside Hospital	Macon	8	478
Coliseum Medical Center	Macon	10	500
Fairview Park Hospital	Dublin	10	451
Flint River Hospital	Montezuma	10	291
Doctors Hospital	Augusta	12	514
Northside Hospital Forsyth	Cumming	14	432
Crisp Regional Hospital	Cordele	15	462
Dorminy Medical Center	Fitzgerald	15	444
Taylor Regional Hospital	Hawkinsville	15	432
Northside Hospital	Atlanta	16	422
Redmond Regional Medical Center	Rome	17	492
Fannin Regional Hospital	Blue Ridge	18	406
Eastside Medical Center	Snellville	19	533
Saint Mary's Good Samaritan Hospital[3]	Greensboro	20	229
Elbert Memorial Hospital	Elberton	21	485
Donalsonville Hospital	Donalsonville	22	413
Evans Memorial Hospital	Claxton	22	354
Barrow Regional Medical Center	Winder	23	473
Habersham County Medical Center	Demorest	23	504
North Fulton Hospital	Roswell	23	373
Northside Hospital Cherokee	Canton	23	440
Emory - Adventist Hospital	Smyrna	24	378
Athens Regional Medical Center	Athens	25	332
Hutcheson Medical Center	Fort Oglethorpe	25	448
Trinity Hospital of Augusta	Augusta	25	416
Burke Medical Center	Waynesboro	26	457
Liberty Regional Medical Center	Hinesville	26	240
Stephens County Hospital	Toccoa	27	349
Ty Cobb Regional Medical Center	Lavonia	27	387
Clearview Regional Medical Center	Monroe	28	551
Cook Medical Center	Adel	28	412
Chatuge Regional Hospital	Hiawassee	29	475
Chestatee Regional Hospital	Dahlonega	29	426
Phoebe Putney Memorial Hospital	Albany	29	854
Polk Medical Center	Cedartown	29	240
Saint Mary's Hospital	Athens	29	412
Dekalb Medical Center at Hillandale	Lithonia	30	430
Dodge County Hospital	Eastman	30	453
Phoebe Sumter Medical Center	Americus	30	437
Tanner Medical Center - Carrollton	Carrollton	30	236
Upson Regional Medical Center	Thomaston	30	296
Washington County Regional Medical Center	Sandersville	30	418
Effingham County Hospital	Springfield	31	459
Meadows Regional Medical Center	Vidalia	31	402
Northridge Medical Center	Commerce	31	485
Perry Hospital	Perry	31	348
Union General Hospital	Blairsville	31	312
Atlanta Medical Center	Atlanta	32	486
Bacon County Hospital	Alma	32	401
Oconee Regional Medical Center	Milledgeville	32	462
Wayne Memorial Hospital	Jesup	32	403
Piedmont Mountainside Hospital	Jasper	33	412
Univ McDuffie Co Reg Med Ctr	Thomson	33	461
East Georgia Regional Medical Center	Statesboro	34	735
Floyd Medical Center	Rome	34	215
North Georgia Medical Center	Ellijay	34	426
Emory Johns Creek Hospital	Johns Creek	35	423
Rockdale Medical Center	Conyers	35	547
Coffee Regional Medical Center	Douglas	36	313
Colquitt Regional Medical Center	Moultrie	36	375
Wellstar Paulding Hospital	Hiram	36	391
Emanuel County Hospital Authority	Swainsboro	37	655
Gordon Hospital	Calhoun	37	466
Grady General Hospital	Cairo	37	462
Northeast Georgia Medical Center	Gainesville	37	430
Memorial Health Univ Medical Center	Savannah	38	395
Higgins General Hospital	Bremen	39	216
Houston Medical Center	Warner Robins	39	397
Piedmont Newnan Hospital	Newnan	39	435
Memorial Hospital & Manor	Bainbridge	40	329
Midtown Medical Center	Columbus	40	513

NOTE: Hospital profiles are in alphabetical order by state, then city, then hospital within the city; Rankings exclude hospitals with less than 25 cases except for patient surveys which excludes hospitals with less than 100 cases; (a) 100-299 cases; (1) The number of cases/patients is too few to report; (2) Data submitted were based on a sample of cases/patients; (3) Results are based on a shorter time period than required; (4) Data suppressed by CMS for one or more quarters; (5) Results are not available for this reporting period; (6) Fewer than 100 patients completed the HCAHPS survey; (7) No cases met the criteria for this measure; (8) The lower limit of the confidence interval cannot be calculated if the number of observed infections equals zero; (9) No data are available from the state/territory for this reporting period; (10) The scores shown reflect fewer than 50 completed surveys; (11) There were discrepancies in the data collection process; (12) This measure does not apply to this hospital for this reporting period; (13) Results cannot be calculated for this reporting period; (14) The results for this state are combined with nearby states to protect confidentiality; Please refer to the User's Guide for a full explanation of data.

Newton Medical Center	Covington	40	442
South Georgia Medical Center	Valdosta	40	452
Tanner Medical Center Villa Rica	Villa Rica	40	306
West Georgia Medical Center	Lagrange	41	383
Dekalb Medical Center	Decatur	42	388
Mayo Clinic Health System - Waycross	Waycross	42	471
Saint Joseph's Hospital - Savannah	Savannah	44	318
Gwinnett Medical Center	Lawrenceville	45	768
Saint Joseph's Hospital of Atlanta	Atlanta	45	337
Wellstar Cobb Hospital	Austell	46	330
Murray Medical Center	Chatsworth	48	378
Piedmont Fayette Hospital	Fayetteville	48	430
Spalding Regional Hospital	Griffin	48	486
Wellstar Douglas Hospital	Douglasville	48	279
Hamilton Medical Center	Dalton	49	213
Wellstar Kennestone Hospital	Marietta	49	419
Jefferson Hospital	Louisville	50	323
University Hospital	Augusta	50	302
Candler Hospital	Savannah	51	331
Medical Center of Central Georgia	Macon	52	376
Tift Regional Medical Center	Tifton	52	500
SE Georgia Health Sys-Brunswick	Brunswick	54	473
SE Georgia Health Sys-Camden Campus	Saint Marys	58	460
Irwin County Hospital	Ocilla	60	236
Piedmont Hospital	Atlanta	69	339
John D Archbold Memorial Hospital	Thomasville	70	448
Med College of Georgia Hosps	Augusta	71	223
Piedmont Henry Hospital	Stockbridge	73	428
Saint Francis Hospital	Columbus	79	425
Emory University Hospital	Atlanta	86	365
Southern Regional Medical Center	Riverdale	91	883
Emory University Hospital Midtown	Atlanta	132	374
Grady Memorial Hospital	Atlanta	160	335

Time to Pain Meds for Bone Fractures (minutes)

Hospital Name	City	Min.	Cases
Taylor Regional Hospital	Hawkinsville	34	39
Coliseum Northside Hospital	Macon	42	70
Washington County Regional Medical Center	Sandersville	42	55
Ty Cobb Regional Medical Center	Lavonia	43	77
Bacon County Hospital	Alma	44	36
North Fulton Hospital	Roswell	44	228
Northside Hospital	Atlanta	44	69
Northside Hospital Forsyth	Cumming	45	228
Doctors Hospital	Augusta	46	215
Grady General Hospital	Cairo	46	46
Clearview Regional Medical Center	Monroe	47	113
Cook Medical Center	Adel	48	28
Evans Memorial Hospital	Claxton	48	42
Meadows Regional Medical Center	Vidalia	48	73
Putnam General Hospital	Eatonton	49	35
Chestatee Regional Hospital	Dahlonega	50	41
Upson Regional Medical Center	Thomaston	50	98
Polk Medical Center	Cedartown	51	50
Emory - Adventist Hospital	Smyrna	52	70
Gwinnett Medical Center	Lawrenceville	52	457
Rockdale Medical Center	Conyers	52	142
Athens Regional Medical Center	Athens	53	189
Northside Hospital Cherokee	Canton	53	142
Coffee Regional Medical Center	Douglas	54	141
East Georgia Regional Medical Center	Statesboro	54	122
Hutcheson Medical Center	Fort Oglethorpe	54	94
Phoebe Putney Memorial Hospital	Albany	54	164
Piedmont Mountainside Hospital	Jasper	54	144
Union General Hospital	Blairsville	54	69
Cartersville Medical Center	Cartersville	55	133
Burke Medical Center	Waynesboro	57	30
Crisp Regional Hospital	Cordele	57	85
Saint Joseph's Hospital - Savannah	Savannah	58	130
Barrow Regional Medical Center	Winder	59	88
Eastside Medical Center	Snellville	60	119
Emory Johns Creek Hospital	Johns Creek	60	116
Fairview Park Hospital	Dublin	60	127
Fannin Regional Hospital	Blue Ridge	60	64
Gordon Hospital	Calhoun	60	118
Habersham County Medical Center	Demorest	60	108
Memorial Health Univ Medical Center	Savannah	60	175
Saint Mary's Hospital	Athens	60	93
Wellstar Kennestone Hospital	Marietta	60	362
Trinity Hospital of Augusta	Augusta	61	50
Atlanta Medical Center	Atlanta	62	133
Northridge Medical Center	Commerce	62	48
Tanner Medical Center - Carrollton	Carrollton	63	190
Univ McDuffie Co Reg Med Ctr	Thomson	64	36
Dekalb Medical Center at Hillandale	Lithonia	66	101
Dodge County Hospital	Eastman	66	43
Med College of Georgia Hosps	Augusta	66	265
Saint Joseph's Hospital of Atlanta	Atlanta	66	56
Tift Regional Medical Center	Tifton	66	127
Wellstar Paulding Hospital	Hiram	66	112
Colquitt Regional Medical Center	Moultrie	67	47
Floyd Medical Center	Rome	67	158
Oconee Regional Medical Center	Milledgeville	67	81
Hamilton Medical Center	Dalton	68	222
Midtown Medical Center	Columbus	68	181
Piedmont Newnan Hospital	Newnan	68	204
South Georgia Medical Center	Valdosta	68	206
Emanuel County Hospital Authority	Swainsboro	70	55
Redmond Regional Medical Center	Rome	71	76
Tanner Medical Center Villa Rica	Villa Rica	71	118
Wellstar Cobb Hospital	Austell	71	244
Northeast Georgia Medical Center	Gainesville	72	319
West Georgia Medical Center	Lagrange	72	162
Mayo Clinic Health System - Waycross	Waycross	74	123
Newton Medical Center	Covington	74	124
Phoebe Sumter Medical Center	Americus	74	92
SE Georgia Health Sys-Brunswick	Brunswick	74	190
Spalding Regional Hospital	Griffin	74	164
Stephens County Hospital	Toccoa	74	78
Wayne Memorial Hospital	Jesup	75	113
Elbert Memorial Hospital	Elberton	76	33
Grady Memorial Hospital	Atlanta	76	130
Piedmont Hospital	Atlanta	76	138
Wellstar Douglas Hospital	Douglasville	76	143
Candler Hospital	Savannah	77	113
Piedmont Henry Hospital	Stockbridge	77	233
Coliseum Medical Center	Macon	78	29
Higgins General Hospital	Bremen	80	126
North Georgia Medical Center	Ellijay	81	62
Medical Center of Central Georgia	Macon	82	111
SE Georgia Health Sys-Camden Campus	Saint Marys	82	94
Piedmont Fayette Hospital	Fayetteville	84	257
Houston Medical Center	Warner Robins	85	101
University Hospital	Augusta	86	232
Dekalb Medical Center	Decatur	88	105
Saint Francis Hospital	Columbus	88	138
John D Archbold Memorial Hospital	Thomasville	90	134
Emory University Hospital Midtown	Atlanta	94	36
Memorial Hospital & Manor	Bainbridge	97	61
Southern Regional Medical Center	Riverdale	109	152
Emory University Hospital	Atlanta	117	29

Heart Attack Care

Aspirin Given at Discharge

Hospital Name	City	Rate	Cases
Athens Regional Medical Center[2]	Athens	100%	277
Atlanta Medical Center	Atlanta	100%	112
Augusta VA Medical Center	Augusta	100%	32
Cartersville Medical Center	Cartersville	100%	112
Coliseum Medical Center	Macon	100%	225
Doctors Hospital	Augusta	100%	93
Eastside Medical Center	Snellville	100%	134
Emory Johns Creek Hospital	Johns Creek	100%	117
Emory University Hospital[2]	Atlanta	100%	271
Emory University Hospital Midtown[2]	Atlanta	100%	280
Fairview Park Hospital	Dublin	100%	118
John D Archbold Memorial Hospital	Thomasville	100%	194
Meadows Regional Medical Center	Vidalia	100%	117
Med College of Georgia Hosps[2]	Augusta	100%	204
Memorial Health Univ Medical Center[2]	Savannah	100%	263
Newton Medical Center[2]	Covington	100%	35
Northeast Georgia Medical Center[2]	Gainesville	100%	333
Northside Hospital	Atlanta	100%	148
Northside Hospital Cherokee	Canton	100%	131
Northside Hospital Forsyth	Cumming	100%	234
Phoebe Putney Memorial Hospital	Albany	100%	486
Piedmont Fayette Hospital[2]	Fayetteville	100%	261
Piedmont Newnan Hospital	Newnan	100%	25
Redmond Regional Medical Center	Rome	100%	570
Rockdale Medical Center	Conyers	100%	29
Saint Francis Hospital	Columbus	100%	378
Saint Mary's Hospital	Athens	100%	144
South Georgia Medical Center	Valdosta	100%	331
Tanner Medical Center - Carrollton	Carrollton	100%	228
Trinity Hospital of Augusta	Augusta	100%	34
University Hospital	Augusta	100%	538
Wellstar Cobb Hospital[2]	Austell	100%	220
Wellstar Douglas Hospital[2]	Douglasville	100%	126
Wellstar Kennestone Hospital[2]	Marietta	100%	556
Gwinnett Medical Center	Lawrenceville	99%	502
Hamilton Medical Center	Dalton	99%	220
Piedmont Henry Hospital	Stockbridge	99%	176
Piedmont Hospital[2]	Atlanta	99%	505
Saint Joseph's Hospital - Savannah	Savannah	99%	304
Saint Joseph's Hospital of Atlanta[2]	Atlanta	99%	299
Spalding Regional Hospital	Griffin	99%	180
West Georgia Medical Center	Lagrange	99%	153
Dekalb Medical Center[2]	Decatur	98%	224
Grady Memorial Hospital	Atlanta	98%	155
Houston Medical Center	Warner Robins	98%	155
Midtown Medical Center	Columbus	98%	46
Southern Regional Medical Center	Riverdale	98%	166
Tift Regional Medical Center	Tifton	98%	159
Crisp Regional Hospital	Cordele	97%	33
Decatur VA Medical Center	Decatur	97%	65
Floyd Medical Center	Rome	97%	198
Mayo Clinic Health System - Waycross[2]	Waycross	97%	93
Medical Center of Central Georgia	Macon	97%	771
SE Georgia Health Sys-Brunswick[2]	Brunswick	96%	139
East Georgia Regional Medical Center	Statesboro	94%	86

PCI Within 90 Minutes of Arrival

Hospital Name	City	Rate	Cases
Athens Regional Medical Center[2]	Athens	100%	45
Emory University Hospital[2]	Atlanta	100%	26
Fairview Park Hospital	Dublin	100%	32
Gwinnett Medical Center	Lawrenceville	100%	119
Hamilton Medical Center	Dalton	100%	53
Northeast Georgia Medical Center[2]	Gainesville	100%	62
Northside Hospital Cherokee	Canton	100%	26
Piedmont Henry Hospital	Stockbridge	100%	30
Saint Joseph's Hospital - Savannah	Savannah	100%	42
Saint Joseph's Hospital of Atlanta[2]	Atlanta	100%	43
South Georgia Medical Center	Valdosta	100%	58
Tanner Medical Center - Carrollton	Carrollton	100%	36
Redmond Regional Medical Center	Rome	99%	71
Eastside Medical Center	Snellville	98%	53
Coliseum Medical Center	Macon	97%	29
Piedmont Hospital[2]	Atlanta	97%	29
West Georgia Medical Center	Lagrange	97%	31
Emory Johns Creek Hospital	Johns Creek	96%	26
Mayo Clinic Health System - Waycross[2]	Waycross	96%	26
Northside Hospital Forsyth	Cumming	96%	53
Spalding Regional Hospital	Griffin	96%	50
Tift Regional Medical Center	Tifton	96%	27
Medical Center of Central Georgia	Macon	95%	77
Saint Francis Hospital	Columbus	95%	88
Cartersville Medical Center	Cartersville	94%	35
University Hospital	Augusta	94%	85
Wellstar Kennestone Hospital[2]	Marietta	94%	137
Memorial Health Univ Medical Center[2]	Savannah	93%	44
Wellstar Cobb Hospital[2]	Austell	92%	39
Houston Medical Center	Warner Robins	91%	33
John D Archbold Memorial Hospital	Thomasville	91%	35
Dekalb Medical Center[2]	Decatur	89%	35
Phoebe Putney Memorial Hospital	Albany	88%	56
Southern Regional Medical Center	Riverdale	88%	48
Wellstar Douglas Hospital[2]	Douglasville	88%	40
Atlanta Medical Center	Atlanta	82%	28
SE Georgia Health Sys-Brunswick[2]	Brunswick	78%	27

Statin Prescribed at Discharge

Hospital Name	City	Rate	Cases
Athens Regional Medical Center[2]	Athens	100%	273
Augusta VA Medical Center	Augusta	100%	31
Coliseum Medical Center	Macon	100%	231
Doctors Hospital	Augusta	100%	88
Eastside Medical Center	Snellville	100%	132
Emory Johns Creek Hospital	Johns Creek	100%	116
Emory University Hospital[2]	Atlanta	100%	256
Emory University Hospital Midtown[2]	Atlanta	100%	267
Fairview Park Hospital	Dublin	100%	120
John D Archbold Memorial Hospital	Thomasville	100%	192
Memorial Health Univ Medical Center[2]	Savannah	100%	260
Midtown Medical Center	Columbus	100%	48
Northeast Georgia Medical Center[2]	Gainesville	100%	314
Northside Hospital	Atlanta	100%	141
Northside Hospital Cherokee	Canton	100%	115
Northside Hospital Forsyth	Cumming	100%	222
Phoebe Putney Memorial Hospital	Albany	100%	479
Saint Mary's Hospital	Athens	100%	141
South Georgia Medical Center	Valdosta	100%	322
Tanner Medical Center - Carrollton	Carrollton	100%	210
Trinity Hospital of Augusta	Augusta	100%	33
University Hospital	Augusta	100%	521
Wellstar Douglas Hospital[2]	Douglasville	100%	126
Cartersville Medical Center	Cartersville	99%	108
Gwinnett Medical Center	Lawrenceville	99%	490
Hamilton Medical Center	Dalton	99%	216
Mayo Clinic Health System - Waycross[2]	Waycross	99%	92
Med College of Georgia Hosps[2]	Augusta	99%	204
Redmond Regional Medical Center	Rome	99%	535
Saint Francis Hospital	Columbus	99%	366
Saint Joseph's Hospital of Atlanta[2]	Atlanta	99%	287
Spalding Regional Hospital	Griffin	99%	178
Wellstar Cobb Hospital[2]	Austell	99%	205
Wellstar Kennestone Hospital[2]	Marietta	99%	551
West Georgia Medical Center	Lagrange	99%	133
Atlanta Medical Center	Atlanta	98%	115
Decatur VA Medical Center	Decatur	98%	63

NOTE: Hospital profiles are in alphabetical order by state, then city, then hospital within the city; Rankings exclude hospitals with less than 25 cases except for patient surveys which excludes hospitals with less than 100 cases; (a) 100-299 cases; (1) The number of cases/patients is too few to report; (2) Data submitted were based on a sample of cases/patients; (3) Results are based on a shorter time period than required; (4) Data suppressed by CMS for one or more quarters; (5) Results are not available for this reporting period; (6) Fewer than 100 patients completed the HCAHPS survey; (7) No cases met the criteria for this measure; (8) The lower limit of the confidence interval cannot be calculated if the number of observed infections equals zero; (9) No data are available from the state/territory for this reporting period; (10) The scores shown reflect fewer than 50 completed surveys; (11) There were discrepancies in the data collection process; (12) This measure does not apply to this hospital for this reporting period; (13) Results cannot be calculated for this reporting period; (14) The results for this state are combined with nearby states to protect confidentiality; Please refer to the User's Guide for a full explanation of data.

Piedmont Fayette Hospital[2]	Fayetteville	98%	258
Piedmont Hospital[2]	Atlanta	98%	481
Saint Joseph's Hospital - Savannah	Savannah	98%	317
Tift Regional Medical Center	Tifton	98%	155
Grady Memorial Hospital	Atlanta	97%	156
Medical Center of Central Georgia	Macon	97%	744
Newton Medical Center[2]	Covington	97%	33
Dekalb Medical Center[2]	Decatur	96%	214
Floyd Medical Center	Rome	96%	192
Southern Regional Medical Center	Riverdale	96%	160
Houston Medical Center	Warner Robins	95%	144
Piedmont Henry Hospital	Stockbridge	95%	173
Crisp Regional Hospital	Cordele	94%	33
Meadows Regional Medical Center	Vidalia	93%	107
East Georgia Regional Medical Center	Statesboro	92%	74
SE Georgia Health Sys-Brunswick[2]	Brunswick	92%	132
Rockdale Medical Center	Conyers	88%	26

Heart Failure Care

ACE Inhibitor or ARB for LVSD

Hospital Name	City	Rate	Cases
Atlanta Medical Center	Atlanta	100%	227
Candler Hospital	Savannah	100%	67
Cartersville Medical Center	Cartersville	100%	46
Coffee Regional Medical Center[2]	Douglas	100%	40
Coliseum Medical Center	Macon	100%	136
Colquitt Regional Medical Center	Moultrie	100%	55
Crisp Regional Hospital	Cordele	100%	45
Doctors Hospital	Augusta	100%	61
Eastside Medical Center	Snellville	100%	59
Emory - Adventist Hospital	Smyrna	100%	26
Emory Johns Creek Hospital	Johns Creek	100%	47
Emory University Hospital[2]	Atlanta	100%	70
Fairview Park Hospital	Dublin	100%	97
John D Archbold Memorial Hospital	Thomasville	100%	103
Northside Hospital	Atlanta	100%	43
Northside Hospital Cherokee	Canton	100%	34
Northside Hospital Forsyth	Cumming	100%	69
Perry Hospital	Perry	100%	26
Saint Mary's Hospital	Athens	100%	48
Spalding Regional Hospital	Griffin	100%	109
University Hospital[2]	Augusta	100%	125
Dekalb Medical Center at Hillandale	Lithonia	99%	135
Emory University Hospital Midtown[2]	Atlanta	99%	102
Gwinnett Medical Center	Lawrenceville	99%	254
Medical Center of Central Georgia[2]	Macon	99%	140
Saint Joseph's Hospital - Savannah	Savannah	99%	109
Saint Joseph's Hospital of Atlanta[2]	Atlanta	99%	87
South Georgia Medical Center	Valdosta	99%	165
Wellstar Douglas Hospital[2]	Douglasville	99%	77
Wellstar Kennestone Hospital[2]	Marietta	99%	209
West Georgia Medical Center	Lagrange	99%	69
Dekalb Medical Center[2]	Decatur	98%	130
Floyd Medical Center	Rome	98%	101
Med College of Georgia Hosps[2]	Augusta	98%	122
Northeast Georgia Medical Center[2]	Gainesville	98%	49
Piedmont Fayette Hospital[2]	Fayetteville	98%	85
Piedmont Newnan Hospital[2]	Newnan	98%	62
Redmond Regional Medical Center	Rome	98%	163
Tanner Medical Center - Carrollton	Carrollton	98%	57
Wellstar Cobb Hospital[2]	Austell	98%	174
Gordon Hospital	Calhoun	97%	31
Hamilton Medical Center	Dalton	97%	76
Midtown Medical Center	Columbus	97%	150
North Fulton Hospital	Roswell	97%	37
Rockdale Medical Center[2]	Conyers	97%	94
SE Georgia Health Sys-Brunswick[2]	Brunswick	97%	107
Trinity Hospital of Augusta	Augusta	97%	39
Upson Regional Medical Center	Thomaston	97%	76
Athens Regional Medical Center[2]	Athens	96%	67
Grady Memorial Hospital[2]	Atlanta	96%	141
Houston Medical Center[2]	Warner Robins	96%	105
Memorial Hospital & Manor[2]	Bainbridge	96%	28
Northridge Medical Center[2]	Commerce	96%	25
Phoebe Sumter Medical Center	Americus	96%	49
Saint Francis Hospital[2]	Columbus	96%	184
Mayo Clinic Health System - Waycross[2]	Waycross	95%	77
Memorial Health Univ Medical Center[2]	Savannah	95%	96
Phoebe Putney Memorial Hospital	Albany	95%	261
Piedmont Hospital[2]	Atlanta	95%	111
Southern Regional Medical Center[2]	Riverdale	95%	133
Tift Regional Medical Center	Tifton	95%	112
Decatur VA Medical Center	Decatur	93%	216
Newton Medical Center[2]	Covington	92%	78
Oconee Regional Medical Center	Milledgeville	91%	44
Augusta VA Medical Center	Augusta	90%	72
Meadows Regional Medical Center	Vidalia	90%	59
Piedmont Henry Hospital[2]	Stockbridge	90%	104
East Georgia Regional Medical Center	Statesboro	86%	86
Dodge County Hospital[2]	Eastman	85%	27
Piedmont Mountainside Hospital	Jasper	85%	27
Wayne Memorial Hospital	Jesup	78%	45

Discharge Instructions Given

Hospital Name	City	Rate	Cases
Candler Hospital	Savannah	100%	262
Coffee Regional Medical Center[2]	Douglas	100%	177
Coliseum Medical Center	Macon	100%	367
Colquitt Regional Medical Center	Moultrie	100%	156
Doctors Hospital	Augusta	100%	175
Dodge County Hospital[2]	Eastman	100%	50
Eastside Medical Center	Snellville	100%	218
Emanuel County Hospital Authority[2]	Swainsboro	100%	30
Emory - Adventist Hospital	Smyrna	100%	57
Grady General Hospital	Cairo	100%	58
Higgins General Hospital	Bremen	100%	28
John D Archbold Memorial Hospital	Thomasville	100%	284
Mayo Clinic Health System - Waycross[2]	Waycross	100%	200
Medical Center of Central Georgia[2]	Macon	100%	243
Memorial Hospital & Manor[2]	Bainbridge	100%	48
Northside Hospital Forsyth	Cumming	100%	220
Saint Joseph's Hospital - Savannah	Savannah	100%	329
Spalding Regional Hospital	Griffin	100%	255
Stephens County Hospital[2]	Toccoa	100%	40
Wills Memorial Hospital	Washington	100%	33
Crisp Regional Hospital	Cordele	99%	134
Emory University Hospital[2]	Atlanta	99%	242
Fairview Park Hospital	Dublin	99%	152
Gordon Hospital	Calhoun	99%	84
North Fulton Hospital	Roswell	99%	151
Northside Hospital	Atlanta	99%	178
Tanner Medical Center - Carrollton	Carrollton	99%	203
Tanner Medical Center Villa Rica	Villa Rica	99%	99
Clearview Regional Medical Center	Monroe	98%	96
Coliseum Northside Hospital	Macon	98%	52
Decatur VA Medical Center	Decatur	98%	403
Dublin VA Medical Center	Dublin	98%	51
Grady Memorial Hospital[2]	Atlanta	98%	259
Memorial Health Univ Medical Center[2]	Savannah	98%	256
Midtown Medical Center	Columbus	98%	228
Piedmont Fayette Hospital[2]	Fayetteville	98%	276
Rockdale Medical Center[2]	Conyers	98%	254
Saint Mary's Hospital	Athens	98%	150
Tift Regional Medical Center	Tifton	98%	257
Atlanta Medical Center	Atlanta	97%	460
Augusta VA Medical Center	Augusta	97%	161
Dekalb Medical Center[2]	Decatur	97%	270
Donalsonville Hospital	Donalsonville	97%	29
Dorminy Medical Center	Fitzgerald	97%	39
Emory Johns Creek Hospital	Johns Creek	97%	191
Emory University Hospital Midtown[2]	Atlanta	97%	235
Liberty Regional Medical Center	Hinesville	97%	36
Northside Hospital Cherokee	Canton	97%	66
Phoebe Sumter Medical Center	Americus	97%	131
Trinity Hospital of Augusta	Augusta	97%	76
East Georgia Regional Medical Center	Statesboro	96%	227
Fannin Regional Hospital	Blue Ridge	96%	26
Hamilton Medical Center	Dalton	96%	279
Wayne Memorial Hospital	Jesup	96%	110
Newton Medical Center[2]	Covington	95%	198
South Georgia Medical Center	Valdosta	95%	403
SE Georgia Health Sys-Brunswick[2]	Brunswick	95%	237
Dekalb Medical Center at Hillandale	Lithonia	93%	262
Doctors Specialty Hospital	Columbus	93%	44
West Georgia Medical Center	Lagrange	93%	202
Barrow Regional Medical Center	Winder	92%	90
Cook Medical Center	Adel	91%	32
Meadows Regional Medical Center	Vidalia	91%	172
Northridge Medical Center[2]	Commerce	91%	65
Oconee Regional Medical Center	Milledgeville	91%	105
University Hospital[2]	Augusta	91%	269
Wellstar Kennestone Hospital[2]	Marietta	91%	707
Northeast Georgia Medical Center[2]	Gainesville	90%	282
Piedmont Mountainside Hospital	Jasper	90%	70
Piedmont Henry Hospital[2]	Stockbridge	89%	309
Redmond Regional Medical Center	Rome	89%	455
Elbert Memorial Hospital	Elberton	88%	58
Evans Memorial Hospital[2]	Claxton	88%	26
Floyd Medical Center	Rome	88%	252
Houston Medical Center[2]	Warner Robins	88%	299
Hutcheson Medical Center[2]	Fort Oglethorpe	88%	60
Jefferson Hospital[2]	Louisville	88%	40
Taylor Regional Hospital[2]	Hawkinsville	88%	25
Upson Regional Medical Center	Thomaston	88%	116
Cartersville Medical Center	Cartersville	87%	193
Southern Regional Medical Center[2]	Riverdale	87%	272
Athens Regional Medical Center[2]	Athens	86%	256
Saint Joseph's Hospital of Atlanta[2]	Atlanta	86%	257
Union General Hospital[2]	Blairsville	85%	46
Perry Hospital	Perry	84%	55
Gwinnett Medical Center	Lawrenceville	83%	812
Piedmont Newnan Hospital[2]	Newnan	83%	241
Saint Francis Hospital[2]	Columbus	83%	411
Med College of Georgia Hosps[2]	Augusta	82%	226
Putnam General Hospital	Eatonton	81%	47
North Georgia Medical Center[2]	Ellijay	80%	35
Washington County Regional Medical Center	Sandersville	80%	35
Wellstar Cobb Hospital[2]	Austell	80%	536
Wellstar Paulding Hospital	Hiram	80%	40
The Medical Center of Peach County[2]	Byron	79%	29
Appling Hospital	Baxley	78%	41
Piedmont Hospital[2]	Atlanta	78%	286
Phoebe Putney Memorial Hospital	Albany	73%	626
Ty Cobb Regional Medical Center	Lavonia	70%	43
Wellstar Douglas Hospital[2]	Douglasville	70%	278
Habersham County Medical Center[2]	Demorest	66%	41

Evaluation of LVS Function

Hospital Name	City	Rate	Cases
Athens Regional Medical Center[2]	Athens	100%	287
Atlanta Medical Center	Atlanta	100%	517
Candler Hospital	Savannah	100%	319
Cartersville Medical Center	Cartersville	100%	210
Clearview Regional Medical Center	Monroe	100%	114
Coffee Regional Medical Center[2]	Douglas	100%	192
Coliseum Medical Center	Macon	100%	410
Colquitt Regional Medical Center	Moultrie	100%	189
Crisp Regional Hospital	Cordele	100%	153
Decatur VA Medical Center	Decatur	100%	422
Dekalb Medical Center[2]	Decatur	100%	308
Dekalb Medical Center at Hillandale	Lithonia	100%	284
Doctors Hospital	Augusta	100%	207
Doctors Specialty Hospital	Columbus	100%	46
Dublin VA Medical Center	Dublin	100%	55
Eastside Medical Center	Snellville	100%	249
Emory - Adventist Hospital	Smyrna	100%	66
Emory Johns Creek Hospital	Johns Creek	100%	204
Emory University Hospital[2]	Atlanta	100%	272
Emory University Hospital Midtown[2]	Atlanta	100%	266
Evans Memorial Hospital[2]	Claxton	100%	28
Fairview Park Hospital	Dublin	100%	181
Fannin Regional Hospital	Blue Ridge	100%	33
Floyd Medical Center	Rome	100%	306
Gordon Hospital	Calhoun	100%	100
Grady Memorial Hospital[2]	Atlanta	100%	286
Gwinnett Medical Center	Lawrenceville	100%	930
Hamilton Medical Center	Dalton	100%	346
Higgins General Hospital	Bremen	100%	35
Houston Medical Center[2]	Warner Robins	100%	340
Hutcheson Medical Center[2]	Fort Oglethorpe	100%	80
John D Archbold Memorial Hospital	Thomasville	100%	334
Liberty Regional Medical Center	Hinesville	100%	40
Mayo Clinic Health System - Waycross[2]	Waycross	100%	256
Medical Center of Central Georgia[2]	Macon	100%	282
Med College of Georgia Hosps[2]	Augusta	100%	251
Memorial Health Univ Medical Center[2]	Savannah	100%	282
Midtown Medical Center	Columbus	100%	271
Northeast Georgia Medical Center[2]	Gainesville	100%	326
Northridge Medical Center[2]	Commerce	100%	72
Northside Hospital Cherokee	Canton	100%	87
Northside Hospital Forsyth	Cumming	100%	252
Oconee Regional Medical Center	Milledgeville	100%	123
Perry Hospital	Perry	100%	74
Phoebe Putney Memorial Hospital	Albany	100%	690
Piedmont Fayette Hospital[2]	Fayetteville	100%	328
Piedmont Hospital[2]	Atlanta	100%	322
Piedmont Newnan Hospital[2]	Newnan	100%	267
Putnam General Hospital	Eatonton	100%	53
Redmond Regional Medical Center	Rome	100%	520
Rockdale Medical Center[2]	Conyers	100%	279
Saint Francis Hospital[2]	Columbus	100%	472
Saint Joseph's Hospital - Savannah	Savannah	100%	375
Saint Joseph's Hospital of Atlanta[2]	Atlanta	100%	292
Saint Mary's Good Samaritan Hospital	Greensboro	100%	28
Saint Mary's Hospital	Athens	100%	165
South Georgia Medical Center	Valdosta	100%	425
SE Georgia Health Sys-Camden Campus[2]	Saint Marys	100%	27
Spalding Regional Hospital	Griffin	100%	287
Stephens County Hospital[2]	Toccoa	100%	49
Tanner Medical Center Villa Rica	Villa Rica	100%	105
Tift Regional Medical Center	Tifton	100%	289
Trinity Hospital of Augusta	Augusta	100%	100
University Hospital[2]	Augusta	100%	326
Wellstar Cobb Hospital[2]	Austell	100%	597
Wellstar Douglas Hospital[2]	Douglasville	100%	298
Wellstar Kennestone Hospital[2]	Marietta	100%	801
Wellstar Paulding Hospital	Hiram	100%	44
West Georgia Medical Center	Lagrange	100%	246
Augusta VA Medical Center	Augusta	99%	170
Barrow Regional Medical Center	Winder	99%	103
East Georgia Regional Medical Center	Statesboro	99%	247

NOTE: Hospital profiles are in alphabetical order by state, then city, then hospital within the city; Rankings exclude hospitals with less than 25 cases except for patient surveys which excludes hospitals with less than 100 cases; (a) 100-299 cases; (1) The number of cases/patients is too few to report; (2) Data submitted were based on a sample of cases/patients; (3) Results are based on a shorter time period than required; (4) Data suppressed by CMS for one or more quarters; (5) Results are not available for this reporting period; (6) Fewer than 100 patients completed the HCAHPS survey; (7) No cases met the criteria for this measure; (8) The lower limit of the confidence interval cannot be calculated if the number of observed infections equals zero; (9) No data are available from the state/territory for this reporting period; (10) The scores shown reflect fewer than 50 completed surveys; (11) There were discrepancies in the data collection process; (12) This measure does not apply to this hospital for this reporting period; (13) Results cannot be calculated for this reporting period; (14) The results for this state are combined with nearby states to protect confidentiality; Please refer to the User's Guide for a full explanation of data.

Hospital Name	City	Rate	Cases
Grady General Hospital	Cairo	99%	71
North Fulton Hospital	Roswell	99%	165
Northside Hospital	Atlanta	99%	203
Phoebe Sumter Medical Center	Americus	99%	145
Piedmont Mountainside Hospital	Jasper	99%	80
SE Georgia Health Sys-Brunswick[2]	Brunswick	99%	267
Southern Regional Medical Center[2]	Riverdale	99%	301
Tanner Medical Center - Carrollton	Carrollton	99%	238
Upson Regional Medical Center	Thomaston	99%	130
Coliseum Northside Hospital	Macon	98%	55
Dorminy Medical Center	Fitzgerald	98%	54
Meadows Regional Medical Center	Vidalia	98%	184
Piedmont Henry Hospital[2]	Stockbridge	98%	341
Union General Hospital[2]	Blairsville	98%	55
Elbert Memorial Hospital	Elberton	97%	67
Taylor Regional Hospital[2]	Hawkinsville	97%	29
Chestatee Regional Hospital[2]	Dahlonega	96%	26
Habersham County Medical Center[2]	Demorest	96%	53
Newton Medical Center[2]	Covington	96%	228
Wills Memorial Hospital	Washington	96%	48
Memorial Hospital & Manor[2]	Bainbridge	95%	57
Ty Cobb Regional Medical Center	Lavonia	95%	57
Dodge County Hospital[2]	Eastman	94%	63
Donalsonville Hospital	Donalsonville	94%	31
The Medical Center of Peach County[2]	Byron	94%	32
Washington County Regional Medical Center	Sandersville	92%	48
Wayne Memorial Hospital	Jesup	91%	114
Cook Medical Center	Adel	89%	36
Emanuel County Hospital Authority[2]	Swainsboro	87%	46
North Georgia Medical Center[2]	Ellijay	80%	46
Jefferson Hospital[2]	Louisville	79%	47
Jeff Davis Hospital	Hazlehurst	72%	25
Appling Hospital	Baxley	71%	42

Medicare Spending

Medicare Spending per Patient (ratio)

Hospital Name	City	Ratio	Cases
Donalsonville Hospital	Donalsonville	0.78	-
Murray Medical Center	Chatsworth	0.79	-
Union General Hospital	Blairsville	0.82	-
Appling Hospital	Baxley	0.83	-
Jefferson Hospital	Louisville	0.83	-
Burke Medical Center	Waynesboro	0.84	-
Elbert Memorial Hospital	Elberton	0.84	-
Grady General Hospital	Cairo	0.85	-
Evans Memorial Hospital	Claxton	0.86	-
Wellstar Paulding Hospital	Hiram	0.86	-
Cook Medical Center	Adel	0.87	-
Crisp Regional Hospital	Cordele	0.87	-
Dorminy Medical Center	Fitzgerald	0.87	-
Tift Regional Medical Center	Tifton	0.87	-
Washington County Regional Medical Center	Sandersville	0.87	-
Coffee Regional Medical Center	Douglas	0.88	-
Memorial Hospital & Manor	Bainbridge	0.88	-
Chestatee Regional Hospital	Dahlonega	0.89	-
Habersham County Medical Center	Demorest	0.89	-
Northridge Medical Center	Commerce	0.89	-
Fairview Park Hospital	Dublin	0.90	-
Hamilton Medical Center	Dalton	0.91	-
Northeast Georgia Medical Center	Gainesville	0.91	-
Perry Hospital	Perry	0.91	-
Athens Regional Medical Center	Athens	0.92	-
Emanuel County Hospital Authority	Swainsboro	0.92	-
Gordon Hospital	Calhoun	0.92	-
Ty Cobb Regional Medical Center	Lavonia	0.92	-
Piedmont Mountainside Hospital	Jasper	0.93	-
Redmond Regional Medical Center	Rome	0.93	-
West Georgia Medical Center	Lagrange	0.93	-
Barrow Regional Medical Center	Winder	0.94	-
Cartersville Medical Center	Cartersville	0.94	-
Emory University Hospital Midtown	Atlanta	0.94	-
Fannin Regional Hospital	Blue Ridge	0.94	-
Hutcheson Medical Center	Fort Oglethorpe	0.94	-
Oconee Regional Medical Center	Milledgeville	0.94	-
Phoebe Putney Memorial Hospital	Albany	0.94	-
Piedmont Newnan Hospital	Newnan	0.94	-
SE Georgia Health Sys-Camden Campus	Saint Marys	0.94	-
Tanner Medical Center - Carrollton	Carrollton	0.94	-
Upson Regional Medical Center	Thomaston	0.94	-
Colquitt Regional Medical Center	Moultrie	0.95	-
East Georgia Regional Medical Center	Statesboro	0.95	-
Grady Memorial Hospital	Atlanta	0.95	-
Meadows Regional Medical Center	Vidalia	0.95	-
Phoebe Sumter Medical Center	Americus	0.95	-
Saint Joseph's Hospital - Savannah	Savannah	0.95	-
Saint Mary's Hospital	Athens	0.95	-
SE Georgia Health Sys-Brunswick	Brunswick	0.95	-
Tanner Medical Center Villa Rica	Villa Rica	0.95	-
Wayne Memorial Hospital	Jesup	0.95	-
Dodge County Hospital	Eastman	0.96	-
Emory Johns Creek Hospital	Johns Creek	0.96	-
Emory University Hospital	Atlanta	0.96	-
Memorial Health Univ Medical Center	Savannah	0.96	-
Saint Joseph's Hospital of Atlanta	Atlanta	0.96	-
South Georgia Medical Center	Valdosta	0.96	-
University Hospital	Augusta	0.96	-
Dekalb Medical Center at Hillandale	Lithonia	0.97	-
John D Archbold Memorial Hospital	Thomasville	0.97	-
Mayo Clinic Health System - Waycross	Waycross	0.97	-
Newton Medical Center	Covington	0.97	-
Northside Hospital Forsyth	Cumming	0.97	-
Northside Medical Center	Columbus	0.97	-
Piedmont Fayette Hospital	Fayetteville	0.97	-
Piedmont Henry Hospital	Stockbridge	0.97	-
Piedmont Hospital	Atlanta	0.97	-
Stephens County Hospital	Toccoa	0.97	-
Wellstar Douglas Hospital	Douglasville	0.97	-
Doctors Specialty Hospital	Columbus	0.98	-
Flint River Hospital	Montezuma	0.98	-
Gwinnett Medical Center	Lawrenceville	0.98	-
Houston Medical Center	Warner Robins	0.98	-
Irwin County Hospital	Ocilla	0.98	-
Medical Center of Central Georgia	Macon	0.98	-
North Georgia Medical Center	Ellijay	0.98	-
Southern Regional Medical Center	Riverdale	0.98	-
Spalding Regional Hospital	Griffin	0.98	-
Wellstar Cobb Hospital	Austell	0.98	-
Wellstar Kennestone Hospital	Marietta	0.98	-
Clearview Regional Medical Center	Monroe	0.99	-
Coliseum Medical Center	Macon	0.99	-
Coliseum Northside Hospital	Macon	0.99	-
Emory - Adventist Hospital	Smyrna	0.99	-
Northside Hospital	Atlanta	0.99	-
Rockdale Medical Center	Conyers	0.99	-
Doctors Hospital	Augusta	1.00	-
Floyd Medical Center	Rome	1.00	-
Med College of Georgia Hosps	Augusta	1.00	-
North Fulton Hospital	Roswell	1.00	-
Taylor Regional Hospital	Hawkinsville	1.01	-
Trinity Hospital of Augusta	Augusta	1.01	-
Dekalb Medical Center	Decatur	1.02	-
Eastside Medical Center	Snellville	1.02	-
Saint Francis Hospital	Columbus	1.03	-
Midtown Medical Center	Columbus	1.04	-
Northside Hospital Cherokee	Canton	1.04	-
Univ McDuffie Co Reg Med Ctr	Thomson	1.04	-
Atlanta Medical Center	Atlanta	1.05	-
Candler Hospital	Savannah	1.05	-
Turning Point Hospital	Moultrie	1.25	-

Pneumonia Care

Appropriate Initial Antibiotic Given

Hospital Name	City	Rate	Cases
Chatuge Regional Hospital	Hiawassee	100%	30
Coffee Regional Medical Center	Douglas	100%	93
Coliseum Northside Hospital	Macon	100%	43
Crisp Regional Hospital	Cordele	100%	84
Doctors Hospital	Augusta	100%	110
Emory - Adventist Hospital	Smyrna	100%	85
Emory Johns Creek Hospital	Johns Creek	100%	90
Fairview Park Hospital	Dublin	100%	115
Fannin Regional Hospital	Blue Ridge	100%	34
Northside Hospital	Atlanta	100%	141
Northside Hospital Cherokee	Canton	100%	126
Putnam General Hospital[2]	Eatonton	100%	51
Saint Mary's Good Samaritan Hospital	Greensboro	100%	26
Saint Mary's Hospital	Athens	100%	73
Coliseum Medical Center	Macon	99%	108
Dekalb Medical Center[2]	Decatur	99%	82
Hamilton Medical Center	Dalton	99%	213
Midtown Medical Center	Columbus	99%	115
Saint Joseph's Hospital - Savannah	Savannah	99%	115
Tift Regional Medical Center	Tifton	99%	118
Athens Regional Medical Center[2]	Athens	98%	89
Emory University Hospital[2]	Atlanta	98%	42
Gordon Hospital	Calhoun	98%	127
Gwinnett Medical Center[2]	Lawrenceville	98%	331
Med College of Georgia Hosps[2]	Augusta	98%	44
Northside Hospital Forsyth	Cumming	98%	197
Oconee Regional Medical Center	Milledgeville	98%	100
Redmond Regional Medical Center	Rome	98%	181
Tanner Medical Center - Carrollton	Carrollton	98%	158
Wellstar Cobb Hospital[2]	Austell	98%	197
Atlanta Medical Center[2]	Atlanta	97%	171
Barrow Regional Medical Center	Winder	97%	58
Candler Hospital	Savannah	97%	148
Colquitt Regional Medical Center	Moultrie	97%	102
Dublin VA Medical Center	Dublin	97%	29
East Georgia Regional Medical Center	Statesboro	97%	119
Higgins General Hospital	Bremen	97%	34
Newton Medical Center[2]	Covington	97%	107
Perry Hospital	Perry	97%	37
Piedmont Fayette Hospital[2]	Fayetteville	97%	89
Piedmont Henry Hospital[2]	Stockbridge	97%	117
Piedmont Hospital[2]	Atlanta	97%	96
Rockdale Medical Center[2]	Conyers	97%	98
Saint Francis Hospital[2]	Columbus	97%	195
Tanner Medical Center Villa Rica	Villa Rica	97%	78
Wellstar Douglas Hospital[2]	Douglasville	97%	123
Wellstar Paulding Hospital	Hiram	97%	63
Cook Medical Center[2]	Adel	96%	26
Decatur VA Medical Center	Decatur	96%	72
Dekalb Medical Center at Hillandale[2]	Lithonia	96%	107
Eastside Medical Center[2]	Snellville	96%	100
Grady Memorial Hospital[2]	Atlanta	96%	50
Houston Medical Center[2]	Warner Robins	96%	102
Hutcheson Medical Center[2]	Fort Oglethorpe	96%	83
Meadows Regional Medical Center	Vidalia	96%	92
Northeast Georgia Medical Center[2]	Gainesville	96%	113
SE Georgia Health Sys-Brunswick[2]	Brunswick	96%	75
Trinity Hospital of Augusta	Augusta	96%	51
University Hospital[2]	Augusta	96%	84
Wellstar Kennestone Hospital[2]	Marietta	96%	280
Floyd Medical Center	Rome	95%	261
John D Archbold Memorial Hospital	Thomasville	95%	129
Memorial Health Univ Medical Center[2]	Savannah	95%	74
North Fulton Hospital[2]	Roswell	95%	110
Piedmont Mountainside Hospital[2]	Jasper	95%	86
South Georgia Medical Center	Valdosta	95%	218
Taylor Regional Hospital[2]	Hawkinsville	95%	42
Upson Regional Medical Center[2]	Thomaston	95%	97
West Georgia Medical Center	Lagrange	95%	105
Cartersville Medical Center[2]	Cartersville	94%	82
Clearview Regional Medical Center	Monroe	94%	49
Emory University Hospital Midtown[2]	Atlanta	94%	68
Pioneer Community Hospital of Early	Blakely	94%	31
Augusta VA Medical Center	Augusta	93%	54
Spalding Regional Hospital	Griffin	93%	166
Northridge Medical Center[2]	Commerce	92%	50
Phoebe Putney Memorial Hospital	Albany	92%	240
Piedmont Newnan Hospital[2]	Newnan	92%	116
Southern Regional Medical Center[2]	Riverdale	92%	98
Stephens County Hospital[2]	Toccoa	92%	93
Union General Hospital[2]	Blairsville	92%	83
Chestatee Regional Hospital	Dahlonega	91%	55
Evans Memorial Hospital[2]	Claxton	91%	45
Saint Joseph's Hospital of Atlanta[2]	Atlanta	90%	116
Bacon County Hospital	Alma	89%	44
Elbert Memorial Hospital	Elberton	89%	65
Burke Medical Center	Waynesboro	88%	26
Phoebe Sumter Medical Center	Americus	88%	33
Habersham County Medical Center[2]	Demorest	87%	133
Mayo Clinic Health System - Waycross[2]	Waycross	87%	135
Memorial Hospital & Manor[2]	Bainbridge	87%	55
Dodge County Hospital[2]	Eastman	86%	36
Jeff Davis Hospital	Hazlehurst	86%	50
SE Georgia Health Sys-Camden Campus[2]	Saint Marys	86%	36
Emanuel County Hospital Authority	Swainsboro	85%	34
Wayne Memorial Hospital[2]	Jesup	85%	173
Donalsonville Hospital	Donalsonville	84%	25
Medical Center of Central Georgia[2]	Macon	84%	76
Ty Cobb Regional Medical Center[2]	Lavonia	79%	33
Irwin County Hospital[2]	Ocilla	78%	27
Appling Hospital[2]	Baxley	76%	33
Washington County Regional Medical Center	Sandersville	74%	43
Liberty Regional Medical Center[2]	Hinesville	70%	44
Candler County Hospital	Metter	68%	28
Wills Memorial Hospital	Washington	64%	44
North Georgia Medical Center[2]	Ellijay	58%	48

Blood Culture Timing

Hospital Name	City	Rate	Cases
Candler County Hospital	Metter	100%	51
Chatuge Regional Hospital	Hiawassee	100%	42
Coffee Regional Medical Center	Douglas	100%	132
Coliseum Medical Center	Macon	100%	230
Colquitt Regional Medical Center	Moultrie	100%	206
Doctors Hospital	Augusta	100%	260
East Georgia Regional Medical Center	Statesboro	100%	154
Fannin Regional Hospital	Blue Ridge	100%	70
Gordon Hospital	Calhoun	100%	222
Higgins General Hospital	Bremen	100%	67
Monroe County Hospital	Forsyth	100%	27
Mountain Lakes Medical Center[2]	Clayton	100%	30
Northside Hospital	Atlanta	100%	185
Northside Hospital Cherokee	Canton	100%	193
Northside Hospital Forsyth	Cumming	100%	259
Putnam General Hospital[2]	Eatonton	100%	37
Saint Mary's Good Samaritan Hospital	Greensboro	100%	25

NOTE: Hospital profiles are in alphabetical order by state, then city, then hospital within the city; Rankings exclude hospitals with less than 25 cases except for patient surveys which excludes hospitals with less than 100 cases; (a) 100-299 cases; (1) The number of cases/patients is too few to report; (2) Data submitted were based on a sample of cases/patients; (3) Results are based on a shorter time period than required; (4) Data suppressed by CMS for one or more quarters; (5) Results are not available for this reporting period; (6) Fewer than 100 patients completed the HCAHPS survey; (7) No cases met the criteria for this measure; (8) The lower limit of the confidence interval cannot be calculated if the number of observed infections equals zero; (9) No data are available from the state/territory for this reporting period; (10) The scores shown reflect fewer than 50 completed surveys; (11) There were discrepancies in the data collection process; (12) This measure does not apply to this hospital for this reporting period; (13) Results cannot be calculated for this reporting period; (14) The results for this state are combined with nearby states to protect confidentiality; Please refer to the User's Guide for a full explanation of data.

SE Georgia Health Sys-Brunswick[2]	Brunswick	100%	98
Tift Regional Medical Center	Tifton	100%	219
University Hospital[2]	Augusta	100%	136
Wellstar Douglas Hospital[2]	Douglasville	100%	271
Athens Regional Medical Center[2]	Athens	99%	95
Atlanta Medical Center[2]	Atlanta	99%	252
Cartersville Medical Center[2]	Cartersville	99%	146
Clearview Regional Medical Center	Monroe	99%	85
Coliseum Northside Hospital	Macon	99%	73
Crisp Regional Hospital	Cordele	99%	120
Decatur VA Medical Center	Decatur	99%	141
Eastside Medical Center[2]	Snellville	99%	162
Emory - Adventist Hospital	Smyrna	99%	123
Emory University Hospital Midtown[2]	Atlanta	99%	131
Fairview Park Hospital	Dublin	99%	220
Floyd Medical Center	Rome	99%	470
Hutcheson Medical Center[2]	Fort Oglethorpe	99%	105
Med College of Georgia Hosps[2]	Augusta	99%	129
Northridge Medical Center[2]	Commerce	99%	68
Saint Joseph's Hospital - Savannah	Savannah	99%	168
Saint Mary's Hospital	Athens	99%	137
Spalding Regional Hospital	Griffin	99%	263
Stephens County Hospital[2]	Toccoa	99%	152
Union General Hospital[2]	Blairsville	99%	102
Wellstar Cobb Hospital[2]	Austell	99%	348
Wellstar Kennestone Hospital[2]	Marietta	99%	402
Wellstar Paulding Hospital	Hiram	99%	121
West Georgia Medical Center	Lagrange	99%	219
Candler Hospital	Savannah	98%	191
Dekalb Medical Center[2]	Decatur	98%	120
Dekalb Medical Center at Hillandale[2]	Lithonia	98%	114
Dublin VA Medical Center	Dublin	98%	41
Habersham County Medical Center[2]	Demorest	98%	205
Midtown Medical Center	Columbus	98%	230
North Fulton Hospital[2]	Roswell	98%	131
North Georgia Medical Center[2]	Ellijay	98%	46
Oconee Regional Medical Center	Milledgeville	98%	197
Phoebe Putney Memorial Hospital	Albany	98%	403
Piedmont Mountainside Hospital[2]	Jasper	98%	148
Redmond Regional Medical Center	Rome	98%	279
Rockdale Medical Center[2]	Conyers	98%	165
Trinity Hospital of Augusta	Augusta	98%	113
Upson Regional Medical Center[2]	Thomaston	98%	124
Barrow Regional Medical Center	Winder	97%	105
Chestatee Regional Hospital	Dahlonega	97%	74
Emory Johns Creek Hospital	Johns Creek	97%	159
Emory University Hospital[2]	Atlanta	97%	90
Gwinnett Medical Center[2]	Lawrenceville	97%	315
Hamilton Medical Center	Dalton	97%	385
Liberty Regional Medical Center[2]	Hinesville	97%	37
Lower Oconee Community Hospital	Glenwood	97%	29
Northeast Georgia Medical Center[2]	Gainesville	97%	215
Phoebe Sumter Medical Center	Americus	97%	58
Piedmont Henry Hospital[2]	Stockbridge	97%	145
Saint Francis Hospital[2]	Columbus	97%	286
South Georgia Medical Center	Valdosta	97%	292
Tanner Medical Center - Carrollton	Carrollton	97%	239
Elbert Memorial Hospital	Elberton	96%	56
Houston Medical Center[2]	Warner Robins	96%	138
Memorial Health Univ Medical Center[2]	Savannah	96%	93
Newton Medical Center[2]	Covington	96%	187
Piedmont Fayette Hospital[2]	Fayetteville	96%	179
SE Georgia Health Sys-Camden Campus[2]	Saint Marys	96%	46
Southern Regional Medical Center[2]	Riverdale	96%	148
Tanner Medical Center Villa Rica	Villa Rica	96%	106
Augusta VA Medical Center	Augusta	95%	92
Jeff Davis Hospital	Hazlehurst	95%	39
John D Archbold Memorial Hospital	Thomasville	95%	226
Evans Memorial Hospital[2]	Claxton	94%	54
Grady Memorial Hospital[2]	Atlanta	94%	86
Mayo Clinic Health System - Waycross[2]	Waycross	94%	221
Perry Hospital	Perry	94%	47
Piedmont Hospital[2]	Atlanta	94%	166
Piedmont Newnan Hospital[2]	Newnan	94%	190
Taylor Regional Hospital[2]	Hawkinsville	94%	51
Emanuel County Hospital Authority	Swainsboro	92%	40
Meadows Regional Medical Center	Vidalia	92%	143
Medical Center of Central Georgia[2]	Macon	92%	110
Murray Medical Center	Chatsworth	92%	40
Memorial Hospital & Manor[2]	Bainbridge	91%	67
Saint Joseph's Hospital of Atlanta[2]	Atlanta	91%	183
Ty Cobb Regional Medical Center[2]	Lavonia	91%	44
Dodge County Hospital[2]	Eastman	90%	40
Washington County Regional Medical Center	Sandersville	90%	67
Burke Medical Center	Waynesboro	87%	31
Dorminy Medical Center[2]	Fitzgerald	86%	73
Wayne Memorial Hospital[2]	Jesup	86%	164
Bacon County Hospital	Alma	83%	36

Pregnancy and Delivery Care

Newborns whose Deliveries were Scheduled Early

Hospital Name	City	Rate	Cases
Cartersville Medical Center[2]	Cartersville	0%	47
Coliseum Medical Center[2]	Macon	0%	38
Crisp Regional Hospital[2]	Cordele	0%	52
Dekalb Medical Center[2]	Decatur	0%	81
Doctors Hospital[2]	Augusta	0%	37
Fannin Regional Hospital[2]	Blue Ridge	0%	35
Habersham County Medical Center	Demorest	0%	58
Meadows Regional Medical Center	Vidalia	0%	72
Memorial Health Univ Medical Center[2]	Savannah	0%	37
Memorial Hospital & Manor	Bainbridge	0%	51
Oconee Regional Medical Center	Milledgeville	0%	109
Phoebe Sumter Medical Center	Americus	0%	34
Piedmont Hospital[2]	Atlanta	0%	43
SE Georgia Health Sys-Brunswick	Brunswick	0%	286
SE Georgia Health Sys-Camden Campus	Saint Marys	0%	66
Tanner Medical Center Villa Rica	Villa Rica	0%	48
Trinity Hospital of Augusta[2]	Augusta	0%	28
Northside Hospital[2]	Atlanta	1%	329
Southern Regional Medical Center[2]	Riverdale	1%	159
Tanner Medical Center - Carrollton	Carrollton	1%	111
Northside Hospital Cherokee	Canton	2%	93
Northside Hospital Forsyth	Cumming	2%	202
Piedmont Fayette Hospital[2]	Fayetteville	2%	49
Piedmont Newnan Hospital[2]	Newnan	2%	60
Rockdale Medical Center[2]	Conyers	2%	45
Spalding Regional Hospital[2]	Griffin	2%	54
Wellstar Cobb Hospital[2]	Austell	2%	56
Atlanta Medical Center[2]	Atlanta	3%	79
Emory University Hospital Midtown[2]	Atlanta	3%	67
Grady Memorial Hospital[2]	Atlanta	3%	59
Med College of Georgia Hosps[2]	Augusta	3%	65
Northeast Georgia Medical Center[2]	Gainesville	3%	69
Saint Mary's Hospital	Athens	3%	101
Coffee Regional Medical Center[2]	Douglas	4%	54
Eastside Medical Center[2]	Snellville	4%	27
Gwinnett Medical Center[2]	Lawrenceville	4%	80
Houston Medical Center[2]	Warner Robins	4%	46
Irwin County Hospital	Ocilla	4%	79
John D Archbold Memorial Hospital[2]	Thomasville	4%	79
Midtown Medical Center[2]	Columbus	5%	604
Piedmont Henry Hospital	Stockbridge	5%	210
Wellstar Kennestone Hospital[2]	Marietta	5%	87
Emory Johns Creek Hospital[2]	Johns Creek	6%	36
Floyd Medical Center[2]	Rome	6%	399
South Georgia Medical Center[2]	Valdosta	6%	51
Donalsonville Hospital	Donalsonville	7%	42
Ty Cobb Regional Medical Center	Lavonia	7%	29
Candler Hospital[2]	Savannah	8%	74
East Georgia Regional Medical Center	Statesboro	8%	153
Fairview Park Hospital[2]	Dublin	8%	26
Mayo Clinic Health System - Waycross	Waycross	8%	89
Medical Center of Central Georgia[2]	Macon	8%	40
Wellstar Douglas Hospital[2]	Douglasville	8%	26
West Georgia Medical Center[2]	Lagrange	8%	40
Colquitt Regional Medical Center[2]	Moultrie	9%	67
Hamilton Medical Center[2]	Dalton	9%	34
Washington County Regional Medical Center[2]	Sandersville	11%	36
Upson Regional Medical Center[2]	Thomaston	13%	39
Wayne Memorial Hospital	Jesup	13%	94
Athens Regional Medical Center	Athens	14%	218
Stephens County Hospital	Toccoa	14%	73
Doctors Specialty Hospital[2]	Columbus	16%	180
Union General Hospital[2]	Blairsville	19%	36
Phoebe Putney Memorial Hospital	Albany	24%	214
Gordon Hospital[2]	Calhoun	25%	68
University Hospital	Augusta	26%	325
Hutcheson Medical Center[2]	Fort Oglethorpe	27%	30
Barrow Regional Medical Center	Winder	41%	27
Newton Medical Center[2]	Covington	45%	104
Dodge County Hospital	Eastman	46%	28
Piedmont Mountainside Hospital[2]	Jasper	47%	36
Taylor Regional Hospital	Hawkinsville	82%	61

Preventive Care

Immunization for Influenza

Hospital Name	City	Rate	Cases
Fannin Regional Hospital[2]	Blue Ridge	100%	277
Jeff Davis Hospital[3]	Hazlehurst	100%	31
Oconee Regional Medical Center[2]	Milledgeville	100%	539
Trinity Hospital of Augusta[2]	Augusta	100%	468
Barrow Regional Medical Center[2]	Winder	99%	406
Clearview Regional Medical Center[2]	Monroe	99%	348
Coliseum Northside Hospital[2]	Macon	99%	328
Doctors Specialty Hospital[2]	Columbus	99%	398
Emory University Hospital Midtown[2]	Atlanta	99%	609
Fairview Park Hospital[2]	Dublin	99%	526
Floyd Medical Center[2]	Rome	99%	497
Hamilton Medical Center[2]	Dalton	99%	492
Higgins General Hospital[2]	Bremen	99%	327
SE Georgia Health Sys-Brunswick[2]	Brunswick	99%	541
Stephens County Hospital[2]	Toccoa	99%	301
Cartersville Medical Center[2]	Cartersville	98%	532
Coffee Regional Medical Center[2]	Douglas	98%	590
Coliseum Medical Center[2]	Macon	98%	597
Doctors Hospital[2]	Augusta	98%	597
Eastside Medical Center[2]	Snellville	98%	567
Emory - Adventist Hospital[2]	Smyrna	98%	290
Emory Johns Creek Hospital[2]	Johns Creek	98%	530
Gordon Hospital[2]	Calhoun	98%	678
Jefferson Hospital[2]	Louisville	98%	245
Mountain Lakes Medical Center[2]	Clayton	98%	153
Northridge Medical Center[2]	Commerce	98%	333
Northside Hospital[2]	Atlanta	98%	440
Northside Hospital Forsyth[2]	Cumming	98%	522
Northside Medical Center[2]	Columbus	98%	312
Putnam General Hospital[2,3]	Eatonton	98%	146
SE Georgia Health Sys-Camden Campus[2]	Saint Marys	98%	215
Tanner Medical Center - Carrollton[2]	Carrollton	98%	525
Wellstar Paulding Hospital[2]	Hiram	98%	317
Candler Hospital[2]	Savannah	97%	481
East Georgia Regional Medical Center[2]	Statesboro	97%	608
Emory University Hospital[2]	Atlanta	97%	591
Northside Hospital Cherokee[2]	Canton	97%	487
Perry Hospital[2]	Perry	97%	301
Redmond Regional Medical Center[2]	Rome	97%	617
Saint Joseph's Hospital - Savannah[2]	Savannah	97%	587
Southern Regional Medical Center[2]	Riverdale	97%	755
Spalding Regional Hospital[2]	Griffin	97%	590
Tift Regional Medical Center[2]	Tifton	97%	573
Hutcheson Medical Center[2]	Fort Oglethorpe	96%	525
Med College of Georgia Hosps[2]	Augusta	96%	535
North Fulton Hospital[2]	Roswell	96%	524
Rockdale Medical Center[2]	Conyers	96%	527
Tanner Medical Center Villa Rica[2]	Villa Rica	96%	235
Wellstar Cobb Hospital[2]	Austell	96%	516
Wellstar Douglas Hospital[2]	Douglasville	96%	574
Jasper Memorial Hospital	Monticello	95%	37
Meadows Regional Medical Center[2]	Vidalia	95%	471
Saint Mary's Hospital[2]	Athens	95%	540
West Georgia Medical Center[2]	Lagrange	95%	539
Saint Mary's Good Samaritan Hospital[2,3]	Greensboro	94%	84
Chatuge Regional Hospital	Hiawassee	93%	121
Effingham County Hospital	Springfield	93%	68
Gwinnett Medical Center[2]	Lawrenceville	93%	709
Northeast Georgia Medical Center[2]	Gainesville	93%	529
Memorial Health Univ Medical Center[2]	Savannah	92%	523
Piedmont Henry Hospital[2]	Stockbridge	92%	522
Chestatee Regional Hospital[2]	Dahlonega	91%	333
Dorminy Medical Center[2]	Fitzgerald	91%	280
Murray Medical Center[2]	Chatsworth	91%	193
Saint Francis Hospital[2]	Columbus	91%	755
Union General Hospital[2]	Blairsville	91%	275
Phoebe Putney Memorial Hospital[2]	Albany	90%	576
Wellstar Kennestone Hospital[2]	Marietta	90%	576
Grady Memorial Hospital[2]	Atlanta	89%	550
Houston Medical Center[2]	Warner Robins	89%	531
Midtown Medical Center[2]	Columbus	89%	531
Phoebe Sumter Medical Center[2]	Americus	89%	410
Saint Joseph's Hospital of Atlanta[2]	Atlanta	89%	628
Taylor Regional Hospital[2]	Hawkinsville	89%	266
Ty Cobb Regional Medical Center[2]	Lavonia	89%	380
Dekalb Medical Center at Hillandale[2]	Lithonia	88%	524
Southeastern Regional Medical Center[2,3]	Newnan	88%	114
Elbert Memorial Hospital[2]	Elberton	87%	517
Colquitt Regional Medical Center[2]	Moultrie	86%	456
Crisp Regional Hospital[2]	Cordele	86%	554
South Georgia Medical Center[2]	Valdosta	86%	670
Dekalb Medical Center[2]	Decatur	85%	492
Emanuel County Hospital Authority[2]	Swainsboro	85%	352
Polk Medical Center[3]	Cedartown	85%	41
Evans Memorial Hospital[2]	Claxton	84%	300
Habersham County Medical Center[2]	Demorest	84%	362
Newton Medical Center[2]	Covington	84%	719
Atlanta Medical Center[2]	Atlanta	83%	505
Mayo Clinic Health System - Waycross[2]	Waycross	83%	980
Piedmont Mountainside Hospital[2]	Jasper	82%	305
Cook Medical Center[2]	Adel	80%	320
Dublin VA Medical Center[2,3]	Dublin	80%	129
Irwin County Hospital[2]	Ocilla	80%	311
Appling Hospital[2]	Baxley	79%	277
Donalsonville Hospital[2]	Donalsonville	78%	415
Morgan Memorial Hospital	Madison	78%	79
John D Archbold Memorial Hospital[2]	Thomasville	77%	644
Bacon County Hospital[2]	Alma	76%	378
University Hospital[2]	Augusta	76%	532
Athens Regional Medical Center[2]	Athens	75%	505

NOTE: Hospital profiles are in alphabetical order by state, then city, then hospital within the city; Rankings exclude hospitals with less than 25 cases except for patient surveys which excludes hospitals with less than 100 cases; (a) 100-299 cases; (1) The number of cases/patients is too few to report; (2) Data submitted were based on a sample of cases/patients; (3) Results are based on a shorter time period than required; (4) Data suppressed by CMS for one or more quarters; (5) Results are not available for this reporting period; (6) Fewer than 100 patients completed the HCAHPS survey; (7) No cases met the criteria for this measure; (8) The lower limit of the confidence interval cannot be calculated if the number of observed infections equals zero; (9) No data are available from the state/territory for this reporting period; (10) The scores shown reflect fewer than 50 completed surveys; (11) There were discrepancies in the data collection process; (12) This measure does not apply to this hospital for this reporting period; (13) Results cannot be calculated for this reporting period; (14) The results for this state are combined with nearby states to protect confidentiality; Please refer to the User's Guide for a full explanation of data.

Hospital Name	City	Rate	Cases
Grady General Hospital[2]	Cairo	72%	265
Washington County Regional Medical Center[2]	Sandersville	71%	340
Piedmont Newnan Hospital[2]	Newnan	68%	569
Piedmont Fayette Hospital[2]	Fayetteville	67%	517
Liberty Regional Medical Center[2]	Hinesville	64%	64
Wills Memorial Hospital[2]	Washington	64%	279
Piedmont Hospital[2]	Atlanta	62%	594
Medical Center of Central Georgia[2]	Macon	60%	531
Memorial Hospital & Manor[2]	Bainbridge	60%	278
Univ McDuffie Co Reg Med Ctr[2]	Thomson	59%	207
North Georgia Medical Center[2]	Ellijay	56%	308
Upson Regional Medical Center[2]	Thomaston	48%	368
Dodge County Hospital[2]	Eastman	45%	313
Wayne Memorial Hospital[2]	Jesup	45%	372
Flint River Hospital[2]	Montezuma	39%	296
Burke Medical Center[2]	Waynesboro	34%	157
Turning Point Hospital[2]	Moultrie	0%	314

Immunization for Pneumonia

Hospital Name	City	Rate	Cases
Fannin Regional Hospital[2]	Blue Ridge	100%	351
Higgins General Hospital[2]	Bremen	100%	582
Jeff Davis Hospital[3]	Hazlehurst	100%	53
Oconee Regional Medical Center[2]	Milledgeville	100%	590
SE Georgia Health Sys-Brunswick[2]	Brunswick	100%	646
SE Georgia Health Sys-Camden Campus[2]	Saint Marys	100%	151
Trinity Hospital of Augusta[2]	Augusta	100%	503
Barrow Regional Medical Center[2]	Winder	99%	436
Candler Hospital[2]	Savannah	99%	516
Coffee Regional Medical Center[2]	Douglas	99%	811
Emory - Adventist Hospital[2]	Smyrna	99%	378
Floyd Medical Center[2]	Rome	99%	604
Hamilton Medical Center[2]	Dalton	99%	569
Perry Hospital[2]	Perry	99%	476
Saint Joseph's Hospital - Savannah[2]	Savannah	99%	888
Stephens County Hospital[2]	Toccoa	99%	469
Cartersville Medical Center[2]	Cartersville	98%	704
Clearview Regional Medical Center[2]	Monroe	98%	450
Doctors Hospital[2]	Augusta	98%	585
Emory University Hospital Midtown[2]	Atlanta	98%	690
Fairview Park Hospital[2]	Dublin	98%	588
Northside Hospital Cherokee[2]	Canton	98%	478
Northside Hospital Forsyth[2]	Cumming	98%	580
Tanner Medical Center - Carrollton[2]	Carrollton	98%	665
Coliseum Medical Center[2]	Macon	97%	824
Emory University Hospital[2]	Atlanta	97%	703
Med College of Georgia Hosps[2]	Augusta	97%	531
Putnam General Hospital[2,3]	Eatonton	97%	307
Redmond Regional Medical Center[2]	Rome	97%	1041
Rockdale Medical Center[2]	Conyers	97%	641
Spalding Regional Hospital[2]	Griffin	97%	776
Tanner Medical Center Villa Rica[2]	Villa Rica	97%	279
Tift Regional Medical Center[2]	Tifton	97%	705
Wellstar Paulding Hospital[2]	Hiram	97%	447
East Georgia Regional Medical Center[2]	Statesboro	96%	633
Emory Johns Creek Hospital[2]	Johns Creek	96%	590
Northridge Medical Center[2]	Commerce	96%	558
West Georgia Medical Center[2]	Lagrange	96%	681
Chestatee Regional Hospital[2]	Dahlonega	95%	448
Doctors Specialty Hospital[2]	Columbus	95%	436
Eastside Medical Center[2]	Snellville	95%	686
Habersham County Medical Center[2]	Demorest	95%	418
Houston Medical Center[2]	Warner Robins	95%	623
Jefferson Hospital[2]	Louisville	95%	462
Meadows Regional Medical Center[2]	Vidalia	95%	551
Wellstar Cobb Hospital[2]	Austell	95%	546
Wellstar Douglas Hospital[2]	Douglasville	95%	772
Coliseum Northside Hospital[2]	Macon	94%	442
Colquitt Regional Medical Center[2]	Moultrie	94%	524
Elbert Memorial Hospital[2]	Elberton	94%	685
Gordon Hospital[2]	Calhoun	94%	905
Memorial Health Univ Medical Center[2]	Savannah	94%	524
Memorial Hospital & Manor[2]	Bainbridge	94%	307
Midtown Medical Center[2]	Columbus	94%	458
North Fulton Hospital[2]	Roswell	94%	570
Northside Hospital[2]	Atlanta	94%	227
Union General Hospital[2]	Blairsville	94%	329
Chatuge Regional Hospital	Hiawassee	93%	214
Crisp Regional Hospital[2]	Cordele	93%	589
Jasper Memorial Hospital	Monticello	93%	58
Mountain Lakes Medical Center[2]	Clayton	93%	216
Murray Medical Center[2]	Chatsworth	93%	289
Northside Medical Center[2]	Columbus	93%	482
Phoebe Putney Memorial Hospital[2]	Albany	93%	722
Saint Mary's Hospital[2]	Athens	93%	675
Southern Regional Medical Center[2]	Riverdale	93%	733
Taylor Regional Hospital[2]	Hawkinsville	93%	341
Effingham County Hospital	Springfield	92%	75
Emanuel County Hospital Authority[2]	Swainsboro	92%	510
Saint Mary's Good Samaritan Hospital[2,3]	Greensboro	92%	74
Dorminy Medical Center[2]	Fitzgerald	91%	431
Grady General Hospital[2]	Cairo	91%	295
Hutcheson Medical Center[2]	Fort Oglethorpe	91%	471
Saint Francis Hospital[2]	Columbus	91%	1086
Saint Joseph's Hospital of Atlanta[2]	Atlanta	91%	937
Southeastern Regional Medical Center[2,3]	Newnan	91%	117
Ty Cobb Regional Medical Center[2]	Lavonia	91%	396
Atlanta Medical Center[2]	Atlanta	90%	472
Dublin VA Medical Center[2,3]	Dublin	90%	334
Gwinnett Medical Center[2]	Lawrenceville	90%	869
Piedmont Henry Hospital[2]	Stockbridge	90%	647
Bacon County Hospital[2]	Alma	89%	465
Northeast Georgia Medical Center[2]	Gainesville	89%	698
Wellstar Kennestone Hospital[2]	Marietta	89%	608
Evans Memorial Hospital[2]	Claxton	88%	475
Grady Memorial Hospital[2]	Atlanta	88%	529
Phoebe Sumter Medical Center[2]	Americus	88%	449
Cook Medical Center[2]	Adel	87%	376
South Georgia Medical Center[2]	Valdosta	87%	757
Athens Regional Medical Center[2]	Athens	86%	679
Newton Medical Center[2]	Covington	86%	884
Dekalb Medical Center at Hillandale[2]	Lithonia	85%	726
John D Archbold Memorial Hospital[2]	Thomasville	85%	757
Polk Medical Center[2,3]	Cedartown	85%	71
Washington County Regional Medical Center[2]	Sandersville	85%	373
Dekalb Medical Center[2]	Decatur	82%	492
Donalsonville Hospital[2]	Donalsonville	82%	395
Piedmont Newnan Hospital[2]	Newnan	82%	731
Appling Hospital[2]	Baxley	80%	375
Piedmont Mountainside Hospital[2]	Jasper	80%	440
Mayo Clinic Health System - Waycross[2]	Waycross	79%	1222
University Hospital[2]	Augusta	79%	694
Morgan Memorial Hospital	Madison	78%	120
Piedmont Fayette Hospital[2]	Fayetteville	78%	643
North Georgia Medical Center[2]	Ellijay	75%	456
Irwin County Hospital[2]	Ocilla	69%	261
Piedmont Hospital[2]	Atlanta	69%	673
Liberty Regional Medical Center[2]	Hinesville	68%	154
Upson Regional Medical Center[2]	Thomaston	68%	454
Wayne Memorial Hospital[2]	Jesup	67%	436
Medical Center of Central Georgia[2]	Macon	66%	646
Dodge County Hospital[2]	Eastman	60%	371
Wills Memorial Hospital[2]	Washington	58%	456
Flint River Hospital[2]	Montezuma	56%	288
Univ McDuffie Co Reg Med Ctr[2]	Thomson	53%	320
Burke Medical Center[2]	Waynesboro	43%	138
Turning Point Hospital[2]	Moultrie	2%	65

Stroke Care

Anticoagulation Therapy for Atrial Fibrillation

Hospital Name	City	Rate	Cases
Memorial Health Univ Medical Center	Savannah	100%	42
Northside Hospital Forsyth	Cumming	100%	25
Redmond Regional Medical Center	Rome	100%	27
Gwinnett Medical Center	Lawrenceville	97%	38
Medical Center of Central Georgia[2]	Macon	97%	36
University Hospital	Augusta	97%	39
Saint Joseph's Hospital - Savannah	Savannah	96%	28
Northeast Georgia Medical Center	Gainesville	93%	68

Antithrombotic Therapy Timing

Hospital Name	City	Rate	Cases
Cartersville Medical Center[2]	Cartersville	100%	62
Clearview Regional Medical Center	Monroe	100%	37
Dekalb Medical Center	Decatur	100%	169
Dekalb Medical Center at Hillandale	Lithonia	100%	64
Doctors Hospital[2]	Augusta	100%	68
Eastside Medical Center[2]	Snellville	100%	100
Gordon Hospital	Calhoun	100%	35
Grady Memorial Hospital[2]	Atlanta	100%	71
Gwinnett Medical Center	Lawrenceville	100%	271
Hamilton Medical Center[2]	Dalton	100%	81
Memorial Hospital & Manor	Bainbridge	100%	40
Midtown Medical Center	Columbus	100%	174
Newton Medical Center[2]	Covington	100%	81
Northside Hospital Cherokee	Canton	100%	28
Piedmont Newnan Hospital	Newnan	100%	75
Redmond Regional Medical Center	Rome	100%	107
Rockdale Medical Center[2]	Conyers	100%	73
Saint Francis Hospital	Columbus	100%	208
Tanner Medical Center - Carrollton	Carrollton	100%	61
Wellstar Kennestone Hospital[2]	Marietta	100%	89
West Georgia Medical Center	Lagrange	100%	82
Athens Regional Medical Center[2]	Athens	99%	74
Fairview Park Hospital[2]	Dublin	99%	67
Floyd Medical Center	Rome	99%	115
John D Archbold Memorial Hospital	Thomasville	99%	155
Memorial Health Univ Medical Center	Savannah	99%	225
Northside Hospital	Atlanta	99%	108
Northside Hospital Forsyth	Cumming	99%	135
South Georgia Medical Center	Valdosta	99%	153
Southern Regional Medical Center	Riverdale	99%	204
University Hospital	Augusta	99%	269
Wellstar Cobb Hospital[2]	Austell	99%	106
Atlanta Medical Center[2]	Atlanta	98%	171
Emory Johns Creek Hospital	Johns Creek	98%	59
Piedmont Fayette Hospital	Fayetteville	98%	84
Piedmont Hospital[2]	Atlanta	98%	82
Saint Joseph's Hospital of Atlanta[2]	Atlanta	98%	66
SE Georgia Health Sys-Brunswick[2]	Brunswick	98%	98
Wellstar Douglas Hospital[2]	Douglasville	98%	86
Crisp Regional Hospital	Cordele	97%	31
East Georgia Regional Medical Center	Statesboro	97%	74
Northeast Georgia Medical Center	Gainesville	97%	274
Tift Regional Medical Center	Tifton	97%	119
Coliseum Medical Center[2]	Macon	96%	74
Emory University Hospital[2]	Atlanta	96%	48
Emory University Hospital Midtown[2]	Atlanta	96%	78
Mayo Clinic Health System - Waycross	Waycross	96%	76
Medical Center of Central Georgia[2]	Macon	96%	327
Phoebe Sumter Medical Center[2]	Americus	96%	54
Habersham County Medical Center	Demorest	95%	37
Spalding Regional Hospital	Griffin	95%	127
Candler Hospital	Savannah	94%	82
Coffee Regional Medical Center[2]	Douglas	94%	32
Med College of Georgia Hosps	Augusta	94%	153
North Fulton Hospital	Roswell	94%	72
Oconee Regional Medical Center	Milledgeville	93%	27
Saint Joseph's Hospital - Savannah	Savannah	93%	174
Tanner Medical Center Villa Rica	Villa Rica	93%	29
Upson Regional Medical Center	Thomaston	93%	30
Saint Mary's Hospital	Athens	91%	135
Phoebe Putney Memorial Hospital[2]	Albany	90%	140
Meadows Regional Medical Center	Vidalia	89%	47
Houston Medical Center	Warner Robins	88%	89
Piedmont Henry Hospital	Stockbridge	87%	144
Colquitt Regional Medical Center	Moultrie	85%	34
Wayne Memorial Hospital	Jesup	84%	31

Assessed for Rehabilitation

Hospital Name	City	Rate	Cases
Athens Regional Medical Center[2]	Athens	100%	94
Cartersville Medical Center[2]	Cartersville	100%	52
Dekalb Medical Center	Decatur	100%	170
Doctors Hospital[2]	Augusta	100%	75
Eastside Medical Center[2]	Snellville	100%	107
Fairview Park Hospital[2]	Dublin	100%	68
Gwinnett Medical Center	Lawrenceville	100%	344
Habersham County Medical Center	Demorest	100%	40
Memorial Health Univ Medical Center	Savannah	100%	354
Midtown Medical Center	Columbus	100%	226
Northside Hospital	Atlanta	100%	147
Northside Hospital Cherokee	Canton	100%	27
Piedmont Fayette Hospital	Fayetteville	100%	89
Rockdale Medical Center[2]	Conyers	100%	75
Saint Francis Hospital	Columbus	100%	226
University Hospital	Augusta	100%	314
Wellstar Kennestone Hospital[2]	Marietta	100%	98
West Georgia Medical Center	Lagrange	100%	82
Atlanta Medical Center[2]	Atlanta	99%	230
Emory Johns Creek Hospital	Johns Creek	99%	80
Emory University Hospital[2]	Atlanta	99%	127
Floyd Medical Center	Rome	99%	141
John D Archbold Memorial Hospital	Thomasville	99%	180
Piedmont Newnan Hospital	Newnan	99%	74
Saint Mary's Hospital	Athens	99%	156
South Georgia Medical Center	Valdosta	99%	190
Spalding Regional Hospital	Griffin	99%	134
Dekalb Medical Center at Hillandale	Lithonia	98%	65
Grady Memorial Hospital[2]	Atlanta	98%	106
Medical Center of Central Georgia[2]	Macon	98%	458
Med College of Georgia Hosps	Augusta	98%	258
Northside Hospital Forsyth	Cumming	98%	147
Phoebe Sumter Medical Center[2]	Americus	98%	63
Redmond Regional Medical Center	Rome	98%	123
Saint Joseph's Hospital of Atlanta[2]	Atlanta	98%	88
Tift Regional Medical Center	Tifton	98%	123
Wellstar Douglas Hospital[2]	Douglasville	98%	87
Candler Hospital	Savannah	97%	89
Coffee Regional Medical Center[2]	Douglas	97%	37
Emory University Hospital Midtown[2]	Atlanta	97%	102
Gordon Hospital	Calhoun	97%	34
Hamilton Medical Center[2]	Dalton	97%	99
Newton Medical Center[2]	Covington	97%	98
North Fulton Hospital	Roswell	97%	105
Saint Joseph's Hospital - Savannah	Savannah	97%	232
Tanner Medical Center Villa Rica	Villa Rica	97%	30
Coliseum Medical Center[2]	Macon	96%	83
Piedmont Hospital[2]	Atlanta	96%	104
Southern Regional Medical Center	Riverdale	96%	269
Wellstar Cobb Hospital[2]	Austell	96%	112

NOTE: Hospital profiles are in alphabetical order by state, then city, then hospital within the city; Rankings exclude hospitals with less than 25 cases except for patient surveys which excludes hospitals with less than 100 cases; (a) 100-299 cases; (1) The number of cases/patients is too few to report; (2) Data submitted were based on a sample of cases/patients; (3) Results are based on a shorter time period than required; (4) Data suppressed by CMS for one or more quarters; (5) Results are not available for this reporting period; (6) Fewer than 100 patients completed the HCAHPS survey; (7) No cases met the criteria for this measure; (8) The lower limit of the confidence interval cannot be calculated if the number of observed infections equals zero; (9) No data are available from the state/territory for this reporting period; (10) The scores shown reflect fewer than 50 completed surveys; (11) There were discrepancies in the data collection process; (12) This measure does not apply to this hospital for this reporting period; (13) Results cannot be calculated for this reporting period; (14) The results for this state are combined with nearby states to protect confidentiality; Please refer to the User's Guide for a full explanation of data.

Hospital Name	City	Rate	Cases
Northeast Georgia Medical Center	Gainesville	95%	360
Phoebe Putney Memorial Hospital[2]	Albany	95%	151
Piedmont Henry Hospital	Stockbridge	95%	148
Meadows Regional Medical Center	Vidalia	94%	52
Memorial Hospital & Manor	Bainbridge	93%	42
East Georgia Regional Medical Center	Statesboro	92%	80
SE Georgia Health Sys-Brunswick[2]	Brunswick	92%	118
Houston Medical Center	Warner Robins	91%	74
Clearview Regional Medical Center	Monroe	90%	39
Crisp Regional Hospital	Cordele	90%	42
Tanner Medical Center - Carrollton	Carrollton	90%	62
Mayo Clinic Health System - Waycross	Waycross	86%	94
Colquitt Regional Medical Center	Moultrie	84%	45
Upson Regional Medical Center	Thomaston	84%	37

Discharged on Antithrombotic Therapy

Hospital Name	City	Rate	Cases
Athens Regional Medical Center[2]	Athens	100%	81
Cartersville Medical Center[2]	Cartersville	100%	52
Clearview Regional Medical Center	Monroe	100%	37
Crisp Regional Hospital	Cordele	100%	37
Dekalb Medical Center at Hillandale	Lithonia	100%	61
Doctors Hospital[2]	Augusta	100%	68
East Georgia Regional Medical Center	Statesboro	100%	80
Eastside Medical Center[2]	Snellville	100%	97
Emory Johns Creek Hospital	Johns Creek	100%	73
Emory University Hospital[2]	Atlanta	100%	61
Fairview Park Hospital[2]	Dublin	100%	66
Grady Memorial Hospital[2]	Atlanta	100%	93
Gwinnett Medical Center	Lawrenceville	100%	306
John D Archbold Memorial Hospital	Thomasville	100%	154
Memorial Health Univ Medical Center	Savannah	100%	281
Memorial Hospital & Manor	Bainbridge	100%	38
Midtown Medical Center	Columbus	100%	181
Newton Medical Center[2]	Covington	100%	94
North Fulton Hospital	Roswell	100%	78
Northside Hospital	Atlanta	100%	125
Northside Hospital Cherokee	Canton	100%	27
Northside Hospital Forsyth	Cumming	100%	131
Phoebe Sumter Medical Center[2]	Americus	100%	61
Piedmont Newnan Hospital	Newnan	100%	70
Redmond Regional Medical Center	Rome	100%	109
Saint Francis Hospital	Columbus	100%	208
University Hospital	Augusta	100%	281
Wellstar Cobb Hospital[2]	Austell	100%	108
Wellstar Douglas Hospital[2]	Douglasville	100%	87
Wellstar Kennestone Hospital[2]	Marietta	100%	84
West Georgia Medical Center	Lagrange	100%	80
Atlanta Medical Center[2]	Atlanta	99%	178
Emory University Hospital Midtown[2]	Atlanta	99%	79
Piedmont Fayette Hospital	Fayetteville	99%	85
Rockdale Medical Center[2]	Conyers	99%	74
Saint Joseph's Hospital - Savannah	Savannah	99%	199
Saint Joseph's Hospital of Atlanta[2]	Atlanta	99%	76
South Georgia Medical Center	Valdosta	99%	175
Southern Regional Medical Center	Riverdale	99%	220
Spalding Regional Hospital	Griffin	99%	131
Tift Regional Medical Center	Tifton	99%	122
Candler Hospital	Savannah	98%	87
Floyd Medical Center	Rome	98%	124
Hamilton Medical Center[2]	Dalton	98%	88
Medical Center of Central Georgia[2]	Macon	98%	343
Med College of Georgia Hosps	Augusta	98%	187
Saint Mary's Hospital	Athens	98%	133
SE Georgia Health Sys-Brunswick[2]	Brunswick	98%	96
Dekalb Medical Center	Decatur	97%	155
Habersham County Medical Center	Demorest	97%	39
Northeast Georgia Medical Center	Gainesville	97%	317
Piedmont Henry Hospital	Stockbridge	97%	140
Piedmont Hospital[2]	Atlanta	97%	90
Tanner Medical Center - Carrollton	Carrollton	97%	61
Coliseum Medical Center[2]	Macon	96%	82
Phoebe Putney Memorial Hospital[2]	Albany	96%	134
Gordon Hospital	Calhoun	94%	34
Mayo Clinic Health System - Waycross	Waycross	94%	83
Coffee Regional Medical Center[2]	Douglas	93%	30
Houston Medical Center	Warner Robins	92%	71
Meadows Regional Medical Center	Vidalia	92%	50
Tanner Medical Center Villa Rica	Villa Rica	90%	30
Colquitt Regional Medical Center	Moultrie	86%	37
Upson Regional Medical Center	Thomaston	86%	36

Discharged on Statin Medication

Hospital Name	City	Rate	Cases
Cartersville Medical Center[2]	Cartersville	100%	41
Doctors Hospital[2]	Augusta	100%	58
Eastside Medical Center[2]	Snellville	100%	65
Emory Johns Creek Hospital	Johns Creek	100%	62
Midtown Medical Center	Columbus	100%	148
Northside Hospital Forsyth	Cumming	100%	97
Saint Joseph's Hospital of Atlanta[2]	Atlanta	100%	69
University Hospital	Augusta	100%	219
Wellstar Kennestone Hospital[2]	Marietta	100%	58
Atlanta Medical Center[2]	Atlanta	99%	132
Memorial Health Univ Medical Center	Savannah	99%	215
Northside Hospital	Atlanta	99%	90
South Georgia Medical Center	Valdosta	99%	144
Spalding Regional Hospital	Griffin	99%	99
Athens Regional Medical Center[2]	Athens	98%	64
Emory University Hospital[2]	Atlanta	98%	44
Fairview Park Hospital[2]	Dublin	98%	52
Med College of Georgia Hosps	Augusta	98%	137
North Fulton Hospital	Roswell	98%	54
Rockdale Medical Center[2]	Conyers	98%	60
Tift Regional Medical Center	Tifton	98%	99
Dekalb Medical Center	Decatur	97%	126
East Georgia Regional Medical Center	Statesboro	97%	61
Piedmont Fayette Hospital	Fayetteville	97%	72
Saint Joseph's Hospital - Savannah	Savannah	97%	156
Wellstar Cobb Hospital[2]	Austell	97%	78
Wellstar Douglas Hospital[2]	Douglasville	97%	67
Emory University Hospital Midtown[2]	Atlanta	96%	52
Gwinnett Medical Center	Lawrenceville	96%	220
Northeast Georgia Medical Center	Gainesville	96%	254
Redmond Regional Medical Center	Rome	96%	98
West Georgia Medical Center	Lagrange	96%	67
Candler Hospital	Savannah	95%	63
Hamilton Medical Center[2]	Dalton	95%	62
John D Archbold Memorial Hospital	Thomasville	95%	130
Medical Center of Central Georgia[2]	Macon	95%	275
Tanner Medical Center - Carrollton	Carrollton	95%	42
Crisp Regional Hospital	Cordele	94%	31
Floyd Medical Center	Rome	94%	78
Grady Memorial Hospital[2]	Atlanta	94%	64
Habersham County Medical Center	Demorest	94%	34
Memorial Hospital & Manor	Bainbridge	94%	32
Piedmont Hospital[2]	Atlanta	94%	77
Saint Francis Hospital	Columbus	94%	161
Southern Regional Medical Center	Riverdale	94%	177
Gordon Hospital	Calhoun	93%	28
Meadows Regional Medical Center	Vidalia	93%	43
Saint Mary's Hospital	Athens	93%	104
Dekalb Medical Center at Hillandale	Lithonia	92%	49
Phoebe Sumter Medical Center[2]	Americus	92%	53
Piedmont Newnan Hospital	Newnan	92%	63
Coliseum Medical Center[2]	Macon	91%	69
Newton Medical Center[2]	Covington	91%	82
Phoebe Putney Memorial Hospital[2]	Albany	90%	114
Houston Medical Center	Warner Robins	87%	60
SE Georgia Health Sys-Brunswick[2]	Brunswick	87%	79
Colquitt Regional Medical Center	Moultrie	85%	34
Piedmont Henry Hospital	Stockbridge	85%	113
Clearview Regional Medical Center	Monroe	83%	30
Coffee Regional Medical Center[2]	Douglas	81%	27
Mayo Clinic Health System - Waycross	Waycross	78%	74
Upson Regional Medical Center	Thomaston	50%	34

Thrombolytic Therapy Timing

Hospital Name	City	Rate	Cases
South Georgia Medical Center	Valdosta	97%	39
Medical Center of Central Georgia[2]	Macon	93%	29
Memorial Health Univ Medical Center	Savannah	88%	26
Northeast Georgia Medical Center	Gainesville	77%	35
Southern Regional Medical Center	Riverdale	63%	38
Piedmont Hospital[2]	Atlanta	4%	25
SE Georgia Health Sys-Brunswick[2]	Brunswick	0%	25

Venous Thromboembolism (VTE) Prophylaxis

Hospital Name	City	Rate	Cases
Cartersville Medical Center[2]	Cartersville	100%	61
Dekalb Medical Center at Hillandale	Lithonia	100%	67
Doctors Hospital[2]	Augusta	100%	85
Eastside Medical Center[2]	Snellville	100%	117
Gordon Hospital	Calhoun	100%	28
Gwinnett Medical Center	Lawrenceville	100%	338
Northside Hospital Cherokee	Canton	100%	27
Tanner Medical Center Villa Rica	Villa Rica	100%	31
Dekalb Medical Center	Decatur	99%	183
Emory Johns Creek Hospital	Johns Creek	99%	73
Northside Hospital	Atlanta	99%	152
South Georgia Medical Center	Valdosta	99%	200
West Georgia Medical Center	Lagrange	99%	85
Atlanta Medical Center[2]	Atlanta	98%	259
Crisp Regional Hospital	Cordele	98%	42
Emory University Hospital[2]	Atlanta	98%	129
Med College of Georgia Hosps	Augusta	98%	273
Northside Hospital Forsyth	Cumming	98%	168
Redmond Regional Medical Center	Rome	98%	120
Rockdale Medical Center[2]	Conyers	98%	62
Tanner Medical Center - Carrollton	Carrollton	98%	62
University Hospital	Augusta	98%	327
Midtown Medical Center	Columbus	97%	229
Saint Joseph's Hospital of Atlanta[2]	Atlanta	97%	88
Athens Regional Medical Center[2]	Athens	96%	80
Emory University Hospital Midtown[2]	Atlanta	96%	112
Fairview Park Hospital[2]	Dublin	96%	69
Hamilton Medical Center[2]	Dalton	96%	83
John D Archbold Memorial Hospital	Thomasville	96%	202
North Fulton Hospital	Roswell	96%	106
Saint Mary's Hospital	Athens	96%	162
Coliseum Medical Center[2]	Macon	95%	84
Grady Memorial Hospital[2]	Atlanta	95%	112
Memorial Health Univ Medical Center	Savannah	95%	359
Saint Francis Hospital	Columbus	95%	242
Saint Joseph's Hospital - Savannah	Savannah	95%	254
Tift Regional Medical Center	Tifton	95%	116
Wellstar Douglas Hospital[2]	Douglasville	95%	82
Wellstar Kennestone Hospital[2]	Marietta	95%	106
Piedmont Newnan Hospital	Newnan	94%	78
Wellstar Cobb Hospital[2]	Austell	94%	117
Floyd Medical Center	Rome	93%	142
Medical Center of Central Georgia[2]	Macon	93%	512
Newton Medical Center[2]	Covington	92%	93
Clearview Regional Medical Center	Monroe	91%	33
Southern Regional Medical Center	Riverdale	91%	292
Spalding Regional Hospital	Griffin	91%	136
Candler Hospital	Savannah	87%	87
Northeast Georgia Medical Center	Gainesville	87%	334
Piedmont Hospital[2]	Atlanta	87%	107
Memorial Hospital & Manor	Bainbridge	85%	41
Piedmont Henry Hospital	Stockbridge	85%	156
Piedmont Fayette Hospital	Fayetteville	84%	90
East Georgia Regional Medical Center	Statesboro	81%	75
SE Georgia Health Sys-Brunswick[2]	Brunswick	81%	122
Phoebe Sumter Medical Center[2]	Americus	80%	60
Phoebe Putney Memorial Hospital[2]	Albany	79%	164
Habersham County Medical Center	Demorest	76%	41
Mayo Clinic Health System - Waycross	Waycross	73%	90
Wayne Memorial Hospital	Jesup	72%	32
Colquitt Regional Medical Center	Moultrie	71%	41
Oconee Regional Medical Center	Milledgeville	70%	27
Meadows Regional Medical Center	Vidalia	69%	48
Houston Medical Center	Warner Robins	64%	96
Coffee Regional Medical Center[2]	Douglas	62%	40
Upson Regional Medical Center	Thomaston	50%	30

Written Stroke Educational Materials Given

Hospital Name	City	Rate	Cases
Coliseum Medical Center[2]	Macon	100%	49
Dekalb Medical Center at Hillandale	Lithonia	100%	47
Doctors Hospital[2]	Augusta	100%	43
Fairview Park Hospital[2]	Dublin	100%	40
Memorial Health Univ Medical Center	Savannah	100%	196
West Georgia Medical Center	Lagrange	100%	41
Dekalb Medical Center	Decatur	99%	105
Med College of Georgia Hosps	Augusta	99%	152
Midtown Medical Center	Columbus	99%	133
Saint Francis Hospital	Columbus	99%	113
Floyd Medical Center	Rome	98%	85
Eastside Medical Center[2]	Snellville	97%	69
Emory University Hospital Midtown[2]	Atlanta	97%	68
North Fulton Hospital	Roswell	97%	72
Northside Hospital	Atlanta	97%	102
Candler Hospital	Savannah	96%	53
Crisp Regional Hospital	Cordele	96%	28
Cartersville Medical Center[2]	Cartersville	95%	38
Northside Hospital Forsyth	Cumming	95%	117
Saint Mary's Hospital	Athens	95%	77
Emory Johns Creek Hospital	Johns Creek	94%	62
Saint Joseph's Hospital - Savannah	Savannah	94%	119
Spalding Regional Hospital	Griffin	94%	80
Medical Center of Central Georgia[2]	Macon	93%	269
University Hospital	Augusta	93%	177
Athens Regional Medical Center[2]	Athens	92%	62
Emory University Hospital[2]	Atlanta	91%	75
Gwinnett Medical Center	Lawrenceville	91%	246
Wellstar Kennestone Hospital[2]	Marietta	91%	54
Grady Memorial Hospital[2]	Atlanta	90%	58
Piedmont Hospital[2]	Atlanta	90%	63
Wellstar Douglas Hospital[2]	Douglasville	90%	71
Atlanta Medical Center[2]	Atlanta	89%	145
South Georgia Medical Center	Valdosta	89%	122
Colquitt Regional Medical Center	Moultrie	88%	26
Hamilton Medical Center[2]	Dalton	88%	66
Northeast Georgia Medical Center	Gainesville	88%	248
Piedmont Henry Hospital	Stockbridge	88%	94
Rockdale Medical Center[2]	Conyers	85%	61
Tift Regional Medical Center	Tifton	83%	95
Wellstar Cobb Hospital[2]	Austell	79%	66
SE Georgia Health Sys-Brunswick[2]	Brunswick	75%	83
Tanner Medical Center - Carrollton	Carrollton	74%	39

NOTE: Hospital profiles are in alphabetical order by state, then city, then hospital within the city; Rankings exclude hospitals with less than 25 cases except for patient surveys which excludes hospitals with less than 100 cases; (a) 100-299 cases; (1) The number of cases/patients is too few to report; (2) Data submitted were based on a sample of cases/patients; (3) Results are based on a shorter time period than required; (4) Data suppressed by CMS for one or more quarters; (5) Results are not available for this reporting period; (6) Fewer than 100 patients completed the HCAHPS survey; (7) No cases met the criteria for this measure; (8) The lower limit of the confidence interval cannot be calculated if the number of observed infections equals zero; (9) No data are available from the state/territory for this reporting period; (10) The scores shown reflect fewer than 50 completed surveys; (11) There were discrepancies in the data collection process; (12) This measure does not apply to this hospital for this reporting period; (13) Results cannot be calculated for this reporting period; (14) The results for this state are combined with nearby states to protect confidentiality; Please refer to the User's Guide for a full explanation of data.

Hospital Name	City	Rate	Cases
Piedmont Fayette Hospital	Fayetteville	73%	60
Southern Regional Medical Center	Riverdale	73%	168
Redmond Regional Medical Center	Rome	69%	75
East Georgia Regional Medical Center	Statesboro	67%	60
John D Archbold Memorial Hospital	Thomasville	65%	81
Mayo Clinic Health System - Waycross	Waycross	65%	54
Piedmont Newnan Hospital	Newnan	62%	48
Saint Joseph's Hospital of Atlanta[2]	Atlanta	61%	64
Memorial Hospital & Manor	Bainbridge	60%	25
Upson Regional Medical Center	Thomaston	46%	26
Phoebe Sumter Medical Center[2]	Americus	29%	41
Phoebe Putney Memorial Hospital[2]	Albany	21%	89
Newton Medical Center[2]	Covington	20%	61
Coffee Regional Medical Center[2]	Douglas	18%	28
Houston Medical Center	Warner Robins	14%	49
Meadows Regional Medical Center	Vidalia	0%	35

Surgical Care Improvement Project

Appropriate Beta Blocker Usage

Hospital Name	City	Rate	Cases
Coffee Regional Medical Center[2]	Douglas	100%	42
Coliseum Medical Center[2]	Macon	100%	169
Colquitt Regional Medical Center	Moultrie	100%	53
Doctors Hospital[2]	Augusta	100%	116
Fairview Park Hospital	Dublin	100%	89
Fannin Regional Hospital	Blue Ridge	100%	48
Floyd Medical Center[2]	Rome	100%	219
Northside Hospital[2]	Atlanta	100%	121
Northside Hospital Cherokee	Canton	100%	122
Northside Hospital Forsyth[2]	Cumming	100%	114
Northside Medical Center	Columbus	100%	160
Oconee Regional Medical Center	Milledgeville	100%	29
Phoebe Sumter Medical Center	Americus	100%	44
Piedmont Henry Hospital[2]	Stockbridge	100%	153
SE Georgia Health Sys-Brunswick[2]	Brunswick	100%	93
Tanner Medical Center - Carrollton	Carrollton	100%	209
University Hospital[2]	Augusta	100%	251
Wellstar Paulding Hospital[2]	Hiram	100%	40
West Georgia Medical Center	Lagrange	100%	91
Coliseum Northside Hospital[2]	Macon	99%	67
Emory Johns Creek Hospital	Johns Creek	99%	83
Emory University Hospital Midtown[2]	Atlanta	99%	201
Gordon Hospital	Calhoun	99%	88
Hamilton Medical Center[2]	Dalton	99%	79
Redmond Regional Medical Center	Rome	99%	526
Rockdale Medical Center[2]	Conyers	99%	75
Saint Joseph's Hospital - Savannah[2]	Savannah	99%	479
Wellstar Cobb Hospital[2]	Austell	99%	282
Wellstar Douglas Hospital[2]	Douglasville	99%	102
Wellstar Kennestone Hospital[2]	Marietta	99%	498
Atlanta Medical Center[2]	Atlanta	98%	119
Cartersville Medical Center[2]	Cartersville	98%	100
Dekalb Medical Center[2]	Decatur	98%	191
Eastside Medical Center[2]	Snellville	98%	101
Emory University Hospital[2]	Atlanta	98%	199
Gwinnett Medical Center[2]	Lawrenceville	98%	283
Houston Medical Center[2]	Warner Robins	98%	130
Northeast Georgia Medical Center[2]	Gainesville	98%	285
Piedmont Fayette Hospital[2]	Fayetteville	98%	115
Piedmont Hospital[2]	Atlanta	98%	229
Piedmont Mountainside Hospital[2]	Jasper	98%	66
Saint Joseph's Hospital of Atlanta[2]	Atlanta	98%	239
Southern Regional Medical Center[2]	Riverdale	98%	90
Tift Regional Medical Center	Tifton	98%	208
Doctors Specialty Hospital	Columbus	97%	33
East Georgia Regional Medical Center	Statesboro	97%	129
John D Archbold Memorial Hospital[2]	Thomasville	97%	174
Mayo Clinic Health System - Waycross	Waycross	97%	109
Meadows Regional Medical Center	Vidalia	97%	63
Med College of Georgia Hosps[2]	Augusta	97%	146
Saint Francis Hospital[2]	Columbus	97%	205
Spalding Regional Hospital	Griffin	97%	77
Athens Regional Medical Center[2]	Athens	96%	214
North Fulton Hospital[2]	Roswell	96%	74
Phoebe Putney Memorial Hospital[2]	Albany	96%	266
Piedmont Newnan Hospital[2]	Newnan	96%	119
South Georgia Medical Center	Valdosta	96%	377
Trinity Hospital of Augusta	Augusta	96%	113
Candler Hospital[2]	Savannah	95%	55
Clearview Regional Medical Center	Monroe	95%	79
Medical Center of Central Georgia[2]	Macon	95%	222
Memorial Health Univ Medical Center[2]	Savannah	94%	197
Saint Mary's Hospital[2]	Athens	94%	172
Chestatee Regional Hospital[2]	Dahlonega	93%	43
Taylor Regional Hospital[2]	Hawkinsville	93%	27
Newton Medical Center[2]	Covington	92%	92
Augusta VA Medical Center[2]	Augusta	91%	79
Wayne Memorial Hospital	Jesup	91%	34
Decatur VA Medical Center[2]	Decatur	90%	48

Hospital Name	City	Rate	Cases
Habersham County Medical Center[2]	Demorest	89%	36
Midtown Medical Center[2]	Columbus	89%	72
Grady Memorial Hospital[2]	Atlanta	85%	55
Upson Regional Medical Center[2]	Thomaston	85%	48

Appropriate VTP Within 24 Hours

Hospital Name	City	Rate	Cases
Coffee Regional Medical Center[2]	Douglas	100%	150
Crisp Regional Hospital	Cordele	100%	89
Doctors Hospital[2]	Augusta	100%	456
Emory University Hospital[2]	Atlanta	100%	417
Fairview Park Hospital	Dublin	100%	274
Fannin Regional Hospital	Blue Ridge	100%	131
Gordon Hospital	Calhoun	100%	239
Northside Hospital[2]	Atlanta	100%	543
Northside Hospital Cherokee	Canton	100%	323
Northside Hospital Forsyth[2]	Cumming	100%	320
Northside Medical Center	Columbus	100%	597
Perry Hospital[2]	Perry	100%	72
Saint Francis Hospital[2]	Columbus	100%	442
SE Georgia Health Sys-Brunswick[2]	Brunswick	100%	361
SE Georgia Health Sys-Camden Campus	Saint Marys	100%	103
Southern Regional Medical Center[2]	Riverdale	100%	369
Tanner Medical Center - Carrollton	Carrollton	100%	556
Tanner Medical Center Villa Rica	Villa Rica	100%	34
University Hospital[2]	Augusta	100%	453
Wellstar Douglas Hospital[2]	Douglasville	100%	300
Wellstar Paulding Hospital[2]	Hiram	100%	142
West Georgia Medical Center	Lagrange	100%	323
Atlanta Medical Center[2]	Atlanta	99%	427
Coliseum Northside Hospital[2]	Macon	99%	210
Colquitt Regional Medical Center	Moultrie	99%	146
Dekalb Medical Center[2]	Decatur	99%	732
Dekalb Medical Center at Hillandale	Lithonia	99%	102
Doctors Specialty Hospital	Columbus	99%	177
East Georgia Regional Medical Center	Statesboro	99%	336
Eastside Medical Center[2]	Snellville	99%	415
Emory Johns Creek Hospital	Johns Creek	99%	302
Floyd Medical Center[2]	Rome	99%	693
Hamilton Medical Center[2]	Dalton	99%	236
John D Archbold Memorial Hospital[2]	Thomasville	99%	463
Meadows Regional Medical Center	Vidalia	99%	189
Medical Center of Central Georgia[2]	Macon	99%	437
Med College of Georgia Hosps[2]	Augusta	99%	276
Memorial Health Univ Medical Center[2]	Savannah	99%	326
Memorial Hospital & Manor	Bainbridge	99%	69
Phoebe Putney Memorial Hospital[2]	Albany	99%	553
Phoebe Sumter Medical Center	Americus	99%	165
Redmond Regional Medical Center	Rome	99%	617
Rockdale Medical Center[2]	Conyers	99%	285
Southeastern Regional Medical Center[3]	Newnan	99%	77
Taylor Regional Hospital[2]	Hawkinsville	99%	76
Trinity Hospital of Augusta	Augusta	99%	432
Wellstar Cobb Hospital[2]	Austell	99%	726
Barrow Regional Medical Center	Winder	98%	80
Cartersville Medical Center[2]	Cartersville	98%	276
Coliseum Medical Center[2]	Macon	98%	250
Grady Memorial Hospital[2]	Atlanta	98%	271
Habersham County Medical Center[2]	Demorest	98%	99
Irwin County Hospital[2]	Ocilla	98%	57
Midtown Medical Center[2]	Columbus	98%	241
North Fulton Hospital[2]	Roswell	98%	304
Piedmont Fayette Hospital[2]	Fayetteville	98%	425
Saint Joseph's Hospital - Savannah[2]	Savannah	98%	917
Spalding Regional Hospital	Griffin	98%	357
Tift Regional Medical Center	Tifton	98%	575
Wellstar Kennestone Hospital[2]	Marietta	98%	809
Augusta VA Medical Center[2]	Augusta	97%	176
Houston Medical Center[2]	Warner Robins	97%	414
Northeast Georgia Medical Center[2]	Gainesville	97%	384
Saint Mary's Hospital[2]	Athens	97%	500
South Georgia Medical Center	Valdosta	97%	760
Upson Regional Medical Center[2]	Thomaston	97%	184
Candler Hospital[2]	Savannah	96%	225
Emory - Adventist Hospital	Smyrna	96%	55
Emory University Hospital Midtown[2]	Atlanta	96%	338
Gwinnett Medical Center[2]	Lawrenceville	96%	596
Mayo Clinic Health System - Waycross	Waycross	96%	231
Oconee Regional Medical Center	Milledgeville	96%	108
Piedmont Henry Hospital[2]	Stockbridge	96%	499
Piedmont Newnan Hospital[2]	Newnan	96%	392
Stephens County Hospital	Toccoa	96%	95
Univ McDuffie Co Reg Med Ctr	Thomson	96%	76
Athens Regional Medical Center[2]	Athens	95%	383
Chestatee Regional Hospital[2]	Dahlonega	95%	106
Clearview Regional Medical Center	Monroe	95%	197
Decatur VA Medical Center[2]	Decatur	95%	194
Hutcheson Medical Center	Fort Oglethorpe	95%	86
Piedmont Mountainside Hospital[2]	Jasper	94%	178
Saint Joseph's Hospital of Atlanta[2]	Atlanta	94%	242
Washington County Regional Medical Center	Sandersville	94%	52

Hospital Name	City	Rate	Cases
Newton Medical Center[2]	Covington	93%	302
Union General Hospital[2]	Blairsville	93%	58
Dodge County Hospital	Eastman	92%	77
Piedmont Hospital[2]	Atlanta	92%	464
Liberty Regional Medical Center	Hinesville	84%	50
Ty Cobb Regional Medical Center[2]	Lavonia	77%	53
Wayne Memorial Hospital	Jesup	77%	101
North Georgia Medical Center[2]	Ellijay	46%	41

Controlled Postoperative Blood Glucose

Hospital Name	City	Rate	Cases
Gwinnett Medical Center[2]	Lawrenceville	100%	169
Medical Center of Central Georgia[2]	Macon	100%	128
Coliseum Medical Center[2]	Macon	98%	119
Emory University Hospital[2]	Atlanta	98%	90
Saint Joseph's Hospital - Savannah[2]	Savannah	98%	276
South Georgia Medical Center	Valdosta	98%	195
University Hospital[2]	Augusta	98%	179
Wellstar Kennestone Hospital[2]	Marietta	98%	248
Saint Francis Hospital[2]	Columbus	97%	103
Athens Regional Medical Center[2]	Athens	96%	111
Northeast Georgia Medical Center[2]	Gainesville	96%	180
Redmond Regional Medical Center	Rome	96%	335
Piedmont Hospital[2]	Atlanta	95%	173
Emory University Hospital Midtown[2]	Atlanta	94%	109
Phoebe Putney Memorial Hospital[2]	Albany	94%	139
Saint Joseph's Hospital of Atlanta[2]	Atlanta	93%	156
Med College of Georgia Hosps[2]	Augusta	92%	96
Memorial Health Univ Medical Center[2]	Savannah	91%	122
Atlanta Medical Center[2]	Atlanta	89%	28

Perioperative Temperature Management

Hospital Name	City	Rate	Cases
Athens Regional Medical Center[2]	Athens	100%	492
Atlanta Medical Center[2]	Atlanta	100%	557
Bacon County Hospital	Alma	100%	75
Barrow Regional Medical Center	Winder	100%	90
Candler Hospital[2]	Savannah	100%	254
Cartersville Medical Center[2]	Cartersville	100%	308
Chestatee Regional Hospital[2]	Dahlonega	100%	126
Clearview Regional Medical Center	Monroe	100%	285
Coffee Regional Medical Center[2]	Douglas	100%	185
Coliseum Medical Center[2]	Macon	100%	356
Coliseum Northside Hospital[2]	Macon	100%	233
Colquitt Regional Medical Center	Moultrie	100%	176
Crisp Regional Hospital	Cordele	100%	97
Decatur VA Medical Center[2]	Decatur	100%	232
Dekalb Medical Center[2]	Decatur	100%	852
Dekalb Medical Center at Hillandale	Lithonia	100%	106
Doctors Hospital[2]	Augusta	100%	512
Doctors Specialty Hospital	Columbus	100%	196
Dodge County Hospital	Eastman	100%	27
Dorminy Medical Center	Fitzgerald	100%	27
East Georgia Regional Medical Center	Statesboro	100%	378
Eastside Medical Center[2]	Snellville	100%	453
Emory - Adventist Hospital	Smyrna	100%	58
Emory Johns Creek Hospital	Johns Creek	100%	339
Emory University Hospital[2]	Atlanta	100%	600
Emory University Hospital Midtown[2]	Atlanta	100%	475
Fairview Park Hospital	Dublin	100%	335
Fannin Regional Hospital	Blue Ridge	100%	154
Floyd Medical Center[2]	Rome	100%	841
Gordon Hospital	Calhoun	100%	259
Habersham County Medical Center[2]	Demorest	100%	102
Hamilton Medical Center[2]	Dalton	100%	276
Houston Medical Center[2]	Warner Robins	100%	447
Hutcheson Medical Center	Fort Oglethorpe	100%	94
Irwin County Hospital[2]	Ocilla	100%	66
John D Archbold Memorial Hospital[2]	Thomasville	100%	600
Liberty Regional Medical Center	Hinesville	100%	53
Mayo Clinic Health System - Waycross	Waycross	100%	285
Medical Center of Central Georgia[2]	Macon	100%	558
Med College of Georgia Hosps[2]	Augusta	100%	349
Memorial Health Univ Medical Center[2]	Savannah	100%	443
Midtown Medical Center[2]	Columbus	100%	278
Newton Medical Center[2]	Covington	100%	324
North Fulton Hospital[2]	Roswell	100%	348
Northeast Georgia Medical Center[2]	Gainesville	100%	555
Northside Hospital[2]	Atlanta	100%	609
Northside Hospital Cherokee	Canton	100%	363
Northside Hospital Forsyth[2]	Cumming	100%	464
Northside Medical Center	Columbus	100%	616
Oconee Regional Medical Center	Milledgeville	100%	117
Perry Hospital[2]	Perry	100%	75
Phoebe Putney Memorial Hospital[2]	Albany	100%	660
Phoebe Sumter Medical Center	Americus	100%	171
Piedmont Fayette Hospital[2]	Fayetteville	100%	499
Piedmont Henry Hospital[2]	Stockbridge	100%	542
Piedmont Mountainside Hospital[2]	Jasper	100%	224
Piedmont Newnan Hospital[2]	Newnan	100%	441

NOTE: Hospital profiles are in alphabetical order by state, then city, then hospital within the city; Rankings exclude hospitals with less than 25 cases except for patient surveys which excludes hospitals with less than 100 cases; (a) 100-299 cases; (1) The number of cases/patients is too few to report; (2) Data submitted were based on a sample of cases/patients; (3) Results are based on a shorter time period than required; (4) Data suppressed by CMS for one or more quarters; (5) Results are not available for this reporting period; (6) Fewer than 100 patients completed the HCAHPS survey; (7) No cases met the criteria for this measure; (8) The lower limit of the confidence interval cannot be calculated if the number of observed infections equals zero; (9) No data are available from the state/territory for this reporting period; (10) The scores shown reflect fewer than 50 completed surveys; (11) There were discrepancies in the data collection process; (12) This measure does not apply to this hospital for this reporting period; (13) Results cannot be calculated for this reporting period; (14) The results for this state are combined with nearby states to protect confidentiality; Please refer to the User's Guide for a full explanation of data.

Redmond Regional Medical Center	Rome	100%	782
Rockdale Medical Center[2]	Conyers	100%	316
Saint Francis Hospital[2]	Columbus	100%	511
Saint Joseph's Hospital - Savannah[2]	Savannah	100%	1152
Saint Joseph's Hospital of Atlanta[2]	Atlanta	100%	559
Saint Mary's Hospital[2]	Athens	100%	554
South Georgia Medical Center	Valdosta	100%	857
SE Georgia Health Sys-Brunswick[2]	Brunswick	100%	422
SE Georgia Health Sys-Camden Campus	Saint Marys	100%	113
Southeastern Regional Medical Center[3]	Newnan	100%	78
Southern Regional Medical Center[2]	Riverdale	100%	404
Spalding Regional Hospital	Griffin	100%	400
Stephens County Hospital	Toccoa	100%	103
Tanner Medical Center - Carrollton	Carrollton	100%	646
Tanner Medical Center Villa Rica	Villa Rica	100%	41
Taylor Regional Hospital[2]	Hawkinsville	100%	84
Tift Regional Medical Center	Tifton	100%	637
Trinity Hospital of Augusta	Augusta	100%	477
Union General Hospital[2]	Blairsville	100%	63
University Hospital[2]	Augusta	100%	590
Washington County Regional Medical Center	Sandersville	100%	54
Wayne Memorial Hospital	Jesup	100%	114
Wellstar Cobb Hospital[2]	Austell	100%	908
Wellstar Douglas Hospital[2]	Douglasville	100%	328
Wellstar Kennestone Hospital[2]	Marietta	100%	1194
Wellstar Paulding Hospital[2]	Hiram	100%	153
West Georgia Medical Center	Lagrange	100%	342
Augusta VA Medical Center[2]	Augusta	99%	224
Grady Memorial Hospital[2]	Atlanta	99%	339
Meadows Regional Medical Center	Vidalia	99%	212
Piedmont Hospital[2]	Atlanta	99%	633
Ty Cobb Regional Medical Center[2]	Lavonia	99%	67
Upson Regional Medical Center[2]	Thomaston	99%	207
Gwinnett Medical Center[2]	Lawrenceville	98%	747
Univ McDuffie Co Reg Med Ctr	Thomson	98%	80
North Georgia Medical Center[2]	Ellijay	95%	42
Memorial Hospital & Manor	Bainbridge	94%	81

Prophylactic Antibiotic Selection

Hospital Name	City	Rate	Cases
Cartersville Medical Center[2]	Cartersville	100%	193
Coffee Regional Medical Center[2]	Douglas	100%	137
Coliseum Northside Hospital[2]	Macon	100%	185
Colquitt Regional Medical Center	Moultrie	100%	91
Crisp Regional Hospital	Cordele	100%	51
Dekalb Medical Center[2]	Decatur	100%	537
Doctors Hospital[2]	Augusta	100%	341
Doctors Specialty Hospital	Columbus	100%	140
Eastside Medical Center[2]	Snellville	100%	281
Emory - Adventist Hospital	Smyrna	100%	27
Fairview Park Hospital	Dublin	100%	239
Fannin Regional Hospital	Blue Ridge	100%	117
Floyd Medical Center[2]	Rome	100%	460
Gordon Hospital	Calhoun	100%	185
Grady Memorial Hospital[2]	Atlanta	100%	207
Habersham County Medical Center[2]	Demorest	100%	53
Hamilton Medical Center[2]	Dalton	100%	162
Irwin County Hospital[2]	Ocilla	100%	52
Med College of Georgia Hosps[2]	Augusta	100%	289
Memorial Health Univ Medical Center[2]	Savannah	100%	407
North Fulton Hospital[2]	Roswell	100%	252
Northside Hospital[2]	Atlanta	100%	427
Northside Hospital Cherokee	Canton	100%	206
Northside Hospital Forsyth[2]	Cumming	100%	287
Northside Medical Center	Columbus	100%	492
Piedmont Fayette Hospital[2]	Fayetteville	100%	323
Piedmont Henry Hospital[2]	Stockbridge	100%	381
Piedmont Newnan Hospital[2]	Newnan	100%	322
Saint Joseph's Hospital - Savannah[2]	Savannah	100%	1285
SE Georgia Health Sys-Brunswick[2]	Brunswick	100%	258
Stephens County Hospital	Toccoa	100%	66
Tanner Medical Center - Carrollton	Carrollton	100%	492
Taylor Regional Hospital[2]	Hawkinsville	100%	64
Tift Regional Medical Center	Tifton	100%	375
Trinity Hospital of Augusta	Augusta	100%	298
University Hospital[2]	Augusta	100%	602
Univ McDuffie Co Reg Med Ctr	Thomson	100%	62
Upson Regional Medical Center[2]	Thomaston	100%	138
Wellstar Paulding Hospital[2]	Hiram	100%	103
West Georgia Medical Center	Lagrange	100%	200
Athens Regional Medical Center[2]	Athens	99%	362
Atlanta Medical Center[2]	Atlanta	99%	355
Augusta VA Medical Center	Augusta	99%	106
Candler Hospital[2]	Savannah	99%	152
Clearview Regional Medical Center	Monroe	99%	173
Coliseum Medical Center[2]	Macon	99%	269
East Georgia Regional Medical Center	Statesboro	99%	245
Emory University Hospital[2]	Atlanta	99%	364
Emory University Hospital Midtown[2]	Atlanta	99%	367
Gwinnett Medical Center[2]	Lawrenceville	99%	675
John D Archbold Memorial Hospital[2]	Thomasville	99%	403
Medical Center of Central Georgia[2]	Macon	99%	513
Midtown Medical Center[2]	Columbus	99%	111
Oconee Regional Medical Center	Milledgeville	99%	69
Phoebe Putney Memorial Hospital[2]	Albany	99%	576
Piedmont Mountainside Hospital[2]	Jasper	99%	177
Redmond Regional Medical Center	Rome	99%	766
Rockdale Medical Center[2]	Conyers	99%	185
Saint Francis Hospital[2]	Columbus	99%	462
Saint Joseph's Hospital of Atlanta[2]	Atlanta	99%	499
Saint Mary's Hospital[2]	Athens	99%	392
Spalding Regional Hospital	Griffin	99%	268
Wellstar Cobb Hospital[2]	Austell	99%	578
Wellstar Douglas Hospital[2]	Douglasville	99%	196
Wellstar Kennestone Hospital[2]	Marietta	99%	852
Barrow Regional Medical Center	Winder	98%	55
Decatur VA Medical Center	Decatur	98%	104
Emory Johns Creek Hospital	Johns Creek	98%	178
Houston Medical Center[2]	Warner Robins	98%	254
Hutcheson Medical Center	Fort Oglethorpe	98%	48
Mayo Clinic Health System - Waycross	Waycross	98%	196
Newton Medical Center[2]	Covington	98%	252
Northeast Georgia Medical Center[2]	Gainesville	98%	504
South Georgia Medical Center	Valdosta	98%	728
Southern Regional Medical Center[2]	Riverdale	98%	261
Dekalb Medical Center at Hillandale	Lithonia	97%	38
Perry Hospital[2]	Perry	97%	60
Phoebe Sumter Medical Center	Americus	97%	121
SE Georgia Health Sys-Camden Campus	Saint Marys	97%	72
Wayne Memorial Hospital	Jesup	97%	92
Piedmont Hospital[2]	Atlanta	96%	547
Meadows Regional Medical Center	Vidalia	94%	142
Dodge County Hospital	Eastman	93%	46
Chestatee Regional Hospital[2]	Dahlonega	92%	99
Union General Hospital[2]	Blairsville	92%	52
Memorial Hospital & Manor	Bainbridge	90%	29
Liberty Regional Medical Center	Hinesville	88%	32

Prophylactic Antibiotic Selection (Outpatient)

Hospital Name	City	Rate	Cases
Candler Hospital	Savannah	100%	528
Cartersville Medical Center	Cartersville	100%	284
Clearview Regional Medical Center	Monroe	100%	36
Coffee Regional Medical Center	Douglas	100%	84
Coliseum Northside Hospital	Macon	100%	38
Crisp Regional Hospital	Cordele	100%	33
Doctors Hospital	Augusta	100%	381
Doctors Specialty Hospital	Columbus	100%	288
Fairview Park Hospital	Dublin	100%	111
Fannin Regional Hospital	Blue Ridge	100%	42
Hutcheson Medical Center	Fort Oglethorpe	100%	37
Med College of Georgia Hosps	Augusta	100%	450
Memorial Hospital & Manor	Bainbridge	100%	29
Midtown Medical Center	Columbus	100%	274
Northside Hospital	Atlanta	100%	870
Northside Hospital Cherokee	Canton	100%	307
Northside Hospital Forsyth	Cumming	100%	347
Redmond Regional Medical Center	Rome	100%	474
Rockdale Medical Center	Conyers	100%	272
Saint Joseph's Hospital - Savannah	Savannah	100%	416
Trinity Hospital of Augusta	Augusta	100%	165
Upson Regional Medical Center	Thomaston	100%	72
West Georgia Medical Center	Lagrange	100%	103
Atlanta Medical Center	Atlanta	99%	202
Coliseum Medical Center	Macon	99%	697
Dekalb Medical Center	Decatur	99%	350
Eastside Medical Center	Snellville	99%	286
Emory Johns Creek Hospital	Johns Creek	99%	293
Emory University Hospital	Atlanta	99%	550
Hamilton Medical Center	Dalton	99%	423
Meadows Regional Medical Center	Vidalia	99%	246
Northside Medical Center	Columbus	99%	159
Piedmont Newnan Hospital	Newnan	99%	82
Saint Mary's Hospital	Athens	99%	389
Tanner Medical Center - Carrollton	Carrollton	99%	356
Tift Regional Medical Center	Tifton	99%	356
Wellstar Cobb Hospital	Austell	99%	548
Wellstar Kennestone Hospital	Marietta	99%	841
East Georgia Regional Medical Center	Statesboro	98%	247
Floyd Medical Center	Rome	98%	413
Gwinnett Medical Center	Lawrenceville	98%	718
Habersham County Medical Center	Demorest	98%	54
John D Archbold Memorial Hospital	Thomasville	98%	319
Mayo Clinic Health System - Waycross	Waycross	98%	129
Medical Center of Central Georgia	Macon	98%	700
Memorial Health Univ Medical Center	Savannah	98%	487
Northeast Georgia Medical Center	Gainesville	98%	774
Northridge Medical Center	Commerce	98%	58
Oconee Regional Medical Center	Milledgeville	98%	54
Piedmont Henry Hospital	Stockbridge	98%	495
Saint Joseph's Hospital of Atlanta	Atlanta	98%	569
SE Georgia Health Sys-Brunswick	Brunswick	98%	624
Spalding Regional Hospital	Griffin	98%	205
University Hospital	Augusta	98%	536
Athens Regional Medical Center	Athens	97%	465
Emory University Hospital Midtown	Atlanta	97%	535
Gordon Hospital	Calhoun	97%	150
North Fulton Hospital	Roswell	97%	187
Phoebe Putney Memorial Hospital	Albany	97%	643
Piedmont Fayette Hospital	Fayetteville	97%	413
Piedmont Hospital	Atlanta	97%	801
Saint Francis Hospital	Columbus	97%	558
SE Georgia Health Sys-Camden Campus	Saint Marys	97%	34
Chestatee Regional Hospital	Dahlonega	96%	57
Higgins General Hospital	Bremen	96%	28
Houston Medical Center	Warner Robins	96%	230
Phoebe Sumter Medical Center	Americus	96%	82
Piedmont Mountainside Hospital	Jasper	96%	100
Southern Regional Medical Center	Riverdale	95%	260
Stephens County Hospital	Toccoa	95%	119
Irwin County Hospital	Ocilla	94%	48
Newton Medical Center	Covington	94%	117
South Georgia Medical Center	Valdosta	94%	543
Union General Hospital	Blairsville	94%	63
Wayne Memorial Hospital	Jesup	94%	125
Emory - Adventist Hospital	Smyrna	93%	28
Grady Memorial Hospital	Atlanta	92%	90

Prophylactic Antibiotic Stopped

Hospital Name	City	Rate	Cases
Coffee Regional Medical Center[2]	Douglas	100%	136
Crisp Regional Hospital	Cordele	100%	48
Doctors Hospital[2]	Augusta	100%	331
Dodge County Hospital	Eastman	100%	44
Fairview Park Hospital	Dublin	100%	236
Fannin Regional Hospital	Blue Ridge	100%	115
Habersham County Medical Center[2]	Demorest	100%	53
Liberty Regional Medical Center	Hinesville	100%	31
Memorial Hospital & Manor	Bainbridge	100%	29
Northside Hospital[2]	Atlanta	100%	407
Northside Hospital Cherokee	Canton	100%	200
Northside Hospital Forsyth[2]	Cumming	100%	281
Northside Medical Center	Columbus	100%	490
Perry Hospital[2]	Perry	100%	54
Piedmont Mountainside Hospital[2]	Jasper	100%	177
Saint Joseph's Hospital - Savannah[2]	Savannah	100%	1274
SE Georgia Health Sys-Brunswick[2]	Brunswick	100%	247
SE Georgia Health Sys-Camden Campus	Saint Marys	100%	69
Tanner Medical Center - Carrollton	Carrollton	100%	491
Univ McDuffie Co Reg Med Ctr	Thomson	100%	62
West Georgia Medical Center	Lagrange	100%	196
Coliseum Medical Center[2]	Macon	99%	257
Colquitt Regional Medical Center	Moultrie	99%	90
Dekalb Medical Center[2]	Decatur	99%	529
Doctors Specialty Hospital	Columbus	99%	138
Eastside Medical Center[2]	Snellville	99%	278
Emory Johns Creek Hospital	Johns Creek	99%	168
Emory University Hospital[2]	Atlanta	99%	350
Emory University Hospital Midtown[2]	Atlanta	99%	344
Floyd Medical Center[2]	Rome	99%	446
Gordon Hospital	Calhoun	99%	178
Hamilton Medical Center[2]	Dalton	99%	156
John D Archbold Memorial Hospital[2]	Thomasville	99%	395
Phoebe Putney Memorial Hospital[2]	Albany	99%	540
Saint Francis Hospital[2]	Columbus	99%	440
University Hospital[2]	Augusta	99%	589
Wellstar Kennestone Hospital[2]	Marietta	99%	832
Wellstar Paulding Hospital[2]	Hiram	99%	100
Barrow Regional Medical Center	Winder	98%	53
Cartersville Medical Center[2]	Cartersville	98%	184
Gwinnett Medical Center[2]	Lawrenceville	98%	646
Hutcheson Medical Center	Fort Oglethorpe	98%	47
Med College of Georgia Hosps[2]	Augusta	98%	247
Midtown Medical Center[2]	Columbus	98%	107
North Fulton Hospital[2]	Roswell	98%	251
Northeast Georgia Medical Center[2]	Gainesville	98%	492
Piedmont Fayette Hospital[2]	Fayetteville	98%	317
Piedmont Henry Hospital[2]	Stockbridge	98%	375
Piedmont Hospital[2]	Atlanta	98%	539
Redmond Regional Medical Center	Rome	98%	746
Southern Regional Medical Center[2]	Riverdale	98%	259
Tift Regional Medical Center	Tifton	98%	356
Trinity Hospital of Augusta	Augusta	98%	287
Wayne Memorial Hospital	Jesup	98%	92
Wellstar Douglas Hospital[2]	Douglasville	98%	189
Atlanta Medical Center[2]	Atlanta	97%	344
Clearview Regional Medical Center	Monroe	97%	168
Coliseum Northside Hospital[2]	Macon	97%	182
Dekalb Medical Center at Hillandale	Lithonia	97%	36
Newton Medical Center[2]	Covington	97%	250
Saint Mary's Hospital[2]	Athens	97%	384
Spalding Regional Hospital	Griffin	97%	257
Wellstar Cobb Hospital[2]	Austell	97%	563

NOTE: Hospital profiles are in alphabetical order by state, then city, then hospital within the city; Rankings exclude hospitals with less than 25 cases except for patient surveys which excludes hospitals with less than 100 cases; (a) 100-299 cases; (1) The number of cases/patients is too few to report; (2) Data submitted were based on a sample of cases/patients; (3) Results are based on a shorter time period than required; (4) Data suppressed by CMS for one or more quarters; (5) Results are not available for this reporting period; (6) Fewer than 100 patients completed the HCAHPS survey; (7) No cases met the criteria for this measure; (8) The lower limit of the confidence interval cannot be calculated if the number of observed infections equals zero; (9) No data are available from the state/territory for this reporting period; (10) The scores shown reflect fewer than 50 completed surveys; (11) There were discrepancies in the data collection process; (12) This measure does not apply to this hospital for this reporting period; (13) Results cannot be calculated for this reporting period; (14) The results for this state are combined with nearby states to protect confidentiality; Please refer to the User's Guide for a full explanation of data.

Athens Regional Medical Center[2]	Athens	96%	346
Augusta VA Medical Center	Augusta	96%	104
Candler Hospital[2]	Savannah	96%	149
Emory - Adventist Hospital	Smyrna	96%	25
Grady Memorial Hospital[2]	Atlanta	96%	202
Meadows Regional Medical Center	Vidalia	96%	132
Medical Center of Central Georgia[2]	Macon	96%	499
Rockdale Medical Center[2]	Conyers	96%	174
Saint Joseph's Hospital of Atlanta[2]	Atlanta	96%	487
East Georgia Regional Medical Center	Statesboro	95%	232
Mayo Clinic Health System - Waycross	Waycross	95%	187
Memorial Health Univ Medical Center[2]	Savannah	95%	396
Oconee Regional Medical Center	Milledgeville	95%	63
Phoebe Sumter Medical Center	Americus	95%	116
Piedmont Newnan Hospital[2]	Newnan	95%	316
South Georgia Medical Center	Valdosta	94%	713
Union General Hospital[2]	Blairsville	94%	52
Upson Regional Medical Center[2]	Thomaston	93%	135
Houston Medical Center[2]	Warner Robins	92%	244
Stephens County Hospital	Toccoa	92%	59
Chestatee Regional Hospital[2]	Dahlonega	91%	94
Taylor Regional Hospital[2]	Hawkinsville	91%	64
Decatur VA Medical Center	Decatur	87%	103
Irwin County Hospital[2]	Ocilla	62%	52

Prophylactic Antibiotic Timing

Hospital Name	City	Rate	Cases
Barrow Regional Medical Center	Winder	100%	55
Cartersville Medical Center[2]	Cartersville	100%	193
Coliseum Northside Hospital[2]	Macon	100%	185
Crisp Regional Hospital	Cordele	100%	51
Dekalb Medical Center[2]	Decatur	100%	537
Dekalb Medical Center at Hillandale	Lithonia	100%	38
Doctors Hospital[2]	Augusta	100%	341
Dodge County Hospital	Eastman	100%	46
Emory - Adventist Hospital	Smyrna	100%	27
Fairview Park Hospital	Dublin	100%	239
Habersham County Medical Center[2]	Demorest	100%	53
Hamilton Medical Center[2]	Dalton	100%	162
Houston Medical Center[2]	Warner Robins	100%	254
Hutcheson Medical Center	Fort Oglethorpe	100%	48
John D Archbold Memorial Hospital[2]	Thomasville	100%	403
Northside Hospital[2]	Atlanta	100%	427
Northside Hospital Cherokee	Canton	100%	206
Northside Hospital Forsyth[2]	Cumming	100%	287
Perry Hospital[2]	Perry	100%	60
Piedmont Mountainside Hospital[2]	Jasper	100%	177
Rockdale Medical Center[2]	Conyers	100%	186
Saint Joseph's Hospital - Savannah[2]	Savannah	100%	1289
SE Georgia Health Sys-Brunswick[2]	Brunswick	100%	259
SE Georgia Health Sys-Camden Campus	Saint Marys	100%	72
Tanner Medical Center - Carrollton	Carrollton	100%	492
Taylor Regional Hospital[2]	Hawkinsville	100%	64
Trinity Hospital of Augusta	Augusta	100%	298
University Hospital[2]	Augusta	100%	602
Univ McDuffie Co Reg Med Ctr	Thomson	100%	62
Wellstar Douglas Hospital[2]	Douglasville	100%	196
West Georgia Medical Center	Lagrange	100%	201
Athens Regional Medical Center[2]	Athens	99%	362
Atlanta Medical Center[2]	Atlanta	99%	355
Candler Hospital[2]	Savannah	99%	152
Chestatee Regional Hospital[2]	Dahlonega	99%	99
Clearview Regional Medical Center	Monroe	99%	173
Coffee Regional Medical Center[2]	Douglas	99%	137
Coliseum Medical Center[2]	Macon	99%	269
Doctors Specialty Hospital	Columbus	99%	141
East Georgia Regional Medical Center	Statesboro	99%	245
Eastside Medical Center[2]	Snellville	99%	281
Emory Johns Creek Hospital	Johns Creek	99%	178
Emory University Hospital[2]	Atlanta	99%	364
Fannin Regional Hospital	Blue Ridge	99%	117
Floyd Medical Center[2]	Rome	99%	460
Gordon Hospital	Calhoun	99%	185
Mayo Clinic Health System - Waycross	Waycross	99%	196
Medical Center of Central Georgia[2]	Macon	99%	513
Med College of Georgia Hosps[2]	Augusta	99%	291
Midtown Medical Center[2]	Columbus	99%	111
North Fulton Hospital[2]	Roswell	99%	252
Northeast Georgia Medical Center[2]	Gainesville	99%	504
Northside Medical Center	Columbus	99%	492
Oconee Regional Medical Center	Milledgeville	99%	69
Phoebe Putney Memorial Hospital[2]	Albany	99%	576
Piedmont Henry Hospital[2]	Stockbridge	99%	381
Redmond Regional Medical Center	Rome	99%	766
Saint Francis Hospital[2]	Columbus	99%	462
Saint Mary's Hospital[2]	Athens	99%	392
Southern Regional Medical Center[2]	Riverdale	99%	263
Spalding Regional Hospital	Griffin	99%	268
Tift Regional Medical Center	Tifton	99%	375
Upson Regional Medical Center[2]	Thomaston	99%	138
Wellstar Cobb Hospital[2]	Austell	99%	578
Wellstar Kennestone Hospital[2]	Marietta	99%	853
Wellstar Paulding Hospital[2]	Hiram	99%	103
Colquitt Regional Medical Center	Moultrie	98%	91
Emory University Hospital Midtown[2]	Atlanta	98%	368
Grady Memorial Hospital[2]	Atlanta	98%	209
Gwinnett Medical Center[2]	Lawrenceville	98%	677
Meadows Regional Medical Center	Vidalia	98%	142
Newton Medical Center[2]	Covington	98%	252
Phoebe Sumter Medical Center	Americus	98%	121
Piedmont Fayette Hospital[2]	Fayetteville	98%	326
Piedmont Newnan Hospital[2]	Newnan	98%	324
Saint Joseph's Hospital of Atlanta[2]	Atlanta	98%	499
South Georgia Medical Center	Valdosta	98%	729
Stephens County Hospital	Toccoa	98%	66
Augusta VA Medical Center	Augusta	97%	106
Decatur VA Medical Center	Decatur	97%	104
Irwin County Hospital[2]	Ocilla	96%	52
Memorial Health Univ Medical Center[2]	Savannah	96%	408
Piedmont Hospital[2]	Atlanta	96%	560
Wayne Memorial Hospital	Jesup	90%	92
Liberty Regional Medical Center	Hinesville	88%	32
Memorial Hospital & Manor	Bainbridge	86%	29
Union General Hospital[2]	Blairsville	81%	53

Prophylactic Antibiotic Timing (Outpatient)

Hospital Name	City	Rate	Cases
Candler Hospital	Savannah	100%	528
Chestatee Regional Hospital	Dahlonega	100%	57
Clearview Regional Medical Center	Monroe	100%	36
Coliseum Northside Hospital	Macon	100%	38
Doctors Hospital	Augusta	100%	381
Doctors Specialty Hospital	Columbus	100%	289
Eastside Medical Center	Snellville	100%	286
Emory - Adventist Hospital	Smyrna	100%	28
Fannin Regional Hospital	Blue Ridge	100%	42
Higgins General Hospital	Bremen	100%	27
John D Archbold Memorial Hospital	Thomasville	100%	319
Med College of Georgia Hosps	Augusta	100%	415
Midtown Medical Center	Columbus	100%	275
Northside Hospital Cherokee	Canton	100%	307
Northside Hospital Forsyth	Cumming	100%	347
Rockdale Medical Center	Conyers	100%	270
SE Georgia Health Sys-Camden Campus	Saint Marys	100%	34
West Georgia Medical Center	Lagrange	100%	102
Cartersville Medical Center	Cartersville	99%	286
Coliseum Medical Center	Macon	99%	698
Dekalb Medical Center	Decatur	99%	335
Emory Johns Creek Hospital	Johns Creek	99%	293
Fairview Park Hospital	Dublin	99%	112
Gordon Hospital	Calhoun	99%	150
Gwinnett Medical Center	Lawrenceville	99%	723
Hamilton Medical Center	Dalton	99%	422
Mayo Clinic Health System - Waycross	Waycross	99%	124
Medical Center of Central Georgia	Macon	99%	701
Newton Medical Center	Covington	99%	118
Northeast Georgia Regional Medical Center	Gainesville	99%	774
Northside Hospital	Atlanta	99%	872
Northside Medical Center	Columbus	99%	159
Piedmont Fayette Hospital	Fayetteville	99%	414
Piedmont Henry Hospital	Stockbridge	99%	496
Saint Francis Hospital	Columbus	99%	560
Saint Mary's Hospital	Athens	99%	392
Southern Regional Medical Center	Riverdale	99%	260
Tanner Medical Center - Carrollton	Carrollton	99%	358
Tift Regional Medical Center	Tifton	99%	358
Trinity Hospital of Augusta	Augusta	99%	166
Upson Regional Medical Center	Thomaston	99%	73
Wellstar Cobb Hospital	Austell	99%	550
Wellstar Kennestone Hospital	Marietta	99%	844
Atlanta Medical Center	Atlanta	98%	203
Coffee Regional Medical Center	Douglas	98%	85
Meadows Regional Medical Center	Vidalia	98%	247
North Fulton Hospital	Roswell	98%	187
Northridge Medical Center	Commerce	98%	58
Oconee Regional Medical Center	Milledgeville	98%	54
Piedmont Mountainside Hospital	Jasper	98%	102
Redmond Regional Medical Center	Rome	98%	477
Saint Joseph's Hospital - Savannah	Savannah	98%	416
Saint Joseph's Hospital of Atlanta	Atlanta	98%	572
South Georgia Medical Center	Valdosta	98%	547
SE Georgia Health Sys-Brunswick	Brunswick	98%	626
Spalding Regional Hospital	Griffin	98%	207
University Hospital	Augusta	98%	541
Wayne Memorial Hospital	Jesup	98%	127
East Georgia Regional Medical Center	Statesboro	97%	251
Memorial Health Univ Medical Center	Savannah	97%	490
Stephens County Hospital	Toccoa	97%	117
Emory University Hospital	Atlanta	96%	557
Emory University Hospital Midtown	Atlanta	96%	545
Floyd Medical Center	Rome	96%	427
Habersham County Medical Center	Demorest	96%	56
Irwin County Hospital	Ocilla	96%	49
Athens Regional Medical Center	Athens	95%	467
Piedmont Newnan Hospital	Newnan	95%	84
Crisp Regional Hospital	Cordele	94%	34
Phoebe Putney Memorial Hospital	Albany	94%	662
Houston Medical Center	Warner Robins	93%	237
Hutcheson Medical Center	Fort Oglethorpe	90%	39
Memorial Hospital & Manor	Bainbridge	90%	31
Phoebe Sumter Medical Center	Americus	90%	69
Piedmont Hospital	Atlanta	90%	841
Union General Hospital	Blairsville	89%	62
Grady Memorial Hospital	Atlanta	82%	67

Urinary Catheter Removal

Hospital Name	City	Rate	Cases
Coffee Regional Medical Center[2]	Douglas	100%	82
Coliseum Medical Center[2]	Macon	100%	194
Colquitt Regional Medical Center	Moultrie	100%	81
Doctors Hospital[2]	Augusta	100%	307
Doctors Specialty Hospital	Columbus	100%	25
Dodge County Hospital	Eastman	100%	52
Emory - Adventist Hospital	Smyrna	100%	50
Fannin Regional Hospital	Blue Ridge	100%	113
Gordon Hospital	Calhoun	100%	101
Hutcheson Medical Center	Fort Oglethorpe	100%	36
Northside Hospital[2]	Atlanta	100%	379
Northside Hospital Cherokee	Canton	100%	237
Northside Hospital Forsyth[2]	Cumming	100%	215
Northside Medical Center	Columbus	100%	532
Perry Hospital[2]	Perry	100%	67
Rockdale Medical Center[2]	Conyers	100%	142
SE Georgia Health Sys-Camden Campus	Saint Marys	100%	72
Tanner Medical Center - Carrollton	Carrollton	100%	507
Wellstar Douglas Hospital[2]	Douglasville	100%	222
West Georgia Medical Center	Lagrange	100%	176
Dekalb Medical Center[2]	Decatur	99%	203
Emory University Hospital Midtown[2]	Atlanta	99%	228
Fairview Park Hospital	Dublin	99%	154
Grady Memorial Hospital[2]	Atlanta	99%	155
Hamilton Medical Center[2]	Dalton	99%	217
Piedmont Henry Hospital[2]	Stockbridge	99%	191
South Georgia Medical Center	Valdosta	99%	636
SE Georgia Health Sys-Brunswick[2]	Brunswick	99%	258
University Hospital[2]	Augusta	99%	259
Wellstar Paulding Hospital[2]	Hiram	99%	118
Crisp Regional Hospital	Cordele	98%	41
East Georgia Regional Medical Center	Statesboro	98%	245
Emory Johns Creek Hospital	Johns Creek	98%	124
Habersham County Medical Center[2]	Demorest	98%	81
Medical Center of Central Georgia[2]	Macon	98%	358
Northeast Georgia Medical Center[2]	Gainesville	98%	437
Phoebe Putney Memorial Hospital[2]	Albany	98%	533
Tift Regional Medical Center	Tifton	98%	439
Trinity Hospital of Augusta	Augusta	98%	192
Wellstar Cobb Hospital[2]	Austell	98%	492
Atlanta Medical Center[2]	Atlanta	97%	235
Emory University Hospital[2]	Atlanta	97%	233
Floyd Medical Center[2]	Rome	97%	475
Gwinnett Medical Center[2]	Lawrenceville	97%	470
Med College of Georgia Hosps[2]	Augusta	97%	230
Midtown Medical Center[2]	Columbus	97%	129
Piedmont Mountainside Hospital[2]	Jasper	97%	145
Redmond Regional Medical Center	Rome	97%	717
Southern Regional Medical Center[2]	Riverdale	97%	180
Spalding Regional Hospital	Griffin	97%	164
Wellstar Kennestone Hospital[2]	Marietta	97%	612
Augusta VA Medical Center[2]	Augusta	96%	114
Coliseum Northside Hospital[2]	Macon	96%	103
Dekalb Medical Center at Hillandale	Lithonia	96%	51
Eastside Medical Center[2]	Snellville	96%	134
John D Archbold Memorial Hospital[2]	Thomasville	96%	368
Mayo Clinic Health System - Waycross	Waycross	96%	113
North Fulton Hospital[2]	Roswell	96%	223
Saint Francis Hospital[2]	Columbus	96%	441
Saint Joseph's Hospital of Atlanta[2]	Atlanta	96%	293
Union General Hospital[2]	Blairsville	96%	27
Athens Regional Medical Center[2]	Athens	95%	299
Cartersville Medical Center[2]	Cartersville	95%	86
Saint Joseph's Hospital - Savannah[2]	Savannah	95%	364
Clearview Regional Medical Center	Monroe	94%	151
Meadows Regional Medical Center	Vidalia	94%	133
Decatur VA Medical Center[2]	Decatur	93%	106
Houston Medical Center[2]	Warner Robins	93%	190
Memorial Health Univ Medical Center[2]	Savannah	93%	235
Phoebe Sumter Medical Center	Americus	93%	126
Piedmont Hospital[2]	Atlanta	93%	427
Chestatee Regional Hospital[2]	Dahlonega	92%	83
Piedmont Newnan Hospital[2]	Newnan	92%	338
Memorial Hospital & Manor	Bainbridge	91%	54
Stephens County Hospital	Toccoa	91%	34
Oconee Regional Medical Center	Milledgeville	90%	29

NOTE: Hospital profiles are in alphabetical order by state, then city, then hospital within the city; Rankings exclude hospitals with less than 25 cases except for patient surveys which excludes hospitals with less than 100 cases; (a) 100-299 cases; (1) The number of cases/patients is too few to report; (2) Data submitted were based on a sample of cases/patients; (3) Results are based on a shorter time period than required; (4) Data suppressed by CMS for one or more quarters; (5) Results are not available for this reporting period; (6) Fewer than 100 patients completed the HCAHPS survey; (7) No cases met the criteria for this measure; (8) The lower limit of the confidence interval cannot be calculated if the number of observed infections equals zero; (9) No data are available from the state/territory for this reporting period; (10) The scores shown reflect fewer than 50 completed surveys; (11) There were discrepancies in the data collection process; (12) This measure does not apply to this hospital for this reporting period; (13) Results cannot be calculated for this reporting period; (14) The results for this state are combined with nearby states to protect confidentiality; Please refer to the User's Guide for a full explanation of data.

Saint Mary's Hospital[2]	Athens	90%	100
Piedmont Fayette Hospital[2]	Fayetteville	89%	295
Upson Regional Medical Center[2]	Thomaston	87%	70
Univ McDuffie Co Reg Med Ctr	Thomson	86%	49
Wayne Memorial Hospital	Jesup	80%	54
Newton Medical Center[2]	Covington	79%	73
Ty Cobb Regional Medical Center[2]	Lavonia	74%	31
Candler Hospital[2]	Savannah	71%	62
North Georgia Medical Center[2]	Ellijay	61%	36

Survey of Patients' Hospital Experiences

Area Around Room 'Always' Quiet at Night

Hospital Name	City	Rate	Cases
Northside Medical Center	Columbus	87%	300+
Bacon County Hospital	Alma	78%	(a)
Phoebe Sumter Medical Center	Americus	78%	300+
Dekalb Medical Center at Hillandale	Lithonia	76%	300+
Coffee Regional Medical Center	Douglas	73%	300+
Coliseum Northside Hospital	Macon	73%	300+
Doctors Specialty Hospital	Columbus	73%	300+
Dodge County Hospital	Eastman	73%	(a)
Donalsonville Hospital	Donalsonville	73%	300+
Emanuel County Hospital Authority	Swainsboro	73%	(a)
Ty Cobb Regional Medical Center	Lavonia	73%	300+
Meadows Regional Medical Center	Vidalia	72%	300+
Piedmont Newnan Hospital	Newnan	72%	300+
Tanner Medical Center Villa Rica	Villa Rica	72%	300+
Upson Regional Medical Center	Thomaston	72%	300+
Emory University Hospital	Atlanta	71%	300+
John D Archbold Memorial Hospital	Thomasville	71%	300+
Union General Hospital	Blairsville	71%	300+
Emory Johns Creek Hospital	Johns Creek	70%	300+
Fairview Park Hospital	Dublin	70%	300+
Gordon Hospital[11]	Calhoun	70%	300+
Phoebe Putney Memorial Hospital	Albany	70%	300+
Stephens County Hospital	Toccoa	70%	300+
Washington County Regional Medical Center	Sandersville	70%	300+
Wayne Memorial Hospital	Jesup	70%	300+
Appling Hospital	Baxley	69%	(a)
Coliseum Medical Center	Macon	69%	300+
Cook Medical Center	Adel	69%	(a)
Grady General Hospital	Cairo	69%	(a)
Northridge Medical Center	Commerce	69%	(a)
Redmond Regional Medical Center	Rome	69%	300+
Tanner Medical Center - Carrollton	Carrollton	69%	300+
Taylor Regional Hospital	Hawkinsville	69%	(a)
Tift Regional Medical Center	Tifton	69%	300+
Irwin County Hospital	Ocilla	68%	(a)
Memorial Hospital & Manor	Bainbridge	68%	300+
Perry Hospital	Perry	68%	300+
Saint Mary's Hospital	Athens	68%	300+
Athens Regional Medical Center	Athens	67%	300+
Hutcheson Medical Center[11]	Fort Oglethorpe	67%	(a)
Oconee Regional Medical Center	Milledgeville	67%	300+
Rockdale Medical Center	Conyers	67%	300+
Trinity Hospital of Augusta	Augusta	67%	300+
University Hospital	Augusta	67%	300+
Clearview Regional Medical Center	Monroe	66%	300+
Emory - Adventist Hospital[11]	Smyrna	66%	(a)
Evans Memorial Hospital	Claxton	66%	(a)
Gwinnett Medical Center	Lawrenceville	66%	300+
Habersham County Medical Center	Demorest	66%	300+
Brooks County Hospital	Quitman	65%	(a)
Dekalb Medical Center	Decatur	65%	300+
Mayo Clinic Health System - Waycross	Waycross	65%	300+
South Georgia Medical Center	Valdosta	65%	300+
Colquitt Regional Medical Center	Moultrie	64%	300+
Floyd Medical Center	Rome	64%	300+
Hamilton Medical Center	Dalton	64%	300+
Houston Medical Center	Warner Robins	64%	300+
Northeast Georgia Medical Center	Gainesville	64%	300+
Piedmont Fayette Hospital	Fayetteville	64%	300+
Wellstar Douglas Hospital	Douglasville	64%	300+
Wellstar Kennestone Hospital	Marietta	64%	300+
Atlanta Medical Center	Atlanta	63%	300+
Chestatee Regional Hospital	Dahlonega	63%	(a)
Grady Memorial Hospital	Atlanta	63%	300+
Medical Center of Central Georgia	Macon	63%	300+
Piedmont Hospital	Atlanta	63%	300+
SE Georgia Health Sys-Brunswick	Brunswick	63%	300+
West Georgia Medical Center	Lagrange	63%	300+
Crisp Regional Hospital	Cordele	62%	300+
Dorminy Medical Center	Fitzgerald	62%	(a)
Med College of Georgia Hosps	Augusta	62%	300+
Northside Hospital	Atlanta	62%	300+
Piedmont Mountainside Hospital	Jasper	62%	300+
Saint Francis Hospital	Columbus	62%	300+
Doctors Hospital	Augusta	61%	300+
Elbert Memorial Hospital	Elberton	61%	(a)
Fannin Regional Hospital	Blue Ridge	61%	300+
Northside Hospital Forsyth	Cumming	61%	300+
East Georgia Regional Medical Center	Statesboro	60%	300+
Eastside Medical Center	Snellville	60%	300+
Emory University Hospital Midtown	Atlanta	60%	300+
Newton Medical Center	Covington	60%	300+
Saint Joseph's Hospital - Savannah	Savannah	60%	300+
Southern Regional Medical Center	Riverdale	60%	300+
Spalding Regional Hospital	Griffin	60%	300+
Wellstar Paulding Hospital	Hiram	59%	300+
Cartersville Medical Center	Cartersville	58%	300+
North Georgia Medical Center	Ellijay	58%	(a)
Wellstar Cobb Hospital	Austell	58%	300+
Barrow Regional Medical Center	Winder	57%	300+
Memorial Health Univ Medical Center	Savannah	57%	300+
Piedmont Henry Hospital	Stockbridge	57%	300+
Candler Hospital	Savannah	56%	300+
Northside Hospital Cherokee	Canton	56%	300+
SE Georgia Health Sys-Camden Campus	Saint Marys	56%	(a)
North Fulton Hospital	Roswell	53%	300+
Saint Joseph's Hospital of Atlanta	Atlanta	53%	300+
Midtown Medical Center	Columbus	52%	300+

Doctors 'Always' Communicated Well

Hospital Name	City	Rate	Cases
Evans Memorial Hospital	Claxton	94%	(a)
Donalsonville Hospital	Donalsonville	91%	300+
Emanuel County Hospital Authority	Swainsboro	90%	(a)
Perry Hospital	Perry	90%	300+
Bacon County Hospital	Alma	89%	(a)
Grady General Hospital	Cairo	89%	(a)
Upson Regional Medical Center	Thomaston	89%	300+
Northside Medical Center	Columbus	88%	300+
Brooks County Hospital	Quitman	87%	(a)
Coffee Regional Medical Center	Douglas	87%	300+
Dodge County Hospital	Eastman	87%	(a)
Elbert Memorial Hospital	Elberton	87%	(a)
John D Archbold Memorial Hospital	Thomasville	87%	300+
Stephens County Hospital	Toccoa	87%	300+
Tanner Medical Center - Carrollton	Carrollton	87%	300+
Taylor Regional Hospital	Hawkinsville	87%	(a)
Appling Hospital	Baxley	86%	(a)
Cook Medical Center	Adel	86%	(a)
Emory University Hospital	Atlanta	86%	300+
Fannin Regional Hospital	Blue Ridge	86%	300+
Gordon Hospital[11]	Calhoun	86%	300+
Irwin County Hospital	Ocilla	86%	(a)
Ty Cobb Regional Medical Center	Lavonia	86%	300+
Union General Hospital	Blairsville	86%	300+
Meadows Regional Medical Center	Vidalia	85%	300+
Oconee Regional Medical Center	Milledgeville	85%	300+
Tanner Medical Center Villa Rica	Villa Rica	85%	300+
Doctors Specialty Hospital	Columbus	84%	300+
Emory Johns Creek Hospital	Johns Creek	83%	300+
Floyd Medical Center	Rome	83%	300+
Hutcheson Medical Center[11]	Fort Oglethorpe	83%	(a)
Memorial Hospital & Manor	Bainbridge	83%	300+
Northridge Medical Center	Commerce	83%	(a)
Phoebe Putney Memorial Hospital	Albany	83%	300+
Piedmont Hospital	Atlanta	83%	300+
Redmond Regional Medical Center	Rome	83%	300+
Saint Francis Hospital	Columbus	83%	300+
Spalding Regional Hospital	Griffin	83%	300+
Tift Regional Medical Center	Tifton	83%	300+
Trinity Hospital of Augusta	Augusta	83%	300+
University Hospital	Augusta	83%	300+
Washington County Regional Medical Center	Sandersville	83%	300+
Athens Regional Medical Center	Athens	82%	300+
Coliseum Medical Center	Macon	82%	300+
Emory University Hospital Midtown	Atlanta	82%	300+
Fairview Park Hospital	Dublin	82%	300+
Grady Memorial Hospital	Atlanta	82%	300+
Habersham County Medical Center	Demorest	82%	300+
Mayo Clinic Health System - Waycross	Waycross	82%	300+
Memorial Health Univ Medical Center	Savannah	82%	300+
Phoebe Sumter Medical Center	Americus	82%	300+
South Georgia Medical Center	Valdosta	82%	300+
SE Georgia Health Sys-Brunswick	Brunswick	82%	300+
Wellstar Douglas Hospital	Douglasville	82%	300+
Candler Hospital	Savannah	81%	300+
Clearview Regional Medical Center	Monroe	81%	300+
Doctors Hospital	Augusta	81%	300+
Dorminy Medical Center	Fitzgerald	81%	(a)
Emory - Adventist Hospital[11]	Smyrna	81%	(a)
Northeast Georgia Medical Center	Gainesville	81%	300+
Piedmont Fayette Hospital	Fayetteville	81%	300+
Rockdale Medical Center	Conyers	81%	300+
Saint Joseph's Hospital - Savannah	Savannah	81%	300+
Saint Mary's Hospital	Athens	81%	300+
Wayne Memorial Hospital	Jesup	81%	300+
Wellstar Paulding Hospital	Hiram	81%	300+
West Georgia Medical Center	Lagrange	81%	300+
Atlanta Medical Center	Atlanta	80%	300+
Chestatee Regional Hospital	Dahlonega	80%	(a)
Colquitt Regional Medical Center	Moultrie	80%	300+
Crisp Regional Hospital	Cordele	80%	300+
Houston Medical Center	Warner Robins	80%	300+
Medical Center of Central Georgia	Macon	80%	300+
Northside Hospital	Atlanta	80%	300+
Piedmont Newnan Hospital	Newnan	80%	300+
SE Georgia Health Sys-Camden Campus	Saint Marys	80%	(a)
Wellstar Cobb Hospital	Austell	80%	300+
Coliseum Northside Hospital	Macon	79%	300+
Gwinnett Medical Center	Lawrenceville	79%	300+
Hamilton Medical Center	Dalton	79%	300+
North Fulton Hospital	Roswell	79%	300+
North Georgia Medical Center	Ellijay	79%	(a)
Northside Hospital Cherokee	Canton	79%	300+
Northside Hospital Forsyth	Cumming	79%	300+
Piedmont Mountainside Hospital	Jasper	79%	300+
Wellstar Kennestone Hospital	Marietta	79%	300+
Newton Medical Center	Covington	78%	300+
Saint Joseph's Hospital of Atlanta	Atlanta	78%	300+
Dekalb Medical Center at Hillandale	Lithonia	77%	300+
East Georgia Regional Medical Center	Statesboro	77%	300+
Med College of Georgia Hosps	Augusta	77%	300+
Midtown Medical Center	Columbus	77%	300+
Eastside Medical Center	Snellville	76%	300+
Piedmont Henry Hospital	Stockbridge	76%	300+
Barrow Regional Medical Center	Winder	75%	300+
Cartersville Medical Center	Cartersville	75%	300+
Dekalb Medical Center	Decatur	75%	300+
Southern Regional Medical Center	Riverdale	75%	300+

Home Recovery Information Given

Hospital Name	City	Rate	Cases
Northside Medical Center	Columbus	92%	300+
Emanuel County Hospital Authority	Swainsboro	91%	(a)
Perry Hospital	Perry	90%	300+
Elbert Memorial Hospital	Elberton	89%	(a)
Grady General Hospital	Cairo	89%	(a)
Stephens County Hospital	Toccoa	89%	300+
Gordon Hospital[11]	Calhoun	88%	300+
John D Archbold Memorial Hospital	Thomasville	88%	300+
Northeast Georgia Medical Center	Gainesville	88%	300+
Saint Mary's Hospital	Athens	88%	300+
Tanner Medical Center - Carrollton	Carrollton	88%	300+
Union General Hospital	Blairsville	88%	300+
Brooks County Hospital	Quitman	87%	(a)
Doctors Specialty Hospital	Columbus	87%	300+
Dodge County Hospital	Eastman	87%	(a)
Fannin Regional Hospital	Blue Ridge	87%	300+
Habersham County Medical Center	Demorest	87%	300+
Northside Hospital Cherokee	Canton	87%	300+
Ty Cobb Regional Medical Center	Lavonia	87%	300+
Coffee Regional Medical Center	Douglas	86%	300+
Cook Medical Center	Adel	86%	(a)
Emory University Hospital	Atlanta	86%	300+
Saint Joseph's Hospital of Atlanta	Atlanta	86%	300+
Appling Hospital	Baxley	85%	(a)
Athens Regional Medical Center	Athens	85%	300+
Bacon County Hospital	Alma	85%	(a)
Candler Hospital	Savannah	85%	300+
Coliseum Medical Center	Macon	85%	300+
Fairview Park Hospital	Dublin	85%	300+
Gwinnett Medical Center	Lawrenceville	85%	300+
Houston Medical Center	Warner Robins	85%	300+
Hutcheson Medical Center[11]	Fort Oglethorpe	85%	(a)
Mayo Clinic Health System - Waycross	Waycross	85%	300+
Northside Hospital	Atlanta	85%	300+
Northside Hospital Forsyth	Cumming	85%	300+
Oconee Regional Medical Center	Milledgeville	85%	300+
Trinity Hospital of Augusta	Augusta	85%	300+
Wayne Memorial Hospital	Jesup	85%	300+
Wellstar Douglas Hospital	Douglasville	85%	300+
West Georgia Medical Center	Lagrange	85%	300+
Colquitt Regional Medical Center	Moultrie	84%	300+
Doctors Hospital	Augusta	84%	300+
Meadows Regional Medical Center	Vidalia	84%	300+
Memorial Health Univ Medical Center	Savannah	84%	300+
Memorial Hospital & Manor	Bainbridge	84%	300+
Northridge Medical Center	Commerce	84%	(a)
Piedmont Hospital	Atlanta	84%	300+
Redmond Regional Medical Center	Rome	84%	300+
Saint Francis Hospital	Columbus	84%	300+
Saint Joseph's Hospital - Savannah	Savannah	84%	300+
SE Georgia Health Sys-Brunswick	Brunswick	84%	300+
SE Georgia Health Sys-Camden Campus	Saint Marys	84%	(a)
Tanner Medical Center Villa Rica	Villa Rica	84%	300+
Taylor Regional Hospital	Hawkinsville	84%	(a)
University Hospital	Augusta	84%	300+
Wellstar Paulding Hospital	Hiram	84%	300+

NOTE: Hospital profiles are in alphabetical order by state, then city, then hospital within the city; Rankings exclude hospitals with less than 25 cases except for patient surveys which excludes hospitals with less than 100 cases; (a) 100-299 cases; (1) The number of cases/patients is too few to report; (2) Data submitted were based on a sample of cases/patients; (3) Results are based on a shorter time period than required; (4) Data suppressed by CMS for one or more quarters; (5) Results are not available for this reporting period; (6) Fewer than 100 patients completed the HCAHPS survey; (7) No cases met the criteria for this measure; (8) The lower limit of the confidence interval cannot be calculated if the number of observed infections equals zero; (9) No data are available from the state/territory for this reporting period; (10) The scores shown reflect fewer than 50 completed surveys; (11) There were discrepancies in the data collection process; (12) This measure does not apply to this hospital for this reporting period; (13) Results cannot be calculated for this reporting period; (14) The results for this state are combined with nearby states to protect confidentiality; Please refer to the User's Guide for a full explanation of data.

Hospital Name	City	Rate	Cases
Cartersville Medical Center	Cartersville	83%	300+
Emory Johns Creek Hospital	Johns Creek	83%	300+
Evans Memorial Hospital	Claxton	83%	(a)
Med College of Georgia Hosps	Augusta	83%	300+
Phoebe Putney Memorial Hospital	Albany	83%	300+
Spalding Regional Hospital	Griffin	83%	300+
Tift Regional Medical Center	Tifton	83%	300+
Upson Regional Medical Center	Thomaston	83%	300+
Washington County Regional Medical Center	Sandersville	83%	300+
Wellstar Kennestone Hospital	Marietta	83%	300+
Clearview Regional Medical Center	Monroe	82%	300+
Coliseum Northside Hospital	Macon	82%	300+
Dekalb Medical Center	Decatur	82%	300+
Eastside Medical Center	Snellville	82%	300+
Floyd Medical Center	Rome	82%	300+
Medical Center of Central Georgia	Macon	82%	300+
North Fulton Hospital	Roswell	82%	300+
Piedmont Fayette Hospital	Fayetteville	82%	300+
Piedmont Mountainside Hospital	Jasper	82%	300+
Piedmont Newnan Hospital	Newnan	82%	300+
Rockdale Medical Center	Conyers	82%	300+
South Georgia Medical Center	Valdosta	82%	300+
Atlanta Medical Center	Atlanta	81%	300+
Chestatee Regional Hospital	Dahlonega	81%	(a)
Emory University Hospital Midtown	Atlanta	81%	300+
Hamilton Medical Center	Dalton	81%	300+
Irwin County Hospital	Ocilla	81%	(a)
Midtown Medical Center	Columbus	81%	300+
North Georgia Medical Center	Ellijay	81%	(a)
Newton Medical Center	Covington	80%	300+
Dekalb Medical Center at Hillandale	Lithonia	79%	300+
Dorminy Medical Center	Fitzgerald	79%	(a)
East Georgia Regional Medical Center	Statesboro	79%	300+
Phoebe Sumter Medical Center	Americus	79%	300+
Piedmont Henry Hospital	Stockbridge	79%	300+
Crisp Regional Hospital	Cordele	78%	300+
Emory - Adventist Hospital[11]	Smyrna	78%	(a)
Grady Memorial Hospital	Atlanta	78%	300+
Wellstar Cobb Hospital	Austell	78%	300+
Barrow Regional Medical Center	Winder	76%	300+
Donalsonville Hospital	Donalsonville	75%	300+
Southern Regional Medical Center	Riverdale	75%	300+

Hospital Given 9 or 10 on 10 Point Scale

Hospital Name	City	Rate	Cases
Northside Medical Center	Columbus	91%	300+
Emory University Hospital	Atlanta	82%	300+
Tanner Medical Center - Carrollton	Carrollton	82%	300+
Bacon County Hospital	Alma	79%	(a)
Tanner Medical Center Villa Rica	Villa Rica	79%	300+
Grady General Hospital	Cairo	78%	(a)
Northside Hospital	Atlanta	78%	300+
Emory Johns Creek Hospital	Johns Creek	77%	300+
Gordon Hospital[11]	Calhoun	77%	300+
Northside Hospital Forsyth	Cumming	77%	300+
Saint Mary's Hospital	Athens	77%	300+
Athens Regional Medical Center	Athens	76%	300+
Doctors Specialty Hospital	Columbus	76%	300+
Gwinnett Medical Center	Lawrenceville	76%	300+
John D Archbold Memorial Hospital	Thomasville	76%	300+
Meadows Regional Medical Center	Vidalia	76%	300+
Perry Hospital	Perry	76%	300+
Redmond Regional Medical Center	Rome	76%	300+
University Hospital	Augusta	76%	300+
Coffee Regional Medical Center	Douglas	75%	300+
Northeast Georgia Medical Center	Gainesville	75%	300+
Brooks County Hospital	Quitman	74%	(a)
Donalsonville Hospital	Donalsonville	74%	300+
Piedmont Fayette Hospital	Fayetteville	74%	300+
Saint Joseph's Hospital - Savannah	Savannah	74%	300+
Tift Regional Medical Center	Tifton	74%	300+
Union General Hospital	Blairsville	74%	300+
Upson Regional Medical Center	Thomaston	74%	300+
Emory University Hospital Midtown	Atlanta	73%	300+
Fannin Regional Hospital	Blue Ridge	73%	300+
Floyd Medical Center	Rome	73%	300+
Phoebe Sumter Medical Center	Americus	73%	300+
Ty Cobb Regional Medical Center	Lavonia	73%	300+
Emanuel County Hospital Authority	Swainsboro	72%	(a)
Irwin County Hospital	Ocilla	72%	(a)
Saint Joseph's Hospital of Atlanta	Atlanta	72%	300+
Wellstar Douglas Hospital	Douglasville	72%	300+
Wellstar Kennestone Hospital	Marietta	72%	300+
Doctors Hospital	Augusta	71%	300+
Hamilton Medical Center	Dalton	71%	300+
Houston Medical Center	Warner Robins	71%	300+
Hutcheson Medical Center[11]	Fort Oglethorpe	71%	(a)
Piedmont Hospital	Atlanta	71%	300+
Piedmont Mountainside Hospital	Jasper	71%	300+
Saint Francis Hospital	Columbus	71%	300+
South Georgia Medical Center	Valdosta	71%	300+
Candler Hospital	Savannah	70%	300+
Coliseum Northside Hospital	Macon	70%	300+
Dekalb Medical Center at Hillandale	Lithonia	70%	300+
Memorial Health Univ Medical Center	Savannah	70%	300+
Piedmont Newnan Hospital	Newnan	70%	300+
Stephens County Hospital	Toccoa	70%	300+
Trinity Hospital of Augusta	Augusta	70%	300+
Wellstar Paulding Hospital	Hiram	70%	300+
West Georgia Medical Center	Lagrange	70%	300+
Coliseum Medical Center	Macon	69%	300+
Evans Memorial Hospital	Claxton	69%	(a)
Mayo Clinic Health System - Waycross	Waycross	69%	300+
Medical Center of Central Georgia	Macon	69%	300+
Med College of Georgia Hosps	Augusta	69%	300+
Newton Medical Center	Covington	69%	300+
Rockdale Medical Center	Conyers	69%	300+
Wayne Memorial Hospital	Jesup	69%	300+
Colquitt Regional Medical Center	Moultrie	68%	300+
Dodge County Hospital	Eastman	68%	(a)
Habersham County Medical Center	Demorest	68%	300+
Northridge Medical Center	Commerce	68%	(a)
Taylor Regional Hospital	Hawkinsville	68%	(a)
Fairview Park Hospital	Dublin	67%	300+
Wellstar Cobb Hospital	Austell	67%	300+
Grady Memorial Hospital	Atlanta	66%	300+
Phoebe Putney Memorial Hospital	Albany	66%	300+
Spalding Regional Hospital	Griffin	66%	300+
Cook Medical Center	Adel	65%	(a)
Emory - Adventist Hospital[11]	Smyrna	65%	(a)
North Fulton Hospital	Roswell	65%	300+
SE Georgia Health Sys-Brunswick	Brunswick	65%	300+
SE Georgia Health Sys-Camden Campus	Saint Marys	65%	(a)
Northside Hospital Cherokee	Canton	64%	300+
Oconee Regional Medical Center	Milledgeville	64%	300+
Clearview Regional Medical Center	Monroe	63%	300+
Dorminy Medical Center	Fitzgerald	63%	(a)
Memorial Hospital & Manor	Bainbridge	63%	300+
Atlanta Medical Center	Atlanta	62%	300+
Elbert Memorial Hospital	Elberton	62%	(a)
Dekalb Medical Center	Decatur	61%	300+
Eastside Medical Center	Snellville	61%	300+
Midtown Medical Center	Columbus	61%	300+
Crisp Regional Hospital	Cordele	60%	300+
Washington County Regional Medical Center	Sandersville	59%	300+
Piedmont Henry Hospital	Stockbridge	58%	300+
Chestatee Regional Hospital	Dahlonega	57%	(a)
Cartersville Medical Center	Cartersville	56%	300+
Southern Regional Medical Center	Riverdale	56%	300+
East Georgia Regional Medical Center	Statesboro	54%	300+
North Georgia Medical Center	Ellijay	52%	(a)
Appling Hospital	Baxley	51%	(a)
Barrow Regional Medical Center	Winder	46%	300+

Meds 'Always' Explained Before Given

Hospital Name	City	Rate	Cases
Northside Medical Center	Columbus	77%	300+
Upson Regional Medical Center	Thomaston	73%	300+
Gordon Hospital[11]	Calhoun	72%	300+
Elbert Memorial Hospital	Elberton	71%	(a)
Perry Hospital	Perry	71%	300+
Stephens County Hospital	Toccoa	71%	300+
Tanner Medical Center - Carrollton	Carrollton	71%	300+
Cook Medical Center	Adel	70%	(a)
Emory University Hospital	Atlanta	70%	300+
Bacon County Hospital	Alma	69%	(a)
Tanner Medical Center Villa Rica	Villa Rica	69%	300+
Taylor Regional Hospital	Hawkinsville	69%	(a)
Dodge County Hospital	Eastman	68%	(a)
Donalsonville Hospital	Donalsonville	68%	300+
Hamilton Medical Center	Dalton	68%	300+
Saint Mary's Hospital	Athens	68%	300+
Ty Cobb Regional Medical Center	Lavonia	68%	(a)
Mayo Clinic Health System - Waycross	Waycross	67%	300+
Wellstar Paulding Hospital	Hiram	67%	300+
West Georgia Medical Center	Lagrange	67%	300+
Doctors Specialty Hospital	Columbus	66%	300+
Irwin County Hospital	Ocilla	66%	(a)
Northridge Medical Center	Commerce	66%	(a)
Washington County Regional Medical Center	Sandersville	66%	300+
Evans Memorial Hospital	Claxton	65%	(a)
Grady General Hospital	Cairo	65%	(a)
John D Archbold Memorial Hospital	Thomasville	65%	300+
Phoebe Sumter Medical Center	Americus	65%	300+
Wellstar Douglas Hospital	Douglasville	65%	300+
Emanuel County Hospital Authority	Swainsboro	64%	(a)
Emory - Adventist Hospital[11]	Smyrna	64%	(a)
Fairview Park Hospital	Dublin	64%	300+
Meadows Regional Medical Center	Vidalia	64%	300+
North Georgia Medical Center	Ellijay	64%	(a)
Phoebe Putney Memorial Hospital	Albany	64%	300+
Saint Joseph's Hospital - Savannah	Savannah	64%	300+
South Georgia Medical Center	Valdosta	64%	300+
SE Georgia Health Sys-Brunswick	Brunswick	64%	300+
Union General Hospital	Blairsville	64%	300+
University Hospital	Augusta	64%	300+
Athens Regional Medical Center	Athens	63%	300+
Brooks County Hospital	Quitman	63%	(a)
Coliseum Northside Hospital	Macon	63%	300+
Fannin Regional Hospital	Blue Ridge	63%	300+
Floyd Medical Center	Rome	63%	300+
Northeast Georgia Medical Center	Gainesville	63%	300+
Northside Hospital	Atlanta	63%	300+
Oconee Regional Medical Center	Milledgeville	63%	300+
Tift Regional Medical Center	Tifton	63%	300+
Coffee Regional Medical Center	Douglas	62%	300+
Coliseum Medical Center	Macon	62%	300+
Doctors Hospital	Augusta	62%	300+
Grady Memorial Hospital	Atlanta	62%	300+
Gwinnett Medical Center	Lawrenceville	62%	300+
Habersham County Medical Center	Demorest	62%	300+
Houston Medical Center	Warner Robins	62%	300+
Memorial Hospital & Manor	Bainbridge	62%	300+
Piedmont Mountainside Hospital	Jasper	62%	300+
Redmond Regional Medical Center	Rome	62%	300+
Saint Francis Hospital	Columbus	62%	300+
Wellstar Cobb Hospital	Austell	62%	300+
Med College of Georgia Hosps	Augusta	61%	300+
Newton Medical Center	Covington	61%	300+
Northside Hospital Forsyth	Cumming	61%	300+
Piedmont Fayette Hospital	Fayetteville	61%	300+
Piedmont Newnan Hospital	Newnan	61%	300+
Wellstar Kennestone Hospital	Marietta	61%	300+
Appling Hospital	Baxley	60%	(a)
Atlanta Medical Center	Atlanta	60%	300+
Candler Hospital	Savannah	60%	300+
Clearview Regional Medical Center	Monroe	60%	300+
Dekalb Medical Center at Hillandale	Lithonia	60%	300+
Memorial Health Univ Medical Center	Savannah	60%	300+
Rockdale Medical Center	Conyers	60%	300+
SE Georgia Health Sys-Camden Campus	Saint Marys	60%	(a)
Trinity Hospital of Augusta	Augusta	60%	300+
Wayne Memorial Hospital	Jesup	60%	300+
Chestatee Regional Hospital	Dahlonega	59%	(a)
Colquitt Regional Medical Center	Moultrie	59%	300+
Emory Johns Creek Hospital	Johns Creek	59%	300+
Emory University Hospital Midtown	Atlanta	59%	300+
North Fulton Hospital	Roswell	59%	300+
Piedmont Hospital	Atlanta	59%	300+
Cartersville Medical Center	Cartersville	58%	300+
Hutcheson Medical Center[11]	Fort Oglethorpe	58%	(a)
Northside Hospital Cherokee	Canton	58%	300+
Spalding Regional Hospital	Griffin	58%	300+
Crisp Regional Hospital	Cordele	57%	300+
Saint Joseph's Hospital of Atlanta	Atlanta	57%	300+
Dekalb Medical Center	Decatur	56%	300+
Dorminy Medical Center	Fitzgerald	55%	(a)
East Georgia Regional Medical Center	Statesboro	55%	300+
Medical Center of Central Georgia	Macon	55%	300+
Midtown Medical Center	Columbus	55%	300+
Piedmont Henry Hospital	Stockbridge	55%	300+
Eastside Medical Center	Snellville	54%	300+
Barrow Regional Medical Center	Winder	52%	300+
Southern Regional Medical Center	Riverdale	52%	300+

Nurses 'Always' Communicated Well

Hospital Name	City	Rate	Cases
Northside Medical Center	Columbus	90%	300+
Tanner Medical Center - Carrollton	Carrollton	87%	300+
Upson Regional Medical Center	Thomaston	87%	300+
Coffee Regional Medical Center	Douglas	86%	300+
Bacon County Hospital	Alma	85%	(a)
Brooks County Hospital	Quitman	84%	(a)
Gordon Hospital[11]	Calhoun	84%	300+
Grady General Hospital	Cairo	84%	(a)
Tanner Medical Center Villa Rica	Villa Rica	84%	300+
Athens Regional Medical Center	Athens	83%	300+
Dodge County Hospital	Eastman	83%	(a)
Emanuel County Hospital Authority	Swainsboro	83%	(a)
Donalsonville Hospital	Donalsonville	82%	300+
Perry Hospital	Perry	82%	300+
Taylor Regional Hospital	Hawkinsville	82%	(a)
Tift Regional Medical Center	Tifton	82%	300+
West Georgia Medical Center	Lagrange	82%	300+
Doctors Specialty Hospital	Columbus	81%	300+
Emory University Hospital	Atlanta	81%	300+
Mayo Clinic Health System - Waycross	Waycross	81%	300+
Meadows Regional Medical Center	Vidalia	81%	300+
Phoebe Putney Memorial Hospital	Albany	81%	300+
Phoebe Sumter Medical Center	Americus	81%	300+
Ty Cobb Regional Medical Center	Lavonia	81%	300+
Wellstar Paulding Hospital	Hiram	81%	300+
Evans Memorial Hospital	Claxton	80%	(a)

NOTE: Hospital profiles are in alphabetical order by state, then city, then hospital within the city; Rankings exclude hospitals with less than 25 cases except for patient surveys which excludes hospitals with less than 100 cases; (a) 100-299 cases; (1) The number of cases/patients is too few to report; (2) Data submitted were based on a sample of cases/patients; (3) Results are based on a shorter time period than required; (4) Data suppressed by CMS for one or more quarters; (5) Results are not available for this reporting period; (6) Fewer than 100 patients completed the HCAHPS survey; (7) No cases met the criteria for this measure; (8) The lower limit of the confidence interval cannot be calculated if the number of observed infections equals zero; (9) No data are available from the state/territory for this reporting period; (10) The scores shown reflect fewer than 50 completed surveys; (11) There were discrepancies in the data collection process; (12) This measure does not apply to this hospital for this reporting period; (13) Results cannot be calculated for this reporting period; (14) The results for this state are combined with nearby states to protect confidentiality; Please refer to the User's Guide for a full explanation of data.

Fannin Regional Hospital	Blue Ridge	80%	300+
Hamilton Medical Center	Dalton	80%	300+
John D Archbold Memorial Hospital	Thomasville	80%	300+
Memorial Hospital & Manor	Bainbridge	80%	300+
Northside Hospital	Atlanta	80%	300+
Redmond Regional Medical Center	Rome	80%	300+
Saint Francis Hospital	Columbus	80%	300+
Stephens County Hospital	Toccoa	80%	300+
Union General Hospital	Blairsville	80%	300+
Wellstar Douglas Hospital	Douglasville	80%	300+
Elbert Memorial Hospital	Elberton	79%	(a)
Fairview Park Hospital	Dublin	79%	300+
Floyd Medical Center	Rome	79%	300+
Saint Mary's Hospital	Athens	79%	300+
South Georgia Medical Center	Valdosta	79%	300+
Trinity Hospital of Augusta	Augusta	79%	300+
University Hospital	Augusta	79%	300+
Washington County Regional Medical Center	Sandersville	79%	300+
Colquitt Regional Medical Center	Moultrie	78%	300+
Cook Medical Center	Adel	78%	(a)
Gwinnett Medical Center	Lawrenceville	78%	300+
Habersham County Medical Center	Demorest	78%	300+
Oconee Regional Medical Center	Milledgeville	78%	300+
Piedmont Fayette Hospital	Fayetteville	78%	300+
Piedmont Newnan Hospital	Newnan	78%	300+
SE Georgia Health Sys-Camden Campus	Saint Marys	78%	(a)
Wellstar Kennestone Hospital	Marietta	78%	300+
Candler Hospital	Savannah	77%	300+
Emory University Hospital Midtown	Atlanta	77%	300+
Houston Medical Center	Warner Robins	77%	300+
Hutcheson Medical Center[11]	Fort Oglethorpe	77%	(a)
Irwin County Hospital	Ocilla	77%	(a)
Memorial Health Univ Medical Center	Savannah	77%	300+
Newton Medical Center	Covington	77%	300+
North Georgia Medical Center	Ellijay	77%	(a)
Northeast Georgia Medical Center	Gainesville	77%	300+
Northside Hospital Forsyth	Cumming	77%	300+
Piedmont Mountainside Hospital	Jasper	77%	300+
Saint Joseph's Hospital - Savannah	Savannah	77%	300+
Wayne Memorial Hospital	Jesup	77%	300+
Coliseum Medical Center	Macon	76%	300+
Crisp Regional Hospital	Cordele	76%	300+
Doctors Hospital	Augusta	76%	300+
Emory Johns Creek Hospital	Johns Creek	76%	300+
Northridge Medical Center	Commerce	76%	(a)
SE Georgia Health Sys-Brunswick	Brunswick	76%	300+
Spalding Regional Hospital	Griffin	76%	300+
Atlanta Medical Center	Atlanta	75%	300+
Coliseum Northside Hospital	Macon	75%	300+
Dekalb Medical Center at Hillandale	Lithonia	75%	300+
Med College of Georgia Hosps	Augusta	75%	300+
Piedmont Hospital	Atlanta	75%	300+
Wellstar Cobb Hospital	Austell	75%	300+
Appling Hospital	Baxley	74%	(a)
Grady Memorial Hospital	Atlanta	74%	300+
Midtown Medical Center	Columbus	74%	300+
North Fulton Hospital	Roswell	74%	300+
Rockdale Medical Center	Conyers	74%	300+
Saint Joseph's Hospital of Atlanta	Atlanta	74%	300+
Dekalb Medical Center	Decatur	73%	300+
Emory - Adventist Hospital[11]	Smyrna	73%	(a)
Medical Center of Central Georgia	Macon	73%	300+
Dorminy Medical Center	Fitzgerald	72%	(a)
East Georgia Regional Medical Center	Statesboro	72%	300+
Northside Hospital Cherokee	Canton	72%	300+
Chestatee Regional Hospital	Dahlonega	71%	(a)
Clearview Regional Medical Center	Monroe	70%	300+
Cartersville Medical Center	Cartersville	69%	300+
Piedmont Henry Hospital	Stockbridge	69%	300+
Eastside Medical Center	Snellville	68%	300+
Barrow Regional Medical Center	Winder	66%	300+
Southern Regional Medical Center	Riverdale	66%	300+

Pain 'Always' Well Controlled

Hospital Name	City	Rate	Cases
Grady General Hospital	Cairo	79%	(a)
Northside Medical Center	Columbus	79%	300+
Bacon County Hospital	Alma	77%	(a)
Gordon Hospital[11]	Calhoun	77%	300+
Dodge County Hospital	Eastman	76%	(a)
Upson Regional Medical Center	Thomaston	76%	300+
Doctors Specialty Hospital	Columbus	75%	300+
Emory University Hospital	Atlanta	75%	300+
Saint Joseph's Hospital of Atlanta	Atlanta	75%	300+
Stephens County Hospital	Toccoa	75%	300+
Tanner Medical Center - Carrollton	Carrollton	75%	300+
Tanner Medical Center Villa Rica	Villa Rica	75%	300+
Wellstar Douglas Hospital	Douglasville	75%	300+
Coffee Regional Medical Center	Douglas	74%	300+
Perry Hospital	Perry	74%	300+
Saint Mary's Hospital	Athens	74%	300+
Tift Regional Medical Center	Tifton	74%	300+
Donalsonville Hospital	Donalsonville	73%	300+
Emory University Hospital Midtown	Atlanta	73%	300+
Fairview Park Hospital	Dublin	73%	300+
Fannin Regional Hospital	Blue Ridge	73%	300+
Memorial Health Univ Medical Center	Savannah	73%	300+
Northside Hospital	Atlanta	73%	300+
Redmond Regional Medical Center	Rome	73%	300+
Athens Regional Medical Center	Athens	72%	300+
Brooks County Hospital	Quitman	72%	(a)
Candler Hospital	Savannah	72%	300+
Hamilton Medical Center	Dalton	72%	300+
John D Archbold Memorial Hospital	Thomasville	72%	300+
Mayo Clinic Health System - Waycross	Waycross	72%	300+
Northside Hospital Forsyth	Cumming	72%	300+
Phoebe Putney Memorial Hospital	Albany	72%	300+
Saint Joseph's Hospital - Savannah	Savannah	72%	300+
South Georgia Medical Center	Valdosta	72%	300+
Ty Cobb Regional Medical Center	Lavonia	72%	300+
Doctors Hospital	Augusta	71%	300+
Elbert Memorial Hospital	Elberton	71%	(a)
Emanuel County Hospital Authority	Swainsboro	71%	(a)
Emory Johns Creek Hospital	Johns Creek	71%	300+
Floyd Medical Center	Rome	71%	300+
Gwinnett Medical Center	Lawrenceville	71%	300+
Habersham County Medical Center	Demorest	71%	300+
Northeast Georgia Medical Center	Gainesville	71%	300+
Phoebe Sumter Medical Center	Americus	71%	300+
Piedmont Newnan Hospital	Newnan	71%	300+
Taylor Regional Hospital	Hawkinsville	71%	(a)
University Hospital	Augusta	71%	300+
Washington County Regional Medical Center	Sandersville	71%	300+
Wellstar Kennestone Hospital	Marietta	71%	300+
Wellstar Paulding Hospital	Hiram	71%	300+
West Georgia Medical Center	Lagrange	71%	300+
Atlanta Medical Center	Atlanta	70%	300+
Coliseum Medical Center	Macon	70%	300+
Coliseum Northside Hospital	Macon	70%	300+
Hutcheson Medical Center[11]	Fort Oglethorpe	70%	(a)
Meadows Regional Medical Center	Vidalia	70%	300+
Piedmont Fayette Hospital	Fayetteville	70%	300+
Piedmont Mountainside Hospital	Jasper	70%	300+
Saint Francis Hospital	Columbus	70%	300+
Trinity Hospital of Augusta	Augusta	70%	300+
Appling Hospital	Baxley	69%	(a)
Colquitt Regional Medical Center	Moultrie	69%	300+
Northridge Medical Center	Commerce	69%	(a)
Oconee Regional Medical Center	Milledgeville	69%	300+
Rockdale Medical Center	Conyers	69%	300+
SE Georgia Health Sys-Brunswick	Brunswick	69%	300+
Spalding Regional Hospital	Griffin	69%	300+
Union General Hospital	Blairsville	69%	300+
Chestatee Regional Hospital	Dahlonega	68%	(a)
Cook Medical Center	Adel	68%	(a)
Houston Medical Center	Warner Robins	68%	300+
Memorial Hospital & Manor	Bainbridge	68%	300+
Piedmont Hospital	Atlanta	68%	300+
Wayne Memorial Hospital	Jesup	68%	300+
Dekalb Medical Center at Hillandale	Lithonia	67%	300+
Dorminy Medical Center	Fitzgerald	67%	(a)
Medical Center of Central Georgia	Macon	67%	300+
Med College of Georgia Hosps	Augusta	67%	300+
Midtown Medical Center	Columbus	67%	300+
Newton Medical Center	Covington	67%	300+
Northside Hospital Cherokee	Canton	67%	300+
Wellstar Cobb Hospital	Austell	67%	300+
Crisp Regional Hospital	Cordele	66%	300+
Grady Memorial Hospital	Atlanta	66%	300+
SE Georgia Health Sys-Camden Campus	Saint Marys	66%	(a)
Dekalb Medical Center	Decatur	65%	300+
Emory - Adventist Hospital[11]	Smyrna	65%	(a)
Evans Memorial Hospital	Claxton	65%	(a)
Irwin County Hospital	Ocilla	65%	(a)
North Fulton Hospital	Roswell	65%	300+
Piedmont Henry Hospital	Stockbridge	65%	300+
East Georgia Regional Medical Center	Statesboro	64%	300+
Clearview Regional Medical Center	Monroe	63%	300+
Eastside Medical Center	Snellville	63%	300+
North Georgia Medical Center	Ellijay	63%	(a)
Southern Regional Medical Center	Riverdale	63%	300+
Cartersville Medical Center	Cartersville	61%	300+
Barrow Regional Medical Center	Winder	56%	300+

Room and Bathroom 'Always' Clean

Hospital Name	City	Rate	Cases
Northside Medical Center	Columbus	84%	300+
Brooks County Hospital	Quitman	81%	(a)
Gordon Hospital[11]	Calhoun	81%	300+
Upson Regional Medical Center	Thomaston	81%	300+
Coffee Regional Medical Center	Douglas	80%	300+
Emanuel County Hospital Authority	Swainsboro	80%	(a)
Grady General Hospital	Cairo	80%	(a)
Tanner Medical Center - Carrollton	Carrollton	80%	300+
Meadows Regional Medical Center	Vidalia	79%	300+
SE Georgia Health Sys-Camden Campus	Saint Marys	79%	(a)
Tanner Medical Center Villa Rica	Villa Rica	79%	300+
Clearview Regional Medical Center	Monroe	78%	300+
Donalsonville Hospital	Donalsonville	78%	300+
Dodge County Hospital	Eastman	77%	(a)
Northside Hospital	Atlanta	77%	300+
Phoebe Sumter Medical Center	Americus	77%	300+
Bacon County Hospital	Alma	76%	(a)
Evans Memorial Hospital	Claxton	76%	(a)
Fannin Regional Hospital	Blue Ridge	76%	300+
Perry Hospital	Perry	76%	300+
Tift Regional Medical Center	Tifton	76%	300+
Emory University Hospital	Atlanta	75%	300+
Northside Hospital Forsyth	Cumming	75%	300+
Redmond Regional Medical Center	Rome	75%	300+
Union General Hospital	Blairsville	75%	300+
West Georgia Medical Center	Lagrange	75%	300+
Athens Regional Medical Center	Athens	74%	300+
Mayo Clinic Health System - Waycross	Waycross	74%	300+
Piedmont Newnan Hospital	Newnan	74%	300+
Taylor Regional Hospital	Hawkinsville	74%	(a)
Wellstar Kennestone Hospital	Marietta	74%	300+
Crisp Regional Hospital	Cordele	73%	300+
Doctors Specialty Hospital	Columbus	73%	300+
Elbert Memorial Hospital	Elberton	73%	(a)
Stephens County Hospital	Toccoa	73%	300+
Ty Cobb Regional Medical Center	Lavonia	73%	300+
Emory Johns Creek Hospital	Johns Creek	72%	300+
Fairview Park Hospital	Dublin	72%	300+
Gwinnett Medical Center	Lawrenceville	72%	300+
John D Archbold Memorial Hospital	Thomasville	72%	300+
Phoebe Putney Memorial Hospital	Albany	72%	300+
SE Georgia Health Sys-Brunswick	Brunswick	72%	300+
University Hospital	Augusta	72%	300+
Wellstar Douglas Hospital	Douglasville	72%	300+
Coliseum Northside Hospital	Macon	71%	300+
Emory - Adventist Hospital[11]	Smyrna	71%	(a)
Emory University Hospital Midtown	Atlanta	71%	300+
Hutcheson Medical Center[11]	Fort Oglethorpe	71%	(a)
Irwin County Hospital	Ocilla	71%	(a)
Piedmont Mountainside Hospital	Jasper	71%	300+
Wayne Memorial Hospital	Jesup	71%	300+
Colquitt Regional Medical Center	Moultrie	70%	300+
Doctors Hospital	Augusta	70%	300+
Dorminy Medical Center	Fitzgerald	70%	(a)
Memorial Hospital & Manor	Bainbridge	70%	300+
Saint Mary's Hospital	Athens	70%	300+
Dekalb Medical Center at Hillandale	Lithonia	69%	300+
Northridge Medical Center	Commerce	69%	(a)
Piedmont Fayette Hospital	Fayetteville	69%	300+
Saint Francis Hospital	Columbus	69%	300+
Saint Joseph's Hospital - Savannah	Savannah	69%	300+
Saint Joseph's Hospital of Atlanta	Atlanta	69%	300+
South Georgia Medical Center	Valdosta	69%	300+
Southern Regional Medical Center	Riverdale	69%	300+
Atlanta Medical Center	Atlanta	68%	300+
Med College of Georgia Hosps	Augusta	68%	300+
North Fulton Hospital	Roswell	68%	300+
Northeast Georgia Medical Center	Gainesville	68%	300+
Wellstar Cobb Hospital	Austell	68%	300+
Eastside Medical Center	Snellville	67%	300+
Habersham County Medical Center	Demorest	67%	300+
Medical Center of Central Georgia	Macon	67%	300+
Midtown Medical Center	Columbus	67%	300+
Rockdale Medical Center	Conyers	67%	300+
Coliseum Medical Center	Macon	66%	300+
Floyd Medical Center	Rome	66%	300+
Hamilton Medical Center	Dalton	66%	300+
Houston Medical Center	Warner Robins	66%	300+
Northside Hospital Cherokee	Canton	66%	300+
Cartersville Medical Center	Cartersville	65%	300+
Dekalb Medical Center	Decatur	65%	300+
East Georgia Regional Medical Center	Statesboro	65%	300+
Grady Memorial Hospital	Atlanta	65%	300+
Newton Medical Center	Covington	65%	300+
Spalding Regional Hospital	Griffin	64%	300+
Trinity Hospital of Augusta	Augusta	64%	300+
Wellstar Paulding Hospital	Hiram	64%	300+
Candler Hospital	Savannah	63%	300+
Oconee Regional Medical Center	Milledgeville	63%	300+
Piedmont Hospital	Atlanta	63%	300+
Barrow Regional Medical Center	Winder	62%	300+
Chestatee Regional Hospital	Dahlonega	62%	(a)
Cook Medical Center	Adel	62%	(a)
Piedmont Henry Hospital	Stockbridge	61%	300+
Memorial Health Univ Medical Center	Savannah	58%	300+
Washington County Regional Medical Center	Sandersville	58%	300+
North Georgia Medical Center	Ellijay	57%	(a)

NOTE: Hospital profiles are in alphabetical order by state, then city, then hospital within the city; Rankings exclude hospitals with less than 25 cases except for patient surveys which excludes hospitals with less than 100 cases; (a) 100-299 cases; (1) The number of cases/patients is too few to report; (2) Data submitted were based on a sample of cases/patients; (3) Results are based on a shorter time period than required; (4) Data suppressed by CMS for one or more quarters; (5) Results are not available for this reporting period; (6) Fewer than 100 patients completed the HCAHPS survey; (7) No cases met the criteria for this measure; (8) The lower limit of the confidence interval cannot be calculated if the number of observed infections equals zero; (9) No data are available from the state/territory for this reporting period; (10) The scores shown reflect fewer than 50 completed surveys; (11) There were discrepancies in the data collection process; (12) This measure does not apply to this hospital for this reporting period; (13) Results cannot be calculated for this reporting period; (14) The results for this state are combined with nearby states to protect confidentiality; Please refer to the User's Guide for a full explanation of data.

Hospital Name	City	Rate	Cases
Appling Hospital	Baxley	56%	(a)

Timely Help 'Always' Received

Hospital Name	City	Rate	Cases
Northside Medical Center	Columbus	79%	300+
Coffee Regional Medical Center	Douglas	77%	300+
Tanner Medical Center - Carrollton	Carrollton	77%	300+
Upson Regional Medical Center	Thomaston	76%	300+
North Georgia Medical Center	Ellijay	75%	(a)
Tanner Medical Center Villa Rica	Villa Rica	75%	300+
Union General Hospital	Blairsville	75%	300+
Emanuel County Hospital Authority	Swainsboro	74%	(a)
Evans Memorial Hospital	Claxton	73%	(a)
Bacon County Hospital	Alma	72%	(a)
Gordon Hospital[11]	Calhoun	72%	300+
Stephens County Hospital	Toccoa	72%	300+
Ty Cobb Regional Medical Center	Lavonia	72%	300+
Emory University Hospital	Atlanta	71%	300+
Grady General Hospital	Cairo	71%	(a)
Tift Regional Medical Center	Tifton	71%	300+
Colquitt Regional Medical Center	Moultrie	69%	300+
Doctors Specialty Hospital	Columbus	69%	300+
Fannin Regional Hospital	Blue Ridge	69%	300+
Hutcheson Medical Center[11]	Fort Oglethorpe	69%	(a)
Mayo Clinic Health System - Waycross	Waycross	69%	300+
Meadows Regional Medical Center	Vidalia	69%	300+
Redmond Regional Medical Center	Rome	69%	300+
Spalding Regional Hospital	Griffin	69%	300+
Donalsonville Hospital	Donalsonville	68%	300+
Perry Hospital	Perry	68%	300+
Hamilton Medical Center	Dalton	67%	300+
Memorial Hospital & Manor	Bainbridge	67%	300+
Piedmont Mountainside Hospital	Jasper	67%	300+
Piedmont Newnan Hospital	Newnan	67%	300+
South Georgia Medical Center	Valdosta	67%	300+
Taylor Regional Hospital	Hawkinsville	67%	(a)
West Georgia Medical Center	Lagrange	67%	300+
Athens Regional Medical Center	Athens	66%	300+
Cook Medical Center	Adel	66%	(a)
Elbert Memorial Hospital	Elberton	66%	(a)
Fairview Park Hospital	Dublin	66%	300+
Newton Medical Center	Covington	66%	300+
SE Georgia Health Sys-Camden Campus	Saint Marys	66%	(a)
Dodge County Hospital	Eastman	65%	(a)
Floyd Medical Center	Rome	65%	300+
Northridge Medical Center	Commerce	65%	(a)
Northside Hospital	Atlanta	65%	300+
Northside Hospital Forsyth	Cumming	65%	300+
Phoebe Putney Memorial Hospital	Albany	65%	300+
Wellstar Kennestone Hospital	Marietta	65%	300+
Brooks County Hospital	Quitman	64%	(a)
Habersham County Medical Center	Demorest	64%	300+
Houston Medical Center	Warner Robins	64%	300+
John D Archbold Memorial Hospital	Thomasville	64%	300+
Northeast Georgia Medical Center	Gainesville	64%	300+
Saint Joseph's Hospital - Savannah	Savannah	64%	300+
Saint Joseph's Hospital of Atlanta	Atlanta	64%	300+
Saint Mary's Hospital	Athens	64%	300+
Wellstar Douglas Hospital	Douglasville	64%	300+
Wellstar Paulding Hospital	Hiram	64%	300+
Gwinnett Medical Center	Lawrenceville	63%	300+
Memorial Health Univ Medical Center	Savannah	63%	300+
Oconee Regional Medical Center	Milledgeville	63%	300+
Phoebe Sumter Medical Center	Americus	63%	300+
Piedmont Fayette Hospital	Fayetteville	63%	300+
Washington County Regional Medical Center	Sandersville	63%	300+
Coliseum Northside Hospital	Macon	62%	300+
Northside Hospital Cherokee	Canton	62%	300+
Trinity Hospital of Augusta	Augusta	62%	300+
Wayne Memorial Hospital	Jesup	62%	300+
Chestatee Regional Hospital	Dahlonega	61%	(a)
Doctors Hospital	Augusta	61%	300+
Emory Johns Creek Hospital	Johns Creek	61%	300+
Emory University Hospital Midtown	Atlanta	61%	300+
Irwin County Hospital	Ocilla	61%	(a)
Saint Francis Hospital	Columbus	61%	300+
SE Georgia Health Sys-Brunswick	Brunswick	61%	300+
University Hospital	Augusta	61%	300+
Coliseum Medical Center	Macon	60%	300+
Piedmont Hospital	Atlanta	60%	300+
Appling Hospital	Baxley	59%	(a)
Dorminy Medical Center	Fitzgerald	59%	(a)
East Georgia Regional Medical Center	Statesboro	59%	300+
Atlanta Medical Center	Atlanta	58%	300+
Candler Hospital	Savannah	58%	300+
Medical Center of Central Georgia	Macon	58%	300+
North Fulton Hospital	Roswell	58%	300+
Rockdale Medical Center	Conyers	58%	300+
Wellstar Cobb Hospital	Austell	58%	300+
Crisp Regional Hospital	Cordele	57%	300+
Dekalb Medical Center at Hillandale	Lithonia	56%	300+
Midtown Medical Center	Columbus	56%	300+
Emory - Adventist Hospital[11]	Smyrna	55%	(a)
Grady Memorial Hospital	Atlanta	55%	300+
Med College of Georgia Hosps	Augusta	55%	300+
Cartersville Medical Center	Cartersville	54%	300+
Piedmont Henry Hospital	Stockbridge	54%	300+
Barrow Regional Medical Center	Winder	53%	300+
Clearview Regional Medical Center	Monroe	53%	300+
Dekalb Medical Center	Decatur	53%	300+
Eastside Medical Center	Snellville	50%	300+
Southern Regional Medical Center	Riverdale	50%	300+

Would Definitely Recommend Hospital

Hospital Name	City	Rate	Cases
Northside Medical Center	Columbus	93%	300+
Emory University Hospital	Atlanta	86%	300+
Emory Johns Creek Hospital	Johns Creek	81%	300+
Northside Hospital	Atlanta	81%	300+
Northside Hospital Forsyth	Cumming	81%	300+
Piedmont Fayette Hospital	Fayetteville	81%	300+
Saint Mary's Hospital	Athens	81%	300+
University Hospital	Augusta	81%	300+
Athens Regional Medical Center	Athens	80%	300+
Northeast Georgia Medical Center	Gainesville	80%	300+
Redmond Regional Medical Center	Rome	80%	300+
Tanner Medical Center - Carrollton	Carrollton	80%	300+
Doctors Specialty Hospital	Columbus	79%	300+
Gwinnett Medical Center	Lawrenceville	79%	300+
Perry Hospital	Perry	79%	300+
Saint Joseph's Hospital of Atlanta	Atlanta	79%	300+
Union General Hospital	Blairsville	79%	300+
John D Archbold Memorial Hospital	Thomasville	78%	300+
Saint Francis Hospital	Columbus	78%	300+
Tanner Medical Center Villa Rica	Villa Rica	78%	300+
Bacon County Hospital	Alma	77%	(a)
Piedmont Hospital	Atlanta	77%	300+
Piedmont Mountainside Hospital	Jasper	77%	300+
Saint Joseph's Hospital - Savannah	Savannah	77%	300+
Floyd Medical Center	Rome	76%	300+
Gordon Hospital[11]	Calhoun	76%	300+
Candler Hospital	Savannah	75%	300+
Emory University Hospital Midtown	Atlanta	75%	300+
South Georgia Medical Center	Valdosta	75%	300+
Taylor Regional Hospital	Hawkinsville	75%	(a)
Grady General Hospital	Cairo	74%	(a)
Meadows Regional Medical Center	Vidalia	74%	300+
Medical Center of Central Georgia	Macon	74%	300+
Piedmont Newnan Hospital	Newnan	74%	300+
Upson Regional Medical Center	Thomaston	74%	300+
Wellstar Kennestone Hospital	Marietta	74%	300+
Coliseum Northside Hospital	Macon	73%	300+
Fannin Regional Hospital	Blue Ridge	73%	300+
Memorial Health Univ Medical Center	Savannah	73%	300+
Wellstar Douglas Hospital	Douglasville	73%	300+
Coliseum Medical Center	Macon	72%	300+
Doctors Hospital	Augusta	72%	300+
Donalsonville Hospital	Donalsonville	72%	300+
Tift Regional Medical Center	Tifton	72%	300+
Ty Cobb Regional Medical Center	Lavonia	72%	300+
Grady Memorial Hospital	Atlanta	71%	300+
Habersham County Medical Center	Demorest	71%	300+
Houston Medical Center	Warner Robins	71%	300+
Irwin County Hospital	Ocilla	71%	(a)
Med College of Georgia Hosps	Augusta	71%	300+
Phoebe Sumter Medical Center	Americus	71%	300+
Emanuel County Hospital Authority	Swainsboro	70%	(a)
Emory - Adventist Hospital[11]	Smyrna	70%	(a)
North Fulton Hospital	Roswell	70%	300+
Trinity Hospital of Augusta	Augusta	70%	300+
Wellstar Paulding Hospital	Hiram	70%	300+
Coffee Regional Medical Center	Douglas	68%	300+
Hutcheson Medical Center[11]	Fort Oglethorpe	68%	(a)
Phoebe Putney Memorial Hospital	Albany	68%	300+
Stephens County Hospital	Toccoa	68%	300+
Wellstar Cobb Hospital	Austell	68%	300+
Dekalb Medical Center at Hillandale	Lithonia	67%	300+
Hamilton Medical Center	Dalton	67%	300+
Rockdale Medical Center	Conyers	67%	300+
West Georgia Medical Center	Lagrange	67%	300+
Brooks County Hospital	Quitman	66%	(a)
Elbert Memorial Hospital	Elberton	66%	(a)
Northside Hospital Cherokee	Canton	66%	300+
SE Georgia Health Sys-Brunswick	Brunswick	66%	300+
Eastside Medical Center	Snellville	65%	300+
Evans Memorial Hospital	Claxton	65%	(a)
Fairview Park Hospital	Dublin	65%	300+
Mayo Clinic Health System - Waycross	Waycross	65%	300+
Newton Medical Center	Covington	65%	300+
SE Georgia Health Sys-Camden Campus	Saint Marys	65%	(a)
Wayne Memorial Hospital	Jesup	65%	300+
Midtown Medical Center	Columbus	64%	300+
Atlanta Medical Center	Atlanta	63%	300+
Dekalb Medical Center	Decatur	63%	300+
Colquitt Regional Medical Center	Moultrie	62%	300+
Dodge County Hospital	Eastman	62%	(a)
Oconee Regional Medical Center	Milledgeville	62%	300+
Spalding Regional Hospital	Griffin	62%	300+
Clearview Regional Medical Center	Monroe	61%	300+
Cook Medical Center	Adel	61%	(a)
Northridge Medical Center	Commerce	61%	(a)
Piedmont Henry Hospital	Stockbridge	61%	300+
Chestatee Regional Hospital	Dahlonega	60%	(a)
Memorial Hospital & Manor	Bainbridge	59%	300+
Washington County Regional Medical Center	Sandersville	57%	300+
East Georgia Regional Medical Center	Statesboro	56%	300+
North Georgia Medical Center	Ellijay	56%	(a)
Crisp Regional Hospital	Cordele	55%	300+
Dorminy Medical Center	Fitzgerald	53%	(a)
Appling Hospital	Baxley	52%	(a)
Cartersville Medical Center	Cartersville	52%	300+
Southern Regional Medical Center	Riverdale	50%	300+
Barrow Regional Medical Center	Winder	49%	300+

Use of Medical Imaging

Cardiac Imaging Stress Test before OP Surgery

Hospital Name	City	Rate	Cases
Saint Francis Hospital	Columbus	1.2%	81
Fannin Regional Hospital	Blue Ridge	1.8%	219
Higgins General Hospital	Bremen	2.0%	49
Appling Hospital	Baxley	2.2%	46
SE Georgia Health Sys-Camden Campus	Saint Marys	3.1%	96
Candler Hospital	Savannah	3.7%	82
Grady Memorial Hospital	Atlanta	3.8%	371
Memorial Health Univ Medical Center	Savannah	3.8%	235
North Georgia Medical Center	Ellijay	3.8%	53
Dekalb Medical Center	Decatur	3.9%	254
Habersham County Medical Center	Demorest	3.9%	205
Fairview Park Hospital	Dublin	4.0%	100
Tanner Medical Center Villa Rica	Villa Rica	4.2%	119
Dekalb Medical Center at Hillandale	Lithonia	4.4%	135
Upson Regional Medical Center	Thomaston	4.4%	204
Wayne Memorial Hospital	Jesup	4.4%	91
Wellstar Kennestone Hospital	Marietta	4.4%	2242
East Georgia Regional Medical Center	Statesboro	4.5%	155
Taylor Regional Hospital	Hawkinsville	4.5%	134
University Hospital	Augusta	4.5%	2451
Saint Joseph's Hospital of Atlanta	Atlanta	4.6%	1650
Southern Regional Medical Center	Riverdale	4.6%	216
Mayo Clinic Health System - Waycross	Waycross	4.7%	425
Meadows Regional Medical Center	Vidalia	4.7%	341
Ty Cobb Regional Medical Center	Lavonia	4.7%	211
Emory University Hospital Midtown	Atlanta	4.8%	764
Hamilton Medical Center	Dalton	4.8%	748
Crisp Regional Hospital	Cordele	5.0%	120
Piedmont Mountainside Hospital	Jasper	5.0%	743
Stephens County Hospital	Toccoa	5.0%	202
Colquitt Regional Medical Center	Moultrie	5.1%	313
Gordon Hospital	Calhoun	5.1%	195
Gwinnett Medical Center	Lawrenceville	5.1%	682
Tift Regional Medical Center	Tifton	5.1%	570
Northeast Georgia Medical Center	Gainesville	5.2%	909
Phoebe Putney Memorial Hospital	Albany	5.2%	897
Saint Mary's Hospital	Athens	5.4%	626
Wellstar Paulding Hospital	Hiram	5.4%	185
Midtown Medical Center	Columbus	5.5%	55
Piedmont Hospital	Atlanta	5.5%	2524
Doctors Hospital	Augusta	5.6%	231
Oconee Regional Medical Center	Milledgeville	5.6%	178
Tanner Medical Center - Carrollton	Carrollton	5.6%	394
Wellstar Cobb Hospital	Austell	5.6%	444
Floyd Medical Center	Rome	5.7%	580
Clearview Regional Medical Center	Monroe	5.8%	69
Eastside Medical Center	Snellville	5.9%	238
Dorminy Medical Center	Fitzgerald	6.0%	117
Medical Center of Central Georgia	Macon	6.1%	358
Piedmont Newnan Hospital	Newnan	6.1%	772
West Georgia Medical Center	Lagrange	6.1%	343
Redmond Regional Medical Center	Rome	6.2%	356
South Georgia Medical Center	Valdosta	6.2%	402
Med College of Georgia Hosps	Augusta	6.4%	405
Northside Hospital Cherokee	Canton	6.4%	157
Atlanta Medical Center	Atlanta	6.5%	155
SE Georgia Health Sys-Brunswick	Brunswick	6.5%	107
Piedmont Fayette Hospital	Fayetteville	6.6%	971
Wellstar Douglas Hospital	Douglasville	6.6%	273
Saint Joseph's Hospital - Savannah	Savannah	6.7%	75
Athens Regional Medical Center	Athens	6.8%	409
John D Archbold Memorial Hospital	Thomasville	6.8%	311
Northside Hospital	Atlanta	7.0%	114
Emory University Hospital	Atlanta	7.4%	842

NOTE: Hospital profiles are in alphabetical order by state, then city, then hospital within the city; Rankings exclude hospitals with less than 25 cases except for patient surveys which excludes hospitals with less than 100 cases; (a) 100-299 cases; (1) The number of cases/patients is too few to report; (2) Data submitted were based on a sample of cases/patients; (3) Results are based on a shorter time period than required; (4) Data suppressed by CMS for one or more quarters; (5) Results are not available for this reporting period; (6) Fewer than 100 patients completed the HCAHPS survey; (7) No cases met the criteria for this measure; (8) The lower limit of the confidence interval cannot be calculated if the number of observed infections equals zero; (9) No data are available from the state/territory for this reporting period; (10) The scores shown reflect fewer than 50 completed surveys; (11) There were discrepancies in the data collection process; (12) This measure does not apply to this hospital for this reporting period; (13) Results cannot be calculated for this reporting period; (14) The results for this state are combined with nearby states to protect confidentiality; Please refer to the User's Guide for a full explanation of data.

Hospital Name	City	Rate	Cases
Rockdale Medical Center	Conyers	7.5%	173
Northside Hospital Forsyth	Cumming	7.7%	326
Hutcheson Medical Center	Fort Oglethorpe	7.8%	141
North Fulton Hospital	Roswell	8.0%	100
Spalding Regional Hospital	Griffin	8.2%	256
Coffee Regional Medical Center	Douglas	8.3%	314
Piedmont Henry Hospital	Stockbridge	8.8%	251
Cartersville Medical Center	Cartersville	9.4%	224
Trinity Hospital of Augusta	Augusta	9.4%	85
Union General Hospital	Blairsville	9.6%	177
Emory Johns Creek Hospital	Johns Creek	10.4%	211

Combination Abdominal CT Scan

Hospital Name	City	Rate	Cases
Polk Medical Center	Cedartown	0.0%	107
Coliseum Medical Center	Macon	1.1%	633
Monroe County Hospital	Forsyth	1.3%	149
Floyd Medical Center	Rome	1.4%	699
Flint River Hospital	Montezuma	1.7%	119
Mayo Clinic Health System - Waycross	Waycross	1.7%	954
Emory Johns Creek Hospital	Johns Creek	1.8%	438
Saint Mary's Hospital	Athens	1.9%	431
Phoebe Sumter Medical Center	Americus	2.0%	345
Grady General Hospital	Cairo	2.3%	222
North Fulton Hospital	Roswell	2.3%	556
Bleckley Memorial Hospital	Cochran	2.7%	75
Barrow Regional Medical Center	Winder	2.8%	431
Tift Regional Medical Center	Tifton	3.0%	951
Northridge Medical Center	Commerce	3.2%	155
Coliseum Northside Hospital	Macon	3.3%	275
Habersham County Medical Center	Demorest	3.3%	514
Midtown Medical Center	Columbus	3.3%	705
Doctors Specialty Hospital	Columbus	3.4%	148
Fairview Park Hospital	Dublin	3.7%	543
Doctors Hospital	Augusta	3.8%	505
Northeast Georgia Medical Center	Gainesville	3.8%	1975
Southwest Georgia Regional Medical Center	Cuthbert	3.8%	80
Dekalb Medical Center at Hillandale	Lithonia	3.9%	492
Piedmont Fayette Hospital	Fayetteville	3.9%	1196
Jasper Memorial Hospital	Monticello	4.0%	50
West Georgia Medical Center	Lagrange	4.0%	708
Emory - Adventist Hospital	Smyrna	4.7%	274
Piedmont Newnan Hospital	Newnan	4.7%	789
Spalding Regional Hospital	Griffin	4.7%	590
Liberty Regional Medical Center	Hinesville	4.8%	289
Redmond Regional Medical Center	Rome	4.8%	625
Saint Joseph's Hospital of Atlanta	Atlanta	4.8%	1371
Union General Hospital	Blairsville	4.8%	643
Hutcheson Medical Center	Fort Oglethorpe	4.9%	307
Atlanta Medical Center	Atlanta	5.1%	431
Northside Hospital Forsyth	Cumming	5.1%	1379
Jefferson Hospital	Louisville	5.2%	58
Bacon County Hospital	Alma	5.4%	130
Gwinnett Medical Center	Lawrenceville	5.6%	2650
Athens Regional Medical Center	Athens	5.7%	1625
Chestatee Regional Hospital	Dahlonega	5.7%	159
Burke Medical Center	Waynesboro	5.8%	103
Higgins General Hospital	Bremen	5.9%	427
Wellstar Paulding Hospital	Hiram	5.9%	733
Dekalb Medical Center	Decatur	6.0%	1000
Eastside Medical Center	Snellville	6.0%	728
Phoebe Putney Memorial Hospital	Albany	6.1%	1386
Southern Regional Medical Center	Riverdale	6.1%	932
University Hospital	Augusta	6.1%	1188
Cartersville Medical Center	Cartersville	6.2%	697
Colquitt Regional Medical Center	Moultrie	6.4%	423
Rockdale Medical Center	Conyers	7.0%	719
Murray Medical Center	Chatsworth	7.1%	182
Taylor Regional Hospital	Hawkinsville	7.2%	293
Morgan Memorial Hospital	Madison	7.3%	109
Clearview Regional Medical Center	Monroe	7.4%	458
Northside Hospital Cherokee	Canton	7.4%	685
SE Georgia Health Sys-Brunswick	Brunswick	7.5%	1091
Hamilton Medical Center	Dalton	7.7%	1272
Piedmont Henry Hospital	Stockbridge	7.7%	957
Tanner Medical Center - Carrollton	Carrollton	7.7%	945
Wellstar Kennestone Hospital	Marietta	7.8%	2809
Emory University Hospital Midtown	Atlanta	7.9%	1122
Trinity Hospital of Augusta	Augusta	7.9%	328
Piedmont Hospital	Atlanta	8.4%	1721
Wellstar Cobb Hospital	Austell	8.5%	1135
Tanner Medical Center Villa Rica	Villa Rica	8.8%	486
Stephens County Hospital	Toccoa	9.0%	400
Grady Memorial Hospital	Atlanta	9.1%	638
Northside Hospital	Atlanta	9.2%	1873
Chatuge Regional Hospital	Hiawassee	9.3%	259
Oconee Regional Medical Center	Milledgeville	9.6%	561
Saint Francis Hospital	Columbus	9.9%	1049
Upson Regional Medical Center	Thomaston	9.9%	393
Crisp Regional Hospital	Cordele	10.3%	351
Fannin Regional Hospital	Blue Ridge	10.4%	288
Medical Center of Central Georgia	Macon	10.4%	882
Ty Cobb Regional Medical Center	Lavonia	10.8%	351
Wayne Memorial Hospital	Jesup	11.1%	451
John D Archbold Memorial Hospital	Thomasville	11.4%	948
SE Georgia Health Sys-Camden Campus	Saint Marys	11.7%	420
Wellstar Douglas Hospital	Douglasville	12.0%	849
Meadows Regional Medical Center	Vidalia	12.6%	795
Univ McDuffie Co Reg Med Ctr	Thomson	12.8%	172
Miller County Hospital	Colquitt	13.7%	117
Emory University Hospital	Atlanta	14.2%	1944
Saint Mary's Good Samaritan Hospital	Greensboro	14.4%	181
North Georgia Medical Center	Ellijay	15.1%	139
Lower Oconee Community Hospital	Glenwood	15.2%	92
Med College of Georgia Hosps	Augusta	15.2%	896
Gordon Hospital	Calhoun	16.0%	349
Newton Medical Center	Covington	16.1%	766
Jeff Davis Hospital	Hazlehurst	16.4%	116
Putnam General Hospital	Eatonton	16.4%	287
Coffee Regional Medical Center	Douglas	17.0%	600
Piedmont Mountainside Hospital	Jasper	17.1%	814
Memorial Hospital & Manor	Bainbridge	18.1%	332
Donalsonville Hospital	Donalsonville	20.1%	149
Saint Joseph's Hospital - Savannah	Savannah	20.8%	615
Washington County Regional Medical Center	Sandersville	20.9%	211
Dodge County Hospital	Eastman	21.0%	248
Appling Hospital	Baxley	21.8%	165
Houston Medical Center	Warner Robins	22.1%	1198
Elbert Memorial Hospital	Elberton	23.5%	153
The Medical Center of Peach County	Byron	23.8%	126
Perry Hospital	Perry	23.8%	269
Irwin County Hospital	Ocilla	25.0%	64
Effingham County Hospital	Springfield	25.1%	223
South Georgia Medical Center	Valdosta	25.4%	1694
Emanuel County Hospital Authority	Swainsboro	26.1%	184
Evans Memorial Hospital	Claxton	29.1%	148
Cook Medical Center	Adel	29.7%	74
Memorial Health Univ Medical Center	Savannah	34.6%	1123
Clinch Memorial Hospital	Homerville	34.8%	66
Dorminy Medical Center	Fitzgerald	36.7%	180
Candler Hospital	Savannah	38.0%	1437
Wills Memorial Hospital	Washington	39.2%	97
East Georgia Regional Medical Center	Statesboro	42.4%	733

Combination Brain/Sinus CT Scan

Hospital Name	City	Rate	Cases
Jasper Memorial Hospital	Monticello	0.0%	59
Morgan Memorial Hospital	Madison	0.0%	155
Hamilton Medical Center	Dalton	0.4%	1279
Med College of Georgia Hosps	Augusta	0.5%	816
North Fulton Hospital	Roswell	0.6%	642
Athens Regional Medical Center	Athens	0.8%	1219
Gwinnett Medical Center	Lawrenceville	0.8%	1869
Spalding Regional Hospital	Griffin	0.8%	866
Union General Hospital	Blairsville	0.8%	596
Eastside Medical Center	Snellville	1.0%	778
Univ McDuffie Co Reg Med Ctr	Thomson	1.0%	200
Atlanta Medical Center	Atlanta	1.1%	466
Donalsonville Hospital	Donalsonville	1.1%	175
Gordon Hospital	Calhoun	1.1%	441
Southern Regional Medical Center	Riverdale	1.1%	851
University Hospital	Augusta	1.1%	1318
Grady Memorial Hospital	Atlanta	1.2%	837
Tanner Medical Center Villa Rica	Villa Rica	1.2%	343
Piedmont Hospital	Atlanta	1.3%	1239
Doctors Hospital	Augusta	1.4%	491
Midtown Medical Center	Columbus	1.4%	731
Northside Hospital	Atlanta	1.4%	736
Piedmont Fayette Hospital	Fayetteville	1.4%	1184
Saint Francis Hospital	Columbus	1.4%	1336
Saint Joseph's Hospital of Atlanta	Atlanta	1.4%	974
Upson Regional Medical Center	Thomaston	1.4%	564
Northside Hospital Cherokee	Canton	1.5%	792
Emory - Adventist Hospital	Smyrna	1.6%	375
Emory University Hospital	Atlanta	1.6%	867
John D Archbold Memorial Hospital	Thomasville	1.6%	632
Tanner Medical Center - Carrollton	Carrollton	1.6%	933
Piedmont Newnan Hospital	Newnan	1.7%	770
Fairview Park Hospital	Dublin	1.8%	664
Wellstar Cobb Hospital	Austell	2.0%	1037
West Georgia Medical Center	Lagrange	2.0%	863
Piedmont Mountainside Hospital	Jasper	2.1%	575
Wellstar Kennestone Hospital	Marietta	2.1%	1963
Floyd Medical Center	Rome	2.2%	872
Medical Center of Central Georgia	Macon	2.2%	1009
Northeast Georgia Medical Center	Gainesville	2.2%	1835
Piedmont Henry Hospital	Stockbridge	2.2%	854
Saint Mary's Hospital	Athens	2.2%	465
South Georgia Medical Center	Valdosta	2.2%	1326
Oconee Regional Medical Center	Milledgeville	2.3%	524
Redmond Regional Medical Center	Rome	2.3%	820
Tift Regional Medical Center	Tifton	2.3%	957
Emory University Hospital Midtown	Atlanta	2.4%	776
Memorial Health Univ Medical Center	Savannah	2.5%	966
Houston Medical Center	Warner Robins	2.6%	1097
Coliseum Medical Center	Macon	2.7%	847
Meadows Regional Medical Center	Vidalia	2.7%	620
Rockdale Medical Center	Conyers	2.8%	726
Saint Joseph's Hospital - Savannah	Savannah	2.9%	765
East Georgia Regional Medical Center	Statesboro	3.0%	742
Candler Hospital	Savannah	3.2%	721
Newton Medical Center	Covington	3.2%	807
Phoebe Putney Memorial Hospital	Albany	3.3%	1107
Northside Hospital Forsyth	Cumming	3.4%	1112
Ty Cobb Regional Medical Center	Lavonia	3.9%	459
Habersham County Medical Center	Demorest	4.1%	588
Clearview Regional Medical Center	Monroe	4.3%	465
Barrow Regional Medical Center	Winder	4.4%	341
Cartersville Medical Center	Cartersville	4.5%	558
Dekalb Medical Center	Decatur	4.6%	910
Mayo Clinic Health System - Waycross	Waycross	4.6%	865
Crisp Regional Hospital	Cordele	4.7%	426
SE Georgia Health Sys-Brunswick	Brunswick	4.7%	876
Coffee Regional Medical Center	Douglas	5.0%	580
Jefferson Hospital	Louisville	5.7%	157
Phoebe Sumter Medical Center	Americus	6.2%	406

Combination Chest CT Scan

Hospital Name	City	Rate	Cases
Colquitt Regional Medical Center	Moultrie	0.0%	374
Dekalb Medical Center	Decatur	0.0%	758
Dekalb Medical Center at Hillandale	Lithonia	0.0%	144
Doctors Specialty Hospital	Columbus	0.0%	92
Emory Johns Creek Hospital	Johns Creek	0.0%	378
Emory University Hospital Midtown	Atlanta	0.0%	1377
Floyd Medical Center	Rome	0.0%	394
Lower Oconee Community Hospital	Glenwood	0.0%	73
Mayo Clinic Health System - Waycross	Waycross	0.0%	657
Med College of Georgia Hosps	Augusta	0.0%	509
North Fulton Hospital	Roswell	0.0%	395
Phoebe Sumter Medical Center	Americus	0.0%	221
Saint Mary's Hospital	Athens	0.0%	240
Athens Regional Medical Center	Athens	0.1%	1557
Emory University Hospital	Atlanta	0.1%	3002
Northside Hospital	Atlanta	0.1%	1615
Tift Regional Medical Center	Tifton	0.1%	719
Piedmont Newnan Hospital	Newnan	0.3%	346
Saint Joseph's Hospital of Atlanta	Atlanta	0.3%	1378
Liberty Regional Medical Center	Hinesville	0.4%	231
Fairview Park Hospital	Dublin	0.5%	194
Northside Hospital Forsyth	Cumming	0.5%	1201
Taylor Regional Hospital	Hawkinsville	0.5%	182
Wellstar Kennestone Hospital	Marietta	0.5%	2704
Doctors Hospital	Augusta	0.6%	165
Northeast Georgia Medical Center	Gainesville	0.6%	827
Piedmont Fayette Hospital	Fayetteville	0.6%	647
Saint Joseph's Hospital - Savannah	Savannah	0.6%	322
Wellstar Cobb Hospital	Austell	0.6%	682
Coliseum Medical Center	Macon	0.7%	290
Piedmont Hospital	Atlanta	0.7%	1188
Midtown Medical Center	Columbus	0.8%	636
Wellstar Paulding Hospital	Hiram	0.8%	780
Piedmont Henry Hospital	Stockbridge	0.9%	327
Habersham County Medical Center	Demorest	1.0%	208
Wellstar Douglas Hospital	Douglasville	1.1%	648
Grady General Hospital	Cairo	1.2%	81
Medical Center of Central Georgia	Macon	1.3%	754
Phoebe Putney Memorial Hospital	Albany	1.3%	1187
Eastside Medical Center	Snellville	1.4%	346
Meadows Regional Medical Center	Vidalia	1.4%	622
Cartersville Medical Center	Cartersville	1.5%	523
Crisp Regional Hospital	Cordele	1.5%	134
Union General Hospital	Blairsville	1.6%	387
Saint Francis Hospital	Columbus	1.7%	657
Spalding Regional Hospital	Griffin	1.8%	167
John D Archbold Memorial Hospital	Thomasville	1.9%	636
Northside Hospital Cherokee	Canton	1.9%	311
Monroe County Hospital	Forsyth	2.0%	98
Rockdale Medical Center	Conyers	2.4%	420
Gwinnett Medical Center	Lawrenceville	3.0%	1692
Tanner Medical Center - Carrollton	Carrollton	3.0%	630
Flint River Hospital	Montezuma	3.1%	64
Redmond Regional Medical Center	Rome	3.2%	311
Candler Hospital	Savannah	3.3%	1198
Northridge Medical Center	Commerce	3.6%	56
Southern Regional Medical Center	Riverdale	3.6%	362
Tanner Medical Center Villa Rica	Villa Rica	3.7%	245
Morgan Memorial Hospital	Madison	3.9%	51
Atlanta Medical Center	Atlanta	4.0%	150
Grady Memorial Hospital	Atlanta	4.0%	649
Barrow Regional Medical Center	Winder	4.1%	193
Chatuge Regional Hospital	Hiawassee	4.4%	137
SE Georgia Health Sys-Brunswick	Brunswick	4.7%	613

NOTE: Hospital profiles are in alphabetical order by state, then city, then hospital within the city; Rankings exclude hospitals with less than 25 cases except for patient surveys which excludes hospitals with less than 100 cases; (a) 100-299 cases; (1) The number of cases/patients is too few to report; (2) Data submitted were based on a sample of cases/patients; (3) Results are based on a shorter time period than required; (4) Data suppressed by CMS for one or more quarters; (5) Results are not available for this reporting period; (6) Fewer than 100 patients completed the HCAHPS survey; (7) No cases met the criteria for this measure; (8) The lower limit of the confidence interval cannot be calculated if the number of observed infections equals zero; (9) No data are available from the state/territory for this reporting period; (10) The scores shown reflect fewer than 50 completed surveys; (11) There were discrepancies in the data collection process; (12) This measure does not apply to this hospital for this reporting period; (13) Results cannot be calculated for this reporting period; (14) The results for this state are combined with nearby states to protect confidentiality; Please refer to the User's Guide for a full explanation of data.

Higgins General Hospital	Bremen	4.8%	166
Hamilton Medical Center	Dalton	5.4%	700
Hutcheson Medical Center	Fort Oglethorpe	6.3%	111
University Hospital	Augusta	6.3%	459
Ty Cobb Regional Medical Center	Lavonia	6.6%	166
West Georgia Medical Center	Lagrange	6.6%	166
Clearview Regional Medical Center	Monroe	7.0%	227
South Georgia Medical Center	Valdosta	7.6%	986
Fannin Regional Hospital	Blue Ridge	7.9%	152
Murray Medical Center	Chatsworth	8.0%	125
Gordon Hospital	Calhoun	8.3%	157
Stephens County Hospital	Toccoa	8.7%	149
Houston Medical Center	Warner Robins	8.8%	782
Memorial Hospital & Manor	Bainbridge	9.7%	144
Upson Regional Medical Center	Thomaston	10.1%	119
Piedmont Mountainside Hospital	Jasper	11.6%	327
Trinity Hospital of Augusta	Augusta	11.6%	86
Newton Medical Center	Covington	11.8%	348
Perry Hospital	Perry	11.9%	176
Putnam General Hospital	Eatonton	11.9%	160
Evans Memorial Hospital	Claxton	12.1%	140
Saint Mary's Good Samaritan Hospital	Greensboro	12.7%	110
Oconee Regional Medical Center	Milledgeville	13.1%	336
Wayne Memorial Hospital	Jesup	14.8%	283
Appling Hospital	Baxley	15.4%	104
SE Georgia Health Sys-Camden Campus	Saint Marys	18.1%	210
Univ McDuffie Co Reg Med Ctr	Thomson	18.8%	69
Washington County Regional Medical Center	Sandersville	19.4%	103
Effingham County Hospital	Springfield	21.0%	62
Coffee Regional Medical Center	Douglas	21.2%	293
Dodge County Hospital	Eastman	21.5%	135
Memorial Health Univ Medical Center	Savannah	22.3%	963
Cook Medical Center	Adel	30.8%	52
Miller County Hospital	Colquitt	31.0%	71
Wills Memorial Hospital	Washington	33.3%	54
Emanuel County Hospital Authority	Swainsboro	35.7%	70
Bacon County Hospital	Alma	36.1%	83
Dorminy Medical Center	Fitzgerald	40.2%	117
East Georgia Regional Medical Center	Statesboro	45.5%	369

Follow-up Mammogram/Ultrasound

A follow-up rate near zero may indicate missed cancer; a rate higher than 14% may mean there is unnecessary follow up.

Hospital Name	City	Rate	Cases
The Medical Center of Peach County	Byron	1.5%	338
Monroe County Hospital	Forsyth	2.5%	277
Liberty Regional Medical Center	Hinesville	3.0%	471
Memorial Hospital & Manor	Bainbridge	3.0%	567
SE Georgia Health Sys-Camden Campus	Saint Marys	3.0%	728
Med College of Georgia Hosps	Augusta	3.4%	989
SE Georgia Health Sys-Brunswick	Brunswick	3.5%	2860
Fairview Park Hospital	Dublin	4.1%	845
Perry Hospital	Perry	4.1%	370
Atlanta Medical Center	Atlanta	4.2%	765
Dodge County Hospital	Eastman	4.2%	263
Saint Joseph's Hospital - Savannah	Savannah	4.2%	381
Midtown Medical Center	Columbus	4.3%	2725
Houston Medical Center	Warner Robins	4.4%	1542
Medical Center of Central Georgia	Macon	4.4%	2673
Elbert Memorial Hospital	Elberton	4.6%	285
Crisp Regional Hospital	Cordele	4.7%	571
Fannin Regional Hospital	Blue Ridge	5.1%	469
Donalsonville Hospital	Donalsonville	5.2%	230
Coliseum Northside Hospital	Macon	5.6%	270
Emory Johns Creek Hospital	Johns Creek	5.7%	318
Washington County Regional Medical Center	Sandersville	5.8%	395
North Georgia Medical Center	Ellijay	6.0%	149
Phoebe Putney Memorial Hospital	Albany	6.1%	3212
Piedmont Newnan Hospital	Newnan	6.1%	1186
Spalding Regional Hospital	Griffin	6.1%	1046
West Georgia Medical Center	Lagrange	6.1%	413
Saint Mary's Good Samaritan Hospital	Greensboro	6.2%	241
Saint Mary's Hospital	Athens	6.4%	1836
Grady Memorial Hospital	Atlanta	6.5%	1824
Candler Hospital	Savannah	6.6%	4013
Tanner Medical Center - Carrollton	Carrollton	6.6%	1342
Dekalb Medical Center	Decatur	6.7%	3451
Hamilton Medical Center	Dalton	6.7%	1814
Upson Regional Medical Center	Thomaston	6.7%	579
Clinch Memorial Hospital	Homerville	6.8%	117
Piedmont Fayette Hospital	Fayetteville	6.8%	2509
Athens Regional Medical Center	Athens	6.9%	2887
Mayo Clinic Health System - Waycross	Waycross	6.9%	1305
Morgan Memorial Hospital	Madison	6.9%	216
Grady General Hospital	Cairo	7.0%	457
Taylor Regional Hospital	Hawkinsville	7.0%	497
Higgins General Hospital	Bremen	7.2%	319
Saint Joseph's Hospital of Atlanta	Atlanta	7.2%	1563
Tanner Medical Center Villa Rica	Villa Rica	7.2%	511
Coliseum Medical Center	Macon	7.4%	1729
North Fulton Hospital	Roswell	7.5%	843
Newton Medical Center	Covington	7.6%	1758
Saint Francis Hospital	Columbus	7.8%	2123
Union General Hospital	Blairsville	7.8%	1340
Piedmont Mountainside Hospital	Jasper	8.1%	970
Dekalb Medical Center at Hillandale	Lithonia	8.2%	970
Emory - Adventist Hospital	Smyrna	8.3%	337
Meadows Regional Medical Center	Vidalia	8.7%	812
Piedmont Henry Hospital	Stockbridge	8.7%	941
Barrow Regional Medical Center	Winder	8.8%	468
Colquitt Regional Medical Center	Moultrie	8.8%	704
Northeast Georgia Medical Center	Gainesville	8.8%	3007
Oconee Regional Medical Center	Milledgeville	8.8%	566
South Georgia Medical Center	Valdosta	8.8%	2147
Eastside Medical Center	Snellville	8.9%	1948
Jefferson Hospital	Louisville	8.9%	236
Memorial Health Univ Medical Center	Savannah	8.9%	1616
Emory University Hospital Midtown	Atlanta	9.0%	1538
Northside Hospital	Atlanta	9.0%	4634
Chatuge Regional Hospital	Hiawassee	9.1%	252
Chestatee Regional Hospital	Dahlonega	9.1%	275
Polk Medical Center	Cedartown	9.1%	132
Emory University Hospital	Atlanta	9.2%	2385
John D Archbold Memorial Hospital	Thomasville	9.4%	1847
Putnam General Hospital	Eatonton	9.4%	480
Bacon County Hospital	Alma	9.5%	190
Effingham County Hospital	Springfield	9.6%	333
Irwin County Hospital	Ocilla	9.6%	104
Floyd Medical Center	Rome	9.7%	2921
Piedmont Hospital	Atlanta	9.7%	2536
University Hospital	Augusta	9.7%	854
Jeff Davis Hospital	Hazlehurst	10.1%	169
Northside Hospital Cherokee	Canton	10.1%	1502
East Georgia Regional Medical Center	Statesboro	10.2%	1264
Coffee Regional Medical Center	Douglas	10.5%	648
Gordon Hospital	Calhoun	10.5%	731
Doctors Hospital	Augusta	10.8%	1594
Rockdale Medical Center	Conyers	10.9%	1625
Univ McDuffie Co Reg Med Ctr	Thomson	10.9%	485
Southern Regional Medical Center	Riverdale	11.0%	1515
Appling Hospital	Baxley	11.1%	243
Murray Medical Center	Chatsworth	11.5%	174
Northside Hospital Forsyth	Cumming	11.6%	2032
Wellstar Paulding Hospital	Hiram	11.6%	952
Clearview Regional Medical Center	Monroe	11.9%	471
Evans Memorial Hospital	Claxton	12.1%	257
Phoebe Sumter Medical Center	Americus	12.3%	693
Cartersville Medical Center	Cartersville	12.4%	669
Stephens County Hospital	Toccoa	12.8%	760
Dorminy Medical Center	Fitzgerald	12.9%	147
Wellstar Cobb Hospital	Austell	12.9%	1529
Trinity Hospital of Augusta	Augusta	13.0%	430
Wayne Memorial Hospital	Jesup	13.4%	397
Burke Medical Center	Waynesboro	13.7%	299
Habersham County Medical Center	Demorest	14.2%	760
Emanuel County Hospital Authority	Swainsboro	14.9%	362
Cook Medical Center	Adel	15.0%	140
Redmond Regional Medical Center	Rome	15.2%	886
Gwinnett Medical Center	Lawrenceville	16.0%	3726
Wellstar Douglas Hospital	Douglasville	16.0%	1264
Wellstar Kennestone Hospital	Marietta	16.5%	4941
Tift Regional Medical Center	Tifton	16.6%	2003
Ty Cobb Regional Medical Center	Lavonia	23.7%	317
Northridge Medical Center	Commerce	39.5%	223

Lumbar Spine MRI for Low Back Pain

Hospital Name	City	Rate	Cases
Northside Medical Center	Columbus	27.1%	59
Wellstar Kennestone Hospital	Marietta	27.3%	187
North Fulton Hospital	Roswell	27.6%	87
University Hospital	Augusta	27.7%	213
SE Georgia Health Sys-Brunswick	Brunswick	27.9%	179
Gordon Hospital	Calhoun	29.1%	127
Saint Mary's Hospital	Athens	29.4%	68
Piedmont Fayette Hospital	Fayetteville	30.4%	112
Grady Memorial Hospital	Atlanta	30.9%	68
Piedmont Mountainside Hospital	Jasper	30.9%	139
Colquitt Regional Medical Center	Moultrie	31.4%	102
Med College of Georgia Hosps	Augusta	32.7%	110
Saint Joseph's Hospital of Atlanta	Atlanta	32.7%	55
Saint Francis Hospital	Columbus	33.5%	203
Phoebe Putney Memorial Hospital	Albany	33.9%	121
Tift Regional Medical Center	Tifton	34.2%	152
Floyd Medical Center	Rome	34.3%	137
Memorial Hospital & Manor	Bainbridge	34.7%	72
Gwinnett Medical Center	Lawrenceville	34.8%	247
John D Archbold Memorial Hospital	Thomasville	35.0%	100
Wellstar Paulding Hospital	Hiram	35.2%	71
Northeast Georgia Medical Center	Gainesville	35.3%	300
Crisp Regional Hospital	Cordele	35.8%	53
Barrow Regional Medical Center	Winder	36.2%	47
Emory University Hospital	Atlanta	36.3%	422
Athens Regional Medical Center	Athens	36.6%	175
Mayo Clinic Health System - Waycross	Waycross	36.7%	188
Tanner Medical Center - Carrollton	Carrollton	36.7%	128
Meadows Regional Medical Center	Vidalia	37.2%	218
Coffee Regional Medical Center	Douglas	37.4%	99
Houston Medical Center	Warner Robins	37.8%	82
Piedmont Hospital	Atlanta	37.8%	127
Cartersville Medical Center	Cartersville	38.0%	50
Northside Hospital	Atlanta	38.0%	166
Upson Regional Medical Center	Thomaston	38.2%	55
South Georgia Medical Center	Valdosta	38.5%	104
Piedmont Henry Hospital	Stockbridge	39.0%	41
Hamilton Medical Center	Dalton	39.4%	180
Eastside Medical Center	Snellville	40.0%	110
Union General Hospital	Blairsville	40.3%	144
Northside Hospital Forsyth	Cumming	40.4%	109
Doctors Hospital	Augusta	40.7%	59
Atlanta Medical Center	Atlanta	40.9%	44
Redmond Regional Medical Center	Rome	40.9%	44
Effingham County Hospital	Springfield	41.0%	39
Newton Medical Center	Covington	41.0%	78
Rockdale Medical Center	Conyers	41.4%	70
Emory University Hospital Midtown	Atlanta	41.9%	62
Memorial Health Univ Medical Center	Savannah	42.0%	131
SE Georgia Health Sys-Camden Campus	Saint Marys	42.9%	42
Grady General Hospital	Cairo	43.2%	44
Wayne Memorial Hospital	Jesup	43.2%	37
Wellstar Douglas Hospital	Douglasville	43.5%	46
Midtown Medical Center	Columbus	43.7%	151
Taylor Regional Hospital	Hawkinsville	45.0%	60
Candler Hospital	Savannah	45.5%	55
Appling Hospital	Baxley	47.5%	40
Dekalb Medical Center	Decatur	47.9%	94
East Georgia Regional Medical Center	Statesboro	48.8%	129
Bacon County Hospital	Alma	50.0%	36
Ty Cobb Regional Medical Center	Lavonia	50.0%	54
Habersham County Medical Center	Demorest	55.6%	45

NOTE: Hospital profiles are in alphabetical order by state, then city, then hospital within the city; Rankings exclude hospitals with less than 25 cases except for patient surveys which excludes hospitals with less than 100 cases; (a) 100-299 cases; (1) The number of cases/patients is too few to report; (2) Data submitted were based on a sample of cases/patients; (3) Results are based on a shorter time period than required; (4) Data suppressed by CMS for one or more quarters; (5) Results are not available for this reporting period; (6) Fewer than 100 patients completed the HCAHPS survey; (7) No cases met the criteria for this measure; (8) The lower limit of the confidence interval cannot be calculated if the number of observed infections equals zero; (9) No data are available from the state/territory for this reporting period; (10) The scores shown reflect fewer than 50 completed surveys; (11) There were discrepancies in the data collection process; (12) This measure does not apply to this hospital for this reporting period; (13) Results cannot be calculated for this reporting period; (14) The results for this state are combined with nearby states to protect confidentiality; Please refer to the User's Guide for a full explanation of data.

Cook Medical Center

706 N Parrish Ave
Adel, GA 31620
Phone: 229-896-8077
Fax: 229-896-8001
Type: Acute Care Hospitals
Emergency Services: Yes
Ownership: Proprietary
Beds: 60

Key Personnel:

Intensive Care Unit. . . . . Bonnie Cronin, RN
Emergency Room . . . . Jimmy Dickerson, RN
Chief of Medical Staff. . . . . William Guest, MD
Infection Control. . . . . Sandi Martin
Quality Assurance . . . . Julie Ratts
CEO/President. . . . . William T. Richardson
Operating Room. . . . . Karen Spires, RN

Measure	Cases	This Hosp.	State Avg.	U.S. Avg.
Blood Clot Prevention and Treatment				
Anticoagulation Overlap Therapy[1,2]	-	-	90%	93%
ICU Venous Thromboembolism Prophylaxis[1,2]	-	-	90%	92%
Incidence of Potentially Preventable VTE[2,7]	-	-	13%	10%
UFH with Dosages/Platelet Monitoring[2,7]	-	-	99%	97%
Venous Thromboembolism Prophylaxis[2]	118	47%	80%	85%
Warfarin Therapy Discharge Instructions[1,2]	-	-	78%	75%
Chest Pain/Possible Heart Attack Care				
Aspirin Given Within 24 Hours of Arrival	20	80%	94%	96%
Fibrinolytic Meds Within 30 Min. of Arrival[7]	-	-	35%	58%
Average Time to ECG (minutes)	20	11	8	7
Average Time to Transfer (minutes)[7]	-	-	73	60
Children's Asthma Care				
Received Home Management Plan of Care	-	-	-	88%
Received Reliever Medication	-	-	-	100%
Received Systemic Corticosteroids	-	-	-	100%
Emergency Department				
Admittance Decision Time (minutes)[2]	203	53	100	98
Head CT Results Within 45 Min. of Arrival[1,3]	-	-	45%	57%
Patients Who Left ER Before Being Seen	9,999	1%	3%	2%
Time from ER Arrival to Admit. (minutes)[2]	233	172	286	274
Time from ER Arrival to Discharge (minutes)[11]	414	94	140	134
Time in ER Before Being Evaluated (minutes)	412	28	32	26
Time to Pain Meds for Fractures (minutes)	28	48	64	57
Heart Attack Care				
Aspirin Given at Discharge[1,3]	-	-	99%	99%
Fibrinolytic Meds Within 30 Min. of Arrival[3,7]	-	-	80%	54%
PCI Within 90 Minutes of Arrival[3,7]	-	-	95%	96%
Statin Prescribed at Discharge[1,3]	-	-	98%	98%
Heart Failure Care				
ACE Inhibitor or ARB for LVSD[1]	-	-	97%	97%
Discharge Instructions Given	32	91%	92%	94%
Evaluation of LVS Function	36	89%	99%	99%
Medicare Spending				
Medicare Spending per Patient (ratio)	-	0.87	0.95	0.98
Pneumonia Care				
Appropriate Initial Antibiotic Given[2]	26	96%	95%	95%
Blood Culture Timing[2]	12	92%	97%	98%
Pregnancy and Delivery Care				
Newborn Deliveries Scheduled Early[1]	-	-	8%	6%
Preventive Care				
Immunization for Influenza[2]	320	80%	88%	90%
Immunization for Pneumonia[2]	376	87%	90%	92%
Stroke Care				
Anticoagulation Therapy for Atrial Fibrillation[2,3]	-	-	94%	95%
Antithrombotic Therapy Timing[1,2]	-	-	97%	98%
Assessed for Rehabilitation[1,2]	-	-	97%	97%
Discharged on Antithrombotic Therapy[1,2]	-	-	98%	99%
Discharged on Statin Medication[1,2]	-	-	94%	94%
Thrombolytic Therapy Timing[2,3]	-	-	58%	66%
Venous Thromboembolism Prophylaxis[1,2]	-	-	92%	94%
Written Stroke Educational Materials Given[1,2]	-	-	84%	88%
Surgical Care Improvement Project				
Appropriate Beta Blocker Usage[5]	-	-	97%	98%
Appropriate VTP Within 24 Hours[5]	-	-	98%	98%
Controlled Postoperative Blood Glucose[5]	-	-	96%	97%
Perioperative Temperature Management[5]	-	-	100%	100%
Prophylactic Antibiotic Selection[5]	-	-	99%	99%
Prophylactic Antibiotic Selection (Outpatient)[3,7]	-	-	98%	98%
Prophylactic Antibiotic Stopped[5]	-	-	98%	98%
Prophylactic Antibiotic Timing[5]	-	-	99%	99%
Prophylactic Antibiotic Timing (Outpatient)[1,3]	-	-	98%	98%
Urinary Catheter Removal[5]	-	-	97%	97%
Survey of Patients' Hospital Experiences				
Area Around Room 'Always' Quiet at Night	(a)	69%	66%	61%
Doctors 'Always' Communicated Well	(a)	86%	83%	82%
Home Recovery Information Given	(a)	86%	84%	85%
Hospital Given 9 or 10 on 10 Point Scale	(a)	65%	69%	71%
Meds 'Always' Explained Before Given	(a)	70%	63%	64%
Nurses 'Always' Communicated Well	(a)	78%	78%	79%
Pain 'Always' Well Controlled	(a)	68%	71%	71%
Room and Bathroom 'Always' Clean	(a)	62%	71%	73%
Timely Help 'Always' Received	(a)	66%	65%	68%
Would Definitely Recommend Hospital	(a)	61%	70%	71%
Use of Medical Imaging				
Cardiac Imaging Stress Test before Surgery[1]	-	-	5.5%	5.3%
Combination Abdominal CT Scan	74	29.7%	10.1%	10.5%
Combination Brain/Sinus CT Scan[1]	-	-	2.3%	2.7%
Combination Chest CT Scan	52	30.8%	3.7%	2.7%
Follow-up Mammogram/Ultrasound	140	15.0%	8.9%	8.8%
Lumbar Spine MRI for Low Back Pain[1]	-	-	36.6%	37.2%

Phoebe Putney Memorial Hospital

417 Third Avenue
Albany, GA 31703
Phone: 229-312-4068
Fax: 229-312-7100
URL: www.phoebeputney.com
Type: Acute Care Hospitals
Emergency Services: Yes
Ownership: Govt - Hospital Dist/Auth
Beds: 691

Key Personnel:

Infection Control. . . . . Patsy Crosson
Quality Assurance . . . . Bob Farr
Pediatric In-Patient Care . . . . Jewel Farr
Radiology. . . . . Suresh Lakhanpal, MD
Chief of Medical Staff . . . . Frank Middleon
Pediatric Ambulatory Care . . . . . . Bruce Smith, MD
CEO/President. . . . . Joel Wernick
Operating Room. . . . . Carol Wright

Measure	Cases	This Hosp.	State Avg.	U.S. Avg.
Blood Clot Prevention and Treatment				
Anticoagulation Overlap Therapy[2]	160	92%	90%	93%
ICU Venous Thromboembolism Prophylaxis[2]	97	79%	90%	92%
Incidence of Potentially Preventable VTE[2]	34	21%	13%	10%
UFH with Dosages/Platelet Monitoring[2]	70	97%	99%	97%
Venous Thromboembolism Prophylaxis[2]	316	74%	80%	85%
Warfarin Therapy Discharge Instructions[2]	130	30%	78%	75%
Chest Pain/Possible Heart Attack Care				
Aspirin Given Within 24 Hours of Arrival[1,3]	-	-	94%	96%
Fibrinolytic Meds Within 30 Min. of Arrival[5]	-	-	35%	58%
Average Time to ECG (minutes)[1,3]	-	-	8	7
Average Time to Transfer (minutes)[5]	-	-	73	60
Children's Asthma Care				
Received Home Management Plan of Care	-	-	-	88%
Received Reliever Medication	-	-	-	100%
Received Systemic Corticosteroids	-	-	-	100%
Emergency Department				
Admittance Decision Time (minutes)[2]	550	138	100	98
Head CT Results Within 45 Min. of Arrival[1]	-	-	45%	57%
Patients Who Left ER Before Being Seen	76,537	3%	3%	2%
Time from ER Arrival to Admit. (minutes)[2]	574	340	286	274
Time from ER Arrival to Discharge (minutes)	827	150	140	134
Time in ER Before Being Evaluated (minutes)	854	29	32	26
Time to Pain Meds for Fractures (minutes)	164	54	64	57
Heart Attack Care				
Aspirin Given at Discharge	486	100%	99%	99%
Fibrinolytic Meds Within 30 Min. of Arrival[7]	-	-	80%	54%
PCI Within 90 Minutes of Arrival	56	88%	95%	96%
Statin Prescribed at Discharge	479	100%	98%	98%
Heart Failure Care				
ACE Inhibitor or ARB for LVSD	261	95%	97%	97%
Discharge Instructions Given	626	73%	92%	94%
Evaluation of LVS Function	690	100%	99%	99%
Medicare Spending				
Medicare Spending per Patient (ratio)	-	0.94	0.95	0.98
Pneumonia Care				
Appropriate Initial Antibiotic Given	240	92%	95%	95%
Blood Culture Timing	403	98%	97%	98%
Pregnancy and Delivery Care				
Newborn Deliveries Scheduled Early	214	24%	8%	6%
Preventive Care				
Immunization for Influenza[2]	576	90%	88%	90%
Immunization for Pneumonia[2]	722	93%	90%	92%
Stroke Care				
Anticoagulation Therapy for Atrial Fibrillation[2]	12	100%	94%	95%
Antithrombotic Therapy Timing[2]	140	90%	97%	98%
Assessed for Rehabilitation[2]	151	95%	97%	97%
Discharged on Antithrombotic Therapy[2]	134	96%	98%	99%
Discharged on Statin Medication[2]	114	90%	94%	94%
Thrombolytic Therapy Timing[1,2]	-	-	58%	66%
Venous Thromboembolism Prophylaxis[2]	164	79%	92%	94%
Written Stroke Educational Materials Given[2]	89	21%	84%	88%
Surgical Care Improvement Project				
Appropriate Beta Blocker Usage[2]	266	96%	97%	98%
Appropriate VTP Within 24 Hours[2]	553	99%	98%	98%
Controlled Postoperative Blood Glucose[2]	139	94%	96%	97%
Perioperative Temperature Management[2]	660	100%	100%	100%
Prophylactic Antibiotic Selection[2]	576	99%	99%	99%
Prophylactic Antibiotic Selection (Outpatient)	643	97%	98%	98%
Prophylactic Antibiotic Stopped[2]	540	99%	98%	98%
Prophylactic Antibiotic Timing[2]	576	99%	99%	99%
Prophylactic Antibiotic Timing (Outpatient)	662	94%	98%	98%
Urinary Catheter Removal[2]	533	98%	97%	97%
Survey of Patients' Hospital Experiences				
Area Around Room 'Always' Quiet at Night	300+	70%	66%	61%
Doctors 'Always' Communicated Well	300+	83%	83%	82%
Home Recovery Information Given	300+	83%	84%	85%
Hospital Given 9 or 10 on 10 Point Scale	300+	66%	69%	71%
Meds 'Always' Explained Before Given	300+	64%	63%	64%
Nurses 'Always' Communicated Well	300+	81%	78%	79%
Pain 'Always' Well Controlled	300+	72%	71%	71%
Room and Bathroom 'Always' Clean	300+	72%	71%	73%
Timely Help 'Always' Received	300+	65%	65%	68%
Would Definitely Recommend Hospital	300+	68%	70%	71%
Use of Medical Imaging				
Cardiac Imaging Stress Test before Surgery	897	5.2%	5.5%	5.3%
Combination Abdominal CT Scan	1,386	6.1%	10.1%	10.5%
Combination Brain/Sinus CT Scan	1,107	3.3%	2.3%	2.7%
Combination Chest CT Scan	1,187	1.3%	3.7%	2.7%
Follow-up Mammogram/Ultrasound	3,212	6.1%	8.9%	8.8%
Lumbar Spine MRI for Low Back Pain	121	33.9%	36.6%	37.2%

Bacon County Hospital

302 South Wayne Street
Alma, GA 31510
Phone: 912-632-8961
Fax: 912-632-5000
E-mail: administration@bchsi.org
URL: www.baconcountyhospital.com
Type: Critical Access Hospitals
Emergency Services: Yes
Ownership: Voluntary non-profit - Other
Beds: 50

Key Personnel:

CEO/President. . . . . O J Booker
Quality Assurance . . . . Deanne Flanders
CEO . . . . Cindy R. Turner

Measure	Cases	This Hosp.	State Avg.	U.S. Avg.
Blood Clot Prevention and Treatment				
Anticoagulation Overlap Therapy[5]	-	-	90%	93%
ICU Venous Thromboembolism Prophylaxis[5]	-	-	90%	92%
Incidence of Potentially Preventable VTE[5]	-	-	13%	10%
UFH with Dosages/Platelet Monitoring[5]	-	-	99%	97%
Venous Thromboembolism Prophylaxis[5]	-	-	80%	85%
Warfarin Therapy Discharge Instructions[5]	-	-	78%	75%
Chest Pain/Possible Heart Attack Care				
Aspirin Given Within 24 Hours of Arrival	21	100%	94%	96%
Fibrinolytic Meds Within 30 Min. of Arrival[1]	-	-	35%	58%
Average Time to ECG (minutes)	26	17	8	7
Average Time to Transfer (minutes)[1]	-	-	73	60
Children's Asthma Care				
Received Home Management Plan of Care	-	-	-	88%
Received Reliever Medication	-	-	-	100%

NOTE: Hospital profiles are in alphabetical order by state, then city, then hospital within the city; Rankings exclude hospitals with less than 25 cases except for patient surveys which excludes hospitals with less than 100 cases; (a) 100-299 cases; (1) The number of cases/patients is too few to report; (2) Data submitted were based on a sample of cases/patients; (3) Results are based on a shorter time period than required; (4) Data suppressed by CMS for one or more quarters; (5) Results are not available for this reporting period; (6) Fewer than 100 patients completed the HCAHPS survey; (7) No cases met the criteria for this measure; (8) The lower limit of the confidence interval cannot be calculated if the number of observed infections equals zero; (9) No data are available from the state/territory for this reporting period; (10) The scores shown reflect fewer than 50 completed surveys; (11) There were discrepancies in the data collection process; (12) This measure does not apply to this hospital for this reporting period; (13) Results cannot be calculated for this reporting period; (14) The results for this state are combined with nearby states to protect confidentiality; Please refer to the User's Guide for a full explanation of data.

Measure	Cases	This Hosp.	State Avg.	U.S. Avg.
Received Systemic Corticosteroids	-	-	-	100%
Emergency Department				
Admittance Decision Time (minutes)[2]	235	49	100	98
Head CT Results Within 45 Min. of Arrival[1]	-	-	45%	57%
Patients Who Left ER Before Being Seen	7,994	1%	3%	2%
Time from ER Arrival to Admit. (minutes)[2]	257	208	286	274
Time from ER Arrival to Discharge (minutes)	411	112	140	134
Time in ER Before Being Evaluated (minutes)	401	32	32	26
Time to Pain Meds for Fractures (minutes)	36	44	64	57
Heart Attack Care				
Aspirin Given at Discharge[5]	-	-	99%	99%
Fibrinolytic Meds Within 30 Min. of Arrival[5]	-	-	80%	54%
PCI Within 90 Minutes of Arrival[5]	-	-	95%	96%
Statin Prescribed at Discharge[5]	-	-	98%	98%
Heart Failure Care				
ACE Inhibitor or ARB for LVSD[1,3]	-	-	97%	97%
Discharge Instructions Given[3]	13	100%	92%	94%
Evaluation of LVS Function[3]	14	100%	99%	99%
Medicare Spending				
Medicare Spending per Patient (ratio)	-	-	0.95	0.98
Pneumonia Care				
Appropriate Initial Antibiotic Given	44	89%	95%	95%
Blood Culture Timing	36	83%	97%	98%
Pregnancy and Delivery Care				
Newborn Deliveries Scheduled Early[5]	-	-	8%	6%
Preventive Care				
Immunization for Influenza[2]	378	76%	88%	90%
Immunization for Pneumonia[2]	465	89%	90%	92%
Stroke Care				
Anticoagulation Therapy for Atrial Fibrillation[5]	-	-	94%	95%
Antithrombotic Therapy Timing[5]	-	-	97%	98%
Assessed for Rehabilitation[5]	-	-	97%	97%
Discharged on Antithrombotic Therapy[5]	-	-	98%	99%
Discharged on Statin Medication[5]	-	-	94%	94%
Thrombolytic Therapy Timing[5]	-	-	58%	66%
Venous Thromboembolism Prophylaxis[5]	-	-	92%	94%
Written Stroke Educational Materials Given[5]	-	-	84%	88%
Surgical Care Improvement Project				
Appropriate Beta Blocker Usage	24	100%	97%	98%
Appropriate VTP Within 24 Hours[3]	14	100%	98%	98%
Controlled Postoperative Blood Glucose[7]	-	-	96%	97%
Perioperative Temperature Management	75	100%	100%	100%
Prophylactic Antibiotic Selection[3]	11	100%	99%	99%
Prophylactic Antibiotic Selection (Outpatient)	13	100%	98%	98%
Prophylactic Antibiotic Stopped[3]	11	100%	98%	98%
Prophylactic Antibiotic Timing[3]	11	91%	99%	99%
Prophylactic Antibiotic Timing (Outpatient)	15	87%	98%	98%
Urinary Catheter Removal	14	86%	97%	97%
Survey of Patients' Hospital Experiences				
Area Around Room 'Always' Quiet at Night	(a)	78%	66%	61%
Doctors 'Always' Communicated Well	(a)	89%	83%	82%
Home Recovery Information Given	(a)	85%	84%	85%
Hospital Given 9 or 10 on 10 Point Scale	(a)	79%	69%	71%
Meds 'Always' Explained Before Given	(a)	69%	63%	64%
Nurses 'Always' Communicated Well	(a)	85%	78%	79%
Pain 'Always' Well Controlled	(a)	77%	71%	71%
Room and Bathroom 'Always' Clean	(a)	76%	71%	73%
Timely Help 'Always' Received	(a)	72%	65%	68%
Would Definitely Recommend Hospital	(a)	77%	70%	71%
Use of Medical Imaging				
Cardiac Imaging Stress Test before Surgery[7]	-	-	5.5%	5.3%
Combination Abdominal CT Scan	130	5.4%	10.1%	10.5%
Combination Brain/Sinus CT Scan[1]	-	-	2.3%	2.7%
Combination Chest CT Scan	83	36.1%	3.7%	2.7%
Follow-up Mammogram/Ultrasound	190	9.5%	8.9%	8.8%
Lumbar Spine MRI for Low Back Pain	36	50.0%	36.6%	37.2%

Phoebe Sumter Medical Center

126 Highway 280 W
Americus, GA 31719
Phone: 229-931-1280
Fax: 229-931-1125
Type: Acute Care Hospitals
Emergency Services: Yes
Ownership: Govt - Hospital Dist/Auth
Beds: 143

Key Personnel:

Radiology. . . . . Timothy Baker, MD
Pediatric Ambulatory Care . . . . . . Andrew Carlson, MD
Pediatric In-Patient Care . . . . Andrew Carlson, MD
Chairman/CEO . . . . John Culbreath
Chief of Medical Staff. . . . . Frank Middleton, MD
Operating Room. . . . . Fran Parker
Quality Assurance . . . . Rebecca Smith
CEO/President. . . . . Joel Wernick

Measure	Cases	This Hosp.	State Avg.	U.S. Avg.
Blood Clot Prevention and Treatment				
Anticoagulation Overlap Therapy[2]	15	87%	90%	93%
ICU Venous Thromboembolism Prophylaxis[2]	93	95%	90%	92%
Incidence of Potentially Preventable VTE[1,2]	-	-	13%	10%
UFH with Dosages/Platelet Monitoring[1,2]	-	-	99%	97%
Venous Thromboembolism Prophylaxis[2]	213	85%	80%	85%
Warfarin Therapy Discharge Instructions[2]	13	38%	78%	75%
Chest Pain/Possible Heart Attack Care				
Aspirin Given Within 24 Hours of Arrival	52	94%	94%	96%
Fibrinolytic Meds Within 30 Min. of Arrival[1]	-	-	35%	58%
Average Time to ECG (minutes)	53	10	8	7
Average Time to Transfer (minutes)[1]	-	-	73	60
Children's Asthma Care				
Received Home Management Plan of Care	-	-	-	88%
Received Reliever Medication	-	-	-	100%
Received Systemic Corticosteroids	-	-	-	100%
Emergency Department				
Admittance Decision Time (minutes)[2]	510	125	100	98
Head CT Results Within 45 Min. of Arrival[1]	-	-	45%	57%
Patients Who Left ER Before Being Seen	23,329	2%	3%	2%
Time from ER Arrival to Admit. (minutes)[2]	516	298	286	274
Time from ER Arrival to Discharge (minutes)	419	148	140	134
Time in ER Before Being Evaluated (minutes)	437	30	32	26
Time to Pain Meds for Fractures (minutes)	92	74	64	57
Heart Attack Care				
Aspirin Given at Discharge[1]	-	-	99%	99%
Fibrinolytic Meds Within 30 Min. of Arrival[7]	-	-	80%	54%
PCI Within 90 Minutes of Arrival[7]	-	-	95%	96%
Statin Prescribed at Discharge[1]	-	-	98%	98%
Heart Failure Care				
ACE Inhibitor or ARB for LVSD	49	96%	97%	97%
Discharge Instructions Given	131	97%	92%	94%
Evaluation of LVS Function	145	99%	99%	99%
Medicare Spending				
Medicare Spending per Patient (ratio)	-	0.95	0.95	0.98
Pneumonia Care				
Appropriate Initial Antibiotic Given	33	88%	95%	95%
Blood Culture Timing	58	97%	97%	98%
Pregnancy and Delivery Care				
Newborn Deliveries Scheduled Early	34	0%	8%	6%
Preventive Care				
Immunization for Influenza[2]	410	89%	88%	90%
Immunization for Pneumonia[2]	449	88%	90%	92%
Stroke Care				
Anticoagulation Therapy for Atrial Fibrillation[1,2]	-	-	94%	95%
Antithrombotic Therapy Timing[2]	54	96%	97%	98%
Assessed for Rehabilitation[2]	63	98%	97%	97%
Discharged on Antithrombotic Therapy[2]	61	100%	98%	99%
Discharged on Statin Medication[2]	53	92%	94%	94%
Thrombolytic Therapy Timing[1,2]	-	-	58%	66%
Venous Thromboembolism Prophylaxis[2]	60	80%	92%	94%
Written Stroke Educational Materials Given[2]	41	29%	84%	88%
Surgical Care Improvement Project				
Appropriate Beta Blocker Usage	44	100%	97%	98%
Appropriate VTP Within 24 Hours	165	99%	98%	98%
Controlled Postoperative Blood Glucose[7]	-	-	96%	97%
Perioperative Temperature Management	171	100%	100%	100%
Prophylactic Antibiotic Selection	121	97%	99%	99%
Prophylactic Antibiotic Selection (Outpatient)	82	96%	98%	98%
Prophylactic Antibiotic Stopped	116	95%	98%	98%
Prophylactic Antibiotic Timing	121	98%	99%	99%
Prophylactic Antibiotic Timing (Outpatient)	69	90%	98%	98%
Urinary Catheter Removal	126	93%	97%	97%
Survey of Patients' Hospital Experiences				
Area Around Room 'Always' Quiet at Night	300+	78%	66%	61%
Doctors 'Always' Communicated Well	300+	82%	83%	82%
Home Recovery Information Given	300+	79%	84%	85%
Hospital Given 9 or 10 on 10 Point Scale	300+	73%	69%	71%
Meds 'Always' Explained Before Given	300+	65%	63%	64%
Nurses 'Always' Communicated Well	300+	81%	78%	79%
Pain 'Always' Well Controlled	300+	71%	71%	71%
Room and Bathroom 'Always' Clean	300+	77%	71%	73%
Timely Help 'Always' Received	300+	63%	65%	68%
Would Definitely Recommend Hospital	300+	71%	70%	71%
Use of Medical Imaging				
Cardiac Imaging Stress Test before Surgery[1]	-	-	5.5%	5.3%
Combination Abdominal CT Scan	345	2.0%	10.1%	10.5%
Combination Brain/Sinus CT Scan	406	6.2%	2.3%	2.7%
Combination Chest CT Scan	221	0.0%	3.7%	2.7%
Follow-up Mammogram/Ultrasound	693	12.3%	8.9%	8.8%
Lumbar Spine MRI for Low Back Pain[1]	-	-	36.6%	37.2%

Athens Regional Medical Center

1199 Prince Avenue
Athens, GA 30606
Phone: 706-475-7000
Fax: 706-475-3305
URL: www.armc.org
Type: Acute Care Hospitals
Emergency Services: Yes
Ownership: Voluntary non-profit - Other
Beds: 315

Key Personnel:

Intensive Care Unit. . . . . Antonio Ararta
Radiology. . . . . Bill Ashley
CEO/President. . . . . John A Drew
Emergency Room . . . . Carolann Eisnhart, MD
Pediatric In-Patient Care . . . . Pat Nielson
Anesthesiology. . . . . Lisa Remedis, MD
Quality Assurance . . . . Diane Todd
Patient Relations . . . . Brian Williams

Measure	Cases	This Hosp.	State Avg.	U.S. Avg.
Blood Clot Prevention and Treatment				
Anticoagulation Overlap Therapy[2]	140	99%	90%	93%
ICU Venous Thromboembolism Prophylaxis[2]	92	84%	90%	92%
Incidence of Potentially Preventable VTE[2]	22	9%	13%	10%
UFH with Dosages/Platelet Monitoring[2]	115	100%	99%	97%
Venous Thromboembolism Prophylaxis[2]	316	77%	80%	85%
Warfarin Therapy Discharge Instructions[2]	111	9%	78%	75%
Chest Pain/Possible Heart Attack Care				
Aspirin Given Within 24 Hours of Arrival[5]	-	-	94%	96%
Fibrinolytic Meds Within 30 Min. of Arrival[5]	-	-	35%	58%
Average Time to ECG (minutes)[5]	-	-	8	7
Average Time to Transfer (minutes)[5]	-	-	73	60
Children's Asthma Care				
Received Home Management Plan of Care	-	-	-	88%
Received Reliever Medication	-	-	-	100%
Received Systemic Corticosteroids	-	-	-	100%
Emergency Department				
Admittance Decision Time (minutes)[2]	478	115	100	98
Head CT Results Within 45 Min. of Arrival	16	31%	45%	57%
Patients Who Left ER Before Being Seen	78,426	2%	3%	2%
Time from ER Arrival to Admit. (minutes)[2]	482	270	286	274
Time from ER Arrival to Discharge (minutes)	305	161	140	134
Time in ER Before Being Evaluated (minutes)	332	25	32	26
Time to Pain Meds for Fractures (minutes)	189	53	64	57
Heart Attack Care				
Aspirin Given at Discharge[2]	277	100%	99%	99%
Fibrinolytic Meds Within 30 Min. of Arrival[2,7]	-	-	80%	54%
PCI Within 90 Minutes of Arrival[2]	45	100%	95%	96%
Statin Prescribed at Discharge[2]	273	100%	98%	98%
Heart Failure Care				
ACE Inhibitor or ARB for LVSD[2]	67	96%	97%	97%
Discharge Instructions Given[2]	256	86%	92%	94%
Evaluation of LVS Function[2]	287	100%	99%	99%
Medicare Spending				
Medicare Spending per Patient (ratio)	-	0.92	0.95	0.98
Pneumonia Care				
Appropriate Initial Antibiotic Given[2]	89	98%	95%	95%
Blood Culture Timing[2]	95	99%	97%	98%
Pregnancy and Delivery Care				
Newborn Deliveries Scheduled Early	218	14%	8%	6%
Preventive Care				

NOTE: Hospital profiles are in alphabetical order by state, then city, then hospital within the city; Rankings exclude hospitals with less than 25 cases except for patient surveys which excludes hospitals with less than 100 cases; (a) 100-299 cases; (1) The number of cases/patients is too few to report; (2) Data submitted were based on a sample of cases/patients; (3) Results are based on a shorter time period than required; (4) Data suppressed by CMS for one or more quarters; (5) Results are not available for this reporting period; (6) Fewer than 100 patients completed the HCAHPS survey; (7) No cases met the criteria for this measure; (8) The lower limit of the confidence interval cannot be calculated if the number of observed infections equals zero; (9) No data are available from the state/territory for this reporting period; (10) The scores shown reflect fewer than 50 completed surveys; (11) There were discrepancies in the data collection process; (12) This measure does not apply to this hospital for this reporting period; (13) Results cannot be calculated for this reporting period; (14) The results for this state are combined with nearby states to protect confidentiality; Please refer to the User's Guide for a full explanation of data.

Measure	Cases	This Hosp.	State Avg.	U.S. Avg.
Immunization for Influenza[2]	505	75%	88%	90%
Immunization for Pneumonia[2]	679	86%	90%	92%
Stroke Care				
Anticoagulation Therapy for Atrial Fibrillation[1,2]	-	-	94%	95%
Antithrombotic Therapy Timing[2]	74	99%	97%	98%
Assessed for Rehabilitation[2]	94	100%	97%	97%
Discharged on Antithrombotic Therapy[2]	81	100%	98%	99%
Discharged on Statin Medication[2]	64	98%	94%	94%
Thrombolytic Therapy Timing[1,2]	-	-	58%	66%
Venous Thromboembolism Prophylaxis[2]	80	96%	92%	94%
Written Stroke Educational Materials Given[2]	62	92%	84%	88%
Surgical Care Improvement Project				
Appropriate Beta Blocker Usage[2]	214	96%	97%	98%
Appropriate VTP Within 24 Hours[2]	383	95%	98%	98%
Controlled Postoperative Blood Glucose[2]	111	96%	96%	97%
Perioperative Temperature Management[2]	492	100%	100%	100%
Prophylactic Antibiotic Selection[2]	362	99%	99%	99%
Prophylactic Antibiotic Selection (Outpatient)	465	97%	98%	98%
Prophylactic Antibiotic Stopped[2]	346	96%	98%	98%
Prophylactic Antibiotic Timing[2]	362	99%	99%	99%
Prophylactic Antibiotic Timing (Outpatient)	467	95%	98%	98%
Urinary Catheter Removal[2]	299	95%	97%	97%
Survey of Patients' Hospital Experiences				
Area Around Room 'Always' Quiet at Night	300+	67%	66%	61%
Doctors 'Always' Communicated Well	300+	82%	83%	82%
Home Recovery Information Given	300+	85%	84%	85%
Hospital Given 9 or 10 on 10 Point Scale	300+	76%	69%	71%
Meds 'Always' Explained Before Given	300+	63%	63%	64%
Nurses 'Always' Communicated Well	300+	83%	78%	79%
Pain 'Always' Well Controlled	300+	72%	71%	71%
Room and Bathroom 'Always' Clean	300+	74%	71%	73%
Timely Help 'Always' Received	300+	66%	65%	68%
Would Definitely Recommend Hospital	300+	80%	70%	71%
Use of Medical Imaging				
Cardiac Imaging Stress Test before Surgery	409	6.8%	5.5%	5.3%
Combination Abdominal CT Scan	1,625	5.7%	10.1%	10.5%
Combination Brain/Sinus CT Scan	1,219	0.8%	2.3%	2.7%
Combination Chest CT Scan	1,557	0.1%	3.7%	2.7%
Follow-up Mammogram/Ultrasound	2,887	6.9%	8.9%	8.8%
Lumbar Spine MRI for Low Back Pain	175	36.6%	36.6%	37.2%

Saint Mary's Hospital

1230 Baxter Street
Athens, GA 30606
Phone: 706-389-3930
Fax: 706-354-3197
Type: Acute Care Hospitals
Emergency Services: Yes
Ownership: Voluntary non-profit - Private
Beds: 196

Key Personnel:

Radiology. . . . . Jimmy Deason, MD
Quality Assurance . . . . Jeff Freshe
President/CEO. . . . . Don McKenna, FACHE
Operating Room. . . . . Pat Thaler
Emergency Room . . . . Maelene Vacquez

Measure	Cases	This Hosp.	State Avg.	U.S. Avg.
Blood Clot Prevention and Treatment				
Anticoagulation Overlap Therapy[2]	54	96%	90%	93%
ICU Venous Thromboembolism Prophylaxis[2]	73	93%	90%	92%
Incidence of Potentially Preventable VTE[1,2]	-	-	13%	10%
UFH with Dosages/Platelet Monitoring[2]	39	100%	99%	97%
Venous Thromboembolism Prophylaxis[2]	248	89%	80%	85%
Warfarin Therapy Discharge Instructions[2]	37	65%	78%	75%
Chest Pain/Possible Heart Attack Care				
Aspirin Given Within 24 Hours of Arrival[1,3]	-	-	94%	96%
Fibrinolytic Meds Within 30 Min. of Arrival[3,7]	-	-	35%	58%
Average Time to ECG (minutes)[1,3]	-	-	8	7
Average Time to Transfer (minutes)[3,7]	-	-	73	60
Children's Asthma Care				
Received Home Management Plan of Care	-	-	-	88%
Received Reliever Medication	-	-	-	100%
Received Systemic Corticosteroids	-	-	-	100%
Emergency Department				
Admittance Decision Time (minutes)[2]	452	118	100	98
Head CT Results Within 45 Min. of Arrival[1]	-	-	45%	57%
Patients Who Left ER Before Being Seen	40,033	2%	3%	2%
Time from ER Arrival to Admit. (minutes)[2]	463	254	286	274
Time from ER Arrival to Discharge (minutes)	407	134	140	134
Time in ER Before Being Evaluated (minutes)	412	29	32	26
Time to Pain Meds for Fractures (minutes)	93	60	64	57
Heart Attack Care				
Aspirin Given at Discharge	144	100%	99%	99%
Fibrinolytic Meds Within 30 Min. of Arrival[7]	-	-	80%	54%
PCI Within 90 Minutes of Arrival	23	96%	95%	96%
Statin Prescribed at Discharge	141	100%	98%	98%
Heart Failure Care				
ACE Inhibitor or ARB for LVSD	48	100%	97%	97%
Discharge Instructions Given	150	98%	92%	94%
Evaluation of LVS Function	165	100%	99%	99%
Medicare Spending				
Medicare Spending per Patient (ratio)	-	0.95	0.95	0.98
Pneumonia Care				
Appropriate Initial Antibiotic Given	73	100%	95%	95%
Blood Culture Timing	137	99%	97%	98%
Pregnancy and Delivery Care				
Newborn Deliveries Scheduled Early	101	3%	8%	6%
Preventive Care				
Immunization for Influenza[2]	540	95%	88%	90%
Immunization for Pneumonia[2]	675	93%	90%	92%
Stroke Care				
Anticoagulation Therapy for Atrial Fibrillation	16	100%	94%	95%
Antithrombotic Therapy Timing	135	91%	97%	98%
Assessed for Rehabilitation	156	99%	97%	97%
Discharged on Antithrombotic Therapy	133	98%	98%	99%
Discharged on Statin Medication	104	93%	94%	94%
Thrombolytic Therapy Timing	11	73%	58%	66%
Venous Thromboembolism Prophylaxis	162	96%	92%	94%
Written Stroke Educational Materials Given	77	95%	84%	88%
Surgical Care Improvement Project				
Appropriate Beta Blocker Usage[2]	172	94%	97%	98%
Appropriate VTP Within 24 Hours[2]	500	97%	98%	98%
Controlled Postoperative Blood Glucose[2,7]	-	-	96%	97%
Perioperative Temperature Management[2]	554	100%	100%	100%
Prophylactic Antibiotic Selection[2]	392	99%	99%	99%
Prophylactic Antibiotic Selection (Outpatient)	389	99%	98%	98%
Prophylactic Antibiotic Stopped[2]	384	97%	98%	98%
Prophylactic Antibiotic Timing[2]	392	99%	99%	99%
Prophylactic Antibiotic Timing (Outpatient)	392	99%	98%	98%
Urinary Catheter Removal[2]	100	90%	97%	97%
Survey of Patients' Hospital Experiences				
Area Around Room 'Always' Quiet at Night	300+	68%	66%	61%
Doctors 'Always' Communicated Well	300+	81%	83%	82%
Home Recovery Information Given	300+	88%	84%	85%
Hospital Given 9 or 10 on 10 Point Scale	300+	77%	69%	71%
Meds 'Always' Explained Before Given	300+	68%	63%	64%
Nurses 'Always' Communicated Well	300+	79%	78%	79%
Pain 'Always' Well Controlled	300+	74%	71%	71%
Room and Bathroom 'Always' Clean	300+	70%	71%	73%
Timely Help 'Always' Received	300+	64%	65%	68%
Would Definitely Recommend Hospital	300+	81%	70%	71%
Use of Medical Imaging				
Cardiac Imaging Stress Test before Surgery	626	5.4%	5.5%	5.3%
Combination Abdominal CT Scan	431	1.9%	10.1%	10.5%
Combination Brain/Sinus CT Scan	465	2.2%	2.3%	2.7%
Combination Chest CT Scan	240	0.0%	3.7%	2.7%
Follow-up Mammogram/Ultrasound	1,836	6.4%	8.9%	8.8%
Lumbar Spine MRI for Low Back Pain	68	29.4%	36.6%	37.2%

Atlanta Medical Center

303 Parkway Dr Ne
Atlanta, GA 30312
Phone: 404-265-4000
Fax: 404-265-3903
URL: www.atlantamedcenter.com
Type: Acute Care Hospitals
Emergency Services: Yes
Ownership: Proprietary
Beds: 403

Key Personnel:

Quality Assurance . . . . Deena Allen
Operating Room. . . . . Barbara Comer
CEO/President. . . . . Trevor Fetter
Anesthesiology. . . . . Julius Hill, III, MD
Chief of Medical Staff. . . . . Paul Krissman
Intensive Care Unit. . . . . Julie Lewis
Radiology. . . . . Larry Ray, MD
Emergency Room . . . . Mark Waterman

Measure	Cases	This Hosp.	State Avg.	U.S. Avg.
Blood Clot Prevention and Treatment				
Anticoagulation Overlap Therapy[2]	91	87%	90%	93%
ICU Venous Thromboembolism Prophylaxis[2]	149	89%	90%	92%
Incidence of Potentially Preventable VTE[2]	29	3%	13%	10%
UFH with Dosages/Platelet Monitoring[2]	66	97%	99%	97%
Venous Thromboembolism Prophylaxis[2]	280	75%	80%	85%
Warfarin Therapy Discharge Instructions[2]	67	55%	78%	75%
Chest Pain/Possible Heart Attack Care				
Aspirin Given Within 24 Hours of Arrival[1,3]	-	-	94%	96%
Fibrinolytic Meds Within 30 Min. of Arrival[3,7]	-	-	35%	58%
Average Time to ECG (minutes)[1,3]	-	-	8	7
Average Time to Transfer (minutes)[3,7]	-	-	73	60
Children's Asthma Care				
Received Home Management Plan of Care	-	-	-	88%
Received Reliever Medication	-	-	-	100%
Received Systemic Corticosteroids	-	-	-	100%
Emergency Department				
Admittance Decision Time (minutes)[2]	568	207	100	98
Head CT Results Within 45 Min. of Arrival[1]	-	-	45%	57%
Patients Who Left ER Before Being Seen	58,630	3%	3%	2%
Time from ER Arrival to Admit. (minutes)[2]	573	417	286	274
Time from ER Arrival to Discharge (minutes)	458	147	140	134
Time in ER Before Being Evaluated (minutes)	486	32	32	26
Time to Pain Meds for Fractures (minutes)	133	62	64	57
Heart Attack Care				
Aspirin Given at Discharge	112	100%	99%	99%
Fibrinolytic Meds Within 30 Min. of Arrival[1]	-	-	80%	54%
PCI Within 90 Minutes of Arrival	28	82%	95%	96%
Statin Prescribed at Discharge	115	98%	98%	98%
Heart Failure Care				
ACE Inhibitor or ARB for LVSD	227	100%	97%	97%
Discharge Instructions Given	460	97%	92%	94%
Evaluation of LVS Function	517	100%	99%	99%
Medicare Spending				
Medicare Spending per Patient (ratio)	-	1.05	0.95	0.98
Pneumonia Care				
Appropriate Initial Antibiotic Given[2]	171	97%	95%	95%
Blood Culture Timing[2]	252	99%	97%	98%
Pregnancy and Delivery Care				
Newborn Deliveries Scheduled Early[2]	79	3%	8%	6%
Preventive Care				
Immunization for Influenza[2]	505	83%	88%	90%
Immunization for Pneumonia[2]	472	90%	90%	92%
Stroke Care				
Anticoagulation Therapy for Atrial Fibrillation[2]	20	100%	94%	95%
Antithrombotic Therapy Timing[2]	171	98%	97%	98%
Assessed for Rehabilitation[2]	230	99%	97%	97%
Discharged on Antithrombotic Therapy[2]	178	99%	98%	99%
Discharged on Statin Medication[2]	132	99%	94%	94%
Thrombolytic Therapy Timing[2]	17	94%	58%	66%
Venous Thromboembolism Prophylaxis[2]	259	98%	92%	94%
Written Stroke Educational Materials Given[2]	145	89%	84%	88%
Surgical Care Improvement Project				
Appropriate Beta Blocker Usage[2]	119	98%	97%	98%
Appropriate VTP Within 24 Hours[2]	427	99%	98%	98%
Controlled Postoperative Blood Glucose[2]	28	89%	96%	97%
Perioperative Temperature Management[2]	557	100%	100%	100%
Prophylactic Antibiotic Selection[2]	355	99%	99%	99%
Prophylactic Antibiotic Selection (Outpatient)	202	99%	98%	98%
Prophylactic Antibiotic Stopped[2]	344	97%	98%	98%
Prophylactic Antibiotic Timing[2]	355	99%	99%	99%
Prophylactic Antibiotic Timing (Outpatient)	203	98%	98%	98%
Urinary Catheter Removal[2]	235	97%	97%	97%
Survey of Patients' Hospital Experiences				
Area Around Room 'Always' Quiet at Night	300+	63%	66%	61%
Doctors 'Always' Communicated Well	300+	80%	83%	82%
Home Recovery Information Given	300+	81%	84%	85%
Hospital Given 9 or 10 on 10 Point Scale	300+	62%	69%	71%
Meds 'Always' Explained Before Given	300+	60%	63%	64%

NOTE: Hospital profiles are in alphabetical order by state, then city, then hospital within the city; Rankings exclude hospitals with less than 25 cases except for patient surveys which excludes hospitals with less than 100 cases; (a) 100-299 cases; (1) The number of cases/patients is too few to report; (2) Data submitted were based on a sample of cases/patients; (3) Results are based on a shorter time period than required; (4) Data suppressed by CMS for one or more quarters; (5) Results are not available for this reporting period; (6) Fewer than 100 patients completed the HCAHPS survey; (7) No cases met the criteria for this measure; (8) The lower limit of the confidence interval cannot be calculated if the number of observed infections equals zero; (9) No data are available from the state/territory for this reporting period; (10) The scores shown reflect fewer than 50 completed surveys; (11) There were discrepancies in the data collection process; (12) This measure does not apply to this hospital for this reporting period; (13) Results cannot be calculated for this reporting period; (14) The results for this state are combined with nearby states to protect confidentiality; Please refer to the User's Guide for a full explanation of data.

Measure	Cases	This Hosp.	State Avg.	U.S. Avg.
Nurses 'Always' Communicated Well	300+	75%	78%	79%
Pain 'Always' Well Controlled	300+	70%	71%	71%
Room and Bathroom 'Always' Clean	300+	68%	71%	73%
Timely Help 'Always' Received	300+	58%	65%	68%
Would Definitely Recommend Hospital	300+	63%	70%	71%
Use of Medical Imaging				
Cardiac Imaging Stress Test before Surgery	155	6.5%	5.5%	5.3%
Combination Abdominal CT Scan	431	5.1%	10.1%	10.5%
Combination Brain/Sinus CT Scan	466	1.1%	2.3%	2.7%
Combination Chest CT Scan	150	4.0%	3.7%	2.7%
Follow-up Mammogram/Ultrasound	765	4.2%	8.9%	8.8%
Lumbar Spine MRI for Low Back Pain	44	40.9%	36.6%	37.2%

Emory University Hospital

1364 Clifton Road, Ne
Atlanta, GA 30322
Phone: 404-686-8500
Fax: 404-778-7327
URL: www.emoryhealthcare.org
Type: Acute Care Hospitals
Emergency Services: Yes
Ownership: Voluntary non-profit - Private
Beds: 587

Key Personnel:

Cardiac Laboratory............ June Connor
CEO/President................ John T Fox
Infection Control.............. Betsy Hackman
Quality Assurance .... Babs Hargett
Radiology.................. Sanjay Saini, MD
Chief of Medical Staff.......... Robert B Smith III, MD
Pediatric In-Patient Care .... Barbara Stoll, MD
Operating Room.............. Jane Vosloh

Measure	Cases	This Hosp.	State Avg.	U.S. Avg.
Blood Clot Prevention and Treatment				
Anticoagulation Overlap Therapy[2]	164	91%	90%	93%
ICU Venous Thromboembolism Prophylaxis[2]	78	94%	90%	92%
Incidence of Potentially Preventable VTE[2]	71	7%	13%	10%
UFH with Dosages/Platelet Monitoring[2]	157	100%	99%	97%
Venous Thromboembolism Prophylaxis[2]	309	93%	80%	85%
Warfarin Therapy Discharge Instructions[2]	121	61%	78%	75%
Chest Pain/Possible Heart Attack Care				
Aspirin Given Within 24 Hours of Arrival[1,3]	-	-	94%	96%
Fibrinolytic Meds Within 30 Min. of Arrival[3,7]	-	-	35%	58%
Average Time to ECG (minutes)[1,3]	-	-	8	7
Average Time to Transfer (minutes)[3,7]	-	-	73	60
Children's Asthma Care				
Received Home Management Plan of Care	-	-	-	88%
Received Reliever Medication	-	-	-	100%
Received Systemic Corticosteroids	-	-	-	100%
Emergency Department				
Admittance Decision Time (minutes)[2]	364	152	100	98
Head CT Results Within 45 Min. of Arrival[1]	-	-	45%	57%
Patients Who Left ER Before Being Seen	37,754	2%	3%	2%
Time from ER Arrival to Admit. (minutes)[2]	378	408	286	274
Time from ER Arrival to Discharge (minutes)	347	324	140	134
Time in ER Before Being Evaluated (minutes)	365	86	32	26
Time to Pain Meds for Fractures (minutes)	29	117	64	57
Heart Attack Care				
Aspirin Given at Discharge[2]	271	100%	99%	99%
Fibrinolytic Meds Within 30 Min. of Arrival[2,7]	-	-	80%	54%
PCI Within 90 Minutes of Arrival[2]	26	100%	95%	96%
Statin Prescribed at Discharge[2]	256	100%	98%	98%
Heart Failure Care				
ACE Inhibitor or ARB for LVSD[2]	70	100%	97%	97%
Discharge Instructions Given[2]	242	99%	92%	94%
Evaluation of LVS Function[2]	272	100%	99%	99%
Medicare Spending				
Medicare Spending per Patient (ratio)	-	0.96	0.95	0.98
Pneumonia Care				
Appropriate Initial Antibiotic Given[2]	42	98%	95%	95%
Blood Culture Timing[2]	90	97%	97%	98%
Pregnancy and Delivery Care				
Newborn Deliveries Scheduled Early[7]	-	-	8%	6%
Preventive Care				
Immunization for Influenza[2]	591	97%	88%	90%
Immunization for Pneumonia[2]	703	97%	90%	92%
Stroke Care				
Anticoagulation Therapy for Atrial Fibrillation[1,2]	-	-	94%	95%
Antithrombotic Therapy Timing[2]	48	96%	97%	98%
Assessed for Rehabilitation[2]	127	99%	97%	97%
Discharged on Antithrombotic Therapy[2]	61	100%	98%	99%
Discharged on Statin Medication[2]	44	98%	94%	94%
Thrombolytic Therapy Timing[1,2]	-	-	58%	66%
Venous Thromboembolism Prophylaxis[2]	129	98%	92%	94%
Written Stroke Educational Materials Given[2]	75	91%	84%	88%
Surgical Care Improvement Project				
Appropriate Beta Blocker Usage[2]	199	98%	97%	98%
Appropriate VTP Within 24 Hours[2]	417	100%	98%	98%
Controlled Postoperative Blood Glucose[2]	90	98%	96%	97%
Perioperative Temperature Management[2]	600	100%	100%	100%
Prophylactic Antibiotic Selection[2]	364	99%	99%	99%
Prophylactic Antibiotic Selection (Outpatient)	550	99%	98%	98%
Prophylactic Antibiotic Stopped[2]	350	99%	98%	98%
Prophylactic Antibiotic Timing[2]	364	99%	99%	99%
Prophylactic Antibiotic Timing (Outpatient)	557	96%	98%	98%
Urinary Catheter Removal[2]	233	97%	97%	97%
Survey of Patients' Hospital Experiences				
Area Around Room 'Always' Quiet at Night	300+	71%	66%	61%
Doctors 'Always' Communicated Well	300+	86%	83%	82%
Home Recovery Information Given	300+	86%	84%	85%
Hospital Given 9 or 10 on 10 Point Scale	300+	82%	69%	71%
Meds 'Always' Explained Before Given	300+	70%	63%	64%
Nurses 'Always' Communicated Well	300+	81%	78%	79%
Pain 'Always' Well Controlled	300+	75%	71%	71%
Room and Bathroom 'Always' Clean	300+	75%	71%	73%
Timely Help 'Always' Received	300+	71%	65%	68%
Would Definitely Recommend Hospital	300+	86%	70%	71%
Use of Medical Imaging				
Cardiac Imaging Stress Test before Surgery	842	7.4%	5.5%	5.3%
Combination Abdominal CT Scan	1,944	14.2%	10.1%	10.5%
Combination Brain/Sinus CT Scan	867	1.6%	2.3%	2.7%
Combination Chest CT Scan	3,002	0.1%	3.7%	2.7%
Follow-up Mammogram/Ultrasound	2,385	9.2%	8.9%	8.8%
Lumbar Spine MRI for Low Back Pain	422	36.3%	36.6%	37.2%

Emory University Hospital Midtown

550 Peachtree Saint Ne
Atlanta, GA 30308
Phone: 404-686-4411
Fax: 404-686-4619
URL: www.emoryhealthcare.org
Type: Acute Care Hospitals
Emergency Services: Yes
Ownership: Voluntary non-profit - Private
Beds: 430

Key Personnel:

Quality Assurance .... William A Bornstein
Intensive Care Unit............ June Connor, RN
Radiology.................. Lawrence Davis, MD
CEO/President............... John T Fox
Chief of Medical Staff.......... Roland H Ingram, MD
Emergency Room .... Arthur Kellerman, MD
Infection Control.............. James Steinberg, MD
Operating Room.............. Carol Turpin, RN

Measure	Cases	This Hosp.	State Avg.	U.S. Avg.
Blood Clot Prevention and Treatment				
Anticoagulation Overlap Therapy[2]	196	96%	90%	93%
ICU Venous Thromboembolism Prophylaxis[2]	130	99%	90%	92%
Incidence of Potentially Preventable VTE[2]	69	10%	13%	10%
UFH with Dosages/Platelet Monitoring[2]	207	100%	99%	97%
Venous Thromboembolism Prophylaxis[2]	351	93%	80%	85%
Warfarin Therapy Discharge Instructions[2]	156	56%	78%	75%
Chest Pain/Possible Heart Attack Care				
Aspirin Given Within 24 Hours of Arrival[1,3]	-	-	94%	96%
Fibrinolytic Meds Within 30 Min. of Arrival[3,7]	-	-	35%	58%
Average Time to ECG (minutes)[1,3]	-	-	8	7
Average Time to Transfer (minutes)[3,7]	-	-	73	60
Children's Asthma Care				
Received Home Management Plan of Care	-	-	-	88%
Received Reliever Medication	-	-	-	100%
Received Systemic Corticosteroids	-	-	-	100%
Emergency Department				
Admittance Decision Time (minutes)[2]	396	128	100	98
Head CT Results Within 45 Min. of Arrival[1]	-	-	45%	57%
Patients Who Left ER Before Being Seen	59,922	5%	3%	2%
Time from ER Arrival to Admit. (minutes)[2]	407	374	286	274
Time from ER Arrival to Discharge (minutes)	355	302	140	134
Time in ER Before Being Evaluated (minutes)	374	132	32	26
Time to Pain Meds for Fractures (minutes)	36	94	64	57
Heart Attack Care				
Aspirin Given at Discharge[2]	280	100%	99%	99%
Fibrinolytic Meds Within 30 Min. of Arrival[2,7]	-	-	80%	54%
PCI Within 90 Minutes of Arrival[2]	18	100%	95%	96%
Statin Prescribed at Discharge[2]	267	100%	98%	98%
Heart Failure Care				
ACE Inhibitor or ARB for LVSD[2]	102	99%	97%	97%
Discharge Instructions Given[2]	235	97%	92%	94%
Evaluation of LVS Function[2]	266	100%	99%	99%
Medicare Spending				
Medicare Spending per Patient (ratio)	-	0.94	0.95	0.98
Pneumonia Care				
Appropriate Initial Antibiotic Given[2]	68	94%	95%	95%
Blood Culture Timing[2]	131	99%	97%	98%
Pregnancy and Delivery Care				
Newborn Deliveries Scheduled Early[2]	67	3%	8%	6%
Preventive Care				
Immunization for Influenza[2]	609	99%	88%	90%
Immunization for Pneumonia[2]	690	98%	90%	92%
Stroke Care				
Anticoagulation Therapy for Atrial Fibrillation[1,2]	-	-	94%	95%
Antithrombotic Therapy Timing[2]	78	96%	97%	98%
Assessed for Rehabilitation[2]	102	97%	97%	97%
Discharged on Antithrombotic Therapy[2]	79	99%	98%	99%
Discharged on Statin Medication[2]	52	96%	94%	94%
Thrombolytic Therapy Timing[1,2]	-	-	58%	66%
Venous Thromboembolism Prophylaxis[2]	112	96%	92%	94%
Written Stroke Educational Materials Given[2]	68	97%	84%	88%
Surgical Care Improvement Project				
Appropriate Beta Blocker Usage[2]	201	99%	97%	98%
Appropriate VTP Within 24 Hours[2]	338	96%	98%	98%
Controlled Postoperative Blood Glucose[2]	109	94%	96%	97%
Perioperative Temperature Management[2]	475	100%	100%	100%
Prophylactic Antibiotic Selection[2]	367	99%	99%	99%
Prophylactic Antibiotic Selection (Outpatient)	535	97%	98%	98%
Prophylactic Antibiotic Stopped[2]	344	99%	98%	98%
Prophylactic Antibiotic Timing[2]	368	98%	99%	99%
Prophylactic Antibiotic Timing (Outpatient)	545	96%	98%	98%
Urinary Catheter Removal[2]	228	99%	97%	97%
Survey of Patients' Hospital Experiences				
Area Around Room 'Always' Quiet at Night	300+	60%	66%	61%
Doctors 'Always' Communicated Well	300+	82%	83%	82%
Home Recovery Information Given	300+	81%	84%	85%
Hospital Given 9 or 10 on 10 Point Scale	300+	73%	69%	71%
Meds 'Always' Explained Before Given	300+	59%	63%	64%
Nurses 'Always' Communicated Well	300+	77%	78%	79%
Pain 'Always' Well Controlled	300+	73%	71%	71%
Room and Bathroom 'Always' Clean	300+	71%	71%	73%
Timely Help 'Always' Received	300+	61%	65%	68%
Would Definitely Recommend Hospital	300+	75%	70%	71%
Use of Medical Imaging				
Cardiac Imaging Stress Test before Surgery	764	4.8%	5.5%	5.3%
Combination Abdominal CT Scan	1,122	7.9%	10.1%	10.5%
Combination Brain/Sinus CT Scan	776	2.4%	2.3%	2.7%
Combination Chest CT Scan	1,377	0.0%	3.7%	2.7%
Follow-up Mammogram/Ultrasound	1,538	9.0%	8.9%	8.8%
Lumbar Spine MRI for Low Back Pain	62	41.9%	36.6%	37.2%

Grady Memorial Hospital

80 Jesse Hill, Jr Drive Se
Atlanta, GA 30303
Phone: 404-616-4252
Fax: 404-616-6033
URL: www.gradyhealthsystem.org
Type: Acute Care Hospitals
Emergency Services: Yes
Ownership: Voluntary non-profit - Other
Beds: 953

Key Personnel:

Operating Room.............. Betty C Blake
Ambulatory Care .... Chris Cintron, MPA
Cardiac Laboratory............ David Harrison, MD
CEO .... John M. Haupert, FACHE
Emergency Room .... Arthur Kellerman, MD
Chief of Medical Staff.......... Curtis Lewis, MD, MBA
Pediatric In-Patient Care .... William Sexson, MD

NOTE: Hospital profiles are in alphabetical order by state, then city, then hospital within the city; Rankings exclude hospitals with less than 25 cases except for patient surveys which excludes hospitals with less than 100 cases; (a) 100-299 cases; (1) The number of cases/patients is too few to report; (2) Data submitted were based on a sample of cases/patients; (3) Results are based on a shorter time period than required; (4) Data suppressed by CMS for one or more quarters; (5) Results are not available for this reporting period; (6) Fewer than 100 patients completed the HCAHPS survey; (7) No cases met the criteria for this measure; (8) The lower limit of the confidence interval cannot be calculated if the number of observed infections equals zero; (9) No data are available from the state/territory for this reporting period; (10) The scores shown reflect fewer than 50 completed surveys; (11) There were discrepancies in the data collection process; (12) This measure does not apply to this hospital for this reporting period; (13) Results cannot be calculated for this reporting period; (14) The results for this state are combined with nearby states to protect confidentiality; Please refer to the User's Guide for a full explanation of data.

Radiology. . . . . William Small, MD

Measure	Cases	This Hosp.	State Avg.	U.S. Avg.
Blood Clot Prevention and Treatment				
Anticoagulation Overlap Therapy[2]	196	98%	90%	93%
ICU Venous Thromboembolism Prophylaxis[2]	93	95%	90%	92%
Incidence of Potentially Preventable VTE[2]	64	16%	13%	10%
UFH with Dosages/Platelet Monitoring[2]	177	100%	99%	97%
Venous Thromboembolism Prophylaxis[2]	334	89%	80%	85%
Warfarin Therapy Discharge Instructions[2]	160	90%	78%	75%
Chest Pain/Possible Heart Attack Care				
Aspirin Given Within 24 Hours of Arrival[1]	-	-	94%	96%
Fibrinolytic Meds Within 30 Min. of Arrival[3,7]	-	-	35%	58%
Average Time to ECG (minutes)[1]	-	-	8	7
Average Time to Transfer (minutes)[3,7]	-	-	73	60
Children's Asthma Care				
Received Home Management Plan of Care	-	-	-	88%
Received Reliever Medication	-	-	-	100%
Received Systemic Corticosteroids	-	-	-	100%
Emergency Department				
Admittance Decision Time (minutes)[2]	381	136	100	98
Head CT Results Within 45 Min. of Arrival[1]	-	-	45%	57%
Patients Who Left ER Before Being Seen	>100k	10%	3%	2%
Time from ER Arrival to Admit. (minutes)[2]	403	511	286	274
Time from ER Arrival to Discharge (minutes)	299	477	140	134
Time in ER Before Being Evaluated (minutes)	335	160	32	26
Time to Pain Meds for Fractures (minutes)	130	76	64	57
Heart Attack Care				
Aspirin Given at Discharge	155	98%	99%	99%
Fibrinolytic Meds Within 30 Min. of Arrival[7]	-	-	80%	54%
PCI Within 90 Minutes of Arrival[1]	-	-	95%	96%
Statin Prescribed at Discharge	156	97%	98%	98%
Heart Failure Care				
ACE Inhibitor or ARB for LVSD[2]	141	96%	97%	97%
Discharge Instructions Given[2]	259	98%	92%	94%
Evaluation of LVS Function[2]	286	100%	99%	99%
Medicare Spending				
Medicare Spending per Patient (ratio)	-	0.95	0.95	0.98
Pneumonia Care				
Appropriate Initial Antibiotic Given[2]	50	96%	95%	95%
Blood Culture Timing[2]	86	94%	97%	98%
Pregnancy and Delivery Care				
Newborn Deliveries Scheduled Early[2]	59	3%	8%	6%
Preventive Care				
Immunization for Influenza[2]	550	89%	88%	90%
Immunization for Pneumonia[2]	529	88%	90%	92%
Stroke Care				
Anticoagulation Therapy for Atrial Fibrillation[2]	13	100%	94%	95%
Antithrombotic Therapy Timing[2]	71	100%	97%	98%
Assessed for Rehabilitation[2]	106	98%	97%	97%
Discharged on Antithrombotic Therapy[2]	93	100%	98%	99%
Discharged on Statin Medication[2]	64	94%	94%	94%
Thrombolytic Therapy Timing[2]	14	86%	58%	66%
Venous Thromboembolism Prophylaxis[2]	112	95%	92%	94%
Written Stroke Educational Materials Given[2]	58	90%	84%	88%
Surgical Care Improvement Project				
Appropriate Beta Blocker Usage[2]	55	85%	97%	98%
Appropriate VTP Within 24 Hours[2]	271	98%	98%	98%
Controlled Postoperative Blood Glucose[2]	17	100%	96%	97%
Perioperative Temperature Management[2]	339	99%	100%	100%
Prophylactic Antibiotic Selection[2]	207	100%	99%	99%
Prophylactic Antibiotic Selection (Outpatient)	90	92%	98%	98%
Prophylactic Antibiotic Stopped[2]	202	96%	98%	98%
Prophylactic Antibiotic Timing[2]	209	98%	99%	99%
Prophylactic Antibiotic Timing (Outpatient)	67	82%	98%	98%
Urinary Catheter Removal[2]	155	99%	97%	97%
Survey of Patients' Hospital Experiences				
Area Around Room 'Always' Quiet at Night	300+	63%	66%	61%
Doctors 'Always' Communicated Well	300+	82%	83%	82%
Home Recovery Information Given	300+	78%	84%	85%
Hospital Given 9 or 10 on 10 Point Scale	300+	66%	69%	71%
Meds 'Always' Explained Before Given	300+	62%	63%	64%
Nurses 'Always' Communicated Well	300+	74%	78%	79%
Pain 'Always' Well Controlled	300+	66%	71%	71%
Room and Bathroom 'Always' Clean	300+	65%	71%	73%
Timely Help 'Always' Received	300+	55%	65%	68%
Would Definitely Recommend Hospital	300+	71%	70%	71%
Use of Medical Imaging				
Cardiac Imaging Stress Test before Surgery	371	3.8%	5.5%	5.3%
Combination Abdominal CT Scan	638	9.1%	10.1%	10.5%
Combination Brain/Sinus CT Scan	837	1.2%	2.3%	2.7%
Combination Chest CT Scan	649	4.0%	3.7%	2.7%
Follow-up Mammogram/Ultrasound	1,824	6.5%	8.9%	8.8%
Lumbar Spine MRI for Low Back Pain	68	30.9%	36.6%	37.2%

Northside Hospital

1000 Johnson Ferry Road, Ne
Atlanta, GA 30342
Phone: 404-851-8000
Fax: 404-250-1317
URL: www.northside.com

Type: Acute Care Hospitals
Emergency Services: Yes
Ownership: Voluntary non-profit - Private
Beds: 537

Key Personnel:

Chief of Medical Staff. . . . . Wayne Ambroze
Quality Assurance . . . . Ora Douglass
Operating Room. . . . . Judy Esserwein
Infection Control. . . . . Janice Fetter
Pediatric In-Patient Care . . . . Margaret Moore
CEO/President. . . . . Robert Quattrochi
Radiology. . . . . James Zakem, MD

Measure	Cases	This Hosp.	State Avg.	U.S. Avg.
Blood Clot Prevention and Treatment				
Anticoagulation Overlap Therapy[2]	136	100%	90%	93%
ICU Venous Thromboembolism Prophylaxis[2]	44	100%	90%	92%
Incidence of Potentially Preventable VTE[2]	48	0%	13%	10%
UFH with Dosages/Platelet Monitoring[2]	121	100%	99%	97%
Venous Thromboembolism Prophylaxis[2]	413	97%	80%	85%
Warfarin Therapy Discharge Instructions[2]	105	100%	78%	75%
Chest Pain/Possible Heart Attack Care				
Aspirin Given Within 24 Hours of Arrival[1]	-	-	94%	96%
Fibrinolytic Meds Within 30 Min. of Arrival[7]	-	-	35%	58%
Average Time to ECG (minutes)[1]	-	-	8	7
Average Time to Transfer (minutes)[7]	-	-	73	60
Children's Asthma Care				
Received Home Management Plan of Care	-	-	-	88%
Received Reliever Medication	-	-	-	100%
Received Systemic Corticosteroids	-	-	-	100%
Emergency Department				
Admittance Decision Time (minutes)[2]	146	106	100	98
Head CT Results Within 45 Min. of Arrival[1]	-	-	45%	57%
Patients Who Left ER Before Being Seen	26,545	1%	3%	2%
Time from ER Arrival to Admit. (minutes)[2]	151	256	286	274
Time from ER Arrival to Discharge (minutes)	402	145	140	134
Time in ER Before Being Evaluated (minutes)	422	16	32	26
Time to Pain Meds for Fractures (minutes)	69	44	64	57
Heart Attack Care				
Aspirin Given at Discharge	148	100%	99%	99%
Fibrinolytic Meds Within 30 Min. of Arrival[7]	-	-	80%	54%
PCI Within 90 Minutes of Arrival	24	96%	95%	96%
Statin Prescribed at Discharge	141	100%	98%	98%
Heart Failure Care				
ACE Inhibitor or ARB for LVSD	43	100%	97%	97%
Discharge Instructions Given	178	99%	92%	94%
Evaluation of LVS Function	203	99%	99%	99%
Medicare Spending				
Medicare Spending per Patient (ratio)	-	0.99	0.95	0.98
Pneumonia Care				
Appropriate Initial Antibiotic Given	141	100%	95%	95%
Blood Culture Timing	185	100%	97%	98%
Pregnancy and Delivery Care				
Newborn Deliveries Scheduled Early[2]	329	1%	8%	6%
Preventive Care				
Immunization for Influenza[2]	440	98%	88%	90%
Immunization for Pneumonia[2]	227	94%	90%	92%
Stroke Care				
Anticoagulation Therapy for Atrial Fibrillation	15	100%	94%	95%
Antithrombotic Therapy Timing	108	99%	97%	98%
Assessed for Rehabilitation	147	100%	97%	97%
Discharged on Antithrombotic Therapy	125	100%	98%	99%
Discharged on Statin Medication	90	99%	94%	94%
Thrombolytic Therapy Timing[1]	-	-	58%	66%
Venous Thromboembolism Prophylaxis	152	99%	92%	94%
Written Stroke Educational Materials Given	102	97%	84%	88%
Surgical Care Improvement Project				
Appropriate Beta Blocker Usage[2]	121	100%	97%	98%
Appropriate VTP Within 24 Hours[2]	543	100%	98%	98%
Controlled Postoperative Blood Glucose[2,7]	-	-	96%	97%
Perioperative Temperature Management[2]	609	100%	100%	100%
Prophylactic Antibiotic Selection[2]	427	100%	99%	99%
Prophylactic Antibiotic Selection (Outpatient)	870	100%	98%	98%
Prophylactic Antibiotic Stopped[2]	407	100%	98%	98%
Prophylactic Antibiotic Timing[2]	427	100%	99%	99%
Prophylactic Antibiotic Timing (Outpatient)	872	99%	98%	98%
Urinary Catheter Removal[2]	379	100%	97%	97%
Survey of Patients' Hospital Experiences				
Area Around Room 'Always' Quiet at Night	300+	62%	66%	61%
Doctors 'Always' Communicated Well	300+	80%	83%	82%
Home Recovery Information Given	300+	85%	84%	85%
Hospital Given 9 or 10 on 10 Point Scale	300+	78%	69%	71%
Meds 'Always' Explained Before Given	300+	63%	63%	64%
Nurses 'Always' Communicated Well	300+	80%	78%	79%
Pain 'Always' Well Controlled	300+	73%	71%	71%
Room and Bathroom 'Always' Clean	300+	77%	71%	73%
Timely Help 'Always' Received	300+	65%	65%	68%
Would Definitely Recommend Hospital	300+	81%	70%	71%
Use of Medical Imaging				
Cardiac Imaging Stress Test before Surgery	114	7.0%	5.5%	5.3%
Combination Abdominal CT Scan	1,873	9.2%	10.1%	10.5%
Combination Brain/Sinus CT Scan	736	1.4%	2.3%	2.7%
Combination Chest CT Scan	1,615	0.1%	3.7%	2.7%
Follow-up Mammogram/Ultrasound	4,634	9.0%	8.9%	8.8%
Lumbar Spine MRI for Low Back Pain	166	38.0%	36.6%	37.2%

Piedmont Hospital

1968 Peachtree Rd Nw
Atlanta, GA 30309
Phone: 404-605-5000
Fax: 404-367-3551
URL: www.piedmonthospital.org

Type: Acute Care Hospitals
Emergency Services: Yes
Ownership: Voluntary non-profit - Private
Beds: 488

Key Personnel:

Operating Room. . . . . Shelly J Ahmann, RN
Radiology. . . . . Jeffrey Allen
Anesthesiology. . . . . Walter Butler, MD
Chief of Medical Staff. . . . . Mark Cohen, MD
CEO/President. . . . . Leslie A. Donahue, DO
Infection Control. . . . . Carol Mims
Emergency Room . . . . Leah Tolly

Measure	Cases	This Hosp.	State Avg.	U.S. Avg.
Blood Clot Prevention and Treatment				
Anticoagulation Overlap Therapy[2]	198	93%	90%	93%
ICU Venous Thromboembolism Prophylaxis[2]	86	93%	90%	92%
Incidence of Potentially Preventable VTE[2]	62	10%	13%	10%
UFH with Dosages/Platelet Monitoring[2]	213	95%	99%	97%
Venous Thromboembolism Prophylaxis[2]	372	77%	80%	85%
Warfarin Therapy Discharge Instructions[2]	135	90%	78%	75%
Chest Pain/Possible Heart Attack Care				
Aspirin Given Within 24 Hours of Arrival[1,3]	-	-	94%	96%
Fibrinolytic Meds Within 30 Min. of Arrival[5]	-	-	35%	58%
Average Time to ECG (minutes)[1,3]	-	-	8	7
Average Time to Transfer (minutes)[5]	-	-	73	60
Children's Asthma Care				
Received Home Management Plan of Care	-	-	-	88%
Received Reliever Medication	-	-	-	100%
Received Systemic Corticosteroids	-	-	-	100%
Emergency Department				
Admittance Decision Time (minutes)[2]	446	159	100	98
Head CT Results Within 45 Min. of Arrival	23	9%	45%	57%
Patients Who Left ER Before Being Seen	50,506	2%	3%	2%
Time from ER Arrival to Admit. (minutes)[2]	456	398	286	274
Time from ER Arrival to Discharge (minutes)	401	219	140	134
Time in ER Before Being Evaluated (minutes)	339	69	32	26

NOTE: Hospital profiles are in alphabetical order by state, then city, then hospital within the city; Rankings exclude hospitals with less than 25 cases except for patient surveys which excludes hospitals with less than 100 cases; (a) 100-299 cases; (1) The number of cases/patients is too few to report; (2) Data submitted were based on a sample of cases/patients; (3) Results are based on a shorter time period than required; (4) Data suppressed by CMS for one or more quarters; (5) Results are not available for this reporting period; (6) Fewer than 100 patients completed the HCAHPS survey; (7) No cases met the criteria for this measure; (8) The lower limit of the confidence interval cannot be calculated if the number of observed infections equals zero; (9) No data are available from the state/territory for this reporting period; (10) The scores shown reflect fewer than 50 completed surveys; (11) There were discrepancies in the data collection process; (12) This measure does not apply to this hospital for this reporting period; (13) Results cannot be calculated for this reporting period; (14) The results for this state are combined with nearby states to protect confidentiality; Please refer to the User's Guide for a full explanation of data.

Measure	Cases	This Hosp.	State Avg.	U.S. Avg.
Time to Pain Meds for Fractures (minutes)	138	76	64	57
Heart Attack Care				
Aspirin Given at Discharge[2]	505	99%	99%	99%
Fibrinolytic Meds Within 30 Min. of Arrival[2,7]	-	-	80%	54%
PCI Within 90 Minutes of Arrival[2]	29	97%	95%	96%
Statin Prescribed at Discharge[2]	481	98%	98%	98%
Heart Failure Care				
ACE Inhibitor or ARB for LVSD[2]	111	95%	97%	97%
Discharge Instructions Given[2]	286	78%	92%	94%
Evaluation of LVS Function[2]	322	100%	99%	99%
Medicare Spending				
Medicare Spending per Patient (ratio)	-	0.97	0.95	0.98
Pneumonia Care				
Appropriate Initial Antibiotic Given[2]	96	97%	95%	95%
Blood Culture Timing[2]	166	94%	97%	98%
Pregnancy and Delivery Care				
Newborn Deliveries Scheduled Early[2]	43	0%	8%	6%
Preventive Care				
Immunization for Influenza[2]	594	62%	88%	90%
Immunization for Pneumonia[2]	673	69%	90%	92%
Stroke Care				
Anticoagulation Therapy for Atrial Fibrillation[2]	11	82%	94%	95%
Antithrombotic Therapy Timing[2]	82	98%	97%	98%
Assessed for Rehabilitation[2]	104	96%	97%	97%
Discharged on Antithrombotic Therapy[2]	90	97%	98%	99%
Discharged on Statin Medication[2]	77	94%	94%	94%
Thrombolytic Therapy Timing[2]	25	4%	58%	66%
Venous Thromboembolism Prophylaxis[2]	107	87%	92%	94%
Written Stroke Educational Materials Given[2]	63	90%	84%	88%
Surgical Care Improvement Project				
Appropriate Beta Blocker Usage[2]	229	98%	97%	98%
Appropriate VTP Within 24 Hours[2]	464	92%	98%	98%
Controlled Postoperative Blood Glucose[2]	173	95%	96%	97%
Perioperative Temperature Management[2]	633	99%	100%	100%
Prophylactic Antibiotic Selection[2]	547	96%	99%	99%
Prophylactic Antibiotic Selection (Outpatient)	801	97%	98%	98%
Prophylactic Antibiotic Stopped[2]	539	98%	98%	98%
Prophylactic Antibiotic Timing[2]	560	96%	99%	99%
Prophylactic Antibiotic Timing (Outpatient)	841	90%	98%	98%
Urinary Catheter Removal[2]	427	93%	97%	97%
Survey of Patients' Hospital Experiences				
Area Around Room 'Always' Quiet at Night	300+	63%	66%	61%
Doctors 'Always' Communicated Well	300+	83%	83%	82%
Home Recovery Information Given	300+	84%	84%	85%
Hospital Given 9 or 10 on 10 Point Scale	300+	71%	69%	71%
Meds 'Always' Explained Before Given	300+	59%	63%	64%
Nurses 'Always' Communicated Well	300+	75%	78%	79%
Pain 'Always' Well Controlled	300+	68%	71%	71%
Room and Bathroom 'Always' Clean	300+	63%	71%	73%
Timely Help 'Always' Received	300+	60%	65%	68%
Would Definitely Recommend Hospital	300+	77%	70%	71%
Use of Medical Imaging				
Cardiac Imaging Stress Test before Surgery	2,524	5.5%	5.5%	5.3%
Combination Abdominal CT Scan	1,721	8.4%	10.1%	10.5%
Combination Brain/Sinus CT Scan	1,239	1.3%	2.3%	2.7%
Combination Chest CT Scan	1,188	0.7%	3.7%	2.7%
Follow-up Mammogram/Ultrasound	2,536	9.7%	8.9%	8.8%
Lumbar Spine MRI for Low Back Pain	127	37.8%	36.6%	37.2%

Saint Joseph's Hospital of Atlanta

5665 Peachtree Dunwoody Road Phone: 678-843-5720
Atlanta, GA 30342 Fax: 404-851-7938
URL: www.stjosephsatlanta.org
Type: Acute Care Hospitals Emergency Services: Yes
Ownership: Voluntary non-profit - Private Beds: 410
Key Personnel:
CEO/President. . . . . Craig McCoy
Chief of Medical Staff. . . . . Paul Scheinberg, MD
Quality Assurance . . . . Robin Spiegel

Measure	Cases	This Hosp.	State Avg.	U.S. Avg.
Blood Clot Prevention and Treatment				
Anticoagulation Overlap Therapy[2]	104	97%	90%	93%
ICU Venous Thromboembolism Prophylaxis[2]	112	82%	90%	92%
Incidence of Potentially Preventable VTE[2]	15	27%	13%	10%
UFH with Dosages/Platelet Monitoring[2]	108	100%	99%	97%
Venous Thromboembolism Prophylaxis[2]	318	81%	80%	85%
Warfarin Therapy Discharge Instructions[2]	77	60%	78%	75%
Chest Pain/Possible Heart Attack Care				
Aspirin Given Within 24 Hours of Arrival[1,3]	-	-	94%	96%
Fibrinolytic Meds Within 30 Min. of Arrival[5]	-	-	35%	58%
Average Time to ECG (minutes)[1,3]	-	-	8	7
Average Time to Transfer (minutes)[5]	-	-	73	60
Children's Asthma Care				
Received Home Management Plan of Care	-	-	-	88%
Received Reliever Medication	-	-	-	100%
Received Systemic Corticosteroids	-	-	-	100%
Emergency Department				
Admittance Decision Time (minutes)[2]	503	135	100	98
Head CT Results Within 45 Min. of Arrival	13	77%	45%	57%
Patients Who Left ER Before Being Seen	33,790	1%	3%	2%
Time from ER Arrival to Admit. (minutes)[2]	535	311	286	274
Time from ER Arrival to Discharge (minutes)	395	197	140	134
Time in ER Before Being Evaluated (minutes)	337	45	32	26
Time to Pain Meds for Fractures (minutes)	56	66	64	57
Heart Attack Care				
Aspirin Given at Discharge[2]	299	99%	99%	99%
Fibrinolytic Meds Within 30 Min. of Arrival[2,7]	-	-	80%	54%
PCI Within 90 Minutes of Arrival[2]	43	100%	95%	96%
Statin Prescribed at Discharge[2]	287	99%	98%	98%
Heart Failure Care				
ACE Inhibitor or ARB for LVSD[2]	87	99%	97%	97%
Discharge Instructions Given[2]	257	86%	92%	94%
Evaluation of LVS Function[2]	292	100%	99%	99%
Medicare Spending				
Medicare Spending per Patient (ratio)	-	0.96	0.95	0.98
Pneumonia Care				
Appropriate Initial Antibiotic Given[2]	116	90%	95%	95%
Blood Culture Timing[2]	183	91%	97%	98%
Pregnancy and Delivery Care				
Newborn Deliveries Scheduled Early[7]	-	-	8%	6%
Preventive Care				
Immunization for Influenza[2]	628	89%	88%	90%
Immunization for Pneumonia[2]	937	91%	90%	92%
Stroke Care				
Anticoagulation Therapy for Atrial Fibrillation[2]	20	95%	94%	95%
Antithrombotic Therapy Timing[2]	66	98%	97%	98%
Assessed for Rehabilitation[2]	88	98%	97%	97%
Discharged on Antithrombotic Therapy[2]	76	99%	98%	99%
Discharged on Statin Medication[2]	69	100%	94%	94%
Thrombolytic Therapy Timing[2]	13	85%	58%	66%
Venous Thromboembolism Prophylaxis[2]	88	97%	92%	94%
Written Stroke Educational Materials Given[2]	64	61%	84%	88%
Surgical Care Improvement Project				
Appropriate Beta Blocker Usage[2]	239	98%	97%	98%
Appropriate VTP Within 24 Hours[2]	242	94%	98%	98%
Controlled Postoperative Blood Glucose[2]	156	93%	96%	97%
Perioperative Temperature Management[2]	559	100%	100%	100%
Prophylactic Antibiotic Selection[2]	499	99%	99%	99%
Prophylactic Antibiotic Selection (Outpatient)	569	98%	98%	98%
Prophylactic Antibiotic Stopped[2]	487	96%	98%	98%
Prophylactic Antibiotic Timing[2]	499	98%	99%	99%
Prophylactic Antibiotic Timing (Outpatient)	572	98%	98%	98%
Urinary Catheter Removal[2]	293	96%	97%	97%
Survey of Patients' Hospital Experiences				
Area Around Room 'Always' Quiet at Night	300+	53%	66%	61%
Doctors 'Always' Communicated Well	300+	78%	83%	82%
Home Recovery Information Given	300+	86%	84%	85%
Hospital Given 9 or 10 on 10 Point Scale	300+	72%	69%	71%
Meds 'Always' Explained Before Given	300+	57%	63%	64%
Nurses 'Always' Communicated Well	300+	74%	78%	79%
Pain 'Always' Well Controlled	300+	75%	71%	71%
Room and Bathroom 'Always' Clean	300+	69%	71%	73%
Timely Help 'Always' Received	300+	64%	65%	68%
Would Definitely Recommend Hospital	300+	79%	70%	71%
Use of Medical Imaging				
Cardiac Imaging Stress Test before Surgery	1,650	4.6%	5.5%	5.3%
Combination Abdominal CT Scan	1,371	4.8%	10.1%	10.5%
Combination Brain/Sinus CT Scan	974	1.4%	2.3%	2.7%
Combination Chest CT Scan	1,378	0.3%	3.7%	2.7%
Follow-up Mammogram/Ultrasound	1,563	7.2%	8.9%	8.8%
Lumbar Spine MRI for Low Back Pain	55	32.7%	36.6%	37.2%

Wesley Woods Geriatric Hospital

1821 Clifton Road, Ne Phone: 404-728-6250
Atlanta, GA 30329 Fax: 404-728-6558
E-mail: peter_basler@emoryhealthcare.org
Type: Acute Care Hospitals Emergency Services: No
Ownership: Voluntary non-profit - Private Beds: 100
Key Personnel:
Quality Assurance . . . . Valerie Bender
Chief of Medical Staff . . . . Joseph Ouslander, MD
Patient Relations . . . . Jennifer Schuck
Infection Control. . . . . Kathy Westmoreland

Measure	Cases	This Hosp.	State Avg.	U.S. Avg.
Blood Clot Prevention and Treatment				
Anticoagulation Overlap Therapy[3,7]	-	-	90%	93%
ICU Venous Thromboembolism Prophylaxis[3,7]	-	-	90%	92%
Incidence of Potentially Preventable VTE[3,7]	-	-	13%	10%
UFH with Dosages/Platelet Monitoring[3,7]	-	-	99%	97%
Venous Thromboembolism Prophylaxis[1,3]	-	-	80%	85%
Warfarin Therapy Discharge Instructions[3,7]	-	-	78%	75%
Chest Pain/Possible Heart Attack Care				
Aspirin Given Within 24 Hours of Arrival[5]	-	-	94%	96%
Fibrinolytic Meds Within 30 Min. of Arrival[5]	-	-	35%	58%
Average Time to ECG (minutes)[5]	-	-	8	7
Average Time to Transfer (minutes)[5]	-	-	73	60
Children's Asthma Care				
Received Home Management Plan of Care	-	-	-	88%
Received Reliever Medication	-	-	-	100%
Received Systemic Corticosteroids	-	-	-	100%
Emergency Department				
Admittance Decision Time (minutes)[3,7]	-	-	100	98
Head CT Results Within 45 Min. of Arrival[5]	-	-	45%	57%
Patients Who Left ER Before Being Seen[5]	-	-	3%	2%
Time from ER Arrival to Admit. (minutes)[3,7]	-	-	286	274
Time from ER Arrival to Discharge (minutes)[5]	-	-	140	134
Time in ER Before Being Evaluated (minutes)[5]	-	-	32	26
Time to Pain Meds for Fractures (minutes)[5]	-	-	64	57
Heart Attack Care				
Aspirin Given at Discharge[5]	-	-	99%	99%
Fibrinolytic Meds Within 30 Min. of Arrival[5]	-	-	80%	54%
PCI Within 90 Minutes of Arrival[5]	-	-	95%	96%
Statin Prescribed at Discharge[5]	-	-	98%	98%
Heart Failure Care				
ACE Inhibitor or ARB for LVSD[1,3]	-	-	97%	97%
Discharge Instructions Given[1,3]	-	-	92%	94%
Evaluation of LVS Function[1,3]	-	-	99%	99%
Medicare Spending				
Medicare Spending per Patient (ratio)[1]	-	-	0.95	0.98
Pneumonia Care				
Appropriate Initial Antibiotic Given[5]	-	-	95%	95%
Blood Culture Timing[5]	-	-	97%	98%
Pregnancy and Delivery Care				
Newborn Deliveries Scheduled Early[7]	-	-	8%	6%
Preventive Care				
Immunization for Influenza[1,3]	-	-	88%	90%
Immunization for Pneumonia[1,3]	-	-	90%	92%
Stroke Care				
Anticoagulation Therapy for Atrial Fibrillation[5]	-	-	94%	95%
Antithrombotic Therapy Timing[5]	-	-	97%	98%
Assessed for Rehabilitation[5]	-	-	97%	97%
Discharged on Antithrombotic Therapy[5]	-	-	98%	99%
Discharged on Statin Medication[5]	-	-	94%	94%
Thrombolytic Therapy Timing[5]	-	-	58%	66%
Venous Thromboembolism Prophylaxis[5]	-	-	92%	94%
Written Stroke Educational Materials Given[5]	-	-	84%	88%
Surgical Care Improvement Project				
Appropriate Beta Blocker Usage[5]	-	-	97%	98%

NOTE: Hospital profiles are in alphabetical order by state, then city, then hospital within the city; Rankings exclude hospitals with less than 25 cases except for patient surveys which excludes hospitals with less than 100 cases; (a) 100-299 cases; (1) The number of cases/patients is too few to report; (2) Data submitted were based on a sample of cases/patients; (3) Results are based on a shorter time period than required; (4) Data suppressed by CMS for one or more quarters; (5) Results are not available for this reporting period; (6) Fewer than 100 patients completed the HCAHPS survey; (7) No cases met the criteria for this measure; (8) The lower limit of the confidence interval cannot be calculated if the number of observed infections equals zero; (9) No data are available from the state/territory for this reporting period; (10) The scores shown reflect fewer than 50 completed surveys; (11) There were discrepancies in the data collection process; (12) This measure does not apply to this hospital for this reporting period; (13) Results cannot be calculated for this reporting period; (14) The results for this state are combined with nearby states to protect confidentiality; Please refer to the User's Guide for a full explanation of data.

Measure	Cases	This Hosp.	State Avg.	U.S. Avg.
Appropriate VTP Within 24 Hours[5]	-	-	98%	98%
Controlled Postoperative Blood Glucose[5]	-	-	96%	97%
Perioperative Temperature Management[5]	-	-	100%	100%
Prophylactic Antibiotic Selection[5]	-	-	99%	99%
Prophylactic Antibiotic Selection (Outpatient)[5]	-	-	98%	98%
Prophylactic Antibiotic Stopped[5]	-	-	98%	98%
Prophylactic Antibiotic Timing[5]	-	-	99%	99%
Prophylactic Antibiotic Timing (Outpatient)[5]	-	-	98%	98%
Urinary Catheter Removal[5]	-	-	97%	97%
Survey of Patients' Hospital Experiences				
Area Around Room 'Always' Quiet at Night[1]	-	-	66%	61%
Doctors 'Always' Communicated Well[1]	-	-	83%	82%
Home Recovery Information Given[1]	-	-	84%	85%
Hospital Given 9 or 10 on 10 Point Scale[1]	-	-	69%	71%
Meds 'Always' Explained Before Given[1]	-	-	63%	64%
Nurses 'Always' Communicated Well[1]	-	-	78%	79%
Pain 'Always' Well Controlled[1]	-	-	71%	71%
Room and Bathroom 'Always' Clean[1]	-	-	71%	73%
Timely Help 'Always' Received[1]	-	-	65%	68%
Would Definitely Recommend Hospital[1]	-	-	70%	71%
Use of Medical Imaging				
Cardiac Imaging Stress Test before Surgery[7]	-	-	5.5%	5.3%
Combination Abdominal CT Scan[1]	-	-	10.1%	10.5%
Combination Brain/Sinus CT Scan[1]	-	-	2.3%	2.7%
Combination Chest CT Scan[1]	-	-	3.7%	2.7%
Follow-up Mammogram/Ultrasound[7]	-	-	8.9%	8.8%
Lumbar Spine MRI for Low Back Pain[7]	-	-	36.6%	37.2%

Augusta VA Medical Center

950 15th Street
Augusta, GA 30901
Phone: 706-823-2201
Fax: 706-823-3978
URL: www.va.gov
Type: Acute Care - VA
Emergency Services: No
Ownership: Government Federal
Beds: 440

Key Personnel:
Infection Control. . . . . Brian A Catto, MD
Coronary Care . . . . Joyce Coleman, RN
Operating Room. . . . . Jorge I Cue, MD
Quality Assurance . . . . Ellen W Harbeson
Chief of Medical Staff . . . . Michael A. Spencer, MD
Radiology. . . . . Suzanne M Thigpen, MD

Measure	Cases	This Hosp.	State Avg.	U.S. Avg.
Blood Clot Prevention and Treatment				
Anticoagulation Overlap Therapy	-	-	90%	93%
ICU Venous Thromboembolism Prophylaxis	-	-	90%	92%
Incidence of Potentially Preventable VTE	-	-	13%	10%
UFH with Dosages/Platelet Monitoring	-	-	99%	97%
Venous Thromboembolism Prophylaxis	-	-	80%	85%
Warfarin Therapy Discharge Instructions	-	-	78%	75%
Chest Pain/Possible Heart Attack Care				
Aspirin Given Within 24 Hours of Arrival	-	-	94%	96%
Fibrinolytic Meds Within 30 Min. of Arrival	-	-	35%	58%
Average Time to ECG (minutes)	-	-	8	7
Average Time to Transfer (minutes)	-	-	73	60
Children's Asthma Care				
Received Home Management Plan of Care	-	-	-	88%
Received Reliever Medication	-	-	-	100%
Received Systemic Corticosteroids	-	-	-	100%
Emergency Department				
Admittance Decision Time (minutes)	-	-	100	98
Head CT Results Within 45 Min. of Arrival	-	-	45%	57%
Patients Who Left ER Before Being Seen	-	-	3%	2%
Time from ER Arrival to Admit. (minutes)	-	-	286	274
Time from ER Arrival to Discharge (minutes)	-	-	140	134
Time in ER Before Being Evaluated (minutes)	-	-	32	26
Time to Pain Meds for Fractures (minutes)	-	-	64	57
Heart Attack Care				
Aspirin Given at Discharge	32	100%	99%	99%
Fibrinolytic Meds Within 30 Min. of Arrival[5]	-	-	80%	54%
PCI Within 90 Minutes of Arrival[1]	-	-	95%	96%
Statin Prescribed at Discharge	31	100%	98%	98%
Heart Failure Care				
ACE Inhibitor or ARB for LVSD	72	90%	97%	97%
Discharge Instructions Given	161	97%	92%	94%
Evaluation of LVS Function	170	99%	99%	99%
Medicare Spending				
Medicare Spending per Patient (ratio)	-	-	0.95	0.98
Pneumonia Care				
Appropriate Initial Antibiotic Given	54	93%	95%	95%
Blood Culture Timing	92	95%	97%	98%
Pregnancy and Delivery Care				
Newborn Deliveries Scheduled Early	-	-	8%	6%
Preventive Care				
Immunization for Influenza[5]	-	-	88%	90%
Immunization for Pneumonia[5]	-	-	90%	92%
Stroke Care				
Anticoagulation Therapy for Atrial Fibrillation	-	-	94%	95%
Antithrombotic Therapy Timing	-	-	97%	98%
Assessed for Rehabilitation	-	-	97%	97%
Discharged on Antithrombotic Therapy	-	-	98%	99%
Discharged on Statin Medication	-	-	94%	94%
Thrombolytic Therapy Timing	-	-	58%	66%
Venous Thromboembolism Prophylaxis	-	-	92%	94%
Written Stroke Educational Materials Given	-	-	84%	88%
Surgical Care Improvement Project				
Appropriate Beta Blocker Usage[2]	79	91%	97%	98%
Appropriate VTP Within 24 Hours[2]	176	97%	98%	98%
Controlled Postoperative Blood Glucose[5]	-	-	96%	97%
Perioperative Temperature Management[2]	224	99%	100%	100%
Prophylactic Antibiotic Selection	106	99%	99%	99%
Prophylactic Antibiotic Selection (Outpatient)	-	-	98%	98%
Prophylactic Antibiotic Stopped	104	96%	98%	98%
Prophylactic Antibiotic Timing	106	97%	99%	99%
Prophylactic Antibiotic Timing (Outpatient)	-	-	98%	98%
Urinary Catheter Removal[2]	114	96%	97%	97%
Survey of Patients' Hospital Experiences				
Area Around Room 'Always' Quiet at Night	-	-	66%	61%
Doctors 'Always' Communicated Well	-	-	83%	82%
Home Recovery Information Given	-	-	84%	85%
Hospital Given 9 or 10 on 10 Point Scale	-	-	69%	71%
Meds 'Always' Explained Before Given	-	-	63%	64%
Nurses 'Always' Communicated Well	-	-	78%	79%
Pain 'Always' Well Controlled	-	-	71%	71%
Room and Bathroom 'Always' Clean	-	-	71%	73%
Timely Help 'Always' Received	-	-	65%	68%
Would Definitely Recommend Hospital	-	-	70%	71%
Use of Medical Imaging				
Cardiac Imaging Stress Test before Surgery	-	-	5.5%	5.3%
Combination Abdominal CT Scan	-	-	10.1%	10.5%
Combination Brain/Sinus CT Scan	-	-	2.3%	2.7%
Combination Chest CT Scan	-	-	3.7%	2.7%
Follow-up Mammogram/Ultrasound	-	-	8.9%	8.8%
Lumbar Spine MRI for Low Back Pain	-	-	36.6%	37.2%

Doctors Hospital

3651 Wheeler Road
Augusta, GA 30909
Phone: 706-651-6008
Fax: 706-651-2041
URL: www.doctors-hospital.net
Type: Acute Care Hospitals
Emergency Services: Yes
Ownership: Proprietary
Beds: 244

Key Personnel:
Intensive Care Unit. . . . . Charles Butcher
Operating Room. . . . . Kevin Cochran
CEO/President. . . . . C Shayne George
Radiology. . . . . William Johnson
Quality Assurance . . . . Teresa Mills
Chief of Medical Staff. . . . . Cristian Thome

Measure	Cases	This Hosp.	State Avg.	U.S. Avg.
Blood Clot Prevention and Treatment				
Anticoagulation Overlap Therapy[2]	51	100%	90%	93%
ICU Venous Thromboembolism Prophylaxis[2]	78	97%	90%	92%
Incidence of Potentially Preventable VTE[2]	35	9%	13%	10%
UFH with Dosages/Platelet Monitoring[2]	21	100%	99%	97%
Venous Thromboembolism Prophylaxis[2]	330	98%	80%	85%
Warfarin Therapy Discharge Instructions[2]	42	100%	78%	75%
Chest Pain/Possible Heart Attack Care				
Aspirin Given Within 24 Hours of Arrival[5]	-	-	94%	96%
Fibrinolytic Meds Within 30 Min. of Arrival[5]	-	-	35%	58%
Average Time to ECG (minutes)[5]	-	-	8	7
Average Time to Transfer (minutes)[5]	-	-	73	60
Children's Asthma Care				
Received Home Management Plan of Care	-	-	-	88%
Received Reliever Medication	-	-	-	100%
Received Systemic Corticosteroids	-	-	-	100%
Emergency Department				
Admittance Decision Time (minutes)[2]	553	57	100	98
Head CT Results Within 45 Min. of Arrival[1]	-	-	45%	57%
Patients Who Left ER Before Being Seen	48,685	1%	3%	2%
Time from ER Arrival to Admit. (minutes)[2]	553	203	286	274
Time from ER Arrival to Discharge (minutes)	486	106	140	134
Time in ER Before Being Evaluated (minutes)	514	12	32	26
Time to Pain Meds for Fractures (minutes)	215	46	64	57
Heart Attack Care				
Aspirin Given at Discharge	93	100%	99%	99%
Fibrinolytic Meds Within 30 Min. of Arrival[7]	-	-	80%	54%
PCI Within 90 Minutes of Arrival	23	100%	95%	96%
Statin Prescribed at Discharge	88	100%	98%	98%
Heart Failure Care				
ACE Inhibitor or ARB for LVSD	61	100%	97%	97%
Discharge Instructions Given	175	100%	92%	94%
Evaluation of LVS Function	207	100%	99%	99%
Medicare Spending				
Medicare Spending per Patient (ratio)	-	1.00	0.95	0.98
Pneumonia Care				
Appropriate Initial Antibiotic Given	110	100%	95%	95%
Blood Culture Timing	260	100%	97%	98%
Pregnancy and Delivery Care				
Newborn Deliveries Scheduled Early[2]	37	0%	8%	6%
Preventive Care				
Immunization for Influenza[2]	597	98%	88%	90%
Immunization for Pneumonia[2]	585	98%	90%	92%
Stroke Care				
Anticoagulation Therapy for Atrial Fibrillation[1,2]	-	-	94%	95%
Antithrombotic Therapy Timing[2]	68	100%	97%	98%
Assessed for Rehabilitation[2]	75	100%	97%	97%
Discharged on Antithrombotic Therapy[2]	68	100%	98%	99%
Discharged on Statin Medication[2]	58	100%	94%	94%
Thrombolytic Therapy Timing[1,2]	-	-	58%	66%
Venous Thromboembolism Prophylaxis[2]	85	100%	92%	94%
Written Stroke Educational Materials Given[2]	43	100%	84%	88%
Surgical Care Improvement Project				
Appropriate Beta Blocker Usage[2]	116	100%	97%	98%
Appropriate VTP Within 24 Hours[2]	456	100%	98%	98%
Controlled Postoperative Blood Glucose[2,7]	-	-	96%	97%
Perioperative Temperature Management[2]	512	100%	100%	100%
Prophylactic Antibiotic Selection[2]	341	100%	99%	99%
Prophylactic Antibiotic Selection (Outpatient)	381	100%	98%	98%
Prophylactic Antibiotic Stopped[2]	331	100%	98%	98%
Prophylactic Antibiotic Timing[2]	341	100%	99%	99%
Prophylactic Antibiotic Timing (Outpatient)	381	100%	98%	98%
Urinary Catheter Removal[2]	307	100%	97%	97%
Survey of Patients' Hospital Experiences				
Area Around Room 'Always' Quiet at Night	300+	61%	66%	61%
Doctors 'Always' Communicated Well	300+	81%	83%	82%
Home Recovery Information Given	300+	84%	84%	85%
Hospital Given 9 or 10 on 10 Point Scale	300+	71%	69%	71%
Meds 'Always' Explained Before Given	300+	62%	63%	64%
Nurses 'Always' Communicated Well	300+	76%	78%	79%
Pain 'Always' Well Controlled	300+	71%	71%	71%
Room and Bathroom 'Always' Clean	300+	70%	71%	73%
Timely Help 'Always' Received	300+	61%	65%	68%
Would Definitely Recommend Hospital	300+	72%	70%	71%
Use of Medical Imaging				
Cardiac Imaging Stress Test before Surgery	231	5.6%	5.5%	5.3%
Combination Abdominal CT Scan	505	3.8%	10.1%	10.5%
Combination Brain/Sinus CT Scan	491	1.4%	2.3%	2.7%
Combination Chest CT Scan	165	0.6%	3.7%	2.7%
Follow-up Mammogram/Ultrasound	1,594	10.8%	8.9%	8.8%
Lumbar Spine MRI for Low Back Pain	59	40.7%	36.6%	37.2%

NOTE: Hospital profiles are in alphabetical order by state, then city, then hospital within the city; Rankings exclude hospitals with less than 25 cases except for patient surveys which excludes hospitals with less than 100 cases; (a) 100-299 cases; (1) The number of cases/patients is too few to report; (2) Data submitted were based on a sample of cases/patients; (3) Results are based on a shorter time period than required; (4) Data suppressed by CMS for one or more quarters; (5) Results are not available for this reporting period; (6) Fewer than 100 patients completed the HCAHPS survey; (7) No cases met the criteria for this measure; (8) The lower limit of the confidence interval cannot be calculated if the number of observed infections equals zero; (9) No data are available from the state/territory for this reporting period; (10) The scores shown reflect fewer than 50 completed surveys; (11) There were discrepancies in the data collection process; (12) This measure does not apply to this hospital for this reporting period; (13) Results cannot be calculated for this reporting period; (14) The results for this state are combined with nearby states to protect confidentiality; Please refer to the User's Guide for a full explanation of data.

Medical College of Georgia Hospitals & Clinics

1120 15th Street — Phone: 706-721-6569
Augusta, GA 30912 — Fax: 706-721-5735
URL: www.mcghealth.org
Type: Acute Care Hospitals — Emergency Services: Yes
Ownership: Voluntary non-profit - Other — Beds: 632

Key Personnel:
Infection Control. . . . . Cyndra Bystrom
Pediatric Ambulatory Care . . . . . . Chris Lee
CEO/President. . . . . Sandra I McVicker, RN, MSN
Pediatric In-Patient Care . . . . Barbara D Meeks, RN, MSN, MBA
Operating Room. . . . . Angeline Pratt, RN, CNOR, MHA
Radiology. . . . . Jim Rawson, MD
Quality Assurance . . . . David A Snyder, MD
Coronary Care . . . . John W Thornton III, MD

Measure	Cases	This Hosp.	State Avg.	U.S. Avg.
Blood Clot Prevention and Treatment				
Anticoagulation Overlap Therapy[2]	82	98%	90%	93%
ICU Venous Thromboembolism Prophylaxis[2]	124	97%	90%	92%
Incidence of Potentially Preventable VTE[2]	67	3%	13%	10%
UFH with Dosages/Platelet Monitoring[2]	73	99%	99%	97%
Venous Thromboembolism Prophylaxis[2]	269	86%	80%	85%
Warfarin Therapy Discharge Instructions[2]	48	58%	78%	75%
Chest Pain/Possible Heart Attack Care				
Aspirin Given Within 24 Hours of Arrival[5]	-	-	94%	96%
Fibrinolytic Meds Within 30 Min. of Arrival[5]	-	-	35%	58%
Average Time to ECG (minutes)[5]	-	-	8	7
Average Time to Transfer (minutes)[5]	-	-	73	60
Children's Asthma Care				
Received Home Management Plan of Care[2]	167	88%	-	88%
Received Reliever Medication[2]	167	100%	-	100%
Received Systemic Corticosteroids[2]	167	100%	-	100%
Emergency Department				
Admittance Decision Time (minutes)[2]	530	192	100	98
Head CT Results Within 45 Min. of Arrival[1,3]	-	-	45%	57%
Patients Who Left ER Before Being Seen	88,653	4%	3%	2%
Time from ER Arrival to Admit. (minutes)[2]	534	374	286	274
Time from ER Arrival to Discharge (minutes)	335	181	140	134
Time in ER Before Being Evaluated (minutes)	223	71	32	26
Time to Pain Meds for Fractures (minutes)	265	66	64	57
Heart Attack Care				
Aspirin Given at Discharge[2]	204	100%	99%	99%
Fibrinolytic Meds Within 30 Min. of Arrival[2,7]	-	-	80%	54%
PCI Within 90 Minutes of Arrival[2]	21	95%	95%	96%
Statin Prescribed at Discharge[2]	204	99%	98%	98%
Heart Failure Care				
ACE Inhibitor or ARB for LVSD[2]	122	98%	97%	97%
Discharge Instructions Given[2]	226	82%	92%	94%
Evaluation of LVS Function[2]	251	100%	99%	99%
Medicare Spending				
Medicare Spending per Patient (ratio)	-	1.00	0.95	0.98
Pneumonia Care				
Appropriate Initial Antibiotic Given[2]	44	98%	95%	95%
Blood Culture Timing[2]	129	99%	97%	98%
Pregnancy and Delivery Care				
Newborn Deliveries Scheduled Early[2]	65	3%	8%	6%
Preventive Care				
Immunization for Influenza[2]	535	96%	88%	90%
Immunization for Pneumonia[2]	531	97%	90%	92%
Stroke Care				
Anticoagulation Therapy for Atrial Fibrillation	24	92%	94%	95%
Antithrombotic Therapy Timing	153	94%	97%	98%
Assessed for Rehabilitation	258	98%	97%	97%
Discharged on Antithrombotic Therapy	187	98%	98%	99%
Discharged on Statin Medication	137	98%	94%	94%
Thrombolytic Therapy Timing	20	85%	58%	66%
Venous Thromboembolism Prophylaxis	273	98%	92%	94%
Written Stroke Educational Materials Given	152	99%	84%	88%
Surgical Care Improvement Project				
Appropriate Beta Blocker Usage[2]	146	97%	97%	98%
Appropriate VTP Within 24 Hours[2]	276	99%	98%	98%
Controlled Postoperative Blood Glucose[2]	96	92%	96%	97%
Perioperative Temperature Management[2]	349	100%	100%	100%
Prophylactic Antibiotic Selection[2]	289	100%	99%	99%
Prophylactic Antibiotic Selection (Outpatient)	450	100%	98%	98%
Prophylactic Antibiotic Stopped[2]	247	98%	98%	98%
Prophylactic Antibiotic Timing[2]	291	99%	99%	99%
Prophylactic Antibiotic Timing (Outpatient)	415	100%	98%	98%
Urinary Catheter Removal[2]	230	97%	97%	97%
Survey of Patients' Hospital Experiences				
Area Around Room 'Always' Quiet at Night	300+	62%	66%	61%
Doctors 'Always' Communicated Well	300+	77%	83%	82%
Home Recovery Information Given	300+	83%	84%	85%
Hospital Given 9 or 10 on 10 Point Scale	300+	69%	69%	71%
Meds 'Always' Explained Before Given	300+	61%	63%	64%
Nurses 'Always' Communicated Well	300+	75%	78%	79%
Pain 'Always' Well Controlled	300+	67%	71%	71%
Room and Bathroom 'Always' Clean	300+	68%	71%	73%
Timely Help 'Always' Received	300+	55%	65%	68%
Would Definitely Recommend Hospital	300+	71%	70%	71%
Use of Medical Imaging				
Cardiac Imaging Stress Test before Surgery	405	6.4%	5.5%	5.3%
Combination Abdominal CT Scan	896	15.2%	10.1%	10.5%
Combination Brain/Sinus CT Scan	816	0.5%	2.3%	2.7%
Combination Chest CT Scan	509	0.0%	3.7%	2.7%
Follow-up Mammogram/Ultrasound	989	3.4%	8.9%	8.8%
Lumbar Spine MRI for Low Back Pain	110	32.7%	36.6%	37.2%

Trinity Hospital of Augusta

2260 Wrightsboro Rd — Phone: 706-481-7000
Augusta, GA 30904 — Fax: 706-481-7863
URL: www.trinityofaugusta.com
Type: Acute Care Hospitals — Emergency Services: Yes
Ownership: Proprietary — Beds: 107

Key Personnel:
Emergency Room . . . . Walter Hardwood
CEO/President. . . . . Andrew A Lasser
Operating Room. . . . . Ann McCarty
Quality Assurance . . . . Peggy McClintock

Measure	Cases	This Hosp.	State Avg.	U.S. Avg.
Blood Clot Prevention and Treatment				
Anticoagulation Overlap Therapy[2]	12	100%	90%	93%
ICU Venous Thromboembolism Prophylaxis[2]	55	100%	90%	92%
Incidence of Potentially Preventable VTE[1,2]	-	-	13%	10%
UFH with Dosages/Platelet Monitoring[1,2]	-	-	99%	97%
Venous Thromboembolism Prophylaxis[2]	272	100%	80%	85%
Warfarin Therapy Discharge Instructions[2]	12	100%	78%	75%
Chest Pain/Possible Heart Attack Care				
Aspirin Given Within 24 Hours of Arrival[1,3]	-	-	94%	96%
Fibrinolytic Meds Within 30 Min. of Arrival[3,7]	-	-	35%	58%
Average Time to ECG (minutes)[1,3]	-	-	8	7
Average Time to Transfer (minutes)[3,7]	-	-	73	60
Children's Asthma Care				
Received Home Management Plan of Care	-	-	-	88%
Received Reliever Medication	-	-	-	100%
Received Systemic Corticosteroids	-	-	-	100%
Emergency Department				
Admittance Decision Time (minutes)[2]	368	68	100	98
Head CT Results Within 45 Min. of Arrival[1]	-	-	45%	57%
Patients Who Left ER Before Being Seen	18,138	1%	3%	2%
Time from ER Arrival to Admit. (minutes)[2]	392	240	286	274
Time from ER Arrival to Discharge (minutes)	400	122	140	134
Time in ER Before Being Evaluated (minutes)	416	25	32	26
Time to Pain Meds for Fractures (minutes)	50	61	64	57
Heart Attack Care				
Aspirin Given at Discharge	34	100%	99%	99%
Fibrinolytic Meds Within 30 Min. of Arrival[7]	-	-	80%	54%
PCI Within 90 Minutes of Arrival[1]	-	-	95%	96%
Statin Prescribed at Discharge	33	100%	98%	98%
Heart Failure Care				
ACE Inhibitor or ARB for LVSD	39	97%	97%	97%
Discharge Instructions Given	76	97%	92%	94%
Evaluation of LVS Function	100	100%	99%	99%
Medicare Spending				
Medicare Spending per Patient (ratio)	-	1.01	0.95	0.98
Pneumonia Care				
Appropriate Initial Antibiotic Given	51	96%	95%	95%
Blood Culture Timing	113	98%	97%	98%
Pregnancy and Delivery Care				
Newborn Deliveries Scheduled Early[2]	28	0%	8%	6%
Preventive Care				
Immunization for Influenza[2]	468	100%	88%	90%
Immunization for Pneumonia[2]	503	100%	90%	92%
Stroke Care				
Anticoagulation Therapy for Atrial Fibrillation[1]	-	-	94%	95%
Antithrombotic Therapy Timing	14	100%	97%	98%
Assessed for Rehabilitation	14	100%	97%	97%
Discharged on Antithrombotic Therapy	12	100%	98%	99%
Discharged on Statin Medication	11	100%	94%	94%
Thrombolytic Therapy Timing[7]	-	-	58%	66%
Venous Thromboembolism Prophylaxis	13	100%	92%	94%
Written Stroke Educational Materials Given[1]	-	-	84%	88%
Surgical Care Improvement Project				
Appropriate Beta Blocker Usage	113	96%	97%	98%
Appropriate VTP Within 24 Hours	432	99%	98%	98%
Controlled Postoperative Blood Glucose[7]	-	-	96%	97%
Perioperative Temperature Management	477	100%	100%	100%
Prophylactic Antibiotic Selection	298	100%	99%	99%
Prophylactic Antibiotic Selection (Outpatient)	165	100%	98%	98%
Prophylactic Antibiotic Stopped	287	98%	98%	98%
Prophylactic Antibiotic Timing	298	100%	99%	99%
Prophylactic Antibiotic Timing (Outpatient)	166	99%	98%	98%
Urinary Catheter Removal	192	98%	97%	97%
Survey of Patients' Hospital Experiences				
Area Around Room 'Always' Quiet at Night	300+	67%	66%	61%
Doctors 'Always' Communicated Well	300+	83%	83%	82%
Home Recovery Information Given	300+	85%	84%	85%
Hospital Given 9 or 10 on 10 Point Scale	300+	70%	69%	71%
Meds 'Always' Explained Before Given	300+	60%	63%	64%
Nurses 'Always' Communicated Well	300+	79%	78%	79%
Pain 'Always' Well Controlled	300+	70%	71%	71%
Room and Bathroom 'Always' Clean	300+	64%	71%	73%
Timely Help 'Always' Received	300+	62%	65%	68%
Would Definitely Recommend Hospital	300+	70%	70%	71%
Use of Medical Imaging				
Cardiac Imaging Stress Test before Surgery	85	9.4%	5.5%	5.3%
Combination Abdominal CT Scan	328	7.9%	10.1%	10.5%
Combination Brain/Sinus CT Scan[1]	-	-	2.3%	2.7%
Combination Chest CT Scan	86	11.6%	3.7%	2.7%
Follow-up Mammogram/Ultrasound	430	13.0%	8.9%	8.8%
Lumbar Spine MRI for Low Back Pain[1]	-	-	36.6%	37.2%

University Hospital

1350 Walton Way — Phone: 706-722-9011
Augusta, GA 30901 — Fax: 706-774-8699
URL: www.universityhealth.org
Type: Acute Care Hospitals — Emergency Services: Yes
Ownership: Voluntary non-profit - Other — Beds: 612

Key Personnel:
Radiology. . . . . Henry Alperin, MD
Infection Control. . . . . Vivian Ashline
CEO/President. . . . . James R. Davis
Emergency Room . . . . Richard Eckert, MD
Chief of Medical Staff . . . . William Farr, MD
Quality Assurance . . . . John B Swihart
Pediatric Ambulatory Care . . . . . . Julian Tanenbaum, MD
Pediatric In-Patient Care . . . . Julian Tanenbaum, MD

Measure	Cases	This Hosp.	State Avg.	U.S. Avg.
Blood Clot Prevention and Treatment				
Anticoagulation Overlap Therapy[2]	176	81%	90%	93%
ICU Venous Thromboembolism Prophylaxis[2]	58	97%	90%	92%
Incidence of Potentially Preventable VTE[2]	39	23%	13%	10%
UFH with Dosages/Platelet Monitoring[2]	81	99%	99%	97%
Venous Thromboembolism Prophylaxis[2]	372	88%	80%	85%
Warfarin Therapy Discharge Instructions[2]	134	72%	78%	75%
Chest Pain/Possible Heart Attack Care				
Aspirin Given Within 24 Hours of Arrival[5]	-	-	94%	96%
Fibrinolytic Meds Within 30 Min. of Arrival[5]	-	-	35%	58%
Average Time to ECG (minutes)[5]	-	-	8	7
Average Time to Transfer (minutes)[5]	-	-	73	60
Children's Asthma Care				

NOTE: Hospital profiles are in alphabetical order by state, then city, then hospital within the city; Rankings exclude hospitals with less than 25 cases except for patient surveys which excludes hospitals with less than 100 cases; (a) 100-299 cases; (1) The number of cases/patients is too few to report; (2) Data submitted were based on a sample of cases/patients; (3) Results are based on a shorter time period than required; (4) Data suppressed by CMS for one or more quarters; (5) Results are not available for this reporting period; (6) Fewer than 100 patients completed the HCAHPS survey; (7) No cases met the criteria for this measure; (8) The lower limit of the confidence interval cannot be calculated if the number of observed infections equals zero; (9) No data are available from the state/territory for this reporting period; (10) The scores shown reflect fewer than 50 completed surveys; (11) There were discrepancies in the data collection process; (12) This measure does not apply to this hospital for this reporting period; (13) Results cannot be calculated for this reporting period; (14) The results for this state are combined with nearby states to protect confidentiality; Please refer to the User's Guide for a full explanation of data.

Measure	Cases	This Hosp.	State Avg.	U.S. Avg.
Received Home Management Plan of Care	-	-	-	88%
Received Reliever Medication	-	-	-	100%
Received Systemic Corticosteroids	-	-	-	100%
Emergency Department				
Admittance Decision Time (minutes)[2]	494	116	100	98
Head CT Results Within 45 Min. of Arrival[3]	15	40%	45%	57%
Patients Who Left ER Before Being Seen	80,877	5%	3%	2%
Time from ER Arrival to Admit. (minutes)[2]	498	318	286	274
Time from ER Arrival to Discharge (minutes)	400	170	140	134
Time in ER Before Being Evaluated (minutes)	302	50	32	26
Time to Pain Meds for Fractures (minutes)	232	86	64	57
Heart Attack Care				
Aspirin Given at Discharge	538	100%	99%	99%
Fibrinolytic Meds Within 30 Min. of Arrival[7]	-	-	80%	54%
PCI Within 90 Minutes of Arrival	85	94%	95%	96%
Statin Prescribed at Discharge	521	100%	98%	98%
Heart Failure Care				
ACE Inhibitor or ARB for LVSD[2]	125	100%	97%	97%
Discharge Instructions Given[2]	269	91%	92%	94%
Evaluation of LVS Function[2]	326	100%	99%	99%
Medicare Spending				
Medicare Spending per Patient (ratio)	-	0.96	0.95	0.98
Pneumonia Care				
Appropriate Initial Antibiotic Given[2]	84	96%	95%	95%
Blood Culture Timing[2]	136	100%	97%	98%
Pregnancy and Delivery Care				
Newborn Deliveries Scheduled Early	325	26%	8%	6%
Preventive Care				
Immunization for Influenza[2]	532	76%	88%	90%
Immunization for Pneumonia[2]	694	79%	90%	92%
Stroke Care				
Anticoagulation Therapy for Atrial Fibrillation	39	97%	94%	95%
Antithrombotic Therapy Timing	269	99%	97%	98%
Assessed for Rehabilitation	314	100%	97%	97%
Discharged on Antithrombotic Therapy	281	100%	98%	99%
Discharged on Statin Medication	219	100%	94%	94%
Thrombolytic Therapy Timing	22	68%	58%	66%
Venous Thromboembolism Prophylaxis	327	98%	92%	94%
Written Stroke Educational Materials Given	177	93%	84%	88%
Surgical Care Improvement Project				
Appropriate Beta Blocker Usage[2]	251	100%	97%	98%
Appropriate VTP Within 24 Hours[2]	453	100%	98%	98%
Controlled Postoperative Blood Glucose[2]	179	98%	96%	97%
Perioperative Temperature Management[2]	590	100%	100%	100%
Prophylactic Antibiotic Selection[2]	602	100%	99%	99%
Prophylactic Antibiotic Selection (Outpatient)	536	98%	98%	98%
Prophylactic Antibiotic Stopped[2]	589	99%	98%	98%
Prophylactic Antibiotic Timing[2]	602	100%	99%	99%
Prophylactic Antibiotic Timing (Outpatient)	541	98%	98%	98%
Urinary Catheter Removal[2]	259	99%	97%	97%
Survey of Patients' Hospital Experiences				
Area Around Room 'Always' Quiet at Night	300+	67%	66%	61%
Doctors 'Always' Communicated Well	300+	83%	83%	82%
Home Recovery Information Given	300+	84%	84%	85%
Hospital Given 9 or 10 on 10 Point Scale	300+	76%	69%	71%
Meds 'Always' Explained Before Given	300+	64%	63%	64%
Nurses 'Always' Communicated Well	300+	79%	78%	79%
Pain 'Always' Well Controlled	300+	71%	71%	71%
Room and Bathroom 'Always' Clean	300+	72%	71%	73%
Timely Help 'Always' Received	300+	61%	65%	68%
Would Definitely Recommend Hospital	300+	81%	70%	71%
Use of Medical Imaging				
Cardiac Imaging Stress Test before Surgery	2,451	4.5%	5.5%	5.3%
Combination Abdominal CT Scan	1,188	6.1%	10.1%	10.5%
Combination Brain/Sinus CT Scan	1,318	1.1%	2.3%	2.7%
Combination Chest CT Scan	459	6.3%	3.7%	2.7%
Follow-up Mammogram/Ultrasound	854	9.7%	8.9%	8.8%
Lumbar Spine MRI for Low Back Pain	213	27.7%	36.6%	37.2%

Wellstar Cobb Hospital

3950 Austell Rd | Phone: 770-732-4000
Austell, GA 30106 | Fax: 770-732-4015
E-mail: generalinfo@wellstar.org
URL: www.wellstar.org
Type: Acute Care Hospitals | Emergency Services: Yes
Ownership: Voluntary non-profit - Other | Beds: 322

Key Personnel:
Emergency Room . . . . Renee Akins
CEO/President. . . . . Randy Cook
Patient Relations . . . . George Fleming
Radiology. . . . . Lynn Hanks
Operating Room. . . . . Michael Jackson
Chair/CEO . . . . Gary A. Miller
Chief of Medical Staff . . . . Dr Odom

Measure	Cases	This Hosp.	State Avg.	U.S. Avg.
Blood Clot Prevention and Treatment				
Anticoagulation Overlap Therapy[2]	127	94%	90%	93%
ICU Venous Thromboembolism Prophylaxis[2]	88	98%	90%	92%
Incidence of Potentially Preventable VTE[2]	23	17%	13%	10%
UFH with Dosages/Platelet Monitoring[2]	129	100%	99%	97%
Venous Thromboembolism Prophylaxis[2]	350	82%	80%	85%
Warfarin Therapy Discharge Instructions[2]	90	80%	78%	75%
Chest Pain/Possible Heart Attack Care				
Aspirin Given Within 24 Hours of Arrival	33	85%	94%	96%
Fibrinolytic Meds Within 30 Min. of Arrival[3,7]	-	-	35%	58%
Average Time to ECG (minutes)	34	4	8	7
Average Time to Transfer (minutes)[3,7]	-	-	73	60
Children's Asthma Care				
Received Home Management Plan of Care	-	-	-	88%
Received Reliever Medication	-	-	-	100%
Received Systemic Corticosteroids	-	-	-	100%
Emergency Department				
Admittance Decision Time (minutes)[2]	333	110	100	98
Head CT Results Within 45 Min. of Arrival	16	69%	45%	57%
Patients Who Left ER Before Being Seen	>100k	1%	3%	2%
Time from ER Arrival to Admit. (minutes)[2]	372	335	286	274
Time from ER Arrival to Discharge (minutes)	400	135	140	134
Time in ER Before Being Evaluated (minutes)	330	46	32	26
Time to Pain Meds for Fractures (minutes)	244	71	64	57
Heart Attack Care				
Aspirin Given at Discharge[2]	220	100%	99%	99%
Fibrinolytic Meds Within 30 Min. of Arrival[2,7]	-	-	80%	54%
PCI Within 90 Minutes of Arrival[2]	39	92%	95%	96%
Statin Prescribed at Discharge[2]	205	99%	98%	98%
Heart Failure Care				
ACE Inhibitor or ARB for LVSD[2]	174	98%	97%	97%
Discharge Instructions Given[2]	536	80%	92%	94%
Evaluation of LVS Function[2]	597	100%	99%	99%
Medicare Spending				
Medicare Spending per Patient (ratio)	-	0.98	0.95	0.98
Pneumonia Care				
Appropriate Initial Antibiotic Given[2]	197	98%	95%	95%
Blood Culture Timing[2]	348	99%	97%	98%
Pregnancy and Delivery Care				
Newborn Deliveries Scheduled Early[2]	56	2%	8%	6%
Preventive Care				
Immunization for Influenza[2]	516	96%	88%	90%
Immunization for Pneumonia[2]	546	95%	90%	92%
Stroke Care				
Anticoagulation Therapy for Atrial Fibrillation[2]	12	83%	94%	95%
Antithrombotic Therapy Timing[2]	106	99%	97%	98%
Assessed for Rehabilitation[2]	112	96%	97%	97%
Discharged on Antithrombotic Therapy[2]	108	100%	98%	99%
Discharged on Statin Medication[2]	78	97%	94%	94%
Thrombolytic Therapy Timing[1,2]	-	-	58%	66%
Venous Thromboembolism Prophylaxis[2]	117	94%	92%	94%
Written Stroke Educational Materials Given[2]	66	79%	84%	88%
Surgical Care Improvement Project				
Appropriate Beta Blocker Usage[2]	282	99%	97%	98%
Appropriate VTP Within 24 Hours[2]	726	99%	98%	98%
Controlled Postoperative Blood Glucose[2,7]	-	-	96%	97%
Perioperative Temperature Management[2]	908	100%	100%	100%
Prophylactic Antibiotic Selection[2]	578	99%	99%	99%
Prophylactic Antibiotic Selection (Outpatient)	548	99%	98%	98%
Prophylactic Antibiotic Stopped[2]	563	97%	98%	98%
Prophylactic Antibiotic Timing[2]	578	99%	99%	99%
Prophylactic Antibiotic Timing (Outpatient)	550	99%	98%	98%
Urinary Catheter Removal[2]	492	98%	97%	97%
Survey of Patients' Hospital Experiences				
Area Around Room 'Always' Quiet at Night	300+	58%	66%	61%
Doctors 'Always' Communicated Well	300+	80%	83%	82%
Home Recovery Information Given	300+	78%	84%	85%
Hospital Given 9 or 10 on 10 Point Scale	300+	67%	69%	71%
Meds 'Always' Explained Before Given	300+	62%	63%	64%
Nurses 'Always' Communicated Well	300+	75%	78%	79%
Pain 'Always' Well Controlled	300+	67%	71%	71%
Room and Bathroom 'Always' Clean	300+	68%	71%	73%
Timely Help 'Always' Received	300+	58%	65%	68%
Would Definitely Recommend Hospital	300+	68%	70%	71%
Use of Medical Imaging				
Cardiac Imaging Stress Test before Surgery	444	5.6%	5.5%	5.3%
Combination Abdominal CT Scan	1,135	8.5%	10.1%	10.5%
Combination Brain/Sinus CT Scan	1,037	2.0%	2.3%	2.7%
Combination Chest CT Scan	682	0.6%	3.7%	2.7%
Follow-up Mammogram/Ultrasound	1,529	12.9%	8.9%	8.8%
Lumbar Spine MRI for Low Back Pain[1]	-	-	36.6%	37.2%

Memorial Hospital & Manor

1500 E Shotwell Street | Phone: 229-246-3500
Bainbridge, GA 39819 | Fax: 229-243-3338
URL: www.mh-m.org
Type: Acute Care Hospitals | Emergency Services: Yes
Ownership: Govt - Hospital Dist/Auth | Beds: 80

Key Personnel:
Radiology. . . . . Jerjis Thomas Alajaji
Emergency Room . . . . Michael Hancock
Quality Assurance . . . . Teresa McMillan
Cardiology . . . . Gordon C Miller, RN
Intensive Care Unit. . . . . Cindy Newton, RN
Anesthesiology. . . . . Thomas H Parker
CEO/President. . . . . James G Peak
Radiology. . . . . Jerjis Thomas, MD

Measure	Cases	This Hosp.	State Avg.	U.S. Avg.
Blood Clot Prevention and Treatment				
Anticoagulation Overlap Therapy[1,2]	-	-	90%	93%
ICU Venous Thromboembolism Prophylaxis[2]	67	81%	90%	92%
Incidence of Potentially Preventable VTE[2,7]	-	-	13%	10%
UFH with Dosages/Platelet Monitoring[2,7]	-	-	99%	97%
Venous Thromboembolism Prophylaxis[2]	208	79%	80%	85%
Warfarin Therapy Discharge Instructions[1,2]	-	-	78%	75%
Chest Pain/Possible Heart Attack Care				
Aspirin Given Within 24 Hours of Arrival	27	89%	94%	96%
Fibrinolytic Meds Within 30 Min. of Arrival[1]	-	-	35%	58%
Average Time to ECG (minutes)	20	14	8	7
Average Time to Transfer (minutes)[7]	-	-	73	60
Children's Asthma Care				
Received Home Management Plan of Care	-	-	-	88%
Received Reliever Medication	-	-	-	100%
Received Systemic Corticosteroids	-	-	-	100%
Emergency Department				
Admittance Decision Time (minutes)[2]	271	44	100	98
Head CT Results Within 45 Min. of Arrival[1]	-	-	45%	57%
Patients Who Left ER Before Being Seen	18,000	1%	3%	2%
Time from ER Arrival to Admit. (minutes)[2]	276	214	286	274
Time from ER Arrival to Discharge (minutes)[3]	311	145	140	134
Time in ER Before Being Evaluated (minutes)	329	40	32	26
Time to Pain Meds for Fractures (minutes)	61	97	64	57
Heart Attack Care				
Aspirin Given at Discharge[1,3]	-	-	99%	99%
Fibrinolytic Meds Within 30 Min. of Arrival[3,7]	-	-	80%	54%
PCI Within 90 Minutes of Arrival[3,7]	-	-	95%	96%
Statin Prescribed at Discharge[1,3]	-	-	98%	98%
Heart Failure Care				
ACE Inhibitor or ARB for LVSD[2]	28	96%	97%	97%
Discharge Instructions Given[2]	48	100%	92%	94%
Evaluation of LVS Function[2]	57	95%	99%	99%
Medicare Spending				

NOTE: Hospital profiles are in alphabetical order by state, then city, then hospital within the city; Rankings exclude hospitals with less than 25 cases except for patient surveys which excludes hospitals with less than 100 cases; (a) 100-299 cases; (1) The number of cases/patients is too few to report; (2) Data submitted were based on a sample of cases/patients; (3) Results are based on a shorter time period than required; (4) Data suppressed by CMS for one or more quarters; (5) Results are not available for this reporting period; (6) Fewer than 100 patients completed the HCAHPS survey; (7) No cases met the criteria for this measure; (8) The lower limit of the confidence interval cannot be calculated if the number of observed infections equals zero; (9) No data are available from the state/territory for this reporting period; (10) The scores shown reflect fewer than 50 completed surveys; (11) There were discrepancies in the data collection process; (12) This measure does not apply to this hospital for this reporting period; (13) Results cannot be calculated for this reporting period; (14) The results for this state are combined with nearby states to protect confidentiality; Please refer to the User's Guide for a full explanation of data.

Medicare Spending per Patient (ratio)	-	0.88	0.95	0.98
Pneumonia Care				
Appropriate Initial Antibiotic Given[2]	55	87%	95%	95%
Blood Culture Timing[2]	67	91%	97%	98%
Pregnancy and Delivery Care				
Newborn Deliveries Scheduled Early	51	0%	8%	6%
Preventive Care				
Immunization for Influenza[2]	278	60%	88%	90%
Immunization for Pneumonia[2]	307	94%	90%	92%
Stroke Care				
Anticoagulation Therapy for Atrial Fibrillation[1]	-	-	94%	95%
Antithrombotic Therapy Timing	40	100%	97%	98%
Assessed for Rehabilitation	42	93%	97%	97%
Discharged on Antithrombotic Therapy	38	100%	98%	99%
Discharged on Statin Medication	32	94%	94%	94%
Thrombolytic Therapy Timing[7]	-	-	58%	66%
Venous Thromboembolism Prophylaxis	41	85%	92%	94%
Written Stroke Educational Materials Given	25	60%	84%	88%
Surgical Care Improvement Project				
Appropriate Beta Blocker Usage[1]	-	-	97%	98%
Appropriate VTP Within 24 Hours	69	99%	98%	98%
Controlled Postoperative Blood Glucose[7]	-	-	96%	97%
Perioperative Temperature Management	81	94%	100%	100%
Prophylactic Antibiotic Selection	29	90%	99%	99%
Prophylactic Antibiotic Selection (Outpatient)	29	100%	98%	98%
Prophylactic Antibiotic Stopped	29	100%	98%	98%
Prophylactic Antibiotic Timing	29	86%	99%	99%
Prophylactic Antibiotic Timing (Outpatient)	31	90%	98%	98%
Urinary Catheter Removal	54	91%	97%	97%
Survey of Patients' Hospital Experiences				
Area Around Room 'Always' Quiet at Night	300+	68%	66%	61%
Doctors 'Always' Communicated Well	300+	83%	83%	82%
Home Recovery Information Given	300+	84%	84%	85%
Hospital Given 9 or 10 on 10 Point Scale	300+	63%	69%	71%
Meds 'Always' Explained Before Given	300+	62%	63%	64%
Nurses 'Always' Communicated Well	300+	80%	78%	79%
Pain 'Always' Well Controlled	300+	68%	71%	71%
Room and Bathroom 'Always' Clean	300+	70%	71%	73%
Timely Help 'Always' Received	300+	67%	65%	68%
Would Definitely Recommend Hospital	300+	59%	70%	71%
Use of Medical Imaging				
Cardiac Imaging Stress Test before Surgery[1]	-	-	5.5%	5.3%
Combination Abdominal CT Scan	332	18.1%	10.1%	10.5%
Combination Brain/Sinus CT Scan[1]	-	-	2.3%	2.7%
Combination Chest CT Scan	144	9.7%	3.7%	2.7%
Follow-up Mammogram/Ultrasound	567	3.0%	8.9%	8.8%
Lumbar Spine MRI for Low Back Pain	72	34.7%	36.6%	37.2%

Appling Hospital

163 E Tollison Street
Baxley, GA 31513
URL: www.appling-hospital.org
Phone: 912-367-9841
Fax: 912-367-7203
Type: Acute Care Hospitals
Emergency Services: Yes
Ownership: Govt - Hospital Dist/Auth
Beds: 39

Key Personnel:

Operating Room. . . . . Shirley Duie
Chief of Medical Staff. . . . . Debbie Griffis
CEO/President. . . . . Dale Spell
Quality Assurance . . . . Dale Spell

Measure	Cases	This Hosp.	State Avg.	U.S. Avg.
Blood Clot Prevention and Treatment				
Anticoagulation Overlap Therapy[1,2]	-	-	90%	93%
ICU Venous Thromboembolism Prophylaxis[2]	40	52%	90%	92%
Incidence of Potentially Preventable VTE[1,2]	-	-	13%	10%
UFH with Dosages/Platelet Monitoring[1,2]	-	-	99%	97%
Venous Thromboembolism Prophylaxis[2]	232	56%	80%	85%
Warfarin Therapy Discharge Instructions[1,2]	-	-	78%	75%
Chest Pain/Possible Heart Attack Care				
Aspirin Given Within 24 Hours of Arrival[5]	-	-	94%	96%
Fibrinolytic Meds Within 30 Min. of Arrival[5]	-	-	35%	58%
Average Time to ECG (minutes)[5]	-	-	8	7
Average Time to Transfer (minutes)[5]	-	-	73	60
Children's Asthma Care				
Received Home Management Plan of Care	-	-	-	88%
Received Reliever Medication	-	-	-	100%
Received Systemic Corticosteroids	-	-	-	100%
Emergency Department				
Admittance Decision Time (minutes)[2]	233	79	100	98
Head CT Results Within 45 Min. of Arrival[1,3]	-	-	45%	57%
Patients Who Left ER Before Being Seen	8,987	1%	3%	2%
Time from ER Arrival to Admit. (minutes)[2]	249	255	286	274
Time from ER Arrival to Discharge (minutes)	240	115	140	134
Time in ER Before Being Evaluated (minutes)	249	8	32	26
Time to Pain Meds for Fractures (minutes)[1,3]	-	-	64	57
Heart Attack Care				
Aspirin Given at Discharge[3,7]	-	-	99%	99%
Fibrinolytic Meds Within 30 Min. of Arrival[3,7]	-	-	80%	54%
PCI Within 90 Minutes of Arrival[3,7]	-	-	95%	96%
Statin Prescribed at Discharge[3,7]	-	-	98%	98%
Heart Failure Care				
ACE Inhibitor or ARB for LVSD	14	71%	97%	97%
Discharge Instructions Given	41	78%	92%	94%
Evaluation of LVS Function	42	71%	99%	99%
Medicare Spending				
Medicare Spending per Patient (ratio)	-	0.83	0.95	0.98
Pneumonia Care				
Appropriate Initial Antibiotic Given[2]	33	76%	95%	95%
Blood Culture Timing[2]	23	87%	97%	98%
Pregnancy and Delivery Care				
Newborn Deliveries Scheduled Early[1]	-	-	8%	6%
Preventive Care				
Immunization for Influenza[2]	277	79%	88%	90%
Immunization for Pneumonia[2]	375	80%	90%	92%
Stroke Care				
Anticoagulation Therapy for Atrial Fibrillation[1]	-	-	94%	95%
Antithrombotic Therapy Timing[1]	-	-	97%	98%
Assessed for Rehabilitation	11	82%	97%	97%
Discharged on Antithrombotic Therapy[1]	-	-	98%	99%
Discharged on Statin Medication[1]	-	-	94%	94%
Thrombolytic Therapy Timing[1]	-	-	58%	66%
Venous Thromboembolism Prophylaxis	12	58%	92%	94%
Written Stroke Educational Materials Given[1]	-	-	84%	88%
Surgical Care Improvement Project				
Appropriate Beta Blocker Usage[1]	-	-	97%	98%
Appropriate VTP Within 24 Hours[1]	-	-	98%	98%
Controlled Postoperative Blood Glucose[7]	-	-	96%	97%
Perioperative Temperature Management[1]	-	-	100%	100%
Prophylactic Antibiotic Selection[1]	-	-	99%	99%
Prophylactic Antibiotic Selection (Outpatient)[3,7]	-	-	98%	98%
Prophylactic Antibiotic Stopped[1]	-	-	98%	98%
Prophylactic Antibiotic Timing[1]	-	-	99%	99%
Prophylactic Antibiotic Timing (Outpatient)[1,3]	-	-	98%	98%
Urinary Catheter Removal[1]	-	-	97%	97%
Survey of Patients' Hospital Experiences				
Area Around Room 'Always' Quiet at Night	(a)	69%	66%	61%
Doctors 'Always' Communicated Well	(a)	86%	83%	82%
Home Recovery Information Given	(a)	85%	84%	85%
Hospital Given 9 or 10 on 10 Point Scale	(a)	51%	69%	71%
Meds 'Always' Explained Before Given	(a)	60%	63%	64%
Nurses 'Always' Communicated Well	(a)	74%	78%	79%
Pain 'Always' Well Controlled	(a)	69%	71%	71%
Room and Bathroom 'Always' Clean	(a)	56%	71%	73%
Timely Help 'Always' Received	(a)	59%	65%	68%
Would Definitely Recommend Hospital	(a)	52%	70%	71%
Use of Medical Imaging				
Cardiac Imaging Stress Test before Surgery	46	2.2%	5.5%	5.3%
Combination Abdominal CT Scan	165	21.8%	10.1%	10.5%
Combination Brain/Sinus CT Scan[1]	-	-	2.3%	2.7%
Combination Chest CT Scan	104	15.4%	3.7%	2.7%
Follow-up Mammogram/Ultrasound	243	11.1%	8.9%	8.8%
Lumbar Spine MRI for Low Back Pain	40	47.5%	36.6%	37.2%

Union General Hospital

35 Hospital Road
Blairsville, GA 30512
URL: www.uniongeneralhospital.com
Phone: 706-745-2111
Fax: 706-745-7677
Type: Acute Care Hospitals
Emergency Services: Yes
Ownership: Govt - Hospital Dist/Auth
Beds: 45

Key Personnel:

Cardiology . . . . William Blincoe, MD
Operating Room. . . . . Susan Brown
CEO/President. . . . . Rebecca T Dyer
Quality Assurance . . . . Catherine Hammock

Measure	Cases	This Hosp.	State Avg.	U.S. Avg.
Blood Clot Prevention and Treatment				
Anticoagulation Overlap Therapy[2]	11	55%	90%	93%
ICU Venous Thromboembolism Prophylaxis[2]	38	100%	90%	92%
Incidence of Potentially Preventable VTE[1,2]	-	-	13%	10%
UFH with Dosages/Platelet Monitoring[1,2]	-	-	99%	97%
Venous Thromboembolism Prophylaxis[2]	178	94%	80%	85%
Warfarin Therapy Discharge Instructions[1,2]	-	-	78%	75%
Chest Pain/Possible Heart Attack Care				
Aspirin Given Within 24 Hours of Arrival	100	92%	94%	96%
Fibrinolytic Meds Within 30 Min. of Arrival[7]	-	-	35%	58%
Average Time to ECG (minutes)	100	6	8	7
Average Time to Transfer (minutes)	11	64	73	60
Children's Asthma Care				
Received Home Management Plan of Care	-	-	-	88%
Received Reliever Medication	-	-	-	100%
Received Systemic Corticosteroids	-	-	-	100%
Emergency Department				
Admittance Decision Time (minutes)[2]	256	56	100	98
Head CT Results Within 45 Min. of Arrival[1]	-	-	45%	57%
Patients Who Left ER Before Being Seen	19,268	0%	3%	2%
Time from ER Arrival to Admit. (minutes)[2]	300	232	286	274
Time from ER Arrival to Discharge (minutes)	410	146	140	134
Time in ER Before Being Evaluated (minutes)	312	31	32	26
Time to Pain Meds for Fractures (minutes)	69	54	64	57
Heart Attack Care				
Aspirin Given at Discharge[1,2]	-	-	99%	99%
Fibrinolytic Meds Within 30 Min. of Arrival[2,7]	-	-	80%	54%
PCI Within 90 Minutes of Arrival[2,7]	-	-	95%	96%
Statin Prescribed at Discharge[1,2]	-	-	98%	98%
Heart Failure Care				
ACE Inhibitor or ARB for LVSD[2]	16	94%	97%	97%
Discharge Instructions Given[2]	46	85%	92%	94%
Evaluation of LVS Function[2]	55	98%	99%	99%
Medicare Spending				
Medicare Spending per Patient (ratio)	-	0.82	0.95	0.98
Pneumonia Care				
Appropriate Initial Antibiotic Given[2]	83	92%	95%	95%
Blood Culture Timing[2]	102	99%	97%	98%
Pregnancy and Delivery Care				
Newborn Deliveries Scheduled Early[2]	36	19%	8%	6%
Preventive Care				
Immunization for Influenza[2]	275	91%	88%	90%
Immunization for Pneumonia[2]	329	94%	90%	92%
Stroke Care				
Anticoagulation Therapy for Atrial Fibrillation[1]	-	-	94%	95%
Antithrombotic Therapy Timing	22	91%	97%	98%
Assessed for Rehabilitation	24	100%	97%	97%
Discharged on Antithrombotic Therapy	23	100%	98%	99%
Discharged on Statin Medication	18	83%	94%	94%
Thrombolytic Therapy Timing[1]	-	-	58%	66%
Venous Thromboembolism Prophylaxis	23	83%	92%	94%
Written Stroke Educational Materials Given[1]	-	-	84%	88%
Surgical Care Improvement Project				
Appropriate Beta Blocker Usage[2]	16	94%	97%	98%
Appropriate VTP Within 24 Hours[2]	58	93%	98%	98%
Controlled Postoperative Blood Glucose[2,7]	-	-	96%	97%
Perioperative Temperature Management[2]	63	100%	100%	100%
Prophylactic Antibiotic Selection[2]	52	92%	99%	99%
Prophylactic Antibiotic Selection (Outpatient)	63	94%	98%	98%
Prophylactic Antibiotic Stopped[2]	52	94%	98%	98%
Prophylactic Antibiotic Timing[2]	53	81%	99%	99%

NOTE: Hospital profiles are in alphabetical order by state, then city, then hospital within the city; Rankings exclude hospitals with less than 25 cases except for patient surveys which excludes hospitals with less than 100 cases; (a) 100-299 cases; (1) The number of cases/patients is too few to report; (2) Data submitted were based on a sample of cases/patients; (3) Results are based on a shorter time period than required; (4) Data suppressed by CMS for one or more quarters; (5) Results are not available for this reporting period; (6) Fewer than 100 patients completed the HCAHPS survey; (7) No cases met the criteria for this measure; (8) The lower limit of the confidence interval cannot be calculated if the number of observed infections equals zero; (9) No data are available from the state/territory for this reporting period; (10) The scores shown reflect fewer than 50 completed surveys; (11) There were discrepancies in the data collection process; (12) This measure does not apply to this hospital for this reporting period; (13) Results cannot be calculated for this reporting period; (14) The results for this state are combined with nearby states to protect confidentiality; Please refer to the User's Guide for a full explanation of data.

Measure	Cases	This Hosp.	State Avg.	U.S. Avg.
Prophylactic Antibiotic Timing (Outpatient)	62	89%	98%	98%
Urinary Catheter Removal[2]	27	96%	97%	97%
Survey of Patients' Hospital Experiences				
Area Around Room 'Always' Quiet at Night	300+	71%	66%	61%
Doctors 'Always' Communicated Well	300+	86%	83%	82%
Home Recovery Information Given	300+	88%	84%	85%
Hospital Given 9 or 10 on 10 Point Scale	300+	74%	69%	71%
Meds 'Always' Explained Before Given	300+	64%	63%	64%
Nurses 'Always' Communicated Well	300+	80%	78%	79%
Pain 'Always' Well Controlled	300+	69%	71%	71%
Room and Bathroom 'Always' Clean	300+	75%	71%	73%
Timely Help 'Always' Received	300+	75%	65%	68%
Would Definitely Recommend Hospital	300+	79%	70%	71%
Use of Medical Imaging				
Cardiac Imaging Stress Test before Surgery	177	9.6%	5.5%	5.3%
Combination Abdominal CT Scan	643	4.8%	10.1%	10.5%
Combination Brain/Sinus CT Scan	596	0.8%	2.3%	2.7%
Combination Chest CT Scan	387	1.6%	3.7%	2.7%
Follow-up Mammogram/Ultrasound	1,340	7.8%	8.9%	8.8%
Lumbar Spine MRI for Low Back Pain	144	40.3%	36.6%	37.2%

Pioneer Community Hospital of Early

11740 Columbia Street Phone: 229-723-4241
Blakely, GA 39823 Fax: 229-723-5558
Type: Critical Access Hospitals Emergency Services: Yes
Ownership: Voluntary non-profit - Private Beds: 52

Key Personnel:
Operating Room. . . . . Stephanie Crawford
Radiology. . . . . Danny Everson
CEO . . . . Allen Gamble
CEO/President. . . . . James Storey, MD
Quality Assurance . . . . Jannie Thomas
Chief of Medical Staff. . . . . Almas Yousuf

Measure	Cases	This Hosp.	State Avg.	U.S. Avg.
Blood Clot Prevention and Treatment				
Anticoagulation Overlap Therapy[5]	-	-	90%	93%
ICU Venous Thromboembolism Prophylaxis[5]	-	-	90%	92%
Incidence of Potentially Preventable VTE[5]	-	-	13%	10%
UFH with Dosages/Platelet Monitoring[5]	-	-	99%	97%
Venous Thromboembolism Prophylaxis[5]	-	-	80%	85%
Warfarin Therapy Discharge Instructions[5]	-	-	78%	75%
Chest Pain/Possible Heart Attack Care				
Aspirin Given Within 24 Hours of Arrival	-	-	94%	96%
Fibrinolytic Meds Within 30 Min. of Arrival	-	-	35%	58%
Average Time to ECG (minutes)	-	-	8	7
Average Time to Transfer (minutes)	-	-	73	60
Children's Asthma Care				
Received Home Management Plan of Care	-	-	-	88%
Received Reliever Medication	-	-	-	100%
Received Systemic Corticosteroids	-	-	-	100%
Emergency Department				
Admittance Decision Time (minutes)[5]	-	-	100	98
Head CT Results Within 45 Min. of Arrival	-	-	45%	57%
Patients Who Left ER Before Being Seen	-	-	3%	2%
Time from ER Arrival to Admit. (minutes)[5]	-	-	286	274
Time from ER Arrival to Discharge (minutes)	-	-	140	134
Time in ER Before Being Evaluated (minutes)	-	-	32	26
Time to Pain Meds for Fractures (minutes)	-	-	64	57
Heart Attack Care				
Aspirin Given at Discharge[5]	-	-	99%	99%
Fibrinolytic Meds Within 30 Min. of Arrival[5]	-	-	80%	54%
PCI Within 90 Minutes of Arrival[5]	-	-	95%	96%
Statin Prescribed at Discharge[5]	-	-	98%	98%
Heart Failure Care				
ACE Inhibitor or ARB for LVSD[1]	-	-	97%	97%
Discharge Instructions Given	13	100%	92%	94%
Evaluation of LVS Function	22	95%	99%	99%
Medicare Spending				
Medicare Spending per Patient (ratio)	-	-	0.95	0.98
Pneumonia Care				
Appropriate Initial Antibiotic Given	31	94%	95%	95%
Blood Culture Timing	18	100%	97%	98%
Pregnancy and Delivery Care				
Newborn Deliveries Scheduled Early[5]	-	-	8%	6%
Preventive Care				
Immunization for Influenza[5]	-	-	88%	90%
Immunization for Pneumonia[5]	-	-	90%	92%
Stroke Care				
Anticoagulation Therapy for Atrial Fibrillation[5]	-	-	94%	95%
Antithrombotic Therapy Timing[5]	-	-	97%	98%
Assessed for Rehabilitation[5]	-	-	97%	97%
Discharged on Antithrombotic Therapy[5]	-	-	98%	99%
Discharged on Statin Medication[5]	-	-	94%	94%
Thrombolytic Therapy Timing[5]	-	-	58%	66%
Venous Thromboembolism Prophylaxis[5]	-	-	92%	94%
Written Stroke Educational Materials Given[5]	-	-	84%	88%
Surgical Care Improvement Project				
Appropriate Beta Blocker Usage[5]	-	-	97%	98%
Appropriate VTP Within 24 Hours[5]	-	-	98%	98%
Controlled Postoperative Blood Glucose[5]	-	-	96%	97%
Perioperative Temperature Management[5]	-	-	100%	100%
Prophylactic Antibiotic Selection[5]	-	-	99%	99%
Prophylactic Antibiotic Selection (Outpatient)	-	-	98%	98%
Prophylactic Antibiotic Stopped[5]	-	-	98%	98%
Prophylactic Antibiotic Timing[5]	-	-	99%	99%
Prophylactic Antibiotic Timing (Outpatient)	-	-	98%	98%
Urinary Catheter Removal[5]	-	-	97%	97%
Survey of Patients' Hospital Experiences				
Area Around Room 'Always' Quiet at Night[5]	-	-	66%	61%
Doctors 'Always' Communicated Well[5]	-	-	83%	82%
Home Recovery Information Given[5]	-	-	84%	85%
Hospital Given 9 or 10 on 10 Point Scale[5]	-	-	69%	71%
Meds 'Always' Explained Before Given[5]	-	-	63%	64%
Nurses 'Always' Communicated Well[5]	-	-	78%	79%
Pain 'Always' Well Controlled[5]	-	-	71%	71%
Room and Bathroom 'Always' Clean[5]	-	-	71%	73%
Timely Help 'Always' Received[5]	-	-	65%	68%
Would Definitely Recommend Hospital[5]	-	-	70%	71%
Use of Medical Imaging				
Cardiac Imaging Stress Test before Surgery	-	-	5.5%	5.3%
Combination Abdominal CT Scan	-	-	10.1%	10.5%
Combination Brain/Sinus CT Scan	-	-	2.3%	2.7%
Combination Chest CT Scan	-	-	3.7%	2.7%
Follow-up Mammogram/Ultrasound	-	-	8.9%	8.8%
Lumbar Spine MRI for Low Back Pain	-	-	36.6%	37.2%

Fannin Regional Hospital

2855 Old Highway 5 North Phone: 706-632-3711
Blue Ridge, GA 30513 Fax: 706-632-9722
URL: www.fanninregionalhospital.com
Type: Acute Care Hospitals Emergency Services: Yes
Ownership: Proprietary Beds: 34

Key Personnel:
Anesthesiology. . . . . Kathy Mann
Intensive Care Unit. . . . . Lori Patterson
CEO/President. . . . . David Sanders
Operating Room. . . . . Carol Voorhees, RN

Measure	Cases	This Hosp.	State Avg.	U.S. Avg.
Blood Clot Prevention and Treatment				
Anticoagulation Overlap Therapy[1,2]	-	-	90%	93%
ICU Venous Thromboembolism Prophylaxis[2]	34	100%	90%	92%
Incidence of Potentially Preventable VTE[1,2]	-	-	13%	10%
UFH with Dosages/Platelet Monitoring[2,7]	-	-	99%	97%
Venous Thromboembolism Prophylaxis[2]	146	99%	80%	85%
Warfarin Therapy Discharge Instructions[1,2]	-	-	78%	75%
Chest Pain/Possible Heart Attack Care				
Aspirin Given Within 24 Hours of Arrival	34	97%	94%	96%
Fibrinolytic Meds Within 30 Min. of Arrival[1]	-	-	35%	58%
Average Time to ECG (minutes)	37	5	8	7
Average Time to Transfer (minutes)[1]	-	-	73	60
Children's Asthma Care				
Received Home Management Plan of Care	-	-	-	88%
Received Reliever Medication	-	-	-	100%
Received Systemic Corticosteroids	-	-	-	100%
Emergency Department				
Admittance Decision Time (minutes)[2]	244	92	100	98
Head CT Results Within 45 Min. of Arrival[1]	-	-	45%	57%
Patients Who Left ER Before Being Seen	10,945	2%	3%	2%
Time from ER Arrival to Admit. (minutes)[2]	298	212	286	274
Time from ER Arrival to Discharge (minutes)	362	96	140	134
Time in ER Before Being Evaluated (minutes)	406	18	32	26
Time to Pain Meds for Fractures (minutes)	64	60	64	57
Heart Attack Care				
Aspirin Given at Discharge[1]	-	-	99%	99%
Fibrinolytic Meds Within 30 Min. of Arrival[7]	-	-	80%	54%
PCI Within 90 Minutes of Arrival[7]	-	-	95%	96%
Statin Prescribed at Discharge[1]	-	-	98%	98%
Heart Failure Care				
ACE Inhibitor or ARB for LVSD[1]	-	-	97%	97%
Discharge Instructions Given	26	96%	92%	94%
Evaluation of LVS Function	33	100%	99%	99%
Medicare Spending				
Medicare Spending per Patient (ratio)	-	0.94	0.95	0.98
Pneumonia Care				
Appropriate Initial Antibiotic Given	34	100%	95%	95%
Blood Culture Timing	70	100%	97%	98%
Pregnancy and Delivery Care				
Newborn Deliveries Scheduled Early[2]	35	0%	8%	6%
Preventive Care				
Immunization for Influenza[2]	277	100%	88%	90%
Immunization for Pneumonia[2]	351	100%	90%	92%
Stroke Care				
Anticoagulation Therapy for Atrial Fibrillation[1]	-	-	94%	95%
Antithrombotic Therapy Timing[1]	-	-	97%	98%
Assessed for Rehabilitation[1]	-	-	97%	97%
Discharged on Antithrombotic Therapy[1]	-	-	98%	99%
Discharged on Statin Medication[1]	-	-	94%	94%
Thrombolytic Therapy Timing[7]	-	-	58%	66%
Venous Thromboembolism Prophylaxis[1]	-	-	92%	94%
Written Stroke Educational Materials Given[1]	-	-	84%	88%
Surgical Care Improvement Project				
Appropriate Beta Blocker Usage	48	100%	97%	98%
Appropriate VTP Within 24 Hours	131	100%	98%	98%
Controlled Postoperative Blood Glucose[7]	-	-	96%	97%
Perioperative Temperature Management	154	100%	100%	100%
Prophylactic Antibiotic Selection	117	100%	99%	99%
Prophylactic Antibiotic Selection (Outpatient)	42	100%	98%	98%
Prophylactic Antibiotic Stopped	115	100%	98%	98%
Prophylactic Antibiotic Timing	117	99%	99%	99%
Prophylactic Antibiotic Timing (Outpatient)	42	100%	98%	98%
Urinary Catheter Removal	113	100%	97%	97%
Survey of Patients' Hospital Experiences				
Area Around Room 'Always' Quiet at Night	300+	61%	66%	61%
Doctors 'Always' Communicated Well	300+	86%	83%	82%
Home Recovery Information Given	300+	87%	84%	85%
Hospital Given 9 or 10 on 10 Point Scale	300+	73%	69%	71%
Meds 'Always' Explained Before Given	300+	63%	63%	64%
Nurses 'Always' Communicated Well	300+	80%	78%	79%
Pain 'Always' Well Controlled	300+	73%	71%	71%
Room and Bathroom 'Always' Clean	300+	76%	71%	73%
Timely Help 'Always' Received	300+	69%	65%	68%
Would Definitely Recommend Hospital	300+	73%	70%	71%
Use of Medical Imaging				
Cardiac Imaging Stress Test before Surgery	219	1.8%	5.5%	5.3%
Combination Abdominal CT Scan	288	10.4%	10.1%	10.5%
Combination Brain/Sinus CT Scan[1]	-	-	2.3%	2.7%
Combination Chest CT Scan	152	7.9%	3.7%	2.7%
Follow-up Mammogram/Ultrasound	469	5.1%	8.9%	8.8%
Lumbar Spine MRI for Low Back Pain[1]	-	-	36.6%	37.2%

Higgins General Hospital

200 Allen Memorial Drive Phone: 770-824-2210
Bremen, GA 30110 Fax: 770-836-9870
Type: Critical Access Hospitals Emergency Services: Yes
Ownership: Govt - Hospital Dist/Auth Beds: 57

Key Personnel:
Radiology. . . . . Monohar Ariband
Chief of Medical Staff. . . . . Benjamin J. Camp, MD
CEO/President. . . . . Loy Howard
Operating Room. . . . . Eloise Whitten

NOTE: Hospital profiles are in alphabetical order by state, then city, then hospital within the city; Rankings exclude hospitals with less than 25 cases except for patient surveys which excludes hospitals with less than 100 cases; (a) 100-299 cases; (1) The number of cases/patients is too few to report; (2) Data submitted were based on a sample of cases/patients; (3) Results are based on a shorter time period than required; (4) Data suppressed by CMS for one or more quarters; (5) Results are not available for this reporting period; (6) Fewer than 100 patients completed the HCAHPS survey; (7) No cases met the criteria for this measure; (8) The lower limit of the confidence interval cannot be calculated if the number of observed infections equals zero; (9) No data are available from the state/territory for this reporting period; (10) The scores shown reflect fewer than 50 completed surveys; (11) There were discrepancies in the data collection process; (12) This measure does not apply to this hospital for this reporting period; (13) Results cannot be calculated for this reporting period; (14) The results for this state are combined with nearby states to protect confidentiality; Please refer to the User's Guide for a full explanation of data.

Measure	Cases	This Hosp.	State Avg.	U.S. Avg.
Blood Clot Prevention and Treatment				
Anticoagulation Overlap Therapy[2]	16	100%	90%	93%
ICU Venous Thromboembolism Prophylaxis[1,2]	-	-	90%	92%
Incidence of Potentially Preventable VTE[2,7]	-	-	13%	10%
UFH with Dosages/Platelet Monitoring[2]	11	100%	99%	97%
Venous Thromboembolism Prophylaxis[2]	138	95%	80%	85%
Warfarin Therapy Discharge Instructions[2]	11	100%	78%	75%
Chest Pain/Possible Heart Attack Care				
Aspirin Given Within 24 Hours of Arrival	60	97%	94%	96%
Fibrinolytic Meds Within 30 Min. of Arrival[7]	-	-	35%	58%
Average Time to ECG (minutes)	62	8	8	7
Average Time to Transfer (minutes)[1]	-	-	73	60
Children's Asthma Care				
Received Home Management Plan of Care	-	-	-	88%
Received Reliever Medication	-	-	-	100%
Received Systemic Corticosteroids	-	-	-	100%
Emergency Department				
Admittance Decision Time (minutes)[2]	339	67	100	98
Head CT Results Within 45 Min. of Arrival[1,3]	-	-	45%	57%
Patients Who Left ER Before Being Seen	23,880	5%	3%	2%
Time from ER Arrival to Admit. (minutes)[2]	339	264	286	274
Time from ER Arrival to Discharge (minutes)	369	116	140	134
Time in ER Before Being Evaluated (minutes)	216	39	32	26
Time to Pain Meds for Fractures (minutes)	126	80	64	57
Heart Attack Care				
Aspirin Given at Discharge[5]	-	-	99%	99%
Fibrinolytic Meds Within 30 Min. of Arrival[5]	-	-	80%	54%
PCI Within 90 Minutes of Arrival[5]	-	-	95%	96%
Statin Prescribed at Discharge[5]	-	-	98%	98%
Heart Failure Care				
ACE Inhibitor or ARB for LVSD	12	100%	97%	97%
Discharge Instructions Given	28	100%	92%	94%
Evaluation of LVS Function	35	100%	99%	99%
Medicare Spending				
Medicare Spending per Patient (ratio)	-	-	0.95	0.98
Pneumonia Care				
Appropriate Initial Antibiotic Given	34	97%	95%	95%
Blood Culture Timing	67	100%	97%	98%
Pregnancy and Delivery Care				
Newborn Deliveries Scheduled Early[3,7]	-	-	8%	6%
Preventive Care				
Immunization for Influenza[2]	327	99%	88%	90%
Immunization for Pneumonia[2]	582	100%	90%	92%
Stroke Care				
Anticoagulation Therapy for Atrial Fibrillation[3,7]	-	-	94%	95%
Antithrombotic Therapy Timing[3,7]	-	-	97%	98%
Assessed for Rehabilitation[1,3]	-	-	97%	97%
Discharged on Antithrombotic Therapy[1,3]	-	-	98%	99%
Discharged on Statin Medication[1,3]	-	-	94%	94%
Thrombolytic Therapy Timing[3,7]	-	-	58%	66%
Venous Thromboembolism Prophylaxis[3,7]	-	-	92%	94%
Written Stroke Educational Materials Given[1,3]	-	-	84%	88%
Surgical Care Improvement Project				
Appropriate Beta Blocker Usage[5]	-	-	97%	98%
Appropriate VTP Within 24 Hours[5]	-	-	98%	98%
Controlled Postoperative Blood Glucose[5]	-	-	96%	97%
Perioperative Temperature Management[5]	-	-	100%	100%
Prophylactic Antibiotic Selection[5]	-	-	99%	99%
Prophylactic Antibiotic Selection (Outpatient)	28	96%	98%	98%
Prophylactic Antibiotic Stopped[5]	-	-	98%	98%
Prophylactic Antibiotic Timing[5]	-	-	99%	99%
Prophylactic Antibiotic Timing (Outpatient)	27	100%	98%	98%
Urinary Catheter Removal[5]	-	-	97%	97%
Survey of Patients' Hospital Experiences				
Area Around Room 'Always' Quiet at Night[6]	<100	67%	66%	61%
Doctors 'Always' Communicated Well[6]	<100	84%	83%	82%
Home Recovery Information Given[6]	<100	86%	84%	85%
Hospital Given 9 or 10 on 10 Point Scale[6]	<100	73%	69%	71%
Meds 'Always' Explained Before Given[6]	<100	68%	63%	64%
Nurses 'Always' Communicated Well[6]	<100	86%	78%	79%
Pain 'Always' Well Controlled[6]	<100	81%	71%	71%
Room and Bathroom 'Always' Clean[6]	<100	79%	71%	73%
Timely Help 'Always' Received[6]	<100	79%	65%	68%
Would Definitely Recommend Hospital[6]	<100	72%	70%	71%
Use of Medical Imaging				
Cardiac Imaging Stress Test before Surgery	49	2.0%	5.5%	5.3%
Combination Abdominal CT Scan	427	5.9%	10.1%	10.5%
Combination Brain/Sinus CT Scan[1]	-	-	2.3%	2.7%
Combination Chest CT Scan	166	4.8%	3.7%	2.7%
Follow-up Mammogram/Ultrasound	319	7.2%	8.9%	8.8%
Lumbar Spine MRI for Low Back Pain[1]	-	-	36.6%	37.2%

Southeast Georgia Health System - Brunswick Campus

2415 Parkwood Drive
Brunswick, GA 31520
Phone: 912-466-7000
Fax: 912-466-7013
E-mail: dritchi@sghs.org
URL: www.sghs.org
Type: Acute Care Hospitals
Emergency Services: Yes
Ownership: Govt - Hospital Dist/Auth
Beds: 278

Key Personnel:
Patient Relations . . . . Sharon Blach
CEO/President. . . . . Gary R Colberg, FACHE
Radiology. . . . . Patrick Ebri
Infection Control. . . . . Marge Gallagher
Operating Room. . . . . Ellen Hamilton
Chair/CEO . . . . Mitchell T. Jones, MD
Cardiac Laboratory. . . . . Gerald Kilroy
Chief of Medical Staff. . . . . Wayne Rentz

Measure	Cases	This Hosp.	State Avg.	U.S. Avg.
Blood Clot Prevention and Treatment				
Anticoagulation Overlap Therapy[2]	72	93%	90%	93%
ICU Venous Thromboembolism Prophylaxis[2]	98	94%	90%	92%
Incidence of Potentially Preventable VTE[1,2]	-	-	13%	10%
UFH with Dosages/Platelet Monitoring[2]	52	100%	99%	97%
Venous Thromboembolism Prophylaxis[2]	338	82%	80%	85%
Warfarin Therapy Discharge Instructions[2]	54	94%	78%	75%
Chest Pain/Possible Heart Attack Care				
Aspirin Given Within 24 Hours of Arrival	11	100%	94%	96%
Fibrinolytic Meds Within 30 Min. of Arrival[3,7]	-	-	35%	58%
Average Time to ECG (minutes)	11	16	8	7
Average Time to Transfer (minutes)[3,7]	-	-	73	60
Children's Asthma Care				
Received Home Management Plan of Care	-	-	-	88%
Received Reliever Medication	-	-	-	100%
Received Systemic Corticosteroids	-	-	-	100%
Emergency Department				
Admittance Decision Time (minutes)[2]	519	103	100	98
Head CT Results Within 45 Min. of Arrival[1]	-	-	45%	57%
Patients Who Left ER Before Being Seen	55,965	6%	3%	2%
Time from ER Arrival to Admit. (minutes)[2]	533	294	286	274
Time from ER Arrival to Discharge (minutes)[11]	445	166	140	134
Time in ER Before Being Evaluated (minutes)	473	54	32	26
Time to Pain Meds for Fractures (minutes)	190	74	64	57
Heart Attack Care				
Aspirin Given at Discharge[2]	139	96%	99%	99%
Fibrinolytic Meds Within 30 Min. of Arrival[2,7]	-	-	80%	54%
PCI Within 90 Minutes of Arrival[2]	27	78%	95%	96%
Statin Prescribed at Discharge[2]	132	92%	98%	98%
Heart Failure Care				
ACE Inhibitor or ARB for LVSD[2]	107	97%	97%	97%
Discharge Instructions Given[2]	237	95%	92%	94%
Evaluation of LVS Function[2]	267	99%	99%	99%
Medicare Spending				
Medicare Spending per Patient (ratio)	-	0.95	0.95	0.98
Pneumonia Care				
Appropriate Initial Antibiotic Given[2]	75	96%	95%	95%
Blood Culture Timing[2]	98	100%	97%	98%
Pregnancy and Delivery Care				
Newborn Deliveries Scheduled Early	286	0%	8%	6%
Preventive Care				
Immunization for Influenza[2]	541	99%	88%	90%
Immunization for Pneumonia[2]	646	100%	90%	92%
Stroke Care				
Anticoagulation Therapy for Atrial Fibrillation[1,2]	-	-	94%	95%
Antithrombotic Therapy Timing[2]	98	98%	97%	98%
Assessed for Rehabilitation[2]	118	92%	97%	97%
Discharged on Antithrombotic Therapy[2]	96	98%	98%	99%
Discharged on Statin Medication[2]	79	87%	94%	94%
Thrombolytic Therapy Timing[2]	25	0%	58%	66%
Venous Thromboembolism Prophylaxis[2]	122	81%	92%	94%
Written Stroke Educational Materials Given[2]	83	75%	84%	88%
Surgical Care Improvement Project				
Appropriate Beta Blocker Usage[2]	93	100%	97%	98%
Appropriate VTP Within 24 Hours[2]	361	100%	98%	98%
Controlled Postoperative Blood Glucose[2,7]	-	-	96%	97%
Perioperative Temperature Management[2]	422	100%	100%	100%
Prophylactic Antibiotic Selection[2]	258	100%	99%	99%
Prophylactic Antibiotic Selection (Outpatient)	624	98%	98%	98%
Prophylactic Antibiotic Stopped[2]	247	100%	98%	98%
Prophylactic Antibiotic Timing[2]	259	100%	99%	99%
Prophylactic Antibiotic Timing (Outpatient)	626	98%	98%	98%
Urinary Catheter Removal[2]	258	99%	97%	97%
Survey of Patients' Hospital Experiences				
Area Around Room 'Always' Quiet at Night	300+	63%	66%	61%
Doctors 'Always' Communicated Well	300+	82%	83%	82%
Home Recovery Information Given	300+	84%	84%	85%
Hospital Given 9 or 10 on 10 Point Scale	300+	65%	69%	71%
Meds 'Always' Explained Before Given	300+	64%	63%	64%
Nurses 'Always' Communicated Well	300+	76%	78%	79%
Pain 'Always' Well Controlled	300+	69%	71%	71%
Room and Bathroom 'Always' Clean	300+	72%	71%	73%
Timely Help 'Always' Received	300+	61%	65%	68%
Would Definitely Recommend Hospital	300+	66%	70%	71%
Use of Medical Imaging				
Cardiac Imaging Stress Test before Surgery	107	6.5%	5.5%	5.3%
Combination Abdominal CT Scan	1,091	7.5%	10.1%	10.5%
Combination Brain/Sinus CT Scan	876	4.7%	2.3%	2.7%
Combination Chest CT Scan	613	4.7%	3.7%	2.7%
Follow-up Mammogram/Ultrasound	2,860	3.5%	8.9%	8.8%
Lumbar Spine MRI for Low Back Pain	179	27.9%	36.6%	37.2%

The Medical Center of Peach County

1960 Highway 247 Connector
Byron, GA 31008
Phone: 478-654-2000
Fax: 478-825-4444
Type: Critical Access Hospitals
Emergency Services: Yes
Ownership: Govt - Hospital Dist/Auth
Beds: 15

Key Personnel:
Cardiology . . . . Mueez Ahmed
Pulmonology . . . . Hatem Asad
Emergency Room . . . . Chris Hobbs, RN
CEO/President. . . . . Nancy Peed
Quality Assurance . . . . Nancy Peed
Radiology. . . . . Gary M Suhr, MD

Measure	Cases	This Hosp.	State Avg.	U.S. Avg.
Blood Clot Prevention and Treatment				
Anticoagulation Overlap Therapy[5]	-	-	90%	93%
ICU Venous Thromboembolism Prophylaxis[5]	-	-	90%	92%
Incidence of Potentially Preventable VTE[5]	-	-	13%	10%
UFH with Dosages/Platelet Monitoring[5]	-	-	99%	97%
Venous Thromboembolism Prophylaxis[5]	-	-	80%	85%
Warfarin Therapy Discharge Instructions[5]	-	-	78%	75%
Chest Pain/Possible Heart Attack Care				
Aspirin Given Within 24 Hours of Arrival[1,3]	-	-	94%	96%
Fibrinolytic Meds Within 30 Min. of Arrival[5]	-	-	35%	58%
Average Time to ECG (minutes)[1,3]	-	-	8	7
Average Time to Transfer (minutes)[5]	-	-	73	60
Children's Asthma Care				
Received Home Management Plan of Care	-	-	-	88%
Received Reliever Medication	-	-	-	100%
Received Systemic Corticosteroids	-	-	-	100%
Emergency Department				
Admittance Decision Time (minutes)[5]	-	-	100	98
Head CT Results Within 45 Min. of Arrival[5]	-	-	45%	57%
Patients Who Left ER Before Being Seen	12,970	3%	3%	2%
Time from ER Arrival to Admit. (minutes)[5]	-	-	286	274
Time from ER Arrival to Discharge (minutes)[5]	-	-	140	134
Time in ER Before Being Evaluated (minutes)[5]	-	-	32	26
Time to Pain Meds for Fractures (minutes)[5]	-	-	64	57

NOTE: Hospital profiles are in alphabetical order by state, then city, then hospital within the city; Rankings exclude hospitals with less than 25 cases except for patient surveys which excludes hospitals with less than 100 cases; (a) 100-299 cases; (1) The number of cases/patients is too few to report; (2) Data submitted were based on a sample of cases/patients; (3) Results are based on a shorter time period than required; (4) Data suppressed by CMS for one or more quarters; (5) Results are not available for this reporting period; (6) Fewer than 100 patients completed the HCAHPS survey; (7) No cases met the criteria for this measure; (8) The lower limit of the confidence interval cannot be calculated if the number of observed infections equals zero; (9) No data are available from the state/territory for this reporting period; (10) The scores shown reflect fewer than 50 completed surveys; (11) There were discrepancies in the data collection process; (12) This measure does not apply to this hospital for this reporting period; (13) Results cannot be calculated for this reporting period; (14) The results for this state are combined with nearby states to protect confidentiality; Please refer to the User's Guide for a full explanation of data.

Heart Attack Care				
Aspirin Given at Discharge[5]	-	-	99%	99%
Fibrinolytic Meds Within 30 Min. of Arrival[5]	-	-	80%	54%
PCI Within 90 Minutes of Arrival[5]	-	-	95%	96%
Statin Prescribed at Discharge[5]	-	-	98%	98%
Heart Failure Care				
ACE Inhibitor or ARB for LVSD[1,2]	-	-	97%	97%
Discharge Instructions Given[2]	29	79%	92%	94%
Evaluation of LVS Function[2]	32	94%	99%	99%
Medicare Spending				
Medicare Spending per Patient (ratio)	-	-	0.95	0.98
Pneumonia Care				
Appropriate Initial Antibiotic Given[2]	19	95%	95%	95%
Blood Culture Timing[2]	24	100%	97%	98%
Pregnancy and Delivery Care				
Newborn Deliveries Scheduled Early[5]	-	-	8%	6%
Preventive Care				
Immunization for Influenza[5]	-	-	88%	90%
Immunization for Pneumonia[5]	-	-	90%	92%
Stroke Care				
Anticoagulation Therapy for Atrial Fibrillation[5]	-	-	94%	95%
Antithrombotic Therapy Timing[5]	-	-	97%	98%
Assessed for Rehabilitation[5]	-	-	97%	97%
Discharged on Antithrombotic Therapy[5]	-	-	98%	99%
Discharged on Statin Medication[5]	-	-	94%	94%
Thrombolytic Therapy Timing[5]	-	-	58%	66%
Venous Thromboembolism Prophylaxis[5]	-	-	92%	94%
Written Stroke Educational Materials Given[5]	-	-	84%	88%
Surgical Care Improvement Project				
Appropriate Beta Blocker Usage[5]	-	-	97%	98%
Appropriate VTP Within 24 Hours[5]	-	-	98%	98%
Controlled Postoperative Blood Glucose[5]	-	-	96%	97%
Perioperative Temperature Management[5]	-	-	100%	100%
Prophylactic Antibiotic Selection[5]	-	-	99%	99%
Prophylactic Antibiotic Selection (Outpatient)[3]	11	100%	98%	98%
Prophylactic Antibiotic Stopped[5]	-	-	98%	98%
Prophylactic Antibiotic Timing[5]	-	-	99%	99%
Prophylactic Antibiotic Timing (Outpatient)[3]	11	100%	98%	98%
Urinary Catheter Removal[5]	-	-	97%	97%
Survey of Patients' Hospital Experiences				
Area Around Room 'Always' Quiet at Night[5]	-	-	66%	61%
Doctors 'Always' Communicated Well[5]	-	-	83%	82%
Home Recovery Information Given[5]	-	-	84%	85%
Hospital Given 9 or 10 on 10 Point Scale[5]	-	-	69%	71%
Meds 'Always' Explained Before Given[5]	-	-	63%	64%
Nurses 'Always' Communicated Well[5]	-	-	78%	79%
Pain 'Always' Well Controlled[5]	-	-	71%	71%
Room and Bathroom 'Always' Clean[5]	-	-	71%	73%
Timely Help 'Always' Received[5]	-	-	65%	68%
Would Definitely Recommend Hospital[5]	-	-	70%	71%
Use of Medical Imaging				
Cardiac Imaging Stress Test before Surgery[7]	-	-	5.5%	5.3%
Combination Abdominal CT Scan	126	23.8%	10.1%	10.5%
Combination Brain/Sinus CT Scan[1]	-	-	2.3%	2.7%
Combination Chest CT Scan[1]	-	-	3.7%	2.7%
Follow-up Mammogram/Ultrasound	338	1.5%	8.9%	8.8%
Lumbar Spine MRI for Low Back Pain[1]	-	-	36.6%	37.2%

Grady General Hospital

1155 5th Street, Se
Cairo, GA 39828
Phone: 229-377-0251
Fax: 229-377-7953
Type: Acute Care Hospitals
Emergency Services: Yes
Ownership: Voluntary non-profit - Private
Beds: 60

Key Personnel:
Operating Room. . . . . Margie Beane
CEO/President. . . . . Glen C Davis
Administrator . . . . Ken Rhudy
Chief of Medical Staff. . . . . Linda Walden

Measure	Cases	This Hosp.	State Avg.	U.S. Avg.
Blood Clot Prevention and Treatment				
Anticoagulation Overlap Therapy[1,2]	-	-	90%	93%
ICU Venous Thromboembolism Prophylaxis[2]	14	86%	90%	92%
Incidence of Potentially Preventable VTE[2,7]	-	-	13%	10%
UFH with Dosages/Platelet Monitoring[2,7]	-	-	99%	97%
Venous Thromboembolism Prophylaxis[2]	123	76%	80%	85%
Warfarin Therapy Discharge Instructions[1,2]	-	-	78%	75%
Chest Pain/Possible Heart Attack Care				
Aspirin Given Within 24 Hours of Arrival[5]	-	-	94%	96%
Fibrinolytic Meds Within 30 Min. of Arrival[5]	-	-	35%	58%
Average Time to ECG (minutes)[5]	-	-	8	7
Average Time to Transfer (minutes)[5]	-	-	73	60
Children's Asthma Care				
Received Home Management Plan of Care	-	-	-	88%
Received Reliever Medication	-	-	-	100%
Received Systemic Corticosteroids	-	-	-	100%
Emergency Department				
Admittance Decision Time (minutes)[2]	281	60	100	98
Head CT Results Within 45 Min. of Arrival[3,7]	-	-	45%	57%
Patients Who Left ER Before Being Seen	11,215	1%	3%	2%
Time from ER Arrival to Admit. (minutes)[2]	281	180	286	274
Time from ER Arrival to Discharge (minutes)	451	97	140	134
Time in ER Before Being Evaluated (minutes)	462	37	32	26
Time to Pain Meds for Fractures (minutes)	46	46	64	57
Heart Attack Care				
Aspirin Given at Discharge[1]	-	-	99%	99%
Fibrinolytic Meds Within 30 Min. of Arrival[7]	-	-	80%	54%
PCI Within 90 Minutes of Arrival[7]	-	-	95%	96%
Statin Prescribed at Discharge[1]	-	-	98%	98%
Heart Failure Care				
ACE Inhibitor or ARB for LVSD	19	100%	97%	97%
Discharge Instructions Given	58	100%	92%	94%
Evaluation of LVS Function	71	99%	99%	99%
Medicare Spending				
Medicare Spending per Patient (ratio)	-	0.85	0.95	0.98
Pneumonia Care				
Appropriate Initial Antibiotic Given	24	100%	95%	95%
Blood Culture Timing	22	95%	97%	98%
Pregnancy and Delivery Care				
Newborn Deliveries Scheduled Early	24	0%	8%	6%
Preventive Care				
Immunization for Influenza[2]	265	72%	88%	90%
Immunization for Pneumonia[2]	295	91%	90%	92%
Stroke Care				
Anticoagulation Therapy for Atrial Fibrillation[7]	-	-	94%	95%
Antithrombotic Therapy Timing[1]	-	-	97%	98%
Assessed for Rehabilitation	11	82%	97%	97%
Discharged on Antithrombotic Therapy[1]	-	-	98%	99%
Discharged on Statin Medication[1]	-	-	94%	94%
Thrombolytic Therapy Timing[7]	-	-	58%	66%
Venous Thromboembolism Prophylaxis	11	82%	92%	94%
Written Stroke Educational Materials Given[1]	-	-	84%	88%
Surgical Care Improvement Project				
Appropriate Beta Blocker Usage[1]	-	-	97%	98%
Appropriate VTP Within 24 Hours	13	92%	98%	98%
Controlled Postoperative Blood Glucose[7]	-	-	96%	97%
Perioperative Temperature Management	15	100%	100%	100%
Prophylactic Antibiotic Selection[1]	-	-	99%	99%
Prophylactic Antibiotic Selection (Outpatient)[3,7]	-	-	98%	98%
Prophylactic Antibiotic Stopped[1]	-	-	98%	98%
Prophylactic Antibiotic Timing[1]	-	-	99%	99%
Prophylactic Antibiotic Timing (Outpatient)[3,7]	-	-	98%	98%
Urinary Catheter Removal[1]	-	-	97%	97%
Survey of Patients' Hospital Experiences				
Area Around Room 'Always' Quiet at Night	(a)	69%	66%	61%
Doctors 'Always' Communicated Well	(a)	89%	83%	82%
Home Recovery Information Given	(a)	89%	84%	85%
Hospital Given 9 or 10 on 10 Point Scale	(a)	78%	69%	71%
Meds 'Always' Explained Before Given	(a)	65%	63%	64%
Nurses 'Always' Communicated Well	(a)	84%	78%	79%
Pain 'Always' Well Controlled	(a)	79%	71%	71%
Room and Bathroom 'Always' Clean	(a)	80%	71%	73%
Timely Help 'Always' Received	(a)	71%	65%	68%
Would Definitely Recommend Hospital	(a)	74%	70%	71%
Use of Medical Imaging				
Cardiac Imaging Stress Test before Surgery[7]	-	-	5.5%	5.3%
Combination Abdominal CT Scan	222	2.3%	10.1%	10.5%
Combination Brain/Sinus CT Scan[1]	-	-	2.3%	2.7%
Combination Chest CT Scan	81	1.2%	3.7%	2.7%
Follow-up Mammogram/Ultrasound	457	7.0%	8.9%	8.8%
Lumbar Spine MRI for Low Back Pain	44	43.2%	36.6%	37.2%

Gordon Hospital

1035 Red Bud Road
Calhoun, GA 30701
Phone: 706-629-2895
Fax: 706-629-4842
URL: www.gordonhospital.com
Type: Acute Care Hospitals
Emergency Services: Yes
Ownership: Voluntary non-profit - Church
Beds: 65

Key Personnel:
Intensive Care Unit. . . . . Cindy Bankhead
Radiology. . . . . William Butt
Operating Room. . . . . Beth Crew
Emergency Room . . . . Gary Moore, MD
CEO/President. . . . . Pete Weber

Measure	Cases	This Hosp.	State Avg.	U.S. Avg.
Blood Clot Prevention and Treatment				
Anticoagulation Overlap Therapy[2]	28	82%	90%	93%
ICU Venous Thromboembolism Prophylaxis[2]	142	100%	90%	92%
Incidence of Potentially Preventable VTE[1,2]	-	-	13%	10%
UFH with Dosages/Platelet Monitoring[1,2]	-	-	99%	97%
Venous Thromboembolism Prophylaxis[2]	388	98%	80%	85%
Warfarin Therapy Discharge Instructions[2]	25	96%	78%	75%
Chest Pain/Possible Heart Attack Care				
Aspirin Given Within 24 Hours of Arrival	51	100%	94%	96%
Fibrinolytic Meds Within 30 Min. of Arrival[7]	-	-	35%	58%
Average Time to ECG (minutes)	50	6	8	7
Average Time to Transfer (minutes)	14	42	73	60
Children's Asthma Care				
Received Home Management Plan of Care	-	-	-	88%
Received Reliever Medication	-	-	-	100%
Received Systemic Corticosteroids	-	-	-	100%
Emergency Department				
Admittance Decision Time (minutes)[2]	1,122	81	100	98
Head CT Results Within 45 Min. of Arrival[1]	-	-	45%	57%
Patients Who Left ER Before Being Seen	39,036	2%	3%	2%
Time from ER Arrival to Admit. (minutes)[2]	1,129	239	286	274
Time from ER Arrival to Discharge (minutes)	454	108	140	134
Time in ER Before Being Evaluated (minutes)	466	37	32	26
Time to Pain Meds for Fractures (minutes)	118	60	64	57
Heart Attack Care				
Aspirin Given at Discharge	20	95%	99%	99%
Fibrinolytic Meds Within 30 Min. of Arrival[7]	-	-	80%	54%
PCI Within 90 Minutes of Arrival[7]	-	-	95%	96%
Statin Prescribed at Discharge	17	100%	98%	98%
Heart Failure Care				
ACE Inhibitor or ARB for LVSD	31	97%	97%	97%
Discharge Instructions Given	84	99%	92%	94%
Evaluation of LVS Function	100	100%	99%	99%
Medicare Spending				
Medicare Spending per Patient (ratio)	-	0.92	0.95	0.98
Pneumonia Care				
Appropriate Initial Antibiotic Given	127	98%	95%	95%
Blood Culture Timing	222	100%	97%	98%
Pregnancy and Delivery Care				
Newborn Deliveries Scheduled Early[2]	68	25%	8%	6%
Preventive Care				
Immunization for Influenza[2]	678	98%	88%	90%
Immunization for Pneumonia[2]	905	94%	90%	92%
Stroke Care				
Anticoagulation Therapy for Atrial Fibrillation[1]	-	-	94%	95%
Antithrombotic Therapy Timing	35	100%	97%	98%
Assessed for Rehabilitation	34	97%	97%	97%
Discharged on Antithrombotic Therapy	34	94%	98%	99%
Discharged on Statin Medication	28	93%	94%	94%
Thrombolytic Therapy Timing[1]	-	-	58%	66%
Venous Thromboembolism Prophylaxis	28	100%	92%	94%
Written Stroke Educational Materials Given	23	96%	84%	88%
Surgical Care Improvement Project				
Appropriate Beta Blocker Usage	88	99%	97%	98%
Appropriate VTP Within 24 Hours	239	100%	98%	98%

NOTE: Hospital profiles are in alphabetical order by state, then city, then hospital within the city; Rankings exclude hospitals with less than 25 cases except for patient surveys which excludes hospitals with less than 100 cases; (a) 100-299 cases; (1) The number of cases/patients is too few to report; (2) Data submitted were based on a sample of cases/patients; (3) Results are based on a shorter time period than required; (4) Data suppressed by CMS for one or more quarters; (5) Results are not available for this reporting period; (6) Fewer than 100 patients completed the HCAHPS survey; (7) No cases met the criteria for this measure; (8) The lower limit of the confidence interval cannot be calculated if the number of observed infections equals zero; (9) No data are available from the state/territory for this reporting period; (10) The scores shown reflect fewer than 50 completed surveys; (11) There were discrepancies in the data collection process; (12) This measure does not apply to this hospital for this reporting period; (13) Results cannot be calculated for this reporting period; (14) The results for this state are combined with nearby states to protect confidentiality; Please refer to the User's Guide for a full explanation of data.

Measure	Cases	This Hosp.	State Avg.	U.S. Avg.
Controlled Postoperative Blood Glucose[7]	-	-	96%	97%
Perioperative Temperature Management	259	100%	100%	100%
Prophylactic Antibiotic Selection	185	100%	99%	99%
Prophylactic Antibiotic Selection (Outpatient)	150	97%	98%	98%
Prophylactic Antibiotic Stopped	178	99%	98%	98%
Prophylactic Antibiotic Timing	185	99%	99%	99%
Prophylactic Antibiotic Timing (Outpatient)	150	99%	98%	98%
Urinary Catheter Removal	101	100%	97%	97%
Survey of Patients' Hospital Experiences				
Area Around Room 'Always' Quiet at Night[11]	300+	70%	66%	61%
Doctors 'Always' Communicated Well[11]	300+	86%	83%	82%
Home Recovery Information Given[11]	300+	88%	84%	85%
Hospital Given 9 or 10 on 10 Point Scale[11]	300+	77%	69%	71%
Meds 'Always' Explained Before Given[11]	300+	72%	63%	64%
Nurses 'Always' Communicated Well[11]	300+	84%	78%	79%
Pain 'Always' Well Controlled[11]	300+	77%	71%	71%
Room and Bathroom 'Always' Clean[11]	300+	81%	71%	73%
Timely Help 'Always' Received[11]	300+	72%	65%	68%
Would Definitely Recommend Hospital[11]	300+	76%	70%	71%
Use of Medical Imaging				
Cardiac Imaging Stress Test before Surgery	195	5.1%	5.5%	5.3%
Combination Abdominal CT Scan	349	16.0%	10.1%	10.5%
Combination Brain/Sinus CT Scan	441	1.1%	2.3%	2.7%
Combination Chest CT Scan	157	8.3%	3.7%	2.7%
Follow-up Mammogram/Ultrasound	731	10.5%	8.9%	8.8%
Lumbar Spine MRI for Low Back Pain	127	29.1%	36.6%	37.2%

Mitchell County Hospital

90 Stephens Street
Camilla, GA 31730
URL: www.archbold.org
Type: Critical Access Hospitals
Ownership: Govt - Hospital Dist/Auth
Phone: 229-336-5284
Fax: 229-336-4682
Emergency Services: Yes
Beds: 25

Key Personnel:
Emergency Room .... Carla Beasley, RN BSN
Infection Control.............. Pam Cornwell, RN
Quality Assurance .... Pam Cornwell, RN
CEO .... Robbie Dewberry
Radiology................... Brooks Holton
Chief of Medical Staff.......... Dinesh Patel, MD
Pediatric Ambulatory Care ...... Dinesh Patel, MD

Measure	Cases	This Hosp.	State Avg.	U.S. Avg.
Blood Clot Prevention and Treatment				
Anticoagulation Overlap Therapy[5]	-	-	90%	93%
ICU Venous Thromboembolism Prophylaxis[5]	-	-	90%	92%
Incidence of Potentially Preventable VTE[5]	-	-	13%	10%
UFH with Dosages/Platelet Monitoring[5]	-	-	99%	97%
Venous Thromboembolism Prophylaxis[5]	-	-	80%	85%
Warfarin Therapy Discharge Instructions[5]	-	-	78%	75%
Chest Pain/Possible Heart Attack Care				
Aspirin Given Within 24 Hours of Arrival	-	-	94%	96%
Fibrinolytic Meds Within 30 Min. of Arrival	-	-	35%	58%
Average Time to ECG (minutes)	-	-	8	7
Average Time to Transfer (minutes)	-	-	73	60
Children's Asthma Care				
Received Home Management Plan of Care	-	-	-	88%
Received Reliever Medication	-	-	-	100%
Received Systemic Corticosteroids	-	-	-	100%
Emergency Department				
Admittance Decision Time (minutes)[5]	-	-	100	98
Head CT Results Within 45 Min. of Arrival	-	-	45%	57%
Patients Who Left ER Before Being Seen	-	-	3%	2%
Time from ER Arrival to Admit. (minutes)[5]	-	-	286	274
Time from ER Arrival to Discharge (minutes)	-	-	140	134
Time in ER Before Being Evaluated (minutes)	-	-	32	26
Time to Pain Meds for Fractures (minutes)	-	-	64	57
Heart Attack Care				
Aspirin Given at Discharge[5]	-	-	99%	99%
Fibrinolytic Meds Within 30 Min. of Arrival[5]	-	-	80%	54%
PCI Within 90 Minutes of Arrival[5]	-	-	95%	96%
Statin Prescribed at Discharge[5]	-	-	98%	98%
Heart Failure Care				
ACE Inhibitor or ARB for LVSD[1]	-	-	97%	97%
Discharge Instructions Given[1]	-	-	92%	94%
Evaluation of LVS Function	13	100%	99%	99%
Medicare Spending				
Medicare Spending per Patient (ratio)	-	-	0.95	0.98
Pneumonia Care				
Appropriate Initial Antibiotic Given[1]	-	-	95%	95%
Blood Culture Timing[1]	-	-	97%	98%
Pregnancy and Delivery Care				
Newborn Deliveries Scheduled Early[5]	-	-	8%	6%
Preventive Care				
Immunization for Influenza[5]	-	-	88%	90%
Immunization for Pneumonia[5]	-	-	90%	92%
Stroke Care				
Anticoagulation Therapy for Atrial Fibrillation[5]	-	-	94%	95%
Antithrombotic Therapy Timing[5]	-	-	97%	98%
Assessed for Rehabilitation[5]	-	-	97%	97%
Discharged on Antithrombotic Therapy[5]	-	-	98%	99%
Discharged on Statin Medication[5]	-	-	94%	94%
Thrombolytic Therapy Timing[5]	-	-	58%	66%
Venous Thromboembolism Prophylaxis[5]	-	-	92%	94%
Written Stroke Educational Materials Given[5]	-	-	84%	88%
Surgical Care Improvement Project				
Appropriate Beta Blocker Usage[5]	-	-	97%	98%
Appropriate VTP Within 24 Hours[5]	-	-	98%	98%
Controlled Postoperative Blood Glucose[5]	-	-	96%	97%
Perioperative Temperature Management[5]	-	-	100%	100%
Prophylactic Antibiotic Selection[5]	-	-	99%	99%
Prophylactic Antibiotic Selection (Outpatient)	-	-	98%	98%
Prophylactic Antibiotic Stopped[5]	-	-	98%	98%
Prophylactic Antibiotic Timing[5]	-	-	99%	99%
Prophylactic Antibiotic Timing (Outpatient)	-	-	98%	98%
Urinary Catheter Removal[5]	-	-	97%	97%
Survey of Patients' Hospital Experiences				
Area Around Room 'Always' Quiet at Night[6]	<100	70%	66%	61%
Doctors 'Always' Communicated Well[6]	<100	90%	83%	82%
Home Recovery Information Given[6]	<100	87%	84%	85%
Hospital Given 9 or 10 on 10 Point Scale[6]	<100	71%	69%	71%
Meds 'Always' Explained Before Given[6]	<100	67%	63%	64%
Nurses 'Always' Communicated Well[6]	<100	78%	78%	79%
Pain 'Always' Well Controlled[6]	<100	79%	71%	71%
Room and Bathroom 'Always' Clean[6]	<100	78%	71%	73%
Timely Help 'Always' Received[6]	<100	64%	65%	68%
Would Definitely Recommend Hospital[6]	<100	65%	70%	71%
Use of Medical Imaging				
Cardiac Imaging Stress Test before Surgery	-	-	5.5%	5.3%
Combination Abdominal CT Scan	-	-	10.1%	10.5%
Combination Brain/Sinus CT Scan	-	-	2.3%	2.7%
Combination Chest CT Scan	-	-	3.7%	2.7%
Follow-up Mammogram/Ultrasound	-	-	8.9%	8.8%
Lumbar Spine MRI for Low Back Pain	-	-	36.6%	37.2%

Northside Hospital Cherokee

201 Hospital Road
Canton, GA 30114
E-mail: janiceb@northside.com
URL: www.northside.com/cherokee
Type: Acute Care Hospitals
Ownership: Voluntary non-profit - Other
Phone: 770-720-5298
Fax: 770-720-5101
Emergency Services: Yes
Beds: 84

Key Personnel:
Radiology.................... J Richard Amerson
Emergency Room .... David Asrael
Infection Control.............. Angela Bijens
Operating Room.............. Anuj Dua
Chief of Medical Staff.......... David Edwards, MD
Intensive Care Unit........... Janice Laleck
Quality Assurance .... Brenda Miller
CEO/President............... Douglas Parker

Measure	Cases	This Hosp.	State Avg.	U.S. Avg.
Blood Clot Prevention and Treatment				
Anticoagulation Overlap Therapy[2]	59	100%	90%	93%
ICU Venous Thromboembolism Prophylaxis[2]	88	100%	90%	92%
Incidence of Potentially Preventable VTE[1,2]	-	-	13%	10%
UFH with Dosages/Platelet Monitoring[2]	38	100%	99%	97%
Venous Thromboembolism Prophylaxis[2]	370	99%	80%	85%
Warfarin Therapy Discharge Instructions[2]	44	100%	78%	75%
Chest Pain/Possible Heart Attack Care				
Aspirin Given Within 24 Hours of Arrival	31	97%	94%	96%
Fibrinolytic Meds Within 30 Min. of Arrival[7]	-	-	35%	58%
Average Time to ECG (minutes)	33	2	8	7
Average Time to Transfer (minutes)[7]	-	-	73	60
Children's Asthma Care				
Received Home Management Plan of Care	-	-	-	88%
Received Reliever Medication	-	-	-	100%
Received Systemic Corticosteroids	-	-	-	100%
Emergency Department				
Admittance Decision Time (minutes)[2]	361	98	100	98
Head CT Results Within 45 Min. of Arrival	15	80%	45%	57%
Patients Who Left ER Before Being Seen	18,896	1%	3%	2%
Time from ER Arrival to Admit. (minutes)[2]	375	306	286	274
Time from ER Arrival to Discharge (minutes)	420	161	140	134
Time in ER Before Being Evaluated (minutes)	440	23	32	26
Time to Pain Meds for Fractures (minutes)	142	53	64	57
Heart Attack Care				
Aspirin Given at Discharge	131	100%	99%	99%
Fibrinolytic Meds Within 30 Min. of Arrival[7]	-	-	80%	54%
PCI Within 90 Minutes of Arrival	26	100%	95%	96%
Statin Prescribed at Discharge	115	100%	98%	98%
Heart Failure Care				
ACE Inhibitor or ARB for LVSD	34	100%	97%	97%
Discharge Instructions Given	66	97%	92%	94%
Evaluation of LVS Function	87	100%	99%	99%
Medicare Spending				
Medicare Spending per Patient (ratio)	-	1.04	0.95	0.98
Pneumonia Care				
Appropriate Initial Antibiotic Given	126	100%	95%	95%
Blood Culture Timing	193	100%	97%	98%
Pregnancy and Delivery Care				
Newborn Deliveries Scheduled Early	93	2%	8%	6%
Preventive Care				
Immunization for Influenza[2]	487	97%	88%	90%
Immunization for Pneumonia[2]	478	98%	90%	92%
Stroke Care				
Anticoagulation Therapy for Atrial Fibrillation[1]	-	-	94%	95%
Antithrombotic Therapy Timing	28	100%	97%	98%
Assessed for Rehabilitation	27	100%	97%	97%
Discharged on Antithrombotic Therapy	27	100%	98%	99%
Discharged on Statin Medication	17	100%	94%	94%
Thrombolytic Therapy Timing[1]	-	-	58%	66%
Venous Thromboembolism Prophylaxis	27	100%	92%	94%
Written Stroke Educational Materials Given	14	93%	84%	88%
Surgical Care Improvement Project				
Appropriate Beta Blocker Usage	122	100%	97%	98%
Appropriate VTP Within 24 Hours	323	100%	98%	98%
Controlled Postoperative Blood Glucose[7]	-	-	96%	97%
Perioperative Temperature Management	363	100%	100%	100%
Prophylactic Antibiotic Selection	206	100%	99%	99%
Prophylactic Antibiotic Selection (Outpatient)	307	100%	98%	98%
Prophylactic Antibiotic Stopped	200	100%	98%	98%
Prophylactic Antibiotic Timing	206	100%	99%	99%
Prophylactic Antibiotic Timing (Outpatient)	307	100%	98%	98%
Urinary Catheter Removal	237	100%	97%	97%
Survey of Patients' Hospital Experiences				
Area Around Room 'Always' Quiet at Night	300+	56%	66%	61%
Doctors 'Always' Communicated Well	300+	79%	83%	82%
Home Recovery Information Given	300+	87%	84%	85%
Hospital Given 9 or 10 on 10 Point Scale	300+	64%	69%	71%
Meds 'Always' Explained Before Given	300+	58%	63%	64%
Nurses 'Always' Communicated Well	300+	72%	78%	79%
Pain 'Always' Well Controlled	300+	67%	71%	71%
Room and Bathroom 'Always' Clean	300+	66%	71%	73%
Timely Help 'Always' Received	300+	62%	65%	68%
Would Definitely Recommend Hospital	300+	66%	70%	71%
Use of Medical Imaging				
Cardiac Imaging Stress Test before Surgery	157	6.4%	5.5%	5.3%
Combination Abdominal CT Scan	685	7.4%	10.1%	10.5%
Combination Brain/Sinus CT Scan	792	1.5%	2.3%	2.7%
Combination Chest CT Scan	311	1.9%	3.7%	2.7%

NOTE: Hospital profiles are in alphabetical order by state, then city, then hospital within the city; Rankings exclude hospitals with less than 25 cases except for patient surveys which excludes hospitals with less than 100 cases; (a) 100-299 cases; (1) The number of cases/patients is too few to report; (2) Data submitted were based on a sample of cases/patients; (3) Results are based on a shorter time period than required; (4) Data suppressed by CMS for one or more quarters; (5) Results are not available for this reporting period; (6) Fewer than 100 patients completed the HCAHPS survey; (7) No cases met the criteria for this measure; (8) The lower limit of the confidence interval cannot be calculated if the number of observed infections equals zero; (9) No data are available from the state/territory for this reporting period; (10) The scores shown reflect fewer than 50 completed surveys; (11) There were discrepancies in the data collection process; (12) This measure does not apply to this hospital for this reporting period; (13) Results cannot be calculated for this reporting period; (14) The results for this state are combined with nearby states to protect confidentiality; Please refer to the User's Guide for a full explanation of data.

Follow-up Mammogram/Ultrasound	1,502	10.1%	8.9%	8.8%
Lumbar Spine MRI for Low Back Pain[1]	-	-	36.6%	37.2%

Tanner Medical Center - Carrollton

705 Dixie Street
Carrollton, GA 30117
URL: www.tanner.org
Type: Acute Care Hospitals
Ownership: Govt - Hospital Dist/Auth

Phone: 770-836-9580
Fax: 770-836-9897
Emergency Services: Yes
Beds: 202

Key Personnel:
Quality Assurance . . . . Beth Allen, RN
Radiology. . . . . Monohar Ariband
Operating Room. . . . . Brian E Barden
Chief of Medical Staff. . . . . Taylor Gordon, MD
President/CEO. . . . . Loy M Howard
Administrator . . . . Larry Steed

Measure	Cases	This Hosp.	State Avg.	U.S. Avg.
Blood Clot Prevention and Treatment				
Anticoagulation Overlap Therapy[2]	75	80%	90%	93%
ICU Venous Thromboembolism Prophylaxis[2]	83	96%	90%	92%
Incidence of Potentially Preventable VTE[2]	14	29%	13%	10%
UFH with Dosages/Platelet Monitoring[2]	69	99%	99%	97%
Venous Thromboembolism Prophylaxis[2]	326	94%	80%	85%
Warfarin Therapy Discharge Instructions[2]	60	53%	78%	75%
Chest Pain/Possible Heart Attack Care				
Aspirin Given Within 24 Hours of Arrival	14	100%	94%	96%
Fibrinolytic Meds Within 30 Min. of Arrival[3,7]	-	-	35%	58%
Average Time to ECG (minutes)	14	5	8	7
Average Time to Transfer (minutes)[3,7]	-	-	73	60
Children's Asthma Care				
Received Home Management Plan of Care	-	-	-	88%
Received Reliever Medication	-	-	-	100%
Received Systemic Corticosteroids	-	-	-	100%
Emergency Department				
Admittance Decision Time (minutes)[2]	391	48	100	98
Head CT Results Within 45 Min. of Arrival[1]	-	-	45%	57%
Patients Who Left ER Before Being Seen	48,291	2%	3%	2%
Time from ER Arrival to Admit. (minutes)[2]	474	226	286	274
Time from ER Arrival to Discharge (minutes)	390	128	140	134
Time in ER Before Being Evaluated (minutes)	236	30	32	26
Time to Pain Meds for Fractures (minutes)	190	63	64	57
Heart Attack Care				
Aspirin Given at Discharge	228	100%	99%	99%
Fibrinolytic Meds Within 30 Min. of Arrival[7]	-	-	80%	54%
PCI Within 90 Minutes of Arrival	36	100%	95%	96%
Statin Prescribed at Discharge	210	100%	98%	98%
Heart Failure Care				
ACE Inhibitor or ARB for LVSD	57	98%	97%	97%
Discharge Instructions Given	203	99%	92%	94%
Evaluation of LVS Function	238	99%	99%	99%
Medicare Spending				
Medicare Spending per Patient (ratio)	-	0.94	0.95	0.98
Pneumonia Care				
Appropriate Initial Antibiotic Given	158	98%	95%	95%
Blood Culture Timing	239	97%	97%	98%
Pregnancy and Delivery Care				
Newborn Deliveries Scheduled Early	111	1%	8%	6%
Preventive Care				
Immunization for Influenza[2]	525	98%	88%	90%
Immunization for Pneumonia[2]	665	98%	90%	92%
Stroke Care				
Anticoagulation Therapy for Atrial Fibrillation[1]	-	-	94%	95%
Antithrombotic Therapy Timing	61	100%	97%	98%
Assessed for Rehabilitation	62	90%	97%	97%
Discharged on Antithrombotic Therapy	61	97%	98%	99%
Discharged on Statin Medication	42	95%	94%	94%
Thrombolytic Therapy Timing[1]	-	-	58%	66%
Venous Thromboembolism Prophylaxis	62	98%	92%	94%
Written Stroke Educational Materials Given	39	74%	84%	88%
Surgical Care Improvement Project				
Appropriate Beta Blocker Usage	209	100%	97%	98%
Appropriate VTP Within 24 Hours	556	100%	98%	98%
Controlled Postoperative Blood Glucose[7]	-	-	96%	97%
Perioperative Temperature Management	646	100%	100%	100%
Prophylactic Antibiotic Selection	492	100%	99%	99%
Prophylactic Antibiotic Selection (Outpatient)	356	99%	98%	98%
Prophylactic Antibiotic Stopped	491	100%	98%	98%
Prophylactic Antibiotic Timing	492	100%	99%	99%
Prophylactic Antibiotic Timing (Outpatient)	358	99%	98%	98%
Urinary Catheter Removal	507	100%	97%	97%
Survey of Patients' Hospital Experiences				
Area Around Room 'Always' Quiet at Night	300+	69%	66%	61%
Doctors 'Always' Communicated Well	300+	87%	83%	82%
Home Recovery Information Given	300+	88%	84%	85%
Hospital Given 9 or 10 on 10 Point Scale	300+	82%	69%	71%
Meds 'Always' Explained Before Given	300+	71%	63%	64%
Nurses 'Always' Communicated Well	300+	87%	78%	79%
Pain 'Always' Well Controlled	300+	75%	71%	71%
Room and Bathroom 'Always' Clean	300+	80%	71%	73%
Timely Help 'Always' Received	300+	77%	65%	68%
Would Definitely Recommend Hospital	300+	80%	70%	71%
Use of Medical Imaging				
Cardiac Imaging Stress Test before Surgery	394	5.6%	5.5%	5.3%
Combination Abdominal CT Scan	945	7.7%	10.1%	10.5%
Combination Brain/Sinus CT Scan	933	1.6%	2.3%	2.7%
Combination Chest CT Scan	630	3.0%	3.7%	2.7%
Follow-up Mammogram/Ultrasound	1,342	6.6%	8.9%	8.8%
Lumbar Spine MRI for Low Back Pain	128	36.7%	36.6%	37.2%

Cartersville Medical Center

960 Joe Frank Harris Parkway
Cartersville, GA 30120
URL: www.emorycartersville.com
Type: Acute Care Hospitals
Ownership: Proprietary

Phone: 770-387-8182
Fax: 770-606-2127
Emergency Services: Yes
Beds: 112

Key Personnel:
Operating Room. . . . . Cammy Boardman
Patient Relations . . . . Kathy Davis
Cardiac Laboratory. . . . . Donna Roberts
President/CEO. . . . . Keith Sandlin
Quality Assurance . . . . Tim Thompson
Emergency Room . . . . Mary Ellen Womack

Measure	Cases	This Hosp.	State Avg.	U.S. Avg.
Blood Clot Prevention and Treatment				
Anticoagulation Overlap Therapy[2]	46	100%	90%	93%
ICU Venous Thromboembolism Prophylaxis[2]	111	100%	90%	92%
Incidence of Potentially Preventable VTE[1,2]	-	-	13%	10%
UFH with Dosages/Platelet Monitoring[2]	57	100%	99%	97%
Venous Thromboembolism Prophylaxis[2]	307	96%	80%	85%
Warfarin Therapy Discharge Instructions[2]	41	90%	78%	75%
Chest Pain/Possible Heart Attack Care				
Aspirin Given Within 24 Hours of Arrival	11	100%	94%	96%
Fibrinolytic Meds Within 30 Min. of Arrival[7]	-	-	35%	58%
Average Time to ECG (minutes)	14	12	8	7
Average Time to Transfer (minutes)[1]	-	-	73	60
Children's Asthma Care				
Received Home Management Plan of Care	-	-	-	88%
Received Reliever Medication	-	-	-	100%
Received Systemic Corticosteroids	-	-	-	100%
Emergency Department				
Admittance Decision Time (minutes)[2]	599	100	100	98
Head CT Results Within 45 Min. of Arrival	11	100%	45%	57%
Patients Who Left ER Before Being Seen	49,298	2%	3%	2%
Time from ER Arrival to Admit. (minutes)[2]	600	284	286	274
Time from ER Arrival to Discharge (minutes)	430	173	140	134
Time in ER Before Being Evaluated (minutes)	510	7	32	26
Time to Pain Meds for Fractures (minutes)	133	55	64	57
Heart Attack Care				
Aspirin Given at Discharge	112	100%	99%	99%
Fibrinolytic Meds Within 30 Min. of Arrival[7]	-	-	80%	54%
PCI Within 90 Minutes of Arrival	35	94%	95%	96%
Statin Prescribed at Discharge	108	99%	98%	98%
Heart Failure Care				
ACE Inhibitor or ARB for LVSD	46	100%	97%	97%
Discharge Instructions Given	193	87%	92%	94%
Evaluation of LVS Function	210	100%	99%	99%
Medicare Spending				
Medicare Spending per Patient (ratio)	-	0.94	0.95	0.98
Pneumonia Care				
Appropriate Initial Antibiotic Given[2]	82	94%	95%	95%
Blood Culture Timing[2]	146	99%	97%	98%
Pregnancy and Delivery Care				
Newborn Deliveries Scheduled Early[2]	47	0%	8%	6%
Preventive Care				
Immunization for Influenza[2]	532	98%	88%	90%
Immunization for Pneumonia[2]	704	98%	90%	92%
Stroke Care				
Anticoagulation Therapy for Atrial Fibrillation[1,2]	-	-	94%	95%
Antithrombotic Therapy Timing[2]	62	100%	97%	98%
Assessed for Rehabilitation[2]	52	100%	97%	97%
Discharged on Antithrombotic Therapy[2]	52	100%	98%	99%
Discharged on Statin Medication[2]	41	100%	94%	94%
Thrombolytic Therapy Timing[1,2]	-	-	58%	66%
Venous Thromboembolism Prophylaxis[2]	61	100%	92%	94%
Written Stroke Educational Materials Given[2]	38	95%	84%	88%
Surgical Care Improvement Project				
Appropriate Beta Blocker Usage[2]	100	98%	97%	98%
Appropriate VTP Within 24 Hours[2]	276	98%	98%	98%
Controlled Postoperative Blood Glucose[2,7]	-	-	96%	97%
Perioperative Temperature Management[2]	308	100%	100%	100%
Prophylactic Antibiotic Selection[2]	193	100%	99%	99%
Prophylactic Antibiotic Selection (Outpatient)	284	100%	98%	98%
Prophylactic Antibiotic Stopped[2]	184	98%	98%	98%
Prophylactic Antibiotic Timing[2]	193	100%	99%	99%
Prophylactic Antibiotic Timing (Outpatient)	286	99%	98%	98%
Urinary Catheter Removal[2]	86	95%	97%	97%
Survey of Patients' Hospital Experiences				
Area Around Room 'Always' Quiet at Night	300+	58%	66%	61%
Doctors 'Always' Communicated Well	300+	75%	83%	82%
Home Recovery Information Given	300+	83%	84%	85%
Hospital Given 9 or 10 on 10 Point Scale	300+	56%	69%	71%
Meds 'Always' Explained Before Given	300+	58%	63%	64%
Nurses 'Always' Communicated Well	300+	69%	78%	79%
Pain 'Always' Well Controlled	300+	61%	71%	71%
Room and Bathroom 'Always' Clean	300+	65%	71%	73%
Timely Help 'Always' Received	300+	54%	65%	68%
Would Definitely Recommend Hospital	300+	52%	70%	71%
Use of Medical Imaging				
Cardiac Imaging Stress Test before Surgery	224	9.4%	5.5%	5.3%
Combination Abdominal CT Scan	697	6.2%	10.1%	10.5%
Combination Brain/Sinus CT Scan	558	4.5%	2.3%	2.7%
Combination Chest CT Scan	523	1.5%	3.7%	2.7%
Follow-up Mammogram/Ultrasound	669	12.4%	8.9%	8.8%
Lumbar Spine MRI for Low Back Pain	50	38.0%	36.6%	37.2%

Polk Medical Center

424 N Main Street
Cedartown, GA 30125
Type: Critical Access Hospitals
Ownership: Govt - Hospital Dist/Auth

Phone: 770-748-2500
Fax: 770-749-9904
Emergency Services: Yes
Beds: 25

Key Personnel:
Chief of Medical Staff. . . . . Neil Gordon, MD
Cardiac Laboratory. . . . . Suzy Hubbard
Quality Assurance . . . . Jill McElwee
Infection Control. . . . . Martine Osselaer
Emergency Room . . . . Missy Puckett
Patient Relations . . . . Missy Puckett
CEO/President. . . . . Kim Scoggins
Radiology. . . . . Maria Treadwell

Measure	Cases	This Hosp.	State Avg.	U.S. Avg.
Blood Clot Prevention and Treatment				
Anticoagulation Overlap Therapy[2,7]	-	-	90%	93%
ICU Venous Thromboembolism Prophylaxis[2,7]	-	-	90%	92%
Incidence of Potentially Preventable VTE[2,7]	-	-	13%	10%
UFH with Dosages/Platelet Monitoring[2,7]	-	-	99%	97%
Venous Thromboembolism Prophylaxis[2]	71	63%	80%	85%
Warfarin Therapy Discharge Instructions[2,7]	-	-	78%	75%
Chest Pain/Possible Heart Attack Care				
Aspirin Given Within 24 Hours of Arrival	171	92%	94%	96%
Fibrinolytic Meds Within 30 Min. of Arrival[7]	-	-	35%	58%
Average Time to ECG (minutes)	171	8	8	7
Average Time to Transfer (minutes)[1]	-	-	73	60

NOTE: Hospital profiles are in alphabetical order by state, then city, then hospital within the city; Rankings exclude hospitals with less than 25 cases except for patient surveys which excludes hospitals with less than 100 cases; (a) 100-299 cases; (1) The number of cases/patients is too few to report; (2) Data submitted were based on a sample of cases/patients; (3) Results are based on a shorter time period than required; (4) Data suppressed by CMS for one or more quarters; (5) Results are not available for this reporting period; (6) Fewer than 100 patients completed the HCAHPS survey; (7) No cases met the criteria for this measure; (8) The lower limit of the confidence interval cannot be calculated if the number of observed infections equals zero; (9) No data are available from the state/territory for this reporting period; (10) The scores shown reflect fewer than 50 completed surveys; (11) There were discrepancies in the data collection process; (12) This measure does not apply to this hospital for this reporting period; (13) Results cannot be calculated for this reporting period; (14) The results for this state are combined with nearby states to protect confidentiality; Please refer to the User's Guide for a full explanation of data.

Measure	Cases	This Hosp.	State Avg.	U.S. Avg.
Children's Asthma Care				
Received Home Management Plan of Care	-	-	-	88%
Received Reliever Medication	-	-	-	100%
Received Systemic Corticosteroids	-	-	-	100%
Emergency Department				
Admittance Decision Time (minutes)[2]	31	25	100	98
Head CT Results Within 45 Min. of Arrival[1]	-	-	45%	57%
Patients Who Left ER Before Being Seen	23,258	4%	3%	2%
Time from ER Arrival to Admit. (minutes)[2]	33	131	286	274
Time from ER Arrival to Discharge (minutes)	396	72	140	134
Time in ER Before Being Evaluated (minutes)	240	29	32	26
Time to Pain Meds for Fractures (minutes)	50	51	64	57
Heart Attack Care				
Aspirin Given at Discharge[3,7]	-	-	99%	99%
Fibrinolytic Meds Within 30 Min. of Arrival[3,7]	-	-	80%	54%
PCI Within 90 Minutes of Arrival[3,7]	-	-	95%	96%
Statin Prescribed at Discharge[3,7]	-	-	98%	98%
Heart Failure Care				
ACE Inhibitor or ARB for LVSD[3,7]	-	-	97%	97%
Discharge Instructions Given[1,3]	-	-	92%	94%
Evaluation of LVS Function[1,3]	-	-	99%	99%
Medicare Spending				
Medicare Spending per Patient (ratio)	-	-	0.95	0.98
Pneumonia Care				
Appropriate Initial Antibiotic Given[2]	20	90%	95%	95%
Blood Culture Timing[2]	19	95%	97%	98%
Pregnancy and Delivery Care				
Newborn Deliveries Scheduled Early[5]	-	-	8%	6%
Preventive Care				
Immunization for Influenza[3]	41	85%	88%	90%
Immunization for Pneumonia[2,3]	71	85%	90%	92%
Stroke Care				
Anticoagulation Therapy for Atrial Fibrillation[5]	-	-	94%	95%
Antithrombotic Therapy Timing[5]	-	-	97%	98%
Assessed for Rehabilitation[5]	-	-	97%	97%
Discharged on Antithrombotic Therapy[5]	-	-	98%	99%
Discharged on Statin Medication[5]	-	-	94%	94%
Thrombolytic Therapy Timing[5]	-	-	58%	66%
Venous Thromboembolism Prophylaxis[5]	-	-	92%	94%
Written Stroke Educational Materials Given[5]	-	-	84%	88%
Surgical Care Improvement Project				
Appropriate Beta Blocker Usage[5]	-	-	97%	98%
Appropriate VTP Within 24 Hours[5]	-	-	98%	98%
Controlled Postoperative Blood Glucose[5]	-	-	96%	97%
Perioperative Temperature Management[5]	-	-	100%	100%
Prophylactic Antibiotic Selection[5]	-	-	99%	99%
Prophylactic Antibiotic Selection (Outpatient)[5]	-	-	98%	98%
Prophylactic Antibiotic Stopped[5]	-	-	98%	98%
Prophylactic Antibiotic Timing[5]	-	-	99%	99%
Prophylactic Antibiotic Timing (Outpatient)[5]	-	-	98%	98%
Urinary Catheter Removal[5]	-	-	97%	97%
Survey of Patients' Hospital Experiences				
Area Around Room 'Always' Quiet at Night[10]	<100	85%	66%	61%
Doctors 'Always' Communicated Well[10]	<100	82%	83%	82%
Home Recovery Information Given[10]	<100	85%	84%	85%
Hospital Given 9 or 10 on 10 Point Scale[10]	<100	70%	69%	71%
Meds 'Always' Explained Before Given[10]	<100	73%	63%	64%
Nurses 'Always' Communicated Well[10]	<100	89%	78%	79%
Pain 'Always' Well Controlled[10]	<100	94%	71%	71%
Room and Bathroom 'Always' Clean[10]	<100	87%	71%	73%
Timely Help 'Always' Received[10]	<100	90%	65%	68%
Would Definitely Recommend Hospital[10]	<100	80%	70%	71%
Use of Medical Imaging				
Cardiac Imaging Stress Test before Surgery[7]	-	-	5.5%	5.3%
Combination Abdominal CT Scan	107	0.0%	10.1%	10.5%
Combination Brain/Sinus CT Scan[1]	-	-	2.3%	2.7%
Combination Chest CT Scan[1]	-	-	3.7%	2.7%
Follow-up Mammogram/Ultrasound	132	9.1%	8.9%	8.8%
Lumbar Spine MRI for Low Back Pain[1]	-	-	36.6%	37.2%

Murray Medical Center

707 Old Dalton Ellijay Road, PO Box 1406 Phone: 706-517-2031
Chatsworth, GA 30705
Type: Acute Care Hospitals Emergency Services: Yes
Ownership: Voluntary non-profit - Private Beds: 42

Key Personnel:

Infection Control.............. Kerri Cofeild
Anesthesiology................ Susan Longley
Operating Room............... Susan Longley
Quality Assurance .... Corey Parrish
Radiology..................... Wayne Straw
Emergency Room .... Michelle Vandergriff
Chief of Medical Staff.......... Michael A Witt, MD
CEO/President................ Donny Wright

Measure	Cases	This Hosp.	State Avg.	U.S. Avg.
Blood Clot Prevention and Treatment				
Anticoagulation Overlap Therapy[1,2]	-	-	90%	93%
ICU Venous Thromboembolism Prophylaxis[2,7]	-	-	90%	92%
Incidence of Potentially Preventable VTE[1,2]	-	-	13%	10%
UFH with Dosages/Platelet Monitoring[2,7]	-	-	99%	97%
Venous Thromboembolism Prophylaxis[2]	128	46%	80%	85%
Warfarin Therapy Discharge Instructions[1,2]	-	-	78%	75%
Chest Pain/Possible Heart Attack Care				
Aspirin Given Within 24 Hours of Arrival[3]	20	95%	94%	96%
Fibrinolytic Meds Within 30 Min. of Arrival[3,7]	-	-	35%	58%
Average Time to ECG (minutes)[3]	24	13	8	7
Average Time to Transfer (minutes)[1,3]	-	-	73	60
Children's Asthma Care				
Received Home Management Plan of Care	-	-	-	88%
Received Reliever Medication	-	-	-	100%
Received Systemic Corticosteroids	-	-	-	100%
Emergency Department				
Admittance Decision Time (minutes)	130	50	100	98
Head CT Results Within 45 Min. of Arrival[5]	-	-	45%	57%
Patients Who Left ER Before Being Seen	18,076	5%	3%	2%
Time from ER Arrival to Admit. (minutes)	136	246	286	274
Time from ER Arrival to Discharge (minutes)	341	135	140	134
Time in ER Before Being Evaluated (minutes)	378	48	32	26
Time to Pain Meds for Fractures (minutes)[1,3]	-	-	64	57
Heart Attack Care				
Aspirin Given at Discharge[5]	-	-	99%	99%
Fibrinolytic Meds Within 30 Min. of Arrival[5]	-	-	80%	54%
PCI Within 90 Minutes of Arrival[5]	-	-	95%	96%
Statin Prescribed at Discharge[5]	-	-	98%	98%
Heart Failure Care				
ACE Inhibitor or ARB for LVSD[1,3]	-	-	97%	97%
Discharge Instructions Given[1,3]	-	-	92%	94%
Evaluation of LVS Function[3]	11	100%	99%	99%
Medicare Spending				
Medicare Spending per Patient (ratio)	-	0.79	0.95	0.98
Pneumonia Care				
Appropriate Initial Antibiotic Given	22	73%	95%	95%
Blood Culture Timing	40	92%	97%	98%
Pregnancy and Delivery Care				
Newborn Deliveries Scheduled Early[7]	-	-	8%	6%
Preventive Care				
Immunization for Influenza[2]	193	91%	88%	90%
Immunization for Pneumonia[2]	289	93%	90%	92%
Stroke Care				
Anticoagulation Therapy for Atrial Fibrillation[5]	-	-	94%	95%
Antithrombotic Therapy Timing[5]	-	-	97%	98%
Assessed for Rehabilitation[5]	-	-	97%	97%
Discharged on Antithrombotic Therapy[5]	-	-	98%	99%
Discharged on Statin Medication[5]	-	-	94%	94%
Thrombolytic Therapy Timing[5]	-	-	58%	66%
Venous Thromboembolism Prophylaxis[5]	-	-	92%	94%
Written Stroke Educational Materials Given[5]	-	-	84%	88%
Surgical Care Improvement Project				
Appropriate Beta Blocker Usage[5]	-	-	97%	98%
Appropriate VTP Within 24 Hours[5]	-	-	98%	98%
Controlled Postoperative Blood Glucose[5]	-	-	96%	97%
Perioperative Temperature Management[5]	-	-	100%	100%
Prophylactic Antibiotic Selection[5]	-	-	99%	99%
Prophylactic Antibiotic Selection (Outpatient)[5]	-	-	98%	98%
Prophylactic Antibiotic Stopped[5]	-	-	98%	98%
Prophylactic Antibiotic Timing[5]	-	-	99%	99%
Prophylactic Antibiotic Timing (Outpatient)[5]	-	-	98%	98%
Urinary Catheter Removal[5]	-	-	97%	97%
Survey of Patients' Hospital Experiences				
Area Around Room 'Always' Quiet at Night[6]	<100	73%	66%	61%
Doctors 'Always' Communicated Well[6]	<100	82%	83%	82%
Home Recovery Information Given[6]	<100	81%	84%	85%
Hospital Given 9 or 10 on 10 Point Scale[6]	<100	63%	69%	71%
Meds 'Always' Explained Before Given[6]	<100	68%	63%	64%
Nurses 'Always' Communicated Well[6]	<100	85%	78%	79%
Pain 'Always' Well Controlled[6]	<100	64%	71%	71%
Room and Bathroom 'Always' Clean[6]	<100	69%	71%	73%
Timely Help 'Always' Received[6]	<100	73%	65%	68%
Would Definitely Recommend Hospital[6]	<100	66%	70%	71%
Use of Medical Imaging				
Cardiac Imaging Stress Test before Surgery[7]	-	-	5.5%	5.3%
Combination Abdominal CT Scan	182	7.1%	10.1%	10.5%
Combination Brain/Sinus CT Scan[1]	-	-	2.3%	2.7%
Combination Chest CT Scan	125	8.0%	3.7%	2.7%
Follow-up Mammogram/Ultrasound	174	11.5%	8.9%	8.8%
Lumbar Spine MRI for Low Back Pain[1]	-	-	36.6%	37.2%

Evans Memorial Hospital

200 N River Street Phone: 912-739-5105
Claxton, GA 30417 Fax: 912-739-5101
URL: www.evansmemorialhospital.org
Type: Acute Care Hospitals Emergency Services: Yes
Ownership: Govt - Hospital Dist/Auth Beds: 49

Key Personnel:

Anesthesiology................ Donald Aliffi, CRNA
Chief of Medical Staff.......... Glenn J Dasher, MD
Emergency Room .... Mark Lewis, MD
CEO/President................ Eston Price, Jr
Cardiac Laboratory............ Michelle Sapp, RRT
Quality Assurance .... Donna Sellers, RN
CEO .... Martha F. Tatum
Infection Control.............. Martha Tucker

Measure	Cases	This Hosp.	State Avg.	U.S. Avg.
Blood Clot Prevention and Treatment				
Anticoagulation Overlap Therapy[1,2]	-	-	90%	93%
ICU Venous Thromboembolism Prophylaxis[2,7]	-	-	90%	92%
Incidence of Potentially Preventable VTE[2,7]	-	-	13%	10%
UFH with Dosages/Platelet Monitoring[2,7]	-	-	99%	97%
Venous Thromboembolism Prophylaxis[2]	222	18%	80%	85%
Warfarin Therapy Discharge Instructions[1,2]	-	-	78%	75%
Chest Pain/Possible Heart Attack Care				
Aspirin Given Within 24 Hours of Arrival	27	100%	94%	96%
Fibrinolytic Meds Within 30 Min. of Arrival[1,3]	-	-	35%	58%
Average Time to ECG (minutes)	30	22	8	7
Average Time to Transfer (minutes)[3,7]	-	-	73	60
Children's Asthma Care				
Received Home Management Plan of Care	-	-	-	88%
Received Reliever Medication	-	-	-	100%
Received Systemic Corticosteroids	-	-	-	100%
Emergency Department				
Admittance Decision Time (minutes)[2]	362	42	100	98
Head CT Results Within 45 Min. of Arrival[1]	-	-	45%	57%
Patients Who Left ER Before Being Seen	9,773	1%	3%	2%
Time from ER Arrival to Admit. (minutes)[2]	362	183	286	274
Time from ER Arrival to Discharge (minutes)	295	90	140	134
Time in ER Before Being Evaluated (minutes)	354	22	32	26
Time to Pain Meds for Fractures (minutes)	42	48	64	57
Heart Attack Care				
Aspirin Given at Discharge[1,3]	-	-	99%	99%
Fibrinolytic Meds Within 30 Min. of Arrival[3,7]	-	-	80%	54%
PCI Within 90 Minutes of Arrival[3,7]	-	-	95%	96%
Statin Prescribed at Discharge[1,3]	-	-	98%	98%
Heart Failure Care				
ACE Inhibitor or ARB for LVSD[1,2]	-	-	97%	97%
Discharge Instructions Given[2]	26	88%	92%	94%
Evaluation of LVS Function[2]	28	100%	99%	99%
Medicare Spending				
Medicare Spending per Patient (ratio)	-	0.86	0.95	0.98

NOTE: Hospital profiles are in alphabetical order by state, then city, then hospital within the city; Rankings exclude hospitals with less than 25 cases except for patient surveys which excludes hospitals with less than 100 cases; (a) 100-299 cases; (1) The number of cases/patients is too few to report; (2) Data submitted were based on a sample of cases/patients; (3) Results are based on a shorter time period than required; (4) Data suppressed by CMS for one or more quarters; (5) Results are not available for this reporting period; (6) Fewer than 100 patients completed the HCAHPS survey; (7) No cases met the criteria for this measure; (8) The lower limit of the confidence interval cannot be calculated if the number of observed infections equals zero; (9) No data are available from the state/territory for this reporting period; (10) The scores shown reflect fewer than 50 completed surveys; (11) There were discrepancies in the data collection process; (12) This measure does not apply to this hospital for this reporting period; (13) Results cannot be calculated for this reporting period; (14) The results for this state are combined with nearby states to protect confidentiality; Please refer to the User's Guide for a full explanation of data.

Measure	Cases	This Hosp.	State Avg.	U.S. Avg.
Pneumonia Care				
Appropriate Initial Antibiotic Given[2]	45	91%	95%	95%
Blood Culture Timing[2]	54	94%	97%	98%
Pregnancy and Delivery Care				
Newborn Deliveries Scheduled Early[7]	-	-	8%	6%
Preventive Care				
Immunization for Influenza[2]	300	84%	88%	90%
Immunization for Pneumonia[2]	475	88%	90%	92%
Stroke Care				
Anticoagulation Therapy for Atrial Fibrillation[7]	-	-	94%	95%
Antithrombotic Therapy Timing[1]	-	-	97%	98%
Assessed for Rehabilitation[1]	-	-	97%	97%
Discharged on Antithrombotic Therapy[1]	-	-	98%	99%
Discharged on Statin Medication[1]	-	-	94%	94%
Thrombolytic Therapy Timing[1]	-	-	58%	66%
Venous Thromboembolism Prophylaxis[1]	-	-	92%	94%
Written Stroke Educational Materials Given[1]	-	-	84%	88%
Surgical Care Improvement Project				
Appropriate Beta Blocker Usage[5]	-	-	97%	98%
Appropriate VTP Within 24 Hours[5]	-	-	98%	98%
Controlled Postoperative Blood Glucose[5]	-	-	96%	97%
Perioperative Temperature Management[5]	-	-	100%	100%
Prophylactic Antibiotic Selection[5]	-	-	99%	99%
Prophylactic Antibiotic Selection (Outpatient)[1,3]	-	-	98%	98%
Prophylactic Antibiotic Stopped[5]	-	-	98%	98%
Prophylactic Antibiotic Timing[5]	-	-	99%	99%
Prophylactic Antibiotic Timing (Outpatient)[1,3]	-	-	98%	98%
Urinary Catheter Removal[5]	-	-	97%	97%
Survey of Patients' Hospital Experiences				
Area Around Room 'Always' Quiet at Night	(a)	66%	66%	61%
Doctors 'Always' Communicated Well	(a)	94%	83%	82%
Home Recovery Information Given	(a)	83%	84%	85%
Hospital Given 9 or 10 on 10 Point Scale	(a)	69%	69%	71%
Meds 'Always' Explained Before Given	(a)	65%	63%	64%
Nurses 'Always' Communicated Well	(a)	80%	78%	79%
Pain 'Always' Well Controlled	(a)	65%	71%	71%
Room and Bathroom 'Always' Clean	(a)	76%	71%	73%
Timely Help 'Always' Received	(a)	73%	65%	68%
Would Definitely Recommend Hospital	(a)	65%	70%	71%
Use of Medical Imaging				
Cardiac Imaging Stress Test before Surgery[1]	-	-	5.5%	5.3%
Combination Abdominal CT Scan	148	29.1%	10.1%	10.5%
Combination Brain/Sinus CT Scan[1]	-	-	2.3%	2.7%
Combination Chest CT Scan	140	12.1%	3.7%	2.7%
Follow-up Mammogram/Ultrasound	257	12.1%	8.9%	8.8%
Lumbar Spine MRI for Low Back Pain[1]	-	-	36.6%	37.2%

Mountain Lakes Medical Center

196 Ridgecrest Circle Phone: 706-782-0400
Clayton, GA 30525
Type: Critical Access Hospitals Emergency Services: Yes
Ownership: Proprietary

Measure	Cases	This Hosp.	State Avg.	U.S. Avg.
Blood Clot Prevention and Treatment				
Anticoagulation Overlap Therapy[1,2]	-	-	90%	93%
ICU Venous Thromboembolism Prophylaxis[1,2]	-	-	90%	92%
Incidence of Potentially Preventable VTE[2,7]	-	-	13%	10%
UFH with Dosages/Platelet Monitoring[1,2]	-	-	99%	97%
Venous Thromboembolism Prophylaxis[2]	173	61%	80%	85%
Warfarin Therapy Discharge Instructions[1,2]	-	-	78%	75%
Chest Pain/Possible Heart Attack Care				
Aspirin Given Within 24 Hours of Arrival	-	-	94%	96%
Fibrinolytic Meds Within 30 Min. of Arrival	-	-	35%	58%
Average Time to ECG (minutes)	-	-	8	7
Average Time to Transfer (minutes)	-	-	73	60
Children's Asthma Care				
Received Home Management Plan of Care	-	-	-	88%
Received Reliever Medication	-	-	-	100%
Received Systemic Corticosteroids	-	-	-	100%
Emergency Department				
Admittance Decision Time (minutes)[2]	225	62	100	98
Head CT Results Within 45 Min. of Arrival	-	-	45%	57%
Patients Who Left ER Before Being Seen	-	-	3%	2%
Time from ER Arrival to Admit. (minutes)[2]	226	248	286	274
Time from ER Arrival to Discharge (minutes)	-	-	140	134
Time in ER Before Being Evaluated (minutes)	-	-	32	26
Time to Pain Meds for Fractures (minutes)	-	-	64	57
Heart Attack Care				
Aspirin Given at Discharge[1,3]	-	-	99%	99%
Fibrinolytic Meds Within 30 Min. of Arrival[3,7]	-	-	80%	54%
PCI Within 90 Minutes of Arrival[3,7]	-	-	95%	96%
Statin Prescribed at Discharge[1,3]	-	-	98%	98%
Heart Failure Care				
ACE Inhibitor or ARB for LVSD[1]	-	-	97%	97%
Discharge Instructions Given	22	82%	92%	94%
Evaluation of LVS Function	24	100%	99%	99%
Medicare Spending				
Medicare Spending per Patient (ratio)	-	-	0.95	0.98
Pneumonia Care				
Appropriate Initial Antibiotic Given[2]	18	78%	95%	95%
Blood Culture Timing[2]	30	100%	97%	98%
Pregnancy and Delivery Care				
Newborn Deliveries Scheduled Early[5]	-	-	8%	6%
Preventive Care				
Immunization for Influenza[2]	153	98%	88%	90%
Immunization for Pneumonia[2]	216	93%	90%	92%
Stroke Care				
Anticoagulation Therapy for Atrial Fibrillation[3,7]	-	-	94%	95%
Antithrombotic Therapy Timing[1,3]	-	-	97%	98%
Assessed for Rehabilitation[3,7]	-	-	97%	97%
Discharged on Antithrombotic Therapy[3,7]	-	-	98%	99%
Discharged on Statin Medication[3,7]	-	-	94%	94%
Thrombolytic Therapy Timing[1,3]	-	-	58%	66%
Venous Thromboembolism Prophylaxis[1,3]	-	-	92%	94%
Written Stroke Educational Materials Given[3,7]	-	-	84%	88%
Surgical Care Improvement Project				
Appropriate Beta Blocker Usage[5]	-	-	97%	98%
Appropriate VTP Within 24 Hours[5]	-	-	98%	98%
Controlled Postoperative Blood Glucose[5]	-	-	96%	97%
Perioperative Temperature Management[5]	-	-	100%	100%
Prophylactic Antibiotic Selection[5]	-	-	99%	99%
Prophylactic Antibiotic Selection (Outpatient)	-	-	98%	98%
Prophylactic Antibiotic Stopped[5]	-	-	98%	98%
Prophylactic Antibiotic Timing[5]	-	-	99%	99%
Prophylactic Antibiotic Timing (Outpatient)	-	-	98%	98%
Urinary Catheter Removal[5]	-	-	97%	97%
Survey of Patients' Hospital Experiences				
Area Around Room 'Always' Quiet at Night[6]	<100	63%	66%	61%
Doctors 'Always' Communicated Well[6]	<100	85%	83%	82%
Home Recovery Information Given[6]	<100	84%	84%	85%
Hospital Given 9 or 10 on 10 Point Scale[6]	<100	55%	69%	71%
Meds 'Always' Explained Before Given[6]	<100	73%	63%	64%
Nurses 'Always' Communicated Well[6]	<100	81%	78%	79%
Pain 'Always' Well Controlled[6]	<100	68%	71%	71%
Room and Bathroom 'Always' Clean[6]	<100	72%	71%	73%
Timely Help 'Always' Received[6]	<100	72%	65%	68%
Would Definitely Recommend Hospital[6]	<100	56%	70%	71%
Use of Medical Imaging				
Cardiac Imaging Stress Test before Surgery	-	-	5.5%	5.3%
Combination Abdominal CT Scan	-	-	10.1%	10.5%
Combination Brain/Sinus CT Scan	-	-	2.3%	2.7%
Combination Chest CT Scan	-	-	3.7%	2.7%
Follow-up Mammogram/Ultrasound	-	-	8.9%	8.8%
Lumbar Spine MRI for Low Back Pain	-	-	36.6%	37.2%

Bleckley Memorial Hospital

145 East Peacock Street Phone: 478-934-6211
Cochran, GA 31014
Type: Critical Access Hospitals Emergency Services: Yes
Ownership: Govt - Hospital Dist/Auth
Key Personnel:
Radiology. . . . . Anne Brown

Measure	Cases	This Hosp.	State Avg.	U.S. Avg.
Blood Clot Prevention and Treatment				
Anticoagulation Overlap Therapy[5]	-	-	90%	93%
ICU Venous Thromboembolism Prophylaxis[5]	-	-	90%	92%
Incidence of Potentially Preventable VTE[5]	-	-	13%	10%
UFH with Dosages/Platelet Monitoring[5]	-	-	99%	97%
Venous Thromboembolism Prophylaxis[5]	-	-	80%	85%
Warfarin Therapy Discharge Instructions[5]	-	-	78%	75%
Chest Pain/Possible Heart Attack Care				
Aspirin Given Within 24 Hours of Arrival[1,3]	-	-	94%	96%
Fibrinolytic Meds Within 30 Min. of Arrival[3,7]	-	-	35%	58%
Average Time to ECG (minutes)[1,3]	-	-	8	7
Average Time to Transfer (minutes)[3,7]	-	-	73	60
Children's Asthma Care				
Received Home Management Plan of Care	-	-	-	88%
Received Reliever Medication	-	-	-	100%
Received Systemic Corticosteroids	-	-	-	100%
Emergency Department				
Admittance Decision Time (minutes)[5]	-	-	100	98
Head CT Results Within 45 Min. of Arrival[5]	-	-	45%	57%
Patients Who Left ER Before Being Seen	4,946	1%	3%	2%
Time from ER Arrival to Admit. (minutes)[5]	-	-	286	274
Time from ER Arrival to Discharge (minutes)[5]	-	-	140	134
Time in ER Before Being Evaluated (minutes)[5]	-	-	32	26
Time to Pain Meds for Fractures (minutes)[5]	-	-	64	57
Heart Attack Care				
Aspirin Given at Discharge[5]	-	-	99%	99%
Fibrinolytic Meds Within 30 Min. of Arrival[5]	-	-	80%	54%
PCI Within 90 Minutes of Arrival[5]	-	-	95%	96%
Statin Prescribed at Discharge[5]	-	-	98%	98%
Heart Failure Care				
ACE Inhibitor or ARB for LVSD[1]	-	-	97%	97%
Discharge Instructions Given[1]	-	-	92%	94%
Evaluation of LVS Function[1]	-	-	99%	99%
Medicare Spending				
Medicare Spending per Patient (ratio)	-	-	0.95	0.98
Pneumonia Care				
Appropriate Initial Antibiotic Given	13	85%	95%	95%
Blood Culture Timing	15	93%	97%	98%
Pregnancy and Delivery Care				
Newborn Deliveries Scheduled Early[5]	-	-	8%	6%
Preventive Care				
Immunization for Influenza[5]	-	-	88%	90%
Immunization for Pneumonia[5]	-	-	90%	92%
Stroke Care				
Anticoagulation Therapy for Atrial Fibrillation[5]	-	-	94%	95%
Antithrombotic Therapy Timing[5]	-	-	97%	98%
Assessed for Rehabilitation[5]	-	-	97%	97%
Discharged on Antithrombotic Therapy[5]	-	-	98%	99%
Discharged on Statin Medication[5]	-	-	94%	94%
Thrombolytic Therapy Timing[5]	-	-	58%	66%
Venous Thromboembolism Prophylaxis[5]	-	-	92%	94%
Written Stroke Educational Materials Given[5]	-	-	84%	88%
Surgical Care Improvement Project				
Appropriate Beta Blocker Usage[5]	-	-	97%	98%
Appropriate VTP Within 24 Hours[5]	-	-	98%	98%
Controlled Postoperative Blood Glucose[5]	-	-	96%	97%
Perioperative Temperature Management[5]	-	-	100%	100%
Prophylactic Antibiotic Selection[5]	-	-	99%	99%
Prophylactic Antibiotic Selection (Outpatient)[5]	-	-	98%	98%
Prophylactic Antibiotic Stopped[5]	-	-	98%	98%
Prophylactic Antibiotic Timing[5]	-	-	99%	99%
Prophylactic Antibiotic Timing (Outpatient)[5]	-	-	98%	98%
Urinary Catheter Removal[5]	-	-	97%	97%
Survey of Patients' Hospital Experiences				
Area Around Room 'Always' Quiet at Night[5]	-	-	66%	61%
Doctors 'Always' Communicated Well[5]	-	-	83%	82%
Home Recovery Information Given[5]	-	-	84%	85%
Hospital Given 9 or 10 on 10 Point Scale[5]	-	-	69%	71%
Meds 'Always' Explained Before Given[5]	-	-	63%	64%
Nurses 'Always' Communicated Well[5]	-	-	78%	79%
Pain 'Always' Well Controlled[5]	-	-	71%	71%
Room and Bathroom 'Always' Clean[5]	-	-	71%	73%
Timely Help 'Always' Received[5]	-	-	65%	68%

NOTE: Hospital profiles are in alphabetical order by state, then city, then hospital within the city; Rankings exclude hospitals with less than 25 cases except for patient surveys which excludes hospitals with less than 100 cases; (a) 100-299 cases; (1) The number of cases/patients is too few to report; (2) Data submitted were based on a sample of cases/patients; (3) Results are based on a shorter time period than required; (4) Data suppressed by CMS for one or more quarters; (5) Results are not available for this reporting period; (6) Fewer than 100 patients completed the HCAHPS survey; (7) No cases met the criteria for this measure; (8) The lower limit of the confidence interval cannot be calculated if the number of observed infections equals zero; (9) No data are available from the state/territory for this reporting period; (10) The scores shown reflect fewer than 50 completed surveys; (11) There were discrepancies in the data collection process; (12) This measure does not apply to this hospital for this reporting period; (13) Results cannot be calculated for this reporting period; (14) The results for this state are combined with nearby states to protect confidentiality; Please refer to the User's Guide for a full explanation of data.

Measure	Cases	This Hosp.	State Avg.	U.S. Avg.
Would Definitely Recommend Hospital[5]	-	-	70%	71%
Use of Medical Imaging				
Cardiac Imaging Stress Test before Surgery[7]	-	-	5.5%	5.3%
Combination Abdominal CT Scan	75	2.7%	10.1%	10.5%
Combination Brain/Sinus CT Scan[1]	-	-	2.3%	2.7%
Combination Chest CT Scan[1]	-	-	3.7%	2.7%
Follow-up Mammogram/Ultrasound[7]	-	-	8.9%	8.8%
Lumbar Spine MRI for Low Back Pain[7]	-	-	36.6%	37.2%

Miller County Hospital

209 N Cuthbert Street
Colquitt, GA 39837
Type: Critical Access Hospitals
Ownership: Govt - Hospital Dist/Auth
Phone: 229-758-4231
Fax: 229-758-5198
Emergency Services: Yes
Beds: 38

Key Personnel:
Quality Assurance .... Sandy Rathel
Operating Room............... Deb Smith
CEO/President............... Harley Smith

Measure	Cases	This Hosp.	State Avg.	U.S. Avg.
Blood Clot Prevention and Treatment				
Anticoagulation Overlap Therapy[5]	-	-	90%	93%
ICU Venous Thromboembolism Prophylaxis[5]	-	-	90%	92%
Incidence of Potentially Preventable VTE[5]	-	-	13%	10%
UFH with Dosages/Platelet Monitoring[5]	-	-	99%	97%
Venous Thromboembolism Prophylaxis[5]	-	-	80%	85%
Warfarin Therapy Discharge Instructions[5]	-	-	78%	75%
Chest Pain/Possible Heart Attack Care				
Aspirin Given Within 24 Hours of Arrival[1,3]	-	-	94%	96%
Fibrinolytic Meds Within 30 Min. of Arrival[3,7]	-	-	35%	58%
Average Time to ECG (minutes)[1,3]	-	-	8	7
Average Time to Transfer (minutes)[1,3]	-	-	73	60
Children's Asthma Care				
Received Home Management Plan of Care	-	-	-	88%
Received Reliever Medication	-	-	-	100%
Received Systemic Corticosteroids	-	-	-	100%
Emergency Department				
Admittance Decision Time (minutes)[5]	-	-	100	98
Head CT Results Within 45 Min. of Arrival[5]	-	-	45%	57%
Patients Who Left ER Before Being Seen	4,731	0%	3%	2%
Time from ER Arrival to Admit. (minutes)[5]	-	-	286	274
Time from ER Arrival to Discharge (minutes)[5]	-	-	140	134
Time in ER Before Being Evaluated (minutes)[5]	-	-	32	26
Time to Pain Meds for Fractures (minutes)[5]	-	-	64	57
Heart Attack Care				
Aspirin Given at Discharge[5]	-	-	99%	99%
Fibrinolytic Meds Within 30 Min. of Arrival[5]	-	-	80%	54%
PCI Within 90 Minutes of Arrival[5]	-	-	95%	96%
Statin Prescribed at Discharge[5]	-	-	98%	98%
Heart Failure Care				
ACE Inhibitor or ARB for LVSD[1,2]	-	-	97%	97%
Discharge Instructions Given[2]	18	100%	92%	94%
Evaluation of LVS Function[2]	21	100%	99%	99%
Medicare Spending				
Medicare Spending per Patient (ratio)	-	-	0.95	0.98
Pneumonia Care				
Appropriate Initial Antibiotic Given[1,2]	-	-	95%	95%
Blood Culture Timing[2]	11	100%	97%	98%
Pregnancy and Delivery Care				
Newborn Deliveries Scheduled Early[5]	-	-	8%	6%
Preventive Care				
Immunization for Influenza[5]	-	-	88%	90%
Immunization for Pneumonia[5]	-	-	90%	92%
Stroke Care				
Anticoagulation Therapy for Atrial Fibrillation[5]	-	-	94%	95%
Antithrombotic Therapy Timing[5]	-	-	97%	98%
Assessed for Rehabilitation[5]	-	-	97%	97%
Discharged on Antithrombotic Therapy[5]	-	-	98%	99%
Discharged on Statin Medication[5]	-	-	94%	94%
Thrombolytic Therapy Timing[5]	-	-	58%	66%
Venous Thromboembolism Prophylaxis[5]	-	-	92%	94%
Written Stroke Educational Materials Given[5]	-	-	84%	88%
Surgical Care Improvement Project				
Appropriate Beta Blocker Usage[5]	-	-	97%	98%
Appropriate VTP Within 24 Hours[5]	-	-	98%	98%
Controlled Postoperative Blood Glucose[5]	-	-	96%	97%
Perioperative Temperature Management[5]	-	-	100%	100%
Prophylactic Antibiotic Selection[5]	-	-	99%	99%
Prophylactic Antibiotic Selection (Outpatient)[5]	-	-	98%	98%
Prophylactic Antibiotic Stopped[5]	-	-	98%	98%
Prophylactic Antibiotic Timing[5]	-	-	99%	99%
Prophylactic Antibiotic Timing (Outpatient)[5]	-	-	98%	98%
Urinary Catheter Removal[5]	-	-	97%	97%
Survey of Patients' Hospital Experiences				
Area Around Room 'Always' Quiet at Night[5]	-	-	66%	61%
Doctors 'Always' Communicated Well[5]	-	-	83%	82%
Home Recovery Information Given[5]	-	-	84%	85%
Hospital Given 9 or 10 on 10 Point Scale[5]	-	-	69%	71%
Meds 'Always' Explained Before Given[5]	-	-	63%	64%
Nurses 'Always' Communicated Well[5]	-	-	78%	79%
Pain 'Always' Well Controlled[5]	-	-	71%	71%
Room and Bathroom 'Always' Clean[5]	-	-	71%	73%
Timely Help 'Always' Received[5]	-	-	65%	68%
Would Definitely Recommend Hospital[5]	-	-	70%	71%
Use of Medical Imaging				
Cardiac Imaging Stress Test before Surgery[1]	-	-	5.5%	5.3%
Combination Abdominal CT Scan	117	13.7%	10.1%	10.5%
Combination Brain/Sinus CT Scan[1]	-	-	2.3%	2.7%
Combination Chest CT Scan	71	31.0%	3.7%	2.7%
Follow-up Mammogram/Ultrasound[7]	-	-	8.9%	8.8%
Lumbar Spine MRI for Low Back Pain[7]	-	-	36.6%	37.2%

Doctors Specialty Hospital

616 19th Street
Columbus, GA 31901
URL: www.doctorshspt.com
Type: Acute Care Hospitals
Ownership: Govt - Hospital Dist/Auth
Phone: 706-494-4262
Fax: 706-327-0131
Emergency Services: Yes
Beds: 219

Key Personnel:
Chief of Medical Staff.......... Donna Burrell, MD
Cardiac Laboratory............ Chris Doods
President/CEO................ ScottHill Duke, FACHE
Pediatric Ambulatory Care ...... David Flowers, MD
Pediatric In-Patient Care .... David Flowers, MD
Emergency Room .... Annie Garrard, RN
Quality Assurance .... Renee Gridley
Operating Room.............. Margaret Webb, RN

Measure	Cases	This Hosp.	State Avg.	U.S. Avg.
Blood Clot Prevention and Treatment				
Anticoagulation Overlap Therapy[1,2]	-	-	90%	93%
ICU Venous Thromboembolism Prophylaxis[2]	48	94%	90%	92%
Incidence of Potentially Preventable VTE[1,2]	-	-	13%	10%
UFH with Dosages/Platelet Monitoring[2,7]	-	-	99%	97%
Venous Thromboembolism Prophylaxis[2]	348	85%	80%	85%
Warfarin Therapy Discharge Instructions[1,2]	-	-	78%	75%
Chest Pain/Possible Heart Attack Care				
Aspirin Given Within 24 Hours of Arrival[5]	-	-	94%	96%
Fibrinolytic Meds Within 30 Min. of Arrival[5]	-	-	35%	58%
Average Time to ECG (minutes)[5]	-	-	8	7
Average Time to Transfer (minutes)[5]	-	-	73	60
Children's Asthma Care				
Received Home Management Plan of Care	-	-	-	88%
Received Reliever Medication	-	-	-	100%
Received Systemic Corticosteroids	-	-	-	100%
Emergency Department				
Admittance Decision Time (minutes)[2,7]	-	-	100	98
Head CT Results Within 45 Min. of Arrival[5]	-	-	45%	57%
Patients Who Left ER Before Being Seen	9,577	6%	3%	2%
Time from ER Arrival to Admit. (minutes)[2,7]	-	-	286	274
Time from ER Arrival to Discharge (minutes)[5]	-	-	140	134
Time in ER Before Being Evaluated (minutes)[5]	-	-	32	26
Time to Pain Meds for Fractures (minutes)[5]	-	-	64	57
Heart Attack Care				
Aspirin Given at Discharge[1,3]	-	-	99%	99%
Fibrinolytic Meds Within 30 Min. of Arrival[3,7]	-	-	80%	54%
PCI Within 90 Minutes of Arrival[3,7]	-	-	95%	96%
Statin Prescribed at Discharge[1,3]	-	-	98%	98%
Heart Failure Care				
ACE Inhibitor or ARB for LVSD	15	100%	97%	97%
Discharge Instructions Given	44	93%	92%	94%
Evaluation of LVS Function	46	100%	99%	99%
Medicare Spending				
Medicare Spending per Patient (ratio)	-	0.98	0.95	0.98
Pneumonia Care				
Appropriate Initial Antibiotic Given	17	94%	95%	95%
Blood Culture Timing[7]	-	-	97%	98%
Pregnancy and Delivery Care				
Newborn Deliveries Scheduled Early[2]	180	16%	8%	6%
Preventive Care				
Immunization for Influenza[2]	398	99%	88%	90%
Immunization for Pneumonia[2]	436	95%	90%	92%
Stroke Care				
Anticoagulation Therapy for Atrial Fibrillation[3,7]	-	-	94%	95%
Antithrombotic Therapy Timing[1,3]	-	-	97%	98%
Assessed for Rehabilitation[1,3]	-	-	97%	97%
Discharged on Antithrombotic Therapy[1,3]	-	-	98%	99%
Discharged on Statin Medication[1,3]	-	-	94%	94%
Thrombolytic Therapy Timing[3,7]	-	-	58%	66%
Venous Thromboembolism Prophylaxis[1,3]	-	-	92%	94%
Written Stroke Educational Materials Given[3,7]	-	-	84%	88%
Surgical Care Improvement Project				
Appropriate Beta Blocker Usage	33	97%	97%	98%
Appropriate VTP Within 24 Hours	177	99%	98%	98%
Controlled Postoperative Blood Glucose[7]	-	-	96%	97%
Perioperative Temperature Management	196	100%	100%	100%
Prophylactic Antibiotic Selection	140	100%	99%	99%
Prophylactic Antibiotic Selection (Outpatient)	288	100%	98%	98%
Prophylactic Antibiotic Stopped	138	99%	98%	98%
Prophylactic Antibiotic Timing	141	99%	99%	99%
Prophylactic Antibiotic Timing (Outpatient)	289	100%	98%	98%
Urinary Catheter Removal	25	100%	97%	97%
Survey of Patients' Hospital Experiences				
Area Around Room 'Always' Quiet at Night	300+	73%	66%	61%
Doctors 'Always' Communicated Well	300+	84%	83%	82%
Home Recovery Information Given	300+	87%	84%	85%
Hospital Given 9 or 10 on 10 Point Scale	300+	76%	69%	71%
Meds 'Always' Explained Before Given	300+	66%	63%	64%
Nurses 'Always' Communicated Well	300+	81%	78%	79%
Pain 'Always' Well Controlled	300+	75%	71%	71%
Room and Bathroom 'Always' Clean	300+	73%	71%	73%
Timely Help 'Always' Received	300+	69%	65%	68%
Would Definitely Recommend Hospital	300+	79%	70%	71%
Use of Medical Imaging				
Cardiac Imaging Stress Test before Surgery[1]	-	-	5.5%	5.3%
Combination Abdominal CT Scan	148	3.4%	10.1%	10.5%
Combination Brain/Sinus CT Scan[1]	-	-	2.3%	2.7%
Combination Chest CT Scan	92	0.0%	3.7%	2.7%
Follow-up Mammogram/Ultrasound[7]	-	-	8.9%	8.8%
Lumbar Spine MRI for Low Back Pain[1]	-	-	36.6%	37.2%

Midtown Medical Center

710 Center Saint Box 951
Columbus, GA 31901
E-mail: info@crhs.net
URL: www.columbusregional.com
Type: Acute Care Hospitals
Ownership: Voluntary non-profit - Other
Phone: 706-571-1000
Fax: 706-571-1216
Emergency Services: Yes
Beds: 537

Key Personnel:
Chief of Medical Staff.......... Ryan Chandler
Quality Assurance .... Karon Dederewicz
Anesthesiology................ James Evans, MD
Infection Control.............. Susan Harp
Pediatric In-Patient Care .... Stanley Levine, MD
Emergency Room .... Dale Miller
Intensive Care Unit............ Sharon Nicks
Operating Room.............. Pat Owens

Measure	Cases	This Hosp.	State Avg.	U.S. Avg.
Blood Clot Prevention and Treatment				
Anticoagulation Overlap Therapy[2]	77	91%	90%	93%
ICU Venous Thromboembolism Prophylaxis[2]	56	93%	90%	92%
Incidence of Potentially Preventable VTE[2]	19	21%	13%	10%
UFH with Dosages/Platelet Monitoring[2]	38	100%	99%	97%

NOTE: Hospital profiles are in alphabetical order by state, then city, then hospital within the city; Rankings exclude hospitals with less than 25 cases except for patient surveys which excludes hospitals with less than 100 cases; (a) 100-299 cases; (1) The number of cases/patients is too few to report; (2) Data submitted were based on a sample of cases/patients; (3) Results are based on a shorter time period than required; (4) Data suppressed by CMS for one or more quarters; (5) Results are not available for this reporting period; (6) Fewer than 100 patients completed the HCAHPS survey; (7) No cases met the criteria for this measure; (8) The lower limit of the confidence interval cannot be calculated if the number of observed infections equals zero; (9) No data are available from the state/territory for this reporting period; (10) The scores shown reflect fewer than 50 completed surveys; (11) There were discrepancies in the data collection process; (12) This measure does not apply to this hospital for this reporting period; (13) Results cannot be calculated for this reporting period; (14) The results for this state are combined with nearby states to protect confidentiality; Please refer to the User's Guide for a full explanation of data.

Measure	Cases	This Hosp.	State Avg.	U.S. Avg.
Venous Thromboembolism Prophylaxis[2]	377	91%	80%	85%
Warfarin Therapy Discharge Instructions[2]	61	98%	78%	75%
Chest Pain/Possible Heart Attack Care				
Aspirin Given Within 24 Hours of Arrival	16	100%	94%	96%
Fibrinolytic Meds Within 30 Min. of Arrival[7]	-	-	35%	58%
Average Time to ECG (minutes)[1]	-	-	8	7
Average Time to Transfer (minutes)[1]	-	-	73	60
Children's Asthma Care				
Received Home Management Plan of Care	-	-	-	88%
Received Reliever Medication	-	-	-	100%
Received Systemic Corticosteroids	-	-	-	100%
Emergency Department				
Admittance Decision Time (minutes)[2]	350	315	100	98
Head CT Results Within 45 Min. of Arrival[1]	-	-	45%	57%
Patients Who Left ER Before Being Seen	66,781	9%	3%	2%
Time from ER Arrival to Admit. (minutes)[2]	376	602	286	274
Time from ER Arrival to Discharge (minutes)	507	169	140	134
Time in ER Before Being Evaluated (minutes)	513	40	32	26
Time to Pain Meds for Fractures (minutes)	181	68	64	57
Heart Attack Care				
Aspirin Given at Discharge	46	98%	99%	99%
Fibrinolytic Meds Within 30 Min. of Arrival[7]	-	-	80%	54%
PCI Within 90 Minutes of Arrival[7]	-	-	95%	96%
Statin Prescribed at Discharge	48	100%	98%	98%
Heart Failure Care				
ACE Inhibitor or ARB for LVSD	150	97%	97%	97%
Discharge Instructions Given	228	98%	92%	94%
Evaluation of LVS Function	271	100%	99%	99%
Medicare Spending				
Medicare Spending per Patient (ratio)	-	1.04	0.95	0.98
Pneumonia Care				
Appropriate Initial Antibiotic Given	115	99%	95%	95%
Blood Culture Timing	230	98%	97%	98%
Pregnancy and Delivery Care				
Newborn Deliveries Scheduled Early[2]	604	5%	8%	6%
Preventive Care				
Immunization for Influenza[2]	531	89%	88%	90%
Immunization for Pneumonia[2]	458	94%	90%	92%
Stroke Care				
Anticoagulation Therapy for Atrial Fibrillation[1]	-	-	94%	95%
Antithrombotic Therapy Timing	174	100%	97%	98%
Assessed for Rehabilitation	226	100%	97%	97%
Discharged on Antithrombotic Therapy	181	100%	98%	99%
Discharged on Statin Medication	148	100%	94%	94%
Thrombolytic Therapy Timing	15	100%	58%	66%
Venous Thromboembolism Prophylaxis	229	97%	92%	94%
Written Stroke Educational Materials Given	133	99%	84%	88%
Surgical Care Improvement Project				
Appropriate Beta Blocker Usage[2]	72	89%	97%	98%
Appropriate VTP Within 24 Hours[2]	241	98%	98%	98%
Controlled Postoperative Blood Glucose[2,7]	-	-	96%	97%
Perioperative Temperature Management[2]	278	100%	100%	100%
Prophylactic Antibiotic Selection[2]	111	99%	99%	99%
Prophylactic Antibiotic Selection (Outpatient)	274	100%	98%	98%
Prophylactic Antibiotic Stopped[2]	107	98%	98%	98%
Prophylactic Antibiotic Timing[2]	111	99%	99%	99%
Prophylactic Antibiotic Timing (Outpatient)	275	100%	98%	98%
Urinary Catheter Removal[2]	129	97%	97%	97%
Survey of Patients' Hospital Experiences				
Area Around Room 'Always' Quiet at Night	300+	52%	66%	61%
Doctors 'Always' Communicated Well	300+	77%	83%	82%
Home Recovery Information Given	300+	81%	84%	85%
Hospital Given 9 or 10 on 10 Point Scale	300+	61%	69%	71%
Meds 'Always' Explained Before Given	300+	55%	63%	64%
Nurses 'Always' Communicated Well	300+	74%	78%	79%
Pain 'Always' Well Controlled	300+	67%	71%	71%
Room and Bathroom 'Always' Clean	300+	67%	71%	73%
Timely Help 'Always' Received	300+	56%	65%	68%
Would Definitely Recommend Hospital	300+	64%	70%	71%
Use of Medical Imaging				
Cardiac Imaging Stress Test before Surgery	55	5.5%	5.5%	5.3%
Combination Abdominal CT Scan	705	3.3%	10.1%	10.5%
Combination Brain/Sinus CT Scan	731	1.4%	2.3%	2.7%
Combination Chest CT Scan	636	0.8%	3.7%	2.7%
Follow-up Mammogram/Ultrasound	2,725	4.3%	8.9%	8.8%
Lumbar Spine MRI for Low Back Pain	151	43.7%	36.6%	37.2%

Northside Medical Center

100 Frist Court
Columbus, GA 31909
Phone: 706-494-2100
Fax: 706-494-2446
URL: www.hughstonsports.com
Type: Acute Care Hospitals
Emergency Services: No
Ownership: Proprietary
Beds: 100

Key Personnel:
CEO/President. . . . . Donald Avery
Chief of Medical Staff . . . . John Burkun, MD
Operating Room. . . . . Susan Garrett, RN
Radiology. . . . . Michael Postma, MD
Quality Assurance . . . . Elaine Sheecs

Measure	Cases	This Hosp.	State Avg.	U.S. Avg.
Blood Clot Prevention and Treatment				
Anticoagulation Overlap Therapy[1,2]	-	-	90%	93%
ICU Venous Thromboembolism Prophylaxis[2]	50	100%	90%	92%
Incidence of Potentially Preventable VTE[1,2]	-	-	13%	10%
UFH with Dosages/Platelet Monitoring[2,7]	-	-	99%	97%
Venous Thromboembolism Prophylaxis[2]	110	98%	80%	85%
Warfarin Therapy Discharge Instructions[1,2]	-	-	78%	75%
Chest Pain/Possible Heart Attack Care				
Aspirin Given Within 24 Hours of Arrival[5]	-	-	94%	96%
Fibrinolytic Meds Within 30 Min. of Arrival[5]	-	-	35%	58%
Average Time to ECG (minutes)[5]	-	-	8	7
Average Time to Transfer (minutes)[5]	-	-	73	60
Children's Asthma Care				
Received Home Management Plan of Care	-	-	-	88%
Received Reliever Medication	-	-	-	100%
Received Systemic Corticosteroids	-	-	-	100%
Emergency Department				
Admittance Decision Time (minutes)[2,7]	-	-	100	98
Head CT Results Within 45 Min. of Arrival[5]	-	-	45%	57%
Patients Who Left ER Before Being Seen[5]	-	-	3%	2%
Time from ER Arrival to Admit. (minutes)[2,7]	-	-	286	274
Time from ER Arrival to Discharge (minutes)[5]	-	-	140	134
Time in ER Before Being Evaluated (minutes)[5]	-	-	32	26
Time to Pain Meds for Fractures (minutes)[5]	-	-	64	57
Heart Attack Care				
Aspirin Given at Discharge[5]	-	-	99%	99%
Fibrinolytic Meds Within 30 Min. of Arrival[5]	-	-	80%	54%
PCI Within 90 Minutes of Arrival[5]	-	-	95%	96%
Statin Prescribed at Discharge[5]	-	-	98%	98%
Heart Failure Care				
ACE Inhibitor or ARB for LVSD[3,7]	-	-	97%	97%
Discharge Instructions Given[3,7]	-	-	92%	94%
Evaluation of LVS Function[1,3]	-	-	99%	99%
Medicare Spending				
Medicare Spending per Patient (ratio)	-	0.97	0.95	0.98
Pneumonia Care				
Appropriate Initial Antibiotic Given[5]	-	-	95%	95%
Blood Culture Timing[5]	-	-	97%	98%
Pregnancy and Delivery Care				
Newborn Deliveries Scheduled Early[7]	-	-	8%	6%
Preventive Care				
Immunization for Influenza[2]	312	98%	88%	90%
Immunization for Pneumonia[2]	482	93%	90%	92%
Stroke Care				
Anticoagulation Therapy for Atrial Fibrillation[5]	-	-	94%	95%
Antithrombotic Therapy Timing[5]	-	-	97%	98%
Assessed for Rehabilitation[5]	-	-	97%	97%
Discharged on Antithrombotic Therapy[5]	-	-	98%	99%
Discharged on Statin Medication[5]	-	-	94%	94%
Thrombolytic Therapy Timing[5]	-	-	58%	66%
Venous Thromboembolism Prophylaxis[5]	-	-	92%	94%
Written Stroke Educational Materials Given[5]	-	-	84%	88%
Surgical Care Improvement Project				
Appropriate Beta Blocker Usage	160	100%	97%	98%
Appropriate VTP Within 24 Hours	597	100%	98%	98%
Controlled Postoperative Blood Glucose[7]	-	-	96%	97%
Perioperative Temperature Management	616	100%	100%	100%
Prophylactic Antibiotic Selection	492	100%	99%	99%
Prophylactic Antibiotic Selection (Outpatient)	159	99%	98%	98%
Prophylactic Antibiotic Stopped	490	100%	98%	98%
Prophylactic Antibiotic Timing	492	99%	99%	99%
Prophylactic Antibiotic Timing (Outpatient)	159	99%	98%	98%
Urinary Catheter Removal	532	100%	97%	97%
Survey of Patients' Hospital Experiences				
Area Around Room 'Always' Quiet at Night	300+	87%	66%	61%
Doctors 'Always' Communicated Well	300+	88%	83%	82%
Home Recovery Information Given	300+	92%	84%	85%
Hospital Given 9 or 10 on 10 Point Scale	300+	91%	69%	71%
Meds 'Always' Explained Before Given	300+	77%	63%	64%
Nurses 'Always' Communicated Well	300+	90%	78%	79%
Pain 'Always' Well Controlled	300+	79%	71%	71%
Room and Bathroom 'Always' Clean	300+	84%	71%	73%
Timely Help 'Always' Received	300+	79%	65%	68%
Would Definitely Recommend Hospital	300+	93%	70%	71%
Use of Medical Imaging				
Cardiac Imaging Stress Test before Surgery[7]	-	-	5.5%	5.3%
Combination Abdominal CT Scan[1]	-	-	10.1%	10.5%
Combination Brain/Sinus CT Scan[1]	-	-	2.3%	2.7%
Combination Chest CT Scan[1]	-	-	3.7%	2.7%
Follow-up Mammogram/Ultrasound[7]	-	-	8.9%	8.8%
Lumbar Spine MRI for Low Back Pain	59	27.1%	36.6%	37.2%

Saint Francis Hospital

2122 Manchester Expressway
Columbus, GA 31995
Phone: 706-596-4020
Fax: 706-596-4481
URL: www.wecareforlife.com
Type: Acute Care Hospitals
Emergency Services: Yes
Ownership: Voluntary non-profit - Private
Beds: 376

Key Personnel:
Radiology. . . . . John Abernathy, MD
Operating Room. . . . . Nancy Daughety
Quality Assurance . . . . Andrew Dickens, MD
Emergency Room . . . . Tammy Driver
Chief of Medical Staff . . . . Bobbi A. Farber, MD
CEO/President. . . . . Robert P Granger
Anesthesiology. . . . . Gary Rogers, MD
Surgery . . . . Charles Scarborough, MD

Measure	Cases	This Hosp.	State Avg.	U.S. Avg.
Blood Clot Prevention and Treatment				
Anticoagulation Overlap Therapy[2]	119	89%	90%	93%
ICU Venous Thromboembolism Prophylaxis[2]	87	77%	90%	92%
Incidence of Potentially Preventable VTE[2]	23	22%	13%	10%
UFH with Dosages/Platelet Monitoring[2]	41	100%	99%	97%
Venous Thromboembolism Prophylaxis[2]	338	76%	80%	85%
Warfarin Therapy Discharge Instructions[2]	97	78%	78%	75%
Chest Pain/Possible Heart Attack Care				
Aspirin Given Within 24 Hours of Arrival[1,3]	-	-	94%	96%
Fibrinolytic Meds Within 30 Min. of Arrival[5]	-	-	35%	58%
Average Time to ECG (minutes)[1,3]	-	-	8	7
Average Time to Transfer (minutes)[5]	-	-	73	60
Children's Asthma Care				
Received Home Management Plan of Care	-	-	-	88%
Received Reliever Medication	-	-	-	100%
Received Systemic Corticosteroids	-	-	-	100%
Emergency Department				
Admittance Decision Time (minutes)[2]	1,004	195	100	98
Head CT Results Within 45 Min. of Arrival[1]	-	-	45%	57%
Patients Who Left ER Before Being Seen	58,011	5%	3%	2%
Time from ER Arrival to Admit. (minutes)[2]	1,004	430	286	274
Time from ER Arrival to Discharge (minutes)	408	196	140	134
Time in ER Before Being Evaluated (minutes)	425	79	32	26
Time to Pain Meds for Fractures (minutes)	138	88	64	57
Heart Attack Care				
Aspirin Given at Discharge	378	100%	99%	99%
Fibrinolytic Meds Within 30 Min. of Arrival[7]	-	-	80%	54%
PCI Within 90 Minutes of Arrival	88	95%	95%	96%
Statin Prescribed at Discharge	366	99%	98%	98%
Heart Failure Care				
ACE Inhibitor or ARB for LVSD[2]	184	96%	97%	97%
Discharge Instructions Given[2]	411	83%	92%	94%

NOTE: Hospital profiles are in alphabetical order by state, then city, then hospital within the city; Rankings exclude hospitals with less than 25 cases except for patient surveys which excludes hospitals with less than 100 cases; (a) 100-299 cases; (1) The number of cases/patients is too few to report; (2) Data submitted were based on a sample of cases/patients; (3) Results are based on a shorter time period than required; (4) Data suppressed by CMS for one or more quarters; (5) Results are not available for this reporting period; (6) Fewer than 100 patients completed the HCAHPS survey; (7) No cases met the criteria for this measure; (8) The lower limit of the confidence interval cannot be calculated if the number of observed infections equals zero; (9) No data are available from the state/territory for this reporting period; (10) The scores shown reflect fewer than 50 completed surveys; (11) There were discrepancies in the data collection process; (12) This measure does not apply to this hospital for this reporting period; (13) Results cannot be calculated for this reporting period; (14) The results for this state are combined with nearby states to protect confidentiality; Please refer to the User's Guide for a full explanation of data.

Measure	Cases	This Hosp.	State Avg.	U.S. Avg.
Evaluation of LVS Function[2]	472	100%	99%	99%
Medicare Spending				
Medicare Spending per Patient (ratio)	-	1.03	0.95	0.98
Pneumonia Care				
Appropriate Initial Antibiotic Given[2]	195	97%	95%	95%
Blood Culture Timing[2]	286	97%	97%	98%
Pregnancy and Delivery Care				
Newborn Deliveries Scheduled Early[7]	-	-	8%	6%
Preventive Care				
Immunization for Influenza[2]	755	91%	88%	90%
Immunization for Pneumonia[2]	1,086	91%	90%	92%
Stroke Care				
Anticoagulation Therapy for Atrial Fibrillation	22	100%	94%	95%
Antithrombotic Therapy Timing	208	100%	97%	98%
Assessed for Rehabilitation	226	100%	97%	97%
Discharged on Antithrombotic Therapy	208	100%	98%	99%
Discharged on Statin Medication	161	94%	94%	94%
Thrombolytic Therapy Timing	11	64%	58%	66%
Venous Thromboembolism Prophylaxis	242	95%	92%	94%
Written Stroke Educational Materials Given	113	99%	84%	88%
Surgical Care Improvement Project				
Appropriate Beta Blocker Usage[2]	205	97%	97%	98%
Appropriate VTP Within 24 Hours[2]	442	100%	98%	98%
Controlled Postoperative Blood Glucose[2]	103	97%	96%	97%
Perioperative Temperature Management[2]	511	100%	100%	100%
Prophylactic Antibiotic Selection[2]	462	99%	99%	99%
Prophylactic Antibiotic Selection (Outpatient)	558	97%	98%	98%
Prophylactic Antibiotic Stopped[2]	440	99%	98%	98%
Prophylactic Antibiotic Timing[2]	462	99%	99%	99%
Prophylactic Antibiotic Timing (Outpatient)	560	99%	98%	98%
Urinary Catheter Removal[2]	441	96%	97%	97%
Survey of Patients' Hospital Experiences				
Area Around Room 'Always' Quiet at Night	300+	62%	66%	61%
Doctors 'Always' Communicated Well	300+	83%	83%	82%
Home Recovery Information Given	300+	84%	84%	85%
Hospital Given 9 or 10 on 10 Point Scale	300+	71%	69%	71%
Meds 'Always' Explained Before Given	300+	62%	63%	64%
Nurses 'Always' Communicated Well	300+	80%	78%	79%
Pain 'Always' Well Controlled	300+	70%	71%	71%
Room and Bathroom 'Always' Clean	300+	69%	71%	73%
Timely Help 'Always' Received	300+	61%	65%	68%
Would Definitely Recommend Hospital	300+	78%	70%	71%
Use of Medical Imaging				
Cardiac Imaging Stress Test before Surgery	81	1.2%	5.5%	5.3%
Combination Abdominal CT Scan	1,049	9.9%	10.1%	10.5%
Combination Brain/Sinus CT Scan	1,336	1.4%	2.3%	2.7%
Combination Chest CT Scan	657	1.7%	3.7%	2.7%
Follow-up Mammogram/Ultrasound	2,123	7.8%	8.9%	8.8%
Lumbar Spine MRI for Low Back Pain	203	33.5%	36.6%	37.2%

Northridge Medical Center

70 Medical Center Drive
Commerce, GA 30529
Phone: 706-335-1100
Fax: 706-335-7701
Type: Acute Care Hospitals
Emergency Services: Yes
Ownership: Govt - Hospital Dist/Auth
Beds: 257

Key Personnel:
Operating Room. . . . . Robin Duffey, RN
Emergency Room . . . . Becky Hambrick, RN
Radiology. . . . . Ron McEver
Chief of Medical Staff . . . . Peter Mirkav
Infection Control. . . . . Patricia Morrison
Quality Assurance . . . . Patricia Morrison, RN
Pediatric Ambulatory Care . . . . . NS Shetty, MD
CEO/President. . . . . James Yarboraugh

Measure	Cases	This Hosp.	State Avg.	U.S. Avg.
Blood Clot Prevention and Treatment				
Anticoagulation Overlap Therapy[1,2]	-	-	90%	93%
ICU Venous Thromboembolism Prophylaxis[2]	19	95%	90%	92%
Incidence of Potentially Preventable VTE[1,2]	-	-	13%	10%
UFH with Dosages/Platelet Monitoring[1,2]	-	-	99%	97%
Venous Thromboembolism Prophylaxis[2]	112	96%	80%	85%
Warfarin Therapy Discharge Instructions[1,2]	-	-	78%	75%
Chest Pain/Possible Heart Attack Care				
Aspirin Given Within 24 Hours of Arrival	16	88%	94%	96%
Fibrinolytic Meds Within 30 Min. of Arrival[7]	-	-	35%	58%
Average Time to ECG (minutes)	16	7	8	7
Average Time to Transfer (minutes)[1]	-	-	73	60
Children's Asthma Care				
Received Home Management Plan of Care	-	-	-	88%
Received Reliever Medication	-	-	-	100%
Received Systemic Corticosteroids	-	-	-	100%
Emergency Department				
Admittance Decision Time (minutes)[2]	429	65	100	98
Head CT Results Within 45 Min. of Arrival[1]	-	-	45%	57%
Patients Who Left ER Before Being Seen	12,699	2%	3%	2%
Time from ER Arrival to Admit. (minutes)[2]	429	225	286	274
Time from ER Arrival to Discharge (minutes)	426	115	140	134
Time in ER Before Being Evaluated (minutes)	485	31	32	26
Time to Pain Meds for Fractures (minutes)	48	62	64	57
Heart Attack Care				
Aspirin Given at Discharge[1]	-	-	99%	99%
Fibrinolytic Meds Within 30 Min. of Arrival[7]	-	-	80%	54%
PCI Within 90 Minutes of Arrival[7]	-	-	95%	96%
Statin Prescribed at Discharge[1]	-	-	98%	98%
Heart Failure Care				
ACE Inhibitor or ARB for LVSD[2]	25	96%	97%	97%
Discharge Instructions Given[2]	65	91%	92%	94%
Evaluation of LVS Function[2]	72	100%	99%	99%
Medicare Spending				
Medicare Spending per Patient (ratio)	-	0.89	0.95	0.98
Pneumonia Care				
Appropriate Initial Antibiotic Given[2]	50	92%	95%	95%
Blood Culture Timing[2]	68	99%	97%	98%
Pregnancy and Delivery Care				
Newborn Deliveries Scheduled Early[7]	-	-	8%	6%
Preventive Care				
Immunization for Influenza[2]	333	98%	88%	90%
Immunization for Pneumonia[2]	558	96%	90%	92%
Stroke Care				
Anticoagulation Therapy for Atrial Fibrillation[7]	-	-	94%	95%
Antithrombotic Therapy Timing	14	93%	97%	98%
Assessed for Rehabilitation	12	100%	97%	97%
Discharged on Antithrombotic Therapy	11	100%	98%	99%
Discharged on Statin Medication[1]	-	-	94%	94%
Thrombolytic Therapy Timing	13	0%	58%	66%
Venous Thromboembolism Prophylaxis	14	93%	92%	94%
Written Stroke Educational Materials Given[1]	-	-	84%	88%
Surgical Care Improvement Project				
Appropriate Beta Blocker Usage	12	92%	97%	98%
Appropriate VTP Within 24 Hours	17	88%	98%	98%
Controlled Postoperative Blood Glucose[7]	-	-	96%	97%
Perioperative Temperature Management	21	100%	100%	100%
Prophylactic Antibiotic Selection	13	100%	99%	99%
Prophylactic Antibiotic Selection (Outpatient)	58	98%	98%	98%
Prophylactic Antibiotic Stopped	13	85%	98%	98%
Prophylactic Antibiotic Timing	13	92%	99%	99%
Prophylactic Antibiotic Timing (Outpatient)	58	98%	98%	98%
Urinary Catheter Removal[1]	-	-	97%	97%
Survey of Patients' Hospital Experiences				
Area Around Room 'Always' Quiet at Night	(a)	69%	66%	61%
Doctors 'Always' Communicated Well	(a)	83%	83%	82%
Home Recovery Information Given	(a)	84%	84%	85%
Hospital Given 9 or 10 on 10 Point Scale	(a)	68%	69%	71%
Meds 'Always' Explained Before Given	(a)	66%	63%	64%
Nurses 'Always' Communicated Well	(a)	76%	78%	79%
Pain 'Always' Well Controlled	(a)	69%	71%	71%
Room and Bathroom 'Always' Clean	(a)	69%	71%	73%
Timely Help 'Always' Received	(a)	65%	65%	68%
Would Definitely Recommend Hospital	(a)	61%	70%	71%
Use of Medical Imaging				
Cardiac Imaging Stress Test before Surgery[1]	-	-	5.5%	5.3%
Combination Abdominal CT Scan	155	3.2%	10.1%	10.5%
Combination Brain/Sinus CT Scan[1]	-	-	2.3%	2.7%
Combination Chest CT Scan	56	3.6%	3.7%	2.7%
Follow-up Mammogram/Ultrasound	223	39.5%	8.9%	8.8%
Lumbar Spine MRI for Low Back Pain[1]	-	-	36.6%	37.2%

Rockdale Medical Center

1412 Milstead Avenue, Ne
Conyers, GA 30012
Phone: 770-918-3000
Fax: 770-918-3104
E-mail: lholbrook@rockdale.org
URL: www.rockdalehospital.org
Type: Acute Care Hospitals
Emergency Services: Yes
Ownership: Proprietary
Beds: 107

Key Personnel:
Quality Assurance . . . . Susan Hallman
CEO/President. . . . . David Huber, MD
Radiology. . . . . Alan Johnson, MD
Emergency Room . . . . Kay Neal, RN
Chief of Medical Staff . . . . Frank Patton, MD
Operating Room. . . . . Nan Wadsworth

Measure	Cases	This Hosp.	State Avg.	U.S. Avg.
Blood Clot Prevention and Treatment				
Anticoagulation Overlap Therapy[2]	92	100%	90%	93%
ICU Venous Thromboembolism Prophylaxis[2]	86	100%	90%	92%
Incidence of Potentially Preventable VTE[1,2]	-	-	13%	10%
UFH with Dosages/Platelet Monitoring[2]	25	100%	99%	97%
Venous Thromboembolism Prophylaxis[2]	356	97%	80%	85%
Warfarin Therapy Discharge Instructions[2]	80	98%	78%	75%
Chest Pain/Possible Heart Attack Care				
Aspirin Given Within 24 Hours of Arrival	49	98%	94%	96%
Fibrinolytic Meds Within 30 Min. of Arrival[1]	-	-	35%	58%
Average Time to ECG (minutes)	49	8	8	7
Average Time to Transfer (minutes)[1]	-	-	73	60
Children's Asthma Care				
Received Home Management Plan of Care	-	-	-	88%
Received Reliever Medication	-	-	-	100%
Received Systemic Corticosteroids	-	-	-	100%
Emergency Department				
Admittance Decision Time (minutes)[2]	665	116	100	98
Head CT Results Within 45 Min. of Arrival[1]	-	-	45%	57%
Patients Who Left ER Before Being Seen	49,002	2%	3%	2%
Time from ER Arrival to Admit. (minutes)[2]	666	304	286	274
Time from ER Arrival to Discharge (minutes)	470	180	140	134
Time in ER Before Being Evaluated (minutes)	547	35	32	26
Time to Pain Meds for Fractures (minutes)	142	52	64	57
Heart Attack Care				
Aspirin Given at Discharge	29	100%	99%	99%
Fibrinolytic Meds Within 30 Min. of Arrival[7]	-	-	80%	54%
PCI Within 90 Minutes of Arrival[7]	-	-	95%	96%
Statin Prescribed at Discharge	26	88%	98%	98%
Heart Failure Care				
ACE Inhibitor or ARB for LVSD[2]	94	97%	97%	97%
Discharge Instructions Given[2]	254	98%	92%	94%
Evaluation of LVS Function[2]	279	100%	99%	99%
Medicare Spending				
Medicare Spending per Patient (ratio)	-	0.99	0.95	0.98
Pneumonia Care				
Appropriate Initial Antibiotic Given[2]	98	97%	95%	95%
Blood Culture Timing[2]	165	98%	97%	98%
Pregnancy and Delivery Care				
Newborn Deliveries Scheduled Early[2]	45	2%	8%	6%
Preventive Care				
Immunization for Influenza[2]	527	96%	88%	90%
Immunization for Pneumonia[2]	641	97%	90%	92%
Stroke Care				
Anticoagulation Therapy for Atrial Fibrillation[2]	12	92%	94%	95%
Antithrombotic Therapy Timing[2]	73	100%	97%	98%
Assessed for Rehabilitation[2]	75	100%	97%	97%
Discharged on Antithrombotic Therapy[2]	74	99%	98%	99%
Discharged on Statin Medication[2]	60	98%	94%	94%
Thrombolytic Therapy Timing[1,2]	-	-	58%	66%
Venous Thromboembolism Prophylaxis[2]	62	98%	92%	94%
Written Stroke Educational Materials Given[2]	61	85%	84%	88%
Surgical Care Improvement Project				
Appropriate Beta Blocker Usage[2]	75	99%	97%	98%
Appropriate VTP Within 24 Hours[2]	285	99%	98%	98%
Controlled Postoperative Blood Glucose[2,7]	-	-	96%	97%
Perioperative Temperature Management[2]	316	100%	100%	100%
Prophylactic Antibiotic Selection[2]	185	99%	99%	99%
Prophylactic Antibiotic Selection (Outpatient)	272	100%	98%	98%

NOTE: Hospital profiles are in alphabetical order by state, then city, then hospital within the city; Rankings exclude hospitals with less than 25 cases except for patient surveys which excludes hospitals with less than 100 cases; (a) 100-299 cases; (1) The number of cases/patients is too few to report; (2) Data submitted were based on a sample of cases/patients; (3) Results are based on a shorter time period than required; (4) Data suppressed by CMS for one or more quarters; (5) Results are not available for this reporting period; (6) Fewer than 100 patients completed the HCAHPS survey; (7) No cases met the criteria for this measure; (8) The lower limit of the confidence interval cannot be calculated if the number of observed infections equals zero; (9) No data are available from the state/territory for this reporting period; (10) The scores shown reflect fewer than 50 completed surveys; (11) There were discrepancies in the data collection process; (12) This measure does not apply to this hospital for this reporting period; (13) Results cannot be calculated for this reporting period; (14) The results for this state are combined with nearby states to protect confidentiality; Please refer to the User's Guide for a full explanation of data.

Measure	Cases	This Hosp.	State Avg.	U.S. Avg.
Prophylactic Antibiotic Stopped[2]	174	96%	98%	98%
Prophylactic Antibiotic Timing[2]	186	100%	99%	99%
Prophylactic Antibiotic Timing (Outpatient)	270	100%	98%	98%
Urinary Catheter Removal[2]	142	100%	97%	97%
Survey of Patients' Hospital Experiences				
Area Around Room 'Always' Quiet at Night	300+	67%	66%	61%
Doctors 'Always' Communicated Well	300+	81%	83%	82%
Home Recovery Information Given	300+	82%	84%	85%
Hospital Given 9 or 10 on 10 Point Scale	300+	69%	69%	71%
Meds 'Always' Explained Before Given	300+	60%	63%	64%
Nurses 'Always' Communicated Well	300+	74%	78%	79%
Pain 'Always' Well Controlled	300+	69%	71%	71%
Room and Bathroom 'Always' Clean	300+	67%	71%	73%
Timely Help 'Always' Received	300+	58%	65%	68%
Would Definitely Recommend Hospital	300+	67%	70%	71%
Use of Medical Imaging				
Cardiac Imaging Stress Test before Surgery	173	7.5%	5.5%	5.3%
Combination Abdominal CT Scan	719	7.0%	10.1%	10.5%
Combination Brain/Sinus CT Scan	726	2.8%	2.3%	2.7%
Combination Chest CT Scan	420	2.4%	3.7%	2.7%
Follow-up Mammogram/Ultrasound	1,625	10.9%	8.9%	8.8%
Lumbar Spine MRI for Low Back Pain	70	41.4%	36.6%	37.2%

Crisp Regional Hospital

902 7th Street North
Cordele, GA 31015
Phone: 229-276-3100
Fax: 229-276-3211
E-mail: mdhartin@hotbot.com
URL: www.crispregional.org
Type: Acute Care Hospitals
Emergency Services: Yes
Ownership: Govt - Hospital Dist/Auth
Beds: 65

Key Personnel:

Emergency Room . . . . Kenneth Benjamin, MD
Quality Assurance . . . . Melody Brown
Radiology. . . . . Deborah Charles, MD
Chairman/CEO . . . . Roe Davis
CEO/President. . . . . Steve Gautney
Chief of Medical Staff. . . . . Cristen Rischar, MD
Pediatrics. . . . . Amelia Stevens, MD
Operating Room. . . . . Sandy Washington

Measure	Cases	This Hosp.	State Avg.	U.S. Avg.
Blood Clot Prevention and Treatment				
Anticoagulation Overlap Therapy[2]	40	95%	90%	93%
ICU Venous Thromboembolism Prophylaxis[2]	135	74%	90%	92%
Incidence of Potentially Preventable VTE[1,2]	-	-	13%	10%
UFH with Dosages/Platelet Monitoring[1,2]	-	-	99%	97%
Venous Thromboembolism Prophylaxis[2]	184	70%	80%	85%
Warfarin Therapy Discharge Instructions[2]	25	100%	78%	75%
Chest Pain/Possible Heart Attack Care				
Aspirin Given Within 24 Hours of Arrival	62	100%	94%	96%
Fibrinolytic Meds Within 30 Min. of Arrival[1]	-	-	35%	58%
Average Time to ECG (minutes)	64	8	8	7
Average Time to Transfer (minutes)[1]	-	-	73	60
Children's Asthma Care				
Received Home Management Plan of Care	-	-	-	88%
Received Reliever Medication	-	-	-	100%
Received Systemic Corticosteroids	-	-	-	100%
Emergency Department				
Admittance Decision Time (minutes)[2]	563	82	100	98
Head CT Results Within 45 Min. of Arrival[1]	-	-	45%	57%
Patients Who Left ER Before Being Seen	18,499	4%	3%	2%
Time from ER Arrival to Admit. (minutes)[2]	614	297	286	274
Time from ER Arrival to Discharge (minutes)	434	190	140	134
Time in ER Before Being Evaluated (minutes)	462	15	32	26
Time to Pain Meds for Fractures (minutes)	85	57	64	57
Heart Attack Care				
Aspirin Given at Discharge	33	97%	99%	99%
Fibrinolytic Meds Within 30 Min. of Arrival[7]	-	-	80%	54%
PCI Within 90 Minutes of Arrival[7]	-	-	95%	96%
Statin Prescribed at Discharge	33	94%	98%	98%
Heart Failure Care				
ACE Inhibitor or ARB for LVSD	45	100%	97%	97%
Discharge Instructions Given	134	99%	92%	94%
Evaluation of LVS Function	153	100%	99%	99%
Medicare Spending				
Medicare Spending per Patient (ratio)	-	0.87	0.95	0.98
Pneumonia Care				
Appropriate Initial Antibiotic Given	84	100%	95%	95%
Blood Culture Timing	120	99%	97%	98%
Pregnancy and Delivery Care				
Newborn Deliveries Scheduled Early[2]	52	0%	8%	6%
Preventive Care				
Immunization for Influenza[2]	554	86%	88%	90%
Immunization for Pneumonia[2]	589	93%	90%	92%
Stroke Care				
Anticoagulation Therapy for Atrial Fibrillation[1]	-	-	94%	95%
Antithrombotic Therapy Timing	31	97%	97%	98%
Assessed for Rehabilitation	42	90%	97%	97%
Discharged on Antithrombotic Therapy	37	100%	98%	99%
Discharged on Statin Medication	31	94%	94%	94%
Thrombolytic Therapy Timing[1]	-	-	58%	66%
Venous Thromboembolism Prophylaxis	42	98%	92%	94%
Written Stroke Educational Materials Given	28	96%	84%	88%
Surgical Care Improvement Project				
Appropriate Beta Blocker Usage	17	100%	97%	98%
Appropriate VTP Within 24 Hours	89	100%	98%	98%
Controlled Postoperative Blood Glucose[7]	-	-	96%	97%
Perioperative Temperature Management	97	100%	100%	100%
Prophylactic Antibiotic Selection	51	100%	99%	99%
Prophylactic Antibiotic Selection (Outpatient)	33	100%	98%	98%
Prophylactic Antibiotic Stopped	48	100%	98%	98%
Prophylactic Antibiotic Timing	51	100%	99%	99%
Prophylactic Antibiotic Timing (Outpatient)	34	94%	98%	98%
Urinary Catheter Removal	41	98%	97%	97%
Survey of Patients' Hospital Experiences				
Area Around Room 'Always' Quiet at Night	300+	62%	66%	61%
Doctors 'Always' Communicated Well	300+	80%	83%	82%
Home Recovery Information Given	300+	78%	84%	85%
Hospital Given 9 or 10 on 10 Point Scale	300+	60%	69%	71%
Meds 'Always' Explained Before Given	300+	57%	63%	64%
Nurses 'Always' Communicated Well	300+	76%	78%	79%
Pain 'Always' Well Controlled	300+	66%	71%	71%
Room and Bathroom 'Always' Clean	300+	73%	71%	73%
Timely Help 'Always' Received	300+	57%	65%	68%
Would Definitely Recommend Hospital	300+	55%	70%	71%
Use of Medical Imaging				
Cardiac Imaging Stress Test before Surgery	120	5.0%	5.5%	5.3%
Combination Abdominal CT Scan	351	10.3%	10.1%	10.5%
Combination Brain/Sinus CT Scan	426	4.7%	2.3%	2.7%
Combination Chest CT Scan	134	1.5%	3.7%	2.7%
Follow-up Mammogram/Ultrasound	571	4.7%	8.9%	8.8%
Lumbar Spine MRI for Low Back Pain	53	35.8%	36.6%	37.2%

Newton Medical Center

5126 Hospital Drive Ne
Covington, GA 30014
Phone: 770-786-7053
Fax: 770-787-9059
URL: www.ngh.org
Type: Acute Care Hospitals
Emergency Services: Yes
Ownership: Voluntary non-profit - Private
Beds: 90

Key Personnel:

Radiology. . . . . Jacob Abraham
Infection Control. . . . . Judy Carman, RN
Quality Assurance . . . . Linda Davis, RN
Coronary Care . . . . Amy Frizzell, RN
Emergency Room . . . . Anthony T Gonter, MD
Chief of Medical Staff. . . . . Doug Nolen
Operating Room. . . . . Fran Offott, RN
Intensive Care Unit. . . . . Donna Persinger, RN

Measure	Cases	This Hosp.	State Avg.	U.S. Avg.
Blood Clot Prevention and Treatment				
Anticoagulation Overlap Therapy[2]	45	89%	90%	93%
ICU Venous Thromboembolism Prophylaxis[2]	94	98%	90%	92%
Incidence of Potentially Preventable VTE[1,2]	-	-	13%	10%
UFH with Dosages/Platelet Monitoring[2]	12	100%	99%	97%
Venous Thromboembolism Prophylaxis[2]	350	85%	80%	85%
Warfarin Therapy Discharge Instructions[2]	43	72%	78%	75%
Chest Pain/Possible Heart Attack Care				
Aspirin Given Within 24 Hours of Arrival	74	97%	94%	96%
Fibrinolytic Meds Within 30 Min. of Arrival	14	50%	35%	58%
Average Time to ECG (minutes)	79	5	8	7
Average Time to Transfer (minutes)[1]	-	-	73	60
Children's Asthma Care				
Received Home Management Plan of Care	-	-	-	88%
Received Reliever Medication	-	-	-	100%
Received Systemic Corticosteroids	-	-	-	100%
Emergency Department				
Admittance Decision Time (minutes)[2]	897	62	100	98
Head CT Results Within 45 Min. of Arrival	16	56%	45%	57%
Patients Who Left ER Before Being Seen	50,687	5%	3%	2%
Time from ER Arrival to Admit. (minutes)[2]	962	260	286	274
Time from ER Arrival to Discharge (minutes)[11]	420	151	140	134
Time in ER Before Being Evaluated (minutes)	442	40	32	26
Time to Pain Meds for Fractures (minutes)	124	74	64	57
Heart Attack Care				
Aspirin Given at Discharge[2]	35	100%	99%	99%
Fibrinolytic Meds Within 30 Min. of Arrival[2,7]	-	-	80%	54%
PCI Within 90 Minutes of Arrival[2,7]	-	-	95%	96%
Statin Prescribed at Discharge[2]	33	97%	98%	98%
Heart Failure Care				
ACE Inhibitor or ARB for LVSD[2]	78	92%	97%	97%
Discharge Instructions Given[2]	198	95%	92%	94%
Evaluation of LVS Function[2]	228	96%	99%	99%
Medicare Spending				
Medicare Spending per Patient (ratio)	-	0.97	0.95	0.98
Pneumonia Care				
Appropriate Initial Antibiotic Given[2]	107	97%	95%	95%
Blood Culture Timing[2]	187	96%	97%	98%
Pregnancy and Delivery Care				
Newborn Deliveries Scheduled Early[2]	104	45%	8%	6%
Preventive Care				
Immunization for Influenza[2]	719	84%	88%	90%
Immunization for Pneumonia[2]	884	86%	90%	92%
Stroke Care				
Anticoagulation Therapy for Atrial Fibrillation[1,2]	-	-	94%	95%
Antithrombotic Therapy Timing[2]	81	100%	97%	98%
Assessed for Rehabilitation[2]	98	97%	97%	97%
Discharged on Antithrombotic Therapy[2]	94	100%	98%	99%
Discharged on Statin Medication[2]	82	91%	94%	94%
Thrombolytic Therapy Timing[2]	15	27%	58%	66%
Venous Thromboembolism Prophylaxis[2]	93	92%	92%	94%
Written Stroke Educational Materials Given[2]	61	20%	84%	88%
Surgical Care Improvement Project				
Appropriate Beta Blocker Usage[2]	92	92%	97%	98%
Appropriate VTP Within 24 Hours[2]	302	93%	98%	98%
Controlled Postoperative Blood Glucose[2,7]	-	-	96%	97%
Perioperative Temperature Management[2]	324	100%	100%	100%
Prophylactic Antibiotic Selection[2]	252	98%	99%	99%
Prophylactic Antibiotic Selection (Outpatient)	117	94%	98%	98%
Prophylactic Antibiotic Stopped[2]	250	97%	98%	98%
Prophylactic Antibiotic Timing[2]	252	98%	99%	99%
Prophylactic Antibiotic Timing (Outpatient)	118	99%	98%	98%
Urinary Catheter Removal[2]	73	79%	97%	97%
Survey of Patients' Hospital Experiences				
Area Around Room 'Always' Quiet at Night	300+	60%	66%	61%
Doctors 'Always' Communicated Well	300+	78%	83%	82%
Home Recovery Information Given	300+	80%	84%	85%
Hospital Given 9 or 10 on 10 Point Scale	300+	69%	69%	71%
Meds 'Always' Explained Before Given	300+	61%	63%	64%
Nurses 'Always' Communicated Well	300+	77%	78%	79%
Pain 'Always' Well Controlled	300+	67%	71%	71%
Room and Bathroom 'Always' Clean	300+	65%	71%	73%
Timely Help 'Always' Received	300+	66%	65%	68%
Would Definitely Recommend Hospital	300+	65%	70%	71%
Use of Medical Imaging				
Cardiac Imaging Stress Test before Surgery[1]	-	-	5.5%	5.3%
Combination Abdominal CT Scan	766	16.1%	10.1%	10.5%
Combination Brain/Sinus CT Scan	807	3.2%	2.3%	2.7%
Combination Chest CT Scan	348	11.8%	3.7%	2.7%
Follow-up Mammogram/Ultrasound	1,758	7.6%	8.9%	8.8%
Lumbar Spine MRI for Low Back Pain	78	41.0%	36.6%	37.2%

NOTE: Hospital profiles are in alphabetical order by state, then city, then hospital within the city; Rankings exclude hospitals with less than 25 cases except for patient surveys which excludes hospitals with less than 100 cases; (a) 100-299 cases; (1) The number of cases/patients is too few to report; (2) Data submitted were based on a sample of cases/patients; (3) Results are based on a shorter time period than required; (4) Data suppressed by CMS for one or more quarters; (5) Results are not available for this reporting period; (6) Fewer than 100 patients completed the HCAHPS survey; (7) No cases met the criteria for this measure; (8) The lower limit of the confidence interval cannot be calculated if the number of observed infections equals zero; (9) No data are available from the state/territory for this reporting period; (10) The scores shown reflect fewer than 50 completed surveys; (11) There were discrepancies in the data collection process; (12) This measure does not apply to this hospital for this reporting period; (13) Results cannot be calculated for this reporting period; (14) The results for this state are combined with nearby states to protect confidentiality; Please refer to the User's Guide for a full explanation of data.

Northside Hospital Forsyth

1200 Northside Forsyth Drive Phone: 404-851-8700
Cumming, GA 30041 Fax: 404-851-6283
URL: www.gbhcs.org
Type: Acute Care Hospitals Emergency Services: Yes
Ownership: Voluntary non-profit - Private Beds: 41

Key Personnel:
Radiology. Huntley J Alper
Operating Room. . . . . Glenda Lane
CEO/President. . . . . Jim Litchford
Emergency Room . . . . Cynthia Miller
Chief of Medical Staff . . . . Shannon Mize, MD

Measure	Cases	This Hosp.	State Avg.	U.S. Avg.
Blood Clot Prevention and Treatment				
Anticoagulation Overlap Therapy[2]	66	100%	90%	93%
ICU Venous Thromboembolism Prophylaxis[2]	88	99%	90%	92%
Incidence of Potentially Preventable VTE[2]	20	0%	13%	10%
UFH with Dosages/Platelet Monitoring[2]	80	100%	99%	97%
Venous Thromboembolism Prophylaxis[2]	377	99%	80%	85%
Warfarin Therapy Discharge Instructions[2]	50	100%	78%	75%
Chest Pain/Possible Heart Attack Care				
Aspirin Given Within 24 Hours of Arrival	25	100%	94%	96%
Fibrinolytic Meds Within 30 Min. of Arrival[7]	-	-	35%	58%
Average Time to ECG (minutes)	27	0	8	7
Average Time to Transfer (minutes)[7]	-	-	73	60
Children's Asthma Care				
Received Home Management Plan of Care	-	-	-	88%
Received Reliever Medication	-	-	-	100%
Received Systemic Corticosteroids	-	-	-	100%
Emergency Department				
Admittance Decision Time (minutes)[2]	517	92	100	98
Head CT Results Within 45 Min. of Arrival[1]	-	-	45%	57%
Patients Who Left ER Before Being Seen	27,752	1%	3%	2%
Time from ER Arrival to Admit. (minutes)[2]	517	238	286	274
Time from ER Arrival to Discharge (minutes)	406	144	140	134
Time in ER Before Being Evaluated (minutes)	432	14	32	26
Time to Pain Meds for Fractures (minutes)	228	45	64	57
Heart Attack Care				
Aspirin Given at Discharge	234	100%	99%	99%
Fibrinolytic Meds Within 30 Min. of Arrival[7]	-	-	80%	54%
PCI Within 90 Minutes of Arrival	53	96%	95%	96%
Statin Prescribed at Discharge	222	100%	98%	98%
Heart Failure Care				
ACE Inhibitor or ARB for LVSD	69	100%	97%	97%
Discharge Instructions Given	220	100%	92%	94%
Evaluation of LVS Function	252	100%	99%	99%
Medicare Spending				
Medicare Spending per Patient (ratio)	-	0.97	0.95	0.98
Pneumonia Care				
Appropriate Initial Antibiotic Given	197	98%	95%	95%
Blood Culture Timing	259	100%	97%	98%
Pregnancy and Delivery Care				
Newborn Deliveries Scheduled Early	202	2%	8%	6%
Preventive Care				
Immunization for Influenza[2]	522	98%	88%	90%
Immunization for Pneumonia[2]	580	98%	90%	92%
Stroke Care				
Anticoagulation Therapy for Atrial Fibrillation	25	100%	94%	95%
Antithrombotic Therapy Timing	135	99%	97%	98%
Assessed for Rehabilitation	147	98%	97%	97%
Discharged on Antithrombotic Therapy	131	100%	98%	99%
Discharged on Statin Medication	97	100%	94%	94%
Thrombolytic Therapy Timing[1]	-	-	58%	66%
Venous Thromboembolism Prophylaxis	168	98%	92%	94%
Written Stroke Educational Materials Given	117	95%	84%	88%
Surgical Care Improvement Project				
Appropriate Beta Blocker Usage[2]	114	100%	97%	98%
Appropriate VTP Within 24 Hours[2]	320	100%	98%	98%
Controlled Postoperative Blood Glucose[2,7]	-	-	96%	97%
Perioperative Temperature Management[2]	464	100%	100%	100%
Prophylactic Antibiotic Selection[2]	287	100%	99%	99%
Prophylactic Antibiotic Selection (Outpatient)	347	100%	98%	98%
Prophylactic Antibiotic Stopped[2]	281	100%	98%	98%
Prophylactic Antibiotic Timing[2]	287	100%	99%	99%
Prophylactic Antibiotic Timing (Outpatient)	347	100%	98%	98%
Urinary Catheter Removal[2]	215	100%	97%	97%
Survey of Patients' Hospital Experiences				
Area Around Room 'Always' Quiet at Night	300+	61%	66%	61%
Doctors 'Always' Communicated Well	300+	79%	83%	82%
Home Recovery Information Given	300+	85%	84%	85%
Hospital Given 9 or 10 on 10 Point Scale	300+	77%	69%	71%
Meds 'Always' Explained Before Given	300+	61%	63%	64%
Nurses 'Always' Communicated Well	300+	77%	78%	79%
Pain 'Always' Well Controlled	300+	72%	71%	71%
Room and Bathroom 'Always' Clean	300+	75%	71%	73%
Timely Help 'Always' Received	300+	65%	65%	68%
Would Definitely Recommend Hospital	300+	81%	70%	71%
Use of Medical Imaging				
Cardiac Imaging Stress Test before Surgery	326	7.7%	5.5%	5.3%
Combination Abdominal CT Scan	1,379	5.1%	10.1%	10.5%
Combination Brain/Sinus CT Scan	1,112	3.4%	2.3%	2.7%
Combination Chest CT Scan	1,201	0.5%	3.7%	2.7%
Follow-up Mammogram/Ultrasound	2,032	11.6%	8.9%	8.8%
Lumbar Spine MRI for Low Back Pain	109	40.4%	36.6%	37.2%

Southwest Georgia Regional Medical Center

361 Randolph Street Phone: 229-732-2181
Cuthbert, GA 39840 Fax: 229-732-6759
Type: Critical Access Hospitals Emergency Services: Yes
Ownership: Govt - Hospital Dist/Auth Beds: 25

Key Personnel:
Emergency Room . . . . Sherri Cartwright
Operating Room. . . . . Sherri Cartwright, RN
Radiology. . . . . Shannon Chapman
Chief of Medical Staff . . . . Oneil Culves, MD
Infection Control . . . . Deborah Jackson
CEO/President. . . . . Keith Peterson
Quality Assurance . . . . Brent Rigsby

Measure	Cases	This Hosp.	State Avg.	U.S. Avg.
Blood Clot Prevention and Treatment				
Anticoagulation Overlap Therapy[5]	-	-	90%	93%
ICU Venous Thromboembolism Prophylaxis[5]	-	-	90%	92%
Incidence of Potentially Preventable VTE[5]	-	-	13%	10%
UFH with Dosages/Platelet Monitoring[5]	-	-	99%	97%
Venous Thromboembolism Prophylaxis[5]	-	-	80%	85%
Warfarin Therapy Discharge Instructions[5]	-	-	78%	75%
Chest Pain/Possible Heart Attack Care				
Aspirin Given Within 24 Hours of Arrival[5]	-	-	94%	96%
Fibrinolytic Meds Within 30 Min. of Arrival[5]	-	-	35%	58%
Average Time to ECG (minutes)[5]	-	-	8	7
Average Time to Transfer (minutes)[5]	-	-	73	60
Children's Asthma Care				
Received Home Management Plan of Care	-	-	-	88%
Received Reliever Medication	-	-	-	100%
Received Systemic Corticosteroids	-	-	-	100%
Emergency Department				
Admittance Decision Time (minutes)[5]	-	-	100	98
Head CT Results Within 45 Min. of Arrival[3,7]	-	-	45%	57%
Patients Who Left ER Before Being Seen	5,560	2%	3%	2%
Time from ER Arrival to Admit. (minutes)[5]	-	-	286	274
Time from ER Arrival to Discharge (minutes)[5]	-	-	140	134
Time in ER Before Being Evaluated (minutes)[5]	-	-	32	26
Time to Pain Meds for Fractures (minutes)[5]	-	-	64	57
Heart Attack Care				
Aspirin Given at Discharge[5]	-	-	99%	99%
Fibrinolytic Meds Within 30 Min. of Arrival[5]	-	-	80%	54%
PCI Within 90 Minutes of Arrival[5]	-	-	95%	96%
Statin Prescribed at Discharge[5]	-	-	98%	98%
Heart Failure Care				
ACE Inhibitor or ARB for LVSD[1]	-	-	97%	97%
Discharge Instructions Given[1,2]	-	-	92%	94%
Evaluation of LVS Function[2,3]	11	100%	99%	99%
Medicare Spending				
Medicare Spending per Patient (ratio)	-	-	0.95	0.98
Pneumonia Care				
Appropriate Initial Antibiotic Given[1,2]	-	-	95%	95%
Blood Culture Timing[1,2]	-	-	97%	98%
Pregnancy and Delivery Care				
Newborn Deliveries Scheduled Early[5]	-	-	8%	6%
Preventive Care				
Immunization for Influenza[5]	-	-	88%	90%
Immunization for Pneumonia[5]	-	-	90%	92%
Stroke Care				
Anticoagulation Therapy for Atrial Fibrillation[5]	-	-	94%	95%
Antithrombotic Therapy Timing[5]	-	-	97%	98%
Assessed for Rehabilitation[5]	-	-	97%	97%
Discharged on Antithrombotic Therapy[5]	-	-	98%	99%
Discharged on Statin Medication[5]	-	-	94%	94%
Thrombolytic Therapy Timing[5]	-	-	58%	66%
Venous Thromboembolism Prophylaxis[5]	-	-	92%	94%
Written Stroke Educational Materials Given[5]	-	-	84%	88%
Surgical Care Improvement Project				
Appropriate Beta Blocker Usage[5]	-	-	97%	98%
Appropriate VTP Within 24 Hours[5]	-	-	98%	98%
Controlled Postoperative Blood Glucose[5]	-	-	96%	97%
Perioperative Temperature Management[5]	-	-	100%	100%
Prophylactic Antibiotic Selection[5]	-	-	99%	99%
Prophylactic Antibiotic Selection (Outpatient)[5]	-	-	98%	98%
Prophylactic Antibiotic Stopped[5]	-	-	98%	98%
Prophylactic Antibiotic Timing[5]	-	-	99%	99%
Prophylactic Antibiotic Timing (Outpatient)[5]	-	-	98%	98%
Urinary Catheter Removal[5]	-	-	97%	97%
Survey of Patients' Hospital Experiences				
Area Around Room 'Always' Quiet at Night[5]	-	-	66%	61%
Doctors 'Always' Communicated Well[5]	-	-	83%	82%
Home Recovery Information Given[5]	-	-	84%	85%
Hospital Given 9 or 10 on 10 Point Scale[5]	-	-	69%	71%
Meds 'Always' Explained Before Given[5]	-	-	63%	64%
Nurses 'Always' Communicated Well[5]	-	-	78%	79%
Pain 'Always' Well Controlled[5]	-	-	71%	71%
Room and Bathroom 'Always' Clean[5]	-	-	71%	73%
Timely Help 'Always' Received[5]	-	-	65%	68%
Would Definitely Recommend Hospital[5]	-	-	70%	71%
Use of Medical Imaging				
Cardiac Imaging Stress Test before Surgery[7]	-	-	5.5%	5.3%
Combination Abdominal CT Scan	80	3.8%	10.1%	10.5%
Combination Brain/Sinus CT Scan[1]	-	-	2.3%	2.7%
Combination Chest CT Scan[1]	-	-	3.7%	2.7%
Follow-up Mammogram/Ultrasound[1]	-	-	8.9%	8.8%
Lumbar Spine MRI for Low Back Pain[7]	-	-	36.6%	37.2%

Chestatee Regional Hospital

227 Mountain Dr Phone: 706-864-6136
Dahlonega, GA 30533 Fax: 706-864-1356
Type: Acute Care Hospitals Emergency Services: Yes
Ownership: Proprietary Beds: 51

Key Personnel:
Coronary Care . . . . Stanley Arnold
Emergency Room . . . . Christopher Atkins
Operating Room. . . . . Frank Creegan
CEO/President. . . . . Robert Follwell
Chief of Medical Staff . . . . Lawrence Kulish
Chairman/CEO . . . . Larry Odom
Radiology. Raul E Paralíticci
Quality Assurance . . . . Cathy Sanford

Measure	Cases	This Hosp.	State Avg.	U.S. Avg.
Blood Clot Prevention and Treatment				
Anticoagulation Overlap Therapy[1,2]	-	-	90%	93%
ICU Venous Thromboembolism Prophylaxis[2]	25	88%	90%	92%
Incidence of Potentially Preventable VTE[1,2]	-	-	13%	10%
UFH with Dosages/Platelet Monitoring[1,2]	-	-	99%	97%
Venous Thromboembolism Prophylaxis[2]	123	77%	80%	85%
Warfarin Therapy Discharge Instructions[1,2]	-	-	78%	75%
Chest Pain/Possible Heart Attack Care				
Aspirin Given Within 24 Hours of Arrival	31	94%	94%	96%
Fibrinolytic Meds Within 30 Min. of Arrival[7]	-	-	35%	58%
Average Time to ECG (minutes)	31	19	8	7
Average Time to Transfer (minutes)[1]	-	-	73	60
Children's Asthma Care				
Received Home Management Plan of Care	-	-	-	88%
Received Reliever Medication	-	-	-	100%

NOTE: Hospital profiles are in alphabetical order by state, then city, then hospital within the city; Rankings exclude hospitals with less than 25 cases except for patient surveys which excludes hospitals with less than 100 cases; (a) 100-299 cases; (1) The number of cases/patients is too few to report; (2) Data submitted were based on a sample of cases/patients; (3) Results are based on a shorter time period than required; (4) Data suppressed by CMS for one or more quarters; (5) Results are not available for this reporting period; (6) Fewer than 100 patients completed the HCAHPS survey; (7) No cases met the criteria for this measure; (8) The lower limit of the confidence interval cannot be calculated if the number of observed infections equals zero; (9) No data are available from the state/territory for this reporting period; (10) The scores shown reflect fewer than 50 completed surveys; (11) There were discrepancies in the data collection process; (12) This measure does not apply to this hospital for this reporting period; (13) Results cannot be calculated for this reporting period; (14) The results for this state are combined with nearby states to protect confidentiality; Please refer to the User's Guide for a full explanation of data.

Measure	Cases	This Hosp.	State Avg.	U.S. Avg.
Received Systemic Corticosteroids	-	-	-	100%
Emergency Department				
Admittance Decision Time (minutes)[2]	364	70	100	98
Head CT Results Within 45 Min. of Arrival[1]	-	-	45%	57%
Patients Who Left ER Before Being Seen	11,636	2%	3%	2%
Time from ER Arrival to Admit. (minutes)[2]	366	244	286	274
Time from ER Arrival to Discharge (minutes)	412	107	140	134
Time in ER Before Being Evaluated (minutes)	426	29	32	26
Time to Pain Meds for Fractures (minutes)	41	50	64	57
Heart Attack Care				
Aspirin Given at Discharge[3,7]	-	-	99%	99%
Fibrinolytic Meds Within 30 Min. of Arrival[3,7]	-	-	80%	54%
PCI Within 90 Minutes of Arrival[3,7]	-	-	95%	96%
Statin Prescribed at Discharge[1,3]	-	-	98%	98%
Heart Failure Care				
ACE Inhibitor or ARB for LVSD[1,2]	-	-	97%	97%
Discharge Instructions Given[2]	24	83%	92%	94%
Evaluation of LVS Function[2]	26	96%	99%	99%
Medicare Spending				
Medicare Spending per Patient (ratio)	-	0.89	0.95	0.98
Pneumonia Care				
Appropriate Initial Antibiotic Given	55	91%	95%	95%
Blood Culture Timing	74	97%	97%	98%
Pregnancy and Delivery Care				
Newborn Deliveries Scheduled Early[1,2]	-	-	8%	6%
Preventive Care				
Immunization for Influenza[2]	333	91%	88%	90%
Immunization for Pneumonia[2]	448	95%	90%	92%
Stroke Care				
Anticoagulation Therapy for Atrial Fibrillation[7]	-	-	94%	95%
Antithrombotic Therapy Timing[1]	-	-	97%	98%
Assessed for Rehabilitation[1]	-	-	97%	97%
Discharged on Antithrombotic Therapy[1]	-	-	98%	99%
Discharged on Statin Medication[1]	-	-	94%	94%
Thrombolytic Therapy Timing[7]	-	-	58%	66%
Venous Thromboembolism Prophylaxis[1]	-	-	92%	94%
Written Stroke Educational Materials Given[1]	-	-	84%	88%
Surgical Care Improvement Project				
Appropriate Beta Blocker Usage[2]	43	93%	97%	98%
Appropriate VTP Within 24 Hours[2]	106	95%	98%	98%
Controlled Postoperative Blood Glucose[2,7]	-	-	96%	97%
Perioperative Temperature Management[2]	126	100%	100%	100%
Prophylactic Antibiotic Selection[2]	99	92%	99%	99%
Prophylactic Antibiotic Selection (Outpatient)	57	96%	98%	98%
Prophylactic Antibiotic Stopped[2]	94	91%	98%	98%
Prophylactic Antibiotic Timing[2]	99	99%	99%	99%
Prophylactic Antibiotic Timing (Outpatient)	57	100%	98%	98%
Urinary Catheter Removal[2]	83	92%	97%	97%
Survey of Patients' Hospital Experiences				
Area Around Room 'Always' Quiet at Night	(a)	63%	66%	61%
Doctors 'Always' Communicated Well	(a)	80%	83%	82%
Home Recovery Information Given	(a)	81%	84%	85%
Hospital Given 9 or 10 on 10 Point Scale	(a)	57%	69%	71%
Meds 'Always' Explained Before Given	(a)	59%	63%	64%
Nurses 'Always' Communicated Well	(a)	71%	78%	79%
Pain 'Always' Well Controlled	(a)	68%	71%	71%
Room and Bathroom 'Always' Clean	(a)	62%	71%	73%
Timely Help 'Always' Received	(a)	61%	65%	68%
Would Definitely Recommend Hospital	(a)	60%	70%	71%
Use of Medical Imaging				
Cardiac Imaging Stress Test before Surgery[1]	-	-	5.5%	5.3%
Combination Abdominal CT Scan	159	5.7%	10.1%	10.5%
Combination Brain/Sinus CT Scan[1]	-	-	2.3%	2.7%
Combination Chest CT Scan[1]	-	-	3.7%	2.7%
Follow-up Mammogram/Ultrasound	275	9.1%	8.9%	8.8%
Lumbar Spine MRI for Low Back Pain[1]	-	-	36.6%	37.2%

Hamilton Medical Center

1200 Memorial Drive
Dalton, GA 30720
Phone: 706-272-6105
Fax: 706-272-6477
URL: www.hamiltonhealth.com
Type: Acute Care Hospitals
Emergency Services: Yes
Ownership: Voluntary non-profit - Private
Beds: 282

Key Personnel:
CEO/President. . . . . John Bowling
Radiology. . . . . William Brammer, MD
Emergency Room . . . . Cathy Ferguson, MD
Pediatric In-Patient Care . . . . Janice Keyes, RN
Chief of Medical Staff. . . . . Paula McManus
Operating Room. . . . . Sandra Moutcastle
Quality Assurance . . . . Pam Stelmack

Measure	Cases	This Hosp.	State Avg.	U.S. Avg.
Blood Clot Prevention and Treatment				
Anticoagulation Overlap Therapy[2]	58	98%	90%	93%
ICU Venous Thromboembolism Prophylaxis[2]	81	93%	90%	92%
Incidence of Potentially Preventable VTE[1,2]	-	-	13%	10%
UFH with Dosages/Platelet Monitoring[2]	47	100%	99%	97%
Venous Thromboembolism Prophylaxis[2]	302	97%	80%	85%
Warfarin Therapy Discharge Instructions[2]	45	84%	78%	75%
Chest Pain/Possible Heart Attack Care				
Aspirin Given Within 24 Hours of Arrival	14	100%	94%	96%
Fibrinolytic Meds Within 30 Min. of Arrival[7]	-	-	35%	58%
Average Time to ECG (minutes)	14	6	8	7
Average Time to Transfer (minutes)[7]	-	-	73	60
Children's Asthma Care				
Received Home Management Plan of Care	-	-	-	88%
Received Reliever Medication	-	-	-	100%
Received Systemic Corticosteroids	-	-	-	100%
Emergency Department				
Admittance Decision Time (minutes)[2]	406	100	100	98
Head CT Results Within 45 Min. of Arrival	21	62%	45%	57%
Patients Who Left ER Before Being Seen	65,492	4%	3%	2%
Time from ER Arrival to Admit. (minutes)[2]	440	286	286	274
Time from ER Arrival to Discharge (minutes)	351	129	140	134
Time in ER Before Being Evaluated (minutes)	213	49	32	26
Time to Pain Meds for Fractures (minutes)	222	68	64	57
Heart Attack Care				
Aspirin Given at Discharge	220	99%	99%	99%
Fibrinolytic Meds Within 30 Min. of Arrival[7]	-	-	80%	54%
PCI Within 90 Minutes of Arrival	53	100%	95%	96%
Statin Prescribed at Discharge	216	99%	98%	98%
Heart Failure Care				
ACE Inhibitor or ARB for LVSD	76	97%	97%	97%
Discharge Instructions Given	279	96%	92%	94%
Evaluation of LVS Function	346	100%	99%	99%
Medicare Spending				
Medicare Spending per Patient (ratio)	-	0.91	0.95	0.98
Pneumonia Care				
Appropriate Initial Antibiotic Given	213	99%	95%	95%
Blood Culture Timing	385	97%	97%	98%
Pregnancy and Delivery Care				
Newborn Deliveries Scheduled Early[2]	34	9%	8%	6%
Preventive Care				
Immunization for Influenza[2]	492	99%	88%	90%
Immunization for Pneumonia[2]	569	99%	90%	92%
Stroke Care				
Anticoagulation Therapy for Atrial Fibrillation[2]	12	92%	94%	95%
Antithrombotic Therapy Timing[2]	81	100%	97%	98%
Assessed for Rehabilitation[2]	99	97%	97%	97%
Discharged on Antithrombotic Therapy[2]	88	98%	98%	99%
Discharged on Statin Medication[2]	62	95%	94%	94%
Thrombolytic Therapy Timing[1,2]	-	-	58%	66%
Venous Thromboembolism Prophylaxis[2]	83	96%	92%	94%
Written Stroke Educational Materials Given[2]	66	88%	84%	88%
Surgical Care Improvement Project				
Appropriate Beta Blocker Usage[2]	79	99%	97%	98%
Appropriate VTP Within 24 Hours[2]	236	99%	98%	98%
Controlled Postoperative Blood Glucose[2,7]	-	-	96%	97%
Perioperative Temperature Management[2]	276	100%	100%	100%
Prophylactic Antibiotic Selection[2]	162	100%	99%	99%
Prophylactic Antibiotic Selection (Outpatient)	423	99%	98%	98%
Prophylactic Antibiotic Stopped[2]	156	99%	98%	98%
Prophylactic Antibiotic Timing[2]	162	100%	99%	99%
Prophylactic Antibiotic Timing (Outpatient)	422	99%	98%	98%
Urinary Catheter Removal[2]	217	99%	97%	97%
Survey of Patients' Hospital Experiences				
Area Around Room 'Always' Quiet at Night	300+	64%	66%	61%
Doctors 'Always' Communicated Well	300+	79%	83%	82%
Home Recovery Information Given	300+	81%	84%	85%
Hospital Given 9 or 10 on 10 Point Scale	300+	71%	69%	71%
Meds 'Always' Explained Before Given	300+	68%	63%	64%
Nurses 'Always' Communicated Well	300+	80%	78%	79%
Pain 'Always' Well Controlled	300+	72%	71%	71%
Room and Bathroom 'Always' Clean	300+	66%	71%	73%
Timely Help 'Always' Received	300+	67%	65%	68%
Would Definitely Recommend Hospital	300+	67%	70%	71%
Use of Medical Imaging				
Cardiac Imaging Stress Test before Surgery	748	4.8%	5.5%	5.3%
Combination Abdominal CT Scan	1,272	7.7%	10.1%	10.5%
Combination Brain/Sinus CT Scan	1,279	0.4%	2.3%	2.7%
Combination Chest CT Scan	700	5.4%	3.7%	2.7%
Follow-up Mammogram/Ultrasound	1,814	6.7%	8.9%	8.8%
Lumbar Spine MRI for Low Back Pain	180	39.4%	36.6%	37.2%

Decatur VA Medical Center

1670 Clairmont Road
Decatur, GA 30033
Phone: 404-321-6111
Fax: 404-728-7733
URL: www1.va.gov/atlanta
Type: Acute Care - VA
Emergency Services: No
Ownership: Government Federal
Beds: 441

Key Personnel:
Chief of Medical Staff. . . . . David J Bower, MD
Quality Assurance . . . . Virgil Brown, MD
Coronary Care. . . . . Samuel Dudley, MD
Patient Relations . . . . Raquel Moore
Operating Room. . . . . Bob Wennegren

Measure	Cases	This Hosp.	State Avg.	U.S. Avg.
Blood Clot Prevention and Treatment				
Anticoagulation Overlap Therapy	-	-	90%	93%
ICU Venous Thromboembolism Prophylaxis	-	-	90%	92%
Incidence of Potentially Preventable VTE	-	-	13%	10%
UFH with Dosages/Platelet Monitoring	-	-	99%	97%
Venous Thromboembolism Prophylaxis	-	-	80%	85%
Warfarin Therapy Discharge Instructions	-	-	78%	75%
Chest Pain/Possible Heart Attack Care				
Aspirin Given Within 24 Hours of Arrival	-	-	94%	96%
Fibrinolytic Meds Within 30 Min. of Arrival	-	-	35%	58%
Average Time to ECG (minutes)	-	-	8	7
Average Time to Transfer (minutes)	-	-	73	60
Children's Asthma Care				
Received Home Management Plan of Care	-	-	-	88%
Received Reliever Medication	-	-	-	100%
Received Systemic Corticosteroids	-	-	-	100%
Emergency Department				
Admittance Decision Time (minutes)	-	-	100	98
Head CT Results Within 45 Min. of Arrival	-	-	45%	57%
Patients Who Left ER Before Being Seen	-	-	3%	2%
Time from ER Arrival to Admit. (minutes)	-	-	286	274
Time from ER Arrival to Discharge (minutes)	-	-	140	134
Time in ER Before Being Evaluated (minutes)	-	-	32	26
Time to Pain Meds for Fractures (minutes)	-	-	64	57
Heart Attack Care				
Aspirin Given at Discharge	65	97%	99%	99%
Fibrinolytic Meds Within 30 Min. of Arrival[5]	-	-	80%	54%
PCI Within 90 Minutes of Arrival[5]	-	-	95%	96%
Statin Prescribed at Discharge	63	98%	98%	98%
Heart Failure Care				
ACE Inhibitor or ARB for LVSD	216	93%	97%	97%
Discharge Instructions Given	403	98%	92%	94%
Evaluation of LVS Function	422	100%	99%	99%
Medicare Spending				
Medicare Spending per Patient (ratio)	-	-	0.95	0.98
Pneumonia Care				
Appropriate Initial Antibiotic Given	72	96%	95%	95%

NOTE: Hospital profiles are in alphabetical order by state, then city, then hospital within the city; Rankings exclude hospitals with less than 25 cases except for patient surveys which excludes hospitals with less than 100 cases; (a) 100-299 cases; (1) The number of cases/patients is too few to report; (2) Data submitted were based on a sample of cases/patients; (3) Results are based on a shorter time period than required; (4) Data suppressed by CMS for one or more quarters; (5) Results are not available for this reporting period; (6) Fewer than 100 patients completed the HCAHPS survey; (7) No cases met the criteria for this measure; (8) The lower limit of the confidence interval cannot be calculated if the number of observed infections equals zero; (9) No data are available from the state/territory for this reporting period; (10) The scores shown reflect fewer than 50 completed surveys; (11) There were discrepancies in the data collection process; (12) This measure does not apply to this hospital for this reporting period; (13) Results cannot be calculated for this reporting period; (14) The results for this state are combined with nearby states to protect confidentiality; Please refer to the User's Guide for a full explanation of data.

Measure	Cases	This Hosp.	State Avg.	U.S. Avg.
Blood Culture Timing	141	99%	97%	98%
Pregnancy and Delivery Care				
Newborn Deliveries Scheduled Early	-	-	8%	6%
Preventive Care				
Immunization for Influenza[5]	-	-	88%	90%
Immunization for Pneumonia[5]	-	-	90%	92%
Stroke Care				
Anticoagulation Therapy for Atrial Fibrillation	-	-	94%	95%
Antithrombotic Therapy Timing	-	-	97%	98%
Assessed for Rehabilitation	-	-	97%	97%
Discharged on Antithrombotic Therapy	-	-	98%	99%
Discharged on Statin Medication	-	-	94%	94%
Thrombolytic Therapy Timing	-	-	58%	66%
Venous Thromboembolism Prophylaxis	-	-	92%	94%
Written Stroke Educational Materials Given	-	-	84%	88%
Surgical Care Improvement Project				
Appropriate Beta Blocker Usage[2]	48	90%	97%	98%
Appropriate VTP Within 24 Hours[2]	194	95%	98%	98%
Controlled Postoperative Blood Glucose[5]	-	-	96%	97%
Perioperative Temperature Management[2]	232	100%	100%	100%
Prophylactic Antibiotic Selection	104	98%	99%	99%
Prophylactic Antibiotic Selection (Outpatient)	-	-	98%	98%
Prophylactic Antibiotic Stopped	103	87%	98%	98%
Prophylactic Antibiotic Timing	104	97%	99%	99%
Prophylactic Antibiotic Timing (Outpatient)	-	-	98%	98%
Urinary Catheter Removal[2]	106	93%	97%	97%
Survey of Patients' Hospital Experiences				
Area Around Room 'Always' Quiet at Night	-	-	66%	61%
Doctors 'Always' Communicated Well	-	-	83%	82%
Home Recovery Information Given	-	-	84%	85%
Hospital Given 9 or 10 on 10 Point Scale	-	-	69%	71%
Meds 'Always' Explained Before Given	-	-	63%	64%
Nurses 'Always' Communicated Well	-	-	78%	79%
Pain 'Always' Well Controlled	-	-	71%	71%
Room and Bathroom 'Always' Clean	-	-	71%	73%
Timely Help 'Always' Received	-	-	65%	68%
Would Definitely Recommend Hospital	-	-	70%	71%
Use of Medical Imaging				
Cardiac Imaging Stress Test before Surgery	-	-	5.5%	5.3%
Combination Abdominal CT Scan	-	-	10.1%	10.5%
Combination Brain/Sinus CT Scan	-	-	2.3%	2.7%
Combination Chest CT Scan	-	-	3.7%	2.7%
Follow-up Mammogram/Ultrasound	-	-	8.9%	8.8%
Lumbar Spine MRI for Low Back Pain	-	-	36.6%	37.2%

Dekalb Medical Center

2701 N Decatur Road
Decatur, GA 30033
Phone: 404-501-1000
Fax: 404-501-5147
URL: www.dekalbmedicalcenter.org
Type: Acute Care Hospitals
Emergency Services: Yes
Ownership: Voluntary non-profit - Private
Beds: 628

Key Personnel:
Infection Control. . . . . Helen Ebaugh, RN
Radiology. . . . . Gary Laskey, MD
Operating Room. . . . . Gwen Lyon, RN
Quality Assurance . . . . Steve Mayfield
CEO/President. . . . . John A. Shelton, Jr., FACHE
Pediatric In-Patient Care . . . . Jacqueline Sulton, MD
Chief of Medical Staff. . . . . Rose M Taylor, MD

Measure	Cases	This Hosp.	State Avg.	U.S. Avg.
Blood Clot Prevention and Treatment				
Anticoagulation Overlap Therapy[2]	196	93%	90%	93%
ICU Venous Thromboembolism Prophylaxis[2]	87	97%	90%	92%
Incidence of Potentially Preventable VTE[2]	26	0%	13%	10%
UFH with Dosages/Platelet Monitoring[2]	165	100%	99%	97%
Venous Thromboembolism Prophylaxis[2]	321	93%	80%	85%
Warfarin Therapy Discharge Instructions[2]	143	84%	78%	75%
Chest Pain/Possible Heart Attack Care				
Aspirin Given Within 24 Hours of Arrival[1]	-	-	94%	96%
Fibrinolytic Meds Within 30 Min. of Arrival[3,7]	-	-	35%	58%
Average Time to ECG (minutes)[1]	-	-	8	7
Average Time to Transfer (minutes)[1,3]	-	-	73	60
Children's Asthma Care				
Received Home Management Plan of Care	-	-	-	88%
Received Reliever Medication	-	-	-	100%
Received Systemic Corticosteroids	-	-	-	100%
Emergency Department				
Admittance Decision Time (minutes)[2]	503	162	100	98
Head CT Results Within 45 Min. of Arrival[1]	-	-	45%	57%
Patients Who Left ER Before Being Seen	66,193	2%	3%	2%
Time from ER Arrival to Admit. (minutes)[2]	505	405	286	274
Time from ER Arrival to Discharge (minutes)	357	209	140	134
Time in ER Before Being Evaluated (minutes)	388	42	32	26
Time to Pain Meds for Fractures (minutes)	105	88	64	57
Heart Attack Care				
Aspirin Given at Discharge[2]	224	98%	99%	99%
Fibrinolytic Meds Within 30 Min. of Arrival[2,7]	-	-	80%	54%
PCI Within 90 Minutes of Arrival[2]	35	89%	95%	96%
Statin Prescribed at Discharge[2]	214	96%	98%	98%
Heart Failure Care				
ACE Inhibitor or ARB for LVSD[2]	130	98%	97%	97%
Discharge Instructions Given[2]	270	97%	92%	94%
Evaluation of LVS Function[2]	308	100%	99%	99%
Medicare Spending				
Medicare Spending per Patient (ratio)	-	1.02	0.95	0.98
Pneumonia Care				
Appropriate Initial Antibiotic Given[2]	82	99%	95%	95%
Blood Culture Timing[2]	120	98%	97%	98%
Pregnancy and Delivery Care				
Newborn Deliveries Scheduled Early[2]	81	0%	8%	6%
Preventive Care				
Immunization for Influenza[2]	492	85%	88%	90%
Immunization for Pneumonia[2]	492	82%	90%	92%
Stroke Care				
Anticoagulation Therapy for Atrial Fibrillation	16	100%	94%	95%
Antithrombotic Therapy Timing	169	100%	97%	98%
Assessed for Rehabilitation	170	100%	97%	97%
Discharged on Antithrombotic Therapy	155	97%	98%	99%
Discharged on Statin Medication	126	97%	94%	94%
Thrombolytic Therapy Timing[1]	-	-	58%	66%
Venous Thromboembolism Prophylaxis	183	99%	92%	94%
Written Stroke Educational Materials Given	105	99%	84%	88%
Surgical Care Improvement Project				
Appropriate Beta Blocker Usage[2]	191	98%	97%	98%
Appropriate VTP Within 24 Hours[2]	732	99%	98%	98%
Controlled Postoperative Blood Glucose[2,7]	-	-	96%	97%
Perioperative Temperature Management[2]	852	100%	100%	100%
Prophylactic Antibiotic Selection[2]	537	100%	99%	99%
Prophylactic Antibiotic Selection (Outpatient)	350	99%	98%	98%
Prophylactic Antibiotic Stopped[2]	529	99%	98%	98%
Prophylactic Antibiotic Timing[2]	537	100%	99%	99%
Prophylactic Antibiotic Timing (Outpatient)	335	99%	98%	98%
Urinary Catheter Removal[2]	203	99%	97%	97%
Survey of Patients' Hospital Experiences				
Area Around Room 'Always' Quiet at Night	300+	65%	66%	61%
Doctors 'Always' Communicated Well	300+	75%	83%	82%
Home Recovery Information Given	300+	82%	84%	85%
Hospital Given 9 or 10 on 10 Point Scale	300+	61%	69%	71%
Meds 'Always' Explained Before Given	300+	56%	63%	64%
Nurses 'Always' Communicated Well	300+	73%	78%	79%
Pain 'Always' Well Controlled	300+	65%	71%	71%
Room and Bathroom 'Always' Clean	300+	65%	71%	73%
Timely Help 'Always' Received	300+	53%	65%	68%
Would Definitely Recommend Hospital	300+	63%	70%	71%
Use of Medical Imaging				
Cardiac Imaging Stress Test before Surgery	254	3.9%	5.5%	5.3%
Combination Abdominal CT Scan	1,000	6.0%	10.1%	10.5%
Combination Brain/Sinus CT Scan	910	4.6%	2.3%	2.7%
Combination Chest CT Scan	758	0.0%	3.7%	2.7%
Follow-up Mammogram/Ultrasound	3,451	6.7%	8.9%	8.8%
Lumbar Spine MRI for Low Back Pain	94	47.9%	36.6%	37.2%

Habersham County Medical Center

541 Historic Highway 441 - North
Demorest, GA 30535
Phone: 706-754-2161
Fax: 706-754-7300
E-mail: tellus@hcmcmed.or
URL: www.hcmcmed.org
Type: Acute Care Hospitals
Emergency Services: Yes
Ownership: Govt - Hospital Dist/Auth
Beds: 137

Key Personnel:
Radiology. . . . . Robert J Balotin
Emergency Room . . . . Marc Chetta, MD
CEO/President. . . . . C Richard Dwozan
Quality Assurance . . . . Jeanne Heintz
Patient Relations . . . . Gaylon Palmer
Chief of Medical Staff. . . . . Wanda Perry
Operating Room. . . . . Evelyn Waugh, RN

Measure	Cases	This Hosp.	State Avg.	U.S. Avg.
Blood Clot Prevention and Treatment				
Anticoagulation Overlap Therapy[2]	12	67%	90%	93%
ICU Venous Thromboembolism Prophylaxis[2]	58	83%	90%	92%
Incidence of Potentially Preventable VTE[2,7]	-	-	13%	10%
UFH with Dosages/Platelet Monitoring[1,2]	-	-	99%	97%
Venous Thromboembolism Prophylaxis[2]	238	77%	80%	85%
Warfarin Therapy Discharge Instructions[1,2]	-	-	78%	75%
Chest Pain/Possible Heart Attack Care				
Aspirin Given Within 24 Hours of Arrival	101	100%	94%	96%
Fibrinolytic Meds Within 30 Min. of Arrival[7]	-	-	35%	58%
Average Time to ECG (minutes)	101	9	8	7
Average Time to Transfer (minutes)	18	63	73	60
Children's Asthma Care				
Received Home Management Plan of Care	-	-	-	88%
Received Reliever Medication	-	-	-	100%
Received Systemic Corticosteroids	-	-	-	100%
Emergency Department				
Admittance Decision Time (minutes)[2]	479	79	100	98
Head CT Results Within 45 Min. of Arrival	16	88%	45%	57%
Patients Who Left ER Before Being Seen	13,503	1%	3%	2%
Time from ER Arrival to Admit. (minutes)[2]	482	228	286	274
Time from ER Arrival to Discharge (minutes)	469	121	140	134
Time in ER Before Being Evaluated (minutes)	504	23	32	26
Time to Pain Meds for Fractures (minutes)	108	60	64	57
Heart Attack Care				
Aspirin Given at Discharge[1]	-	-	99%	99%
Fibrinolytic Meds Within 30 Min. of Arrival[7]	-	-	80%	54%
PCI Within 90 Minutes of Arrival[7]	-	-	95%	96%
Statin Prescribed at Discharge[1]	-	-	98%	98%
Heart Failure Care				
ACE Inhibitor or ARB for LVSD[1,2]	-	-	97%	97%
Discharge Instructions Given[2]	41	66%	92%	94%
Evaluation of LVS Function[2]	53	96%	99%	99%
Medicare Spending				
Medicare Spending per Patient (ratio)	-	0.89	0.95	0.98
Pneumonia Care				
Appropriate Initial Antibiotic Given[2]	133	87%	95%	95%
Blood Culture Timing[2]	205	98%	97%	98%
Pregnancy and Delivery Care				
Newborn Deliveries Scheduled Early	58	0%	8%	6%
Preventive Care				
Immunization for Influenza[2]	362	84%	88%	90%
Immunization for Pneumonia[2]	418	95%	90%	92%
Stroke Care				
Anticoagulation Therapy for Atrial Fibrillation[1]	-	-	94%	95%
Antithrombotic Therapy Timing	37	95%	97%	98%
Assessed for Rehabilitation	40	100%	97%	97%
Discharged on Antithrombotic Therapy	39	97%	98%	99%
Discharged on Statin Medication	34	94%	94%	94%
Thrombolytic Therapy Timing[1]	-	-	58%	66%
Venous Thromboembolism Prophylaxis	41	76%	92%	94%
Written Stroke Educational Materials Given	19	100%	84%	88%
Surgical Care Improvement Project				
Appropriate Beta Blocker Usage[2]	36	89%	97%	98%
Appropriate VTP Within 24 Hours[2]	99	98%	98%	98%
Controlled Postoperative Blood Glucose[2,7]	-	-	96%	97%
Perioperative Temperature Management[2]	102	100%	100%	100%
Prophylactic Antibiotic Selection[2]	53	100%	99%	99%

NOTE: Hospital profiles are in alphabetical order by state, then city, then hospital within the city; Rankings exclude hospitals with less than 25 cases except for patient surveys which excludes hospitals with less than 100 cases; (a) 100-299 cases; (1) The number of cases/patients is too few to report; (2) Data submitted were based on a sample of cases/patients; (3) Results are based on a shorter time period than required; (4) Data suppressed by CMS for one or more quarters; (5) Results are not available for this reporting period; (6) Fewer than 100 patients completed the HCAHPS survey; (7) No cases met the criteria for this measure; (8) The lower limit of the confidence interval cannot be calculated if the number of observed infections equals zero; (9) No data are available from the state/territory for this reporting period; (10) The scores shown reflect fewer than 50 completed surveys; (11) There were discrepancies in the data collection process; (12) This measure does not apply to this hospital for this reporting period; (13) Results cannot be calculated for this reporting period; (14) The results for this state are combined with nearby states to protect confidentiality; Please refer to the User's Guide for a full explanation of data.

Measure	Cases	This Hosp.	State Avg.	U.S. Avg.
Prophylactic Antibiotic Selection (Outpatient)	54	98%	98%	98%
Prophylactic Antibiotic Stopped[2]	53	100%	98%	98%
Prophylactic Antibiotic Timing[2]	53	100%	99%	99%
Prophylactic Antibiotic Timing (Outpatient)	56	96%	98%	98%
Urinary Catheter Removal[2]	81	98%	97%	97%
Survey of Patients' Hospital Experiences				
Area Around Room 'Always' Quiet at Night	300+	66%	66%	61%
Doctors 'Always' Communicated Well	300+	82%	83%	82%
Home Recovery Information Given	300+	87%	84%	85%
Hospital Given 9 or 10 on 10 Point Scale	300+	68%	69%	71%
Meds 'Always' Explained Before Given	300+	62%	63%	64%
Nurses 'Always' Communicated Well	300+	78%	78%	79%
Pain 'Always' Well Controlled	300+	71%	71%	71%
Room and Bathroom 'Always' Clean	300+	67%	71%	73%
Timely Help 'Always' Received	300+	64%	65%	68%
Would Definitely Recommend Hospital	300+	71%	70%	71%
Use of Medical Imaging				
Cardiac Imaging Stress Test before Surgery	205	3.9%	5.5%	5.3%
Combination Abdominal CT Scan	514	3.3%	10.1%	10.5%
Combination Brain/Sinus CT Scan	588	4.1%	2.3%	2.7%
Combination Chest CT Scan	208	1.0%	3.7%	2.7%
Follow-up Mammogram/Ultrasound	760	14.2%	8.9%	8.8%
Lumbar Spine MRI for Low Back Pain	45	55.6%	36.6%	37.2%

Donalsonville Hospital

102 Hospital Cir
Donalsonville, GA 39845
Phone: 229-524-5217
Fax: 229-524-8217
E-mail: jmoody@surfsouth.com
Type: Acute Care Hospitals
Emergency Services: Yes
Ownership: Voluntary non-profit - Private
Beds: 65

Key Personnel:

Quality Assurance .... Susan Brookins, RN
Pediatric In-Patient Care .... Dion Nicole Martin, MD
CEO/President............... Charles Orrick
Pediatric Ambulatory Care ...... Kristen P. DeWeese, MD
Operating Room............. Chrystal Smith, RN
Surgery .... Charles O. Walker, Jr., MD
Emergency Room .... Dale Whitaker, RN

Measure	Cases	This Hosp.	State Avg.	U.S. Avg.
Blood Clot Prevention and Treatment				
Anticoagulation Overlap Therapy[1,2]	-	-	90%	93%
ICU Venous Thromboembolism Prophylaxis[2,7]	-	-	90%	92%
Incidence of Potentially Preventable VTE[2,7]	-	-	13%	10%
UFH with Dosages/Platelet Monitoring[2,7]	-	-	99%	97%
Venous Thromboembolism Prophylaxis[2]	336	31%	80%	85%
Warfarin Therapy Discharge Instructions[1,2]	-	-	78%	75%
Chest Pain/Possible Heart Attack Care				
Aspirin Given Within 24 Hours of Arrival	13	100%	94%	96%
Fibrinolytic Meds Within 30 Min. of Arrival[1,3]	-	-	35%	58%
Average Time to ECG (minutes)	13	20	8	7
Average Time to Transfer (minutes)[3,7]	-	-	73	60
Children's Asthma Care				
Received Home Management Plan of Care	-	-	-	88%
Received Reliever Medication	-	-	-	100%
Received Systemic Corticosteroids	-	-	-	100%
Emergency Department				
Admittance Decision Time (minutes)[2]	79	40	100	98
Head CT Results Within 45 Min. of Arrival[1,3]	-	-	45%	57%
Patients Who Left ER Before Being Seen	6,784	3%	3%	2%
Time from ER Arrival to Admit. (minutes)[2]	79	205	286	274
Time from ER Arrival to Discharge (minutes)	433	119	140	134
Time in ER Before Being Evaluated (minutes)	413	22	32	26
Time to Pain Meds for Fractures (minutes)	11	75	64	57
Heart Attack Care				
Aspirin Given at Discharge[1,3]	-	-	99%	99%
Fibrinolytic Meds Within 30 Min. of Arrival[3,7]	-	-	80%	54%
PCI Within 90 Minutes of Arrival[3,7]	-	-	95%	96%
Statin Prescribed at Discharge[1,3]	-	-	98%	98%
Heart Failure Care				
ACE Inhibitor or ARB for LVSD	15	100%	97%	97%
Discharge Instructions Given	29	97%	92%	94%
Evaluation of LVS Function	31	94%	99%	99%
Medicare Spending				
Medicare Spending per Patient (ratio)	-	0.78	0.95	0.98
Pneumonia Care				
Appropriate Initial Antibiotic Given	25	84%	95%	95%
Blood Culture Timing[1]	-	-	97%	98%
Pregnancy and Delivery Care				
Newborn Deliveries Scheduled Early	42	7%	8%	6%
Preventive Care				
Immunization for Influenza[2]	415	78%	88%	90%
Immunization for Pneumonia[2]	395	82%	90%	92%
Stroke Care				
Anticoagulation Therapy for Atrial Fibrillation[7]	-	-	94%	95%
Antithrombotic Therapy Timing[1]	-	-	97%	98%
Assessed for Rehabilitation[1]	-	-	97%	97%
Discharged on Antithrombotic Therapy[1]	-	-	98%	99%
Discharged on Statin Medication[1]	-	-	94%	94%
Thrombolytic Therapy Timing[7]	-	-	58%	66%
Venous Thromboembolism Prophylaxis[1]	-	-	92%	94%
Written Stroke Educational Materials Given[1]	-	-	84%	88%
Surgical Care Improvement Project				
Appropriate Beta Blocker Usage[1]	-	-	97%	98%
Appropriate VTP Within 24 Hours	19	79%	98%	98%
Controlled Postoperative Blood Glucose[7]	-	-	96%	97%
Perioperative Temperature Management	19	89%	100%	100%
Prophylactic Antibiotic Selection	12	58%	99%	99%
Prophylactic Antibiotic Selection (Outpatient)[1]	-	-	98%	98%
Prophylactic Antibiotic Stopped[1]	-	-	98%	98%
Prophylactic Antibiotic Timing	12	83%	99%	99%
Prophylactic Antibiotic Timing (Outpatient)[1]	-	-	98%	98%
Urinary Catheter Removal[1]	-	-	97%	97%
Survey of Patients' Hospital Experiences				
Area Around Room 'Always' Quiet at Night	300+	73%	66%	61%
Doctors 'Always' Communicated Well	300+	91%	83%	82%
Home Recovery Information Given	300+	75%	84%	85%
Hospital Given 9 or 10 on 10 Point Scale	300+	74%	69%	71%
Meds 'Always' Explained Before Given	300+	68%	63%	64%
Nurses 'Always' Communicated Well	300+	82%	78%	79%
Pain 'Always' Well Controlled	300+	73%	71%	71%
Room and Bathroom 'Always' Clean	300+	78%	71%	73%
Timely Help 'Always' Received	300+	68%	65%	68%
Would Definitely Recommend Hospital	300+	72%	70%	71%
Use of Medical Imaging				
Cardiac Imaging Stress Test before Surgery[7]	-	-	5.5%	5.3%
Combination Abdominal CT Scan	149	20.1%	10.1%	10.5%
Combination Brain/Sinus CT Scan	175	1.1%	2.3%	2.7%
Combination Chest CT Scan[1]	-	-	3.7%	2.7%
Follow-up Mammogram/Ultrasound	230	5.2%	8.9%	8.8%
Lumbar Spine MRI for Low Back Pain[1]	-	-	36.6%	37.2%

Coffee Regional Medical Center

1101 Ocilla Road
Douglas, GA 31533
Phone: 229-384-1900
Fax: 912-389-2112
URL: www.coffeeregional.org
Type: Acute Care Hospitals
Emergency Services: Yes
Ownership: Govt - Hospital Dist/Auth
Beds: 88

Key Personnel:

Chief of Medical Staff.......... Eric Anderson
Operating Room.............. Doyle Baker
Pediatric In-Patient Care .... Olivia Daya
CEO/President............... George Heck
Radiology.................. Nirandr Inthachak
Infection Control............. Rudean Long
Intensive Care Unit........... Betty Smith
Quality Assurance .... Beth Sumner

Measure	Cases	This Hosp.	State Avg.	U.S. Avg.
Blood Clot Prevention and Treatment				
Anticoagulation Overlap Therapy[2]	35	97%	90%	93%
ICU Venous Thromboembolism Prophylaxis[2]	93	74%	90%	92%
Incidence of Potentially Preventable VTE[1,2]	-	-	13%	10%
UFH with Dosages/Platelet Monitoring[2]	25	100%	99%	97%
Venous Thromboembolism Prophylaxis[2]	377	54%	80%	85%
Warfarin Therapy Discharge Instructions[2]	30	83%	78%	75%
Chest Pain/Possible Heart Attack Care				
Aspirin Given Within 24 Hours of Arrival	57	96%	94%	96%
Fibrinolytic Meds Within 30 Min. of Arrival[1]	-	-	35%	58%
Average Time to ECG (minutes)	58	4	8	7
Average Time to Transfer (minutes)[1]	-	-	73	60
Children's Asthma Care				
Received Home Management Plan of Care	-	-	-	88%
Received Reliever Medication	-	-	-	100%
Received Systemic Corticosteroids	-	-	-	100%
Emergency Department				
Admittance Decision Time (minutes)[2]	427	55	100	98
Head CT Results Within 45 Min. of Arrival	12	83%	45%	57%
Patients Who Left ER Before Being Seen	33,332	3%	3%	2%
Time from ER Arrival to Admit. (minutes)[2]	437	203	286	274
Time from ER Arrival to Discharge (minutes)	444	102	140	134
Time in ER Before Being Evaluated (minutes)	313	36	32	26
Time to Pain Meds for Fractures (minutes)	141	54	64	57
Heart Attack Care				
Aspirin Given at Discharge[1]	-	-	99%	99%
Fibrinolytic Meds Within 30 Min. of Arrival[7]	-	-	80%	54%
PCI Within 90 Minutes of Arrival[7]	-	-	95%	96%
Statin Prescribed at Discharge[1]	-	-	98%	98%
Heart Failure Care				
ACE Inhibitor or ARB for LVSD[2]	40	100%	97%	97%
Discharge Instructions Given[2]	177	100%	92%	94%
Evaluation of LVS Function[2]	192	100%	99%	99%
Medicare Spending				
Medicare Spending per Patient (ratio)	-	0.88	0.95	0.98
Pneumonia Care				
Appropriate Initial Antibiotic Given	93	100%	95%	95%
Blood Culture Timing	132	100%	97%	98%
Pregnancy and Delivery Care				
Newborn Deliveries Scheduled Early[2]	54	4%	8%	6%
Preventive Care				
Immunization for Influenza[2]	590	98%	88%	90%
Immunization for Pneumonia[2]	811	99%	90%	92%
Stroke Care				
Anticoagulation Therapy for Atrial Fibrillation[1,2]	-	-	94%	95%
Antithrombotic Therapy Timing[2]	32	94%	97%	98%
Assessed for Rehabilitation[2]	37	97%	97%	97%
Discharged on Antithrombotic Therapy[2]	30	93%	98%	99%
Discharged on Statin Medication[2]	27	81%	94%	94%
Thrombolytic Therapy Timing[2,7]	-	-	58%	66%
Venous Thromboembolism Prophylaxis[2]	40	62%	92%	94%
Written Stroke Educational Materials Given[2]	28	18%	84%	88%
Surgical Care Improvement Project				
Appropriate Beta Blocker Usage[2]	42	100%	97%	98%
Appropriate VTP Within 24 Hours[2]	150	100%	98%	98%
Controlled Postoperative Blood Glucose[2,7]	-	-	96%	97%
Perioperative Temperature Management[2]	185	100%	100%	100%
Prophylactic Antibiotic Selection[2]	137	100%	99%	99%
Prophylactic Antibiotic Selection (Outpatient)	84	100%	98%	98%
Prophylactic Antibiotic Stopped[2]	136	100%	98%	98%
Prophylactic Antibiotic Timing[2]	137	99%	99%	99%
Prophylactic Antibiotic Timing (Outpatient)	85	98%	98%	98%
Urinary Catheter Removal[2]	82	100%	97%	97%
Survey of Patients' Hospital Experiences				
Area Around Room 'Always' Quiet at Night	300+	73%	66%	61%
Doctors 'Always' Communicated Well	300+	87%	83%	82%
Home Recovery Information Given	300+	86%	84%	85%
Hospital Given 9 or 10 on 10 Point Scale	300+	75%	69%	71%
Meds 'Always' Explained Before Given	300+	62%	63%	64%
Nurses 'Always' Communicated Well	300+	86%	78%	79%
Pain 'Always' Well Controlled	300+	74%	71%	71%
Room and Bathroom 'Always' Clean	300+	80%	71%	73%
Timely Help 'Always' Received	300+	77%	65%	68%
Would Definitely Recommend Hospital	300+	68%	70%	71%
Use of Medical Imaging				
Cardiac Imaging Stress Test before Surgery	314	8.3%	5.5%	5.3%
Combination Abdominal CT Scan	600	17.0%	10.1%	10.5%
Combination Brain/Sinus CT Scan	580	5.0%	2.3%	2.7%
Combination Chest CT Scan	293	21.2%	3.7%	2.7%
Follow-up Mammogram/Ultrasound	648	10.5%	8.9%	8.8%
Lumbar Spine MRI for Low Back Pain	99	37.4%	36.6%	37.2%

NOTE: Hospital profiles are in alphabetical order by state, then city, then hospital within the city; Rankings exclude hospitals with less than 25 cases except for patient surveys which excludes hospitals with less than 100 cases; (a) 100-299 cases; (1) The number of cases/patients is too few to report; (2) Data submitted were based on a sample of cases/patients; (3) Results are based on a shorter time period than required; (4) Data suppressed by CMS for one or more quarters; (5) Results are not available for this reporting period; (6) Fewer than 100 patients completed the HCAHPS survey; (7) No cases met the criteria for this measure; (8) The lower limit of the confidence interval cannot be calculated if the number of observed infections equals zero; (9) No data are available from the state/territory for this reporting period; (10) The scores shown reflect fewer than 50 completed surveys; (11) There were discrepancies in the data collection process; (12) This measure does not apply to this hospital for this reporting period; (13) Results cannot be calculated for this reporting period; (14) The results for this state are combined with nearby states to protect confidentiality; Please refer to the User's Guide for a full explanation of data.

Wellstar Douglas Hospital

8954 Hospital Drive Phone: 770-949-1500
Douglasville, GA 30134 Fax: 770-920-6354
URL: www.wellstar.org
Type: Acute Care Hospitals Emergency Services: Yes
Ownership: Voluntary non-profit - Private Beds: 71

Key Personnel:
Chief of Medical Staff. . . . . Barbara Tennill Lewis
CEO/President. . . . . Michael Poore

Measure	Cases	This Hosp.	State Avg.	U.S. Avg.
Blood Clot Prevention and Treatment				
Anticoagulation Overlap Therapy[2]	65	98%	90%	93%
ICU Venous Thromboembolism Prophylaxis[2]	80	95%	90%	92%
Incidence of Potentially Preventable VTE[1,2]	-	-	13%	10%
UFH with Dosages/Platelet Monitoring[2]	35	100%	99%	97%
Venous Thromboembolism Prophylaxis[2]	379	77%	80%	85%
Warfarin Therapy Discharge Instructions[2]	55	98%	78%	75%
Chest Pain/Possible Heart Attack Care				
Aspirin Given Within 24 Hours of Arrival	29	93%	94%	96%
Fibrinolytic Meds Within 30 Min. of Arrival[3,7]	-	-	35%	58%
Average Time to ECG (minutes)	31	3	8	7
Average Time to Transfer (minutes)[1,3]	-	-	73	60
Children's Asthma Care				
Received Home Management Plan of Care	-	-	-	88%
Received Reliever Medication	-	-	-	100%
Received Systemic Corticosteroids	-	-	-	100%
Emergency Department				
Admittance Decision Time (minutes)[2]	354	98	100	98
Head CT Results Within 45 Min. of Arrival[1,3]	-	-	45%	57%
Patients Who Left ER Before Being Seen	64,011	3%	3%	2%
Time from ER Arrival to Admit. (minutes)[2]	396	323	286	274
Time from ER Arrival to Discharge (minutes)	399	150	140	134
Time in ER Before Being Evaluated (minutes)	279	48	32	26
Time to Pain Meds for Fractures (minutes)	143	76	64	57
Heart Attack Care				
Aspirin Given at Discharge[2]	126	100%	99%	99%
Fibrinolytic Meds Within 30 Min. of Arrival[2,7]	-	-	80%	54%
PCI Within 90 Minutes of Arrival[2]	40	88%	95%	96%
Statin Prescribed at Discharge[2]	126	100%	98%	98%
Heart Failure Care				
ACE Inhibitor or ARB for LVSD[2]	77	99%	97%	97%
Discharge Instructions Given[2]	278	70%	92%	94%
Evaluation of LVS Function[2]	298	100%	99%	99%
Medicare Spending				
Medicare Spending per Patient (ratio)	-	0.97	0.95	0.98
Pneumonia Care				
Appropriate Initial Antibiotic Given[2]	123	97%	95%	95%
Blood Culture Timing[2]	271	100%	97%	98%
Pregnancy and Delivery Care				
Newborn Deliveries Scheduled Early[2]	26	8%	8%	6%
Preventive Care				
Immunization for Influenza[2]	574	96%	88%	90%
Immunization for Pneumonia[2]	772	95%	90%	92%
Stroke Care				
Anticoagulation Therapy for Atrial Fibrillation[1,2]	-	-	94%	95%
Antithrombotic Therapy Timing[2]	86	98%	97%	98%
Assessed for Rehabilitation[2]	87	98%	97%	97%
Discharged on Antithrombotic Therapy[2]	87	100%	98%	99%
Discharged on Statin Medication[2]	67	97%	94%	94%
Thrombolytic Therapy Timing[1,2]	-	-	58%	66%
Venous Thromboembolism Prophylaxis[2]	82	95%	92%	94%
Written Stroke Educational Materials Given[2]	71	90%	84%	88%
Surgical Care Improvement Project				
Appropriate Beta Blocker Usage[2]	102	99%	97%	98%
Appropriate VTP Within 24 Hours[2]	300	100%	98%	98%
Controlled Postoperative Blood Glucose[2,7]	-	-	96%	97%
Perioperative Temperature Management[2]	328	100%	100%	100%
Prophylactic Antibiotic Selection[2]	196	99%	99%	99%
Prophylactic Antibiotic Selection (Outpatient)	22	100%	98%	98%
Prophylactic Antibiotic Stopped[2]	189	98%	98%	98%
Prophylactic Antibiotic Timing[2]	196	100%	99%	99%
Prophylactic Antibiotic Timing (Outpatient)	22	82%	98%	98%
Urinary Catheter Removal[2]	222	100%	97%	97%
Survey of Patients' Hospital Experiences				
Area Around Room 'Always' Quiet at Night	300+	64%	66%	61%
Doctors 'Always' Communicated Well	300+	82%	83%	82%
Home Recovery Information Given	300+	85%	84%	85%
Hospital Given 9 or 10 on 10 Point Scale	300+	72%	69%	71%
Meds 'Always' Explained Before Given	300+	65%	63%	64%
Nurses 'Always' Communicated Well	300+	80%	78%	79%
Pain 'Always' Well Controlled	300+	75%	71%	71%
Room and Bathroom 'Always' Clean	300+	72%	71%	73%
Timely Help 'Always' Received	300+	64%	65%	68%
Would Definitely Recommend Hospital	300+	73%	70%	71%
Use of Medical Imaging				
Cardiac Imaging Stress Test before Surgery	273	6.6%	5.5%	5.3%
Combination Abdominal CT Scan	849	12.0%	10.1%	10.5%
Combination Brain/Sinus CT Scan[1]	-	-	2.3%	2.7%
Combination Chest CT Scan	648	1.1%	3.7%	2.7%
Follow-up Mammogram/Ultrasound	1,264	16.0%	8.9%	8.8%
Lumbar Spine MRI for Low Back Pain	46	43.5%	36.6%	37.2%

Dublin VA Medical Center

1826 Veterans Boulevard Phone: 478-277-2701
Dublin, GA 31021 Fax: 478-277-2717
Type: Acute Care - VA Emergency Services: No
Ownership: Government Federal Beds: 796

Key Personnel:
Infection Control. . . . . Terry Avant, RN
Chief of Medical Staff. . . . . Nomie Finn, MD
CEO/President. . . . . James L Robinson III
Patient Relations . . . . Drema Sutphin
Emergency Room . . . . K J Upadhya, MD

Measure	Cases	This Hosp.	State Avg.	U.S. Avg.
Blood Clot Prevention and Treatment				
Anticoagulation Overlap Therapy	-	-	90%	93%
ICU Venous Thromboembolism Prophylaxis	-	-	90%	92%
Incidence of Potentially Preventable VTE	-	-	13%	10%
UFH with Dosages/Platelet Monitoring	-	-	99%	97%
Venous Thromboembolism Prophylaxis	-	-	80%	85%
Warfarin Therapy Discharge Instructions	-	-	78%	75%
Chest Pain/Possible Heart Attack Care				
Aspirin Given Within 24 Hours of Arrival	-	-	94%	96%
Fibrinolytic Meds Within 30 Min. of Arrival	-	-	35%	58%
Average Time to ECG (minutes)	-	-	8	7
Average Time to Transfer (minutes)	-	-	73	60
Children's Asthma Care				
Received Home Management Plan of Care	-	-	-	88%
Received Reliever Medication	-	-	-	100%
Received Systemic Corticosteroids	-	-	-	100%
Emergency Department				
Admittance Decision Time (minutes)	-	-	100	98
Head CT Results Within 45 Min. of Arrival	-	-	45%	57%
Patients Who Left ER Before Being Seen	-	-	3%	2%
Time from ER Arrival to Admit. (minutes)	-	-	286	274
Time from ER Arrival to Discharge (minutes)	-	-	140	134
Time in ER Before Being Evaluated (minutes)	-	-	32	26
Time to Pain Meds for Fractures (minutes)	-	-	64	57
Heart Attack Care				
Aspirin Given at Discharge[5]	-	-	99%	99%
Fibrinolytic Meds Within 30 Min. of Arrival[5]	-	-	80%	54%
PCI Within 90 Minutes of Arrival[5]	-	-	95%	96%
Statin Prescribed at Discharge[5]	-	-	98%	98%
Heart Failure Care				
ACE Inhibitor or ARB for LVSD[1]	23	96%	97%	97%
Discharge Instructions Given	51	98%	92%	94%
Evaluation of LVS Function	55	100%	99%	99%
Medicare Spending				
Medicare Spending per Patient (ratio)	-	-	0.95	0.98
Pneumonia Care				
Appropriate Initial Antibiotic Given	29	97%	95%	95%
Blood Culture Timing	41	98%	97%	98%
Pregnancy and Delivery Care				
Newborn Deliveries Scheduled Early	-	-	8%	6%
Preventive Care				
Immunization for Influenza[2,3]	129	80%	88%	90%
Immunization for Pneumonia[2,3]	334	90%	90%	92%
Stroke Care				
Anticoagulation Therapy for Atrial Fibrillation	-	-	94%	95%
Antithrombotic Therapy Timing	-	-	97%	98%
Assessed for Rehabilitation	-	-	97%	97%
Discharged on Antithrombotic Therapy	-	-	98%	99%
Discharged on Statin Medication	-	-	94%	94%
Thrombolytic Therapy Timing	-	-	58%	66%
Venous Thromboembolism Prophylaxis	-	-	92%	94%
Written Stroke Educational Materials Given	-	-	84%	88%
Surgical Care Improvement Project				
Appropriate Beta Blocker Usage[5]	-	-	97%	98%
Appropriate VTP Within 24 Hours[5]	-	-	98%	98%
Controlled Postoperative Blood Glucose[5]	-	-	96%	97%
Perioperative Temperature Management[5]	-	-	100%	100%
Prophylactic Antibiotic Selection[5]	-	-	99%	99%
Prophylactic Antibiotic Selection (Outpatient)	-	-	98%	98%
Prophylactic Antibiotic Stopped[5]	-	-	98%	98%
Prophylactic Antibiotic Timing[5]	-	-	99%	99%
Prophylactic Antibiotic Timing (Outpatient)	-	-	98%	98%
Urinary Catheter Removal[5]	-	-	97%	97%
Survey of Patients' Hospital Experiences				
Area Around Room 'Always' Quiet at Night	-	-	66%	61%
Doctors 'Always' Communicated Well	-	-	83%	82%
Home Recovery Information Given	-	-	84%	85%
Hospital Given 9 or 10 on 10 Point Scale	-	-	69%	71%
Meds 'Always' Explained Before Given	-	-	63%	64%
Nurses 'Always' Communicated Well	-	-	78%	79%
Pain 'Always' Well Controlled	-	-	71%	71%
Room and Bathroom 'Always' Clean	-	-	71%	73%
Timely Help 'Always' Received	-	-	65%	68%
Would Definitely Recommend Hospital	-	-	70%	71%
Use of Medical Imaging				
Cardiac Imaging Stress Test before Surgery	-	-	5.5%	5.3%
Combination Abdominal CT Scan	-	-	10.1%	10.5%
Combination Brain/Sinus CT Scan	-	-	2.3%	2.7%
Combination Chest CT Scan	-	-	3.7%	2.7%
Follow-up Mammogram/Ultrasound	-	-	8.9%	8.8%
Lumbar Spine MRI for Low Back Pain	-	-	36.6%	37.2%

Fairview Park Hospital

200 Industrial Boulevard Phone: 478-274-3100
Dublin, GA 31021 Fax: 478-274-3673
URL: www.fairviewparkhospital.com
Type: Acute Care Hospitals Emergency Services: Yes
Ownership: Proprietary Beds: 190

Key Personnel:
CEO . . . . Don Avery
Operating Room. . . . . Debra Batey, RN
Quality Assurance . . . . Sandra Campbell
Pediatric Ambulatory Care . . . . . . Nelson Carswell, MD
Pediatric In-Patient Care . . . . Nelson Carswell, MD
Radiology. . . . . George Paul Forsyth, MD
Chief of Medical Staff. . . . . Berry Parker
Emergency Room . . . . Berry Parker

Measure	Cases	This Hosp.	State Avg.	U.S. Avg.
Blood Clot Prevention and Treatment				
Anticoagulation Overlap Therapy[2]	45	91%	90%	93%
ICU Venous Thromboembolism Prophylaxis[2]	185	98%	90%	92%
Incidence of Potentially Preventable VTE[1,2]	-	-	13%	10%
UFH with Dosages/Platelet Monitoring[2]	45	100%	99%	97%
Venous Thromboembolism Prophylaxis[2]	286	98%	80%	85%
Warfarin Therapy Discharge Instructions[2]	36	100%	78%	75%
Chest Pain/Possible Heart Attack Care				
Aspirin Given Within 24 Hours of Arrival	20	100%	94%	96%
Fibrinolytic Meds Within 30 Min. of Arrival[3,7]	-	-	35%	58%
Average Time to ECG (minutes)	20	6	8	7
Average Time to Transfer (minutes)[1,3]	-	-	73	60
Children's Asthma Care				
Received Home Management Plan of Care	-	-	-	88%
Received Reliever Medication	-	-	-	100%
Received Systemic Corticosteroids	-	-	-	100%
Emergency Department				
Admittance Decision Time (minutes)[2]	713	90	100	98

NOTE: Hospital profiles are in alphabetical order by state, then city, then hospital within the city; Rankings exclude hospitals with less than 25 cases except for patient surveys which excludes hospitals with less than 100 cases; (a) 100-299 cases; (1) The number of cases/patients is too few to report; (2) Data submitted were based on a sample of cases/patients; (3) Results are based on a shorter time period than required; (4) Data suppressed by CMS for one or more quarters; (5) Results are not available for this reporting period; (6) Fewer than 100 patients completed the HCAHPS survey; (7) No cases met the criteria for this measure; (8) The lower limit of the confidence interval cannot be calculated if the number of observed infections equals zero; (9) No data are available from the state/territory for this reporting period; (10) The scores shown reflect fewer than 50 completed surveys; (11) There were discrepancies in the data collection process; (12) This measure does not apply to this hospital for this reporting period; (13) Results cannot be calculated for this reporting period; (14) The results for this state are combined with nearby states to protect confidentiality; Please refer to the User's Guide for a full explanation of data.

Measure	Cases	This Hosp.	State Avg.	U.S. Avg.
Head CT Results Within 45 Min. of Arrival[1]	-	-	45%	57%
Patients Who Left ER Before Being Seen	37,598	0%	3%	2%
Time from ER Arrival to Admit. (minutes)[2]	713	255	286	274
Time from ER Arrival to Discharge (minutes)	426	140	140	134
Time in ER Before Being Evaluated (minutes)	451	10	32	26
Time to Pain Meds for Fractures (minutes)	127	60	64	57
Heart Attack Care				
Aspirin Given at Discharge	118	100%	99%	99%
Fibrinolytic Meds Within 30 Min. of Arrival[7]	-	-	80%	54%
PCI Within 90 Minutes of Arrival	32	100%	95%	96%
Statin Prescribed at Discharge	120	100%	98%	98%
Heart Failure Care				
ACE Inhibitor or ARB for LVSD	97	100%	97%	97%
Discharge Instructions Given	152	99%	92%	94%
Evaluation of LVS Function	181	100%	99%	99%
Medicare Spending				
Medicare Spending per Patient (ratio)	-	0.90	0.95	0.98
Pneumonia Care				
Appropriate Initial Antibiotic Given	115	100%	95%	95%
Blood Culture Timing	220	99%	97%	98%
Pregnancy and Delivery Care				
Newborn Deliveries Scheduled Early[2]	26	8%	8%	6%
Preventive Care				
Immunization for Influenza[2]	526	99%	88%	90%
Immunization for Pneumonia[2]	588	98%	90%	92%
Stroke Care				
Anticoagulation Therapy for Atrial Fibrillation[2]	15	100%	94%	95%
Antithrombotic Therapy Timing[2]	67	99%	97%	98%
Assessed for Rehabilitation[2]	68	100%	97%	97%
Discharged on Antithrombotic Therapy[2]	66	100%	98%	99%
Discharged on Statin Medication[2]	52	98%	94%	94%
Thrombolytic Therapy Timing[1,2]	-	-	58%	66%
Venous Thromboembolism Prophylaxis[2]	69	96%	92%	94%
Written Stroke Educational Materials Given[2]	40	100%	84%	88%
Surgical Care Improvement Project				
Appropriate Beta Blocker Usage	89	100%	97%	98%
Appropriate VTP Within 24 Hours	274	100%	98%	98%
Controlled Postoperative Blood Glucose[7]	-	-	96%	97%
Perioperative Temperature Management	335	100%	100%	100%
Prophylactic Antibiotic Selection	239	100%	99%	99%
Prophylactic Antibiotic Selection (Outpatient)	111	100%	98%	98%
Prophylactic Antibiotic Stopped	236	100%	98%	98%
Prophylactic Antibiotic Timing	239	100%	99%	99%
Prophylactic Antibiotic Timing (Outpatient)	112	99%	98%	98%
Urinary Catheter Removal	154	99%	97%	97%
Survey of Patients' Hospital Experiences				
Area Around Room 'Always' Quiet at Night	300+	70%	66%	61%
Doctors 'Always' Communicated Well	300+	82%	83%	82%
Home Recovery Information Given	300+	85%	84%	85%
Hospital Given 9 or 10 on 10 Point Scale	300+	67%	69%	71%
Meds 'Always' Explained Before Given	300+	64%	63%	64%
Nurses 'Always' Communicated Well	300+	79%	78%	79%
Pain 'Always' Well Controlled	300+	73%	71%	71%
Room and Bathroom 'Always' Clean	300+	72%	71%	73%
Timely Help 'Always' Received	300+	66%	65%	68%
Would Definitely Recommend Hospital	300+	65%	70%	71%
Use of Medical Imaging				
Cardiac Imaging Stress Test before Surgery	100	4.0%	5.5%	5.3%
Combination Abdominal CT Scan	543	3.7%	10.1%	10.5%
Combination Brain/Sinus CT Scan	664	1.8%	2.3%	2.7%
Combination Chest CT Scan	194	0.5%	3.7%	2.7%
Follow-up Mammogram/Ultrasound	845	4.1%	8.9%	8.8%
Lumbar Spine MRI for Low Back Pain[1]	-	-	36.6%	37.2%

Dodge County Hospital

901 Griffin Ave
Eastman, GA 31023
Phone: 478-448-4067
Fax: 478-374-9411
URL: www.dodgecountyhospital.com
Type: Acute Care Hospitals
Emergency Services: Yes
Ownership: Govt - Hospital Dist/Auth
Beds: 94

Key Personnel:

CEO/President. . . . . Kevin Bierschenk
Operating Room. . . . . Carole Bundick
Quality Assurance . . . . Carole Bundick
Emergency Room . . . . Christopher Davis
Radiology. . . . . Tommy Meadows
Pediatric Ambulatory Care . . . . . . Johnny Peeples, MD
Pediatric In-Patient Care . . . . Johnny Peeples, MD
Chief of Medical Staff. . . . . James Tison

Measure	Cases	This Hosp.	State Avg.	U.S. Avg.
Blood Clot Prevention and Treatment				
Anticoagulation Overlap Therapy[1,2]	-	-	90%	93%
ICU Venous Thromboembolism Prophylaxis[2]	41	73%	90%	92%
Incidence of Potentially Preventable VTE[2,7]	-	-	13%	10%
UFH with Dosages/Platelet Monitoring[1,2]	-	-	99%	97%
Venous Thromboembolism Prophylaxis[2]	159	68%	80%	85%
Warfarin Therapy Discharge Instructions[1,2]	-	-	78%	75%
Chest Pain/Possible Heart Attack Care				
Aspirin Given Within 24 Hours of Arrival	37	81%	94%	96%
Fibrinolytic Meds Within 30 Min. of Arrival[1]	-	-	35%	58%
Average Time to ECG (minutes)	42	10	8	7
Average Time to Transfer (minutes)[1]	-	-	73	60
Children's Asthma Care				
Received Home Management Plan of Care	-	-	-	88%
Received Reliever Medication	-	-	-	100%
Received Systemic Corticosteroids	-	-	-	100%
Emergency Department				
Admittance Decision Time (minutes)[2]	280	60	100	98
Head CT Results Within 45 Min. of Arrival	13	8%	45%	57%
Patients Who Left ER Before Being Seen	13,602	3%	3%	2%
Time from ER Arrival to Admit. (minutes)[2]	291	250	286	274
Time from ER Arrival to Discharge (minutes)	414	133	140	134
Time in ER Before Being Evaluated (minutes)	453	30	32	26
Time to Pain Meds for Fractures (minutes)	43	66	64	57
Heart Attack Care				
Aspirin Given at Discharge[1,3]	-	-	99%	99%
Fibrinolytic Meds Within 30 Min. of Arrival[3,7]	-	-	80%	54%
PCI Within 90 Minutes of Arrival[3,7]	-	-	95%	96%
Statin Prescribed at Discharge[1,3]	-	-	98%	98%
Heart Failure Care				
ACE Inhibitor or ARB for LVSD[2]	27	85%	97%	97%
Discharge Instructions Given[2]	50	100%	92%	94%
Evaluation of LVS Function[2]	63	94%	99%	99%
Medicare Spending				
Medicare Spending per Patient (ratio)	-	0.96	0.95	0.98
Pneumonia Care				
Appropriate Initial Antibiotic Given[2]	36	86%	95%	95%
Blood Culture Timing[2]	40	90%	97%	98%
Pregnancy and Delivery Care				
Newborn Deliveries Scheduled Early	28	46%	8%	6%
Preventive Care				
Immunization for Influenza[2]	313	45%	88%	90%
Immunization for Pneumonia[2]	371	60%	90%	92%
Stroke Care				
Anticoagulation Therapy for Atrial Fibrillation[2,7]	-	-	94%	95%
Antithrombotic Therapy Timing[1,2]	-	-	97%	98%
Assessed for Rehabilitation[1,2]	-	-	97%	97%
Discharged on Antithrombotic Therapy[1,2]	-	-	98%	99%
Discharged on Statin Medication[1,2]	-	-	94%	94%
Thrombolytic Therapy Timing[1,2]	-	-	58%	66%
Venous Thromboembolism Prophylaxis[1,2]	-	-	92%	94%
Written Stroke Educational Materials Given[1,2]	-	-	84%	88%
Surgical Care Improvement Project				
Appropriate Beta Blocker Usage	21	90%	97%	98%
Appropriate VTP Within 24 Hours	77	92%	98%	98%
Controlled Postoperative Blood Glucose[7]	-	-	96%	97%
Perioperative Temperature Management	27	100%	100%	100%
Prophylactic Antibiotic Selection	46	93%	99%	99%
Prophylactic Antibiotic Selection (Outpatient)[1,3]	-	-	98%	98%
Prophylactic Antibiotic Stopped	44	100%	98%	98%
Prophylactic Antibiotic Timing	46	100%	99%	99%
Prophylactic Antibiotic Timing (Outpatient)[3,7]	-	-	98%	98%
Urinary Catheter Removal	52	100%	97%	97%
Survey of Patients' Hospital Experiences				
Area Around Room 'Always' Quiet at Night	(a)	73%	66%	61%
Doctors 'Always' Communicated Well	(a)	87%	83%	82%
Home Recovery Information Given	(a)	87%	84%	85%
Hospital Given 9 or 10 on 10 Point Scale	(a)	68%	69%	71%
Meds 'Always' Explained Before Given	(a)	68%	63%	64%
Nurses 'Always' Communicated Well	(a)	83%	78%	79%
Pain 'Always' Well Controlled	(a)	76%	71%	71%
Room and Bathroom 'Always' Clean	(a)	77%	71%	73%
Timely Help 'Always' Received	(a)	65%	65%	68%
Would Definitely Recommend Hospital	(a)	62%	70%	71%
Use of Medical Imaging				
Cardiac Imaging Stress Test before Surgery[1]	-	-	5.5%	5.3%
Combination Abdominal CT Scan	248	21.0%	10.1%	10.5%
Combination Brain/Sinus CT Scan[1]	-	-	2.3%	2.7%
Combination Chest CT Scan	135	21.5%	3.7%	2.7%
Follow-up Mammogram/Ultrasound	263	4.2%	8.9%	8.8%
Lumbar Spine MRI for Low Back Pain[1]	-	-	36.6%	37.2%

Putnam General Hospital

101 Lake Oconee Parkway
Eatonton, GA 31024
Phone: 706-485-2711
Fax: 706-485-6770
URL: www.putnamgeneral.com
Type: Critical Access Hospitals
Emergency Services: Yes
Ownership: Govt - Hospital Dist/Auth
Beds: 50

Key Personnel:

Operating Room. . . . . Pam Douglas
CEO . . . . Alan Horton
Chief of Medical Staff. . . . . Susan Jones, MD
Quality Assurance . . . . Cheryl Kimbrell
Emergency Room . . . . Rakesh Kumar, MD
CEO/President. . . . . Darrell Oglesby

Measure	Cases	This Hosp.	State Avg.	U.S. Avg.
Blood Clot Prevention and Treatment				
Anticoagulation Overlap Therapy[1,2]	-	-	90%	93%
ICU Venous Thromboembolism Prophylaxis[2,3]	-	-	90%	92%
Incidence of Potentially Preventable VTE[1,2]	-	-	13%	10%
UFH with Dosages/Platelet Monitoring[2,3]	-	-	99%	97%
Venous Thromboembolism Prophylaxis[2,3]	34	88%	80%	85%
Warfarin Therapy Discharge Instructions[1,2]	-	-	78%	75%
Chest Pain/Possible Heart Attack Care				
Aspirin Given Within 24 Hours of Arrival	78	95%	94%	96%
Fibrinolytic Meds Within 30 Min. of Arrival[1]	-	-	35%	58%
Average Time to ECG (minutes)	81	9	8	7
Average Time to Transfer (minutes)[1]	-	-	73	60
Children's Asthma Care				
Received Home Management Plan of Care	-	-	-	88%
Received Reliever Medication	-	-	-	100%
Received Systemic Corticosteroids	-	-	-	100%
Emergency Department				
Admittance Decision Time (minutes)[2]	295	65	100	98
Head CT Results Within 45 Min. of Arrival[5]	-	-	45%	57%
Patients Who Left ER Before Being Seen	11,507	2%	3%	2%
Time from ER Arrival to Admit. (minutes)[2]	388	206	286	274
Time from ER Arrival to Discharge (minutes)[5]	-	-	140	134
Time in ER Before Being Evaluated (minutes)[5]	-	-	32	26
Time to Pain Meds for Fractures (minutes)	35	49	64	57
Heart Attack Care				
Aspirin Given at Discharge[1]	-	-	99%	99%
Fibrinolytic Meds Within 30 Min. of Arrival[7]	-	-	80%	54%
PCI Within 90 Minutes of Arrival[7]	-	-	95%	96%
Statin Prescribed at Discharge[3,7]	-	-	98%	98%
Heart Failure Care				
ACE Inhibitor or ARB for LVSD	24	100%	97%	97%
Discharge Instructions Given	47	81%	92%	94%
Evaluation of LVS Function	53	100%	99%	99%
Medicare Spending				
Medicare Spending per Patient (ratio)	-	-	0.95	0.98
Pneumonia Care				
Appropriate Initial Antibiotic Given[2]	51	100%	95%	95%
Blood Culture Timing[2]	37	100%	97%	98%
Pregnancy and Delivery Care				
Newborn Deliveries Scheduled Early[5]	-	-	8%	6%
Preventive Care				
Immunization for Influenza[2,3]	146	98%	88%	90%
Immunization for Pneumonia[2,3]	307	97%	90%	92%
Stroke Care				

NOTE: Hospital profiles are in alphabetical order by state, then city, then hospital within the city; Rankings exclude hospitals with less than 25 cases except for patient surveys which excludes hospitals with less than 100 cases; (a) 100-299 cases; (1) The number of cases/patients is too few to report; (2) Data submitted were based on a sample of cases/patients; (3) Results are based on a shorter time period than required; (4) Data suppressed by CMS for one or more quarters; (5) Results are not available for this reporting period; (6) Fewer than 100 patients completed the HCAHPS survey; (7) No cases met the criteria for this measure; (8) The lower limit of the confidence interval cannot be calculated if the number of observed infections equals zero; (9) No data are available from the state/territory for this reporting period; (10) The scores shown reflect fewer than 50 completed surveys; (11) There were discrepancies in the data collection process; (12) This measure does not apply to this hospital for this reporting period; (13) Results cannot be calculated for this reporting period; (14) The results for this state are combined with nearby states to protect confidentiality; Please refer to the User's Guide for a full explanation of data.

Measure	Cases	This Hosp.	State Avg.	U.S. Avg.
Anticoagulation Therapy for Atrial Fibrillation[5]	-	-	94%	95%
Antithrombotic Therapy Timing[5]	-	-	97%	98%
Assessed for Rehabilitation[5]	-	-	97%	97%
Discharged on Antithrombotic Therapy[5]	-	-	98%	99%
Discharged on Statin Medication[5]	-	-	94%	94%
Thrombolytic Therapy Timing[5]	-	-	58%	66%
Venous Thromboembolism Prophylaxis[5]	-	-	92%	94%
Written Stroke Educational Materials Given[5]	-	-	84%	88%
Surgical Care Improvement Project				
Appropriate Beta Blocker Usage[5]	-	-	97%	98%
Appropriate VTP Within 24 Hours[5]	-	-	98%	98%
Controlled Postoperative Blood Glucose[5]	-	-	96%	97%
Perioperative Temperature Management[5]	-	-	100%	100%
Prophylactic Antibiotic Selection[5]	-	-	99%	99%
Prophylactic Antibiotic Selection (Outpatient)[1,3]	-	-	98%	98%
Prophylactic Antibiotic Stopped[5]	-	-	98%	98%
Prophylactic Antibiotic Timing[5]	-	-	99%	99%
Prophylactic Antibiotic Timing (Outpatient)[1,3]	-	-	98%	98%
Urinary Catheter Removal[5]	-	-	97%	97%
Survey of Patients' Hospital Experiences				
Area Around Room 'Always' Quiet at Night[5]	-	-	66%	61%
Doctors 'Always' Communicated Well[5]	-	-	83%	82%
Home Recovery Information Given[5]	-	-	84%	85%
Hospital Given 9 or 10 on 10 Point Scale[5]	-	-	69%	71%
Meds 'Always' Explained Before Given[5]	-	-	63%	64%
Nurses 'Always' Communicated Well[5]	-	-	78%	79%
Pain 'Always' Well Controlled[5]	-	-	71%	71%
Room and Bathroom 'Always' Clean[5]	-	-	71%	73%
Timely Help 'Always' Received[5]	-	-	65%	68%
Would Definitely Recommend Hospital[5]	-	-	70%	71%
Use of Medical Imaging				
Cardiac Imaging Stress Test before Surgery[7]	-	-	5.5%	5.3%
Combination Abdominal CT Scan	287	16.4%	10.1%	10.5%
Combination Brain/Sinus CT Scan[1]	-	-	2.3%	2.7%
Combination Chest CT Scan	160	11.9%	3.7%	2.7%
Follow-up Mammogram/Ultrasound	480	9.4%	8.9%	8.8%
Lumbar Spine MRI for Low Back Pain[1]	-	-	36.6%	37.2%

Elbert Memorial Hospital

4 Medical Drive
Elberton, GA 30635
Type: Acute Care Hospitals
Ownership: Govt - Hospital Dist/Auth
Phone: 706-213-2535
Fax: 706-213-2578
Emergency Services: Yes
Beds: 52

Key Personnel:
Chief of Medical Staff.......... William K. Haley, MD
Operating Room............ William R Haley
Chair/CEO.................. Jim Lloyd
Quality Assurance .... Janna Sanders
CEO/President............... Nancy Seymour

Measure	Cases	This Hosp.	State Avg.	U.S. Avg.
Blood Clot Prevention and Treatment				
Anticoagulation Overlap Therapy[2]	16	88%	90%	93%
ICU Venous Thromboembolism Prophylaxis[2]	32	66%	90%	92%
Incidence of Potentially Preventable VTE[1,2]	-	-	13%	10%
UFH with Dosages/Platelet Monitoring[1,2]	-	-	99%	97%
Venous Thromboembolism Prophylaxis[2]	140	56%	80%	85%
Warfarin Therapy Discharge Instructions[2]	13	100%	78%	75%
Chest Pain/Possible Heart Attack Care				
Aspirin Given Within 24 Hours of Arrival[1,3]	-	-	94%	96%
Fibrinolytic Meds Within 30 Min. of Arrival[3,7]	-	-	35%	58%
Average Time to ECG (minutes)[1,3]	-	-	8	7
Average Time to Transfer (minutes)[1,3]	-	-	73	60
Children's Asthma Care				
Received Home Management Plan of Care	-	-	-	88%
Received Reliever Medication	-	-	-	100%
Received Systemic Corticosteroids	-	-	-	100%
Emergency Department				
Admittance Decision Time (minutes)[2]	410	40	100	98
Head CT Results Within 45 Min. of Arrival[1]	-	-	45%	57%
Patients Who Left ER Before Being Seen	8,356	2%	3%	2%
Time from ER Arrival to Admit. (minutes)[2]	414	200	286	274
Time from ER Arrival to Discharge (minutes)	443	112	140	134
Time in ER Before Being Evaluated (minutes)	485	21	32	26
Time to Pain Meds for Fractures (minutes)	33	76	64	57
Heart Attack Care				
Aspirin Given at Discharge[1,3]	-	-	99%	99%
Fibrinolytic Meds Within 30 Min. of Arrival[3,7]	-	-	80%	54%
PCI Within 90 Minutes of Arrival[3,7]	-	-	95%	96%
Statin Prescribed at Discharge[1,3]	-	-	98%	98%
Heart Failure Care				
ACE Inhibitor or ARB for LVSD[1]	-	-	97%	97%
Discharge Instructions Given	58	88%	92%	94%
Evaluation of LVS Function	67	97%	99%	99%
Medicare Spending				
Medicare Spending per Patient (ratio)	-	0.84	0.95	0.98
Pneumonia Care				
Appropriate Initial Antibiotic Given	65	89%	95%	95%
Blood Culture Timing	56	96%	97%	98%
Pregnancy and Delivery Care				
Newborn Deliveries Scheduled Early[7]	-	-	8%	6%
Preventive Care				
Immunization for Influenza[2]	517	87%	88%	90%
Immunization for Pneumonia[2]	685	94%	90%	92%
Stroke Care				
Anticoagulation Therapy for Atrial Fibrillation[7]	-	-	94%	95%
Antithrombotic Therapy Timing[1]	-	-	97%	98%
Assessed for Rehabilitation[1]	-	-	97%	97%
Discharged on Antithrombotic Therapy[1]	-	-	98%	99%
Discharged on Statin Medication[1]	-	-	94%	94%
Thrombolytic Therapy Timing[7]	-	-	58%	66%
Venous Thromboembolism Prophylaxis[1]	-	-	92%	94%
Written Stroke Educational Materials Given[1]	-	-	84%	88%
Surgical Care Improvement Project				
Appropriate Beta Blocker Usage[1]	-	-	97%	98%
Appropriate VTP Within 24 Hours	15	93%	98%	98%
Controlled Postoperative Blood Glucose[7]	-	-	96%	97%
Perioperative Temperature Management	17	100%	100%	100%
Prophylactic Antibiotic Selection	11	100%	99%	99%
Prophylactic Antibiotic Selection (Outpatient)[3]	16	94%	98%	98%
Prophylactic Antibiotic Stopped	11	100%	98%	98%
Prophylactic Antibiotic Timing	11	100%	99%	99%
Prophylactic Antibiotic Timing (Outpatient)[3]	16	100%	98%	98%
Urinary Catheter Removal[7]	-	-	97%	97%
Survey of Patients' Hospital Experiences				
Area Around Room 'Always' Quiet at Night	(a)	61%	66%	61%
Doctors 'Always' Communicated Well	(a)	87%	83%	82%
Home Recovery Information Given	(a)	89%	84%	85%
Hospital Given 9 or 10 on 10 Point Scale	(a)	62%	69%	71%
Meds 'Always' Explained Before Given	(a)	71%	63%	64%
Nurses 'Always' Communicated Well	(a)	79%	78%	79%
Pain 'Always' Well Controlled	(a)	71%	71%	71%
Room and Bathroom 'Always' Clean	(a)	73%	71%	73%
Timely Help 'Always' Received	(a)	66%	65%	68%
Would Definitely Recommend Hospital	(a)	66%	70%	71%
Use of Medical Imaging				
Cardiac Imaging Stress Test before Surgery[7]	-	-	5.5%	5.3%
Combination Abdominal CT Scan	153	23.5%	10.1%	10.5%
Combination Brain/Sinus CT Scan[1]	-	-	2.3%	2.7%
Combination Chest CT Scan[1]	-	-	3.7%	2.7%
Follow-up Mammogram/Ultrasound	285	4.6%	8.9%	8.8%
Lumbar Spine MRI for Low Back Pain[1]	-	-	36.6%	37.2%

North Georgia Medical Center

1362 South Main Street
Ellijay, GA 30540
Type: Acute Care Hospitals
Ownership: Proprietary
Phone: 706-276-4741
Fax: 706-276-3698
Emergency Services: Yes
Beds: 49

Key Personnel:
CEO/President.............. Carol Burrell
Infection Control............ Cindy Ensley, RN
Quality Assurance .... Cindy Ensley, RN
Chief of Medical Staff.......... Sam Johnson, MD
Radiology.................. Cynthia Jones
Emergency Room .... Michael Mudrey, DO
Operating Room............. Makisha Watson, RN
Intensive Care Unit........... Vansessa Wilbanks, RN

Measure	Cases	This Hosp.	State Avg.	U.S. Avg.
Blood Clot Prevention and Treatment				
Anticoagulation Overlap Therapy[1,2]	-	-	90%	93%
ICU Venous Thromboembolism Prophylaxis[2]	66	27%	90%	92%
Incidence of Potentially Preventable VTE[1,2]	-	-	13%	10%
UFH with Dosages/Platelet Monitoring[1,2]	-	-	99%	97%
Venous Thromboembolism Prophylaxis[2]	126	30%	80%	85%
Warfarin Therapy Discharge Instructions[1,2]	-	-	78%	75%
Chest Pain/Possible Heart Attack Care				
Aspirin Given Within 24 Hours of Arrival	27	63%	94%	96%
Fibrinolytic Meds Within 30 Min. of Arrival[1]	-	-	35%	58%
Average Time to ECG (minutes)	26	14	8	7
Average Time to Transfer (minutes)[1]	-	-	73	60
Children's Asthma Care				
Received Home Management Plan of Care	-	-	-	88%
Received Reliever Medication	-	-	-	100%
Received Systemic Corticosteroids	-	-	-	100%
Emergency Department				
Admittance Decision Time (minutes)[2]	469	61	100	98
Head CT Results Within 45 Min. of Arrival[1]	-	-	45%	57%
Patients Who Left ER Before Being Seen	10,647	3%	3%	2%
Time from ER Arrival to Admit. (minutes)[2]	518	227	286	274
Time from ER Arrival to Discharge (minutes)[11]	383	133	140	134
Time in ER Before Being Evaluated (minutes)	426	34	32	26
Time to Pain Meds for Fractures (minutes)	62	81	64	57
Heart Attack Care				
Aspirin Given at Discharge[7]	-	-	99%	99%
Fibrinolytic Meds Within 30 Min. of Arrival[7]	-	-	80%	54%
PCI Within 90 Minutes of Arrival[7]	-	-	95%	96%
Statin Prescribed at Discharge[7]	-	-	98%	98%
Heart Failure Care				
ACE Inhibitor or ARB for LVSD[2]	11	82%	97%	97%
Discharge Instructions Given[2]	35	80%	92%	94%
Evaluation of LVS Function[2]	46	80%	99%	99%
Medicare Spending				
Medicare Spending per Patient (ratio)	-	0.98	0.95	0.98
Pneumonia Care				
Appropriate Initial Antibiotic Given[2]	48	58%	95%	95%
Blood Culture Timing[2]	46	98%	97%	98%
Pregnancy and Delivery Care				
Newborn Deliveries Scheduled Early[7]	-	-	8%	6%
Preventive Care				
Immunization for Influenza[2]	308	56%	88%	90%
Immunization for Pneumonia[2]	456	75%	90%	92%
Stroke Care				
Anticoagulation Therapy for Atrial Fibrillation[2,7]	-	-	94%	95%
Antithrombotic Therapy Timing[1,2]	-	-	97%	98%
Assessed for Rehabilitation[1,2]	-	-	97%	97%
Discharged on Antithrombotic Therapy[1,2]	-	-	98%	99%
Discharged on Statin Medication[1,2]	-	-	94%	94%
Thrombolytic Therapy Timing[2,7]	-	-	58%	66%
Venous Thromboembolism Prophylaxis[1,2]	-	-	92%	94%
Written Stroke Educational Materials Given[1,2]	-	-	84%	88%
Surgical Care Improvement Project				
Appropriate Beta Blocker Usage[1,2]	-	-	97%	98%
Appropriate VTP Within 24 Hours[2]	41	46%	98%	98%
Controlled Postoperative Blood Glucose[2,7]	-	-	96%	97%
Perioperative Temperature Management[2]	42	95%	100%	100%
Prophylactic Antibiotic Selection[1,2]	-	-	99%	99%
Prophylactic Antibiotic Selection (Outpatient)[1]	-	-	98%	98%
Prophylactic Antibiotic Stopped[1,2]	-	-	98%	98%
Prophylactic Antibiotic Timing[1,2]	-	-	99%	99%
Prophylactic Antibiotic Timing (Outpatient)[1]	-	-	98%	98%
Urinary Catheter Removal[2]	36	61%	97%	97%
Survey of Patients' Hospital Experiences				
Area Around Room 'Always' Quiet at Night	(a)	58%	66%	61%
Doctors 'Always' Communicated Well	(a)	79%	83%	82%
Home Recovery Information Given	(a)	81%	84%	85%
Hospital Given 9 or 10 on 10 Point Scale	(a)	52%	69%	71%
Meds 'Always' Explained Before Given	(a)	64%	63%	64%
Nurses 'Always' Communicated Well	(a)	77%	78%	79%
Pain 'Always' Well Controlled	(a)	63%	71%	71%
Room and Bathroom 'Always' Clean	(a)	57%	71%	73%

NOTE: Hospital profiles are in alphabetical order by state, then city, then hospital within the city; Rankings exclude hospitals with less than 25 cases except for patient surveys which excludes hospitals with less than 100 cases; (a) 100-299 cases; (1) The number of cases/patients is too few to report; (2) Data submitted were based on a sample of cases/patients; (3) Results are based on a shorter time period than required; (4) Data suppressed by CMS for one or more quarters; (5) Results are not available for this reporting period; (6) Fewer than 100 patients completed the HCAHPS survey; (7) No cases met the criteria for this measure; (8) The lower limit of the confidence interval cannot be calculated if the number of observed infections equals zero; (9) No data are available from the state/territory for this reporting period; (10) The scores shown reflect fewer than 50 completed surveys; (11) There were discrepancies in the data collection process; (12) This measure does not apply to this hospital for this reporting period; (13) Results cannot be calculated for this reporting period; (14) The results for this state are combined with nearby states to protect confidentiality; Please refer to the User's Guide for a full explanation of data.

Measure	Cases	This Hosp.	State Avg.	U.S. Avg.
Timely Help 'Always' Received	(a)	75%	65%	68%
Would Definitely Recommend Hospital	(a)	56%	70%	71%
Use of Medical Imaging				
Cardiac Imaging Stress Test before Surgery	53	3.8%	5.5%	5.3%
Combination Abdominal CT Scan	139	15.1%	10.1%	10.5%
Combination Brain/Sinus CT Scan[1]	-	-	2.3%	2.7%
Combination Chest CT Scan[1]	-	-	3.7%	2.7%
Follow-up Mammogram/Ultrasound	149	6.0%	8.9%	8.8%
Lumbar Spine MRI for Low Back Pain[1]	-	-	36.6%	37.2%

Piedmont Fayette Hospital

1255 Highway 54 West Phone: 770-719-7071
Fayetteville, GA 30214 Fax: 770-719-7092
URL: www.fayettehospital.org
Type: Acute Care Hospitals Emergency Services: Yes
Ownership: Voluntary non-profit - Private Beds: 100

Key Personnel:

Chief of Medical Staff. . . . . Frederick Willms
Anesthesiology. . . . . Chad M Achilles
Radiology. . . . . Jeffrey D Allen
Radiology. . . . . Timothy W Baker
CEO/President. . . . . J. Michael Burnett

Measure	Cases	This Hosp.	State Avg.	U.S. Avg.
Blood Clot Prevention and Treatment				
Anticoagulation Overlap Therapy[2]	109	98%	90%	93%
ICU Venous Thromboembolism Prophylaxis[2]	54	94%	90%	92%
Incidence of Potentially Preventable VTE[2]	16	12%	13%	10%
UFH with Dosages/Platelet Monitoring[2]	104	100%	99%	97%
Venous Thromboembolism Prophylaxis[2]	389	87%	80%	85%
Warfarin Therapy Discharge Instructions[2]	89	85%	78%	75%
Chest Pain/Possible Heart Attack Care				
Aspirin Given Within 24 Hours of Arrival	37	100%	94%	96%
Fibrinolytic Meds Within 30 Min. of Arrival[7]	-	-	35%	58%
Average Time to ECG (minutes)	39	3	8	7
Average Time to Transfer (minutes)[7]	-	-	73	60
Children's Asthma Care				
Received Home Management Plan of Care	-	-	-	88%
Received Reliever Medication	-	-	-	100%
Received Systemic Corticosteroids	-	-	-	100%
Emergency Department				
Admittance Decision Time (minutes)[2]	624	188	100	98
Head CT Results Within 45 Min. of Arrival	21	62%	45%	57%
Patients Who Left ER Before Being Seen	63,594	2%	3%	2%
Time from ER Arrival to Admit. (minutes)[2]	630	414	286	274
Time from ER Arrival to Discharge (minutes)	411	188	140	134
Time in ER Before Being Evaluated (minutes)	430	48	32	26
Time to Pain Meds for Fractures (minutes)	257	84	64	57
Heart Attack Care				
Aspirin Given at Discharge[2]	261	100%	99%	99%
Fibrinolytic Meds Within 30 Min. of Arrival[2,7]	-	-	80%	54%
PCI Within 90 Minutes of Arrival[2]	19	95%	95%	96%
Statin Prescribed at Discharge[2]	258	98%	98%	98%
Heart Failure Care				
ACE Inhibitor or ARB for LVSD[2]	85	98%	97%	97%
Discharge Instructions Given[2]	276	98%	92%	94%
Evaluation of LVS Function[2]	328	100%	99%	99%
Medicare Spending				
Medicare Spending per Patient (ratio)	-	0.97	0.95	0.98
Pneumonia Care				
Appropriate Initial Antibiotic Given[2]	89	97%	95%	95%
Blood Culture Timing[2]	179	96%	97%	98%
Pregnancy and Delivery Care				
Newborn Deliveries Scheduled Early[2]	49	2%	8%	6%
Preventive Care				
Immunization for Influenza[2]	517	67%	88%	90%
Immunization for Pneumonia[2]	643	78%	90%	92%
Stroke Care				
Anticoagulation Therapy for Atrial Fibrillation[1]	-	-	94%	95%
Antithrombotic Therapy Timing	84	98%	97%	98%
Assessed for Rehabilitation	89	100%	97%	97%
Discharged on Antithrombotic Therapy	85	99%	98%	99%
Discharged on Statin Medication	72	97%	94%	94%
Thrombolytic Therapy Timing	11	0%	58%	66%
Venous Thromboembolism Prophylaxis	90	84%	92%	94%
Written Stroke Educational Materials Given	60	73%	84%	88%
Surgical Care Improvement Project				
Appropriate Beta Blocker Usage[2]	115	98%	97%	98%
Appropriate VTP Within 24 Hours[2]	425	98%	98%	98%
Controlled Postoperative Blood Glucose[2,7]	-	-	96%	97%
Perioperative Temperature Management[2]	499	100%	100%	100%
Prophylactic Antibiotic Selection[2]	323	100%	99%	99%
Prophylactic Antibiotic Selection (Outpatient)	413	97%	98%	98%
Prophylactic Antibiotic Stopped[2]	317	98%	98%	98%
Prophylactic Antibiotic Timing[2]	326	98%	99%	99%
Prophylactic Antibiotic Timing (Outpatient)	414	99%	98%	98%
Urinary Catheter Removal[2]	295	89%	97%	97%
Survey of Patients' Hospital Experiences				
Area Around Room 'Always' Quiet at Night	300+	64%	66%	61%
Doctors 'Always' Communicated Well	300+	81%	83%	82%
Home Recovery Information Given	300+	82%	84%	85%
Hospital Given 9 or 10 on 10 Point Scale	300+	74%	69%	71%
Meds 'Always' Explained Before Given	300+	61%	63%	64%
Nurses 'Always' Communicated Well	300+	78%	78%	79%
Pain 'Always' Well Controlled	300+	70%	71%	71%
Room and Bathroom 'Always' Clean	300+	69%	71%	73%
Timely Help 'Always' Received	300+	63%	65%	68%
Would Definitely Recommend Hospital	300+	81%	70%	71%
Use of Medical Imaging				
Cardiac Imaging Stress Test before Surgery	971	6.6%	5.5%	5.3%
Combination Abdominal CT Scan	1,196	3.9%	10.1%	10.5%
Combination Brain/Sinus CT Scan	1,184	1.4%	2.3%	2.7%
Combination Chest CT Scan	647	0.6%	3.7%	2.7%
Follow-up Mammogram/Ultrasound	2,509	6.8%	8.9%	8.8%
Lumbar Spine MRI for Low Back Pain	112	30.4%	36.6%	37.2%

Dorminy Medical Center

200 Perry House Road, Box 1447 Phone: 229-424-7100
Fitzgerald, GA 31750 Fax: 229-424-7281
URL: www.dorminymedical.org
Type: Acute Care Hospitals Emergency Services: Yes
Ownership: Govt - Hospital Dist/Auth Beds: 75

Key Personnel:

Quality Assurance . . . . Beth Bryant
Anesthesiology. . . . . Dr Phillips Grooms
CEO/President. . . . . Warren Manley
Patient Relations . . . . Jenny McCranie
Infection Control. . . . . Dot O'Scott
Intensive Care Unit. . . . . Dot O'Scott, RN
Chief of Medical Staff. . . . . Dr Don T Smith Jr, MD
Emergency Room . . . . Paul Webb, RN

Measure	Cases	This Hosp.	State Avg.	U.S. Avg.
Blood Clot Prevention and Treatment				
Anticoagulation Overlap Therapy[1,2]	-	-	90%	93%
ICU Venous Thromboembolism Prophylaxis[2]	44	86%	90%	92%
Incidence of Potentially Preventable VTE[2,7]	-	-	13%	10%
UFH with Dosages/Platelet Monitoring[1,2]	-	-	99%	97%
Venous Thromboembolism Prophylaxis[2]	126	70%	80%	85%
Warfarin Therapy Discharge Instructions[1,2]	-	-	78%	75%
Chest Pain/Possible Heart Attack Care				
Aspirin Given Within 24 Hours of Arrival	35	97%	94%	96%
Fibrinolytic Meds Within 30 Min. of Arrival[1]	-	-	35%	58%
Average Time to ECG (minutes)	38	14	8	7
Average Time to Transfer (minutes)[1]	-	-	73	60
Children's Asthma Care				
Received Home Management Plan of Care	-	-	-	88%
Received Reliever Medication	-	-	-	100%
Received Systemic Corticosteroids	-	-	-	100%
Emergency Department				
Admittance Decision Time (minutes)[2]	508	48	100	98
Head CT Results Within 45 Min. of Arrival[1,3]	-	-	45%	57%
Patients Who Left ER Before Being Seen	11,111	2%	3%	2%
Time from ER Arrival to Admit. (minutes)[2]	514	218	286	274
Time from ER Arrival to Discharge (minutes)	419	117	140	134
Time in ER Before Being Evaluated (minutes)	444	15	32	26
Time to Pain Meds for Fractures (minutes)[1]	-	-	64	57
Heart Attack Care				
Aspirin Given at Discharge[1]	-	-	99%	99%
Fibrinolytic Meds Within 30 Min. of Arrival[7]	-	-	80%	54%
PCI Within 90 Minutes of Arrival[7]	-	-	95%	96%
Statin Prescribed at Discharge[1]	-	-	98%	98%
Heart Failure Care				
ACE Inhibitor or ARB for LVSD	19	100%	97%	97%
Discharge Instructions Given	39	97%	92%	94%
Evaluation of LVS Function	54	98%	99%	99%
Medicare Spending				
Medicare Spending per Patient (ratio)	-	0.87	0.95	0.98
Pneumonia Care				
Appropriate Initial Antibiotic Given[2]	24	88%	95%	95%
Blood Culture Timing[2]	73	86%	97%	98%
Pregnancy and Delivery Care				
Newborn Deliveries Scheduled Early	14	14%	8%	6%
Preventive Care				
Immunization for Influenza[2]	280	91%	88%	90%
Immunization for Pneumonia[2]	431	91%	90%	92%
Stroke Care				
Anticoagulation Therapy for Atrial Fibrillation[1]	-	-	94%	95%
Antithrombotic Therapy Timing[1]	-	-	97%	98%
Assessed for Rehabilitation[1]	-	-	97%	97%
Discharged on Antithrombotic Therapy[1]	-	-	98%	99%
Discharged on Statin Medication[1]	-	-	94%	94%
Thrombolytic Therapy Timing[1]	-	-	58%	66%
Venous Thromboembolism Prophylaxis	11	45%	92%	94%
Written Stroke Educational Materials Given[1]	-	-	84%	88%
Surgical Care Improvement Project				
Appropriate Beta Blocker Usage[1]	-	-	97%	98%
Appropriate VTP Within 24 Hours	21	86%	98%	98%
Controlled Postoperative Blood Glucose[7]	-	-	96%	97%
Perioperative Temperature Management	27	100%	100%	100%
Prophylactic Antibiotic Selection	13	92%	99%	99%
Prophylactic Antibiotic Selection (Outpatient)	11	100%	98%	98%
Prophylactic Antibiotic Stopped	12	100%	98%	98%
Prophylactic Antibiotic Timing	13	100%	99%	99%
Prophylactic Antibiotic Timing (Outpatient)	11	100%	98%	98%
Urinary Catheter Removal[1]	-	-	97%	97%
Survey of Patients' Hospital Experiences				
Area Around Room 'Always' Quiet at Night	(a)	62%	66%	61%
Doctors 'Always' Communicated Well	(a)	81%	83%	82%
Home Recovery Information Given	(a)	79%	84%	85%
Hospital Given 9 or 10 on 10 Point Scale	(a)	63%	69%	71%
Meds 'Always' Explained Before Given	(a)	55%	63%	64%
Nurses 'Always' Communicated Well	(a)	72%	78%	79%
Pain 'Always' Well Controlled	(a)	67%	71%	71%
Room and Bathroom 'Always' Clean	(a)	70%	71%	73%
Timely Help 'Always' Received	(a)	59%	65%	68%
Would Definitely Recommend Hospital	(a)	53%	70%	71%
Use of Medical Imaging				
Cardiac Imaging Stress Test before Surgery	117	6.0%	5.5%	5.3%
Combination Abdominal CT Scan	180	36.7%	10.1%	10.5%
Combination Brain/Sinus CT Scan[1]	-	-	2.3%	2.7%
Combination Chest CT Scan	117	40.2%	3.7%	2.7%
Follow-up Mammogram/Ultrasound	147	12.9%	8.9%	8.8%
Lumbar Spine MRI for Low Back Pain[1]	-	-	36.6%	37.2%

Monroe County Hospital

88 Martin Luther King Jr Drive Phone: 478-994-2521
Forsyth, GA 31029 Fax: 478-994-8798
E-mail: e.sowell@monroehospital.org
URL: www.monroehospital.org
Type: Critical Access Hospitals Emergency Services: Yes
Ownership: Govt - Hospital Dist/Auth Beds: 25

Key Personnel:

Surgery . . . . Doug Brewer
Chief of Medical Staff. . . . . Craig Caldwell, MD
Operating Room. . . . . Cassie Davis
CEO/President. . . . . Kay Floyd
Quality Assurance . . . . Kathy Louth
Cardiology . . . . Carmine Oddis
Infection Control. . . . . Jean Riley
Emergency Room . . . . Nancy Waller

Measure	Cases	This Hosp.	State Avg.	U.S. Avg.
Blood Clot Prevention and Treatment				
Anticoagulation Overlap Therapy[5]	-	-	90%	93%

NOTE: Hospital profiles are in alphabetical order by state, then city, then hospital within the city; Rankings exclude hospitals with less than 25 cases except for patient surveys which excludes hospitals with less than 100 cases; (a) 100-299 cases; (1) The number of cases/patients is too few to report; (2) Data submitted were based on a sample of cases/patients; (3) Results are based on a shorter time period than required; (4) Data suppressed by CMS for one or more quarters; (5) Results are not available for this reporting period; (6) Fewer than 100 patients completed the HCAHPS survey; (7) No cases met the criteria for this measure; (8) The lower limit of the confidence interval cannot be calculated if the number of observed infections equals zero; (9) No data are available from the state/territory for this reporting period; (10) The scores shown reflect fewer than 50 completed surveys; (11) There were discrepancies in the data collection process; (12) This measure does not apply to this hospital for this reporting period; (13) Results cannot be calculated for this reporting period; (14) The results for this state are combined with nearby states to protect confidentiality; Please refer to the User's Guide for a full explanation of data.

Measure	Cases	This Hosp.	State Avg.	U.S. Avg.
ICU Venous Thromboembolism Prophylaxis[5]	-	-	90%	92%
Incidence of Potentially Preventable VTE[5]	-	-	13%	10%
UFH with Dosages/Platelet Monitoring[5]	-	-	99%	97%
Venous Thromboembolism Prophylaxis[5]	-	-	80%	85%
Warfarin Therapy Discharge Instructions[5]	-	-	78%	75%
Chest Pain/Possible Heart Attack Care				
Aspirin Given Within 24 Hours of Arrival	13	92%	94%	96%
Fibrinolytic Meds Within 30 Min. of Arrival[7]	-	-	35%	58%
Average Time to ECG (minutes)	14	14	8	7
Average Time to Transfer (minutes)[1]	-	-	73	60
Children's Asthma Care				
Received Home Management Plan of Care	-	-	-	88%
Received Reliever Medication	-	-	-	100%
Received Systemic Corticosteroids	-	-	-	100%
Emergency Department				
Admittance Decision Time (minutes)[5]	-	-	100	98
Head CT Results Within 45 Min. of Arrival[5]	-	-	45%	57%
Patients Who Left ER Before Being Seen	8,726	2%	3%	2%
Time from ER Arrival to Admit. (minutes)[5]	-	-	286	274
Time from ER Arrival to Discharge (minutes)[5]	-	-	140	134
Time in ER Before Being Evaluated (minutes)[5]	-	-	32	26
Time to Pain Meds for Fractures (minutes)[5]	-	-	64	57
Heart Attack Care				
Aspirin Given at Discharge[5]	-	-	99%	99%
Fibrinolytic Meds Within 30 Min. of Arrival[5]	-	-	80%	54%
PCI Within 90 Minutes of Arrival[5]	-	-	95%	96%
Statin Prescribed at Discharge[5]	-	-	98%	98%
Heart Failure Care				
ACE Inhibitor or ARB for LVSD[2]	11	91%	97%	97%
Discharge Instructions Given[2]	21	81%	92%	94%
Evaluation of LVS Function[2]	24	96%	99%	99%
Medicare Spending				
Medicare Spending per Patient (ratio)	-	-	0.95	0.98
Pneumonia Care				
Appropriate Initial Antibiotic Given	24	100%	95%	95%
Blood Culture Timing	27	100%	97%	98%
Pregnancy and Delivery Care				
Newborn Deliveries Scheduled Early[3,7]	-	-	8%	6%
Preventive Care				
Immunization for Influenza[5]	-	-	88%	90%
Immunization for Pneumonia[5]	-	-	90%	92%
Stroke Care				
Anticoagulation Therapy for Atrial Fibrillation[5]	-	-	94%	95%
Antithrombotic Therapy Timing[5]	-	-	97%	98%
Assessed for Rehabilitation[5]	-	-	97%	97%
Discharged on Antithrombotic Therapy[5]	-	-	98%	99%
Discharged on Statin Medication[5]	-	-	94%	94%
Thrombolytic Therapy Timing[5]	-	-	58%	66%
Venous Thromboembolism Prophylaxis[5]	-	-	92%	94%
Written Stroke Educational Materials Given[5]	-	-	84%	88%
Surgical Care Improvement Project				
Appropriate Beta Blocker Usage[5]	-	-	97%	98%
Appropriate VTP Within 24 Hours[5]	-	-	98%	98%
Controlled Postoperative Blood Glucose[5]	-	-	96%	97%
Perioperative Temperature Management[5]	-	-	100%	100%
Prophylactic Antibiotic Selection[5]	-	-	99%	99%
Prophylactic Antibiotic Selection (Outpatient)[5]	-	-	98%	98%
Prophylactic Antibiotic Stopped[5]	-	-	98%	98%
Prophylactic Antibiotic Timing[5]	-	-	99%	99%
Prophylactic Antibiotic Timing (Outpatient)[5]	-	-	98%	98%
Urinary Catheter Removal[5]	-	-	97%	97%
Survey of Patients' Hospital Experiences				
Area Around Room 'Always' Quiet at Night[5]	-	-	66%	61%
Doctors 'Always' Communicated Well[5]	-	-	83%	82%
Home Recovery Information Given[5]	-	-	84%	85%
Hospital Given 9 or 10 on 10 Point Scale[5]	-	-	69%	71%
Meds 'Always' Explained Before Given[5]	-	-	63%	64%
Nurses 'Always' Communicated Well[5]	-	-	78%	79%
Pain 'Always' Well Controlled[5]	-	-	71%	71%
Room and Bathroom 'Always' Clean[5]	-	-	71%	73%
Timely Help 'Always' Received[5]	-	-	65%	68%
Would Definitely Recommend Hospital[5]	-	-	70%	71%
Use of Medical Imaging				
Cardiac Imaging Stress Test before Surgery[7]	-	-	5.5%	5.3%
Combination Abdominal CT Scan	149	1.3%	10.1%	10.5%
Combination Brain/Sinus CT Scan[1]	-	-	2.3%	2.7%
Combination Chest CT Scan	98	2.0%	3.7%	2.7%
Follow-up Mammogram/Ultrasound	277	2.5%	8.9%	8.8%
Lumbar Spine MRI for Low Back Pain[1]	-	-	36.6%	37.2%

Hutcheson Medical Center

100 Gross Crescent
Fort Oglethorpe, GA 30742
E-mail: dhardin@hutcheson.org
Phone: 706-858-2101
Fax: 706-858-2028
Type: Acute Care Hospitals
Ownership: Govt - Hospital Dist/Auth
Emergency Services: Yes
Beds: 179

Key Personnel:
Radiology. . . . . Brett Austin, MD
Emergency Room . . . . Debbie Doran, RN
Quality Assurance . . . . Nan Dyer
CEO/President. . . . . Farrell Hayes
Operating Room. . . . . Judy Holder, RN
Chief of Medical Staff. . . . . Melissa Phillips, MD

Measure	Cases	This Hosp.	State Avg.	U.S. Avg.
Blood Clot Prevention and Treatment				
Anticoagulation Overlap Therapy[2]	11	100%	90%	93%
ICU Venous Thromboembolism Prophylaxis[2]	133	88%	90%	92%
Incidence of Potentially Preventable VTE[1,2]	-	-	13%	10%
UFH with Dosages/Platelet Monitoring[1,2]	-	-	99%	97%
Venous Thromboembolism Prophylaxis[2]	324	76%	80%	85%
Warfarin Therapy Discharge Instructions[1,2]	-	-	78%	75%
Chest Pain/Possible Heart Attack Care				
Aspirin Given Within 24 Hours of Arrival	36	97%	94%	96%
Fibrinolytic Meds Within 30 Min. of Arrival[7]	-	-	35%	58%
Average Time to ECG (minutes)	36	8	8	7
Average Time to Transfer (minutes)[1]	-	-	73	60
Children's Asthma Care				
Received Home Management Plan of Care	-	-	-	88%
Received Reliever Medication	-	-	-	100%
Received Systemic Corticosteroids	-	-	-	100%
Emergency Department				
Admittance Decision Time (minutes)[2]	461	64	100	98
Head CT Results Within 45 Min. of Arrival[1]	-	-	45%	57%
Patients Who Left ER Before Being Seen	34,410	2%	3%	2%
Time from ER Arrival to Admit. (minutes)[2]	496	226	286	274
Time from ER Arrival to Discharge (minutes)	431	114	140	134
Time in ER Before Being Evaluated (minutes)	448	25	32	26
Time to Pain Meds for Fractures (minutes)	94	54	64	57
Heart Attack Care				
Aspirin Given at Discharge	12	100%	99%	99%
Fibrinolytic Meds Within 30 Min. of Arrival[7]	-	-	80%	54%
PCI Within 90 Minutes of Arrival[7]	-	-	95%	96%
Statin Prescribed at Discharge	12	100%	98%	98%
Heart Failure Care				
ACE Inhibitor or ARB for LVSD[2]	24	100%	97%	97%
Discharge Instructions Given[2]	60	88%	92%	94%
Evaluation of LVS Function[2]	80	100%	99%	99%
Medicare Spending				
Medicare Spending per Patient (ratio)	-	0.94	0.95	0.98
Pneumonia Care				
Appropriate Initial Antibiotic Given[2]	83	96%	95%	95%
Blood Culture Timing[2]	105	99%	97%	98%
Pregnancy and Delivery Care				
Newborn Deliveries Scheduled Early[2]	30	27%	8%	6%
Preventive Care				
Immunization for Influenza[2]	525	96%	88%	90%
Immunization for Pneumonia[2]	471	91%	90%	92%
Stroke Care				
Anticoagulation Therapy for Atrial Fibrillation[7]	-	-	94%	95%
Antithrombotic Therapy Timing[1]	-	-	97%	98%
Assessed for Rehabilitation[1]	-	-	97%	97%
Discharged on Antithrombotic Therapy[1]	-	-	98%	99%
Discharged on Statin Medication[1]	-	-	94%	94%
Thrombolytic Therapy Timing[7]	-	-	58%	66%
Venous Thromboembolism Prophylaxis[1]	-	-	92%	94%
Written Stroke Educational Materials Given[1]	-	-	84%	88%
Surgical Care Improvement Project				
Appropriate Beta Blocker Usage	18	100%	97%	98%
Appropriate VTP Within 24 Hours	86	95%	98%	98%
Controlled Postoperative Blood Glucose[7]	-	-	96%	97%
Perioperative Temperature Management	94	100%	100%	100%
Prophylactic Antibiotic Selection	48	98%	99%	99%
Prophylactic Antibiotic Selection (Outpatient)	37	100%	98%	98%
Prophylactic Antibiotic Stopped	47	98%	98%	98%
Prophylactic Antibiotic Timing	48	100%	99%	99%
Prophylactic Antibiotic Timing (Outpatient)	39	90%	98%	98%
Urinary Catheter Removal	36	100%	97%	97%
Survey of Patients' Hospital Experiences				
Area Around Room 'Always' Quiet at Night[11]	(a)	67%	66%	61%
Doctors 'Always' Communicated Well[11]	(a)	83%	83%	82%
Home Recovery Information Given[11]	(a)	85%	84%	85%
Hospital Given 9 or 10 on 10 Point Scale[11]	(a)	71%	69%	71%
Meds 'Always' Explained Before Given[11]	(a)	58%	63%	64%
Nurses 'Always' Communicated Well[11]	(a)	77%	78%	79%
Pain 'Always' Well Controlled[11]	(a)	70%	71%	71%
Room and Bathroom 'Always' Clean[11]	(a)	71%	71%	73%
Timely Help 'Always' Received[11]	(a)	69%	65%	68%
Would Definitely Recommend Hospital[11]	(a)	68%	70%	71%
Use of Medical Imaging				
Cardiac Imaging Stress Test before Surgery	141	7.8%	5.5%	5.3%
Combination Abdominal CT Scan	307	4.9%	10.1%	10.5%
Combination Brain/Sinus CT Scan[1]	-	-	2.3%	2.7%
Combination Chest CT Scan	111	6.3%	3.7%	2.7%
Follow-up Mammogram/Ultrasound[7]	-	-	8.9%	8.8%
Lumbar Spine MRI for Low Back Pain[1]	-	-	36.6%	37.2%

Northeast Georgia Medical Center

743 Spring Street
Gainesville, GA 30501
URL: www.nghs.com
Phone: 770-535-3553
Fax: 770-538-7128
Type: Acute Care Hospitals
Ownership: Government - Local
Emergency Services: Yes
Beds: 557

Key Personnel:
Chief of Medical Staff. . . . . James Bailey, MD
CEO/President. . . . . Carol Burrell
Hemotology Center . . . . Tom Enright
Coronary Care . . . . Heather Home
Infection Control. . . . . Bette Meisch
Cardiac Laboratory. . . . . Daniel Tarte

Measure	Cases	This Hosp.	State Avg.	U.S. Avg.
Blood Clot Prevention and Treatment				
Anticoagulation Overlap Therapy[2]	192	91%	90%	93%
ICU Venous Thromboembolism Prophylaxis[2]	155	83%	90%	92%
Incidence of Potentially Preventable VTE[2]	37	22%	13%	10%
UFH with Dosages/Platelet Monitoring[2]	191	100%	99%	97%
Venous Thromboembolism Prophylaxis[2]	296	72%	80%	85%
Warfarin Therapy Discharge Instructions[2]	149	100%	78%	75%
Chest Pain/Possible Heart Attack Care				
Aspirin Given Within 24 Hours of Arrival[1,3]	-	-	94%	96%
Fibrinolytic Meds Within 30 Min. of Arrival[5]	-	-	35%	58%
Average Time to ECG (minutes)[1,3]	-	-	8	7
Average Time to Transfer (minutes)[5]	-	-	73	60
Children's Asthma Care				
Received Home Management Plan of Care	-	-	-	88%
Received Reliever Medication	-	-	-	100%
Received Systemic Corticosteroids	-	-	-	100%
Emergency Department				
Admittance Decision Time (minutes)[2]	541	113	100	98
Head CT Results Within 45 Min. of Arrival[1]	-	-	45%	57%
Patients Who Left ER Before Being Seen	>100k	1%	3%	2%
Time from ER Arrival to Admit. (minutes)[2]	549	281	286	274
Time from ER Arrival to Discharge (minutes)	395	150	140	134
Time in ER Before Being Evaluated (minutes)	430	37	32	26
Time to Pain Meds for Fractures (minutes)	319	72	64	57
Heart Attack Care				
Aspirin Given at Discharge[2]	333	100%	99%	99%
Fibrinolytic Meds Within 30 Min. of Arrival[1,2]	-	-	80%	54%
PCI Within 90 Minutes of Arrival[2]	62	100%	95%	96%
Statin Prescribed at Discharge[2]	314	100%	98%	98%
Heart Failure Care				

NOTE: Hospital profiles are in alphabetical order by state, then city, then hospital within the city; Rankings exclude hospitals with less than 25 cases except for patient surveys which excludes hospitals with less than 100 cases; (a) 100-299 cases; (1) The number of cases/patients is too few to report; (2) Data submitted were based on a sample of cases/patients; (3) Results are based on a shorter time period than required; (4) Data suppressed by CMS for one or more quarters; (5) Results are not available for this reporting period; (6) Fewer than 100 patients completed the HCAHPS survey; (7) No cases met the criteria for this measure; (8) The lower limit of the confidence interval cannot be calculated if the number of observed infections equals zero; (9) No data are available from the state/territory for this reporting period; (10) The scores shown reflect fewer than 50 completed surveys; (11) There were discrepancies in the data collection process; (12) This measure does not apply to this hospital for this reporting period; (13) Results cannot be calculated for this reporting period; (14) The results for this state are combined with nearby states to protect confidentiality; Please refer to the User's Guide for a full explanation of data.

Measure	Cases	This Hosp.	State Avg.	U.S. Avg.
ACE Inhibitor or ARB for LVSD[2]	49	98%	97%	97%
Discharge Instructions Given[2]	282	90%	92%	94%
Evaluation of LVS Function[2]	326	100%	99%	99%
Medicare Spending				
Medicare Spending per Patient (ratio)	-	0.91	0.95	0.98
Pneumonia Care				
Appropriate Initial Antibiotic Given[2]	113	96%	95%	95%
Blood Culture Timing[2]	215	97%	97%	98%
Pregnancy and Delivery Care				
Newborn Deliveries Scheduled Early[2]	69	3%	8%	6%
Preventive Care				
Immunization for Influenza[2]	529	93%	88%	90%
Immunization for Pneumonia[2]	698	89%	90%	92%
Stroke Care				
Anticoagulation Therapy for Atrial Fibrillation	68	93%	94%	95%
Antithrombotic Therapy Timing	274	97%	97%	98%
Assessed for Rehabilitation	360	95%	97%	97%
Discharged on Antithrombotic Therapy	317	97%	98%	99%
Discharged on Statin Medication	254	96%	94%	94%
Thrombolytic Therapy Timing	35	77%	58%	66%
Venous Thromboembolism Prophylaxis	334	87%	92%	94%
Written Stroke Educational Materials Given	248	88%	84%	88%
Surgical Care Improvement Project				
Appropriate Beta Blocker Usage[2]	285	98%	97%	98%
Appropriate VTP Within 24 Hours[2]	384	97%	98%	98%
Controlled Postoperative Blood Glucose[2]	180	96%	96%	97%
Perioperative Temperature Management[2]	555	100%	100%	100%
Prophylactic Antibiotic Selection[2]	504	98%	99%	99%
Prophylactic Antibiotic Selection (Outpatient)	774	98%	98%	98%
Prophylactic Antibiotic Stopped[2]	492	98%	98%	98%
Prophylactic Antibiotic Timing[2]	504	99%	99%	99%
Prophylactic Antibiotic Timing (Outpatient)	774	99%	98%	98%
Urinary Catheter Removal[2]	437	98%	97%	97%
Survey of Patients' Hospital Experiences				
Area Around Room 'Always' Quiet at Night	300+	64%	66%	61%
Doctors 'Always' Communicated Well	300+	81%	83%	82%
Home Recovery Information Given	300+	88%	84%	85%
Hospital Given 9 or 10 on 10 Point Scale	300+	75%	69%	71%
Meds 'Always' Explained Before Given	300+	63%	63%	64%
Nurses 'Always' Communicated Well	300+	77%	78%	79%
Pain 'Always' Well Controlled	300+	71%	71%	71%
Room and Bathroom 'Always' Clean	300+	68%	71%	73%
Timely Help 'Always' Received	300+	64%	65%	68%
Would Definitely Recommend Hospital	300+	80%	70%	71%
Use of Medical Imaging				
Cardiac Imaging Stress Test before Surgery	909	5.2%	5.5%	5.3%
Combination Abdominal CT Scan	1,975	3.8%	10.1%	10.5%
Combination Brain/Sinus CT Scan	1,835	2.2%	2.3%	2.7%
Combination Chest CT Scan	827	0.6%	3.7%	2.7%
Follow-up Mammogram/Ultrasound	3,007	8.8%	8.9%	8.8%
Lumbar Spine MRI for Low Back Pain	300	35.3%	36.6%	37.2%

Lower Oconee Community Hospital

111 N Third Street Phone: 912-523-5113
Glenwood, GA 30428
Type: Critical Access Hospitals Emergency Services: Yes
Ownership: Proprietary

Measure	Cases	This Hosp.	State Avg.	U.S. Avg.
Blood Clot Prevention and Treatment				
Anticoagulation Overlap Therapy[5]	-	-	90%	93%
ICU Venous Thromboembolism Prophylaxis[5]	-	-	90%	92%
Incidence of Potentially Preventable VTE[5]	-	-	13%	10%
UFH with Dosages/Platelet Monitoring[5]	-	-	99%	97%
Venous Thromboembolism Prophylaxis[5]	-	-	80%	85%
Warfarin Therapy Discharge Instructions[5]	-	-	78%	75%
Chest Pain/Possible Heart Attack Care				
Aspirin Given Within 24 Hours of Arrival[1,3]	-	-	94%	96%
Fibrinolytic Meds Within 30 Min. of Arrival[3,7]	-	-	35%	58%
Average Time to ECG (minutes)[1,3]	-	-	8	7
Average Time to Transfer (minutes)[3,7]	-	-	73	60
Children's Asthma Care				
Received Home Management Plan of Care	-	-	-	88%
Received Reliever Medication	-	-	-	100%
Received Systemic Corticosteroids	-	-	-	100%
Emergency Department				
Admittance Decision Time (minutes)[5]	-	-	100	98
Head CT Results Within 45 Min. of Arrival[5]	-	-	45%	57%
Patients Who Left ER Before Being Seen[5]	-	-	3%	2%
Time from ER Arrival to Admit. (minutes)[5]	-	-	286	274
Time from ER Arrival to Discharge (minutes)[5]	-	-	140	134
Time in ER Before Being Evaluated (minutes)[5]	-	-	32	26
Time to Pain Meds for Fractures (minutes)[5]	-	-	64	57
Heart Attack Care				
Aspirin Given at Discharge[5]	-	-	99%	99%
Fibrinolytic Meds Within 30 Min. of Arrival[5]	-	-	80%	54%
PCI Within 90 Minutes of Arrival[5]	-	-	95%	96%
Statin Prescribed at Discharge[5]	-	-	98%	98%
Heart Failure Care				
ACE Inhibitor or ARB for LVSD[1,3]	-	-	97%	97%
Discharge Instructions Given[3]	18	100%	92%	94%
Evaluation of LVS Function[3]	22	100%	99%	99%
Medicare Spending				
Medicare Spending per Patient (ratio)	-	-	0.95	0.98
Pneumonia Care				
Appropriate Initial Antibiotic Given	19	100%	95%	95%
Blood Culture Timing	29	97%	97%	98%
Pregnancy and Delivery Care				
Newborn Deliveries Scheduled Early[5]	-	-	8%	6%
Preventive Care				
Immunization for Influenza[5]	-	-	88%	90%
Immunization for Pneumonia[5]	-	-	90%	92%
Stroke Care				
Anticoagulation Therapy for Atrial Fibrillation[5]	-	-	94%	95%
Antithrombotic Therapy Timing[5]	-	-	97%	98%
Assessed for Rehabilitation[5]	-	-	97%	97%
Discharged on Antithrombotic Therapy[5]	-	-	98%	99%
Discharged on Statin Medication[5]	-	-	94%	94%
Thrombolytic Therapy Timing[5]	-	-	58%	66%
Venous Thromboembolism Prophylaxis[5]	-	-	92%	94%
Written Stroke Educational Materials Given[5]	-	-	84%	88%
Surgical Care Improvement Project				
Appropriate Beta Blocker Usage[5]	-	-	97%	98%
Appropriate VTP Within 24 Hours[5]	-	-	98%	98%
Controlled Postoperative Blood Glucose[5]	-	-	96%	97%
Perioperative Temperature Management[5]	-	-	100%	100%
Prophylactic Antibiotic Selection[5]	-	-	99%	99%
Prophylactic Antibiotic Selection (Outpatient)[5]	-	-	98%	98%
Prophylactic Antibiotic Stopped[5]	-	-	98%	98%
Prophylactic Antibiotic Timing[5]	-	-	99%	99%
Prophylactic Antibiotic Timing (Outpatient)[5]	-	-	98%	98%
Urinary Catheter Removal[5]	-	-	97%	97%
Survey of Patients' Hospital Experiences				
Area Around Room 'Always' Quiet at Night[5]	-	-	66%	61%
Doctors 'Always' Communicated Well[5]	-	-	83%	82%
Home Recovery Information Given[5]	-	-	84%	85%
Hospital Given 9 or 10 on 10 Point Scale[5]	-	-	69%	71%
Meds 'Always' Explained Before Given[5]	-	-	63%	64%
Nurses 'Always' Communicated Well[5]	-	-	78%	79%
Pain 'Always' Well Controlled[5]	-	-	71%	71%
Room and Bathroom 'Always' Clean[5]	-	-	71%	73%
Timely Help 'Always' Received[5]	-	-	65%	68%
Would Definitely Recommend Hospital[5]	-	-	70%	71%
Use of Medical Imaging				
Cardiac Imaging Stress Test before Surgery[7]	-	-	5.5%	5.3%
Combination Abdominal CT Scan	92	15.2%	10.1%	10.5%
Combination Brain/Sinus CT Scan[1]	-	-	2.3%	2.7%
Combination Chest CT Scan	73	0.0%	3.7%	2.7%
Follow-up Mammogram/Ultrasound[7]	-	-	8.9%	8.8%
Lumbar Spine MRI for Low Back Pain[1]	-	-	36.6%	37.2%

Saint Mary's Good Samaritan Hospital

5401 Lake Oconee Parkway Phone: 706-453-7331
Greensboro, GA 30642
URL: www.stmarysgoodsam.org
Type: Critical Access Hospitals Emergency Services: Yes
Ownership: Proprietary

Measure	Cases	This Hosp.	State Avg.	U.S. Avg.
Blood Clot Prevention and Treatment				
Anticoagulation Overlap Therapy[5]	-	-	90%	93%
ICU Venous Thromboembolism Prophylaxis[5]	-	-	90%	92%
Incidence of Potentially Preventable VTE[5]	-	-	13%	10%
UFH with Dosages/Platelet Monitoring[5]	-	-	99%	97%
Venous Thromboembolism Prophylaxis[5]	-	-	80%	85%
Warfarin Therapy Discharge Instructions[5]	-	-	78%	75%
Chest Pain/Possible Heart Attack Care				
Aspirin Given Within 24 Hours of Arrival[1,3]	-	-	94%	96%
Fibrinolytic Meds Within 30 Min. of Arrival[3,7]	-	-	35%	58%
Average Time to ECG (minutes)[1,3]	-	-	8	7
Average Time to Transfer (minutes)[1,3]	-	-	73	60
Children's Asthma Care				
Received Home Management Plan of Care	-	-	-	88%
Received Reliever Medication	-	-	-	100%
Received Systemic Corticosteroids	-	-	-	100%
Emergency Department				
Admittance Decision Time (minutes)[2,3]	47	70	100	98
Head CT Results Within 45 Min. of Arrival[1,3]	-	-	45%	57%
Patients Who Left ER Before Being Seen	8,698	1%	3%	2%
Time from ER Arrival to Admit. (minutes)[2,3]	48	248	286	274
Time from ER Arrival to Discharge (minutes)[3]	209	90	140	134
Time in ER Before Being Evaluated (minutes)[3]	229	20	32	26
Time to Pain Meds for Fractures (minutes)[3]	22	58	64	57
Heart Attack Care				
Aspirin Given at Discharge[5]	-	-	99%	99%
Fibrinolytic Meds Within 30 Min. of Arrival[5]	-	-	80%	54%
PCI Within 90 Minutes of Arrival[5]	-	-	95%	96%
Statin Prescribed at Discharge[5]	-	-	98%	98%
Heart Failure Care				
ACE Inhibitor or ARB for LVSD[1]	-	-	97%	97%
Discharge Instructions Given	19	89%	92%	94%
Evaluation of LVS Function	28	100%	99%	99%
Medicare Spending				
Medicare Spending per Patient (ratio)	-	-	0.95	0.98
Pneumonia Care				
Appropriate Initial Antibiotic Given	26	100%	95%	95%
Blood Culture Timing	25	100%	97%	98%
Pregnancy and Delivery Care				
Newborn Deliveries Scheduled Early[5]	-	-	8%	6%
Preventive Care				
Immunization for Influenza[2,3]	84	94%	88%	90%
Immunization for Pneumonia[2,3]	74	92%	90%	92%
Stroke Care				
Anticoagulation Therapy for Atrial Fibrillation[5]	-	-	94%	95%
Antithrombotic Therapy Timing[5]	-	-	97%	98%
Assessed for Rehabilitation[5]	-	-	97%	97%
Discharged on Antithrombotic Therapy[5]	-	-	98%	99%
Discharged on Statin Medication[5]	-	-	94%	94%
Thrombolytic Therapy Timing[5]	-	-	58%	66%
Venous Thromboembolism Prophylaxis[5]	-	-	92%	94%
Written Stroke Educational Materials Given[5]	-	-	84%	88%
Surgical Care Improvement Project				
Appropriate Beta Blocker Usage[5]	-	-	97%	98%
Appropriate VTP Within 24 Hours[5]	-	-	98%	98%
Controlled Postoperative Blood Glucose[5]	-	-	96%	97%
Perioperative Temperature Management[5]	-	-	100%	100%
Prophylactic Antibiotic Selection[5]	-	-	99%	99%
Prophylactic Antibiotic Selection (Outpatient)[3,7]	-	-	98%	98%
Prophylactic Antibiotic Stopped[5]	-	-	98%	98%
Prophylactic Antibiotic Timing[5]	-	-	99%	99%
Prophylactic Antibiotic Timing (Outpatient)[3,7]	-	-	98%	98%
Urinary Catheter Removal[5]	-	-	97%	97%
Survey of Patients' Hospital Experiences				
Area Around Room 'Always' Quiet at Night[5]	-	-	66%	61%

NOTE: Hospital profiles are in alphabetical order by state, then city, then hospital within the city; Rankings exclude hospitals with less than 25 cases except for patient surveys which excludes hospitals with less than 100 cases; (a) 100-299 cases; (1) The number of cases/patients is too few to report; (2) Data submitted were based on a sample of cases/patients; (3) Results are based on a shorter time period than required; (4) Data suppressed by CMS for one or more quarters; (5) Results are not available for this reporting period; (6) Fewer than 100 patients completed the HCAHPS survey; (7) No cases met the criteria for this measure; (8) The lower limit of the confidence interval cannot be calculated if the number of observed infections equals zero; (9) No data are available from the state/territory for this reporting period; (10) The scores shown reflect fewer than 50 completed surveys; (11) There were discrepancies in the data collection process; (12) This measure does not apply to this hospital for this reporting period; (13) Results cannot be calculated for this reporting period; (14) The results for this state are combined with nearby states to protect confidentiality; Please refer to the User's Guide for a full explanation of data.

Measure	Cases	This Hosp.	State Avg.	U.S. Avg.
Doctors 'Always' Communicated Well[5]	-	-	83%	82%
Home Recovery Information Given[5]	-	-	84%	85%
Hospital Given 9 or 10 on 10 Point Scale[5]	-	-	69%	71%
Meds 'Always' Explained Before Given[5]	-	-	63%	64%
Nurses 'Always' Communicated Well[5]	-	-	78%	79%
Pain 'Always' Well Controlled[5]	-	-	71%	71%
Room and Bathroom 'Always' Clean[5]	-	-	71%	73%
Timely Help 'Always' Received[5]	-	-	65%	68%
Would Definitely Recommend Hospital[5]	-	-	70%	71%
Use of Medical Imaging				
Cardiac Imaging Stress Test before Surgery[7]	-	-	5.5%	5.3%
Combination Abdominal CT Scan	181	14.4%	10.1%	10.5%
Combination Brain/Sinus CT Scan[1]	-	-	2.3%	2.7%
Combination Chest CT Scan	110	12.7%	3.7%	2.7%
Follow-up Mammogram/Ultrasound	241	6.2%	8.9%	8.8%
Lumbar Spine MRI for Low Back Pain[1]	-	-	36.6%	37.2%

Spalding Regional Hospital

601 South 8th Street
Griffin, GA 30223
Phone: 770-228-2721
Fax: 770-229-6953
URL: www.spaldingregional.com
Type: Acute Care Hospitals
Emergency Services: Yes
Ownership: Proprietary
Beds: 160

Key Personnel:
Pediatric Ambulatory Care . . . . . . Bill Colvin
Pediatric In-Patient Care . . . . Bill Colvin
Quality Assurance . . . . Nancy Franklin
Chief of Medical Staff . . . . Vinod C Mehta
CEO/President . . . . John Quinn
Emergency Room . . . . Howard Stirne

Measure	Cases	This Hosp.	State Avg.	U.S. Avg.
Blood Clot Prevention and Treatment				
Anticoagulation Overlap Therapy[2]	78	96%	90%	93%
ICU Venous Thromboembolism Prophylaxis[2]	116	94%	90%	92%
Incidence of Potentially Preventable VTE[1,2]	-	-	13%	10%
UFH with Dosages/Platelet Monitoring[2]	57	100%	99%	97%
Venous Thromboembolism Prophylaxis[2]	350	91%	80%	85%
Warfarin Therapy Discharge Instructions[2]	56	100%	78%	75%
Chest Pain/Possible Heart Attack Care				
Aspirin Given Within 24 Hours of Arrival	16	94%	94%	96%
Fibrinolytic Meds Within 30 Min. of Arrival[3,7]	-	-	35%	58%
Average Time to ECG (minutes)	16	6	8	7
Average Time to Transfer (minutes)[3,7]	-	-	73	60
Children's Asthma Care				
Received Home Management Plan of Care	-	-	-	88%
Received Reliever Medication	-	-	-	100%
Received Systemic Corticosteroids	-	-	-	100%
Emergency Department				
Admittance Decision Time (minutes)[2]	530	106	100	98
Head CT Results Within 45 Min. of Arrival	25	92%	45%	57%
Patients Who Left ER Before Being Seen	54,365	2%	3%	2%
Time from ER Arrival to Admit. (minutes)[2]	598	286	286	274
Time from ER Arrival to Discharge (minutes)	446	162	140	134
Time in ER Before Being Evaluated (minutes)	486	48	32	26
Time to Pain Meds for Fractures (minutes)	164	74	64	57
Heart Attack Care				
Aspirin Given at Discharge	180	99%	99%	99%
Fibrinolytic Meds Within 30 Min. of Arrival[7]	-	-	80%	54%
PCI Within 90 Minutes of Arrival	50	96%	95%	96%
Statin Prescribed at Discharge	178	99%	98%	98%
Heart Failure Care				
ACE Inhibitor or ARB for LVSD	109	100%	97%	97%
Discharge Instructions Given	255	100%	92%	94%
Evaluation of LVS Function	287	100%	99%	99%
Medicare Spending				
Medicare Spending per Patient (ratio)	-	0.98	0.95	0.98
Pneumonia Care				
Appropriate Initial Antibiotic Given	166	93%	95%	95%
Blood Culture Timing	263	99%	97%	98%
Pregnancy and Delivery Care				
Newborn Deliveries Scheduled Early[2]	54	2%	8%	6%
Preventive Care				
Immunization for Influenza[2]	590	97%	88%	90%
Immunization for Pneumonia[2]	776	97%	90%	92%
Stroke Care				
Anticoagulation Therapy for Atrial Fibrillation	13	100%	94%	95%
Antithrombotic Therapy Timing	127	95%	97%	98%
Assessed for Rehabilitation	134	99%	97%	97%
Discharged on Antithrombotic Therapy	131	99%	98%	99%
Discharged on Statin Medication	99	99%	94%	94%
Thrombolytic Therapy Timing[1]	-	-	58%	66%
Venous Thromboembolism Prophylaxis	136	91%	92%	94%
Written Stroke Educational Materials Given	80	94%	84%	88%
Surgical Care Improvement Project				
Appropriate Beta Blocker Usage	77	97%	97%	98%
Appropriate VTP Within 24 Hours	357	98%	98%	98%
Controlled Postoperative Blood Glucose[7]	-	-	96%	97%
Perioperative Temperature Management	400	100%	100%	100%
Prophylactic Antibiotic Selection	268	99%	99%	99%
Prophylactic Antibiotic Selection (Outpatient)	205	98%	98%	98%
Prophylactic Antibiotic Stopped	257	97%	98%	98%
Prophylactic Antibiotic Timing	268	99%	99%	99%
Prophylactic Antibiotic Timing (Outpatient)	207	98%	98%	98%
Urinary Catheter Removal	164	97%	97%	97%
Survey of Patients' Hospital Experiences				
Area Around Room 'Always' Quiet at Night	300+	60%	66%	61%
Doctors 'Always' Communicated Well	300+	83%	83%	82%
Home Recovery Information Given	300+	83%	84%	85%
Hospital Given 9 or 10 on 10 Point Scale	300+	66%	69%	71%
Meds 'Always' Explained Before Given	300+	58%	63%	64%
Nurses 'Always' Communicated Well	300+	76%	78%	79%
Pain 'Always' Well Controlled	300+	69%	71%	71%
Room and Bathroom 'Always' Clean	300+	64%	71%	73%
Timely Help 'Always' Received	300+	69%	65%	68%
Would Definitely Recommend Hospital	300+	62%	70%	71%
Use of Medical Imaging				
Cardiac Imaging Stress Test before Surgery	256	8.2%	5.5%	5.3%
Combination Abdominal CT Scan	590	4.7%	10.1%	10.5%
Combination Brain/Sinus CT Scan	866	0.8%	2.3%	2.7%
Combination Chest CT Scan	167	1.8%	3.7%	2.7%
Follow-up Mammogram/Ultrasound	1,046	6.1%	8.9%	8.8%
Lumbar Spine MRI for Low Back Pain[1]	-	-	36.6%	37.2%

Taylor Regional Hospital

222 Perry Hwy
Hawkinsville, GA 31036
Phone: 478-783-0200
Fax: 478-783-2731
URL: www.taylorregional.org
Type: Acute Care Hospitals
Emergency Services: Yes
Ownership: Voluntary non-profit - Private
Beds: 55

Key Personnel:
Quality Assurance . . . . Karen Brown
Emergency Room . . . . William Cirillo, MD
Cardiac Laboratory. . . . . Helen Laster
CEO/President. . . . . Dan Maddock
Operating Room. . . . . Patricia Mayo
Chief of Medical Staff . . . . Nikki Paulk

Measure	Cases	This Hosp.	State Avg.	U.S. Avg.
Blood Clot Prevention and Treatment				
Anticoagulation Overlap Therapy[1,2]	-	-	90%	93%
ICU Venous Thromboembolism Prophylaxis[2]	60	93%	90%	92%
Incidence of Potentially Preventable VTE[1,2]	-	-	13%	10%
UFH with Dosages/Platelet Monitoring[1,2]	-	-	99%	97%
Venous Thromboembolism Prophylaxis[2]	128	69%	80%	85%
Warfarin Therapy Discharge Instructions[1,2]	-	-	78%	75%
Chest Pain/Possible Heart Attack Care				
Aspirin Given Within 24 Hours of Arrival	32	94%	94%	96%
Fibrinolytic Meds Within 30 Min. of Arrival[7]	-	-	35%	58%
Average Time to ECG (minutes)	30	5	8	7
Average Time to Transfer (minutes)[1]	-	-	73	60
Children's Asthma Care				
Received Home Management Plan of Care	-	-	-	88%
Received Reliever Medication	-	-	-	100%
Received Systemic Corticosteroids	-	-	-	100%
Emergency Department				
Admittance Decision Time (minutes)[2]	298	75	100	98
Head CT Results Within 45 Min. of Arrival[1,3]	-	-	45%	57%
Patients Who Left ER Before Being Seen	10,099	1%	3%	2%
Time from ER Arrival to Admit. (minutes)[2]	318	222	286	274
Time from ER Arrival to Discharge (minutes)	391	104	140	134
Time in ER Before Being Evaluated (minutes)	432	15	32	26
Time to Pain Meds for Fractures (minutes)	39	34	64	57
Heart Attack Care				
Aspirin Given at Discharge[3,7]	-	-	99%	99%
Fibrinolytic Meds Within 30 Min. of Arrival[3,7]	-	-	80%	54%
PCI Within 90 Minutes of Arrival[3,7]	-	-	95%	96%
Statin Prescribed at Discharge[3,7]	-	-	98%	98%
Heart Failure Care				
ACE Inhibitor or ARB for LVSD[2]	12	100%	97%	97%
Discharge Instructions Given[2]	25	88%	92%	94%
Evaluation of LVS Function[2]	29	97%	99%	99%
Medicare Spending				
Medicare Spending per Patient (ratio)	-	1.01	0.95	0.98
Pneumonia Care				
Appropriate Initial Antibiotic Given[2]	42	95%	95%	95%
Blood Culture Timing[2]	51	94%	97%	98%
Pregnancy and Delivery Care				
Newborn Deliveries Scheduled Early	61	82%	8%	6%
Preventive Care				
Immunization for Influenza[2]	266	89%	88%	90%
Immunization for Pneumonia[2]	341	93%	90%	92%
Stroke Care				
Anticoagulation Therapy for Atrial Fibrillation[2,7]	-	-	94%	95%
Antithrombotic Therapy Timing[1,2]	-	-	97%	98%
Assessed for Rehabilitation[1,2]	-	-	97%	97%
Discharged on Antithrombotic Therapy[1,2]	-	-	98%	99%
Discharged on Statin Medication[1,2]	-	-	94%	94%
Thrombolytic Therapy Timing[1,2]	-	-	58%	66%
Venous Thromboembolism Prophylaxis[1,2]	-	-	92%	94%
Written Stroke Educational Materials Given[1,2]	-	-	84%	88%
Surgical Care Improvement Project				
Appropriate Beta Blocker Usage[2]	27	93%	97%	98%
Appropriate VTP Within 24 Hours[2]	76	99%	98%	98%
Controlled Postoperative Blood Glucose[2,7]	-	-	96%	97%
Perioperative Temperature Management[2]	84	100%	100%	100%
Prophylactic Antibiotic Selection[2]	64	100%	99%	99%
Prophylactic Antibiotic Selection (Outpatient)[1,3]	-	-	98%	98%
Prophylactic Antibiotic Stopped[2]	64	91%	98%	98%
Prophylactic Antibiotic Timing[2]	64	100%	99%	99%
Prophylactic Antibiotic Timing (Outpatient)[1,3]	-	-	98%	98%
Urinary Catheter Removal[2]	12	92%	97%	97%
Survey of Patients' Hospital Experiences				
Area Around Room 'Always' Quiet at Night	(a)	69%	66%	61%
Doctors 'Always' Communicated Well	(a)	87%	83%	82%
Home Recovery Information Given	(a)	84%	84%	85%
Hospital Given 9 or 10 on 10 Point Scale	(a)	68%	69%	71%
Meds 'Always' Explained Before Given	(a)	69%	63%	64%
Nurses 'Always' Communicated Well	(a)	82%	78%	79%
Pain 'Always' Well Controlled	(a)	71%	71%	71%
Room and Bathroom 'Always' Clean	(a)	74%	71%	73%
Timely Help 'Always' Received	(a)	67%	65%	68%
Would Definitely Recommend Hospital	(a)	75%	70%	71%
Use of Medical Imaging				
Cardiac Imaging Stress Test before Surgery	134	4.5%	5.5%	5.3%
Combination Abdominal CT Scan	293	7.2%	10.1%	10.5%
Combination Brain/Sinus CT Scan[1]	-	-	2.3%	2.7%
Combination Chest CT Scan	182	0.5%	3.7%	2.7%
Follow-up Mammogram/Ultrasound	497	7.0%	8.9%	8.8%
Lumbar Spine MRI for Low Back Pain	60	45.0%	36.6%	37.2%

Jeff Davis Hospital

163 South Tallahassee Street, PO Box 1690
Phone: 912-375-7781
Hazlehurst, GA 31539
Fax: 912-375-4055
URL: www.jeffdavishospital.org
Type: Critical Access Hospitals
Emergency Services: Yes
Ownership: Govt - Hospital Dist/Auth
Beds: 50

Key Personnel:
Operating Room. . . . . Rosa Bowen, RN
Quality Assurance . . . . Shirley McIver, RN
CEO . . . . Jerry Schoendienst
Chief of Medical Staff . . . . Kyle Smith
CEO/President. . . . . Oreta L Williams
Emergency Room . . . . Paula Wilzoa

NOTE: Hospital profiles are in alphabetical order by state, then city, then hospital within the city; Rankings exclude hospitals with less than 25 cases except for patient surveys which excludes hospitals with less than 100 cases; (a) 100-299 cases; (1) The number of cases/patients is too few to report; (2) Data submitted were based on a sample of cases/patients; (3) Results are based on a shorter time period than required; (4) Data suppressed by CMS for one or more quarters; (5) Results are not available for this reporting period; (6) Fewer than 100 patients completed the HCAHPS survey; (7) No cases met the criteria for this measure; (8) The lower limit of the confidence interval cannot be calculated if the number of observed infections equals zero; (9) No data are available from the state/territory for this reporting period; (10) The scores shown reflect fewer than 50 completed surveys; (11) There were discrepancies in the data collection process; (12) This measure does not apply to this hospital for this reporting period; (13) Results cannot be calculated for this reporting period; (14) The results for this state are combined with nearby states to protect confidentiality; Please refer to the User's Guide for a full explanation of data.

Measure	Cases	This Hosp.	State Avg.	U.S. Avg.
Blood Clot Prevention and Treatment				
Anticoagulation Overlap Therapy[3,7]	-	-	90%	93%
ICU Venous Thromboembolism Prophylaxis[1,3]	-	-	90%	92%
Incidence of Potentially Preventable VTE[3,7]	-	-	13%	10%
UFH with Dosages/Platelet Monitoring[3,7]	-	-	99%	97%
Venous Thromboembolism Prophylaxis[3]	15	73%	80%	85%
Warfarin Therapy Discharge Instructions[3,7]	-	-	78%	75%
Chest Pain/Possible Heart Attack Care				
Aspirin Given Within 24 Hours of Arrival	17	94%	94%	96%
Fibrinolytic Meds Within 30 Min. of Arrival[1,3]	-	-	35%	58%
Average Time to ECG (minutes)[7]	-	-	8	7
Average Time to Transfer (minutes)[3,7]	-	-	73	60
Children's Asthma Care				
Received Home Management Plan of Care	-	-	-	88%
Received Reliever Medication	-	-	-	100%
Received Systemic Corticosteroids	-	-	-	100%
Emergency Department				
Admittance Decision Time (minutes)[2]	78	56	100	98
Head CT Results Within 45 Min. of Arrival	13	0%	45%	57%
Patients Who Left ER Before Being Seen	8,794	6%	3%	2%
Time from ER Arrival to Admit. (minutes)[2]	78	198	286	274
Time from ER Arrival to Discharge (minutes)[11]	-	-	140	134
Time in ER Before Being Evaluated (minutes)[7]	-	-	32	26
Time to Pain Meds for Fractures (minutes)[3,7]	-	-	64	57
Heart Attack Care				
Aspirin Given at Discharge[3,7]	-	-	99%	99%
Fibrinolytic Meds Within 30 Min. of Arrival[3,7]	-	-	80%	54%
PCI Within 90 Minutes of Arrival[3,7]	-	-	95%	96%
Statin Prescribed at Discharge[3,7]	-	-	98%	98%
Heart Failure Care				
ACE Inhibitor or ARB for LVSD[1]	-	-	97%	97%
Discharge Instructions Given	22	100%	92%	94%
Evaluation of LVS Function	25	72%	99%	99%
Medicare Spending				
Medicare Spending per Patient (ratio)	-	-	0.95	0.98
Pneumonia Care				
Appropriate Initial Antibiotic Given	50	86%	95%	95%
Blood Culture Timing	39	95%	97%	98%
Pregnancy and Delivery Care				
Newborn Deliveries Scheduled Early[5]	-	-	8%	6%
Preventive Care				
Immunization for Influenza[3]	31	100%	88%	90%
Immunization for Pneumonia[3]	53	100%	90%	92%
Stroke Care				
Anticoagulation Therapy for Atrial Fibrillation[5]	-	-	94%	95%
Antithrombotic Therapy Timing[5]	-	-	97%	98%
Assessed for Rehabilitation[5]	-	-	97%	97%
Discharged on Antithrombotic Therapy[5]	-	-	98%	99%
Discharged on Statin Medication[5]	-	-	94%	94%
Thrombolytic Therapy Timing[5]	-	-	58%	66%
Venous Thromboembolism Prophylaxis[5]	-	-	92%	94%
Written Stroke Educational Materials Given[5]	-	-	84%	88%
Surgical Care Improvement Project				
Appropriate Beta Blocker Usage[5]	-	-	97%	98%
Appropriate VTP Within 24 Hours[5]	-	-	98%	98%
Controlled Postoperative Blood Glucose[5]	-	-	96%	97%
Perioperative Temperature Management[5]	-	-	100%	100%
Prophylactic Antibiotic Selection[5]	-	-	99%	99%
Prophylactic Antibiotic Selection (Outpatient)[1,3]	-	-	98%	98%
Prophylactic Antibiotic Stopped[5]	-	-	98%	98%
Prophylactic Antibiotic Timing[5]	-	-	99%	99%
Prophylactic Antibiotic Timing (Outpatient)[1,3]	-	-	98%	98%
Urinary Catheter Removal[5]	-	-	97%	97%
Survey of Patients' Hospital Experiences				
Area Around Room 'Always' Quiet at Night[5]	-	-	66%	61%
Doctors 'Always' Communicated Well[5]	-	-	83%	82%
Home Recovery Information Given[5]	-	-	84%	85%
Hospital Given 9 or 10 on 10 Point Scale[5]	-	-	69%	71%
Meds 'Always' Explained Before Given[5]	-	-	63%	64%
Nurses 'Always' Communicated Well[5]	-	-	78%	79%
Pain 'Always' Well Controlled[5]	-	-	71%	71%
Room and Bathroom 'Always' Clean[5]	-	-	71%	73%
Timely Help 'Always' Received[5]	-	-	65%	68%
Would Definitely Recommend Hospital[5]	-	-	70%	71%
Use of Medical Imaging				
Cardiac Imaging Stress Test before Surgery[7]	-	-	5.5%	5.3%
Combination Abdominal CT Scan	116	16.4%	10.1%	10.5%
Combination Brain/Sinus CT Scan[1]	-	-	2.3%	2.7%
Combination Chest CT Scan[1]	-	-	3.7%	2.7%
Follow-up Mammogram/Ultrasound	169	10.1%	8.9%	8.8%
Lumbar Spine MRI for Low Back Pain[1]	-	-	36.6%	37.2%

Chatuge Regional Hospital

110 East Main Street
Hiawassee, GA 30546
Phone: 706-896-2222
Fax: 706-745-7677
URL: www.chatugeregionalhospital.org
Type: Critical Access Hospitals
Emergency Services: Yes
Ownership: Govt - Hospital Dist/Auth
Beds: 25

Key Personnel:
Emergency Room . . . . Paul Conrad
Administrator . . . . Lewis Kelley
Ambulatory Care . . . . Ricky Mathis
Radiology. . . . . Israel Rogers
Quality Assurance . . . . Dexter Shook
Chief of Medical Staff. . . . . Robert F Stahlkuppe

Measure	Cases	This Hosp.	State Avg.	U.S. Avg.
Blood Clot Prevention and Treatment				
Anticoagulation Overlap Therapy[1,2]	-	-	90%	93%
ICU Venous Thromboembolism Prophylaxis[1,2]	-	-	90%	92%
Incidence of Potentially Preventable VTE[2,7]	-	-	13%	10%
UFH with Dosages/Platelet Monitoring[2,7]	-	-	99%	97%
Venous Thromboembolism Prophylaxis[2]	79	100%	80%	85%
Warfarin Therapy Discharge Instructions[2,7]	-	-	78%	75%
Chest Pain/Possible Heart Attack Care				
Aspirin Given Within 24 Hours of Arrival	37	95%	94%	96%
Fibrinolytic Meds Within 30 Min. of Arrival[1]	-	-	35%	58%
Average Time to ECG (minutes)	38	21	8	7
Average Time to Transfer (minutes)[1]	-	-	73	60
Children's Asthma Care				
Received Home Management Plan of Care	-	-	-	88%
Received Reliever Medication	-	-	-	100%
Received Systemic Corticosteroids	-	-	-	100%
Emergency Department				
Admittance Decision Time (minutes)	51	68	100	98
Head CT Results Within 45 Min. of Arrival[1]	-	-	45%	57%
Patients Who Left ER Before Being Seen	5,491	0%	3%	2%
Time from ER Arrival to Admit. (minutes)	52	255	286	274
Time from ER Arrival to Discharge (minutes)[11]	395	105	140	134
Time in ER Before Being Evaluated (minutes)	475	29	32	26
Time to Pain Meds for Fractures (minutes)	24	57	64	57
Heart Attack Care				
Aspirin Given at Discharge[1,3]	-	-	99%	99%
Fibrinolytic Meds Within 30 Min. of Arrival[3,7]	-	-	80%	54%
PCI Within 90 Minutes of Arrival[3,7]	-	-	95%	96%
Statin Prescribed at Discharge[1,3]	-	-	98%	98%
Heart Failure Care				
ACE Inhibitor or ARB for LVSD[1]	-	-	97%	97%
Discharge Instructions Given[1]	-	-	92%	94%
Evaluation of LVS Function	11	91%	99%	99%
Medicare Spending				
Medicare Spending per Patient (ratio)	-	-	0.95	0.98
Pneumonia Care				
Appropriate Initial Antibiotic Given	30	100%	95%	95%
Blood Culture Timing	42	100%	97%	98%
Pregnancy and Delivery Care				
Newborn Deliveries Scheduled Early[5]	-	-	8%	6%
Preventive Care				
Immunization for Influenza	121	93%	88%	90%
Immunization for Pneumonia	214	93%	90%	92%
Stroke Care				
Anticoagulation Therapy for Atrial Fibrillation[1]	-	-	94%	95%
Antithrombotic Therapy Timing[1]	-	-	97%	98%
Assessed for Rehabilitation[1]	-	-	97%	97%
Discharged on Antithrombotic Therapy[1]	-	-	98%	99%
Discharged on Statin Medication[1]	-	-	94%	94%
Thrombolytic Therapy Timing[7]	-	-	58%	66%
Venous Thromboembolism Prophylaxis[1]	-	-	92%	94%
Written Stroke Educational Materials Given[1]	-	-	84%	88%
Surgical Care Improvement Project				
Appropriate Beta Blocker Usage[5]	-	-	97%	98%
Appropriate VTP Within 24 Hours[5]	-	-	98%	98%
Controlled Postoperative Blood Glucose[5]	-	-	96%	97%
Perioperative Temperature Management[5]	-	-	100%	100%
Prophylactic Antibiotic Selection[5]	-	-	99%	99%
Prophylactic Antibiotic Selection (Outpatient)[5]	-	-	98%	98%
Prophylactic Antibiotic Stopped[5]	-	-	98%	98%
Prophylactic Antibiotic Timing[5]	-	-	99%	99%
Prophylactic Antibiotic Timing (Outpatient)[5]	-	-	98%	98%
Urinary Catheter Removal[5]	-	-	97%	97%
Survey of Patients' Hospital Experiences				
Area Around Room 'Always' Quiet at Night[5]	-	-	66%	61%
Doctors 'Always' Communicated Well[5]	-	-	83%	82%
Home Recovery Information Given[5]	-	-	84%	85%
Hospital Given 9 or 10 on 10 Point Scale[5]	-	-	69%	71%
Meds 'Always' Explained Before Given[5]	-	-	63%	64%
Nurses 'Always' Communicated Well[5]	-	-	78%	79%
Pain 'Always' Well Controlled[5]	-	-	71%	71%
Room and Bathroom 'Always' Clean[5]	-	-	71%	73%
Timely Help 'Always' Received[5]	-	-	65%	68%
Would Definitely Recommend Hospital[5]	-	-	70%	71%
Use of Medical Imaging				
Cardiac Imaging Stress Test before Surgery[7]	-	-	5.5%	5.3%
Combination Abdominal CT Scan	259	9.3%	10.1%	10.5%
Combination Brain/Sinus CT Scan[1]	-	-	2.3%	2.7%
Combination Chest CT Scan	137	4.4%	3.7%	2.7%
Follow-up Mammogram/Ultrasound	252	9.1%	8.9%	8.8%
Lumbar Spine MRI for Low Back Pain[1]	-	-	36.6%	37.2%

Liberty Regional Medical Center

462 E G Miles Parkway
Hinesville, GA 31310
Phone: 912-369-9438
Fax: 912-369-3653
E-mail: jcampbell@libertyregional.org
URL: www.libertyregional.org
Type: Critical Access Hospitals
Emergency Services: Yes
Ownership: Govt - Hospital Dist/Auth
Beds: 25

Key Personnel:
Radiology. . . . . Sanford Berens, MD
Chief of Medical Staff. . . . . Chris Blasy, MD
Patient Relations . . . . Joyce Campbell
Operating Room. . . . . Lori Campbell, RN
Emergency Room . . . . Kathy Donaldson
CEO . . . . Scott Kroell
Infection Control. . . . . Peggy McGee
Quality Assurance . . . . Lisa Pearson

Measure	Cases	This Hosp.	State Avg.	U.S. Avg.
Blood Clot Prevention and Treatment				
Anticoagulation Overlap Therapy[1,2]	-	-	90%	93%
ICU Venous Thromboembolism Prophylaxis[2,3]	-	-	90%	92%
Incidence of Potentially Preventable VTE[2,3]	-	-	13%	10%
UFH with Dosages/Platelet Monitoring[2,3]	-	-	99%	97%
Venous Thromboembolism Prophylaxis[2,3]	89	83%	80%	85%
Warfarin Therapy Discharge Instructions[1,2]	-	-	78%	75%
Chest Pain/Possible Heart Attack Care				
Aspirin Given Within 24 Hours of Arrival	52	94%	94%	96%
Fibrinolytic Meds Within 30 Min. of Arrival[1]	-	-	35%	58%
Average Time to ECG (minutes)	25	7	8	7
Average Time to Transfer (minutes)[1]	-	-	73	60
Children's Asthma Care				
Received Home Management Plan of Care	-	-	-	88%
Received Reliever Medication	-	-	-	100%
Received Systemic Corticosteroids	-	-	-	100%
Emergency Department				
Admittance Decision Time (minutes)[2]	125	72	100	98
Head CT Results Within 45 Min. of Arrival	14	0%	45%	57%
Patients Who Left ER Before Being Seen	23,987	1%	3%	2%
Time from ER Arrival to Admit. (minutes)[2]	125	274	286	274
Time from ER Arrival to Discharge (minutes)	214	110	140	134
Time in ER Before Being Evaluated (minutes)	240	26	32	26
Time to Pain Meds for Fractures (minutes)[1]	-	-	64	57

NOTE: Hospital profiles are in alphabetical order by state, then city, then hospital within the city; Rankings exclude hospitals with less than 25 cases except for patient surveys which excludes hospitals with less than 100 cases; (a) 100-299 cases; (1) The number of cases/patients is too few to report; (2) Data submitted were based on a sample of cases/patients; (3) Results are based on a shorter time period than required; (4) Data suppressed by CMS for one or more quarters; (5) Results are not available for this reporting period; (6) Fewer than 100 patients completed the HCAHPS survey; (7) No cases met the criteria for this measure; (8) The lower limit of the confidence interval cannot be calculated if the number of observed infections equals zero; (9) No data are available from the state/territory for this reporting period; (10) The scores shown reflect fewer than 50 completed surveys; (11) There were discrepancies in the data collection process; (12) This measure does not apply to this hospital for this reporting period; (13) Results cannot be calculated for this reporting period; (14) The results for this state are combined with nearby states to protect confidentiality; Please refer to the User's Guide for a full explanation of data.

Measure	Cases	This Hosp.	State Avg.	U.S. Avg.
Heart Attack Care				
Aspirin Given at Discharge[1,3]	-	-	99%	99%
Fibrinolytic Meds Within 30 Min. of Arrival[3,7]	-	-	80%	54%
PCI Within 90 Minutes of Arrival[3,7]	-	-	95%	96%
Statin Prescribed at Discharge[1,3]	-	-	98%	98%
Heart Failure Care				
ACE Inhibitor or ARB for LVSD	13	92%	97%	97%
Discharge Instructions Given	36	97%	92%	94%
Evaluation of LVS Function	40	100%	99%	99%
Medicare Spending				
Medicare Spending per Patient (ratio)	-	-	0.95	0.98
Pneumonia Care				
Appropriate Initial Antibiotic Given[2]	44	70%	95%	95%
Blood Culture Timing[2]	37	97%	97%	98%
Pregnancy and Delivery Care				
Newborn Deliveries Scheduled Early[5]	-	-	8%	6%
Preventive Care				
Immunization for Influenza[2]	64	64%	88%	90%
Immunization for Pneumonia[2]	154	68%	90%	92%
Stroke Care				
Anticoagulation Therapy for Atrial Fibrillation[3,7]	-	-	94%	95%
Antithrombotic Therapy Timing[3,7]	-	-	97%	98%
Assessed for Rehabilitation[1,3]	-	-	97%	97%
Discharged on Antithrombotic Therapy[3,7]	-	-	98%	99%
Discharged on Statin Medication[3,7]	-	-	94%	94%
Thrombolytic Therapy Timing[1,3]	-	-	58%	66%
Venous Thromboembolism Prophylaxis[1,3]	-	-	92%	94%
Written Stroke Educational Materials Given[1,3]	-	-	84%	88%
Surgical Care Improvement Project				
Appropriate Beta Blocker Usage[1]	-	-	97%	98%
Appropriate VTP Within 24 Hours	50	84%	98%	98%
Controlled Postoperative Blood Glucose[7]	-	-	96%	97%
Perioperative Temperature Management	53	100%	100%	100%
Prophylactic Antibiotic Selection	32	88%	99%	99%
Prophylactic Antibiotic Selection (Outpatient)	11	91%	98%	98%
Prophylactic Antibiotic Stopped	31	100%	98%	98%
Prophylactic Antibiotic Timing	32	88%	99%	99%
Prophylactic Antibiotic Timing (Outpatient)	13	77%	98%	98%
Urinary Catheter Removal	22	100%	97%	97%
Survey of Patients' Hospital Experiences				
Area Around Room 'Always' Quiet at Night[5]	-	-	66%	61%
Doctors 'Always' Communicated Well[5]	-	-	83%	82%
Home Recovery Information Given[5]	-	-	84%	85%
Hospital Given 9 or 10 on 10 Point Scale[5]	-	-	69%	71%
Meds 'Always' Explained Before Given[5]	-	-	63%	64%
Nurses 'Always' Communicated Well[5]	-	-	78%	79%
Pain 'Always' Well Controlled[5]	-	-	71%	71%
Room and Bathroom 'Always' Clean[5]	-	-	71%	73%
Timely Help 'Always' Received[5]	-	-	65%	68%
Would Definitely Recommend Hospital[5]	-	-	70%	71%
Use of Medical Imaging				
Cardiac Imaging Stress Test before Surgery[1]	-	-	5.5%	5.3%
Combination Abdominal CT Scan	289	4.8%	10.1%	10.5%
Combination Brain/Sinus CT Scan[1]	-	-	2.3%	2.7%
Combination Chest CT Scan	231	0.4%	3.7%	2.7%
Follow-up Mammogram/Ultrasound	471	3.0%	8.9%	8.8%
Lumbar Spine MRI for Low Back Pain[1]	-	-	36.6%	37.2%

Wellstar Paulding Hospital

148 Bill Carruth Parkway
Hiram, GA 30141
URL: www.wellstar.org
Phone: 470-644-7000
Fax: 770-443-7057
Type: Acute Care Hospitals
Ownership: Voluntary non-profit - Other
Emergency Services: Yes
Beds: 219

Key Personnel:
CEO/President. . . . . Rob Lipson
Emergency Room . . . . Okiki Louis
Operating Room. . . . . Anne Medlin
Chief of Medical Staff. . . . . Charles Pesson, MD
Pediatric Ambulatory Care . . . . . . Abolhassan Yamin, MD
Pediatric In-Patient Care . . . . Abolhassan Yamin, MD

Measure	Cases	This Hosp.	State Avg.	U.S. Avg.
Blood Clot Prevention and Treatment				
Anticoagulation Overlap Therapy[2]	20	95%	90%	93%
ICU Venous Thromboembolism Prophylaxis[2]	25	92%	90%	92%
Incidence of Potentially Preventable VTE[1,2]	-	-	13%	10%
UFH with Dosages/Platelet Monitoring[2]	12	100%	99%	97%
Venous Thromboembolism Prophylaxis[2]	184	88%	80%	85%
Warfarin Therapy Discharge Instructions[2]	13	100%	78%	75%
Chest Pain/Possible Heart Attack Care				
Aspirin Given Within 24 Hours of Arrival	150	94%	94%	96%
Fibrinolytic Meds Within 30 Min. of Arrival[7]	-	-	35%	58%
Average Time to ECG (minutes)	152	0	8	7
Average Time to Transfer (minutes)	18	32	73	60
Children's Asthma Care				
Received Home Management Plan of Care	-	-	-	88%
Received Reliever Medication	-	-	-	100%
Received Systemic Corticosteroids	-	-	-	100%
Emergency Department				
Admittance Decision Time (minutes)[2]	388	55	100	98
Head CT Results Within 45 Min. of Arrival[7]	-	-	45%	57%
Patients Who Left ER Before Being Seen	42,324	3%	3%	2%
Time from ER Arrival to Admit. (minutes)[2]	412	257	286	274
Time from ER Arrival to Discharge (minutes)	402	132	140	134
Time in ER Before Being Evaluated (minutes)	391	36	32	26
Time to Pain Meds for Fractures (minutes)	112	66	64	57
Heart Attack Care				
Aspirin Given at Discharge[3,7]	-	-	99%	99%
Fibrinolytic Meds Within 30 Min. of Arrival[3,7]	-	-	80%	54%
PCI Within 90 Minutes of Arrival[3,7]	-	-	95%	96%
Statin Prescribed at Discharge[3,7]	-	-	98%	98%
Heart Failure Care				
ACE Inhibitor or ARB for LVSD[1]	-	-	97%	97%
Discharge Instructions Given	40	80%	92%	94%
Evaluation of LVS Function	44	100%	99%	99%
Medicare Spending				
Medicare Spending per Patient (ratio)	-	0.86	0.95	0.98
Pneumonia Care				
Appropriate Initial Antibiotic Given	63	97%	95%	95%
Blood Culture Timing	121	99%	97%	98%
Pregnancy and Delivery Care				
Newborn Deliveries Scheduled Early[7]	-	-	8%	6%
Preventive Care				
Immunization for Influenza[2]	317	98%	88%	90%
Immunization for Pneumonia[2]	447	97%	90%	92%
Stroke Care				
Anticoagulation Therapy for Atrial Fibrillation[2,7]	-	-	94%	95%
Antithrombotic Therapy Timing[1,2]	-	-	97%	98%
Assessed for Rehabilitation[1,2]	-	-	97%	97%
Discharged on Antithrombotic Therapy[1,2]	-	-	98%	99%
Discharged on Statin Medication[1,2]	-	-	94%	94%
Thrombolytic Therapy Timing[2,7]	-	-	58%	66%
Venous Thromboembolism Prophylaxis[1,2]	-	-	92%	94%
Written Stroke Educational Materials Given[2,7]	-	-	84%	88%
Surgical Care Improvement Project				
Appropriate Beta Blocker Usage[2]	40	100%	97%	98%
Appropriate VTP Within 24 Hours[2]	142	100%	98%	98%
Controlled Postoperative Blood Glucose[2,7]	-	-	96%	97%
Perioperative Temperature Management[2]	153	100%	100%	100%
Prophylactic Antibiotic Selection[2]	103	100%	99%	99%
Prophylactic Antibiotic Selection (Outpatient)	13	92%	98%	98%
Prophylactic Antibiotic Stopped[2]	100	99%	98%	98%
Prophylactic Antibiotic Timing[2]	103	99%	99%	99%
Prophylactic Antibiotic Timing (Outpatient)	13	100%	98%	98%
Urinary Catheter Removal[2]	118	99%	97%	97%
Survey of Patients' Hospital Experiences				
Area Around Room 'Always' Quiet at Night	300+	59%	66%	61%
Doctors 'Always' Communicated Well	300+	81%	83%	82%
Home Recovery Information Given	300+	84%	84%	85%
Hospital Given 9 or 10 on 10 Point Scale	300+	70%	69%	71%
Meds 'Always' Explained Before Given	300+	67%	63%	64%
Nurses 'Always' Communicated Well	300+	81%	78%	79%
Pain 'Always' Well Controlled	300+	71%	71%	71%
Room and Bathroom 'Always' Clean	300+	64%	71%	73%
Timely Help 'Always' Received	300+	64%	65%	68%
Would Definitely Recommend Hospital	300+	70%	70%	71%
Use of Medical Imaging				
Cardiac Imaging Stress Test before Surgery	185	5.4%	5.5%	5.3%
Combination Abdominal CT Scan	733	5.9%	10.1%	10.5%
Combination Brain/Sinus CT Scan[1]	-	-	2.3%	2.7%
Combination Chest CT Scan	780	0.8%	3.7%	2.7%
Follow-up Mammogram/Ultrasound	952	11.6%	8.9%	8.8%
Lumbar Spine MRI for Low Back Pain	71	35.2%	36.6%	37.2%

Clinch Memorial Hospital

1050 Valdosta Highway
Homerville, GA 31634
Phone: 912-487-5211
Fax: 912-487-3769
Type: Critical Access Hospitals
Ownership: Govt - Hospital Dist/Auth
Emergency Services: Yes
Beds: 25

Key Personnel:
Chief of Medical Staff. . . . . Sam B Cobarrubias, MD
CEO/President. . . . . Phillip C Cook
Ambulatory Care . . . . Wallace Hodge
Emergency Room . . . . Roger Huelsnitz, MD
Radiology. . . . . Sheila Rogers
Quality Assurance . . . . Patricia Stalzey
Operating Room. . . . . Beverly Tippins

Measure	Cases	This Hosp.	State Avg.	U.S. Avg.
Blood Clot Prevention and Treatment				
Anticoagulation Overlap Therapy[5]	-	-	90%	93%
ICU Venous Thromboembolism Prophylaxis[5]	-	-	90%	92%
Incidence of Potentially Preventable VTE[5]	-	-	13%	10%
UFH with Dosages/Platelet Monitoring[5]	-	-	99%	97%
Venous Thromboembolism Prophylaxis[5]	-	-	80%	85%
Warfarin Therapy Discharge Instructions[5]	-	-	78%	75%
Chest Pain/Possible Heart Attack Care				
Aspirin Given Within 24 Hours of Arrival[1,3]	-	-	94%	96%
Fibrinolytic Meds Within 30 Min. of Arrival[3,7]	-	-	35%	58%
Average Time to ECG (minutes)[1,3]	-	-	8	7
Average Time to Transfer (minutes)[3,7]	-	-	73	60
Children's Asthma Care				
Received Home Management Plan of Care	-	-	-	88%
Received Reliever Medication	-	-	-	100%
Received Systemic Corticosteroids	-	-	-	100%
Emergency Department				
Admittance Decision Time (minutes)[5]	-	-	100	98
Head CT Results Within 45 Min. of Arrival[5]	-	-	45%	57%
Patients Who Left ER Before Being Seen	5,902	0%	3%	2%
Time from ER Arrival to Admit. (minutes)[5]	-	-	286	274
Time from ER Arrival to Discharge (minutes)[5]	-	-	140	134
Time in ER Before Being Evaluated (minutes)[5]	-	-	32	26
Time to Pain Meds for Fractures (minutes)[5]	-	-	64	57
Heart Attack Care				
Aspirin Given at Discharge[5]	-	-	99%	99%
Fibrinolytic Meds Within 30 Min. of Arrival[5]	-	-	80%	54%
PCI Within 90 Minutes of Arrival[5]	-	-	95%	96%
Statin Prescribed at Discharge[5]	-	-	98%	98%
Heart Failure Care				
ACE Inhibitor or ARB for LVSD[1]	-	-	97%	97%
Discharge Instructions Given	13	100%	92%	94%
Evaluation of LVS Function	14	93%	99%	99%
Medicare Spending				
Medicare Spending per Patient (ratio)	-	-	0.95	0.98
Pneumonia Care				
Appropriate Initial Antibiotic Given[1]	-	-	95%	95%
Blood Culture Timing	11	82%	97%	98%
Pregnancy and Delivery Care				
Newborn Deliveries Scheduled Early[5]	-	-	8%	6%
Preventive Care				
Immunization for Influenza[5]	-	-	88%	90%
Immunization for Pneumonia[5]	-	-	90%	92%
Stroke Care				
Anticoagulation Therapy for Atrial Fibrillation[5]	-	-	94%	95%
Antithrombotic Therapy Timing[5]	-	-	97%	98%
Assessed for Rehabilitation[5]	-	-	97%	97%
Discharged on Antithrombotic Therapy[5]	-	-	98%	99%
Discharged on Statin Medication[5]	-	-	94%	94%
Thrombolytic Therapy Timing[5]	-	-	58%	66%
Venous Thromboembolism Prophylaxis[5]	-	-	92%	94%
Written Stroke Educational Materials Given[5]	-	-	84%	88%

NOTE: Hospital profiles are in alphabetical order by state, then city, then hospital within the city; Rankings exclude hospitals with less than 25 cases except for patient surveys which excludes hospitals with less than 100 cases; (a) 100-299 cases; (1) The number of cases/patients is too few to report; (2) Data submitted were based on a sample of cases/patients; (3) Results are based on a shorter time period than required; (4) Data suppressed by CMS for one or more quarters; (5) Results are not available for this reporting period; (6) Fewer than 100 patients completed the HCAHPS survey; (7) No cases met the criteria for this measure; (8) The lower limit of the confidence interval cannot be calculated if the number of observed infections equals zero; (9) No data are available from the state/territory for this reporting period; (10) The scores shown reflect fewer than 50 completed surveys; (11) There were discrepancies in the data collection process; (12) This measure does not apply to this hospital for this reporting period; (13) Results cannot be calculated for this reporting period; (14) The results for this state are combined with nearby states to protect confidentiality; Please refer to the User's Guide for a full explanation of data.

Surgical Care Improvement Project				
Appropriate Beta Blocker Usage[5]	-	-	97%	98%
Appropriate VTP Within 24 Hours[5]	-	-	98%	98%
Controlled Postoperative Blood Glucose[5]	-	-	96%	97%
Perioperative Temperature Management[5]	-	-	100%	100%
Prophylactic Antibiotic Selection[5]	-	-	99%	99%
Prophylactic Antibiotic Selection (Outpatient)[5]	-	-	98%	98%
Prophylactic Antibiotic Stopped[5]	-	-	98%	98%
Prophylactic Antibiotic Timing[5]	-	-	99%	99%
Prophylactic Antibiotic Timing (Outpatient)[5]	-	-	98%	98%
Urinary Catheter Removal[5]	-	-	97%	97%
Survey of Patients' Hospital Experiences				
Area Around Room 'Always' Quiet at Night[6]	<100	77%	66%	61%
Doctors 'Always' Communicated Well[6]	<100	86%	83%	82%
Home Recovery Information Given[6]	<100	82%	84%	85%
Hospital Given 9 or 10 on 10 Point Scale[6]	<100	78%	69%	71%
Meds 'Always' Explained Before Given[6]	<100	80%	63%	64%
Nurses 'Always' Communicated Well[6]	<100	91%	78%	79%
Pain 'Always' Well Controlled[6]	<100	78%	71%	71%
Room and Bathroom 'Always' Clean[6]	<100	88%	71%	73%
Timely Help 'Always' Received[6]	<100	83%	65%	68%
Would Definitely Recommend Hospital[6]	<100	79%	70%	71%
Use of Medical Imaging				
Cardiac Imaging Stress Test before Surgery[7]	-	-	5.5%	5.3%
Combination Abdominal CT Scan	66	34.8%	10.1%	10.5%
Combination Brain/Sinus CT Scan[1]	-	-	2.3%	2.7%
Combination Chest CT Scan[1]	-	-	3.7%	2.7%
Follow-up Mammogram/Ultrasound	117	6.8%	8.9%	8.8%
Lumbar Spine MRI for Low Back Pain[7]	-	-	36.6%	37.2%

Sylvan Grove Hospital

1050 Mcdonough Road
Jackson, GA 30233
Phone: 770-775-7861
Fax: 770-775-4478
URL: www.sylvangrovehospital.com
Type: Critical Access Hospitals
Emergency Services: Yes
Ownership: Govt - Hospital Dist/Auth
Beds: 25

Key Personnel:
CEO/President. . . . . Jean Dodson
Chief of Medical Staff. . . . . Shashi Madan, MD
Emergency Room . . . . Bernardo Maldonado, MD
Quality Assurance . . . . Bobby Roberts
Ambulatory Care . . . . Edward Whitehouse
Radiology. . . . . James Zimmerman

Measure	Cases	This Hosp.	State Avg.	U.S. Avg.
Blood Clot Prevention and Treatment				
Anticoagulation Overlap Therapy[5]	-	-	90%	93%
ICU Venous Thromboembolism Prophylaxis[5]	-	-	90%	92%
Incidence of Potentially Preventable VTE[5]	-	-	13%	10%
UFH with Dosages/Platelet Monitoring[5]	-	-	99%	97%
Venous Thromboembolism Prophylaxis[5]	-	-	80%	85%
Warfarin Therapy Discharge Instructions[5]	-	-	78%	75%
Chest Pain/Possible Heart Attack Care				
Aspirin Given Within 24 Hours of Arrival	-	-	94%	96%
Fibrinolytic Meds Within 30 Min. of Arrival	-	-	35%	58%
Average Time to ECG (minutes)	-	-	8	7
Average Time to Transfer (minutes)	-	-	73	60
Children's Asthma Care				
Received Home Management Plan of Care	-	-	-	88%
Received Reliever Medication	-	-	-	100%
Received Systemic Corticosteroids	-	-	-	100%
Emergency Department				
Admittance Decision Time (minutes)[5]	-	-	100	98
Head CT Results Within 45 Min. of Arrival	-	-	45%	57%
Patients Who Left ER Before Being Seen	-	-	3%	2%
Time from ER Arrival to Admit. (minutes)[5]	-	-	286	274
Time from ER Arrival to Discharge (minutes)	-	-	140	134
Time in ER Before Being Evaluated (minutes)	-	-	32	26
Time to Pain Meds for Fractures (minutes)	-	-	64	57
Heart Attack Care				
Aspirin Given at Discharge[5]	-	-	99%	99%
Fibrinolytic Meds Within 30 Min. of Arrival[5]	-	-	80%	54%
PCI Within 90 Minutes of Arrival[5]	-	-	95%	96%
Statin Prescribed at Discharge[5]	-	-	98%	98%
Heart Failure Care				
ACE Inhibitor or ARB for LVSD[3,7]	-	-	97%	97%
Discharge Instructions Given[1,3]	-	-	92%	94%
Evaluation of LVS Function[1,3]	-	-	99%	99%
Medicare Spending				
Medicare Spending per Patient (ratio)	-	-	0.95	0.98
Pneumonia Care				
Appropriate Initial Antibiotic Given[1]	-	-	95%	95%
Blood Culture Timing[1]	-	-	97%	98%
Pregnancy and Delivery Care				
Newborn Deliveries Scheduled Early[5]	-	-	8%	6%
Preventive Care				
Immunization for Influenza[5]	-	-	88%	90%
Immunization for Pneumonia[5]	-	-	90%	92%
Stroke Care				
Anticoagulation Therapy for Atrial Fibrillation[5]	-	-	94%	95%
Antithrombotic Therapy Timing[5]	-	-	97%	98%
Assessed for Rehabilitation[5]	-	-	97%	97%
Discharged on Antithrombotic Therapy[5]	-	-	98%	99%
Discharged on Statin Medication[5]	-	-	94%	94%
Thrombolytic Therapy Timing[5]	-	-	58%	66%
Venous Thromboembolism Prophylaxis[5]	-	-	92%	94%
Written Stroke Educational Materials Given[5]	-	-	84%	88%
Surgical Care Improvement Project				
Appropriate Beta Blocker Usage[5]	-	-	97%	98%
Appropriate VTP Within 24 Hours[5]	-	-	98%	98%
Controlled Postoperative Blood Glucose[5]	-	-	96%	97%
Perioperative Temperature Management[5]	-	-	100%	100%
Prophylactic Antibiotic Selection[5]	-	-	99%	99%
Prophylactic Antibiotic Selection (Outpatient)	-	-	98%	98%
Prophylactic Antibiotic Stopped[5]	-	-	98%	98%
Prophylactic Antibiotic Timing[5]	-	-	99%	99%
Prophylactic Antibiotic Timing (Outpatient)	-	-	98%	98%
Urinary Catheter Removal[5]	-	-	97%	97%
Survey of Patients' Hospital Experiences				
Area Around Room 'Always' Quiet at Night[5]	-	-	66%	61%
Doctors 'Always' Communicated Well[5]	-	-	83%	82%
Home Recovery Information Given[5]	-	-	84%	85%
Hospital Given 9 or 10 on 10 Point Scale[5]	-	-	69%	71%
Meds 'Always' Explained Before Given[5]	-	-	63%	64%
Nurses 'Always' Communicated Well[5]	-	-	78%	79%
Pain 'Always' Well Controlled[5]	-	-	71%	71%
Room and Bathroom 'Always' Clean[5]	-	-	71%	73%
Timely Help 'Always' Received[5]	-	-	65%	68%
Would Definitely Recommend Hospital[5]	-	-	70%	71%
Use of Medical Imaging				
Cardiac Imaging Stress Test before Surgery	-	-	5.5%	5.3%
Combination Abdominal CT Scan	-	-	10.1%	10.5%
Combination Brain/Sinus CT Scan	-	-	2.3%	2.7%
Combination Chest CT Scan	-	-	3.7%	2.7%
Follow-up Mammogram/Ultrasound	-	-	8.9%	8.8%
Lumbar Spine MRI for Low Back Pain	-	-	36.6%	37.2%

Piedmont Mountainside Hospital

1266 Highway 515 South
Jasper, GA 30143
Phone: 706-301-5269
Fax: 706-692-0939
URL: www.piedmontmountainsidehospital.org
Type: Acute Care Hospitals
Emergency Services: Yes
Ownership: Voluntary non-profit - Other

Key Personnel:
Radiology. . . . . Roly Alvarez
Operating Room. . . . . Cindy Connelly, RN
Infection Control. . . . . Marianne Gaeland, RN
Quality Assurance . . . . Paula Huszar, RN
Pediatric Ambulatory Care . . . . . . K Raza Mahmood, MD
Chief of Medical Staff. . . . . Folsom C Proctor III, MD
CEO . . . . Denise Ray, RN, BSN, MBA

Measure	Cases	This Hosp.	State Avg.	U.S. Avg.
Blood Clot Prevention and Treatment				
Anticoagulation Overlap Therapy[2]	21	71%	90%	93%
ICU Venous Thromboembolism Prophylaxis[2]	50	88%	90%	92%
Incidence of Potentially Preventable VTE[1,2]	-	-	13%	10%
UFH with Dosages/Platelet Monitoring[2]	13	100%	99%	97%
Venous Thromboembolism Prophylaxis[2]	246	85%	80%	85%
Warfarin Therapy Discharge Instructions[2]	18	89%	78%	75%
Chest Pain/Possible Heart Attack Care				
Aspirin Given Within 24 Hours of Arrival	75	87%	94%	96%
Fibrinolytic Meds Within 30 Min. of Arrival[1]	-	-	35%	58%
Average Time to ECG (minutes)	73	7	8	7
Average Time to Transfer (minutes)[1]	-	-	73	60
Children's Asthma Care				
Received Home Management Plan of Care	-	-	-	88%
Received Reliever Medication	-	-	-	100%
Received Systemic Corticosteroids	-	-	-	100%
Emergency Department				
Admittance Decision Time (minutes)[1,2]	-	-	100	98
Head CT Results Within 45 Min. of Arrival	21	19%	45%	57%
Patients Who Left ER Before Being Seen	22,131	4%	3%	2%
Time from ER Arrival to Admit. (minutes)[1,2]	-	-	286	274
Time from ER Arrival to Discharge (minutes)	393	145	140	134
Time in ER Before Being Evaluated (minutes)	412	33	32	26
Time to Pain Meds for Fractures (minutes)	144	54	64	57
Heart Attack Care				
Aspirin Given at Discharge	18	94%	99%	99%
Fibrinolytic Meds Within 30 Min. of Arrival[7]	-	-	80%	54%
PCI Within 90 Minutes of Arrival[7]	-	-	95%	96%
Statin Prescribed at Discharge	14	93%	98%	98%
Heart Failure Care				
ACE Inhibitor or ARB for LVSD	27	85%	97%	97%
Discharge Instructions Given	70	90%	92%	94%
Evaluation of LVS Function	80	99%	99%	99%
Medicare Spending				
Medicare Spending per Patient (ratio)	-	0.93	0.95	0.98
Pneumonia Care				
Appropriate Initial Antibiotic Given[2]	86	95%	95%	95%
Blood Culture Timing[2]	148	98%	97%	98%
Pregnancy and Delivery Care				
Newborn Deliveries Scheduled Early[2]	36	47%	8%	6%
Preventive Care				
Immunization for Influenza[2]	305	82%	88%	90%
Immunization for Pneumonia[2]	440	80%	90%	92%
Stroke Care				
Anticoagulation Therapy for Atrial Fibrillation[1]	-	-	94%	95%
Antithrombotic Therapy Timing[1]	-	-	97%	98%
Assessed for Rehabilitation	13	69%	97%	97%
Discharged on Antithrombotic Therapy	11	100%	98%	99%
Discharged on Statin Medication	11	73%	94%	94%
Thrombolytic Therapy Timing[1]	-	-	58%	66%
Venous Thromboembolism Prophylaxis	11	73%	92%	94%
Written Stroke Educational Materials Given[1]	-	-	84%	88%
Surgical Care Improvement Project				
Appropriate Beta Blocker Usage[2]	66	98%	97%	98%
Appropriate VTP Within 24 Hours[2]	178	94%	98%	98%
Controlled Postoperative Blood Glucose[2,7]	-	-	96%	97%
Perioperative Temperature Management[2]	224	100%	100%	100%
Prophylactic Antibiotic Selection[2]	177	99%	99%	99%
Prophylactic Antibiotic Selection (Outpatient)	100	96%	98%	98%
Prophylactic Antibiotic Stopped[2]	177	100%	98%	98%
Prophylactic Antibiotic Timing[2]	177	100%	99%	99%
Prophylactic Antibiotic Timing (Outpatient)	102	98%	98%	98%
Urinary Catheter Removal[2]	145	97%	97%	97%
Survey of Patients' Hospital Experiences				
Area Around Room 'Always' Quiet at Night	300+	62%	66%	61%
Doctors 'Always' Communicated Well	300+	79%	83%	82%
Home Recovery Information Given	300+	82%	84%	85%
Hospital Given 9 or 10 on 10 Point Scale	300+	71%	69%	71%
Meds 'Always' Explained Before Given	300+	62%	63%	64%
Nurses 'Always' Communicated Well	300+	77%	78%	79%
Pain 'Always' Well Controlled	300+	70%	71%	71%
Room and Bathroom 'Always' Clean	300+	71%	71%	73%
Timely Help 'Always' Received	300+	67%	65%	68%
Would Definitely Recommend Hospital	300+	77%	70%	71%
Use of Medical Imaging				
Cardiac Imaging Stress Test before Surgery	743	5.0%	5.5%	5.3%
Combination Abdominal CT Scan	814	17.1%	10.1%	10.5%
Combination Brain/Sinus CT Scan	575	2.1%	2.3%	2.7%
Combination Chest CT Scan	327	11.6%	3.7%	2.7%

NOTE: Hospital profiles are in alphabetical order by state, then city, then hospital within the city; Rankings exclude hospitals with less than 25 cases except for patient surveys which excludes hospitals with less than 100 cases; (a) 100-299 cases; (1) The number of cases/patients is too few to report; (2) Data submitted were based on a sample of cases/patients; (3) Results are based on a shorter time period than required; (4) Data suppressed by CMS for one or more quarters; (5) Results are not available for this reporting period; (6) Fewer than 100 patients completed the HCAHPS survey; (7) No cases met the criteria for this measure; (8) The lower limit of the confidence interval cannot be calculated if the number of observed infections equals zero; (9) No data are available from the state/territory for this reporting period; (10) The scores shown reflect fewer than 50 completed surveys; (11) There were discrepancies in the data collection process; (12) This measure does not apply to this hospital for this reporting period; (13) Results cannot be calculated for this reporting period; (14) The results for this state are combined with nearby states to protect confidentiality; Please refer to the User's Guide for a full explanation of data.

Follow-up Mammogram/Ultrasound	970	8.1%	8.9%	8.8%
Lumbar Spine MRI for Low Back Pain	139	30.9%	36.6%	37.2%

Wayne Memorial Hospital

865 South First Street Phone: 912-530-3302
Jesup, GA 31545 Fax: 912-530-3495
URL: www.wmhweb.com
Type: Acute Care Hospitals Emergency Services: Yes
Ownership: Govt - Hospital Dist/Auth Beds: 85

Key Personnel:
Quality Assurance . . . . Sharon Boathright, RN
Radiology. . . . . Charles W Brown
Anesthesiology. . . . . Robert S Diamant, MD
Patient Relations . . . . Tina Hinson
CEO/President. . . . . Charles R Morgan, III
Coronary Care. . . . . Deborah Wasdin, RN
Operating Room. . . . . Pam White, RN
Infection Control. . . . . Sue Williamson, RN

Measure	Cases	This Hosp.	State Avg.	U.S. Avg.
Blood Clot Prevention and Treatment				
Anticoagulation Overlap Therapy[2]	13	69%	90%	93%
ICU Venous Thromboembolism Prophylaxis[2]	120	93%	90%	92%
Incidence of Potentially Preventable VTE[1,2]	-	-	13%	10%
UFH with Dosages/Platelet Monitoring[1,2]	-	-	99%	97%
Venous Thromboembolism Prophylaxis[2]	314	91%	80%	85%
Warfarin Therapy Discharge Instructions[2]	11	100%	78%	75%
Chest Pain/Possible Heart Attack Care				
Aspirin Given Within 24 Hours of Arrival	50	94%	94%	96%
Fibrinolytic Meds Within 30 Min. of Arrival	13	23%	35%	58%
Average Time to ECG (minutes)	53	12	8	7
Average Time to Transfer (minutes)[1]	-	-	73	60
Children's Asthma Care				
Received Home Management Plan of Care	-	-	-	88%
Received Reliever Medication	-	-	-	100%
Received Systemic Corticosteroids	-	-	-	100%
Emergency Department				
Admittance Decision Time (minutes)[2]	403	59	100	98
Head CT Results Within 45 Min. of Arrival	19	26%	45%	57%
Patients Who Left ER Before Being Seen	29,320	0%	3%	2%
Time from ER Arrival to Admit. (minutes)[2]	405	215	286	274
Time from ER Arrival to Discharge (minutes)	429	117	140	134
Time in ER Before Being Evaluated (minutes)	403	32	32	26
Time to Pain Meds for Fractures (minutes)	113	75	64	57
Heart Attack Care				
Aspirin Given at Discharge[1,2]	-	-	99%	99%
Fibrinolytic Meds Within 30 Min. of Arrival[2,7]	-	-	80%	54%
PCI Within 90 Minutes of Arrival[2,7]	-	-	95%	96%
Statin Prescribed at Discharge[1,2]	-	-	98%	98%
Heart Failure Care				
ACE Inhibitor or ARB for LVSD	45	78%	97%	97%
Discharge Instructions Given	110	96%	92%	94%
Evaluation of LVS Function	114	91%	99%	99%
Medicare Spending				
Medicare Spending per Patient (ratio)	-	0.95	0.95	0.98
Pneumonia Care				
Appropriate Initial Antibiotic Given[2]	173	85%	95%	95%
Blood Culture Timing[2]	164	86%	97%	98%
Pregnancy and Delivery Care				
Newborn Deliveries Scheduled Early	94	13%	8%	6%
Preventive Care				
Immunization for Influenza[2]	372	45%	88%	90%
Immunization for Pneumonia[2]	436	67%	90%	92%
Stroke Care				
Anticoagulation Therapy for Atrial Fibrillation[1]	-	-	94%	95%
Antithrombotic Therapy Timing	31	84%	97%	98%
Assessed for Rehabilitation	20	95%	97%	97%
Discharged on Antithrombotic Therapy	19	89%	98%	99%
Discharged on Statin Medication	18	61%	94%	94%
Thrombolytic Therapy Timing[1]	-	-	58%	66%
Venous Thromboembolism Prophylaxis	32	72%	92%	94%
Written Stroke Educational Materials Given	19	89%	84%	88%
Surgical Care Improvement Project				
Appropriate Beta Blocker Usage	34	91%	97%	98%
Appropriate VTP Within 24 Hours	101	77%	98%	98%
Controlled Postoperative Blood Glucose[7]	-	-	96%	97%
Perioperative Temperature Management	114	100%	100%	100%
Prophylactic Antibiotic Selection	92	97%	99%	99%
Prophylactic Antibiotic Selection (Outpatient)	125	94%	98%	98%
Prophylactic Antibiotic Stopped	92	98%	98%	98%
Prophylactic Antibiotic Timing	92	90%	99%	99%
Prophylactic Antibiotic Timing (Outpatient)	127	98%	98%	98%
Urinary Catheter Removal	54	80%	97%	97%
Survey of Patients' Hospital Experiences				
Area Around Room 'Always' Quiet at Night	300+	70%	66%	61%
Doctors 'Always' Communicated Well	300+	81%	83%	82%
Home Recovery Information Given	300+	85%	84%	85%
Hospital Given 9 or 10 on 10 Point Scale	300+	69%	69%	71%
Meds 'Always' Explained Before Given	300+	60%	63%	64%
Nurses 'Always' Communicated Well	300+	77%	78%	79%
Pain 'Always' Well Controlled	300+	68%	71%	71%
Room and Bathroom 'Always' Clean	300+	71%	71%	73%
Timely Help 'Always' Received	300+	62%	65%	68%
Would Definitely Recommend Hospital	300+	65%	70%	71%
Use of Medical Imaging				
Cardiac Imaging Stress Test before Surgery	91	4.4%	5.5%	5.3%
Combination Abdominal CT Scan	451	11.1%	10.1%	10.5%
Combination Brain/Sinus CT Scan[1]	-	-	2.3%	2.7%
Combination Chest CT Scan	283	14.8%	3.7%	2.7%
Follow-up Mammogram/Ultrasound	397	13.4%	8.9%	8.8%
Lumbar Spine MRI for Low Back Pain	37	43.2%	36.6%	37.2%

Emory Johns Creek Hospital

6325 Hospital Parkway Phone: 678-474-7000
Johns Creek, GA 30097
Type: Acute Care Hospitals Emergency Services: Yes
Ownership: Proprietary

Measure	Cases	This Hosp.	State Avg.	U.S. Avg.
Blood Clot Prevention and Treatment				
Anticoagulation Overlap Therapy[2]	39	95%	90%	93%
ICU Venous Thromboembolism Prophylaxis[2]	91	96%	90%	92%
Incidence of Potentially Preventable VTE[1,2]	-	-	13%	10%
UFH with Dosages/Platelet Monitoring[2]	24	100%	99%	97%
Venous Thromboembolism Prophylaxis[2]	326	95%	80%	85%
Warfarin Therapy Discharge Instructions[2]	27	48%	78%	75%
Chest Pain/Possible Heart Attack Care				
Aspirin Given Within 24 Hours of Arrival[1,3]	-	-	94%	96%
Fibrinolytic Meds Within 30 Min. of Arrival[5]	-	-	35%	58%
Average Time to ECG (minutes)[1,3]	-	-	8	7
Average Time to Transfer (minutes)[5]	-	-	73	60
Children's Asthma Care				
Received Home Management Plan of Care	-	-	-	88%
Received Reliever Medication	-	-	-	100%
Received Systemic Corticosteroids	-	-	-	100%
Emergency Department				
Admittance Decision Time (minutes)[2]	683	119	100	98
Head CT Results Within 45 Min. of Arrival[1]	-	-	45%	57%
Patients Who Left ER Before Being Seen	24,292	1%	3%	2%
Time from ER Arrival to Admit. (minutes)[2]	683	322	286	274
Time from ER Arrival to Discharge (minutes)	380	172	140	134
Time in ER Before Being Evaluated (minutes)	423	35	32	26
Time to Pain Meds for Fractures (minutes)	116	60	64	57
Heart Attack Care				
Aspirin Given at Discharge	117	100%	99%	99%
Fibrinolytic Meds Within 30 Min. of Arrival[7]	-	-	80%	54%
PCI Within 90 Minutes of Arrival	26	96%	95%	96%
Statin Prescribed at Discharge	116	100%	98%	98%
Heart Failure Care				
ACE Inhibitor or ARB for LVSD	47	100%	97%	97%
Discharge Instructions Given	191	97%	92%	94%
Evaluation of LVS Function	204	100%	99%	99%
Medicare Spending				
Medicare Spending per Patient (ratio)	-	0.96	0.95	0.98
Pneumonia Care				
Appropriate Initial Antibiotic Given	90	100%	95%	95%
Blood Culture Timing	159	97%	97%	98%
Pregnancy and Delivery Care				
Newborn Deliveries Scheduled Early[2]	36	6%	8%	6%
Preventive Care				
Immunization for Influenza[2]	530	98%	88%	90%
Immunization for Pneumonia[2]	590	96%	90%	92%
Stroke Care				
Anticoagulation Therapy for Atrial Fibrillation[1]	-	-	94%	95%
Antithrombotic Therapy Timing	59	98%	97%	98%
Assessed for Rehabilitation	80	99%	97%	97%
Discharged on Antithrombotic Therapy	73	100%	98%	99%
Discharged on Statin Medication	62	100%	94%	94%
Thrombolytic Therapy Timing[1]	-	-	58%	66%
Venous Thromboembolism Prophylaxis	73	99%	92%	94%
Written Stroke Educational Materials Given	62	94%	84%	88%
Surgical Care Improvement Project				
Appropriate Beta Blocker Usage	83	99%	97%	98%
Appropriate VTP Within 24 Hours	302	99%	98%	98%
Controlled Postoperative Blood Glucose[7]	-	-	96%	97%
Perioperative Temperature Management	339	100%	100%	100%
Prophylactic Antibiotic Selection	178	98%	99%	99%
Prophylactic Antibiotic Selection (Outpatient)	293	99%	98%	98%
Prophylactic Antibiotic Stopped	168	99%	98%	98%
Prophylactic Antibiotic Timing	178	99%	99%	99%
Prophylactic Antibiotic Timing (Outpatient)	293	99%	98%	98%
Urinary Catheter Removal	124	98%	97%	97%
Survey of Patients' Hospital Experiences				
Area Around Room 'Always' Quiet at Night	300+	70%	66%	61%
Doctors 'Always' Communicated Well	300+	83%	83%	82%
Home Recovery Information Given	300+	83%	84%	85%
Hospital Given 9 or 10 on 10 Point Scale	300+	77%	69%	71%
Meds 'Always' Explained Before Given	300+	59%	63%	64%
Nurses 'Always' Communicated Well	300+	76%	78%	79%
Pain 'Always' Well Controlled	300+	71%	71%	71%
Room and Bathroom 'Always' Clean	300+	72%	71%	73%
Timely Help 'Always' Received	300+	61%	65%	68%
Would Definitely Recommend Hospital	300+	81%	70%	71%
Use of Medical Imaging				
Cardiac Imaging Stress Test before Surgery	211	10.4%	5.5%	5.3%
Combination Abdominal CT Scan	438	1.8%	10.1%	10.5%
Combination Brain/Sinus CT Scan[1]	-	-	2.3%	2.7%
Combination Chest CT Scan	378	0.0%	3.7%	2.7%
Follow-up Mammogram/Ultrasound	318	5.7%	8.9%	8.8%
Lumbar Spine MRI for Low Back Pain[1]	-	-	36.6%	37.2%

West Georgia Medical Center

1514 Vernon Road Phone: 706-882-1411
Lagrange, GA 30240 Fax: 706-845-8918
E-mail: info@wghs.org
URL: www.wghealth.org
Type: Acute Care Hospitals Emergency Services: Yes
Ownership: Govt - Hospital Dist/Auth Beds: 276

Key Personnel:
Coronary Care . . . . Sue Brown
Radiology. . . . . Joe Calhoun, MD
Quality Assurance . . . . Liza Fritchley
CEO/President. . . . . Gerald N Fulks, FACHE
Pediatric Ambulatory Care . . . . . . Tracy Gynther, RN
Pediatric In-Patient Care . . . . Tracy Gynther, RN
Operating Room. . . . . Tracey Stribling, RN

Measure	Cases	This Hosp.	State Avg.	U.S. Avg.
Blood Clot Prevention and Treatment				
Anticoagulation Overlap Therapy[2]	75	100%	90%	93%
ICU Venous Thromboembolism Prophylaxis[2]	120	98%	90%	92%
Incidence of Potentially Preventable VTE[1,2]	-	-	13%	10%
UFH with Dosages/Platelet Monitoring[2]	68	100%	99%	97%
Venous Thromboembolism Prophylaxis[2]	292	98%	80%	85%
Warfarin Therapy Discharge Instructions[2]	61	100%	78%	75%
Chest Pain/Possible Heart Attack Care				
Aspirin Given Within 24 Hours of Arrival[1]	-	-	94%	96%
Fibrinolytic Meds Within 30 Min. of Arrival[3,7]	-	-	35%	58%
Average Time to ECG (minutes)[1]	-	-	8	7
Average Time to Transfer (minutes)[3,7]	-	-	73	60
Children's Asthma Care				
Received Home Management Plan of Care	-	-	-	88%
Received Reliever Medication	-	-	-	100%

NOTE: Hospital profiles are in alphabetical order by state, then city, then hospital within the city; Rankings exclude hospitals with less than 25 cases except for patient surveys which excludes hospitals with less than 100 cases; (a) 100-299 cases; (1) The number of cases/patients is too few to report; (2) Data submitted were based on a sample of cases/patients; (3) Results are based on a shorter time period than required; (4) Data suppressed by CMS for one or more quarters; (5) Results are not available for this reporting period; (6) Fewer than 100 patients completed the HCAHPS survey; (7) No cases met the criteria for this measure; (8) The lower limit of the confidence interval cannot be calculated if the number of observed infections equals zero; (9) No data are available from the state/territory for this reporting period; (10) The scores shown reflect fewer than 50 completed surveys; (11) There were discrepancies in the data collection process; (12) This measure does not apply to this hospital for this reporting period; (13) Results cannot be calculated for this reporting period; (14) The results for this state are combined with nearby states to protect confidentiality; Please refer to the User's Guide for a full explanation of data.

Measure	Cases	This Hosp.	State Avg.	U.S. Avg.
Received Systemic Corticosteroids	-	-	-	100%
Emergency Department				
Admittance Decision Time (minutes)[2]	625	88	100	98
Head CT Results Within 45 Min. of Arrival[1]	-	-	45%	57%
Patients Who Left ER Before Being Seen	66,895	1%	3%	2%
Time from ER Arrival to Admit. (minutes)[2]	626	212	286	274
Time from ER Arrival to Discharge (minutes)	357	106	140	134
Time in ER Before Being Evaluated (minutes)	383	41	32	26
Time to Pain Meds for Fractures (minutes)	162	72	64	57
Heart Attack Care				
Aspirin Given at Discharge	153	99%	99%	99%
Fibrinolytic Meds Within 30 Min. of Arrival[7]	-	-	80%	54%
PCI Within 90 Minutes of Arrival	31	97%	95%	96%
Statin Prescribed at Discharge	133	99%	98%	98%
Heart Failure Care				
ACE Inhibitor or ARB for LVSD	69	99%	97%	97%
Discharge Instructions Given	202	93%	92%	94%
Evaluation of LVS Function	246	100%	99%	99%
Medicare Spending				
Medicare Spending per Patient (ratio)	-	0.93	0.95	0.98
Pneumonia Care				
Appropriate Initial Antibiotic Given	105	95%	95%	95%
Blood Culture Timing	219	99%	97%	98%
Pregnancy and Delivery Care				
Newborn Deliveries Scheduled Early[2]	40	8%	8%	6%
Preventive Care				
Immunization for Influenza[2]	539	95%	88%	90%
Immunization for Pneumonia[2]	681	96%	90%	92%
Stroke Care				
Anticoagulation Therapy for Atrial Fibrillation[1]	-	-	94%	95%
Antithrombotic Therapy Timing	82	100%	97%	98%
Assessed for Rehabilitation	82	100%	97%	97%
Discharged on Antithrombotic Therapy	80	100%	98%	99%
Discharged on Statin Medication	67	96%	94%	94%
Thrombolytic Therapy Timing[1]	-	-	58%	66%
Venous Thromboembolism Prophylaxis	85	99%	92%	94%
Written Stroke Educational Materials Given	41	100%	84%	88%
Surgical Care Improvement Project				
Appropriate Beta Blocker Usage	91	100%	97%	98%
Appropriate VTP Within 24 Hours	323	100%	98%	98%
Controlled Postoperative Blood Glucose[7]	-	-	96%	97%
Perioperative Temperature Management	342	100%	100%	100%
Prophylactic Antibiotic Selection	200	100%	99%	99%
Prophylactic Antibiotic Selection (Outpatient)	103	100%	98%	98%
Prophylactic Antibiotic Stopped	196	100%	98%	98%
Prophylactic Antibiotic Timing	201	100%	99%	99%
Prophylactic Antibiotic Timing (Outpatient)	102	100%	98%	98%
Urinary Catheter Removal	176	100%	97%	97%
Survey of Patients' Hospital Experiences				
Area Around Room 'Always' Quiet at Night	300+	63%	66%	61%
Doctors 'Always' Communicated Well	300+	81%	83%	82%
Home Recovery Information Given	300+	85%	84%	85%
Hospital Given 9 or 10 on 10 Point Scale	300+	70%	69%	71%
Meds 'Always' Explained Before Given	300+	67%	63%	64%
Nurses 'Always' Communicated Well	300+	82%	78%	79%
Pain 'Always' Well Controlled	300+	71%	71%	71%
Room and Bathroom 'Always' Clean	300+	75%	71%	73%
Timely Help 'Always' Received	300+	67%	65%	68%
Would Definitely Recommend Hospital	300+	67%	70%	71%
Use of Medical Imaging				
Cardiac Imaging Stress Test before Surgery	343	6.1%	5.5%	5.3%
Combination Abdominal CT Scan	708	4.0%	10.1%	10.5%
Combination Brain/Sinus CT Scan	863	2.0%	2.3%	2.7%
Combination Chest CT Scan	166	6.6%	3.7%	2.7%
Follow-up Mammogram/Ultrasound	413	6.1%	8.9%	8.8%
Lumbar Spine MRI for Low Back Pain[1]	-	-	36.6%	37.2%

Louis Smith Memorial Hospital

116 West Thigpen Avenue Phone: 229-482-8402
Lakeland, GA 31635
Type: Critical Access Hospitals Emergency Services: Yes
Ownership: Voluntary non-profit - Private

Measure	Cases	This Hosp.	State Avg.	U.S. Avg.
Blood Clot Prevention and Treatment				
Anticoagulation Overlap Therapy[5]	-	-	90%	93%
ICU Venous Thromboembolism Prophylaxis[5]	-	-	90%	92%
Incidence of Potentially Preventable VTE[5]	-	-	13%	10%
UFH with Dosages/Platelet Monitoring[5]	-	-	99%	97%
Venous Thromboembolism Prophylaxis[5]	-	-	80%	85%
Warfarin Therapy Discharge Instructions[5]	-	-	78%	75%
Chest Pain/Possible Heart Attack Care				
Aspirin Given Within 24 Hours of Arrival	-	-	94%	96%
Fibrinolytic Meds Within 30 Min. of Arrival	-	-	35%	58%
Average Time to ECG (minutes)	-	-	8	7
Average Time to Transfer (minutes)	-	-	73	60
Children's Asthma Care				
Received Home Management Plan of Care	-	-	-	88%
Received Reliever Medication	-	-	-	100%
Received Systemic Corticosteroids	-	-	-	100%
Emergency Department				
Admittance Decision Time (minutes)[5]	-	-	100	98
Head CT Results Within 45 Min. of Arrival	-	-	45%	57%
Patients Who Left ER Before Being Seen	-	-	3%	2%
Time from ER Arrival to Admit. (minutes)[5]	-	-	286	274
Time from ER Arrival to Discharge (minutes)	-	-	140	134
Time in ER Before Being Evaluated (minutes)	-	-	32	26
Time to Pain Meds for Fractures (minutes)	-	-	64	57
Heart Attack Care				
Aspirin Given at Discharge[5]	-	-	99%	99%
Fibrinolytic Meds Within 30 Min. of Arrival[5]	-	-	80%	54%
PCI Within 90 Minutes of Arrival[5]	-	-	95%	96%
Statin Prescribed at Discharge[5]	-	-	98%	98%
Heart Failure Care				
ACE Inhibitor or ARB for LVSD[1]	-	-	97%	97%
Discharge Instructions Given	16	94%	92%	94%
Evaluation of LVS Function	16	94%	99%	99%
Medicare Spending				
Medicare Spending per Patient (ratio)	-	-	0.95	0.98
Pneumonia Care				
Appropriate Initial Antibiotic Given	16	50%	95%	95%
Blood Culture Timing[1]	-	-	97%	98%
Pregnancy and Delivery Care				
Newborn Deliveries Scheduled Early[5]	-	-	8%	6%
Preventive Care				
Immunization for Influenza[5]	-	-	88%	90%
Immunization for Pneumonia[5]	-	-	90%	92%
Stroke Care				
Anticoagulation Therapy for Atrial Fibrillation[5]	-	-	94%	95%
Antithrombotic Therapy Timing[5]	-	-	97%	98%
Assessed for Rehabilitation[5]	-	-	97%	97%
Discharged on Antithrombotic Therapy[5]	-	-	98%	99%
Discharged on Statin Medication[5]	-	-	94%	94%
Thrombolytic Therapy Timing[5]	-	-	58%	66%
Venous Thromboembolism Prophylaxis[5]	-	-	92%	94%
Written Stroke Educational Materials Given[5]	-	-	84%	88%
Surgical Care Improvement Project				
Appropriate Beta Blocker Usage[5]	-	-	97%	98%
Appropriate VTP Within 24 Hours[5]	-	-	98%	98%
Controlled Postoperative Blood Glucose[5]	-	-	96%	97%
Perioperative Temperature Management[5]	-	-	100%	100%
Prophylactic Antibiotic Selection[5]	-	-	99%	99%
Prophylactic Antibiotic Selection (Outpatient)	-	-	98%	98%
Prophylactic Antibiotic Stopped[5]	-	-	98%	98%
Prophylactic Antibiotic Timing[5]	-	-	99%	99%
Prophylactic Antibiotic Timing (Outpatient)	-	-	98%	98%
Urinary Catheter Removal[5]	-	-	97%	97%
Survey of Patients' Hospital Experiences				
Area Around Room 'Always' Quiet at Night[6]	<100	65%	66%	61%
Doctors 'Always' Communicated Well[6]	<100	80%	83%	82%
Home Recovery Information Given[6]	<100	81%	84%	85%
Hospital Given 9 or 10 on 10 Point Scale[6]	<100	73%	69%	71%
Meds 'Always' Explained Before Given[6]	<100	71%	63%	64%
Nurses 'Always' Communicated Well[6]	<100	78%	78%	79%
Pain 'Always' Well Controlled[6]	<100	71%	71%	71%
Room and Bathroom 'Always' Clean[6]	<100	82%	71%	73%
Timely Help 'Always' Received[6]	<100	82%	65%	68%
Would Definitely Recommend Hospital[6]	<100	68%	70%	71%
Use of Medical Imaging				
Cardiac Imaging Stress Test before Surgery	-	-	5.5%	5.3%
Combination Abdominal CT Scan	-	-	10.1%	10.5%
Combination Brain/Sinus CT Scan	-	-	2.3%	2.7%
Combination Chest CT Scan	-	-	3.7%	2.7%
Follow-up Mammogram/Ultrasound	-	-	8.9%	8.8%
Lumbar Spine MRI for Low Back Pain	-	-	36.6%	37.2%

Ty Cobb Regional Medical Center

367 Clear Creek Parkway Phone: 706-356-7800
Lavonia, GA 30553 Fax: 706-245-1831
Type: Acute Care Hospitals Emergency Services: Yes
Ownership: Voluntary non-profit - Private Beds: 71

Key Personnel:
Emergency Room . . . . Debbie Barlett
CEO . . . . Gregory K. Hearn, CPA

Measure	Cases	This Hosp.	State Avg.	U.S. Avg.
Blood Clot Prevention and Treatment				
Anticoagulation Overlap Therapy[2]	12	75%	90%	93%
ICU Venous Thromboembolism Prophylaxis[2]	34	56%	90%	92%
Incidence of Potentially Preventable VTE[2,7]	-	-	13%	10%
UFH with Dosages/Platelet Monitoring[1,2]	-	-	99%	97%
Venous Thromboembolism Prophylaxis[2]	108	44%	80%	85%
Warfarin Therapy Discharge Instructions[1,2]	-	-	78%	75%
Chest Pain/Possible Heart Attack Care				
Aspirin Given Within 24 Hours of Arrival	52	92%	94%	96%
Fibrinolytic Meds Within 30 Min. of Arrival[1]	-	-	35%	58%
Average Time to ECG (minutes)	48	13	8	7
Average Time to Transfer (minutes)[1]	-	-	73	60
Children's Asthma Care				
Received Home Management Plan of Care	-	-	-	88%
Received Reliever Medication	-	-	-	100%
Received Systemic Corticosteroids	-	-	-	100%
Emergency Department				
Admittance Decision Time (minutes)[2]	291	50	100	98
Head CT Results Within 45 Min. of Arrival[1]	-	-	45%	57%
Patients Who Left ER Before Being Seen	17,186	2%	3%	2%
Time from ER Arrival to Admit. (minutes)[2]	393	229	286	274
Time from ER Arrival to Discharge (minutes)	417	118	140	134
Time in ER Before Being Evaluated (minutes)	387	27	32	26
Time to Pain Meds for Fractures (minutes)	77	43	64	57
Heart Attack Care				
Aspirin Given at Discharge[1]	-	-	99%	99%
Fibrinolytic Meds Within 30 Min. of Arrival[7]	-	-	80%	54%
PCI Within 90 Minutes of Arrival[7]	-	-	95%	96%
Statin Prescribed at Discharge[1]	-	-	98%	98%
Heart Failure Care				
ACE Inhibitor or ARB for LVSD	23	96%	97%	97%
Discharge Instructions Given	43	70%	92%	94%
Evaluation of LVS Function	57	95%	99%	99%
Medicare Spending				
Medicare Spending per Patient (ratio)	-	0.92	0.95	0.98
Pneumonia Care				
Appropriate Initial Antibiotic Given[2]	33	79%	95%	95%
Blood Culture Timing[2]	44	91%	97%	98%
Pregnancy and Delivery Care				
Newborn Deliveries Scheduled Early	29	7%	8%	6%
Preventive Care				
Immunization for Influenza[2]	380	89%	88%	90%
Immunization for Pneumonia[2]	396	91%	90%	92%
Stroke Care				
Anticoagulation Therapy for Atrial Fibrillation[1]	-	-	94%	95%
Antithrombotic Therapy Timing	13	46%	97%	98%
Assessed for Rehabilitation	14	100%	97%	97%
Discharged on Antithrombotic Therapy	14	86%	98%	99%

NOTE: Hospital profiles are in alphabetical order by state, then city, then hospital within the city; Rankings exclude hospitals with less than 25 cases except for patient surveys which excludes hospitals with less than 100 cases; (a) 100-299 cases; (1) The number of cases/patients is too few to report; (2) Data submitted were based on a sample of cases/patients; (3) Results are based on a shorter time period than required; (4) Data suppressed by CMS for one or more quarters; (5) Results are not available for this reporting period; (6) Fewer than 100 patients completed the HCAHPS survey; (7) No cases met the criteria for this measure; (8) The lower limit of the confidence interval cannot be calculated if the number of observed infections equals zero; (9) No data are available from the state/territory for this reporting period; (10) The scores shown reflect fewer than 50 completed surveys; (11) There were discrepancies in the data collection process; (12) This measure does not apply to this hospital for this reporting period; (13) Results cannot be calculated for this reporting period; (14) The results for this state are combined with nearby states to protect confidentiality; Please refer to the User's Guide for a full explanation of data.

Measure	Cases	This Hosp.	State Avg.	U.S. Avg.
Discharged on Statin Medication[1]	-	-	94%	94%
Thrombolytic Therapy Timing[1]	-	-	58%	66%
Venous Thromboembolism Prophylaxis	18	39%	92%	94%
Written Stroke Educational Materials Given[1]	-	-	84%	88%
Surgical Care Improvement Project				
Appropriate Beta Blocker Usage[2]	19	68%	97%	98%
Appropriate VTP Within 24 Hours[2]	53	77%	98%	98%
Controlled Postoperative Blood Glucose[2,7]	-	-	96%	97%
Perioperative Temperature Management[2]	67	99%	100%	100%
Prophylactic Antibiotic Selection[2]	23	96%	99%	99%
Prophylactic Antibiotic Selection (Outpatient)	11	82%	98%	98%
Prophylactic Antibiotic Stopped[2]	23	91%	98%	98%
Prophylactic Antibiotic Timing[2]	24	88%	99%	99%
Prophylactic Antibiotic Timing (Outpatient)	17	59%	98%	98%
Urinary Catheter Removal[2]	31	74%	97%	97%
Survey of Patients' Hospital Experiences				
Area Around Room 'Always' Quiet at Night	300+	73%	66%	61%
Doctors 'Always' Communicated Well	300+	86%	83%	82%
Home Recovery Information Given	300+	87%	84%	85%
Hospital Given 9 or 10 on 10 Point Scale	300+	73%	69%	71%
Meds 'Always' Explained Before Given	300+	68%	63%	64%
Nurses 'Always' Communicated Well	300+	81%	78%	79%
Pain 'Always' Well Controlled	300+	72%	71%	71%
Room and Bathroom 'Always' Clean	300+	73%	71%	73%
Timely Help 'Always' Received	300+	72%	65%	68%
Would Definitely Recommend Hospital	300+	72%	70%	71%
Use of Medical Imaging				
Cardiac Imaging Stress Test before Surgery	211	4.7%	5.5%	5.3%
Combination Abdominal CT Scan	351	10.8%	10.1%	10.5%
Combination Brain/Sinus CT Scan	459	3.9%	2.3%	2.7%
Combination Chest CT Scan	166	6.6%	3.7%	2.7%
Follow-up Mammogram/Ultrasound	317	23.7%	8.9%	8.8%
Lumbar Spine MRI for Low Back Pain	54	50.0%	36.6%	37.2%

Gwinnett Medical Center

1000 Medical Center Boulevard — Phone: 678-312-1000
Lawrenceville, GA 30045 — Fax: 770-682-2257
URL: www.gwinnettmedicalcenter.org
Type: Acute Care Hospitals — Emergency Services: Yes
Ownership: Govt - Hospital Dist/Auth — Beds: 350

Key Personnel:
Chief of Medical Staff.......... Alan Bier, MD
Radiology.................... Patrick Green
Emergency Room .... Judy Keller
Chairman/CEO .... David McCleskey
Operating Room.............. Mary Nash
Quality Assurance .... Wendy Solberg
Coronary Care .... Chip Wheeler
CEO/President................ Philip R Wolfe

Measure	Cases	This Hosp.	State Avg.	U.S. Avg.
Blood Clot Prevention and Treatment				
Anticoagulation Overlap Therapy[2]	263	96%	90%	93%
ICU Venous Thromboembolism Prophylaxis[2]	59	97%	90%	92%
Incidence of Potentially Preventable VTE[2]	32	0%	13%	10%
UFH with Dosages/Platelet Monitoring[2]	173	100%	99%	97%
Venous Thromboembolism Prophylaxis[2]	378	90%	80%	85%
Warfarin Therapy Discharge Instructions[2]	203	88%	78%	75%
Chest Pain/Possible Heart Attack Care				
Aspirin Given Within 24 Hours of Arrival[1]	-	-	94%	96%
Fibrinolytic Meds Within 30 Min. of Arrival[3,7]	-	-	35%	58%
Average Time to ECG (minutes)[1]	-	-	8	7
Average Time to Transfer (minutes)[1,3]	-	-	73	60
Children's Asthma Care				
Received Home Management Plan of Care	-	-	-	88%
Received Reliever Medication	-	-	-	100%
Received Systemic Corticosteroids	-	-	-	100%
Emergency Department				
Admittance Decision Time (minutes)[2]	884	181	100	98
Head CT Results Within 45 Min. of Arrival	39	72%	45%	57%
Patients Who Left ER Before Being Seen	>100k	3%	3%	2%
Time from ER Arrival to Admit. (minutes)[2]	922	378	286	274
Time from ER Arrival to Discharge (minutes)	811	177	140	134
Time in ER Before Being Evaluated (minutes)	768	45	32	26
Time to Pain Meds for Fractures (minutes)	457	52	64	57
Heart Attack Care				
Aspirin Given at Discharge	502	99%	99%	99%
Fibrinolytic Meds Within 30 Min. of Arrival[7]	-	-	80%	54%
PCI Within 90 Minutes of Arrival	119	100%	95%	96%
Statin Prescribed at Discharge	490	99%	98%	98%
Heart Failure Care				
ACE Inhibitor or ARB for LVSD	254	99%	97%	97%
Discharge Instructions Given	812	83%	92%	94%
Evaluation of LVS Function	930	100%	99%	99%
Medicare Spending				
Medicare Spending per Patient (ratio)	-	0.98	0.95	0.98
Pneumonia Care				
Appropriate Initial Antibiotic Given[2]	331	98%	95%	95%
Blood Culture Timing[2]	315	97%	97%	98%
Pregnancy and Delivery Care				
Newborn Deliveries Scheduled Early[2]	80	4%	8%	6%
Preventive Care				
Immunization for Influenza[2]	709	93%	88%	90%
Immunization for Pneumonia[2]	869	90%	90%	92%
Stroke Care				
Anticoagulation Therapy for Atrial Fibrillation	38	97%	94%	95%
Antithrombotic Therapy Timing	271	100%	97%	98%
Assessed for Rehabilitation	344	100%	97%	97%
Discharged on Antithrombotic Therapy	306	100%	98%	99%
Discharged on Statin Medication	220	96%	94%	94%
Thrombolytic Therapy Timing	22	86%	58%	66%
Venous Thromboembolism Prophylaxis	338	100%	92%	94%
Written Stroke Educational Materials Given	246	91%	84%	88%
Surgical Care Improvement Project				
Appropriate Beta Blocker Usage[2]	283	98%	97%	98%
Appropriate VTP Within 24 Hours[2]	596	96%	98%	98%
Controlled Postoperative Blood Glucose[2]	169	100%	96%	97%
Perioperative Temperature Management[2]	747	98%	100%	100%
Prophylactic Antibiotic Selection[2]	675	99%	99%	99%
Prophylactic Antibiotic Selection (Outpatient)	718	98%	98%	98%
Prophylactic Antibiotic Stopped[2]	646	98%	98%	98%
Prophylactic Antibiotic Timing[2]	677	98%	99%	99%
Prophylactic Antibiotic Timing (Outpatient)	723	99%	98%	98%
Urinary Catheter Removal[2]	470	97%	97%	97%
Survey of Patients' Hospital Experiences				
Area Around Room 'Always' Quiet at Night	300+	66%	66%	61%
Doctors 'Always' Communicated Well	300+	79%	83%	82%
Home Recovery Information Given	300+	85%	84%	85%
Hospital Given 9 or 10 on 10 Point Scale	300+	76%	69%	71%
Meds 'Always' Explained Before Given	300+	62%	63%	64%
Nurses 'Always' Communicated Well	300+	78%	78%	79%
Pain 'Always' Well Controlled	300+	71%	71%	71%
Room and Bathroom 'Always' Clean	300+	72%	71%	73%
Timely Help 'Always' Received	300+	63%	65%	68%
Would Definitely Recommend Hospital	300+	79%	70%	71%
Use of Medical Imaging				
Cardiac Imaging Stress Test before Surgery	682	5.1%	5.5%	5.3%
Combination Abdominal CT Scan	2,650	5.6%	10.1%	10.5%
Combination Brain/Sinus CT Scan	1,869	0.8%	2.3%	2.7%
Combination Chest CT Scan	1,692	3.0%	3.7%	2.7%
Follow-up Mammogram/Ultrasound	3,726	16.0%	8.9%	8.8%
Lumbar Spine MRI for Low Back Pain	247	34.8%	36.6%	37.2%

Dekalb Medical Center at Hillandale

2801 Dekalb Medical Parkway — Phone: 404-501-8040
Lithonia, GA 30058
URL: www.deklabmedicalcenter.org
Type: Acute Care Hospitals — Emergency Services: Yes
Ownership: Govt - Hospital Dist/Auth

Key Personnel:
Patient Relations .... Lynne Anderson
CEO/President................ Eric P Norwood
Quality Assurance .... Cathleen Wheatley

Measure	Cases	This Hosp.	State Avg.	U.S. Avg.
Blood Clot Prevention and Treatment				
Anticoagulation Overlap Therapy[2]	92	97%	90%	93%
ICU Venous Thromboembolism Prophylaxis[2]	68	91%	90%	92%
Incidence of Potentially Preventable VTE[1,2]	-	-	13%	10%
UFH with Dosages/Platelet Monitoring[2]	72	100%	99%	97%
Venous Thromboembolism Prophylaxis[2]	398	93%	80%	85%
Warfarin Therapy Discharge Instructions[2]	80	92%	78%	75%
Chest Pain/Possible Heart Attack Care				
Aspirin Given Within 24 Hours of Arrival	51	98%	94%	96%
Fibrinolytic Meds Within 30 Min. of Arrival[7]	-	-	35%	58%
Average Time to ECG (minutes)	52	10	8	7
Average Time to Transfer (minutes)	15	55	73	60
Children's Asthma Care				
Received Home Management Plan of Care	-	-	-	88%
Received Reliever Medication	-	-	-	100%
Received Systemic Corticosteroids	-	-	-	100%
Emergency Department				
Admittance Decision Time (minutes)[2]	1,060	227	100	98
Head CT Results Within 45 Min. of Arrival[1]	-	-	45%	57%
Patients Who Left ER Before Being Seen	60,407	2%	3%	2%
Time from ER Arrival to Admit. (minutes)[2]	1,061	465	286	274
Time from ER Arrival to Discharge (minutes)	398	162	140	134
Time in ER Before Being Evaluated (minutes)	430	30	32	26
Time to Pain Meds for Fractures (minutes)	101	66	64	57
Heart Attack Care				
Aspirin Given at Discharge	20	95%	99%	99%
Fibrinolytic Meds Within 30 Min. of Arrival[7]	-	-	80%	54%
PCI Within 90 Minutes of Arrival[7]	-	-	95%	96%
Statin Prescribed at Discharge	21	90%	98%	98%
Heart Failure Care				
ACE Inhibitor or ARB for LVSD	135	99%	97%	97%
Discharge Instructions Given	262	93%	92%	94%
Evaluation of LVS Function	284	100%	99%	99%
Medicare Spending				
Medicare Spending per Patient (ratio)	-	0.97	0.95	0.98
Pneumonia Care				
Appropriate Initial Antibiotic Given[2]	107	96%	95%	95%
Blood Culture Timing[2]	114	98%	97%	98%
Pregnancy and Delivery Care				
Newborn Deliveries Scheduled Early[2,7]	-	-	8%	6%
Preventive Care				
Immunization for Influenza[2]	524	88%	88%	90%
Immunization for Pneumonia[2]	726	85%	90%	92%
Stroke Care				
Anticoagulation Therapy for Atrial Fibrillation[1]	-	-	94%	95%
Antithrombotic Therapy Timing	64	100%	97%	98%
Assessed for Rehabilitation	65	98%	97%	97%
Discharged on Antithrombotic Therapy	61	100%	98%	99%
Discharged on Statin Medication	49	92%	94%	94%
Thrombolytic Therapy Timing[7]	-	-	58%	66%
Venous Thromboembolism Prophylaxis	67	100%	92%	94%
Written Stroke Educational Materials Given	47	100%	84%	88%
Surgical Care Improvement Project				
Appropriate Beta Blocker Usage	17	88%	97%	98%
Appropriate VTP Within 24 Hours	102	99%	98%	98%
Controlled Postoperative Blood Glucose[7]	-	-	96%	97%
Perioperative Temperature Management	106	100%	100%	100%
Prophylactic Antibiotic Selection	38	97%	99%	99%
Prophylactic Antibiotic Selection (Outpatient)	13	100%	98%	98%
Prophylactic Antibiotic Stopped	36	97%	98%	98%
Prophylactic Antibiotic Timing	38	100%	99%	99%
Prophylactic Antibiotic Timing (Outpatient)	13	100%	98%	98%
Urinary Catheter Removal	51	96%	97%	97%
Survey of Patients' Hospital Experiences				
Area Around Room 'Always' Quiet at Night	300+	76%	66%	61%
Doctors 'Always' Communicated Well	300+	77%	83%	82%
Home Recovery Information Given	300+	79%	84%	85%
Hospital Given 9 or 10 on 10 Point Scale	300+	70%	69%	71%
Meds 'Always' Explained Before Given	300+	60%	63%	64%
Nurses 'Always' Communicated Well	300+	75%	78%	79%
Pain 'Always' Well Controlled	300+	67%	71%	71%
Room and Bathroom 'Always' Clean	300+	69%	71%	73%
Timely Help 'Always' Received	300+	56%	65%	68%
Would Definitely Recommend Hospital	300+	67%	70%	71%
Use of Medical Imaging				
Cardiac Imaging Stress Test before Surgery	135	4.4%	5.5%	5.3%

NOTE: Hospital profiles are in alphabetical order by state, then city, then hospital within the city; Rankings exclude hospitals with less than 25 cases except for patient surveys which excludes hospitals with less than 100 cases; (a) 100-299 cases; (1) The number of cases/patients is too few to report; (2) Data submitted were based on a sample of cases/patients; (3) Results are based on a shorter time period than required; (4) Data suppressed by CMS for one or more quarters; (5) Results are not available for this reporting period; (6) Fewer than 100 patients completed the HCAHPS survey; (7) No cases met the criteria for this measure; (8) The lower limit of the confidence interval cannot be calculated if the number of observed infections equals zero; (9) No data are available from the state/territory for this reporting period; (10) The scores shown reflect fewer than 50 completed surveys; (11) There were discrepancies in the data collection process; (12) This measure does not apply to this hospital for this reporting period; (13) Results cannot be calculated for this reporting period; (14) The results for this state are combined with nearby states to protect confidentiality; Please refer to the User's Guide for a full explanation of data.

Measure	Cases	This Hosp.	State Avg.	U.S. Avg.
Combination Abdominal CT Scan	492	3.9%	10.1%	10.5%
Combination Brain/Sinus CT Scan[1]	-	-	2.3%	2.7%
Combination Chest CT Scan	144	0.0%	3.7%	2.7%
Follow-up Mammogram/Ultrasound	970	8.2%	8.9%	8.8%
Lumbar Spine MRI for Low Back Pain[1]	-	-	36.6%	37.2%

Jefferson Hospital

1067 Peachtree St
Louisville, GA 30434
Type: Acute Care Hospitals
Ownership: Govt - Hospital Dist/Auth
Phone: 478-625-7000
Fax: 478-625-7446
Emergency Services: Yes
Beds: 37

Measure	Cases	This Hosp.	State Avg.	U.S. Avg.
Blood Clot Prevention and Treatment				
Anticoagulation Overlap Therapy[1,2]	-	-	90%	93%
ICU Venous Thromboembolism Prophylaxis[1,2]	-	-	90%	92%
Incidence of Potentially Preventable VTE[1,2]	-	-	13%	10%
UFH with Dosages/Platelet Monitoring[2,7]	-	-	99%	97%
Venous Thromboembolism Prophylaxis[2]	126	40%	80%	85%
Warfarin Therapy Discharge Instructions[1,2]	-	-	78%	75%
Chest Pain/Possible Heart Attack Care				
Aspirin Given Within 24 Hours of Arrival	45	91%	94%	96%
Fibrinolytic Meds Within 30 Min. of Arrival[7]	-	-	35%	58%
Average Time to ECG (minutes)	44	9	8	7
Average Time to Transfer (minutes)[1]	-	-	73	60
Children's Asthma Care				
Received Home Management Plan of Care	-	-	-	88%
Received Reliever Medication	-	-	-	100%
Received Systemic Corticosteroids	-	-	-	100%
Emergency Department				
Admittance Decision Time (minutes)[2]	263	65	100	98
Head CT Results Within 45 Min. of Arrival[1,3]	-	-	45%	57%
Patients Who Left ER Before Being Seen	4,983	2%	3%	2%
Time from ER Arrival to Admit. (minutes)[2]	283	215	286	274
Time from ER Arrival to Discharge (minutes)	338	125	140	134
Time in ER Before Being Evaluated (minutes)	323	50	32	26
Time to Pain Meds for Fractures (minutes)	21	62	64	57
Heart Attack Care				
Aspirin Given at Discharge[1,3]	-	-	99%	99%
Fibrinolytic Meds Within 30 Min. of Arrival[3,7]	-	-	80%	54%
PCI Within 90 Minutes of Arrival[3,7]	-	-	95%	96%
Statin Prescribed at Discharge[1,3]	-	-	98%	98%
Heart Failure Care				
ACE Inhibitor or ARB for LVSD[1,2]	-	-	97%	97%
Discharge Instructions Given[2]	40	88%	92%	94%
Evaluation of LVS Function[2]	47	79%	99%	99%
Medicare Spending				
Medicare Spending per Patient (ratio)	-	0.83	0.95	0.98
Pneumonia Care				
Appropriate Initial Antibiotic Given[1,2]	-	-	95%	95%
Blood Culture Timing[1,2]	-	-	97%	98%
Pregnancy and Delivery Care				
Newborn Deliveries Scheduled Early[2,7]	-	-	8%	6%
Preventive Care				
Immunization for Influenza[2]	245	98%	88%	90%
Immunization for Pneumonia[2]	462	95%	90%	92%
Stroke Care				
Anticoagulation Therapy for Atrial Fibrillation[2,3]	-	-	94%	95%
Antithrombotic Therapy Timing[1,2]	-	-	97%	98%
Assessed for Rehabilitation[1,2]	-	-	97%	97%
Discharged on Antithrombotic Therapy[1,2]	-	-	98%	99%
Discharged on Statin Medication[1,2]	-	-	94%	94%
Thrombolytic Therapy Timing[1,2]	-	-	58%	66%
Venous Thromboembolism Prophylaxis[1,2]	-	-	92%	94%
Written Stroke Educational Materials Given[1,2]	-	-	84%	88%
Surgical Care Improvement Project				
Appropriate Beta Blocker Usage[5]	-	-	97%	98%
Appropriate VTP Within 24 Hours[5]	-	-	98%	98%
Controlled Postoperative Blood Glucose[5]	-	-	96%	97%
Perioperative Temperature Management[5]	-	-	100%	100%
Prophylactic Antibiotic Selection[5]	-	-	99%	99%
Prophylactic Antibiotic Selection (Outpatient)[1,3]	-	-	98%	98%
Prophylactic Antibiotic Stopped[5]	-	-	98%	98%
Prophylactic Antibiotic Timing[5]	-	-	99%	99%
Prophylactic Antibiotic Timing (Outpatient)[1,3]	-	-	98%	98%
Urinary Catheter Removal[5]	-	-	97%	97%
Survey of Patients' Hospital Experiences				
Area Around Room 'Always' Quiet at Night[6]	<100	73%	66%	61%
Doctors 'Always' Communicated Well[6]	<100	88%	83%	82%
Home Recovery Information Given[6]	<100	80%	84%	85%
Hospital Given 9 or 10 on 10 Point Scale[6]	<100	77%	69%	71%
Meds 'Always' Explained Before Given[6]	<100	63%	63%	64%
Nurses 'Always' Communicated Well[6]	<100	79%	78%	79%
Pain 'Always' Well Controlled[6]	<100	71%	71%	71%
Room and Bathroom 'Always' Clean[6]	<100	81%	71%	73%
Timely Help 'Always' Received[6]	<100	69%	65%	68%
Would Definitely Recommend Hospital[6]	<100	71%	70%	71%
Use of Medical Imaging				
Cardiac Imaging Stress Test before Surgery[7]	-	-	5.5%	5.3%
Combination Abdominal CT Scan	58	5.2%	10.1%	10.5%
Combination Brain/Sinus CT Scan	157	5.7%	2.3%	2.7%
Combination Chest CT Scan[1]	-	-	3.7%	2.7%
Follow-up Mammogram/Ultrasound	236	8.9%	8.9%	8.8%
Lumbar Spine MRI for Low Back Pain[7]	-	-	36.6%	37.2%

Coliseum Medical Center

350 Hospital Drive
Macon, GA 31217
URL: www.coliseumhealthsystem.com
Type: Acute Care Hospitals
Ownership: Voluntary non-profit - Private
Phone: 478-765-4100
Fax: 478-751-0424
Emergency Services: Yes
Beds: 250

Key Personnel:
CEO/President. . . . . Timothy C Tobin
Emergency Room . . . . Dan Weathers, MD

Measure	Cases	This Hosp.	State Avg.	U.S. Avg.
Blood Clot Prevention and Treatment				
Anticoagulation Overlap Therapy[2]	71	77%	90%	93%
ICU Venous Thromboembolism Prophylaxis[2]	108	96%	90%	92%
Incidence of Potentially Preventable VTE[1,2]	-	-	13%	10%
UFH with Dosages/Platelet Monitoring[2]	80	100%	99%	97%
Venous Thromboembolism Prophylaxis[2]	333	86%	80%	85%
Warfarin Therapy Discharge Instructions[2]	57	100%	78%	75%
Chest Pain/Possible Heart Attack Care				
Aspirin Given Within 24 Hours of Arrival[1,3]	-	-	94%	96%
Fibrinolytic Meds Within 30 Min. of Arrival[5]	-	-	35%	58%
Average Time to ECG (minutes)[1,3]	-	-	8	7
Average Time to Transfer (minutes)[5]	-	-	73	60
Children's Asthma Care				
Received Home Management Plan of Care	-	-	-	88%
Received Reliever Medication	-	-	-	100%
Received Systemic Corticosteroids	-	-	-	100%
Emergency Department				
Admittance Decision Time (minutes)[2]	641	78	100	98
Head CT Results Within 45 Min. of Arrival	12	50%	45%	57%
Patients Who Left ER Before Being Seen	41,650	1%	3%	2%
Time from ER Arrival to Admit. (minutes)[2]	641	239	286	274
Time from ER Arrival to Discharge (minutes)	455	162	140	134
Time in ER Before Being Evaluated (minutes)	500	10	32	26
Time to Pain Meds for Fractures (minutes)	29	78	64	57
Heart Attack Care				
Aspirin Given at Discharge	225	100%	99%	99%
Fibrinolytic Meds Within 30 Min. of Arrival[7]	-	-	80%	54%
PCI Within 90 Minutes of Arrival	29	97%	95%	96%
Statin Prescribed at Discharge	231	100%	98%	98%
Heart Failure Care				
ACE Inhibitor or ARB for LVSD	136	100%	97%	97%
Discharge Instructions Given	367	100%	92%	94%
Evaluation of LVS Function	410	100%	99%	99%
Medicare Spending				
Medicare Spending per Patient (ratio)	-	0.99	0.95	0.98
Pneumonia Care				
Appropriate Initial Antibiotic Given	108	99%	95%	95%
Blood Culture Timing	230	100%	97%	98%
Pregnancy and Delivery Care				
Newborn Deliveries Scheduled Early[2]	38	0%	8%	6%
Preventive Care				
Immunization for Influenza[2]	597	98%	88%	90%
Immunization for Pneumonia[2]	824	97%	90%	92%
Stroke Care				
Anticoagulation Therapy for Atrial Fibrillation[1,2]	-	-	94%	95%
Antithrombotic Therapy Timing[2]	74	96%	97%	98%
Assessed for Rehabilitation[2]	83	96%	97%	97%
Discharged on Antithrombotic Therapy[2]	82	96%	98%	99%
Discharged on Statin Medication[2]	69	91%	94%	94%
Thrombolytic Therapy Timing[1,2]	-	-	58%	66%
Venous Thromboembolism Prophylaxis[2]	84	95%	92%	94%
Written Stroke Educational Materials Given[2]	49	100%	84%	88%
Surgical Care Improvement Project				
Appropriate Beta Blocker Usage[2]	169	100%	97%	98%
Appropriate VTP Within 24 Hours[2]	250	98%	98%	98%
Controlled Postoperative Blood Glucose[2]	119	98%	96%	97%
Perioperative Temperature Management[2]	356	100%	100%	100%
Prophylactic Antibiotic Selection[2]	269	99%	99%	99%
Prophylactic Antibiotic Selection (Outpatient)	697	99%	98%	98%
Prophylactic Antibiotic Stopped[2]	257	99%	98%	98%
Prophylactic Antibiotic Timing[2]	269	99%	99%	99%
Prophylactic Antibiotic Timing (Outpatient)	698	99%	98%	98%
Urinary Catheter Removal[2]	194	100%	97%	97%
Survey of Patients' Hospital Experiences				
Area Around Room 'Always' Quiet at Night	300+	69%	66%	61%
Doctors 'Always' Communicated Well	300+	82%	83%	82%
Home Recovery Information Given	300+	85%	84%	85%
Hospital Given 9 or 10 on 10 Point Scale	300+	69%	69%	71%
Meds 'Always' Explained Before Given	300+	62%	63%	64%
Nurses 'Always' Communicated Well	300+	76%	78%	79%
Pain 'Always' Well Controlled	300+	70%	71%	71%
Room and Bathroom 'Always' Clean	300+	66%	71%	73%
Timely Help 'Always' Received	300+	60%	65%	68%
Would Definitely Recommend Hospital	300+	72%	70%	71%
Use of Medical Imaging				
Cardiac Imaging Stress Test before Surgery[1]	-	-	5.5%	5.3%
Combination Abdominal CT Scan	633	1.1%	10.1%	10.5%
Combination Brain/Sinus CT Scan	847	2.7%	2.3%	2.7%
Combination Chest CT Scan	290	0.7%	3.7%	2.7%
Follow-up Mammogram/Ultrasound	1,729	7.4%	8.9%	8.8%
Lumbar Spine MRI for Low Back Pain[1]	-	-	36.6%	37.2%

Coliseum Northside Hospital

400 Charter Boulevard
Macon, GA 31210
Type: Acute Care Hospitals
Ownership: Proprietary
Phone: 478-757-5990
Fax: 478-751-0424
Emergency Services: Yes
Beds: 103

Key Personnel:
Operating Room. . . . . Frank Arnold
Radiology. . . . . Thomas Butler, MD
CEO . . . . Steve Daugherty
Quality Assurance . . . . Karen Henneberry
Chief of Medical Staff. . . . . Susan Oliver, MD
Emergency Room . . . . Mary Stone, RN

Measure	Cases	This Hosp.	State Avg.	U.S. Avg.
Blood Clot Prevention and Treatment				
Anticoagulation Overlap Therapy[2]	22	68%	90%	93%
ICU Venous Thromboembolism Prophylaxis[2]	55	100%	90%	92%
Incidence of Potentially Preventable VTE[1,2]	-	-	13%	10%
UFH with Dosages/Platelet Monitoring[2]	23	100%	99%	97%
Venous Thromboembolism Prophylaxis[2]	204	92%	80%	85%
Warfarin Therapy Discharge Instructions[2]	17	100%	78%	75%
Chest Pain/Possible Heart Attack Care				
Aspirin Given Within 24 Hours of Arrival	33	94%	94%	96%
Fibrinolytic Meds Within 30 Min. of Arrival[7]	-	-	35%	58%
Average Time to ECG (minutes)	33	12	8	7
Average Time to Transfer (minutes)[1]	-	-	73	60
Children's Asthma Care				
Received Home Management Plan of Care	-	-	-	88%
Received Reliever Medication	-	-	-	100%
Received Systemic Corticosteroids	-	-	-	100%
Emergency Department				
Admittance Decision Time (minutes)[2]	410	62	100	98
Head CT Results Within 45 Min. of Arrival[1]	-	-	45%	57%

NOTE: Hospital profiles are in alphabetical order by state, then city, then hospital within the city; Rankings exclude hospitals with less than 25 cases except for patient surveys which excludes hospitals with less than 100 cases; (a) 100-299 cases; (1) The number of cases/patients is too few to report; (2) Data submitted were based on a sample of cases/patients; (3) Results are based on a shorter time period than required; (4) Data suppressed by CMS for one or more quarters; (5) Results are not available for this reporting period; (6) Fewer than 100 patients completed the HCAHPS survey; (7) No cases met the criteria for this measure; (8) The lower limit of the confidence interval cannot be calculated if the number of observed infections equals zero; (9) No data are available from the state/territory for this reporting period; (10) The scores shown reflect fewer than 50 completed surveys; (11) There were discrepancies in the data collection process; (12) This measure does not apply to this hospital for this reporting period; (13) Results cannot be calculated for this reporting period; (14) The results for this state are combined with nearby states to protect confidentiality; Please refer to the User's Guide for a full explanation of data.

Measure	Cases	This Hosp.	State Avg.	U.S. Avg.
Patients Who Left ER Before Being Seen	23,478	1%	3%	2%
Time from ER Arrival to Admit. (minutes)[2]	410	224	286	274
Time from ER Arrival to Discharge (minutes)	453	114	140	134
Time in ER Before Being Evaluated (minutes)	478	8	32	26
Time to Pain Meds for Fractures (minutes)	70	42	64	57
Heart Attack Care				
Aspirin Given at Discharge[1]	-	-	99%	99%
Fibrinolytic Meds Within 30 Min. of Arrival[7]	-	-	80%	54%
PCI Within 90 Minutes of Arrival[7]	-	-	95%	96%
Statin Prescribed at Discharge[1]	-	-	98%	98%
Heart Failure Care				
ACE Inhibitor or ARB for LVSD	16	94%	97%	97%
Discharge Instructions Given	52	98%	92%	94%
Evaluation of LVS Function	55	98%	99%	99%
Medicare Spending				
Medicare Spending per Patient (ratio)	-	0.99	0.95	0.98
Pneumonia Care				
Appropriate Initial Antibiotic Given	43	100%	95%	95%
Blood Culture Timing	73	99%	97%	98%
Pregnancy and Delivery Care				
Newborn Deliveries Scheduled Early[2,7]	-	-	8%	6%
Preventive Care				
Immunization for Influenza[2]	328	99%	88%	90%
Immunization for Pneumonia[2]	442	94%	90%	92%
Stroke Care				
Anticoagulation Therapy for Atrial Fibrillation[1,2]	-	-	94%	95%
Antithrombotic Therapy Timing[2]	12	100%	97%	98%
Assessed for Rehabilitation[2]	12	100%	97%	97%
Discharged on Antithrombotic Therapy[2]	12	100%	98%	99%
Discharged on Statin Medication[1,2]	-	-	94%	94%
Thrombolytic Therapy Timing[2,7]	-	-	58%	66%
Venous Thromboembolism Prophylaxis[2]	11	91%	92%	94%
Written Stroke Educational Materials Given[1,2]	-	-	84%	88%
Surgical Care Improvement Project				
Appropriate Beta Blocker Usage[2]	67	99%	97%	98%
Appropriate VTP Within 24 Hours[2]	210	99%	98%	98%
Controlled Postoperative Blood Glucose[2,7]	-	-	96%	97%
Perioperative Temperature Management[2]	233	100%	100%	100%
Prophylactic Antibiotic Selection[2]	185	100%	99%	99%
Prophylactic Antibiotic Selection (Outpatient)	38	100%	98%	98%
Prophylactic Antibiotic Stopped[2]	182	97%	98%	98%
Prophylactic Antibiotic Timing[2]	185	100%	99%	99%
Prophylactic Antibiotic Timing (Outpatient)	38	100%	98%	98%
Urinary Catheter Removal[2]	103	96%	97%	97%
Survey of Patients' Hospital Experiences				
Area Around Room 'Always' Quiet at Night	300+	73%	66%	61%
Doctors 'Always' Communicated Well	300+	79%	83%	82%
Home Recovery Information Given	300+	82%	84%	85%
Hospital Given 9 or 10 on 10 Point Scale	300+	70%	69%	71%
Meds 'Always' Explained Before Given	300+	63%	63%	64%
Nurses 'Always' Communicated Well	300+	75%	78%	79%
Pain 'Always' Well Controlled	300+	70%	71%	71%
Room and Bathroom 'Always' Clean	300+	71%	71%	73%
Timely Help 'Always' Received	300+	62%	65%	68%
Would Definitely Recommend Hospital	300+	73%	70%	71%
Use of Medical Imaging				
Cardiac Imaging Stress Test before Surgery[1]	-	-	5.5%	5.3%
Combination Abdominal CT Scan	275	3.3%	10.1%	10.5%
Combination Brain/Sinus CT Scan[1]	-	-	2.3%	2.7%
Combination Chest CT Scan[1]	-	-	3.7%	2.7%
Follow-up Mammogram/Ultrasound	270	5.6%	8.9%	8.8%
Lumbar Spine MRI for Low Back Pain[1]	-	-	36.6%	37.2%

Medical Center of Central Georgia

777 Hemlock Street Phone: 478-633-6805
Macon, GA 31201 Fax: 478-633-1772
URL: www.mccg.org
Type: Acute Care Hospitals Emergency Services: Yes
Ownership: Govt - Hospital Dist/Auth Beds: 603

Key Personnel:
Pediatric In-Patient Care . . . . Frank Bowyer
Anesthesiology. . . . . Manuel Castrosana
Infection Control. . . . . Nancy Dunham
Operating Room. . . . . Mary Freeman, RN
Radiology. . . . . Lee H Hall
Chairman/CEO . . . . A. Kenneth Harper, MD
Chief of Medical Staff. . . . . Dr. Ninfa Saunders, FACHE
Quality Assurance . . . . Lisa Smitha

Measure	Cases	This Hosp.	State Avg.	U.S. Avg.
Blood Clot Prevention and Treatment				
Anticoagulation Overlap Therapy[2]	188	64%	90%	93%
ICU Venous Thromboembolism Prophylaxis[2]	87	98%	90%	92%
Incidence of Potentially Preventable VTE[2]	51	6%	13%	10%
UFH with Dosages/Platelet Monitoring[2]	199	99%	99%	97%
Venous Thromboembolism Prophylaxis[2]	312	81%	80%	85%
Warfarin Therapy Discharge Instructions[2]	148	61%	78%	75%
Chest Pain/Possible Heart Attack Care				
Aspirin Given Within 24 Hours of Arrival[1,3]	-	-	94%	96%
Fibrinolytic Meds Within 30 Min. of Arrival[5]	-	-	35%	58%
Average Time to ECG (minutes)[1,3]	-	-	8	7
Average Time to Transfer (minutes)[5]	-	-	73	60
Children's Asthma Care				
Received Home Management Plan of Care	-	-	-	88%
Received Reliever Medication	-	-	-	100%
Received Systemic Corticosteroids	-	-	-	100%
Emergency Department				
Admittance Decision Time (minutes)[2]	528	218	100	98
Head CT Results Within 45 Min. of Arrival	14	21%	45%	57%
Patients Who Left ER Before Being Seen	66,546	5%	3%	2%
Time from ER Arrival to Admit. (minutes)[2]	530	482	286	274
Time from ER Arrival to Discharge (minutes)	359	243	140	134
Time in ER Before Being Evaluated (minutes)	376	52	32	26
Time to Pain Meds for Fractures (minutes)	111	82	64	57
Heart Attack Care				
Aspirin Given at Discharge	771	97%	99%	99%
Fibrinolytic Meds Within 30 Min. of Arrival[7]	-	-	80%	54%
PCI Within 90 Minutes of Arrival	77	95%	95%	96%
Statin Prescribed at Discharge	744	97%	98%	98%
Heart Failure Care				
ACE Inhibitor or ARB for LVSD[2]	140	99%	97%	97%
Discharge Instructions Given[2]	243	100%	92%	94%
Evaluation of LVS Function[2]	282	100%	99%	99%
Medicare Spending				
Medicare Spending per Patient (ratio)	-	0.98	0.95	0.98
Pneumonia Care				
Appropriate Initial Antibiotic Given[2]	76	84%	95%	95%
Blood Culture Timing[2]	110	92%	97%	98%
Pregnancy and Delivery Care				
Newborn Deliveries Scheduled Early[2]	40	8%	8%	6%
Preventive Care				
Immunization for Influenza[2]	531	60%	88%	90%
Immunization for Pneumonia[2]	646	66%	90%	92%
Stroke Care				
Anticoagulation Therapy for Atrial Fibrillation[2]	36	97%	94%	95%
Antithrombotic Therapy Timing[2]	327	96%	97%	98%
Assessed for Rehabilitation[2]	458	98%	97%	97%
Discharged on Antithrombotic Therapy[2]	343	98%	98%	99%
Discharged on Statin Medication[2]	275	95%	94%	94%
Thrombolytic Therapy Timing[2]	29	93%	58%	66%
Venous Thromboembolism Prophylaxis[2]	512	93%	92%	94%
Written Stroke Educational Materials Given[2]	269	93%	84%	88%
Surgical Care Improvement Project				
Appropriate Beta Blocker Usage[2]	222	95%	97%	98%
Appropriate VTP Within 24 Hours[2]	437	99%	98%	98%
Controlled Postoperative Blood Glucose[2]	128	100%	96%	97%
Perioperative Temperature Management[2]	558	100%	100%	100%
Prophylactic Antibiotic Selection[2]	513	99%	99%	99%
Prophylactic Antibiotic Selection (Outpatient)	700	98%	98%	98%
Prophylactic Antibiotic Stopped[2]	499	96%	98%	98%
Prophylactic Antibiotic Timing[2]	513	99%	99%	99%
Prophylactic Antibiotic Timing (Outpatient)	701	99%	98%	98%
Urinary Catheter Removal[2]	358	98%	97%	97%
Survey of Patients' Hospital Experiences				
Area Around Room 'Always' Quiet at Night	300+	63%	66%	61%
Doctors 'Always' Communicated Well	300+	80%	83%	82%
Home Recovery Information Given	300+	82%	84%	85%
Hospital Given 9 or 10 on 10 Point Scale	300+	69%	69%	71%
Meds 'Always' Explained Before Given	300+	55%	63%	64%
Nurses 'Always' Communicated Well	300+	73%	78%	79%
Pain 'Always' Well Controlled	300+	67%	71%	71%
Room and Bathroom 'Always' Clean	300+	67%	71%	73%
Timely Help 'Always' Received	300+	58%	65%	68%
Would Definitely Recommend Hospital	300+	74%	70%	71%
Use of Medical Imaging				
Cardiac Imaging Stress Test before Surgery	358	6.1%	5.5%	5.3%
Combination Abdominal CT Scan	882	10.4%	10.1%	10.5%
Combination Brain/Sinus CT Scan	1,009	2.2%	2.3%	2.7%
Combination Chest CT Scan	754	1.3%	3.7%	2.7%
Follow-up Mammogram/Ultrasound	2,673	4.4%	8.9%	8.8%
Lumbar Spine MRI for Low Back Pain[1]	-	-	36.6%	37.2%

Morgan Memorial Hospital

1077 South Main Street Phone: 706-342-1667
Madison, GA 30650
Type: Critical Access Hospitals Emergency Services: Yes
Ownership: Govt - Hospital Dist/Auth

Measure	Cases	This Hosp.	State Avg.	U.S. Avg.
Blood Clot Prevention and Treatment				
Anticoagulation Overlap Therapy[5]	-	-	90%	93%
ICU Venous Thromboembolism Prophylaxis[5]	-	-	90%	92%
Incidence of Potentially Preventable VTE[5]	-	-	13%	10%
UFH with Dosages/Platelet Monitoring[5]	-	-	99%	97%
Venous Thromboembolism Prophylaxis[5]	-	-	80%	85%
Warfarin Therapy Discharge Instructions[5]	-	-	78%	75%
Chest Pain/Possible Heart Attack Care				
Aspirin Given Within 24 Hours of Arrival[1,3]	-	-	94%	96%
Fibrinolytic Meds Within 30 Min. of Arrival[5]	-	-	35%	58%
Average Time to ECG (minutes)[1,3]	-	-	8	7
Average Time to Transfer (minutes)[5]	-	-	73	60
Children's Asthma Care				
Received Home Management Plan of Care	-	-	-	88%
Received Reliever Medication	-	-	-	100%
Received Systemic Corticosteroids	-	-	-	100%
Emergency Department				
Admittance Decision Time (minutes)	86	56	100	98
Head CT Results Within 45 Min. of Arrival[5]	-	-	45%	57%
Patients Who Left ER Before Being Seen	7,375	1%	3%	2%
Time from ER Arrival to Admit. (minutes)	91	216	286	274
Time from ER Arrival to Discharge (minutes)	363	79	140	134
Time in ER Before Being Evaluated (minutes)[7]	-	-	32	26
Time to Pain Meds for Fractures (minutes)[1,3]	-	-	64	57
Heart Attack Care				
Aspirin Given at Discharge[3,7]	-	-	99%	99%
Fibrinolytic Meds Within 30 Min. of Arrival[3,7]	-	-	80%	54%
PCI Within 90 Minutes of Arrival[3,7]	-	-	95%	96%
Statin Prescribed at Discharge[3,7]	-	-	98%	98%
Heart Failure Care				
ACE Inhibitor or ARB for LVSD[1]	-	-	97%	97%
Discharge Instructions Given[1]	-	-	92%	94%
Evaluation of LVS Function[1]	-	-	99%	99%
Medicare Spending				
Medicare Spending per Patient (ratio)	-	-	0.95	0.98
Pneumonia Care				
Appropriate Initial Antibiotic Given	13	69%	95%	95%
Blood Culture Timing	14	100%	97%	98%
Pregnancy and Delivery Care				
Newborn Deliveries Scheduled Early[5]	-	-	8%	6%
Preventive Care				
Immunization for Influenza	79	78%	88%	90%
Immunization for Pneumonia	120	78%	90%	92%
Stroke Care				
Anticoagulation Therapy for Atrial Fibrillation[5]	-	-	94%	95%
Antithrombotic Therapy Timing[5]	-	-	97%	98%
Assessed for Rehabilitation[5]	-	-	97%	97%
Discharged on Antithrombotic Therapy[5]	-	-	98%	99%
Discharged on Statin Medication[5]	-	-	94%	94%
Thrombolytic Therapy Timing[5]	-	-	58%	66%
Venous Thromboembolism Prophylaxis[5]	-	-	92%	94%
Written Stroke Educational Materials Given[5]	-	-	84%	88%

NOTE: Hospital profiles are in alphabetical order by state, then city, then hospital within the city; Rankings exclude hospitals with less than 25 cases except for patient surveys which excludes hospitals with less than 100 cases; (a) 100-299 cases; (1) The number of cases/patients is too few to report; (2) Data submitted were based on a sample of cases/patients; (3) Results are based on a shorter time period than required; (4) Data suppressed by CMS for one or more quarters; (5) Results are not available for this reporting period; (6) Fewer than 100 patients completed the HCAHPS survey; (7) No cases met the criteria for this measure; (8) The lower limit of the confidence interval cannot be calculated if the number of observed infections equals zero; (9) No data are available from the state/territory for this reporting period; (10) The scores shown reflect fewer than 50 completed surveys; (11) There were discrepancies in the data collection process; (12) This measure does not apply to this hospital for this reporting period; (13) Results cannot be calculated for this reporting period; (14) The results for this state are combined with nearby states to protect confidentiality; Please refer to the User's Guide for a full explanation of data.

Measure	Cases	This Hosp.	State Avg.	U.S. Avg.
Surgical Care Improvement Project				
Appropriate Beta Blocker Usage[5]	-	-	97%	98%
Appropriate VTP Within 24 Hours[5]	-	-	98%	98%
Controlled Postoperative Blood Glucose[5]	-	-	96%	97%
Perioperative Temperature Management[5]	-	-	100%	100%
Prophylactic Antibiotic Selection[5]	-	-	99%	99%
Prophylactic Antibiotic Selection (Outpatient)[5]	-	-	98%	98%
Prophylactic Antibiotic Stopped[5]	-	-	98%	98%
Prophylactic Antibiotic Timing[5]	-	-	99%	99%
Prophylactic Antibiotic Timing (Outpatient)[5]	-	-	98%	98%
Urinary Catheter Removal[5]	-	-	97%	97%
Survey of Patients' Hospital Experiences				
Area Around Room 'Always' Quiet at Night[5]	-	-	66%	61%
Doctors 'Always' Communicated Well[5]	-	-	83%	82%
Home Recovery Information Given[5]	-	-	84%	85%
Hospital Given 9 or 10 on 10 Point Scale[5]	-	-	69%	71%
Meds 'Always' Explained Before Given[5]	-	-	63%	64%
Nurses 'Always' Communicated Well[5]	-	-	78%	79%
Pain 'Always' Well Controlled[5]	-	-	71%	71%
Room and Bathroom 'Always' Clean[5]	-	-	71%	73%
Timely Help 'Always' Received[5]	-	-	65%	68%
Would Definitely Recommend Hospital[5]	-	-	70%	71%
Use of Medical Imaging				
Cardiac Imaging Stress Test before Surgery[1]	-	-	5.5%	5.3%
Combination Abdominal CT Scan	109	7.3%	10.1%	10.5%
Combination Brain/Sinus CT Scan	155	0.0%	2.3%	2.7%
Combination Chest CT Scan	51	3.9%	3.7%	2.7%
Follow-up Mammogram/Ultrasound	216	6.9%	8.9%	8.8%
Lumbar Spine MRI for Low Back Pain[1]	-	-	36.6%	37.2%

Wellstar Kennestone Hospital

677 Church Street
Marietta, GA 30060
Phone: 770-793-5000
URL: www.wellstar.org
Type: Acute Care Hospitals
Emergency Services: Yes
Ownership: Voluntary non-profit - Other
Beds: 633

Key Personnel:
Administrator . . . . Candice Saunders
Radiology. . . . . Gerry Sharp

Measure	Cases	This Hosp.	State Avg.	U.S. Avg.
Blood Clot Prevention and Treatment				
Anticoagulation Overlap Therapy[2]	229	98%	90%	93%
ICU Venous Thromboembolism Prophylaxis[2]	97	98%	90%	92%
Incidence of Potentially Preventable VTE[2]	67	15%	13%	10%
UFH with Dosages/Platelet Monitoring[2]	199	100%	99%	97%
Venous Thromboembolism Prophylaxis[2]	332	83%	80%	85%
Warfarin Therapy Discharge Instructions[2]	154	84%	78%	75%
Chest Pain/Possible Heart Attack Care				
Aspirin Given Within 24 Hours of Arrival	37	89%	94%	96%
Fibrinolytic Meds Within 30 Min. of Arrival[5]	-	-	35%	58%
Average Time to ECG (minutes)	38	0	8	7
Average Time to Transfer (minutes)[5]	-	-	73	60
Children's Asthma Care				
Received Home Management Plan of Care	-	-	-	88%
Received Reliever Medication	-	-	-	100%
Received Systemic Corticosteroids	-	-	-	100%
Emergency Department				
Admittance Decision Time (minutes)[2]	540	125	100	98
Head CT Results Within 45 Min. of Arrival	31	55%	45%	57%
Patients Who Left ER Before Being Seen	>100k	3%	3%	2%
Time from ER Arrival to Admit. (minutes)[2]	570	312	286	274
Time from ER Arrival to Discharge (minutes)	384	201	140	134
Time in ER Before Being Evaluated (minutes)	419	49	32	26
Time to Pain Meds for Fractures (minutes)	362	60	64	57
Heart Attack Care				
Aspirin Given at Discharge[2]	556	100%	99%	99%
Fibrinolytic Meds Within 30 Min. of Arrival[2,7]	-	-	80%	54%
PCI Within 90 Minutes of Arrival[2]	137	94%	95%	96%
Statin Prescribed at Discharge[2]	551	99%	98%	98%
Heart Failure Care				
ACE Inhibitor or ARB for LVSD[2]	209	99%	97%	97%
Discharge Instructions Given[2]	707	91%	92%	94%
Evaluation of LVS Function[2]	801	100%	99%	99%
Medicare Spending				
Medicare Spending per Patient (ratio)	-	0.98	0.95	0.98
Pneumonia Care				
Appropriate Initial Antibiotic Given[2]	280	96%	95%	95%
Blood Culture Timing[2]	402	99%	97%	98%
Pregnancy and Delivery Care				
Newborn Deliveries Scheduled Early[2]	87	5%	8%	6%
Preventive Care				
Immunization for Influenza[2]	576	90%	88%	90%
Immunization for Pneumonia[2]	608	89%	90%	92%
Stroke Care				
Anticoagulation Therapy for Atrial Fibrillation[2]	12	92%	94%	95%
Antithrombotic Therapy Timing[2]	89	100%	97%	98%
Assessed for Rehabilitation[2]	98	100%	97%	97%
Discharged on Antithrombotic Therapy[2]	84	100%	98%	99%
Discharged on Statin Medication[2]	58	100%	94%	94%
Thrombolytic Therapy Timing[1,2]	-	-	58%	66%
Venous Thromboembolism Prophylaxis[2]	106	95%	92%	94%
Written Stroke Educational Materials Given[2]	54	91%	84%	88%
Surgical Care Improvement Project				
Appropriate Beta Blocker Usage[2]	498	99%	97%	98%
Appropriate VTP Within 24 Hours[2]	809	98%	98%	98%
Controlled Postoperative Blood Glucose[2]	248	98%	96%	97%
Perioperative Temperature Management[2]	1,194	100%	100%	100%
Prophylactic Antibiotic Selection[2]	852	99%	99%	99%
Prophylactic Antibiotic Selection (Outpatient)	841	99%	98%	98%
Prophylactic Antibiotic Stopped[2]	832	99%	98%	98%
Prophylactic Antibiotic Timing[2]	853	99%	99%	99%
Prophylactic Antibiotic Timing (Outpatient)	844	99%	98%	98%
Urinary Catheter Removal[2]	612	97%	97%	97%
Survey of Patients' Hospital Experiences				
Area Around Room 'Always' Quiet at Night	300+	64%	66%	61%
Doctors 'Always' Communicated Well	300+	79%	83%	82%
Home Recovery Information Given	300+	83%	84%	85%
Hospital Given 9 or 10 on 10 Point Scale	300+	72%	69%	71%
Meds 'Always' Explained Before Given	300+	61%	63%	64%
Nurses 'Always' Communicated Well	300+	78%	78%	79%
Pain 'Always' Well Controlled	300+	71%	71%	71%
Room and Bathroom 'Always' Clean	300+	74%	71%	73%
Timely Help 'Always' Received	300+	65%	65%	68%
Would Definitely Recommend Hospital	300+	74%	70%	71%
Use of Medical Imaging				
Cardiac Imaging Stress Test before Surgery	2,242	4.4%	5.5%	5.3%
Combination Abdominal CT Scan	2,809	7.8%	10.1%	10.5%
Combination Brain/Sinus CT Scan	1,963	2.1%	2.3%	2.7%
Combination Chest CT Scan	2,704	0.5%	3.7%	2.7%
Follow-up Mammogram/Ultrasound	4,941	16.5%	8.9%	8.8%
Lumbar Spine MRI for Low Back Pain	187	27.3%	36.6%	37.2%

Candler County Hospital

400 Cedar Street
Metter, GA 30439
Phone: 912-685-5741
Fax: 912-685-3905
E-mail: cchospital@pineland.net
URL: www.candlercountyhospital.com
Type: Critical Access Hospitals
Emergency Services: Yes
Ownership: Govt - Hospital Dist/Auth
Beds: 60

Key Personnel:
Chief of Medical Staff. . . . . Roger G Branch, MD
Chairman/CEO . . . . Dale Fordham
Infection Control. . . . . Teal Jeffers, RN
CEO/President. . . . . Damien Scott, PT MS OCS
Emergency Room . . . . Dorsey Smith, MD
Radiology. . . . . Courtney Waters
Quality Assurance . . . . Linda Whitfeild
Operating Room. . . . . Nancy Wrenn, RN

Measure	Cases	This Hosp.	State Avg.	U.S. Avg.
Blood Clot Prevention and Treatment				
Anticoagulation Overlap Therapy[5]	-	-	90%	93%
ICU Venous Thromboembolism Prophylaxis[5]	-	-	90%	92%
Incidence of Potentially Preventable VTE[5]	-	-	13%	10%
UFH with Dosages/Platelet Monitoring[5]	-	-	99%	97%
Venous Thromboembolism Prophylaxis[5]	-	-	80%	85%
Warfarin Therapy Discharge Instructions[5]	-	-	78%	75%
Chest Pain/Possible Heart Attack Care				
Aspirin Given Within 24 Hours of Arrival	-	-	94%	96%
Fibrinolytic Meds Within 30 Min. of Arrival	-	-	35%	58%
Average Time to ECG (minutes)	-	-	8	7
Average Time to Transfer (minutes)	-	-	73	60
Children's Asthma Care				
Received Home Management Plan of Care	-	-	-	88%
Received Reliever Medication	-	-	-	100%
Received Systemic Corticosteroids	-	-	-	100%
Emergency Department				
Admittance Decision Time (minutes)[5]	-	-	100	98
Head CT Results Within 45 Min. of Arrival	-	-	45%	57%
Patients Who Left ER Before Being Seen	-	-	3%	2%
Time from ER Arrival to Admit. (minutes)[5]	-	-	286	274
Time from ER Arrival to Discharge (minutes)	-	-	140	134
Time in ER Before Being Evaluated (minutes)	-	-	32	26
Time to Pain Meds for Fractures (minutes)	-	-	64	57
Heart Attack Care				
Aspirin Given at Discharge[1,3]	-	-	99%	99%
Fibrinolytic Meds Within 30 Min. of Arrival[3,7]	-	-	80%	54%
PCI Within 90 Minutes of Arrival[3,7]	-	-	95%	96%
Statin Prescribed at Discharge[1,3]	-	-	98%	98%
Heart Failure Care				
ACE Inhibitor or ARB for LVSD[1]	-	-	97%	97%
Discharge Instructions Given	15	100%	92%	94%
Evaluation of LVS Function	24	96%	99%	99%
Medicare Spending				
Medicare Spending per Patient (ratio)	-	-	0.95	0.98
Pneumonia Care				
Appropriate Initial Antibiotic Given	28	68%	95%	95%
Blood Culture Timing	51	100%	97%	98%
Pregnancy and Delivery Care				
Newborn Deliveries Scheduled Early[5]	-	-	8%	6%
Preventive Care				
Immunization for Influenza[5]	-	-	88%	90%
Immunization for Pneumonia[5]	-	-	90%	92%
Stroke Care				
Anticoagulation Therapy for Atrial Fibrillation[5]	-	-	94%	95%
Antithrombotic Therapy Timing[5]	-	-	97%	98%
Assessed for Rehabilitation[5]	-	-	97%	97%
Discharged on Antithrombotic Therapy[5]	-	-	98%	99%
Discharged on Statin Medication[5]	-	-	94%	94%
Thrombolytic Therapy Timing[5]	-	-	58%	66%
Venous Thromboembolism Prophylaxis[5]	-	-	92%	94%
Written Stroke Educational Materials Given[5]	-	-	84%	88%
Surgical Care Improvement Project				
Appropriate Beta Blocker Usage[5]	-	-	97%	98%
Appropriate VTP Within 24 Hours[5]	-	-	98%	98%
Controlled Postoperative Blood Glucose[5]	-	-	96%	97%
Perioperative Temperature Management[5]	-	-	100%	100%
Prophylactic Antibiotic Selection[5]	-	-	99%	99%
Prophylactic Antibiotic Selection (Outpatient)	-	-	98%	98%
Prophylactic Antibiotic Stopped[5]	-	-	98%	98%
Prophylactic Antibiotic Timing[5]	-	-	99%	99%
Prophylactic Antibiotic Timing (Outpatient)	-	-	98%	98%
Urinary Catheter Removal[5]	-	-	97%	97%
Survey of Patients' Hospital Experiences				
Area Around Room 'Always' Quiet at Night[5]	-	-	66%	61%
Doctors 'Always' Communicated Well[5]	-	-	83%	82%
Home Recovery Information Given[5]	-	-	84%	85%
Hospital Given 9 or 10 on 10 Point Scale[5]	-	-	69%	71%
Meds 'Always' Explained Before Given[5]	-	-	63%	64%
Nurses 'Always' Communicated Well[5]	-	-	78%	79%
Pain 'Always' Well Controlled[5]	-	-	71%	71%
Room and Bathroom 'Always' Clean[5]	-	-	71%	73%
Timely Help 'Always' Received[5]	-	-	65%	68%
Would Definitely Recommend Hospital[5]	-	-	70%	71%
Use of Medical Imaging				
Cardiac Imaging Stress Test before Surgery	-	-	5.5%	5.3%
Combination Abdominal CT Scan	-	-	10.1%	10.5%
Combination Brain/Sinus CT Scan	-	-	2.3%	2.7%
Combination Chest CT Scan	-	-	3.7%	2.7%
Follow-up Mammogram/Ultrasound	-	-	8.9%	8.8%

NOTE: Hospital profiles are in alphabetical order by state, then city, then hospital within the city; Rankings exclude hospitals with less than 25 cases except for patient surveys which excludes hospitals with less than 100 cases; (a) 100-299 cases; (1) The number of cases/patients is too few to report; (2) Data submitted were based on a sample of cases/patients; (3) Results are based on a shorter time period than required; (4) Data suppressed by CMS for one or more quarters; (5) Results are not available for this reporting period; (6) Fewer than 100 patients completed the HCAHPS survey; (7) No cases met the criteria for this measure; (8) The lower limit of the confidence interval cannot be calculated if the number of observed infections equals zero; (9) No data are available from the state/territory for this reporting period; (10) The scores shown reflect fewer than 50 completed surveys; (11) There were discrepancies in the data collection process; (12) This measure does not apply to this hospital for this reporting period; (13) Results cannot be calculated for this reporting period; (14) The results for this state are combined with nearby states to protect confidentiality; Please refer to the User's Guide for a full explanation of data.

Measure	Cases	This Hosp.	State Avg.	U.S. Avg.
Lumbar Spine MRI for Low Back Pain		-	36.6%	37.2%

Oconee Regional Medical Center

821 N Cobb Street Post Office Box 690 Phone: 478-454-3550
Milledgeville, GA 31061 Fax: 478-454-3555
URL: www.oconeeregional.com
Type: Acute Care Hospitals Emergency Services: Yes
Ownership: Voluntary non-profit - Private Beds: 160
Key Personnel:
CEO/President. . . . . Jean Aycock
Operating Room. . . . . Dianne Franklin
Quality Assurance . . . . Mollie Thomas

Measure	Cases	This Hosp.	State Avg.	U.S. Avg.
Blood Clot Prevention and Treatment				
Anticoagulation Overlap Therapy[2]	41	68%	90%	93%
ICU Venous Thromboembolism Prophylaxis[2]	122	90%	90%	92%
Incidence of Potentially Preventable VTE[1,2]	-	-	13%	10%
UFH with Dosages/Platelet Monitoring[2]	29	100%	99%	97%
Venous Thromboembolism Prophylaxis[2]	384	81%	80%	85%
Warfarin Therapy Discharge Instructions[2]	30	50%	78%	75%
Chest Pain/Possible Heart Attack Care				
Aspirin Given Within 24 Hours of Arrival	105	100%	94%	96%
Fibrinolytic Meds Within 30 Min. of Arrival[7]	-	-	35%	58%
Average Time to ECG (minutes)	107	8	8	7
Average Time to Transfer (minutes)[1]	-	-	73	60
Children's Asthma Care				
Received Home Management Plan of Care	-	-	-	88%
Received Reliever Medication	-	-	-	100%
Received Systemic Corticosteroids	-	-	-	100%
Emergency Department				
Admittance Decision Time (minutes)[2]	690	130	100	98
Head CT Results Within 45 Min. of Arrival[1]	-	-	45%	57%
Patients Who Left ER Before Being Seen	31,175	2%	3%	2%
Time from ER Arrival to Admit. (minutes)[2]	690	385	286	274
Time from ER Arrival to Discharge (minutes)	404	198	140	134
Time in ER Before Being Evaluated (minutes)	462	32	32	26
Time to Pain Meds for Fractures (minutes)	81	67	64	57
Heart Attack Care				
Aspirin Given at Discharge[1]	-	-	99%	99%
Fibrinolytic Meds Within 30 Min. of Arrival[7]	-	-	80%	54%
PCI Within 90 Minutes of Arrival[7]	-	-	95%	96%
Statin Prescribed at Discharge[1]	-	-	98%	98%
Heart Failure Care				
ACE Inhibitor or ARB for LVSD	44	91%	97%	97%
Discharge Instructions Given	105	91%	92%	94%
Evaluation of LVS Function	123	100%	99%	99%
Medicare Spending				
Medicare Spending per Patient (ratio)	-	0.94	0.95	0.98
Pneumonia Care				
Appropriate Initial Antibiotic Given	100	98%	95%	95%
Blood Culture Timing	197	98%	97%	98%
Pregnancy and Delivery Care				
Newborn Deliveries Scheduled Early	109	0%	8%	6%
Preventive Care				
Immunization for Influenza[2]	539	100%	88%	90%
Immunization for Pneumonia[2]	590	100%	90%	92%
Stroke Care				
Anticoagulation Therapy for Atrial Fibrillation[1]	-	-	94%	95%
Antithrombotic Therapy Timing	27	93%	97%	98%
Assessed for Rehabilitation	23	87%	97%	97%
Discharged on Antithrombotic Therapy	23	96%	98%	99%
Discharged on Statin Medication	21	90%	94%	94%
Thrombolytic Therapy Timing[1]	-	-	58%	66%
Venous Thromboembolism Prophylaxis	27	70%	92%	94%
Written Stroke Educational Materials Given	13	0%	84%	88%
Surgical Care Improvement Project				
Appropriate Beta Blocker Usage	29	100%	97%	98%
Appropriate VTP Within 24 Hours	108	96%	98%	98%
Controlled Postoperative Blood Glucose[7]	-	-	96%	97%
Perioperative Temperature Management	117	100%	100%	100%
Prophylactic Antibiotic Selection	69	99%	99%	99%
Prophylactic Antibiotic Selection (Outpatient)	54	98%	98%	98%
Prophylactic Antibiotic Stopped	63	95%	98%	98%
Prophylactic Antibiotic Timing	69	99%	99%	99%
Prophylactic Antibiotic Timing (Outpatient)	54	98%	98%	98%
Urinary Catheter Removal	29	90%	97%	97%
Survey of Patients' Hospital Experiences				
Area Around Room 'Always' Quiet at Night	300+	67%	66%	61%
Doctors 'Always' Communicated Well	300+	85%	83%	82%
Home Recovery Information Given	300+	85%	84%	85%
Hospital Given 9 or 10 on 10 Point Scale	300+	64%	69%	71%
Meds 'Always' Explained Before Given	300+	63%	63%	64%
Nurses 'Always' Communicated Well	300+	78%	78%	79%
Pain 'Always' Well Controlled	300+	69%	71%	71%
Room and Bathroom 'Always' Clean	300+	63%	71%	73%
Timely Help 'Always' Received	300+	63%	65%	68%
Would Definitely Recommend Hospital	300+	62%	70%	71%
Use of Medical Imaging				
Cardiac Imaging Stress Test before Surgery	178	5.6%	5.5%	5.3%
Combination Abdominal CT Scan	561	9.6%	10.1%	10.5%
Combination Brain/Sinus CT Scan	524	2.3%	2.3%	2.7%
Combination Chest CT Scan	336	13.1%	3.7%	2.7%
Follow-up Mammogram/Ultrasound	566	8.8%	8.9%	8.8%
Lumbar Spine MRI for Low Back Pain[1]	-	-	36.6%	37.2%

Clearview Regional Medical Center

2151 West Spring Street Phone: 770-267-1792
Monroe, GA 30655 Fax: 770-267-1888
URL: www.clearviewregionalmedicalcenter.com
Type: Acute Care Hospitals Emergency Services: Yes
Ownership: Proprietary Beds: 77
Key Personnel:
Emergency Room . . . . Norman Baker
Radiology. . . . . David Causey
CEO/President. . . . . Alen E George
Quality Assurance . . . . John Martz
Chief of Medical Staff. . . . . Mark Shaffer
Operating Room. . . . . Dawn Smith, RN

Measure	Cases	This Hosp.	State Avg.	U.S. Avg.
Blood Clot Prevention and Treatment				
Anticoagulation Overlap Therapy[2]	22	86%	90%	93%
ICU Venous Thromboembolism Prophylaxis[2]	83	90%	90%	92%
Incidence of Potentially Preventable VTE[1,2]	-	-	13%	10%
UFH with Dosages/Platelet Monitoring[2]	23	100%	99%	97%
Venous Thromboembolism Prophylaxis[2]	247	84%	80%	85%
Warfarin Therapy Discharge Instructions[2]	15	100%	78%	75%
Chest Pain/Possible Heart Attack Care				
Aspirin Given Within 24 Hours of Arrival	36	97%	94%	96%
Fibrinolytic Meds Within 30 Min. of Arrival[1]	-	-	35%	58%
Average Time to ECG (minutes)	39	4	8	7
Average Time to Transfer (minutes)[1]	-	-	73	60
Children's Asthma Care				
Received Home Management Plan of Care	-	-	-	88%
Received Reliever Medication	-	-	-	100%
Received Systemic Corticosteroids	-	-	-	100%
Emergency Department				
Admittance Decision Time (minutes)[2]	512	106	100	98
Head CT Results Within 45 Min. of Arrival[7]	-	-	45%	57%
Patients Who Left ER Before Being Seen	32,076	3%	3%	2%
Time from ER Arrival to Admit. (minutes)[2]	515	303	286	274
Time from ER Arrival to Discharge (minutes)	529	128	140	134
Time in ER Before Being Evaluated (minutes)	551	28	32	26
Time to Pain Meds for Fractures (minutes)	113	47	64	57
Heart Attack Care				
Aspirin Given at Discharge[1]	-	-	99%	99%
Fibrinolytic Meds Within 30 Min. of Arrival[7]	-	-	80%	54%
PCI Within 90 Minutes of Arrival[7]	-	-	95%	96%
Statin Prescribed at Discharge[1]	-	-	98%	98%
Heart Failure Care				
ACE Inhibitor or ARB for LVSD	19	100%	97%	97%
Discharge Instructions Given	96	98%	92%	94%
Evaluation of LVS Function	114	100%	99%	99%
Medicare Spending				
Medicare Spending per Patient (ratio)	-	0.99	0.95	0.98
Pneumonia Care				
Appropriate Initial Antibiotic Given	49	94%	95%	95%
Blood Culture Timing	85	99%	97%	98%
Pregnancy and Delivery Care				
Newborn Deliveries Scheduled Early	12	0%	8%	6%
Preventive Care				
Immunization for Influenza[2]	348	99%	88%	90%
Immunization for Pneumonia[2]	450	98%	90%	92%
Stroke Care				
Anticoagulation Therapy for Atrial Fibrillation[1]	-	-	94%	95%
Antithrombotic Therapy Timing	37	100%	97%	98%
Assessed for Rehabilitation	39	90%	97%	97%
Discharged on Antithrombotic Therapy	37	100%	98%	99%
Discharged on Statin Medication	30	83%	94%	94%
Thrombolytic Therapy Timing[1]	-	-	58%	66%
Venous Thromboembolism Prophylaxis	33	91%	92%	94%
Written Stroke Educational Materials Given	24	83%	84%	88%
Surgical Care Improvement Project				
Appropriate Beta Blocker Usage	79	95%	97%	98%
Appropriate VTP Within 24 Hours	197	95%	98%	98%
Controlled Postoperative Blood Glucose[7]	-	-	96%	97%
Perioperative Temperature Management	285	100%	100%	100%
Prophylactic Antibiotic Selection	173	99%	99%	99%
Prophylactic Antibiotic Selection (Outpatient)	36	100%	98%	98%
Prophylactic Antibiotic Stopped	168	97%	98%	98%
Prophylactic Antibiotic Timing	173	99%	99%	99%
Prophylactic Antibiotic Timing (Outpatient)	36	100%	98%	98%
Urinary Catheter Removal	151	94%	97%	97%
Survey of Patients' Hospital Experiences				
Area Around Room 'Always' Quiet at Night	300+	66%	66%	61%
Doctors 'Always' Communicated Well	300+	81%	83%	82%
Home Recovery Information Given	300+	82%	84%	85%
Hospital Given 9 or 10 on 10 Point Scale	300+	63%	69%	71%
Meds 'Always' Explained Before Given	300+	60%	63%	64%
Nurses 'Always' Communicated Well	300+	70%	78%	79%
Pain 'Always' Well Controlled	300+	63%	71%	71%
Room and Bathroom 'Always' Clean	300+	78%	71%	73%
Timely Help 'Always' Received	300+	53%	65%	68%
Would Definitely Recommend Hospital	300+	61%	70%	71%
Use of Medical Imaging				
Cardiac Imaging Stress Test before Surgery	69	5.8%	5.5%	5.3%
Combination Abdominal CT Scan	458	7.4%	10.1%	10.5%
Combination Brain/Sinus CT Scan	465	4.3%	2.3%	2.7%
Combination Chest CT Scan	227	7.0%	3.7%	2.7%
Follow-up Mammogram/Ultrasound	471	11.9%	8.9%	8.8%
Lumbar Spine MRI for Low Back Pain[1]	-	-	36.6%	37.2%

Flint River Hospital

509 Sumter Street, Box 770 Phone: 478-472-3100
Montezuma, GA 31063 Fax: 478-472-2412
URL: www.resurgencehealthgroup.com
Type: Acute Care Hospitals Emergency Services: Yes
Ownership: Proprietary Beds: 49
Key Personnel:
Chief of Medical Staff. . . . . WM Michael McDonald, DO
CEO/President. . . . . Curt Roberts

Measure	Cases	This Hosp.	State Avg.	U.S. Avg.
Blood Clot Prevention and Treatment				
Anticoagulation Overlap Therapy[2,7]	-	-	90%	93%
ICU Venous Thromboembolism Prophylaxis[2,7]	-	-	90%	92%
Incidence of Potentially Preventable VTE[2,7]	-	-	13%	10%
UFH with Dosages/Platelet Monitoring[2,7]	-	-	99%	97%
Venous Thromboembolism Prophylaxis[2]	68	19%	80%	85%
Warfarin Therapy Discharge Instructions[2,7]	-	-	78%	75%
Chest Pain/Possible Heart Attack Care				
Aspirin Given Within 24 Hours of Arrival[3]	21	71%	94%	96%
Fibrinolytic Meds Within 30 Min. of Arrival[3,7]	-	-	35%	58%
Average Time to ECG (minutes)[1,3]	-	-	8	7
Average Time to Transfer (minutes)[1,3]	-	-	73	60
Children's Asthma Care				
Received Home Management Plan of Care	-	-	-	88%
Received Reliever Medication	-	-	-	100%
Received Systemic Corticosteroids	-	-	-	100%
Emergency Department				
Admittance Decision Time (minutes)[2]	160	56	100	98
Head CT Results Within 45 Min. of Arrival[3,7]	-	-	45%	57%

NOTE: Hospital profiles are in alphabetical order by state, then city, then hospital within the city; Rankings exclude hospitals with less than 25 cases except for patient surveys which excludes hospitals with less than 100 cases; (a) 100-299 cases; (1) The number of cases/patients is too few to report; (2) Data submitted were based on a sample of cases/patients; (3) Results are based on a shorter time period than required; (4) Data suppressed by CMS for one or more quarters; (5) Results are not available for this reporting period; (6) Fewer than 100 patients completed the HCAHPS survey; (7) No cases met the criteria for this measure; (8) The lower limit of the confidence interval cannot be calculated if the number of observed infections equals zero; (9) No data are available from the state/territory for this reporting period; (10) The scores shown reflect fewer than 50 completed surveys; (11) There were discrepancies in the data collection process; (12) This measure does not apply to this hospital for this reporting period; (13) Results cannot be calculated for this reporting period; (14) The results for this state are combined with nearby states to protect confidentiality; Please refer to the User's Guide for a full explanation of data.

Measure	Cases	This Hosp.	State Avg.	U.S. Avg.
Patients Who Left ER Before Being Seen[5]	-	-	3%	2%
Time from ER Arrival to Admit. (minutes)[2]	174	274	286	274
Time from ER Arrival to Discharge (minutes)	188	150	140	134
Time in ER Before Being Evaluated (minutes)	291	10	32	26
Time to Pain Meds for Fractures (minutes)[1,3]	-	-	64	57
Heart Attack Care				
Aspirin Given at Discharge[1,2]	-	-	99%	99%
Fibrinolytic Meds Within 30 Min. of Arrival[2,3]	-	-	80%	54%
PCI Within 90 Minutes of Arrival[2,3]	-	-	95%	96%
Statin Prescribed at Discharge[1,2]	-	-	98%	98%
Heart Failure Care				
ACE Inhibitor or ARB for LVSD[1,2]	-	-	97%	97%
Discharge Instructions Given[2,3]	11	0%	92%	94%
Evaluation of LVS Function[2,3]	17	24%	99%	99%
Medicare Spending				
Medicare Spending per Patient (ratio)	-	0.98	0.95	0.98
Pneumonia Care				
Appropriate Initial Antibiotic Given[1,2]	-	-	95%	95%
Blood Culture Timing[1,2]	-	-	97%	98%
Pregnancy and Delivery Care				
Newborn Deliveries Scheduled Early[7]	-	-	8%	6%
Preventive Care				
Immunization for Influenza[2]	296	39%	88%	90%
Immunization for Pneumonia[2]	288	56%	90%	92%
Stroke Care				
Anticoagulation Therapy for Atrial Fibrillation[3,7]	-	-	94%	95%
Antithrombotic Therapy Timing[1,3]	-	-	97%	98%
Assessed for Rehabilitation[1,3]	-	-	97%	97%
Discharged on Antithrombotic Therapy[1,3]	-	-	98%	99%
Discharged on Statin Medication[1,3]	-	-	94%	94%
Thrombolytic Therapy Timing[3,7]	-	-	58%	66%
Venous Thromboembolism Prophylaxis[1,3]	-	-	92%	94%
Written Stroke Educational Materials Given[3,7]	-	-	84%	88%
Surgical Care Improvement Project				
Appropriate Beta Blocker Usage[3,7]	-	-	97%	98%
Appropriate VTP Within 24 Hours[1,3]	-	-	98%	98%
Controlled Postoperative Blood Glucose[3,7]	-	-	96%	97%
Perioperative Temperature Management[1,3]	-	-	100%	100%
Prophylactic Antibiotic Selection[3,7]	-	-	99%	99%
Prophylactic Antibiotic Selection (Outpatient)[3,7]	-	-	98%	98%
Prophylactic Antibiotic Stopped[3,7]	-	-	98%	98%
Prophylactic Antibiotic Timing[3,7]	-	-	99%	99%
Prophylactic Antibiotic Timing (Outpatient)[1,3]	-	-	98%	98%
Urinary Catheter Removal[3,7]	-	-	97%	97%
Survey of Patients' Hospital Experiences				
Area Around Room 'Always' Quiet at Night[6]	<100	73%	66%	61%
Doctors 'Always' Communicated Well[6]	<100	87%	83%	82%
Home Recovery Information Given[6]	<100	81%	84%	85%
Hospital Given 9 or 10 on 10 Point Scale[6]	<100	74%	69%	71%
Meds 'Always' Explained Before Given[6]	<100	58%	63%	64%
Nurses 'Always' Communicated Well[6]	<100	79%	78%	79%
Pain 'Always' Well Controlled[6]	<100	65%	71%	71%
Room and Bathroom 'Always' Clean[6]	<100	64%	71%	73%
Timely Help 'Always' Received[6]	<100	60%	65%	68%
Would Definitely Recommend Hospital[6]	<100	72%	70%	71%
Use of Medical Imaging				
Cardiac Imaging Stress Test before Surgery[7]	-	-	5.5%	5.3%
Combination Abdominal CT Scan	119	1.7%	10.1%	10.5%
Combination Brain/Sinus CT Scan[1]	-	-	2.3%	2.7%
Combination Chest CT Scan	64	3.1%	3.7%	2.7%
Follow-up Mammogram/Ultrasound[7]	-	-	8.9%	8.8%
Lumbar Spine MRI for Low Back Pain[7]	-	-	36.6%	37.2%

Jasper Memorial Hospital

898 College Street
Monticello, GA 31064
Phone: 706-468-6411
Fax: 706-468-8289
Type: Critical Access Hospitals
Emergency Services: Yes
Ownership: Voluntary non-profit - Private
Beds: 75

Key Personnel:

Chief of Medical Staff.......... Kerry Blake, MD
Pediatrics.................... Muneer-Al Hakeem, MD
CEO/President............... David Owens
Radiology.................... John Penuel

Measure	Cases	This Hosp.	State Avg.	U.S. Avg.
Blood Clot Prevention and Treatment				
Anticoagulation Overlap Therapy[5]	-	-	90%	93%
ICU Venous Thromboembolism Prophylaxis[5]	-	-	90%	92%
Incidence of Potentially Preventable VTE[5]	-	-	13%	10%
UFH with Dosages/Platelet Monitoring[5]	-	-	99%	97%
Venous Thromboembolism Prophylaxis[5]	-	-	80%	85%
Warfarin Therapy Discharge Instructions[5]	-	-	78%	75%
Chest Pain/Possible Heart Attack Care				
Aspirin Given Within 24 Hours of Arrival[3]	14	100%	94%	96%
Fibrinolytic Meds Within 30 Min. of Arrival[5]	-	-	35%	58%
Average Time to ECG (minutes)[3]	14	2	8	7
Average Time to Transfer (minutes)[5]	-	-	73	60
Children's Asthma Care				
Received Home Management Plan of Care	-	-	-	88%
Received Reliever Medication	-	-	-	100%
Received Systemic Corticosteroids	-	-	-	100%
Emergency Department				
Admittance Decision Time (minutes)	37	55	100	98
Head CT Results Within 45 Min. of Arrival[5]	-	-	45%	57%
Patients Who Left ER Before Being Seen	4,842	1%	3%	2%
Time from ER Arrival to Admit. (minutes)	46	232	286	274
Time from ER Arrival to Discharge (minutes)[5]	-	-	140	134
Time in ER Before Being Evaluated (minutes)[5]	-	-	32	26
Time to Pain Meds for Fractures (minutes)[5]	-	-	64	57
Heart Attack Care				
Aspirin Given at Discharge[5]	-	-	99%	99%
Fibrinolytic Meds Within 30 Min. of Arrival[5]	-	-	80%	54%
PCI Within 90 Minutes of Arrival[5]	-	-	95%	96%
Statin Prescribed at Discharge[5]	-	-	98%	98%
Heart Failure Care				
ACE Inhibitor or ARB for LVSD[1,3]	-	-	97%	97%
Discharge Instructions Given[1,3]	-	-	92%	94%
Evaluation of LVS Function[1,3]	-	-	99%	99%
Medicare Spending				
Medicare Spending per Patient (ratio)	-	-	0.95	0.98
Pneumonia Care				
Appropriate Initial Antibiotic Given[1]	-	-	95%	95%
Blood Culture Timing[1]	-	-	97%	98%
Pregnancy and Delivery Care				
Newborn Deliveries Scheduled Early[5]	-	-	8%	6%
Preventive Care				
Immunization for Influenza	37	95%	88%	90%
Immunization for Pneumonia	58	93%	90%	92%
Stroke Care				
Anticoagulation Therapy for Atrial Fibrillation[5]	-	-	94%	95%
Antithrombotic Therapy Timing[5]	-	-	97%	98%
Assessed for Rehabilitation[5]	-	-	97%	97%
Discharged on Antithrombotic Therapy[5]	-	-	98%	99%
Discharged on Statin Medication[5]	-	-	94%	94%
Thrombolytic Therapy Timing[5]	-	-	58%	66%
Venous Thromboembolism Prophylaxis[5]	-	-	92%	94%
Written Stroke Educational Materials Given[5]	-	-	84%	88%
Surgical Care Improvement Project				
Appropriate Beta Blocker Usage[5]	-	-	97%	98%
Appropriate VTP Within 24 Hours[5]	-	-	98%	98%
Controlled Postoperative Blood Glucose[5]	-	-	96%	97%
Perioperative Temperature Management[5]	-	-	100%	100%
Prophylactic Antibiotic Selection[5]	-	-	99%	99%
Prophylactic Antibiotic Selection (Outpatient)[5]	-	-	98%	98%
Prophylactic Antibiotic Stopped[5]	-	-	98%	98%
Prophylactic Antibiotic Timing[5]	-	-	99%	99%
Prophylactic Antibiotic Timing (Outpatient)[5]	-	-	98%	98%
Urinary Catheter Removal[5]	-	-	97%	97%
Survey of Patients' Hospital Experiences				
Area Around Room 'Always' Quiet at Night[5]	-	-	66%	61%
Doctors 'Always' Communicated Well[5]	-	-	83%	82%
Home Recovery Information Given[5]	-	-	84%	85%
Hospital Given 9 or 10 on 10 Point Scale[5]	-	-	69%	71%
Meds 'Always' Explained Before Given[5]	-	-	63%	64%
Nurses 'Always' Communicated Well[5]	-	-	78%	79%
Pain 'Always' Well Controlled[5]	-	-	71%	71%
Room and Bathroom 'Always' Clean[5]	-	-	71%	73%
Timely Help 'Always' Received[5]	-	-	65%	68%
Would Definitely Recommend Hospital[5]	-	-	70%	71%
Use of Medical Imaging				
Cardiac Imaging Stress Test before Surgery[7]	-	-	5.5%	5.3%
Combination Abdominal CT Scan	50	4.0%	10.1%	10.5%
Combination Brain/Sinus CT Scan	59	0.0%	2.3%	2.7%
Combination Chest CT Scan[1]	-	-	3.7%	2.7%
Follow-up Mammogram/Ultrasound[7]	-	-	8.9%	8.8%
Lumbar Spine MRI for Low Back Pain[1]	-	-	36.6%	37.2%

Colquitt Regional Medical Center

3131 Thomasville Hwy Box 40
Moultrie, GA 31768
Phone: 229-985-3420
Fax: 229-890-2173
E-mail: crmc@colquittregional.com
URL: www.colquittregionad.com
Type: Acute Care Hospitals
Emergency Services: Yes
Ownership: Govt - Hospital Dist/Auth
Beds: 99

Key Personnel:

Radiology.................. Mark Blanchard
Operating Room............. Beth Bridges
Pediatric Ambulatory Care...... Patricia Lee June, MD
Pediatric In-Patient Care....... Patricia Lee June, MD
CEO/President............... James R Lowry, FACHE
Chief of Medical Staff.......... Howard Nelton
Quality Assurance............ Cathy Rovel
Infection Control.............. Gail Sparkman, RN

Measure	Cases	This Hosp.	State Avg.	U.S. Avg.
Blood Clot Prevention and Treatment				
Anticoagulation Overlap Therapy[2]	28	86%	90%	93%
ICU Venous Thromboembolism Prophylaxis[2]	77	84%	90%	92%
Incidence of Potentially Preventable VTE[1,2]	-	-	13%	10%
UFH with Dosages/Platelet Monitoring[1,2]	-	-	99%	97%
Venous Thromboembolism Prophylaxis[2]	326	71%	80%	85%
Warfarin Therapy Discharge Instructions[2]	18	89%	78%	75%
Chest Pain/Possible Heart Attack Care				
Aspirin Given Within 24 Hours of Arrival	54	100%	94%	96%
Fibrinolytic Meds Within 30 Min. of Arrival	11	36%	35%	58%
Average Time to ECG (minutes)	60	18	8	7
Average Time to Transfer (minutes)[1]	-	-	73	60
Children's Asthma Care				
Received Home Management Plan of Care	-	-	-	88%
Received Reliever Medication	-	-	-	100%
Received Systemic Corticosteroids	-	-	-	100%
Emergency Department				
Admittance Decision Time (minutes)[2]	545	70	100	98
Head CT Results Within 45 Min. of Arrival[1]	-	-	45%	57%
Patients Who Left ER Before Being Seen	27,825	3%	3%	2%
Time from ER Arrival to Admit. (minutes)[2]	562	265	286	274
Time from ER Arrival to Discharge (minutes)	341	136	140	134
Time in ER Before Being Evaluated (minutes)	375	36	32	26
Time to Pain Meds for Fractures (minutes)	47	67	64	57
Heart Attack Care				
Aspirin Given at Discharge[1]	-	-	99%	99%
Fibrinolytic Meds Within 30 Min. of Arrival[7]	-	-	80%	54%
PCI Within 90 Minutes of Arrival[7]	-	-	95%	96%
Statin Prescribed at Discharge	12	100%	98%	98%
Heart Failure Care				
ACE Inhibitor or ARB for LVSD	55	100%	97%	97%
Discharge Instructions Given	156	100%	92%	94%
Evaluation of LVS Function	189	100%	99%	99%
Medicare Spending				
Medicare Spending per Patient (ratio)	-	0.95	0.95	0.98
Pneumonia Care				
Appropriate Initial Antibiotic Given	102	97%	95%	95%
Blood Culture Timing	206	100%	97%	98%
Pregnancy and Delivery Care				
Newborn Deliveries Scheduled Early[2]	67	9%	8%	6%
Preventive Care				
Immunization for Influenza[2]	456	86%	88%	90%
Immunization for Pneumonia[2]	524	94%	90%	92%
Stroke Care				
Anticoagulation Therapy for Atrial Fibrillation[1]	-	-	94%	95%
Antithrombotic Therapy Timing	34	85%	97%	98%

NOTE: Hospital profiles are in alphabetical order by state, then city, then hospital within the city; Rankings exclude hospitals with less than 25 cases except for patient surveys which excludes hospitals with less than 100 cases; (a) 100-299 cases; (1) The number of cases/patients is too few to report; (2) Data submitted were based on a sample of cases/patients; (3) Results are based on a shorter time period than required; (4) Data suppressed by CMS for one or more quarters; (5) Results are not available for this reporting period; (6) Fewer than 100 patients completed the HCAHPS survey; (7) No cases met the criteria for this measure; (8) The lower limit of the confidence interval cannot be calculated if the number of observed infections equals zero; (9) No data are available from the state/territory for this reporting period; (10) The scores shown reflect fewer than 50 completed surveys; (11) There were discrepancies in the data collection process; (12) This measure does not apply to this hospital for this reporting period; (13) Results cannot be calculated for this reporting period; (14) The results for this state are combined with nearby states to protect confidentiality; Please refer to the User's Guide for a full explanation of data.

Measure	Cases	This Hosp.	State Avg.	U.S. Avg.
Assessed for Rehabilitation	45	84%	97%	97%
Discharged on Antithrombotic Therapy	37	86%	98%	99%
Discharged on Statin Medication	34	85%	94%	94%
Thrombolytic Therapy Timing[1]	-	-	58%	66%
Venous Thromboembolism Prophylaxis	41	71%	92%	94%
Written Stroke Educational Materials Given	26	88%	84%	88%
Surgical Care Improvement Project				
Appropriate Beta Blocker Usage	53	100%	97%	98%
Appropriate VTP Within 24 Hours	146	99%	98%	98%
Controlled Postoperative Blood Glucose[7]	-	-	96%	97%
Perioperative Temperature Management	176	100%	100%	100%
Prophylactic Antibiotic Selection	91	100%	99%	99%
Prophylactic Antibiotic Selection (Outpatient)	21	90%	98%	98%
Prophylactic Antibiotic Stopped	90	99%	98%	98%
Prophylactic Antibiotic Timing	91	98%	99%	99%
Prophylactic Antibiotic Timing (Outpatient)	21	100%	98%	98%
Urinary Catheter Removal	81	100%	97%	97%
Survey of Patients' Hospital Experiences				
Area Around Room 'Always' Quiet at Night	300+	64%	66%	61%
Doctors 'Always' Communicated Well	300+	80%	83%	82%
Home Recovery Information Given	300+	84%	84%	85%
Hospital Given 9 or 10 on 10 Point Scale	300+	68%	69%	71%
Meds 'Always' Explained Before Given	300+	59%	63%	64%
Nurses 'Always' Communicated Well	300+	78%	78%	79%
Pain 'Always' Well Controlled	300+	69%	71%	71%
Room and Bathroom 'Always' Clean	300+	70%	71%	73%
Timely Help 'Always' Received	300+	69%	65%	68%
Would Definitely Recommend Hospital	300+	62%	70%	71%
Use of Medical Imaging				
Cardiac Imaging Stress Test before Surgery	313	5.1%	5.5%	5.3%
Combination Abdominal CT Scan	423	6.4%	10.1%	10.5%
Combination Brain/Sinus CT Scan[1]	-	-	2.3%	2.7%
Combination Chest CT Scan	374	0.0%	3.7%	2.7%
Follow-up Mammogram/Ultrasound	704	8.8%	8.9%	8.8%
Lumbar Spine MRI for Low Back Pain	102	31.4%	36.6%	37.2%

Turning Point Hospital

3015 Veterans Parkway
Moultrie, GA 31788
Phone: 229-985-4815
Fax: 229-890-1614
E-mail: tpservices@turningpointcare.com
URL: www.turningpointcare.com
Type: Acute Care Hospitals
Emergency Services: No
Ownership: Proprietary
Beds: 70

Key Personnel:
CEO/President. . . . . Ben Marion
Quality Assurance . . . . Lila Seay

Measure	Cases	This Hosp.	State Avg.	U.S. Avg.
Blood Clot Prevention and Treatment				
Anticoagulation Overlap Therapy[2,7]	-	-	90%	93%
ICU Venous Thromboembolism Prophylaxis[2,7]	-	-	90%	92%
Incidence of Potentially Preventable VTE[2,7]	-	-	13%	10%
UFH with Dosages/Platelet Monitoring[2,7]	-	-	99%	97%
Venous Thromboembolism Prophylaxis[2,7]	-	-	80%	85%
Warfarin Therapy Discharge Instructions[2,7]	-	-	78%	75%
Chest Pain/Possible Heart Attack Care				
Aspirin Given Within 24 Hours of Arrival[5]	-	-	94%	96%
Fibrinolytic Meds Within 30 Min. of Arrival[5]	-	-	35%	58%
Average Time to ECG (minutes)[5]	-	-	8	7
Average Time to Transfer (minutes)[5]	-	-	73	60
Children's Asthma Care				
Received Home Management Plan of Care	-	-	-	88%
Received Reliever Medication	-	-	-	100%
Received Systemic Corticosteroids	-	-	-	100%
Emergency Department				
Admittance Decision Time (minutes)[2,7]	-	-	100	98
Head CT Results Within 45 Min. of Arrival[5]	-	-	45%	57%
Patients Who Left ER Before Being Seen[5]	-	-	3%	2%
Time from ER Arrival to Admit. (minutes)[2,7]	-	-	286	274
Time from ER Arrival to Discharge (minutes)[5]	-	-	140	134
Time in ER Before Being Evaluated (minutes)[5]	-	-	32	26
Time to Pain Meds for Fractures (minutes)[5]	-	-	64	57
Heart Attack Care				
Aspirin Given at Discharge[5]	-	-	99%	99%
Fibrinolytic Meds Within 30 Min. of Arrival[5]	-	-	80%	54%
PCI Within 90 Minutes of Arrival[5]	-	-	95%	96%
Statin Prescribed at Discharge[5]	-	-	98%	98%
Heart Failure Care				
ACE Inhibitor or ARB for LVSD[5]	-	-	97%	97%
Discharge Instructions Given[5]	-	-	92%	94%
Evaluation of LVS Function[5]	-	-	99%	99%
Medicare Spending				
Medicare Spending per Patient (ratio)	-	1.25	0.95	0.98
Pneumonia Care				
Appropriate Initial Antibiotic Given[5]	-	-	95%	95%
Blood Culture Timing[5]	-	-	97%	98%
Pregnancy and Delivery Care				
Newborn Deliveries Scheduled Early[7]	-	-	8%	6%
Preventive Care				
Immunization for Influenza[2]	314	0%	88%	90%
Immunization for Pneumonia[2]	65	2%	90%	92%
Stroke Care				
Anticoagulation Therapy for Atrial Fibrillation[5]	-	-	94%	95%
Antithrombotic Therapy Timing[5]	-	-	97%	98%
Assessed for Rehabilitation[5]	-	-	97%	97%
Discharged on Antithrombotic Therapy[5]	-	-	98%	99%
Discharged on Statin Medication[5]	-	-	94%	94%
Thrombolytic Therapy Timing[5]	-	-	58%	66%
Venous Thromboembolism Prophylaxis[5]	-	-	92%	94%
Written Stroke Educational Materials Given[5]	-	-	84%	88%
Surgical Care Improvement Project				
Appropriate Beta Blocker Usage[5]	-	-	97%	98%
Appropriate VTP Within 24 Hours[5]	-	-	98%	98%
Controlled Postoperative Blood Glucose[5]	-	-	96%	97%
Perioperative Temperature Management[5]	-	-	100%	100%
Prophylactic Antibiotic Selection[5]	-	-	99%	99%
Prophylactic Antibiotic Selection (Outpatient)[5]	-	-	98%	98%
Prophylactic Antibiotic Stopped[5]	-	-	98%	98%
Prophylactic Antibiotic Timing[5]	-	-	99%	99%
Prophylactic Antibiotic Timing (Outpatient)[5]	-	-	98%	98%
Urinary Catheter Removal[5]	-	-	97%	97%
Survey of Patients' Hospital Experiences				
Area Around Room 'Always' Quiet at Night[1]	-	-	66%	61%
Doctors 'Always' Communicated Well[1]	-	-	83%	82%
Home Recovery Information Given[1]	-	-	84%	85%
Hospital Given 9 or 10 on 10 Point Scale[1]	-	-	69%	71%
Meds 'Always' Explained Before Given[1]	-	-	63%	64%
Nurses 'Always' Communicated Well[1]	-	-	78%	79%
Pain 'Always' Well Controlled[1]	-	-	71%	71%
Room and Bathroom 'Always' Clean[1]	-	-	71%	73%
Timely Help 'Always' Received[1]	-	-	65%	68%
Would Definitely Recommend Hospital[1]	-	-	70%	71%
Use of Medical Imaging				
Cardiac Imaging Stress Test before Surgery[7]	-	-	5.5%	5.3%
Combination Abdominal CT Scan[7]	-	-	10.1%	10.5%
Combination Brain/Sinus CT Scan[7]	-	-	2.3%	2.7%
Combination Chest CT Scan[7]	-	-	3.7%	2.7%
Follow-up Mammogram/Ultrasound[7]	-	-	8.9%	8.8%
Lumbar Spine MRI for Low Back Pain[7]	-	-	36.6%	37.2%

Sgmc Berrien Campus

1221 E Mcpherson Avenue
Nashville, GA 31639
Phone: 229-543-7100
Type: Acute Care Hospitals
Emergency Services: Yes
Ownership: Govt - Hospital Dist/Auth

Measure	Cases	This Hosp.	State Avg.	U.S. Avg.
Blood Clot Prevention and Treatment				
Anticoagulation Overlap Therapy[5]	-	-	90%	93%
ICU Venous Thromboembolism Prophylaxis[5]	-	-	90%	92%
Incidence of Potentially Preventable VTE[5]	-	-	13%	10%
UFH with Dosages/Platelet Monitoring[5]	-	-	99%	97%
Venous Thromboembolism Prophylaxis[5]	-	-	80%	85%
Warfarin Therapy Discharge Instructions[5]	-	-	78%	75%
Chest Pain/Possible Heart Attack Care				
Aspirin Given Within 24 Hours of Arrival[5]	-	-	94%	96%
Fibrinolytic Meds Within 30 Min. of Arrival[5]	-	-	35%	58%
Average Time to ECG (minutes)[5]	-	-	8	7
Average Time to Transfer (minutes)[5]	-	-	73	60
Children's Asthma Care				
Received Home Management Plan of Care	-	-	-	88%
Received Reliever Medication	-	-	-	100%
Received Systemic Corticosteroids	-	-	-	100%
Emergency Department				
Admittance Decision Time (minutes)[5]	-	-	100	98
Head CT Results Within 45 Min. of Arrival[5]	-	-	45%	57%
Patients Who Left ER Before Being Seen[5]	-	-	3%	2%
Time from ER Arrival to Admit. (minutes)[5]	-	-	286	274
Time from ER Arrival to Discharge (minutes)[5]	-	-	140	134
Time in ER Before Being Evaluated (minutes)[5]	-	-	32	26
Time to Pain Meds for Fractures (minutes)[5]	-	-	64	57
Heart Attack Care				
Aspirin Given at Discharge[5]	-	-	99%	99%
Fibrinolytic Meds Within 30 Min. of Arrival[5]	-	-	80%	54%
PCI Within 90 Minutes of Arrival[5]	-	-	95%	96%
Statin Prescribed at Discharge[5]	-	-	98%	98%
Heart Failure Care				
ACE Inhibitor or ARB for LVSD[5]	-	-	97%	97%
Discharge Instructions Given[5]	-	-	92%	94%
Evaluation of LVS Function[5]	-	-	99%	99%
Medicare Spending				
Medicare Spending per Patient (ratio)	-	-	0.95	0.98
Pneumonia Care				
Appropriate Initial Antibiotic Given[5]	-	-	95%	95%
Blood Culture Timing[5]	-	-	97%	98%
Pregnancy and Delivery Care				
Newborn Deliveries Scheduled Early[5]	-	-	8%	6%
Preventive Care				
Immunization for Influenza[5]	-	-	88%	90%
Immunization for Pneumonia[5]	-	-	90%	92%
Stroke Care				
Anticoagulation Therapy for Atrial Fibrillation[5]	-	-	94%	95%
Antithrombotic Therapy Timing[5]	-	-	97%	98%
Assessed for Rehabilitation[5]	-	-	97%	97%
Discharged on Antithrombotic Therapy[5]	-	-	98%	99%
Discharged on Statin Medication[5]	-	-	94%	94%
Thrombolytic Therapy Timing[5]	-	-	58%	66%
Venous Thromboembolism Prophylaxis[5]	-	-	92%	94%
Written Stroke Educational Materials Given[5]	-	-	84%	88%
Surgical Care Improvement Project				
Appropriate Beta Blocker Usage[5]	-	-	97%	98%
Appropriate VTP Within 24 Hours[5]	-	-	98%	98%
Controlled Postoperative Blood Glucose[5]	-	-	96%	97%
Perioperative Temperature Management[5]	-	-	100%	100%
Prophylactic Antibiotic Selection[5]	-	-	99%	99%
Prophylactic Antibiotic Selection (Outpatient)[5]	-	-	98%	98%
Prophylactic Antibiotic Stopped[5]	-	-	98%	98%
Prophylactic Antibiotic Timing[5]	-	-	99%	99%
Prophylactic Antibiotic Timing (Outpatient)[5]	-	-	98%	98%
Urinary Catheter Removal[5]	-	-	97%	97%
Survey of Patients' Hospital Experiences				
Area Around Room 'Always' Quiet at Night[5]	-	-	66%	61%
Doctors 'Always' Communicated Well[5]	-	-	83%	82%
Home Recovery Information Given[5]	-	-	84%	85%
Hospital Given 9 or 10 on 10 Point Scale[5]	-	-	69%	71%
Meds 'Always' Explained Before Given[5]	-	-	63%	64%
Nurses 'Always' Communicated Well[5]	-	-	78%	79%
Pain 'Always' Well Controlled[5]	-	-	71%	71%
Room and Bathroom 'Always' Clean[5]	-	-	71%	73%
Timely Help 'Always' Received[5]	-	-	65%	68%
Would Definitely Recommend Hospital[5]	-	-	70%	71%
Use of Medical Imaging				
Cardiac Imaging Stress Test before Surgery[7]	-	-	5.5%	5.3%
Combination Abdominal CT Scan[7]	-	-	10.1%	10.5%
Combination Brain/Sinus CT Scan[7]	-	-	2.3%	2.7%
Combination Chest CT Scan[7]	-	-	3.7%	2.7%
Follow-up Mammogram/Ultrasound[7]	-	-	8.9%	8.8%
Lumbar Spine MRI for Low Back Pain[7]	-	-	36.6%	37.2%

NOTE: Hospital profiles are in alphabetical order by state, then city, then hospital within the city; Rankings exclude hospitals with less than 25 cases except for patient surveys which excludes hospitals with less than 100 cases; (a) 100-299 cases; (1) The number of cases/patients is too few to report; (2) Data submitted were based on a sample of cases/patients; (3) Results are based on a shorter time period than required; (4) Data suppressed by CMS for one or more quarters; (5) Results are not available for this reporting period; (6) Fewer than 100 patients completed the HCAHPS survey; (7) No cases met the criteria for this measure; (8) The lower limit of the confidence interval cannot be calculated if the number of observed infections equals zero; (9) No data are available from the state/territory for this reporting period; (10) The scores shown reflect fewer than 50 completed surveys; (11) There were discrepancies in the data collection process; (12) This measure does not apply to this hospital for this reporting period; (13) Results cannot be calculated for this reporting period; (14) The results for this state are combined with nearby states to protect confidentiality; Please refer to the User's Guide for a full explanation of data.

Piedmont Newnan Hospital

745 Poplar Road | Phone: 770-400-2300
Newnan, GA 30265 | Fax: 770-253-8845
E-mail: info@newnanhospital.org
URL: www.newnanhospital.org
Type: Acute Care Hospitals | Emergency Services: Yes
Ownership: Voluntary non-profit - Private | Beds: 100

Key Personnel:
Radiology. . . . . Timothy W Baker, MD
Chief of Medical Staff . . . . Cleland Child
Operating Room. . . . . Garnet R Craddock, RN
CEO/President. . . . . Richard Hubbard
Pediatric Ambulatory Care . . . . . . Lewis Jackson, MD
Pediatric In-Patient Care . . . . Lewis Jackson, MD
Quality Assurance . . . . Brent Price
Cardiac Laboratory. . . . . George Suji Vellanikaran

Measure	Cases	This Hosp.	State Avg.	U.S. Avg.
Blood Clot Prevention and Treatment				
Anticoagulation Overlap Therapy[2]	50	92%	90%	93%
ICU Venous Thromboembolism Prophylaxis[2]	80	89%	90%	92%
Incidence of Potentially Preventable VTE[1,2]	-	-	13%	10%
UFH with Dosages/Platelet Monitoring[2]	46	100%	99%	97%
Venous Thromboembolism Prophylaxis[2]	389	86%	80%	85%
Warfarin Therapy Discharge Instructions[2]	43	91%	78%	75%
Chest Pain/Possible Heart Attack Care				
Aspirin Given Within 24 Hours of Arrival	41	98%	94%	96%
Fibrinolytic Meds Within 30 Min. of Arrival[7]	-	-	35%	58%
Average Time to ECG (minutes)	42	2	8	7
Average Time to Transfer (minutes)[1]	-	-	73	60
Children's Asthma Care				
Received Home Management Plan of Care	-	-	-	88%
Received Reliever Medication	-	-	-	100%
Received Systemic Corticosteroids	-	-	-	100%
Emergency Department				
Admittance Decision Time (minutes)[2]	706	126	100	98
Head CT Results Within 45 Min. of Arrival[1]	-	-	45%	57%
Patients Who Left ER Before Being Seen	47,951	3%	3%	2%
Time from ER Arrival to Admit. (minutes)[2]	714	335	286	274
Time from ER Arrival to Discharge (minutes)	470	203	140	134
Time in ER Before Being Evaluated (minutes)	435	39	32	26
Time to Pain Meds for Fractures (minutes)	204	68	64	57
Heart Attack Care				
Aspirin Given at Discharge	25	100%	99%	99%
Fibrinolytic Meds Within 30 Min. of Arrival[7]	-	-	80%	54%
PCI Within 90 Minutes of Arrival[7]	-	-	95%	96%
Statin Prescribed at Discharge	20	100%	98%	98%
Heart Failure Care				
ACE Inhibitor or ARB for LVSD[2]	62	98%	97%	97%
Discharge Instructions Given[2]	241	83%	92%	94%
Evaluation of LVS Function[2]	267	100%	99%	99%
Medicare Spending				
Medicare Spending per Patient (ratio)	-	0.94	0.95	0.98
Pneumonia Care				
Appropriate Initial Antibiotic Given[2]	116	92%	95%	95%
Blood Culture Timing[2]	190	94%	97%	98%
Pregnancy and Delivery Care				
Newborn Deliveries Scheduled Early[2]	60	2%	8%	6%
Preventive Care				
Immunization for Influenza[2]	569	68%	88%	90%
Immunization for Pneumonia[2]	731	82%	90%	92%
Stroke Care				
Anticoagulation Therapy for Atrial Fibrillation[1]	-	-	94%	95%
Antithrombotic Therapy Timing	75	100%	97%	98%
Assessed for Rehabilitation	74	99%	97%	97%
Discharged on Antithrombotic Therapy	70	100%	98%	99%
Discharged on Statin Medication	63	92%	94%	94%
Thrombolytic Therapy Timing	12	0%	58%	66%
Venous Thromboembolism Prophylaxis	78	94%	92%	94%
Written Stroke Educational Materials Given	48	62%	84%	88%
Surgical Care Improvement Project				
Appropriate Beta Blocker Usage[2]	119	96%	97%	98%
Appropriate VTP Within 24 Hours[2]	392	96%	98%	98%
Controlled Postoperative Blood Glucose[2,7]	-	-	96%	97%
Perioperative Temperature Management[2]	441	100%	100%	100%
Prophylactic Antibiotic Selection[2]	322	100%	99%	99%
Prophylactic Antibiotic Selection (Outpatient)	82	99%	98%	98%
Prophylactic Antibiotic Stopped[2]	316	95%	98%	98%
Prophylactic Antibiotic Timing[2]	324	98%	99%	99%
Prophylactic Antibiotic Timing (Outpatient)	84	95%	98%	98%
Urinary Catheter Removal[2]	338	92%	97%	97%
Survey of Patients' Hospital Experiences				
Area Around Room 'Always' Quiet at Night	300+	72%	66%	61%
Doctors 'Always' Communicated Well	300+	80%	83%	82%
Home Recovery Information Given	300+	82%	84%	85%
Hospital Given 9 or 10 on 10 Point Scale	300+	70%	69%	71%
Meds 'Always' Explained Before Given	300+	61%	63%	64%
Nurses 'Always' Communicated Well	300+	78%	78%	79%
Pain 'Always' Well Controlled	300+	71%	71%	71%
Room and Bathroom 'Always' Clean	300+	74%	71%	73%
Timely Help 'Always' Received	300+	67%	65%	68%
Would Definitely Recommend Hospital	300+	74%	70%	71%
Use of Medical Imaging				
Cardiac Imaging Stress Test before Surgery	772	6.1%	5.5%	5.3%
Combination Abdominal CT Scan	789	4.7%	10.1%	10.5%
Combination Brain/Sinus CT Scan	770	1.7%	2.3%	2.7%
Combination Chest CT Scan	346	0.3%	3.7%	2.7%
Follow-up Mammogram/Ultrasound	1,186	6.1%	8.9%	8.8%
Lumbar Spine MRI for Low Back Pain[1]	-	-	36.6%	37.2%

Southeastern Regional Medical Center

600 Parkway North | Phone: 404-844-8334
Newnan, GA 30265
Type: Acute Care Hospitals | Emergency Services: No
Ownership: Proprietary

Measure	Cases	This Hosp.	State Avg.	U.S. Avg.
Blood Clot Prevention and Treatment				
Anticoagulation Overlap Therapy[1,2]	-	-	90%	93%
ICU Venous Thromboembolism Prophylaxis[1,2]	-	-	90%	92%
Incidence of Potentially Preventable VTE[2,7]	-	-	13%	10%
UFH with Dosages/Platelet Monitoring[1,2]	-	-	99%	97%
Venous Thromboembolism Prophylaxis[2]	89	97%	80%	85%
Warfarin Therapy Discharge Instructions[1,2]	-	-	78%	75%
Chest Pain/Possible Heart Attack Care				
Aspirin Given Within 24 Hours of Arrival[5]	-	-	94%	96%
Fibrinolytic Meds Within 30 Min. of Arrival[5]	-	-	35%	58%
Average Time to ECG (minutes)[5]	-	-	8	7
Average Time to Transfer (minutes)[5]	-	-	73	60
Children's Asthma Care				
Received Home Management Plan of Care	-	-	-	88%
Received Reliever Medication	-	-	-	100%
Received Systemic Corticosteroids	-	-	-	100%
Emergency Department				
Admittance Decision Time (minutes)[2,3]	-	-	100	98
Head CT Results Within 45 Min. of Arrival[5]	-	-	45%	57%
Patients Who Left ER Before Being Seen[5]	-	-	3%	2%
Time from ER Arrival to Admit. (minutes)[2,3]	-	-	286	274
Time from ER Arrival to Discharge (minutes)[5]	-	-	140	134
Time in ER Before Being Evaluated (minutes)[5]	-	-	32	26
Time to Pain Meds for Fractures (minutes)[5]	-	-	64	57
Heart Attack Care				
Aspirin Given at Discharge[5]	-	-	99%	99%
Fibrinolytic Meds Within 30 Min. of Arrival[5]	-	-	80%	54%
PCI Within 90 Minutes of Arrival[5]	-	-	95%	96%
Statin Prescribed at Discharge[5]	-	-	98%	98%
Heart Failure Care				
ACE Inhibitor or ARB for LVSD[5]	-	-	97%	97%
Discharge Instructions Given[5]	-	-	92%	94%
Evaluation of LVS Function[5]	-	-	99%	99%
Medicare Spending				
Medicare Spending per Patient (ratio)	-	-	0.95	0.98
Pneumonia Care				
Appropriate Initial Antibiotic Given[1,3]	-	-	95%	95%
Blood Culture Timing[3,7]	-	-	97%	98%
Pregnancy and Delivery Care				
Newborn Deliveries Scheduled Early[7]	-	-	8%	6%
Preventive Care				
Immunization for Influenza[2,3]	114	88%	88%	90%
Immunization for Pneumonia[2,3]	117	91%	90%	92%
Stroke Care				
Anticoagulation Therapy for Atrial Fibrillation[5]	-	-	94%	95%
Antithrombotic Therapy Timing[5]	-	-	97%	98%
Assessed for Rehabilitation[5]	-	-	97%	97%
Discharged on Antithrombotic Therapy[5]	-	-	98%	99%
Discharged on Statin Medication[5]	-	-	94%	94%
Thrombolytic Therapy Timing[5]	-	-	58%	66%
Venous Thromboembolism Prophylaxis[5]	-	-	92%	94%
Written Stroke Educational Materials Given[5]	-	-	84%	88%
Surgical Care Improvement Project				
Appropriate Beta Blocker Usage[3]	18	72%	97%	98%
Appropriate VTP Within 24 Hours[3]	77	99%	98%	98%
Controlled Postoperative Blood Glucose[3,7]	-	-	96%	97%
Perioperative Temperature Management[3]	78	100%	100%	100%
Prophylactic Antibiotic Selection[3]	12	100%	99%	99%
Prophylactic Antibiotic Selection (Outpatient)[3]	15	93%	98%	98%
Prophylactic Antibiotic Stopped[1,3]	-	-	98%	98%
Prophylactic Antibiotic Timing[3]	12	100%	99%	99%
Prophylactic Antibiotic Timing (Outpatient)[3]	15	93%	98%	98%
Urinary Catheter Removal[3]	13	46%	97%	97%
Survey of Patients' Hospital Experiences				
Area Around Room 'Always' Quiet at Night[5]	-	-	66%	61%
Doctors 'Always' Communicated Well[5]	-	-	83%	82%
Home Recovery Information Given[5]	-	-	84%	85%
Hospital Given 9 or 10 on 10 Point Scale[5]	-	-	69%	71%
Meds 'Always' Explained Before Given[5]	-	-	63%	64%
Nurses 'Always' Communicated Well[5]	-	-	78%	79%
Pain 'Always' Well Controlled[5]	-	-	71%	71%
Room and Bathroom 'Always' Clean[5]	-	-	71%	73%
Timely Help 'Always' Received[5]	-	-	65%	68%
Would Definitely Recommend Hospital[5]	-	-	70%	71%
Use of Medical Imaging				
Cardiac Imaging Stress Test before Surgery[7]	-	-	5.5%	5.3%
Combination Abdominal CT Scan[1]	-	-	10.1%	10.5%
Combination Brain/Sinus CT Scan[7]	-	-	2.3%	2.7%
Combination Chest CT Scan[1]	-	-	3.7%	2.7%
Follow-up Mammogram/Ultrasound[7]	-	-	8.9%	8.8%
Lumbar Spine MRI for Low Back Pain[7]	-	-	36.6%	37.2%

Irwin County Hospital

710 N Irwin Avenue | Phone: 229-468-3845
Ocilla, GA 31774 | Fax: 229-468-3880
Type: Acute Care Hospitals | Emergency Services: No
Ownership: Govt - Hospital Dist/Auth | Beds: 34

Key Personnel:
Operating Room. . . . . Michelle Brown
Emergency Room . . . . Becky Cook
Radiology. . . . . Pankaj Patel
CEO/President. . . . . Sue Spivei
Quality Assurance . . . . Jenny Tucker

Measure	Cases	This Hosp.	State Avg.	U.S. Avg.
Blood Clot Prevention and Treatment				
Anticoagulation Overlap Therapy[1,2]	-	-	90%	93%
ICU Venous Thromboembolism Prophylaxis[2,7]	-	-	90%	92%
Incidence of Potentially Preventable VTE[2,7]	-	-	13%	10%
UFH with Dosages/Platelet Monitoring[2,7]	-	-	99%	97%
Venous Thromboembolism Prophylaxis[2]	126	5%	80%	85%
Warfarin Therapy Discharge Instructions[1,2]	-	-	78%	75%
Chest Pain/Possible Heart Attack Care				
Aspirin Given Within 24 Hours of Arrival	22	86%	94%	96%
Fibrinolytic Meds Within 30 Min. of Arrival[1,3]	-	-	35%	58%
Average Time to ECG (minutes)	22	9	8	7
Average Time to Transfer (minutes)[1,3]	-	-	73	60
Children's Asthma Care				
Received Home Management Plan of Care	-	-	-	88%
Received Reliever Medication	-	-	-	100%
Received Systemic Corticosteroids	-	-	-	100%
Emergency Department				
Admittance Decision Time (minutes)[1,2]	-	-	100	98
Head CT Results Within 45 Min. of Arrival[3,7]	-	-	45%	57%
Patients Who Left ER Before Being Seen	4,661	2%	3%	2%

NOTE: Hospital profiles are in alphabetical order by state, then city, then hospital within the city; Rankings exclude hospitals with less than 25 cases except for patient surveys which excludes hospitals with less than 100 cases; (a) 100-299 cases; (1) The number of cases/patients is too few to report; (2) Data submitted were based on a sample of cases/patients; (3) Results are based on a shorter time period than required; (4) Data suppressed by CMS for one or more quarters; (5) Results are not available for this reporting period; (6) Fewer than 100 patients completed the HCAHPS survey; (7) No cases met the criteria for this measure; (8) The lower limit of the confidence interval cannot be calculated if the number of observed infections equals zero; (9) No data are available from the state/territory for this reporting period; (10) The scores shown reflect fewer than 50 completed surveys; (11) There were discrepancies in the data collection process; (12) This measure does not apply to this hospital for this reporting period; (13) Results cannot be calculated for this reporting period; (14) The results for this state are combined with nearby states to protect confidentiality; Please refer to the User's Guide for a full explanation of data.

Time from ER Arrival to Admit. (minutes)[1,2]	-	-	286	274
Time from ER Arrival to Discharge (minutes)	396	105	140	134
Time in ER Before Being Evaluated (minutes)	236	60	32	26
Time to Pain Meds for Fractures (minutes)	13	50	64	57
Heart Attack Care				
Aspirin Given at Discharge[1,3]	-	-	99%	99%
Fibrinolytic Meds Within 30 Min. of Arrival[3,7]	-	-	80%	54%
PCI Within 90 Minutes of Arrival[3,7]	-	-	95%	96%
Statin Prescribed at Discharge[1,3]	-	-	98%	98%
Heart Failure Care				
ACE Inhibitor or ARB for LVSD[1,2]	-	-	97%	97%
Discharge Instructions Given[1,2]	-	-	92%	94%
Evaluation of LVS Function[1,2]	-	-	99%	99%
Medicare Spending				
Medicare Spending per Patient (ratio)	-	0.98	0.95	0.98
Pneumonia Care				
Appropriate Initial Antibiotic Given[2]	27	78%	95%	95%
Blood Culture Timing[1,2]	-	-	97%	98%
Pregnancy and Delivery Care				
Newborn Deliveries Scheduled Early	79	4%	8%	6%
Preventive Care				
Immunization for Influenza[2]	311	80%	88%	90%
Immunization for Pneumonia[2]	261	69%	90%	92%
Stroke Care				
Anticoagulation Therapy for Atrial Fibrillation[3,7]	-	-	94%	95%
Antithrombotic Therapy Timing[1,3]	-	-	97%	98%
Assessed for Rehabilitation[3,7]	-	-	97%	97%
Discharged on Antithrombotic Therapy[3,7]	-	-	98%	99%
Discharged on Statin Medication[3,7]	-	-	94%	94%
Thrombolytic Therapy Timing[1,3]	-	-	58%	66%
Venous Thromboembolism Prophylaxis[1,3]	-	-	92%	94%
Written Stroke Educational Materials Given[3,7]	-	-	84%	88%
Surgical Care Improvement Project				
Appropriate Beta Blocker Usage[1,2]	-	-	97%	98%
Appropriate VTP Within 24 Hours[2]	57	98%	98%	98%
Controlled Postoperative Blood Glucose[2,7]	-	-	96%	97%
Perioperative Temperature Management[2]	66	100%	100%	100%
Prophylactic Antibiotic Selection[2]	52	100%	99%	99%
Prophylactic Antibiotic Selection (Outpatient)	48	94%	98%	98%
Prophylactic Antibiotic Stopped[2]	52	62%	98%	98%
Prophylactic Antibiotic Timing[2]	52	96%	99%	99%
Prophylactic Antibiotic Timing (Outpatient)	49	96%	98%	98%
Urinary Catheter Removal[1,2]	-	-	97%	97%
Survey of Patients' Hospital Experiences				
Area Around Room 'Always' Quiet at Night	(a)	68%	66%	61%
Doctors 'Always' Communicated Well	(a)	86%	83%	82%
Home Recovery Information Given	(a)	81%	84%	85%
Hospital Given 9 or 10 on 10 Point Scale	(a)	72%	69%	71%
Meds 'Always' Explained Before Given	(a)	66%	63%	64%
Nurses 'Always' Communicated Well	(a)	77%	78%	79%
Pain 'Always' Well Controlled	(a)	65%	71%	71%
Room and Bathroom 'Always' Clean	(a)	71%	71%	73%
Timely Help 'Always' Received	(a)	61%	65%	68%
Would Definitely Recommend Hospital	(a)	71%	70%	71%
Use of Medical Imaging				
Cardiac Imaging Stress Test before Surgery[1]	-	-	5.5%	5.3%
Combination Abdominal CT Scan	64	25.0%	10.1%	10.5%
Combination Brain/Sinus CT Scan[1]	-	-	2.3%	2.7%
Combination Chest CT Scan[1]	-	-	3.7%	2.7%
Follow-up Mammogram/Ultrasound	104	9.6%	8.9%	8.8%
Lumbar Spine MRI for Low Back Pain[1]	-	-	36.6%	37.2%

Perry Hospital

1120 Morningside Dr
Perry, GA 31069
URL: www.hhc.org
Phone: 478-987-3600
Fax: 478-988-1613
Type: Acute Care Hospitals
Ownership: Voluntary non-profit - Private
Emergency Services: Yes
Beds: 45

Key Personnel:
Emergency Room . . . . Horatio V Cabasares, MD
Chief of Medical Staff. . . . . Jefferson U. Davis, D.D.S., M.D
CEO/President. . . . . Lora Davis
Operating Room. . . . . Jesselyn Lacefield, RN
Radiology. . . . . Richard Macarin, MD
Quality Assurance . . . . Rose Reilly, RN
Pediatric Ambulatory Care . . . . . . Larry D Stewart, MD
Pediatric In-Patient Care . . . . Larry D Stewart, MD

Measure	Cases	This Hosp.	State Avg.	U.S. Avg.
Blood Clot Prevention and Treatment				
Anticoagulation Overlap Therapy[2]	19	53%	90%	93%
ICU Venous Thromboembolism Prophylaxis[2]	22	73%	90%	92%
Incidence of Potentially Preventable VTE[1,2]	-	-	13%	10%
UFH with Dosages/Platelet Monitoring[2]	12	75%	99%	97%
Venous Thromboembolism Prophylaxis[2]	153	64%	80%	85%
Warfarin Therapy Discharge Instructions[2]	15	40%	78%	75%
Chest Pain/Possible Heart Attack Care				
Aspirin Given Within 24 Hours of Arrival[5]	-	-	94%	96%
Fibrinolytic Meds Within 30 Min. of Arrival[5]	-	-	35%	58%
Average Time to ECG (minutes)[5]	-	-	8	7
Average Time to Transfer (minutes)[5]	-	-	73	60
Children's Asthma Care				
Received Home Management Plan of Care	-	-	-	88%
Received Reliever Medication	-	-	-	100%
Received Systemic Corticosteroids	-	-	-	100%
Emergency Department				
Admittance Decision Time (minutes)[2]	353	85	100	98
Head CT Results Within 45 Min. of Arrival[1,3]	-	-	45%	57%
Patients Who Left ER Before Being Seen	15,116	2%	3%	2%
Time from ER Arrival to Admit. (minutes)[2]	354	298	286	274
Time from ER Arrival to Discharge (minutes)	401	137	140	134
Time in ER Before Being Evaluated (minutes)	348	31	32	26
Time to Pain Meds for Fractures (minutes)	21	55	64	57
Heart Attack Care				
Aspirin Given at Discharge[1]	-	-	99%	99%
Fibrinolytic Meds Within 30 Min. of Arrival[7]	-	-	80%	54%
PCI Within 90 Minutes of Arrival[7]	-	-	95%	96%
Statin Prescribed at Discharge[1]	-	-	98%	98%
Heart Failure Care				
ACE Inhibitor or ARB for LVSD	26	100%	97%	97%
Discharge Instructions Given	55	84%	92%	94%
Evaluation of LVS Function	74	100%	99%	99%
Medicare Spending				
Medicare Spending per Patient (ratio)	-	0.91	0.95	0.98
Pneumonia Care				
Appropriate Initial Antibiotic Given	37	97%	95%	95%
Blood Culture Timing	47	94%	97%	98%
Pregnancy and Delivery Care				
Newborn Deliveries Scheduled Early[7]	-	-	8%	6%
Preventive Care				
Immunization for Influenza[2]	301	97%	88%	90%
Immunization for Pneumonia[2]	476	99%	90%	92%
Stroke Care				
Anticoagulation Therapy for Atrial Fibrillation[7]	-	-	94%	95%
Antithrombotic Therapy Timing[1]	-	-	97%	98%
Assessed for Rehabilitation[1]	-	-	97%	97%
Discharged on Antithrombotic Therapy[1]	-	-	98%	99%
Discharged on Statin Medication[1]	-	-	94%	94%
Thrombolytic Therapy Timing[7]	-	-	58%	66%
Venous Thromboembolism Prophylaxis[1]	-	-	92%	94%
Written Stroke Educational Materials Given[1]	-	-	84%	88%
Surgical Care Improvement Project				
Appropriate Beta Blocker Usage[2]	23	100%	97%	98%
Appropriate VTP Within 24 Hours[2]	72	100%	98%	98%
Controlled Postoperative Blood Glucose[2,7]	-	-	96%	97%
Perioperative Temperature Management[2]	75	100%	100%	100%
Prophylactic Antibiotic Selection[2]	60	97%	99%	99%
Prophylactic Antibiotic Selection (Outpatient)[5]	-	-	98%	98%
Prophylactic Antibiotic Stopped[2]	54	100%	98%	98%
Prophylactic Antibiotic Timing[2]	60	100%	99%	99%
Prophylactic Antibiotic Timing (Outpatient)[5]	-	-	98%	98%
Urinary Catheter Removal[2]	67	100%	97%	97%
Survey of Patients' Hospital Experiences				
Area Around Room 'Always' Quiet at Night	300+	68%	66%	61%
Doctors 'Always' Communicated Well	300+	90%	83%	82%
Home Recovery Information Given	300+	90%	84%	85%
Hospital Given 9 or 10 on 10 Point Scale	300+	76%	69%	71%
Meds 'Always' Explained Before Given	300+	71%	63%	64%
Nurses 'Always' Communicated Well	300+	82%	78%	79%
Pain 'Always' Well Controlled	300+	74%	71%	71%
Room and Bathroom 'Always' Clean	300+	76%	71%	73%
Timely Help 'Always' Received	300+	68%	65%	68%
Would Definitely Recommend Hospital	300+	79%	70%	71%
Use of Medical Imaging				
Cardiac Imaging Stress Test before Surgery[7]	-	-	5.5%	5.3%
Combination Abdominal CT Scan	269	23.8%	10.1%	10.5%
Combination Brain/Sinus CT Scan[1]	-	-	2.3%	2.7%
Combination Chest CT Scan	176	11.9%	3.7%	2.7%
Follow-up Mammogram/Ultrasound	370	4.1%	8.9%	8.8%
Lumbar Spine MRI for Low Back Pain[1]	-	-	36.6%	37.2%

Brooks County Hospital

903 N Court St
Quitman, GA 31643
Phone: 912-263-6309
Fax: 229-263-6318
Type: Critical Access Hospitals
Ownership: Voluntary non-profit - Other
Emergency Services: Yes
Beds: 35

Key Personnel:
Emergency Room . . . . June Furney, RN
Infection Control. . . . . Patricia Johnson
CEO/President. . . . . LaDon Toole
Quality Assurance . . . . Nancy Williams, RN

Measure	Cases	This Hosp.	State Avg.	U.S. Avg.
Blood Clot Prevention and Treatment				
Anticoagulation Overlap Therapy[5]	-	-	90%	93%
ICU Venous Thromboembolism Prophylaxis[5]	-	-	90%	92%
Incidence of Potentially Preventable VTE[5]	-	-	13%	10%
UFH with Dosages/Platelet Monitoring[5]	-	-	99%	97%
Venous Thromboembolism Prophylaxis[5]	-	-	80%	85%
Warfarin Therapy Discharge Instructions[5]	-	-	78%	75%
Chest Pain/Possible Heart Attack Care				
Aspirin Given Within 24 Hours of Arrival	-	-	94%	96%
Fibrinolytic Meds Within 30 Min. of Arrival	-	-	35%	58%
Average Time to ECG (minutes)	-	-	8	7
Average Time to Transfer (minutes)	-	-	73	60
Children's Asthma Care				
Received Home Management Plan of Care	-	-	-	88%
Received Reliever Medication	-	-	-	100%
Received Systemic Corticosteroids	-	-	-	100%
Emergency Department				
Admittance Decision Time (minutes)[5]	-	-	100	98
Head CT Results Within 45 Min. of Arrival	-	-	45%	57%
Patients Who Left ER Before Being Seen	-	-	3%	2%
Time from ER Arrival to Admit. (minutes)[5]	-	-	286	274
Time from ER Arrival to Discharge (minutes)	-	-	140	134
Time in ER Before Being Evaluated (minutes)	-	-	32	26
Time to Pain Meds for Fractures (minutes)	-	-	64	57
Heart Attack Care				
Aspirin Given at Discharge[5]	-	-	99%	99%
Fibrinolytic Meds Within 30 Min. of Arrival[5]	-	-	80%	54%
PCI Within 90 Minutes of Arrival[5]	-	-	95%	96%
Statin Prescribed at Discharge[5]	-	-	98%	98%
Heart Failure Care				
ACE Inhibitor or ARB for LVSD[1]	-	-	97%	97%
Discharge Instructions Given	11	100%	92%	94%
Evaluation of LVS Function	19	89%	99%	99%
Medicare Spending				
Medicare Spending per Patient (ratio)	-	-	0.95	0.98
Pneumonia Care				
Appropriate Initial Antibiotic Given	12	92%	95%	95%
Blood Culture Timing	21	100%	97%	98%
Pregnancy and Delivery Care				
Newborn Deliveries Scheduled Early[5]	-	-	8%	6%
Preventive Care				
Immunization for Influenza[5]	-	-	88%	90%
Immunization for Pneumonia[5]	-	-	90%	92%
Stroke Care				
Anticoagulation Therapy for Atrial Fibrillation[5]	-	-	94%	95%
Antithrombotic Therapy Timing[5]	-	-	97%	98%
Assessed for Rehabilitation[5]	-	-	97%	97%
Discharged on Antithrombotic Therapy[5]	-	-	98%	99%
Discharged on Statin Medication[5]	-	-	94%	94%

NOTE: Hospital profiles are in alphabetical order by state, then city, then hospital within the city; Rankings exclude hospitals with less than 25 cases except for patient surveys which excludes hospitals with less than 100 cases; (a) 100-299 cases; (1) The number of cases/patients is too few to report; (2) Data submitted were based on a sample of cases/patients; (3) Results are based on a shorter time period than required; (4) Data suppressed by CMS for one or more quarters; (5) Results are not available for this reporting period; (6) Fewer than 100 patients completed the HCAHPS survey; (7) No cases met the criteria for this measure; (8) The lower limit of the confidence interval cannot be calculated if the number of observed infections equals zero; (9) No data are available from the state/territory for this reporting period; (10) The scores shown reflect fewer than 50 completed surveys; (11) There were discrepancies in the data collection process; (12) This measure does not apply to this hospital for this reporting period; (13) Results cannot be calculated for this reporting period; (14) The results for this state are combined with nearby states to protect confidentiality; Please refer to the User's Guide for a full explanation of data.

Measure	Cases	This Hosp.	State Avg.	U.S. Avg.
Thrombolytic Therapy Timing[5]	-	-	58%	66%
Venous Thromboembolism Prophylaxis[5]	-	-	92%	94%
Written Stroke Educational Materials Given[5]	-	-	84%	88%
Surgical Care Improvement Project				
Appropriate Beta Blocker Usage[5]	-	-	97%	98%
Appropriate VTP Within 24 Hours[5]	-	-	98%	98%
Controlled Postoperative Blood Glucose[5]	-	-	96%	97%
Perioperative Temperature Management[5]	-	-	100%	100%
Prophylactic Antibiotic Selection[5]	-	-	99%	99%
Prophylactic Antibiotic Selection (Outpatient)	-	-	98%	98%
Prophylactic Antibiotic Stopped[5]	-	-	98%	98%
Prophylactic Antibiotic Timing[5]	-	-	99%	99%
Prophylactic Antibiotic Timing (Outpatient)	-	-	98%	98%
Urinary Catheter Removal[5]	-	-	97%	97%
Survey of Patients' Hospital Experiences				
Area Around Room 'Always' Quiet at Night	(a)	65%	66%	61%
Doctors 'Always' Communicated Well	(a)	87%	83%	82%
Home Recovery Information Given	(a)	87%	84%	85%
Hospital Given 9 or 10 on 10 Point Scale	(a)	74%	69%	71%
Meds 'Always' Explained Before Given	(a)	63%	63%	64%
Nurses 'Always' Communicated Well	(a)	84%	78%	79%
Pain 'Always' Well Controlled	(a)	72%	71%	71%
Room and Bathroom 'Always' Clean	(a)	81%	71%	73%
Timely Help 'Always' Received	(a)	64%	65%	68%
Would Definitely Recommend Hospital	(a)	66%	70%	71%
Use of Medical Imaging				
Cardiac Imaging Stress Test before Surgery	-	-	5.5%	5.3%
Combination Abdominal CT Scan	-	-	10.1%	10.5%
Combination Brain/Sinus CT Scan	-	-	2.3%	2.7%
Combination Chest CT Scan	-	-	3.7%	2.7%
Follow-up Mammogram/Ultrasound	-	-	8.9%	8.8%
Lumbar Spine MRI for Low Back Pain	-	-	36.6%	37.2%

Southern Regional Medical Center

11 Upper Riverdale Road, Sw | Phone: 770-991-8160
Riverdale, GA 30274 | Fax: 770-991-8595
E-mail: srhs.website@southernregional.org
URL: www.southernregional.org
Type: Acute Care Hospitals | Emergency Services: Yes
Ownership: Voluntary non-profit - Private | Beds: 331

Key Personnel:
Quality Assurance . . . . Paul Casbergue
Chief of Medical Staff . . . . Willie Cochran Jr, MD
CEO/President . . . . James E. Crissey
Patient Relations . . . . Maria Kulma
Operating Room . . . . Patricia Middleton
Emergency Room . . . . Linda Power, RN
Radiology . . . . Danial Whitt

Measure	Cases	This Hosp.	State Avg.	U.S. Avg.
Blood Clot Prevention and Treatment				
Anticoagulation Overlap Therapy[2]	120	90%	90%	93%
ICU Venous Thromboembolism Prophylaxis[2]	120	89%	90%	92%
Incidence of Potentially Preventable VTE[1,2]	-	-	13%	10%
UFH with Dosages/Platelet Monitoring[2]	79	100%	99%	97%
Venous Thromboembolism Prophylaxis[2]	382	71%	80%	85%
Warfarin Therapy Discharge Instructions[2]	99	65%	78%	75%
Chest Pain/Possible Heart Attack Care				
Aspirin Given Within 24 Hours of Arrival[5]	-	-	94%	96%
Fibrinolytic Meds Within 30 Min. of Arrival[5]	-	-	35%	58%
Average Time to ECG (minutes)[5]	-	-	8	7
Average Time to Transfer (minutes)[5]	-	-	73	60
Children's Asthma Care				
Received Home Management Plan of Care	-	-	-	88%
Received Reliever Medication	-	-	-	100%
Received Systemic Corticosteroids	-	-	-	100%
Emergency Department				
Admittance Decision Time (minutes)[2]	669	175	100	98
Head CT Results Within 45 Min. of Arrival	14	64%	45%	57%
Patients Who Left ER Before Being Seen	85,352	6%	3%	2%
Time from ER Arrival to Admit. (minutes)[2]	850	415	286	274
Time from ER Arrival to Discharge (minutes)	1,010	186	140	134
Time in ER Before Being Evaluated (minutes)	883	91	32	26
Time to Pain Meds for Fractures (minutes)	152	109	64	57
Heart Attack Care				
Aspirin Given at Discharge	166	98%	99%	99%
Fibrinolytic Meds Within 30 Min. of Arrival[7]	-	-	80%	54%
PCI Within 90 Minutes of Arrival	48	88%	95%	96%
Statin Prescribed at Discharge	160	96%	98%	98%
Heart Failure Care				
ACE Inhibitor or ARB for LVSD[2]	133	95%	97%	97%
Discharge Instructions Given[2]	272	87%	92%	94%
Evaluation of LVS Function[2]	301	99%	99%	99%
Medicare Spending				
Medicare Spending per Patient (ratio)	-	0.98	0.95	0.98
Pneumonia Care				
Appropriate Initial Antibiotic Given[2]	98	92%	95%	95%
Blood Culture Timing[2]	148	96%	97%	98%
Pregnancy and Delivery Care				
Newborn Deliveries Scheduled Early[2]	159	1%	8%	6%
Preventive Care				
Immunization for Influenza[2]	755	97%	88%	90%
Immunization for Pneumonia[2]	733	93%	90%	92%
Stroke Care				
Anticoagulation Therapy for Atrial Fibrillation	22	100%	94%	95%
Antithrombotic Therapy Timing	204	99%	97%	98%
Assessed for Rehabilitation	269	96%	97%	97%
Discharged on Antithrombotic Therapy	220	99%	98%	99%
Discharged on Statin Medication	177	94%	94%	94%
Thrombolytic Therapy Timing	38	63%	58%	66%
Venous Thromboembolism Prophylaxis	292	91%	92%	94%
Written Stroke Educational Materials Given	168	73%	84%	88%
Surgical Care Improvement Project				
Appropriate Beta Blocker Usage[2]	90	98%	97%	98%
Appropriate VTP Within 24 Hours[2]	369	100%	98%	98%
Controlled Postoperative Blood Glucose[2,7]	-	-	96%	97%
Perioperative Temperature Management[2]	404	100%	100%	100%
Prophylactic Antibiotic Selection[2]	261	98%	99%	99%
Prophylactic Antibiotic Selection (Outpatient)	260	95%	98%	98%
Prophylactic Antibiotic Stopped[2]	259	98%	98%	98%
Prophylactic Antibiotic Timing[2]	263	99%	99%	99%
Prophylactic Antibiotic Timing (Outpatient)	260	99%	98%	98%
Urinary Catheter Removal[2]	180	97%	97%	97%
Survey of Patients' Hospital Experiences				
Area Around Room 'Always' Quiet at Night	300+	60%	66%	61%
Doctors 'Always' Communicated Well	300+	75%	83%	82%
Home Recovery Information Given	300+	75%	84%	85%
Hospital Given 9 or 10 on 10 Point Scale	300+	56%	69%	71%
Meds 'Always' Explained Before Given	300+	52%	63%	64%
Nurses 'Always' Communicated Well	300+	66%	78%	79%
Pain 'Always' Well Controlled	300+	63%	71%	71%
Room and Bathroom 'Always' Clean	300+	69%	71%	73%
Timely Help 'Always' Received	300+	50%	65%	68%
Would Definitely Recommend Hospital	300+	50%	70%	71%
Use of Medical Imaging				
Cardiac Imaging Stress Test before Surgery	216	4.6%	5.5%	5.3%
Combination Abdominal CT Scan	932	6.1%	10.1%	10.5%
Combination Brain/Sinus CT Scan	851	1.1%	2.3%	2.7%
Combination Chest CT Scan	362	3.6%	3.7%	2.7%
Follow-up Mammogram/Ultrasound	1,515	11.0%	8.9%	8.8%
Lumbar Spine MRI for Low Back Pain[1]	-	-	36.6%	37.2%

Floyd Medical Center

304 Turner Mccall Blvd PO Box 233 | Phone: 706-509-6900
Rome, GA 30162 | Fax: 706-509-5771
E-mail: dnighten@floydmed.org
URL: www.floydmed.org
Type: Acute Care Hospitals | Emergency Services: Yes
Ownership: Govt - Hospital Dist/Auth | Beds: 304

Key Personnel:
Radiology . . . . Joseph Burch, MD
Cardiac Laboratory . . . . Mike Cornwell
Coronary Care . . . . Mike Cornwell
Operating Room . . . . Jackie Eschbaugh
Pediatric Ambulatory Care . . . . . . Tami Hincy
Quality Assurance . . . . Jackie Newby
CEO/President . . . . Kurt Stuenkel, FACHE

Measure	Cases	This Hosp.	State Avg.	U.S. Avg.
Blood Clot Prevention and Treatment				
Anticoagulation Overlap Therapy[2]	78	91%	90%	93%
ICU Venous Thromboembolism Prophylaxis[2]	71	96%	90%	92%
Incidence of Potentially Preventable VTE[1,2]	-	-	13%	10%
UFH with Dosages/Platelet Monitoring[2]	31	100%	99%	97%
Venous Thromboembolism Prophylaxis[2]	319	94%	80%	85%
Warfarin Therapy Discharge Instructions[2]	65	89%	78%	75%
Chest Pain/Possible Heart Attack Care				
Aspirin Given Within 24 Hours of Arrival[1,3]	-	-	94%	96%
Fibrinolytic Meds Within 30 Min. of Arrival[3,7]	-	-	35%	58%
Average Time to ECG (minutes)[1,3]	-	-	8	7
Average Time to Transfer (minutes)[1,3]	-	-	73	60
Children's Asthma Care				
Received Home Management Plan of Care	-	-	-	88%
Received Reliever Medication	-	-	-	100%
Received Systemic Corticosteroids	-	-	-	100%
Emergency Department				
Admittance Decision Time (minutes)[2]	450	84	100	98
Head CT Results Within 45 Min. of Arrival[1]	-	-	45%	57%
Patients Who Left ER Before Being Seen	79,941	2%	3%	2%
Time from ER Arrival to Admit. (minutes)[2]	509	238	286	274
Time from ER Arrival to Discharge (minutes)	338	146	140	134
Time in ER Before Being Evaluated (minutes)	215	34	32	26
Time to Pain Meds for Fractures (minutes)	158	67	64	57
Heart Attack Care				
Aspirin Given at Discharge	198	97%	99%	99%
Fibrinolytic Meds Within 30 Min. of Arrival[7]	-	-	80%	54%
PCI Within 90 Minutes of Arrival	22	100%	95%	96%
Statin Prescribed at Discharge	192	96%	98%	98%
Heart Failure Care				
ACE Inhibitor or ARB for LVSD	101	98%	97%	97%
Discharge Instructions Given	252	88%	92%	94%
Evaluation of LVS Function	306	100%	99%	99%
Medicare Spending				
Medicare Spending per Patient (ratio)	-	1.00	0.95	0.98
Pneumonia Care				
Appropriate Initial Antibiotic Given	261	95%	95%	95%
Blood Culture Timing	470	99%	97%	98%
Pregnancy and Delivery Care				
Newborn Deliveries Scheduled Early[2]	399	6%	8%	6%
Preventive Care				
Immunization for Influenza[2]	497	99%	88%	90%
Immunization for Pneumonia[2]	604	99%	90%	92%
Stroke Care				
Anticoagulation Therapy for Atrial Fibrillation	16	100%	94%	95%
Antithrombotic Therapy Timing	115	99%	97%	98%
Assessed for Rehabilitation	141	99%	97%	97%
Discharged on Antithrombotic Therapy	124	98%	98%	99%
Discharged on Statin Medication	78	94%	94%	94%
Thrombolytic Therapy Timing[1]	-	-	58%	66%
Venous Thromboembolism Prophylaxis	142	93%	92%	94%
Written Stroke Educational Materials Given	85	98%	84%	88%
Surgical Care Improvement Project				
Appropriate Beta Blocker Usage[2]	219	100%	97%	98%
Appropriate VTP Within 24 Hours[2]	693	99%	98%	98%
Controlled Postoperative Blood Glucose[2,7]	-	-	96%	97%
Perioperative Temperature Management[2]	841	100%	100%	100%
Prophylactic Antibiotic Selection[2]	460	100%	99%	99%
Prophylactic Antibiotic Selection (Outpatient)	413	98%	98%	98%
Prophylactic Antibiotic Stopped[2]	446	99%	98%	98%
Prophylactic Antibiotic Timing[2]	460	99%	99%	99%
Prophylactic Antibiotic Timing (Outpatient)	427	96%	98%	98%
Urinary Catheter Removal[2]	475	97%	97%	97%
Survey of Patients' Hospital Experiences				
Area Around Room 'Always' Quiet at Night	300+	64%	66%	61%
Doctors 'Always' Communicated Well	300+	83%	83%	82%
Home Recovery Information Given	300+	82%	84%	85%
Hospital Given 9 or 10 on 10 Point Scale	300+	73%	69%	71%
Meds 'Always' Explained Before Given	300+	63%	63%	64%
Nurses 'Always' Communicated Well	300+	79%	78%	79%
Pain 'Always' Well Controlled	300+	71%	71%	71%
Room and Bathroom 'Always' Clean	300+	66%	71%	73%
Timely Help 'Always' Received	300+	65%	65%	68%

NOTE: Hospital profiles are in alphabetical order by state, then city, then hospital within the city; Rankings exclude hospitals with less than 25 cases except for patient surveys which excludes hospitals with less than 100 cases; (a) 100-299 cases; (1) The number of cases/patients is too few to report; (2) Data submitted were based on a sample of cases/patients; (3) Results are based on a shorter time period than required; (4) Data suppressed by CMS for one or more quarters; (5) Results are not available for this reporting period; (6) Fewer than 100 patients completed the HCAHPS survey; (7) No cases met the criteria for this measure; (8) The lower limit of the confidence interval cannot be calculated if the number of observed infections equals zero; (9) No data are available from the state/territory for this reporting period; (10) The scores shown reflect fewer than 50 completed surveys; (11) There were discrepancies in the data collection process; (12) This measure does not apply to this hospital for this reporting period; (13) Results cannot be calculated for this reporting period; (14) The results for this state are combined with nearby states to protect confidentiality; Please refer to the User's Guide for a full explanation of data.

Would Definitely Recommend Hospital	300+	76%	70%	71%
Use of Medical Imaging				
Cardiac Imaging Stress Test before Surgery	580	5.7%	5.5%	5.3%
Combination Abdominal CT Scan	699	1.4%	10.1%	10.5%
Combination Brain/Sinus CT Scan	872	2.2%	2.3%	2.7%
Combination Chest CT Scan	394	0.0%	3.7%	2.7%
Follow-up Mammogram/Ultrasound	2,921	9.7%	8.9%	8.8%
Lumbar Spine MRI for Low Back Pain	137	34.3%	36.6%	37.2%

Redmond Regional Medical Center

501 Redmond Road Phone: 706-802-3012
Rome, GA 30165 Fax: 706-291-0971
URL: www.redmondregional.com
Type: Acute Care Hospitals Emergency Services: Yes
Ownership: Proprietary Beds: 201

Key Personnel:
Radiology. . . . . J C Abdou
Quality Assurance . . . . Deborah Branton, RN
Chief of Medical Staff. . . . . Louis Lataif, MD
Operating Room. . . . . Melanie H Mccary, RN
Emergency Room . . . . Jean Miller, RN
CEO . . . . John Quinlivan

Measure	Cases	This Hosp.	State Avg.	U.S. Avg.
Blood Clot Prevention and Treatment				
Anticoagulation Overlap Therapy[2]	97	94%	90%	93%
ICU Venous Thromboembolism Prophylaxis[2]	122	90%	90%	92%
Incidence of Potentially Preventable VTE[2]	17	6%	13%	10%
UFH with Dosages/Platelet Monitoring[2]	39	100%	99%	97%
Venous Thromboembolism Prophylaxis[2]	339	88%	80%	85%
Warfarin Therapy Discharge Instructions[2]	75	97%	78%	75%
Chest Pain/Possible Heart Attack Care				
Aspirin Given Within 24 Hours of Arrival[5]	-	-	94%	96%
Fibrinolytic Meds Within 30 Min. of Arrival[5]	-	-	35%	58%
Average Time to ECG (minutes)[5]	-	-	8	7
Average Time to Transfer (minutes)[5]	-	-	73	60
Children's Asthma Care				
Received Home Management Plan of Care	-	-	-	88%
Received Reliever Medication	-	-	-	100%
Received Systemic Corticosteroids	-	-	-	100%
Emergency Department				
Admittance Decision Time (minutes)[2]	678	98	100	98
Head CT Results Within 45 Min. of Arrival[1]	-	-	45%	57%
Patients Who Left ER Before Being Seen	39,685	1%	3%	2%
Time from ER Arrival to Admit. (minutes)[2]	680	201	286	274
Time from ER Arrival to Discharge (minutes)	458	140	140	134
Time in ER Before Being Evaluated (minutes)	492	17	32	26
Time to Pain Meds for Fractures (minutes)	76	71	64	57
Heart Attack Care				
Aspirin Given at Discharge	570	100%	99%	99%
Fibrinolytic Meds Within 30 Min. of Arrival[7]	-	-	80%	54%
PCI Within 90 Minutes of Arrival	71	99%	95%	96%
Statin Prescribed at Discharge	535	99%	98%	98%
Heart Failure Care				
ACE Inhibitor or ARB for LVSD	163	98%	97%	97%
Discharge Instructions Given	455	89%	92%	94%
Evaluation of LVS Function	520	100%	99%	99%
Medicare Spending				
Medicare Spending per Patient (ratio)	-	0.93	0.95	0.98
Pneumonia Care				
Appropriate Initial Antibiotic Given	181	98%	95%	95%
Blood Culture Timing	279	98%	97%	98%
Pregnancy and Delivery Care				
Newborn Deliveries Scheduled Early[2,7]	-	-	8%	6%
Preventive Care				
Immunization for Influenza[2]	617	97%	88%	90%
Immunization for Pneumonia[2]	1,041	97%	90%	92%
Stroke Care				
Anticoagulation Therapy for Atrial Fibrillation	27	100%	94%	95%
Antithrombotic Therapy Timing	107	100%	97%	98%
Assessed for Rehabilitation	123	98%	97%	97%
Discharged on Antithrombotic Therapy	109	100%	98%	99%
Discharged on Statin Medication	98	96%	94%	94%
Thrombolytic Therapy Timing[1]	-	-	58%	66%
Venous Thromboembolism Prophylaxis	120	98%	92%	94%
Written Stroke Educational Materials Given	75	69%	84%	88%
Surgical Care Improvement Project				
Appropriate Beta Blocker Usage	526	99%	97%	98%
Appropriate VTP Within 24 Hours	617	99%	98%	98%
Controlled Postoperative Blood Glucose	335	96%	96%	97%
Perioperative Temperature Management	782	100%	100%	100%
Prophylactic Antibiotic Selection	766	99%	99%	99%
Prophylactic Antibiotic Selection (Outpatient)	474	100%	98%	98%
Prophylactic Antibiotic Stopped	746	98%	98%	98%
Prophylactic Antibiotic Timing	766	99%	99%	99%
Prophylactic Antibiotic Timing (Outpatient)	477	98%	98%	98%
Urinary Catheter Removal	717	97%	97%	97%
Survey of Patients' Hospital Experiences				
Area Around Room 'Always' Quiet at Night	300+	69%	66%	61%
Doctors 'Always' Communicated Well	300+	83%	83%	82%
Home Recovery Information Given	300+	84%	84%	85%
Hospital Given 9 or 10 on 10 Point Scale	300+	76%	69%	71%
Meds 'Always' Explained Before Given	300+	62%	63%	64%
Nurses 'Always' Communicated Well	300+	80%	78%	79%
Pain 'Always' Well Controlled	300+	73%	71%	71%
Room and Bathroom 'Always' Clean	300+	75%	71%	73%
Timely Help 'Always' Received	300+	69%	65%	68%
Would Definitely Recommend Hospital	300+	80%	70%	71%
Use of Medical Imaging				
Cardiac Imaging Stress Test before Surgery	356	6.2%	5.5%	5.3%
Combination Abdominal CT Scan	625	4.8%	10.1%	10.5%
Combination Brain/Sinus CT Scan	820	2.3%	2.3%	2.7%
Combination Chest CT Scan	311	3.2%	3.7%	2.7%
Follow-up Mammogram/Ultrasound	886	15.2%	8.9%	8.8%
Lumbar Spine MRI for Low Back Pain	44	40.9%	36.6%	37.2%

North Fulton Hospital

3000 Hospital Boulevard Phone: 770-751-2500
Roswell, GA 30076 Fax: 770-751-2899
URL: www.northfultonregional.com
Type: Acute Care Hospitals Emergency Services: Yes
Ownership: Proprietary Beds: 167

Key Personnel:
Emergency Room . . . . Ann Abrams
Radiology. . . . . Boyd Bird
Quality Assurance . . . . Courtney Brodley
Chief of Medical Staff. . . . . John Harvey
CEO/President. . . . . John Holland
Pediatric Ambulatory Care . . . . . . Edward Salzberg, MD
Pediatric In-Patient Care . . . . Edward Salzberg, MD

Measure	Cases	This Hosp.	State Avg.	U.S. Avg.
Blood Clot Prevention and Treatment				
Anticoagulation Overlap Therapy[2]	42	81%	90%	93%
ICU Venous Thromboembolism Prophylaxis[2]	125	96%	90%	92%
Incidence of Potentially Preventable VTE[1,2]	-	-	13%	10%
UFH with Dosages/Platelet Monitoring[2]	43	100%	99%	97%
Venous Thromboembolism Prophylaxis[2]	279	87%	80%	85%
Warfarin Therapy Discharge Instructions[2]	30	97%	78%	75%
Chest Pain/Possible Heart Attack Care				
Aspirin Given Within 24 Hours of Arrival	88	100%	94%	96%
Fibrinolytic Meds Within 30 Min. of Arrival[7]	-	-	35%	58%
Average Time to ECG (minutes)	88	7	8	7
Average Time to Transfer (minutes)	25	77	73	60
Children's Asthma Care				
Received Home Management Plan of Care	-	-	-	88%
Received Reliever Medication	-	-	-	100%
Received Systemic Corticosteroids	-	-	-	100%
Emergency Department				
Admittance Decision Time (minutes)[2]	681	110	100	98
Head CT Results Within 45 Min. of Arrival[1]	-	-	45%	57%
Patients Who Left ER Before Being Seen	40,016	2%	3%	2%
Time from ER Arrival to Admit. (minutes)[2]	682	274	286	274
Time from ER Arrival to Discharge (minutes)	346	135	140	134
Time in ER Before Being Evaluated (minutes)	373	23	32	26
Time to Pain Meds for Fractures (minutes)	228	44	64	57
Heart Attack Care				
Aspirin Given at Discharge	14	100%	99%	99%
Fibrinolytic Meds Within 30 Min. of Arrival[7]	-	-	80%	54%
PCI Within 90 Minutes of Arrival[7]	-	-	95%	96%
Statin Prescribed at Discharge	17	100%	98%	98%
Heart Failure Care				
ACE Inhibitor or ARB for LVSD	37	97%	97%	97%
Discharge Instructions Given	151	99%	92%	94%
Evaluation of LVS Function	165	99%	99%	99%
Medicare Spending				
Medicare Spending per Patient (ratio)	-	1.00	0.95	0.98
Pneumonia Care				
Appropriate Initial Antibiotic Given[2]	110	95%	95%	95%
Blood Culture Timing[2]	131	98%	97%	98%
Pregnancy and Delivery Care				
Newborn Deliveries Scheduled Early[2]	23	4%	8%	6%
Preventive Care				
Immunization for Influenza[2]	524	96%	88%	90%
Immunization for Pneumonia[2]	570	94%	90%	92%
Stroke Care				
Anticoagulation Therapy for Atrial Fibrillation	16	100%	94%	95%
Antithrombotic Therapy Timing	72	94%	97%	98%
Assessed for Rehabilitation	105	97%	97%	97%
Discharged on Antithrombotic Therapy	78	100%	98%	99%
Discharged on Statin Medication	54	98%	94%	94%
Thrombolytic Therapy Timing	13	85%	58%	66%
Venous Thromboembolism Prophylaxis	106	96%	92%	94%
Written Stroke Educational Materials Given	72	97%	84%	88%
Surgical Care Improvement Project				
Appropriate Beta Blocker Usage[2]	74	96%	97%	98%
Appropriate VTP Within 24 Hours[2]	304	98%	98%	98%
Controlled Postoperative Blood Glucose[2,7]	-	-	96%	97%
Perioperative Temperature Management[2]	348	100%	100%	100%
Prophylactic Antibiotic Selection[2]	252	100%	99%	99%
Prophylactic Antibiotic Selection (Outpatient)	187	97%	98%	98%
Prophylactic Antibiotic Stopped[2]	251	98%	98%	98%
Prophylactic Antibiotic Timing[2]	252	99%	99%	99%
Prophylactic Antibiotic Timing (Outpatient)	187	98%	98%	98%
Urinary Catheter Removal[2]	223	96%	97%	97%
Survey of Patients' Hospital Experiences				
Area Around Room 'Always' Quiet at Night	300+	53%	66%	61%
Doctors 'Always' Communicated Well	300+	79%	83%	82%
Home Recovery Information Given	300+	82%	84%	85%
Hospital Given 9 or 10 on 10 Point Scale	300+	65%	69%	71%
Meds 'Always' Explained Before Given	300+	59%	63%	64%
Nurses 'Always' Communicated Well	300+	74%	78%	79%
Pain 'Always' Well Controlled	300+	65%	71%	71%
Room and Bathroom 'Always' Clean	300+	68%	71%	73%
Timely Help 'Always' Received	300+	58%	65%	68%
Would Definitely Recommend Hospital	300+	70%	70%	71%
Use of Medical Imaging				
Cardiac Imaging Stress Test before Surgery	100	8.0%	5.5%	5.3%
Combination Abdominal CT Scan	556	2.3%	10.1%	10.5%
Combination Brain/Sinus CT Scan	642	0.6%	2.3%	2.7%
Combination Chest CT Scan	395	0.0%	3.7%	2.7%
Follow-up Mammogram/Ultrasound	843	7.5%	8.9%	8.8%
Lumbar Spine MRI for Low Back Pain	87	27.6%	36.6%	37.2%

Southeast Georgia Health System - Camden Campus

2000 Dan Proctor Drive Phone: 912-576-6401
Saint Marys, GA 31558
Type: Acute Care Hospitals Emergency Services: Yes
Ownership: Govt - Hospital Dist/Auth

Key Personnel:
CEO/President. . . . . Gary R. Colberg, FACHE

Measure	Cases	This Hosp.	State Avg.	U.S. Avg.
Blood Clot Prevention and Treatment				
Anticoagulation Overlap Therapy[1,2]	-	-	90%	93%
ICU Venous Thromboembolism Prophylaxis[2]	37	76%	90%	92%
Incidence of Potentially Preventable VTE[2,7]	-	-	13%	10%
UFH with Dosages/Platelet Monitoring[2,7]	-	-	99%	97%
Venous Thromboembolism Prophylaxis[2]	130	78%	80%	85%
Warfarin Therapy Discharge Instructions[1,2]	-	-	78%	75%
Chest Pain/Possible Heart Attack Care				
Aspirin Given Within 24 Hours of Arrival	64	100%	94%	96%
Fibrinolytic Meds Within 30 Min. of Arrival[1]	-	-	35%	58%

NOTE: Hospital profiles are in alphabetical order by state, then city, then hospital within the city; Rankings exclude hospitals with less than 25 cases except for patient surveys which excludes hospitals with less than 100 cases; (a) 100-299 cases; (1) The number of cases/patients is too few to report; (2) Data submitted were based on a sample of cases/patients; (3) Results are based on a shorter time period than required; (4) Data suppressed by CMS for one or more quarters; (5) Results are not available for this reporting period; (6) Fewer than 100 patients completed the HCAHPS survey; (7) No cases met the criteria for this measure; (8) The lower limit of the confidence interval cannot be calculated if the number of observed infections equals zero; (9) No data are available from the state/territory for this reporting period; (10) The scores shown reflect fewer than 50 completed surveys; (11) There were discrepancies in the data collection process; (12) This measure does not apply to this hospital for this reporting period; (13) Results cannot be calculated for this reporting period; (14) The results for this state are combined with nearby states to protect confidentiality; Please refer to the User's Guide for a full explanation of data.

Measure	Cases	This Hosp.	State Avg.	U.S. Avg.
Average Time to ECG (minutes)	67	20	8	7
Average Time to Transfer (minutes)[1]	-	-	73	60
Children's Asthma Care				
Received Home Management Plan of Care	-	-	-	88%
Received Reliever Medication	-	-	-	100%
Received Systemic Corticosteroids	-	-	-	100%
Emergency Department				
Admittance Decision Time (minutes)[2]	164	83	100	98
Head CT Results Within 45 Min. of Arrival	11	55%	45%	57%
Patients Who Left ER Before Being Seen	30,511	5%	3%	2%
Time from ER Arrival to Admit. (minutes)[2]	165	284	286	274
Time from ER Arrival to Discharge (minutes)[11]	437	147	140	134
Time in ER Before Being Evaluated (minutes)	460	58	32	26
Time to Pain Meds for Fractures (minutes)	94	82	64	57
Heart Attack Care				
Aspirin Given at Discharge[1,3]	-	-	99%	99%
Fibrinolytic Meds Within 30 Min. of Arrival[3,7]	-	-	80%	54%
PCI Within 90 Minutes of Arrival[3,7]	-	-	95%	96%
Statin Prescribed at Discharge[1,3]	-	-	98%	98%
Heart Failure Care				
ACE Inhibitor or ARB for LVSD[1,2]	-	-	97%	97%
Discharge Instructions Given[2]	20	100%	92%	94%
Evaluation of LVS Function[2]	27	100%	99%	99%
Medicare Spending				
Medicare Spending per Patient (ratio)	-	0.94	0.95	0.98
Pneumonia Care				
Appropriate Initial Antibiotic Given[2]	36	86%	95%	95%
Blood Culture Timing[2]	46	96%	97%	98%
Pregnancy and Delivery Care				
Newborn Deliveries Scheduled Early	66	0%	8%	6%
Preventive Care				
Immunization for Influenza[2]	215	98%	88%	90%
Immunization for Pneumonia[2]	151	100%	90%	92%
Stroke Care				
Anticoagulation Therapy for Atrial Fibrillation[1,2]	-	-	94%	95%
Antithrombotic Therapy Timing[1,2]	-	-	97%	98%
Assessed for Rehabilitation[1,2]	-	-	97%	97%
Discharged on Antithrombotic Therapy[1,2]	-	-	98%	99%
Discharged on Statin Medication[1,2]	-	-	94%	94%
Thrombolytic Therapy Timing[1,2]	-	-	58%	66%
Venous Thromboembolism Prophylaxis[1,2]	-	-	92%	94%
Written Stroke Educational Materials Given[1,2]	-	-	84%	88%
Surgical Care Improvement Project				
Appropriate Beta Blocker Usage	22	95%	97%	98%
Appropriate VTP Within 24 Hours	103	100%	98%	98%
Controlled Postoperative Blood Glucose[7]	-	-	96%	97%
Perioperative Temperature Management	113	100%	100%	100%
Prophylactic Antibiotic Selection	72	97%	99%	99%
Prophylactic Antibiotic Selection (Outpatient)	34	97%	98%	98%
Prophylactic Antibiotic Stopped	69	100%	98%	98%
Prophylactic Antibiotic Timing	72	100%	99%	99%
Prophylactic Antibiotic Timing (Outpatient)	34	100%	98%	98%
Urinary Catheter Removal	72	100%	97%	97%
Survey of Patients' Hospital Experiences				
Area Around Room 'Always' Quiet at Night	(a)	56%	66%	61%
Doctors 'Always' Communicated Well	(a)	80%	83%	82%
Home Recovery Information Given	(a)	84%	84%	85%
Hospital Given 9 or 10 on 10 Point Scale	(a)	65%	69%	71%
Meds 'Always' Explained Before Given	(a)	60%	63%	64%
Nurses 'Always' Communicated Well	(a)	78%	78%	79%
Pain 'Always' Well Controlled	(a)	66%	71%	71%
Room and Bathroom 'Always' Clean	(a)	79%	71%	73%
Timely Help 'Always' Received	(a)	66%	65%	68%
Would Definitely Recommend Hospital	(a)	65%	70%	71%
Use of Medical Imaging				
Cardiac Imaging Stress Test before Surgery	96	3.1%	5.5%	5.3%
Combination Abdominal CT Scan	420	11.7%	10.1%	10.5%
Combination Brain/Sinus CT Scan[1]	-	-	2.3%	2.7%
Combination Chest CT Scan	210	18.1%	3.7%	2.7%
Follow-up Mammogram/Ultrasound	728	3.0%	8.9%	8.8%
Lumbar Spine MRI for Low Back Pain	42	42.9%	36.6%	37.2%

Washington County Regional Medical Center

610 Sparta Road
Sandersville, GA 31082
Phone: 478-240-2100
Fax: 478-240-2390
Type: Acute Care Hospitals
Emergency Services: Yes
Ownership: Govt - Hospital Dist/Auth
Beds: 116

Key Personnel:

Chief of Medical Staff. . . . . Oberto Baga
Radiology. . . . . Sheri Black
CEO/President. . . . . Tom Brown
Quality Assurance . . . . Gloria Evans
Pediatric Ambulatory Care . . . . . Sandra Tinley, MD
Pediatric In-Patient Care . . . . Sandra Tinley, MD
Operating Room. . . . . Cheryl Wright, RN
Coronary Care . . . . Robert Wright

Measure	Cases	This Hosp.	State Avg.	U.S. Avg.
Blood Clot Prevention and Treatment				
Anticoagulation Overlap Therapy[1,2]	-	-	90%	93%
ICU Venous Thromboembolism Prophylaxis[2]	44	68%	90%	92%
Incidence of Potentially Preventable VTE[1,2]	-	-	13%	10%
UFH with Dosages/Platelet Monitoring[2,7]	-	-	99%	97%
Venous Thromboembolism Prophylaxis[2]	282	73%	80%	85%
Warfarin Therapy Discharge Instructions[1,2]	-	-	78%	75%
Chest Pain/Possible Heart Attack Care				
Aspirin Given Within 24 Hours of Arrival	55	85%	94%	96%
Fibrinolytic Meds Within 30 Min. of Arrival[1]	-	-	35%	58%
Average Time to ECG (minutes)	59	9	8	7
Average Time to Transfer (minutes)[1]	-	-	73	60
Children's Asthma Care				
Received Home Management Plan of Care	-	-	-	88%
Received Reliever Medication	-	-	-	100%
Received Systemic Corticosteroids	-	-	-	100%
Emergency Department				
Admittance Decision Time (minutes)[2]	302	44	100	98
Head CT Results Within 45 Min. of Arrival	15	53%	45%	57%
Patients Who Left ER Before Being Seen	12,095	2%	3%	2%
Time from ER Arrival to Admit. (minutes)[2]	302	228	286	274
Time from ER Arrival to Discharge (minutes)	379	107	140	134
Time in ER Before Being Evaluated (minutes)	418	30	32	26
Time to Pain Meds for Fractures (minutes)	55	42	64	57
Heart Attack Care				
Aspirin Given at Discharge[1,3]	-	-	99%	99%
Fibrinolytic Meds Within 30 Min. of Arrival[3,7]	-	-	80%	54%
PCI Within 90 Minutes of Arrival[3,7]	-	-	95%	96%
Statin Prescribed at Discharge[1,3]	-	-	98%	98%
Heart Failure Care				
ACE Inhibitor or ARB for LVSD[1]	-	-	97%	97%
Discharge Instructions Given	35	80%	92%	94%
Evaluation of LVS Function	48	92%	99%	99%
Medicare Spending				
Medicare Spending per Patient (ratio)	-	0.87	0.95	0.98
Pneumonia Care				
Appropriate Initial Antibiotic Given	43	74%	95%	95%
Blood Culture Timing	67	90%	97%	98%
Pregnancy and Delivery Care				
Newborn Deliveries Scheduled Early[2]	36	11%	8%	6%
Preventive Care				
Immunization for Influenza[2]	340	71%	88%	90%
Immunization for Pneumonia[2]	373	85%	90%	92%
Stroke Care				
Anticoagulation Therapy for Atrial Fibrillation[7]	-	-	94%	95%
Antithrombotic Therapy Timing	13	92%	97%	98%
Assessed for Rehabilitation	13	92%	97%	97%
Discharged on Antithrombotic Therapy[1]	-	-	98%	99%
Discharged on Statin Medication	11	36%	94%	94%
Thrombolytic Therapy Timing[1]	-	-	58%	66%
Venous Thromboembolism Prophylaxis	15	60%	92%	94%
Written Stroke Educational Materials Given[1]	-	-	84%	88%
Surgical Care Improvement Project				
Appropriate Beta Blocker Usage[1]	-	-	97%	98%
Appropriate VTP Within 24 Hours	52	94%	98%	98%
Controlled Postoperative Blood Glucose[7]	-	-	96%	97%
Perioperative Temperature Management	54	100%	100%	100%
Prophylactic Antibiotic Selection[1]	-	-	99%	99%
Prophylactic Antibiotic Selection (Outpatient)[1]	-	-	98%	98%
Prophylactic Antibiotic Stopped[1]	-	-	98%	98%
Prophylactic Antibiotic Timing[1]	-	-	99%	99%
Prophylactic Antibiotic Timing (Outpatient)[1]	-	-	98%	98%
Urinary Catheter Removal[1]	-	-	97%	97%
Survey of Patients' Hospital Experiences				
Area Around Room 'Always' Quiet at Night	300+	70%	66%	61%
Doctors 'Always' Communicated Well	300+	83%	83%	82%
Home Recovery Information Given	300+	83%	84%	85%
Hospital Given 9 or 10 on 10 Point Scale	300+	59%	69%	71%
Meds 'Always' Explained Before Given	300+	66%	63%	64%
Nurses 'Always' Communicated Well	300+	79%	78%	79%
Pain 'Always' Well Controlled	300+	71%	71%	71%
Room and Bathroom 'Always' Clean	300+	58%	71%	73%
Timely Help 'Always' Received	300+	63%	65%	68%
Would Definitely Recommend Hospital	300+	57%	70%	71%
Use of Medical Imaging				
Cardiac Imaging Stress Test before Surgery[1]	-	-	5.5%	5.3%
Combination Abdominal CT Scan	211	20.9%	10.1%	10.5%
Combination Brain/Sinus CT Scan[1]	-	-	2.3%	2.7%
Combination Chest CT Scan	103	19.4%	3.7%	2.7%
Follow-up Mammogram/Ultrasound	395	5.8%	8.9%	8.8%
Lumbar Spine MRI for Low Back Pain[1]	-	-	36.6%	37.2%

Candler Hospital

5353 Reynolds Street
Savannah, GA 31412
Phone: 912-819-6000
Type: Acute Care Hospitals
Emergency Services: Yes
Ownership: Voluntary non-profit - Other

Key Personnel:

Radiology. . . . . Vivian Austin
Emergency Room . . . . Vicky Butler
CEO/President. . . . . Paul P Hinchey

Measure	Cases	This Hosp.	State Avg.	U.S. Avg.
Blood Clot Prevention and Treatment				
Anticoagulation Overlap Therapy[2]	95	96%	90%	93%
ICU Venous Thromboembolism Prophylaxis[2]	60	92%	90%	92%
Incidence of Potentially Preventable VTE[2]	19	21%	13%	10%
UFH with Dosages/Platelet Monitoring[2]	15	100%	99%	97%
Venous Thromboembolism Prophylaxis[2]	396	79%	80%	85%
Warfarin Therapy Discharge Instructions[2]	65	95%	78%	75%
Chest Pain/Possible Heart Attack Care				
Aspirin Given Within 24 Hours of Arrival	42	98%	94%	96%
Fibrinolytic Meds Within 30 Min. of Arrival[7]	-	-	35%	58%
Average Time to ECG (minutes)	42	18	8	7
Average Time to Transfer (minutes)[1]	-	-	73	60
Children's Asthma Care				
Received Home Management Plan of Care	-	-	-	88%
Received Reliever Medication	-	-	-	100%
Received Systemic Corticosteroids	-	-	-	100%
Emergency Department				
Admittance Decision Time (minutes)[2]	340	230	100	98
Head CT Results Within 45 Min. of Arrival[1,3]	-	-	45%	57%
Patients Who Left ER Before Being Seen	54,486	2%	3%	2%
Time from ER Arrival to Admit. (minutes)[2]	341	538	286	274
Time from ER Arrival to Discharge (minutes)	370	154	140	134
Time in ER Before Being Evaluated (minutes)	331	51	32	26
Time to Pain Meds for Fractures (minutes)	113	77	64	57
Heart Attack Care				
Aspirin Given at Discharge[1,3]	-	-	99%	99%
Fibrinolytic Meds Within 30 Min. of Arrival[3,7]	-	-	80%	54%
PCI Within 90 Minutes of Arrival[3,7]	-	-	95%	96%
Statin Prescribed at Discharge[1,3]	-	-	98%	98%
Heart Failure Care				
ACE Inhibitor or ARB for LVSD	67	100%	97%	97%
Discharge Instructions Given	262	100%	92%	94%
Evaluation of LVS Function	319	100%	99%	99%
Medicare Spending				
Medicare Spending per Patient (ratio)	-	1.05	0.95	0.98
Pneumonia Care				
Appropriate Initial Antibiotic Given	148	97%	95%	95%
Blood Culture Timing	191	98%	97%	98%
Pregnancy and Delivery Care				
Newborn Deliveries Scheduled Early[2]	74	8%	8%	6%

NOTE: Hospital profiles are in alphabetical order by state, then city, then hospital within the city; Rankings exclude hospitals with less than 25 cases except for patient surveys which excludes hospitals with less than 100 cases; (a) 100-299 cases; (1) The number of cases/patients is too few to report; (2) Data submitted were based on a sample of cases/patients; (3) Results are based on a shorter time period than required; (4) Data suppressed by CMS for one or more quarters; (5) Results are not available for this reporting period; (6) Fewer than 100 patients completed the HCAHPS survey; (7) No cases met the criteria for this measure; (8) The lower limit of the confidence interval cannot be calculated if the number of observed infections equals zero; (9) No data are available from the state/territory for this reporting period; (10) The scores shown reflect fewer than 50 completed surveys; (11) There were discrepancies in the data collection process; (12) This measure does not apply to this hospital for this reporting period; (13) Results cannot be calculated for this reporting period; (14) The results for this state are combined with nearby states to protect confidentiality; Please refer to the User's Guide for a full explanation of data.

Measure	Cases	This Hosp.	State Avg.	U.S. Avg.
Preventive Care				
Immunization for Influenza[2]	481	97%	88%	90%
Immunization for Pneumonia[2]	516	99%	90%	92%
Stroke Care				
Anticoagulation Therapy for Atrial Fibrillation[1]	-	-	94%	95%
Antithrombotic Therapy Timing	82	94%	97%	98%
Assessed for Rehabilitation	89	97%	97%	97%
Discharged on Antithrombotic Therapy	87	98%	98%	99%
Discharged on Statin Medication	63	95%	94%	94%
Thrombolytic Therapy Timing[1]	-	-	58%	66%
Venous Thromboembolism Prophylaxis	87	87%	92%	94%
Written Stroke Educational Materials Given	53	96%	84%	88%
Surgical Care Improvement Project				
Appropriate Beta Blocker Usage[2]	55	95%	97%	98%
Appropriate VTP Within 24 Hours[2]	225	96%	98%	98%
Controlled Postoperative Blood Glucose[2,7]	-	-	96%	97%
Perioperative Temperature Management[2]	254	100%	100%	100%
Prophylactic Antibiotic Selection[2]	152	99%	99%	99%
Prophylactic Antibiotic Selection (Outpatient)	528	100%	98%	98%
Prophylactic Antibiotic Stopped[2]	149	96%	98%	98%
Prophylactic Antibiotic Timing[2]	152	99%	99%	99%
Prophylactic Antibiotic Timing (Outpatient)	528	100%	98%	98%
Urinary Catheter Removal[2]	62	71%	97%	97%
Survey of Patients' Hospital Experiences				
Area Around Room 'Always' Quiet at Night	300+	56%	66%	61%
Doctors 'Always' Communicated Well	300+	81%	83%	82%
Home Recovery Information Given	300+	85%	84%	85%
Hospital Given 9 or 10 on 10 Point Scale	300+	70%	69%	71%
Meds 'Always' Explained Before Given	300+	60%	63%	64%
Nurses 'Always' Communicated Well	300+	77%	78%	79%
Pain 'Always' Well Controlled	300+	72%	71%	71%
Room and Bathroom 'Always' Clean	300+	63%	71%	73%
Timely Help 'Always' Received	300+	58%	65%	68%
Would Definitely Recommend Hospital	300+	75%	70%	71%
Use of Medical Imaging				
Cardiac Imaging Stress Test before Surgery	82	3.7%	5.5%	5.3%
Combination Abdominal CT Scan	1,437	38.0%	10.1%	10.5%
Combination Brain/Sinus CT Scan	721	3.2%	2.3%	2.7%
Combination Chest CT Scan	1,198	3.3%	3.7%	2.7%
Follow-up Mammogram/Ultrasound	4,013	6.6%	8.9%	8.8%
Lumbar Spine MRI for Low Back Pain	55	45.5%	36.6%	37.2%

Memorial Health Univ Medical Center

4700 Waters Avenue
Savannah, GA 31403
Phone: 912-350-8000
Fax: 912-350-7073
URL: www.memorialhealth.com
Type: Acute Care Hospitals
Emergency Services: Yes
Ownership: Voluntary non-profit - Other
Beds: 530

Key Personnel:

Coronary Care . . . . Maria Davis, RN
Cardiac Laboratory. . . . . Linda Dominey
Patient Relations . . . . Joseph Gardner
CEO/President. . . . . Margaret Gill, MBA
Infection Control . . . . Mary McNally
Chief of Medical Staff. . . . . Ramon V. Meguiar, MD
Radiology. . . . . Steve Stanic
Anesthesiology. . . . . Kathy Sydow

Measure	Cases	This Hosp.	State Avg.	U.S. Avg.
Blood Clot Prevention and Treatment				
Anticoagulation Overlap Therapy[2]	155	89%	90%	93%
ICU Venous Thromboembolism Prophylaxis[2]	66	92%	90%	92%
Incidence of Potentially Preventable VTE[2]	45	7%	13%	10%
UFH with Dosages/Platelet Monitoring[2]	30	100%	99%	97%
Venous Thromboembolism Prophylaxis[2]	307	80%	80%	85%
Warfarin Therapy Discharge Instructions[2]	96	70%	78%	75%
Chest Pain/Possible Heart Attack Care				
Aspirin Given Within 24 Hours of Arrival[5]	-	-	94%	96%
Fibrinolytic Meds Within 30 Min. of Arrival[5]	-	-	35%	58%
Average Time to ECG (minutes)[5]	-	-	8	7
Average Time to Transfer (minutes)[5]	-	-	73	60
Children's Asthma Care				
Received Home Management Plan of Care	-	-	-	88%
Received Reliever Medication	-	-	-	100%
Received Systemic Corticosteroids	-	-	-	100%
Emergency Department				
Admittance Decision Time (minutes)[2]	562	277	100	98
Head CT Results Within 45 Min. of Arrival[1]	-	-	45%	57%
Patients Who Left ER Before Being Seen	>100k	1%	3%	2%
Time from ER Arrival to Admit. (minutes)[2]	575	521	286	274
Time from ER Arrival to Discharge (minutes)	334	130	140	134
Time in ER Before Being Evaluated (minutes)	395	38	32	26
Time to Pain Meds for Fractures (minutes)	175	60	64	57
Heart Attack Care				
Aspirin Given at Discharge[2]	263	100%	99%	99%
Fibrinolytic Meds Within 30 Min. of Arrival[2,7]	-	-	80%	54%
PCI Within 90 Minutes of Arrival[2]	44	93%	95%	96%
Statin Prescribed at Discharge[2]	260	100%	98%	98%
Heart Failure Care				
ACE Inhibitor or ARB for LVSD[2]	96	95%	97%	97%
Discharge Instructions Given[2]	256	98%	92%	94%
Evaluation of LVS Function[2]	282	100%	99%	99%
Medicare Spending				
Medicare Spending per Patient (ratio)	-	0.96	0.95	0.98
Pneumonia Care				
Appropriate Initial Antibiotic Given[2]	74	95%	95%	95%
Blood Culture Timing[2]	93	96%	97%	98%
Pregnancy and Delivery Care				
Newborn Deliveries Scheduled Early[2]	37	0%	8%	6%
Preventive Care				
Immunization for Influenza[2]	523	92%	88%	90%
Immunization for Pneumonia[2]	524	94%	90%	92%
Stroke Care				
Anticoagulation Therapy for Atrial Fibrillation	42	100%	94%	95%
Antithrombotic Therapy Timing	225	99%	97%	98%
Assessed for Rehabilitation	354	100%	97%	97%
Discharged on Antithrombotic Therapy	281	100%	98%	99%
Discharged on Statin Medication	215	99%	94%	94%
Thrombolytic Therapy Timing	26	88%	58%	66%
Venous Thromboembolism Prophylaxis	359	95%	92%	94%
Written Stroke Educational Materials Given	196	100%	84%	88%
Surgical Care Improvement Project				
Appropriate Beta Blocker Usage[2]	197	94%	97%	98%
Appropriate VTP Within 24 Hours[2]	326	99%	98%	98%
Controlled Postoperative Blood Glucose[2]	122	91%	96%	97%
Perioperative Temperature Management[2]	443	100%	100%	100%
Prophylactic Antibiotic Selection[2]	407	100%	99%	99%
Prophylactic Antibiotic Selection (Outpatient)	487	98%	98%	98%
Prophylactic Antibiotic Stopped[2]	396	95%	98%	98%
Prophylactic Antibiotic Timing[2]	408	96%	99%	99%
Prophylactic Antibiotic Timing (Outpatient)	490	97%	98%	98%
Urinary Catheter Removal[2]	235	93%	97%	97%
Survey of Patients' Hospital Experiences				
Area Around Room 'Always' Quiet at Night	300+	57%	66%	61%
Doctors 'Always' Communicated Well	300+	82%	83%	82%
Home Recovery Information Given	300+	84%	84%	85%
Hospital Given 9 or 10 on 10 Point Scale	300+	70%	69%	71%
Meds 'Always' Explained Before Given	300+	60%	63%	64%
Nurses 'Always' Communicated Well	300+	77%	78%	79%
Pain 'Always' Well Controlled	300+	73%	71%	71%
Room and Bathroom 'Always' Clean	300+	58%	71%	73%
Timely Help 'Always' Received	300+	63%	65%	68%
Would Definitely Recommend Hospital	300+	73%	70%	71%
Use of Medical Imaging				
Cardiac Imaging Stress Test before Surgery	235	3.8%	5.5%	5.3%
Combination Abdominal CT Scan	1,123	34.6%	10.1%	10.5%
Combination Brain/Sinus CT Scan	966	2.5%	2.3%	2.7%
Combination Chest CT Scan	963	22.3%	3.7%	2.7%
Follow-up Mammogram/Ultrasound	1,616	8.9%	8.9%	8.8%
Lumbar Spine MRI for Low Back Pain	131	42.0%	36.6%	37.2%

Saint Joseph's Hospital - Savannah

11705 Mercy Boulevard
Savannah, GA 31419
Phone: 912-819-4100
Fax: 912-819-8039
URL: www.sjchs.org
Type: Acute Care Hospitals
Emergency Services: Yes
Ownership: Voluntary non-profit - Private
Beds: 305

Key Personnel:

Chairman/CEO . . . . William E. Bill Johnston
Quality Assurance . . . . Mary Christain
Radiology. . . . . TA Hetherington, MD
CEO/President. . . . . Paul P Hinchey
Pediatric Ambulatory Care . . . . . . Cliphane McLeod, MD
Pediatric In-Patient Care . . . . Cliphane McLeod, MD
Chief of Medical Staff. . . . . J Allen Meadows, MD
Operating Room. . . . . Martha Stratton, RN

Measure	Cases	This Hosp.	State Avg.	U.S. Avg.
Blood Clot Prevention and Treatment				
Anticoagulation Overlap Therapy[2]	138	96%	90%	93%
ICU Venous Thromboembolism Prophylaxis[2]	108	83%	90%	92%
Incidence of Potentially Preventable VTE[2]	35	9%	13%	10%
UFH with Dosages/Platelet Monitoring[2]	46	100%	99%	97%
Venous Thromboembolism Prophylaxis[2]	310	76%	80%	85%
Warfarin Therapy Discharge Instructions[2]	118	87%	78%	75%
Chest Pain/Possible Heart Attack Care				
Aspirin Given Within 24 Hours of Arrival[5]	-	-	94%	96%
Fibrinolytic Meds Within 30 Min. of Arrival[5]	-	-	35%	58%
Average Time to ECG (minutes)[5]	-	-	8	7
Average Time to Transfer (minutes)[5]	-	-	73	60
Children's Asthma Care				
Received Home Management Plan of Care	-	-	-	88%
Received Reliever Medication	-	-	-	100%
Received Systemic Corticosteroids	-	-	-	100%
Emergency Department				
Admittance Decision Time (minutes)[2]	516	122	100	98
Head CT Results Within 45 Min. of Arrival[5]	-	-	45%	57%
Patients Who Left ER Before Being Seen	36,124	2%	3%	2%
Time from ER Arrival to Admit. (minutes)[2]	516	356	286	274
Time from ER Arrival to Discharge (minutes)	367	157	140	134
Time in ER Before Being Evaluated (minutes)	318	44	32	26
Time to Pain Meds for Fractures (minutes)	130	58	64	57
Heart Attack Care				
Aspirin Given at Discharge	304	99%	99%	99%
Fibrinolytic Meds Within 30 Min. of Arrival[7]	-	-	80%	54%
PCI Within 90 Minutes of Arrival	42	100%	95%	96%
Statin Prescribed at Discharge	317	98%	98%	98%
Heart Failure Care				
ACE Inhibitor or ARB for LVSD	109	99%	97%	97%
Discharge Instructions Given	329	100%	92%	94%
Evaluation of LVS Function	375	100%	99%	99%
Medicare Spending				
Medicare Spending per Patient (ratio)	-	0.95	0.95	0.98
Pneumonia Care				
Appropriate Initial Antibiotic Given	115	99%	95%	95%
Blood Culture Timing	168	99%	97%	98%
Pregnancy and Delivery Care				
Newborn Deliveries Scheduled Early[7]	-	-	8%	6%
Preventive Care				
Immunization for Influenza[2]	587	97%	88%	90%
Immunization for Pneumonia[2]	888	99%	90%	92%
Stroke Care				
Anticoagulation Therapy for Atrial Fibrillation	28	96%	94%	95%
Antithrombotic Therapy Timing	174	93%	97%	98%
Assessed for Rehabilitation	232	97%	97%	97%
Discharged on Antithrombotic Therapy	199	99%	98%	99%
Discharged on Statin Medication	156	97%	94%	94%
Thrombolytic Therapy Timing[1]	-	-	58%	66%
Venous Thromboembolism Prophylaxis	254	95%	92%	94%
Written Stroke Educational Materials Given	119	94%	84%	88%
Surgical Care Improvement Project				
Appropriate Beta Blocker Usage[2]	479	99%	97%	98%
Appropriate VTP Within 24 Hours[2]	917	98%	98%	98%
Controlled Postoperative Blood Glucose[2]	276	98%	96%	97%
Perioperative Temperature Management[2]	1,152	100%	100%	100%
Prophylactic Antibiotic Selection[2]	1,285	100%	99%	99%
Prophylactic Antibiotic Selection (Outpatient)	416	100%	98%	98%
Prophylactic Antibiotic Stopped[2]	1,274	100%	98%	98%
Prophylactic Antibiotic Timing[2]	1,289	100%	99%	99%
Prophylactic Antibiotic Timing (Outpatient)	416	98%	98%	98%
Urinary Catheter Removal[2]	364	95%	97%	97%
Survey of Patients' Hospital Experiences				
Area Around Room 'Always' Quiet at Night	300+	60%	66%	61%

NOTE: Hospital profiles are in alphabetical order by state, then city, then hospital within the city; Rankings exclude hospitals with less than 25 cases except for patient surveys which excludes hospitals with less than 100 cases; (a) 100-299 cases; (1) The number of cases/patients is too few to report; (2) Data submitted were based on a sample of cases/patients; (3) Results are based on a shorter time period than required; (4) Data suppressed by CMS for one or more quarters; (5) Results are not available for this reporting period; (6) Fewer than 100 patients completed the HCAHPS survey; (7) No cases met the criteria for this measure; (8) The lower limit of the confidence interval cannot be calculated if the number of observed infections equals zero; (9) No data are available from the state/territory for this reporting period; (10) The scores shown reflect fewer than 50 completed surveys; (11) There were discrepancies in the data collection process; (12) This measure does not apply to this hospital for this reporting period; (13) Results cannot be calculated for this reporting period; (14) The results for this state are combined with nearby states to protect confidentiality; Please refer to the User's Guide for a full explanation of data.

Doctors 'Always' Communicated Well	300+	81%	83%	82%
Home Recovery Information Given	300+	84%	84%	85%
Hospital Given 9 or 10 on 10 Point Scale	300+	74%	69%	71%
Meds 'Always' Explained Before Given	300+	64%	63%	64%
Nurses 'Always' Communicated Well	300+	77%	78%	79%
Pain 'Always' Well Controlled	300+	72%	71%	71%
Room and Bathroom 'Always' Clean	300+	69%	71%	73%
Timely Help 'Always' Received	300+	64%	65%	68%
Would Definitely Recommend Hospital	300+	77%	70%	71%
Use of Medical Imaging				
Cardiac Imaging Stress Test before Surgery	75	6.7%	5.5%	5.3%
Combination Abdominal CT Scan	615	20.8%	10.1%	10.5%
Combination Brain/Sinus CT Scan	765	2.9%	2.3%	2.7%
Combination Chest CT Scan	322	0.6%	3.7%	2.7%
Follow-up Mammogram/Ultrasound	381	4.2%	8.9%	8.8%
Lumbar Spine MRI for Low Back Pain[1]	-	-	36.6%	37.2%

Emory - Adventist Hospital

3949 South Cobb Drive
Smyrna, GA 30080
Phone: 770-434-0710
Fax: 770-432-4260
URL: www.ahss.org
Type: Acute Care Hospitals
Emergency Services: Yes
Ownership: Voluntary non-profit - Church
Beds: 100

Key Personnel:
Emergency Room . . . . Eric Deal, MD
Infection Control. . . . . Susan Hebert
Quality Assurance . . . . Susan Hebert
CEO/President. . . . . Donald L Jernigan
Intensive Care Unit. . . . . Beth Lingerfelt
Anesthesiology. . . . . Dale Meyer, MD
Patient Relations . . . . Gerry Minerva
Ambulatory Care . . . . Tim Welch

Measure	Cases	This Hosp.	State Avg.	U.S. Avg.
Blood Clot Prevention and Treatment				
Anticoagulation Overlap Therapy[2]	25	100%	90%	93%
ICU Venous Thromboembolism Prophylaxis[2]	32	100%	90%	92%
Incidence of Potentially Preventable VTE[2,7]	-	-	13%	10%
UFH with Dosages/Platelet Monitoring[1,2]	-	-	99%	97%
Venous Thromboembolism Prophylaxis[2]	159	99%	80%	85%
Warfarin Therapy Discharge Instructions[2]	24	100%	78%	75%
Chest Pain/Possible Heart Attack Care				
Aspirin Given Within 24 Hours of Arrival	19	100%	94%	96%
Fibrinolytic Meds Within 30 Min. of Arrival[7]	-	-	35%	58%
Average Time to ECG (minutes)	22	5	8	7
Average Time to Transfer (minutes)[7]	-	-	73	60
Children's Asthma Care				
Received Home Management Plan of Care	-	-	-	88%
Received Reliever Medication	-	-	-	100%
Received Systemic Corticosteroids	-	-	-	100%
Emergency Department				
Admittance Decision Time (minutes)[2]	463	55	100	98
Head CT Results Within 45 Min. of Arrival[1]	-	-	45%	57%
Patients Who Left ER Before Being Seen	28,429	2%	3%	2%
Time from ER Arrival to Admit. (minutes)[2]	506	214	286	274
Time from ER Arrival to Discharge (minutes)	350	120	140	134
Time in ER Before Being Evaluated (minutes)	378	24	32	26
Time to Pain Meds for Fractures (minutes)	70	52	64	57
Heart Attack Care				
Aspirin Given at Discharge[1]	-	-	99%	99%
Fibrinolytic Meds Within 30 Min. of Arrival[7]	-	-	80%	54%
PCI Within 90 Minutes of Arrival[7]	-	-	95%	96%
Statin Prescribed at Discharge[1]	-	-	98%	98%
Heart Failure Care				
ACE Inhibitor or ARB for LVSD	26	100%	97%	97%
Discharge Instructions Given	57	100%	92%	94%
Evaluation of LVS Function	66	100%	99%	99%
Medicare Spending				
Medicare Spending per Patient (ratio)	-	0.99	0.95	0.98
Pneumonia Care				
Appropriate Initial Antibiotic Given	85	100%	95%	95%
Blood Culture Timing	123	99%	97%	98%
Pregnancy and Delivery Care				
Newborn Deliveries Scheduled Early[2,7]	-	-	8%	6%
Preventive Care				
Immunization for Influenza[2]	290	98%	88%	90%
Immunization for Pneumonia[2]	378	99%	90%	92%
Stroke Care				
Anticoagulation Therapy for Atrial Fibrillation[1,2]	-	-	94%	95%
Antithrombotic Therapy Timing[2]	16	100%	97%	98%
Assessed for Rehabilitation[2]	19	100%	97%	97%
Discharged on Antithrombotic Therapy[2]	19	100%	98%	99%
Discharged on Statin Medication[2]	12	100%	94%	94%
Thrombolytic Therapy Timing[1,2]	-	-	58%	66%
Venous Thromboembolism Prophylaxis[2]	18	94%	92%	94%
Written Stroke Educational Materials Given[2]	16	100%	84%	88%
Surgical Care Improvement Project				
Appropriate Beta Blocker Usage[1]	-	-	97%	98%
Appropriate VTP Within 24 Hours	55	96%	98%	98%
Controlled Postoperative Blood Glucose[7]	-	-	96%	97%
Perioperative Temperature Management	58	100%	100%	100%
Prophylactic Antibiotic Selection	27	100%	99%	99%
Prophylactic Antibiotic Selection (Outpatient)	28	93%	98%	98%
Prophylactic Antibiotic Stopped	25	96%	98%	98%
Prophylactic Antibiotic Timing	27	100%	99%	99%
Prophylactic Antibiotic Timing (Outpatient)	28	100%	98%	98%
Urinary Catheter Removal	50	100%	97%	97%
Survey of Patients' Hospital Experiences				
Area Around Room 'Always' Quiet at Night[11]	(a)	66%	66%	61%
Doctors 'Always' Communicated Well[11]	(a)	81%	83%	82%
Home Recovery Information Given[11]	(a)	78%	84%	85%
Hospital Given 9 or 10 on 10 Point Scale[11]	(a)	65%	69%	71%
Meds 'Always' Explained Before Given[11]	(a)	64%	63%	64%
Nurses 'Always' Communicated Well[11]	(a)	73%	78%	79%
Pain 'Always' Well Controlled[11]	(a)	65%	71%	71%
Room and Bathroom 'Always' Clean[11]	(a)	71%	71%	73%
Timely Help 'Always' Received[11]	(a)	55%	65%	68%
Would Definitely Recommend Hospital[11]	(a)	70%	70%	71%
Use of Medical Imaging				
Cardiac Imaging Stress Test before Surgery[1]	-	-	5.5%	5.3%
Combination Abdominal CT Scan	274	4.7%	10.1%	10.5%
Combination Brain/Sinus CT Scan	375	1.6%	2.3%	2.7%
Combination Chest CT Scan[1]	-	-	3.7%	2.7%
Follow-up Mammogram/Ultrasound	337	8.3%	8.9%	8.8%
Lumbar Spine MRI for Low Back Pain[1]	-	-	36.6%	37.2%

Eastside Medical Center

1700 Medical Way
Snellville, GA 30078
Phone: 770-736-2498
Fax: 770-736-2395
Type: Acute Care Hospitals
Emergency Services: Yes
Ownership: Proprietary
Beds: 131

Key Personnel:
CEO/President. . . . . Les Beard
Radiology. . . . . Gregory Berkey, MD
Quality Assurance . . . . Amy Everheart
Emergency Room . . . . Tim Grubbs
Cardiac Laboratory. . . . . Richard Harrison
CEO . . . . Kim Ryan
Operating Room. . . . . Dixon Savage

Measure	Cases	This Hosp.	State Avg.	U.S. Avg.
Blood Clot Prevention and Treatment				
Anticoagulation Overlap Therapy[2]	92	98%	90%	93%
ICU Venous Thromboembolism Prophylaxis[2]	91	98%	90%	92%
Incidence of Potentially Preventable VTE[1,2]	-	-	13%	10%
UFH with Dosages/Platelet Monitoring[2]	41	100%	99%	97%
Venous Thromboembolism Prophylaxis[2]	359	98%	80%	85%
Warfarin Therapy Discharge Instructions[2]	68	100%	78%	75%
Chest Pain/Possible Heart Attack Care				
Aspirin Given Within 24 Hours of Arrival[1,3]	-	-	94%	96%
Fibrinolytic Meds Within 30 Min. of Arrival[3,7]	-	-	35%	58%
Average Time to ECG (minutes)[1,3]	-	-	8	7
Average Time to Transfer (minutes)[3,7]	-	-	73	60
Children's Asthma Care				
Received Home Management Plan of Care	-	-	-	88%
Received Reliever Medication	-	-	-	100%
Received Systemic Corticosteroids	-	-	-	100%
Emergency Department				
Admittance Decision Time (minutes)[2]	577	197	100	98
Head CT Results Within 45 Min. of Arrival[1]	-	-	45%	57%
Patients Who Left ER Before Being Seen	61,866	1%	3%	2%
Time from ER Arrival to Admit. (minutes)[2]	607	340	286	274
Time from ER Arrival to Discharge (minutes)	491	195	140	134
Time in ER Before Being Evaluated (minutes)	533	19	32	26
Time to Pain Meds for Fractures (minutes)	119	60	64	57
Heart Attack Care				
Aspirin Given at Discharge	134	100%	99%	99%
Fibrinolytic Meds Within 30 Min. of Arrival[7]	-	-	80%	54%
PCI Within 90 Minutes of Arrival	53	98%	95%	96%
Statin Prescribed at Discharge	132	100%	98%	98%
Heart Failure Care				
ACE Inhibitor or ARB for LVSD	59	100%	97%	97%
Discharge Instructions Given	218	100%	92%	94%
Evaluation of LVS Function	249	100%	99%	99%
Medicare Spending				
Medicare Spending per Patient (ratio)	-	1.02	0.95	0.98
Pneumonia Care				
Appropriate Initial Antibiotic Given[2]	100	96%	95%	95%
Blood Culture Timing[2]	162	99%	97%	98%
Pregnancy and Delivery Care				
Newborn Deliveries Scheduled Early[2]	27	4%	8%	6%
Preventive Care				
Immunization for Influenza[2]	567	98%	88%	90%
Immunization for Pneumonia[2]	686	95%	90%	92%
Stroke Care				
Anticoagulation Therapy for Atrial Fibrillation[1,2]	-	-	94%	95%
Antithrombotic Therapy Timing[2]	100	100%	97%	98%
Assessed for Rehabilitation[2]	107	100%	97%	97%
Discharged on Antithrombotic Therapy[2]	97	100%	98%	99%
Discharged on Statin Medication[2]	65	100%	94%	94%
Thrombolytic Therapy Timing[1,2]	-	-	58%	66%
Venous Thromboembolism Prophylaxis[2]	117	100%	92%	94%
Written Stroke Educational Materials Given[2]	69	97%	84%	88%
Surgical Care Improvement Project				
Appropriate Beta Blocker Usage[2]	101	98%	97%	98%
Appropriate VTP Within 24 Hours[2]	415	99%	98%	98%
Controlled Postoperative Blood Glucose[2,7]	-	-	96%	97%
Perioperative Temperature Management[2]	453	100%	100%	100%
Prophylactic Antibiotic Selection[2]	281	100%	99%	99%
Prophylactic Antibiotic Selection (Outpatient)	286	99%	98%	98%
Prophylactic Antibiotic Stopped[2]	278	99%	98%	98%
Prophylactic Antibiotic Timing[2]	281	99%	99%	99%
Prophylactic Antibiotic Timing (Outpatient)	286	100%	98%	98%
Urinary Catheter Removal[2]	134	96%	97%	97%
Survey of Patients' Hospital Experiences				
Area Around Room 'Always' Quiet at Night	300+	60%	66%	61%
Doctors 'Always' Communicated Well	300+	76%	83%	82%
Home Recovery Information Given	300+	82%	84%	85%
Hospital Given 9 or 10 on 10 Point Scale	300+	61%	69%	71%
Meds 'Always' Explained Before Given	300+	54%	63%	64%
Nurses 'Always' Communicated Well	300+	68%	78%	79%
Pain 'Always' Well Controlled	300+	63%	71%	71%
Room and Bathroom 'Always' Clean	300+	67%	71%	73%
Timely Help 'Always' Received	300+	50%	65%	68%
Would Definitely Recommend Hospital	300+	65%	70%	71%
Use of Medical Imaging				
Cardiac Imaging Stress Test before Surgery	238	5.9%	5.5%	5.3%
Combination Abdominal CT Scan	728	6.0%	10.1%	10.5%
Combination Brain/Sinus CT Scan	778	1.0%	2.3%	2.7%
Combination Chest CT Scan	346	1.4%	3.7%	2.7%
Follow-up Mammogram/Ultrasound	1,948	8.9%	8.9%	8.8%
Lumbar Spine MRI for Low Back Pain	110	40.0%	36.6%	37.2%

Effingham County Hospital

459 Ga Highway 119 South
Springfield, GA 31329
Phone: 912-754-0160
Fax: 912-754-9901
E-mail: gelowkr1@memorialhealth.com
URL: www.effinghamhospital.com
Type: Critical Access Hospitals
Emergency Services: Yes
Ownership: Govt - Hospital Dist/Auth
Beds: 45

Key Personnel:
Quality Assurance . . . . James Edwards
CEO/President. . . . . Norma Jean Morgan
Chief of Medical Staff . . . . Chris Mathews
Infection Control. . . . . Jane Miller

NOTE: Hospital profiles are in alphabetical order by state, then city, then hospital within the city; Rankings exclude hospitals with less than 25 cases except for patient surveys which excludes hospitals with less than 100 cases; (a) 100-299 cases; (1) The number of cases/patients is too few to report; (2) Data submitted were based on a sample of cases/patients; (3) Results are based on a shorter time period than required; (4) Data suppressed by CMS for one or more quarters; (5) Results are not available for this reporting period; (6) Fewer than 100 patients completed the HCAHPS survey; (7) No cases met the criteria for this measure; (8) The lower limit of the confidence interval cannot be calculated if the number of observed infections equals zero; (9) No data are available from the state/territory for this reporting period; (10) The scores shown reflect fewer than 50 completed surveys; (11) There were discrepancies in the data collection process; (12) This measure does not apply to this hospital for this reporting period; (13) Results cannot be calculated for this reporting period; (14) The results for this state are combined with nearby states to protect confidentiality; Please refer to the User's Guide for a full explanation of data.

Operating Room. . . . . Patricia Parrish
Radiology. . . . . Kenneth Wimmer

Measure	Cases	This Hosp.	State Avg.	U.S. Avg.
Blood Clot Prevention and Treatment				
Anticoagulation Overlap Therapy[7]	-	-	90%	93%
ICU Venous Thromboembolism Prophylaxis[7]	-	-	90%	92%
Incidence of Potentially Preventable VTE[7]	-	-	13%	10%
UFH with Dosages/Platelet Monitoring[7]	-	-	99%	97%
Venous Thromboembolism Prophylaxis	60	38%	80%	85%
Warfarin Therapy Discharge Instructions[7]	-	-	78%	75%
Chest Pain/Possible Heart Attack Care				
Aspirin Given Within 24 Hours of Arrival[1,3]	-	-	94%	96%
Fibrinolytic Meds Within 30 Min. of Arrival[1,3]	-	-	35%	58%
Average Time to ECG (minutes)[1,3]	-	-	8	7
Average Time to Transfer (minutes)[1,3]	-	-	73	60
Children's Asthma Care				
Received Home Management Plan of Care	-	-	-	88%
Received Reliever Medication	-	-	-	100%
Received Systemic Corticosteroids	-	-	-	100%
Emergency Department				
Admittance Decision Time (minutes)	91	68	100	98
Head CT Results Within 45 Min. of Arrival[1,3]	-	-	45%	57%
Patients Who Left ER Before Being Seen	13,410	1%	3%	2%
Time from ER Arrival to Admit. (minutes)	91	259	286	274
Time from ER Arrival to Discharge (minutes)	426	106	140	134
Time in ER Before Being Evaluated (minutes)	459	31	32	26
Time to Pain Meds for Fractures (minutes)	12	70	64	57
Heart Attack Care				
Aspirin Given at Discharge[5]	-	-	99%	99%
Fibrinolytic Meds Within 30 Min. of Arrival[5]	-	-	80%	54%
PCI Within 90 Minutes of Arrival[5]	-	-	95%	96%
Statin Prescribed at Discharge[5]	-	-	98%	98%
Heart Failure Care				
ACE Inhibitor or ARB for LVSD[1,3]	-	-	97%	97%
Discharge Instructions Given[1,3]	-	-	92%	94%
Evaluation of LVS Function[1,3]	-	-	99%	99%
Medicare Spending				
Medicare Spending per Patient (ratio)	-	-	0.95	0.98
Pneumonia Care				
Appropriate Initial Antibiotic Given[1]	-	-	95%	95%
Blood Culture Timing[1]	-	-	97%	98%
Pregnancy and Delivery Care				
Newborn Deliveries Scheduled Early[5]	-	-	8%	6%
Preventive Care				
Immunization for Influenza	68	93%	88%	90%
Immunization for Pneumonia	75	92%	90%	92%
Stroke Care				
Anticoagulation Therapy for Atrial Fibrillation[3,7]	-	-	94%	95%
Antithrombotic Therapy Timing[1,3]	-	-	97%	98%
Assessed for Rehabilitation[3,7]	-	-	97%	97%
Discharged on Antithrombotic Therapy[3,7]	-	-	98%	99%
Discharged on Statin Medication[3,7]	-	-	94%	94%
Thrombolytic Therapy Timing[1,3]	-	-	58%	66%
Venous Thromboembolism Prophylaxis[3,7]	-	-	92%	94%
Written Stroke Educational Materials Given[3,7]	-	-	84%	88%
Surgical Care Improvement Project				
Appropriate Beta Blocker Usage[1]	-	-	97%	98%
Appropriate VTP Within 24 Hours[1]	-	-	98%	98%
Controlled Postoperative Blood Glucose[7]	-	-	96%	97%
Perioperative Temperature Management[1]	-	-	100%	100%
Prophylactic Antibiotic Selection[1]	-	-	99%	99%
Prophylactic Antibiotic Selection (Outpatient)[1,3]	-	-	98%	98%
Prophylactic Antibiotic Stopped[1]	-	-	98%	98%
Prophylactic Antibiotic Timing[1]	-	-	99%	99%
Prophylactic Antibiotic Timing (Outpatient)[1,3]	-	-	98%	98%
Urinary Catheter Removal[1]	-	-	97%	97%
Survey of Patients' Hospital Experiences				
Area Around Room 'Always' Quiet at Night[6]	<100	74%	66%	61%
Doctors 'Always' Communicated Well[6]	<100	84%	83%	82%
Home Recovery Information Given[6]	<100	94%	84%	85%
Hospital Given 9 or 10 on 10 Point Scale[6]	<100	74%	69%	71%
Meds 'Always' Explained Before Given[6]	<100	73%	63%	64%
Nurses 'Always' Communicated Well[6]	<100	84%	78%	79%
Pain 'Always' Well Controlled[6]	<100	77%	71%	71%
Room and Bathroom 'Always' Clean[6]	<100	79%	71%	73%
Timely Help 'Always' Received[6]	<100	78%	65%	68%
Would Definitely Recommend Hospital[6]	<100	71%	70%	71%
Use of Medical Imaging				
Cardiac Imaging Stress Test before Surgery[7]	-	-	5.5%	5.3%
Combination Abdominal CT Scan	223	25.1%	10.1%	10.5%
Combination Brain/Sinus CT Scan[1]	-	-	2.3%	2.7%
Combination Chest CT Scan	62	21.0%	3.7%	2.7%
Follow-up Mammogram/Ultrasound	333	9.6%	8.9%	8.8%
Lumbar Spine MRI for Low Back Pain	39	41.0%	36.6%	37.2%

East Georgia Regional Medical Center

1499 Fair Road
Statesboro, GA 30458
URL: www.egrmc.com
Type: Acute Care Hospitals
Ownership: Proprietary
Phone: 912-486-1500
Fax: 912-871-2363
Emergency Services: Yes
Beds: 150

Key Personnel:
Chief of Medical Staff. . . . . Robert M Benson
Hemotology Center . . . . Harsh Bhushan, MD
CEO/President. . . . . Bob Bigley
Surgery . . . . Akram Hassanyeh, MD
Cardiology . . . . Ajay Jain, MD
Cardiac Laboratory. . . . . Stanley Shin, MD

Measure	Cases	This Hosp.	State Avg.	U.S. Avg.
Blood Clot Prevention and Treatment				
Anticoagulation Overlap Therapy[2]	81	79%	90%	93%
ICU Venous Thromboembolism Prophylaxis[2]	81	84%	90%	92%
Incidence of Potentially Preventable VTE[1,2]	-	-	13%	10%
UFH with Dosages/Platelet Monitoring[2]	28	100%	99%	97%
Venous Thromboembolism Prophylaxis[2]	389	78%	80%	85%
Warfarin Therapy Discharge Instructions[2]	70	67%	78%	75%
Chest Pain/Possible Heart Attack Care				
Aspirin Given Within 24 Hours of Arrival[3]	47	100%	94%	96%
Fibrinolytic Meds Within 30 Min. of Arrival[3,7]	-	-	35%	58%
Average Time to ECG (minutes)[3]	50	11	8	7
Average Time to Transfer (minutes)[3,7]	-	-	73	60
Children's Asthma Care				
Received Home Management Plan of Care	-	-	-	88%
Received Reliever Medication	-	-	-	100%
Received Systemic Corticosteroids	-	-	-	100%
Emergency Department				
Admittance Decision Time (minutes)[2]	563	129	100	98
Head CT Results Within 45 Min. of Arrival[1]	-	-	45%	57%
Patients Who Left ER Before Being Seen	41,075	4%	3%	2%
Time from ER Arrival to Admit. (minutes)[2]	563	328	286	274
Time from ER Arrival to Discharge (minutes)	665	151	140	134
Time in ER Before Being Evaluated (minutes)	735	34	32	26
Time to Pain Meds for Fractures (minutes)	122	54	64	57
Heart Attack Care				
Aspirin Given at Discharge	86	94%	99%	99%
Fibrinolytic Meds Within 30 Min. of Arrival[7]	-	-	80%	54%
PCI Within 90 Minutes of Arrival	17	88%	95%	96%
Statin Prescribed at Discharge	74	92%	98%	98%
Heart Failure Care				
ACE Inhibitor or ARB for LVSD	86	86%	97%	97%
Discharge Instructions Given	227	96%	92%	94%
Evaluation of LVS Function	247	99%	99%	99%
Medicare Spending				
Medicare Spending per Patient (ratio)	-	0.95	0.95	0.98
Pneumonia Care				
Appropriate Initial Antibiotic Given	119	97%	95%	95%
Blood Culture Timing	154	100%	97%	98%
Pregnancy and Delivery Care				
Newborn Deliveries Scheduled Early	153	8%	8%	6%
Preventive Care				
Immunization for Influenza[2]	608	97%	88%	90%
Immunization for Pneumonia[2]	633	96%	90%	92%
Stroke Care				
Anticoagulation Therapy for Atrial Fibrillation[1]	-	-	94%	95%
Antithrombotic Therapy Timing	74	97%	97%	98%
Assessed for Rehabilitation	80	92%	97%	97%
Discharged on Antithrombotic Therapy	80	100%	98%	99%
Discharged on Statin Medication	61	97%	94%	94%
Thrombolytic Therapy Timing[1]	-	-	58%	66%
Venous Thromboembolism Prophylaxis	75	81%	92%	94%
Written Stroke Educational Materials Given	60	67%	84%	88%
Surgical Care Improvement Project				
Appropriate Beta Blocker Usage	129	97%	97%	98%
Appropriate VTP Within 24 Hours	336	99%	98%	98%
Controlled Postoperative Blood Glucose[7]	-	-	96%	97%
Perioperative Temperature Management	378	100%	100%	100%
Prophylactic Antibiotic Selection	245	99%	99%	99%
Prophylactic Antibiotic Selection (Outpatient)	247	98%	98%	98%
Prophylactic Antibiotic Stopped	232	95%	98%	98%
Prophylactic Antibiotic Timing	245	99%	99%	99%
Prophylactic Antibiotic Timing (Outpatient)	251	97%	98%	98%
Urinary Catheter Removal	245	98%	97%	97%
Survey of Patients' Hospital Experiences				
Area Around Room 'Always' Quiet at Night	300+	60%	66%	61%
Doctors 'Always' Communicated Well	300+	77%	83%	82%
Home Recovery Information Given	300+	79%	84%	85%
Hospital Given 9 or 10 on 10 Point Scale	300+	54%	69%	71%
Meds 'Always' Explained Before Given	300+	55%	63%	64%
Nurses 'Always' Communicated Well	300+	72%	78%	79%
Pain 'Always' Well Controlled	300+	64%	71%	71%
Room and Bathroom 'Always' Clean	300+	65%	71%	73%
Timely Help 'Always' Received	300+	59%	65%	68%
Would Definitely Recommend Hospital	300+	56%	70%	71%
Use of Medical Imaging				
Cardiac Imaging Stress Test before Surgery	155	4.5%	5.5%	5.3%
Combination Abdominal CT Scan	733	42.4%	10.1%	10.5%
Combination Brain/Sinus CT Scan	742	3.0%	2.3%	2.7%
Combination Chest CT Scan	369	45.5%	3.7%	2.7%
Follow-up Mammogram/Ultrasound	1,264	10.2%	8.9%	8.8%
Lumbar Spine MRI for Low Back Pain	129	48.8%	36.6%	37.2%

Piedmont Henry Hospital

1133 Eagle's Landing Parkway
Stockbridge, GA 30281
URL: www.henrymedical.com
Type: Acute Care Hospitals
Ownership: Govt - Hospital Dist/Auth
Phone: 678-604-1000
Fax: 770-389-2093
Emergency Services: Yes
Beds: 124

Key Personnel:
Quality Assurance . . . . Sandy Broder
Radiology. . . . . Dwight Fancher
Chair/CEO . . . . Gregory A. Hurst
Pediatric In-Patient Care . . . . Pat McAfee
Operating Room. . . . . Freda D McCarter
Emergency Room . . . . Cheryl Minor, RN
CEO/President. . . . . Charles F. Scott
Chief of Medical Staff . . . . Jagdeep Singh, MD

Measure	Cases	This Hosp.	State Avg.	U.S. Avg.
Blood Clot Prevention and Treatment				
Anticoagulation Overlap Therapy[2]	132	96%	90%	93%
ICU Venous Thromboembolism Prophylaxis[2]	82	99%	90%	92%
Incidence of Potentially Preventable VTE[1,2]	-	-	13%	10%
UFH with Dosages/Platelet Monitoring[2]	92	100%	99%	97%
Venous Thromboembolism Prophylaxis[2]	347	95%	80%	85%
Warfarin Therapy Discharge Instructions[2]	106	95%	78%	75%
Chest Pain/Possible Heart Attack Care				
Aspirin Given Within 24 Hours of Arrival[5]	-	-	94%	96%
Fibrinolytic Meds Within 30 Min. of Arrival[5]	-	-	35%	58%
Average Time to ECG (minutes)[5]	-	-	8	7
Average Time to Transfer (minutes)[5]	-	-	73	60
Children's Asthma Care				
Received Home Management Plan of Care	-	-	-	88%
Received Reliever Medication	-	-	-	100%
Received Systemic Corticosteroids	-	-	-	100%
Emergency Department				
Admittance Decision Time (minutes)[2]	671	177	100	98
Head CT Results Within 45 Min. of Arrival[1]	-	-	45%	57%
Patients Who Left ER Before Being Seen	79,978	4%	3%	2%
Time from ER Arrival to Admit. (minutes)[2]	671	402	286	274
Time from ER Arrival to Discharge (minutes)	413	192	140	134
Time in ER Before Being Evaluated (minutes)	428	73	32	26

NOTE: Hospital profiles are in alphabetical order by state, then city, then hospital within the city; Rankings exclude hospitals with less than 25 cases except for patient surveys which excludes hospitals with less than 100 cases; (a) 100-299 cases; (1) The number of cases/patients is too few to report; (2) Data submitted were based on a sample of cases/patients; (3) Results are based on a shorter time period than required; (4) Data suppressed by CMS for one or more quarters; (5) Results are not available for this reporting period; (6) Fewer than 100 patients completed the HCAHPS survey; (7) No cases met the criteria for this measure; (8) The lower limit of the confidence interval cannot be calculated if the number of observed infections equals zero; (9) No data are available from the state/territory for this reporting period; (10) The scores shown reflect fewer than 50 completed surveys; (11) There were discrepancies in the data collection process; (12) This measure does not apply to this hospital for this reporting period; (13) Results cannot be calculated for this reporting period; (14) The results for this state are combined with nearby states to protect confidentiality; Please refer to the User's Guide for a full explanation of data.

Measure	Cases	This Hosp.	State Avg.	U.S. Avg.
Time to Pain Meds for Fractures (minutes)	233	77	64	57
Heart Attack Care				
Aspirin Given at Discharge	176	99%	99%	99%
Fibrinolytic Meds Within 30 Min. of Arrival[7]	-	-	80%	54%
PCI Within 90 Minutes of Arrival	30	100%	95%	96%
Statin Prescribed at Discharge	173	95%	98%	98%
Heart Failure Care				
ACE Inhibitor or ARB for LVSD[2]	104	90%	97%	97%
Discharge Instructions Given[2]	309	89%	92%	94%
Evaluation of LVS Function[2]	341	98%	99%	99%
Medicare Spending				
Medicare Spending per Patient (ratio)	-	0.97	0.95	0.98
Pneumonia Care				
Appropriate Initial Antibiotic Given[2]	117	97%	95%	95%
Blood Culture Timing[2]	145	97%	97%	98%
Pregnancy and Delivery Care				
Newborn Deliveries Scheduled Early	210	5%	8%	6%
Preventive Care				
Immunization for Influenza[2]	522	92%	88%	90%
Immunization for Pneumonia[2]	647	90%	90%	92%
Stroke Care				
Anticoagulation Therapy for Atrial Fibrillation	12	100%	94%	95%
Antithrombotic Therapy Timing	144	87%	97%	98%
Assessed for Rehabilitation	148	95%	97%	97%
Discharged on Antithrombotic Therapy	140	97%	98%	99%
Discharged on Statin Medication	113	85%	94%	94%
Thrombolytic Therapy Timing[1]	-	-	58%	66%
Venous Thromboembolism Prophylaxis	156	85%	92%	94%
Written Stroke Educational Materials Given	94	88%	84%	88%
Surgical Care Improvement Project				
Appropriate Beta Blocker Usage[2]	153	100%	97%	98%
Appropriate VTP Within 24 Hours[2]	499	96%	98%	98%
Controlled Postoperative Blood Glucose[2,7]	-	-	96%	97%
Perioperative Temperature Management[2]	542	100%	100%	100%
Prophylactic Antibiotic Selection[2]	381	100%	99%	99%
Prophylactic Antibiotic Selection (Outpatient)	495	98%	98%	98%
Prophylactic Antibiotic Stopped[2]	375	98%	98%	98%
Prophylactic Antibiotic Timing[2]	381	99%	99%	99%
Prophylactic Antibiotic Timing (Outpatient)	496	99%	98%	98%
Urinary Catheter Removal[2]	191	99%	99%	97%
Survey of Patients' Hospital Experiences				
Area Around Room 'Always' Quiet at Night	300+	57%	66%	61%
Doctors 'Always' Communicated Well	300+	76%	83%	82%
Home Recovery Information Given	300+	79%	84%	85%
Hospital Given 9 or 10 on 10 Point Scale	300+	58%	69%	71%
Meds 'Always' Explained Before Given	300+	55%	63%	64%
Nurses 'Always' Communicated Well	300+	69%	78%	79%
Pain 'Always' Well Controlled	300+	65%	71%	71%
Room and Bathroom 'Always' Clean	300+	61%	71%	73%
Timely Help 'Always' Received	300+	54%	65%	68%
Would Definitely Recommend Hospital	300+	61%	70%	71%
Use of Medical Imaging				
Cardiac Imaging Stress Test before Surgery	251	8.8%	5.5%	5.3%
Combination Abdominal CT Scan	957	7.7%	10.1%	10.5%
Combination Brain/Sinus CT Scan	854	2.2%	2.3%	2.7%
Combination Chest CT Scan	327	0.9%	3.7%	2.7%
Follow-up Mammogram/Ultrasound	941	8.7%	8.9%	8.8%
Lumbar Spine MRI for Low Back Pain	41	39.0%	36.6%	37.2%

Emanuel County Hospital Authority

117 Kite Road　　Phone: 478-289-1304
Swainsboro, GA 30401　　Fax: 478-289-1300
Type: Acute Care Hospitals　　Emergency Services: Yes
Ownership: Govt - Hospital Dist/Auth　　Beds: 120

Key Personnel:
Quality Assurance . . . . Gail Dillard
Operating Room. . . . . Brad Headley
CEO . . . . Mel Pyne

Measure	Cases	This Hosp.	State Avg.	U.S. Avg.
Blood Clot Prevention and Treatment				
Anticoagulation Overlap Therapy[2]	11	82%	90%	93%
ICU Venous Thromboembolism Prophylaxis[2]	40	48%	90%	92%
Incidence of Potentially Preventable VTE[1,2]	-	-	13%	10%
UFH with Dosages/Platelet Monitoring[2,7]	-	-	99%	97%
Venous Thromboembolism Prophylaxis[2]	118	26%	80%	85%
Warfarin Therapy Discharge Instructions[1,2]	-	-	78%	75%
Chest Pain/Possible Heart Attack Care				
Aspirin Given Within 24 Hours of Arrival[3]	25	92%	94%	96%
Fibrinolytic Meds Within 30 Min. of Arrival[1,3]	-	-	35%	58%
Average Time to ECG (minutes)[3]	16	4	8	7
Average Time to Transfer (minutes)[1,3]	-	-	73	60
Children's Asthma Care				
Received Home Management Plan of Care	-	-	-	88%
Received Reliever Medication	-	-	-	100%
Received Systemic Corticosteroids	-	-	-	100%
Emergency Department				
Admittance Decision Time (minutes)[2]	489	90	100	98
Head CT Results Within 45 Min. of Arrival	23	13%	45%	57%
Patients Who Left ER Before Being Seen	12,922	3%	3%	2%
Time from ER Arrival to Admit. (minutes)[2]	493	268	286	274
Time from ER Arrival to Discharge (minutes)	561	145	140	134
Time in ER Before Being Evaluated (minutes)	655	37	32	26
Time to Pain Meds for Fractures (minutes)	55	70	64	57
Heart Attack Care				
Aspirin Given at Discharge[1,3]	-	-	99%	99%
Fibrinolytic Meds Within 30 Min. of Arrival[3,7]	-	-	80%	54%
PCI Within 90 Minutes of Arrival[3,7]	-	-	95%	96%
Statin Prescribed at Discharge[1,3]	-	-	98%	98%
Heart Failure Care				
ACE Inhibitor or ARB for LVSD[2]	14	86%	97%	97%
Discharge Instructions Given[2]	30	100%	92%	94%
Evaluation of LVS Function[2]	46	87%	99%	99%
Medicare Spending				
Medicare Spending per Patient (ratio)	-	0.92	0.95	0.98
Pneumonia Care				
Appropriate Initial Antibiotic Given	34	85%	95%	95%
Blood Culture Timing	40	92%	97%	98%
Pregnancy and Delivery Care				
Newborn Deliveries Scheduled Early	19	0%	8%	6%
Preventive Care				
Immunization for Influenza[2]	352	85%	88%	90%
Immunization for Pneumonia[2]	510	92%	90%	92%
Stroke Care				
Anticoagulation Therapy for Atrial Fibrillation[7]	-	-	94%	95%
Antithrombotic Therapy Timing	18	11%	97%	98%
Assessed for Rehabilitation	19	53%	97%	97%
Discharged on Antithrombotic Therapy	19	53%	98%	99%
Discharged on Statin Medication	19	58%	94%	94%
Thrombolytic Therapy Timing[1]	-	-	58%	66%
Venous Thromboembolism Prophylaxis	18	39%	92%	94%
Written Stroke Educational Materials Given[1]	-	-	84%	88%
Surgical Care Improvement Project				
Appropriate Beta Blocker Usage[1]	-	-	97%	98%
Appropriate VTP Within 24 Hours[1]	-	-	98%	98%
Controlled Postoperative Blood Glucose[7]	-	-	96%	97%
Perioperative Temperature Management[1]	-	-	100%	100%
Prophylactic Antibiotic Selection[1]	-	-	99%	99%
Prophylactic Antibiotic Selection (Outpatient)[5]	-	-	98%	98%
Prophylactic Antibiotic Stopped[1]	-	-	98%	98%
Prophylactic Antibiotic Timing[1]	-	-	99%	99%
Prophylactic Antibiotic Timing (Outpatient)[5]	-	-	98%	98%
Urinary Catheter Removal[1]	-	-	97%	97%
Survey of Patients' Hospital Experiences				
Area Around Room 'Always' Quiet at Night	(a)	73%	66%	61%
Doctors 'Always' Communicated Well	(a)	90%	83%	82%
Home Recovery Information Given	(a)	91%	84%	85%
Hospital Given 9 or 10 on 10 Point Scale	(a)	72%	69%	71%
Meds 'Always' Explained Before Given	(a)	64%	63%	64%
Nurses 'Always' Communicated Well	(a)	83%	78%	79%
Pain 'Always' Well Controlled	(a)	71%	71%	71%
Room and Bathroom 'Always' Clean	(a)	80%	71%	73%
Timely Help 'Always' Received	(a)	74%	65%	68%
Would Definitely Recommend Hospital	(a)	70%	70%	71%
Use of Medical Imaging				
Cardiac Imaging Stress Test before Surgery[1]	-	-	5.5%	5.3%
Combination Abdominal CT Scan	184	26.1%	10.1%	10.5%
Combination Brain/Sinus CT Scan[1]	-	-	2.3%	2.7%
Combination Chest CT Scan	70	35.7%	3.7%	2.7%
Follow-up Mammogram/Ultrasound	362	14.9%	8.9%	8.8%
Lumbar Spine MRI for Low Back Pain[1]	-	-	36.6%	37.2%

Phoebe Worth Medical Center

807 South Isabella Street　　Phone: 229-777-3851
Sylvester, GA 31791　　Fax: 229-777-0517
Type: Critical Access Hospitals　　Emergency Services: Yes
Ownership: Voluntary non-profit - Private　　Beds: 25

Key Personnel:
CEO . . . . Kim Gilman

Measure	Cases	This Hosp.	State Avg.	U.S. Avg.
Blood Clot Prevention and Treatment				
Anticoagulation Overlap Therapy[5]	-	-	90%	93%
ICU Venous Thromboembolism Prophylaxis[5]	-	-	90%	92%
Incidence of Potentially Preventable VTE[5]	-	-	13%	10%
UFH with Dosages/Platelet Monitoring[5]	-	-	99%	97%
Venous Thromboembolism Prophylaxis[5]	-	-	80%	85%
Warfarin Therapy Discharge Instructions[5]	-	-	78%	75%
Chest Pain/Possible Heart Attack Care				
Aspirin Given Within 24 Hours of Arrival	-	-	94%	96%
Fibrinolytic Meds Within 30 Min. of Arrival	-	-	35%	58%
Average Time to ECG (minutes)	-	-	8	7
Average Time to Transfer (minutes)	-	-	73	60
Children's Asthma Care				
Received Home Management Plan of Care	-	-	-	88%
Received Reliever Medication	-	-	-	100%
Received Systemic Corticosteroids	-	-	-	100%
Emergency Department				
Admittance Decision Time (minutes)[5]	-	-	100	98
Head CT Results Within 45 Min. of Arrival	-	-	45%	57%
Patients Who Left ER Before Being Seen	-	-	3%	2%
Time from ER Arrival to Admit. (minutes)[5]	-	-	286	274
Time from ER Arrival to Discharge (minutes)	-	-	140	134
Time in ER Before Being Evaluated (minutes)	-	-	32	26
Time to Pain Meds for Fractures (minutes)	-	-	64	57
Heart Attack Care				
Aspirin Given at Discharge[5]	-	-	99%	99%
Fibrinolytic Meds Within 30 Min. of Arrival[5]	-	-	80%	54%
PCI Within 90 Minutes of Arrival[5]	-	-	95%	96%
Statin Prescribed at Discharge[5]	-	-	98%	98%
Heart Failure Care				
ACE Inhibitor or ARB for LVSD[1]	-	-	97%	97%
Discharge Instructions Given[1]	-	-	92%	94%
Evaluation of LVS Function	14	50%	99%	99%
Medicare Spending				
Medicare Spending per Patient (ratio)	-	-	0.95	0.98
Pneumonia Care				
Appropriate Initial Antibiotic Given[1]	-	-	95%	95%
Blood Culture Timing	20	90%	97%	98%
Pregnancy and Delivery Care				
Newborn Deliveries Scheduled Early[5]	-	-	8%	6%
Preventive Care				
Immunization for Influenza[5]	-	-	88%	90%
Immunization for Pneumonia[5]	-	-	90%	92%
Stroke Care				
Anticoagulation Therapy for Atrial Fibrillation[5]	-	-	94%	95%
Antithrombotic Therapy Timing[5]	-	-	97%	98%
Assessed for Rehabilitation[5]	-	-	97%	97%
Discharged on Antithrombotic Therapy[5]	-	-	98%	99%
Discharged on Statin Medication[5]	-	-	94%	94%
Thrombolytic Therapy Timing[5]	-	-	58%	66%
Venous Thromboembolism Prophylaxis[5]	-	-	92%	94%
Written Stroke Educational Materials Given[5]	-	-	84%	88%
Surgical Care Improvement Project				
Appropriate Beta Blocker Usage[5]	-	-	97%	98%
Appropriate VTP Within 24 Hours[5]	-	-	98%	98%
Controlled Postoperative Blood Glucose[5]	-	-	96%	97%
Perioperative Temperature Management[5]	-	-	100%	100%
Prophylactic Antibiotic Selection[5]	-	-	99%	99%
Prophylactic Antibiotic Selection (Outpatient)	-	-	98%	98%

NOTE: Hospital profiles are in alphabetical order by state, then city, then hospital within the city; Rankings exclude hospitals with less than 25 cases except for patient surveys which excludes hospitals with less than 100 cases; (a) 100-299 cases; (1) The number of cases/patients is too few to report; (2) Data submitted were based on a sample of cases/patients; (3) Results are based on a shorter time period than required; (4) Data suppressed by CMS for one or more quarters; (5) Results are not available for this reporting period; (6) Fewer than 100 patients completed the HCAHPS survey; (7) No cases met the criteria for this measure; (8) The lower limit of the confidence interval cannot be calculated if the number of observed infections equals zero; (9) No data are available from the state/territory for this reporting period; (10) The scores shown reflect fewer than 50 completed surveys; (11) There were discrepancies in the data collection process; (12) This measure does not apply to this hospital for this reporting period; (13) Results cannot be calculated for this reporting period; (14) The results for this state are combined with nearby states to protect confidentiality; Please refer to the User's Guide for a full explanation of data.

Measure	Cases	This Hosp.	State Avg.	U.S. Avg.
Prophylactic Antibiotic Stopped[5]	-	-	98%	98%
Prophylactic Antibiotic Timing[5]	-	-	99%	99%
Prophylactic Antibiotic Timing (Outpatient)	-	-	98%	98%
Urinary Catheter Removal[5]	-	-	97%	97%
Survey of Patients' Hospital Experiences				
Area Around Room 'Always' Quiet at Night[5]	-	-	66%	61%
Doctors 'Always' Communicated Well[5]	-	-	83%	82%
Home Recovery Information Given[5]	-	-	84%	85%
Hospital Given 9 or 10 on 10 Point Scale[5]	-	-	69%	71%
Meds 'Always' Explained Before Given[5]	-	-	63%	64%
Nurses 'Always' Communicated Well[5]	-	-	78%	79%
Pain 'Always' Well Controlled[5]	-	-	71%	71%
Room and Bathroom 'Always' Clean[5]	-	-	71%	73%
Timely Help 'Always' Received[5]	-	-	65%	68%
Would Definitely Recommend Hospital[5]	-	-	70%	71%
Use of Medical Imaging				
Cardiac Imaging Stress Test before Surgery	-	-	5.5%	5.3%
Combination Abdominal CT Scan	-	-	10.1%	10.5%
Combination Brain/Sinus CT Scan	-	-	2.3%	2.7%
Combination Chest CT Scan	-	-	3.7%	2.7%
Follow-up Mammogram/Ultrasound	-	-	8.9%	8.8%
Lumbar Spine MRI for Low Back Pain	-	-	36.6%	37.2%

Upson Regional Medical Center

801 W Gordon Street
Thomaston, GA 30286
Phone: 706-647-8111
Fax: 706-646-3310
URL: www.urmc.org
Type: Acute Care Hospitals
Emergency Services: Yes
Ownership: Voluntary non-profit - Other
Beds: 115

Key Personnel:
Pediatric In-Patient Care .... Donna Anderson, RN
Operating Room.............. Phillip Brown, RN
Chief of Medical Staff.......... Chris Colby, MD
Radiology.................. Alan J Helrich
President.................. William H. Hightower, IV
Coronary Care.............. Trish Morway, RN
Quality Assurance .... Suzanne Streetman, RN
Infection Control............. Glenda Van Houten, RN

Measure	Cases	This Hosp.	State Avg.	U.S. Avg.
Blood Clot Prevention and Treatment				
Anticoagulation Overlap Therapy[2]	22	45%	90%	93%
ICU Venous Thromboembolism Prophylaxis[2]	48	71%	90%	92%
Incidence of Potentially Preventable VTE[1,2]	-	-	13%	10%
UFH with Dosages/Platelet Monitoring[1,2]	-	-	99%	97%
Venous Thromboembolism Prophylaxis[2]	339	49%	80%	85%
Warfarin Therapy Discharge Instructions[2]	15	100%	78%	75%
Chest Pain/Possible Heart Attack Care				
Aspirin Given Within 24 Hours of Arrival	97	88%	94%	96%
Fibrinolytic Meds Within 30 Min. of Arrival[7]	-	-	35%	58%
Average Time to ECG (minutes)	102	8	8	7
Average Time to Transfer (minutes)[1]	-	-	73	60
Children's Asthma Care				
Received Home Management Plan of Care	-	-	-	88%
Received Reliever Medication	-	-	-	100%
Received Systemic Corticosteroids	-	-	-	100%
Emergency Department				
Admittance Decision Time (minutes)[2]	400	68	100	98
Head CT Results Within 45 Min. of Arrival	14	0%	45%	57%
Patients Who Left ER Before Being Seen	33,329	1%	3%	2%
Time from ER Arrival to Admit. (minutes)[2]	423	258	286	274
Time from ER Arrival to Discharge (minutes)	372	137	140	134
Time in ER Before Being Evaluated (minutes)	296	30	32	26
Time to Pain Meds for Fractures (minutes)	98	50	64	57
Heart Attack Care				
Aspirin Given at Discharge[1]	-	-	99%	99%
Fibrinolytic Meds Within 30 Min. of Arrival[7]	-	-	80%	54%
PCI Within 90 Minutes of Arrival[7]	-	-	95%	96%
Statin Prescribed at Discharge[1]	-	-	98%	98%
Heart Failure Care				
ACE Inhibitor or ARB for LVSD	76	97%	97%	97%
Discharge Instructions Given	116	88%	92%	94%
Evaluation of LVS Function	130	99%	99%	99%
Medicare Spending				
Medicare Spending per Patient (ratio)	-	0.94	0.95	0.98
Pneumonia Care				
Appropriate Initial Antibiotic Given[2]	97	95%	95%	95%
Blood Culture Timing[2]	124	98%	97%	98%
Pregnancy and Delivery Care				
Newborn Deliveries Scheduled Early[2]	39	13%	8%	6%
Preventive Care				
Immunization for Influenza[2]	368	48%	88%	90%
Immunization for Pneumonia[2]	454	68%	90%	92%
Stroke Care				
Anticoagulation Therapy for Atrial Fibrillation[1]	-	-	94%	95%
Antithrombotic Therapy Timing	30	93%	97%	98%
Assessed for Rehabilitation	37	84%	97%	97%
Discharged on Antithrombotic Therapy	36	86%	98%	99%
Discharged on Statin Medication	34	50%	94%	94%
Thrombolytic Therapy Timing[1]	-	-	58%	66%
Venous Thromboembolism Prophylaxis	30	50%	92%	94%
Written Stroke Educational Materials Given	26	46%	84%	88%
Surgical Care Improvement Project				
Appropriate Beta Blocker Usage[2]	48	85%	97%	98%
Appropriate VTP Within 24 Hours[2]	184	97%	98%	98%
Controlled Postoperative Blood Glucose[2,7]	-	-	96%	97%
Perioperative Temperature Management[2]	207	99%	100%	100%
Prophylactic Antibiotic Selection[2]	138	100%	99%	99%
Prophylactic Antibiotic Selection (Outpatient)	72	100%	98%	98%
Prophylactic Antibiotic Stopped[2]	135	93%	98%	98%
Prophylactic Antibiotic Timing[2]	138	99%	99%	99%
Prophylactic Antibiotic Timing (Outpatient)	73	99%	98%	98%
Urinary Catheter Removal[2]	70	87%	97%	97%
Survey of Patients' Hospital Experiences				
Area Around Room 'Always' Quiet at Night	300+	72%	66%	61%
Doctors 'Always' Communicated Well	300+	89%	83%	82%
Home Recovery Information Given	300+	83%	84%	85%
Hospital Given 9 or 10 on 10 Point Scale	300+	74%	69%	71%
Meds 'Always' Explained Before Given	300+	73%	63%	64%
Nurses 'Always' Communicated Well	300+	87%	78%	79%
Pain 'Always' Well Controlled	300+	76%	71%	71%
Room and Bathroom 'Always' Clean	300+	81%	71%	73%
Timely Help 'Always' Received	300+	76%	65%	68%
Would Definitely Recommend Hospital	300+	74%	70%	71%
Use of Medical Imaging				
Cardiac Imaging Stress Test before Surgery	204	4.4%	5.5%	5.3%
Combination Abdominal CT Scan	393	9.9%	10.1%	10.5%
Combination Brain/Sinus CT Scan	564	1.4%	2.3%	2.7%
Combination Chest CT Scan	119	10.1%	3.7%	2.7%
Follow-up Mammogram/Ultrasound	579	6.7%	8.9%	8.8%
Lumbar Spine MRI for Low Back Pain	55	38.2%	36.6%	37.2%

John D Archbold Memorial Hospital

915 Gordon Avenue & Mimosa Drive
Thomasville, GA 31792
Phone: 229-228-2880
Fax: 229-228-8591
E-mail: customerservice@archbold.org
URL: www.archbold.org
Type: Acute Care Hospitals
Emergency Services: Yes
Ownership: Voluntary non-profit - Private
Beds: 800

Key Personnel:
Cardiac Laboratory............ Sally Bain
Radiology.................. Paul Carpenter, MD
Operating Room.............. David Grantham
CEO/President............... Perry Mustain, MD
Pediatric In-Patient Care .... Jose Peralta, MD
Chief of Medical Staff.......... Wesley Simmes
Emergency Room .... Mark Swicord

Measure	Cases	This Hosp.	State Avg.	U.S. Avg.
Blood Clot Prevention and Treatment				
Anticoagulation Overlap Therapy[2]	76	99%	90%	93%
ICU Venous Thromboembolism Prophylaxis[2]	63	95%	90%	92%
Incidence of Potentially Preventable VTE[1,2]	-	-	13%	10%
UFH with Dosages/Platelet Monitoring[2]	63	100%	99%	97%
Venous Thromboembolism Prophylaxis[2]	326	94%	80%	85%
Warfarin Therapy Discharge Instructions[2]	67	97%	78%	75%
Chest Pain/Possible Heart Attack Care				
Aspirin Given Within 24 Hours of Arrival[5]	-	-	94%	96%
Fibrinolytic Meds Within 30 Min. of Arrival[5]	-	-	35%	58%
Average Time to ECG (minutes)[5]	-	-	8	7
Average Time to Transfer (minutes)[5]	-	-	73	60
Children's Asthma Care				
Received Home Management Plan of Care	-	-	-	88%
Received Reliever Medication	-	-	-	100%
Received Systemic Corticosteroids	-	-	-	100%
Emergency Department				
Admittance Decision Time (minutes)[2]	622	163	100	98
Head CT Results Within 45 Min. of Arrival[7]	-	-	45%	57%
Patients Who Left ER Before Being Seen	32,335	7%	3%	2%
Time from ER Arrival to Admit. (minutes)[2]	622	356	286	274
Time from ER Arrival to Discharge (minutes)[11]	452	167	140	134
Time in ER Before Being Evaluated (minutes)	448	70	32	26
Time to Pain Meds for Fractures (minutes)	134	90	64	57
Heart Attack Care				
Aspirin Given at Discharge	194	100%	99%	99%
Fibrinolytic Meds Within 30 Min. of Arrival[7]	-	-	80%	54%
PCI Within 90 Minutes of Arrival	35	91%	95%	96%
Statin Prescribed at Discharge	192	100%	98%	98%
Heart Failure Care				
ACE Inhibitor or ARB for LVSD	103	100%	97%	97%
Discharge Instructions Given	284	100%	92%	94%
Evaluation of LVS Function	334	100%	99%	99%
Medicare Spending				
Medicare Spending per Patient (ratio)	-	0.97	0.95	0.98
Pneumonia Care				
Appropriate Initial Antibiotic Given	129	95%	95%	95%
Blood Culture Timing	226	95%	97%	98%
Pregnancy and Delivery Care				
Newborn Deliveries Scheduled Early[2]	79	4%	8%	6%
Preventive Care				
Immunization for Influenza[2]	644	77%	88%	90%
Immunization for Pneumonia[2]	757	85%	90%	92%
Stroke Care				
Anticoagulation Therapy for Atrial Fibrillation	23	100%	94%	95%
Antithrombotic Therapy Timing	155	99%	97%	98%
Assessed for Rehabilitation	180	99%	97%	97%
Discharged on Antithrombotic Therapy	154	100%	98%	99%
Discharged on Statin Medication	130	95%	94%	94%
Thrombolytic Therapy Timing	13	77%	58%	66%
Venous Thromboembolism Prophylaxis	202	96%	92%	94%
Written Stroke Educational Materials Given	81	65%	84%	88%
Surgical Care Improvement Project				
Appropriate Beta Blocker Usage[2]	174	97%	97%	98%
Appropriate VTP Within 24 Hours[2]	463	99%	98%	98%
Controlled Postoperative Blood Glucose[2,7]	-	-	96%	97%
Perioperative Temperature Management[2]	600	100%	100%	100%
Prophylactic Antibiotic Selection[2]	403	99%	99%	99%
Prophylactic Antibiotic Selection (Outpatient)	319	98%	98%	98%
Prophylactic Antibiotic Stopped[2]	395	99%	98%	98%
Prophylactic Antibiotic Timing[2]	403	100%	99%	99%
Prophylactic Antibiotic Timing (Outpatient)	319	100%	98%	98%
Urinary Catheter Removal[2]	368	96%	97%	97%
Survey of Patients' Hospital Experiences				
Area Around Room 'Always' Quiet at Night	300+	71%	66%	61%
Doctors 'Always' Communicated Well	300+	87%	83%	82%
Home Recovery Information Given	300+	88%	84%	85%
Hospital Given 9 or 10 on 10 Point Scale	300+	76%	69%	71%
Meds 'Always' Explained Before Given	300+	65%	63%	64%
Nurses 'Always' Communicated Well	300+	80%	78%	79%
Pain 'Always' Well Controlled	300+	72%	71%	71%
Room and Bathroom 'Always' Clean	300+	72%	71%	73%
Timely Help 'Always' Received	300+	64%	65%	68%
Would Definitely Recommend Hospital	300+	78%	70%	71%
Use of Medical Imaging				
Cardiac Imaging Stress Test before Surgery	311	6.8%	5.5%	5.3%
Combination Abdominal CT Scan	948	11.4%	10.1%	10.5%
Combination Brain/Sinus CT Scan	632	1.6%	2.3%	2.7%
Combination Chest CT Scan	636	1.9%	3.7%	2.7%
Follow-up Mammogram/Ultrasound	1,847	9.4%	8.9%	8.8%
Lumbar Spine MRI for Low Back Pain	100	35.0%	36.6%	37.2%

NOTE: Hospital profiles are in alphabetical order by state, then city, then hospital within the city; Rankings exclude hospitals with less than 25 cases except for patient surveys which excludes hospitals with less than 100 cases; (a) 100-299 cases; (1) The number of cases/patients is too few to report; (2) Data submitted were based on a sample of cases/patients; (3) Results are based on a shorter time period than required; (4) Data suppressed by CMS for one or more quarters; (5) Results are not available for this reporting period; (6) Fewer than 100 patients completed the HCAHPS survey; (7) No cases met the criteria for this measure; (8) The lower limit of the confidence interval cannot be calculated if the number of observed infections equals zero; (9) No data are available from the state/territory for this reporting period; (10) The scores shown reflect fewer than 50 completed surveys; (11) There were discrepancies in the data collection process; (12) This measure does not apply to this hospital for this reporting period; (13) Results cannot be calculated for this reporting period; (14) The results for this state are combined with nearby states to protect confidentiality; Please refer to the User's Guide for a full explanation of data.

University Mcduffie County Regional Medical Center

521 Hill Street, Sw
Thomson, GA 30824
Phone: 706-595-1411
Fax: 706-597-5377
URL: www.mrmc.org
Type: Acute Care Hospitals
Emergency Services: Yes
Ownership: Govt - Hospital Dist/Auth
Beds: 47

Key Personnel:

Quality Assurance . . . . Belinda Campbell
Operating Room. . . . . Michael A Edwards, RN
Pediatrics. . . . . Nargis Husainy, MD
CEO/President. . . . . Douglas C Keir
Infection Control. . . . . Rande Maynard
Chief of Medical Staff. . . . . M Frank Powell
Radiology. . . . . Sharon Rutkowski
Emergency Room . . . . Harry Wingate

Measure	Cases	This Hosp.	State Avg.	U.S. Avg.
Blood Clot Prevention and Treatment				
Anticoagulation Overlap Therapy[2,7]	-	-	90%	93%
ICU Venous Thromboembolism Prophylaxis[2,7]	-	-	90%	92%
Incidence of Potentially Preventable VTE[2,7]	-	-	13%	10%
UFH with Dosages/Platelet Monitoring[2,7]	-	-	99%	97%
Venous Thromboembolism Prophylaxis[2]	145	34%	80%	85%
Warfarin Therapy Discharge Instructions[2,7]	-	-	78%	75%
Chest Pain/Possible Heart Attack Care				
Aspirin Given Within 24 Hours of Arrival	60	87%	94%	96%
Fibrinolytic Meds Within 30 Min. of Arrival[1]	-	-	35%	58%
Average Time to ECG (minutes)	61	17	8	7
Average Time to Transfer (minutes)[1]	-	-	73	60
Children's Asthma Care				
Received Home Management Plan of Care	-	-	-	88%
Received Reliever Medication	-	-	-	100%
Received Systemic Corticosteroids	-	-	-	100%
Emergency Department				
Admittance Decision Time (minutes)[2]	168	73	100	98
Head CT Results Within 45 Min. of Arrival[1,3]	-	-	45%	57%
Patients Who Left ER Before Being Seen	13,649	3%	3%	2%
Time from ER Arrival to Admit. (minutes)[2]	172	256	286	274
Time from ER Arrival to Discharge (minutes)[11]	412	116	140	134
Time in ER Before Being Evaluated (minutes)	461	33	32	26
Time to Pain Meds for Fractures (minutes)	36	64	64	57
Heart Attack Care				
Aspirin Given at Discharge[5]	-	-	99%	99%
Fibrinolytic Meds Within 30 Min. of Arrival[5]	-	-	80%	54%
PCI Within 90 Minutes of Arrival[5]	-	-	95%	96%
Statin Prescribed at Discharge[5]	-	-	98%	98%
Heart Failure Care				
ACE Inhibitor or ARB for LVSD[1,3]	-	-	97%	97%
Discharge Instructions Given[1,3]	-	-	92%	94%
Evaluation of LVS Function[3]	12	92%	99%	99%
Medicare Spending				
Medicare Spending per Patient (ratio)	-	1.04	0.95	0.98
Pneumonia Care				
Appropriate Initial Antibiotic Given	19	84%	95%	95%
Blood Culture Timing	18	94%	97%	98%
Pregnancy and Delivery Care				
Newborn Deliveries Scheduled Early[7]	-	-	8%	6%
Preventive Care				
Immunization for Influenza[2]	207	59%	88%	90%
Immunization for Pneumonia[2]	320	53%	90%	92%
Stroke Care				
Anticoagulation Therapy for Atrial Fibrillation[5]	-	-	94%	95%
Antithrombotic Therapy Timing[5]	-	-	97%	98%
Assessed for Rehabilitation[5]	-	-	97%	97%
Discharged on Antithrombotic Therapy[5]	-	-	98%	99%
Discharged on Statin Medication[5]	-	-	94%	94%
Thrombolytic Therapy Timing[5]	-	-	58%	66%
Venous Thromboembolism Prophylaxis[5]	-	-	92%	94%
Written Stroke Educational Materials Given[5]	-	-	84%	88%
Surgical Care Improvement Project				
Appropriate Beta Blocker Usage	20	95%	97%	98%
Appropriate VTP Within 24 Hours	76	96%	98%	98%
Controlled Postoperative Blood Glucose[7]	-	-	96%	97%
Perioperative Temperature Management	80	98%	100%	100%
Prophylactic Antibiotic Selection	62	100%	99%	99%
Prophylactic Antibiotic Selection (Outpatient)[1,3]	-	-	98%	98%
Prophylactic Antibiotic Stopped	62	100%	98%	98%
Prophylactic Antibiotic Timing	62	100%	99%	99%
Prophylactic Antibiotic Timing (Outpatient)[1,3]	-	-	98%	98%
Urinary Catheter Removal	49	86%	97%	97%
Survey of Patients' Hospital Experiences				
Area Around Room 'Always' Quiet at Night[6]	<100	75%	66%	61%
Doctors 'Always' Communicated Well[6]	<100	82%	83%	82%
Home Recovery Information Given[6]	<100	87%	84%	85%
Hospital Given 9 or 10 on 10 Point Scale[6]	<100	67%	69%	71%
Meds 'Always' Explained Before Given[6]	<100	64%	63%	64%
Nurses 'Always' Communicated Well[6]	<100	80%	78%	79%
Pain 'Always' Well Controlled[6]	<100	68%	71%	71%
Room and Bathroom 'Always' Clean[6]	<100	60%	71%	73%
Timely Help 'Always' Received[6]	<100	77%	65%	68%
Would Definitely Recommend Hospital[6]	<100	68%	70%	71%
Use of Medical Imaging				
Cardiac Imaging Stress Test before Surgery[7]	-	-	5.5%	5.3%
Combination Abdominal CT Scan	172	12.8%	10.1%	10.5%
Combination Brain/Sinus CT Scan	200	1.0%	2.3%	2.7%
Combination Chest CT Scan	69	18.8%	3.7%	2.7%
Follow-up Mammogram/Ultrasound	485	10.9%	8.9%	8.8%
Lumbar Spine MRI for Low Back Pain[7]	-	-	36.6%	37.2%

Tift Regional Medical Center

901 E 18th Street
Tifton, GA 31793
Phone: 229-382-7120
Fax: 229-353-6192
E-mail: hrdept@surfsouth.com
URL: www.tiftregional.com
Type: Acute Care Hospitals
Emergency Services: Yes
Ownership: Govt - Hospital Dist/Auth
Beds: 191

Key Personnel:

Emergency Room . . . . Ed Bryan
Radiology. . . . . Patrick Crimmin
Operating Room. . . . . William H Davis
Quality Assurance . . . . Angela King, RN
Chief of Medical Staff. . . . . Ray Moreno, MD
CEO . . . . Michael Purvis
President/CEO. . . . . William T Richardson, FACHE

Measure	Cases	This Hosp.	State Avg.	U.S. Avg.
Blood Clot Prevention and Treatment				
Anticoagulation Overlap Therapy[2]	75	85%	90%	93%
ICU Venous Thromboembolism Prophylaxis[2]	62	100%	90%	92%
Incidence of Potentially Preventable VTE[2]	12	0%	13%	10%
UFH with Dosages/Platelet Monitoring[2]	38	100%	99%	97%
Venous Thromboembolism Prophylaxis[2]	336	90%	80%	85%
Warfarin Therapy Discharge Instructions[2]	63	6%	78%	75%
Chest Pain/Possible Heart Attack Care				
Aspirin Given Within 24 Hours of Arrival[1,3]	-	-	94%	96%
Fibrinolytic Meds Within 30 Min. of Arrival[5]	-	-	35%	58%
Average Time to ECG (minutes)[1,3]	-	-	8	7
Average Time to Transfer (minutes)[5]	-	-	73	60
Children's Asthma Care				
Received Home Management Plan of Care	27	78%	-	88%
Received Reliever Medication	28	100%	-	100%
Received Systemic Corticosteroids	27	100%	-	100%
Emergency Department				
Admittance Decision Time (minutes)[2]	624	146	100	98
Head CT Results Within 45 Min. of Arrival	13	31%	45%	57%
Patients Who Left ER Before Being Seen	55,045	2%	3%	2%
Time from ER Arrival to Admit. (minutes)[2]	626	326	286	274
Time from ER Arrival to Discharge (minutes)	454	160	140	134
Time in ER Before Being Evaluated (minutes)	500	52	32	26
Time to Pain Meds for Fractures (minutes)	127	66	64	57
Heart Attack Care				
Aspirin Given at Discharge	159	98%	99%	99%
Fibrinolytic Meds Within 30 Min. of Arrival[7]	-	-	80%	54%
PCI Within 90 Minutes of Arrival	27	96%	95%	96%
Statin Prescribed at Discharge	155	98%	98%	98%
Heart Failure Care				
ACE Inhibitor or ARB for LVSD	112	95%	97%	97%
Discharge Instructions Given	257	98%	92%	94%
Evaluation of LVS Function	289	100%	99%	99%
Medicare Spending				
Medicare Spending per Patient (ratio)	-	0.87	0.95	0.98
Pneumonia Care				
Appropriate Initial Antibiotic Given	118	99%	95%	95%
Blood Culture Timing	219	100%	97%	98%
Pregnancy and Delivery Care				
Newborn Deliveries Scheduled Early[2]	23	4%	8%	6%
Preventive Care				
Immunization for Influenza[2]	573	97%	88%	90%
Immunization for Pneumonia[2]	705	97%	90%	92%
Stroke Care				
Anticoagulation Therapy for Atrial Fibrillation	15	93%	94%	95%
Antithrombotic Therapy Timing	119	97%	97%	98%
Assessed for Rehabilitation	123	98%	97%	97%
Discharged on Antithrombotic Therapy	122	99%	98%	99%
Discharged on Statin Medication	99	98%	94%	94%
Thrombolytic Therapy Timing	16	50%	58%	66%
Venous Thromboembolism Prophylaxis	116	95%	92%	94%
Written Stroke Educational Materials Given	95	83%	84%	88%
Surgical Care Improvement Project				
Appropriate Beta Blocker Usage	208	98%	97%	98%
Appropriate VTP Within 24 Hours	575	98%	98%	98%
Controlled Postoperative Blood Glucose[7]	-	-	96%	97%
Perioperative Temperature Management	637	100%	100%	100%
Prophylactic Antibiotic Selection	375	100%	99%	99%
Prophylactic Antibiotic Selection (Outpatient)	356	99%	98%	98%
Prophylactic Antibiotic Stopped	356	98%	98%	98%
Prophylactic Antibiotic Timing	375	99%	99%	99%
Prophylactic Antibiotic Timing (Outpatient)	358	99%	98%	98%
Urinary Catheter Removal	439	98%	97%	97%
Survey of Patients' Hospital Experiences				
Area Around Room 'Always' Quiet at Night	300+	69%	66%	61%
Doctors 'Always' Communicated Well	300+	83%	83%	82%
Home Recovery Information Given	300+	83%	84%	85%
Hospital Given 9 or 10 on 10 Point Scale	300+	74%	69%	71%
Meds 'Always' Explained Before Given	300+	63%	63%	64%
Nurses 'Always' Communicated Well	300+	82%	78%	79%
Pain 'Always' Well Controlled	300+	74%	71%	71%
Room and Bathroom 'Always' Clean	300+	76%	71%	73%
Timely Help 'Always' Received	300+	71%	65%	68%
Would Definitely Recommend Hospital	300+	72%	70%	71%
Use of Medical Imaging				
Cardiac Imaging Stress Test before Surgery	570	5.1%	5.5%	5.3%
Combination Abdominal CT Scan	951	3.0%	10.1%	10.5%
Combination Brain/Sinus CT Scan	957	2.3%	2.3%	2.7%
Combination Chest CT Scan	719	0.1%	3.7%	2.7%
Follow-up Mammogram/Ultrasound	2,003	16.6%	8.9%	8.8%
Lumbar Spine MRI for Low Back Pain	152	34.2%	36.6%	37.2%

Stephens County Hospital

163 Hospital Drive
Toccoa, GA 30577
Phone: 706-282-4250
Fax: 706-886-8045
URL: www.stephenscountyhospital.com
Type: Acute Care Hospitals
Emergency Services: Yes
Ownership: Govt - Hospital Dist/Auth
Beds: 96

Key Personnel:

Emergency Room . . . . Vickie Ansley, RN
Operating Room. . . . . Robert Buchanan
Quality Assurance . . . . Tina Debord
Chief of Medical Staff. . . . . Paul Easley
Radiology. . . . . Mary Eline
CEO/President. . . . . Ed Gambrell, Jr

Measure	Cases	This Hosp.	State Avg.	U.S. Avg.
Blood Clot Prevention and Treatment				
Anticoagulation Overlap Therapy[2]	17	71%	90%	93%
ICU Venous Thromboembolism Prophylaxis[2]	29	83%	90%	92%
Incidence of Potentially Preventable VTE[1,2]	-	-	13%	10%
UFH with Dosages/Platelet Monitoring[2]	15	100%	99%	97%
Venous Thromboembolism Prophylaxis[2]	202	68%	80%	85%
Warfarin Therapy Discharge Instructions[2]	12	100%	78%	75%
Chest Pain/Possible Heart Attack Care				
Aspirin Given Within 24 Hours of Arrival	70	100%	94%	96%
Fibrinolytic Meds Within 30 Min. of Arrival[7]	-	-	35%	58%
Average Time to ECG (minutes)	70	7	8	7
Average Time to Transfer (minutes)[1]	-	-	73	60

NOTE: Hospital profiles are in alphabetical order by state, then city, then hospital within the city; Rankings exclude hospitals with less than 25 cases except for patient surveys which excludes hospitals with less than 100 cases; (a) 100-299 cases; (1) The number of cases/patients is too few to report; (2) Data submitted were based on a sample of cases/patients; (3) Results are based on a shorter time period than required; (4) Data suppressed by CMS for one or more quarters; (5) Results are not available for this reporting period; (6) Fewer than 100 patients completed the HCAHPS survey; (7) No cases met the criteria for this measure; (8) The lower limit of the confidence interval cannot be calculated if the number of observed infections equals zero; (9) No data are available from the state/territory for this reporting period; (10) The scores shown reflect fewer than 50 completed surveys; (11) There were discrepancies in the data collection process; (12) This measure does not apply to this hospital for this reporting period; (13) Results cannot be calculated for this reporting period; (14) The results for this state are combined with nearby states to protect confidentiality; Please refer to the User's Guide for a full explanation of data.

Measure	Cases	This Hosp.	State Avg.	U.S. Avg.
Children's Asthma Care				
Received Home Management Plan of Care	-	-	-	88%
Received Reliever Medication	-	-	-	100%
Received Systemic Corticosteroids	-	-	-	100%
Emergency Department				
Admittance Decision Time (minutes)[2]	510	34	100	98
Head CT Results Within 45 Min. of Arrival[1]	-	-	45%	57%
Patients Who Left ER Before Being Seen	21,444	1%	3%	2%
Time from ER Arrival to Admit. (minutes)[2]	510	181	286	274
Time from ER Arrival to Discharge (minutes)	371	95	140	134
Time in ER Before Being Evaluated (minutes)	349	27	32	26
Time to Pain Meds for Fractures (minutes)	78	74	64	57
Heart Attack Care				
Aspirin Given at Discharge[1,2]	-	-	99%	99%
Fibrinolytic Meds Within 30 Min. of Arrival[2,7]	-	-	80%	54%
PCI Within 90 Minutes of Arrival[2,7]	-	-	95%	96%
Statin Prescribed at Discharge[1,2]	-	-	98%	98%
Heart Failure Care				
ACE Inhibitor or ARB for LVSD[1,2]	-	-	97%	97%
Discharge Instructions Given[2]	40	100%	92%	94%
Evaluation of LVS Function[2]	49	100%	99%	99%
Medicare Spending				
Medicare Spending per Patient (ratio)	-	0.97	0.95	0.98
Pneumonia Care				
Appropriate Initial Antibiotic Given[2]	93	92%	95%	95%
Blood Culture Timing[2]	152	99%	97%	98%
Pregnancy and Delivery Care				
Newborn Deliveries Scheduled Early	73	14%	8%	6%
Preventive Care				
Immunization for Influenza[2]	301	99%	88%	90%
Immunization for Pneumonia[2]	469	99%	90%	92%
Stroke Care				
Anticoagulation Therapy for Atrial Fibrillation[1]	-	-	94%	95%
Antithrombotic Therapy Timing	22	77%	97%	98%
Assessed for Rehabilitation	19	100%	97%	97%
Discharged on Antithrombotic Therapy	19	100%	98%	99%
Discharged on Statin Medication	16	69%	94%	94%
Thrombolytic Therapy Timing[1]	-	-	58%	66%
Venous Thromboembolism Prophylaxis	21	76%	92%	94%
Written Stroke Educational Materials Given[1]	-	-	84%	88%
Surgical Care Improvement Project				
Appropriate Beta Blocker Usage	21	100%	97%	98%
Appropriate VTP Within 24 Hours	95	96%	98%	98%
Controlled Postoperative Blood Glucose[7]	-	-	96%	97%
Perioperative Temperature Management	103	100%	100%	100%
Prophylactic Antibiotic Selection	66	100%	99%	99%
Prophylactic Antibiotic Selection (Outpatient)	119	95%	98%	98%
Prophylactic Antibiotic Stopped	59	92%	98%	98%
Prophylactic Antibiotic Timing	66	98%	99%	99%
Prophylactic Antibiotic Timing (Outpatient)	117	97%	98%	98%
Urinary Catheter Removal	34	91%	97%	97%
Survey of Patients' Hospital Experiences				
Area Around Room 'Always' Quiet at Night	300+	70%	66%	61%
Doctors 'Always' Communicated Well	300+	87%	83%	82%
Home Recovery Information Given	300+	89%	84%	85%
Hospital Given 9 or 10 on 10 Point Scale	300+	70%	69%	71%
Meds 'Always' Explained Before Given	300+	71%	63%	64%
Nurses 'Always' Communicated Well	300+	80%	78%	79%
Pain 'Always' Well Controlled	300+	75%	71%	71%
Room and Bathroom 'Always' Clean	300+	73%	71%	73%
Timely Help 'Always' Received	300+	72%	65%	68%
Would Definitely Recommend Hospital	300+	68%	70%	71%
Use of Medical Imaging				
Cardiac Imaging Stress Test before Surgery	202	5.0%	5.5%	5.3%
Combination Abdominal CT Scan	400	9.0%	10.1%	10.5%
Combination Brain/Sinus CT Scan[1]	-	-	2.3%	2.7%
Combination Chest CT Scan	149	8.7%	3.7%	2.7%
Follow-up Mammogram/Ultrasound	760	12.8%	8.9%	8.8%
Lumbar Spine MRI for Low Back Pain[1]	-	-	36.6%	37.2%

South Georgia Medical Center

2501 North Patterson Street, PO Box 1727 Phone: 229-333-1020
Valdosta, GA 31603 Fax: 229-259-4423
URL: www.sgmc.org
Type: Acute Care Hospitals Emergency Services: Yes
Ownership: Govt - Hospital Dist/Auth Beds: 330

Key Personnel:
Chairman/CEO . . . . William S. Cowart
Quality Assurance . . . . Susan Hurley, RN
Chief of Medical Staff . . . . Kim Megow, MD
Radiology . . . . William Querin, MD
Pediatric Ambulatory Care . . . . . . Maria Ranola, MD
CEO/President . . . . Randy Sauls
Surgery . . . . Timothy J. Schlairet, DO
Emergency Room . . . . Andre Shackleford

Measure	Cases	This Hosp.	State Avg.	U.S. Avg.
Blood Clot Prevention and Treatment				
Anticoagulation Overlap Therapy[2]	103	61%	90%	93%
ICU Venous Thromboembolism Prophylaxis[2]	192	69%	90%	92%
Incidence of Potentially Preventable VTE[2]	13	23%	13%	10%
UFH with Dosages/Platelet Monitoring[2]	30	67%	99%	97%
Venous Thromboembolism Prophylaxis[2]	438	72%	80%	85%
Warfarin Therapy Discharge Instructions[2]	82	74%	78%	75%
Chest Pain/Possible Heart Attack Care				
Aspirin Given Within 24 Hours of Arrival[3,7]	-	-	94%	96%
Fibrinolytic Meds Within 30 Min. of Arrival[5]	-	-	35%	58%
Average Time to ECG (minutes)[3,7]	-	-	8	7
Average Time to Transfer (minutes)[5]	-	-	73	60
Children's Asthma Care				
Received Home Management Plan of Care	-	-	-	88%
Received Reliever Medication	-	-	-	100%
Received Systemic Corticosteroids	-	-	-	100%
Emergency Department				
Admittance Decision Time (minutes)[2]	636	150	100	98
Head CT Results Within 45 Min. of Arrival	15	47%	45%	57%
Patients Who Left ER Before Being Seen	74,751	4%	3%	2%
Time from ER Arrival to Admit. (minutes)[2]	650	366	286	274
Time from ER Arrival to Discharge (minutes)	432	164	140	134
Time in ER Before Being Evaluated (minutes)	452	40	32	26
Time to Pain Meds for Fractures (minutes)	206	68	64	57
Heart Attack Care				
Aspirin Given at Discharge	331	100%	99%	99%
Fibrinolytic Meds Within 30 Min. of Arrival[1]	-	-	80%	54%
PCI Within 90 Minutes of Arrival	58	100%	95%	96%
Statin Prescribed at Discharge	322	100%	98%	98%
Heart Failure Care				
ACE Inhibitor or ARB for LVSD	165	99%	97%	97%
Discharge Instructions Given	403	95%	92%	94%
Evaluation of LVS Function	425	100%	99%	99%
Medicare Spending				
Medicare Spending per Patient (ratio)	-	0.96	0.95	0.98
Pneumonia Care				
Appropriate Initial Antibiotic Given	218	95%	95%	95%
Blood Culture Timing	292	97%	97%	98%
Pregnancy and Delivery Care				
Newborn Deliveries Scheduled Early[2]	51	6%	8%	6%
Preventive Care				
Immunization for Influenza[2]	670	86%	88%	90%
Immunization for Pneumonia[2]	757	87%	90%	92%
Stroke Care				
Anticoagulation Therapy for Atrial Fibrillation	17	94%	94%	95%
Antithrombotic Therapy Timing	153	99%	97%	98%
Assessed for Rehabilitation	190	99%	97%	97%
Discharged on Antithrombotic Therapy	175	99%	98%	99%
Discharged on Statin Medication	144	99%	94%	94%
Thrombolytic Therapy Timing	39	97%	58%	66%
Venous Thromboembolism Prophylaxis	200	99%	92%	94%
Written Stroke Educational Materials Given	122	89%	84%	88%
Surgical Care Improvement Project				
Appropriate Beta Blocker Usage	377	96%	97%	98%
Appropriate VTP Within 24 Hours	760	97%	98%	98%
Controlled Postoperative Blood Glucose	195	98%	96%	97%
Perioperative Temperature Management	857	100%	100%	100%
Prophylactic Antibiotic Selection	728	98%	99%	99%
Prophylactic Antibiotic Selection (Outpatient)	543	94%	98%	98%
Prophylactic Antibiotic Stopped	713	94%	98%	98%
Prophylactic Antibiotic Timing	729	98%	99%	99%
Prophylactic Antibiotic Timing (Outpatient)	547	98%	98%	98%
Urinary Catheter Removal	636	99%	97%	97%
Survey of Patients' Hospital Experiences				
Area Around Room 'Always' Quiet at Night	300+	65%	66%	61%
Doctors 'Always' Communicated Well	300+	82%	83%	82%
Home Recovery Information Given	300+	82%	84%	85%
Hospital Given 9 or 10 on 10 Point Scale	300+	71%	69%	71%
Meds 'Always' Explained Before Given	300+	64%	63%	64%
Nurses 'Always' Communicated Well	300+	79%	78%	79%
Pain 'Always' Well Controlled	300+	72%	71%	71%
Room and Bathroom 'Always' Clean	300+	69%	71%	73%
Timely Help 'Always' Received	300+	67%	65%	68%
Would Definitely Recommend Hospital	300+	75%	70%	71%
Use of Medical Imaging				
Cardiac Imaging Stress Test before Surgery	402	6.2%	5.5%	5.3%
Combination Abdominal CT Scan	1,694	25.4%	10.1%	10.5%
Combination Brain/Sinus CT Scan	1,326	2.2%	2.3%	2.7%
Combination Chest CT Scan	986	7.6%	3.7%	2.7%
Follow-up Mammogram/Ultrasound	2,147	8.8%	8.9%	8.8%
Lumbar Spine MRI for Low Back Pain	104	38.5%	36.6%	37.2%

Meadows Regional Medical Center

One Meadows Parkway Phone: 912-535-5828
Vidalia, GA 30474 Fax: 912-538-5529
Type: Acute Care Hospitals Emergency Services: Yes
Ownership: Voluntary non-profit - Other Beds: 122

Key Personnel:
Radiology . . . . David T Estle
Quality Assurance . . . . Mebny Jacobs
CEO/President . . . . Alan Kent
Emergency Room . . . . Marie Smith
Chairman/CEO . . . . Ronnie Stewart

Measure	Cases	This Hosp.	State Avg.	U.S. Avg.
Blood Clot Prevention and Treatment				
Anticoagulation Overlap Therapy[2]	38	84%	90%	93%
ICU Venous Thromboembolism Prophylaxis[2]	96	80%	90%	92%
Incidence of Potentially Preventable VTE[2]	14	43%	13%	10%
UFH with Dosages/Platelet Monitoring[2]	23	100%	99%	97%
Venous Thromboembolism Prophylaxis[2]	345	66%	80%	85%
Warfarin Therapy Discharge Instructions[2]	27	26%	78%	75%
Chest Pain/Possible Heart Attack Care				
Aspirin Given Within 24 Hours of Arrival	18	94%	94%	96%
Fibrinolytic Meds Within 30 Min. of Arrival[1,3]	-	-	35%	58%
Average Time to ECG (minutes)	18	7	8	7
Average Time to Transfer (minutes)[3,7]	-	-	73	60
Children's Asthma Care				
Received Home Management Plan of Care	-	-	-	88%
Received Reliever Medication	-	-	-	100%
Received Systemic Corticosteroids	-	-	-	100%
Emergency Department				
Admittance Decision Time (minutes)[2]	465	93	100	98
Head CT Results Within 45 Min. of Arrival	21	52%	45%	57%
Patients Who Left ER Before Being Seen	30,298	1%	3%	2%
Time from ER Arrival to Admit. (minutes)[2]	485	277	286	274
Time from ER Arrival to Discharge (minutes)	396	142	140	134
Time in ER Before Being Evaluated (minutes)	402	31	32	26
Time to Pain Meds for Fractures (minutes)	73	48	64	57
Heart Attack Care				
Aspirin Given at Discharge	117	100%	99%	99%
Fibrinolytic Meds Within 30 Min. of Arrival[1]	-	-	80%	54%
PCI Within 90 Minutes of Arrival	19	89%	95%	96%
Statin Prescribed at Discharge	107	93%	98%	98%
Heart Failure Care				
ACE Inhibitor or ARB for LVSD	59	90%	97%	97%
Discharge Instructions Given	172	91%	92%	94%
Evaluation of LVS Function	184	98%	99%	99%
Medicare Spending				
Medicare Spending per Patient (ratio)	-	0.95	0.95	0.98
Pneumonia Care				
Appropriate Initial Antibiotic Given	92	96%	95%	95%

NOTE: Hospital profiles are in alphabetical order by state, then city, then hospital within the city; Rankings exclude hospitals with less than 25 cases except for patient surveys which excludes hospitals with less than 100 cases; (a) 100-299 cases; (1) The number of cases/patients is too few to report; (2) Data submitted were based on a sample of cases/patients; (3) Results are based on a shorter time period than required; (4) Data suppressed by CMS for one or more quarters; (5) Results are not available for this reporting period; (6) Fewer than 100 patients completed the HCAHPS survey; (7) No cases met the criteria for this measure; (8) The lower limit of the confidence interval cannot be calculated if the number of observed infections equals zero; (9) No data are available from the state/territory for this reporting period; (10) The scores shown reflect fewer than 50 completed surveys; (11) There were discrepancies in the data collection process; (12) This measure does not apply to this hospital for this reporting period; (13) Results cannot be calculated for this reporting period; (14) The results for this state are combined with nearby states to protect confidentiality; Please refer to the User's Guide for a full explanation of data.

Measure	Cases	This Hosp.	State Avg.	U.S. Avg.
Blood Culture Timing	143	92%	97%	98%
Pregnancy and Delivery Care				
Newborn Deliveries Scheduled Early	72	0%	8%	6%
Preventive Care				
Immunization for Influenza[2]	471	95%	88%	90%
Immunization for Pneumonia[2]	551	95%	90%	92%
Stroke Care				
Anticoagulation Therapy for Atrial Fibrillation[1]	-	-	94%	95%
Antithrombotic Therapy Timing	47	89%	97%	98%
Assessed for Rehabilitation	52	94%	97%	97%
Discharged on Antithrombotic Therapy	50	92%	98%	99%
Discharged on Statin Medication	43	93%	94%	94%
Thrombolytic Therapy Timing[1]	-	-	58%	66%
Venous Thromboembolism Prophylaxis	48	69%	92%	94%
Written Stroke Educational Materials Given	35	0%	84%	88%
Surgical Care Improvement Project				
Appropriate Beta Blocker Usage	63	97%	97%	98%
Appropriate VTP Within 24 Hours	189	99%	98%	98%
Controlled Postoperative Blood Glucose[7]	-	-	96%	97%
Perioperative Temperature Management	212	99%	100%	100%
Prophylactic Antibiotic Selection	142	94%	99%	99%
Prophylactic Antibiotic Selection (Outpatient)	246	99%	98%	98%
Prophylactic Antibiotic Stopped	132	96%	98%	98%
Prophylactic Antibiotic Timing	142	98%	99%	99%
Prophylactic Antibiotic Timing (Outpatient)	247	98%	98%	98%
Urinary Catheter Removal	133	94%	97%	97%
Survey of Patients' Hospital Experiences				
Area Around Room 'Always' Quiet at Night	300+	72%	66%	61%
Doctors 'Always' Communicated Well	300+	85%	83%	82%
Home Recovery Information Given	300+	84%	84%	85%
Hospital Given 9 or 10 on 10 Point Scale	300+	76%	69%	71%
Meds 'Always' Explained Before Given	300+	64%	63%	64%
Nurses 'Always' Communicated Well	300+	81%	78%	79%
Pain 'Always' Well Controlled	300+	70%	71%	71%
Room and Bathroom 'Always' Clean	300+	79%	71%	73%
Timely Help 'Always' Received	300+	69%	65%	68%
Would Definitely Recommend Hospital	300+	74%	70%	71%
Use of Medical Imaging				
Cardiac Imaging Stress Test before Surgery	341	4.7%	5.5%	5.3%
Combination Abdominal CT Scan	795	12.6%	10.1%	10.5%
Combination Brain/Sinus CT Scan	620	2.7%	2.3%	2.7%
Combination Chest CT Scan	622	1.4%	3.7%	2.7%
Follow-up Mammogram/Ultrasound	812	8.7%	8.9%	8.8%
Lumbar Spine MRI for Low Back Pain	218	37.2%	36.6%	37.2%

Tanner Medical Center Villa Rica

601 Dallas Highway
Villa Rica, GA 30180
Phone: 770-456-3101
Fax: 770-456-7214
Type: Acute Care Hospitals
Emergency Services: Yes
Ownership: Govt - Hospital Dist/Auth
Beds: 52

Key Personnel:

Emergency Room . . . . Ben J Camp
Chief of Medical Staff. . . . . Benjamin J. Camp
Radiology. . . . . Eric Elder
Anesthesiology. . . . . Tunicia Girion
Quality Assurance . . . . Lea Hicks
President/CEO. . . . . Loy Howard
Infection Control. . . . . Lynne Valenti

Measure	Cases	This Hosp.	State Avg.	U.S. Avg.
Blood Clot Prevention and Treatment				
Anticoagulation Overlap Therapy[2]	27	85%	90%	93%
ICU Venous Thromboembolism Prophylaxis[2]	51	96%	90%	92%
Incidence of Potentially Preventable VTE[1,2]	-	-	13%	10%
UFH with Dosages/Platelet Monitoring[2]	29	97%	99%	97%
Venous Thromboembolism Prophylaxis[2]	137	93%	80%	85%
Warfarin Therapy Discharge Instructions[2]	27	81%	78%	75%
Chest Pain/Possible Heart Attack Care				
Aspirin Given Within 24 Hours of Arrival	52	100%	94%	96%
Fibrinolytic Meds Within 30 Min. of Arrival[7]	-	-	35%	58%
Average Time to ECG (minutes)	54	3	8	7
Average Time to Transfer (minutes)[1]	-	-	73	60
Children's Asthma Care				
Received Home Management Plan of Care	-	-	-	88%
Received Reliever Medication	-	-	-	100%
Received Systemic Corticosteroids	-	-	-	100%
Emergency Department				
Admittance Decision Time (minutes)[2]	246	52	100	98
Head CT Results Within 45 Min. of Arrival[1]	-	-	45%	57%
Patients Who Left ER Before Being Seen	39,689	3%	3%	2%
Time from ER Arrival to Admit. (minutes)[2]	257	235	286	274
Time from ER Arrival to Discharge (minutes)	385	139	140	134
Time in ER Before Being Evaluated (minutes)	306	40	32	26
Time to Pain Meds for Fractures (minutes)	118	71	64	57
Heart Attack Care				
Aspirin Given at Discharge	19	100%	99%	99%
Fibrinolytic Meds Within 30 Min. of Arrival[7]	-	-	80%	54%
PCI Within 90 Minutes of Arrival[7]	-	-	95%	96%
Statin Prescribed at Discharge	19	100%	98%	98%
Heart Failure Care				
ACE Inhibitor or ARB for LVSD	21	100%	97%	97%
Discharge Instructions Given	99	99%	92%	94%
Evaluation of LVS Function	105	100%	99%	99%
Medicare Spending				
Medicare Spending per Patient (ratio)	-	0.95	0.95	0.98
Pneumonia Care				
Appropriate Initial Antibiotic Given	78	97%	95%	95%
Blood Culture Timing	106	96%	97%	98%
Pregnancy and Delivery Care				
Newborn Deliveries Scheduled Early	48	0%	8%	6%
Preventive Care				
Immunization for Influenza[2]	235	96%	88%	90%
Immunization for Pneumonia[2]	279	97%	90%	92%
Stroke Care				
Anticoagulation Therapy for Atrial Fibrillation[1]	-	-	94%	95%
Antithrombotic Therapy Timing	29	93%	97%	98%
Assessed for Rehabilitation	30	97%	97%	97%
Discharged on Antithrombotic Therapy	30	90%	98%	99%
Discharged on Statin Medication	23	100%	94%	94%
Thrombolytic Therapy Timing[1]	-	-	58%	66%
Venous Thromboembolism Prophylaxis	31	100%	92%	94%
Written Stroke Educational Materials Given	22	95%	84%	88%
Surgical Care Improvement Project				
Appropriate Beta Blocker Usage[1]	-	-	97%	98%
Appropriate VTP Within 24 Hours	34	100%	98%	98%
Controlled Postoperative Blood Glucose[7]	-	-	96%	97%
Perioperative Temperature Management	41	100%	100%	100%
Prophylactic Antibiotic Selection	13	92%	99%	99%
Prophylactic Antibiotic Selection (Outpatient)	20	90%	98%	98%
Prophylactic Antibiotic Stopped	11	100%	98%	98%
Prophylactic Antibiotic Timing	13	92%	99%	99%
Prophylactic Antibiotic Timing (Outpatient)	20	100%	98%	98%
Urinary Catheter Removal	14	100%	97%	97%
Survey of Patients' Hospital Experiences				
Area Around Room 'Always' Quiet at Night	300+	72%	66%	61%
Doctors 'Always' Communicated Well	300+	85%	83%	82%
Home Recovery Information Given	300+	84%	84%	85%
Hospital Given 9 or 10 on 10 Point Scale	300+	79%	69%	71%
Meds 'Always' Explained Before Given	300+	69%	63%	64%
Nurses 'Always' Communicated Well	300+	84%	78%	79%
Pain 'Always' Well Controlled	300+	75%	71%	71%
Room and Bathroom 'Always' Clean	300+	79%	71%	73%
Timely Help 'Always' Received	300+	75%	65%	68%
Would Definitely Recommend Hospital	300+	78%	70%	71%
Use of Medical Imaging				
Cardiac Imaging Stress Test before Surgery	119	4.2%	5.5%	5.3%
Combination Abdominal CT Scan	486	8.8%	10.1%	10.5%
Combination Brain/Sinus CT Scan	343	1.2%	2.3%	2.7%
Combination Chest CT Scan	245	3.7%	3.7%	2.7%
Follow-up Mammogram/Ultrasound	511	7.2%	8.9%	8.8%
Lumbar Spine MRI for Low Back Pain[1]	-	-	36.6%	37.2%

Warm Springs Medical Center

5995 Spring Street
Warm Springs, GA 31830
Phone: 706-655-9351
Fax: 706-655-9233
Type: Critical Access Hospitals
Emergency Services: Yes
Ownership: Voluntary non-profit - Other
Beds: 25

Key Personnel:

CEO/President. . . . . John Dixon
Quality Assurance . . . . Anne Hudgins
Operating Room. . . . . Brooke Jones
Emergency Room . . . . James Ragan, MD
Cardiology . . . . Angampally Rajeev, MD
Chief of Medical Staff . . . . George E Thompson

Measure	Cases	This Hosp.	State Avg.	U.S. Avg.
Blood Clot Prevention and Treatment				
Anticoagulation Overlap Therapy[5]	-	-	90%	93%
ICU Venous Thromboembolism Prophylaxis[5]	-	-	90%	92%
Incidence of Potentially Preventable VTE[5]	-	-	13%	10%
UFH with Dosages/Platelet Monitoring[5]	-	-	99%	97%
Venous Thromboembolism Prophylaxis[5]	-	-	80%	85%
Warfarin Therapy Discharge Instructions[5]	-	-	78%	75%
Chest Pain/Possible Heart Attack Care				
Aspirin Given Within 24 Hours of Arrival	-	-	94%	96%
Fibrinolytic Meds Within 30 Min. of Arrival	-	-	35%	58%
Average Time to ECG (minutes)	-	-	8	7
Average Time to Transfer (minutes)	-	-	73	60
Children's Asthma Care				
Received Home Management Plan of Care	-	-	-	88%
Received Reliever Medication	-	-	-	100%
Received Systemic Corticosteroids	-	-	-	100%
Emergency Department				
Admittance Decision Time (minutes)[5]	-	-	100	98
Head CT Results Within 45 Min. of Arrival	-	-	45%	57%
Patients Who Left ER Before Being Seen	-	-	3%	2%
Time from ER Arrival to Admit. (minutes)[5]	-	-	286	274
Time from ER Arrival to Discharge (minutes)	-	-	140	134
Time in ER Before Being Evaluated (minutes)	-	-	32	26
Time to Pain Meds for Fractures (minutes)	-	-	64	57
Heart Attack Care				
Aspirin Given at Discharge[5]	-	-	99%	99%
Fibrinolytic Meds Within 30 Min. of Arrival[5]	-	-	80%	54%
PCI Within 90 Minutes of Arrival[5]	-	-	95%	96%
Statin Prescribed at Discharge[5]	-	-	98%	98%
Heart Failure Care				
ACE Inhibitor or ARB for LVSD[1,3]	-	-	97%	97%
Discharge Instructions Given[3]	14	79%	92%	94%
Evaluation of LVS Function[3]	15	87%	99%	99%
Medicare Spending				
Medicare Spending per Patient (ratio)	-	-	0.95	0.98
Pneumonia Care				
Appropriate Initial Antibiotic Given[1,3]	-	-	95%	95%
Blood Culture Timing[1,3]	-	-	97%	98%
Pregnancy and Delivery Care				
Newborn Deliveries Scheduled Early[5]	-	-	8%	6%
Preventive Care				
Immunization for Influenza[5]	-	-	88%	90%
Immunization for Pneumonia[5]	-	-	90%	92%
Stroke Care				
Anticoagulation Therapy for Atrial Fibrillation[5]	-	-	94%	95%
Antithrombotic Therapy Timing[5]	-	-	97%	98%
Assessed for Rehabilitation[5]	-	-	97%	97%
Discharged on Antithrombotic Therapy[5]	-	-	98%	99%
Discharged on Statin Medication[5]	-	-	94%	94%
Thrombolytic Therapy Timing[5]	-	-	58%	66%
Venous Thromboembolism Prophylaxis[5]	-	-	92%	94%
Written Stroke Educational Materials Given[5]	-	-	84%	88%
Surgical Care Improvement Project				
Appropriate Beta Blocker Usage[5]	-	-	97%	98%
Appropriate VTP Within 24 Hours[5]	-	-	98%	98%
Controlled Postoperative Blood Glucose[5]	-	-	96%	97%
Perioperative Temperature Management[5]	-	-	100%	100%
Prophylactic Antibiotic Selection[5]	-	-	99%	99%
Prophylactic Antibiotic Selection (Outpatient)	-	-	98%	98%
Prophylactic Antibiotic Stopped[5]	-	-	98%	98%
Prophylactic Antibiotic Timing[5]	-	-	99%	99%
Prophylactic Antibiotic Timing (Outpatient)	-	-	98%	98%
Urinary Catheter Removal[5]	-	-	97%	97%
Survey of Patients' Hospital Experiences				
Area Around Room 'Always' Quiet at Night[5]	-	-	66%	61%
Doctors 'Always' Communicated Well[5]	-	-	83%	82%

NOTE: Hospital profiles are in alphabetical order by state, then city, then hospital within the city; Rankings exclude hospitals with less than 25 cases except for patient surveys which excludes hospitals with less than 100 cases; (a) 100-299 cases; (1) The number of cases/patients is too few to report; (2) Data submitted were based on a sample of cases/patients; (3) Results are based on a shorter time period than required; (4) Data suppressed by CMS for one or more quarters; (5) Results are not available for this reporting period; (6) Fewer than 100 patients completed the HCAHPS survey; (7) No cases met the criteria for this measure; (8) The lower limit of the confidence interval cannot be calculated if the number of observed infections equals zero; (9) No data are available from the state/territory for this reporting period; (10) The scores shown reflect fewer than 50 completed surveys; (11) There were discrepancies in the data collection process; (12) This measure does not apply to this hospital for this reporting period; (13) Results cannot be calculated for this reporting period; (14) The results for this state are combined with nearby states to protect confidentiality; Please refer to the User's Guide for a full explanation of data.

Measure	Cases	This Hosp.	State Avg.	U.S. Avg.
Home Recovery Information Given[5]	-	-	84%	85%
Hospital Given 9 or 10 on 10 Point Scale[5]	-	-	69%	71%
Meds 'Always' Explained Before Given[5]	-	-	63%	64%
Nurses 'Always' Communicated Well[5]	-	-	78%	79%
Pain 'Always' Well Controlled[5]	-	-	71%	71%
Room and Bathroom 'Always' Clean[5]	-	-	71%	73%
Timely Help 'Always' Received[5]	-	-	65%	68%
Would Definitely Recommend Hospital[5]	-	-	70%	71%
Use of Medical Imaging				
Cardiac Imaging Stress Test before Surgery	-	-	5.5%	5.3%
Combination Abdominal CT Scan	-	-	10.1%	10.5%
Combination Brain/Sinus CT Scan	-	-	2.3%	2.7%
Combination Chest CT Scan	-	-	3.7%	2.7%
Follow-up Mammogram/Ultrasound	-	-	8.9%	8.8%
Lumbar Spine MRI for Low Back Pain	-	-	36.6%	37.2%

Houston Medical Center

1601 Watson Boulevard
Warner Robins, GA 31093
URL: www.hhc.org
Type: Acute Care Hospitals
Ownership: Voluntary non-profit - Private

Phone: 478-922-4281
Fax: 478-542-7955
Emergency Services: Yes
Beds: 198

Key Personnel:
Radiology. . . . . Maher A Abdulla, MD
Pediatric In-Patient Care . . . . David N Harvey, MD
Chief of Medical Staff. . . . . Samuel O Johnson, MD
CEO/President. . . . . Grady W Philips III, MBA
Cardiac Laboratory. . . . . Karen Talton
Operating Room. . . . . Diane Taylor
Quality Assurance . . . . Elisabeth Walker
Emergency Room . . . . Carla Weese

Measure	Cases	This Hosp.	State Avg.	U.S. Avg.
Blood Clot Prevention and Treatment				
Anticoagulation Overlap Therapy[2]	113	69%	90%	93%
ICU Venous Thromboembolism Prophylaxis[2]	25	72%	90%	92%
Incidence of Potentially Preventable VTE[2]	19	63%	13%	10%
UFH with Dosages/Platelet Monitoring[2]	49	94%	99%	97%
Venous Thromboembolism Prophylaxis[2]	381	52%	80%	85%
Warfarin Therapy Discharge Instructions[2]	88	34%	78%	75%
Chest Pain/Possible Heart Attack Care				
Aspirin Given Within 24 Hours of Arrival	28	96%	94%	96%
Fibrinolytic Meds Within 30 Min. of Arrival[3,7]	-	-	35%	58%
Average Time to ECG (minutes)	28	0	8	7
Average Time to Transfer (minutes)[3,7]	-	-	73	60
Children's Asthma Care				
Received Home Management Plan of Care	-	-	-	88%
Received Reliever Medication	-	-	-	100%
Received Systemic Corticosteroids	-	-	-	100%
Emergency Department				
Admittance Decision Time (minutes)[2]	627	130	100	98
Head CT Results Within 45 Min. of Arrival[1,3]	-	-	45%	57%
Patients Who Left ER Before Being Seen	26,978	10%	3%	2%
Time from ER Arrival to Admit. (minutes)[2]	640	380	286	274
Time from ER Arrival to Discharge (minutes)	380	206	140	134
Time in ER Before Being Evaluated (minutes)	397	39	32	26
Time to Pain Meds for Fractures (minutes)	101	85	64	57
Heart Attack Care				
Aspirin Given at Discharge	155	98%	99%	99%
Fibrinolytic Meds Within 30 Min. of Arrival[7]	-	-	80%	54%
PCI Within 90 Minutes of Arrival	33	91%	95%	96%
Statin Prescribed at Discharge	144	95%	98%	98%
Heart Failure Care				
ACE Inhibitor or ARB for LVSD[2]	105	96%	97%	97%
Discharge Instructions Given[2]	299	88%	92%	94%
Evaluation of LVS Function[2]	340	100%	99%	99%
Medicare Spending				
Medicare Spending per Patient (ratio)	-	0.98	0.95	0.98
Pneumonia Care				
Appropriate Initial Antibiotic Given[2]	102	96%	95%	95%
Blood Culture Timing[2]	138	96%	97%	98%
Pregnancy and Delivery Care				
Newborn Deliveries Scheduled Early[2]	46	4%	8%	6%
Preventive Care				
Immunization for Influenza[2]	531	89%	88%	90%
Immunization for Pneumonia[2]	623	95%	90%	92%
Stroke Care				
Anticoagulation Therapy for Atrial Fibrillation[1]	-	-	94%	95%
Antithrombotic Therapy Timing	89	88%	97%	98%
Assessed for Rehabilitation	74	91%	97%	97%
Discharged on Antithrombotic Therapy	71	92%	98%	99%
Discharged on Statin Medication	60	87%	94%	94%
Thrombolytic Therapy Timing[1]	-	-	58%	66%
Venous Thromboembolism Prophylaxis	96	64%	92%	94%
Written Stroke Educational Materials Given	49	14%	84%	88%
Surgical Care Improvement Project				
Appropriate Beta Blocker Usage[2]	130	98%	97%	98%
Appropriate VTP Within 24 Hours[2]	414	97%	98%	98%
Controlled Postoperative Blood Glucose[2,7]	-	-	96%	97%
Perioperative Temperature Management[2]	447	100%	100%	100%
Prophylactic Antibiotic Selection[2]	254	98%	99%	99%
Prophylactic Antibiotic Selection (Outpatient)	230	96%	98%	98%
Prophylactic Antibiotic Stopped[2]	244	92%	98%	98%
Prophylactic Antibiotic Timing[2]	254	100%	99%	99%
Prophylactic Antibiotic Timing (Outpatient)	237	93%	98%	98%
Urinary Catheter Removal[2]	190	93%	97%	97%
Survey of Patients' Hospital Experiences				
Area Around Room 'Always' Quiet at Night	300+	64%	66%	61%
Doctors 'Always' Communicated Well	300+	80%	83%	82%
Home Recovery Information Given	300+	85%	84%	85%
Hospital Given 9 or 10 on 10 Point Scale	300+	71%	69%	71%
Meds 'Always' Explained Before Given	300+	62%	63%	64%
Nurses 'Always' Communicated Well	300+	77%	78%	79%
Pain 'Always' Well Controlled	300+	68%	71%	71%
Room and Bathroom 'Always' Clean	300+	66%	71%	73%
Timely Help 'Always' Received	300+	64%	65%	68%
Would Definitely Recommend Hospital	300+	71%	70%	71%
Use of Medical Imaging				
Cardiac Imaging Stress Test before Surgery[1]	-	-	5.5%	5.3%
Combination Abdominal CT Scan	1,198	22.1%	10.1%	10.5%
Combination Brain/Sinus CT Scan	1,097	2.6%	2.3%	2.7%
Combination Chest CT Scan	782	8.8%	3.7%	2.7%
Follow-up Mammogram/Ultrasound	1,542	4.4%	8.9%	8.8%
Lumbar Spine MRI for Low Back Pain	82	37.8%	36.6%	37.2%

Wills Memorial Hospital

120 Gordon Street
Washington, GA 30673
URL: www.willsmemorialhospital.com
Type: Critical Access Hospitals
Ownership: Govt - Hospital Dist/Auth

Phone: 706-678-9212
Fax: 706-678-4051
Emergency Services: Yes
Beds: 25

Key Personnel:
Emergency Room . . . . Kristi Bradford, RN
Intensive Care Unit. . . . . Kristi Bradford, RN
CEO/President. . . . . T Marvin Goldman
Operating Room. . . . . D Scott Lind, RN
Quality Assurance . . . . Phil S Robb
Infection Control. . . . . Laurie Sargent
Chief of Medical Staff . . . . Robert J Williams, MD

Measure	Cases	This Hosp.	State Avg.	U.S. Avg.
Blood Clot Prevention and Treatment				
Anticoagulation Overlap Therapy[5]	-	-	90%	93%
ICU Venous Thromboembolism Prophylaxis[5]	-	-	90%	92%
Incidence of Potentially Preventable VTE[5]	-	-	13%	10%
UFH with Dosages/Platelet Monitoring[5]	-	-	99%	97%
Venous Thromboembolism Prophylaxis[5]	-	-	80%	85%
Warfarin Therapy Discharge Instructions[5]	-	-	78%	75%
Chest Pain/Possible Heart Attack Care				
Aspirin Given Within 24 Hours of Arrival[5]	-	-	94%	96%
Fibrinolytic Meds Within 30 Min. of Arrival[5]	-	-	35%	58%
Average Time to ECG (minutes)[5]	-	-	8	7
Average Time to Transfer (minutes)[5]	-	-	73	60
Children's Asthma Care				
Received Home Management Plan of Care	-	-	-	88%
Received Reliever Medication	-	-	-	100%
Received Systemic Corticosteroids	-	-	-	100%
Emergency Department				
Admittance Decision Time (minutes)[2]	286	40	100	98
Head CT Results Within 45 Min. of Arrival[5]	-	-	45%	57%
Patients Who Left ER Before Being Seen	5,521	0%	3%	2%
Time from ER Arrival to Admit. (minutes)[2]	286	150	286	274
Time from ER Arrival to Discharge (minutes)[5]	-	-	140	134
Time in ER Before Being Evaluated (minutes)[5]	-	-	32	26
Time to Pain Meds for Fractures (minutes)[5]	-	-	64	57
Heart Attack Care				
Aspirin Given at Discharge[1]	-	-	99%	99%
Fibrinolytic Meds Within 30 Min. of Arrival[7]	-	-	80%	54%
PCI Within 90 Minutes of Arrival[7]	-	-	95%	96%
Statin Prescribed at Discharge[1]	-	-	98%	98%
Heart Failure Care				
ACE Inhibitor or ARB for LVSD	13	92%	97%	97%
Discharge Instructions Given	33	100%	92%	94%
Evaluation of LVS Function	48	96%	99%	99%
Medicare Spending				
Medicare Spending per Patient (ratio)	-	-	0.95	0.98
Pneumonia Care				
Appropriate Initial Antibiotic Given	44	64%	95%	95%
Blood Culture Timing	13	100%	97%	98%
Pregnancy and Delivery Care				
Newborn Deliveries Scheduled Early[7]	-	-	8%	6%
Preventive Care				
Immunization for Influenza[2]	279	64%	88%	90%
Immunization for Pneumonia[2]	456	58%	90%	92%
Stroke Care				
Anticoagulation Therapy for Atrial Fibrillation[5]	-	-	94%	95%
Antithrombotic Therapy Timing[5]	-	-	97%	98%
Assessed for Rehabilitation[5]	-	-	97%	97%
Discharged on Antithrombotic Therapy[5]	-	-	98%	99%
Discharged on Statin Medication[5]	-	-	94%	94%
Thrombolytic Therapy Timing[5]	-	-	58%	66%
Venous Thromboembolism Prophylaxis[5]	-	-	92%	94%
Written Stroke Educational Materials Given[5]	-	-	84%	88%
Surgical Care Improvement Project				
Appropriate Beta Blocker Usage[5]	-	-	97%	98%
Appropriate VTP Within 24 Hours[5]	-	-	98%	98%
Controlled Postoperative Blood Glucose[5]	-	-	96%	97%
Perioperative Temperature Management[5]	-	-	100%	100%
Prophylactic Antibiotic Selection[5]	-	-	99%	99%
Prophylactic Antibiotic Selection (Outpatient)[5]	-	-	98%	98%
Prophylactic Antibiotic Stopped[5]	-	-	98%	98%
Prophylactic Antibiotic Timing[5]	-	-	99%	99%
Prophylactic Antibiotic Timing (Outpatient)[5]	-	-	98%	98%
Urinary Catheter Removal[5]	-	-	97%	97%
Survey of Patients' Hospital Experiences				
Area Around Room 'Always' Quiet at Night[5]	-	-	66%	61%
Doctors 'Always' Communicated Well[5]	-	-	83%	82%
Home Recovery Information Given[5]	-	-	84%	85%
Hospital Given 9 or 10 on 10 Point Scale[5]	-	-	69%	71%
Meds 'Always' Explained Before Given[5]	-	-	63%	64%
Nurses 'Always' Communicated Well[5]	-	-	78%	79%
Pain 'Always' Well Controlled[5]	-	-	71%	71%
Room and Bathroom 'Always' Clean[5]	-	-	71%	73%
Timely Help 'Always' Received[5]	-	-	65%	68%
Would Definitely Recommend Hospital[5]	-	-	70%	71%
Use of Medical Imaging				
Cardiac Imaging Stress Test before Surgery[7]	-	-	5.5%	5.3%
Combination Abdominal CT Scan	97	39.2%	10.1%	10.5%
Combination Brain/Sinus CT Scan[1]	-	-	2.3%	2.7%
Combination Chest CT Scan	54	33.3%	3.7%	2.7%
Follow-up Mammogram/Ultrasound[7]	-	-	8.9%	8.8%
Lumbar Spine MRI for Low Back Pain[1]	-	-	36.6%	37.2%

Mayo Clinic Health System - Waycross

1900 Tebeau Street
Waycross, GA 31501
E-mail: info@satilla.org
URL: www.satilla.org
Type: Acute Care Hospitals
Ownership: Voluntary non-profit - Private

Phone: 912-287-2500
Fax: 912-287-2505
Emergency Services: Yes
Beds: 231

Key Personnel:
Radiology. . . . . Richard Clinton
Chief of Medical Staff . . . . Wade Dye, MD
Emergency Room . . . . James Hagen Bottom, MD
Operating Room. . . . . Dubose Medlock

NOTE: Hospital profiles are in alphabetical order by state, then city, then hospital within the city; Rankings exclude hospitals with less than 25 cases except for patient surveys which excludes hospitals with less than 100 cases; (a) 100-299 cases; (1) The number of cases/patients is too few to report; (2) Data submitted were based on a sample of cases/patients; (3) Results are based on a shorter time period than required; (4) Data suppressed by CMS for one or more quarters; (5) Results are not available for this reporting period; (6) Fewer than 100 patients completed the HCAHPS survey; (7) No cases met the criteria for this measure; (8) The lower limit of the confidence interval cannot be calculated if the number of observed infections equals zero; (9) No data are available from the state/territory for this reporting period; (10) The scores shown reflect fewer than 50 completed surveys; (11) There were discrepancies in the data collection process; (12) This measure does not apply to this hospital for this reporting period; (13) Results cannot be calculated for this reporting period; (14) The results for this state are combined with nearby states to protect confidentiality; Please refer to the User's Guide for a full explanation of data.

CEO/President. . . . . Robert M Trimm
Quality Assurance . . . . Linda Wilson

Measure	Cases	This Hosp.	State Avg.	U.S. Avg.
Blood Clot Prevention and Treatment				
Anticoagulation Overlap Therapy[2]	75	79%	90%	93%
ICU Venous Thromboembolism Prophylaxis[2]	95	85%	90%	92%
Incidence of Potentially Preventable VTE[2]	13	15%	13%	10%
UFH with Dosages/Platelet Monitoring[2]	43	100%	99%	97%
Venous Thromboembolism Prophylaxis[2]	382	74%	80%	85%
Warfarin Therapy Discharge Instructions[2]	58	93%	78%	75%
Chest Pain/Possible Heart Attack Care				
Aspirin Given Within 24 Hours of Arrival	34	94%	94%	96%
Fibrinolytic Meds Within 30 Min. of Arrival[7]	-	-	35%	58%
Average Time to ECG (minutes)	37	9	8	7
Average Time to Transfer (minutes)[1]	-	-	73	60
Children's Asthma Care				
Received Home Management Plan of Care	-	-	-	88%
Received Reliever Medication	-	-	-	100%
Received Systemic Corticosteroids	-	-	-	100%
Emergency Department				
Admittance Decision Time (minutes)[2]	993	82	100	98
Head CT Results Within 45 Min. of Arrival[1]	-	-	45%	57%
Patients Who Left ER Before Being Seen	48,775	3%	3%	2%
Time from ER Arrival to Admit. (minutes)[2]	995	244	286	274
Time from ER Arrival to Discharge (minutes)	443	136	140	134
Time in ER Before Being Evaluated (minutes)	471	42	32	26
Time to Pain Meds for Fractures (minutes)	123	74	64	57
Heart Attack Care				
Aspirin Given at Discharge[2]	93	97%	99%	99%
Fibrinolytic Meds Within 30 Min. of Arrival[2,7]	-	-	80%	54%
PCI Within 90 Minutes of Arrival[2]	26	96%	95%	96%
Statin Prescribed at Discharge[2]	92	99%	98%	98%
Heart Failure Care				
ACE Inhibitor or ARB for LVSD[2]	77	95%	97%	97%
Discharge Instructions Given[2]	200	100%	92%	94%
Evaluation of LVS Function[2]	256	100%	99%	99%
Medicare Spending				
Medicare Spending per Patient (ratio)	-	0.97	0.95	0.98
Pneumonia Care				
Appropriate Initial Antibiotic Given[2]	135	87%	95%	95%
Blood Culture Timing[2]	221	94%	97%	98%
Pregnancy and Delivery Care				
Newborn Deliveries Scheduled Early	89	8%	8%	6%
Preventive Care				
Immunization for Influenza[2]	980	83%	88%	90%
Immunization for Pneumonia[2]	1,222	79%	90%	92%
Stroke Care				
Anticoagulation Therapy for Atrial Fibrillation	16	69%	94%	95%
Antithrombotic Therapy Timing	76	96%	97%	98%
Assessed for Rehabilitation	94	86%	97%	97%
Discharged on Antithrombotic Therapy	83	94%	98%	99%
Discharged on Statin Medication	74	78%	94%	94%
Thrombolytic Therapy Timing	12	50%	58%	66%
Venous Thromboembolism Prophylaxis	90	73%	92%	94%
Written Stroke Educational Materials Given	54	65%	84%	88%
Surgical Care Improvement Project				
Appropriate Beta Blocker Usage	109	97%	97%	98%
Appropriate VTP Within 24 Hours	231	96%	98%	98%
Controlled Postoperative Blood Glucose[7]	-	-	96%	97%
Perioperative Temperature Management	285	100%	100%	100%
Prophylactic Antibiotic Selection	196	98%	99%	99%
Prophylactic Antibiotic Selection (Outpatient)	129	98%	98%	98%
Prophylactic Antibiotic Stopped	187	95%	98%	98%
Prophylactic Antibiotic Timing	196	99%	99%	99%
Prophylactic Antibiotic Timing (Outpatient)	124	99%	98%	98%
Urinary Catheter Removal	113	96%	97%	97%
Survey of Patients' Hospital Experiences				
Area Around Room 'Always' Quiet at Night	300+	65%	66%	61%
Doctors 'Always' Communicated Well	300+	82%	83%	82%
Home Recovery Information Given	300+	85%	84%	85%
Hospital Given 9 or 10 on 10 Point Scale	300+	69%	69%	71%
Meds 'Always' Explained Before Given	300+	67%	63%	64%
Nurses 'Always' Communicated Well	300+	81%	78%	79%
Pain 'Always' Well Controlled	300+	72%	71%	71%
Room and Bathroom 'Always' Clean	300+	74%	71%	73%
Timely Help 'Always' Received	300+	69%	65%	68%
Would Definitely Recommend Hospital	300+	65%	70%	71%
Use of Medical Imaging				
Cardiac Imaging Stress Test before Surgery	425	4.7%	5.5%	5.3%
Combination Abdominal CT Scan	954	1.7%	10.1%	10.5%
Combination Brain/Sinus CT Scan	865	4.6%	2.3%	2.7%
Combination Chest CT Scan	657	0.0%	3.7%	2.7%
Follow-up Mammogram/Ultrasound	1,305	6.9%	8.9%	8.8%
Lumbar Spine MRI for Low Back Pain	188	36.7%	36.6%	37.2%

Burke Medical Center

351 Liberty Street
Waynesboro, GA 30830
E-mail: dhighsmith@burke.net
Type: Acute Care Hospitals
Ownership: Proprietary

Phone: 706-554-4435
Fax: 706-554-4854
Emergency Services: Yes
Beds: 40

Key Personnel:
Anesthesiology. . . . . Herb Dingbaum, CRNA
Pediatrics. . . . . Shelley Griffin, MD
Emergency Room . . . . Julie Herrmann, RN
Operating Room. . . . . Cheryl Hollingsworth, RN
Chief of Medical Staff. . . . . Doug Keir
Infection Control. . . . . Mary Owens, RN
Radiology. . . . . Tammie Salter
Quality Assurance . . . . Liz Walker

Measure	Cases	This Hosp.	State Avg.	U.S. Avg.
Blood Clot Prevention and Treatment				
Anticoagulation Overlap Therapy[1,2]	-	-	90%	93%
ICU Venous Thromboembolism Prophylaxis[2,7]	-	-	90%	92%
Incidence of Potentially Preventable VTE[2,7]	-	-	13%	10%
UFH with Dosages/Platelet Monitoring[2,7]	-	-	99%	97%
Venous Thromboembolism Prophylaxis[2]	114	38%	80%	85%
Warfarin Therapy Discharge Instructions[2,7]	-	-	78%	75%
Chest Pain/Possible Heart Attack Care				
Aspirin Given Within 24 Hours of Arrival	22	100%	94%	96%
Fibrinolytic Meds Within 30 Min. of Arrival[7]	-	-	35%	58%
Average Time to ECG (minutes)	24	17	8	7
Average Time to Transfer (minutes)[7]	-	-	73	60
Children's Asthma Care				
Received Home Management Plan of Care	-	-	-	88%
Received Reliever Medication	-	-	-	100%
Received Systemic Corticosteroids	-	-	-	100%
Emergency Department				
Admittance Decision Time (minutes)[2]	95	83	100	98
Head CT Results Within 45 Min. of Arrival[1]	-	-	45%	57%
Patients Who Left ER Before Being Seen	8,729	1%	3%	2%
Time from ER Arrival to Admit. (minutes)[2]	108	234	286	274
Time from ER Arrival to Discharge (minutes)[11]	407	89	140	134
Time in ER Before Being Evaluated (minutes)	457	26	32	26
Time to Pain Meds for Fractures (minutes)	30	57	64	57
Heart Attack Care				
Aspirin Given at Discharge[3,7]	-	-	99%	99%
Fibrinolytic Meds Within 30 Min. of Arrival[3,7]	-	-	80%	54%
PCI Within 90 Minutes of Arrival[3,7]	-	-	95%	96%
Statin Prescribed at Discharge[3,7]	-	-	98%	98%
Heart Failure Care				
ACE Inhibitor or ARB for LVSD[1]	-	-	97%	97%
Discharge Instructions Given[1]	-	-	92%	94%
Evaluation of LVS Function[1]	-	-	99%	99%
Medicare Spending				
Medicare Spending per Patient (ratio)	-	0.84	0.95	0.98
Pneumonia Care				
Appropriate Initial Antibiotic Given	26	88%	95%	95%
Blood Culture Timing	31	87%	97%	98%
Pregnancy and Delivery Care				
Newborn Deliveries Scheduled Early[7]	-	-	8%	6%
Preventive Care				
Immunization for Influenza[2]	157	34%	88%	90%
Immunization for Pneumonia[2]	138	43%	90%	92%
Stroke Care				
Anticoagulation Therapy for Atrial Fibrillation[3,7]	-	-	94%	95%
Antithrombotic Therapy Timing[3,7]	-	-	97%	98%
Assessed for Rehabilitation[3,7]	-	-	97%	97%
Discharged on Antithrombotic Therapy[3,7]	-	-	98%	99%
Discharged on Statin Medication[3,7]	-	-	94%	94%
Thrombolytic Therapy Timing[3,7]	-	-	58%	66%
Venous Thromboembolism Prophylaxis[3,7]	-	-	92%	94%
Written Stroke Educational Materials Given[3,7]	-	-	84%	88%
Surgical Care Improvement Project				
Appropriate Beta Blocker Usage[3,7]	-	-	97%	98%
Appropriate VTP Within 24 Hours[1,3]	-	-	98%	98%
Controlled Postoperative Blood Glucose[3,7]	-	-	96%	97%
Perioperative Temperature Management[1,3]	-	-	100%	100%
Prophylactic Antibiotic Selection[3,7]	-	-	99%	99%
Prophylactic Antibiotic Selection (Outpatient)[1,3]	-	-	98%	98%
Prophylactic Antibiotic Stopped[3,7]	-	-	98%	98%
Prophylactic Antibiotic Timing[3,7]	-	-	99%	99%
Prophylactic Antibiotic Timing (Outpatient)[1,3]	-	-	98%	98%
Urinary Catheter Removal[3,7]	-	-	97%	97%
Survey of Patients' Hospital Experiences				
Area Around Room 'Always' Quiet at Night[6]	<100	79%	66%	61%
Doctors 'Always' Communicated Well[6]	<100	90%	83%	82%
Home Recovery Information Given[6]	<100	84%	84%	85%
Hospital Given 9 or 10 on 10 Point Scale[6]	<100	67%	69%	71%
Meds 'Always' Explained Before Given[6]	<100	53%	63%	64%
Nurses 'Always' Communicated Well[6]	<100	85%	78%	79%
Pain 'Always' Well Controlled[6]	<100	73%	71%	71%
Room and Bathroom 'Always' Clean[6]	<100	77%	71%	73%
Timely Help 'Always' Received[6]	<100	76%	65%	68%
Would Definitely Recommend Hospital[6]	<100	67%	70%	71%
Use of Medical Imaging				
Cardiac Imaging Stress Test before Surgery[7]	-	-	5.5%	5.3%
Combination Abdominal CT Scan	103	5.8%	10.1%	10.5%
Combination Brain/Sinus CT Scan[1]	-	-	2.3%	2.7%
Combination Chest CT Scan[1]	-	-	3.7%	2.7%
Follow-up Mammogram/Ultrasound	299	13.7%	8.9%	8.8%
Lumbar Spine MRI for Low Back Pain[7]	-	-	36.6%	37.2%

Barrow Regional Medical Center

316 North Broad Street
Winder, GA 30680
URL: www.barrowmedical.com
Type: Acute Care Hospitals
Ownership: Proprietary

Phone: 770-307-5210
Fax: 770-307-5215
Emergency Services: Yes
Beds: 56

Key Personnel:
Operating Room. . . . . Christopher J Brandys, RN
Radiology. . . . . David A Causey, MD
Quality Assurance . . . . Kathy Haymon
CEO/President. . . . . Randy Mills

Measure	Cases	This Hosp.	State Avg.	U.S. Avg.
Blood Clot Prevention and Treatment				
Anticoagulation Overlap Therapy[2]	28	96%	90%	93%
ICU Venous Thromboembolism Prophylaxis[2]	77	96%	90%	92%
Incidence of Potentially Preventable VTE[1,2]	-	-	13%	10%
UFH with Dosages/Platelet Monitoring[2]	25	100%	99%	97%
Venous Thromboembolism Prophylaxis[2]	225	91%	80%	85%
Warfarin Therapy Discharge Instructions[2]	23	91%	78%	75%
Chest Pain/Possible Heart Attack Care				
Aspirin Given Within 24 Hours of Arrival	43	95%	94%	96%
Fibrinolytic Meds Within 30 Min. of Arrival[1]	-	-	35%	58%
Average Time to ECG (minutes)	46	10	8	7
Average Time to Transfer (minutes)[1]	-	-	73	60
Children's Asthma Care				
Received Home Management Plan of Care	-	-	-	88%
Received Reliever Medication	-	-	-	100%
Received Systemic Corticosteroids	-	-	-	100%
Emergency Department				
Admittance Decision Time (minutes)[2]	548	161	100	98
Head CT Results Within 45 Min. of Arrival[1]	-	-	45%	57%
Patients Who Left ER Before Being Seen	23,213	3%	3%	2%
Time from ER Arrival to Admit. (minutes)[2]	550	316	286	274
Time from ER Arrival to Discharge (minutes)	437	120	140	134
Time in ER Before Being Evaluated (minutes)	473	23	32	26
Time to Pain Meds for Fractures (minutes)	88	59	64	57

NOTE: Hospital profiles are in alphabetical order by state, then city, then hospital within the city; Rankings exclude hospitals with less than 25 cases except for patient surveys which excludes hospitals with less than 100 cases; (a) 100-299 cases; (1) The number of cases/patients is too few to report; (2) Data submitted were based on a sample of cases/patients; (3) Results are based on a shorter time period than required; (4) Data suppressed by CMS for one or more quarters; (5) Results are not available for this reporting period; (6) Fewer than 100 patients completed the HCAHPS survey; (7) No cases met the criteria for this measure; (8) The lower limit of the confidence interval cannot be calculated if the number of observed infections equals zero; (9) No data are available from the state/territory for this reporting period; (10) The scores shown reflect fewer than 50 completed surveys; (11) There were discrepancies in the data collection process; (12) This measure does not apply to this hospital for this reporting period; (13) Results cannot be calculated for this reporting period; (14) The results for this state are combined with nearby states to protect confidentiality; Please refer to the User's Guide for a full explanation of data.

Heart Attack Care				
Aspirin Given at Discharge[1]	-	-	99%	99%
Fibrinolytic Meds Within 30 Min. of Arrival[7]	-	-	80%	54%
PCI Within 90 Minutes of Arrival[7]	-	-	95%	96%
Statin Prescribed at Discharge[1]	-	-	98%	98%
Heart Failure Care				
ACE Inhibitor or ARB for LVSD	20	95%	97%	97%
Discharge Instructions Given	90	92%	92%	94%
Evaluation of LVS Function	103	99%	99%	99%
Medicare Spending				
Medicare Spending per Patient (ratio)	-	0.94	0.95	0.98
Pneumonia Care				
Appropriate Initial Antibiotic Given	58	97%	95%	95%
Blood Culture Timing	105	97%	97%	98%
Pregnancy and Delivery Care				
Newborn Deliveries Scheduled Early	27	41%	8%	6%
Preventive Care				
Immunization for Influenza[2]	406	99%	88%	90%
Immunization for Pneumonia[2]	436	99%	90%	92%
Stroke Care				
Anticoagulation Therapy for Atrial Fibrillation[7]	-	-	94%	95%
Antithrombotic Therapy Timing	14	100%	97%	98%
Assessed for Rehabilitation	17	88%	97%	97%
Discharged on Antithrombotic Therapy	15	100%	98%	99%
Discharged on Statin Medication	13	100%	94%	94%
Thrombolytic Therapy Timing[7]	-	-	58%	66%
Venous Thromboembolism Prophylaxis	16	100%	92%	94%
Written Stroke Educational Materials Given	11	45%	84%	88%
Surgical Care Improvement Project				
Appropriate Beta Blocker Usage	21	100%	97%	98%
Appropriate VTP Within 24 Hours	80	98%	98%	98%
Controlled Postoperative Blood Glucose[7]	-	-	96%	97%
Perioperative Temperature Management	90	100%	100%	100%
Prophylactic Antibiotic Selection	55	98%	99%	99%
Prophylactic Antibiotic Selection (Outpatient)	20	100%	98%	98%
Prophylactic Antibiotic Stopped	53	98%	98%	98%
Prophylactic Antibiotic Timing	55	100%	99%	99%
Prophylactic Antibiotic Timing (Outpatient)	20	100%	98%	98%
Urinary Catheter Removal	16	100%	97%	97%
Survey of Patients' Hospital Experiences				
Area Around Room 'Always' Quiet at Night	300+	57%	66%	61%
Doctors 'Always' Communicated Well	300+	75%	83%	82%
Home Recovery Information Given	300+	76%	84%	85%
Hospital Given 9 or 10 on 10 Point Scale	300+	46%	69%	71%
Meds 'Always' Explained Before Given	300+	52%	63%	64%
Nurses 'Always' Communicated Well	300+	66%	78%	79%
Pain 'Always' Well Controlled	300+	56%	71%	71%
Room and Bathroom 'Always' Clean	300+	62%	71%	73%
Timely Help 'Always' Received	300+	53%	65%	68%
Would Definitely Recommend Hospital	300+	49%	70%	71%
Use of Medical Imaging				
Cardiac Imaging Stress Test before Surgery[1]	-	-	5.5%	5.3%
Combination Abdominal CT Scan	431	2.8%	10.1%	10.5%
Combination Brain/Sinus CT Scan	341	4.4%	2.3%	2.7%
Combination Chest CT Scan	193	4.1%	3.7%	2.7%
Follow-up Mammogram/Ultrasound	468	8.8%	8.9%	8.8%
Lumbar Spine MRI for Low Back Pain	47	36.2%	36.6%	37.2%

NOTE: Hospital profiles are in alphabetical order by state, then city, then hospital within the city; Rankings exclude hospitals with less than 25 cases except for patient surveys which excludes hospitals with less than 100 cases; (a) 100-299 cases; (1) The number of cases/patients is too few to report; (2) Data submitted were based on a sample of cases/patients; (3) Results are based on a shorter time period than required; (4) Data suppressed by CMS for one or more quarters; (5) Results are not available for this reporting period; (6) Fewer than 100 patients completed the HCAHPS survey; (7) No cases met the criteria for this measure; (8) The lower limit of the confidence interval cannot be calculated if the number of observed infections equals zero; (9) No data are available from the state/territory for this reporting period; (10) The scores shown reflect fewer than 50 completed surveys; (11) There were discrepancies in the data collection process; (12) This measure does not apply to this hospital for this reporting period; (13) Results cannot be calculated for this reporting period; (14) The results for this state are combined with nearby states to protect confidentiality; Please refer to the User's Guide for a full explanation of data.

Blood Clot Prevention and Treatment

Anticoagulation Overlap Therapy

Hospital Name	City	Rate	Cases
East Jefferson General Hospital[2]	Metairie	100%	72
Lake Charles Memorial Hospital[2]	Lake Charles	100%	43
Lakeview Regional Medical Center[2]	Covington	100%	27
Minden Medical Center[2]	Minden	100%	26
Northern Louisiana Medical Center[2]	Ruston	100%	36
Rapides Regional Medical Center[2]	Alexandria	100%	89
Saint Elizabeth Hospital[2]	Gonzales	100%	28
Slidell Memorial Hospital[2]	Slidell	100%	50
Thibodaux Regional Medical Center[2]	Thibodaux	100%	42
University Hospital & Clinics[2]	Lafayette	100%	32
West Jefferson Medical Center[2]	Marrero	100%	53
Tulane Medical Center[2]	New Orleans	99%	75
Touro Infirmary[2]	New Orleans	98%	56
Ochsner Medical Center - Baton Rouge[2]	Baton Rouge	97%	35
Terrebonne General Medical Center[2]	Houma	97%	34
Baton Rouge General Medical Center[2]	Baton Rouge	96%	139
Lafayette General Medical Center[2]	Lafayette	96%	69
North Oaks Medical Center[2]	Hammond	95%	55
Charity Hosp & Med Ctr of Louisiana[2]	New Orleans	94%	48
Christus Saint Frances Cabrini Hospital[2]	Alexandria	94%	99
Ochsner Medical Center - Kenner[2]	Kenner	93%	29
Ochsner Medical Center - Northshore[2]	Slidell	93%	41
Our Lady of the Lake Reg Med Ctr[2]	Baton Rouge	93%	169
Christus Health Shreveport - Bossier[2]	Shreveport	92%	50
Willis Knighton Medical Center[2]	Shreveport	90%	178
Leonard J Chabert Medical Center[2]	Houma	89%	27
Saint Tammany Parish Hospital[2]	Covington	89%	61
Glenwood Regional Medical Center[2]	West Monroe	87%	70
Ochsner Medical Center[2]	New Orleans	87%	195
B R F Hospital Holdings[2]	Shreveport	85%	55
Iberia General Hospital & Medical Center[2]	New Iberia	85%	27
Opelousas General Health System[2]	Opelousas	78%	41
Lane Regional Medical Center[2]	Zachary	76%	25
Our Lady of Lourdes Reg Med Ctr[2]	Lafayette	75%	57
Saint Francis Medical Center[2]	Monroe	73%	105
Willis Knighton Bossier Health Center[2]	Bossier City	67%	58
Christus Saint Patrick Hospital[2]	Lake Charles	57%	58
West Calcasieu Cameron Hospital[2]	Sulphur	48%	33

ICU Venous Thromboembolism Prophylaxis

Hospital Name	City	Rate	Cases
Dauterive Hospital[2]	New Iberia	100%	56
Lakeview Regional Medical Center[2]	Covington	100%	84
Minden Medical Center[2]	Minden	100%	76
Northern Louisiana Medical Center[2]	Ruston	100%	165
Rapides Regional Medical Center[2]	Alexandria	100%	162
The Regional Medical Center of Acadiana[2]	Lafayette	100%	104
Saint Elizabeth Hospital[2]	Gonzales	100%	63
Slidell Memorial Hospital[2]	Slidell	100%	106
Teche Regional Medical Center[2]	Morgan City	100%	40
Tulane Medical Center[2]	New Orleans	100%	208
West Jefferson Medical Center[2]	Marrero	99%	134
Leonard J Chabert Medical Center[2]	Houma	98%	45
Touro Infirmary[2]	New Orleans	98%	117
Lafayette General Medical Center[2]	Lafayette	97%	73
Mercy Regional Medical Center[2]	Ville Platte	97%	88
B R F Hospital Holdings[2]	Shreveport	96%	93
Charity Hosp & Med Ctr of Louisiana[2]	New Orleans	96%	121
Thibodaux Regional Medical Center[2]	Thibodaux	96%	109
Baton Rouge General Medical Center[2]	Baton Rouge	95%	58
Beauregard Memorial Hospital[2]	Deridder	95%	41
Heart Hospital of Lafayette[2]	Lafayette	95%	73
Our Lady of Lourdes Reg Med Ctr[2]	Lafayette	95%	63
Byrd Regional Hospital[2]	Leesville	94%	79
Louisiana Heart Hospital[2]	Lacombe	94%	110
Our Lady of the Lake Reg Med Ctr[2]	Baton Rouge	94%	99
Christus Saint Frances Cabrini Hospital[2]	Alexandria	93%	132
Ochsner Medical Center - Baton Rouge[2]	Baton Rouge	93%	105
University Hospital & Clinics[2]	Lafayette	93%	43
Iberia General Hospital & Medical Center[2]	New Iberia	92%	65
American Legion Hospital[2]	Crowley	91%	43
Saint Francis Medical Center[2]	Monroe	91%	105
Ochsner Medical Center - Kenner[2]	Kenner	90%	124
Ochsner Medical Center - Northshore[2]	Slidell	89%	122
Lallie Kemp Medical Center	Independence	88%	86
Jennings American Legion Hospital[2]	Jennings	87%	52
North Oaks Medical Center[2]	Hammond	87%	52
Ochsner Medical Center[2]	New Orleans	87%	69
E A Conway Medical Center[2]	Monroe	86%	81
Terrebonne General Medical Center[2]	Houma	86%	114
West Calcasieu Cameron Hospital[2]	Sulphur	85%	78
East Jefferson General Hospital[2]	Metairie	83%	102
Winn Parish Medical Center[2]	Winnfield	83%	87
Lake Charles Memorial Hospital[2]	Lake Charles	82%	74
Morehouse General Hospital[2]	Bastrop	82%	33
Saint Tammany Parish Hospital[2]	Covington	81%	85
Willis Knighton Medical Center[2]	Shreveport	81%	238
Saint Bernard Parish Hospital[3]	Chalmette	80%	80
Homer Memorial Hospital[2]	Homer	77%	43
Opelousas General Health System[2]	Opelousas	77%	98
Glenwood Regional Medical Center[2]	West Monroe	76%	102
Natchitoches Regional Medical Center[2]	Natchitoches	75%	61
Washington St Tammany Reg Med Ctr[2]	Bogalusa	75%	72
River Parishes Hospital[2]	Laplace	73%	56
Richardson Medical Center[2]	Rayville	72%	25
Christus Saint Patrick Hospital[2]	Lake Charles	70%	98
Willis Knighton Bossier Health Center[2]	Bossier City	70%	80
Christus Health Shreveport - Bossier[2]	Shreveport	68%	56
Springhill Medical Center[2]	Springhill	61%	46
Savoy Medical Center[2]	Mamou	59%	37
Lane Regional Medical Center[2]	Zachary	58%	66
Saint Charles Parish Hospital[2]	Luling	57%	65
Franklin Medical Center[2]	Winnsboro	54%	37

Incidence of Potentially Preventable VTE

Hospital Name	City	Rate	Cases
Tulane Medical Center[2]	New Orleans	0%	41
Baton Rouge General Medical Center[2]	Baton Rouge	5%	40
B R F Hospital Holdings[2]	Shreveport	10%	29
Our Lady of the Lake Reg Med Ctr[2]	Baton Rouge	11%	35
East Jefferson General Hospital[2]	Metairie	15%	27
Ochsner Medical Center[2]	New Orleans	19%	48
Saint Francis Medical Center[2]	Monroe	22%	32
Willis Knighton Medical Center[2]	Shreveport	39%	51

UFH with Dosages/Platelet Count Monitoring

Hospital Name	City	Rate	Cases
B R F Hospital Holdings[2]	Shreveport	100%	32
Ochsner Medical Center - Baton Rouge[2]	Baton Rouge	100%	27
Rapides Regional Medical Center[2]	Alexandria	100%	37
Saint Francis Medical Center[2]	Monroe	100%	26
Terrebonne General Medical Center[2]	Houma	100%	29
Thibodaux Regional Medical Center[2]	Thibodaux	100%	36
Tulane Medical Center[2]	New Orleans	100%	67
Willis Knighton Medical Center[2]	Shreveport	100%	42
Charity Hosp & Med Ctr of Louisiana[2]	New Orleans	97%	32
Christus Saint Frances Cabrini Hospital[2]	Alexandria	95%	66
Our Lady of the Lake Reg Med Ctr[2]	Baton Rouge	88%	25
Ochsner Medical Center[2]	New Orleans	49%	51

Venous Thromboembolism Prophylaxis

Hospital Name	City	Rate	Cases
Central Louisiana Surgical Hospital[2]	Alexandria	100%	51
Dauterive Hospital[2]	New Iberia	100%	133
Fairway Medical Center[2]	Covington	100%	49
Lakeview Regional Medical Center[2]	Covington	100%	367
Minden Medical Center[2]	Minden	100%	255
The Neuromedical Center Hospital[2]	Baton Rouge	100%	193
Northern Louisiana Medical Center[2]	Ruston	100%	360
The Regional Medical Center of Acadiana[2]	Lafayette	100%	329
Southern Surgical Hospital[2]	Slidell	100%	45
Rapides Regional Medical Center[2]	Alexandria	99%	390
Tulane Medical Center[2]	New Orleans	99%	247
Teche Regional Medical Center[2]	Morgan City	98%	225
West Jefferson Medical Center[2]	Marrero	98%	269
Lake Area Medical Center[2]	Lake Charles	97%	93
Slidell Memorial Hospital[2]	Slidell	97%	291
Thibodaux Regional Medical Center[2]	Thibodaux	97%	330
Specialists Hospital Shreveport[2]	Shreveport	96%	108
Lafayette Surgical Specialty Hospital	Lafayette	95%	243
Winn Parish Medical Center[2]	Winnfield	95%	92
Touro Infirmary[2]	New Orleans	94%	305
E A Conway Medical Center[2]	Monroe	92%	246
Green Clinic Surgical Hospital	Ruston	92%	154
Leonard J Chabert Medical Center[2]	Houma	92%	245
Mercy Regional Medical Center[2]	Ville Platte	92%	308
Louisiana Heart Hospital[2]	Lacombe	90%	198
Saint Elizabeth Hospital[2]	Gonzales	89%	264
Beauregard Memorial Hospital[2]	Deridder	88%	174
Iberia General Hospital & Medical Center[2]	New Iberia	88%	301
Our Lady of Lourdes Reg Med Ctr[2]	Lafayette	88%	356
Ochsner Medical Center - Baton Rouge[2]	Baton Rouge	86%	325
Byrd Regional Hospital[2]	Leesville	85%	322
Avoyelles Hospital[2]	Marksville	84%	136
Ochsner Medical Center - Northshore[2]	Slidell	84%	338
Saint Francis Medical Center[2]	Monroe	84%	347
Charity Hosp & Med Ctr of Louisiana[2]	New Orleans	83%	252
University Hospital & Clinics[2]	Lafayette	83%	163
B R F Hospital Holdings[2]	Shreveport	82%	299
Lafayette General Medical Center[2]	Lafayette	82%	327
Monroe Surgical Hospital[2]	Monroe	82%	33
Our Lady of the Lake Reg Med Ctr[2]	Baton Rouge	82%	304
Ochsner Medical Center - Kenner[2]	Kenner	81%	290
Lallie Kemp Medical Center	Independence	80%	284
P & S Surgical Hospital[2]	Monroe	80%	85
American Legion Hospital[2]	Crowley	78%	313
Baton Rouge General Medical Center[2]	Baton Rouge	77%	346
West Calcasieu Cameron Hospital[2]	Sulphur	77%	265
Lake Charles Memorial Hospital[2]	Lake Charles	76%	367
Jennings American Legion Hospital[2]	Jennings	75%	281
Physicians Medical Center	Houma	75%	88
Homer Memorial Hospital[2]	Homer	74%	196
Terrebonne General Medical Center[2]	Houma	74%	315
Ochsner Medical Center[2]	New Orleans	73%	347
Abbeville General Hospital[2]	Abbeville	72%	104
Saint Tammany Parish Hospital[2]	Covington	72%	320
Christus Saint Frances Cabrini Hospital[2]	Alexandria	71%	351
Morehouse General Hospital[2]	Bastrop	71%	104
Opelousas General Health System[2]	Opelousas	71%	318
North Oaks Medical Center[2]	Hammond	70%	403
Surgical Specialty Center of Baton Rouge	Baton Rouge	70%	79
Christus Health Shreveport - Bossier[2]	Shreveport	69%	377
Cypress Pointe Surgical Hospital	Hammond	69%	169
Saint Bernard Parish Hospital[3]	Chalmette	68%	292
Woman's Hospital[2]	Baton Rouge	68%	57
Natchitoches Regional Medical Center[2]	Natchitoches	66%	152
East Jefferson General Hospital[2]	Metairie	65%	310
Heart Hospital of Lafayette[2]	Lafayette	65%	120
Saint Charles Parish Hospital[2]	Luling	64%	127
Richardson Medical Center[2]	Rayville	63%	181
Willis Knighton Medical Center[2]	Shreveport	62%	1393
Christus Saint Patrick Hospital[2]	Lake Charles	61%	382
Glenwood Regional Medical Center[2]	West Monroe	61%	385
Washington St Tammany Reg Med Ctr[2]	Bogalusa	61%	142
Huey P Long Medical Center[2]	Pineville	60%	148
Willis Knighton Bossier Health Center[2]	Bossier City	60%	737
East Carroll Parish Hospital[2]	Lake Providence	51%	257
Savoy Medical Center[2]	Mamou	50%	107
River Parishes Hospital[2]	Laplace	48%	120
Lasalle General Hospital[2]	Jena	47%	173
Oakdale Community Hospital[2]	Oakdale	47%	108
Franklin Medical Center[2]	Winnsboro	45%	350
Springhill Medical Center[2]	Springhill	40%	67
Lane Regional Medical Center[2]	Zachary	38%	402
Citizens Medical Center[2]	Columbia	35%	139
Desoto Regional Health System[2]	Mansfield	29%	287
Sabine Medical Center[2]	Many	28%	122
Doctors Hospital at Deer Creek	Leesville	21%	192
Allen Parish Hospital	Kinder	14%	58
West Carroll Memorial Hospital[2]	Oak Grove	9%	410
Caldwell Memorial Hospital[2]	Columbia	0%	221

Warfarin Therapy Discharge Instructions

Hospital Name	City	Rate	Cases
Glenwood Regional Medical Center[2]	West Monroe	100%	42
Northern Louisiana Medical Center[2]	Ruston	100%	25
Ochsner Medical Center - Baton Rouge[2]	Baton Rouge	100%	26
Rapides Regional Medical Center[2]	Alexandria	100%	69
Touro Infirmary[2]	New Orleans	100%	37
Slidell Memorial Hospital[2]	Slidell	98%	43
Tulane Medical Center[2]	New Orleans	98%	49
Saint Tammany Parish Hospital[2]	Covington	96%	46
Lake Charles Memorial Hospital[2]	Lake Charles	93%	27
Ochsner Medical Center - Northshore[2]	Slidell	93%	28
B R F Hospital Holdings[2]	Shreveport	91%	46
Our Lady of Lourdes Reg Med Ctr[2]	Lafayette	90%	39
Christus Health Shreveport - Bossier[2]	Shreveport	89%	35
Willis Knighton Bossier Health Center[2]	Bossier City	89%	45
Willis Knighton Medical Center[2]	Shreveport	89%	119
Our Lady of the Lake Reg Med Ctr[2]	Baton Rouge	88%	140
West Jefferson Medical Center[2]	Marrero	88%	33
Charity Hosp & Med Ctr of Louisiana[2]	New Orleans	86%	36
Ochsner Medical Center[2]	New Orleans	85%	156
East Jefferson General Hospital[2]	Metairie	84%	51
Opelousas General Health System[2]	Opelousas	83%	30
Lafayette General Medical Center[2]	Lafayette	79%	43
Baton Rouge General Medical Center[2]	Baton Rouge	74%	101
Christus Saint Patrick Hospital[2]	Lake Charles	74%	46
Saint Francis Medical Center[2]	Monroe	69%	85
Christus Saint Frances Cabrini Hospital[2]	Alexandria	52%	65
University Hospital & Clinics[2]	Lafayette	40%	30
North Oaks Medical Center[2]	Hammond	39%	31

Chest Pain/Possible Heart Attack Care

Aspirin Given Within 24 Hours of Arrival

Hospital Name	City	Rate	Cases
Jennings American Legion Hospital	Jennings	100%	38
Minden Medical Center	Minden	100%	27
Morehouse General Hospital	Bastrop	100%	35
Oakdale Community Hospital	Oakdale	100%	50
Saint Elizabeth Hospital	Gonzales	100%	58
Saint James Parish Hospital	Lutcher	100%	55
Teche Regional Medical Center	Morgan City	100%	45
Union General Hospital	Farmerville	100%	37
Washington St Tammany Reg Med Ctr	Bogalusa	100%	118

NOTE: Hospital profiles are in alphabetical order by state, then city, then hospital within the city; Rankings exclude hospitals with less than 25 cases except for patient surveys which excludes hospitals with less than 100 cases; (a) 100-299 cases; (1) The number of cases/patients is too few to report; (2) Data submitted were based on a sample of cases/patients; (3) Results are based on a shorter time period than required; (4) Data suppressed by CMS for one or more quarters; (5) Results are not available for this reporting period; (6) Fewer than 100 patients completed the HCAHPS survey; (7) No cases met the criteria for this measure; (8) The lower limit of the confidence interval cannot be calculated if the number of observed infections equals zero; (9) No data are available from the state/territory for this reporting period; (10) The scores shown reflect fewer than 50 completed surveys; (11) There were discrepancies in the data collection process; (12) This measure does not apply to this hospital for this reporting period; (13) Results cannot be calculated for this reporting period; (14) The results for this state are combined with nearby states to protect confidentiality; Please refer to the User's Guide for a full explanation of data.

Hospital Name	City	Rate	Cases
Franklin Medical Center	Winnsboro	97%	101
Natchitoches Regional Medical Center	Natchitoches	97%	30
Willis Knighton Medical Center	Shreveport	96%	49
E A Conway Medical Center	Monroe	95%	63
Springhill Medical Center	Springhill	95%	38
Winn Parish Medical Center	Winnfield	95%	44
Saint Charles Parish Hospital	Luling	94%	33
Byrd Regional Hospital	Leesville	93%	41
Mercy Regional Medical Center	Ville Platte	93%	58
River Parishes Hospital	Laplace	93%	29
West Carroll Memorial Hospital	Oak Grove	93%	27
Ochsner Saint Anne General Hospital	Raceland	92%	38
Lasalle General Hospital	Jena	91%	55
Beauregard Memorial Hospital	Deridder	88%	32
Avoyelles Hospital	Marksville	86%	49
Sabine Medical Center	Many	81%	54
American Legion Hospital	Crowley	80%	44

Average Time to ECG (minutes)

Hospital Name	City	Min.	Cases
Mercy Regional Medical Center	Ville Platte	1	62
Minden Medical Center	Minden	4	27
Springhill Medical Center	Springhill	4	36
Union General Hospital	Farmerville	4	40
West Feliciana Parish Hospital	Saint Francisville	5	26
River Parishes Hospital	Laplace	6	29
Byrd Regional Hospital	Leesville	7	40
Franklin Medical Center	Winnsboro	7	104
Jennings American Legion Hospital	Jennings	7	38
Avoyelles Hospital	Marksville	8	50
Morehouse General Hospital	Bastrop	8	35
Sabine Medical Center	Many	8	56
Saint Charles Parish Hospital	Luling	8	34
Teche Regional Medical Center	Morgan City	8	47
Ochsner Saint Anne General Hospital	Raceland	9	41
Winn Parish Medical Center	Winnfield	9	45
Natchitoches Regional Medical Center	Natchitoches	10	30
Oakdale Community Hospital	Oakdale	10	52
Saint James Parish Hospital	Lutcher	10	58
Willis Knighton Medical Center	Shreveport	10	51
Citizens Medical Center	Columbia	11	27
Lasalle General Hospital	Jena	12	57
Saint Elizabeth Hospital	Gonzales	13	60
Beauregard Memorial Hospital	Deridder	14	34
Washington St Tammany Reg Med Ctr	Bogalusa	15	120
American Legion Hospital	Crowley	20	43
E A Conway Medical Center	Monroe	22	64
West Carroll Memorial Hospital	Oak Grove	51	27

Children's Asthma Care

Received Home Management Plan of Care

Hospital Name	City	Rate	Cases
Saint Francis Medical Center	Monroe	94%	47

Received Reliever Medication

Hospital Name	City	Rate	Cases
Saint Francis Medical Center	Monroe	100%	47

Received Systemic Corticosteroids

Hospital Name	City	Rate	Cases
Saint Francis Medical Center	Monroe	100%	46

Emergency Department

Admittance Decision Time (minutes)

Hospital Name	City	Min.	Cases
Allen Parish Hospital[2]	Kinder	0	49
West Carroll Memorial Hospital[2,3]	Oak Grove	0	360
Woman's Hospital[2]	Baton Rouge	14	250
Citizens Medical Center[2]	Columbia	25	118
East Carroll Parish Hospital[2]	Lake Providence	34	128
Winn Parish Medical Center[2]	Winnfield	40	527
Lake Area Medical Center[2]	Lake Charles	43	153
Desoto Regional Health System[2]	Mansfield	45	460
Heart Hospital of Lafayette[2]	Lafayette	46	114
Franklin Medical Center[2]	Winnsboro	48	260
Mercy Regional Medical Center[2]	Ville Platte	48	282
American Legion Hospital[2]	Crowley	52	599
Springhill Medical Center[2]	Springhill	53	595
Oakdale Community Hospital[2]	Oakdale	55	347
The Regional Medical Center of Acadiana[2]	Lafayette	55	478
Sabine Medical Center[2]	Many	58	384
Avoyelles Hospital[2]	Marksville	60	445
Lallie Kemp Regional Medical Center[2]	Independence	60	293
Lakeview Regional Medical Center[2]	Covington	61	558
Dauterive Hospital[2]	New Iberia	62	345
Jennings American Legion Hospital[2]	Jennings	64	296
Saint James Parish Hospital	Lutcher	64	68
Homer Memorial Hospital[2]	Homer	65	481
Lafayette General Medical Center[2]	Lafayette	67	654
Saint Tammany Parish Hospital[2]	Covington	67	315
West Calcasieu Cameron Hospital[2]	Sulphur	68	436
Beauregard Memorial Hospital[2]	Deridder	69	189
Morehouse General Hospital[2]	Bastrop	70	150
Richardson Medical Center[2]	Rayville	70	252
Savoy Medical Center[2]	Mamou	70	184
Thibodaux Regional Medical Center[2]	Thibodaux	70	614
Union General Hospital	Farmerville	70	300
Saint Bernard Parish Hospital[3]	Chalmette	72	153
Iberia General Hospital & Medical Center[2]	New Iberia	75	316
Natchitoches Regional Medical Center[2]	Natchitoches	75	165
Minden Medical Center[2]	Minden	76	376
Abbeville General Hospital[2]	Abbeville	80	225
Franklin Foundation Hospital[3]	Franklin	80	256
Ochsner Medical Center - Northshore[2]	Slidell	81	441
Saint Charles Parish Hospital[2]	Luling	81	428
Lane Regional Medical Center[2]	Zachary	83	494
Louisiana Heart Hospital[2]	Lacombe	84	204
River Parishes Hospital[2]	Laplace	84	374
Terrebonne General Medical Center[2]	Houma	86	588
Lasalle General Hospital[2]	Jena	90	352
Our Lady of the Lake Reg Med Ctr[2]	Baton Rouge	90	491
Willis Knighton Medical Center[2]	Shreveport	90	1305
Byrd Regional Hospital[2]	Leesville	92	423
Saint Elizabeth Hospital[2]	Gonzales	92	518
Northern Louisiana Medical Center[2]	Ruston	95	623
Christus Saint Patrick Hospital[2]	Lake Charles	96	855
Rapides Regional Medical Center[2]	Alexandria	100	816
East Jefferson General Hospital[2]	Metairie	101	664
Willis Knighton Bossier Health Center[2]	Bossier City	101	874
Touro Infirmary[2]	New Orleans	104	380
Lake Charles Memorial Hospital[2]	Lake Charles	106	487
Saint Francis Medical Center[2]	Monroe	110	401
Christus Health Shreveport - Bossier[2]	Shreveport	111	505
Our Lady of Lourdes Reg Med Ctr[2]	Lafayette	111	616
Opelousas General Health System[2]	Opelousas	118	449
Teche Regional Medical Center[2]	Morgan City	119	252
Slidell Memorial Hospital[2]	Slidell	120	302
West Jefferson Medical Center[2]	Marrero	123	546
Glenwood Regional Medical Center[2]	West Monroe	124	697
Ochsner Medical Center - Baton Rouge[2]	Baton Rouge	131	603
Tulane Medical Center[2]	New Orleans	132	644
B R F Hospital Holdings[2]	Shreveport	133	448
North Oaks Medical Center[2]	Hammond	138	644
Washington St Tammany Reg Med Ctr[2]	Bogalusa	140	226
Ochsner Medical Center[2]	New Orleans	144	558
E A Conway Medical Center[2]	Monroe	145	255
Huey P Long Medical Center[2]	Pineville	148	306
Ochsner Medical Center - Kenner[2]	Kenner	155	370
Leonard J Chabert Medical Center[2]	Houma	165	249
University Hospital & Clinics[2]	Lafayette	165	195
Christus Saint Frances Cabrini Hospital[2]	Alexandria	187	432
Baton Rouge General Medical Center[2]	Baton Rouge	192	816
Charity Hosp & Med Ctr of Louisiana[2]	New Orleans	293	625

Head CT Results Within 45 Minutes of Arrival

Hospital Name	City	Rate	Cases
Ochsner Medical Center - Northshore	Slidell	86%	28

Patients Who Left ER Before Being Seen

Hospital Name	City	Rate	Cases
Heart Hospital of Lafayette	Lafayette	0%	2503
Ochsner Saint Anne General Hospital	Raceland	0%	14266
Reeves Memorial Medical Center	Bernice	0%	1680
Richland Parish Hospital - Delhi	Delhi	0%	4593
South Cameron Memorial Hospital	Cameron	0%	1108
Allen Parish Hospital	Kinder	1%	5456
Assumption Community Hospital	Napoleonville	1%	6735
Christus Health Shreveport - Bossier	Shreveport	1%	63722
Christus Saint Frances Cabrini Hospital	Alexandria	1%	49380
Christus Saint Patrick Hospital	Lake Charles	1%	25980
Citizens Medical Center	Columbia	1%	5484
Dauterive Hospital	New Iberia	1%	23601
Desoto Regional Health System	Mansfield	1%	8361
East Carroll Parish Hospital	Lake Providence	1%	4597
Hardtner Medical Center	Olla	1%	4883
Homer Memorial Hospital	Homer	1%	11524
Jackson Parish Hospital	Jonesboro	1%	7796
Lasalle General Hospital	Jena	1%	9971
Louisiana Heart Hospital	Lacombe	1%	9861
Mercy Regional Medical Center	Ville Platte	1%	24942
Minden Medical Center	Minden	1%	20982
Ochsner Medical Center - Baton Rouge	Baton Rouge	1%	54149
Ochsner Medical Center - Kenner	Kenner	1%	38425
The Regional Medical Center of Acadiana	Lafayette	1%	53400
Saint Charles Parish Hospital	Luling	1%	13680
Saint Elizabeth Hospital	Gonzales	1%	36848
Saint James Parish Hospital	Lutcher	1%	13180
Savoy Medical Center	Mamou	1%	7997
Tulane Medical Center	New Orleans	1%	65582
Union General Hospital	Farmerville	1%	6108
West Carroll Memorial Hospital	Oak Grove	1%	5065
West Feliciana Parish Hospital	Saint Francisville	1%	5229
Winn Parish Medical Center	Winnfield	1%	9369
Avoyelles Hospital	Marksville	2%	14472
Baton Rouge General Medical Center	Baton Rouge	2%	101495
East Jefferson General Hospital	Metairie	2%	52494
Lady of the Sea General Hospital	Cut Off	2%	10794
Lake Area Medical Center	Lake Charles	2%	24873
Lake Charles Memorial Hospital	Lake Charles	2%	36463
Lakeview Regional Medical Center	Covington	2%	21979
Lane Regional Medical Center	Zachary	2%	32940
Morehouse General Hospital	Bastrop	2%	14718
Opelousas General Health System	Opelousas	2%	54605
Our Lady of Lourdes Reg Med Ctr	Lafayette	2%	33942
Rapides Regional Medical Center	Alexandria	2%	65862
Sabine Medical Center	Many	2%	9195
Saint Francis Medical Center	Monroe	2%	61829
Saint Tammany Parish Hospital	Covington	2%	37984
Slidell Memorial Hospital	Slidell	2%	29007
Springhill Medical Center	Springhill	2%	9148
Thibodaux Regional Medical Center	Thibodaux	2%	34425
Acadia Saint Landry	Church Point	3%	3952
Byrd Regional Hospital	Leesville	3%	16294
Franklin Medical Center	Winnsboro	3%	10287
Glenwood Regional Medical Center	West Monroe	3%	28120
Iberia General Hospital & Medical Center	New Iberia	3%	26606
Leonard J Chabert Medical Center	Houma	3%	36360
Northern Louisiana Medical Center	Ruston	3%	27358
Oakdale Community Hospital	Oakdale	3%	9585
Ochsner Medical Center - Northshore	Slidell	3%	26312
Our Lady of the Lake Reg Med Ctr	Baton Rouge	3%	112723
River Parishes Hospital	Laplace	3%	17806
West Calcasieu Cameron Hospital	Sulphur	3%	25898
Abbeville General Hospital	Abbeville	4%	14088
Beauregard Memorial Hospital	Deridder	4%	18187
Ochsner Medical Center	New Orleans	4%	126583
Richardson Medical Center	Rayville	4%	6030
Saint Bernard Parish Hospital	Chalmette	4%	6593
Teche Regional Medical Center	Morgan City	4%	29621
Terrebonne General Medical Center	Houma	4%	53393
Washington St Tammany Reg Med Ctr	Bogalusa	4%	30115
West Jefferson Medical Center	Marrero	4%	58687
Willis Knighton Medical Center	Shreveport	4%	109659
Woman's Hospital	Baton Rouge	4%	9196
Lafayette General Medical Center	Lafayette	5%	62271
Touro Infirmary	New Orleans	5%	33561
Willis Knighton Bossier Health Center	Bossier City	5%	46881
Natchitoches Regional Medical Center	Natchitoches	6%	20151
Jennings American Legion Hospital	Jennings	7%	15272
North Oaks Medical Center	Hammond	7%	72361
E A Conway Medical Center	Monroe	8%	30831
Huey P Long Medical Center	Pineville	8%	29558
American Legion Hospital	Crowley	10%	16603
B R F Hospital Holdings	Shreveport	10%	59614
Charity Hosp & Med Ctr of Louisiana	New Orleans	10%	52517
University Hospital & Clinics	Lafayette	13%	42258

Time from ER Arrival to Being Admitted (minutes)

Hospital Name	City	Min.	Cases
Woman's Hospital[2]	Baton Rouge	62	253
Springhill Medical Center[2]	Springhill	130	604
East Carroll Parish Hospital[2]	Lake Providence	144	128
Winn Parish Medical Center[2]	Winnfield	154	588
Desoto Regional Health System[2]	Mansfield	160	473
Saint James Parish Hospital	Lutcher	160	68
Avoyelles Hospital[2]	Marksville	165	449
Heart Hospital of Lafayette[2]	Lafayette	167	114
Homer Memorial Hospital[2]	Homer	176	481
Mercy Regional Medical Center[2]	Ville Platte	184	310
The Regional Medical Center of Acadiana[2]	Lafayette	188	478
Citizens Medical Center[2]	Columbia	195	118
Richardson Medical Center[2]	Rayville	195	259
Dauterive Hospital[2]	New Iberia	198	349
West Carroll Memorial Hospital[2,3]	Oak Grove	205	485
Sabine Medical Center[2]	Many	206	388
Savoy Medical Center[2]	Mamou	206	185
Lake Area Medical Center[2]	Lake Charles	207	153
West Calcasieu Cameron Hospital[2]	Sulphur	210	448
Morehouse General Hospital[2]	Bastrop	211	171
Saint Charles Parish Hospital[2]	Luling	218	431
Allen Parish Hospital[2]	Kinder	220	49
Oakdale Community Hospital[2]	Oakdale	225	349
Union General Hospital	Farmerville	226	300
Byrd Regional Hospital[2]	Leesville	227	439
Minden Medical Center[2]	Minden	228	376
Jennings American Legion Hospital[2]	Jennings	229	299
Willis Knighton Medical Center[2]	Shreveport	230	1428

NOTE: Hospital profiles are in alphabetical order by state, then city, then hospital within the city; Rankings exclude hospitals with less than 25 cases except for patient surveys which excludes hospitals with less than 100 cases; (a) 100-299 cases; (1) The number of cases/patients is too few to report; (2) Data submitted were based on a sample of cases/patients; (3) Results are based on a shorter time period than required; (4) Data suppressed by CMS for one or more quarters; (5) Results are not available for this reporting period; (6) Fewer than 100 patients completed the HCAHPS survey; (7) No cases met the criteria for this measure; (8) The lower limit of the confidence interval cannot be calculated if the number of observed infections equals zero; (9) No data are available from the state/territory for this reporting period; (10) The scores shown reflect fewer than 50 completed surveys; (11) There were discrepancies in the data collection process; (12) This measure does not apply to this hospital for this reporting period; (13) Results cannot be calculated for this reporting period; (14) The results for this state are combined with nearby states to protect confidentiality; Please refer to the User's Guide for a full explanation of data.

American Legion Hospital[2]	Crowley	234	601
Lafayette General Medical Center[2]	Lafayette	234	668
Franklin Foundation Hospital[3]	Franklin	235	265
Beauregard Memorial Hospital[2]	Deridder	236	189
Lane Regional Medical Center[2]	Zachary	236	528
Lakeview Regional Medical Center[2]	Covington	243	558
Franklin Medical Center[2]	Winnsboro	244	282
Willis Knighton Bossier Health Center[2]	Bossier City	245	972
Saint Tammany Parish Hospital[2]	Covington	248	365
Louisiana Heart Hospital[2]	Lacombe	250	349
Northern Louisiana Medical Center[2]	Ruston	250	623
Ochsner Medical Center - Northshore[2]	Slidell	250	442
Our Lady of Lourdes Reg Med Ctr[2]	Lafayette	256	628
River Parishes Hospital[2]	Laplace	256	374
Saint Elizabeth Hospital[2]	Gonzales	257	525
Teche Regional Medical Center[2]	Morgan City	257	253
Abbeville General Hospital[2]	Abbeville	258	228
Lasalle General Hospital[2]	Jena	260	353
Christus Health Shreveport - Bossier[2]	Shreveport	265	507
Thibodaux Regional Medical Center[2]	Thibodaux	265	617
Saint Bernard Parish Hospital[3]	Chalmette	267	160
Christus Saint Patrick Hospital[2]	Lake Charles	270	895
Iberia General Hospital & Medical Center[2]	New Iberia	270	324
North Oaks Medical Center[2]	Hammond	272	649
Opelousas General Health System[2]	Opelousas	272	452
Terrebonne General Medical Center[2]	Houma	276	592
Natchitoches Regional Medical Center[2]	Natchitoches	285	190
Lallie Kemp Medical Center[2]	Independence	286	354
Glenwood Regional Medical Center[2]	West Monroe	291	702
Rapides Regional Medical Center[2]	Alexandria	291	816
Lake Charles Memorial Hospital[2]	Lake Charles	293	510
West Jefferson Medical Center[2]	Marrero	293	546
Slidell Memorial Hospital[2]	Slidell	296	312
East Jefferson General Hospital[2]	Metairie	299	683
Our Lady of the Lake Reg Med Ctr[2]	Baton Rouge	301	513
Touro Infirmary[2]	New Orleans	301	384
Ochsner Medical Center - Baton Rouge[2]	Baton Rouge	309	611
Washington St Tammany Reg Med Ctr[2]	Bogalusa	315	303
Saint Francis Medical Center[2]	Monroe	325	437
Ochsner Medical Center - Kenner[2]	Kenner	350	370
Christus Saint Frances Cabrini Hospital[2]	Alexandria	382	582
Baton Rouge General Medical Center[2]	Baton Rouge	388	817
B R F Hospital Holdings[2]	Shreveport	389	449
Tulane Medical Center[2]	New Orleans	402	644
University Hospital & Clinics[2]	Lafayette	410	215
Ochsner Medical Center[2]	New Orleans	417	587
Leonard J Chabert Medical Center[2]	Houma	494	258
E A Conway Medical Center[2]	Monroe	508	258
Huey P Long Medical Center[2]	Pineville	538	308
Charity Hosp & Med Ctr of Louisiana[2]	New Orleans	654	642

Time from ER Arrival to Discharge (minutes)

Hospital Name	City	Min.	Cases
East Carroll Parish Hospital	Lake Providence	67	385
Avoyelles Hospital	Marksville	75	341
Richardson Medical Center	Rayville	75	382
Teche Regional Medical Center	Morgan City	77	392
Springhill Medical Center	Springhill	79	1159
Mercy Regional Medical Center	Ville Platte	80	354
Winn Parish Medical Center	Winnfield	85	297
Homer Memorial Hospital	Homer	88	644
Oakdale Community Hospital	Oakdale	88	351
Dauterive Hospital	New Iberia	90	552
Ochsner Medical Center - Baton Rouge	Baton Rouge	90	362
Saint Charles Parish Hospital	Luling	93	365
Savoy Medical Center	Mamou	94	414
Reeves Memorial Medical Center[3]	Bernice	95	867
West Calcasieu Cameron Hospital	Sulphur	96	512
Lake Area Medical Center	Lake Charles	98	398
Minden Medical Center	Minden	98	370
Northern Louisiana Medical Center	Ruston	98	385
Jackson Parish Hospital	Jonesboro	99	288
Desoto Regional Health System	Mansfield	100	166
Sabine Medical Center	Many	102	287
River Parishes Hospital	Laplace	104	366
Byrd Regional Hospital	Leesville	105	265
Lasalle General Hospital	Jena	109	289
Allen Parish Hospital[3]	Kinder	110	608
Lane Regional Medical Center	Zachary	112	479
Morehouse General Hospital	Bastrop	112	330
Abbeville General Hospital	Abbeville	114	546
Opelousas General Health System	Opelousas	115	385
The Regional Medical Center of Acadiana	Lafayette	116	494
Saint Elizabeth Hospital	Gonzales	116	360
Lafayette General Medical Center	Lafayette	118	397
Washington St Tammany Reg Med Ctr	Bogalusa	120	421
Iberia General Hospital & Medical Center	New Iberia	121	369
Ochsner Medical Center - Kenner	Kenner	122	350
Christus Health Shreveport - Bossier	Shreveport	123	394
Citizens Medical Center	Columbia	126	699
Ochsner Medical Center - Northshore	Slidell	126	333
Saint Tammany Parish Hospital	Covington	127	366
Lake Charles Memorial Hospital	Lake Charles	129	348
Jennings American Legion Hospital	Jennings	130	373
Terrebonne General Medical Center	Houma	131	372
West Carroll Memorial Hospital	Oak Grove	133	770
Willis Knighton Medical Center	Shreveport	133	2305
Beauregard Memorial Hospital	Deridder	135	360
Christus Saint Patrick Hospital	Lake Charles	135	363
Heart Hospital of Lafayette	Lafayette	135	234
Saint Bernard Parish Hospital[3]	Chalmette	138	200
Louisiana Heart Hospital	Lacombe	140	387
American Legion Hospital	Crowley	143	389
Franklin Medical Center	Winnsboro	144	313
Glenwood Regional Medical Center	West Monroe	148	473
Thibodaux Regional Medical Center	Thibodaux	148	409
Our Lady of Lourdes Reg Med Ctr	Lafayette	149	333
Saint Francis Medical Center	Monroe	149	279
East Jefferson General Hospital	Metairie	150	362
Willis Knighton Bossier Health Center	Bossier City	150	1240
West Jefferson Medical Center	Marrero	156	366
Slidell Memorial Hospital	Slidell	157	331
Rapides Regional Medical Center	Alexandria	159	536
Baton Rouge General Medical Center	Baton Rouge	160	365
Ochsner Medical Center	New Orleans	165	354
Touro Infirmary	New Orleans	166	394
Natchitoches Regional Medical Center	Natchitoches	168	344
Lakeview Regional Medical Center	Covington	169	429
North Oaks Medical Center	Hammond	169	374
Tulane Medical Center	New Orleans	172	509
Our Lady of the Lake Reg Med Ctr	Baton Rouge	186	323
Woman's Hospital	Baton Rouge	190	320
University Hospital & Clinics	Lafayette	200	336
E A Conway Medical Center	Monroe	212	300
Christus Saint Frances Cabrini Hospital	Alexandria	216	405
Leonard J Chabert Medical Center	Houma	231	433
Huey P Long Medical Center	Pineville	262	342
B R F Hospital Holdings	Shreveport	271	322
Charity Hosp & Med Ctr of Louisiana	New Orleans	375	397

Time in ER Before Being Evaluated (minutes)

Hospital Name	City	Min.	Cases
Allen Parish Hospital[3]	Kinder	0	694
Heart Hospital of Lafayette	Lafayette	5	308
Minden Medical Center	Minden	5	399
Saint James Parish Hospital	Lutcher	5	68
Saint Charles Parish Hospital	Luling	6	402
Ochsner Medical Center - Baton Rouge	Baton Rouge	8	381
Richardson Medical Center	Rayville	9	384
Mercy Regional Medical Center	Ville Platte	12	409
Teche Regional Medical Center	Morgan City	12	408
Winn Parish Medical Center	Winnfield	13	412
Dauterive Hospital	New Iberia	15	591
Desoto Regional Health System	Mansfield	15	356
River Parishes Hospital	Laplace	15	396
Tulane Medical Center	New Orleans	15	568
Avoyelles Hospital	Marksville	16	392
Baton Rouge General Medical Center	Baton Rouge	18	404
Byrd Regional Hospital	Leesville	18	423
East Carroll Parish Hospital	Lake Providence	18	439
Oakdale Community Hospital	Oakdale	18	379
Ochsner Medical Center - Kenner	Kenner	18	380
Ochsner Medical Center - Northshore	Slidell	18	383
Louisiana Heart Hospital	Lacombe	19	385
Northern Louisiana Medical Center	Ruston	19	417
Citizens Medical Center	Columbia	20	580
Reeves Memorial Medical Center[3]	Bernice	20	901
Savoy Medical Center	Mamou	21	486
Springhill Medical Center	Springhill	21	1107
Lakeview Regional Medical Center	Covington	22	472
Lasalle General Hospital	Jena	22	424
The Regional Medical Center of Acadiana	Lafayette	22	523
American Legion Hospital	Crowley	23	392
Morehouse General Hospital	Bastrop	23	351
Opelousas General Health System	Opelousas	23	408
Christus Saint Patrick Hospital	Lake Charles	24	300
Beauregard Memorial Hospital	Deridder	25	385
Lake Area Medical Center	Lake Charles	25	415
Lane Regional Medical Center	Zachary	25	393
West Carroll Memorial Hospital	Oak Grove	25	863
Lafayette General Medical Center	Lafayette	26	407
Abbeville General Hospital	Abbeville	27	600
Jennings American Legion Hospital	Jennings	27	363
Iberia General Hospital & Medical Center	New Iberia	28	404
Jackson Parish Hospital	Jonesboro	28	321
Saint Elizabeth Hospital	Gonzales	28	379
Homer Memorial Hospital	Homer	30	657
Touro Infirmary	New Orleans	30	417
Christus Health Shreveport - Bossier	Shreveport	31	395
Slidell Memorial Hospital	Slidell	31	371
West Calcasieu Cameron Hospital	Sulphur	31	518
Washington St Tammany Reg Med Ctr	Bogalusa	32	438
Franklin Medical Center	Winnsboro	37	331
University Hospital & Clinics	Lafayette	38	378
Glenwood Regional Medical Center	West Monroe	40	532
Leonard J Chabert Medical Center	Houma	40	465
Rapides Regional Medical Center	Alexandria	41	576
Sabine Medical Center	Many	41	391
Saint Tammany Parish Hospital	Covington	41	366
Thibodaux Regional Medical Center	Thibodaux	42	439
Ochsner Medical Center	New Orleans	43	350
Willis Knighton Bossier Health Center	Bossier City	46	1310
Natchitoches Regional Medical Center	Natchitoches	48	370
Saint Francis Medical Center	Monroe	48	384
Our Lady of Lourdes Reg Med Ctr	Lafayette	49	348
West Jefferson Medical Center	Marrero	49	396
East Jefferson General Hospital	Metairie	50	82
Lake Charles Memorial Hospital	Lake Charles	50	340
Our Lady of the Lake Reg Med Ctr	Baton Rouge	51	361
Terrebonne General Medical Center	Houma	51	380
Willis Knighton Medical Center	Shreveport	52	2434
Saint Bernard Parish Hospital[3]	Chalmette	54	209
North Oaks Medical Center	Hammond	63	394
Christus Saint Frances Cabrini Hospital	Alexandria	95	417
B R F Hospital Holdings	Shreveport	96	352
Huey P Long Medical Center	Pineville	115	351
Charity Hosp & Med Ctr of Louisiana	New Orleans	117	267
Woman's Hospital	Baton Rouge	118	356

Time to Pain Meds for Bone Fractures (minutes)

Hospital Name	City	Min.	Cases
Saint Tammany Parish Hospital	Covington	18	139
Minden Medical Center	Minden	26	66
Teche Regional Medical Center	Morgan City	27	82
West Jefferson Medical Center	Marrero	30	78
Dauterive Hospital	New Iberia	31	57
Mercy Regional Medical Center	Ville Platte	36	64
Springhill Medical Center	Springhill	38	47
River Parishes Hospital	Laplace	39	34
Saint Charles Parish Hospital	Luling	41	52
Avoyelles Hospital	Marksville	45	67
Christus Saint Patrick Hospital	Lake Charles	46	78
West Calcasieu Cameron Hospital	Sulphur	46	156
Byrd Regional Hospital	Leesville	47	77
Oakdale Community Hospital	Oakdale	48	60
Lane Regional Medical Center	Zachary	50	107
Ochsner Medical Center - Baton Rouge	Baton Rouge	50	122
Ochsner Medical Center - Northshore	Slidell	50	115
The Regional Medical Center of Acadiana	Lafayette	50	197
Touro Infirmary	New Orleans	50	55
Saint Elizabeth Hospital	Gonzales	51	135
Winn Parish Medical Center	Winnfield	51	31
Jennings American Legion Hospital	Jennings	52	56
Northern Louisiana Medical Center	Ruston	52	95
Ochsner Medical Center - Kenner	Kenner	53	88
Willis Knighton Bossier Health Center	Bossier City	55	145
East Jefferson General Hospital	Metairie	56	142
Lake Area Medical Center	Lake Charles	56	127
Morehouse General Hospital	Bastrop	57	42
Lafayette General Medical Center	Lafayette	60	178
Our Lady of Lourdes Reg Med Ctr	Lafayette	60	145
Sabine Medical Center	Many	60	38
Franklin Medical Center	Winnsboro	61	48
Iberia General Hospital & Medical Center	New Iberia	61	90
Lasalle General Hospital	Jena	61	53
Beauregard Memorial Hospital	Deridder	62	96
Our Lady of the Lake Reg Med Ctr	Baton Rouge	62	284
Christus Health Shreveport - Bossier	Shreveport	63	109
Opelousas General Health System	Opelousas	64	164
Slidell Memorial Hospital	Slidell	64	109
Willis Knighton Medical Center	Shreveport	64	237
Abbeville General Hospital	Abbeville	65	59
Baton Rouge General Medical Center	Baton Rouge	66	184
North Oaks Medical Center	Hammond	67	174
Glenwood Regional Medical Center	West Monroe	68	105
American Legion Hospital	Crowley	69	44
Tulane Medical Center	New Orleans	70	184
Thibodaux Regional Medical Center	Thibodaux	72	122
Lake Charles Memorial Hospital	Lake Charles	74	85
Saint Francis Medical Center	Monroe	75	188
Lakeview Regional Medical Center	Covington	79	70
Louisiana Heart Hospital	Lacombe	79	29
Rapides Regional Medical Center	Alexandria	79	159
Ochsner Medical Center	New Orleans	80	352
Christus Saint Frances Cabrini Hospital	Alexandria	85	121
Terrebonne General Medical Center	Houma	85	143
Washington St Tammany Reg Med Ctr	Bogalusa	93	47
Charity Hosp & Med Ctr of Louisiana	New Orleans	97	70
Natchitoches Regional Medical Center	Natchitoches	102	54
University Hospital & Clinics	Lafayette	132	54
B R F Hospital Holdings	Shreveport	188	154

NOTE: Hospital profiles are in alphabetical order by state, then city, then hospital within the city; Rankings exclude hospitals with less than 25 cases except for patient surveys which excludes hospitals with less than 100 cases; (a) 100-299 cases; (1) The number of cases/patients is too few to report; (2) Data submitted were based on a sample of cases/patients; (3) Results are based on a shorter time period than required; (4) Data suppressed by CMS for one or more quarters; (5) Results are not available for this reporting period; (6) Fewer than 100 patients completed the HCAHPS survey; (7) No cases met the criteria for this measure; (8) The lower limit of the confidence interval cannot be calculated if the number of observed infections equals zero; (9) No data are available from the state/territory for this reporting period; (10) The scores shown reflect fewer than 50 completed surveys; (11) There were discrepancies in the data collection process; (12) This measure does not apply to this hospital for this reporting period; (13) Results cannot be calculated for this reporting period; (14) The results for this state are combined with nearby states to protect confidentiality; Please refer to the User's Guide for a full explanation of data.

Heart Attack Care

Aspirin Given at Discharge

Hospital Name	City	Rate	Cases
Charity Hosp & Med Ctr of Louisiana	New Orleans	100%	114
Christus Saint Frances Cabrini Hospital	Alexandria	100%	286
Christus Saint Patrick Hospital	Lake Charles	100%	155
Dauterive Hospital	New Iberia	100%	31
Glenwood Regional Medical Center	West Monroe	100%	376
Heart Hospital of Lafayette	Lafayette	100%	265
Lafayette General Medical Center	Lafayette	100%	200
Lakeview Regional Medical Center	Covington	100%	83
Louisiana Heart Hospital	Lacombe	100%	92
Minden Medical Center	Minden	100%	26
North Oaks Medical Center	Hammond	100%	230
Northern Louisiana Medical Center	Ruston	100%	49
Rapides Regional Medical Center	Alexandria	100%	294
The Regional Medical Center of Acadiana[2]	Lafayette	100%	61
Saint Francis Medical Center	Monroe	100%	208
Slidell Memorial Hospital	Slidell	100%	126
Thibodaux Regional Medical Center	Thibodaux	100%	194
Tulane Medical Center	New Orleans	100%	206
West Calcasieu Cameron Hospital	Sulphur	100%	70
Baton Rouge General Medical Center	Baton Rouge	99%	327
East Jefferson General Hospital[2]	Metairie	99%	257
Iberia General Hospital & Medical Center	New Iberia	99%	74
Lane Regional Medical Center	Zachary	99%	89
Ochsner Medical Center[2]	New Orleans	99%	323
Ochsner Medical Center - Northshore	Slidell	99%	94
Opelousas General Health System	Opelousas	99%	89
Our Lady of the Lake Reg Med Ctr[2]	Baton Rouge	99%	377
Terrebonne General Medical Center	Houma	99%	240
Willis Knighton Medical Center	Shreveport	99%	486
B R F Hospital Holdings[2]	Shreveport	98%	215
Ochsner Medical Center - Baton Rouge	Baton Rouge	98%	116
Ochsner Medical Center - Kenner[2]	Kenner	98%	198
Our Lady of Lourdes Reg Med Ctr	Lafayette	98%	122
Overton Brooks VA Med Ctr-Shreveport	Shreveport	98%	62
Saint Tammany Parish Hospital	Covington	98%	197
West Jefferson Medical Center	Marrero	98%	246
Christus Health Shreveport - Bossier	Shreveport	97%	117
Touro Infirmary	New Orleans	97%	112
Willis Knighton Bossier Health Center	Bossier City	97%	115
Lake Charles Memorial Hospital	Lake Charles	95%	142
Leonard J Chabert Medical Center	Houma	93%	45

PCI Within 90 Minutes of Arrival

Hospital Name	City	Rate	Cases
East Jefferson General Hospital[2]	Metairie	100%	44
Lafayette General Medical Center	Lafayette	100%	58
Lane Regional Medical Center	Zachary	100%	33
Ochsner Medical Center - Kenner[2]	Kenner	100%	32
Our Lady of Lourdes Reg Med Ctr	Lafayette	100%	34
Rapides Regional Medical Center	Alexandria	100%	38
Saint Tammany Parish Hospital	Covington	100%	30
West Jefferson Medical Center	Marrero	100%	43
Our Lady of the Lake Reg Med Ctr[2]	Baton Rouge	99%	73
Terrebonne General Medical Center	Houma	98%	47
Christus Saint Frances Cabrini Hospital	Alexandria	96%	27
Glenwood Regional Medical Center	West Monroe	96%	27
Willis Knighton Bossier Health Center	Bossier City	96%	46
Willis Knighton Medical Center	Shreveport	96%	48
Baton Rouge General Medical Center	Baton Rouge	95%	61
North Oaks Medical Center	Hammond	93%	45
Thibodaux Regional Medical Center	Thibodaux	93%	30
Ochsner Medical Center[2]	New Orleans	92%	36
Tulane Medical Center	New Orleans	92%	52
Saint Francis Medical Center	Monroe	91%	33
Christus Saint Patrick Hospital	Lake Charles	89%	46
Ochsner Medical Center - Northshore	Slidell	88%	26
B R F Hospital Holdings[2]	Shreveport	52%	25

Statin Prescribed at Discharge

Hospital Name	City	Rate	Cases
Christus Saint Frances Cabrini Hospital	Alexandria	100%	268
Christus Saint Patrick Hospital	Lake Charles	100%	153
Dauterive Hospital	New Iberia	100%	28
Lakeview Regional Medical Center	Covington	100%	77
Northern Louisiana Medical Center	Ruston	100%	45
Ochsner Medical Center - Baton Rouge	Baton Rouge	100%	117
Ochsner Medical Center - Northshore	Slidell	100%	98
Overton Brooks VA Med Ctr-Shreveport	Shreveport	100%	63
Rapides Regional Medical Center	Alexandria	100%	269
The Regional Medical Center of Acadiana[2]	Lafayette	100%	57
Saint Francis Medical Center	Monroe	100%	195
Slidell Memorial Hospital	Slidell	100%	123
Terrebonne General Medical Center	Houma	100%	249
Thibodaux Regional Medical Center	Thibodaux	100%	194
Tulane Medical Center	New Orleans	100%	205
West Jefferson Medical Center	Marrero	100%	245
Glenwood Regional Medical Center	West Monroe	99%	340
Lafayette General Medical Center	Lafayette	99%	187
Lane Regional Medical Center	Zachary	99%	89
Louisiana Heart Hospital	Lacombe	99%	94
Charity Hosp & Med Ctr of Louisiana	New Orleans	98%	115
East Jefferson General Hospital[2]	Metairie	98%	231
Heart Hospital of Lafayette	Lafayette	98%	240
Lake Charles Memorial Hospital	Lake Charles	98%	135
Ochsner Medical Center[2]	New Orleans	98%	314
Our Lady of Lourdes Reg Med Ctr	Lafayette	98%	123
Our Lady of the Lake Reg Med Ctr[2]	Baton Rouge	98%	360
Touro Infirmary	New Orleans	98%	109
Baton Rouge General Medical Center	Baton Rouge	97%	316
Ochsner Medical Center - Kenner[2]	Kenner	97%	194
West Calcasieu Cameron Hospital	Sulphur	97%	71
B R F Hospital Holdings[2]	Shreveport	96%	210
Saint Tammany Parish Hospital	Covington	96%	192
Leonard J Chabert Medical Center	Houma	95%	42
North Oaks Medical Center	Hammond	95%	224
Willis Knighton Medical Center	Shreveport	95%	465
Iberia General Hospital & Medical Center	New Iberia	94%	77
Christus Health Shreveport - Bossier	Shreveport	93%	110
Opelousas General Health System	Opelousas	93%	89
Willis Knighton Bossier Health Center	Bossier City	89%	116

Heart Failure Care

ACE Inhibitor or ARB for LVSD

Hospital Name	City	Rate	Cases
Beauregard Memorial Hospital	Deridder	100%	38
Christus Saint Frances Cabrini Hospital	Alexandria	100%	137
Christus Saint Patrick Hospital	Lake Charles	100%	103
Dauterive Hospital	New Iberia	100%	29
E A Conway Medical Center	Monroe	100%	76
Heart Hospital of Lafayette	Lafayette	100%	31
Jennings American Legion Hospital	Jennings	100%	45
Lafayette General Medical Center	Lafayette	100%	127
Lakeview Regional Medical Center	Covington	100%	70
Leonard J Chabert Medical Center	Houma	100%	54
Minden Medical Center	Minden	100%	59
Northern Louisiana Medical Center	Ruston	100%	65
Ochsner Medical Center - Kenner[2]	Kenner	100%	96
Rapides Regional Medical Center[2]	Alexandria	100%	132
The Regional Medical Center of Acadiana[2]	Lafayette	100%	35
Saint Charles Parish Hospital	Luling	100%	25
Saint Francis Medical Center	Monroe	100%	153
Slidell Memorial Hospital	Slidell	100%	67
Terrebonne General Medical Center	Houma	100%	120
Tulane Medical Center	New Orleans	100%	204
Baton Rouge General Medical Center[2]	Baton Rouge	99%	106
Glenwood Regional Medical Center	West Monroe	99%	106
North Oaks Medical Center[2]	Hammond	99%	94
Our Lady of Lourdes Reg Med Ctr	Lafayette	99%	86
Overton Brooks VA Med Ctr-Shreveport	Shreveport	99%	110
Thibodaux Regional Medical Center	Thibodaux	99%	67
Lane Regional Medical Center	Zachary	98%	60
Ochsner Medical Center - Northshore	Slidell	98%	63
River Parishes Hospital	Laplace	98%	57
East Jefferson General Hospital[2]	Metairie	97%	71
Touro Infirmary	New Orleans	97%	192
University Hospital & Clinics	Lafayette	97%	38
B R F Hospital Holdings[2]	Shreveport	96%	168
Byrd Regional Hospital	Leesville	96%	48
Charity Hosp & Med Ctr of Louisiana	New Orleans	96%	117
West Jefferson Medical Center	Marrero	96%	150
Iberia General Hospital & Medical Center	New Iberia	95%	58
Ochsner Medical Center - Baton Rouge[2]	Baton Rouge	95%	66
Washington St Tammany Reg Med Ctr	Bogalusa	95%	39
Mercy Regional Medical Center	Ville Platte	94%	54
Saint Elizabeth Hospital	Gonzales	94%	35
Louisiana Heart Hospital	Lacombe	92%	60
Our Lady of the Lake Reg Med Ctr[2]	Baton Rouge	92%	119
Saint Tammany Parish Hospital[2]	Covington	92%	85
Willis Knighton Bossier Health Center[2]	Bossier City	90%	88
Ochsner Medical Center[2]	New Orleans	88%	145
Christus Health Shreveport - Bossier[2]	Shreveport	87%	107
Lake Charles Memorial Hospital[2]	Lake Charles	86%	118
Opelousas General Health System[2]	Opelousas	86%	70
Natchitoches Regional Medical Center	Natchitoches	85%	26
Willis Knighton Medical Center[2]	Shreveport	83%	208
Desoto Regional Health System[2]	Mansfield	68%	41
American Legion Hospital[2]	Crowley	63%	30

Discharge Instructions Given

Hospital Name	City	Rate	Cases
Abbeville General Hospital	Abbeville	100%	49
Alexandria VA Medical Center	Pineville	100%	52
Christus Saint Frances Cabrini Hospital	Alexandria	100%	361
Heart Hospital of Lafayette	Lafayette	100%	99
Iberia General Hospital & Medical Center	New Iberia	100%	147
Jennings American Legion Hospital	Jennings	100%	102
Lady of the Sea General Hospital	Cut Off	100%	36
Lakeview Regional Medical Center	Covington	100%	162
Mercy Regional Medical Center	Ville Platte	100%	119
Minden Medical Center	Minden	100%	126
Ochsner Medical Center - Baton Rouge[2]	Baton Rouge	100%	206
Ochsner Medical Center - Northshore	Slidell	100%	173
Saint Charles Parish Hospital	Luling	100%	68
Saint Elizabeth Hospital	Gonzales	100%	101
Saint James Parish Hospital	Lutcher	100%	25
Terrebonne General Medical Center	Houma	100%	370
Thibodaux Regional Medical Center	Thibodaux	100%	233
Washington St Tammany Reg Med Ctr	Bogalusa	100%	68
Charity Hosp & Med Ctr of Louisiana	New Orleans	99%	191
Glenwood Regional Medical Center	West Monroe	99%	305
Homer Memorial Hospital[2]	Homer	98%	42
Lafayette General Medical Center	Lafayette	98%	369
Ochsner Medical Center - Kenner[2]	Kenner	98%	183
Rapides Regional Medical Center[2]	Alexandria	98%	254
Saint Tammany Parish Hospital[2]	Covington	98%	236
Teche Regional Medical Center	Morgan City	98%	87
Christus Saint Patrick Hospital	Lake Charles	97%	255
E A Conway Medical Center	Monroe	97%	117
Lane Regional Medical Center	Zachary	97%	161
Leonard J Chabert Medical Center	Houma	97%	87
Louisiana Heart Hospital	Lacombe	97%	157
Northern Louisiana Medical Center	Ruston	97%	163
Ochsner Medical Center[2]	New Orleans	97%	293
Overton Brooks VA Med Ctr-Shreveport	Shreveport	97%	205
Springhill Medical Center	Springhill	97%	32
West Jefferson Medical Center	Marrero	97%	443
Baton Rouge General Medical Center[2]	Baton Rouge	96%	281
Byrd Regional Hospital	Leesville	96%	165
Opelousas General Health System[2]	Opelousas	96%	208
American Legion Hospital[2]	Crowley	95%	73
Our Lady of the Lake Reg Med Ctr[2]	Baton Rouge	95%	353
Savoy Medical Center	Mamou	95%	38
Tulane Medical Center	New Orleans	95%	316
Dauterive Hospital	New Iberia	94%	69
Our Lady of Lourdes Reg Med Ctr	Lafayette	93%	218
River Parishes Hospital	Laplace	93%	97
Winn Parish Medical Center[2]	Winnfield	93%	27
Franklin Medical Center	Winnsboro	92%	39
Ochsner Saint Anne General Hospital	Raceland	92%	26
The Regional Medical Center of Acadiana[2]	Lafayette	92%	88
Willis Knighton Bossier Health Center[2]	Bossier City	92%	219
Oakdale Community Hospital	Oakdale	91%	33
North Oaks Medical Center[2]	Hammond	90%	242
Saint Francis Medical Center	Monroe	90%	308
Desoto Regional Health System[2]	Mansfield	89%	38
East Jefferson General Hospital[2]	Metairie	89%	236
University Hospital & Clinics	Lafayette	89%	65
Richland Parish Hospital - Delhi	Delhi	88%	26
Willis Knighton Medical Center[2]	Shreveport	88%	481
Avoyelles Hospital	Marksville	87%	47
Slidell Memorial Hospital	Slidell	87%	205
Christus Health Shreveport - Bossier[2]	Shreveport	86%	228
Lake Charles Memorial Hospital[2]	Lake Charles	85%	263
Natchitoches Regional Medical Center	Natchitoches	85%	53
B R F Hospital Holdings[2]	Shreveport	84%	273
Touro Infirmary	New Orleans	84%	320
West Calcasieu Cameron Hospital	Sulphur	81%	91
Beauregard Memorial Hospital	Deridder	78%	58
East Carroll Parish Hospital	Lake Providence	61%	36
Morehouse General Hospital	Bastrop	61%	44
Caldwell Memorial Hospital[2]	Columbia	60%	87
Saint Bernard Parish Hospital[3]	Chalmette	55%	29
Sabine Medical Center[2]	Many	47%	38

Evaluation of LVS Function

Hospital Name	City	Rate	Cases
Alexandria VA Medical Center	Pineville	100%	60
B R F Hospital Holdings[2]	Shreveport	100%	293
Baton Rouge General Medical Center[2]	Baton Rouge	100%	314
Beauregard Memorial Hospital	Deridder	100%	74
Byrd Regional Hospital	Leesville	100%	191
Christus Saint Frances Cabrini Hospital	Alexandria	100%	431
Christus Saint Patrick Hospital	Lake Charles	100%	299
Dauterive Hospital	New Iberia	100%	77
East Jefferson General Hospital[2]	Metairie	100%	296
Glenwood Regional Medical Center	West Monroe	100%	408
Jennings American Legion Hospital	Jennings	100%	137
Lady of the Sea General Hospital	Cut Off	100%	46
Lafayette General Medical Center	Lafayette	100%	442
Lakeview Regional Medical Center	Covington	100%	199
Leonard J Chabert Medical Center	Houma	100%	90
Louisiana Heart Hospital	Lacombe	100%	169
Minden Medical Center	Minden	100%	150
North Oaks Medical Center[2]	Hammond	100%	290
Northern Louisiana Medical Center	Ruston	100%	223
Ochsner Medical Center - Baton Rouge[2]	Baton Rouge	100%	234

NOTE: Hospital profiles are in alphabetical order by state, then city, then hospital within the city; Rankings exclude hospitals with less than 25 cases except for patient surveys which excludes hospitals with less than 100 cases; (a) 100-299 cases; (1) The number of cases/patients is too few to report; (2) Data submitted were based on a sample of cases/patients; (3) Results are based on a shorter time period than required; (4) Data suppressed by CMS for one or more quarters; (5) Results are not available for this reporting period; (6) Fewer than 100 patients completed the HCAHPS survey; (7) No cases met the criteria for this measure; (8) The lower limit of the confidence interval cannot be calculated if the number of observed infections equals zero; (9) No data are available from the state/territory for this reporting period; (10) The scores shown reflect fewer than 50 completed surveys; (11) There were discrepancies in the data collection process; (12) This measure does not apply to this hospital for this reporting period; (13) Results cannot be calculated for this reporting period; (14) The results for this state are combined with nearby states to protect confidentiality; Please refer to the User's Guide for a full explanation of data.

Hospital Name	City	Rate	Cases
Ochsner Medical Center - Kenner[2]	Kenner	100%	215
Ochsner Saint Anne General Hospital	Raceland	100%	28
Overton Brooks VA Med Ctr-Shreveport	Shreveport	100%	221
Pointe Coupee General Hospital	New Roads	100%	36
Rapides Regional Medical Center[2]	Alexandria	100%	299
The Regional Medical Center of Acadiana[2]	Lafayette	100%	103
River Parishes Hospital	Laplace	100%	111
Saint Francis Medical Center	Monroe	100%	377
Saint Tammany Parish Hospital[2]	Covington	100%	279
Slidell Memorial Hospital	Slidell	100%	226
Thibodaux Regional Medical Center	Thibodaux	100%	294
Tulane Medical Center	New Orleans	100%	336
University Hospital & Clinics	Lafayette	100%	69
Washington St Tammany Reg Med Ctr	Bogalusa	100%	81
West Calcasieu Cameron Hospital	Sulphur	100%	105
West Jefferson Medical Center	Marrero	100%	523
Christus Health Shreveport - Bossier[2]	Shreveport	99%	283
E A Conway Medical Center	Monroe	99%	123
Iberia General Hospital & Medical Center	New Iberia	99%	183
Lake Charles Memorial Hospital[2]	Lake Charles	99%	313
Lane Regional Medical Center	Zachary	99%	197
Mercy Regional Medical Center	Ville Platte	99%	167
Ochsner Medical Center[2]	New Orleans	99%	328
Ochsner Medical Center - Northshore	Slidell	99%	194
Our Lady of the Lake Reg Med Ctr[2]	Baton Rouge	99%	378
Saint Elizabeth Hospital	Gonzales	99%	124
Terrebonne General Medical Center	Houma	99%	416
Touro Infirmary	New Orleans	99%	380
Willis Knighton Bossier Health Center[2]	Bossier City	99%	277
Willis Knighton Medical Center[2]	Shreveport	99%	587
Abbeville General Hospital	Abbeville	98%	66
Charity Hosp & Med Ctr of Louisiana	New Orleans	98%	198
Springhill Medical Center	Springhill	98%	44
Teche Regional Medical Center	Morgan City	98%	104
Opelousas General Health System[2]	Opelousas	97%	249
Our Lady of Lourdes Reg Med Ctr	Lafayette	97%	299
Heart Hospital of Lafayette	Lafayette	96%	113
Savoy Medical Center	Mamou	96%	72
Avoyelles Hospital	Marksville	95%	79
Morehouse General Hospital	Bastrop	95%	61
Natchitoches Regional Medical Center	Natchitoches	95%	74
Oakdale Community Hospital	Oakdale	94%	47
Saint Bernard Parish Hospital[3]	Chalmette	93%	29
Winn Parish Medical Center[2]	Winnfield	93%	42
Saint Charles Parish Hospital	Luling	92%	80
Richland Parish Hospital - Delhi	Delhi	91%	34
Saint James Parish Hospital	Lutcher	91%	32
Franklin Medical Center	Winnsboro	89%	53
American Legion Hospital[2]	Crowley	88%	101
Desoto Regional Health System[2]	Mansfield	88%	72
Homer Memorial Hospital[2]	Homer	62%	76
Abrom Kaplan Memorial Hospital	Kaplan	61%	28
Sabine Medical Center[2]	Many	55%	51
Richardson Medical Center	Rayville	48%	33
Caldwell Memorial Hospital[2]	Columbia	46%	90
West Carroll Memorial Hospital[3]	Oak Grove	3%	31
East Carroll Parish Hospital	Lake Providence	2%	45

Medicare Spending

Medicare Spending per Patient (ratio)

Hospital Name	City	Ratio	Cases
Monroe Surgical Hospital	Monroe	0.81	-
Caldwell Memorial Hospital	Columbia	0.84	-
East Carroll Parish Hospital	Lake Providence	0.87	-
Lasalle General Hospital	Jena	0.88	-
Leonard J Chabert Medical Center	Houma	0.88	-
Huey P Long Medical Center	Pineville	0.90	-
E A Conway Medical Center	Monroe	0.91	-
Surgical Specialty Center of Baton Rouge	Baton Rouge	0.91	-
Tulane Medical Center	New Orleans	0.91	-
Beauregard Memorial Hospital	Deridder	0.94	-
Charity Hosp & Med Ctr of Louisiana	New Orleans	0.94	-
Fairway Medical Center	Covington	0.94	-
Southern Surgical Hospital	Slidell	0.94	-
Doctors Hospital at Deer Creek	Leesville	0.95	-
Ochsner Medical Center	New Orleans	0.95	-
B R F Hospital Holdings	Shreveport	0.96	-
Lake Area Medical Center	Lake Charles	0.96	-
Woman's Hospital	Baton Rouge	0.96	-
Heart Hospital of Lafayette	Lafayette	0.97	-
Ochsner Medical Center - Kenner	Kenner	0.97	-
University Hospital & Clinics	Lafayette	0.97	-
Baton Rouge General Medical Center	Baton Rouge	0.98	-
Louisiana Heart Hospital	Lacombe	0.98	-
Oakdale Community Hospital	Oakdale	0.98	-
West Carroll Memorial Hospital	Oak Grove	0.98	-
The Neuromedical Center Hospital	Baton Rouge	0.99	-
Specialists Hospital Shreveport	Shreveport	0.99	-
Abbeville General Hospital	Abbeville	1.00	-
Central Louisiana Surgical Hospital	Alexandria	1.00	-
Citizens Medical Center	Columbia	1.00	-
Dauterive Hospital	New Iberia	1.00	-
East Jefferson General Hospital	Metairie	1.00	-
Lake Charles Memorial Hospital	Lake Charles	1.00	-
Ochsner Medical Center - Northshore	Slidell	1.00	-
P & S Surgical Hospital	Monroe	1.00	-
Sabine Medical Center	Many	1.00	-
Terrebonne General Medical Center	Houma	1.00	-
Allen Parish Hospital	Kinder	1.01	-
Thibodaux Regional Medical Center	Thibodaux	1.01	-
American Legion Hospital	Crowley	1.02	-
Christus Saint Frances Cabrini Hospital	Alexandria	1.02	-
Christus Saint Patrick Hospital	Lake Charles	1.02	-
Lafayette General Medical Center	Lafayette	1.02	-
Our Lady of the Lake Reg Med Ctr	Baton Rouge	1.02	-
Minden Medical Center	Minden	1.03	-
Physicians Medical Center	Houma	1.03	-
Rapides Regional Medical Center	Alexandria	1.03	-
Slidell Memorial Hospital	Slidell	1.03	-
Touro Infirmary	New Orleans	1.03	-
West Calcasieu Cameron Hospital	Sulphur	1.03	-
Jennings American Legion Hospital	Jennings	1.04	-
Richardson Medical Center	Rayville	1.04	-
Saint Francis Medical Center	Monroe	1.04	-
Christus Health Shreveport - Bossier	Shreveport	1.05	-
Green Clinic Surgical Hospital	Ruston	1.05	-
Franklin Medical Center	Winnsboro	1.06	-
Opelousas General Health System	Opelousas	1.06	-
Saint Charles Parish Hospital	Luling	1.06	-
Saint Tammany Parish Hospital	Covington	1.06	-
Avoyelles Hospital	Marksville	1.07	-
Desoto Regional Health System	Mansfield	1.07	-
Glenwood Regional Medical Center	West Monroe	1.07	-
Lakeview Regional Medical Center	Covington	1.07	-
Our Lady of Lourdes Reg Med Ctr	Lafayette	1.07	-
Springhill Medical Center	Springhill	1.07	-
Byrd Regional Hospital	Leesville	1.08	-
The Regional Medical Center of Acadiana	Lafayette	1.08	-
West Jefferson Medical Center	Marrero	1.08	-
Ochsner Medical Center - Baton Rouge	Baton Rouge	1.09	-
Willis Knighton Medical Center	Shreveport	1.09	-
Iberia General Hospital & Medical Center	New Iberia	1.10	-
Lafayette Surgical Specialty Hospital	Lafayette	1.10	-
Lane Regional Medical Center	Zachary	1.10	-
Teche Regional Medical Center	Morgan City	1.10	-
River Parishes Hospital	Laplace	1.12	-
Mercy Regional Medical Center	Ville Platte	1.13	-
Northern Louisiana Medical Center	Ruston	1.13	-
North Oaks Medical Center	Hammond	1.14	-
Homer Memorial Hospital	Homer	1.17	-
Saint Elizabeth Hospital	Gonzales	1.18	-
Willis Knighton Bossier Health Center	Bossier City	1.19	-
Morehouse General Hospital	Bastrop	1.22	-
Winn Parish Medical Center	Winnfield	1.23	-
Natchitoches Regional Medical Center	Natchitoches	1.24	-
Savoy Medical Center	Mamou	1.24	-
Washington St Tammany Reg Med Ctr	Bogalusa	1.30	-
Cypress Pointe Surgical Hospital	Hammond	1.34	-

Pneumonia Care

Appropriate Initial Antibiotic Given

Hospital Name	City	Rate	Cases
Dauterive Hospital	New Iberia	100%	30
Jennings American Legion Hospital	Jennings	100%	88
Lakeview Regional Medical Center	Covington	100%	103
Lallie Kemp Medical Center	Independence	100%	25
Leonard J Chabert Medical Center	Houma	100%	46
Minden Medical Center	Minden	100%	78
Overton Brooks VA Med Ctr-Shreveport	Shreveport	100%	29
Rapides Regional Medical Center[2]	Alexandria	100%	52
The Regional Medical Center of Acadiana[2]	Lafayette	100%	37
River Parishes Hospital	Laplace	100%	44
Union General Hospital	Farmerville	100%	32
Ochsner Medical Center - Baton Rouge[2]	Baton Rouge	99%	67
Terrebonne General Medical Center	Houma	99%	106
Abbeville General Hospital	Abbeville	98%	42
Byrd Regional Hospital	Leesville	98%	52
Christus Saint Frances Cabrini Hospital	Alexandria	98%	152
Lafayette General Medical Center	Lafayette	98%	134
Mercy Regional Medical Center	Ville Platte	98%	132
Northern Louisiana Medical Center	Ruston	98%	58
Ochsner Medical Center - Kenner[2]	Kenner	98%	51
Ochsner Medical Center - Northshore	Slidell	98%	99
Our Lady of the Lake Reg Med Ctr[2]	Baton Rouge	98%	61
Touro Infirmary	New Orleans	98%	81
Tulane Medical Center	New Orleans	98%	51
West Jefferson Medical Center	Marrero	98%	122
Saint Elizabeth Hospital	Gonzales	97%	93
Saint Francis Medical Center	Monroe	97%	151
Alexandria VA Medical Center	Pineville	96%	52
Avoyelles Hospital	Marksville	96%	51
Iberia General Hospital & Medical Center[2]	New Iberia	96%	102
Ochsner Medical Center[2]	New Orleans	96%	68
Opelousas General Health System[2]	Opelousas	96%	73
Our Lady of Lourdes Reg Med Ctr	Lafayette	96%	167
Saint Tammany Parish Hospital[2]	Covington	96%	71
Thibodaux Regional Medical Center	Thibodaux	96%	71
University Hospital & Clinics	Lafayette	96%	27
West Calcasieu Cameron Hospital	Sulphur	96%	67
Charity Hosp & Med Ctr of Louisiana	New Orleans	95%	38
East Jefferson General Hospital[2]	Metairie	95%	63
Glenwood Regional Medical Center	West Monroe	95%	110
Lane Regional Medical Center[2]	Zachary	95%	93
Slidell Memorial Hospital	Slidell	95%	83
Washington St Tammany Reg Med Ctr	Bogalusa	95%	61
Willis Knighton Bossier Health Center[2]	Bossier City	95%	108
American Legion Hospital[2]	Crowley	94%	112
E A Conway Medical Center	Monroe	94%	77
Baton Rouge General Medical Center[2]	Baton Rouge	93%	76
Christus Saint Patrick Hospital	Lake Charles	93%	72
Lady of the Sea General Hospital	Cut Off	93%	42
Louisiana Heart Hospital	Lacombe	93%	44
Willis Knighton Medical Center[2]	Shreveport	92%	158
Winn Parish Medical Center[2]	Winnfield	92%	36
North Oaks Medical Center[2]	Hammond	91%	105
Saint James Parish Hospital	Lutcher	91%	34
Lasalle General Hospital	Jena	90%	62
Morehouse General Hospital	Bastrop	90%	40
Springhill Medical Center	Springhill	90%	42
Saint Charles Parish Hospital	Luling	89%	37
Lake Charles Memorial Hospital[2]	Lake Charles	88%	59
Savoy Medical Center	Mamou	88%	52
Christus Health Shreveport - Bossier[2]	Shreveport	87%	67
Jackson Parish Hospital	Jonesboro	87%	53
Natchitoches Regional Medical Center	Natchitoches	86%	69
Teche Regional Medical Center	Morgan City	85%	48
Huey P Long Medical Center	Pineville	84%	51
Sabine Medical Center[2]	Many	84%	55
Richland Parish Hospital - Delhi[2]	Delhi	83%	41
Franklin Medical Center	Winnsboro	80%	54
Homer Memorial Hospital[2]	Homer	79%	53
Beauregard Memorial Hospital	Deridder	76%	42
Citizens Medical Center[2]	Columbia	73%	41
Desoto Regional Health System[2]	Mansfield	73%	37
West Carroll Memorial Hospital[2,3]	Oak Grove	64%	53

Blood Culture Timing

Hospital Name	City	Rate	Cases
Abbeville General Hospital	Abbeville	100%	67
Baton Rouge General Medical Center[2]	Baton Rouge	100%	160
Glenwood Regional Medical Center	West Monroe	100%	208
Jennings American Legion Hospital	Jennings	100%	91
Lafayette General Medical Center	Lafayette	100%	241
Lakeview Regional Medical Center	Covington	100%	177
Minden Medical Center	Minden	100%	118
Ochsner Medical Center - Baton Rouge[2]	Baton Rouge	100%	156
Ochsner Saint Anne General Hospital	Raceland	100%	30
Our Lady of the Lake Reg Med Ctr	Lafayette	100%	181
Overton Brooks VA Med Ctr-Shreveport	Shreveport	100%	59
Pointe Coupee General Hospital	New Roads	100%	25
Rapides Regional Medical Center[2]	Alexandria	100%	148
Richardson Medical Center	Rayville	100%	31
River Parishes Hospital	Laplace	100%	72
Saint Tammany Parish Hospital[2]	Covington	100%	137
Savoy Medical Center	Mamou	100%	100
Christus Saint Frances Cabrini Hospital	Alexandria	99%	356
E A Conway Medical Center	Monroe	99%	92
East Jefferson General Hospital[2]	Metairie	99%	153
Leonard J Chabert Medical Center	Houma	99%	101
Louisiana Heart Hospital	Lacombe	99%	69
Mercy Regional Medical Center	Ville Platte	99%	174
Northern Louisiana Medical Center	Ruston	99%	133
Ochsner Medical Center - Kenner[2]	Kenner	99%	141
Opelousas General Health System[2]	Opelousas	99%	110
The Regional Medical Center of Acadiana[2]	Lafayette	99%	72
Saint Elizabeth Hospital	Gonzales	99%	177
Slidell Memorial Hospital	Slidell	99%	190
West Calcasieu Cameron Hospital	Sulphur	99%	100
Dauterive Hospital	New Iberia	98%	59
Oakdale Community Hospital	Oakdale	98%	43
Our Lady of the Lake Reg Med Ctr[2]	Baton Rouge	98%	121
Saint Francis Medical Center	Monroe	98%	355
Springhill Medical Center	Springhill	98%	59
Terrebonne General Medical Center	Houma	98%	219
Thibodaux Regional Medical Center	Thibodaux	98%	142
Touro Infirmary	New Orleans	98%	240
Tulane Medical Center	New Orleans	98%	137
West Jefferson Medical Center	Marrero	98%	190
Winn Parish Medical Center[2]	Winnfield	98%	62

NOTE: Hospital profiles are in alphabetical order by state, then city, then hospital within the city; Rankings exclude hospitals with less than 25 cases except for patient surveys which excludes hospitals with less than 100 cases; (a) 100-299 cases; (1) The number of cases/patients is too few to report; (2) Data submitted were based on a sample of cases/patients; (3) Results are based on a shorter time period than required; (4) Data suppressed by CMS for one or more quarters; (5) Results are not available for this reporting period; (6) Fewer than 100 patients completed the HCAHPS survey; (7) No cases met the criteria for this measure; (8) The lower limit of the confidence interval cannot be calculated if the number of observed infections equals zero; (9) No data are available from the state/territory for this reporting period; (10) The scores shown reflect fewer than 50 completed surveys; (11) There were discrepancies in the data collection process; (12) This measure does not apply to this hospital for this reporting period; (13) Results cannot be calculated for this reporting period; (14) The results for this state are combined with nearby states to protect confidentiality; Please refer to the User's Guide for a full explanation of data.

Byrd Regional Hospital	Leesville	97%	91
Christus Saint Patrick Hospital	Lake Charles	97%	155
Iberia General Hospital & Medical Center[2]	New Iberia	97%	182
Lady of the Sea General Hospital	Cut Off	97%	60
Lasalle General Hospital	Jena	97%	96
Morehouse General Hospital	Bastrop	97%	59
Natchitoches Regional Medical Center	Natchitoches	97%	76
North Oaks Medical Center[2]	Hammond	97%	136
Ochsner Medical Center - Northshore	Slidell	97%	236
Saint James Parish Hospital	Lutcher	97%	39
Teche Regional Medical Center	Morgan City	97%	63
American Legion Hospital[2]	Crowley	96%	142
Beauregard Memorial Hospital	Deridder	96%	74
Lane Regional Medical Center[2]	Zachary	96%	153
University Hospital & Clinics	Lafayette	96%	46
Willis Knighton Bossier Health Center[2]	Bossier City	96%	137
Willis Knighton Medical Center[2]	Shreveport	96%	226
Lake Area Medical Center	Lake Charles	95%	38
Union General Hospital	Farmerville	95%	74
Washington St Tammany Reg Med Ctr	Bogalusa	95%	87
Charity Hosp & Med Ctr of Louisiana	New Orleans	94%	114
Christus Health Shreveport - Bossier[2]	Shreveport	94%	107
Ochsner Medical Center[2]	New Orleans	93%	191
Sabine Medical Center[2]	Many	93%	58
Huey P Long Medical Center	Pineville	92%	48
Desoto Regional Health System[2]	Mansfield	91%	33
Franklin Medical Center	Winnsboro	91%	56
Lake Charles Memorial Hospital[2]	Lake Charles	91%	152
Alexandria VA Medical Center	Pineville	89%	95
Homer Memorial Hospital[2]	Homer	89%	61
Lallie Kemp Medical Center	Independence	89%	36
Avoyelles Hospital	Marksville	83%	29
B R F Hospital Holdings[2]	Shreveport	83%	54
Saint Charles Parish Hospital	Luling	83%	41
Saint Martin Hospital	Breaux Bridge	80%	25
Jackson Parish Hospital	Jonesboro	58%	38

Pregnancy and Delivery Care

Newborns whose Deliveries were Scheduled Early

Hospital Name	City	Rate	Cases
B R F Hospital Holdings[2]	Shreveport	0%	28
Byrd Regional Hospital[2]	Leesville	0%	34
Dauterive Hospital[2]	New Iberia	0%	40
E A Conway Medical Center[2]	Monroe	0%	39
Lafayette General Medical Center[2]	Lafayette	0%	34
Lake Area Medical Center[2]	Lake Charles	0%	50
Lake Charles Memorial Hospital[2]	Lake Charles	0%	33
Lakeview Regional Medical Center	Covington	0%	115
Natchitoches Regional Medical Center[2]	Natchitoches	0%	37
North Oaks Medical Center[2]	Hammond	0%	29
Ochsner Medical Center - Northshore[2]	Slidell	0%	32
Rapides Regional Medical Center[2]	Alexandria	0%	75
Touro Infirmary[2]	New Orleans	0%	57
Christus Health Shreveport - Bossier	Shreveport	1%	305
Lane Regional Medical Center	Zachary	1%	68
West Jefferson Medical Center[2]	Marrero	1%	208
Woman's Hospital[2]	Baton Rouge	1%	130
East Jefferson General Hospital[2]	Metairie	2%	316
Iberia General Hospital & Medical Center[2]	New Iberia	2%	50
The Regional Medical Center of Acadiana[2]	Lafayette	2%	52
Saint Tammany Parish Hospital[2]	Covington	2%	44
Tulane Medical Center[2]	New Orleans	2%	45
Jennings American Legion Hospital	Jennings	3%	32
Ochsner Medical Center - Baton Rouge[2]	Baton Rouge	3%	33
Northern Louisiana Medical Center[2]	Ruston	4%	45
Ochsner Medical Center[2]	New Orleans	4%	53
Ochsner Medical Center - Kenner[2]	Kenner	4%	26
Mercy Regional Medical Center[2]	Ville Platte	5%	55
Minden Medical Center[2]	Minden	5%	42
Baton Rouge General Medical Center[2]	Baton Rouge	7%	27
Terrebonne General Medical Center	Houma	7%	135
Thibodaux Regional Medical Center[2]	Thibodaux	7%	71
Willis Knighton Bossier Health Center[2]	Bossier City	7%	56
Willis Knighton Medical Center[2]	Shreveport	7%	109
Morehouse General Hospital[2]	Bastrop	8%	26
Opelousas General Health System[2]	Opelousas	9%	43
Slidell Memorial Hospital[2]	Slidell	9%	80
American Legion Hospital	Crowley	10%	102
Washington St Tammany Reg Med Ctr	Bogalusa	10%	30
Saint Francis Medical Center[2]	Monroe	12%	50
Teche Regional Medical Center[2]	Morgan City	14%	49
Glenwood Regional Medical Center[2]	West Monroe	31%	59
Beauregard Memorial Hospital[2]	Deridder	41%	91

Preventive Care

Immunization for Influenza

Hospital Name	City	Rate	Cases
Byrd Regional Hospital[2]	Leesville	100%	422
Central Louisiana Surgical Hospital[2]	Alexandria	100%	333
Cypress Pointe Hospital East[2]	Slidell	100%	39
Lakeview Regional Medical Center[2]	Covington	100%	542
Minden Medical Center[2]	Minden	100%	371
Northern Louisiana Medical Center[2]	Ruston	100%	573
Rapides Regional Medical Center[2]	Alexandria	100%	640
The Regional Medical Center of Acadiana[2]	Lafayette	100%	456
Teche Regional Medical Center[2]	Morgan City	100%	228
Tulane Medical Center[2]	New Orleans	100%	598
Dauterive Hospital[2]	New Iberia	99%	306
Mercy Regional Medical Center[2]	Ville Platte	99%	415
West Jefferson Medical Center[2]	Marrero	99%	549
Baton Rouge General Medical Center[2]	Baton Rouge	98%	583
Iberia General Hospital & Medical Center[2]	New Iberia	98%	413
Lake Area Medical Center[2]	Lake Charles	98%	307
Saint Elizabeth Hospital[2]	Gonzales	98%	290
Saint Tammany Parish Hospital[2]	Covington	98%	527
Slidell Memorial Hospital[2]	Slidell	98%	523
Touro Infirmary[2]	New Orleans	98%	508
West Feliciana Parish Hospital	Saint Francisville	98%	44
Glenwood Regional Medical Center[2]	West Monroe	97%	548
Lallie Kemp Medical Center[2]	Independence	97%	279
Thibodaux Regional Medical Center[2]	Thibodaux	97%	587
Union General Hospital	Farmerville	97%	198
Willis Knighton Bossier Health Center[2]	Bossier City	97%	851
Lafayette General Surgical Hospital	Lafayette	96%	28
Our Lady of the Lake Reg Med Ctr[2]	Baton Rouge	96%	573
P & S Surgical Hospital[2]	Monroe	96%	281
West Calcasieu Cameron Hospital[2]	Sulphur	96%	400
Our Lady of Lourdes Reg Med Ctr[2]	Lafayette	95%	591
Springhill Medical Center[2]	Springhill	95%	436
Willis Knighton Medical Center[2]	Shreveport	95%	1356
Heart Hospital of Lafayette[2]	Lafayette	94%	323
Louisiana Heart Hospital[2]	Lacombe	94%	326
Terrebonne General Medical Center[2]	Houma	94%	521
Beauregard Memorial Hospital[2]	Deridder	93%	258
Christus Health Shreveport - Bossier[2]	Shreveport	93%	507
Jennings American Legion Hospital[2]	Jennings	93%	318
Christus Saint Patrick Hospital[2]	Lake Charles	92%	579
Lafayette General Medical Center[2]	Lafayette	92%	545
Lasalle General Hospital[2]	Jena	92%	232
North Oaks Medical Center[2]	Hammond	91%	521
River Parishes Hospital[2]	Laplace	91%	254
Saint Francis Medical Center[2]	Monroe	91%	504
Saint James Parish Hospital	Lutcher	91%	45
Winn Parish Medical Center[2]	Winnfield	91%	332
Citizens Medical Center[2]	Columbia	90%	135
Franklin Medical Center[2]	Winnsboro	90%	325
Leonard J Chabert Medical Center[2]	Houma	90%	378
American Legion Hospital[2]	Crowley	88%	320
Green Clinic Surgical Hospital	Ruston	88%	180
Ochsner Medical Center - Baton Rouge[2]	Baton Rouge	88%	496
Park Place Surgical Hospital	Lafayette	88%	33
University Hospital & Clinics[2]	Lafayette	88%	303
Homer Memorial Hospital[2]	Homer	87%	297
Physicians Medical Center	Houma	87%	151
Abbeville General Hospital[2]	Abbeville	86%	249
Avoyelles Hospital[2]	Marksville	86%	295
Christus Saint Frances Cabrini Hospital[2]	Alexandria	86%	534
Lane Regional Medical Center[2]	Zachary	86%	458
Washington St Tammany Reg Med Ctr[2]	Bogalusa	86%	310
Lake Charles Memorial Hospital[2]	Lake Charles	85%	486
Ochsner Medical Center - Kenner[2]	Kenner	84%	482
Ochsner Medical Center - Northshore[2]	Slidell	83%	444
Oakdale Community Hospital[2]	Oakdale	80%	293
East Jefferson General Hospital[2]	Metairie	79%	581
Saint Charles Parish Hospital[2]	Luling	79%	370
Cypress Pointe Surgical Hospital	Hammond	78%	326
Opelousas General Health System[2]	Opelousas	74%	530
Savoy Medical Center[2]	Mamou	74%	361
Franklin Foundation Hospital	Franklin	71%	285
Lafayette Surgical Specialty Hospital	Lafayette	70%	376
Allen Parish Hospital[2]	Kinder	69%	81
Desoto Regional Health System[2]	Mansfield	69%	295
E A Conway Medical Center[2]	Monroe	69%	394
Ochsner Medical Center[2]	New Orleans	69%	720
Alexandria VA Medical Center[2,3]	Pineville	68%	140
West Carroll Memorial Hospital[2,3]	Oak Grove	68%	209
Morehouse General Hospital[2]	Bastrop	66%	238
Natchitoches Regional Medical Center[2]	Natchitoches	64%	245
Ouachita Community Hospital[2]	West Monroe	64%	39
East Carroll Parish Hospital[2]	Lake Providence	62%	250
B R F Hospital Holdings[2]	Shreveport	60%	512
Richardson Medical Center	Rayville	59%	164
Fairway Medical Center	Covington	56%	189
Charity Hosp & Med Ctr of Louisiana[2]	New Orleans	54%	619
Huey P Long Medical Center[2]	Pineville	54%	295
Southern Surgical Hospital[2]	Slidell	53%	301
Sabine Medical Center[2]	Many	47%	276
Woman's Hospital[2]	Baton Rouge	47%	352
Monroe Surgical Hospital[2]	Monroe	45%	109
The Neuromedical Center Hospital[2]	Baton Rouge	43%	424
Doctors Hospital at Deer Creek[2]	Leesville	39%	244
Surgical Specialty Center of Baton Rouge	Baton Rouge	23%	141
Specialists Hospital Shreveport[2]	Shreveport	15%	307
Caldwell Memorial Hospital[2]	Columbia	12%	297

Immunization for Pneumonia

Hospital Name	City	Rate	Cases
Byrd Regional Hospital[2]	Leesville	100%	525
Cypress Pointe Hospital East[2]	Slidell	100%	27
Lakeview Regional Medical Center[2]	Covington	100%	689
Minden Medical Center[2]	Minden	100%	392
Northern Louisiana Medical Center[2]	Ruston	100%	693
Rapides Regional Medical Center[2]	Alexandria	100%	689
The Regional Medical Center of Acadiana[2]	Lafayette	100%	264
West Feliciana Parish Hospital	Saint Francisville	100%	42
West Jefferson Medical Center[2]	Marrero	100%	675
Dauterive Hospital[2]	New Iberia	99%	300
Iberia General Hospital & Medical Center[2]	New Iberia	99%	475
Lake Area Medical Center[2]	Lake Charles	99%	142
Lane Regional Medical Center[2]	Zachary	99%	607
Lasalle General Hospital[2]	Jena	99%	367
Tulane Medical Center[2]	New Orleans	99%	574
Baton Rouge General Medical Center[2]	Baton Rouge	98%	779
Beauregard Memorial Hospital[2]	Deridder	98%	288
Glenwood Regional Medical Center[2]	West Monroe	98%	762
Mercy Regional Medical Center[2]	Ville Platte	98%	470
Saint Tammany Parish Hospital[2]	Covington	98%	607
Slidell Memorial Hospital[2]	Slidell	98%	645
Teche Regional Medical Center[2]	Morgan City	98%	241
Thibodaux Regional Medical Center[2]	Thibodaux	98%	736
Union General Hospital	Farmerville	98%	304
Central Louisiana Surgical Hospital[2]	Alexandria	97%	442
Saint Elizabeth Hospital[2]	Gonzales	97%	424
Springhill Medical Center[2]	Springhill	97%	634
West Calcasieu Cameron Hospital[2]	Sulphur	97%	545
Willis Knighton Bossier Health Center[2]	Bossier City	97%	1093
Lallie Kemp Medical Center[2]	Independence	96%	341
P & S Surgical Hospital[2]	Monroe	96%	391
Saint James Parish Hospital	Lutcher	96%	72
Willis Knighton Medical Center[2]	Shreveport	96%	1891
American Legion Hospital[2]	Crowley	95%	500
Avoyelles Hospital[2]	Marksville	95%	449
Franklin Medical Center[2]	Winnsboro	95%	493
Green Clinic Surgical Hospital	Ruston	95%	217
Homer Memorial Hospital[2]	Homer	95%	387
Jennings American Legion Hospital[2]	Jennings	95%	401
Physicians Medical Center	Houma	95%	64
Touro Infirmary[2]	New Orleans	95%	502
Winn Parish Medical Center[2]	Winnfield	95%	507
Christus Health Shreveport - Bossier[2]	Shreveport	94%	561
Christus Saint Patrick Hospital[2]	Lake Charles	94%	901
Lake Charles Memorial Hospital[2]	Lake Charles	94%	531
Savoy Medical Center[2]	Mamou	94%	270
Abbeville General Hospital[2]	Abbeville	92%	293
Leonard J Chabert Medical Center[2]	Houma	92%	327
Saint Francis Medical Center[2]	Monroe	92%	638
Terrebonne General Medical Center[2]	Houma	92%	749
Alexandria VA Medical Center[2,3]	Pineville	91%	255
River Parishes Hospital[2]	Laplace	91%	419
Christus Saint Frances Cabrini Hospital[2]	Alexandria	90%	741
Heart Hospital of Lafayette[2]	Lafayette	90%	493
Lafayette General Medical Center[2]	Lafayette	90%	632
Louisiana Heart Hospital[2]	Lacombe	90%	516
Ochsner Medical Center - Baton Rouge[2]	Baton Rouge	89%	586
Our Lady of the Lake Reg Med Ctr[2]	Baton Rouge	89%	694
Christus Coushatta Health Care Center[3]	Coushatta	88%	25
East Jefferson General Hospital[2]	Metairie	88%	786
Oakdale Community Hospital[2]	Oakdale	88%	445
Ochsner Medical Center - Kenner[2]	Kenner	88%	505
North Oaks Medical Center[2]	Hammond	87%	666
Saint Charles Parish Hospital[2]	Luling	87%	352
Washington St Tammany Reg Med Ctr[2]	Bogalusa	87%	278
Natchitoches Regional Medical Center[2]	Natchitoches	85%	236
Ochsner Medical Center - Northshore[2]	Slidell	83%	567
Our Lady of Lourdes Reg Med Ctr[2]	Lafayette	83%	798
Franklin Foundation Hospital[3]	Franklin	82%	250
Opelousas General Health System[2]	Opelousas	81%	579
Cypress Pointe Surgical Hospital	Hammond	80%	327
Desoto Regional Health System[2]	Mansfield	78%	530
Morehouse General Hospital[2]	Bastrop	78%	226
University Hospital & Clinics[2]	Lafayette	78%	294
Citizens Medical Center[2]	Columbia	77%	221
Lafayette Surgical Specialty Hospital[2]	Lafayette	73%	308
B R F Hospital Holdings[2]	Shreveport	72%	427
Ochsner Medical Center[2]	New Orleans	72%	776
Allen Parish Hospital[2]	Kinder	71%	78
Saint Bernard Parish Hospital[3]	Chalmette	71%	325
Sabine Medical Center[2]	Many	68%	341
Surgical Specialty Center of Baton Rouge	Baton Rouge	67%	42
Doctors Hospital at Deer Creek[2]	Leesville	65%	217

NOTE: Hospital profiles are in alphabetical order by state, then city, then hospital within the city; Rankings exclude hospitals with less than 25 cases except for patient surveys which excludes hospitals with less than 100 cases; (a) 100-299 cases; (1) The number of cases/patients is too few to report; (2) Data submitted were based on a sample of cases/patients; (3) Results are based on a shorter time period than required; (4) Data suppressed by CMS for one or more quarters; (5) Results are not available for this reporting period; (6) Fewer than 100 patients completed the HCAHPS survey; (7) No cases met the criteria for this measure; (8) The lower limit of the confidence interval cannot be calculated if the number of observed infections equals zero; (9) No data are available from the state/territory for this reporting period; (10) The scores shown reflect fewer than 50 completed surveys; (11) There were discrepancies in the data collection process; (12) This measure does not apply to this hospital for this reporting period; (13) Results cannot be calculated for this reporting period; (14) The results for this state are combined with nearby states to protect confidentiality; Please refer to the User's Guide for a full explanation of data.

Richardson Medical Center[2]	Rayville	62%	268
Fairway Medical Center[2]	Covington	60%	168
Monroe Surgical Hospital[2]	Monroe	59%	104
Charity Hosp & Med Ctr of Louisiana[2]	New Orleans	58%	480
E A Conway Medical Center[2]	Monroe	56%	284
Huey P Long Medical Center[2]	Pineville	53%	229
Southern Surgical Hospital[2]	Slidell	52%	263
The Neuromedical Center Hospital[2]	Baton Rouge	51%	275
West Carroll Memorial Hospital[2,3]	Oak Grove	50%	309
East Carroll Parish Hospital[2]	Lake Providence	47%	373
Ouachita Community Hospital[2]	West Monroe	46%	26
Woman's Hospital[2]	Baton Rouge	37%	27
Specialists Hospital Shreveport[2]	Shreveport	29%	368
Caldwell Memorial Hospital[2]	Columbia	4%	472

Stroke Care

Anticoagulation Therapy for Atrial Fibrillation

Hospital Name	City	Rate	Cases
Baton Rouge General Medical Center	Baton Rouge	100%	31
Lafayette General Medical Center	Lafayette	100%	44
Our Lady of Lourdes Reg Med Ctr	Lafayette	100%	29
Ochsner Medical Center[2]	New Orleans	94%	34
Willis Knighton Medical Center[2]	Shreveport	84%	31

Antithrombotic Therapy Timing

Hospital Name	City	Rate	Cases
Dauterive Hospital	New Iberia	100%	25
Iberia General Hospital & Medical Center	New Iberia	100%	36
Lakeview Regional Medical Center	Covington	100%	45
Lane Regional Medical Center	Zachary	100%	34
Leonard J Chabert Medical Center	Houma	100%	30
Louisiana Heart Hospital	Lacombe	100%	30
Minden Medical Center	Minden	100%	43
Northern Louisiana Medical Center	Ruston	100%	49
Ochsner Medical Center - Baton Rouge	Baton Rouge	100%	47
Ochsner Medical Center - Northshore	Slidell	100%	48
Rapides Regional Medical Center[2]	Alexandria	100%	75
Saint Tammany Parish Hospital[2]	Covington	100%	81
Slidell Memorial Hospital	Slidell	100%	43
Terrebonne General Medical Center	Houma	100%	79
Thibodaux Regional Medical Center	Thibodaux	100%	83
Touro Infirmary	New Orleans	100%	88
West Calcasieu Cameron Hospital	Sulphur	100%	34
East Jefferson General Hospital[2]	Metairie	99%	147
Lafayette General Medical Center	Lafayette	99%	190
Our Lady of Lourdes Reg Med Ctr	Lafayette	99%	149
Tulane Medical Center[2]	New Orleans	99%	78
Willis Knighton Bossier Health Center[2]	Bossier City	99%	91
Lake Charles Memorial Hospital[2]	Lake Charles	98%	81
West Jefferson Medical Center	Marrero	98%	142
Baton Rouge General Medical Center	Baton Rouge	97%	216
Charity Hosp & Med Ctr of Louisiana	New Orleans	97%	67
Christus Health Shreveport - Bossier[2]	Shreveport	97%	93
Christus Saint Frances Cabrini Hospital	Alexandria	97%	102
Ochsner Medical Center - Kenner	Kenner	97%	37
Ochsner Medical Center[2]	New Orleans	96%	154
Our Lady of the Lake Reg Med Ctr[2]	Baton Rouge	96%	80
Saint Francis Medical Center[2]	Monroe	96%	76
Christus Saint Patrick Hospital	Lake Charles	95%	110
E A Conway Medical Center	Monroe	95%	61
Willis Knighton Medical Center[2]	Shreveport	95%	167
Jennings American Legion Hospital	Jennings	94%	34
B R F Hospital Holdings[2]	Shreveport	93%	43
Opelousas General Health System	Opelousas	93%	55
North Oaks Medical Center[2]	Hammond	92%	89
Glenwood Regional Medical Center	West Monroe	87%	112

Assessed for Rehabilitation

Hospital Name	City	Rate	Cases
Dauterive Hospital	New Iberia	100%	25
Lakeview Regional Medical Center	Covington	100%	60
Minden Medical Center	Minden	100%	44
Northern Louisiana Medical Center	Ruston	100%	53
Ochsner Medical Center[2]	New Orleans	100%	265
Ochsner Medical Center - Kenner	Kenner	100%	40
Our Lady of Lourdes Reg Med Ctr	Lafayette	100%	213
Rapides Regional Medical Center[2]	Alexandria	100%	111
The Regional Medical Center of Acadiana[2]	Lafayette	100%	33
Thibodaux Regional Medical Center	Thibodaux	100%	99
West Jefferson Medical Center	Marrero	100%	222
Charity Hosp & Med Ctr of Louisiana	New Orleans	99%	116
East Jefferson General Hospital[2]	Metairie	99%	182
Lafayette General Medical Center	Lafayette	99%	295
Touro Infirmary	New Orleans	99%	100
Tulane Medical Center[2]	New Orleans	99%	132
Baton Rouge General Medical Center	Baton Rouge	98%	262
Saint Tammany Parish Hospital[2]	Covington	98%	93
Slidell Memorial Hospital	Slidell	98%	60
Terrebonne General Medical Center	Houma	98%	84
Ochsner Medical Center - Baton Rouge	Baton Rouge	97%	58
Christus Saint Frances Cabrini Hospital	Alexandria	96%	122
Ochsner Medical Center - Northshore	Slidell	96%	52
B R F Hospital Holdings[2]	Shreveport	95%	93
Iberia General Hospital & Medical Center	New Iberia	95%	40
Our Lady of the Lake Reg Med Ctr[2]	Baton Rouge	95%	116
Leonard J Chabert Medical Center	Houma	94%	31
Opelousas General Health System	Opelousas	94%	50
West Calcasieu Cameron Hospital	Sulphur	94%	35
North Oaks Medical Center[2]	Hammond	93%	98
Jennings American Legion Hospital	Jennings	92%	39
Lake Charles Memorial Hospital[2]	Lake Charles	92%	79
Christus Saint Patrick Hospital	Lake Charles	91%	127
Lane Regional Medical Center	Zachary	91%	33
Christus Health Shreveport - Bossier[2]	Shreveport	90%	110
Saint Francis Medical Center[2]	Monroe	90%	103
Willis Knighton Medical Center[2]	Shreveport	90%	173
Glenwood Regional Medical Center	West Monroe	88%	115
Willis Knighton Bossier Health Center[2]	Bossier City	88%	106
Louisiana Heart Hospital	Lacombe	84%	31
E A Conway Medical Center	Monroe	79%	58

Discharged on Antithrombotic Therapy

Hospital Name	City	Rate	Cases
Baton Rouge General Medical Center	Baton Rouge	100%	250
Christus Saint Frances Cabrini Hospital	Alexandria	100%	108
Lafayette General Medical Center	Lafayette	100%	217
Lakeview Regional Medical Center	Covington	100%	50
Leonard J Chabert Medical Center	Houma	100%	31
Louisiana Heart Hospital	Lacombe	100%	31
Minden Medical Center	Minden	100%	42
Northern Louisiana Medical Center	Ruston	100%	47
Ochsner Medical Center - Baton Rouge	Baton Rouge	100%	57
Ochsner Medical Center - Kenner	Kenner	100%	38
Rapides Regional Medical Center[2]	Alexandria	100%	82
The Regional Medical Center of Acadiana[2]	Lafayette	100%	27
Saint Tammany Parish Hospital[2]	Covington	100%	84
Thibodaux Regional Medical Center	Thibodaux	100%	85
Tulane Medical Center[2]	New Orleans	100%	114
West Calcasieu Cameron Hospital	Sulphur	100%	33
Willis Knighton Bossier Health Center[2]	Bossier City	100%	96
Willis Knighton Medical Center[2]	Shreveport	100%	160
Christus Health Shreveport - Bossier[2]	Shreveport	99%	95
East Jefferson General Hospital[2]	Metairie	99%	160
Lake Charles Memorial Hospital[2]	Lake Charles	99%	73
Our Lady of Lourdes Reg Med Ctr	Lafayette	99%	174
Terrebonne General Medical Center	Houma	99%	80
West Jefferson Medical Center	Marrero	99%	165
B R F Hospital Holdings[2]	Shreveport	98%	53
Charity Hosp & Med Ctr of Louisiana	New Orleans	98%	98
Ochsner Medical Center - Northshore	Slidell	98%	51
Slidell Memorial Hospital	Slidell	98%	50
Touro Infirmary	New Orleans	98%	96
Iberia General Hospital & Medical Center	New Iberia	97%	38
Jennings American Legion Hospital	Jennings	97%	34
Lane Regional Medical Center	Zachary	97%	31
Our Lady of the Lake Reg Med Ctr[2]	Baton Rouge	97%	86
E A Conway Medical Center	Monroe	96%	57
Ochsner Medical Center[2]	New Orleans	96%	226
Christus Saint Patrick Hospital	Lake Charles	95%	113
Saint Francis Medical Center[2]	Monroe	95%	87
Glenwood Regional Medical Center	West Monroe	93%	108
North Oaks Medical Center[2]	Hammond	92%	89
Opelousas General Health System	Opelousas	88%	49

Discharged on Statin Medication

Hospital Name	City	Rate	Cases
Lakeview Regional Medical Center	Covington	100%	40
Minden Medical Center	Minden	100%	26
Northern Louisiana Medical Center	Ruston	100%	29
Ochsner Medical Center - Northshore	Slidell	100%	35
Our Lady of Lourdes Reg Med Ctr	Lafayette	100%	137
Tulane Medical Center[2]	New Orleans	100%	83
Charity Hosp & Med Ctr of Louisiana	New Orleans	99%	81
Thibodaux Regional Medical Center	Thibodaux	99%	69
Slidell Memorial Hospital	Slidell	98%	40
Terrebonne General Medical Center	Houma	98%	64
Lafayette General Medical Center	Lafayette	97%	177
Ochsner Medical Center - Kenner	Kenner	97%	33
Rapides Regional Medical Center[2]	Alexandria	97%	69
West Jefferson Medical Center	Marrero	97%	124
Louisiana Heart Hospital	Lacombe	96%	28
E A Conway Medical Center	Monroe	95%	44
Ochsner Medical Center[2]	New Orleans	95%	183
Our Lady of the Lake Reg Med Ctr[2]	Baton Rouge	95%	74
East Jefferson General Hospital[2]	Metairie	94%	126
Baton Rouge General Medical Center	Baton Rouge	93%	189
Ochsner Medical Center - Baton Rouge	Baton Rouge	93%	45
Saint Tammany Parish Hospital[2]	Covington	93%	73
Touro Infirmary	New Orleans	93%	67
B R F Hospital Holdings[2]	Shreveport	92%	49
Leonard J Chabert Medical Center	Houma	92%	26
Christus Saint Frances Cabrini Hospital	Alexandria	90%	90
Iberia General Hospital & Medical Center	New Iberia	87%	31
Jennings American Legion Hospital	Jennings	86%	29
Saint Francis Medical Center[2]	Monroe	85%	68
Christus Saint Patrick Hospital	Lake Charles	84%	96
North Oaks Medical Center[2]	Hammond	81%	67
Glenwood Regional Medical Center	West Monroe	78%	93
Christus Health Shreveport - Bossier[2]	Shreveport	77%	82
Willis Knighton Bossier Health Center[2]	Bossier City	75%	76
Willis Knighton Medical Center[2]	Shreveport	69%	133
Lake Charles Memorial Hospital[2]	Lake Charles	68%	71
Lane Regional Medical Center	Zachary	68%	28
Opelousas General Health System	Opelousas	62%	45

Thrombolytic Therapy Timing

Hospital Name	City	Rate	Cases
West Jefferson Medical Center	Marrero	88%	25

Venous Thromboembolism (VTE) Prophylaxis

Hospital Name	City	Rate	Cases
Dauterive Hospital	New Iberia	100%	25
Lakeview Regional Medical Center	Covington	100%	64
Minden Medical Center	Minden	100%	44
Northern Louisiana Medical Center	Ruston	100%	53
Our Lady of Lourdes Reg Med Ctr	Lafayette	100%	226
Rapides Regional Medical Center[2]	Alexandria	100%	123
The Regional Medical Center of Acadiana[2]	Lafayette	100%	28
Slidell Memorial Hospital	Slidell	100%	47
Tulane Medical Center[2]	New Orleans	100%	134
Thibodaux Regional Medical Center	Thibodaux	99%	101
Touro Infirmary	New Orleans	99%	95
West Jefferson Medical Center	Marrero	99%	243
East Jefferson General Hospital[2]	Metairie	98%	172
Leonard J Chabert Medical Center	Houma	96%	26
Louisiana Heart Hospital	Lacombe	96%	27
B R F Hospital Holdings[2]	Shreveport	95%	107
Charity Hosp & Med Ctr of Louisiana	New Orleans	95%	110
Ochsner Medical Center - Baton Rouge	Baton Rouge	95%	56
Lafayette General Medical Center	Lafayette	93%	308
Baton Rouge General Medical Center	Baton Rouge	92%	254
Iberia General Hospital & Medical Center	New Iberia	92%	38
Ochsner Medical Center - Kenner	Kenner	92%	38
Ochsner Medical Center - Northshore	Slidell	92%	50
Our Lady of the Lake Reg Med Ctr[2]	Baton Rouge	92%	118
Saint Francis Medical Center[2]	Monroe	92%	104
Terrebonne General Medical Center	Houma	89%	84
West Calcasieu Cameron Hospital	Sulphur	89%	38
Saint Tammany Parish Hospital[2]	Covington	88%	88
Jennings American Legion Hospital	Jennings	87%	38
Lake Charles Memorial Hospital[2]	Lake Charles	85%	88
Christus Saint Frances Cabrini Hospital	Alexandria	84%	128
E A Conway Medical Center	Monroe	83%	63
Ochsner Medical Center[2]	New Orleans	77%	257
Opelousas General Health System	Opelousas	75%	55
Glenwood Regional Medical Center	West Monroe	73%	115
North Oaks Medical Center[2]	Hammond	73%	104
Christus Health Shreveport - Bossier[2]	Shreveport	67%	111
Willis Knighton Bossier Health Center[2]	Bossier City	67%	97
Christus Saint Patrick Hospital	Lake Charles	63%	123
Willis Knighton Medical Center[2]	Shreveport	59%	179
Lane Regional Medical Center	Zachary	47%	36

Written Stroke Educational Materials Given

Hospital Name	City	Rate	Cases
Lakeview Regional Medical Center	Covington	100%	35
Ochsner Medical Center[2]	New Orleans	100%	181
Ochsner Medical Center - Northshore	Slidell	100%	33
Rapides Regional Medical Center[2]	Alexandria	100%	53
Thibodaux Regional Medical Center	Thibodaux	100%	54
West Jefferson Medical Center	Marrero	100%	114
Our Lady of Lourdes Reg Med Ctr	Lafayette	99%	111
Lafayette General Medical Center	Lafayette	98%	184
Northern Louisiana Medical Center	Ruston	97%	35
Ochsner Medical Center - Baton Rouge	Baton Rouge	97%	37
Terrebonne General Medical Center	Houma	96%	48
East Jefferson General Hospital[2]	Metairie	95%	116
Slidell Memorial Hospital	Slidell	95%	39
Saint Tammany Parish Hospital[2]	Covington	94%	63
Tulane Medical Center[2]	New Orleans	93%	76
Glenwood Regional Medical Center	West Monroe	91%	56
Our Lady of the Lake Reg Med Ctr[2]	Baton Rouge	91%	68
Charity Hosp & Med Ctr of Louisiana	New Orleans	89%	80
Ochsner Medical Center - Kenner	Kenner	86%	29
Touro Infirmary	New Orleans	85%	65
Baton Rouge General Medical Center	Baton Rouge	79%	130
E A Conway Medical Center	Monroe	69%	49
Saint Francis Medical Center[2]	Monroe	67%	48

NOTE: Hospital profiles are in alphabetical order by state, then city, then hospital within the city; Rankings exclude hospitals with less than 25 cases except for patient surveys which excludes hospitals with less than 100 cases; (a) 100-299 cases; (1) The number of cases/patients is too few to report; (2) Data submitted were based on a sample of cases/patients; (3) Results are based on a shorter time period than required; (4) Data suppressed by CMS for one or more quarters; (5) Results are not available for this reporting period; (6) Fewer than 100 patients completed the HCAHPS survey; (7) No cases met the criteria for this measure; (8) The lower limit of the confidence interval cannot be calculated if the number of observed infections equals zero; (9) No data are available from the state/territory for this reporting period; (10) The scores shown reflect fewer than 50 completed surveys; (11) There were discrepancies in the data collection process; (12) This measure does not apply to this hospital for this reporting period; (13) Results cannot be calculated for this reporting period; (14) The results for this state are combined with nearby states to protect confidentiality; Please refer to the User's Guide for a full explanation of data.

Willis Knighton Bossier Health Center[2]	Bossier City	63%	68
Christus Saint Patrick Hospital	Lake Charles	59%	68
B R F Hospital Holdings[2]	Shreveport	58%	55
Christus Saint Frances Cabrini Hospital	Alexandria	58%	62
Willis Knighton Medical Center[2]	Shreveport	57%	87
North Oaks Medical Center[2]	Hammond	53%	53
Lake Charles Memorial Hospital[2]	Lake Charles	52%	52
Leonard J Chabert Medical Center	Houma	32%	25
Christus Health Shreveport - Bossier[2]	Shreveport	18%	49

Surgical Care Improvement Project

Appropriate Beta Blocker Usage

Hospital Name	City	Rate	Cases
Baton Rouge General Medical Center[2]	Baton Rouge	100%	224
Central Louisiana Surgical Hospital[2]	Alexandria	100%	109
Christus Saint Patrick Hospital	Lake Charles	100%	147
Dauterive Hospital	New Iberia	100%	45
Heart Hospital of Lafayette	Lafayette	100%	234
Lakeview Regional Medical Center	Covington	100%	165
Leonard J Chabert Medical Center	Houma	100%	76
Minden Medical Center	Minden	100%	65
Ochsner Medical Center - Northshore	Slidell	100%	78
P & S Surgical Hospital[2]	Monroe	100%	79
Rapides Regional Medical Center[2]	Alexandria	100%	210
The Regional Medical Center of Acadiana[2]	Lafayette	100%	144
Saint Elizabeth Hospital	Gonzales	100%	69
Saint Francis Medical Center[2]	Monroe	100%	183
Southern Surgical Hospital[2]	Slidell	100%	32
Terrebonne General Medical Center[2]	Houma	100%	229
Tulane Medical Center[2]	New Orleans	100%	147
West Jefferson Medical Center[2]	Marrero	100%	200
Christus Saint Frances Cabrini Hospital	Alexandria	99%	326
East Jefferson General Hospital[2]	Metairie	99%	205
Ochsner Medical Center[2]	New Orleans	99%	210
Our Lady of Lourdes Reg Med Ctr[2]	Lafayette	99%	110
Our Lady of the Lake Reg Med Ctr[2]	Baton Rouge	99%	483
Thibodaux Regional Medical Center	Thibodaux	99%	237
Byrd Regional Hospital	Leesville	98%	46
Glenwood Regional Medical Center	West Monroe	98%	170
Jennings American Legion Hospital	Jennings	98%	43
Lafayette General Medical Center[2]	Lafayette	98%	236
Louisiana Heart Hospital[2]	Lacombe	98%	163
Ochsner Medical Center - Baton Rouge[2]	Baton Rouge	98%	124
Ochsner Medical Center - Kenner[2]	Kenner	98%	60
River Parishes Hospital[2]	Laplace	98%	43
Slidell Memorial Hospital	Slidell	98%	182
B R F Hospital Holdings[2]	Shreveport	97%	149
Christus Health Shreveport - Bossier[2]	Shreveport	97%	144
Lane Regional Medical Center	Zachary	97%	104
North Oaks Medical Center[2]	Hammond	97%	191
Northern Louisiana Medical Center	Ruston	97%	39
Saint Tammany Parish Hospital[2]	Covington	97%	145
Willis Knighton Medical Center[2]	Shreveport	97%	579
Charity Hosp & Med Ctr of Louisiana[2]	New Orleans	96%	164
Lake Area Medical Center	Lake Charles	96%	45
Natchitoches Regional Medical Center	Natchitoches	96%	26
Touro Infirmary[2]	New Orleans	96%	228
West Calcasieu Cameron Hospital	Sulphur	96%	127
Willis Knighton Bossier Health Center[2]	Bossier City	94%	172
Iberia General Hospital & Medical Center	New Iberia	93%	67
Lake Charles Memorial Hospital[2]	Lake Charles	93%	241
Physicians Medical Center	Houma	93%	28
Lafayette Surgical Specialty Hospital[2]	Lafayette	92%	38
Opelousas General Health System[2]	Opelousas	90%	109
Overton Brooks VA Med Ctr-Shreveport[2]	Shreveport	90%	71
Mercy Regional Medical Center	Ville Platte	87%	31
Cypress Pointe Surgical Hospital	Hammond	85%	33
University Hospital & Clinics[2]	Lafayette	84%	49
Fairway Medical Center[2]	Covington	81%	26
Specialists Hospital Shreveport[2]	Shreveport	81%	53

Appropriate VTP Within 24 Hours

Hospital Name	City	Rate	Cases
Abbeville General Hospital	Abbeville	100%	43
Christus Saint Patrick Hospital	Lake Charles	100%	227
Dauterive Hospital	New Iberia	100%	121
Franklin Foundation Hospital[3]	Franklin	100%	44
Green Clinic Surgical Hospital	Ruston	100%	100
Iberia General Hospital & Medical Center	New Iberia	100%	237
Lakeview Regional Medical Center	Covington	100%	340
Minden Medical Center	Minden	100%	196
Ouachita Community Hospital[2]	West Monroe	100%	36
P & S Surgical Hospital[2]	Monroe	100%	288
Rapides Regional Medical Center[2]	Alexandria	100%	365
The Regional Medical Center of Acadiana[2]	Lafayette	100%	153
Richardson Medical Center	Rayville	100%	45
Saint Elizabeth Hospital	Gonzales	100%	188
Saint Francis Medical Center[2]	Monroe	100%	257
Savoy Medical Center	Mamou	100%	27
Baton Rouge General Medical Center[2]	Baton Rouge	99%	405
Central Louisiana Surgical Hospital[2]	Alexandria	99%	322
Christus Saint Frances Cabrini Hospital	Alexandria	99%	385
Jennings American Legion Hospital	Jennings	99%	138
Lafayette Surgical Specialty Hospital[2]	Lafayette	99%	160
Lane Regional Medical Center	Zachary	99%	285
Ochsner Medical Center - Northshore	Slidell	99%	223
Slidell Memorial Hospital	Slidell	99%	389
Southern Surgical Hospital[2]	Slidell	99%	166
Specialists Hospital Shreveport[2]	Shreveport	99%	204
Terrebonne General Medical Center[2]	Houma	99%	358
Thibodaux Regional Medical Center	Thibodaux	99%	434
Touro Infirmary[2]	New Orleans	99%	635
Tulane Medical Center[2]	New Orleans	99%	340
West Jefferson Medical Center[2]	Marrero	99%	389
Byrd Regional Hospital	Leesville	98%	98
Charity Hosp & Med Ctr of Louisiana[2]	New Orleans	98%	360
Lake Area Medical Center	Lake Charles	98%	196
Monroe Surgical Hospital[2]	Monroe	98%	81
Natchitoches Regional Medical Center	Natchitoches	98%	97
Northern Louisiana Medical Center	Ruston	98%	121
Our Lady of Lourdes Reg Med Ctr[2]	Lafayette	98%	253
River Parishes Hospital[2]	Laplace	98%	106
West Calcasieu Cameron Hospital	Sulphur	98%	432
Willis Knighton Bossier Health Center[2]	Bossier City	98%	333
Willis Knighton Medical Center[2]	Shreveport	98%	1002
Doctors Hospital at Deer Creek[2]	Leesville	97%	29
East Jefferson General Hospital[2]	Metairie	97%	356
Glenwood Regional Medical Center	West Monroe	97%	221
Lafayette General Medical Center[2]	Lafayette	97%	422
Leonard J Chabert Medical Center	Houma	97%	299
Louisiana Heart Hospital[2]	Lacombe	97%	62
Ochsner Medical Center - Kenner[2]	Kenner	97%	245
Our Lady of the Lake Reg Med Ctr[2]	Baton Rouge	97%	659
Overton Brooks VA Med Ctr-Shreveport[2]	Shreveport	97%	157
University Hospital & Clinics[2]	Lafayette	97%	150
Washington St Tammany Reg Med Ctr	Bogalusa	97%	79
Woman's Hospital[2]	Baton Rouge	97%	102
Fairway Medical Center[2]	Covington	96%	83
Mercy Regional Medical Center	Ville Platte	96%	121
Saint Charles Parish Hospital	Luling	96%	25
Saint Tammany Parish Hospital[2]	Covington	96%	300
E A Conway Medical Center	Monroe	95%	110
Lallie Kemp Medical Center	Independence	95%	66
Ochsner Medical Center[2]	New Orleans	95%	418
Ochsner Medical Center - Baton Rouge[2]	Baton Rouge	95%	196
Physicians Medical Center	Houma	95%	75
Opelousas General Health System[2]	Opelousas	94%	303
B R F Hospital Holdings[2]	Shreveport	92%	283
Christus Health Shreveport - Bossier[2]	Shreveport	92%	369
Lake Charles Memorial Hospital[2]	Lake Charles	92%	492
Teche Regional Medical Center	Morgan City	92%	65
Beauregard Memorial Hospital	Deridder	91%	76
Morehouse General Hospital	Bastrop	91%	34
Cypress Pointe Surgical Hospital	Hammond	90%	102
Huey P Long Medical Center	Pineville	90%	61
North Oaks Medical Center[2]	Hammond	89%	390
American Legion Hospital[2]	Crowley	79%	86

Controlled Postoperative Blood Glucose

Hospital Name	City	Rate	Cases
The Regional Medical Center of Acadiana[2]	Lafayette	100%	139
Saint Francis Medical Center[2]	Monroe	100%	91
Tulane Medical Center[2]	New Orleans	100%	47
Willis Knighton Bossier Health Center[2]	Bossier City	100%	47
Baton Rouge General Medical Center[2]	Baton Rouge	99%	146
Glenwood Regional Medical Center	West Monroe	99%	123
Lafayette General Medical Center[2]	Lafayette	99%	156
Our Lady of the Lake Reg Med Ctr[2]	Baton Rouge	99%	313
Rapides Regional Medical Center[2]	Alexandria	98%	131
Slidell Memorial Hospital	Slidell	98%	96
Touro Infirmary[2]	New Orleans	98%	65
Christus Saint Patrick Hospital	Lake Charles	97%	60
North Oaks Medical Center[2]	Hammond	97%	78
Heart Hospital of Lafayette	Lafayette	96%	343
Lakeview Regional Medical Center	Covington	96%	82
Willis Knighton Medical Center[2]	Shreveport	96%	289
Ochsner Medical Center[2]	New Orleans	95%	122
Saint Tammany Parish Hospital[2]	Covington	95%	80
Terrebonne General Medical Center[2]	Houma	95%	81
Thibodaux Regional Medical Center	Thibodaux	95%	81
East Jefferson General Hospital[2]	Metairie	94%	110
B R F Hospital Holdings[2]	Shreveport	93%	87
Ochsner Medical Center - Baton Rouge[2]	Baton Rouge	93%	60
West Jefferson Medical Center[2]	Marrero	93%	57
Louisiana Heart Hospital[2]	Lacombe	92%	181
Christus Saint Frances Cabrini Hospital	Alexandria	91%	270
Lake Charles Memorial Hospital[2]	Lake Charles	90%	101
Our Lady of Lourdes Reg Med Ctr[2]	Lafayette	90%	40
Charity Hosp & Med Ctr of Louisiana[2]	New Orleans	83%	144

Perioperative Temperature Management

Hospital Name	City	Rate	Cases
Abbeville General Hospital	Abbeville	100%	64
American Legion Hospital[2]	Crowley	100%	90
B R F Hospital Holdings[2]	Shreveport	100%	359
Baton Rouge General Medical Center[2]	Baton Rouge	100%	596
Central Louisiana Surgical Hospital[2]	Alexandria	100%	356
Charity Hosp & Med Ctr of Louisiana[2]	New Orleans	100%	469
Christus Health Shreveport - Bossier[2]	Shreveport	100%	440
Christus Saint Patrick Hospital	Lake Charles	100%	298
Cypress Pointe Surgical Hospital	Hammond	100%	130
Dauterive Hospital	New Iberia	100%	149
E A Conway Medical Center	Monroe	100%	159
Franklin Foundation Hospital[3]	Franklin	100%	52
Glenwood Regional Medical Center	West Monroe	100%	309
Green Clinic Surgical Hospital	Ruston	100%	114
Heart Hospital of Lafayette	Lafayette	100%	419
Iberia General Hospital & Medical Center	New Iberia	100%	281
Jennings American Legion Hospital	Jennings	100%	154
Lafayette General Medical Center[2]	Lafayette	100%	581
Lafayette General Surgical Hospital	Lafayette	100%	26
Lake Area Medical Center	Lake Charles	100%	279
Lake Charles Memorial Hospital[2]	Lake Charles	100%	545
Lakeview Regional Medical Center	Covington	100%	410
Lallie Kemp Medical Center	Independence	100%	91
Lane Regional Medical Center	Zachary	100%	322
Leonard J Chabert Medical Center	Houma	100%	330
Louisiana Heart Hospital[2]	Lacombe	100%	137
Mercy Regional Medical Center	Ville Platte	100%	139
Minden Medical Center	Minden	100%	244
Monroe Surgical Hospital[2]	Monroe	100%	90
Morehouse General Hospital	Bastrop	100%	48
Natchitoches Regional Medical Center	Natchitoches	100%	103
Northern Louisiana Medical Center	Ruston	100%	139
Ochsner Medical Center[2]	New Orleans	100%	591
Ochsner Medical Center - Baton Rouge[2]	Baton Rouge	100%	236
Ochsner Medical Center - Kenner[2]	Kenner	100%	284
Ochsner Medical Center - Northshore	Slidell	100%	250
Opelousas General Health System[2]	Opelousas	100%	356
Our Lady of Lourdes Reg Med Ctr[2]	Lafayette	100%	317
Our Lady of the Lake Reg Med Ctr[2]	Baton Rouge	100%	1088
Overton Brooks VA Med Ctr-Shreveport[2]	Shreveport	100%	174
P & S Surgical Hospital[2]	Monroe	100%	303
Physicians Medical Center	Houma	100%	82
Rapides Regional Medical Center[2]	Alexandria	100%	429
The Regional Medical Center of Acadiana[2]	Lafayette	100%	292
Richardson Medical Center	Rayville	100%	54
River Parishes Hospital[2]	Laplace	100%	111
Saint Charles Parish Hospital	Luling	100%	29
Saint Elizabeth Hospital	Gonzales	100%	196
Saint Francis Medical Center[2]	Monroe	100%	327
Saint Tammany Parish Hospital[2]	Covington	100%	372
Savoy Medical Center	Mamou	100%	30
Slidell Memorial Hospital	Slidell	100%	436
Southern Surgical Hospital[2]	Slidell	100%	188
Specialists Hospital Shreveport[2]	Shreveport	100%	214
Surgical Specialty Center of Baton Rouge	Baton Rouge	100%	38
Teche Regional Medical Center	Morgan City	100%	77
Terrebonne General Medical Center[2]	Houma	100%	412
Thibodaux Regional Medical Center	Thibodaux	100%	498
Touro Infirmary[2]	New Orleans	100%	735
Tulane Medical Center[2]	New Orleans	100%	426
University Hospital & Clinics[2]	Lafayette	100%	202
Washington St Tammany Reg Med Ctr	Bogalusa	100%	84
West Calcasieu Cameron Hospital	Sulphur	100%	488
West Jefferson Medical Center[2]	Marrero	100%	491
Willis Knighton Bossier Health Center[2]	Bossier City	100%	394
Willis Knighton Medical Center[2]	Shreveport	100%	1155
Woman's Hospital[2]	Baton Rouge	100%	149
Beauregard Memorial Hospital	Deridder	99%	93
Byrd Regional Hospital	Leesville	99%	122
Christus Saint Frances Cabrini Hospital	Alexandria	99%	655
East Jefferson General Hospital[2]	Metairie	99%	471
Fairway Medical Center[2]	Covington	99%	95
Huey P Long Medical Center	Pineville	99%	80
Lafayette Surgical Specialty Hospital[2]	Lafayette	99%	171
North Oaks Medical Center[2]	Hammond	99%	470
Ochsner Saint Anne General Hospital	Raceland	97%	36
Ouachita Community Hospital[2]	West Monroe	95%	37
Doctors Hospital at Deer Creek[2]	Leesville	86%	37

Prophylactic Antibiotic Selection

Hospital Name	City	Rate	Cases
Central Louisiana Surgical Hospital[2]	Alexandria	100%	252
Christus Saint Patrick Hospital	Lake Charles	100%	164
Dauterive Hospital	New Iberia	100%	90
Franklin Foundation Hospital[3]	Franklin	100%	40
Heart Hospital of Lafayette	Lafayette	100%	361
Huey P Long Medical Center	Pineville	100%	42
Jennings American Legion Hospital	Jennings	100%	128

NOTE: Hospital profiles are in alphabetical order by state, then city, then hospital within the city; Rankings exclude hospitals with less than 25 cases except for patient surveys which excludes hospitals with less than 100 cases; (a) 100-299 cases; (1) The number of cases/patients is too few to report; (2) Data submitted were based on a sample of cases/patients; (3) Results are based on a shorter time period than required; (4) Data suppressed by CMS for one or more quarters; (5) Results are not available for this reporting period; (6) Fewer than 100 patients completed the HCAHPS survey; (7) No cases met the criteria for this measure; (8) The lower limit of the confidence interval cannot be calculated if the number of observed infections equals zero; (9) No data are available from the state/territory for this reporting period; (10) The scores shown reflect fewer than 50 completed surveys; (11) There were discrepancies in the data collection process; (12) This measure does not apply to this hospital for this reporting period; (13) Results cannot be calculated for this reporting period; (14) The results for this state are combined with nearby states to protect confidentiality; Please refer to the User's Guide for a full explanation of data.

Lafayette Surgical Specialty Hospital[2]	Lafayette	100%	158
Lake Area Medical Center	Lake Charles	100%	222
Lakeview Regional Medical Center	Covington	100%	324
Lallie Kemp Medical Center	Independence	100%	67
Leonard J Chabert Medical Center	Houma	100%	224
Louisiana Heart Hospital[2]	Lacombe	100%	212
Our Lady of Lourdes Reg Med Ctr[2]	Lafayette	100%	238
Our Lady of the Lake Reg Med Ctr[2]	Baton Rouge	100%	788
Overton Brooks VA Med Ctr-Shreveport	Shreveport	100%	79
P & S Surgical Hospital[2]	Monroe	100%	242
Physicians Medical Center	Houma	100%	62
Rapides Regional Medical Center[2]	Alexandria	100%	341
The Regional Medical Center of Acadiana[2]	Lafayette	100%	284
Saint Elizabeth Hospital	Gonzales	100%	137
Saint Francis Medical Center[2]	Monroe	100%	279
Specialists Hospital Shreveport[2]	Shreveport	100%	195
Terrebonne General Medical Center[2]	Houma	100%	383
Thibodaux Regional Medical Center	Thibodaux	100%	411
Touro Infirmary[2]	New Orleans	100%	627
Tulane Medical Center[2]	New Orleans	100%	257
Washington St Tammany Reg Med Ctr	Bogalusa	100%	46
Willis Knighton Bossier Health Center[2]	Bossier City	100%	250
Woman's Hospital[2]	Baton Rouge	100%	77
Christus Saint Frances Cabrini Hospital	Alexandria	99%	504
East Jefferson General Hospital[2]	Metairie	99%	438
Fairway Medical Center[2]	Covington	99%	70
Green Clinic Surgical Hospital	Ruston	99%	92
Lake Charles Memorial Hospital[2]	Lake Charles	99%	480
Lane Regional Medical Center	Zachary	99%	236
Mercy Regional Medical Center	Ville Platte	99%	79
Minden Medical Center	Minden	99%	128
Natchitoches Regional Medical Center	Natchitoches	99%	84
Northern Louisiana Medical Center	Ruston	99%	92
Ochsner Medical Center[2]	New Orleans	99%	404
Ochsner Medical Center - Kenner[2]	Kenner	99%	196
Ochsner Medical Center - Northshore	Slidell	99%	176
Saint Tammany Parish Hospital[2]	Covington	99%	304
Slidell Memorial Hospital	Slidell	99%	315
West Calcasieu Cameron Hospital	Sulphur	99%	353
West Jefferson Medical Center[2]	Marrero	99%	398
Byrd Regional Hospital	Leesville	98%	89
Charity Hosp & Med Ctr of Louisiana[2]	New Orleans	98%	363
Glenwood Regional Medical Center	West Monroe	98%	210
Iberia General Hospital & Medical Center	New Iberia	98%	194
Lafayette General Medical Center[2]	Lafayette	98%	551
Monroe Surgical Hospital[2]	Monroe	98%	65
North Oaks Medical Center[2]	Hammond	98%	328
Ochsner Medical Center - Baton Rouge[2]	Baton Rouge	98%	187
Opelousas General Health System[2]	Opelousas	98%	254
University Hospital & Clinics[2]	Lafayette	98%	100
Willis Knighton Medical Center[2]	Shreveport	98%	753
Baton Rouge General Medical Center[2]	Baton Rouge	97%	476
Doctors Hospital at Deer Creek[2]	Leesville	97%	32
Ouachita Community Hospital[2]	West Monroe	97%	34
River Parishes Hospital[2]	Laplace	97%	75
Southern Surgical Hospital[2]	Slidell	97%	142
B R F Hospital Holdings[2]	Shreveport	96%	311
Beauregard Memorial Hospital	Deridder	96%	73
Christus Health Shreveport - Bossier[2]	Shreveport	96%	335
E A Conway Medical Center	Monroe	95%	106
Morehouse General Hospital	Bastrop	95%	40
Abbeville General Hospital	Abbeville	93%	46
Cypress Pointe Surgical Hospital	Hammond	93%	75
Teche Regional Medical Center	Morgan City	90%	31
Richardson Medical Center	Rayville	76%	38

Prophylactic Antibiotic Selection (Outpatient)

Hospital Name	City	Rate	Cases
Abbeville General Hospital	Abbeville	100%	39
Byrd Regional Hospital	Leesville	100%	44
Central Louisiana Surgical Hospital	Alexandria	100%	271
Christus Saint Patrick Hospital	Lake Charles	100%	490
Heart Hospital of Lafayette	Lafayette	100%	241
Lakeview Regional Medical Center	Covington	100%	218
Lane Regional Medical Center	Zachary	100%	64
The Neuromedical Center Hospital	Baton Rouge	100%	358
Northern Louisiana Medical Center	Ruston	100%	35
Ochsner Saint Anne General Hospital	Raceland	100%	25
Rapides Regional Medical Center	Alexandria	100%	214
The Regional Medical Center of Acadiana	Lafayette	100%	191
Specialists Hospital Shreveport	Shreveport	100%	408
University Hospital & Clinics	Lafayette	100%	97
Dauterive Hospital	New Iberia	99%	95
Green Clinic Surgical Hospital	Ruston	99%	85
Jennings American Legion Hospital	Jennings	99%	89
Lafayette General Medical Center	Lafayette	99%	244
Lake Area Medical Center	Lake Charles	99%	203
Leonard J Chabert Medical Center	Houma	99%	193
Ochsner Medical Center - Kenner	Kenner	99%	86
P & S Surgical Hospital	Monroe	99%	462
Touro Infirmary	New Orleans	99%	347
Tulane Medical Center	New Orleans	99%	389
East Jefferson General Hospital	Metairie	98%	500
Glenwood Regional Medical Center	West Monroe	98%	213
Iberia General Hospital & Medical Center	New Iberia	98%	88
Lafayette General Surgical Hospital	Lafayette	98%	54
Lafayette Surgical Specialty Hospital	Lafayette	98%	370
Louisiana Heart Hospital	Lacombe	98%	195
Ochsner Medical Center - Baton Rouge	Baton Rouge	98%	243
Our Lady of the Lake Reg Med Ctr	Baton Rouge	98%	561
Southern Surgical Hospital	Slidell	98%	50
Terrebonne General Medical Center	Houma	98%	410
Thibodaux Regional Medical Center	Thibodaux	98%	361
West Jefferson Medical Center	Marrero	98%	446
Willis Knighton Bossier Health Center	Bossier City	98%	260
Woman's Hospital	Baton Rouge	98%	189
Baton Rouge General Medical Center	Baton Rouge	97%	304
Christus Saint Frances Cabrini Hospital	Alexandria	97%	318
Natchitoches Regional Medical Center	Natchitoches	97%	30
Opelousas General Health System	Opelousas	97%	174
Physicians Medical Center	Houma	97%	101
Saint Tammany Parish Hospital	Covington	97%	341
Surgical Specialty Center of Baton Rouge	Baton Rouge	97%	191
West Calcasieu Cameron Hospital	Sulphur	97%	31
B R F Hospital Holdings	Shreveport	96%	113
Morehouse General Hospital	Bastrop	96%	27
North Oaks Medical Center	Hammond	96%	371
Ochsner Medical Center	New Orleans	96%	676
Park Place Surgical Hospital	Lafayette	96%	74
Willis Knighton Medical Center	Shreveport	96%	1044
Charity Hosp & Med Ctr of Louisiana	New Orleans	95%	265
Christus Health Shreveport - Bossier	Shreveport	95%	213
Mercy Regional Medical Center	Ville Platte	95%	76
Saint Francis Medical Center	Monroe	95%	267
Lake Charles Memorial Hospital	Lake Charles	94%	306
Our Lady of Lourdes Reg Med Ctr	Lafayette	94%	277
Slidell Memorial Hospital	Slidell	94%	143
Cypress Pointe Surgical Hospital	Hammond	92%	182
Ochsner Medical Center - Northshore	Slidell	92%	84
American Legion Hospital	Crowley	91%	85
Monroe Surgical Hospital	Monroe	91%	33
River Parishes Hospital	Laplace	90%	29
Teche Regional Medical Center	Morgan City	90%	52
Beauregard Memorial Hospital	Deridder	85%	88

Prophylactic Antibiotic Stopped

Hospital Name	City	Rate	Cases
Byrd Regional Hospital	Leesville	100%	82
Central Louisiana Surgical Hospital[2]	Alexandria	100%	252
Dauterive Hospital	New Iberia	100%	82
E A Conway Medical Center	Monroe	100%	105
Franklin Foundation Hospital[3]	Franklin	100%	39
Green Clinic Surgical Hospital	Ruston	100%	92
Heart Hospital of Lafayette	Lafayette	100%	359
Lakeview Regional Medical Center	Covington	100%	314
Minden Medical Center	Minden	100%	116
Morehouse General Hospital	Bastrop	100%	40
Ouachita Community Hospital[2]	West Monroe	100%	34
P & S Surgical Hospital[2]	Monroe	100%	240
Richardson Medical Center	Rayville	100%	38
Saint Francis Medical Center[2]	Monroe	100%	253
Thibodaux Regional Medical Center	Thibodaux	100%	403
Washington St Tammany Reg Med Ctr	Bogalusa	100%	46
Christus Saint Patrick Hospital	Lake Charles	99%	147
Lake Area Medical Center	Lake Charles	99%	217
Lallie Kemp Medical Center	Independence	99%	67
Leonard J Chabert Medical Center	Houma	99%	216
Northern Louisiana Medical Center	Ruston	99%	85
Rapides Regional Medical Center[2]	Alexandria	99%	324
The Regional Medical Center of Acadiana[2]	Lafayette	99%	272
Terrebonne General Medical Center[2]	Houma	99%	381
West Calcasieu Cameron Hospital	Sulphur	99%	349
West Jefferson Medical Center[2]	Marrero	99%	392
Baton Rouge General Medical Center[2]	Baton Rouge	98%	463
Charity Hosp & Med Ctr of Louisiana[2]	New Orleans	98%	347
Christus Saint Frances Cabrini Hospital	Alexandria	98%	491
Huey P Long Medical Center	Pineville	98%	42
Iberia General Hospital & Medical Center	New Iberia	98%	189
Jennings American Legion Hospital	Jennings	98%	127
North Oaks Medical Center[2]	Hammond	98%	320
Ochsner Medical Center - Northshore	Slidell	98%	164
Saint Elizabeth Hospital	Gonzales	98%	130
Specialists Hospital Shreveport[2]	Shreveport	98%	194
Tulane Medical Center[2]	New Orleans	98%	251
University Hospital & Clinics[2]	Lafayette	98%	100
Cypress Pointe Surgical Hospital	Hammond	97%	75
Fairway Medical Center[2]	Covington	97%	70
Lafayette General Medical Center[2]	Lafayette	97%	546
Lane Regional Medical Center	Zachary	97%	225
Ochsner Medical Center - Kenner[2]	Kenner	97%	181
Our Lady of Lourdes Reg Med Ctr[2]	Lafayette	97%	234
Our Lady of the Lake Reg Med Ctr[2]	Baton Rouge	97%	770
River Parishes Hospital[2]	Laplace	97%	73
Slidell Memorial Hospital	Slidell	97%	304
Touro Infirmary[2]	New Orleans	97%	620
Woman's Hospital[2]	Baton Rouge	97%	74
Abbeville General Hospital	Abbeville	96%	46
Christus Health Shreveport - Bossier[2]	Shreveport	96%	315
East Jefferson General Hospital[2]	Metairie	96%	423
Glenwood Regional Medical Center	West Monroe	96%	183
Lake Charles Memorial Hospital[2]	Lake Charles	96%	472
Mercy Regional Medical Center	Ville Platte	96%	72
Ochsner Medical Center - Baton Rouge[2]	Baton Rouge	96%	183
Lafayette Surgical Specialty Hospital[2]	Lafayette	95%	158
Ochsner Medical Center[2]	New Orleans	95%	394
Saint Tammany Parish Hospital[2]	Covington	95%	301
Willis Knighton Bossier Health Center[2]	Bossier City	95%	244
B R F Hospital Holdings[2]	Shreveport	94%	299
Monroe Surgical Hospital[2]	Monroe	94%	65
Overton Brooks VA Med Ctr-Shreveport	Shreveport	94%	77
Louisiana Heart Hospital[2]	Lacombe	93%	211
Opelousas General Health System[2]	Opelousas	93%	246
Willis Knighton Medical Center[2]	Shreveport	93%	724
Physicians Medical Center	Houma	92%	59
Southern Surgical Hospital[2]	Slidell	91%	142
Natchitoches Regional Medical Center	Natchitoches	89%	80
Doctors Hospital at Deer Creek[2]	Leesville	88%	32
Beauregard Memorial Hospital	Deridder	85%	72
Teche Regional Medical Center	Morgan City	84%	25

Prophylactic Antibiotic Timing

Hospital Name	City	Rate	Cases
Abbeville General Hospital	Abbeville	100%	46
Baton Rouge General Medical Center[2]	Baton Rouge	100%	478
Byrd Regional Hospital	Leesville	100%	89
Christus Saint Patrick Hospital	Lake Charles	100%	166
Dauterive Hospital	New Iberia	100%	90
Green Clinic Surgical Hospital	Ruston	100%	92
Heart Hospital of Lafayette	Lafayette	100%	366
Lakeview Regional Medical Center	Covington	100%	324
Leonard J Chabert Medical Center	Houma	100%	224
Louisiana Heart Hospital[2]	Lacombe	100%	212
Mercy Regional Medical Center	Ville Platte	100%	79
Minden Medical Center	Minden	100%	128
Morehouse General Hospital	Bastrop	100%	40
Our Lady of Lourdes Reg Med Ctr[2]	Lafayette	100%	239
Our Lady of the Lake Reg Med Ctr[2]	Baton Rouge	100%	790
Overton Brooks VA Med Ctr-Shreveport	Shreveport	100%	79
P & S Surgical Hospital[2]	Monroe	100%	242
Physicians Medical Center	Houma	100%	62
Rapides Regional Medical Center[2]	Alexandria	100%	341
The Regional Medical Center of Acadiana[2]	Lafayette	100%	286
Richardson Medical Center	Rayville	100%	38
River Parishes Hospital[2]	Laplace	100%	75
Saint Francis Medical Center[2]	Monroe	100%	279
Teche Regional Medical Center	Morgan City	100%	31
Terrebonne General Medical Center[2]	Houma	100%	384
Thibodaux Regional Medical Center	Thibodaux	100%	411
Touro Infirmary[2]	New Orleans	100%	628
Tulane Medical Center[2]	New Orleans	100%	257
Washington St Tammany Reg Med Ctr	Bogalusa	100%	46
Woman's Hospital[2]	Baton Rouge	100%	77
Central Louisiana Surgical Hospital[2]	Alexandria	99%	252
Christus Saint Frances Cabrini Hospital	Alexandria	99%	504
Glenwood Regional Medical Center	West Monroe	99%	210
Iberia General Hospital & Medical Center	New Iberia	99%	194
Lane Regional Medical Center	Zachary	99%	236
Northern Louisiana Medical Center	Ruston	99%	92
Ochsner Medical Center - Baton Rouge[2]	Baton Rouge	99%	187
Ochsner Medical Center - Kenner[2]	Kenner	99%	197
Ochsner Medical Center - Northshore	Slidell	99%	177
Saint Elizabeth Hospital	Gonzales	99%	138
Saint Tammany Parish Hospital[2]	Covington	99%	305
Slidell Memorial Hospital	Slidell	99%	315
Southern Surgical Hospital[2]	Slidell	99%	142
West Calcasieu Cameron Hospital	Sulphur	99%	353
West Jefferson Medical Center[2]	Marrero	99%	398
Willis Knighton Bossier Health Center[2]	Bossier City	99%	250
Christus Health Shreveport - Bossier[2]	Shreveport	98%	337
Franklin Foundation Hospital[3]	Franklin	98%	40
Jennings American Legion Hospital	Jennings	98%	128
Lafayette Surgical Specialty Hospital[2]	Lafayette	98%	158
Lake Area Medical Center	Lake Charles	98%	221
Lake Charles Memorial Hospital[2]	Lake Charles	98%	482
University Hospital & Clinics[2]	Lafayette	98%	101
Beauregard Memorial Hospital	Deridder	97%	73
Cypress Pointe Surgical Hospital	Hammond	97%	75
East Jefferson General Hospital[2]	Metairie	97%	440
North Oaks Medical Center[2]	Hammond	97%	329
Willis Knighton Medical Center[2]	Shreveport	97%	758
Lafayette General Medical Center[2]	Lafayette	96%	560
Lallie Kemp Medical Center	Independence	96%	67
Natchitoches Regional Medical Center	Natchitoches	96%	84

NOTE: Hospital profiles are in alphabetical order by state, then city, then hospital within the city; Rankings exclude hospitals with less than 25 cases except for patient surveys which excludes hospitals with less than 100 cases; (a) 100-299 cases; (1) The number of cases/patients is too few to report; (2) Data submitted were based on a sample of cases/patients; (3) Results are based on a shorter time period than required; (4) Data suppressed by CMS for one or more quarters; (5) Results are not available for this reporting period; (6) Fewer than 100 patients completed the HCAHPS survey; (7) No cases met the criteria for this measure; (8) The lower limit of the confidence interval cannot be calculated if the number of observed infections equals zero; (9) No data are available from the state/territory for this reporting period; (10) The scores shown reflect fewer than 50 completed surveys; (11) There were discrepancies in the data collection process; (12) This measure does not apply to this hospital for this reporting period; (13) Results cannot be calculated for this reporting period; (14) The results for this state are combined with nearby states to protect confidentiality; Please refer to the User's Guide for a full explanation of data.

Ochsner Medical Center[2]	New Orleans	96%	406
Opelousas General Health System[2]	Opelousas	96%	256
Specialists Hospital Shreveport[2]	Shreveport	96%	195
Monroe Surgical Hospital[2]	Monroe	95%	65
Charity Hosp & Med Ctr of Louisiana[2]	New Orleans	94%	370
Fairway Medical Center[2]	Covington	94%	70
Ouachita Community Hospital[2]	West Monroe	94%	34
E A Conway Medical Center	Monroe	92%	106
B R F Hospital Holdings[2]	Shreveport	89%	320
Huey P Long Medical Center	Pineville	89%	44
Doctors Hospital at Deer Creek[2]	Leesville	79%	33

Prophylactic Antibiotic Timing (Outpatient)

Hospital Name	City	Rate	Cases
Christus Saint Patrick Hospital	Lake Charles	100%	491
Dauterive Hospital	New Iberia	100%	94
Glenwood Regional Medical Center	West Monroe	100%	213
Heart Hospital of Lafayette	Lafayette	100%	241
Jennings American Legion Hospital	Jennings	100%	89
Lake Area Medical Center	Lake Charles	100%	204
Lakeview Regional Medical Center	Covington	100%	218
Morehouse General Hospital	Bastrop	100%	27
The Neuromedical Center Hospital	Baton Rouge	100%	358
Northern Louisiana Medical Center	Ruston	100%	35
Physicians Medical Center	Houma	100%	101
Rapides Regional Medical Center	Alexandria	100%	214
Slidell Memorial Hospital	Slidell	100%	143
Southern Surgical Hospital	Slidell	100%	50
Terrebonne General Medical Center	Houma	100%	409
Touro Infirmary	New Orleans	100%	346
Christus Saint Frances Cabrini Hospital	Alexandria	99%	318
East Jefferson General Hospital	Metairie	99%	501
Green Clinic Surgical Hospital	Ruston	99%	85
Leonard J Chabert Medical Center	Houma	99%	194
Mercy Regional Medical Center	Ville Platte	99%	77
P & S Surgical Hospital	Monroe	99%	464
Park Place Surgical Hospital	Lafayette	99%	74
The Regional Medical Center of Acadiana	Lafayette	99%	192
Saint Francis Medical Center	Monroe	99%	269
Thibodaux Regional Medical Center	Thibodaux	99%	357
Tulane Medical Center	New Orleans	99%	282
West Jefferson Medical Center	Marrero	99%	447
Abbeville General Hospital	Abbeville	98%	40
American Legion Hospital	Crowley	98%	85
Byrd Regional Hospital	Leesville	98%	44
Central Louisiana Surgical Hospital	Alexandria	98%	271
Lake Charles Memorial Hospital	Lake Charles	98%	310
Ochsner Medical Center - Baton Rouge	Baton Rouge	98%	247
Ochsner Medical Center - Kenner	Kenner	98%	88
Ochsner Medical Center - Northshore	Slidell	98%	86
Our Lady of the Lake Reg Med Ctr	Baton Rouge	98%	561
Surgical Specialty Center of Baton Rouge	Baton Rouge	98%	191
Teche Regional Medical Center	Morgan City	98%	52
Woman's Hospital	Baton Rouge	98%	189
B R F Hospital Holdings	Shreveport	97%	66
Baton Rouge General Medical Center	Baton Rouge	97%	308
Lane Regional Medical Center	Zachary	97%	65
Natchitoches Regional Medical Center	Natchitoches	97%	30
Opelousas General Health System	Opelousas	97%	179
River Parishes Hospital	Laplace	97%	30
Saint Tammany Parish Hospital	Covington	97%	347
West Calcasieu Cameron Hospital	Sulphur	97%	30
Willis Knighton Medical Center	Shreveport	97%	1034
North Oaks Medical Center	Hammond	96%	377
Willis Knighton Bossier Health Center	Bossier City	96%	257
Our Lady of Lourdes Reg Med Ctr	Lafayette	95%	285
Lafayette General Medical Center	Lafayette	94%	254
Lafayette Surgical Specialty Hospital	Lafayette	94%	371
Monroe Surgical Hospital	Monroe	94%	34
Specialists Hospital Shreveport	Shreveport	94%	420
Christus Health Shreveport - Bossier	Shreveport	93%	216
Lafayette General Surgical Hospital	Lafayette	93%	56
Ochsner Medical Center	New Orleans	93%	600
Cypress Pointe Hospital East[3]	Slidell	92%	25
Louisiana Heart Hospital	Lacombe	92%	201
Cypress Pointe Surgical Hospital	Hammond	91%	184
Iberia General Hospital & Medical Center	New Iberia	91%	95
University Hospital & Clinics	Lafayette	90%	71
Beauregard Memorial Hospital	Deridder	89%	70
Charity Hosp & Med Ctr of Louisiana	New Orleans	85%	189

Urinary Catheter Removal

Hospital Name	City	Rate	Cases
Central Louisiana Surgical Hospital[2]	Alexandria	100%	273
Christus Saint Patrick Hospital	Lake Charles	100%	119
Dauterive Hospital	New Iberia	100%	30
Green Clinic Surgical Hospital	Ruston	100%	27
Heart Hospital of Lafayette	Lafayette	100%	314
Lafayette Surgical Specialty Hospital[2]	Lafayette	100%	120
Lakeview Regional Medical Center	Covington	100%	253
Leonard J Chabert Medical Center	Houma	100%	165
Mercy Regional Medical Center	Ville Platte	100%	50
Minden Medical Center	Minden	100%	146
Northern Louisiana Medical Center	Ruston	100%	35
Our Lady of Lourdes Reg Med Ctr[2]	Lafayette	100%	226
Overton Brooks VA Med Ctr-Shreveport[2]	Shreveport	100%	93
Rapides Regional Medical Center[2]	Alexandria	100%	288
The Regional Medical Center of Acadiana[2]	Lafayette	100%	191
Saint Francis Medical Center[2]	Monroe	100%	289
Slidell Memorial Hospital	Slidell	100%	336
Thibodaux Regional Medical Center	Thibodaux	100%	398
Tulane Medical Center[2]	New Orleans	100%	253
East Jefferson General Hospital[2]	Metairie	99%	361
Glenwood Regional Medical Center	West Monroe	99%	145
Ochsner Medical Center - Kenner[2]	Kenner	99%	165
Saint Elizabeth Hospital	Gonzales	99%	172
Terrebonne General Medical Center[2]	Houma	99%	315
West Calcasieu Cameron Hospital	Sulphur	99%	314
West Jefferson Medical Center[2]	Marrero	99%	282
Baton Rouge General Medical Center[2]	Baton Rouge	98%	452
Jennings American Legion Hospital	Jennings	98%	64
Natchitoches Regional Medical Center	Natchitoches	98%	62
Ochsner Medical Center - Baton Rouge[2]	Baton Rouge	98%	209
Ochsner Medical Center - Northshore	Slidell	98%	152
Touro Infirmary[2]	New Orleans	98%	586
Byrd Regional Hospital	Leesville	97%	78
Cypress Pointe Surgical Hospital	Hammond	97%	96
Fairway Medical Center[2]	Covington	97%	60
P & S Surgical Hospital[2]	Monroe	97%	236
Franklin Foundation Hospital[3]	Franklin	96%	26
Lafayette General Medical Center[2]	Lafayette	96%	492
Iberia General Hospital & Medical Center	New Iberia	95%	169
Lane Regional Medical Center	Zachary	95%	240
Louisiana Heart Hospital[2]	Lacombe	95%	232
Our Lady of the Lake Reg Med Ctr[2]	Baton Rouge	95%	847
B R F Hospital Holdings[2]	Shreveport	94%	246
Lake Charles Memorial Hospital[2]	Lake Charles	94%	320
Monroe Surgical Hospital[2]	Monroe	94%	50
Specialists Hospital Shreveport[2]	Shreveport	94%	62
University Hospital & Clinics[2]	Lafayette	94%	67
Christus Health Shreveport - Bossier[2]	Shreveport	93%	281
North Oaks Medical Center[2]	Hammond	93%	283
Ochsner Medical Center[2]	New Orleans	93%	355
Willis Knighton Medical Center[2]	Shreveport	93%	760
Charity Hosp & Med Ctr of Louisiana[2]	New Orleans	92%	279
E A Conway Medical Center	Monroe	91%	33
Opelousas General Health System[2]	Opelousas	91%	213
Teche Regional Medical Center	Morgan City	91%	34
Saint Tammany Parish Hospital[2]	Covington	90%	242
Southern Surgical Hospital[2]	Slidell	90%	125
Christus Saint Frances Cabrini Hospital	Alexandria	88%	326
Ouachita Community Hospital[2]	West Monroe	88%	26
Physicians Medical Center	Houma	87%	52
Willis Knighton Bossier Health Center[2]	Bossier City	87%	176
Morehouse General Hospital	Bastrop	84%	25
American Legion Hospital[2]	Crowley	70%	44

Survey of Patients' Hospital Experiences

Area Around Room 'Always' Quiet at Night

Hospital Name	City	Rate	Cases
Surgical Specialty Center of Baton Rouge	Baton Rouge	95%	(a)
P & S Surgical Hospital	Monroe	93%	(a)
Physicians Medical Center	Houma	92%	(a)
Central Louisiana Surgical Hospital	Alexandria	91%	300+
The Neuromedical Center Hospital	Baton Rouge	91%	300+
Fairway Medical Center	Covington	90%	(a)
Southern Surgical Hospital	Slidell	90%	300+
Citizens Medical Center	Columbia	89%	(a)
Lafayette Surgical Specialty Hospital	Lafayette	87%	300+
Ouachita Community Hospital	West Monroe	87%	(a)
Specialists Hospital Shreveport	Shreveport	86%	300+
Doctors Hospital at Deer Creek	Leesville	84%	(a)
Green Clinic Surgical Hospital	Ruston	83%	(a)
Heart Hospital of Lafayette	Lafayette	82%	300+
Cypress Pointe Surgical Hospital	Hammond	81%	(a)
Lady of the Sea General Hospital	Cut Off	81%	(a)
Caldwell Memorial Hospital	Columbia	78%	(a)
Our Lady of Lourdes Reg Med Ctr	Lafayette	78%	300+
Saint James Parish Hospital	Lutcher	78%	(a)
Savoy Medical Center	Mamou	78%	(a)
Thibodaux Regional Medical Center	Thibodaux	78%	300+
Abbeville General Hospital	Abbeville	76%	(a)
Lallie Kemp Medical Center	Independence	76%	(a)
North Oaks Medical Center	Hammond	76%	300+
Saint Elizabeth Hospital	Gonzales	76%	300+
Jennings American Legion Hospital	Jennings	75%	300+
Morehouse General Hospital	Bastrop	75%	(a)
Richardson Medical Center	Rayville	75%	(a)
Baton Rouge General Medical Center	Baton Rouge	74%	300+
East Carroll Parish Hospital	Lake Providence	74%	(a)
Lafayette General Medical Center	Lafayette	74%	300+
Richland Parish Hospital - Delhi	Delhi	74%	(a)
Avoyelles Hospital	Marksville	73%	(a)
Iberia General Hospital & Medical Center	New Iberia	73%	300+
Saint Charles Parish Hospital	Luling	73%	(a)
Springhill Medical Center	Springhill	73%	(a)
University Hospital & Clinics	Lafayette	73%	300+
Sabine Medical Center	Many	72%	(a)
Willis Knighton Bossier Health Center	Bossier City	72%	300+
Willis Knighton Medical Center	Shreveport	72%	300+
Winn Parish Medical Center	Winnfield	72%	(a)
Lake Charles Memorial Hospital	Lake Charles	71%	300+
Leonard J Chabert Medical Center	Houma	71%	300+
Louisiana Heart Hospital	Lacombe	71%	300+
Minden Medical Center	Minden	71%	300+
Ochsner Medical Center - Northshore	Slidell	71%	300+
West Calcasieu Cameron Hospital	Sulphur	71%	300+
Beauregard Memorial Hospital	Deridder	70%	300+
Franklin Medical Center	Winnsboro	70%	(a)
Oakdale Community Hospital	Oakdale	70%	(a)
Desoto Regional Health System	Mansfield	69%	(a)
E A Conway Medical Center	Monroe	69%	300+
Lake Area Medical Center	Lake Charles	69%	300+
Our Lady of the Lake Reg Med Ctr	Baton Rouge	69%	300+
Dauterive Hospital	New Iberia	68%	300+
Glenwood Regional Medical Center	West Monroe	68%	300+
Ochsner Saint Anne General Hospital	Raceland	68%	(a)
Rapides Regional Medical Center	Alexandria	68%	300+
The Regional Medical Center of Acadiana	Lafayette	68%	300+
River Parishes Hospital	Laplace	68%	(a)
Saint Francis Medical Center	Monroe	68%	300+
Byrd Regional Hospital	Leesville	67%	300+
Lakeview Regional Medical Center	Covington	67%	300+
Mercy Regional Medical Center	Ville Platte	67%	300+
Natchitoches Regional Medical Center	Natchitoches	67%	300+
Touro Infirmary	New Orleans	67%	300+
West Jefferson Medical Center	Marrero	67%	300+
Jackson Parish Hospital	Jonesboro	66%	(a)
Saint Tammany Parish Hospital	Covington	66%	300+
Washington St Tammany Reg Med Ctr	Bogalusa	66%	(a)
Woman's Hospital	Baton Rouge	66%	300+
Homer Memorial Hospital	Homer	65%	(a)
Ochsner Medical Center - Baton Rouge	Baton Rouge	65%	300+
Opelousas General Health System	Opelousas	65%	300+
Teche Regional Medical Center	Morgan City	65%	300+
West Carroll Memorial Hospital	Oak Grove	65%	(a)
Christus Health Shreveport - Bossier	Shreveport	64%	300+
Christus Saint Frances Cabrini Hospital	Alexandria	64%	300+
East Jefferson General Hospital	Metairie	64%	300+
Huey P Long Medical Center	Pineville	64%	(a)
Christus Saint Patrick Hospital	Lake Charles	63%	300+
Terrebonne General Medical Center	Houma	63%	300+
Tulane Medical Center	New Orleans	63%	300+
American Legion Hospital	Crowley	62%	300+
Northern Louisiana Medical Center	Ruston	62%	300+
Charity Hosp & Med Ctr of Louisiana	New Orleans	61%	300+
B R F Hospital Holdings	Shreveport	60%	300+
Lane Regional Medical Center	Zachary	60%	300+
Ochsner Medical Center	New Orleans	60%	300+
Slidell Memorial Hospital	Slidell	60%	300+
Ochsner Medical Center - Kenner	Kenner	57%	300+

Doctors 'Always' Communicated Well

Hospital Name	City	Rate	Cases
Caldwell Memorial Hospital	Columbia	97%	(a)
Citizens Medical Center	Columbia	96%	(a)
Lady of the Sea General Hospital	Cut Off	96%	(a)
East Carroll Parish Hospital	Lake Providence	95%	(a)
Green Clinic Surgical Hospital	Ruston	95%	(a)
Oakdale Community Hospital	Oakdale	94%	(a)
Richardson Medical Center	Rayville	94%	(a)
Surgical Specialty Center of Baton Rouge	Baton Rouge	94%	(a)
Richland Parish Hospital - Delhi	Delhi	92%	(a)
Savoy Medical Center	Mamou	92%	(a)
West Carroll Memorial Hospital	Oak Grove	92%	(a)
Homer Memorial Hospital	Homer	91%	(a)
Ouachita Community Hospital	West Monroe	91%	(a)
Doctors Hospital at Deer Creek	Leesville	90%	(a)
Fairway Medical Center	Covington	90%	(a)
Heart Hospital of Lafayette	Lafayette	90%	300+
Lafayette Surgical Specialty Hospital	Lafayette	90%	300+
River Parishes Hospital	Laplace	90%	(a)
Sabine Medical Center	Many	90%	(a)
Beauregard Memorial Hospital	Deridder	89%	300+
Central Louisiana Surgical Hospital	Alexandria	89%	300+
Cypress Pointe Surgical Hospital	Hammond	89%	(a)
Franklin Medical Center	Winnsboro	89%	(a)
P & S Surgical Hospital	Monroe	89%	(a)
Physicians Medical Center	Houma	89%	(a)
Thibodaux Regional Medical Center	Thibodaux	89%	300+

NOTE: Hospital profiles are in alphabetical order by state, then city, then hospital within the city; Rankings exclude hospitals with less than 25 cases except for patient surveys which excludes hospitals with less than 100 cases; (a) 100-299 cases; (1) The number of cases/patients is too few to report; (2) Data submitted were based on a sample of cases/patients; (3) Results are based on a shorter time period than required; (4) Data suppressed by CMS for one or more quarters; (5) Results are not available for this reporting period; (6) Fewer than 100 patients completed the HCAHPS survey; (7) No cases met the criteria for this measure; (8) The lower limit of the confidence interval cannot be calculated if the number of observed infections equals zero; (9) No data are available from the state/territory for this reporting period; (10) The scores shown reflect fewer than 50 completed surveys; (11) There were discrepancies in the data collection process; (12) This measure does not apply to this hospital for this reporting period; (13) Results cannot be calculated for this reporting period; (14) The results for this state are combined with nearby states to protect confidentiality; Please refer to the User's Guide for a full explanation of data.

Hospital Name	City	Rate	Cases
Desoto Regional Health System	Mansfield	88%	(a)
Iberia General Hospital & Medical Center	New Iberia	88%	300+
Jennings American Legion Hospital	Jennings	88%	300+
Lafayette General Medical Center	Lafayette	88%	300+
Southern Surgical Hospital	Slidell	88%	300+
Specialists Hospital Shreveport	Shreveport	88%	300+
American Legion Hospital	Crowley	87%	300+
Dauterive Hospital	New Iberia	87%	300+
Mercy Regional Medical Center	Ville Platte	87%	300+
Our Lady of the Lake Reg Med Ctr	Baton Rouge	87%	300+
Lake Charles Memorial Hospital	Lake Charles	86%	300+
Lane Regional Medical Center	Zachary	86%	300+
Leonard J Chabert Medical Center	Houma	86%	300+
Minden Medical Center	Minden	86%	300+
Morehouse General Hospital	Bastrop	86%	(a)
The Neuromedical Center Hospital	Baton Rouge	86%	300+
Our Lady of Lourdes Reg Med Ctr	Lafayette	86%	300+
Saint Elizabeth Hospital	Gonzales	86%	300+
Saint Francis Medical Center	Monroe	86%	300+
Springhill Medical Center	Springhill	86%	(a)
Abbeville General Hospital	Abbeville	85%	(a)
Christus Health Shreveport - Bossier	Shreveport	85%	300+
Glenwood Regional Medical Center	West Monroe	85%	300+
Lake Area Medical Center	Lake Charles	85%	300+
Natchitoches Regional Medical Center	Natchitoches	85%	300+
Saint James Parish Hospital	Lutcher	85%	(a)
Saint Tammany Parish Hospital	Covington	85%	300+
Teche Regional Medical Center	Morgan City	85%	300+
University Hospital & Clinics	Lafayette	85%	(a)
Willis Knighton Bossier Health Center	Bossier City	85%	300+
Willis Knighton Medical Center	Shreveport	85%	300+
Woman's Hospital	Baton Rouge	85%	300+
Baton Rouge General Medical Center	Baton Rouge	84%	300+
Christus Saint Patrick Hospital	Lake Charles	84%	300+
East Jefferson General Hospital	Metairie	84%	300+
Jackson Parish Hospital	Jonesboro	84%	(a)
Ochsner Saint Anne General Hospital	Raceland	84%	(a)
The Regional Medical Center of Acadiana	Lafayette	84%	300+
Terrebonne General Medical Center	Houma	84%	300+
Touro Infirmary	New Orleans	84%	300+
Byrd Regional Hospital	Leesville	83%	(a)
E A Conway Medical Center	Monroe	83%	300+
Louisiana Heart Hospital	Lacombe	83%	300+
Opelousas General Health System	Opelousas	83%	300+
Saint Charles Parish Hospital	Luling	83%	(a)
Tulane Medical Center	New Orleans	83%	300+
Washington St Tammany Reg Med Ctr	Bogalusa	83%	(a)
West Calcasieu Cameron Hospital	Sulphur	83%	300+
Avoyelles Hospital	Marksville	82%	(a)
Lallie Kemp Medical Center	Independence	82%	(a)
North Oaks Medical Center	Hammond	82%	300+
Northern Louisiana Medical Center	Ruston	82%	300+
Slidell Memorial Hospital	Slidell	82%	300+
West Jefferson Medical Center	Marrero	82%	300+
Christus Saint Frances Cabrini Hospital	Alexandria	81%	300+
Lakeview Regional Medical Center	Covington	81%	300+
Rapides Regional Medical Center	Alexandria	81%	300+
Charity Hosp & Med Ctr of Louisiana	New Orleans	80%	300+
Ochsner Medical Center - Kenner	Kenner	80%	300+
Ochsner Medical Center - Northshore	Slidell	80%	300+
Huey P Long Medical Center	Pineville	79%	(a)
Ochsner Medical Center	New Orleans	79%	300+
B R F Hospital Holdings	Shreveport	78%	300+
Ochsner Medical Center - Baton Rouge	Baton Rouge	78%	300+
Winn Parish Medical Center	Winnfield	76%	(a)

Home Recovery Information Given

Hospital Name	City	Rate	Cases
Ouachita Community Hospital	West Monroe	92%	(a)
Specialists Hospital Shreveport	Shreveport	92%	300+
Woman's Hospital	Baton Rouge	92%	300+
Fairway Medical Center	Covington	91%	(a)
Doctors Hospital at Deer Creek	Leesville	90%	(a)
Lafayette Surgical Specialty Hospital	Lafayette	90%	300+
Physicians Medical Center	Houma	90%	(a)
Surgical Specialty Center of Baton Rouge	Baton Rouge	90%	(a)
Beauregard Memorial Hospital	Deridder	89%	300+
Citizens Medical Center	Columbia	89%	(a)
Lady of the Sea General Hospital	Cut Off	89%	(a)
The Neuromedical Center Hospital	Baton Rouge	89%	300+
Ochsner Saint Anne General Hospital	Raceland	89%	(a)
Saint Tammany Parish Hospital	Covington	89%	300+
Central Louisiana Surgical Hospital	Alexandria	88%	300+
Cypress Pointe Surgical Hospital	Hammond	88%	(a)
Green Clinic Surgical Hospital	Ruston	88%	(a)
Heart Hospital of Lafayette	Lafayette	88%	300+
Jennings American Legion Hospital	Jennings	88%	(a)
Lake Area Medical Center	Lake Charles	88%	300+
Saint James Parish Hospital	Lutcher	88%	(a)
Southern Surgical Hospital	Slidell	88%	300+
West Jefferson Medical Center	Marrero	88%	300+
Lakeview Regional Medical Center	Covington	87%	300+
Mercy Regional Medical Center	Ville Platte	87%	300+
Our Lady of the Lake Reg Med Ctr	Baton Rouge	87%	300+
P & S Surgical Hospital	Monroe	87%	(a)
River Parishes Hospital	Laplace	87%	(a)
Savoy Medical Center	Mamou	87%	(a)
Thibodaux Regional Medical Center	Thibodaux	87%	300+
Touro Infirmary	New Orleans	87%	300+
Franklin Medical Center	Winnsboro	86%	(a)
Lafayette General Medical Center	Lafayette	86%	300+
Lane Regional Medical Center	Zachary	86%	300+
Louisiana Heart Hospital	Lacombe	86%	300+
North Oaks Medical Center	Hammond	86%	300+
Ochsner Medical Center - Baton Rouge	Baton Rouge	86%	300+
The Regional Medical Center of Acadiana	Lafayette	86%	300+
Saint Charles Parish Hospital	Luling	86%	(a)
Saint Elizabeth Hospital	Gonzales	86%	300+
West Calcasieu Cameron Hospital	Sulphur	86%	300+
Willis Knighton Bossier Health Center	Bossier City	86%	300+
Willis Knighton Medical Center	Shreveport	86%	300+
Christus Health Shreveport - Bossier	Shreveport	85%	300+
Homer Memorial Hospital	Homer	85%	(a)
Minden Medical Center	Minden	85%	300+
Northern Louisiana Medical Center	Ruston	85%	300+
Ochsner Medical Center - Kenner	Kenner	85%	300+
Our Lady of Lourdes Reg Med Ctr	Lafayette	85%	300+
Richland Parish Hospital - Delhi	Delhi	85%	(a)
Slidell Memorial Hospital	Slidell	85%	300+
Springhill Medical Center	Springhill	85%	(a)
Terrebonne General Medical Center	Houma	85%	300+
Tulane Medical Center	New Orleans	85%	300+
Washington St Tammany Reg Med Ctr	Bogalusa	85%	(a)
Baton Rouge General Medical Center	Baton Rouge	84%	300+
Byrd Regional Hospital	Leesville	84%	300+
Caldwell Memorial Hospital	Columbia	84%	(a)
Desoto Regional Health System	Mansfield	84%	(a)
East Jefferson General Hospital	Metairie	84%	300+
Huey P Long Medical Center	Pineville	84%	(a)
Lake Charles Memorial Hospital	Lake Charles	84%	300+
Oakdale Community Hospital	Oakdale	84%	(a)
Ochsner Medical Center - Northshore	Slidell	84%	300+
Rapides Regional Medical Center	Alexandria	84%	300+
Sabine Medical Center	Many	84%	(a)
Teche Regional Medical Center	Morgan City	84%	300+
Abbeville General Hospital	Abbeville	83%	(a)
Dauterive Hospital	New Iberia	83%	300+
Iberia General Hospital & Medical Center	New Iberia	83%	300+
Lallie Kemp Medical Center	Independence	83%	(a)
Ochsner Medical Center	New Orleans	83%	300+
West Carroll Memorial Hospital	Oak Grove	83%	(a)
Christus Saint Patrick Hospital	Lake Charles	82%	300+
East Carroll Parish Hospital	Lake Providence	82%	(a)
Natchitoches Regional Medical Center	Natchitoches	82%	300+
Opelousas General Health System	Opelousas	82%	300+
B R F Hospital Holdings	Shreveport	81%	300+
Leonard J Chabert Medical Center	Houma	81%	300+
Charity Hosp & Med Ctr of Louisiana	New Orleans	80%	300+
Christus Saint Frances Cabrini Hospital	Alexandria	80%	300+
E A Conway Medical Center	Monroe	80%	300+
Jackson Parish Hospital	Jonesboro	80%	(a)
Saint Francis Medical Center	Monroe	80%	300+
Richardson Medical Center	Rayville	79%	(a)
American Legion Hospital	Crowley	78%	300+
Glenwood Regional Medical Center	West Monroe	78%	300+
Morehouse General Hospital	Bastrop	78%	(a)
Winn Parish Medical Center	Winnfield	76%	(a)
Avoyelles Hospital	Marksville	75%	(a)
University Hospital & Clinics	Lafayette	75%	(a)

Hospital Given 9 or 10 on 10 Point Scale

Hospital Name	City	Rate	Cases
Surgical Specialty Center of Baton Rouge	Baton Rouge	96%	(a)
Green Clinic Surgical Hospital	Ruston	93%	(a)
Cypress Pointe Surgical Hospital	Hammond	92%	(a)
Heart Hospital of Lafayette	Lafayette	92%	300+
Central Louisiana Surgical Hospital	Alexandria	91%	300+
P & S Surgical Hospital	Monroe	89%	(a)
Specialists Hospital Shreveport	Shreveport	89%	300+
Doctors Hospital at Deer Creek	Leesville	88%	(a)
Lafayette Surgical Specialty Hospital	Lafayette	88%	300+
Ouachita Community Hospital	West Monroe	88%	(a)
Southern Surgical Hospital	Slidell	88%	300+
Fairway Medical Center	Covington	87%	(a)
The Neuromedical Center Hospital	Baton Rouge	87%	300+
Physicians Medical Center	Houma	86%	(a)
Lady of the Sea General Hospital	Cut Off	85%	(a)
Louisiana Heart Hospital	Lacombe	83%	300+
Richland Parish Hospital - Delhi	Delhi	83%	(a)
Woman's Hospital	Baton Rouge	83%	300+
Caldwell Memorial Hospital	Columbia	82%	(a)
Lafayette General Medical Center	Lafayette	82%	300+
Saint Tammany Parish Hospital	Covington	82%	300+
Saint James Parish Hospital	Lutcher	81%	(a)
Lake Area Medical Center	Lake Charles	80%	300+
Our Lady of Lourdes Reg Med Ctr	Lafayette	80%	300+
Citizens Medical Center	Columbia	79%	(a)
Thibodaux Regional Medical Center	Thibodaux	78%	300+
Saint Elizabeth Hospital	Gonzales	76%	300+
Savoy Medical Center	Mamou	76%	(a)
Willis Knighton Bossier Health Center	Bossier City	76%	300+
Minden Medical Center	Minden	75%	300+
Our Lady of the Lake Reg Med Ctr	Baton Rouge	75%	300+
West Jefferson Medical Center	Marrero	75%	300+
Baton Rouge General Medical Center	Baton Rouge	74%	300+
Desoto Regional Health System	Mansfield	74%	(a)
East Jefferson General Hospital	Metairie	73%	300+
Homer Memorial Hospital	Homer	73%	(a)
Jennings American Legion Hospital	Jennings	73%	300+
Lallie Kemp Medical Center	Independence	73%	(a)
Richardson Medical Center	Rayville	73%	(a)
Saint Francis Medical Center	Monroe	73%	300+
West Calcasieu Cameron Hospital	Sulphur	73%	300+
Lake Charles Memorial Hospital	Lake Charles	72%	300+
Leonard J Chabert Medical Center	Houma	72%	300+
North Oaks Medical Center	Hammond	72%	300+
Touro Infirmary	New Orleans	72%	300+
University Hospital & Clinics	Lafayette	72%	(a)
Washington St Tammany Reg Med Ctr	Bogalusa	72%	(a)
Willis Knighton Medical Center	Shreveport	72%	300+
Beauregard Memorial Hospital	Deridder	71%	300+
Christus Health Shreveport - Bossier	Shreveport	71%	300+
Springhill Medical Center	Springhill	71%	(a)
West Carroll Memorial Hospital	Oak Grove	71%	(a)
Abbeville General Hospital	Abbeville	70%	(a)
Glenwood Regional Medical Center	West Monroe	70%	300+
Ochsner Medical Center - Baton Rouge	Baton Rouge	70%	300+
The Regional Medical Center of Acadiana	Lafayette	70%	300+
Saint Charles Parish Hospital	Luling	70%	(a)
East Carroll Parish Hospital	Lake Providence	69%	(a)
Iberia General Hospital & Medical Center	New Iberia	69%	300+
Lakeview Regional Medical Center	Covington	69%	300+
Terrebonne General Medical Center	Houma	69%	300+
Tulane Medical Center	New Orleans	69%	300+
Christus Saint Frances Cabrini Hospital	Alexandria	68%	300+
Christus Saint Patrick Hospital	Lake Charles	68%	300+
Franklin Medical Center	Winnsboro	68%	(a)
Huey P Long Medical Center	Pineville	68%	(a)
Jackson Parish Hospital	Jonesboro	68%	(a)
Mercy Regional Medical Center	Ville Platte	68%	300+
Rapides Regional Medical Center	Alexandria	68%	300+
Dauterive Hospital	New Iberia	67%	300+
Ochsner Saint Anne General Hospital	Raceland	67%	(a)
Slidell Memorial Hospital	Slidell	67%	300+
E A Conway Medical Center	Monroe	66%	300+
Lane Regional Medical Center	Zachary	66%	300+
Morehouse General Hospital	Bastrop	66%	(a)
Ochsner Medical Center - Kenner	Kenner	66%	300+
Ochsner Medical Center - Northshore	Slidell	66%	300+
Opelousas General Health System	Opelousas	66%	300+
Sabine Medical Center	Many	66%	(a)
Ochsner Medical Center	New Orleans	65%	300+
River Parishes Hospital	Laplace	65%	(a)
Northern Louisiana Medical Center	Ruston	64%	300+
Byrd Regional Hospital	Leesville	63%	300+
Winn Parish Medical Center	Winnfield	63%	(a)
B R F Hospital Holdings	Shreveport	62%	300+
Teche Regional Medical Center	Morgan City	62%	300+
Avoyelles Hospital	Marksville	59%	(a)
Natchitoches Regional Medical Center	Natchitoches	58%	300+
Charity Hosp & Med Ctr of Louisiana	New Orleans	57%	300+
American Legion Hospital	Crowley	53%	300+
Oakdale Community Hospital	Oakdale	53%	(a)

Meds 'Always' Explained Before Given

Hospital Name	City	Rate	Cases
Lady of the Sea General Hospital	Cut Off	88%	(a)
Green Clinic Surgical Hospital	Ruston	85%	(a)
Richland Parish Hospital - Delhi	Delhi	83%	(a)
Central Louisiana Surgical Hospital	Alexandria	82%	300+
Heart Hospital of Lafayette	Lafayette	82%	300+
Richardson Medical Center	Rayville	82%	(a)
Lafayette Surgical Specialty Hospital	Lafayette	81%	300+
Ouachita Community Hospital	West Monroe	81%	(a)
P & S Surgical Hospital	Monroe	80%	(a)
Physicians Medical Center	Houma	80%	(a)
Fairway Medical Center	Covington	78%	(a)
Cypress Pointe Surgical Hospital	Hammond	77%	(a)
Specialists Hospital Shreveport	Shreveport	77%	300+
Citizens Medical Center	Columbia	76%	(a)
Doctors Hospital at Deer Creek	Leesville	74%	(a)
Savoy Medical Center	Mamou	74%	(a)
Surgical Specialty Center of Baton Rouge	Baton Rouge	73%	(a)

NOTE: Hospital profiles are in alphabetical order by state, then city, then hospital within the city; Rankings exclude hospitals with less than 25 cases except for patient surveys which excludes hospitals with less than 100 cases; (a) 100-299 cases; (1) The number of cases/patients is too few to report; (2) Data submitted were based on a sample of cases/patients; (3) Results are based on a shorter time period than required; (4) Data suppressed by CMS for one or more quarters; (5) Results are not available for this reporting period; (6) Fewer than 100 patients completed the HCAHPS survey; (7) No cases met the criteria for this measure; (8) The lower limit of the confidence interval cannot be calculated if the number of observed infections equals zero; (9) No data are available from the state/territory for this reporting period; (10) The scores shown reflect fewer than 50 completed surveys; (11) There were discrepancies in the data collection process; (12) This measure does not apply to this hospital for this reporting period; (13) Results cannot be calculated for this reporting period; (14) The results for this state are combined with nearby states to protect confidentiality; Please refer to the User's Guide for a full explanation of data.

Hospital Name	City	Rate	Cases
East Carroll Parish Hospital	Lake Providence	71%	(a)
Jennings American Legion Hospital	Jennings	71%	300+
Lafayette General Medical Center	Lafayette	71%	300+
The Neuromedical Center Hospital	Baton Rouge	71%	300+
Ochsner Saint Anne General Hospital	Raceland	71%	(a)
Caldwell Memorial Hospital	Columbia	70%	(a)
Franklin Medical Center	Winnsboro	70%	(a)
Springhill Medical Center	Springhill	70%	(a)
West Carroll Memorial Hospital	Oak Grove	70%	(a)
Lake Area Medical Center	Lake Charles	69%	300+
Leonard J Chabert Medical Center	Houma	69%	300+
North Oaks Medical Center	Hammond	69%	300+
Saint James Parish Hospital	Lutcher	69%	(a)
West Calcasieu Cameron Hospital	Sulphur	69%	300+
Huey P Long Medical Center	Pineville	68%	(a)
Natchitoches Regional Medical Center	Natchitoches	68%	300+
River Parishes Hospital	Laplace	68%	(a)
Saint Elizabeth Hospital	Gonzales	68%	300+
Southern Surgical Hospital	Slidell	68%	300+
Thibodaux Regional Medical Center	Thibodaux	68%	300+
Abbeville General Hospital	Abbeville	67%	(a)
Christus Health Shreveport - Bossier	Shreveport	67%	300+
E A Conway Medical Center	Monroe	67%	300+
Louisiana Heart Hospital	Lacombe	67%	300+
Oakdale Community Hospital	Oakdale	67%	(a)
Saint Francis Medical Center	Monroe	67%	300+
Avoyelles Hospital	Marksville	66%	(a)
Byrd Regional Hospital	Leesville	66%	300+
Lake Charles Memorial Hospital	Lake Charles	66%	300+
Ochsner Medical Center - Baton Rouge	Baton Rouge	66%	300+
Our Lady of Lourdes Reg Med Ctr	Lafayette	66%	300+
Our Lady of the Lake Reg Med Ctr	Baton Rouge	66%	300+
Saint Tammany Parish Hospital	Covington	66%	300+
Terrebonne General Medical Center	Houma	66%	300+
Washington St Tammany Reg Med Ctr	Bogalusa	66%	(a)
Willis Knighton Bossier Health Center	Bossier City	66%	300+
Winn Parish Medical Center	Winnfield	66%	(a)
Woman's Hospital	Baton Rouge	66%	300+
Glenwood Regional Medical Center	West Monroe	65%	300+
Homer Memorial Hospital	Homer	65%	(a)
Lane Regional Medical Center	Zachary	65%	300+
Minden Medical Center	Minden	65%	300+
West Jefferson Medical Center	Marrero	65%	300+
Baton Rouge General Medical Center	Baton Rouge	64%	300+
Mercy Regional Medical Center	Ville Platte	64%	300+
Tulane Medical Center	New Orleans	64%	300+
Beauregard Memorial Hospital	Deridder	63%	300+
Desoto Regional Health System	Mansfield	63%	(a)
Northern Louisiana Medical Center	Ruston	63%	300+
Rapides Regional Medical Center	Alexandria	63%	300+
Willis Knighton Medical Center	Shreveport	63%	300+
American Legion Hospital	Crowley	62%	300+
East Jefferson General Hospital	Metairie	62%	300+
Lakeview Regional Medical Center	Covington	62%	300+
The Regional Medical Center of Acadiana	Lafayette	62%	300+
Sabine Medical Center	Many	62%	(a)
Christus Saint Patrick Hospital	Lake Charles	61%	300+
Iberia General Hospital & Medical Center	New Iberia	61%	300+
Jackson Parish Hospital	Jonesboro	61%	(a)
Lallie Kemp Medical Center	Independence	61%	(a)
Touro Infirmary	New Orleans	61%	300+
B R F Hospital Holdings	Shreveport	60%	300+
Christus Saint Frances Cabrini Hospital	Alexandria	60%	300+
Teche Regional Medical Center	Morgan City	60%	300+
University Hospital & Clinics	Lafayette	60%	(a)
Charity Hosp & Med Ctr of Louisiana	New Orleans	59%	300+
Dauterive Hospital	New Iberia	59%	300+
Ochsner Medical Center	New Orleans	59%	300+
Slidell Memorial Hospital	Slidell	59%	300+
Morehouse General Hospital	Bastrop	58%	(a)
Ochsner Medical Center - Kenner	Kenner	58%	300+
Ochsner Medical Center - Northshore	Slidell	58%	300+
Opelousas General Health System	Opelousas	58%	300+
Saint Charles Parish Hospital	Luling	52%	(a)

Nurses 'Always' Communicated Well

Hospital Name	City	Rate	Cases
Citizens Medical Center	Columbia	96%	(a)
Central Louisiana Surgical Hospital	Alexandria	94%	300+
Heart Hospital of Lafayette	Lafayette	94%	300+
P & S Surgical Hospital	Monroe	93%	(a)
Surgical Specialty Center of Baton Rouge	Baton Rouge	93%	(a)
Cypress Pointe Surgical Hospital	Hammond	92%	(a)
Green Clinic Surgical Hospital	Ruston	92%	(a)
Lady of the Sea General Hospital	Cut Off	92%	(a)
Southern Surgical Hospital	Slidell	92%	300+
Fairway Medical Center	Covington	90%	(a)
Lafayette Surgical Specialty Hospital	Lafayette	90%	300+
Physicians Medical Center	Houma	90%	(a)
Lafayette General Medical Center	Lafayette	89%	300+
The Neuromedical Center Hospital	Baton Rouge	89%	300+
Specialists Hospital Shreveport	Shreveport	89%	300+
Ouachita Community Hospital	West Monroe	87%	(a)
Richardson Medical Center	Rayville	87%	(a)
Richland Parish Hospital - Delhi	Delhi	87%	(a)
Thibodaux Regional Medical Center	Thibodaux	87%	300+
Caldwell Memorial Hospital	Columbia	86%	(a)
Doctors Hospital at Deer Creek	Leesville	86%	(a)
Abbeville General Hospital	Abbeville	85%	(a)
Springhill Medical Center	Springhill	85%	(a)
East Carroll Parish Hospital	Lake Providence	84%	(a)
Iberia General Hospital & Medical Center	New Iberia	84%	300+
Lake Area Medical Center	Lake Charles	84%	300+
Louisiana Heart Hospital	Lacombe	84%	300+
Our Lady of Lourdes Reg Med Ctr	Lafayette	84%	300+
Saint Elizabeth Hospital	Gonzales	84%	300+
Saint Francis Medical Center	Monroe	84%	300+
Saint Tammany Parish Hospital	Covington	84%	300+
University Hospital & Clinics	Lafayette	84%	(a)
Franklin Medical Center	Winnsboro	83%	(a)
Jennings American Legion Hospital	Jennings	83%	300+
North Oaks Medical Center	Hammond	83%	300+
Our Lady of the Lake Reg Med Ctr	Baton Rouge	83%	300+
River Parishes Hospital	Laplace	83%	(a)
Terrebonne General Medical Center	Houma	83%	300+
Beauregard Memorial Hospital	Deridder	82%	300+
Lake Charles Memorial Hospital	Lake Charles	82%	300+
Lallie Kemp Medical Center	Independence	82%	(a)
Lane Regional Medical Center	Zachary	82%	300+
Leonard J Chabert Medical Center	Houma	82%	300+
Ochsner Medical Center - Baton Rouge	Baton Rouge	82%	300+
Saint James Parish Hospital	Lutcher	82%	(a)
West Carroll Memorial Hospital	Oak Grove	82%	(a)
Winn Parish Medical Center	Winnfield	82%	(a)
East Jefferson General Hospital	Metairie	81%	300+
Homer Memorial Hospital	Homer	81%	(a)
Jackson Parish Hospital	Jonesboro	81%	(a)
Ochsner Saint Anne General Hospital	Raceland	81%	(a)
Sabine Medical Center	Many	81%	(a)
Washington St Tammany Reg Med Ctr	Bogalusa	81%	(a)
West Calcasieu Cameron Hospital	Sulphur	81%	300+
West Jefferson Medical Center	Marrero	81%	300+
Willis Knighton Bossier Health Center	Bossier City	81%	300+
Baton Rouge General Medical Center	Baton Rouge	80%	300+
Desoto Regional Health System	Mansfield	80%	(a)
Minden Medical Center	Minden	80%	300+
Saint Charles Parish Hospital	Luling	80%	(a)
Savoy Medical Center	Mamou	80%	(a)
Willis Knighton Medical Center	Shreveport	80%	300+
Woman's Hospital	Baton Rouge	80%	300+
Christus Health Shreveport - Bossier	Shreveport	79%	300+
Glenwood Regional Medical Center	West Monroe	79%	300+
Christus Saint Frances Cabrini Hospital	Alexandria	78%	300+
Christus Saint Patrick Hospital	Lake Charles	78%	300+
E A Conway Medical Center	Monroe	78%	300+
Morehouse General Hospital	Bastrop	78%	(a)
Northern Louisiana Medical Center	Ruston	78%	300+
Ochsner Medical Center - Northshore	Slidell	78%	300+
Slidell Memorial Hospital	Slidell	78%	300+
Touro Infirmary	New Orleans	78%	300+
Avoyelles Hospital	Marksville	77%	(a)
Huey P Long Medical Center	Pineville	77%	(a)
Lakeview Regional Medical Center	Covington	77%	300+
Mercy Regional Medical Center	Ville Platte	77%	300+
Natchitoches Regional Medical Center	Natchitoches	77%	300+
Opelousas General Health System	Opelousas	77%	300+
The Regional Medical Center of Acadiana	Lafayette	77%	300+
Tulane Medical Center	New Orleans	77%	300+
Byrd Regional Hospital	Leesville	76%	300+
Dauterive Hospital	New Iberia	76%	300+
Oakdale Community Hospital	Oakdale	76%	(a)
Ochsner Medical Center - Kenner	Kenner	76%	300+
Rapides Regional Medical Center	Alexandria	76%	300+
Teche Regional Medical Center	Morgan City	76%	300+
American Legion Hospital	Crowley	75%	300+
B R F Hospital Holdings	Shreveport	75%	300+
Ochsner Medical Center	New Orleans	75%	300+
Charity Hosp & Med Ctr of Louisiana	New Orleans	70%	300+

Pain 'Always' Well Controlled

Hospital Name	City	Rate	Cases
Doctors Hospital at Deer Creek	Leesville	88%	(a)
Green Clinic Surgical Hospital	Ruston	86%	(a)
Heart Hospital of Lafayette	Lafayette	85%	300+
P & S Surgical Hospital	Monroe	85%	(a)
Ouachita Community Hospital	West Monroe	84%	(a)
Physicians Medical Center	Houma	84%	(a)
Caldwell Memorial Hospital	Columbia	83%	(a)
Central Louisiana Surgical Hospital	Alexandria	83%	300+
Lady of the Sea General Hospital	Cut Off	83%	(a)
Saint James Parish Hospital	Lutcher	83%	(a)
Springhill Medical Center	Springhill	83%	(a)
Southern Surgical Hospital	Slidell	82%	300+
Surgical Specialty Center of Baton Rouge	Baton Rouge	82%	(a)
Citizens Medical Center	Columbia	81%	(a)
Fairway Medical Center	Covington	81%	(a)
Lafayette Surgical Specialty Hospital	Lafayette	81%	300+
Cypress Pointe Surgical Hospital	Hammond	79%	(a)
Lafayette General Medical Center	Lafayette	79%	300+
Richardson Medical Center	Rayville	79%	(a)
Specialists Hospital Shreveport	Shreveport	79%	300+
Desoto Regional Health System	Mansfield	78%	(a)
The Neuromedical Center Hospital	Baton Rouge	78%	300+
West Carroll Memorial Hospital	Oak Grove	78%	(a)
Beauregard Memorial Hospital	Deridder	77%	300+
East Carroll Parish Hospital	Lake Providence	77%	(a)
Jennings American Legion Hospital	Jennings	77%	300+
Lake Area Medical Center	Lake Charles	77%	300+
Louisiana Heart Hospital	Lacombe	77%	300+
Our Lady of Lourdes Reg Med Ctr	Lafayette	77%	300+
Abbeville General Hospital	Abbeville	76%	(a)
Richland Parish Hospital - Delhi	Delhi	76%	(a)
Saint Tammany Parish Hospital	Covington	76%	300+
West Calcasieu Cameron Hospital	Sulphur	76%	300+
Iberia General Hospital & Medical Center	New Iberia	75%	300+
Lane Regional Medical Center	Zachary	75%	300+
Our Lady of the Lake Reg Med Ctr	Baton Rouge	75%	300+
Savoy Medical Center	Mamou	75%	(a)
Willis Knighton Medical Center	Shreveport	75%	300+
Woman's Hospital	Baton Rouge	75%	300+
Lake Charles Memorial Hospital	Lake Charles	74%	300+
Minden Medical Center	Minden	74%	300+
North Oaks Medical Center	Hammond	74%	300+
Thibodaux Regional Medical Center	Thibodaux	74%	300+
Washington St Tammany Reg Med Ctr	Bogalusa	74%	(a)
Willis Knighton Bossier Health Center	Bossier City	74%	300+
Byrd Regional Hospital	Leesville	73%	300+
Dauterive Hospital	New Iberia	73%	300+
Leonard J Chabert Medical Center	Houma	73%	300+
Saint Francis Medical Center	Monroe	73%	300+
Terrebonne General Medical Center	Houma	73%	300+
West Jefferson Medical Center	Marrero	73%	300+
Christus Health Shreveport - Bossier	Shreveport	72%	300+
East Jefferson General Hospital	Metairie	72%	300+
Franklin Medical Center	Winnsboro	72%	(a)
Homer Memorial Hospital	Homer	72%	(a)
Lakeview Regional Medical Center	Covington	72%	300+
Northern Louisiana Medical Center	Ruston	72%	300+
University Hospital & Clinics	Lafayette	72%	(a)
Baton Rouge General Medical Center	Baton Rouge	71%	300+
Christus Saint Frances Cabrini Hospital	Alexandria	71%	300+
Glenwood Regional Medical Center	West Monroe	71%	300+
Huey P Long Medical Center	Pineville	71%	(a)
Lallie Kemp Medical Center	Independence	71%	(a)
Morehouse General Hospital	Bastrop	71%	(a)
Ochsner Medical Center - Baton Rouge	Baton Rouge	71%	300+
Ochsner Medical Center - Northshore	Slidell	71%	300+
Saint Elizabeth Hospital	Gonzales	71%	300+
Slidell Memorial Hospital	Slidell	71%	300+
Mercy Regional Medical Center	Ville Platte	70%	300+
Ochsner Saint Anne General Hospital	Raceland	70%	(a)
The Regional Medical Center of Acadiana	Lafayette	70%	300+
Tulane Medical Center	New Orleans	70%	300+
Christus Saint Patrick Hospital	Lake Charles	69%	300+
Jackson Parish Hospital	Jonesboro	69%	(a)
Opelousas General Health System	Opelousas	69%	300+
River Parishes Hospital	Laplace	69%	(a)
Teche Regional Medical Center	Morgan City	69%	300+
Touro Infirmary	New Orleans	69%	300+
Natchitoches Regional Medical Center	Natchitoches	68%	300+
Rapides Regional Medical Center	Alexandria	68%	300+
E A Conway Medical Center	Monroe	67%	300+
Oakdale Community Hospital	Oakdale	67%	(a)
Ochsner Medical Center - Kenner	Kenner	67%	300+
Saint Charles Parish Hospital	Luling	67%	(a)
Sabine Medical Center	Many	66%	(a)
Avoyelles Hospital	Marksville	65%	(a)
B R F Hospital Holdings	Shreveport	65%	300+
Winn Parish Medical Center	Winnfield	65%	(a)
American Legion Hospital	Crowley	64%	300+
Ochsner Medical Center	New Orleans	64%	300+
Charity Hosp & Med Ctr of Louisiana	New Orleans	63%	300+

Room and Bathroom 'Always' Clean

Hospital Name	City	Rate	Cases
Citizens Medical Center	Columbia	96%	(a)
Cypress Pointe Surgical Hospital	Hammond	91%	(a)
Lady of the Sea General Hospital	Cut Off	90%	(a)
Physicians Medical Center	Houma	90%	(a)
Fairway Medical Center	Covington	89%	(a)
P & S Surgical Hospital	Monroe	88%	(a)
Richardson Medical Center	Rayville	87%	(a)
Central Louisiana Surgical Hospital	Alexandria	86%	300+

NOTE: Hospital profiles are in alphabetical order by state, then city, then hospital within the city; Rankings exclude hospitals with less than 25 cases except for patient surveys which excludes hospitals with less than 100 cases; (a) 100-299 cases; (1) The number of cases/patients is too few to report; (2) Data submitted were based on a sample of cases/patients; (3) Results are based on a shorter time period than required; (4) Data suppressed by CMS for one or more quarters; (5) Results are not available for this reporting period; (6) Fewer than 100 patients completed the HCAHPS survey; (7) No cases met the criteria for this measure; (8) The lower limit of the confidence interval cannot be calculated if the number of observed infections equals zero; (9) No data are available from the state/territory for this reporting period; (10) The scores shown reflect fewer than 50 completed surveys; (11) There were discrepancies in the data collection process; (12) This measure does not apply to this hospital for this reporting period; (13) Results cannot be calculated for this reporting period; (14) The results for this state are combined with nearby states to protect confidentiality; Please refer to the User's Guide for a full explanation of data.

Heart Hospital of Lafayette	Lafayette	86%	300+
Lallie Kemp Medical Center	Independence	85%	(a)
The Neuromedical Center Hospital	Baton Rouge	85%	300+
Saint James Parish Hospital	Lutcher	85%	(a)
Surgical Specialty Center of Baton Rouge	Baton Rouge	85%	(a)
Lafayette Surgical Specialty Hospital	Lafayette	84%	300+
Savoy Medical Center	Mamou	84%	(a)
Green Clinic Surgical Hospital	Ruston	83%	(a)
Southern Surgical Hospital	Slidell	83%	300+
Ouachita Community Hospital	West Monroe	82%	(a)
Specialists Hospital Shreveport	Shreveport	82%	300+
Doctors Hospital at Deer Creek	Leesville	80%	(a)
Our Lady of Lourdes Reg Med Ctr	Lafayette	80%	300+
Abbeville General Hospital	Abbeville	79%	(a)
Saint Charles Parish Hospital	Luling	79%	(a)
Saint Elizabeth Hospital	Gonzales	79%	300+
Thibodaux Regional Medical Center	Thibodaux	79%	300+
North Oaks Medical Center	Hammond	78%	300+
E A Conway Medical Center	Monroe	77%	300+
Lafayette General Medical Center	Lafayette	77%	300+
Desoto Regional Health System	Mansfield	76%	(a)
Franklin Medical Center	Winnsboro	76%	(a)
Iberia General Hospital & Medical Center	New Iberia	76%	300+
Washington St Tammany Reg Med Ctr	Bogalusa	76%	(a)
Winn Parish Medical Center	Winnfield	76%	(a)
Caldwell Memorial Hospital	Columbia	75%	(a)
Dauterive Hospital	New Iberia	75%	300+
Jennings American Legion Hospital	Jennings	75%	300+
Ochsner Saint Anne General Hospital	Raceland	75%	(a)
Springhill Medical Center	Springhill	75%	(a)
University Hospital & Clinics	Lafayette	75%	(a)
Woman's Hospital	Baton Rouge	75%	300+
Avoyelles Hospital	Marksville	74%	(a)
Louisiana Heart Hospital	Lacombe	74%	300+
Richland Parish Hospital - Delhi	Delhi	74%	(a)
East Carroll Parish Hospital	Lake Providence	73%	(a)
Saint Francis Medical Center	Monroe	73%	300+
Willis Knighton Bossier Health Center	Bossier City	73%	300+
Morehouse General Hospital	Bastrop	72%	(a)
Terrebonne General Medical Center	Houma	72%	300+
West Calcasieu Cameron Hospital	Sulphur	72%	300+
Homer Memorial Hospital	Homer	71%	(a)
Leonard J Chabert Medical Center	Houma	71%	300+
Mercy Regional Medical Center	Ville Platte	71%	300+
Opelousas General Health System	Opelousas	71%	300+
West Jefferson Medical Center	Marrero	71%	300+
Baton Rouge General Medical Center	Baton Rouge	70%	300+
Christus Health Shreveport - Bossier	Shreveport	70%	300+
Jackson Parish Hospital	Jonesboro	70%	(a)
Lake Area Medical Center	Lake Charles	70%	300+
Lake Charles Memorial Hospital	Lake Charles	70%	300+
Natchitoches Regional Medical Center	Natchitoches	70%	300+
Oakdale Community Hospital	Oakdale	70%	(a)
Sabine Medical Center	Many	70%	(a)
Saint Tammany Parish Hospital	Covington	70%	300+
Willis Knighton Medical Center	Shreveport	70%	300+
Beauregard Memorial Hospital	Deridder	69%	300+
Glenwood Regional Medical Center	West Monroe	69%	300+
Northern Louisiana Medical Center	Ruston	69%	300+
The Regional Medical Center of Acadiana	Lafayette	69%	300+
West Carroll Memorial Hospital	Oak Grove	69%	(a)
Christus Saint Frances Cabrini Hospital	Alexandria	67%	300+
Christus Saint Patrick Hospital	Lake Charles	67%	300+
Our Lady of the Lake Reg Med Ctr	Baton Rouge	67%	300+
East Jefferson General Hospital	Metairie	66%	300+
Lakeview Regional Medical Center	Covington	66%	300+
Minden Medical Center	Minden	66%	300+
Ochsner Medical Center - Baton Rouge	Baton Rouge	66%	300+
Slidell Memorial Hospital	Slidell	66%	300+
American Legion Hospital	Crowley	64%	300+
Rapides Regional Medical Center	Alexandria	64%	300+
Teche Regional Medical Center	Morgan City	64%	300+
Touro Infirmary	New Orleans	64%	300+
Lane Regional Medical Center	Zachary	63%	300+
Ochsner Medical Center - Northshore	Slidell	63%	300+
River Parishes Hospital	Laplace	63%	(a)
Tulane Medical Center	New Orleans	63%	300+
Byrd Regional Hospital	Leesville	62%	300+
Huey P Long Medical Center	Pineville	62%	(a)
Ochsner Medical Center - Kenner	Kenner	62%	300+
Ochsner Medical Center	New Orleans	60%	300+
Charity Hosp & Med Ctr of Louisiana	New Orleans	58%	300+
B R F Hospital Holdings	Shreveport	56%	300+

Timely Help 'Always' Received

Hospital Name	City	Rate	Cases
P & S Surgical Hospital	Monroe	92%	(a)
Surgical Specialty Center of Baton Rouge	Baton Rouge	90%	(a)
Citizens Medical Center	Columbia	89%	(a)
Fairway Medical Center	Covington	89%	(a)
Heart Hospital of Lafayette	Lafayette	89%	300+
Cypress Pointe Surgical Hospital	Hammond	87%	(a)
Green Clinic Surgical Hospital	Ruston	87%	(a)
Specialists Hospital Shreveport	Shreveport	86%	300+
Ouachita Community Hospital	West Monroe	85%	(a)
Southern Surgical Hospital	Slidell	85%	300+
Central Louisiana Surgical Hospital	Alexandria	84%	300+
Lady of the Sea General Hospital	Cut Off	84%	(a)
Lafayette Surgical Specialty Hospital	Lafayette	84%	300+
Physicians Medical Center	Houma	84%	(a)
The Neuromedical Center Hospital	Baton Rouge	82%	300+
Richland Parish Hospital - Delhi	Delhi	80%	(a)
Doctors Hospital at Deer Creek	Leesville	78%	(a)
Richardson Medical Center	Rayville	78%	(a)
East Carroll Parish Hospital	Lake Providence	77%	(a)
West Carroll Memorial Hospital	Oak Grove	77%	(a)
Abbeville General Hospital	Abbeville	76%	(a)
Desoto Regional Health System	Mansfield	76%	(a)
Franklin Medical Center	Winnsboro	76%	(a)
Lafayette General Medical Center	Lafayette	76%	300+
Caldwell Memorial Hospital	Columbia	75%	(a)
Springhill Medical Center	Springhill	75%	(a)
Jennings American Legion Hospital	Jennings	73%	300+
Lake Area Medical Center	Lake Charles	73%	300+
Lallie Kemp Medical Center	Independence	73%	(a)
Louisiana Heart Hospital	Lacombe	73%	300+
Savoy Medical Center	Mamou	73%	(a)
Saint Elizabeth Hospital	Gonzales	72%	300+
Thibodaux Regional Medical Center	Thibodaux	72%	300+
Washington St Tammany Reg Med Ctr	Bogalusa	72%	(a)
Jackson Parish Hospital	Jonesboro	71%	(a)
North Oaks Medical Center	Hammond	71%	300+
Saint Charles Parish Hospital	Luling	71%	(a)
Saint Tammany Parish Hospital	Covington	71%	300+
Sabine Medical Center	Many	70%	(a)
West Calcasieu Cameron Hospital	Sulphur	70%	300+
Willis Knighton Bossier Health Center	Bossier City	70%	300+
Iberia General Hospital & Medical Center	New Iberia	69%	300+
Morehouse General Hospital	Bastrop	69%	(a)
Saint James Parish Hospital	Lutcher	69%	(a)
University Hospital & Clinics	Lafayette	69%	(a)
Minden Medical Center	Minden	68%	300+
West Jefferson Medical Center	Marrero	68%	300+
Winn Parish Medical Center	Winnfield	68%	(a)
Woman's Hospital	Baton Rouge	68%	300+
Beauregard Memorial Hospital	Deridder	67%	300+
Glenwood Regional Medical Center	West Monroe	67%	300+
Our Lady of Lourdes Reg Med Ctr	Lafayette	67%	300+
Willis Knighton Medical Center	Shreveport	67%	300+
Natchitoches Regional Medical Center	Natchitoches	66%	300+
Baton Rouge General Medical Center	Baton Rouge	65%	300+
Byrd Regional Hospital	Leesville	65%	300+
Dauterive Hospital	New Iberia	65%	300+
Ochsner Saint Anne General Hospital	Raceland	65%	(a)
River Parishes Hospital	Laplace	65%	(a)
Saint Francis Medical Center	Monroe	65%	300+
Terrebonne General Medical Center	Houma	65%	300+
Homer Memorial Hospital	Homer	64%	(a)
Lane Regional Medical Center	Zachary	64%	300+
Mercy Regional Medical Center	Ville Platte	64%	300+
Ochsner Medical Center - Northshore	Slidell	64%	300+
Christus Health Shreveport - Bossier	Shreveport	63%	300+
Lake Charles Memorial Hospital	Lake Charles	63%	300+
Lakeview Regional Medical Center	Covington	63%	300+
Ochsner Medical Center - Baton Rouge	Baton Rouge	63%	300+
Our Lady of the Lake Reg Med Ctr	Baton Rouge	63%	300+
The Regional Medical Center of Acadiana	Lafayette	63%	300+
Slidell Memorial Hospital	Slidell	63%	300+
Tulane Medical Center	New Orleans	63%	300+
Christus Saint Patrick Hospital	Lake Charles	62%	300+
Huey P Long Medical Center	Pineville	62%	(a)
Oakdale Community Hospital	Oakdale	62%	(a)
B R F Hospital Holdings	Shreveport	60%	300+
Leonard J Chabert Medical Center	Houma	60%	300+
Northern Louisiana Medical Center	Ruston	60%	300+
Ochsner Medical Center - Kenner	Kenner	60%	300+
Opelousas General Health System	Opelousas	60%	300+
Teche Regional Medical Center	Morgan City	60%	300+
East Jefferson General Hospital	Metairie	59%	300+
Touro Infirmary	New Orleans	59%	300+
Christus Saint Frances Cabrini Hospital	Alexandria	58%	300+
Rapides Regional Medical Center	Alexandria	58%	300+
E A Conway Medical Center	Monroe	56%	300+
Ochsner Medical Center	New Orleans	56%	300+
American Legion Hospital	Crowley	55%	300+
Avoyelles Hospital	Marksville	55%	(a)
Charity Hosp & Med Ctr of Louisiana	New Orleans	49%	300+

Would Definitely Recommend Hospital

Hospital Name	City	Rate	Cases
Surgical Specialty Center of Baton Rouge	Baton Rouge	94%	(a)
Central Louisiana Surgical Hospital	Alexandria	93%	300+
Cypress Pointe Surgical Hospital	Hammond	92%	(a)
Green Clinic Surgical Hospital	Ruston	92%	(a)
Heart Hospital of Lafayette	Lafayette	92%	300+
P & S Surgical Hospital	Monroe	92%	(a)
Fairway Medical Center	Covington	90%	(a)
Southern Surgical Hospital	Slidell	90%	300+
Specialists Hospital Shreveport	Shreveport	90%	300+
Doctors Hospital at Deer Creek	Leesville	89%	(a)
Lafayette Surgical Specialty Hospital	Lafayette	88%	300+
The Neuromedical Center Hospital	Baton Rouge	87%	300+
Louisiana Heart Hospital	Lacombe	86%	300+
Saint Tammany Parish Hospital	Covington	86%	300+
Woman's Hospital	Baton Rouge	86%	300+
Caldwell Memorial Hospital	Columbia	85%	(a)
Lafayette General Medical Center	Lafayette	85%	300+
Ouachita Community Hospital	West Monroe	85%	(a)
Physicians Medical Center	Houma	85%	(a)
Citizens Medical Center	Columbia	83%	(a)
Our Lady of Lourdes Reg Med Ctr	Lafayette	83%	300+
Thibodaux Regional Medical Center	Thibodaux	83%	300+
Willis Knighton Bossier Health Center	Bossier City	83%	300+
Lake Area Medical Center	Lake Charles	82%	300+
Richland Parish Hospital - Delhi	Delhi	82%	(a)
Willis Knighton Medical Center	Shreveport	82%	300+
Lady of the Sea General Hospital	Cut Off	80%	(a)
Saint Elizabeth Hospital	Gonzales	80%	300+
Saint Francis Medical Center	Monroe	79%	300+
Saint James Parish Hospital	Lutcher	79%	(a)
Baton Rouge General Medical Center	Baton Rouge	78%	300+
Lake Charles Memorial Hospital	Lake Charles	78%	300+
Savoy Medical Center	Mamou	78%	(a)
Leonard J Chabert Medical Center	Houma	77%	300+
East Jefferson General Hospital	Metairie	76%	300+
Iberia General Hospital & Medical Center	New Iberia	76%	300+
Our Lady of the Lake Reg Med Ctr	Baton Rouge	76%	300+
West Jefferson Medical Center	Marrero	76%	300+
Christus Health Shreveport - Bossier	Shreveport	75%	300+
Lallie Kemp Medical Center	Independence	75%	(a)
Christus Saint Frances Cabrini Hospital	Alexandria	74%	300+
Minden Medical Center	Minden	74%	300+
University Hospital & Clinics	Lafayette	74%	(a)
Beauregard Memorial Hospital	Deridder	72%	300+
Christus Saint Patrick Hospital	Lake Charles	72%	300+
Rapides Regional Medical Center	Alexandria	72%	300+
Slidell Memorial Hospital	Slidell	72%	300+
West Calcasieu Cameron Hospital	Sulphur	72%	300+
Glenwood Regional Medical Center	West Monroe	71%	300+
The Regional Medical Center of Acadiana	Lafayette	71%	300+
Lakeview Regional Medical Center	Covington	70%	300+
Mercy Regional Medical Center	Ville Platte	70%	300+
Ochsner Medical Center	New Orleans	70%	300+
Ochsner Medical Center - Baton Rouge	Baton Rouge	70%	300+
Touro Infirmary	New Orleans	70%	300+
Lane Regional Medical Center	Zachary	69%	300+
Terrebonne General Medical Center	Houma	69%	300+
B R F Hospital Holdings	Shreveport	68%	300+
Dauterive Hospital	New Iberia	68%	300+
East Carroll Parish Hospital	Lake Providence	68%	(a)
Huey P Long Medical Center	Pineville	68%	(a)
Jennings American Legion Hospital	Jennings	68%	300+
Tulane Medical Center	New Orleans	68%	300+
Washington St Tammany Reg Med Ctr	Bogalusa	68%	(a)
E A Conway Medical Center	Monroe	67%	300+
North Oaks Medical Center	Hammond	67%	300+
Ochsner Medical Center - Northshore	Slidell	67%	300+
Ochsner Saint Anne General Hospital	Raceland	67%	(a)
Saint Charles Parish Hospital	Luling	67%	(a)
Abbeville General Hospital	Abbeville	66%	(a)
Homer Memorial Hospital	Homer	66%	(a)
Desoto Regional Health System	Mansfield	64%	(a)
Springhill Medical Center	Springhill	64%	(a)
West Carroll Memorial Hospital	Oak Grove	64%	(a)
Franklin Medical Center	Winnsboro	63%	(a)
Ochsner Medical Center - Kenner	Kenner	63%	300+
Opelousas General Health System	Opelousas	63%	300+
Byrd Regional Hospital	Leesville	62%	300+
Jackson Parish Hospital	Jonesboro	62%	(a)
Sabine Medical Center	Many	62%	(a)
Teche Regional Medical Center	Morgan City	62%	300+
Charity Hosp & Med Ctr of Louisiana	New Orleans	61%	300+
Northern Louisiana Medical Center	Ruston	61%	300+
Morehouse General Hospital	Bastrop	60%	(a)
River Parishes Hospital	Laplace	60%	(a)
Richardson Medical Center	Rayville	59%	(a)
Natchitoches Regional Medical Center	Natchitoches	57%	300+
Oakdale Community Hospital	Oakdale	57%	(a)
Avoyelles Hospital	Marksville	55%	(a)
Winn Parish Medical Center	Winnfield	52%	(a)
American Legion Hospital	Crowley	51%	300+

NOTE: Hospital profiles are in alphabetical order by state, then city, then hospital within the city; Rankings exclude hospitals with less than 25 cases except for patient surveys which excludes hospitals with less than 100 cases; (a) 100-299 cases; (1) The number of cases/patients is too few to report; (2) Data submitted were based on a sample of cases/patients; (3) Results are based on a shorter time period than required; (4) Data suppressed by CMS for one or more quarters; (5) Results are not available for this reporting period; (6) Fewer than 100 patients completed the HCAHPS survey; (7) No cases met the criteria for this measure; (8) The lower limit of the confidence interval cannot be calculated if the number of observed infections equals zero; (9) No data are available from the state/territory for this reporting period; (10) The scores shown reflect fewer than 50 completed surveys; (11) There were discrepancies in the data collection process; (12) This measure does not apply to this hospital for this reporting period; (13) Results cannot be calculated for this reporting period; (14) The results for this state are combined with nearby states to protect confidentiality; Please refer to the User's Guide for a full explanation of data.

Use of Medical Imaging

Cardiac Imaging Stress Test before OP Surgery

Hospital Name	City	Rate	Cases
Washington St Tammany Reg Med Ctr	Bogalusa	1.0%	97
Byrd Regional Hospital	Leesville	1.2%	86
B R F Hospital Holdings	Shreveport	1.7%	173
West Calcasieu Cameron Hospital	Sulphur	2.1%	189
Huey P Long Medical Center	Pineville	2.2%	45
Heart Hospital of Lafayette	Lafayette	2.7%	150
Lasalle General Hospital	Jena	2.8%	71
Winn Parish Medical Center	Winnfield	2.8%	72
Terrebonne General Medical Center	Houma	2.9%	140
E A Conway Medical Center	Monroe	3.8%	53
Christus Health Shreveport - Bossier	Shreveport	3.9%	597
Monroe Surgical Hospital	Monroe	3.9%	152
Northern Louisiana Medical Center	Ruston	3.9%	103
University Hospital & Clinics	Lafayette	4.0%	126
Louisiana Heart Hospital	Lacombe	4.1%	585
Jennings American Legion Hospital	Jennings	4.2%	142
Rapides Regional Medical Center	Alexandria	4.3%	187
Mercy Regional Medical Center	Ville Platte	4.5%	202
Baton Rouge General Medical Center	Baton Rouge	4.8%	62
Christus Saint Frances Cabrini Hospital	Alexandria	4.8%	186
East Jefferson General Hospital	Metairie	4.8%	913
Lakeview Regional Medical Center	Covington	4.8%	62
Touro Infirmary	New Orleans	5.0%	320
River Parishes Hospital	Laplace	5.1%	59
West Jefferson Medical Center	Marrero	5.1%	273
Charity Hosp & Med Ctr of Louisiana	New Orleans	5.4%	92
Desoto Regional Health System	Mansfield	5.5%	127
Leonard J Chabert Medical Center	Houma	5.5%	181
Iberia General Hospital & Medical Center	New Iberia	5.7%	315
North Oaks Medical Center	Hammond	5.7%	315
Ochsner Medical Center - Northshore	Slidell	6.0%	201
Willis Knighton Bossier Health Center	Bossier City	6.0%	84
Ochsner Medical Center - Kenner	Kenner	6.1%	98
Natchitoches Regional Medical Center	Natchitoches	6.6%	182
Our Lady of the Lake Reg Med Ctr	Baton Rouge	6.6%	762
Lady of the Sea General Hospital	Cut Off	6.7%	89
Ochsner Medical Center	New Orleans	7.0%	614
Saint Francis Medical Center	Monroe	7.1%	98
Lake Charles Memorial Hospital	Lake Charles	7.2%	152
Christus Saint Patrick Hospital	Lake Charles	7.4%	148
Willis Knighton Medical Center	Shreveport	8.3%	217
Saint Tammany Parish Hospital	Covington	8.4%	107
Tulane Medical Center	New Orleans	8.8%	182
Glenwood Regional Medical Center	West Monroe	10.8%	130
Slidell Memorial Hospital	Slidell	12.0%	175

Combination Abdominal CT Scan

Hospital Name	City	Rate	Cases
Huey P Long Medical Center	Pineville	1.1%	94
E A Conway Medical Center	Monroe	1.4%	142
Lasalle General Hospital	Jena	1.4%	141
Minden Medical Center	Minden	1.4%	277
Christus Health Shreveport - Bossier	Shreveport	1.7%	1147
Lake Area Medical Center	Lake Charles	2.6%	114
The Regional Medical Center of Acadiana	Lafayette	4.1%	220
Union General Hospital	Farmerville	4.5%	89
Lady of the Sea General Hospital	Cut Off	5.2%	172
North Oaks Medical Center	Hammond	5.8%	669
Desoto Regional Health System	Mansfield	6.1%	163
Ochsner Medical Center - Baton Rouge	Baton Rouge	6.6%	333
Physicians Medical Center	Houma	7.3%	123
Rapides Regional Medical Center	Alexandria	8.7%	823
Terrebonne General Medical Center	Houma	9.4%	1089
Charity Hosp & Med Ctr of Louisiana	New Orleans	10.9%	239
Ochsner Medical Center - Northshore	Slidell	12.2%	237
Franklin Medical Center	Winnsboro	12.8%	289
Our Lady of the Lake Reg Med Ctr	Baton Rouge	13.2%	1231
Saint Elizabeth Hospital	Gonzales	13.2%	357
Ochsner Medical Center	New Orleans	13.8%	1869
Ochsner Saint Anne General Hospital	Raceland	14.3%	203
Teche Regional Medical Center	Morgan City	14.3%	356
B R F Hospital Holdings	Shreveport	15.3%	379
Christus Saint Patrick Hospital	Lake Charles	15.5%	815
Louisiana Heart Hospital	Lacombe	15.9%	113
Jackson Parish Hospital	Jonesboro	16.5%	133
Leonard J Chabert Medical Center	Houma	16.5%	309
Homer Memorial Hospital	Homer	16.8%	107
Lake Charles Memorial Hospital	Lake Charles	16.8%	928
West Calcasieu Cameron Hospital	Sulphur	17.0%	376
Willis Knighton Bossier Health Center	Bossier City	18.9%	856
Saint Charles Parish Hospital	Luling	19.0%	84
Our Lady of Lourdes Reg Med Ctr	Lafayette	19.2%	1159
River Parishes Hospital	Laplace	19.4%	103
Saint Francis Medical Center	Monroe	19.7%	1065
Saint James Parish Hospital	Lutcher	20.7%	145
Touro Infirmary	New Orleans	20.7%	536
Lane Regional Medical Center	Zachary	21.1%	303
Richardson Medical Center	Rayville	21.4%	112
Opelousas General Health System	Opelousas	21.7%	701
Baton Rouge General Medical Center	Baton Rouge	22.1%	706
Citizens Medical Center	Columbia	22.7%	97
West Jefferson Medical Center	Marrero	23.1%	329
East Carroll Parish Hospital	Lake Providence	23.4%	64
Willis Knighton Medical Center	Shreveport	23.9%	1690
Richland Parish Hospital - Delhi	Delhi	24.0%	100
Abbeville General Hospital	Abbeville	24.2%	330
Springhill Medical Center	Springhill	25.4%	126
Lakeview Regional Medical Center	Covington	25.7%	261
Ochsner Medical Center - Kenner	Kenner	26.5%	339
Christus Saint Frances Cabrini Hospital	Alexandria	27.1%	1326
Washington St Tammany Reg Med Ctr	Bogalusa	27.5%	233
Lafayette General Medical Center	Lafayette	27.8%	1265
Tulane Medical Center	New Orleans	30.9%	450
Northern Louisiana Medical Center	Ruston	32.0%	172
Winn Parish Medical Center	Winnfield	33.6%	107
Byrd Regional Hospital	Leesville	33.7%	407
Beauregard Memorial Hospital	Deridder	34.0%	379
Morehouse General Hospital	Bastrop	34.4%	218
West Carroll Memorial Hospital	Oak Grove	35.4%	96
University Hospital & Clinics	Lafayette	36.4%	305
Avoyelles Hospital	Marksville	36.7%	177
Allen Parish Hospital	Kinder	40.4%	52
Monroe Surgical Hospital	Monroe	40.9%	203
Dauterive Hospital	New Iberia	41.2%	226
East Jefferson General Hospital	Metairie	42.5%	1193
Thibodaux Regional Medical Center	Thibodaux	42.7%	758
Slidell Memorial Hospital	Slidell	44.5%	605
Iberia General Hospital & Medical Center	New Iberia	44.7%	752
Mercy Regional Medical Center	Ville Platte	45.3%	534
Sabine Medical Center	Many	47.3%	241
Saint Tammany Parish Hospital	Covington	48.2%	649
Savoy Medical Center	Mamou	48.9%	135
Central Louisiana Surgical Hospital	Alexandria	50.2%	219
Acadia Saint Landry	Church Point	51.2%	41
West Feliciana Parish Hospital	Saint Francisville	52.8%	53
Natchitoches Regional Medical Center	Natchitoches	53.0%	334
Hardtner Medical Center	Olla	60.8%	171
American Legion Hospital	Crowley	61.8%	275
Glenwood Regional Medical Center	West Monroe	65.1%	568
Oakdale Community Hospital	Oakdale	68.8%	112
Cypress Pointe Surgical Hospital	Hammond	73.6%	87

Combination Brain/Sinus CT Scan

Hospital Name	City	Rate	Cases
Caldwell Memorial Hospital	Columbia	0.0%	32
Central Louisiana Surgical Hospital	Alexandria	0.0%	68
Lafayette Surgical Specialty Hospital	Lafayette	0.0%	46
Monroe Surgical Hospital	Monroe	0.0%	64
The Neuromedical Center Hospital	Baton Rouge	0.0%	115
P & S Surgical Hospital	Monroe	0.0%	32
Reeves Memorial Medical Center	Bernice	0.0%	51
Ochsner Medical Center - Northshore	Slidell	0.4%	229
Savoy Medical Center	Mamou	0.6%	158
Citizens Medical Center	Columbia	0.7%	144
Franklin Medical Center	Winnsboro	0.7%	434
Thibodaux Regional Medical Center	Thibodaux	0.7%	547
West Jefferson Medical Center	Marrero	0.8%	516
Lasalle General Hospital	Jena	0.9%	222
Hardtner Medical Center	Olla	1.0%	191
North Oaks Medical Center	Hammond	1.1%	757
Lake Charles Memorial Hospital	Lake Charles	1.2%	988
West Carroll Memorial Hospital	Oak Grove	1.2%	167
Opelousas General Health System	Opelousas	1.3%	896
Morehouse General Hospital	Bastrop	1.7%	348
East Jefferson General Hospital	Metairie	1.8%	1029
Mercy Regional Medical Center	Ville Platte	1.8%	566
Willis Knighton Medical Center	Shreveport	1.8%	1730
Christus Health Shreveport - Bossier	Shreveport	1.9%	904
Minden Medical Center	Minden	1.9%	475
Northern Louisiana Medical Center	Ruston	2.0%	446
Our Lady of Lourdes Reg Med Ctr	Lafayette	2.0%	998
Ochsner Medical Center	New Orleans	2.2%	1279
Terrebonne General Medical Center	Houma	2.2%	820
Christus Saint Frances Cabrini Hospital	Alexandria	2.5%	1115
Christus Saint Patrick Hospital	Lake Charles	2.6%	691
Lafayette General Medical Center	Lafayette	2.6%	1242
Willis Knighton Bossier Health Center	Bossier City	2.6%	737
Slidell Memorial Hospital	Slidell	2.7%	523
Saint Tammany Parish Hospital	Covington	2.8%	647
Rapides Regional Medical Center	Alexandria	2.9%	1005
Our Lady of the Lake Reg Med Ctr	Baton Rouge	3.3%	1497
Saint Francis Medical Center	Monroe	3.4%	1488
Baton Rouge General Medical Center	Baton Rouge	3.5%	1156
Glenwood Regional Medical Center	West Monroe	4.0%	756
American Legion Hospital	Crowley	4.3%	326
Byrd Regional Hospital	Leesville	4.5%	354
West Calcasieu Cameron Hospital	Sulphur	4.9%	411
Sabine Medical Center	Many	5.4%	258
Lane Regional Medical Center	Zachary	5.7%	460
Jackson Parish Hospital	Jonesboro	6.9%	233
Saint Charles Parish Hospital	Luling	7.5%	106
Lake Area Medical Center	Lake Charles	9.3%	108

Combination Chest CT Scan

Hospital Name	City	Rate	Cases
Christus Health Shreveport - Bossier	Shreveport	0.0%	710
E A Conway Medical Center	Monroe	0.0%	128
Hardtner Medical Center	Olla	0.0%	87
Huey P Long Medical Center	Pineville	0.0%	52
Minden Medical Center	Minden	0.0%	150
Ochsner Medical Center	New Orleans	0.0%	1346
Ochsner Medical Center - Northshore	Slidell	0.0%	49
Physicians Medical Center	Houma	0.0%	58
Saint Elizabeth Hospital	Gonzales	0.0%	113
Saint Francis Medical Center	Monroe	0.0%	811
Thibodaux Regional Medical Center	Thibodaux	0.0%	401
Willis Knighton Bossier Health Center	Bossier City	0.0%	564
Iberia General Hospital & Medical Center	New Iberia	0.2%	441
Willis Knighton Medical Center	Shreveport	0.2%	1235
B R F Hospital Holdings	Shreveport	0.3%	391
Slidell Memorial Hospital	Slidell	0.3%	374
Glenwood Regional Medical Center	West Monroe	0.6%	330
Dauterive Hospital	New Iberia	0.8%	126
Lakeview Regional Medical Center	Covington	0.8%	125
Ochsner Medical Center - Baton Rouge	Baton Rouge	0.8%	127
Charity Hosp & Med Ctr of Louisiana	New Orleans	1.2%	172
Christus Saint Frances Cabrini Hospital	Alexandria	1.4%	1158
Ochsner Medical Center - Kenner	Kenner	1.4%	144
Lady of the Sea General Hospital	Cut Off	1.8%	57
Springhill Medical Center	Springhill	2.0%	50
Lasalle General Hospital	Jena	2.1%	48
East Jefferson General Hospital	Metairie	2.2%	924
North Oaks Medical Center	Hammond	2.6%	418
Louisiana Heart Hospital	Lacombe	2.9%	70
Lake Charles Memorial Hospital	Lake Charles	3.0%	366
Leonard J Chabert Medical Center	Houma	3.1%	160
Our Lady of Lourdes Reg Med Ctr	Lafayette	3.2%	873
Rapides Regional Medical Center	Alexandria	3.3%	845
The Regional Medical Center of Acadiana	Lafayette	3.3%	91
Ochsner Saint Anne General Hospital	Raceland	3.9%	77
University Hospital & Clinics	Lafayette	4.5%	177
Byrd Regional Hospital	Leesville	4.7%	192
Monroe Surgical Hospital	Monroe	4.7%	107
Terrebonne General Medical Center	Houma	5.1%	546
Heart Hospital of Lafayette	Lafayette	5.7%	123
Our Lady of the Lake Reg Med Ctr	Baton Rouge	5.8%	711
Winn Parish Medical Center	Winnfield	6.3%	80
Abbeville General Hospital	Abbeville	7.0%	158
Tulane Medical Center	New Orleans	8.0%	286
Saint Tammany Parish Hospital	Covington	8.4%	357
Jackson Parish Hospital	Jonesboro	9.2%	109
Desoto Regional Health System	Mansfield	9.9%	71
Touro Infirmary	New Orleans	10.6%	423
West Calcasieu Cameron Hospital	Sulphur	11.4%	264
Teche Regional Medical Center	Morgan City	14.5%	110
Lane Regional Medical Center	Zachary	14.9%	202
Franklin Medical Center	Winnsboro	16.0%	106
Washington St Tammany Reg Med Ctr	Bogalusa	19.5%	154
Opelousas General Health System	Opelousas	20.2%	430
Christus Saint Patrick Hospital	Lake Charles	23.2%	367
Lafayette General Medical Center	Lafayette	23.7%	998
Sabine Medical Center	Many	25.0%	104
Baton Rouge General Medical Center	Baton Rouge	26.0%	312
West Jefferson Medical Center	Marrero	27.1%	210
Mercy Regional Medical Center	Ville Platte	28.1%	310
American Legion Hospital	Crowley	31.3%	217
Central Louisiana Surgical Hospital	Alexandria	34.5%	55
Morehouse General Hospital	Bastrop	35.8%	106
West Carroll Memorial Hospital	Oak Grove	36.5%	63
Beauregard Memorial Hospital	Deridder	38.1%	181
Natchitoches Regional Medical Center	Natchitoches	38.6%	207
Avoyelles Hospital	Marksville	39.2%	51
Oakdale Community Hospital	Oakdale	44.1%	59
Savoy Medical Center	Mamou	45.7%	92

Follow-up Mammogram/Ultrasound

A follow-up rate near zero may indicate missed cancer; a rate higher than 14% may mean there is unnecessary follow up.

Hospital Name	City	Rate	Cases
Huey P Long Medical Center	Pineville	2.1%	390
Leonard J Chabert Medical Center	Houma	2.2%	778
B R F Hospital Holdings	Shreveport	2.5%	1197
Richland Parish Hospital - Delhi	Delhi	2.7%	375
Springhill Medical Center	Springhill	3.0%	299
Lake Charles Memorial Hospital	Lake Charles	3.7%	1859
E A Conway Medical Center	Monroe	3.9%	356
Morehouse General Hospital	Bastrop	4.0%	347

NOTE: Hospital profiles are in alphabetical order by state, then city, then hospital within the city; Rankings exclude hospitals with less than 25 cases except for patient surveys which excludes hospitals with less than 100 cases; (a) 100-299 cases; (1) The number of cases/patients is too few to report; (2) Data submitted were based on a sample of cases/patients; (3) Results are based on a shorter time period than required; (4) Data suppressed by CMS for one or more quarters; (5) Results are not available for this reporting period; (6) Fewer than 100 patients completed the HCAHPS survey; (7) No cases met the criteria for this measure; (8) The lower limit of the confidence interval cannot be calculated if the number of observed infections equals zero; (9) No data are available from the state/territory for this reporting period; (10) The scores shown reflect fewer than 50 completed surveys; (11) There were discrepancies in the data collection process; (12) This measure does not apply to this hospital for this reporting period; (13) Results cannot be calculated for this reporting period; (14) The results for this state are combined with nearby states to protect confidentiality; Please refer to the User's Guide for a full explanation of data.

Thibodaux Regional Medical Center	Thibodaux	4.5%	1458
Jackson Parish Hospital	Jonesboro	4.6%	153
American Legion Hospital	Crowley	4.8%	947
Minden Medical Center	Minden	4.8%	671
Beauregard Memorial Hospital	Deridder	5.1%	467
Ochsner Medical Center - Kenner	Kenner	5.3%	301
Natchitoches Regional Medical Center	Natchitoches	5.4%	392
Rapides Regional Medical Center	Alexandria	5.4%	1771
Ochsner Saint Anne General Hospital	Raceland	5.5%	366
Byrd Regional Hospital	Leesville	5.9%	444
Ochsner Medical Center	New Orleans	6.1%	3124
Terrebonne General Medical Center	Houma	6.2%	1092
Touro Infirmary	New Orleans	6.3%	939
Charity Hosp & Med Ctr of Louisiana	New Orleans	6.4%	344
Richardson Medical Center	Rayville	6.5%	184
North Oaks Medical Center	Hammond	7.0%	1169
Lane Regional Medical Center	Zachary	7.1%	310
Lady of the Sea General Hospital	Cut Off	7.2%	97
River Parishes Hospital	Laplace	7.2%	279
Savoy Medical Center	Mamou	7.2%	180
Lafayette General Medical Center	Lafayette	7.3%	1131
Glenwood Regional Medical Center	West Monroe	7.4%	1654
Teche Regional Medical Center	Morgan City	7.6%	381
Christus Health Shreveport - Bossier	Shreveport	8.0%	3083
Physicians Medical Center	Houma	8.0%	402
West Jefferson Medical Center	Marrero	8.1%	1180
Dauterive Hospital	New Iberia	8.3%	338
Lake Area Medical Center	Lake Charles	8.3%	496
Ochsner Medical Center - Northshore	Slidell	8.5%	130
Our Lady of the Lake Reg Med Ctr	Baton Rouge	8.5%	246
Willis Knighton Medical Center	Shreveport	8.7%	3325
Saint James Parish Hospital	Lutcher	8.8%	171
Homer Memorial Hospital	Homer	9.0%	266
Monroe Surgical Hospital	Monroe	9.2%	273
West Carroll Memorial Hospital	Oak Grove	9.2%	185
Christus Saint Frances Cabrini Hospital	Alexandria	9.4%	2255
Desoto Regional Health System	Mansfield	9.4%	276
Sabine Medical Center	Many	9.5%	147
Abbeville General Hospital	Abbeville	9.6%	366
Avoyelles Hospital	Marksville	9.6%	386
Iberia General Hospital & Medical Center	New Iberia	9.7%	671
Slidell Memorial Hospital	Slidell	9.7%	999
Northern Louisiana Medical Center	Ruston	10.2%	235
Saint Francis Medical Center	Monroe	10.2%	2088
Christus Saint Patrick Hospital	Lake Charles	10.3%	1079
Oakdale Community Hospital	Oakdale	10.3%	232
University Hospital & Clinics	Lafayette	10.9%	598
Saint Elizabeth Hospital	Gonzales	11.4%	360
Saint Tammany Parish Hospital	Covington	11.4%	1013
Opelousas General Health System	Opelousas	11.6%	1280
Willis Knighton Bossier Health Center	Bossier City	11.7%	1738
West Calcasieu Cameron Hospital	Sulphur	12.1%	846
Our Lady of Lourdes Reg Med Ctr	Lafayette	12.2%	1811
Woman's Hospital	Baton Rouge	12.3%	2501
Lasalle General Hospital	Jena	12.7%	173
Mercy Regional Medical Center	Ville Platte	12.8%	822
Tulane Medical Center	New Orleans	13.8%	516
Washington St Tammany Reg Med Ctr	Bogalusa	13.8%	210
The Regional Medical Center of Acadiana	Lafayette	14.2%	950
Franklin Medical Center	Winnsboro	14.7%	150
Saint Charles Parish Hospital	Luling	16.1%	155
Baton Rouge General Medical Center	Baton Rouge	16.6%	745
Lakeview Regional Medical Center	Covington	26.2%	275
East Jefferson General Hospital	Metairie	47.9%	1446

Lumbar Spine MRI for Low Back Pain

Hospital Name	City	Rate	Cases
West Calcasieu Cameron Hospital	Sulphur	29.8%	124
Minden Medical Center	Minden	31.7%	63
Lafayette Surgical Specialty Hospital	Lafayette	35.5%	76
Our Lady of Lourdes Reg Med Ctr	Lafayette	37.3%	201
West Jefferson Medical Center	Marrero	37.3%	75
Monroe Surgical Hospital	Monroe	37.8%	45
Thibodaux Regional Medical Center	Thibodaux	37.8%	111
Saint Francis Medical Center	Monroe	38.1%	281
Southern Surgical Hospital	Slidell	38.6%	44
Willis Knighton Medical Center	Shreveport	39.4%	292
P & S Surgical Hospital	Monroe	39.5%	119
Cypress Pointe Surgical Hospital	Hammond	40.1%	137
Opelousas General Health System	Opelousas	40.6%	101
Christus Health Shreveport - Bossier	Shreveport	41.2%	68
Touro Infirmary	New Orleans	41.3%	75
East Jefferson General Hospital	Metairie	41.9%	129
Abbeville General Hospital	Abbeville	42.0%	69
Central Louisiana Surgical Hospital	Alexandria	42.6%	155
Saint Tammany Parish Hospital	Covington	42.7%	75
Christus Saint Frances Cabrini Hospital	Alexandria	42.8%	271
Terrebonne General Medical Center	Houma	44.1%	227
Morehouse General Hospital	Bastrop	44.6%	65
Glenwood Regional Medical Center	West Monroe	44.8%	125
Lafayette General Medical Center	Lafayette	45.0%	131
Teche Regional Medical Center	Morgan City	45.0%	60
Northern Louisiana Medical Center	Ruston	45.1%	82
Willis Knighton Bossier Health Center	Bossier City	45.6%	147
Mercy Regional Medical Center	Ville Platte	45.7%	140
Our Lady of the Lake Reg Med Ctr	Baton Rouge	45.8%	48
Richardson Medical Center	Rayville	45.8%	83
Slidell Memorial Hospital	Slidell	46.5%	185
North Oaks Medical Center	Hammond	46.9%	143
Rapides Regional Medical Center	Alexandria	47.2%	72
Ochsner Medical Center	New Orleans	48.4%	248

NOTE: Hospital profiles are in alphabetical order by state, then city, then hospital within the city; Rankings exclude hospitals with less than 25 cases except for patient surveys which excludes hospitals with less than 100 cases; (a) 100-299 cases; (1) The number of cases/patients is too few to report; (2) Data submitted were based on a sample of cases/patients; (3) Results are based on a shorter time period than required; (4) Data suppressed by CMS for one or more quarters; (5) Results are not available for this reporting period; (6) Fewer than 100 patients completed the HCAHPS survey; (7) No cases met the criteria for this measure; (8) The lower limit of the confidence interval cannot be calculated if the number of observed infections equals zero; (9) No data are available from the state/territory for this reporting period; (10) The scores shown reflect fewer than 50 completed surveys; (11) There were discrepancies in the data collection process; (12) This measure does not apply to this hospital for this reporting period; (13) Results cannot be calculated for this reporting period; (14) The results for this state are combined with nearby states to protect confidentiality; Please refer to the User's Guide for a full explanation of data.

Abbeville General Hospital

118 N Hospital Dr
Abbeville, LA 70510
Phone: 337-893-5466
Fax: 337-893-2801
E-mail: info@abbgen.net
URL: www.abgen.net
Type: Acute Care Hospitals
Emergency Services: Yes
Ownership: Govt - Hospital Dist/Auth
Beds: 60

Key Personnel:
CEO/President. . . . . Ray Landry, FACHE
Chairman/CEO . . . . Robert J. LeBlanc
Quality Assurance . . . . Lou LeMaire
Chief of Medical Staff. . . . . Claude Meeks, MD
Patient Relations . . . . Denise Noel

Measure	Cases	This Hosp.	State Avg.	U.S. Avg.
Blood Clot Prevention and Treatment				
Anticoagulation Overlap Therapy[1,2]	-	-	89%	93%
ICU Venous Thromboembolism Prophylaxis[2]	20	75%	88%	92%
Incidence of Potentially Preventable VTE[1,2]	-	-	16%	10%
UFH with Dosages/Platelet Monitoring[1,2]	-	-	94%	97%
Venous Thromboembolism Prophylaxis[2]	104	72%	74%	85%
Warfarin Therapy Discharge Instructions[1,2]	-	-	85%	75%
Chest Pain/Possible Heart Attack Care				
Aspirin Given Within 24 Hours of Arrival	17	88%	94%	96%
Fibrinolytic Meds Within 30 Min. of Arrival[7]	-	-	54%	58%
Average Time to ECG (minutes)	18	10	10	7
Average Time to Transfer (minutes)[1]	-	-	94	60
Children's Asthma Care				
Received Home Management Plan of Care	-	-	-	88%
Received Reliever Medication	-	-	-	100%
Received Systemic Corticosteroids	-	-	-	100%
Emergency Department				
Admittance Decision Time (minutes)[2]	225	80	86	98
Head CT Results Within 45 Min. of Arrival[1]	-	-	49%	57%
Patients Who Left ER Before Being Seen	14,088	4%	3%	2%
Time from ER Arrival to Admit. (minutes)[2]	228	258	256	274
Time from ER Arrival to Discharge (minutes)	546	114	125	134
Time in ER Before Being Evaluated (minutes)	600	27	27	26
Time to Pain Meds for Fractures (minutes)	59	65	61	57
Heart Attack Care				
Aspirin Given at Discharge[1,3]	-	-	99%	99%
Fibrinolytic Meds Within 30 Min. of Arrival[3,7]	-	-	71%	54%
PCI Within 90 Minutes of Arrival[3,7]	-	-	94%	96%
Statin Prescribed at Discharge[1,3]	-	-	98%	98%
Heart Failure Care				
ACE Inhibitor or ARB for LVSD	11	100%	95%	97%
Discharge Instructions Given	49	100%	94%	94%
Evaluation of LVS Function	66	98%	97%	99%
Medicare Spending				
Medicare Spending per Patient (ratio)	-	1.00	1.04	0.98
Pneumonia Care				
Appropriate Initial Antibiotic Given	42	98%	93%	95%
Blood Culture Timing	67	100%	97%	98%
Pregnancy and Delivery Care				
Newborn Deliveries Scheduled Early	17	0%	5%	6%
Preventive Care				
Immunization for Influenza[2]	249	86%	85%	90%
Immunization for Pneumonia[2]	293	92%	88%	92%
Stroke Care				
Anticoagulation Therapy for Atrial Fibrillation[7]	-	-	93%	95%
Antithrombotic Therapy Timing[1]	-	-	96%	98%
Assessed for Rehabilitation[1]	-	-	95%	97%
Discharged on Antithrombotic Therapy[1]	-	-	97%	99%
Discharged on Statin Medication[1]	-	-	89%	94%
Thrombolytic Therapy Timing[1]	-	-	53%	66%
Venous Thromboembolism Prophylaxis[1]	-	-	87%	94%
Written Stroke Educational Materials Given[1]	-	-	83%	88%
Surgical Care Improvement Project				
Appropriate Beta Blocker Usage[1]	-	-	97%	98%
Appropriate VTP Within 24 Hours	43	100%	97%	98%
Controlled Postoperative Blood Glucose[7]	-	-	96%	97%
Perioperative Temperature Management	64	100%	100%	100%
Prophylactic Antibiotic Selection	46	93%	99%	99%
Prophylactic Antibiotic Selection (Outpatient)	39	100%	97%	98%
Prophylactic Antibiotic Stopped	46	96%	97%	98%
Prophylactic Antibiotic Timing	46	100%	98%	99%
Prophylactic Antibiotic Timing (Outpatient)	40	98%	97%	98%
Urinary Catheter Removal[1]	-	-	96%	97%
Survey of Patients' Hospital Experiences				
Area Around Room 'Always' Quiet at Night	(a)	76%	74%	61%
Doctors 'Always' Communicated Well	(a)	85%	87%	82%
Home Recovery Information Given	(a)	83%	85%	85%
Hospital Given 9 or 10 on 10 Point Scale	(a)	70%	75%	71%
Meds 'Always' Explained Before Given	(a)	67%	69%	64%
Nurses 'Always' Communicated Well	(a)	85%	83%	79%
Pain 'Always' Well Controlled	(a)	76%	75%	71%
Room and Bathroom 'Always' Clean	(a)	79%	75%	73%
Timely Help 'Always' Received	(a)	76%	71%	68%
Would Definitely Recommend Hospital	(a)	66%	75%	71%
Use of Medical Imaging				
Cardiac Imaging Stress Test before Surgery[7]	-	-	5.3%	5.3%
Combination Abdominal CT Scan	330	24.2%	24.5%	10.5%
Combination Brain/Sinus CT Scan[1]	-	-	2.6%	2.7%
Combination Chest CT Scan	158	7.0%	7.6%	2.7%
Follow-up Mammogram/Ultrasound	366	9.6%	9.4%	8.8%
Lumbar Spine MRI for Low Back Pain	69	42.0%	42.7%	37.2%

Central Louisiana Surgical Hospital

651 North Bolton Ave
Alexandria, LA 71301
Phone: 318-449-6400
URL: www.clshospital.com
Type: Acute Care Hospitals
Emergency Services: No
Ownership: Physician

Measure	Cases	This Hosp.	State Avg.	U.S. Avg.
Blood Clot Prevention and Treatment				
Anticoagulation Overlap Therapy[2,7]	-	-	89%	93%
ICU Venous Thromboembolism Prophylaxis[2,7]	-	-	88%	92%
Incidence of Potentially Preventable VTE[2,7]	-	-	16%	10%
UFH with Dosages/Platelet Monitoring[2,7]	-	-	94%	97%
Venous Thromboembolism Prophylaxis[2]	51	100%	74%	85%
Warfarin Therapy Discharge Instructions[2,7]	-	-	85%	75%
Chest Pain/Possible Heart Attack Care				
Aspirin Given Within 24 Hours of Arrival[5]	-	-	94%	96%
Fibrinolytic Meds Within 30 Min. of Arrival[5]	-	-	54%	58%
Average Time to ECG (minutes)[5]	-	-	10	7
Average Time to Transfer (minutes)[5]	-	-	94	60
Children's Asthma Care				
Received Home Management Plan of Care	-	-	-	88%
Received Reliever Medication	-	-	-	100%
Received Systemic Corticosteroids	-	-	-	100%
Emergency Department				
Admittance Decision Time (minutes)[2,7]	-	-	86	98
Head CT Results Within 45 Min. of Arrival[5]	-	-	49%	57%
Patients Who Left ER Before Being Seen[5]	-	-	3%	2%
Time from ER Arrival to Admit. (minutes)[2,7]	-	-	256	274
Time from ER Arrival to Discharge (minutes)[5]	-	-	125	134
Time in ER Before Being Evaluated (minutes)[5]	-	-	27	26
Time to Pain Meds for Fractures (minutes)[5]	-	-	61	57
Heart Attack Care				
Aspirin Given at Discharge[5]	-	-	99%	99%
Fibrinolytic Meds Within 30 Min. of Arrival[5]	-	-	71%	54%
PCI Within 90 Minutes of Arrival[5]	-	-	94%	96%
Statin Prescribed at Discharge[5]	-	-	98%	98%
Heart Failure Care				
ACE Inhibitor or ARB for LVSD[5]	-	-	95%	97%
Discharge Instructions Given[5]	-	-	94%	94%
Evaluation of LVS Function[5]	-	-	97%	99%
Medicare Spending				
Medicare Spending per Patient (ratio)	-	1.00	1.04	0.98
Pneumonia Care				
Appropriate Initial Antibiotic Given[5]	-	-	93%	95%
Blood Culture Timing[5]	-	-	97%	98%
Pregnancy and Delivery Care				
Newborn Deliveries Scheduled Early[7]	-	-	5%	6%
Preventive Care				
Immunization for Influenza[2]	333	100%	85%	90%
Immunization for Pneumonia[2]	442	97%	88%	92%
Stroke Care				
Anticoagulation Therapy for Atrial Fibrillation[5]	-	-	93%	95%
Antithrombotic Therapy Timing[5]	-	-	96%	98%
Assessed for Rehabilitation[5]	-	-	95%	97%
Discharged on Antithrombotic Therapy[5]	-	-	97%	99%
Discharged on Statin Medication[5]	-	-	89%	94%
Thrombolytic Therapy Timing[5]	-	-	53%	66%
Venous Thromboembolism Prophylaxis[5]	-	-	87%	94%
Written Stroke Educational Materials Given[5]	-	-	83%	88%
Surgical Care Improvement Project				
Appropriate Beta Blocker Usage[2]	109	100%	97%	98%
Appropriate VTP Within 24 Hours[2]	322	99%	97%	98%
Controlled Postoperative Blood Glucose[2,7]	-	-	96%	97%
Perioperative Temperature Management[2]	356	100%	100%	100%
Prophylactic Antibiotic Selection[2]	252	100%	99%	99%
Prophylactic Antibiotic Selection (Outpatient)	271	100%	97%	98%
Prophylactic Antibiotic Stopped[2]	252	100%	97%	98%
Prophylactic Antibiotic Timing[2]	252	99%	98%	99%
Prophylactic Antibiotic Timing (Outpatient)	271	98%	97%	98%
Urinary Catheter Removal[2]	273	100%	96%	97%
Survey of Patients' Hospital Experiences				
Area Around Room 'Always' Quiet at Night	300+	91%	74%	61%
Doctors 'Always' Communicated Well	300+	89%	87%	82%
Home Recovery Information Given	300+	88%	85%	85%
Hospital Given 9 or 10 on 10 Point Scale	300+	91%	75%	71%
Meds 'Always' Explained Before Given	300+	82%	69%	64%
Nurses 'Always' Communicated Well	300+	94%	83%	79%
Pain 'Always' Well Controlled	300+	83%	75%	71%
Room and Bathroom 'Always' Clean	300+	86%	75%	73%
Timely Help 'Always' Received	300+	84%	71%	68%
Would Definitely Recommend Hospital	300+	93%	75%	71%
Use of Medical Imaging				
Cardiac Imaging Stress Test before Surgery[7]	-	-	5.3%	5.3%
Combination Abdominal CT Scan	219	50.2%	24.5%	10.5%
Combination Brain/Sinus CT Scan	68	0.0%	2.6%	2.7%
Combination Chest CT Scan	55	34.5%	7.6%	2.7%
Follow-up Mammogram/Ultrasound[7]	-	-	9.4%	8.8%
Lumbar Spine MRI for Low Back Pain	155	42.6%	42.7%	37.2%

Christus Saint Frances Cabrini Hospital

3330 Masonic Drive
Alexandria, LA 71301
Phone: 318-487-1122
Fax: 318-448-6755
URL: www.cabrini.org
Type: Acute Care Hospitals
Emergency Services: Yes
Ownership: Voluntary non-profit - Church
Beds: 232

Key Personnel:
Radiology. . . . . Michael Allen, MD
Quality Assurance . . . . Bruce Tassin
CEO/President. . . . . Steven F Wright

Measure	Cases	This Hosp.	State Avg.	U.S. Avg.
Blood Clot Prevention and Treatment				
Anticoagulation Overlap Therapy[2]	99	94%	89%	93%
ICU Venous Thromboembolism Prophylaxis[2]	132	93%	88%	92%
Incidence of Potentially Preventable VTE[2]	17	12%	16%	10%
UFH with Dosages/Platelet Monitoring[2]	66	95%	94%	97%
Venous Thromboembolism Prophylaxis[2]	351	71%	74%	85%
Warfarin Therapy Discharge Instructions[2]	65	52%	85%	75%
Chest Pain/Possible Heart Attack Care				
Aspirin Given Within 24 Hours of Arrival[5]	-	-	94%	96%
Fibrinolytic Meds Within 30 Min. of Arrival[5]	-	-	54%	58%
Average Time to ECG (minutes)[5]	-	-	10	7
Average Time to Transfer (minutes)[5]	-	-	94	60
Children's Asthma Care				
Received Home Management Plan of Care	-	-	-	88%
Received Reliever Medication	-	-	-	100%
Received Systemic Corticosteroids	-	-	-	100%
Emergency Department				
Admittance Decision Time (minutes)[2]	432	187	86	98
Head CT Results Within 45 Min. of Arrival	11	82%	49%	57%
Patients Who Left ER Before Being Seen	49,380	1%	3%	2%
Time from ER Arrival to Admit. (minutes)[2]	582	382	256	274
Time from ER Arrival to Discharge (minutes)	405	216	125	134
Time in ER Before Being Evaluated (minutes)	417	95	27	26

NOTE: Hospital profiles are in alphabetical order by state, then city, then hospital within the city; Rankings exclude hospitals with less than 25 cases except for patient surveys which excludes hospitals with less than 100 cases; (a) 100-299 cases; (1) The number of cases/patients is too few to report; (2) Data submitted were based on a sample of cases/patients; (3) Results are based on a shorter time period than required; (4) Data suppressed by CMS for one or more quarters; (5) Results are not available for this reporting period; (6) Fewer than 100 patients completed the HCAHPS survey; (7) No cases met the criteria for this measure; (8) The lower limit of the confidence interval cannot be calculated if the number of observed infections equals zero; (9) No data are available from the state/territory for this reporting period; (10) The scores shown reflect fewer than 50 completed surveys; (11) There were discrepancies in the data collection process; (12) This measure does not apply to this hospital for this reporting period; (13) Results cannot be calculated for this reporting period; (14) The results for this state are combined with nearby states to protect confidentiality; Please refer to the User's Guide for a full explanation of data.

Time to Pain Meds for Fractures (minutes)	121	85	61	57
Heart Attack Care				
Aspirin Given at Discharge	286	100%	99%	99%
Fibrinolytic Meds Within 30 Min. of Arrival[7]	-	-	71%	54%
PCI Within 90 Minutes of Arrival	27	96%	94%	96%
Statin Prescribed at Discharge	268	100%	98%	98%
Heart Failure Care				
ACE Inhibitor or ARB for LVSD	137	100%	95%	97%
Discharge Instructions Given	361	100%	94%	94%
Evaluation of LVS Function	431	100%	97%	99%
Medicare Spending				
Medicare Spending per Patient (ratio)	-	1.02	1.04	0.98
Pneumonia Care				
Appropriate Initial Antibiotic Given	152	98%	93%	95%
Blood Culture Timing	356	99%	97%	98%
Pregnancy and Delivery Care				
Newborn Deliveries Scheduled Early[1,2]	-	-	5%	6%
Preventive Care				
Immunization for Influenza[2]	534	86%	85%	90%
Immunization for Pneumonia[2]	741	90%	88%	92%
Stroke Care				
Anticoagulation Therapy for Atrial Fibrillation	13	100%	93%	95%
Antithrombotic Therapy Timing	102	97%	96%	98%
Assessed for Rehabilitation	122	96%	95%	97%
Discharged on Antithrombotic Therapy	108	100%	97%	99%
Discharged on Statin Medication	90	90%	89%	94%
Thrombolytic Therapy Timing	15	20%	53%	66%
Venous Thromboembolism Prophylaxis	128	84%	87%	94%
Written Stroke Educational Materials Given	62	58%	83%	88%
Surgical Care Improvement Project				
Appropriate Beta Blocker Usage	326	99%	97%	98%
Appropriate VTP Within 24 Hours	385	99%	97%	98%
Controlled Postoperative Blood Glucose	270	91%	96%	97%
Perioperative Temperature Management	655	99%	100%	100%
Prophylactic Antibiotic Selection	504	99%	99%	99%
Prophylactic Antibiotic Selection (Outpatient)	318	97%	97%	98%
Prophylactic Antibiotic Stopped	491	98%	97%	98%
Prophylactic Antibiotic Timing	504	99%	98%	99%
Prophylactic Antibiotic Timing (Outpatient)	318	99%	97%	98%
Urinary Catheter Removal	326	88%	96%	97%
Survey of Patients' Hospital Experiences				
Area Around Room 'Always' Quiet at Night	300+	64%	74%	61%
Doctors 'Always' Communicated Well	300+	81%	87%	82%
Home Recovery Information Given	300+	80%	85%	85%
Hospital Given 9 or 10 on 10 Point Scale	300+	68%	75%	71%
Meds 'Always' Explained Before Given	300+	60%	69%	64%
Nurses 'Always' Communicated Well	300+	78%	83%	79%
Pain 'Always' Well Controlled	300+	71%	75%	71%
Room and Bathroom 'Always' Clean	300+	67%	75%	73%
Timely Help 'Always' Received	300+	58%	71%	68%
Would Definitely Recommend Hospital	300+	74%	75%	71%
Use of Medical Imaging				
Cardiac Imaging Stress Test before Surgery	186	4.8%	5.3%	5.3%
Combination Abdominal CT Scan	1,326	27.1%	24.5%	10.5%
Combination Brain/Sinus CT Scan	1,115	2.5%	2.6%	2.7%
Combination Chest CT Scan	1,158	1.4%	7.6%	2.7%
Follow-up Mammogram/Ultrasound	2,255	9.4%	9.4%	8.8%
Lumbar Spine MRI for Low Back Pain	271	42.8%	42.7%	37.2%

Rapides Regional Medical Center

211 4th Street
Alexandria, LA 71301
Phone: 318-769-3000
Fax: 318-449-7575
URL: www.rapidesregional.com
Type: Acute Care Hospitals
Emergency Services: Yes
Ownership: Voluntary non-profit - Other
Beds: 314

Key Personnel:

CEO/President. . . . . Jason E. Cobb
Quality Assurance . . . . Jessie Futrell
Infection Control. . . . . Grace Luneau
Radiology. . . . . Alfred A Mansour, MD
Operating Room. . . . . Charlotte Pato
Pediatric Ambulatory Care . . . . . . John N Rhodes, MD
Pediatric In-Patient Care . . . . John N Rhodes, MD

Measure	Cases	This Hosp.	State Avg.	U.S. Avg.
Blood Clot Prevention and Treatment				
Anticoagulation Overlap Therapy[2]	89	100%	89%	93%
ICU Venous Thromboembolism Prophylaxis[2]	162	100%	88%	92%
Incidence of Potentially Preventable VTE[2]	18	0%	16%	10%
UFH with Dosages/Platelet Monitoring[2]	37	100%	94%	97%
Venous Thromboembolism Prophylaxis[2]	390	99%	74%	85%
Warfarin Therapy Discharge Instructions[2]	69	100%	85%	75%
Chest Pain/Possible Heart Attack Care				
Aspirin Given Within 24 Hours of Arrival[3,7]	-	-	94%	96%
Fibrinolytic Meds Within 30 Min. of Arrival[5]	-	-	54%	58%
Average Time to ECG (minutes)[3,7]	-	-	10	7
Average Time to Transfer (minutes)[5]	-	-	94	60
Children's Asthma Care				
Received Home Management Plan of Care	-	-	-	88%
Received Reliever Medication	-	-	-	100%
Received Systemic Corticosteroids	-	-	-	100%
Emergency Department				
Admittance Decision Time (minutes)[2]	816	100	86	98
Head CT Results Within 45 Min. of Arrival[1]	-	-	49%	57%
Patients Who Left ER Before Being Seen	65,862	2%	3%	2%
Time from ER Arrival to Admit. (minutes)[2]	816	291	256	274
Time from ER Arrival to Discharge (minutes)	536	159	125	134
Time in ER Before Being Evaluated (minutes)	576	41	27	26
Time to Pain Meds for Fractures (minutes)	159	79	61	57
Heart Attack Care				
Aspirin Given at Discharge	294	100%	99%	99%
Fibrinolytic Meds Within 30 Min. of Arrival[7]	-	-	71%	54%
PCI Within 90 Minutes of Arrival	38	100%	94%	96%
Statin Prescribed at Discharge	269	100%	98%	98%
Heart Failure Care				
ACE Inhibitor or ARB for LVSD[2]	132	100%	95%	97%
Discharge Instructions Given[2]	254	98%	94%	94%
Evaluation of LVS Function[2]	299	100%	97%	99%
Medicare Spending				
Medicare Spending per Patient (ratio)	-	1.03	1.04	0.98
Pneumonia Care				
Appropriate Initial Antibiotic Given[2]	52	100%	93%	95%
Blood Culture Timing[2]	148	100%	97%	98%
Pregnancy and Delivery Care				
Newborn Deliveries Scheduled Early[2]	75	0%	5%	6%
Preventive Care				
Immunization for Influenza[2]	640	100%	85%	90%
Immunization for Pneumonia[2]	689	100%	88%	92%
Stroke Care				
Anticoagulation Therapy for Atrial Fibrillation[2]	11	100%	93%	95%
Antithrombotic Therapy Timing[2]	75	100%	96%	98%
Assessed for Rehabilitation[2]	111	100%	95%	97%
Discharged on Antithrombotic Therapy[2]	82	100%	97%	99%
Discharged on Statin Medication[2]	69	97%	89%	94%
Thrombolytic Therapy Timing[1,2]	-	-	53%	66%
Venous Thromboembolism Prophylaxis[2]	123	100%	87%	94%
Written Stroke Educational Materials Given[2]	53	100%	83%	88%
Surgical Care Improvement Project				
Appropriate Beta Blocker Usage[2]	210	100%	97%	98%
Appropriate VTP Within 24 Hours[2]	365	100%	97%	98%
Controlled Postoperative Blood Glucose[2]	131	98%	96%	97%
Perioperative Temperature Management[2]	429	100%	100%	100%
Prophylactic Antibiotic Selection[2]	341	100%	99%	99%
Prophylactic Antibiotic Selection (Outpatient)	214	100%	97%	98%
Prophylactic Antibiotic Stopped[2]	324	99%	97%	98%
Prophylactic Antibiotic Timing[2]	341	100%	98%	99%
Prophylactic Antibiotic Timing (Outpatient)	214	100%	97%	98%
Urinary Catheter Removal[2]	288	100%	96%	97%
Survey of Patients' Hospital Experiences				
Area Around Room 'Always' Quiet at Night	300+	68%	74%	61%
Doctors 'Always' Communicated Well	300+	81%	87%	82%
Home Recovery Information Given	300+	84%	85%	85%
Hospital Given 9 or 10 on 10 Point Scale	300+	68%	75%	71%
Meds 'Always' Explained Before Given	300+	63%	69%	64%
Nurses 'Always' Communicated Well	300+	76%	83%	79%
Pain 'Always' Well Controlled	300+	68%	75%	71%
Room and Bathroom 'Always' Clean	300+	64%	75%	73%
Timely Help 'Always' Received	300+	58%	71%	68%
Would Definitely Recommend Hospital	300+	72%	75%	71%
Use of Medical Imaging				
Cardiac Imaging Stress Test before Surgery	187	4.3%	5.3%	5.3%
Combination Abdominal CT Scan	823	8.7%	24.5%	10.5%
Combination Brain/Sinus CT Scan	1,005	2.9%	2.6%	2.7%
Combination Chest CT Scan	845	3.3%	7.6%	2.7%
Follow-up Mammogram/Ultrasound	1,771	5.4%	9.4%	8.8%
Lumbar Spine MRI for Low Back Pain	72	47.2%	42.7%	37.2%

Hood Memorial Hospital

301 W Walnut Street
Amite, LA 70422
Phone: 985-748-9485
Type: Critical Access Hospitals
Emergency Services: Yes
Ownership: Govt - Hospital Dist/Auth

Measure	Cases	This Hosp.	State Avg.	U.S. Avg.
Blood Clot Prevention and Treatment				
Anticoagulation Overlap Therapy[5]	-	-	89%	93%
ICU Venous Thromboembolism Prophylaxis[5]	-	-	88%	92%
Incidence of Potentially Preventable VTE[5]	-	-	16%	10%
UFH with Dosages/Platelet Monitoring[5]	-	-	94%	97%
Venous Thromboembolism Prophylaxis[5]	-	-	74%	85%
Warfarin Therapy Discharge Instructions[5]	-	-	85%	75%
Chest Pain/Possible Heart Attack Care				
Aspirin Given Within 24 Hours of Arrival	-	-	94%	96%
Fibrinolytic Meds Within 30 Min. of Arrival	-	-	54%	58%
Average Time to ECG (minutes)	-	-	10	7
Average Time to Transfer (minutes)	-	-	94	60
Children's Asthma Care				
Received Home Management Plan of Care	-	-	-	88%
Received Reliever Medication	-	-	-	100%
Received Systemic Corticosteroids	-	-	-	100%
Emergency Department				
Admittance Decision Time (minutes)[5]	-	-	86	98
Head CT Results Within 45 Min. of Arrival	-	-	49%	57%
Patients Who Left ER Before Being Seen	-	-	3%	2%
Time from ER Arrival to Admit. (minutes)[5]	-	-	256	274
Time from ER Arrival to Discharge (minutes)	-	-	125	134
Time in ER Before Being Evaluated (minutes)	-	-	27	26
Time to Pain Meds for Fractures (minutes)	-	-	61	57
Heart Attack Care				
Aspirin Given at Discharge[5]	-	-	99%	99%
Fibrinolytic Meds Within 30 Min. of Arrival[5]	-	-	71%	54%
PCI Within 90 Minutes of Arrival[5]	-	-	94%	96%
Statin Prescribed at Discharge[5]	-	-	98%	98%
Heart Failure Care				
ACE Inhibitor or ARB for LVSD[5]	-	-	95%	97%
Discharge Instructions Given[5]	-	-	94%	94%
Evaluation of LVS Function[5]	-	-	97%	99%
Medicare Spending				
Medicare Spending per Patient (ratio)	-	-	1.04	0.98
Pneumonia Care				
Appropriate Initial Antibiotic Given[5]	-	-	93%	95%
Blood Culture Timing[5]	-	-	97%	98%
Pregnancy and Delivery Care				
Newborn Deliveries Scheduled Early[5]	-	-	5%	6%
Preventive Care				
Immunization for Influenza[5]	-	-	85%	90%
Immunization for Pneumonia[5]	-	-	88%	92%
Stroke Care				
Anticoagulation Therapy for Atrial Fibrillation[5]	-	-	93%	95%
Antithrombotic Therapy Timing[5]	-	-	96%	98%
Assessed for Rehabilitation[5]	-	-	95%	97%
Discharged on Antithrombotic Therapy[5]	-	-	97%	99%
Discharged on Statin Medication[5]	-	-	89%	94%
Thrombolytic Therapy Timing[5]	-	-	53%	66%
Venous Thromboembolism Prophylaxis[5]	-	-	87%	94%
Written Stroke Educational Materials Given[5]	-	-	83%	88%
Surgical Care Improvement Project				
Appropriate Beta Blocker Usage[5]	-	-	97%	98%
Appropriate VTP Within 24 Hours[5]	-	-	97%	98%
Controlled Postoperative Blood Glucose[5]	-	-	96%	97%

NOTE: Hospital profiles are in alphabetical order by state, then city, then hospital within the city; Rankings exclude hospitals with less than 25 cases except for patient surveys which excludes hospitals with less than 100 cases; (a) 100-299 cases; (1) The number of cases/patients is too few to report; (2) Data submitted were based on a sample of cases/patients; (3) Results are based on a shorter time period than required; (4) Data suppressed by CMS for one or more quarters; (5) Results are not available for this reporting period; (6) Fewer than 100 patients completed the HCAHPS survey; (7) No cases met the criteria for this measure; (8) The lower limit of the confidence interval cannot be calculated if the number of observed infections equals zero; (9) No data are available from the state/territory for this reporting period; (10) The scores shown reflect fewer than 50 completed surveys; (11) There were discrepancies in the data collection process; (12) This measure does not apply to this hospital for this reporting period; (13) Results cannot be calculated for this reporting period; (14) The results for this state are combined with nearby states to protect confidentiality; Please refer to the User's Guide for a full explanation of data.

Measure	Cases	This Hosp.	State Avg.	U.S. Avg.
Perioperative Temperature Management[5]	-	-	100%	100%
Prophylactic Antibiotic Selection[5]	-	-	99%	99%
Prophylactic Antibiotic Selection (Outpatient)	-	-	97%	98%
Prophylactic Antibiotic Stopped[5]	-	-	97%	98%
Prophylactic Antibiotic Timing[5]	-	-	98%	99%
Prophylactic Antibiotic Timing (Outpatient)	-	-	97%	98%
Urinary Catheter Removal[5]	-	-	96%	97%
Survey of Patients' Hospital Experiences				
Area Around Room 'Always' Quiet at Night[6]	<100	73%	74%	61%
Doctors 'Always' Communicated Well[6]	<100	93%	87%	82%
Home Recovery Information Given[6]	<100	81%	85%	85%
Hospital Given 9 or 10 on 10 Point Scale[6]	<100	79%	75%	71%
Meds 'Always' Explained Before Given[6]	<100	66%	69%	64%
Nurses 'Always' Communicated Well[6]	<100	86%	83%	79%
Pain 'Always' Well Controlled[6]	<100	84%	75%	71%
Room and Bathroom 'Always' Clean[6]	<100	82%	75%	73%
Timely Help 'Always' Received[6]	<100	76%	71%	68%
Would Definitely Recommend Hospital[6]	<100	74%	75%	71%
Use of Medical Imaging				
Cardiac Imaging Stress Test before Surgery	-	-	5.3%	5.3%
Combination Abdominal CT Scan	-	-	24.5%	10.5%
Combination Brain/Sinus CT Scan	-	-	2.6%	2.7%
Combination Chest CT Scan	-	-	7.6%	2.7%
Follow-up Mammogram/Ultrasound	-	-	9.4%	8.8%
Lumbar Spine MRI for Low Back Pain	-	-	42.7%	37.2%

Bienville Medical Center

1175 Pine Street Phone: 318-263-4700
Arcadia, LA 71001
Type: Critical Access Hospitals Emergency Services: Yes
Ownership: Proprietary

Measure	Cases	This Hosp.	State Avg.	U.S. Avg.
Blood Clot Prevention and Treatment				
Anticoagulation Overlap Therapy[5]	-	-	89%	93%
ICU Venous Thromboembolism Prophylaxis[5]	-	-	88%	92%
Incidence of Potentially Preventable VTE[5]	-	-	16%	10%
UFH with Dosages/Platelet Monitoring[5]	-	-	94%	97%
Venous Thromboembolism Prophylaxis[5]	-	-	74%	85%
Warfarin Therapy Discharge Instructions[5]	-	-	85%	75%
Chest Pain/Possible Heart Attack Care				
Aspirin Given Within 24 Hours of Arrival	-	-	94%	96%
Fibrinolytic Meds Within 30 Min. of Arrival	-	-	54%	58%
Average Time to ECG (minutes)	-	-	10	7
Average Time to Transfer (minutes)	-	-	94	60
Children's Asthma Care				
Received Home Management Plan of Care	-	-	-	88%
Received Reliever Medication	-	-	-	100%
Received Systemic Corticosteroids	-	-	-	100%
Emergency Department				
Admittance Decision Time (minutes)[5]	-	-	86	98
Head CT Results Within 45 Min. of Arrival[5]	-	-	49%	57%
Patients Who Left ER Before Being Seen	-	-	3%	2%
Time from ER Arrival to Admit. (minutes)[5]	-	-	256	274
Time from ER Arrival to Discharge (minutes)	-	-	125	134
Time in ER Before Being Evaluated (minutes)	-	-	27	26
Time to Pain Meds for Fractures (minutes)	-	-	61	57
Heart Attack Care				
Aspirin Given at Discharge[5]	-	-	99%	99%
Fibrinolytic Meds Within 30 Min. of Arrival[5]	-	-	71%	54%
PCI Within 90 Minutes of Arrival[5]	-	-	94%	96%
Statin Prescribed at Discharge[5]	-	-	98%	98%
Heart Failure Care				
ACE Inhibitor or ARB for LVSD[5]	-	-	95%	97%
Discharge Instructions Given[5]	-	-	94%	94%
Evaluation of LVS Function[5]	-	-	97%	99%
Medicare Spending				
Medicare Spending per Patient (ratio)	-	-	1.04	0.98
Pneumonia Care				
Appropriate Initial Antibiotic Given[5]	-	-	93%	95%
Blood Culture Timing[5]	-	-	97%	98%
Pregnancy and Delivery Care				
Newborn Deliveries Scheduled Early[5]	-	-	5%	6%
Preventive Care				
Immunization for Influenza[5]	-	-	85%	90%
Immunization for Pneumonia[5]	-	-	88%	92%
Stroke Care				
Anticoagulation Therapy for Atrial Fibrillation[5]	-	-	93%	95%
Antithrombotic Therapy Timing[5]	-	-	96%	98%
Assessed for Rehabilitation[5]	-	-	95%	97%
Discharged on Antithrombotic Therapy[5]	-	-	97%	99%
Discharged on Statin Medication[5]	-	-	89%	94%
Thrombolytic Therapy Timing[5]	-	-	53%	66%
Venous Thromboembolism Prophylaxis[5]	-	-	87%	94%
Written Stroke Educational Materials Given[5]	-	-	83%	88%
Surgical Care Improvement Project				
Appropriate Beta Blocker Usage[5]	-	-	97%	98%
Appropriate VTP Within 24 Hours[5]	-	-	97%	98%
Controlled Postoperative Blood Glucose[5]	-	-	96%	97%
Perioperative Temperature Management[5]	-	-	100%	100%
Prophylactic Antibiotic Selection[5]	-	-	99%	99%
Prophylactic Antibiotic Selection (Outpatient)	-	-	97%	98%
Prophylactic Antibiotic Stopped[5]	-	-	97%	98%
Prophylactic Antibiotic Timing[5]	-	-	98%	99%
Prophylactic Antibiotic Timing (Outpatient)	-	-	97%	98%
Urinary Catheter Removal[5]	-	-	96%	97%
Survey of Patients' Hospital Experiences				
Area Around Room 'Always' Quiet at Night[5]	-	-	74%	61%
Doctors 'Always' Communicated Well[5]	-	-	87%	82%
Home Recovery Information Given[5]	-	-	85%	85%
Hospital Given 9 or 10 on 10 Point Scale[5]	-	-	75%	71%
Meds 'Always' Explained Before Given[5]	-	-	69%	64%
Nurses 'Always' Communicated Well[5]	-	-	83%	79%
Pain 'Always' Well Controlled[5]	-	-	75%	71%
Room and Bathroom 'Always' Clean[5]	-	-	75%	73%
Timely Help 'Always' Received[5]	-	-	71%	68%
Would Definitely Recommend Hospital[5]	-	-	75%	71%
Use of Medical Imaging				
Cardiac Imaging Stress Test before Surgery	-	-	5.3%	5.3%
Combination Abdominal CT Scan	-	-	24.5%	10.5%
Combination Brain/Sinus CT Scan	-	-	2.6%	2.7%
Combination Chest CT Scan	-	-	7.6%	2.7%
Follow-up Mammogram/Ultrasound	-	-	9.4%	8.8%
Lumbar Spine MRI for Low Back Pain	-	-	42.7%	37.2%

Morehouse General Hospital

323 W Walnut Phone: 318-283-3600
Bastrop, LA 71220 Fax: 318-283-3663
URL: www.mghospital.com
Type: Acute Care Hospitals Emergency Services: Yes
Ownership: Govt - Hospital Dist/Auth Beds: 60

Key Personnel:
Coronary Care . . . . Pam Chambers, RN
Intensive Care Unit. . . . . Pam Chambers, RN
Emergency Room . . . . EL Chorette, MD
Anesthesiology. . . . . Amy Douglas-McVay, MDA
Operating Room. . . . . Teresa Hankins, RN
Infection Control. . . . . Melinda Jones, RN
Hemotology Center . . . . Peggy Skains, RN
Chief of Medical Staff . . . . J M Smith, MD

Measure	Cases	This Hosp.	State Avg.	U.S. Avg.
Blood Clot Prevention and Treatment				
Anticoagulation Overlap Therapy[1,2]	-	-	89%	93%
ICU Venous Thromboembolism Prophylaxis[2]	33	82%	88%	92%
Incidence of Potentially Preventable VTE[1,2]	-	-	16%	10%
UFH with Dosages/Platelet Monitoring[2,7]	-	-	94%	97%
Venous Thromboembolism Prophylaxis[2]	104	71%	74%	85%
Warfarin Therapy Discharge Instructions[1,2]	-	-	85%	75%
Chest Pain/Possible Heart Attack Care				
Aspirin Given Within 24 Hours of Arrival	35	100%	94%	96%
Fibrinolytic Meds Within 30 Min. of Arrival	14	43%	54%	58%
Average Time to ECG (minutes)	35	8	10	7
Average Time to Transfer (minutes)[1]	-	-	94	60
Children's Asthma Care				
Received Home Management Plan of Care	-	-	-	88%
Received Reliever Medication	-	-	-	100%
Received Systemic Corticosteroids	-	-	-	100%
Emergency Department				
Admittance Decision Time (minutes)[2]	150	70	86	98
Head CT Results Within 45 Min. of Arrival[1]	-	-	49%	57%
Patients Who Left ER Before Being Seen	14,718	2%	3%	2%
Time from ER Arrival to Admit. (minutes)[2]	171	211	256	274
Time from ER Arrival to Discharge (minutes)	330	112	125	134
Time in ER Before Being Evaluated (minutes)	351	23	27	26
Time to Pain Meds for Fractures (minutes)	42	57	61	57
Heart Attack Care				
Aspirin Given at Discharge[1,3]	-	-	99%	99%
Fibrinolytic Meds Within 30 Min. of Arrival[3,7]	-	-	71%	54%
PCI Within 90 Minutes of Arrival[3,7]	-	-	94%	96%
Statin Prescribed at Discharge[1,3]	-	-	98%	98%
Heart Failure Care				
ACE Inhibitor or ARB for LVSD	21	86%	95%	97%
Discharge Instructions Given	44	61%	94%	94%
Evaluation of LVS Function	61	95%	97%	99%
Medicare Spending				
Medicare Spending per Patient (ratio)	-	1.22	1.04	0.98
Pneumonia Care				
Appropriate Initial Antibiotic Given	40	90%	93%	95%
Blood Culture Timing	59	97%	97%	98%
Pregnancy and Delivery Care				
Newborn Deliveries Scheduled Early[2]	26	8%	5%	6%
Preventive Care				
Immunization for Influenza[2]	238	66%	85%	90%
Immunization for Pneumonia[2]	226	78%	88%	92%
Stroke Care				
Anticoagulation Therapy for Atrial Fibrillation[1]	-	-	93%	95%
Antithrombotic Therapy Timing	12	67%	96%	98%
Assessed for Rehabilitation[1]	-	-	95%	97%
Discharged on Antithrombotic Therapy[1]	-	-	97%	99%
Discharged on Statin Medication[1]	-	-	89%	94%
Thrombolytic Therapy Timing[7]	-	-	53%	66%
Venous Thromboembolism Prophylaxis	15	80%	87%	94%
Written Stroke Educational Materials Given[1]	-	-	83%	88%
Surgical Care Improvement Project				
Appropriate Beta Blocker Usage[1]	-	-	97%	98%
Appropriate VTP Within 24 Hours	34	91%	97%	98%
Controlled Postoperative Blood Glucose[7]	-	-	96%	97%
Perioperative Temperature Management	48	100%	100%	100%
Prophylactic Antibiotic Selection	40	95%	99%	99%
Prophylactic Antibiotic Selection (Outpatient)	27	96%	97%	98%
Prophylactic Antibiotic Stopped	40	100%	97%	98%
Prophylactic Antibiotic Timing	40	100%	98%	99%
Prophylactic Antibiotic Timing (Outpatient)	27	100%	97%	98%
Urinary Catheter Removal	25	84%	96%	97%
Survey of Patients' Hospital Experiences				
Area Around Room 'Always' Quiet at Night	(a)	75%	74%	61%
Doctors 'Always' Communicated Well	(a)	86%	87%	82%
Home Recovery Information Given	(a)	78%	85%	85%
Hospital Given 9 or 10 on 10 Point Scale	(a)	66%	75%	71%
Meds 'Always' Explained Before Given	(a)	58%	69%	64%
Nurses 'Always' Communicated Well	(a)	78%	83%	79%
Pain 'Always' Well Controlled	(a)	71%	75%	71%
Room and Bathroom 'Always' Clean	(a)	72%	75%	73%
Timely Help 'Always' Received	(a)	69%	71%	68%
Would Definitely Recommend Hospital	(a)	60%	75%	71%
Use of Medical Imaging				
Cardiac Imaging Stress Test before Surgery[1]	-	-	5.3%	5.3%
Combination Abdominal CT Scan	218	34.4%	24.5%	10.5%
Combination Brain/Sinus CT Scan	348	1.7%	2.6%	2.7%
Combination Chest CT Scan	106	35.8%	7.6%	2.7%
Follow-up Mammogram/Ultrasound	347	4.0%	9.4%	8.8%
Lumbar Spine MRI for Low Back Pain	65	44.6%	42.7%	37.2%

Baton Rouge General Medical Center

3600 Florida Street Phone: 225-387-7767
Baton Rouge, LA 70806
URL: www.brgeneral.org
Type: Acute Care Hospitals Emergency Services: Yes
Ownership: Voluntary non-profit - Private

Key Personnel:
Chief of Medical Staff . . . . Floyd Roberts, MD

NOTE: Hospital profiles are in alphabetical order by state, then city, then hospital within the city; Rankings exclude hospitals with less than 25 cases except for patient surveys which excludes hospitals with less than 100 cases; (a) 100-299 cases; (1) The number of cases/patients is too few to report; (2) Data submitted were based on a sample of cases/patients; (3) Results are based on a shorter time period than required; (4) Data suppressed by CMS for one or more quarters; (5) Results are not available for this reporting period; (6) Fewer than 100 patients completed the HCAHPS survey; (7) No cases met the criteria for this measure; (8) The lower limit of the confidence interval cannot be calculated if the number of observed infections equals zero; (9) No data are available from the state/territory for this reporting period; (10) The scores shown reflect fewer than 50 completed surveys; (11) There were discrepancies in the data collection process; (12) This measure does not apply to this hospital for this reporting period; (13) Results cannot be calculated for this reporting period; (14) The results for this state are combined with nearby states to protect confidentiality; Please refer to the User's Guide for a full explanation of data.

President/CEO. . . . . Mark F. Slyter, FACHE

Measure	Cases	This Hosp.	State Avg.	U.S. Avg.
Blood Clot Prevention and Treatment				
Anticoagulation Overlap Therapy[2]	139	96%	89%	93%
ICU Venous Thromboembolism Prophylaxis[2]	58	95%	88%	92%
Incidence of Potentially Preventable VTE[2]	40	5%	16%	10%
UFH with Dosages/Platelet Monitoring[2]	11	100%	94%	97%
Venous Thromboembolism Prophylaxis[2]	346	77%	74%	85%
Warfarin Therapy Discharge Instructions[2]	101	74%	85%	75%
Chest Pain/Possible Heart Attack Care				
Aspirin Given Within 24 Hours of Arrival[5]	-	-	94%	96%
Fibrinolytic Meds Within 30 Min. of Arrival[5]	-	-	54%	58%
Average Time to ECG (minutes)[5]	-	-	10	7
Average Time to Transfer (minutes)[5]	-	-	94	60
Children's Asthma Care				
Received Home Management Plan of Care	-	-	-	88%
Received Reliever Medication	-	-	-	100%
Received Systemic Corticosteroids	-	-	-	100%
Emergency Department				
Admittance Decision Time (minutes)[2]	816	192	86	98
Head CT Results Within 45 Min. of Arrival[1]	-	-	49%	57%
Patients Who Left ER Before Being Seen	>100k	2%	3%	2%
Time from ER Arrival to Admit. (minutes)[2]	817	388	256	274
Time from ER Arrival to Discharge (minutes)	365	160	125	134
Time in ER Before Being Evaluated (minutes)	404	18	27	26
Time to Pain Meds for Fractures (minutes)	184	66	61	57
Heart Attack Care				
Aspirin Given at Discharge	327	99%	99%	99%
Fibrinolytic Meds Within 30 Min. of Arrival[7]	-	-	71%	54%
PCI Within 90 Minutes of Arrival	61	95%	94%	96%
Statin Prescribed at Discharge	316	97%	98%	98%
Heart Failure Care				
ACE Inhibitor or ARB for LVSD[2]	106	99%	95%	97%
Discharge Instructions Given[2]	281	96%	94%	94%
Evaluation of LVS Function[2]	314	100%	97%	99%
Medicare Spending				
Medicare Spending per Patient (ratio)	-	0.98	1.04	0.98
Pneumonia Care				
Appropriate Initial Antibiotic Given[2]	76	93%	93%	95%
Blood Culture Timing[2]	160	100%	97%	98%
Pregnancy and Delivery Care				
Newborn Deliveries Scheduled Early[2]	27	7%	5%	6%
Preventive Care				
Immunization for Influenza[2]	583	98%	85%	90%
Immunization for Pneumonia[2]	779	98%	88%	92%
Stroke Care				
Anticoagulation Therapy for Atrial Fibrillation	31	100%	93%	95%
Antithrombotic Therapy Timing	216	97%	96%	98%
Assessed for Rehabilitation	262	98%	95%	97%
Discharged on Antithrombotic Therapy	250	100%	97%	99%
Discharged on Statin Medication	189	93%	89%	94%
Thrombolytic Therapy Timing	14	86%	53%	66%
Venous Thromboembolism Prophylaxis	254	92%	87%	94%
Written Stroke Educational Materials Given	130	79%	83%	88%
Surgical Care Improvement Project				
Appropriate Beta Blocker Usage[2]	224	100%	97%	98%
Appropriate VTP Within 24 Hours[2]	405	99%	97%	98%
Controlled Postoperative Blood Glucose[2]	146	99%	96%	97%
Perioperative Temperature Management[2]	596	100%	100%	100%
Prophylactic Antibiotic Selection[2]	476	97%	99%	99%
Prophylactic Antibiotic Selection (Outpatient)	304	97%	97%	98%
Prophylactic Antibiotic Stopped[2]	463	98%	97%	98%
Prophylactic Antibiotic Timing[2]	478	100%	98%	99%
Prophylactic Antibiotic Timing (Outpatient)	308	97%	97%	98%
Urinary Catheter Removal[2]	452	98%	96%	97%
Survey of Patients' Hospital Experiences				
Area Around Room 'Always' Quiet at Night	300+	74%	74%	61%
Doctors 'Always' Communicated Well	300+	84%	87%	82%
Home Recovery Information Given	300+	84%	85%	85%
Hospital Given 9 or 10 on 10 Point Scale	300+	74%	75%	71%
Meds 'Always' Explained Before Given	300+	64%	69%	64%
Nurses 'Always' Communicated Well	300+	80%	83%	79%
Pain 'Always' Well Controlled	300+	71%	75%	71%
Room and Bathroom 'Always' Clean	300+	70%	75%	73%
Timely Help 'Always' Received	300+	65%	71%	68%
Would Definitely Recommend Hospital	300+	78%	75%	71%
Use of Medical Imaging				
Cardiac Imaging Stress Test before Surgery	62	4.8%	5.3%	5.3%
Combination Abdominal CT Scan	706	22.1%	24.5%	10.5%
Combination Brain/Sinus CT Scan	1,156	3.5%	2.6%	2.7%
Combination Chest CT Scan	312	26.0%	7.6%	2.7%
Follow-up Mammogram/Ultrasound	745	16.6%	9.4%	8.8%
Lumbar Spine MRI for Low Back Pain[1]	-	-	42.7%	37.2%

The Neuromedical Center Hospital

10105 Park Row Circle Phone: 225-763-9900
Baton Rouge, LA 70810
URL: www.theneuromedicalcenter.com
Type: Acute Care Hospitals Emergency Services: No
Ownership: Proprietary
Key Personnel:
CEO . . . . Nancy M. Kelly
President . . . . Kelly J. Scrantz, M.D.

Measure	Cases	This Hosp.	State Avg.	U.S. Avg.
Blood Clot Prevention and Treatment				
Anticoagulation Overlap Therapy[2,7]	-	-	89%	93%
ICU Venous Thromboembolism Prophylaxis[2,7]	-	-	88%	92%
Incidence of Potentially Preventable VTE[2,7]	-	-	16%	10%
UFH with Dosages/Platelet Monitoring[2,7]	-	-	94%	97%
Venous Thromboembolism Prophylaxis[2]	193	100%	74%	85%
Warfarin Therapy Discharge Instructions[2,7]	-	-	85%	75%
Chest Pain/Possible Heart Attack Care				
Aspirin Given Within 24 Hours of Arrival[5]	-	-	94%	96%
Fibrinolytic Meds Within 30 Min. of Arrival[5]	-	-	54%	58%
Average Time to ECG (minutes)[5]	-	-	10	7
Average Time to Transfer (minutes)[5]	-	-	94	60
Children's Asthma Care				
Received Home Management Plan of Care	-	-	-	88%
Received Reliever Medication	-	-	-	100%
Received Systemic Corticosteroids	-	-	-	100%
Emergency Department				
Admittance Decision Time (minutes)[2,7]	-	-	86	98
Head CT Results Within 45 Min. of Arrival[5]	-	-	49%	57%
Patients Who Left ER Before Being Seen[5]	-	-	3%	2%
Time from ER Arrival to Admit. (minutes)[2,7]	-	-	256	274
Time from ER Arrival to Discharge (minutes)[5]	-	-	125	134
Time in ER Before Being Evaluated (minutes)[5]	-	-	27	26
Time to Pain Meds for Fractures (minutes)[5]	-	-	61	57
Heart Attack Care				
Aspirin Given at Discharge[5]	-	-	99%	99%
Fibrinolytic Meds Within 30 Min. of Arrival[5]	-	-	71%	54%
PCI Within 90 Minutes of Arrival[5]	-	-	94%	96%
Statin Prescribed at Discharge[5]	-	-	98%	98%
Heart Failure Care				
ACE Inhibitor or ARB for LVSD[5]	-	-	95%	97%
Discharge Instructions Given[5]	-	-	94%	94%
Evaluation of LVS Function[5]	-	-	97%	99%
Medicare Spending				
Medicare Spending per Patient (ratio)	-	0.99	1.04	0.98
Pneumonia Care				
Appropriate Initial Antibiotic Given[5]	-	-	93%	95%
Blood Culture Timing[5]	-	-	97%	98%
Pregnancy and Delivery Care				
Newborn Deliveries Scheduled Early[7]	-	-	5%	6%
Preventive Care				
Immunization for Influenza[2]	424	43%	85%	90%
Immunization for Pneumonia[2]	275	51%	88%	92%
Stroke Care				
Anticoagulation Therapy for Atrial Fibrillation[5]	-	-	93%	95%
Antithrombotic Therapy Timing[5]	-	-	96%	98%
Assessed for Rehabilitation[5]	-	-	95%	97%
Discharged on Antithrombotic Therapy[5]	-	-	97%	99%
Discharged on Statin Medication[5]	-	-	89%	94%
Thrombolytic Therapy Timing[5]	-	-	53%	66%
Venous Thromboembolism Prophylaxis[5]	-	-	87%	94%
Written Stroke Educational Materials Given[5]	-	-	83%	88%
Surgical Care Improvement Project				
Appropriate Beta Blocker Usage[5]	-	-	97%	98%
Appropriate VTP Within 24 Hours[5]	-	-	97%	98%
Controlled Postoperative Blood Glucose[5]	-	-	96%	97%
Perioperative Temperature Management[5]	-	-	100%	100%
Prophylactic Antibiotic Selection[5]	-	-	99%	99%
Prophylactic Antibiotic Selection (Outpatient)	358	100%	97%	98%
Prophylactic Antibiotic Stopped[5]	-	-	97%	98%
Prophylactic Antibiotic Timing[5]	-	-	98%	99%
Prophylactic Antibiotic Timing (Outpatient)	358	100%	97%	98%
Urinary Catheter Removal[5]	-	-	96%	97%
Survey of Patients' Hospital Experiences				
Area Around Room 'Always' Quiet at Night	300+	91%	74%	61%
Doctors 'Always' Communicated Well	300+	86%	87%	82%
Home Recovery Information Given	300+	89%	85%	85%
Hospital Given 9 or 10 on 10 Point Scale	300+	87%	75%	71%
Meds 'Always' Explained Before Given	300+	71%	69%	64%
Nurses 'Always' Communicated Well	300+	89%	83%	79%
Pain 'Always' Well Controlled	300+	78%	75%	71%
Room and Bathroom 'Always' Clean	300+	85%	75%	73%
Timely Help 'Always' Received	300+	82%	71%	68%
Would Definitely Recommend Hospital	300+	87%	75%	71%
Use of Medical Imaging				
Cardiac Imaging Stress Test before Surgery[7]	-	-	5.3%	5.3%
Combination Abdominal CT Scan[7]	-	-	24.5%	10.5%
Combination Brain/Sinus CT Scan	115	0.0%	2.6%	2.7%
Combination Chest CT Scan[1]	-	-	7.6%	2.7%
Follow-up Mammogram/Ultrasound[7]	-	-	9.4%	8.8%
Lumbar Spine MRI for Low Back Pain[7]	-	-	42.7%	37.2%

Ochsner Medical Center - Baton Rouge

17000 Medical Center Dr Phone: 225-755-4876
Baton Rouge, LA 70816 Fax: 225-755-4883
Type: Acute Care Hospitals Emergency Services: Yes
Ownership: Voluntary non-profit - Private Beds: 201
Key Personnel:
Quality Assurance . . . . Rose Crespo
Chief of Medical Staff. . . . . Robert Elliott, MD
Cardiac Laboratory. . . . . Mark Green
Radiology. . . . . Mark Green
CEO/President. . . . . Robert Jernigan, CHE
Coronary Care . . . . Mary Johnson, MSN, RN
Infection Control. . . . . Bonnie Rosenthal, RN
Operating Room. . . . . Louise Ryals, RN

Measure	Cases	This Hosp.	State Avg.	U.S. Avg.
Blood Clot Prevention and Treatment				
Anticoagulation Overlap Therapy[2]	35	97%	89%	93%
ICU Venous Thromboembolism Prophylaxis[2]	105	93%	88%	92%
Incidence of Potentially Preventable VTE[1,2]	-	-	16%	10%
UFH with Dosages/Platelet Monitoring[2]	27	100%	94%	97%
Venous Thromboembolism Prophylaxis[2]	325	86%	74%	85%
Warfarin Therapy Discharge Instructions[2]	26	100%	85%	75%
Chest Pain/Possible Heart Attack Care				
Aspirin Given Within 24 Hours of Arrival[1,3]	-	-	94%	96%
Fibrinolytic Meds Within 30 Min. of Arrival[5]	-	-	54%	58%
Average Time to ECG (minutes)[1,3]	-	-	10	7
Average Time to Transfer (minutes)[5]	-	-	94	60
Children's Asthma Care				
Received Home Management Plan of Care	-	-	-	88%
Received Reliever Medication	-	-	-	100%
Received Systemic Corticosteroids	-	-	-	100%
Emergency Department				
Admittance Decision Time (minutes)[2]	603	131	86	98
Head CT Results Within 45 Min. of Arrival[1]	-	-	49%	57%
Patients Who Left ER Before Being Seen	54,149	1%	3%	2%
Time from ER Arrival to Admit. (minutes)[2]	611	309	256	274
Time from ER Arrival to Discharge (minutes)	362	90	125	134
Time in ER Before Being Evaluated (minutes)	381	8	27	26
Time to Pain Meds for Fractures (minutes)	122	50	61	57
Heart Attack Care				
Aspirin Given at Discharge	116	98%	99%	99%
Fibrinolytic Meds Within 30 Min. of Arrival[7]	-	-	71%	54%

NOTE: Hospital profiles are in alphabetical order by state, then city, then hospital within the city; Rankings exclude hospitals with less than 25 cases except for patient surveys which excludes hospitals with less than 100 cases; (a) 100-299 cases; (1) The number of cases/patients is too few to report; (2) Data submitted were based on a sample of cases/patients; (3) Results are based on a shorter time period than required; (4) Data suppressed by CMS for one or more quarters; (5) Results are not available for this reporting period; (6) Fewer than 100 patients completed the HCAHPS survey; (7) No cases met the criteria for this measure; (8) The lower limit of the confidence interval cannot be calculated if the number of observed infections equals zero; (9) No data are available from the state/territory for this reporting period; (10) The scores shown reflect fewer than 50 completed surveys; (11) There were discrepancies in the data collection process; (12) This measure does not apply to this hospital for this reporting period; (13) Results cannot be calculated for this reporting period; (14) The results for this state are combined with nearby states to protect confidentiality; Please refer to the User's Guide for a full explanation of data.

Measure	Cases	This Hosp.	State Avg.	U.S. Avg.
PCI Within 90 Minutes of Arrival	16	81%	94%	96%
Statin Prescribed at Discharge	117	100%	98%	98%
Heart Failure Care				
ACE Inhibitor or ARB for LVSD[2]	66	95%	95%	97%
Discharge Instructions Given[2]	206	100%	94%	94%
Evaluation of LVS Function[2]	234	100%	97%	99%
Medicare Spending				
Medicare Spending per Patient (ratio)	-	1.09	1.04	0.98
Pneumonia Care				
Appropriate Initial Antibiotic Given[2]	67	99%	93%	95%
Blood Culture Timing[2]	156	100%	97%	98%
Pregnancy and Delivery Care				
Newborn Deliveries Scheduled Early[2]	33	3%	5%	6%
Preventive Care				
Immunization for Influenza[2]	496	88%	85%	90%
Immunization for Pneumonia[2]	586	89%	88%	92%
Stroke Care				
Anticoagulation Therapy for Atrial Fibrillation[1]	-	-	93%	95%
Antithrombotic Therapy Timing	47	100%	96%	98%
Assessed for Rehabilitation	58	97%	95%	97%
Discharged on Antithrombotic Therapy	57	100%	97%	99%
Discharged on Statin Medication	45	93%	89%	94%
Thrombolytic Therapy Timing[1]	-	-	53%	66%
Venous Thromboembolism Prophylaxis	56	95%	87%	94%
Written Stroke Educational Materials Given	37	97%	83%	88%
Surgical Care Improvement Project				
Appropriate Beta Blocker Usage[2]	124	98%	97%	98%
Appropriate VTP Within 24 Hours[2]	196	95%	97%	98%
Controlled Postoperative Blood Glucose[2]	60	93%	96%	97%
Perioperative Temperature Management[2]	236	100%	100%	100%
Prophylactic Antibiotic Selection[2]	187	98%	99%	99%
Prophylactic Antibiotic Selection (Outpatient)	243	98%	97%	98%
Prophylactic Antibiotic Stopped[2]	183	96%	97%	98%
Prophylactic Antibiotic Timing[2]	187	99%	98%	99%
Prophylactic Antibiotic Timing (Outpatient)	247	98%	97%	98%
Urinary Catheter Removal[2]	209	98%	96%	97%
Survey of Patients' Hospital Experiences				
Area Around Room 'Always' Quiet at Night	300+	65%	74%	61%
Doctors 'Always' Communicated Well	300+	78%	87%	82%
Home Recovery Information Given	300+	86%	85%	85%
Hospital Given 9 or 10 on 10 Point Scale	300+	70%	75%	71%
Meds 'Always' Explained Before Given	300+	66%	69%	64%
Nurses 'Always' Communicated Well	300+	82%	83%	79%
Pain 'Always' Well Controlled	300+	71%	75%	71%
Room and Bathroom 'Always' Clean	300+	66%	75%	73%
Timely Help 'Always' Received	300+	63%	71%	68%
Would Definitely Recommend Hospital	300+	70%	75%	71%
Use of Medical Imaging				
Cardiac Imaging Stress Test before Surgery[1]	-	-	5.3%	5.3%
Combination Abdominal CT Scan	333	6.6%	24.5%	10.5%
Combination Brain/Sinus CT Scan[1]	-	-	2.6%	2.7%
Combination Chest CT Scan	127	0.8%	7.6%	2.7%
Follow-up Mammogram/Ultrasound[1]	-	-	9.4%	8.8%
Lumbar Spine MRI for Low Back Pain[1]	-	-	42.7%	37.2%

Our Lady of the Lake Regional Medical Center

5000 Hennessy Blvd — Phone: 225-765-6565
Baton Rouge, LA 70808 — Fax: 225-769-3659
URL: www.ololrmc.com
Type: Acute Care Hospitals — Emergency Services: Yes
Ownership: Voluntary non-profit - Church — Beds: 763

Key Personnel:
Quality Assurance .... Adelaide Currier
Pediatric In-Patient Care .... Faith Hansbrough, MD
Operating Room.............. Mark Hausmann, MD
Radiology.................. Robert F Hayden, MD
Infection Control............. Darlene J Picoci
Cardiac Laboratory............ Andrew Rees, MD
Chief of Medical Staff.......... Richard Vath, MD
CEO/President............... K Scott Wester

Measure	Cases	This Hosp.	State Avg.	U.S. Avg.
Blood Clot Prevention and Treatment				
Anticoagulation Overlap Therapy[2]	169	93%	89%	93%
ICU Venous Thromboembolism Prophylaxis[2]	99	94%	88%	92%
Incidence of Potentially Preventable VTE[2]	35	11%	16%	10%
UFH with Dosages/Platelet Monitoring[2]	25	88%	94%	97%
Venous Thromboembolism Prophylaxis[2]	304	82%	74%	85%
Warfarin Therapy Discharge Instructions[2]	140	88%	85%	75%
Chest Pain/Possible Heart Attack Care				
Aspirin Given Within 24 Hours of Arrival[1]	-	-	94%	96%
Fibrinolytic Meds Within 30 Min. of Arrival[3,7]	-	-	54%	58%
Average Time to ECG (minutes)[1]	-	-	10	7
Average Time to Transfer (minutes)[3,7]	-	-	94	60
Children's Asthma Care				
Received Home Management Plan of Care	-	-	-	88%
Received Reliever Medication	-	-	-	100%
Received Systemic Corticosteroids	-	-	-	100%
Emergency Department				
Admittance Decision Time (minutes)[2]	491	90	86	98
Head CT Results Within 45 Min. of Arrival[1]	-	-	49%	57%
Patients Who Left ER Before Being Seen	>100k	3%	3%	2%
Time from ER Arrival to Admit. (minutes)[2]	513	301	256	274
Time from ER Arrival to Discharge (minutes)	323	186	125	134
Time in ER Before Being Evaluated (minutes)	361	51	27	26
Time to Pain Meds for Fractures (minutes)	284	62	61	57
Heart Attack Care				
Aspirin Given at Discharge[2]	377	99%	99%	99%
Fibrinolytic Meds Within 30 Min. of Arrival[2,7]	-	-	71%	54%
PCI Within 90 Minutes of Arrival[2]	73	99%	94%	96%
Statin Prescribed at Discharge[2]	360	98%	98%	98%
Heart Failure Care				
ACE Inhibitor or ARB for LVSD[2]	119	92%	95%	97%
Discharge Instructions Given[2]	353	95%	94%	94%
Evaluation of LVS Function[2]	378	99%	97%	99%
Medicare Spending				
Medicare Spending per Patient (ratio)	-	1.02	1.04	0.98
Pneumonia Care				
Appropriate Initial Antibiotic Given[2]	61	98%	93%	95%
Blood Culture Timing[2]	121	98%	97%	98%
Pregnancy and Delivery Care				
Newborn Deliveries Scheduled Early[7]	-	-	5%	6%
Preventive Care				
Immunization for Influenza[2]	573	96%	85%	90%
Immunization for Pneumonia[2]	694	89%	88%	92%
Stroke Care				
Anticoagulation Therapy for Atrial Fibrillation[1,2]	-	-	93%	95%
Antithrombotic Therapy Timing[2]	80	96%	96%	98%
Assessed for Rehabilitation[2]	116	95%	95%	97%
Discharged on Antithrombotic Therapy[2]	86	97%	97%	99%
Discharged on Statin Medication[2]	74	95%	89%	94%
Thrombolytic Therapy Timing[1,2]	-	-	53%	66%
Venous Thromboembolism Prophylaxis[2]	118	92%	87%	94%
Written Stroke Educational Materials Given[2]	68	91%	83%	88%
Surgical Care Improvement Project				
Appropriate Beta Blocker Usage[2]	483	99%	97%	98%
Appropriate VTP Within 24 Hours[2]	659	97%	97%	98%
Controlled Postoperative Blood Glucose[2]	313	99%	96%	97%
Perioperative Temperature Management[2]	1,088	100%	100%	100%
Prophylactic Antibiotic Selection[2]	788	100%	99%	99%
Prophylactic Antibiotic Selection (Outpatient)	561	98%	97%	98%
Prophylactic Antibiotic Stopped[2]	770	97%	97%	98%
Prophylactic Antibiotic Timing[2]	790	100%	98%	99%
Prophylactic Antibiotic Timing (Outpatient)	561	98%	97%	98%
Urinary Catheter Removal[2]	847	95%	96%	97%
Survey of Patients' Hospital Experiences				
Area Around Room 'Always' Quiet at Night	300+	69%	74%	61%
Doctors 'Always' Communicated Well	300+	87%	87%	82%
Home Recovery Information Given	300+	87%	85%	85%
Hospital Given 9 or 10 on 10 Point Scale	300+	75%	75%	71%
Meds 'Always' Explained Before Given	300+	66%	69%	64%
Nurses 'Always' Communicated Well	300+	83%	83%	79%
Pain 'Always' Well Controlled	300+	75%	75%	71%
Room and Bathroom 'Always' Clean	300+	67%	75%	73%
Timely Help 'Always' Received	300+	63%	71%	68%
Would Definitely Recommend Hospital	300+	76%	75%	71%
Use of Medical Imaging				
Cardiac Imaging Stress Test before Surgery	762	6.6%	5.3%	5.3%
Combination Abdominal CT Scan	1,231	13.2%	24.5%	10.5%
Combination Brain/Sinus CT Scan	1,497	3.3%	2.6%	2.7%
Combination Chest CT Scan	711	5.8%	7.6%	2.7%
Follow-up Mammogram/Ultrasound	246	8.5%	9.4%	8.8%
Lumbar Spine MRI for Low Back Pain	48	45.8%	42.7%	37.2%

Surgical Specialty Center of Baton Rouge

8080 Bluebonnet Blvd — Phone: 225-408-5730
Baton Rouge, LA 70810
URL: www.sscbr.com
Type: Acute Care Hospitals — Emergency Services: No
Ownership: Physician

Key Personnel:
Chief of Medical Staff.......... Brent Bankston, MD
Radiology.................. Robert Branstetter, MD
CEO .... Craig Hume
Operating Room.............. William Loe, MD

Measure	Cases	This Hosp.	State Avg.	U.S. Avg.
Blood Clot Prevention and Treatment				
Anticoagulation Overlap Therapy[7]	-	-	89%	93%
ICU Venous Thromboembolism Prophylaxis[7]	-	-	88%	92%
Incidence of Potentially Preventable VTE[7]	-	-	16%	10%
UFH with Dosages/Platelet Monitoring[7]	-	-	94%	97%
Venous Thromboembolism Prophylaxis	79	70%	74%	85%
Warfarin Therapy Discharge Instructions[7]	-	-	85%	75%
Chest Pain/Possible Heart Attack Care				
Aspirin Given Within 24 Hours of Arrival[5]	-	-	94%	96%
Fibrinolytic Meds Within 30 Min. of Arrival[5]	-	-	54%	58%
Average Time to ECG (minutes)[5]	-	-	10	7
Average Time to Transfer (minutes)[5]	-	-	94	60
Children's Asthma Care				
Received Home Management Plan of Care	-	-	-	88%
Received Reliever Medication	-	-	-	100%
Received Systemic Corticosteroids	-	-	-	100%
Emergency Department				
Admittance Decision Time (minutes)[7]	-	-	86	98
Head CT Results Within 45 Min. of Arrival[5]	-	-	49%	57%
Patients Who Left ER Before Being Seen[5]	-	-	3%	2%
Time from ER Arrival to Admit. (minutes)[7]	-	-	256	274
Time from ER Arrival to Discharge (minutes)[5]	-	-	125	134
Time in ER Before Being Evaluated (minutes)[5]	-	-	27	26
Time to Pain Meds for Fractures (minutes)[5]	-	-	61	57
Heart Attack Care				
Aspirin Given at Discharge[5]	-	-	99%	99%
Fibrinolytic Meds Within 30 Min. of Arrival[5]	-	-	71%	54%
PCI Within 90 Minutes of Arrival[5]	-	-	94%	96%
Statin Prescribed at Discharge[5]	-	-	98%	98%
Heart Failure Care				
ACE Inhibitor or ARB for LVSD[5]	-	-	95%	97%
Discharge Instructions Given[5]	-	-	94%	94%
Evaluation of LVS Function[5]	-	-	97%	99%
Medicare Spending				
Medicare Spending per Patient (ratio)	-	0.91	1.04	0.98
Pneumonia Care				
Appropriate Initial Antibiotic Given[5]	-	-	93%	95%
Blood Culture Timing[5]	-	-	97%	98%
Pregnancy and Delivery Care				
Newborn Deliveries Scheduled Early[7]	-	-	5%	6%
Preventive Care				
Immunization for Influenza	141	23%	85%	90%
Immunization for Pneumonia	42	67%	88%	92%
Stroke Care				
Anticoagulation Therapy for Atrial Fibrillation[5]	-	-	93%	95%
Antithrombotic Therapy Timing[5]	-	-	96%	98%
Assessed for Rehabilitation[5]	-	-	95%	97%
Discharged on Antithrombotic Therapy[5]	-	-	97%	99%
Discharged on Statin Medication[5]	-	-	89%	94%
Thrombolytic Therapy Timing[5]	-	-	53%	66%
Venous Thromboembolism Prophylaxis[5]	-	-	87%	94%
Written Stroke Educational Materials Given[5]	-	-	83%	88%
Surgical Care Improvement Project				
Appropriate Beta Blocker Usage[1]	-	-	97%	98%

NOTE: Hospital profiles are in alphabetical order by state, then city, then hospital within the city; Rankings exclude hospitals with less than 25 cases except for patient surveys which excludes hospitals with less than 100 cases; (a) 100-299 cases; (1) The number of cases/patients is too few to report; (2) Data submitted were based on a sample of cases/patients; (3) Results are based on a shorter time period than required; (4) Data suppressed by CMS for one or more quarters; (5) Results are not available for this reporting period; (6) Fewer than 100 patients completed the HCAHPS survey; (7) No cases met the criteria for this measure; (8) The lower limit of the confidence interval cannot be calculated if the number of observed infections equals zero; (9) No data are available from the state/territory for this reporting period; (10) The scores shown reflect fewer than 50 completed surveys; (11) There were discrepancies in the data collection process; (12) This measure does not apply to this hospital for this reporting period; (13) Results cannot be calculated for this reporting period; (14) The results for this state are combined with nearby states to protect confidentiality; Please refer to the User's Guide for a full explanation of data.

Measure	Cases	This Hosp.	State Avg.	U.S. Avg.
Appropriate VTP Within 24 Hours	16	100%	97%	98%
Controlled Postoperative Blood Glucose[7]	-	-	96%	97%
Perioperative Temperature Management	38	100%	100%	100%
Prophylactic Antibiotic Selection[1]	-	-	99%	99%
Prophylactic Antibiotic Selection (Outpatient)	191	97%	97%	98%
Prophylactic Antibiotic Stopped[1]	-	-	97%	98%
Prophylactic Antibiotic Timing[1]	-	-	98%	99%
Prophylactic Antibiotic Timing (Outpatient)	191	98%	97%	98%
Urinary Catheter Removal[7]	-	-	96%	97%
Survey of Patients' Hospital Experiences				
Area Around Room 'Always' Quiet at Night	(a)	95%	74%	61%
Doctors 'Always' Communicated Well	(a)	94%	87%	82%
Home Recovery Information Given	(a)	90%	85%	85%
Hospital Given 9 or 10 on 10 Point Scale	(a)	96%	75%	71%
Meds 'Always' Explained Before Given	(a)	73%	69%	64%
Nurses 'Always' Communicated Well	(a)	93%	83%	79%
Pain 'Always' Well Controlled	(a)	82%	75%	71%
Room and Bathroom 'Always' Clean	(a)	85%	75%	73%
Timely Help 'Always' Received	(a)	90%	71%	68%
Would Definitely Recommend Hospital	(a)	94%	75%	71%
Use of Medical Imaging				
Cardiac Imaging Stress Test before Surgery[7]	-	-	5.3%	5.3%
Combination Abdominal CT Scan[1]	-	-	24.5%	10.5%
Combination Brain/Sinus CT Scan[1]	-	-	2.6%	2.7%
Combination Chest CT Scan[1]	-	-	7.6%	2.7%
Follow-up Mammogram/Ultrasound[7]	-	-	9.4%	8.8%
Lumbar Spine MRI for Low Back Pain[1]	-	-	42.7%	37.2%

Woman's Hospital

100 Woman's Way
Baton Rouge, LA 70817
URL: www.womans.com
Phone: 225-927-1300
Fax: 225-924-8233
Type: Acute Care Hospitals
Emergency Services: Yes
Ownership: Voluntary non-profit - Other
Beds: 225

Key Personnel:
Radiology. . . . . Chester Coles, MD
CEO/President. . . . . Teri G Fontenot
Pediatric Ambulatory Care . . . . . . Patricia Schneider, MD
Pediatric In-Patient Care . . . . Patricia Schneider, MD
Chief of Medical Staff. . . . . Edward Schwartzenbur, MD

Measure	Cases	This Hosp.	State Avg.	U.S. Avg.
Blood Clot Prevention and Treatment				
Anticoagulation Overlap Therapy[1,2]	-	-	89%	93%
ICU Venous Thromboembolism Prophylaxis[2]	11	100%	88%	92%
Incidence of Potentially Preventable VTE[1,2]	-	-	16%	10%
UFH with Dosages/Platelet Monitoring[1,2]	-	-	94%	97%
Venous Thromboembolism Prophylaxis[2]	57	68%	74%	85%
Warfarin Therapy Discharge Instructions[1,2]	-	-	85%	75%
Chest Pain/Possible Heart Attack Care				
Aspirin Given Within 24 Hours of Arrival[1,3]	-	-	94%	96%
Fibrinolytic Meds Within 30 Min. of Arrival[5]	-	-	54%	58%
Average Time to ECG (minutes)[1,3]	-	-	10	7
Average Time to Transfer (minutes)[5]	-	-	94	60
Children's Asthma Care				
Received Home Management Plan of Care	-	-	-	88%
Received Reliever Medication	-	-	-	100%
Received Systemic Corticosteroids	-	-	-	100%
Emergency Department				
Admittance Decision Time (minutes)[2]	250	14	86	98
Head CT Results Within 45 Min. of Arrival[5]	-	-	49%	57%
Patients Who Left ER Before Being Seen	9,196	4%	3%	2%
Time from ER Arrival to Admit. (minutes)[2]	253	62	256	274
Time from ER Arrival to Discharge (minutes)	320	190	125	134
Time in ER Before Being Evaluated (minutes)	356	118	27	26
Time to Pain Meds for Fractures (minutes)[5]	-	-	61	57
Heart Attack Care				
Aspirin Given at Discharge[5]	-	-	99%	99%
Fibrinolytic Meds Within 30 Min. of Arrival[5]	-	-	71%	54%
PCI Within 90 Minutes of Arrival[5]	-	-	94%	96%
Statin Prescribed at Discharge[5]	-	-	98%	98%
Heart Failure Care				
ACE Inhibitor or ARB for LVSD[5]	-	-	95%	97%
Discharge Instructions Given[5]	-	-	94%	94%
Evaluation of LVS Function[5]	-	-	97%	99%
Medicare Spending				
Medicare Spending per Patient (ratio)	-	0.96	1.04	0.98
Pneumonia Care				
Appropriate Initial Antibiotic Given[5]	-	-	93%	95%
Blood Culture Timing[5]	-	-	97%	98%
Pregnancy and Delivery Care				
Newborn Deliveries Scheduled Early[2]	130	1%	5%	6%
Preventive Care				
Immunization for Influenza[2]	352	47%	85%	90%
Immunization for Pneumonia[2]	27	37%	88%	92%
Stroke Care				
Anticoagulation Therapy for Atrial Fibrillation[5]	-	-	93%	95%
Antithrombotic Therapy Timing[5]	-	-	96%	98%
Assessed for Rehabilitation[5]	-	-	95%	97%
Discharged on Antithrombotic Therapy[5]	-	-	97%	99%
Discharged on Statin Medication[5]	-	-	89%	94%
Thrombolytic Therapy Timing[5]	-	-	53%	66%
Venous Thromboembolism Prophylaxis[5]	-	-	87%	94%
Written Stroke Educational Materials Given[5]	-	-	83%	88%
Surgical Care Improvement Project				
Appropriate Beta Blocker Usage[2]	13	100%	97%	98%
Appropriate VTP Within 24 Hours[2]	102	97%	97%	98%
Controlled Postoperative Blood Glucose[2,7]	-	-	96%	97%
Perioperative Temperature Management[2]	149	100%	100%	100%
Prophylactic Antibiotic Selection[2]	77	100%	99%	99%
Prophylactic Antibiotic Selection (Outpatient)	189	98%	97%	98%
Prophylactic Antibiotic Stopped[2]	74	97%	97%	98%
Prophylactic Antibiotic Timing[2]	77	100%	98%	99%
Prophylactic Antibiotic Timing (Outpatient)	189	98%	97%	98%
Urinary Catheter Removal[1,2]	-	-	96%	97%
Survey of Patients' Hospital Experiences				
Area Around Room 'Always' Quiet at Night	300+	66%	74%	61%
Doctors 'Always' Communicated Well	300+	85%	87%	82%
Home Recovery Information Given	300+	92%	85%	85%
Hospital Given 9 or 10 on 10 Point Scale	300+	83%	75%	71%
Meds 'Always' Explained Before Given	300+	66%	69%	64%
Nurses 'Always' Communicated Well	300+	80%	83%	79%
Pain 'Always' Well Controlled	300+	75%	75%	71%
Room and Bathroom 'Always' Clean	300+	75%	75%	73%
Timely Help 'Always' Received	300+	68%	71%	68%
Would Definitely Recommend Hospital	300+	86%	75%	71%
Use of Medical Imaging				
Cardiac Imaging Stress Test before Surgery[7]	-	-	5.3%	5.3%
Combination Abdominal CT Scan[1]	-	-	24.5%	10.5%
Combination Brain/Sinus CT Scan[7]	-	-	2.6%	2.7%
Combination Chest CT Scan[1]	-	-	7.6%	2.7%
Follow-up Mammogram/Ultrasound	2,501	12.3%	9.4%	8.8%
Lumbar Spine MRI for Low Back Pain[1]	-	-	42.7%	37.2%

Reeves Memorial Medical Center

409 First Street
Bernice, LA 71222
Phone: 318-285-9066
Fax: 318-285-9039
Type: Critical Access Hospitals
Emergency Services: Yes
Ownership: Govt - Hospital Dist/Auth
Beds: 11

Key Personnel:
Chief of Medical Staff. . . . . Brian Harris, MD
Emergency Room . . . . Barbara B Jones
Quality Assurance . . . . Barbara B Jones
CEO/President. . . . . Charolette Thompson
Infection Control. . . . . Iram Zando, MD

Measure	Cases	This Hosp.	State Avg.	U.S. Avg.
Blood Clot Prevention and Treatment				
Anticoagulation Overlap Therapy[5]	-	-	89%	93%
ICU Venous Thromboembolism Prophylaxis[5]	-	-	88%	92%
Incidence of Potentially Preventable VTE[5]	-	-	16%	10%
UFH with Dosages/Platelet Monitoring[5]	-	-	94%	97%
Venous Thromboembolism Prophylaxis[5]	-	-	74%	85%
Warfarin Therapy Discharge Instructions[5]	-	-	85%	75%
Chest Pain/Possible Heart Attack Care				
Aspirin Given Within 24 Hours of Arrival[1,3]	-	-	94%	96%
Fibrinolytic Meds Within 30 Min. of Arrival[1,3]	-	-	54%	58%
Average Time to ECG (minutes)[1,3]	-	-	10	7
Average Time to Transfer (minutes)[3,7]	-	-	94	60
Children's Asthma Care				
Received Home Management Plan of Care	-	-	-	88%
Received Reliever Medication	-	-	-	100%
Received Systemic Corticosteroids	-	-	-	100%
Emergency Department				
Admittance Decision Time (minutes)[3]	21	0	86	98
Head CT Results Within 45 Min. of Arrival[1]	-	-	49%	57%
Patients Who Left ER Before Being Seen	1,680	0%	3%	2%
Time from ER Arrival to Admit. (minutes)[3]	21	150	256	274
Time from ER Arrival to Discharge (minutes)[3]	867	95	125	134
Time in ER Before Being Evaluated (minutes)[3]	901	20	27	26
Time to Pain Meds for Fractures (minutes)[1,3]	-	-	61	57
Heart Attack Care				
Aspirin Given at Discharge[3,7]	-	-	99%	99%
Fibrinolytic Meds Within 30 Min. of Arrival[3,7]	-	-	71%	54%
PCI Within 90 Minutes of Arrival[3,7]	-	-	94%	96%
Statin Prescribed at Discharge[3,7]	-	-	98%	98%
Heart Failure Care				
ACE Inhibitor or ARB for LVSD[1,3]	-	-	95%	97%
Discharge Instructions Given[1,3]	-	-	94%	94%
Evaluation of LVS Function[1,3]	-	-	97%	99%
Medicare Spending				
Medicare Spending per Patient (ratio)	-	-	1.04	0.98
Pneumonia Care				
Appropriate Initial Antibiotic Given	16	100%	93%	95%
Blood Culture Timing[1]	-	-	97%	98%
Pregnancy and Delivery Care				
Newborn Deliveries Scheduled Early[5]	-	-	5%	6%
Preventive Care				
Immunization for Influenza[5]	-	-	85%	90%
Immunization for Pneumonia[5]	-	-	88%	92%
Stroke Care				
Anticoagulation Therapy for Atrial Fibrillation[3,7]	-	-	93%	95%
Antithrombotic Therapy Timing[1,3]	-	-	96%	98%
Assessed for Rehabilitation[1,3]	-	-	95%	97%
Discharged on Antithrombotic Therapy[1,3]	-	-	97%	99%
Discharged on Statin Medication[1,3]	-	-	89%	94%
Thrombolytic Therapy Timing[1,3]	-	-	53%	66%
Venous Thromboembolism Prophylaxis[1,3]	-	-	87%	94%
Written Stroke Educational Materials Given[3,7]	-	-	83%	88%
Surgical Care Improvement Project				
Appropriate Beta Blocker Usage[5]	-	-	97%	98%
Appropriate VTP Within 24 Hours[5]	-	-	97%	98%
Controlled Postoperative Blood Glucose[5]	-	-	96%	97%
Perioperative Temperature Management[5]	-	-	100%	100%
Prophylactic Antibiotic Selection[5]	-	-	99%	99%
Prophylactic Antibiotic Selection (Outpatient)[5]	-	-	97%	98%
Prophylactic Antibiotic Stopped[5]	-	-	97%	98%
Prophylactic Antibiotic Timing[5]	-	-	98%	99%
Prophylactic Antibiotic Timing (Outpatient)[5]	-	-	97%	98%
Urinary Catheter Removal[5]	-	-	96%	97%
Survey of Patients' Hospital Experiences				
Area Around Room 'Always' Quiet at Night[5]	-	-	74%	61%
Doctors 'Always' Communicated Well[5]	-	-	87%	82%
Home Recovery Information Given[5]	-	-	85%	85%
Hospital Given 9 or 10 on 10 Point Scale[5]	-	-	75%	71%
Meds 'Always' Explained Before Given[5]	-	-	69%	64%
Nurses 'Always' Communicated Well[5]	-	-	83%	79%
Pain 'Always' Well Controlled[5]	-	-	75%	71%
Room and Bathroom 'Always' Clean[5]	-	-	75%	73%
Timely Help 'Always' Received[5]	-	-	71%	68%
Would Definitely Recommend Hospital[5]	-	-	75%	71%
Use of Medical Imaging				
Cardiac Imaging Stress Test before Surgery[7]	-	-	5.3%	5.3%
Combination Abdominal CT Scan[1]	-	-	24.5%	10.5%
Combination Brain/Sinus CT Scan	51	0.0%	2.6%	2.7%
Combination Chest CT Scan[1]	-	-	7.6%	2.7%
Follow-up Mammogram/Ultrasound[7]	-	-	9.4%	8.8%
Lumbar Spine MRI for Low Back Pain[7]	-	-	42.7%	37.2%

NOTE: Hospital profiles are in alphabetical order by state, then city, then hospital within the city; Rankings exclude hospitals with less than 25 cases except for patient surveys which excludes hospitals with less than 100 cases; (a) 100-299 cases; (1) The number of cases/patients is too few to report; (2) Data submitted were based on a sample of cases/patients; (3) Results are based on a shorter time period than required; (4) Data suppressed by CMS for one or more quarters; (5) Results are not available for this reporting period; (6) Fewer than 100 patients completed the HCAHPS survey; (7) No cases met the criteria for this measure; (8) The lower limit of the confidence interval cannot be calculated if the number of observed infections equals zero; (9) No data are available from the state/territory for this reporting period; (10) The scores shown reflect fewer than 50 completed surveys; (11) There were discrepancies in the data collection process; (12) This measure does not apply to this hospital for this reporting period; (13) Results cannot be calculated for this reporting period; (14) The results for this state are combined with nearby states to protect confidentiality; Please refer to the User's Guide for a full explanation of data.

Washington Saint Tammany Regional Medical Center

433 Plaza St Phone: 985-730-6700
Bogalusa, LA 70427 Fax: 985-730-6709
Type: Acute Care Hospitals Emergency Services: Yes
Ownership: Government - State Beds: 66

Key Personnel:
Infection Control. . . . . Janice Augustine, RN
Patient Relations . . . . Katherine Goux
Chief of Medical Staff. . . . . Dr Lee Roy Joyner
Operating Room. . . . . Anna Peters, RN
Radiology. . . . . Gary Pierce
CEO/President. . . . . Kurt M Scott

Measure	Cases	This Hosp.	State Avg.	U.S. Avg.
Blood Clot Prevention and Treatment				
Anticoagulation Overlap Therapy[2]	17	59%	89%	93%
ICU Venous Thromboembolism Prophylaxis[2]	72	75%	88%	92%
Incidence of Potentially Preventable VTE[1,2]	-	-	16%	10%
UFH with Dosages/Platelet Monitoring[1,2]	-	-	94%	97%
Venous Thromboembolism Prophylaxis[2]	142	61%	74%	85%
Warfarin Therapy Discharge Instructions[1,2]	-	-	85%	75%
Chest Pain/Possible Heart Attack Care				
Aspirin Given Within 24 Hours of Arrival	118	100%	94%	96%
Fibrinolytic Meds Within 30 Min. of Arrival[1]	-	-	54%	58%
Average Time to ECG (minutes)	120	15	10	7
Average Time to Transfer (minutes)	20	69	94	60
Children's Asthma Care				
Received Home Management Plan of Care	-	-	-	88%
Received Reliever Medication	-	-	-	100%
Received Systemic Corticosteroids	-	-	-	100%
Emergency Department				
Admittance Decision Time (minutes)[2]	226	140	86	98
Head CT Results Within 45 Min. of Arrival	13	62%	49%	57%
Patients Who Left ER Before Being Seen	30,115	4%	3%	2%
Time from ER Arrival to Admit. (minutes)[2]	303	315	256	274
Time from ER Arrival to Discharge (minutes)	421	120	125	134
Time in ER Before Being Evaluated (minutes)	438	32	27	26
Time to Pain Meds for Fractures (minutes)	47	93	61	57
Heart Attack Care				
Aspirin Given at Discharge[1,3]	-	-	99%	99%
Fibrinolytic Meds Within 30 Min. of Arrival[3,7]	-	-	71%	54%
PCI Within 90 Minutes of Arrival[3,7]	-	-	94%	96%
Statin Prescribed at Discharge[1,3]	-	-	98%	98%
Heart Failure Care				
ACE Inhibitor or ARB for LVSD	39	95%	95%	97%
Discharge Instructions Given	68	100%	94%	94%
Evaluation of LVS Function	81	100%	97%	99%
Medicare Spending				
Medicare Spending per Patient (ratio)	-	1.30	1.04	0.98
Pneumonia Care				
Appropriate Initial Antibiotic Given	61	95%	93%	95%
Blood Culture Timing	87	95%	97%	98%
Pregnancy and Delivery Care				
Newborn Deliveries Scheduled Early	30	10%	5%	6%
Preventive Care				
Immunization for Influenza[2]	310	86%	85%	90%
Immunization for Pneumonia[2]	278	87%	88%	92%
Stroke Care				
Anticoagulation Therapy for Atrial Fibrillation[1]	-	-	93%	95%
Antithrombotic Therapy Timing	12	100%	96%	98%
Assessed for Rehabilitation	12	100%	95%	97%
Discharged on Antithrombotic Therapy	12	92%	97%	99%
Discharged on Statin Medication	11	82%	89%	94%
Thrombolytic Therapy Timing[1]	-	-	53%	66%
Venous Thromboembolism Prophylaxis	13	77%	87%	94%
Written Stroke Educational Materials Given[1]	-	-	83%	88%
Surgical Care Improvement Project				
Appropriate Beta Blocker Usage	22	91%	97%	98%
Appropriate VTP Within 24 Hours	79	97%	97%	98%
Controlled Postoperative Blood Glucose[7]	-	-	96%	97%
Perioperative Temperature Management	84	100%	100%	100%
Prophylactic Antibiotic Selection	46	100%	99%	99%
Prophylactic Antibiotic Selection (Outpatient)	24	83%	97%	98%
Prophylactic Antibiotic Stopped	46	100%	97%	98%
Prophylactic Antibiotic Timing	46	100%	98%	99%
Prophylactic Antibiotic Timing (Outpatient)	13	62%	97%	98%
Urinary Catheter Removal	20	95%	96%	97%
Survey of Patients' Hospital Experiences				
Area Around Room 'Always' Quiet at Night	(a)	66%	74%	61%
Doctors 'Always' Communicated Well	(a)	83%	87%	82%
Home Recovery Information Given	(a)	85%	85%	85%
Hospital Given 9 or 10 on 10 Point Scale	(a)	72%	75%	71%
Meds 'Always' Explained Before Given	(a)	66%	69%	64%
Nurses 'Always' Communicated Well	(a)	81%	83%	79%
Pain 'Always' Well Controlled	(a)	74%	75%	71%
Room and Bathroom 'Always' Clean	(a)	76%	75%	73%
Timely Help 'Always' Received	(a)	72%	71%	68%
Would Definitely Recommend Hospital	(a)	68%	75%	71%
Use of Medical Imaging				
Cardiac Imaging Stress Test before Surgery	97	1.0%	5.3%	5.3%
Combination Abdominal CT Scan	233	27.5%	24.5%	10.5%
Combination Brain/Sinus CT Scan[1]	-	-	2.6%	2.7%
Combination Chest CT Scan	154	19.5%	7.6%	2.7%
Follow-up Mammogram/Ultrasound	210	13.8%	9.4%	8.8%
Lumbar Spine MRI for Low Back Pain[1]	-	-	42.7%	37.2%

Willis Knighton Bossier Health Center

2400 Hospital Dr Phone: 318-212-7000
Bossier City, LA 71111
URL: www.wkhs.com/locations/bossier.aspx
Type: Acute Care Hospitals Emergency Services: Yes
Ownership: Voluntary non-profit - Private

Key Personnel:
Emergency Room . . . . Susan Cash

Measure	Cases	This Hosp.	State Avg.	U.S. Avg.
Blood Clot Prevention and Treatment				
Anticoagulation Overlap Therapy[2]	58	67%	89%	93%
ICU Venous Thromboembolism Prophylaxis[2]	80	70%	88%	92%
Incidence of Potentially Preventable VTE[2]	11	45%	16%	10%
UFH with Dosages/Platelet Monitoring[2]	11	100%	94%	97%
Venous Thromboembolism Prophylaxis[2]	737	60%	74%	85%
Warfarin Therapy Discharge Instructions[2]	45	89%	85%	75%
Chest Pain/Possible Heart Attack Care				
Aspirin Given Within 24 Hours of Arrival[1,3]	-	-	94%	96%
Fibrinolytic Meds Within 30 Min. of Arrival[5]	-	-	54%	58%
Average Time to ECG (minutes)[1,3]	-	-	10	7
Average Time to Transfer (minutes)[5]	-	-	94	60
Children's Asthma Care				
Received Home Management Plan of Care	-	-	-	88%
Received Reliever Medication	-	-	-	100%
Received Systemic Corticosteroids	-	-	-	100%
Emergency Department				
Admittance Decision Time (minutes)[2]	874	101	86	98
Head CT Results Within 45 Min. of Arrival[1]	-	-	49%	57%
Patients Who Left ER Before Being Seen	46,881	5%	3%	2%
Time from ER Arrival to Admit. (minutes)[2]	972	245	256	274
Time from ER Arrival to Discharge (minutes)	1,240	150	125	134
Time in ER Before Being Evaluated (minutes)	1,310	46	27	26
Time to Pain Meds for Fractures (minutes)	145	55	61	57
Heart Attack Care				
Aspirin Given at Discharge	115	97%	99%	99%
Fibrinolytic Meds Within 30 Min. of Arrival[7]	-	-	71%	54%
PCI Within 90 Minutes of Arrival	46	96%	94%	96%
Statin Prescribed at Discharge	116	89%	98%	98%
Heart Failure Care				
ACE Inhibitor or ARB for LVSD[2]	88	90%	95%	97%
Discharge Instructions Given[2]	219	92%	94%	94%
Evaluation of LVS Function[2]	277	99%	97%	99%
Medicare Spending				
Medicare Spending per Patient (ratio)	-	1.19	1.04	0.98
Pneumonia Care				
Appropriate Initial Antibiotic Given[2]	108	95%	93%	95%
Blood Culture Timing[2]	137	96%	97%	98%
Pregnancy and Delivery Care				
Newborn Deliveries Scheduled Early[2]	56	7%	5%	6%
Preventive Care				
Immunization for Influenza[2]	851	97%	85%	90%
Immunization for Pneumonia[2]	1,093	97%	88%	92%
Stroke Care				
Anticoagulation Therapy for Atrial Fibrillation[1,2]	-	-	93%	95%
Antithrombotic Therapy Timing[2]	91	99%	96%	98%
Assessed for Rehabilitation[2]	106	88%	95%	97%
Discharged on Antithrombotic Therapy[2]	96	100%	97%	99%
Discharged on Statin Medication[2]	76	75%	89%	94%
Thrombolytic Therapy Timing[1,2]	-	-	53%	66%
Venous Thromboembolism Prophylaxis[2]	97	67%	87%	94%
Written Stroke Educational Materials Given[2]	68	63%	83%	88%
Surgical Care Improvement Project				
Appropriate Beta Blocker Usage[2]	172	94%	97%	98%
Appropriate VTP Within 24 Hours[2]	333	98%	97%	98%
Controlled Postoperative Blood Glucose[2]	47	100%	96%	97%
Perioperative Temperature Management[2]	394	100%	100%	100%
Prophylactic Antibiotic Selection[2]	250	100%	99%	99%
Prophylactic Antibiotic Selection (Outpatient)	260	98%	97%	98%
Prophylactic Antibiotic Stopped[2]	244	95%	97%	98%
Prophylactic Antibiotic Timing[2]	250	99%	98%	99%
Prophylactic Antibiotic Timing (Outpatient)	257	96%	97%	98%
Urinary Catheter Removal[2]	176	87%	96%	97%
Survey of Patients' Hospital Experiences				
Area Around Room 'Always' Quiet at Night	300+	72%	74%	61%
Doctors 'Always' Communicated Well	300+	85%	87%	82%
Home Recovery Information Given	300+	86%	85%	85%
Hospital Given 9 or 10 on 10 Point Scale	300+	76%	75%	71%
Meds 'Always' Explained Before Given	300+	66%	69%	64%
Nurses 'Always' Communicated Well	300+	81%	83%	79%
Pain 'Always' Well Controlled	300+	74%	75%	71%
Room and Bathroom 'Always' Clean	300+	73%	75%	73%
Timely Help 'Always' Received	300+	70%	71%	68%
Would Definitely Recommend Hospital	300+	83%	75%	71%
Use of Medical Imaging				
Cardiac Imaging Stress Test before Surgery	84	6.0%	5.3%	5.3%
Combination Abdominal CT Scan	856	18.9%	24.5%	10.5%
Combination Brain/Sinus CT Scan	737	2.6%	2.6%	2.7%
Combination Chest CT Scan	564	0.0%	7.6%	2.7%
Follow-up Mammogram/Ultrasound	1,738	11.7%	9.4%	8.8%
Lumbar Spine MRI for Low Back Pain	147	45.6%	42.7%	37.2%

Saint Martin Hospital

210 Champagne Boulevard Phone: 337-332-2178
Breaux Bridge, LA 70517
Type: Critical Access Hospitals Emergency Services: Yes
Ownership: Voluntary non-profit - Private

Measure	Cases	This Hosp.	State Avg.	U.S. Avg.
Blood Clot Prevention and Treatment				
Anticoagulation Overlap Therapy[5]	-	-	89%	93%
ICU Venous Thromboembolism Prophylaxis[5]	-	-	88%	92%
Incidence of Potentially Preventable VTE[5]	-	-	16%	10%
UFH with Dosages/Platelet Monitoring[5]	-	-	94%	97%
Venous Thromboembolism Prophylaxis[5]	-	-	74%	85%
Warfarin Therapy Discharge Instructions[5]	-	-	85%	75%
Chest Pain/Possible Heart Attack Care				
Aspirin Given Within 24 Hours of Arrival	-	-	94%	96%
Fibrinolytic Meds Within 30 Min. of Arrival	-	-	54%	58%
Average Time to ECG (minutes)	-	-	10	7
Average Time to Transfer (minutes)	-	-	94	60
Children's Asthma Care				
Received Home Management Plan of Care	-	-	-	88%
Received Reliever Medication	-	-	-	100%
Received Systemic Corticosteroids	-	-	-	100%
Emergency Department				
Admittance Decision Time (minutes)[5]	-	-	86	98
Head CT Results Within 45 Min. of Arrival	-	-	49%	57%
Patients Who Left ER Before Being Seen	-	-	3%	2%
Time from ER Arrival to Admit. (minutes)[5]	-	-	256	274
Time from ER Arrival to Discharge (minutes)	-	-	125	134
Time in ER Before Being Evaluated (minutes)	-	-	27	26
Time to Pain Meds for Fractures (minutes)	-	-	61	57
Heart Attack Care				
Aspirin Given at Discharge[3,7]	-	-	99%	99%

NOTE: Hospital profiles are in alphabetical order by state, then city, then hospital within the city; Rankings exclude hospitals with less than 25 cases except for patient surveys which excludes hospitals with less than 100 cases; (a) 100-299 cases; (1) The number of cases/patients is too few to report; (2) Data submitted were based on a sample of cases/patients; (3) Results are based on a shorter time period than required; (4) Data suppressed by CMS for one or more quarters; (5) Results are not available for this reporting period; (6) Fewer than 100 patients completed the HCAHPS survey; (7) No cases met the criteria for this measure; (8) The lower limit of the confidence interval cannot be calculated if the number of observed infections equals zero; (9) No data are available from the state/territory for this reporting period; (10) The scores shown reflect fewer than 50 completed surveys; (11) There were discrepancies in the data collection process; (12) This measure does not apply to this hospital for this reporting period; (13) Results cannot be calculated for this reporting period; (14) The results for this state are combined with nearby states to protect confidentiality; Please refer to the User's Guide for a full explanation of data.

Measure	Cases	This Hosp.	State Avg.	U.S. Avg.
Fibrinolytic Meds Within 30 Min. of Arrival[3,7]	-	-	71%	54%
PCI Within 90 Minutes of Arrival[3,7]	-	-	94%	96%
Statin Prescribed at Discharge[3,7]	-	-	98%	98%
Heart Failure Care				
ACE Inhibitor or ARB for LVSD[1]	-	-	95%	97%
Discharge Instructions Given[1]	-	-	94%	94%
Evaluation of LVS Function[1]	-	-	97%	99%
Medicare Spending				
Medicare Spending per Patient (ratio)	-	-	1.04	0.98
Pneumonia Care				
Appropriate Initial Antibiotic Given	17	88%	93%	95%
Blood Culture Timing	25	80%	97%	98%
Pregnancy and Delivery Care				
Newborn Deliveries Scheduled Early[5]	-	-	5%	6%
Preventive Care				
Immunization for Influenza[5]	-	-	85%	90%
Immunization for Pneumonia[5]	-	-	88%	92%
Stroke Care				
Anticoagulation Therapy for Atrial Fibrillation[5]	-	-	93%	95%
Antithrombotic Therapy Timing[5]	-	-	96%	98%
Assessed for Rehabilitation[5]	-	-	95%	97%
Discharged on Antithrombotic Therapy[5]	-	-	97%	99%
Discharged on Statin Medication[5]	-	-	89%	94%
Thrombolytic Therapy Timing[5]	-	-	53%	66%
Venous Thromboembolism Prophylaxis[5]	-	-	87%	94%
Written Stroke Educational Materials Given[5]	-	-	83%	88%
Surgical Care Improvement Project				
Appropriate Beta Blocker Usage[5]	-	-	97%	98%
Appropriate VTP Within 24 Hours[5]	-	-	97%	98%
Controlled Postoperative Blood Glucose[5]	-	-	96%	97%
Perioperative Temperature Management[5]	-	-	100%	100%
Prophylactic Antibiotic Selection[5]	-	-	99%	99%
Prophylactic Antibiotic Selection (Outpatient)	-	-	97%	98%
Prophylactic Antibiotic Stopped[5]	-	-	97%	98%
Prophylactic Antibiotic Timing[5]	-	-	98%	99%
Prophylactic Antibiotic Timing (Outpatient)	-	-	97%	98%
Urinary Catheter Removal[5]	-	-	96%	97%
Survey of Patients' Hospital Experiences				
Area Around Room 'Always' Quiet at Night[5]	-	-	74%	61%
Doctors 'Always' Communicated Well[5]	-	-	87%	82%
Home Recovery Information Given[5]	-	-	85%	85%
Hospital Given 9 or 10 on 10 Point Scale[5]	-	-	75%	71%
Meds 'Always' Explained Before Given[5]	-	-	69%	64%
Nurses 'Always' Communicated Well[5]	-	-	83%	79%
Pain 'Always' Well Controlled[5]	-	-	75%	71%
Room and Bathroom 'Always' Clean[5]	-	-	75%	73%
Timely Help 'Always' Received[5]	-	-	71%	68%
Would Definitely Recommend Hospital[5]	-	-	75%	71%
Use of Medical Imaging				
Cardiac Imaging Stress Test before Surgery	-	-	5.3%	5.3%
Combination Abdominal CT Scan	-	-	24.5%	10.5%
Combination Brain/Sinus CT Scan	-	-	2.6%	2.7%
Combination Chest CT Scan	-	-	7.6%	2.7%
Follow-up Mammogram/Ultrasound	-	-	9.4%	8.8%
Lumbar Spine MRI for Low Back Pain	-	-	42.7%	37.2%

South Cameron Memorial Hospital

5360 West Creole Hwy — Phone: 337-542-4111
Cameron, LA 70631
Type: Acute Care Hospitals — Emergency Services: Yes
Ownership: Proprietary

Measure	Cases	This Hosp.	State Avg.	U.S. Avg.
Blood Clot Prevention and Treatment				
Anticoagulation Overlap Therapy[5]	-	-	89%	93%
ICU Venous Thromboembolism Prophylaxis[5]	-	-	88%	92%
Incidence of Potentially Preventable VTE[5]	-	-	16%	10%
UFH with Dosages/Platelet Monitoring[5]	-	-	94%	97%
Venous Thromboembolism Prophylaxis[5]	-	-	74%	85%
Warfarin Therapy Discharge Instructions[5]	-	-	85%	75%
Chest Pain/Possible Heart Attack Care				
Aspirin Given Within 24 Hours of Arrival[5]	-	-	94%	96%
Fibrinolytic Meds Within 30 Min. of Arrival[5]	-	-	54%	58%
Average Time to ECG (minutes)[5]	-	-	10	7
Average Time to Transfer (minutes)[5]	-	-	94	60
Children's Asthma Care				
Received Home Management Plan of Care	-	-	-	88%
Received Reliever Medication	-	-	-	100%
Received Systemic Corticosteroids	-	-	-	100%
Emergency Department				
Admittance Decision Time (minutes)[5]	-	-	86	98
Head CT Results Within 45 Min. of Arrival[5]	-	-	49%	57%
Patients Who Left ER Before Being Seen	1,108	0%	3%	2%
Time from ER Arrival to Admit. (minutes)[5]	-	-	256	274
Time from ER Arrival to Discharge (minutes)[5]	-	-	125	134
Time in ER Before Being Evaluated (minutes)[3,7]	-	-	27	26
Time to Pain Meds for Fractures (minutes)[5]	-	-	61	57
Heart Attack Care				
Aspirin Given at Discharge[5]	-	-	99%	99%
Fibrinolytic Meds Within 30 Min. of Arrival[5]	-	-	71%	54%
PCI Within 90 Minutes of Arrival[5]	-	-	94%	96%
Statin Prescribed at Discharge[5]	-	-	98%	98%
Heart Failure Care				
ACE Inhibitor or ARB for LVSD[5]	-	-	95%	97%
Discharge Instructions Given[5]	-	-	94%	94%
Evaluation of LVS Function[5]	-	-	97%	99%
Medicare Spending				
Medicare Spending per Patient (ratio)[1]	-	-	1.04	0.98
Pneumonia Care				
Appropriate Initial Antibiotic Given[5]	-	-	93%	95%
Blood Culture Timing[5]	-	-	97%	98%
Pregnancy and Delivery Care				
Newborn Deliveries Scheduled Early[7]	-	-	5%	6%
Preventive Care				
Immunization for Influenza[5]	-	-	85%	90%
Immunization for Pneumonia[5]	-	-	88%	92%
Stroke Care				
Anticoagulation Therapy for Atrial Fibrillation[5]	-	-	93%	95%
Antithrombotic Therapy Timing[5]	-	-	96%	98%
Assessed for Rehabilitation[5]	-	-	95%	97%
Discharged on Antithrombotic Therapy[5]	-	-	97%	99%
Discharged on Statin Medication[5]	-	-	89%	94%
Thrombolytic Therapy Timing[5]	-	-	53%	66%
Venous Thromboembolism Prophylaxis[5]	-	-	87%	94%
Written Stroke Educational Materials Given[5]	-	-	83%	88%
Surgical Care Improvement Project				
Appropriate Beta Blocker Usage[5]	-	-	97%	98%
Appropriate VTP Within 24 Hours[5]	-	-	97%	98%
Controlled Postoperative Blood Glucose[5]	-	-	96%	97%
Perioperative Temperature Management[5]	-	-	100%	100%
Prophylactic Antibiotic Selection[5]	-	-	99%	99%
Prophylactic Antibiotic Selection (Outpatient)[5]	-	-	97%	98%
Prophylactic Antibiotic Stopped[5]	-	-	97%	98%
Prophylactic Antibiotic Timing[5]	-	-	98%	99%
Prophylactic Antibiotic Timing (Outpatient)[5]	-	-	97%	98%
Urinary Catheter Removal[5]	-	-	96%	97%
Survey of Patients' Hospital Experiences				
Area Around Room 'Always' Quiet at Night[1]	-	-	74%	61%
Doctors 'Always' Communicated Well[1]	-	-	87%	82%
Home Recovery Information Given[1]	-	-	85%	85%
Hospital Given 9 or 10 on 10 Point Scale[1]	-	-	75%	71%
Meds 'Always' Explained Before Given[1]	-	-	69%	64%
Nurses 'Always' Communicated Well[1]	-	-	83%	79%
Pain 'Always' Well Controlled[1]	-	-	75%	71%
Room and Bathroom 'Always' Clean[1]	-	-	75%	73%
Timely Help 'Always' Received[1]	-	-	71%	68%
Would Definitely Recommend Hospital[1]	-	-	75%	71%
Use of Medical Imaging				
Cardiac Imaging Stress Test before Surgery[7]	-	-	5.3%	5.3%
Combination Abdominal CT Scan[1]	-	-	24.5%	10.5%
Combination Brain/Sinus CT Scan[1]	-	-	2.6%	2.7%
Combination Chest CT Scan[1]	-	-	7.6%	2.7%
Follow-up Mammogram/Ultrasound[7]	-	-	9.4%	8.8%
Lumbar Spine MRI for Low Back Pain[7]	-	-	42.7%	37.2%

Saint Bernard Parish Hospital

8000 West Judge Perez Drive — Phone: 504-826-9500
Chalmette, LA 70043
Type: Acute Care Hospitals — Emergency Services: Yes
Ownership: Govt - Hospital Dist/Auth

Measure	Cases	This Hosp.	State Avg.	U.S. Avg.
Blood Clot Prevention and Treatment				
Anticoagulation Overlap Therapy[1,3]	-	-	89%	93%
ICU Venous Thromboembolism Prophylaxis[3]	80	80%	88%	92%
Incidence of Potentially Preventable VTE[3,7]	-	-	16%	10%
UFH with Dosages/Platelet Monitoring[1,3]	-	-	94%	97%
Venous Thromboembolism Prophylaxis[3]	292	68%	74%	85%
Warfarin Therapy Discharge Instructions[1,3]	-	-	85%	75%
Chest Pain/Possible Heart Attack Care				
Aspirin Given Within 24 Hours of Arrival[1,3]	-	-	94%	96%
Fibrinolytic Meds Within 30 Min. of Arrival[3,7]	-	-	54%	58%
Average Time to ECG (minutes)[1,3]	-	-	10	7
Average Time to Transfer (minutes)[1,3]	-	-	94	60
Children's Asthma Care				
Received Home Management Plan of Care	-	-	-	88%
Received Reliever Medication	-	-	-	100%
Received Systemic Corticosteroids	-	-	-	100%
Emergency Department				
Admittance Decision Time (minutes)[3]	153	72	86	98
Head CT Results Within 45 Min. of Arrival[1,3]	-	-	49%	57%
Patients Who Left ER Before Being Seen	6,593	4%	3%	2%
Time from ER Arrival to Admit. (minutes)[3]	160	267	256	274
Time from ER Arrival to Discharge (minutes)[3]	200	138	125	134
Time in ER Before Being Evaluated (minutes)[3]	209	54	27	26
Time to Pain Meds for Fractures (minutes)[3]	15	73	61	57
Heart Attack Care				
Aspirin Given at Discharge[1,3]	-	-	99%	99%
Fibrinolytic Meds Within 30 Min. of Arrival[3,7]	-	-	71%	54%
PCI Within 90 Minutes of Arrival[3,7]	-	-	94%	96%
Statin Prescribed at Discharge[1,3]	-	-	98%	98%
Heart Failure Care				
ACE Inhibitor or ARB for LVSD[1,3]	-	-	95%	97%
Discharge Instructions Given[3]	29	55%	94%	94%
Evaluation of LVS Function[3]	29	93%	97%	99%
Medicare Spending				
Medicare Spending per Patient (ratio)	-	-	1.04	0.98
Pneumonia Care				
Appropriate Initial Antibiotic Given[3]	14	64%	93%	95%
Blood Culture Timing[3]	23	91%	97%	98%
Pregnancy and Delivery Care				
Newborn Deliveries Scheduled Early[7]	-	-	5%	6%
Preventive Care				
Immunization for Influenza[5]	-	-	85%	90%
Immunization for Pneumonia[3]	325	71%	88%	92%
Stroke Care				
Anticoagulation Therapy for Atrial Fibrillation[3,7]	-	-	93%	95%
Antithrombotic Therapy Timing[1,3]	-	-	96%	98%
Assessed for Rehabilitation[1,3]	-	-	95%	97%
Discharged on Antithrombotic Therapy[1,3]	-	-	97%	99%
Discharged on Statin Medication[1,3]	-	-	89%	94%
Thrombolytic Therapy Timing[3,7]	-	-	53%	66%
Venous Thromboembolism Prophylaxis[1,3]	-	-	87%	94%
Written Stroke Educational Materials Given[1,3]	-	-	83%	88%
Surgical Care Improvement Project				
Appropriate Beta Blocker Usage[1,3]	-	-	97%	98%
Appropriate VTP Within 24 Hours[1,3]	-	-	97%	98%
Controlled Postoperative Blood Glucose[3,7]	-	-	96%	97%
Perioperative Temperature Management[1,3]	-	-	100%	100%
Prophylactic Antibiotic Selection[1,3]	-	-	99%	99%
Prophylactic Antibiotic Selection (Outpatient)[5]	-	-	97%	98%
Prophylactic Antibiotic Stopped[1,3]	-	-	97%	98%
Prophylactic Antibiotic Timing[1,3]	-	-	98%	99%
Prophylactic Antibiotic Timing (Outpatient)[5]	-	-	97%	98%
Urinary Catheter Removal[1,3]	-	-	96%	97%
Survey of Patients' Hospital Experiences				
Area Around Room 'Always' Quiet at Night[5]	-	-	74%	61%
Doctors 'Always' Communicated Well[5]	-	-	87%	82%

NOTE: Hospital profiles are in alphabetical order by state, then city, then hospital within the city; Rankings exclude hospitals with less than 25 cases except for patient surveys which excludes hospitals with less than 100 cases; (a) 100-299 cases; (1) The number of cases/patients is too few to report; (2) Data submitted were based on a sample of cases/patients; (3) Results are based on a shorter time period than required; (4) Data suppressed by CMS for one or more quarters; (5) Results are not available for this reporting period; (6) Fewer than 100 patients completed the HCAHPS survey; (7) No cases met the criteria for this measure; (8) The lower limit of the confidence interval cannot be calculated if the number of observed infections equals zero; (9) No data are available from the state/territory for this reporting period; (10) The scores shown reflect fewer than 50 completed surveys; (11) There were discrepancies in the data collection process; (12) This measure does not apply to this hospital for this reporting period; (13) Results cannot be calculated for this reporting period; (14) The results for this state are combined with nearby states to protect confidentiality; Please refer to the User's Guide for a full explanation of data.

Measure	Cases	This Hosp.	State Avg.	U.S. Avg.
Home Recovery Information Given[5]	-	-	85%	85%
Hospital Given 9 or 10 on 10 Point Scale[5]	-	-	75%	71%
Meds 'Always' Explained Before Given[5]	-	-	69%	64%
Nurses 'Always' Communicated Well[5]	-	-	83%	79%
Pain 'Always' Well Controlled[5]	-	-	75%	71%
Room and Bathroom 'Always' Clean[5]	-	-	75%	73%
Timely Help 'Always' Received[5]	-	-	71%	68%
Would Definitely Recommend Hospital[5]	-	-	75%	71%
Use of Medical Imaging				
Cardiac Imaging Stress Test before Surgery[1]	-	-	5.3%	5.3%
Combination Abdominal CT Scan[1]	-	-	24.5%	10.5%
Combination Brain/Sinus CT Scan[1]	-	-	2.6%	2.7%
Combination Chest CT Scan[1]	-	-	7.6%	2.7%
Follow-up Mammogram/Ultrasound[1]	-	-	9.4%	8.8%
Lumbar Spine MRI for Low Back Pain[1]	-	-	42.7%	37.2%

Acadia Saint Landry

810 South Broadway Street
Church Point, LA 70525
Phone: 337-684-5435
Type: Critical Access Hospitals
Emergency Services: Yes
Ownership: Govt - Hospital Dist/Auth

Measure	Cases	This Hosp.	State Avg.	U.S. Avg.
Blood Clot Prevention and Treatment				
Anticoagulation Overlap Therapy	-	-	89%	93%
ICU Venous Thromboembolism Prophylaxis	-	-	88%	92%
Incidence of Potentially Preventable VTE	-	-	16%	10%
UFH with Dosages/Platelet Monitoring	-	-	94%	97%
Venous Thromboembolism Prophylaxis	-	-	74%	85%
Warfarin Therapy Discharge Instructions	-	-	85%	75%
Chest Pain/Possible Heart Attack Care				
Aspirin Given Within 24 Hours of Arrival[5]	-	-	94%	96%
Fibrinolytic Meds Within 30 Min. of Arrival[5]	-	-	54%	58%
Average Time to ECG (minutes)[5]	-	-	10	7
Average Time to Transfer (minutes)[5]	-	-	94	60
Children's Asthma Care				
Received Home Management Plan of Care	-	-	-	88%
Received Reliever Medication	-	-	-	100%
Received Systemic Corticosteroids	-	-	-	100%
Emergency Department				
Admittance Decision Time (minutes)	-	-	86	98
Head CT Results Within 45 Min. of Arrival[5]	-	-	49%	57%
Patients Who Left ER Before Being Seen	3,952	3%	3%	2%
Time from ER Arrival to Admit. (minutes)	-	-	256	274
Time from ER Arrival to Discharge (minutes)[5]	-	-	125	134
Time in ER Before Being Evaluated (minutes)[5]	-	-	27	26
Time to Pain Meds for Fractures (minutes)[5]	-	-	61	57
Heart Attack Care				
Aspirin Given at Discharge	-	-	99%	99%
Fibrinolytic Meds Within 30 Min. of Arrival	-	-	71%	54%
PCI Within 90 Minutes of Arrival	-	-	94%	96%
Statin Prescribed at Discharge	-	-	98%	98%
Heart Failure Care				
ACE Inhibitor or ARB for LVSD	-	-	95%	97%
Discharge Instructions Given	-	-	94%	94%
Evaluation of LVS Function	-	-	97%	99%
Medicare Spending				
Medicare Spending per Patient (ratio)	-	-	1.04	0.98
Pneumonia Care				
Appropriate Initial Antibiotic Given	-	-	93%	95%
Blood Culture Timing	-	-	97%	98%
Pregnancy and Delivery Care				
Newborn Deliveries Scheduled Early	-	-	5%	6%
Preventive Care				
Immunization for Influenza	-	-	85%	90%
Immunization for Pneumonia	-	-	88%	92%
Stroke Care				
Anticoagulation Therapy for Atrial Fibrillation	-	-	93%	95%
Antithrombotic Therapy Timing	-	-	96%	98%
Assessed for Rehabilitation	-	-	95%	97%
Discharged on Antithrombotic Therapy	-	-	97%	99%
Discharged on Statin Medication	-	-	89%	94%
Thrombolytic Therapy Timing	-	-	53%	66%
Venous Thromboembolism Prophylaxis	-	-	87%	94%
Written Stroke Educational Materials Given	-	-	83%	88%
Surgical Care Improvement Project				
Appropriate Beta Blocker Usage	-	-	97%	98%
Appropriate VTP Within 24 Hours	-	-	97%	98%
Controlled Postoperative Blood Glucose	-	-	96%	97%
Perioperative Temperature Management	-	-	100%	100%
Prophylactic Antibiotic Selection	-	-	99%	99%
Prophylactic Antibiotic Selection (Outpatient)[5]	-	-	97%	98%
Prophylactic Antibiotic Stopped	-	-	97%	98%
Prophylactic Antibiotic Timing	-	-	98%	99%
Prophylactic Antibiotic Timing (Outpatient)[5]	-	-	97%	98%
Urinary Catheter Removal	-	-	96%	97%
Survey of Patients' Hospital Experiences				
Area Around Room 'Always' Quiet at Night	-	-	74%	61%
Doctors 'Always' Communicated Well	-	-	87%	82%
Home Recovery Information Given	-	-	85%	85%
Hospital Given 9 or 10 on 10 Point Scale	-	-	75%	71%
Meds 'Always' Explained Before Given	-	-	69%	64%
Nurses 'Always' Communicated Well	-	-	83%	79%
Pain 'Always' Well Controlled	-	-	75%	71%
Room and Bathroom 'Always' Clean	-	-	75%	73%
Timely Help 'Always' Received	-	-	71%	68%
Would Definitely Recommend Hospital	-	-	75%	71%
Use of Medical Imaging				
Cardiac Imaging Stress Test before Surgery[7]	-	-	5.3%	5.3%
Combination Abdominal CT Scan	41	51.2%	24.5%	10.5%
Combination Brain/Sinus CT Scan[1]	-	-	2.6%	2.7%
Combination Chest CT Scan[1]	-	-	7.6%	2.7%
Follow-up Mammogram/Ultrasound[7]	-	-	9.4%	8.8%
Lumbar Spine MRI for Low Back Pain[1]	-	-	42.7%	37.2%

Caldwell Memorial Hospital

411 Main Street
Columbia, LA 71418
Phone: 318-649-6111
Fax: 318-649-8908
Type: Acute Care Hospitals
Emergency Services: No
Ownership: Proprietary
Beds: 22

Key Personnel:
CEO/President. . . . . Heather Clark
Infection Control. . . . . Mel Hart
Chief of Medical Staff. . . . . Salman Shafig, MD

Measure	Cases	This Hosp.	State Avg.	U.S. Avg.
Blood Clot Prevention and Treatment				
Anticoagulation Overlap Therapy[1,2]	-	-	89%	93%
ICU Venous Thromboembolism Prophylaxis[2,7]	-	-	88%	92%
Incidence of Potentially Preventable VTE[1,2]	-	-	16%	10%
UFH with Dosages/Platelet Monitoring[2,7]	-	-	94%	97%
Venous Thromboembolism Prophylaxis[2]	221	0%	74%	85%
Warfarin Therapy Discharge Instructions[2,7]	-	-	85%	75%
Chest Pain/Possible Heart Attack Care				
Aspirin Given Within 24 Hours of Arrival[5]	-	-	94%	96%
Fibrinolytic Meds Within 30 Min. of Arrival[5]	-	-	54%	58%
Average Time to ECG (minutes)[5]	-	-	10	7
Average Time to Transfer (minutes)[5]	-	-	94	60
Children's Asthma Care				
Received Home Management Plan of Care	-	-	-	88%
Received Reliever Medication	-	-	-	100%
Received Systemic Corticosteroids	-	-	-	100%
Emergency Department				
Admittance Decision Time (minutes)[2,7]	-	-	86	98
Head CT Results Within 45 Min. of Arrival[5]	-	-	49%	57%
Patients Who Left ER Before Being Seen[5]	-	-	3%	2%
Time from ER Arrival to Admit. (minutes)[2,7]	-	-	256	274
Time from ER Arrival to Discharge (minutes)[5]	-	-	125	134
Time in ER Before Being Evaluated (minutes)[5]	-	-	27	26
Time to Pain Meds for Fractures (minutes)[5]	-	-	61	57
Heart Attack Care				
Aspirin Given at Discharge[5]	-	-	99%	99%
Fibrinolytic Meds Within 30 Min. of Arrival[5]	-	-	71%	54%
PCI Within 90 Minutes of Arrival[5]	-	-	94%	96%
Statin Prescribed at Discharge[5]	-	-	98%	98%
Heart Failure Care				
ACE Inhibitor or ARB for LVSD[2]	11	64%	95%	97%
Discharge Instructions Given[2]	87	60%	94%	94%
Evaluation of LVS Function[2]	90	46%	97%	99%
Medicare Spending				
Medicare Spending per Patient (ratio)	-	0.84	1.04	0.98
Pneumonia Care				
Appropriate Initial Antibiotic Given	16	75%	93%	95%
Blood Culture Timing[7]	-	-	97%	98%
Pregnancy and Delivery Care				
Newborn Deliveries Scheduled Early[2,7]	-	-	5%	6%
Preventive Care				
Immunization for Influenza[2]	297	12%	85%	90%
Immunization for Pneumonia[2]	472	4%	88%	92%
Stroke Care				
Anticoagulation Therapy for Atrial Fibrillation[7]	-	-	93%	95%
Antithrombotic Therapy Timing[1]	-	-	96%	98%
Assessed for Rehabilitation[1]	-	-	95%	97%
Discharged on Antithrombotic Therapy[1]	-	-	97%	99%
Discharged on Statin Medication[1]	-	-	89%	94%
Thrombolytic Therapy Timing[7]	-	-	53%	66%
Venous Thromboembolism Prophylaxis[1]	-	-	87%	94%
Written Stroke Educational Materials Given[1]	-	-	83%	88%
Surgical Care Improvement Project				
Appropriate Beta Blocker Usage[5]	-	-	97%	98%
Appropriate VTP Within 24 Hours[5]	-	-	97%	98%
Controlled Postoperative Blood Glucose[5]	-	-	96%	97%
Perioperative Temperature Management[5]	-	-	100%	100%
Prophylactic Antibiotic Selection[5]	-	-	99%	99%
Prophylactic Antibiotic Selection (Outpatient)[5]	-	-	97%	98%
Prophylactic Antibiotic Stopped[5]	-	-	97%	98%
Prophylactic Antibiotic Timing[5]	-	-	98%	99%
Prophylactic Antibiotic Timing (Outpatient)[5]	-	-	97%	98%
Urinary Catheter Removal[5]	-	-	96%	97%
Survey of Patients' Hospital Experiences				
Area Around Room 'Always' Quiet at Night	(a)	78%	74%	61%
Doctors 'Always' Communicated Well	(a)	97%	87%	82%
Home Recovery Information Given	(a)	84%	85%	85%
Hospital Given 9 or 10 on 10 Point Scale	(a)	82%	75%	71%
Meds 'Always' Explained Before Given	(a)	70%	69%	64%
Nurses 'Always' Communicated Well	(a)	86%	83%	79%
Pain 'Always' Well Controlled	(a)	83%	75%	71%
Room and Bathroom 'Always' Clean	(a)	75%	75%	73%
Timely Help 'Always' Received	(a)	75%	71%	68%
Would Definitely Recommend Hospital	(a)	85%	75%	71%
Use of Medical Imaging				
Cardiac Imaging Stress Test before Surgery[7]	-	-	5.3%	5.3%
Combination Abdominal CT Scan[1]	-	-	24.5%	10.5%
Combination Brain/Sinus CT Scan	32	0.0%	2.6%	2.7%
Combination Chest CT Scan[1]	-	-	7.6%	2.7%
Follow-up Mammogram/Ultrasound[7]	-	-	9.4%	8.8%
Lumbar Spine MRI for Low Back Pain[1]	-	-	42.7%	37.2%

Citizens Medical Center

7939 U S Hwy 165 South
Columbia, LA 71418
Phone: 318-649-6106
Fax: 318-649-2080
URL: www.citizensmedcenter.com
Type: Acute Care Hospitals
Emergency Services: Yes
Ownership: Govt - Hospital Dist/Auth
Beds: 40

Key Personnel:
CEO/President. . . . . Steve Barbo
Chief of Medical Staff. . . . . Glynda Mason
Quality Assurance . . . . Sharon Silverthorne
Infection Control. . . . . Debbie Volentine
Operating Room. . . . . Debbie Volentine, RN

Measure	Cases	This Hosp.	State Avg.	U.S. Avg.
Blood Clot Prevention and Treatment				
Anticoagulation Overlap Therapy[1,2]	-	-	89%	93%
ICU Venous Thromboembolism Prophylaxis[2,7]	-	-	88%	92%
Incidence of Potentially Preventable VTE[1,2]	-	-	16%	10%
UFH with Dosages/Platelet Monitoring[1,2]	-	-	94%	97%
Venous Thromboembolism Prophylaxis[2]	139	35%	74%	85%
Warfarin Therapy Discharge Instructions[1,2]	-	-	85%	75%
Chest Pain/Possible Heart Attack Care				
Aspirin Given Within 24 Hours of Arrival	23	100%	94%	96%

NOTE: Hospital profiles are in alphabetical order by state, then city, then hospital within the city; Rankings exclude hospitals with less than 25 cases except for patient surveys which excludes hospitals with less than 100 cases; (a) 100-299 cases; (1) The number of cases/patients is too few to report; (2) Data submitted were based on a sample of cases/patients; (3) Results are based on a shorter time period than required; (4) Data suppressed by CMS for one or more quarters; (5) Results are not available for this reporting period; (6) Fewer than 100 patients completed the HCAHPS survey; (7) No cases met the criteria for this measure; (8) The lower limit of the confidence interval cannot be calculated if the number of observed infections equals zero; (9) No data are available from the state/territory for this reporting period; (10) The scores shown reflect fewer than 50 completed surveys; (11) There were discrepancies in the data collection process; (12) This measure does not apply to this hospital for this reporting period; (13) Results cannot be calculated for this reporting period; (14) The results for this state are combined with nearby states to protect confidentiality; Please refer to the User's Guide for a full explanation of data.

Measure	Cases	This Hosp.	State Avg.	U.S. Avg.
Fibrinolytic Meds Within 30 Min. of Arrival[1]	-	-	54%	58%
Average Time to ECG (minutes)	27	11	10	7
Average Time to Transfer (minutes)[1]	-	-	94	60
Children's Asthma Care				
Received Home Management Plan of Care	-	-	-	88%
Received Reliever Medication	-	-	-	100%
Received Systemic Corticosteroids	-	-	-	100%
Emergency Department				
Admittance Decision Time (minutes)[2]	118	25	86	98
Head CT Results Within 45 Min. of Arrival[1]	-	-	49%	57%
Patients Who Left ER Before Being Seen	5,484	1%	3%	2%
Time from ER Arrival to Admit. (minutes)[2]	118	195	256	274
Time from ER Arrival to Discharge (minutes)	699	126	125	134
Time in ER Before Being Evaluated (minutes)	580	20	27	26
Time to Pain Meds for Fractures (minutes)[1]	-	-	61	57
Heart Attack Care				
Aspirin Given at Discharge[2,3]	-	-	99%	99%
Fibrinolytic Meds Within 30 Min. of Arrival[2,3]	-	-	71%	54%
PCI Within 90 Minutes of Arrival[2,3]	-	-	94%	96%
Statin Prescribed at Discharge[2,3]	-	-	98%	98%
Heart Failure Care				
ACE Inhibitor or ARB for LVSD[1,2]	-	-	95%	97%
Discharge Instructions Given[2]	18	100%	94%	94%
Evaluation of LVS Function[2]	20	70%	97%	99%
Medicare Spending				
Medicare Spending per Patient (ratio)	-	1.00	1.04	0.98
Pneumonia Care				
Appropriate Initial Antibiotic Given[2]	41	73%	93%	95%
Blood Culture Timing[2]	22	86%	97%	98%
Pregnancy and Delivery Care				
Newborn Deliveries Scheduled Early[2,7]	-	-	5%	6%
Preventive Care				
Immunization for Influenza[2]	135	90%	85%	90%
Immunization for Pneumonia[2]	221	77%	88%	92%
Stroke Care				
Anticoagulation Therapy for Atrial Fibrillation[5]	-	-	93%	95%
Antithrombotic Therapy Timing[5]	-	-	96%	98%
Assessed for Rehabilitation[5]	-	-	95%	97%
Discharged on Antithrombotic Therapy[5]	-	-	97%	99%
Discharged on Statin Medication[5]	-	-	89%	94%
Thrombolytic Therapy Timing[5]	-	-	53%	66%
Venous Thromboembolism Prophylaxis[5]	-	-	87%	94%
Written Stroke Educational Materials Given[5]	-	-	83%	88%
Surgical Care Improvement Project				
Appropriate Beta Blocker Usage[1,2]	-	-	97%	98%
Appropriate VTP Within 24 Hours[2]	13	100%	97%	98%
Controlled Postoperative Blood Glucose[2,7]	-	-	96%	97%
Perioperative Temperature Management[2]	15	100%	100%	100%
Prophylactic Antibiotic Selection[2]	15	7%	99%	99%
Prophylactic Antibiotic Selection (Outpatient)[5]	-	-	97%	98%
Prophylactic Antibiotic Stopped[2]	15	0%	97%	98%
Prophylactic Antibiotic Timing[2]	15	7%	98%	99%
Prophylactic Antibiotic Timing (Outpatient)[5]	-	-	97%	98%
Urinary Catheter Removal[1,2]	-	-	96%	97%
Survey of Patients' Hospital Experiences				
Area Around Room 'Always' Quiet at Night	(a)	89%	74%	61%
Doctors 'Always' Communicated Well	(a)	96%	87%	82%
Home Recovery Information Given	(a)	89%	85%	85%
Hospital Given 9 or 10 on 10 Point Scale	(a)	79%	75%	71%
Meds 'Always' Explained Before Given	(a)	76%	69%	64%
Nurses 'Always' Communicated Well	(a)	96%	83%	79%
Pain 'Always' Well Controlled	(a)	81%	75%	71%
Room and Bathroom 'Always' Clean	(a)	96%	75%	73%
Timely Help 'Always' Received	(a)	89%	71%	68%
Would Definitely Recommend Hospital	(a)	83%	75%	71%
Use of Medical Imaging				
Cardiac Imaging Stress Test before Surgery[7]	-	-	5.3%	5.3%
Combination Abdominal CT Scan	97	22.7%	24.5%	10.5%
Combination Brain/Sinus CT Scan	144	0.7%	2.6%	2.7%
Combination Chest CT Scan[1]	-	-	7.6%	2.7%
Follow-up Mammogram/Ultrasound[7]	-	-	9.4%	8.8%
Lumbar Spine MRI for Low Back Pain[1]	-	-	42.7%	37.2%

Christus Coushatta Health Care Center

1635 Marvel Street Phone: 318-932-2000
Coushatta, LA 71019
Type: Critical Access Hospitals Emergency Services: Yes
Ownership: Voluntary non-profit - Church

Measure	Cases	This Hosp.	State Avg.	U.S. Avg.
Blood Clot Prevention and Treatment				
Anticoagulation Overlap Therapy[5]	-	-	89%	93%
ICU Venous Thromboembolism Prophylaxis[5]	-	-	88%	92%
Incidence of Potentially Preventable VTE[5]	-	-	16%	10%
UFH with Dosages/Platelet Monitoring[5]	-	-	94%	97%
Venous Thromboembolism Prophylaxis[5]	-	-	74%	85%
Warfarin Therapy Discharge Instructions[5]	-	-	85%	75%
Chest Pain/Possible Heart Attack Care				
Aspirin Given Within 24 Hours of Arrival	-	-	94%	96%
Fibrinolytic Meds Within 30 Min. of Arrival	-	-	54%	58%
Average Time to ECG (minutes)	-	-	10	7
Average Time to Transfer (minutes)	-	-	94	60
Children's Asthma Care				
Received Home Management Plan of Care	-	-	-	88%
Received Reliever Medication	-	-	-	100%
Received Systemic Corticosteroids	-	-	-	100%
Emergency Department				
Admittance Decision Time (minutes)[5]	-	-	86	98
Head CT Results Within 45 Min. of Arrival	-	-	49%	57%
Patients Who Left ER Before Being Seen	-	-	3%	2%
Time from ER Arrival to Admit. (minutes)[5]	-	-	256	274
Time from ER Arrival to Discharge (minutes)	-	-	125	134
Time in ER Before Being Evaluated (minutes)	-	-	27	26
Time to Pain Meds for Fractures (minutes)	-	-	61	57
Heart Attack Care				
Aspirin Given at Discharge[3,7]	-	-	99%	99%
Fibrinolytic Meds Within 30 Min. of Arrival[3,7]	-	-	71%	54%
PCI Within 90 Minutes of Arrival[3,7]	-	-	94%	96%
Statin Prescribed at Discharge[3,7]	-	-	98%	98%
Heart Failure Care				
ACE Inhibitor or ARB for LVSD[1,3]	-	-	95%	97%
Discharge Instructions Given[3]	13	69%	94%	94%
Evaluation of LVS Function[3]	23	87%	97%	99%
Medicare Spending				
Medicare Spending per Patient (ratio)	-	-	1.04	0.98
Pneumonia Care				
Appropriate Initial Antibiotic Given[3]	12	83%	93%	95%
Blood Culture Timing[1,3]	-	-	97%	98%
Pregnancy and Delivery Care				
Newborn Deliveries Scheduled Early[5]	-	-	5%	6%
Preventive Care				
Immunization for Influenza[3]	17	88%	85%	90%
Immunization for Pneumonia[3]	25	88%	88%	92%
Stroke Care				
Anticoagulation Therapy for Atrial Fibrillation[5]	-	-	93%	95%
Antithrombotic Therapy Timing[5]	-	-	96%	98%
Assessed for Rehabilitation[5]	-	-	95%	97%
Discharged on Antithrombotic Therapy[5]	-	-	97%	99%
Discharged on Statin Medication[5]	-	-	89%	94%
Thrombolytic Therapy Timing[5]	-	-	53%	66%
Venous Thromboembolism Prophylaxis[5]	-	-	87%	94%
Written Stroke Educational Materials Given[5]	-	-	83%	88%
Surgical Care Improvement Project				
Appropriate Beta Blocker Usage[5]	-	-	97%	98%
Appropriate VTP Within 24 Hours[5]	-	-	97%	98%
Controlled Postoperative Blood Glucose[5]	-	-	96%	97%
Perioperative Temperature Management[5]	-	-	100%	100%
Prophylactic Antibiotic Selection[5]	-	-	99%	99%
Prophylactic Antibiotic Selection (Outpatient)	-	-	97%	98%
Prophylactic Antibiotic Stopped[5]	-	-	97%	98%
Prophylactic Antibiotic Timing[5]	-	-	98%	99%
Prophylactic Antibiotic Timing (Outpatient)	-	-	97%	98%
Urinary Catheter Removal[5]	-	-	96%	97%
Survey of Patients' Hospital Experiences				
Area Around Room 'Always' Quiet at Night[5]	-	-	74%	61%
Doctors 'Always' Communicated Well[5]	-	-	87%	82%
Home Recovery Information Given[5]	-	-	85%	85%
Hospital Given 9 or 10 on 10 Point Scale[5]	-	-	75%	71%
Meds 'Always' Explained Before Given[5]	-	-	69%	64%
Nurses 'Always' Communicated Well[5]	-	-	83%	79%
Pain 'Always' Well Controlled[5]	-	-	75%	71%
Room and Bathroom 'Always' Clean[5]	-	-	75%	73%
Timely Help 'Always' Received[5]	-	-	71%	68%
Would Definitely Recommend Hospital[5]	-	-	75%	71%
Use of Medical Imaging				
Cardiac Imaging Stress Test before Surgery	-	-	5.3%	5.3%
Combination Abdominal CT Scan	-	-	24.5%	10.5%
Combination Brain/Sinus CT Scan	-	-	2.6%	2.7%
Combination Chest CT Scan	-	-	7.6%	2.7%
Follow-up Mammogram/Ultrasound	-	-	9.4%	8.8%
Lumbar Spine MRI for Low Back Pain	-	-	42.7%	37.2%

Fairway Medical Center

67252 Industry Lane Phone: 985-801-3010
Covington, LA 70433
URL: www.fairwaymedical.com
Type: Acute Care Hospitals Emergency Services: No
Ownership: Physician
Key Personnel:
Anesthesiology. . . . . Scott Branting, MD
Cardiology . . . . Martha Carr, MD
CEO . . . . David Guzen
Radiology. . . . . Michael Hall, MD

Measure	Cases	This Hosp.	State Avg.	U.S. Avg.
Blood Clot Prevention and Treatment				
Anticoagulation Overlap Therapy[2,7]	-	-	89%	93%
ICU Venous Thromboembolism Prophylaxis[2,7]	-	-	88%	92%
Incidence of Potentially Preventable VTE[2,7]	-	-	16%	10%
UFH with Dosages/Platelet Monitoring[2,7]	-	-	94%	97%
Venous Thromboembolism Prophylaxis[2]	49	100%	74%	85%
Warfarin Therapy Discharge Instructions[2,7]	-	-	85%	75%
Chest Pain/Possible Heart Attack Care				
Aspirin Given Within 24 Hours of Arrival[5]	-	-	94%	96%
Fibrinolytic Meds Within 30 Min. of Arrival[5]	-	-	54%	58%
Average Time to ECG (minutes)[5]	-	-	10	7
Average Time to Transfer (minutes)[5]	-	-	94	60
Children's Asthma Care				
Received Home Management Plan of Care	-	-	-	88%
Received Reliever Medication	-	-	-	100%
Received Systemic Corticosteroids	-	-	-	100%
Emergency Department				
Admittance Decision Time (minutes)[2,7]	-	-	86	98
Head CT Results Within 45 Min. of Arrival[5]	-	-	49%	57%
Patients Who Left ER Before Being Seen[5]	-	-	3%	2%
Time from ER Arrival to Admit. (minutes)[2,7]	-	-	256	274
Time from ER Arrival to Discharge (minutes)[5]	-	-	125	134
Time in ER Before Being Evaluated (minutes)[5]	-	-	27	26
Time to Pain Meds for Fractures (minutes)[5]	-	-	61	57
Heart Attack Care				
Aspirin Given at Discharge[5]	-	-	99%	99%
Fibrinolytic Meds Within 30 Min. of Arrival[5]	-	-	71%	54%
PCI Within 90 Minutes of Arrival[5]	-	-	94%	96%
Statin Prescribed at Discharge[5]	-	-	98%	98%
Heart Failure Care				
ACE Inhibitor or ARB for LVSD[5]	-	-	95%	97%
Discharge Instructions Given[5]	-	-	94%	94%
Evaluation of LVS Function[5]	-	-	97%	99%
Medicare Spending				
Medicare Spending per Patient (ratio)	-	0.94	1.04	0.98
Pneumonia Care				
Appropriate Initial Antibiotic Given[5]	-	-	93%	95%
Blood Culture Timing[5]	-	-	97%	98%
Pregnancy and Delivery Care				
Newborn Deliveries Scheduled Early[7]	-	-	5%	6%
Preventive Care				
Immunization for Influenza	189	56%	85%	90%
Immunization for Pneumonia[2]	168	60%	88%	92%
Stroke Care				
Anticoagulation Therapy for Atrial Fibrillation[5]	-	-	93%	95%

NOTE: Hospital profiles are in alphabetical order by state, then city, then hospital within the city; Rankings exclude hospitals with less than 25 cases except for patient surveys which excludes hospitals with less than 100 cases; (a) 100-299 cases; (1) The number of cases/patients is too few to report; (2) Data submitted were based on a sample of cases/patients; (3) Results are based on a shorter time period than required; (4) Data suppressed by CMS for one or more quarters; (5) Results are not available for this reporting period; (6) Fewer than 100 patients completed the HCAHPS survey; (7) No cases met the criteria for this measure; (8) The lower limit of the confidence interval cannot be calculated if the number of observed infections equals zero; (9) No data are available from the state/territory for this reporting period; (10) The scores shown reflect fewer than 50 completed surveys; (11) There were discrepancies in the data collection process; (12) This measure does not apply to this hospital for this reporting period; (13) Results cannot be calculated for this reporting period; (14) The results for this state are combined with nearby states to protect confidentiality; Please refer to the User's Guide for a full explanation of data.

Measure	Cases	This Hosp.	State Avg.	U.S. Avg.
Antithrombotic Therapy Timing[5]	-	-	96%	98%
Assessed for Rehabilitation[5]	-	-	95%	97%
Discharged on Antithrombotic Therapy[5]	-	-	97%	99%
Discharged on Statin Medication[5]	-	-	89%	94%
Thrombolytic Therapy Timing[5]	-	-	53%	66%
Venous Thromboembolism Prophylaxis[5]	-	-	87%	94%
Written Stroke Educational Materials Given[5]	-	-	83%	88%
Surgical Care Improvement Project				
Appropriate Beta Blocker Usage[2]	26	81%	97%	98%
Appropriate VTP Within 24 Hours[2]	83	96%	97%	98%
Controlled Postoperative Blood Glucose[2,7]	-	-	96%	97%
Perioperative Temperature Management[2]	95	99%	100%	100%
Prophylactic Antibiotic Selection[2]	70	99%	99%	99%
Prophylactic Antibiotic Selection (Outpatient)	24	100%	97%	98%
Prophylactic Antibiotic Stopped[2]	70	97%	97%	98%
Prophylactic Antibiotic Timing[2]	70	94%	98%	99%
Prophylactic Antibiotic Timing (Outpatient)	24	100%	97%	98%
Urinary Catheter Removal[2]	60	97%	96%	97%
Survey of Patients' Hospital Experiences				
Area Around Room 'Always' Quiet at Night	(a)	90%	74%	61%
Doctors 'Always' Communicated Well	(a)	90%	87%	82%
Home Recovery Information Given	(a)	91%	85%	85%
Hospital Given 9 or 10 on 10 Point Scale	(a)	87%	75%	71%
Meds 'Always' Explained Before Given	(a)	78%	69%	64%
Nurses 'Always' Communicated Well	(a)	90%	83%	79%
Pain 'Always' Well Controlled	(a)	81%	75%	71%
Room and Bathroom 'Always' Clean	(a)	89%	75%	73%
Timely Help 'Always' Received	(a)	89%	71%	68%
Would Definitely Recommend Hospital	(a)	90%	75%	71%
Use of Medical Imaging				
Cardiac Imaging Stress Test before Surgery[7]	-	-	5.3%	5.3%
Combination Abdominal CT Scan[1]	-	-	24.5%	10.5%
Combination Brain/Sinus CT Scan[1]	-	-	2.6%	2.7%
Combination Chest CT Scan[1]	-	-	7.6%	2.7%
Follow-up Mammogram/Ultrasound[7]	-	-	9.4%	8.8%
Lumbar Spine MRI for Low Back Pain[7]	-	-	42.7%	37.2%

Lakeview Regional Medical Center

95 Judge Tanner Boulevard
Covington, LA 70433
Phone: 985-867-4443
Fax: 985-867-3879
URL: www.lakeviewregional.com
Type: Acute Care Hospitals
Ownership: Proprietary
Emergency Services: Yes
Beds: 178

Key Personnel:
Radiology. . . . . Michael D Hall
CEO/President. . . . . Max Lauderdale
Pediatrics. . . . . Joshua LeBlanc
Cardiology . . . . Naveed Malik
Chief of Medical Staff. . . . . Chad Muntan

Measure	Cases	This Hosp.	State Avg.	U.S. Avg.
Blood Clot Prevention and Treatment				
Anticoagulation Overlap Therapy[2]	27	100%	89%	93%
ICU Venous Thromboembolism Prophylaxis[2]	84	100%	88%	92%
Incidence of Potentially Preventable VTE[1,2]	-	-	16%	10%
UFH with Dosages/Platelet Monitoring[1,2]	-	-	94%	97%
Venous Thromboembolism Prophylaxis[2]	367	100%	74%	85%
Warfarin Therapy Discharge Instructions[2]	24	100%	85%	75%
Chest Pain/Possible Heart Attack Care				
Aspirin Given Within 24 Hours of Arrival[5]	-	-	94%	96%
Fibrinolytic Meds Within 30 Min. of Arrival[5]	-	-	54%	58%
Average Time to ECG (minutes)[5]	-	-	10	7
Average Time to Transfer (minutes)[5]	-	-	94	60
Children's Asthma Care				
Received Home Management Plan of Care	-	-	-	88%
Received Reliever Medication	-	-	-	100%
Received Systemic Corticosteroids	-	-	-	100%
Emergency Department				
Admittance Decision Time (minutes)[2]	558	61	86	98
Head CT Results Within 45 Min. of Arrival[1]	-	-	49%	57%
Patients Who Left ER Before Being Seen	21,979	2%	3%	2%
Time from ER Arrival to Admit. (minutes)[2]	558	243	256	274
Time from ER Arrival to Discharge (minutes)	429	169	125	134
Time in ER Before Being Evaluated (minutes)	472	22	27	26
Time to Pain Meds for Fractures (minutes)	70	79	61	57
Heart Attack Care				
Aspirin Given at Discharge	83	100%	99%	99%
Fibrinolytic Meds Within 30 Min. of Arrival[7]	-	-	71%	54%
PCI Within 90 Minutes of Arrival	16	100%	94%	96%
Statin Prescribed at Discharge	77	100%	98%	98%
Heart Failure Care				
ACE Inhibitor or ARB for LVSD	70	100%	95%	97%
Discharge Instructions Given	162	100%	94%	94%
Evaluation of LVS Function	199	100%	97%	99%
Medicare Spending				
Medicare Spending per Patient (ratio)	-	1.07	1.04	0.98
Pneumonia Care				
Appropriate Initial Antibiotic Given	103	100%	93%	95%
Blood Culture Timing	177	100%	97%	98%
Pregnancy and Delivery Care				
Newborn Deliveries Scheduled Early	115	0%	5%	6%
Preventive Care				
Immunization for Influenza[2]	542	100%	85%	90%
Immunization for Pneumonia[2]	689	100%	88%	92%
Stroke Care				
Anticoagulation Therapy for Atrial Fibrillation[1]	-	-	93%	95%
Antithrombotic Therapy Timing	45	100%	96%	98%
Assessed for Rehabilitation	60	100%	95%	97%
Discharged on Antithrombotic Therapy	50	100%	97%	99%
Discharged on Statin Medication	40	100%	89%	94%
Thrombolytic Therapy Timing[1]	-	-	53%	66%
Venous Thromboembolism Prophylaxis	64	100%	87%	94%
Written Stroke Educational Materials Given	35	100%	83%	88%
Surgical Care Improvement Project				
Appropriate Beta Blocker Usage	165	100%	97%	98%
Appropriate VTP Within 24 Hours	340	100%	97%	98%
Controlled Postoperative Blood Glucose	82	96%	96%	97%
Perioperative Temperature Management	410	100%	100%	100%
Prophylactic Antibiotic Selection	324	100%	99%	99%
Prophylactic Antibiotic Selection (Outpatient)	218	100%	97%	98%
Prophylactic Antibiotic Stopped	314	100%	97%	98%
Prophylactic Antibiotic Timing	324	100%	98%	99%
Prophylactic Antibiotic Timing (Outpatient)	218	100%	97%	98%
Urinary Catheter Removal	253	100%	96%	97%
Survey of Patients' Hospital Experiences				
Area Around Room 'Always' Quiet at Night	300+	67%	74%	61%
Doctors 'Always' Communicated Well	300+	81%	87%	82%
Home Recovery Information Given	300+	87%	85%	85%
Hospital Given 9 or 10 on 10 Point Scale	300+	69%	75%	71%
Meds 'Always' Explained Before Given	300+	62%	69%	64%
Nurses 'Always' Communicated Well	300+	77%	83%	79%
Pain 'Always' Well Controlled	300+	72%	75%	71%
Room and Bathroom 'Always' Clean	300+	66%	75%	73%
Timely Help 'Always' Received	300+	63%	71%	68%
Would Definitely Recommend Hospital	300+	70%	75%	71%
Use of Medical Imaging				
Cardiac Imaging Stress Test before Surgery	62	4.8%	5.3%	5.3%
Combination Abdominal CT Scan	261	25.7%	24.5%	10.5%
Combination Brain/Sinus CT Scan[1]	-	-	2.6%	2.7%
Combination Chest CT Scan	125	0.8%	7.6%	2.7%
Follow-up Mammogram/Ultrasound	275	26.2%	9.4%	8.8%
Lumbar Spine MRI for Low Back Pain[1]	-	-	42.7%	37.2%

Saint Tammany Parish Hospital

1202 S Tyler Street
Covington, LA 70433
Phone: 985-898-4000
Fax: 985-898-4679
E-mail: marketing@stph.com
URL: www.stph.org
Type: Acute Care Hospitals
Ownership: Govt - Hospital Dist/Auth
Emergency Services: Yes
Beds: 203

Key Personnel:
Radiology. . . . . Vikas Bhushan
Chief of Medical Staff. . . . . Robert Capitelli, MD
Hemotology Center . . . . Chryl Corizzo
Emergency Room . . . . Joan Curtis, MD
President/CEO. . . . . Patti Ellish, FACHE
Infection Control. . . . . Karen Moise

Measure	Cases	This Hosp.	State Avg.	U.S. Avg.
Blood Clot Prevention and Treatment				
Anticoagulation Overlap Therapy[2]	61	89%	89%	93%
ICU Venous Thromboembolism Prophylaxis[2]	85	81%	88%	92%
Incidence of Potentially Preventable VTE[1,2]	-	-	16%	10%
UFH with Dosages/Platelet Monitoring[1,2]	-	-	94%	97%
Venous Thromboembolism Prophylaxis[2]	320	72%	74%	85%
Warfarin Therapy Discharge Instructions[2]	46	96%	85%	75%
Chest Pain/Possible Heart Attack Care				
Aspirin Given Within 24 Hours of Arrival[1,3]	-	-	94%	96%
Fibrinolytic Meds Within 30 Min. of Arrival[5]	-	-	54%	58%
Average Time to ECG (minutes)[1,3]	-	-	10	7
Average Time to Transfer (minutes)[5]	-	-	94	60
Children's Asthma Care				
Received Home Management Plan of Care	-	-	-	88%
Received Reliever Medication	-	-	-	100%
Received Systemic Corticosteroids	-	-	-	100%
Emergency Department				
Admittance Decision Time (minutes)[2]	315	67	86	98
Head CT Results Within 45 Min. of Arrival	16	100%	49%	57%
Patients Who Left ER Before Being Seen	37,984	2%	3%	2%
Time from ER Arrival to Admit. (minutes)[2]	365	248	256	274
Time from ER Arrival to Discharge (minutes)	366	127	125	134
Time in ER Before Being Evaluated (minutes)	366	41	27	26
Time to Pain Meds for Fractures (minutes)	139	18	61	57
Heart Attack Care				
Aspirin Given at Discharge	197	98%	99%	99%
Fibrinolytic Meds Within 30 Min. of Arrival[7]	-	-	71%	54%
PCI Within 90 Minutes of Arrival	30	100%	94%	96%
Statin Prescribed at Discharge	192	96%	98%	98%
Heart Failure Care				
ACE Inhibitor or ARB for LVSD[2]	85	92%	95%	97%
Discharge Instructions Given[2]	236	98%	94%	94%
Evaluation of LVS Function[2]	279	100%	97%	99%
Medicare Spending				
Medicare Spending per Patient (ratio)	-	1.06	1.04	0.98
Pneumonia Care				
Appropriate Initial Antibiotic Given[2]	71	96%	93%	95%
Blood Culture Timing[2]	137	100%	97%	98%
Pregnancy and Delivery Care				
Newborn Deliveries Scheduled Early[2]	44	2%	5%	6%
Preventive Care				
Immunization for Influenza[2]	527	98%	85%	90%
Immunization for Pneumonia[2]	607	98%	88%	92%
Stroke Care				
Anticoagulation Therapy for Atrial Fibrillation[2]	18	100%	93%	95%
Antithrombotic Therapy Timing[2]	81	100%	96%	98%
Assessed for Rehabilitation[2]	93	98%	95%	97%
Discharged on Antithrombotic Therapy[2]	84	100%	97%	99%
Discharged on Statin Medication[2]	73	93%	89%	94%
Thrombolytic Therapy Timing[1,2]	-	-	53%	66%
Venous Thromboembolism Prophylaxis[2]	88	88%	87%	94%
Written Stroke Educational Materials Given[2]	63	94%	83%	88%
Surgical Care Improvement Project				
Appropriate Beta Blocker Usage[2]	145	97%	97%	98%
Appropriate VTP Within 24 Hours[2]	300	96%	97%	98%
Controlled Postoperative Blood Glucose[2]	80	95%	96%	97%
Perioperative Temperature Management[2]	372	100%	100%	100%
Prophylactic Antibiotic Selection[2]	304	99%	99%	99%
Prophylactic Antibiotic Selection (Outpatient)	341	97%	97%	98%
Prophylactic Antibiotic Stopped[2]	301	95%	97%	98%
Prophylactic Antibiotic Timing[2]	305	99%	98%	99%
Prophylactic Antibiotic Timing (Outpatient)	347	97%	97%	98%
Urinary Catheter Removal[2]	242	90%	96%	97%
Survey of Patients' Hospital Experiences				
Area Around Room 'Always' Quiet at Night	300+	66%	74%	61%
Doctors 'Always' Communicated Well	300+	85%	87%	82%
Home Recovery Information Given	300+	89%	85%	85%
Hospital Given 9 or 10 on 10 Point Scale	300+	82%	75%	71%
Meds 'Always' Explained Before Given	300+	66%	69%	64%
Nurses 'Always' Communicated Well	300+	84%	83%	79%
Pain 'Always' Well Controlled	300+	76%	75%	71%
Room and Bathroom 'Always' Clean	300+	70%	75%	73%

NOTE: Hospital profiles are in alphabetical order by state, then city, then hospital within the city; Rankings exclude hospitals with less than 25 cases except for patient surveys which excludes hospitals with less than 100 cases; (a) 100-299 cases; (1) The number of cases/patients is too few to report; (2) Data submitted were based on a sample of cases/patients; (3) Results are based on a shorter time period than required; (4) Data suppressed by CMS for one or more quarters; (5) Results are not available for this reporting period; (6) Fewer than 100 patients completed the HCAHPS survey; (7) No cases met the criteria for this measure; (8) The lower limit of the confidence interval cannot be calculated if the number of observed infections equals zero; (9) No data are available from the state/territory for this reporting period; (10) The scores shown reflect fewer than 50 completed surveys; (11) There were discrepancies in the data collection process; (12) This measure does not apply to this hospital for this reporting period; (13) Results cannot be calculated for this reporting period; (14) The results for this state are combined with nearby states to protect confidentiality; Please refer to the User's Guide for a full explanation of data.

Measure	Cases	This Hosp.	State Avg.	U.S. Avg.
Timely Help 'Always' Received	300+	71%	71%	68%
Would Definitely Recommend Hospital	300+	86%	75%	71%
Use of Medical Imaging				
Cardiac Imaging Stress Test before Surgery	107	8.4%	5.3%	5.3%
Combination Abdominal CT Scan	649	48.2%	24.5%	10.5%
Combination Brain/Sinus CT Scan	647	2.8%	2.6%	2.7%
Combination Chest CT Scan	357	8.4%	7.6%	2.7%
Follow-up Mammogram/Ultrasound	1,013	11.4%	9.4%	8.8%
Lumbar Spine MRI for Low Back Pain	75	42.7%	42.7%	37.2%

American Legion Hospital

1305 Crowley Rayne Highway Phone: 337-783-3222
Crowley, LA 70526
Type: Acute Care Hospitals Emergency Services: Yes
Ownership: Voluntary non-profit - Private Beds: 178
Key Personnel:
Radiology. . . . . Glenn Dailey

Measure	Cases	This Hosp.	State Avg.	U.S. Avg.
Blood Clot Prevention and Treatment				
Anticoagulation Overlap Therapy[1,2]	-	-	89%	93%
ICU Venous Thromboembolism Prophylaxis[2]	43	91%	88%	92%
Incidence of Potentially Preventable VTE[2,7]	-	-	16%	10%
UFH with Dosages/Platelet Monitoring[1,2]	-	-	94%	97%
Venous Thromboembolism Prophylaxis[2]	313	78%	74%	85%
Warfarin Therapy Discharge Instructions[1,2]	-	-	85%	75%
Chest Pain/Possible Heart Attack Care				
Aspirin Given Within 24 Hours of Arrival	44	80%	94%	96%
Fibrinolytic Meds Within 30 Min. of Arrival[7]	-	-	54%	58%
Average Time to ECG (minutes)	43	20	10	7
Average Time to Transfer (minutes)[1]	-	-	94	60
Children's Asthma Care				
Received Home Management Plan of Care	-	-	-	88%
Received Reliever Medication	-	-	-	100%
Received Systemic Corticosteroids	-	-	-	100%
Emergency Department				
Admittance Decision Time (minutes)[2]	599	52	86	98
Head CT Results Within 45 Min. of Arrival[1]	-	-	49%	57%
Patients Who Left ER Before Being Seen	16,603	10%	3%	2%
Time from ER Arrival to Admit. (minutes)[2]	601	234	256	274
Time from ER Arrival to Discharge (minutes)	389	143	125	134
Time in ER Before Being Evaluated (minutes)	392	23	27	26
Time to Pain Meds for Fractures (minutes)	44	69	61	57
Heart Attack Care				
Aspirin Given at Discharge[2,7]	-	-	99%	99%
Fibrinolytic Meds Within 30 Min. of Arrival[2,7]	-	-	71%	54%
PCI Within 90 Minutes of Arrival[2,7]	-	-	94%	96%
Statin Prescribed at Discharge[2,7]	-	-	98%	98%
Heart Failure Care				
ACE Inhibitor or ARB for LVSD[2]	30	63%	95%	97%
Discharge Instructions Given[2]	73	95%	94%	94%
Evaluation of LVS Function[2]	101	88%	97%	99%
Medicare Spending				
Medicare Spending per Patient (ratio)	-	1.02	1.04	0.98
Pneumonia Care				
Appropriate Initial Antibiotic Given[2]	112	94%	93%	95%
Blood Culture Timing[2]	142	96%	97%	98%
Pregnancy and Delivery Care				
Newborn Deliveries Scheduled Early	102	10%	5%	6%
Preventive Care				
Immunization for Influenza[2]	320	88%	85%	90%
Immunization for Pneumonia[2]	500	95%	88%	92%
Stroke Care				
Anticoagulation Therapy for Atrial Fibrillation[1,2]	-	-	93%	95%
Antithrombotic Therapy Timing[2]	15	80%	96%	98%
Assessed for Rehabilitation[2]	15	80%	95%	97%
Discharged on Antithrombotic Therapy[2]	15	73%	97%	99%
Discharged on Statin Medication[2]	14	71%	89%	94%
Thrombolytic Therapy Timing[2,7]	-	-	53%	66%
Venous Thromboembolism Prophylaxis[2]	13	69%	87%	94%
Written Stroke Educational Materials Given[1,2]	-	-	83%	88%
Surgical Care Improvement Project				
Appropriate Beta Blocker Usage[2]	19	74%	97%	98%
Appropriate VTP Within 24 Hours[2]	86	79%	97%	98%
Controlled Postoperative Blood Glucose[2,7]	-	-	96%	97%
Perioperative Temperature Management[2]	90	100%	100%	100%
Prophylactic Antibiotic Selection[2]	17	65%	99%	99%
Prophylactic Antibiotic Selection (Outpatient)	85	91%	97%	98%
Prophylactic Antibiotic Stopped[2]	17	82%	97%	98%
Prophylactic Antibiotic Timing[2]	17	100%	98%	99%
Prophylactic Antibiotic Timing (Outpatient)	85	98%	97%	98%
Urinary Catheter Removal[2]	44	70%	96%	97%
Survey of Patients' Hospital Experiences				
Area Around Room 'Always' Quiet at Night	300+	62%	74%	61%
Doctors 'Always' Communicated Well	300+	87%	87%	82%
Home Recovery Information Given	300+	78%	85%	85%
Hospital Given 9 or 10 on 10 Point Scale	300+	53%	75%	71%
Meds 'Always' Explained Before Given	300+	62%	69%	64%
Nurses 'Always' Communicated Well	300+	75%	83%	79%
Pain 'Always' Well Controlled	300+	64%	75%	71%
Room and Bathroom 'Always' Clean	300+	64%	75%	73%
Timely Help 'Always' Received	300+	55%	71%	68%
Would Definitely Recommend Hospital	300+	51%	75%	71%
Use of Medical Imaging				
Cardiac Imaging Stress Test before Surgery[1]	-	-	5.3%	5.3%
Combination Abdominal CT Scan	275	61.8%	24.5%	10.5%
Combination Brain/Sinus CT Scan	326	4.3%	2.6%	2.7%
Combination Chest CT Scan	217	31.3%	7.6%	2.7%
Follow-up Mammogram/Ultrasound	947	4.8%	9.4%	8.8%
Lumbar Spine MRI for Low Back Pain[7]	-	-	42.7%	37.2%

Lady of the Sea General Hospital

200 West 134th Place Phone: 985-632-6401
Cut Off, LA 70345 Fax: 985-632-8310
URL: www.losgh.org
Type: Critical Access Hospitals Emergency Services: Yes
Ownership: Govt - Hospital Dist/Auth Beds: 49
Key Personnel:
Emergency Room . . . . William Crenshaw, LVN
Chairman/CEO . . . . Darren Duet, MD
Patient Relations . . . . Gayle Duet
Infection Control. . . . . Helene Durham, RN
CEO/President. . . . . Don Werner

Measure	Cases	This Hosp.	State Avg.	U.S. Avg.
Blood Clot Prevention and Treatment				
Anticoagulation Overlap Therapy[5]	-	-	89%	93%
ICU Venous Thromboembolism Prophylaxis[5]	-	-	88%	92%
Incidence of Potentially Preventable VTE[5]	-	-	16%	10%
UFH with Dosages/Platelet Monitoring[5]	-	-	94%	97%
Venous Thromboembolism Prophylaxis[5]	-	-	74%	85%
Warfarin Therapy Discharge Instructions[5]	-	-	85%	75%
Chest Pain/Possible Heart Attack Care				
Aspirin Given Within 24 Hours of Arrival[5]	-	-	94%	96%
Fibrinolytic Meds Within 30 Min. of Arrival[5]	-	-	54%	58%
Average Time to ECG (minutes)[5]	-	-	10	7
Average Time to Transfer (minutes)[5]	-	-	94	60
Children's Asthma Care				
Received Home Management Plan of Care	-	-	-	88%
Received Reliever Medication	-	-	-	100%
Received Systemic Corticosteroids	-	-	-	100%
Emergency Department				
Admittance Decision Time (minutes)[5]	-	-	86	98
Head CT Results Within 45 Min. of Arrival[5]	-	-	49%	57%
Patients Who Left ER Before Being Seen	10,794	2%	3%	2%
Time from ER Arrival to Admit. (minutes)[5]	-	-	256	274
Time from ER Arrival to Discharge (minutes)[5]	-	-	125	134
Time in ER Before Being Evaluated (minutes)[5]	-	-	27	26
Time to Pain Meds for Fractures (minutes)[5]	-	-	61	57
Heart Attack Care				
Aspirin Given at Discharge[5]	-	-	99%	99%
Fibrinolytic Meds Within 30 Min. of Arrival[5]	-	-	71%	54%
PCI Within 90 Minutes of Arrival[5]	-	-	94%	96%
Statin Prescribed at Discharge[5]	-	-	98%	98%
Heart Failure Care				
ACE Inhibitor or ARB for LVSD[1]	-	-	95%	97%
Discharge Instructions Given	36	100%	94%	94%
Evaluation of LVS Function	46	100%	97%	99%
Medicare Spending				
Medicare Spending per Patient (ratio)	-	-	1.04	0.98
Pneumonia Care				
Appropriate Initial Antibiotic Given	42	93%	93%	95%
Blood Culture Timing	60	97%	97%	98%
Pregnancy and Delivery Care				
Newborn Deliveries Scheduled Early[5]	-	-	5%	6%
Preventive Care				
Immunization for Influenza[5]	-	-	85%	90%
Immunization for Pneumonia[5]	-	-	88%	92%
Stroke Care				
Anticoagulation Therapy for Atrial Fibrillation[5]	-	-	93%	95%
Antithrombotic Therapy Timing[5]	-	-	96%	98%
Assessed for Rehabilitation[5]	-	-	95%	97%
Discharged on Antithrombotic Therapy[5]	-	-	97%	99%
Discharged on Statin Medication[5]	-	-	89%	94%
Thrombolytic Therapy Timing[5]	-	-	53%	66%
Venous Thromboembolism Prophylaxis[5]	-	-	87%	94%
Written Stroke Educational Materials Given[5]	-	-	83%	88%
Surgical Care Improvement Project				
Appropriate Beta Blocker Usage[5]	-	-	97%	98%
Appropriate VTP Within 24 Hours[5]	-	-	97%	98%
Controlled Postoperative Blood Glucose[5]	-	-	96%	97%
Perioperative Temperature Management[5]	-	-	100%	100%
Prophylactic Antibiotic Selection[5]	-	-	99%	99%
Prophylactic Antibiotic Selection (Outpatient)[5]	-	-	97%	98%
Prophylactic Antibiotic Stopped[5]	-	-	97%	98%
Prophylactic Antibiotic Timing[5]	-	-	98%	99%
Prophylactic Antibiotic Timing (Outpatient)[5]	-	-	97%	98%
Urinary Catheter Removal[5]	-	-	96%	97%
Survey of Patients' Hospital Experiences				
Area Around Room 'Always' Quiet at Night	(a)	81%	74%	61%
Doctors 'Always' Communicated Well	(a)	96%	87%	82%
Home Recovery Information Given	(a)	89%	85%	85%
Hospital Given 9 or 10 on 10 Point Scale	(a)	85%	75%	71%
Meds 'Always' Explained Before Given	(a)	88%	69%	64%
Nurses 'Always' Communicated Well	(a)	92%	83%	79%
Pain 'Always' Well Controlled	(a)	83%	75%	71%
Room and Bathroom 'Always' Clean	(a)	90%	75%	73%
Timely Help 'Always' Received	(a)	84%	71%	68%
Would Definitely Recommend Hospital	(a)	80%	75%	71%
Use of Medical Imaging				
Cardiac Imaging Stress Test before Surgery	89	6.7%	5.3%	5.3%
Combination Abdominal CT Scan	172	5.2%	24.5%	10.5%
Combination Brain/Sinus CT Scan[1]	-	-	2.6%	2.7%
Combination Chest CT Scan	57	1.8%	7.6%	2.7%
Follow-up Mammogram/Ultrasound	97	7.2%	9.4%	8.8%
Lumbar Spine MRI for Low Back Pain[1]	-	-	42.7%	37.2%

Richland Parish Hospital - Delhi

407 Cincinnati Street Phone: 318-878-5171
Delhi, LA 71232 Fax: 318-878-6363
E-mail: bquince@delhihospital.com
URL: www.delhihospital.com
Type: Critical Access Hospitals Emergency Services: Yes
Ownership: Govt - Hospital Dist/Auth Beds: 42
Key Personnel:
CEO/President. . . . . Michael W Carroll
Chief of Medical Staff . . . . Laura Free
Administrator . . . . Michael W. Carroll

Measure	Cases	This Hosp.	State Avg.	U.S. Avg.
Blood Clot Prevention and Treatment				
Anticoagulation Overlap Therapy[5]	-	-	89%	93%
ICU Venous Thromboembolism Prophylaxis[5]	-	-	88%	92%
Incidence of Potentially Preventable VTE[5]	-	-	16%	10%
UFH with Dosages/Platelet Monitoring[5]	-	-	94%	97%
Venous Thromboembolism Prophylaxis[5]	-	-	74%	85%
Warfarin Therapy Discharge Instructions[5]	-	-	85%	75%
Chest Pain/Possible Heart Attack Care				
Aspirin Given Within 24 Hours of Arrival[5]	-	-	94%	96%
Fibrinolytic Meds Within 30 Min. of Arrival[5]	-	-	54%	58%
Average Time to ECG (minutes)[5]	-	-	10	7
Average Time to Transfer (minutes)[5]	-	-	94	60

NOTE: Hospital profiles are in alphabetical order by state, then city, then hospital within the city; Rankings exclude hospitals with less than 25 cases except for patient surveys which excludes hospitals with less than 100 cases; (a) 100-299 cases; (1) The number of cases/patients is too few to report; (2) Data submitted were based on a sample of cases/patients; (3) Results are based on a shorter time period than required; (4) Data suppressed by CMS for one or more quarters; (5) Results are not available for this reporting period; (6) Fewer than 100 patients completed the HCAHPS survey; (7) No cases met the criteria for this measure; (8) The lower limit of the confidence interval cannot be calculated if the number of observed infections equals zero; (9) No data are available from the state/territory for this reporting period; (10) The scores shown reflect fewer than 50 completed surveys; (11) There were discrepancies in the data collection process; (12) This measure does not apply to this hospital for this reporting period; (13) Results cannot be calculated for this reporting period; (14) The results for this state are combined with nearby states to protect confidentiality; Please refer to the User's Guide for a full explanation of data.

Measure	Cases	This Hosp.	State Avg.	U.S. Avg.
Children's Asthma Care				
Received Home Management Plan of Care	-	-	-	88%
Received Reliever Medication	-	-	-	100%
Received Systemic Corticosteroids	-	-	-	100%
Emergency Department				
Admittance Decision Time (minutes)[5]	-	-	86	98
Head CT Results Within 45 Min. of Arrival[5]	-	-	49%	57%
Patients Who Left ER Before Being Seen	4,593	0%	3%	2%
Time from ER Arrival to Admit. (minutes)[5]	-	-	256	274
Time from ER Arrival to Discharge (minutes)[5]	-	-	125	134
Time in ER Before Being Evaluated (minutes)[5]	-	-	27	26
Time to Pain Meds for Fractures (minutes)[5]	-	-	61	57
Heart Attack Care				
Aspirin Given at Discharge[5]	-	-	99%	99%
Fibrinolytic Meds Within 30 Min. of Arrival[5]	-	-	71%	54%
PCI Within 90 Minutes of Arrival[5]	-	-	94%	96%
Statin Prescribed at Discharge[5]	-	-	98%	98%
Heart Failure Care				
ACE Inhibitor or ARB for LVSD[1]	-	-	95%	97%
Discharge Instructions Given	26	88%	94%	94%
Evaluation of LVS Function	34	91%	97%	99%
Medicare Spending				
Medicare Spending per Patient (ratio)	-	-	1.04	0.98
Pneumonia Care				
Appropriate Initial Antibiotic Given[2]	41	83%	93%	95%
Blood Culture Timing[2]	21	71%	97%	98%
Pregnancy and Delivery Care				
Newborn Deliveries Scheduled Early[5]	-	-	5%	6%
Preventive Care				
Immunization for Influenza[5]	-	-	85%	90%
Immunization for Pneumonia[5]	-	-	88%	92%
Stroke Care				
Anticoagulation Therapy for Atrial Fibrillation[5]	-	-	93%	95%
Antithrombotic Therapy Timing[5]	-	-	96%	98%
Assessed for Rehabilitation[5]	-	-	95%	97%
Discharged on Antithrombotic Therapy[5]	-	-	97%	99%
Discharged on Statin Medication[5]	-	-	89%	94%
Thrombolytic Therapy Timing[5]	-	-	53%	66%
Venous Thromboembolism Prophylaxis[5]	-	-	87%	94%
Written Stroke Educational Materials Given[5]	-	-	83%	88%
Surgical Care Improvement Project				
Appropriate Beta Blocker Usage[5]	-	-	97%	98%
Appropriate VTP Within 24 Hours[5]	-	-	97%	98%
Controlled Postoperative Blood Glucose[5]	-	-	96%	97%
Perioperative Temperature Management[5]	-	-	100%	100%
Prophylactic Antibiotic Selection[5]	-	-	99%	99%
Prophylactic Antibiotic Selection (Outpatient)[5]	-	-	97%	98%
Prophylactic Antibiotic Stopped[5]	-	-	97%	98%
Prophylactic Antibiotic Timing[5]	-	-	98%	99%
Prophylactic Antibiotic Timing (Outpatient)[5]	-	-	97%	98%
Urinary Catheter Removal[5]	-	-	96%	97%
Survey of Patients' Hospital Experiences				
Area Around Room 'Always' Quiet at Night	(a)	74%	74%	61%
Doctors 'Always' Communicated Well	(a)	92%	87%	82%
Home Recovery Information Given	(a)	85%	85%	85%
Hospital Given 9 or 10 on 10 Point Scale	(a)	83%	75%	71%
Meds 'Always' Explained Before Given	(a)	83%	69%	64%
Nurses 'Always' Communicated Well	(a)	87%	83%	79%
Pain 'Always' Well Controlled	(a)	76%	75%	71%
Room and Bathroom 'Always' Clean	(a)	74%	75%	73%
Timely Help 'Always' Received	(a)	80%	71%	68%
Would Definitely Recommend Hospital	(a)	82%	75%	71%
Use of Medical Imaging				
Cardiac Imaging Stress Test before Surgery[7]	-	-	5.3%	5.3%
Combination Abdominal CT Scan	100	24.0%	24.5%	10.5%
Combination Brain/Sinus CT Scan[1]	-	-	2.6%	2.7%
Combination Chest CT Scan[1]	-	-	7.6%	2.7%
Follow-up Mammogram/Ultrasound	375	2.7%	9.4%	8.8%
Lumbar Spine MRI for Low Back Pain[7]	-	-	42.7%	37.2%

Beauregard Memorial Hospital

600 S Pine Street
Deridder, LA 70634
Phone: 337-462-7100
Fax: 337-462-7479
URL: www.beauregard.org
Type: Acute Care Hospitals
Emergency Services: Yes
Ownership: Govt - Hospital Dist/Auth
Beds: 60

Key Personnel:

Infection Control. . . . . Jo Blankenship
Chief of Medical Staff . . . . David Brown, MD
CEO/President. . . . . Bob Charron
Patient Relations . . . . Jill Cooper
Pediatric In-Patient Care . . . . Vic Gray, RN
Emergency Room . . . . Sharon Manitzas, RN
Anesthesiology. . . . . Pete Peterson
Intensive Care Unit. . . . . Lee Pinkley, RN

Measure	Cases	This Hosp.	State Avg.	U.S. Avg.
Blood Clot Prevention and Treatment				
Anticoagulation Overlap Therapy[2]	21	71%	89%	93%
ICU Venous Thromboembolism Prophylaxis[2]	41	95%	88%	92%
Incidence of Potentially Preventable VTE[1,2]	-	-	16%	10%
UFH with Dosages/Platelet Monitoring[2]	19	100%	94%	97%
Venous Thromboembolism Prophylaxis[2]	174	88%	74%	85%
Warfarin Therapy Discharge Instructions[2]	17	76%	85%	75%
Chest Pain/Possible Heart Attack Care				
Aspirin Given Within 24 Hours of Arrival	32	88%	94%	96%
Fibrinolytic Meds Within 30 Min. of Arrival[1]	-	-	54%	58%
Average Time to ECG (minutes)	34	14	10	7
Average Time to Transfer (minutes)[7]	-	-	94	60
Children's Asthma Care				
Received Home Management Plan of Care	-	-	-	88%
Received Reliever Medication	-	-	-	100%
Received Systemic Corticosteroids	-	-	-	100%
Emergency Department				
Admittance Decision Time (minutes)[2]	189	69	86	98
Head CT Results Within 45 Min. of Arrival[1]	-	-	49%	57%
Patients Who Left ER Before Being Seen	18,187	4%	3%	2%
Time from ER Arrival to Admit. (minutes)[2]	189	236	256	274
Time from ER Arrival to Discharge (minutes)	360	135	125	134
Time in ER Before Being Evaluated (minutes)	385	25	27	26
Time to Pain Meds for Fractures (minutes)	96	62	61	57
Heart Attack Care				
Aspirin Given at Discharge	15	100%	99%	99%
Fibrinolytic Meds Within 30 Min. of Arrival[1]	-	-	71%	54%
PCI Within 90 Minutes of Arrival[7]	-	-	94%	96%
Statin Prescribed at Discharge	15	93%	98%	98%
Heart Failure Care				
ACE Inhibitor or ARB for LVSD	38	100%	95%	97%
Discharge Instructions Given	58	78%	94%	94%
Evaluation of LVS Function	74	100%	97%	99%
Medicare Spending				
Medicare Spending per Patient (ratio)	-	0.94	1.04	0.98
Pneumonia Care				
Appropriate Initial Antibiotic Given	42	76%	93%	95%
Blood Culture Timing	74	96%	97%	98%
Pregnancy and Delivery Care				
Newborn Deliveries Scheduled Early[2]	91	41%	5%	6%
Preventive Care				
Immunization for Influenza[2]	258	93%	85%	90%
Immunization for Pneumonia[2]	288	98%	88%	92%
Stroke Care				
Anticoagulation Therapy for Atrial Fibrillation[1]	-	-	93%	95%
Antithrombotic Therapy Timing	14	86%	96%	98%
Assessed for Rehabilitation	13	92%	95%	97%
Discharged on Antithrombotic Therapy	13	92%	97%	99%
Discharged on Statin Medication	11	82%	89%	94%
Thrombolytic Therapy Timing[7]	-	-	53%	66%
Venous Thromboembolism Prophylaxis[1]	-	-	87%	94%
Written Stroke Educational Materials Given[1]	-	-	83%	88%
Surgical Care Improvement Project				
Appropriate Beta Blocker Usage	18	78%	97%	98%
Appropriate VTP Within 24 Hours	76	91%	97%	98%
Controlled Postoperative Blood Glucose[7]	-	-	96%	97%
Perioperative Temperature Management	93	99%	100%	100%
Prophylactic Antibiotic Selection	73	96%	99%	99%
Prophylactic Antibiotic Selection (Outpatient)	88	85%	97%	98%
Prophylactic Antibiotic Stopped	72	85%	97%	98%
Prophylactic Antibiotic Timing	73	97%	98%	99%
Prophylactic Antibiotic Timing (Outpatient)	70	89%	97%	98%
Urinary Catheter Removal	13	100%	96%	97%
Survey of Patients' Hospital Experiences				
Area Around Room 'Always' Quiet at Night	300+	70%	74%	61%
Doctors 'Always' Communicated Well	300+	89%	87%	82%
Home Recovery Information Given	300+	89%	85%	85%
Hospital Given 9 or 10 on 10 Point Scale	300+	71%	75%	71%
Meds 'Always' Explained Before Given	300+	63%	69%	64%
Nurses 'Always' Communicated Well	300+	82%	83%	79%
Pain 'Always' Well Controlled	300+	77%	75%	71%
Room and Bathroom 'Always' Clean	300+	69%	75%	73%
Timely Help 'Always' Received	300+	67%	71%	68%
Would Definitely Recommend Hospital	300+	72%	75%	71%
Use of Medical Imaging				
Cardiac Imaging Stress Test before Surgery[1]	-	-	5.3%	5.3%
Combination Abdominal CT Scan	379	34.0%	24.5%	10.5%
Combination Brain/Sinus CT Scan[1]	-	-	2.6%	2.7%
Combination Chest CT Scan	181	38.1%	7.6%	2.7%
Follow-up Mammogram/Ultrasound	467	5.1%	9.4%	8.8%
Lumbar Spine MRI for Low Back Pain[1]	-	-	42.7%	37.2%

Union General Hospital

901 James Ave
Farmerville, LA 71241
Phone: 318-368-9751
URL: www.uniongen.org
Type: Critical Access Hospitals
Emergency Services: Yes
Ownership: Voluntary non-profit - Private

Measure	Cases	This Hosp.	State Avg.	U.S. Avg.
Blood Clot Prevention and Treatment				
Anticoagulation Overlap Therapy[5]	-	-	89%	93%
ICU Venous Thromboembolism Prophylaxis[5]	-	-	88%	92%
Incidence of Potentially Preventable VTE[5]	-	-	16%	10%
UFH with Dosages/Platelet Monitoring[5]	-	-	94%	97%
Venous Thromboembolism Prophylaxis[5]	-	-	74%	85%
Warfarin Therapy Discharge Instructions[5]	-	-	85%	75%
Chest Pain/Possible Heart Attack Care				
Aspirin Given Within 24 Hours of Arrival	37	100%	94%	96%
Fibrinolytic Meds Within 30 Min. of Arrival[1]	-	-	54%	58%
Average Time to ECG (minutes)	40	4	10	7
Average Time to Transfer (minutes)[1]	-	-	94	60
Children's Asthma Care				
Received Home Management Plan of Care	-	-	-	88%
Received Reliever Medication	-	-	-	100%
Received Systemic Corticosteroids	-	-	-	100%
Emergency Department				
Admittance Decision Time (minutes)	300	70	86	98
Head CT Results Within 45 Min. of Arrival[5]	-	-	49%	57%
Patients Who Left ER Before Being Seen	6,108	1%	3%	2%
Time from ER Arrival to Admit. (minutes)	300	226	256	274
Time from ER Arrival to Discharge (minutes)[5]	-	-	125	134
Time in ER Before Being Evaluated (minutes)[5]	-	-	27	26
Time to Pain Meds for Fractures (minutes)[5]	-	-	61	57
Heart Attack Care				
Aspirin Given at Discharge[1,3]	-	-	99%	99%
Fibrinolytic Meds Within 30 Min. of Arrival[3,7]	-	-	71%	54%
PCI Within 90 Minutes of Arrival[3,7]	-	-	94%	96%
Statin Prescribed at Discharge[1,3]	-	-	98%	98%
Heart Failure Care				
ACE Inhibitor or ARB for LVSD[1]	-	-	95%	97%
Discharge Instructions Given	16	100%	94%	94%
Evaluation of LVS Function	22	100%	97%	99%
Medicare Spending				
Medicare Spending per Patient (ratio)	-	-	1.04	0.98
Pneumonia Care				
Appropriate Initial Antibiotic Given	32	100%	93%	95%
Blood Culture Timing	74	95%	97%	98%
Pregnancy and Delivery Care				
Newborn Deliveries Scheduled Early[5]	-	-	5%	6%
Preventive Care				

NOTE: Hospital profiles are in alphabetical order by state, then city, then hospital within the city; Rankings exclude hospitals with less than 25 cases except for patient surveys which excludes hospitals with less than 100 cases; (a) 100-299 cases; (1) The number of cases/patients is too few to report; (2) Data submitted were based on a sample of cases/patients; (3) Results are based on a shorter time period than required; (4) Data suppressed by CMS for one or more quarters; (5) Results are not available for this reporting period; (6) Fewer than 100 patients completed the HCAHPS survey; (7) No cases met the criteria for this measure; (8) The lower limit of the confidence interval cannot be calculated if the number of observed infections equals zero; (9) No data are available from the state/territory for this reporting period; (10) The scores shown reflect fewer than 50 completed surveys; (11) There were discrepancies in the data collection process; (12) This measure does not apply to this hospital for this reporting period; (13) Results cannot be calculated for this reporting period; (14) The results for this state are combined with nearby states to protect confidentiality; Please refer to the User's Guide for a full explanation of data.

Measure	Cases	This Hosp.	State Avg.	U.S. Avg.
Immunization for Influenza	198	97%	85%	90%
Immunization for Pneumonia	304	98%	88%	92%
Stroke Care				
Anticoagulation Therapy for Atrial Fibrillation[5]	-	-	93%	95%
Antithrombotic Therapy Timing[5]	-	-	96%	98%
Assessed for Rehabilitation[5]	-	-	95%	97%
Discharged on Antithrombotic Therapy[5]	-	-	97%	99%
Discharged on Statin Medication[5]	-	-	89%	94%
Thrombolytic Therapy Timing[5]	-	-	53%	66%
Venous Thromboembolism Prophylaxis[5]	-	-	87%	94%
Written Stroke Educational Materials Given[5]	-	-	83%	88%
Surgical Care Improvement Project				
Appropriate Beta Blocker Usage[5]	-	-	97%	98%
Appropriate VTP Within 24 Hours[5]	-	-	97%	98%
Controlled Postoperative Blood Glucose[5]	-	-	96%	97%
Perioperative Temperature Management[5]	-	-	100%	100%
Prophylactic Antibiotic Selection[5]	-	-	99%	99%
Prophylactic Antibiotic Selection (Outpatient)[5]	-	-	97%	98%
Prophylactic Antibiotic Stopped[5]	-	-	97%	98%
Prophylactic Antibiotic Timing[5]	-	-	98%	99%
Prophylactic Antibiotic Timing (Outpatient)[5]	-	-	97%	98%
Urinary Catheter Removal[5]	-	-	96%	97%
Survey of Patients' Hospital Experiences				
Area Around Room 'Always' Quiet at Night[10]	<100	95%	74%	61%
Doctors 'Always' Communicated Well[10]	<100	95%	87%	82%
Home Recovery Information Given[10]	<100	76%	85%	85%
Hospital Given 9 or 10 on 10 Point Scale[10]	<100	77%	75%	71%
Meds 'Always' Explained Before Given[10]	<100	76%	69%	64%
Nurses 'Always' Communicated Well[10]	<100	87%	83%	79%
Pain 'Always' Well Controlled[10]	<100	70%	75%	71%
Room and Bathroom 'Always' Clean[10]	<100	97%	75%	73%
Timely Help 'Always' Received[10]	<100	69%	71%	68%
Would Definitely Recommend Hospital[10]	<100	76%	75%	71%
Use of Medical Imaging				
Cardiac Imaging Stress Test before Surgery[7]			5.3%	5.3%
Combination Abdominal CT Scan	89	4.5%	24.5%	10.5%
Combination Brain/Sinus CT Scan[1]			2.6%	2.7%
Combination Chest CT Scan[1]			7.6%	2.7%
Follow-up Mammogram/Ultrasound[7]			9.4%	8.8%
Lumbar Spine MRI for Low Back Pain[7]	-	-	42.7%	37.2%

Riverland Medical Center

1700 Wallace Blvd — Phone: 318-757-6551
Ferriday, LA 71334
Type: Critical Access Hospitals — Emergency Services: Yes
Ownership: Govt - Hospital Dist/Auth

Measure	Cases	This Hosp.	State Avg.	U.S. Avg.
Blood Clot Prevention and Treatment				
Anticoagulation Overlap Therapy[5]	-	-	89%	93%
ICU Venous Thromboembolism Prophylaxis[5]	-	-	88%	92%
Incidence of Potentially Preventable VTE[5]	-	-	16%	10%
UFH with Dosages/Platelet Monitoring[5]	-	-	94%	97%
Venous Thromboembolism Prophylaxis[5]	-	-	74%	85%
Warfarin Therapy Discharge Instructions[5]	-	-	85%	75%
Chest Pain/Possible Heart Attack Care				
Aspirin Given Within 24 Hours of Arrival	-	-	94%	96%
Fibrinolytic Meds Within 30 Min. of Arrival	-	-	54%	58%
Average Time to ECG (minutes)	-	-	10	7
Average Time to Transfer (minutes)	-	-	94	60
Children's Asthma Care				
Received Home Management Plan of Care	-	-	-	88%
Received Reliever Medication	-	-	-	100%
Received Systemic Corticosteroids	-	-	-	100%
Emergency Department				
Admittance Decision Time (minutes)[5]	-	-	86	98
Head CT Results Within 45 Min. of Arrival	-	-	49%	57%
Patients Who Left ER Before Being Seen	-	-	3%	2%
Time from ER Arrival to Admit. (minutes)[5]	-	-	256	274
Time from ER Arrival to Discharge (minutes)	-	-	125	134
Time in ER Before Being Evaluated (minutes)	-	-	27	26
Time to Pain Meds for Fractures (minutes)	-	-	61	57
Heart Attack Care				
Aspirin Given at Discharge[5]	-	-	99%	99%
Fibrinolytic Meds Within 30 Min. of Arrival[5]	-	-	71%	54%
PCI Within 90 Minutes of Arrival[5]	-	-	94%	96%
Statin Prescribed at Discharge[5]	-	-	98%	98%
Heart Failure Care				
ACE Inhibitor or ARB for LVSD[1,2]	-	-	95%	97%
Discharge Instructions Given[1,2]	-	-	94%	94%
Evaluation of LVS Function[1,2]	-	-	97%	99%
Medicare Spending				
Medicare Spending per Patient (ratio)	-	-	1.04	0.98
Pneumonia Care				
Appropriate Initial Antibiotic Given[1,2]	-	-	93%	95%
Blood Culture Timing[1,2]	-	-	97%	98%
Pregnancy and Delivery Care				
Newborn Deliveries Scheduled Early[5]	-	-	5%	6%
Preventive Care				
Immunization for Influenza[5]	-	-	85%	90%
Immunization for Pneumonia[5]	-	-	88%	92%
Stroke Care				
Anticoagulation Therapy for Atrial Fibrillation[5]	-	-	93%	95%
Antithrombotic Therapy Timing[5]	-	-	96%	98%
Assessed for Rehabilitation[5]	-	-	95%	97%
Discharged on Antithrombotic Therapy[5]	-	-	97%	99%
Discharged on Statin Medication[5]	-	-	89%	94%
Thrombolytic Therapy Timing[5]	-	-	53%	66%
Venous Thromboembolism Prophylaxis[5]	-	-	87%	94%
Written Stroke Educational Materials Given[5]	-	-	83%	88%
Surgical Care Improvement Project				
Appropriate Beta Blocker Usage[5]	-	-	97%	98%
Appropriate VTP Within 24 Hours[5]	-	-	97%	98%
Controlled Postoperative Blood Glucose[5]	-	-	96%	97%
Perioperative Temperature Management[5]	-	-	100%	100%
Prophylactic Antibiotic Selection[5]	-	-	99%	99%
Prophylactic Antibiotic Selection (Outpatient)	-	-	97%	98%
Prophylactic Antibiotic Stopped[5]	-	-	97%	98%
Prophylactic Antibiotic Timing[5]	-	-	98%	99%
Prophylactic Antibiotic Timing (Outpatient)	-	-	97%	98%
Urinary Catheter Removal[5]	-	-	96%	97%
Survey of Patients' Hospital Experiences				
Area Around Room 'Always' Quiet at Night[5]	-	-	74%	61%
Doctors 'Always' Communicated Well[5]	-	-	87%	82%
Home Recovery Information Given[5]	-	-	85%	85%
Hospital Given 9 or 10 on 10 Point Scale[5]	-	-	75%	71%
Meds 'Always' Explained Before Given[5]	-	-	69%	64%
Nurses 'Always' Communicated Well[5]	-	-	83%	79%
Pain 'Always' Well Controlled[5]	-	-	75%	71%
Room and Bathroom 'Always' Clean[5]	-	-	75%	73%
Timely Help 'Always' Received[5]	-	-	71%	68%
Would Definitely Recommend Hospital[5]	-	-	75%	71%
Use of Medical Imaging				
Cardiac Imaging Stress Test before Surgery	-	-	5.3%	5.3%
Combination Abdominal CT Scan	-	-	24.5%	10.5%
Combination Brain/Sinus CT Scan	-	-	2.6%	2.7%
Combination Chest CT Scan	-	-	7.6%	2.7%
Follow-up Mammogram/Ultrasound	-	-	9.4%	8.8%
Lumbar Spine MRI for Low Back Pain	-	-	42.7%	37.2%

Franklin Foundation Hospital

1097 Northwest Blvd — Phone: 337-828-0760
Franklin, LA 70538
Type: Critical Access Hospitals — Emergency Services: Yes
Ownership: Voluntary non-profit - Other

Measure	Cases	This Hosp.	State Avg.	U.S. Avg.
Blood Clot Prevention and Treatment				
Anticoagulation Overlap Therapy[5]	-	-	89%	93%
ICU Venous Thromboembolism Prophylaxis[5]	-	-	88%	92%
Incidence of Potentially Preventable VTE[5]	-	-	16%	10%
UFH with Dosages/Platelet Monitoring[5]	-	-	94%	97%
Venous Thromboembolism Prophylaxis[5]	-	-	74%	85%
Warfarin Therapy Discharge Instructions[5]	-	-	85%	75%
Chest Pain/Possible Heart Attack Care				
Aspirin Given Within 24 Hours of Arrival	-	-	94%	96%
Fibrinolytic Meds Within 30 Min. of Arrival	-	-	54%	58%
Average Time to ECG (minutes)	-	-	10	7
Average Time to Transfer (minutes)	-	-	94	60
Children's Asthma Care				
Received Home Management Plan of Care	-	-	-	88%
Received Reliever Medication	-	-	-	100%
Received Systemic Corticosteroids	-	-	-	100%
Emergency Department				
Admittance Decision Time (minutes)[3]	256	80	86	98
Head CT Results Within 45 Min. of Arrival	-	-	49%	57%
Patients Who Left ER Before Being Seen	-	-	3%	2%
Time from ER Arrival to Admit. (minutes)[3]	265	235	256	274
Time from ER Arrival to Discharge (minutes)	-	-	125	134
Time in ER Before Being Evaluated (minutes)	-	-	27	26
Time to Pain Meds for Fractures (minutes)	-	-	61	57
Heart Attack Care				
Aspirin Given at Discharge[3,7]	-	-	99%	99%
Fibrinolytic Meds Within 30 Min. of Arrival[3,7]	-	-	71%	54%
PCI Within 90 Minutes of Arrival[3,7]	-	-	94%	96%
Statin Prescribed at Discharge[3,7]	-	-	98%	98%
Heart Failure Care				
ACE Inhibitor or ARB for LVSD[1,3]	-	-	95%	97%
Discharge Instructions Given[1,3]	-	-	94%	94%
Evaluation of LVS Function[3]	16	100%	97%	99%
Medicare Spending				
Medicare Spending per Patient (ratio)	-	-	1.04	0.98
Pneumonia Care				
Appropriate Initial Antibiotic Given[3]	14	86%	93%	95%
Blood Culture Timing[3]	24	96%	97%	98%
Pregnancy and Delivery Care				
Newborn Deliveries Scheduled Early[5]	-	-	5%	6%
Preventive Care				
Immunization for Influenza	285	71%	85%	90%
Immunization for Pneumonia[3]	250	82%	88%	92%
Stroke Care				
Anticoagulation Therapy for Atrial Fibrillation[5]	-	-	93%	95%
Antithrombotic Therapy Timing[5]	-	-	96%	98%
Assessed for Rehabilitation[5]	-	-	95%	97%
Discharged on Antithrombotic Therapy[5]	-	-	97%	99%
Discharged on Statin Medication[5]	-	-	89%	94%
Thrombolytic Therapy Timing[5]	-	-	53%	66%
Venous Thromboembolism Prophylaxis[5]	-	-	87%	94%
Written Stroke Educational Materials Given[5]	-	-	83%	88%
Surgical Care Improvement Project				
Appropriate Beta Blocker Usage[3]	13	92%	97%	98%
Appropriate VTP Within 24 Hours[3]	44	100%	97%	98%
Controlled Postoperative Blood Glucose[3,7]	-	-	96%	97%
Perioperative Temperature Management[3]	52	100%	100%	100%
Prophylactic Antibiotic Selection[3]	40	100%	99%	99%
Prophylactic Antibiotic Selection (Outpatient)	-	-	97%	98%
Prophylactic Antibiotic Stopped[3]	39	100%	97%	98%
Prophylactic Antibiotic Timing[3]	40	98%	98%	99%
Prophylactic Antibiotic Timing (Outpatient)	-	-	97%	98%
Urinary Catheter Removal[3]	26	96%	96%	97%
Survey of Patients' Hospital Experiences				
Area Around Room 'Always' Quiet at Night[6]	<100	76%	74%	61%
Doctors 'Always' Communicated Well[6]	<100	89%	87%	82%
Home Recovery Information Given[6]	<100	90%	85%	85%
Hospital Given 9 or 10 on 10 Point Scale[6]	<100	84%	75%	71%
Meds 'Always' Explained Before Given[6]	<100	72%	69%	64%
Nurses 'Always' Communicated Well[6]	<100	88%	83%	79%
Pain 'Always' Well Controlled[6]	<100	82%	75%	71%
Room and Bathroom 'Always' Clean[6]	<100	86%	75%	73%
Timely Help 'Always' Received[6]	<100	81%	71%	68%
Would Definitely Recommend Hospital[6]	<100	76%	75%	71%
Use of Medical Imaging				
Cardiac Imaging Stress Test before Surgery	-	-	5.3%	5.3%
Combination Abdominal CT Scan	-	-	24.5%	10.5%
Combination Brain/Sinus CT Scan	-	-	2.6%	2.7%
Combination Chest CT Scan	-	-	7.6%	2.7%
Follow-up Mammogram/Ultrasound	-	-	9.4%	8.8%
Lumbar Spine MRI for Low Back Pain	-	-	42.7%	37.2%

NOTE: Hospital profiles are in alphabetical order by state, then city, then hospital within the city; Rankings exclude hospitals with less than 25 cases except for patient surveys which excludes hospitals with less than 100 cases; (a) 100-299 cases; (1) The number of cases/patients is too few to report; (2) Data submitted were based on a sample of cases/patients; (3) Results are based on a shorter time period than required; (4) Data suppressed by CMS for one or more quarters; (5) Results are not available for this reporting period; (6) Fewer than 100 patients completed the HCAHPS survey; (7) No cases met the criteria for this measure; (8) The lower limit of the confidence interval cannot be calculated if the number of observed infections equals zero; (9) No data are available from the state/territory for this reporting period; (10) The scores shown reflect fewer than 50 completed surveys; (11) There were discrepancies in the data collection process; (12) This measure does not apply to this hospital for this reporting period; (13) Results cannot be calculated for this reporting period; (14) The results for this state are combined with nearby states to protect confidentiality; Please refer to the User's Guide for a full explanation of data.

Riverside Medical Center

1900 South Main St
Franklinton, LA 70438
Phone: 985-795-4431
Type: Critical Access Hospitals
Emergency Services: Yes
Ownership: Govt - Hospital Dist/Auth

Measure	Cases	This Hosp.	State Avg.	U.S. Avg.
Blood Clot Prevention and Treatment				
Anticoagulation Overlap Therapy[5]	-	-	89%	93%
ICU Venous Thromboembolism Prophylaxis[5]	-	-	88%	92%
Incidence of Potentially Preventable VTE[5]	-	-	16%	10%
UFH with Dosages/Platelet Monitoring[5]	-	-	94%	97%
Venous Thromboembolism Prophylaxis[5]	-	-	74%	85%
Warfarin Therapy Discharge Instructions[5]	-	-	85%	75%
Chest Pain/Possible Heart Attack Care				
Aspirin Given Within 24 Hours of Arrival	-	-	94%	96%
Fibrinolytic Meds Within 30 Min. of Arrival	-	-	54%	58%
Average Time to ECG (minutes)	-	-	10	7
Average Time to Transfer (minutes)	-	-	94	60
Children's Asthma Care				
Received Home Management Plan of Care	-	-	-	88%
Received Reliever Medication	-	-	-	100%
Received Systemic Corticosteroids	-	-	-	100%
Emergency Department				
Admittance Decision Time (minutes)[5]	-	-	86	98
Head CT Results Within 45 Min. of Arrival	-	-	49%	57%
Patients Who Left ER Before Being Seen	-	-	3%	2%
Time from ER Arrival to Admit. (minutes)[5]	-	-	256	274
Time from ER Arrival to Discharge (minutes)	-	-	125	134
Time in ER Before Being Evaluated (minutes)	-	-	27	26
Time to Pain Meds for Fractures (minutes)	-	-	61	57
Heart Attack Care				
Aspirin Given at Discharge[5]	-	-	99%	99%
Fibrinolytic Meds Within 30 Min. of Arrival[5]	-	-	71%	54%
PCI Within 90 Minutes of Arrival[5]	-	-	94%	96%
Statin Prescribed at Discharge[5]	-	-	98%	98%
Heart Failure Care				
ACE Inhibitor or ARB for LVSD[5]	-	-	95%	97%
Discharge Instructions Given[5]	-	-	94%	94%
Evaluation of LVS Function[5]	-	-	97%	99%
Medicare Spending				
Medicare Spending per Patient (ratio)	-	-	1.04	0.98
Pneumonia Care				
Appropriate Initial Antibiotic Given[5]	-	-	93%	95%
Blood Culture Timing[5]	-	-	97%	98%
Pregnancy and Delivery Care				
Newborn Deliveries Scheduled Early[5]	-	-	5%	6%
Preventive Care				
Immunization for Influenza[5]	-	-	85%	90%
Immunization for Pneumonia[5]	-	-	88%	92%
Stroke Care				
Anticoagulation Therapy for Atrial Fibrillation[5]	-	-	93%	95%
Antithrombotic Therapy Timing[5]	-	-	96%	98%
Assessed for Rehabilitation[5]	-	-	95%	97%
Discharged on Antithrombotic Therapy[5]	-	-	97%	99%
Discharged on Statin Medication[5]	-	-	89%	94%
Thrombolytic Therapy Timing[5]	-	-	53%	66%
Venous Thromboembolism Prophylaxis[5]	-	-	87%	94%
Written Stroke Educational Materials Given[5]	-	-	83%	88%
Surgical Care Improvement Project				
Appropriate Beta Blocker Usage[5]	-	-	97%	98%
Appropriate VTP Within 24 Hours[5]	-	-	97%	98%
Controlled Postoperative Blood Glucose[5]	-	-	96%	97%
Perioperative Temperature Management[5]	-	-	100%	100%
Prophylactic Antibiotic Selection[5]	-	-	99%	99%
Prophylactic Antibiotic Selection (Outpatient)	-	-	97%	98%
Prophylactic Antibiotic Stopped[5]	-	-	97%	98%
Prophylactic Antibiotic Timing[5]	-	-	98%	99%
Prophylactic Antibiotic Timing (Outpatient)	-	-	97%	98%
Urinary Catheter Removal[5]	-	-	96%	97%
Survey of Patients' Hospital Experiences				
Area Around Room 'Always' Quiet at Night[5]	-	-	74%	61%
Doctors 'Always' Communicated Well[5]	-	-	87%	82%
Home Recovery Information Given[5]	-	-	85%	85%
Hospital Given 9 or 10 on 10 Point Scale[5]	-	-	75%	71%
Meds 'Always' Explained Before Given[5]	-	-	69%	64%
Nurses 'Always' Communicated Well[5]	-	-	83%	79%
Pain 'Always' Well Controlled[5]	-	-	75%	71%
Room and Bathroom 'Always' Clean[5]	-	-	75%	73%
Timely Help 'Always' Received[5]	-	-	71%	68%
Would Definitely Recommend Hospital[5]	-	-	75%	71%
Use of Medical Imaging				
Cardiac Imaging Stress Test before Surgery	-	-	5.3%	5.3%
Combination Abdominal CT Scan	-	-	24.5%	10.5%
Combination Brain/Sinus CT Scan	-	-	2.6%	2.7%
Combination Chest CT Scan	-	-	7.6%	2.7%
Follow-up Mammogram/Ultrasound	-	-	9.4%	8.8%
Lumbar Spine MRI for Low Back Pain	-	-	42.7%	37.2%

Saint Elizabeth Hospital

1125 West Highway 30
Gonzales, LA 70737
Phone: 225-647-5000
Fax: 225-647-7408
URL: www.steh.com
Type: Acute Care Hospitals
Emergency Services: Yes
Ownership: Voluntary non-profit - Private
Beds: 95

Key Personnel:
Radiology. . . . . Albert Alexander
Emergency Room . . . . Jamie Broussard
President/CEO. . . . . Robert Burgess
Chair/CEO . . . . Teri Casso
Chief of Medical Staff. . . . . John Knapp, MD
Operating Room. . . . . Jill Lee
Infection Control. . . . . Susan Waguespack
Patient Relations . . . . Kristin Wolkart

Measure	Cases	This Hosp.	State Avg.	U.S. Avg.
Blood Clot Prevention and Treatment				
Anticoagulation Overlap Therapy[2]	28	100%	89%	93%
ICU Venous Thromboembolism Prophylaxis[2]	63	100%	88%	92%
Incidence of Potentially Preventable VTE[1,2]	-	-	16%	10%
UFH with Dosages/Platelet Monitoring[1,2]	-	-	94%	97%
Venous Thromboembolism Prophylaxis[2]	264	89%	74%	85%
Warfarin Therapy Discharge Instructions[2]	20	90%	85%	75%
Chest Pain/Possible Heart Attack Care				
Aspirin Given Within 24 Hours of Arrival	58	100%	94%	96%
Fibrinolytic Meds Within 30 Min. of Arrival[7]	-	-	54%	58%
Average Time to ECG (minutes)	60	13	10	7
Average Time to Transfer (minutes)[7]	-	-	94	60
Children's Asthma Care				
Received Home Management Plan of Care	-	-	-	88%
Received Reliever Medication	-	-	-	100%
Received Systemic Corticosteroids	-	-	-	100%
Emergency Department				
Admittance Decision Time (minutes)[2]	518	92	86	98
Head CT Results Within 45 Min. of Arrival	12	42%	49%	57%
Patients Who Left ER Before Being Seen	36,848	1%	3%	2%
Time from ER Arrival to Admit. (minutes)[2]	525	257	256	274
Time from ER Arrival to Discharge (minutes)	360	116	125	134
Time in ER Before Being Evaluated (minutes)	379	28	27	26
Time to Pain Meds for Fractures (minutes)	135	51	61	57
Heart Attack Care				
Aspirin Given at Discharge	11	100%	99%	99%
Fibrinolytic Meds Within 30 Min. of Arrival[7]	-	-	71%	54%
PCI Within 90 Minutes of Arrival[7]	-	-	94%	96%
Statin Prescribed at Discharge[1]	-	-	98%	98%
Heart Failure Care				
ACE Inhibitor or ARB for LVSD	35	94%	95%	97%
Discharge Instructions Given	101	100%	94%	94%
Evaluation of LVS Function	124	99%	97%	99%
Medicare Spending				
Medicare Spending per Patient (ratio)	-	1.18	1.04	0.98
Pneumonia Care				
Appropriate Initial Antibiotic Given	93	97%	93%	95%
Blood Culture Timing	177	99%	97%	98%
Pregnancy and Delivery Care				
Newborn Deliveries Scheduled Early[7]	-	-	5%	6%
Preventive Care				
Immunization for Influenza[2]	290	98%	85%	90%
Immunization for Pneumonia[2]	424	97%	88%	92%
Stroke Care				
Anticoagulation Therapy for Atrial Fibrillation[1]	-	-	93%	95%
Antithrombotic Therapy Timing	20	95%	96%	98%
Assessed for Rehabilitation	22	91%	95%	97%
Discharged on Antithrombotic Therapy	22	95%	97%	99%
Discharged on Statin Medication	20	90%	89%	94%
Thrombolytic Therapy Timing[1]	-	-	53%	66%
Venous Thromboembolism Prophylaxis	21	95%	87%	94%
Written Stroke Educational Materials Given	15	87%	83%	88%
Surgical Care Improvement Project				
Appropriate Beta Blocker Usage	69	100%	97%	98%
Appropriate VTP Within 24 Hours	188	100%	97%	98%
Controlled Postoperative Blood Glucose[7]	-	-	96%	97%
Perioperative Temperature Management	196	100%	100%	100%
Prophylactic Antibiotic Selection	137	100%	99%	99%
Prophylactic Antibiotic Selection (Outpatient)	11	73%	97%	98%
Prophylactic Antibiotic Stopped	130	98%	97%	98%
Prophylactic Antibiotic Timing	138	99%	98%	99%
Prophylactic Antibiotic Timing (Outpatient)	14	43%	97%	98%
Urinary Catheter Removal	172	99%	96%	97%
Survey of Patients' Hospital Experiences				
Area Around Room 'Always' Quiet at Night	300+	76%	74%	61%
Doctors 'Always' Communicated Well	300+	86%	87%	82%
Home Recovery Information Given	300+	86%	85%	85%
Hospital Given 9 or 10 on 10 Point Scale	300+	76%	75%	71%
Meds 'Always' Explained Before Given	300+	68%	69%	64%
Nurses 'Always' Communicated Well	300+	84%	83%	79%
Pain 'Always' Well Controlled	300+	71%	75%	71%
Room and Bathroom 'Always' Clean	300+	79%	75%	73%
Timely Help 'Always' Received	300+	72%	71%	68%
Would Definitely Recommend Hospital	300+	80%	75%	71%
Use of Medical Imaging				
Cardiac Imaging Stress Test before Surgery[1]	-	-	5.3%	5.3%
Combination Abdominal CT Scan	357	13.2%	24.5%	10.5%
Combination Brain/Sinus CT Scan[1]	-	-	2.6%	2.7%
Combination Chest CT Scan	113	0.0%	7.6%	2.7%
Follow-up Mammogram/Ultrasound	360	11.4%	9.4%	8.8%
Lumbar Spine MRI for Low Back Pain[1]	-	-	42.7%	37.2%

Saint Helena Parish Hospital

16874 Highway 43
Greensburg, LA 70441
Phone: 225-222-6111
Type: Critical Access Hospitals
Emergency Services: Yes
Ownership: Govt - Hospital Dist/Auth

Measure	Cases	This Hosp.	State Avg.	U.S. Avg.
Blood Clot Prevention and Treatment				
Anticoagulation Overlap Therapy[5]	-	-	89%	93%
ICU Venous Thromboembolism Prophylaxis[5]	-	-	88%	92%
Incidence of Potentially Preventable VTE[5]	-	-	16%	10%
UFH with Dosages/Platelet Monitoring[5]	-	-	94%	97%
Venous Thromboembolism Prophylaxis[5]	-	-	74%	85%
Warfarin Therapy Discharge Instructions[5]	-	-	85%	75%
Chest Pain/Possible Heart Attack Care				
Aspirin Given Within 24 Hours of Arrival	-	-	94%	96%
Fibrinolytic Meds Within 30 Min. of Arrival	-	-	54%	58%
Average Time to ECG (minutes)	-	-	10	7
Average Time to Transfer (minutes)	-	-	94	60
Children's Asthma Care				
Received Home Management Plan of Care	-	-	-	88%
Received Reliever Medication	-	-	-	100%
Received Systemic Corticosteroids	-	-	-	100%
Emergency Department				
Admittance Decision Time (minutes)[5]	-	-	86	98
Head CT Results Within 45 Min. of Arrival	-	-	49%	57%
Patients Who Left ER Before Being Seen	-	-	3%	2%
Time from ER Arrival to Admit. (minutes)[5]	-	-	256	274
Time from ER Arrival to Discharge (minutes)	-	-	125	134
Time in ER Before Being Evaluated (minutes)	-	-	27	26
Time to Pain Meds for Fractures (minutes)	-	-	61	57
Heart Attack Care				
Aspirin Given at Discharge[5]	-	-	99%	99%

NOTE: Hospital profiles are in alphabetical order by state, then city, then hospital within the city; Rankings exclude hospitals with less than 25 cases except for patient surveys which excludes hospitals with less than 100 cases; (a) 100-299 cases; (1) The number of cases/patients is too few to report; (2) Data submitted were based on a sample of cases/patients; (3) Results are based on a shorter time period than required; (4) Data suppressed by CMS for one or more quarters; (5) Results are not available for this reporting period; (6) Fewer than 100 patients completed the HCAHPS survey; (7) No cases met the criteria for this measure; (8) The lower limit of the confidence interval cannot be calculated if the number of observed infections equals zero; (9) No data are available from the state/territory for this reporting period; (10) The scores shown reflect fewer than 50 completed surveys; (11) There were discrepancies in the data collection process; (12) This measure does not apply to this hospital for this reporting period; (13) Results cannot be calculated for this reporting period; (14) The results for this state are combined with nearby states to protect confidentiality; Please refer to the User's Guide for a full explanation of data.

Measure	Cases	This Hosp.	State Avg.	U.S. Avg.
Fibrinolytic Meds Within 30 Min. of Arrival[5]	-	-	71%	54%
PCI Within 90 Minutes of Arrival[5]	-	-	94%	96%
Statin Prescribed at Discharge[5]	-	-	98%	98%
Heart Failure Care				
ACE Inhibitor or ARB for LVSD[3,7]	-	-	95%	97%
Discharge Instructions Given[1,3]	-	-	94%	94%
Evaluation of LVS Function[1,3]	-	-	97%	99%
Medicare Spending				
Medicare Spending per Patient (ratio)	-	-	1.04	0.98
Pneumonia Care				
Appropriate Initial Antibiotic Given[5]	-	-	93%	95%
Blood Culture Timing[5]	-	-	97%	98%
Pregnancy and Delivery Care				
Newborn Deliveries Scheduled Early[5]	-	-	5%	6%
Preventive Care				
Immunization for Influenza[5]	-	-	85%	90%
Immunization for Pneumonia[5]	-	-	88%	92%
Stroke Care				
Anticoagulation Therapy for Atrial Fibrillation[5]	-	-	93%	95%
Antithrombotic Therapy Timing[5]	-	-	96%	98%
Assessed for Rehabilitation[5]	-	-	95%	97%
Discharged on Antithrombotic Therapy[5]	-	-	97%	99%
Discharged on Statin Medication[5]	-	-	89%	94%
Thrombolytic Therapy Timing[5]	-	-	53%	66%
Venous Thromboembolism Prophylaxis[5]	-	-	87%	94%
Written Stroke Educational Materials Given[5]	-	-	83%	88%
Surgical Care Improvement Project				
Appropriate Beta Blocker Usage[5]	-	-	97%	98%
Appropriate VTP Within 24 Hours[5]	-	-	97%	98%
Controlled Postoperative Blood Glucose[5]	-	-	96%	97%
Perioperative Temperature Management[5]	-	-	100%	100%
Prophylactic Antibiotic Selection[5]	-	-	99%	99%
Prophylactic Antibiotic Selection (Outpatient)	-	-	97%	98%
Prophylactic Antibiotic Stopped[5]	-	-	97%	98%
Prophylactic Antibiotic Timing[5]	-	-	98%	99%
Prophylactic Antibiotic Timing (Outpatient)	-	-	97%	98%
Urinary Catheter Removal[5]	-	-	96%	97%
Survey of Patients' Hospital Experiences				
Area Around Room 'Always' Quiet at Night[5]	-	-	74%	61%
Doctors 'Always' Communicated Well[5]	-	-	87%	82%
Home Recovery Information Given[5]	-	-	85%	85%
Hospital Given 9 or 10 on 10 Point Scale[5]	-	-	75%	71%
Meds 'Always' Explained Before Given[5]	-	-	69%	64%
Nurses 'Always' Communicated Well[5]	-	-	83%	79%
Pain 'Always' Well Controlled[5]	-	-	75%	71%
Room and Bathroom 'Always' Clean[5]	-	-	75%	73%
Timely Help 'Always' Received[5]	-	-	71%	68%
Would Definitely Recommend Hospital[5]	-	-	75%	71%
Use of Medical Imaging				
Cardiac Imaging Stress Test before Surgery	-	-	5.3%	5.3%
Combination Abdominal CT Scan	-	-	24.5%	10.5%
Combination Brain/Sinus CT Scan	-	-	2.6%	2.7%
Combination Chest CT Scan	-	-	7.6%	2.7%
Follow-up Mammogram/Ultrasound	-	-	9.4%	8.8%
Lumbar Spine MRI for Low Back Pain	-	-	42.7%	37.2%

Cypress Pointe Surgical Hospital

42570 South Airport Rd Phone: 985-510-6200
Hammond, LA 70403
URL: www.cpsh.org
Type: Acute Care Hospitals Emergency Services: No
Ownership: Proprietary

Measure	Cases	This Hosp.	State Avg.	U.S. Avg.
Blood Clot Prevention and Treatment				
Anticoagulation Overlap Therapy[1]	-	-	89%	93%
ICU Venous Thromboembolism Prophylaxis[7]	-	-	88%	92%
Incidence of Potentially Preventable VTE[1]	-	-	16%	10%
UFH with Dosages/Platelet Monitoring[7]	-	-	94%	97%
Venous Thromboembolism Prophylaxis	169	69%	74%	85%
Warfarin Therapy Discharge Instructions[7]	-	-	85%	75%
Chest Pain/Possible Heart Attack Care				
Aspirin Given Within 24 Hours of Arrival[5]	-	-	94%	96%
Fibrinolytic Meds Within 30 Min. of Arrival[5]	-	-	54%	58%
Average Time to ECG (minutes)[5]	-	-	10	7
Average Time to Transfer (minutes)[5]	-	-	94	60
Children's Asthma Care				
Received Home Management Plan of Care	-	-	-	88%
Received Reliever Medication	-	-	-	100%
Received Systemic Corticosteroids	-	-	-	100%
Emergency Department				
Admittance Decision Time (minutes)[2,7]	-	-	86	98
Head CT Results Within 45 Min. of Arrival[5]	-	-	49%	57%
Patients Who Left ER Before Being Seen[5]	-	-	3%	2%
Time from ER Arrival to Admit. (minutes)[2,7]	-	-	256	274
Time from ER Arrival to Discharge (minutes)[5]	-	-	125	134
Time in ER Before Being Evaluated (minutes)[5]	-	-	27	26
Time to Pain Meds for Fractures (minutes)[5]	-	-	61	57
Heart Attack Care				
Aspirin Given at Discharge[5]	-	-	99%	99%
Fibrinolytic Meds Within 30 Min. of Arrival[5]	-	-	71%	54%
PCI Within 90 Minutes of Arrival[5]	-	-	94%	96%
Statin Prescribed at Discharge[5]	-	-	98%	98%
Heart Failure Care				
ACE Inhibitor or ARB for LVSD[5]	-	-	95%	97%
Discharge Instructions Given[5]	-	-	94%	94%
Evaluation of LVS Function[5]	-	-	97%	99%
Medicare Spending				
Medicare Spending per Patient (ratio)	-	1.34	1.04	0.98
Pneumonia Care				
Appropriate Initial Antibiotic Given[5]	-	-	93%	95%
Blood Culture Timing[5]	-	-	97%	98%
Pregnancy and Delivery Care				
Newborn Deliveries Scheduled Early[7]	-	-	5%	6%
Preventive Care				
Immunization for Influenza	326	78%	85%	90%
Immunization for Pneumonia	327	80%	88%	92%
Stroke Care				
Anticoagulation Therapy for Atrial Fibrillation[5]	-	-	93%	95%
Antithrombotic Therapy Timing[5]	-	-	96%	98%
Assessed for Rehabilitation[5]	-	-	95%	97%
Discharged on Antithrombotic Therapy[5]	-	-	97%	99%
Discharged on Statin Medication[5]	-	-	89%	94%
Thrombolytic Therapy Timing[5]	-	-	53%	66%
Venous Thromboembolism Prophylaxis[5]	-	-	87%	94%
Written Stroke Educational Materials Given[5]	-	-	83%	88%
Surgical Care Improvement Project				
Appropriate Beta Blocker Usage	33	85%	97%	98%
Appropriate VTP Within 24 Hours	102	90%	97%	98%
Controlled Postoperative Blood Glucose[7]	-	-	96%	97%
Perioperative Temperature Management	130	100%	100%	100%
Prophylactic Antibiotic Selection	75	93%	99%	99%
Prophylactic Antibiotic Selection (Outpatient)	182	92%	97%	98%
Prophylactic Antibiotic Stopped	75	97%	97%	98%
Prophylactic Antibiotic Timing	75	97%	98%	99%
Prophylactic Antibiotic Timing (Outpatient)	184	91%	97%	98%
Urinary Catheter Removal	96	97%	96%	97%
Survey of Patients' Hospital Experiences				
Area Around Room 'Always' Quiet at Night	(a)	81%	74%	61%
Doctors 'Always' Communicated Well	(a)	89%	87%	82%
Home Recovery Information Given	(a)	88%	85%	85%
Hospital Given 9 or 10 on 10 Point Scale	(a)	92%	75%	71%
Meds 'Always' Explained Before Given	(a)	77%	69%	64%
Nurses 'Always' Communicated Well	(a)	92%	83%	79%
Pain 'Always' Well Controlled	(a)	79%	75%	71%
Room and Bathroom 'Always' Clean	(a)	91%	75%	73%
Timely Help 'Always' Received	(a)	87%	71%	68%
Would Definitely Recommend Hospital	(a)	92%	75%	71%
Use of Medical Imaging				
Cardiac Imaging Stress Test before Surgery[7]	-	-	5.3%	5.3%
Combination Abdominal CT Scan	87	73.6%	24.5%	10.5%
Combination Brain/Sinus CT Scan[1]	-	-	2.6%	2.7%
Combination Chest CT Scan[1]	-	-	7.6%	2.7%
Follow-up Mammogram/Ultrasound[7]	-	-	9.4%	8.8%
Lumbar Spine MRI for Low Back Pain	137	40.1%	42.7%	37.2%

North Oaks Medical Center

15790 Paul Vega Md Drive Phone: 985-345-2700
Hammond, LA 70403 Fax: 985-230-6482
E-mail: nohs@northoaks.org
URL: www.northoaks.org
Type: Acute Care Hospitals Emergency Services: Yes
Ownership: Govt - Hospital Dist/Auth Beds: 354
Key Personnel:
Radiology. John Braud
CEO/President. . . . . James E Cathey Jr
Chief of Medical Staff. . . . . Robert Peltier, MD

Measure	Cases	This Hosp.	State Avg.	U.S. Avg.
Blood Clot Prevention and Treatment				
Anticoagulation Overlap Therapy[2]	55	95%	89%	93%
ICU Venous Thromboembolism Prophylaxis[2]	52	87%	88%	92%
Incidence of Potentially Preventable VTE[1,2]	-	-	16%	10%
UFH with Dosages/Platelet Monitoring[1,2]	-	-	94%	97%
Venous Thromboembolism Prophylaxis[2]	403	70%	74%	85%
Warfarin Therapy Discharge Instructions[2]	31	39%	85%	75%
Chest Pain/Possible Heart Attack Care				
Aspirin Given Within 24 Hours of Arrival[1,3]	-	-	94%	96%
Fibrinolytic Meds Within 30 Min. of Arrival[3,7]	-	-	54%	58%
Average Time to ECG (minutes)[1,3]	-	-	10	7
Average Time to Transfer (minutes)[3,7]	-	-	94	60
Children's Asthma Care				
Received Home Management Plan of Care	-	-	-	88%
Received Reliever Medication	-	-	-	100%
Received Systemic Corticosteroids	-	-	-	100%
Emergency Department				
Admittance Decision Time (minutes)[2]	644	138	86	98
Head CT Results Within 45 Min. of Arrival[1]	-	-	49%	57%
Patients Who Left ER Before Being Seen	72,361	7%	3%	2%
Time from ER Arrival to Admit. (minutes)[2]	649	272	256	274
Time from ER Arrival to Discharge (minutes)	374	169	125	134
Time in ER Before Being Evaluated (minutes)	394	63	27	26
Time to Pain Meds for Fractures (minutes)	174	67	61	57
Heart Attack Care				
Aspirin Given at Discharge	230	100%	99%	99%
Fibrinolytic Meds Within 30 Min. of Arrival[7]	-	-	71%	54%
PCI Within 90 Minutes of Arrival	45	93%	94%	96%
Statin Prescribed at Discharge	224	95%	98%	98%
Heart Failure Care				
ACE Inhibitor or ARB for LVSD[2]	94	99%	95%	97%
Discharge Instructions Given[2]	242	90%	94%	94%
Evaluation of LVS Function[2]	290	100%	97%	99%
Medicare Spending				
Medicare Spending per Patient (ratio)	-	1.14	1.04	0.98
Pneumonia Care				
Appropriate Initial Antibiotic Given[2]	105	91%	93%	95%
Blood Culture Timing[2]	136	97%	97%	98%
Pregnancy and Delivery Care				
Newborn Deliveries Scheduled Early[2]	29	0%	5%	6%
Preventive Care				
Immunization for Influenza[2]	521	91%	85%	90%
Immunization for Pneumonia[2]	666	87%	88%	92%
Stroke Care				
Anticoagulation Therapy for Atrial Fibrillation[2]	15	80%	93%	95%
Antithrombotic Therapy Timing[2]	89	92%	96%	98%
Assessed for Rehabilitation[2]	98	93%	95%	97%
Discharged on Antithrombotic Therapy[2]	89	92%	97%	99%
Discharged on Statin Medication[2]	67	81%	89%	94%
Thrombolytic Therapy Timing[1,2]	-	-	53%	66%
Venous Thromboembolism Prophylaxis[2]	104	73%	87%	94%
Written Stroke Educational Materials Given[2]	53	53%	83%	88%
Surgical Care Improvement Project				
Appropriate Beta Blocker Usage[2]	191	97%	97%	98%
Appropriate VTP Within 24 Hours[2]	390	89%	97%	98%
Controlled Postoperative Blood Glucose[2]	78	97%	96%	97%
Perioperative Temperature Management[2]	470	99%	100%	100%
Prophylactic Antibiotic Selection[2]	328	98%	99%	99%
Prophylactic Antibiotic Selection (Outpatient)	371	96%	97%	98%
Prophylactic Antibiotic Stopped[2]	320	98%	97%	98%
Prophylactic Antibiotic Timing[2]	329	97%	98%	99%

NOTE: Hospital profiles are in alphabetical order by state, then city, then hospital within the city; Rankings exclude hospitals with less than 25 cases except for patient surveys which excludes hospitals with less than 100 cases; (a) 100-299 cases; (1) The number of cases/patients is too few to report; (2) Data submitted were based on a sample of cases/patients; (3) Results are based on a shorter time period than required; (4) Data suppressed by CMS for one or more quarters; (5) Results are not available for this reporting period; (6) Fewer than 100 patients completed the HCAHPS survey; (7) No cases met the criteria for this measure; (8) The lower limit of the confidence interval cannot be calculated if the number of observed infections equals zero; (9) No data are available from the state/territory for this reporting period; (10) The scores shown reflect fewer than 50 completed surveys; (11) There were discrepancies in the data collection process; (12) This measure does not apply to this hospital for this reporting period; (13) Results cannot be calculated for this reporting period; (14) The results for this state are combined with nearby states to protect confidentiality; Please refer to the User's Guide for a full explanation of data.

Prophylactic Antibiotic Timing (Outpatient)	377	96%	97%	98%
Urinary Catheter Removal[2]	283	93%	96%	97%
Survey of Patients' Hospital Experiences				
Area Around Room 'Always' Quiet at Night	300+	76%	74%	61%
Doctors 'Always' Communicated Well	300+	82%	87%	82%
Home Recovery Information Given	300+	86%	85%	85%
Hospital Given 9 or 10 on 10 Point Scale	300+	72%	75%	71%
Meds 'Always' Explained Before Given	300+	69%	69%	64%
Nurses 'Always' Communicated Well	300+	83%	83%	79%
Pain 'Always' Well Controlled	300+	74%	75%	71%
Room and Bathroom 'Always' Clean	300+	78%	75%	73%
Timely Help 'Always' Received	300+	71%	71%	68%
Would Definitely Recommend Hospital	300+	67%	75%	71%
Use of Medical Imaging				
Cardiac Imaging Stress Test before Surgery	315	5.7%	5.3%	5.3%
Combination Abdominal CT Scan	669	5.8%	24.5%	10.5%
Combination Brain/Sinus CT Scan	757	1.1%	2.6%	2.7%
Combination Chest CT Scan	418	2.6%	7.6%	2.7%
Follow-up Mammogram/Ultrasound	1,169	7.0%	9.4%	8.8%
Lumbar Spine MRI for Low Back Pain	143	46.9%	42.7%	37.2%

Homer Memorial Hospital

620 East College Street
Homer, LA 71040
Phone: 318-927-2024
Fax: 318-927-3158
Type: Acute Care Hospitals
Emergency Services: Yes
Ownership: Government - Local
Beds: 50

Key Personnel:
CEO/President . . . . Doug Efferson
Emergency Room . . . . Larry Ezell, MD
Surgery . . . . John D. Gladney, MD
Chief of Medical Staff . . . . DK Haynes
Cardiology . . . . William Haynie, MD

Measure	Cases	This Hosp.	State Avg.	U.S. Avg.
Blood Clot Prevention and Treatment				
Anticoagulation Overlap Therapy[2,7]	-	-	89%	93%
ICU Venous Thromboembolism Prophylaxis[2]	43	77%	88%	92%
Incidence of Potentially Preventable VTE[1,2]	-	-	16%	10%
UFH with Dosages/Platelet Monitoring[2,7]	-	-	94%	97%
Venous Thromboembolism Prophylaxis[2]	196	74%	74%	85%
Warfarin Therapy Discharge Instructions[2,7]	-	-	85%	75%
Chest Pain/Possible Heart Attack Care				
Aspirin Given Within 24 Hours of Arrival[1,3]	-	-	94%	96%
Fibrinolytic Meds Within 30 Min. of Arrival[1,3]	-	-	54%	58%
Average Time to ECG (minutes)[1,3]	-	-	10	7
Average Time to Transfer (minutes)[3,7]	-	-	94	60
Children's Asthma Care				
Received Home Management Plan of Care	-	-	-	88%
Received Reliever Medication	-	-	-	100%
Received Systemic Corticosteroids	-	-	-	100%
Emergency Department				
Admittance Decision Time (minutes)[2]	481	65	86	98
Head CT Results Within 45 Min. of Arrival[1]	-	-	49%	57%
Patients Who Left ER Before Being Seen	11,524	1%	3%	2%
Time from ER Arrival to Admit. (minutes)[2]	481	176	256	274
Time from ER Arrival to Discharge (minutes)	644	88	125	134
Time in ER Before Being Evaluated (minutes)	657	30	27	26
Time to Pain Meds for Fractures (minutes)	22	55	61	57
Heart Attack Care				
Aspirin Given at Discharge[1,2]	-	-	99%	99%
Fibrinolytic Meds Within 30 Min. of Arrival[2,3]	-	-	71%	54%
PCI Within 90 Minutes of Arrival[2,3]	-	-	94%	96%
Statin Prescribed at Discharge[1,2]	-	-	98%	98%
Heart Failure Care				
ACE Inhibitor or ARB for LVSD[2]	13	100%	95%	97%
Discharge Instructions Given[2]	42	98%	94%	94%
Evaluation of LVS Function[2]	76	62%	97%	99%
Medicare Spending				
Medicare Spending per Patient (ratio)	-	1.17	1.04	0.98
Pneumonia Care				
Appropriate Initial Antibiotic Given[2]	53	79%	93%	95%
Blood Culture Timing[2]	61	89%	97%	98%
Pregnancy and Delivery Care				
Newborn Deliveries Scheduled Early[7]	-	-	5%	6%
Preventive Care				
Immunization for Influenza[2]	297	87%	85%	90%
Immunization for Pneumonia[2]	387	95%	88%	92%
Stroke Care				
Anticoagulation Therapy for Atrial Fibrillation[1,2]	-	-	93%	95%
Antithrombotic Therapy Timing[1,2]	-	-	96%	98%
Assessed for Rehabilitation[1,2]	-	-	95%	97%
Discharged on Antithrombotic Therapy[1,2]	-	-	97%	99%
Discharged on Statin Medication[1,2]	-	-	89%	94%
Thrombolytic Therapy Timing[1,2]	-	-	53%	66%
Venous Thromboembolism Prophylaxis[2]	12	100%	87%	94%
Written Stroke Educational Materials Given[1,2]	-	-	83%	88%
Surgical Care Improvement Project				
Appropriate Beta Blocker Usage[1,2]	-	-	97%	98%
Appropriate VTP Within 24 Hours[1,2]	-	-	97%	98%
Controlled Postoperative Blood Glucose[2,3]	-	-	96%	97%
Perioperative Temperature Management[1,2]	-	-	100%	100%
Prophylactic Antibiotic Selection[1,2]	-	-	99%	99%
Prophylactic Antibiotic Selection (Outpatient)[7]	-	-	97%	98%
Prophylactic Antibiotic Stopped[1,2]	-	-	97%	98%
Prophylactic Antibiotic Timing[1,2]	-	-	98%	99%
Prophylactic Antibiotic Timing (Outpatient)[1]	-	-	97%	98%
Urinary Catheter Removal[1,2]	-	-	96%	97%
Survey of Patients' Hospital Experiences				
Area Around Room 'Always' Quiet at Night	(a)	65%	74%	61%
Doctors 'Always' Communicated Well	(a)	91%	87%	82%
Home Recovery Information Given	(a)	85%	85%	85%
Hospital Given 9 or 10 on 10 Point Scale	(a)	73%	75%	71%
Meds 'Always' Explained Before Given	(a)	65%	69%	64%
Nurses 'Always' Communicated Well	(a)	81%	83%	79%
Pain 'Always' Well Controlled	(a)	72%	75%	71%
Room and Bathroom 'Always' Clean	(a)	71%	75%	73%
Timely Help 'Always' Received	(a)	64%	71%	68%
Would Definitely Recommend Hospital	(a)	66%	75%	71%
Use of Medical Imaging				
Cardiac Imaging Stress Test before Surgery[1]	-	-	5.3%	5.3%
Combination Abdominal CT Scan	107	16.8%	24.5%	10.5%
Combination Brain/Sinus CT Scan[1]	-	-	2.6%	2.7%
Combination Chest CT Scan[1]	-	-	7.6%	2.7%
Follow-up Mammogram/Ultrasound	266	9.0%	9.4%	8.8%
Lumbar Spine MRI for Low Back Pain[1]	-	-	42.7%	37.2%

Leonard J Chabert Medical Center

1978 Industrial Blvd
Houma, LA 70363
Phone: 985-873-1285
Fax: 985-873-1262
E-mail: trahanda@cmc.lhca.state.la.us
URL: www.lsuhsc.edu/hcsd
Type: Acute Care Hospitals
Emergency Services: Yes
Ownership: Government - State
Beds: 147

Key Personnel:
Cardiology . . . . Lee Arcement, MD
Quality Assurance . . . . Mildred Dampeer
CEO . . . . Ritchie Dupre
Chief of Medical Staff . . . . Michael Garcia, MD
CEO/President . . . . Donald R Smithburg

Measure	Cases	This Hosp.	State Avg.	U.S. Avg.
Blood Clot Prevention and Treatment				
Anticoagulation Overlap Therapy[2]	27	89%	89%	93%
ICU Venous Thromboembolism Prophylaxis[2]	45	98%	88%	92%
Incidence of Potentially Preventable VTE[1,2]	-	-	16%	10%
UFH with Dosages/Platelet Monitoring[2]	16	100%	94%	97%
Venous Thromboembolism Prophylaxis[2]	245	92%	74%	85%
Warfarin Therapy Discharge Instructions[2]	23	100%	85%	75%
Chest Pain/Possible Heart Attack Care				
Aspirin Given Within 24 Hours of Arrival	21	100%	94%	96%
Fibrinolytic Meds Within 30 Min. of Arrival[7]	-	-	54%	58%
Average Time to ECG (minutes)	22	5	10	7
Average Time to Transfer (minutes)[1]	-	-	94	60
Children's Asthma Care				
Received Home Management Plan of Care	-	-	-	88%
Received Reliever Medication	-	-	-	100%
Received Systemic Corticosteroids	-	-	-	100%
Emergency Department				
Admittance Decision Time (minutes)[2]	249	165	86	98
Head CT Results Within 45 Min. of Arrival[1,3]	-	-	49%	57%
Patients Who Left ER Before Being Seen	36,360	3%	3%	2%
Time from ER Arrival to Admit. (minutes)[2]	258	494	256	274
Time from ER Arrival to Discharge (minutes)	433	231	125	134
Time in ER Before Being Evaluated (minutes)	465	40	27	26
Time to Pain Meds for Fractures (minutes)	14	95	61	57
Heart Attack Care				
Aspirin Given at Discharge	45	93%	99%	99%
Fibrinolytic Meds Within 30 Min. of Arrival[7]	-	-	71%	54%
PCI Within 90 Minutes of Arrival[7]	-	-	94%	96%
Statin Prescribed at Discharge	42	95%	98%	98%
Heart Failure Care				
ACE Inhibitor or ARB for LVSD	54	100%	95%	97%
Discharge Instructions Given	87	97%	94%	94%
Evaluation of LVS Function	90	100%	97%	99%
Medicare Spending				
Medicare Spending per Patient (ratio)	-	0.88	1.04	0.98
Pneumonia Care				
Appropriate Initial Antibiotic Given	46	100%	93%	95%
Blood Culture Timing	101	99%	97%	98%
Pregnancy and Delivery Care				
Newborn Deliveries Scheduled Early[7]	-	-	5%	6%
Preventive Care				
Immunization for Influenza[2]	378	90%	85%	90%
Immunization for Pneumonia[2]	327	92%	88%	92%
Stroke Care				
Anticoagulation Therapy for Atrial Fibrillation[7]	-	-	93%	95%
Antithrombotic Therapy Timing	30	100%	96%	98%
Assessed for Rehabilitation	31	94%	95%	97%
Discharged on Antithrombotic Therapy	31	100%	97%	99%
Discharged on Statin Medication	26	92%	89%	94%
Thrombolytic Therapy Timing[1]	-	-	53%	66%
Venous Thromboembolism Prophylaxis	26	96%	87%	94%
Written Stroke Educational Materials Given	25	32%	83%	88%
Surgical Care Improvement Project				
Appropriate Beta Blocker Usage	76	100%	97%	98%
Appropriate VTP Within 24 Hours	299	97%	97%	98%
Controlled Postoperative Blood Glucose[7]	-	-	96%	97%
Perioperative Temperature Management	330	100%	100%	100%
Prophylactic Antibiotic Selection	224	100%	99%	99%
Prophylactic Antibiotic Selection (Outpatient)	193	99%	97%	98%
Prophylactic Antibiotic Stopped	216	99%	97%	98%
Prophylactic Antibiotic Timing	224	100%	98%	99%
Prophylactic Antibiotic Timing (Outpatient)	194	99%	97%	98%
Urinary Catheter Removal	165	100%	96%	97%
Survey of Patients' Hospital Experiences				
Area Around Room 'Always' Quiet at Night	300+	71%	74%	61%
Doctors 'Always' Communicated Well	300+	86%	87%	82%
Home Recovery Information Given	300+	81%	85%	85%
Hospital Given 9 or 10 on 10 Point Scale	300+	72%	75%	71%
Meds 'Always' Explained Before Given	300+	69%	69%	64%
Nurses 'Always' Communicated Well	300+	82%	83%	79%
Pain 'Always' Well Controlled	300+	73%	75%	71%
Room and Bathroom 'Always' Clean	300+	71%	75%	73%
Timely Help 'Always' Received	300+	60%	71%	68%
Would Definitely Recommend Hospital	300+	77%	75%	71%
Use of Medical Imaging				
Cardiac Imaging Stress Test before Surgery	181	5.5%	5.3%	5.3%
Combination Abdominal CT Scan	309	16.5%	24.5%	10.5%
Combination Brain/Sinus CT Scan[1]	-	-	2.6%	2.7%
Combination Chest CT Scan	160	3.1%	7.6%	2.7%
Follow-up Mammogram/Ultrasound	778	2.2%	9.4%	8.8%
Lumbar Spine MRI for Low Back Pain[1]	-	-	42.7%	37.2%

Physicians Medical Center

218 Corporate Drive
Houma, LA 70360
Phone: 985-853-1390
URL: www.physicianshouma.com
Type: Acute Care Hospitals
Emergency Services: No
Ownership: Proprietary
Beds: 30

Measure	Cases	This Hosp.	State Avg.	U.S. Avg.
Blood Clot Prevention and Treatment				

NOTE: Hospital profiles are in alphabetical order by state, then city, then hospital within the city; Rankings exclude hospitals with less than 25 cases except for patient surveys which excludes hospitals with less than 100 cases; (a) 100-299 cases; (1) The number of cases/patients is too few to report; (2) Data submitted were based on a sample of cases/patients; (3) Results are based on a shorter time period than required; (4) Data suppressed by CMS for one or more quarters; (5) Results are not available for this reporting period; (6) Fewer than 100 patients completed the HCAHPS survey; (7) No cases met the criteria for this measure; (8) The lower limit of the confidence interval cannot be calculated if the number of observed infections equals zero; (9) No data are available from the state/territory for this reporting period; (10) The scores shown reflect fewer than 50 completed surveys; (11) There were discrepancies in the data collection process; (12) This measure does not apply to this hospital for this reporting period; (13) Results cannot be calculated for this reporting period; (14) The results for this state are combined with nearby states to protect confidentiality; Please refer to the User's Guide for a full explanation of data.

Measure	Cases	This Hosp.	State Avg.	U.S. Avg.
Anticoagulation Overlap Therapy[7]	-	-	89%	93%
ICU Venous Thromboembolism Prophylaxis[7]	-	-	88%	92%
Incidence of Potentially Preventable VTE[7]	-	-	16%	10%
UFH with Dosages/Platelet Monitoring[7]	-	-	94%	97%
Venous Thromboembolism Prophylaxis	88	75%	74%	85%
Warfarin Therapy Discharge Instructions[7]	-	-	85%	75%
Chest Pain/Possible Heart Attack Care				
Aspirin Given Within 24 Hours of Arrival[5]	-	-	94%	96%
Fibrinolytic Meds Within 30 Min. of Arrival[5]	-	-	54%	58%
Average Time to ECG (minutes)[5]	-	-	10	7
Average Time to Transfer (minutes)[5]	-	-	94	60
Children's Asthma Care				
Received Home Management Plan of Care	-	-	-	88%
Received Reliever Medication	-	-	-	100%
Received Systemic Corticosteroids	-	-	-	100%
Emergency Department				
Admittance Decision Time (minutes)[7]	-	-	86	98
Head CT Results Within 45 Min. of Arrival[5]	-	-	49%	57%
Patients Who Left ER Before Being Seen[5]	-	-	3%	2%
Time from ER Arrival to Admit. (minutes)[7]	-	-	256	274
Time from ER Arrival to Discharge (minutes)[5]	-	-	125	134
Time in ER Before Being Evaluated (minutes)[5]	-	-	27	26
Time to Pain Meds for Fractures (minutes)[5]	-	-	61	57
Heart Attack Care				
Aspirin Given at Discharge[5]	-	-	99%	99%
Fibrinolytic Meds Within 30 Min. of Arrival[5]	-	-	71%	54%
PCI Within 90 Minutes of Arrival[5]	-	-	94%	96%
Statin Prescribed at Discharge[5]	-	-	98%	98%
Heart Failure Care				
ACE Inhibitor or ARB for LVSD[5]	-	-	95%	97%
Discharge Instructions Given[5]	-	-	94%	94%
Evaluation of LVS Function[5]	-	-	97%	99%
Medicare Spending				
Medicare Spending per Patient (ratio)	-	1.03	1.04	0.98
Pneumonia Care				
Appropriate Initial Antibiotic Given[5]	-	-	93%	95%
Blood Culture Timing[5]	-	-	97%	98%
Pregnancy and Delivery Care				
Newborn Deliveries Scheduled Early[7]	-	-	5%	6%
Preventive Care				
Immunization for Influenza	151	87%	85%	90%
Immunization for Pneumonia	64	95%	88%	92%
Stroke Care				
Anticoagulation Therapy for Atrial Fibrillation[5]	-	-	93%	95%
Antithrombotic Therapy Timing[5]	-	-	96%	98%
Assessed for Rehabilitation[5]	-	-	95%	97%
Discharged on Antithrombotic Therapy[5]	-	-	97%	99%
Discharged on Statin Medication[5]	-	-	89%	94%
Thrombolytic Therapy Timing[5]	-	-	53%	66%
Venous Thromboembolism Prophylaxis[5]	-	-	87%	94%
Written Stroke Educational Materials Given[5]	-	-	83%	88%
Surgical Care Improvement Project				
Appropriate Beta Blocker Usage	28	93%	97%	98%
Appropriate VTP Within 24 Hours	75	95%	97%	98%
Controlled Postoperative Blood Glucose[7]	-	-	96%	97%
Perioperative Temperature Management	82	100%	100%	100%
Prophylactic Antibiotic Selection	62	100%	99%	99%
Prophylactic Antibiotic Selection (Outpatient)	101	97%	97%	98%
Prophylactic Antibiotic Stopped	59	92%	97%	98%
Prophylactic Antibiotic Timing	62	100%	98%	99%
Prophylactic Antibiotic Timing (Outpatient)	101	100%	97%	98%
Urinary Catheter Removal	52	87%	96%	97%
Survey of Patients' Hospital Experiences				
Area Around Room 'Always' Quiet at Night	(a)	92%	74%	61%
Doctors 'Always' Communicated Well	(a)	89%	87%	82%
Home Recovery Information Given	(a)	90%	85%	85%
Hospital Given 9 or 10 on 10 Point Scale	(a)	86%	75%	71%
Meds 'Always' Explained Before Given	(a)	80%	69%	64%
Nurses 'Always' Communicated Well	(a)	90%	83%	79%
Pain 'Always' Well Controlled	(a)	84%	75%	71%
Room and Bathroom 'Always' Clean	(a)	90%	75%	73%
Timely Help 'Always' Received	(a)	84%	71%	68%
Would Definitely Recommend Hospital	(a)	85%	75%	71%
Use of Medical Imaging				
Cardiac Imaging Stress Test before Surgery[7]	-	-	5.3%	5.3%
Combination Abdominal CT Scan	123	7.3%	24.5%	10.5%
Combination Brain/Sinus CT Scan[1]	-	-	2.6%	2.7%
Combination Chest CT Scan	58	0.0%	7.6%	2.7%
Follow-up Mammogram/Ultrasound	402	8.0%	9.4%	8.8%
Lumbar Spine MRI for Low Back Pain[7]	-	-	42.7%	37.2%

Terrebonne General Medical Center

8166 Main Street
Houma, LA 70360
Phone: 985-873-4141
Fax: 985-873-4215
E-mail: comrelations@cajunnet.com
URL: www.tgmc.com
Type: Acute Care Hospitals
Emergency Services: Yes
Ownership: Govt - Hospital Dist/Auth
Beds: 321

Key Personnel:

Pediatric Ambulatory Care . . . . . . Robert Clark, MD
Chief of Medical Staff . . . . Robert Davis, MD
Radiology. . . . . Joe Fontenot, MD
Infection Control. . . . . Gustavia Growe
Chairman/CEO . . . . Morris Hebert
Intensive Care Unit. . . . . Teresita Melancon, RN
Anesthesiology. . . . . Mohammad Naraghi
CEO/President. . . . . Phyllis Peoples

Measure	Cases	This Hosp.	State Avg.	U.S. Avg.
Blood Clot Prevention and Treatment				
Anticoagulation Overlap Therapy[2]	34	97%	89%	93%
ICU Venous Thromboembolism Prophylaxis[2]	114	86%	88%	92%
Incidence of Potentially Preventable VTE[1,2]	-	-	16%	10%
UFH with Dosages/Platelet Monitoring[2]	29	100%	94%	97%
Venous Thromboembolism Prophylaxis[2]	315	74%	74%	85%
Warfarin Therapy Discharge Instructions[2]	24	92%	85%	75%
Chest Pain/Possible Heart Attack Care				
Aspirin Given Within 24 Hours of Arrival[5]	-	-	94%	96%
Fibrinolytic Meds Within 30 Min. of Arrival[5]	-	-	54%	58%
Average Time to ECG (minutes)[5]	-	-	10	7
Average Time to Transfer (minutes)[5]	-	-	94	60
Children's Asthma Care				
Received Home Management Plan of Care	-	-	-	88%
Received Reliever Medication	-	-	-	100%
Received Systemic Corticosteroids	-	-	-	100%
Emergency Department				
Admittance Decision Time (minutes)[2]	588	86	86	98
Head CT Results Within 45 Min. of Arrival	18	33%	49%	57%
Patients Who Left ER Before Being Seen	53,393	4%	3%	2%
Time from ER Arrival to Admit. (minutes)[2]	592	276	256	274
Time from ER Arrival to Discharge (minutes)	372	131	125	134
Time in ER Before Being Evaluated (minutes)	380	51	27	26
Time to Pain Meds for Fractures (minutes)	143	85	61	57
Heart Attack Care				
Aspirin Given at Discharge	240	99%	99%	99%
Fibrinolytic Meds Within 30 Min. of Arrival[7]	-	-	71%	54%
PCI Within 90 Minutes of Arrival	47	98%	94%	96%
Statin Prescribed at Discharge	249	100%	98%	98%
Heart Failure Care				
ACE Inhibitor or ARB for LVSD	120	100%	95%	97%
Discharge Instructions Given	370	100%	94%	94%
Evaluation of LVS Function	416	99%	97%	99%
Medicare Spending				
Medicare Spending per Patient (ratio)	-	1.00	1.04	0.98
Pneumonia Care				
Appropriate Initial Antibiotic Given	106	99%	93%	95%
Blood Culture Timing	219	98%	97%	98%
Pregnancy and Delivery Care				
Newborn Deliveries Scheduled Early	135	7%	5%	6%
Preventive Care				
Immunization for Influenza[2]	521	94%	85%	90%
Immunization for Pneumonia[2]	749	92%	88%	92%
Stroke Care				
Anticoagulation Therapy for Atrial Fibrillation[1]	-	-	93%	95%
Antithrombotic Therapy Timing	79	100%	96%	98%
Assessed for Rehabilitation	84	98%	95%	97%
Discharged on Antithrombotic Therapy	80	99%	97%	99%
Discharged on Statin Medication	64	98%	89%	94%
Thrombolytic Therapy Timing[7]	-	-	53%	66%
Venous Thromboembolism Prophylaxis	84	89%	87%	94%
Written Stroke Educational Materials Given	48	96%	83%	88%
Surgical Care Improvement Project				
Appropriate Beta Blocker Usage[2]	229	100%	97%	98%
Appropriate VTP Within 24 Hours[2]	358	99%	97%	98%
Controlled Postoperative Blood Glucose[2]	81	95%	96%	97%
Perioperative Temperature Management[2]	412	100%	100%	100%
Prophylactic Antibiotic Selection[2]	383	100%	99%	99%
Prophylactic Antibiotic Selection (Outpatient)	410	98%	97%	98%
Prophylactic Antibiotic Stopped[2]	381	99%	97%	98%
Prophylactic Antibiotic Timing[2]	384	100%	98%	99%
Prophylactic Antibiotic Timing (Outpatient)	409	100%	97%	98%
Urinary Catheter Removal[2]	315	99%	96%	97%
Survey of Patients' Hospital Experiences				
Area Around Room 'Always' Quiet at Night	300+	63%	74%	61%
Doctors 'Always' Communicated Well	300+	84%	87%	82%
Home Recovery Information Given	300+	85%	85%	85%
Hospital Given 9 or 10 on 10 Point Scale	300+	69%	75%	71%
Meds 'Always' Explained Before Given	300+	66%	69%	64%
Nurses 'Always' Communicated Well	300+	83%	83%	79%
Pain 'Always' Well Controlled	300+	73%	75%	71%
Room and Bathroom 'Always' Clean	300+	72%	75%	73%
Timely Help 'Always' Received	300+	65%	71%	68%
Would Definitely Recommend Hospital	300+	69%	75%	71%
Use of Medical Imaging				
Cardiac Imaging Stress Test before Surgery	140	2.9%	5.3%	5.3%
Combination Abdominal CT Scan	1,089	9.4%	24.5%	10.5%
Combination Brain/Sinus CT Scan	820	2.2%	2.6%	2.7%
Combination Chest CT Scan	546	5.1%	7.6%	2.7%
Follow-up Mammogram/Ultrasound	1,092	6.2%	9.4%	8.8%
Lumbar Spine MRI for Low Back Pain	227	44.1%	42.7%	37.2%

Lallie Kemp Medical Center

52579 Highway 21 South
Independence, LA 70443
Phone: 985-878-9421
Fax: 985-878-1306
URL: www.lsuhospitals.org
Type: Critical Access Hospitals
Emergency Services: Yes
Ownership: Government - State
Beds: 90

Key Personnel:

Quality Assurance . . . . Tonia Canale
Pediatric Ambulatory Care . . . . . . Irwin Cohen
Pediatric In-Patient Care . . . . Irwin Cohen
Emergency Room. . . . . Michael Kotler
Anesthesiology. . . . . Jeff Lausteau
CEO/President. . . . . Sherre Pack-Hookfin
Chief of Medical Staff . . . . Kathleen Willis

Measure	Cases	This Hosp.	State Avg.	U.S. Avg.
Blood Clot Prevention and Treatment				
Anticoagulation Overlap Therapy[1]	-	-	89%	93%
ICU Venous Thromboembolism Prophylaxis	86	88%	88%	92%
Incidence of Potentially Preventable VTE[7]	-	-	16%	10%
UFH with Dosages/Platelet Monitoring[1]	-	-	94%	97%
Venous Thromboembolism Prophylaxis	284	80%	74%	85%
Warfarin Therapy Discharge Instructions[1]	-	-	85%	75%
Chest Pain/Possible Heart Attack Care				
Aspirin Given Within 24 Hours of Arrival	-	-	94%	96%
Fibrinolytic Meds Within 30 Min. of Arrival	-	-	54%	58%
Average Time to ECG (minutes)	-	-	10	7
Average Time to Transfer (minutes)	-	-	94	60
Children's Asthma Care				
Received Home Management Plan of Care	-	-	-	88%
Received Reliever Medication	-	-	-	100%
Received Systemic Corticosteroids	-	-	-	100%
Emergency Department				
Admittance Decision Time (minutes)[2]	293	60	86	98
Head CT Results Within 45 Min. of Arrival	-	-	49%	57%
Patients Who Left ER Before Being Seen	-	-	3%	2%
Time from ER Arrival to Admit. (minutes)[2]	354	286	256	274
Time from ER Arrival to Discharge (minutes)	-	-	125	134
Time in ER Before Being Evaluated (minutes)	-	-	27	26
Time to Pain Meds for Fractures (minutes)	-	-	61	57
Heart Attack Care				

NOTE: Hospital profiles are in alphabetical order by state, then city, then hospital within the city; Rankings exclude hospitals with less than 25 cases except for patient surveys which excludes hospitals with less than 100 cases; (a) 100-299 cases; (1) The number of cases/patients is too few to report; (2) Data submitted were based on a sample of cases/patients; (3) Results are based on a shorter time period than required; (4) Data suppressed by CMS for one or more quarters; (5) Results are not available for this reporting period; (6) Fewer than 100 patients completed the HCAHPS survey; (7) No cases met the criteria for this measure; (8) The lower limit of the confidence interval cannot be calculated if the number of observed infections equals zero; (9) No data are available from the state/territory for this reporting period; (10) The scores shown reflect fewer than 50 completed surveys; (11) There were discrepancies in the data collection process; (12) This measure does not apply to this hospital for this reporting period; (13) Results cannot be calculated for this reporting period; (14) The results for this state are combined with nearby states to protect confidentiality; Please refer to the User's Guide for a full explanation of data.

Measure	Cases	This Hosp.	State Avg.	U.S. Avg.
Aspirin Given at Discharge[3,7]	-	-	99%	99%
Fibrinolytic Meds Within 30 Min. of Arrival[3,7]	-	-	71%	54%
PCI Within 90 Minutes of Arrival[3,7]	-	-	94%	96%
Statin Prescribed at Discharge[3,7]	-	-	98%	98%
Heart Failure Care				
ACE Inhibitor or ARB for LVSD[1]	-	-	95%	97%
Discharge Instructions Given	19	95%	94%	94%
Evaluation of LVS Function	19	100%	97%	99%
Medicare Spending				
Medicare Spending per Patient (ratio)	-	-	1.04	0.98
Pneumonia Care				
Appropriate Initial Antibiotic Given	25	100%	93%	95%
Blood Culture Timing	36	89%	97%	98%
Pregnancy and Delivery Care				
Newborn Deliveries Scheduled Early[7]	-	-	5%	6%
Preventive Care				
Immunization for Influenza[2]	279	97%	85%	90%
Immunization for Pneumonia[2]	341	96%	88%	92%
Stroke Care				
Anticoagulation Therapy for Atrial Fibrillation[5]	-	-	93%	95%
Antithrombotic Therapy Timing[5]	-	-	96%	98%
Assessed for Rehabilitation[5]	-	-	95%	97%
Discharged on Antithrombotic Therapy[5]	-	-	97%	99%
Discharged on Statin Medication[5]	-	-	89%	94%
Thrombolytic Therapy Timing[5]	-	-	53%	66%
Venous Thromboembolism Prophylaxis[5]	-	-	87%	94%
Written Stroke Educational Materials Given[5]	-	-	83%	88%
Surgical Care Improvement Project				
Appropriate Beta Blocker Usage[1]	-	-	97%	98%
Appropriate VTP Within 24 Hours	66	95%	97%	98%
Controlled Postoperative Blood Glucose[3,7]	-	-	96%	97%
Perioperative Temperature Management	91	100%	100%	100%
Prophylactic Antibiotic Selection	67	100%	99%	99%
Prophylactic Antibiotic Selection (Outpatient)	-	-	97%	98%
Prophylactic Antibiotic Stopped	67	99%	97%	98%
Prophylactic Antibiotic Timing	67	96%	98%	99%
Prophylactic Antibiotic Timing (Outpatient)	-	-	97%	98%
Urinary Catheter Removal	17	94%	96%	97%
Survey of Patients' Hospital Experiences				
Area Around Room 'Always' Quiet at Night	(a)	76%	74%	61%
Doctors 'Always' Communicated Well	(a)	82%	87%	82%
Home Recovery Information Given	(a)	83%	85%	85%
Hospital Given 9 or 10 on 10 Point Scale	(a)	73%	75%	71%
Meds 'Always' Explained Before Given	(a)	61%	69%	64%
Nurses 'Always' Communicated Well	(a)	82%	83%	79%
Pain 'Always' Well Controlled	(a)	71%	75%	71%
Room and Bathroom 'Always' Clean	(a)	85%	75%	73%
Timely Help 'Always' Received	(a)	73%	71%	68%
Would Definitely Recommend Hospital	(a)	75%	75%	71%
Use of Medical Imaging				
Cardiac Imaging Stress Test before Surgery	-	-	5.3%	5.3%
Combination Abdominal CT Scan	-	-	24.5%	10.5%
Combination Brain/Sinus CT Scan	-	-	2.6%	2.7%
Combination Chest CT Scan	-	-	7.6%	2.7%
Follow-up Mammogram/Ultrasound	-	-	9.4%	8.8%
Lumbar Spine MRI for Low Back Pain	-	-	42.7%	37.2%

Villa Feliciana Medical Complex

5002 Highway 10 Phone: 225-634-4010
Jackson, LA 70748 Fax: 225-634-4191
Type: Acute Care Hospitals Emergency Services: No
Ownership: Government - State Beds: 225
Key Personnel:
Infection Control. . . . . Jessica Holden
Hemotology Center . . . . Ann McDaniel-Echols
Chief of Medical Staff. . . . . John Piker

Measure	Cases	This Hosp.	State Avg.	U.S. Avg.
Blood Clot Prevention and Treatment				
Anticoagulation Overlap Therapy[5]	-	-	89%	93%
ICU Venous Thromboembolism Prophylaxis[5]	-	-	88%	92%
Incidence of Potentially Preventable VTE[5]	-	-	16%	10%
UFH with Dosages/Platelet Monitoring[5]	-	-	94%	97%
Venous Thromboembolism Prophylaxis[5]	-	-	74%	85%
Warfarin Therapy Discharge Instructions[5]	-	-	85%	75%
Chest Pain/Possible Heart Attack Care				
Aspirin Given Within 24 Hours of Arrival	-	-	94%	96%
Fibrinolytic Meds Within 30 Min. of Arrival	-	-	54%	58%
Average Time to ECG (minutes)	-	-	10	7
Average Time to Transfer (minutes)	-	-	94	60
Children's Asthma Care				
Received Home Management Plan of Care	-	-	-	88%
Received Reliever Medication	-	-	-	100%
Received Systemic Corticosteroids	-	-	-	100%
Emergency Department				
Admittance Decision Time (minutes)[2,3]	-	-	86	98
Head CT Results Within 45 Min. of Arrival	-	-	49%	57%
Patients Who Left ER Before Being Seen	-	-	3%	2%
Time from ER Arrival to Admit. (minutes)[2,3]	-	-	256	274
Time from ER Arrival to Discharge (minutes)	-	-	125	134
Time in ER Before Being Evaluated (minutes)	-	-	27	26
Time to Pain Meds for Fractures (minutes)	-	-	61	57
Heart Attack Care				
Aspirin Given at Discharge[5]	-	-	99%	99%
Fibrinolytic Meds Within 30 Min. of Arrival[5]	-	-	71%	54%
PCI Within 90 Minutes of Arrival[5]	-	-	94%	96%
Statin Prescribed at Discharge[5]	-	-	98%	98%
Heart Failure Care				
ACE Inhibitor or ARB for LVSD[5]	-	-	95%	97%
Discharge Instructions Given[5]	-	-	94%	94%
Evaluation of LVS Function[5]	-	-	97%	99%
Medicare Spending				
Medicare Spending per Patient (ratio)[1]	-	-	1.04	0.98
Pneumonia Care				
Appropriate Initial Antibiotic Given[5]	-	-	93%	95%
Blood Culture Timing[5]	-	-	97%	98%
Pregnancy and Delivery Care				
Newborn Deliveries Scheduled Early[2,7]	-	-	5%	6%
Preventive Care				
Immunization for Influenza[1,2]	-	-	85%	90%
Immunization for Pneumonia[1,2]	-	-	88%	92%
Stroke Care				
Anticoagulation Therapy for Atrial Fibrillation[5]	-	-	93%	95%
Antithrombotic Therapy Timing[5]	-	-	96%	98%
Assessed for Rehabilitation[5]	-	-	95%	97%
Discharged on Antithrombotic Therapy[5]	-	-	97%	99%
Discharged on Statin Medication[5]	-	-	89%	94%
Thrombolytic Therapy Timing[5]	-	-	53%	66%
Venous Thromboembolism Prophylaxis[5]	-	-	87%	94%
Written Stroke Educational Materials Given[5]	-	-	83%	88%
Surgical Care Improvement Project				
Appropriate Beta Blocker Usage[5]	-	-	97%	98%
Appropriate VTP Within 24 Hours[5]	-	-	97%	98%
Controlled Postoperative Blood Glucose[5]	-	-	96%	97%
Perioperative Temperature Management[5]	-	-	100%	100%
Prophylactic Antibiotic Selection[5]	-	-	99%	99%
Prophylactic Antibiotic Selection (Outpatient)	-	-	97%	98%
Prophylactic Antibiotic Stopped[5]	-	-	97%	98%
Prophylactic Antibiotic Timing[5]	-	-	98%	99%
Prophylactic Antibiotic Timing (Outpatient)	-	-	97%	98%
Urinary Catheter Removal[5]	-	-	96%	97%
Survey of Patients' Hospital Experiences				
Area Around Room 'Always' Quiet at Night[1]	-	-	74%	61%
Doctors 'Always' Communicated Well[1]	-	-	87%	82%
Home Recovery Information Given[1]	-	-	85%	85%
Hospital Given 9 or 10 on 10 Point Scale[1]	-	-	75%	71%
Meds 'Always' Explained Before Given[1]	-	-	69%	64%
Nurses 'Always' Communicated Well[1]	-	-	83%	79%
Pain 'Always' Well Controlled[1]	-	-	75%	71%
Room and Bathroom 'Always' Clean[1]	-	-	75%	73%
Timely Help 'Always' Received[1]	-	-	71%	68%
Would Definitely Recommend Hospital[1]	-	-	75%	71%
Use of Medical Imaging				
Cardiac Imaging Stress Test before Surgery	-	-	5.3%	5.3%
Combination Abdominal CT Scan	-	-	24.5%	10.5%
Combination Brain/Sinus CT Scan	-	-	2.6%	2.7%
Combination Chest CT Scan	-	-	7.6%	2.7%
Follow-up Mammogram/Ultrasound	-	-	9.4%	8.8%
Lumbar Spine MRI for Low Back Pain	-	-	42.7%	37.2%

Lasalle General Hospital

187 Ninth St/hwy 84 West Phone: 318-992-9200
Jena, LA 71342 Fax: 318-992-9245
E-mail: information@lasallegeneralhospital.com
URL: www.lasallegeneralhospital.com
Type: Acute Care Hospitals Emergency Services: Yes
Ownership: Govt - Hospital Dist/Auth Beds: 60
Key Personnel:
CEO/President. . . . . Douglas A. Newman
Quality Assurance . . . . Jane Paul
Emergency Room . . . . Gabriela Rohr
Chief of Medical Staff. . . . . Sinit Srookul

Measure	Cases	This Hosp.	State Avg.	U.S. Avg.
Blood Clot Prevention and Treatment				
Anticoagulation Overlap Therapy[2]	12	75%	89%	93%
ICU Venous Thromboembolism Prophylaxis[2,7]	-	-	88%	92%
Incidence of Potentially Preventable VTE[2,7]	-	-	16%	10%
UFH with Dosages/Platelet Monitoring[1,2]	-	-	94%	97%
Venous Thromboembolism Prophylaxis[2]	173	47%	74%	85%
Warfarin Therapy Discharge Instructions[1,2]	-	-	85%	75%
Chest Pain/Possible Heart Attack Care				
Aspirin Given Within 24 Hours of Arrival	55	91%	94%	96%
Fibrinolytic Meds Within 30 Min. of Arrival[1]	-	-	54%	58%
Average Time to ECG (minutes)	57	12	10	7
Average Time to Transfer (minutes)[7]	-	-	94	60
Children's Asthma Care				
Received Home Management Plan of Care	-	-	-	88%
Received Reliever Medication	-	-	-	100%
Received Systemic Corticosteroids	-	-	-	100%
Emergency Department				
Admittance Decision Time (minutes)[2]	352	90	86	98
Head CT Results Within 45 Min. of Arrival[1]	-	-	49%	57%
Patients Who Left ER Before Being Seen	9,971	1%	3%	2%
Time from ER Arrival to Admit. (minutes)[2]	353	260	256	274
Time from ER Arrival to Discharge (minutes)	289	109	125	134
Time in ER Before Being Evaluated (minutes)	424	22	27	26
Time to Pain Meds for Fractures (minutes)	53	61	61	57
Heart Attack Care				
Aspirin Given at Discharge[5]	-	-	99%	99%
Fibrinolytic Meds Within 30 Min. of Arrival[5]	-	-	71%	54%
PCI Within 90 Minutes of Arrival[5]	-	-	94%	96%
Statin Prescribed at Discharge[5]	-	-	98%	98%
Heart Failure Care				
ACE Inhibitor or ARB for LVSD[1]	-	-	95%	97%
Discharge Instructions Given	12	100%	94%	94%
Evaluation of LVS Function	16	100%	97%	99%
Medicare Spending				
Medicare Spending per Patient (ratio)	-	0.88	1.04	0.98
Pneumonia Care				
Appropriate Initial Antibiotic Given	62	90%	93%	95%
Blood Culture Timing	96	97%	97%	98%
Pregnancy and Delivery Care				
Newborn Deliveries Scheduled Early[7]	-	-	5%	6%
Preventive Care				
Immunization for Influenza[2]	232	92%	85%	90%
Immunization for Pneumonia[2]	367	99%	88%	92%
Stroke Care				
Anticoagulation Therapy for Atrial Fibrillation[7]	-	-	93%	95%
Antithrombotic Therapy Timing[1]	-	-	96%	98%
Assessed for Rehabilitation[1]	-	-	95%	97%
Discharged on Antithrombotic Therapy[1]	-	-	97%	99%
Discharged on Statin Medication[1]	-	-	89%	94%
Thrombolytic Therapy Timing[1]	-	-	53%	66%
Venous Thromboembolism Prophylaxis[1]	-	-	87%	94%
Written Stroke Educational Materials Given[1]	-	-	83%	88%
Surgical Care Improvement Project				
Appropriate Beta Blocker Usage[3,7]	-	-	97%	98%
Appropriate VTP Within 24 Hours[3,7]	-	-	97%	98%
Controlled Postoperative Blood Glucose[3,7]	-	-	96%	97%
Perioperative Temperature Management[1,3]	-	-	100%	100%

NOTE: Hospital profiles are in alphabetical order by state, then city, then hospital within the city; Rankings exclude hospitals with less than 25 cases except for patient surveys which excludes hospitals with less than 100 cases; (a) 100-299 cases; (1) The number of cases/patients is too few to report; (2) Data submitted were based on a sample of cases/patients; (3) Results are based on a shorter time period than required; (4) Data suppressed by CMS for one or more quarters; (5) Results are not available for this reporting period; (6) Fewer than 100 patients completed the HCAHPS survey; (7) No cases met the criteria for this measure; (8) The lower limit of the confidence interval cannot be calculated if the number of observed infections equals zero; (9) No data are available from the state/territory for this reporting period; (10) The scores shown reflect fewer than 50 completed surveys; (11) There were discrepancies in the data collection process; (12) This measure does not apply to this hospital for this reporting period; (13) Results cannot be calculated for this reporting period; (14) The results for this state are combined with nearby states to protect confidentiality; Please refer to the User's Guide for a full explanation of data.

Measure	Cases	This Hosp.	State Avg.	U.S. Avg.
Prophylactic Antibiotic Selection[1,3]	-	-	99%	99%
Prophylactic Antibiotic Selection (Outpatient)[1,3]	-	-	97%	98%
Prophylactic Antibiotic Stopped[1,3]	-	-	97%	98%
Prophylactic Antibiotic Timing[1,3]	-	-	98%	99%
Prophylactic Antibiotic Timing (Outpatient)[1,3]	-	-	97%	98%
Urinary Catheter Removal[3,7]	-	-	96%	97%
Survey of Patients' Hospital Experiences				
Area Around Room 'Always' Quiet at Night[6]	<100	69%	74%	61%
Doctors 'Always' Communicated Well[6]	<100	87%	87%	82%
Home Recovery Information Given[6]	<100	88%	85%	85%
Hospital Given 9 or 10 on 10 Point Scale[6]	<100	72%	75%	71%
Meds 'Always' Explained Before Given[6]	<100	72%	69%	64%
Nurses 'Always' Communicated Well[6]	<100	88%	83%	79%
Pain 'Always' Well Controlled[6]	<100	80%	75%	71%
Room and Bathroom 'Always' Clean[6]	<100	84%	75%	73%
Timely Help 'Always' Received[6]	<100	85%	71%	68%
Would Definitely Recommend Hospital[6]	<100	73%	75%	71%
Use of Medical Imaging				
Cardiac Imaging Stress Test before Surgery	71	2.8%	5.3%	5.3%
Combination Abdominal CT Scan	141	1.4%	24.5%	10.5%
Combination Brain/Sinus CT Scan	222	0.9%	2.6%	2.7%
Combination Chest CT Scan	48	2.1%	7.6%	2.7%
Follow-up Mammogram/Ultrasound	173	12.7%	9.4%	8.8%
Lumbar Spine MRI for Low Back Pain[1]	-	-	42.7%	37.2%

Jennings American Legion Hospital

1634 Elton Road
Jennings, LA 70546
Phone: 337-616-7000
Fax: 337-616-7044
E-mail: webmail@jalh.com
URL: www.jalh.com
Type: Acute Care Hospitals
Emergency Services: Yes
Ownership: Voluntary non-profit - Private
Beds: 178

Key Personnel:
Operating Room. . . . . Nell Freed
Emergency Room . . . . Faye Kershaw
Quality Assurance . . . . Gary LaCaze
Anesthesiology. . . . . Arshavir Michael, MD
Chief of Medical Staff. . . . . Arshavir Michael, MD
Intensive Care Unit. . . . . Tricia Semar
Infection Control. . . . . Connie Sittig
CEO/President. . . . . Terry Terrebonne

Measure	Cases	This Hosp.	State Avg.	U.S. Avg.
Blood Clot Prevention and Treatment				
Anticoagulation Overlap Therapy[2]	19	89%	89%	93%
ICU Venous Thromboembolism Prophylaxis[2]	52	87%	88%	92%
Incidence of Potentially Preventable VTE[2,7]	-	-	16%	10%
UFH with Dosages/Platelet Monitoring[1,2]	-	-	94%	97%
Venous Thromboembolism Prophylaxis[2]	281	75%	74%	85%
Warfarin Therapy Discharge Instructions[2]	11	82%	85%	75%
Chest Pain/Possible Heart Attack Care				
Aspirin Given Within 24 Hours of Arrival	38	100%	94%	96%
Fibrinolytic Meds Within 30 Min. of Arrival[1]	-	-	54%	58%
Average Time to ECG (minutes)	38	7	10	7
Average Time to Transfer (minutes)[1]	-	-	94	60
Children's Asthma Care				
Received Home Management Plan of Care	-	-	-	88%
Received Reliever Medication	-	-	-	100%
Received Systemic Corticosteroids	-	-	-	100%
Emergency Department				
Admittance Decision Time (minutes)[2]	296	64	86	98
Head CT Results Within 45 Min. of Arrival[1]	-	-	49%	57%
Patients Who Left ER Before Being Seen	15,272	7%	3%	2%
Time from ER Arrival to Admit. (minutes)[2]	299	229	256	274
Time from ER Arrival to Discharge (minutes)	373	130	125	134
Time in ER Before Being Evaluated (minutes)	363	27	27	26
Time to Pain Meds for Fractures (minutes)	56	52	61	57
Heart Attack Care				
Aspirin Given at Discharge	17	100%	99%	99%
Fibrinolytic Meds Within 30 Min. of Arrival[1]	-	-	71%	54%
PCI Within 90 Minutes of Arrival[7]	-	-	94%	96%
Statin Prescribed at Discharge	17	100%	98%	98%
Heart Failure Care				
ACE Inhibitor or ARB for LVSD	45	100%	95%	97%
Discharge Instructions Given	102	100%	94%	94%
Evaluation of LVS Function	137	100%	97%	99%
Medicare Spending				
Medicare Spending per Patient (ratio)	-	1.04	1.04	0.98
Pneumonia Care				
Appropriate Initial Antibiotic Given	88	100%	93%	95%
Blood Culture Timing	91	100%	97%	98%
Pregnancy and Delivery Care				
Newborn Deliveries Scheduled Early	32	3%	5%	6%
Preventive Care				
Immunization for Influenza[2]	318	93%	85%	90%
Immunization for Pneumonia[2]	401	95%	88%	92%
Stroke Care				
Anticoagulation Therapy for Atrial Fibrillation[1]	-	-	93%	95%
Antithrombotic Therapy Timing	34	94%	96%	98%
Assessed for Rehabilitation	39	92%	95%	97%
Discharged on Antithrombotic Therapy	34	97%	97%	99%
Discharged on Statin Medication	29	86%	89%	94%
Thrombolytic Therapy Timing[1]	-	-	53%	66%
Venous Thromboembolism Prophylaxis	38	87%	87%	94%
Written Stroke Educational Materials Given[1]	-	-	83%	88%
Surgical Care Improvement Project				
Appropriate Beta Blocker Usage	43	98%	97%	98%
Appropriate VTP Within 24 Hours	138	99%	97%	98%
Controlled Postoperative Blood Glucose[7]	-	-	96%	97%
Perioperative Temperature Management	154	100%	100%	100%
Prophylactic Antibiotic Selection	128	100%	99%	99%
Prophylactic Antibiotic Selection (Outpatient)	89	99%	97%	98%
Prophylactic Antibiotic Stopped	127	98%	97%	98%
Prophylactic Antibiotic Timing	128	98%	98%	99%
Prophylactic Antibiotic Timing (Outpatient)	89	100%	97%	98%
Urinary Catheter Removal	64	98%	96%	97%
Survey of Patients' Hospital Experiences				
Area Around Room 'Always' Quiet at Night	300+	75%	74%	61%
Doctors 'Always' Communicated Well	300+	88%	87%	82%
Home Recovery Information Given	300+	88%	85%	85%
Hospital Given 9 or 10 on 10 Point Scale	300+	73%	75%	71%
Meds 'Always' Explained Before Given	300+	71%	69%	64%
Nurses 'Always' Communicated Well	300+	83%	83%	79%
Pain 'Always' Well Controlled	300+	77%	75%	71%
Room and Bathroom 'Always' Clean	300+	75%	75%	73%
Timely Help 'Always' Received	300+	73%	71%	68%
Would Definitely Recommend Hospital	300+	68%	75%	71%
Use of Medical Imaging				
Cardiac Imaging Stress Test before Surgery	142	4.2%	5.3%	5.3%
Combination Abdominal CT Scan[1]	-	-	24.5%	10.5%
Combination Brain/Sinus CT Scan[1]	-	-	2.6%	2.7%
Combination Chest CT Scan[1]	-	-	7.6%	2.7%
Follow-up Mammogram/Ultrasound[7]	-	-	9.4%	8.8%
Lumbar Spine MRI for Low Back Pain[1]	-	-	42.7%	37.2%

Jackson Parish Hospital

165 Beech Springs Road
Jonesboro, LA 71251
Phone: 318-259-4435
Fax: 318-395-4259
E-mail: nashw@stfran.com
URL: www.jacksonparishhospital.com
Type: Critical Access Hospitals
Emergency Services: Yes
Ownership: Govt - Hospital Dist/Auth
Beds: 49

Key Personnel:
Operating Room. . . . . Bonita Caskey
Chief of Medical Staff. . . . . Rebecca Crouch, MD
Infection Control. . . . . Mary Lynn McBride
CEO/President. . . . . LJ Pecot
Emergency Room . . . . Ann Standley

Measure	Cases	This Hosp.	State Avg.	U.S. Avg.
Blood Clot Prevention and Treatment				
Anticoagulation Overlap Therapy[5]	-	-	89%	93%
ICU Venous Thromboembolism Prophylaxis[5]	-	-	88%	92%
Incidence of Potentially Preventable VTE[5]	-	-	16%	10%
UFH with Dosages/Platelet Monitoring[5]	-	-	94%	97%
Venous Thromboembolism Prophylaxis[5]	-	-	74%	85%
Warfarin Therapy Discharge Instructions[5]	-	-	85%	75%
Chest Pain/Possible Heart Attack Care				
Aspirin Given Within 24 Hours of Arrival[1,3]	-	-	94%	96%
Fibrinolytic Meds Within 30 Min. of Arrival[3,7]	-	-	54%	58%
Average Time to ECG (minutes)[1,3]	-	-	10	7
Average Time to Transfer (minutes)[3,7]	-	-	94	60
Children's Asthma Care				
Received Home Management Plan of Care	-	-	-	88%
Received Reliever Medication	-	-	-	100%
Received Systemic Corticosteroids	-	-	-	100%
Emergency Department				
Admittance Decision Time (minutes)[5]	-	-	86	98
Head CT Results Within 45 Min. of Arrival[1,3]	-	-	49%	57%
Patients Who Left ER Before Being Seen	7,796	1%	3%	2%
Time from ER Arrival to Admit. (minutes)[5]	-	-	256	274
Time from ER Arrival to Discharge (minutes)	288	99	125	134
Time in ER Before Being Evaluated (minutes)	321	28	27	26
Time to Pain Meds for Fractures (minutes)[3,7]	-	-	61	57
Heart Attack Care				
Aspirin Given at Discharge[5]	-	-	99%	99%
Fibrinolytic Meds Within 30 Min. of Arrival[5]	-	-	71%	54%
PCI Within 90 Minutes of Arrival[5]	-	-	94%	96%
Statin Prescribed at Discharge[5]	-	-	98%	98%
Heart Failure Care				
ACE Inhibitor or ARB for LVSD[1]	-	-	95%	97%
Discharge Instructions Given	22	18%	94%	94%
Evaluation of LVS Function	24	83%	97%	99%
Medicare Spending				
Medicare Spending per Patient (ratio)	-	-	1.04	0.98
Pneumonia Care				
Appropriate Initial Antibiotic Given	53	87%	93%	95%
Blood Culture Timing	38	58%	97%	98%
Pregnancy and Delivery Care				
Newborn Deliveries Scheduled Early[5]	-	-	5%	6%
Preventive Care				
Immunization for Influenza[5]	-	-	85%	90%
Immunization for Pneumonia[5]	-	-	88%	92%
Stroke Care				
Anticoagulation Therapy for Atrial Fibrillation[5]	-	-	93%	95%
Antithrombotic Therapy Timing[5]	-	-	96%	98%
Assessed for Rehabilitation[5]	-	-	95%	97%
Discharged on Antithrombotic Therapy[5]	-	-	97%	99%
Discharged on Statin Medication[5]	-	-	89%	94%
Thrombolytic Therapy Timing[5]	-	-	53%	66%
Venous Thromboembolism Prophylaxis[5]	-	-	87%	94%
Written Stroke Educational Materials Given[5]	-	-	83%	88%
Surgical Care Improvement Project				
Appropriate Beta Blocker Usage[5]	-	-	97%	98%
Appropriate VTP Within 24 Hours[5]	-	-	97%	98%
Controlled Postoperative Blood Glucose[5]	-	-	96%	97%
Perioperative Temperature Management[5]	-	-	100%	100%
Prophylactic Antibiotic Selection[5]	-	-	99%	99%
Prophylactic Antibiotic Selection (Outpatient)[5]	-	-	97%	98%
Prophylactic Antibiotic Stopped[5]	-	-	97%	98%
Prophylactic Antibiotic Timing[5]	-	-	98%	99%
Prophylactic Antibiotic Timing (Outpatient)[5]	-	-	97%	98%
Urinary Catheter Removal[5]	-	-	96%	97%
Survey of Patients' Hospital Experiences				
Area Around Room 'Always' Quiet at Night	(a)	66%	74%	61%
Doctors 'Always' Communicated Well	(a)	84%	87%	82%
Home Recovery Information Given	(a)	80%	85%	85%
Hospital Given 9 or 10 on 10 Point Scale	(a)	68%	75%	71%
Meds 'Always' Explained Before Given	(a)	61%	69%	64%
Nurses 'Always' Communicated Well	(a)	81%	83%	79%
Pain 'Always' Well Controlled	(a)	69%	75%	71%
Room and Bathroom 'Always' Clean	(a)	70%	75%	73%
Timely Help 'Always' Received	(a)	71%	71%	68%
Would Definitely Recommend Hospital	(a)	62%	75%	71%
Use of Medical Imaging				
Cardiac Imaging Stress Test before Surgery[7]	-	-	5.3%	5.3%
Combination Abdominal CT Scan	133	16.5%	24.5%	10.5%
Combination Brain/Sinus CT Scan	233	6.9%	2.6%	2.7%
Combination Chest CT Scan	109	9.2%	7.6%	2.7%
Follow-up Mammogram/Ultrasound	153	4.6%	9.4%	8.8%
Lumbar Spine MRI for Low Back Pain[1]	-	-	42.7%	37.2%

NOTE: Hospital profiles are in alphabetical order by state, then city, then hospital within the city; Rankings exclude hospitals with less than 25 cases except for patient surveys which excludes hospitals with less than 100 cases; (a) 100-299 cases; (1) The number of cases/patients is too few to report; (2) Data submitted were based on a sample of cases/patients; (3) Results are based on a shorter time period than required; (4) Data suppressed by CMS for one or more quarters; (5) Results are not available for this reporting period; (6) Fewer than 100 patients completed the HCAHPS survey; (7) No cases met the criteria for this measure; (8) The lower limit of the confidence interval cannot be calculated if the number of observed infections equals zero; (9) No data are available from the state/territory for this reporting period; (10) The scores shown reflect fewer than 50 completed surveys; (11) There were discrepancies in the data collection process; (12) This measure does not apply to this hospital for this reporting period; (13) Results cannot be calculated for this reporting period; (14) The results for this state are combined with nearby states to protect confidentiality; Please refer to the User's Guide for a full explanation of data.

Abrom Kaplan Memorial Hospital

1310 West Seventh Street Phone: 337-643-8300
Kaplan, LA 70548 Fax: 337-643-5309
URL: www.compasshealthcare.com/site78.php
Type: Critical Access Hospitals Emergency Services: Yes
Ownership: Govt - Hospital Dist/Auth Beds: 50

Key Personnel:
Quality Assurance . . . . Danny Faulk
Chief of Medical Staff. . . . . Randell Faulk
Emergency Room . . . . Kitty Lormand, RN
CEO . . . . Bryce Quebodeaux
Infection Control. . . . . Terry Williams
Operating Room. . . . . Terry Williams

Measure	Cases	This Hosp.	State Avg.	U.S. Avg.
Blood Clot Prevention and Treatment				
Anticoagulation Overlap Therapy[1,3]	-	-	89%	93%
ICU Venous Thromboembolism Prophylaxis[3,7]	-	-	88%	92%
Incidence of Potentially Preventable VTE[3,7]	-	-	16%	10%
UFH with Dosages/Platelet Monitoring[3,7]	-	-	94%	97%
Venous Thromboembolism Prophylaxis[3,7]	-	-	74%	85%
Warfarin Therapy Discharge Instructions[1,3]	-	-	85%	75%
Chest Pain/Possible Heart Attack Care				
Aspirin Given Within 24 Hours of Arrival	-	-	94%	96%
Fibrinolytic Meds Within 30 Min. of Arrival	-	-	54%	58%
Average Time to ECG (minutes)	-	-	10	7
Average Time to Transfer (minutes)	-	-	94	60
Children's Asthma Care				
Received Home Management Plan of Care	-	-	-	88%
Received Reliever Medication	-	-	-	100%
Received Systemic Corticosteroids	-	-	-	100%
Emergency Department				
Admittance Decision Time (minutes)[5]	-	-	86	98
Head CT Results Within 45 Min. of Arrival	-	-	49%	57%
Patients Who Left ER Before Being Seen	-	-	3%	2%
Time from ER Arrival to Admit. (minutes)[5]	-	-	256	274
Time from ER Arrival to Discharge (minutes)	-	-	125	134
Time in ER Before Being Evaluated (minutes)	-	-	27	26
Time to Pain Meds for Fractures (minutes)	-	-	61	57
Heart Attack Care				
Aspirin Given at Discharge[5]	-	-	99%	99%
Fibrinolytic Meds Within 30 Min. of Arrival[5]	-	-	71%	54%
PCI Within 90 Minutes of Arrival[5]	-	-	94%	96%
Statin Prescribed at Discharge[5]	-	-	98%	98%
Heart Failure Care				
ACE Inhibitor or ARB for LVSD[1]	-	-	95%	97%
Discharge Instructions Given	17	71%	94%	94%
Evaluation of LVS Function	28	61%	97%	99%
Medicare Spending				
Medicare Spending per Patient (ratio)	-	-	1.04	0.98
Pneumonia Care				
Appropriate Initial Antibiotic Given	18	94%	93%	95%
Blood Culture Timing	16	88%	97%	98%
Pregnancy and Delivery Care				
Newborn Deliveries Scheduled Early[5]	-	-	5%	6%
Preventive Care				
Immunization for Influenza[5]	-	-	85%	90%
Immunization for Pneumonia[5]	-	-	88%	92%
Stroke Care				
Anticoagulation Therapy for Atrial Fibrillation[3,7]	-	-	93%	95%
Antithrombotic Therapy Timing[1,3]	-	-	96%	98%
Assessed for Rehabilitation[1,3]	-	-	95%	97%
Discharged on Antithrombotic Therapy[1,3]	-	-	97%	99%
Discharged on Statin Medication[1,3]	-	-	89%	94%
Thrombolytic Therapy Timing[3,7]	-	-	53%	66%
Venous Thromboembolism Prophylaxis[1,3]	-	-	87%	94%
Written Stroke Educational Materials Given[3,7]	-	-	83%	88%
Surgical Care Improvement Project				
Appropriate Beta Blocker Usage[1,3]	-	-	97%	98%
Appropriate VTP Within 24 Hours[1,3]	-	-	97%	98%
Controlled Postoperative Blood Glucose[3,7]	-	-	96%	97%
Perioperative Temperature Management[1,3]	-	-	100%	100%
Prophylactic Antibiotic Selection[3,7]	-	-	99%	99%
Prophylactic Antibiotic Selection (Outpatient)	-	-	97%	98%
Prophylactic Antibiotic Stopped[3,7]	-	-	97%	98%
Prophylactic Antibiotic Timing[3,7]	-	-	98%	99%
Prophylactic Antibiotic Timing (Outpatient)	-	-	97%	98%
Urinary Catheter Removal[1,3]	-	-	96%	97%
Survey of Patients' Hospital Experiences				
Area Around Room 'Always' Quiet at Night[5]	-	-	74%	61%
Doctors 'Always' Communicated Well[5]	-	-	87%	82%
Home Recovery Information Given[5]	-	-	85%	85%
Hospital Given 9 or 10 on 10 Point Scale[5]	-	-	75%	71%
Meds 'Always' Explained Before Given[5]	-	-	69%	64%
Nurses 'Always' Communicated Well[5]	-	-	83%	79%
Pain 'Always' Well Controlled[5]	-	-	75%	71%
Room and Bathroom 'Always' Clean[5]	-	-	75%	73%
Timely Help 'Always' Received[5]	-	-	71%	68%
Would Definitely Recommend Hospital[5]	-	-	75%	71%
Use of Medical Imaging				
Cardiac Imaging Stress Test before Surgery	-	-	5.3%	5.3%
Combination Abdominal CT Scan	-	-	24.5%	10.5%
Combination Brain/Sinus CT Scan	-	-	2.6%	2.7%
Combination Chest CT Scan	-	-	7.6%	2.7%
Follow-up Mammogram/Ultrasound	-	-	9.4%	8.8%
Lumbar Spine MRI for Low Back Pain	-	-	42.7%	37.2%

Ochsner Medical Center - Kenner

180 West Esplanade Avenue Phone: 504-464-8065
Kenner, LA 70065 Fax: 504-464-8139
URL: www.kenneregional.com
Type: Acute Care Hospitals Emergency Services: Yes
Ownership: Voluntary non-profit - Private Beds: 203

Key Personnel:
Emergency Room . . . . Elizabeth Allen, RN
Chief of Medical Staff. . . . . Melissa Ponthieux
CEO/President. . . . . Paolo Zambito, RN

Measure	Cases	This Hosp.	State Avg.	U.S. Avg.
Blood Clot Prevention and Treatment				
Anticoagulation Overlap Therapy[2]	29	93%	89%	93%
ICU Venous Thromboembolism Prophylaxis[2]	124	90%	88%	92%
Incidence of Potentially Preventable VTE[2]	11	45%	16%	10%
UFH with Dosages/Platelet Monitoring[2]	16	94%	94%	97%
Venous Thromboembolism Prophylaxis[2]	290	81%	74%	85%
Warfarin Therapy Discharge Instructions[2]	16	81%	85%	75%
Chest Pain/Possible Heart Attack Care				
Aspirin Given Within 24 Hours of Arrival[3,7]	-	-	94%	96%
Fibrinolytic Meds Within 30 Min. of Arrival[5]	-	-	54%	58%
Average Time to ECG (minutes)[3,7]	-	-	10	7
Average Time to Transfer (minutes)[5]	-	-	94	60
Children's Asthma Care				
Received Home Management Plan of Care	-	-	-	88%
Received Reliever Medication	-	-	-	100%
Received Systemic Corticosteroids	-	-	-	100%
Emergency Department				
Admittance Decision Time (minutes)[2]	370	155	86	98
Head CT Results Within 45 Min. of Arrival	18	56%	49%	57%
Patients Who Left ER Before Being Seen	38,425	1%	3%	2%
Time from ER Arrival to Admit. (minutes)[2]	370	350	256	274
Time from ER Arrival to Discharge (minutes)	350	122	125	134
Time in ER Before Being Evaluated (minutes)	380	18	27	26
Time to Pain Meds for Fractures (minutes)	88	53	61	57
Heart Attack Care				
Aspirin Given at Discharge[2]	198	98%	99%	99%
Fibrinolytic Meds Within 30 Min. of Arrival[2,7]	-	-	71%	54%
PCI Within 90 Minutes of Arrival[2]	32	100%	94%	96%
Statin Prescribed at Discharge[2]	194	97%	98%	98%
Heart Failure Care				
ACE Inhibitor or ARB for LVSD[2]	96	100%	95%	97%
Discharge Instructions Given[2]	183	98%	94%	94%
Evaluation of LVS Function[2]	215	100%	97%	99%
Medicare Spending				
Medicare Spending per Patient (ratio)	-	0.97	1.04	0.98
Pneumonia Care				
Appropriate Initial Antibiotic Given[2]	51	98%	93%	95%
Blood Culture Timing[2]	141	99%	97%	98%
Pregnancy and Delivery Care				
Newborn Deliveries Scheduled Early[2]	26	4%	5%	6%
Preventive Care				
Immunization for Influenza[2]	482	84%	85%	90%
Immunization for Pneumonia[2]	505	88%	88%	92%
Stroke Care				
Anticoagulation Therapy for Atrial Fibrillation[1]	-	-	93%	95%
Antithrombotic Therapy Timing	37	97%	96%	98%
Assessed for Rehabilitation	40	100%	95%	97%
Discharged on Antithrombotic Therapy	38	100%	97%	99%
Discharged on Statin Medication	33	97%	89%	94%
Thrombolytic Therapy Timing[7]	-	-	53%	66%
Venous Thromboembolism Prophylaxis	38	92%	87%	94%
Written Stroke Educational Materials Given	29	86%	83%	88%
Surgical Care Improvement Project				
Appropriate Beta Blocker Usage[2]	60	98%	97%	98%
Appropriate VTP Within 24 Hours[2]	245	97%	97%	98%
Controlled Postoperative Blood Glucose[1,2]	-	-	96%	97%
Perioperative Temperature Management[2]	284	100%	100%	100%
Prophylactic Antibiotic Selection[2]	196	99%	99%	99%
Prophylactic Antibiotic Selection (Outpatient)	86	99%	97%	98%
Prophylactic Antibiotic Stopped[2]	181	97%	97%	98%
Prophylactic Antibiotic Timing[2]	197	99%	98%	99%
Prophylactic Antibiotic Timing (Outpatient)	88	98%	97%	98%
Urinary Catheter Removal[2]	165	99%	96%	97%
Survey of Patients' Hospital Experiences				
Area Around Room 'Always' Quiet at Night	300+	57%	74%	61%
Doctors 'Always' Communicated Well	300+	80%	87%	82%
Home Recovery Information Given	300+	85%	85%	85%
Hospital Given 9 or 10 on 10 Point Scale	300+	66%	75%	71%
Meds 'Always' Explained Before Given	300+	58%	69%	64%
Nurses 'Always' Communicated Well	300+	76%	83%	79%
Pain 'Always' Well Controlled	300+	67%	75%	71%
Room and Bathroom 'Always' Clean	300+	62%	75%	73%
Timely Help 'Always' Received	300+	60%	71%	68%
Would Definitely Recommend Hospital	300+	63%	75%	71%
Use of Medical Imaging				
Cardiac Imaging Stress Test before Surgery	98	6.1%	5.3%	5.3%
Combination Abdominal CT Scan	339	26.5%	24.5%	10.5%
Combination Brain/Sinus CT Scan[1]	-	-	2.6%	2.7%
Combination Chest CT Scan	144	1.4%	7.6%	2.7%
Follow-up Mammogram/Ultrasound	301	5.3%	9.4%	8.8%
Lumbar Spine MRI for Low Back Pain[1]	-	-	42.7%	37.2%

Allen Parish Hospital

108 6th Avenue Phone: 337-738-2527
Kinder, LA 70648 Fax: 337-738-2901
E-mail: allenph@yahoo.com
Type: Acute Care Hospitals Emergency Services: Yes
Ownership: Govt - Hospital Dist/Auth Beds: 49

Key Personnel:
Chief of Medical Staff. . . . . Peggy Allemand, MD
CEO/President. . . . . Scott G Barrilleaux
Quality Assurance . . . . Deidra Dunagan
Infection Control. . . . . Paige Fontenot
Emergency Room . . . . Levie Johnson
CEO . . . . Don Kannady
Radiology. . . . . Terry Robin

Measure	Cases	This Hosp.	State Avg.	U.S. Avg.
Blood Clot Prevention and Treatment				
Anticoagulation Overlap Therapy[7]	-	-	89%	93%
ICU Venous Thromboembolism Prophylaxis[7]	-	-	88%	92%
Incidence of Potentially Preventable VTE[7]	-	-	16%	10%
UFH with Dosages/Platelet Monitoring[7]	-	-	94%	97%
Venous Thromboembolism Prophylaxis	58	14%	74%	85%
Warfarin Therapy Discharge Instructions[7]	-	-	85%	75%
Chest Pain/Possible Heart Attack Care				
Aspirin Given Within 24 Hours of Arrival[1,3]	-	-	94%	96%
Fibrinolytic Meds Within 30 Min. of Arrival[3,7]	-	-	54%	58%
Average Time to ECG (minutes)[1,3]	-	-	10	7
Average Time to Transfer (minutes)[3,7]	-	-	94	60
Children's Asthma Care				
Received Home Management Plan of Care	-	-	-	88%
Received Reliever Medication	-	-	-	100%
Received Systemic Corticosteroids	-	-	-	100%
Emergency Department				

NOTE: Hospital profiles are in alphabetical order by state, then city, then hospital within the city; Rankings exclude hospitals with less than 25 cases except for patient surveys which excludes hospitals with less than 100 cases; (a) 100-299 cases; (1) The number of cases/patients is too few to report; (2) Data submitted were based on a sample of cases/patients; (3) Results are based on a shorter time period than required; (4) Data suppressed by CMS for one or more quarters; (5) Results are not available for this reporting period; (6) Fewer than 100 patients completed the HCAHPS survey; (7) No cases met the criteria for this measure; (8) The lower limit of the confidence interval cannot be calculated if the number of observed infections equals zero; (9) No data are available from the state/territory for this reporting period; (10) The scores shown reflect fewer than 50 completed surveys; (11) There were discrepancies in the data collection process; (12) This measure does not apply to this hospital for this reporting period; (13) Results cannot be calculated for this reporting period; (14) The results for this state are combined with nearby states to protect confidentiality; Please refer to the User's Guide for a full explanation of data.

Measure	Cases	This Hosp.	State Avg.	U.S. Avg.
Admittance Decision Time (minutes)[2]	49	0	86	98
Head CT Results Within 45 Min. of Arrival[5]	-	-	49%	57%
Patients Who Left ER Before Being Seen	5,456	1%	3%	2%
Time from ER Arrival to Admit. (minutes)[2]	49	220	256	274
Time from ER Arrival to Discharge (minutes)[3]	608	110	125	134
Time in ER Before Being Evaluated (minutes)[3]	694	0	27	26
Time to Pain Meds for Fractures (minutes)[1,3]	-	-	61	57
Heart Attack Care				
Aspirin Given at Discharge[5]	-	-	99%	99%
Fibrinolytic Meds Within 30 Min. of Arrival[5]	-	-	71%	54%
PCI Within 90 Minutes of Arrival[5]	-	-	94%	96%
Statin Prescribed at Discharge[5]	-	-	98%	98%
Heart Failure Care				
ACE Inhibitor or ARB for LVSD[2,3]	-	-	95%	97%
Discharge Instructions Given[1,2]	-	-	94%	94%
Evaluation of LVS Function[2,3]	11	100%	97%	99%
Medicare Spending				
Medicare Spending per Patient (ratio)	-	1.01	1.04	0.98
Pneumonia Care				
Appropriate Initial Antibiotic Given[2]	12	83%	93%	95%
Blood Culture Timing[1,2]	-	-	97%	98%
Pregnancy and Delivery Care				
Newborn Deliveries Scheduled Early[7]	-	-	5%	6%
Preventive Care				
Immunization for Influenza[2]	81	69%	85%	90%
Immunization for Pneumonia[2]	78	71%	88%	92%
Stroke Care				
Anticoagulation Therapy for Atrial Fibrillation[5]	-	-	93%	95%
Antithrombotic Therapy Timing[5]	-	-	96%	98%
Assessed for Rehabilitation[5]	-	-	95%	97%
Discharged on Antithrombotic Therapy[5]	-	-	97%	99%
Discharged on Statin Medication[5]	-	-	89%	94%
Thrombolytic Therapy Timing[5]	-	-	53%	66%
Venous Thromboembolism Prophylaxis[5]	-	-	87%	94%
Written Stroke Educational Materials Given[5]	-	-	83%	88%
Surgical Care Improvement Project				
Appropriate Beta Blocker Usage[5]	-	-	97%	98%
Appropriate VTP Within 24 Hours[5]	-	-	97%	98%
Controlled Postoperative Blood Glucose[5]	-	-	96%	97%
Perioperative Temperature Management[5]	-	-	100%	100%
Prophylactic Antibiotic Selection[5]	-	-	99%	99%
Prophylactic Antibiotic Selection (Outpatient)[5]	-	-	97%	98%
Prophylactic Antibiotic Stopped[5]	-	-	97%	98%
Prophylactic Antibiotic Timing[5]	-	-	98%	99%
Prophylactic Antibiotic Timing (Outpatient)[5]	-	-	97%	98%
Urinary Catheter Removal[5]	-	-	96%	97%
Survey of Patients' Hospital Experiences				
Area Around Room 'Always' Quiet at Night[10]	<100	86%	74%	61%
Doctors 'Always' Communicated Well[10]	<100	96%	87%	82%
Home Recovery Information Given[10]	<100	90%	85%	85%
Hospital Given 9 or 10 on 10 Point Scale[10]	<100	80%	75%	71%
Meds 'Always' Explained Before Given[10]	<100	80%	69%	64%
Nurses 'Always' Communicated Well[10]	<100	89%	83%	79%
Pain 'Always' Well Controlled[10]	<100	76%	75%	71%
Room and Bathroom 'Always' Clean[10]	<100	86%	75%	73%
Timely Help 'Always' Received[10]	<100	85%	71%	68%
Would Definitely Recommend Hospital[10]	<100	76%	75%	71%
Use of Medical Imaging				
Cardiac Imaging Stress Test before Surgery[7]	-	-	5.3%	5.3%
Combination Abdominal CT Scan	52	40.4%	24.5%	10.5%
Combination Brain/Sinus CT Scan[1]	-	-	2.6%	2.7%
Combination Chest CT Scan[1]	-	-	7.6%	2.7%
Follow-up Mammogram/Ultrasound[7]	-	-	9.4%	8.8%
Lumbar Spine MRI for Low Back Pain[7]	-	-	42.7%	37.2%

Louisiana Heart Hospital

64030 Highway 434
Lacombe, LA 70445
Phone: 985-690-7500
Fax: 985-690-7530
E-mail: info@louisianahearthospital.com
URL: www.louisianahearthospital.com
Type: Acute Care Hospitals
Emergency Services: Yes
Ownership: Proprietary
Beds: 137

Key Personnel:

Radiology. . . . . Sean Behlar
Quality Assurance . . . . Donna Breaux
Intensive Care Unit. . . . . Julie Diodene
CEO/President. . . . . Donnie Frederic, FACHE
Surgery . . . . Cary Gray, MD
Emergency Room . . . . Tania Loumiet
Operating Room. . . . . Claire Manuel
Cardiology . . . . Lisa Mejia, APRN

Measure	Cases	This Hosp.	State Avg.	U.S. Avg.
Blood Clot Prevention and Treatment				
Anticoagulation Overlap Therapy[2]	15	80%	89%	93%
ICU Venous Thromboembolism Prophylaxis[2]	110	94%	88%	92%
Incidence of Potentially Preventable VTE[1,2]	-	-	16%	10%
UFH with Dosages/Platelet Monitoring[1,2]	-	-	94%	97%
Venous Thromboembolism Prophylaxis[2]	198	90%	74%	85%
Warfarin Therapy Discharge Instructions[1,2]	-	-	85%	75%
Chest Pain/Possible Heart Attack Care				
Aspirin Given Within 24 Hours of Arrival[1,3]	-	-	94%	96%
Fibrinolytic Meds Within 30 Min. of Arrival[5]	-	-	54%	58%
Average Time to ECG (minutes)[1,3]	-	-	10	7
Average Time to Transfer (minutes)[5]	-	-	94	60
Children's Asthma Care				
Received Home Management Plan of Care	-	-	-	88%
Received Reliever Medication	-	-	-	100%
Received Systemic Corticosteroids	-	-	-	100%
Emergency Department				
Admittance Decision Time (minutes)[2]	204	84	86	98
Head CT Results Within 45 Min. of Arrival[1]	-	-	49%	57%
Patients Who Left ER Before Being Seen	9,861	1%	3%	2%
Time from ER Arrival to Admit. (minutes)[2]	349	250	256	274
Time from ER Arrival to Discharge (minutes)	387	140	125	134
Time in ER Before Being Evaluated (minutes)	385	19	27	26
Time to Pain Meds for Fractures (minutes)	29	79	61	57
Heart Attack Care				
Aspirin Given at Discharge	92	100%	99%	99%
Fibrinolytic Meds Within 30 Min. of Arrival[7]	-	-	71%	54%
PCI Within 90 Minutes of Arrival	13	85%	94%	96%
Statin Prescribed at Discharge	94	99%	98%	98%
Heart Failure Care				
ACE Inhibitor or ARB for LVSD	60	92%	95%	97%
Discharge Instructions Given	157	97%	94%	94%
Evaluation of LVS Function	169	100%	97%	99%
Medicare Spending				
Medicare Spending per Patient (ratio)	-	0.98	1.04	0.98
Pneumonia Care				
Appropriate Initial Antibiotic Given	44	93%	93%	95%
Blood Culture Timing	69	99%	97%	98%
Pregnancy and Delivery Care				
Newborn Deliveries Scheduled Early[7]	-	-	5%	6%
Preventive Care				
Immunization for Influenza[2]	326	94%	85%	90%
Immunization for Pneumonia[2]	516	90%	88%	92%
Stroke Care				
Anticoagulation Therapy for Atrial Fibrillation[1]	-	-	93%	95%
Antithrombotic Therapy Timing	30	100%	96%	98%
Assessed for Rehabilitation	31	84%	95%	97%
Discharged on Antithrombotic Therapy	31	100%	97%	99%
Discharged on Statin Medication	28	96%	89%	94%
Thrombolytic Therapy Timing[1]	-	-	53%	66%
Venous Thromboembolism Prophylaxis	27	96%	87%	94%
Written Stroke Educational Materials Given	22	91%	83%	88%
Surgical Care Improvement Project				
Appropriate Beta Blocker Usage[2]	163	98%	97%	98%
Appropriate VTP Within 24 Hours[2]	62	97%	97%	98%
Controlled Postoperative Blood Glucose[2]	181	92%	96%	97%
Perioperative Temperature Management[2]	137	100%	100%	100%
Prophylactic Antibiotic Selection[2]	212	100%	99%	99%
Prophylactic Antibiotic Selection (Outpatient)	195	98%	97%	98%
Prophylactic Antibiotic Stopped[2]	211	93%	97%	98%
Prophylactic Antibiotic Timing[2]	212	100%	98%	99%
Prophylactic Antibiotic Timing (Outpatient)	201	92%	97%	98%
Urinary Catheter Removal[2]	232	95%	96%	97%
Survey of Patients' Hospital Experiences				
Area Around Room 'Always' Quiet at Night	300+	71%	74%	61%
Doctors 'Always' Communicated Well	300+	83%	87%	82%
Home Recovery Information Given	300+	86%	85%	85%
Hospital Given 9 or 10 on 10 Point Scale	300+	83%	75%	71%
Meds 'Always' Explained Before Given	300+	67%	69%	64%
Nurses 'Always' Communicated Well	300+	84%	83%	79%
Pain 'Always' Well Controlled	300+	77%	75%	71%
Room and Bathroom 'Always' Clean	300+	74%	75%	73%
Timely Help 'Always' Received	300+	73%	71%	68%
Would Definitely Recommend Hospital	300+	86%	75%	71%
Use of Medical Imaging				
Cardiac Imaging Stress Test before Surgery	585	4.1%	5.3%	5.3%
Combination Abdominal CT Scan	113	15.9%	24.5%	10.5%
Combination Brain/Sinus CT Scan[1]	-	-	2.6%	2.7%
Combination Chest CT Scan	70	2.9%	7.6%	2.7%
Follow-up Mammogram/Ultrasound[7]	-	-	9.4%	8.8%
Lumbar Spine MRI for Low Back Pain[1]	-	-	42.7%	37.2%

Heart Hospital of Lafayette

1105 Kaliste Saloom Road
Lafayette, LA 70508
Phone: 337-521-1000
Fax: 337-521-1006
E-mail: info@hearthospitaloflafayette.com
URL: www.hearthospitaloflafayette.com
Type: Acute Care Hospitals
Emergency Services: Yes
Ownership: Proprietary
Beds: 24

Key Personnel:

Chief of Medical Staff . . . . Edgar Feinberg, MD
Operating Room. . . . . John Horn
Infection Control. . . . . Vicky Manuel
Cardiac Laboratory. . . . . Elizabeth Reinhardt
CEO/President. . . . . Karen Wyble

Measure	Cases	This Hosp.	State Avg.	U.S. Avg.
Blood Clot Prevention and Treatment				
Anticoagulation Overlap Therapy[1,2]	-	-	89%	93%
ICU Venous Thromboembolism Prophylaxis[2]	73	95%	88%	92%
Incidence of Potentially Preventable VTE[1,2]	-	-	16%	10%
UFH with Dosages/Platelet Monitoring[1,2]	-	-	94%	97%
Venous Thromboembolism Prophylaxis[2]	120	65%	74%	85%
Warfarin Therapy Discharge Instructions[1,2]	-	-	85%	75%
Chest Pain/Possible Heart Attack Care				
Aspirin Given Within 24 Hours of Arrival[5]	-	-	94%	96%
Fibrinolytic Meds Within 30 Min. of Arrival[5]	-	-	54%	58%
Average Time to ECG (minutes)[5]	-	-	10	7
Average Time to Transfer (minutes)[5]	-	-	94	60
Children's Asthma Care				
Received Home Management Plan of Care	-	-	-	88%
Received Reliever Medication	-	-	-	100%
Received Systemic Corticosteroids	-	-	-	100%
Emergency Department				
Admittance Decision Time (minutes)[2]	114	46	86	98
Head CT Results Within 45 Min. of Arrival[5]	-	-	49%	57%
Patients Who Left ER Before Being Seen	2,503	0%	3%	2%
Time from ER Arrival to Admit. (minutes)[2]	114	167	256	274
Time from ER Arrival to Discharge (minutes)	234	135	125	134
Time in ER Before Being Evaluated (minutes)	308	5	27	26
Time to Pain Meds for Fractures (minutes)[5]	-	-	61	57
Heart Attack Care				
Aspirin Given at Discharge	265	100%	99%	99%
Fibrinolytic Meds Within 30 Min. of Arrival[7]	-	-	71%	54%
PCI Within 90 Minutes of Arrival	14	93%	94%	96%
Statin Prescribed at Discharge	240	98%	98%	98%
Heart Failure Care				
ACE Inhibitor or ARB for LVSD	31	100%	95%	97%
Discharge Instructions Given	99	100%	94%	94%
Evaluation of LVS Function	113	96%	97%	99%
Medicare Spending				
Medicare Spending per Patient (ratio)	-	0.97	1.04	0.98
Pneumonia Care				
Appropriate Initial Antibiotic Given[1]	-	-	93%	95%
Blood Culture Timing	16	100%	97%	98%
Pregnancy and Delivery Care				
Newborn Deliveries Scheduled Early[7]	-	-	5%	6%
Preventive Care				
Immunization for Influenza[2]	323	94%	85%	90%
Immunization for Pneumonia[2]	493	90%	88%	92%

NOTE: Hospital profiles are in alphabetical order by state, then city, then hospital within the city; Rankings exclude hospitals with less than 25 cases except for patient surveys which excludes hospitals with less than 100 cases; (a) 100-299 cases; (1) The number of cases/patients is too few to report; (2) Data submitted were based on a sample of cases/patients; (3) Results are based on a shorter time period than required; (4) Data suppressed by CMS for one or more quarters; (5) Results are not available for this reporting period; (6) Fewer than 100 patients completed the HCAHPS survey; (7) No cases met the criteria for this measure; (8) The lower limit of the confidence interval cannot be calculated if the number of observed infections equals zero; (9) No data are available from the state/territory for this reporting period; (10) The scores shown reflect fewer than 50 completed surveys; (11) There were discrepancies in the data collection process; (12) This measure does not apply to this hospital for this reporting period; (13) Results cannot be calculated for this reporting period; (14) The results for this state are combined with nearby states to protect confidentiality; Please refer to the User's Guide for a full explanation of data.

Measure	Cases	This Hosp.	State Avg.	U.S. Avg.
Stroke Care				
Anticoagulation Therapy for Atrial Fibrillation[1]	-	-	93%	95%
Antithrombotic Therapy Timing[1]	-	-	96%	98%
Assessed for Rehabilitation[1]	-	-	95%	97%
Discharged on Antithrombotic Therapy[1]	-	-	97%	99%
Discharged on Statin Medication[1]	-	-	89%	94%
Thrombolytic Therapy Timing[1]	-	-	53%	66%
Venous Thromboembolism Prophylaxis[1]	-	-	87%	94%
Written Stroke Educational Materials Given[1]	-	-	83%	88%
Surgical Care Improvement Project				
Appropriate Beta Blocker Usage	234	100%	97%	98%
Appropriate VTP Within 24 Hours	16	94%	97%	98%
Controlled Postoperative Blood Glucose	343	96%	96%	97%
Perioperative Temperature Management	419	100%	100%	100%
Prophylactic Antibiotic Selection	361	100%	99%	99%
Prophylactic Antibiotic Selection (Outpatient)	241	100%	97%	98%
Prophylactic Antibiotic Stopped	359	100%	97%	98%
Prophylactic Antibiotic Timing	366	100%	98%	99%
Prophylactic Antibiotic Timing (Outpatient)	241	100%	97%	98%
Urinary Catheter Removal	314	100%	96%	97%
Survey of Patients' Hospital Experiences				
Area Around Room 'Always' Quiet at Night	300+	82%	74%	61%
Doctors 'Always' Communicated Well	300+	90%	87%	82%
Home Recovery Information Given	300+	88%	85%	85%
Hospital Given 9 or 10 on 10 Point Scale	300+	92%	75%	71%
Meds 'Always' Explained Before Given	300+	82%	69%	64%
Nurses 'Always' Communicated Well	300+	94%	83%	79%
Pain 'Always' Well Controlled	300+	85%	75%	71%
Room and Bathroom 'Always' Clean	300+	86%	75%	73%
Timely Help 'Always' Received	300+	89%	71%	68%
Would Definitely Recommend Hospital	300+	92%	75%	71%
Use of Medical Imaging				
Cardiac Imaging Stress Test before Surgery	150	2.7%	5.3%	5.3%
Combination Abdominal CT Scan[1]	-	-	24.5%	10.5%
Combination Brain/Sinus CT Scan[1]	-	-	2.6%	2.7%
Combination Chest CT Scan	123	5.7%	7.6%	2.7%
Follow-up Mammogram/Ultrasound[7]	-	-	9.4%	8.8%
Lumbar Spine MRI for Low Back Pain[7]	-	-	42.7%	37.2%

Lafayette General Medical Center

1214 Coolidge Avenue
Lafayette, LA 70503
Phone: 337-289-7991
Fax: 337-289-8466
URL: www.lafayettegeneral.org
Type: Acute Care Hospitals
Emergency Services: Yes
Ownership: Voluntary non-profit - Private
Beds: 377

Key Personnel:

CEO/President. . . . . Patrick W. Gandy, Jr.
Operating Room. . . . . Dani Marine
Pediatric In-Patient Care . . . . Sylvia Oats
Cardiac Laboratory. . . . . Charlie Olinger
Chief of Medical Staff . . . . Juan Perez Ruiz, MD
Radiology. . . . . Paul Thibodeaux
Emergency Room . . . . Karen Wible

Measure	Cases	This Hosp.	State Avg.	U.S. Avg.
Blood Clot Prevention and Treatment				
Anticoagulation Overlap Therapy[2]	69	96%	89%	93%
ICU Venous Thromboembolism Prophylaxis[2]	73	97%	88%	92%
Incidence of Potentially Preventable VTE[2]	12	8%	16%	10%
UFH with Dosages/Platelet Monitoring[1,2]	-	-	94%	97%
Venous Thromboembolism Prophylaxis[2]	327	82%	74%	85%
Warfarin Therapy Discharge Instructions[2]	43	79%	85%	75%
Chest Pain/Possible Heart Attack Care				
Aspirin Given Within 24 Hours of Arrival[5]	-	-	94%	96%
Fibrinolytic Meds Within 30 Min. of Arrival[5]	-	-	54%	58%
Average Time to ECG (minutes)[5]	-	-	10	7
Average Time to Transfer (minutes)[5]	-	-	94	60
Children's Asthma Care				
Received Home Management Plan of Care	23	91%	-	88%
Received Reliever Medication	23	100%	-	100%
Received Systemic Corticosteroids	23	96%	-	100%
Emergency Department				
Admittance Decision Time (minutes)[2]	654	67	86	98
Head CT Results Within 45 Min. of Arrival[7]	-	-	49%	57%
Patients Who Left ER Before Being Seen	62,271	5%	3%	2%
Time from ER Arrival to Admit. (minutes)[2]	668	234	256	274
Time from ER Arrival to Discharge (minutes)	397	118	125	134
Time in ER Before Being Evaluated (minutes)	407	26	27	26
Time to Pain Meds for Fractures (minutes)	178	60	61	57
Heart Attack Care				
Aspirin Given at Discharge	200	100%	99%	99%
Fibrinolytic Meds Within 30 Min. of Arrival[7]	-	-	71%	54%
PCI Within 90 Minutes of Arrival	58	100%	94%	96%
Statin Prescribed at Discharge	187	99%	98%	98%
Heart Failure Care				
ACE Inhibitor or ARB for LVSD	127	100%	95%	97%
Discharge Instructions Given	369	98%	94%	94%
Evaluation of LVS Function	442	100%	97%	99%
Medicare Spending				
Medicare Spending per Patient (ratio)	-	1.02	1.04	0.98
Pneumonia Care				
Appropriate Initial Antibiotic Given	134	98%	93%	95%
Blood Culture Timing	241	100%	97%	98%
Pregnancy and Delivery Care				
Newborn Deliveries Scheduled Early[2]	34	0%	5%	6%
Preventive Care				
Immunization for Influenza[2]	545	92%	85%	90%
Immunization for Pneumonia[2]	632	90%	88%	92%
Stroke Care				
Anticoagulation Therapy for Atrial Fibrillation	44	100%	93%	95%
Antithrombotic Therapy Timing	190	99%	96%	98%
Assessed for Rehabilitation	295	99%	95%	97%
Discharged on Antithrombotic Therapy	217	100%	97%	99%
Discharged on Statin Medication	177	97%	89%	94%
Thrombolytic Therapy Timing	17	88%	53%	66%
Venous Thromboembolism Prophylaxis	308	93%	87%	94%
Written Stroke Educational Materials Given	184	98%	83%	88%
Surgical Care Improvement Project				
Appropriate Beta Blocker Usage[2]	236	98%	97%	98%
Appropriate VTP Within 24 Hours[2]	422	97%	97%	98%
Controlled Postoperative Blood Glucose[2]	156	99%	96%	97%
Perioperative Temperature Management[2]	581	100%	100%	100%
Prophylactic Antibiotic Selection[2]	551	98%	99%	99%
Prophylactic Antibiotic Selection (Outpatient)	244	99%	97%	98%
Prophylactic Antibiotic Stopped[2]	546	97%	97%	98%
Prophylactic Antibiotic Timing[2]	560	96%	98%	99%
Prophylactic Antibiotic Timing (Outpatient)	254	94%	97%	98%
Urinary Catheter Removal[2]	492	96%	96%	97%
Survey of Patients' Hospital Experiences				
Area Around Room 'Always' Quiet at Night	300+	74%	74%	61%
Doctors 'Always' Communicated Well	300+	88%	87%	82%
Home Recovery Information Given	300+	86%	85%	85%
Hospital Given 9 or 10 on 10 Point Scale	300+	82%	75%	71%
Meds 'Always' Explained Before Given	300+	71%	69%	64%
Nurses 'Always' Communicated Well	300+	89%	83%	79%
Pain 'Always' Well Controlled	300+	79%	75%	71%
Room and Bathroom 'Always' Clean	300+	77%	75%	73%
Timely Help 'Always' Received	300+	76%	71%	68%
Would Definitely Recommend Hospital	300+	85%	75%	71%
Use of Medical Imaging				
Cardiac Imaging Stress Test before Surgery[1]	-	-	5.3%	5.3%
Combination Abdominal CT Scan	1,265	27.8%	24.5%	10.5%
Combination Brain/Sinus CT Scan	1,242	2.6%	2.6%	2.7%
Combination Chest CT Scan	998	23.7%	7.6%	2.7%
Follow-up Mammogram/Ultrasound	1,131	7.3%	9.4%	8.8%
Lumbar Spine MRI for Low Back Pain	131	45.0%	42.7%	37.2%

Lafayette General Surgical Hospital

1000 W Pinhook Rd Suite 100
Lafayette, LA 70503
Phone: 337-289-8095
URL: www.lgsh.us
Type: Acute Care Hospitals
Emergency Services: No
Ownership: Voluntary non-profit - Private
Beds: 10

Measure	Cases	This Hosp.	State Avg.	U.S. Avg.
Blood Clot Prevention and Treatment				
Anticoagulation Overlap Therapy[7]	-	-	89%	93%
ICU Venous Thromboembolism Prophylaxis[7]	-	-	88%	92%
Incidence of Potentially Preventable VTE[7]	-	-	16%	10%
UFH with Dosages/Platelet Monitoring[7]	-	-	94%	97%
Venous Thromboembolism Prophylaxis[1]	-	-	74%	85%
Warfarin Therapy Discharge Instructions[7]	-	-	85%	75%
Chest Pain/Possible Heart Attack Care				
Aspirin Given Within 24 Hours of Arrival[5]	-	-	94%	96%
Fibrinolytic Meds Within 30 Min. of Arrival[5]	-	-	54%	58%
Average Time to ECG (minutes)[5]	-	-	10	7
Average Time to Transfer (minutes)[5]	-	-	94	60
Children's Asthma Care				
Received Home Management Plan of Care	-	-	-	88%
Received Reliever Medication	-	-	-	100%
Received Systemic Corticosteroids	-	-	-	100%
Emergency Department				
Admittance Decision Time (minutes)[7]	-	-	86	98
Head CT Results Within 45 Min. of Arrival[5]	-	-	49%	57%
Patients Who Left ER Before Being Seen[5]	-	-	3%	2%
Time from ER Arrival to Admit. (minutes)[7]	-	-	256	274
Time from ER Arrival to Discharge (minutes)[5]	-	-	125	134
Time in ER Before Being Evaluated (minutes)[5]	-	-	27	26
Time to Pain Meds for Fractures (minutes)[5]	-	-	61	57
Heart Attack Care				
Aspirin Given at Discharge[5]	-	-	99%	99%
Fibrinolytic Meds Within 30 Min. of Arrival[5]	-	-	71%	54%
PCI Within 90 Minutes of Arrival[5]	-	-	94%	96%
Statin Prescribed at Discharge[5]	-	-	98%	98%
Heart Failure Care				
ACE Inhibitor or ARB for LVSD[5]	-	-	95%	97%
Discharge Instructions Given[5]	-	-	94%	94%
Evaluation of LVS Function[5]	-	-	97%	99%
Medicare Spending				
Medicare Spending per Patient (ratio)[1]	-	-	1.04	0.98
Pneumonia Care				
Appropriate Initial Antibiotic Given[5]	-	-	93%	95%
Blood Culture Timing[5]	-	-	97%	98%
Pregnancy and Delivery Care				
Newborn Deliveries Scheduled Early[7]	-	-	5%	6%
Preventive Care				
Immunization for Influenza	28	96%	85%	90%
Immunization for Pneumonia	20	100%	88%	92%
Stroke Care				
Anticoagulation Therapy for Atrial Fibrillation[5]	-	-	93%	95%
Antithrombotic Therapy Timing[5]	-	-	96%	98%
Assessed for Rehabilitation[5]	-	-	95%	97%
Discharged on Antithrombotic Therapy[5]	-	-	97%	99%
Discharged on Statin Medication[5]	-	-	89%	94%
Thrombolytic Therapy Timing[5]	-	-	53%	66%
Venous Thromboembolism Prophylaxis[5]	-	-	87%	94%
Written Stroke Educational Materials Given[5]	-	-	83%	88%
Surgical Care Improvement Project				
Appropriate Beta Blocker Usage[1]	-	-	97%	98%
Appropriate VTP Within 24 Hours	22	100%	97%	98%
Controlled Postoperative Blood Glucose[7]	-	-	96%	97%
Perioperative Temperature Management	26	100%	100%	100%
Prophylactic Antibiotic Selection	24	100%	99%	99%
Prophylactic Antibiotic Selection (Outpatient)	54	98%	97%	98%
Prophylactic Antibiotic Stopped	24	100%	97%	98%
Prophylactic Antibiotic Timing	24	96%	98%	99%
Prophylactic Antibiotic Timing (Outpatient)	56	93%	97%	98%
Urinary Catheter Removal	23	100%	96%	97%
Survey of Patients' Hospital Experiences				
Area Around Room 'Always' Quiet at Night[10]	<100	94%	74%	61%
Doctors 'Always' Communicated Well[10]	<100	98%	87%	82%
Home Recovery Information Given[10]	<100	96%	85%	85%
Hospital Given 9 or 10 on 10 Point Scale[10]	<100	99%	75%	71%
Meds 'Always' Explained Before Given[10]	<100	97%	69%	64%
Nurses 'Always' Communicated Well[10]	<100	97%	83%	79%
Pain 'Always' Well Controlled[10]	<100	84%	75%	71%
Room and Bathroom 'Always' Clean[10]	<100	93%	75%	73%
Timely Help 'Always' Received[10]	<100	89%	71%	68%
Would Definitely Recommend Hospital[10]	<100	99%	75%	71%
Use of Medical Imaging				

NOTE: Hospital profiles are in alphabetical order by state, then city, then hospital within the city; Rankings exclude hospitals with less than 25 cases except for patient surveys which excludes hospitals with less than 100 cases; (a) 100-299 cases; (1) The number of cases/patients is too few to report; (2) Data submitted were based on a sample of cases/patients; (3) Results are based on a shorter time period than required; (4) Data suppressed by CMS for one or more quarters; (5) Results are not available for this reporting period; (6) Fewer than 100 patients completed the HCAHPS survey; (7) No cases met the criteria for this measure; (8) The lower limit of the confidence interval cannot be calculated if the number of observed infections equals zero; (9) No data are available from the state/territory for this reporting period; (10) The scores shown reflect fewer than 50 completed surveys; (11) There were discrepancies in the data collection process; (12) This measure does not apply to this hospital for this reporting period; (13) Results cannot be calculated for this reporting period; (14) The results for this state are combined with nearby states to protect confidentiality; Please refer to the User's Guide for a full explanation of data.

Measure	Cases	This Hosp.	State Avg.	U.S. Avg.
Cardiac Imaging Stress Test before Surgery[7]	-	-	5.3%	5.3%
Combination Abdominal CT Scan[7]	-	-	24.5%	10.5%
Combination Brain/Sinus CT Scan[7]	-	-	2.6%	2.7%
Combination Chest CT Scan[7]	-	-	7.6%	2.7%
Follow-up Mammogram/Ultrasound[7]	-	-	9.4%	8.8%
Lumbar Spine MRI for Low Back Pain[7]	-	-	42.7%	37.2%

Lafayette Surgical Specialty Hospital

1101 Kaliste Saloom Rd Phone: 337-769-4100
Lafayette, LA 70508 Fax: 337-769-4100
URL: www.lafayettesurgical.com
Type: Acute Care Hospitals Emergency Services: No
Ownership: Voluntary non-profit - Private Beds: 20
Key Personnel:
Chief of Medical Staff.......... Thomas Bertuccini
CEO .... Buffy Domingue
Operating Room.............. James S Garcelon, MD, FACS

Measure	Cases	This Hosp.	State Avg.	U.S. Avg.
Blood Clot Prevention and Treatment				
Anticoagulation Overlap Therapy[7]	-	-	89%	93%
ICU Venous Thromboembolism Prophylaxis[7]	-	-	88%	92%
Incidence of Potentially Preventable VTE[7]	-	-	16%	10%
UFH with Dosages/Platelet Monitoring[7]	-	-	94%	97%
Venous Thromboembolism Prophylaxis	243	95%	74%	85%
Warfarin Therapy Discharge Instructions[7]	-	-	85%	75%
Chest Pain/Possible Heart Attack Care				
Aspirin Given Within 24 Hours of Arrival[5]	-	-	94%	96%
Fibrinolytic Meds Within 30 Min. of Arrival[5]	-	-	54%	58%
Average Time to ECG (minutes)[5]	-	-	10	7
Average Time to Transfer (minutes)[5]	-	-	94	60
Children's Asthma Care				
Received Home Management Plan of Care	-	-	-	88%
Received Reliever Medication	-	-	-	100%
Received Systemic Corticosteroids	-	-	-	100%
Emergency Department				
Admittance Decision Time (minutes)[7]	-	-	86	98
Head CT Results Within 45 Min. of Arrival[5]	-	-	49%	57%
Patients Who Left ER Before Being Seen[5]	-	-	3%	2%
Time from ER Arrival to Admit. (minutes)[7]	-	-	256	274
Time from ER Arrival to Discharge (minutes)[5]	-	-	125	134
Time in ER Before Being Evaluated (minutes)[5]	-	-	27	26
Time to Pain Meds for Fractures (minutes)[5]	-	-	61	57
Heart Attack Care				
Aspirin Given at Discharge[5]	-	-	99%	99%
Fibrinolytic Meds Within 30 Min. of Arrival[5]	-	-	71%	54%
PCI Within 90 Minutes of Arrival[5]	-	-	94%	96%
Statin Prescribed at Discharge[5]	-	-	98%	98%
Heart Failure Care				
ACE Inhibitor or ARB for LVSD[5]	-	-	95%	97%
Discharge Instructions Given[5]	-	-	94%	94%
Evaluation of LVS Function[5]	-	-	97%	99%
Medicare Spending				
Medicare Spending per Patient (ratio)	-	1.10	1.04	0.98
Pneumonia Care				
Appropriate Initial Antibiotic Given[5]	-	-	93%	95%
Blood Culture Timing[5]	-	-	97%	98%
Pregnancy and Delivery Care				
Newborn Deliveries Scheduled Early[7]	-	-	5%	6%
Preventive Care				
Immunization for Influenza	376	70%	85%	90%
Immunization for Pneumonia[2]	308	73%	88%	92%
Stroke Care				
Anticoagulation Therapy for Atrial Fibrillation[5]	-	-	93%	95%
Antithrombotic Therapy Timing[5]	-	-	96%	98%
Assessed for Rehabilitation[5]	-	-	95%	97%
Discharged on Antithrombotic Therapy[5]	-	-	97%	99%
Discharged on Statin Medication[5]	-	-	89%	94%
Thrombolytic Therapy Timing[5]	-	-	53%	66%
Venous Thromboembolism Prophylaxis[5]	-	-	87%	94%
Written Stroke Educational Materials Given[5]	-	-	83%	88%
Surgical Care Improvement Project				
Appropriate Beta Blocker Usage[2]	38	92%	97%	98%
Appropriate VTP Within 24 Hours[2]	160	99%	97%	98%
Controlled Postoperative Blood Glucose[2,7]	-	-	96%	97%
Perioperative Temperature Management[2]	171	99%	100%	100%
Prophylactic Antibiotic Selection[2]	158	100%	99%	99%
Prophylactic Antibiotic Selection (Outpatient)	370	98%	97%	98%
Prophylactic Antibiotic Stopped[2]	158	95%	97%	98%
Prophylactic Antibiotic Timing[2]	158	98%	98%	99%
Prophylactic Antibiotic Timing (Outpatient)	371	94%	97%	98%
Urinary Catheter Removal[2]	120	100%	96%	97%
Survey of Patients' Hospital Experiences				
Area Around Room 'Always' Quiet at Night	300+	87%	74%	61%
Doctors 'Always' Communicated Well	300+	90%	87%	82%
Home Recovery Information Given	300+	90%	85%	85%
Hospital Given 9 or 10 on 10 Point Scale	300+	88%	75%	71%
Meds 'Always' Explained Before Given	300+	81%	69%	64%
Nurses 'Always' Communicated Well	300+	90%	83%	79%
Pain 'Always' Well Controlled	300+	81%	75%	71%
Room and Bathroom 'Always' Clean	300+	84%	75%	73%
Timely Help 'Always' Received	300+	84%	71%	68%
Would Definitely Recommend Hospital	300+	88%	75%	71%
Use of Medical Imaging				
Cardiac Imaging Stress Test before Surgery[7]	-	-	5.3%	5.3%
Combination Abdominal CT Scan[1]	-	-	24.5%	10.5%
Combination Brain/Sinus CT Scan	46	0.0%	2.6%	2.7%
Combination Chest CT Scan[1]	-	-	7.6%	2.7%
Follow-up Mammogram/Ultrasound[7]	-	-	9.4%	8.8%
Lumbar Spine MRI for Low Back Pain	76	35.5%	42.7%	37.2%

Our Lady of Lourdes Regional Medical Center

4801 Ambassador Caffery Parkway Phone: 337-470-2000
Lafayette, LA 70508 Fax: 337-289-2796
E-mail: info@lourdes.net
URL: www.lourdes.net
Type: Acute Care Hospitals Emergency Services: Yes
Ownership: Voluntary non-profit - Church Beds: 293
Key Personnel:
CEO/President.............. William F Barrow
Chairman/CEO .... John L. Indest
Chief of Medical Staff.......... Henry J. Kaufman, MD
Emergency Room .... Michael Odinet, MD
Anesthesiology.............. Robert Theard, MD
Radiology................... Joan Wojak, MD

Measure	Cases	This Hosp.	State Avg.	U.S. Avg.
Blood Clot Prevention and Treatment				
Anticoagulation Overlap Therapy[2]	57	75%	89%	93%
ICU Venous Thromboembolism Prophylaxis[2]	63	95%	88%	92%
Incidence of Potentially Preventable VTE[2]	18	6%	16%	10%
UFH with Dosages/Platelet Monitoring[1,2]	-	-	94%	97%
Venous Thromboembolism Prophylaxis[2]	356	88%	74%	85%
Warfarin Therapy Discharge Instructions[2]	39	90%	85%	75%
Chest Pain/Possible Heart Attack Care				
Aspirin Given Within 24 Hours of Arrival[5]	-	-	94%	96%
Fibrinolytic Meds Within 30 Min. of Arrival[5]	-	-	54%	58%
Average Time to ECG (minutes)[5]	-	-	10	7
Average Time to Transfer (minutes)[5]	-	-	94	60
Children's Asthma Care				
Received Home Management Plan of Care	-	-	-	88%
Received Reliever Medication	-	-	-	100%
Received Systemic Corticosteroids	-	-	-	100%
Emergency Department				
Admittance Decision Time (minutes)[2]	616	111	86	98
Head CT Results Within 45 Min. of Arrival[1]	-	-	49%	57%
Patients Who Left ER Before Being Seen	33,942	2%	3%	2%
Time from ER Arrival to Admit. (minutes)[2]	628	256	256	274
Time from ER Arrival to Discharge (minutes)	333	149	125	134
Time in ER Before Being Evaluated (minutes)	348	49	27	26
Time to Pain Meds for Fractures (minutes)	145	60	61	57
Heart Attack Care				
Aspirin Given at Discharge	122	98%	99%	99%
Fibrinolytic Meds Within 30 Min. of Arrival[7]	-	-	71%	54%
PCI Within 90 Minutes of Arrival	34	100%	94%	96%
Statin Prescribed at Discharge	123	98%	98%	98%
Heart Failure Care				
ACE Inhibitor or ARB for LVSD	86	99%	95%	97%
Discharge Instructions Given	218	93%	94%	94%
Evaluation of LVS Function	299	97%	97%	99%
Medicare Spending				
Medicare Spending per Patient (ratio)	-	1.07	1.04	0.98
Pneumonia Care				
Appropriate Initial Antibiotic Given	167	96%	93%	95%
Blood Culture Timing	181	100%	97%	98%
Pregnancy and Delivery Care				
Newborn Deliveries Scheduled Early[7]	-	-	5%	6%
Preventive Care				
Immunization for Influenza[2]	591	95%	85%	90%
Immunization for Pneumonia[2]	798	83%	88%	92%
Stroke Care				
Anticoagulation Therapy for Atrial Fibrillation	29	100%	93%	95%
Antithrombotic Therapy Timing	149	99%	96%	98%
Assessed for Rehabilitation	213	100%	95%	97%
Discharged on Antithrombotic Therapy	174	99%	97%	99%
Discharged on Statin Medication	137	100%	89%	94%
Thrombolytic Therapy Timing	13	100%	53%	66%
Venous Thromboembolism Prophylaxis	226	100%	87%	94%
Written Stroke Educational Materials Given	111	99%	83%	88%
Surgical Care Improvement Project				
Appropriate Beta Blocker Usage[2]	110	99%	97%	98%
Appropriate VTP Within 24 Hours[2]	253	98%	97%	98%
Controlled Postoperative Blood Glucose[2]	40	90%	96%	97%
Perioperative Temperature Management[2]	317	100%	100%	100%
Prophylactic Antibiotic Selection[2]	238	100%	99%	99%
Prophylactic Antibiotic Selection (Outpatient)	277	94%	97%	98%
Prophylactic Antibiotic Stopped[2]	234	97%	97%	98%
Prophylactic Antibiotic Timing[2]	239	100%	98%	99%
Prophylactic Antibiotic Timing (Outpatient)	285	95%	97%	98%
Urinary Catheter Removal[2]	226	100%	96%	97%
Survey of Patients' Hospital Experiences				
Area Around Room 'Always' Quiet at Night	300+	78%	74%	61%
Doctors 'Always' Communicated Well	300+	86%	87%	82%
Home Recovery Information Given	300+	85%	85%	85%
Hospital Given 9 or 10 on 10 Point Scale	300+	80%	75%	71%
Meds 'Always' Explained Before Given	300+	66%	69%	64%
Nurses 'Always' Communicated Well	300+	84%	83%	79%
Pain 'Always' Well Controlled	300+	77%	75%	71%
Room and Bathroom 'Always' Clean	300+	80%	75%	73%
Timely Help 'Always' Received	300+	67%	71%	68%
Would Definitely Recommend Hospital	300+	83%	75%	71%
Use of Medical Imaging				
Cardiac Imaging Stress Test before Surgery[1]	-	-	5.3%	5.3%
Combination Abdominal CT Scan	1,159	19.2%	24.5%	10.5%
Combination Brain/Sinus CT Scan	998	2.0%	2.6%	2.7%
Combination Chest CT Scan	873	3.2%	7.6%	2.7%
Follow-up Mammogram/Ultrasound	1,811	12.2%	9.4%	8.8%
Lumbar Spine MRI for Low Back Pain	201	37.3%	42.7%	37.2%

Park Place Surgical Hospital

901 Wilson Street Phone: 337-237-8119
Lafayette, LA 70503 Fax: 337-267-4182
E-mail: info@parkplacesurgery.com
URL: www.parkplacesurgery.com
Type: Acute Care Hospitals Emergency Services: No
Ownership: Proprietary Beds: 10
Key Personnel:
Anesthesiology.............. Reginald Ardoin, MD
Pediatric In-Patient Care .... Sanjiv Jindia
CEO/President............... James Moore

Measure	Cases	This Hosp.	State Avg.	U.S. Avg.
Blood Clot Prevention and Treatment				
Anticoagulation Overlap Therapy[7]	-	-	89%	93%
ICU Venous Thromboembolism Prophylaxis[7]	-	-	88%	92%
Incidence of Potentially Preventable VTE[7]	-	-	16%	10%
UFH with Dosages/Platelet Monitoring[7]	-	-	94%	97%
Venous Thromboembolism Prophylaxis	13	100%	74%	85%
Warfarin Therapy Discharge Instructions[7]	-	-	85%	75%
Chest Pain/Possible Heart Attack Care				
Aspirin Given Within 24 Hours of Arrival[5]	-	-	94%	96%
Fibrinolytic Meds Within 30 Min. of Arrival[5]	-	-	54%	58%
Average Time to ECG (minutes)[5]	-	-	10	7

NOTE: Hospital profiles are in alphabetical order by state, then city, then hospital within the city; Rankings exclude hospitals with less than 25 cases except for patient surveys which excludes hospitals with less than 100 cases; (a) 100-299 cases; (1) The number of cases/patients is too few to report; (2) Data submitted were based on a sample of cases/patients; (3) Results are based on a shorter time period than required; (4) Data suppressed by CMS for one or more quarters; (5) Results are not available for this reporting period; (6) Fewer than 100 patients completed the HCAHPS survey; (7) No cases met the criteria for this measure; (8) The lower limit of the confidence interval cannot be calculated if the number of observed infections equals zero; (9) No data are available from the state/territory for this reporting period; (10) The scores shown reflect fewer than 50 completed surveys; (11) There were discrepancies in the data collection process; (12) This measure does not apply to this hospital for this reporting period; (13) Results cannot be calculated for this reporting period; (14) The results for this state are combined with nearby states to protect confidentiality; Please refer to the User's Guide for a full explanation of data.

Measure	Cases	This Hosp.	State Avg.	U.S. Avg.
Average Time to Transfer (minutes)[5]	-	-	94	60
Children's Asthma Care				
Received Home Management Plan of Care	-	-	-	88%
Received Reliever Medication	-	-	-	100%
Received Systemic Corticosteroids	-	-	-	100%
Emergency Department				
Admittance Decision Time (minutes)[7]	-	-	86	98
Head CT Results Within 45 Min. of Arrival[5]	-	-	49%	57%
Patients Who Left ER Before Being Seen[5]	-	-	3%	2%
Time from ER Arrival to Admit. (minutes)[7]	-	-	256	274
Time from ER Arrival to Discharge (minutes)[5]	-	-	125	134
Time in ER Before Being Evaluated (minutes)[5]	-	-	27	26
Time to Pain Meds for Fractures (minutes)[5]	-	-	61	57
Heart Attack Care				
Aspirin Given at Discharge[5]	-	-	99%	99%
Fibrinolytic Meds Within 30 Min. of Arrival[5]	-	-	71%	54%
PCI Within 90 Minutes of Arrival[5]	-	-	94%	96%
Statin Prescribed at Discharge[5]	-	-	98%	98%
Heart Failure Care				
ACE Inhibitor or ARB for LVSD[5]	-	-	95%	97%
Discharge Instructions Given[5]	-	-	94%	94%
Evaluation of LVS Function[5]	-	-	97%	99%
Medicare Spending				
Medicare Spending per Patient (ratio)[1]	-	-	1.04	0.98
Pneumonia Care				
Appropriate Initial Antibiotic Given[5]	-	-	93%	95%
Blood Culture Timing[5]	-	-	97%	98%
Pregnancy and Delivery Care				
Newborn Deliveries Scheduled Early[7]	-	-	5%	6%
Preventive Care				
Immunization for Influenza	33	88%	85%	90%
Immunization for Pneumonia[1]	-	-	88%	92%
Stroke Care				
Anticoagulation Therapy for Atrial Fibrillation[5]	-	-	93%	95%
Antithrombotic Therapy Timing[5]	-	-	96%	98%
Assessed for Rehabilitation[5]	-	-	95%	97%
Discharged on Antithrombotic Therapy[5]	-	-	97%	99%
Discharged on Statin Medication[5]	-	-	89%	94%
Thrombolytic Therapy Timing[5]	-	-	53%	66%
Venous Thromboembolism Prophylaxis[5]	-	-	87%	94%
Written Stroke Educational Materials Given[5]	-	-	83%	88%
Surgical Care Improvement Project				
Appropriate Beta Blocker Usage[7]	-	-	97%	98%
Appropriate VTP Within 24 Hours	16	100%	97%	98%
Controlled Postoperative Blood Glucose[7]	-	-	96%	97%
Perioperative Temperature Management	19	100%	100%	100%
Prophylactic Antibiotic Selection	14	100%	99%	99%
Prophylactic Antibiotic Selection (Outpatient)	74	96%	97%	98%
Prophylactic Antibiotic Stopped	13	92%	97%	98%
Prophylactic Antibiotic Timing	14	100%	98%	99%
Prophylactic Antibiotic Timing (Outpatient)	74	99%	97%	98%
Urinary Catheter Removal[7]	-	-	96%	97%
Survey of Patients' Hospital Experiences				
Area Around Room 'Always' Quiet at Night[10]	<100	88%	74%	61%
Doctors 'Always' Communicated Well[10]	<100	87%	87%	82%
Home Recovery Information Given[10]	<100	90%	85%	85%
Hospital Given 9 or 10 on 10 Point Scale[10]	<100	92%	75%	71%
Meds 'Always' Explained Before Given[10]	<100	85%	69%	64%
Nurses 'Always' Communicated Well[10]	<100	93%	83%	79%
Pain 'Always' Well Controlled[10]	<100	84%	75%	71%
Room and Bathroom 'Always' Clean[10]	<100	84%	75%	73%
Timely Help 'Always' Received[10]	<100	90%	71%	68%
Would Definitely Recommend Hospital[10]	<100	92%	75%	71%
Use of Medical Imaging				
Cardiac Imaging Stress Test before Surgery[7]	-	-	5.3%	5.3%
Combination Abdominal CT Scan[7]	-	-	24.5%	10.5%
Combination Brain/Sinus CT Scan[7]	-	-	2.6%	2.7%
Combination Chest CT Scan[7]	-	-	7.6%	2.7%
Follow-up Mammogram/Ultrasound[7]	-	-	9.4%	8.8%
Lumbar Spine MRI for Low Back Pain[7]	-	-	42.7%	37.2%

The Regional Medical Center of Acadiana

2810 Ambassador Caffery Parkway — Phone: 337-981-2949
Lafayette, LA 70506 — Fax: 337-989-6781
URL: www.medicalcentersw.com
Type: Acute Care Hospitals — Emergency Services: Yes
Ownership: Proprietary — Beds: 142

Key Personnel:
Anesthesiology. . . . . Scott Gamel, MD
Emergency Room . . . . Michael Glassinger, MD
CEO/President. . . . . Kyle J Viator

Measure	Cases	This Hosp.	State Avg.	U.S. Avg.
Blood Clot Prevention and Treatment				
Anticoagulation Overlap Therapy[2]	21	100%	89%	93%
ICU Venous Thromboembolism Prophylaxis[2]	104	100%	88%	92%
Incidence of Potentially Preventable VTE[1,2]	-	-	16%	10%
UFH with Dosages/Platelet Monitoring[2]	11	100%	94%	97%
Venous Thromboembolism Prophylaxis[2]	329	100%	74%	85%
Warfarin Therapy Discharge Instructions[2]	17	100%	85%	75%
Chest Pain/Possible Heart Attack Care				
Aspirin Given Within 24 Hours of Arrival[3,7]	-	-	94%	96%
Fibrinolytic Meds Within 30 Min. of Arrival[5]	-	-	54%	58%
Average Time to ECG (minutes)[3,7]	-	-	10	7
Average Time to Transfer (minutes)[5]	-	-	94	60
Children's Asthma Care				
Received Home Management Plan of Care	-	-	-	88%
Received Reliever Medication	-	-	-	100%
Received Systemic Corticosteroids	-	-	-	100%
Emergency Department				
Admittance Decision Time (minutes)[2]	478	55	86	98
Head CT Results Within 45 Min. of Arrival[1]	-	-	49%	57%
Patients Who Left ER Before Being Seen	53,400	1%	3%	2%
Time from ER Arrival to Admit. (minutes)[2]	478	188	256	274
Time from ER Arrival to Discharge (minutes)	494	116	125	134
Time in ER Before Being Evaluated (minutes)	523	22	27	26
Time to Pain Meds for Fractures (minutes)	197	50	61	57
Heart Attack Care				
Aspirin Given at Discharge[2]	61	100%	99%	99%
Fibrinolytic Meds Within 30 Min. of Arrival[2,7]	-	-	71%	54%
PCI Within 90 Minutes of Arrival[2]	14	100%	94%	96%
Statin Prescribed at Discharge[2]	57	100%	98%	98%
Heart Failure Care				
ACE Inhibitor or ARB for LVSD[2]	35	100%	95%	97%
Discharge Instructions Given[2]	88	92%	94%	94%
Evaluation of LVS Function[2]	103	100%	97%	99%
Medicare Spending				
Medicare Spending per Patient (ratio)	-	1.08	1.04	0.98
Pneumonia Care				
Appropriate Initial Antibiotic Given[2]	37	100%	93%	95%
Blood Culture Timing[2]	72	99%	97%	98%
Pregnancy and Delivery Care				
Newborn Deliveries Scheduled Early[2]	52	2%	5%	6%
Preventive Care				
Immunization for Influenza[2]	456	100%	85%	90%
Immunization for Pneumonia[2]	264	100%	88%	92%
Stroke Care				
Anticoagulation Therapy for Atrial Fibrillation[1,2]	-	-	93%	95%
Antithrombotic Therapy Timing[2]	21	100%	96%	98%
Assessed for Rehabilitation[2]	33	100%	95%	97%
Discharged on Antithrombotic Therapy[2]	27	100%	97%	99%
Discharged on Statin Medication[2]	22	100%	89%	94%
Thrombolytic Therapy Timing[1,2]	-	-	53%	66%
Venous Thromboembolism Prophylaxis[2]	28	100%	87%	94%
Written Stroke Educational Materials Given[2]	22	100%	83%	88%
Surgical Care Improvement Project				
Appropriate Beta Blocker Usage[2]	144	100%	97%	98%
Appropriate VTP Within 24 Hours[2]	153	100%	97%	98%
Controlled Postoperative Blood Glucose[2]	139	100%	96%	97%
Perioperative Temperature Management[2]	292	100%	100%	100%
Prophylactic Antibiotic Selection[2]	284	100%	99%	99%
Prophylactic Antibiotic Selection (Outpatient)	191	100%	97%	98%
Prophylactic Antibiotic Stopped[2]	272	99%	97%	98%
Prophylactic Antibiotic Timing[2]	286	100%	98%	99%
Prophylactic Antibiotic Timing (Outpatient)	192	99%	97%	98%
Urinary Catheter Removal[2]	191	100%	96%	97%
Survey of Patients' Hospital Experiences				
Area Around Room 'Always' Quiet at Night	300+	68%	74%	61%
Doctors 'Always' Communicated Well	300+	84%	87%	82%
Home Recovery Information Given	300+	86%	85%	85%
Hospital Given 9 or 10 on 10 Point Scale	300+	70%	75%	71%
Meds 'Always' Explained Before Given	300+	62%	69%	64%
Nurses 'Always' Communicated Well	300+	77%	83%	79%
Pain 'Always' Well Controlled	300+	70%	75%	71%
Room and Bathroom 'Always' Clean	300+	69%	75%	73%
Timely Help 'Always' Received	300+	63%	71%	68%
Would Definitely Recommend Hospital	300+	71%	75%	71%
Use of Medical Imaging				
Cardiac Imaging Stress Test before Surgery[7]	-	-	5.3%	5.3%
Combination Abdominal CT Scan	220	4.1%	24.5%	10.5%
Combination Brain/Sinus CT Scan[1]	-	-	2.6%	2.7%
Combination Chest CT Scan	91	3.3%	7.6%	2.7%
Follow-up Mammogram/Ultrasound	950	14.2%	9.4%	8.8%
Lumbar Spine MRI for Low Back Pain[1]	-	-	42.7%	37.2%

University Hospital & Clinics

2390 West Congress — Phone: 337-261-6000
Lafayette, LA 70506 — Fax: 337-261-6660
E-mail: ldorse1@lsuhsc.edu
URL: www.umcip.lsumc.edu
Type: Acute Care Hospitals — Emergency Services: Yes
Ownership: Government - State — Beds: 208

Key Personnel:
Operating Room. . . . . Kitty Bell, RN
Pediatric In-Patient Care . . . . Mary Dell Berard, RN
Quality Assurance . . . . Kathy Colgin, RN
CEO/President. . . . . Larry Dorsey
Chief of Medical Staff . . . . Dr James Falterman Jr, MD
Pediatric Ambulatory Care . . . . . . Richard Howes, MD
Infection Control. . . . . Becky McNeese, RN
Cardiac Laboratory. . . . . Carolyn Pons

Measure	Cases	This Hosp.	State Avg.	U.S. Avg.
Blood Clot Prevention and Treatment				
Anticoagulation Overlap Therapy[2]	32	100%	89%	93%
ICU Venous Thromboembolism Prophylaxis[2]	43	93%	88%	92%
Incidence of Potentially Preventable VTE[1,2]	-	-	16%	10%
UFH with Dosages/Platelet Monitoring[2]	23	91%	94%	97%
Venous Thromboembolism Prophylaxis[2]	163	83%	74%	85%
Warfarin Therapy Discharge Instructions[2]	30	40%	85%	75%
Chest Pain/Possible Heart Attack Care				
Aspirin Given Within 24 Hours of Arrival	17	100%	94%	96%
Fibrinolytic Meds Within 30 Min. of Arrival[3,7]	-	-	54%	58%
Average Time to ECG (minutes)	17	19	10	7
Average Time to Transfer (minutes)[1,3]	-	-	94	60
Children's Asthma Care				
Received Home Management Plan of Care	-	-	-	88%
Received Reliever Medication	-	-	-	100%
Received Systemic Corticosteroids	-	-	-	100%
Emergency Department				
Admittance Decision Time (minutes)[2]	195	165	86	98
Head CT Results Within 45 Min. of Arrival[1]	-	-	49%	57%
Patients Who Left ER Before Being Seen	42,258	13%	3%	2%
Time from ER Arrival to Admit. (minutes)[2]	215	410	256	274
Time from ER Arrival to Discharge (minutes)	336	200	125	134
Time in ER Before Being Evaluated (minutes)	378	38	27	26
Time to Pain Meds for Fractures (minutes)	54	132	61	57
Heart Attack Care				
Aspirin Given at Discharge[1,2]	-	-	99%	99%
Fibrinolytic Meds Within 30 Min. of Arrival[2,7]	-	-	71%	54%
PCI Within 90 Minutes of Arrival[2,7]	-	-	94%	96%
Statin Prescribed at Discharge[2]	11	100%	98%	98%
Heart Failure Care				
ACE Inhibitor or ARB for LVSD	38	97%	95%	97%
Discharge Instructions Given	65	89%	94%	94%
Evaluation of LVS Function	69	100%	97%	99%
Medicare Spending				
Medicare Spending per Patient (ratio)	-	0.97	1.04	0.98
Pneumonia Care				
Appropriate Initial Antibiotic Given	27	96%	93%	95%

NOTE: Hospital profiles are in alphabetical order by state, then city, then hospital within the city; Rankings exclude hospitals with less than 25 cases except for patient surveys which excludes hospitals with less than 100 cases; (a) 100-299 cases; (1) The number of cases/patients is too few to report; (2) Data submitted were based on a sample of cases/patients; (3) Results are based on a shorter time period than required; (4) Data suppressed by CMS for one or more quarters; (5) Results are not available for this reporting period; (6) Fewer than 100 patients completed the HCAHPS survey; (7) No cases met the criteria for this measure; (8) The lower limit of the confidence interval cannot be calculated if the number of observed infections equals zero; (9) No data are available from the state/territory for this reporting period; (10) The scores shown reflect fewer than 50 completed surveys; (11) There were discrepancies in the data collection process; (12) This measure does not apply to this hospital for this reporting period; (13) Results cannot be calculated for this reporting period; (14) The results for this state are combined with nearby states to protect confidentiality; Please refer to the User's Guide for a full explanation of data.

Measure	Cases	This Hosp.	State Avg.	U.S. Avg.
Blood Culture Timing	46	96%	97%	98%
Pregnancy and Delivery Care				
Newborn Deliveries Scheduled Early[1,2]	-	-	5%	6%
Preventive Care				
Immunization for Influenza[2]	303	88%	85%	90%
Immunization for Pneumonia[2]	294	78%	88%	92%
Stroke Care				
Anticoagulation Therapy for Atrial Fibrillation[7]	-	-	93%	95%
Antithrombotic Therapy Timing	14	100%	96%	98%
Assessed for Rehabilitation	13	85%	95%	97%
Discharged on Antithrombotic Therapy	13	100%	97%	99%
Discharged on Statin Medication[1]	-	-	89%	94%
Thrombolytic Therapy Timing[7]	-	-	53%	66%
Venous Thromboembolism Prophylaxis	12	83%	87%	94%
Written Stroke Educational Materials Given	12	17%	83%	88%
Surgical Care Improvement Project				
Appropriate Beta Blocker Usage[2]	49	84%	97%	98%
Appropriate VTP Within 24 Hours[2]	150	97%	97%	98%
Controlled Postoperative Blood Glucose[2,7]	-	-	96%	97%
Perioperative Temperature Management[2]	202	100%	100%	100%
Prophylactic Antibiotic Selection[2]	100	98%	99%	99%
Prophylactic Antibiotic Selection (Outpatient)	97	100%	97%	98%
Prophylactic Antibiotic Stopped[2]	100	98%	97%	98%
Prophylactic Antibiotic Timing[2]	101	98%	98%	99%
Prophylactic Antibiotic Timing (Outpatient)	71	90%	97%	98%
Urinary Catheter Removal[2]	67	94%	96%	97%
Survey of Patients' Hospital Experiences				
Area Around Room 'Always' Quiet at Night	(a)	73%	74%	61%
Doctors 'Always' Communicated Well	(a)	85%	87%	82%
Home Recovery Information Given	(a)	75%	85%	85%
Hospital Given 9 or 10 on 10 Point Scale	(a)	72%	75%	71%
Meds 'Always' Explained Before Given	(a)	60%	69%	64%
Nurses 'Always' Communicated Well	(a)	84%	83%	79%
Pain 'Always' Well Controlled	(a)	72%	75%	71%
Room and Bathroom 'Always' Clean	(a)	75%	75%	73%
Timely Help 'Always' Received	(a)	69%	71%	68%
Would Definitely Recommend Hospital	(a)	74%	75%	71%
Use of Medical Imaging				
Cardiac Imaging Stress Test before Surgery	126	4.0%	5.3%	5.3%
Combination Abdominal CT Scan	305	36.4%	24.5%	10.5%
Combination Brain/Sinus CT Scan[1]	-	-	2.6%	2.7%
Combination Chest CT Scan	177	4.5%	7.6%	2.7%
Follow-up Mammogram/Ultrasound	598	10.9%	9.4%	8.8%
Lumbar Spine MRI for Low Back Pain[1]	-	-	42.7%	37.2%

Christus Saint Patrick Hospital

524 Dr Michael Debakey Street
Lake Charles, LA 70601
Phone: 337-436-2511
Fax: 337-491-7798
URL: www.christushealth.org
Type: Acute Care Hospitals
Emergency Services: Yes
Ownership: Voluntary non-profit - Private
Beds: 392
Key Personnel:
Pediatric In-Patient Care .... Yoko Broussard
Chief of Medical Staff.......... Walter Divers, MD
Anesthesiology............... James Eddy, MD
CEO/President............... Ellen Jones
Emergency Room .... Howard Rigg, MD
Radiology.................... John R Romero, III, DP
Infection Control.............. Carol Spence

Measure	Cases	This Hosp.	State Avg.	U.S. Avg.
Blood Clot Prevention and Treatment				
Anticoagulation Overlap Therapy[2]	58	57%	89%	93%
ICU Venous Thromboembolism Prophylaxis[2]	98	70%	88%	92%
Incidence of Potentially Preventable VTE[1,2]	-	-	16%	10%
UFH with Dosages/Platelet Monitoring[1,2]	-	-	94%	97%
Venous Thromboembolism Prophylaxis[2]	382	61%	74%	85%
Warfarin Therapy Discharge Instructions[2]	46	74%	85%	75%
Chest Pain/Possible Heart Attack Care				
Aspirin Given Within 24 Hours of Arrival[3,7]	-	-	94%	96%
Fibrinolytic Meds Within 30 Min. of Arrival[5]	-	-	54%	58%
Average Time to ECG (minutes)[3,7]	-	-	10	7
Average Time to Transfer (minutes)[5]	-	-	94	60
Children's Asthma Care				
Received Home Management Plan of Care	-	-	-	88%
Received Reliever Medication	-	-	-	100%
Received Systemic Corticosteroids	-	-	-	100%
Emergency Department				
Admittance Decision Time (minutes)[2]	855	96	86	98
Head CT Results Within 45 Min. of Arrival[1]	-	-	49%	57%
Patients Who Left ER Before Being Seen	25,980	1%	3%	2%
Time from ER Arrival to Admit. (minutes)[2]	895	270	256	274
Time from ER Arrival to Discharge (minutes)	363	135	125	134
Time in ER Before Being Evaluated (minutes)	300	24	27	26
Time to Pain Meds for Fractures (minutes)	78	46	61	57
Heart Attack Care				
Aspirin Given at Discharge	155	100%	99%	99%
Fibrinolytic Meds Within 30 Min. of Arrival[7]	-	-	71%	54%
PCI Within 90 Minutes of Arrival	46	89%	94%	96%
Statin Prescribed at Discharge	153	100%	98%	98%
Heart Failure Care				
ACE Inhibitor or ARB for LVSD	103	100%	95%	97%
Discharge Instructions Given	255	97%	94%	94%
Evaluation of LVS Function	299	100%	97%	99%
Medicare Spending				
Medicare Spending per Patient (ratio)	-	1.02	1.04	0.98
Pneumonia Care				
Appropriate Initial Antibiotic Given	72	93%	93%	95%
Blood Culture Timing	155	97%	97%	98%
Pregnancy and Delivery Care				
Newborn Deliveries Scheduled Early[7]	-	-	5%	6%
Preventive Care				
Immunization for Influenza[2]	579	92%	85%	90%
Immunization for Pneumonia[2]	901	94%	88%	92%
Stroke Care				
Anticoagulation Therapy for Atrial Fibrillation	19	84%	93%	95%
Antithrombotic Therapy Timing	110	95%	96%	98%
Assessed for Rehabilitation	127	91%	95%	97%
Discharged on Antithrombotic Therapy	113	95%	97%	99%
Discharged on Statin Medication	96	84%	89%	94%
Thrombolytic Therapy Timing[1]	-	-	53%	66%
Venous Thromboembolism Prophylaxis	123	63%	87%	94%
Written Stroke Educational Materials Given	68	59%	83%	88%
Surgical Care Improvement Project				
Appropriate Beta Blocker Usage	147	100%	97%	98%
Appropriate VTP Within 24 Hours	227	100%	97%	98%
Controlled Postoperative Blood Glucose	60	97%	96%	97%
Perioperative Temperature Management	298	100%	100%	100%
Prophylactic Antibiotic Selection	164	100%	99%	99%
Prophylactic Antibiotic Selection (Outpatient)	490	100%	97%	98%
Prophylactic Antibiotic Stopped	147	99%	97%	98%
Prophylactic Antibiotic Timing	166	100%	98%	99%
Prophylactic Antibiotic Timing (Outpatient)	491	100%	97%	98%
Urinary Catheter Removal	119	100%	96%	97%
Survey of Patients' Hospital Experiences				
Area Around Room 'Always' Quiet at Night	300+	63%	74%	61%
Doctors 'Always' Communicated Well	300+	84%	87%	82%
Home Recovery Information Given	300+	82%	85%	85%
Hospital Given 9 or 10 on 10 Point Scale	300+	68%	75%	71%
Meds 'Always' Explained Before Given	300+	61%	69%	64%
Nurses 'Always' Communicated Well	300+	78%	83%	79%
Pain 'Always' Well Controlled	300+	69%	75%	71%
Room and Bathroom 'Always' Clean	300+	67%	75%	73%
Timely Help 'Always' Received	300+	62%	71%	68%
Would Definitely Recommend Hospital	300+	72%	75%	71%
Use of Medical Imaging				
Cardiac Imaging Stress Test before Surgery	148	7.4%	5.3%	5.3%
Combination Abdominal CT Scan	815	15.5%	24.5%	10.5%
Combination Brain/Sinus CT Scan	691	2.6%	2.6%	2.7%
Combination Chest CT Scan	367	23.2%	7.6%	2.7%
Follow-up Mammogram/Ultrasound	1,079	10.3%	9.4%	8.8%
Lumbar Spine MRI for Low Back Pain[1]	-	-	42.7%	37.2%

Lake Area Medical Center

4200 Nelson Road
Lake Charles, LA 70605
Phone: 337-474-6370
Fax: 337-475-4750
E-mail: info@women-childrens.com
URL: www.women-childrens.com
Type: Acute Care Hospitals
Emergency Services: Yes
Ownership: Proprietary
Beds: 80
Key Personnel:
Radiology.................... Dawn Matte
CEO/President............... Rich Robinson

Measure	Cases	This Hosp.	State Avg.	U.S. Avg.
Blood Clot Prevention and Treatment				
Anticoagulation Overlap Therapy[1,2]	-	-	89%	93%
ICU Venous Thromboembolism Prophylaxis[2]	17	100%	88%	92%
Incidence of Potentially Preventable VTE[2,7]	-	-	16%	10%
UFH with Dosages/Platelet Monitoring[1,2]	-	-	94%	97%
Venous Thromboembolism Prophylaxis[2]	93	97%	74%	85%
Warfarin Therapy Discharge Instructions[1,2]	-	-	85%	75%
Chest Pain/Possible Heart Attack Care				
Aspirin Given Within 24 Hours of Arrival	12	100%	94%	96%
Fibrinolytic Meds Within 30 Min. of Arrival[3,7]	-	-	54%	58%
Average Time to ECG (minutes)	13	15	10	7
Average Time to Transfer (minutes)[1,3]	-	-	94	60
Children's Asthma Care				
Received Home Management Plan of Care	-	-	-	88%
Received Reliever Medication	-	-	-	100%
Received Systemic Corticosteroids	-	-	-	100%
Emergency Department				
Admittance Decision Time (minutes)[2]	153	43	86	98
Head CT Results Within 45 Min. of Arrival[1]	-	-	49%	57%
Patients Who Left ER Before Being Seen	24,873	2%	3%	2%
Time from ER Arrival to Admit. (minutes)[2]	153	207	256	274
Time from ER Arrival to Discharge (minutes)	398	98	125	134
Time in ER Before Being Evaluated (minutes)	415	25	27	26
Time to Pain Meds for Fractures (minutes)	127	56	61	57
Heart Attack Care				
Aspirin Given at Discharge[3,7]	-	-	99%	99%
Fibrinolytic Meds Within 30 Min. of Arrival[3,7]	-	-	71%	54%
PCI Within 90 Minutes of Arrival[3,7]	-	-	94%	96%
Statin Prescribed at Discharge[3,7]	-	-	98%	98%
Heart Failure Care				
ACE Inhibitor or ARB for LVSD[1]	-	-	95%	97%
Discharge Instructions Given	17	94%	94%	94%
Evaluation of LVS Function	17	100%	97%	99%
Medicare Spending				
Medicare Spending per Patient (ratio)	-	0.96	1.04	0.98
Pneumonia Care				
Appropriate Initial Antibiotic Given	23	100%	93%	95%
Blood Culture Timing	38	95%	97%	98%
Pregnancy and Delivery Care				
Newborn Deliveries Scheduled Early[2]	50	0%	5%	6%
Preventive Care				
Immunization for Influenza[2]	307	98%	85%	90%
Immunization for Pneumonia[2]	142	99%	88%	92%
Stroke Care				
Anticoagulation Therapy for Atrial Fibrillation[7]	-	-	93%	95%
Antithrombotic Therapy Timing[1]	-	-	96%	98%
Assessed for Rehabilitation[1]	-	-	95%	97%
Discharged on Antithrombotic Therapy[1]	-	-	97%	99%
Discharged on Statin Medication[1]	-	-	89%	94%
Thrombolytic Therapy Timing[7]	-	-	53%	66%
Venous Thromboembolism Prophylaxis[1]	-	-	87%	94%
Written Stroke Educational Materials Given[1]	-	-	83%	88%
Surgical Care Improvement Project				
Appropriate Beta Blocker Usage	45	96%	97%	98%
Appropriate VTP Within 24 Hours	196	98%	97%	98%
Controlled Postoperative Blood Glucose[7]	-	-	96%	97%
Perioperative Temperature Management	279	100%	100%	100%
Prophylactic Antibiotic Selection	222	100%	99%	99%
Prophylactic Antibiotic Selection (Outpatient)	203	99%	97%	98%
Prophylactic Antibiotic Stopped	217	99%	97%	98%
Prophylactic Antibiotic Timing	221	98%	98%	99%
Prophylactic Antibiotic Timing (Outpatient)	204	100%	97%	98%

NOTE: Hospital profiles are in alphabetical order by state, then city, then hospital within the city; Rankings exclude hospitals with less than 25 cases except for patient surveys which excludes hospitals with less than 100 cases; (a) 100-299 cases; (1) The number of cases/patients is too few to report; (2) Data submitted were based on a sample of cases/patients; (3) Results are based on a shorter time period than required; (4) Data suppressed by CMS for one or more quarters; (5) Results are not available for this reporting period; (6) Fewer than 100 patients completed the HCAHPS survey; (7) No cases met the criteria for this measure; (8) The lower limit of the confidence interval cannot be calculated if the number of observed infections equals zero; (9) No data are available from the state/territory for this reporting period; (10) The scores shown reflect fewer than 50 completed surveys; (11) There were discrepancies in the data collection process; (12) This measure does not apply to this hospital for this reporting period; (13) Results cannot be calculated for this reporting period; (14) The results for this state are combined with nearby states to protect confidentiality; Please refer to the User's Guide for a full explanation of data.

Measure	Cases	This Hosp.	State Avg.	U.S. Avg.
Urinary Catheter Removal	21	95%	96%	97%
Survey of Patients' Hospital Experiences				
Area Around Room 'Always' Quiet at Night	300+	69%	74%	61%
Doctors 'Always' Communicated Well	300+	85%	87%	82%
Home Recovery Information Given	300+	88%	85%	85%
Hospital Given 9 or 10 on 10 Point Scale	300+	80%	75%	71%
Meds 'Always' Explained Before Given	300+	69%	69%	64%
Nurses 'Always' Communicated Well	300+	84%	83%	79%
Pain 'Always' Well Controlled	300+	77%	75%	71%
Room and Bathroom 'Always' Clean	300+	70%	75%	73%
Timely Help 'Always' Received	300+	73%	71%	68%
Would Definitely Recommend Hospital	300+	82%	75%	71%
Use of Medical Imaging				
Cardiac Imaging Stress Test before Surgery[1]	-	-	5.3%	5.3%
Combination Abdominal CT Scan	114	2.6%	24.5%	10.5%
Combination Brain/Sinus CT Scan	108	9.3%	2.6%	2.7%
Combination Chest CT Scan[1]	-	-	7.6%	2.7%
Follow-up Mammogram/Ultrasound	496	8.3%	9.4%	8.8%
Lumbar Spine MRI for Low Back Pain[7]	-	-	42.7%	37.2%

Lake Charles Memorial Hospital

1701 Oak Park Blvd
Lake Charles, LA 70601
Phone: 337-494-3200
Fax: 337-494-3299
URL: www.lcmh.com
Type: Acute Care Hospitals
Emergency Services: Yes
Ownership: Voluntary non-profit - Private
Beds: 324

Key Personnel:
Emergency Room . . . . Robert M Anderson, MD
Chief of Medical Staff . . . . Alan Le Le Bato, MD
Intensive Care Unit. . . . . Denise Collett
Radiology. . . . . Scott Daigle
Chair/CEO . . . . Denise Emerson Rau
Infection Control. . . . . Belinda Fitzgerald
President/CEO. . . . . Larry M. Graham
Quality Assurance . . . . David Usher

Measure	Cases	This Hosp.	State Avg.	U.S. Avg.
Blood Clot Prevention and Treatment				
Anticoagulation Overlap Therapy[2]	43	100%	89%	93%
ICU Venous Thromboembolism Prophylaxis[2]	74	82%	88%	92%
Incidence of Potentially Preventable VTE[1,2]	-	-	16%	10%
UFH with Dosages/Platelet Monitoring[1,2]	-	-	94%	97%
Venous Thromboembolism Prophylaxis[2]	367	76%	74%	85%
Warfarin Therapy Discharge Instructions[2]	27	93%	85%	75%
Chest Pain/Possible Heart Attack Care				
Aspirin Given Within 24 Hours of Arrival[5]	-	-	94%	96%
Fibrinolytic Meds Within 30 Min. of Arrival[5]	-	-	54%	58%
Average Time to ECG (minutes)[5]	-	-	10	7
Average Time to Transfer (minutes)[5]	-	-	94	60
Children's Asthma Care				
Received Home Management Plan of Care	-	-	-	88%
Received Reliever Medication	-	-	-	100%
Received Systemic Corticosteroids	-	-	-	100%
Emergency Department				
Admittance Decision Time (minutes)[2]	487	106	86	98
Head CT Results Within 45 Min. of Arrival[1]	-	-	49%	57%
Patients Who Left ER Before Being Seen	36,463	2%	3%	2%
Time from ER Arrival to Admit. (minutes)[2]	510	293	256	274
Time from ER Arrival to Discharge (minutes)	348	129	125	134
Time in ER Before Being Evaluated (minutes)	340	50	27	26
Time to Pain Meds for Fractures (minutes)	85	74	61	57
Heart Attack Care				
Aspirin Given at Discharge	142	95%	99%	99%
Fibrinolytic Meds Within 30 Min. of Arrival[7]	-	-	71%	54%
PCI Within 90 Minutes of Arrival	19	79%	94%	96%
Statin Prescribed at Discharge	135	98%	98%	98%
Heart Failure Care				
ACE Inhibitor or ARB for LVSD[2]	118	86%	95%	97%
Discharge Instructions Given[2]	263	85%	94%	94%
Evaluation of LVS Function[2]	313	99%	97%	99%
Medicare Spending				
Medicare Spending per Patient (ratio)	-	1.00	1.04	0.98
Pneumonia Care				
Appropriate Initial Antibiotic Given[2]	59	88%	93%	95%
Blood Culture Timing[2]	152	91%	97%	98%
Pregnancy and Delivery Care				
Newborn Deliveries Scheduled Early[2]	33	0%	5%	6%
Preventive Care				
Immunization for Influenza[2]	486	85%	85%	90%
Immunization for Pneumonia[2]	531	94%	88%	92%
Stroke Care				
Anticoagulation Therapy for Atrial Fibrillation[2]	13	85%	93%	95%
Antithrombotic Therapy Timing[2]	81	98%	96%	98%
Assessed for Rehabilitation[2]	79	92%	95%	97%
Discharged on Antithrombotic Therapy[2]	73	99%	97%	99%
Discharged on Statin Medication[2]	71	68%	89%	94%
Thrombolytic Therapy Timing[2]	19	5%	53%	66%
Venous Thromboembolism Prophylaxis[2]	88	85%	87%	94%
Written Stroke Educational Materials Given[2]	52	52%	83%	88%
Surgical Care Improvement Project				
Appropriate Beta Blocker Usage[2]	241	93%	97%	98%
Appropriate VTP Within 24 Hours[2]	492	92%	97%	98%
Controlled Postoperative Blood Glucose[2]	101	90%	96%	97%
Perioperative Temperature Management[2]	545	100%	100%	100%
Prophylactic Antibiotic Selection[2]	480	99%	99%	99%
Prophylactic Antibiotic Selection (Outpatient)	306	94%	97%	98%
Prophylactic Antibiotic Stopped[2]	472	96%	97%	98%
Prophylactic Antibiotic Timing[2]	482	98%	98%	99%
Prophylactic Antibiotic Timing (Outpatient)	310	98%	97%	98%
Urinary Catheter Removal[2]	320	94%	96%	97%
Survey of Patients' Hospital Experiences				
Area Around Room 'Always' Quiet at Night	300+	71%	74%	61%
Doctors 'Always' Communicated Well	300+	86%	87%	82%
Home Recovery Information Given	300+	84%	85%	85%
Hospital Given 9 or 10 on 10 Point Scale	300+	72%	75%	71%
Meds 'Always' Explained Before Given	300+	66%	69%	64%
Nurses 'Always' Communicated Well	300+	82%	83%	79%
Pain 'Always' Well Controlled	300+	74%	75%	71%
Room and Bathroom 'Always' Clean	300+	70%	75%	73%
Timely Help 'Always' Received	300+	63%	71%	68%
Would Definitely Recommend Hospital	300+	78%	75%	71%
Use of Medical Imaging				
Cardiac Imaging Stress Test before Surgery	152	7.2%	5.3%	5.3%
Combination Abdominal CT Scan	928	16.8%	24.5%	10.5%
Combination Brain/Sinus CT Scan	988	1.2%	2.6%	2.7%
Combination Chest CT Scan	366	3.0%	7.6%	2.7%
Follow-up Mammogram/Ultrasound	1,859	3.7%	9.4%	8.8%
Lumbar Spine MRI for Low Back Pain[1]	-	-	42.7%	37.2%

East Carroll Parish Hospital

336 North Hood Street
Lake Providence, LA 71254
Phone: 318-559-4023
Fax: 318-559-3761
Type: Acute Care Hospitals
Emergency Services: Yes
Ownership: Govt - Hospital Dist/Auth
Beds: 23

Key Personnel:
CEO/President. . . . . Ladonna Benglerth

Measure	Cases	This Hosp.	State Avg.	U.S. Avg.
Blood Clot Prevention and Treatment				
Anticoagulation Overlap Therapy[2,7]	-	-	89%	93%
ICU Venous Thromboembolism Prophylaxis[2,7]	-	-	88%	92%
Incidence of Potentially Preventable VTE[2,7]	-	-	16%	10%
UFH with Dosages/Platelet Monitoring[2,7]	-	-	94%	97%
Venous Thromboembolism Prophylaxis[2]	257	51%	74%	85%
Warfarin Therapy Discharge Instructions[2,7]	-	-	85%	75%
Chest Pain/Possible Heart Attack Care				
Aspirin Given Within 24 Hours of Arrival[3]	17	94%	94%	96%
Fibrinolytic Meds Within 30 Min. of Arrival[3,7]	-	-	54%	58%
Average Time to ECG (minutes)[3]	17	21	10	7
Average Time to Transfer (minutes)[1,3]	-	-	94	60
Children's Asthma Care				
Received Home Management Plan of Care	-	-	-	88%
Received Reliever Medication	-	-	-	100%
Received Systemic Corticosteroids	-	-	-	100%
Emergency Department				
Admittance Decision Time (minutes)[2]	128	34	86	98
Head CT Results Within 45 Min. of Arrival[5]	-	-	49%	57%
Patients Who Left ER Before Being Seen	4,597	1%	3%	2%
Time from ER Arrival to Admit. (minutes)[2]	128	144	256	274
Time from ER Arrival to Discharge (minutes)	385	67	125	134
Time in ER Before Being Evaluated (minutes)	439	18	27	26
Time to Pain Meds for Fractures (minutes)[1,3]	-	-	61	57
Heart Attack Care				
Aspirin Given at Discharge[5]	-	-	99%	99%
Fibrinolytic Meds Within 30 Min. of Arrival[5]	-	-	71%	54%
PCI Within 90 Minutes of Arrival[5]	-	-	94%	96%
Statin Prescribed at Discharge[5]	-	-	98%	98%
Heart Failure Care				
ACE Inhibitor or ARB for LVSD[7]	-	-	95%	97%
Discharge Instructions Given	36	61%	94%	94%
Evaluation of LVS Function	45	2%	97%	99%
Medicare Spending				
Medicare Spending per Patient (ratio)	-	0.87	1.04	0.98
Pneumonia Care				
Appropriate Initial Antibiotic Given	17	65%	93%	95%
Blood Culture Timing[1]	-	-	97%	98%
Pregnancy and Delivery Care				
Newborn Deliveries Scheduled Early[7]	-	-	5%	6%
Preventive Care				
Immunization for Influenza[2]	250	62%	85%	90%
Immunization for Pneumonia[2]	373	47%	88%	92%
Stroke Care				
Anticoagulation Therapy for Atrial Fibrillation[3,7]	-	-	93%	95%
Antithrombotic Therapy Timing[1,3]	-	-	96%	98%
Assessed for Rehabilitation[3,7]	-	-	95%	97%
Discharged on Antithrombotic Therapy[3,7]	-	-	97%	99%
Discharged on Statin Medication[3,7]	-	-	89%	94%
Thrombolytic Therapy Timing[3,7]	-	-	53%	66%
Venous Thromboembolism Prophylaxis[1,3]	-	-	87%	94%
Written Stroke Educational Materials Given[3,7]	-	-	83%	88%
Surgical Care Improvement Project				
Appropriate Beta Blocker Usage[5]	-	-	97%	98%
Appropriate VTP Within 24 Hours[5]	-	-	97%	98%
Controlled Postoperative Blood Glucose[5]	-	-	96%	97%
Perioperative Temperature Management[5]	-	-	100%	100%
Prophylactic Antibiotic Selection[5]	-	-	99%	99%
Prophylactic Antibiotic Selection (Outpatient)[5]	-	-	97%	98%
Prophylactic Antibiotic Stopped[5]	-	-	97%	98%
Prophylactic Antibiotic Timing[5]	-	-	98%	99%
Prophylactic Antibiotic Timing (Outpatient)[5]	-	-	97%	98%
Urinary Catheter Removal[5]	-	-	96%	97%
Survey of Patients' Hospital Experiences				
Area Around Room 'Always' Quiet at Night	(a)	74%	74%	61%
Doctors 'Always' Communicated Well	(a)	95%	87%	82%
Home Recovery Information Given	(a)	82%	85%	85%
Hospital Given 9 or 10 on 10 Point Scale	(a)	69%	75%	71%
Meds 'Always' Explained Before Given	(a)	71%	69%	64%
Nurses 'Always' Communicated Well	(a)	84%	83%	79%
Pain 'Always' Well Controlled	(a)	77%	75%	71%
Room and Bathroom 'Always' Clean	(a)	73%	75%	73%
Timely Help 'Always' Received	(a)	77%	71%	68%
Would Definitely Recommend Hospital	(a)	68%	75%	71%
Use of Medical Imaging				
Cardiac Imaging Stress Test before Surgery[7]	-	-	5.3%	5.3%
Combination Abdominal CT Scan	64	23.4%	24.5%	10.5%
Combination Brain/Sinus CT Scan[1]	-	-	2.6%	2.7%
Combination Chest CT Scan[1]	-	-	7.6%	2.7%
Follow-up Mammogram/Ultrasound[7]	-	-	9.4%	8.8%
Lumbar Spine MRI for Low Back Pain[7]	-	-	42.7%	37.2%

River Parishes Hospital

500 Rue De Sante
Laplace, LA 70068
Phone: 985-652-7000
Fax: 985-652-5161
URL: www.riverparisheshospital.com
Type: Acute Care Hospitals
Emergency Services: Yes
Ownership: Proprietary
Beds: 102

Key Personnel:
CEO/President. . . . . Charlotte Dupre
Radiology. . . . . Julian B Foreman
Chief of Medical Staff . . . . Majit Wadhwa

Measure	Cases	This Hosp.	State Avg.	U.S. Avg.

NOTE: Hospital profiles are in alphabetical order by state, then city, then hospital within the city; Rankings exclude hospitals with less than 25 cases except for patient surveys which excludes hospitals with less than 100 cases; (a) 100-299 cases; (1) The number of cases/patients is too few to report; (2) Data submitted were based on a sample of cases/patients; (3) Results are based on a shorter time period than required; (4) Data suppressed by CMS for one or more quarters; (5) Results are not available for this reporting period; (6) Fewer than 100 patients completed the HCAHPS survey; (7) No cases met the criteria for this measure; (8) The lower limit of the confidence interval cannot be calculated if the number of observed infections equals zero; (9) No data are available from the state/territory for this reporting period; (10) The scores shown reflect fewer than 50 completed surveys; (11) There were discrepancies in the data collection process; (12) This measure does not apply to this hospital for this reporting period; (13) Results cannot be calculated for this reporting period; (14) The results for this state are combined with nearby states to protect confidentiality; Please refer to the User's Guide for a full explanation of data.

Measure	Cases	This Hosp.	State Avg.	U.S. Avg.
Blood Clot Prevention and Treatment				
Anticoagulation Overlap Therapy[2]	19	68%	89%	93%
ICU Venous Thromboembolism Prophylaxis[2]	56	73%	88%	92%
Incidence of Potentially Preventable VTE[1,2]	-	-	16%	10%
UFH with Dosages/Platelet Monitoring[1,2]	-	-	94%	97%
Venous Thromboembolism Prophylaxis[2]	120	48%	74%	85%
Warfarin Therapy Discharge Instructions[2]	11	100%	85%	75%
Chest Pain/Possible Heart Attack Care				
Aspirin Given Within 24 Hours of Arrival	29	93%	94%	96%
Fibrinolytic Meds Within 30 Min. of Arrival[7]	-	-	54%	58%
Average Time to ECG (minutes)	29	6	10	7
Average Time to Transfer (minutes)[1]	-	-	94	60
Children's Asthma Care				
Received Home Management Plan of Care	-	-	-	88%
Received Reliever Medication	-	-	-	100%
Received Systemic Corticosteroids	-	-	-	100%
Emergency Department				
Admittance Decision Time (minutes)[2]	374	84	86	98
Head CT Results Within 45 Min. of Arrival[1]	-	-	49%	57%
Patients Who Left ER Before Being Seen	17,806	3%	3%	2%
Time from ER Arrival to Admit. (minutes)[2]	374	256	256	274
Time from ER Arrival to Discharge (minutes)	366	104	125	134
Time in ER Before Being Evaluated (minutes)	396	15	27	26
Time to Pain Meds for Fractures (minutes)	34	39	61	57
Heart Attack Care				
Aspirin Given at Discharge	14	71%	99%	99%
Fibrinolytic Meds Within 30 Min. of Arrival[7]	-	-	71%	54%
PCI Within 90 Minutes of Arrival[7]	-	-	94%	96%
Statin Prescribed at Discharge	12	83%	98%	98%
Heart Failure Care				
ACE Inhibitor or ARB for LVSD	57	98%	95%	97%
Discharge Instructions Given	97	93%	94%	94%
Evaluation of LVS Function	111	100%	97%	99%
Medicare Spending				
Medicare Spending per Patient (ratio)	-	1.12	1.04	0.98
Pneumonia Care				
Appropriate Initial Antibiotic Given	44	100%	93%	95%
Blood Culture Timing	72	100%	97%	98%
Pregnancy and Delivery Care				
Newborn Deliveries Scheduled Early[2,7]	-	-	5%	6%
Preventive Care				
Immunization for Influenza[2]	254	91%	85%	90%
Immunization for Pneumonia[2]	419	91%	88%	92%
Stroke Care				
Anticoagulation Therapy for Atrial Fibrillation[7]	-	-	93%	95%
Antithrombotic Therapy Timing	14	100%	96%	98%
Assessed for Rehabilitation	16	94%	95%	97%
Discharged on Antithrombotic Therapy	15	93%	97%	99%
Discharged on Statin Medication	14	93%	89%	94%
Thrombolytic Therapy Timing[1]	-	-	53%	66%
Venous Thromboembolism Prophylaxis	13	62%	87%	94%
Written Stroke Educational Materials Given[1]	-	-	83%	88%
Surgical Care Improvement Project				
Appropriate Beta Blocker Usage[2]	43	98%	97%	98%
Appropriate VTP Within 24 Hours[2]	106	98%	97%	98%
Controlled Postoperative Blood Glucose[2,7]	-	-	96%	97%
Perioperative Temperature Management[2]	111	100%	100%	100%
Prophylactic Antibiotic Selection[2]	75	97%	99%	99%
Prophylactic Antibiotic Selection (Outpatient)	29	90%	97%	98%
Prophylactic Antibiotic Stopped[2]	73	97%	97%	98%
Prophylactic Antibiotic Timing[2]	75	100%	98%	99%
Prophylactic Antibiotic Timing (Outpatient)	30	97%	97%	98%
Urinary Catheter Removal[2]	15	93%	96%	97%
Survey of Patients' Hospital Experiences				
Area Around Room 'Always' Quiet at Night	(a)	68%	74%	61%
Doctors 'Always' Communicated Well	(a)	90%	87%	82%
Home Recovery Information Given	(a)	87%	85%	85%
Hospital Given 9 or 10 on 10 Point Scale	(a)	65%	75%	71%
Meds 'Always' Explained Before Given	(a)	68%	69%	64%
Nurses 'Always' Communicated Well	(a)	83%	83%	79%
Pain 'Always' Well Controlled	(a)	69%	75%	71%
Room and Bathroom 'Always' Clean	(a)	63%	75%	73%
Timely Help 'Always' Received	(a)	65%	71%	68%
Would Definitely Recommend Hospital	(a)	60%	75%	71%
Use of Medical Imaging				
Cardiac Imaging Stress Test before Surgery	59	5.1%	5.3%	5.3%
Combination Abdominal CT Scan	103	19.4%	24.5%	10.5%
Combination Brain/Sinus CT Scan[1]	-	-	2.6%	2.7%
Combination Chest CT Scan[1]	-	-	7.6%	2.7%
Follow-up Mammogram/Ultrasound	279	7.2%	9.4%	8.8%
Lumbar Spine MRI for Low Back Pain[1]	-	-	42.7%	37.2%

Byrd Regional Hospital

1020 Fertitta Blvd
Leesville, LA 71446
Phone: 337-239-9041
Fax: 337-239-6541
E-mail: lmaricle@hq.chs.net
URL: www.chs.net
Type: Acute Care Hospitals
Emergency Services: Yes
Ownership: Proprietary
Beds: 70

Key Personnel:
Emergency Room . . . . Angie Dixon, RN
Ambulatory Care . . . . Fran Gibson
Pediatric Ambulatory Care . . . . . . Naila Khateeb
CEO/President. . . . . Roger LeDoux
Chief of Medical Staff . . . . Hanna Lubbos, MD
Radiology. . . . . Joe Rankin
Intensive Care Unit. . . . . Chuck Weaver, RN

Measure	Cases	This Hosp.	State Avg.	U.S. Avg.
Blood Clot Prevention and Treatment				
Anticoagulation Overlap Therapy[1,2]	-	-	89%	93%
ICU Venous Thromboembolism Prophylaxis[2]	79	94%	88%	92%
Incidence of Potentially Preventable VTE[2,7]	-	-	16%	10%
UFH with Dosages/Platelet Monitoring[1,2]	-	-	94%	97%
Venous Thromboembolism Prophylaxis[2]	322	85%	74%	85%
Warfarin Therapy Discharge Instructions[1,2]	-	-	85%	75%
Chest Pain/Possible Heart Attack Care				
Aspirin Given Within 24 Hours of Arrival	41	93%	94%	96%
Fibrinolytic Meds Within 30 Min. of Arrival[1]	-	-	54%	58%
Average Time to ECG (minutes)	40	7	10	7
Average Time to Transfer (minutes)[1]	-	-	94	60
Children's Asthma Care				
Received Home Management Plan of Care	-	-	-	88%
Received Reliever Medication	-	-	-	100%
Received Systemic Corticosteroids	-	-	-	100%
Emergency Department				
Admittance Decision Time (minutes)[2]	423	92	86	98
Head CT Results Within 45 Min. of Arrival	14	57%	49%	57%
Patients Who Left ER Before Being Seen	16,294	3%	3%	2%
Time from ER Arrival to Admit. (minutes)[2]	439	227	256	274
Time from ER Arrival to Discharge (minutes)	265	105	125	134
Time in ER Before Being Evaluated (minutes)	423	18	27	26
Time to Pain Meds for Fractures (minutes)	77	47	61	57
Heart Attack Care				
Aspirin Given at Discharge[1]	-	-	99%	99%
Fibrinolytic Meds Within 30 Min. of Arrival[7]	-	-	71%	54%
PCI Within 90 Minutes of Arrival[7]	-	-	94%	96%
Statin Prescribed at Discharge[1]	-	-	98%	98%
Heart Failure Care				
ACE Inhibitor or ARB for LVSD	48	96%	95%	97%
Discharge Instructions Given	165	96%	94%	94%
Evaluation of LVS Function	191	100%	97%	99%
Medicare Spending				
Medicare Spending per Patient (ratio)	-	1.08	1.04	0.98
Pneumonia Care				
Appropriate Initial Antibiotic Given	52	98%	93%	95%
Blood Culture Timing	91	97%	97%	98%
Pregnancy and Delivery Care				
Newborn Deliveries Scheduled Early[2]	34	0%	5%	6%
Preventive Care				
Immunization for Influenza[2]	422	100%	85%	90%
Immunization for Pneumonia[2]	525	100%	88%	92%
Stroke Care				
Anticoagulation Therapy for Atrial Fibrillation[1]	-	-	93%	95%
Antithrombotic Therapy Timing	12	100%	96%	98%
Assessed for Rehabilitation	13	100%	95%	97%
Discharged on Antithrombotic Therapy	11	100%	97%	99%
Discharged on Statin Medication	11	73%	89%	94%
Thrombolytic Therapy Timing[7]	-	-	53%	66%
Venous Thromboembolism Prophylaxis	12	75%	87%	94%
Written Stroke Educational Materials Given[1]	-	-	83%	88%
Surgical Care Improvement Project				
Appropriate Beta Blocker Usage	46	98%	97%	98%
Appropriate VTP Within 24 Hours	98	98%	97%	98%
Controlled Postoperative Blood Glucose[7]	-	-	96%	97%
Perioperative Temperature Management	122	99%	100%	100%
Prophylactic Antibiotic Selection	89	98%	99%	99%
Prophylactic Antibiotic Selection (Outpatient)	44	100%	97%	98%
Prophylactic Antibiotic Stopped	82	100%	97%	98%
Prophylactic Antibiotic Timing	89	100%	98%	99%
Prophylactic Antibiotic Timing (Outpatient)	44	98%	97%	98%
Urinary Catheter Removal	78	97%	96%	97%
Survey of Patients' Hospital Experiences				
Area Around Room 'Always' Quiet at Night	300+	67%	74%	61%
Doctors 'Always' Communicated Well	300+	83%	87%	82%
Home Recovery Information Given	300+	84%	85%	85%
Hospital Given 9 or 10 on 10 Point Scale	300+	63%	75%	71%
Meds 'Always' Explained Before Given	300+	66%	69%	64%
Nurses 'Always' Communicated Well	300+	76%	83%	79%
Pain 'Always' Well Controlled	300+	73%	75%	71%
Room and Bathroom 'Always' Clean	300+	62%	75%	73%
Timely Help 'Always' Received	300+	65%	71%	68%
Would Definitely Recommend Hospital	300+	62%	75%	71%
Use of Medical Imaging				
Cardiac Imaging Stress Test before Surgery	86	1.2%	5.3%	5.3%
Combination Abdominal CT Scan	407	33.7%	24.5%	10.5%
Combination Brain/Sinus CT Scan	354	4.5%	2.6%	2.7%
Combination Chest CT Scan	192	4.7%	7.6%	2.7%
Follow-up Mammogram/Ultrasound	444	5.9%	9.4%	8.8%
Lumbar Spine MRI for Low Back Pain[1]	-	-	42.7%	37.2%

Doctors Hospital at Deer Creek

815 South 10th Street
Leesville, LA 71446
Phone: 337-392-5088
URL: www.dhdc.md
Type: Acute Care Hospitals
Emergency Services: No
Ownership: Physician

Measure	Cases	This Hosp.	State Avg.	U.S. Avg.
Blood Clot Prevention and Treatment				
Anticoagulation Overlap Therapy[1]	-	-	89%	93%
ICU Venous Thromboembolism Prophylaxis[7]	-	-	88%	92%
Incidence of Potentially Preventable VTE[1]	-	-	16%	10%
UFH with Dosages/Platelet Monitoring[7]	-	-	94%	97%
Venous Thromboembolism Prophylaxis	192	21%	74%	85%
Warfarin Therapy Discharge Instructions[7]	-	-	85%	75%
Chest Pain/Possible Heart Attack Care				
Aspirin Given Within 24 Hours of Arrival[5]	-	-	94%	96%
Fibrinolytic Meds Within 30 Min. of Arrival[5]	-	-	54%	58%
Average Time to ECG (minutes)[5]	-	-	10	7
Average Time to Transfer (minutes)[5]	-	-	94	60
Children's Asthma Care				
Received Home Management Plan of Care	-	-	-	88%
Received Reliever Medication	-	-	-	100%
Received Systemic Corticosteroids	-	-	-	100%
Emergency Department				
Admittance Decision Time (minutes)[2,7]	-	-	86	98
Head CT Results Within 45 Min. of Arrival[5]	-	-	49%	57%
Patients Who Left ER Before Being Seen[5]	-	-	3%	2%
Time from ER Arrival to Admit. (minutes)[2,7]	-	-	256	274
Time from ER Arrival to Discharge (minutes)[5]	-	-	125	134
Time in ER Before Being Evaluated (minutes)[5]	-	-	27	26
Time to Pain Meds for Fractures (minutes)[5]	-	-	61	57
Heart Attack Care				
Aspirin Given at Discharge[5]	-	-	99%	99%
Fibrinolytic Meds Within 30 Min. of Arrival[5]	-	-	71%	54%
PCI Within 90 Minutes of Arrival[5]	-	-	94%	96%
Statin Prescribed at Discharge[5]	-	-	98%	98%
Heart Failure Care				
ACE Inhibitor or ARB for LVSD[2,7]	-	-	95%	97%

NOTE: Hospital profiles are in alphabetical order by state, then city, then hospital within the city; Rankings exclude hospitals with less than 25 cases except for patient surveys which excludes hospitals with less than 100 cases; (a) 100-299 cases; (1) The number of cases/patients is too few to report; (2) Data submitted were based on a sample of cases/patients; (3) Results are based on a shorter time period than required; (4) Data suppressed by CMS for one or more quarters; (5) Results are not available for this reporting period; (6) Fewer than 100 patients completed the HCAHPS survey; (7) No cases met the criteria for this measure; (8) The lower limit of the confidence interval cannot be calculated if the number of observed infections equals zero; (9) No data are available from the state/territory for this reporting period; (10) The scores shown reflect fewer than 50 completed surveys; (11) There were discrepancies in the data collection process; (12) This measure does not apply to this hospital for this reporting period; (13) Results cannot be calculated for this reporting period; (14) The results for this state are combined with nearby states to protect confidentiality; Please refer to the User's Guide for a full explanation of data.

Measure	Cases	This Hosp.	State Avg.	U.S. Avg.
Discharge Instructions Given[1,2]	-	-	94%	94%
Evaluation of LVS Function[1,2]	-	-	97%	99%
Medicare Spending				
Medicare Spending per Patient (ratio)	-	0.95	1.04	0.98
Pneumonia Care				
Appropriate Initial Antibiotic Given[2]	22	91%	93%	95%
Blood Culture Timing[1,2]	-	-	97%	98%
Pregnancy and Delivery Care				
Newborn Deliveries Scheduled Early[7]	-	-	5%	6%
Preventive Care				
Immunization for Influenza[2]	244	39%	85%	90%
Immunization for Pneumonia[2]	217	65%	88%	92%
Stroke Care				
Anticoagulation Therapy for Atrial Fibrillation[5]	-	-	93%	95%
Antithrombotic Therapy Timing[5]	-	-	96%	98%
Assessed for Rehabilitation[5]	-	-	95%	97%
Discharged on Antithrombotic Therapy[5]	-	-	97%	99%
Discharged on Statin Medication[5]	-	-	89%	94%
Thrombolytic Therapy Timing[5]	-	-	53%	66%
Venous Thromboembolism Prophylaxis[5]	-	-	87%	94%
Written Stroke Educational Materials Given[5]	-	-	83%	88%
Surgical Care Improvement Project				
Appropriate Beta Blocker Usage[2]	12	83%	97%	98%
Appropriate VTP Within 24 Hours[2]	29	97%	97%	98%
Controlled Postoperative Blood Glucose[2,7]	-	-	96%	97%
Perioperative Temperature Management[2]	37	86%	100%	100%
Prophylactic Antibiotic Selection[2]	32	97%	99%	99%
Prophylactic Antibiotic Selection (Outpatient)[1,3]	-	-	97%	98%
Prophylactic Antibiotic Stopped[2]	32	88%	97%	98%
Prophylactic Antibiotic Timing[2]	33	79%	98%	99%
Prophylactic Antibiotic Timing (Outpatient)[1,3]	-	-	97%	98%
Urinary Catheter Removal[2]	21	76%	96%	97%
Survey of Patients' Hospital Experiences				
Area Around Room 'Always' Quiet at Night	(a)	84%	74%	61%
Doctors 'Always' Communicated Well	(a)	90%	87%	82%
Home Recovery Information Given	(a)	90%	85%	85%
Hospital Given 9 or 10 on 10 Point Scale	(a)	88%	75%	71%
Meds 'Always' Explained Before Given	(a)	74%	69%	64%
Nurses 'Always' Communicated Well	(a)	86%	83%	79%
Pain 'Always' Well Controlled	(a)	88%	75%	71%
Room and Bathroom 'Always' Clean	(a)	80%	75%	73%
Timely Help 'Always' Received	(a)	78%	71%	68%
Would Definitely Recommend Hospital	(a)	89%	75%	71%
Use of Medical Imaging				
Cardiac Imaging Stress Test before Surgery[7]	-	-	5.3%	5.3%
Combination Abdominal CT Scan[1]	-	-	24.5%	10.5%
Combination Brain/Sinus CT Scan[1]	-	-	2.6%	2.7%
Combination Chest CT Scan[1]	-	-	7.6%	2.7%
Follow-up Mammogram/Ultrasound[7]	-	-	9.4%	8.8%
Lumbar Spine MRI for Low Back Pain[7]	-	-	42.7%	37.2%

Saint Charles Parish Hospital

1057 Paul Maillard Road
Luling, LA 70070
URL: www.stch.net
Type: Acute Care Hospitals
Ownership: Govt - Hospital Dist/Auth

Phone: 985-785-6242
Fax: 985-785-3642
Emergency Services: Yes
Beds: 56

Key Personnel:
Chief of Medical Staff.......... Martin Belanger
Infection Control.............. Donna Bologna
Radiology.................... Thomas Efrid, MD
Emergency Room .... Cris Mandry, MD
Operating Room............. W Kenneth Mann
CEO/President............... Federico Martin, Jr
Quality Assurance .... Ilene Nicklas
Anesthesiology............... Manjit Wadhwa, MD

Measure	Cases	This Hosp.	State Avg.	U.S. Avg.
Blood Clot Prevention and Treatment				
Anticoagulation Overlap Therapy[1,2]	-	-	89%	93%
ICU Venous Thromboembolism Prophylaxis[2]	65	57%	88%	92%
Incidence of Potentially Preventable VTE[2,7]	-	-	16%	10%
UFH with Dosages/Platelet Monitoring[1,2]	-	-	94%	97%
Venous Thromboembolism Prophylaxis[2]	127	64%	74%	85%
Warfarin Therapy Discharge Instructions[1,2]	-	-	85%	75%
Chest Pain/Possible Heart Attack Care				
Aspirin Given Within 24 Hours of Arrival	33	94%	94%	96%
Fibrinolytic Meds Within 30 Min. of Arrival[3,7]	-	-	54%	58%
Average Time to ECG (minutes)	34	8	10	7
Average Time to Transfer (minutes)[3,7]	-	-	94	60
Children's Asthma Care				
Received Home Management Plan of Care	-	-	-	88%
Received Reliever Medication	-	-	-	100%
Received Systemic Corticosteroids	-	-	-	100%
Emergency Department				
Admittance Decision Time (minutes)[2]	428	81	86	98
Head CT Results Within 45 Min. of Arrival[1]	-	-	49%	57%
Patients Who Left ER Before Being Seen	13,680	1%	3%	2%
Time from ER Arrival to Admit. (minutes)[2]	431	218	256	274
Time from ER Arrival to Discharge (minutes)	365	93	125	134
Time in ER Before Being Evaluated (minutes)	402	6	27	26
Time to Pain Meds for Fractures (minutes)	52	41	61	57
Heart Attack Care				
Aspirin Given at Discharge[1]	-	-	99%	99%
Fibrinolytic Meds Within 30 Min. of Arrival[7]	-	-	71%	54%
PCI Within 90 Minutes of Arrival[7]	-	-	94%	96%
Statin Prescribed at Discharge[1]	-	-	98%	98%
Heart Failure Care				
ACE Inhibitor or ARB for LVSD	25	100%	95%	97%
Discharge Instructions Given	68	100%	94%	94%
Evaluation of LVS Function	80	92%	97%	99%
Medicare Spending				
Medicare Spending per Patient (ratio)	-	1.06	1.04	0.98
Pneumonia Care				
Appropriate Initial Antibiotic Given	37	89%	93%	95%
Blood Culture Timing	41	83%	97%	98%
Pregnancy and Delivery Care				
Newborn Deliveries Scheduled Early[7]	-	-	5%	6%
Preventive Care				
Immunization for Influenza[2]	370	79%	85%	90%
Immunization for Pneumonia[2]	352	87%	88%	92%
Stroke Care				
Anticoagulation Therapy for Atrial Fibrillation[7]	-	-	93%	95%
Antithrombotic Therapy Timing[1]	-	-	96%	98%
Assessed for Rehabilitation[1]	-	-	95%	97%
Discharged on Antithrombotic Therapy[1]	-	-	97%	99%
Discharged on Statin Medication[1]	-	-	89%	94%
Thrombolytic Therapy Timing[7]	-	-	53%	66%
Venous Thromboembolism Prophylaxis[1]	-	-	87%	94%
Written Stroke Educational Materials Given[1]	-	-	83%	88%
Surgical Care Improvement Project				
Appropriate Beta Blocker Usage[1]	-	-	97%	98%
Appropriate VTP Within 24 Hours	25	96%	97%	98%
Controlled Postoperative Blood Glucose[7]	-	-	96%	97%
Perioperative Temperature Management	29	100%	100%	100%
Prophylactic Antibiotic Selection[1]	-	-	99%	99%
Prophylactic Antibiotic Selection (Outpatient)	21	95%	97%	98%
Prophylactic Antibiotic Stopped[1]	-	-	97%	98%
Prophylactic Antibiotic Timing[1]	-	-	98%	99%
Prophylactic Antibiotic Timing (Outpatient)	21	100%	97%	98%
Urinary Catheter Removal[1]	-	-	96%	97%
Survey of Patients' Hospital Experiences				
Area Around Room 'Always' Quiet at Night	(a)	73%	74%	61%
Doctors 'Always' Communicated Well	(a)	83%	87%	82%
Home Recovery Information Given	(a)	86%	85%	85%
Hospital Given 9 or 10 on 10 Point Scale	(a)	70%	75%	71%
Meds 'Always' Explained Before Given	(a)	52%	69%	64%
Nurses 'Always' Communicated Well	(a)	80%	83%	79%
Pain 'Always' Well Controlled	(a)	67%	75%	71%
Room and Bathroom 'Always' Clean	(a)	79%	75%	73%
Timely Help 'Always' Received	(a)	71%	71%	68%
Would Definitely Recommend Hospital	(a)	67%	75%	71%
Use of Medical Imaging				
Cardiac Imaging Stress Test before Surgery[1]	-	-	5.3%	5.3%
Combination Abdominal CT Scan	84	19.0%	24.5%	10.5%
Combination Brain/Sinus CT Scan	106	7.5%	2.6%	2.7%
Combination Chest CT Scan[1]	-	-	7.6%	2.7%
Follow-up Mammogram/Ultrasound	155	16.1%	9.4%	8.8%
Lumbar Spine MRI for Low Back Pain[1]	-	-	42.7%	37.2%

Specialty Rehabilitation Hospital of Luling

1125 Paul Maillard Rd
Luling, LA 70070
Type: Acute Care Hospitals
Ownership: Proprietary

Phone: 985-785-5233
Emergency Services: No

Measure	Cases	This Hosp.	State Avg.	U.S. Avg.
Blood Clot Prevention and Treatment				
Anticoagulation Overlap Therapy[5]	-	-	89%	93%
ICU Venous Thromboembolism Prophylaxis[5]	-	-	88%	92%
Incidence of Potentially Preventable VTE[5]	-	-	16%	10%
UFH with Dosages/Platelet Monitoring[5]	-	-	94%	97%
Venous Thromboembolism Prophylaxis[5]	-	-	74%	85%
Warfarin Therapy Discharge Instructions[5]	-	-	85%	75%
Chest Pain/Possible Heart Attack Care				
Aspirin Given Within 24 Hours of Arrival[5]	-	-	94%	96%
Fibrinolytic Meds Within 30 Min. of Arrival[5]	-	-	54%	58%
Average Time to ECG (minutes)[5]	-	-	10	7
Average Time to Transfer (minutes)[5]	-	-	94	60
Children's Asthma Care				
Received Home Management Plan of Care	-	-	-	88%
Received Reliever Medication	-	-	-	100%
Received Systemic Corticosteroids	-	-	-	100%
Emergency Department				
Admittance Decision Time (minutes)[5]	-	-	86	98
Head CT Results Within 45 Min. of Arrival[5]	-	-	49%	57%
Patients Who Left ER Before Being Seen[5]	-	-	3%	2%
Time from ER Arrival to Admit. (minutes)[5]	-	-	256	274
Time from ER Arrival to Discharge (minutes)[5]	-	-	125	134
Time in ER Before Being Evaluated (minutes)[5]	-	-	27	26
Time to Pain Meds for Fractures (minutes)[5]	-	-	61	57
Heart Attack Care				
Aspirin Given at Discharge[5]	-	-	99%	99%
Fibrinolytic Meds Within 30 Min. of Arrival[5]	-	-	71%	54%
PCI Within 90 Minutes of Arrival[5]	-	-	94%	96%
Statin Prescribed at Discharge[5]	-	-	98%	98%
Heart Failure Care				
ACE Inhibitor or ARB for LVSD[5]	-	-	95%	97%
Discharge Instructions Given[5]	-	-	94%	94%
Evaluation of LVS Function[5]	-	-	97%	99%
Medicare Spending				
Medicare Spending per Patient (ratio)	-	-	1.04	0.98
Pneumonia Care				
Appropriate Initial Antibiotic Given[5]	-	-	93%	95%
Blood Culture Timing[5]	-	-	97%	98%
Pregnancy and Delivery Care				
Newborn Deliveries Scheduled Early[5]	-	-	5%	6%
Preventive Care				
Immunization for Influenza[5]	-	-	85%	90%
Immunization for Pneumonia[5]	-	-	88%	92%
Stroke Care				
Anticoagulation Therapy for Atrial Fibrillation[5]	-	-	93%	95%
Antithrombotic Therapy Timing[5]	-	-	96%	98%
Assessed for Rehabilitation[5]	-	-	95%	97%
Discharged on Antithrombotic Therapy[5]	-	-	97%	99%
Discharged on Statin Medication[5]	-	-	89%	94%
Thrombolytic Therapy Timing[5]	-	-	53%	66%
Venous Thromboembolism Prophylaxis[5]	-	-	87%	94%
Written Stroke Educational Materials Given[5]	-	-	83%	88%
Surgical Care Improvement Project				
Appropriate Beta Blocker Usage[5]	-	-	97%	98%
Appropriate VTP Within 24 Hours[5]	-	-	97%	98%
Controlled Postoperative Blood Glucose[5]	-	-	96%	97%
Perioperative Temperature Management[5]	-	-	100%	100%
Prophylactic Antibiotic Selection[5]	-	-	99%	99%
Prophylactic Antibiotic Selection (Outpatient)[5]	-	-	97%	98%
Prophylactic Antibiotic Stopped[5]	-	-	97%	98%
Prophylactic Antibiotic Timing[5]	-	-	98%	99%
Prophylactic Antibiotic Timing (Outpatient)[5]	-	-	97%	98%
Urinary Catheter Removal[5]	-	-	96%	97%

NOTE: Hospital profiles are in alphabetical order by state, then city, then hospital within the city; Rankings exclude hospitals with less than 25 cases except for patient surveys which excludes hospitals with less than 100 cases; (a) 100-299 cases; (1) The number of cases/patients is too few to report; (2) Data submitted were based on a sample of cases/patients; (3) Results are based on a shorter time period than required; (4) Data suppressed by CMS for one or more quarters; (5) Results are not available for this reporting period; (6) Fewer than 100 patients completed the HCAHPS survey; (7) No cases met the criteria for this measure; (8) The lower limit of the confidence interval cannot be calculated if the number of observed infections equals zero; (9) No data are available from the state/territory for this reporting period; (10) The scores shown reflect fewer than 50 completed surveys; (11) There were discrepancies in the data collection process; (12) This measure does not apply to this hospital for this reporting period; (13) Results cannot be calculated for this reporting period; (14) The results for this state are combined with nearby states to protect confidentiality; Please refer to the User's Guide for a full explanation of data.

Measure	Cases	This Hosp.	State Avg.	U.S. Avg.
Survey of Patients' Hospital Experiences				
Area Around Room 'Always' Quiet at Night[5]	-	-	74%	61%
Doctors 'Always' Communicated Well[5]	-	-	87%	82%
Home Recovery Information Given[5]	-	-	85%	85%
Hospital Given 9 or 10 on 10 Point Scale[5]	-	-	75%	71%
Meds 'Always' Explained Before Given[5]	-	-	69%	64%
Nurses 'Always' Communicated Well[5]	-	-	83%	79%
Pain 'Always' Well Controlled[5]	-	-	75%	71%
Room and Bathroom 'Always' Clean[5]	-	-	75%	73%
Timely Help 'Always' Received[5]	-	-	71%	68%
Would Definitely Recommend Hospital[5]	-	-	75%	71%
Use of Medical Imaging				
Cardiac Imaging Stress Test before Surgery[7]	-	-	5.3%	5.3%
Combination Abdominal CT Scan[7]	-	-	24.5%	10.5%
Combination Brain/Sinus CT Scan[7]	-	-	2.6%	2.7%
Combination Chest CT Scan[7]	-	-	7.6%	2.7%
Follow-up Mammogram/Ultrasound[7]	-	-	9.4%	8.8%
Lumbar Spine MRI for Low Back Pain[7]	-	-	42.7%	37.2%

Saint James Parish Hospital

1645 Lutcher Avenue
Lutcher, LA 70071
Phone: 225-869-5512
Fax: 225-869-4956
URL: www.sjph.org
Type: Critical Access Hospitals
Emergency Services: Yes
Ownership: Govt - Hospital Dist/Auth
Beds: 25

Key Personnel:

Radiology. . . . . Bryan Landry
Infection Control. . . . . Lizette Lougue, RN
Pediatric In-Patient Care . . . . Leya Mathew
Chief of Medical Staff. . . . . Charles Mc Gaff, MD
CEO/President. . . . . Mary Ellen Pratt
Cardiac Laboratory. . . . . Louis Siegel

Measure	Cases	This Hosp.	State Avg.	U.S. Avg.
Blood Clot Prevention and Treatment				
Anticoagulation Overlap Therapy[1,3]	-	-	89%	93%
ICU Venous Thromboembolism Prophylaxis[5]	-	-	88%	92%
Incidence of Potentially Preventable VTE[3,7]	-	-	16%	10%
UFH with Dosages/Platelet Monitoring[5]	-	-	94%	97%
Venous Thromboembolism Prophylaxis[3,7]	-	-	74%	85%
Warfarin Therapy Discharge Instructions[1,3]	-	-	85%	75%
Chest Pain/Possible Heart Attack Care				
Aspirin Given Within 24 Hours of Arrival	55	100%	94%	96%
Fibrinolytic Meds Within 30 Min. of Arrival[1]	-	-	54%	58%
Average Time to ECG (minutes)	58	10	10	7
Average Time to Transfer (minutes)[1]	-	-	94	60
Children's Asthma Care				
Received Home Management Plan of Care	-	-	-	88%
Received Reliever Medication	-	-	-	100%
Received Systemic Corticosteroids	-	-	-	100%
Emergency Department				
Admittance Decision Time (minutes)	68	64	86	98
Head CT Results Within 45 Min. of Arrival[1,3]	-	-	49%	57%
Patients Who Left ER Before Being Seen	13,180	1%	3%	2%
Time from ER Arrival to Admit. (minutes)	68	160	256	274
Time from ER Arrival to Discharge (minutes)[7]	-	-	125	134
Time in ER Before Being Evaluated (minutes)	68	5	27	26
Time to Pain Meds for Fractures (minutes)[5]	-	-	61	57
Heart Attack Care				
Aspirin Given at Discharge[1,3]	-	-	99%	99%
Fibrinolytic Meds Within 30 Min. of Arrival[3,7]	-	-	71%	54%
PCI Within 90 Minutes of Arrival[5]	-	-	94%	96%
Statin Prescribed at Discharge[1,3]	-	-	98%	98%
Heart Failure Care				
ACE Inhibitor or ARB for LVSD	19	84%	95%	97%
Discharge Instructions Given	25	100%	94%	94%
Evaluation of LVS Function	32	91%	97%	99%
Medicare Spending				
Medicare Spending per Patient (ratio)	-	-	1.04	0.98
Pneumonia Care				
Appropriate Initial Antibiotic Given	34	91%	93%	95%
Blood Culture Timing	39	97%	97%	98%
Pregnancy and Delivery Care				
Newborn Deliveries Scheduled Early[5]	-	-	5%	6%
Preventive Care				
Immunization for Influenza	45	91%	85%	90%
Immunization for Pneumonia	72	96%	88%	92%
Stroke Care				
Anticoagulation Therapy for Atrial Fibrillation[3,7]	-	-	93%	95%
Antithrombotic Therapy Timing[1,3]	-	-	96%	98%
Assessed for Rehabilitation[1,3]	-	-	95%	97%
Discharged on Antithrombotic Therapy[1,3]	-	-	97%	99%
Discharged on Statin Medication[1,3]	-	-	89%	94%
Thrombolytic Therapy Timing[3,7]	-	-	53%	66%
Venous Thromboembolism Prophylaxis[1,3]	-	-	87%	94%
Written Stroke Educational Materials Given[3,7]	-	-	83%	88%
Surgical Care Improvement Project				
Appropriate Beta Blocker Usage[5]	-	-	97%	98%
Appropriate VTP Within 24 Hours[1,3]	-	-	97%	98%
Controlled Postoperative Blood Glucose[5]	-	-	96%	97%
Perioperative Temperature Management[1,3]	-	-	100%	100%
Prophylactic Antibiotic Selection[3,7]	-	-	99%	99%
Prophylactic Antibiotic Selection (Outpatient)[1,3]	-	-	97%	98%
Prophylactic Antibiotic Stopped[3,7]	-	-	97%	98%
Prophylactic Antibiotic Timing[3,7]	-	-	98%	99%
Prophylactic Antibiotic Timing (Outpatient)[1,3]	-	-	97%	98%
Urinary Catheter Removal[3,7]	-	-	96%	97%
Survey of Patients' Hospital Experiences				
Area Around Room 'Always' Quiet at Night	(a)	78%	74%	61%
Doctors 'Always' Communicated Well	(a)	85%	87%	82%
Home Recovery Information Given	(a)	88%	85%	85%
Hospital Given 9 or 10 on 10 Point Scale	(a)	81%	75%	71%
Meds 'Always' Explained Before Given	(a)	69%	69%	64%
Nurses 'Always' Communicated Well	(a)	82%	83%	79%
Pain 'Always' Well Controlled	(a)	83%	75%	71%
Room and Bathroom 'Always' Clean	(a)	85%	75%	73%
Timely Help 'Always' Received	(a)	69%	71%	68%
Would Definitely Recommend Hospital	(a)	79%	75%	71%
Use of Medical Imaging				
Cardiac Imaging Stress Test before Surgery[1]	-	-	5.3%	5.3%
Combination Abdominal CT Scan	145	20.7%	24.5%	10.5%
Combination Brain/Sinus CT Scan[1]	-	-	2.6%	2.7%
Combination Chest CT Scan[1]	-	-	7.6%	2.7%
Follow-up Mammogram/Ultrasound	171	8.8%	9.4%	8.8%
Lumbar Spine MRI for Low Back Pain[1]	-	-	42.7%	37.2%

Savoy Medical Center

801 Poinciana Avenue
Mamou, LA 70554
Phone: 337-468-5261
Fax: 337-468-0348
URL: www.savorymedical.com
Type: Acute Care Hospitals
Emergency Services: Yes
Ownership: Govt - Hospital Dist/Auth
Beds: 25

Key Personnel:

Pediatric In-Patient Care . . . . Meena A Bakare, MD
Intensive Care Unit. . . . . Greg Blood
Radiology. . . . . Keith Daigle
Emergency Room . . . . Larry T Leblanc
CEO/President. . . . . Jim Schuessler

Measure	Cases	This Hosp.	State Avg.	U.S. Avg.
Blood Clot Prevention and Treatment				
Anticoagulation Overlap Therapy[1,2]	-	-	89%	93%
ICU Venous Thromboembolism Prophylaxis[2]	37	59%	88%	92%
Incidence of Potentially Preventable VTE[1,2]	-	-	16%	10%
UFH with Dosages/Platelet Monitoring[1,2]	-	-	94%	97%
Venous Thromboembolism Prophylaxis[2]	107	50%	74%	85%
Warfarin Therapy Discharge Instructions[1,2]	-	-	85%	75%
Chest Pain/Possible Heart Attack Care				
Aspirin Given Within 24 Hours of Arrival	14	71%	94%	96%
Fibrinolytic Meds Within 30 Min. of Arrival[3,7]	-	-	54%	58%
Average Time to ECG (minutes)	15	14	10	7
Average Time to Transfer (minutes)[1,3]	-	-	94	60
Children's Asthma Care				
Received Home Management Plan of Care	-	-	-	88%
Received Reliever Medication	-	-	-	100%
Received Systemic Corticosteroids	-	-	-	100%
Emergency Department				
Admittance Decision Time (minutes)[2]	184	70	86	98
Head CT Results Within 45 Min. of Arrival[1,3]	-	-	49%	57%
Patients Who Left ER Before Being Seen	7,997	1%	3%	2%
Time from ER Arrival to Admit. (minutes)[2]	185	206	256	274
Time from ER Arrival to Discharge (minutes)	414	94	125	134
Time in ER Before Being Evaluated (minutes)	486	21	27	26
Time to Pain Meds for Fractures (minutes)	18	43	61	57
Heart Attack Care				
Aspirin Given at Discharge[1,3]	-	-	99%	99%
Fibrinolytic Meds Within 30 Min. of Arrival[3,7]	-	-	71%	54%
PCI Within 90 Minutes of Arrival[3,7]	-	-	94%	96%
Statin Prescribed at Discharge[1,3]	-	-	98%	98%
Heart Failure Care				
ACE Inhibitor or ARB for LVSD[1]	-	-	95%	97%
Discharge Instructions Given	38	95%	94%	94%
Evaluation of LVS Function	72	96%	97%	99%
Medicare Spending				
Medicare Spending per Patient (ratio)	-	1.24	1.04	0.98
Pneumonia Care				
Appropriate Initial Antibiotic Given	52	88%	93%	95%
Blood Culture Timing	100	100%	97%	98%
Pregnancy and Delivery Care				
Newborn Deliveries Scheduled Early[7]	-	-	5%	6%
Preventive Care				
Immunization for Influenza[2]	361	74%	85%	90%
Immunization for Pneumonia[2]	270	94%	88%	92%
Stroke Care				
Anticoagulation Therapy for Atrial Fibrillation[1]	-	-	93%	95%
Antithrombotic Therapy Timing[1]	-	-	96%	98%
Assessed for Rehabilitation[1]	-	-	95%	97%
Discharged on Antithrombotic Therapy[1]	-	-	97%	99%
Discharged on Statin Medication[1]	-	-	89%	94%
Thrombolytic Therapy Timing[1]	-	-	53%	66%
Venous Thromboembolism Prophylaxis[1]	-	-	87%	94%
Written Stroke Educational Materials Given[1]	-	-	83%	88%
Surgical Care Improvement Project				
Appropriate Beta Blocker Usage[1]	-	-	97%	98%
Appropriate VTP Within 24 Hours	27	100%	97%	98%
Controlled Postoperative Blood Glucose[7]	-	-	96%	97%
Perioperative Temperature Management	30	100%	100%	100%
Prophylactic Antibiotic Selection	18	94%	99%	99%
Prophylactic Antibiotic Selection (Outpatient)[1,3]	-	-	97%	98%
Prophylactic Antibiotic Stopped	17	88%	97%	98%
Prophylactic Antibiotic Timing	18	94%	98%	99%
Prophylactic Antibiotic Timing (Outpatient)[1,3]	-	-	97%	98%
Urinary Catheter Removal[1]	-	-	96%	97%
Survey of Patients' Hospital Experiences				
Area Around Room 'Always' Quiet at Night	(a)	78%	74%	61%
Doctors 'Always' Communicated Well	(a)	92%	87%	82%
Home Recovery Information Given	(a)	87%	85%	85%
Hospital Given 9 or 10 on 10 Point Scale	(a)	76%	75%	71%
Meds 'Always' Explained Before Given	(a)	74%	69%	64%
Nurses 'Always' Communicated Well	(a)	80%	83%	79%
Pain 'Always' Well Controlled	(a)	75%	75%	71%
Room and Bathroom 'Always' Clean	(a)	84%	75%	73%
Timely Help 'Always' Received	(a)	73%	71%	68%
Would Definitely Recommend Hospital	(a)	78%	75%	71%
Use of Medical Imaging				
Cardiac Imaging Stress Test before Surgery[1]	-	-	5.3%	5.3%
Combination Abdominal CT Scan	135	48.9%	24.5%	10.5%
Combination Brain/Sinus CT Scan	158	0.6%	2.6%	2.7%
Combination Chest CT Scan	92	45.7%	7.6%	2.7%
Follow-up Mammogram/Ultrasound	180	7.2%	9.4%	8.8%
Lumbar Spine MRI for Low Back Pain[7]	-	-	42.7%	37.2%

Desoto Regional Health System

207 Jefferson Street
Mansfield, LA 71052
Phone: 318-872-4610
Fax: 318-871-1884
E-mail: lhishaw@bellsouth.net
URL: www.desotoregional.com
Type: Acute Care Hospitals
Emergency Services: Yes
Ownership: Proprietary
Beds: 57

Key Personnel:

Radiology. . . . . Md Campbell
Chief of Medical Staff . . . . W L Dillard, MD
CEO/President. . . . . Todd Eppler, FACHE, CEO
Emergency Room . . . . Shane Goodman

NOTE: Hospital profiles are in alphabetical order by state, then city, then hospital within the city; Rankings exclude hospitals with less than 25 cases except for patient surveys which excludes hospitals with less than 100 cases; (a) 100-299 cases; (1) The number of cases/patients is too few to report; (2) Data submitted were based on a sample of cases/patients; (3) Results are based on a shorter time period than required; (4) Data suppressed by CMS for one or more quarters; (5) Results are not available for this reporting period; (6) Fewer than 100 patients completed the HCAHPS survey; (7) No cases met the criteria for this measure; (8) The lower limit of the confidence interval cannot be calculated if the number of observed infections equals zero; (9) No data are available from the state/territory for this reporting period; (10) The scores shown reflect fewer than 50 completed surveys; (11) There were discrepancies in the data collection process; (12) This measure does not apply to this hospital for this reporting period; (13) Results cannot be calculated for this reporting period; (14) The results for this state are combined with nearby states to protect confidentiality; Please refer to the User's Guide for a full explanation of data.

Infection Control. . . . . Jean P Hall

Measure	Cases	This Hosp.	State Avg.	U.S. Avg.
Blood Clot Prevention and Treatment				
Anticoagulation Overlap Therapy[1,2]	-	-	89%	93%
ICU Venous Thromboembolism Prophylaxis[2,7]	-	-	88%	92%
Incidence of Potentially Preventable VTE[2,7]	-	-	16%	10%
UFH with Dosages/Platelet Monitoring[1,2]	-	-	94%	97%
Venous Thromboembolism Prophylaxis[2]	287	29%	74%	85%
Warfarin Therapy Discharge Instructions[1,2]	-	-	85%	75%
Chest Pain/Possible Heart Attack Care				
Aspirin Given Within 24 Hours of Arrival	13	85%	94%	96%
Fibrinolytic Meds Within 30 Min. of Arrival[3,7]	-	-	54%	58%
Average Time to ECG (minutes)	19	12	10	7
Average Time to Transfer (minutes)[3,7]	-	-	94	60
Children's Asthma Care				
Received Home Management Plan of Care	-	-	-	88%
Received Reliever Medication	-	-	-	100%
Received Systemic Corticosteroids	-	-	-	100%
Emergency Department				
Admittance Decision Time (minutes)[2]	460	45	86	98
Head CT Results Within 45 Min. of Arrival[1]	-	-	49%	57%
Patients Who Left ER Before Being Seen	8,361	1%	3%	2%
Time from ER Arrival to Admit. (minutes)[2]	473	160	256	274
Time from ER Arrival to Discharge (minutes)	166	100	125	134
Time in ER Before Being Evaluated (minutes)	356	15	27	26
Time to Pain Meds for Fractures (minutes)[1]	-	-	61	57
Heart Attack Care				
Aspirin Given at Discharge[1,2]	-	-	99%	99%
Fibrinolytic Meds Within 30 Min. of Arrival[2,3]	-	-	71%	54%
PCI Within 90 Minutes of Arrival[2,3]	-	-	94%	96%
Statin Prescribed at Discharge[1,2]	-	-	98%	98%
Heart Failure Care				
ACE Inhibitor or ARB for LVSD[2]	41	68%	95%	97%
Discharge Instructions Given[2]	38	89%	94%	94%
Evaluation of LVS Function[2]	72	88%	97%	99%
Medicare Spending				
Medicare Spending per Patient (ratio)	-	1.07	1.04	0.98
Pneumonia Care				
Appropriate Initial Antibiotic Given[2]	37	73%	93%	95%
Blood Culture Timing[2]	33	91%	97%	98%
Pregnancy and Delivery Care				
Newborn Deliveries Scheduled Early[2,7]	-	-	5%	6%
Preventive Care				
Immunization for Influenza[2]	295	69%	85%	90%
Immunization for Pneumonia[2]	530	78%	88%	92%
Stroke Care				
Anticoagulation Therapy for Atrial Fibrillation[1,2]	-	-	93%	95%
Antithrombotic Therapy Timing[1,2]	-	-	96%	98%
Assessed for Rehabilitation[1,2]	-	-	95%	97%
Discharged on Antithrombotic Therapy[1,2]	-	-	97%	99%
Discharged on Statin Medication[1,2]	-	-	89%	94%
Thrombolytic Therapy Timing[1,2]	-	-	53%	66%
Venous Thromboembolism Prophylaxis[1,2]	-	-	87%	94%
Written Stroke Educational Materials Given[1,2]	-	-	83%	88%
Surgical Care Improvement Project				
Appropriate Beta Blocker Usage[5]	-	-	97%	98%
Appropriate VTP Within 24 Hours[5]	-	-	97%	98%
Controlled Postoperative Blood Glucose[5]	-	-	96%	97%
Perioperative Temperature Management[5]	-	-	100%	100%
Prophylactic Antibiotic Selection[5]	-	-	99%	99%
Prophylactic Antibiotic Selection (Outpatient)[1,3]	-	-	97%	98%
Prophylactic Antibiotic Stopped[5]	-	-	97%	98%
Prophylactic Antibiotic Timing[5]	-	-	98%	99%
Prophylactic Antibiotic Timing (Outpatient)[1,3]	-	-	97%	98%
Urinary Catheter Removal[5]	-	-	96%	97%
Survey of Patients' Hospital Experiences				
Area Around Room 'Always' Quiet at Night	(a)	69%	74%	61%
Doctors 'Always' Communicated Well	(a)	88%	87%	82%
Home Recovery Information Given	(a)	84%	85%	85%
Hospital Given 9 or 10 on 10 Point Scale	(a)	74%	75%	71%
Meds 'Always' Explained Before Given	(a)	63%	69%	64%
Nurses 'Always' Communicated Well	(a)	80%	83%	79%
Pain 'Always' Well Controlled	(a)	78%	75%	71%
Room and Bathroom 'Always' Clean	(a)	76%	75%	73%
Timely Help 'Always' Received	(a)	76%	71%	68%
Would Definitely Recommend Hospital	(a)	64%	75%	71%
Use of Medical Imaging				
Cardiac Imaging Stress Test before Surgery	127	5.5%	5.3%	5.3%
Combination Abdominal CT Scan	163	6.1%	24.5%	10.5%
Combination Brain/Sinus CT Scan[1]	-	-	2.6%	2.7%
Combination Chest CT Scan	71	9.9%	7.6%	2.7%
Follow-up Mammogram/Ultrasound	276	9.4%	9.4%	8.8%
Lumbar Spine MRI for Low Back Pain[1]	-	-	42.7%	37.2%

Sabine Medical Center

240 Highland Drive
Many, LA 71449
URL: www.sabinemedicalcenter.net
Type: Acute Care Hospitals
Ownership: Proprietary
Phone: 318-256-1232
Fax: 318-256-1298
Emergency Services: Yes
Beds: 48

Key Personnel:

CEO/President. . . . . Chris Beddle
Cardiology . . . . Anil Chhabra, MD
Chief of Medical Staff . . . . Willie Corley, MD
Surgery . . . . Khaled Ghorab, MD
Emergency Room . . . . Charles R Pearson
Radiology. . . . . Benny Ramsey
Pediatrics. . . . . Husam Sukerek, MD
Quality Assurance . . . . Cathy Troquille

Measure	Cases	This Hosp.	State Avg.	U.S. Avg.
Blood Clot Prevention and Treatment				
Anticoagulation Overlap Therapy[1,2]	-	-	89%	93%
ICU Venous Thromboembolism Prophylaxis[2]	11	18%	88%	92%
Incidence of Potentially Preventable VTE[1,2]	-	-	16%	10%
UFH with Dosages/Platelet Monitoring[2,7]	-	-	94%	97%
Venous Thromboembolism Prophylaxis[2]	122	28%	74%	85%
Warfarin Therapy Discharge Instructions[1,2]	-	-	85%	75%
Chest Pain/Possible Heart Attack Care				
Aspirin Given Within 24 Hours of Arrival	54	81%	94%	96%
Fibrinolytic Meds Within 30 Min. of Arrival[1]	-	-	54%	58%
Average Time to ECG (minutes)	56	8	10	7
Average Time to Transfer (minutes)[7]	-	-	94	60
Children's Asthma Care				
Received Home Management Plan of Care	-	-	-	88%
Received Reliever Medication	-	-	-	100%
Received Systemic Corticosteroids	-	-	-	100%
Emergency Department				
Admittance Decision Time (minutes)[2]	384	58	86	98
Head CT Results Within 45 Min. of Arrival[1,3]	-	-	49%	57%
Patients Who Left ER Before Being Seen	9,195	2%	3%	2%
Time from ER Arrival to Admit. (minutes)[2]	388	206	256	274
Time from ER Arrival to Discharge (minutes)	287	102	125	134
Time in ER Before Being Evaluated (minutes)	391	41	27	26
Time to Pain Meds for Fractures (minutes)	38	60	61	57
Heart Attack Care				
Aspirin Given at Discharge[5]	-	-	99%	99%
Fibrinolytic Meds Within 30 Min. of Arrival[5]	-	-	71%	54%
PCI Within 90 Minutes of Arrival[5]	-	-	94%	96%
Statin Prescribed at Discharge[5]	-	-	98%	98%
Heart Failure Care				
ACE Inhibitor or ARB for LVSD[1,2]	-	-	95%	97%
Discharge Instructions Given[2]	38	47%	94%	94%
Evaluation of LVS Function[2]	51	55%	97%	99%
Medicare Spending				
Medicare Spending per Patient (ratio)	-	1.00	1.04	0.98
Pneumonia Care				
Appropriate Initial Antibiotic Given[2]	55	84%	93%	95%
Blood Culture Timing[2]	58	93%	97%	98%
Pregnancy and Delivery Care				
Newborn Deliveries Scheduled Early[7]	-	-	5%	6%
Preventive Care				
Immunization for Influenza[2]	276	47%	85%	90%
Immunization for Pneumonia[2]	341	68%	88%	92%
Stroke Care				
Anticoagulation Therapy for Atrial Fibrillation[5]	-	-	93%	95%
Antithrombotic Therapy Timing[5]	-	-	96%	98%
Assessed for Rehabilitation[5]	-	-	95%	97%
Discharged on Antithrombotic Therapy[5]	-	-	97%	99%
Discharged on Statin Medication[5]	-	-	89%	94%
Thrombolytic Therapy Timing[5]	-	-	53%	66%
Venous Thromboembolism Prophylaxis[5]	-	-	87%	94%
Written Stroke Educational Materials Given[5]	-	-	83%	88%
Surgical Care Improvement Project				
Appropriate Beta Blocker Usage[5]	-	-	97%	98%
Appropriate VTP Within 24 Hours[5]	-	-	97%	98%
Controlled Postoperative Blood Glucose[5]	-	-	96%	97%
Perioperative Temperature Management[5]	-	-	100%	100%
Prophylactic Antibiotic Selection[5]	-	-	99%	99%
Prophylactic Antibiotic Selection (Outpatient)[5]	-	-	97%	98%
Prophylactic Antibiotic Stopped[5]	-	-	97%	98%
Prophylactic Antibiotic Timing[5]	-	-	98%	99%
Prophylactic Antibiotic Timing (Outpatient)[5]	-	-	97%	98%
Urinary Catheter Removal[5]	-	-	96%	97%
Survey of Patients' Hospital Experiences				
Area Around Room 'Always' Quiet at Night	(a)	72%	74%	61%
Doctors 'Always' Communicated Well	(a)	90%	87%	82%
Home Recovery Information Given	(a)	84%	85%	85%
Hospital Given 9 or 10 on 10 Point Scale	(a)	66%	75%	71%
Meds 'Always' Explained Before Given	(a)	62%	69%	64%
Nurses 'Always' Communicated Well	(a)	81%	83%	79%
Pain 'Always' Well Controlled	(a)	66%	75%	71%
Room and Bathroom 'Always' Clean	(a)	70%	75%	73%
Timely Help 'Always' Received	(a)	70%	71%	68%
Would Definitely Recommend Hospital	(a)	62%	75%	71%
Use of Medical Imaging				
Cardiac Imaging Stress Test before Surgery[7]	-	-	5.3%	5.3%
Combination Abdominal CT Scan	241	47.3%	24.5%	10.5%
Combination Brain/Sinus CT Scan	258	5.4%	2.6%	2.7%
Combination Chest CT Scan	104	25.0%	7.6%	2.7%
Follow-up Mammogram/Ultrasound	147	9.5%	9.4%	8.8%
Lumbar Spine MRI for Low Back Pain[1]	-	-	42.7%	37.2%

Avoyelles Hospital

4231 Highway 1192
Marksville, LA 71351
URL: www.avoyelleshospital.com
Type: Acute Care Hospitals
Ownership: Proprietary
Phone: 318-253-8611
Fax: 318-240-6077
Emergency Services: Yes
Beds: 51

Key Personnel:

Emergency Room . . . . Kenny Bordelon, RN
Chief of Medical Staff . . . . Fernando Garcia, MD
Anesthesiology. . . . . Mark Gremillion, CRNA
Quality Assurance . . . . Cindy Juneau
Operating Room. . . . . Rachel Laborde
CEO/President. . . . . David M Mitchel
Intensive Care Unit. . . . . Jenny Nugent
Infection Control. . . . . Jeanie Tessin

Measure	Cases	This Hosp.	State Avg.	U.S. Avg.
Blood Clot Prevention and Treatment				
Anticoagulation Overlap Therapy[2]	14	100%	89%	93%
ICU Venous Thromboembolism Prophylaxis[2]	14	100%	88%	92%
Incidence of Potentially Preventable VTE[2,7]	-	-	16%	10%
UFH with Dosages/Platelet Monitoring[1,2]	-	-	94%	97%
Venous Thromboembolism Prophylaxis[2]	136	84%	74%	85%
Warfarin Therapy Discharge Instructions[1,2]	-	-	85%	75%
Chest Pain/Possible Heart Attack Care				
Aspirin Given Within 24 Hours of Arrival	49	86%	94%	96%
Fibrinolytic Meds Within 30 Min. of Arrival[1]	-	-	54%	58%
Average Time to ECG (minutes)	50	8	10	7
Average Time to Transfer (minutes)[1]	-	-	94	60
Children's Asthma Care				
Received Home Management Plan of Care	-	-	-	88%
Received Reliever Medication	-	-	-	100%
Received Systemic Corticosteroids	-	-	-	100%
Emergency Department				
Admittance Decision Time (minutes)[2]	445	60	86	98
Head CT Results Within 45 Min. of Arrival[1]	-	-	49%	57%
Patients Who Left ER Before Being Seen	14,472	2%	3%	2%
Time from ER Arrival to Admit. (minutes)[2]	449	165	256	274

NOTE: Hospital profiles are in alphabetical order by state, then city, then hospital within the city; Rankings exclude hospitals with less than 25 cases except for patient surveys which excludes hospitals with less than 100 cases; (a) 100-299 cases; (1) The number of cases/patients is too few to report; (2) Data submitted were based on a sample of cases/patients; (3) Results are based on a shorter time period than required; (4) Data suppressed by CMS for one or more quarters; (5) Results are not available for this reporting period; (6) Fewer than 100 patients completed the HCAHPS survey; (7) No cases met the criteria for this measure; (8) The lower limit of the confidence interval cannot be calculated if the number of observed infections equals zero; (9) No data are available from the state/territory for this reporting period; (10) The scores shown reflect fewer than 50 completed surveys; (11) There were discrepancies in the data collection process; (12) This measure does not apply to this hospital for this reporting period; (13) Results cannot be calculated for this reporting period; (14) The results for this state are combined with nearby states to protect confidentiality; Please refer to the User's Guide for a full explanation of data.

Measure	Cases	This Hosp.	State Avg.	U.S. Avg.
Time from ER Arrival to Discharge (minutes)	341	75	125	134
Time in ER Before Being Evaluated (minutes)	392	16	27	26
Time to Pain Meds for Fractures (minutes)	67	45	61	57
Heart Attack Care				
Aspirin Given at Discharge[1]	-	-	99%	99%
Fibrinolytic Meds Within 30 Min. of Arrival[7]	-	-	71%	54%
PCI Within 90 Minutes of Arrival[7]	-	-	94%	96%
Statin Prescribed at Discharge[1]	-	-	98%	98%
Heart Failure Care				
ACE Inhibitor or ARB for LVSD	13	77%	95%	97%
Discharge Instructions Given	47	87%	94%	94%
Evaluation of LVS Function	79	95%	97%	99%
Medicare Spending				
Medicare Spending per Patient (ratio)	-	1.07	1.04	0.98
Pneumonia Care				
Appropriate Initial Antibiotic Given	51	96%	93%	95%
Blood Culture Timing	29	83%	97%	98%
Pregnancy and Delivery Care				
Newborn Deliveries Scheduled Early[7]	-	-	5%	6%
Preventive Care				
Immunization for Influenza[2]	295	86%	85%	90%
Immunization for Pneumonia[2]	449	95%	88%	92%
Stroke Care				
Anticoagulation Therapy for Atrial Fibrillation[7]	-	-	93%	95%
Antithrombotic Therapy Timing[1]	-	-	96%	98%
Assessed for Rehabilitation[1]	-	-	95%	97%
Discharged on Antithrombotic Therapy[1]	-	-	97%	99%
Discharged on Statin Medication[1]	-	-	89%	94%
Thrombolytic Therapy Timing[1]	-	-	53%	66%
Venous Thromboembolism Prophylaxis[1]	-	-	87%	94%
Written Stroke Educational Materials Given[1]	-	-	83%	88%
Surgical Care Improvement Project				
Appropriate Beta Blocker Usage[1]	-	-	97%	98%
Appropriate VTP Within 24 Hours	22	100%	97%	98%
Controlled Postoperative Blood Glucose[7]	-	-	96%	97%
Perioperative Temperature Management	21	90%	100%	100%
Prophylactic Antibiotic Selection[1]	-	-	99%	99%
Prophylactic Antibiotic Selection (Outpatient)[1]	-	-	97%	98%
Prophylactic Antibiotic Stopped[1]	-	-	97%	98%
Prophylactic Antibiotic Timing[1]	-	-	98%	99%
Prophylactic Antibiotic Timing (Outpatient)[1]	-	-	97%	98%
Urinary Catheter Removal	11	73%	96%	97%
Survey of Patients' Hospital Experiences				
Area Around Room 'Always' Quiet at Night	(a)	73%	74%	61%
Doctors 'Always' Communicated Well	(a)	82%	87%	82%
Home Recovery Information Given	(a)	75%	85%	85%
Hospital Given 9 or 10 on 10 Point Scale	(a)	59%	75%	71%
Meds 'Always' Explained Before Given	(a)	66%	69%	64%
Nurses 'Always' Communicated Well	(a)	77%	83%	79%
Pain 'Always' Well Controlled	(a)	65%	75%	71%
Room and Bathroom 'Always' Clean	(a)	74%	75%	73%
Timely Help 'Always' Received	(a)	55%	71%	68%
Would Definitely Recommend Hospital	(a)	55%	75%	71%
Use of Medical Imaging				
Cardiac Imaging Stress Test before Surgery[7]	-	-	5.3%	5.3%
Combination Abdominal CT Scan	177	36.7%	24.5%	10.5%
Combination Brain/Sinus CT Scan[1]	-	-	2.6%	2.7%
Combination Chest CT Scan	51	39.2%	7.6%	2.7%
Follow-up Mammogram/Ultrasound	386	9.6%	9.4%	8.8%
Lumbar Spine MRI for Low Back Pain[7]	-	-	42.7%	37.2%

West Jefferson Medical Center

1101 Medical Center Blvd
Marrero, LA 70072
Phone: 504-347-5511
Fax: 504-349-6299
URL: www.wjmc.org
Type: Acute Care Hospitals
Emergency Services: Yes
Ownership: Govt - Hospital Dist/Auth
Beds: 462

Key Personnel:
Chief of Medical Staff .... Alfred Abaunza, MD
Quality Assurance .... Larry E Barbe
Infection Control............. Toni Bergeron
CEO/President................ Nancy Cassagne
Pediatric In-Patient Care .... Dean Edell, RN
Cardiac Laboratory............ Louis Glade
Patient Relations .... Mitchell Leckelt
Radiology.................... Jimmy Mains, MD

Measure	Cases	This Hosp.	State Avg.	U.S. Avg.
Blood Clot Prevention and Treatment				
Anticoagulation Overlap Therapy[2]	53	100%	89%	93%
ICU Venous Thromboembolism Prophylaxis[2]	134	99%	88%	92%
Incidence of Potentially Preventable VTE[2]	16	0%	16%	10%
UFH with Dosages/Platelet Monitoring[2]	16	100%	94%	97%
Venous Thromboembolism Prophylaxis[2]	269	98%	74%	85%
Warfarin Therapy Discharge Instructions[2]	33	88%	85%	75%
Chest Pain/Possible Heart Attack Care				
Aspirin Given Within 24 Hours of Arrival[1,3]	-	-	94%	96%
Fibrinolytic Meds Within 30 Min. of Arrival[5]	-	-	54%	58%
Average Time to ECG (minutes)[1,3]	-	-	10	7
Average Time to Transfer (minutes)[5]	-	-	94	60
Children's Asthma Care				
Received Home Management Plan of Care	-	-	-	88%
Received Reliever Medication	-	-	-	100%
Received Systemic Corticosteroids	-	-	-	100%
Emergency Department				
Admittance Decision Time (minutes)[2]	546	123	86	98
Head CT Results Within 45 Min. of Arrival[1]	-	-	49%	57%
Patients Who Left ER Before Being Seen	58,687	4%	3%	2%
Time from ER Arrival to Admit. (minutes)[2]	546	293	256	274
Time from ER Arrival to Discharge (minutes)	366	156	125	134
Time in ER Before Being Evaluated (minutes)	396	49	27	26
Time to Pain Meds for Fractures (minutes)	78	30	61	57
Heart Attack Care				
Aspirin Given at Discharge	246	98%	99%	99%
Fibrinolytic Meds Within 30 Min. of Arrival[7]	-	-	71%	54%
PCI Within 90 Minutes of Arrival	43	100%	94%	96%
Statin Prescribed at Discharge	245	100%	98%	98%
Heart Failure Care				
ACE Inhibitor or ARB for LVSD	150	96%	95%	97%
Discharge Instructions Given	443	97%	94%	94%
Evaluation of LVS Function	523	100%	97%	99%
Medicare Spending				
Medicare Spending per Patient (ratio)	-	1.08	1.04	0.98
Pneumonia Care				
Appropriate Initial Antibiotic Given	122	98%	93%	95%
Blood Culture Timing	190	98%	97%	98%
Pregnancy and Delivery Care				
Newborn Deliveries Scheduled Early[2]	208	1%	5%	6%
Preventive Care				
Immunization for Influenza[2]	549	99%	85%	90%
Immunization for Pneumonia[2]	675	100%	88%	92%
Stroke Care				
Anticoagulation Therapy for Atrial Fibrillation	21	100%	93%	95%
Antithrombotic Therapy Timing	142	98%	96%	98%
Assessed for Rehabilitation	222	100%	95%	97%
Discharged on Antithrombotic Therapy	165	99%	97%	99%
Discharged on Statin Medication	124	97%	89%	94%
Thrombolytic Therapy Timing	25	88%	53%	66%
Venous Thromboembolism Prophylaxis	243	99%	87%	94%
Written Stroke Educational Materials Given	114	100%	83%	88%
Surgical Care Improvement Project				
Appropriate Beta Blocker Usage[2]	200	100%	97%	98%
Appropriate VTP Within 24 Hours[2]	389	99%	97%	98%
Controlled Postoperative Blood Glucose[2]	57	93%	96%	97%
Perioperative Temperature Management[2]	491	100%	100%	100%
Prophylactic Antibiotic Selection[2]	398	99%	99%	99%
Prophylactic Antibiotic Selection (Outpatient)	446	98%	97%	98%
Prophylactic Antibiotic Stopped[2]	392	99%	97%	98%
Prophylactic Antibiotic Timing[2]	398	99%	98%	99%
Prophylactic Antibiotic Timing (Outpatient)	447	99%	97%	98%
Urinary Catheter Removal[2]	282	99%	96%	97%
Survey of Patients' Hospital Experiences				
Area Around Room 'Always' Quiet at Night	300+	67%	74%	61%
Doctors 'Always' Communicated Well	300+	82%	87%	82%
Home Recovery Information Given	300+	88%	85%	85%
Hospital Given 9 or 10 on 10 Point Scale	300+	75%	75%	71%
Meds 'Always' Explained Before Given	300+	65%	69%	64%
Nurses 'Always' Communicated Well	300+	81%	83%	79%
Pain 'Always' Well Controlled	300+	73%	75%	71%
Room and Bathroom 'Always' Clean	300+	71%	75%	73%
Timely Help 'Always' Received	300+	68%	71%	68%
Would Definitely Recommend Hospital	300+	76%	75%	71%
Use of Medical Imaging				
Cardiac Imaging Stress Test before Surgery	273	5.1%	5.3%	5.3%
Combination Abdominal CT Scan	329	23.1%	24.5%	10.5%
Combination Brain/Sinus CT Scan	516	0.8%	2.6%	2.7%
Combination Chest CT Scan	210	27.1%	7.6%	2.7%
Follow-up Mammogram/Ultrasound	1,180	8.1%	9.4%	8.8%
Lumbar Spine MRI for Low Back Pain	75	37.3%	42.7%	37.2%

East Jefferson General Hospital

4200 Houma Blvd
Metairie, LA 70006
Phone: 504-454-4000
Fax: 504-456-8151
URL: www.eastjeffhospital.org
Type: Acute Care Hospitals
Emergency Services: Yes
Ownership: Govt - Hospital Dist/Auth
Beds: 448

Key Personnel:
Radiology.................. Ricky Arbuckle
Emergency Room .... Cheryl Carter
Chief of Medical Staff.......... Raymond DeCorte, MD
Cardiac Laboratory............ Clement C Eisworth
Infection Control............. Cathy Lopez
CEO/President............... Mark J. Peters, MD, CPE
Operating Room............. Ann Seal
Intensive Care Unit............ Lynn Strain

Measure	Cases	This Hosp.	State Avg.	U.S. Avg.
Blood Clot Prevention and Treatment				
Anticoagulation Overlap Therapy[2]	72	100%	89%	93%
ICU Venous Thromboembolism Prophylaxis[2]	102	83%	88%	92%
Incidence of Potentially Preventable VTE[2]	27	15%	16%	10%
UFH with Dosages/Platelet Monitoring[2]	22	100%	94%	97%
Venous Thromboembolism Prophylaxis[2]	310	65%	74%	85%
Warfarin Therapy Discharge Instructions[2]	51	84%	85%	75%
Chest Pain/Possible Heart Attack Care				
Aspirin Given Within 24 Hours of Arrival[5]	-	-	94%	96%
Fibrinolytic Meds Within 30 Min. of Arrival[5]	-	-	54%	58%
Average Time to ECG (minutes)[5]	-	-	10	7
Average Time to Transfer (minutes)[5]	-	-	94	60
Children's Asthma Care				
Received Home Management Plan of Care	-	-	-	88%
Received Reliever Medication	-	-	-	100%
Received Systemic Corticosteroids	-	-	-	100%
Emergency Department				
Admittance Decision Time (minutes)[2]	664	101	86	98
Head CT Results Within 45 Min. of Arrival	16	38%	49%	57%
Patients Who Left ER Before Being Seen	52,494	2%	3%	2%
Time from ER Arrival to Admit. (minutes)[2]	683	299	256	274
Time from ER Arrival to Discharge (minutes)	362	150	125	134
Time in ER Before Being Evaluated (minutes)	82	50	27	26
Time to Pain Meds for Fractures (minutes)	142	56	61	57
Heart Attack Care				
Aspirin Given at Discharge[2]	257	99%	99%	99%
Fibrinolytic Meds Within 30 Min. of Arrival[2,7]	-	-	71%	54%
PCI Within 90 Minutes of Arrival[2]	44	100%	94%	96%
Statin Prescribed at Discharge[2]	231	98%	98%	98%
Heart Failure Care				
ACE Inhibitor or ARB for LVSD[2]	71	97%	95%	97%
Discharge Instructions Given[2]	236	89%	94%	94%
Evaluation of LVS Function[2]	296	100%	97%	99%
Medicare Spending				
Medicare Spending per Patient (ratio)	-	1.00	1.04	0.98
Pneumonia Care				
Appropriate Initial Antibiotic Given[2]	63	95%	93%	95%
Blood Culture Timing[2]	153	99%	97%	98%
Pregnancy and Delivery Care				
Newborn Deliveries Scheduled Early[2]	316	2%	5%	6%
Preventive Care				
Immunization for Influenza[2]	581	79%	85%	90%
Immunization for Pneumonia[2]	786	88%	88%	92%
Stroke Care				
Anticoagulation Therapy for Atrial Fibrillation[2]	21	100%	93%	95%

NOTE: Hospital profiles are in alphabetical order by state, then city, then hospital within the city; Rankings exclude hospitals with less than 25 cases except for patient surveys which excludes hospitals with less than 100 cases; (a) 100-299 cases; (1) The number of cases/patients is too few to report; (2) Data submitted were based on a sample of cases/patients; (3) Results are based on a shorter time period than required; (4) Data suppressed by CMS for one or more quarters; (5) Results are not available for this reporting period; (6) Fewer than 100 patients completed the HCAHPS survey; (7) No cases met the criteria for this measure; (8) The lower limit of the confidence interval cannot be calculated if the number of observed infections equals zero; (9) No data are available from the state/territory for this reporting period; (10) The scores shown reflect fewer than 50 completed surveys; (11) There were discrepancies in the data collection process; (12) This measure does not apply to this hospital for this reporting period; (13) Results cannot be calculated for this reporting period; (14) The results for this state are combined with nearby states to protect confidentiality; Please refer to the User's Guide for a full explanation of data.

Measure	Cases	This Hosp.	State Avg.	U.S. Avg.
Antithrombotic Therapy Timing[2]	147	99%	96%	98%
Assessed for Rehabilitation[2]	182	99%	95%	97%
Discharged on Antithrombotic Therapy[2]	160	99%	97%	99%
Discharged on Statin Medication[2]	126	94%	89%	94%
Thrombolytic Therapy Timing[1,2]	-	-	53%	66%
Venous Thromboembolism Prophylaxis[2]	172	98%	87%	94%
Written Stroke Educational Materials Given[2]	116	95%	83%	88%
Surgical Care Improvement Project				
Appropriate Beta Blocker Usage[2]	205	99%	97%	98%
Appropriate VTP Within 24 Hours[2]	356	97%	97%	98%
Controlled Postoperative Blood Glucose[2]	110	94%	96%	97%
Perioperative Temperature Management[2]	471	99%	100%	100%
Prophylactic Antibiotic Selection[2]	438	99%	99%	99%
Prophylactic Antibiotic Selection (Outpatient)	500	98%	97%	98%
Prophylactic Antibiotic Stopped[2]	423	96%	97%	98%
Prophylactic Antibiotic Timing[2]	440	97%	98%	99%
Prophylactic Antibiotic Timing (Outpatient)	501	99%	97%	98%
Urinary Catheter Removal[2]	361	99%	96%	97%
Survey of Patients' Hospital Experiences				
Area Around Room 'Always' Quiet at Night	300+	64%	74%	61%
Doctors 'Always' Communicated Well	300+	84%	87%	82%
Home Recovery Information Given	300+	84%	85%	85%
Hospital Given 9 or 10 on 10 Point Scale	300+	73%	75%	71%
Meds 'Always' Explained Before Given	300+	62%	69%	64%
Nurses 'Always' Communicated Well	300+	81%	83%	79%
Pain 'Always' Well Controlled	300+	72%	75%	71%
Room and Bathroom 'Always' Clean	300+	66%	75%	73%
Timely Help 'Always' Received	300+	59%	71%	68%
Would Definitely Recommend Hospital	300+	76%	75%	71%
Use of Medical Imaging				
Cardiac Imaging Stress Test before Surgery	913	4.8%	5.3%	5.3%
Combination Abdominal CT Scan	1,193	42.5%	24.5%	10.5%
Combination Brain/Sinus CT Scan	1,029	1.8%	2.6%	2.7%
Combination Chest CT Scan	924	2.2%	7.6%	2.7%
Follow-up Mammogram/Ultrasound	1,446	47.9%	9.4%	8.8%
Lumbar Spine MRI for Low Back Pain	129	41.9%	42.7%	37.2%

Minden Medical Center

No 1 Medical Plaza
Minden, LA 71055
Phone: 318-377-2321
Fax: 318-371-5606
URL: www.mindenmedicalcenter.com
Type: Acute Care Hospitals
Emergency Services: Yes
Ownership: Proprietary
Beds: 159

Key Personnel:
CEO . . . . George E French III, III
Chief of Medical Staff . . . . James O Hudson
Quality Assurance . . . . Lynn Maynor
Operating Room. . . . . Christy Owen
Radiology. . . . . Webster R Stewart, MD

Measure	Cases	This Hosp.	State Avg.	U.S. Avg.
Blood Clot Prevention and Treatment				
Anticoagulation Overlap Therapy[2]	26	100%	89%	93%
ICU Venous Thromboembolism Prophylaxis[2]	76	100%	88%	92%
Incidence of Potentially Preventable VTE[1,2]	-	-	16%	10%
UFH with Dosages/Platelet Monitoring[1,2]	-	-	94%	97%
Venous Thromboembolism Prophylaxis[2]	255	100%	74%	85%
Warfarin Therapy Discharge Instructions[2]	17	100%	85%	75%
Chest Pain/Possible Heart Attack Care				
Aspirin Given Within 24 Hours of Arrival	27	100%	94%	96%
Fibrinolytic Meds Within 30 Min. of Arrival[1,3]	-	-	54%	58%
Average Time to ECG (minutes)	27	4	10	7
Average Time to Transfer (minutes)[3,7]	-	-	94	60
Children's Asthma Care				
Received Home Management Plan of Care	-	-	-	88%
Received Reliever Medication	-	-	-	100%
Received Systemic Corticosteroids	-	-	-	100%
Emergency Department				
Admittance Decision Time (minutes)[2]	376	76	86	98
Head CT Results Within 45 Min. of Arrival	12	92%	49%	57%
Patients Who Left ER Before Being Seen	20,982	1%	3%	2%
Time from ER Arrival to Admit. (minutes)[2]	376	228	256	274
Time from ER Arrival to Discharge (minutes)	370	98	125	134
Time in ER Before Being Evaluated (minutes)	399	5	27	26
Time to Pain Meds for Fractures (minutes)	66	26	61	57
Heart Attack Care				
Aspirin Given at Discharge	26	100%	99%	99%
Fibrinolytic Meds Within 30 Min. of Arrival[1]	-	-	71%	54%
PCI Within 90 Minutes of Arrival[1]	-	-	94%	96%
Statin Prescribed at Discharge	21	100%	98%	98%
Heart Failure Care				
ACE Inhibitor or ARB for LVSD	59	100%	95%	97%
Discharge Instructions Given	126	100%	94%	94%
Evaluation of LVS Function	150	100%	97%	99%
Medicare Spending				
Medicare Spending per Patient (ratio)	-	1.03	1.04	0.98
Pneumonia Care				
Appropriate Initial Antibiotic Selection	78	100%	93%	95%
Blood Culture Timing	118	100%	97%	98%
Pregnancy and Delivery Care				
Newborn Deliveries Scheduled Early[2]	42	5%	5%	6%
Preventive Care				
Immunization for Influenza[2]	371	100%	85%	90%
Immunization for Pneumonia[2]	392	100%	88%	92%
Stroke Care				
Anticoagulation Therapy for Atrial Fibrillation[1]	-	-	93%	95%
Antithrombotic Therapy Timing	43	100%	96%	98%
Assessed for Rehabilitation	44	100%	95%	97%
Discharged on Antithrombotic Therapy	42	100%	97%	99%
Discharged on Statin Medication	26	100%	89%	94%
Thrombolytic Therapy Timing[7]	-	-	53%	66%
Venous Thromboembolism Prophylaxis	44	100%	87%	94%
Written Stroke Educational Materials Given	21	100%	83%	88%
Surgical Care Improvement Project				
Appropriate Beta Blocker Usage	65	100%	97%	98%
Appropriate VTP Within 24 Hours	196	100%	97%	98%
Controlled Postoperative Blood Glucose[7]	-	-	96%	97%
Perioperative Temperature Management	244	100%	100%	100%
Prophylactic Antibiotic Selection	128	99%	99%	99%
Prophylactic Antibiotic Selection (Outpatient)	21	100%	97%	98%
Prophylactic Antibiotic Stopped	116	100%	97%	98%
Prophylactic Antibiotic Timing	128	100%	98%	99%
Prophylactic Antibiotic Timing (Outpatient)	22	95%	97%	98%
Urinary Catheter Removal	146	100%	96%	97%
Survey of Patients' Hospital Experiences				
Area Around Room 'Always' Quiet at Night	300+	71%	74%	61%
Doctors 'Always' Communicated Well	300+	86%	87%	82%
Home Recovery Information Given	300+	85%	85%	85%
Hospital Given 9 or 10 on 10 Point Scale	300+	75%	75%	71%
Meds 'Always' Explained Before Given	300+	65%	69%	64%
Nurses 'Always' Communicated Well	300+	80%	83%	79%
Pain 'Always' Well Controlled	300+	74%	75%	71%
Room and Bathroom 'Always' Clean	300+	66%	75%	73%
Timely Help 'Always' Received	300+	68%	71%	68%
Would Definitely Recommend Hospital	300+	74%	75%	71%
Use of Medical Imaging				
Cardiac Imaging Stress Test before Surgery[1]	-	-	5.3%	5.3%
Combination Abdominal CT Scan	277	1.4%	24.5%	10.5%
Combination Brain/Sinus CT Scan	475	1.9%	2.6%	2.7%
Combination Chest CT Scan	150	0.0%	7.6%	2.7%
Follow-up Mammogram/Ultrasound	671	4.8%	9.4%	8.8%
Lumbar Spine MRI for Low Back Pain	63	31.7%	42.7%	37.2%

E A Conway Medical Center

4864 Jackson Street
Monroe, LA 71202
Phone: 318-330-7000
Fax: 318-330-7446
URL: www.conway.lsuhsc.edu
Type: Acute Care Hospitals
Emergency Services: Yes
Ownership: Government - State
Beds: 158

Key Personnel:
Chief of Medical Staff . . . . LaDonna Ford

Measure	Cases	This Hosp.	State Avg.	U.S. Avg.
Blood Clot Prevention and Treatment				
Anticoagulation Overlap Therapy[2]	15	100%	89%	93%
ICU Venous Thromboembolism Prophylaxis[2]	81	86%	88%	92%
Incidence of Potentially Preventable VTE[1,2]	-	-	16%	10%
UFH with Dosages/Platelet Monitoring[1,2]	-	-	94%	97%
Venous Thromboembolism Prophylaxis[2]	246	92%	74%	85%
Warfarin Therapy Discharge Instructions[2]	14	57%	85%	75%
Chest Pain/Possible Heart Attack Care				
Aspirin Given Within 24 Hours of Arrival	63	95%	94%	96%
Fibrinolytic Meds Within 30 Min. of Arrival[1]	-	-	54%	58%
Average Time to ECG (minutes)	64	22	10	7
Average Time to Transfer (minutes)[1]	-	-	94	60
Children's Asthma Care				
Received Home Management Plan of Care	-	-	-	88%
Received Reliever Medication	-	-	-	100%
Received Systemic Corticosteroids	-	-	-	100%
Emergency Department				
Admittance Decision Time (minutes)[2]	255	145	86	98
Head CT Results Within 45 Min. of Arrival[7]	-	-	49%	57%
Patients Who Left ER Before Being Seen	30,831	8%	3%	2%
Time from ER Arrival to Admit. (minutes)[2]	258	508	256	274
Time from ER Arrival to Discharge (minutes)	300	212	125	134
Time in ER Before Being Evaluated (minutes)[1]	-	-	27	26
Time to Pain Meds for Fractures (minutes)	11	110	61	57
Heart Attack Care				
Aspirin Given at Discharge[1]	-	-	99%	99%
Fibrinolytic Meds Within 30 Min. of Arrival[7]	-	-	71%	54%
PCI Within 90 Minutes of Arrival[7]	-	-	94%	96%
Statin Prescribed at Discharge[1]	-	-	98%	98%
Heart Failure Care				
ACE Inhibitor or ARB for LVSD	76	100%	95%	97%
Discharge Instructions Given	117	97%	94%	94%
Evaluation of LVS Function	123	99%	97%	99%
Medicare Spending				
Medicare Spending per Patient (ratio)	-	0.91	1.04	0.98
Pneumonia Care				
Appropriate Initial Antibiotic Selection	77	94%	93%	95%
Blood Culture Timing	92	99%	97%	98%
Pregnancy and Delivery Care				
Newborn Deliveries Scheduled Early[2]	39	0%	5%	6%
Preventive Care				
Immunization for Influenza[2]	394	69%	85%	90%
Immunization for Pneumonia[2]	284	56%	88%	92%
Stroke Care				
Anticoagulation Therapy for Atrial Fibrillation[1]	-	-	93%	95%
Antithrombotic Therapy Timing	61	95%	96%	98%
Assessed for Rehabilitation	58	79%	95%	97%
Discharged on Antithrombotic Therapy	57	96%	97%	99%
Discharged on Statin Medication	44	95%	89%	94%
Thrombolytic Therapy Timing	16	0%	53%	66%
Venous Thromboembolism Prophylaxis	63	83%	87%	94%
Written Stroke Educational Materials Given	49	69%	83%	88%
Surgical Care Improvement Project				
Appropriate Beta Blocker Usage	22	77%	97%	98%
Appropriate VTP Within 24 Hours	110	95%	97%	98%
Controlled Postoperative Blood Glucose[7]	-	-	96%	97%
Perioperative Temperature Management	159	100%	100%	100%
Prophylactic Antibiotic Selection	106	95%	99%	99%
Prophylactic Antibiotic Selection (Outpatient)[1,3]	-	-	97%	98%
Prophylactic Antibiotic Stopped	105	100%	97%	98%
Prophylactic Antibiotic Timing	106	92%	98%	99%
Prophylactic Antibiotic Timing (Outpatient)[1,3]	-	-	97%	98%
Urinary Catheter Removal	33	91%	96%	97%
Survey of Patients' Hospital Experiences				
Area Around Room 'Always' Quiet at Night	300+	69%	74%	61%
Doctors 'Always' Communicated Well	300+	83%	87%	82%
Home Recovery Information Given	300+	80%	85%	85%
Hospital Given 9 or 10 on 10 Point Scale	300+	66%	75%	71%
Meds 'Always' Explained Before Given	300+	67%	69%	64%
Nurses 'Always' Communicated Well	300+	78%	83%	79%
Pain 'Always' Well Controlled	300+	67%	75%	71%
Room and Bathroom 'Always' Clean	300+	77%	75%	73%
Timely Help 'Always' Received	300+	56%	71%	68%
Would Definitely Recommend Hospital	300+	67%	75%	71%
Use of Medical Imaging				
Cardiac Imaging Stress Test before Surgery	53	3.8%	5.3%	5.3%
Combination Abdominal CT Scan	142	1.4%	24.5%	10.5%

NOTE: Hospital profiles are in alphabetical order by state, then city, then hospital within the city; Rankings exclude hospitals with less than 25 cases except for patient surveys which excludes hospitals with less than 100 cases; (a) 100-299 cases; (1) The number of cases/patients is too few to report; (2) Data submitted were based on a sample of cases/patients; (3) Results are based on a shorter time period than required; (4) Data suppressed by CMS for one or more quarters; (5) Results are not available for this reporting period; (6) Fewer than 100 patients completed the HCAHPS survey; (7) No cases met the criteria for this measure; (8) The lower limit of the confidence interval cannot be calculated if the number of observed infections equals zero; (9) No data are available from the state/territory for this reporting period; (10) The scores shown reflect fewer than 50 completed surveys; (11) There were discrepancies in the data collection process; (12) This measure does not apply to this hospital for this reporting period; (13) Results cannot be calculated for this reporting period; (14) The results for this state are combined with nearby states to protect confidentiality; Please refer to the User's Guide for a full explanation of data.

Measure	Cases	This Hosp.	State Avg.	U.S. Avg.
Combination Brain/Sinus CT Scan[1]	-	-	2.6%	2.7%
Combination Chest CT Scan	128	0.0%	7.6%	2.7%
Follow-up Mammogram/Ultrasound	356	3.9%	9.4%	8.8%
Lumbar Spine MRI for Low Back Pain[1]	-	-	42.7%	37.2%

Monroe Surgical Hospital

2408 Broadmoor Blvd Phone: 318-410-0002
Monroe, LA 71201
Type: Acute Care Hospitals Emergency Services: No
Ownership: Proprietary
Key Personnel:
CEO/President. . . . . Garland McCarty, MD
Radiology. . . . . John McGibbonney

Measure	Cases	This Hosp.	State Avg.	U.S. Avg.
Blood Clot Prevention and Treatment				
Anticoagulation Overlap Therapy[1,2]	-	-	89%	93%
ICU Venous Thromboembolism Prophylaxis[2,7]	-	-	88%	92%
Incidence of Potentially Preventable VTE[2,7]	-	-	16%	10%
UFH with Dosages/Platelet Monitoring[2,7]	-	-	94%	97%
Venous Thromboembolism Prophylaxis[2]	33	82%	74%	85%
Warfarin Therapy Discharge Instructions[1,2]	-	-	85%	75%
Chest Pain/Possible Heart Attack Care				
Aspirin Given Within 24 Hours of Arrival[5]	-	-	94%	96%
Fibrinolytic Meds Within 30 Min. of Arrival[5]	-	-	54%	58%
Average Time to ECG (minutes)[5]	-	-	10	7
Average Time to Transfer (minutes)[5]	-	-	94	60
Children's Asthma Care				
Received Home Management Plan of Care	-	-	-	88%
Received Reliever Medication	-	-	-	100%
Received Systemic Corticosteroids	-	-	-	100%
Emergency Department				
Admittance Decision Time (minutes)[2,7]	-	-	86	98
Head CT Results Within 45 Min. of Arrival[5]	-	-	49%	57%
Patients Who Left ER Before Being Seen[5]	-	-	3%	2%
Time from ER Arrival to Admit. (minutes)[2,7]	-	-	256	274
Time from ER Arrival to Discharge (minutes)[5]	-	-	125	134
Time in ER Before Being Evaluated (minutes)[5]	-	-	27	26
Time to Pain Meds for Fractures (minutes)[5]	-	-	61	57
Heart Attack Care				
Aspirin Given at Discharge[5]	-	-	99%	99%
Fibrinolytic Meds Within 30 Min. of Arrival[5]	-	-	71%	54%
PCI Within 90 Minutes of Arrival[5]	-	-	94%	96%
Statin Prescribed at Discharge[5]	-	-	98%	98%
Heart Failure Care				
ACE Inhibitor or ARB for LVSD[5]	-	-	95%	97%
Discharge Instructions Given[5]	-	-	94%	94%
Evaluation of LVS Function[5]	-	-	97%	99%
Medicare Spending				
Medicare Spending per Patient (ratio)	-	0.81	1.04	0.98
Pneumonia Care				
Appropriate Initial Antibiotic Given[5]	-	-	93%	95%
Blood Culture Timing[5]	-	-	97%	98%
Pregnancy and Delivery Care				
Newborn Deliveries Scheduled Early[7]	-	-	5%	6%
Preventive Care				
Immunization for Influenza[2]	109	45%	85%	90%
Immunization for Pneumonia[2]	104	59%	88%	92%
Stroke Care				
Anticoagulation Therapy for Atrial Fibrillation[5]	-	-	93%	95%
Antithrombotic Therapy Timing[5]	-	-	96%	98%
Assessed for Rehabilitation[5]	-	-	95%	97%
Discharged on Antithrombotic Therapy[5]	-	-	97%	99%
Discharged on Statin Medication[5]	-	-	89%	94%
Thrombolytic Therapy Timing[5]	-	-	53%	66%
Venous Thromboembolism Prophylaxis[5]	-	-	87%	94%
Written Stroke Educational Materials Given[5]	-	-	83%	88%
Surgical Care Improvement Project				
Appropriate Beta Blocker Usage[2]	24	83%	97%	98%
Appropriate VTP Within 24 Hours[2]	81	98%	97%	98%
Controlled Postoperative Blood Glucose[2,7]	-	-	96%	97%
Perioperative Temperature Management[2]	90	100%	100%	100%
Prophylactic Antibiotic Selection[2]	65	98%	99%	99%
Prophylactic Antibiotic Selection (Outpatient)	33	91%	97%	98%
Prophylactic Antibiotic Stopped[2]	65	94%	97%	98%
Prophylactic Antibiotic Timing[2]	65	95%	98%	99%
Prophylactic Antibiotic Timing (Outpatient)	34	94%	97%	98%
Urinary Catheter Removal[2]	50	94%	96%	97%
Survey of Patients' Hospital Experiences				
Area Around Room 'Always' Quiet at Night[6]	<100	91%	74%	61%
Doctors 'Always' Communicated Well[6]	<100	90%	87%	82%
Home Recovery Information Given[6]	<100	86%	85%	85%
Hospital Given 9 or 10 on 10 Point Scale[6]	<100	87%	75%	71%
Meds 'Always' Explained Before Given[6]	<100	79%	69%	64%
Nurses 'Always' Communicated Well[6]	<100	89%	83%	79%
Pain 'Always' Well Controlled[6]	<100	79%	75%	71%
Room and Bathroom 'Always' Clean[6]	<100	81%	75%	73%
Timely Help 'Always' Received[6]	<100	89%	71%	68%
Would Definitely Recommend Hospital[6]	<100	85%	75%	71%
Use of Medical Imaging				
Cardiac Imaging Stress Test before Surgery	152	3.9%	5.3%	5.3%
Combination Abdominal CT Scan	203	40.9%	24.5%	10.5%
Combination Brain/Sinus CT Scan	64	0.0%	2.6%	2.7%
Combination Chest CT Scan	107	4.7%	7.6%	2.7%
Follow-up Mammogram/Ultrasound	273	9.2%	9.4%	8.8%
Lumbar Spine MRI for Low Back Pain	45	37.8%	42.7%	37.2%

P & S Surgical Hospital

312 Grammont Saint Suite 101 Phone: 318-388-4040
Monroe, LA 71201
URL: www.pssurgery.com
Type: Acute Care Hospitals Emergency Services: No
Ownership: Physician

Measure	Cases	This Hosp.	State Avg.	U.S. Avg.
Blood Clot Prevention and Treatment				
Anticoagulation Overlap Therapy[2,7]	-	-	89%	93%
ICU Venous Thromboembolism Prophylaxis[2,7]	-	-	88%	92%
Incidence of Potentially Preventable VTE[2,7]	-	-	16%	10%
UFH with Dosages/Platelet Monitoring[2,7]	-	-	94%	97%
Venous Thromboembolism Prophylaxis[2]	85	80%	74%	85%
Warfarin Therapy Discharge Instructions[2,7]	-	-	85%	75%
Chest Pain/Possible Heart Attack Care				
Aspirin Given Within 24 Hours of Arrival[5]	-	-	94%	96%
Fibrinolytic Meds Within 30 Min. of Arrival[5]	-	-	54%	58%
Average Time to ECG (minutes)[5]	-	-	10	7
Average Time to Transfer (minutes)[5]	-	-	94	60
Children's Asthma Care				
Received Home Management Plan of Care	-	-	-	88%
Received Reliever Medication	-	-	-	100%
Received Systemic Corticosteroids	-	-	-	100%
Emergency Department				
Admittance Decision Time (minutes)[2,7]	-	-	86	98
Head CT Results Within 45 Min. of Arrival[5]	-	-	49%	57%
Patients Who Left ER Before Being Seen[5]	-	-	3%	2%
Time from ER Arrival to Admit. (minutes)[2,7]	-	-	256	274
Time from ER Arrival to Discharge (minutes)[5]	-	-	125	134
Time in ER Before Being Evaluated (minutes)[5]	-	-	27	26
Time to Pain Meds for Fractures (minutes)[5]	-	-	61	57
Heart Attack Care				
Aspirin Given at Discharge[5]	-	-	99%	99%
Fibrinolytic Meds Within 30 Min. of Arrival[5]	-	-	71%	54%
PCI Within 90 Minutes of Arrival[5]	-	-	94%	96%
Statin Prescribed at Discharge[5]	-	-	98%	98%
Heart Failure Care				
ACE Inhibitor or ARB for LVSD[2,3]	-	-	95%	97%
Discharge Instructions Given[2,3]	-	-	94%	94%
Evaluation of LVS Function[2,3]	-	-	97%	99%
Medicare Spending				
Medicare Spending per Patient (ratio)	-	1.00	1.04	0.98
Pneumonia Care				
Appropriate Initial Antibiotic Given[5]	-	-	93%	95%
Blood Culture Timing[5]	-	-	97%	98%
Pregnancy and Delivery Care				
Newborn Deliveries Scheduled Early[7]	-	-	5%	6%
Preventive Care				
Immunization for Influenza[2]	281	96%	85%	90%
Immunization for Pneumonia[2]	391	96%	88%	92%
Stroke Care				
Anticoagulation Therapy for Atrial Fibrillation[2,7]	-	-	93%	95%
Antithrombotic Therapy Timing[2,7]	-	-	96%	98%
Assessed for Rehabilitation[2,7]	-	-	95%	97%
Discharged on Antithrombotic Therapy[2,7]	-	-	97%	99%
Discharged on Statin Medication[2,7]	-	-	89%	94%
Thrombolytic Therapy Timing[2,7]	-	-	53%	66%
Venous Thromboembolism Prophylaxis[2,7]	-	-	87%	94%
Written Stroke Educational Materials Given[2,7]	-	-	83%	88%
Surgical Care Improvement Project				
Appropriate Beta Blocker Usage[2]	79	100%	97%	98%
Appropriate VTP Within 24 Hours[2]	288	100%	97%	98%
Controlled Postoperative Blood Glucose[2,7]	-	-	96%	97%
Perioperative Temperature Management[2]	303	100%	100%	100%
Prophylactic Antibiotic Selection[2]	242	100%	99%	99%
Prophylactic Antibiotic Selection (Outpatient)	462	99%	97%	98%
Prophylactic Antibiotic Stopped[2]	240	100%	97%	98%
Prophylactic Antibiotic Timing[2]	242	100%	98%	99%
Prophylactic Antibiotic Timing (Outpatient)	464	99%	97%	98%
Urinary Catheter Removal[2]	236	97%	96%	97%
Survey of Patients' Hospital Experiences				
Area Around Room 'Always' Quiet at Night	(a)	93%	74%	61%
Doctors 'Always' Communicated Well	(a)	89%	87%	82%
Home Recovery Information Given	(a)	87%	85%	85%
Hospital Given 9 or 10 on 10 Point Scale	(a)	89%	75%	71%
Meds 'Always' Explained Before Given	(a)	80%	69%	64%
Nurses 'Always' Communicated Well	(a)	93%	83%	79%
Pain 'Always' Well Controlled	(a)	85%	75%	71%
Room and Bathroom 'Always' Clean	(a)	88%	75%	73%
Timely Help 'Always' Received	(a)	92%	71%	68%
Would Definitely Recommend Hospital	(a)	92%	75%	71%
Use of Medical Imaging				
Cardiac Imaging Stress Test before Surgery[7]	-	-	5.3%	5.3%
Combination Abdominal CT Scan[1]	-	-	24.5%	10.5%
Combination Brain/Sinus CT Scan	32	0.0%	2.6%	2.7%
Combination Chest CT Scan[1]	-	-	7.6%	2.7%
Follow-up Mammogram/Ultrasound[7]	-	-	9.4%	8.8%
Lumbar Spine MRI for Low Back Pain	119	39.5%	42.7%	37.2%

Saint Francis Medical Center

309 Jackson Street Phone: 318-966-4000
Monroe, LA 71201 Fax: 318-327-4142
URL: www.stfran.com
Type: Acute Care Hospitals Emergency Services: Yes
Ownership: Voluntary non-profit - Private Beds: 339
Key Personnel:
Anesthesiology. . . . . Dr. Johnathan Beebe
CEO/President. . . . . Louis H. Bremer, Jr., FACHE
Radiology. . . . . Dr. John Davis
Chairman/CEO . . . . J. Stewart Gentry
Surgery . . . . Dr. Lee Miller
Pediatrics. . . . . Dr. Joaquin Rosales
Chief of Medical Staff . . . . Bob Seegers, MD
Emergency Room . . . . Dr. Edward Shaheen

Measure	Cases	This Hosp.	State Avg.	U.S. Avg.
Blood Clot Prevention and Treatment				
Anticoagulation Overlap Therapy[2]	105	73%	89%	93%
ICU Venous Thromboembolism Prophylaxis[2]	105	91%	88%	92%
Incidence of Potentially Preventable VTE[2]	32	22%	16%	10%
UFH with Dosages/Platelet Monitoring[2]	26	100%	94%	97%
Venous Thromboembolism Prophylaxis[2]	347	84%	74%	85%
Warfarin Therapy Discharge Instructions[2]	85	69%	85%	75%
Chest Pain/Possible Heart Attack Care				
Aspirin Given Within 24 Hours of Arrival[1,3]	-	-	94%	96%
Fibrinolytic Meds Within 30 Min. of Arrival[5]	-	-	54%	58%
Average Time to ECG (minutes)[1,3]	-	-	10	7
Average Time to Transfer (minutes)[5]	-	-	94	60
Children's Asthma Care				
Received Home Management Plan of Care	47	94%	-	88%
Received Reliever Medication	47	100%	-	100%
Received Systemic Corticosteroids	46	100%	-	100%
Emergency Department				
Admittance Decision Time (minutes)[2]	401	110	86	98

NOTE: Hospital profiles are in alphabetical order by state, then city, then hospital within the city; Rankings exclude hospitals with less than 25 cases except for patient surveys which excludes hospitals with less than 100 cases; (a) 100-299 cases; (1) The number of cases/patients is too few to report; (2) Data submitted were based on a sample of cases/patients; (3) Results are based on a shorter time period than required; (4) Data suppressed by CMS for one or more quarters; (5) Results are not available for this reporting period; (6) Fewer than 100 patients completed the HCAHPS survey; (7) No cases met the criteria for this measure; (8) The lower limit of the confidence interval cannot be calculated if the number of observed infections equals zero; (9) No data are available from the state/territory for this reporting period; (10) The scores shown reflect fewer than 50 completed surveys; (11) There were discrepancies in the data collection process; (12) This measure does not apply to this hospital for this reporting period; (13) Results cannot be calculated for this reporting period; (14) The results for this state are combined with nearby states to protect confidentiality; Please refer to the User's Guide for a full explanation of data.

Measure	Cases	This Hosp.	State Avg.	U.S. Avg.
Head CT Results Within 45 Min. of Arrival[1]	-	-	49%	57%
Patients Who Left ER Before Being Seen	61,829	2%	3%	2%
Time from ER Arrival to Admit. (minutes)[2]	437	325	256	274
Time from ER Arrival to Discharge (minutes)	279	149	125	134
Time in ER Before Being Evaluated (minutes)	384	48	27	26
Time to Pain Meds for Fractures (minutes)	188	75	61	57
Heart Attack Care				
Aspirin Given at Discharge	208	100%	99%	99%
Fibrinolytic Meds Within 30 Min. of Arrival[7]	-	-	71%	54%
PCI Within 90 Minutes of Arrival	33	91%	94%	96%
Statin Prescribed at Discharge	195	100%	98%	98%
Heart Failure Care				
ACE Inhibitor or ARB for LVSD	153	100%	95%	97%
Discharge Instructions Given	308	90%	94%	94%
Evaluation of LVS Function	377	100%	97%	99%
Medicare Spending				
Medicare Spending per Patient (ratio)	-	1.04	1.04	0.98
Pneumonia Care				
Appropriate Initial Antibiotic Given	151	97%	93%	95%
Blood Culture Timing	355	98%	97%	98%
Pregnancy and Delivery Care				
Newborn Deliveries Scheduled Early[2]	50	12%	5%	6%
Preventive Care				
Immunization for Influenza[2]	504	91%	85%	90%
Immunization for Pneumonia[2]	638	92%	88%	92%
Stroke Care				
Anticoagulation Therapy for Atrial Fibrillation[2]	15	80%	93%	95%
Antithrombotic Therapy Timing[2]	76	96%	96%	98%
Assessed for Rehabilitation[2]	103	90%	95%	97%
Discharged on Antithrombotic Therapy[2]	87	95%	97%	99%
Discharged on Statin Medication[2]	68	85%	89%	94%
Thrombolytic Therapy Timing[2]	14	57%	53%	66%
Venous Thromboembolism Prophylaxis[2]	104	92%	87%	94%
Written Stroke Educational Materials Given[2]	48	67%	83%	88%
Surgical Care Improvement Project				
Appropriate Beta Blocker Usage[2]	183	100%	97%	98%
Appropriate VTP Within 24 Hours[2]	257	100%	97%	98%
Controlled Postoperative Blood Glucose[2]	91	100%	96%	97%
Perioperative Temperature Management[2]	327	100%	100%	100%
Prophylactic Antibiotic Selection[2]	279	100%	99%	99%
Prophylactic Antibiotic Selection (Outpatient)	267	95%	97%	98%
Prophylactic Antibiotic Stopped[2]	253	100%	97%	98%
Prophylactic Antibiotic Timing[2]	279	100%	98%	99%
Prophylactic Antibiotic Timing (Outpatient)	269	99%	97%	98%
Urinary Catheter Removal[2]	289	100%	96%	97%
Survey of Patients' Hospital Experiences				
Area Around Room 'Always' Quiet at Night	300+	68%	74%	61%
Doctors 'Always' Communicated Well	300+	86%	87%	82%
Home Recovery Information Given	300+	80%	85%	85%
Hospital Given 9 or 10 on 10 Point Scale	300+	73%	75%	71%
Meds 'Always' Explained Before Given	300+	67%	69%	64%
Nurses 'Always' Communicated Well	300+	84%	83%	79%
Pain 'Always' Well Controlled	300+	73%	75%	71%
Room and Bathroom 'Always' Clean	300+	73%	75%	73%
Timely Help 'Always' Received	300+	65%	71%	68%
Would Definitely Recommend Hospital	300+	79%	75%	71%
Use of Medical Imaging				
Cardiac Imaging Stress Test before Surgery	98	7.1%	5.3%	5.3%
Combination Abdominal CT Scan	1,065	19.7%	24.5%	10.5%
Combination Brain/Sinus CT Scan	1,488	3.4%	2.6%	2.7%
Combination Chest CT Scan	811	0.0%	7.6%	2.7%
Follow-up Mammogram/Ultrasound	2,088	10.2%	9.4%	8.8%
Lumbar Spine MRI for Low Back Pain	281	38.1%	42.7%	37.2%

Teche Regional Medical Center

1125 Marguerite Street
Morgan City, LA 70380
URL: www.techeregional.com
Type: Acute Care Hospitals
Ownership: Proprietary

Phone: 985-384-2200
Fax: 985-380-4546
Emergency Services: No
Beds: 149

Key Personnel:
Operating Room. . . . . Tomas Birriel
Chief of Medical Staff. . . . . Natalie Dishman
Emergency Room . . . . Cerri Gianluca, MD
CEO/President. . . . . Scott Smith
Infection Control. . . . . Brenda Topham
Quality Assurance . . . . Verna Whealley

Measure	Cases	This Hosp.	State Avg.	U.S. Avg.
Blood Clot Prevention and Treatment				
Anticoagulation Overlap Therapy[2]	16	81%	89%	93%
ICU Venous Thromboembolism Prophylaxis[2]	40	100%	88%	92%
Incidence of Potentially Preventable VTE[1,2]	-	-	16%	10%
UFH with Dosages/Platelet Monitoring[1,2]	-	-	94%	97%
Venous Thromboembolism Prophylaxis[2]	225	98%	74%	85%
Warfarin Therapy Discharge Instructions[2]	14	100%	85%	75%
Chest Pain/Possible Heart Attack Care				
Aspirin Given Within 24 Hours of Arrival	45	100%	94%	96%
Fibrinolytic Meds Within 30 Min. of Arrival[1]	-	-	54%	58%
Average Time to ECG (minutes)	47	8	10	7
Average Time to Transfer (minutes)[1]	-	-	94	60
Children's Asthma Care				
Received Home Management Plan of Care	-	-	-	88%
Received Reliever Medication	-	-	-	100%
Received Systemic Corticosteroids	-	-	-	100%
Emergency Department				
Admittance Decision Time (minutes)[2]	252	119	86	98
Head CT Results Within 45 Min. of Arrival[1]	-	-	49%	57%
Patients Who Left ER Before Being Seen	29,621	4%	3%	2%
Time from ER Arrival to Admit. (minutes)[2]	253	257	256	274
Time from ER Arrival to Discharge (minutes)	392	77	125	134
Time in ER Before Being Evaluated (minutes)	408	12	27	26
Time to Pain Meds for Fractures (minutes)	82	27	61	57
Heart Attack Care				
Aspirin Given at Discharge	21	90%	99%	99%
Fibrinolytic Meds Within 30 Min. of Arrival[1]	-	-	71%	54%
PCI Within 90 Minutes of Arrival[7]	-	-	94%	96%
Statin Prescribed at Discharge	19	89%	98%	98%
Heart Failure Care				
ACE Inhibitor or ARB for LVSD	20	85%	95%	97%
Discharge Instructions Given	87	98%	94%	94%
Evaluation of LVS Function	104	98%	97%	99%
Medicare Spending				
Medicare Spending per Patient (ratio)	-	1.10	1.04	0.98
Pneumonia Care				
Appropriate Initial Antibiotic Given	48	85%	93%	95%
Blood Culture Timing	63	97%	97%	98%
Pregnancy and Delivery Care				
Newborn Deliveries Scheduled Early[2]	49	14%	5%	6%
Preventive Care				
Immunization for Influenza[2]	228	100%	85%	90%
Immunization for Pneumonia[2]	241	98%	88%	92%
Stroke Care				
Anticoagulation Therapy for Atrial Fibrillation[1]	-	-	93%	95%
Antithrombotic Therapy Timing	20	100%	96%	98%
Assessed for Rehabilitation	22	100%	95%	97%
Discharged on Antithrombotic Therapy	21	100%	97%	99%
Discharged on Statin Medication	19	100%	89%	94%
Thrombolytic Therapy Timing[7]	-	-	53%	66%
Venous Thromboembolism Prophylaxis	22	100%	87%	94%
Written Stroke Educational Materials Given	14	100%	83%	88%
Surgical Care Improvement Project				
Appropriate Beta Blocker Usage	20	90%	97%	98%
Appropriate VTP Within 24 Hours	65	92%	97%	98%
Controlled Postoperative Blood Glucose[7]	-	-	96%	97%
Perioperative Temperature Management	77	100%	100%	100%
Prophylactic Antibiotic Selection	31	90%	99%	99%
Prophylactic Antibiotic Selection (Outpatient)	52	90%	97%	98%
Prophylactic Antibiotic Stopped	25	84%	97%	98%
Prophylactic Antibiotic Timing	31	100%	98%	99%
Prophylactic Antibiotic Timing (Outpatient)	52	98%	97%	98%
Urinary Catheter Removal	34	91%	96%	97%
Survey of Patients' Hospital Experiences				
Area Around Room 'Always' Quiet at Night	300+	65%	74%	61%
Doctors 'Always' Communicated Well	300+	85%	87%	82%
Home Recovery Information Given	300+	84%	85%	85%
Hospital Given 9 or 10 on 10 Point Scale	300+	62%	75%	71%
Meds 'Always' Explained Before Given	300+	60%	69%	64%
Nurses 'Always' Communicated Well	300+	76%	83%	79%
Pain 'Always' Well Controlled	300+	69%	75%	71%
Room and Bathroom 'Always' Clean	300+	64%	75%	73%
Timely Help 'Always' Received	300+	60%	71%	68%
Would Definitely Recommend Hospital	300+	62%	75%	71%
Use of Medical Imaging				
Cardiac Imaging Stress Test before Surgery[1]	-	-	5.3%	5.3%
Combination Abdominal CT Scan	356	14.3%	24.5%	10.5%
Combination Brain/Sinus CT Scan[1]	-	-	2.6%	2.7%
Combination Chest CT Scan	110	14.5%	7.6%	2.7%
Follow-up Mammogram/Ultrasound	381	7.6%	9.4%	8.8%
Lumbar Spine MRI for Low Back Pain	60	45.0%	42.7%	37.2%

Assumption Community Hospital

135 Highway 402
Napoleonville, LA 70390
Type: Critical Access Hospitals
Ownership: Voluntary non-profit - Private

Phone: 985-369-3600
Fax: 985-369-4271
Emergency Services: Yes
Beds: 15

Key Personnel:
CEO/President. . . . . Wayne M Arboneaux
Chief of Medical Staff. . . . . Tony Sun, MD

Measure	Cases	This Hosp.	State Avg.	U.S. Avg.
Blood Clot Prevention and Treatment				
Anticoagulation Overlap Therapy[5]	-	-	89%	93%
ICU Venous Thromboembolism Prophylaxis[5]	-	-	88%	92%
Incidence of Potentially Preventable VTE[5]	-	-	16%	10%
UFH with Dosages/Platelet Monitoring[5]	-	-	94%	97%
Venous Thromboembolism Prophylaxis[5]	-	-	74%	85%
Warfarin Therapy Discharge Instructions[5]	-	-	85%	75%
Chest Pain/Possible Heart Attack Care				
Aspirin Given Within 24 Hours of Arrival[5]	-	-	94%	96%
Fibrinolytic Meds Within 30 Min. of Arrival[5]	-	-	54%	58%
Average Time to ECG (minutes)[5]	-	-	10	7
Average Time to Transfer (minutes)[5]	-	-	94	60
Children's Asthma Care				
Received Home Management Plan of Care	-	-	-	88%
Received Reliever Medication	-	-	-	100%
Received Systemic Corticosteroids	-	-	-	100%
Emergency Department				
Admittance Decision Time (minutes)[5]	-	-	86	98
Head CT Results Within 45 Min. of Arrival[5]	-	-	49%	57%
Patients Who Left ER Before Being Seen	6,735	1%	3%	2%
Time from ER Arrival to Admit. (minutes)[5]	-	-	256	274
Time from ER Arrival to Discharge (minutes)[5]	-	-	125	134
Time in ER Before Being Evaluated (minutes)[5]	-	-	27	26
Time to Pain Meds for Fractures (minutes)[5]	-	-	61	57
Heart Attack Care				
Aspirin Given at Discharge[5]	-	-	99%	99%
Fibrinolytic Meds Within 30 Min. of Arrival[5]	-	-	71%	54%
PCI Within 90 Minutes of Arrival[5]	-	-	94%	96%
Statin Prescribed at Discharge[5]	-	-	98%	98%
Heart Failure Care				
ACE Inhibitor or ARB for LVSD[1,2]	-	-	95%	97%
Discharge Instructions Given[1,2]	-	-	94%	94%
Evaluation of LVS Function[1,2]	-	-	97%	99%
Medicare Spending				
Medicare Spending per Patient (ratio)	-	-	1.04	0.98
Pneumonia Care				
Appropriate Initial Antibiotic Given[1,2]	-	-	93%	95%
Blood Culture Timing[1,2]	-	-	97%	98%
Pregnancy and Delivery Care				
Newborn Deliveries Scheduled Early[5]	-	-	5%	6%
Preventive Care				
Immunization for Influenza[5]	-	-	85%	90%
Immunization for Pneumonia[5]	-	-	88%	92%
Stroke Care				
Anticoagulation Therapy for Atrial Fibrillation[5]	-	-	93%	95%
Antithrombotic Therapy Timing[5]	-	-	96%	98%
Assessed for Rehabilitation[5]	-	-	95%	97%
Discharged on Antithrombotic Therapy[5]	-	-	97%	99%
Discharged on Statin Medication[5]	-	-	89%	94%
Thrombolytic Therapy Timing[5]	-	-	53%	66%

NOTE: Hospital profiles are in alphabetical order by state, then city, then hospital within the city; Rankings exclude hospitals with less than 25 cases except for patient surveys which excludes hospitals with less than 100 cases; (a) 100-299 cases; (1) The number of cases/patients is too few to report; (2) Data submitted were based on a sample of cases/patients; (3) Results are based on a shorter time period than required; (4) Data suppressed by CMS for one or more quarters; (5) Results are not available for this reporting period; (6) Fewer than 100 patients completed the HCAHPS survey; (7) No cases met the criteria for this measure; (8) The lower limit of the confidence interval cannot be calculated if the number of observed infections equals zero; (9) No data are available from the state/territory for this reporting period; (10) The scores shown reflect fewer than 50 completed surveys; (11) There were discrepancies in the data collection process; (12) This measure does not apply to this hospital for this reporting period; (13) Results cannot be calculated for this reporting period; (14) The results for this state are combined with nearby states to protect confidentiality; Please refer to the User's Guide for a full explanation of data.

Measure	Cases	This Hosp.	State Avg.	U.S. Avg.
Venous Thromboembolism Prophylaxis[5]	-	-	87%	94%
Written Stroke Educational Materials Given[5]	-	-	83%	88%
Surgical Care Improvement Project				
Appropriate Beta Blocker Usage[5]	-	-	97%	98%
Appropriate VTP Within 24 Hours[5]	-	-	97%	98%
Controlled Postoperative Blood Glucose[5]	-	-	96%	97%
Perioperative Temperature Management[5]	-	-	100%	100%
Prophylactic Antibiotic Selection[5]	-	-	99%	99%
Prophylactic Antibiotic Selection (Outpatient)[5]	-	-	97%	98%
Prophylactic Antibiotic Stopped[5]	-	-	97%	98%
Prophylactic Antibiotic Timing[5]	-	-	98%	99%
Prophylactic Antibiotic Timing (Outpatient)[5]	-	-	97%	98%
Urinary Catheter Removal[5]	-	-	96%	97%
Survey of Patients' Hospital Experiences				
Area Around Room 'Always' Quiet at Night[10]	<100	92%	74%	61%
Doctors 'Always' Communicated Well[10]	<100	99%	87%	82%
Home Recovery Information Given[10]	<100	98%	85%	85%
Hospital Given 9 or 10 on 10 Point Scale[10]	<100	92%	75%	71%
Meds 'Always' Explained Before Given[10]	<100	93%	69%	64%
Nurses 'Always' Communicated Well[10]	<100	97%	83%	79%
Pain 'Always' Well Controlled[10]	<100	87%	75%	71%
Room and Bathroom 'Always' Clean[10]	<100	96%	75%	73%
Timely Help 'Always' Received[10]	<100	100%	71%	68%
Would Definitely Recommend Hospital[10]	<100	91%	75%	71%
Use of Medical Imaging				
Cardiac Imaging Stress Test before Surgery[7]	-	-	5.3%	5.3%
Combination Abdominal CT Scan[7]	-	-	24.5%	10.5%
Combination Brain/Sinus CT Scan[7]	-	-	2.6%	2.7%
Combination Chest CT Scan[7]	-	-	7.6%	2.7%
Follow-up Mammogram/Ultrasound[1]	-	-	9.4%	8.8%
Lumbar Spine MRI for Low Back Pain[7]	-	-	42.7%	37.2%

Natchitoches Regional Medical Center

501 Keyser Ave — Phone: 318-214-4200
Natchitoches, LA 71457 — Fax: 318-214-4354
URL: www.natchitocheshospital.org
Type: Acute Care Hospitals — Emergency Services: Yes
Ownership: Govt - Hospital Dist/Auth — Beds: 99

Key Personnel:
Operating Room. . . . . William Ball
Chief of Medical Staff. . . . . Otis Barnum
Patient Relations . . . . Merry Jo Grayson
CEO/President. . . . . Mark Marley
Radiology. . . . . Edna McLeod

Measure	Cases	This Hosp.	State Avg.	U.S. Avg.
Blood Clot Prevention and Treatment				
Anticoagulation Overlap Therapy[2]	14	43%	89%	93%
ICU Venous Thromboembolism Prophylaxis[2]	61	75%	88%	92%
Incidence of Potentially Preventable VTE[1,2]	-	-	16%	10%
UFH with Dosages/Platelet Monitoring[2,7]	-	-	94%	97%
Venous Thromboembolism Prophylaxis[2]	152	66%	74%	85%
Warfarin Therapy Discharge Instructions[1,2]	-	-	85%	75%
Chest Pain/Possible Heart Attack Care				
Aspirin Given Within 24 Hours of Arrival	30	97%	94%	96%
Fibrinolytic Meds Within 30 Min. of Arrival[1]	-	-	54%	58%
Average Time to ECG (minutes)	30	10	10	7
Average Time to Transfer (minutes)[1]	-	-	94	60
Children's Asthma Care				
Received Home Management Plan of Care	-	-	-	88%
Received Reliever Medication	-	-	-	100%
Received Systemic Corticosteroids	-	-	-	100%
Emergency Department				
Admittance Decision Time (minutes)[2]	165	75	86	98
Head CT Results Within 45 Min. of Arrival[1]	-	-	49%	57%
Patients Who Left ER Before Being Seen	20,151	6%	3%	2%
Time from ER Arrival to Admit. (minutes)[2]	190	285	256	274
Time from ER Arrival to Discharge (minutes)	344	168	125	134
Time in ER Before Being Evaluated (minutes)	370	48	27	26
Time to Pain Meds for Fractures (minutes)	54	102	61	57
Heart Attack Care				
Aspirin Given at Discharge[1]	-	-	99%	99%
Fibrinolytic Meds Within 30 Min. of Arrival[7]	-	-	71%	54%
PCI Within 90 Minutes of Arrival[7]	-	-	94%	96%
Statin Prescribed at Discharge[1]	-	-	98%	98%
Heart Failure Care				
ACE Inhibitor or ARB for LVSD	26	85%	95%	97%
Discharge Instructions Given	53	85%	94%	94%
Evaluation of LVS Function	74	95%	97%	99%
Medicare Spending				
Medicare Spending per Patient (ratio)	-	1.24	1.04	0.98
Pneumonia Care				
Appropriate Initial Antibiotic Given	69	86%	93%	95%
Blood Culture Timing	76	97%	97%	98%
Pregnancy and Delivery Care				
Newborn Deliveries Scheduled Early[2]	37	0%	5%	6%
Preventive Care				
Immunization for Influenza[2]	245	64%	85%	90%
Immunization for Pneumonia[2]	236	85%	88%	92%
Stroke Care				
Anticoagulation Therapy for Atrial Fibrillation[7]	-	-	93%	95%
Antithrombotic Therapy Timing	13	100%	96%	98%
Assessed for Rehabilitation	13	77%	95%	97%
Discharged on Antithrombotic Therapy	13	100%	97%	99%
Discharged on Statin Medication	11	73%	89%	94%
Thrombolytic Therapy Timing[1]	-	-	53%	66%
Venous Thromboembolism Prophylaxis	14	57%	87%	94%
Written Stroke Educational Materials Given[1]	-	-	83%	88%
Surgical Care Improvement Project				
Appropriate Beta Blocker Usage	26	96%	97%	98%
Appropriate VTP Within 24 Hours	97	98%	97%	98%
Controlled Postoperative Blood Glucose[7]	-	-	96%	97%
Perioperative Temperature Management	103	100%	100%	100%
Prophylactic Antibiotic Selection	84	99%	99%	99%
Prophylactic Antibiotic Selection (Outpatient)	30	97%	97%	98%
Prophylactic Antibiotic Stopped	80	89%	97%	98%
Prophylactic Antibiotic Timing	84	96%	98%	99%
Prophylactic Antibiotic Timing (Outpatient)	30	97%	97%	98%
Urinary Catheter Removal	62	98%	96%	97%
Survey of Patients' Hospital Experiences				
Area Around Room 'Always' Quiet at Night	300+	67%	74%	61%
Doctors 'Always' Communicated Well	300+	85%	87%	82%
Home Recovery Information Given	300+	82%	85%	85%
Hospital Given 9 or 10 on 10 Point Scale	300+	58%	75%	71%
Meds 'Always' Explained Before Given	300+	68%	69%	64%
Nurses 'Always' Communicated Well	300+	77%	83%	79%
Pain 'Always' Well Controlled	300+	68%	75%	71%
Room and Bathroom 'Always' Clean	300+	70%	75%	73%
Timely Help 'Always' Received	300+	66%	71%	68%
Would Definitely Recommend Hospital	300+	57%	75%	71%
Use of Medical Imaging				
Cardiac Imaging Stress Test before Surgery	182	6.6%	5.3%	5.3%
Combination Abdominal CT Scan	334	53.0%	24.5%	10.5%
Combination Brain/Sinus CT Scan[1]	-	-	2.6%	2.7%
Combination Chest CT Scan	207	38.6%	7.6%	2.7%
Follow-up Mammogram/Ultrasound	392	5.4%	9.4%	8.8%
Lumbar Spine MRI for Low Back Pain[7]	-	-	42.7%	37.2%

Dauterive Hospital

600 North Lewis Street — Phone: 337-365-7311
New Iberia, LA 70563 — Fax: 337-374-4104
URL: www.dauterivehospital.com
Type: Acute Care Hospitals — Emergency Services: Yes
Ownership: Proprietary — Beds: 107

Key Personnel:
Pediatric Ambulatory Care . . . . . . Mounaf Ahmad, MD
Pediatric In-Patient Care . . . . . . Mounaf Ahmad, MD
Chief of Medical Staff. . . . . Michael Alvarez, MD
Operating Room. . . . . Thomas Borland
Radiology. . . . . Jaime Boudreaux
Infection Control. . . . . Tara Dubois, RN
CEO/President. . . . . Alan Fabian
Emergency Room . . . . Craig Frederick, MD

Measure	Cases	This Hosp.	State Avg.	U.S. Avg.
Blood Clot Prevention and Treatment				
Anticoagulation Overlap Therapy[2]	14	100%	89%	93%
ICU Venous Thromboembolism Prophylaxis[2]	56	100%	88%	92%
Incidence of Potentially Preventable VTE[1,2]	-	-	16%	10%
UFH with Dosages/Platelet Monitoring[1,2]	-	-	94%	97%
Venous Thromboembolism Prophylaxis[2]	133	100%	74%	85%
Warfarin Therapy Discharge Instructions[2]	13	100%	85%	75%
Chest Pain/Possible Heart Attack Care				
Aspirin Given Within 24 Hours of Arrival[1,3]	-	-	94%	96%
Fibrinolytic Meds Within 30 Min. of Arrival[5]	-	-	54%	58%
Average Time to ECG (minutes)[1,3]	-	-	10	7
Average Time to Transfer (minutes)[5]	-	-	94	60
Children's Asthma Care				
Received Home Management Plan of Care	-	-	-	88%
Received Reliever Medication	-	-	-	100%
Received Systemic Corticosteroids	-	-	-	100%
Emergency Department				
Admittance Decision Time (minutes)[2]	345	62	86	98
Head CT Results Within 45 Min. of Arrival[1]	-	-	49%	57%
Patients Who Left ER Before Being Seen	23,601	1%	3%	2%
Time from ER Arrival to Admit. (minutes)[2]	349	198	256	274
Time from ER Arrival to Discharge (minutes)	552	90	125	134
Time in ER Before Being Evaluated (minutes)	591	15	27	26
Time to Pain Meds for Fractures (minutes)	57	31	61	57
Heart Attack Care				
Aspirin Given at Discharge	31	100%	99%	99%
Fibrinolytic Meds Within 30 Min. of Arrival[7]	-	-	71%	54%
PCI Within 90 Minutes of Arrival[1]	-	-	94%	96%
Statin Prescribed at Discharge	28	100%	98%	98%
Heart Failure Care				
ACE Inhibitor or ARB for LVSD	29	100%	95%	97%
Discharge Instructions Given	69	94%	94%	94%
Evaluation of LVS Function	77	100%	97%	99%
Medicare Spending				
Medicare Spending per Patient (ratio)	-	1.00	1.04	0.98
Pneumonia Care				
Appropriate Initial Antibiotic Given	30	100%	93%	95%
Blood Culture Timing	59	98%	97%	98%
Pregnancy and Delivery Care				
Newborn Deliveries Scheduled Early[2]	40	0%	5%	6%
Preventive Care				
Immunization for Influenza[2]	306	99%	85%	90%
Immunization for Pneumonia[2]	300	99%	88%	92%
Stroke Care				
Anticoagulation Therapy for Atrial Fibrillation[1]	-	-	93%	95%
Antithrombotic Therapy Timing	25	100%	96%	98%
Assessed for Rehabilitation	25	100%	95%	97%
Discharged on Antithrombotic Therapy	24	100%	97%	99%
Discharged on Statin Medication	17	100%	89%	94%
Thrombolytic Therapy Timing[7]	-	-	53%	66%
Venous Thromboembolism Prophylaxis	25	100%	87%	94%
Written Stroke Educational Materials Given[1]	-	-	83%	88%
Surgical Care Improvement Project				
Appropriate Beta Blocker Usage	45	100%	97%	98%
Appropriate VTP Within 24 Hours	121	100%	97%	98%
Controlled Postoperative Blood Glucose[7]	-	-	96%	97%
Perioperative Temperature Management	149	100%	100%	100%
Prophylactic Antibiotic Selection	90	100%	99%	99%
Prophylactic Antibiotic Selection (Outpatient)	95	99%	97%	98%
Prophylactic Antibiotic Stopped	82	100%	97%	98%
Prophylactic Antibiotic Timing	90	100%	98%	99%
Prophylactic Antibiotic Timing (Outpatient)	94	100%	97%	98%
Urinary Catheter Removal	30	100%	96%	97%
Survey of Patients' Hospital Experiences				
Area Around Room 'Always' Quiet at Night	300+	68%	74%	61%
Doctors 'Always' Communicated Well	300+	87%	87%	82%
Home Recovery Information Given	300+	83%	85%	85%
Hospital Given 9 or 10 on 10 Point Scale	300+	67%	75%	71%
Meds 'Always' Explained Before Given	300+	59%	69%	64%
Nurses 'Always' Communicated Well	300+	76%	83%	79%
Pain 'Always' Well Controlled	300+	73%	75%	71%
Room and Bathroom 'Always' Clean	300+	75%	75%	73%
Timely Help 'Always' Received	300+	65%	71%	68%
Would Definitely Recommend Hospital	300+	68%	75%	71%
Use of Medical Imaging				
Cardiac Imaging Stress Test before Surgery[1]	-	-	5.3%	5.3%

NOTE: Hospital profiles are in alphabetical order by state, then city, then hospital within the city; Rankings exclude hospitals with less than 25 cases except for patient surveys which excludes hospitals with less than 100 cases; (a) 100-299 cases; (1) The number of cases/patients is too few to report; (2) Data submitted were based on a sample of cases/patients; (3) Results are based on a shorter time period than required; (4) Data suppressed by CMS for one or more quarters; (5) Results are not available for this reporting period; (6) Fewer than 100 patients completed the HCAHPS survey; (7) No cases met the criteria for this measure; (8) The lower limit of the confidence interval cannot be calculated if the number of observed infections equals zero; (9) No data are available from the state/territory for this reporting period; (10) The scores shown reflect fewer than 50 completed surveys; (11) There were discrepancies in the data collection process; (12) This measure does not apply to this hospital for this reporting period; (13) Results cannot be calculated for this reporting period; (14) The results for this state are combined with nearby states to protect confidentiality; Please refer to the User's Guide for a full explanation of data.

Combination Abdominal CT Scan	226	41.2%	24.5%	10.5%
Combination Brain/Sinus CT Scan[1]	-	-	2.6%	2.7%
Combination Chest CT Scan	126	0.8%	7.6%	2.7%
Follow-up Mammogram/Ultrasound	338	8.3%	9.4%	8.8%
Lumbar Spine MRI for Low Back Pain[1]	-	-	42.7%	37.2%

Iberia General Hospital & Medical Center

2315 E Main Street Phone: 337-364-0441
New Iberia, LA 70562 Fax: 337-374-7641
URL: www.iberiamedicalcenter.com
Type: Acute Care Hospitals Emergency Services: Yes
Ownership: Govt - Hospital Dist/Auth Beds: 101

Key Personnel:
Surgery . . . . Thomas Borland
Radiology. . . . . David Fontenot
Cardiology . . . . Paul Gulotta, Jr
Pulmonology . . . . Moses Kitakule
Cardiology. . . . . Eli Levine
Chief of Medical Staff . . . . Shane Myers
Quality Assurance . . . . Mary Taylor, RN
CEO/President. . . . . John Tucker

Measure	Cases	This Hosp.	State Avg.	U.S. Avg.
Blood Clot Prevention and Treatment				
Anticoagulation Overlap Therapy[2]	27	85%	89%	93%
ICU Venous Thromboembolism Prophylaxis[2]	65	92%	88%	92%
Incidence of Potentially Preventable VTE[1,2]	-	-	16%	10%
UFH with Dosages/Platelet Monitoring[1,2]	-	-	94%	97%
Venous Thromboembolism Prophylaxis[2]	301	88%	74%	85%
Warfarin Therapy Discharge Instructions[2]	19	100%	85%	75%
Chest Pain/Possible Heart Attack Care				
Aspirin Given Within 24 Hours of Arrival[1,3]	-	-	94%	96%
Fibrinolytic Meds Within 30 Min. of Arrival[3,7]	-	-	54%	58%
Average Time to ECG (minutes)[1,3]	-	-	10	7
Average Time to Transfer (minutes)[3,7]	-	-	94	60
Children's Asthma Care				
Received Home Management Plan of Care	-	-	-	88%
Received Reliever Medication	-	-	-	100%
Received Systemic Corticosteroids	-	-	-	100%
Emergency Department				
Admittance Decision Time (minutes)[2]	316	75	86	98
Head CT Results Within 45 Min. of Arrival	15	40%	49%	57%
Patients Who Left ER Before Being Seen	26,606	3%	3%	2%
Time from ER Arrival to Admit. (minutes)[2]	324	270	256	274
Time from ER Arrival to Discharge (minutes)	369	121	125	134
Time in ER Before Being Evaluated (minutes)	404	28	27	26
Time to Pain Meds for Fractures (minutes)	90	61	61	57
Heart Attack Care				
Aspirin Given at Discharge	74	99%	99%	99%
Fibrinolytic Meds Within 30 Min. of Arrival[7]	-	-	71%	54%
PCI Within 90 Minutes of Arrival	17	71%	94%	96%
Statin Prescribed at Discharge	77	94%	98%	98%
Heart Failure Care				
ACE Inhibitor or ARB for LVSD	58	95%	95%	97%
Discharge Instructions Given	147	100%	94%	94%
Evaluation of LVS Function	183	99%	97%	99%
Medicare Spending				
Medicare Spending per Patient (ratio)	-	1.10	1.04	0.98
Pneumonia Care				
Appropriate Initial Antibiotic Given[2]	102	96%	93%	95%
Blood Culture Timing[2]	182	97%	97%	98%
Pregnancy and Delivery Care				
Newborn Deliveries Scheduled Early[2]	50	2%	5%	6%
Preventive Care				
Immunization for Influenza[2]	413	98%	85%	90%
Immunization for Pneumonia[2]	475	99%	88%	92%
Stroke Care				
Anticoagulation Therapy for Atrial Fibrillation[1]	-	-	93%	95%
Antithrombotic Therapy Timing	36	100%	96%	98%
Assessed for Rehabilitation	40	95%	95%	97%
Discharged on Antithrombotic Therapy	38	97%	97%	99%
Discharged on Statin Medication	31	87%	89%	94%
Thrombolytic Therapy Timing[1]	-	-	53%	66%
Venous Thromboembolism Prophylaxis	38	92%	87%	94%
Written Stroke Educational Materials Given	20	95%	83%	88%
Surgical Care Improvement Project				
Appropriate Beta Blocker Usage	67	93%	97%	98%
Appropriate VTP Within 24 Hours	237	100%	97%	98%
Controlled Postoperative Blood Glucose[7]	-	-	96%	97%
Perioperative Temperature Management	281	100%	100%	100%
Prophylactic Antibiotic Selection	194	98%	99%	99%
Prophylactic Antibiotic Selection (Outpatient)	88	98%	97%	98%
Prophylactic Antibiotic Stopped	189	98%	97%	98%
Prophylactic Antibiotic Timing	194	99%	98%	99%
Prophylactic Antibiotic Timing (Outpatient)	95	91%	97%	98%
Urinary Catheter Removal	169	95%	96%	97%
Survey of Patients' Hospital Experiences				
Area Around Room 'Always' Quiet at Night	300+	73%	74%	61%
Doctors 'Always' Communicated Well	300+	88%	87%	82%
Home Recovery Information Given	300+	83%	85%	85%
Hospital Given 9 or 10 on 10 Point Scale	300+	69%	75%	71%
Meds 'Always' Explained Before Given	300+	61%	69%	64%
Nurses 'Always' Communicated Well	300+	84%	83%	79%
Pain 'Always' Well Controlled	300+	75%	75%	71%
Room and Bathroom 'Always' Clean	300+	76%	75%	73%
Timely Help 'Always' Received	300+	69%	71%	68%
Would Definitely Recommend Hospital	300+	76%	75%	71%
Use of Medical Imaging				
Cardiac Imaging Stress Test before Surgery	315	5.7%	5.3%	5.3%
Combination Abdominal CT Scan	752	44.7%	24.5%	10.5%
Combination Brain/Sinus CT Scan[1]	-	-	2.6%	2.7%
Combination Chest CT Scan	441	0.2%	7.6%	2.7%
Follow-up Mammogram/Ultrasound	671	9.7%	9.4%	8.8%
Lumbar Spine MRI for Low Back Pain[7]	-	-	42.7%	37.2%

Iberia Rehabilitation Hospital

532 Jefferson Terrace Street Phone: 337-364-6923
New Iberia, LA 70560
Type: Acute Care Hospitals Emergency Services: No
Ownership: Proprietary

Measure	Cases	This Hosp.	State Avg.	U.S. Avg.
Blood Clot Prevention and Treatment				
Anticoagulation Overlap Therapy[2,3]	-	-	89%	93%
ICU Venous Thromboembolism Prophylaxis[2,3]	-	-	88%	92%
Incidence of Potentially Preventable VTE[2,3]	-	-	16%	10%
UFH with Dosages/Platelet Monitoring[2,3]	-	-	94%	97%
Venous Thromboembolism Prophylaxis[1,2]	-	-	74%	85%
Warfarin Therapy Discharge Instructions[2,3]	-	-	85%	75%
Chest Pain/Possible Heart Attack Care				
Aspirin Given Within 24 Hours of Arrival	-	-	94%	96%
Fibrinolytic Meds Within 30 Min. of Arrival	-	-	54%	58%
Average Time to ECG (minutes)	-	-	10	7
Average Time to Transfer (minutes)	-	-	94	60
Children's Asthma Care				
Received Home Management Plan of Care	-	-	-	88%
Received Reliever Medication	-	-	-	100%
Received Systemic Corticosteroids	-	-	-	100%
Emergency Department				
Admittance Decision Time (minutes)[2,3]	-	-	86	98
Head CT Results Within 45 Min. of Arrival	-	-	49%	57%
Patients Who Left ER Before Being Seen	-	-	3%	2%
Time from ER Arrival to Admit. (minutes)[2,3]	-	-	256	274
Time from ER Arrival to Discharge (minutes)	-	-	125	134
Time in ER Before Being Evaluated (minutes)	-	-	27	26
Time to Pain Meds for Fractures (minutes)	-	-	61	57
Heart Attack Care				
Aspirin Given at Discharge[5]	-	-	99%	99%
Fibrinolytic Meds Within 30 Min. of Arrival[5]	-	-	71%	54%
PCI Within 90 Minutes of Arrival[5]	-	-	94%	96%
Statin Prescribed at Discharge[5]	-	-	98%	98%
Heart Failure Care				
ACE Inhibitor or ARB for LVSD[5]	-	-	95%	97%
Discharge Instructions Given[5]	-	-	94%	94%
Evaluation of LVS Function[5]	-	-	97%	99%
Medicare Spending				
Medicare Spending per Patient (ratio)[1]	-	-	1.04	0.98
Pneumonia Care				
Appropriate Initial Antibiotic Given[5]	-	-	93%	95%
Blood Culture Timing[5]	-	-	97%	98%
Pregnancy and Delivery Care				
Newborn Deliveries Scheduled Early[2,7]	-	-	5%	6%
Preventive Care				
Immunization for Influenza[2]	11	73%	85%	90%
Immunization for Pneumonia[1,2]	-	-	88%	92%
Stroke Care				
Anticoagulation Therapy for Atrial Fibrillation[5]	-	-	93%	95%
Antithrombotic Therapy Timing[5]	-	-	96%	98%
Assessed for Rehabilitation[5]	-	-	95%	97%
Discharged on Antithrombotic Therapy[5]	-	-	97%	99%
Discharged on Statin Medication[5]	-	-	89%	94%
Thrombolytic Therapy Timing[5]	-	-	53%	66%
Venous Thromboembolism Prophylaxis[5]	-	-	87%	94%
Written Stroke Educational Materials Given[5]	-	-	83%	88%
Surgical Care Improvement Project				
Appropriate Beta Blocker Usage[5]	-	-	97%	98%
Appropriate VTP Within 24 Hours[5]	-	-	97%	98%
Controlled Postoperative Blood Glucose[5]	-	-	96%	97%
Perioperative Temperature Management[5]	-	-	100%	100%
Prophylactic Antibiotic Selection[5]	-	-	99%	99%
Prophylactic Antibiotic Selection (Outpatient)	-	-	97%	98%
Prophylactic Antibiotic Stopped[5]	-	-	97%	98%
Prophylactic Antibiotic Timing[5]	-	-	98%	99%
Prophylactic Antibiotic Timing (Outpatient)	-	-	97%	98%
Urinary Catheter Removal[5]	-	-	96%	97%
Survey of Patients' Hospital Experiences				
Area Around Room 'Always' Quiet at Night[1]	-	-	74%	61%
Doctors 'Always' Communicated Well[1]	-	-	87%	82%
Home Recovery Information Given[1]	-	-	85%	85%
Hospital Given 9 or 10 on 10 Point Scale[1]	-	-	75%	71%
Meds 'Always' Explained Before Given[1]	-	-	69%	64%
Nurses 'Always' Communicated Well[1]	-	-	83%	79%
Pain 'Always' Well Controlled[1]	-	-	75%	71%
Room and Bathroom 'Always' Clean[1]	-	-	75%	73%
Timely Help 'Always' Received[1]	-	-	71%	68%
Would Definitely Recommend Hospital[1]	-	-	75%	71%
Use of Medical Imaging				
Cardiac Imaging Stress Test before Surgery	-	-	5.3%	5.3%
Combination Abdominal CT Scan	-	-	24.5%	10.5%
Combination Brain/Sinus CT Scan	-	-	2.6%	2.7%
Combination Chest CT Scan	-	-	7.6%	2.7%
Follow-up Mammogram/Ultrasound	-	-	9.4%	8.8%
Lumbar Spine MRI for Low Back Pain	-	-	42.7%	37.2%

Charity Hospital & Medical Center of Louisiana

2021 Perdido St Phone: 504-903-3000
New Orleans, LA 70112
URL: www.lsuhospitals.org/hospitals/mclno
Type: Acute Care Hospitals Emergency Services: Yes
Ownership: Voluntary non-profit - Private Beds: 714

Key Personnel:
Chief of Medical Staff . . . . Cathi Fontenot, MD
Patient Relations . . . . Pam McVey RN MSN
CEO/President. . . . . Cindy Nuesslein, RN, MBA, FACHE

Measure	Cases	This Hosp.	State Avg.	U.S. Avg.
Blood Clot Prevention and Treatment				
Anticoagulation Overlap Therapy[2]	48	94%	89%	93%
ICU Venous Thromboembolism Prophylaxis[2]	121	96%	88%	92%
Incidence of Potentially Preventable VTE[2]	13	8%	16%	10%
UFH with Dosages/Platelet Monitoring[2]	32	97%	94%	97%
Venous Thromboembolism Prophylaxis[2]	252	83%	74%	85%
Warfarin Therapy Discharge Instructions[2]	36	86%	85%	75%
Chest Pain/Possible Heart Attack Care				
Aspirin Given Within 24 Hours of Arrival[5]	-	-	94%	96%
Fibrinolytic Meds Within 30 Min. of Arrival[5]	-	-	54%	58%
Average Time to ECG (minutes)[5]	-	-	10	7
Average Time to Transfer (minutes)[5]	-	-	94	60
Children's Asthma Care				
Received Home Management Plan of Care	-	-	-	88%
Received Reliever Medication	-	-	-	100%

NOTE: Hospital profiles are in alphabetical order by state, then city, then hospital within the city; Rankings exclude hospitals with less than 25 cases except for patient surveys which excludes hospitals with less than 100 cases; (a) 100-299 cases; (1) The number of cases/patients is too few to report; (2) Data submitted were based on a sample of cases/patients; (3) Results are based on a shorter time period than required; (4) Data suppressed by CMS for one or more quarters; (5) Results are not available for this reporting period; (6) Fewer than 100 patients completed the HCAHPS survey; (7) No cases met the criteria for this measure; (8) The lower limit of the confidence interval cannot be calculated if the number of observed infections equals zero; (9) No data are available from the state/territory for this reporting period; (10) The scores shown reflect fewer than 50 completed surveys; (11) There were discrepancies in the data collection process; (12) This measure does not apply to this hospital for this reporting period; (13) Results cannot be calculated for this reporting period; (14) The results for this state are combined with nearby states to protect confidentiality; Please refer to the User's Guide for a full explanation of data.

Measure	Cases	This Hosp.	State Avg.	U.S. Avg.
Received Systemic Corticosteroids	-	-	-	100%
Emergency Department				
Admittance Decision Time (minutes)[2]	625	293	86	98
Head CT Results Within 45 Min. of Arrival[1,3]	-	-	49%	57%
Patients Who Left ER Before Being Seen	52,517	10%	3%	2%
Time from ER Arrival to Admit. (minutes)[2]	642	654	256	274
Time from ER Arrival to Discharge (minutes)	397	375	125	134
Time in ER Before Being Evaluated (minutes)	267	117	27	26
Time to Pain Meds for Fractures (minutes)	70	97	61	57
Heart Attack Care				
Aspirin Given at Discharge	114	100%	99%	99%
Fibrinolytic Meds Within 30 Min. of Arrival[7]	-	-	71%	54%
PCI Within 90 Minutes of Arrival	13	85%	94%	96%
Statin Prescribed at Discharge	115	98%	98%	98%
Heart Failure Care				
ACE Inhibitor or ARB for LVSD	117	96%	95%	97%
Discharge Instructions Given	191	99%	94%	94%
Evaluation of LVS Function	198	98%	97%	99%
Medicare Spending				
Medicare Spending per Patient (ratio)	-	0.94	1.04	0.98
Pneumonia Care				
Appropriate Initial Antibiotic Given	38	95%	93%	95%
Blood Culture Timing	114	94%	97%	98%
Pregnancy and Delivery Care				
Newborn Deliveries Scheduled Early[7]	-	-	5%	6%
Preventive Care				
Immunization for Influenza[2]	619	54%	85%	90%
Immunization for Pneumonia[2]	480	58%	88%	92%
Stroke Care				
Anticoagulation Therapy for Atrial Fibrillation[1]	-	-	93%	95%
Antithrombotic Therapy Timing	67	97%	96%	98%
Assessed for Rehabilitation	116	99%	95%	97%
Discharged on Antithrombotic Therapy	98	98%	97%	99%
Discharged on Statin Medication	81	99%	89%	94%
Thrombolytic Therapy Timing	16	88%	53%	66%
Venous Thromboembolism Prophylaxis	110	95%	87%	94%
Written Stroke Educational Materials Given	80	89%	83%	88%
Surgical Care Improvement Project				
Appropriate Beta Blocker Usage[2]	164	96%	97%	98%
Appropriate VTP Within 24 Hours[2]	360	98%	97%	98%
Controlled Postoperative Blood Glucose[2]	144	83%	96%	97%
Perioperative Temperature Management[2]	469	100%	100%	100%
Prophylactic Antibiotic Selection[2]	363	98%	99%	99%
Prophylactic Antibiotic Selection (Outpatient)	265	95%	97%	98%
Prophylactic Antibiotic Stopped[2]	347	98%	97%	98%
Prophylactic Antibiotic Timing[2]	370	94%	98%	99%
Prophylactic Antibiotic Timing (Outpatient)	189	85%	97%	98%
Urinary Catheter Removal[2]	279	92%	96%	97%
Survey of Patients' Hospital Experiences				
Area Around Room 'Always' Quiet at Night	300+	61%	74%	61%
Doctors 'Always' Communicated Well	300+	80%	87%	82%
Home Recovery Information Given	300+	80%	85%	85%
Hospital Given 9 or 10 on 10 Point Scale	300+	57%	75%	71%
Meds 'Always' Explained Before Given	300+	59%	69%	64%
Nurses 'Always' Communicated Well	300+	70%	83%	79%
Pain 'Always' Well Controlled	300+	63%	75%	71%
Room and Bathroom 'Always' Clean	300+	58%	75%	73%
Timely Help 'Always' Received	300+	49%	71%	68%
Would Definitely Recommend Hospital	300+	61%	75%	71%
Use of Medical Imaging				
Cardiac Imaging Stress Test before Surgery	92	5.4%	5.3%	5.3%
Combination Abdominal CT Scan	239	10.9%	24.5%	10.5%
Combination Brain/Sinus CT Scan[1]	-	-	2.6%	2.7%
Combination Chest CT Scan	172	1.2%	7.6%	2.7%
Follow-up Mammogram/Ultrasound	344	6.4%	9.4%	8.8%
Lumbar Spine MRI for Low Back Pain[1]	-	-	42.7%	37.2%

Ochsner Medical Center

1516 Jefferson Hwy
New Orleans, LA 70121
Phone: 504-842-3000
Fax: 504-842-5856
URL: www.ochsner.org
Type: Acute Care Hospitals
Emergency Services: Yes
Ownership: Voluntary non-profit - Private
Beds: 460

Key Personnel:
Pediatric Ambulatory Care . . . . . . Connie Bellone
Chief of Medical Staff . . . . Joseph E. Bisordi, MD, FACP
Cardiac Laboratory. . . . . Mark French
Coronary Care . . . . Mark French
Infection Control . . . . Eric McMillen
Radiology. . . . . Eric McMillen
CEO/President . . . . Warner L. Thomas, MD
Operating Room. . . . . Paul Waguespack

Measure	Cases	This Hosp.	State Avg.	U.S. Avg.
Blood Clot Prevention and Treatment				
Anticoagulation Overlap Therapy[2]	195	87%	89%	93%
ICU Venous Thromboembolism Prophylaxis[2]	69	87%	88%	92%
Incidence of Potentially Preventable VTE[2]	48	19%	16%	10%
UFH with Dosages/Platelet Monitoring[2]	51	49%	94%	97%
Venous Thromboembolism Prophylaxis[2]	347	73%	74%	85%
Warfarin Therapy Discharge Instructions[2]	156	85%	85%	75%
Chest Pain/Possible Heart Attack Care				
Aspirin Given Within 24 Hours of Arrival[1,3]	-	-	94%	96%
Fibrinolytic Meds Within 30 Min. of Arrival[5]	-	-	54%	58%
Average Time to ECG (minutes)[1,3]	-	-	10	7
Average Time to Transfer (minutes)[5]	-	-	94	60
Children's Asthma Care				
Received Home Management Plan of Care	-	-	-	88%
Received Reliever Medication	-	-	-	100%
Received Systemic Corticosteroids	-	-	-	100%
Emergency Department				
Admittance Decision Time (minutes)[2]	558	144	86	98
Head CT Results Within 45 Min. of Arrival[1]	-	-	49%	57%
Patients Who Left ER Before Being Seen	>100k	4%	3%	2%
Time from ER Arrival to Admit. (minutes)[2]	587	417	256	274
Time from ER Arrival to Discharge (minutes)	354	165	125	134
Time in ER Before Being Evaluated (minutes)	350	43	27	26
Time to Pain Meds for Fractures (minutes)	352	80	61	57
Heart Attack Care				
Aspirin Given at Discharge[2]	323	99%	99%	99%
Fibrinolytic Meds Within 30 Min. of Arrival[2,7]	-	-	71%	54%
PCI Within 90 Minutes of Arrival[2]	36	92%	94%	96%
Statin Prescribed at Discharge[2]	314	98%	98%	98%
Heart Failure Care				
ACE Inhibitor or ARB for LVSD[2]	145	88%	95%	97%
Discharge Instructions Given[2]	293	97%	94%	94%
Evaluation of LVS Function[2]	328	99%	97%	99%
Medicare Spending				
Medicare Spending per Patient (ratio)	-	0.95	1.04	0.98
Pneumonia Care				
Appropriate Initial Antibiotic Given[2]	68	96%	93%	95%
Blood Culture Timing[2]	191	93%	97%	98%
Pregnancy and Delivery Care				
Newborn Deliveries Scheduled Early[2]	53	4%	5%	6%
Preventive Care				
Immunization for Influenza[2]	720	69%	85%	90%
Immunization for Pneumonia[2]	776	72%	88%	92%
Stroke Care				
Anticoagulation Therapy for Atrial Fibrillation[2]	34	94%	93%	95%
Antithrombotic Therapy Timing[2]	154	96%	96%	98%
Assessed for Rehabilitation[2]	265	100%	95%	97%
Discharged on Antithrombotic Therapy[2]	226	96%	97%	99%
Discharged on Statin Medication[2]	183	95%	89%	94%
Thrombolytic Therapy Timing[2]	16	88%	53%	66%
Venous Thromboembolism Prophylaxis[2]	257	77%	87%	94%
Written Stroke Educational Materials Given[2]	181	100%	83%	88%
Surgical Care Improvement Project				
Appropriate Beta Blocker Usage[2]	210	99%	97%	98%
Appropriate VTP Within 24 Hours[2]	418	95%	97%	98%
Controlled Postoperative Blood Glucose[2]	122	95%	96%	97%
Perioperative Temperature Management[2]	591	100%	100%	100%
Prophylactic Antibiotic Selection[2]	404	99%	99%	99%
Prophylactic Antibiotic Selection (Outpatient)	676	96%	97%	98%
Prophylactic Antibiotic Stopped[2]	394	95%	97%	98%
Prophylactic Antibiotic Timing[2]	406	96%	98%	99%
Prophylactic Antibiotic Timing (Outpatient)	600	93%	97%	98%
Urinary Catheter Removal[2]	355	93%	96%	97%
Survey of Patients' Hospital Experiences				
Area Around Room 'Always' Quiet at Night	300+	60%	74%	61%
Doctors 'Always' Communicated Well	300+	79%	87%	82%
Home Recovery Information Given	300+	83%	85%	85%
Hospital Given 9 or 10 on 10 Point Scale	300+	65%	75%	71%
Meds 'Always' Explained Before Given	300+	59%	69%	64%
Nurses 'Always' Communicated Well	300+	75%	83%	79%
Pain 'Always' Well Controlled	300+	64%	75%	71%
Room and Bathroom 'Always' Clean	300+	60%	75%	73%
Timely Help 'Always' Received	300+	56%	71%	68%
Would Definitely Recommend Hospital	300+	70%	75%	71%
Use of Medical Imaging				
Cardiac Imaging Stress Test before Surgery	614	7.0%	5.3%	5.3%
Combination Abdominal CT Scan	1,869	13.8%	24.5%	10.5%
Combination Brain/Sinus CT Scan	1,279	2.2%	2.6%	2.7%
Combination Chest CT Scan	1,346	0.0%	7.6%	2.7%
Follow-up Mammogram/Ultrasound	3,124	6.1%	9.4%	8.8%
Lumbar Spine MRI for Low Back Pain	248	48.4%	42.7%	37.2%

Touro Infirmary

1401 Foucher Street
New Orleans, LA 70115
Phone: 504-897-7011
Fax: 504-897-8106
E-mail: rhodesd@touro.com
URL: www.touro.com
Type: Acute Care Hospitals
Emergency Services: Yes
Ownership: Voluntary non-profit - Private
Beds: 465

Key Personnel:
Pediatric Ambulatory Care . . . . . . Dianne Albrecht, MD
Pediatric In-Patient Care . . . . Dianne Albrecht, MD
Chief of Medical Staff . . . . Sal Caputto, MD
Quality Assurance . . . . Marie Everitt
Radiology. . . . . Robert Karl, MD
CEO/President . . . . James T. Montgomery
Coronary Care . . . . Judy Mysing
Infection Control . . . . Carol Scioneaux

Measure	Cases	This Hosp.	State Avg.	U.S. Avg.
Blood Clot Prevention and Treatment				
Anticoagulation Overlap Therapy[2]	56	98%	89%	93%
ICU Venous Thromboembolism Prophylaxis[2]	117	98%	88%	92%
Incidence of Potentially Preventable VTE[2]	22	9%	16%	10%
UFH with Dosages/Platelet Monitoring[2]	23	100%	94%	97%
Venous Thromboembolism Prophylaxis[2]	305	94%	74%	85%
Warfarin Therapy Discharge Instructions[2]	37	100%	85%	75%
Chest Pain/Possible Heart Attack Care				
Aspirin Given Within 24 Hours of Arrival[5]	-	-	94%	96%
Fibrinolytic Meds Within 30 Min. of Arrival[5]	-	-	54%	58%
Average Time to ECG (minutes)[5]	-	-	10	7
Average Time to Transfer (minutes)[5]	-	-	94	60
Children's Asthma Care				
Received Home Management Plan of Care	-	-	-	88%
Received Reliever Medication	-	-	-	100%
Received Systemic Corticosteroids	-	-	-	100%
Emergency Department				
Admittance Decision Time (minutes)[2]	380	104	86	98
Head CT Results Within 45 Min. of Arrival[1]	-	-	49%	57%
Patients Who Left ER Before Being Seen	33,561	5%	3%	2%
Time from ER Arrival to Admit. (minutes)[2]	384	301	256	274
Time from ER Arrival to Discharge (minutes)	394	166	125	134
Time in ER Before Being Evaluated (minutes)	417	30	27	26
Time to Pain Meds for Fractures (minutes)	55	50	61	57
Heart Attack Care				
Aspirin Given at Discharge	112	97%	99%	99%
Fibrinolytic Meds Within 30 Min. of Arrival[7]	-	-	71%	54%
PCI Within 90 Minutes of Arrival	18	94%	94%	96%
Statin Prescribed at Discharge	109	98%	98%	98%
Heart Failure Care				
ACE Inhibitor or ARB for LVSD	192	97%	95%	97%
Discharge Instructions Given	320	84%	94%	94%
Evaluation of LVS Function	380	99%	97%	99%

NOTE: Hospital profiles are in alphabetical order by state, then city, then hospital within the city; Rankings exclude hospitals with less than 25 cases except for patient surveys which excludes hospitals with less than 100 cases; (a) 100-299 cases; (1) The number of cases/patients is too few to report; (2) Data submitted were based on a sample of cases/patients; (3) Results are based on a shorter time period than required; (4) Data suppressed by CMS for one or more quarters; (5) Results are not available for this reporting period; (6) Fewer than 100 patients completed the HCAHPS survey; (7) No cases met the criteria for this measure; (8) The lower limit of the confidence interval cannot be calculated if the number of observed infections equals zero; (9) No data are available from the state/territory for this reporting period; (10) The scores shown reflect fewer than 50 completed surveys; (11) There were discrepancies in the data collection process; (12) This measure does not apply to this hospital for this reporting period; (13) Results cannot be calculated for this reporting period; (14) The results for this state are combined with nearby states to protect confidentiality; Please refer to the User's Guide for a full explanation of data.

Measure	Cases	This Hosp.	State Avg.	U.S. Avg.
Medicare Spending				
Medicare Spending per Patient (ratio)	-	1.03	1.04	0.98
Pneumonia Care				
Appropriate Initial Antibiotic Given	81	98%	93%	95%
Blood Culture Timing	240	98%	97%	98%
Pregnancy and Delivery Care				
Newborn Deliveries Scheduled Early[2]	57	0%	5%	6%
Preventive Care				
Immunization for Influenza[2]	508	98%	85%	90%
Immunization for Pneumonia[2]	502	95%	88%	92%
Stroke Care				
Anticoagulation Therapy for Atrial Fibrillation	14	100%	93%	95%
Antithrombotic Therapy Timing	88	100%	96%	98%
Assessed for Rehabilitation	100	99%	95%	97%
Discharged on Antithrombotic Therapy	96	98%	97%	99%
Discharged on Statin Medication	67	93%	89%	94%
Thrombolytic Therapy Timing[1]	-	-	53%	66%
Venous Thromboembolism Prophylaxis	95	99%	87%	94%
Written Stroke Educational Materials Given	65	85%	83%	88%
Surgical Care Improvement Project				
Appropriate Beta Blocker Usage[2]	228	96%	97%	98%
Appropriate VTP Within 24 Hours[2]	635	99%	97%	98%
Controlled Postoperative Blood Glucose[2]	65	98%	96%	97%
Perioperative Temperature Management[2]	735	100%	100%	100%
Prophylactic Antibiotic Selection[2]	627	100%	99%	99%
Prophylactic Antibiotic Selection (Outpatient)	347	99%	97%	98%
Prophylactic Antibiotic Stopped[2]	620	97%	97%	98%
Prophylactic Antibiotic Timing[2]	628	100%	98%	99%
Prophylactic Antibiotic Timing (Outpatient)	346	100%	97%	98%
Urinary Catheter Removal[2]	586	98%	96%	97%
Survey of Patients' Hospital Experiences				
Area Around Room 'Always' Quiet at Night	300+	67%	74%	61%
Doctors 'Always' Communicated Well	300+	84%	87%	82%
Home Recovery Information Given	300+	87%	85%	85%
Hospital Given 9 or 10 on 10 Point Scale	300+	72%	75%	71%
Meds 'Always' Explained Before Given	300+	61%	69%	64%
Nurses 'Always' Communicated Well	300+	78%	83%	79%
Pain 'Always' Well Controlled	300+	69%	75%	71%
Room and Bathroom 'Always' Clean	300+	64%	75%	73%
Timely Help 'Always' Received	300+	59%	71%	68%
Would Definitely Recommend Hospital	300+	70%	75%	71%
Use of Medical Imaging				
Cardiac Imaging Stress Test before Surgery	320	5.0%	5.3%	5.3%
Combination Abdominal CT Scan	536	20.7%	24.5%	10.5%
Combination Brain/Sinus CT Scan[1]	-	-	2.6%	2.7%
Combination Chest CT Scan	423	10.6%	7.6%	2.7%
Follow-up Mammogram/Ultrasound	939	6.3%	9.4%	8.8%
Lumbar Spine MRI for Low Back Pain	75	41.3%	42.7%	37.2%

Tulane Medical Center

1415 Tulane Ave
New Orleans, LA 70112
Phone: 504-988-1900
Fax: 504-988-6077
URL: www.tuhc.com
Type: Acute Care Hospitals
Emergency Services: Yes
Ownership: Proprietary
Beds: 341

Key Personnel:

Cardiac Laboratory. . . . . Patricie Delafontaine
Anesthesiology. . . . . Melissa Guidry
Operating Room. . . . . Daryl Miller
Hemotology Center . . . . Vicki Miller
CEO/President. . . . . Jim Montgomery
Radiology. . . . . Abraham Morris
Pediatric In-Patient Care . . . . . . Nancy Schryer
Emergency Room . . . . Tom Serviss

Measure	Cases	This Hosp.	State Avg.	U.S. Avg.
Blood Clot Prevention and Treatment				
Anticoagulation Overlap Therapy[2]	75	99%	89%	93%
ICU Venous Thromboembolism Prophylaxis[2]	208	100%	88%	92%
Incidence of Potentially Preventable VTE[2]	41	0%	16%	10%
UFH with Dosages/Platelet Monitoring[2]	67	100%	94%	97%
Venous Thromboembolism Prophylaxis[2]	247	99%	74%	85%
Warfarin Therapy Discharge Instructions[2]	49	98%	85%	75%
Chest Pain/Possible Heart Attack Care				
Aspirin Given Within 24 Hours of Arrival[5]	-	-	94%	96%
Fibrinolytic Meds Within 30 Min. of Arrival[5]	-	-	54%	58%
Average Time to ECG (minutes)[5]	-	-	10	7
Average Time to Transfer (minutes)[5]	-	-	94	60
Children's Asthma Care				
Received Home Management Plan of Care	-	-	-	88%
Received Reliever Medication	-	-	-	100%
Received Systemic Corticosteroids	-	-	-	100%
Emergency Department				
Admittance Decision Time (minutes)[2]	644	132	86	98
Head CT Results Within 45 Min. of Arrival[3,7]	-	-	49%	57%
Patients Who Left ER Before Being Seen	65,582	1%	3%	2%
Time from ER Arrival to Admit. (minutes)[2]	644	402	256	274
Time from ER Arrival to Discharge (minutes)	509	172	125	134
Time in ER Before Being Evaluated (minutes)	568	15	27	26
Time to Pain Meds for Fractures (minutes)	184	70	61	57
Heart Attack Care				
Aspirin Given at Discharge	206	100%	99%	99%
Fibrinolytic Meds Within 30 Min. of Arrival[7]	-	-	71%	54%
PCI Within 90 Minutes of Arrival	52	92%	94%	96%
Statin Prescribed at Discharge	205	100%	98%	98%
Heart Failure Care				
ACE Inhibitor or ARB for LVSD	204	100%	95%	97%
Discharge Instructions Given	316	95%	94%	94%
Evaluation of LVS Function	336	100%	97%	99%
Medicare Spending				
Medicare Spending per Patient (ratio)	-	0.91	1.04	0.98
Pneumonia Care				
Appropriate Initial Antibiotic Given	51	98%	93%	95%
Blood Culture Timing	137	98%	97%	98%
Pregnancy and Delivery Care				
Newborn Deliveries Scheduled Early[2]	45	2%	5%	6%
Preventive Care				
Immunization for Influenza[2]	598	100%	85%	90%
Immunization for Pneumonia[2]	574	99%	88%	92%
Stroke Care				
Anticoagulation Therapy for Atrial Fibrillation[2]	15	100%	93%	95%
Antithrombotic Therapy Timing[2]	78	99%	96%	98%
Assessed for Rehabilitation[2]	132	99%	95%	97%
Discharged on Antithrombotic Therapy[2]	114	100%	97%	99%
Discharged on Statin Medication[2]	83	100%	89%	94%
Thrombolytic Therapy Timing[2]	23	100%	53%	66%
Venous Thromboembolism Prophylaxis[2]	134	100%	87%	94%
Written Stroke Educational Materials Given[2]	76	93%	83%	88%
Surgical Care Improvement Project				
Appropriate Beta Blocker Usage[2]	147	100%	97%	98%
Appropriate VTP Within 24 Hours[2]	340	99%	97%	98%
Controlled Postoperative Blood Glucose[2]	47	100%	96%	97%
Perioperative Temperature Management[2]	426	100%	100%	100%
Prophylactic Antibiotic Selection[2]	257	100%	99%	99%
Prophylactic Antibiotic Selection (Outpatient)	389	99%	97%	98%
Prophylactic Antibiotic Stopped[2]	251	98%	97%	98%
Prophylactic Antibiotic Timing[2]	257	100%	98%	99%
Prophylactic Antibiotic Timing (Outpatient)	282	99%	97%	98%
Urinary Catheter Removal[2]	253	100%	96%	97%
Survey of Patients' Hospital Experiences				
Area Around Room 'Always' Quiet at Night	300+	63%	74%	61%
Doctors 'Always' Communicated Well	300+	83%	87%	82%
Home Recovery Information Given	300+	85%	85%	85%
Hospital Given 9 or 10 on 10 Point Scale	300+	69%	75%	71%
Meds 'Always' Explained Before Given	300+	64%	69%	64%
Nurses 'Always' Communicated Well	300+	77%	83%	79%
Pain 'Always' Well Controlled	300+	70%	75%	71%
Room and Bathroom 'Always' Clean	300+	63%	75%	73%
Timely Help 'Always' Received	300+	63%	71%	68%
Would Definitely Recommend Hospital	300+	68%	75%	71%
Use of Medical Imaging				
Cardiac Imaging Stress Test before Surgery	182	8.8%	5.3%	5.3%
Combination Abdominal CT Scan	450	30.9%	24.5%	10.5%
Combination Brain/Sinus CT Scan[1]	-	-	2.6%	2.7%
Combination Chest CT Scan	286	8.0%	7.6%	2.7%
Follow-up Mammogram/Ultrasound	516	13.8%	9.4%	8.8%
Lumbar Spine MRI for Low Back Pain[1]	-	-	42.7%	37.2%

Pointe Coupee General Hospital

2202 False River Drive
New Roads, LA 70760
Phone: 225-638-6331
Fax: 225-638-5785
URL: www.pcgh.org
Type: Critical Access Hospitals
Emergency Services: Yes
Ownership: Govt - Hospital Dist/Auth
Beds: 45

Key Personnel:

Infection Control. . . . . Traci Achad
Quality Assurance . . . . Maggie Jarreau
Chairman/CEO . . . . Carl McLemore, MD
CEO . . . . Chad Olinde, CPA, MBA
CEO/President. . . . . Chad Olinde
Chief of Medical Staff . . . . Paul Rachal, MD

Measure	Cases	This Hosp.	State Avg.	U.S. Avg.
Blood Clot Prevention and Treatment				
Anticoagulation Overlap Therapy[5]	-	-	89%	93%
ICU Venous Thromboembolism Prophylaxis[5]	-	-	88%	92%
Incidence of Potentially Preventable VTE[5]	-	-	16%	10%
UFH with Dosages/Platelet Monitoring[5]	-	-	94%	97%
Venous Thromboembolism Prophylaxis[5]	-	-	74%	85%
Warfarin Therapy Discharge Instructions[5]	-	-	85%	75%
Chest Pain/Possible Heart Attack Care				
Aspirin Given Within 24 Hours of Arrival[5]	-	-	94%	96%
Fibrinolytic Meds Within 30 Min. of Arrival[5]	-	-	54%	58%
Average Time to ECG (minutes)[5]	-	-	10	7
Average Time to Transfer (minutes)[5]	-	-	94	60
Children's Asthma Care				
Received Home Management Plan of Care	-	-	-	88%
Received Reliever Medication	-	-	-	100%
Received Systemic Corticosteroids	-	-	-	100%
Emergency Department				
Admittance Decision Time (minutes)[5]	-	-	86	98
Head CT Results Within 45 Min. of Arrival[5]	-	-	49%	57%
Patients Who Left ER Before Being Seen[5]	-	-	3%	2%
Time from ER Arrival to Admit. (minutes)[5]	-	-	256	274
Time from ER Arrival to Discharge (minutes)[5]	-	-	125	134
Time in ER Before Being Evaluated (minutes)[5]	-	-	27	26
Time to Pain Meds for Fractures (minutes)[5]	-	-	61	57
Heart Attack Care				
Aspirin Given at Discharge[5]	-	-	99%	99%
Fibrinolytic Meds Within 30 Min. of Arrival[5]	-	-	71%	54%
PCI Within 90 Minutes of Arrival[5]	-	-	94%	96%
Statin Prescribed at Discharge[5]	-	-	98%	98%
Heart Failure Care				
ACE Inhibitor or ARB for LVSD	14	100%	95%	97%
Discharge Instructions Given	24	100%	94%	94%
Evaluation of LVS Function	36	100%	97%	99%
Medicare Spending				
Medicare Spending per Patient (ratio)	-	-	1.04	0.98
Pneumonia Care				
Appropriate Initial Antibiotic Given	18	100%	93%	95%
Blood Culture Timing	25	100%	97%	98%
Pregnancy and Delivery Care				
Newborn Deliveries Scheduled Early[5]	-	-	5%	6%
Preventive Care				
Immunization for Influenza[5]	-	-	85%	90%
Immunization for Pneumonia[5]	-	-	88%	92%
Stroke Care				
Anticoagulation Therapy for Atrial Fibrillation[5]	-	-	93%	95%
Antithrombotic Therapy Timing[5]	-	-	96%	98%
Assessed for Rehabilitation[5]	-	-	95%	97%
Discharged on Antithrombotic Therapy[5]	-	-	97%	99%
Discharged on Statin Medication[5]	-	-	89%	94%
Thrombolytic Therapy Timing[5]	-	-	53%	66%
Venous Thromboembolism Prophylaxis[5]	-	-	87%	94%
Written Stroke Educational Materials Given[5]	-	-	83%	88%
Surgical Care Improvement Project				
Appropriate Beta Blocker Usage[5]	-	-	97%	98%
Appropriate VTP Within 24 Hours[5]	-	-	97%	98%
Controlled Postoperative Blood Glucose[5]	-	-	96%	97%
Perioperative Temperature Management[5]	-	-	100%	100%
Prophylactic Antibiotic Selection[5]	-	-	99%	99%
Prophylactic Antibiotic Selection (Outpatient)[5]	-	-	97%	98%
Prophylactic Antibiotic Stopped[5]	-	-	97%	98%

NOTE: Hospital profiles are in alphabetical order by state, then city, then hospital within the city; Rankings exclude hospitals with less than 25 cases except for patient surveys which excludes hospitals with less than 100 cases; (a) 100-299 cases; (1) The number of cases/patients is too few to report; (2) Data submitted were based on a sample of cases/patients; (3) Results are based on a shorter time period than required; (4) Data suppressed by CMS for one or more quarters; (5) Results are not available for this reporting period; (6) Fewer than 100 patients completed the HCAHPS survey; (7) No cases met the criteria for this measure; (8) The lower limit of the confidence interval cannot be calculated if the number of observed infections equals zero; (9) No data are available from the state/territory for this reporting period; (10) The scores shown reflect fewer than 50 completed surveys; (11) There were discrepancies in the data collection process; (12) This measure does not apply to this hospital for this reporting period; (13) Results cannot be calculated for this reporting period; (14) The results for this state are combined with nearby states to protect confidentiality; Please refer to the User's Guide for a full explanation of data.

Prophylactic Antibiotic Timing[5]	-	-	98%	99%
Prophylactic Antibiotic Timing (Outpatient)[5]	-	-	97%	98%
Urinary Catheter Removal[5]	-	-	96%	97%
Survey of Patients' Hospital Experiences				
Area Around Room 'Always' Quiet at Night[5]	-	-	74%	61%
Doctors 'Always' Communicated Well[5]	-	-	87%	82%
Home Recovery Information Given[5]	-	-	85%	85%
Hospital Given 9 or 10 on 10 Point Scale[5]	-	-	75%	71%
Meds 'Always' Explained Before Given[5]	-	-	69%	64%
Nurses 'Always' Communicated Well[5]	-	-	83%	79%
Pain 'Always' Well Controlled[5]	-	-	75%	71%
Room and Bathroom 'Always' Clean[5]	-	-	75%	73%
Timely Help 'Always' Received[5]	-	-	71%	68%
Would Definitely Recommend Hospital[5]	-	-	75%	71%
Use of Medical Imaging				
Cardiac Imaging Stress Test before Surgery[5]	-	-	5.3%	5.3%
Combination Abdominal CT Scan[5]	-	-	24.5%	10.5%
Combination Brain/Sinus CT Scan[5]	-	-	2.6%	2.7%
Combination Chest CT Scan[5]	-	-	7.6%	2.7%
Follow-up Mammogram/Ultrasound[5]	-	-	9.4%	8.8%
Lumbar Spine MRI for Low Back Pain[5]	-	-	42.7%	37.2%

West Carroll Memorial Hospital

706 Ross Street
Oak Grove, LA 71263
Phone: 318-428-3237
Fax: 318-428-6180
Type: Acute Care Hospitals
Emergency Services: Yes
Ownership: Proprietary
Beds: 29

Key Personnel:

Patient Relations . . . . Diane Ainsworth
CEO/President. . . . . Randall Morris

Measure	Cases	This Hosp.	State Avg.	U.S. Avg.
Blood Clot Prevention and Treatment				
Anticoagulation Overlap Therapy[1,2]	-	-	89%	93%
ICU Venous Thromboembolism Prophylaxis[2,7]	-	-	88%	92%
Incidence of Potentially Preventable VTE[2,7]	-	-	16%	10%
UFH with Dosages/Platelet Monitoring[2,7]	-	-	94%	97%
Venous Thromboembolism Prophylaxis[2]	410	9%	74%	85%
Warfarin Therapy Discharge Instructions[1,2]	-	-	85%	75%
Chest Pain/Possible Heart Attack Care				
Aspirin Given Within 24 Hours of Arrival	27	93%	94%	96%
Fibrinolytic Meds Within 30 Min. of Arrival[1]	-	-	54%	58%
Average Time to ECG (minutes)	27	51	10	7
Average Time to Transfer (minutes)[1]	-	-	94	60
Children's Asthma Care				
Received Home Management Plan of Care	-	-	-	88%
Received Reliever Medication	-	-	-	100%
Received Systemic Corticosteroids	-	-	-	100%
Emergency Department				
Admittance Decision Time (minutes)[2,3]	360	0	86	98
Head CT Results Within 45 Min. of Arrival[1]	-	-	49%	57%
Patients Who Left ER Before Being Seen	5,065	1%	3%	2%
Time from ER Arrival to Admit. (minutes)[2,3]	485	205	256	274
Time from ER Arrival to Discharge (minutes)	770	133	125	134
Time in ER Before Being Evaluated (minutes)	863	25	27	26
Time to Pain Meds for Fractures (minutes)	22	78	61	57
Heart Attack Care				
Aspirin Given at Discharge[1,3]	-	-	99%	99%
Fibrinolytic Meds Within 30 Min. of Arrival[3,7]	-	-	71%	54%
PCI Within 90 Minutes of Arrival[3,7]	-	-	94%	96%
Statin Prescribed at Discharge[1,3]	-	-	98%	98%
Heart Failure Care				
ACE Inhibitor or ARB for LVSD[3,7]	-	-	95%	97%
Discharge Instructions Given[3]	22	73%	94%	94%
Evaluation of LVS Function[3]	31	3%	97%	99%
Medicare Spending				
Medicare Spending per Patient (ratio)	-	0.98	1.04	0.98
Pneumonia Care				
Appropriate Initial Antibiotic Given[2,3]	53	64%	93%	95%
Blood Culture Timing[1,2]	-	-	97%	98%
Pregnancy and Delivery Care				
Newborn Deliveries Scheduled Early[7]	-	-	5%	6%
Preventive Care				
Immunization for Influenza[2,3]	209	68%	85%	90%
Immunization for Pneumonia[2,3]	309	50%	88%	92%
Stroke Care				
Anticoagulation Therapy for Atrial Fibrillation[1]	-	-	93%	95%
Antithrombotic Therapy Timing[1]	-	-	96%	98%
Assessed for Rehabilitation[1]	-	-	95%	97%
Discharged on Antithrombotic Therapy[1]	-	-	97%	99%
Discharged on Statin Medication[1]	-	-	89%	94%
Thrombolytic Therapy Timing[1]	-	-	53%	66%
Venous Thromboembolism Prophylaxis[1]	-	-	87%	94%
Written Stroke Educational Materials Given[1]	-	-	83%	88%
Surgical Care Improvement Project				
Appropriate Beta Blocker Usage[5]	-	-	97%	98%
Appropriate VTP Within 24 Hours[5]	-	-	97%	98%
Controlled Postoperative Blood Glucose[5]	-	-	96%	97%
Perioperative Temperature Management[5]	-	-	100%	100%
Prophylactic Antibiotic Selection[5]	-	-	99%	99%
Prophylactic Antibiotic Selection (Outpatient)[5]	-	-	97%	98%
Prophylactic Antibiotic Stopped[5]	-	-	97%	98%
Prophylactic Antibiotic Timing[5]	-	-	98%	99%
Prophylactic Antibiotic Timing (Outpatient)[5]	-	-	97%	98%
Urinary Catheter Removal[5]	-	-	96%	97%
Survey of Patients' Hospital Experiences				
Area Around Room 'Always' Quiet at Night	(a)	65%	74%	61%
Doctors 'Always' Communicated Well	(a)	92%	87%	82%
Home Recovery Information Given	(a)	83%	85%	85%
Hospital Given 9 or 10 on 10 Point Scale	(a)	71%	75%	71%
Meds 'Always' Explained Before Given	(a)	70%	69%	64%
Nurses 'Always' Communicated Well	(a)	82%	83%	79%
Pain 'Always' Well Controlled	(a)	78%	75%	71%
Room and Bathroom 'Always' Clean	(a)	69%	75%	73%
Timely Help 'Always' Received	(a)	77%	71%	68%
Would Definitely Recommend Hospital	(a)	64%	75%	71%
Use of Medical Imaging				
Cardiac Imaging Stress Test before Surgery[7]	-	-	5.3%	5.3%
Combination Abdominal CT Scan	96	35.4%	24.5%	10.5%
Combination Brain/Sinus CT Scan	167	1.2%	2.6%	2.7%
Combination Chest CT Scan	63	36.5%	7.6%	2.7%
Follow-up Mammogram/Ultrasound	185	9.2%	9.4%	8.8%
Lumbar Spine MRI for Low Back Pain[7]	-	-	42.7%	37.2%

Oakdale Community Hospital

130 N Hospital Dr
Oakdale, LA 71463
Phone: 318-335-3700
Fax: 318-215-3024
URL: www.oakdalecommunityhospital.com
Type: Acute Care Hospitals
Emergency Services: Yes
Ownership: Proprietary
Beds: 60

Key Personnel:

Emergency Room . . . . Joshua Burton
Infection Control. . . . . Paula Carter, RN
Operating Room. . . . . Paula Carter
Pediatric Ambulatory Care . . . . . . MR Ghanta, MD
Pediatric In-Patient Care . . . . MR Ghanta, MD
CEO/President. . . . . John W Stigall
Quality Assurance . . . . Melissa Welch
Intensive Care Unit. . . . . Anette Wyble

Measure	Cases	This Hosp.	State Avg.	U.S. Avg.
Blood Clot Prevention and Treatment				
Anticoagulation Overlap Therapy[1,2]	-	-	89%	93%
ICU Venous Thromboembolism Prophylaxis[2]	13	54%	88%	92%
Incidence of Potentially Preventable VTE[2,7]	-	-	16%	10%
UFH with Dosages/Platelet Monitoring[1,2]	-	-	94%	97%
Venous Thromboembolism Prophylaxis[2]	108	47%	74%	85%
Warfarin Therapy Discharge Instructions[1,2]	-	-	85%	75%
Chest Pain/Possible Heart Attack Care				
Aspirin Given Within 24 Hours of Arrival	50	100%	94%	96%
Fibrinolytic Meds Within 30 Min. of Arrival[1,3]	-	-	54%	58%
Average Time to ECG (minutes)	52	10	10	7
Average Time to Transfer (minutes)[1,3]	-	-	94	60
Children's Asthma Care				
Received Home Management Plan of Care	-	-	-	88%
Received Reliever Medication	-	-	-	100%
Received Systemic Corticosteroids	-	-	-	100%
Emergency Department				
Admittance Decision Time (minutes)[2]	347	55	86	98
Head CT Results Within 45 Min. of Arrival[1,3]	-	-	49%	57%
Patients Who Left ER Before Being Seen	9,585	3%	3%	2%
Time from ER Arrival to Admit. (minutes)[2]	349	225	256	274
Time from ER Arrival to Discharge (minutes)	351	88	125	134
Time in ER Before Being Evaluated (minutes)	379	18	27	26
Time to Pain Meds for Fractures (minutes)	60	48	61	57
Heart Attack Care				
Aspirin Given at Discharge[3,7]	-	-	99%	99%
Fibrinolytic Meds Within 30 Min. of Arrival[3,7]	-	-	71%	54%
PCI Within 90 Minutes of Arrival[3,7]	-	-	94%	96%
Statin Prescribed at Discharge[3,7]	-	-	98%	98%
Heart Failure Care				
ACE Inhibitor or ARB for LVSD	15	93%	95%	97%
Discharge Instructions Given	33	91%	94%	94%
Evaluation of LVS Function	47	94%	97%	99%
Medicare Spending				
Medicare Spending per Patient (ratio)	-	0.98	1.04	0.98
Pneumonia Care				
Appropriate Initial Antibiotic Given[1]	-	-	93%	95%
Blood Culture Timing	43	98%	97%	98%
Pregnancy and Delivery Care				
Newborn Deliveries Scheduled Early[7]	-	-	5%	6%
Preventive Care				
Immunization for Influenza[2]	293	80%	85%	90%
Immunization for Pneumonia[2]	445	88%	88%	92%
Stroke Care				
Anticoagulation Therapy for Atrial Fibrillation[3,7]	-	-	93%	95%
Antithrombotic Therapy Timing[1,3]	-	-	96%	98%
Assessed for Rehabilitation[1,3]	-	-	95%	97%
Discharged on Antithrombotic Therapy[1,3]	-	-	97%	99%
Discharged on Statin Medication[1,3]	-	-	89%	94%
Thrombolytic Therapy Timing[1,3]	-	-	53%	66%
Venous Thromboembolism Prophylaxis[1,3]	-	-	87%	94%
Written Stroke Educational Materials Given[1,3]	-	-	83%	88%
Surgical Care Improvement Project				
Appropriate Beta Blocker Usage[1]	-	-	97%	98%
Appropriate VTP Within 24 Hours	22	86%	97%	98%
Controlled Postoperative Blood Glucose[7]	-	-	96%	97%
Perioperative Temperature Management	22	100%	100%	100%
Prophylactic Antibiotic Selection[1]	-	-	99%	99%
Prophylactic Antibiotic Selection (Outpatient)[1,3]	-	-	97%	98%
Prophylactic Antibiotic Stopped[1]	-	-	97%	98%
Prophylactic Antibiotic Timing[1]	-	-	98%	99%
Prophylactic Antibiotic Timing (Outpatient)[1,3]	-	-	97%	98%
Urinary Catheter Removal[1]	-	-	96%	97%
Survey of Patients' Hospital Experiences				
Area Around Room 'Always' Quiet at Night	(a)	70%	74%	61%
Doctors 'Always' Communicated Well	(a)	94%	87%	82%
Home Recovery Information Given	(a)	84%	85%	85%
Hospital Given 9 or 10 on 10 Point Scale	(a)	53%	75%	71%
Meds 'Always' Explained Before Given	(a)	67%	69%	64%
Nurses 'Always' Communicated Well	(a)	76%	83%	79%
Pain 'Always' Well Controlled	(a)	67%	75%	71%
Room and Bathroom 'Always' Clean	(a)	70%	75%	73%
Timely Help 'Always' Received	(a)	62%	71%	68%
Would Definitely Recommend Hospital	(a)	57%	75%	71%
Use of Medical Imaging				
Cardiac Imaging Stress Test before Surgery[1]	-	-	5.3%	5.3%
Combination Abdominal CT Scan	112	68.8%	24.5%	10.5%
Combination Brain/Sinus CT Scan[1]	-	-	2.6%	2.7%
Combination Chest CT Scan	59	44.1%	7.6%	2.7%
Follow-up Mammogram/Ultrasound	232	10.3%	9.4%	8.8%
Lumbar Spine MRI for Low Back Pain[1]	-	-	42.7%	37.2%

Hardtner Medical Center

1102 N Pine Road
Olla, LA 71465
Phone: 318-495-3131
Fax: 318-495-3229
E-mail: admin@hardtnermedical.com
URL: www.hardtnermedical.com
Type: Critical Access Hospitals
Emergency Services: Yes
Ownership: Govt - Hospital Dist/Auth
Beds: 41

Key Personnel:

Emergency Room . . . . Roy Braswell, MD
Infection Control. . . . . Genae Butler, RN

NOTE: Hospital profiles are in alphabetical order by state, then city, then hospital within the city; Rankings exclude hospitals with less than 25 cases except for patient surveys which excludes hospitals with less than 100 cases; (a) 100-299 cases; (1) The number of cases/patients is too few to report; (2) Data submitted were based on a sample of cases/patients; (3) Results are based on a shorter time period than required; (4) Data suppressed by CMS for one or more quarters; (5) Results are not available for this reporting period; (6) Fewer than 100 patients completed the HCAHPS survey; (7) No cases met the criteria for this measure; (8) The lower limit of the confidence interval cannot be calculated if the number of observed infections equals zero; (9) No data are available from the state/territory for this reporting period; (10) The scores shown reflect fewer than 50 completed surveys; (11) There were discrepancies in the data collection process; (12) This measure does not apply to this hospital for this reporting period; (13) Results cannot be calculated for this reporting period; (14) The results for this state are combined with nearby states to protect confidentiality; Please refer to the User's Guide for a full explanation of data.

Quality Assurance . . . . Genae Butler, RN
CEO/President. . . . . Paul G Mathews, FHFMA, CPA
Chief of Medical Staff . . . . Kenneth P Mauterer, MD

Measure	Cases	This Hosp.	State Avg.	U.S. Avg.
Blood Clot Prevention and Treatment				
Anticoagulation Overlap Therapy[5]	-	-	89%	93%
ICU Venous Thromboembolism Prophylaxis[5]	-	-	88%	92%
Incidence of Potentially Preventable VTE[5]	-	-	16%	10%
UFH with Dosages/Platelet Monitoring[5]	-	-	94%	97%
Venous Thromboembolism Prophylaxis[5]	-	-	74%	85%
Warfarin Therapy Discharge Instructions[5]	-	-	85%	75%
Chest Pain/Possible Heart Attack Care				
Aspirin Given Within 24 Hours of Arrival	12	83%	94%	96%
Fibrinolytic Meds Within 30 Min. of Arrival[1]	-	-	54%	58%
Average Time to ECG (minutes)	12	26	10	7
Average Time to Transfer (minutes)[7]	-	-	94	60
Children's Asthma Care				
Received Home Management Plan of Care	-	-	-	88%
Received Reliever Medication	-	-	-	100%
Received Systemic Corticosteroids	-	-	-	100%
Emergency Department				
Admittance Decision Time (minutes)[5]	-	-	86	98
Head CT Results Within 45 Min. of Arrival[5]	-	-	49%	57%
Patients Who Left ER Before Being Seen	4,883	1%	3%	2%
Time from ER Arrival to Admit. (minutes)[5]	-	-	256	274
Time from ER Arrival to Discharge (minutes)[5]	-	-	125	134
Time in ER Before Being Evaluated (minutes)[5]	-	-	27	26
Time to Pain Meds for Fractures (minutes)[5]	-	-	61	57
Heart Attack Care				
Aspirin Given at Discharge[5]	-	-	99%	99%
Fibrinolytic Meds Within 30 Min. of Arrival[5]	-	-	71%	54%
PCI Within 90 Minutes of Arrival[5]	-	-	94%	96%
Statin Prescribed at Discharge[5]	-	-	98%	98%
Heart Failure Care				
ACE Inhibitor or ARB for LVSD[1,3]	-	-	95%	97%
Discharge Instructions Given[1,3]	-	-	94%	94%
Evaluation of LVS Function[3]	19	68%	97%	99%
Medicare Spending				
Medicare Spending per Patient (ratio)	-	-	1.04	0.98
Pneumonia Care				
Appropriate Initial Antibiotic Given[5]	-	-	93%	95%
Blood Culture Timing[5]	-	-	97%	98%
Pregnancy and Delivery Care				
Newborn Deliveries Scheduled Early[5]	-	-	5%	6%
Preventive Care				
Immunization for Influenza[5]	-	-	85%	90%
Immunization for Pneumonia[5]	-	-	88%	92%
Stroke Care				
Anticoagulation Therapy for Atrial Fibrillation[5]	-	-	93%	95%
Antithrombotic Therapy Timing[5]	-	-	96%	98%
Assessed for Rehabilitation[5]	-	-	95%	97%
Discharged on Antithrombotic Therapy[5]	-	-	97%	99%
Discharged on Statin Medication[5]	-	-	89%	94%
Thrombolytic Therapy Timing[5]	-	-	53%	66%
Venous Thromboembolism Prophylaxis[5]	-	-	87%	94%
Written Stroke Educational Materials Given[5]	-	-	83%	88%
Surgical Care Improvement Project				
Appropriate Beta Blocker Usage[5]	-	-	97%	98%
Appropriate VTP Within 24 Hours[5]	-	-	97%	98%
Controlled Postoperative Blood Glucose[5]	-	-	96%	97%
Perioperative Temperature Management[5]	-	-	100%	100%
Prophylactic Antibiotic Selection[5]	-	-	99%	99%
Prophylactic Antibiotic Selection (Outpatient)[5]	-	-	97%	98%
Prophylactic Antibiotic Stopped[5]	-	-	97%	98%
Prophylactic Antibiotic Timing[5]	-	-	98%	99%
Prophylactic Antibiotic Timing (Outpatient)[5]	-	-	97%	98%
Urinary Catheter Removal[5]	-	-	96%	97%
Survey of Patients' Hospital Experiences				
Area Around Room 'Always' Quiet at Night[5]	-	-	74%	61%
Doctors 'Always' Communicated Well[5]	-	-	87%	82%
Home Recovery Information Given[5]	-	-	85%	85%
Hospital Given 9 or 10 on 10 Point Scale[5]	-	-	75%	71%
Meds 'Always' Explained Before Given[5]	-	-	69%	64%
Nurses 'Always' Communicated Well[5]	-	-	83%	79%
Pain 'Always' Well Controlled[5]	-	-	75%	71%
Room and Bathroom 'Always' Clean[5]	-	-	75%	73%
Timely Help 'Always' Received[5]	-	-	71%	68%
Would Definitely Recommend Hospital[5]	-	-	75%	71%
Use of Medical Imaging				
Cardiac Imaging Stress Test before Surgery[7]	-	-	5.3%	5.3%
Combination Abdominal CT Scan	171	60.8%	24.5%	10.5%
Combination Brain/Sinus CT Scan	191	1.0%	2.6%	2.7%
Combination Chest CT Scan	87	0.0%	7.6%	2.7%
Follow-up Mammogram/Ultrasound[7]	-	-	9.4%	8.8%
Lumbar Spine MRI for Low Back Pain[1]	-	-	42.7%	37.2%

Opelousas General Health System

539 East Prudhomme Street
Opelousas, LA 70570
Phone: 337-948-3011
Fax: 337-948-5126
URL: www.opelousasgeneral.com
Type: Acute Care Hospitals
Emergency Services: Yes
Ownership: Govt - Hospital Dist/Auth
Beds: 180

Key Personnel:
Radiology. . . . . Gerard A Ballanco
Chief of Medical Staff . . . . Gary Blanchard, MD
Infection Control . . . . Laurie Going
Operating Room. . . . . Lynda Innes
CEO/President. . . . . Mark E. Marley, FACHE
Pediatric Ambulatory Care . . . . . . Ann Ruffino
Pediatric In-Patient Care . . . . Ann Ruffino

Measure	Cases	This Hosp.	State Avg.	U.S. Avg.
Blood Clot Prevention and Treatment				
Anticoagulation Overlap Therapy[2]	41	78%	89%	93%
ICU Venous Thromboembolism Prophylaxis[2]	98	77%	88%	92%
Incidence of Potentially Preventable VTE[1,2]	-	-	16%	10%
UFH with Dosages/Platelet Monitoring[2]	24	96%	94%	97%
Venous Thromboembolism Prophylaxis[2]	318	71%	74%	85%
Warfarin Therapy Discharge Instructions[2]	30	83%	85%	75%
Chest Pain/Possible Heart Attack Care				
Aspirin Given Within 24 Hours of Arrival[1]	-	-	94%	96%
Fibrinolytic Meds Within 30 Min. of Arrival[5]	-	-	54%	58%
Average Time to ECG (minutes)[1]	-	-	10	7
Average Time to Transfer (minutes)[5]	-	-	94	60
Children's Asthma Care				
Received Home Management Plan of Care	-	-	-	88%
Received Reliever Medication	-	-	-	100%
Received Systemic Corticosteroids	-	-	-	100%
Emergency Department				
Admittance Decision Time (minutes)[2]	449	118	86	98
Head CT Results Within 45 Min. of Arrival	20	85%	49%	57%
Patients Who Left ER Before Being Seen	54,605	2%	3%	2%
Time from ER Arrival to Admit. (minutes)[2]	452	272	256	274
Time from ER Arrival to Discharge (minutes)	385	115	125	134
Time in ER Before Being Evaluated (minutes)	408	23	27	26
Time to Pain Meds for Fractures (minutes)	164	64	61	57
Heart Attack Care				
Aspirin Given at Discharge	89	99%	99%	99%
Fibrinolytic Meds Within 30 Min. of Arrival[7]	-	-	71%	54%
PCI Within 90 Minutes of Arrival	13	100%	94%	96%
Statin Prescribed at Discharge	89	93%	98%	98%
Heart Failure Care				
ACE Inhibitor or ARB for LVSD[2]	70	86%	95%	97%
Discharge Instructions Given[2]	208	96%	94%	94%
Evaluation of LVS Function[2]	249	97%	97%	99%
Medicare Spending				
Medicare Spending per Patient (ratio)	-	1.06	1.04	0.98
Pneumonia Care				
Appropriate Initial Antibiotic Given[2]	73	96%	93%	95%
Blood Culture Timing[2]	110	99%	97%	98%
Pregnancy and Delivery Care				
Newborn Deliveries Scheduled Early[2]	43	9%	5%	6%
Preventive Care				
Immunization for Influenza[2]	530	74%	85%	90%
Immunization for Pneumonia[2]	579	81%	88%	92%
Stroke Care				
Anticoagulation Therapy for Atrial Fibrillation	12	92%	93%	95%
Antithrombotic Therapy Timing	55	93%	96%	98%
Assessed for Rehabilitation	50	94%	95%	97%
Discharged on Antithrombotic Therapy	49	88%	97%	99%
Discharged on Statin Medication	45	62%	89%	94%
Thrombolytic Therapy Timing[1]	-	-	53%	66%
Venous Thromboembolism Prophylaxis	55	75%	87%	94%
Written Stroke Educational Materials Given	19	95%	83%	88%
Surgical Care Improvement Project				
Appropriate Beta Blocker Usage[2]	109	90%	97%	98%
Appropriate VTP Within 24 Hours[2]	303	94%	97%	98%
Controlled Postoperative Blood Glucose[2,7]	-	-	96%	97%
Perioperative Temperature Management[2]	356	100%	100%	100%
Prophylactic Antibiotic Selection[2]	254	98%	99%	99%
Prophylactic Antibiotic Selection (Outpatient)	174	97%	97%	98%
Prophylactic Antibiotic Stopped[2]	246	93%	97%	98%
Prophylactic Antibiotic Timing[2]	256	96%	98%	99%
Prophylactic Antibiotic Timing (Outpatient)	179	97%	97%	98%
Urinary Catheter Removal[2]	213	91%	96%	97%
Survey of Patients' Hospital Experiences				
Area Around Room 'Always' Quiet at Night	300+	65%	74%	61%
Doctors 'Always' Communicated Well	300+	83%	87%	82%
Home Recovery Information Given	300+	82%	85%	85%
Hospital Given 9 or 10 on 10 Point Scale	300+	66%	75%	71%
Meds 'Always' Explained Before Given	300+	58%	69%	64%
Nurses 'Always' Communicated Well	300+	77%	83%	79%
Pain 'Always' Well Controlled	300+	69%	75%	71%
Room and Bathroom 'Always' Clean	300+	71%	75%	73%
Timely Help 'Always' Received	300+	60%	71%	68%
Would Definitely Recommend Hospital	300+	63%	75%	71%
Use of Medical Imaging				
Cardiac Imaging Stress Test before Surgery[1]	-	-	5.3%	5.3%
Combination Abdominal CT Scan	701	21.7%	24.5%	10.5%
Combination Brain/Sinus CT Scan	896	1.3%	2.6%	2.7%
Combination Chest CT Scan	430	20.2%	7.6%	2.7%
Follow-up Mammogram/Ultrasound	1,280	11.6%	9.4%	8.8%
Lumbar Spine MRI for Low Back Pain	101	40.6%	42.7%	37.2%

Alexandria VA Medical Center

2495 Shreveport Highway 71 N
Pineville, LA 71360
Phone: 318-473-0010
Fax: 318-483-5029
URL: www.alexandria.med.va.gov
Type: Acute Care - VA
Emergency Services: No
Ownership: Government Federal
Beds: 401

Key Personnel:
Emergency Room . . . . Jose Andino
Infection Control. . . . . Ouida Hawkins, RN
Quality Assurance . . . . Portia McDaniel
Operating Room. . . . . Mary Phillips, RN
Radiology. . . . . James Ponthier
Chief of Medical Staff . . . . Jose N. Rivera, MD
Patient Relations . . . . Dale Walker
CEO/President. . . . . Barbara C Watkins

Measure	Cases	This Hosp.	State Avg.	U.S. Avg.
Blood Clot Prevention and Treatment				
Anticoagulation Overlap Therapy	-	-	89%	93%
ICU Venous Thromboembolism Prophylaxis	-	-	88%	92%
Incidence of Potentially Preventable VTE	-	-	16%	10%
UFH with Dosages/Platelet Monitoring	-	-	94%	97%
Venous Thromboembolism Prophylaxis	-	-	74%	85%
Warfarin Therapy Discharge Instructions	-	-	85%	75%
Chest Pain/Possible Heart Attack Care				
Aspirin Given Within 24 Hours of Arrival	-	-	94%	96%
Fibrinolytic Meds Within 30 Min. of Arrival	-	-	54%	58%
Average Time to ECG (minutes)	-	-	10	7
Average Time to Transfer (minutes)	-	-	94	60
Children's Asthma Care				
Received Home Management Plan of Care	-	-	-	88%
Received Reliever Medication	-	-	-	100%
Received Systemic Corticosteroids	-	-	-	100%
Emergency Department				
Admittance Decision Time (minutes)	-	-	86	98
Head CT Results Within 45 Min. of Arrival	-	-	49%	57%
Patients Who Left ER Before Being Seen	-	-	3%	2%
Time from ER Arrival to Admit. (minutes)	-	-	256	274

NOTE: Hospital profiles are in alphabetical order by state, then city, then hospital within the city; Rankings exclude hospitals with less than 25 cases except for patient surveys which excludes hospitals with less than 100 cases; (a) 100-299 cases; (1) The number of cases/patients is too few to report; (2) Data submitted were based on a sample of cases/patients; (3) Results are based on a shorter time period than required; (4) Data suppressed by CMS for one or more quarters; (5) Results are not available for this reporting period; (6) Fewer than 100 patients completed the HCAHPS survey; (7) No cases met the criteria for this measure; (8) The lower limit of the confidence interval cannot be calculated if the number of observed infections equals zero; (9) No data are available from the state/territory for this reporting period; (10) The scores shown reflect fewer than 50 completed surveys; (11) There were discrepancies in the data collection process; (12) This measure does not apply to this hospital for this reporting period; (13) Results cannot be calculated for this reporting period; (14) The results for this state are combined with nearby states to protect confidentiality; Please refer to the User's Guide for a full explanation of data.

Measure	Cases	This Hosp.	State Avg.	U.S. Avg.
Time from ER Arrival to Discharge (minutes)	-	-	125	134
Time in ER Before Being Evaluated (minutes)	-	-	27	26
Time to Pain Meds for Fractures (minutes)	-	-	61	57
Heart Attack Care				
Aspirin Given at Discharge[5]	-	-	99%	99%
Fibrinolytic Meds Within 30 Min. of Arrival[5]	-	-	71%	54%
PCI Within 90 Minutes of Arrival[5]	-	-	94%	96%
Statin Prescribed at Discharge[5]	-	-	98%	98%
Heart Failure Care				
ACE Inhibitor or ARB for LVSD[1]	19	100%	95%	97%
Discharge Instructions Given	52	100%	94%	94%
Evaluation of LVS Function	60	100%	97%	99%
Medicare Spending				
Medicare Spending per Patient (ratio)	-	-	1.04	0.98
Pneumonia Care				
Appropriate Initial Antibiotic Given	52	96%	93%	95%
Blood Culture Timing	95	89%	97%	98%
Pregnancy and Delivery Care				
Newborn Deliveries Scheduled Early	-	-	5%	6%
Preventive Care				
Immunization for Influenza[2,3]	140	68%	85%	90%
Immunization for Pneumonia[2,3]	255	91%	88%	92%
Stroke Care				
Anticoagulation Therapy for Atrial Fibrillation	-	-	93%	95%
Antithrombotic Therapy Timing	-	-	96%	98%
Assessed for Rehabilitation	-	-	95%	97%
Discharged on Antithrombotic Therapy	-	-	97%	99%
Discharged on Statin Medication	-	-	89%	94%
Thrombolytic Therapy Timing	-	-	53%	66%
Venous Thromboembolism Prophylaxis	-	-	87%	94%
Written Stroke Educational Materials Given	-	-	83%	88%
Surgical Care Improvement Project				
Appropriate Beta Blocker Usage[5]	-	-	97%	98%
Appropriate VTP Within 24 Hours[5]	-	-	97%	98%
Controlled Postoperative Blood Glucose[5]	-	-	96%	97%
Perioperative Temperature Management[5]	-	-	100%	100%
Prophylactic Antibiotic Selection[5]	-	-	99%	99%
Prophylactic Antibiotic Selection (Outpatient)	-	-	97%	98%
Prophylactic Antibiotic Stopped[5]	-	-	97%	98%
Prophylactic Antibiotic Timing[5]	-	-	98%	99%
Prophylactic Antibiotic Timing (Outpatient)	-	-	97%	98%
Urinary Catheter Removal[5]	-	-	96%	97%
Survey of Patients' Hospital Experiences				
Area Around Room 'Always' Quiet at Night	-	-	74%	61%
Doctors 'Always' Communicated Well	-	-	87%	82%
Home Recovery Information Given	-	-	85%	85%
Hospital Given 9 or 10 on 10 Point Scale	-	-	75%	71%
Meds 'Always' Explained Before Given	-	-	69%	64%
Nurses 'Always' Communicated Well	-	-	83%	79%
Pain 'Always' Well Controlled	-	-	75%	71%
Room and Bathroom 'Always' Clean	-	-	75%	73%
Timely Help 'Always' Received	-	-	71%	68%
Would Definitely Recommend Hospital	-	-	75%	71%
Use of Medical Imaging				
Cardiac Imaging Stress Test before Surgery	-	-	5.3%	5.3%
Combination Abdominal CT Scan	-	-	24.5%	10.5%
Combination Brain/Sinus CT Scan	-	-	2.6%	2.7%
Combination Chest CT Scan	-	-	7.6%	2.7%
Follow-up Mammogram/Ultrasound	-	-	9.4%	8.8%
Lumbar Spine MRI for Low Back Pain	-	-	42.7%	37.2%

Huey P Long Medical Center

352 Hospital Blvd
Pineville, LA 71360
Phone: 318-448-0811
Fax: 318-473-6360
E-mail: j.morga2@lsumc.edu
URL: www.lsuhsc.edu/hcsd
Type: Acute Care Hospitals
Emergency Services: Yes
Ownership: Government - State
Beds: 137
Key Personnel:
Chief of Medical Staff.......... Margaret Brummett, MD
CEO/President............... Gary Crockett

Measure	Cases	This Hosp.	State Avg.	U.S. Avg.
Blood Clot Prevention and Treatment				
Anticoagulation Overlap Therapy[1,2]	-	-	89%	93%
ICU Venous Thromboembolism Prophylaxis[1,2]	-	-	88%	92%
Incidence of Potentially Preventable VTE[2,7]	-	-	16%	10%
UFH with Dosages/Platelet Monitoring[1,2]	-	-	94%	97%
Venous Thromboembolism Prophylaxis[2]	148	60%	74%	85%
Warfarin Therapy Discharge Instructions[1,2]	-	-	85%	75%
Chest Pain/Possible Heart Attack Care				
Aspirin Given Within 24 Hours of Arrival[1,3]	-	-	94%	96%
Fibrinolytic Meds Within 30 Min. of Arrival[3,7]	-	-	54%	58%
Average Time to ECG (minutes)[1,3]	-	-	10	7
Average Time to Transfer (minutes)[1,3]	-	-	94	60
Children's Asthma Care				
Received Home Management Plan of Care	-	-	-	88%
Received Reliever Medication	-	-	-	100%
Received Systemic Corticosteroids	-	-	-	100%
Emergency Department				
Admittance Decision Time (minutes)[2]	306	148	86	98
Head CT Results Within 45 Min. of Arrival[1]	-	-	49%	57%
Patients Who Left ER Before Being Seen	29,558	8%	3%	2%
Time from ER Arrival to Admit. (minutes)[2]	308	538	256	274
Time from ER Arrival to Discharge (minutes)	342	262	125	134
Time in ER Before Being Evaluated (minutes)	351	115	27	26
Time to Pain Meds for Fractures (minutes)[1]	-	-	61	57
Heart Attack Care				
Aspirin Given at Discharge[3,7]	-	-	99%	99%
Fibrinolytic Meds Within 30 Min. of Arrival[3,7]	-	-	71%	54%
PCI Within 90 Minutes of Arrival[3,7]	-	-	94%	96%
Statin Prescribed at Discharge[3,7]	-	-	98%	98%
Heart Failure Care				
ACE Inhibitor or ARB for LVSD[1]	-	-	95%	97%
Discharge Instructions Given	19	89%	94%	94%
Evaluation of LVS Function	19	89%	97%	99%
Medicare Spending				
Medicare Spending per Patient (ratio)	-	0.90	1.04	0.98
Pneumonia Care				
Appropriate Initial Antibiotic Given	51	84%	93%	95%
Blood Culture Timing	48	92%	97%	98%
Pregnancy and Delivery Care				
Newborn Deliveries Scheduled Early[7]	-	-	5%	6%
Preventive Care				
Immunization for Influenza[2]	295	54%	85%	90%
Immunization for Pneumonia[2]	229	53%	88%	92%
Stroke Care				
Anticoagulation Therapy for Atrial Fibrillation[1,3]	-	-	93%	95%
Antithrombotic Therapy Timing[1,3]	-	-	96%	98%
Assessed for Rehabilitation[1,3]	-	-	95%	97%
Discharged on Antithrombotic Therapy[1,3]	-	-	97%	99%
Discharged on Statin Medication[1,3]	-	-	89%	94%
Thrombolytic Therapy Timing[3,7]	-	-	53%	66%
Venous Thromboembolism Prophylaxis[1,3]	-	-	87%	94%
Written Stroke Educational Materials Given[1,3]	-	-	83%	88%
Surgical Care Improvement Project				
Appropriate Beta Blocker Usage	18	67%	97%	98%
Appropriate VTP Within 24 Hours	61	90%	97%	98%
Controlled Postoperative Blood Glucose[7]	-	-	96%	97%
Perioperative Temperature Management	80	99%	100%	100%
Prophylactic Antibiotic Selection	42	100%	99%	99%
Prophylactic Antibiotic Selection (Outpatient)[5]	-	-	97%	98%
Prophylactic Antibiotic Stopped	42	98%	97%	98%
Prophylactic Antibiotic Timing	44	89%	98%	99%
Prophylactic Antibiotic Timing (Outpatient)[5]	-	-	97%	98%
Urinary Catheter Removal	12	50%	96%	97%
Survey of Patients' Hospital Experiences				
Area Around Room 'Always' Quiet at Night	(a)	64%	74%	61%
Doctors 'Always' Communicated Well	(a)	79%	87%	82%
Home Recovery Information Given	(a)	84%	85%	85%
Hospital Given 9 or 10 on 10 Point Scale	(a)	68%	75%	71%
Meds 'Always' Explained Before Given	(a)	68%	69%	64%
Nurses 'Always' Communicated Well	(a)	77%	83%	79%
Pain 'Always' Well Controlled	(a)	71%	75%	71%
Room and Bathroom 'Always' Clean	(a)	62%	75%	73%
Timely Help 'Always' Received	(a)	62%	71%	68%
Would Definitely Recommend Hospital	(a)	68%	75%	71%
Use of Medical Imaging				
Cardiac Imaging Stress Test before Surgery	45	2.2%	5.3%	5.3%
Combination Abdominal CT Scan	94	1.1%	24.5%	10.5%
Combination Brain/Sinus CT Scan[1]	-	-	2.6%	2.7%
Combination Chest CT Scan	52	0.0%	7.6%	2.7%
Follow-up Mammogram/Ultrasound	390	2.1%	9.4%	8.8%
Lumbar Spine MRI for Low Back Pain[1]	-	-	42.7%	37.2%

Ochsner Saint Anne General Hospital

4608 Highway 1
Raceland, LA 70394
Phone: 985-537-8377
Fax: 985-537-8272
E-mail: jechampagne@oschner.org
URL: www.ochsnerstanne.com
Type: Critical Access Hospitals
Emergency Services: Yes
Ownership: Voluntary non-profit - Private
Beds: 45
Key Personnel:
CEO........................ Tim Allen
CEO/President............... Milton Bourgeoi, Jr
Emergency Room............ Adele Dantin
Radiology.................. John Flannery

Measure	Cases	This Hosp.	State Avg.	U.S. Avg.
Blood Clot Prevention and Treatment				
Anticoagulation Overlap Therapy[5]	-	-	89%	93%
ICU Venous Thromboembolism Prophylaxis[5]	-	-	88%	92%
Incidence of Potentially Preventable VTE[5]	-	-	16%	10%
UFH with Dosages/Platelet Monitoring[5]	-	-	94%	97%
Venous Thromboembolism Prophylaxis[5]	-	-	74%	85%
Warfarin Therapy Discharge Instructions[5]	-	-	85%	75%
Chest Pain/Possible Heart Attack Care				
Aspirin Given Within 24 Hours of Arrival	38	92%	94%	96%
Fibrinolytic Meds Within 30 Min. of Arrival[1]	-	-	54%	58%
Average Time to ECG (minutes)	41	9	10	7
Average Time to Transfer (minutes)[1]	-	-	94	60
Children's Asthma Care				
Received Home Management Plan of Care	-	-	-	88%
Received Reliever Medication	-	-	-	100%
Received Systemic Corticosteroids	-	-	-	100%
Emergency Department				
Admittance Decision Time (minutes)[5]	-	-	86	98
Head CT Results Within 45 Min. of Arrival[5]	-	-	49%	57%
Patients Who Left ER Before Being Seen	14,266	0%	3%	2%
Time from ER Arrival to Admit. (minutes)[5]	-	-	256	274
Time from ER Arrival to Discharge (minutes)[5]	-	-	125	134
Time in ER Before Being Evaluated (minutes)[5]	-	-	27	26
Time to Pain Meds for Fractures (minutes)[5]	-	-	61	57
Heart Attack Care				
Aspirin Given at Discharge[1]	-	-	99%	99%
Fibrinolytic Meds Within 30 Min. of Arrival[7]	-	-	71%	54%
PCI Within 90 Minutes of Arrival[7]	-	-	94%	96%
Statin Prescribed at Discharge[1]	-	-	98%	98%
Heart Failure Care				
ACE Inhibitor or ARB for LVSD[1]	-	-	95%	97%
Discharge Instructions Given	26	92%	94%	94%
Evaluation of LVS Function	28	100%	97%	99%
Medicare Spending				
Medicare Spending per Patient (ratio)	-	-	1.04	0.98
Pneumonia Care				
Appropriate Initial Antibiotic Given	21	81%	93%	95%
Blood Culture Timing	30	100%	97%	98%
Pregnancy and Delivery Care				
Newborn Deliveries Scheduled Early[5]	-	-	5%	6%
Preventive Care				
Immunization for Influenza[5]	-	-	85%	90%
Immunization for Pneumonia[5]	-	-	88%	92%
Stroke Care				
Anticoagulation Therapy for Atrial Fibrillation[5]	-	-	93%	95%
Antithrombotic Therapy Timing[5]	-	-	96%	98%
Assessed for Rehabilitation[5]	-	-	95%	97%
Discharged on Antithrombotic Therapy[5]	-	-	97%	99%
Discharged on Statin Medication[5]	-	-	89%	94%
Thrombolytic Therapy Timing[5]	-	-	53%	66%
Venous Thromboembolism Prophylaxis[5]	-	-	87%	94%
Written Stroke Educational Materials Given[5]	-	-	83%	88%

NOTE: Hospital profiles are in alphabetical order by state, then city, then hospital within the city; Rankings exclude hospitals with less than 25 cases except for patient surveys which excludes hospitals with less than 100 cases; (a) 100-299 cases; (1) The number of cases/patients is too few to report; (2) Data submitted were based on a sample of cases/patients; (3) Results are based on a shorter time period than required; (4) Data suppressed by CMS for one or more quarters; (5) Results are not available for this reporting period; (6) Fewer than 100 patients completed the HCAHPS survey; (7) No cases met the criteria for this measure; (8) The lower limit of the confidence interval cannot be calculated if the number of observed infections equals zero; (9) No data are available from the state/territory for this reporting period; (10) The scores shown reflect fewer than 50 completed surveys; (11) There were discrepancies in the data collection process; (12) This measure does not apply to this hospital for this reporting period; (13) Results cannot be calculated for this reporting period; (14) The results for this state are combined with nearby states to protect confidentiality; Please refer to the User's Guide for a full explanation of data.

Measure	Cases	This Hosp.	State Avg.	U.S. Avg.
Surgical Care Improvement Project				
Appropriate Beta Blocker Usage[1]	-	-	97%	98%
Appropriate VTP Within 24 Hours	12	100%	97%	98%
Controlled Postoperative Blood Glucose[7]	-	-	96%	97%
Perioperative Temperature Management	36	97%	100%	100%
Prophylactic Antibiotic Selection	21	100%	99%	99%
Prophylactic Antibiotic Selection (Outpatient)	25	100%	97%	98%
Prophylactic Antibiotic Stopped	21	100%	97%	98%
Prophylactic Antibiotic Timing	21	100%	98%	99%
Prophylactic Antibiotic Timing (Outpatient)	13	100%	97%	98%
Urinary Catheter Removal[1]	-	-	96%	97%
Survey of Patients' Hospital Experiences				
Area Around Room 'Always' Quiet at Night	(a)	68%	74%	61%
Doctors 'Always' Communicated Well	(a)	84%	87%	82%
Home Recovery Information Given	(a)	89%	85%	85%
Hospital Given 9 or 10 on 10 Point Scale	(a)	67%	75%	71%
Meds 'Always' Explained Before Given	(a)	71%	69%	64%
Nurses 'Always' Communicated Well	(a)	81%	83%	79%
Pain 'Always' Well Controlled	(a)	70%	75%	71%
Room and Bathroom 'Always' Clean	(a)	75%	75%	73%
Timely Help 'Always' Received	(a)	65%	71%	68%
Would Definitely Recommend Hospital	(a)	67%	75%	71%
Use of Medical Imaging				
Cardiac Imaging Stress Test before Surgery[1]	-	-	5.3%	5.3%
Combination Abdominal CT Scan	203	14.3%	24.5%	10.5%
Combination Brain/Sinus CT Scan[1]	-	-	2.6%	2.7%
Combination Chest CT Scan	77	3.9%	7.6%	2.7%
Follow-up Mammogram/Ultrasound	366	5.5%	9.4%	8.8%
Lumbar Spine MRI for Low Back Pain[1]	-	-	42.7%	37.2%

Richardson Medical Center

254 Highway 3048
Rayville, LA 71269
Phone: 318-728-4181
Fax: 318-728-8248
E-mail: info@richardsonmed.org
URL: www.richardsonmedicalcenter.org
Type: Acute Care Hospitals
Emergency Services: Yes
Ownership: Govt - Hospital Dist/Auth
Beds: 49

Key Personnel:
Intensive Care Unit. . . . . Carolyn Arnold, RN
Radiology. . . . . Edward Brown, MD
Cardiology . . . . Imran Chaudry, MD
Infection Control. . . . . Betty Hill, RN
Chief of Medical Staff . . . . Dan LaFleur, MD
Emergency Room . . . . Gordon B Massengale, MD
Quality Assurance . . . . Charles Parker
Surgery . . . . Addison Thompson, MD

Measure	Cases	This Hosp.	State Avg.	U.S. Avg.
Blood Clot Prevention and Treatment				
Anticoagulation Overlap Therapy[1,2]	-	-	89%	93%
ICU Venous Thromboembolism Prophylaxis[2]	25	72%	88%	92%
Incidence of Potentially Preventable VTE[1,2]	-	-	16%	10%
UFH with Dosages/Platelet Monitoring[1,2]	-	-	94%	97%
Venous Thromboembolism Prophylaxis[2]	181	63%	74%	85%
Warfarin Therapy Discharge Instructions[1,2]	-	-	85%	75%
Chest Pain/Possible Heart Attack Care				
Aspirin Given Within 24 Hours of Arrival[1,3]	-	-	94%	96%
Fibrinolytic Meds Within 30 Min. of Arrival[3,7]	-	-	54%	58%
Average Time to ECG (minutes)[1,3]	-	-	10	7
Average Time to Transfer (minutes)[3,7]	-	-	94	60
Children's Asthma Care				
Received Home Management Plan of Care	-	-	-	88%
Received Reliever Medication	-	-	-	100%
Received Systemic Corticosteroids	-	-	-	100%
Emergency Department				
Admittance Decision Time (minutes)[2]	252	70	86	98
Head CT Results Within 45 Min. of Arrival[1,3]	-	-	49%	57%
Patients Who Left ER Before Being Seen	6,030	4%	3%	2%
Time from ER Arrival to Admit. (minutes)[2]	259	195	256	274
Time from ER Arrival to Discharge (minutes)	382	75	125	134
Time in ER Before Being Evaluated (minutes)	384	9	27	26
Time to Pain Meds for Fractures (minutes)[1,3]	-	-	61	57
Heart Attack Care				
Aspirin Given at Discharge[1,2]	-	-	99%	99%
Fibrinolytic Meds Within 30 Min. of Arrival[2,3]	-	-	71%	54%
PCI Within 90 Minutes of Arrival[2,3]	-	-	94%	96%
Statin Prescribed at Discharge[1,2]	-	-	98%	98%
Heart Failure Care				
ACE Inhibitor or ARB for LVSD[1]	-	-	95%	97%
Discharge Instructions Given	21	95%	94%	94%
Evaluation of LVS Function	33	48%	97%	99%
Medicare Spending				
Medicare Spending per Patient (ratio)	-	1.04	1.04	0.98
Pneumonia Care				
Appropriate Initial Antibiotic Given[1]	-	-	93%	95%
Blood Culture Timing	31	100%	97%	98%
Pregnancy and Delivery Care				
Newborn Deliveries Scheduled Early[7]	-	-	5%	6%
Preventive Care				
Immunization for Influenza	164	59%	85%	90%
Immunization for Pneumonia[2]	268	62%	88%	92%
Stroke Care				
Anticoagulation Therapy for Atrial Fibrillation[1]	-	-	93%	95%
Antithrombotic Therapy Timing[1]	-	-	96%	98%
Assessed for Rehabilitation[1]	-	-	95%	97%
Discharged on Antithrombotic Therapy[1]	-	-	97%	99%
Discharged on Statin Medication[1]	-	-	89%	94%
Thrombolytic Therapy Timing[7]	-	-	53%	66%
Venous Thromboembolism Prophylaxis[1]	-	-	87%	94%
Written Stroke Educational Materials Given[1]	-	-	83%	88%
Surgical Care Improvement Project				
Appropriate Beta Blocker Usage[1]	-	-	97%	98%
Appropriate VTP Within 24 Hours	45	100%	97%	98%
Controlled Postoperative Blood Glucose[7]	-	-	96%	97%
Perioperative Temperature Management	54	100%	100%	100%
Prophylactic Antibiotic Selection	38	76%	99%	99%
Prophylactic Antibiotic Selection (Outpatient)[3]	15	100%	97%	98%
Prophylactic Antibiotic Stopped	38	100%	97%	98%
Prophylactic Antibiotic Timing	38	100%	98%	99%
Prophylactic Antibiotic Timing (Outpatient)[3]	16	94%	97%	98%
Urinary Catheter Removal	15	100%	96%	97%
Survey of Patients' Hospital Experiences				
Area Around Room 'Always' Quiet at Night	(a)	75%	74%	61%
Doctors 'Always' Communicated Well	(a)	94%	87%	82%
Home Recovery Information Given	(a)	79%	85%	85%
Hospital Given 9 or 10 on 10 Point Scale	(a)	73%	75%	71%
Meds 'Always' Explained Before Given	(a)	82%	69%	64%
Nurses 'Always' Communicated Well	(a)	87%	83%	79%
Pain 'Always' Well Controlled	(a)	79%	75%	71%
Room and Bathroom 'Always' Clean	(a)	87%	75%	73%
Timely Help 'Always' Received	(a)	78%	71%	68%
Would Definitely Recommend Hospital	(a)	59%	75%	71%
Use of Medical Imaging				
Cardiac Imaging Stress Test before Surgery[1]	-	-	5.3%	5.3%
Combination Abdominal CT Scan	112	21.4%	24.5%	10.5%
Combination Brain/Sinus CT Scan[1]	-	-	2.6%	2.7%
Combination Chest CT Scan[1]	-	-	7.6%	2.7%
Follow-up Mammogram/Ultrasound	184	6.5%	9.4%	8.8%
Lumbar Spine MRI for Low Back Pain	83	45.8%	42.7%	37.2%

Green Clinic Surgical Hospital

1118 Farmerville Street
Ruston, LA 71270
Phone: 318-232-7700
Fax: 318-255-4360
URL: www.green-clinic.com
Type: Acute Care Hospitals
Emergency Services: No
Ownership: Physician

Key Personnel:
Pediatrics. . . . . Marlene Daher, M.D.
CEO/President. . . . . Robert Goodwill
Pulmonary Disease . . . . Thomas P. Smith, M.D.
Radiology. . . . . Jeff Weeks, M.D.

Measure	Cases	This Hosp.	State Avg.	U.S. Avg.
Blood Clot Prevention and Treatment				
Anticoagulation Overlap Therapy[1]	-	-	89%	93%
ICU Venous Thromboembolism Prophylaxis[1]	-	-	88%	92%
Incidence of Potentially Preventable VTE[7]	-	-	16%	10%
UFH with Dosages/Platelet Monitoring[1]	-	-	94%	97%
Venous Thromboembolism Prophylaxis	154	92%	74%	85%
Warfarin Therapy Discharge Instructions[1]	-	-	85%	75%
Chest Pain/Possible Heart Attack Care				
Aspirin Given Within 24 Hours of Arrival[5]	-	-	94%	96%
Fibrinolytic Meds Within 30 Min. of Arrival[5]	-	-	54%	58%
Average Time to ECG (minutes)[5]	-	-	10	7
Average Time to Transfer (minutes)[5]	-	-	94	60
Children's Asthma Care				
Received Home Management Plan of Care	-	-	-	88%
Received Reliever Medication	-	-	-	100%
Received Systemic Corticosteroids	-	-	-	100%
Emergency Department				
Admittance Decision Time (minutes)[7]	-	-	86	98
Head CT Results Within 45 Min. of Arrival[5]	-	-	49%	57%
Patients Who Left ER Before Being Seen[5]	-	-	3%	2%
Time from ER Arrival to Admit. (minutes)[7]	-	-	256	274
Time from ER Arrival to Discharge (minutes)[5]	-	-	125	134
Time in ER Before Being Evaluated (minutes)[5]	-	-	27	26
Time to Pain Meds for Fractures (minutes)[5]	-	-	61	57
Heart Attack Care				
Aspirin Given at Discharge[5]	-	-	99%	99%
Fibrinolytic Meds Within 30 Min. of Arrival[5]	-	-	71%	54%
PCI Within 90 Minutes of Arrival[5]	-	-	94%	96%
Statin Prescribed at Discharge[5]	-	-	98%	98%
Heart Failure Care				
ACE Inhibitor or ARB for LVSD[1,3]	-	-	95%	97%
Discharge Instructions Given[3]	18	94%	94%	94%
Evaluation of LVS Function[3]	18	100%	97%	99%
Medicare Spending				
Medicare Spending per Patient (ratio)	-	1.05	1.04	0.98
Pneumonia Care				
Appropriate Initial Antibiotic Given[1]	-	-	93%	95%
Blood Culture Timing[7]	-	-	97%	98%
Pregnancy and Delivery Care				
Newborn Deliveries Scheduled Early[7]	-	-	5%	6%
Preventive Care				
Immunization for Influenza	180	88%	85%	90%
Immunization for Pneumonia	217	95%	88%	92%
Stroke Care				
Anticoagulation Therapy for Atrial Fibrillation[3,7]	-	-	93%	95%
Antithrombotic Therapy Timing[3,7]	-	-	96%	98%
Assessed for Rehabilitation[3,7]	-	-	95%	97%
Discharged on Antithrombotic Therapy[3,7]	-	-	97%	99%
Discharged on Statin Medication[3,7]	-	-	89%	94%
Thrombolytic Therapy Timing[3,7]	-	-	53%	66%
Venous Thromboembolism Prophylaxis[3,7]	-	-	87%	94%
Written Stroke Educational Materials Given[3,7]	-	-	83%	88%
Surgical Care Improvement Project				
Appropriate Beta Blocker Usage	23	96%	97%	98%
Appropriate VTP Within 24 Hours	100	100%	97%	98%
Controlled Postoperative Blood Glucose[7]	-	-	96%	97%
Perioperative Temperature Management	114	100%	100%	100%
Prophylactic Antibiotic Selection	92	99%	99%	99%
Prophylactic Antibiotic Selection (Outpatient)	85	99%	97%	98%
Prophylactic Antibiotic Stopped	92	100%	97%	98%
Prophylactic Antibiotic Timing	92	100%	98%	99%
Prophylactic Antibiotic Timing (Outpatient)	85	99%	97%	98%
Urinary Catheter Removal	27	100%	96%	97%
Survey of Patients' Hospital Experiences				
Area Around Room 'Always' Quiet at Night	(a)	83%	74%	61%
Doctors 'Always' Communicated Well	(a)	95%	87%	82%
Home Recovery Information Given	(a)	88%	85%	85%
Hospital Given 9 or 10 on 10 Point Scale	(a)	93%	75%	71%
Meds 'Always' Explained Before Given	(a)	85%	69%	64%
Nurses 'Always' Communicated Well	(a)	92%	83%	79%
Pain 'Always' Well Controlled	(a)	86%	75%	71%
Room and Bathroom 'Always' Clean	(a)	83%	75%	73%
Timely Help 'Always' Received	(a)	87%	71%	68%
Would Definitely Recommend Hospital	(a)	92%	75%	71%
Use of Medical Imaging				
Cardiac Imaging Stress Test before Surgery[7]	-	-	5.3%	5.3%
Combination Abdominal CT Scan[7]	-	-	24.5%	10.5%
Combination Brain/Sinus CT Scan[7]	-	-	2.6%	2.7%

NOTE: Hospital profiles are in alphabetical order by state, then city, then hospital within the city; Rankings exclude hospitals with less than 25 cases except for patient surveys which excludes hospitals with less than 100 cases; (a) 100-299 cases; (1) The number of cases/patients is too few to report; (2) Data submitted were based on a sample of cases/patients; (3) Results are based on a shorter time period than required; (4) Data suppressed by CMS for one or more quarters; (5) Results are not available for this reporting period; (6) Fewer than 100 patients completed the HCAHPS survey; (7) No cases met the criteria for this measure; (8) The lower limit of the confidence interval cannot be calculated if the number of observed infections equals zero; (9) No data are available from the state/territory for this reporting period; (10) The scores shown reflect fewer than 50 completed surveys; (11) There were discrepancies in the data collection process; (12) This measure does not apply to this hospital for this reporting period; (13) Results cannot be calculated for this reporting period; (14) The results for this state are combined with nearby states to protect confidentiality; Please refer to the User's Guide for a full explanation of data.

Combination Chest CT Scan[7]	-	-	7.6%	2.7%
Follow-up Mammogram/Ultrasound[7]	-	-	9.4%	8.8%
Lumbar Spine MRI for Low Back Pain[7]	-	-	42.7%	37.2%

Northern Louisiana Medical Center

401 East Vaughn Avenue — Phone: 318-254-2100
Ruston, LA 71270 — Fax: 318-254-2728
URL: www.lincolnhealth.com
Type: Acute Care Hospitals — Emergency Services: Yes
Ownership: Proprietary — Beds: 160

Key Personnel:
Cardiac Laboratory. . . . . Alan Brazzell
Quality Assurance . . . . Kandy Easley
Intensive Care Unit. . . . . Belinda Gray
Infection Control. . . . . Carrie McCullin, RNC
Emergency Room . . . . Eva Morris
CEO/President. . . . . Doug Sills
Operating Room. . . . . Gayle Smith, RN
Chief of Medical Staff . . . . William Tanner, MD

Measure	Cases	This Hosp.	State Avg.	U.S. Avg.
Blood Clot Prevention and Treatment				
Anticoagulation Overlap Therapy[2]	36	100%	89%	93%
ICU Venous Thromboembolism Prophylaxis[2]	165	100%	88%	92%
Incidence of Potentially Preventable VTE[1,2]	-	-	16%	10%
UFH with Dosages/Platelet Monitoring[2]	21	100%	94%	97%
Venous Thromboembolism Prophylaxis[2]	360	100%	74%	85%
Warfarin Therapy Discharge Instructions[2]	25	100%	85%	75%
Chest Pain/Possible Heart Attack Care				
Aspirin Given Within 24 Hours of Arrival	13	100%	94%	96%
Fibrinolytic Meds Within 30 Min. of Arrival[1,3]	-	-	54%	58%
Average Time to ECG (minutes)	13	2	10	7
Average Time to Transfer (minutes)[3,7]	-	-	94	60
Children's Asthma Care				
Received Home Management Plan of Care	-	-	-	88%
Received Reliever Medication	-	-	-	100%
Received Systemic Corticosteroids	-	-	-	100%
Emergency Department				
Admittance Decision Time (minutes)[2]	623	95	86	98
Head CT Results Within 45 Min. of Arrival[1]	-	-	49%	57%
Patients Who Left ER Before Being Seen	27,358	3%	3%	2%
Time from ER Arrival to Admit. (minutes)[2]	623	250	256	274
Time from ER Arrival to Discharge (minutes)	385	98	125	134
Time in ER Before Being Evaluated (minutes)	417	19	27	26
Time to Pain Meds for Fractures (minutes)	95	52	61	57
Heart Attack Care				
Aspirin Given at Discharge	49	100%	99%	99%
Fibrinolytic Meds Within 30 Min. of Arrival[7]	-	-	71%	54%
PCI Within 90 Minutes of Arrival[1]	-	-	94%	96%
Statin Prescribed at Discharge	45	100%	98%	98%
Heart Failure Care				
ACE Inhibitor or ARB for LVSD	65	100%	95%	97%
Discharge Instructions Given	163	97%	94%	94%
Evaluation of LVS Function	223	100%	97%	99%
Medicare Spending				
Medicare Spending per Patient (ratio)	-	1.13	1.04	0.98
Pneumonia Care				
Appropriate Initial Antibiotic Given	58	98%	93%	95%
Blood Culture Timing	133	99%	97%	98%
Pregnancy and Delivery Care				
Newborn Deliveries Scheduled Early[2]	45	4%	5%	6%
Preventive Care				
Immunization for Influenza[2]	573	100%	85%	90%
Immunization for Pneumonia[2]	693	100%	88%	92%
Stroke Care				
Anticoagulation Therapy for Atrial Fibrillation[1]	-	-	93%	95%
Antithrombotic Therapy Timing	49	100%	96%	98%
Assessed for Rehabilitation	53	100%	95%	97%
Discharged on Antithrombotic Therapy	47	100%	97%	99%
Discharged on Statin Medication	29	100%	89%	94%
Thrombolytic Therapy Timing[1]	-	-	53%	66%
Venous Thromboembolism Prophylaxis	53	100%	87%	94%
Written Stroke Educational Materials Given	35	97%	83%	88%
Surgical Care Improvement Project				
Appropriate Beta Blocker Usage	39	97%	97%	98%
Appropriate VTP Within 24 Hours	121	98%	97%	98%
Controlled Postoperative Blood Glucose[7]	-	-	96%	97%
Perioperative Temperature Management	139	100%	100%	100%
Prophylactic Antibiotic Selection	92	99%	99%	99%
Prophylactic Antibiotic Selection (Outpatient)	35	100%	97%	98%
Prophylactic Antibiotic Stopped	85	99%	97%	98%
Prophylactic Antibiotic Timing	92	99%	98%	99%
Prophylactic Antibiotic Timing (Outpatient)	35	100%	97%	98%
Urinary Catheter Removal	35	100%	96%	97%
Survey of Patients' Hospital Experiences				
Area Around Room 'Always' Quiet at Night	300+	62%	74%	61%
Doctors 'Always' Communicated Well	300+	82%	87%	82%
Home Recovery Information Given	300+	85%	85%	85%
Hospital Given 9 or 10 on 10 Point Scale	300+	64%	75%	71%
Meds 'Always' Explained Before Given	300+	63%	69%	64%
Nurses 'Always' Communicated Well	300+	78%	83%	79%
Pain 'Always' Well Controlled	300+	72%	75%	71%
Room and Bathroom 'Always' Clean	300+	69%	75%	73%
Timely Help 'Always' Received	300+	60%	71%	68%
Would Definitely Recommend Hospital	300+	61%	75%	71%
Use of Medical Imaging				
Cardiac Imaging Stress Test before Surgery	103	3.9%	5.3%	5.3%
Combination Abdominal CT Scan	172	32.0%	24.5%	10.5%
Combination Brain/Sinus CT Scan	446	2.0%	2.6%	2.7%
Combination Chest CT Scan[1]	-	-	7.6%	2.7%
Follow-up Mammogram/Ultrasound	235	10.2%	9.4%	8.8%
Lumbar Spine MRI for Low Back Pain	82	45.1%	42.7%	37.2%

West Feliciana Parish Hospital

5266 Commerce Street — Phone: 225-635-3811
Saint Francisville, LA 70775 — Fax: 225-635-2435
URL: www.wfph.org
Type: Critical Access Hospitals — Emergency Services: Yes
Ownership: Govt - Hospital Dist/Auth — Beds: 22

Key Personnel:
Cardiology . . . . Jeffrey D. Hyde, MD, FACC
Chief of Medical Staff. . . . . Nnamdi Nwabueze, MD
Emergency Room . . . . Nnamdi Nwabueze, MD
Infection Control. . . . . Mary Weller

Measure	Cases	This Hosp.	State Avg.	U.S. Avg.
Blood Clot Prevention and Treatment				
Anticoagulation Overlap Therapy[5]	-	-	89%	93%
ICU Venous Thromboembolism Prophylaxis[5]	-	-	88%	92%
Incidence of Potentially Preventable VTE[5]	-	-	16%	10%
UFH with Dosages/Platelet Monitoring[5]	-	-	94%	97%
Venous Thromboembolism Prophylaxis[5]	-	-	74%	85%
Warfarin Therapy Discharge Instructions[5]	-	-	85%	75%
Chest Pain/Possible Heart Attack Care				
Aspirin Given Within 24 Hours of Arrival	24	96%	94%	96%
Fibrinolytic Meds Within 30 Min. of Arrival[7]	-	-	54%	58%
Average Time to ECG (minutes)	26	5	10	7
Average Time to Transfer (minutes)[1]	-	-	94	60
Children's Asthma Care				
Received Home Management Plan of Care	-	-	-	88%
Received Reliever Medication	-	-	-	100%
Received Systemic Corticosteroids	-	-	-	100%
Emergency Department				
Admittance Decision Time (minutes)[1]	-	-	86	98
Head CT Results Within 45 Min. of Arrival[1,3]	-	-	49%	57%
Patients Who Left ER Before Being Seen	5,229	1%	3%	2%
Time from ER Arrival to Admit. (minutes)[1]	-	-	256	274
Time from ER Arrival to Discharge (minutes)[5]	-	-	125	134
Time in ER Before Being Evaluated (minutes)[5]	-	-	27	26
Time to Pain Meds for Fractures (minutes)[1,3]	-	-	61	57
Heart Attack Care				
Aspirin Given at Discharge[5]	-	-	99%	99%
Fibrinolytic Meds Within 30 Min. of Arrival[5]	-	-	71%	54%
PCI Within 90 Minutes of Arrival[5]	-	-	94%	96%
Statin Prescribed at Discharge[5]	-	-	98%	98%
Heart Failure Care				
ACE Inhibitor or ARB for LVSD[1,3]	-	-	95%	97%
Discharge Instructions Given[1,3]	-	-	94%	94%
Evaluation of LVS Function[1,3]	-	-	97%	99%
Medicare Spending				
Medicare Spending per Patient (ratio)	-	-	1.04	0.98
Pneumonia Care				
Appropriate Initial Antibiotic Given[1,3]	-	-	93%	95%
Blood Culture Timing[1,3]	-	-	97%	98%
Pregnancy and Delivery Care				
Newborn Deliveries Scheduled Early[5]	-	-	5%	6%
Preventive Care				
Immunization for Influenza	44	98%	85%	90%
Immunization for Pneumonia	42	100%	88%	92%
Stroke Care				
Anticoagulation Therapy for Atrial Fibrillation[5]	-	-	93%	95%
Antithrombotic Therapy Timing[5]	-	-	96%	98%
Assessed for Rehabilitation[5]	-	-	95%	97%
Discharged on Antithrombotic Therapy[5]	-	-	97%	99%
Discharged on Statin Medication[5]	-	-	89%	94%
Thrombolytic Therapy Timing[5]	-	-	53%	66%
Venous Thromboembolism Prophylaxis[5]	-	-	87%	94%
Written Stroke Educational Materials Given[5]	-	-	83%	88%
Surgical Care Improvement Project				
Appropriate Beta Blocker Usage[5]	-	-	97%	98%
Appropriate VTP Within 24 Hours[5]	-	-	97%	98%
Controlled Postoperative Blood Glucose[5]	-	-	96%	97%
Perioperative Temperature Management[5]	-	-	100%	100%
Prophylactic Antibiotic Selection[5]	-	-	99%	99%
Prophylactic Antibiotic Selection (Outpatient)[5]	-	-	97%	98%
Prophylactic Antibiotic Stopped[5]	-	-	97%	98%
Prophylactic Antibiotic Timing[5]	-	-	98%	99%
Prophylactic Antibiotic Timing (Outpatient)[5]	-	-	97%	98%
Urinary Catheter Removal[5]	-	-	96%	97%
Survey of Patients' Hospital Experiences				
Area Around Room 'Always' Quiet at Night[10]	<100	81%	74%	61%
Doctors 'Always' Communicated Well[10]	<100	96%	87%	82%
Home Recovery Information Given[10]	<100	89%	85%	85%
Hospital Given 9 or 10 on 10 Point Scale[10]	<100	88%	75%	71%
Meds 'Always' Explained Before Given[10]	<100	68%	69%	64%
Nurses 'Always' Communicated Well[10]	<100	86%	83%	79%
Pain 'Always' Well Controlled[10]	<100	83%	75%	71%
Room and Bathroom 'Always' Clean[10]	<100	90%	75%	73%
Timely Help 'Always' Received[10]	<100	82%	71%	68%
Would Definitely Recommend Hospital[10]	<100	73%	75%	71%
Use of Medical Imaging				
Cardiac Imaging Stress Test before Surgery[7]	-	-	5.3%	5.3%
Combination Abdominal CT Scan	53	52.8%	24.5%	10.5%
Combination Brain/Sinus CT Scan[1]	-	-	2.6%	2.7%
Combination Chest CT Scan[1]	-	-	7.6%	2.7%
Follow-up Mammogram/Ultrasound[7]	-	-	9.4%	8.8%
Lumbar Spine MRI for Low Back Pain[1]	-	-	42.7%	37.2%

B R F Hospital Holdings

1541 Kings Highway — Phone: 318-675-5000
Shreveport, LA 71130 — Fax: 318-675-5666
URL: www.lsumc.edu
Type: Acute Care Hospitals — Emergency Services: Yes
Ownership: Voluntary non-profit - Private — Beds: 650

Key Personnel:
Pediatric Ambulatory Care . . . . . . Joseph Bocchini, MD
Pediatric In-Patient Care . . . . Joseph Bocchini, MD
Quality Assurance . . . . Ann Ford
Chief of Medical Staff. . . . . Ronald George
Radiology. . . . . James Lecky, MD
Infection Control. . . . . Robert Penn
CEO/President. . . . . Benjamin Rush, MD

Measure	Cases	This Hosp.	State Avg.	U.S. Avg.
Blood Clot Prevention and Treatment				
Anticoagulation Overlap Therapy[2]	55	85%	89%	93%
ICU Venous Thromboembolism Prophylaxis[2]	93	96%	88%	92%
Incidence of Potentially Preventable VTE[2]	29	10%	16%	10%
UFH with Dosages/Platelet Monitoring[2]	32	100%	94%	97%
Venous Thromboembolism Prophylaxis[2]	299	82%	74%	85%
Warfarin Therapy Discharge Instructions[2]	46	91%	85%	75%
Chest Pain/Possible Heart Attack Care				
Aspirin Given Within 24 Hours of Arrival[5]	-	-	94%	96%
Fibrinolytic Meds Within 30 Min. of Arrival[5]	-	-	54%	58%

NOTE: Hospital profiles are in alphabetical order by state, then city, then hospital within the city; Rankings exclude hospitals with less than 25 cases except for patient surveys which excludes hospitals with less than 100 cases; (a) 100-299 cases; (1) The number of cases/patients is too few to report; (2) Data submitted were based on a sample of cases/patients; (3) Results are based on a shorter time period than required; (4) Data suppressed by CMS for one or more quarters; (5) Results are not available for this reporting period; (6) Fewer than 100 patients completed the HCAHPS survey; (7) No cases met the criteria for this measure; (8) The lower limit of the confidence interval cannot be calculated if the number of observed infections equals zero; (9) No data are available from the state/territory for this reporting period; (10) The scores shown reflect fewer than 50 completed surveys; (11) There were discrepancies in the data collection process; (12) This measure does not apply to this hospital for this reporting period; (13) Results cannot be calculated for this reporting period; (14) The results for this state are combined with nearby states to protect confidentiality; Please refer to the User's Guide for a full explanation of data.

Measure	Cases	This Hosp.	State Avg.	U.S. Avg.
Average Time to ECG (minutes)[5]	-	-	10	7
Average Time to Transfer (minutes)[5]	-	-	94	60
Children's Asthma Care				
Received Home Management Plan of Care	-	-	-	88%
Received Reliever Medication	-	-	-	100%
Received Systemic Corticosteroids	-	-	-	100%
Emergency Department				
Admittance Decision Time (minutes)[2]	448	133	86	98
Head CT Results Within 45 Min. of Arrival[1,3]	-	-	49%	57%
Patients Who Left ER Before Being Seen	59,614	10%	3%	2%
Time from ER Arrival to Admit. (minutes)[2]	449	389	256	274
Time from ER Arrival to Discharge (minutes)	322	271	125	134
Time in ER Before Being Evaluated (minutes)	352	96	27	26
Time to Pain Meds for Fractures (minutes)	154	188	61	57
Heart Attack Care				
Aspirin Given at Discharge[2]	215	98%	99%	99%
Fibrinolytic Meds Within 30 Min. of Arrival[2,7]	-	-	71%	54%
PCI Within 90 Minutes of Arrival[2]	25	52%	94%	96%
Statin Prescribed at Discharge[2]	210	96%	98%	98%
Heart Failure Care				
ACE Inhibitor or ARB for LVSD[2]	168	96%	95%	97%
Discharge Instructions Given[2]	273	84%	94%	94%
Evaluation of LVS Function[2]	293	100%	97%	99%
Medicare Spending				
Medicare Spending per Patient (ratio)	-	0.96	1.04	0.98
Pneumonia Care				
Appropriate Initial Antibiotic Given[2]	22	86%	93%	95%
Blood Culture Timing[2]	54	83%	97%	98%
Pregnancy and Delivery Care				
Newborn Deliveries Scheduled Early[2]	28	0%	5%	6%
Preventive Care				
Immunization for Influenza[2]	512	60%	85%	90%
Immunization for Pneumonia[2]	427	72%	88%	92%
Stroke Care				
Anticoagulation Therapy for Atrial Fibrillation[1,2]	-	-	93%	95%
Antithrombotic Therapy Timing[2]	43	93%	96%	98%
Assessed for Rehabilitation[2]	93	95%	95%	97%
Discharged on Antithrombotic Therapy[2]	53	98%	97%	99%
Discharged on Statin Medication[2]	49	92%	89%	94%
Thrombolytic Therapy Timing[2,7]	-	-	53%	66%
Venous Thromboembolism Prophylaxis[2]	107	95%	87%	94%
Written Stroke Educational Materials Given[2]	55	58%	83%	88%
Surgical Care Improvement Project				
Appropriate Beta Blocker Usage[2]	149	97%	97%	98%
Appropriate VTP Within 24 Hours[2]	283	92%	97%	98%
Controlled Postoperative Blood Glucose[2]	87	93%	96%	97%
Perioperative Temperature Management[2]	359	100%	100%	100%
Prophylactic Antibiotic Selection[2]	311	96%	99%	99%
Prophylactic Antibiotic Selection (Outpatient)	113	96%	97%	98%
Prophylactic Antibiotic Stopped[2]	299	94%	97%	98%
Prophylactic Antibiotic Timing[2]	320	89%	98%	99%
Prophylactic Antibiotic Timing (Outpatient)	66	97%	97%	98%
Urinary Catheter Removal[2]	246	94%	96%	97%
Survey of Patients' Hospital Experiences				
Area Around Room 'Always' Quiet at Night	300+	60%	74%	61%
Doctors 'Always' Communicated Well	300+	78%	87%	82%
Home Recovery Information Given	300+	81%	85%	85%
Hospital Given 9 or 10 on 10 Point Scale	300+	62%	75%	71%
Meds 'Always' Explained Before Given	300+	60%	69%	64%
Nurses 'Always' Communicated Well	300+	75%	83%	79%
Pain 'Always' Well Controlled	300+	65%	75%	71%
Room and Bathroom 'Always' Clean	300+	56%	75%	73%
Timely Help 'Always' Received	300+	60%	71%	68%
Would Definitely Recommend Hospital	300+	68%	75%	71%
Use of Medical Imaging				
Cardiac Imaging Stress Test before Surgery	173	1.7%	5.3%	5.3%
Combination Abdominal CT Scan	379	15.3%	24.5%	10.5%
Combination Brain/Sinus CT Scan[1]	-	-	2.6%	2.7%
Combination Chest CT Scan	391	0.3%	7.6%	2.7%
Follow-up Mammogram/Ultrasound	1,197	2.5%	9.4%	8.8%
Lumbar Spine MRI for Low Back Pain[1]	-	-	42.7%	37.2%

Christus Health Shreveport - Bossier

1453 E Bert Kouns Industrial Drive Phone: 318-681-5000
Shreveport, LA 71105 Fax: 318-681-4424
E-mail: sally.croom@christushealth.org
URL: www.christusschumpert.org
Type: Acute Care Hospitals Emergency Services: Yes
Ownership: Voluntary non-profit - Church Beds: 601

Measure	Cases	This Hosp.	State Avg.	U.S. Avg.
Blood Clot Prevention and Treatment				
Anticoagulation Overlap Therapy[2]	50	92%	89%	93%
ICU Venous Thromboembolism Prophylaxis[2]	56	68%	88%	92%
Incidence of Potentially Preventable VTE[2]	20	40%	16%	10%
UFH with Dosages/Platelet Monitoring[1,2]	-	-	94%	97%
Venous Thromboembolism Prophylaxis[2]	377	69%	74%	85%
Warfarin Therapy Discharge Instructions[2]	35	89%	85%	75%
Chest Pain/Possible Heart Attack Care				
Aspirin Given Within 24 Hours of Arrival[1,3]	-	-	94%	96%
Fibrinolytic Meds Within 30 Min. of Arrival[3,7]	-	-	54%	58%
Average Time to ECG (minutes)[1,3]	-	-	10	7
Average Time to Transfer (minutes)[1,3]	-	-	94	60
Children's Asthma Care				
Received Home Management Plan of Care	-	-	-	88%
Received Reliever Medication	-	-	-	100%
Received Systemic Corticosteroids	-	-	-	100%
Emergency Department				
Admittance Decision Time (minutes)[2]	505	111	86	98
Head CT Results Within 45 Min. of Arrival[1]	-	-	49%	57%
Patients Who Left ER Before Being Seen	63,722	1%	3%	2%
Time from ER Arrival to Admit. (minutes)[2]	507	265	256	274
Time from ER Arrival to Discharge (minutes)	394	123	125	134
Time in ER Before Being Evaluated (minutes)	395	31	27	26
Time to Pain Meds for Fractures (minutes)	109	63	61	57
Heart Attack Care				
Aspirin Given at Discharge	117	97%	99%	99%
Fibrinolytic Meds Within 30 Min. of Arrival[7]	-	-	71%	54%
PCI Within 90 Minutes of Arrival[1]	-	-	94%	96%
Statin Prescribed at Discharge	110	93%	98%	98%
Heart Failure Care				
ACE Inhibitor or ARB for LVSD[2]	107	87%	95%	97%
Discharge Instructions Given[2]	228	86%	94%	94%
Evaluation of LVS Function[2]	283	99%	97%	99%
Medicare Spending				
Medicare Spending per Patient (ratio)	-	1.05	1.04	0.98
Pneumonia Care				
Appropriate Initial Antibiotic Given[2]	67	87%	93%	95%
Blood Culture Timing[2]	107	94%	97%	98%
Pregnancy and Delivery Care				
Newborn Deliveries Scheduled Early	305	1%	5%	6%
Preventive Care				
Immunization for Influenza[2]	507	93%	85%	90%
Immunization for Pneumonia[2]	561	94%	88%	92%
Stroke Care				
Anticoagulation Therapy for Atrial Fibrillation[2]	13	100%	93%	95%
Antithrombotic Therapy Timing[2]	93	97%	96%	98%
Assessed for Rehabilitation[2]	110	90%	95%	97%
Discharged on Antithrombotic Therapy[2]	95	99%	97%	99%
Discharged on Statin Medication[2]	82	77%	89%	94%
Thrombolytic Therapy Timing[2]	13	15%	53%	66%
Venous Thromboembolism Prophylaxis[2]	111	67%	87%	94%
Written Stroke Educational Materials Given[2]	49	18%	83%	88%
Surgical Care Improvement Project				
Appropriate Beta Blocker Usage[2]	144	97%	97%	98%
Appropriate VTP Within 24 Hours[2]	369	92%	97%	98%
Controlled Postoperative Blood Glucose[2]	24	83%	96%	97%
Perioperative Temperature Management[2]	440	100%	100%	100%
Prophylactic Antibiotic Selection[2]	335	96%	99%	99%
Prophylactic Antibiotic Selection (Outpatient)	213	95%	97%	98%
Prophylactic Antibiotic Stopped[2]	315	96%	97%	98%
Prophylactic Antibiotic Timing[2]	337	98%	98%	99%
Prophylactic Antibiotic Timing (Outpatient)	216	93%	97%	98%
Urinary Catheter Removal[2]	281	93%	96%	97%
Survey of Patients' Hospital Experiences				
Area Around Room 'Always' Quiet at Night	300+	64%	74%	61%
Doctors 'Always' Communicated Well	300+	85%	87%	82%
Home Recovery Information Given	300+	85%	85%	85%
Hospital Given 9 or 10 on 10 Point Scale	300+	71%	75%	71%
Meds 'Always' Explained Before Given	300+	67%	69%	64%
Nurses 'Always' Communicated Well	300+	79%	83%	79%
Pain 'Always' Well Controlled	300+	72%	75%	71%
Room and Bathroom 'Always' Clean	300+	70%	75%	73%
Timely Help 'Always' Received	300+	63%	71%	68%
Would Definitely Recommend Hospital	300+	75%	75%	71%
Use of Medical Imaging				
Cardiac Imaging Stress Test before Surgery	597	3.9%	5.3%	5.3%
Combination Abdominal CT Scan	1,147	1.7%	24.5%	10.5%
Combination Brain/Sinus CT Scan	904	1.9%	2.6%	2.7%
Combination Chest CT Scan	710	0.0%	7.6%	2.7%
Follow-up Mammogram/Ultrasound	3,083	8.0%	9.4%	8.8%
Lumbar Spine MRI for Low Back Pain	68	41.2%	42.7%	37.2%

Overton Brooks VA Medical Center - Shreveport

510 East Stoner Avenue Phone: 318-424-6037
Shreveport, LA 71101 Fax: 318-424-6156
E-mail: patricia.kim@med.va.gov
URL: www.va.gov/sta/guide/home.asp
Type: Acute Care - VA Emergency Services: No
Ownership: Government Federal Beds: 112

Key Personnel:

Patient Relations . . . . Bill Callahan
Radiology. . . . . Hong Chin, MD
Operating Room. . . . . Jeanne Niell, RN
Chief of Medical Staff . . . . Virginia W Short, MD
Anesthesiology. . . . . Praful Vakil, MD

Measure	Cases	This Hosp.	State Avg.	U.S. Avg.
Blood Clot Prevention and Treatment				
Anticoagulation Overlap Therapy	-	-	89%	93%
ICU Venous Thromboembolism Prophylaxis	-	-	88%	92%
Incidence of Potentially Preventable VTE	-	-	16%	10%
UFH with Dosages/Platelet Monitoring	-	-	94%	97%
Venous Thromboembolism Prophylaxis	-	-	74%	85%
Warfarin Therapy Discharge Instructions	-	-	85%	75%
Chest Pain/Possible Heart Attack Care				
Aspirin Given Within 24 Hours of Arrival	-	-	94%	96%
Fibrinolytic Meds Within 30 Min. of Arrival	-	-	54%	58%
Average Time to ECG (minutes)	-	-	10	7
Average Time to Transfer (minutes)	-	-	94	60
Children's Asthma Care				
Received Home Management Plan of Care	-	-	-	88%
Received Reliever Medication	-	-	-	100%
Received Systemic Corticosteroids	-	-	-	100%
Emergency Department				
Admittance Decision Time (minutes)	-	-	86	98
Head CT Results Within 45 Min. of Arrival	-	-	49%	57%
Patients Who Left ER Before Being Seen	-	-	3%	2%
Time from ER Arrival to Admit. (minutes)	-	-	256	274
Time from ER Arrival to Discharge (minutes)	-	-	125	134
Time in ER Before Being Evaluated (minutes)	-	-	27	26
Time to Pain Meds for Fractures (minutes)	-	-	61	57
Heart Attack Care				
Aspirin Given at Discharge	62	98%	99%	99%
Fibrinolytic Meds Within 30 Min. of Arrival[5]	-	-	71%	54%
PCI Within 90 Minutes of Arrival[1]	11	45%	94%	96%
Statin Prescribed at Discharge	63	100%	98%	98%
Heart Failure Care				
ACE Inhibitor or ARB for LVSD	110	99%	95%	97%
Discharge Instructions Given	205	97%	94%	94%
Evaluation of LVS Function	221	100%	97%	99%
Medicare Spending				
Medicare Spending per Patient (ratio)	-	-	1.04	0.98
Pneumonia Care				
Appropriate Initial Antibiotic Given	29	100%	93%	95%
Blood Culture Timing	59	100%	97%	98%
Pregnancy and Delivery Care				
Newborn Deliveries Scheduled Early	-	-	5%	6%
Preventive Care				
Immunization for Influenza[5]	-	-	85%	90%

NOTE: Hospital profiles are in alphabetical order by state, then city, then hospital within the city; Rankings exclude hospitals with less than 25 cases except for patient surveys which excludes hospitals with less than 100 cases; (a) 100-299 cases; (1) The number of cases/patients is too few to report; (2) Data submitted were based on a sample of cases/patients; (3) Results are based on a shorter time period than required; (4) Data suppressed by CMS for one or more quarters; (5) Results are not available for this reporting period; (6) Fewer than 100 patients completed the HCAHPS survey; (7) No cases met the criteria for this measure; (8) The lower limit of the confidence interval cannot be calculated if the number of observed infections equals zero; (9) No data are available from the state/territory for this reporting period; (10) The scores shown reflect fewer than 50 completed surveys; (11) There were discrepancies in the data collection process; (12) This measure does not apply to this hospital for this reporting period; (13) Results cannot be calculated for this reporting period; (14) The results for this state are combined with nearby states to protect confidentiality; Please refer to the User's Guide for a full explanation of data.

Measure	Cases	This Hosp.	State Avg.	U.S. Avg.
Immunization for Pneumonia[5]	-	-	88%	92%
Stroke Care				
Anticoagulation Therapy for Atrial Fibrillation	-	-	93%	95%
Antithrombotic Therapy Timing	-	-	96%	98%
Assessed for Rehabilitation	-	-	95%	97%
Discharged on Antithrombotic Therapy	-	-	97%	99%
Discharged on Statin Medication	-	-	89%	94%
Thrombolytic Therapy Timing	-	-	53%	66%
Venous Thromboembolism Prophylaxis	-	-	87%	94%
Written Stroke Educational Materials Given	-	-	83%	88%
Surgical Care Improvement Project				
Appropriate Beta Blocker Usage[2]	71	90%	97%	98%
Appropriate VTP Within 24 Hours[2]	157	97%	97%	98%
Controlled Postoperative Blood Glucose[5]	-	-	96%	97%
Perioperative Temperature Management[2]	174	100%	100%	100%
Prophylactic Antibiotic Selection	79	100%	99%	99%
Prophylactic Antibiotic Selection (Outpatient)	-	-	97%	98%
Prophylactic Antibiotic Stopped	77	94%	97%	98%
Prophylactic Antibiotic Timing	79	100%	98%	99%
Prophylactic Antibiotic Timing (Outpatient)	-	-	97%	98%
Urinary Catheter Removal[2]	93	100%	96%	97%
Survey of Patients' Hospital Experiences				
Area Around Room 'Always' Quiet at Night	-	-	74%	61%
Doctors 'Always' Communicated Well	-	-	87%	82%
Home Recovery Information Given	-	-	85%	85%
Hospital Given 9 or 10 on 10 Point Scale	-	-	75%	71%
Meds 'Always' Explained Before Given	-	-	69%	64%
Nurses 'Always' Communicated Well	-	-	83%	79%
Pain 'Always' Well Controlled	-	-	75%	71%
Room and Bathroom 'Always' Clean	-	-	75%	73%
Timely Help 'Always' Received	-	-	71%	68%
Would Definitely Recommend Hospital	-	-	75%	71%
Use of Medical Imaging				
Cardiac Imaging Stress Test before Surgery	-	-	5.3%	5.3%
Combination Abdominal CT Scan	-	-	24.5%	10.5%
Combination Brain/Sinus CT Scan	-	-	2.6%	2.7%
Combination Chest CT Scan	-	-	7.6%	2.7%
Follow-up Mammogram/Ultrasound	-	-	9.4%	8.8%
Lumbar Spine MRI for Low Back Pain	-	-	42.7%	37.2%

Specialists Hospital Shreveport

1500 Line Avenue
Shreveport, LA 71101
Phone: 318-213-3800
URL: www.specialistshospitalshreveport.com
Type: Acute Care Hospitals
Emergency Services: No
Ownership: Physician
Key Personnel:
CEO .... Kandi Moore

Measure	Cases	This Hosp.	State Avg.	U.S. Avg.
Blood Clot Prevention and Treatment				
Anticoagulation Overlap Therapy[2,7]	-	-	89%	93%
ICU Venous Thromboembolism Prophylaxis[2,7]	-	-	88%	92%
Incidence of Potentially Preventable VTE[2,7]	-	-	16%	10%
UFH with Dosages/Platelet Monitoring[2,7]	-	-	94%	97%
Venous Thromboembolism Prophylaxis[2]	108	96%	74%	85%
Warfarin Therapy Discharge Instructions[2,7]	-	-	85%	75%
Chest Pain/Possible Heart Attack Care				
Aspirin Given Within 24 Hours of Arrival[5]	-	-	94%	96%
Fibrinolytic Meds Within 30 Min. of Arrival[5]	-	-	54%	58%
Average Time to ECG (minutes)[5]	-	-	10	7
Average Time to Transfer (minutes)[5]	-	-	94	60
Children's Asthma Care				
Received Home Management Plan of Care	-	-	-	88%
Received Reliever Medication	-	-	-	100%
Received Systemic Corticosteroids	-	-	-	100%
Emergency Department				
Admittance Decision Time (minutes)[2,7]	-	-	86	98
Head CT Results Within 45 Min. of Arrival[5]	-	-	49%	57%
Patients Who Left ER Before Being Seen[5]	-	-	3%	2%
Time from ER Arrival to Admit. (minutes)[2,7]	-	-	256	274
Time from ER Arrival to Discharge (minutes)[5]	-	-	125	134
Time in ER Before Being Evaluated (minutes)[5]	-	-	27	26
Time to Pain Meds for Fractures (minutes)[5]	-	-	61	57
Heart Attack Care				
Aspirin Given at Discharge[5]	-	-	99%	99%
Fibrinolytic Meds Within 30 Min. of Arrival[5]	-	-	71%	54%
PCI Within 90 Minutes of Arrival[5]	-	-	94%	96%
Statin Prescribed at Discharge[5]	-	-	98%	98%
Heart Failure Care				
ACE Inhibitor or ARB for LVSD[5]	-	-	95%	97%
Discharge Instructions Given[5]	-	-	94%	94%
Evaluation of LVS Function[5]	-	-	97%	99%
Medicare Spending				
Medicare Spending per Patient (ratio)	-	0.99	1.04	0.98
Pneumonia Care				
Appropriate Initial Antibiotic Given[5]	-	-	93%	95%
Blood Culture Timing[5]	-	-	97%	98%
Pregnancy and Delivery Care				
Newborn Deliveries Scheduled Early[7]	-	-	5%	6%
Preventive Care				
Immunization for Influenza[2]	307	15%	85%	90%
Immunization for Pneumonia[2]	368	29%	88%	92%
Stroke Care				
Anticoagulation Therapy for Atrial Fibrillation[5]	-	-	93%	95%
Antithrombotic Therapy Timing[5]	-	-	96%	98%
Assessed for Rehabilitation[5]	-	-	95%	97%
Discharged on Antithrombotic Therapy[5]	-	-	97%	99%
Discharged on Statin Medication[5]	-	-	89%	94%
Thrombolytic Therapy Timing[5]	-	-	53%	66%
Venous Thromboembolism Prophylaxis[5]	-	-	87%	94%
Written Stroke Educational Materials Given[5]	-	-	83%	88%
Surgical Care Improvement Project				
Appropriate Beta Blocker Usage[2]	53	81%	97%	98%
Appropriate VTP Within 24 Hours[2]	204	99%	97%	98%
Controlled Postoperative Blood Glucose[2,7]	-	-	96%	97%
Perioperative Temperature Management[2]	214	100%	100%	100%
Prophylactic Antibiotic Selection[2]	195	100%	99%	99%
Prophylactic Antibiotic Selection (Outpatient)	408	100%	97%	98%
Prophylactic Antibiotic Stopped[2]	194	98%	97%	98%
Prophylactic Antibiotic Timing[2]	195	96%	98%	99%
Prophylactic Antibiotic Timing (Outpatient)	420	94%	97%	98%
Urinary Catheter Removal[2]	62	94%	96%	97%
Survey of Patients' Hospital Experiences				
Area Around Room 'Always' Quiet at Night	300+	86%	74%	61%
Doctors 'Always' Communicated Well	300+	88%	87%	82%
Home Recovery Information Given	300+	92%	85%	85%
Hospital Given 9 or 10 on 10 Point Scale	300+	89%	75%	71%
Meds 'Always' Explained Before Given	300+	77%	69%	64%
Nurses 'Always' Communicated Well	300+	89%	83%	79%
Pain 'Always' Well Controlled	300+	79%	75%	71%
Room and Bathroom 'Always' Clean	300+	82%	75%	73%
Timely Help 'Always' Received	300+	86%	71%	68%
Would Definitely Recommend Hospital	300+	90%	75%	71%
Use of Medical Imaging				
Cardiac Imaging Stress Test before Surgery[7]	-	-	5.3%	5.3%
Combination Abdominal CT Scan[7]	-	-	24.5%	10.5%
Combination Brain/Sinus CT Scan[1]	-	-	2.6%	2.7%
Combination Chest CT Scan[7]	-	-	7.6%	2.7%
Follow-up Mammogram/Ultrasound[7]	-	-	9.4%	8.8%
Lumbar Spine MRI for Low Back Pain[7]	-	-	42.7%	37.2%

Willis Knighton Medical Center

2600 Greenwood Road
Shreveport, LA 71103
Phone: 318-212-4000
URL: www.wkhs.com//locations/medicalcenter.aspx
Type: Acute Care Hospitals
Emergency Services: Yes
Ownership: Voluntary non-profit - Private
Key Personnel:
CEO/President............... James Elrod

Measure	Cases	This Hosp.	State Avg.	U.S. Avg.
Blood Clot Prevention and Treatment				
Anticoagulation Overlap Therapy[2]	178	90%	89%	93%
ICU Venous Thromboembolism Prophylaxis[2]	238	81%	88%	92%
Incidence of Potentially Preventable VTE[2]	51	39%	16%	10%
UFH with Dosages/Platelet Monitoring[2]	42	100%	94%	97%
Venous Thromboembolism Prophylaxis[2]	1,393	62%	74%	85%
Warfarin Therapy Discharge Instructions[2]	119	89%	85%	75%
Chest Pain/Possible Heart Attack Care				
Aspirin Given Within 24 Hours of Arrival	49	96%	94%	96%
Fibrinolytic Meds Within 30 Min. of Arrival[7]	-	-	54%	58%
Average Time to ECG (minutes)	51	10	10	7
Average Time to Transfer (minutes)[1]	-	-	94	60
Children's Asthma Care				
Received Home Management Plan of Care	-	-	-	88%
Received Reliever Medication	-	-	-	100%
Received Systemic Corticosteroids	-	-	-	100%
Emergency Department				
Admittance Decision Time (minutes)[2]	1,305	90	86	98
Head CT Results Within 45 Min. of Arrival	12	42%	49%	57%
Patients Who Left ER Before Being Seen	>100k	4%	3%	2%
Time from ER Arrival to Admit. (minutes)[2]	1,428	230	256	274
Time from ER Arrival to Discharge (minutes)	2,305	133	125	134
Time in ER Before Being Evaluated (minutes)	2,434	52	27	26
Time to Pain Meds for Fractures (minutes)	237	64	61	57
Heart Attack Care				
Aspirin Given at Discharge	486	99%	99%	99%
Fibrinolytic Meds Within 30 Min. of Arrival[7]	-	-	71%	54%
PCI Within 90 Minutes of Arrival	48	96%	94%	96%
Statin Prescribed at Discharge	465	95%	98%	98%
Heart Failure Care				
ACE Inhibitor or ARB for LVSD[2]	208	83%	95%	97%
Discharge Instructions Given[2]	481	88%	94%	94%
Evaluation of LVS Function[2]	587	99%	97%	99%
Medicare Spending				
Medicare Spending per Patient (ratio)	-	1.09	1.04	0.98
Pneumonia Care				
Appropriate Initial Antibiotic Given[2]	158	92%	93%	95%
Blood Culture Timing[2]	226	96%	97%	98%
Pregnancy and Delivery Care				
Newborn Deliveries Scheduled Early[2]	109	7%	5%	6%
Preventive Care				
Immunization for Influenza[2]	1,356	95%	85%	90%
Immunization for Pneumonia[2]	1,891	96%	88%	92%
Stroke Care				
Anticoagulation Therapy for Atrial Fibrillation[2]	31	84%	93%	95%
Antithrombotic Therapy Timing[2]	167	95%	96%	98%
Assessed for Rehabilitation[2]	173	90%	95%	97%
Discharged on Antithrombotic Therapy[2]	160	100%	97%	99%
Discharged on Statin Medication[2]	133	69%	89%	94%
Thrombolytic Therapy Timing[2]	13	31%	53%	66%
Venous Thromboembolism Prophylaxis[2]	179	59%	87%	94%
Written Stroke Educational Materials Given[2]	87	57%	83%	88%
Surgical Care Improvement Project				
Appropriate Beta Blocker Usage[2]	579	97%	97%	98%
Appropriate VTP Within 24 Hours[2]	1,002	98%	97%	98%
Controlled Postoperative Blood Glucose[2]	289	96%	96%	97%
Perioperative Temperature Management[2]	1,155	100%	100%	100%
Prophylactic Antibiotic Selection[2]	753	98%	99%	99%
Prophylactic Antibiotic Selection (Outpatient)	1,044	96%	97%	98%
Prophylactic Antibiotic Stopped[2]	724	93%	97%	98%
Prophylactic Antibiotic Timing[2]	758	97%	98%	99%
Prophylactic Antibiotic Timing (Outpatient)	1,034	97%	97%	98%
Urinary Catheter Removal[2]	760	93%	96%	97%
Survey of Patients' Hospital Experiences				
Area Around Room 'Always' Quiet at Night	300+	72%	74%	61%
Doctors 'Always' Communicated Well	300+	85%	87%	82%
Home Recovery Information Given	300+	86%	85%	85%
Hospital Given 9 or 10 on 10 Point Scale	300+	72%	75%	71%
Meds 'Always' Explained Before Given	300+	63%	69%	64%
Nurses 'Always' Communicated Well	300+	80%	83%	79%
Pain 'Always' Well Controlled	300+	75%	75%	71%
Room and Bathroom 'Always' Clean	300+	70%	75%	73%
Timely Help 'Always' Received	300+	67%	71%	68%
Would Definitely Recommend Hospital	300+	82%	75%	71%
Use of Medical Imaging				
Cardiac Imaging Stress Test before Surgery	217	8.3%	5.3%	5.3%
Combination Abdominal CT Scan	1,690	23.9%	24.5%	10.5%
Combination Brain/Sinus CT Scan	1,730	1.8%	2.6%	2.7%

NOTE: Hospital profiles are in alphabetical order by state, then city, then hospital within the city; Rankings exclude hospitals with less than 25 cases except for patient surveys which excludes hospitals with less than 100 cases; (a) 100-299 cases; (1) The number of cases/patients is too few to report; (2) Data submitted were based on a sample of cases/patients; (3) Results are based on a shorter time period than required; (4) Data suppressed by CMS for one or more quarters; (5) Results are not available for this reporting period; (6) Fewer than 100 patients completed the HCAHPS survey; (7) No cases met the criteria for this measure; (8) The lower limit of the confidence interval cannot be calculated if the number of observed infections equals zero; (9) No data are available from the state/territory for this reporting period; (10) The scores shown reflect fewer than 50 completed surveys; (11) There were discrepancies in the data collection process; (12) This measure does not apply to this hospital for this reporting period; (13) Results cannot be calculated for this reporting period; (14) The results for this state are combined with nearby states to protect confidentiality; Please refer to the User's Guide for a full explanation of data.

Combination Chest CT Scan	1,235	0.2%	7.6%	2.7%
Follow-up Mammogram/Ultrasound	3,325	8.7%	9.4%	8.8%
Lumbar Spine MRI for Low Back Pain	292	39.4%	42.7%	37.2%

Cypress Pointe Hospital East

989 Robert Blvd — Phone: 504-690-8200
Slidell, LA 70458
Type: Acute Care Hospitals — Emergency Services: No
Ownership: Proprietary

Measure	Cases	This Hosp.	State Avg.	U.S. Avg.
Blood Clot Prevention and Treatment				
Anticoagulation Overlap Therapy[2,7]	-	-	89%	93%
ICU Venous Thromboembolism Prophylaxis[2,7]	-	-	88%	92%
Incidence of Potentially Preventable VTE[2,7]	-	-	16%	10%
UFH with Dosages/Platelet Monitoring[2,7]	-	-	94%	97%
Venous Thromboembolism Prophylaxis[2]	11	73%	74%	85%
Warfarin Therapy Discharge Instructions[2,7]	-	-	85%	75%
Chest Pain/Possible Heart Attack Care				
Aspirin Given Within 24 Hours of Arrival[5]	-	-	94%	96%
Fibrinolytic Meds Within 30 Min. of Arrival[5]	-	-	54%	58%
Average Time to ECG (minutes)[5]	-	-	10	7
Average Time to Transfer (minutes)[5]	-	-	94	60
Children's Asthma Care				
Received Home Management Plan of Care	-	-	-	88%
Received Reliever Medication	-	-	-	100%
Received Systemic Corticosteroids	-	-	-	100%
Emergency Department				
Admittance Decision Time (minutes)[2,7]	-	-	86	98
Head CT Results Within 45 Min. of Arrival[5]	-	-	49%	57%
Patients Who Left ER Before Being Seen[5]	-	-	3%	2%
Time from ER Arrival to Admit. (minutes)[2,7]	-	-	256	274
Time from ER Arrival to Discharge (minutes)[5]	-	-	125	134
Time in ER Before Being Evaluated (minutes)[5]	-	-	27	26
Time to Pain Meds for Fractures (minutes)[5]	-	-	61	57
Heart Attack Care				
Aspirin Given at Discharge[5]	-	-	99%	99%
Fibrinolytic Meds Within 30 Min. of Arrival[5]	-	-	71%	54%
PCI Within 90 Minutes of Arrival[5]	-	-	94%	96%
Statin Prescribed at Discharge[5]	-	-	98%	98%
Heart Failure Care				
ACE Inhibitor or ARB for LVSD[5]	-	-	95%	97%
Discharge Instructions Given[5]	-	-	94%	94%
Evaluation of LVS Function[5]	-	-	97%	99%
Medicare Spending				
Medicare Spending per Patient (ratio)[1]	-	-	1.04	0.98
Pneumonia Care				
Appropriate Initial Antibiotic Given[5]	-	-	93%	95%
Blood Culture Timing[5]	-	-	97%	98%
Pregnancy and Delivery Care				
Newborn Deliveries Scheduled Early[7]	-	-	5%	6%
Preventive Care				
Immunization for Influenza[2]	39	100%	85%	90%
Immunization for Pneumonia[2]	27	100%	88%	92%
Stroke Care				
Anticoagulation Therapy for Atrial Fibrillation[5]	-	-	93%	95%
Antithrombotic Therapy Timing[5]	-	-	96%	98%
Assessed for Rehabilitation[5]	-	-	95%	97%
Discharged on Antithrombotic Therapy[5]	-	-	97%	99%
Discharged on Statin Medication[5]	-	-	89%	94%
Thrombolytic Therapy Timing[5]	-	-	53%	66%
Venous Thromboembolism Prophylaxis[5]	-	-	87%	94%
Written Stroke Educational Materials Given[5]	-	-	83%	88%
Surgical Care Improvement Project				
Appropriate Beta Blocker Usage[1,2]	-	-	97%	98%
Appropriate VTP Within 24 Hours[2]	19	89%	97%	98%
Controlled Postoperative Blood Glucose[2,7]	-	-	96%	97%
Perioperative Temperature Management[2]	23	100%	100%	100%
Prophylactic Antibiotic Selection[2]	15	93%	99%	99%
Prophylactic Antibiotic Selection (Outpatient)[3]	23	96%	97%	98%
Prophylactic Antibiotic Stopped[2]	15	100%	97%	98%
Prophylactic Antibiotic Timing[2]	15	93%	98%	99%
Prophylactic Antibiotic Timing (Outpatient)[3]	25	92%	97%	98%
Urinary Catheter Removal[2]	16	100%	96%	97%
Survey of Patients' Hospital Experiences				
Area Around Room 'Always' Quiet at Night[10]	<100	86%	74%	61%
Doctors 'Always' Communicated Well[10]	<100	89%	87%	82%
Home Recovery Information Given[10]	<100	84%	85%	85%
Hospital Given 9 or 10 on 10 Point Scale[10]	<100	73%	75%	71%
Meds 'Always' Explained Before Given[10]	<100	59%	69%	64%
Nurses 'Always' Communicated Well[10]	<100	85%	83%	79%
Pain 'Always' Well Controlled[10]	<100	81%	75%	71%
Room and Bathroom 'Always' Clean[10]	<100	77%	75%	73%
Timely Help 'Always' Received[10]	<100	80%	71%	68%
Would Definitely Recommend Hospital[10]	<100	82%	75%	71%
Use of Medical Imaging				
Cardiac Imaging Stress Test before Surgery[7]	-	-	5.3%	5.3%
Combination Abdominal CT Scan[1]	-	-	24.5%	10.5%
Combination Brain/Sinus CT Scan[1]	-	-	2.6%	2.7%
Combination Chest CT Scan[1]	-	-	7.6%	2.7%
Follow-up Mammogram/Ultrasound[7]	-	-	9.4%	8.8%
Lumbar Spine MRI for Low Back Pain[7]	-	-	42.7%	37.2%

Ochsner Medical Center - Northshore

100 Medical Center Drive — Phone: 985-649-7070
Slidell, LA 70461 — Fax: 985-646-5552
E-mail: rita.koder@tenethealth.com
URL: www.northshoremedctr.com
Type: Acute Care Hospitals — Emergency Services: Yes
Ownership: Voluntary non-profit - Private — Beds: 58

Key Personnel:
CEO/President. . . . . Alan R Cason
Radiology. . . . . David Jr
Quality Assurance . . . . Anglie Lolie

Measure	Cases	This Hosp.	State Avg.	U.S. Avg.
Blood Clot Prevention and Treatment				
Anticoagulation Overlap Therapy[2]	41	93%	89%	93%
ICU Venous Thromboembolism Prophylaxis[2]	122	89%	88%	92%
Incidence of Potentially Preventable VTE[1,2]	-	-	16%	10%
UFH with Dosages/Platelet Monitoring[1,2]	-	-	94%	97%
Venous Thromboembolism Prophylaxis[2]	338	84%	74%	85%
Warfarin Therapy Discharge Instructions[2]	28	93%	85%	75%
Chest Pain/Possible Heart Attack Care				
Aspirin Given Within 24 Hours of Arrival[3,7]	-	-	94%	96%
Fibrinolytic Meds Within 30 Min. of Arrival[5]	-	-	54%	58%
Average Time to ECG (minutes)[1,3]	-	-	10	7
Average Time to Transfer (minutes)[5]	-	-	94	60
Children's Asthma Care				
Received Home Management Plan of Care	-	-	-	88%
Received Reliever Medication	-	-	-	100%
Received Systemic Corticosteroids	-	-	-	100%
Emergency Department				
Admittance Decision Time (minutes)[2]	441	81	86	98
Head CT Results Within 45 Min. of Arrival	28	86%	49%	57%
Patients Who Left ER Before Being Seen	26,312	3%	3%	2%
Time from ER Arrival to Admit. (minutes)[2]	442	250	256	274
Time from ER Arrival to Discharge (minutes)	333	126	125	134
Time in ER Before Being Evaluated (minutes)	383	18	27	26
Time to Pain Meds for Fractures (minutes)	115	50	61	57
Heart Attack Care				
Aspirin Given at Discharge	94	99%	99%	99%
Fibrinolytic Meds Within 30 Min. of Arrival[7]	-	-	71%	54%
PCI Within 90 Minutes of Arrival	26	88%	94%	96%
Statin Prescribed at Discharge	98	100%	98%	98%
Heart Failure Care				
ACE Inhibitor or ARB for LVSD	63	98%	95%	97%
Discharge Instructions Given	173	100%	94%	94%
Evaluation of LVS Function	194	99%	97%	99%
Medicare Spending				
Medicare Spending per Patient (ratio)	-	1.00	1.04	0.98
Pneumonia Care				
Appropriate Initial Antibiotic Given	99	98%	93%	95%
Blood Culture Timing	236	97%	97%	98%
Pregnancy and Delivery Care				
Newborn Deliveries Scheduled Early[2]	32	0%	5%	6%
Preventive Care				
Immunization for Influenza[2]	444	83%	85%	90%
Immunization for Pneumonia[2]	567	83%	88%	92%
Stroke Care				
Anticoagulation Therapy for Atrial Fibrillation[1]	-	-	93%	95%
Antithrombotic Therapy Timing	48	100%	96%	98%
Assessed for Rehabilitation	52	96%	95%	97%
Discharged on Antithrombotic Therapy	51	98%	97%	99%
Discharged on Statin Medication	35	100%	89%	94%
Thrombolytic Therapy Timing[7]	-	-	53%	66%
Venous Thromboembolism Prophylaxis	50	92%	87%	94%
Written Stroke Educational Materials Given	33	100%	83%	88%
Surgical Care Improvement Project				
Appropriate Beta Blocker Usage	78	100%	97%	98%
Appropriate VTP Within 24 Hours	223	99%	97%	98%
Controlled Postoperative Blood Glucose	24	96%	96%	97%
Perioperative Temperature Management	250	100%	100%	100%
Prophylactic Antibiotic Selection	176	99%	99%	99%
Prophylactic Antibiotic Selection (Outpatient)	84	92%	97%	98%
Prophylactic Antibiotic Stopped	164	98%	97%	98%
Prophylactic Antibiotic Timing	177	99%	98%	99%
Prophylactic Antibiotic Timing (Outpatient)	86	98%	97%	98%
Urinary Catheter Removal	152	98%	96%	97%
Survey of Patients' Hospital Experiences				
Area Around Room 'Always' Quiet at Night	300+	71%	74%	61%
Doctors 'Always' Communicated Well	300+	80%	87%	82%
Home Recovery Information Given	300+	84%	85%	85%
Hospital Given 9 or 10 on 10 Point Scale	300+	66%	75%	71%
Meds 'Always' Explained Before Given	300+	58%	69%	64%
Nurses 'Always' Communicated Well	300+	78%	83%	79%
Pain 'Always' Well Controlled	300+	71%	75%	71%
Room and Bathroom 'Always' Clean	300+	63%	75%	73%
Timely Help 'Always' Received	300+	64%	71%	68%
Would Definitely Recommend Hospital	300+	67%	75%	71%
Use of Medical Imaging				
Cardiac Imaging Stress Test before Surgery	201	6.0%	5.3%	5.3%
Combination Abdominal CT Scan	237	12.2%	24.5%	10.5%
Combination Brain/Sinus CT Scan	229	0.4%	2.6%	2.7%
Combination Chest CT Scan	49	0.0%	7.6%	2.7%
Follow-up Mammogram/Ultrasound	130	8.5%	9.4%	8.8%
Lumbar Spine MRI for Low Back Pain[1]	-	-	42.7%	37.2%

Slidell Memorial Hospital

1001 Gause Blvd — Phone: 985-643-2200
Slidell, LA 70458 — Fax: 985-649-8778
URL: www.slidelmemorial.org
Type: Acute Care Hospitals — Emergency Services: Yes
Ownership: Govt - Hospital Dist/Auth — Beds: 182

Key Personnel:
Emergency Room . . . . Kumar Amaraneni, MD
Radiology. . . . . Dean Batten
Quality Assurance . . . . Jenny Bell
Coronary Care . . . . Tom Cook
CEO . . . . Bill Davis
Operating Room. . . . . Cary Gray
Chief of Medical Staff . . . . Robert Shafor, MD

Measure	Cases	This Hosp.	State Avg.	U.S. Avg.
Blood Clot Prevention and Treatment				
Anticoagulation Overlap Therapy[2]	50	100%	89%	93%
ICU Venous Thromboembolism Prophylaxis[2]	106	100%	88%	92%
Incidence of Potentially Preventable VTE[1,2]	-	-	16%	10%
UFH with Dosages/Platelet Monitoring[1,2]	-	-	94%	97%
Venous Thromboembolism Prophylaxis[2]	291	97%	74%	85%
Warfarin Therapy Discharge Instructions[2]	43	98%	85%	75%
Chest Pain/Possible Heart Attack Care				
Aspirin Given Within 24 Hours of Arrival[1,3]	-	-	94%	96%
Fibrinolytic Meds Within 30 Min. of Arrival[3,7]	-	-	54%	58%
Average Time to ECG (minutes)[1,3]	-	-	10	7
Average Time to Transfer (minutes)[3,7]	-	-	94	60
Children's Asthma Care				
Received Home Management Plan of Care	-	-	-	88%
Received Reliever Medication	-	-	-	100%
Received Systemic Corticosteroids	-	-	-	100%
Emergency Department				
Admittance Decision Time (minutes)[2]	302	120	86	98

NOTE: Hospital profiles are in alphabetical order by state, then city, then hospital within the city; Rankings exclude hospitals with less than 25 cases except for patient surveys which excludes hospitals with less than 100 cases; (a) 100-299 cases; (1) The number of cases/patients is too few to report; (2) Data submitted were based on a sample of cases/patients; (3) Results are based on a shorter time period than required; (4) Data suppressed by CMS for one or more quarters; (5) Results are not available for this reporting period; (6) Fewer than 100 patients completed the HCAHPS survey; (7) No cases met the criteria for this measure; (8) The lower limit of the confidence interval cannot be calculated if the number of observed infections equals zero; (9) No data are available from the state/territory for this reporting period; (10) The scores shown reflect fewer than 50 completed surveys; (11) There were discrepancies in the data collection process; (12) This measure does not apply to this hospital for this reporting period; (13) Results cannot be calculated for this reporting period; (14) The results for this state are combined with nearby states to protect confidentiality; Please refer to the User's Guide for a full explanation of data.

Measure	Cases	This Hosp.	State Avg.	U.S. Avg.
Head CT Results Within 45 Min. of Arrival[1]	-	-	49%	57%
Patients Who Left ER Before Being Seen	29,007	2%	3%	2%
Time from ER Arrival to Admit. (minutes)[2]	312	296	256	274
Time from ER Arrival to Discharge (minutes)	331	157	125	134
Time in ER Before Being Evaluated (minutes)	371	31	27	26
Time to Pain Meds for Fractures (minutes)	109	64	61	57
Heart Attack Care				
Aspirin Given at Discharge	126	100%	99%	99%
Fibrinolytic Meds Within 30 Min. of Arrival[7]	-	-	71%	54%
PCI Within 90 Minutes of Arrival	13	85%	94%	96%
Statin Prescribed at Discharge	123	100%	98%	98%
Heart Failure Care				
ACE Inhibitor or ARB for LVSD	67	100%	95%	97%
Discharge Instructions Given	205	87%	94%	94%
Evaluation of LVS Function	226	100%	97%	99%
Medicare Spending				
Medicare Spending per Patient (ratio)	-	1.03	1.04	0.98
Pneumonia Care				
Appropriate Initial Antibiotic Given	83	95%	93%	95%
Blood Culture Timing	190	99%	97%	98%
Pregnancy and Delivery Care				
Newborn Deliveries Scheduled Early[2]	80	9%	5%	6%
Preventive Care				
Immunization for Influenza[2]	523	98%	85%	90%
Immunization for Pneumonia[2]	645	98%	88%	92%
Stroke Care				
Anticoagulation Therapy for Atrial Fibrillation[1]	-	-	93%	95%
Antithrombotic Therapy Timing	43	100%	96%	98%
Assessed for Rehabilitation	60	98%	95%	97%
Discharged on Antithrombotic Therapy	50	98%	97%	99%
Discharged on Statin Medication	40	98%	89%	94%
Thrombolytic Therapy Timing[1]	-	-	53%	66%
Venous Thromboembolism Prophylaxis	47	100%	87%	94%
Written Stroke Educational Materials Given	39	95%	83%	88%
Surgical Care Improvement Project				
Appropriate Beta Blocker Usage	182	98%	97%	98%
Appropriate VTP Within 24 Hours	389	99%	97%	98%
Controlled Postoperative Blood Glucose	96	98%	96%	97%
Perioperative Temperature Management	436	100%	100%	100%
Prophylactic Antibiotic Selection	315	99%	99%	99%
Prophylactic Antibiotic Selection (Outpatient)	143	94%	97%	98%
Prophylactic Antibiotic Stopped	304	97%	97%	98%
Prophylactic Antibiotic Timing	315	99%	98%	99%
Prophylactic Antibiotic Timing (Outpatient)	143	100%	97%	98%
Urinary Catheter Removal	336	100%	96%	97%
Survey of Patients' Hospital Experiences				
Area Around Room 'Always' Quiet at Night	300+	60%	74%	61%
Doctors 'Always' Communicated Well	300+	82%	87%	82%
Home Recovery Information Given	300+	85%	85%	85%
Hospital Given 9 or 10 on 10 Point Scale	300+	67%	75%	71%
Meds 'Always' Explained Before Given	300+	59%	69%	64%
Nurses 'Always' Communicated Well	300+	78%	83%	79%
Pain 'Always' Well Controlled	300+	71%	75%	71%
Room and Bathroom 'Always' Clean	300+	66%	75%	73%
Timely Help 'Always' Received	300+	63%	71%	68%
Would Definitely Recommend Hospital	300+	72%	75%	71%
Use of Medical Imaging				
Cardiac Imaging Stress Test before Surgery	175	12.0%	5.3%	5.3%
Combination Abdominal CT Scan	605	44.5%	24.5%	10.5%
Combination Brain/Sinus CT Scan	523	2.7%	2.6%	2.7%
Combination Chest CT Scan	374	0.3%	7.6%	2.7%
Follow-up Mammogram/Ultrasound	999	9.7%	9.4%	8.8%
Lumbar Spine MRI for Low Back Pain	185	46.5%	42.7%	37.2%

Southern Surgical Hospital

1700 W Lindberg Drive
Slidell, LA 70458
Phone: 985-641-0600
URL: www.sshla.com
Type: Acute Care Hospitals
Emergency Services: No
Ownership: Physician
Key Personnel:
CEO .... Michael Pisciotta

Measure	Cases	This Hosp.	State Avg.	U.S. Avg.
Blood Clot Prevention and Treatment				
Anticoagulation Overlap Therapy[2,7]	-	-	89%	93%
ICU Venous Thromboembolism Prophylaxis[2,7]	-	-	88%	92%
Incidence of Potentially Preventable VTE[2,7]	-	-	16%	10%
UFH with Dosages/Platelet Monitoring[2,7]	-	-	94%	97%
Venous Thromboembolism Prophylaxis[2]	45	100%	74%	85%
Warfarin Therapy Discharge Instructions[2,7]	-	-	85%	75%
Chest Pain/Possible Heart Attack Care				
Aspirin Given Within 24 Hours of Arrival[5]	-	-	94%	96%
Fibrinolytic Meds Within 30 Min. of Arrival[5]	-	-	54%	58%
Average Time to ECG (minutes)[5]	-	-	10	7
Average Time to Transfer (minutes)[5]	-	-	94	60
Children's Asthma Care				
Received Home Management Plan of Care	-	-	-	88%
Received Reliever Medication	-	-	-	100%
Received Systemic Corticosteroids	-	-	-	100%
Emergency Department				
Admittance Decision Time (minutes)[2,7]	-	-	86	98
Head CT Results Within 45 Min. of Arrival[5]	-	-	49%	57%
Patients Who Left ER Before Being Seen[5]	-	-	3%	2%
Time from ER Arrival to Admit. (minutes)[2,7]	-	-	256	274
Time from ER Arrival to Discharge (minutes)[5]	-	-	125	134
Time in ER Before Being Evaluated (minutes)[5]	-	-	27	26
Time to Pain Meds for Fractures (minutes)[5]	-	-	61	57
Heart Attack Care				
Aspirin Given at Discharge[5]	-	-	99%	99%
Fibrinolytic Meds Within 30 Min. of Arrival[5]	-	-	71%	54%
PCI Within 90 Minutes of Arrival[5]	-	-	94%	96%
Statin Prescribed at Discharge[5]	-	-	98%	98%
Heart Failure Care				
ACE Inhibitor or ARB for LVSD[3,7]	-	-	95%	97%
Discharge Instructions Given[1,3]	-	-	94%	94%
Evaluation of LVS Function[1,3]	-	-	97%	99%
Medicare Spending				
Medicare Spending per Patient (ratio)	-	0.94	1.04	0.98
Pneumonia Care				
Appropriate Initial Antibiotic Given[5]	-	-	93%	95%
Blood Culture Timing[5]	-	-	97%	98%
Pregnancy and Delivery Care				
Newborn Deliveries Scheduled Early[7]	-	-	5%	6%
Preventive Care				
Immunization for Influenza[2]	301	53%	85%	90%
Immunization for Pneumonia[2]	263	52%	88%	92%
Stroke Care				
Anticoagulation Therapy for Atrial Fibrillation[5]	-	-	93%	95%
Antithrombotic Therapy Timing[5]	-	-	96%	98%
Assessed for Rehabilitation[5]	-	-	95%	97%
Discharged on Antithrombotic Therapy[5]	-	-	97%	99%
Discharged on Statin Medication[5]	-	-	89%	94%
Thrombolytic Therapy Timing[5]	-	-	53%	66%
Venous Thromboembolism Prophylaxis[5]	-	-	87%	94%
Written Stroke Educational Materials Given[5]	-	-	83%	88%
Surgical Care Improvement Project				
Appropriate Beta Blocker Usage[2]	32	100%	97%	98%
Appropriate VTP Within 24 Hours[2]	166	99%	97%	98%
Controlled Postoperative Blood Glucose[2,7]	-	-	96%	97%
Perioperative Temperature Management[2]	188	100%	100%	100%
Prophylactic Antibiotic Selection[2]	142	97%	99%	99%
Prophylactic Antibiotic Selection (Outpatient)	50	98%	97%	98%
Prophylactic Antibiotic Stopped[2]	142	91%	97%	98%
Prophylactic Antibiotic Timing[2]	142	99%	98%	99%
Prophylactic Antibiotic Timing (Outpatient)	50	100%	97%	98%
Urinary Catheter Removal[2]	125	90%	96%	97%
Survey of Patients' Hospital Experiences				
Area Around Room 'Always' Quiet at Night	300+	90%	74%	61%
Doctors 'Always' Communicated Well	300+	88%	87%	82%
Home Recovery Information Given	300+	88%	85%	85%
Hospital Given 9 or 10 on 10 Point Scale	300+	88%	75%	71%
Meds 'Always' Explained Before Given	300+	68%	69%	64%
Nurses 'Always' Communicated Well	300+	92%	83%	79%
Pain 'Always' Well Controlled	300+	82%	75%	71%
Room and Bathroom 'Always' Clean	300+	83%	75%	73%
Timely Help 'Always' Received	300+	85%	71%	68%
Would Definitely Recommend Hospital	300+	90%	75%	71%
Use of Medical Imaging				
Cardiac Imaging Stress Test before Surgery[7]	-	-	5.3%	5.3%
Combination Abdominal CT Scan[1]	-	-	24.5%	10.5%
Combination Brain/Sinus CT Scan[1]	-	-	2.6%	2.7%
Combination Chest CT Scan[1]	-	-	7.6%	2.7%
Follow-up Mammogram/Ultrasound[7]	-	-	9.4%	8.8%
Lumbar Spine MRI for Low Back Pain	44	38.6%	42.7%	37.2%

Springhill Medical Center

2001 Doctors Drive
Springhill, LA 71075
Phone: 318-539-1000
Fax: 318-539-4085
E-mail: derek.melancon@emailsmc.com
URL: www.smccare.com
Type: Acute Care Hospitals
Emergency Services: Yes
Ownership: Voluntary non-profit - Private
Beds: 60
Key Personnel:
Chairman/CEO .... David Anderson
Chief of Medical Staff.......... Luke Baudoin
Cardiac Laboratory............ Albert N Krause, MD
Quality Assurance .... Marilyn Mow
CEO/President............... Vincent Sedminik, BSHM
Pediatric In-Patient Care .... Christian Smith, DPM

Measure	Cases	This Hosp.	State Avg.	U.S. Avg.
Blood Clot Prevention and Treatment				
Anticoagulation Overlap Therapy[2]	16	75%	89%	93%
ICU Venous Thromboembolism Prophylaxis[2]	46	61%	88%	92%
Incidence of Potentially Preventable VTE[2,7]	-	-	16%	10%
UFH with Dosages/Platelet Monitoring[1,2]	-	-	94%	97%
Venous Thromboembolism Prophylaxis[2]	67	40%	74%	85%
Warfarin Therapy Discharge Instructions[1,2]	-	-	85%	75%
Chest Pain/Possible Heart Attack Care				
Aspirin Given Within 24 Hours of Arrival	38	95%	94%	96%
Fibrinolytic Meds Within 30 Min. of Arrival[1]	-	-	54%	58%
Average Time to ECG (minutes)	36	4	10	7
Average Time to Transfer (minutes)[7]	-	-	94	60
Children's Asthma Care				
Received Home Management Plan of Care	-	-	-	88%
Received Reliever Medication	-	-	-	100%
Received Systemic Corticosteroids	-	-	-	100%
Emergency Department				
Admittance Decision Time (minutes)[2]	595	53	86	98
Head CT Results Within 45 Min. of Arrival[1]	-	-	49%	57%
Patients Who Left ER Before Being Seen	9,148	2%	3%	2%
Time from ER Arrival to Admit. (minutes)[2]	604	130	256	274
Time from ER Arrival to Discharge (minutes)	1,159	79	125	134
Time in ER Before Being Evaluated (minutes)	1,107	21	27	26
Time to Pain Meds for Fractures (minutes)	47	38	61	57
Heart Attack Care				
Aspirin Given at Discharge[1,3]	-	-	99%	99%
Fibrinolytic Meds Within 30 Min. of Arrival[3,7]	-	-	71%	54%
PCI Within 90 Minutes of Arrival[3,7]	-	-	94%	96%
Statin Prescribed at Discharge[1,3]	-	-	98%	98%
Heart Failure Care				
ACE Inhibitor or ARB for LVSD[1]	-	-	95%	97%
Discharge Instructions Given	32	97%	94%	94%
Evaluation of LVS Function	44	98%	97%	99%
Medicare Spending				
Medicare Spending per Patient (ratio)	-	1.07	1.04	0.98
Pneumonia Care				
Appropriate Initial Antibiotic Given	42	90%	93%	95%
Blood Culture Timing	59	98%	97%	98%
Pregnancy and Delivery Care				
Newborn Deliveries Scheduled Early[7]	-	-	5%	6%
Preventive Care				
Immunization for Influenza[2]	436	95%	85%	90%
Immunization for Pneumonia[2]	634	97%	88%	92%
Stroke Care				
Anticoagulation Therapy for Atrial Fibrillation[1]	-	-	93%	95%
Antithrombotic Therapy Timing	14	93%	96%	98%
Assessed for Rehabilitation	15	93%	95%	97%
Discharged on Antithrombotic Therapy	13	92%	97%	99%
Discharged on Statin Medication	13	54%	89%	94%

NOTE: Hospital profiles are in alphabetical order by state, then city, then hospital within the city; Rankings exclude hospitals with less than 25 cases except for patient surveys which excludes hospitals with less than 100 cases; (a) 100-299 cases; (1) The number of cases/patients is too few to report; (2) Data submitted were based on a sample of cases/patients; (3) Results are based on a shorter time period than required; (4) Data suppressed by CMS for one or more quarters; (5) Results are not available for this reporting period; (6) Fewer than 100 patients completed the HCAHPS survey; (7) No cases met the criteria for this measure; (8) The lower limit of the confidence interval cannot be calculated if the number of observed infections equals zero; (9) No data are available from the state/territory for this reporting period; (10) The scores shown reflect fewer than 50 completed surveys; (11) There were discrepancies in the data collection process; (12) This measure does not apply to this hospital for this reporting period; (13) Results cannot be calculated for this reporting period; (14) The results for this state are combined with nearby states to protect confidentiality; Please refer to the User's Guide for a full explanation of data.

Measure	Cases	This Hosp.	State Avg.	U.S. Avg.
Thrombolytic Therapy Timing[1]	-	-	53%	66%
Venous Thromboembolism Prophylaxis	14	21%	87%	94%
Written Stroke Educational Materials Given[1]	-	-	83%	88%
Surgical Care Improvement Project				
Appropriate Beta Blocker Usage[1,3]	-	-	97%	98%
Appropriate VTP Within 24 Hours[1,3]	-	-	97%	98%
Controlled Postoperative Blood Glucose[3,7]	-	-	96%	97%
Perioperative Temperature Management[1,3]	-	-	100%	100%
Prophylactic Antibiotic Selection[1,3]	-	-	99%	99%
Prophylactic Antibiotic Selection (Outpatient)[3,7]	-	-	97%	98%
Prophylactic Antibiotic Stopped[3,7]	-	-	97%	98%
Prophylactic Antibiotic Timing[1,3]	-	-	98%	99%
Prophylactic Antibiotic Timing (Outpatient)[3,7]	-	-	97%	98%
Urinary Catheter Removal[1,3]	-	-	96%	97%
Survey of Patients' Hospital Experiences				
Area Around Room 'Always' Quiet at Night	(a)	73%	74%	61%
Doctors 'Always' Communicated Well	(a)	86%	87%	82%
Home Recovery Information Given	(a)	85%	85%	85%
Hospital Given 9 or 10 on 10 Point Scale	(a)	71%	75%	71%
Meds 'Always' Explained Before Given	(a)	70%	69%	64%
Nurses 'Always' Communicated Well	(a)	85%	83%	79%
Pain 'Always' Well Controlled	(a)	83%	75%	71%
Room and Bathroom 'Always' Clean	(a)	75%	75%	73%
Timely Help 'Always' Received	(a)	75%	71%	68%
Would Definitely Recommend Hospital	(a)	64%	75%	71%
Use of Medical Imaging				
Cardiac Imaging Stress Test before Surgery[1]	-	-	5.3%	5.3%
Combination Abdominal CT Scan	126	25.4%	24.5%	10.5%
Combination Brain/Sinus CT Scan[1]	-	-	2.6%	2.7%
Combination Chest CT Scan	50	2.0%	7.6%	2.7%
Follow-up Mammogram/Ultrasound	299	3.0%	9.4%	8.8%
Lumbar Spine MRI for Low Back Pain[1]	-	-	42.7%	37.2%

West Calcasieu Cameron Hospital

701 East Cypress Street
Sulphur, LA 70663
E-mail: info@wcch.com
URL: www.wcch.com
Phone: 337-527-7034
Fax: 337-527-4163
Type: Acute Care Hospitals
Ownership: Govt - Hospital Dist/Auth
Emergency Services: Yes
Beds: 120

Key Personnel:
Anesthesiology. . . . . Syd Dyer, MD
Chief of Medical Staff . . . . Josen Gonzales
CEO/President. . . . . Bill Hankins
Intensive Care Unit. . . . . Beth Hundley
Infection Control. . . . . Jolie Khoury
Operating Room. . . . . Walter P Ledet Jr
Quality Assurance . . . . Reta Manuel, RN
Emergency Room . . . . Tim Quattrone, MD

Measure	Cases	This Hosp.	State Avg.	U.S. Avg.
Blood Clot Prevention and Treatment				
Anticoagulation Overlap Therapy[2]	33	48%	89%	93%
ICU Venous Thromboembolism Prophylaxis[2]	78	85%	88%	92%
Incidence of Potentially Preventable VTE[1,2]	-	-	16%	10%
UFH with Dosages/Platelet Monitoring[2]	14	100%	94%	97%
Venous Thromboembolism Prophylaxis[2]	265	77%	74%	85%
Warfarin Therapy Discharge Instructions[2]	22	100%	85%	75%
Chest Pain/Possible Heart Attack Care				
Aspirin Given Within 24 Hours of Arrival[1,3]	-	-	94%	96%
Fibrinolytic Meds Within 30 Min. of Arrival[3,7]	-	-	54%	58%
Average Time to ECG (minutes)[1,3]	-	-	10	7
Average Time to Transfer (minutes)[3,7]	-	-	94	60
Children's Asthma Care				
Received Home Management Plan of Care	-	-	-	88%
Received Reliever Medication	-	-	-	100%
Received Systemic Corticosteroids	-	-	-	100%
Emergency Department				
Admittance Decision Time (minutes)[2]	436	68	86	98
Head CT Results Within 45 Min. of Arrival[1]	-	-	49%	57%
Patients Who Left ER Before Being Seen	25,898	3%	3%	2%
Time from ER Arrival to Admit. (minutes)[2]	448	210	256	274
Time from ER Arrival to Discharge (minutes)	512	96	125	134
Time in ER Before Being Evaluated (minutes)	518	31	27	26
Time to Pain Meds for Fractures (minutes)	156	46	61	57
Heart Attack Care				
Aspirin Given at Discharge	70	100%	99%	99%
Fibrinolytic Meds Within 30 Min. of Arrival[7]	-	-	71%	54%
PCI Within 90 Minutes of Arrival	24	92%	94%	96%
Statin Prescribed at Discharge	71	97%	98%	98%
Heart Failure Care				
ACE Inhibitor or ARB for LVSD	14	100%	95%	97%
Discharge Instructions Given	91	81%	94%	94%
Evaluation of LVS Function	105	100%	97%	99%
Medicare Spending				
Medicare Spending per Patient (ratio)	-	1.03	1.04	0.98
Pneumonia Care				
Appropriate Initial Antibiotic Given	67	96%	93%	95%
Blood Culture Timing	100	99%	97%	98%
Pregnancy and Delivery Care				
Newborn Deliveries Scheduled Early[2]	24	4%	5%	6%
Preventive Care				
Immunization for Influenza[2]	400	96%	85%	90%
Immunization for Pneumonia[2]	545	97%	88%	92%
Stroke Care				
Anticoagulation Therapy for Atrial Fibrillation	11	64%	93%	95%
Antithrombotic Therapy Timing	34	100%	96%	98%
Assessed for Rehabilitation	35	94%	95%	97%
Discharged on Antithrombotic Therapy	33	100%	97%	99%
Discharged on Statin Medication	24	83%	89%	94%
Thrombolytic Therapy Timing[1]	-	-	53%	66%
Venous Thromboembolism Prophylaxis	38	89%	87%	94%
Written Stroke Educational Materials Given	17	76%	83%	88%
Surgical Care Improvement Project				
Appropriate Beta Blocker Usage	127	96%	97%	98%
Appropriate VTP Within 24 Hours	432	98%	97%	98%
Controlled Postoperative Blood Glucose[7]	-	-	96%	97%
Perioperative Temperature Management	488	100%	100%	100%
Prophylactic Antibiotic Selection	353	99%	99%	99%
Prophylactic Antibiotic Selection (Outpatient)	31	97%	97%	98%
Prophylactic Antibiotic Stopped	349	99%	97%	98%
Prophylactic Antibiotic Timing	353	99%	98%	99%
Prophylactic Antibiotic Timing (Outpatient)	30	97%	97%	98%
Urinary Catheter Removal	314	99%	96%	97%
Survey of Patients' Hospital Experiences				
Area Around Room 'Always' Quiet at Night	300+	71%	74%	61%
Doctors 'Always' Communicated Well	300+	83%	87%	82%
Home Recovery Information Given	300+	86%	85%	85%
Hospital Given 9 or 10 on 10 Point Scale	300+	73%	75%	71%
Meds 'Always' Explained Before Given	300+	69%	69%	64%
Nurses 'Always' Communicated Well	300+	81%	83%	79%
Pain 'Always' Well Controlled	300+	76%	75%	71%
Room and Bathroom 'Always' Clean	300+	72%	75%	73%
Timely Help 'Always' Received	300+	70%	71%	68%
Would Definitely Recommend Hospital	300+	72%	75%	71%
Use of Medical Imaging				
Cardiac Imaging Stress Test before Surgery	189	2.1%	5.3%	5.3%
Combination Abdominal CT Scan	376	17.0%	24.5%	10.5%
Combination Brain/Sinus CT Scan	411	4.9%	2.6%	2.7%
Combination Chest CT Scan	264	11.4%	7.6%	2.7%
Follow-up Mammogram/Ultrasound	846	12.1%	9.4%	8.8%
Lumbar Spine MRI for Low Back Pain	124	29.8%	42.7%	37.2%

Thibodaux Regional Medical Center

602 N Acadia Road
Thibodaux, LA 70301
E-mail: info@thibodaux.com
URL: www.thibodaux.com
Phone: 985-447-5500
Fax: 985-449-2533
Type: Acute Care Hospitals
Ownership: Govt - Hospital Dist/Auth
Emergency Services: Yes
Beds: 185

Key Personnel:
Radiology. . . . . Blain Arthurs, MD
Infection Control. . . . . Rita Cade
Chief of Medical Staff . . . . Leo Hebert
Emergency Room . . . . Missy Keiffe
Intensive Care Unit. . . . . Missy Keiffe
Pediatric Ambulatory Care . . . . . . Henry Peltier
Pediatric In-Patient Care . . . . Henry Peltier
CEO/President. . . . . Greg Stock

Measure	Cases	This Hosp.	State Avg.	U.S. Avg.
Blood Clot Prevention and Treatment				
Anticoagulation Overlap Therapy[2]	42	100%	89%	93%
ICU Venous Thromboembolism Prophylaxis[2]	109	96%	88%	92%
Incidence of Potentially Preventable VTE[1,2]	-	-	16%	10%
UFH with Dosages/Platelet Monitoring[2]	36	100%	94%	97%
Venous Thromboembolism Prophylaxis[2]	330	97%	74%	85%
Warfarin Therapy Discharge Instructions[2]	21	95%	85%	75%
Chest Pain/Possible Heart Attack Care				
Aspirin Given Within 24 Hours of Arrival[1,3]	-	-	94%	96%
Fibrinolytic Meds Within 30 Min. of Arrival[5]	-	-	54%	58%
Average Time to ECG (minutes)[1,3]	-	-	10	7
Average Time to Transfer (minutes)[5]	-	-	94	60
Children's Asthma Care				
Received Home Management Plan of Care	-	-	-	88%
Received Reliever Medication	-	-	-	100%
Received Systemic Corticosteroids	-	-	-	100%
Emergency Department				
Admittance Decision Time (minutes)[2]	614	70	86	98
Head CT Results Within 45 Min. of Arrival[1]	-	-	49%	57%
Patients Who Left ER Before Being Seen	34,425	2%	3%	2%
Time from ER Arrival to Admit. (minutes)[2]	617	265	256	274
Time from ER Arrival to Discharge (minutes)	409	148	125	134
Time in ER Before Being Evaluated (minutes)	439	42	27	26
Time to Pain Meds for Fractures (minutes)	122	72	61	57
Heart Attack Care				
Aspirin Given at Discharge	194	100%	99%	99%
Fibrinolytic Meds Within 30 Min. of Arrival[7]	-	-	71%	54%
PCI Within 90 Minutes of Arrival	30	93%	94%	96%
Statin Prescribed at Discharge	194	100%	98%	98%
Heart Failure Care				
ACE Inhibitor or ARB for LVSD	67	99%	95%	97%
Discharge Instructions Given	233	100%	94%	94%
Evaluation of LVS Function	294	100%	97%	99%
Medicare Spending				
Medicare Spending per Patient (ratio)	-	1.01	1.04	0.98
Pneumonia Care				
Appropriate Initial Antibiotic Given	71	96%	93%	95%
Blood Culture Timing	142	98%	97%	98%
Pregnancy and Delivery Care				
Newborn Deliveries Scheduled Early[2]	71	7%	5%	6%
Preventive Care				
Immunization for Influenza[2]	587	97%	85%	90%
Immunization for Pneumonia[2]	736	98%	88%	92%
Stroke Care				
Anticoagulation Therapy for Atrial Fibrillation[1]	-	-	93%	95%
Antithrombotic Therapy Timing	83	100%	96%	98%
Assessed for Rehabilitation	99	100%	95%	97%
Discharged on Antithrombotic Therapy	85	100%	97%	99%
Discharged on Statin Medication	69	99%	89%	94%
Thrombolytic Therapy Timing[1]	-	-	53%	66%
Venous Thromboembolism Prophylaxis	101	99%	87%	94%
Written Stroke Educational Materials Given	54	100%	83%	88%
Surgical Care Improvement Project				
Appropriate Beta Blocker Usage	237	99%	97%	98%
Appropriate VTP Within 24 Hours	434	99%	97%	98%
Controlled Postoperative Blood Glucose	81	95%	96%	97%
Perioperative Temperature Management	498	100%	100%	100%
Prophylactic Antibiotic Selection	411	100%	99%	99%
Prophylactic Antibiotic Selection (Outpatient)	361	98%	97%	98%
Prophylactic Antibiotic Stopped	403	100%	97%	98%
Prophylactic Antibiotic Timing	411	100%	98%	99%
Prophylactic Antibiotic Timing (Outpatient)	357	99%	97%	98%
Urinary Catheter Removal	398	100%	96%	97%
Survey of Patients' Hospital Experiences				
Area Around Room 'Always' Quiet at Night	300+	78%	74%	61%
Doctors 'Always' Communicated Well	300+	89%	87%	82%
Home Recovery Information Given	300+	87%	85%	85%
Hospital Given 9 or 10 on 10 Point Scale	300+	78%	75%	71%
Meds 'Always' Explained Before Given	300+	68%	69%	64%
Nurses 'Always' Communicated Well	300+	87%	83%	79%
Pain 'Always' Well Controlled	300+	74%	75%	71%

NOTE: Hospital profiles are in alphabetical order by state, then city, then hospital within the city; Rankings exclude hospitals with less than 25 cases except for patient surveys which excludes hospitals with less than 100 cases; (a) 100-299 cases; (1) The number of cases/patients is too few to report; (2) Data submitted were based on a sample of cases/patients; (3) Results are based on a shorter time period than required; (4) Data suppressed by CMS for one or more quarters; (5) Results are not available for this reporting period; (6) Fewer than 100 patients completed the HCAHPS survey; (7) No cases met the criteria for this measure; (8) The lower limit of the confidence interval cannot be calculated if the number of observed infections equals zero; (9) No data are available from the state/territory for this reporting period; (10) The scores shown reflect fewer than 50 completed surveys; (11) There were discrepancies in the data collection process; (12) This measure does not apply to this hospital for this reporting period; (13) Results cannot be calculated for this reporting period; (14) The results for this state are combined with nearby states to protect confidentiality; Please refer to the User's Guide for a full explanation of data.

Room and Bathroom 'Always' Clean	300+	79%	75%	73%
Timely Help 'Always' Received	300+	72%	71%	68%
Would Definitely Recommend Hospital	300+	83%	75%	71%
Use of Medical Imaging				
Cardiac Imaging Stress Test before Surgery[7]	-	-	5.3%	5.3%
Combination Abdominal CT Scan	758	42.7%	24.5%	10.5%
Combination Brain/Sinus CT Scan	547	0.7%	2.6%	2.7%
Combination Chest CT Scan	401	0.0%	7.6%	2.7%
Follow-up Mammogram/Ultrasound	1,458	4.5%	9.4%	8.8%
Lumbar Spine MRI for Low Back Pain	111	37.8%	42.7%	37.2%

Mercy Regional Medical Center

800 E Main
Ville Platte, LA 70586
Phone: 337-363-5684
Fax: 337-363-9488
E-mail: dana.mcdaniel@lpnt.net
URL: www.vpmc.com
Type: Acute Care Hospitals
Emergency Services: Yes
Ownership: Proprietary
Beds: 102

Key Personnel:
Quality Assurance . . . . Gene Amons, RN
President/CEO. . . . . Thomas D. Gessel, FACHE
Cardiac Laboratory. . . . . Jeanett LeDay, RN
Chief of Medical Staff . . . . Charles Monier, MD
Radiology. . . . . Steven Pitre
Operating Room. . . . . Michelle Reed, RN
Infection Control. . . . . Melissa Soileau, RN

Measure	Cases	This Hosp.	State Avg.	U.S. Avg.
Blood Clot Prevention and Treatment				
Anticoagulation Overlap Therapy[2]	23	96%	89%	93%
ICU Venous Thromboembolism Prophylaxis[2]	88	97%	88%	92%
Incidence of Potentially Preventable VTE[1,2]	-	-	16%	10%
UFH with Dosages/Platelet Monitoring[2,7]	-	-	94%	97%
Venous Thromboembolism Prophylaxis[2]	308	92%	74%	85%
Warfarin Therapy Discharge Instructions[2]	14	93%	85%	75%
Chest Pain/Possible Heart Attack Care				
Aspirin Given Within 24 Hours of Arrival	58	93%	94%	96%
Fibrinolytic Meds Within 30 Min. of Arrival[1]	-	-	54%	58%
Average Time to ECG (minutes)	62	1	10	7
Average Time to Transfer (minutes)[1]	-	-	94	60
Children's Asthma Care				
Received Home Management Plan of Care	-	-	-	88%
Received Reliever Medication	-	-	-	100%
Received Systemic Corticosteroids	-	-	-	100%
Emergency Department				
Admittance Decision Time (minutes)[2]	282	48	86	98
Head CT Results Within 45 Min. of Arrival[1]	-	-	49%	57%
Patients Who Left ER Before Being Seen	24,942	1%	3%	2%
Time from ER Arrival to Admit. (minutes)[2]	310	184	256	274
Time from ER Arrival to Discharge (minutes)	354	80	125	134
Time in ER Before Being Evaluated (minutes)	409	12	27	26
Time to Pain Meds for Fractures (minutes)	64	36	61	57
Heart Attack Care				
Aspirin Given at Discharge	18	89%	99%	99%
Fibrinolytic Meds Within 30 Min. of Arrival[7]	-	-	71%	54%
PCI Within 90 Minutes of Arrival[7]	-	-	94%	96%
Statin Prescribed at Discharge	18	94%	98%	98%
Heart Failure Care				
ACE Inhibitor or ARB for LVSD	54	94%	95%	97%
Discharge Instructions Given	119	100%	94%	94%
Evaluation of LVS Function	167	99%	97%	99%
Medicare Spending				
Medicare Spending per Patient (ratio)	-	1.13	1.04	0.98
Pneumonia Care				
Appropriate Initial Antibiotic Given	132	98%	93%	95%
Blood Culture Timing	174	99%	97%	98%
Pregnancy and Delivery Care				
Newborn Deliveries Scheduled Early[2]	55	5%	5%	6%
Preventive Care				
Immunization for Influenza[2]	415	99%	85%	90%
Immunization for Pneumonia[2]	470	98%	88%	92%
Stroke Care				
Anticoagulation Therapy for Atrial Fibrillation[7]	-	-	93%	95%
Antithrombotic Therapy Timing	24	100%	96%	98%
Assessed for Rehabilitation	22	100%	95%	97%
Discharged on Antithrombotic Therapy	21	100%	97%	99%
Discharged on Statin Medication	17	100%	89%	94%
Thrombolytic Therapy Timing[1]	-	-	53%	66%
Venous Thromboembolism Prophylaxis	24	100%	87%	94%
Written Stroke Educational Materials Given[1]	-	-	83%	88%
Surgical Care Improvement Project				
Appropriate Beta Blocker Usage	31	87%	97%	98%
Appropriate VTP Within 24 Hours	121	96%	97%	98%
Controlled Postoperative Blood Glucose[7]	-	-	96%	97%
Perioperative Temperature Management	139	100%	100%	100%
Prophylactic Antibiotic Selection	79	99%	99%	99%
Prophylactic Antibiotic Selection (Outpatient)	76	95%	97%	98%
Prophylactic Antibiotic Stopped	72	96%	97%	98%
Prophylactic Antibiotic Timing	79	100%	98%	99%
Prophylactic Antibiotic Timing (Outpatient)	77	99%	97%	98%
Urinary Catheter Removal	50	100%	96%	97%
Survey of Patients' Hospital Experiences				
Area Around Room 'Always' Quiet at Night	300+	67%	74%	61%
Doctors 'Always' Communicated Well	300+	87%	87%	82%
Home Recovery Information Given	300+	87%	85%	85%
Hospital Given 9 or 10 on 10 Point Scale	300+	68%	75%	71%
Meds 'Always' Explained Before Given	300+	64%	69%	64%
Nurses 'Always' Communicated Well	300+	77%	83%	79%
Pain 'Always' Well Controlled	300+	70%	75%	71%
Room and Bathroom 'Always' Clean	300+	71%	75%	73%
Timely Help 'Always' Received	300+	64%	71%	68%
Would Definitely Recommend Hospital	300+	70%	75%	71%
Use of Medical Imaging				
Cardiac Imaging Stress Test before Surgery	202	4.5%	5.3%	5.3%
Combination Abdominal CT Scan	534	45.3%	24.5%	10.5%
Combination Brain/Sinus CT Scan	566	1.8%	2.6%	2.7%
Combination Chest CT Scan	310	28.1%	7.6%	2.7%
Follow-up Mammogram/Ultrasound	822	12.8%	9.4%	8.8%
Lumbar Spine MRI for Low Back Pain	140	45.7%	42.7%	37.2%

North Caddo Medical Center

1000 South Spruce St
Vivian, LA 71082
Phone: 318-375-3235
Type: Critical Access Hospitals
Emergency Services: Yes
Ownership: Govt - Hospital Dist/Auth

Measure	Cases	This Hosp.	State Avg.	U.S. Avg.
Blood Clot Prevention and Treatment				
Anticoagulation Overlap Therapy[5]	-	-	89%	93%
ICU Venous Thromboembolism Prophylaxis[5]	-	-	88%	92%
Incidence of Potentially Preventable VTE[5]	-	-	16%	10%
UFH with Dosages/Platelet Monitoring[5]	-	-	94%	97%
Venous Thromboembolism Prophylaxis[5]	-	-	74%	85%
Warfarin Therapy Discharge Instructions[5]	-	-	85%	75%
Chest Pain/Possible Heart Attack Care				
Aspirin Given Within 24 Hours of Arrival	-	-	94%	96%
Fibrinolytic Meds Within 30 Min. of Arrival	-	-	54%	58%
Average Time to ECG (minutes)	-	-	10	7
Average Time to Transfer (minutes)	-	-	94	60
Children's Asthma Care				
Received Home Management Plan of Care	-	-	-	88%
Received Reliever Medication	-	-	-	100%
Received Systemic Corticosteroids	-	-	-	100%
Emergency Department				
Admittance Decision Time (minutes)[5]	-	-	86	98
Head CT Results Within 45 Min. of Arrival	-	-	49%	57%
Patients Who Left ER Before Being Seen	-	-	3%	2%
Time from ER Arrival to Admit. (minutes)[5]	-	-	256	274
Time from ER Arrival to Discharge (minutes)	-	-	125	134
Time in ER Before Being Evaluated (minutes)	-	-	27	26
Time to Pain Meds for Fractures (minutes)	-	-	61	57
Heart Attack Care				
Aspirin Given at Discharge[1,3]	-	-	99%	99%
Fibrinolytic Meds Within 30 Min. of Arrival[3,7]	-	-	71%	54%
PCI Within 90 Minutes of Arrival[3,7]	-	-	94%	96%
Statin Prescribed at Discharge[1,3]	-	-	98%	98%
Heart Failure Care				
ACE Inhibitor or ARB for LVSD[3]	13	92%	95%	97%
Discharge Instructions Given[3]	12	100%	94%	94%
Evaluation of LVS Function[3]	17	100%	97%	99%
Medicare Spending				
Medicare Spending per Patient (ratio)	-	-	1.04	0.98
Pneumonia Care				
Appropriate Initial Antibiotic Given[3]	20	95%	93%	95%
Blood Culture Timing[3]	19	89%	97%	98%
Pregnancy and Delivery Care				
Newborn Deliveries Scheduled Early[5]	-	-	5%	6%
Preventive Care				
Immunization for Influenza[5]	-	-	85%	90%
Immunization for Pneumonia[5]	-	-	88%	92%
Stroke Care				
Anticoagulation Therapy for Atrial Fibrillation[5]	-	-	93%	95%
Antithrombotic Therapy Timing[5]	-	-	96%	98%
Assessed for Rehabilitation[5]	-	-	95%	97%
Discharged on Antithrombotic Therapy[5]	-	-	97%	99%
Discharged on Statin Medication[5]	-	-	89%	94%
Thrombolytic Therapy Timing[5]	-	-	53%	66%
Venous Thromboembolism Prophylaxis[5]	-	-	87%	94%
Written Stroke Educational Materials Given[5]	-	-	83%	88%
Surgical Care Improvement Project				
Appropriate Beta Blocker Usage[5]	-	-	97%	98%
Appropriate VTP Within 24 Hours[5]	-	-	97%	98%
Controlled Postoperative Blood Glucose[5]	-	-	96%	97%
Perioperative Temperature Management[5]	-	-	100%	100%
Prophylactic Antibiotic Selection[5]	-	-	99%	99%
Prophylactic Antibiotic Selection (Outpatient)	-	-	97%	98%
Prophylactic Antibiotic Stopped[5]	-	-	97%	98%
Prophylactic Antibiotic Timing[5]	-	-	98%	99%
Prophylactic Antibiotic Timing (Outpatient)	-	-	97%	98%
Urinary Catheter Removal[5]	-	-	96%	97%
Survey of Patients' Hospital Experiences				
Area Around Room 'Always' Quiet at Night[5]	-	-	74%	61%
Doctors 'Always' Communicated Well[5]	-	-	87%	82%
Home Recovery Information Given[5]	-	-	85%	85%
Hospital Given 9 or 10 on 10 Point Scale[5]	-	-	75%	71%
Meds 'Always' Explained Before Given[5]	-	-	69%	64%
Nurses 'Always' Communicated Well[5]	-	-	83%	79%
Pain 'Always' Well Controlled[5]	-	-	75%	71%
Room and Bathroom 'Always' Clean[5]	-	-	75%	73%
Timely Help 'Always' Received[5]	-	-	71%	68%
Would Definitely Recommend Hospital[5]	-	-	75%	71%
Use of Medical Imaging				
Cardiac Imaging Stress Test before Surgery	-	-	5.3%	5.3%
Combination Abdominal CT Scan	-	-	24.5%	10.5%
Combination Brain/Sinus CT Scan	-	-	2.6%	2.7%
Combination Chest CT Scan	-	-	7.6%	2.7%
Follow-up Mammogram/Ultrasound	-	-	9.4%	8.8%
Lumbar Spine MRI for Low Back Pain	-	-	42.7%	37.2%

Glenwood Regional Medical Center

503 Mcmillan Road
West Monroe, LA 71291
Phone: 318-329-4600
Fax: 318-329-4710
URL: www.grmc.com
Type: Acute Care Hospitals
Emergency Services: Yes
Ownership: Proprietary
Beds: 244

Key Personnel:
Coronary Care. . . . . Michael Ballinger
Pediatric In-Patient Care . . . . Naomi Bamburg
Radiology. . . . . Sandy Caselo
CEO/President. . . . . Ron Elder
Quality Assurance . . . . Charlene Jackson
Operating Room. . . . . Mandy Nolan
Chief of Medical Staff. . . . . Joe Travis, MD
Infection Control. . . . . Brandi Vaughn

Measure	Cases	This Hosp.	State Avg.	U.S. Avg.
Blood Clot Prevention and Treatment				
Anticoagulation Overlap Therapy[2]	70	87%	89%	93%
ICU Venous Thromboembolism Prophylaxis[2]	102	76%	88%	92%
Incidence of Potentially Preventable VTE[2]	24	21%	16%	10%
UFH with Dosages/Platelet Monitoring[2]	13	100%	94%	97%
Venous Thromboembolism Prophylaxis[2]	385	61%	74%	85%
Warfarin Therapy Discharge Instructions[2]	42	100%	85%	75%

NOTE: Hospital profiles are in alphabetical order by state, then city, then hospital within the city; Rankings exclude hospitals with less than 25 cases except for patient surveys which excludes hospitals with less than 100 cases; (a) 100-299 cases; (1) The number of cases/patients is too few to report; (2) Data submitted were based on a sample of cases/patients; (3) Results are based on a shorter time period than required; (4) Data suppressed by CMS for one or more quarters; (5) Results are not available for this reporting period; (6) Fewer than 100 patients completed the HCAHPS survey; (7) No cases met the criteria for this measure; (8) The lower limit of the confidence interval cannot be calculated if the number of observed infections equals zero; (9) No data are available from the state/territory for this reporting period; (10) The scores shown reflect fewer than 50 completed surveys; (11) There were discrepancies in the data collection process; (12) This measure does not apply to this hospital for this reporting period; (13) Results cannot be calculated for this reporting period; (14) The results for this state are combined with nearby states to protect confidentiality; Please refer to the User's Guide for a full explanation of data.

Measure	Cases	This Hosp.	State Avg.	U.S. Avg.
Chest Pain/Possible Heart Attack Care				
Aspirin Given Within 24 Hours of Arrival[1,3]	-	-	94%	96%
Fibrinolytic Meds Within 30 Min. of Arrival[3,7]	-	-	54%	58%
Average Time to ECG (minutes)[1,3]	-	-	10	7
Average Time to Transfer (minutes)[3,7]	-	-	94	60
Children's Asthma Care				
Received Home Management Plan of Care	-	-	-	88%
Received Reliever Medication	-	-	-	100%
Received Systemic Corticosteroids	-	-	-	100%
Emergency Department				
Admittance Decision Time (minutes)[2]	697	124	86	98
Head CT Results Within 45 Min. of Arrival[1,3]	-	-	49%	57%
Patients Who Left ER Before Being Seen	28,120	3%	3%	2%
Time from ER Arrival to Admit. (minutes)[2]	702	291	256	274
Time from ER Arrival to Discharge (minutes)	473	148	125	134
Time in ER Before Being Evaluated (minutes)	532	40	27	26
Time to Pain Meds for Fractures (minutes)	105	68	61	57
Heart Attack Care				
Aspirin Given at Discharge	376	100%	99%	99%
Fibrinolytic Meds Within 30 Min. of Arrival[7]	-	-	71%	54%
PCI Within 90 Minutes of Arrival	27	96%	94%	96%
Statin Prescribed at Discharge	340	99%	98%	98%
Heart Failure Care				
ACE Inhibitor or ARB for LVSD	106	99%	95%	97%
Discharge Instructions Given	305	99%	94%	94%
Evaluation of LVS Function	408	100%	97%	99%
Medicare Spending				
Medicare Spending per Patient (ratio)	-	1.07	1.04	0.98
Pneumonia Care				
Appropriate Initial Antibiotic Given	110	95%	93%	95%
Blood Culture Timing	208	100%	97%	98%
Pregnancy and Delivery Care				
Newborn Deliveries Scheduled Early[2]	59	31%	5%	6%
Preventive Care				
Immunization for Influenza[2]	548	97%	85%	90%
Immunization for Pneumonia[2]	762	98%	88%	92%
Stroke Care				
Anticoagulation Therapy for Atrial Fibrillation	15	60%	93%	95%
Antithrombotic Therapy Timing	112	87%	96%	98%
Assessed for Rehabilitation	115	88%	95%	97%
Discharged on Antithrombotic Therapy	108	93%	97%	99%
Discharged on Statin Medication	93	78%	89%	94%
Thrombolytic Therapy Timing[1]	-	-	53%	66%
Venous Thromboembolism Prophylaxis	115	73%	87%	94%
Written Stroke Educational Materials Given	56	91%	83%	88%
Surgical Care Improvement Project				
Appropriate Beta Blocker Usage	170	98%	97%	98%
Appropriate VTP Within 24 Hours	221	97%	97%	98%
Controlled Postoperative Blood Glucose	123	99%	96%	97%
Perioperative Temperature Management	309	100%	100%	100%
Prophylactic Antibiotic Selection	210	98%	99%	99%
Prophylactic Antibiotic Selection (Outpatient)	213	98%	97%	98%
Prophylactic Antibiotic Stopped	183	96%	97%	98%
Prophylactic Antibiotic Timing	210	99%	98%	99%
Prophylactic Antibiotic Timing (Outpatient)	213	100%	97%	98%
Urinary Catheter Removal	145	99%	96%	97%
Survey of Patients' Hospital Experiences				
Area Around Room 'Always' Quiet at Night	300+	68%	74%	61%
Doctors 'Always' Communicated Well	300+	85%	87%	82%
Home Recovery Information Given	300+	78%	85%	85%
Hospital Given 9 or 10 on 10 Point Scale	300+	70%	75%	71%
Meds 'Always' Explained Before Given	300+	65%	69%	64%
Nurses 'Always' Communicated Well	300+	79%	83%	79%
Pain 'Always' Well Controlled	300+	71%	75%	71%
Room and Bathroom 'Always' Clean	300+	69%	75%	73%
Timely Help 'Always' Received	300+	67%	71%	68%
Would Definitely Recommend Hospital	300+	71%	75%	71%
Use of Medical Imaging				
Cardiac Imaging Stress Test before Surgery	130	10.8%	5.3%	5.3%
Combination Abdominal CT Scan	568	65.1%	24.5%	10.5%
Combination Brain/Sinus CT Scan	756	4.0%	2.6%	2.7%
Combination Chest CT Scan	330	0.6%	7.6%	2.7%
Follow-up Mammogram/Ultrasound	1,654	7.4%	9.4%	8.8%
Lumbar Spine MRI for Low Back Pain	125	44.8%	42.7%	37.2%

Ouachita Community Hospital

1275 Glennwood Drive
West Monroe, LA 71291
URL: www.ouachitahospital.com
Type: Acute Care Hospitals
Ownership: Proprietary

Phone: 318-322-1339
Fax: 318-322-1693
Emergency Services: No

Measure	Cases	This Hosp.	State Avg.	U.S. Avg.
Blood Clot Prevention and Treatment				
Anticoagulation Overlap Therapy[3,7]	-	-	89%	93%
ICU Venous Thromboembolism Prophylaxis[3,7]	-	-	88%	92%
Incidence of Potentially Preventable VTE[3,7]	-	-	16%	10%
UFH with Dosages/Platelet Monitoring[3,7]	-	-	94%	97%
Venous Thromboembolism Prophylaxis[3]	13	100%	74%	85%
Warfarin Therapy Discharge Instructions[3,7]	-	-	85%	75%
Chest Pain/Possible Heart Attack Care				
Aspirin Given Within 24 Hours of Arrival[5]	-	-	94%	96%
Fibrinolytic Meds Within 30 Min. of Arrival[5]	-	-	54%	58%
Average Time to ECG (minutes)[5]	-	-	10	7
Average Time to Transfer (minutes)[5]	-	-	94	60
Children's Asthma Care				
Received Home Management Plan of Care	-	-	-	88%
Received Reliever Medication	-	-	-	100%
Received Systemic Corticosteroids	-	-	-	100%
Emergency Department				
Admittance Decision Time (minutes)[2,7]	-	-	86	98
Head CT Results Within 45 Min. of Arrival[5]	-	-	49%	57%
Patients Who Left ER Before Being Seen[5]	-	-	3%	2%
Time from ER Arrival to Admit. (minutes)[2,7]	-	-	256	274
Time from ER Arrival to Discharge (minutes)[5]	-	-	125	134
Time in ER Before Being Evaluated (minutes)[5]	-	-	27	26
Time to Pain Meds for Fractures (minutes)[5]	-	-	61	57
Heart Attack Care				
Aspirin Given at Discharge[5]	-	-	99%	99%
Fibrinolytic Meds Within 30 Min. of Arrival[5]	-	-	71%	54%
PCI Within 90 Minutes of Arrival[5]	-	-	94%	96%
Statin Prescribed at Discharge[5]	-	-	98%	98%
Heart Failure Care				
ACE Inhibitor or ARB for LVSD[5]	-	-	95%	97%
Discharge Instructions Given[5]	-	-	94%	94%
Evaluation of LVS Function[5]	-	-	97%	99%
Medicare Spending				
Medicare Spending per Patient (ratio)[1]	-	-	1.04	0.98
Pneumonia Care				
Appropriate Initial Antibiotic Given[5]	-	-	93%	95%
Blood Culture Timing[5]	-	-	97%	98%
Pregnancy and Delivery Care				
Newborn Deliveries Scheduled Early[2,3]	-	-	5%	6%
Preventive Care				
Immunization for Influenza[2]	39	64%	85%	90%
Immunization for Pneumonia[2]	26	46%	88%	92%
Stroke Care				
Anticoagulation Therapy for Atrial Fibrillation[5]	-	-	93%	95%
Antithrombotic Therapy Timing[5]	-	-	96%	98%
Assessed for Rehabilitation[5]	-	-	95%	97%
Discharged on Antithrombotic Therapy[5]	-	-	97%	99%
Discharged on Statin Medication[5]	-	-	89%	94%
Thrombolytic Therapy Timing[5]	-	-	53%	66%
Venous Thromboembolism Prophylaxis[5]	-	-	87%	94%
Written Stroke Educational Materials Given[5]	-	-	83%	88%
Surgical Care Improvement Project				
Appropriate Beta Blocker Usage[1,2]	-	-	97%	98%
Appropriate VTP Within 24 Hours[2]	36	100%	97%	98%
Controlled Postoperative Blood Glucose[2,7]	-	-	96%	97%
Perioperative Temperature Management[2]	37	95%	100%	100%
Prophylactic Antibiotic Selection[2]	34	97%	99%	99%
Prophylactic Antibiotic Selection (Outpatient)[5]	-	-	97%	98%
Prophylactic Antibiotic Stopped[2]	34	100%	97%	98%
Prophylactic Antibiotic Timing[2]	34	94%	98%	99%
Prophylactic Antibiotic Timing (Outpatient)[5]	-	-	97%	98%
Urinary Catheter Removal[2]	26	88%	96%	97%
Survey of Patients' Hospital Experiences				
Area Around Room 'Always' Quiet at Night	(a)	87%	74%	61%
Doctors 'Always' Communicated Well	(a)	91%	87%	82%
Home Recovery Information Given	(a)	92%	85%	85%
Hospital Given 9 or 10 on 10 Point Scale	(a)	88%	75%	71%
Meds 'Always' Explained Before Given	(a)	81%	69%	64%
Nurses 'Always' Communicated Well	(a)	87%	83%	79%
Pain 'Always' Well Controlled	(a)	84%	75%	71%
Room and Bathroom 'Always' Clean	(a)	82%	75%	73%
Timely Help 'Always' Received	(a)	85%	71%	68%
Would Definitely Recommend Hospital	(a)	85%	75%	71%
Use of Medical Imaging				
Cardiac Imaging Stress Test before Surgery[7]	-	-	5.3%	5.3%
Combination Abdominal CT Scan[7]	-	-	24.5%	10.5%
Combination Brain/Sinus CT Scan[7]	-	-	2.6%	2.7%
Combination Chest CT Scan[7]	-	-	7.6%	2.7%
Follow-up Mammogram/Ultrasound[7]	-	-	9.4%	8.8%
Lumbar Spine MRI for Low Back Pain[7]	-	-	42.7%	37.2%

Winn Parish Medical Center

301 W Boundary Street
Winnfield, LA 71483
URL: www.winnparishmedical.com
Type: Acute Care Hospitals
Ownership: Proprietary

Phone: 318-648-3000
Fax: 318-628-2035
Emergency Services: Yes
Beds: 60

Key Personnel:
CEO/President. . . . . Bobby Jordan

Measure	Cases	This Hosp.	State Avg.	U.S. Avg.
Blood Clot Prevention and Treatment				
Anticoagulation Overlap Therapy[1,2]	-	-	89%	93%
ICU Venous Thromboembolism Prophylaxis[2]	87	83%	88%	92%
Incidence of Potentially Preventable VTE[2,7]	-	-	16%	10%
UFH with Dosages/Platelet Monitoring[2,7]	-	-	94%	97%
Venous Thromboembolism Prophylaxis[2]	92	95%	74%	85%
Warfarin Therapy Discharge Instructions[1,2]	-	-	85%	75%
Chest Pain/Possible Heart Attack Care				
Aspirin Given Within 24 Hours of Arrival	44	95%	94%	96%
Fibrinolytic Meds Within 30 Min. of Arrival[1]	-	-	54%	58%
Average Time to ECG (minutes)	45	9	10	7
Average Time to Transfer (minutes)[1]	-	-	94	60
Children's Asthma Care				
Received Home Management Plan of Care	-	-	-	88%
Received Reliever Medication	-	-	-	100%
Received Systemic Corticosteroids	-	-	-	100%
Emergency Department				
Admittance Decision Time (minutes)[2]	527	40	86	98
Head CT Results Within 45 Min. of Arrival[1,3]	-	-	49%	57%
Patients Who Left ER Before Being Seen	9,369	1%	3%	2%
Time from ER Arrival to Admit. (minutes)[2]	588	154	256	274
Time from ER Arrival to Discharge (minutes)	297	85	125	134
Time in ER Before Being Evaluated (minutes)	412	13	27	26
Time to Pain Meds for Fractures (minutes)	31	51	61	57
Heart Attack Care				
Aspirin Given at Discharge[1,2]	-	-	99%	99%
Fibrinolytic Meds Within 30 Min. of Arrival[2,3]	-	-	71%	54%
PCI Within 90 Minutes of Arrival[2,3]	-	-	94%	96%
Statin Prescribed at Discharge[1,2]	-	-	98%	98%
Heart Failure Care				
ACE Inhibitor or ARB for LVSD[1,2]	-	-	95%	97%
Discharge Instructions Given[2]	27	93%	94%	94%
Evaluation of LVS Function[2]	42	93%	97%	99%
Medicare Spending				
Medicare Spending per Patient (ratio)	-	1.23	1.04	0.98
Pneumonia Care				
Appropriate Initial Antibiotic Given[2]	36	92%	93%	95%
Blood Culture Timing[2]	62	98%	97%	98%
Pregnancy and Delivery Care				
Newborn Deliveries Scheduled Early[7]	-	-	5%	6%
Preventive Care				
Immunization for Influenza[2]	332	91%	85%	90%
Immunization for Pneumonia[2]	507	95%	88%	92%
Stroke Care				

NOTE: Hospital profiles are in alphabetical order by state, then city, then hospital within the city; Rankings exclude hospitals with less than 25 cases except for patient surveys which excludes hospitals with less than 100 cases; (a) 100-299 cases; (1) The number of cases/patients is too few to report; (2) Data submitted were based on a sample of cases/patients; (3) Results are based on a shorter time period than required; (4) Data suppressed by CMS for one or more quarters; (5) Results are not available for this reporting period; (6) Fewer than 100 patients completed the HCAHPS survey; (7) No cases met the criteria for this measure; (8) The lower limit of the confidence interval cannot be calculated if the number of observed infections equals zero; (9) No data are available from the state/territory for this reporting period; (10) The scores shown reflect fewer than 50 completed surveys; (11) There were discrepancies in the data collection process; (12) This measure does not apply to this hospital for this reporting period; (13) Results cannot be calculated for this reporting period; (14) The results for this state are combined with nearby states to protect confidentiality; Please refer to the User's Guide for a full explanation of data.

Measure	Cases	This Hosp.	State Avg.	U.S. Avg.
Anticoagulation Therapy for Atrial Fibrillation[3,7]	-	-	93%	95%
Antithrombotic Therapy Timing[1,3]	-	-	96%	98%
Assessed for Rehabilitation[1,3]	-	-	95%	97%
Discharged on Antithrombotic Therapy[1,3]	-	-	97%	99%
Discharged on Statin Medication[1,3]	-	-	89%	94%
Thrombolytic Therapy Timing[3,7]	-	-	53%	66%
Venous Thromboembolism Prophylaxis[1,3]	-	-	87%	94%
Written Stroke Educational Materials Given[3,7]	-	-	83%	88%
Surgical Care Improvement Project				
Appropriate Beta Blocker Usage[3,7]	-	-	97%	98%
Appropriate VTP Within 24 Hours[3,7]	-	-	97%	98%
Controlled Postoperative Blood Glucose[3,7]	-	-	96%	97%
Perioperative Temperature Management[1,3]	-	-	100%	100%
Prophylactic Antibiotic Selection[3,7]	-	-	99%	99%
Prophylactic Antibiotic Selection (Outpatient)[3,7]	-	-	97%	98%
Prophylactic Antibiotic Stopped[3,7]	-	-	97%	98%
Prophylactic Antibiotic Timing[3,7]	-	-	98%	99%
Prophylactic Antibiotic Timing (Outpatient)[3,7]	-	-	97%	98%
Urinary Catheter Removal[3,7]	-	-	96%	97%
Survey of Patients' Hospital Experiences				
Area Around Room 'Always' Quiet at Night	(a)	72%	74%	61%
Doctors 'Always' Communicated Well	(a)	76%	87%	82%
Home Recovery Information Given	(a)	76%	85%	85%
Hospital Given 9 or 10 on 10 Point Scale	(a)	63%	75%	71%
Meds 'Always' Explained Before Given	(a)	66%	69%	64%
Nurses 'Always' Communicated Well	(a)	82%	83%	79%
Pain 'Always' Well Controlled	(a)	65%	75%	71%
Room and Bathroom 'Always' Clean	(a)	76%	75%	73%
Timely Help 'Always' Received	(a)	68%	71%	68%
Would Definitely Recommend Hospital	(a)	52%	75%	71%
Use of Medical Imaging				
Cardiac Imaging Stress Test before Surgery	72	2.8%	5.3%	5.3%
Combination Abdominal CT Scan	107	33.6%	24.5%	10.5%
Combination Brain/Sinus CT Scan[1]	-	-	2.6%	2.7%
Combination Chest CT Scan	80	6.3%	7.6%	2.7%
Follow-up Mammogram/Ultrasound[7]	-	-	9.4%	8.8%
Lumbar Spine MRI for Low Back Pain[1]	-	-	42.7%	37.2%

Franklin Medical Center

2106 Loop Road
Winnsboro, LA 71295
Phone: 318-435-9411
Fax: 318-435-3842
URL: www.fmc-cares.com
Type: Acute Care Hospitals
Emergency Services: Yes
Ownership: Govt - Hospital Dist/Auth
Beds: 59

Key Personnel:
Chief of Medical Staff. . . . . Vernon T Baldwin
Quality Assurance . . . . Dwaine Boothe
CEO/President. . . . . Robert Boullion
Radiology. . . . . Julie Collins
Infection Control. . . . . Debi Elrod
Operating Room. . . . . Derrick Frazier
Cardiac Laboratory. . . . . Dr Roger Smith

Measure	Cases	This Hosp.	State Avg.	U.S. Avg.
Blood Clot Prevention and Treatment				
Anticoagulation Overlap Therapy[1,2]	-	-	89%	93%
ICU Venous Thromboembolism Prophylaxis[2]	37	54%	88%	92%
Incidence of Potentially Preventable VTE[2,7]	-	-	16%	10%
UFH with Dosages/Platelet Monitoring[1,2]	-	-	94%	97%
Venous Thromboembolism Prophylaxis[2]	350	45%	74%	85%
Warfarin Therapy Discharge Instructions[1,2]	-	-	85%	75%
Chest Pain/Possible Heart Attack Care				
Aspirin Given Within 24 Hours of Arrival	101	97%	94%	96%
Fibrinolytic Meds Within 30 Min. of Arrival[1]	-	-	54%	58%
Average Time to ECG (minutes)	104	7	10	7
Average Time to Transfer (minutes)[7]	-	-	94	60
Children's Asthma Care				
Received Home Management Plan of Care	-	-	-	88%
Received Reliever Medication	-	-	-	100%
Received Systemic Corticosteroids	-	-	-	100%
Emergency Department				
Admittance Decision Time (minutes)[2]	260	48	86	98
Head CT Results Within 45 Min. of Arrival[1]	-	-	49%	57%
Patients Who Left ER Before Being Seen	10,287	3%	3%	2%
Time from ER Arrival to Admit. (minutes)[2]	282	244	256	274
Time from ER Arrival to Discharge (minutes)	313	144	125	134
Time in ER Before Being Evaluated (minutes)	331	37	27	26
Time to Pain Meds for Fractures (minutes)	48	61	61	57
Heart Attack Care				
Aspirin Given at Discharge[1,3]	-	-	99%	99%
Fibrinolytic Meds Within 30 Min. of Arrival[3,7]	-	-	71%	54%
PCI Within 90 Minutes of Arrival[3,7]	-	-	94%	96%
Statin Prescribed at Discharge[1,3]	-	-	98%	98%
Heart Failure Care				
ACE Inhibitor or ARB for LVSD[1]	-	-	95%	97%
Discharge Instructions Given	39	92%	94%	94%
Evaluation of LVS Function	53	89%	97%	99%
Medicare Spending				
Medicare Spending per Patient (ratio)	-	1.06	1.04	0.98
Pneumonia Care				
Appropriate Initial Antibiotic Given	54	80%	93%	95%
Blood Culture Timing	56	91%	97%	98%
Pregnancy and Delivery Care				
Newborn Deliveries Scheduled Early[7]	-	-	5%	6%
Preventive Care				
Immunization for Influenza[2]	325	90%	85%	90%
Immunization for Pneumonia[2]	493	95%	88%	92%
Stroke Care				
Anticoagulation Therapy for Atrial Fibrillation[3,7]	-	-	93%	95%
Antithrombotic Therapy Timing[1,3]	-	-	96%	98%
Assessed for Rehabilitation[1,3]	-	-	95%	97%
Discharged on Antithrombotic Therapy[1,3]	-	-	97%	99%
Discharged on Statin Medication[1,3]	-	-	89%	94%
Thrombolytic Therapy Timing[3,7]	-	-	53%	66%
Venous Thromboembolism Prophylaxis[1,3]	-	-	87%	94%
Written Stroke Educational Materials Given[1,3]	-	-	83%	88%
Surgical Care Improvement Project				
Appropriate Beta Blocker Usage[5]	-	-	97%	98%
Appropriate VTP Within 24 Hours[5]	-	-	97%	98%
Controlled Postoperative Blood Glucose[5]	-	-	96%	97%
Perioperative Temperature Management[5]	-	-	100%	100%
Prophylactic Antibiotic Selection[5]	-	-	99%	99%
Prophylactic Antibiotic Selection (Outpatient)[5]	-	-	97%	98%
Prophylactic Antibiotic Stopped[5]	-	-	97%	98%
Prophylactic Antibiotic Timing[5]	-	-	98%	99%
Prophylactic Antibiotic Timing (Outpatient)[5]	-	-	97%	98%
Urinary Catheter Removal[5]	-	-	96%	97%
Survey of Patients' Hospital Experiences				
Area Around Room 'Always' Quiet at Night	(a)	70%	74%	61%
Doctors 'Always' Communicated Well	(a)	89%	87%	82%
Home Recovery Information Given	(a)	86%	85%	85%
Hospital Given 9 or 10 on 10 Point Scale	(a)	68%	75%	71%
Meds 'Always' Explained Before Given	(a)	70%	69%	64%
Nurses 'Always' Communicated Well	(a)	83%	83%	79%
Pain 'Always' Well Controlled	(a)	72%	75%	71%
Room and Bathroom 'Always' Clean	(a)	76%	75%	73%
Timely Help 'Always' Received	(a)	76%	71%	68%
Would Definitely Recommend Hospital	(a)	63%	75%	71%
Use of Medical Imaging				
Cardiac Imaging Stress Test before Surgery[1]	-	-	5.3%	5.3%
Combination Abdominal CT Scan	289	12.8%	24.5%	10.5%
Combination Brain/Sinus CT Scan	434	0.7%	2.6%	2.7%
Combination Chest CT Scan	106	16.0%	7.6%	2.7%
Follow-up Mammogram/Ultrasound	150	14.7%	9.4%	8.8%
Lumbar Spine MRI for Low Back Pain[1]	-	-	42.7%	37.2%

Lane Regional Medical Center

6300 Main Street
Zachary, LA 70791
Phone: 225-658-4000
Fax: 225-658-4287
URL: www.lanehospital.org
Type: Acute Care Hospitals
Emergency Services: Yes
Ownership: Govt - Hospital Dist/Auth
Beds: 137

Key Personnel:
Intensive Care Unit. . . . . Billy Conerly, RN
Radiology. . . . . Charles Greeson
CEO . . . . Randall Olson
Chief of Medical Staff. . . . . Brad Smith, MD

Measure	Cases	This Hosp.	State Avg.	U.S. Avg.
Blood Clot Prevention and Treatment				
Anticoagulation Overlap Therapy[2]	25	76%	89%	93%
ICU Venous Thromboembolism Prophylaxis[2]	66	58%	88%	92%
Incidence of Potentially Preventable VTE[1,2]	-	-	16%	10%
UFH with Dosages/Platelet Monitoring[1,2]	-	-	94%	97%
Venous Thromboembolism Prophylaxis[2]	402	38%	74%	85%
Warfarin Therapy Discharge Instructions[2]	18	89%	85%	75%
Chest Pain/Possible Heart Attack Care				
Aspirin Given Within 24 Hours of Arrival[1]	-	-	94%	96%
Fibrinolytic Meds Within 30 Min. of Arrival[3,7]	-	-	54%	58%
Average Time to ECG (minutes)[1]	-	-	10	7
Average Time to Transfer (minutes)[3,7]	-	-	94	60
Children's Asthma Care				
Received Home Management Plan of Care	-	-	-	88%
Received Reliever Medication	-	-	-	100%
Received Systemic Corticosteroids	-	-	-	100%
Emergency Department				
Admittance Decision Time (minutes)[2]	494	83	86	98
Head CT Results Within 45 Min. of Arrival[1]	-	-	49%	57%
Patients Who Left ER Before Being Seen	32,940	2%	3%	2%
Time from ER Arrival to Admit. (minutes)[2]	528	236	256	274
Time from ER Arrival to Discharge (minutes)	479	112	125	134
Time in ER Before Being Evaluated (minutes)	393	25	27	26
Time to Pain Meds for Fractures (minutes)	107	50	61	57
Heart Attack Care				
Aspirin Given at Discharge	89	99%	99%	99%
Fibrinolytic Meds Within 30 Min. of Arrival[7]	-	-	71%	54%
PCI Within 90 Minutes of Arrival	33	100%	94%	96%
Statin Prescribed at Discharge	89	99%	98%	98%
Heart Failure Care				
ACE Inhibitor or ARB for LVSD	60	98%	95%	97%
Discharge Instructions Given	161	97%	94%	94%
Evaluation of LVS Function	197	99%	97%	99%
Medicare Spending				
Medicare Spending per Patient (ratio)	-	1.10	1.04	0.98
Pneumonia Care				
Appropriate Initial Antibiotic Given[2]	93	95%	93%	95%
Blood Culture Timing[2]	153	96%	97%	98%
Pregnancy and Delivery Care				
Newborn Deliveries Scheduled Early	68	1%	5%	6%
Preventive Care				
Immunization for Influenza[2]	458	86%	85%	90%
Immunization for Pneumonia[2]	607	99%	88%	92%
Stroke Care				
Anticoagulation Therapy for Atrial Fibrillation[1]	-	-	93%	95%
Antithrombotic Therapy Timing	34	100%	96%	98%
Assessed for Rehabilitation	33	91%	95%	97%
Discharged on Antithrombotic Therapy	31	97%	97%	99%
Discharged on Statin Medication	28	68%	89%	94%
Thrombolytic Therapy Timing[1]	-	-	53%	66%
Venous Thromboembolism Prophylaxis	36	47%	87%	94%
Written Stroke Educational Materials Given	16	38%	83%	88%
Surgical Care Improvement Project				
Appropriate Beta Blocker Usage	104	97%	97%	98%
Appropriate VTP Within 24 Hours	285	99%	97%	98%
Controlled Postoperative Blood Glucose[7]	-	-	96%	97%
Perioperative Temperature Management	322	100%	100%	100%
Prophylactic Antibiotic Selection	236	99%	99%	99%
Prophylactic Antibiotic Selection (Outpatient)	64	100%	97%	98%
Prophylactic Antibiotic Stopped	225	97%	97%	98%
Prophylactic Antibiotic Timing	236	99%	98%	99%
Prophylactic Antibiotic Timing (Outpatient)	65	97%	97%	98%
Urinary Catheter Removal	240	95%	96%	97%
Survey of Patients' Hospital Experiences				
Area Around Room 'Always' Quiet at Night	300+	60%	74%	61%
Doctors 'Always' Communicated Well	300+	86%	87%	82%
Home Recovery Information Given	300+	86%	85%	85%
Hospital Given 9 or 10 on 10 Point Scale	300+	66%	75%	71%
Meds 'Always' Explained Before Given	300+	65%	69%	64%
Nurses 'Always' Communicated Well	300+	82%	83%	79%
Pain 'Always' Well Controlled	300+	75%	75%	71%
Room and Bathroom 'Always' Clean	300+	63%	75%	73%

NOTE: Hospital profiles are in alphabetical order by state, then city, then hospital within the city; Rankings exclude hospitals with less than 25 cases except for patient surveys which excludes hospitals with less than 100 cases; (a) 100-299 cases; (1) The number of cases/patients is too few to report; (2) Data submitted were based on a sample of cases/patients; (3) Results are based on a shorter time period than required; (4) Data suppressed by CMS for one or more quarters; (5) Results are not available for this reporting period; (6) Fewer than 100 patients completed the HCAHPS survey; (7) No cases met the criteria for this measure; (8) The lower limit of the confidence interval cannot be calculated if the number of observed infections equals zero; (9) No data are available from the state/territory for this reporting period; (10) The scores shown reflect fewer than 50 completed surveys; (11) There were discrepancies in the data collection process; (12) This measure does not apply to this hospital for this reporting period; (13) Results cannot be calculated for this reporting period; (14) The results for this state are combined with nearby states to protect confidentiality; Please refer to the User's Guide for a full explanation of data.

Timely Help 'Always' Received	300+	64%	71%	68%
Would Definitely Recommend Hospital	300+	69%	75%	71%
Use of Medical Imaging				
Cardiac Imaging Stress Test before Surgery[1]	-	-	5.3%	5.3%
Combination Abdominal CT Scan	303	21.1%	24.5%	10.5%
Combination Brain/Sinus CT Scan	460	5.7%	2.6%	2.7%
Combination Chest CT Scan	202	14.9%	7.6%	2.7%
Follow-up Mammogram/Ultrasound	310	7.1%	9.4%	8.8%
Lumbar Spine MRI for Low Back Pain[1]	-	-	42.7%	37.2%

NOTE: Hospital profiles are in alphabetical order by state, then city, then hospital within the city; Rankings exclude hospitals with less than 25 cases except for patient surveys which excludes hospitals with less than 100 cases; (a) 100-299 cases; (1) The number of cases/patients is too few to report; (2) Data submitted were based on a sample of cases/patients; (3) Results are based on a shorter time period than required; (4) Data suppressed by CMS for one or more quarters; (5) Results are not available for this reporting period; (6) Fewer than 100 patients completed the HCAHPS survey; (7) No cases met the criteria for this measure; (8) The lower limit of the confidence interval cannot be calculated if the number of observed infections equals zero; (9) No data are available from the state/territory for this reporting period; (10) The scores shown reflect fewer than 50 completed surveys; (11) There were discrepancies in the data collection process; (12) This measure does not apply to this hospital for this reporting period; (13) Results cannot be calculated for this reporting period; (14) The results for this state are combined with nearby states to protect confidentiality; Please refer to the User's Guide for a full explanation of data.

Blood Clot Prevention and Treatment

Anticoagulation Overlap Therapy

Hospital Name	City	Rate	Cases
Baptist Memorial Hospital/Golden Triangle[2]	Columbus	100%	50
Garden Park Medical Center[2]	Gulfport	100%	25
Magnolia Regional Health Center[2]	Corinth	100%	35
River Oaks Hospital[2]	Flowood	100%	25
River Region Health System[2]	Vicksburg	100%	39
Wesley Medical Center[2]	Hattiesburg	100%	41
Rush Foundation Hospital[2]	Meridian	98%	62
Baptist Memorial Hospital Desoto[2]	Southaven	97%	132
Greenwood Leflore Hospital[2]	Greenwood	95%	41
Forrest General Hospital[2]	Hattiesburg	94%	118
North Mississippi Medical Center[2]	Tupelo	94%	126
Saint Dominic - Jackson Memorial Hospital[2]	Jackson	93%	229
Anderson Regional Medical Center[2]	Meridian	92%	76
University of Mississippi Medical Center[2]	Jackson	87%	119
Mississippi Baptist Medical Center[2]	Jackson	86%	182
Singing River Hospital[2]	Pascagoula	85%	73
Memorial Hospital at Gulfport[2]	Gulfport	83%	76
Baptist Mem Hosp North Mississippi[2]	Oxford	81%	43
Och Regional Medical Center[2]	Starkville	74%	27
South Central Regional Medical Center[2]	Laurel	74%	69
Delta Regional Medical Center[2]	Greenville	61%	59
Southwest Ms Regional Medical Center[2]	Mccomb	49%	53
Grenada Lake Medical Center[2]	Grenada	28%	32

ICU Venous Thromboembolism Prophylaxis

Hospital Name	City	Rate	Cases
Baptist Memorial Hospital Union County[2]	New Albany	100%	36
Garden Park Medical Center[2]	Gulfport	100%	66
King's Daughters Med Ctr-Brookhaven[2]	Brookhaven	100%	27
Magnolia Regional Health Center[2]	Corinth	100%	147
River Oaks Hospital[2]	Flowood	100%	32
Wesley Medical Center[2]	Hattiesburg	100%	96
Gilmore Memorial Regional Medical Center[2]	Amory	98%	40
River Region Health System[2]	Vicksburg	98%	86
Baptist Memorial Hospital Desoto[2]	Southaven	97%	139
Baptist Memorial Hospital/Golden Triangle[2]	Columbus	97%	118
Biloxi Regional Medical Center[2]	Biloxi	97%	64
Saint Dominic - Jackson Memorial Hospital[2]	Jackson	97%	74
North Mississippi Medical Center[2]	Tupelo	96%	90
Southwest Ms Regional Medical Center[2]	Mccomb	96%	116
Baptist Mem Hosp North Mississippi[2]	Oxford	93%	109
Forrest General Hospital[2]	Hattiesburg	93%	57
Memorial Hospital at Gulfport[2]	Gulfport	93%	85
Singing River Hospital[2]	Pascagoula	92%	120
Central Mississippi Medical Center[2]	Jackson	91%	87
Madison River Oaks Medical Center[2]	Canton	91%	43
Northwest Mississippi Reg Med Ctr[2]	Clarksdale	89%	94
Baptist Memorial Hospital Booneville[2]	Booneville	88%	50
Crossgates River Oaks Hospital[2]	Brandon	88%	33
Hancock Medical Center[2]	Bay Saint Louis	86%	37
George County Hospital[2]	Lucedale	85%	40
Greenwood Leflore Hospital[2]	Greenwood	85%	95
Rush Foundation Hospital[2]	Meridian	85%	124
Tri Lakes Medical Center[2]	Batesville	81%	32
University of Mississippi Medical Center[2]	Jackson	80%	138
Grenada Lake Medical Center[2]	Grenada	79%	230
Mississippi Baptist Medical Center[2]	Jackson	76%	67
Bolivar Medical Center[2]	Cleveland	75%	61
Natchez Community Hospital[2]	Natchez	72%	36
Anderson Regional Medical Center[2]	Meridian	68%	96
South Central Regional Medical Center[2]	Laurel	68%	59
Highland Community Hospital[2]	Picayune	64%	96
Delta Regional Medical Center[2]	Greenville	58%	132
South Sunflower County Hospital[2]	Indianola	55%	65
Och Regional Medical Center[2]	Starkville	53%	34
Natchez Regional Medical Center[2]	Natchez	52%	25

Incidence of Potentially Preventable VTE

Hospital Name	City	Rate	Cases
University of Mississippi Medical Center[2]	Jackson	6%	78
Forrest General Hospital[2]	Hattiesburg	8%	25
Saint Dominic - Jackson Memorial Hospital[2]	Jackson	12%	84
Memorial Hospital at Gulfport[2]	Gulfport	18%	28
Mississippi Baptist Medical Center[2]	Jackson	24%	37

UFH with Dosages/Platelet Count Monitoring

Hospital Name	City	Rate	Cases
Baptist Memorial Hospital Desoto[2]	Southaven	100%	117
Saint Dominic - Jackson Memorial Hospital[2]	Jackson	100%	58
University of Mississippi Medical Center[2]	Jackson	98%	84
Memorial Hospital at Gulfport[2]	Gulfport	97%	31
Mississippi Baptist Medical Center[2]	Jackson	97%	36
Anderson Regional Medical Center[2]	Meridian	96%	27
Singing River Hospital[2]	Pascagoula	0%	28

Venous Thromboembolism Prophylaxis

Hospital Name	City	Rate	Cases
Garden Park Medical Center[2]	Gulfport	100%	271
Baptist Memorial Hospital Union County[2]	New Albany	99%	239
Woman's Hospital at River Oaks[2]	Flowood	99%	79
Magnolia Regional Health Center[2]	Corinth	97%	268
Wesley Medical Center[2]	Hattiesburg	97%	348
Baptist Memorial Hospital Desoto[2]	Southaven	96%	392
Baptist Mem Hosp North Mississippi[2]	Oxford	96%	340
Baptist Memorial Hospital/Golden Triangle[2]	Columbus	94%	348
King's Daughters Med Ctr-Brookhaven[2]	Brookhaven	94%	215
Pontotoc Health Service[2]	Pontotoc	94%	130
River Oaks Hospital[2]	Flowood	94%	196
River Region Health System[2]	Vicksburg	94%	422
Calhoun Health Services	Calhoun City	92%	176
Gilmore Memorial Regional Medical Center[2]	Amory	92%	198
Southwest Ms Regional Medical Center[2]	Mccomb	91%	282
Whitfield Medical Surgical Hospital[2]	Whitfield	91%	79
George County Hospital[2]	Lucedale	89%	90
Tishomingo Health Services[2]	Iuka	89%	114
Biloxi Regional Medical Center[2]	Biloxi	87%	307
Magee General Hospital[2]	Magee	87%	222
Singing River Hospital[2]	Pascagoula	85%	299
Forrest General Hospital[2]	Hattiesburg	82%	285
North Mississippi Medical Center[2]	Tupelo	81%	379
University of Mississippi Medical Center[2]	Jackson	79%	305
Baptist Memorial Hospital Booneville[2]	Booneville	78%	89
Memorial Hospital at Gulfport[2]	Gulfport	77%	357
Rush Foundation Hospital[2]	Meridian	77%	332
Central Mississippi Medical Center[2]	Jackson	76%	319
Northwest Mississippi Reg Med Ctr[2]	Clarksdale	75%	375
Marion General Hospital[2]	Columbia	73%	426
North Oak Regional Medical Center[2]	Senatobia	72%	280
Natchez Community Hospital[2]	Natchez	71%	292
Webster General Hospital/Swing Bed[2]	Eupora	71%	182
Greenwood Leflore Hospital[2]	Greenwood	69%	296
Hancock Medical Center[2]	Bay Saint Louis	69%	127
Grenada Lake Medical Center[2]	Grenada	65%	807
Madison River Oaks Medical Center[2]	Canton	65%	91
Bolivar Medical Center[2]	Cleveland	63%	290
South Central Regional Medical Center[2]	Laurel	63%	332
Saint Dominic - Jackson Memorial Hospital[2]	Jackson	62%	408
Tri Lakes Medical Center[2]	Batesville	57%	96
Mississippi Baptist Medical Center[2]	Jackson	56%	383
Clay County Medical Center[2]	West Point	53%	189
Crossgates River Oaks Hospital[2]	Brandon	52%	236
Natchez Regional Medical Center[2]	Natchez	49%	195
South Sunflower County Hospital[2]	Indianola	49%	165
Wayne General Hospital[2]	Waynesboro	49%	209
Anderson Regional Medical Center[2]	Meridian	48%	363
Winston Medical Center & Swingbed[2]	Louisville	44%	126
Highland Community Hospital[2]	Picayune	42%	263
Och Regional Medical Center[2]	Starkville	39%	123
Delta Regional Medical Center[2]	Greenville	32%	351
Tippah County Hospital[2,3]	Ripley	25%	88
Trace Regional Hospital & Swing Bed[2,3]	Houston	23%	139
Yalobusha General Hospital[2]	Water Valley	16%	131
Beacham Memorial Hospital[2]	Magnolia	14%	133
Alliance Healthcare System[2]	Holly Springs	6%	134
Montfort Jones Memorial Hospital[2]	Kosciusko	1%	288
Neshoba County General Hospital[2]	Philadelphia	1%	118
Jefferson County Hospital[2]	Fayette	0%	25

Warfarin Therapy Discharge Instructions

Hospital Name	City	Rate	Cases
Baptist Mem Hosp North Mississippi[2]	Oxford	100%	37
North Mississippi Medical Center[2]	Tupelo	99%	87
Greenwood Leflore Hospital[2]	Greenwood	97%	29
River Region Health System[2]	Vicksburg	97%	31
Wesley Medical Center[2]	Hattiesburg	97%	33
Baptist Memorial Hospital/Golden Triangle[2]	Columbus	92%	40
Saint Dominic - Jackson Memorial Hospital[2]	Jackson	92%	169
Baptist Memorial Hospital Desoto[2]	Southaven	91%	92
Southwest Ms Regional Medical Center[2]	Mccomb	90%	41
Delta Regional Medical Center[2]	Greenville	82%	44
Forrest General Hospital[2]	Hattiesburg	77%	93
Anderson Regional Medical Center[2]	Meridian	74%	58
Singing River Hospital[2]	Pascagoula	74%	58
Memorial Hospital at Gulfport[2]	Gulfport	68%	56
University of Mississippi Medical Center[2]	Jackson	63%	93
Rush Foundation Hospital[2]	Meridian	56%	43
Mississippi Baptist Medical Center[2]	Jackson	48%	153
South Central Regional Medical Center[2]	Laurel	24%	58
Grenada Lake Medical Center[2]	Grenada	6%	31

Chest Pain/Possible Heart Attack Care

Aspirin Given Within 24 Hours of Arrival

Hospital Name	City	Rate	Cases
Baptist Memorial Hospital Union County	New Albany	100%	74
Bolivar Medical Center	Cleveland	100%	29
Calhoun Health Services	Calhoun City	100%	42
Clay County Medical Center	West Point	100%	26
Crossgates River Oaks Hospital	Brandon	100%	33
Highland Community Hospital	Picayune	100%	65
Magee General Hospital	Magee	100%	54
Natchez Regional Medical Center	Natchez	100%	66
Pontotoc Health Service	Pontotoc	100%	42
Baptist Memorial Hospital Booneville	Booneville	99%	79
Tri Lakes Medical Center	Batesville	99%	71
Biloxi Regional Medical Center	Biloxi	98%	45
Baptist Mem Hosp North Mississippi	Oxford	97%	36
Field Memorial Community Hospital	Centreville	97%	29
Gilmore Memorial Regional Medical Center	Amory	97%	59
River Oaks Hospital	Flowood	97%	36
Holmes County Hospital & Clinics	Lexington	96%	27
Och Regional Medical Center	Starkville	95%	60
King's Daughters Med Ctr-Brookhaven	Brookhaven	94%	79
Madison River Oaks Medical Center	Canton	94%	70
South Central Regional Medical Center	Laurel	94%	35
Trace Regional Hospital & Swing Bed	Houston	94%	33
George County Hospital	Lucedale	93%	137
Grenada Lake Medical Center	Grenada	92%	39
Montfort Jones Memorial Hospital	Kosciusko	91%	33
North Oak Regional Medical Center	Senatobia	91%	44
Northwest Mississippi Reg Med Ctr	Clarksdale	91%	35
Tippah County Hospital	Ripley	90%	31
Greene County Hospital[3]	Leakesville	86%	42
Marion General Hospital	Columbia	86%	28
Hardy Wilson Memorial Hospital	Hazlehurst	85%	26
H C Watkins Memorial Hospital	Quitman	71%	41
Neshoba County General Hospital	Philadelphia	70%	44

Average Time to ECG (minutes)

Hospital Name	City	Min.	Cases
Gilmore Memorial Regional Medical Center	Amory	0	59
Biloxi Regional Medical Center	Biloxi	3	46
Greene County Hospital[3]	Leakesville	3	43
Baptist Memorial Hospital Union County	New Albany	4	72
Field Memorial Community Hospital	Centreville	4	29
Natchez Regional Medical Center	Natchez	4	72
Magee General Hospital	Magee	5	58
H C Watkins Memorial Hospital	Quitman	6	41
Crossgates River Oaks Hospital	Brandon	7	36
South Central Regional Medical Center	Laurel	7	36
Clay County Medical Center	West Point	8	26
Madison River Oaks Medical Center	Canton	8	71
Pontotoc Health Service	Pontotoc	8	43
River Oaks Hospital	Flowood	8	40
Tippah County Hospital	Ripley	8	30
Highland Community Hospital	Picayune	9	68
Baptist Mem Hosp North Mississippi	Oxford	10	38
Marion General Hospital	Columbia	10	28
Neshoba County General Hospital	Philadelphia	10	44
Tri Lakes Medical Center	Batesville	10	73
Calhoun Health Services	Calhoun City	11	42
Montfort Jones Memorial Hospital	Kosciusko	11	35
North Oak Regional Medical Center	Senatobia	11	46
Hardy Wilson Memorial Hospital	Hazlehurst	12	27
Bolivar Medical Center	Cleveland	13	29
Holmes County Hospital & Clinics	Lexington	13	28
King's Daughters Med Ctr-Brookhaven	Brookhaven	13	81
Trace Regional Hospital & Swing Bed	Houston	13	32
Baptist Memorial Hospital Booneville	Booneville	15	79
George County Hospital	Lucedale	16	144
Northwest Mississippi Reg Med Ctr	Clarksdale	18	38
Grenada Lake Medical Center	Grenada	20	40
Och Regional Medical Center	Starkville	24	62
South Sunflower County Hospital	Indianola	35	25

Children's Asthma Care

Received Home Management Plan of Care

Hospital Name	City	Rate	Cases
University of Mississippi Medical Center[2]	Jackson	89%	208

Received Reliever Medication

Hospital Name	City	Rate	Cases
University of Mississippi Medical Center[2]	Jackson	100%	209

Received Systemic Corticosteroids

Hospital Name	City	Rate	Cases
University of Mississippi Medical Center[2]	Jackson	100%	209

NOTE: Hospital profiles are in alphabetical order by state, then city, then hospital within the city; Rankings exclude hospitals with less than 25 cases except for patient surveys which excludes hospitals with less than 100 cases; (a) 100-299 cases; (1) The number of cases/patients is too few to report; (2) Data submitted were based on a sample of cases/patients; (3) Results are based on a shorter time period than required; (4) Data suppressed by CMS for one or more quarters; (5) Results are not available for this reporting period; (6) Fewer than 100 patients completed the HCAHPS survey; (7) No cases met the criteria for this measure; (8) The lower limit of the confidence interval cannot be calculated if the number of observed infections equals zero; (9) No data are available from the state/territory for this reporting period; (10) The scores shown reflect fewer than 50 completed surveys; (11) There were discrepancies in the data collection process; (12) This measure does not apply to this hospital for this reporting period; (13) Results cannot be calculated for this reporting period; (14) The results for this state are combined with nearby states to protect confidentiality; Please refer to the User's Guide for a full explanation of data.

Emergency Department

Admittance Decision Time (minutes)

Hospital Name	City	Min.	Cases
Clay County Medical Center[2]	West Point	20	263
Calhoun Health Services	Calhoun City	21	237
Walthall County General Hospital	Tylertown	25	78
Pontotoc Health Service[2]	Pontotoc	29	226
Baptist Memorial Hospital Union County[2]	New Albany	30	297
Webster General Hospital/Swing Bed[2]	Eupora	31	274
Greenwood Leflore Hospital[2]	Greenwood	34	370
Montfort Jones Memorial Hospital[2]	Kosciusko	35	484
South Sunflower County Hospital[2]	Indianola	35	113
Tishomingo Health Services[2]	Iuka	38	359
Baptist Memorial Hospital Booneville[2]	Booneville	40	302
Grenada Lake Medical Center[2]	Grenada	40	1309
Jefferson Davis Community Hospital[2]	Prentiss	40	127
Neshoba County General Hospital[2]	Philadelphia	40	294
South Central Regional Medical Center[2]	Laurel	46	506
Natchez Community Hospital[2]	Natchez	47	467
Magee General Hospital[2]	Magee	48	206
Trace Regional Hospital & Swing Bed[2]	Houston	50	230
Baptist Mem Hosp North Mississippi[2]	Oxford	52	436
Memorial Hospital at Gulfport[2]	Gulfport	53	648
Och Regional Medical Center[2]	Starkville	56	151
Wayne General Hospital[2]	Waynesboro	57	423
Forrest General Hospital[2]	Hattiesburg	58	594
North Mississippi Medical Center[2]	Tupelo	58	520
River Oaks Hospital[2]	Flowood	58	235
Tri Lakes Medical Center[2]	Batesville	58	224
Wesley Medical Center[2]	Hattiesburg	58	558
Marion General Hospital[2]	Columbia	60	434
Southwest Ms Regional Medical Center[2]	Mccomb	61	753
Winston Medical Center & Swingbed[2]	Louisville	62	259
Northwest Mississippi Reg Med Ctr[2]	Clarksdale	64	778
Anderson Regional Medical Center[2]	Meridian	65	530
Gilmore Memorial Regional Medical Center[2]	Amory	68	315
Baptist Memorial Hospital Desoto[2]	Southaven	70	522
Covington County Hospital CAH	Collins	70	208
Hancock Medical Center[2]	Bay Saint Louis	70	275
King's Daughters Med Ctr-Brookhaven[2]	Brookhaven	71	339
Madison River Oaks Medical Center[2]	Canton	71	304
Magnolia Regional Health Center[2]	Corinth	71	684
Biloxi Regional Medical Center[2]	Biloxi	72	462
Crossgates River Oaks Hospital[2]	Brandon	72	481
Tippah County Hospital[2]	Ripley	72	126
North Oak Regional Medical Center[2]	Senatobia	73	417
George County Hospital[2]	Lucedale	74	309
Baptist Memorial Hospital/Golden Triangle[2]	Columbus	77	493
Alliance Healthcare System[2]	Holly Springs	78	106
Highland Community Hospital[2]	Picayune	78	481
Rush Foundation Hospital[2]	Meridian	79	348
Mississippi Baptist Medical Center[2]	Jackson	82	583
Bolivar Medical Center[2]	Cleveland	86	325
Garden Park Medical Center[2]	Gulfport	87	456
Saint Dominic - Jackson Memorial Hospital[2]	Jackson	93	678
Delta Regional Medical Center[2]	Greenville	95	521
River Region Health System[2]	Vicksburg	98	739
Central Mississippi Medical Center[2]	Jackson	112	752
Natchez Regional Medical Center[2]	Natchez	115	235
Singing River Hospital[2]	Pascagoula	133	647
University of Mississippi Medical Center[2]	Jackson	146	290

Head CT Results Within 45 Minutes of Arrival

Hospital Name	City	Rate	Cases
Baptist Memorial Hospital Desoto	Southaven	52%	40
Southwest Ms Regional Medical Center	Mccomb	4%	26

Patients Who Left ER Before Being Seen

Hospital Name	City	Rate	Cases
North Sunflower Medical Center	Ruleville	0%	5365
Southwest Ms Regional Medical Center	Mccomb	0%	42594
Alliance Healthcare System	Holly Springs	1%	4400
Baptist Memorial Hospital/Golden Triangle	Columbus	1%	58026
Biloxi Regional Medical Center	Biloxi	1%	36586
Calhoun Health Services	Calhoun City	1%	5530
Clay County Medical Center	West Point	1%	16639
Field Memorial Community Hospital	Centreville	1%	5330
King's Daughters Med Ctr-Brookhaven	Brookhaven	1%	29794
Madison River Oaks Medical Center	Canton	1%	21769
Pearl River County Hospital	Poplarville	1%	2458
Perry County General Hospital	Richton	1%	2835
Pontotoc Health Service	Pontotoc	1%	11214
River Oaks Hospital	Flowood	1%	21272
Rush Foundation Hospital	Meridian	1%	31153
Scott Regional Hospital	Morton	1%	5764
Tishomingo Health Services	Iuka	1%	10585
Trace Regional Hospital & Swing Bed	Houston	1%	7312
Tyler Holmes Memorial Hospital	Winona	1%	6858
Webster General Hospital/Swing Bed	Eupora	1%	8890
Winston Medical Center & Swingbed	Louisville	1%	11177
Baptist Memorial Hospital Desoto	Southaven	2%	63833
Baptist Mem Hosp North Mississippi	Oxford	2%	35802
Baptist Memorial Hospital Union County	New Albany	2%	23912
Garden Park Medical Center	Gulfport	2%	38430
Gilmore Memorial Regional Medical Center	Amory	2%	20648
Greenwood Leflore Hospital	Greenwood	2%	43911
Grenada Lake Medical Center	Grenada	2%	18392
Memorial Hospital at Gulfport	Gulfport	2%	75247
Montfort Jones Memorial Hospital	Kosciusko	2%	14919
Natchez Community Hospital	Natchez	2%	16551
River Region Health System	Vicksburg	2%	34579
Singing River Hospital	Pascagoula	2%	108515
South Central Regional Medical Center	Laurel	2%	36959
Tri Lakes Medical Center	Batesville	2%	16034
Wayne General Hospital	Waynesboro	2%	15500
Anderson Regional Medical Center	Meridian	3%	32232
Baptist Memorial Hospital Booneville	Booneville	3%	15814
Bolivar Medical Center	Cleveland	3%	17934
Central Mississippi Medical Center	Jackson	3%	47816
Mississippi Baptist Medical Center	Jackson	3%	51001
Natchez Regional Medical Center	Natchez	3%	13676
Neshoba County General Hospital	Philadelphia	3%	19446
North Mississippi Medical Center	Tupelo	3%	89284
Northwest Mississippi Reg Med Ctr	Clarksdale	3%	6540
Saint Dominic - Jackson Memorial Hospital	Jackson	3%	51855
Crossgates River Oaks Hospital	Brandon	4%	24211
George County Hospital	Lucedale	4%	14574
H C Watkins Memorial Hospital	Quitman	4%	4933
Highland Community Hospital	Picayune	4%	22095
Magnolia Regional Health Center	Corinth	4%	35740
Marion General Hospital	Columbia	4%	18404
North Oak Regional Medical Center	Senatobia	4%	10222
University of Mississippi Medical Center	Jackson	4%	122018
Wesley Medical Center	Hattiesburg	4%	36445
Forrest General Hospital	Hattiesburg	5%	83340
Hancock Medical Center	Bay Saint Louis	5%	20690
Holmes County Hospital & Clinics	Lexington	5%	7042
Magee General Hospital	Magee	5%	11056
Kings Daughters Hospital	Yazoo City	7%	4749
Delta Regional Medical Center	Greenville	8%	40541
Greene County Hospital	Leakesville	100%	47

Time from ER Arrival to Being Admitted (minutes)

Hospital Name	City	Min.	Cases
Greenwood Leflore Hospital[2]	Greenwood	142	370
Calhoun Health Services	Calhoun City	154	239
Webster General Hospital/Swing Bed[2]	Eupora	155	309
Clay County Medical Center[2]	West Point	156	276
Tishomingo Health Services[2]	Iuka	161	377
South Sunflower County Hospital[2]	Indianola	162	155
Neshoba County General Hospital[2]	Philadelphia	169	324
Walthall County General Hospital	Tylertown	173	79
Baptist Memorial Hospital Union County[2]	New Albany	174	297
Och Regional Medical Center[2]	Starkville	182	151
Gilmore Memorial Regional Medical Center[2]	Amory	184	315
Jefferson Davis Community Hospital[2]	Prentiss	184	132
Trace Regional Hospital & Swing Bed[2]	Houston	185	236
Wayne General Hospital[2]	Waynesboro	186	449
Magee General Hospital[2]	Magee	190	210
Southwest Ms Regional Medical Center[2]	Mccomb	190	794
Alliance Healthcare System[2]	Holly Springs	195	114
Grenada Lake Medical Center[2]	Grenada	196	1328
Madison River Oaks Medical Center[2]	Canton	197	304
Anderson Regional Medical Center[2]	Meridian	200	550
North Oak Regional Medical Center[2]	Senatobia	200	417
Natchez Community Hospital[2]	Natchez	203	467
Pontotoc Health Service[2]	Pontotoc	203	236
South Central Regional Medical Center[2]	Laurel	203	528
River Oaks Hospital[2]	Flowood	205	237
Marion General Hospital[2]	Columbia	208	488
Tippah County Hospital[2]	Ripley	208	168
Wesley Medical Center[2]	Hattiesburg	209	565
Baptist Mem Hosp North Mississippi[2]	Oxford	210	483
Crossgates River Oaks Hospital[2]	Brandon	210	482
King's Daughters Med Ctr-Brookhaven[2]	Brookhaven	217	351
Montfort Jones Memorial Hospital[2]	Kosciusko	217	525
Garden Park Medical Center[2]	Gulfport	218	456
Bolivar Medical Center[2]	Cleveland	220	329
Baptist Memorial Hospital Booneville[2]	Booneville	222	312
Biloxi Regional Medical Center[2]	Biloxi	223	514
Rush Foundation Hospital[2]	Meridian	227	568
Northwest Mississippi Reg Med Ctr[2]	Clarksdale	231	781
North Mississippi Medical Center[2]	Tupelo	239	542
River Region Health System[2]	Vicksburg	242	748
Covington County Hospital CAH	Collins	243	215
Magnolia Regional Health Center[2]	Corinth	243	684
Winston Medical Center & Swingbed[2]	Louisville	243	272
Tri Lakes Medical Center[2]	Batesville	244	227
Baptist Memorial Hospital/Golden Triangle[2]	Columbus	254	519
Memorial Hospital at Gulfport[2]	Gulfport	255	650
George County Hospital[2]	Lucedale	256	329
Singing River Hospital[2]	Pascagoula	258	669
Forrest General Hospital[2]	Hattiesburg	261	627
Highland Community Hospital[2]	Picayune	263	480
Central Mississippi Medical Center[2]	Jackson	265	753
Hancock Medical Center[2]	Bay Saint Louis	274	284
Saint Dominic - Jackson Memorial Hospital[2]	Jackson	286	695
Natchez Regional Medical Center[2]	Natchez	300	244
Mississippi Baptist Medical Center[2]	Jackson	304	611
Delta Regional Medical Center[2]	Greenville	313	570
Baptist Memorial Hospital Desoto[2]	Southaven	324	541
University of Mississippi Medical Center[2]	Jackson	363	295

Time from ER Arrival to Discharge (minutes)

Hospital Name	City	Min.	Cases
Pearl River County Hospital[3]	Poplarville	60	49
Trace Regional Hospital & Swing Bed	Houston	73	403
Webster General Hospital/Swing Bed	Eupora	75	379
Jefferson County Hospital[3]	Fayette	78	304
Alliance Healthcare System	Holly Springs	80	273
Perry County General Hospital	Richton	80	229
Pioneer Community Hospital of Aberdeen[3]	Aberdeen	82	1056
Lackey Memorial Hospital	Forest	89	392
Madison River Oaks Medical Center	Canton	89	1037
Biloxi Regional Medical Center	Biloxi	90	460
Central Mississippi Medical Center	Jackson	94	742
Tishomingo Health Services	Iuka	94	406
Garden Park Medical Center	Gulfport	96	517
Calhoun Health Services	Calhoun City	97	435
Gilmore Memorial Regional Medical Center	Amory	97	369
Neshoba County General Hospital	Philadelphia	97	121
Pioneer Health Services of Newton	Newton	97	1087
Tallahatchie Critical Access Hospital	Charleston	100	1268
Clay County Medical Center	West Point	103	382
Greenwood Leflore Hospital	Greenwood	106	410
Och Regional Medical Center	Starkville	107	439
Singing River Hospital	Pascagoula	107	470
Winston Medical Center & Swingbed	Louisville	107	353
River Oaks Hospital	Flowood	108	517
Baptist Memorial Hospital Union County	New Albany	110	382
Southwest Ms Regional Medical Center	Mccomb	110	450
Tippah County Hospital	Ripley	111	364
Covington County Hospital CAH	Collins	112	312
Crossgates River Oaks Hospital	Brandon	112	349
Grenada Lake Medical Center	Grenada	112	14526
Natchez Community Hospital	Natchez	112	489
Wayne General Hospital	Waynesboro	112	362
Marion General Hospital	Columbia	113	475
Pontotoc Health Service	Pontotoc	113	389
South Sunflower County Hospital	Indianola	113	355
River Region Health System	Vicksburg	115	393
South Central Regional Medical Center	Laurel	116	372
Anderson Regional Medical Center	Meridian	117	359
Magee General Hospital	Magee	120	496
George County Hospital	Lucedale	121	395
Hancock Medical Center	Bay Saint Louis	121	344
Bolivar Medical Center	Cleveland	122	362
North Oak Regional Medical Center	Senatobia	122	1414
Northwest Mississippi Reg Med Ctr	Clarksdale	123	678
Hardy Wilson Memorial Hospital	Hazlehurst	124	353
Baptist Memorial Hospital Booneville	Booneville	125	377
King's Daughters Med Ctr-Brookhaven	Brookhaven	126	352
Tri Lakes Medical Center	Batesville	126	444
Highland Community Hospital	Picayune	127	506
Wesley Medical Center	Hattiesburg	127	404
Rush Foundation Hospital	Meridian	129	361
Baptist Mem Hosp North Mississippi	Oxford	130	344
Montfort Jones Memorial Hospital	Kosciusko	130	361
Magnolia Regional Health Center	Corinth	137	526
Memorial Hospital at Gulfport	Gulfport	143	393
University of Mississippi Medical Center	Jackson	144	366
Baptist Memorial Hospital/Golden Triangle	Columbus	150	368
Natchez Regional Medical Center	Natchez	157	392
Mississippi Baptist Medical Center	Jackson	181	451
North Mississippi Medical Center	Tupelo	186	417
Saint Dominic - Jackson Memorial Hospital	Jackson	197	361
Delta Regional Medical Center	Greenville	201	361
Baptist Memorial Hospital Desoto	Southaven	235	337
Forrest General Hospital	Hattiesburg	236	430

Time in ER Before Being Evaluated (minutes)

Hospital Name	City	Min.	Cases
Alliance Healthcare System	Holly Springs	10	321
Jefferson County Hospital[3]	Fayette	10	331
Neshoba County General Hospital	Philadelphia	10	308
Perry County General Hospital	Richton	10	247
Pioneer Health Services of Newton	Newton	15	1119
Tallahatchie Critical Access Hospital	Charleston	15	1236
Memorial Hospital at Gulfport	Gulfport	16	424
Pearl River County Hospital[3]	Poplarville	16	62

NOTE: Hospital profiles are in alphabetical order by state, then city, then hospital within the city; Rankings exclude hospitals with less than 25 cases except for patient surveys which excludes hospitals with less than 100 cases; (a) 100-299 cases; (1) The number of cases/patients is too few to report; (2) Data submitted were based on a sample of cases/patients; (3) Results are based on a shorter time period than required; (4) Data suppressed by CMS for one or more quarters; (5) Results are not available for this reporting period; (6) Fewer than 100 patients completed the HCAHPS survey; (7) No cases met the criteria for this measure; (8) The lower limit of the confidence interval cannot be calculated if the number of observed infections equals zero; (9) No data are available from the state/territory for this reporting period; (10) The scores shown reflect fewer than 50 completed surveys; (11) There were discrepancies in the data collection process; (12) This measure does not apply to this hospital for this reporting period; (13) Results cannot be calculated for this reporting period; (14) The results for this state are combined with nearby states to protect confidentiality; Please refer to the User's Guide for a full explanation of data.

Pioneer Community Hospital of Aberdeen[3]	Aberdeen	17	988
Southwest Ms Regional Medical Center	Mccomb	17	389
Biloxi Regional Medical Center	Biloxi	18	509
Bolivar Medical Center	Cleveland	18	437
Montfort Jones Memorial Hospital	Kosciusko	19	312
Trace Regional Hospital & Swing Bed	Houston	19	415
Garden Park Medical Center	Gulfport	20	541
Gilmore Memorial Regional Medical Center	Amory	20	389
Lackey Memorial Hospital	Forest	20	401
Natchez Community Hospital	Natchez	20	517
Natchez Regional Medical Center	Natchez	20	418
Webster General Hospital/Swing Bed	Eupora	20	394
Calhoun Health Services	Calhoun City	22	444
Highland Community Hospital	Picayune	22	625
King's Daughters Med Ctr-Brookhaven	Brookhaven	22	378
South Central Regional Medical Center	Laurel	22	386
Tri Lakes Medical Center	Batesville	22	507
Covington County Hospital CAH	Collins	23	308
Greenwood Leflore Hospital	Greenwood	25	435
Tishomingo Health Services	Iuka	27	418
Madison River Oaks Medical Center	Canton	28	1115
Wesley Medical Center	Hattiesburg	28	415
Winston Medical Center & Swingbed	Louisville	28	369
Baptist Memorial Hospital Union County	New Albany	29	407
Central Mississippi Medical Center	Jackson	29	789
Grenada Lake Medical Center	Grenada	30	14972
Tippah County Hospital	Ripley	30	377
Marion General Hospital	Columbia	31	547
Hancock Medical Center	Bay Saint Louis	34	381
University of Mississippi Medical Center	Jackson	34	152
Anderson Regional Medical Center	Meridian	35	402
Baptist Mem Hosp North Mississippi	Oxford	35	372
River Region Health System	Vicksburg	35	408
Baptist Memorial Hospital Booneville	Booneville	36	392
Hardy Wilson Memorial Hospital	Hazlehurst	36	349
Pontotoc Health Service	Pontotoc	37	414
Magee General Hospital	Magee	39	563
Northwest Mississippi Reg Med Ctr	Clarksdale	39	733
Rush Foundation Hospital	Meridian	39	394
George County Hospital	Lucedale	40	294
North Oak Regional Medical Center	Senatobia	40	1564
Singing River Hospital	Pascagoula	40	314
River Oaks Hospital	Flowood	41	534
Clay County Medical Center	West Point	43	410
Wayne General Hospital	Waynesboro	43	371
Crossgates River Oaks Hospital	Brandon	45	378
Magnolia Regional Health Center	Corinth	47	541
Baptist Memorial Hospital/Golden Triangle	Columbus	54	384
North Mississippi Medical Center	Tupelo	60	429
Och Regional Medical Center	Starkville	60	453
South Sunflower County Hospital	Indianola	62	199
Saint Dominic - Jackson Memorial Hospital	Jackson	65	401
Forrest General Hospital	Hattiesburg	72	241
Baptist Memorial Hospital Desoto	Southaven	76	398
Delta Regional Medical Center	Greenville	79	172
Mississippi Baptist Medical Center	Jackson	90	478

Time to Pain Meds for Bone Fractures (minutes)

Hospital Name	City	Min.	Cases
Neshoba County General Hospital	Philadelphia	38	60
Rush Foundation Hospital	Meridian	44	94
Madison River Oaks Medical Center	Canton	47	79
Garden Park Medical Center	Gulfport	52	96
Southwest Ms Regional Medical Center	Mccomb	52	83
Bolivar Medical Center	Cleveland	53	43
River Region Health System	Vicksburg	53	75
Calhoun Health Services	Calhoun City	54	25
Clay County Medical Center	West Point	55	31
Magee General Hospital	Magee	55	44
Trace Regional Hospital & Swing Bed	Houston	55	29
Biloxi Regional Medical Center	Biloxi	56	83
George County Hospital	Lucedale	56	40
River Oaks Hospital	Flowood	56	76
Tippah County Hospital	Ripley	56	34
Baptist Mem Hosp North Mississippi	Oxford	57	114
Crossgates River Oaks Hospital	Brandon	57	77
Memorial Hospital at Gulfport	Gulfport	58	125
King's Daughters Med Ctr-Brookhaven	Brookhaven	59	52
Central Mississippi Medical Center	Jackson	60	71
Highland Community Hospital	Picayune	60	99
South Central Regional Medical Center	Laurel	60	126
Greenwood Leflore Hospital	Greenwood	61	63
Winston Medical Center & Swingbed	Louisville	62	40
Natchez Community Hospital	Natchez	64	41
Och Regional Medical Center	Starkville	64	68
Wesley Medical Center	Hattiesburg	64	104
Anderson Regional Medical Center	Meridian	65	129
Gilmore Memorial Regional Medical Center	Amory	65	59
Northwest Mississippi Reg Med Ctr	Clarksdale	66	42
University of Mississippi Medical Center	Jackson	66	306
Montfort Jones Memorial Hospital	Kosciusko	67	37

Baptist Memorial Hospital Booneville	Booneville	68	41
Baptist Memorial Hospital Union County	New Albany	68	100
Pontotoc Health Service	Pontotoc	68	52
Covington County Hospital CAH	Collins	69	29
Grenada Lake Medical Center	Grenada	70	91
Singing River Hospital	Pascagoula	70	231
Tishomingo Health Services	Iuka	72	29
Wayne General Hospital	Waynesboro	72	50
Magnolia Regional Health Center	Corinth	73	120
Saint Dominic - Jackson Memorial Hospital	Jackson	77	83
Baptist Memorial Hospital/Golden Triangle	Columbus	78	121
Forrest General Hospital	Hattiesburg	79	253
Hancock Medical Center	Bay Saint Louis	79	71
Marion General Hospital	Columbia	82	57
North Mississippi Medical Center	Tupelo	84	308
Tri Lakes Medical Center	Batesville	84	52
Baptist Memorial Hospital Desoto	Southaven	86	190
Mississippi Baptist Medical Center	Jackson	90	170
North Oak Regional Medical Center	Senatobia	90	51
Natchez Regional Medical Center	Natchez	92	41
Delta Regional Medical Center	Greenville	114	110

Heart Attack Care

Aspirin Given at Discharge

Hospital Name	City	Rate	Cases
Anderson Regional Medical Center	Meridian	100%	231
Baptist Memorial Hospital Desoto	Southaven	100%	530
Baptist Mem Hosp North Mississippi	Oxford	100%	215
Baptist Memorial Hospital/Golden Triangle	Columbus	100%	143
GV (Sonny) Montgomery VA Med Ctr	Jackson	100%	59
Magnolia Regional Health Center	Corinth	100%	188
Memorial Hospital at Gulfport[2]	Gulfport	100%	295
North Mississippi Medical Center[2]	Tupelo	100%	513
Singing River Hospital[2]	Pascagoula	100%	301
University of Mississippi Medical Center[2]	Jackson	100%	267
Forrest General Hospital	Hattiesburg	99%	493
River Region Health System	Vicksburg	99%	120
Rush Foundation Hospital	Meridian	99%	171
Mississippi Baptist Medical Center	Jackson	98%	264
Saint Dominic - Jackson Memorial Hospital	Jackson	98%	568
Southwest Ms Regional Medical Center	Mccomb	98%	132
Wesley Medical Center	Hattiesburg	98%	106
Greenwood Leflore Hospital	Greenwood	97%	65
Delta Regional Medical Center	Greenville	95%	144
Northwest Mississippi Reg Med Ctr	Clarksdale	91%	44
Central Mississippi Medical Center	Jackson	90%	104
South Central Regional Medical Center	Laurel	86%	29

PCI Within 90 Minutes of Arrival

Hospital Name	City	Rate	Cases
Baptist Mem Hosp North Mississippi	Oxford	100%	26
Baptist Memorial Hospital/Golden Triangle	Columbus	100%	41
Forrest General Hospital	Hattiesburg	100%	47
Magnolia Regional Health Center	Corinth	100%	28
Saint Dominic - Jackson Memorial Hospital	Jackson	100%	63
Baptist Memorial Hospital Desoto	Southaven	99%	67
Mississippi Baptist Medical Center	Jackson	98%	46
North Mississippi Medical Center[2]	Tupelo	98%	52
Singing River Hospital[2]	Pascagoula	98%	45
Memorial Hospital at Gulfport[2]	Gulfport	89%	54
University of Mississippi Medical Center[2]	Jackson	89%	28

Statin Prescribed at Discharge

Hospital Name	City	Rate	Cases
Baptist Mem Hosp North Mississippi	Oxford	100%	206
Baptist Memorial Hospital/Golden Triangle	Columbus	100%	137
North Mississippi Medical Center[2]	Tupelo	100%	516
University of Mississippi Medical Center[2]	Jackson	100%	263
Wesley Medical Center	Hattiesburg	100%	93
Baptist Memorial Hospital Desoto	Southaven	99%	512
Magnolia Regional Health Center	Corinth	99%	173
Singing River Hospital[2]	Pascagoula	99%	302
Anderson Regional Medical Center	Meridian	98%	229
Forrest General Hospital	Hattiesburg	98%	472
GV (Sonny) Montgomery VA Med Ctr	Jackson	98%	60
River Region Health System	Vicksburg	98%	98
Southwest Ms Regional Medical Center	Mccomb	98%	124
Mississippi Baptist Medical Center	Jackson	97%	259
Saint Dominic - Jackson Memorial Hospital	Jackson	97%	561
Rush Foundation Hospital	Meridian	96%	171
Central Mississippi Medical Center	Jackson	95%	86
Memorial Hospital at Gulfport[2]	Gulfport	95%	277
Northwest Mississippi Reg Med Ctr	Clarksdale	95%	43
Greenwood Leflore Hospital	Greenwood	94%	65
Delta Regional Medical Center	Greenville	92%	133
South Central Regional Medical Center	Laurel	69%	26

Heart Failure Care

ACE Inhibitor or ARB for LVSD

Hospital Name	City	Rate	Cases
Anderson Regional Medical Center[2]	Meridian	100%	90
Baptist Mem Hosp North Mississippi	Oxford	100%	95
Baptist Memorial Hospital Union County	New Albany	100%	32
Baptist Memorial Hospital/Golden Triangle	Columbus	100%	86
Biloxi Regional Medical Center	Biloxi	100%	37
Bolivar Medical Center	Cleveland	100%	32
Garden Park Medical Center[2]	Gulfport	100%	34
Gilmore Memorial Regional Medical Center	Amory	100%	31
GV (Sonny) Montgomery VA Med Ctr	Jackson	100%	102
Highland Community Hospital	Picayune	100%	26
Wesley Medical Center	Hattiesburg	100%	72
Baptist Memorial Hospital Desoto	Southaven	99%	193
Greenwood Leflore Hospital	Greenwood	99%	84
Memorial Hospital at Gulfport[2]	Gulfport	99%	98
Singing River Hospital	Pascagoula	99%	172
University of Mississippi Medical Center[2]	Jackson	99%	137
Forrest General Hospital	Hattiesburg	98%	244
Magnolia Regional Health Center	Corinth	98%	84
North Mississippi Medical Center[2]	Tupelo	98%	136
River Region Health System	Vicksburg	98%	128
Clay County Medical Center	West Point	97%	33
Delta Regional Medical Center	Greenville	97%	161
Northwest Mississippi Reg Med Ctr	Clarksdale	97%	100
Central Mississippi Medical Center	Jackson	95%	93
King's Daughters Med Ctr-Brookhaven	Brookhaven	95%	40
Saint Dominic - Jackson Memorial Hospital[2]	Jackson	95%	105
Natchez Community Hospital	Natchez	93%	45
Rush Foundation Hospital	Meridian	92%	97
Southwest Ms Regional Medical Center	Mccomb	89%	98
Wayne General Hospital	Waynesboro	84%	45
Grenada Lake Medical Center[2]	Grenada	81%	37
Mississippi Baptist Medical Center	Jackson	81%	163
Natchez Regional Medical Center	Natchez	76%	41
South Central Regional Medical Center	Laurel	61%	101

Discharge Instructions Given

Hospital Name	City	Rate	Cases
Baptist Memorial Hospital Desoto	Southaven	100%	618
Baptist Memorial Hospital Union County	New Albany	100%	73
Biloxi Regional Medical Center	Biloxi	100%	116
Bolivar Medical Center	Cleveland	100%	121
Crossgates River Oaks Hospital	Brandon	100%	58
Forrest General Hospital	Hattiesburg	100%	603
Garden Park Medical Center[2]	Gulfport	100%	97
Wayne General Hospital	Waynesboro	100%	96
Webster General Hospital/Swing Bed	Eupora	100%	34
Greenwood Leflore Hospital	Greenwood	99%	159
GV (Sonny) Montgomery VA Med Ctr	Jackson	99%	199
Magnolia Regional Health Center	Corinth	99%	191
North Mississippi Medical Center[2]	Tupelo	99%	274
River Region Health System	Vicksburg	99%	283
Singing River Hospital	Pascagoula	99%	403
University of Mississippi Medical Center[2]	Jackson	99%	256
Wesley Medical Center	Hattiesburg	99%	176
Baptist Memorial Hospital/Golden Triangle	Columbus	98%	184
Hancock Medical Center	Bay Saint Louis	98%	50
River Oaks Hospital	Flowood	98%	40
Delta Regional Medical Center	Greenville	97%	435
King's Daughters Med Ctr-Brookhaven	Brookhaven	97%	101
Madison River Oaks Medical Center	Canton	95%	84
Neshoba County General Hospital[2]	Philadelphia	95%	65
Saint Dominic - Jackson Memorial Hospital[2]	Jackson	95%	280
Anderson Regional Medical Center[2]	Meridian	94%	267
Baptist Mem Hosp North Mississippi	Oxford	94%	231
Montfort Jones Memorial Hospital[2]	Kosciusko	93%	45
Magee General Hospital	Magee	92%	26
Memorial Hospital at Gulfport[2]	Gulfport	92%	262
Natchez Regional Medical Center	Natchez	92%	92
Tri Lakes Medical Center	Batesville	92%	59
Northwest Mississippi Reg Med Ctr	Clarksdale	91%	218
Rush Foundation Hospital	Meridian	91%	160
North Sunflower Medical Center	Ruleville	90%	29
Och Regional Medical Center	Starkville	90%	41
Gilmore Memorial Regional Medical Center	Amory	89%	37
Highland Community Hospital	Picayune	88%	60
Southwest Ms Regional Medical Center	Mccomb	88%	185
Clay County Medical Center	West Point	86%	66
Natchez Community Hospital	Natchez	86%	99
VA Gulf Coast Healthcare System	Biloxi	85%	41
Central Mississippi Medical Center	Jackson	84%	195
George County Hospital[2]	Lucedale	83%	41
South Central Regional Medical Center	Laurel	79%	210
Grenada Lake Medical Center[2]	Grenada	72%	80
Mississippi Baptist Medical Center	Jackson	63%	461
South Sunflower County Hospital[2]	Indianola	60%	45
Kings Daughters Hospital	Yazoo City	59%	34

NOTE: Hospital profiles are in alphabetical order by state, then city, then hospital within the city; Rankings exclude hospitals with less than 25 cases except for patient surveys which excludes hospitals with less than 100 cases; (a) 100-299 cases; (1) The number of cases/patients is too few to report; (2) Data submitted were based on a sample of cases/patients; (3) Results are based on a shorter time period than required; (4) Data suppressed by CMS for one or more quarters; (5) Results are not available for this reporting period; (6) Fewer than 100 patients completed the HCAHPS survey; (7) No cases met the criteria for this measure; (8) The lower limit of the confidence interval cannot be calculated if the number of observed infections equals zero; (9) No data are available from the state/territory for this reporting period; (10) The scores shown reflect fewer than 50 completed surveys; (11) There were discrepancies in the data collection process; (12) This measure does not apply to this hospital for this reporting period; (13) Results cannot be calculated for this reporting period; (14) The results for this state are combined with nearby states to protect confidentiality; Please refer to the User's Guide for a full explanation of data.

Marion General Hospital[2]	Columbia	56%	50
Hardy Wilson Memorial Hospital[2]	Hazlehurst	19%	27

Evaluation of LVS Function

Hospital Name	City	Rate	Cases
Anderson Regional Medical Center[2]	Meridian	100%	327
Baptist Memorial Hospital Desoto	Southaven	100%	740
Baptist Mem Hosp North Mississippi	Oxford	100%	276
Baptist Memorial Hospital Union County	New Albany	100%	102
Baptist Memorial Hospital/Golden Triangle	Columbus	100%	212
Biloxi Regional Medical Center	Biloxi	100%	144
Bolivar Medical Center	Cleveland	100%	133
Forrest General Hospital	Hattiesburg	100%	717
Garden Park Medical Center[2]	Gulfport	100%	101
Gilmore Memorial Regional Medical Center	Amory	100%	65
GV (Sonny) Montgomery VA Med Ctr	Jackson	100%	208
King's Daughters Med Ctr-Brookhaven	Brookhaven	100%	128
Magnolia Regional Health Center	Corinth	100%	238
Memorial Hospital at Gulfport[2]	Gulfport	100%	306
North Mississippi Medical Center[2]	Tupelo	100%	315
Northwest Mississippi Reg Med Ctr	Clarksdale	100%	238
River Oaks Hospital	Flowood	100%	48
River Region Health System	Vicksburg	100%	324
Singing River Hospital	Pascagoula	100%	460
Tishomingo Health Services	Iuka	100%	35
VA Gulf Coast Healthcare System	Biloxi	100%	49
Webster General Hospital/Swing Bed	Eupora	100%	43
Wesley Medical Center	Hattiesburg	100%	205
Clay County Medical Center	West Point	99%	92
Crossgates River Oaks Hospital	Brandon	99%	94
Natchez Community Hospital	Natchez	99%	116
University of Mississippi Medical Center[2]	Jackson	99%	275
Baptist Memorial Hospital Booneville	Booneville	98%	42
Central Mississippi Medical Center	Jackson	98%	214
Greenwood Leflore Hospital	Greenwood	98%	191
Madison River Oaks Medical Center	Canton	98%	93
Marion General Hospital[2]	Columbia	98%	63
Natchez Regional Medical Center	Natchez	98%	112
Och Regional Medical Center	Starkville	98%	49
Saint Dominic - Jackson Memorial Hospital[2]	Jackson	98%	326
Delta Regional Medical Center	Greenville	97%	487
Hancock Medical Center	Bay Saint Louis	97%	60
Highland Community Hospital	Picayune	97%	69
Rush Foundation Hospital	Meridian	97%	190
Grenada Lake Medical Center[2]	Grenada	96%	101
Montfort Jones Memorial Hospital[2]	Kosciusko	96%	68
North Sunflower Medical Center	Ruleville	96%	49
Tri Lakes Medical Center	Batesville	96%	76
Wayne General Hospital	Waynesboro	96%	111
Mississippi Baptist Medical Center	Jackson	95%	549
George County Hospital[2]	Lucedale	94%	54
Southwest Ms Regional Medical Center	Mccomb	94%	211
Magee General Hospital	Magee	92%	37
Scott Regional Hospital	Morton	92%	25
North Oak Regional Medical Center	Senatobia	91%	32
South Central Regional Medical Center	Laurel	91%	264
Tyler Holmes Memorial Hospital	Winona	88%	34
Beacham Memorial Hospital[2]	Magnolia	83%	30
South Sunflower County Hospital[2]	Indianola	82%	57
Kings Daughters Hospital	Yazoo City	80%	44
Tippah County Hospital	Ripley	44%	25
Pioneer Health Services of Newton[2,3]	Newton	42%	26
Neshoba County General Hospital[2]	Philadelphia	34%	65
Hardy Wilson Memorial Hospital[2]	Hazlehurst	31%	32

Medicare Spending

Medicare Spending per Patient (ratio)

Hospital Name	City	Ratio	Cases
Whitfield Medical Surgical Hospital	Whitfield	0.54	-
Yalobusha General Hospital	Water Valley	0.75	-
Kilmichael Hospital	Kilmichael	0.82	-
Neshoba County General Hospital	Philadelphia	0.84	-
Wayne General Hospital	Waynesboro	0.86	-
South Sunflower County Hospital	Indianola	0.87	-
Beacham Memorial Hospital	Magnolia	0.89	-
Winston Medical Center & Swingbed	Louisville	0.90	-
Trace Regional Hospital & Swing Bed	Houston	0.91	-
Montfort Jones Memorial Hospital	Kosciusko	0.92	-
Northwest Mississippi Reg Med Ctr	Clarksdale	0.92	-
Tishomingo Health Services	Iuka	0.92	-
Webster General Hospital/Swing Bed	Eupora	0.92	-
Baptist Memorial Hospital Union County	New Albany	0.93	-
Marion General Hospital	Columbia	0.93	-
South Central Regional Medical Center	Laurel	0.93	-
North Oak Regional Medical Center	Senatobia	0.94	-
Tippah County Hospital	Ripley	0.95	-
Baptist Memorial Hospital Desoto	Southaven	0.96	-
Baptist Mem Hosp North Mississippi	Oxford	0.96	-
Clay County Medical Center	West Point	0.96	-
Gilmore Memorial Regional Medical Center	Amory	0.96	-
Magnolia Regional Health Center	Corinth	0.96	-
Jefferson County Hospital	Fayette	0.97	-
North Mississippi Medical Center	Tupelo	0.97	-
River Oaks Hospital	Flowood	0.97	-
Sharkey Issaquena Community Hospital	Rolling Fork	0.97	-
Baptist Memorial Hospital Booneville	Booneville	0.98	-
Baptist Memorial Hospital/Golden Triangle	Columbus	0.98	-
Grenada Lake Medical Center	Grenada	0.98	-
Hancock Medical Center	Bay Saint Louis	0.98	-
Och Regional Medical Center	Starkville	0.98	-
Forrest General Hospital	Hattiesburg	0.99	-
Garden Park Medical Center	Gulfport	0.99	-
George County Hospital	Lucedale	0.99	-
Highland Community Hospital	Picayune	0.99	-
King's Daughters Med Ctr-Brookhaven	Brookhaven	0.99	-
Saint Dominic - Jackson Memorial Hospital	Jackson	0.99	-
Wesley Medical Center	Hattiesburg	0.99	-
Anderson Regional Medical Center	Meridian	1.00	-
Madison River Oaks Medical Center	Canton	1.00	-
Memorial Hospital at Gulfport	Gulfport	1.00	-
Singing River Hospital	Pascagoula	1.00	-
Southwest Ms Regional Medical Center	Mccomb	1.00	-
Woman's Hospital at River Oaks	Flowood	1.00	-
Mississippi Baptist Medical Center	Jackson	1.01	-
Biloxi Regional Medical Center	Biloxi	1.02	-
Bolivar Medical Center	Cleveland	1.02	-
Tri Lakes Medical Center	Batesville	1.02	-
University of Mississippi Medical Center	Jackson	1.02	-
Central Mississippi Medical Center	Jackson	1.03	-
Magee General Hospital	Magee	1.03	-
Alliance Healthcare System	Holly Springs	1.04	-
Greenwood Leflore Hospital	Greenwood	1.04	-
Crossgates River Oaks Hospital	Brandon	1.05	-
Delta Regional Medical Center	Greenville	1.06	-
Natchez Regional Medical Center	Natchez	1.07	-
River Region Health System	Vicksburg	1.07	-
Natchez Community Hospital	Natchez	1.09	-
Alliance Health Center	Meridian	1.12	-
Rush Foundation Hospital	Meridian	1.13	-

Pneumonia Care

Appropriate Initial Antibiotic Given

Hospital Name	City	Rate	Cases
Baptist Mem Hosp North Mississippi	Oxford	100%	111
Bolivar Medical Center	Cleveland	100%	42
Crossgates River Oaks Hospital	Brandon	100%	48
Garden Park Medical Center[2]	Gulfport	100%	60
George County Hospital	Lucedale	100%	31
Gilmore Memorial Regional Medical Center	Amory	100%	72
Northwest Mississippi Reg Med Ctr	Clarksdale	100%	29
Pontotoc Health Service	Pontotoc	100%	40
Singing River Hospital[2]	Pascagoula	100%	88
Baptist Memorial Hospital Union County	New Albany	99%	82
Baptist Memorial Hospital/Golden Triangle	Columbus	99%	74
GV (Sonny) Montgomery VA Med Ctr	Jackson	99%	69
North Mississippi Medical Center[2]	Tupelo	99%	212
River Oaks Hospital	Flowood	99%	68
Wesley Medical Center	Hattiesburg	99%	94
Baptist Memorial Hospital Desoto	Southaven	98%	350
Tishomingo Health Services	Iuka	98%	47
Tri Lakes Medical Center	Batesville	98%	42
Baptist Memorial Hospital Booneville	Booneville	97%	90
Central Mississippi Medical Center	Jackson	97%	58
King's Daughters Med Ctr-Brookhaven	Brookhaven	97%	100
Biloxi Regional Medical Center	Biloxi	96%	83
South Sunflower County Hospital[2]	Indianola	96%	26
University of Mississippi Medical Center[2]	Jackson	96%	28
Highland Community Hospital[2]	Picayune	95%	74
Natchez Regional Medical Center	Natchez	95%	55
Scott Regional Hospital	Morton	95%	43
Wayne General Hospital	Waynesboro	95%	62
Greenwood Leflore Hospital	Greenwood	94%	77
Magnolia Regional Health Center	Corinth	94%	162
Marion General Hospital[2]	Columbia	94%	48
Natchez Community Hospital	Natchez	94%	67
Forrest General Hospital	Hattiesburg	93%	214
Madison River Oaks Medical Center	Canton	93%	45
Memorial Hospital at Gulfport[2]	Gulfport	93%	87
River Region Health System	Vicksburg	93%	128
Rush Foundation Hospital	Meridian	93%	69
Delta Regional Medical Center	Greenville	92%	95
Clay County Medical Center	West Point	91%	79
Och Regional Medical Center	Starkville	91%	65
Mississippi Baptist Medical Center[2]	Jackson	90%	124
South Central Regional Medical Center	Laurel	90%	191
North Sunflower Medical Center	Ruleville	89%	35
Southwest Ms Regional Medical Center[2]	Mccomb	89%	108
Anderson Regional Medical Center[2]	Meridian	88%	66
Hancock Medical Center[2]	Bay Saint Louis	86%	51
Saint Dominic - Jackson Memorial Hospital[2]	Jackson	86%	113
Lackey Memorial Hospital	Forest	85%	34
Webster General Hospital/Swing Bed	Eupora	85%	88
Magee General Hospital	Magee	84%	99
Trace Regional Hospital & Swing Bed[2]	Houston	81%	26
Hardy Wilson Memorial Hospital[2]	Hazlehurst	80%	25
North Oak Regional Medical Center	Senatobia	79%	28
Tippah County Hospital	Ripley	76%	33
Grenada Lake Medical Center[2]	Grenada	73%	49
Montfort Jones Memorial Hospital[2]	Kosciusko	72%	46
Pioneer Health Services of Newton[2,3]	Newton	65%	26
Tallahatchie Critical Access Hospital	Charleston	63%	27
Beacham Memorial Hospital[2]	Magnolia	36%	90

Blood Culture Timing

Hospital Name	City	Rate	Cases
Anderson Regional Medical Center[2]	Meridian	100%	103
Baptist Memorial Hospital Booneville	Booneville	100%	84
Baptist Mem Hosp North Mississippi	Oxford	100%	235
Biloxi Regional Medical Center	Biloxi	100%	126
Bolivar Medical Center	Cleveland	100%	97
Garden Park Medical Center[2]	Gulfport	100%	86
Greenwood Leflore Hospital	Greenwood	100%	108
Natchez Community Hospital	Natchez	100%	99
River Oaks Hospital	Flowood	100%	59
Singing River Hospital[2]	Pascagoula	100%	152
Tishomingo Health Services	Iuka	100%	53
Tri Lakes Medical Center	Batesville	100%	38
VA Gulf Coast Healthcare System	Biloxi	100%	62
Baptist Memorial Hospital Desoto	Southaven	99%	523
Baptist Memorial Hospital Union County	New Albany	99%	102
Baptist Memorial Hospital/Golden Triangle	Columbus	99%	191
Crossgates River Oaks Hospital	Brandon	99%	91
Gilmore Memorial Regional Medical Center	Amory	99%	94
GV (Sonny) Montgomery VA Med Ctr	Jackson	99%	192
King's Daughters Med Ctr-Brookhaven	Brookhaven	99%	146
Magnolia Regional Health Center	Corinth	99%	197
Mississippi Baptist Medical Center[2]	Jackson	99%	210
River Region Health System	Vicksburg	99%	198
Wesley Medical Center	Hattiesburg	99%	140
Central Mississippi Medical Center	Jackson	98%	94
Highland Community Hospital[2]	Picayune	98%	129
North Mississippi Medical Center[2]	Tupelo	98%	329
Och Regional Medical Center	Starkville	98%	66
Pontotoc Health Service	Pontotoc	98%	51
Rush Foundation Hospital	Meridian	98%	97
Saint Dominic - Jackson Memorial Hospital[2]	Jackson	98%	163
Webster General Hospital/Swing Bed	Eupora	98%	84
Marion General Hospital[2]	Columbia	97%	62
Memorial Hospital at Gulfport[2]	Gulfport	97%	169
Natchez Regional Medical Center	Natchez	97%	63
Northwest Mississippi Reg Med Ctr	Clarksdale	97%	31
South Central Regional Medical Center	Laurel	97%	219
Southwest Ms Regional Medical Center[2]	Mccomb	97%	179
Forrest General Hospital	Hattiesburg	95%	352
George County Hospital	Lucedale	95%	57
University of Mississippi Medical Center[2]	Jackson	95%	103
Calhoun Health Services[2]	Calhoun City	94%	34
Clay County Medical Center	West Point	94%	81
Grenada Lake Medical Center[2]	Grenada	94%	80
Wayne General Hospital	Waynesboro	94%	66
Delta Regional Medical Center	Greenville	93%	127
Hardy Wilson Memorial Hospital[2]	Hazlehurst	93%	29
Madison River Oaks Medical Center	Canton	93%	57
Montfort Jones Memorial Hospital[2]	Kosciusko	92%	49
Scott Regional Hospital	Morton	92%	26
Hancock Medical Center[2]	Bay Saint Louis	91%	47
Magee General Hospital	Magee	91%	86
Tippah County Hospital	Ripley	90%	31
Trace Regional Hospital & Swing Bed[2]	Houston	90%	29
North Oak Regional Medical Center	Senatobia	88%	32
North Sunflower Medical Center	Ruleville	75%	51

Pregnancy and Delivery Care

Newborns whose Deliveries were Scheduled Early

Hospital Name	City	Rate	Cases
Baptist Memorial Hospital Union County[2]	New Albany	0%	31
Bolivar Medical Center[2]	Cleveland	0%	27
Garden Park Medical Center[2]	Gulfport	0%	42
Madison River Oaks Medical Center	Canton	0%	42
Wesley Medical Center[2]	Hattiesburg	0%	41
Greenwood Leflore Hospital	Greenwood	1%	74
King's Daughters Med Ctr-Brookhaven	Brookhaven	6%	66
River Oaks Hospital[2]	Flowood	6%	50
Magee General Hospital	Magee	7%	82
Magnolia Regional Health Center	Corinth	7%	70
North Mississippi Medical Center[2]	Tupelo	7%	55
Baptist Mem Hosp North Mississippi[2]	Oxford	9%	33

NOTE: Hospital profiles are in alphabetical order by state, then city, then hospital within the city; Rankings exclude hospitals with less than 25 cases except for patient surveys which excludes hospitals with less than 100 cases; (a) 100-299 cases; (1) The number of cases/patients is too few to report; (2) Data submitted were based on a sample of cases/patients; (3) Results are based on a shorter time period than required; (4) Data suppressed by CMS for one or more quarters; (5) Results are not available for this reporting period; (6) Fewer than 100 patients completed the HCAHPS survey; (7) No cases met the criteria for this measure; (8) The lower limit of the confidence interval cannot be calculated if the number of observed infections equals zero; (9) No data are available from the state/territory for this reporting period; (10) The scores shown reflect fewer than 50 completed surveys; (11) There were discrepancies in the data collection process; (12) This measure does not apply to this hospital for this reporting period; (13) Results cannot be calculated for this reporting period; (14) The results for this state are combined with nearby states to protect confidentiality; Please refer to the User's Guide for a full explanation of data.

Memorial Hospital at Gulfport[2]	Gulfport	10%	52
Och Regional Medical Center[2]	Starkville	11%	57
Singing River Hospital[2]	Pascagoula	14%	58
Southwest Ms Regional Medical Center[2]	Mccomb	14%	37
South Central Regional Medical Center[2]	Laurel	16%	32
George County Hospital	Lucedale	17%	64
Delta Regional Medical Center	Greenville	19%	147
Natchez Community Hospital	Natchez	19%	47
Forrest General Hospital	Hattiesburg	20%	313
Natchez Regional Medical Center	Natchez	20%	35
Rush Foundation Hospital[2]	Meridian	20%	45
Central Mississippi Medical Center	Jackson	21%	89
Anderson Regional Medical Center[2]	Meridian	22%	27
Gilmore Memorial Regional Medical Center	Amory	24%	83
Mississippi Baptist Medical Center	Jackson	24%	140
Biloxi Regional Medical Center[2]	Biloxi	29%	63
Northwest Mississippi Reg Med Ctr	Clarksdale	32%	112
Saint Dominic - Jackson Memorial Hospital[2]	Jackson	38%	60
Grenada Lake Medical Center	Grenada	39%	84
Baptist Memorial Hospital Desoto[2]	Southaven	40%	436
Highland Community Hospital[2]	Picayune	43%	100
Woman's Hospital at River Oaks[2]	Flowood	45%	29
Clay County Medical Center[2]	West Point	51%	43

Preventive Care

Immunization for Influenza

Hospital Name	City	Rate	Cases
Biloxi Regional Medical Center[2]	Biloxi	100%	566
Calhoun Health Services[2]	Calhoun City	100%	145
Central Mississippi Medical Center[2]	Jackson	100%	752
Garden Park Medical Center[2]	Gulfport	100%	486
Greenwood Leflore Hospital[2]	Greenwood	100%	509
Baptist Memorial Hospital Booneville[2]	Booneville	99%	307
Baptist Memorial Hospital Union County[2]	New Albany	99%	382
Crossgates River Oaks Hospital[2]	Brandon	99%	379
Natchez Community Hospital[2]	Natchez	99%	357
River Oaks Hospital[2]	Flowood	99%	475
River Region Health System[2]	Vicksburg	99%	646
Anderson Regional Medical Center[2]	Meridian	98%	542
Baptist Memorial Hospital Desoto[2]	Southaven	98%	566
Baptist Memorial Hospital/Golden Triangle[2]	Columbus	98%	559
Forrest General Hospital[2]	Hattiesburg	98%	584
King's Daughters Med Ctr-Brookhaven[2]	Brookhaven	98%	313
Magnolia Regional Health Center[2]	Corinth	98%	696
Pontotoc Health Service[2]	Pontotoc	98%	181
North Mississippi Medical Center[2]	Tupelo	97%	589
Webster General Hospital/Swing Bed[2]	Eupora	97%	319
Baptist Mem Hosp North Mississippi[2]	Oxford	96%	552
Bolivar Medical Center[2]	Cleveland	96%	355
Gilmore Memorial Regional Medical Center[2]	Amory	96%	338
Northwest Mississippi Reg Med Ctr[2]	Clarksdale	96%	913
Memorial Hospital at Gulfport[2]	Gulfport	95%	570
Wesley Medical Center[2]	Hattiesburg	95%	548
Hancock Medical Center[2]	Bay Saint Louis	94%	262
Tishomingo Health Services[2]	Iuka	94%	299
Marion General Hospital[2]	Columbia	92%	352
Rush Foundation Hospital[2]	Meridian	92%	558
Madison River Oaks Medical Center[2]	Canton	91%	246
Natchez Regional Medical Center[2]	Natchez	91%	256
Mississippi Baptist Medical Center[2]	Jackson	89%	625
Singing River Hospital[2]	Pascagoula	89%	634
Magee General Hospital[2]	Magee	88%	253
Delta Regional Medical Center[2]	Greenville	87%	513
Grenada Lake Medical Center[2]	Grenada	87%	1258
Saint Dominic - Jackson Memorial Hospital[2]	Jackson	87%	578
Tippah County Hospital[2]	Ripley	87%	216
Tri Lakes Medical Center[2]	Batesville	87%	319
Woman's Hospital at River Oaks[2]	Flowood	86%	170
Montfort Jones Memorial Hospital[2]	Kosciusko	82%	267
George County Hospital[2]	Lucedale	79%	278
Southwest Ms Regional Medical Center[2]	Mccomb	79%	531
Highland Community Hospital[2]	Picayune	78%	362
University of Mississippi Medical Center[2]	Jackson	77%	502
Whitfield Medical Surgical Hospital	Whitfield	77%	93
North Oak Regional Medical Center[2]	Senatobia	76%	315
Walthall County General Hospital[2]	Tylertown	73%	88
Alliance Healthcare System[2]	Holly Springs	69%	117
Trace Regional Hospital & Swing Bed[2]	Houston	65%	181
Winston Medical Center & Swingbed	Louisville	65%	207
Covington County Hospital CAH	Collins	61%	75
Clay County Medical Center[2]	West Point	59%	287
Beacham Memorial Hospital[2]	Magnolia	58%	330
South Sunflower County Hospital[2]	Indianola	55%	269
Neshoba County General Hospital[2]	Philadelphia	51%	203
Och Regional Medical Center[2]	Starkville	48%	246
Wayne General Hospital[2]	Waynesboro	43%	265
Yalobusha General Hospital[2]	Water Valley	41%	148
Kilmichael Hospital	Kilmichael	39%	59
South Central Regional Medical Center[2]	Laurel	37%	606
Jefferson Davis Community Hospital[2]	Prentiss	33%	110
Jefferson County Hospital[2]	Fayette	11%	35
Alliance Health Center[2]	Meridian	1%	172

Immunization for Pneumonia

Hospital Name	City	Rate	Cases
Biloxi Regional Medical Center[2]	Biloxi	100%	526
Bolivar Medical Center[2]	Cleveland	100%	355
Calhoun Health Services[2]	Calhoun City	100%	200
Central Mississippi Medical Center[2]	Jackson	100%	738
Garden Park Medical Center[2]	Gulfport	100%	490
Pontotoc Health Service[2]	Pontotoc	100%	252
Baptist Memorial Hospital Booneville[2]	Booneville	99%	501
Baptist Memorial Hospital Union County[2]	New Albany	99%	311
Greenwood Leflore Hospital[2]	Greenwood	99%	585
River Region Health System[2]	Vicksburg	99%	774
Anderson Regional Medical Center[2]	Meridian	98%	704
Baptist Memorial Hospital/Golden Triangle[2]	Columbus	98%	698
King's Daughters Med Ctr-Brookhaven[2]	Brookhaven	98%	295
Natchez Community Hospital[2]	Natchez	98%	383
North Mississippi Medical Center[2]	Tupelo	98%	688
Webster General Hospital/Swing Bed[2]	Eupora	98%	495
Wesley Medical Center[2]	Hattiesburg	98%	614
Baptist Memorial Hospital Desoto[2]	Southaven	97%	660
Crossgates River Oaks Hospital[2]	Brandon	97%	415
Forrest General Hospital[2]	Hattiesburg	97%	652
Magnolia Regional Health Center[2]	Corinth	97%	874
Memorial Hospital at Gulfport[2]	Gulfport	97%	734
River Oaks Hospital[2]	Flowood	97%	359
Gilmore Memorial Regional Medical Center[2]	Amory	96%	297
Tishomingo Health Services[2]	Iuka	96%	446
Northwest Mississippi Reg Med Ctr[2]	Clarksdale	95%	742
Delta Regional Medical Center[2]	Greenville	94%	631
Natchez Regional Medical Center[2]	Natchez	94%	279
Rush Foundation Hospital[2]	Meridian	94%	653
Grenada Lake Medical Center[2]	Grenada	93%	1311
Madison River Oaks Medical Center[2]	Canton	93%	230
Magee General Hospital[2]	Magee	93%	269
Marion General Hospital[2]	Columbia	93%	538
Baptist Mem Hosp North Mississippi[2]	Oxford	92%	678
Tri Lakes Medical Center[2]	Batesville	92%	305
Hancock Medical Center[2]	Bay Saint Louis	91%	265
Singing River Hospital[2]	Pascagoula	91%	737
Tippah County Hospital[2]	Ripley	91%	369
George County Hospital[2]	Lucedale	88%	323
Mississippi Baptist Medical Center[2]	Jackson	88%	831
University of Mississippi Medical Center[2]	Jackson	86%	428
Wayne General Hospital[2]	Waynesboro	86%	374
Montfort Jones Memorial Hospital[2]	Kosciusko	84%	404
Saint Dominic - Jackson Memorial Hospital[2]	Jackson	84%	782
Southwest Ms Regional Medical Center[2]	Mccomb	84%	716
North Oak Regional Medical Center[2]	Senatobia	83%	420
Whitfield Medical Surgical Hospital	Whitfield	82%	115
Highland Community Hospital[2]	Picayune	81%	573
Walthall County General Hospital[2]	Tylertown	79%	91
Winston Medical Center & Swingbed[2]	Louisville	72%	288
Neshoba County General Hospital[2]	Philadelphia	71%	291
Trace Regional Hospital & Swing Bed[2]	Houston	70%	268
Alliance Healthcare System[2]	Holly Springs	67%	183
Och Regional Medical Center[2]	Starkville	64%	209
Clay County Medical Center[2]	West Point	61%	276
Yalobusha General Hospital[2]	Water Valley	61%	205
South Central Regional Medical Center[2]	Laurel	59%	598
South Sunflower County Hospital[2]	Indianola	52%	296
Jefferson Davis Community Hospital[2]	Prentiss	49%	191
Beacham Memorial Hospital[2]	Magnolia	48%	563
Woman's Hospital at River Oaks[2]	Flowood	45%	29
Alliance Health Center[2]	Meridian	40%	70
Covington County Hospital CAH	Collins	40%	201
Kilmichael Hospital	Kilmichael	31%	55
Jefferson County Hospital[2]	Fayette	11%	47

Stroke Care

Anticoagulation Therapy for Atrial Fibrillation

Hospital Name	City	Rate	Cases
Singing River Hospital	Pascagoula	100%	31
Baptist Memorial Hospital Desoto	Southaven	97%	30
Saint Dominic - Jackson Memorial Hospital	Jackson	97%	38
Mississippi Baptist Medical Center	Jackson	92%	38

Antithrombotic Therapy Timing

Hospital Name	City	Rate	Cases
Baptist Mem Hosp North Mississippi	Oxford	100%	82
Baptist Memorial Hospital Union County	New Albany	100%	28
Baptist Memorial Hospital/Golden Triangle	Columbus	100%	96
Central Mississippi Medical Center	Jackson	100%	53
Magnolia Regional Health Center	Corinth	100%	94
Rush Foundation Hospital[2]	Meridian	100%	106
Wesley Medical Center	Hattiesburg	100%	58
Memorial Hospital at Gulfport[2]	Gulfport	99%	83
Singing River Hospital	Pascagoula	99%	174
South Central Regional Medical Center	Laurel	99%	92
Mississippi Baptist Medical Center	Jackson	98%	250
North Mississippi Medical Center[2]	Tupelo	98%	84
Southwest Ms Regional Medical Center	Mccomb	98%	53
Baptist Memorial Hospital Desoto	Southaven	97%	242
Northwest Mississippi Reg Med Ctr	Clarksdale	97%	39
Anderson Regional Medical Center[2]	Meridian	96%	104
Biloxi Regional Medical Center	Biloxi	96%	27
Forrest General Hospital[2]	Hattiesburg	96%	77
Grenada Lake Medical Center[2]	Grenada	96%	28
Highland Community Hospital	Picayune	96%	26
Natchez Regional Medical Center	Natchez	96%	26
Saint Dominic - Jackson Memorial Hospital	Jackson	96%	294
Webster General Hospital/Swing Bed[2]	Eupora	96%	27
Greenwood Leflore Hospital	Greenwood	95%	85
River Region Health System	Vicksburg	95%	64
Delta Regional Medical Center	Greenville	94%	80
University of Mississippi Medical Center[2]	Jackson	93%	59
Clay County Medical Center[2]	West Point	88%	25

Assessed for Rehabilitation

Hospital Name	City	Rate	Cases
Baptist Memorial Hospital Union County	New Albany	100%	34
Baptist Memorial Hospital/Golden Triangle	Columbus	100%	109
Forrest General Hospital[2]	Hattiesburg	100%	92
Magnolia Regional Health Center	Corinth	100%	98
Baptist Mem Hosp North Mississippi	Oxford	99%	79
Mississippi Baptist Medical Center	Jackson	99%	296
North Mississippi Medical Center[2]	Tupelo	99%	97
River Region Health System	Vicksburg	99%	68
Rush Foundation Hospital[2]	Meridian	99%	113
Singing River Hospital	Pascagoula	99%	214
Wesley Medical Center	Hattiesburg	99%	69
Saint Dominic - Jackson Memorial Hospital	Jackson	98%	441
Baptist Memorial Hospital Desoto	Southaven	96%	241
South Central Regional Medical Center	Laurel	96%	96
University of Mississippi Medical Center[2]	Jackson	96%	112
Central Mississippi Medical Center	Jackson	95%	64
Anderson Regional Medical Center[2]	Meridian	94%	122
Highland Community Hospital	Picayune	94%	31
Memorial Hospital at Gulfport[2]	Gulfport	93%	100
Webster General Hospital/Swing Bed[2]	Eupora	93%	28
Greenwood Leflore Hospital	Greenwood	92%	95
Delta Regional Medical Center	Greenville	91%	82
Natchez Regional Medical Center	Natchez	89%	27
Northwest Mississippi Reg Med Ctr	Clarksdale	87%	39
Natchez Community Hospital	Natchez	86%	29
Grenada Lake Medical Center[2]	Grenada	85%	26
Biloxi Regional Medical Center	Biloxi	82%	34
Southwest Ms Regional Medical Center	Mccomb	56%	52

Discharged on Antithrombotic Therapy

Hospital Name	City	Rate	Cases
Baptist Memorial Hospital Desoto	Southaven	100%	237
Baptist Mem Hosp North Mississippi	Oxford	100%	74
Baptist Memorial Hospital Union County	New Albany	100%	29
Baptist Memorial Hospital/Golden Triangle	Columbus	100%	105
Magnolia Regional Health Center	Corinth	100%	91
Natchez Regional Medical Center	Natchez	100%	27
North Mississippi Medical Center[2]	Tupelo	100%	85
Wesley Medical Center	Hattiesburg	100%	64
Anderson Regional Medical Center[2]	Meridian	99%	109
Forrest General Hospital[2]	Hattiesburg	99%	83
Memorial Hospital at Gulfport[2]	Gulfport	99%	80
Mississippi Baptist Medical Center	Jackson	99%	275
Rush Foundation Hospital[2]	Meridian	99%	107
Saint Dominic - Jackson Memorial Hospital	Jackson	99%	341
Singing River Hospital	Pascagoula	99%	192
Greenwood Leflore Hospital	Greenwood	97%	89
Highland Community Hospital	Picayune	97%	30
River Region Health System	Vicksburg	97%	65
South Central Regional Medical Center	Laurel	97%	89
University of Mississippi Medical Center[2]	Jackson	97%	75
Biloxi Regional Medical Center	Biloxi	96%	26
Natchez Community Hospital	Natchez	96%	28
Southwest Ms Regional Medical Center	Mccomb	96%	51
Central Mississippi Medical Center	Jackson	95%	57
Webster General Hospital/Swing Bed[2]	Eupora	93%	27
Delta Regional Medical Center	Greenville	92%	78
Grenada Lake Medical Center[2]	Grenada	92%	26
Northwest Mississippi Reg Med Ctr	Clarksdale	92%	37

Discharged on Statin Medication

Hospital Name	City	Rate	Cases
Baptist Mem Hosp North Mississippi	Oxford	100%	61
Baptist Memorial Hospital/Golden Triangle	Columbus	100%	73
Magnolia Regional Health Center	Corinth	100%	75

NOTE: Hospital profiles are in alphabetical order by state, then city, then hospital within the city; Rankings exclude hospitals with less than 25 cases except for patient surveys which excludes hospitals with less than 100 cases; (a) 100-299 cases; (1) The number of cases/patients is too few to report; (2) Data submitted were based on a sample of cases/patients; (3) Results are based on a shorter time period than required; (4) Data suppressed by CMS for one or more quarters; (5) Results are not available for this reporting period; (6) Fewer than 100 patients completed the HCAHPS survey; (7) No cases met the criteria for this measure; (8) The lower limit of the confidence interval cannot be calculated if the number of observed infections equals zero; (9) No data are available from the state/territory for this reporting period; (10) The scores shown reflect fewer than 50 completed surveys; (11) There were discrepancies in the data collection process; (12) This measure does not apply to this hospital for this reporting period; (13) Results cannot be calculated for this reporting period; (14) The results for this state are combined with nearby states to protect confidentiality; Please refer to the User's Guide for a full explanation of data.

Hospital Name	City	Rate	Cases
Memorial Hospital at Gulfport[2]	Gulfport	100%	64
North Mississippi Medical Center[2]	Tupelo	100%	74
Wesley Medical Center	Hattiesburg	100%	51
University of Mississippi Medical Center[2]	Jackson	98%	51
Baptist Memorial Hospital Desoto	Southaven	96%	200
Singing River Hospital	Pascagoula	96%	154
Mississippi Baptist Medical Center	Jackson	95%	201
Forrest General Hospital[2]	Hattiesburg	94%	63
Rush Foundation Hospital[2]	Meridian	94%	82
River Region Health System	Vicksburg	91%	44
Saint Dominic - Jackson Memorial Hospital	Jackson	91%	280
Central Mississippi Medical Center	Jackson	90%	40
Northwest Mississippi Reg Med Ctr	Clarksdale	88%	33
Grenada Lake Medical Center[2]	Grenada	85%	26
Anderson Regional Medical Center[2]	Meridian	78%	91
Southwest Ms Regional Medical Center	Mccomb	78%	40
Delta Regional Medical Center	Greenville	70%	60
Greenwood Leflore Hospital	Greenwood	66%	80
South Central Regional Medical Center	Laurel	60%	83

Thrombolytic Therapy Timing

Hospital Name	City	Rate	Cases
Central Mississippi Medical Center	Jackson	0%	27
South Central Regional Medical Center	Laurel	0%	41

Venous Thromboembolism (VTE) Prophylaxis

Hospital Name	City	Rate	Cases
Singing River Hospital	Pascagoula	100%	215
Baptist Mem Hosp North Mississippi	Oxford	99%	77
Baptist Memorial Hospital Desoto	Southaven	98%	246
Baptist Memorial Hospital/Golden Triangle	Columbus	98%	97
Magnolia Regional Health Center	Corinth	98%	108
North Mississippi Medical Center[2]	Tupelo	98%	102
Baptist Memorial Hospital Union County	New Albany	97%	32
Memorial Hospital at Gulfport[2]	Gulfport	95%	104
University of Mississippi Medical Center[2]	Jackson	95%	125
Grenada Lake Medical Center[2]	Grenada	94%	31
Southwest Ms Regional Medical Center	Mccomb	94%	54
River Region Health System	Vicksburg	92%	76
Mississippi Baptist Medical Center	Jackson	91%	292
Wesley Medical Center	Hattiesburg	91%	66
Saint Dominic - Jackson Memorial Hospital	Jackson	89%	455
Forrest General Hospital[2]	Hattiesburg	88%	81
Central Mississippi Medical Center	Jackson	82%	65
Rush Foundation Hospital[2]	Meridian	82%	114
Webster General Hospital/Swing Bed[2]	Eupora	82%	28
Biloxi Regional Medical Center	Biloxi	79%	39
Delta Regional Medical Center	Greenville	78%	92
Greenwood Leflore Hospital	Greenwood	78%	95
Natchez Community Hospital	Natchez	77%	26
Northwest Mississippi Reg Med Ctr	Clarksdale	74%	43
Anderson Regional Medical Center[2]	Meridian	67%	126
South Central Regional Medical Center	Laurel	67%	100
Natchez Regional Medical Center	Natchez	63%	27
Och Regional Medical Center	Starkville	56%	25
Highland Community Hospital	Picayune	48%	25
Clay County Medical Center[2]	West Point	38%	26

Written Stroke Educational Materials Given

Hospital Name	City	Rate	Cases
Singing River Hospital	Pascagoula	100%	125
Baptist Mem Hosp North Mississippi	Oxford	98%	47
Baptist Memorial Hospital/Golden Triangle	Columbus	98%	62
North Mississippi Medical Center[2]	Tupelo	98%	52
University of Mississippi Medical Center[2]	Jackson	98%	56
Wesley Medical Center	Hattiesburg	98%	44
River Region Health System	Vicksburg	97%	38
Saint Dominic - Jackson Memorial Hospital	Jackson	97%	253
Baptist Memorial Hospital Desoto	Southaven	91%	144
Central Mississippi Medical Center	Jackson	89%	45
Biloxi Regional Medical Center	Biloxi	86%	28
Mississippi Baptist Medical Center	Jackson	83%	175
Southwest Ms Regional Medical Center	Mccomb	83%	35
Forrest General Hospital[2]	Hattiesburg	82%	44
Magnolia Regional Health Center	Corinth	82%	56
Delta Regional Medical Center	Greenville	81%	42
Greenwood Leflore Hospital	Greenwood	77%	43
Memorial Hospital at Gulfport[2]	Gulfport	62%	58
Rush Foundation Hospital[2]	Meridian	58%	62
Anderson Regional Medical Center[2]	Meridian	55%	58
South Central Regional Medical Center	Laurel	46%	61

Surgical Care Improvement Project

Appropriate Beta Blocker Usage

Hospital Name	City	Rate	Cases
Baptist Memorial Hospital Desoto[2]	Southaven	100%	206
Baptist Mem Hosp North Mississippi	Oxford	100%	218
Baptist Memorial Hospital Union County	New Albany	100%	33
Biloxi Regional Medical Center	Biloxi	100%	58
Garden Park Medical Center[2]	Gulfport	100%	71
North Mississippi Medical Center[2]	Tupelo	100%	611
Northwest Mississippi Reg Med Ctr	Clarksdale	100%	28
River Oaks Hospital[2]	Flowood	100%	111
River Region Health System	Vicksburg	100%	94
Wesley Medical Center	Hattiesburg	100%	261
Baptist Memorial Hospital/Golden Triangle	Columbus	99%	198
Magnolia Regional Health Center	Corinth	99%	261
Mississippi Baptist Medical Center[2]	Jackson	98%	398
Singing River Hospital[2]	Pascagoula	98%	227
Anderson Regional Medical Center[2]	Meridian	97%	156
Forrest General Hospital[2]	Hattiesburg	97%	253
Rush Foundation Hospital[2]	Meridian	97%	165
University of Mississippi Medical Center[2]	Jackson	97%	135
Memorial Hospital at Gulfport[2]	Gulfport	96%	228
Saint Dominic - Jackson Memorial Hospital[2]	Jackson	96%	205
Central Mississippi Medical Center[2]	Jackson	95%	87
GV (Sonny) Montgomery VA Med Ctr[2]	Jackson	95%	39
Delta Regional Medical Center	Greenville	94%	78
VA Gulf Coast Healthcare System[2]	Biloxi	94%	34
Greenwood Leflore Hospital	Greenwood	90%	80
South Central Regional Medical Center	Laurel	86%	92
Natchez Regional Medical Center	Natchez	81%	26
Southwest Ms Regional Medical Center	Mccomb	76%	125
Och Regional Medical Center	Starkville	73%	48

Appropriate VTP Within 24 Hours

Hospital Name	City	Rate	Cases
Baptist Mem Hosp North Mississippi	Oxford	100%	523
Baptist Memorial Hospital Union County	New Albany	100%	162
Baptist Memorial Hospital/Golden Triangle	Columbus	100%	582
Biloxi Regional Medical Center	Biloxi	100%	304
Bolivar Medical Center	Cleveland	100%	103
Crossgates River Oaks Hospital	Brandon	100%	48
Garden Park Medical Center[2]	Gulfport	100%	304
Gilmore Memorial Regional Medical Center	Amory	100%	79
GV (Sonny) Montgomery VA Med Ctr[2]	Jackson	100%	127
North Mississippi Medical Center[2]	Tupelo	100%	784
River Oaks Hospital[2]	Flowood	100%	552
River Region Health System	Vicksburg	100%	221
Magnolia Regional Health Center	Corinth	99%	450
Natchez Community Hospital	Natchez	99%	79
Singing River Hospital[2]	Pascagoula	99%	433
Wesley Medical Center	Hattiesburg	99%	578
Greenwood Leflore Hospital	Greenwood	98%	293
Mississippi Baptist Medical Center[2]	Jackson	98%	949
Northwest Mississippi Reg Med Ctr	Clarksdale	98%	90
University of Mississippi Medical Center[2]	Jackson	98%	300
Anderson Regional Medical Center[2]	Meridian	97%	386
Baptist Memorial Hospital Desoto[2]	Southaven	97%	332
Clay County Medical Center	West Point	97%	68
Forrest General Hospital[2]	Hattiesburg	97%	367
Highland Community Hospital[2]	Picayune	97%	72
Rush Foundation Hospital[2]	Meridian	97%	389
Saint Dominic - Jackson Memorial Hospital[2]	Jackson	97%	485
Central Mississippi Medical Center[2]	Jackson	95%	219
South Central Regional Medical Center	Laurel	95%	359
Woman's Hospital at River Oaks	Flowood	95%	42
Delta Regional Medical Center	Greenville	94%	312
Natchez Regional Medical Center	Natchez	94%	93
Hancock Medical Center	Bay Saint Louis	93%	46
Madison River Oaks Medical Center	Canton	93%	72
Memorial Hospital at Gulfport[2]	Gulfport	93%	398
VA Gulf Coast Healthcare System[2]	Biloxi	90%	86
King's Daughters Med Ctr-Brookhaven	Brookhaven	89%	47
Och Regional Medical Center	Starkville	88%	206
Grenada Lake Medical Center[2]	Grenada	87%	55
North Oak Regional Medical Center	Senatobia	83%	30
Southwest Ms Regional Medical Center	Mccomb	83%	253

Controlled Postoperative Blood Glucose

Hospital Name	City	Rate	Cases
Mississippi Baptist Medical Center[2]	Jackson	100%	204
North Mississippi Medical Center[2]	Tupelo	100%	501
Wesley Medical Center	Hattiesburg	100%	119
Memorial Hospital at Gulfport[2]	Gulfport	99%	107
River Region Health System	Vicksburg	99%	70
Baptist Mem Hosp North Mississippi	Oxford	98%	54
Rush Foundation Hospital[2]	Meridian	98%	60
Singing River Hospital[2]	Pascagoula	97%	140
Baptist Memorial Hospital Desoto[2]	Southaven	96%	107
Central Mississippi Medical Center[2]	Jackson	96%	51
Saint Dominic - Jackson Memorial Hospital[2]	Jackson	95%	146
Baptist Memorial Hospital/Golden Triangle	Columbus	94%	47
Anderson Regional Medical Center[2]	Meridian	93%	89
University of Mississippi Medical Center[2]	Jackson	92%	61
Forrest General Hospital[2]	Hattiesburg	91%	174
Southwest Ms Regional Medical Center	Mccomb	91%	32
Magnolia Regional Health Center	Corinth	89%	153

Perioperative Temperature Management

Hospital Name	City	Rate	Cases
Anderson Regional Medical Center[2]	Meridian	100%	427
Baptist Memorial Hospital Desoto[2]	Southaven	100%	446
Baptist Mem Hosp North Mississippi	Oxford	100%	599
Baptist Memorial Hospital Union County	New Albany	100%	182
Baptist Memorial Hospital/Golden Triangle	Columbus	100%	627
Biloxi Regional Medical Center	Biloxi	100%	393
Bolivar Medical Center	Cleveland	100%	112
Clay County Medical Center	West Point	100%	78
Crossgates River Oaks Hospital	Brandon	100%	60
Delta Regional Medical Center	Greenville	100%	357
Forrest General Hospital[2]	Hattiesburg	100%	474
Garden Park Medical Center[2]	Gulfport	100%	319
George County Hospital[3]	Lucedale	100%	25
Gilmore Memorial Regional Medical Center	Amory	100%	98
Greenwood Leflore Hospital	Greenwood	100%	339
GV (Sonny) Montgomery VA Med Ctr[2]	Jackson	100%	148
Hancock Medical Center	Bay Saint Louis	100%	50
Highland Community Hospital[2]	Picayune	100%	71
King's Daughters Med Ctr-Brookhaven	Brookhaven	100%	55
Madison River Oaks Medical Center	Canton	100%	78
Magnolia Regional Health Center	Corinth	100%	601
Memorial Hospital at Gulfport[2]	Gulfport	100%	507
Mississippi Baptist Medical Center[2]	Jackson	100%	1159
Natchez Community Hospital	Natchez	100%	89
Natchez Regional Medical Center	Natchez	100%	120
North Mississippi Medical Center[2]	Tupelo	100%	920
North Oak Regional Medical Center	Senatobia	100%	34
Northwest Mississippi Reg Med Ctr	Clarksdale	100%	96
River Oaks Hospital[2]	Flowood	100%	590
River Region Health System	Vicksburg	100%	352
Rush Foundation Hospital[2]	Meridian	100%	500
Saint Dominic - Jackson Memorial Hospital[2]	Jackson	100%	545
Singing River Hospital[2]	Pascagoula	100%	521
South Central Regional Medical Center	Laurel	100%	392
VA Gulf Coast Healthcare System[2]	Biloxi	100%	113
Wesley Medical Center	Hattiesburg	100%	641
Woman's Hospital at River Oaks	Flowood	100%	45
Central Mississippi Medical Center[2]	Jackson	99%	265
Southwest Ms Regional Medical Center	Mccomb	99%	311
Och Regional Medical Center	Starkville	98%	224
University of Mississippi Medical Center[2]	Jackson	96%	458
Grenada Lake Medical Center[2]	Grenada	95%	87

Prophylactic Antibiotic Selection

Hospital Name	City	Rate	Cases
Anderson Regional Medical Center[2]	Meridian	100%	362
Baptist Memorial Hospital/Golden Triangle	Columbus	100%	467
Biloxi Regional Medical Center	Biloxi	100%	242
Bolivar Medical Center	Cleveland	100%	59
Central Mississippi Medical Center[2]	Jackson	100%	202
Crossgates River Oaks Hospital	Brandon	100%	25
Garden Park Medical Center[2]	Gulfport	100%	221
GV (Sonny) Montgomery VA Med Ctr	Jackson	100%	51
Magnolia Regional Health Center	Corinth	100%	551
North Mississippi Medical Center[2]	Tupelo	100%	1146
River Oaks Hospital[2]	Flowood	100%	490
Wesley Medical Center	Hattiesburg	100%	484
Woman's Hospital at River Oaks	Flowood	100%	32
Baptist Memorial Hospital Desoto[2]	Southaven	99%	368
Baptist Mem Hosp North Mississippi	Oxford	99%	390
Baptist Memorial Hospital Union County	New Albany	99%	136
Greenwood Leflore Hospital	Greenwood	99%	242
Mississippi Baptist Medical Center[2]	Jackson	99%	1083
River Region Health System	Vicksburg	99%	236
Rush Foundation Hospital[2]	Meridian	99%	340
Saint Dominic - Jackson Memorial Hospital[2]	Jackson	99%	504
Singing River Hospital[2]	Pascagoula	99%	455
Gilmore Memorial Regional Medical Center	Amory	98%	40
Madison River Oaks Medical Center	Canton	98%	66
Northwest Mississippi Reg Med Ctr	Clarksdale	98%	54
Och Regional Medical Center	Starkville	98%	147
VA Gulf Coast Healthcare System	Biloxi	98%	54
Delta Regional Medical Center	Greenville	97%	260
Forrest General Hospital[2]	Hattiesburg	97%	497
Memorial Hospital at Gulfport[2]	Gulfport	97%	384
University of Mississippi Medical Center[2]	Jackson	97%	315
Hancock Medical Center	Bay Saint Louis	96%	27
Natchez Community Hospital	Natchez	96%	55
North Oak Regional Medical Center	Senatobia	96%	26
Southwest Ms Regional Medical Center	Mccomb	95%	212
Clay County Medical Center	West Point	94%	50
Natchez Regional Medical Center	Natchez	94%	85
Highland Community Hospital[2]	Picayune	91%	46
South Central Regional Medical Center	Laurel	90%	290
Grenada Lake Medical Center[2]	Grenada	88%	41

NOTE: Hospital profiles are in alphabetical order by state, then city, then hospital within the city; Rankings exclude hospitals with less than 25 cases except for patient surveys which excludes hospitals with less than 100 cases; (a) 100-299 cases; (1) The number of cases/patients is too few to report; (2) Data submitted were based on a sample of cases/patients; (3) Results are based on a shorter time period than required; (4) Data suppressed by CMS for one or more quarters; (5) Results are not available for this reporting period; (6) Fewer than 100 patients completed the HCAHPS survey; (7) No cases met the criteria for this measure; (8) The lower limit of the confidence interval cannot be calculated if the number of observed infections equals zero; (9) No data are available from the state/territory for this reporting period; (10) The scores shown reflect fewer than 50 completed surveys; (11) There were discrepancies in the data collection process; (12) This measure does not apply to this hospital for this reporting period; (13) Results cannot be calculated for this reporting period; (14) The results for this state are combined with nearby states to protect confidentiality; Please refer to the User's Guide for a full explanation of data.

Prophylactic Antibiotic Selection (Outpatient)

Hospital Name	City	Rate	Cases
Baptist Memorial Hospital Union County	New Albany	100%	94
Baptist Memorial Hospital/Golden Triangle	Columbus	100%	334
Bolivar Medical Center	Cleveland	100%	46
Central Mississippi Medical Center	Jackson	100%	258
Garden Park Medical Center	Gulfport	100%	145
Magee General Hospital	Magee	100%	36
North Mississippi Medical Center	Tupelo	100%	740
Woman's Hospital at River Oaks	Flowood	100%	510
Baptist Memorial Hospital Desoto	Southaven	99%	318
Biloxi Regional Medical Center	Biloxi	99%	222
Mississippi Baptist Medical Center	Jackson	99%	798
Natchez Community Hospital	Natchez	99%	130
River Oaks Hospital	Flowood	99%	820
River Region Health System	Vicksburg	99%	211
Wesley Medical Center	Hattiesburg	99%	382
Gilmore Memorial Regional Medical Center	Amory	98%	80
Magnolia Regional Health Center	Corinth	98%	245
Singing River Hospital	Pascagoula	98%	230
Anderson Regional Medical Center	Meridian	97%	402
Baptist Mem Hosp North Mississippi	Oxford	97%	496
Forrest General Hospital	Hattiesburg	97%	555
Memorial Hospital at Gulfport	Gulfport	97%	461
Northwest Mississippi Reg Med Ctr	Clarksdale	97%	156
Saint Dominic - Jackson Memorial Hospital	Jackson	97%	582
University of Mississippi Medical Center	Jackson	97%	245
Clay County Medical Center	West Point	96%	97
Greenwood Leflore Hospital	Greenwood	95%	197
Rush Foundation Hospital	Meridian	95%	471
Southwest Ms Regional Medical Center	Mccomb	95%	199
Delta Regional Medical Center	Greenville	94%	87
King's Daughters Med Ctr-Brookhaven	Brookhaven	94%	180
Grenada Lake Medical Center	Grenada	92%	37
Madison River Oaks Medical Center	Canton	92%	37
South Central Regional Medical Center	Laurel	92%	62
Och Regional Medical Center	Starkville	89%	158

Prophylactic Antibiotic Stopped

Hospital Name	City	Rate	Cases
Baptist Mem Hosp North Mississippi	Oxford	100%	376
Biloxi Regional Medical Center	Biloxi	100%	226
Bolivar Medical Center	Cleveland	100%	56
Garden Park Medical Center[2]	Gulfport	100%	217
GV (Sonny) Montgomery VA Med Ctr	Jackson	100%	51
River Oaks Hospital[2]	Flowood	100%	488
River Region Health System	Vicksburg	100%	226
VA Gulf Coast Healthcare System	Biloxi	100%	52
Wesley Medical Center	Hattiesburg	100%	377
Baptist Memorial Hospital Union County	New Albany	99%	133
Baptist Memorial Hospital/Golden Triangle	Columbus	99%	450
Mississippi Baptist Medical Center[2]	Jackson	99%	1069
North Mississippi Medical Center[2]	Tupelo	99%	1120
Singing River Hospital[2]	Pascagoula	99%	439
Central Mississippi Medical Center[2]	Jackson	98%	199
Gilmore Memorial Regional Medical Center	Amory	98%	40
Magnolia Regional Health Center	Corinth	98%	541
Northwest Mississippi Reg Med Ctr	Clarksdale	98%	52
Saint Dominic - Jackson Memorial Hospital[2]	Jackson	98%	492
Baptist Memorial Hospital Desoto[2]	Southaven	97%	349
Madison River Oaks Medical Center	Canton	97%	66
Memorial Hospital at Gulfport[2]	Gulfport	97%	362
Woman's Hospital at River Oaks	Flowood	97%	32
Anderson Regional Medical Center[2]	Meridian	96%	355
Crossgates River Oaks Hospital	Brandon	96%	25
Delta Regional Medical Center	Greenville	96%	257
South Central Regional Medical Center	Laurel	96%	285
Forrest General Hospital[2]	Hattiesburg	95%	472
University of Mississippi Medical Center[2]	Jackson	95%	308
Clay County Medical Center	West Point	94%	48
Greenwood Leflore Hospital	Greenwood	93%	238
Rush Foundation Hospital[2]	Meridian	93%	321
Och Regional Medical Center	Starkville	92%	142
Natchez Community Hospital	Natchez	91%	54
Southwest Ms Regional Medical Center	Mccomb	91%	207
Natchez Regional Medical Center	Natchez	90%	82
Hancock Medical Center	Bay Saint Louis	89%	27
Grenada Lake Medical Center[2]	Grenada	85%	41
Highland Community Hospital[2]	Picayune	85%	46

Prophylactic Antibiotic Timing

Hospital Name	City	Rate	Cases
Anderson Regional Medical Center[2]	Meridian	100%	363
Baptist Memorial Hospital Union County	New Albany	100%	136
Baptist Memorial Hospital/Golden Triangle	Columbus	100%	467
Biloxi Regional Medical Center	Biloxi	100%	242
Bolivar Medical Center	Cleveland	100%	59
Clay County Medical Center	West Point	100%	50
Crossgates River Oaks Hospital	Brandon	100%	25
Garden Park Medical Center[2]	Gulfport	100%	222
Hancock Medical Center	Bay Saint Louis	100%	27
Magnolia Regional Health Center	Corinth	100%	563
Mississippi Baptist Medical Center[2]	Jackson	100%	1088
Natchez Community Hospital	Natchez	100%	55
North Mississippi Medical Center[2]	Tupelo	100%	1149
River Oaks Hospital[2]	Flowood	100%	490
River Region Health System	Vicksburg	100%	236
Rush Foundation Hospital[2]	Meridian	100%	341
Singing River Hospital[2]	Pascagoula	100%	457
VA Gulf Coast Healthcare System	Biloxi	100%	54
Woman's Hospital at River Oaks	Flowood	100%	32
Baptist Memorial Hospital Desoto[2]	Southaven	99%	370
Delta Regional Medical Center	Greenville	99%	260
Greenwood Leflore Hospital	Greenwood	99%	244
Memorial Hospital at Gulfport[2]	Gulfport	99%	385
Wesley Medical Center	Hattiesburg	99%	484
Forrest General Hospital[2]	Hattiesburg	98%	498
Gilmore Memorial Regional Medical Center	Amory	98%	40
GV (Sonny) Montgomery VA Med Ctr	Jackson	98%	51
Highland Community Hospital[2]	Picayune	98%	46
Madison River Oaks Medical Center	Canton	98%	66
Saint Dominic - Jackson Memorial Hospital[2]	Jackson	98%	505
Baptist Mem Hosp North Mississippi	Oxford	97%	390
Central Mississippi Medical Center[2]	Jackson	96%	202
North Oak Regional Medical Center	Senatobia	96%	26
South Central Regional Medical Center	Laurel	96%	292
Natchez Regional Medical Center	Natchez	95%	85
Southwest Ms Regional Medical Center	Mccomb	93%	215
University of Mississippi Medical Center[2]	Jackson	93%	324
Grenada Lake Medical Center[2]	Grenada	91%	43
Northwest Mississippi Reg Med Ctr	Clarksdale	91%	54
Och Regional Medical Center	Starkville	91%	147

Prophylactic Antibiotic Timing (Outpatient)

Hospital Name	City	Rate	Cases
Baptist Memorial Hospital Union County	New Albany	100%	94
Bolivar Medical Center	Cleveland	100%	46
Gilmore Memorial Regional Medical Center	Amory	100%	80
Madison River Oaks Medical Center	Canton	100%	37
Magee General Hospital	Magee	100%	36
North Mississippi Medical Center	Tupelo	100%	740
River Oaks Hospital	Flowood	100%	821
River Region Health System	Vicksburg	100%	211
Singing River Hospital	Pascagoula	100%	230
Woman's Hospital at River Oaks	Flowood	100%	510
Baptist Memorial Hospital Desoto	Southaven	99%	318
Baptist Memorial Hospital/Golden Triangle	Columbus	99%	334
Biloxi Regional Medical Center	Biloxi	99%	224
Clay County Medical Center	West Point	99%	97
Garden Park Medical Center	Gulfport	99%	146
King's Daughters Med Ctr-Brookhaven	Brookhaven	99%	180
Magnolia Regional Health Center	Corinth	99%	246
Memorial Hospital at Gulfport	Gulfport	99%	457
Mississippi Baptist Medical Center	Jackson	99%	801
Natchez Community Hospital	Natchez	99%	131
Northwest Mississippi Reg Med Ctr	Clarksdale	99%	158
Rush Foundation Hospital	Meridian	99%	471
Wesley Medical Center	Hattiesburg	99%	383
Anderson Regional Medical Center	Meridian	98%	403
Baptist Mem Hosp North Mississippi	Oxford	98%	501
Greenwood Leflore Hospital	Greenwood	98%	157
Southwest Ms Regional Medical Center	Mccomb	98%	200
Central Mississippi Medical Center	Jackson	97%	259
Forrest General Hospital	Hattiesburg	97%	561
Saint Dominic - Jackson Memorial Hospital	Jackson	94%	595
University of Mississippi Medical Center	Jackson	92%	259
Delta Regional Medical Center	Greenville	90%	94
Och Regional Medical Center	Starkville	86%	160
South Central Regional Medical Center	Laurel	86%	70
Grenada Lake Medical Center	Grenada	78%	46

Urinary Catheter Removal

Hospital Name	City	Rate	Cases
Baptist Mem Hosp North Mississippi	Oxford	100%	388
Baptist Memorial Hospital Union County	New Albany	100%	108
Garden Park Medical Center[2]	Gulfport	100%	262
GV (Sonny) Montgomery VA Med Ctr[2]	Jackson	100%	54
Magnolia Regional Health Center	Corinth	100%	202
North Mississippi Medical Center[2]	Tupelo	100%	585
River Oaks Hospital[2]	Flowood	100%	291
Saint Dominic - Jackson Memorial Hospital[2]	Jackson	100%	418
Wesley Medical Center	Hattiesburg	100%	411
Biloxi Regional Medical Center	Biloxi	99%	117
River Region Health System	Vicksburg	99%	153
Baptist Memorial Hospital/Golden Triangle	Columbus	98%	164
Bolivar Medical Center	Cleveland	98%	53
Mississippi Baptist Medical Center[2]	Jackson	98%	890
Singing River Hospital[2]	Pascagoula	98%	346
Anderson Regional Medical Center[2]	Meridian	97%	236
Central Mississippi Medical Center[2]	Jackson	97%	139
Northwest Mississippi Reg Med Ctr	Clarksdale	97%	31
Och Regional Medical Center	Starkville	97%	143
Memorial Hospital at Gulfport[2]	Gulfport	96%	348
VA Gulf Coast Healthcare System[2]	Biloxi	96%	79
Forrest General Hospital[2]	Hattiesburg	95%	441
Madison River Oaks Medical Center	Canton	95%	66
Natchez Community Hospital	Natchez	95%	63
Rush Foundation Hospital[2]	Meridian	95%	390
Baptist Memorial Hospital Desoto[2]	Southaven	94%	224
Delta Regional Medical Center	Greenville	94%	178
Greenwood Leflore Hospital	Greenwood	94%	194
Southwest Ms Regional Medical Center	Mccomb	94%	170
Crossgates River Oaks Hospital	Brandon	93%	30
South Central Regional Medical Center	Laurel	92%	207
Gilmore Memorial Regional Medical Center	Amory	89%	45
University of Mississippi Medical Center[2]	Jackson	87%	277
Natchez Regional Medical Center	Natchez	63%	30

Survey of Patients' Hospital Experiences

Area Around Room 'Always' Quiet at Night

Hospital Name	City	Rate	Cases
Tishomingo Health Services	Iuka	81%	(a)
Montfort Jones Memorial Hospital	Kosciusko	79%	(a)
King's Daughters Med Ctr-Brookhaven	Brookhaven	78%	300+
Lawrence County Hospital	Monticello	78%	(a)
Madison River Oaks Medical Center	Canton	78%	(a)
Magnolia Regional Health Center	Corinth	78%	300+
Neshoba County General Hospital	Philadelphia	78%	300+
George County Hospital	Lucedale	77%	(a)
Och Regional Medical Center	Starkville	77%	300+
Beacham Memorial Hospital	Magnolia	76%	(a)
Gilmore Memorial Regional Medical Center	Amory	76%	300+
Mississippi Baptist Medical Center[11]	Jackson	76%	300+
Wayne General Hospital	Waynesboro	76%	300+
Baptist Mem Hosp North Mississippi	Oxford	75%	300+
Baptist Memorial Hospital Union County	New Albany	75%	300+
Hancock Medical Center	Bay Saint Louis	75%	300+
Saint Dominic - Jackson Memorial Hospital	Jackson	75%	300+
Baptist Memorial Hospital/Golden Triangle	Columbus	74%	300+
Magee General Hospital	Magee	74%	(a)
North Mississippi Medical Center	Tupelo	74%	300+
Rush Foundation Hospital	Meridian	74%	300+
Central Mississippi Medical Center	Jackson	73%	300+
North Oak Regional Medical Center	Senatobia	73%	(a)
Delta Regional Medical Center	Greenville	72%	300+
River Oaks Hospital	Flowood	72%	300+
South Central Regional Medical Center	Laurel	72%	300+
Tri Lakes Medical Center	Batesville	72%	(a)
Webster General Hospital/Swing Bed	Eupora	72%	(a)
Wesley Medical Center	Hattiesburg	72%	300+
Forrest General Hospital	Hattiesburg	71%	300+
Garden Park Medical Center	Gulfport	71%	300+
Grenada Lake Medical Center	Grenada	71%	300+
Highland Community Hospital	Picayune	71%	(a)
River Region Health System	Vicksburg	71%	300+
Southwest Ms Regional Medical Center	Mccomb	71%	300+
Baptist Memorial Hospital Booneville	Booneville	70%	(a)
Clay County Medical Center	West Point	70%	300+
Anderson Regional Medical Center	Meridian	69%	300+
Greenwood Leflore Hospital	Greenwood	69%	300+
South Sunflower County Hospital	Indianola	69%	(a)
Woman's Hospital at River Oaks	Flowood	69%	300+
Bolivar Medical Center	Cleveland	68%	300+
Marion General Hospital	Columbia	68%	(a)
Singing River Hospital	Pascagoula	67%	300+
University of Mississippi Medical Center	Jackson	67%	300+
Crossgates River Oaks Hospital	Brandon	66%	300+
Natchez Regional Medical Center[11]	Natchez	66%	300+
Baptist Memorial Hospital Desoto	Southaven	65%	300+
Northwest Mississippi Reg Med Ctr	Clarksdale	61%	300+
Memorial Hospital at Gulfport	Gulfport	60%	300+
Natchez Community Hospital	Natchez	60%	300+
Biloxi Regional Medical Center	Biloxi	59%	300+

Doctors 'Always' Communicated Well

Hospital Name	City	Rate	Cases
Beacham Memorial Hospital	Magnolia	96%	(a)
Lawrence County Hospital	Monticello	96%	(a)
Webster General Hospital/Swing Bed	Eupora	95%	(a)
Magee General Hospital	Magee	94%	(a)
Tishomingo Health Services	Iuka	94%	(a)
Baptist Memorial Hospital Booneville	Booneville	91%	(a)
Clay County Medical Center	West Point	91%	300+
South Sunflower County Hospital	Indianola	91%	(a)
Wayne General Hospital	Waynesboro	91%	300+
Gilmore Memorial Regional Medical Center	Amory	90%	300+
Grenada Lake Medical Center	Grenada	90%	300+
Neshoba County General Hospital	Philadelphia	90%	300+

NOTE: Hospital profiles are in alphabetical order by state, then city, then hospital within the city; Rankings exclude hospitals with less than 25 cases except for patient surveys which excludes hospitals with less than 100 cases; (a) 100-299 cases; (1) The number of cases/patients is too few to report; (2) Data submitted were based on a sample of cases/patients; (3) Results are based on a shorter time period than required; (4) Data suppressed by CMS for one or more quarters; (5) Results are not available for this reporting period; (6) Fewer than 100 patients completed the HCAHPS survey; (7) No cases met the criteria for this measure; (8) The lower limit of the confidence interval cannot be calculated if the number of observed infections equals zero; (9) No data are available from the state/territory for this reporting period; (10) The scores shown reflect fewer than 50 completed surveys; (11) There were discrepancies in the data collection process; (12) This measure does not apply to this hospital for this reporting period; (13) Results cannot be calculated for this reporting period; (14) The results for this state are combined with nearby states to protect confidentiality; Please refer to the User's Guide for a full explanation of data.

George County Hospital	Lucedale	89%	(a)
Baptist Memorial Hospital Union County	New Albany	88%	300+
King's Daughters Med Ctr-Brookhaven	Brookhaven	87%	300+
Och Regional Medical Center	Starkville	87%	300+
South Central Regional Medical Center	Laurel	87%	300+
Woman's Hospital at River Oaks	Flowood	87%	300+
Greenwood Leflore Hospital	Greenwood	86%	300+
Magnolia Regional Health Center	Corinth	86%	300+
Mississippi Baptist Medical Center[11]	Jackson	86%	300+
North Mississippi Medical Center	Tupelo	86%	300+
River Region Health System	Vicksburg	86%	300+
Wesley Medical Center	Hattiesburg	86%	300+
Anderson Regional Medical Center	Meridian	85%	300+
Bolivar Medical Center	Cleveland	85%	300+
River Oaks Hospital	Flowood	85%	300+
Baptist Memorial Hospital/Golden Triangle	Columbus	84%	300+
Delta Regional Medical Center	Greenville	84%	300+
Garden Park Medical Center	Gulfport	84%	300+
Hancock Medical Center	Bay Saint Louis	84%	300+
Montfort Jones Memorial Hospital	Kosciusko	84%	(a)
Natchez Regional Medical Center[11]	Natchez	84%	300+
Northwest Mississippi Reg Med Ctr	Clarksdale	84%	300+
Saint Dominic - Jackson Memorial Hospital	Jackson	84%	300+
Madison River Oaks Medical Center	Canton	83%	(a)
Rush Foundation Hospital	Meridian	83%	300+
Baptist Mem Hosp North Mississippi	Oxford	82%	300+
Forrest General Hospital	Hattiesburg	82%	300+
Marion General Hospital	Columbia	82%	(a)
University of Mississippi Medical Center	Jackson	82%	300+
Memorial Hospital at Gulfport	Gulfport	81%	300+
Natchez Community Hospital	Natchez	81%	300+
Singing River Hospital	Pascagoula	81%	300+
Biloxi Regional Medical Center	Biloxi	80%	300+
Highland Community Hospital	Picayune	80%	(a)
Southwest Ms Regional Medical Center	Mccomb	80%	300+
Central Mississippi Medical Center	Jackson	79%	300+
Crossgates River Oaks Hospital	Brandon	79%	300+
Tri Lakes Medical Center	Batesville	79%	(a)
North Oak Regional Medical Center	Senatobia	77%	(a)
Baptist Memorial Hospital Desoto	Southaven	76%	300+

Home Recovery Information Given

Hospital Name	City	Rate	Cases
King's Daughters Med Ctr-Brookhaven	Brookhaven	90%	300+
Magnolia Regional Health Center	Corinth	90%	300+
Woman's Hospital at River Oaks	Flowood	90%	300+
Anderson Regional Medical Center	Meridian	88%	300+
Rush Foundation Hospital	Meridian	88%	300+
George County Hospital	Lucedale	87%	(a)
Mississippi Baptist Medical Center[11]	Jackson	87%	300+
Tishomingo Health Services	Iuka	87%	(a)
Wesley Medical Center	Hattiesburg	87%	300+
Baptist Memorial Hospital Union County	New Albany	86%	300+
Garden Park Medical Center	Gulfport	86%	300+
Greenwood Leflore Hospital	Greenwood	86%	300+
Neshoba County General Hospital	Philadelphia	86%	300+
Saint Dominic - Jackson Memorial Hospital	Jackson	86%	300+
Gilmore Memorial Regional Medical Center	Amory	85%	300+
Grenada Lake Medical Center	Grenada	85%	300+
North Mississippi Medical Center	Tupelo	85%	300+
Och Regional Medical Center	Starkville	85%	300+
Webster General Hospital/Swing Bed	Eupora	85%	(a)
Clay County Medical Center	West Point	84%	300+
Hancock Medical Center	Bay Saint Louis	84%	300+
Highland Community Hospital	Picayune	84%	(a)
Memorial Hospital at Gulfport	Gulfport	84%	300+
River Oaks Hospital	Flowood	84%	300+
Southwest Ms Regional Medical Center	Mccomb	84%	300+
Wayne General Hospital	Waynesboro	84%	300+
Baptist Mem Hosp North Mississippi	Oxford	83%	300+
Biloxi Regional Medical Center	Biloxi	83%	300+
Lawrence County Hospital	Monticello	83%	(a)
River Region Health System	Vicksburg	83%	300+
Magee General Hospital	Magee	82%	(a)
Singing River Hospital	Pascagoula	82%	300+
Baptist Memorial Hospital Booneville	Booneville	81%	(a)
Baptist Memorial Hospital/Golden Triangle	Columbus	81%	300+
Bolivar Medical Center	Cleveland	81%	300+
South Central Regional Medical Center	Laurel	81%	300+
University of Mississippi Medical Center	Jackson	81%	300+
Baptist Memorial Hospital Desoto	Southaven	80%	300+
Forrest General Hospital	Hattiesburg	80%	300+
Madison River Oaks Medical Center	Canton	80%	(a)
Marion General Hospital	Columbia	80%	(a)
North Oak Regional Medical Center	Senatobia	80%	(a)
Central Mississippi Medical Center	Jackson	79%	300+
Natchez Community Hospital	Natchez	79%	300+
Natchez Regional Medical Center[11]	Natchez	79%	300+
Montfort Jones Memorial Hospital	Kosciusko	78%	(a)
Delta Regional Medical Center	Greenville	77%	300+
Tri Lakes Medical Center	Batesville	77%	(a)
Crossgates River Oaks Hospital	Brandon	76%	300+
Northwest Mississippi Reg Med Ctr	Clarksdale	76%	300+
Beacham Memorial Hospital	Magnolia	73%	(a)
South Sunflower County Hospital	Indianola	68%	(a)

Hospital Given 9 or 10 on 10 Point Scale

Hospital Name	City	Rate	Cases
King's Daughters Med Ctr-Brookhaven	Brookhaven	83%	300+
Tishomingo Health Services	Iuka	82%	(a)
Woman's Hospital at River Oaks	Flowood	82%	300+
George County Hospital	Lucedale	81%	(a)
Baptist Memorial Hospital Booneville	Booneville	80%	(a)
Mississippi Baptist Medical Center[11]	Jackson	80%	300+
North Mississippi Medical Center	Tupelo	80%	300+
Lawrence County Hospital	Monticello	79%	(a)
Baptist Memorial Hospital Union County	New Albany	78%	300+
Magnolia Regional Health Center	Corinth	77%	300+
Neshoba County General Hospital	Philadelphia	77%	300+
Och Regional Medical Center	Starkville	77%	300+
Saint Dominic - Jackson Memorial Hospital	Jackson	76%	300+
Webster General Hospital/Swing Bed	Eupora	76%	(a)
Wesley Medical Center	Hattiesburg	75%	300+
Forrest General Hospital	Hattiesburg	74%	300+
Garden Park Medical Center	Gulfport	74%	300+
Gilmore Memorial Regional Medical Center	Amory	74%	300+
Hancock Medical Center	Bay Saint Louis	74%	300+
Highland Community Hospital	Picayune	74%	(a)
Magee General Hospital	Magee	74%	(a)
South Central Regional Medical Center	Laurel	74%	300+
Anderson Regional Medical Center	Meridian	73%	300+
Beacham Memorial Hospital	Magnolia	72%	(a)
Clay County Medical Center	West Point	72%	300+
Grenada Lake Medical Center	Grenada	71%	300+
River Oaks Hospital	Flowood	71%	300+
University of Mississippi Medical Center	Jackson	71%	300+
Baptist Memorial Hospital Desoto	Southaven	70%	300+
Baptist Mem Hosp North Mississippi	Oxford	70%	300+
Singing River Hospital	Pascagoula	70%	300+
Baptist Memorial Hospital/Golden Triangle	Columbus	69%	300+
Greenwood Leflore Hospital	Greenwood	69%	300+
Memorial Hospital at Gulfport	Gulfport	69%	300+
Montfort Jones Memorial Hospital	Kosciusko	68%	(a)
Madison River Oaks Medical Center	Canton	67%	(a)
South Sunflower County Hospital	Indianola	67%	(a)
Southwest Ms Regional Medical Center	Mccomb	67%	300+
Wayne General Hospital	Waynesboro	67%	300+
River Region Health System	Vicksburg	66%	300+
Rush Foundation Hospital	Meridian	66%	300+
North Oak Regional Medical Center	Senatobia	65%	(a)
Bolivar Medical Center	Cleveland	62%	300+
Natchez Community Hospital	Natchez	61%	300+
Central Mississippi Medical Center	Jackson	60%	300+
Crossgates River Oaks Hospital	Brandon	60%	300+
Delta Regional Medical Center	Greenville	60%	300+
Marion General Hospital	Columbia	60%	(a)
Biloxi Regional Medical Center	Biloxi	58%	300+
Natchez Regional Medical Center[11]	Natchez	56%	300+
Tri Lakes Medical Center	Batesville	55%	(a)
Northwest Mississippi Reg Med Ctr	Clarksdale	48%	300+

Meds 'Always' Explained Before Given

Hospital Name	City	Rate	Cases
Lawrence County Hospital	Monticello	80%	(a)
Tishomingo Health Services	Iuka	78%	(a)
Neshoba County General Hospital	Philadelphia	75%	300+
Webster General Hospital/Swing Bed	Eupora	75%	(a)
Beacham Memorial Hospital	Magnolia	74%	(a)
Wayne General Hospital	Waynesboro	74%	300+
Montfort Jones Memorial Hospital	Kosciusko	73%	(a)
King's Daughters Med Ctr-Brookhaven	Brookhaven	72%	300+
Baptist Memorial Hospital Booneville	Booneville	71%	(a)
Baptist Memorial Hospital Union County	New Albany	71%	300+
Magnolia Regional Health Center	Corinth	71%	300+
George County Hospital	Lucedale	70%	(a)
Memorial Hospital at Gulfport	Gulfport	68%	300+
Mississippi Baptist Medical Center[11]	Jackson	68%	300+
Gilmore Memorial Regional Medical Center	Amory	67%	300+
Greenwood Leflore Hospital	Greenwood	67%	300+
Grenada Lake Medical Center	Grenada	67%	300+
North Mississippi Medical Center	Tupelo	67%	300+
Baptist Memorial Hospital/Golden Triangle	Columbus	66%	300+
Magee General Hospital	Magee	66%	(a)
Och Regional Medical Center	Starkville	66%	300+
Singing River Hospital	Pascagoula	66%	300+
South Sunflower County Hospital	Indianola	66%	(a)
Clay County Medical Center	West Point	65%	300+
Garden Park Medical Center	Gulfport	65%	300+
Hancock Medical Center	Bay Saint Louis	65%	300+
Northwest Mississippi Reg Med Ctr	Clarksdale	65%	300+
Rush Foundation Hospital	Meridian	65%	300+
South Central Regional Medical Center	Laurel	65%	300+
Wesley Medical Center	Hattiesburg	65%	300+
Anderson Regional Medical Center	Meridian	64%	300+
Saint Dominic - Jackson Memorial Hospital	Jackson	64%	300+
Woman's Hospital at River Oaks	Flowood	64%	300+
Bolivar Medical Center	Cleveland	63%	300+
Delta Regional Medical Center	Greenville	63%	300+
Forrest General Hospital	Hattiesburg	63%	300+
University of Mississippi Medical Center	Jackson	63%	300+
Marion General Hospital	Columbia	62%	(a)
North Oak Regional Medical Center	Senatobia	62%	(a)
Baptist Mem Hosp North Mississippi	Oxford	61%	300+
Natchez Community Hospital	Natchez	61%	300+
Natchez Regional Medical Center[11]	Natchez	61%	300+
River Oaks Hospital	Flowood	61%	300+
River Region Health System	Vicksburg	61%	300+
Baptist Memorial Hospital Desoto	Southaven	60%	300+
Madison River Oaks Medical Center	Canton	60%	(a)
Tri Lakes Medical Center	Batesville	59%	(a)
Southwest Ms Regional Medical Center	Mccomb	58%	300+
Central Mississippi Medical Center	Jackson	57%	300+
Highland Community Hospital	Picayune	57%	(a)
Biloxi Regional Medical Center	Biloxi	56%	300+
Crossgates River Oaks Hospital	Brandon	54%	300+

Nurses 'Always' Communicated Well

Hospital Name	City	Rate	Cases
King's Daughters Med Ctr-Brookhaven	Brookhaven	89%	300+
Tishomingo Health Services	Iuka	89%	(a)
Woman's Hospital at River Oaks	Flowood	88%	300+
Beacham Memorial Hospital	Magnolia	87%	(a)
Lawrence County Hospital	Monticello	87%	(a)
Magee General Hospital	Magee	87%	(a)
Neshoba County General Hospital	Philadelphia	87%	300+
Webster General Hospital/Swing Bed	Eupora	87%	(a)
Baptist Memorial Hospital Union County	New Albany	86%	300+
North Mississippi Medical Center	Tupelo	86%	300+
Magnolia Regional Health Center	Corinth	85%	300+
Baptist Memorial Hospital Booneville	Booneville	84%	(a)
Och Regional Medical Center	Starkville	84%	300+
Clay County Medical Center	West Point	83%	300+
George County Hospital	Lucedale	83%	(a)
Gilmore Memorial Regional Medical Center	Amory	83%	300+
Hancock Medical Center	Bay Saint Louis	83%	300+
Grenada Lake Medical Center	Grenada	82%	300+
Mississippi Baptist Medical Center[11]	Jackson	82%	300+
Singing River Hospital	Pascagoula	82%	300+
Wayne General Hospital	Waynesboro	82%	300+
Montfort Jones Memorial Hospital	Kosciusko	81%	(a)
Baptist Memorial Hospital/Golden Triangle	Columbus	80%	300+
Forrest General Hospital	Hattiesburg	80%	300+
Memorial Hospital at Gulfport	Gulfport	80%	300+
North Oak Regional Medical Center	Senatobia	80%	(a)
River Oaks Hospital	Flowood	80%	300+
South Central Regional Medical Center	Laurel	80%	300+
South Sunflower County Hospital	Indianola	80%	(a)
Wesley Medical Center	Hattiesburg	80%	300+
Anderson Regional Medical Center	Meridian	79%	300+
Baptist Mem Hosp North Mississippi	Oxford	79%	300+
Greenwood Leflore Hospital	Greenwood	79%	300+
Saint Dominic - Jackson Memorial Hospital	Jackson	79%	300+
Baptist Memorial Hospital Desoto	Southaven	78%	300+
Garden Park Medical Center	Gulfport	78%	300+
Highland Community Hospital	Picayune	78%	(a)
Madison River Oaks Medical Center	Canton	78%	(a)
Natchez Community Hospital	Natchez	78%	300+
Rush Foundation Hospital	Meridian	78%	300+
University of Mississippi Medical Center	Jackson	78%	300+
Bolivar Medical Center	Cleveland	77%	300+
River Region Health System	Vicksburg	77%	300+
Southwest Ms Regional Medical Center	Mccomb	77%	300+
Northwest Mississippi Reg Med Ctr	Clarksdale	76%	300+
Central Mississippi Medical Center	Jackson	75%	300+
Delta Regional Medical Center	Greenville	75%	300+
Tri Lakes Medical Center	Batesville	75%	(a)
Marion General Hospital	Columbia	74%	(a)
Biloxi Regional Medical Center	Biloxi	73%	300+
Natchez Regional Medical Center[11]	Natchez	73%	300+
Crossgates River Oaks Hospital	Brandon	70%	300+

Pain 'Always' Well Controlled

Hospital Name	City	Rate	Cases
Lawrence County Hospital	Monticello	86%	(a)
King's Daughters Med Ctr-Brookhaven	Brookhaven	82%	300+
Webster General Hospital/Swing Bed	Eupora	81%	(a)
Woman's Hospital at River Oaks	Flowood	81%	300+
George County Hospital	Lucedale	79%	(a)
Magee General Hospital	Magee	79%	(a)
Magnolia Regional Health Center	Corinth	78%	300+
South Sunflower County Hospital	Indianola	78%	(a)

NOTE: Hospital profiles are in alphabetical order by state, then city, then hospital within the city; Rankings exclude hospitals with less than 25 cases except for patient surveys which excludes hospitals with less than 100 cases; (a) 100-299 cases; (1) The number of cases/patients is too few to report; (2) Data submitted were based on a sample of cases/patients; (3) Results are based on a shorter time period than required; (4) Data suppressed by CMS for one or more quarters; (5) Results are not available for this reporting period; (6) Fewer than 100 patients completed the HCAHPS survey; (7) No cases met the criteria for this measure; (8) The lower limit of the confidence interval cannot be calculated if the number of observed infections equals zero; (9) No data are available from the state/territory for this reporting period; (10) The scores shown reflect fewer than 50 completed surveys; (11) There were discrepancies in the data collection process; (12) This measure does not apply to this hospital for this reporting period; (13) Results cannot be calculated for this reporting period; (14) The results for this state are combined with nearby states to protect confidentiality; Please refer to the User's Guide for a full explanation of data.

Hospital Name	City	Rate	Cases
Beacham Memorial Hospital	Magnolia	77%	(a)
North Mississippi Medical Center	Tupelo	77%	300+
Gilmore Memorial Regional Medical Center	Amory	76%	300+
Neshoba County General Hospital	Philadelphia	76%	300+
Och Regional Medical Center	Starkville	76%	300+
Grenada Lake Medical Center	Grenada	75%	300+
Memorial Hospital at Gulfport	Gulfport	75%	300+
Mississippi Baptist Medical Center[11]	Jackson	75%	300+
Wayne General Hospital	Waynesboro	75%	300+
Anderson Regional Medical Center	Meridian	74%	300+
Baptist Memorial Hospital/Golden Triangle	Columbus	74%	300+
Clay County Medical Center	West Point	74%	300+
Wesley Medical Center	Hattiesburg	74%	300+
Greenwood Leflore Hospital	Greenwood	73%	300+
Hancock Medical Center	Bay Saint Louis	73%	300+
Tishomingo Health Services	Iuka	73%	(a)
Baptist Memorial Hospital Union County	New Albany	72%	300+
Madison River Oaks Medical Center	Canton	72%	(a)
River Oaks Hospital	Flowood	72%	300+
Southwest Ms Regional Medical Center	Mccomb	72%	300+
Baptist Mem Hosp North Mississippi	Oxford	71%	300+
Delta Regional Medical Center	Greenville	71%	300+
Forrest General Hospital	Hattiesburg	71%	300+
Saint Dominic - Jackson Memorial Hospital	Jackson	71%	300+
South Central Regional Medical Center	Laurel	71%	300+
Garden Park Medical Center	Gulfport	70%	300+
River Region Health System	Vicksburg	70%	300+
Singing River Hospital	Pascagoula	70%	300+
Baptist Memorial Hospital Booneville	Booneville	69%	(a)
Bolivar Medical Center	Cleveland	69%	300+
North Oak Regional Medical Center	Senatobia	69%	(a)
Northwest Mississippi Reg Med Ctr	Clarksdale	69%	300+
Rush Foundation Hospital	Meridian	69%	300+
University of Mississippi Medical Center	Jackson	69%	300+
Baptist Memorial Hospital Desoto	Southaven	68%	300+
Natchez Community Hospital	Natchez	68%	300+
Natchez Regional Medical Center[11]	Natchez	68%	300+
Biloxi Regional Medical Center	Biloxi	67%	300+
Central Mississippi Medical Center	Jackson	67%	300+
Montfort Jones Memorial Hospital	Kosciusko	67%	(a)
Crossgates River Oaks Hospital	Brandon	65%	300+
Highland Community Hospital	Picayune	65%	(a)
Marion General Hospital	Columbia	62%	(a)
Tri Lakes Medical Center	Batesville	59%	(a)

Room and Bathroom 'Always' Clean

Hospital Name	City	Rate	Cases
Webster General Hospital/Swing Bed	Eupora	88%	(a)
George County Hospital	Lucedale	84%	(a)
Neshoba County General Hospital	Philadelphia	83%	300+
Och Regional Medical Center	Starkville	82%	300+
Clay County Medical Center	West Point	81%	300+
Lawrence County Hospital	Monticello	80%	(a)
Magnolia Regional Health Center	Corinth	79%	300+
North Mississippi Medical Center	Tupelo	79%	300+
Baptist Memorial Hospital Booneville	Booneville	78%	(a)
Gilmore Memorial Regional Medical Center	Amory	78%	300+
Grenada Lake Medical Center	Grenada	78%	300+
King's Daughters Med Ctr-Brookhaven	Brookhaven	77%	300+
North Oak Regional Medical Center	Senatobia	76%	(a)
Tri Lakes Medical Center	Batesville	76%	(a)
Hancock Medical Center	Bay Saint Louis	75%	300+
Highland Community Hospital	Picayune	75%	(a)
River Region Health System	Vicksburg	75%	300+
Baptist Memorial Hospital Union County	New Albany	74%	300+
Baptist Memorial Hospital/Golden Triangle	Columbus	74%	300+
Magee General Hospital	Magee	74%	(a)
Tishomingo Health Services	Iuka	74%	(a)
Baptist Mem Hosp North Mississippi	Oxford	73%	300+
Beacham Memorial Hospital	Magnolia	73%	(a)
Woman's Hospital at River Oaks	Flowood	73%	300+
Montfort Jones Memorial Hospital	Kosciusko	72%	(a)
Wesley Medical Center	Hattiesburg	72%	300+
Anderson Regional Medical Center	Meridian	71%	300+
Baptist Memorial Hospital Desoto	Southaven	70%	300+
Delta Regional Medical Center	Greenville	70%	300+
Forrest General Hospital	Hattiesburg	70%	300+
Rush Foundation Hospital	Meridian	70%	300+
Singing River Hospital	Pascagoula	70%	300+
Southwest Ms Regional Medical Center	Mccomb	70%	300+
Greenwood Leflore Hospital	Greenwood	69%	300+
Northwest Mississippi Reg Med Ctr	Clarksdale	69%	300+
South Central Regional Medical Center	Laurel	69%	300+
Natchez Community Hospital	Natchez	68%	300+
Central Mississippi Medical Center	Jackson	67%	300+
Garden Park Medical Center	Gulfport	67%	300+
Madison River Oaks Medical Center	Canton	67%	(a)
Memorial Hospital at Gulfport	Gulfport	67%	300+
Natchez Regional Medical Center[11]	Natchez	67%	300+
Mississippi Baptist Medical Center[11]	Jackson	66%	300+
Saint Dominic - Jackson Memorial Hospital	Jackson	66%	300+
University of Mississippi Medical Center	Jackson	66%	300+
Wayne General Hospital	Waynesboro	66%	300+
River Oaks Hospital	Flowood	65%	300+
Crossgates River Oaks Hospital	Brandon	64%	300+
South Sunflower County Hospital	Indianola	63%	(a)
Bolivar Medical Center	Cleveland	59%	300+
Marion General Hospital	Columbia	59%	(a)
Biloxi Regional Medical Center	Biloxi	56%	300+

Timely Help 'Always' Received

Hospital Name	City	Rate	Cases
Baptist Memorial Hospital Booneville	Booneville	83%	(a)
Lawrence County Hospital	Monticello	81%	(a)
King's Daughters Med Ctr-Brookhaven	Brookhaven	80%	300+
Montfort Jones Memorial Hospital	Kosciusko	79%	(a)
Neshoba County General Hospital	Philadelphia	77%	300+
Beacham Memorial Hospital	Magnolia	76%	(a)
Tishomingo Health Services	Iuka	76%	(a)
Clay County Medical Center	West Point	75%	300+
George County Hospital	Lucedale	75%	(a)
Grenada Lake Medical Center	Grenada	75%	300+
Hancock Medical Center	Bay Saint Louis	75%	300+
Magnolia Regional Health Center	Corinth	74%	300+
Och Regional Medical Center	Starkville	74%	300+
Woman's Hospital at River Oaks	Flowood	74%	300+
Baptist Memorial Hospital Union County	New Albany	73%	300+
North Mississippi Medical Center	Tupelo	73%	300+
Garden Park Medical Center	Gulfport	70%	300+
Magee General Hospital	Magee	70%	(a)
South Central Regional Medical Center	Laurel	70%	300+
Wesley Medical Center	Hattiesburg	70%	300+
River Oaks Hospital	Flowood	69%	300+
Singing River Hospital	Pascagoula	69%	300+
Wayne General Hospital	Waynesboro	69%	300+
Memorial Hospital at Gulfport	Gulfport	68%	300+
Southwest Ms Regional Medical Center	Mccomb	68%	300+
Anderson Regional Medical Center	Meridian	67%	300+
Greenwood Leflore Hospital	Greenwood	67%	300+
Mississippi Baptist Medical Center[11]	Jackson	67%	300+
North Oak Regional Medical Center	Senatobia	67%	(a)
Gilmore Memorial Regional Medical Center	Amory	66%	300+
Saint Dominic - Jackson Memorial Hospital	Jackson	66%	300+
Webster General Hospital/Swing Bed	Eupora	66%	(a)
Highland Community Hospital	Picayune	65%	(a)
Northwest Mississippi Reg Med Ctr	Clarksdale	65%	300+
South Sunflower County Hospital	Indianola	65%	(a)
Baptist Mem Hosp North Mississippi	Oxford	64%	300+
Baptist Memorial Hospital/Golden Triangle	Columbus	64%	300+
Rush Foundation Hospital	Meridian	64%	300+
Bolivar Medical Center	Cleveland	63%	300+
Delta Regional Medical Center	Greenville	63%	300+
Forrest General Hospital	Hattiesburg	63%	300+
Madison River Oaks Medical Center	Canton	62%	(a)
River Region Health System	Vicksburg	61%	300+
University of Mississippi Medical Center	Jackson	59%	300+
Baptist Memorial Hospital Desoto	Southaven	58%	300+
Biloxi Regional Medical Center	Biloxi	57%	300+
Natchez Community Hospital	Natchez	57%	300+
Marion General Hospital	Columbia	56%	(a)
Tri Lakes Medical Center	Batesville	56%	(a)
Central Mississippi Medical Center	Jackson	55%	300+
Crossgates River Oaks Hospital	Brandon	55%	300+
Natchez Regional Medical Center[11]	Natchez	55%	300+

Would Definitely Recommend Hospital

Hospital Name	City	Rate	Cases
Woman's Hospital at River Oaks	Flowood	85%	300+
King's Daughters Med Ctr-Brookhaven	Brookhaven	84%	300+
Mississippi Baptist Medical Center[11]	Jackson	81%	300+
North Mississippi Medical Center	Tupelo	81%	300+
Magnolia Regional Health Center	Corinth	80%	300+
Saint Dominic - Jackson Memorial Hospital	Jackson	80%	300+
Tishomingo Health Services	Iuka	80%	(a)
Anderson Regional Medical Center	Meridian	78%	300+
Wesley Medical Center	Hattiesburg	78%	300+
Baptist Memorial Hospital Union County	New Albany	77%	300+
Beacham Memorial Hospital	Magnolia	77%	(a)
Forrest General Hospital	Hattiesburg	77%	300+
Memorial Hospital at Gulfport	Gulfport	76%	300+
Garden Park Medical Center	Gulfport	75%	300+
Och Regional Medical Center	Starkville	75%	300+
University of Mississippi Medical Center	Jackson	75%	300+
Gilmore Memorial Regional Medical Center	Amory	74%	300+
River Oaks Hospital	Flowood	74%	300+
Webster General Hospital/Swing Bed	Eupora	74%	(a)
Baptist Mem Hosp North Mississippi	Oxford	73%	300+
Singing River Hospital	Pascagoula	73%	300+
Lawrence County Hospital	Monticello	72%	(a)
Rush Foundation Hospital	Meridian	72%	300+
Magee General Hospital	Magee	71%	(a)
Neshoba County General Hospital	Philadelphia	71%	300+
Baptist Memorial Hospital Booneville	Booneville	70%	(a)
Baptist Memorial Hospital Desoto	Southaven	70%	300+
George County Hospital	Lucedale	70%	(a)
Hancock Medical Center	Bay Saint Louis	69%	300+
Natchez Community Hospital	Natchez	69%	300+
South Central Regional Medical Center	Laurel	69%	300+
Clay County Medical Center	West Point	68%	300+
Highland Community Hospital	Picayune	68%	(a)
Madison River Oaks Medical Center	Canton	67%	(a)
Baptist Memorial Hospital/Golden Triangle	Columbus	66%	300+
Greenwood Leflore Hospital	Greenwood	66%	300+
Grenada Lake Medical Center	Grenada	66%	300+
South Sunflower County Hospital	Indianola	66%	(a)
Southwest Ms Regional Medical Center	Mccomb	64%	300+
Wayne General Hospital	Waynesboro	64%	300+
River Region Health System	Vicksburg	62%	300+
Montfort Jones Memorial Hospital	Kosciusko	61%	(a)
Natchez Regional Medical Center[11]	Natchez	60%	300+
Biloxi Regional Medical Center	Biloxi	59%	300+
Marion General Hospital	Columbia	59%	(a)
North Oak Regional Medical Center	Senatobia	59%	(a)
Central Mississippi Medical Center	Jackson	58%	300+
Crossgates River Oaks Hospital	Brandon	58%	300+
Bolivar Medical Center	Cleveland	57%	300+
Delta Regional Medical Center	Greenville	55%	300+
Tri Lakes Medical Center	Batesville	51%	(a)
Northwest Mississippi Reg Med Ctr	Clarksdale	47%	300+

Use of Medical Imaging

Cardiac Imaging Stress Test before OP Surgery

Hospital Name	City	Rate	Cases
Delta Regional Medical Center	Greenville	2.5%	161
Central Mississippi Medical Center	Jackson	2.9%	103
George County Hospital	Lucedale	2.9%	102
Highland Community Hospital	Picayune	3.1%	129
Hancock Medical Center	Bay Saint Louis	3.3%	90
River Region Health System	Vicksburg	4.0%	376
Singing River Hospital	Pascagoula	4.5%	243
Southwest Ms Regional Medical Center	Mccomb	4.5%	398
Greenwood Leflore Hospital	Greenwood	5.1%	216
University of Mississippi Medical Center	Jackson	5.1%	513
Magnolia Regional Health Center	Corinth	5.4%	957
Baptist Memorial Hospital Desoto	Southaven	5.6%	1462
Wesley Medical Center	Hattiesburg	5.7%	279
North Mississippi Medical Center	Tupelo	5.8%	482
Biloxi Regional Medical Center	Biloxi	5.9%	153
Forrest General Hospital	Hattiesburg	6.1%	478
Baptist Memorial Hospital Booneville	Booneville	6.4%	94
Natchez Regional Medical Center	Natchez	6.4%	233
Baptist Mem Hosp North Mississippi	Oxford	6.6%	211
Memorial Hospital at Gulfport	Gulfport	6.8%	338
Anderson Regional Medical Center	Meridian	7.0%	142
Rush Foundation Hospital	Meridian	7.2%	600
Garden Park Medical Center	Gulfport	7.5%	67
Baptist Memorial Hospital Union County	New Albany	8.0%	113
Gilmore Memorial Regional Medical Center	Amory	8.0%	112
Saint Dominic - Jackson Memorial Hospital	Jackson	8.0%	176
Mississippi Baptist Medical Center	Jackson	8.1%	335
King's Daughters Med Ctr-Brookhaven	Brookhaven	8.5%	117
Field Memorial Community Hospital	Centreville	9.4%	64

Combination Abdominal CT Scan

Hospital Name	City	Rate	Cases
Walthall County General Hospital	Tylertown	1.0%	105
Forrest General Hospital	Hattiesburg	1.1%	963
Covington County Hospital CAH	Collins	1.4%	140
Pioneer Health Services of Newton	Newton	1.5%	68
Tyler Holmes Memorial Hospital	Winona	1.6%	184
Marion General Hospital	Columbia	2.0%	201
Baptist Memorial Hospital Booneville	Booneville	2.3%	438
North Mississippi Medical Center	Tupelo	2.3%	2381
Tippah County Hospital	Ripley	2.4%	209
Pontotoc Health Service	Pontotoc	2.5%	237
Saint Dominic - Jackson Memorial Hospital	Jackson	2.6%	1816
Central Mississippi Medical Center	Jackson	2.9%	315
Magnolia Regional Health Center	Corinth	3.3%	1814
Yalobusha General Hospital	Water Valley	3.7%	82
Baptist Memorial Hospital Desoto	Southaven	3.9%	1348
Mississippi Baptist Medical Center	Jackson	4.0%	1966
Crossgates River Oaks Hospital	Brandon	4.1%	217
Wesley Medical Center	Hattiesburg	4.2%	643
Hardy Wilson Memorial Hospital	Hazlehurst	4.3%	162
Baptist Medical Center - Leake	Carthage	4.7%	107
Holmes County Hospital & Clinics	Lexington	4.7%	127
Madison River Oaks Medical Center	Canton	4.8%	189
Baptist Memorial Hospital Union County	New Albany	5.0%	681
Southwest Ms Regional Medical Center	Mccomb	5.2%	949
River Region Health System	Vicksburg	5.6%	498

NOTE: Hospital profiles are in alphabetical order by state, then city, then hospital within the city; Rankings exclude hospitals with less than 25 cases except for patient surveys which excludes hospitals with less than 100 cases; (a) 100-299 cases; (1) The number of cases/patients is too few to report; (2) Data submitted were based on a sample of cases/patients; (3) Results are based on a shorter time period than required; (4) Data suppressed by CMS for one or more quarters; (5) Results are not available for this reporting period; (6) Fewer than 100 patients completed the HCAHPS survey; (7) No cases met the criteria for this measure; (8) The lower limit of the confidence interval cannot be calculated if the number of observed infections equals zero; (9) No data are available from the state/territory for this reporting period; (10) The scores shown reflect fewer than 50 completed surveys; (11) There were discrepancies in the data collection process; (12) This measure does not apply to this hospital for this reporting period; (13) Results cannot be calculated for this reporting period; (14) The results for this state are combined with nearby states to protect confidentiality; Please refer to the User's Guide for a full explanation of data.

Hospital Name	City	Rate	Cases
Montfort Jones Memorial Hospital	Kosciusko	6.0%	248
Hancock Medical Center	Bay Saint Louis	6.2%	243
Natchez Community Hospital	Natchez	6.3%	382
Kings Daughters Hospital	Yazoo City	6.9%	159
Bolivar Medical Center	Cleveland	7.7%	234
Pioneer Community Hospital of Choctaw	Ackerman	7.8%	77
Laird Hospital	Union	8.3%	109
Singing River Hospital	Pascagoula	8.3%	1610
Stone County Hospital	Wiggins	8.6%	139
Tri Lakes Medical Center	Batesville	9.2%	251
George County Hospital	Lucedale	9.4%	266
Tishomingo Health Services	Iuka	9.7%	300
University of Mississippi Medical Center	Jackson	9.7%	1264
Gilmore Memorial Regional Medical Center	Amory	10.0%	478
Highland Community Hospital	Picayune	10.0%	291
King's Daughters Med Ctr-Brookhaven	Brookhaven	10.0%	608
River Oaks Hospital	Flowood	10.2%	391
H C Watkins Memorial Hospital	Quitman	10.9%	92
Wayne General Hospital	Waynesboro	11.0%	155
Neshoba County General Hospital	Philadelphia	11.1%	262
Clay County Medical Center	West Point	11.3%	150
Rush Foundation Hospital	Meridian	11.4%	641
Webster General Hospital/Swing Bed	Eupora	12.8%	250
Baptist Mem Hosp North Mississippi	Oxford	13.8%	745
Och Regional Medical Center	Starkville	15.0%	642
Delta Regional Medical Center	Greenville	16.6%	766
Baptist Memorial Hospital/Golden Triangle	Columbus	17.1%	1712
Franklin County Memorial Hospital	Meadville	17.1%	76
Winston Medical Center & Swingbed	Louisville	17.3%	127
Pioneer Community Hospital of Aberdeen	Aberdeen	17.4%	184
Anderson Regional Medical Center	Meridian	19.8%	1243
Grenada Lake Medical Center	Grenada	19.8%	222
Calhoun Health Services	Calhoun City	20.8%	149
South Central Regional Medical Center	Laurel	20.9%	549
Scott Regional Hospital	Morton	21.7%	69
Anderson Rmc South	Meridian	22.2%	72
North Sunflower Medical Center	Ruleville	30.4%	207
Biloxi Regional Medical Center	Biloxi	31.4%	423
Natchez Regional Medical Center	Natchez	31.4%	392
Greenwood Leflore Hospital	Greenwood	36.6%	489
Lackey Memorial Hospital	Forest	36.6%	153
Northwest Mississippi Reg Med Ctr	Clarksdale	37.5%	355
South Sunflower County Hospital	Indianola	41.4%	186
Garden Park Medical Center	Gulfport	43.1%	360
Field Memorial Community Hospital	Centreville	43.6%	101
Trace Regional Hospital & Swing Bed	Houston	48.0%	150
North Oak Regional Medical Center	Senatobia	48.1%	81
Sharkey Issaquena Community Hospital	Rolling Fork	59.4%	64
Memorial Hospital at Gulfport	Gulfport	64.8%	1270
Magee General Hospital	Magee	67.2%	268

Combination Brain/Sinus CT Scan

Hospital Name	City	Rate	Cases
Beacham Memorial Hospital	Magnolia	0.0%	33
John C Stennis Memorial Hospital	De Kalb	0.0%	128
Perry County General Hospital	Richton	0.0%	99
Quitman County Hospital	Marks	0.0%	31
George County Hospital	Lucedale	0.4%	284
Och Regional Medical Center	Starkville	1.1%	436
South Sunflower County Hospital	Indianola	1.1%	270
Baptist Memorial Hospital Desoto	Southaven	1.7%	1395
Grenada Lake Medical Center	Grenada	1.7%	462
Memorial Hospital at Gulfport	Gulfport	1.7%	1300
Baptist Memorial Hospital Union County	New Albany	2.0%	554
University of Mississippi Medical Center	Jackson	2.3%	744
River Region Health System	Vicksburg	2.4%	533
Saint Dominic - Jackson Memorial Hospital	Jackson	2.4%	1730
Mississippi Baptist Medical Center	Jackson	2.5%	942
Singing River Hospital	Pascagoula	2.5%	1247
King's Daughters Med Ctr-Brookhaven	Brookhaven	2.7%	639
Baptist Memorial Hospital/Golden Triangle	Columbus	3.1%	977
Forrest General Hospital	Hattiesburg	3.1%	1680
North Mississippi Medical Center	Tupelo	3.3%	2094
Rush Foundation Hospital	Meridian	3.3%	748
Tishomingo Health Services	Iuka	3.9%	412
Anderson Regional Medical Center	Meridian	4.1%	1356
Delta Regional Medical Center	Greenville	4.1%	724
Northwest Mississippi Reg Med Ctr	Clarksdale	4.1%	461
Biloxi Regional Medical Center	Biloxi	4.3%	468
Greenwood Leflore Hospital	Greenwood	4.4%	685
Crossgates River Oaks Hospital	Brandon	4.5%	267
Southwest Ms Regional Medical Center	Mccomb	4.5%	776
Gilmore Memorial Regional Medical Center	Amory	4.6%	456
South Central Regional Medical Center	Laurel	4.6%	658
Baptist Mem Hosp North Mississippi	Oxford	5.0%	761
Calhoun Health Services	Calhoun City	5.0%	202
River Oaks Hospital	Flowood	5.0%	417
Baptist Medical Center - Leake	Carthage	5.1%	214
Bolivar Medical Center	Cleveland	5.1%	370
Hardy Wilson Memorial Hospital	Hazlehurst	5.1%	294
Marion General Hospital	Columbia	5.1%	373
Madison River Oaks Medical Center	Canton	5.3%	374
Baptist Memorial Hospital Booneville	Booneville	5.5%	433
Magnolia Regional Health Center	Corinth	5.5%	1108
Kings Daughters Hospital	Yazoo City	5.7%	316
Central Mississippi Medical Center	Jackson	5.9%	322
Natchez Regional Medical Center	Natchez	7.7%	456
North Oak Regional Medical Center	Senatobia	7.7%	143
Sharkey Issaquena Community Hospital	Rolling Fork	12.4%	89

Combination Chest CT Scan

Hospital Name	City	Rate	Cases
Baptist Memorial Hospital Booneville	Booneville	0.0%	254
Baptist Memorial Hospital Union County	New Albany	0.0%	213
George County Hospital	Lucedale	0.0%	138
Highland Community Hospital	Picayune	0.0%	114
Marion General Hospital	Columbia	0.0%	96
Tippah County Hospital	Ripley	0.0%	65
Baptist Memorial Hospital/Golden Triangle	Columbus	0.1%	938
Magnolia Regional Health Center	Corinth	0.2%	1074
University of Mississippi Medical Center	Jackson	0.4%	1279
Tri Lakes Medical Center	Batesville	0.6%	169
North Mississippi Medical Center	Tupelo	0.7%	1639
South Central Regional Medical Center	Laurel	1.1%	179
Singing River Hospital	Pascagoula	1.2%	1187
Forrest General Hospital	Hattiesburg	1.3%	299
Saint Dominic - Jackson Memorial Hospital	Jackson	1.3%	1300
Crossgates River Oaks Hospital	Brandon	1.4%	71
Laird Hospital	Union	1.4%	74
Baptist Memorial Hospital Desoto	Southaven	1.8%	726
Wayne General Hospital	Waynesboro	1.9%	52
Baptist Mem Hosp North Mississippi	Oxford	2.0%	356
Rush Foundation Hospital	Meridian	2.0%	497
Central Mississippi Medical Center	Jackson	2.3%	129
Bolivar Medical Center	Cleveland	2.4%	84
Tyler Holmes Memorial Hospital	Winona	2.5%	79
Garden Park Medical Center	Gulfport	2.8%	141
Wesley Medical Center	Hattiesburg	2.9%	341
Memorial Hospital at Gulfport	Gulfport	3.2%	1149
King's Daughters Med Ctr-Brookhaven	Brookhaven	3.3%	180
Hancock Medical Center	Bay Saint Louis	4.0%	99
River Region Health System	Vicksburg	4.2%	289
Hardy Wilson Memorial Hospital	Hazlehurst	4.5%	88
Tishomingo Health Services	Iuka	4.8%	125
Webster General Hospital/Swing Bed	Eupora	5.2%	77
Stone County Hospital	Wiggins	5.3%	76
Natchez Community Hospital	Natchez	6.0%	117
Gilmore Memorial Regional Medical Center	Amory	6.7%	120
Anderson Regional Medical Center	Meridian	7.2%	953
Madison River Oaks Medical Center	Canton	7.2%	97
Southwest Ms Regional Medical Center	Mccomb	7.6%	380
Mississippi Baptist Medical Center	Jackson	7.8%	1535
Montfort Jones Memorial Hospital	Kosciusko	7.9%	63
Och Regional Medical Center	Starkville	13.1%	336
River Oaks Hospital	Flowood	17.1%	164
Grenada Lake Medical Center	Grenada	20.2%	124
Northwest Mississippi Reg Med Ctr	Clarksdale	20.5%	166
Delta Regional Medical Center	Greenville	20.7%	363
Pioneer Community Hospital of Aberdeen	Aberdeen	24.3%	74
Kings Daughters Hospital	Yazoo City	27.4%	73
Magee General Hospital	Magee	27.7%	112
Biloxi Regional Medical Center	Biloxi	28.4%	236
South Sunflower County Hospital	Indianola	36.1%	72
Neshoba County General Hospital	Philadelphia	39.0%	82
Lackey Memorial Hospital	Forest	39.1%	69
Natchez Regional Medical Center	Natchez	44.8%	306
Greenwood Leflore Hospital	Greenwood	47.1%	276
Field Memorial Community Hospital	Centreville	52.2%	46

Follow-up Mammogram/Ultrasound

A follow-up rate near zero may indicate missed cancer; a rate higher than 14% may mean there is unnecessary follow up.

Hospital Name	City	Rate	Cases
Clay County Medical Center	West Point	1.1%	362
Winston Medical Center & Swingbed	Louisville	1.2%	421
Hardy Wilson Memorial Hospital	Hazlehurst	1.9%	206
Grenada Lake Medical Center	Grenada	2.5%	1011
Baptist Memorial Hospital/Golden Triangle	Columbus	3.2%	1263
Southwest Ms Regional Medical Center	Mccomb	3.5%	993
Field Memorial Community Hospital	Centreville	3.6%	197
Trace Regional Hospital & Swing Bed	Houston	4.2%	264
South Central Regional Medical Center	Laurel	4.3%	1293
Greenwood Leflore Hospital	Greenwood	4.4%	1149
Magee General Hospital	Magee	4.6%	478
River Oaks Hospital	Flowood	4.9%	632
South Sunflower County Hospital	Indianola	5.0%	181
Baptist Memorial Hospital Union County	New Albany	5.3%	869
Laird Hospital	Union	5.6%	215
Saint Dominic - Jackson Memorial Hospital	Jackson	5.6%	1622
King's Daughters Med Ctr-Brookhaven	Brookhaven	5.9%	610
Crossgates River Oaks Hospital	Brandon	6.2%	465
Lackey Memorial Hospital	Forest	6.2%	242
Tri Lakes Medical Center	Batesville	6.2%	305
Baptist Mem Hosp North Mississippi	Oxford	6.3%	95
Delta Regional Medical Center	Greenville	6.5%	1369
North Mississippi Medical Center	Tupelo	6.6%	3661
River Region Health System	Vicksburg	6.6%	1058
Madison River Oaks Medical Center	Canton	6.7%	268
Forrest General Hospital	Hattiesburg	7.4%	190
Northwest Mississippi Reg Med Ctr	Clarksdale	7.6%	315
Woman's Hospital at River Oaks	Flowood	7.6%	675
George County Hospital	Lucedale	7.8%	345
Mississippi Baptist Medical Center	Jackson	7.8%	1952
Holmes County Hospital & Clinics	Lexington	8.9%	90
Natchez Regional Medical Center	Natchez	8.9%	797
Tippah County Hospital	Ripley	9.0%	156
Central Mississippi Medical Center	Jackson	9.3%	713
Highland Community Hospital	Picayune	9.3%	420
Singing River Hospital	Pascagoula	9.3%	2743
Baptist Memorial Hospital Desoto	Southaven	9.4%	1529
Anderson Regional Medical Center	Meridian	9.8%	1811
Alliance Healthcare System	Holly Springs	10.5%	152
Wesley Medical Center	Hattiesburg	10.6%	1226
Hancock Medical Center	Bay Saint Louis	11.0%	281
Rush Foundation Hospital	Meridian	11.2%	2627
Kings Daughters Hospital	Yazoo City	11.7%	145
Anderson Rmc South	Meridian	11.8%	161
Och Regional Medical Center	Starkville	11.8%	1224
Garden Park Medical Center	Gulfport	12.0%	401
Magnolia Regional Health Center	Corinth	12.6%	1022
Wayne General Hospital	Waynesboro	12.9%	163
Memorial Hospital at Gulfport	Gulfport	13.0%	1883
Baptist Memorial Hospital Booneville	Booneville	13.5%	260
University of Mississippi Medical Center	Jackson	13.6%	968
Montfort Jones Memorial Hospital	Kosciusko	14.7%	619
Bolivar Medical Center	Cleveland	15.2%	335
Gilmore Memorial Regional Medical Center	Amory	19.7%	529
Biloxi Regional Medical Center	Biloxi	19.8%	803

Lumbar Spine MRI for Low Back Pain

Hospital Name	City	Rate	Cases
Highland Community Hospital	Picayune	29.9%	87
Garden Park Medical Center	Gulfport	30.8%	78
Biloxi Regional Medical Center	Biloxi	33.3%	81
Trace Regional Hospital & Swing Bed	Houston	33.3%	60
River Oaks Hospital	Flowood	33.5%	215
South Central Regional Medical Center	Laurel	34.8%	69
Magnolia Regional Health Center	Corinth	35.4%	302
Wesley Medical Center	Hattiesburg	35.4%	82
Webster General Hospital/Swing Bed	Eupora	35.6%	101
Baptist Memorial Hospital Desoto	Southaven	37.2%	164
Och Regional Medical Center	Starkville	37.2%	78
Saint Dominic - Jackson Memorial Hospital	Jackson	37.3%	475
North Mississippi Medical Center	Tupelo	37.9%	480
Southwest Ms Regional Medical Center	Mccomb	38.9%	90
University of Mississippi Medical Center	Jackson	39.2%	143
Bolivar Medical Center	Cleveland	40.4%	57
Tishomingo Health Services	Iuka	40.4%	104
Singing River Hospital	Pascagoula	40.5%	311
Greenwood Leflore Hospital	Greenwood	41.1%	146
Crossgates River Oaks Hospital	Brandon	41.3%	46
Forrest General Hospital	Hattiesburg	41.4%	70
Baptist Memorial Hospital/Golden Triangle	Columbus	41.9%	117
Memorial Hospital at Gulfport	Gulfport	42.0%	257
Anderson Regional Medical Center	Meridian	42.7%	199
Grenada Lake Medical Center	Grenada	43.0%	114
River Region Health System	Vicksburg	43.6%	140
Baptist Memorial Hospital Booneville	Booneville	44.4%	108
Baptist Memorial Hospital Union County	New Albany	45.6%	180
Laird Hospital	Union	45.7%	35
Tri Lakes Medical Center	Batesville	46.3%	67
Mississippi Baptist Medical Center	Jackson	46.4%	265
Delta Regional Medical Center	Greenville	46.5%	127
Clay County Medical Center	West Point	46.7%	45
Central Mississippi Medical Center	Jackson	47.0%	115
Kings Daughters Hospital	Yazoo City	47.1%	34
Gilmore Memorial Regional Medical Center	Amory	48.1%	77
King's Daughters Med Ctr-Brookhaven	Brookhaven	50.0%	114
Neshoba County General Hospital	Philadelphia	54.2%	48
George County Hospital	Lucedale	55.6%	36
Northwest Mississippi Reg Med Ctr	Clarksdale	57.4%	54

NOTE: Hospital profiles are in alphabetical order by state, then city, then hospital within the city; Rankings exclude hospitals with less than 25 cases except for patient surveys which excludes hospitals with less than 100 cases; (a) 100-299 cases; (1) The number of cases/patients is too few to report; (2) Data submitted were based on a sample of cases/patients; (3) Results are based on a shorter time period than required; (4) Data suppressed by CMS for one or more quarters; (5) Results are not available for this reporting period; (6) Fewer than 100 patients completed the HCAHPS survey; (7) No cases met the criteria for this measure; (8) The lower limit of the confidence interval cannot be calculated if the number of observed infections equals zero; (9) No data are available from the state/territory for this reporting period; (10) The scores shown reflect fewer than 50 completed surveys; (11) There were discrepancies in the data collection process; (12) This measure does not apply to this hospital for this reporting period; (13) Results cannot be calculated for this reporting period; (14) The results for this state are combined with nearby states to protect confidentiality; Please refer to the User's Guide for a full explanation of data.

Pioneer Community Hospital of Aberdeen

400 S Chestnut Street   Phone: 662-369-2455
Aberdeen, MS 39730
Type: Critical Access Hospitals   Emergency Services: Yes
Ownership: Voluntary non-profit - Private

Measure	Cases	This Hosp.	State Avg.	U.S. Avg.
Blood Clot Prevention and Treatment				
Anticoagulation Overlap Therapy	-	-	86%	93%
ICU Venous Thromboembolism Prophylaxis	-	-	86%	92%
Incidence of Potentially Preventable VTE	-	-	15%	10%
UFH with Dosages/Platelet Monitoring	-	-	94%	97%
Venous Thromboembolism Prophylaxis	-	-	70%	85%
Warfarin Therapy Discharge Instructions	-	-	77%	75%
Chest Pain/Possible Heart Attack Care				
Aspirin Given Within 24 Hours of Arrival[5]	-	-	94%	96%
Fibrinolytic Meds Within 30 Min. of Arrival[5]	-	-	40%	58%
Average Time to ECG (minutes)[5]	-	-	10	7
Average Time to Transfer (minutes)[5]	-	-	77	60
Children's Asthma Care				
Received Home Management Plan of Care	-	-	-	88%
Received Reliever Medication	-	-	-	100%
Received Systemic Corticosteroids	-	-	-	100%
Emergency Department				
Admittance Decision Time (minutes)	-	-	61	98
Head CT Results Within 45 Min. of Arrival[3,7]	-	-	42%	57%
Patients Who Left ER Before Being Seen[5]	-	-	3%	2%
Time from ER Arrival to Admit. (minutes)	-	-	223	274
Time from ER Arrival to Discharge (minutes)[3]	1,056	82	112	134
Time in ER Before Being Evaluated (minutes)[3]	988	17	29	26
Time to Pain Meds for Fractures (minutes)[5]	-	-	68	57
Heart Attack Care				
Aspirin Given at Discharge	-	-	99%	99%
Fibrinolytic Meds Within 30 Min. of Arrival	-	-	50%	54%
PCI Within 90 Minutes of Arrival	-	-	96%	96%
Statin Prescribed at Discharge	-	-	97%	98%
Heart Failure Care				
ACE Inhibitor or ARB for LVSD	-	-	93%	97%
Discharge Instructions Given	-	-	91%	94%
Evaluation of LVS Function	-	-	96%	99%
Medicare Spending				
Medicare Spending per Patient (ratio)	-	-	0.95	0.98
Pneumonia Care				
Appropriate Initial Antibiotic Given	-	-	91%	95%
Blood Culture Timing	-	-	97%	98%
Pregnancy and Delivery Care				
Newborn Deliveries Scheduled Early	-	-	22%	6%
Preventive Care				
Immunization for Influenza	-	-	87%	90%
Immunization for Pneumonia	-	-	89%	92%
Stroke Care				
Anticoagulation Therapy for Atrial Fibrillation	-	-	93%	95%
Antithrombotic Therapy Timing	-	-	96%	98%
Assessed for Rehabilitation	-	-	95%	97%
Discharged on Antithrombotic Therapy	-	-	97%	99%
Discharged on Statin Medication	-	-	88%	94%
Thrombolytic Therapy Timing	-	-	25%	66%
Venous Thromboembolism Prophylaxis	-	-	87%	94%
Written Stroke Educational Materials Given	-	-	84%	88%
Surgical Care Improvement Project				
Appropriate Beta Blocker Usage	-	-	97%	98%
Appropriate VTP Within 24 Hours	-	-	97%	98%
Controlled Postoperative Blood Glucose	-	-	97%	97%
Perioperative Temperature Management	-	-	100%	100%
Prophylactic Antibiotic Selection	-	-	99%	99%
Prophylactic Antibiotic Selection (Outpatient)[5]	-	-	98%	98%
Prophylactic Antibiotic Stopped	-	-	97%	98%
Prophylactic Antibiotic Timing	-	-	99%	99%
Prophylactic Antibiotic Timing (Outpatient)[5]	-	-	98%	98%
Urinary Catheter Removal	-	-	97%	97%
Survey of Patients' Hospital Experiences				
Area Around Room 'Always' Quiet at Night	-	-	72%	61%
Doctors 'Always' Communicated Well	-	-	86%	82%
Home Recovery Information Given	-	-	83%	85%
Hospital Given 9 or 10 on 10 Point Scale	-	-	71%	71%
Meds 'Always' Explained Before Given	-	-	67%	64%
Nurses 'Always' Communicated Well	-	-	81%	79%
Pain 'Always' Well Controlled	-	-	72%	71%
Room and Bathroom 'Always' Clean	-	-	74%	73%
Timely Help 'Always' Received	-	-	69%	68%
Would Definitely Recommend Hospital	-	-	69%	71%
Use of Medical Imaging				
Cardiac Imaging Stress Test before Surgery[7]	-	-	5.7%	5.3%
Combination Abdominal CT Scan	184	17.4%	12.9%	10.5%
Combination Brain/Sinus CT Scan[1]	-	-	3.3%	2.7%
Combination Chest CT Scan	74	24.3%	6.1%	2.7%
Follow-up Mammogram/Ultrasound[7]	-	-	8.4%	8.8%
Lumbar Spine MRI for Low Back Pain[1]	-	-	41.1%	37.2%

Pioneer Community Hospital of Choctaw

8613 Ms Highway 12   Phone: 662-285-6235
Ackerman, MS 39735
Type: Critical Access Hospitals   Emergency Services: No
Ownership: Voluntary non-profit - Other

Measure	Cases	This Hosp.	State Avg.	U.S. Avg.
Blood Clot Prevention and Treatment				
Anticoagulation Overlap Therapy[5]	-	-	86%	93%
ICU Venous Thromboembolism Prophylaxis[5]	-	-	86%	92%
Incidence of Potentially Preventable VTE[5]	-	-	15%	10%
UFH with Dosages/Platelet Monitoring[5]	-	-	94%	97%
Venous Thromboembolism Prophylaxis[5]	-	-	70%	85%
Warfarin Therapy Discharge Instructions[5]	-	-	77%	75%
Chest Pain/Possible Heart Attack Care				
Aspirin Given Within 24 Hours of Arrival[1,3]	-	-	94%	96%
Fibrinolytic Meds Within 30 Min. of Arrival[3,7]	-	-	40%	58%
Average Time to ECG (minutes)[1,3]	-	-	10	7
Average Time to Transfer (minutes)[1,3]	-	-	77	60
Children's Asthma Care				
Received Home Management Plan of Care	-	-	-	88%
Received Reliever Medication	-	-	-	100%
Received Systemic Corticosteroids	-	-	-	100%
Emergency Department				
Admittance Decision Time (minutes)[5]	-	-	61	98
Head CT Results Within 45 Min. of Arrival[3,7]	-	-	42%	57%
Patients Who Left ER Before Being Seen[5]	-	-	3%	2%
Time from ER Arrival to Admit. (minutes)[5]	-	-	223	274
Time from ER Arrival to Discharge (minutes)[5]	-	-	112	134
Time in ER Before Being Evaluated (minutes)[5]	-	-	29	26
Time to Pain Meds for Fractures (minutes)[1]	-	-	68	57
Heart Attack Care				
Aspirin Given at Discharge[5]	-	-	99%	99%
Fibrinolytic Meds Within 30 Min. of Arrival[5]	-	-	50%	54%
PCI Within 90 Minutes of Arrival[5]	-	-	96%	96%
Statin Prescribed at Discharge[5]	-	-	97%	98%
Heart Failure Care				
ACE Inhibitor or ARB for LVSD[1,3]	-	-	93%	97%
Discharge Instructions Given[1,3]	-	-	91%	94%
Evaluation of LVS Function[1,3]	-	-	96%	99%
Medicare Spending				
Medicare Spending per Patient (ratio)	-	-	0.95	0.98
Pneumonia Care				
Appropriate Initial Antibiotic Given[1,3]	-	-	91%	95%
Blood Culture Timing[1,3]	-	-	97%	98%
Pregnancy and Delivery Care				
Newborn Deliveries Scheduled Early[5]	-	-	22%	6%
Preventive Care				
Immunization for Influenza[1,3]	-	-	87%	90%
Immunization for Pneumonia[1,3]	-	-	89%	92%
Stroke Care				
Anticoagulation Therapy for Atrial Fibrillation[5]	-	-	93%	95%
Antithrombotic Therapy Timing[5]	-	-	96%	98%
Assessed for Rehabilitation[5]	-	-	95%	97%
Discharged on Antithrombotic Therapy[5]	-	-	97%	99%
Discharged on Statin Medication[5]	-	-	88%	94%
Thrombolytic Therapy Timing[5]	-	-	25%	66%
Venous Thromboembolism Prophylaxis[5]	-	-	87%	94%
Written Stroke Educational Materials Given[5]	-	-	84%	88%
Surgical Care Improvement Project				
Appropriate Beta Blocker Usage[5]	-	-	97%	98%
Appropriate VTP Within 24 Hours[5]	-	-	97%	98%
Controlled Postoperative Blood Glucose[5]	-	-	97%	97%
Perioperative Temperature Management[5]	-	-	100%	100%
Prophylactic Antibiotic Selection[5]	-	-	99%	99%
Prophylactic Antibiotic Selection (Outpatient)[5]	-	-	98%	98%
Prophylactic Antibiotic Stopped[5]	-	-	97%	98%
Prophylactic Antibiotic Timing[5]	-	-	99%	99%
Prophylactic Antibiotic Timing (Outpatient)[5]	-	-	98%	98%
Urinary Catheter Removal[5]	-	-	97%	97%
Survey of Patients' Hospital Experiences				
Area Around Room 'Always' Quiet at Night[5]	-	-	72%	61%
Doctors 'Always' Communicated Well[5]	-	-	86%	82%
Home Recovery Information Given[5]	-	-	83%	85%
Hospital Given 9 or 10 on 10 Point Scale[5]	-	-	71%	71%
Meds 'Always' Explained Before Given[5]	-	-	67%	64%
Nurses 'Always' Communicated Well[5]	-	-	81%	79%
Pain 'Always' Well Controlled[5]	-	-	72%	71%
Room and Bathroom 'Always' Clean[5]	-	-	74%	73%
Timely Help 'Always' Received[5]	-	-	69%	68%
Would Definitely Recommend Hospital[5]	-	-	69%	71%
Use of Medical Imaging				
Cardiac Imaging Stress Test before Surgery[7]	-	-	5.7%	5.3%
Combination Abdominal CT Scan	77	7.8%	12.9%	10.5%
Combination Brain/Sinus CT Scan[1]	-	-	3.3%	2.7%
Combination Chest CT Scan[1]	-	-	6.1%	2.7%
Follow-up Mammogram/Ultrasound[7]	-	-	8.4%	8.8%
Lumbar Spine MRI for Low Back Pain[7]	-	-	41.1%	37.2%

Gilmore Memorial Regional Medical Center

1105 Earl Frye Blvd   Phone: 662-256-7111
Amory, MS 38821   Fax: 662-256-6007
URL: www.gilmorehealth.com
Type: Acute Care Hospitals   Emergency Services: Yes
Ownership: Proprietary   Beds: 95

Key Personnel:
CEO/President. . . . . Dwayne Blaylock
Chief of Medical Staff. . . . . Woodrow W Brand III, MD
Emergency Room . . . . Tammy Lyle
Anesthesiology. . . . . David McKinney, MD
Cardiac Laboratory. . . . . Bert Mize
Operating Room. . . . . Curtis Rainey
Quality Assurance . . . . Myrna Summerford

Measure	Cases	This Hosp.	State Avg.	U.S. Avg.
Blood Clot Prevention and Treatment				
Anticoagulation Overlap Therapy[2]	14	100%	86%	93%
ICU Venous Thromboembolism Prophylaxis[2]	40	98%	86%	92%
Incidence of Potentially Preventable VTE[1,2]	-	-	15%	10%
UFH with Dosages/Platelet Monitoring[1,2]	-	-	94%	97%
Venous Thromboembolism Prophylaxis[2]	198	92%	70%	85%
Warfarin Therapy Discharge Instructions[1,2]	-	-	77%	75%
Chest Pain/Possible Heart Attack Care				
Aspirin Given Within 24 Hours of Arrival	59	97%	94%	96%
Fibrinolytic Meds Within 30 Min. of Arrival[7]	-	-	40%	58%
Average Time to ECG (minutes)	59	0	10	7
Average Time to Transfer (minutes)[7]	-	-	77	60
Children's Asthma Care				
Received Home Management Plan of Care	-	-	-	88%
Received Reliever Medication	-	-	-	100%
Received Systemic Corticosteroids	-	-	-	100%
Emergency Department				
Admittance Decision Time (minutes)[2]	315	68	61	98
Head CT Results Within 45 Min. of Arrival[1]	-	-	42%	57%
Patients Who Left ER Before Being Seen	20,648	2%	3%	2%
Time from ER Arrival to Admit. (minutes)[2]	315	184	223	274
Time from ER Arrival to Discharge (minutes)	369	97	112	134
Time in ER Before Being Evaluated (minutes)	389	20	29	26
Time to Pain Meds for Fractures (minutes)	59	65	68	57
Heart Attack Care				
Aspirin Given at Discharge[1,3]	-	-	99%	99%
Fibrinolytic Meds Within 30 Min. of Arrival[3,7]	-	-	50%	54%

NOTE: Hospital profiles are in alphabetical order by state, then city, then hospital within the city; Rankings exclude hospitals with less than 25 cases except for patient surveys which excludes hospitals with less than 100 cases; (a) 100-299 cases; (1) The number of cases/patients is too few to report; (2) Data submitted were based on a sample of cases/patients; (3) Results are based on a shorter time period than required; (4) Data suppressed by CMS for one or more quarters; (5) Results are not available for this reporting period; (6) Fewer than 100 patients completed the HCAHPS survey; (7) No cases met the criteria for this measure; (8) The lower limit of the confidence interval cannot be calculated if the number of observed infections equals zero; (9) No data are available from the state/territory for this reporting period; (10) The scores shown reflect fewer than 50 completed surveys; (11) There were discrepancies in the data collection process; (12) This measure does not apply to this hospital for this reporting period; (13) Results cannot be calculated for this reporting period; (14) The results for this state are combined with nearby states to protect confidentiality; Please refer to the User's Guide for a full explanation of data.

Measure	Cases	This Hosp.	State Avg.	U.S. Avg.
PCI Within 90 Minutes of Arrival[3,7]	-	-	96%	96%
Statin Prescribed at Discharge[1,3]	-	-	97%	98%
Heart Failure Care				
ACE Inhibitor or ARB for LVSD	31	100%	93%	97%
Discharge Instructions Given	37	89%	91%	94%
Evaluation of LVS Function	65	100%	96%	99%
Medicare Spending				
Medicare Spending per Patient (ratio)	-	0.96	0.95	0.98
Pneumonia Care				
Appropriate Initial Antibiotic Given	72	100%	91%	95%
Blood Culture Timing	94	99%	97%	98%
Pregnancy and Delivery Care				
Newborn Deliveries Scheduled Early	83	24%	22%	6%
Preventive Care				
Immunization for Influenza[2]	338	96%	87%	90%
Immunization for Pneumonia[2]	297	96%	89%	92%
Stroke Care				
Anticoagulation Therapy for Atrial Fibrillation[1]	-	-	93%	95%
Antithrombotic Therapy Timing	22	95%	96%	98%
Assessed for Rehabilitation	21	100%	95%	97%
Discharged on Antithrombotic Therapy	20	100%	97%	99%
Discharged on Statin Medication	20	75%	88%	94%
Thrombolytic Therapy Timing[1]	-	-	25%	66%
Venous Thromboembolism Prophylaxis	22	91%	87%	94%
Written Stroke Educational Materials Given[1]	-	-	84%	88%
Surgical Care Improvement Project				
Appropriate Beta Blocker Usage	20	95%	97%	98%
Appropriate VTP Within 24 Hours	79	100%	97%	98%
Controlled Postoperative Blood Glucose[7]	-	-	97%	97%
Perioperative Temperature Management	98	100%	100%	100%
Prophylactic Antibiotic Selection	40	98%	99%	99%
Prophylactic Antibiotic Selection (Outpatient)	80	98%	98%	98%
Prophylactic Antibiotic Stopped	40	98%	97%	98%
Prophylactic Antibiotic Timing	40	98%	99%	99%
Prophylactic Antibiotic Timing (Outpatient)	80	100%	98%	98%
Urinary Catheter Removal	45	89%	97%	97%
Survey of Patients' Hospital Experiences				
Area Around Room 'Always' Quiet at Night	300+	76%	72%	61%
Doctors 'Always' Communicated Well	300+	90%	86%	82%
Home Recovery Information Given	300+	85%	83%	85%
Hospital Given 9 or 10 on 10 Point Scale	300+	74%	71%	71%
Meds 'Always' Explained Before Given	300+	67%	67%	64%
Nurses 'Always' Communicated Well	300+	83%	81%	79%
Pain 'Always' Well Controlled	300+	76%	72%	71%
Room and Bathroom 'Always' Clean	300+	78%	74%	73%
Timely Help 'Always' Received	300+	66%	69%	68%
Would Definitely Recommend Hospital	300+	74%	69%	71%
Use of Medical Imaging				
Cardiac Imaging Stress Test before Surgery	112	8.0%	5.7%	5.3%
Combination Abdominal CT Scan	478	10.0%	12.9%	10.5%
Combination Brain/Sinus CT Scan	456	4.6%	3.3%	2.7%
Combination Chest CT Scan	120	6.7%	6.1%	2.7%
Follow-up Mammogram/Ultrasound	529	19.7%	8.4%	8.8%
Lumbar Spine MRI for Low Back Pain	77	48.1%	41.1%	37.2%

Tri Lakes Medical Center

303 Medical Center Drive
Batesville, MS 38606
Phone: 662-563-5611
Fax: 662-563-0155
URL: www.trilakesmedical.com
Type: Acute Care Hospitals
Emergency Services: Yes
Ownership: Proprietary
Beds: 110

Key Personnel:
Radiology. . . . . Falon Harris
CEO/President. . . . . Barry Morrison

Measure	Cases	This Hosp.	State Avg.	U.S. Avg.
Blood Clot Prevention and Treatment				
Anticoagulation Overlap Therapy[1,2]	-	-	86%	93%
ICU Venous Thromboembolism Prophylaxis[2]	32	81%	86%	92%
Incidence of Potentially Preventable VTE[2,7]	-	-	15%	10%
UFH with Dosages/Platelet Monitoring[2,7]	-	-	94%	97%
Venous Thromboembolism Prophylaxis[2]	96	57%	70%	85%
Warfarin Therapy Discharge Instructions[1,2]	-	-	77%	75%
Chest Pain/Possible Heart Attack Care				
Aspirin Given Within 24 Hours of Arrival	71	99%	94%	96%
Fibrinolytic Meds Within 30 Min. of Arrival[7]	-	-	40%	58%
Average Time to ECG (minutes)	73	10	10	7
Average Time to Transfer (minutes)	15	179	77	60
Children's Asthma Care				
Received Home Management Plan of Care	-	-	-	88%
Received Reliever Medication	-	-	-	100%
Received Systemic Corticosteroids	-	-	-	100%
Emergency Department				
Admittance Decision Time (minutes)[2]	224	58	61	98
Head CT Results Within 45 Min. of Arrival[1]	-	-	42%	57%
Patients Who Left ER Before Being Seen	16,034	2%	3%	2%
Time from ER Arrival to Admit. (minutes)[2]	227	244	223	274
Time from ER Arrival to Discharge (minutes)	444	126	112	134
Time in ER Before Being Evaluated (minutes)	507	22	29	26
Time to Pain Meds for Fractures (minutes)	52	84	68	57
Heart Attack Care				
Aspirin Given at Discharge[1,3]	-	-	99%	99%
Fibrinolytic Meds Within 30 Min. of Arrival[3,7]	-	-	50%	54%
PCI Within 90 Minutes of Arrival[3,7]	-	-	96%	96%
Statin Prescribed at Discharge[1,3]	-	-	97%	98%
Heart Failure Care				
ACE Inhibitor or ARB for LVSD	21	100%	93%	97%
Discharge Instructions Given	59	92%	91%	94%
Evaluation of LVS Function	76	96%	96%	99%
Medicare Spending				
Medicare Spending per Patient (ratio)	-	1.02	0.95	0.98
Pneumonia Care				
Appropriate Initial Antibiotic Given	42	98%	91%	95%
Blood Culture Timing	38	100%	97%	98%
Pregnancy and Delivery Care				
Newborn Deliveries Scheduled Early	21	5%	22%	6%
Preventive Care				
Immunization for Influenza[2]	319	87%	87%	90%
Immunization for Pneumonia[2]	305	92%	89%	92%
Stroke Care				
Anticoagulation Therapy for Atrial Fibrillation[1]	-	-	93%	95%
Antithrombotic Therapy Timing[1]	-	-	96%	98%
Assessed for Rehabilitation[1]	-	-	95%	97%
Discharged on Antithrombotic Therapy[1]	-	-	97%	99%
Discharged on Statin Medication[1]	-	-	88%	94%
Thrombolytic Therapy Timing[7]	-	-	25%	66%
Venous Thromboembolism Prophylaxis[1]	-	-	87%	94%
Written Stroke Educational Materials Given[1]	-	-	84%	88%
Surgical Care Improvement Project				
Appropriate Beta Blocker Usage[1]	-	-	97%	98%
Appropriate VTP Within 24 Hours[1]	-	-	97%	98%
Controlled Postoperative Blood Glucose[7]	-	-	97%	97%
Perioperative Temperature Management[1]	-	-	100%	100%
Prophylactic Antibiotic Selection[1]	-	-	99%	99%
Prophylactic Antibiotic Selection (Outpatient)[1]	-	-	98%	98%
Prophylactic Antibiotic Stopped[1]	-	-	97%	98%
Prophylactic Antibiotic Timing[1]	-	-	99%	99%
Prophylactic Antibiotic Timing (Outpatient)	11	64%	98%	98%
Urinary Catheter Removal[1]	-	-	97%	97%
Survey of Patients' Hospital Experiences				
Area Around Room 'Always' Quiet at Night	(a)	72%	72%	61%
Doctors 'Always' Communicated Well	(a)	79%	86%	82%
Home Recovery Information Given	(a)	77%	83%	85%
Hospital Given 9 or 10 on 10 Point Scale	(a)	55%	71%	71%
Meds 'Always' Explained Before Given	(a)	59%	67%	64%
Nurses 'Always' Communicated Well	(a)	75%	81%	79%
Pain 'Always' Well Controlled	(a)	59%	72%	71%
Room and Bathroom 'Always' Clean	(a)	76%	74%	73%
Timely Help 'Always' Received	(a)	56%	69%	68%
Would Definitely Recommend Hospital	(a)	51%	69%	71%
Use of Medical Imaging				
Cardiac Imaging Stress Test before Surgery[1]	-	-	5.7%	5.3%
Combination Abdominal CT Scan	251	9.2%	12.9%	10.5%
Combination Brain/Sinus CT Scan[1]	-	-	3.3%	2.7%
Combination Chest CT Scan	169	0.6%	6.1%	2.7%
Follow-up Mammogram/Ultrasound	305	6.2%	8.4%	8.8%
Lumbar Spine MRI for Low Back Pain	67	46.3%	41.1%	37.2%

Hancock Medical Center

149 Drinkwater Blvd
Bay Saint Louis, MS 39521
Phone: 228-467-8600
Fax: 228-467-8799
E-mail: hmcmkt@bellsouth.net
URL: www.hmc.org
Type: Acute Care Hospitals
Emergency Services: Yes
Ownership: Government - Local
Beds: 104

Key Personnel:
Infection Control. . . . . Cecilia Burke, RN
Chief of Medical Staff. . . . . Tad Carter
Emergency Room . . . . Jeffrey Giddins, MD
Operating Room. . . . . Virginia Kenny, RN
Cardiac Laboratory. . . . . Jay J Libys
Anesthesiology. . . . . Dale Loiacano
Quality Assurance . . . . Susan Stevens
Radiology. . . . . Raymond Tipton, MD

Measure	Cases	This Hosp.	State Avg.	U.S. Avg.
Blood Clot Prevention and Treatment				
Anticoagulation Overlap Therapy[2]	20	70%	86%	93%
ICU Venous Thromboembolism Prophylaxis[2]	37	86%	86%	92%
Incidence of Potentially Preventable VTE[1,2]	-	-	15%	10%
UFH with Dosages/Platelet Monitoring[1,2]	-	-	94%	97%
Venous Thromboembolism Prophylaxis[2]	127	69%	70%	85%
Warfarin Therapy Discharge Instructions[2]	15	20%	77%	75%
Chest Pain/Possible Heart Attack Care				
Aspirin Given Within 24 Hours of Arrival[1,3]	-	-	94%	96%
Fibrinolytic Meds Within 30 Min. of Arrival[3,7]	-	-	40%	58%
Average Time to ECG (minutes)[1,3]	-	-	10	7
Average Time to Transfer (minutes)[1,3]	-	-	77	60
Children's Asthma Care				
Received Home Management Plan of Care	-	-	-	88%
Received Reliever Medication	-	-	-	100%
Received Systemic Corticosteroids	-	-	-	100%
Emergency Department				
Admittance Decision Time (minutes)[2]	275	70	61	98
Head CT Results Within 45 Min. of Arrival[7]	-	-	42%	57%
Patients Who Left ER Before Being Seen	20,690	5%	3%	2%
Time from ER Arrival to Admit. (minutes)[2]	284	274	223	274
Time from ER Arrival to Discharge (minutes)	344	121	112	134
Time in ER Before Being Evaluated (minutes)	381	34	29	26
Time to Pain Meds for Fractures (minutes)	71	79	68	57
Heart Attack Care				
Aspirin Given at Discharge[1]	-	-	99%	99%
Fibrinolytic Meds Within 30 Min. of Arrival[7]	-	-	50%	54%
PCI Within 90 Minutes of Arrival[7]	-	-	96%	96%
Statin Prescribed at Discharge[1]	-	-	97%	98%
Heart Failure Care				
ACE Inhibitor or ARB for LVSD	24	92%	93%	97%
Discharge Instructions Given	50	98%	91%	94%
Evaluation of LVS Function	60	97%	96%	99%
Medicare Spending				
Medicare Spending per Patient (ratio)	-	0.98	0.95	0.98
Pneumonia Care				
Appropriate Initial Antibiotic Given[2]	51	86%	91%	95%
Blood Culture Timing[2]	47	91%	97%	98%
Pregnancy and Delivery Care				
Newborn Deliveries Scheduled Early	20	40%	22%	6%
Preventive Care				
Immunization for Influenza[2]	262	94%	87%	90%
Immunization for Pneumonia[2]	265	91%	89%	92%
Stroke Care				
Anticoagulation Therapy for Atrial Fibrillation[7]	-	-	93%	95%
Antithrombotic Therapy Timing[1]	-	-	96%	98%
Assessed for Rehabilitation[1]	-	-	95%	97%
Discharged on Antithrombotic Therapy[1]	-	-	97%	99%
Discharged on Statin Medication[1]	-	-	88%	94%
Thrombolytic Therapy Timing[1]	-	-	25%	66%
Venous Thromboembolism Prophylaxis[1]	-	-	87%	94%
Written Stroke Educational Materials Given[1]	-	-	84%	88%
Surgical Care Improvement Project				
Appropriate Beta Blocker Usage[1]	-	-	97%	98%
Appropriate VTP Within 24 Hours	46	93%	97%	98%

NOTE: Hospital profiles are in alphabetical order by state, then city, then hospital within the city; Rankings exclude hospitals with less than 25 cases except for patient surveys which excludes hospitals with less than 100 cases; (a) 100-299 cases; (1) The number of cases/patients is too few to report; (2) Data submitted were based on a sample of cases/patients; (3) Results are based on a shorter time period than required; (4) Data suppressed by CMS for one or more quarters; (5) Results are not available for this reporting period; (6) Fewer than 100 patients completed the HCAHPS survey; (7) No cases met the criteria for this measure; (8) The lower limit of the confidence interval cannot be calculated if the number of observed infections equals zero; (9) No data are available from the state/territory for this reporting period; (10) The scores shown reflect fewer than 50 completed surveys; (11) There were discrepancies in the data collection process; (12) This measure does not apply to this hospital for this reporting period; (13) Results cannot be calculated for this reporting period; (14) The results for this state are combined with nearby states to protect confidentiality; Please refer to the User's Guide for a full explanation of data.

Measure	Cases	This Hosp.	State Avg.	U.S. Avg.
Controlled Postoperative Blood Glucose[7]	-	-	97%	97%
Perioperative Temperature Management	50	100%	100%	100%
Prophylactic Antibiotic Selection	27	96%	99%	99%
Prophylactic Antibiotic Selection (Outpatient)[1,3]	-	-	98%	98%
Prophylactic Antibiotic Stopped	27	89%	97%	98%
Prophylactic Antibiotic Timing	27	100%	99%	99%
Prophylactic Antibiotic Timing (Outpatient)[1,3]	-	-	98%	98%
Urinary Catheter Removal	14	93%	97%	97%
Survey of Patients' Hospital Experiences				
Area Around Room 'Always' Quiet at Night	300+	75%	72%	61%
Doctors 'Always' Communicated Well	300+	84%	86%	82%
Home Recovery Information Given	300+	84%	83%	85%
Hospital Given 9 or 10 on 10 Point Scale	300+	74%	71%	71%
Meds 'Always' Explained Before Given	300+	65%	67%	64%
Nurses 'Always' Communicated Well	300+	83%	81%	79%
Pain 'Always' Well Controlled	300+	73%	72%	71%
Room and Bathroom 'Always' Clean	300+	75%	74%	73%
Timely Help 'Always' Received	300+	75%	69%	68%
Would Definitely Recommend Hospital	300+	69%	69%	71%
Use of Medical Imaging				
Cardiac Imaging Stress Test before Surgery	90	3.3%	5.7%	5.3%
Combination Abdominal CT Scan	243	6.2%	12.9%	10.5%
Combination Brain/Sinus CT Scan[1]	-	-	3.3%	2.7%
Combination Chest CT Scan	99	4.0%	6.1%	2.7%
Follow-up Mammogram/Ultrasound	281	11.0%	8.4%	8.8%
Lumbar Spine MRI for Low Back Pain[1]	-	-	41.1%	37.2%

Jasper General Hospital

15 South 6th Street
Bay Springs, MS 39422
Type: Acute Care Hospitals
Ownership: Government - Local
Phone: 601-764-2101
Fax: 601-764-4789
Emergency Services: No
Beds: 22

Key Personnel:
Quality Assurance .... Posha Patson
Administrator .... Ken Posey
CEO/President................ Kenneth Posey

Measure	Cases	This Hosp.	State Avg.	U.S. Avg.
Blood Clot Prevention and Treatment				
Anticoagulation Overlap Therapy	-	-	86%	93%
ICU Venous Thromboembolism Prophylaxis	-	-	86%	92%
Incidence of Potentially Preventable VTE	-	-	15%	10%
UFH with Dosages/Platelet Monitoring	-	-	94%	97%
Venous Thromboembolism Prophylaxis	-	-	70%	85%
Warfarin Therapy Discharge Instructions	-	-	77%	75%
Chest Pain/Possible Heart Attack Care				
Aspirin Given Within 24 Hours of Arrival[5]	-	-	94%	96%
Fibrinolytic Meds Within 30 Min. of Arrival[5]	-	-	40%	58%
Average Time to ECG (minutes)[5]	-	-	10	7
Average Time to Transfer (minutes)[5]	-	-	77	60
Children's Asthma Care				
Received Home Management Plan of Care	-	-	-	88%
Received Reliever Medication	-	-	-	100%
Received Systemic Corticosteroids	-	-	-	100%
Emergency Department				
Admittance Decision Time (minutes)	-	-	61	98
Head CT Results Within 45 Min. of Arrival[5]	-	-	42%	57%
Patients Who Left ER Before Being Seen[5]	-	-	3%	2%
Time from ER Arrival to Admit. (minutes)	-	-	223	274
Time from ER Arrival to Discharge (minutes)[5]	-	-	112	134
Time in ER Before Being Evaluated (minutes)[5]	-	-	29	26
Time to Pain Meds for Fractures (minutes)[5]	-	-	68	57
Heart Attack Care				
Aspirin Given at Discharge	-	-	99%	99%
Fibrinolytic Meds Within 30 Min. of Arrival	-	-	50%	54%
PCI Within 90 Minutes of Arrival	-	-	96%	96%
Statin Prescribed at Discharge	-	-	97%	98%
Heart Failure Care				
ACE Inhibitor or ARB for LVSD	-	-	93%	97%
Discharge Instructions Given	-	-	91%	94%
Evaluation of LVS Function	-	-	96%	99%
Medicare Spending				
Medicare Spending per Patient (ratio)	-	-	0.95	0.98
Pneumonia Care				
Appropriate Initial Antibiotic Given	-	-	91%	95%
Blood Culture Timing	-	-	97%	98%
Pregnancy and Delivery Care				
Newborn Deliveries Scheduled Early	-	-	22%	6%
Preventive Care				
Immunization for Influenza	-	-	87%	90%
Immunization for Pneumonia	-	-	89%	92%
Stroke Care				
Anticoagulation Therapy for Atrial Fibrillation	-	-	93%	95%
Antithrombotic Therapy Timing	-	-	96%	98%
Assessed for Rehabilitation	-	-	95%	97%
Discharged on Antithrombotic Therapy	-	-	97%	99%
Discharged on Statin Medication	-	-	88%	94%
Thrombolytic Therapy Timing	-	-	25%	66%
Venous Thromboembolism Prophylaxis	-	-	87%	94%
Written Stroke Educational Materials Given	-	-	84%	88%
Surgical Care Improvement Project				
Appropriate Beta Blocker Usage	-	-	97%	98%
Appropriate VTP Within 24 Hours	-	-	97%	98%
Controlled Postoperative Blood Glucose	-	-	97%	97%
Perioperative Temperature Management	-	-	100%	100%
Prophylactic Antibiotic Selection	-	-	99%	99%
Prophylactic Antibiotic Selection (Outpatient)[5]	-	-	98%	98%
Prophylactic Antibiotic Stopped	-	-	97%	98%
Prophylactic Antibiotic Timing	-	-	99%	99%
Prophylactic Antibiotic Timing (Outpatient)[5]	-	-	98%	98%
Urinary Catheter Removal	-	-	97%	97%
Survey of Patients' Hospital Experiences				
Area Around Room 'Always' Quiet at Night	-	-	72%	61%
Doctors 'Always' Communicated Well	-	-	86%	82%
Home Recovery Information Given	-	-	83%	85%
Hospital Given 9 or 10 on 10 Point Scale	-	-	71%	71%
Meds 'Always' Explained Before Given	-	-	67%	64%
Nurses 'Always' Communicated Well	-	-	81%	79%
Pain 'Always' Well Controlled	-	-	72%	71%
Room and Bathroom 'Always' Clean	-	-	74%	73%
Timely Help 'Always' Received	-	-	69%	68%
Would Definitely Recommend Hospital	-	-	69%	71%
Use of Medical Imaging				
Cardiac Imaging Stress Test before Surgery[7]	-	-	5.7%	5.3%
Combination Abdominal CT Scan[7]	-	-	12.9%	10.5%
Combination Brain/Sinus CT Scan[7]	-	-	3.3%	2.7%
Combination Chest CT Scan[7]	-	-	6.1%	2.7%
Follow-up Mammogram/Ultrasound[7]	-	-	8.4%	8.8%
Lumbar Spine MRI for Low Back Pain[7]	-	-	41.1%	37.2%

Biloxi Regional Medical Center

150 Reynoir Street
Biloxi, MS 39530
URL: www.hmabrmc.com
Type: Acute Care Hospitals
Ownership: Proprietary
Phone: 228-436-1104
Fax: 228-436-1205
Emergency Services: Yes
Beds: 153

Key Personnel:
CEO .... Monte Bostwick
Operating Room............. Robert Brunston
Quality Assurance .... Jean Cooper
Radiology.................. Douglas G Cosentino
Pediatric Ambulatory Care ...... Cathy Dailey, DO
Infection Control............. Pam McVey
Pediatric In-Patient Care .... Beth Mellish
Chief of Medical Staff......... Edward Shumski, MD

Measure	Cases	This Hosp.	State Avg.	U.S. Avg.
Blood Clot Prevention and Treatment				
Anticoagulation Overlap Therapy[2]	19	89%	86%	93%
ICU Venous Thromboembolism Prophylaxis[2]	64	97%	86%	92%
Incidence of Potentially Preventable VTE[1,2]	-	-	15%	10%
UFH with Dosages/Platelet Monitoring[1,2]	-	-	94%	97%
Venous Thromboembolism Prophylaxis[2]	307	87%	70%	85%
Warfarin Therapy Discharge Instructions[2]	17	94%	77%	75%
Chest Pain/Possible Heart Attack Care				
Aspirin Given Within 24 Hours of Arrival	45	98%	94%	96%
Fibrinolytic Meds Within 30 Min. of Arrival[7]	-	-	40%	58%
Average Time to ECG (minutes)	46	3	10	7
Average Time to Transfer (minutes)	13	51	77	60
Children's Asthma Care				
Received Home Management Plan of Care	-	-	-	88%
Received Reliever Medication	-	-	-	100%
Received Systemic Corticosteroids	-	-	-	100%
Emergency Department				
Admittance Decision Time (minutes)[2]	462	72	61	98
Head CT Results Within 45 Min. of Arrival[3,7]	-	-	42%	57%
Patients Who Left ER Before Being Seen	36,586	1%	3%	2%
Time from ER Arrival to Admit. (minutes)[2]	514	223	223	274
Time from ER Arrival to Discharge (minutes)	460	90	112	134
Time in ER Before Being Evaluated (minutes)	509	18	29	26
Time to Pain Meds for Fractures (minutes)	83	56	68	57
Heart Attack Care				
Aspirin Given at Discharge[1]	-	-	99%	99%
Fibrinolytic Meds Within 30 Min. of Arrival[7]	-	-	50%	54%
PCI Within 90 Minutes of Arrival[7]	-	-	96%	96%
Statin Prescribed at Discharge[1]	-	-	97%	98%
Heart Failure Care				
ACE Inhibitor or ARB for LVSD	37	100%	93%	97%
Discharge Instructions Given	116	100%	91%	94%
Evaluation of LVS Function	144	100%	96%	99%
Medicare Spending				
Medicare Spending per Patient (ratio)	-	1.02	0.95	0.98
Pneumonia Care				
Appropriate Initial Antibiotic Given	83	96%	91%	95%
Blood Culture Timing	126	100%	97%	98%
Pregnancy and Delivery Care				
Newborn Deliveries Scheduled Early[2]	63	29%	22%	6%
Preventive Care				
Immunization for Influenza[2]	566	100%	87%	90%
Immunization for Pneumonia[2]	526	100%	89%	92%
Stroke Care				
Anticoagulation Therapy for Atrial Fibrillation[1]	-	-	93%	95%
Antithrombotic Therapy Timing	27	96%	96%	98%
Assessed for Rehabilitation	34	82%	95%	97%
Discharged on Antithrombotic Therapy	26	96%	97%	99%
Discharged on Statin Medication	18	94%	88%	94%
Thrombolytic Therapy Timing[1]	-	-	25%	66%
Venous Thromboembolism Prophylaxis	39	79%	87%	94%
Written Stroke Educational Materials Given	28	86%	84%	88%
Surgical Care Improvement Project				
Appropriate Beta Blocker Usage	58	100%	97%	98%
Appropriate VTP Within 24 Hours	304	100%	97%	98%
Controlled Postoperative Blood Glucose[7]	-	-	97%	97%
Perioperative Temperature Management	393	100%	100%	100%
Prophylactic Antibiotic Selection	242	100%	99%	99%
Prophylactic Antibiotic Selection (Outpatient)	222	99%	98%	98%
Prophylactic Antibiotic Stopped	226	100%	97%	98%
Prophylactic Antibiotic Timing	242	100%	99%	99%
Prophylactic Antibiotic Timing (Outpatient)	224	99%	98%	98%
Urinary Catheter Removal	117	99%	97%	97%
Survey of Patients' Hospital Experiences				
Area Around Room 'Always' Quiet at Night	300+	59%	72%	61%
Doctors 'Always' Communicated Well	300+	80%	86%	82%
Home Recovery Information Given	300+	83%	83%	85%
Hospital Given 9 or 10 on 10 Point Scale	300+	58%	71%	71%
Meds 'Always' Explained Before Given	300+	56%	67%	64%
Nurses 'Always' Communicated Well	300+	73%	81%	79%
Pain 'Always' Well Controlled	300+	67%	72%	71%
Room and Bathroom 'Always' Clean	300+	56%	74%	73%
Timely Help 'Always' Received	300+	57%	69%	68%
Would Definitely Recommend Hospital	300+	59%	69%	71%
Use of Medical Imaging				
Cardiac Imaging Stress Test before Surgery	153	5.9%	5.7%	5.3%
Combination Abdominal CT Scan	423	31.4%	12.9%	10.5%
Combination Brain/Sinus CT Scan	468	4.3%	3.3%	2.7%
Combination Chest CT Scan	236	28.4%	6.1%	2.7%
Follow-up Mammogram/Ultrasound	803	19.8%	8.4%	8.8%
Lumbar Spine MRI for Low Back Pain	81	33.3%	41.1%	37.2%

NOTE: Hospital profiles are in alphabetical order by state, then city, then hospital within the city; Rankings exclude hospitals with less than 25 cases except for patient surveys which excludes hospitals with less than 100 cases; (a) 100-299 cases; (1) The number of cases/patients is too few to report; (2) Data submitted were based on a sample of cases/patients; (3) Results are based on a shorter time period than required; (4) Data suppressed by CMS for one or more quarters; (5) Results are not available for this reporting period; (6) Fewer than 100 patients completed the HCAHPS survey; (7) No cases met the criteria for this measure; (8) The lower limit of the confidence interval cannot be calculated if the number of observed infections equals zero; (9) No data are available from the state/territory for this reporting period; (10) The scores shown reflect fewer than 50 completed surveys; (11) There were discrepancies in the data collection process; (12) This measure does not apply to this hospital for this reporting period; (13) Results cannot be calculated for this reporting period; (14) The results for this state are combined with nearby states to protect confidentiality; Please refer to the User's Guide for a full explanation of data.

VA Gulf Coast Healthcare System

400 Veterans Avenue
Biloxi, MS 39531
URL: www.va.gov
Type: Acute Care - VA
Ownership: Government Federal

Phone: 228-523-5000
Fax: 228-523-5719
Emergency Services: No
Beds: 380

Key Personnel:
Patient Relations . . . . Mary Cook
Operating Room. . . . . A Letch Kline, MD
Infection Control. . . . . Linda Morton, RN
Quality Assurance . . . . Linda Morton, RN MSN
Chief of Medical Staff . . . . Kenneth Simon, MD, MBA, FACS
Radiology. . . . . Paul Watson, MD

Measure	Cases	This Hosp.	State Avg.	U.S. Avg.
Blood Clot Prevention and Treatment				
Anticoagulation Overlap Therapy	-	-	86%	93%
ICU Venous Thromboembolism Prophylaxis	-	-	86%	92%
Incidence of Potentially Preventable VTE	-	-	15%	10%
UFH with Dosages/Platelet Monitoring	-	-	94%	97%
Venous Thromboembolism Prophylaxis	-	-	70%	85%
Warfarin Therapy Discharge Instructions	-	-	77%	75%
Chest Pain/Possible Heart Attack Care				
Aspirin Given Within 24 Hours of Arrival	-	-	94%	96%
Fibrinolytic Meds Within 30 Min. of Arrival	-	-	40%	58%
Average Time to ECG (minutes)	-	-	10	7
Average Time to Transfer (minutes)	-	-	77	60
Children's Asthma Care				
Received Home Management Plan of Care	-	-	-	88%
Received Reliever Medication	-	-	-	100%
Received Systemic Corticosteroids	-	-	-	100%
Emergency Department				
Admittance Decision Time (minutes)	-	-	61	98
Head CT Results Within 45 Min. of Arrival	-	-	42%	57%
Patients Who Left ER Before Being Seen	-	-	3%	2%
Time from ER Arrival to Admit. (minutes)	-	-	223	274
Time from ER Arrival to Discharge (minutes)	-	-	112	134
Time in ER Before Being Evaluated (minutes)	-	-	29	26
Time to Pain Meds for Fractures (minutes)	-	-	68	57
Heart Attack Care				
Aspirin Given at Discharge[5]	-	-	99%	99%
Fibrinolytic Meds Within 30 Min. of Arrival[5]	-	-	50%	54%
PCI Within 90 Minutes of Arrival[5]	-	-	96%	96%
Statin Prescribed at Discharge[5]	-	-	97%	98%
Heart Failure Care				
ACE Inhibitor or ARB for LVSD[1]	13	92%	93%	97%
Discharge Instructions Given	41	85%	91%	94%
Evaluation of LVS Function	49	100%	96%	99%
Medicare Spending				
Medicare Spending per Patient (ratio)	-	-	0.95	0.98
Pneumonia Care				
Appropriate Initial Antibiotic Given[1]	20	95%	91%	95%
Blood Culture Timing	62	100%	97%	98%
Pregnancy and Delivery Care				
Newborn Deliveries Scheduled Early	-	-	22%	6%
Preventive Care				
Immunization for Influenza[5]	-	-	87%	90%
Immunization for Pneumonia[5]	-	-	89%	92%
Stroke Care				
Anticoagulation Therapy for Atrial Fibrillation	-	-	93%	95%
Antithrombotic Therapy Timing	-	-	96%	98%
Assessed for Rehabilitation	-	-	95%	97%
Discharged on Antithrombotic Therapy	-	-	97%	99%
Discharged on Statin Medication	-	-	88%	94%
Thrombolytic Therapy Timing	-	-	25%	66%
Venous Thromboembolism Prophylaxis	-	-	87%	94%
Written Stroke Educational Materials Given	-	-	84%	88%
Surgical Care Improvement Project				
Appropriate Beta Blocker Usage[2]	34	94%	97%	98%
Appropriate VTP Within 24 Hours[2]	86	90%	97%	98%
Controlled Postoperative Blood Glucose[5]	-	-	97%	97%
Perioperative Temperature Management[2]	113	100%	100%	100%
Prophylactic Antibiotic Selection	54	98%	99%	99%
Prophylactic Antibiotic Selection (Outpatient)	-	-	98%	98%
Prophylactic Antibiotic Stopped	52	100%	97%	98%
Prophylactic Antibiotic Timing	54	100%	99%	99%
Prophylactic Antibiotic Timing (Outpatient)	-	-	98%	98%
Urinary Catheter Removal[2]	79	96%	97%	97%
Survey of Patients' Hospital Experiences				
Area Around Room 'Always' Quiet at Night	-	-	72%	61%
Doctors 'Always' Communicated Well	-	-	86%	82%
Home Recovery Information Given	-	-	83%	85%
Hospital Given 9 or 10 on 10 Point Scale	-	-	71%	71%
Meds 'Always' Explained Before Given	-	-	67%	64%
Nurses 'Always' Communicated Well	-	-	81%	79%
Pain 'Always' Well Controlled	-	-	72%	71%
Room and Bathroom 'Always' Clean	-	-	74%	73%
Timely Help 'Always' Received	-	-	69%	68%
Would Definitely Recommend Hospital	-	-	69%	71%
Use of Medical Imaging				
Cardiac Imaging Stress Test before Surgery	-	-	5.7%	5.3%
Combination Abdominal CT Scan	-	-	12.9%	10.5%
Combination Brain/Sinus CT Scan	-	-	3.3%	2.7%
Combination Chest CT Scan	-	-	6.1%	2.7%
Follow-up Mammogram/Ultrasound	-	-	8.4%	8.8%
Lumbar Spine MRI for Low Back Pain	-	-	41.1%	37.2%

Baptist Memorial Hospital Booneville

100 Hospital Drive
Booneville, MS 38829
URL: www.baptistonline.org/facilities/booneville
Type: Acute Care Hospitals
Ownership: Voluntary non-profit - Church

Phone: 662-720-5000
Fax: 662-720-5005
Emergency Services: Yes
Beds: 114

Key Personnel:
Radiology. . . . . Jacob Abraham
Emergency Room . . . . John Adams, RN
Infection Control. . . . . Doris Box, RN
Quality Assurance . . . . Linda Chaffin
President/CEO. . . . . Jason Little, Jr
Intensive Care Unit. . . . . Jean Pannell, RN
Operating Room. . . . . Mary Rhodes
Anesthesiology. . . . . Wayne Thomas, CRNA

Measure	Cases	This Hosp.	State Avg.	U.S. Avg.
Blood Clot Prevention and Treatment				
Anticoagulation Overlap Therapy[2]	12	83%	86%	93%
ICU Venous Thromboembolism Prophylaxis[2]	50	88%	86%	92%
Incidence of Potentially Preventable VTE[2,7]	-	-	15%	10%
UFH with Dosages/Platelet Monitoring[2,7]	-	-	94%	97%
Venous Thromboembolism Prophylaxis[2]	89	78%	70%	85%
Warfarin Therapy Discharge Instructions[1,2]	-	-	77%	75%
Chest Pain/Possible Heart Attack Care				
Aspirin Given Within 24 Hours of Arrival	79	99%	94%	96%
Fibrinolytic Meds Within 30 Min. of Arrival[1]	-	-	40%	58%
Average Time to ECG (minutes)	79	15	10	7
Average Time to Transfer (minutes)[1]	-	-	77	60
Children's Asthma Care				
Received Home Management Plan of Care	-	-	-	88%
Received Reliever Medication	-	-	-	100%
Received Systemic Corticosteroids	-	-	-	100%
Emergency Department				
Admittance Decision Time (minutes)[2]	302	40	61	98
Head CT Results Within 45 Min. of Arrival[1]	-	-	42%	57%
Patients Who Left ER Before Being Seen	15,814	3%	3%	2%
Time from ER Arrival to Admit. (minutes)[2]	312	222	223	274
Time from ER Arrival to Discharge (minutes)	377	125	112	134
Time in ER Before Being Evaluated (minutes)	392	36	29	26
Time to Pain Meds for Fractures (minutes)	41	68	68	57
Heart Attack Care				
Aspirin Given at Discharge[1,3]	-	-	99%	99%
Fibrinolytic Meds Within 30 Min. of Arrival[3,7]	-	-	50%	54%
PCI Within 90 Minutes of Arrival[3,7]	-	-	96%	96%
Statin Prescribed at Discharge[1,3]	-	-	97%	98%
Heart Failure Care				
ACE Inhibitor or ARB for LVSD[1]	-	-	93%	97%
Discharge Instructions Given	23	96%	91%	94%
Evaluation of LVS Function	42	98%	96%	99%
Medicare Spending				
Medicare Spending per Patient (ratio)	-	0.98	0.95	0.98
Pneumonia Care				
Appropriate Initial Antibiotic Given	90	97%	91%	95%
Blood Culture Timing	84	100%	97%	98%
Pregnancy and Delivery Care				
Newborn Deliveries Scheduled Early[7]	-	-	22%	6%
Preventive Care				
Immunization for Influenza[2]	307	99%	87%	90%
Immunization for Pneumonia[2]	501	99%	89%	92%
Stroke Care				
Anticoagulation Therapy for Atrial Fibrillation[1]	-	-	93%	95%
Antithrombotic Therapy Timing[1]	-	-	96%	98%
Assessed for Rehabilitation[1]	-	-	95%	97%
Discharged on Antithrombotic Therapy[1]	-	-	97%	99%
Discharged on Statin Medication[1]	-	-	88%	94%
Thrombolytic Therapy Timing[7]	-	-	25%	66%
Venous Thromboembolism Prophylaxis[1]	-	-	87%	94%
Written Stroke Educational Materials Given[1]	-	-	84%	88%
Surgical Care Improvement Project				
Appropriate Beta Blocker Usage[3,7]	-	-	97%	98%
Appropriate VTP Within 24 Hours[1,3]	-	-	97%	98%
Controlled Postoperative Blood Glucose[3,7]	-	-	97%	97%
Perioperative Temperature Management[1,3]	-	-	100%	100%
Prophylactic Antibiotic Selection[1,3]	-	-	99%	99%
Prophylactic Antibiotic Selection (Outpatient)[3,7]	-	-	98%	98%
Prophylactic Antibiotic Stopped[1,3]	-	-	97%	98%
Prophylactic Antibiotic Timing[1,3]	-	-	99%	99%
Prophylactic Antibiotic Timing (Outpatient)[3,7]	-	-	98%	98%
Urinary Catheter Removal[1,3]	-	-	97%	97%
Survey of Patients' Hospital Experiences				
Area Around Room 'Always' Quiet at Night	(a)	70%	72%	61%
Doctors 'Always' Communicated Well	(a)	91%	86%	82%
Home Recovery Information Given	(a)	81%	83%	85%
Hospital Given 9 or 10 on 10 Point Scale	(a)	80%	71%	71%
Meds 'Always' Explained Before Given	(a)	71%	67%	64%
Nurses 'Always' Communicated Well	(a)	84%	81%	79%
Pain 'Always' Well Controlled	(a)	69%	72%	71%
Room and Bathroom 'Always' Clean	(a)	78%	74%	73%
Timely Help 'Always' Received	(a)	83%	69%	68%
Would Definitely Recommend Hospital	(a)	70%	69%	71%
Use of Medical Imaging				
Cardiac Imaging Stress Test before Surgery	94	6.4%	5.7%	5.3%
Combination Abdominal CT Scan	438	2.3%	12.9%	10.5%
Combination Brain/Sinus CT Scan	433	5.5%	3.3%	2.7%
Combination Chest CT Scan	254	0.0%	6.1%	2.7%
Follow-up Mammogram/Ultrasound	260	13.5%	8.4%	8.8%
Lumbar Spine MRI for Low Back Pain	108	44.4%	41.1%	37.2%

Crossgates River Oaks Hospital

350 Crossgates Blvd
Brandon, MS 39042
URL: www.rankinmedcenter.com
Type: Acute Care Hospitals
Ownership: Proprietary

Phone: 601-825-2811
Fax: 601-824-8530
Emergency Services: Yes
Beds: 134

Key Personnel:
Infection Control. . . . . Marie Bagwell
Radiology. . . . . Nancy W Burrow
Pediatric In-Patient Care . . . . Kim Byrd
Chief of Medical Staff . . . . James A Jefferson
CEO . . . . Glen M. Silverman
Operating Room. . . . . Diane Smith
Quality Assurance . . . . Margaret Stubblefield
CEO/President. . . . . J Allen Tyra

Measure	Cases	This Hosp.	State Avg.	U.S. Avg.
Blood Clot Prevention and Treatment				
Anticoagulation Overlap Therapy[2]	19	100%	86%	93%
ICU Venous Thromboembolism Prophylaxis[2]	33	88%	86%	92%
Incidence of Potentially Preventable VTE[1,2]	-	-	15%	10%
UFH with Dosages/Platelet Monitoring[2]	11	100%	94%	97%
Venous Thromboembolism Prophylaxis[2]	236	52%	70%	85%
Warfarin Therapy Discharge Instructions[1,2]	-	-	77%	75%
Chest Pain/Possible Heart Attack Care				
Aspirin Given Within 24 Hours of Arrival	33	100%	94%	96%
Fibrinolytic Meds Within 30 Min. of Arrival[7]	-	-	40%	58%
Average Time to ECG (minutes)	36	7	10	7
Average Time to Transfer (minutes)	12	54	77	60

NOTE: Hospital profiles are in alphabetical order by state, then city, then hospital within the city; Rankings exclude hospitals with less than 25 cases except for patient surveys which excludes hospitals with less than 100 cases; (a) 100-299 cases; (1) The number of cases/patients is too few to report; (2) Data submitted were based on a sample of cases/patients; (3) Results are based on a shorter time period than required; (4) Data suppressed by CMS for one or more quarters; (5) Results are not available for this reporting period; (6) Fewer than 100 patients completed the HCAHPS survey; (7) No cases met the criteria for this measure; (8) The lower limit of the confidence interval cannot be calculated if the number of observed infections equals zero; (9) No data are available from the state/territory for this reporting period; (10) The scores shown reflect fewer than 50 completed surveys; (11) There were discrepancies in the data collection process; (12) This measure does not apply to this hospital for this reporting period; (13) Results cannot be calculated for this reporting period; (14) The results for this state are combined with nearby states to protect confidentiality; Please refer to the User's Guide for a full explanation of data.

Measure	Cases	This Hosp.	State Avg.	U.S. Avg.
Children's Asthma Care				
Received Home Management Plan of Care	-	-	-	88%
Received Reliever Medication	-	-	-	100%
Received Systemic Corticosteroids	-	-	-	100%
Emergency Department				
Admittance Decision Time (minutes)[2]	481	72	61	98
Head CT Results Within 45 Min. of Arrival[1]	-	-	42%	57%
Patients Who Left ER Before Being Seen	24,211	4%	3%	2%
Time from ER Arrival to Admit. (minutes)[2]	482	210	223	274
Time from ER Arrival to Discharge (minutes)	349	112	112	134
Time in ER Before Being Evaluated (minutes)	378	45	29	26
Time to Pain Meds for Fractures (minutes)	77	57	68	57
Heart Attack Care				
Aspirin Given at Discharge[1]	-	-	99%	99%
Fibrinolytic Meds Within 30 Min. of Arrival[7]	-	-	50%	54%
PCI Within 90 Minutes of Arrival[7]	-	-	96%	96%
Statin Prescribed at Discharge[1]	-	-	97%	98%
Heart Failure Care				
ACE Inhibitor or ARB for LVSD	15	100%	93%	97%
Discharge Instructions Given	58	100%	91%	94%
Evaluation of LVS Function	94	99%	96%	99%
Medicare Spending				
Medicare Spending per Patient (ratio)	-	1.05	0.95	0.98
Pneumonia Care				
Appropriate Initial Antibiotic Given	48	100%	91%	95%
Blood Culture Timing	91	99%	97%	98%
Pregnancy and Delivery Care				
Newborn Deliveries Scheduled Early[7]	-	-	22%	6%
Preventive Care				
Immunization for Influenza[2]	379	99%	87%	90%
Immunization for Pneumonia[2]	415	97%	89%	92%
Stroke Care				
Anticoagulation Therapy for Atrial Fibrillation[1]	-	-	93%	95%
Antithrombotic Therapy Timing	14	100%	96%	98%
Assessed for Rehabilitation	14	100%	95%	97%
Discharged on Antithrombotic Therapy	14	100%	97%	99%
Discharged on Statin Medication	14	79%	88%	94%
Thrombolytic Therapy Timing[1]	-	-	25%	66%
Venous Thromboembolism Prophylaxis	15	67%	87%	94%
Written Stroke Educational Materials Given[1]	-	-	84%	88%
Surgical Care Improvement Project				
Appropriate Beta Blocker Usage	13	92%	97%	98%
Appropriate VTP Within 24 Hours	48	100%	97%	98%
Controlled Postoperative Blood Glucose[7]	-	-	97%	97%
Perioperative Temperature Management	60	100%	100%	100%
Prophylactic Antibiotic Selection	25	100%	99%	99%
Prophylactic Antibiotic Selection (Outpatient)	14	100%	98%	98%
Prophylactic Antibiotic Stopped	25	96%	97%	98%
Prophylactic Antibiotic Timing	25	100%	99%	99%
Prophylactic Antibiotic Timing (Outpatient)	15	93%	98%	98%
Urinary Catheter Removal	30	93%	97%	97%
Survey of Patients' Hospital Experiences				
Area Around Room 'Always' Quiet at Night	300+	66%	72%	61%
Doctors 'Always' Communicated Well	300+	79%	86%	82%
Home Recovery Information Given	300+	76%	83%	85%
Hospital Given 9 or 10 on 10 Point Scale	300+	60%	71%	71%
Meds 'Always' Explained Before Given	300+	54%	67%	64%
Nurses 'Always' Communicated Well	300+	70%	81%	79%
Pain 'Always' Well Controlled	300+	65%	72%	71%
Room and Bathroom 'Always' Clean	300+	64%	74%	73%
Timely Help 'Always' Received	300+	55%	69%	68%
Would Definitely Recommend Hospital	300+	58%	69%	71%
Use of Medical Imaging				
Cardiac Imaging Stress Test before Surgery[1]	-	-	5.7%	5.3%
Combination Abdominal CT Scan	217	4.1%	12.9%	10.5%
Combination Brain/Sinus CT Scan	267	4.5%	3.3%	2.7%
Combination Chest CT Scan	71	1.4%	6.1%	2.7%
Follow-up Mammogram/Ultrasound	465	6.2%	8.4%	8.8%
Lumbar Spine MRI for Low Back Pain	46	41.3%	41.1%	37.2%

King's Daughters Medical Center - Brookhaven

PO Box 948/427 Highway 51 North Phone: 601-833-6011
Brookhaven, MS 39601 Fax: 601-833-2791
E-mail: ccraig@kdmc.org
URL: www.kdmc.org
Type: Acute Care Hospitals Emergency Services: Yes
Ownership: Voluntary non-profit - Other Beds: 122

Key Personnel:
Infection Control.............. Cathy Bridge, RN
Quality Assurance .... Cathy Bridge
Operating Room............... Cathy Davis
CEO/President................ Phillip Gradey
Emergency Room .... Jane Jones
Chief of Medical Staff.......... Jeffrey Ross

Measure	Cases	This Hosp.	State Avg.	U.S. Avg.
Blood Clot Prevention and Treatment				
Anticoagulation Overlap Therapy[2]	24	92%	86%	93%
ICU Venous Thromboembolism Prophylaxis[2]	27	100%	86%	92%
Incidence of Potentially Preventable VTE[1,2]	-	-	15%	10%
UFH with Dosages/Platelet Monitoring[1,2]	-	-	94%	97%
Venous Thromboembolism Prophylaxis[2]	215	94%	70%	85%
Warfarin Therapy Discharge Instructions[2]	20	100%	77%	75%
Chest Pain/Possible Heart Attack Care				
Aspirin Given Within 24 Hours of Arrival	79	94%	94%	96%
Fibrinolytic Meds Within 30 Min. of Arrival[7]	-	-	40%	58%
Average Time to ECG (minutes)	81	13	10	7
Average Time to Transfer (minutes)[7]	-	-	77	60
Children's Asthma Care				
Received Home Management Plan of Care	-	-	-	88%
Received Reliever Medication	-	-	-	100%
Received Systemic Corticosteroids	-	-	-	100%
Emergency Department				
Admittance Decision Time (minutes)[2]	339	71	61	98
Head CT Results Within 45 Min. of Arrival	17	47%	42%	57%
Patients Who Left ER Before Being Seen	29,794	1%	3%	2%
Time from ER Arrival to Admit. (minutes)[2]	351	217	223	274
Time from ER Arrival to Discharge (minutes)	352	126	112	134
Time in ER Before Being Evaluated (minutes)	378	22	29	26
Time to Pain Meds for Fractures (minutes)	52	59	68	57
Heart Attack Care				
Aspirin Given at Discharge[1]	-	-	99%	99%
Fibrinolytic Meds Within 30 Min. of Arrival[7]	-	-	50%	54%
PCI Within 90 Minutes of Arrival[7]	-	-	96%	96%
Statin Prescribed at Discharge[1]	-	-	97%	98%
Heart Failure Care				
ACE Inhibitor or ARB for LVSD	40	95%	93%	97%
Discharge Instructions Given	101	97%	91%	94%
Evaluation of LVS Function	128	100%	96%	99%
Medicare Spending				
Medicare Spending per Patient (ratio)	-	0.99	0.95	0.98
Pneumonia Care				
Appropriate Initial Antibiotic Given	100	97%	91%	95%
Blood Culture Timing	146	99%	97%	98%
Pregnancy and Delivery Care				
Newborn Deliveries Scheduled Early	66	6%	22%	6%
Preventive Care				
Immunization for Influenza[2]	313	98%	87%	90%
Immunization for Pneumonia[2]	295	98%	89%	92%
Stroke Care				
Anticoagulation Therapy for Atrial Fibrillation[1]	-	-	93%	95%
Antithrombotic Therapy Timing	20	100%	96%	98%
Assessed for Rehabilitation	24	92%	95%	97%
Discharged on Antithrombotic Therapy	22	100%	97%	99%
Discharged on Statin Medication	17	100%	88%	94%
Thrombolytic Therapy Timing[7]	-	-	25%	66%
Venous Thromboembolism Prophylaxis	23	100%	87%	94%
Written Stroke Educational Materials Given	13	100%	84%	88%
Surgical Care Improvement Project				
Appropriate Beta Blocker Usage[1]	-	-	97%	98%
Appropriate VTP Within 24 Hours	47	89%	97%	98%
Controlled Postoperative Blood Glucose[7]	-	-	97%	97%
Perioperative Temperature Management	55	100%	100%	100%
Prophylactic Antibiotic Selection	23	96%	99%	99%
Prophylactic Antibiotic Selection (Outpatient)	180	94%	98%	98%
Prophylactic Antibiotic Stopped	23	91%	97%	98%
Prophylactic Antibiotic Timing	23	100%	99%	99%
Prophylactic Antibiotic Timing (Outpatient)	180	99%	98%	98%
Urinary Catheter Removal	19	95%	97%	97%
Survey of Patients' Hospital Experiences				
Area Around Room 'Always' Quiet at Night	300+	78%	72%	61%
Doctors 'Always' Communicated Well	300+	87%	86%	82%
Home Recovery Information Given	300+	90%	83%	85%
Hospital Given 9 or 10 on 10 Point Scale	300+	83%	71%	71%
Meds 'Always' Explained Before Given	300+	72%	67%	64%
Nurses 'Always' Communicated Well	300+	89%	81%	79%
Pain 'Always' Well Controlled	300+	82%	72%	71%
Room and Bathroom 'Always' Clean	300+	77%	74%	73%
Timely Help 'Always' Received	300+	80%	69%	68%
Would Definitely Recommend Hospital	300+	84%	69%	71%
Use of Medical Imaging				
Cardiac Imaging Stress Test before Surgery	117	8.5%	5.7%	5.3%
Combination Abdominal CT Scan	608	10.0%	12.9%	10.5%
Combination Brain/Sinus CT Scan	639	2.7%	3.3%	2.7%
Combination Chest CT Scan	180	3.3%	6.1%	2.7%
Follow-up Mammogram/Ultrasound	610	5.9%	8.4%	8.8%
Lumbar Spine MRI for Low Back Pain	114	50.0%	41.1%	37.2%

Calhoun Health Services

140 Burke - Calhoun City Road Phone: 662-628-6611
Calhoun City, MS 38916
URL: www.nmhs.net
Type: Critical Access Hospitals Emergency Services: Yes
Ownership: Government - Local

Measure	Cases	This Hosp.	State Avg.	U.S. Avg.
Blood Clot Prevention and Treatment				
Anticoagulation Overlap Therapy[1]	-	-	86%	93%
ICU Venous Thromboembolism Prophylaxis[7]	-	-	86%	92%
Incidence of Potentially Preventable VTE[7]	-	-	15%	10%
UFH with Dosages/Platelet Monitoring[7]	-	-	94%	97%
Venous Thromboembolism Prophylaxis	176	92%	70%	85%
Warfarin Therapy Discharge Instructions[1]	-	-	77%	75%
Chest Pain/Possible Heart Attack Care				
Aspirin Given Within 24 Hours of Arrival	42	100%	94%	96%
Fibrinolytic Meds Within 30 Min. of Arrival[7]	-	-	40%	58%
Average Time to ECG (minutes)	42	11	10	7
Average Time to Transfer (minutes)[7]	-	-	77	60
Children's Asthma Care				
Received Home Management Plan of Care	-	-	-	88%
Received Reliever Medication	-	-	-	100%
Received Systemic Corticosteroids	-	-	-	100%
Emergency Department				
Admittance Decision Time (minutes)	237	21	61	98
Head CT Results Within 45 Min. of Arrival[1]	-	-	42%	57%
Patients Who Left ER Before Being Seen	5,530	1%	3%	2%
Time from ER Arrival to Admit. (minutes)	239	154	223	274
Time from ER Arrival to Discharge (minutes)	435	97	112	134
Time in ER Before Being Evaluated (minutes)	444	22	29	26
Time to Pain Meds for Fractures (minutes)	25	54	68	57
Heart Attack Care				
Aspirin Given at Discharge[3,7]	-	-	99%	99%
Fibrinolytic Meds Within 30 Min. of Arrival[3,7]	-	-	50%	54%
PCI Within 90 Minutes of Arrival[5]	-	-	96%	96%
Statin Prescribed at Discharge[3,7]	-	-	97%	98%
Heart Failure Care				
ACE Inhibitor or ARB for LVSD[1]	-	-	93%	97%
Discharge Instructions Given	13	100%	91%	94%
Evaluation of LVS Function	14	93%	96%	99%
Medicare Spending				
Medicare Spending per Patient (ratio)	-	-	0.95	0.98
Pneumonia Care				
Appropriate Initial Antibiotic Given[2]	19	95%	91%	95%
Blood Culture Timing[2]	34	94%	97%	98%
Pregnancy and Delivery Care				
Newborn Deliveries Scheduled Early[7]	-	-	22%	6%
Preventive Care				
Immunization for Influenza[2]	145	100%	87%	90%

NOTE: Hospital profiles are in alphabetical order by state, then city, then hospital within the city; Rankings exclude hospitals with less than 25 cases except for patient surveys which excludes hospitals with less than 100 cases; (a) 100-299 cases; (1) The number of cases/patients is too few to report; (2) Data submitted were based on a sample of cases/patients; (3) Results are based on a shorter time period than required; (4) Data suppressed by CMS for one or more quarters; (5) Results are not available for this reporting period; (6) Fewer than 100 patients completed the HCAHPS survey; (7) No cases met the criteria for this measure; (8) The lower limit of the confidence interval cannot be calculated if the number of observed infections equals zero; (9) No data are available from the state/territory for this reporting period; (10) The scores shown reflect fewer than 50 completed surveys; (11) There were discrepancies in the data collection process; (12) This measure does not apply to this hospital for this reporting period; (13) Results cannot be calculated for this reporting period; (14) The results for this state are combined with nearby states to protect confidentiality; Please refer to the User's Guide for a full explanation of data.

Measure	Cases	This Hosp.	State Avg.	U.S. Avg.
Immunization for Pneumonia[2]	200	100%	89%	92%
Stroke Care				
Anticoagulation Therapy for Atrial Fibrillation[1,3]	-	-	93%	95%
Antithrombotic Therapy Timing[3,7]	-	-	96%	98%
Assessed for Rehabilitation[1,3]	-	-	95%	97%
Discharged on Antithrombotic Therapy[1,3]	-	-	97%	99%
Discharged on Statin Medication[1,3]	-	-	88%	94%
Thrombolytic Therapy Timing[3,7]	-	-	25%	66%
Venous Thromboembolism Prophylaxis[1,3]	-	-	87%	94%
Written Stroke Educational Materials Given[1,3]	-	-	84%	88%
Surgical Care Improvement Project				
Appropriate Beta Blocker Usage[5]	-	-	97%	98%
Appropriate VTP Within 24 Hours[5]	-	-	97%	98%
Controlled Postoperative Blood Glucose[5]	-	-	97%	97%
Perioperative Temperature Management[5]	-	-	100%	100%
Prophylactic Antibiotic Selection[5]	-	-	99%	99%
Prophylactic Antibiotic Selection (Outpatient)[5]	-	-	98%	98%
Prophylactic Antibiotic Stopped[5]	-	-	97%	98%
Prophylactic Antibiotic Timing[5]	-	-	99%	99%
Prophylactic Antibiotic Timing (Outpatient)[5]	-	-	98%	98%
Urinary Catheter Removal[5]	-	-	97%	97%
Survey of Patients' Hospital Experiences				
Area Around Room 'Always' Quiet at Night[6]	<100	75%	72%	61%
Doctors 'Always' Communicated Well[6]	<100	93%	86%	82%
Home Recovery Information Given[6]	<100	89%	83%	85%
Hospital Given 9 or 10 on 10 Point Scale[6]	<100	77%	71%	71%
Meds 'Always' Explained Before Given[6]	<100	87%	67%	64%
Nurses 'Always' Communicated Well[6]	<100	84%	81%	79%
Pain 'Always' Well Controlled[6]	<100	82%	72%	71%
Room and Bathroom 'Always' Clean[6]	<100	92%	74%	73%
Timely Help 'Always' Received[6]	<100	88%	69%	68%
Would Definitely Recommend Hospital[6]	<100	77%	69%	71%
Use of Medical Imaging				
Cardiac Imaging Stress Test before Surgery[7]	-	-	5.7%	5.3%
Combination Abdominal CT Scan	149	20.8%	12.9%	10.5%
Combination Brain/Sinus CT Scan	202	5.0%	3.3%	2.7%
Combination Chest CT Scan[1]	-	-	6.1%	2.7%
Follow-up Mammogram/Ultrasound[7]	-	-	8.4%	8.8%
Lumbar Spine MRI for Low Back Pain[1]	-	-	41.1%	37.2%

Madison River Oaks Medical Center

161 River Oaks Drive
Canton, MS 39046
Phone: 601-855-5323
Fax: 601-855-5100
URL: www.madisonriveroaks.com
Type: Acute Care Hospitals
Emergency Services: Yes
Ownership: Proprietary
Beds: 127

Key Personnel:

Radiology. . . . . Nancy Burrow
Quality Assurance . . . . Beth Harkins, RN
Infection Control. . . . . Brenda Ledbetter, RN
Cardiac Laboratory. . . . . Anurag Mehta, MD
Operating Room. . . . . Carol Newcomb
Chief of Medical Staff . . . . Sanjib Shrestha
Pediatric Ambulatory Care . . . . . Vibha Vig, MD
CEO/President. . . . . Joseph D Weaver

Measure	Cases	This Hosp.	State Avg.	U.S. Avg.
Blood Clot Prevention and Treatment				
Anticoagulation Overlap Therapy[1,2]	-	-	86%	93%
ICU Venous Thromboembolism Prophylaxis[2]	43	91%	86%	92%
Incidence of Potentially Preventable VTE[2,7]	-	-	15%	10%
UFH with Dosages/Platelet Monitoring[1,2]	-	-	94%	97%
Venous Thromboembolism Prophylaxis[2]	91	65%	70%	85%
Warfarin Therapy Discharge Instructions[1,2]	-	-	77%	75%
Chest Pain/Possible Heart Attack Care				
Aspirin Given Within 24 Hours of Arrival	70	94%	94%	96%
Fibrinolytic Meds Within 30 Min. of Arrival[1]	-	-	40%	58%
Average Time to ECG (minutes)	71	8	10	7
Average Time to Transfer (minutes)[7]	-	-	77	60
Children's Asthma Care				
Received Home Management Plan of Care	-	-	-	88%
Received Reliever Medication	-	-	-	100%
Received Systemic Corticosteroids	-	-	-	100%
Emergency Department				
Admittance Decision Time (minutes)[2]	304	71	61	98
Head CT Results Within 45 Min. of Arrival[1]	-	-	42%	57%
Patients Who Left ER Before Being Seen	21,769	1%	3%	2%
Time from ER Arrival to Admit. (minutes)[2]	304	197	223	274
Time from ER Arrival to Discharge (minutes)	1,037	89	112	134
Time in ER Before Being Evaluated (minutes)	1,115	28	29	26
Time to Pain Meds for Fractures (minutes)	79	47	68	57
Heart Attack Care				
Aspirin Given at Discharge[1]	-	-	99%	99%
Fibrinolytic Meds Within 30 Min. of Arrival[7]	-	-	50%	54%
PCI Within 90 Minutes of Arrival[7]	-	-	96%	96%
Statin Prescribed at Discharge[1]	-	-	97%	98%
Heart Failure Care				
ACE Inhibitor or ARB for LVSD	24	100%	93%	97%
Discharge Instructions Given	84	95%	91%	94%
Evaluation of LVS Function	93	98%	96%	99%
Medicare Spending				
Medicare Spending per Patient (ratio)	-	1.00	0.95	0.98
Pneumonia Care				
Appropriate Initial Antibiotic Given	45	93%	91%	95%
Blood Culture Timing	57	93%	97%	98%
Pregnancy and Delivery Care				
Newborn Deliveries Scheduled Early	42	0%	22%	6%
Preventive Care				
Immunization for Influenza[2]	246	91%	87%	90%
Immunization for Pneumonia[2]	230	93%	89%	92%
Stroke Care				
Anticoagulation Therapy for Atrial Fibrillation[7]	-	-	93%	95%
Antithrombotic Therapy Timing[1]	-	-	96%	98%
Assessed for Rehabilitation[1]	-	-	95%	97%
Discharged on Antithrombotic Therapy[1]	-	-	97%	99%
Discharged on Statin Medication[1]	-	-	88%	94%
Thrombolytic Therapy Timing[7]	-	-	25%	66%
Venous Thromboembolism Prophylaxis[1]	-	-	87%	94%
Written Stroke Educational Materials Given[7]	-	-	84%	88%
Surgical Care Improvement Project				
Appropriate Beta Blocker Usage	18	94%	97%	98%
Appropriate VTP Within 24 Hours	72	93%	97%	98%
Controlled Postoperative Blood Glucose[7]	-	-	97%	97%
Perioperative Temperature Management	78	100%	100%	100%
Prophylactic Antibiotic Selection	66	98%	99%	99%
Prophylactic Antibiotic Selection (Outpatient)	37	92%	98%	98%
Prophylactic Antibiotic Stopped	66	97%	97%	98%
Prophylactic Antibiotic Timing	66	98%	99%	99%
Prophylactic Antibiotic Timing (Outpatient)	37	100%	98%	98%
Urinary Catheter Removal	66	95%	97%	97%
Survey of Patients' Hospital Experiences				
Area Around Room 'Always' Quiet at Night	(a)	78%	72%	61%
Doctors 'Always' Communicated Well	(a)	83%	86%	82%
Home Recovery Information Given	(a)	80%	83%	85%
Hospital Given 9 or 10 on 10 Point Scale	(a)	67%	71%	71%
Meds 'Always' Explained Before Given	(a)	60%	67%	64%
Nurses 'Always' Communicated Well	(a)	78%	81%	79%
Pain 'Always' Well Controlled	(a)	72%	72%	71%
Room and Bathroom 'Always' Clean	(a)	67%	74%	73%
Timely Help 'Always' Received	(a)	62%	69%	68%
Would Definitely Recommend Hospital	(a)	67%	69%	71%
Use of Medical Imaging				
Cardiac Imaging Stress Test before Surgery[7]	-	-	5.7%	5.3%
Combination Abdominal CT Scan	189	4.8%	12.9%	10.5%
Combination Brain/Sinus CT Scan	374	5.3%	3.3%	2.7%
Combination Chest CT Scan	97	7.2%	6.1%	2.7%
Follow-up Mammogram/Ultrasound	268	6.7%	8.4%	8.8%
Lumbar Spine MRI for Low Back Pain[7]	-	-	41.1%	37.2%

Baptist Medical Center - Leake

310 Ellis Street
Carthage, MS 39051
Phone: 601-267-1454
Type: Critical Access Hospitals
Emergency Services: Yes
Ownership: Voluntary non-profit - Private

Measure	Cases	This Hosp.	State Avg.	U.S. Avg.
Blood Clot Prevention and Treatment				
Anticoagulation Overlap Therapy[5]	-	-	86%	93%
ICU Venous Thromboembolism Prophylaxis[5]	-	-	86%	92%
Incidence of Potentially Preventable VTE[5]	-	-	15%	10%
UFH with Dosages/Platelet Monitoring[5]	-	-	94%	97%
Venous Thromboembolism Prophylaxis[5]	-	-	70%	85%
Warfarin Therapy Discharge Instructions[5]	-	-	77%	75%
Chest Pain/Possible Heart Attack Care				
Aspirin Given Within 24 Hours of Arrival[1]	-	-	94%	96%
Fibrinolytic Meds Within 30 Min. of Arrival[5]	-	-	40%	58%
Average Time to ECG (minutes)[1]	-	-	10	7
Average Time to Transfer (minutes)[5]	-	-	77	60
Children's Asthma Care				
Received Home Management Plan of Care	-	-	-	88%
Received Reliever Medication	-	-	-	100%
Received Systemic Corticosteroids	-	-	-	100%
Emergency Department				
Admittance Decision Time (minutes)[5]	-	-	61	98
Head CT Results Within 45 Min. of Arrival[5]	-	-	42%	57%
Patients Who Left ER Before Being Seen[5]	-	-	3%	2%
Time from ER Arrival to Admit. (minutes)[5]	-	-	223	274
Time from ER Arrival to Discharge (minutes)[5]	-	-	112	134
Time in ER Before Being Evaluated (minutes)[5]	-	-	29	26
Time to Pain Meds for Fractures (minutes)[5]	-	-	68	57
Heart Attack Care				
Aspirin Given at Discharge[3,7]	-	-	99%	99%
Fibrinolytic Meds Within 30 Min. of Arrival[1,3]	-	-	50%	54%
PCI Within 90 Minutes of Arrival[3,7]	-	-	96%	96%
Statin Prescribed at Discharge[1,3]	-	-	97%	98%
Heart Failure Care				
ACE Inhibitor or ARB for LVSD[1]	-	-	93%	97%
Discharge Instructions Given	12	17%	91%	94%
Evaluation of LVS Function	19	37%	96%	99%
Medicare Spending				
Medicare Spending per Patient (ratio)	-	-	0.95	0.98
Pneumonia Care				
Appropriate Initial Antibiotic Given	14	64%	91%	95%
Blood Culture Timing[1]	-	-	97%	98%
Pregnancy and Delivery Care				
Newborn Deliveries Scheduled Early[5]	-	-	22%	6%
Preventive Care				
Immunization for Influenza[5]	-	-	87%	90%
Immunization for Pneumonia[5]	-	-	89%	92%
Stroke Care				
Anticoagulation Therapy for Atrial Fibrillation[5]	-	-	93%	95%
Antithrombotic Therapy Timing[5]	-	-	96%	98%
Assessed for Rehabilitation[5]	-	-	95%	97%
Discharged on Antithrombotic Therapy[5]	-	-	97%	99%
Discharged on Statin Medication[5]	-	-	88%	94%
Thrombolytic Therapy Timing[5]	-	-	25%	66%
Venous Thromboembolism Prophylaxis[5]	-	-	87%	94%
Written Stroke Educational Materials Given[5]	-	-	84%	88%
Surgical Care Improvement Project				
Appropriate Beta Blocker Usage[5]	-	-	97%	98%
Appropriate VTP Within 24 Hours[5]	-	-	97%	98%
Controlled Postoperative Blood Glucose[5]	-	-	97%	97%
Perioperative Temperature Management[5]	-	-	100%	100%
Prophylactic Antibiotic Selection[5]	-	-	99%	99%
Prophylactic Antibiotic Selection (Outpatient)[5]	-	-	98%	98%
Prophylactic Antibiotic Stopped[5]	-	-	97%	98%
Prophylactic Antibiotic Timing[5]	-	-	99%	99%
Prophylactic Antibiotic Timing (Outpatient)[5]	-	-	98%	98%
Urinary Catheter Removal[5]	-	-	97%	97%
Survey of Patients' Hospital Experiences				
Area Around Room 'Always' Quiet at Night[5]	-	-	72%	61%
Doctors 'Always' Communicated Well[5]	-	-	86%	82%
Home Recovery Information Given[5]	-	-	83%	85%
Hospital Given 9 or 10 on 10 Point Scale[5]	-	-	71%	71%
Meds 'Always' Explained Before Given[5]	-	-	67%	64%
Nurses 'Always' Communicated Well[5]	-	-	81%	79%
Pain 'Always' Well Controlled[5]	-	-	72%	71%
Room and Bathroom 'Always' Clean[5]	-	-	74%	73%
Timely Help 'Always' Received[5]	-	-	69%	68%
Would Definitely Recommend Hospital[5]	-	-	69%	71%

NOTE: Hospital profiles are in alphabetical order by state, then city, then hospital within the city; Rankings exclude hospitals with less than 25 cases except for patient surveys which excludes hospitals with less than 100 cases; (a) 100-299 cases; (1) The number of cases/patients is too few to report; (2) Data submitted were based on a sample of cases/patients; (3) Results are based on a shorter time period than required; (4) Data suppressed by CMS for one or more quarters; (5) Results are not available for this reporting period; (6) Fewer than 100 patients completed the HCAHPS survey; (7) No cases met the criteria for this measure; (8) The lower limit of the confidence interval cannot be calculated if the number of observed infections equals zero; (9) No data are available from the state/territory for this reporting period; (10) The scores shown reflect fewer than 50 completed surveys; (11) There were discrepancies in the data collection process; (12) This measure does not apply to this hospital for this reporting period; (13) Results cannot be calculated for this reporting period; (14) The results for this state are combined with nearby states to protect confidentiality; Please refer to the User's Guide for a full explanation of data.

Use of Medical Imaging				
Cardiac Imaging Stress Test before Surgery[7]	-	-	5.7%	5.3%
Combination Abdominal CT Scan	107	4.7%	12.9%	10.5%
Combination Brain/Sinus CT Scan	214	5.1%	3.3%	2.7%
Combination Chest CT Scan[1]	-	-	6.1%	2.7%
Follow-up Mammogram/Ultrasound[1]	-	-	8.4%	8.8%
Lumbar Spine MRI for Low Back Pain[1]	-	-	41.1%	37.2%

Field Memorial Community Hospital

270 West Main Street PO Box 639
Centreville, MS 39631
Phone: 601-645-5221
Fax: 601-645-5842
Type: Critical Access Hospitals
Emergency Services: Yes
Ownership: Government - Local
Beds: 25

Key Personnel:

Operating Room. . . . . Cheryl Cavin
Anesthesiology. . . . . Sandy Clark
Emergency Room . . . . Dr Rich Field
Chief of Medical Staff . . . . Robert Lewis
Infection Control . . . . LaVerne McDaniel, RN
Quality Assurance . . . . LaVerne McDaniel
CEO/President . . . . Chad Netterville

Measure	Cases	This Hosp.	State Avg.	U.S. Avg.
Blood Clot Prevention and Treatment				
Anticoagulation Overlap Therapy[5]	-	-	86%	93%
ICU Venous Thromboembolism Prophylaxis[5]	-	-	86%	92%
Incidence of Potentially Preventable VTE[5]	-	-	15%	10%
UFH with Dosages/Platelet Monitoring[5]	-	-	94%	97%
Venous Thromboembolism Prophylaxis[5]	-	-	70%	85%
Warfarin Therapy Discharge Instructions[5]	-	-	77%	75%
Chest Pain/Possible Heart Attack Care				
Aspirin Given Within 24 Hours of Arrival	29	97%	94%	96%
Fibrinolytic Meds Within 30 Min. of Arrival[1]	-	-	40%	58%
Average Time to ECG (minutes)	29	4	10	7
Average Time to Transfer (minutes)[1]	-	-	77	60
Children's Asthma Care				
Received Home Management Plan of Care	-	-	-	88%
Received Reliever Medication	-	-	-	100%
Received Systemic Corticosteroids	-	-	-	100%
Emergency Department				
Admittance Decision Time (minutes)[5]	-	-	61	98
Head CT Results Within 45 Min. of Arrival[5]	-	-	42%	57%
Patients Who Left ER Before Being Seen	5,330	1%	3%	2%
Time from ER Arrival to Admit. (minutes)[5]	-	-	223	274
Time from ER Arrival to Discharge (minutes)[5]	-	-	112	134
Time in ER Before Being Evaluated (minutes)[5]	-	-	29	26
Time to Pain Meds for Fractures (minutes)[5]	-	-	68	57
Heart Attack Care				
Aspirin Given at Discharge[1]	-	-	99%	99%
Fibrinolytic Meds Within 30 Min. of Arrival[7]	-	-	50%	54%
PCI Within 90 Minutes of Arrival[3,7]	-	-	96%	96%
Statin Prescribed at Discharge[1]	-	-	97%	98%
Heart Failure Care				
ACE Inhibitor or ARB for LVSD	12	100%	93%	97%
Discharge Instructions Given	20	85%	91%	94%
Evaluation of LVS Function	20	100%	96%	99%
Medicare Spending				
Medicare Spending per Patient (ratio)	-	-	0.95	0.98
Pneumonia Care				
Appropriate Initial Antibiotic Given	14	93%	91%	95%
Blood Culture Timing	13	100%	97%	98%
Pregnancy and Delivery Care				
Newborn Deliveries Scheduled Early[3,7]	-	-	22%	6%
Preventive Care				
Immunization for Influenza[5]	-	-	87%	90%
Immunization for Pneumonia[5]	-	-	89%	92%
Stroke Care				
Anticoagulation Therapy for Atrial Fibrillation[5]	-	-	93%	95%
Antithrombotic Therapy Timing[5]	-	-	96%	98%
Assessed for Rehabilitation[5]	-	-	95%	97%
Discharged on Antithrombotic Therapy[5]	-	-	97%	99%
Discharged on Statin Medication[5]	-	-	88%	94%
Thrombolytic Therapy Timing[5]	-	-	25%	66%
Venous Thromboembolism Prophylaxis[5]	-	-	87%	94%
Written Stroke Educational Materials Given[5]	-	-	84%	88%
Surgical Care Improvement Project				
Appropriate Beta Blocker Usage[1]	-	-	97%	98%
Appropriate VTP Within 24 Hours[1]	-	-	97%	98%
Controlled Postoperative Blood Glucose[7]	-	-	97%	97%
Perioperative Temperature Management[1]	-	-	100%	100%
Prophylactic Antibiotic Selection[1]	-	-	99%	99%
Prophylactic Antibiotic Selection (Outpatient)[5]	-	-	98%	98%
Prophylactic Antibiotic Stopped[1]	-	-	97%	98%
Prophylactic Antibiotic Timing[1]	-	-	99%	99%
Prophylactic Antibiotic Timing (Outpatient)[5]	-	-	98%	98%
Urinary Catheter Removal[1]	-	-	97%	97%
Survey of Patients' Hospital Experiences				
Area Around Room 'Always' Quiet at Night[6]	<100	71%	72%	61%
Doctors 'Always' Communicated Well[6]	<100	91%	86%	82%
Home Recovery Information Given[6]	<100	85%	83%	85%
Hospital Given 9 or 10 on 10 Point Scale[6]	<100	69%	71%	71%
Meds 'Always' Explained Before Given[6]	<100	76%	67%	64%
Nurses 'Always' Communicated Well[6]	<100	87%	81%	79%
Pain 'Always' Well Controlled[6]	<100	71%	72%	71%
Room and Bathroom 'Always' Clean[6]	<100	77%	74%	73%
Timely Help 'Always' Received[6]	<100	66%	69%	68%
Would Definitely Recommend Hospital[6]	<100	68%	69%	71%
Use of Medical Imaging				
Cardiac Imaging Stress Test before Surgery	64	9.4%	5.7%	5.3%
Combination Abdominal CT Scan	101	43.6%	12.9%	10.5%
Combination Brain/Sinus CT Scan[1]	-	-	3.3%	2.7%
Combination Chest CT Scan	46	52.2%	6.1%	2.7%
Follow-up Mammogram/Ultrasound	197	3.6%	8.4%	8.8%
Lumbar Spine MRI for Low Back Pain[7]	-	-	41.1%	37.2%

Tallahatchie Critical Access Hospital

201 South Market Saint / PO Box 230
Charleston, MS 38921
Phone: 662-647-5535
Type: Critical Access Hospitals
Emergency Services: Yes
Ownership: Government - Local

Measure	Cases	This Hosp.	State Avg.	U.S. Avg.
Blood Clot Prevention and Treatment				
Anticoagulation Overlap Therapy[3,7]	-	-	86%	93%
ICU Venous Thromboembolism Prophylaxis[3,7]	-	-	86%	92%
Incidence of Potentially Preventable VTE[3,7]	-	-	15%	10%
UFH with Dosages/Platelet Monitoring[3,7]	-	-	94%	97%
Venous Thromboembolism Prophylaxis[1,3]	-	-	70%	85%
Warfarin Therapy Discharge Instructions[3,7]	-	-	77%	75%
Chest Pain/Possible Heart Attack Care				
Aspirin Given Within 24 Hours of Arrival[1,3]	-	-	94%	96%
Fibrinolytic Meds Within 30 Min. of Arrival[3,7]	-	-	40%	58%
Average Time to ECG (minutes)[1,3]	-	-	10	7
Average Time to Transfer (minutes)[1,3]	-	-	77	60
Children's Asthma Care				
Received Home Management Plan of Care	-	-	-	88%
Received Reliever Medication	-	-	-	100%
Received Systemic Corticosteroids	-	-	-	100%
Emergency Department				
Admittance Decision Time (minutes)[5]	-	-	61	98
Head CT Results Within 45 Min. of Arrival[5]	-	-	42%	57%
Patients Who Left ER Before Being Seen[5]	-	-	3%	2%
Time from ER Arrival to Admit. (minutes)[5]	-	-	223	274
Time from ER Arrival to Discharge (minutes)	1,268	100	112	134
Time in ER Before Being Evaluated (minutes)	1,236	15	29	26
Time to Pain Meds for Fractures (minutes)[5]	-	-	68	57
Heart Attack Care				
Aspirin Given at Discharge[5]	-	-	99%	99%
Fibrinolytic Meds Within 30 Min. of Arrival[5]	-	-	50%	54%
PCI Within 90 Minutes of Arrival[5]	-	-	96%	96%
Statin Prescribed at Discharge[5]	-	-	97%	98%
Heart Failure Care				
ACE Inhibitor or ARB for LVSD[1,3]	-	-	93%	97%
Discharge Instructions Given[1,3]	-	-	91%	94%
Evaluation of LVS Function[1,3]	-	-	96%	99%
Medicare Spending				
Medicare Spending per Patient (ratio)	-	-	0.95	0.98
Pneumonia Care				
Appropriate Initial Antibiotic Given	27	63%	91%	95%
Blood Culture Timing[1]	-	-	97%	98%
Pregnancy and Delivery Care				
Newborn Deliveries Scheduled Early[5]	-	-	22%	6%
Preventive Care				
Immunization for Influenza[5]	-	-	87%	90%
Immunization for Pneumonia[5]	-	-	89%	92%
Stroke Care				
Anticoagulation Therapy for Atrial Fibrillation[3,7]	-	-	93%	95%
Antithrombotic Therapy Timing[1,3]	-	-	96%	98%
Assessed for Rehabilitation[1,3]	-	-	95%	97%
Discharged on Antithrombotic Therapy[1,3]	-	-	97%	99%
Discharged on Statin Medication[1,3]	-	-	88%	94%
Thrombolytic Therapy Timing[1,3]	-	-	25%	66%
Venous Thromboembolism Prophylaxis[1,3]	-	-	87%	94%
Written Stroke Educational Materials Given[1,3]	-	-	84%	88%
Surgical Care Improvement Project				
Appropriate Beta Blocker Usage[5]	-	-	97%	98%
Appropriate VTP Within 24 Hours[5]	-	-	97%	98%
Controlled Postoperative Blood Glucose[5]	-	-	97%	97%
Perioperative Temperature Management[5]	-	-	100%	100%
Prophylactic Antibiotic Selection[5]	-	-	99%	99%
Prophylactic Antibiotic Selection (Outpatient)[5]	-	-	98%	98%
Prophylactic Antibiotic Stopped[5]	-	-	97%	98%
Prophylactic Antibiotic Timing[5]	-	-	99%	99%
Prophylactic Antibiotic Timing (Outpatient)[5]	-	-	98%	98%
Urinary Catheter Removal[5]	-	-	97%	97%
Survey of Patients' Hospital Experiences				
Area Around Room 'Always' Quiet at Night[5]	-	-	72%	61%
Doctors 'Always' Communicated Well[5]	-	-	86%	82%
Home Recovery Information Given[5]	-	-	83%	85%
Hospital Given 9 or 10 on 10 Point Scale[5]	-	-	71%	71%
Meds 'Always' Explained Before Given[5]	-	-	67%	64%
Nurses 'Always' Communicated Well[5]	-	-	81%	79%
Pain 'Always' Well Controlled[5]	-	-	72%	71%
Room and Bathroom 'Always' Clean[5]	-	-	74%	73%
Timely Help 'Always' Received[5]	-	-	69%	68%
Would Definitely Recommend Hospital[5]	-	-	69%	71%
Use of Medical Imaging				
Cardiac Imaging Stress Test before Surgery[7]	-	-	5.7%	5.3%
Combination Abdominal CT Scan[1]	-	-	12.9%	10.5%
Combination Brain/Sinus CT Scan[1]	-	-	3.3%	2.7%
Combination Chest CT Scan[1]	-	-	6.1%	2.7%
Follow-up Mammogram/Ultrasound[7]	-	-	8.4%	8.8%
Lumbar Spine MRI for Low Back Pain[1]	-	-	41.1%	37.2%

Northwest Mississippi Regional Medical Center

1970 Hospital Drive
Clarksdale, MS 38614
Phone: 662-627-3211
Fax: 662-627-5440
URL: www.nwmsregionalmedcenter.com
Type: Acute Care Hospitals
Emergency Services: Yes
Ownership: Proprietary
Beds: 195

Key Personnel:

CEO/President. . . . . W Douglas Arnold
Infection Control. . . . . Mae Bramlett
Operating Room. . . . . Anne Brooks
Radiology. . . . . James Edwards
Quality Assurance . . . . Teresa Gove
Cardiac Laboratory. . . . . Steve Gressmire
Chief of Medical Staff . . . . Vernon Thomas Hughes, DO
Pediatric In-Patient Care . . . . Sherry Metcalf

Measure	Cases	This Hosp.	State Avg.	U.S. Avg.
Blood Clot Prevention and Treatment				
Anticoagulation Overlap Therapy[2]	15	67%	86%	93%
ICU Venous Thromboembolism Prophylaxis[2]	94	89%	86%	92%
Incidence of Potentially Preventable VTE[1,2]	-	-	15%	10%
UFH with Dosages/Platelet Monitoring[1,2]	-	-	94%	97%
Venous Thromboembolism Prophylaxis[2]	375	75%	70%	85%
Warfarin Therapy Discharge Instructions[2]	13	85%	77%	75%
Chest Pain/Possible Heart Attack Care				
Aspirin Given Within 24 Hours of Arrival	35	91%	94%	96%
Fibrinolytic Meds Within 30 Min. of Arrival[7]	-	-	40%	58%
Average Time to ECG (minutes)	38	18	10	7
Average Time to Transfer (minutes)[1]	-	-	77	60

NOTE: Hospital profiles are in alphabetical order by state, then city, then hospital within the city; Rankings exclude hospitals with less than 25 cases except for patient surveys which excludes hospitals with less than 100 cases; (a) 100-299 cases; (1) The number of cases/patients is too few to report; (2) Data submitted were based on a sample of cases/patients; (3) Results are based on a shorter time period than required; (4) Data suppressed by CMS for one or more quarters; (5) Results are not available for this reporting period; (6) Fewer than 100 patients completed the HCAHPS survey; (7) No cases met the criteria for this measure; (8) The lower limit of the confidence interval cannot be calculated if the number of observed infections equals zero; (9) No data are available from the state/territory for this reporting period; (10) The scores shown reflect fewer than 50 completed surveys; (11) There were discrepancies in the data collection process; (12) This measure does not apply to this hospital for this reporting period; (13) Results cannot be calculated for this reporting period; (14) The results for this state are combined with nearby states to protect confidentiality; Please refer to the User's Guide for a full explanation of data.

Children's Asthma Care				
Received Home Management Plan of Care	-	-	-	88%
Received Reliever Medication	-	-	-	100%
Received Systemic Corticosteroids	-	-	-	100%
Emergency Department				
Admittance Decision Time (minutes)[2]	778	64	61	98
Head CT Results Within 45 Min. of Arrival[1]	-	-	42%	57%
Patients Who Left ER Before Being Seen	6,540	3%	3%	2%
Time from ER Arrival to Admit. (minutes)[2]	781	231	223	274
Time from ER Arrival to Discharge (minutes)	678	123	112	134
Time in ER Before Being Evaluated (minutes)	733	39	29	26
Time to Pain Meds for Fractures (minutes)	42	66	68	57
Heart Attack Care				
Aspirin Given at Discharge	44	91%	99%	99%
Fibrinolytic Meds Within 30 Min. of Arrival[1]	-	-	50%	54%
PCI Within 90 Minutes of Arrival[7]	-	-	96%	96%
Statin Prescribed at Discharge	43	95%	97%	98%
Heart Failure Care				
ACE Inhibitor or ARB for LVSD	100	97%	93%	97%
Discharge Instructions Given	218	91%	91%	94%
Evaluation of LVS Function	238	100%	96%	99%
Medicare Spending				
Medicare Spending per Patient (ratio)	-	0.92	0.95	0.98
Pneumonia Care				
Appropriate Initial Antibiotic Given	29	100%	91%	95%
Blood Culture Timing	31	97%	97%	98%
Pregnancy and Delivery Care				
Newborn Deliveries Scheduled Early	112	32%	22%	6%
Preventive Care				
Immunization for Influenza[2]	913	96%	87%	90%
Immunization for Pneumonia[2]	742	95%	89%	92%
Stroke Care				
Anticoagulation Therapy for Atrial Fibrillation[1]	-	-	93%	95%
Antithrombotic Therapy Timing	39	97%	96%	98%
Assessed for Rehabilitation	39	87%	95%	97%
Discharged on Antithrombotic Therapy	37	92%	97%	99%
Discharged on Statin Medication	33	88%	88%	94%
Thrombolytic Therapy Timing[1]	-	-	25%	66%
Venous Thromboembolism Prophylaxis	43	74%	87%	94%
Written Stroke Educational Materials Given	21	52%	84%	88%
Surgical Care Improvement Project				
Appropriate Beta Blocker Usage	28	100%	97%	98%
Appropriate VTP Within 24 Hours	90	98%	97%	98%
Controlled Postoperative Blood Glucose[7]	-	-	97%	97%
Perioperative Temperature Management	96	100%	100%	100%
Prophylactic Antibiotic Selection	54	98%	99%	99%
Prophylactic Antibiotic Selection (Outpatient)	156	97%	98%	98%
Prophylactic Antibiotic Stopped	52	98%	97%	98%
Prophylactic Antibiotic Timing	54	91%	99%	99%
Prophylactic Antibiotic Timing (Outpatient)	158	99%	98%	98%
Urinary Catheter Removal	31	97%	97%	97%
Survey of Patients' Hospital Experiences				
Area Around Room 'Always' Quiet at Night	300+	61%	72%	61%
Doctors 'Always' Communicated Well	300+	84%	86%	82%
Home Recovery Information Given	300+	76%	83%	85%
Hospital Given 9 or 10 on 10 Point Scale	300+	48%	71%	71%
Meds 'Always' Explained Before Given	300+	65%	67%	64%
Nurses 'Always' Communicated Well	300+	76%	81%	79%
Pain 'Always' Well Controlled	300+	69%	72%	71%
Room and Bathroom 'Always' Clean	300+	69%	74%	73%
Timely Help 'Always' Received	300+	65%	69%	68%
Would Definitely Recommend Hospital	300+	47%	69%	71%
Use of Medical Imaging				
Cardiac Imaging Stress Test before Surgery[1]	-	-	5.7%	5.3%
Combination Abdominal CT Scan	355	37.5%	12.9%	10.5%
Combination Brain/Sinus CT Scan	461	4.1%	3.3%	2.7%
Combination Chest CT Scan	166	20.5%	6.1%	2.7%
Follow-up Mammogram/Ultrasound	315	7.6%	8.4%	8.8%
Lumbar Spine MRI for Low Back Pain	54	57.4%	41.1%	37.2%

Bolivar Medical Center

Hwy 8 E
Cleveland, MS 38732
E-mail: barbara.levingston@lpnt.net
URL: www.bolivarmedical.com
Type: Acute Care Hospitals
Ownership: Proprietary

Phone: 662-846-2551
Fax: 662-846-2380
Emergency Services: Yes
Beds: 106

Key Personnel:
CEO . . . . James Atkins
Intensive Care Unit. . . . . Lisa Ellis
Ambulatory Care . . . . Minta Hill
Quality Assurance . . . . Noel Hopper
Emergency Room . . . . Perry Wallace
Radiology. . . . . Jason Williams
Operating Room. . . . . Bennie Wright

Measure	Cases	This Hosp.	State Avg.	U.S. Avg.
Blood Clot Prevention and Treatment				
Anticoagulation Overlap Therapy[2]	17	59%	86%	93%
ICU Venous Thromboembolism Prophylaxis[2]	61	75%	86%	92%
Incidence of Potentially Preventable VTE[1,2]	-	-	15%	10%
UFH with Dosages/Platelet Monitoring[1,2]	-	-	94%	97%
Venous Thromboembolism Prophylaxis[2]	290	63%	70%	85%
Warfarin Therapy Discharge Instructions[2]	11	91%	77%	75%
Chest Pain/Possible Heart Attack Care				
Aspirin Given Within 24 Hours of Arrival	29	100%	94%	96%
Fibrinolytic Meds Within 30 Min. of Arrival[7]	-	-	40%	58%
Average Time to ECG (minutes)	29	13	10	7
Average Time to Transfer (minutes)[1]	-	-	77	60
Children's Asthma Care				
Received Home Management Plan of Care	-	-	-	88%
Received Reliever Medication	-	-	-	100%
Received Systemic Corticosteroids	-	-	-	100%
Emergency Department				
Admittance Decision Time (minutes)[2]	325	86	61	98
Head CT Results Within 45 Min. of Arrival	14	71%	42%	57%
Patients Who Left ER Before Being Seen	17,934	3%	3%	2%
Time from ER Arrival to Admit. (minutes)[2]	329	220	223	274
Time from ER Arrival to Discharge (minutes)	362	122	112	134
Time in ER Before Being Evaluated (minutes)	437	18	29	26
Time to Pain Meds for Fractures (minutes)	43	53	68	57
Heart Attack Care				
Aspirin Given at Discharge[3,7]	-	-	99%	99%
Fibrinolytic Meds Within 30 Min. of Arrival[3,7]	-	-	50%	54%
PCI Within 90 Minutes of Arrival[3,7]	-	-	96%	96%
Statin Prescribed at Discharge[3,7]	-	-	97%	98%
Heart Failure Care				
ACE Inhibitor or ARB for LVSD	32	100%	93%	97%
Discharge Instructions Given	121	100%	91%	94%
Evaluation of LVS Function	133	100%	96%	99%
Medicare Spending				
Medicare Spending per Patient (ratio)	-	1.02	0.95	0.98
Pneumonia Care				
Appropriate Initial Antibiotic Given	42	100%	91%	95%
Blood Culture Timing	97	100%	97%	98%
Pregnancy and Delivery Care				
Newborn Deliveries Scheduled Early[2]	27	0%	22%	6%
Preventive Care				
Immunization for Influenza[2]	355	96%	87%	90%
Immunization for Pneumonia[2]	355	100%	89%	92%
Stroke Care				
Anticoagulation Therapy for Atrial Fibrillation[1]	-	-	93%	95%
Antithrombotic Therapy Timing	19	89%	96%	98%
Assessed for Rehabilitation	14	100%	95%	97%
Discharged on Antithrombotic Therapy	13	85%	97%	99%
Discharged on Statin Medication	11	55%	88%	94%
Thrombolytic Therapy Timing[1]	-	-	25%	66%
Venous Thromboembolism Prophylaxis	20	65%	87%	94%
Written Stroke Educational Materials Given[1]	-	-	84%	88%
Surgical Care Improvement Project				
Appropriate Beta Blocker Usage	14	100%	97%	98%
Appropriate VTP Within 24 Hours	103	100%	97%	98%
Controlled Postoperative Blood Glucose[7]	-	-	97%	97%
Perioperative Temperature Management	112	100%	100%	100%
Prophylactic Antibiotic Selection	59	100%	99%	99%
Prophylactic Antibiotic Selection (Outpatient)	46	100%	98%	98%
Prophylactic Antibiotic Stopped	56	100%	97%	98%
Prophylactic Antibiotic Timing	59	100%	99%	99%
Prophylactic Antibiotic Timing (Outpatient)	46	100%	98%	98%
Urinary Catheter Removal	53	98%	97%	97%
Survey of Patients' Hospital Experiences				
Area Around Room 'Always' Quiet at Night	300+	68%	72%	61%
Doctors 'Always' Communicated Well	300+	85%	86%	82%
Home Recovery Information Given	300+	81%	83%	85%
Hospital Given 9 or 10 on 10 Point Scale	300+	62%	71%	71%
Meds 'Always' Explained Before Given	300+	63%	67%	64%
Nurses 'Always' Communicated Well	300+	77%	81%	79%
Pain 'Always' Well Controlled	300+	69%	72%	71%
Room and Bathroom 'Always' Clean	300+	59%	74%	73%
Timely Help 'Always' Received	300+	63%	69%	68%
Would Definitely Recommend Hospital	300+	57%	69%	71%
Use of Medical Imaging				
Cardiac Imaging Stress Test before Surgery[7]	-	-	5.7%	5.3%
Combination Abdominal CT Scan	234	7.7%	12.9%	10.5%
Combination Brain/Sinus CT Scan	370	5.1%	3.3%	2.7%
Combination Chest CT Scan	84	2.4%	6.1%	2.7%
Follow-up Mammogram/Ultrasound	335	15.2%	8.4%	8.8%
Lumbar Spine MRI for Low Back Pain	57	40.4%	41.1%	37.2%

Covington County Hospital CAH

701 South Holly Avenue
Collins, MS 39428
Type: Critical Access Hospitals
Ownership: Government - Local

Phone: 601-765-6711
Fax: 601-698-0180
Emergency Services: Yes
Beds: 82

Key Personnel:
Quality Assurance . . . . Irving Hitt
CEO/President. . . . . Clay Johnson
Chief of Medical Staff. . . . . Ward Johnson
Infection Control. . . . . Audie Lawson
Emergency Room . . . . Betty Mason, RN
Operating Room. . . . . Lynn Scott, RN

Measure	Cases	This Hosp.	State Avg.	U.S. Avg.
Blood Clot Prevention and Treatment				
Anticoagulation Overlap Therapy[1,3]	-	-	86%	93%
ICU Venous Thromboembolism Prophylaxis[3,7]	-	-	86%	92%
Incidence of Potentially Preventable VTE[3,7]	-	-	15%	10%
UFH with Dosages/Platelet Monitoring[3,7]	-	-	94%	97%
Venous Thromboembolism Prophylaxis[3,7]	-	-	70%	85%
Warfarin Therapy Discharge Instructions[1,3]	-	-	77%	75%
Chest Pain/Possible Heart Attack Care				
Aspirin Given Within 24 Hours of Arrival	22	95%	94%	96%
Fibrinolytic Meds Within 30 Min. of Arrival[3,7]	-	-	40%	58%
Average Time to ECG (minutes)	24	12	10	7
Average Time to Transfer (minutes)[3,7]	-	-	77	60
Children's Asthma Care				
Received Home Management Plan of Care	-	-	-	88%
Received Reliever Medication	-	-	-	100%
Received Systemic Corticosteroids	-	-	-	100%
Emergency Department				
Admittance Decision Time (minutes)	208	70	61	98
Head CT Results Within 45 Min. of Arrival[1]	-	-	42%	57%
Patients Who Left ER Before Being Seen[5]	-	-	3%	2%
Time from ER Arrival to Admit. (minutes)	215	243	223	274
Time from ER Arrival to Discharge (minutes)	312	112	112	134
Time in ER Before Being Evaluated (minutes)	308	23	29	26
Time to Pain Meds for Fractures (minutes)	29	69	68	57
Heart Attack Care				
Aspirin Given at Discharge[5]	-	-	99%	99%
Fibrinolytic Meds Within 30 Min. of Arrival[5]	-	-	50%	54%
PCI Within 90 Minutes of Arrival[5]	-	-	96%	96%
Statin Prescribed at Discharge[5]	-	-	97%	98%
Heart Failure Care				
ACE Inhibitor or ARB for LVSD[1]	-	-	93%	97%
Discharge Instructions Given	14	100%	91%	94%
Evaluation of LVS Function	18	50%	96%	99%
Medicare Spending				
Medicare Spending per Patient (ratio)	-	-	0.95	0.98
Pneumonia Care				

NOTE: Hospital profiles are in alphabetical order by state, then city, then hospital within the city; Rankings exclude hospitals with less than 25 cases except for patient surveys which excludes hospitals with less than 100 cases; (a) 100-299 cases; (1) The number of cases/patients is too few to report; (2) Data submitted were based on a sample of cases/patients; (3) Results are based on a shorter time period than required; (4) Data suppressed by CMS for one or more quarters; (5) Results are not available for this reporting period; (6) Fewer than 100 patients completed the HCAHPS survey; (7) No cases met the criteria for this measure; (8) The lower limit of the confidence interval cannot be calculated if the number of observed infections equals zero; (9) No data are available from the state/territory for this reporting period; (10) The scores shown reflect fewer than 50 completed surveys; (11) There were discrepancies in the data collection process; (12) This measure does not apply to this hospital for this reporting period; (13) Results cannot be calculated for this reporting period; (14) The results for this state are combined with nearby states to protect confidentiality; Please refer to the User's Guide for a full explanation of data.

Appropriate Initial Antibiotic Given	14	57%	91%	95%
Blood Culture Timing	24	92%	97%	98%
Pregnancy and Delivery Care				
Newborn Deliveries Scheduled Early[5]	-	-	22%	6%
Preventive Care				
Immunization for Influenza	75	61%	87%	90%
Immunization for Pneumonia	201	40%	89%	92%
Stroke Care				
Anticoagulation Therapy for Atrial Fibrillation[5]	-	-	93%	95%
Antithrombotic Therapy Timing[5]	-	-	96%	98%
Assessed for Rehabilitation[5]	-	-	95%	97%
Discharged on Antithrombotic Therapy[5]	-	-	97%	99%
Discharged on Statin Medication[5]	-	-	88%	94%
Thrombolytic Therapy Timing[5]	-	-	25%	66%
Venous Thromboembolism Prophylaxis[5]	-	-	87%	94%
Written Stroke Educational Materials Given[5]	-	-	84%	88%
Surgical Care Improvement Project				
Appropriate Beta Blocker Usage[5]	-	-	97%	98%
Appropriate VTP Within 24 Hours[5]	-	-	97%	98%
Controlled Postoperative Blood Glucose[5]	-	-	97%	97%
Perioperative Temperature Management[5]	-	-	100%	100%
Prophylactic Antibiotic Selection[5]	-	-	99%	99%
Prophylactic Antibiotic Selection (Outpatient)[5]	-	-	98%	98%
Prophylactic Antibiotic Stopped[5]	-	-	97%	98%
Prophylactic Antibiotic Timing[5]	-	-	99%	99%
Prophylactic Antibiotic Timing (Outpatient)[5]	-	-	98%	98%
Urinary Catheter Removal[5]	-	-	97%	97%
Survey of Patients' Hospital Experiences				
Area Around Room 'Always' Quiet at Night[5]	-	-	72%	61%
Doctors 'Always' Communicated Well[5]	-	-	86%	82%
Home Recovery Information Given[5]	-	-	83%	85%
Hospital Given 9 or 10 on 10 Point Scale[5]	-	-	71%	71%
Meds 'Always' Explained Before Given[5]	-	-	67%	64%
Nurses 'Always' Communicated Well[5]	-	-	81%	79%
Pain 'Always' Well Controlled[5]	-	-	72%	71%
Room and Bathroom 'Always' Clean[5]	-	-	74%	73%
Timely Help 'Always' Received[5]	-	-	69%	68%
Would Definitely Recommend Hospital[5]	-	-	69%	71%
Use of Medical Imaging				
Cardiac Imaging Stress Test before Surgery[1]	-	-	5.7%	5.3%
Combination Abdominal CT Scan	140	1.4%	12.9%	10.5%
Combination Brain/Sinus CT Scan[1]	-	-	3.3%	2.7%
Combination Chest CT Scan[1]	-	-	6.1%	2.7%
Follow-up Mammogram/Ultrasound[7]	-	-	8.4%	8.8%
Lumbar Spine MRI for Low Back Pain[7]	-	-	41.1%	37.2%

Marion General Hospital

1560 Sumrall Rd — Phone: 601-736-6303
Columbia, MS 39429 — Fax: 601-740-2244
Type: Acute Care Hospitals — Emergency Services: Yes
Ownership: Voluntary non-profit - Other — Beds: 90

Key Personnel:
CEO/President . . . . Jerry Howell
Anesthesiology. . . . . Ronald H Luethje
Radiology. . . . . Rosalind Mikell

Measure	Cases	This Hosp.	State Avg.	U.S. Avg.
Blood Clot Prevention and Treatment				
Anticoagulation Overlap Therapy[2]	14	93%	86%	93%
ICU Venous Thromboembolism Prophylaxis[2,7]	-	-	86%	92%
Incidence of Potentially Preventable VTE[1,2]	-	-	15%	10%
UFH with Dosages/Platelet Monitoring[2,7]	-	-	94%	97%
Venous Thromboembolism Prophylaxis[2]	426	73%	70%	85%
Warfarin Therapy Discharge Instructions[1,2]	-	-	77%	75%
Chest Pain/Possible Heart Attack Care				
Aspirin Given Within 24 Hours of Arrival	28	86%	94%	96%
Fibrinolytic Meds Within 30 Min. of Arrival[7]	-	-	40%	58%
Average Time to ECG (minutes)	28	10	10	7
Average Time to Transfer (minutes)[1]	-	-	77	60
Children's Asthma Care				
Received Home Management Plan of Care	-	-	-	88%
Received Reliever Medication	-	-	-	100%
Received Systemic Corticosteroids	-	-	-	100%
Emergency Department				
Admittance Decision Time (minutes)[2]	434	60	61	98
Head CT Results Within 45 Min. of Arrival[1]	-	-	42%	57%
Patients Who Left ER Before Being Seen	18,404	4%	3%	2%
Time from ER Arrival to Admit. (minutes)[2]	488	208	223	274
Time from ER Arrival to Discharge (minutes)	475	113	112	134
Time in ER Before Being Evaluated (minutes)	547	31	29	26
Time to Pain Meds for Fractures (minutes)	57	82	68	57
Heart Attack Care				
Aspirin Given at Discharge[1]	-	-	99%	99%
Fibrinolytic Meds Within 30 Min. of Arrival[7]	-	-	50%	54%
PCI Within 90 Minutes of Arrival[7]	-	-	96%	96%
Statin Prescribed at Discharge[1]	-	-	97%	98%
Heart Failure Care				
ACE Inhibitor or ARB for LVSD[2]	21	90%	93%	97%
Discharge Instructions Given[2]	50	56%	91%	94%
Evaluation of LVS Function[2]	63	98%	96%	99%
Medicare Spending				
Medicare Spending per Patient (ratio)	-	0.93	0.95	0.98
Pneumonia Care				
Appropriate Initial Antibiotic Given[2]	48	94%	91%	95%
Blood Culture Timing[2]	62	97%	97%	98%
Pregnancy and Delivery Care				
Newborn Deliveries Scheduled Early[7]	-	-	22%	6%
Preventive Care				
Immunization for Influenza[2]	352	92%	87%	90%
Immunization for Pneumonia[2]	538	93%	89%	92%
Stroke Care				
Anticoagulation Therapy for Atrial Fibrillation[1,2]	-	-	93%	95%
Antithrombotic Therapy Timing[1,2]	-	-	96%	98%
Assessed for Rehabilitation[1,2]	-	-	95%	97%
Discharged on Antithrombotic Therapy[1,2]	-	-	97%	99%
Discharged on Statin Medication[1,2]	-	-	88%	94%
Thrombolytic Therapy Timing[1,2]	-	-	25%	66%
Venous Thromboembolism Prophylaxis[1,2]	-	-	87%	94%
Written Stroke Educational Materials Given[1,2]	-	-	84%	88%
Surgical Care Improvement Project				
Appropriate Beta Blocker Usage[5]	-	-	97%	98%
Appropriate VTP Within 24 Hours[5]	-	-	97%	98%
Controlled Postoperative Blood Glucose[5]	-	-	97%	97%
Perioperative Temperature Management[5]	-	-	100%	100%
Prophylactic Antibiotic Selection[5]	-	-	99%	99%
Prophylactic Antibiotic Selection (Outpatient)[5]	-	-	98%	98%
Prophylactic Antibiotic Stopped[5]	-	-	97%	98%
Prophylactic Antibiotic Timing[5]	-	-	99%	99%
Prophylactic Antibiotic Timing (Outpatient)[5]	-	-	98%	98%
Urinary Catheter Removal[5]	-	-	97%	97%
Survey of Patients' Hospital Experiences				
Area Around Room 'Always' Quiet at Night	(a)	68%	72%	61%
Doctors 'Always' Communicated Well	(a)	82%	86%	82%
Home Recovery Information Given	(a)	80%	83%	85%
Hospital Given 9 or 10 on 10 Point Scale	(a)	60%	71%	71%
Meds 'Always' Explained Before Given	(a)	62%	67%	64%
Nurses 'Always' Communicated Well	(a)	74%	81%	79%
Pain 'Always' Well Controlled	(a)	62%	72%	71%
Room and Bathroom 'Always' Clean	(a)	59%	74%	73%
Timely Help 'Always' Received	(a)	56%	69%	68%
Would Definitely Recommend Hospital	(a)	59%	69%	71%
Use of Medical Imaging				
Cardiac Imaging Stress Test before Surgery[1]	-	-	5.7%	5.3%
Combination Abdominal CT Scan	201	2.0%	12.9%	10.5%
Combination Brain/Sinus CT Scan	373	5.1%	3.3%	2.7%
Combination Chest CT Scan	96	0.0%	6.1%	2.7%
Follow-up Mammogram/Ultrasound[7]	-	-	8.4%	8.8%
Lumbar Spine MRI for Low Back Pain[7]	-	-	41.1%	37.2%

Baptist Memorial Hospital/Golden Triangle

2520 5th Saint N — Phone: 662-244-1500
Columbus, MS 39701 — Fax: 662-244-1564
URL: www.bmhcc.org/facilities/goldentriangle
Type: Acute Care Hospitals — Emergency Services: Yes
Ownership: Voluntary non-profit - Private — Beds: 328

Key Personnel:
Administrator . . . . Paul Cade
Chief of Medical Staff. . . . . Michael Duckworth, MD
Operating Room. . . . . Francine Glenn
CEO/President. . . . . Jason Little
Radiology. . . . . Barry McAllister

Measure	Cases	This Hosp.	State Avg.	U.S. Avg.
Blood Clot Prevention and Treatment				
Anticoagulation Overlap Therapy[2]	50	100%	86%	93%
ICU Venous Thromboembolism Prophylaxis[2]	118	97%	86%	92%
Incidence of Potentially Preventable VTE[1,2]	-	-	15%	10%
UFH with Dosages/Platelet Monitoring[2]	14	100%	94%	97%
Venous Thromboembolism Prophylaxis[2]	348	94%	70%	85%
Warfarin Therapy Discharge Instructions[2]	40	92%	77%	75%
Chest Pain/Possible Heart Attack Care				
Aspirin Given Within 24 Hours of Arrival	12	92%	94%	96%
Fibrinolytic Meds Within 30 Min. of Arrival[3,7]	-	-	40%	58%
Average Time to ECG (minutes)	13	14	10	7
Average Time to Transfer (minutes)[3,7]	-	-	77	60
Children's Asthma Care				
Received Home Management Plan of Care	-	-	-	88%
Received Reliever Medication	-	-	-	100%
Received Systemic Corticosteroids	-	-	-	100%
Emergency Department				
Admittance Decision Time (minutes)[2]	493	77	61	98
Head CT Results Within 45 Min. of Arrival	15	60%	42%	57%
Patients Who Left ER Before Being Seen	58,026	1%	3%	2%
Time from ER Arrival to Admit. (minutes)[2]	519	254	223	274
Time from ER Arrival to Discharge (minutes)	368	150	112	134
Time in ER Before Being Evaluated (minutes)	384	54	29	26
Time to Pain Meds for Fractures (minutes)	121	78	68	57
Heart Attack Care				
Aspirin Given at Discharge	143	100%	99%	99%
Fibrinolytic Meds Within 30 Min. of Arrival[7]	-	-	50%	54%
PCI Within 90 Minutes of Arrival	41	100%	96%	96%
Statin Prescribed at Discharge	137	100%	97%	98%
Heart Failure Care				
ACE Inhibitor or ARB for LVSD	86	100%	93%	97%
Discharge Instructions Given	184	98%	91%	94%
Evaluation of LVS Function	212	100%	96%	99%
Medicare Spending				
Medicare Spending per Patient (ratio)	-	0.98	0.95	0.98
Pneumonia Care				
Appropriate Initial Antibiotic Given	74	99%	91%	95%
Blood Culture Timing	191	99%	97%	98%
Pregnancy and Delivery Care				
Newborn Deliveries Scheduled Early[2]	22	23%	22%	6%
Preventive Care				
Immunization for Influenza[2]	559	98%	87%	90%
Immunization for Pneumonia[2]	698	98%	89%	92%
Stroke Care				
Anticoagulation Therapy for Atrial Fibrillation	12	100%	93%	95%
Antithrombotic Therapy Timing	96	100%	96%	98%
Assessed for Rehabilitation	109	100%	95%	97%
Discharged on Antithrombotic Therapy	105	100%	97%	99%
Discharged on Statin Medication	73	100%	88%	94%
Thrombolytic Therapy Timing[1]	-	-	25%	66%
Venous Thromboembolism Prophylaxis	97	98%	87%	94%
Written Stroke Educational Materials Given	62	98%	84%	88%
Surgical Care Improvement Project				
Appropriate Beta Blocker Usage	198	99%	97%	98%
Appropriate VTP Within 24 Hours	582	100%	97%	98%
Controlled Postoperative Blood Glucose	47	94%	97%	97%
Perioperative Temperature Management	627	100%	100%	100%
Prophylactic Antibiotic Selection	467	100%	99%	99%
Prophylactic Antibiotic Selection (Outpatient)	334	100%	98%	98%
Prophylactic Antibiotic Stopped	450	99%	97%	98%
Prophylactic Antibiotic Timing	467	100%	99%	99%
Prophylactic Antibiotic Timing (Outpatient)	334	99%	98%	98%
Urinary Catheter Removal	164	98%	97%	97%
Survey of Patients' Hospital Experiences				
Area Around Room 'Always' Quiet at Night	300+	74%	72%	61%
Doctors 'Always' Communicated Well	300+	84%	86%	82%
Home Recovery Information Given	300+	81%	83%	85%
Hospital Given 9 or 10 on 10 Point Scale	300+	69%	71%	71%

NOTE: Hospital profiles are in alphabetical order by state, then city, then hospital within the city; Rankings exclude hospitals with less than 25 cases except for patient surveys which excludes hospitals with less than 100 cases; (a) 100-299 cases; (1) The number of cases/patients is too few to report; (2) Data submitted were based on a sample of cases/patients; (3) Results are based on a shorter time period than required; (4) Data suppressed by CMS for one or more quarters; (5) Results are not available for this reporting period; (6) Fewer than 100 patients completed the HCAHPS survey; (7) No cases met the criteria for this measure; (8) The lower limit of the confidence interval cannot be calculated if the number of observed infections equals zero; (9) No data are available from the state/territory for this reporting period; (10) The scores shown reflect fewer than 50 completed surveys; (11) There were discrepancies in the data collection process; (12) This measure does not apply to this hospital for this reporting period; (13) Results cannot be calculated for this reporting period; (14) The results for this state are combined with nearby states to protect confidentiality; Please refer to the User's Guide for a full explanation of data.

Meds 'Always' Explained Before Given	300+	66%	67%	64%
Nurses 'Always' Communicated Well	300+	80%	81%	79%
Pain 'Always' Well Controlled	300+	74%	72%	71%
Room and Bathroom 'Always' Clean	300+	74%	74%	73%
Timely Help 'Always' Received	300+	64%	69%	68%
Would Definitely Recommend Hospital	300+	66%	69%	71%
Use of Medical Imaging				
Cardiac Imaging Stress Test before Surgery[1]	-	-	5.7%	5.3%
Combination Abdominal CT Scan	1,712	17.1%	12.9%	10.5%
Combination Brain/Sinus CT Scan	977	3.1%	3.3%	2.7%
Combination Chest CT Scan	938	0.1%	6.1%	2.7%
Follow-up Mammogram/Ultrasound	1,263	3.2%	8.4%	8.8%
Lumbar Spine MRI for Low Back Pain	117	41.9%	41.1%	37.2%

Magnolia Regional Health Center

611 Alcorn Drive
Corinth, MS 38834
Phone: 662-293-7660
Fax: 662-293-4285
E-mail: info@mrhc.org
URL: www.mrhc.org
Type: Acute Care Hospitals
Emergency Services: Yes
Ownership: Voluntary non-profit - Other
Beds: 164

Key Personnel:
Cardiac Laboratory. . . . . Tommy Bain
Chief of Medical Staff. . . . . Chauntay Bradley
Radiology. . . . . Donna Crandell
Coronary Care. . . . . Rick Crane
CEO/President. . . . . Ronny Humes
Quality Assurance . . . . Lydia Linton
Infection Control. . . . . Elwanda Whiteker
Operating Room. . . . . Betsy Wood

Measure	Cases	This Hosp.	State Avg.	U.S. Avg.
Blood Clot Prevention and Treatment				
Anticoagulation Overlap Therapy[2]	35	100%	86%	93%
ICU Venous Thromboembolism Prophylaxis[2]	147	100%	86%	92%
Incidence of Potentially Preventable VTE[2]	11	0%	15%	10%
UFH with Dosages/Platelet Monitoring[2]	23	100%	94%	97%
Venous Thromboembolism Prophylaxis[2]	268	97%	70%	85%
Warfarin Therapy Discharge Instructions[2]	19	100%	77%	75%
Chest Pain/Possible Heart Attack Care				
Aspirin Given Within 24 Hours of Arrival[1]	-	-	94%	96%
Fibrinolytic Meds Within 30 Min. of Arrival[5]	-	-	40%	58%
Average Time to ECG (minutes)[1]	-	-	10	7
Average Time to Transfer (minutes)[5]	-	-	77	60
Children's Asthma Care				
Received Home Management Plan of Care	-	-	-	88%
Received Reliever Medication	-	-	-	100%
Received Systemic Corticosteroids	-	-	-	100%
Emergency Department				
Admittance Decision Time (minutes)[2]	684	71	61	98
Head CT Results Within 45 Min. of Arrival[1]	-	-	42%	57%
Patients Who Left ER Before Being Seen	35,740	4%	3%	2%
Time from ER Arrival to Admit. (minutes)[2]	684	243	223	274
Time from ER Arrival to Discharge (minutes)	526	137	112	134
Time in ER Before Being Evaluated (minutes)	541	47	29	26
Time to Pain Meds for Fractures (minutes)	120	73	68	57
Heart Attack Care				
Aspirin Given at Discharge	188	100%	99%	99%
Fibrinolytic Meds Within 30 Min. of Arrival[1]	-	-	50%	54%
PCI Within 90 Minutes of Arrival	28	100%	96%	96%
Statin Prescribed at Discharge	173	99%	97%	98%
Heart Failure Care				
ACE Inhibitor or ARB for LVSD	84	98%	93%	97%
Discharge Instructions Given	191	99%	91%	94%
Evaluation of LVS Function	238	100%	96%	99%
Medicare Spending				
Medicare Spending per Patient (ratio)	-	0.96	0.95	0.98
Pneumonia Care				
Appropriate Initial Antibiotic Given	162	94%	91%	95%
Blood Culture Timing	197	99%	97%	98%
Pregnancy and Delivery Care				
Newborn Deliveries Scheduled Early	70	7%	22%	6%
Preventive Care				
Immunization for Influenza[2]	696	98%	87%	90%
Immunization for Pneumonia[2]	874	97%	89%	92%
Stroke Care				
Anticoagulation Therapy for Atrial Fibrillation	16	100%	93%	95%
Antithrombotic Therapy Timing	94	100%	96%	98%
Assessed for Rehabilitation	98	100%	95%	97%
Discharged on Antithrombotic Therapy	91	100%	97%	99%
Discharged on Statin Medication	75	100%	88%	94%
Thrombolytic Therapy Timing[1]	-	-	25%	66%
Venous Thromboembolism Prophylaxis	108	98%	87%	94%
Written Stroke Educational Materials Given	56	82%	84%	88%
Surgical Care Improvement Project				
Appropriate Beta Blocker Usage	261	99%	97%	98%
Appropriate VTP Within 24 Hours	450	99%	97%	98%
Controlled Postoperative Blood Glucose	153	89%	97%	97%
Perioperative Temperature Management	601	100%	100%	100%
Prophylactic Antibiotic Selection	551	100%	99%	99%
Prophylactic Antibiotic Selection (Outpatient)	245	98%	98%	98%
Prophylactic Antibiotic Stopped	541	98%	97%	98%
Prophylactic Antibiotic Timing	563	100%	99%	99%
Prophylactic Antibiotic Timing (Outpatient)	246	99%	98%	98%
Urinary Catheter Removal	202	100%	97%	97%
Survey of Patients' Hospital Experiences				
Area Around Room 'Always' Quiet at Night	300+	78%	72%	61%
Doctors 'Always' Communicated Well	300+	86%	86%	82%
Home Recovery Information Given	300+	90%	83%	85%
Hospital Given 9 or 10 on 10 Point Scale	300+	77%	71%	71%
Meds 'Always' Explained Before Given	300+	71%	67%	64%
Nurses 'Always' Communicated Well	300+	85%	81%	79%
Pain 'Always' Well Controlled	300+	78%	72%	71%
Room and Bathroom 'Always' Clean	300+	79%	74%	73%
Timely Help 'Always' Received	300+	74%	69%	68%
Would Definitely Recommend Hospital	300+	80%	69%	71%
Use of Medical Imaging				
Cardiac Imaging Stress Test before Surgery	957	5.4%	5.7%	5.3%
Combination Abdominal CT Scan	1,814	3.3%	12.9%	10.5%
Combination Brain/Sinus CT Scan	1,108	5.5%	3.3%	2.7%
Combination Chest CT Scan	1,074	0.2%	6.1%	2.7%
Follow-up Mammogram/Ultrasound	1,022	12.6%	8.4%	8.8%
Lumbar Spine MRI for Low Back Pain	302	35.4%	41.1%	37.2%

John C Stennis Memorial Hospital

14365 Highway 16 West
De Kalb, MS 39328
Phone: 769-486-1000
Type: Critical Access Hospitals
Emergency Services: Yes
Ownership: Voluntary non-profit - Private

Measure	Cases	This Hosp.	State Avg.	U.S. Avg.
Blood Clot Prevention and Treatment				
Anticoagulation Overlap Therapy[5]	-	-	86%	93%
ICU Venous Thromboembolism Prophylaxis[5]	-	-	86%	92%
Incidence of Potentially Preventable VTE[5]	-	-	15%	10%
UFH with Dosages/Platelet Monitoring[5]	-	-	94%	97%
Venous Thromboembolism Prophylaxis[5]	-	-	70%	85%
Warfarin Therapy Discharge Instructions[5]	-	-	77%	75%
Chest Pain/Possible Heart Attack Care				
Aspirin Given Within 24 Hours of Arrival[1,3]	-	-	94%	96%
Fibrinolytic Meds Within 30 Min. of Arrival[1,3]	-	-	40%	58%
Average Time to ECG (minutes)[1,3]	-	-	10	7
Average Time to Transfer (minutes)[1,3]	-	-	77	60
Children's Asthma Care				
Received Home Management Plan of Care	-	-	-	88%
Received Reliever Medication	-	-	-	100%
Received Systemic Corticosteroids	-	-	-	100%
Emergency Department				
Admittance Decision Time (minutes)[5]	-	-	61	98
Head CT Results Within 45 Min. of Arrival[5]	-	-	42%	57%
Patients Who Left ER Before Being Seen[5]	-	-	3%	2%
Time from ER Arrival to Admit. (minutes)[5]	-	-	223	274
Time from ER Arrival to Discharge (minutes)[5]	-	-	112	134
Time in ER Before Being Evaluated (minutes)[5]	-	-	29	26
Time to Pain Meds for Fractures (minutes)[5]	-	-	68	57
Heart Attack Care				
Aspirin Given at Discharge[5]	-	-	99%	99%
Fibrinolytic Meds Within 30 Min. of Arrival[5]	-	-	50%	54%
PCI Within 90 Minutes of Arrival[5]	-	-	96%	96%
Statin Prescribed at Discharge[5]	-	-	97%	98%
Heart Failure Care				
ACE Inhibitor or ARB for LVSD[2,3]	-	-	93%	97%
Discharge Instructions Given[1,2]	-	-	91%	94%
Evaluation of LVS Function[1,2]	-	-	96%	99%
Medicare Spending				
Medicare Spending per Patient (ratio)	-	-	0.95	0.98
Pneumonia Care				
Appropriate Initial Antibiotic Given[1,2]	-	-	91%	95%
Blood Culture Timing[1,2]	-	-	97%	98%
Pregnancy and Delivery Care				
Newborn Deliveries Scheduled Early[5]	-	-	22%	6%
Preventive Care				
Immunization for Influenza[5]	-	-	87%	90%
Immunization for Pneumonia[5]	-	-	89%	92%
Stroke Care				
Anticoagulation Therapy for Atrial Fibrillation[5]	-	-	93%	95%
Antithrombotic Therapy Timing[5]	-	-	96%	98%
Assessed for Rehabilitation[5]	-	-	95%	97%
Discharged on Antithrombotic Therapy[5]	-	-	97%	99%
Discharged on Statin Medication[5]	-	-	88%	94%
Thrombolytic Therapy Timing[5]	-	-	25%	66%
Venous Thromboembolism Prophylaxis[5]	-	-	87%	94%
Written Stroke Educational Materials Given[5]	-	-	84%	88%
Surgical Care Improvement Project				
Appropriate Beta Blocker Usage[5]	-	-	97%	98%
Appropriate VTP Within 24 Hours[5]	-	-	97%	98%
Controlled Postoperative Blood Glucose[5]	-	-	97%	97%
Perioperative Temperature Management[5]	-	-	100%	100%
Prophylactic Antibiotic Selection[5]	-	-	99%	99%
Prophylactic Antibiotic Selection (Outpatient)[5]	-	-	98%	98%
Prophylactic Antibiotic Stopped[5]	-	-	97%	98%
Prophylactic Antibiotic Timing[5]	-	-	99%	99%
Prophylactic Antibiotic Timing (Outpatient)[5]	-	-	98%	98%
Urinary Catheter Removal[5]	-	-	97%	97%
Survey of Patients' Hospital Experiences				
Area Around Room 'Always' Quiet at Night[10]	<100	86%	72%	61%
Doctors 'Always' Communicated Well[10]	<100	82%	86%	82%
Home Recovery Information Given[10]	<100	91%	83%	85%
Hospital Given 9 or 10 on 10 Point Scale[10]	<100	75%	71%	71%
Meds 'Always' Explained Before Given[10]	<100	45%	67%	64%
Nurses 'Always' Communicated Well[10]	<100	81%	81%	79%
Pain 'Always' Well Controlled[10]	<100	77%	72%	71%
Room and Bathroom 'Always' Clean[10]	<100	80%	74%	73%
Timely Help 'Always' Received[10]	<100	76%	69%	68%
Would Definitely Recommend Hospital[10]	<100	72%	69%	71%
Use of Medical Imaging				
Cardiac Imaging Stress Test before Surgery[1]	-	-	5.7%	5.3%
Combination Abdominal CT Scan[1]	-	-	12.9%	10.5%
Combination Brain/Sinus CT Scan	128	0.0%	3.3%	2.7%
Combination Chest CT Scan[1]	-	-	6.1%	2.7%
Follow-up Mammogram/Ultrasound[7]	-	-	8.4%	8.8%
Lumbar Spine MRI for Low Back Pain[1]	-	-	41.1%	37.2%

Webster General Hospital/Swing Bed

70 Medical Plaza
Eupora, MS 39744
Phone: 662-258-6221
Fax: 662-258-9291
Type: Acute Care Hospitals
Emergency Services: Yes
Ownership: Voluntary non-profit - Other
Beds: 33

Key Personnel:
Quality Assurance . . . . Gaye Bekkering, RN
Operating Room. . . . . James Edward Booth, RN
Emergency Room . . . . Evelyn Easley, RN
Infection Control. . . . . Sherrie Johnson, RN
Chief of Medical Staff. . . . . Charles Ozborn, MD

Measure	Cases	This Hosp.	State Avg.	U.S. Avg.
Blood Clot Prevention and Treatment				
Anticoagulation Overlap Therapy[1,2]	-	-	86%	93%
ICU Venous Thromboembolism Prophylaxis[2,7]	-	-	86%	92%
Incidence of Potentially Preventable VTE[2,7]	-	-	15%	10%
UFH with Dosages/Platelet Monitoring[2,7]	-	-	94%	97%
Venous Thromboembolism Prophylaxis[2]	182	71%	70%	85%

NOTE: Hospital profiles are in alphabetical order by state, then city, then hospital within the city; Rankings exclude hospitals with less than 25 cases except for patient surveys which excludes hospitals with less than 100 cases; (a) 100-299 cases; (1) The number of cases/patients is too few to report; (2) Data submitted were based on a sample of cases/patients; (3) Results are based on a shorter time period than required; (4) Data suppressed by CMS for one or more quarters; (5) Results are not available for this reporting period; (6) Fewer than 100 patients completed the HCAHPS survey; (7) No cases met the criteria for this measure; (8) The lower limit of the confidence interval cannot be calculated if the number of observed infections equals zero; (9) No data are available from the state/territory for this reporting period; (10) The scores shown reflect fewer than 50 completed surveys; (11) There were discrepancies in the data collection process; (12) This measure does not apply to this hospital for this reporting period; (13) Results cannot be calculated for this reporting period; (14) The results for this state are combined with nearby states to protect confidentiality; Please refer to the User's Guide for a full explanation of data.

Measure	Cases	This Hosp.	State Avg.	U.S. Avg.
Warfarin Therapy Discharge Instructions[1,2]	-	-	77%	75%
Chest Pain/Possible Heart Attack Care				
Aspirin Given Within 24 Hours of Arrival	24	96%	94%	96%
Fibrinolytic Meds Within 30 Min. of Arrival[7]	-	-	40%	58%
Average Time to ECG (minutes)	23	8	10	7
Average Time to Transfer (minutes)[1]	-	-	77	60
Children's Asthma Care				
Received Home Management Plan of Care	-	-	-	88%
Received Reliever Medication	-	-	-	100%
Received Systemic Corticosteroids	-	-	-	100%
Emergency Department				
Admittance Decision Time (minutes)[2]	274	31	61	98
Head CT Results Within 45 Min. of Arrival[1]	-	-	42%	57%
Patients Who Left ER Before Being Seen	8,890	1%	3%	2%
Time from ER Arrival to Admit. (minutes)[2]	309	155	223	274
Time from ER Arrival to Discharge (minutes)	379	75	112	134
Time in ER Before Being Evaluated (minutes)	394	20	29	26
Time to Pain Meds for Fractures (minutes)	18	50	68	57
Heart Attack Care				
Aspirin Given at Discharge[1,3]	-	-	99%	99%
Fibrinolytic Meds Within 30 Min. of Arrival[3,7]	-	-	50%	54%
PCI Within 90 Minutes of Arrival[3,7]	-	-	96%	96%
Statin Prescribed at Discharge[1,3]	-	-	97%	98%
Heart Failure Care				
ACE Inhibitor or ARB for LVSD	14	100%	93%	97%
Discharge Instructions Given	34	100%	91%	94%
Evaluation of LVS Function	43	100%	96%	99%
Medicare Spending				
Medicare Spending per Patient (ratio)	-	0.92	0.95	0.98
Pneumonia Care				
Appropriate Initial Antibiotic Given	88	85%	91%	95%
Blood Culture Timing	84	98%	97%	98%
Pregnancy and Delivery Care				
Newborn Deliveries Scheduled Early[7]	-	-	22%	6%
Preventive Care				
Immunization for Influenza[2]	319	97%	87%	90%
Immunization for Pneumonia[2]	495	98%	89%	92%
Stroke Care				
Anticoagulation Therapy for Atrial Fibrillation[1,2]	-	-	93%	95%
Antithrombotic Therapy Timing[2]	27	96%	96%	98%
Assessed for Rehabilitation[2]	28	93%	95%	97%
Discharged on Antithrombotic Therapy[2]	27	93%	97%	99%
Discharged on Statin Medication[2]	21	95%	88%	94%
Thrombolytic Therapy Timing[2,7]	-	-	25%	66%
Venous Thromboembolism Prophylaxis[2]	28	82%	87%	94%
Written Stroke Educational Materials Given[2]	14	86%	84%	88%
Surgical Care Improvement Project				
Appropriate Beta Blocker Usage[5]	-	-	97%	98%
Appropriate VTP Within 24 Hours[5]	-	-	97%	98%
Controlled Postoperative Blood Glucose[5]	-	-	97%	97%
Perioperative Temperature Management[5]	-	-	100%	100%
Prophylactic Antibiotic Selection[5]	-	-	99%	99%
Prophylactic Antibiotic Selection (Outpatient)[5]	-	-	98%	98%
Prophylactic Antibiotic Stopped[5]	-	-	97%	98%
Prophylactic Antibiotic Timing[5]	-	-	99%	99%
Prophylactic Antibiotic Timing (Outpatient)[5]	-	-	98%	98%
Urinary Catheter Removal[5]	-	-	97%	97%
Survey of Patients' Hospital Experiences				
Area Around Room 'Always' Quiet at Night	(a)	72%	72%	61%
Doctors 'Always' Communicated Well	(a)	95%	86%	82%
Home Recovery Information Given	(a)	85%	83%	85%
Hospital Given 9 or 10 on 10 Point Scale	(a)	76%	71%	71%
Meds 'Always' Explained Before Given	(a)	75%	67%	64%
Nurses 'Always' Communicated Well	(a)	87%	81%	79%
Pain 'Always' Well Controlled	(a)	81%	72%	71%
Room and Bathroom 'Always' Clean	(a)	88%	74%	73%
Timely Help 'Always' Received	(a)	66%	69%	68%
Would Definitely Recommend Hospital	(a)	74%	69%	71%
Use of Medical Imaging				
Cardiac Imaging Stress Test before Surgery[7]	-	-	5.7%	5.3%
Combination Abdominal CT Scan	250	12.8%	12.9%	10.5%
Combination Brain/Sinus CT Scan[1]	-	-	3.3%	2.7%
Combination Chest CT Scan	77	5.2%	6.1%	2.7%
Follow-up Mammogram/Ultrasound[7]	-	-	8.4%	8.8%
Lumbar Spine MRI for Low Back Pain	101	35.6%	41.1%	37.2%

Jefferson County Hospital

870 S Main Box 577
Fayette, MS 39069
Phone: 601-786-3401
Fax: 601-786-3400

Type: Acute Care Hospitals
Ownership: Government - Local
Emergency Services: Yes
Beds: 30

Key Personnel:
Quality Assurance . . . . Mary Thomas
Emergency Room . . . . Ado Wilson

Measure	Cases	This Hosp.	State Avg.	U.S. Avg.
Blood Clot Prevention and Treatment				
Anticoagulation Overlap Therapy[2,7]	-	-	86%	93%
ICU Venous Thromboembolism Prophylaxis[2,7]	-	-	86%	92%
Incidence of Potentially Preventable VTE[2,7]	-	-	15%	10%
UFH with Dosages/Platelet Monitoring[2,7]	-	-	94%	97%
Venous Thromboembolism Prophylaxis[2]	25	0%	70%	85%
Warfarin Therapy Discharge Instructions[2,7]	-	-	77%	75%
Chest Pain/Possible Heart Attack Care				
Aspirin Given Within 24 Hours of Arrival[5]	-	-	94%	96%
Fibrinolytic Meds Within 30 Min. of Arrival[5]	-	-	40%	58%
Average Time to ECG (minutes)[5]	-	-	10	7
Average Time to Transfer (minutes)[5]	-	-	77	60
Children's Asthma Care				
Received Home Management Plan of Care	-	-	-	88%
Received Reliever Medication	-	-	-	100%
Received Systemic Corticosteroids	-	-	-	100%
Emergency Department				
Admittance Decision Time (minutes)[1,2]	-	-	61	98
Head CT Results Within 45 Min. of Arrival[5]	-	-	42%	57%
Patients Who Left ER Before Being Seen[5]	-	-	3%	2%
Time from ER Arrival to Admit. (minutes)[1,2]	-	-	223	274
Time from ER Arrival to Discharge (minutes)[3]	304	78	112	134
Time in ER Before Being Evaluated (minutes)[3]	331	10	29	26
Time to Pain Meds for Fractures (minutes)[5]	-	-	68	57
Heart Attack Care				
Aspirin Given at Discharge[5]	-	-	99%	99%
Fibrinolytic Meds Within 30 Min. of Arrival[5]	-	-	50%	54%
PCI Within 90 Minutes of Arrival[5]	-	-	96%	96%
Statin Prescribed at Discharge[5]	-	-	97%	98%
Heart Failure Care				
ACE Inhibitor or ARB for LVSD[2,7]	-	-	93%	97%
Discharge Instructions Given[1,2]	-	-	91%	94%
Evaluation of LVS Function[1,2]	-	-	96%	99%
Medicare Spending				
Medicare Spending per Patient (ratio)	-	0.97	0.95	0.98
Pneumonia Care				
Appropriate Initial Antibiotic Given[1,2]	-	-	91%	95%
Blood Culture Timing[2,3]	-	-	97%	98%
Pregnancy and Delivery Care				
Newborn Deliveries Scheduled Early[7]	-	-	22%	6%
Preventive Care				
Immunization for Influenza[2]	35	11%	87%	90%
Immunization for Pneumonia[2]	47	11%	89%	92%
Stroke Care				
Anticoagulation Therapy for Atrial Fibrillation[5]	-	-	93%	95%
Antithrombotic Therapy Timing[5]	-	-	96%	98%
Assessed for Rehabilitation[5]	-	-	95%	97%
Discharged on Antithrombotic Therapy[5]	-	-	97%	99%
Discharged on Statin Medication[5]	-	-	88%	94%
Thrombolytic Therapy Timing[5]	-	-	25%	66%
Venous Thromboembolism Prophylaxis[5]	-	-	87%	94%
Written Stroke Educational Materials Given[5]	-	-	84%	88%
Surgical Care Improvement Project				
Appropriate Beta Blocker Usage[5]	-	-	97%	98%
Appropriate VTP Within 24 Hours[5]	-	-	97%	98%
Controlled Postoperative Blood Glucose[5]	-	-	97%	97%
Perioperative Temperature Management[5]	-	-	100%	100%
Prophylactic Antibiotic Selection[5]	-	-	99%	99%
Prophylactic Antibiotic Selection (Outpatient)[5]	-	-	98%	98%
Prophylactic Antibiotic Stopped[5]	-	-	97%	98%
Prophylactic Antibiotic Timing[5]	-	-	99%	99%
Prophylactic Antibiotic Timing (Outpatient)[5]	-	-	98%	98%
Urinary Catheter Removal[5]	-	-	97%	97%
Survey of Patients' Hospital Experiences				
Area Around Room 'Always' Quiet at Night[6]	<100	85%	72%	61%
Doctors 'Always' Communicated Well[6]	<100	90%	86%	82%
Home Recovery Information Given[6]	<100	75%	83%	85%
Hospital Given 9 or 10 on 10 Point Scale[6]	<100	67%	71%	71%
Meds 'Always' Explained Before Given[6]	<100	77%	67%	64%
Nurses 'Always' Communicated Well[6]	<100	90%	81%	79%
Pain 'Always' Well Controlled[6]	<100	79%	72%	71%
Room and Bathroom 'Always' Clean[6]	<100	76%	74%	73%
Timely Help 'Always' Received[6]	<100	59%	69%	68%
Would Definitely Recommend Hospital[6]	<100	57%	69%	71%
Use of Medical Imaging				
Cardiac Imaging Stress Test before Surgery[7]	-	-	5.7%	5.3%
Combination Abdominal CT Scan[7]	-	-	12.9%	10.5%
Combination Brain/Sinus CT Scan[7]	-	-	3.3%	2.7%
Combination Chest CT Scan[7]	-	-	6.1%	2.7%
Follow-up Mammogram/Ultrasound[7]	-	-	8.4%	8.8%
Lumbar Spine MRI for Low Back Pain[7]	-	-	41.1%	37.2%

River Oaks Hospital

1030 River Oaks Drive
Flowood, MS 39232
Phone: 601-936-2390
Fax: 601-936-2275
URL: www.riveroakshospital.org

Type: Acute Care Hospitals
Ownership: Proprietary
Emergency Services: Yes
Beds: 110

Key Personnel:
CEO/President. . . . . Dennis R Bruns
Chief of Medical Staff . . . . C Ron Cannon
Radiology. . . . . Beverly Greenhill
Operating Room. . . . . Bob Newton
Infection Control. . . . . Peggy Shute
Quality Assurance . . . . Vicki Striding

Measure	Cases	This Hosp.	State Avg.	U.S. Avg.
Blood Clot Prevention and Treatment				
Anticoagulation Overlap Therapy[2]	25	100%	86%	93%
ICU Venous Thromboembolism Prophylaxis[2]	32	100%	86%	92%
Incidence of Potentially Preventable VTE[1,2]	-	-	15%	10%
UFH with Dosages/Platelet Monitoring[1,2]	-	-	94%	97%
Venous Thromboembolism Prophylaxis[2]	196	94%	70%	85%
Warfarin Therapy Discharge Instructions[2]	24	88%	77%	75%
Chest Pain/Possible Heart Attack Care				
Aspirin Given Within 24 Hours of Arrival	36	97%	94%	96%
Fibrinolytic Meds Within 30 Min. of Arrival[7]	-	-	40%	58%
Average Time to ECG (minutes)	40	8	10	7
Average Time to Transfer (minutes)[1]	-	-	77	60
Children's Asthma Care				
Received Home Management Plan of Care	-	-	-	88%
Received Reliever Medication	-	-	-	100%
Received Systemic Corticosteroids	-	-	-	100%
Emergency Department				
Admittance Decision Time (minutes)[2]	235	58	61	98
Head CT Results Within 45 Min. of Arrival[1]	-	-	42%	57%
Patients Who Left ER Before Being Seen	21,272	1%	3%	2%
Time from ER Arrival to Admit. (minutes)[2]	237	205	223	274
Time from ER Arrival to Discharge (minutes)	517	108	112	134
Time in ER Before Being Evaluated (minutes)	534	41	29	26
Time to Pain Meds for Fractures (minutes)	76	56	68	57
Heart Attack Care				
Aspirin Given at Discharge[1]	-	-	99%	99%
Fibrinolytic Meds Within 30 Min. of Arrival[7]	-	-	50%	54%
PCI Within 90 Minutes of Arrival[7]	-	-	96%	96%
Statin Prescribed at Discharge[1]	-	-	97%	98%
Heart Failure Care				
ACE Inhibitor or ARB for LVSD[1]	-	-	93%	97%
Discharge Instructions Given	40	98%	91%	94%
Evaluation of LVS Function	48	100%	96%	99%
Medicare Spending				
Medicare Spending per Patient (ratio)	-	0.97	0.95	0.98
Pneumonia Care				
Appropriate Initial Antibiotic Given	68	99%	91%	95%
Blood Culture Timing	59	100%	97%	98%

NOTE: Hospital profiles are in alphabetical order by state, then city, then hospital within the city; Rankings exclude hospitals with less than 25 cases except for patient surveys which excludes hospitals with less than 100 cases; (a) 100-299 cases; (1) The number of cases/patients is too few to report; (2) Data submitted were based on a sample of cases/patients; (3) Results are based on a shorter time period than required; (4) Data suppressed by CMS for one or more quarters; (5) Results are not available for this reporting period; (6) Fewer than 100 patients completed the HCAHPS survey; (7) No cases met the criteria for this measure; (8) The lower limit of the confidence interval cannot be calculated if the number of observed infections equals zero; (9) No data are available from the state/territory for this reporting period; (10) The scores shown reflect fewer than 50 completed surveys; (11) There were discrepancies in the data collection process; (12) This measure does not apply to this hospital for this reporting period; (13) Results cannot be calculated for this reporting period; (14) The results for this state are combined with nearby states to protect confidentiality; Please refer to the User's Guide for a full explanation of data.

Measure	Cases	This Hosp.	State Avg.	U.S. Avg.
Pregnancy and Delivery Care				
Newborn Deliveries Scheduled Early[2]	50	6%	22%	6%
Preventive Care				
Immunization for Influenza[2]	475	99%	87%	90%
Immunization for Pneumonia[2]	359	97%	89%	92%
Stroke Care				
Anticoagulation Therapy for Atrial Fibrillation[1]	-	-	93%	95%
Antithrombotic Therapy Timing	18	100%	96%	98%
Assessed for Rehabilitation	19	100%	95%	97%
Discharged on Antithrombotic Therapy	18	100%	97%	99%
Discharged on Statin Medication	11	100%	88%	94%
Thrombolytic Therapy Timing[7]	-	-	25%	66%
Venous Thromboembolism Prophylaxis	17	100%	87%	94%
Written Stroke Educational Materials Given	14	86%	84%	88%
Surgical Care Improvement Project				
Appropriate Beta Blocker Usage[2]	111	100%	97%	98%
Appropriate VTP Within 24 Hours[2]	552	100%	97%	98%
Controlled Postoperative Blood Glucose[2,7]	-	-	97%	97%
Perioperative Temperature Management[2]	590	100%	100%	100%
Prophylactic Antibiotic Selection[2]	490	100%	99%	99%
Prophylactic Antibiotic Selection (Outpatient)	820	99%	98%	98%
Prophylactic Antibiotic Stopped[2]	488	100%	97%	98%
Prophylactic Antibiotic Timing[2]	490	100%	99%	99%
Prophylactic Antibiotic Timing (Outpatient)	821	100%	98%	98%
Urinary Catheter Removal[2]	291	100%	97%	97%
Survey of Patients' Hospital Experiences				
Area Around Room 'Always' Quiet at Night	300+	72%	72%	61%
Doctors 'Always' Communicated Well	300+	85%	86%	82%
Home Recovery Information Given	300+	84%	83%	85%
Hospital Given 9 or 10 on 10 Point Scale	300+	71%	71%	71%
Meds 'Always' Explained Before Given	300+	61%	67%	64%
Nurses 'Always' Communicated Well	300+	80%	81%	79%
Pain 'Always' Well Controlled	300+	72%	72%	71%
Room and Bathroom 'Always' Clean	300+	65%	74%	73%
Timely Help 'Always' Received	300+	69%	69%	68%
Would Definitely Recommend Hospital	300+	74%	69%	71%
Use of Medical Imaging				
Cardiac Imaging Stress Test before Surgery[1]	-	-	5.7%	5.3%
Combination Abdominal CT Scan	391	10.2%	12.9%	10.5%
Combination Brain/Sinus CT Scan	417	5.0%	3.3%	2.7%
Combination Chest CT Scan	164	17.1%	6.1%	2.7%
Follow-up Mammogram/Ultrasound	632	4.9%	8.4%	8.8%
Lumbar Spine MRI for Low Back Pain	215	33.5%	41.1%	37.2%

Woman's Hospital at River Oaks

1026 River Oaks Drive
Flowood, MS 39232
Phone: 601-936-1000
Fax: 601-936-3086
URL: www.womanshospitalone.com
Type: Acute Care Hospitals
Emergency Services: No
Ownership: Proprietary
Beds: 111

Key Personnel:

Radiology. . . . . Ed D Barham
Infection Control. . . . . Jennifer Freeny
Chief of Medical Staff . . . . Edra Kimmel, MD
CEO . . . . Sherry J. Pitts
Operating Room. . . . . Carmen Polk
Quality Assurance . . . . Jan Shannon

Measure	Cases	This Hosp.	State Avg.	U.S. Avg.
Blood Clot Prevention and Treatment				
Anticoagulation Overlap Therapy[1,2]	-	-	86%	93%
ICU Venous Thromboembolism Prophylaxis[2,7]	-	-	86%	92%
Incidence of Potentially Preventable VTE[2,7]	-	-	15%	10%
UFH with Dosages/Platelet Monitoring[2,7]	-	-	94%	97%
Venous Thromboembolism Prophylaxis[2]	79	99%	70%	85%
Warfarin Therapy Discharge Instructions[2,7]	-	-	77%	75%
Chest Pain/Possible Heart Attack Care				
Aspirin Given Within 24 Hours of Arrival[5]	-	-	94%	96%
Fibrinolytic Meds Within 30 Min. of Arrival[5]	-	-	40%	58%
Average Time to ECG (minutes)[5]	-	-	10	7
Average Time to Transfer (minutes)[5]	-	-	77	60
Children's Asthma Care				
Received Home Management Plan of Care	-	-	-	88%
Received Reliever Medication	-	-	-	100%
Received Systemic Corticosteroids	-	-	-	100%
Emergency Department				
Admittance Decision Time (minutes)[2,7]	-	-	61	98
Head CT Results Within 45 Min. of Arrival[5]	-	-	42%	57%
Patients Who Left ER Before Being Seen[5]	-	-	3%	2%
Time from ER Arrival to Admit. (minutes)[2,7]	-	-	223	274
Time from ER Arrival to Discharge (minutes)[5]	-	-	112	134
Time in ER Before Being Evaluated (minutes)[5]	-	-	29	26
Time to Pain Meds for Fractures (minutes)[5]	-	-	68	57
Heart Attack Care				
Aspirin Given at Discharge[5]	-	-	99%	99%
Fibrinolytic Meds Within 30 Min. of Arrival[5]	-	-	50%	54%
PCI Within 90 Minutes of Arrival[5]	-	-	96%	96%
Statin Prescribed at Discharge[5]	-	-	97%	98%
Heart Failure Care				
ACE Inhibitor or ARB for LVSD[5]	-	-	93%	97%
Discharge Instructions Given[5]	-	-	91%	94%
Evaluation of LVS Function[5]	-	-	96%	99%
Medicare Spending				
Medicare Spending per Patient (ratio)	-	1.00	0.95	0.98
Pneumonia Care				
Appropriate Initial Antibiotic Given[5]	-	-	91%	95%
Blood Culture Timing[5]	-	-	97%	98%
Pregnancy and Delivery Care				
Newborn Deliveries Scheduled Early[2]	29	45%	22%	6%
Preventive Care				
Immunization for Influenza[2]	170	86%	87%	90%
Immunization for Pneumonia[2]	29	45%	89%	92%
Stroke Care				
Anticoagulation Therapy for Atrial Fibrillation[5]	-	-	93%	95%
Antithrombotic Therapy Timing[5]	-	-	96%	98%
Assessed for Rehabilitation[5]	-	-	95%	97%
Discharged on Antithrombotic Therapy[5]	-	-	97%	99%
Discharged on Statin Medication[5]	-	-	88%	94%
Thrombolytic Therapy Timing[5]	-	-	25%	66%
Venous Thromboembolism Prophylaxis[5]	-	-	87%	94%
Written Stroke Educational Materials Given[5]	-	-	84%	88%
Surgical Care Improvement Project				
Appropriate Beta Blocker Usage[1]	-	-	97%	98%
Appropriate VTP Within 24 Hours	42	95%	97%	98%
Controlled Postoperative Blood Glucose[7]	-	-	97%	97%
Perioperative Temperature Management	45	100%	100%	100%
Prophylactic Antibiotic Selection	32	100%	99%	99%
Prophylactic Antibiotic Selection (Outpatient)	510	100%	98%	98%
Prophylactic Antibiotic Stopped	32	97%	97%	98%
Prophylactic Antibiotic Timing	32	100%	99%	99%
Prophylactic Antibiotic Timing (Outpatient)	510	100%	98%	98%
Urinary Catheter Removal[1]	-	-	97%	97%
Survey of Patients' Hospital Experiences				
Area Around Room 'Always' Quiet at Night	300+	69%	72%	61%
Doctors 'Always' Communicated Well	300+	87%	86%	82%
Home Recovery Information Given	300+	90%	83%	85%
Hospital Given 9 or 10 on 10 Point Scale	300+	82%	71%	71%
Meds 'Always' Explained Before Given	300+	64%	67%	64%
Nurses 'Always' Communicated Well	300+	88%	81%	79%
Pain 'Always' Well Controlled	300+	81%	72%	71%
Room and Bathroom 'Always' Clean	300+	73%	74%	73%
Timely Help 'Always' Received	300+	74%	69%	68%
Would Definitely Recommend Hospital	300+	85%	69%	71%
Use of Medical Imaging				
Cardiac Imaging Stress Test before Surgery[7]	-	-	5.7%	5.3%
Combination Abdominal CT Scan[7]	-	-	12.9%	10.5%
Combination Brain/Sinus CT Scan[7]	-	-	3.3%	2.7%
Combination Chest CT Scan[7]	-	-	6.1%	2.7%
Follow-up Mammogram/Ultrasound	675	7.6%	8.4%	8.8%
Lumbar Spine MRI for Low Back Pain[7]	-	-	41.1%	37.2%

Lackey Memorial Hospital

330 N Broad Street
Forest, MS 39074
Phone: 601-469-4151
Fax: 601-469-3681
URL: www.selackey.com
Type: Critical Access Hospitals
Emergency Services: Yes
Ownership: Voluntary non-profit - Private
Beds: 74

Key Personnel:

Operating Room. . . . . Judy Henry
Chief of Medical Staff . . . . John Paul Lee, MD
Radiology. . . . . Phillip Lucas
Patient Relations . . . . Sydney Sawyer, RN
Quality Assurance . . . . Dana Watkins

Measure	Cases	This Hosp.	State Avg.	U.S. Avg.
Blood Clot Prevention and Treatment				
Anticoagulation Overlap Therapy[5]	-	-	86%	93%
ICU Venous Thromboembolism Prophylaxis[5]	-	-	86%	92%
Incidence of Potentially Preventable VTE[5]	-	-	15%	10%
UFH with Dosages/Platelet Monitoring[5]	-	-	94%	97%
Venous Thromboembolism Prophylaxis[5]	-	-	70%	85%
Warfarin Therapy Discharge Instructions[5]	-	-	77%	75%
Chest Pain/Possible Heart Attack Care				
Aspirin Given Within 24 Hours of Arrival[1]	-	-	94%	96%
Fibrinolytic Meds Within 30 Min. of Arrival[7]	-	-	40%	58%
Average Time to ECG (minutes)[1]	-	-	10	7
Average Time to Transfer (minutes)[7]	-	-	77	60
Children's Asthma Care				
Received Home Management Plan of Care	-	-	-	88%
Received Reliever Medication	-	-	-	100%
Received Systemic Corticosteroids	-	-	-	100%
Emergency Department				
Admittance Decision Time (minutes)[5]	-	-	61	98
Head CT Results Within 45 Min. of Arrival[1,3]	-	-	42%	57%
Patients Who Left ER Before Being Seen[5]	-	-	3%	2%
Time from ER Arrival to Admit. (minutes)[5]	-	-	223	274
Time from ER Arrival to Discharge (minutes)	392	89	112	134
Time in ER Before Being Evaluated (minutes)	401	20	29	26
Time to Pain Meds for Fractures (minutes)[1,3]	-	-	68	57
Heart Attack Care				
Aspirin Given at Discharge[5]	-	-	99%	99%
Fibrinolytic Meds Within 30 Min. of Arrival[5]	-	-	50%	54%
PCI Within 90 Minutes of Arrival[5]	-	-	96%	96%
Statin Prescribed at Discharge[5]	-	-	97%	98%
Heart Failure Care				
ACE Inhibitor or ARB for LVSD	11	64%	93%	97%
Discharge Instructions Given	23	96%	91%	94%
Evaluation of LVS Function	23	100%	96%	99%
Medicare Spending				
Medicare Spending per Patient (ratio)	-	-	0.95	0.98
Pneumonia Care				
Appropriate Initial Antibiotic Given	34	85%	91%	95%
Blood Culture Timing[1]	-	-	97%	98%
Pregnancy and Delivery Care				
Newborn Deliveries Scheduled Early[5]	-	-	22%	6%
Preventive Care				
Immunization for Influenza[5]	-	-	87%	90%
Immunization for Pneumonia[5]	-	-	89%	92%
Stroke Care				
Anticoagulation Therapy for Atrial Fibrillation[3,7]	-	-	93%	95%
Antithrombotic Therapy Timing[3,7]	-	-	96%	98%
Assessed for Rehabilitation[3,7]	-	-	95%	97%
Discharged on Antithrombotic Therapy[3,7]	-	-	97%	99%
Discharged on Statin Medication[3,7]	-	-	88%	94%
Thrombolytic Therapy Timing[1,3]	-	-	25%	66%
Venous Thromboembolism Prophylaxis[3,7]	-	-	87%	94%
Written Stroke Educational Materials Given[3,7]	-	-	84%	88%
Surgical Care Improvement Project				
Appropriate Beta Blocker Usage[5]	-	-	97%	98%
Appropriate VTP Within 24 Hours[5]	-	-	97%	98%
Controlled Postoperative Blood Glucose[5]	-	-	97%	97%
Perioperative Temperature Management[5]	-	-	100%	100%
Prophylactic Antibiotic Selection[5]	-	-	99%	99%
Prophylactic Antibiotic Selection (Outpatient)[5]	-	-	98%	98%
Prophylactic Antibiotic Stopped[5]	-	-	97%	98%
Prophylactic Antibiotic Timing[5]	-	-	99%	99%
Prophylactic Antibiotic Timing (Outpatient)[5]	-	-	98%	98%
Urinary Catheter Removal[5]	-	-	97%	97%
Survey of Patients' Hospital Experiences				
Area Around Room 'Always' Quiet at Night[5]	-	-	72%	61%
Doctors 'Always' Communicated Well[5]	-	-	86%	82%
Home Recovery Information Given[5]	-	-	83%	85%

NOTE: Hospital profiles are in alphabetical order by state, then city, then hospital within the city; Rankings exclude hospitals with less than 25 cases except for patient surveys which excludes hospitals with less than 100 cases; (a) 100-299 cases; (1) The number of cases/patients is too few to report; (2) Data submitted were based on a sample of cases/patients; (3) Results are based on a shorter time period than required; (4) Data suppressed by CMS for one or more quarters; (5) Results are not available for this reporting period; (6) Fewer than 100 patients completed the HCAHPS survey; (7) No cases met the criteria for this measure; (8) The lower limit of the confidence interval cannot be calculated if the number of observed infections equals zero; (9) No data are available from the state/territory for this reporting period; (10) The scores shown reflect fewer than 50 completed surveys; (11) There were discrepancies in the data collection process; (12) This measure does not apply to this hospital for this reporting period; (13) Results cannot be calculated for this reporting period; (14) The results for this state are combined with nearby states to protect confidentiality; Please refer to the User's Guide for a full explanation of data.

Measure	Cases	This Hosp.	State Avg.	U.S. Avg.
Hospital Given 9 or 10 on 10 Point Scale[5]	-	-	71%	71%
Meds 'Always' Explained Before Given[5]	-	-	67%	64%
Nurses 'Always' Communicated Well[5]	-	-	81%	79%
Pain 'Always' Well Controlled[5]	-	-	72%	71%
Room and Bathroom 'Always' Clean[5]	-	-	74%	73%
Timely Help 'Always' Received[5]	-	-	69%	68%
Would Definitely Recommend Hospital[5]	-	-	69%	71%
Use of Medical Imaging				
Cardiac Imaging Stress Test before Surgery[1]	-	-	5.7%	5.3%
Combination Abdominal CT Scan	153	36.6%	12.9%	10.5%
Combination Brain/Sinus CT Scan[1]	-	-	3.3%	2.7%
Combination Chest CT Scan	69	39.1%	6.1%	2.7%
Follow-up Mammogram/Ultrasound	242	6.2%	8.4%	8.8%
Lumbar Spine MRI for Low Back Pain[1]	-	-	41.1%	37.2%

Delta Regional Medical Center

1400 E Union St
Greenville, MS 38704
Phone: 662-378-3783
Fax: 662-725-2189
URL: www.deltaregional.com
Type: Acute Care Hospitals
Emergency Services: Yes
Ownership: Government - Local
Beds: 398

Key Personnel:
Cardiac Laboratory............ Michelle Britton
CEO/President............... Scott Christensen
Chief of Medical Staff.......... Michael Cirilli, MD
Quality Assurance .... Amy Donoly
Emergency Room .... Melany Graham
Infection Control............. Sharon Henderson
Operating Room............. Sue Peets, RN
Radiology.................. David Wallace

Measure	Cases	This Hosp.	State Avg.	U.S. Avg.
Blood Clot Prevention and Treatment				
Anticoagulation Overlap Therapy[2]	59	61%	86%	93%
ICU Venous Thromboembolism Prophylaxis[2]	132	58%	86%	92%
Incidence of Potentially Preventable VTE[1,2]	-	-	15%	10%
UFH with Dosages/Platelet Monitoring[2]	17	100%	94%	97%
Venous Thromboembolism Prophylaxis[2]	351	32%	70%	85%
Warfarin Therapy Discharge Instructions[2]	44	82%	77%	75%
Chest Pain/Possible Heart Attack Care				
Aspirin Given Within 24 Hours of Arrival[3,7]	-	-	94%	96%
Fibrinolytic Meds Within 30 Min. of Arrival[5]	-	-	40%	58%
Average Time to ECG (minutes)[3,7]	-	-	10	7
Average Time to Transfer (minutes)[5]	-	-	77	60
Children's Asthma Care				
Received Home Management Plan of Care	-	-	-	88%
Received Reliever Medication	-	-	-	100%
Received Systemic Corticosteroids	-	-	-	100%
Emergency Department				
Admittance Decision Time (minutes)[2]	521	95	61	98
Head CT Results Within 45 Min. of Arrival[1]	-	-	42%	57%
Patients Who Left ER Before Being Seen	40,541	8%	3%	2%
Time from ER Arrival to Admit. (minutes)[2]	570	313	223	274
Time from ER Arrival to Discharge (minutes)	361	201	112	134
Time in ER Before Being Evaluated (minutes)	172	79	29	26
Time to Pain Meds for Fractures (minutes)	110	114	68	57
Heart Attack Care				
Aspirin Given at Discharge	144	95%	99%	99%
Fibrinolytic Meds Within 30 Min. of Arrival[1]	-	-	50%	54%
PCI Within 90 Minutes of Arrival[1]	-	-	96%	96%
Statin Prescribed at Discharge	133	92%	97%	98%
Heart Failure Care				
ACE Inhibitor or ARB for LVSD	161	97%	93%	97%
Discharge Instructions Given	435	97%	91%	94%
Evaluation of LVS Function	487	97%	96%	99%
Medicare Spending				
Medicare Spending per Patient (ratio)	-	1.06	0.95	0.98
Pneumonia Care				
Appropriate Initial Antibiotic Given	95	92%	91%	95%
Blood Culture Timing	127	93%	97%	98%
Pregnancy and Delivery Care				
Newborn Deliveries Scheduled Early	147	19%	22%	6%
Preventive Care				
Immunization for Influenza[2]	513	87%	87%	90%
Immunization for Pneumonia[2]	631	94%	89%	92%
Stroke Care				
Anticoagulation Therapy for Atrial Fibrillation[1]	-	-	93%	95%
Antithrombotic Therapy Timing	80	94%	96%	98%
Assessed for Rehabilitation	82	91%	95%	97%
Discharged on Antithrombotic Therapy	78	92%	97%	99%
Discharged on Statin Medication	60	70%	88%	94%
Thrombolytic Therapy Timing[1]	-	-	25%	66%
Venous Thromboembolism Prophylaxis	92	78%	87%	94%
Written Stroke Educational Materials Given	42	81%	84%	88%
Surgical Care Improvement Project				
Appropriate Beta Blocker Usage	78	94%	97%	98%
Appropriate VTP Within 24 Hours	312	94%	97%	98%
Controlled Postoperative Blood Glucose	14	93%	97%	97%
Perioperative Temperature Management	357	100%	100%	100%
Prophylactic Antibiotic Selection	260	97%	99%	99%
Prophylactic Antibiotic Selection (Outpatient)	87	94%	98%	98%
Prophylactic Antibiotic Stopped	257	96%	97%	98%
Prophylactic Antibiotic Timing	260	99%	99%	99%
Prophylactic Antibiotic Timing (Outpatient)	94	90%	98%	98%
Urinary Catheter Removal	178	94%	97%	97%
Survey of Patients' Hospital Experiences				
Area Around Room 'Always' Quiet at Night	300+	72%	72%	61%
Doctors 'Always' Communicated Well	300+	84%	86%	82%
Home Recovery Information Given	300+	77%	83%	85%
Hospital Given 9 or 10 on 10 Point Scale	300+	60%	71%	71%
Meds 'Always' Explained Before Given	300+	63%	67%	64%
Nurses 'Always' Communicated Well	300+	75%	81%	79%
Pain 'Always' Well Controlled	300+	71%	72%	71%
Room and Bathroom 'Always' Clean	300+	70%	74%	73%
Timely Help 'Always' Received	300+	63%	69%	68%
Would Definitely Recommend Hospital	300+	55%	69%	71%
Use of Medical Imaging				
Cardiac Imaging Stress Test before Surgery	161	2.5%	5.7%	5.3%
Combination Abdominal CT Scan	766	16.6%	12.9%	10.5%
Combination Brain/Sinus CT Scan	724	4.1%	3.3%	2.7%
Combination Chest CT Scan	363	20.7%	6.1%	2.7%
Follow-up Mammogram/Ultrasound	1,369	6.5%	8.4%	8.8%
Lumbar Spine MRI for Low Back Pain	127	46.5%	41.1%	37.2%

Greenwood Leflore Hospital

1401 River Rd / PO Box 1410
Greenwood, MS 38930
Phone: 662-459-7000
Fax: 662-459-7117
E-mail: humanresources@glh.org
URL: www.glh.org
Type: Acute Care Hospitals
Emergency Services: Yes
Ownership: Government - Local
Beds: 260

Key Personnel:
Surgery .... Douglas E. Bowden, DO, FACOS
CEO/President............... Jim Jackson
Pediatric Ambulatory Care ...... Melynda McCrimmon, MD
Pediatric In-Patient Care .... Melynda McCrimmon, MD
Quality Assurance .... Karen Upchurch
Chairman/CEO .... Brian Waldrop

Measure	Cases	This Hosp.	State Avg.	U.S. Avg.
Blood Clot Prevention and Treatment				
Anticoagulation Overlap Therapy[2]	41	95%	86%	93%
ICU Venous Thromboembolism Prophylaxis[2]	95	85%	86%	92%
Incidence of Potentially Preventable VTE[2]	15	40%	15%	10%
UFH with Dosages/Platelet Monitoring[1,2]	-	-	94%	97%
Venous Thromboembolism Prophylaxis[2]	296	69%	70%	85%
Warfarin Therapy Discharge Instructions[2]	29	97%	77%	75%
Chest Pain/Possible Heart Attack Care				
Aspirin Given Within 24 Hours of Arrival	19	95%	94%	96%
Fibrinolytic Meds Within 30 Min. of Arrival[7]	-	-	40%	58%
Average Time to ECG (minutes)	21	11	10	7
Average Time to Transfer (minutes)[7]	-	-	77	60
Children's Asthma Care				
Received Home Management Plan of Care	-	-	-	88%
Received Reliever Medication	-	-	-	100%
Received Systemic Corticosteroids	-	-	-	100%
Emergency Department				
Admittance Decision Time (minutes)[2]	370	34	61	98
Head CT Results Within 45 Min. of Arrival[1]	-	-	42%	57%
Patients Who Left ER Before Being Seen	43,911	2%	3%	2%
Time from ER Arrival to Admit. (minutes)[2]	370	142	223	274
Time from ER Arrival to Discharge (minutes)	410	106	112	134
Time in ER Before Being Evaluated (minutes)	435	25	29	26
Time to Pain Meds for Fractures (minutes)	63	61	68	57
Heart Attack Care				
Aspirin Given at Discharge	65	97%	99%	99%
Fibrinolytic Meds Within 30 Min. of Arrival[1]	-	-	50%	54%
PCI Within 90 Minutes of Arrival[7]	-	-	96%	96%
Statin Prescribed at Discharge	65	94%	97%	98%
Heart Failure Care				
ACE Inhibitor or ARB for LVSD	84	99%	93%	97%
Discharge Instructions Given	159	99%	91%	94%
Evaluation of LVS Function	191	98%	96%	99%
Medicare Spending				
Medicare Spending per Patient (ratio)	-	1.04	0.95	0.98
Pneumonia Care				
Appropriate Initial Antibiotic Given	77	94%	91%	95%
Blood Culture Timing	108	100%	97%	98%
Pregnancy and Delivery Care				
Newborn Deliveries Scheduled Early	74	1%	22%	6%
Preventive Care				
Immunization for Influenza[2]	509	100%	87%	90%
Immunization for Pneumonia[2]	585	99%	89%	92%
Stroke Care				
Anticoagulation Therapy for Atrial Fibrillation	16	94%	93%	95%
Antithrombotic Therapy Timing	85	95%	96%	98%
Assessed for Rehabilitation	95	92%	95%	97%
Discharged on Antithrombotic Therapy	89	97%	97%	99%
Discharged on Statin Medication	80	66%	88%	94%
Thrombolytic Therapy Timing[1]	-	-	25%	66%
Venous Thromboembolism Prophylaxis	95	78%	87%	94%
Written Stroke Educational Materials Given	43	77%	84%	88%
Surgical Care Improvement Project				
Appropriate Beta Blocker Usage	80	90%	97%	98%
Appropriate VTP Within 24 Hours	293	98%	97%	98%
Controlled Postoperative Blood Glucose[7]	-	-	97%	97%
Perioperative Temperature Management	339	100%	100%	100%
Prophylactic Antibiotic Selection	242	99%	99%	99%
Prophylactic Antibiotic Selection (Outpatient)	197	95%	98%	98%
Prophylactic Antibiotic Stopped	238	93%	97%	98%
Prophylactic Antibiotic Timing	244	99%	99%	99%
Prophylactic Antibiotic Timing (Outpatient)	157	98%	98%	98%
Urinary Catheter Removal	194	94%	97%	97%
Survey of Patients' Hospital Experiences				
Area Around Room 'Always' Quiet at Night	300+	69%	72%	61%
Doctors 'Always' Communicated Well	300+	86%	86%	82%
Home Recovery Information Given	300+	86%	83%	85%
Hospital Given 9 or 10 on 10 Point Scale	300+	69%	71%	71%
Meds 'Always' Explained Before Given	300+	67%	67%	64%
Nurses 'Always' Communicated Well	300+	79%	81%	79%
Pain 'Always' Well Controlled	300+	73%	72%	71%
Room and Bathroom 'Always' Clean	300+	69%	74%	73%
Timely Help 'Always' Received	300+	67%	69%	68%
Would Definitely Recommend Hospital	300+	66%	69%	71%
Use of Medical Imaging				
Cardiac Imaging Stress Test before Surgery	216	5.1%	5.7%	5.3%
Combination Abdominal CT Scan	489	36.6%	12.9%	10.5%
Combination Brain/Sinus CT Scan	685	4.4%	3.3%	2.7%
Combination Chest CT Scan	276	47.1%	6.1%	2.7%
Follow-up Mammogram/Ultrasound	1,149	4.4%	8.4%	8.8%
Lumbar Spine MRI for Low Back Pain	146	41.1%	41.1%	37.2%

Grenada Lake Medical Center

960 Avent Drive
Grenada, MS 38901
Phone: 662-227-7000
Fax: 662-227-7453
Type: Acute Care Hospitals
Emergency Services: Yes
Ownership: Government - Local
Beds: 156

Key Personnel:
Quality Assurance .... Mabry Bell
Intensive Care Unit........... Mickey Cannon
Operating Room............. Mike Cole
CEO/President.............. Charles L Denton
Emergency Room .... Gayle Harrell
Chief of Medical Staff.......... John Paul Lee
Radiology.................. Phillip Lucas

NOTE: Hospital profiles are in alphabetical order by state, then city, then hospital within the city; Rankings exclude hospitals with less than 25 cases except for patient surveys which excludes hospitals with less than 100 cases; (a) 100-299 cases; (1) The number of cases/patients is too few to report; (2) Data submitted were based on a sample of cases/patients; (3) Results are based on a shorter time period than required; (4) Data suppressed by CMS for one or more quarters; (5) Results are not available for this reporting period; (6) Fewer than 100 patients completed the HCAHPS survey; (7) No cases met the criteria for this measure; (8) The lower limit of the confidence interval cannot be calculated if the number of observed infections equals zero; (9) No data are available from the state/territory for this reporting period; (10) The scores shown reflect fewer than 50 completed surveys; (11) There were discrepancies in the data collection process; (12) This measure does not apply to this hospital for this reporting period; (13) Results cannot be calculated for this reporting period; (14) The results for this state are combined with nearby states to protect confidentiality; Please refer to the User's Guide for a full explanation of data.

Cardiac Laboratory. . . . . John Seibel, MD

Measure	Cases	This Hosp.	State Avg.	U.S. Avg.
Blood Clot Prevention and Treatment				
Anticoagulation Overlap Therapy[2]	32	28%	86%	93%
ICU Venous Thromboembolism Prophylaxis[2]	230	79%	86%	92%
Incidence of Potentially Preventable VTE[1,2]	-	-	15%	10%
UFH with Dosages/Platelet Monitoring[1,2]	-	-	94%	97%
Venous Thromboembolism Prophylaxis[2]	807	65%	70%	85%
Warfarin Therapy Discharge Instructions[2]	31	6%	77%	75%
Chest Pain/Possible Heart Attack Care				
Aspirin Given Within 24 Hours of Arrival	39	92%	94%	96%
Fibrinolytic Meds Within 30 Min. of Arrival[1]	-	-	40%	58%
Average Time to ECG (minutes)	40	20	10	7
Average Time to Transfer (minutes)[1]	-	-	77	60
Children's Asthma Care				
Received Home Management Plan of Care	-	-	-	88%
Received Reliever Medication	-	-	-	100%
Received Systemic Corticosteroids	-	-	-	100%
Emergency Department				
Admittance Decision Time (minutes)[2]	1,309	40	61	98
Head CT Results Within 45 Min. of Arrival	16	38%	42%	57%
Patients Who Left ER Before Being Seen	18,392	2%	3%	2%
Time from ER Arrival to Admit. (minutes)[2]	1,328	196	223	274
Time from ER Arrival to Discharge (minutes)	14,526	112	112	134
Time in ER Before Being Evaluated (minutes)	14,972	30	29	26
Time to Pain Meds for Fractures (minutes)	91	70	68	57
Heart Attack Care				
Aspirin Given at Discharge[2]	18	89%	99%	99%
Fibrinolytic Meds Within 30 Min. of Arrival[2,7]	-	-	50%	54%
PCI Within 90 Minutes of Arrival[2,7]	-	-	96%	96%
Statin Prescribed at Discharge[2]	20	50%	97%	98%
Heart Failure Care				
ACE Inhibitor or ARB for LVSD[2]	37	81%	93%	97%
Discharge Instructions Given[2]	80	72%	91%	94%
Evaluation of LVS Function[2]	101	96%	96%	99%
Medicare Spending				
Medicare Spending per Patient (ratio)	-	0.98	0.95	0.98
Pneumonia Care				
Appropriate Initial Antibiotic Given[2]	49	73%	91%	95%
Blood Culture Timing[2]	80	94%	97%	98%
Pregnancy and Delivery Care				
Newborn Deliveries Scheduled Early	84	39%	22%	6%
Preventive Care				
Immunization for Influenza[2]	1,258	87%	87%	90%
Immunization for Pneumonia[2]	1,311	93%	89%	92%
Stroke Care				
Anticoagulation Therapy for Atrial Fibrillation[1,2]	-	-	93%	95%
Antithrombotic Therapy Timing[2]	28	96%	96%	98%
Assessed for Rehabilitation[2]	26	85%	95%	97%
Discharged on Antithrombotic Therapy[2]	26	92%	97%	99%
Discharged on Statin Medication[2]	26	85%	88%	94%
Thrombolytic Therapy Timing[1,2]	-	-	25%	66%
Venous Thromboembolism Prophylaxis[2]	31	94%	87%	94%
Written Stroke Educational Materials Given[2]	13	85%	84%	88%
Surgical Care Improvement Project				
Appropriate Beta Blocker Usage[2]	16	44%	97%	98%
Appropriate VTP Within 24 Hours[2]	55	87%	97%	98%
Controlled Postoperative Blood Glucose[2,7]	-	-	97%	97%
Perioperative Temperature Management[2]	87	95%	100%	100%
Prophylactic Antibiotic Selection[2]	41	88%	99%	99%
Prophylactic Antibiotic Selection (Outpatient)	37	92%	98%	98%
Prophylactic Antibiotic Stopped[2]	41	85%	97%	98%
Prophylactic Antibiotic Timing[2]	43	91%	99%	99%
Prophylactic Antibiotic Timing (Outpatient)	46	78%	98%	98%
Urinary Catheter Removal[2]	16	62%	97%	97%
Survey of Patients' Hospital Experiences				
Area Around Room 'Always' Quiet at Night	300+	71%	72%	61%
Doctors 'Always' Communicated Well	300+	90%	86%	82%
Home Recovery Information Given	300+	85%	83%	85%
Hospital Given 9 or 10 on 10 Point Scale	300+	71%	71%	71%
Meds 'Always' Explained Before Given	300+	67%	67%	64%
Nurses 'Always' Communicated Well	300+	82%	81%	79%
Pain 'Always' Well Controlled	300+	75%	72%	71%
Room and Bathroom 'Always' Clean	300+	78%	74%	73%
Timely Help 'Always' Received	300+	75%	69%	68%
Would Definitely Recommend Hospital	300+	66%	69%	71%
Use of Medical Imaging				
Cardiac Imaging Stress Test before Surgery[1]	-	-	5.7%	5.3%
Combination Abdominal CT Scan	222	19.8%	12.9%	10.5%
Combination Brain/Sinus CT Scan	462	1.7%	3.3%	2.7%
Combination Chest CT Scan	124	20.2%	6.1%	2.7%
Follow-up Mammogram/Ultrasound	1,011	2.5%	8.4%	8.8%
Lumbar Spine MRI for Low Back Pain	114	43.0%	41.1%	37.2%

Garden Park Medical Center

15200 Community Road
Gulfport, MS 39501
Phone: 228-575-7000
Fax: 228-575-7114
URL: www.gardenparkmedical.com
Type: Acute Care Hospitals
Emergency Services: Yes
Ownership: Proprietary
Beds: 130

Key Personnel:

Chief of Medical Staff. . . . . Lance Johansen
Chairman/CEO . . . . Michael Matthews
CEO/President. . . . . Tim Mcmanus
CEO . . . . Brenda M. Waltz, FACHE

Measure	Cases	This Hosp.	State Avg.	U.S. Avg.
Blood Clot Prevention and Treatment				
Anticoagulation Overlap Therapy[2]	25	100%	86%	93%
ICU Venous Thromboembolism Prophylaxis[2]	66	100%	86%	92%
Incidence of Potentially Preventable VTE[1,2]	-	-	15%	10%
UFH with Dosages/Platelet Monitoring[1,2]	-	-	94%	97%
Venous Thromboembolism Prophylaxis[2]	271	100%	70%	85%
Warfarin Therapy Discharge Instructions[2]	21	100%	77%	75%
Chest Pain/Possible Heart Attack Care				
Aspirin Given Within 24 Hours of Arrival[1,3]	-	-	94%	96%
Fibrinolytic Meds Within 30 Min. of Arrival[3,7]	-	-	40%	58%
Average Time to ECG (minutes)[1,3]	-	-	10	7
Average Time to Transfer (minutes)[3,7]	-	-	77	60
Children's Asthma Care				
Received Home Management Plan of Care	-	-	-	88%
Received Reliever Medication	-	-	-	100%
Received Systemic Corticosteroids	-	-	-	100%
Emergency Department				
Admittance Decision Time (minutes)[2]	456	87	61	98
Head CT Results Within 45 Min. of Arrival[7]	-	-	42%	57%
Patients Who Left ER Before Being Seen	38,430	2%	3%	2%
Time from ER Arrival to Admit. (minutes)[2]	456	218	223	274
Time from ER Arrival to Discharge (minutes)	517	96	112	134
Time in ER Before Being Evaluated (minutes)	541	20	29	26
Time to Pain Meds for Fractures (minutes)	96	52	68	57
Heart Attack Care				
Aspirin Given at Discharge[1]	-	-	99%	99%
Fibrinolytic Meds Within 30 Min. of Arrival[7]	-	-	50%	54%
PCI Within 90 Minutes of Arrival[7]	-	-	96%	96%
Statin Prescribed at Discharge[1]	-	-	97%	98%
Heart Failure Care				
ACE Inhibitor or ARB for LVSD[2]	34	100%	93%	97%
Discharge Instructions Given[2]	97	100%	91%	94%
Evaluation of LVS Function[2]	101	100%	96%	99%
Medicare Spending				
Medicare Spending per Patient (ratio)	-	0.99	0.95	0.98
Pneumonia Care				
Appropriate Initial Antibiotic Given[2]	60	100%	91%	95%
Blood Culture Timing[2]	86	100%	97%	98%
Pregnancy and Delivery Care				
Newborn Deliveries Scheduled Early[2]	42	0%	22%	6%
Preventive Care				
Immunization for Influenza[2]	486	100%	87%	90%
Immunization for Pneumonia[2]	490	100%	89%	92%
Stroke Care				
Anticoagulation Therapy for Atrial Fibrillation[1,2]	-	-	93%	95%
Antithrombotic Therapy Timing[2]	23	100%	96%	98%
Assessed for Rehabilitation[2]	24	100%	95%	97%
Discharged on Antithrombotic Therapy[2]	21	100%	97%	99%
Discharged on Statin Medication[2]	18	100%	88%	94%
Thrombolytic Therapy Timing[1,2]	-	-	25%	66%
Venous Thromboembolism Prophylaxis[2]	24	100%	87%	94%
Written Stroke Educational Materials Given[2]	11	100%	84%	88%
Surgical Care Improvement Project				
Appropriate Beta Blocker Usage[2]	71	100%	97%	98%
Appropriate VTP Within 24 Hours[2]	304	100%	97%	98%
Controlled Postoperative Blood Glucose[2,7]	-	-	97%	97%
Perioperative Temperature Management[2]	319	100%	100%	100%
Prophylactic Antibiotic Selection[2]	221	100%	99%	99%
Prophylactic Antibiotic Selection (Outpatient)	145	100%	98%	98%
Prophylactic Antibiotic Stopped[2]	217	100%	97%	98%
Prophylactic Antibiotic Timing[2]	222	100%	99%	99%
Prophylactic Antibiotic Timing (Outpatient)	146	99%	98%	98%
Urinary Catheter Removal[2]	262	100%	97%	97%
Survey of Patients' Hospital Experiences				
Area Around Room 'Always' Quiet at Night	300+	71%	72%	61%
Doctors 'Always' Communicated Well	300+	84%	86%	82%
Home Recovery Information Given	300+	86%	83%	85%
Hospital Given 9 or 10 on 10 Point Scale	300+	74%	71%	71%
Meds 'Always' Explained Before Given	300+	65%	67%	64%
Nurses 'Always' Communicated Well	300+	78%	81%	79%
Pain 'Always' Well Controlled	300+	70%	72%	71%
Room and Bathroom 'Always' Clean	300+	67%	74%	73%
Timely Help 'Always' Received	300+	70%	69%	68%
Would Definitely Recommend Hospital	300+	75%	69%	71%
Use of Medical Imaging				
Cardiac Imaging Stress Test before Surgery	67	7.5%	5.7%	5.3%
Combination Abdominal CT Scan	360	43.1%	12.9%	10.5%
Combination Brain/Sinus CT Scan[1]	-	-	3.3%	2.7%
Combination Chest CT Scan	141	2.8%	6.1%	2.7%
Follow-up Mammogram/Ultrasound	401	12.0%	8.4%	8.8%
Lumbar Spine MRI for Low Back Pain	78	30.8%	41.1%	37.2%

Memorial Hospital at Gulfport

4500 13th Saint - PO Box 1810
Gulfport, MS 39502
Phone: 228-867-4000
Fax: 228-865-3378
URL: www.gulfportmemorial.com
Type: Acute Care Hospitals
Emergency Services: Yes
Ownership: Government - Local
Beds: 445

Key Personnel:

Hemotology Center . . . . Sandra Bishop
Chief of Medical Staff. . . . . Nancy Downs
Intensive Care Unit. . . . . Kathy Ladner
Quality Assurance . . . . Virginia Ladner
CEO/President. . . . . Gary G. Marchand
Pediatric Ambulatory Care . . . . Shahidur Rahman, MD
Pediatric In-Patient Care . . . . Shahidur Rahman, MD
Emergency Room . . . . George Ward, MD

Measure	Cases	This Hosp.	State Avg.	U.S. Avg.
Blood Clot Prevention and Treatment				
Anticoagulation Overlap Therapy[2]	76	83%	86%	93%
ICU Venous Thromboembolism Prophylaxis[2]	85	93%	86%	92%
Incidence of Potentially Preventable VTE[2]	28	18%	15%	10%
UFH with Dosages/Platelet Monitoring[2]	31	97%	94%	97%
Venous Thromboembolism Prophylaxis[2]	357	77%	70%	85%
Warfarin Therapy Discharge Instructions[2]	56	68%	77%	75%
Chest Pain/Possible Heart Attack Care				
Aspirin Given Within 24 Hours of Arrival[5]	-	-	94%	96%
Fibrinolytic Meds Within 30 Min. of Arrival[5]	-	-	40%	58%
Average Time to ECG (minutes)[5]	-	-	10	7
Average Time to Transfer (minutes)[5]	-	-	77	60
Children's Asthma Care				
Received Home Management Plan of Care	-	-	-	88%
Received Reliever Medication	-	-	-	100%
Received Systemic Corticosteroids	-	-	-	100%
Emergency Department				
Admittance Decision Time (minutes)[2]	648	53	61	98
Head CT Results Within 45 Min. of Arrival[1]	-	-	42%	57%
Patients Who Left ER Before Being Seen	75,247	2%	3%	2%
Time from ER Arrival to Admit. (minutes)[2]	650	255	223	274
Time from ER Arrival to Discharge (minutes)	393	143	112	134
Time in ER Before Being Evaluated (minutes)	424	16	29	26
Time to Pain Meds for Fractures (minutes)	125	58	68	57

NOTE: Hospital profiles are in alphabetical order by state, then city, then hospital within the city; Rankings exclude hospitals with less than 25 cases except for patient surveys which excludes hospitals with less than 100 cases; (a) 100-299 cases; (1) The number of cases/patients is too few to report; (2) Data submitted were based on a sample of cases/patients; (3) Results are based on a shorter time period than required; (4) Data suppressed by CMS for one or more quarters; (5) Results are not available for this reporting period; (6) Fewer than 100 patients completed the HCAHPS survey; (7) No cases met the criteria for this measure; (8) The lower limit of the confidence interval cannot be calculated if the number of observed infections equals zero; (9) No data are available from the state/territory for this reporting period; (10) The scores shown reflect fewer than 50 completed surveys; (11) There were discrepancies in the data collection process; (12) This measure does not apply to this hospital for this reporting period; (13) Results cannot be calculated for this reporting period; (14) The results for this state are combined with nearby states to protect confidentiality; Please refer to the User's Guide for a full explanation of data.

Measure	Cases	This Hosp.	State Avg.	U.S. Avg.
Heart Attack Care				
Aspirin Given at Discharge[2]	295	100%	99%	99%
Fibrinolytic Meds Within 30 Min. of Arrival[2,7]	-	-	50%	54%
PCI Within 90 Minutes of Arrival[2]	54	89%	96%	96%
Statin Prescribed at Discharge[2]	277	95%	97%	98%
Heart Failure Care				
ACE Inhibitor or ARB for LVSD[2]	98	99%	93%	97%
Discharge Instructions Given[2]	262	92%	91%	94%
Evaluation of LVS Function[2]	306	100%	96%	99%
Medicare Spending				
Medicare Spending per Patient (ratio)	-	1.00	0.95	0.98
Pneumonia Care				
Appropriate Initial Antibiotic Given[2]	87	93%	91%	95%
Blood Culture Timing[2]	169	97%	97%	98%
Pregnancy and Delivery Care				
Newborn Deliveries Scheduled Early[2]	52	10%	22%	6%
Preventive Care				
Immunization for Influenza[2]	570	95%	87%	90%
Immunization for Pneumonia[2]	734	97%	89%	92%
Stroke Care				
Anticoagulation Therapy for Atrial Fibrillation[1,2]	-	-	93%	95%
Antithrombotic Therapy Timing[2]	83	99%	96%	98%
Assessed for Rehabilitation[2]	100	93%	95%	97%
Discharged on Antithrombotic Therapy[2]	80	99%	97%	99%
Discharged on Statin Medication[2]	64	100%	88%	94%
Thrombolytic Therapy Timing[1,2]	-	-	25%	66%
Venous Thromboembolism Prophylaxis[2]	104	95%	87%	94%
Written Stroke Educational Materials Given[2]	58	62%	84%	88%
Surgical Care Improvement Project				
Appropriate Beta Blocker Usage[2]	228	96%	97%	98%
Appropriate VTP Within 24 Hours[2]	398	93%	97%	98%
Controlled Postoperative Blood Glucose[2]	107	99%	97%	97%
Perioperative Temperature Management[2]	507	100%	100%	100%
Prophylactic Antibiotic Selection[2]	384	97%	99%	99%
Prophylactic Antibiotic Selection (Outpatient)	461	97%	98%	98%
Prophylactic Antibiotic Stopped[2]	362	97%	97%	98%
Prophylactic Antibiotic Timing[2]	385	99%	99%	99%
Prophylactic Antibiotic Timing (Outpatient)	457	99%	98%	98%
Urinary Catheter Removal[2]	348	96%	97%	97%
Survey of Patients' Hospital Experiences				
Area Around Room 'Always' Quiet at Night	300+	60%	72%	61%
Doctors 'Always' Communicated Well	300+	81%	86%	82%
Home Recovery Information Given	300+	84%	83%	85%
Hospital Given 9 or 10 on 10 Point Scale	300+	69%	71%	71%
Meds 'Always' Explained Before Given	300+	68%	67%	64%
Nurses 'Always' Communicated Well	300+	80%	81%	79%
Pain 'Always' Well Controlled	300+	75%	72%	71%
Room and Bathroom 'Always' Clean	300+	67%	74%	73%
Timely Help 'Always' Received	300+	68%	69%	68%
Would Definitely Recommend Hospital	300+	76%	69%	71%
Use of Medical Imaging				
Cardiac Imaging Stress Test before Surgery	338	6.8%	5.7%	5.3%
Combination Abdominal CT Scan	1,270	64.8%	12.9%	10.5%
Combination Brain/Sinus CT Scan	1,300	1.7%	3.3%	2.7%
Combination Chest CT Scan	1,149	3.2%	6.1%	2.7%
Follow-up Mammogram/Ultrasound	1,883	13.0%	8.4%	8.8%
Lumbar Spine MRI for Low Back Pain	257	42.0%	41.1%	37.2%

Forrest General Hospital

6051 Us Highway 49
Hattiesburg, MS 39404
Phone: 601-288-7000
Fax: 601-288-4441
URL: www.forrestgeneral.com
Type: Acute Care Hospitals
Emergency Services: Yes
Ownership: Government - Local
Beds: 512

Key Personnel:

Infection Control . . . . Cathy Blythe
Quality Assurance . . . . Gayle Curtis
CEO/President. . . . . Evan S. Dillard, MPH, MBA, FACHE
Cardiac Laboratory. . . . . Sandra K Jones
Radiology. . . . . Joe Marcello
Chief of Medical Staff . . . . William H Peters, MD
Pediatric Ambulatory Care . . . . . . Angie Reeves
Operating Room. . . . . Kathryn Russum

Measure	Cases	This Hosp.	State Avg.	U.S. Avg.
Blood Clot Prevention and Treatment				
Anticoagulation Overlap Therapy[2]	118	94%	86%	93%
ICU Venous Thromboembolism Prophylaxis[2]	57	93%	86%	92%
Incidence of Potentially Preventable VTE[2]	25	8%	15%	10%
UFH with Dosages/Platelet Monitoring[2]	21	100%	94%	97%
Venous Thromboembolism Prophylaxis[2]	285	82%	70%	85%
Warfarin Therapy Discharge Instructions[2]	93	77%	77%	75%
Chest Pain/Possible Heart Attack Care				
Aspirin Given Within 24 Hours of Arrival[3,7]	-	-	94%	96%
Fibrinolytic Meds Within 30 Min. of Arrival[5]	-	-	40%	58%
Average Time to ECG (minutes)[3,7]	-	-	10	7
Average Time to Transfer (minutes)[5]	-	-	77	60
Children's Asthma Care				
Received Home Management Plan of Care	-	-	-	88%
Received Reliever Medication	-	-	-	100%
Received Systemic Corticosteroids	-	-	-	100%
Emergency Department				
Admittance Decision Time (minutes)[2]	594	58	61	98
Head CT Results Within 45 Min. of Arrival[1]	-	-	42%	57%
Patients Who Left ER Before Being Seen	83,340	5%	3%	2%
Time from ER Arrival to Admit. (minutes)[2]	627	261	223	274
Time from ER Arrival to Discharge (minutes)	430	236	112	134
Time in ER Before Being Evaluated (minutes)	241	72	29	26
Time to Pain Meds for Fractures (minutes)	253	79	68	57
Heart Attack Care				
Aspirin Given at Discharge	493	99%	99%	99%
Fibrinolytic Meds Within 30 Min. of Arrival[7]	-	-	50%	54%
PCI Within 90 Minutes of Arrival	47	100%	96%	96%
Statin Prescribed at Discharge	472	98%	97%	98%
Heart Failure Care				
ACE Inhibitor or ARB for LVSD	244	98%	93%	97%
Discharge Instructions Given	603	100%	91%	94%
Evaluation of LVS Function	717	100%	96%	99%
Medicare Spending				
Medicare Spending per Patient (ratio)	-	0.99	0.95	0.98
Pneumonia Care				
Appropriate Initial Antibiotic Given	214	93%	91%	95%
Blood Culture Timing	352	95%	97%	98%
Pregnancy and Delivery Care				
Newborn Deliveries Scheduled Early	313	20%	22%	6%
Preventive Care				
Immunization for Influenza[2]	584	98%	87%	90%
Immunization for Pneumonia[2]	652	97%	89%	92%
Stroke Care				
Anticoagulation Therapy for Atrial Fibrillation[1,2]	-	-	93%	95%
Antithrombotic Therapy Timing[2]	77	96%	96%	98%
Assessed for Rehabilitation[2]	92	100%	95%	97%
Discharged on Antithrombotic Therapy[2]	83	99%	97%	99%
Discharged on Statin Medication[2]	63	94%	88%	94%
Thrombolytic Therapy Timing[1,2]	-	-	25%	66%
Venous Thromboembolism Prophylaxis[2]	81	88%	87%	94%
Written Stroke Educational Materials Given[2]	44	82%	84%	88%
Surgical Care Improvement Project				
Appropriate Beta Blocker Usage[2]	253	97%	97%	98%
Appropriate VTP Within 24 Hours[2]	367	97%	97%	98%
Controlled Postoperative Blood Glucose[2]	174	91%	97%	97%
Perioperative Temperature Management[2]	474	100%	100%	100%
Prophylactic Antibiotic Selection[2]	497	97%	99%	99%
Prophylactic Antibiotic Selection (Outpatient)	555	97%	98%	98%
Prophylactic Antibiotic Stopped[2]	472	95%	97%	98%
Prophylactic Antibiotic Timing[2]	498	98%	99%	99%
Prophylactic Antibiotic Timing (Outpatient)	561	97%	98%	98%
Urinary Catheter Removal[2]	441	95%	97%	97%
Survey of Patients' Hospital Experiences				
Area Around Room 'Always' Quiet at Night	300+	71%	72%	61%
Doctors 'Always' Communicated Well	300+	82%	86%	82%
Home Recovery Information Given	300+	80%	83%	85%
Hospital Given 9 or 10 on 10 Point Scale	300+	74%	71%	71%
Meds 'Always' Explained Before Given	300+	63%	67%	64%
Nurses 'Always' Communicated Well	300+	80%	81%	79%
Pain 'Always' Well Controlled	300+	71%	72%	71%
Room and Bathroom 'Always' Clean	300+	70%	74%	73%
Timely Help 'Always' Received	300+	63%	69%	68%
Would Definitely Recommend Hospital	300+	77%	69%	71%
Use of Medical Imaging				
Cardiac Imaging Stress Test before Surgery	478	6.1%	5.7%	5.3%
Combination Abdominal CT Scan	963	1.1%	12.9%	10.5%
Combination Brain/Sinus CT Scan	1,680	3.1%	3.3%	2.7%
Combination Chest CT Scan	299	1.3%	6.1%	2.7%
Follow-up Mammogram/Ultrasound	190	7.4%	8.4%	8.8%
Lumbar Spine MRI for Low Back Pain	70	41.4%	41.1%	37.2%

Wesley Medical Center

5001 W Hardy St
Hattiesburg, MS 39402
Phone: 601-268-8000
Fax: 601-268-5008
URL: www.wesley.com
Type: Acute Care Hospitals
Emergency Services: Yes
Ownership: Voluntary non-profit - Private
Beds: 211

Key Personnel:

Quality Assurance . . . . Debbie Burt
Radiology. . . . . Stephen Cunningham
CEO . . . . Steve Edgar
Chief of Medical Staff . . . . Francie Ekengren
Pediatric Ambulatory Care . . . . . . John Gaudet, MD
Pediatric In-Patient Care . . . . John Gaudet, MD
President/CEO. . . . . Hugh Tappan

Measure	Cases	This Hosp.	State Avg.	U.S. Avg.
Blood Clot Prevention and Treatment				
Anticoagulation Overlap Therapy[2]	41	100%	86%	93%
ICU Venous Thromboembolism Prophylaxis[2]	96	100%	86%	92%
Incidence of Potentially Preventable VTE[1,2]	-	-	15%	10%
UFH with Dosages/Platelet Monitoring[2,7]	-	-	94%	97%
Venous Thromboembolism Prophylaxis[2]	348	97%	70%	85%
Warfarin Therapy Discharge Instructions[2]	33	97%	77%	75%
Chest Pain/Possible Heart Attack Care				
Aspirin Given Within 24 Hours of Arrival[1,3]	-	-	94%	96%
Fibrinolytic Meds Within 30 Min. of Arrival[5]	-	-	40%	58%
Average Time to ECG (minutes)[1,3]	-	-	10	7
Average Time to Transfer (minutes)[5]	-	-	77	60
Children's Asthma Care				
Received Home Management Plan of Care	-	-	-	88%
Received Reliever Medication	-	-	-	100%
Received Systemic Corticosteroids	-	-	-	100%
Emergency Department				
Admittance Decision Time (minutes)[2]	558	58	61	98
Head CT Results Within 45 Min. of Arrival[1]	-	-	42%	57%
Patients Who Left ER Before Being Seen	36,445	4%	3%	2%
Time from ER Arrival to Admit. (minutes)[2]	565	209	223	274
Time from ER Arrival to Discharge (minutes)	404	127	112	134
Time in ER Before Being Evaluated (minutes)	415	28	29	26
Time to Pain Meds for Fractures (minutes)	104	64	68	57
Heart Attack Care				
Aspirin Given at Discharge	106	98%	99%	99%
Fibrinolytic Meds Within 30 Min. of Arrival[7]	-	-	50%	54%
PCI Within 90 Minutes of Arrival[1]	-	-	96%	96%
Statin Prescribed at Discharge	93	100%	97%	98%
Heart Failure Care				
ACE Inhibitor or ARB for LVSD	72	100%	93%	97%
Discharge Instructions Given	176	99%	91%	94%
Evaluation of LVS Function	205	100%	96%	99%
Medicare Spending				
Medicare Spending per Patient (ratio)	-	0.99	0.95	0.98
Pneumonia Care				
Appropriate Initial Antibiotic Given	94	99%	91%	95%
Blood Culture Timing	140	99%	97%	98%
Pregnancy and Delivery Care				
Newborn Deliveries Scheduled Early[2]	41	0%	22%	6%
Preventive Care				
Immunization for Influenza[2]	548	95%	87%	90%
Immunization for Pneumonia[2]	614	98%	89%	92%
Stroke Care				
Anticoagulation Therapy for Atrial Fibrillation[1]	-	-	93%	95%
Antithrombotic Therapy Timing	58	100%	96%	98%
Assessed for Rehabilitation	69	99%	95%	97%
Discharged on Antithrombotic Therapy	64	100%	97%	99%

NOTE: Hospital profiles are in alphabetical order by state, then city, then hospital within the city; Rankings exclude hospitals with less than 25 cases except for patient surveys which excludes hospitals with less than 100 cases; (a) 100-299 cases; (1) The number of cases/patients is too few to report; (2) Data submitted were based on a sample of cases/patients; (3) Results are based on a shorter time period than required; (4) Data suppressed by CMS for one or more quarters; (5) Results are not available for this reporting period; (6) Fewer than 100 patients completed the HCAHPS survey; (7) No cases met the criteria for this measure; (8) The lower limit of the confidence interval cannot be calculated if the number of observed infections equals zero; (9) No data are available from the state/territory for this reporting period; (10) The scores shown reflect fewer than 50 completed surveys; (11) There were discrepancies in the data collection process; (12) This measure does not apply to this hospital for this reporting period; (13) Results cannot be calculated for this reporting period; (14) The results for this state are combined with nearby states to protect confidentiality; Please refer to the User's Guide for a full explanation of data.

Measure	Cases	This Hosp.	State Avg.	U.S. Avg.
Discharged on Statin Medication	51	100%	88%	94%
Thrombolytic Therapy Timing[7]	-	-	25%	66%
Venous Thromboembolism Prophylaxis	66	91%	87%	94%
Written Stroke Educational Materials Given	44	98%	84%	88%
Surgical Care Improvement Project				
Appropriate Beta Blocker Usage	261	100%	97%	98%
Appropriate VTP Within 24 Hours	578	99%	97%	98%
Controlled Postoperative Blood Glucose	119	100%	97%	97%
Perioperative Temperature Management	641	100%	100%	100%
Prophylactic Antibiotic Selection	484	100%	99%	99%
Prophylactic Antibiotic Selection (Outpatient)	382	99%	98%	98%
Prophylactic Antibiotic Stopped	377	100%	97%	98%
Prophylactic Antibiotic Timing	484	99%	99%	99%
Prophylactic Antibiotic Timing (Outpatient)	383	99%	98%	98%
Urinary Catheter Removal	411	100%	97%	97%
Survey of Patients' Hospital Experiences				
Area Around Room 'Always' Quiet at Night	300+	72%	72%	61%
Doctors 'Always' Communicated Well	300+	86%	86%	82%
Home Recovery Information Given	300+	87%	83%	85%
Hospital Given 9 or 10 on 10 Point Scale	300+	75%	71%	71%
Meds 'Always' Explained Before Given	300+	65%	67%	64%
Nurses 'Always' Communicated Well	300+	80%	81%	79%
Pain 'Always' Well Controlled	300+	74%	72%	71%
Room and Bathroom 'Always' Clean	300+	72%	74%	73%
Timely Help 'Always' Received	300+	70%	69%	68%
Would Definitely Recommend Hospital	300+	78%	69%	71%
Use of Medical Imaging				
Cardiac Imaging Stress Test before Surgery	279	5.7%	5.7%	5.3%
Combination Abdominal CT Scan	643	4.2%	12.9%	10.5%
Combination Brain/Sinus CT Scan[1]	-	-	3.3%	2.7%
Combination Chest CT Scan	341	2.9%	6.1%	2.7%
Follow-up Mammogram/Ultrasound	1,226	10.6%	8.4%	8.8%
Lumbar Spine MRI for Low Back Pain	82	35.4%	41.1%	37.2%

Hardy Wilson Memorial Hospital

233 Magnolia Street
Hazlehurst, MS 39083
Type: Critical Access Hospitals
Ownership: Government - Local

Phone: 601-894-4541
Fax: 601-894-6279
Emergency Services: Yes
Beds: 35

Measure	Cases	This Hosp.	State Avg.	U.S. Avg.
Blood Clot Prevention and Treatment				
Anticoagulation Overlap Therapy[5]	-	-	86%	93%
ICU Venous Thromboembolism Prophylaxis[5]	-	-	86%	92%
Incidence of Potentially Preventable VTE[5]	-	-	15%	10%
UFH with Dosages/Platelet Monitoring[5]	-	-	94%	97%
Venous Thromboembolism Prophylaxis[5]	-	-	70%	85%
Warfarin Therapy Discharge Instructions[5]	-	-	77%	75%
Chest Pain/Possible Heart Attack Care				
Aspirin Given Within 24 Hours of Arrival	26	85%	94%	96%
Fibrinolytic Meds Within 30 Min. of Arrival[1]	-	-	40%	58%
Average Time to ECG (minutes)	27	12	10	7
Average Time to Transfer (minutes)[1]	-	-	77	60
Children's Asthma Care				
Received Home Management Plan of Care	-	-	-	88%
Received Reliever Medication	-	-	-	100%
Received Systemic Corticosteroids	-	-	-	100%
Emergency Department				
Admittance Decision Time (minutes)[5]	-	-	61	98
Head CT Results Within 45 Min. of Arrival[5]	-	-	42%	57%
Patients Who Left ER Before Being Seen[5]	-	-	3%	2%
Time from ER Arrival to Admit. (minutes)[5]	-	-	223	274
Time from ER Arrival to Discharge (minutes)	353	124	112	134
Time in ER Before Being Evaluated (minutes)	349	36	29	26
Time to Pain Meds for Fractures (minutes)[5]	-	-	68	57
Heart Attack Care				
Aspirin Given at Discharge[5]	-	-	99%	99%
Fibrinolytic Meds Within 30 Min. of Arrival[5]	-	-	50%	54%
PCI Within 90 Minutes of Arrival[5]	-	-	96%	96%
Statin Prescribed at Discharge[5]	-	-	97%	98%
Heart Failure Care				
ACE Inhibitor or ARB for LVSD[1,2]	-	-	93%	97%
Discharge Instructions Given[2]	27	19%	91%	94%
Evaluation of LVS Function[2]	32	31%	96%	99%
Medicare Spending				
Medicare Spending per Patient (ratio)	-	-	0.95	0.98
Pneumonia Care				
Appropriate Initial Antibiotic Given[2]	25	80%	91%	95%
Blood Culture Timing[2]	29	93%	97%	98%
Pregnancy and Delivery Care				
Newborn Deliveries Scheduled Early[5]	-	-	22%	6%
Preventive Care				
Immunization for Influenza[5]	-	-	87%	90%
Immunization for Pneumonia[5]	-	-	89%	92%
Stroke Care				
Anticoagulation Therapy for Atrial Fibrillation[5]	-	-	93%	95%
Antithrombotic Therapy Timing[5]	-	-	96%	98%
Assessed for Rehabilitation[5]	-	-	95%	97%
Discharged on Antithrombotic Therapy[5]	-	-	97%	99%
Discharged on Statin Medication[5]	-	-	88%	94%
Thrombolytic Therapy Timing[5]	-	-	25%	66%
Venous Thromboembolism Prophylaxis[5]	-	-	87%	94%
Written Stroke Educational Materials Given[5]	-	-	84%	88%
Surgical Care Improvement Project				
Appropriate Beta Blocker Usage[5]	-	-	97%	98%
Appropriate VTP Within 24 Hours[5]	-	-	97%	98%
Controlled Postoperative Blood Glucose[5]	-	-	97%	97%
Perioperative Temperature Management[5]	-	-	100%	100%
Prophylactic Antibiotic Selection[5]	-	-	99%	99%
Prophylactic Antibiotic Selection (Outpatient)[5]	-	-	98%	98%
Prophylactic Antibiotic Stopped[5]	-	-	97%	98%
Prophylactic Antibiotic Timing[5]	-	-	99%	99%
Prophylactic Antibiotic Timing (Outpatient)[5]	-	-	98%	98%
Urinary Catheter Removal[5]	-	-	97%	97%
Survey of Patients' Hospital Experiences				
Area Around Room 'Always' Quiet at Night[5]	-	-	72%	61%
Doctors 'Always' Communicated Well[5]	-	-	86%	82%
Home Recovery Information Given[5]	-	-	83%	85%
Hospital Given 9 or 10 on 10 Point Scale[5]	-	-	71%	71%
Meds 'Always' Explained Before Given[5]	-	-	67%	64%
Nurses 'Always' Communicated Well[5]	-	-	81%	79%
Pain 'Always' Well Controlled[5]	-	-	72%	71%
Room and Bathroom 'Always' Clean[5]	-	-	74%	73%
Timely Help 'Always' Received[5]	-	-	69%	68%
Would Definitely Recommend Hospital[5]	-	-	69%	71%
Use of Medical Imaging				
Cardiac Imaging Stress Test before Surgery[7]	-	-	5.7%	5.3%
Combination Abdominal CT Scan	162	4.3%	12.9%	10.5%
Combination Brain/Sinus CT Scan	294	5.1%	3.3%	2.7%
Combination Chest CT Scan	88	4.5%	6.1%	2.7%
Follow-up Mammogram/Ultrasound	206	1.9%	8.4%	8.8%
Lumbar Spine MRI for Low Back Pain[1]	-	-	41.1%	37.2%

Alliance Healthcare System

1430 Highway 4 East / PO Box 6000
Holly Springs, MS 38635
Type: Acute Care Hospitals
Ownership: Proprietary

Phone: 662-252-1212
Fax: 662-252-5537
Emergency Services: Yes
Beds: 40

Key Personnel:
Chief of Medical Staff. . . . . Joseph Diaz
CEO/President. . . . . Perry E Williams, SR

Measure	Cases	This Hosp.	State Avg.	U.S. Avg.
Blood Clot Prevention and Treatment				
Anticoagulation Overlap Therapy[1,2]	-	-	86%	93%
ICU Venous Thromboembolism Prophylaxis[1,2]	-	-	86%	92%
Incidence of Potentially Preventable VTE[1,2]	-	-	15%	10%
UFH with Dosages/Platelet Monitoring[2,7]	-	-	94%	97%
Venous Thromboembolism Prophylaxis[2]	134	6%	70%	85%
Warfarin Therapy Discharge Instructions[1,2]	-	-	77%	75%
Chest Pain/Possible Heart Attack Care				
Aspirin Given Within 24 Hours of Arrival[1,3]	-	-	94%	96%
Fibrinolytic Meds Within 30 Min. of Arrival[3,7]	-	-	40%	58%
Average Time to ECG (minutes)[1,3]	-	-	10	7
Average Time to Transfer (minutes)[3,7]	-	-	77	60
Children's Asthma Care				
Received Home Management Plan of Care	-	-	-	88%
Received Reliever Medication	-	-	-	100%
Received Systemic Corticosteroids	-	-	-	100%
Emergency Department				
Admittance Decision Time (minutes)[2]	106	78	61	98
Head CT Results Within 45 Min. of Arrival[5]	-	-	42%	57%
Patients Who Left ER Before Being Seen	4,400	1%	3%	2%
Time from ER Arrival to Admit. (minutes)[2]	114	195	223	274
Time from ER Arrival to Discharge (minutes)	273	80	112	134
Time in ER Before Being Evaluated (minutes)	321	10	29	26
Time to Pain Meds for Fractures (minutes)[1,3]	-	-	68	57
Heart Attack Care				
Aspirin Given at Discharge[3,7]	-	-	99%	99%
Fibrinolytic Meds Within 30 Min. of Arrival[3,7]	-	-	50%	54%
PCI Within 90 Minutes of Arrival[3,7]	-	-	96%	96%
Statin Prescribed at Discharge[3,7]	-	-	97%	98%
Heart Failure Care				
ACE Inhibitor or ARB for LVSD[1,2]	-	-	93%	97%
Discharge Instructions Given[1,2]	-	-	91%	94%
Evaluation of LVS Function[1,2]	-	-	96%	99%
Medicare Spending				
Medicare Spending per Patient (ratio)	-	1.04	0.95	0.98
Pneumonia Care				
Appropriate Initial Antibiotic Given[2]	11	82%	91%	95%
Blood Culture Timing[1,2]	-	-	97%	98%
Pregnancy and Delivery Care				
Newborn Deliveries Scheduled Early[2,7]	-	-	22%	6%
Preventive Care				
Immunization for Influenza[2]	117	69%	87%	90%
Immunization for Pneumonia[2]	183	67%	89%	92%
Stroke Care				
Anticoagulation Therapy for Atrial Fibrillation[3,7]	-	-	93%	95%
Antithrombotic Therapy Timing[1,3]	-	-	96%	98%
Assessed for Rehabilitation[1,3]	-	-	95%	97%
Discharged on Antithrombotic Therapy[1,3]	-	-	97%	99%
Discharged on Statin Medication[3,7]	-	-	88%	94%
Thrombolytic Therapy Timing[1,3]	-	-	25%	66%
Venous Thromboembolism Prophylaxis[1,3]	-	-	87%	94%
Written Stroke Educational Materials Given[1,3]	-	-	84%	88%
Surgical Care Improvement Project				
Appropriate Beta Blocker Usage[5]	-	-	97%	98%
Appropriate VTP Within 24 Hours[5]	-	-	97%	98%
Controlled Postoperative Blood Glucose[5]	-	-	97%	97%
Perioperative Temperature Management[5]	-	-	100%	100%
Prophylactic Antibiotic Selection[5]	-	-	99%	99%
Prophylactic Antibiotic Selection (Outpatient)[5]	-	-	98%	98%
Prophylactic Antibiotic Stopped[5]	-	-	97%	98%
Prophylactic Antibiotic Timing[5]	-	-	99%	99%
Prophylactic Antibiotic Timing (Outpatient)[5]	-	-	98%	98%
Urinary Catheter Removal[5]	-	-	97%	97%
Survey of Patients' Hospital Experiences				
Area Around Room 'Always' Quiet at Night[6]	<100	78%	72%	61%
Doctors 'Always' Communicated Well[6]	<100	87%	86%	82%
Home Recovery Information Given[6]	<100	75%	83%	85%
Hospital Given 9 or 10 on 10 Point Scale[6]	<100	51%	71%	71%
Meds 'Always' Explained Before Given[6]	<100	55%	67%	64%
Nurses 'Always' Communicated Well[6]	<100	70%	81%	79%
Pain 'Always' Well Controlled[6]	<100	65%	72%	71%
Room and Bathroom 'Always' Clean[6]	<100	75%	74%	73%
Timely Help 'Always' Received[6]	<100	63%	69%	68%
Would Definitely Recommend Hospital[6]	<100	44%	69%	71%
Use of Medical Imaging				
Cardiac Imaging Stress Test before Surgery[7]	-	-	5.7%	5.3%
Combination Abdominal CT Scan[7]	-	-	12.9%	10.5%
Combination Brain/Sinus CT Scan[7]	-	-	3.3%	2.7%
Combination Chest CT Scan[7]	-	-	6.1%	2.7%
Follow-up Mammogram/Ultrasound	152	10.5%	8.4%	8.8%
Lumbar Spine MRI for Low Back Pain[7]	-	-	41.1%	37.2%

NOTE: Hospital profiles are in alphabetical order by state, then city, then hospital within the city; Rankings exclude hospitals with less than 25 cases except for patient surveys which excludes hospitals with less than 100 cases; (a) 100-299 cases; (1) The number of cases/patients is too few to report; (2) Data submitted were based on a sample of cases/patients; (3) Results are based on a shorter time period than required; (4) Data suppressed by CMS for one or more quarters; (5) Results are not available for this reporting period; (6) Fewer than 100 patients completed the HCAHPS survey; (7) No cases met the criteria for this measure; (8) The lower limit of the confidence interval cannot be calculated if the number of observed infections equals zero; (9) No data are available from the state/territory for this reporting period; (10) The scores shown reflect fewer than 50 completed surveys; (11) There were discrepancies in the data collection process; (12) This measure does not apply to this hospital for this reporting period; (13) Results cannot be calculated for this reporting period; (14) The results for this state are combined with nearby states to protect confidentiality; Please refer to the User's Guide for a full explanation of data.

Trace Regional Hospital & Swing Bed

1004 East Madison Street
Houston, MS 38851
URL: www.traceregional.com
Type: Acute Care Hospitals
Ownership: Proprietary
Phone: 662-456-3700
Fax: 662-456-5417
Emergency Services: Yes
Beds: 125

Key Personnel:
Emergency Room . . . . Curtis Cunningham
CEO . . . . Gary Staten

Measure	Cases	This Hosp.	State Avg.	U.S. Avg.
Blood Clot Prevention and Treatment				
Anticoagulation Overlap Therapy[1,2]	-	-	86%	93%
ICU Venous Thromboembolism Prophylaxis[1,2]	-	-	86%	92%
Incidence of Potentially Preventable VTE[1,2]	-	-	15%	10%
UFH with Dosages/Platelet Monitoring[2,3]	-	-	94%	97%
Venous Thromboembolism Prophylaxis[2,3]	139	23%	70%	85%
Warfarin Therapy Discharge Instructions[1,2]	-	-	77%	75%
Chest Pain/Possible Heart Attack Care				
Aspirin Given Within 24 Hours of Arrival	33	94%	94%	96%
Fibrinolytic Meds Within 30 Min. of Arrival[1]	-	-	40%	58%
Average Time to ECG (minutes)	32	13	10	7
Average Time to Transfer (minutes)[1]	-	-	77	60
Children's Asthma Care				
Received Home Management Plan of Care	-	-	-	88%
Received Reliever Medication	-	-	-	100%
Received Systemic Corticosteroids	-	-	-	100%
Emergency Department				
Admittance Decision Time (minutes)[2]	230	50	61	98
Head CT Results Within 45 Min. of Arrival[1]	-	-	42%	57%
Patients Who Left ER Before Being Seen	7,312	1%	3%	2%
Time from ER Arrival to Admit. (minutes)[2]	236	185	223	274
Time from ER Arrival to Discharge (minutes)	403	73	112	134
Time in ER Before Being Evaluated (minutes)	415	19	29	26
Time to Pain Meds for Fractures (minutes)	29	55	68	57
Heart Attack Care				
Aspirin Given at Discharge[1,3]	-	-	99%	99%
Fibrinolytic Meds Within 30 Min. of Arrival[3,7]	-	-	50%	54%
PCI Within 90 Minutes of Arrival[3,7]	-	-	96%	96%
Statin Prescribed at Discharge[1,3]	-	-	97%	98%
Heart Failure Care				
ACE Inhibitor or ARB for LVSD[1,2]	-	-	93%	97%
Discharge Instructions Given[2]	12	92%	91%	94%
Evaluation of LVS Function[2]	17	76%	96%	99%
Medicare Spending				
Medicare Spending per Patient (ratio)	-	0.91	0.95	0.98
Pneumonia Care				
Appropriate Initial Antibiotic Given[2]	26	81%	91%	95%
Blood Culture Timing[2]	29	90%	97%	98%
Pregnancy and Delivery Care				
Newborn Deliveries Scheduled Early[7]	-	-	22%	6%
Preventive Care				
Immunization for Influenza[2]	181	65%	87%	90%
Immunization for Pneumonia[2]	268	70%	89%	92%
Stroke Care				
Anticoagulation Therapy for Atrial Fibrillation[3,7]	-	-	93%	95%
Antithrombotic Therapy Timing[1,3]	-	-	96%	98%
Assessed for Rehabilitation[1,3]	-	-	95%	97%
Discharged on Antithrombotic Therapy[1,3]	-	-	97%	99%
Discharged on Statin Medication[1,3]	-	-	88%	94%
Thrombolytic Therapy Timing[3,7]	-	-	25%	66%
Venous Thromboembolism Prophylaxis[1,3]	-	-	87%	94%
Written Stroke Educational Materials Given[1,3]	-	-	84%	88%
Surgical Care Improvement Project				
Appropriate Beta Blocker Usage[5]	-	-	97%	98%
Appropriate VTP Within 24 Hours[5]	-	-	97%	98%
Controlled Postoperative Blood Glucose[5]	-	-	97%	97%
Perioperative Temperature Management[5]	-	-	100%	100%
Prophylactic Antibiotic Selection[5]	-	-	99%	99%
Prophylactic Antibiotic Selection (Outpatient)[5]	-	-	98%	98%
Prophylactic Antibiotic Stopped[5]	-	-	97%	98%
Prophylactic Antibiotic Timing[5]	-	-	99%	99%
Prophylactic Antibiotic Timing (Outpatient)[5]	-	-	98%	98%
Urinary Catheter Removal[5]	-	-	97%	97%
Survey of Patients' Hospital Experiences				
Area Around Room 'Always' Quiet at Night[6]	<100	72%	72%	61%
Doctors 'Always' Communicated Well[6]	<100	81%	86%	82%
Home Recovery Information Given[6]	<100	82%	83%	85%
Hospital Given 9 or 10 on 10 Point Scale[6]	<100	52%	71%	71%
Meds 'Always' Explained Before Given[6]	<100	84%	67%	64%
Nurses 'Always' Communicated Well[6]	<100	77%	81%	79%
Pain 'Always' Well Controlled[6]	<100	60%	72%	71%
Room and Bathroom 'Always' Clean[6]	<100	67%	74%	73%
Timely Help 'Always' Received[6]	<100	60%	69%	68%
Would Definitely Recommend Hospital[6]	<100	54%	69%	71%
Use of Medical Imaging				
Cardiac Imaging Stress Test before Surgery[7]	-	-	5.7%	5.3%
Combination Abdominal CT Scan	150	48.0%	12.9%	10.5%
Combination Brain/Sinus CT Scan[1]	-	-	3.3%	2.7%
Combination Chest CT Scan[1]	-	-	6.1%	2.7%
Follow-up Mammogram/Ultrasound	264	4.2%	8.4%	8.8%
Lumbar Spine MRI for Low Back Pain	60	33.3%	41.1%	37.2%

South Sunflower County Hospital

121 E Baker St
Indianola, MS 38751
Type: Acute Care Hospitals
Ownership: Government - Local
Phone: 662-887-5235
Fax: 662-887-4111
Emergency Services: Yes
Beds: 69

Measure	Cases	This Hosp.	State Avg.	U.S. Avg.
Blood Clot Prevention and Treatment				
Anticoagulation Overlap Therapy[1,2]	-	-	86%	93%
ICU Venous Thromboembolism Prophylaxis[2]	65	55%	86%	92%
Incidence of Potentially Preventable VTE[2,7]	-	-	15%	10%
UFH with Dosages/Platelet Monitoring[2,7]	-	-	94%	97%
Venous Thromboembolism Prophylaxis[2]	165	49%	70%	85%
Warfarin Therapy Discharge Instructions[1,2]	-	-	77%	75%
Chest Pain/Possible Heart Attack Care				
Aspirin Given Within 24 Hours of Arrival	24	83%	94%	96%
Fibrinolytic Meds Within 30 Min. of Arrival[1]	-	-	40%	58%
Average Time to ECG (minutes)	25	35	10	7
Average Time to Transfer (minutes)[1]	-	-	77	60
Children's Asthma Care				
Received Home Management Plan of Care	-	-	-	88%
Received Reliever Medication	-	-	-	100%
Received Systemic Corticosteroids	-	-	-	100%
Emergency Department				
Admittance Decision Time (minutes)[2]	113	35	61	98
Head CT Results Within 45 Min. of Arrival[3]	12	8%	42%	57%
Patients Who Left ER Before Being Seen[5]	-	-	3%	2%
Time from ER Arrival to Admit. (minutes)[2]	155	162	223	274
Time from ER Arrival to Discharge (minutes)	355	113	112	134
Time in ER Before Being Evaluated (minutes)	199	62	29	26
Time to Pain Meds for Fractures (minutes)[3]	19	64	68	57
Heart Attack Care				
Aspirin Given at Discharge[1,2]	-	-	99%	99%
Fibrinolytic Meds Within 30 Min. of Arrival[2,3]	-	-	50%	54%
PCI Within 90 Minutes of Arrival[2,3]	-	-	96%	96%
Statin Prescribed at Discharge[1,2]	-	-	97%	98%
Heart Failure Care				
ACE Inhibitor or ARB for LVSD[2]	20	90%	93%	97%
Discharge Instructions Given[2]	45	60%	91%	94%
Evaluation of LVS Function[2]	57	82%	96%	99%
Medicare Spending				
Medicare Spending per Patient (ratio)	-	0.87	0.95	0.98
Pneumonia Care				
Appropriate Initial Antibiotic Given[2]	26	96%	91%	95%
Blood Culture Timing[2]	14	100%	97%	98%
Pregnancy and Delivery Care				
Newborn Deliveries Scheduled Early[2,7]	-	-	22%	6%
Preventive Care				
Immunization for Influenza[2]	269	55%	87%	90%
Immunization for Pneumonia[2]	296	52%	89%	92%
Stroke Care				
Anticoagulation Therapy for Atrial Fibrillation[1,2]	-	-	93%	95%
Antithrombotic Therapy Timing[2]	15	87%	96%	98%
Assessed for Rehabilitation[2]	11	73%	95%	97%
Discharged on Antithrombotic Therapy[2]	11	82%	97%	99%
Discharged on Statin Medication[2]	11	36%	88%	94%
Thrombolytic Therapy Timing[1,2]	-	-	25%	66%
Venous Thromboembolism Prophylaxis[2]	14	64%	87%	94%
Written Stroke Educational Materials Given[1,2]	-	-	84%	88%
Surgical Care Improvement Project				
Appropriate Beta Blocker Usage[2,3]	-	-	97%	98%
Appropriate VTP Within 24 Hours[1,2]	-	-	97%	98%
Controlled Postoperative Blood Glucose[2,3]	-	-	97%	97%
Perioperative Temperature Management[1,2]	-	-	100%	100%
Prophylactic Antibiotic Selection[2,3]	-	-	99%	99%
Prophylactic Antibiotic Selection (Outpatient)[1,3]	-	-	98%	98%
Prophylactic Antibiotic Stopped[2,3]	-	-	97%	98%
Prophylactic Antibiotic Timing[2,3]	-	-	99%	99%
Prophylactic Antibiotic Timing (Outpatient)[1,3]	-	-	98%	98%
Urinary Catheter Removal[2,3]	-	-	97%	97%
Survey of Patients' Hospital Experiences				
Area Around Room 'Always' Quiet at Night	(a)	69%	72%	61%
Doctors 'Always' Communicated Well	(a)	91%	86%	82%
Home Recovery Information Given	(a)	68%	83%	85%
Hospital Given 9 or 10 on 10 Point Scale	(a)	67%	71%	71%
Meds 'Always' Explained Before Given	(a)	66%	67%	64%
Nurses 'Always' Communicated Well	(a)	80%	81%	79%
Pain 'Always' Well Controlled	(a)	78%	72%	71%
Room and Bathroom 'Always' Clean	(a)	63%	74%	73%
Timely Help 'Always' Received	(a)	65%	69%	68%
Would Definitely Recommend Hospital	(a)	66%	69%	71%
Use of Medical Imaging				
Cardiac Imaging Stress Test before Surgery[7]	-	-	5.7%	5.3%
Combination Abdominal CT Scan	186	41.4%	12.9%	10.5%
Combination Brain/Sinus CT Scan	270	1.1%	3.3%	2.7%
Combination Chest CT Scan	72	36.1%	6.1%	2.7%
Follow-up Mammogram/Ultrasound	181	5.0%	8.4%	8.8%
Lumbar Spine MRI for Low Back Pain[1]	-	-	41.1%	37.2%

Tishomingo Health Services

1777 Curtis Drive
Iuka, MS 38852
URL: www.nmhs.net/iuka
Type: Acute Care Hospitals
Ownership: Voluntary non-profit - Private
Phone: 662-423-6051
Fax: 662-423-4515
Emergency Services: Yes
Beds: 48

Key Personnel:
Radiology. . . . . Kirk Haney
CEO/President. . . . . Joe Reppert
Chief of Medical Staff. . . . . Mark Williams

Measure	Cases	This Hosp.	State Avg.	U.S. Avg.
Blood Clot Prevention and Treatment				
Anticoagulation Overlap Therapy[1,2]	-	-	86%	93%
ICU Venous Thromboembolism Prophylaxis[1,2]	-	-	86%	92%
Incidence of Potentially Preventable VTE[2,7]	-	-	15%	10%
UFH with Dosages/Platelet Monitoring[2,7]	-	-	94%	97%
Venous Thromboembolism Prophylaxis[2]	114	89%	70%	85%
Warfarin Therapy Discharge Instructions[1,2]	-	-	77%	75%
Chest Pain/Possible Heart Attack Care				
Aspirin Given Within 24 Hours of Arrival	23	96%	94%	96%
Fibrinolytic Meds Within 30 Min. of Arrival[3,7]	-	-	40%	58%
Average Time to ECG (minutes)	24	8	10	7
Average Time to Transfer (minutes)[1,3]	-	-	77	60
Children's Asthma Care				
Received Home Management Plan of Care	-	-	-	88%
Received Reliever Medication	-	-	-	100%
Received Systemic Corticosteroids	-	-	-	100%
Emergency Department				
Admittance Decision Time (minutes)[2]	359	38	61	98
Head CT Results Within 45 Min. of Arrival[1]	-	-	42%	57%
Patients Who Left ER Before Being Seen	10,585	1%	3%	2%
Time from ER Arrival to Admit. (minutes)[2]	377	161	223	274
Time from ER Arrival to Discharge (minutes)	406	94	112	134
Time in ER Before Being Evaluated (minutes)	418	27	29	26
Time to Pain Meds for Fractures (minutes)	29	72	68	57
Heart Attack Care				
Aspirin Given at Discharge[1,3]	-	-	99%	99%
Fibrinolytic Meds Within 30 Min. of Arrival[3,7]	-	-	50%	54%

NOTE: Hospital profiles are in alphabetical order by state, then city, then hospital within the city; Rankings exclude hospitals with less than 25 cases except for patient surveys which excludes hospitals with less than 100 cases; (a) 100-299 cases; (1) The number of cases/patients is too few to report; (2) Data submitted were based on a sample of cases/patients; (3) Results are based on a shorter time period than required; (4) Data suppressed by CMS for one or more quarters; (5) Results are not available for this reporting period; (6) Fewer than 100 patients completed the HCAHPS survey; (7) No cases met the criteria for this measure; (8) The lower limit of the confidence interval cannot be calculated if the number of observed infections equals zero; (9) No data are available from the state/territory for this reporting period; (10) The scores shown reflect fewer than 50 completed surveys; (11) There were discrepancies in the data collection process; (12) This measure does not apply to this hospital for this reporting period; (13) Results cannot be calculated for this reporting period; (14) The results for this state are combined with nearby states to protect confidentiality; Please refer to the User's Guide for a full explanation of data.

Measure	Cases	This Hosp.	State Avg.	U.S. Avg.
PCI Within 90 Minutes of Arrival[3,7]	-	-	96%	96%
Statin Prescribed at Discharge[1,3]	-	-	97%	98%
Heart Failure Care				
ACE Inhibitor or ARB for LVSD[1]	-	-	93%	97%
Discharge Instructions Given	22	100%	91%	94%
Evaluation of LVS Function	35	100%	96%	99%
Medicare Spending				
Medicare Spending per Patient (ratio)	-	0.92	0.95	0.98
Pneumonia Care				
Appropriate Initial Antibiotic Given	47	98%	91%	95%
Blood Culture Timing	53	100%	97%	98%
Pregnancy and Delivery Care				
Newborn Deliveries Scheduled Early[7]	-	-	22%	6%
Preventive Care				
Immunization for Influenza[2]	299	94%	87%	90%
Immunization for Pneumonia[2]	446	96%	89%	92%
Stroke Care				
Anticoagulation Therapy for Atrial Fibrillation[1,2]	-	-	93%	95%
Antithrombotic Therapy Timing[2]	11	73%	96%	98%
Assessed for Rehabilitation[1,2]	-	-	95%	97%
Discharged on Antithrombotic Therapy[1,2]	-	-	97%	99%
Discharged on Statin Medication[1,2]	-	-	88%	94%
Thrombolytic Therapy Timing[2,7]	-	-	25%	66%
Venous Thromboembolism Prophylaxis[1,2]	-	-	87%	94%
Written Stroke Educational Materials Given[1,2]	-	-	84%	88%
Surgical Care Improvement Project				
Appropriate Beta Blocker Usage[5]	-	-	97%	98%
Appropriate VTP Within 24 Hours[5]	-	-	97%	98%
Controlled Postoperative Blood Glucose[5]	-	-	97%	97%
Perioperative Temperature Management[5]	-	-	100%	100%
Prophylactic Antibiotic Selection[5]	-	-	99%	99%
Prophylactic Antibiotic Selection (Outpatient)[5]	-	-	98%	98%
Prophylactic Antibiotic Stopped[5]	-	-	97%	98%
Prophylactic Antibiotic Timing[5]	-	-	99%	99%
Prophylactic Antibiotic Timing (Outpatient)[5]	-	-	98%	98%
Urinary Catheter Removal[5]	-	-	97%	97%
Survey of Patients' Hospital Experiences				
Area Around Room 'Always' Quiet at Night	(a)	81%	72%	61%
Doctors 'Always' Communicated Well	(a)	94%	86%	82%
Home Recovery Information Given	(a)	87%	83%	85%
Hospital Given 9 or 10 on 10 Point Scale	(a)	82%	71%	71%
Meds 'Always' Explained Before Given	(a)	78%	67%	64%
Nurses 'Always' Communicated Well	(a)	89%	81%	79%
Pain 'Always' Well Controlled	(a)	73%	72%	71%
Room and Bathroom 'Always' Clean	(a)	74%	74%	73%
Timely Help 'Always' Received	(a)	76%	69%	68%
Would Definitely Recommend Hospital	(a)	80%	69%	71%
Use of Medical Imaging				
Cardiac Imaging Stress Test before Surgery[7]	-	-	5.7%	5.3%
Combination Abdominal CT Scan	300	9.7%	12.9%	10.5%
Combination Brain/Sinus CT Scan	412	3.9%	3.3%	2.7%
Combination Chest CT Scan	125	4.8%	6.1%	2.7%
Follow-up Mammogram/Ultrasound[7]	-	-	8.4%	8.8%
Lumbar Spine MRI for Low Back Pain	104	40.4%	41.1%	37.2%

Central Mississippi Medical Center

1850 Chadwick Dr
Jackson, MS 39204
Phone: 601-376-1000
Fax: 601-376-2975
URL: www.centralmississippimedicalcenter.com
Type: Acute Care Hospitals
Emergency Services: Yes
Ownership: Proprietary
Beds: 473

Key Personnel:

CEO/President. . . . . Charlotte W. Dupre
Pediatric Ambulatory Care . . . . . . Charles A Friedman, MD
Pediatric In-Patient Care . . . . Charles A Friedman, MD
Operating Room. . . . . Karen Metz
Quality Assurance . . . . Carole Newell
Chief of Medical Staff. . . . . Barbara J Proctor, MD
Radiology. . . . . Waymond L Rone, MD
Infection Control. . . . . Jo P Wilson, MD

Measure	Cases	This Hosp.	State Avg.	U.S. Avg.
Blood Clot Prevention and Treatment				
Anticoagulation Overlap Therapy[2]	22	82%	86%	93%
ICU Venous Thromboembolism Prophylaxis[2]	87	91%	86%	92%
Incidence of Potentially Preventable VTE[1,2]	-	-	15%	10%
UFH with Dosages/Platelet Monitoring[2]	13	100%	94%	97%
Venous Thromboembolism Prophylaxis[2]	319	76%	70%	85%
Warfarin Therapy Discharge Instructions[2]	17	94%	77%	75%
Chest Pain/Possible Heart Attack Care				
Aspirin Given Within 24 Hours of Arrival[1,3]	-	-	94%	96%
Fibrinolytic Meds Within 30 Min. of Arrival[3,7]	-	-	40%	58%
Average Time to ECG (minutes)[1,3]	-	-	10	7
Average Time to Transfer (minutes)[3,7]	-	-	77	60
Children's Asthma Care				
Received Home Management Plan of Care	-	-	-	88%
Received Reliever Medication	-	-	-	100%
Received Systemic Corticosteroids	-	-	-	100%
Emergency Department				
Admittance Decision Time (minutes)[2]	752	112	61	98
Head CT Results Within 45 Min. of Arrival[1]	-	-	42%	57%
Patients Who Left ER Before Being Seen	47,816	3%	3%	2%
Time from ER Arrival to Admit. (minutes)[2]	753	265	223	274
Time from ER Arrival to Discharge (minutes)	742	94	112	134
Time in ER Before Being Evaluated (minutes)	789	29	29	26
Time to Pain Meds for Fractures (minutes)	71	60	68	57
Heart Attack Care				
Aspirin Given at Discharge	104	90%	99%	99%
Fibrinolytic Meds Within 30 Min. of Arrival[7]	-	-	50%	54%
PCI Within 90 Minutes of Arrival[1]	-	-	96%	96%
Statin Prescribed at Discharge	86	95%	97%	98%
Heart Failure Care				
ACE Inhibitor or ARB for LVSD	93	95%	93%	97%
Discharge Instructions Given	195	84%	91%	94%
Evaluation of LVS Function	214	98%	96%	99%
Medicare Spending				
Medicare Spending per Patient (ratio)	-	1.03	0.95	0.98
Pneumonia Care				
Appropriate Initial Antibiotic Given	58	97%	91%	95%
Blood Culture Timing	94	98%	97%	98%
Pregnancy and Delivery Care				
Newborn Deliveries Scheduled Early	89	21%	22%	6%
Preventive Care				
Immunization for Influenza[2]	752	100%	87%	90%
Immunization for Pneumonia[2]	738	100%	89%	92%
Stroke Care				
Anticoagulation Therapy for Atrial Fibrillation[7]	-	-	93%	95%
Antithrombotic Therapy Timing	53	100%	96%	98%
Assessed for Rehabilitation	64	95%	95%	97%
Discharged on Antithrombotic Therapy	57	95%	97%	99%
Discharged on Statin Medication	40	90%	88%	94%
Thrombolytic Therapy Timing	27	0%	25%	66%
Venous Thromboembolism Prophylaxis	65	82%	87%	94%
Written Stroke Educational Materials Given	45	89%	84%	88%
Surgical Care Improvement Project				
Appropriate Beta Blocker Usage[2]	87	95%	97%	98%
Appropriate VTP Within 24 Hours[2]	219	95%	97%	98%
Controlled Postoperative Blood Glucose[2]	51	96%	97%	97%
Perioperative Temperature Management[2]	265	99%	100%	100%
Prophylactic Antibiotic Selection[2]	202	100%	99%	99%
Prophylactic Antibiotic Selection (Outpatient)	258	100%	98%	98%
Prophylactic Antibiotic Stopped[2]	199	98%	97%	98%
Prophylactic Antibiotic Timing[2]	202	96%	99%	99%
Prophylactic Antibiotic Timing (Outpatient)	259	97%	98%	98%
Urinary Catheter Removal[2]	139	97%	97%	97%
Survey of Patients' Hospital Experiences				
Area Around Room 'Always' Quiet at Night	300+	73%	72%	61%
Doctors 'Always' Communicated Well	300+	79%	86%	82%
Home Recovery Information Given	300+	79%	83%	85%
Hospital Given 9 or 10 on 10 Point Scale	300+	60%	71%	71%
Meds 'Always' Explained Before Given	300+	57%	67%	64%
Nurses 'Always' Communicated Well	300+	75%	81%	79%
Pain 'Always' Well Controlled	300+	67%	72%	71%
Room and Bathroom 'Always' Clean	300+	67%	74%	73%
Timely Help 'Always' Received	300+	55%	69%	68%
Would Definitely Recommend Hospital	300+	58%	69%	71%
Use of Medical Imaging				
Cardiac Imaging Stress Test before Surgery	103	2.9%	5.7%	5.3%
Combination Abdominal CT Scan	315	2.9%	12.9%	10.5%
Combination Brain/Sinus CT Scan	322	5.9%	3.3%	2.7%
Combination Chest CT Scan	129	2.3%	6.1%	2.7%
Follow-up Mammogram/Ultrasound	713	9.3%	8.4%	8.8%
Lumbar Spine MRI for Low Back Pain	115	47.0%	41.1%	37.2%

GV (Sonny) Montgomery VA Medical Center Jackson

1500 E. Woodrow Wilson Drive
Jackson, MS 39216
Phone: 601-362-4471
Fax: 601-364-1359
URL: www.visn16.med.va.gov
Type: Acute Care - VA
Emergency Services: No
Ownership: Government Federal
Beds: 163

Key Personnel:

Quality Assurance . . . . Janet Autry
Radiology. . . . . Wayne Chan, MD
Operating Room. . . . . Charles Clericuzio, MD
Chief of Medical Staff. . . . . Kent Kirchner, MD
Infection Control. . . . . G.v. (sonny) Mo Spruill, RN
Coronary Care . . . . Sara Wirt, RN

Measure	Cases	This Hosp.	State Avg.	U.S. Avg.
Blood Clot Prevention and Treatment				
Anticoagulation Overlap Therapy	-	-	86%	93%
ICU Venous Thromboembolism Prophylaxis	-	-	86%	92%
Incidence of Potentially Preventable VTE	-	-	15%	10%
UFH with Dosages/Platelet Monitoring	-	-	94%	97%
Venous Thromboembolism Prophylaxis	-	-	70%	85%
Warfarin Therapy Discharge Instructions	-	-	77%	75%
Chest Pain/Possible Heart Attack Care				
Aspirin Given Within 24 Hours of Arrival	-	-	94%	96%
Fibrinolytic Meds Within 30 Min. of Arrival	-	-	40%	58%
Average Time to ECG (minutes)	-	-	10	7
Average Time to Transfer (minutes)	-	-	77	60
Children's Asthma Care				
Received Home Management Plan of Care	-	-	-	88%
Received Reliever Medication	-	-	-	100%
Received Systemic Corticosteroids	-	-	-	100%
Emergency Department				
Admittance Decision Time (minutes)	-	-	61	98
Head CT Results Within 45 Min. of Arrival	-	-	42%	57%
Patients Who Left ER Before Being Seen	-	-	3%	2%
Time from ER Arrival to Admit. (minutes)	-	-	223	274
Time from ER Arrival to Discharge (minutes)	-	-	112	134
Time in ER Before Being Evaluated (minutes)	-	-	29	26
Time to Pain Meds for Fractures (minutes)	-	-	68	57
Heart Attack Care				
Aspirin Given at Discharge	59	100%	99%	99%
Fibrinolytic Meds Within 30 Min. of Arrival[5]	-	-	50%	54%
PCI Within 90 Minutes of Arrival[5]	-	-	96%	96%
Statin Prescribed at Discharge	60	98%	97%	98%
Heart Failure Care				
ACE Inhibitor or ARB for LVSD	102	100%	93%	97%
Discharge Instructions Given	199	99%	91%	94%
Evaluation of LVS Function	208	100%	96%	99%
Medicare Spending				
Medicare Spending per Patient (ratio)	-	-	0.95	0.98
Pneumonia Care				
Appropriate Initial Antibiotic Given	69	99%	91%	95%
Blood Culture Timing	192	99%	97%	98%
Pregnancy and Delivery Care				
Newborn Deliveries Scheduled Early	-	-	22%	6%
Preventive Care				
Immunization for Influenza[5]	-	-	87%	90%
Immunization for Pneumonia[5]	-	-	89%	92%
Stroke Care				
Anticoagulation Therapy for Atrial Fibrillation	-	-	93%	95%
Antithrombotic Therapy Timing	-	-	96%	98%
Assessed for Rehabilitation	-	-	95%	97%
Discharged on Antithrombotic Therapy	-	-	97%	99%
Discharged on Statin Medication	-	-	88%	94%
Thrombolytic Therapy Timing	-	-	25%	66%
Venous Thromboembolism Prophylaxis	-	-	87%	94%
Written Stroke Educational Materials Given	-	-	84%	88%

NOTE: Hospital profiles are in alphabetical order by state, then city, then hospital within the city; Rankings exclude hospitals with less than 25 cases except for patient surveys which excludes hospitals with less than 100 cases; (a) 100-299 cases; (1) The number of cases/patients is too few to report; (2) Data submitted were based on a sample of cases/patients; (3) Results are based on a shorter time period than required; (4) Data suppressed by CMS for one or more quarters; (5) Results are not available for this reporting period; (6) Fewer than 100 patients completed the HCAHPS survey; (7) No cases met the criteria for this measure; (8) The lower limit of the confidence interval cannot be calculated if the number of observed infections equals zero; (9) No data are available from the state/territory for this reporting period; (10) The scores shown reflect fewer than 50 completed surveys; (11) There were discrepancies in the data collection process; (12) This measure does not apply to this hospital for this reporting period; (13) Results cannot be calculated for this reporting period; (14) The results for this state are combined with nearby states to protect confidentiality; Please refer to the User's Guide for a full explanation of data.

Surgical Care Improvement Project				
Appropriate Beta Blocker Usage[2]	39	95%	97%	98%
Appropriate VTP Within 24 Hours[2]	127	100%	97%	98%
Controlled Postoperative Blood Glucose[5]	-	-	97%	97%
Perioperative Temperature Management[2]	148	100%	100%	100%
Prophylactic Antibiotic Selection	51	100%	99%	99%
Prophylactic Antibiotic Selection (Outpatient)	-	-	98%	98%
Prophylactic Antibiotic Stopped	51	100%	97%	98%
Prophylactic Antibiotic Timing	51	98%	99%	99%
Prophylactic Antibiotic Timing (Outpatient)	-	-	98%	98%
Urinary Catheter Removal[2]	54	100%	97%	97%
Survey of Patients' Hospital Experiences				
Area Around Room 'Always' Quiet at Night	-	-	72%	61%
Doctors 'Always' Communicated Well	-	-	86%	82%
Home Recovery Information Given	-	-	83%	85%
Hospital Given 9 or 10 on 10 Point Scale	-	-	71%	71%
Meds 'Always' Explained Before Given	-	-	67%	64%
Nurses 'Always' Communicated Well	-	-	81%	79%
Pain 'Always' Well Controlled	-	-	72%	71%
Room and Bathroom 'Always' Clean	-	-	74%	73%
Timely Help 'Always' Received	-	-	69%	68%
Would Definitely Recommend Hospital	-	-	69%	71%
Use of Medical Imaging				
Cardiac Imaging Stress Test before Surgery	-	-	5.7%	5.3%
Combination Abdominal CT Scan	-	-	12.9%	10.5%
Combination Brain/Sinus CT Scan	-	-	3.3%	2.7%
Combination Chest CT Scan	-	-	6.1%	2.7%
Follow-up Mammogram/Ultrasound	-	-	8.4%	8.8%
Lumbar Spine MRI for Low Back Pain	-	-	41.1%	37.2%

Mississippi Baptist Medical Center

1225 N State St
Jackson, MS 39202
URL: www.mbmc.org
Phone: 601-968-1000
Fax: 601-968-1383
Type: Acute Care Hospitals
Emergency Services: Yes
Ownership: Voluntary non-profit - Private
Beds: 564

Key Personnel:
Chief of Medical Staff.......... R Deaver Collins, MD
Quality Assurance .... Roger Harrison
CEO/President................ Kurt Metzer
Operating Room.............. Wynn Norris
Infection Control.............. Carol Pate
Radiology.................... Edward Phillips, MD
Pediatric Ambulatory Care ...... Melinda Ray, MD
Pediatric In-Patient Care .... Melinda Ray, MD

Measure	Cases	This Hosp.	State Avg.	U.S. Avg.
Blood Clot Prevention and Treatment				
Anticoagulation Overlap Therapy[2]	182	86%	86%	93%
ICU Venous Thromboembolism Prophylaxis[2]	67	76%	86%	92%
Incidence of Potentially Preventable VTE[2]	37	24%	15%	10%
UFH with Dosages/Platelet Monitoring[2]	36	97%	94%	97%
Venous Thromboembolism Prophylaxis[2]	383	56%	70%	85%
Warfarin Therapy Discharge Instructions[2]	153	48%	77%	75%
Chest Pain/Possible Heart Attack Care				
Aspirin Given Within 24 Hours of Arrival[3,7]	-	-	94%	96%
Fibrinolytic Meds Within 30 Min. of Arrival[5]	-	-	40%	58%
Average Time to ECG (minutes)[3,7]	-	-	10	7
Average Time to Transfer (minutes)[5]	-	-	77	60
Children's Asthma Care				
Received Home Management Plan of Care	-	-	-	88%
Received Reliever Medication	-	-	-	100%
Received Systemic Corticosteroids	-	-	-	100%
Emergency Department				
Admittance Decision Time (minutes)[2]	583	82	61	98
Head CT Results Within 45 Min. of Arrival[1]	-	-	42%	57%
Patients Who Left ER Before Being Seen	51,001	3%	3%	2%
Time from ER Arrival to Admit. (minutes)[2]	611	304	223	274
Time from ER Arrival to Discharge (minutes)	451	181	112	134
Time in ER Before Being Evaluated (minutes)	478	90	29	26
Time to Pain Meds for Fractures (minutes)	170	90	68	57
Heart Attack Care				
Aspirin Given at Discharge	264	98%	99%	99%
Fibrinolytic Meds Within 30 Min. of Arrival[7]	-	-	50%	54%
PCI Within 90 Minutes of Arrival	46	98%	96%	96%
Statin Prescribed at Discharge	259	97%	97%	98%
Heart Failure Care				
ACE Inhibitor or ARB for LVSD	163	81%	93%	97%
Discharge Instructions Given	461	63%	91%	94%
Evaluation of LVS Function	549	95%	96%	99%
Medicare Spending				
Medicare Spending per Patient (ratio)	-	1.01	0.95	0.98
Pneumonia Care				
Appropriate Initial Antibiotic Given[2]	124	90%	91%	95%
Blood Culture Timing[2]	210	99%	97%	98%
Pregnancy and Delivery Care				
Newborn Deliveries Scheduled Early	140	24%	22%	6%
Preventive Care				
Immunization for Influenza[2]	625	89%	87%	90%
Immunization for Pneumonia[2]	831	88%	89%	92%
Stroke Care				
Anticoagulation Therapy for Atrial Fibrillation	38	92%	93%	95%
Antithrombotic Therapy Timing	250	98%	96%	98%
Assessed for Rehabilitation	296	99%	95%	97%
Discharged on Antithrombotic Therapy	275	99%	97%	99%
Discharged on Statin Medication	201	95%	88%	94%
Thrombolytic Therapy Timing	12	83%	25%	66%
Venous Thromboembolism Prophylaxis	292	91%	87%	94%
Written Stroke Educational Materials Given	175	83%	84%	88%
Surgical Care Improvement Project				
Appropriate Beta Blocker Usage[2]	398	98%	97%	98%
Appropriate VTP Within 24 Hours[2]	949	98%	97%	98%
Controlled Postoperative Blood Glucose[2]	204	100%	97%	97%
Perioperative Temperature Management[2]	1,159	100%	100%	100%
Prophylactic Antibiotic Selection[2]	1,083	99%	99%	99%
Prophylactic Antibiotic Selection (Outpatient)	798	99%	98%	98%
Prophylactic Antibiotic Stopped[2]	1,069	99%	97%	98%
Prophylactic Antibiotic Timing[2]	1,088	100%	99%	99%
Prophylactic Antibiotic Timing (Outpatient)	801	99%	98%	98%
Urinary Catheter Removal[2]	890	98%	97%	97%
Survey of Patients' Hospital Experiences				
Area Around Room 'Always' Quiet at Night[11]	300+	76%	72%	61%
Doctors 'Always' Communicated Well[11]	300+	86%	86%	82%
Home Recovery Information Given[11]	300+	87%	83%	85%
Hospital Given 9 or 10 on 10 Point Scale[11]	300+	80%	71%	71%
Meds 'Always' Explained Before Given[11]	300+	68%	67%	64%
Nurses 'Always' Communicated Well[11]	300+	82%	81%	79%
Pain 'Always' Well Controlled[11]	300+	75%	72%	71%
Room and Bathroom 'Always' Clean[11]	300+	66%	74%	73%
Timely Help 'Always' Received[11]	300+	67%	69%	68%
Would Definitely Recommend Hospital[11]	300+	81%	69%	71%
Use of Medical Imaging				
Cardiac Imaging Stress Test before Surgery	335	8.1%	5.7%	5.3%
Combination Abdominal CT Scan	1,966	4.0%	12.9%	10.5%
Combination Brain/Sinus CT Scan	942	2.5%	3.3%	2.7%
Combination Chest CT Scan	1,535	7.8%	6.1%	2.7%
Follow-up Mammogram/Ultrasound	1,952	7.8%	8.4%	8.8%
Lumbar Spine MRI for Low Back Pain	265	46.4%	41.1%	37.2%

Mississippi Methodist Rehab Center

1350 E Woodrow Wilson Dr
Jackson, MS 39216
Phone: 601-981-2611
Type: Acute Care Hospitals
Emergency Services: No
Ownership: Voluntary non-profit - Private

Key Personnel:
CEO/President................ Mark A Adams
Patient Relations .... Susan B Greco, RN, CRRN

Measure	Cases	This Hosp.	State Avg.	U.S. Avg.
Blood Clot Prevention and Treatment				
Anticoagulation Overlap Therapy	-	-	86%	93%
ICU Venous Thromboembolism Prophylaxis	-	-	86%	92%
Incidence of Potentially Preventable VTE	-	-	15%	10%
UFH with Dosages/Platelet Monitoring	-	-	94%	97%
Venous Thromboembolism Prophylaxis	-	-	70%	85%
Warfarin Therapy Discharge Instructions	-	-	77%	75%
Chest Pain/Possible Heart Attack Care				
Aspirin Given Within 24 Hours of Arrival[5]	-	-	94%	96%
Fibrinolytic Meds Within 30 Min. of Arrival[5]	-	-	40%	58%
Average Time to ECG (minutes)[5]	-	-	10	7
Average Time to Transfer (minutes)[5]	-	-	77	60
Children's Asthma Care				
Received Home Management Plan of Care	-	-	-	88%
Received Reliever Medication	-	-	-	100%
Received Systemic Corticosteroids	-	-	-	100%
Emergency Department				
Admittance Decision Time (minutes)	-	-	61	98
Head CT Results Within 45 Min. of Arrival[5]	-	-	42%	57%
Patients Who Left ER Before Being Seen[5]	-	-	3%	2%
Time from ER Arrival to Admit. (minutes)	-	-	223	274
Time from ER Arrival to Discharge (minutes)[5]	-	-	112	134
Time in ER Before Being Evaluated (minutes)[5]	-	-	29	26
Time to Pain Meds for Fractures (minutes)[5]	-	-	68	57
Heart Attack Care				
Aspirin Given at Discharge	-	-	99%	99%
Fibrinolytic Meds Within 30 Min. of Arrival	-	-	50%	54%
PCI Within 90 Minutes of Arrival	-	-	96%	96%
Statin Prescribed at Discharge	-	-	97%	98%
Heart Failure Care				
ACE Inhibitor or ARB for LVSD	-	-	93%	97%
Discharge Instructions Given	-	-	91%	94%
Evaluation of LVS Function	-	-	96%	99%
Medicare Spending				
Medicare Spending per Patient (ratio)	-	-	0.95	0.98
Pneumonia Care				
Appropriate Initial Antibiotic Given	-	-	91%	95%
Blood Culture Timing	-	-	97%	98%
Pregnancy and Delivery Care				
Newborn Deliveries Scheduled Early	-	-	22%	6%
Preventive Care				
Immunization for Influenza	-	-	87%	90%
Immunization for Pneumonia	-	-	89%	92%
Stroke Care				
Anticoagulation Therapy for Atrial Fibrillation	-	-	93%	95%
Antithrombotic Therapy Timing	-	-	96%	98%
Assessed for Rehabilitation	-	-	95%	97%
Discharged on Antithrombotic Therapy	-	-	97%	99%
Discharged on Statin Medication	-	-	88%	94%
Thrombolytic Therapy Timing	-	-	25%	66%
Venous Thromboembolism Prophylaxis	-	-	87%	94%
Written Stroke Educational Materials Given	-	-	84%	88%
Surgical Care Improvement Project				
Appropriate Beta Blocker Usage	-	-	97%	98%
Appropriate VTP Within 24 Hours	-	-	97%	98%
Controlled Postoperative Blood Glucose	-	-	97%	97%
Perioperative Temperature Management	-	-	100%	100%
Prophylactic Antibiotic Selection	-	-	99%	99%
Prophylactic Antibiotic Selection (Outpatient)[5]	-	-	98%	98%
Prophylactic Antibiotic Stopped	-	-	97%	98%
Prophylactic Antibiotic Timing	-	-	99%	99%
Prophylactic Antibiotic Timing (Outpatient)[5]	-	-	98%	98%
Urinary Catheter Removal	-	-	97%	97%
Survey of Patients' Hospital Experiences				
Area Around Room 'Always' Quiet at Night	-	-	72%	61%
Doctors 'Always' Communicated Well	-	-	86%	82%
Home Recovery Information Given	-	-	83%	85%
Hospital Given 9 or 10 on 10 Point Scale	-	-	71%	71%
Meds 'Always' Explained Before Given	-	-	67%	64%
Nurses 'Always' Communicated Well	-	-	81%	79%
Pain 'Always' Well Controlled	-	-	72%	71%
Room and Bathroom 'Always' Clean	-	-	74%	73%
Timely Help 'Always' Received	-	-	69%	68%
Would Definitely Recommend Hospital	-	-	69%	71%
Use of Medical Imaging				
Cardiac Imaging Stress Test before Surgery[7]	-	-	5.7%	5.3%
Combination Abdominal CT Scan[7]	-	-	12.9%	10.5%
Combination Brain/Sinus CT Scan[7]	-	-	3.3%	2.7%
Combination Chest CT Scan[7]	-	-	6.1%	2.7%
Follow-up Mammogram/Ultrasound[7]	-	-	8.4%	8.8%
Lumbar Spine MRI for Low Back Pain[7]	-	-	41.1%	37.2%

NOTE: Hospital profiles are in alphabetical order by state, then city, then hospital within the city; Rankings exclude hospitals with less than 25 cases except for patient surveys which excludes hospitals with less than 100 cases; (a) 100-299 cases; (1) The number of cases/patients is too few to report; (2) Data submitted were based on a sample of cases/patients; (3) Results are based on a shorter time period than required; (4) Data suppressed by CMS for one or more quarters; (5) Results are not available for this reporting period; (6) Fewer than 100 patients completed the HCAHPS survey; (7) No cases met the criteria for this measure; (8) The lower limit of the confidence interval cannot be calculated if the number of observed infections equals zero; (9) No data are available from the state/territory for this reporting period; (10) The scores shown reflect fewer than 50 completed surveys; (11) There were discrepancies in the data collection process; (12) This measure does not apply to this hospital for this reporting period; (13) Results cannot be calculated for this reporting period; (14) The results for this state are combined with nearby states to protect confidentiality; Please refer to the User's Guide for a full explanation of data.

Saint Dominic - Jackson Memorial Hospital

969 Lakeland Dr Phone: 601-200-2000
Jackson, MS 39216 Fax: 601-200-0890
URL: www.stdom.com
Type: Acute Care Hospitals Emergency Services: Yes
Ownership: Voluntary non-profit - Church Beds: 571

Key Personnel:
CEO/President. . . . . Claude W Harbarger
Patient Relations . . . . Trace Swartzfager

Measure	Cases	This Hosp.	State Avg.	U.S. Avg.
Blood Clot Prevention and Treatment				
Anticoagulation Overlap Therapy[2]	229	93%	86%	93%
ICU Venous Thromboembolism Prophylaxis[2]	74	97%	86%	92%
Incidence of Potentially Preventable VTE[2]	84	12%	15%	10%
UFH with Dosages/Platelet Monitoring[2]	58	100%	94%	97%
Venous Thromboembolism Prophylaxis[2]	408	62%	70%	85%
Warfarin Therapy Discharge Instructions[2]	169	92%	77%	75%
Chest Pain/Possible Heart Attack Care				
Aspirin Given Within 24 Hours of Arrival[5]	-	-	94%	96%
Fibrinolytic Meds Within 30 Min. of Arrival[5]	-	-	40%	58%
Average Time to ECG (minutes)[5]	-	-	10	7
Average Time to Transfer (minutes)[5]	-	-	77	60
Children's Asthma Care				
Received Home Management Plan of Care	-	-	-	88%
Received Reliever Medication	-	-	-	100%
Received Systemic Corticosteroids	-	-	-	100%
Emergency Department				
Admittance Decision Time (minutes)[2]	678	93	61	98
Head CT Results Within 45 Min. of Arrival[3,7]	-	-	42%	57%
Patients Who Left ER Before Being Seen	51,855	3%	3%	2%
Time from ER Arrival to Admit. (minutes)[2]	695	286	223	274
Time from ER Arrival to Discharge (minutes)	361	197	112	134
Time in ER Before Being Evaluated (minutes)	401	65	29	26
Time to Pain Meds for Fractures (minutes)	83	77	68	57
Heart Attack Care				
Aspirin Given at Discharge	568	98%	99%	99%
Fibrinolytic Meds Within 30 Min. of Arrival[7]	-	-	50%	54%
PCI Within 90 Minutes of Arrival	63	100%	96%	96%
Statin Prescribed at Discharge	561	97%	97%	98%
Heart Failure Care				
ACE Inhibitor or ARB for LVSD[2]	105	95%	93%	97%
Discharge Instructions Given[2]	280	95%	91%	94%
Evaluation of LVS Function[2]	326	98%	96%	99%
Medicare Spending				
Medicare Spending per Patient (ratio)	-	0.99	0.95	0.98
Pneumonia Care				
Appropriate Initial Antibiotic Given[2]	113	86%	91%	95%
Blood Culture Timing[2]	163	98%	97%	98%
Pregnancy and Delivery Care				
Newborn Deliveries Scheduled Early[2]	60	38%	22%	6%
Preventive Care				
Immunization for Influenza[2]	578	87%	87%	90%
Immunization for Pneumonia[2]	782	84%	89%	92%
Stroke Care				
Anticoagulation Therapy for Atrial Fibrillation	38	97%	93%	95%
Antithrombotic Therapy Timing	294	96%	96%	98%
Assessed for Rehabilitation	441	98%	95%	97%
Discharged on Antithrombotic Therapy	341	99%	97%	99%
Discharged on Statin Medication	280	91%	88%	94%
Thrombolytic Therapy Timing	16	88%	25%	66%
Venous Thromboembolism Prophylaxis	455	89%	87%	94%
Written Stroke Educational Materials Given	253	97%	84%	88%
Surgical Care Improvement Project				
Appropriate Beta Blocker Usage[2]	205	96%	97%	98%
Appropriate VTP Within 24 Hours[2]	485	97%	97%	98%
Controlled Postoperative Blood Glucose[2]	146	95%	97%	97%
Perioperative Temperature Management[2]	545	100%	100%	100%
Prophylactic Antibiotic Selection[2]	504	99%	99%	99%
Prophylactic Antibiotic Selection (Outpatient)	582	97%	98%	98%
Prophylactic Antibiotic Stopped[2]	492	98%	97%	98%
Prophylactic Antibiotic Timing[2]	505	98%	99%	99%
Prophylactic Antibiotic Timing (Outpatient)	595	94%	98%	98%
Urinary Catheter Removal[2]	418	100%	97%	97%
Survey of Patients' Hospital Experiences				
Area Around Room 'Always' Quiet at Night	300+	75%	72%	61%
Doctors 'Always' Communicated Well	300+	84%	86%	82%
Home Recovery Information Given	300+	86%	83%	85%
Hospital Given 9 or 10 on 10 Point Scale	300+	76%	71%	71%
Meds 'Always' Explained Before Given	300+	64%	67%	64%
Nurses 'Always' Communicated Well	300+	79%	81%	79%
Pain 'Always' Well Controlled	300+	71%	72%	71%
Room and Bathroom 'Always' Clean	300+	66%	74%	73%
Timely Help 'Always' Received	300+	66%	69%	68%
Would Definitely Recommend Hospital	300+	80%	69%	71%
Use of Medical Imaging				
Cardiac Imaging Stress Test before Surgery	176	8.0%	5.7%	5.3%
Combination Abdominal CT Scan	1,816	2.6%	12.9%	10.5%
Combination Brain/Sinus CT Scan	1,730	2.4%	3.3%	2.7%
Combination Chest CT Scan	1,300	1.3%	6.1%	2.7%
Follow-up Mammogram/Ultrasound	1,622	5.6%	8.4%	8.8%
Lumbar Spine MRI for Low Back Pain	475	37.3%	41.1%	37.2%

University of Mississippi Medical Center

2500 N State St Phone: 601-984-4100
Jackson, MS 39216 Fax: 601-984-1973
URL: www.umc.edu
Type: Acute Care Hospitals Emergency Services: Yes
Ownership: Government - State Beds: 665

Key Personnel:
Quality Assurance . . . . Carl Andre
Infection Control. . . . . Stanley Chapman, MD
Emergency Room . . . . Becky Egger
Pediatric Ambulatory Care . . . . . . Owen B Evans, MD
Pediatric In-Patient Care . . . . Owen B Evans, MD
Chief of Medical Staff. . . . . Joe Files, MD
CEO/President. . . . . Daniel Jones

Measure	Cases	This Hosp.	State Avg.	U.S. Avg.
Blood Clot Prevention and Treatment				
Anticoagulation Overlap Therapy[2]	119	87%	86%	93%
ICU Venous Thromboembolism Prophylaxis[2]	138	80%	86%	92%
Incidence of Potentially Preventable VTE[2]	78	6%	15%	10%
UFH with Dosages/Platelet Monitoring[2]	84	98%	94%	97%
Venous Thromboembolism Prophylaxis[2]	305	79%	70%	85%
Warfarin Therapy Discharge Instructions[2]	93	63%	77%	75%
Chest Pain/Possible Heart Attack Care				
Aspirin Given Within 24 Hours of Arrival[5]	-	-	94%	96%
Fibrinolytic Meds Within 30 Min. of Arrival[5]	-	-	40%	58%
Average Time to ECG (minutes)[5]	-	-	10	7
Average Time to Transfer (minutes)[5]	-	-	77	60
Children's Asthma Care				
Received Home Management Plan of Care[2]	208	89%	-	88%
Received Reliever Medication[2]	209	100%	-	100%
Received Systemic Corticosteroids[2]	209	100%	-	100%
Emergency Department				
Admittance Decision Time (minutes)[2]	290	146	61	98
Head CT Results Within 45 Min. of Arrival[1]	-	-	42%	57%
Patients Who Left ER Before Being Seen	>100k	4%	3%	2%
Time from ER Arrival to Admit. (minutes)[2]	295	363	223	274
Time from ER Arrival to Discharge (minutes)	366	144	112	134
Time in ER Before Being Evaluated (minutes)	152	34	29	26
Time to Pain Meds for Fractures (minutes)	306	66	68	57
Heart Attack Care				
Aspirin Given at Discharge[2]	267	100%	99%	99%
Fibrinolytic Meds Within 30 Min. of Arrival[2,7]	-	-	50%	54%
PCI Within 90 Minutes of Arrival[2]	28	89%	96%	96%
Statin Prescribed at Discharge[2]	263	100%	97%	98%
Heart Failure Care				
ACE Inhibitor or ARB for LVSD[2]	137	99%	93%	97%
Discharge Instructions Given[2]	256	99%	91%	94%
Evaluation of LVS Function[2]	275	99%	96%	99%
Medicare Spending				
Medicare Spending per Patient (ratio)	-	1.02	0.95	0.98
Pneumonia Care				
Appropriate Initial Antibiotic Given[2]	28	96%	91%	95%
Blood Culture Timing[2]	103	95%	97%	98%
Pregnancy and Delivery Care				
Newborn Deliveries Scheduled Early[1,2]	-	-	22%	6%
Preventive Care				
Immunization for Influenza[2]	502	77%	87%	90%
Immunization for Pneumonia[2]	428	86%	89%	92%
Stroke Care				
Anticoagulation Therapy for Atrial Fibrillation[1,2]	-	-	93%	95%
Antithrombotic Therapy Timing[2]	59	93%	96%	98%
Assessed for Rehabilitation[2]	112	96%	95%	97%
Discharged on Antithrombotic Therapy[2]	75	97%	97%	99%
Discharged on Statin Medication[2]	51	98%	88%	94%
Thrombolytic Therapy Timing[1,2]	-	-	25%	66%
Venous Thromboembolism Prophylaxis[2]	125	95%	87%	94%
Written Stroke Educational Materials Given[2]	56	98%	84%	88%
Surgical Care Improvement Project				
Appropriate Beta Blocker Usage[2]	135	97%	97%	98%
Appropriate VTP Within 24 Hours[2]	300	98%	97%	98%
Controlled Postoperative Blood Glucose[2]	61	92%	97%	97%
Perioperative Temperature Management[2]	458	96%	100%	100%
Prophylactic Antibiotic Selection[2]	315	97%	99%	99%
Prophylactic Antibiotic Selection (Outpatient)	245	97%	98%	98%
Prophylactic Antibiotic Stopped[2]	308	95%	97%	98%
Prophylactic Antibiotic Timing[2]	324	93%	99%	99%
Prophylactic Antibiotic Timing (Outpatient)	259	92%	98%	98%
Urinary Catheter Removal[2]	277	87%	97%	97%
Survey of Patients' Hospital Experiences				
Area Around Room 'Always' Quiet at Night	300+	67%	72%	61%
Doctors 'Always' Communicated Well	300+	82%	86%	82%
Home Recovery Information Given	300+	81%	83%	85%
Hospital Given 9 or 10 on 10 Point Scale	300+	71%	71%	71%
Meds 'Always' Explained Before Given	300+	63%	67%	64%
Nurses 'Always' Communicated Well	300+	78%	81%	79%
Pain 'Always' Well Controlled	300+	69%	72%	71%
Room and Bathroom 'Always' Clean	300+	66%	74%	73%
Timely Help 'Always' Received	300+	59%	69%	68%
Would Definitely Recommend Hospital	300+	75%	69%	71%
Use of Medical Imaging				
Cardiac Imaging Stress Test before Surgery	513	5.1%	5.7%	5.3%
Combination Abdominal CT Scan	1,264	9.7%	12.9%	10.5%
Combination Brain/Sinus CT Scan	744	2.3%	3.3%	2.7%
Combination Chest CT Scan	1,279	0.4%	6.1%	2.7%
Follow-up Mammogram/Ultrasound	968	13.6%	8.4%	8.8%
Lumbar Spine MRI for Low Back Pain	143	39.2%	41.1%	37.2%

Kilmichael Hospital

301 Lamar Avenue Phone: 662-262-4311
Kilmichael, MS 39747 Fax: 662-262-5586
Type: Acute Care Hospitals Emergency Services: No
Ownership: Government - Local Beds: 19

Key Personnel:
Emergency Room . . . . LC Henson, MD
CEO/President. . . . . Calvin Johnson
Radiology. . . . . Myra M King
Chief of Medical Staff . . . . Katrina Poe, MD

Measure	Cases	This Hosp.	State Avg.	U.S. Avg.
Blood Clot Prevention and Treatment				
Anticoagulation Overlap Therapy[5]	-	-	86%	93%
ICU Venous Thromboembolism Prophylaxis[5]	-	-	86%	92%
Incidence of Potentially Preventable VTE[5]	-	-	15%	10%
UFH with Dosages/Platelet Monitoring[5]	-	-	94%	97%
Venous Thromboembolism Prophylaxis[5]	-	-	70%	85%
Warfarin Therapy Discharge Instructions[5]	-	-	77%	75%
Chest Pain/Possible Heart Attack Care				
Aspirin Given Within 24 Hours of Arrival[5]	-	-	94%	96%
Fibrinolytic Meds Within 30 Min. of Arrival[5]	-	-	40%	58%
Average Time to ECG (minutes)[5]	-	-	10	7
Average Time to Transfer (minutes)[5]	-	-	77	60
Children's Asthma Care				
Received Home Management Plan of Care	-	-	-	88%
Received Reliever Medication	-	-	-	100%
Received Systemic Corticosteroids	-	-	-	100%
Emergency Department				
Admittance Decision Time (minutes)[7]	-	-	61	98
Head CT Results Within 45 Min. of Arrival[5]	-	-	42%	57%
Patients Who Left ER Before Being Seen[5]	-	-	3%	2%

NOTE: Hospital profiles are in alphabetical order by state, then city, then hospital within the city; Rankings exclude hospitals with less than 25 cases except for patient surveys which excludes hospitals with less than 100 cases; (a) 100-299 cases; (1) The number of cases/patients is too few to report; (2) Data submitted were based on a sample of cases/patients; (3) Results are based on a shorter time period than required; (4) Data suppressed by CMS for one or more quarters; (5) Results are not available for this reporting period; (6) Fewer than 100 patients completed the HCAHPS survey; (7) No cases met the criteria for this measure; (8) The lower limit of the confidence interval cannot be calculated if the number of observed infections equals zero; (9) No data are available from the state/territory for this reporting period; (10) The scores shown reflect fewer than 50 completed surveys; (11) There were discrepancies in the data collection process; (12) This measure does not apply to this hospital for this reporting period; (13) Results cannot be calculated for this reporting period; (14) The results for this state are combined with nearby states to protect confidentiality; Please refer to the User's Guide for a full explanation of data.

Measure	Cases	This Hosp.	State Avg.	U.S. Avg.
Time from ER Arrival to Admit. (minutes)[7]	-	-	223	274
Time from ER Arrival to Discharge (minutes)[5]	-	-	112	134
Time in ER Before Being Evaluated (minutes)[5]	-	-	29	26
Time to Pain Meds for Fractures (minutes)[5]	-	-	68	57
Heart Attack Care				
Aspirin Given at Discharge[5]	-	-	99%	99%
Fibrinolytic Meds Within 30 Min. of Arrival[5]	-	-	50%	54%
PCI Within 90 Minutes of Arrival[5]	-	-	96%	96%
Statin Prescribed at Discharge[5]	-	-	97%	98%
Heart Failure Care				
ACE Inhibitor or ARB for LVSD[3,7]	-	-	93%	97%
Discharge Instructions Given[1,3]	-	-	91%	94%
Evaluation of LVS Function[1,3]	-	-	96%	99%
Medicare Spending				
Medicare Spending per Patient (ratio)	-	0.82	0.95	0.98
Pneumonia Care				
Appropriate Initial Antibiotic Given[1,3]	-	-	91%	95%
Blood Culture Timing[3,7]	-	-	97%	98%
Pregnancy and Delivery Care				
Newborn Deliveries Scheduled Early[7]	-	-	22%	6%
Preventive Care				
Immunization for Influenza	59	39%	87%	90%
Immunization for Pneumonia	55	31%	89%	92%
Stroke Care				
Anticoagulation Therapy for Atrial Fibrillation[5]	-	-	93%	95%
Antithrombotic Therapy Timing[5]	-	-	96%	98%
Assessed for Rehabilitation[5]	-	-	95%	97%
Discharged on Antithrombotic Therapy[5]	-	-	97%	99%
Discharged on Statin Medication[5]	-	-	88%	94%
Thrombolytic Therapy Timing[5]	-	-	25%	66%
Venous Thromboembolism Prophylaxis[5]	-	-	87%	94%
Written Stroke Educational Materials Given[5]	-	-	84%	88%
Surgical Care Improvement Project				
Appropriate Beta Blocker Usage[5]	-	-	97%	98%
Appropriate VTP Within 24 Hours[5]	-	-	97%	98%
Controlled Postoperative Blood Glucose[5]	-	-	97%	97%
Perioperative Temperature Management[5]	-	-	100%	100%
Prophylactic Antibiotic Selection[5]	-	-	99%	99%
Prophylactic Antibiotic Selection (Outpatient)[5]	-	-	98%	98%
Prophylactic Antibiotic Stopped[5]	-	-	97%	98%
Prophylactic Antibiotic Timing[5]	-	-	99%	99%
Prophylactic Antibiotic Timing (Outpatient)[5]	-	-	98%	98%
Urinary Catheter Removal[5]	-	-	97%	97%
Survey of Patients' Hospital Experiences				
Area Around Room 'Always' Quiet at Night[10]	<100	82%	72%	61%
Doctors 'Always' Communicated Well[10]	<100	98%	86%	82%
Home Recovery Information Given[10]	<100	99%	83%	85%
Hospital Given 9 or 10 on 10 Point Scale[10]	<100	89%	71%	71%
Meds 'Always' Explained Before Given[10]	<100	66%	67%	64%
Nurses 'Always' Communicated Well[10]	<100	97%	81%	79%
Pain 'Always' Well Controlled[10]	<100	96%	72%	71%
Room and Bathroom 'Always' Clean[10]	<100	89%	74%	73%
Timely Help 'Always' Received[10]	<100	93%	69%	68%
Would Definitely Recommend Hospital[10]	<100	95%	69%	71%
Use of Medical Imaging				
Cardiac Imaging Stress Test before Surgery[7]	-	-	5.7%	5.3%
Combination Abdominal CT Scan[7]	-	-	12.9%	10.5%
Combination Brain/Sinus CT Scan[7]	-	-	3.3%	2.7%
Combination Chest CT Scan[7]	-	-	6.1%	2.7%
Follow-up Mammogram/Ultrasound[7]	-	-	8.4%	8.8%
Lumbar Spine MRI for Low Back Pain[7]	-	-	41.1%	37.2%

Montfort Jones Memorial Hospital

220 Hwy 12 West
Kosciusko, MS 39090
Phone: 662-289-4311
Fax: 662-289-9970
E-mail: cindy@mjmh.com
Type: Acute Care Hospitals
Emergency Services: Yes
Ownership: Voluntary non-profit - Other
Beds: 72

Key Personnel:

Quality Assurance . . . . Thomas Bland
Chief of Medical Staff. . . . . D Stanley Hartness, MD
Emergency Room . . . . Cynthia Lassiter, RN
Operating Room. . . . . Stirling Steen, RN
Radiology. Chris Threadgil, MD

Measure	Cases	This Hosp.	State Avg.	U.S. Avg.
Blood Clot Prevention and Treatment				
Anticoagulation Overlap Therapy[2]	13	85%	86%	93%
ICU Venous Thromboembolism Prophylaxis[1,2]	-	-	86%	92%
Incidence of Potentially Preventable VTE[2,7]	-	-	15%	10%
UFH with Dosages/Platelet Monitoring[1,2]	-	-	94%	97%
Venous Thromboembolism Prophylaxis[2]	288	1%	70%	85%
Warfarin Therapy Discharge Instructions[1,2]	-	-	77%	75%
Chest Pain/Possible Heart Attack Care				
Aspirin Given Within 24 Hours of Arrival	33	91%	94%	96%
Fibrinolytic Meds Within 30 Min. of Arrival[1]	-	-	40%	58%
Average Time to ECG (minutes)	35	11	10	7
Average Time to Transfer (minutes)	21	120	77	60
Children's Asthma Care				
Received Home Management Plan of Care	-	-	-	88%
Received Reliever Medication	-	-	-	100%
Received Systemic Corticosteroids	-	-	-	100%
Emergency Department				
Admittance Decision Time (minutes)[2]	484	35	61	98
Head CT Results Within 45 Min. of Arrival	14	43%	42%	57%
Patients Who Left ER Before Being Seen	14,919	2%	3%	2%
Time from ER Arrival to Admit. (minutes)[2]	525	217	223	274
Time from ER Arrival to Discharge (minutes)	361	130	112	134
Time in ER Before Being Evaluated (minutes)	312	19	29	26
Time to Pain Meds for Fractures (minutes)	37	67	68	57
Heart Attack Care				
Aspirin Given at Discharge[1,3]	-	-	99%	99%
Fibrinolytic Meds Within 30 Min. of Arrival[3,7]	-	-	50%	54%
PCI Within 90 Minutes of Arrival[3,7]	-	-	96%	96%
Statin Prescribed at Discharge[1,3]	-	-	97%	98%
Heart Failure Care				
ACE Inhibitor or ARB for LVSD[1,2]	-	-	93%	97%
Discharge Instructions Given[2]	45	93%	91%	94%
Evaluation of LVS Function[2]	68	96%	96%	99%
Medicare Spending				
Medicare Spending per Patient (ratio)	-	0.92	0.95	0.98
Pneumonia Care				
Appropriate Initial Antibiotic Given[2]	46	72%	91%	95%
Blood Culture Timing[2]	49	92%	97%	98%
Pregnancy and Delivery Care				
Newborn Deliveries Scheduled Early[7]	-	-	22%	6%
Preventive Care				
Immunization for Influenza[2]	267	82%	87%	90%
Immunization for Pneumonia[2]	404	84%	89%	92%
Stroke Care				
Anticoagulation Therapy for Atrial Fibrillation[1]	-	-	93%	95%
Antithrombotic Therapy Timing[1]	-	-	96%	98%
Assessed for Rehabilitation[1]	-	-	95%	97%
Discharged on Antithrombotic Therapy[1]	-	-	97%	99%
Discharged on Statin Medication[1]	-	-	88%	94%
Thrombolytic Therapy Timing[1]	-	-	25%	66%
Venous Thromboembolism Prophylaxis[1]	-	-	87%	94%
Written Stroke Educational Materials Given[1]	-	-	84%	88%
Surgical Care Improvement Project				
Appropriate Beta Blocker Usage[5]	-	-	97%	98%
Appropriate VTP Within 24 Hours[5]	-	-	97%	98%
Controlled Postoperative Blood Glucose[5]	-	-	97%	97%
Perioperative Temperature Management[5]	-	-	100%	100%
Prophylactic Antibiotic Selection[5]	-	-	99%	99%
Prophylactic Antibiotic Selection (Outpatient)[3,7]	-	-	98%	98%
Prophylactic Antibiotic Stopped[5]	-	-	97%	98%
Prophylactic Antibiotic Timing[5]	-	-	99%	99%
Prophylactic Antibiotic Timing (Outpatient)[1,3]	-	-	98%	98%
Urinary Catheter Removal[5]	-	-	97%	97%
Survey of Patients' Hospital Experiences				
Area Around Room 'Always' Quiet at Night	(a)	79%	72%	61%
Doctors 'Always' Communicated Well	(a)	84%	86%	82%
Home Recovery Information Given	(a)	78%	83%	85%
Hospital Given 9 or 10 on 10 Point Scale	(a)	68%	71%	71%
Meds 'Always' Explained Before Given	(a)	73%	67%	64%
Nurses 'Always' Communicated Well	(a)	81%	81%	79%
Pain 'Always' Well Controlled	(a)	67%	72%	71%
Room and Bathroom 'Always' Clean	(a)	72%	74%	73%
Timely Help 'Always' Received	(a)	79%	69%	68%
Would Definitely Recommend Hospital	(a)	61%	69%	71%
Use of Medical Imaging				
Cardiac Imaging Stress Test before Surgery[1]	-	-	5.7%	5.3%
Combination Abdominal CT Scan	248	6.0%	12.9%	10.5%
Combination Brain/Sinus CT Scan[1]	-	-	3.3%	2.7%
Combination Chest CT Scan	63	7.9%	6.1%	2.7%
Follow-up Mammogram/Ultrasound	619	14.7%	8.4%	8.8%
Lumbar Spine MRI for Low Back Pain[7]	-	-	41.1%	37.2%

South Central Regional Medical Center

1220 Jefferson Saint Box 607
Laurel, MS 39440
Phone: 601-649-4000
Fax: 601-426-4729
E-mail: info@scrmc.com
URL: www.scrmc.com
Type: Acute Care Hospitals
Emergency Services: Yes
Ownership: Government - Local
Beds: 285

Key Personnel:

Quality Assurance . . . . Marcia Easterwood
Chief of Medical Staff. . . . . Stephen Johnson, MD
Emergency Room . . . . Michael LaRochelle, DO
Intensive Care Unit. . . . . Pam Ninu, RN
Operating Room. . . . . Paula Prestwood, RN
Radiology. . . . . Kathy Sumrall
Cardiac Laboratory. . . . . Edwin Todd
Pediatric In-Patient Care . . . . Vicki Walters

Measure	Cases	This Hosp.	State Avg.	U.S. Avg.
Blood Clot Prevention and Treatment				
Anticoagulation Overlap Therapy[2]	69	74%	86%	93%
ICU Venous Thromboembolism Prophylaxis[2]	59	68%	86%	92%
Incidence of Potentially Preventable VTE[2]	15	27%	15%	10%
UFH with Dosages/Platelet Monitoring[1,2]	-	-	94%	97%
Venous Thromboembolism Prophylaxis[2]	332	63%	70%	85%
Warfarin Therapy Discharge Instructions[2]	58	24%	77%	75%
Chest Pain/Possible Heart Attack Care				
Aspirin Given Within 24 Hours of Arrival	35	94%	94%	96%
Fibrinolytic Meds Within 30 Min. of Arrival[7]	-	-	40%	58%
Average Time to ECG (minutes)	36	7	10	7
Average Time to Transfer (minutes)	19	33	77	60
Children's Asthma Care				
Received Home Management Plan of Care	-	-	-	88%
Received Reliever Medication	-	-	-	100%
Received Systemic Corticosteroids	-	-	-	100%
Emergency Department				
Admittance Decision Time (minutes)[2]	506	46	61	98
Head CT Results Within 45 Min. of Arrival	19	16%	42%	57%
Patients Who Left ER Before Being Seen	36,959	2%	3%	2%
Time from ER Arrival to Admit. (minutes)[2]	528	203	223	274
Time from ER Arrival to Discharge (minutes)	372	116	112	134
Time in ER Before Being Evaluated (minutes)	386	22	29	26
Time to Pain Meds for Fractures (minutes)	126	60	68	57
Heart Attack Care				
Aspirin Given at Discharge	29	86%	99%	99%
Fibrinolytic Meds Within 30 Min. of Arrival[7]	-	-	50%	54%
PCI Within 90 Minutes of Arrival[7]	-	-	96%	96%
Statin Prescribed at Discharge	26	69%	97%	98%
Heart Failure Care				
ACE Inhibitor or ARB for LVSD	101	61%	93%	97%
Discharge Instructions Given	210	79%	91%	94%
Evaluation of LVS Function	264	91%	96%	99%
Medicare Spending				
Medicare Spending per Patient (ratio)	-	0.93	0.95	0.98
Pneumonia Care				
Appropriate Initial Antibiotic Given	191	90%	91%	95%
Blood Culture Timing	219	97%	97%	98%
Pregnancy and Delivery Care				
Newborn Deliveries Scheduled Early[2]	32	16%	22%	6%
Preventive Care				
Immunization for Influenza[2]	606	37%	87%	90%
Immunization for Pneumonia[2]	598	59%	89%	92%
Stroke Care				
Anticoagulation Therapy for Atrial Fibrillation	15	87%	93%	95%
Antithrombotic Therapy Timing	92	99%	96%	98%

NOTE: Hospital profiles are in alphabetical order by state, then city, then hospital within the city; Rankings exclude hospitals with less than 25 cases except for patient surveys which excludes hospitals with less than 100 cases; (a) 100-299 cases; (1) The number of cases/patients is too few to report; (2) Data submitted were based on a sample of cases/patients; (3) Results are based on a shorter time period than required; (4) Data suppressed by CMS for one or more quarters; (5) Results are not available for this reporting period; (6) Fewer than 100 patients completed the HCAHPS survey; (7) No cases met the criteria for this measure; (8) The lower limit of the confidence interval cannot be calculated if the number of observed infections equals zero; (9) No data are available from the state/territory for this reporting period; (10) The scores shown reflect fewer than 50 completed surveys; (11) There were discrepancies in the data collection process; (12) This measure does not apply to this hospital for this reporting period; (13) Results cannot be calculated for this reporting period; (14) The results for this state are combined with nearby states to protect confidentiality; Please refer to the User's Guide for a full explanation of data.

Measure	Cases	This Hosp.	State Avg.	U.S. Avg.
Assessed for Rehabilitation	96	96%	95%	97%
Discharged on Antithrombotic Therapy	89	97%	97%	99%
Discharged on Statin Medication	83	60%	88%	94%
Thrombolytic Therapy Timing	41	0%	25%	66%
Venous Thromboembolism Prophylaxis	100	67%	87%	94%
Written Stroke Educational Materials Given	61	46%	84%	88%
Surgical Care Improvement Project				
Appropriate Beta Blocker Usage	92	86%	97%	98%
Appropriate VTP Within 24 Hours	359	95%	97%	98%
Controlled Postoperative Blood Glucose[7]	-	-	97%	97%
Perioperative Temperature Management	392	100%	100%	100%
Prophylactic Antibiotic Selection	290	90%	99%	99%
Prophylactic Antibiotic Selection (Outpatient)	62	92%	98%	98%
Prophylactic Antibiotic Stopped	285	96%	97%	98%
Prophylactic Antibiotic Timing	292	96%	99%	99%
Prophylactic Antibiotic Timing (Outpatient)	70	86%	98%	98%
Urinary Catheter Removal	207	92%	97%	97%
Survey of Patients' Hospital Experiences				
Area Around Room 'Always' Quiet at Night	300+	72%	72%	61%
Doctors 'Always' Communicated Well	300+	87%	86%	82%
Home Recovery Information Given	300+	81%	83%	85%
Hospital Given 9 or 10 on 10 Point Scale	300+	74%	71%	71%
Meds 'Always' Explained Before Given	300+	65%	67%	64%
Nurses 'Always' Communicated Well	300+	80%	81%	79%
Pain 'Always' Well Controlled	300+	71%	72%	71%
Room and Bathroom 'Always' Clean	300+	69%	74%	73%
Timely Help 'Always' Received	300+	70%	69%	68%
Would Definitely Recommend Hospital	300+	69%	69%	71%
Use of Medical Imaging				
Cardiac Imaging Stress Test before Surgery[1]	-	-	5.7%	5.3%
Combination Abdominal CT Scan	549	20.9%	12.9%	10.5%
Combination Brain/Sinus CT Scan	658	4.6%	3.3%	2.7%
Combination Chest CT Scan	179	1.1%	6.1%	2.7%
Follow-up Mammogram/Ultrasound	1,293	4.3%	8.4%	8.8%
Lumbar Spine MRI for Low Back Pain	69	34.8%	41.1%	37.2%

Greene County Hospital

1017 Jackson Street
Leakesville, MS 39451
Phone: 601-394-4135
Type: Critical Access Hospitals
Emergency Services: Yes
Ownership: Government - Local

Measure	Cases	This Hosp.	State Avg.	U.S. Avg.
Blood Clot Prevention and Treatment				
Anticoagulation Overlap Therapy[5]	-	-	86%	93%
ICU Venous Thromboembolism Prophylaxis[5]	-	-	86%	92%
Incidence of Potentially Preventable VTE[5]	-	-	15%	10%
UFH with Dosages/Platelet Monitoring[5]	-	-	94%	97%
Venous Thromboembolism Prophylaxis[5]	-	-	70%	85%
Warfarin Therapy Discharge Instructions[5]	-	-	77%	75%
Chest Pain/Possible Heart Attack Care				
Aspirin Given Within 24 Hours of Arrival[3]	42	86%	94%	96%
Fibrinolytic Meds Within 30 Min. of Arrival[5]	-	-	40%	58%
Average Time to ECG (minutes)[3]	43	3	10	7
Average Time to Transfer (minutes)[5]	-	-	77	60
Children's Asthma Care				
Received Home Management Plan of Care	-	-	-	88%
Received Reliever Medication	-	-	-	100%
Received Systemic Corticosteroids	-	-	-	100%
Emergency Department				
Admittance Decision Time (minutes)[5]	-	-	61	98
Head CT Results Within 45 Min. of Arrival[5]	-	-	42%	57%
Patients Who Left ER Before Being Seen	47	100%	3%	2%
Time from ER Arrival to Admit. (minutes)[5]	-	-	223	274
Time from ER Arrival to Discharge (minutes)[5]	-	-	112	134
Time in ER Before Being Evaluated (minutes)[5]	-	-	29	26
Time to Pain Meds for Fractures (minutes)[5]	-	-	68	57
Heart Attack Care				
Aspirin Given at Discharge[5]	-	-	99%	99%
Fibrinolytic Meds Within 30 Min. of Arrival[5]	-	-	50%	54%
PCI Within 90 Minutes of Arrival[5]	-	-	96%	96%
Statin Prescribed at Discharge[5]	-	-	97%	98%
Heart Failure Care				
ACE Inhibitor or ARB for LVSD[5]	-	-	93%	97%
Discharge Instructions Given[5]	-	-	91%	94%
Evaluation of LVS Function[5]	-	-	96%	99%
Medicare Spending				
Medicare Spending per Patient (ratio)	-	-	0.95	0.98
Pneumonia Care				
Appropriate Initial Antibiotic Given[1,3]	-	-	91%	95%
Blood Culture Timing[1,3]	-	-	97%	98%
Pregnancy and Delivery Care				
Newborn Deliveries Scheduled Early[5]	-	-	22%	6%
Preventive Care				
Immunization for Influenza[5]	-	-	87%	90%
Immunization for Pneumonia[5]	-	-	89%	92%
Stroke Care				
Anticoagulation Therapy for Atrial Fibrillation[5]	-	-	93%	95%
Antithrombotic Therapy Timing[5]	-	-	96%	98%
Assessed for Rehabilitation[5]	-	-	95%	97%
Discharged on Antithrombotic Therapy[5]	-	-	97%	99%
Discharged on Statin Medication[5]	-	-	88%	94%
Thrombolytic Therapy Timing[5]	-	-	25%	66%
Venous Thromboembolism Prophylaxis[5]	-	-	87%	94%
Written Stroke Educational Materials Given[5]	-	-	84%	88%
Surgical Care Improvement Project				
Appropriate Beta Blocker Usage[5]	-	-	97%	98%
Appropriate VTP Within 24 Hours[5]	-	-	97%	98%
Controlled Postoperative Blood Glucose[5]	-	-	97%	97%
Perioperative Temperature Management[5]	-	-	100%	100%
Prophylactic Antibiotic Selection[5]	-	-	99%	99%
Prophylactic Antibiotic Selection (Outpatient)[5]	-	-	98%	98%
Prophylactic Antibiotic Stopped[5]	-	-	97%	98%
Prophylactic Antibiotic Timing[5]	-	-	99%	99%
Prophylactic Antibiotic Timing (Outpatient)[5]	-	-	98%	98%
Urinary Catheter Removal[5]	-	-	97%	97%
Survey of Patients' Hospital Experiences				
Area Around Room 'Always' Quiet at Night[5]	-	-	72%	61%
Doctors 'Always' Communicated Well[5]	-	-	86%	82%
Home Recovery Information Given[5]	-	-	83%	85%
Hospital Given 9 or 10 on 10 Point Scale[5]	-	-	71%	71%
Meds 'Always' Explained Before Given[5]	-	-	67%	64%
Nurses 'Always' Communicated Well[5]	-	-	81%	79%
Pain 'Always' Well Controlled[5]	-	-	72%	71%
Room and Bathroom 'Always' Clean[5]	-	-	74%	73%
Timely Help 'Always' Received[5]	-	-	69%	68%
Would Definitely Recommend Hospital[5]	-	-	69%	71%
Use of Medical Imaging				
Cardiac Imaging Stress Test before Surgery[7]	-	-	5.7%	5.3%
Combination Abdominal CT Scan[1]	-	-	12.9%	10.5%
Combination Brain/Sinus CT Scan[1]	-	-	3.3%	2.7%
Combination Chest CT Scan[1]	-	-	6.1%	2.7%
Follow-up Mammogram/Ultrasound[7]	-	-	8.4%	8.8%
Lumbar Spine MRI for Low Back Pain[7]	-	-	41.1%	37.2%

Holmes County Hospital & Clinics

239 Bowling Green Road
Lexington, MS 39095
Phone: 662-834-1321
Fax: 662-834-5172
Type: Critical Access Hospitals
Emergency Services: Yes
Ownership: Government - State
Beds: 84

Key Personnel:
Infection Control.............. Anne Kealhofer
Quality Assurance .... Anne Kealhofer
Chief of Medical Staff.......... James Major, MD
Emergency Room .... Mark Smothers, MD

Measure	Cases	This Hosp.	State Avg.	U.S. Avg.
Blood Clot Prevention and Treatment				
Anticoagulation Overlap Therapy[5]	-	-	86%	93%
ICU Venous Thromboembolism Prophylaxis[5]	-	-	86%	92%
Incidence of Potentially Preventable VTE[5]	-	-	15%	10%
UFH with Dosages/Platelet Monitoring[5]	-	-	94%	97%
Venous Thromboembolism Prophylaxis[5]	-	-	70%	85%
Warfarin Therapy Discharge Instructions[5]	-	-	77%	75%
Chest Pain/Possible Heart Attack Care				
Aspirin Given Within 24 Hours of Arrival	27	96%	94%	96%
Fibrinolytic Meds Within 30 Min. of Arrival[7]	-	-	40%	58%
Average Time to ECG (minutes)	28	13	10	7
Average Time to Transfer (minutes)[1]	-	-	77	60
Children's Asthma Care				
Received Home Management Plan of Care	-	-	-	88%
Received Reliever Medication	-	-	-	100%
Received Systemic Corticosteroids	-	-	-	100%
Emergency Department				
Admittance Decision Time (minutes)[5]	-	-	61	98
Head CT Results Within 45 Min. of Arrival[5]	-	-	42%	57%
Patients Who Left ER Before Being Seen	7,042	5%	3%	2%
Time from ER Arrival to Admit. (minutes)[5]	-	-	223	274
Time from ER Arrival to Discharge (minutes)[5]	-	-	112	134
Time in ER Before Being Evaluated (minutes)[5]	-	-	29	26
Time to Pain Meds for Fractures (minutes)[5]	-	-	68	57
Heart Attack Care				
Aspirin Given at Discharge[3,7]	-	-	99%	99%
Fibrinolytic Meds Within 30 Min. of Arrival[3,7]	-	-	50%	54%
PCI Within 90 Minutes of Arrival[3,7]	-	-	96%	96%
Statin Prescribed at Discharge[3,7]	-	-	97%	98%
Heart Failure Care				
ACE Inhibitor or ARB for LVSD[1]	-	-	93%	97%
Discharge Instructions Given	13	62%	91%	94%
Evaluation of LVS Function	14	71%	96%	99%
Medicare Spending				
Medicare Spending per Patient (ratio)	-	-	0.95	0.98
Pneumonia Care				
Appropriate Initial Antibiotic Given[1]	-	-	91%	95%
Blood Culture Timing[1]	-	-	97%	98%
Pregnancy and Delivery Care				
Newborn Deliveries Scheduled Early[3,7]	-	-	22%	6%
Preventive Care				
Immunization for Influenza[5]	-	-	87%	90%
Immunization for Pneumonia[5]	-	-	89%	92%
Stroke Care				
Anticoagulation Therapy for Atrial Fibrillation[5]	-	-	93%	95%
Antithrombotic Therapy Timing[5]	-	-	96%	98%
Assessed for Rehabilitation[5]	-	-	95%	97%
Discharged on Antithrombotic Therapy[5]	-	-	97%	99%
Discharged on Statin Medication[5]	-	-	88%	94%
Thrombolytic Therapy Timing[5]	-	-	25%	66%
Venous Thromboembolism Prophylaxis[5]	-	-	87%	94%
Written Stroke Educational Materials Given[5]	-	-	84%	88%
Surgical Care Improvement Project				
Appropriate Beta Blocker Usage[5]	-	-	97%	98%
Appropriate VTP Within 24 Hours[5]	-	-	97%	98%
Controlled Postoperative Blood Glucose[5]	-	-	97%	97%
Perioperative Temperature Management[5]	-	-	100%	100%
Prophylactic Antibiotic Selection[5]	-	-	99%	99%
Prophylactic Antibiotic Selection (Outpatient)[5]	-	-	98%	98%
Prophylactic Antibiotic Stopped[5]	-	-	97%	98%
Prophylactic Antibiotic Timing[5]	-	-	99%	99%
Prophylactic Antibiotic Timing (Outpatient)[5]	-	-	98%	98%
Urinary Catheter Removal[5]	-	-	97%	97%
Survey of Patients' Hospital Experiences				
Area Around Room 'Always' Quiet at Night[5]	-	-	72%	61%
Doctors 'Always' Communicated Well[5]	-	-	86%	82%
Home Recovery Information Given[5]	-	-	83%	85%
Hospital Given 9 or 10 on 10 Point Scale[5]	-	-	71%	71%
Meds 'Always' Explained Before Given[5]	-	-	67%	64%
Nurses 'Always' Communicated Well[5]	-	-	81%	79%
Pain 'Always' Well Controlled[5]	-	-	72%	71%
Room and Bathroom 'Always' Clean[5]	-	-	74%	73%
Timely Help 'Always' Received[5]	-	-	69%	68%
Would Definitely Recommend Hospital[5]	-	-	69%	71%
Use of Medical Imaging				
Cardiac Imaging Stress Test before Surgery[7]	-	-	5.7%	5.3%
Combination Abdominal CT Scan	127	4.7%	12.9%	10.5%
Combination Brain/Sinus CT Scan[1]	-	-	3.3%	2.7%
Combination Chest CT Scan[1]	-	-	6.1%	2.7%
Follow-up Mammogram/Ultrasound	90	8.9%	8.4%	8.8%
Lumbar Spine MRI for Low Back Pain[1]	-	-	41.1%	37.2%

NOTE: Hospital profiles are in alphabetical order by state, then city, then hospital within the city; Rankings exclude hospitals with less than 25 cases except for patient surveys which excludes hospitals with less than 100 cases; (a) 100-299 cases; (1) The number of cases/patients is too few to report; (2) Data submitted were based on a sample of cases/patients; (3) Results are based on a shorter time period than required; (4) Data suppressed by CMS for one or more quarters; (5) Results are not available for this reporting period; (6) Fewer than 100 patients completed the HCAHPS survey; (7) No cases met the criteria for this measure; (8) The lower limit of the confidence interval cannot be calculated if the number of observed infections equals zero; (9) No data are available from the state/territory for this reporting period; (10) The scores shown reflect fewer than 50 completed surveys; (11) There were discrepancies in the data collection process; (12) This measure does not apply to this hospital for this reporting period; (13) Results cannot be calculated for this reporting period; (14) The results for this state are combined with nearby states to protect confidentiality; Please refer to the User's Guide for a full explanation of data.

Winston Medical Center & Swingbed

562 East Main Street
Louisville, MS 39339
Phone: 662-773-6211
Fax: 662-773-6223
E-mail: info@winstonmedical.org
URL: www.winstonmedical.org
Type: Acute Care Hospitals
Emergency Services: Yes
Ownership: Government - Local
Beds: 185

Measure	Cases	This Hosp.	State Avg.	U.S. Avg.
Blood Clot Prevention and Treatment				
Anticoagulation Overlap Therapy[1,2]	-	-	86%	93%
ICU Venous Thromboembolism Prophylaxis[2,7]	-	-	86%	92%
Incidence of Potentially Preventable VTE[2,7]	-	-	15%	10%
UFH with Dosages/Platelet Monitoring[2,7]	-	-	94%	97%
Venous Thromboembolism Prophylaxis[2]	126	44%	70%	85%
Warfarin Therapy Discharge Instructions[1,2]	-	-	77%	75%
Chest Pain/Possible Heart Attack Care				
Aspirin Given Within 24 Hours of Arrival[3]	24	96%	94%	96%
Fibrinolytic Meds Within 30 Min. of Arrival[1,3]	-	-	40%	58%
Average Time to ECG (minutes)[3]	24	18	10	7
Average Time to Transfer (minutes)[1,3]	-	-	77	60
Children's Asthma Care				
Received Home Management Plan of Care	-	-	-	88%
Received Reliever Medication	-	-	-	100%
Received Systemic Corticosteroids	-	-	-	100%
Emergency Department				
Admittance Decision Time (minutes)[2]	259	62	61	98
Head CT Results Within 45 Min. of Arrival[1,3]	-	-	42%	57%
Patients Who Left ER Before Being Seen	11,177	1%	3%	2%
Time from ER Arrival to Admit. (minutes)[2]	272	243	223	274
Time from ER Arrival to Discharge (minutes)	353	107	112	134
Time in ER Before Being Evaluated (minutes)	369	28	29	26
Time to Pain Meds for Fractures (minutes)	40	62	68	57
Heart Attack Care				
Aspirin Given at Discharge[5]	-	-	99%	99%
Fibrinolytic Meds Within 30 Min. of Arrival[5]	-	-	50%	54%
PCI Within 90 Minutes of Arrival[5]	-	-	96%	96%
Statin Prescribed at Discharge[5]	-	-	97%	98%
Heart Failure Care				
ACE Inhibitor or ARB for LVSD[1,3]	-	-	93%	97%
Discharge Instructions Given[1,3]	-	-	91%	94%
Evaluation of LVS Function[3]	11	100%	96%	99%
Medicare Spending				
Medicare Spending per Patient (ratio)	-	0.90	0.95	0.98
Pneumonia Care				
Appropriate Initial Antibiotic Given	18	94%	91%	95%
Blood Culture Timing	24	88%	97%	98%
Pregnancy and Delivery Care				
Newborn Deliveries Scheduled Early[7]	-	-	22%	6%
Preventive Care				
Immunization for Influenza	207	65%	87%	90%
Immunization for Pneumonia[2]	288	72%	89%	92%
Stroke Care				
Anticoagulation Therapy for Atrial Fibrillation[5]	-	-	93%	95%
Antithrombotic Therapy Timing[5]	-	-	96%	98%
Assessed for Rehabilitation[5]	-	-	95%	97%
Discharged on Antithrombotic Therapy[5]	-	-	97%	99%
Discharged on Statin Medication[5]	-	-	88%	94%
Thrombolytic Therapy Timing[5]	-	-	25%	66%
Venous Thromboembolism Prophylaxis[5]	-	-	87%	94%
Written Stroke Educational Materials Given[5]	-	-	84%	88%
Surgical Care Improvement Project				
Appropriate Beta Blocker Usage[5]	-	-	97%	98%
Appropriate VTP Within 24 Hours[5]	-	-	97%	98%
Controlled Postoperative Blood Glucose[5]	-	-	97%	97%
Perioperative Temperature Management[5]	-	-	100%	100%
Prophylactic Antibiotic Selection[5]	-	-	99%	99%
Prophylactic Antibiotic Selection (Outpatient)[5]	-	-	98%	98%
Prophylactic Antibiotic Stopped[5]	-	-	97%	98%
Prophylactic Antibiotic Timing[5]	-	-	99%	99%
Prophylactic Antibiotic Timing (Outpatient)[5]	-	-	98%	98%
Urinary Catheter Removal[5]	-	-	97%	97%
Survey of Patients' Hospital Experiences				
Area Around Room 'Always' Quiet at Night[6]	<100	81%	72%	61%
Doctors 'Always' Communicated Well[6]	<100	91%	86%	82%
Home Recovery Information Given[6]	<100	77%	83%	85%
Hospital Given 9 or 10 on 10 Point Scale[6]	<100	65%	71%	71%
Meds 'Always' Explained Before Given[6]	<100	73%	67%	64%
Nurses 'Always' Communicated Well[6]	<100	87%	81%	79%
Pain 'Always' Well Controlled[6]	<100	78%	72%	71%
Room and Bathroom 'Always' Clean[6]	<100	75%	74%	73%
Timely Help 'Always' Received[6]	<100	83%	69%	68%
Would Definitely Recommend Hospital[6]	<100	60%	69%	71%
Use of Medical Imaging				
Cardiac Imaging Stress Test before Surgery[7]	-	-	5.7%	5.3%
Combination Abdominal CT Scan	127	17.3%	12.9%	10.5%
Combination Brain/Sinus CT Scan[1]	-	-	3.3%	2.7%
Combination Chest CT Scan[1]	-	-	6.1%	2.7%
Follow-up Mammogram/Ultrasound	421	1.2%	8.4%	8.8%
Lumbar Spine MRI for Low Back Pain[7]	-	-	41.1%	37.2%

George County Hospital

859 Winter Street
Lucedale, MS 39452
Phone: 601-947-3161
Fax: 601-947-9206
E-mail: hospital@ametro.nrt
URL: www.georgeregional.com
Type: Acute Care Hospitals
Emergency Services: Yes
Ownership: Government - Local
Beds: 53

Key Personnel:

Infection Control.............. Retha Gunter, RN
CEO/President............... Lester Hatcher
Pediatric In-Patient Care .... Tara Mallett, DO
Chief of Medical Staff.......... E Kevin O'Hea
Anesthesiology................ Derrick Scott
Intensive Care Unit............ Mark Scott
Emergency Room .... John Van Derwood, MD
Operating Room.............. Evelyn Vickers

Measure	Cases	This Hosp.	State Avg.	U.S. Avg.
Blood Clot Prevention and Treatment				
Anticoagulation Overlap Therapy[1,2]	-	-	86%	93%
ICU Venous Thromboembolism Prophylaxis[2]	40	85%	86%	92%
Incidence of Potentially Preventable VTE[1,2]	-	-	15%	10%
UFH with Dosages/Platelet Monitoring[2,7]	-	-	94%	97%
Venous Thromboembolism Prophylaxis[2]	90	89%	70%	85%
Warfarin Therapy Discharge Instructions[1,2]	-	-	77%	75%
Chest Pain/Possible Heart Attack Care				
Aspirin Given Within 24 Hours of Arrival	137	93%	94%	96%
Fibrinolytic Meds Within 30 Min. of Arrival[7]	-	-	40%	58%
Average Time to ECG (minutes)	144	16	10	7
Average Time to Transfer (minutes)[1]	-	-	77	60
Children's Asthma Care				
Received Home Management Plan of Care	-	-	-	88%
Received Reliever Medication	-	-	-	100%
Received Systemic Corticosteroids	-	-	-	100%
Emergency Department				
Admittance Decision Time (minutes)[2]	309	74	61	98
Head CT Results Within 45 Min. of Arrival[3,7]	-	-	42%	57%
Patients Who Left ER Before Being Seen	14,574	4%	3%	2%
Time from ER Arrival to Admit. (minutes)[2]	329	256	223	274
Time from ER Arrival to Discharge (minutes)	395	121	112	134
Time in ER Before Being Evaluated (minutes)	294	40	29	26
Time to Pain Meds for Fractures (minutes)	40	56	68	57
Heart Attack Care				
Aspirin Given at Discharge[1,3]	-	-	99%	99%
Fibrinolytic Meds Within 30 Min. of Arrival[3,7]	-	-	50%	54%
PCI Within 90 Minutes of Arrival[3,7]	-	-	96%	96%
Statin Prescribed at Discharge[1,3]	-	-	97%	98%
Heart Failure Care				
ACE Inhibitor or ARB for LVSD[1,2]	-	-	93%	97%
Discharge Instructions Given[2]	41	83%	91%	94%
Evaluation of LVS Function[2]	54	94%	96%	99%
Medicare Spending				
Medicare Spending per Patient (ratio)	-	0.99	0.95	0.98
Pneumonia Care				
Appropriate Initial Antibiotic Given	31	100%	91%	95%
Blood Culture Timing	57	95%	97%	98%
Pregnancy and Delivery Care				
Newborn Deliveries Scheduled Early	64	17%	22%	6%
Preventive Care				
Immunization for Influenza[2]	278	79%	87%	90%
Immunization for Pneumonia[2]	323	88%	89%	92%
Stroke Care				
Anticoagulation Therapy for Atrial Fibrillation[1]	-	-	93%	95%
Antithrombotic Therapy Timing	17	100%	96%	98%
Assessed for Rehabilitation	15	93%	95%	97%
Discharged on Antithrombotic Therapy	15	100%	97%	99%
Discharged on Statin Medication[1]	-	-	88%	94%
Thrombolytic Therapy Timing[1]	-	-	25%	66%
Venous Thromboembolism Prophylaxis	16	94%	87%	94%
Written Stroke Educational Materials Given[1]	-	-	84%	88%
Surgical Care Improvement Project				
Appropriate Beta Blocker Usage[1,3]	-	-	97%	98%
Appropriate VTP Within 24 Hours[3]	23	57%	97%	98%
Controlled Postoperative Blood Glucose[3,7]	-	-	97%	97%
Perioperative Temperature Management[3]	25	100%	100%	100%
Prophylactic Antibiotic Selection[3]	14	57%	99%	99%
Prophylactic Antibiotic Selection (Outpatient)[5]	-	-	98%	98%
Prophylactic Antibiotic Stopped[3]	14	71%	97%	98%
Prophylactic Antibiotic Timing[3]	15	80%	99%	99%
Prophylactic Antibiotic Timing (Outpatient)[5]	-	-	98%	98%
Urinary Catheter Removal[3]	12	83%	97%	97%
Survey of Patients' Hospital Experiences				
Area Around Room 'Always' Quiet at Night	(a)	77%	72%	61%
Doctors 'Always' Communicated Well	(a)	89%	86%	82%
Home Recovery Information Given	(a)	87%	83%	85%
Hospital Given 9 or 10 on 10 Point Scale	(a)	81%	71%	71%
Meds 'Always' Explained Before Given	(a)	70%	67%	64%
Nurses 'Always' Communicated Well	(a)	83%	81%	79%
Pain 'Always' Well Controlled	(a)	79%	72%	71%
Room and Bathroom 'Always' Clean	(a)	84%	74%	73%
Timely Help 'Always' Received	(a)	75%	69%	68%
Would Definitely Recommend Hospital	(a)	70%	69%	71%
Use of Medical Imaging				
Cardiac Imaging Stress Test before Surgery	102	2.9%	5.7%	5.3%
Combination Abdominal CT Scan	266	9.4%	12.9%	10.5%
Combination Brain/Sinus CT Scan	284	0.4%	3.3%	2.7%
Combination Chest CT Scan	138	0.0%	6.1%	2.7%
Follow-up Mammogram/Ultrasound	345	7.8%	8.4%	8.8%
Lumbar Spine MRI for Low Back Pain	36	55.6%	41.1%	37.2%

Magee General Hospital

300 3rd Ave Se
Magee, MS 39111
Phone: 601-849-5070
Fax: 601-849-7397
URL: www.mghosp.org
Type: Acute Care Hospitals
Emergency Services: Yes
Ownership: Voluntary non-profit - Private
Beds: 56

Key Personnel:

Chief of Medical Staff.......... Thomas Blackledge
Operating Room.............. Blair Faulkner, RN
Emergency Room .... RS Runnels, MD

Measure	Cases	This Hosp.	State Avg.	U.S. Avg.
Blood Clot Prevention and Treatment				
Anticoagulation Overlap Therapy[1,2]	-	-	86%	93%
ICU Venous Thromboembolism Prophylaxis[2,7]	-	-	86%	92%
Incidence of Potentially Preventable VTE[2,7]	-	-	15%	10%
UFH with Dosages/Platelet Monitoring[2,7]	-	-	94%	97%
Venous Thromboembolism Prophylaxis[2]	222	87%	70%	85%
Warfarin Therapy Discharge Instructions[1,2]	-	-	77%	75%
Chest Pain/Possible Heart Attack Care				
Aspirin Given Within 24 Hours of Arrival	54	100%	94%	96%
Fibrinolytic Meds Within 30 Min. of Arrival[1]	-	-	40%	58%
Average Time to ECG (minutes)	58	5	10	7
Average Time to Transfer (minutes)	14	79	77	60
Children's Asthma Care				
Received Home Management Plan of Care	-	-	-	88%
Received Reliever Medication	-	-	-	100%
Received Systemic Corticosteroids	-	-	-	100%
Emergency Department				
Admittance Decision Time (minutes)[2]	206	48	61	98
Head CT Results Within 45 Min. of Arrival[1]	-	-	42%	57%

NOTE: Hospital profiles are in alphabetical order by state, then city, then hospital within the city; Rankings exclude hospitals with less than 25 cases except for patient surveys which excludes hospitals with less than 100 cases; (a) 100-299 cases; (1) The number of cases/patients is too few to report; (2) Data submitted were based on a sample of cases/patients; (3) Results are based on a shorter time period than required; (4) Data suppressed by CMS for one or more quarters; (5) Results are not available for this reporting period; (6) Fewer than 100 patients completed the HCAHPS survey; (7) No cases met the criteria for this measure; (8) The lower limit of the confidence interval cannot be calculated if the number of observed infections equals zero; (9) No data are available from the state/territory for this reporting period; (10) The scores shown reflect fewer than 50 completed surveys; (11) There were discrepancies in the data collection process; (12) This measure does not apply to this hospital for this reporting period; (13) Results cannot be calculated for this reporting period; (14) The results for this state are combined with nearby states to protect confidentiality; Please refer to the User's Guide for a full explanation of data.

Measure	Cases	This Hosp.	State Avg.	U.S. Avg.
Patients Who Left ER Before Being Seen	11,056	5%	3%	2%
Time from ER Arrival to Admit. (minutes)[2]	210	190	223	274
Time from ER Arrival to Discharge (minutes)	496	120	112	134
Time in ER Before Being Evaluated (minutes)	563	39	29	26
Time to Pain Meds for Fractures (minutes)	44	55	68	57
Heart Attack Care				
Aspirin Given at Discharge[1,3]	-	-	99%	99%
Fibrinolytic Meds Within 30 Min. of Arrival[3,7]	-	-	50%	54%
PCI Within 90 Minutes of Arrival[3,7]	-	-	96%	96%
Statin Prescribed at Discharge[1,3]	-	-	97%	98%
Heart Failure Care				
ACE Inhibitor or ARB for LVSD[1]	-	-	93%	97%
Discharge Instructions Given	26	92%	91%	94%
Evaluation of LVS Function	37	92%	96%	99%
Medicare Spending				
Medicare Spending per Patient (ratio)	-	1.03	0.95	0.98
Pneumonia Care				
Appropriate Initial Antibiotic Given	99	84%	91%	95%
Blood Culture Timing	86	91%	97%	98%
Pregnancy and Delivery Care				
Newborn Deliveries Scheduled Early	82	7%	22%	6%
Preventive Care				
Immunization for Influenza[2]	253	88%	87%	90%
Immunization for Pneumonia[2]	269	93%	89%	92%
Stroke Care				
Anticoagulation Therapy for Atrial Fibrillation[1]	-	-	93%	95%
Antithrombotic Therapy Timing[1]	-	-	96%	98%
Assessed for Rehabilitation[1]	-	-	95%	97%
Discharged on Antithrombotic Therapy[1]	-	-	97%	99%
Discharged on Statin Medication[1]	-	-	88%	94%
Thrombolytic Therapy Timing[1]	-	-	25%	66%
Venous Thromboembolism Prophylaxis[1]	-	-	87%	94%
Written Stroke Educational Materials Given[1]	-	-	84%	88%
Surgical Care Improvement Project				
Appropriate Beta Blocker Usage[7]	-	-	97%	98%
Appropriate VTP Within 24 Hours[1]	-	-	97%	98%
Controlled Postoperative Blood Glucose[7]	-	-	97%	97%
Perioperative Temperature Management[1]	-	-	100%	100%
Prophylactic Antibiotic Selection[1]	-	-	99%	99%
Prophylactic Antibiotic Selection (Outpatient)	36	100%	98%	98%
Prophylactic Antibiotic Stopped[1]	-	-	97%	98%
Prophylactic Antibiotic Timing[1]	-	-	99%	99%
Prophylactic Antibiotic Timing (Outpatient)	36	100%	98%	98%
Urinary Catheter Removal[1]	-	-	97%	97%
Survey of Patients' Hospital Experiences				
Area Around Room 'Always' Quiet at Night	(a)	74%	72%	61%
Doctors 'Always' Communicated Well	(a)	94%	86%	82%
Home Recovery Information Given	(a)	82%	83%	85%
Hospital Given 9 or 10 on 10 Point Scale	(a)	74%	71%	71%
Meds 'Always' Explained Before Given	(a)	66%	67%	64%
Nurses 'Always' Communicated Well	(a)	87%	81%	79%
Pain 'Always' Well Controlled	(a)	79%	72%	71%
Room and Bathroom 'Always' Clean	(a)	74%	74%	73%
Timely Help 'Always' Received	(a)	70%	69%	68%
Would Definitely Recommend Hospital	(a)	71%	69%	71%
Use of Medical Imaging				
Cardiac Imaging Stress Test before Surgery[1]	-	-	5.7%	5.3%
Combination Abdominal CT Scan	268	67.2%	12.9%	10.5%
Combination Brain/Sinus CT Scan[1]	-	-	3.3%	2.7%
Combination Chest CT Scan	112	27.7%	6.1%	2.7%
Follow-up Mammogram/Ultrasound	478	4.6%	8.4%	8.8%
Lumbar Spine MRI for Low Back Pain[1]	-	-	41.1%	37.2%

Beacham Memorial Hospital

205 N Cherry St
Magnolia, MS 39652
Phone: 601-783-2351
Fax: 601-783-9003
URL: www.beachammemorial.com
Type: Acute Care Hospitals
Emergency Services: No
Ownership: Voluntary non-profit - Private
Beds: 37

Key Personnel:
Radiology. . . . . Alesia Dillon
CEO . . . . Guy Geller
Infection Control. . . . . Debra Hughes, RN
Chief of Medical Staff. . . . . Lucius M Lampton, MD
Quality Assurance . . . . Melanie Weekley, RN

Measure	Cases	This Hosp.	State Avg.	U.S. Avg.
Blood Clot Prevention and Treatment				
Anticoagulation Overlap Therapy[1,2]	-	-	86%	93%
ICU Venous Thromboembolism Prophylaxis[2,7]	-	-	86%	92%
Incidence of Potentially Preventable VTE[1,2]	-	-	15%	10%
UFH with Dosages/Platelet Monitoring[1,2]	-	-	94%	97%
Venous Thromboembolism Prophylaxis[2]	133	14%	70%	85%
Warfarin Therapy Discharge Instructions[1,2]	-	-	77%	75%
Chest Pain/Possible Heart Attack Care				
Aspirin Given Within 24 Hours of Arrival[5]	-	-	94%	96%
Fibrinolytic Meds Within 30 Min. of Arrival[5]	-	-	40%	58%
Average Time to ECG (minutes)[5]	-	-	10	7
Average Time to Transfer (minutes)[5]	-	-	77	60
Children's Asthma Care				
Received Home Management Plan of Care	-	-	-	88%
Received Reliever Medication	-	-	-	100%
Received Systemic Corticosteroids	-	-	-	100%
Emergency Department				
Admittance Decision Time (minutes)[2,7]	-	-	61	98
Head CT Results Within 45 Min. of Arrival[5]	-	-	42%	57%
Patients Who Left ER Before Being Seen[5]	-	-	3%	2%
Time from ER Arrival to Admit. (minutes)[2,7]	-	-	223	274
Time from ER Arrival to Discharge (minutes)[5]	-	-	112	134
Time in ER Before Being Evaluated (minutes)[5]	-	-	29	26
Time to Pain Meds for Fractures (minutes)[5]	-	-	68	57
Heart Attack Care				
Aspirin Given at Discharge[5]	-	-	99%	99%
Fibrinolytic Meds Within 30 Min. of Arrival[5]	-	-	50%	54%
PCI Within 90 Minutes of Arrival[5]	-	-	96%	96%
Statin Prescribed at Discharge[5]	-	-	97%	98%
Heart Failure Care				
ACE Inhibitor or ARB for LVSD[1,2]	-	-	93%	97%
Discharge Instructions Given[2]	19	84%	91%	94%
Evaluation of LVS Function[2]	30	83%	96%	99%
Medicare Spending				
Medicare Spending per Patient (ratio)	-	0.89	0.95	0.98
Pneumonia Care				
Appropriate Initial Antibiotic Given[2]	90	36%	91%	95%
Blood Culture Timing[1,2]	-	-	97%	98%
Pregnancy and Delivery Care				
Newborn Deliveries Scheduled Early[7]	-	-	22%	6%
Preventive Care				
Immunization for Influenza[2]	330	58%	87%	90%
Immunization for Pneumonia[2]	563	48%	89%	92%
Stroke Care				
Anticoagulation Therapy for Atrial Fibrillation[1,2]	-	-	93%	95%
Antithrombotic Therapy Timing[2,3]	13	62%	96%	98%
Assessed for Rehabilitation[2,3]	13	46%	95%	97%
Discharged on Antithrombotic Therapy[2,3]	13	38%	97%	99%
Discharged on Statin Medication[2,3]	12	33%	88%	94%
Thrombolytic Therapy Timing[2,3]	-	-	25%	66%
Venous Thromboembolism Prophylaxis[2,3]	14	14%	87%	94%
Written Stroke Educational Materials Given[1,2]	-	-	84%	88%
Surgical Care Improvement Project				
Appropriate Beta Blocker Usage[5]	-	-	97%	98%
Appropriate VTP Within 24 Hours[5]	-	-	97%	98%
Controlled Postoperative Blood Glucose[5]	-	-	97%	97%
Perioperative Temperature Management[5]	-	-	100%	100%
Prophylactic Antibiotic Selection[5]	-	-	99%	99%
Prophylactic Antibiotic Selection (Outpatient)[5]	-	-	98%	98%
Prophylactic Antibiotic Stopped[5]	-	-	97%	98%
Prophylactic Antibiotic Timing[5]	-	-	99%	99%
Prophylactic Antibiotic Timing (Outpatient)[5]	-	-	98%	98%
Urinary Catheter Removal[5]	-	-	97%	97%
Survey of Patients' Hospital Experiences				
Area Around Room 'Always' Quiet at Night	(a)	76%	72%	61%
Doctors 'Always' Communicated Well	(a)	96%	86%	82%
Home Recovery Information Given	(a)	73%	83%	85%
Hospital Given 9 or 10 on 10 Point Scale	(a)	72%	71%	71%
Meds 'Always' Explained Before Given	(a)	74%	67%	64%
Nurses 'Always' Communicated Well	(a)	87%	81%	79%
Pain 'Always' Well Controlled	(a)	77%	72%	71%
Room and Bathroom 'Always' Clean	(a)	73%	74%	73%
Timely Help 'Always' Received	(a)	76%	69%	68%
Would Definitely Recommend Hospital	(a)	77%	69%	71%
Use of Medical Imaging				
Cardiac Imaging Stress Test before Surgery[7]	-	-	5.7%	5.3%
Combination Abdominal CT Scan[1]	-	-	12.9%	10.5%
Combination Brain/Sinus CT Scan	33	0.0%	3.3%	2.7%
Combination Chest CT Scan[1]	-	-	6.1%	2.7%
Follow-up Mammogram/Ultrasound[7]	-	-	8.4%	8.8%
Lumbar Spine MRI for Low Back Pain[7]	-	-	41.1%	37.2%

Quitman County Hospital

340 Getwell Drive
Marks, MS 38646
Phone: 662-326-8031
Type: Critical Access Hospitals
Emergency Services: Yes
Ownership: Proprietary

Measure	Cases	This Hosp.	State Avg.	U.S. Avg.
Blood Clot Prevention and Treatment				
Anticoagulation Overlap Therapy	-	-	86%	93%
ICU Venous Thromboembolism Prophylaxis	-	-	86%	92%
Incidence of Potentially Preventable VTE	-	-	15%	10%
UFH with Dosages/Platelet Monitoring	-	-	94%	97%
Venous Thromboembolism Prophylaxis	-	-	70%	85%
Warfarin Therapy Discharge Instructions	-	-	77%	75%
Chest Pain/Possible Heart Attack Care				
Aspirin Given Within 24 Hours of Arrival[1,3]	-	-	94%	96%
Fibrinolytic Meds Within 30 Min. of Arrival[1,3]	-	-	40%	58%
Average Time to ECG (minutes)[1,3]	-	-	10	7
Average Time to Transfer (minutes)[3,7]	-	-	77	60
Children's Asthma Care				
Received Home Management Plan of Care	-	-	-	88%
Received Reliever Medication	-	-	-	100%
Received Systemic Corticosteroids	-	-	-	100%
Emergency Department				
Admittance Decision Time (minutes)	-	-	61	98
Head CT Results Within 45 Min. of Arrival[5]	-	-	42%	57%
Patients Who Left ER Before Being Seen[5]	-	-	3%	2%
Time from ER Arrival to Admit. (minutes)	-	-	223	274
Time from ER Arrival to Discharge (minutes)[5]	-	-	112	134
Time in ER Before Being Evaluated (minutes)[5]	-	-	29	26
Time to Pain Meds for Fractures (minutes)[5]	-	-	68	57
Heart Attack Care				
Aspirin Given at Discharge	-	-	99%	99%
Fibrinolytic Meds Within 30 Min. of Arrival	-	-	50%	54%
PCI Within 90 Minutes of Arrival	-	-	96%	96%
Statin Prescribed at Discharge	-	-	97%	98%
Heart Failure Care				
ACE Inhibitor or ARB for LVSD	-	-	93%	97%
Discharge Instructions Given	-	-	91%	94%
Evaluation of LVS Function	-	-	96%	99%
Medicare Spending				
Medicare Spending per Patient (ratio)	-	-	0.95	0.98
Pneumonia Care				
Appropriate Initial Antibiotic Given	-	-	91%	95%
Blood Culture Timing	-	-	97%	98%
Pregnancy and Delivery Care				
Newborn Deliveries Scheduled Early	-	-	22%	6%
Preventive Care				
Immunization for Influenza	-	-	87%	90%
Immunization for Pneumonia	-	-	89%	92%
Stroke Care				
Anticoagulation Therapy for Atrial Fibrillation	-	-	93%	95%
Antithrombotic Therapy Timing	-	-	96%	98%
Assessed for Rehabilitation	-	-	95%	97%
Discharged on Antithrombotic Therapy	-	-	97%	99%
Discharged on Statin Medication	-	-	88%	94%
Thrombolytic Therapy Timing	-	-	25%	66%
Venous Thromboembolism Prophylaxis	-	-	87%	94%
Written Stroke Educational Materials Given	-	-	84%	88%
Surgical Care Improvement Project				
Appropriate Beta Blocker Usage	-	-	97%	98%
Appropriate VTP Within 24 Hours	-	-	97%	98%

NOTE: Hospital profiles are in alphabetical order by state, then city, then hospital within the city; Rankings exclude hospitals with less than 25 cases except for patient surveys which excludes hospitals with less than 100 cases; (a) 100-299 cases; (1) The number of cases/patients is too few to report; (2) Data submitted were based on a sample of cases/patients; (3) Results are based on a shorter time period than required; (4) Data suppressed by CMS for one or more quarters; (5) Results are not available for this reporting period; (6) Fewer than 100 patients completed the HCAHPS survey; (7) No cases met the criteria for this measure; (8) The lower limit of the confidence interval cannot be calculated if the number of observed infections equals zero; (9) No data are available from the state/territory for this reporting period; (10) The scores shown reflect fewer than 50 completed surveys; (11) There were discrepancies in the data collection process; (12) This measure does not apply to this hospital for this reporting period; (13) Results cannot be calculated for this reporting period; (14) The results for this state are combined with nearby states to protect confidentiality; Please refer to the User's Guide for a full explanation of data.

Measure	Cases	This Hosp.	State Avg.	U.S. Avg.
Controlled Postoperative Blood Glucose	-	-	97%	97%
Perioperative Temperature Management	-	-	100%	100%
Prophylactic Antibiotic Selection	-	-	99%	99%
Prophylactic Antibiotic Selection (Outpatient)[5]	-	-	98%	98%
Prophylactic Antibiotic Stopped	-	-	97%	98%
Prophylactic Antibiotic Timing	-	-	99%	99%
Prophylactic Antibiotic Timing (Outpatient)[5]	-	-	98%	98%
Urinary Catheter Removal	-	-	97%	97%
Survey of Patients' Hospital Experiences				
Area Around Room 'Always' Quiet at Night	-	-	72%	61%
Doctors 'Always' Communicated Well	-	-	86%	82%
Home Recovery Information Given	-	-	83%	85%
Hospital Given 9 or 10 on 10 Point Scale	-	-	71%	71%
Meds 'Always' Explained Before Given	-	-	67%	64%
Nurses 'Always' Communicated Well	-	-	81%	79%
Pain 'Always' Well Controlled	-	-	72%	71%
Room and Bathroom 'Always' Clean	-	-	74%	73%
Timely Help 'Always' Received	-	-	69%	68%
Would Definitely Recommend Hospital	-	-	69%	71%
Use of Medical Imaging				
Cardiac Imaging Stress Test before Surgery[7]	-	-	5.7%	5.3%
Combination Abdominal CT Scan[1]	-	-	12.9%	10.5%
Combination Brain/Sinus CT Scan	31	0.0%	3.3%	2.7%
Combination Chest CT Scan[1]	-	-	6.1%	2.7%
Follow-up Mammogram/Ultrasound[7]	-	-	8.4%	8.8%
Lumbar Spine MRI for Low Back Pain[7]	-	-	41.1%	37.2%

Southwest Ms Regional Medical Center

215 Marion Av Box 1307
Mccomb, MS 39649
Phone: 601-249-5500
Fax: 601-249-1748
E-mail: pubrel@smrmc.com
URL: www.smrmc.com
Type: Acute Care Hospitals
Emergency Services: Yes
Ownership: Government - Local
Beds: 160

Key Personnel:
Operating Room. . . . . Lavoyce Boggs, RN
Infection Control. . . . . Charles Dykes, RN
Quality Assurance . . . . Suzonne McLain
CEO . . . . Norman M. Price, FACHE
Radiology. . . . . Charles Regan
Chief of Medical Staff. . . . . Brian Remley, MD
Pediatric Ambulatory Care . . . . . Shelby Smith

Measure	Cases	This Hosp.	State Avg.	U.S. Avg.
Blood Clot Prevention and Treatment				
Anticoagulation Overlap Therapy[2]	53	49%	86%	93%
ICU Venous Thromboembolism Prophylaxis[2]	116	96%	86%	92%
Incidence of Potentially Preventable VTE[1,2]	-	-	15%	10%
UFH with Dosages/Platelet Monitoring[2]	17	100%	94%	97%
Venous Thromboembolism Prophylaxis[2]	282	91%	70%	85%
Warfarin Therapy Discharge Instructions[2]	41	90%	77%	75%
Chest Pain/Possible Heart Attack Care				
Aspirin Given Within 24 Hours of Arrival[1]	-	-	94%	96%
Fibrinolytic Meds Within 30 Min. of Arrival[5]	-	-	40%	58%
Average Time to ECG (minutes)[1]	-	-	10	7
Average Time to Transfer (minutes)[5]	-	-	77	60
Children's Asthma Care				
Received Home Management Plan of Care	-	-	-	88%
Received Reliever Medication	-	-	-	100%
Received Systemic Corticosteroids	-	-	-	100%
Emergency Department				
Admittance Decision Time (minutes)[2]	753	61	61	98
Head CT Results Within 45 Min. of Arrival	26	4%	42%	57%
Patients Who Left ER Before Being Seen	42,594	0%	3%	2%
Time from ER Arrival to Admit. (minutes)[2]	794	190	223	274
Time from ER Arrival to Discharge (minutes)	450	110	112	134
Time in ER Before Being Evaluated (minutes)	389	17	29	26
Time to Pain Meds for Fractures (minutes)	83	52	68	57
Heart Attack Care				
Aspirin Given at Discharge	132	98%	99%	99%
Fibrinolytic Meds Within 30 Min. of Arrival[7]	-	-	50%	54%
PCI Within 90 Minutes of Arrival	18	100%	96%	96%
Statin Prescribed at Discharge	124	98%	97%	98%
Heart Failure Care				
ACE Inhibitor or ARB for LVSD	98	89%	93%	97%
Discharge Instructions Given	185	88%	91%	94%
Evaluation of LVS Function	211	94%	96%	99%
Medicare Spending				
Medicare Spending per Patient (ratio)	-	1.00	0.95	0.98
Pneumonia Care				
Appropriate Initial Antibiotic Given[2]	108	89%	91%	95%
Blood Culture Timing[2]	179	97%	97%	98%
Pregnancy and Delivery Care				
Newborn Deliveries Scheduled Early[2]	37	14%	22%	6%
Preventive Care				
Immunization for Influenza[2]	531	79%	87%	90%
Immunization for Pneumonia[2]	716	84%	89%	92%
Stroke Care				
Anticoagulation Therapy for Atrial Fibrillation[1]	-	-	93%	95%
Antithrombotic Therapy Timing	53	98%	96%	98%
Assessed for Rehabilitation	52	56%	95%	97%
Discharged on Antithrombotic Therapy	51	96%	97%	99%
Discharged on Statin Medication	40	78%	88%	94%
Thrombolytic Therapy Timing[1]	-	-	25%	66%
Venous Thromboembolism Prophylaxis	54	94%	87%	94%
Written Stroke Educational Materials Given	35	83%	84%	88%
Surgical Care Improvement Project				
Appropriate Beta Blocker Usage	125	76%	97%	98%
Appropriate VTP Within 24 Hours	253	83%	97%	98%
Controlled Postoperative Blood Glucose	32	91%	97%	97%
Perioperative Temperature Management	311	99%	100%	100%
Prophylactic Antibiotic Selection	212	95%	99%	99%
Prophylactic Antibiotic Selection (Outpatient)	199	95%	98%	98%
Prophylactic Antibiotic Stopped	207	91%	97%	98%
Prophylactic Antibiotic Timing	215	93%	99%	99%
Prophylactic Antibiotic Timing (Outpatient)	200	98%	98%	98%
Urinary Catheter Removal	170	94%	97%	97%
Survey of Patients' Hospital Experiences				
Area Around Room 'Always' Quiet at Night	300+	71%	72%	61%
Doctors 'Always' Communicated Well	300+	80%	86%	82%
Home Recovery Information Given	300+	84%	83%	85%
Hospital Given 9 or 10 on 10 Point Scale	300+	67%	71%	71%
Meds 'Always' Explained Before Given	300+	58%	67%	64%
Nurses 'Always' Communicated Well	300+	77%	81%	79%
Pain 'Always' Well Controlled	300+	72%	72%	71%
Room and Bathroom 'Always' Clean	300+	70%	74%	73%
Timely Help 'Always' Received	300+	68%	69%	68%
Would Definitely Recommend Hospital	300+	64%	69%	71%
Use of Medical Imaging				
Cardiac Imaging Stress Test before Surgery	398	4.5%	5.7%	5.3%
Combination Abdominal CT Scan	949	5.2%	12.9%	10.5%
Combination Brain/Sinus CT Scan	776	4.5%	3.3%	2.7%
Combination Chest CT Scan	380	7.6%	6.1%	2.7%
Follow-up Mammogram/Ultrasound	993	3.5%	8.4%	8.8%
Lumbar Spine MRI for Low Back Pain	90	38.9%	41.1%	37.2%

Franklin County Memorial Hospital

Hwy 84 Box 636
Meadville, MS 39653
Phone: 601-384-5801
Type: Critical Access Hospitals
Emergency Services: Yes
Ownership: Voluntary non-profit - Other

Measure	Cases	This Hosp.	State Avg.	U.S. Avg.
Blood Clot Prevention and Treatment				
Anticoagulation Overlap Therapy[5]	-	-	86%	93%
ICU Venous Thromboembolism Prophylaxis[5]	-	-	86%	92%
Incidence of Potentially Preventable VTE[5]	-	-	15%	10%
UFH with Dosages/Platelet Monitoring[5]	-	-	94%	97%
Venous Thromboembolism Prophylaxis[5]	-	-	70%	85%
Warfarin Therapy Discharge Instructions[5]	-	-	77%	75%
Chest Pain/Possible Heart Attack Care				
Aspirin Given Within 24 Hours of Arrival[5]	-	-	94%	96%
Fibrinolytic Meds Within 30 Min. of Arrival[5]	-	-	40%	58%
Average Time to ECG (minutes)[5]	-	-	10	7
Average Time to Transfer (minutes)[5]	-	-	77	60
Children's Asthma Care				
Received Home Management Plan of Care	-	-	-	88%
Received Reliever Medication	-	-	-	100%
Received Systemic Corticosteroids	-	-	-	100%
Emergency Department				
Admittance Decision Time (minutes)[5]	-	-	61	98
Head CT Results Within 45 Min. of Arrival[5]	-	-	42%	57%
Patients Who Left ER Before Being Seen[5]	-	-	3%	2%
Time from ER Arrival to Admit. (minutes)[5]	-	-	223	274
Time from ER Arrival to Discharge (minutes)[5]	-	-	112	134
Time in ER Before Being Evaluated (minutes)[5]	-	-	29	26
Time to Pain Meds for Fractures (minutes)[5]	-	-	68	57
Heart Attack Care				
Aspirin Given at Discharge[5]	-	-	99%	99%
Fibrinolytic Meds Within 30 Min. of Arrival[5]	-	-	50%	54%
PCI Within 90 Minutes of Arrival[5]	-	-	96%	96%
Statin Prescribed at Discharge[5]	-	-	97%	98%
Heart Failure Care				
ACE Inhibitor or ARB for LVSD[5]	-	-	93%	97%
Discharge Instructions Given[5]	-	-	91%	94%
Evaluation of LVS Function[5]	-	-	96%	99%
Medicare Spending				
Medicare Spending per Patient (ratio)	-	-	0.95	0.98
Pneumonia Care				
Appropriate Initial Antibiotic Given[3,7]	-	-	91%	95%
Blood Culture Timing[3,7]	-	-	97%	98%
Pregnancy and Delivery Care				
Newborn Deliveries Scheduled Early[5]	-	-	22%	6%
Preventive Care				
Immunization for Influenza[5]	-	-	87%	90%
Immunization for Pneumonia[5]	-	-	89%	92%
Stroke Care				
Anticoagulation Therapy for Atrial Fibrillation[5]	-	-	93%	95%
Antithrombotic Therapy Timing[5]	-	-	96%	98%
Assessed for Rehabilitation[5]	-	-	95%	97%
Discharged on Antithrombotic Therapy[5]	-	-	97%	99%
Discharged on Statin Medication[5]	-	-	88%	94%
Thrombolytic Therapy Timing[5]	-	-	25%	66%
Venous Thromboembolism Prophylaxis[5]	-	-	87%	94%
Written Stroke Educational Materials Given[5]	-	-	84%	88%
Surgical Care Improvement Project				
Appropriate Beta Blocker Usage[5]	-	-	97%	98%
Appropriate VTP Within 24 Hours[5]	-	-	97%	98%
Controlled Postoperative Blood Glucose[5]	-	-	97%	97%
Perioperative Temperature Management[5]	-	-	100%	100%
Prophylactic Antibiotic Selection[5]	-	-	99%	99%
Prophylactic Antibiotic Selection (Outpatient)[5]	-	-	98%	98%
Prophylactic Antibiotic Stopped[5]	-	-	97%	98%
Prophylactic Antibiotic Timing[5]	-	-	99%	99%
Prophylactic Antibiotic Timing (Outpatient)[5]	-	-	98%	98%
Urinary Catheter Removal[5]	-	-	97%	97%
Survey of Patients' Hospital Experiences				
Area Around Room 'Always' Quiet at Night[10]	<100	60%	72%	61%
Doctors 'Always' Communicated Well[10]	<100	92%	86%	82%
Home Recovery Information Given[10]	<100	84%	83%	85%
Hospital Given 9 or 10 on 10 Point Scale[10]	<100	62%	71%	71%
Meds 'Always' Explained Before Given[10]	<100	67%	67%	64%
Nurses 'Always' Communicated Well[10]	<100	88%	81%	79%
Pain 'Always' Well Controlled[10]	<100	86%	72%	71%
Room and Bathroom 'Always' Clean[10]	<100	84%	74%	73%
Timely Help 'Always' Received[10]	<100	61%	69%	68%
Would Definitely Recommend Hospital[10]	<100	71%	69%	71%
Use of Medical Imaging				
Cardiac Imaging Stress Test before Surgery[7]	-	-	5.7%	5.3%
Combination Abdominal CT Scan	76	17.1%	12.9%	10.5%
Combination Brain/Sinus CT Scan[1]	-	-	3.3%	2.7%
Combination Chest CT Scan[1]	-	-	6.1%	2.7%
Follow-up Mammogram/Ultrasound[7]	-	-	8.4%	8.8%
Lumbar Spine MRI for Low Back Pain[7]	-	-	41.1%	37.2%

NOTE: Hospital profiles are in alphabetical order by state, then city, then hospital within the city; Rankings exclude hospitals with less than 25 cases except for patient surveys which excludes hospitals with less than 100 cases; (a) 100-299 cases; (1) The number of cases/patients is too few to report; (2) Data submitted were based on a sample of cases/patients; (3) Results are based on a shorter time period than required; (4) Data suppressed by CMS for one or more quarters; (5) Results are not available for this reporting period; (6) Fewer than 100 patients completed the HCAHPS survey; (7) No cases met the criteria for this measure; (8) The lower limit of the confidence interval cannot be calculated if the number of observed infections equals zero; (9) No data are available from the state/territory for this reporting period; (10) The scores shown reflect fewer than 50 completed surveys; (11) There were discrepancies in the data collection process; (12) This measure does not apply to this hospital for this reporting period; (13) Results cannot be calculated for this reporting period; (14) The results for this state are combined with nearby states to protect confidentiality; Please refer to the User's Guide for a full explanation of data.

Simpson General Hospital

1842 Simpson Highway 149
Mendenhall, MS 39114
Phone: 601-847-2221
Fax: 601-847-5872
URL: www.simpsongeneralhospital.com
Type: Critical Access Hospitals
Emergency Services: Yes
Ownership: Voluntary non-profit - Private
Beds: 25

Key Personnel:

CEO/President . . . . Winnie Grantham
Chief of Medical Staff . . . . Chip Holbrook, MD
Operating Room. . . . . Betsy Osborn
Infection Control . . . . Joyce Pearson, RN
Quality Assurance . . . . Joyce Pearson

Measure	Cases	This Hosp.	State Avg.	U.S. Avg.
Blood Clot Prevention and Treatment				
Anticoagulation Overlap Therapy[5]	-	-	86%	93%
ICU Venous Thromboembolism Prophylaxis[5]	-	-	86%	92%
Incidence of Potentially Preventable VTE[5]	-	-	15%	10%
UFH with Dosages/Platelet Monitoring[5]	-	-	94%	97%
Venous Thromboembolism Prophylaxis[5]	-	-	70%	85%
Warfarin Therapy Discharge Instructions[5]	-	-	77%	75%
Chest Pain/Possible Heart Attack Care				
Aspirin Given Within 24 Hours of Arrival	-	-	94%	96%
Fibrinolytic Meds Within 30 Min. of Arrival	-	-	40%	58%
Average Time to ECG (minutes)	-	-	10	7
Average Time to Transfer (minutes)	-	-	77	60
Children's Asthma Care				
Received Home Management Plan of Care	-	-	-	88%
Received Reliever Medication	-	-	-	100%
Received Systemic Corticosteroids	-	-	-	100%
Emergency Department				
Admittance Decision Time (minutes)[5]	-	-	61	98
Head CT Results Within 45 Min. of Arrival	-	-	42%	57%
Patients Who Left ER Before Being Seen	-	-	3%	2%
Time from ER Arrival to Admit. (minutes)[5]	-	-	223	274
Time from ER Arrival to Discharge (minutes)	-	-	112	134
Time in ER Before Being Evaluated (minutes)	-	-	29	26
Time to Pain Meds for Fractures (minutes)	-	-	68	57
Heart Attack Care				
Aspirin Given at Discharge[5]	-	-	99%	99%
Fibrinolytic Meds Within 30 Min. of Arrival[5]	-	-	50%	54%
PCI Within 90 Minutes of Arrival[5]	-	-	96%	96%
Statin Prescribed at Discharge[5]	-	-	97%	98%
Heart Failure Care				
ACE Inhibitor or ARB for LVSD[1,3]	-	-	93%	97%
Discharge Instructions Given[1,3]	-	-	91%	94%
Evaluation of LVS Function[1,3]	-	-	96%	99%
Medicare Spending				
Medicare Spending per Patient (ratio)	-	-	0.95	0.98
Pneumonia Care				
Appropriate Initial Antibiotic Given	13	31%	91%	95%
Blood Culture Timing[1]	-	-	97%	98%
Pregnancy and Delivery Care				
Newborn Deliveries Scheduled Early[5]	-	-	22%	6%
Preventive Care				
Immunization for Influenza[5]	-	-	87%	90%
Immunization for Pneumonia[5]	-	-	89%	92%
Stroke Care				
Anticoagulation Therapy for Atrial Fibrillation[5]	-	-	93%	95%
Antithrombotic Therapy Timing[5]	-	-	96%	98%
Assessed for Rehabilitation[5]	-	-	95%	97%
Discharged on Antithrombotic Therapy[5]	-	-	97%	99%
Discharged on Statin Medication[5]	-	-	88%	94%
Thrombolytic Therapy Timing[5]	-	-	25%	66%
Venous Thromboembolism Prophylaxis[5]	-	-	87%	94%
Written Stroke Educational Materials Given[5]	-	-	84%	88%
Surgical Care Improvement Project				
Appropriate Beta Blocker Usage[5]	-	-	97%	98%
Appropriate VTP Within 24 Hours[5]	-	-	97%	98%
Controlled Postoperative Blood Glucose[5]	-	-	97%	97%
Perioperative Temperature Management[5]	-	-	100%	100%
Prophylactic Antibiotic Selection[5]	-	-	99%	99%
Prophylactic Antibiotic Selection (Outpatient)	-	-	98%	98%
Prophylactic Antibiotic Stopped[5]	-	-	97%	98%
Prophylactic Antibiotic Timing[5]	-	-	99%	99%
Prophylactic Antibiotic Timing (Outpatient)	-	-	98%	98%
Urinary Catheter Removal[5]	-	-	97%	97%
Survey of Patients' Hospital Experiences				
Area Around Room 'Always' Quiet at Night[5]	-	-	72%	61%
Doctors 'Always' Communicated Well[5]	-	-	86%	82%
Home Recovery Information Given[5]	-	-	83%	85%
Hospital Given 9 or 10 on 10 Point Scale[5]	-	-	71%	71%
Meds 'Always' Explained Before Given[5]	-	-	67%	64%
Nurses 'Always' Communicated Well[5]	-	-	81%	79%
Pain 'Always' Well Controlled[5]	-	-	72%	71%
Room and Bathroom 'Always' Clean[5]	-	-	74%	73%
Timely Help 'Always' Received[5]	-	-	69%	68%
Would Definitely Recommend Hospital[5]	-	-	69%	71%
Use of Medical Imaging				
Cardiac Imaging Stress Test before Surgery	-	-	5.7%	5.3%
Combination Abdominal CT Scan	-	-	12.9%	10.5%
Combination Brain/Sinus CT Scan	-	-	3.3%	2.7%
Combination Chest CT Scan	-	-	6.1%	2.7%
Follow-up Mammogram/Ultrasound	-	-	8.4%	8.8%
Lumbar Spine MRI for Low Back Pain	-	-	41.1%	37.2%

Alliance Health Center

5000 Highway 39 North
Meridian, MS 39301
Phone: 601-483-6211
Fax: 601-696-4898
E-mail: bpatterson@psysolutions.com
URL: www.alliancehealthcenter.com
Type: Acute Care Hospitals
Emergency Services: No
Ownership: Proprietary
Beds: 134

Key Personnel:

Chief of Medical Staff . . . . Terry Jordan, MD
CEO . . . . James Miller
CEO/President . . . . Bill Patterson
Patient Relations . . . . Shannon Smith
Infection Control . . . . Brenda Thompson
Quality Assurance . . . . Brenda Thompson

Measure	Cases	This Hosp.	State Avg.	U.S. Avg.
Blood Clot Prevention and Treatment				
Anticoagulation Overlap Therapy[2,7]	-	-	86%	93%
ICU Venous Thromboembolism Prophylaxis[2,7]	-	-	86%	92%
Incidence of Potentially Preventable VTE[2,7]	-	-	15%	10%
UFH with Dosages/Platelet Monitoring[2,7]	-	-	94%	97%
Venous Thromboembolism Prophylaxis[1,2]	-	-	70%	85%
Warfarin Therapy Discharge Instructions[2,7]	-	-	77%	75%
Chest Pain/Possible Heart Attack Care				
Aspirin Given Within 24 Hours of Arrival[5]	-	-	94%	96%
Fibrinolytic Meds Within 30 Min. of Arrival[5]	-	-	40%	58%
Average Time to ECG (minutes)[5]	-	-	10	7
Average Time to Transfer (minutes)[5]	-	-	77	60
Children's Asthma Care				
Received Home Management Plan of Care	-	-	-	88%
Received Reliever Medication	-	-	-	100%
Received Systemic Corticosteroids	-	-	-	100%
Emergency Department				
Admittance Decision Time (minutes)[2,7]	-	-	61	98
Head CT Results Within 45 Min. of Arrival[5]	-	-	42%	57%
Patients Who Left ER Before Being Seen[5]	-	-	3%	2%
Time from ER Arrival to Admit. (minutes)[2,7]	-	-	223	274
Time from ER Arrival to Discharge (minutes)[5]	-	-	112	134
Time in ER Before Being Evaluated (minutes)[5]	-	-	29	26
Time to Pain Meds for Fractures (minutes)[5]	-	-	68	57
Heart Attack Care				
Aspirin Given at Discharge[5]	-	-	99%	99%
Fibrinolytic Meds Within 30 Min. of Arrival[5]	-	-	50%	54%
PCI Within 90 Minutes of Arrival[5]	-	-	96%	96%
Statin Prescribed at Discharge[5]	-	-	97%	98%
Heart Failure Care				
ACE Inhibitor or ARB for LVSD[5]	-	-	93%	97%
Discharge Instructions Given[5]	-	-	91%	94%
Evaluation of LVS Function[5]	-	-	96%	99%
Medicare Spending				
Medicare Spending per Patient (ratio)	-	1.12	0.95	0.98
Pneumonia Care				
Appropriate Initial Antibiotic Given[5]	-	-	91%	95%
Blood Culture Timing[5]	-	-	97%	98%
Pregnancy and Delivery Care				
Newborn Deliveries Scheduled Early[7]	-	-	22%	6%
Preventive Care				
Immunization for Influenza[2]	172	1%	87%	90%
Immunization for Pneumonia[2]	70	40%	89%	92%
Stroke Care				
Anticoagulation Therapy for Atrial Fibrillation[5]	-	-	93%	95%
Antithrombotic Therapy Timing[5]	-	-	96%	98%
Assessed for Rehabilitation[5]	-	-	95%	97%
Discharged on Antithrombotic Therapy[5]	-	-	97%	99%
Discharged on Statin Medication[5]	-	-	88%	94%
Thrombolytic Therapy Timing[5]	-	-	25%	66%
Venous Thromboembolism Prophylaxis[5]	-	-	87%	94%
Written Stroke Educational Materials Given[5]	-	-	84%	88%
Surgical Care Improvement Project				
Appropriate Beta Blocker Usage[5]	-	-	97%	98%
Appropriate VTP Within 24 Hours[5]	-	-	97%	98%
Controlled Postoperative Blood Glucose[5]	-	-	97%	97%
Perioperative Temperature Management[5]	-	-	100%	100%
Prophylactic Antibiotic Selection[5]	-	-	99%	99%
Prophylactic Antibiotic Selection (Outpatient)[5]	-	-	98%	98%
Prophylactic Antibiotic Stopped[5]	-	-	97%	98%
Prophylactic Antibiotic Timing[5]	-	-	99%	99%
Prophylactic Antibiotic Timing (Outpatient)[5]	-	-	98%	98%
Urinary Catheter Removal[5]	-	-	97%	97%
Survey of Patients' Hospital Experiences				
Area Around Room 'Always' Quiet at Night[1]	-	-	72%	61%
Doctors 'Always' Communicated Well[1]	-	-	86%	82%
Home Recovery Information Given[1]	-	-	83%	85%
Hospital Given 9 or 10 on 10 Point Scale[1]	-	-	71%	71%
Meds 'Always' Explained Before Given[1]	-	-	67%	64%
Nurses 'Always' Communicated Well[1]	-	-	81%	79%
Pain 'Always' Well Controlled[1]	-	-	72%	71%
Room and Bathroom 'Always' Clean[1]	-	-	74%	73%
Timely Help 'Always' Received[1]	-	-	69%	68%
Would Definitely Recommend Hospital[1]	-	-	69%	71%
Use of Medical Imaging				
Cardiac Imaging Stress Test before Surgery[7]	-	-	5.7%	5.3%
Combination Abdominal CT Scan[7]	-	-	12.9%	10.5%
Combination Brain/Sinus CT Scan[7]	-	-	3.3%	2.7%
Combination Chest CT Scan[7]	-	-	6.1%	2.7%
Follow-up Mammogram/Ultrasound[7]	-	-	8.4%	8.8%
Lumbar Spine MRI for Low Back Pain[7]	-	-	41.1%	37.2%

Anderson Regional Medical Center

2124 14 St
Meridian, MS 39301
Phone: 601-553-6000
Fax: 601-553-6834
URL: www.jarmc.org
Type: Acute Care Hospitals
Emergency Services: Yes
Ownership: Voluntary non-profit - Private
Beds: 260

Key Personnel:

CEO/President . . . . John Anderson
Chief of Medical Staff . . . . Scot Bell, MD, JD, MMM, FA
Quality Assurance . . . . Wanda B Cooper
Emergency Room . . . . Ramona Jackson, RN
Pediatric Ambulatory Care . . . . . . William Simmons, MD
Pediatric In-Patient Care . . . . William Simmons, MD

Measure	Cases	This Hosp.	State Avg.	U.S. Avg.
Blood Clot Prevention and Treatment				
Anticoagulation Overlap Therapy[2]	76	92%	86%	93%
ICU Venous Thromboembolism Prophylaxis[2]	96	68%	86%	92%
Incidence of Potentially Preventable VTE[2]	17	53%	15%	10%
UFH with Dosages/Platelet Monitoring[2]	27	96%	94%	97%
Venous Thromboembolism Prophylaxis[2]	363	48%	70%	85%
Warfarin Therapy Discharge Instructions[2]	58	74%	77%	75%
Chest Pain/Possible Heart Attack Care				
Aspirin Given Within 24 Hours of Arrival[1,3]	-	-	94%	96%
Fibrinolytic Meds Within 30 Min. of Arrival[5]	-	-	40%	58%
Average Time to ECG (minutes)[1,3]	-	-	10	7
Average Time to Transfer (minutes)[5]	-	-	77	60
Children's Asthma Care				
Received Home Management Plan of Care	-	-	-	88%
Received Reliever Medication	-	-	-	100%

NOTE: Hospital profiles are in alphabetical order by state, then city, then hospital within the city; Rankings exclude hospitals with less than 25 cases except for patient surveys which excludes hospitals with less than 100 cases; (a) 100-299 cases; (1) The number of cases/patients is too few to report; (2) Data submitted were based on a sample of cases/patients; (3) Results are based on a shorter time period than required; (4) Data suppressed by CMS for one or more quarters; (5) Results are not available for this reporting period; (6) Fewer than 100 patients completed the HCAHPS survey; (7) No cases met the criteria for this measure; (8) The lower limit of the confidence interval cannot be calculated if the number of observed infections equals zero; (9) No data are available from the state/territory for this reporting period; (10) The scores shown reflect fewer than 50 completed surveys; (11) There were discrepancies in the data collection process; (12) This measure does not apply to this hospital for this reporting period; (13) Results cannot be calculated for this reporting period; (14) The results for this state are combined with nearby states to protect confidentiality; Please refer to the User's Guide for a full explanation of data.

Received Systemic Corticosteroids	-	-	-	100%
Emergency Department				
Admittance Decision Time (minutes)[2]	530	65	61	98
Head CT Results Within 45 Min. of Arrival	13	8%	42%	57%
Patients Who Left ER Before Being Seen	32,232	3%	3%	2%
Time from ER Arrival to Admit. (minutes)[2]	550	200	223	274
Time from ER Arrival to Discharge (minutes)	359	117	112	134
Time in ER Before Being Evaluated (minutes)	402	35	29	26
Time to Pain Meds for Fractures (minutes)	129	65	68	57
Heart Attack Care				
Aspirin Given at Discharge	231	100%	99%	99%
Fibrinolytic Meds Within 30 Min. of Arrival[1]	-	-	50%	54%
PCI Within 90 Minutes of Arrival	20	85%	96%	96%
Statin Prescribed at Discharge	229	98%	97%	98%
Heart Failure Care				
ACE Inhibitor or ARB for LVSD[2]	90	100%	93%	97%
Discharge Instructions Given[2]	267	94%	91%	94%
Evaluation of LVS Function[2]	327	100%	96%	99%
Medicare Spending				
Medicare Spending per Patient (ratio)	-	1.00	0.95	0.98
Pneumonia Care				
Appropriate Initial Antibiotic Given[2]	66	88%	91%	95%
Blood Culture Timing[2]	103	100%	97%	98%
Pregnancy and Delivery Care				
Newborn Deliveries Scheduled Early[2]	27	22%	22%	6%
Preventive Care				
Immunization for Influenza[2]	542	98%	87%	90%
Immunization for Pneumonia[2]	704	98%	89%	92%
Stroke Care				
Anticoagulation Therapy for Atrial Fibrillation[2]	14	93%	93%	95%
Antithrombotic Therapy Timing[2]	104	96%	96%	98%
Assessed for Rehabilitation[2]	122	94%	95%	97%
Discharged on Antithrombotic Therapy[2]	109	99%	97%	99%
Discharged on Statin Medication[2]	91	78%	88%	94%
Thrombolytic Therapy Timing[2]	14	14%	25%	66%
Venous Thromboembolism Prophylaxis[2]	126	67%	87%	94%
Written Stroke Educational Materials Given[2]	58	55%	84%	88%
Surgical Care Improvement Project				
Appropriate Beta Blocker Usage[2]	156	97%	97%	98%
Appropriate VTP Within 24 Hours[2]	386	97%	97%	98%
Controlled Postoperative Blood Glucose[2]	89	93%	97%	97%
Perioperative Temperature Management[2]	427	100%	100%	100%
Prophylactic Antibiotic Selection[2]	362	100%	99%	99%
Prophylactic Antibiotic Selection (Outpatient)	402	97%	98%	98%
Prophylactic Antibiotic Stopped[2]	355	96%	97%	98%
Prophylactic Antibiotic Timing[2]	363	100%	99%	99%
Prophylactic Antibiotic Timing (Outpatient)	403	98%	98%	98%
Urinary Catheter Removal[2]	236	97%	97%	97%
Survey of Patients' Hospital Experiences				
Area Around Room 'Always' Quiet at Night	300+	69%	72%	61%
Doctors 'Always' Communicated Well	300+	85%	86%	82%
Home Recovery Information Given	300+	88%	83%	85%
Hospital Given 9 or 10 on 10 Point Scale	300+	73%	71%	71%
Meds 'Always' Explained Before Given	300+	64%	67%	64%
Nurses 'Always' Communicated Well	300+	79%	81%	79%
Pain 'Always' Well Controlled	300+	74%	72%	71%
Room and Bathroom 'Always' Clean	300+	71%	74%	73%
Timely Help 'Always' Received	300+	67%	69%	68%
Would Definitely Recommend Hospital	300+	78%	69%	71%
Use of Medical Imaging				
Cardiac Imaging Stress Test before Surgery	142	7.0%	5.7%	5.3%
Combination Abdominal CT Scan	1,243	19.8%	12.9%	10.5%
Combination Brain/Sinus CT Scan	1,356	4.1%	3.3%	2.7%
Combination Chest CT Scan	953	7.2%	6.1%	2.7%
Follow-up Mammogram/Ultrasound	1,811	9.8%	8.4%	8.8%
Lumbar Spine MRI for Low Back Pain	199	42.7%	41.1%	37.2%

Anderson Rmc South

1102 Constitution Avenue
Meridian, MS 39301
Phone: 601-484-3590
Fax: 601-484-3130
URL: www.rileyhosp.com
Type: Acute Care Hospitals
Emergency Services: Yes
Ownership: Proprietary
Beds: 140

Key Personnel:

Emergency Room . . . . Razee A Ahmad
CEO . . . . John Anderson
Chief of Medical Staff . . . . Jack Andy, MD
Radiology. . . . . William D Armstrong
CEO/President. . . . . Steve Nicholas

Measure	Cases	This Hosp.	State Avg.	U.S. Avg.
Blood Clot Prevention and Treatment				
Anticoagulation Overlap Therapy[3,7]	-	-	86%	93%
ICU Venous Thromboembolism Prophylaxis[3,7]	-	-	86%	92%
Incidence of Potentially Preventable VTE[3,7]	-	-	15%	10%
UFH with Dosages/Platelet Monitoring[3,7]	-	-	94%	97%
Venous Thromboembolism Prophylaxis[1,3]	-	-	70%	85%
Warfarin Therapy Discharge Instructions[3,7]	-	-	77%	75%
Chest Pain/Possible Heart Attack Care				
Aspirin Given Within 24 Hours of Arrival[5]	-	-	94%	96%
Fibrinolytic Meds Within 30 Min. of Arrival[5]	-	-	40%	58%
Average Time to ECG (minutes)[5]	-	-	10	7
Average Time to Transfer (minutes)[5]	-	-	77	60
Children's Asthma Care				
Received Home Management Plan of Care	-	-	-	88%
Received Reliever Medication	-	-	-	100%
Received Systemic Corticosteroids	-	-	-	100%
Emergency Department				
Admittance Decision Time (minutes)[3,7]	-	-	61	98
Head CT Results Within 45 Min. of Arrival[5]	-	-	42%	57%
Patients Who Left ER Before Being Seen[5]	-	-	3%	2%
Time from ER Arrival to Admit. (minutes)[3,7]	-	-	223	274
Time from ER Arrival to Discharge (minutes)[5]	-	-	112	134
Time in ER Before Being Evaluated (minutes)[5]	-	-	29	26
Time to Pain Meds for Fractures (minutes)[5]	-	-	68	57
Heart Attack Care				
Aspirin Given at Discharge[5]	-	-	99%	99%
Fibrinolytic Meds Within 30 Min. of Arrival[5]	-	-	50%	54%
PCI Within 90 Minutes of Arrival[5]	-	-	96%	96%
Statin Prescribed at Discharge[5]	-	-	97%	98%
Heart Failure Care				
ACE Inhibitor or ARB for LVSD[5]	-	-	93%	97%
Discharge Instructions Given[5]	-	-	91%	94%
Evaluation of LVS Function[5]	-	-	96%	99%
Medicare Spending				
Medicare Spending per Patient (ratio)[1]	-	-	0.95	0.98
Pneumonia Care				
Appropriate Initial Antibiotic Given[5]	-	-	91%	95%
Blood Culture Timing[5]	-	-	97%	98%
Pregnancy and Delivery Care				
Newborn Deliveries Scheduled Early[7]	-	-	22%	6%
Preventive Care				
Immunization for Influenza[5]	-	-	87%	90%
Immunization for Pneumonia[1,3]	-	-	89%	92%
Stroke Care				
Anticoagulation Therapy for Atrial Fibrillation[5]	-	-	93%	95%
Antithrombotic Therapy Timing[5]	-	-	96%	98%
Assessed for Rehabilitation[5]	-	-	95%	97%
Discharged on Antithrombotic Therapy[5]	-	-	97%	99%
Discharged on Statin Medication[5]	-	-	88%	94%
Thrombolytic Therapy Timing[5]	-	-	25%	66%
Venous Thromboembolism Prophylaxis[5]	-	-	87%	94%
Written Stroke Educational Materials Given[5]	-	-	84%	88%
Surgical Care Improvement Project				
Appropriate Beta Blocker Usage[5]	-	-	97%	98%
Appropriate VTP Within 24 Hours[5]	-	-	97%	98%
Controlled Postoperative Blood Glucose[5]	-	-	97%	97%
Perioperative Temperature Management[5]	-	-	100%	100%
Prophylactic Antibiotic Selection[5]	-	-	99%	99%
Prophylactic Antibiotic Selection (Outpatient)[1,3]	-	-	98%	98%
Prophylactic Antibiotic Stopped[5]	-	-	97%	98%
Prophylactic Antibiotic Timing[5]	-	-	99%	99%
Prophylactic Antibiotic Timing (Outpatient)[1,3]	-	-	98%	98%
Urinary Catheter Removal[5]	-	-	97%	97%
Survey of Patients' Hospital Experiences				
Area Around Room 'Always' Quiet at Night[10]	<100	88%	72%	61%
Doctors 'Always' Communicated Well[10]	<100	73%	86%	82%
Home Recovery Information Given[10]	<100	92%	83%	85%
Hospital Given 9 or 10 on 10 Point Scale[10]	<100	60%	71%	71%
Meds 'Always' Explained Before Given[10]	<100	92%	67%	64%
Nurses 'Always' Communicated Well[10]	<100	73%	81%	79%
Pain 'Always' Well Controlled[10]	<100	73%	72%	71%
Room and Bathroom 'Always' Clean[10]	<100	74%	74%	73%
Timely Help 'Always' Received[10]	<100	36%	69%	68%
Would Definitely Recommend Hospital[10]	<100	81%	69%	71%
Use of Medical Imaging				
Cardiac Imaging Stress Test before Surgery[7]	-	-	5.7%	5.3%
Combination Abdominal CT Scan	72	22.2%	12.9%	10.5%
Combination Brain/Sinus CT Scan[1]	-	-	3.3%	2.7%
Combination Chest CT Scan[1]	-	-	6.1%	2.7%
Follow-up Mammogram/Ultrasound	161	11.8%	8.4%	8.8%
Lumbar Spine MRI for Low Back Pain[1]	-	-	41.1%	37.2%

Rush Foundation Hospital

1314 19th Ave
Meridian, MS 39301
Phone: 601-483-0011
Fax: 601-485-8079
URL: www.rushhealthsystems.org
Type: Acute Care Hospitals
Emergency Services: Yes
Ownership: Voluntary non-profit - Private
Beds: 215

Key Personnel:

Radiology. . . . . William D Armstrong
Chief of Medical Staff . . . . Scott Bell
Operating Room. . . . . Oscar J Briseno
Pediatric Ambulatory Care . . . . . . Robert Duban, DO
Infection Control. . . . . Cherry Flanigan
Quality Assurance . . . . Ken Purvis
Pediatric In-Patient Care . . . . KJ Reid, MD
CEO/President. . . . . Wallace Strickland

Measure	Cases	This Hosp.	State Avg.	U.S. Avg.
Blood Clot Prevention and Treatment				
Anticoagulation Overlap Therapy[2]	62	98%	86%	93%
ICU Venous Thromboembolism Prophylaxis[2]	124	85%	86%	92%
Incidence of Potentially Preventable VTE[2]	16	0%	15%	10%
UFH with Dosages/Platelet Monitoring[2]	12	92%	94%	97%
Venous Thromboembolism Prophylaxis[2]	332	77%	70%	85%
Warfarin Therapy Discharge Instructions[2]	43	56%	77%	75%
Chest Pain/Possible Heart Attack Care				
Aspirin Given Within 24 Hours of Arrival[1,3]	-	-	94%	96%
Fibrinolytic Meds Within 30 Min. of Arrival[5]	-	-	40%	58%
Average Time to ECG (minutes)[1,3]	-	-	10	7
Average Time to Transfer (minutes)[5]	-	-	77	60
Children's Asthma Care				
Received Home Management Plan of Care	-	-	-	88%
Received Reliever Medication	-	-	-	100%
Received Systemic Corticosteroids	-	-	-	100%
Emergency Department				
Admittance Decision Time (minutes)[2]	348	79	61	98
Head CT Results Within 45 Min. of Arrival[1]	-	-	42%	57%
Patients Who Left ER Before Being Seen	31,153	1%	3%	2%
Time from ER Arrival to Admit. (minutes)[2]	568	227	223	274
Time from ER Arrival to Discharge (minutes)	361	129	112	134
Time in ER Before Being Evaluated (minutes)	394	39	29	26
Time to Pain Meds for Fractures (minutes)	94	44	68	57
Heart Attack Care				
Aspirin Given at Discharge	171	99%	99%	99%
Fibrinolytic Meds Within 30 Min. of Arrival[7]	-	-	50%	54%
PCI Within 90 Minutes of Arrival	15	93%	96%	96%
Statin Prescribed at Discharge	171	96%	97%	98%
Heart Failure Care				
ACE Inhibitor or ARB for LVSD	97	92%	93%	97%
Discharge Instructions Given	160	91%	91%	94%
Evaluation of LVS Function	190	97%	96%	99%
Medicare Spending				
Medicare Spending per Patient (ratio)	-	1.13	0.95	0.98
Pneumonia Care				

NOTE: Hospital profiles are in alphabetical order by state, then city, then hospital within the city; Rankings exclude hospitals with less than 25 cases except for patient surveys which excludes hospitals with less than 100 cases; (a) 100-299 cases; (1) The number of cases/patients is too few to report; (2) Data submitted were based on a sample of cases/patients; (3) Results are based on a shorter time period than required; (4) Data suppressed by CMS for one or more quarters; (5) Results are not available for this reporting period; (6) Fewer than 100 patients completed the HCAHPS survey; (7) No cases met the criteria for this measure; (8) The lower limit of the confidence interval cannot be calculated if the number of observed infections equals zero; (9) No data are available from the state/territory for this reporting period; (10) The scores shown reflect fewer than 50 completed surveys; (11) There were discrepancies in the data collection process; (12) This measure does not apply to this hospital for this reporting period; (13) Results cannot be calculated for this reporting period; (14) The results for this state are combined with nearby states to protect confidentiality; Please refer to the User's Guide for a full explanation of data.

Measure	Cases	This Hosp.	State Avg.	U.S. Avg.
Appropriate Initial Antibiotic Given	69	93%	91%	95%
Blood Culture Timing	97	98%	97%	98%
Pregnancy and Delivery Care				
Newborn Deliveries Scheduled Early[2]	45	20%	22%	6%
Preventive Care				
Immunization for Influenza[2]	558	92%	87%	90%
Immunization for Pneumonia[2]	653	94%	89%	92%
Stroke Care				
Anticoagulation Therapy for Atrial Fibrillation[1,2]	-	-	93%	95%
Antithrombotic Therapy Timing[2]	106	100%	96%	98%
Assessed for Rehabilitation[2]	113	99%	95%	97%
Discharged on Antithrombotic Therapy[2]	107	99%	97%	99%
Discharged on Statin Medication[2]	82	94%	88%	94%
Thrombolytic Therapy Timing[1,2]	-	-	25%	66%
Venous Thromboembolism Prophylaxis[2]	114	82%	87%	94%
Written Stroke Educational Materials Given[2]	62	58%	84%	88%
Surgical Care Improvement Project				
Appropriate Beta Blocker Usage[2]	165	97%	97%	98%
Appropriate VTP Within 24 Hours[2]	389	97%	97%	98%
Controlled Postoperative Blood Glucose[2]	60	98%	97%	97%
Perioperative Temperature Management[2]	500	100%	100%	100%
Prophylactic Antibiotic Selection[2]	340	99%	99%	99%
Prophylactic Antibiotic Selection (Outpatient)	471	95%	98%	98%
Prophylactic Antibiotic Stopped[2]	321	93%	97%	98%
Prophylactic Antibiotic Timing[2]	341	100%	99%	99%
Prophylactic Antibiotic Timing (Outpatient)	471	99%	98%	98%
Urinary Catheter Removal[2]	390	95%	97%	97%
Survey of Patients' Hospital Experiences				
Area Around Room 'Always' Quiet at Night	300+	74%	72%	61%
Doctors 'Always' Communicated Well	300+	83%	86%	82%
Home Recovery Information Given	300+	88%	83%	85%
Hospital Given 9 or 10 on 10 Point Scale	300+	66%	71%	71%
Meds 'Always' Explained Before Given	300+	65%	67%	64%
Nurses 'Always' Communicated Well	300+	78%	81%	79%
Pain 'Always' Well Controlled	300+	69%	72%	71%
Room and Bathroom 'Always' Clean	300+	70%	74%	73%
Timely Help 'Always' Received	300+	64%	69%	68%
Would Definitely Recommend Hospital	300+	72%	69%	71%
Use of Medical Imaging				
Cardiac Imaging Stress Test before Surgery	600	7.2%	5.7%	5.3%
Combination Abdominal CT Scan	641	11.4%	12.9%	10.5%
Combination Brain/Sinus CT Scan	748	3.3%	3.3%	2.7%
Combination Chest CT Scan	497	2.0%	6.1%	2.7%
Follow-up Mammogram/Ultrasound	2,627	11.2%	8.4%	8.8%
Lumbar Spine MRI for Low Back Pain[1]	-	-	41.1%	37.2%

Lawrence County Hospital

1065 East Broad St — Phone: 601-587-4051
Monticello, MS 39654 — Fax: 601-587-0306
URL: www.smrmc.com/index.php
Type: Critical Access Hospitals — Emergency Services: Yes
Ownership: Government - Local — Beds: 25

Measure	Cases	This Hosp.	State Avg.	U.S. Avg.
Blood Clot Prevention and Treatment				
Anticoagulation Overlap Therapy[5]	-	-	86%	93%
ICU Venous Thromboembolism Prophylaxis[5]	-	-	86%	92%
Incidence of Potentially Preventable VTE[5]	-	-	15%	10%
UFH with Dosages/Platelet Monitoring[5]	-	-	94%	97%
Venous Thromboembolism Prophylaxis[5]	-	-	70%	85%
Warfarin Therapy Discharge Instructions[5]	-	-	77%	75%
Chest Pain/Possible Heart Attack Care				
Aspirin Given Within 24 Hours of Arrival	-	-	94%	96%
Fibrinolytic Meds Within 30 Min. of Arrival	-	-	40%	58%
Average Time to ECG (minutes)	-	-	10	7
Average Time to Transfer (minutes)	-	-	77	60
Children's Asthma Care				
Received Home Management Plan of Care	-	-	-	88%
Received Reliever Medication	-	-	-	100%
Received Systemic Corticosteroids	-	-	-	100%
Emergency Department				
Admittance Decision Time (minutes)[5]	-	-	61	98
Head CT Results Within 45 Min. of Arrival	-	-	42%	57%
Patients Who Left ER Before Being Seen	-	-	3%	2%
Time from ER Arrival to Admit. (minutes)[5]	-	-	223	274
Time from ER Arrival to Discharge (minutes)	-	-	112	134
Time in ER Before Being Evaluated (minutes)	-	-	29	26
Time to Pain Meds for Fractures (minutes)	-	-	68	57
Heart Attack Care				
Aspirin Given at Discharge[1,3]	-	-	99%	99%
Fibrinolytic Meds Within 30 Min. of Arrival[3,7]	-	-	50%	54%
PCI Within 90 Minutes of Arrival[3,7]	-	-	96%	96%
Statin Prescribed at Discharge[1,3]	-	-	97%	98%
Heart Failure Care				
ACE Inhibitor or ARB for LVSD[1,3]	-	-	93%	97%
Discharge Instructions Given[1,3]	-	-	91%	94%
Evaluation of LVS Function[1,3]	-	-	96%	99%
Medicare Spending				
Medicare Spending per Patient (ratio)	-	-	0.95	0.98
Pneumonia Care				
Appropriate Initial Antibiotic Given	16	62%	91%	95%
Blood Culture Timing	17	82%	97%	98%
Pregnancy and Delivery Care				
Newborn Deliveries Scheduled Early[5]	-	-	22%	6%
Preventive Care				
Immunization for Influenza[5]	-	-	87%	90%
Immunization for Pneumonia[5]	-	-	89%	92%
Stroke Care				
Anticoagulation Therapy for Atrial Fibrillation[5]	-	-	93%	95%
Antithrombotic Therapy Timing[5]	-	-	96%	98%
Assessed for Rehabilitation[5]	-	-	95%	97%
Discharged on Antithrombotic Therapy[5]	-	-	97%	99%
Discharged on Statin Medication[5]	-	-	88%	94%
Thrombolytic Therapy Timing[5]	-	-	25%	66%
Venous Thromboembolism Prophylaxis[5]	-	-	87%	94%
Written Stroke Educational Materials Given[5]	-	-	84%	88%
Surgical Care Improvement Project				
Appropriate Beta Blocker Usage[5]	-	-	97%	98%
Appropriate VTP Within 24 Hours[5]	-	-	97%	98%
Controlled Postoperative Blood Glucose[5]	-	-	97%	97%
Perioperative Temperature Management[5]	-	-	100%	100%
Prophylactic Antibiotic Selection[5]	-	-	99%	99%
Prophylactic Antibiotic Selection (Outpatient)	-	-	98%	98%
Prophylactic Antibiotic Stopped[5]	-	-	97%	98%
Prophylactic Antibiotic Timing[5]	-	-	99%	99%
Prophylactic Antibiotic Timing (Outpatient)	-	-	98%	98%
Urinary Catheter Removal[5]	-	-	97%	97%
Survey of Patients' Hospital Experiences				
Area Around Room 'Always' Quiet at Night	(a)	78%	72%	61%
Doctors 'Always' Communicated Well	(a)	96%	86%	82%
Home Recovery Information Given	(a)	83%	83%	85%
Hospital Given 9 or 10 on 10 Point Scale	(a)	79%	71%	71%
Meds 'Always' Explained Before Given	(a)	80%	67%	64%
Nurses 'Always' Communicated Well	(a)	87%	81%	79%
Pain 'Always' Well Controlled	(a)	86%	72%	71%
Room and Bathroom 'Always' Clean	(a)	80%	74%	73%
Timely Help 'Always' Received	(a)	81%	69%	68%
Would Definitely Recommend Hospital	(a)	72%	69%	71%
Use of Medical Imaging				
Cardiac Imaging Stress Test before Surgery	-	-	5.7%	5.3%
Combination Abdominal CT Scan	-	-	12.9%	10.5%
Combination Brain/Sinus CT Scan	-	-	3.3%	2.7%
Combination Chest CT Scan	-	-	6.1%	2.7%
Follow-up Mammogram/Ultrasound	-	-	8.4%	8.8%
Lumbar Spine MRI for Low Back Pain	-	-	41.1%	37.2%

Scott Regional Hospital

317 Highway 13 South — Phone: 601-732-6301
Morton, MS 39117 — Fax: 601-732-8970
Type: Critical Access Hospitals — Emergency Services: Yes
Ownership: Voluntary non-profit - Private — Beds: 30
Key Personnel:
CEO/President . . . . Paul Black
Chief of Medical Staff . . . . Michael Edwards

Measure	Cases	This Hosp.	State Avg.	U.S. Avg.
Blood Clot Prevention and Treatment				
Anticoagulation Overlap Therapy[5]	-	-	86%	93%
ICU Venous Thromboembolism Prophylaxis[5]	-	-	86%	92%
Incidence of Potentially Preventable VTE[5]	-	-	15%	10%
UFH with Dosages/Platelet Monitoring[5]	-	-	94%	97%
Venous Thromboembolism Prophylaxis[5]	-	-	70%	85%
Warfarin Therapy Discharge Instructions[5]	-	-	77%	75%
Chest Pain/Possible Heart Attack Care				
Aspirin Given Within 24 Hours of Arrival	14	93%	94%	96%
Fibrinolytic Meds Within 30 Min. of Arrival[3,7]	-	-	40%	58%
Average Time to ECG (minutes)	14	10	10	7
Average Time to Transfer (minutes)[1,3]	-	-	77	60
Children's Asthma Care				
Received Home Management Plan of Care	-	-	-	88%
Received Reliever Medication	-	-	-	100%
Received Systemic Corticosteroids	-	-	-	100%
Emergency Department				
Admittance Decision Time (minutes)[5]	-	-	61	98
Head CT Results Within 45 Min. of Arrival[1,3]	-	-	42%	57%
Patients Who Left ER Before Being Seen	5,764	1%	3%	2%
Time from ER Arrival to Admit. (minutes)[5]	-	-	223	274
Time from ER Arrival to Discharge (minutes)[5]	-	-	112	134
Time in ER Before Being Evaluated (minutes)[5]	-	-	29	26
Time to Pain Meds for Fractures (minutes)	21	47	68	57
Heart Attack Care				
Aspirin Given at Discharge[5]	-	-	99%	99%
Fibrinolytic Meds Within 30 Min. of Arrival[5]	-	-	50%	54%
PCI Within 90 Minutes of Arrival[5]	-	-	96%	96%
Statin Prescribed at Discharge[5]	-	-	97%	98%
Heart Failure Care				
ACE Inhibitor or ARB for LVSD[1]	-	-	93%	97%
Discharge Instructions Given	17	88%	91%	94%
Evaluation of LVS Function	25	92%	96%	99%
Medicare Spending				
Medicare Spending per Patient (ratio)	-	-	0.95	0.98
Pneumonia Care				
Appropriate Initial Antibiotic Given	43	95%	91%	95%
Blood Culture Timing	26	92%	97%	98%
Pregnancy and Delivery Care				
Newborn Deliveries Scheduled Early[5]	-	-	22%	6%
Preventive Care				
Immunization for Influenza[5]	-	-	87%	90%
Immunization for Pneumonia[5]	-	-	89%	92%
Stroke Care				
Anticoagulation Therapy for Atrial Fibrillation[5]	-	-	93%	95%
Antithrombotic Therapy Timing[5]	-	-	96%	98%
Assessed for Rehabilitation[5]	-	-	95%	97%
Discharged on Antithrombotic Therapy[5]	-	-	97%	99%
Discharged on Statin Medication[5]	-	-	88%	94%
Thrombolytic Therapy Timing[5]	-	-	25%	66%
Venous Thromboembolism Prophylaxis[5]	-	-	87%	94%
Written Stroke Educational Materials Given[5]	-	-	84%	88%
Surgical Care Improvement Project				
Appropriate Beta Blocker Usage[5]	-	-	97%	98%
Appropriate VTP Within 24 Hours[5]	-	-	97%	98%
Controlled Postoperative Blood Glucose[5]	-	-	97%	97%
Perioperative Temperature Management[5]	-	-	100%	100%
Prophylactic Antibiotic Selection[5]	-	-	99%	99%
Prophylactic Antibiotic Selection (Outpatient)[5]	-	-	98%	98%
Prophylactic Antibiotic Stopped[5]	-	-	97%	98%
Prophylactic Antibiotic Timing[5]	-	-	99%	99%
Prophylactic Antibiotic Timing (Outpatient)[5]	-	-	98%	98%
Urinary Catheter Removal[5]	-	-	97%	97%
Survey of Patients' Hospital Experiences				
Area Around Room 'Always' Quiet at Night[6]	<100	71%	72%	61%
Doctors 'Always' Communicated Well[6]	<100	89%	86%	82%
Home Recovery Information Given[6]	<100	74%	83%	85%
Hospital Given 9 or 10 on 10 Point Scale[6]	<100	73%	71%	71%
Meds 'Always' Explained Before Given[6]	<100	80%	67%	64%
Nurses 'Always' Communicated Well[6]	<100	77%	81%	79%
Pain 'Always' Well Controlled[6]	<100	64%	72%	71%
Room and Bathroom 'Always' Clean[6]	<100	77%	74%	73%
Timely Help 'Always' Received[6]	<100	70%	69%	68%

NOTE: Hospital profiles are in alphabetical order by state, then city, then hospital within the city; Rankings exclude hospitals with less than 25 cases except for patient surveys which excludes hospitals with less than 100 cases; (a) 100-299 cases; (1) The number of cases/patients is too few to report; (2) Data submitted were based on a sample of cases/patients; (3) Results are based on a shorter time period than required; (4) Data suppressed by CMS for one or more quarters; (5) Results are not available for this reporting period; (6) Fewer than 100 patients completed the HCAHPS survey; (7) No cases met the criteria for this measure; (8) The lower limit of the confidence interval cannot be calculated if the number of observed infections equals zero; (9) No data are available from the state/territory for this reporting period; (10) The scores shown reflect fewer than 50 completed surveys; (11) There were discrepancies in the data collection process; (12) This measure does not apply to this hospital for this reporting period; (13) Results cannot be calculated for this reporting period; (14) The results for this state are combined with nearby states to protect confidentiality; Please refer to the User's Guide for a full explanation of data.

Would Definitely Recommend Hospital[6]	<100	75%	69%	71%
Use of Medical Imaging				
Cardiac Imaging Stress Test before Surgery[1]	-	-	5.7%	5.3%
Combination Abdominal CT Scan	69	21.7%	12.9%	10.5%
Combination Brain/Sinus CT Scan[1]	-	-	3.3%	2.7%
Combination Chest CT Scan[1]	-	-	6.1%	2.7%
Follow-up Mammogram/Ultrasound[7]	-	-	8.4%	8.8%
Lumbar Spine MRI for Low Back Pain[1]	-	-	41.1%	37.2%

Natchez Community Hospital

129 Jefferson Davis Blvd Box 1203 Phone: 601-445-6205
Natchez, MS 39120 Fax: 601-445-6233
URL: www.natchezcommunityhospital.com
Type: Acute Care Hospitals Emergency Services: Yes
Ownership: Proprietary Beds: 101
Key Personnel:
Emergency Room . . . . Tracy Laird
CEO . . . . Eric Robinson
Chief of Medical Staff . . . . Jennifer Russ

Measure	Cases	This Hosp.	State Avg.	U.S. Avg.
Blood Clot Prevention and Treatment				
Anticoagulation Overlap Therapy[2]	13	54%	86%	93%
ICU Venous Thromboembolism Prophylaxis[2]	36	72%	86%	92%
Incidence of Potentially Preventable VTE[1,2]	-	-	15%	10%
UFH with Dosages/Platelet Monitoring[2,7]	-	-	94%	97%
Venous Thromboembolism Prophylaxis[2]	292	71%	70%	85%
Warfarin Therapy Discharge Instructions[2]	12	92%	77%	75%
Chest Pain/Possible Heart Attack Care				
Aspirin Given Within 24 Hours of Arrival	20	90%	94%	96%
Fibrinolytic Meds Within 30 Min. of Arrival[1]	-	-	40%	58%
Average Time to ECG (minutes)	21	6	10	7
Average Time to Transfer (minutes)[7]	-	-	77	60
Children's Asthma Care				
Received Home Management Plan of Care	-	-	-	88%
Received Reliever Medication	-	-	-	100%
Received Systemic Corticosteroids	-	-	-	100%
Emergency Department				
Admittance Decision Time (minutes)[2]	467	47	61	98
Head CT Results Within 45 Min. of Arrival[1]	-	-	42%	57%
Patients Who Left ER Before Being Seen	16,551	2%	3%	2%
Time from ER Arrival to Admit. (minutes)[2]	467	203	223	274
Time from ER Arrival to Discharge (minutes)	489	112	112	134
Time in ER Before Being Evaluated (minutes)	517	20	29	26
Time to Pain Meds for Fractures (minutes)	41	64	68	57
Heart Attack Care				
Aspirin Given at Discharge	20	95%	99%	99%
Fibrinolytic Meds Within 30 Min. of Arrival[1]	-	-	50%	54%
PCI Within 90 Minutes of Arrival[7]	-	-	96%	96%
Statin Prescribed at Discharge	17	88%	97%	98%
Heart Failure Care				
ACE Inhibitor or ARB for LVSD	45	93%	93%	97%
Discharge Instructions Given	99	86%	91%	94%
Evaluation of LVS Function	116	99%	96%	99%
Medicare Spending				
Medicare Spending per Patient (ratio)	-	1.09	0.95	0.98
Pneumonia Care				
Appropriate Initial Antibiotic Given	67	94%	91%	95%
Blood Culture Timing	99	100%	97%	98%
Pregnancy and Delivery Care				
Newborn Deliveries Scheduled Early	47	19%	22%	6%
Preventive Care				
Immunization for Influenza[2]	357	99%	87%	90%
Immunization for Pneumonia[2]	383	98%	89%	92%
Stroke Care				
Anticoagulation Therapy for Atrial Fibrillation[1]	-	-	93%	95%
Antithrombotic Therapy Timing	24	67%	96%	98%
Assessed for Rehabilitation	29	86%	95%	97%
Discharged on Antithrombotic Therapy	28	96%	97%	99%
Discharged on Statin Medication	21	86%	88%	94%
Thrombolytic Therapy Timing[1]	-	-	25%	66%
Venous Thromboembolism Prophylaxis	26	77%	87%	94%
Written Stroke Educational Materials Given	19	74%	84%	88%
Surgical Care Improvement Project				
Appropriate Beta Blocker Usage	23	65%	97%	98%
Appropriate VTP Within 24 Hours	79	99%	97%	98%
Controlled Postoperative Blood Glucose[7]	-	-	97%	97%
Perioperative Temperature Management	89	100%	100%	100%
Prophylactic Antibiotic Selection	55	96%	99%	99%
Prophylactic Antibiotic Selection (Outpatient)	130	99%	98%	98%
Prophylactic Antibiotic Stopped	54	91%	97%	98%
Prophylactic Antibiotic Timing	55	100%	99%	99%
Prophylactic Antibiotic Timing (Outpatient)	131	99%	98%	98%
Urinary Catheter Removal	63	95%	97%	97%
Survey of Patients' Hospital Experiences				
Area Around Room 'Always' Quiet at Night	300+	60%	72%	61%
Doctors 'Always' Communicated Well	300+	81%	86%	82%
Home Recovery Information Given	300+	79%	83%	85%
Hospital Given 9 or 10 on 10 Point Scale	300+	61%	71%	71%
Meds 'Always' Explained Before Given	300+	61%	67%	64%
Nurses 'Always' Communicated Well	300+	78%	81%	79%
Pain 'Always' Well Controlled	300+	68%	72%	71%
Room and Bathroom 'Always' Clean	300+	68%	74%	73%
Timely Help 'Always' Received	300+	57%	69%	68%
Would Definitely Recommend Hospital	300+	69%	69%	71%
Use of Medical Imaging				
Cardiac Imaging Stress Test before Surgery[1]	-	-	5.7%	5.3%
Combination Abdominal CT Scan	382	6.3%	12.9%	10.5%
Combination Brain/Sinus CT Scan[1]	-	-	3.3%	2.7%
Combination Chest CT Scan	117	6.0%	6.1%	2.7%
Follow-up Mammogram/Ultrasound[7]	-	-	8.4%	8.8%
Lumbar Spine MRI for Low Back Pain[7]	-	-	41.1%	37.2%

Natchez Regional Medical Center

52 Seargent Prentiss Drive Phone: 601-443-2100
Natchez, MS 39120 Fax: 601-443-2891
Type: Acute Care Hospitals Emergency Services: Yes
Ownership: Government - Local Beds: 205
Key Personnel:
Radiology. . . . . Raymond Brown
Operating Room. . . . . Geoffrey Flattman
Cardiac Laboratory. . . . . Lisa Moise
Infection Control. . . . . Lana Morgan
Intensive Care Unit. . . . . Catherine Ratcliffe
CEO . . . . Donny Rentfro
Quality Assurance . . . . Terry Stutzman
Emergency Room . . . . Rosie Williams

Measure	Cases	This Hosp.	State Avg.	U.S. Avg.
Blood Clot Prevention and Treatment				
Anticoagulation Overlap Therapy[1,2]	-	-	86%	93%
ICU Venous Thromboembolism Prophylaxis[2]	25	52%	86%	92%
Incidence of Potentially Preventable VTE[1,2]	-	-	15%	10%
UFH with Dosages/Platelet Monitoring[1,2]	-	-	94%	97%
Venous Thromboembolism Prophylaxis[2]	195	49%	70%	85%
Warfarin Therapy Discharge Instructions[1,2]	-	-	77%	75%
Chest Pain/Possible Heart Attack Care				
Aspirin Given Within 24 Hours of Arrival	66	100%	94%	96%
Fibrinolytic Meds Within 30 Min. of Arrival	12	75%	40%	58%
Average Time to ECG (minutes)	72	4	10	7
Average Time to Transfer (minutes)[1]	-	-	77	60
Children's Asthma Care				
Received Home Management Plan of Care	-	-	-	88%
Received Reliever Medication	-	-	-	100%
Received Systemic Corticosteroids	-	-	-	100%
Emergency Department				
Admittance Decision Time (minutes)[2]	235	115	61	98
Head CT Results Within 45 Min. of Arrival[1]	-	-	42%	57%
Patients Who Left ER Before Being Seen	13,676	3%	3%	2%
Time from ER Arrival to Admit. (minutes)[2]	244	300	223	274
Time from ER Arrival to Discharge (minutes)	392	157	112	134
Time in ER Before Being Evaluated (minutes)	418	20	29	26
Time to Pain Meds for Fractures (minutes)	41	92	68	57
Heart Attack Care				
Aspirin Given at Discharge	14	100%	99%	99%
Fibrinolytic Meds Within 30 Min. of Arrival[7]	-	-	50%	54%
PCI Within 90 Minutes of Arrival[7]	-	-	96%	96%
Statin Prescribed at Discharge	16	75%	97%	98%
Heart Failure Care				
ACE Inhibitor or ARB for LVSD	41	76%	93%	97%
Discharge Instructions Given	92	92%	91%	94%
Evaluation of LVS Function	112	98%	96%	99%
Medicare Spending				
Medicare Spending per Patient (ratio)	-	1.07	0.95	0.98
Pneumonia Care				
Appropriate Initial Antibiotic Given	55	95%	91%	95%
Blood Culture Timing	63	97%	97%	98%
Pregnancy and Delivery Care				
Newborn Deliveries Scheduled Early	35	20%	22%	6%
Preventive Care				
Immunization for Influenza[2]	256	91%	87%	90%
Immunization for Pneumonia[2]	279	94%	89%	92%
Stroke Care				
Anticoagulation Therapy for Atrial Fibrillation[1]	-	-	93%	95%
Antithrombotic Therapy Timing	26	96%	96%	98%
Assessed for Rehabilitation	27	89%	95%	97%
Discharged on Antithrombotic Therapy	27	100%	97%	99%
Discharged on Statin Medication	23	65%	88%	94%
Thrombolytic Therapy Timing[1]	-	-	25%	66%
Venous Thromboembolism Prophylaxis	27	63%	87%	94%
Written Stroke Educational Materials Given	23	65%	84%	88%
Surgical Care Improvement Project				
Appropriate Beta Blocker Usage	26	81%	97%	98%
Appropriate VTP Within 24 Hours	93	94%	97%	98%
Controlled Postoperative Blood Glucose[7]	-	-	97%	97%
Perioperative Temperature Management	120	100%	100%	100%
Prophylactic Antibiotic Selection	85	94%	99%	99%
Prophylactic Antibiotic Selection (Outpatient)	14	86%	98%	98%
Prophylactic Antibiotic Stopped	82	90%	97%	98%
Prophylactic Antibiotic Timing	85	95%	99%	99%
Prophylactic Antibiotic Timing (Outpatient)	16	81%	98%	98%
Urinary Catheter Removal	30	63%	97%	97%
Survey of Patients' Hospital Experiences				
Area Around Room 'Always' Quiet at Night[11]	300+	66%	72%	61%
Doctors 'Always' Communicated Well[11]	300+	84%	86%	82%
Home Recovery Information Given[11]	300+	79%	83%	85%
Hospital Given 9 or 10 on 10 Point Scale[11]	300+	56%	71%	71%
Meds 'Always' Explained Before Given[11]	300+	61%	67%	64%
Nurses 'Always' Communicated Well[11]	300+	73%	81%	79%
Pain 'Always' Well Controlled[11]	300+	68%	72%	71%
Room and Bathroom 'Always' Clean[11]	300+	67%	74%	73%
Timely Help 'Always' Received[11]	300+	55%	69%	68%
Would Definitely Recommend Hospital[11]	300+	60%	69%	71%
Use of Medical Imaging				
Cardiac Imaging Stress Test before Surgery	233	6.4%	5.7%	5.3%
Combination Abdominal CT Scan	392	31.4%	12.9%	10.5%
Combination Brain/Sinus CT Scan	456	7.7%	3.3%	2.7%
Combination Chest CT Scan	306	44.8%	6.1%	2.7%
Follow-up Mammogram/Ultrasound	797	8.9%	8.4%	8.8%
Lumbar Spine MRI for Low Back Pain[1]	-	-	41.1%	37.2%

Baptist Memorial Hospital Union County

200 Hwy 30 West Phone: 662-538-7631
New Albany, MS 38652 Fax: 662-538-2572
URL: www.baptistonline.org
Type: Acute Care Hospitals Emergency Services: Yes
Ownership: Voluntary non-profit - Other Beds: 153
Key Personnel:
Emergency Room . . . . Muhammad Abushaer
Radiology. . . . . James D Acker
Infection Control. . . . . Doris Box
Quality Assurance . . . . Paul Cade
Intensive Care Unit. . . . . Barbara Freeman
CEO/President. . . . . Jason Little
Anesthesiology. . . . . Clint Taylor
Ambulatory Care . . . . Philip Whiteside

Measure	Cases	This Hosp.	State Avg.	U.S. Avg.
Blood Clot Prevention and Treatment				
Anticoagulation Overlap Therapy[2]	20	100%	86%	93%
ICU Venous Thromboembolism Prophylaxis[2]	36	100%	86%	92%
Incidence of Potentially Preventable VTE[1,2]	-	-	15%	10%
UFH with Dosages/Platelet Monitoring[1,2]	-	-	94%	97%
Venous Thromboembolism Prophylaxis[2]	239	99%	70%	85%

NOTE: Hospital profiles are in alphabetical order by state, then city, then hospital within the city; Rankings exclude hospitals with less than 25 cases except for patient surveys which excludes hospitals with less than 100 cases; (a) 100-299 cases; (1) The number of cases/patients is too few to report; (2) Data submitted were based on a sample of cases/patients; (3) Results are based on a shorter time period than required; (4) Data suppressed by CMS for one or more quarters; (5) Results are not available for this reporting period; (6) Fewer than 100 patients completed the HCAHPS survey; (7) No cases met the criteria for this measure; (8) The lower limit of the confidence interval cannot be calculated if the number of observed infections equals zero; (9) No data are available from the state/territory for this reporting period; (10) The scores shown reflect fewer than 50 completed surveys; (11) There were discrepancies in the data collection process; (12) This measure does not apply to this hospital for this reporting period; (13) Results cannot be calculated for this reporting period; (14) The results for this state are combined with nearby states to protect confidentiality; Please refer to the User's Guide for a full explanation of data.

Measure	Cases	This Hosp.	State Avg.	U.S. Avg.
Warfarin Therapy Discharge Instructions[2]	11	91%	77%	75%
Chest Pain/Possible Heart Attack Care				
Aspirin Given Within 24 Hours of Arrival	74	100%	94%	96%
Fibrinolytic Meds Within 30 Min. of Arrival[1]	-	-	40%	58%
Average Time to ECG (minutes)	72	4	10	7
Average Time to Transfer (minutes)[7]	-	-	77	60
Children's Asthma Care				
Received Home Management Plan of Care	-	-	-	88%
Received Reliever Medication	-	-	-	100%
Received Systemic Corticosteroids	-	-	-	100%
Emergency Department				
Admittance Decision Time (minutes)[2]	297	30	61	98
Head CT Results Within 45 Min. of Arrival	12	50%	42%	57%
Patients Who Left ER Before Being Seen	23,912	2%	3%	2%
Time from ER Arrival to Admit. (minutes)[2]	297	174	223	274
Time from ER Arrival to Discharge (minutes)	382	110	112	134
Time in ER Before Being Evaluated (minutes)	407	29	29	26
Time to Pain Meds for Fractures (minutes)	100	68	68	57
Heart Attack Care				
Aspirin Given at Discharge[1]	-	-	99%	99%
Fibrinolytic Meds Within 30 Min. of Arrival[7]	-	-	50%	54%
PCI Within 90 Minutes of Arrival[7]	-	-	96%	96%
Statin Prescribed at Discharge[1]	-	-	97%	98%
Heart Failure Care				
ACE Inhibitor or ARB for LVSD	32	100%	93%	97%
Discharge Instructions Given	73	100%	91%	94%
Evaluation of LVS Function	102	100%	96%	99%
Medicare Spending				
Medicare Spending per Patient (ratio)	-	0.93	0.95	0.98
Pneumonia Care				
Appropriate Initial Antibiotic Given	82	99%	91%	95%
Blood Culture Timing	102	99%	97%	98%
Pregnancy and Delivery Care				
Newborn Deliveries Scheduled Early[2]	31	0%	22%	6%
Preventive Care				
Immunization for Influenza[2]	382	99%	87%	90%
Immunization for Pneumonia[2]	311	99%	89%	92%
Stroke Care				
Anticoagulation Therapy for Atrial Fibrillation[1]	-	-	93%	95%
Antithrombotic Therapy Timing	28	100%	96%	98%
Assessed for Rehabilitation	34	100%	95%	97%
Discharged on Antithrombotic Therapy	29	100%	97%	99%
Discharged on Statin Medication	23	100%	88%	94%
Thrombolytic Therapy Timing[7]	-	-	25%	66%
Venous Thromboembolism Prophylaxis	32	97%	87%	94%
Written Stroke Educational Materials Given	18	100%	84%	88%
Surgical Care Improvement Project				
Appropriate Beta Blocker Usage	33	100%	97%	98%
Appropriate VTP Within 24 Hours	162	100%	97%	98%
Controlled Postoperative Blood Glucose[7]	-	-	97%	97%
Perioperative Temperature Management	182	100%	100%	100%
Prophylactic Antibiotic Selection	136	99%	99%	99%
Prophylactic Antibiotic Selection (Outpatient)	94	100%	98%	98%
Prophylactic Antibiotic Stopped	133	99%	97%	98%
Prophylactic Antibiotic Timing	136	100%	99%	99%
Prophylactic Antibiotic Timing (Outpatient)	94	100%	98%	98%
Urinary Catheter Removal	108	100%	97%	97%
Survey of Patients' Hospital Experiences				
Area Around Room 'Always' Quiet at Night	300+	75%	72%	61%
Doctors 'Always' Communicated Well	300+	88%	86%	82%
Home Recovery Information Given	300+	86%	83%	85%
Hospital Given 9 or 10 on 10 Point Scale	300+	78%	71%	71%
Meds 'Always' Explained Before Given	300+	71%	67%	64%
Nurses 'Always' Communicated Well	300+	86%	81%	79%
Pain 'Always' Well Controlled	300+	72%	72%	71%
Room and Bathroom 'Always' Clean	300+	74%	74%	73%
Timely Help 'Always' Received	300+	73%	69%	68%
Would Definitely Recommend Hospital	300+	77%	69%	71%
Use of Medical Imaging				
Cardiac Imaging Stress Test before Surgery	113	8.0%	5.7%	5.3%
Combination Abdominal CT Scan	681	5.0%	12.9%	10.5%
Combination Brain/Sinus CT Scan	554	2.0%	3.3%	2.7%
Combination Chest CT Scan	213	0.0%	6.1%	2.7%
Follow-up Mammogram/Ultrasound	869	5.3%	8.4%	8.8%
Lumbar Spine MRI for Low Back Pain	180	45.6%	41.1%	37.2%

Pioneer Health Services of Newton

9421 East Side Drive Extension, Pob 299 Phone: 601-683-2031
Newton, MS 39345
Type: Critical Access Hospitals Emergency Services: Yes
Ownership: Proprietary

Measure	Cases	This Hosp.	State Avg.	U.S. Avg.
Blood Clot Prevention and Treatment				
Anticoagulation Overlap Therapy[5]	-	-	86%	93%
ICU Venous Thromboembolism Prophylaxis[5]	-	-	86%	92%
Incidence of Potentially Preventable VTE[5]	-	-	15%	10%
UFH with Dosages/Platelet Monitoring[5]	-	-	94%	97%
Venous Thromboembolism Prophylaxis[5]	-	-	70%	85%
Warfarin Therapy Discharge Instructions[5]	-	-	77%	75%
Chest Pain/Possible Heart Attack Care				
Aspirin Given Within 24 Hours of Arrival[1]	-	-	94%	96%
Fibrinolytic Meds Within 30 Min. of Arrival[7]	-	-	40%	58%
Average Time to ECG (minutes)[1]	-	-	10	7
Average Time to Transfer (minutes)[7]	-	-	77	60
Children's Asthma Care				
Received Home Management Plan of Care	-	-	-	88%
Received Reliever Medication	-	-	-	100%
Received Systemic Corticosteroids	-	-	-	100%
Emergency Department				
Admittance Decision Time (minutes)[5]	-	-	61	98
Head CT Results Within 45 Min. of Arrival[1]	-	-	42%	57%
Patients Who Left ER Before Being Seen[5]	-	-	3%	2%
Time from ER Arrival to Admit. (minutes)[5]	-	-	223	274
Time from ER Arrival to Discharge (minutes)	1,087	97	112	134
Time in ER Before Being Evaluated (minutes)	1,119	15	29	26
Time to Pain Meds for Fractures (minutes)	19	65	68	57
Heart Attack Care				
Aspirin Given at Discharge[2,3]	-	-	99%	99%
Fibrinolytic Meds Within 30 Min. of Arrival[2,3]	-	-	50%	54%
PCI Within 90 Minutes of Arrival[2,3]	-	-	96%	96%
Statin Prescribed at Discharge[2,3]	-	-	97%	98%
Heart Failure Care				
ACE Inhibitor or ARB for LVSD[1,2]	-	-	93%	97%
Discharge Instructions Given[2,3]	20	50%	91%	94%
Evaluation of LVS Function[2,3]	26	42%	96%	99%
Medicare Spending				
Medicare Spending per Patient (ratio)	-	-	0.95	0.98
Pneumonia Care				
Appropriate Initial Antibiotic Given[2,3]	26	65%	91%	95%
Blood Culture Timing[2,3]	22	77%	97%	98%
Pregnancy and Delivery Care				
Newborn Deliveries Scheduled Early[5]	-	-	22%	6%
Preventive Care				
Immunization for Influenza[5]	-	-	87%	90%
Immunization for Pneumonia[5]	-	-	89%	92%
Stroke Care				
Anticoagulation Therapy for Atrial Fibrillation[2,3]	-	-	93%	95%
Antithrombotic Therapy Timing[2,3]	-	-	96%	98%
Assessed for Rehabilitation[2,3]	-	-	95%	97%
Discharged on Antithrombotic Therapy[2,3]	-	-	97%	99%
Discharged on Statin Medication[2,3]	-	-	88%	94%
Thrombolytic Therapy Timing[2,3]	-	-	25%	66%
Venous Thromboembolism Prophylaxis[1,2]	-	-	87%	94%
Written Stroke Educational Materials Given[2,3]	-	-	84%	88%
Surgical Care Improvement Project				
Appropriate Beta Blocker Usage[1,3]	-	-	97%	98%
Appropriate VTP Within 24 Hours[1,3]	-	-	97%	98%
Controlled Postoperative Blood Glucose[3,7]	-	-	97%	97%
Perioperative Temperature Management[1,3]	-	-	100%	100%
Prophylactic Antibiotic Selection[3,7]	-	-	99%	99%
Prophylactic Antibiotic Selection (Outpatient)[5]	-	-	98%	98%
Prophylactic Antibiotic Stopped[3,7]	-	-	97%	98%
Prophylactic Antibiotic Timing[3,7]	-	-	99%	99%
Prophylactic Antibiotic Timing (Outpatient)[5]	-	-	98%	98%
Urinary Catheter Removal[1,3]	-	-	97%	97%
Survey of Patients' Hospital Experiences				
Area Around Room 'Always' Quiet at Night[5]	-	-	72%	61%
Doctors 'Always' Communicated Well[5]	-	-	86%	82%
Home Recovery Information Given[5]	-	-	83%	85%
Hospital Given 9 or 10 on 10 Point Scale[5]	-	-	71%	71%
Meds 'Always' Explained Before Given[5]	-	-	67%	64%
Nurses 'Always' Communicated Well[5]	-	-	81%	79%
Pain 'Always' Well Controlled[5]	-	-	72%	71%
Room and Bathroom 'Always' Clean[5]	-	-	74%	73%
Timely Help 'Always' Received[5]	-	-	69%	68%
Would Definitely Recommend Hospital[5]	-	-	69%	71%
Use of Medical Imaging				
Cardiac Imaging Stress Test before Surgery[7]	-	-	5.7%	5.3%
Combination Abdominal CT Scan	68	1.5%	12.9%	10.5%
Combination Brain/Sinus CT Scan[1]	-	-	3.3%	2.7%
Combination Chest CT Scan[1]	-	-	6.1%	2.7%
Follow-up Mammogram/Ultrasound[7]	-	-	8.4%	8.8%
Lumbar Spine MRI for Low Back Pain[1]	-	-	41.1%	37.2%

Methodist Healthcare - Olive Branch Hospital

4250 Bethel Road Phone: 662-932-9000
Olive Branch, MS 38654
Type: Acute Care Hospitals Emergency Services: Yes
Ownership: Voluntary non-profit - Private

Measure	Cases	This Hosp.	State Avg.	U.S. Avg.
Blood Clot Prevention and Treatment				
Anticoagulation Overlap Therapy[5]	-	-	86%	93%
ICU Venous Thromboembolism Prophylaxis[5]	-	-	86%	92%
Incidence of Potentially Preventable VTE[5]	-	-	15%	10%
UFH with Dosages/Platelet Monitoring[5]	-	-	94%	97%
Venous Thromboembolism Prophylaxis[5]	-	-	70%	85%
Warfarin Therapy Discharge Instructions[5]	-	-	77%	75%
Chest Pain/Possible Heart Attack Care				
Aspirin Given Within 24 Hours of Arrival[5]	-	-	94%	96%
Fibrinolytic Meds Within 30 Min. of Arrival[5]	-	-	40%	58%
Average Time to ECG (minutes)[5]	-	-	10	7
Average Time to Transfer (minutes)[5]	-	-	77	60
Children's Asthma Care				
Received Home Management Plan of Care	-	-	-	88%
Received Reliever Medication	-	-	-	100%
Received Systemic Corticosteroids	-	-	-	100%
Emergency Department				
Admittance Decision Time (minutes)[5]	-	-	61	98
Head CT Results Within 45 Min. of Arrival[5]	-	-	42%	57%
Patients Who Left ER Before Being Seen[5]	-	-	3%	2%
Time from ER Arrival to Admit. (minutes)[5]	-	-	223	274
Time from ER Arrival to Discharge (minutes)[5]	-	-	112	134
Time in ER Before Being Evaluated (minutes)[5]	-	-	29	26
Time to Pain Meds for Fractures (minutes)[5]	-	-	68	57
Heart Attack Care				
Aspirin Given at Discharge[5]	-	-	99%	99%
Fibrinolytic Meds Within 30 Min. of Arrival[5]	-	-	50%	54%
PCI Within 90 Minutes of Arrival[5]	-	-	96%	96%
Statin Prescribed at Discharge[5]	-	-	97%	98%
Heart Failure Care				
ACE Inhibitor or ARB for LVSD[5]	-	-	93%	97%
Discharge Instructions Given[5]	-	-	91%	94%
Evaluation of LVS Function[5]	-	-	96%	99%
Medicare Spending				
Medicare Spending per Patient (ratio)	-	-	0.95	0.98
Pneumonia Care				
Appropriate Initial Antibiotic Given[5]	-	-	91%	95%
Blood Culture Timing[5]	-	-	97%	98%
Pregnancy and Delivery Care				
Newborn Deliveries Scheduled Early[5]	-	-	22%	6%
Preventive Care				
Immunization for Influenza[5]	-	-	87%	90%
Immunization for Pneumonia[5]	-	-	89%	92%
Stroke Care				
Anticoagulation Therapy for Atrial Fibrillation[5]	-	-	93%	95%
Antithrombotic Therapy Timing[5]	-	-	96%	98%

NOTE: Hospital profiles are in alphabetical order by state, then city, then hospital within the city; Rankings exclude hospitals with less than 25 cases except for patient surveys which excludes hospitals with less than 100 cases; (a) 100-299 cases; (1) The number of cases/patients is too few to report; (2) Data submitted were based on a sample of cases/patients; (3) Results are based on a shorter time period than required; (4) Data suppressed by CMS for one or more quarters; (5) Results are not available for this reporting period; (6) Fewer than 100 patients completed the HCAHPS survey; (7) No cases met the criteria for this measure; (8) The lower limit of the confidence interval cannot be calculated if the number of observed infections equals zero; (9) No data are available from the state/territory for this reporting period; (10) The scores shown reflect fewer than 50 completed surveys; (11) There were discrepancies in the data collection process; (12) This measure does not apply to this hospital for this reporting period; (13) Results cannot be calculated for this reporting period; (14) The results for this state are combined with nearby states to protect confidentiality; Please refer to the User's Guide for a full explanation of data.

Measure	Cases	This Hosp.	State Avg.	U.S. Avg.
Assessed for Rehabilitation[5]	-	-	95%	97%
Discharged on Antithrombotic Therapy[5]	-	-	97%	99%
Discharged on Statin Medication[5]	-	-	88%	94%
Thrombolytic Therapy Timing[5]	-	-	25%	66%
Venous Thromboembolism Prophylaxis[5]	-	-	87%	94%
Written Stroke Educational Materials Given[5]	-	-	84%	88%
Surgical Care Improvement Project				
Appropriate Beta Blocker Usage[5]	-	-	97%	98%
Appropriate VTP Within 24 Hours[5]	-	-	97%	98%
Controlled Postoperative Blood Glucose[5]	-	-	97%	97%
Perioperative Temperature Management[5]	-	-	100%	100%
Prophylactic Antibiotic Selection[5]	-	-	99%	99%
Prophylactic Antibiotic Selection (Outpatient)[5]	-	-	98%	98%
Prophylactic Antibiotic Stopped[5]	-	-	97%	98%
Prophylactic Antibiotic Timing[5]	-	-	99%	99%
Prophylactic Antibiotic Timing (Outpatient)[5]	-	-	98%	98%
Urinary Catheter Removal[5]	-	-	97%	97%
Survey of Patients' Hospital Experiences				
Area Around Room 'Always' Quiet at Night[5]	-	-	72%	61%
Doctors 'Always' Communicated Well[5]	-	-	86%	82%
Home Recovery Information Given[5]	-	-	83%	85%
Hospital Given 9 or 10 on 10 Point Scale[5]	-	-	71%	71%
Meds 'Always' Explained Before Given[5]	-	-	67%	64%
Nurses 'Always' Communicated Well[5]	-	-	81%	79%
Pain 'Always' Well Controlled[5]	-	-	72%	71%
Room and Bathroom 'Always' Clean[5]	-	-	74%	73%
Timely Help 'Always' Received[5]	-	-	69%	68%
Would Definitely Recommend Hospital[5]	-	-	69%	71%
Use of Medical Imaging				
Cardiac Imaging Stress Test before Surgery[5]	-	-	5.7%	5.3%
Combination Abdominal CT Scan[5]	-	-	12.9%	10.5%
Combination Brain/Sinus CT Scan[5]	-	-	3.3%	2.7%
Combination Chest CT Scan[5]	-	-	6.1%	2.7%
Follow-up Mammogram/Ultrasound[5]	-	-	8.4%	8.8%
Lumbar Spine MRI for Low Back Pain[5]	-	-	41.1%	37.2%

Baptist Memorial Hospital North Mississippi

2301 South Lamar
Oxford, MS 38655
URL: www.baptistonline.org/facilities/oxford
Phone: 662-232-8100
Fax: 662-232-8391
Type: Acute Care Hospitals
Emergency Services: Yes
Ownership: Voluntary non-profit - Private
Beds: 204

Key Personnel:
Chief of Medical Staff.......... Ralph C Armstrong Jr
Radiology.................... Brice Boughner
Administrator .... William C. Hennings
CEO .... William C. Hennings

Measure	Cases	This Hosp.	State Avg.	U.S. Avg.
Blood Clot Prevention and Treatment				
Anticoagulation Overlap Therapy[2]	43	81%	86%	93%
ICU Venous Thromboembolism Prophylaxis[2]	109	93%	86%	92%
Incidence of Potentially Preventable VTE[1,2]	-	-	15%	10%
UFH with Dosages/Platelet Monitoring[1,2]	-	-	94%	97%
Venous Thromboembolism Prophylaxis[2]	340	96%	70%	85%
Warfarin Therapy Discharge Instructions[2]	37	100%	77%	75%
Chest Pain/Possible Heart Attack Care				
Aspirin Given Within 24 Hours of Arrival	36	97%	94%	96%
Fibrinolytic Meds Within 30 Min. of Arrival[1,3]	-	-	40%	58%
Average Time to ECG (minutes)	38	10	10	7
Average Time to Transfer (minutes)[3,7]	-	-	77	60
Children's Asthma Care				
Received Home Management Plan of Care	-	-	-	88%
Received Reliever Medication	-	-	-	100%
Received Systemic Corticosteroids	-	-	-	100%
Emergency Department				
Admittance Decision Time (minutes)[2]	436	52	61	98
Head CT Results Within 45 Min. of Arrival	15	73%	42%	57%
Patients Who Left ER Before Being Seen	35,802	2%	3%	2%
Time from ER Arrival to Admit. (minutes)[2]	483	210	223	274
Time from ER Arrival to Discharge (minutes)	344	130	112	134
Time in ER Before Being Evaluated (minutes)	372	35	29	26
Time to Pain Meds for Fractures (minutes)	114	57	68	57
Heart Attack Care				
Aspirin Given at Discharge	215	100%	99%	99%
Fibrinolytic Meds Within 30 Min. of Arrival[1]	-	-	50%	54%
PCI Within 90 Minutes of Arrival	26	100%	96%	96%
Statin Prescribed at Discharge	206	100%	97%	98%
Heart Failure Care				
ACE Inhibitor or ARB for LVSD	95	100%	93%	97%
Discharge Instructions Given	231	94%	91%	94%
Evaluation of LVS Function	276	100%	96%	99%
Medicare Spending				
Medicare Spending per Patient (ratio)	-	0.96	0.95	0.98
Pneumonia Care				
Appropriate Initial Antibiotic Given	111	100%	91%	95%
Blood Culture Timing	235	100%	97%	98%
Pregnancy and Delivery Care				
Newborn Deliveries Scheduled Early[2]	33	9%	22%	6%
Preventive Care				
Immunization for Influenza[2]	552	96%	87%	90%
Immunization for Pneumonia[2]	678	92%	89%	92%
Stroke Care				
Anticoagulation Therapy for Atrial Fibrillation[1]	-	-	93%	95%
Antithrombotic Therapy Timing	82	100%	96%	98%
Assessed for Rehabilitation	79	99%	95%	97%
Discharged on Antithrombotic Therapy	74	100%	97%	99%
Discharged on Statin Medication	61	100%	88%	94%
Thrombolytic Therapy Timing[7]	-	-	25%	66%
Venous Thromboembolism Prophylaxis	77	99%	87%	94%
Written Stroke Educational Materials Given	47	98%	84%	88%
Surgical Care Improvement Project				
Appropriate Beta Blocker Usage	218	100%	97%	98%
Appropriate VTP Within 24 Hours	523	100%	97%	98%
Controlled Postoperative Blood Glucose	54	98%	97%	97%
Perioperative Temperature Management	599	100%	100%	100%
Prophylactic Antibiotic Selection	390	99%	99%	99%
Prophylactic Antibiotic Selection (Outpatient)	496	97%	98%	98%
Prophylactic Antibiotic Stopped	376	100%	97%	98%
Prophylactic Antibiotic Timing	390	97%	99%	99%
Prophylactic Antibiotic Timing (Outpatient)	501	98%	98%	98%
Urinary Catheter Removal	388	100%	97%	97%
Survey of Patients' Hospital Experiences				
Area Around Room 'Always' Quiet at Night	300+	75%	72%	61%
Doctors 'Always' Communicated Well	300+	82%	86%	82%
Home Recovery Information Given	300+	83%	83%	85%
Hospital Given 9 or 10 on 10 Point Scale	300+	70%	71%	71%
Meds 'Always' Explained Before Given	300+	61%	67%	64%
Nurses 'Always' Communicated Well	300+	79%	81%	79%
Pain 'Always' Well Controlled	300+	71%	72%	71%
Room and Bathroom 'Always' Clean	300+	73%	74%	73%
Timely Help 'Always' Received	300+	64%	69%	68%
Would Definitely Recommend Hospital	300+	73%	69%	71%
Use of Medical Imaging				
Cardiac Imaging Stress Test before Surgery	211	6.6%	5.7%	5.3%
Combination Abdominal CT Scan	745	13.8%	12.9%	10.5%
Combination Brain/Sinus CT Scan	761	5.0%	3.3%	2.7%
Combination Chest CT Scan	356	2.0%	6.1%	2.7%
Follow-up Mammogram/Ultrasound	95	6.3%	8.4%	8.8%
Lumbar Spine MRI for Low Back Pain[1]	-	-	41.1%	37.2%

Singing River Hospital

2809 Denny Av
Pascagoula, MS 39581
URL: www.srhshealth.com
Phone: 228-809-5000
Fax: 228-809-5064
Type: Acute Care Hospitals
Emergency Services: Yes
Ownership: Government - Local
Beds: 378

Key Personnel:
CEO/President.............. Chris Anderson
Operating Room.............. Donna Casey
Radiology.................. Tommy Crawford
Chief of Medical Staff.......... Steve Demetropoulos
Hemotology Center .... Carolyn Freeman
Emergency Room .... Charles Howard
Cardiac Laboratory............ Glenda Smith
Quality Assurance .... June Wood

Measure	Cases	This Hosp.	State Avg.	U.S. Avg.
Blood Clot Prevention and Treatment				
Anticoagulation Overlap Therapy[2]	73	85%	86%	93%
ICU Venous Thromboembolism Prophylaxis[2]	120	92%	86%	92%
Incidence of Potentially Preventable VTE[2]	14	0%	15%	10%
UFH with Dosages/Platelet Monitoring[2]	28	0%	94%	97%
Venous Thromboembolism Prophylaxis[2]	299	85%	70%	85%
Warfarin Therapy Discharge Instructions[2]	58	74%	77%	75%
Chest Pain/Possible Heart Attack Care				
Aspirin Given Within 24 Hours of Arrival[1,3]	-	-	94%	96%
Fibrinolytic Meds Within 30 Min. of Arrival[5]	-	-	40%	58%
Average Time to ECG (minutes)[1,3]	-	-	10	7
Average Time to Transfer (minutes)[5]	-	-	77	60
Children's Asthma Care				
Received Home Management Plan of Care	-	-	-	88%
Received Reliever Medication	-	-	-	100%
Received Systemic Corticosteroids	-	-	-	100%
Emergency Department				
Admittance Decision Time (minutes)[2]	647	133	61	98
Head CT Results Within 45 Min. of Arrival[1,3]	-	-	42%	57%
Patients Who Left ER Before Being Seen	>100k	2%	3%	2%
Time from ER Arrival to Admit. (minutes)[2]	669	258	223	274
Time from ER Arrival to Discharge (minutes)	470	107	112	134
Time in ER Before Being Evaluated (minutes)	314	40	29	26
Time to Pain Meds for Fractures (minutes)	231	70	68	57
Heart Attack Care				
Aspirin Given at Discharge[2]	301	100%	99%	99%
Fibrinolytic Meds Within 30 Min. of Arrival[2,7]	-	-	50%	54%
PCI Within 90 Minutes of Arrival[2]	45	98%	96%	96%
Statin Prescribed at Discharge[2]	302	99%	97%	98%
Heart Failure Care				
ACE Inhibitor or ARB for LVSD	172	99%	93%	97%
Discharge Instructions Given	403	99%	91%	94%
Evaluation of LVS Function	460	100%	96%	99%
Medicare Spending				
Medicare Spending per Patient (ratio)	-	1.00	0.95	0.98
Pneumonia Care				
Appropriate Initial Antibiotic Given[2]	88	100%	91%	95%
Blood Culture Timing[2]	152	100%	97%	98%
Pregnancy and Delivery Care				
Newborn Deliveries Scheduled Early[2]	58	14%	22%	6%
Preventive Care				
Immunization for Influenza[2]	634	89%	87%	90%
Immunization for Pneumonia[2]	737	91%	89%	92%
Stroke Care				
Anticoagulation Therapy for Atrial Fibrillation	31	100%	93%	95%
Antithrombotic Therapy Timing	174	99%	96%	98%
Assessed for Rehabilitation	214	99%	95%	97%
Discharged on Antithrombotic Therapy	192	99%	97%	99%
Discharged on Statin Medication	154	96%	88%	94%
Thrombolytic Therapy Timing	17	94%	25%	66%
Venous Thromboembolism Prophylaxis	215	100%	87%	94%
Written Stroke Educational Materials Given	125	100%	84%	88%
Surgical Care Improvement Project				
Appropriate Beta Blocker Usage[2]	227	98%	97%	98%
Appropriate VTP Within 24 Hours[2]	433	99%	97%	98%
Controlled Postoperative Blood Glucose[2]	140	97%	97%	97%
Perioperative Temperature Management[2]	521	100%	100%	100%
Prophylactic Antibiotic Selection[2]	455	99%	99%	99%
Prophylactic Antibiotic Selection (Outpatient)	230	98%	98%	98%
Prophylactic Antibiotic Stopped[2]	439	99%	97%	98%
Prophylactic Antibiotic Timing[2]	457	100%	99%	99%
Prophylactic Antibiotic Timing (Outpatient)	230	100%	98%	98%
Urinary Catheter Removal[2]	346	98%	97%	97%
Survey of Patients' Hospital Experiences				
Area Around Room 'Always' Quiet at Night	300+	67%	72%	61%
Doctors 'Always' Communicated Well	300+	81%	86%	82%
Home Recovery Information Given	300+	82%	83%	85%
Hospital Given 9 or 10 on 10 Point Scale	300+	70%	71%	71%
Meds 'Always' Explained Before Given	300+	66%	67%	64%
Nurses 'Always' Communicated Well	300+	82%	81%	79%
Pain 'Always' Well Controlled	300+	70%	72%	71%
Room and Bathroom 'Always' Clean	300+	70%	74%	73%
Timely Help 'Always' Received	300+	69%	69%	68%

NOTE: Hospital profiles are in alphabetical order by state, then city, then hospital within the city; Rankings exclude hospitals with less than 25 cases except for patient surveys which excludes hospitals with less than 100 cases; (a) 100-299 cases; (1) The number of cases/patients is too few to report; (2) Data submitted were based on a sample of cases/patients; (3) Results are based on a shorter time period than required; (4) Data suppressed by CMS for one or more quarters; (5) Results are not available for this reporting period; (6) Fewer than 100 patients completed the HCAHPS survey; (7) No cases met the criteria for this measure; (8) The lower limit of the confidence interval cannot be calculated if the number of observed infections equals zero; (9) No data are available from the state/territory for this reporting period; (10) The scores shown reflect fewer than 50 completed surveys; (11) There were discrepancies in the data collection process; (12) This measure does not apply to this hospital for this reporting period; (13) Results cannot be calculated for this reporting period; (14) The results for this state are combined with nearby states to protect confidentiality; Please refer to the User's Guide for a full explanation of data.

Would Definitely Recommend Hospital	300+	73%	69%	71%
Use of Medical Imaging				
Cardiac Imaging Stress Test before Surgery	243	4.5%	5.7%	5.3%
Combination Abdominal CT Scan	1,610	8.3%	12.9%	10.5%
Combination Brain/Sinus CT Scan	1,247	2.5%	3.3%	2.7%
Combination Chest CT Scan	1,187	1.2%	6.1%	2.7%
Follow-up Mammogram/Ultrasound	2,743	9.3%	8.4%	8.8%
Lumbar Spine MRI for Low Back Pain	311	40.5%	41.1%	37.2%

Neshoba County General Hospital

1001 Holland Avenue
Philadelphia, MS 39350
Phone: 601-663-1200
Fax: 601-663-1497
URL: www.neshobageneral.com
Type: Acute Care Hospitals
Emergency Services: Yes
Ownership: Government - Local
Beds: 82

Key Personnel:
Infection Control . . . . Beth Burns
Quality Assurance . . . . Beth Burns
Operating Room. . . . . Andrew P Dabbs
Anesthesiology. . . . . Ron Lackey
Radiology. . . . . Kerry Smith, MD
Chief of Medical Staff . . . . AP Soriano, MD
Emergency Room . . . . Todd Willis, MD

Measure	Cases	This Hosp.	State Avg.	U.S. Avg.
Blood Clot Prevention and Treatment				
Anticoagulation Overlap Therapy[1,2]	-	-	86%	93%
ICU Venous Thromboembolism Prophylaxis[2,7]	-	-	86%	92%
Incidence of Potentially Preventable VTE[1,2]	-	-	15%	10%
UFH with Dosages/Platelet Monitoring[2,7]	-	-	94%	97%
Venous Thromboembolism Prophylaxis[2]	118	1%	70%	85%
Warfarin Therapy Discharge Instructions[1,2]	-	-	77%	75%
Chest Pain/Possible Heart Attack Care				
Aspirin Given Within 24 Hours of Arrival	44	70%	94%	96%
Fibrinolytic Meds Within 30 Min. of Arrival[1]	-	-	40%	58%
Average Time to ECG (minutes)	44	10	10	7
Average Time to Transfer (minutes)[7]	-	-	77	60
Children's Asthma Care				
Received Home Management Plan of Care	-	-	-	88%
Received Reliever Medication	-	-	-	100%
Received Systemic Corticosteroids	-	-	-	100%
Emergency Department				
Admittance Decision Time (minutes)[2]	294	40	61	98
Head CT Results Within 45 Min. of Arrival[3,7]	-	-	42%	57%
Patients Who Left ER Before Being Seen	19,446	3%	3%	2%
Time from ER Arrival to Admit. (minutes)[2]	324	169	223	274
Time from ER Arrival to Discharge (minutes)	121	97	112	134
Time in ER Before Being Evaluated (minutes)	308	10	29	26
Time to Pain Meds for Fractures (minutes)	60	38	68	57
Heart Attack Care				
Aspirin Given at Discharge[2,3]	-	-	99%	99%
Fibrinolytic Meds Within 30 Min. of Arrival[2,3]	-	-	50%	54%
PCI Within 90 Minutes of Arrival[2,3]	-	-	96%	96%
Statin Prescribed at Discharge[2,3]	-	-	97%	98%
Heart Failure Care				
ACE Inhibitor or ARB for LVSD[2]	19	68%	93%	97%
Discharge Instructions Given[2]	65	95%	91%	94%
Evaluation of LVS Function[2]	65	34%	96%	99%
Medicare Spending				
Medicare Spending per Patient (ratio)	-	0.84	0.95	0.98
Pneumonia Care				
Appropriate Initial Antibiotic Given[2,7]	-	-	91%	95%
Blood Culture Timing[2,7]	-	-	97%	98%
Pregnancy and Delivery Care				
Newborn Deliveries Scheduled Early[7]	-	-	22%	6%
Preventive Care				
Immunization for Influenza[2]	203	51%	87%	90%
Immunization for Pneumonia[2]	291	71%	89%	92%
Stroke Care				
Anticoagulation Therapy for Atrial Fibrillation[2,3]	-	-	93%	95%
Antithrombotic Therapy Timing[1,2]	-	-	96%	98%
Assessed for Rehabilitation[1,2]	-	-	95%	97%
Discharged on Antithrombotic Therapy[1,2]	-	-	97%	99%
Discharged on Statin Medication[1,2]	-	-	88%	94%
Thrombolytic Therapy Timing[2,3]	-	-	25%	66%
Venous Thromboembolism Prophylaxis[1,2]	-	-	87%	94%
Written Stroke Educational Materials Given[1,2]	-	-	84%	88%
Surgical Care Improvement Project				
Appropriate Beta Blocker Usage[5]	-	-	97%	98%
Appropriate VTP Within 24 Hours[5]	-	-	97%	98%
Controlled Postoperative Blood Glucose[5]	-	-	97%	97%
Perioperative Temperature Management[5]	-	-	100%	100%
Prophylactic Antibiotic Selection[5]	-	-	99%	99%
Prophylactic Antibiotic Selection (Outpatient)[5]	-	-	98%	98%
Prophylactic Antibiotic Stopped[5]	-	-	97%	98%
Prophylactic Antibiotic Timing[5]	-	-	99%	99%
Prophylactic Antibiotic Timing (Outpatient)[5]	-	-	98%	98%
Urinary Catheter Removal[5]	-	-	97%	97%
Survey of Patients' Hospital Experiences				
Area Around Room 'Always' Quiet at Night	300+	78%	72%	61%
Doctors 'Always' Communicated Well	300+	90%	86%	82%
Home Recovery Information Given	300+	86%	83%	85%
Hospital Given 9 or 10 on 10 Point Scale	300+	77%	71%	71%
Meds 'Always' Explained Before Given	300+	75%	67%	64%
Nurses 'Always' Communicated Well	300+	87%	81%	79%
Pain 'Always' Well Controlled	300+	76%	72%	71%
Room and Bathroom 'Always' Clean	300+	83%	74%	73%
Timely Help 'Always' Received	300+	77%	69%	68%
Would Definitely Recommend Hospital	300+	71%	69%	71%
Use of Medical Imaging				
Cardiac Imaging Stress Test before Surgery[1]	-	-	5.7%	5.3%
Combination Abdominal CT Scan	262	11.1%	12.9%	10.5%
Combination Brain/Sinus CT Scan[1]	-	-	3.3%	2.7%
Combination Chest CT Scan	82	39.0%	6.1%	2.7%
Follow-up Mammogram/Ultrasound[1]	-	-	8.4%	8.8%
Lumbar Spine MRI for Low Back Pain	48	54.2%	41.1%	37.2%

Highland Community Hospital

130 Highland Pkwy
Picayune, MS 39466
Phone: 601-358-9400
Fax: 601-749-3187
URL: www.highlandch.com
Type: Acute Care Hospitals
Emergency Services: Yes
Ownership: Govt - Hospital Dist/Auth
Beds: 95

Key Personnel:
Coronary Care . . . . Shannon Felder
Operating Room. . . . . Debbie Green
Chief of Medical Staff . . . . Ahmad Haidar, MD
Emergency Room . . . . Sandy Spiers
Radiology. . . . . James Turnage
Quality Assurance . . . . Melissa Wise

Measure	Cases	This Hosp.	State Avg.	U.S. Avg.
Blood Clot Prevention and Treatment				
Anticoagulation Overlap Therapy[2]	20	75%	86%	93%
ICU Venous Thromboembolism Prophylaxis[2]	96	64%	86%	92%
Incidence of Potentially Preventable VTE[1,2]	-	-	15%	10%
UFH with Dosages/Platelet Monitoring[2,7]	-	-	94%	97%
Venous Thromboembolism Prophylaxis[2]	263	42%	70%	85%
Warfarin Therapy Discharge Instructions[2]	16	100%	77%	75%
Chest Pain/Possible Heart Attack Care				
Aspirin Given Within 24 Hours of Arrival	65	100%	94%	96%
Fibrinolytic Meds Within 30 Min. of Arrival[1]	-	-	40%	58%
Average Time to ECG (minutes)	68	9	10	7
Average Time to Transfer (minutes)	20	73	77	60
Children's Asthma Care				
Received Home Management Plan of Care	-	-	-	88%
Received Reliever Medication	-	-	-	100%
Received Systemic Corticosteroids	-	-	-	100%
Emergency Department				
Admittance Decision Time (minutes)[2]	481	78	61	98
Head CT Results Within 45 Min. of Arrival[1]	-	-	42%	57%
Patients Who Left ER Before Being Seen	22,095	4%	3%	2%
Time from ER Arrival to Admit. (minutes)[2]	480	263	223	274
Time from ER Arrival to Discharge (minutes)	506	127	112	134
Time in ER Before Being Evaluated (minutes)	625	22	29	26
Time to Pain Meds for Fractures (minutes)	99	60	68	57
Heart Attack Care				
Aspirin Given at Discharge[7]	-	-	99%	99%
Fibrinolytic Meds Within 30 Min. of Arrival[7]	-	-	50%	54%
PCI Within 90 Minutes of Arrival[7]	-	-	96%	96%
Statin Prescribed at Discharge[7]	-	-	97%	98%
Heart Failure Care				
ACE Inhibitor or ARB for LVSD	26	100%	93%	97%
Discharge Instructions Given	60	88%	91%	94%
Evaluation of LVS Function	69	97%	96%	99%
Medicare Spending				
Medicare Spending per Patient (ratio)	-	0.99	0.95	0.98
Pneumonia Care				
Appropriate Initial Antibiotic Given[2]	74	95%	91%	95%
Blood Culture Timing[2]	129	98%	97%	98%
Pregnancy and Delivery Care				
Newborn Deliveries Scheduled Early[2]	100	43%	22%	6%
Preventive Care				
Immunization for Influenza[2]	362	78%	87%	90%
Immunization for Pneumonia[2]	573	81%	89%	92%
Stroke Care				
Anticoagulation Therapy for Atrial Fibrillation[1]	-	-	93%	95%
Antithrombotic Therapy Timing	26	96%	96%	98%
Assessed for Rehabilitation	31	94%	95%	97%
Discharged on Antithrombotic Therapy	30	97%	97%	99%
Discharged on Statin Medication	24	75%	88%	94%
Thrombolytic Therapy Timing	12	0%	25%	66%
Venous Thromboembolism Prophylaxis	25	48%	87%	94%
Written Stroke Educational Materials Given	16	88%	84%	88%
Surgical Care Improvement Project				
Appropriate Beta Blocker Usage[2]	14	100%	97%	98%
Appropriate VTP Within 24 Hours[2]	72	97%	97%	98%
Controlled Postoperative Blood Glucose[2,7]	-	-	97%	97%
Perioperative Temperature Management[2]	71	100%	100%	100%
Prophylactic Antibiotic Selection[2]	46	91%	99%	99%
Prophylactic Antibiotic Selection (Outpatient)[1,3]	-	-	98%	98%
Prophylactic Antibiotic Stopped[2]	46	85%	97%	98%
Prophylactic Antibiotic Timing[2]	46	98%	99%	99%
Prophylactic Antibiotic Timing (Outpatient)[1,3]	-	-	98%	98%
Urinary Catheter Removal[2]	22	100%	97%	97%
Survey of Patients' Hospital Experiences				
Area Around Room 'Always' Quiet at Night	(a)	71%	72%	61%
Doctors 'Always' Communicated Well	(a)	80%	86%	82%
Home Recovery Information Given	(a)	84%	83%	85%
Hospital Given 9 or 10 on 10 Point Scale	(a)	74%	71%	71%
Meds 'Always' Explained Before Given	(a)	57%	67%	64%
Nurses 'Always' Communicated Well	(a)	78%	81%	79%
Pain 'Always' Well Controlled	(a)	65%	72%	71%
Room and Bathroom 'Always' Clean	(a)	75%	74%	73%
Timely Help 'Always' Received	(a)	65%	69%	68%
Would Definitely Recommend Hospital	(a)	68%	69%	71%
Use of Medical Imaging				
Cardiac Imaging Stress Test before Surgery	129	3.1%	5.7%	5.3%
Combination Abdominal CT Scan	291	10.0%	12.9%	10.5%
Combination Brain/Sinus CT Scan[1]	-	-	3.3%	2.7%
Combination Chest CT Scan	114	0.0%	6.1%	2.7%
Follow-up Mammogram/Ultrasound	420	9.3%	8.4%	8.8%
Lumbar Spine MRI for Low Back Pain	87	29.9%	41.1%	37.2%

Pontotoc Health Service

176 South Main Street
Pontotoc, MS 38863
Phone: 662-489-5510
Fax: 662-488-7661
Type: Critical Access Hospitals
Emergency Services: Yes
Ownership: Voluntary non-profit - Private
Beds: 69

Key Personnel:
Emergency Room . . . . Kevin Koehler, MD
Infection Control . . . . Jan Rowan, RN
CEO/President. . . . . Shane Spees
Quality Assurance . . . . Cathy Waldrop, CFNP

Measure	Cases	This Hosp.	State Avg.	U.S. Avg.
Blood Clot Prevention and Treatment				
Anticoagulation Overlap Therapy[1,2]	-	-	86%	93%
ICU Venous Thromboembolism Prophylaxis[2,7]	-	-	86%	92%
Incidence of Potentially Preventable VTE[2,7]	-	-	15%	10%
UFH with Dosages/Platelet Monitoring[2,7]	-	-	94%	97%
Venous Thromboembolism Prophylaxis[2]	130	94%	70%	85%
Warfarin Therapy Discharge Instructions[1,2]	-	-	77%	75%
Chest Pain/Possible Heart Attack Care				

NOTE: Hospital profiles are in alphabetical order by state, then city, then hospital within the city; Rankings exclude hospitals with less than 25 cases except for patient surveys which excludes hospitals with less than 100 cases; (a) 100-299 cases; (1) The number of cases/patients is too few to report; (2) Data submitted were based on a sample of cases/patients; (3) Results are based on a shorter time period than required; (4) Data suppressed by CMS for one or more quarters; (5) Results are not available for this reporting period; (6) Fewer than 100 patients completed the HCAHPS survey; (7) No cases met the criteria for this measure; (8) The lower limit of the confidence interval cannot be calculated if the number of observed infections equals zero; (9) No data are available from the state/territory for this reporting period; (10) The scores shown reflect fewer than 50 completed surveys; (11) There were discrepancies in the data collection process; (12) This measure does not apply to this hospital for this reporting period; (13) Results cannot be calculated for this reporting period; (14) The results for this state are combined with nearby states to protect confidentiality; Please refer to the User's Guide for a full explanation of data.

Measure	Cases	This Hosp.	State Avg.	U.S. Avg.
Aspirin Given Within 24 Hours of Arrival	42	100%	94%	96%
Fibrinolytic Meds Within 30 Min. of Arrival[7]	-	-	40%	58%
Average Time to ECG (minutes)	43	8	10	7
Average Time to Transfer (minutes)[7]	-	-	77	60
Children's Asthma Care				
Received Home Management Plan of Care	-	-	-	88%
Received Reliever Medication	-	-	-	100%
Received Systemic Corticosteroids	-	-	-	100%
Emergency Department				
Admittance Decision Time (minutes)[2]	226	29	61	98
Head CT Results Within 45 Min. of Arrival[1]	-	-	42%	57%
Patients Who Left ER Before Being Seen	11,214	1%	3%	2%
Time from ER Arrival to Admit. (minutes)[2]	236	203	223	274
Time from ER Arrival to Discharge (minutes)	389	113	112	134
Time in ER Before Being Evaluated (minutes)	414	37	29	26
Time to Pain Meds for Fractures (minutes)	52	68	68	57
Heart Attack Care				
Aspirin Given at Discharge[3,7]	-	-	99%	99%
Fibrinolytic Meds Within 30 Min. of Arrival[3,7]	-	-	50%	54%
PCI Within 90 Minutes of Arrival[3,7]	-	-	96%	96%
Statin Prescribed at Discharge[3,7]	-	-	97%	98%
Heart Failure Care				
ACE Inhibitor or ARB for LVSD[1]	-	-	93%	97%
Discharge Instructions Given[1]	-	-	91%	94%
Evaluation of LVS Function[1]	-	-	96%	99%
Medicare Spending				
Medicare Spending per Patient (ratio)	-	-	0.95	0.98
Pneumonia Care				
Appropriate Initial Antibiotic Given	40	100%	91%	95%
Blood Culture Timing	51	98%	97%	98%
Pregnancy and Delivery Care				
Newborn Deliveries Scheduled Early[7]	-	-	22%	6%
Preventive Care				
Immunization for Influenza[2]	181	98%	87%	90%
Immunization for Pneumonia[2]	252	100%	89%	92%
Stroke Care				
Anticoagulation Therapy for Atrial Fibrillation[2,3]	-	-	93%	95%
Antithrombotic Therapy Timing[1,2]	-	-	96%	98%
Assessed for Rehabilitation[2,3]	-	-	95%	97%
Discharged on Antithrombotic Therapy[2,3]	-	-	97%	99%
Discharged on Statin Medication[2,3]	-	-	88%	94%
Thrombolytic Therapy Timing[2,3]	-	-	25%	66%
Venous Thromboembolism Prophylaxis[1,2]	-	-	87%	94%
Written Stroke Educational Materials Given[2,3]	-	-	84%	88%
Surgical Care Improvement Project				
Appropriate Beta Blocker Usage[5]	-	-	97%	98%
Appropriate VTP Within 24 Hours[5]	-	-	97%	98%
Controlled Postoperative Blood Glucose[5]	-	-	97%	97%
Perioperative Temperature Management[5]	-	-	100%	100%
Prophylactic Antibiotic Selection[5]	-	-	99%	99%
Prophylactic Antibiotic Selection (Outpatient)[5]	-	-	98%	98%
Prophylactic Antibiotic Stopped[5]	-	-	97%	98%
Prophylactic Antibiotic Timing[5]	-	-	99%	99%
Prophylactic Antibiotic Timing (Outpatient)[5]	-	-	98%	98%
Urinary Catheter Removal[5]	-	-	97%	97%
Survey of Patients' Hospital Experiences				
Area Around Room 'Always' Quiet at Night[6]	<100	75%	72%	61%
Doctors 'Always' Communicated Well[6]	<100	91%	86%	82%
Home Recovery Information Given[6]	<100	75%	83%	85%
Hospital Given 9 or 10 on 10 Point Scale[6]	<100	73%	71%	71%
Meds 'Always' Explained Before Given[6]	<100	62%	67%	64%
Nurses 'Always' Communicated Well[6]	<100	86%	81%	79%
Pain 'Always' Well Controlled[6]	<100	73%	72%	71%
Room and Bathroom 'Always' Clean[6]	<100	69%	74%	73%
Timely Help 'Always' Received[6]	<100	84%	69%	68%
Would Definitely Recommend Hospital[6]	<100	65%	69%	71%
Use of Medical Imaging				
Cardiac Imaging Stress Test before Surgery[7]	-	-	5.7%	5.3%
Combination Abdominal CT Scan	237	2.5%	12.9%	10.5%
Combination Brain/Sinus CT Scan[1]	-	-	3.3%	2.7%
Combination Chest CT Scan[1]	-	-	6.1%	2.7%
Follow-up Mammogram/Ultrasound[7]	-	-	8.4%	8.8%
Lumbar Spine MRI for Low Back Pain[7]	-	-	41.1%	37.2%

Pearl River County Hospital

305 West Moody Street Phone: 601-795-4543
Poplarville, MS 39470
Type: Critical Access Hospitals Emergency Services: Yes
Ownership: Voluntary non-profit - Other

Measure	Cases	This Hosp.	State Avg.	U.S. Avg.
Blood Clot Prevention and Treatment				
Anticoagulation Overlap Therapy[5]	-	-	86%	93%
ICU Venous Thromboembolism Prophylaxis[5]	-	-	86%	92%
Incidence of Potentially Preventable VTE[5]	-	-	15%	10%
UFH with Dosages/Platelet Monitoring[5]	-	-	94%	97%
Venous Thromboembolism Prophylaxis[5]	-	-	70%	85%
Warfarin Therapy Discharge Instructions[5]	-	-	77%	75%
Chest Pain/Possible Heart Attack Care				
Aspirin Given Within 24 Hours of Arrival[5]	-	-	94%	96%
Fibrinolytic Meds Within 30 Min. of Arrival[5]	-	-	40%	58%
Average Time to ECG (minutes)[5]	-	-	10	7
Average Time to Transfer (minutes)[5]	-	-	77	60
Children's Asthma Care				
Received Home Management Plan of Care	-	-	-	88%
Received Reliever Medication	-	-	-	100%
Received Systemic Corticosteroids	-	-	-	100%
Emergency Department				
Admittance Decision Time (minutes)[5]	-	-	61	98
Head CT Results Within 45 Min. of Arrival[5]	-	-	42%	57%
Patients Who Left ER Before Being Seen	2,458	1%	3%	2%
Time from ER Arrival to Admit. (minutes)[5]	-	-	223	274
Time from ER Arrival to Discharge (minutes)[3]	49	60	112	134
Time in ER Before Being Evaluated (minutes)[3]	62	16	29	26
Time to Pain Meds for Fractures (minutes)[5]	-	-	68	57
Heart Attack Care				
Aspirin Given at Discharge[5]	-	-	99%	99%
Fibrinolytic Meds Within 30 Min. of Arrival[5]	-	-	50%	54%
PCI Within 90 Minutes of Arrival[5]	-	-	96%	96%
Statin Prescribed at Discharge[5]	-	-	97%	98%
Heart Failure Care				
ACE Inhibitor or ARB for LVSD[5]	-	-	93%	97%
Discharge Instructions Given[5]	-	-	91%	94%
Evaluation of LVS Function[5]	-	-	96%	99%
Medicare Spending				
Medicare Spending per Patient (ratio)	-	-	0.95	0.98
Pneumonia Care				
Appropriate Initial Antibiotic Given[5]	-	-	91%	95%
Blood Culture Timing[5]	-	-	97%	98%
Pregnancy and Delivery Care				
Newborn Deliveries Scheduled Early[5]	-	-	22%	6%
Preventive Care				
Immunization for Influenza[5]	-	-	87%	90%
Immunization for Pneumonia[5]	-	-	89%	92%
Stroke Care				
Anticoagulation Therapy for Atrial Fibrillation[5]	-	-	93%	95%
Antithrombotic Therapy Timing[5]	-	-	96%	98%
Assessed for Rehabilitation[5]	-	-	95%	97%
Discharged on Antithrombotic Therapy[5]	-	-	97%	99%
Discharged on Statin Medication[5]	-	-	88%	94%
Thrombolytic Therapy Timing[5]	-	-	25%	66%
Venous Thromboembolism Prophylaxis[5]	-	-	87%	94%
Written Stroke Educational Materials Given[5]	-	-	84%	88%
Surgical Care Improvement Project				
Appropriate Beta Blocker Usage[5]	-	-	97%	98%
Appropriate VTP Within 24 Hours[5]	-	-	97%	98%
Controlled Postoperative Blood Glucose[5]	-	-	97%	97%
Perioperative Temperature Management[5]	-	-	100%	100%
Prophylactic Antibiotic Selection[5]	-	-	99%	99%
Prophylactic Antibiotic Selection (Outpatient)[5]	-	-	98%	98%
Prophylactic Antibiotic Stopped[5]	-	-	97%	98%
Prophylactic Antibiotic Timing[5]	-	-	99%	99%
Prophylactic Antibiotic Timing (Outpatient)[5]	-	-	98%	98%
Urinary Catheter Removal[5]	-	-	97%	97%
Survey of Patients' Hospital Experiences				
Area Around Room 'Always' Quiet at Night[10]	<100	75%	72%	61%
Doctors 'Always' Communicated Well[10]	<100	95%	86%	82%
Home Recovery Information Given[10]	<100	93%	83%	85%
Hospital Given 9 or 10 on 10 Point Scale[10]	<100	81%	71%	71%
Meds 'Always' Explained Before Given[10]	<100	80%	67%	64%
Nurses 'Always' Communicated Well[10]	<100	93%	81%	79%
Pain 'Always' Well Controlled[10]	<100	73%	72%	71%
Room and Bathroom 'Always' Clean[10]	<100	88%	74%	73%
Timely Help 'Always' Received[10]	<100	87%	69%	68%
Would Definitely Recommend Hospital[10]	<100	80%	69%	71%
Use of Medical Imaging				
Cardiac Imaging Stress Test before Surgery[7]	-	-	5.7%	5.3%
Combination Abdominal CT Scan[1]	-	-	12.9%	10.5%
Combination Brain/Sinus CT Scan[1]	-	-	3.3%	2.7%
Combination Chest CT Scan[1]	-	-	6.1%	2.7%
Follow-up Mammogram/Ultrasound[7]	-	-	8.4%	8.8%
Lumbar Spine MRI for Low Back Pain[7]	-	-	41.1%	37.2%

Claiborne County Hospital

123 Mccomb Avenue Phone: 601-437-5141
Port Gibson, MS 39150 Fax: 601-437-5145
Type: Critical Access Hospitals Emergency Services: Yes
Ownership: Government - Local Beds: 32

Key Personnel:

Chief of Medical Staff . . . . Roy Barnes
Quality Assurance . . . . Ginetta Felton
CEO/President. . . . . Wanda Fleming
Infection Control. . . . . Sandra Sampson

Measure	Cases	This Hosp.	State Avg.	U.S. Avg.
Blood Clot Prevention and Treatment				
Anticoagulation Overlap Therapy[5]	-	-	86%	93%
ICU Venous Thromboembolism Prophylaxis[5]	-	-	86%	92%
Incidence of Potentially Preventable VTE[5]	-	-	15%	10%
UFH with Dosages/Platelet Monitoring[5]	-	-	94%	97%
Venous Thromboembolism Prophylaxis[5]	-	-	70%	85%
Warfarin Therapy Discharge Instructions[5]	-	-	77%	75%
Chest Pain/Possible Heart Attack Care				
Aspirin Given Within 24 Hours of Arrival[5]	-	-	94%	96%
Fibrinolytic Meds Within 30 Min. of Arrival[5]	-	-	40%	58%
Average Time to ECG (minutes)[5]	-	-	10	7
Average Time to Transfer (minutes)[5]	-	-	77	60
Children's Asthma Care				
Received Home Management Plan of Care	-	-	-	88%
Received Reliever Medication	-	-	-	100%
Received Systemic Corticosteroids	-	-	-	100%
Emergency Department				
Admittance Decision Time (minutes)[5]	-	-	61	98
Head CT Results Within 45 Min. of Arrival[5]	-	-	42%	57%
Patients Who Left ER Before Being Seen[5]	-	-	3%	2%
Time from ER Arrival to Admit. (minutes)[5]	-	-	223	274
Time from ER Arrival to Discharge (minutes)[5]	-	-	112	134
Time in ER Before Being Evaluated (minutes)[5]	-	-	29	26
Time to Pain Meds for Fractures (minutes)[5]	-	-	68	57
Heart Attack Care				
Aspirin Given at Discharge[5]	-	-	99%	99%
Fibrinolytic Meds Within 30 Min. of Arrival[5]	-	-	50%	54%
PCI Within 90 Minutes of Arrival[5]	-	-	96%	96%
Statin Prescribed at Discharge[5]	-	-	97%	98%
Heart Failure Care				
ACE Inhibitor or ARB for LVSD[5]	-	-	93%	97%
Discharge Instructions Given[5]	-	-	91%	94%
Evaluation of LVS Function[5]	-	-	96%	99%
Medicare Spending				
Medicare Spending per Patient (ratio)	-	-	0.95	0.98
Pneumonia Care				
Appropriate Initial Antibiotic Given[5]	-	-	91%	95%
Blood Culture Timing[5]	-	-	97%	98%
Pregnancy and Delivery Care				
Newborn Deliveries Scheduled Early[3,7]	-	-	22%	6%
Preventive Care				
Immunization for Influenza[5]	-	-	87%	90%
Immunization for Pneumonia[5]	-	-	89%	92%
Stroke Care				

NOTE: Hospital profiles are in alphabetical order by state, then city, then hospital within the city; Rankings exclude hospitals with less than 25 cases except for patient surveys which excludes hospitals with less than 100 cases; (a) 100-299 cases; (1) The number of cases/patients is too few to report; (2) Data submitted were based on a sample of cases/patients; (3) Results are based on a shorter time period than required; (4) Data suppressed by CMS for one or more quarters; (5) Results are not available for this reporting period; (6) Fewer than 100 patients completed the HCAHPS survey; (7) No cases met the criteria for this measure; (8) The lower limit of the confidence interval cannot be calculated if the number of observed infections equals zero; (9) No data are available from the state/territory for this reporting period; (10) The scores shown reflect fewer than 50 completed surveys; (11) There were discrepancies in the data collection process; (12) This measure does not apply to this hospital for this reporting period; (13) Results cannot be calculated for this reporting period; (14) The results for this state are combined with nearby states to protect confidentiality; Please refer to the User's Guide for a full explanation of data.

Measure	Cases	This Hosp.	State Avg.	U.S. Avg.
Anticoagulation Therapy for Atrial Fibrillation[5]	-	-	93%	95%
Antithrombotic Therapy Timing[5]	-	-	96%	98%
Assessed for Rehabilitation[5]	-	-	95%	97%
Discharged on Antithrombotic Therapy[5]	-	-	97%	99%
Discharged on Statin Medication[5]	-	-	88%	94%
Thrombolytic Therapy Timing[5]	-	-	25%	66%
Venous Thromboembolism Prophylaxis[5]	-	-	87%	94%
Written Stroke Educational Materials Given[5]	-	-	84%	88%
Surgical Care Improvement Project				
Appropriate Beta Blocker Usage[5]	-	-	97%	98%
Appropriate VTP Within 24 Hours[5]	-	-	97%	98%
Controlled Postoperative Blood Glucose[5]	-	-	97%	97%
Perioperative Temperature Management[5]	-	-	100%	100%
Prophylactic Antibiotic Selection[5]	-	-	99%	99%
Prophylactic Antibiotic Selection (Outpatient)[5]	-	-	98%	98%
Prophylactic Antibiotic Stopped[5]	-	-	97%	98%
Prophylactic Antibiotic Timing[5]	-	-	99%	99%
Prophylactic Antibiotic Timing (Outpatient)[5]	-	-	98%	98%
Urinary Catheter Removal[5]	-	-	97%	97%
Survey of Patients' Hospital Experiences				
Area Around Room 'Always' Quiet at Night[5]	-	-	72%	61%
Doctors 'Always' Communicated Well[5]	-	-	86%	82%
Home Recovery Information Given[5]	-	-	83%	85%
Hospital Given 9 or 10 on 10 Point Scale[5]	-	-	71%	71%
Meds 'Always' Explained Before Given[5]	-	-	67%	64%
Nurses 'Always' Communicated Well[5]	-	-	81%	79%
Pain 'Always' Well Controlled[5]	-	-	72%	71%
Room and Bathroom 'Always' Clean[5]	-	-	74%	73%
Timely Help 'Always' Received[5]	-	-	69%	68%
Would Definitely Recommend Hospital[5]	-	-	69%	71%
Use of Medical Imaging				
Cardiac Imaging Stress Test before Surgery[7]	-	-	5.7%	5.3%
Combination Abdominal CT Scan[7]	-	-	12.9%	10.5%
Combination Brain/Sinus CT Scan[7]	-	-	3.3%	2.7%
Combination Chest CT Scan[7]	-	-	6.1%	2.7%
Follow-up Mammogram/Ultrasound[7]	-	-	8.4%	8.8%
Lumbar Spine MRI for Low Back Pain[7]	-	-	41.1%	37.2%

Jefferson Davis Community Hospital

1102 Rose Street
Prentiss, MS 39474
Phone: 601-792-4276
Fax: 601-792-2947
Type: Critical Access Hospitals
Emergency Services: Yes
Ownership: Government - Local
Beds: 41

Key Personnel:
Chief of Medical Staff . . . . Calor Berg
Emergency Room . . . . Lisa Berry, RN
CEO/President. . . . . Mary Cardis
Quality Assurance . . . . Melinda Pears

Measure	Cases	This Hosp.	State Avg.	U.S. Avg.
Blood Clot Prevention and Treatment				
Anticoagulation Overlap Therapy[5]	-	-	86%	93%
ICU Venous Thromboembolism Prophylaxis[5]	-	-	86%	92%
Incidence of Potentially Preventable VTE[5]	-	-	15%	10%
UFH with Dosages/Platelet Monitoring[5]	-	-	94%	97%
Venous Thromboembolism Prophylaxis[5]	-	-	70%	85%
Warfarin Therapy Discharge Instructions[5]	-	-	77%	75%
Chest Pain/Possible Heart Attack Care				
Aspirin Given Within 24 Hours of Arrival	-	-	94%	96%
Fibrinolytic Meds Within 30 Min. of Arrival	-	-	40%	58%
Average Time to ECG (minutes)	-	-	10	7
Average Time to Transfer (minutes)	-	-	77	60
Children's Asthma Care				
Received Home Management Plan of Care	-	-	-	88%
Received Reliever Medication	-	-	-	100%
Received Systemic Corticosteroids	-	-	-	100%
Emergency Department				
Admittance Decision Time (minutes)[2]	127	40	61	98
Head CT Results Within 45 Min. of Arrival	-	-	42%	57%
Patients Who Left ER Before Being Seen	-	-	3%	2%
Time from ER Arrival to Admit. (minutes)[2]	132	184	223	274
Time from ER Arrival to Discharge (minutes)	-	-	112	134
Time in ER Before Being Evaluated (minutes)	-	-	29	26
Time to Pain Meds for Fractures (minutes)	-	-	68	57
Heart Attack Care				
Aspirin Given at Discharge[5]	-	-	99%	99%
Fibrinolytic Meds Within 30 Min. of Arrival[5]	-	-	50%	54%
PCI Within 90 Minutes of Arrival[5]	-	-	96%	96%
Statin Prescribed at Discharge[5]	-	-	97%	98%
Heart Failure Care				
ACE Inhibitor or ARB for LVSD[1,2]	-	-	93%	97%
Discharge Instructions Given[2]	22	32%	91%	94%
Evaluation of LVS Function[2]	24	88%	96%	99%
Medicare Spending				
Medicare Spending per Patient (ratio)	-	-	0.95	0.98
Pneumonia Care				
Appropriate Initial Antibiotic Given[2]	21	71%	91%	95%
Blood Culture Timing[1,2]	-	-	97%	98%
Pregnancy and Delivery Care				
Newborn Deliveries Scheduled Early[3,7]	-	-	22%	6%
Preventive Care				
Immunization for Influenza[2]	110	33%	87%	90%
Immunization for Pneumonia[2]	191	49%	89%	92%
Stroke Care				
Anticoagulation Therapy for Atrial Fibrillation[3,7]	-	-	93%	95%
Antithrombotic Therapy Timing[3,7]	-	-	96%	98%
Assessed for Rehabilitation[1,3]	-	-	95%	97%
Discharged on Antithrombotic Therapy[3,7]	-	-	97%	99%
Discharged on Statin Medication[3,7]	-	-	88%	94%
Thrombolytic Therapy Timing[3,7]	-	-	25%	66%
Venous Thromboembolism Prophylaxis[1,3]	-	-	87%	94%
Written Stroke Educational Materials Given[1,3]	-	-	84%	88%
Surgical Care Improvement Project				
Appropriate Beta Blocker Usage[5]	-	-	97%	98%
Appropriate VTP Within 24 Hours[5]	-	-	97%	98%
Controlled Postoperative Blood Glucose[5]	-	-	97%	97%
Perioperative Temperature Management[5]	-	-	100%	100%
Prophylactic Antibiotic Selection[5]	-	-	99%	99%
Prophylactic Antibiotic Selection (Outpatient)	-	-	98%	98%
Prophylactic Antibiotic Stopped[5]	-	-	97%	98%
Prophylactic Antibiotic Timing[5]	-	-	99%	99%
Prophylactic Antibiotic Timing (Outpatient)	-	-	98%	98%
Urinary Catheter Removal[5]	-	-	97%	97%
Survey of Patients' Hospital Experiences				
Area Around Room 'Always' Quiet at Night[6]	<100	81%	72%	61%
Doctors 'Always' Communicated Well[6]	<100	93%	86%	82%
Home Recovery Information Given[6]	<100	85%	83%	85%
Hospital Given 9 or 10 on 10 Point Scale[6]	<100	79%	71%	71%
Meds 'Always' Explained Before Given[6]	<100	67%	67%	64%
Nurses 'Always' Communicated Well[6]	<100	86%	81%	79%
Pain 'Always' Well Controlled[6]	<100	68%	72%	71%
Room and Bathroom 'Always' Clean[6]	<100	81%	74%	73%
Timely Help 'Always' Received[6]	<100	82%	69%	68%
Would Definitely Recommend Hospital[6]	<100	68%	69%	71%
Use of Medical Imaging				
Cardiac Imaging Stress Test before Surgery	-	-	5.7%	5.3%
Combination Abdominal CT Scan	-	-	12.9%	10.5%
Combination Brain/Sinus CT Scan	-	-	3.3%	2.7%
Combination Chest CT Scan	-	-	6.1%	2.7%
Follow-up Mammogram/Ultrasound	-	-	8.4%	8.8%
Lumbar Spine MRI for Low Back Pain	-	-	41.1%	37.2%

H C Watkins Memorial Hospital

605 South Archusa Avenue
Quitman, MS 39355
Phone: 601-776-6925
Fax: 601-776-7158
Type: Critical Access Hospitals
Emergency Services: Yes
Ownership: Voluntary non-profit - Private
Beds: 32

Key Personnel:
Emergency Room . . . . OW Byrd, MD
CEO/President. . . . . Fred Truesdale
Chief of Medical Staff . . . . IV Zamora, MD

Measure	Cases	This Hosp.	State Avg.	U.S. Avg.
Blood Clot Prevention and Treatment				
Anticoagulation Overlap Therapy[5]	-	-	86%	93%
ICU Venous Thromboembolism Prophylaxis[5]	-	-	86%	92%
Incidence of Potentially Preventable VTE[5]	-	-	15%	10%
UFH with Dosages/Platelet Monitoring[5]	-	-	94%	97%
Venous Thromboembolism Prophylaxis[5]	-	-	70%	85%
Warfarin Therapy Discharge Instructions[5]	-	-	77%	75%
Chest Pain/Possible Heart Attack Care				
Aspirin Given Within 24 Hours of Arrival	41	71%	94%	96%
Fibrinolytic Meds Within 30 Min. of Arrival[7]	-	-	40%	58%
Average Time to ECG (minutes)	41	6	10	7
Average Time to Transfer (minutes)[1]	-	-	77	60
Children's Asthma Care				
Received Home Management Plan of Care	-	-	-	88%
Received Reliever Medication	-	-	-	100%
Received Systemic Corticosteroids	-	-	-	100%
Emergency Department				
Admittance Decision Time (minutes)[5]	-	-	61	98
Head CT Results Within 45 Min. of Arrival[5]	-	-	42%	57%
Patients Who Left ER Before Being Seen	4,933	4%	3%	2%
Time from ER Arrival to Admit. (minutes)[5]	-	-	223	274
Time from ER Arrival to Discharge (minutes)[5]	-	-	112	134
Time in ER Before Being Evaluated (minutes)[5]	-	-	29	26
Time to Pain Meds for Fractures (minutes)[5]	-	-	68	57
Heart Attack Care				
Aspirin Given at Discharge[5]	-	-	99%	99%
Fibrinolytic Meds Within 30 Min. of Arrival[5]	-	-	50%	54%
PCI Within 90 Minutes of Arrival[5]	-	-	96%	96%
Statin Prescribed at Discharge[5]	-	-	97%	98%
Heart Failure Care				
ACE Inhibitor or ARB for LVSD[1]	-	-	93%	97%
Discharge Instructions Given[1]	-	-	91%	94%
Evaluation of LVS Function	12	75%	96%	99%
Medicare Spending				
Medicare Spending per Patient (ratio)	-	-	0.95	0.98
Pneumonia Care				
Appropriate Initial Antibiotic Given[1]	-	-	91%	95%
Blood Culture Timing	11	100%	97%	98%
Pregnancy and Delivery Care				
Newborn Deliveries Scheduled Early[5]	-	-	22%	6%
Preventive Care				
Immunization for Influenza[5]	-	-	87%	90%
Immunization for Pneumonia[5]	-	-	89%	92%
Stroke Care				
Anticoagulation Therapy for Atrial Fibrillation[5]	-	-	93%	95%
Antithrombotic Therapy Timing[5]	-	-	96%	98%
Assessed for Rehabilitation[5]	-	-	95%	97%
Discharged on Antithrombotic Therapy[5]	-	-	97%	99%
Discharged on Statin Medication[5]	-	-	88%	94%
Thrombolytic Therapy Timing[5]	-	-	25%	66%
Venous Thromboembolism Prophylaxis[5]	-	-	87%	94%
Written Stroke Educational Materials Given[5]	-	-	84%	88%
Surgical Care Improvement Project				
Appropriate Beta Blocker Usage[5]	-	-	97%	98%
Appropriate VTP Within 24 Hours[5]	-	-	97%	98%
Controlled Postoperative Blood Glucose[5]	-	-	97%	97%
Perioperative Temperature Management[5]	-	-	100%	100%
Prophylactic Antibiotic Selection[5]	-	-	99%	99%
Prophylactic Antibiotic Selection (Outpatient)[5]	-	-	98%	98%
Prophylactic Antibiotic Stopped[5]	-	-	97%	98%
Prophylactic Antibiotic Timing[5]	-	-	99%	99%
Prophylactic Antibiotic Timing (Outpatient)[5]	-	-	98%	98%
Urinary Catheter Removal[5]	-	-	97%	97%
Survey of Patients' Hospital Experiences				
Area Around Room 'Always' Quiet at Night[10]	<100	80%	72%	61%
Doctors 'Always' Communicated Well[10]	<100	93%	86%	82%
Home Recovery Information Given[10]	<100	85%	83%	85%
Hospital Given 9 or 10 on 10 Point Scale[10]	<100	72%	71%	71%
Meds 'Always' Explained Before Given[10]	<100	75%	67%	64%
Nurses 'Always' Communicated Well[10]	<100	79%	81%	79%
Pain 'Always' Well Controlled[10]	<100	72%	72%	71%
Room and Bathroom 'Always' Clean[10]	<100	69%	74%	73%
Timely Help 'Always' Received[10]	<100	77%	69%	68%
Would Definitely Recommend Hospital[10]	<100	71%	69%	71%
Use of Medical Imaging				
Cardiac Imaging Stress Test before Surgery[1]	-	-	5.7%	5.3%
Combination Abdominal CT Scan	92	10.9%	12.9%	10.5%

NOTE: Hospital profiles are in alphabetical order by state, then city, then hospital within the city; Rankings exclude hospitals with less than 25 cases except for patient surveys which excludes hospitals with less than 100 cases; (a) 100-299 cases; (1) The number of cases/patients is too few to report; (2) Data submitted were based on a sample of cases/patients; (3) Results are based on a shorter time period than required; (4) Data suppressed by CMS for one or more quarters; (5) Results are not available for this reporting period; (6) Fewer than 100 patients completed the HCAHPS survey; (7) No cases met the criteria for this measure; (8) The lower limit of the confidence interval cannot be calculated if the number of observed infections equals zero; (9) No data are available from the state/territory for this reporting period; (10) The scores shown reflect fewer than 50 completed surveys; (11) There were discrepancies in the data collection process; (12) This measure does not apply to this hospital for this reporting period; (13) Results cannot be calculated for this reporting period; (14) The results for this state are combined with nearby states to protect confidentiality; Please refer to the User's Guide for a full explanation of data.

Measure	Cases	This Hosp.	State Avg.	U.S. Avg.
Combination Brain/Sinus CT Scan[1]	-	-	3.3%	2.7%
Combination Chest CT Scan[1]	-	-	6.1%	2.7%
Follow-up Mammogram/Ultrasound[7]	-	-	8.4%	8.8%
Lumbar Spine MRI for Low Back Pain[1]	-	-	41.1%	37.2%

Patients Choice Medical Center

347 Magnolia Drive — Phone: 601-782-9997
Raleigh, MS 39153
Type: Acute Care Hospitals — Emergency Services: No
Ownership: Proprietary

Measure	Cases	This Hosp.	State Avg.	U.S. Avg.
Blood Clot Prevention and Treatment				
Anticoagulation Overlap Therapy[5]	-	-	86%	93%
ICU Venous Thromboembolism Prophylaxis[5]	-	-	86%	92%
Incidence of Potentially Preventable VTE[5]	-	-	15%	10%
UFH with Dosages/Platelet Monitoring[5]	-	-	94%	97%
Venous Thromboembolism Prophylaxis[5]	-	-	70%	85%
Warfarin Therapy Discharge Instructions[5]	-	-	77%	75%
Chest Pain/Possible Heart Attack Care				
Aspirin Given Within 24 Hours of Arrival[5]	-	-	94%	96%
Fibrinolytic Meds Within 30 Min. of Arrival[5]	-	-	40%	58%
Average Time to ECG (minutes)[5]	-	-	10	7
Average Time to Transfer (minutes)[5]	-	-	77	60
Children's Asthma Care				
Received Home Management Plan of Care	-	-	-	88%
Received Reliever Medication	-	-	-	100%
Received Systemic Corticosteroids	-	-	-	100%
Emergency Department				
Admittance Decision Time (minutes)[5]	-	-	61	98
Head CT Results Within 45 Min. of Arrival[5]	-	-	42%	57%
Patients Who Left ER Before Being Seen[5]	-	-	3%	2%
Time from ER Arrival to Admit. (minutes)[5]	-	-	223	274
Time from ER Arrival to Discharge (minutes)[5]	-	-	112	134
Time in ER Before Being Evaluated (minutes)[5]	-	-	29	26
Time to Pain Meds for Fractures (minutes)[5]	-	-	68	57
Heart Attack Care				
Aspirin Given at Discharge[5]	-	-	99%	99%
Fibrinolytic Meds Within 30 Min. of Arrival[5]	-	-	50%	54%
PCI Within 90 Minutes of Arrival[5]	-	-	96%	96%
Statin Prescribed at Discharge[5]	-	-	97%	98%
Heart Failure Care				
ACE Inhibitor or ARB for LVSD[5]	-	-	93%	97%
Discharge Instructions Given[5]	-	-	91%	94%
Evaluation of LVS Function[5]	-	-	96%	99%
Medicare Spending				
Medicare Spending per Patient (ratio)	-	-	0.95	0.98
Pneumonia Care				
Appropriate Initial Antibiotic Given[5]	-	-	91%	95%
Blood Culture Timing[5]	-	-	97%	98%
Pregnancy and Delivery Care				
Newborn Deliveries Scheduled Early[2,3]	-	-	22%	6%
Preventive Care				
Immunization for Influenza[5]	-	-	87%	90%
Immunization for Pneumonia[5]	-	-	89%	92%
Stroke Care				
Anticoagulation Therapy for Atrial Fibrillation[5]	-	-	93%	95%
Antithrombotic Therapy Timing[5]	-	-	96%	98%
Assessed for Rehabilitation[5]	-	-	95%	97%
Discharged on Antithrombotic Therapy[5]	-	-	97%	99%
Discharged on Statin Medication[5]	-	-	88%	94%
Thrombolytic Therapy Timing[5]	-	-	25%	66%
Venous Thromboembolism Prophylaxis[5]	-	-	87%	94%
Written Stroke Educational Materials Given[5]	-	-	84%	88%
Surgical Care Improvement Project				
Appropriate Beta Blocker Usage[5]	-	-	97%	98%
Appropriate VTP Within 24 Hours[5]	-	-	97%	98%
Controlled Postoperative Blood Glucose[5]	-	-	97%	97%
Perioperative Temperature Management[5]	-	-	100%	100%
Prophylactic Antibiotic Selection[5]	-	-	99%	99%
Prophylactic Antibiotic Selection (Outpatient)[5]	-	-	98%	98%
Prophylactic Antibiotic Stopped[5]	-	-	97%	98%
Prophylactic Antibiotic Timing[5]	-	-	99%	99%
Prophylactic Antibiotic Timing (Outpatient)[5]	-	-	98%	98%
Urinary Catheter Removal[5]	-	-	97%	97%
Survey of Patients' Hospital Experiences				
Area Around Room 'Always' Quiet at Night[1]	-	-	72%	61%
Doctors 'Always' Communicated Well[1]	-	-	86%	82%
Home Recovery Information Given[1]	-	-	83%	85%
Hospital Given 9 or 10 on 10 Point Scale[1]	-	-	71%	71%
Meds 'Always' Explained Before Given[1]	-	-	67%	64%
Nurses 'Always' Communicated Well[1]	-	-	81%	79%
Pain 'Always' Well Controlled[1]	-	-	72%	71%
Room and Bathroom 'Always' Clean[1]	-	-	74%	73%
Timely Help 'Always' Received[1]	-	-	69%	68%
Would Definitely Recommend Hospital[1]	-	-	69%	71%
Use of Medical Imaging				
Cardiac Imaging Stress Test before Surgery[7]	-	-	5.7%	5.3%
Combination Abdominal CT Scan[7]	-	-	12.9%	10.5%
Combination Brain/Sinus CT Scan[7]	-	-	3.3%	2.7%
Combination Chest CT Scan[7]	-	-	6.1%	2.7%
Follow-up Mammogram/Ultrasound[7]	-	-	8.4%	8.8%
Lumbar Spine MRI for Low Back Pain[7]	-	-	41.1%	37.2%

Perry County General Hospital

206 Bay St — Phone: 601-788-6316
Richton, MS 39476
Type: Critical Access Hospitals — Emergency Services: Yes
Ownership: Proprietary

Measure	Cases	This Hosp.	State Avg.	U.S. Avg.
Blood Clot Prevention and Treatment				
Anticoagulation Overlap Therapy[5]	-	-	86%	93%
ICU Venous Thromboembolism Prophylaxis[5]	-	-	86%	92%
Incidence of Potentially Preventable VTE[5]	-	-	15%	10%
UFH with Dosages/Platelet Monitoring[5]	-	-	94%	97%
Venous Thromboembolism Prophylaxis[5]	-	-	70%	85%
Warfarin Therapy Discharge Instructions[5]	-	-	77%	75%
Chest Pain/Possible Heart Attack Care				
Aspirin Given Within 24 Hours of Arrival	14	93%	94%	96%
Fibrinolytic Meds Within 30 Min. of Arrival[1]	-	-	40%	58%
Average Time to ECG (minutes)	15	6	10	7
Average Time to Transfer (minutes)[7]	-	-	77	60
Children's Asthma Care				
Received Home Management Plan of Care	-	-	-	88%
Received Reliever Medication	-	-	-	100%
Received Systemic Corticosteroids	-	-	-	100%
Emergency Department				
Admittance Decision Time (minutes)[5]	-	-	61	98
Head CT Results Within 45 Min. of Arrival[1,3]	-	-	42%	57%
Patients Who Left ER Before Being Seen	2,835	1%	3%	2%
Time from ER Arrival to Admit. (minutes)[5]	-	-	223	274
Time from ER Arrival to Discharge (minutes)	229	80	112	134
Time in ER Before Being Evaluated (minutes)	247	10	29	26
Time to Pain Meds for Fractures (minutes)[1]	-	-	68	57
Heart Attack Care				
Aspirin Given at Discharge[3,7]	-	-	99%	99%
Fibrinolytic Meds Within 30 Min. of Arrival[3,7]	-	-	50%	54%
PCI Within 90 Minutes of Arrival[3,7]	-	-	96%	96%
Statin Prescribed at Discharge[3,7]	-	-	97%	98%
Heart Failure Care				
ACE Inhibitor or ARB for LVSD[2,7]	-	-	93%	97%
Discharge Instructions Given[1,2]	-	-	91%	94%
Evaluation of LVS Function[1,2]	-	-	96%	99%
Medicare Spending				
Medicare Spending per Patient (ratio)	-	-	0.95	0.98
Pneumonia Care				
Appropriate Initial Antibiotic Given	17	94%	91%	95%
Blood Culture Timing[1]	-	-	97%	98%
Pregnancy and Delivery Care				
Newborn Deliveries Scheduled Early[7]	-	-	22%	6%
Preventive Care				
Immunization for Influenza[5]	-	-	87%	90%
Immunization for Pneumonia[5]	-	-	89%	92%
Stroke Care				
Anticoagulation Therapy for Atrial Fibrillation[3,7]	-	-	93%	95%
Antithrombotic Therapy Timing[1,3]	-	-	96%	98%
Assessed for Rehabilitation[1,3]	-	-	95%	97%
Discharged on Antithrombotic Therapy[1,3]	-	-	97%	99%
Discharged on Statin Medication[1,3]	-	-	88%	94%
Thrombolytic Therapy Timing[3,7]	-	-	25%	66%
Venous Thromboembolism Prophylaxis[1,3]	-	-	87%	94%
Written Stroke Educational Materials Given[3,7]	-	-	84%	88%
Surgical Care Improvement Project				
Appropriate Beta Blocker Usage[5]	-	-	97%	98%
Appropriate VTP Within 24 Hours[5]	-	-	97%	98%
Controlled Postoperative Blood Glucose[5]	-	-	97%	97%
Perioperative Temperature Management[5]	-	-	100%	100%
Prophylactic Antibiotic Selection[5]	-	-	99%	99%
Prophylactic Antibiotic Selection (Outpatient)[5]	-	-	98%	98%
Prophylactic Antibiotic Stopped[5]	-	-	97%	98%
Prophylactic Antibiotic Timing[5]	-	-	99%	99%
Prophylactic Antibiotic Timing (Outpatient)[5]	-	-	98%	98%
Urinary Catheter Removal[5]	-	-	97%	97%
Survey of Patients' Hospital Experiences				
Area Around Room 'Always' Quiet at Night[10]	<100	79%	72%	61%
Doctors 'Always' Communicated Well[10]	<100	89%	86%	82%
Home Recovery Information Given[10]	<100	83%	83%	85%
Hospital Given 9 or 10 on 10 Point Scale[10]	<100	68%	71%	71%
Meds 'Always' Explained Before Given[10]	<100	72%	67%	64%
Nurses 'Always' Communicated Well[10]	<100	85%	81%	79%
Pain 'Always' Well Controlled[10]	<100	69%	72%	71%
Room and Bathroom 'Always' Clean[10]	<100	78%	74%	73%
Timely Help 'Always' Received[10]	<100	75%	69%	68%
Would Definitely Recommend Hospital[10]	<100	62%	69%	71%
Use of Medical Imaging				
Cardiac Imaging Stress Test before Surgery[7]	-	-	5.7%	5.3%
Combination Abdominal CT Scan[1]	-	-	12.9%	10.5%
Combination Brain/Sinus CT Scan	99	0.0%	3.3%	2.7%
Combination Chest CT Scan[1]	-	-	6.1%	2.7%
Follow-up Mammogram/Ultrasound[7]	-	-	8.4%	8.8%
Lumbar Spine MRI for Low Back Pain[7]	-	-	41.1%	37.2%

Tippah County Hospital

1005 Hwy 15 N — Phone: 662-837-9221
Ripley, MS 38663 — Fax: 662-837-2110
Type: Acute Care Hospitals — Emergency Services: Yes
Ownership: Government - Local — Beds: 110

Key Personnel:
Emergency Room . . . . Pam Bates, RN, DON
Intensive Care Unit. . . . . Pam Bates, RN
Chief of Medical Staff. . . . . Charles M Elliot, MD
Infection Control. . . . . Joey Gray, RN
Radiology. . . . . Linda Tomaszewski, RRT
Quality Assurance . . . . Margaret Weeks

Measure	Cases	This Hosp.	State Avg.	U.S. Avg.
Blood Clot Prevention and Treatment				
Anticoagulation Overlap Therapy[1,2]	-	-	86%	93%
ICU Venous Thromboembolism Prophylaxis[2,3]	-	-	86%	92%
Incidence of Potentially Preventable VTE[2,3]	-	-	15%	10%
UFH with Dosages/Platelet Monitoring[2,3]	-	-	94%	97%
Venous Thromboembolism Prophylaxis[2,3]	88	25%	70%	85%
Warfarin Therapy Discharge Instructions[1,2]	-	-	77%	75%
Chest Pain/Possible Heart Attack Care				
Aspirin Given Within 24 Hours of Arrival	31	90%	94%	96%
Fibrinolytic Meds Within 30 Min. of Arrival[1]	-	-	40%	58%
Average Time to ECG (minutes)	30	8	10	7
Average Time to Transfer (minutes)[1]	-	-	77	60
Children's Asthma Care				
Received Home Management Plan of Care	-	-	-	88%
Received Reliever Medication	-	-	-	100%
Received Systemic Corticosteroids	-	-	-	100%
Emergency Department				
Admittance Decision Time (minutes)[2]	126	72	61	98
Head CT Results Within 45 Min. of Arrival[3,7]	-	-	42%	57%
Patients Who Left ER Before Being Seen[5]	-	-	3%	2%
Time from ER Arrival to Admit. (minutes)[2]	168	208	223	274
Time from ER Arrival to Discharge (minutes)	364	111	112	134
Time in ER Before Being Evaluated (minutes)	377	30	29	26

NOTE: Hospital profiles are in alphabetical order by state, then city, then hospital within the city; Rankings exclude hospitals with less than 25 cases except for patient surveys which excludes hospitals with less than 100 cases; (a) 100-299 cases; (1) The number of cases/patients is too few to report; (2) Data submitted were based on a sample of cases/patients; (3) Results are based on a shorter time period than required; (4) Data suppressed by CMS for one or more quarters; (5) Results are not available for this reporting period; (6) Fewer than 100 patients completed the HCAHPS survey; (7) No cases met the criteria for this measure; (8) The lower limit of the confidence interval cannot be calculated if the number of observed infections equals zero; (9) No data are available from the state/territory for this reporting period; (10) The scores shown reflect fewer than 50 completed surveys; (11) There were discrepancies in the data collection process; (12) This measure does not apply to this hospital for this reporting period; (13) Results cannot be calculated for this reporting period; (14) The results for this state are combined with nearby states to protect confidentiality; Please refer to the User's Guide for a full explanation of data.

Measure	Cases	This Hosp.	State Avg.	U.S. Avg.
Time to Pain Meds for Fractures (minutes)	34	56	68	57
Heart Attack Care				
Aspirin Given at Discharge[1,3]	-	-	99%	99%
Fibrinolytic Meds Within 30 Min. of Arrival[3,7]	-	-	50%	54%
PCI Within 90 Minutes of Arrival[3,7]	-	-	96%	96%
Statin Prescribed at Discharge[1,3]	-	-	97%	98%
Heart Failure Care				
ACE Inhibitor or ARB for LVSD[1]	-	-	93%	97%
Discharge Instructions Given	15	53%	91%	94%
Evaluation of LVS Function	25	44%	96%	99%
Medicare Spending				
Medicare Spending per Patient (ratio)	-	0.95	0.95	0.98
Pneumonia Care				
Appropriate Initial Antibiotic Given	33	76%	91%	95%
Blood Culture Timing	31	90%	97%	98%
Pregnancy and Delivery Care				
Newborn Deliveries Scheduled Early[7]	-	-	22%	6%
Preventive Care				
Immunization for Influenza[2]	216	87%	87%	90%
Immunization for Pneumonia[2]	369	91%	89%	92%
Stroke Care				
Anticoagulation Therapy for Atrial Fibrillation[1,3]	-	-	93%	95%
Antithrombotic Therapy Timing[1,3]	-	-	96%	98%
Assessed for Rehabilitation[1,3]	-	-	95%	97%
Discharged on Antithrombotic Therapy[1,3]	-	-	97%	99%
Discharged on Statin Medication[1,3]	-	-	88%	94%
Thrombolytic Therapy Timing[3,7]	-	-	25%	66%
Venous Thromboembolism Prophylaxis[1,3]	-	-	87%	94%
Written Stroke Educational Materials Given[1,3]	-	-	84%	88%
Surgical Care Improvement Project				
Appropriate Beta Blocker Usage[5]	-	-	97%	98%
Appropriate VTP Within 24 Hours[5]	-	-	97%	98%
Controlled Postoperative Blood Glucose[5]	-	-	97%	97%
Perioperative Temperature Management[5]	-	-	100%	100%
Prophylactic Antibiotic Selection[5]	-	-	99%	99%
Prophylactic Antibiotic Selection (Outpatient)[5]	-	-	98%	98%
Prophylactic Antibiotic Stopped[5]	-	-	97%	98%
Prophylactic Antibiotic Timing[5]	-	-	99%	99%
Prophylactic Antibiotic Timing (Outpatient)[5]	-	-	98%	98%
Urinary Catheter Removal[5]	-	-	97%	97%
Survey of Patients' Hospital Experiences				
Area Around Room 'Always' Quiet at Night[6]	<100	77%	72%	61%
Doctors 'Always' Communicated Well[6]	<100	92%	86%	82%
Home Recovery Information Given[6]	<100	76%	83%	85%
Hospital Given 9 or 10 on 10 Point Scale[6]	<100	65%	71%	71%
Meds 'Always' Explained Before Given[6]	<100	62%	67%	64%
Nurses 'Always' Communicated Well[6]	<100	83%	81%	79%
Pain 'Always' Well Controlled[6]	<100	73%	72%	71%
Room and Bathroom 'Always' Clean[6]	<100	84%	74%	73%
Timely Help 'Always' Received[6]	<100	80%	69%	68%
Would Definitely Recommend Hospital[6]	<100	56%	69%	71%
Use of Medical Imaging				
Cardiac Imaging Stress Test before Surgery[7]	-	-	5.7%	5.3%
Combination Abdominal CT Scan	209	2.4%	12.9%	10.5%
Combination Brain/Sinus CT Scan[1]	-	-	3.3%	2.7%
Combination Chest CT Scan	65	0.0%	6.1%	2.7%
Follow-up Mammogram/Ultrasound	156	9.0%	8.4%	8.8%
Lumbar Spine MRI for Low Back Pain[7]	-	-	41.1%	37.2%

Sharkey Issaquena Community Hospital

47 South 4 St
Rolling Fork, MS 39159
Phone: 662-873-4395
Type: Acute Care Hospitals
Ownership: Government - Local
Emergency Services: Yes
Beds: 29

Key Personnel:
CEO/President. . . . . Jerry Keever

Measure	Cases	This Hosp.	State Avg.	U.S. Avg.
Blood Clot Prevention and Treatment				
Anticoagulation Overlap Therapy[5]	-	-	86%	93%
ICU Venous Thromboembolism Prophylaxis[5]	-	-	86%	92%
Incidence of Potentially Preventable VTE[5]	-	-	15%	10%
UFH with Dosages/Platelet Monitoring[5]	-	-	94%	97%
Venous Thromboembolism Prophylaxis[5]	-	-	70%	85%
Warfarin Therapy Discharge Instructions[5]	-	-	77%	75%
Chest Pain/Possible Heart Attack Care				
Aspirin Given Within 24 Hours of Arrival[5]	-	-	94%	96%
Fibrinolytic Meds Within 30 Min. of Arrival[5]	-	-	40%	58%
Average Time to ECG (minutes)[5]	-	-	10	7
Average Time to Transfer (minutes)[5]	-	-	77	60
Children's Asthma Care				
Received Home Management Plan of Care	-	-	-	88%
Received Reliever Medication	-	-	-	100%
Received Systemic Corticosteroids	-	-	-	100%
Emergency Department				
Admittance Decision Time (minutes)[5]	-	-	61	98
Head CT Results Within 45 Min. of Arrival[5]	-	-	42%	57%
Patients Who Left ER Before Being Seen[5]	-	-	3%	2%
Time from ER Arrival to Admit. (minutes)[5]	-	-	223	274
Time from ER Arrival to Discharge (minutes)[5]	-	-	112	134
Time in ER Before Being Evaluated (minutes)[5]	-	-	29	26
Time to Pain Meds for Fractures (minutes)[5]	-	-	68	57
Heart Attack Care				
Aspirin Given at Discharge[2,3]	-	-	99%	99%
Fibrinolytic Meds Within 30 Min. of Arrival[2,3]	-	-	50%	54%
PCI Within 90 Minutes of Arrival[2,3]	-	-	96%	96%
Statin Prescribed at Discharge[2,3]	-	-	97%	98%
Heart Failure Care				
ACE Inhibitor or ARB for LVSD[1,2]	-	-	93%	97%
Discharge Instructions Given[1,2]	-	-	91%	94%
Evaluation of LVS Function[2]	16	0%	96%	99%
Medicare Spending				
Medicare Spending per Patient (ratio)	-	0.97	0.95	0.98
Pneumonia Care				
Appropriate Initial Antibiotic Given[2,7]	-	-	91%	95%
Blood Culture Timing[2,7]	-	-	97%	98%
Pregnancy and Delivery Care				
Newborn Deliveries Scheduled Early[3,7]	-	-	22%	6%
Preventive Care				
Immunization for Influenza[5]	-	-	87%	90%
Immunization for Pneumonia[5]	-	-	89%	92%
Stroke Care				
Anticoagulation Therapy for Atrial Fibrillation[5]	-	-	93%	95%
Antithrombotic Therapy Timing[5]	-	-	96%	98%
Assessed for Rehabilitation[5]	-	-	95%	97%
Discharged on Antithrombotic Therapy[5]	-	-	97%	99%
Discharged on Statin Medication[5]	-	-	88%	94%
Thrombolytic Therapy Timing[5]	-	-	25%	66%
Venous Thromboembolism Prophylaxis[5]	-	-	87%	94%
Written Stroke Educational Materials Given[5]	-	-	84%	88%
Surgical Care Improvement Project				
Appropriate Beta Blocker Usage[5]	-	-	97%	98%
Appropriate VTP Within 24 Hours[5]	-	-	97%	98%
Controlled Postoperative Blood Glucose[5]	-	-	97%	97%
Perioperative Temperature Management[5]	-	-	100%	100%
Prophylactic Antibiotic Selection[5]	-	-	99%	99%
Prophylactic Antibiotic Selection (Outpatient)[5]	-	-	98%	98%
Prophylactic Antibiotic Stopped[5]	-	-	97%	98%
Prophylactic Antibiotic Timing[5]	-	-	99%	99%
Prophylactic Antibiotic Timing (Outpatient)[5]	-	-	98%	98%
Urinary Catheter Removal[5]	-	-	97%	97%
Survey of Patients' Hospital Experiences				
Area Around Room 'Always' Quiet at Night[5]	-	-	72%	61%
Doctors 'Always' Communicated Well[5]	-	-	86%	82%
Home Recovery Information Given[5]	-	-	83%	85%
Hospital Given 9 or 10 on 10 Point Scale[5]	-	-	71%	71%
Meds 'Always' Explained Before Given[5]	-	-	67%	64%
Nurses 'Always' Communicated Well[5]	-	-	81%	79%
Pain 'Always' Well Controlled[5]	-	-	72%	71%
Room and Bathroom 'Always' Clean[5]	-	-	74%	73%
Timely Help 'Always' Received[5]	-	-	69%	68%
Would Definitely Recommend Hospital[5]	-	-	69%	71%
Use of Medical Imaging				
Cardiac Imaging Stress Test before Surgery[7]	-	-	5.7%	5.3%
Combination Abdominal CT Scan	64	59.4%	12.9%	10.5%
Combination Brain/Sinus CT Scan	89	12.4%	3.3%	2.7%
Combination Chest CT Scan[1]	-	-	6.1%	2.7%
Follow-up Mammogram/Ultrasound[7]	-	-	8.4%	8.8%
Lumbar Spine MRI for Low Back Pain[1]	-	-	41.1%	37.2%

North Sunflower Medical Center

840 North Oak Avenue/po Box 369
Ruleville, MS 38771
Phone: 662-756-2711
Fax: 662-756-4114
Type: Critical Access Hospitals
Ownership: Government - Local
Emergency Services: Yes
Beds: 92

Key Personnel:
Chief of Medical Staff. . . . . Adelo Aquino, MD
Infection Control. . . . . Mechelle Barnes
CEO/President. . . . . Billy Marlow

Measure	Cases	This Hosp.	State Avg.	U.S. Avg.
Blood Clot Prevention and Treatment				
Anticoagulation Overlap Therapy[5]	-	-	86%	93%
ICU Venous Thromboembolism Prophylaxis[5]	-	-	86%	92%
Incidence of Potentially Preventable VTE[5]	-	-	15%	10%
UFH with Dosages/Platelet Monitoring[5]	-	-	94%	97%
Venous Thromboembolism Prophylaxis[5]	-	-	70%	85%
Warfarin Therapy Discharge Instructions[5]	-	-	77%	75%
Chest Pain/Possible Heart Attack Care				
Aspirin Given Within 24 Hours of Arrival[5]	-	-	94%	96%
Fibrinolytic Meds Within 30 Min. of Arrival[5]	-	-	40%	58%
Average Time to ECG (minutes)[5]	-	-	10	7
Average Time to Transfer (minutes)[5]	-	-	77	60
Children's Asthma Care				
Received Home Management Plan of Care	-	-	-	88%
Received Reliever Medication	-	-	-	100%
Received Systemic Corticosteroids	-	-	-	100%
Emergency Department				
Admittance Decision Time (minutes)[5]	-	-	61	98
Head CT Results Within 45 Min. of Arrival[3,7]	-	-	42%	57%
Patients Who Left ER Before Being Seen	5,365	0%	3%	2%
Time from ER Arrival to Admit. (minutes)[5]	-	-	223	274
Time from ER Arrival to Discharge (minutes)[5]	-	-	112	134
Time in ER Before Being Evaluated (minutes)[5]	-	-	29	26
Time to Pain Meds for Fractures (minutes)[1,3]	-	-	68	57
Heart Attack Care				
Aspirin Given at Discharge[5]	-	-	99%	99%
Fibrinolytic Meds Within 30 Min. of Arrival[5]	-	-	50%	54%
PCI Within 90 Minutes of Arrival[5]	-	-	96%	96%
Statin Prescribed at Discharge[5]	-	-	97%	98%
Heart Failure Care				
ACE Inhibitor or ARB for LVSD[1]	-	-	93%	97%
Discharge Instructions Given	29	90%	91%	94%
Evaluation of LVS Function	49	96%	96%	99%
Medicare Spending				
Medicare Spending per Patient (ratio)	-	-	0.95	0.98
Pneumonia Care				
Appropriate Initial Antibiotic Given	35	89%	91%	95%
Blood Culture Timing	51	75%	97%	98%
Pregnancy and Delivery Care				
Newborn Deliveries Scheduled Early[5]	-	-	22%	6%
Preventive Care				
Immunization for Influenza[5]	-	-	87%	90%
Immunization for Pneumonia[5]	-	-	89%	92%
Stroke Care				
Anticoagulation Therapy for Atrial Fibrillation[5]	-	-	93%	95%
Antithrombotic Therapy Timing[5]	-	-	96%	98%
Assessed for Rehabilitation[5]	-	-	95%	97%
Discharged on Antithrombotic Therapy[5]	-	-	97%	99%
Discharged on Statin Medication[5]	-	-	88%	94%
Thrombolytic Therapy Timing[5]	-	-	25%	66%
Venous Thromboembolism Prophylaxis[5]	-	-	87%	94%
Written Stroke Educational Materials Given[5]	-	-	84%	88%
Surgical Care Improvement Project				
Appropriate Beta Blocker Usage[5]	-	-	97%	98%
Appropriate VTP Within 24 Hours[5]	-	-	97%	98%
Controlled Postoperative Blood Glucose[5]	-	-	97%	97%
Perioperative Temperature Management[5]	-	-	100%	100%
Prophylactic Antibiotic Selection[5]	-	-	99%	99%

NOTE: Hospital profiles are in alphabetical order by state, then city, then hospital within the city; Rankings exclude hospitals with less than 25 cases except for patient surveys which excludes hospitals with less than 100 cases; (a) 100-299 cases; (1) The number of cases/patients is too few to report; (2) Data submitted were based on a sample of cases/patients; (3) Results are based on a shorter time period than required; (4) Data suppressed by CMS for one or more quarters; (5) Results are not available for this reporting period; (6) Fewer than 100 patients completed the HCAHPS survey; (7) No cases met the criteria for this measure; (8) The lower limit of the confidence interval cannot be calculated if the number of observed infections equals zero; (9) No data are available from the state/territory for this reporting period; (10) The scores shown reflect fewer than 50 completed surveys; (11) There were discrepancies in the data collection process; (12) This measure does not apply to this hospital for this reporting period; (13) Results cannot be calculated for this reporting period; (14) The results for this state are combined with nearby states to protect confidentiality; Please refer to the User's Guide for a full explanation of data.

Measure	Cases	This Hosp.	State Avg.	U.S. Avg.
Prophylactic Antibiotic Selection (Outpatient)[5]	-	-	98%	98%
Prophylactic Antibiotic Stopped[5]	-	-	97%	98%
Prophylactic Antibiotic Timing[5]	-	-	99%	99%
Prophylactic Antibiotic Timing (Outpatient)[5]	-	-	98%	98%
Urinary Catheter Removal[5]	-	-	97%	97%
Survey of Patients' Hospital Experiences				
Area Around Room 'Always' Quiet at Night[10]	<100	43%	72%	61%
Doctors 'Always' Communicated Well[10]	<100	88%	86%	82%
Home Recovery Information Given[10]	<100	93%	83%	85%
Hospital Given 9 or 10 on 10 Point Scale[10]	<100	89%	71%	71%
Meds 'Always' Explained Before Given[10]	<100	36%	67%	64%
Nurses 'Always' Communicated Well[10]	<100	84%	81%	79%
Pain 'Always' Well Controlled[10]	<100	77%	72%	71%
Room and Bathroom 'Always' Clean[10]	<100	98%	74%	73%
Timely Help 'Always' Received[10]	<100	72%	69%	68%
Would Definitely Recommend Hospital[10]	<100	89%	69%	71%
Use of Medical Imaging				
Cardiac Imaging Stress Test before Surgery[1]	-	-	5.7%	5.3%
Combination Abdominal CT Scan	207	30.4%	12.9%	10.5%
Combination Brain/Sinus CT Scan[1]	-	-	3.3%	2.7%
Combination Chest CT Scan[1]	-	-	6.1%	2.7%
Follow-up Mammogram/Ultrasound[7]	-	-	8.4%	8.8%
Lumbar Spine MRI for Low Back Pain[1]	-	-	41.1%	37.2%

North Oak Regional Medical Center

401 Getwell Dr
Senatobia, MS 38668
Phone: 662-562-3100
Fax: 662-560-6295
Type: Acute Care Hospitals
Emergency Services: Yes
Ownership: Proprietary
Beds: 76

Key Personnel:
Radiology. . . . . Vicki Wright

Measure	Cases	This Hosp.	State Avg.	U.S. Avg.
Blood Clot Prevention and Treatment				
Anticoagulation Overlap Therapy[1,2]	-	-	86%	93%
ICU Venous Thromboembolism Prophylaxis[2,7]	-	-	86%	92%
Incidence of Potentially Preventable VTE[2,7]	-	-	15%	10%
UFH with Dosages/Platelet Monitoring[2,7]	-	-	94%	97%
Venous Thromboembolism Prophylaxis[2]	280	72%	70%	85%
Warfarin Therapy Discharge Instructions[1,2]	-	-	77%	75%
Chest Pain/Possible Heart Attack Care				
Aspirin Given Within 24 Hours of Arrival	44	91%	94%	96%
Fibrinolytic Meds Within 30 Min. of Arrival[7]	-	-	40%	58%
Average Time to ECG (minutes)	46	11	10	7
Average Time to Transfer (minutes)[1]	-	-	77	60
Children's Asthma Care				
Received Home Management Plan of Care	-	-	-	88%
Received Reliever Medication	-	-	-	100%
Received Systemic Corticosteroids	-	-	-	100%
Emergency Department				
Admittance Decision Time (minutes)[2]	417	73	61	98
Head CT Results Within 45 Min. of Arrival[1]	-	-	42%	57%
Patients Who Left ER Before Being Seen	10,222	4%	3%	2%
Time from ER Arrival to Admit. (minutes)[2]	417	200	223	274
Time from ER Arrival to Discharge (minutes)	1,414	122	112	134
Time in ER Before Being Evaluated (minutes)	1,564	40	29	26
Time to Pain Meds for Fractures (minutes)	51	90	68	57
Heart Attack Care				
Aspirin Given at Discharge[1,3]	-	-	99%	99%
Fibrinolytic Meds Within 30 Min. of Arrival[3,7]	-	-	50%	54%
PCI Within 90 Minutes of Arrival[3,7]	-	-	96%	96%
Statin Prescribed at Discharge[1,3]	-	-	97%	98%
Heart Failure Care				
ACE Inhibitor or ARB for LVSD[1]	-	-	93%	97%
Discharge Instructions Given	22	91%	91%	94%
Evaluation of LVS Function	32	91%	96%	99%
Medicare Spending				
Medicare Spending per Patient (ratio)	-	0.94	0.95	0.98
Pneumonia Care				
Appropriate Initial Antibiotic Given	28	79%	91%	95%
Blood Culture Timing	32	88%	97%	98%
Pregnancy and Delivery Care				
Newborn Deliveries Scheduled Early[7]	-	-	22%	6%
Preventive Care				
Immunization for Influenza[2]	315	76%	87%	90%
Immunization for Pneumonia[2]	420	83%	89%	92%
Stroke Care				
Anticoagulation Therapy for Atrial Fibrillation[3,7]	-	-	93%	95%
Antithrombotic Therapy Timing[1,3]	-	-	96%	98%
Assessed for Rehabilitation[1,3]	-	-	95%	97%
Discharged on Antithrombotic Therapy[1,3]	-	-	97%	99%
Discharged on Statin Medication[3,7]	-	-	88%	94%
Thrombolytic Therapy Timing[3,7]	-	-	25%	66%
Venous Thromboembolism Prophylaxis[1,3]	-	-	87%	94%
Written Stroke Educational Materials Given[3,7]	-	-	84%	88%
Surgical Care Improvement Project				
Appropriate Beta Blocker Usage[1]	-	-	97%	98%
Appropriate VTP Within 24 Hours	30	83%	97%	98%
Controlled Postoperative Blood Glucose[7]	-	-	97%	97%
Perioperative Temperature Management	34	100%	100%	100%
Prophylactic Antibiotic Selection	26	96%	99%	99%
Prophylactic Antibiotic Selection (Outpatient)[3,7]	-	-	98%	98%
Prophylactic Antibiotic Stopped	24	83%	97%	98%
Prophylactic Antibiotic Timing	26	96%	99%	99%
Prophylactic Antibiotic Timing (Outpatient)[1,3]	-	-	98%	98%
Urinary Catheter Removal[1]	-	-	97%	97%
Survey of Patients' Hospital Experiences				
Area Around Room 'Always' Quiet at Night	(a)	73%	72%	61%
Doctors 'Always' Communicated Well	(a)	77%	86%	82%
Home Recovery Information Given	(a)	80%	83%	85%
Hospital Given 9 or 10 on 10 Point Scale	(a)	65%	71%	71%
Meds 'Always' Explained Before Given	(a)	62%	67%	64%
Nurses 'Always' Communicated Well	(a)	80%	81%	79%
Pain 'Always' Well Controlled	(a)	69%	72%	71%
Room and Bathroom 'Always' Clean	(a)	76%	74%	73%
Timely Help 'Always' Received	(a)	67%	69%	68%
Would Definitely Recommend Hospital	(a)	59%	69%	71%
Use of Medical Imaging				
Cardiac Imaging Stress Test before Surgery[7]	-	-	5.7%	5.3%
Combination Abdominal CT Scan	81	48.1%	12.9%	10.5%
Combination Brain/Sinus CT Scan	143	7.7%	3.3%	2.7%
Combination Chest CT Scan[1]	-	-	6.1%	2.7%
Follow-up Mammogram/Ultrasound[7]	-	-	8.4%	8.8%
Lumbar Spine MRI for Low Back Pain[7]	-	-	41.1%	37.2%

Baptist Memorial Hospital Desoto

7601 Southcrest Parkway
Southaven, MS 38671
Phone: 662-772-4000
Fax: 662-349-4570
URL: www.bmhcc.org/facilities/desoto
Type: Acute Care Hospitals
Emergency Services: Yes
Ownership: Voluntary non-profit - Private
Beds: 339

Key Personnel:
Chief of Medical Staff . . . . JoAnn Phillips Wood
CEO/President. . . . . James Russell Huffman
Emergency Room . . . . Stanley Thomson

Measure	Cases	This Hosp.	State Avg.	U.S. Avg.
Blood Clot Prevention and Treatment				
Anticoagulation Overlap Therapy[2]	132	97%	86%	93%
ICU Venous Thromboembolism Prophylaxis[2]	139	97%	86%	92%
Incidence of Potentially Preventable VTE[2]	14	0%	15%	10%
UFH with Dosages/Platelet Monitoring[2]	117	100%	94%	97%
Venous Thromboembolism Prophylaxis[2]	392	96%	70%	85%
Warfarin Therapy Discharge Instructions[2]	92	91%	77%	75%
Chest Pain/Possible Heart Attack Care				
Aspirin Given Within 24 Hours of Arrival[1]	-	-	94%	96%
Fibrinolytic Meds Within 30 Min. of Arrival[5]	-	-	40%	58%
Average Time to ECG (minutes)[1]	-	-	10	7
Average Time to Transfer (minutes)[5]	-	-	77	60
Children's Asthma Care				
Received Home Management Plan of Care	-	-	-	88%
Received Reliever Medication	-	-	-	100%
Received Systemic Corticosteroids	-	-	-	100%
Emergency Department				
Admittance Decision Time (minutes)[2]	522	70	61	98
Head CT Results Within 45 Min. of Arrival	40	52%	42%	57%
Patients Who Left ER Before Being Seen	63,833	2%	3%	2%
Time from ER Arrival to Admit. (minutes)[2]	541	324	223	274
Time from ER Arrival to Discharge (minutes)	337	235	112	134
Time in ER Before Being Evaluated (minutes)	398	76	29	26
Time to Pain Meds for Fractures (minutes)	190	86	68	57
Heart Attack Care				
Aspirin Given at Discharge	530	100%	99%	99%
Fibrinolytic Meds Within 30 Min. of Arrival[7]	-	-	50%	54%
PCI Within 90 Minutes of Arrival	67	99%	96%	96%
Statin Prescribed at Discharge	512	99%	97%	98%
Heart Failure Care				
ACE Inhibitor or ARB for LVSD	193	99%	93%	97%
Discharge Instructions Given	618	100%	91%	94%
Evaluation of LVS Function	740	100%	96%	99%
Medicare Spending				
Medicare Spending per Patient (ratio)	-	0.96	0.95	0.98
Pneumonia Care				
Appropriate Initial Antibiotic Given	350	98%	91%	95%
Blood Culture Timing	523	99%	97%	98%
Pregnancy and Delivery Care				
Newborn Deliveries Scheduled Early[2]	436	40%	22%	6%
Preventive Care				
Immunization for Influenza[2]	566	98%	87%	90%
Immunization for Pneumonia[2]	660	97%	89%	92%
Stroke Care				
Anticoagulation Therapy for Atrial Fibrillation	30	97%	93%	95%
Antithrombotic Therapy Timing	242	97%	96%	98%
Assessed for Rehabilitation	241	96%	95%	97%
Discharged on Antithrombotic Therapy	237	100%	97%	99%
Discharged on Statin Medication	200	96%	88%	94%
Thrombolytic Therapy Timing[1]	-	-	25%	66%
Venous Thromboembolism Prophylaxis	246	98%	87%	94%
Written Stroke Educational Materials Given	144	91%	84%	88%
Surgical Care Improvement Project				
Appropriate Beta Blocker Usage[2]	206	100%	97%	98%
Appropriate VTP Within 24 Hours[2]	332	97%	97%	98%
Controlled Postoperative Blood Glucose[2]	107	96%	97%	97%
Perioperative Temperature Management[2]	446	100%	100%	100%
Prophylactic Antibiotic Selection[2]	368	99%	99%	99%
Prophylactic Antibiotic Selection (Outpatient)	318	99%	98%	98%
Prophylactic Antibiotic Stopped[2]	349	97%	97%	98%
Prophylactic Antibiotic Timing[2]	370	99%	99%	99%
Prophylactic Antibiotic Timing (Outpatient)	318	99%	98%	98%
Urinary Catheter Removal[2]	224	94%	97%	97%
Survey of Patients' Hospital Experiences				
Area Around Room 'Always' Quiet at Night	300+	65%	72%	61%
Doctors 'Always' Communicated Well	300+	76%	86%	82%
Home Recovery Information Given	300+	80%	83%	85%
Hospital Given 9 or 10 on 10 Point Scale	300+	70%	71%	71%
Meds 'Always' Explained Before Given	300+	60%	67%	64%
Nurses 'Always' Communicated Well	300+	78%	81%	79%
Pain 'Always' Well Controlled	300+	68%	72%	71%
Room and Bathroom 'Always' Clean	300+	70%	74%	73%
Timely Help 'Always' Received	300+	58%	69%	68%
Would Definitely Recommend Hospital	300+	70%	69%	71%
Use of Medical Imaging				
Cardiac Imaging Stress Test before Surgery	1,462	5.6%	5.7%	5.3%
Combination Abdominal CT Scan	1,348	3.9%	12.9%	10.5%
Combination Brain/Sinus CT Scan	1,395	1.7%	3.3%	2.7%
Combination Chest CT Scan	726	1.8%	6.1%	2.7%
Follow-up Mammogram/Ultrasound	1,529	9.4%	8.4%	8.8%
Lumbar Spine MRI for Low Back Pain	164	37.2%	41.1%	37.2%

Och Regional Medical Center

400 Hospital Road
Starkville, MS 39759
Phone: 662-323-4320
Fax: 662-338-3345
URL: www.och.org
Type: Acute Care Hospitals
Emergency Services: Yes
Ownership: Government - Local
Beds: 96

Key Personnel:
Infection Control. . . . . Carolyn Arnold, RN
Chief of Medical Staff . . . . Linda Blake
Radiology. . . . . Michael Buehler
Quality Assurance . . . . Molly Fonderen
Administrator . . . . Richard Hilton
Operating Room. . . . . Pat Holmes, RN
CEO/President. . . . . Arthur C Kelly

NOTE: Hospital profiles are in alphabetical order by state, then city, then hospital within the city; Rankings exclude hospitals with less than 25 cases except for patient surveys which excludes hospitals with less than 100 cases; (a) 100-299 cases; (1) The number of cases/patients is too few to report; (2) Data submitted were based on a sample of cases/patients; (3) Results are based on a shorter time period than required; (4) Data suppressed by CMS for one or more quarters; (5) Results are not available for this reporting period; (6) Fewer than 100 patients completed the HCAHPS survey; (7) No cases met the criteria for this measure; (8) The lower limit of the confidence interval cannot be calculated if the number of observed infections equals zero; (9) No data are available from the state/territory for this reporting period; (10) The scores shown reflect fewer than 50 completed surveys; (11) There were discrepancies in the data collection process; (12) This measure does not apply to this hospital for this reporting period; (13) Results cannot be calculated for this reporting period; (14) The results for this state are combined with nearby states to protect confidentiality; Please refer to the User's Guide for a full explanation of data.

Cardiac Laboratory. . . . . Elizabeth Varco, RN

Measure	Cases	This Hosp.	State Avg.	U.S. Avg.
Blood Clot Prevention and Treatment				
Anticoagulation Overlap Therapy[2]	27	74%	86%	93%
ICU Venous Thromboembolism Prophylaxis[2]	34	53%	86%	92%
Incidence of Potentially Preventable VTE[1,2]	-	-	15%	10%
UFH with Dosages/Platelet Monitoring[1,2]	-	-	94%	97%
Venous Thromboembolism Prophylaxis[2]	123	39%	70%	85%
Warfarin Therapy Discharge Instructions[2]	19	89%	77%	75%
Chest Pain/Possible Heart Attack Care				
Aspirin Given Within 24 Hours of Arrival	60	95%	94%	96%
Fibrinolytic Meds Within 30 Min. of Arrival[1]	-	-	40%	58%
Average Time to ECG (minutes)	62	24	10	7
Average Time to Transfer (minutes)[1]	-	-	77	60
Children's Asthma Care				
Received Home Management Plan of Care	-	-	-	88%
Received Reliever Medication	-	-	-	100%
Received Systemic Corticosteroids	-	-	-	100%
Emergency Department				
Admittance Decision Time (minutes)[2]	151	56	61	98
Head CT Results Within 45 Min. of Arrival[1]	-	-	42%	57%
Patients Who Left ER Before Being Seen[5]	-	-	3%	2%
Time from ER Arrival to Admit. (minutes)[2]	151	182	223	274
Time from ER Arrival to Discharge (minutes)	439	107	112	134
Time in ER Before Being Evaluated (minutes)	453	60	29	26
Time to Pain Meds for Fractures (minutes)	68	64	68	57
Heart Attack Care				
Aspirin Given at Discharge[1]	-	-	99%	99%
Fibrinolytic Meds Within 30 Min. of Arrival[7]	-	-	50%	54%
PCI Within 90 Minutes of Arrival[7]	-	-	96%	96%
Statin Prescribed at Discharge[1]	-	-	97%	98%
Heart Failure Care				
ACE Inhibitor or ARB for LVSD	20	75%	93%	97%
Discharge Instructions Given	41	90%	91%	94%
Evaluation of LVS Function	49	98%	96%	99%
Medicare Spending				
Medicare Spending per Patient (ratio)	-	0.98	0.95	0.98
Pneumonia Care				
Appropriate Initial Antibiotic Given	65	91%	91%	95%
Blood Culture Timing	66	98%	97%	98%
Pregnancy and Delivery Care				
Newborn Deliveries Scheduled Early[2]	57	11%	22%	6%
Preventive Care				
Immunization for Influenza[2]	246	48%	87%	90%
Immunization for Pneumonia[2]	209	64%	89%	92%
Stroke Care				
Anticoagulation Therapy for Atrial Fibrillation[1]	-	-	93%	95%
Antithrombotic Therapy Timing	24	92%	96%	98%
Assessed for Rehabilitation	22	100%	95%	97%
Discharged on Antithrombotic Therapy	22	100%	97%	99%
Discharged on Statin Medication	20	80%	88%	94%
Thrombolytic Therapy Timing[1]	-	-	25%	66%
Venous Thromboembolism Prophylaxis	25	56%	87%	94%
Written Stroke Educational Materials Given	13	77%	84%	88%
Surgical Care Improvement Project				
Appropriate Beta Blocker Usage	48	73%	97%	98%
Appropriate VTP Within 24 Hours	206	88%	97%	98%
Controlled Postoperative Blood Glucose[7]	-	-	97%	97%
Perioperative Temperature Management	224	98%	100%	100%
Prophylactic Antibiotic Selection	147	98%	99%	99%
Prophylactic Antibiotic Selection (Outpatient)	158	89%	98%	98%
Prophylactic Antibiotic Stopped	142	92%	97%	98%
Prophylactic Antibiotic Timing	147	91%	99%	99%
Prophylactic Antibiotic Timing (Outpatient)	160	86%	98%	98%
Urinary Catheter Removal	143	97%	97%	97%
Survey of Patients' Hospital Experiences				
Area Around Room 'Always' Quiet at Night	300+	77%	72%	61%
Doctors 'Always' Communicated Well	300+	87%	86%	82%
Home Recovery Information Given	300+	85%	83%	85%
Hospital Given 9 or 10 on 10 Point Scale	300+	77%	71%	71%
Meds 'Always' Explained Before Given	300+	66%	67%	64%
Nurses 'Always' Communicated Well	300+	84%	81%	79%
Pain 'Always' Well Controlled	300+	76%	72%	71%
Room and Bathroom 'Always' Clean	300+	82%	74%	73%
Timely Help 'Always' Received	300+	74%	69%	68%
Would Definitely Recommend Hospital	300+	75%	69%	71%
Use of Medical Imaging				
Cardiac Imaging Stress Test before Surgery[1]	-	-	5.7%	5.3%
Combination Abdominal CT Scan	642	15.0%	12.9%	10.5%
Combination Brain/Sinus CT Scan	436	1.1%	3.3%	2.7%
Combination Chest CT Scan	336	13.1%	6.1%	2.7%
Follow-up Mammogram/Ultrasound	1,224	11.8%	8.4%	8.8%
Lumbar Spine MRI for Low Back Pain	78	37.2%	41.1%	37.2%

North Mississippi Medical Center

830 S Gloster
Tupelo, MS 38801
Phone: 662-377-3000
Fax: 662-377-3552
URL: www.nmhs.net/nmmc
Type: Acute Care Hospitals
Emergency Services: Yes
Ownership: Voluntary non-profit - Private
Beds: 650
Key Personnel:
Radiology. . . . . Doug Clark, MD
Surgery . . . . Mike Denham, MD
Quality Assurance . . . . Elizabeth C Ford
Cardiology . . . . George Hand
CEO/President. . . . . Shane Spees
Chief of Medical Staff. . . . . Mark Williams, MD

Measure	Cases	This Hosp.	State Avg.	U.S. Avg.
Blood Clot Prevention and Treatment				
Anticoagulation Overlap Therapy[2]	126	94%	86%	93%
ICU Venous Thromboembolism Prophylaxis[2]	90	96%	86%	92%
Incidence of Potentially Preventable VTE[2]	17	12%	15%	10%
UFH with Dosages/Platelet Monitoring[2]	19	100%	94%	97%
Venous Thromboembolism Prophylaxis[2]	379	81%	70%	85%
Warfarin Therapy Discharge Instructions[2]	87	99%	77%	75%
Chest Pain/Possible Heart Attack Care				
Aspirin Given Within 24 Hours of Arrival[1,3]	-	-	94%	96%
Fibrinolytic Meds Within 30 Min. of Arrival[5]	-	-	40%	58%
Average Time to ECG (minutes)[1,3]	-	-	10	7
Average Time to Transfer (minutes)[5]	-	-	77	60
Children's Asthma Care				
Received Home Management Plan of Care	-	-	-	88%
Received Reliever Medication	-	-	-	100%
Received Systemic Corticosteroids	-	-	-	100%
Emergency Department				
Admittance Decision Time (minutes)[2]	520	58	61	98
Head CT Results Within 45 Min. of Arrival[1]	-	-	42%	57%
Patients Who Left ER Before Being Seen	89,284	3%	3%	2%
Time from ER Arrival to Admit. (minutes)[2]	542	239	223	274
Time from ER Arrival to Discharge (minutes)	417	186	112	134
Time in ER Before Being Evaluated (minutes)	429	60	29	26
Time to Pain Meds for Fractures (minutes)	308	84	68	57
Heart Attack Care				
Aspirin Given at Discharge[2]	513	100%	99%	99%
Fibrinolytic Meds Within 30 Min. of Arrival[2,7]	-	-	50%	54%
PCI Within 90 Minutes of Arrival[2]	52	98%	96%	96%
Statin Prescribed at Discharge[2]	516	100%	97%	98%
Heart Failure Care				
ACE Inhibitor or ARB for LVSD[2]	136	98%	93%	97%
Discharge Instructions Given[2]	274	99%	91%	94%
Evaluation of LVS Function[2]	315	100%	96%	99%
Medicare Spending				
Medicare Spending per Patient (ratio)	-	0.97	0.95	0.98
Pneumonia Care				
Appropriate Initial Antibiotic Given[2]	212	99%	91%	95%
Blood Culture Timing[2]	329	98%	97%	98%
Pregnancy and Delivery Care				
Newborn Deliveries Scheduled Early[2]	55	7%	22%	6%
Preventive Care				
Immunization for Influenza[2]	589	97%	87%	90%
Immunization for Pneumonia[2]	688	98%	89%	92%
Stroke Care				
Anticoagulation Therapy for Atrial Fibrillation[1,2]	-	-	93%	95%
Antithrombotic Therapy Timing[2]	84	98%	96%	98%
Assessed for Rehabilitation[2]	97	99%	95%	97%
Discharged on Antithrombotic Therapy[2]	85	100%	97%	99%
Discharged on Statin Medication[2]	74	100%	88%	94%
Thrombolytic Therapy Timing[1,2]	-	-	25%	66%
Venous Thromboembolism Prophylaxis[2]	102	98%	87%	94%
Written Stroke Educational Materials Given[2]	52	98%	84%	88%
Surgical Care Improvement Project				
Appropriate Beta Blocker Usage[2]	611	100%	97%	98%
Appropriate VTP Within 24 Hours[2]	784	100%	97%	98%
Controlled Postoperative Blood Glucose[2]	501	100%	97%	97%
Perioperative Temperature Management[2]	920	100%	100%	100%
Prophylactic Antibiotic Selection[2]	1,146	100%	99%	99%
Prophylactic Antibiotic Selection (Outpatient)	740	100%	98%	98%
Prophylactic Antibiotic Stopped[2]	1,120	99%	97%	98%
Prophylactic Antibiotic Timing[2]	1,149	100%	99%	99%
Prophylactic Antibiotic Timing (Outpatient)	740	100%	98%	98%
Urinary Catheter Removal[2]	585	100%	97%	97%
Survey of Patients' Hospital Experiences				
Area Around Room 'Always' Quiet at Night	300+	74%	72%	61%
Doctors 'Always' Communicated Well	300+	86%	86%	82%
Home Recovery Information Given	300+	85%	83%	85%
Hospital Given 9 or 10 on 10 Point Scale	300+	80%	71%	71%
Meds 'Always' Explained Before Given	300+	67%	67%	64%
Nurses 'Always' Communicated Well	300+	86%	81%	79%
Pain 'Always' Well Controlled	300+	77%	72%	71%
Room and Bathroom 'Always' Clean	300+	79%	74%	73%
Timely Help 'Always' Received	300+	73%	69%	68%
Would Definitely Recommend Hospital	300+	81%	69%	71%
Use of Medical Imaging				
Cardiac Imaging Stress Test before Surgery	482	5.8%	5.7%	5.3%
Combination Abdominal CT Scan	2,381	2.3%	12.9%	10.5%
Combination Brain/Sinus CT Scan	2,094	3.3%	3.3%	2.7%
Combination Chest CT Scan	1,639	0.7%	6.1%	2.7%
Follow-up Mammogram/Ultrasound	3,661	6.6%	8.4%	8.8%
Lumbar Spine MRI for Low Back Pain	480	37.9%	41.1%	37.2%

Walthall County General Hospital

100 Hospital Drive
Tylertown, MS 39667
Phone: 601-876-2122
URL: www.wcghospital.datastar.net
Type: Critical Access Hospitals
Emergency Services: Yes
Ownership: Government - Local
Beds: 49
Key Personnel:
CEO/President. . . . . Jimmy Graves

Measure	Cases	This Hosp.	State Avg.	U.S. Avg.
Blood Clot Prevention and Treatment				
Anticoagulation Overlap Therapy[5]	-	-	86%	93%
ICU Venous Thromboembolism Prophylaxis[5]	-	-	86%	92%
Incidence of Potentially Preventable VTE[5]	-	-	15%	10%
UFH with Dosages/Platelet Monitoring[5]	-	-	94%	97%
Venous Thromboembolism Prophylaxis[5]	-	-	70%	85%
Warfarin Therapy Discharge Instructions[5]	-	-	77%	75%
Chest Pain/Possible Heart Attack Care				
Aspirin Given Within 24 Hours of Arrival[5]	-	-	94%	96%
Fibrinolytic Meds Within 30 Min. of Arrival[5]	-	-	40%	58%
Average Time to ECG (minutes)[5]	-	-	10	7
Average Time to Transfer (minutes)[5]	-	-	77	60
Children's Asthma Care				
Received Home Management Plan of Care	-	-	-	88%
Received Reliever Medication	-	-	-	100%
Received Systemic Corticosteroids	-	-	-	100%
Emergency Department				
Admittance Decision Time (minutes)	78	25	61	98
Head CT Results Within 45 Min. of Arrival[5]	-	-	42%	57%
Patients Who Left ER Before Being Seen[5]	-	-	3%	2%
Time from ER Arrival to Admit. (minutes)	79	173	223	274
Time from ER Arrival to Discharge (minutes)[5]	-	-	112	134
Time in ER Before Being Evaluated (minutes)[5]	-	-	29	26
Time to Pain Meds for Fractures (minutes)[5]	-	-	68	57
Heart Attack Care				
Aspirin Given at Discharge[1,3]	-	-	99%	99%
Fibrinolytic Meds Within 30 Min. of Arrival[3,7]	-	-	50%	54%
PCI Within 90 Minutes of Arrival[3,7]	-	-	96%	96%
Statin Prescribed at Discharge[1,3]	-	-	97%	98%

NOTE: Hospital profiles are in alphabetical order by state, then city, then hospital within the city; Rankings exclude hospitals with less than 25 cases except for patient surveys which excludes hospitals with less than 100 cases; (a) 100-299 cases; (1) The number of cases/patients is too few to report; (2) Data submitted were based on a sample of cases/patients; (3) Results are based on a shorter time period than required; (4) Data suppressed by CMS for one or more quarters; (5) Results are not available for this reporting period; (6) Fewer than 100 patients completed the HCAHPS survey; (7) No cases met the criteria for this measure; (8) The lower limit of the confidence interval cannot be calculated if the number of observed infections equals zero; (9) No data are available from the state/territory for this reporting period; (10) The scores shown reflect fewer than 50 completed surveys; (11) There were discrepancies in the data collection process; (12) This measure does not apply to this hospital for this reporting period; (13) Results cannot be calculated for this reporting period; (14) The results for this state are combined with nearby states to protect confidentiality; Please refer to the User's Guide for a full explanation of data.

Heart Failure Care				
ACE Inhibitor or ARB for LVSD[1]	-	-	93%	97%
Discharge Instructions Given	13	0%	91%	94%
Evaluation of LVS Function	16	56%	96%	99%
Medicare Spending				
Medicare Spending per Patient (ratio)	-	-	0.95	0.98
Pneumonia Care				
Appropriate Initial Antibiotic Given[1,2]	-	-	91%	95%
Blood Culture Timing[2]	11	91%	97%	98%
Pregnancy and Delivery Care				
Newborn Deliveries Scheduled Early[5]	-	-	22%	6%
Preventive Care				
Immunization for Influenza[2]	88	73%	87%	90%
Immunization for Pneumonia[2]	91	79%	89%	92%
Stroke Care				
Anticoagulation Therapy for Atrial Fibrillation[5]	-	-	93%	95%
Antithrombotic Therapy Timing[5]	-	-	96%	98%
Assessed for Rehabilitation[5]	-	-	95%	97%
Discharged on Antithrombotic Therapy[5]	-	-	97%	99%
Discharged on Statin Medication[5]	-	-	88%	94%
Thrombolytic Therapy Timing[5]	-	-	25%	66%
Venous Thromboembolism Prophylaxis[5]	-	-	87%	94%
Written Stroke Educational Materials Given[5]	-	-	84%	88%
Surgical Care Improvement Project				
Appropriate Beta Blocker Usage[5]	-	-	97%	98%
Appropriate VTP Within 24 Hours[5]	-	-	97%	98%
Controlled Postoperative Blood Glucose[5]	-	-	97%	97%
Perioperative Temperature Management[5]	-	-	100%	100%
Prophylactic Antibiotic Selection[5]	-	-	99%	99%
Prophylactic Antibiotic Selection (Outpatient)[5]	-	-	98%	98%
Prophylactic Antibiotic Stopped[5]	-	-	97%	98%
Prophylactic Antibiotic Timing[5]	-	-	99%	99%
Prophylactic Antibiotic Timing (Outpatient)[5]	-	-	98%	98%
Urinary Catheter Removal[5]	-	-	97%	97%
Survey of Patients' Hospital Experiences				
Area Around Room 'Always' Quiet at Night[6]	<100	77%	72%	61%
Doctors 'Always' Communicated Well[6]	<100	89%	86%	82%
Home Recovery Information Given[6]	<100	77%	83%	85%
Hospital Given 9 or 10 on 10 Point Scale[6]	<100	79%	71%	71%
Meds 'Always' Explained Before Given[6]	<100	68%	67%	64%
Nurses 'Always' Communicated Well[6]	<100	82%	81%	79%
Pain 'Always' Well Controlled[6]	<100	78%	72%	71%
Room and Bathroom 'Always' Clean[6]	<100	74%	74%	73%
Timely Help 'Always' Received[6]	<100	61%	69%	68%
Would Definitely Recommend Hospital[6]	<100	67%	69%	71%
Use of Medical Imaging				
Cardiac Imaging Stress Test before Surgery[1]	-	-	5.7%	5.3%
Combination Abdominal CT Scan	105	1.0%	12.9%	10.5%
Combination Brain/Sinus CT Scan[1]	-	-	3.3%	2.7%
Combination Chest CT Scan[1]	-	-	6.1%	2.7%
Follow-up Mammogram/Ultrasound[7]	-	-	8.4%	8.8%
Lumbar Spine MRI for Low Back Pain[7]	-	-	41.1%	37.2%

Laird Hospital

25117 Highway 15
Union, MS 39365
Phone: 601-774-8214
Fax: 601-774-1573
URL: www.rushhealthsystems.org
Type: Critical Access Hospitals
Emergency Services: Yes
Ownership: Voluntary non-profit - Private
Beds: 25

Key Personnel:
CEO/President. . . . . Tomy Bartlett
Emergency Room . . . . OJ Briseno, MD
Emergency Room . . . . Kellie Jones
Operating Room. . . . . Jill Keen, RN
Anesthesiology. . . . . Sheri Luebrecht, MD
Quality Assurance . . . . Noel Palmer, RN

Measure	Cases	This Hosp.	State Avg.	U.S. Avg.
Blood Clot Prevention and Treatment				
Anticoagulation Overlap Therapy[5]	-	-	86%	93%
ICU Venous Thromboembolism Prophylaxis[5]	-	-	86%	92%
Incidence of Potentially Preventable VTE[5]	-	-	15%	10%
UFH with Dosages/Platelet Monitoring[5]	-	-	94%	97%
Venous Thromboembolism Prophylaxis[5]	-	-	70%	85%
Warfarin Therapy Discharge Instructions[5]	-	-	77%	75%
Chest Pain/Possible Heart Attack Care				
Aspirin Given Within 24 Hours of Arrival[5]	-	-	94%	96%
Fibrinolytic Meds Within 30 Min. of Arrival[5]	-	-	40%	58%
Average Time to ECG (minutes)[5]	-	-	10	7
Average Time to Transfer (minutes)[5]	-	-	77	60
Children's Asthma Care				
Received Home Management Plan of Care	-	-	-	88%
Received Reliever Medication	-	-	-	100%
Received Systemic Corticosteroids	-	-	-	100%
Emergency Department				
Admittance Decision Time (minutes)[5]	-	-	61	98
Head CT Results Within 45 Min. of Arrival[5]	-	-	42%	57%
Patients Who Left ER Before Being Seen[5]	-	-	3%	2%
Time from ER Arrival to Admit. (minutes)[5]	-	-	223	274
Time from ER Arrival to Discharge (minutes)[5]	-	-	112	134
Time in ER Before Being Evaluated (minutes)[5]	-	-	29	26
Time to Pain Meds for Fractures (minutes)[5]	-	-	68	57
Heart Attack Care				
Aspirin Given at Discharge[5]	-	-	99%	99%
Fibrinolytic Meds Within 30 Min. of Arrival[5]	-	-	50%	54%
PCI Within 90 Minutes of Arrival[5]	-	-	96%	96%
Statin Prescribed at Discharge[5]	-	-	97%	98%
Heart Failure Care				
ACE Inhibitor or ARB for LVSD[1,3]	-	-	93%	97%
Discharge Instructions Given[1,3]	-	-	91%	94%
Evaluation of LVS Function[1,3]	-	-	96%	99%
Medicare Spending				
Medicare Spending per Patient (ratio)	-	-	0.95	0.98
Pneumonia Care				
Appropriate Initial Antibiotic Given[3]	19	84%	91%	95%
Blood Culture Timing[3]	16	94%	97%	98%
Pregnancy and Delivery Care				
Newborn Deliveries Scheduled Early[5]	-	-	22%	6%
Preventive Care				
Immunization for Influenza[5]	-	-	87%	90%
Immunization for Pneumonia[5]	-	-	89%	92%
Stroke Care				
Anticoagulation Therapy for Atrial Fibrillation[5]	-	-	93%	95%
Antithrombotic Therapy Timing[5]	-	-	96%	98%
Assessed for Rehabilitation[5]	-	-	95%	97%
Discharged on Antithrombotic Therapy[5]	-	-	97%	99%
Discharged on Statin Medication[5]	-	-	88%	94%
Thrombolytic Therapy Timing[5]	-	-	25%	66%
Venous Thromboembolism Prophylaxis[5]	-	-	87%	94%
Written Stroke Educational Materials Given[5]	-	-	84%	88%
Surgical Care Improvement Project				
Appropriate Beta Blocker Usage[5]	-	-	97%	98%
Appropriate VTP Within 24 Hours[5]	-	-	97%	98%
Controlled Postoperative Blood Glucose[5]	-	-	97%	97%
Perioperative Temperature Management[5]	-	-	100%	100%
Prophylactic Antibiotic Selection[5]	-	-	99%	99%
Prophylactic Antibiotic Selection (Outpatient)[5]	-	-	98%	98%
Prophylactic Antibiotic Stopped[5]	-	-	97%	98%
Prophylactic Antibiotic Timing[5]	-	-	99%	99%
Prophylactic Antibiotic Timing (Outpatient)[5]	-	-	98%	98%
Urinary Catheter Removal[5]	-	-	97%	97%
Survey of Patients' Hospital Experiences				
Area Around Room 'Always' Quiet at Night[6]	<100	77%	72%	61%
Doctors 'Always' Communicated Well[6]	<100	88%	86%	82%
Home Recovery Information Given[6]	<100	81%	83%	85%
Hospital Given 9 or 10 on 10 Point Scale[6]	<100	75%	71%	71%
Meds 'Always' Explained Before Given[6]	<100	61%	67%	64%
Nurses 'Always' Communicated Well[6]	<100	86%	81%	79%
Pain 'Always' Well Controlled[6]	<100	72%	72%	71%
Room and Bathroom 'Always' Clean[6]	<100	69%	74%	73%
Timely Help 'Always' Received[6]	<100	74%	69%	68%
Would Definitely Recommend Hospital[6]	<100	65%	69%	71%
Use of Medical Imaging				
Cardiac Imaging Stress Test before Surgery[1]	-	-	5.7%	5.3%
Combination Abdominal CT Scan	109	8.3%	12.9%	10.5%
Combination Brain/Sinus CT Scan[1]	-	-	3.3%	2.7%
Combination Chest CT Scan	74	1.4%	6.1%	2.7%
Follow-up Mammogram/Ultrasound	215	5.6%	8.4%	8.8%
Lumbar Spine MRI for Low Back Pain	35	45.7%	41.1%	37.2%

River Region Health System

2100 Hwy 61 N
Vicksburg, MS 39183
Phone: 601-883-5000
URL: www.riverregion.com
Type: Acute Care Hospitals
Emergency Services: Yes
Ownership: Proprietary
Beds: 372

Key Personnel:
CEO/President. . . . . Vance Reynolds

Measure	Cases	This Hosp.	State Avg.	U.S. Avg.
Blood Clot Prevention and Treatment				
Anticoagulation Overlap Therapy[2]	39	100%	86%	93%
ICU Venous Thromboembolism Prophylaxis[2]	86	98%	86%	92%
Incidence of Potentially Preventable VTE[2]	14	21%	15%	10%
UFH with Dosages/Platelet Monitoring[1,2]	-	-	94%	97%
Venous Thromboembolism Prophylaxis[2]	422	94%	70%	85%
Warfarin Therapy Discharge Instructions[2]	31	97%	77%	75%
Chest Pain/Possible Heart Attack Care				
Aspirin Given Within 24 Hours of Arrival[1,3]	-	-	94%	96%
Fibrinolytic Meds Within 30 Min. of Arrival[3,7]	-	-	40%	58%
Average Time to ECG (minutes)[1,3]	-	-	10	7
Average Time to Transfer (minutes)[3,7]	-	-	77	60
Children's Asthma Care				
Received Home Management Plan of Care	-	-	-	88%
Received Reliever Medication	-	-	-	100%
Received Systemic Corticosteroids	-	-	-	100%
Emergency Department				
Admittance Decision Time (minutes)[2]	739	98	61	98
Head CT Results Within 45 Min. of Arrival	17	65%	42%	57%
Patients Who Left ER Before Being Seen	34,579	2%	3%	2%
Time from ER Arrival to Admit. (minutes)[2]	748	242	223	274
Time from ER Arrival to Discharge (minutes)	393	115	112	134
Time in ER Before Being Evaluated (minutes)	408	35	29	26
Time to Pain Meds for Fractures (minutes)	75	53	68	57
Heart Attack Care				
Aspirin Given at Discharge	120	99%	99%	99%
Fibrinolytic Meds Within 30 Min. of Arrival[7]	-	-	50%	54%
PCI Within 90 Minutes of Arrival	16	100%	96%	96%
Statin Prescribed at Discharge	98	98%	97%	98%
Heart Failure Care				
ACE Inhibitor or ARB for LVSD	128	98%	93%	97%
Discharge Instructions Given	283	99%	91%	94%
Evaluation of LVS Function	324	100%	96%	99%
Medicare Spending				
Medicare Spending per Patient (ratio)	-	1.07	0.95	0.98
Pneumonia Care				
Appropriate Initial Antibiotic Given	128	93%	91%	95%
Blood Culture Timing	198	99%	97%	98%
Pregnancy and Delivery Care				
Newborn Deliveries Scheduled Early[1,2]	-	-	22%	6%
Preventive Care				
Immunization for Influenza[2]	646	99%	87%	90%
Immunization for Pneumonia[2]	774	99%	89%	92%
Stroke Care				
Anticoagulation Therapy for Atrial Fibrillation[1]	-	-	93%	95%
Antithrombotic Therapy Timing	64	95%	96%	98%
Assessed for Rehabilitation	68	99%	95%	97%
Discharged on Antithrombotic Therapy	65	97%	97%	99%
Discharged on Statin Medication	44	91%	88%	94%
Thrombolytic Therapy Timing[7]	-	-	25%	66%
Venous Thromboembolism Prophylaxis	76	92%	87%	94%
Written Stroke Educational Materials Given	38	97%	84%	88%
Surgical Care Improvement Project				
Appropriate Beta Blocker Usage	94	100%	97%	98%
Appropriate VTP Within 24 Hours	221	100%	97%	98%
Controlled Postoperative Blood Glucose	70	99%	97%	97%
Perioperative Temperature Management	352	100%	100%	100%
Prophylactic Antibiotic Selection	236	99%	99%	99%
Prophylactic Antibiotic Selection (Outpatient)	211	99%	98%	98%
Prophylactic Antibiotic Stopped	226	100%	97%	98%
Prophylactic Antibiotic Timing	236	100%	99%	99%

NOTE: Hospital profiles are in alphabetical order by state, then city, then hospital within the city; Rankings exclude hospitals with less than 25 cases except for patient surveys which excludes hospitals with less than 100 cases; (a) 100-299 cases; (1) The number of cases/patients is too few to report; (2) Data submitted were based on a sample of cases/patients; (3) Results are based on a shorter time period than required; (4) Data suppressed by CMS for one or more quarters; (5) Results are not available for this reporting period; (6) Fewer than 100 patients completed the HCAHPS survey; (7) No cases met the criteria for this measure; (8) The lower limit of the confidence interval cannot be calculated if the number of observed infections equals zero; (9) No data are available from the state/territory for this reporting period; (10) The scores shown reflect fewer than 50 completed surveys; (11) There were discrepancies in the data collection process; (12) This measure does not apply to this hospital for this reporting period; (13) Results cannot be calculated for this reporting period; (14) The results for this state are combined with nearby states to protect confidentiality; Please refer to the User's Guide for a full explanation of data.

Measure	Cases	This Hosp.	State Avg.	U.S. Avg.
Prophylactic Antibiotic Timing (Outpatient)	211	100%	98%	98%
Urinary Catheter Removal	153	99%	97%	97%
Survey of Patients' Hospital Experiences				
Area Around Room 'Always' Quiet at Night	300+	71%	72%	61%
Doctors 'Always' Communicated Well	300+	86%	86%	82%
Home Recovery Information Given	300+	83%	83%	85%
Hospital Given 9 or 10 on 10 Point Scale	300+	66%	71%	71%
Meds 'Always' Explained Before Given	300+	61%	67%	64%
Nurses 'Always' Communicated Well	300+	77%	81%	79%
Pain 'Always' Well Controlled	300+	70%	72%	71%
Room and Bathroom 'Always' Clean	300+	75%	74%	73%
Timely Help 'Always' Received	300+	61%	69%	68%
Would Definitely Recommend Hospital	300+	62%	69%	71%
Use of Medical Imaging				
Cardiac Imaging Stress Test before Surgery	376	4.0%	5.7%	5.3%
Combination Abdominal CT Scan	498	5.6%	12.9%	10.5%
Combination Brain/Sinus CT Scan	533	2.4%	3.3%	2.7%
Combination Chest CT Scan	289	4.2%	6.1%	2.7%
Follow-up Mammogram/Ultrasound	1,058	6.6%	8.4%	8.8%
Lumbar Spine MRI for Low Back Pain	140	43.6%	41.1%	37.2%

Yalobusha General Hospital

630 South Main Street
Water Valley, MS 38965
Phone: 662-473-1411
Fax: 662-473-4922
Type: Acute Care Hospitals
Emergency Services: No
Ownership: Government - Local
Beds: 72
Key Personnel:
Chief of Medical Staff.......... Joe Walker

Measure	Cases	This Hosp.	State Avg.	U.S. Avg.
Blood Clot Prevention and Treatment				
Anticoagulation Overlap Therapy[1,2]	-	-	86%	93%
ICU Venous Thromboembolism Prophylaxis[2,7]	-	-	86%	92%
Incidence of Potentially Preventable VTE[2,7]	-	-	15%	10%
UFH with Dosages/Platelet Monitoring[2,7]	-	-	94%	97%
Venous Thromboembolism Prophylaxis[2]	131	16%	70%	85%
Warfarin Therapy Discharge Instructions[2,7]	-	-	77%	75%
Chest Pain/Possible Heart Attack Care				
Aspirin Given Within 24 Hours of Arrival[5]	-	-	94%	96%
Fibrinolytic Meds Within 30 Min. of Arrival[5]	-	-	40%	58%
Average Time to ECG (minutes)[5]	-	-	10	7
Average Time to Transfer (minutes)[5]	-	-	77	60
Children's Asthma Care				
Received Home Management Plan of Care	-	-	-	88%
Received Reliever Medication	-	-	-	100%
Received Systemic Corticosteroids	-	-	-	100%
Emergency Department				
Admittance Decision Time (minutes)[2,7]	-	-	61	98
Head CT Results Within 45 Min. of Arrival[5]	-	-	42%	57%
Patients Who Left ER Before Being Seen[5]	-	-	3%	2%
Time from ER Arrival to Admit. (minutes)[2,7]	-	-	223	274
Time from ER Arrival to Discharge (minutes)[5]	-	-	112	134
Time in ER Before Being Evaluated (minutes)[5]	-	-	29	26
Time to Pain Meds for Fractures (minutes)[5]	-	-	68	57
Heart Attack Care				
Aspirin Given at Discharge[2,3]	-	-	99%	99%
Fibrinolytic Meds Within 30 Min. of Arrival[2,3]	-	-	50%	54%
PCI Within 90 Minutes of Arrival[2,3]	-	-	96%	96%
Statin Prescribed at Discharge[2,3]	-	-	97%	98%
Heart Failure Care				
ACE Inhibitor or ARB for LVSD[1,2]	-	-	93%	97%
Discharge Instructions Given[1,2]	-	-	91%	94%
Evaluation of LVS Function[2]	17	71%	96%	99%
Medicare Spending				
Medicare Spending per Patient (ratio)	-	0.75	0.95	0.98
Pneumonia Care				
Appropriate Initial Antibiotic Given[1,2]	-	-	91%	95%
Blood Culture Timing[2,7]	-	-	97%	98%
Pregnancy and Delivery Care				
Newborn Deliveries Scheduled Early[7]	-	-	22%	6%
Preventive Care				
Immunization for Influenza[2]	148	41%	87%	90%
Immunization for Pneumonia[2]	205	61%	89%	92%
Stroke Care				
Anticoagulation Therapy for Atrial Fibrillation[2,3]	-	-	93%	95%
Antithrombotic Therapy Timing[1,2]	-	-	96%	98%
Assessed for Rehabilitation[1,2]	-	-	95%	97%
Discharged on Antithrombotic Therapy[1,2]	-	-	97%	99%
Discharged on Statin Medication[1,2]	-	-	88%	94%
Thrombolytic Therapy Timing[2,3]	-	-	25%	66%
Venous Thromboembolism Prophylaxis[1,2]	-	-	87%	94%
Written Stroke Educational Materials Given[2,3]	-	-	84%	88%
Surgical Care Improvement Project				
Appropriate Beta Blocker Usage[5]	-	-	97%	98%
Appropriate VTP Within 24 Hours[5]	-	-	97%	98%
Controlled Postoperative Blood Glucose[5]	-	-	97%	97%
Perioperative Temperature Management[5]	-	-	100%	100%
Prophylactic Antibiotic Selection[5]	-	-	99%	99%
Prophylactic Antibiotic Selection (Outpatient)[5]	-	-	98%	98%
Prophylactic Antibiotic Stopped[5]	-	-	97%	98%
Prophylactic Antibiotic Timing[5]	-	-	99%	99%
Prophylactic Antibiotic Timing (Outpatient)[5]	-	-	98%	98%
Urinary Catheter Removal[5]	-	-	97%	97%
Survey of Patients' Hospital Experiences				
Area Around Room 'Always' Quiet at Night[10]	<100	60%	72%	61%
Doctors 'Always' Communicated Well[10]	<100	87%	86%	82%
Home Recovery Information Given[10]	<100	75%	83%	85%
Hospital Given 9 or 10 on 10 Point Scale[10]	<100	71%	71%	71%
Meds 'Always' Explained Before Given[10]	<100	61%	67%	64%
Nurses 'Always' Communicated Well[10]	<100	78%	81%	79%
Pain 'Always' Well Controlled[10]	<100	62%	72%	71%
Room and Bathroom 'Always' Clean[10]	<100	67%	74%	73%
Timely Help 'Always' Received[10]	<100	60%	69%	68%
Would Definitely Recommend Hospital[10]	<100	70%	69%	71%
Use of Medical Imaging				
Cardiac Imaging Stress Test before Surgery[7]	-	-	5.7%	5.3%
Combination Abdominal CT Scan	82	3.7%	12.9%	10.5%
Combination Brain/Sinus CT Scan[1]	-	-	3.3%	2.7%
Combination Chest CT Scan[1]	-	-	6.1%	2.7%
Follow-up Mammogram/Ultrasound[7]	-	-	8.4%	8.8%
Lumbar Spine MRI for Low Back Pain[1]	-	-	41.1%	37.2%

Wayne General Hospital

950 Matthew Dr
Waynesboro, MS 39367
Phone: 601-735-5151
Fax: 601-735-7150
Type: Acute Care Hospitals
Emergency Services: Yes
Ownership: Government - Local
Beds: 80
Key Personnel:
Emergency Room .... Bobbie Cooksey
Infection Control............. Paulette Cooley
Quality Assurance .... Margeret Graham
Chief of Medical Staff.......... Tod Stokley
Operating Room............. Tonda Waller

Measure	Cases	This Hosp.	State Avg.	U.S. Avg.
Blood Clot Prevention and Treatment				
Anticoagulation Overlap Therapy[2]	19	63%	86%	93%
ICU Venous Thromboembolism Prophylaxis[2]	19	58%	86%	92%
Incidence of Potentially Preventable VTE[1,2]	-	-	15%	10%
UFH with Dosages/Platelet Monitoring[1,2]	-	-	94%	97%
Venous Thromboembolism Prophylaxis[2]	209	49%	70%	85%
Warfarin Therapy Discharge Instructions[2]	14	86%	77%	75%
Chest Pain/Possible Heart Attack Care				
Aspirin Given Within 24 Hours of Arrival	18	83%	94%	96%
Fibrinolytic Meds Within 30 Min. of Arrival[1]	-	-	40%	58%
Average Time to ECG (minutes)	19	25	10	7
Average Time to Transfer (minutes)[1]	-	-	77	60
Children's Asthma Care				
Received Home Management Plan of Care	-	-	-	88%
Received Reliever Medication	-	-	-	100%
Received Systemic Corticosteroids	-	-	-	100%
Emergency Department				
Admittance Decision Time (minutes)[2]	423	57	61	98
Head CT Results Within 45 Min. of Arrival[1]	-	-	42%	57%
Patients Who Left ER Before Being Seen	15,500	2%	3%	2%
Time from ER Arrival to Admit. (minutes)[2]	449	186	223	274
Time from ER Arrival to Discharge (minutes)	362	112	112	134
Time in ER Before Being Evaluated (minutes)	371	43	29	26
Time to Pain Meds for Fractures (minutes)	50	72	68	57
Heart Attack Care				
Aspirin Given at Discharge[1]	-	-	99%	99%
Fibrinolytic Meds Within 30 Min. of Arrival[7]	-	-	50%	54%
PCI Within 90 Minutes of Arrival[7]	-	-	96%	96%
Statin Prescribed at Discharge[1]	-	-	97%	98%
Heart Failure Care				
ACE Inhibitor or ARB for LVSD	45	84%	93%	97%
Discharge Instructions Given	96	100%	91%	94%
Evaluation of LVS Function	111	96%	96%	99%
Medicare Spending				
Medicare Spending per Patient (ratio)	-	0.86	0.95	0.98
Pneumonia Care				
Appropriate Initial Antibiotic Given	62	95%	91%	95%
Blood Culture Timing	66	94%	97%	98%
Pregnancy and Delivery Care				
Newborn Deliveries Scheduled Early	24	21%	22%	6%
Preventive Care				
Immunization for Influenza[2]	265	43%	87%	90%
Immunization for Pneumonia[2]	374	86%	89%	92%
Stroke Care				
Anticoagulation Therapy for Atrial Fibrillation[1]	-	-	93%	95%
Antithrombotic Therapy Timing	18	94%	96%	98%
Assessed for Rehabilitation	18	100%	95%	97%
Discharged on Antithrombotic Therapy	17	82%	97%	99%
Discharged on Statin Medication	16	62%	88%	94%
Thrombolytic Therapy Timing	11	0%	25%	66%
Venous Thromboembolism Prophylaxis	18	56%	87%	94%
Written Stroke Educational Materials Given	13	69%	84%	88%
Surgical Care Improvement Project				
Appropriate Beta Blocker Usage[1]	-	-	97%	98%
Appropriate VTP Within 24 Hours	19	79%	97%	98%
Controlled Postoperative Blood Glucose[7]	-	-	97%	97%
Perioperative Temperature Management	20	95%	100%	100%
Prophylactic Antibiotic Selection[1]	-	-	99%	99%
Prophylactic Antibiotic Selection (Outpatient)[1]	-	-	98%	98%
Prophylactic Antibiotic Stopped[1]	-	-	97%	98%
Prophylactic Antibiotic Timing[1]	-	-	99%	99%
Prophylactic Antibiotic Timing (Outpatient)[1]	-	-	98%	98%
Urinary Catheter Removal[1]	-	-	97%	97%
Survey of Patients' Hospital Experiences				
Area Around Room 'Always' Quiet at Night	300+	76%	72%	61%
Doctors 'Always' Communicated Well	300+	91%	86%	82%
Home Recovery Information Given	300+	84%	83%	85%
Hospital Given 9 or 10 on 10 Point Scale	300+	67%	71%	71%
Meds 'Always' Explained Before Given	300+	74%	67%	64%
Nurses 'Always' Communicated Well	300+	82%	81%	79%
Pain 'Always' Well Controlled	300+	75%	72%	71%
Room and Bathroom 'Always' Clean	300+	66%	74%	73%
Timely Help 'Always' Received	300+	69%	69%	68%
Would Definitely Recommend Hospital	300+	64%	69%	71%
Use of Medical Imaging				
Cardiac Imaging Stress Test before Surgery[1]	-	-	5.7%	5.3%
Combination Abdominal CT Scan	155	11.0%	12.9%	10.5%
Combination Brain/Sinus CT Scan[1]	-	-	3.3%	2.7%
Combination Chest CT Scan	52	1.9%	6.1%	2.7%
Follow-up Mammogram/Ultrasound	163	12.9%	8.4%	8.8%
Lumbar Spine MRI for Low Back Pain[1]	-	-	41.1%	37.2%

Clay County Medical Center

835 Medical Center Dr
West Point, MS 39773
Phone: 662-495-2300
Fax: 662-495-2361
URL: www.nmhs.net
Type: Acute Care Hospitals
Emergency Services: Yes
Ownership: Voluntary non-profit - Private
Beds: 60
Key Personnel:
Infection Control............. Paula Bryan
Quality Assurance .... Glenda Colbert
Anesthesiology............... Carlie Godwin, CRNA
Chief of Medical Staff.......... Charlotte Magnussen
Operating Room............. Nancy Turnage, RN

Measure	Cases	This Hosp.	State Avg.	U.S. Avg.
Blood Clot Prevention and Treatment				
Anticoagulation Overlap Therapy[2]	11	45%	86%	93%

NOTE: Hospital profiles are in alphabetical order by state, then city, then hospital within the city; Rankings exclude hospitals with less than 25 cases except for patient surveys which excludes hospitals with less than 100 cases; (a) 100-299 cases; (1) The number of cases/patients is too few to report; (2) Data submitted were based on a sample of cases/patients; (3) Results are based on a shorter time period than required; (4) Data suppressed by CMS for one or more quarters; (5) Results are not available for this reporting period; (6) Fewer than 100 patients completed the HCAHPS survey; (7) No cases met the criteria for this measure; (8) The lower limit of the confidence interval cannot be calculated if the number of observed infections equals zero; (9) No data are available from the state/territory for this reporting period; (10) The scores shown reflect fewer than 50 completed surveys; (11) There were discrepancies in the data collection process; (12) This measure does not apply to this hospital for this reporting period; (13) Results cannot be calculated for this reporting period; (14) The results for this state are combined with nearby states to protect confidentiality; Please refer to the User's Guide for a full explanation of data.

Measure	Cases	This Hosp.	State Avg.	U.S. Avg.
ICU Venous Thromboembolism Prophylaxis[2]	17	82%	86%	92%
Incidence of Potentially Preventable VTE[2,7]	-	-	15%	10%
UFH with Dosages/Platelet Monitoring[2,7]	-	-	94%	97%
Venous Thromboembolism Prophylaxis[2]	189	53%	70%	85%
Warfarin Therapy Discharge Instructions[1,2]	-	-	77%	75%
Chest Pain/Possible Heart Attack Care				
Aspirin Given Within 24 Hours of Arrival	26	100%	94%	96%
Fibrinolytic Meds Within 30 Min. of Arrival[3,7]	-	-	40%	58%
Average Time to ECG (minutes)	26	8	10	7
Average Time to Transfer (minutes)[1,3]	-	-	77	60
Children's Asthma Care				
Received Home Management Plan of Care	-	-	-	88%
Received Reliever Medication	-	-	-	100%
Received Systemic Corticosteroids	-	-	-	100%
Emergency Department				
Admittance Decision Time (minutes)[2]	263	20	61	98
Head CT Results Within 45 Min. of Arrival[1]	-	-	42%	57%
Patients Who Left ER Before Being Seen	16,639	1%	3%	2%
Time from ER Arrival to Admit. (minutes)[2]	276	156	223	274
Time from ER Arrival to Discharge (minutes)	382	103	112	134
Time in ER Before Being Evaluated (minutes)	410	43	29	26
Time to Pain Meds for Fractures (minutes)	31	55	68	57
Heart Attack Care				
Aspirin Given at Discharge[3,7]	-	-	99%	99%
Fibrinolytic Meds Within 30 Min. of Arrival[3,7]	-	-	50%	54%
PCI Within 90 Minutes of Arrival[3,7]	-	-	96%	96%
Statin Prescribed at Discharge[1,3]	-	-	97%	98%
Heart Failure Care				
ACE Inhibitor or ARB for LVSD	33	97%	93%	97%
Discharge Instructions Given	66	86%	91%	94%
Evaluation of LVS Function	92	99%	96%	99%
Medicare Spending				
Medicare Spending per Patient (ratio)	-	0.96	0.95	0.98
Pneumonia Care				
Appropriate Initial Antibiotic Given	79	91%	91%	95%
Blood Culture Timing	81	94%	97%	98%
Pregnancy and Delivery Care				
Newborn Deliveries Scheduled Early[2]	43	51%	22%	6%
Preventive Care				
Immunization for Influenza[2]	287	59%	87%	90%
Immunization for Pneumonia[2]	276	61%	89%	92%
Stroke Care				
Anticoagulation Therapy for Atrial Fibrillation[1,2]	-	-	93%	95%
Antithrombotic Therapy Timing[2]	25	88%	96%	98%
Assessed for Rehabilitation[2]	24	100%	95%	97%
Discharged on Antithrombotic Therapy[2]	24	88%	97%	99%
Discharged on Statin Medication[2]	23	74%	88%	94%
Thrombolytic Therapy Timing[1,2]	-	-	25%	66%
Venous Thromboembolism Prophylaxis[2]	26	38%	87%	94%
Written Stroke Educational Materials Given[2]	11	91%	84%	88%
Surgical Care Improvement Project				
Appropriate Beta Blocker Usage	12	100%	97%	98%
Appropriate VTP Within 24 Hours	68	97%	97%	98%
Controlled Postoperative Blood Glucose[7]	-	-	97%	97%
Perioperative Temperature Management	78	100%	100%	100%
Prophylactic Antibiotic Selection	50	94%	99%	99%
Prophylactic Antibiotic Selection (Outpatient)	97	96%	98%	98%
Prophylactic Antibiotic Stopped	48	94%	97%	98%
Prophylactic Antibiotic Timing	50	100%	99%	99%
Prophylactic Antibiotic Timing (Outpatient)	97	99%	98%	98%
Urinary Catheter Removal[1]	-	-	97%	97%
Survey of Patients' Hospital Experiences				
Area Around Room 'Always' Quiet at Night	300+	70%	72%	61%
Doctors 'Always' Communicated Well	300+	91%	86%	82%
Home Recovery Information Given	300+	84%	83%	85%
Hospital Given 9 or 10 on 10 Point Scale	300+	72%	71%	71%
Meds 'Always' Explained Before Given	300+	65%	67%	64%
Nurses 'Always' Communicated Well	300+	83%	81%	79%
Pain 'Always' Well Controlled	300+	74%	72%	71%
Room and Bathroom 'Always' Clean	300+	81%	74%	73%
Timely Help 'Always' Received	300+	75%	69%	68%
Would Definitely Recommend Hospital	300+	68%	69%	71%
Use of Medical Imaging				
Cardiac Imaging Stress Test before Surgery[1]	-	-	5.7%	5.3%
Combination Abdominal CT Scan	150	11.3%	12.9%	10.5%
Combination Brain/Sinus CT Scan[1]	-	-	3.3%	2.7%
Combination Chest CT Scan[1]	-	-	6.1%	2.7%
Follow-up Mammogram/Ultrasound	362	1.1%	8.4%	8.8%
Lumbar Spine MRI for Low Back Pain	45	46.7%	41.1%	37.2%

Whitfield Medical Surgical Hospital

3550 Hwy 468 W, Bldg 60
Whitfield, MS 39193
E-mail: mikula@msh.state.ms.us
Phone: 601-351-8001
Fax: 601-351-8364
Type: Acute Care Hospitals
Emergency Services: No
Ownership: Government - State
Beds: 43
Key Personnel:
Anesthesiology. . . . . Georgia Coleman
Chief of Medical Staff. . . . . Dan Coughlin, MD
Quality Assurance . . . . Jody Donald
Infection Control. . . . . Judy Pearce
Patient Relations . . . . Clenistine Stewart

Measure	Cases	This Hosp.	State Avg.	U.S. Avg.
Blood Clot Prevention and Treatment				
Anticoagulation Overlap Therapy[2,7]	-	-	86%	93%
ICU Venous Thromboembolism Prophylaxis[2,7]	-	-	86%	92%
Incidence of Potentially Preventable VTE[2,7]	-	-	15%	10%
UFH with Dosages/Platelet Monitoring[2,7]	-	-	94%	97%
Venous Thromboembolism Prophylaxis[2]	79	91%	70%	85%
Warfarin Therapy Discharge Instructions[2,7]	-	-	77%	75%
Chest Pain/Possible Heart Attack Care				
Aspirin Given Within 24 Hours of Arrival[5]	-	-	94%	96%
Fibrinolytic Meds Within 30 Min. of Arrival[5]	-	-	40%	58%
Average Time to ECG (minutes)[5]	-	-	10	7
Average Time to Transfer (minutes)[5]	-	-	77	60
Children's Asthma Care				
Received Home Management Plan of Care	-	-	-	88%
Received Reliever Medication	-	-	-	100%
Received Systemic Corticosteroids	-	-	-	100%
Emergency Department				
Admittance Decision Time (minutes)[7]	-	-	61	98
Head CT Results Within 45 Min. of Arrival[5]	-	-	42%	57%
Patients Who Left ER Before Being Seen[5]	-	-	3%	2%
Time from ER Arrival to Admit. (minutes)[7]	-	-	223	274
Time from ER Arrival to Discharge (minutes)[5]	-	-	112	134
Time in ER Before Being Evaluated (minutes)[5]	-	-	29	26
Time to Pain Meds for Fractures (minutes)[5]	-	-	68	57
Heart Attack Care				
Aspirin Given at Discharge[5]	-	-	99%	99%
Fibrinolytic Meds Within 30 Min. of Arrival[5]	-	-	50%	54%
PCI Within 90 Minutes of Arrival[5]	-	-	96%	96%
Statin Prescribed at Discharge[5]	-	-	97%	98%
Heart Failure Care				
ACE Inhibitor or ARB for LVSD[3,7]	-	-	93%	97%
Discharge Instructions Given[3,7]	-	-	91%	94%
Evaluation of LVS Function[3,7]	-	-	96%	99%
Medicare Spending				
Medicare Spending per Patient (ratio)	-	0.54	0.95	0.98
Pneumonia Care				
Appropriate Initial Antibiotic Given[7]	-	-	91%	95%
Blood Culture Timing[7]	-	-	97%	98%
Pregnancy and Delivery Care				
Newborn Deliveries Scheduled Early[7]	-	-	22%	6%
Preventive Care				
Immunization for Influenza	93	77%	87%	90%
Immunization for Pneumonia	115	82%	89%	92%
Stroke Care				
Anticoagulation Therapy for Atrial Fibrillation[7]	-	-	93%	95%
Antithrombotic Therapy Timing[1]	-	-	96%	98%
Assessed for Rehabilitation[1]	-	-	95%	97%
Discharged on Antithrombotic Therapy[1]	-	-	97%	99%
Discharged on Statin Medication[1]	-	-	88%	94%
Thrombolytic Therapy Timing[7]	-	-	25%	66%
Venous Thromboembolism Prophylaxis[1]	-	-	87%	94%
Written Stroke Educational Materials Given[7]	-	-	84%	88%
Surgical Care Improvement Project				
Appropriate Beta Blocker Usage[5]	-	-	97%	98%
Appropriate VTP Within 24 Hours[5]	-	-	97%	98%
Controlled Postoperative Blood Glucose[5]	-	-	97%	97%
Perioperative Temperature Management[5]	-	-	100%	100%
Prophylactic Antibiotic Selection[5]	-	-	99%	99%
Prophylactic Antibiotic Selection (Outpatient)[5]	-	-	98%	98%
Prophylactic Antibiotic Stopped[5]	-	-	97%	98%
Prophylactic Antibiotic Timing[5]	-	-	99%	99%
Prophylactic Antibiotic Timing (Outpatient)[5]	-	-	98%	98%
Urinary Catheter Removal[5]	-	-	97%	97%
Survey of Patients' Hospital Experiences				
Area Around Room 'Always' Quiet at Night[10]	<100	55%	72%	61%
Doctors 'Always' Communicated Well[10]	<100	70%	86%	82%
Home Recovery Information Given[10]	<100	-	83%	85%
Hospital Given 9 or 10 on 10 Point Scale[10]	<100	92%	71%	71%
Meds 'Always' Explained Before Given[10]	<100	73%	67%	64%
Nurses 'Always' Communicated Well[10]	<100	76%	81%	79%
Pain 'Always' Well Controlled[10]	<100	35%	72%	71%
Room and Bathroom 'Always' Clean[10]	<100	70%	74%	73%
Timely Help 'Always' Received[10]	<100	43%	69%	68%
Would Definitely Recommend Hospital[10]	<100	83%	69%	71%
Use of Medical Imaging				
Cardiac Imaging Stress Test before Surgery[7]	-	-	5.7%	5.3%
Combination Abdominal CT Scan[7]	-	-	12.9%	10.5%
Combination Brain/Sinus CT Scan[1]	-	-	3.3%	2.7%
Combination Chest CT Scan[7]	-	-	6.1%	2.7%
Follow-up Mammogram/Ultrasound[7]	-	-	8.4%	8.8%
Lumbar Spine MRI for Low Back Pain[7]	-	-	41.1%	37.2%

Stone County Hospital

1434 East Central Avenue
Wiggins, MS 39577
URL: www.schospital.net
Phone: 601-928-6600
Type: Critical Access Hospitals
Emergency Services: Yes
Ownership: Proprietary
Key Personnel:
President . . . . James Holmes
Radiology. . . . . Sandy Sellers
CEO . . . . James Williams

Measure	Cases	This Hosp.	State Avg.	U.S. Avg.
Blood Clot Prevention and Treatment				
Anticoagulation Overlap Therapy[5]	-	-	86%	93%
ICU Venous Thromboembolism Prophylaxis[5]	-	-	86%	92%
Incidence of Potentially Preventable VTE[5]	-	-	15%	10%
UFH with Dosages/Platelet Monitoring[5]	-	-	94%	97%
Venous Thromboembolism Prophylaxis[5]	-	-	70%	85%
Warfarin Therapy Discharge Instructions[5]	-	-	77%	75%
Chest Pain/Possible Heart Attack Care				
Aspirin Given Within 24 Hours of Arrival[5]	-	-	94%	96%
Fibrinolytic Meds Within 30 Min. of Arrival[5]	-	-	40%	58%
Average Time to ECG (minutes)[5]	-	-	10	7
Average Time to Transfer (minutes)[5]	-	-	77	60
Children's Asthma Care				
Received Home Management Plan of Care	-	-	-	88%
Received Reliever Medication	-	-	-	100%
Received Systemic Corticosteroids	-	-	-	100%
Emergency Department				
Admittance Decision Time (minutes)[5]	-	-	61	98
Head CT Results Within 45 Min. of Arrival[5]	-	-	42%	57%
Patients Who Left ER Before Being Seen[5]	-	-	3%	2%
Time from ER Arrival to Admit. (minutes)[5]	-	-	223	274
Time from ER Arrival to Discharge (minutes)[5]	-	-	112	134
Time in ER Before Being Evaluated (minutes)[5]	-	-	29	26
Time to Pain Meds for Fractures (minutes)[5]	-	-	68	57
Heart Attack Care				
Aspirin Given at Discharge[5]	-	-	99%	99%
Fibrinolytic Meds Within 30 Min. of Arrival[5]	-	-	50%	54%
PCI Within 90 Minutes of Arrival[5]	-	-	96%	96%
Statin Prescribed at Discharge[5]	-	-	97%	98%
Heart Failure Care				
ACE Inhibitor or ARB for LVSD[1,3]	-	-	93%	97%
Discharge Instructions Given[1,3]	-	-	91%	94%
Evaluation of LVS Function[3]	12	75%	96%	99%

NOTE: Hospital profiles are in alphabetical order by state, then city, then hospital within the city; Rankings exclude hospitals with less than 25 cases except for patient surveys which excludes hospitals with less than 100 cases; (a) 100-299 cases; (1) The number of cases/patients is too few to report; (2) Data submitted were based on a sample of cases/patients; (3) Results are based on a shorter time period than required; (4) Data suppressed by CMS for one or more quarters; (5) Results are not available for this reporting period; (6) Fewer than 100 patients completed the HCAHPS survey; (7) No cases met the criteria for this measure; (8) The lower limit of the confidence interval cannot be calculated if the number of observed infections equals zero; (9) No data are available from the state/territory for this reporting period; (10) The scores shown reflect fewer than 50 completed surveys; (11) There were discrepancies in the data collection process; (12) This measure does not apply to this hospital for this reporting period; (13) Results cannot be calculated for this reporting period; (14) The results for this state are combined with nearby states to protect confidentiality; Please refer to the User's Guide for a full explanation of data.

Measure	Cases	This Hosp.	State Avg.	U.S. Avg.
Medicare Spending				
Medicare Spending per Patient (ratio)	-	-	0.95	0.98
Pneumonia Care				
Appropriate Initial Antibiotic Given[1,3]	-	-	91%	95%
Blood Culture Timing[1,3]	-	-	97%	98%
Pregnancy and Delivery Care				
Newborn Deliveries Scheduled Early[5]	-	-	22%	6%
Preventive Care				
Immunization for Influenza[5]	-	-	87%	90%
Immunization for Pneumonia[5]	-	-	89%	92%
Stroke Care				
Anticoagulation Therapy for Atrial Fibrillation[5]	-	-	93%	95%
Antithrombotic Therapy Timing[5]	-	-	96%	98%
Assessed for Rehabilitation[5]	-	-	95%	97%
Discharged on Antithrombotic Therapy[5]	-	-	97%	99%
Discharged on Statin Medication[5]	-	-	88%	94%
Thrombolytic Therapy Timing[5]	-	-	25%	66%
Venous Thromboembolism Prophylaxis[5]	-	-	87%	94%
Written Stroke Educational Materials Given[5]	-	-	84%	88%
Surgical Care Improvement Project				
Appropriate Beta Blocker Usage[5]	-	-	97%	98%
Appropriate VTP Within 24 Hours[5]	-	-	97%	98%
Controlled Postoperative Blood Glucose[5]	-	-	97%	97%
Perioperative Temperature Management[5]	-	-	100%	100%
Prophylactic Antibiotic Selection[5]	-	-	99%	99%
Prophylactic Antibiotic Selection (Outpatient)[5]	-	-	98%	98%
Prophylactic Antibiotic Stopped[5]	-	-	97%	98%
Prophylactic Antibiotic Timing[5]	-	-	99%	99%
Prophylactic Antibiotic Timing (Outpatient)[5]	-	-	98%	98%
Urinary Catheter Removal[5]	-	-	97%	97%
Survey of Patients' Hospital Experiences				
Area Around Room 'Always' Quiet at Night[6]	<100	66%	72%	61%
Doctors 'Always' Communicated Well[6]	<100	93%	86%	82%
Home Recovery Information Given[6]	<100	80%	83%	85%
Hospital Given 9 or 10 on 10 Point Scale[6]	<100	73%	71%	71%
Meds 'Always' Explained Before Given[6]	<100	79%	67%	64%
Nurses 'Always' Communicated Well[6]	<100	86%	81%	79%
Pain 'Always' Well Controlled[6]	<100	78%	72%	71%
Room and Bathroom 'Always' Clean[6]	<100	75%	74%	73%
Timely Help 'Always' Received[6]	<100	76%	69%	68%
Would Definitely Recommend Hospital[6]	<100	70%	69%	71%
Use of Medical Imaging				
Cardiac Imaging Stress Test before Surgery[1]	-	-	5.7%	5.3%
Combination Abdominal CT Scan	139	8.6%	12.9%	10.5%
Combination Brain/Sinus CT Scan[1]	-	-	3.3%	2.7%
Combination Chest CT Scan	76	5.3%	6.1%	2.7%
Follow-up Mammogram/Ultrasound[7]	-	-	8.4%	8.8%
Lumbar Spine MRI for Low Back Pain[1]	-	-	41.1%	37.2%

Tyler Holmes Memorial Hospital

409 Tyler Holmes Drive
Winona, MS 38967
Phone: 662-283-4114
Fax: 662-283-4640
Type: Critical Access Hospitals
Emergency Services: Yes
Ownership: Government - Local
Beds: 49

Key Personnel:
Infection Control . . . . Latia Crawford

Measure	Cases	This Hosp.	State Avg.	U.S. Avg.
Blood Clot Prevention and Treatment				
Anticoagulation Overlap Therapy[5]	-	-	86%	93%
ICU Venous Thromboembolism Prophylaxis[5]	-	-	86%	92%
Incidence of Potentially Preventable VTE[5]	-	-	15%	10%
UFH with Dosages/Platelet Monitoring[5]	-	-	94%	97%
Venous Thromboembolism Prophylaxis[5]	-	-	70%	85%
Warfarin Therapy Discharge Instructions[5]	-	-	77%	75%
Chest Pain/Possible Heart Attack Care				
Aspirin Given Within 24 Hours of Arrival[5]	-	-	94%	96%
Fibrinolytic Meds Within 30 Min. of Arrival[5]	-	-	40%	58%
Average Time to ECG (minutes)[5]	-	-	10	7
Average Time to Transfer (minutes)[5]	-	-	77	60
Children's Asthma Care				
Received Home Management Plan of Care	-	-	-	88%
Received Reliever Medication	-	-	-	100%
Received Systemic Corticosteroids	-	-	-	100%
Emergency Department				
Admittance Decision Time (minutes)[5]	-	-	61	98
Head CT Results Within 45 Min. of Arrival[5]	-	-	42%	57%
Patients Who Left ER Before Being Seen	6,858	1%	3%	2%
Time from ER Arrival to Admit. (minutes)[5]	-	-	223	274
Time from ER Arrival to Discharge (minutes)[5]	-	-	112	134
Time in ER Before Being Evaluated (minutes)[5]	-	-	29	26
Time to Pain Meds for Fractures (minutes)[5]	-	-	68	57
Heart Attack Care				
Aspirin Given at Discharge[3,7]	-	-	99%	99%
Fibrinolytic Meds Within 30 Min. of Arrival[3,7]	-	-	50%	54%
PCI Within 90 Minutes of Arrival[3,7]	-	-	96%	96%
Statin Prescribed at Discharge[3,7]	-	-	97%	98%
Heart Failure Care				
ACE Inhibitor or ARB for LVSD[1]	-	-	93%	97%
Discharge Instructions Given	21	57%	91%	94%
Evaluation of LVS Function	34	88%	96%	99%
Medicare Spending				
Medicare Spending per Patient (ratio)	-	-	0.95	0.98
Pneumonia Care				
Appropriate Initial Antibiotic Given[2]	20	85%	91%	95%
Blood Culture Timing[2]	19	79%	97%	98%
Pregnancy and Delivery Care				
Newborn Deliveries Scheduled Early[5]	-	-	22%	6%
Preventive Care				
Immunization for Influenza[5]	-	-	87%	90%
Immunization for Pneumonia[5]	-	-	89%	92%
Stroke Care				
Anticoagulation Therapy for Atrial Fibrillation[5]	-	-	93%	95%
Antithrombotic Therapy Timing[5]	-	-	96%	98%
Assessed for Rehabilitation[5]	-	-	95%	97%
Discharged on Antithrombotic Therapy[5]	-	-	97%	99%
Discharged on Statin Medication[5]	-	-	88%	94%
Thrombolytic Therapy Timing[5]	-	-	25%	66%
Venous Thromboembolism Prophylaxis[5]	-	-	87%	94%
Written Stroke Educational Materials Given[5]	-	-	84%	88%
Surgical Care Improvement Project				
Appropriate Beta Blocker Usage[5]	-	-	97%	98%
Appropriate VTP Within 24 Hours[5]	-	-	97%	98%
Controlled Postoperative Blood Glucose[5]	-	-	97%	97%
Perioperative Temperature Management[5]	-	-	100%	100%
Prophylactic Antibiotic Selection[5]	-	-	99%	99%
Prophylactic Antibiotic Selection (Outpatient)[5]	-	-	98%	98%
Prophylactic Antibiotic Stopped[5]	-	-	97%	98%
Prophylactic Antibiotic Timing[5]	-	-	99%	99%
Prophylactic Antibiotic Timing (Outpatient)[5]	-	-	98%	98%
Urinary Catheter Removal[5]	-	-	97%	97%
Survey of Patients' Hospital Experiences				
Area Around Room 'Always' Quiet at Night[6]	<100	68%	72%	61%
Doctors 'Always' Communicated Well[6]	<100	88%	86%	82%
Home Recovery Information Given[6]	<100	87%	83%	85%
Hospital Given 9 or 10 on 10 Point Scale[6]	<100	65%	71%	71%
Meds 'Always' Explained Before Given[6]	<100	61%	67%	64%
Nurses 'Always' Communicated Well[6]	<100	83%	81%	79%
Pain 'Always' Well Controlled[6]	<100	71%	72%	71%
Room and Bathroom 'Always' Clean[6]	<100	76%	74%	73%
Timely Help 'Always' Received[6]	<100	77%	69%	68%
Would Definitely Recommend Hospital[6]	<100	60%	69%	71%
Use of Medical Imaging				
Cardiac Imaging Stress Test before Surgery[1]	-	-	5.7%	5.3%
Combination Abdominal CT Scan	184	1.6%	12.9%	10.5%
Combination Brain/Sinus CT Scan[1]	-	-	3.3%	2.7%
Combination Chest CT Scan	79	2.5%	6.1%	2.7%
Follow-up Mammogram/Ultrasound[7]	-	-	8.4%	8.8%
Lumbar Spine MRI for Low Back Pain[1]	-	-	41.1%	37.2%

Kings Daughters Hospital

823 Grand Avenue
Yazoo City, MS 39194
Phone: 662-746-2261
Type: Critical Access Hospitals
Emergency Services: Yes
Ownership: Voluntary non-profit - Private

Measure	Cases	This Hosp.	State Avg.	U.S. Avg.
Blood Clot Prevention and Treatment				
Anticoagulation Overlap Therapy[5]	-	-	86%	93%
ICU Venous Thromboembolism Prophylaxis[5]	-	-	86%	92%
Incidence of Potentially Preventable VTE[5]	-	-	15%	10%
UFH with Dosages/Platelet Monitoring[5]	-	-	94%	97%
Venous Thromboembolism Prophylaxis[5]	-	-	70%	85%
Warfarin Therapy Discharge Instructions[5]	-	-	77%	75%
Chest Pain/Possible Heart Attack Care				
Aspirin Given Within 24 Hours of Arrival[5]	-	-	94%	96%
Fibrinolytic Meds Within 30 Min. of Arrival[5]	-	-	40%	58%
Average Time to ECG (minutes)[5]	-	-	10	7
Average Time to Transfer (minutes)[5]	-	-	77	60
Children's Asthma Care				
Received Home Management Plan of Care	-	-	-	88%
Received Reliever Medication	-	-	-	100%
Received Systemic Corticosteroids	-	-	-	100%
Emergency Department				
Admittance Decision Time (minutes)[5]	-	-	61	98
Head CT Results Within 45 Min. of Arrival[5]	-	-	42%	57%
Patients Who Left ER Before Being Seen	4,749	7%	3%	2%
Time from ER Arrival to Admit. (minutes)[5]	-	-	223	274
Time from ER Arrival to Discharge (minutes)[5]	-	-	112	134
Time in ER Before Being Evaluated (minutes)[5]	-	-	29	26
Time to Pain Meds for Fractures (minutes)[5]	-	-	68	57
Heart Attack Care				
Aspirin Given at Discharge[5]	-	-	99%	99%
Fibrinolytic Meds Within 30 Min. of Arrival[5]	-	-	50%	54%
PCI Within 90 Minutes of Arrival[5]	-	-	96%	96%
Statin Prescribed at Discharge[5]	-	-	97%	98%
Heart Failure Care				
ACE Inhibitor or ARB for LVSD	20	70%	93%	97%
Discharge Instructions Given	34	59%	91%	94%
Evaluation of LVS Function	44	80%	96%	99%
Medicare Spending				
Medicare Spending per Patient (ratio)	-	-	0.95	0.98
Pneumonia Care				
Appropriate Initial Antibiotic Given[5]	-	-	91%	95%
Blood Culture Timing[5]	-	-	97%	98%
Pregnancy and Delivery Care				
Newborn Deliveries Scheduled Early[5]	-	-	22%	6%
Preventive Care				
Immunization for Influenza[5]	-	-	87%	90%
Immunization for Pneumonia[5]	-	-	89%	92%
Stroke Care				
Anticoagulation Therapy for Atrial Fibrillation[5]	-	-	93%	95%
Antithrombotic Therapy Timing[5]	-	-	96%	98%
Assessed for Rehabilitation[5]	-	-	95%	97%
Discharged on Antithrombotic Therapy[5]	-	-	97%	99%
Discharged on Statin Medication[5]	-	-	88%	94%
Thrombolytic Therapy Timing[5]	-	-	25%	66%
Venous Thromboembolism Prophylaxis[5]	-	-	87%	94%
Written Stroke Educational Materials Given[5]	-	-	84%	88%
Surgical Care Improvement Project				
Appropriate Beta Blocker Usage[5]	-	-	97%	98%
Appropriate VTP Within 24 Hours[5]	-	-	97%	98%
Controlled Postoperative Blood Glucose[5]	-	-	97%	97%
Perioperative Temperature Management[5]	-	-	100%	100%
Prophylactic Antibiotic Selection[5]	-	-	99%	99%
Prophylactic Antibiotic Selection (Outpatient)[5]	-	-	98%	98%
Prophylactic Antibiotic Stopped[5]	-	-	97%	98%
Prophylactic Antibiotic Timing[5]	-	-	99%	99%
Prophylactic Antibiotic Timing (Outpatient)[5]	-	-	98%	98%
Urinary Catheter Removal[5]	-	-	97%	97%
Survey of Patients' Hospital Experiences				
Area Around Room 'Always' Quiet at Night[5]	-	-	72%	61%
Doctors 'Always' Communicated Well[5]	-	-	86%	82%

NOTE: Hospital profiles are in alphabetical order by state, then city, then hospital within the city; Rankings exclude hospitals with less than 25 cases except for patient surveys which excludes hospitals with less than 100 cases; (a) 100-299 cases; (1) The number of cases/patients is too few to report; (2) Data submitted were based on a sample of cases/patients; (3) Results are based on a shorter time period than required; (4) Data suppressed by CMS for one or more quarters; (5) Results are not available for this reporting period; (6) Fewer than 100 patients completed the HCAHPS survey; (7) No cases met the criteria for this measure; (8) The lower limit of the confidence interval cannot be calculated if the number of observed infections equals zero; (9) No data are available from the state/territory for this reporting period; (10) The scores shown reflect fewer than 50 completed surveys; (11) There were discrepancies in the data collection process; (12) This measure does not apply to this hospital for this reporting period; (13) Results cannot be calculated for this reporting period; (14) The results for this state are combined with nearby states to protect confidentiality; Please refer to the User's Guide for a full explanation of data.

Home Recovery Information Given[5]	-	-	83%	85%
Hospital Given 9 or 10 on 10 Point Scale[5]	-	-	71%	71%
Meds 'Always' Explained Before Given[5]	-	-	67%	64%
Nurses 'Always' Communicated Well[5]	-	-	81%	79%
Pain 'Always' Well Controlled[5]	-	-	72%	71%
Room and Bathroom 'Always' Clean[5]	-	-	74%	73%
Timely Help 'Always' Received[5]	-	-	69%	68%
Would Definitely Recommend Hospital[5]	-	-	69%	71%
Use of Medical Imaging				
Cardiac Imaging Stress Test before Surgery[1]	-	-	5.7%	5.3%
Combination Abdominal CT Scan	159	6.9%	12.9%	10.5%
Combination Brain/Sinus CT Scan	316	5.7%	3.3%	2.7%
Combination Chest CT Scan	73	27.4%	6.1%	2.7%
Follow-up Mammogram/Ultrasound	145	11.7%	8.4%	8.8%
Lumbar Spine MRI for Low Back Pain	34	47.1%	41.1%	37.2%

NOTE: Hospital profiles are in alphabetical order by state, then city, then hospital within the city; Rankings exclude hospitals with less than 25 cases except for patient surveys which excludes hospitals with less than 100 cases; (a) 100-299 cases; (1) The number of cases/patients is too few to report; (2) Data submitted were based on a sample of cases/patients; (3) Results are based on a shorter time period than required; (4) Data suppressed by CMS for one or more quarters; (5) Results are not available for this reporting period; (6) Fewer than 100 patients completed the HCAHPS survey; (7) No cases met the criteria for this measure; (8) The lower limit of the confidence interval cannot be calculated if the number of observed infections equals zero; (9) No data are available from the state/territory for this reporting period; (10) The scores shown reflect fewer than 50 completed surveys; (11) There were discrepancies in the data collection process; (12) This measure does not apply to this hospital for this reporting period; (13) Results cannot be calculated for this reporting period; (14) The results for this state are combined with nearby states to protect confidentiality; Please refer to the User's Guide for a full explanation of data.

Blood Clot Prevention and Treatment

Venous Thromboembolism Prophylaxis

Hospital Name	City	Rate	Cases
Hospital Hermanos Melendez[2,3]	Bayamon	100%	36

Chest Pain/Possible Heart Attack Care

No hospitals met the 25 case threshold.

Children's Asthma Care

No hospitals met the 25 case threshold.

Emergency Department

Admittance Decision Time (minutes)

Hospital Name	City	Min.	Cases
Hospital Hermanos Melendez[2]	Bayamon	190	513

Time from ER Arrival to Being Admitted (minutes)

Hospital Name	City	Min.	Cases
Hospital Hermanos Melendez[2]	Bayamon	645	513

Heart Attack Care

Aspirin Given at Discharge

Hospital Name	City	Rate	Cases
Doctors' Center Hospital	Manati	100%	63
Hospital De La Concepcion	San German	100%	147
Hospital Episcopal San Lucas Guayama	Guayama	100%	37
Hospital San Cristobal[2]	Coto Laurel	100%	79
Manati Medical Center Doctor Otero Lopez[3]	Manati	100%	57
Presbyterian Community Hospital	San Juan	100%	55
San Juan VA Medical Center	San Juan	100%	119
Sistema Integrados De Salud Del Sur Oeste	Mayaguez	100%	212
Hospital UPR - Doctor Federico Trilla	Carolina	99%	108
San Luke's Memorial Hospital	Ponce	99%	655
Hima San Pablo Humacao	Humacao	98%	40
Hospital Damas	Ponce	98%	66
Hospital Pavia Santurce	Fernandez Junc	98%	232
Hospital Hermanos Melendez	Bayamon	97%	77
Hospital Hima - San Pablo Bayamon	Bayamon	97%	342
Hospital San Carlos Borromeo	Moca	96%	52
Hima San Pablo - Caguas	Caguas	95%	64
Hospital Menonita Caguas	Caguas	94%	147
Hospital Pavia Hato Rey	Hato Rey	93%	28
Hospital Comunitario Buen Samaritano	Aguadilla	92%	75
Hospital Metropolitano Doctor Pila	Ponce	92%	36
Hospital Metropolitano Doctor Tito Mattei	Yauco	92%	128
Bella Vista Hospital	Mayaguez	90%	39
Auxilio Mutuo Hospital	Hato Rey	89%	114
Centro Cardiovascular	Rio Piedras	89%	383
Hospital Metropolitano San German[2]	San German	89%	63
Mennonite General Hospital	Aibonito	89%	45
Hima - San Pablo Fajardo	Fajardo	88%	32
Hospital Menonita De Cayey	Cayey	85%	133
Ryder Memorial Hospital[3]	Humacao	69%	61
Hospital Doctor Cayetano Coll y Toste	Arecibo	66%	80
Hospital Doctor Susoni[2]	Arecibo	56%	63

PCI Within 90 Minutes of Arrival

Hospital Name	City	Rate	Cases
San Luke's Memorial Hospital	Ponce	58%	36

Statin Prescribed at Discharge

Hospital Name	City	Rate	Cases
Doctors' Center Hospital	Manati	100%	70
Hospital De La Concepcion	San German	100%	163
Hospital Episcopal San Lucas Guayama	Guayama	100%	44
Hospital Hermanos Melendez	Bayamon	100%	85
Hospital Pavia Hato Rey	Hato Rey	100%	26
Hospital San Cristobal[2]	Coto Laurel	100%	76
Manati Medical Center Doctor Otero Lopez[3]	Manati	100%	47
Presbyterian Community Hospital	San Juan	100%	51
Sistema Integrados De Salud Del Sur Oeste	Mayaguez	100%	224
Hima San Pablo - Caguas	Caguas	99%	73
Hospital UPR - Doctor Federico Trilla	Carolina	99%	114
San Juan VA Medical Center	San Juan	98%	128
Hospital Hima - San Pablo Bayamon	Bayamon	96%	390
Hospital Pavia Santurce	Fernandez Junc	96%	237
Hospital Damas	Ponce	94%	68
Hospital Menonita Caguas	Caguas	92%	143
Hospital San Carlos Borromeo	Moca	92%	60
Metropolitan Hospital	San Juan	92%	26
Hospital Comunitario Buen Samaritano	Aguadilla	91%	94
Hima San Pablo Humacao	Humacao	90%	48
Centro Cardiovascular	Rio Piedras	89%	415
Hospital Metropolitano Doctor Tito Mattei	Yauco	88%	140
Mennonite General Hospital	Aibonito	88%	50
San Luke's Memorial Hospital	Ponce	86%	621
Hospital Metropolitano San German[2]	San German	84%	64
Hospital Doctor Cayetano Coll y Toste	Arecibo	83%	87
Hospital Menonita De Cayey	Cayey	81%	150
Bella Vista Hospital	Mayaguez	76%	46
Hospital Metropolitano Doctor Pila	Ponce	73%	33
Auxilio Mutuo Hospital	Hato Rey	63%	115
Hima - San Pablo Fajardo	Fajardo	60%	40
Hospital Doctor Susoni[2]	Arecibo	60%	58
Hospital San Francisco	San Juan	52%	33
Ryder Memorial Hospital[3]	Humacao	25%	57

Heart Failure Care

ACE Inhibitor or ARB for LVSD

Hospital Name	City	Rate	Cases
Asociacion Hospital Del Maestro	San Juan	100%	33
Doctors' Center Hospital	Manati	100%	85
Hima San Pablo - Caguas	Caguas	100%	94
Hospital De La Concepcion	San German	100%	84
Hospital Hermanos Melendez	Bayamon	100%	58
Hospital Menonita De Cayey	Cayey	100%	45
Hospital Pavia Santurce	Fernandez Junc	100%	98
Hospital San Carlos Borromeo[2]	Moca	100%	35
Hospital San Cristobal[2]	Coto Laurel	100%	58
Hospital UPR - Doctor Federico Trilla	Carolina	100%	96
Manati Medical Center Doctor Otero Lopez[3]	Manati	100%	45
Presbyterian Community Hospital	San Juan	100%	27
San Juan Municipal Hospital	Rio Piedras	100%	49
San Juan VA Medical Center	San Juan	100%	95
Sistema Integrados De Salud Del Sur Oeste	Mayaguez	100%	63
Hospital Damas	Ponce	98%	51
Metropolitan Hospital	San Juan	98%	55
San Luke's Memorial Hospital	Ponce	97%	112
Hospital Pavia Hato Rey	Hato Rey	96%	25
Centro Cardiovascular	Rio Piedras	95%	227
Hospital Hima - San Pablo Bayamon[2]	Bayamon	95%	130
Hima - San Pablo Fajardo	Fajardo	94%	50
Mennonite General Hospital	Aibonito	94%	63
Hospital Comunitario Buen Samaritano	Aguadilla	92%	99
Hospital Doctor Cayetano Coll y Toste	Arecibo	89%	80
Hospital Metropolitano Doctor Tito Mattei	Yauco	86%	76
Bella Vista Hospital	Mayaguez	84%	43
Hospital Metropolitano Doctor Pila	Ponce	70%	50
Ryder Memorial Hospital[3]	Humacao	69%	42
Auxilio Mutuo Hospital	Hato Rey	68%	107
Hospital Doctor Susoni[2]	Arecibo	47%	49

Discharge Instructions Given

Hospital Name	City	Rate	Cases
Doctors' Center Hospital	Manati	100%	147
Hima San Pablo - Caguas	Caguas	100%	201
Hima San Pablo Humacao	Humacao	100%	64
Hospital Comunitario Buen Samaritano	Aguadilla	100%	246
Hospital De La Concepcion	San German	100%	151
Hospital Episcopal San Lucas Guayama	Guayama	100%	67
Hospital Hermanos Melendez	Bayamon	100%	273
Hospital Pavia Santurce	Fernandez Junc	100%	260
Hospital Perea[2]	Mayaguez	100%	35
Manati Medical Center Doctor Otero Lopez[3]	Manati	100%	146
Presbyterian Community Hospital	San Juan	100%	94
San Juan Municipal Hospital	Rio Piedras	100%	49
San Juan VA Medical Center	San Juan	100%	256
San Luke's Memorial Hospital	Ponce	100%	401
Sistema Integrados De Salud Del Sur Oeste	Mayaguez	100%	170
Asociacion Hospital Del Maestro	San Juan	99%	147
Hospital Hima - San Pablo Bayamon[2]	Bayamon	99%	300
Hospital San Cristobal[2]	Coto Laurel	99%	75
Centro Cardiovascular	Rio Piedras	97%	388
Centro Medico Wilma N Vazquez[2,3]	Vega Baja	97%	29
Hospital Pavia Hato Rey	Hato Rey	96%	57
Hospital San Carlos Borromeo[2]	Moca	96%	81
Hospital UPR - Doctor Federico Trilla	Carolina	96%	211
Bella Vista Hospital	Mayaguez	94%	136
Hospital Doctor Susoni[2]	Arecibo	93%	86
Hospital Menonita De Cayey	Cayey	93%	170
Mennonite General Hospital	Aibonito	92%	98
Hospital Universitario Doctor Ruiz Arnau	Bayamon	90%	42
Metropolitan Hospital	San Juan	90%	113
Hospital Oriente	Humacao	89%	28
Hospital Damas	Ponce	86%	125
Hima - San Pablo Fajardo	Fajardo	84%	160
Hospital Metropolitano Doctor Tito Mattei	Yauco	82%	184
Santa Rosa Clinic[3]	Guayama	71%	28
Doctors Center Hospital Bayamon[2]	Bayamon	67%	84
Hospital Metropolitano Doctor Pila	Ponce	61%	116
Hospital Metropolitano San German[2]	San German	60%	45
Auxilio Mutuo Hospital	Hato Rey	59%	395
Doctors' Center Hospital San Juan[2]	Fernandez Junc	47%	75
Hospital Doctor Cayetano Coll y Toste	Arecibo	37%	183
Hospital San Francisco	San Juan	37%	49
Ryder Memorial Hospital[3]	Humacao	8%	110

Evaluation of LVS Function

Hospital Name	City	Rate	Cases
Asociacion Hospital Del Maestro	San Juan	100%	149
Centro Medico Wilma N Vazquez[2,3]	Vega Baja	100%	30
Hospital Damas	Ponce	100%	118
Hospital De La Concepcion	San German	100%	150
Hospital Hima - San Pablo Bayamon[2]	Bayamon	100%	302
Hospital Oriente	Humacao	100%	28
Hospital Pavia Santurce	Fernandez Junc	100%	260
Hospital Perea[2]	Mayaguez	100%	35
Hospital UPR - Doctor Federico Trilla	Carolina	100%	211
Presbyterian Community Hospital	San Juan	100%	33
San Juan Municipal Hospital	Rio Piedras	100%	49
San Juan VA Medical Center	San Juan	100%	268
Sistema Integrados De Salud Del Sur Oeste	Mayaguez	100%	171
Doctors' Center Hospital	Manati	99%	150
Hima San Pablo - Caguas	Caguas	99%	204
Manati Medical Center Doctor Otero Lopez[3]	Manati	99%	149
Mennonite General Hospital	Aibonito	99%	98
Metropolitan Hospital	San Juan	99%	112
Hospital Episcopal San Lucas Guayama	Guayama	98%	66
Hospital Menonita De Cayey	Cayey	98%	172
Hospital Pavia Hato Rey	Hato Rey	98%	63
Hospital Hermanos Melendez	Bayamon	97%	274
Hospital San Francisco	San Juan	96%	50
Hospital Universitario Doctor Ruiz Arnau	Bayamon	96%	53
Santa Rosa Clinic[3]	Guayama	96%	28
Centro Cardiovascular	Rio Piedras	95%	389
San Luke's Memorial Hospital	Ponce	95%	401
Hospital Comunitario Buen Samaritano	Aguadilla	93%	246
Hospital San Cristobal[2]	Coto Laurel	93%	76
Bella Vista Hospital	Mayaguez	92%	139
Hima - San Pablo Fajardo	Fajardo	92%	160
Hospital Metropolitano Doctor Pila	Ponce	92%	120
Ryder Memorial Hospital[3]	Humacao	90%	101
Hima San Pablo Humacao	Humacao	89%	65
Hospital Doctor Susoni[2]	Arecibo	88%	86
Hospital Metropolitano Doctor Tito Mattei	Yauco	88%	184
Auxilio Mutuo Hospital	Hato Rey	87%	399
Hospital Doctor Cayetano Coll y Toste	Arecibo	86%	172
Doctors Center Hospital Bayamon[2]	Bayamon	83%	84
Hospital Metropolitano San German[2]	San German	80%	46
Hospital San Carlos Borromeo[2]	Moca	80%	81
Doctors' Center Hospital San Juan[2]	Fernandez Junc	68%	50

Medicare Spending

Data was not available for this measure.

Pneumonia Care

Appropriate Initial Antibiotic Given

Hospital Name	City	Rate	Cases
Hospital Pavia Santurce	Fernandez Junc	100%	63
San Juan VA Medical Center	San Juan	97%	79
Doctors' Center Hospital	Manati	95%	74
Hima San Pablo Humacao	Humacao	95%	74
Hospital Comunitario Buen Samaritano	Aguadilla	93%	140
Hospital De La Concepcion	San German	93%	46
Hospital Hermanos Melendez	Bayamon	93%	116
Metropolitan Hospital	San Juan	93%	158
Manati Medical Center Doctor Otero Lopez[3]	Manati	91%	139
Hospital UPR - Doctor Federico Trilla	Carolina	89%	142
Hospital Episcopal San Lucas Guayama	Guayama	88%	51
Hospital Menonita De Cayey	Cayey	87%	93
Mennonite General Hospital	Aibonito	85%	214
Hospital Hima - San Pablo Bayamon[2]	Bayamon	84%	135
San Luke's Memorial Hospital	Ponce	82%	144
Hima San Pablo - Caguas[2]	Caguas	81%	111
Hospital Pavia Hato Rey	Hato Rey	81%	80
Bella Vista Hospital	Mayaguez	80%	107
Doctors Center Hospital Bayamon[2]	Bayamon	80%	46
Hospital Doctor Susoni[2]	Arecibo	79%	42
Asociacion Hospital Del Maestro	San Juan	78%	88
Auxilio Mutuo Hospital	Hato Rey	76%	88
Hospital Doctor Cayetano Coll y Toste	Arecibo	73%	44
Hospital Metropolitano Doctor Pila	Ponce	73%	106
Hospital Universitario Doctor Ruiz Arnau	Bayamon	72%	93
Hospital Perea[2]	Mayaguez	70%	99
Sistema Integrados De Salud Del Sur Oeste	Mayaguez	69%	94
Hima - San Pablo Fajardo	Fajardo	67%	57
Santa Rosa Clinic	Guayama	56%	25
Hospital San Francisco	San Juan	54%	39
Hospital San Carlos Borromeo[2]	Moca	51%	37
Hospital Menonita Caguas	Caguas	46%	37

NOTE: Hospital profiles are in alphabetical order by state, then city, then hospital within the city; Rankings exclude hospitals with less than 25 cases except for patient surveys which excludes hospitals with less than 100 cases; (a) 100-299 cases; (1) The number of cases/patients is too few to report; (2) Data submitted were based on a sample of cases/patients; (3) Results are based on a shorter time period than required; (4) Data suppressed by CMS for one or more quarters; (5) Results are not available for this reporting period; (6) Fewer than 100 patients completed the HCAHPS survey; (7) No cases met the criteria for this measure; (8) The lower limit of the confidence interval cannot be calculated if the number of observed infections equals zero; (9) No data are available from the state/territory for this reporting period; (10) The scores shown reflect fewer than 50 completed surveys; (11) There were discrepancies in the data collection process; (12) This measure does not apply to this hospital for this reporting period; (13) Results cannot be calculated for this reporting period; (14) The results for this state are combined with nearby states to protect confidentiality; Please refer to the User's Guide for a full explanation of data.

Blood Culture Timing

Hospital Name	City	Rate	Cases
Doctors' Center Hospital	Manati	100%	37
Hospital Pavia Santurce	Fernandez Junc	100%	69
San Juan Municipal Hospital	Rio Piedras	100%	27
San Juan VA Medical Center	San Juan	99%	291
Hospital Comunitario Buen Samaritano	Aguadilla	98%	107
Hospital Pavia Hato Rey	Hato Rey	98%	48
Hospital Hermanos Melendez	Bayamon	94%	106
Hospital Damas	Ponce	92%	26
Hospital Menonita De Cayey	Cayey	90%	128
Hospital Hima - San Pablo Bayamon[2]	Bayamon	89%	166
Metropolitan Hospital	San Juan	89%	186
Hospital Episcopal San Lucas Guayama	Guayama	88%	34
Mennonite General Hospital	Aibonito	88%	215
San Luke's Memorial Hospital	Ponce	88%	77
Manati Medical Center Doctor Otero Lopez[3]	Manati	87%	115
Hima San Pablo - Caguas[2]	Caguas	84%	146
Hospital Metropolitano Doctor Pila	Ponce	84%	77
Hospital Doctor Susoni[2]	Arecibo	83%	35
Hima San Pablo Humacao	Humacao	82%	82
Hospital UPR - Doctor Federico Trilla	Carolina	80%	145
Sistema Integrados De Salud Del Sur Oeste	Mayaguez	80%	178
Asociacion Hospital Del Maestro	San Juan	79%	81
Hima - San Pablo Fajardo	Fajardo	78%	59
Auxilio Mutuo Hospital	Hato Rey	73%	128
Hospital San Carlos Borromeo[2]	Moca	71%	35
Hospital Universitario Doctor Ruiz Arnau	Bayamon	71%	97
Doctors Center Hospital Bayamon[2]	Bayamon	65%	26
Hospital Doctor Cayetano Coll y Toste	Arecibo	64%	28
Bella Vista Hospital	Mayaguez	61%	123
Hospital San Francisco	San Juan	54%	106
Hospital Perea[2]	Mayaguez	45%	29

Pregnancy and Delivery Care

No hospitals met the 25 case threshold.

Preventive Care

Immunization for Influenza

Hospital Name	City	Rate	Cases
Hospital Hermanos Melendez[2]	Bayamon	44%	283

Immunization for Pneumonia

Hospital Name	City	Rate	Cases
Hospital Hermanos Melendez[2]	Bayamon	28%	461

Stroke Care

Antithrombotic Therapy Timing

Hospital Name	City	Rate	Cases
Manati Medical Center Doctor Otero Lopez[3]	Manati	89%	44
Hospital Universitario De Adulto	Rio Piedras	80%	66

Assessed for Rehabilitation

Hospital Name	City	Rate	Cases
Hospital Universitario De Adulto	Rio Piedras	80%	125
Manati Medical Center Doctor Otero Lopez[3]	Manati	39%	62

Discharged on Antithrombotic Therapy

Hospital Name	City	Rate	Cases
Hospital Universitario De Adulto	Rio Piedras	82%	55
Manati Medical Center Doctor Otero Lopez[3]	Manati	44%	59

Discharged on Statin Medication

Hospital Name	City	Rate	Cases
Manati Medical Center Doctor Otero Lopez[3]	Manati	100%	59
Hospital Universitario De Adulto	Rio Piedras	84%	51

Thrombolytic Therapy Timing

Hospital Name	City	Rate	Cases
Hospital Universitario De Adulto	Rio Piedras	0%	64

Venous Thromboembolism (VTE) Prophylaxis

Hospital Name	City	Rate	Cases
Manati Medical Center Doctor Otero Lopez[3]	Manati	82%	60
Hospital Universitario De Adulto	Rio Piedras	34%	150

Written Stroke Educational Materials Given

Hospital Name	City	Rate	Cases
Manati Medical Center Doctor Otero Lopez[3]	Manati	100%	62
Hospital Universitario De Adulto	Rio Piedras	94%	99

Surgical Care Improvement Project

Appropriate Beta Blocker Usage

Hospital Name	City	Rate	Cases
Hospital Damas	Ponce	100%	36
Hospital Metropolitano Doctor Pila	Ponce	100%	25
Manati Medical Center Doctor Otero Lopez[3]	Manati	100%	27
San Juan VA Medical Center[2]	San Juan	94%	66
Sistema Integrados De Salud Del Sur Oeste	Mayaguez	94%	113
Bella Vista Hospital	Mayaguez	85%	192
Auxilio Mutuo Hospital[2]	Hato Rey	84%	203
San Luke's Memorial Hospital	Ponce	81%	42
Centro Cardiovascular[2]	Rio Piedras	79%	298
Hospital Pavia Santurce	Fernandez Junc	65%	110
Hima - San Pablo Fajardo	Fajardo	54%	28
Mennonite General Hospital	Aibonito	51%	73
Hospital San Francisco	San Juan	35%	31

Appropriate VTP Within 24 Hours

Hospital Name	City	Rate	Cases
Doctors' Center Hospital	Manati	100%	170
Hospital De La Concepcion	San German	100%	132
Hospital Hermanos Melendez	Bayamon	100%	57
Manati Medical Center Doctor Otero Lopez[3]	Manati	100%	90
Hospital Damas	Ponce	99%	265
Hospital Doctor Cayetano Coll y Toste	Arecibo	99%	218
Hospital Universitario Doctor Ruiz Arnau	Bayamon	99%	124
Presbyterian Community Hospital	San Juan	99%	796
San Juan VA Medical Center[2]	San Juan	99%	161
Asociacion Hospital Del Maestro	San Juan	98%	145
Dr I Gonzalez Martinez Oncology Hosp[2,3]	San Juan	98%	138
Doctors Center Hospital Bayamon[2]	Bayamon	98%	95
Metropolitan Hospital	San Juan	98%	57
San Luke's Memorial Hospital	Ponce	98%	214
Hospital Menonita De Cayey[2]	Cayey	97%	255
Hospital Episcopal San Lucas Guayama	Guayama	96%	162
Hima San Pablo - Caguas[2]	Caguas	95%	301
Hospital Hima - San Pablo Bayamon[2]	Bayamon	95%	351
Hospital UPR - Doctor Federico Trilla	Carolina	95%	106
Hospital Comunitario Buen Samaritano	Aguadilla	94%	179
San Juan Municipal Hospital	Rio Piedras	93%	107
Auxilio Mutuo Hospital[2]	Hato Rey	92%	689
Hima San Pablo Humacao	Humacao	91%	79
Hospital Metropolitano Doctor Pila	Ponce	91%	129
Hospital Pavia Hato Rey	Hato Rey	90%	88
Hospital Pavia Santurce	Fernandez Junc	89%	303
Hospital Universitario De Adulto	Rio Piedras	89%	189
Bella Vista Hospital	Mayaguez	88%	864
Sistema Integrados De Salud Del Sur Oeste	Mayaguez	86%	37
Hospital Metropolitano Doctor Tito Mattei	Yauco	82%	40
Hima - San Pablo Fajardo	Fajardo	79%	225
Hospital San Francisco	San Juan	78%	137
Mennonite General Hospital	Aibonito	60%	226
Hospital San Cristobal[2]	Coto Laurel	29%	42
Hospital Doctor Susoni[2]	Arecibo	4%	98

Controlled Postoperative Blood Glucose

Hospital Name	City	Rate	Cases
San Juan VA Medical Center[2]	San Juan	98%	57
Hospital Damas	Ponce	97%	69
Hospital Hima - San Pablo Bayamon[2]	Bayamon	97%	129
Centro Cardiovascular[2]	Rio Piedras	83%	928
San Luke's Memorial Hospital	Ponce	81%	79
Hospital Pavia Santurce	Fernandez Junc	71%	196
Auxilio Mutuo Hospital[2]	Hato Rey	70%	103
Sistema Integrados De Salud Del Sur Oeste	Mayaguez	60%	144

Perioperative Temperature Management

Hospital Name	City	Rate	Cases
Asociacion Hospital Del Maestro	San Juan	100%	148
Auxilio Mutuo Hospital[2]	Hato Rey	100%	729
Bella Vista Hospital	Mayaguez	100%	893
Dr I Gonzalez Martinez Oncology Hosp[2,3]	San Juan	100%	205
Doctors Center Hospital Bayamon[2]	Bayamon	100%	100
Doctors' Center Hospital	Manati	100%	175
Hima - San Pablo Fajardo	Fajardo	100%	220
Hima San Pablo - Caguas[2]	Caguas	100%	314
Hima San Pablo Humacao	Humacao	100%	84
Hospital Comunitario Buen Samaritano	Aguadilla	100%	219
Hospital Doctor Cayetano Coll y Toste	Arecibo	100%	255
Hospital Episcopal San Lucas Guayama	Guayama	100%	165
Hospital Hermanos Melendez	Bayamon	100%	66
Hospital Hima - San Pablo Bayamon[2]	Bayamon	100%	391
Hospital Menonita De Cayey[2]	Cayey	100%	286
Hospital Metropolitano Doctor Pila	Ponce	100%	138
Hospital Metropolitano Doctor Tito Mattei	Yauco	100%	75
Hospital Pavia Hato Rey	Hato Rey	100%	90
Hospital Pavia Santurce	Fernandez Junc	100%	375
Hospital San Francisco	San Juan	100%	141
Hospital UPR - Doctor Federico Trilla	Carolina	100%	122
Manati Medical Center Doctor Otero Lopez[3]	Manati	100%	90
Presbyterian Community Hospital	San Juan	100%	846
San Juan Municipal Hospital	Rio Piedras	100%	112
San Luke's Memorial Hospital	Ponce	100%	300
Sistema Integrados De Salud Del Sur Oeste	Mayaguez	100%	262
Hospital Doctor Susoni[2]	Arecibo	99%	104
San Juan VA Medical Center[2]	San Juan	99%	157
Metropolitan Hospital	San Juan	98%	64
Hospital San Cristobal[2]	Coto Laurel	97%	59
Hospital De La Concepcion[3]	San German	96%	27
Mennonite General Hospital	Aibonito	95%	475
Hospital Universitario De Adulto	Rio Piedras	93%	205
Hospital Damas	Ponce	89%	276
Hospital Universitario Doctor Ruiz Arnau	Bayamon	74%	149
Ryder Memorial Hospital[3]	Humacao	15%	82

Prophylactic Antibiotic Selection

Hospital Name	City	Rate	Cases
Centro Cardiovascular[2]	Rio Piedras	100%	938
Hospital San Cristobal[2]	Coto Laurel	100%	59
San Juan VA Medical Center	San Juan	100%	105
Hospital Damas	Ponce	99%	341
Presbyterian Community Hospital	San Juan	99%	615
Bella Vista Hospital	Mayaguez	98%	727
Dr I Gonzalez Martinez Oncology Hosp[2,3]	San Juan	98%	184
Hima - San Pablo Fajardo	Fajardo	98%	213
Hospital De La Concepcion	San German	98%	130
Hospital Episcopal San Lucas Guayama	Guayama	98%	163
Hospital Hima - San Pablo Bayamon[2]	Bayamon	98%	437
Metropolitan Hospital	San Juan	98%	61
San Juan Municipal Hospital	Rio Piedras	98%	109
Auxilio Mutuo Hospital[2]	Hato Rey	97%	738
Doctors' Center Hospital	Manati	97%	154
Hima San Pablo - Caguas[2]	Caguas	97%	301
Hospital Comunitario Buen Samaritano	Aguadilla	97%	116
Sistema Integrados De Salud Del Sur Oeste	Mayaguez	97%	214
Hospital Hermanos Melendez	Bayamon	96%	78
Hospital Menonita De Cayey[2]	Cayey	96%	154
Hospital Metropolitano Doctor Pila	Ponce	96%	136
Hospital Metropolitano Doctor Tito Mattei	Yauco	96%	28
Hospital Universitario Doctor Ruiz Arnau	Bayamon	96%	134
Mennonite General Hospital	Aibonito	96%	396
Hospital UPR - Doctor Federico Trilla	Carolina	95%	111
Hospital Pavia Santurce	Fernandez Junc	94%	388
Hospital Doctor Cayetano Coll y Toste	Arecibo	93%	226
Hospital Pavia Hato Rey	Hato Rey	93%	82
Manati Medical Center Doctor Otero Lopez[3]	Manati	93%	94
Doctors Center Hospital Bayamon[2]	Bayamon	92%	90
San Luke's Memorial Hospital	Ponce	91%	291
Hima San Pablo Humacao	Humacao	88%	73
Hospital San Francisco	San Juan	88%	110
Hospital Universitario De Adulto	Rio Piedras	88%	149
Asociacion Hospital Del Maestro	San Juan	87%	125
Hospital Doctor Susoni[2]	Arecibo	87%	92
Ryder Memorial Hospital[3]	Humacao	38%	52

Prophylactic Antibiotic Stopped

Hospital Name	City	Rate	Cases
Asociacion Hospital Del Maestro	San Juan	100%	125
Hospital Comunitario Buen Samaritano	Aguadilla	100%	116
Hospital Hermanos Melendez	Bayamon	100%	78
Hospital Universitario Doctor Ruiz Arnau	Bayamon	100%	134
Presbyterian Community Hospital	San Juan	100%	615
San Juan Municipal Hospital	Rio Piedras	100%	109
Hospital Episcopal San Lucas Guayama	Guayama	99%	151
Hospital Pavia Hato Rey	Hato Rey	99%	82
Manati Medical Center Doctor Otero Lopez[3]	Manati	99%	93
Mennonite General Hospital	Aibonito	99%	396
Doctors Center Hospital Bayamon[2]	Bayamon	98%	84
Doctors' Center Hospital	Manati	98%	154
Metropolitan Hospital	San Juan	98%	59
Hima San Pablo - Caguas[2]	Caguas	97%	296
Hospital Doctor Susoni[2]	Arecibo	97%	92
San Juan VA Medical Center	San Juan	97%	100
Hospital Menonita De Cayey[2]	Cayey	95%	153
Hospital Metropolitano Doctor Pila	Ponce	95%	130
Centro Cardiovascular[2]	Rio Piedras	92%	934
Hospital Damas	Ponce	91%	338
Hospital Hima - San Pablo Bayamon[2]	Bayamon	87%	421
Hospital San Cristobal[2]	Coto Laurel	85%	59
Hospital UPR - Doctor Federico Trilla	Carolina	85%	110
Auxilio Mutuo Hospital[2]	Hato Rey	83%	723
Dr I Gonzalez Martinez Oncology Hosp[2,3]	San Juan	82%	180
Sistema Integrados De Salud Del Sur Oeste	Mayaguez	81%	210
San Luke's Memorial Hospital	Ponce	80%	287
Hospital Pavia Santurce	Fernandez Junc	75%	355
Hospital Metropolitano Doctor Tito Mattei	Yauco	71%	28
Hospital Doctor Cayetano Coll y Toste	Arecibo	61%	224
Hospital Universitario De Adulto	Rio Piedras	61%	149

NOTE: Hospital profiles are in alphabetical order by state, then city, then hospital within the city; Rankings exclude hospitals with less than 25 cases except for patient surveys which excludes hospitals with less than 100 cases; (a) 100-299 cases; (1) The number of cases/patients is too few to report; (2) Data submitted were based on a sample of cases/patients; (3) Results are based on a shorter time period than required; (4) Data suppressed by CMS for one or more quarters; (5) Results are not available for this reporting period; (6) Fewer than 100 patients completed the HCAHPS survey; (7) No cases met the criteria for this measure; (8) The lower limit of the confidence interval cannot be calculated if the number of observed infections equals zero; (9) No data are available from the state/territory for this reporting period; (10) The scores shown reflect fewer than 50 completed surveys; (11) There were discrepancies in the data collection process; (12) This measure does not apply to this hospital for this reporting period; (13) Results cannot be calculated for this reporting period; (14) The results for this state are combined with nearby states to protect confidentiality; Please refer to the User's Guide for a full explanation of data.

Hospital Name	City	Rate	Cases
Hospital San Francisco	San Juan	54%	109
Hima - San Pablo Fajardo	Fajardo	52%	211
Bella Vista Hospital	Mayaguez	50%	719
Ryder Memorial Hospital[3]	Humacao	38%	52
Hima San Pablo Humacao	Humacao	26%	72

Prophylactic Antibiotic Timing

Hospital Name	City	Rate	Cases
Doctors' Center Hospital	Manati	100%	154
Presbyterian Community Hospital	San Juan	99%	615
San Juan VA Medical Center	San Juan	99%	105
Hospital Episcopal San Lucas Guayama	Guayama	98%	164
Hospital Damas	Ponce	97%	341
Hospital Hima - San Pablo Bayamon[2]	Bayamon	97%	438
Bella Vista Hospital	Mayaguez	95%	729
San Juan Municipal Hospital	Rio Piedras	95%	109
Hospital Hermanos Melendez	Bayamon	94%	79
Asociacion Hospital Del Maestro	San Juan	93%	127
Hospital Comunitario Buen Samaritano	Aguadilla	93%	122
Centro Cardiovascular[2]	Rio Piedras	92%	947
Hospital Metropolitano Doctor Pila	Ponce	92%	136
Hospital Pavia Santurce	Fernandez Junc	92%	392
Hospital Universitario Doctor Ruiz Arnau	Bayamon	92%	135
San Luke's Memorial Hospital	Ponce	91%	292
Hospital Menonita De Cayey[2]	Cayey	90%	154
Metropolitan Hospital	San Juan	90%	61
Hima San Pablo - Caguas[2]	Caguas	89%	302
Hospital UPR - Doctor Federico Trilla	Carolina	89%	113
Auxilio Mutuo Hospital[2]	Hato Rey	88%	740
Hospital De La Concepcion	San German	87%	130
Mennonite General Hospital	Aibonito	87%	397
Manati Medical Center Doctor Otero Lopez[3]	Manati	86%	94
Hima San Pablo Humacao	Humacao	85%	73
Hospital Pavia Hato Rey	Hato Rey	83%	82
Doctors Center Hospital Bayamon[2]	Bayamon	82%	91
Hospital Doctor Cayetano Coll y Toste	Arecibo	79%	230
Hospital Universitario De Adulto	Rio Piedras	79%	151
Dr I Gonzalez Martinez Oncology Hosp[2,3]	San Juan	75%	186
Hima - San Pablo Fajardo	Fajardo	75%	213
Hospital Metropolitano Doctor Tito Mattei	Yauco	75%	28
Hospital San Francisco	San Juan	75%	110
Sistema Integrados De Salud Del Sur Oeste	Mayaguez	63%	222
Hospital San Cristobal[2]	Coto Laurel	62%	60
Hospital Doctor Susoni[2]	Arecibo	61%	106
Ryder Memorial Hospital[3]	Humacao	33%	54

Urinary Catheter Removal

Hospital Name	City	Rate	Cases
Centro Cardiovascular[2]	Rio Piedras	100%	650
Doctors' Center Hospital	Manati	100%	54
Hospital Comunitario Buen Samaritano	Aguadilla	100%	69
Hospital Doctor Cayetano Coll y Toste	Arecibo	100%	71
Presbyterian Community Hospital	San Juan	100%	452
San Juan Municipal Hospital	Rio Piedras	100%	43
Sistema Integrados De Salud Del Sur Oeste	Mayaguez	100%	66
Hospital Pavia Santurce	Fernandez Junc	99%	201
Mennonite General Hospital	Aibonito	99%	147
Hospital Menonita De Cayey[2]	Cayey	97%	140
San Juan VA Medical Center[2]	San Juan	97%	116
San Luke's Memorial Hospital	Ponce	97%	65
Hospital Metropolitano Doctor Pila	Ponce	96%	49
Dr I Gonzalez Martinez Oncology Hosp[2,3]	San Juan	95%	101
Hima San Pablo - Caguas[2]	Caguas	93%	42
Hospital San Francisco	San Juan	93%	61
Hospital Metropolitano Doctor Tito Mattei	Yauco	92%	36
Hospital Universitario Doctor Ruiz Arnau	Bayamon	90%	39
Auxilio Mutuo Hospital[2]	Hato Rey	77%	157
Hospital Universitario De Adulto	Rio Piedras	74%	74
Bella Vista Hospital	Mayaguez	69%	334
Hima - San Pablo Fajardo	Fajardo	63%	41
Ryder Memorial Hospital[3]	Humacao	4%	25

Survey of Patients' Hospital Experiences

No hospitals met the 100 case threshold.

Use of Medical Imaging

No hospitals met the 25 case threshold.

NOTE: Hospital profiles are in alphabetical order by state, then city, then hospital within the city; Rankings exclude hospitals with less than 25 cases except for patient surveys which excludes hospitals with less than 100 cases; (a) 100-299 cases; (1) The number of cases/patients is too few to report; (2) Data submitted were based on a sample of cases/patients; (3) Results are based on a shorter time period than required; (4) Data suppressed by CMS for one or more quarters; (5) Results are not available for this reporting period; (6) Fewer than 100 patients completed the HCAHPS survey; (7) No cases met the criteria for this measure; (8) The lower limit of the confidence interval cannot be calculated if the number of observed infections equals zero; (9) No data are available from the state/territory for this reporting period; (10) The scores shown reflect fewer than 50 completed surveys; (11) There were discrepancies in the data collection process; (12) This measure does not apply to this hospital for this reporting period; (13) Results cannot be calculated for this reporting period; (14) The results for this state are combined with nearby states to protect confidentiality; Please refer to the User's Guide for a full explanation of data.

Hospital Comunitario Buen Samaritano

Carr.2 Km.1.4 Ave. Severiano Cuevas #18 Phone: 787-658-0000
Aguadilla, PR 603 Fax: 787-658-0294
Type: Acute Care Hospitals Emergency Services: Yes
Ownership: Voluntary non-profit - Other
Key Personnel:
CEO/President. . . . . Marco Reyes

Measure	Cases	This Hosp.	State Avg.	U.S. Avg.
Blood Clot Prevention and Treatment				
Anticoagulation Overlap Therapy[5]	-	-	50%	93%
ICU Venous Thromboembolism Prophylaxis[5]	-	-	-	92%
Incidence of Potentially Preventable VTE[5]	-	-	-	10%
UFH with Dosages/Platelet Monitoring[5]	-	-	100%	97%
Venous Thromboembolism Prophylaxis[5]	-	-	98%	85%
Warfarin Therapy Discharge Instructions[5]	-	-	92%	75%
Chest Pain/Possible Heart Attack Care				
Aspirin Given Within 24 Hours of Arrival	-	-	-	96%
Fibrinolytic Meds Within 30 Min. of Arrival	-	-	-	58%
Average Time to ECG (minutes)	-	-	-	7
Average Time to Transfer (minutes)	-	-	-	60
Children's Asthma Care				
Received Home Management Plan of Care	-	-	-	88%
Received Reliever Medication	-	-	-	100%
Received Systemic Corticosteroids	-	-	-	100%
Emergency Department				
Admittance Decision Time (minutes)[5]	-	-	190	98
Head CT Results Within 45 Min. of Arrival	-	-	-	57%
Patients Who Left ER Before Being Seen	-	-	-	2%
Time from ER Arrival to Admit. (minutes)[5]	-	-	635	274
Time from ER Arrival to Discharge (minutes)	-	-	-	134
Time in ER Before Being Evaluated (minutes)	-	-	-	26
Time to Pain Meds for Fractures (minutes)	-	-	-	57
Heart Attack Care				
Aspirin Given at Discharge	75	92%	94%	99%
Fibrinolytic Meds Within 30 Min. of Arrival[1]	-	-	47%	54%
PCI Within 90 Minutes of Arrival[7]	-	-	53%	96%
Statin Prescribed at Discharge	94	91%	89%	98%
Heart Failure Care				
ACE Inhibitor or ARB for LVSD	99	92%	92%	97%
Discharge Instructions Given	246	100%	87%	94%
Evaluation of LVS Function	246	93%	94%	99%
Medicare Spending				
Medicare Spending per Patient (ratio)	-	-	-	0.98
Pneumonia Care				
Appropriate Initial Antibiotic Given	140	93%	82%	95%
Blood Culture Timing	107	98%	82%	98%
Pregnancy and Delivery Care				
Newborn Deliveries Scheduled Early[5]	-	-	-	6%
Preventive Care				
Immunization for Influenza[5]	-	-	42%	90%
Immunization for Pneumonia[5]	-	-	29%	92%
Stroke Care				
Anticoagulation Therapy for Atrial Fibrillation[5]	-	-	60%	95%
Antithrombotic Therapy Timing[5]	-	-	77%	98%
Assessed for Rehabilitation[5]	-	-	59%	97%
Discharged on Antithrombotic Therapy[5]	-	-	63%	99%
Discharged on Statin Medication[5]	-	-	90%	94%
Thrombolytic Therapy Timing[5]	-	-	-	66%
Venous Thromboembolism Prophylaxis[5]	-	-	52%	94%
Written Stroke Educational Materials Given[5]	-	-	95%	88%
Surgical Care Improvement Project				
Appropriate Beta Blocker Usage	15	100%	75%	98%
Appropriate VTP Within 24 Hours	179	94%	90%	98%
Controlled Postoperative Blood Glucose[7]	-	-	81%	97%
Perioperative Temperature Management	219	100%	98%	100%
Prophylactic Antibiotic Selection	116	97%	96%	99%
Prophylactic Antibiotic Selection (Outpatient)	-	-	-	98%
Prophylactic Antibiotic Stopped	116	100%	83%	98%
Prophylactic Antibiotic Timing	122	93%	89%	99%
Prophylactic Antibiotic Timing (Outpatient)	-	-	-	98%
Urinary Catheter Removal	69	100%	91%	97%
Survey of Patients' Hospital Experiences				
Area Around Room 'Always' Quiet at Night[5]	-	-	-	61%
Doctors 'Always' Communicated Well[5]	-	-	-	82%
Home Recovery Information Given[5]	-	-	-	85%
Hospital Given 9 or 10 on 10 Point Scale[5]	-	-	-	71%
Meds 'Always' Explained Before Given[5]	-	-	-	64%
Nurses 'Always' Communicated Well[5]	-	-	-	79%
Pain 'Always' Well Controlled[5]	-	-	-	71%
Room and Bathroom 'Always' Clean[5]	-	-	-	73%
Timely Help 'Always' Received[5]	-	-	-	68%
Would Definitely Recommend Hospital[5]	-	-	-	71%
Use of Medical Imaging				
Cardiac Imaging Stress Test before Surgery	-	-	4.5%	5.3%
Combination Abdominal CT Scan	-	-	7.4%	10.5%
Combination Brain/Sinus CT Scan	-	-	0.8%	2.7%
Combination Chest CT Scan	-	-	6.1%	2.7%
Follow-up Mammogram/Ultrasound	-	-	43.2%	8.8%
Lumbar Spine MRI for Low Back Pain	-	-	44.3%	37.2%

Mennonite General Hospital

Calle Jose C Vasquez Bo. Caonillas Phone: 787-535-1001
Aibonito, PR 705 Fax: 787-735-7111
URL: www.hospitalmenonita.com
Type: Acute Care Hospitals Emergency Services: Yes
Ownership: Voluntary non-profit - Other Beds: 150
Key Personnel:
Chief of Medical Staff. . . . . Roberto Alvaves
Emergency Room . . . . Jorge Calderon
Infection Control. . . . . Ana Amelia Camacho
Radiology. . . . . Juan F Cancio Acevedo
Intensive Care Unit. . . . . Sonia Davila
Cardiac Laboratory. . . . . Orlando Dorres
Pediatric In-Patient Care . . . . Ginnette Marrero
Quality Assurance . . . . Lisbeth Rodriguez

Measure	Cases	This Hosp.	State Avg.	U.S. Avg.
Blood Clot Prevention and Treatment				
Anticoagulation Overlap Therapy[5]	-	-	50%	93%
ICU Venous Thromboembolism Prophylaxis[5]	-	-	-	92%
Incidence of Potentially Preventable VTE[5]	-	-	-	10%
UFH with Dosages/Platelet Monitoring[5]	-	-	100%	97%
Venous Thromboembolism Prophylaxis[5]	-	-	98%	85%
Warfarin Therapy Discharge Instructions[5]	-	-	92%	75%
Chest Pain/Possible Heart Attack Care				
Aspirin Given Within 24 Hours of Arrival	-	-	-	96%
Fibrinolytic Meds Within 30 Min. of Arrival	-	-	-	58%
Average Time to ECG (minutes)	-	-	-	7
Average Time to Transfer (minutes)	-	-	-	60
Children's Asthma Care				
Received Home Management Plan of Care	-	-	-	88%
Received Reliever Medication	-	-	-	100%
Received Systemic Corticosteroids	-	-	-	100%
Emergency Department				
Admittance Decision Time (minutes)[5]	-	-	190	98
Head CT Results Within 45 Min. of Arrival	-	-	-	57%
Patients Who Left ER Before Being Seen	-	-	-	2%
Time from ER Arrival to Admit. (minutes)[5]	-	-	635	274
Time from ER Arrival to Discharge (minutes)	-	-	-	134
Time in ER Before Being Evaluated (minutes)	-	-	-	26
Time to Pain Meds for Fractures (minutes)	-	-	-	57
Heart Attack Care				
Aspirin Given at Discharge	45	89%	94%	99%
Fibrinolytic Meds Within 30 Min. of Arrival[1]	-	-	47%	54%
PCI Within 90 Minutes of Arrival[7]	-	-	53%	96%
Statin Prescribed at Discharge	50	88%	89%	98%
Heart Failure Care				
ACE Inhibitor or ARB for LVSD	63	94%	92%	97%
Discharge Instructions Given	98	92%	87%	94%
Evaluation of LVS Function	98	99%	94%	99%
Medicare Spending				
Medicare Spending per Patient (ratio)	-	-	-	0.98
Pneumonia Care				
Appropriate Initial Antibiotic Given	214	85%	82%	95%
Blood Culture Timing	215	88%	82%	98%
Pregnancy and Delivery Care				
Newborn Deliveries Scheduled Early[5]	-	-	-	6%
Preventive Care				
Immunization for Influenza[5]	-	-	42%	90%
Immunization for Pneumonia[5]	-	-	29%	92%
Stroke Care				
Anticoagulation Therapy for Atrial Fibrillation[5]	-	-	60%	95%
Antithrombotic Therapy Timing[5]	-	-	77%	98%
Assessed for Rehabilitation[5]	-	-	59%	97%
Discharged on Antithrombotic Therapy[5]	-	-	63%	99%
Discharged on Statin Medication[5]	-	-	90%	94%
Thrombolytic Therapy Timing[5]	-	-	-	66%
Venous Thromboembolism Prophylaxis[5]	-	-	52%	94%
Written Stroke Educational Materials Given[5]	-	-	95%	88%
Surgical Care Improvement Project				
Appropriate Beta Blocker Usage	73	51%	75%	98%
Appropriate VTP Within 24 Hours	226	60%	90%	98%
Controlled Postoperative Blood Glucose[7]	-	-	81%	97%
Perioperative Temperature Management	475	95%	98%	100%
Prophylactic Antibiotic Selection	396	96%	96%	99%
Prophylactic Antibiotic Selection (Outpatient)	-	-	-	98%
Prophylactic Antibiotic Stopped	396	99%	83%	98%
Prophylactic Antibiotic Timing	397	87%	89%	99%
Prophylactic Antibiotic Timing (Outpatient)	-	-	-	98%
Urinary Catheter Removal	147	99%	91%	97%
Survey of Patients' Hospital Experiences				
Area Around Room 'Always' Quiet at Night[5]	-	-	-	61%
Doctors 'Always' Communicated Well[5]	-	-	-	82%
Home Recovery Information Given[5]	-	-	-	85%
Hospital Given 9 or 10 on 10 Point Scale[5]	-	-	-	71%
Meds 'Always' Explained Before Given[5]	-	-	-	64%
Nurses 'Always' Communicated Well[5]	-	-	-	79%
Pain 'Always' Well Controlled[5]	-	-	-	71%
Room and Bathroom 'Always' Clean[5]	-	-	-	73%
Timely Help 'Always' Received[5]	-	-	-	68%
Would Definitely Recommend Hospital[5]	-	-	-	71%
Use of Medical Imaging				
Cardiac Imaging Stress Test before Surgery	-	-	4.5%	5.3%
Combination Abdominal CT Scan	-	-	7.4%	10.5%
Combination Brain/Sinus CT Scan	-	-	0.8%	2.7%
Combination Chest CT Scan	-	-	6.1%	2.7%
Follow-up Mammogram/Ultrasound	-	-	43.2%	8.8%
Lumbar Spine MRI for Low Back Pain	-	-	44.3%	37.2%

Hospital Doctor Cayetano Coll y Toste

Carretera 129 Km.1 Avenida San Luis Phone: 787-650-7272
Arecibo, PR 613
Type: Acute Care Hospitals Emergency Services: Yes
Ownership: Proprietary

Measure	Cases	This Hosp.	State Avg.	U.S. Avg.
Blood Clot Prevention and Treatment				
Anticoagulation Overlap Therapy[5]	-	-	50%	93%
ICU Venous Thromboembolism Prophylaxis[5]	-	-	-	92%
Incidence of Potentially Preventable VTE[5]	-	-	-	10%
UFH with Dosages/Platelet Monitoring[5]	-	-	100%	97%
Venous Thromboembolism Prophylaxis[5]	-	-	98%	85%
Warfarin Therapy Discharge Instructions[5]	-	-	92%	75%
Chest Pain/Possible Heart Attack Care				
Aspirin Given Within 24 Hours of Arrival	-	-	-	96%
Fibrinolytic Meds Within 30 Min. of Arrival	-	-	-	58%
Average Time to ECG (minutes)	-	-	-	7
Average Time to Transfer (minutes)	-	-	-	60
Children's Asthma Care				
Received Home Management Plan of Care	-	-	-	88%
Received Reliever Medication	-	-	-	100%
Received Systemic Corticosteroids	-	-	-	100%
Emergency Department				
Admittance Decision Time (minutes)[5]	-	-	190	98
Head CT Results Within 45 Min. of Arrival	-	-	-	57%
Patients Who Left ER Before Being Seen	-	-	-	2%
Time from ER Arrival to Admit. (minutes)[5]	-	-	635	274
Time from ER Arrival to Discharge (minutes)	-	-	-	134
Time in ER Before Being Evaluated (minutes)	-	-	-	26
Time to Pain Meds for Fractures (minutes)	-	-	-	57

NOTE: Hospital profiles are in alphabetical order by state, then city, then hospital within the city; Rankings exclude hospitals with less than 25 cases except for patient surveys which excludes hospitals with less than 100 cases; (a) 100-299 cases; (1) The number of cases/patients is too few to report; (2) Data submitted were based on a sample of cases/patients; (3) Results are based on a shorter time period than required; (4) Data suppressed by CMS for one or more quarters; (5) Results are not available for this reporting period; (6) Fewer than 100 patients completed the HCAHPS survey; (7) No cases met the criteria for this measure; (8) The lower limit of the confidence interval cannot be calculated if the number of observed infections equals zero; (9) No data are available from the state/territory for this reporting period; (10) The scores shown reflect fewer than 50 completed surveys; (11) There were discrepancies in the data collection process; (12) This measure does not apply to this hospital for this reporting period; (13) Results cannot be calculated for this reporting period; (14) The results for this state are combined with nearby states to protect confidentiality; Please refer to the User's Guide for a full explanation of data.

Measure	Cases	This Hosp.	State Avg.	U.S. Avg.
Heart Attack Care				
Aspirin Given at Discharge	80	66%	94%	99%
Fibrinolytic Meds Within 30 Min. of Arrival	12	100%	47%	54%
PCI Within 90 Minutes of Arrival[7]	-	-	53%	96%
Statin Prescribed at Discharge	87	83%	89%	98%
Heart Failure Care				
ACE Inhibitor or ARB for LVSD	80	89%	92%	97%
Discharge Instructions Given	183	37%	87%	94%
Evaluation of LVS Function	172	86%	94%	99%
Medicare Spending				
Medicare Spending per Patient (ratio)	-	-	-	0.98
Pneumonia Care				
Appropriate Initial Antibiotic Given	44	73%	82%	95%
Blood Culture Timing	28	64%	82%	98%
Pregnancy and Delivery Care				
Newborn Deliveries Scheduled Early[5]	-	-	-	6%
Preventive Care				
Immunization for Influenza[5]	-	-	42%	90%
Immunization for Pneumonia[5]	-	-	29%	92%
Stroke Care				
Anticoagulation Therapy for Atrial Fibrillation[5]	-	-	60%	95%
Antithrombotic Therapy Timing[5]	-	-	77%	98%
Assessed for Rehabilitation[5]	-	-	59%	97%
Discharged on Antithrombotic Therapy[5]	-	-	63%	99%
Discharged on Statin Medication[5]	-	-	90%	94%
Thrombolytic Therapy Timing[5]	-	-	-	66%
Venous Thromboembolism Prophylaxis[5]	-	-	52%	94%
Written Stroke Educational Materials Given[5]	-	-	95%	88%
Surgical Care Improvement Project				
Appropriate Beta Blocker Usage[1]	-	-	75%	98%
Appropriate VTP Within 24 Hours	218	99%	90%	98%
Controlled Postoperative Blood Glucose[7]	-	-	81%	97%
Perioperative Temperature Management	255	100%	98%	100%
Prophylactic Antibiotic Selection	226	93%	96%	99%
Prophylactic Antibiotic Selection (Outpatient)	-	-	-	98%
Prophylactic Antibiotic Stopped	224	61%	83%	98%
Prophylactic Antibiotic Timing	230	79%	89%	99%
Prophylactic Antibiotic Timing (Outpatient)	-	-	-	98%
Urinary Catheter Removal	71	100%	91%	97%
Survey of Patients' Hospital Experiences				
Area Around Room 'Always' Quiet at Night[5]	-	-	-	61%
Doctors 'Always' Communicated Well[5]	-	-	-	82%
Home Recovery Information Given[5]	-	-	-	85%
Hospital Given 9 or 10 on 10 Point Scale[5]	-	-	-	71%
Meds 'Always' Explained Before Given[5]	-	-	-	64%
Nurses 'Always' Communicated Well[5]	-	-	-	79%
Pain 'Always' Well Controlled[5]	-	-	-	71%
Room and Bathroom 'Always' Clean[5]	-	-	-	73%
Timely Help 'Always' Received[5]	-	-	-	68%
Would Definitely Recommend Hospital[5]	-	-	-	71%
Use of Medical Imaging				
Cardiac Imaging Stress Test before Surgery	-	-	4.5%	5.3%
Combination Abdominal CT Scan	-	-	7.4%	10.5%
Combination Brain/Sinus CT Scan	-	-	0.8%	2.7%
Combination Chest CT Scan	-	-	6.1%	2.7%
Follow-up Mammogram/Ultrasound	-	-	43.2%	8.8%
Lumbar Spine MRI for Low Back Pain	-	-	44.3%	37.2%

Hospital Doctor Susoni

55 Palm St — Phone: 787-650-1031
Arecibo, PR 614 — Fax: 787-650-1040
Type: Acute Care Hospitals — Emergency Services: Yes
Ownership: Voluntary non-profit - Private — Beds: 185

Key Personnel:
Anesthesiology. . . . . Marciel Buch
Intensive Care Unit. . . . . Francisco Garcia Cortes
CEO/President. . . . . Homer Perez
Operating Room. . . . . Maria Rios
Quality Assurance . . . . Lydia Rodriguez
Chief of Medical Staff . . . . Manuel Somohano, MD

Measure	Cases	This Hosp.	State Avg.	U.S. Avg.
Blood Clot Prevention and Treatment				
Anticoagulation Overlap Therapy[5]	-	-	50%	93%
ICU Venous Thromboembolism Prophylaxis[5]	-	-	-	92%
Incidence of Potentially Preventable VTE[5]	-	-	-	10%
UFH with Dosages/Platelet Monitoring[5]	-	-	100%	97%
Venous Thromboembolism Prophylaxis[5]	-	-	98%	85%
Warfarin Therapy Discharge Instructions[5]	-	-	92%	75%
Chest Pain/Possible Heart Attack Care				
Aspirin Given Within 24 Hours of Arrival	-	-	-	96%
Fibrinolytic Meds Within 30 Min. of Arrival	-	-	-	58%
Average Time to ECG (minutes)	-	-	-	7
Average Time to Transfer (minutes)	-	-	-	60
Children's Asthma Care				
Received Home Management Plan of Care	-	-	-	88%
Received Reliever Medication	-	-	-	100%
Received Systemic Corticosteroids	-	-	-	100%
Emergency Department				
Admittance Decision Time (minutes)[5]	-	-	190	98
Head CT Results Within 45 Min. of Arrival	-	-	-	57%
Patients Who Left ER Before Being Seen	-	-	-	2%
Time from ER Arrival to Admit. (minutes)[5]	-	-	635	274
Time from ER Arrival to Discharge (minutes)	-	-	-	134
Time in ER Before Being Evaluated (minutes)	-	-	-	26
Time to Pain Meds for Fractures (minutes)	-	-	-	57
Heart Attack Care				
Aspirin Given at Discharge[2]	63	56%	94%	99%
Fibrinolytic Meds Within 30 Min. of Arrival[1,2]	-	-	47%	54%
PCI Within 90 Minutes of Arrival[2,7]	-	-	53%	96%
Statin Prescribed at Discharge[2]	58	60%	89%	98%
Heart Failure Care				
ACE Inhibitor or ARB for LVSD[2]	49	47%	92%	97%
Discharge Instructions Given[2]	86	93%	87%	94%
Evaluation of LVS Function[2]	86	88%	94%	99%
Medicare Spending				
Medicare Spending per Patient (ratio)	-	-	-	0.98
Pneumonia Care				
Appropriate Initial Antibiotic Given[2]	42	79%	82%	95%
Blood Culture Timing[2]	35	83%	82%	98%
Pregnancy and Delivery Care				
Newborn Deliveries Scheduled Early[5]	-	-	-	6%
Preventive Care				
Immunization for Influenza[5]	-	-	42%	90%
Immunization for Pneumonia[5]	-	-	29%	92%
Stroke Care				
Anticoagulation Therapy for Atrial Fibrillation[5]	-	-	60%	95%
Antithrombotic Therapy Timing[5]	-	-	77%	98%
Assessed for Rehabilitation[5]	-	-	59%	97%
Discharged on Antithrombotic Therapy[5]	-	-	63%	99%
Discharged on Statin Medication[5]	-	-	90%	94%
Thrombolytic Therapy Timing[5]	-	-	-	66%
Venous Thromboembolism Prophylaxis[5]	-	-	52%	94%
Written Stroke Educational Materials Given[5]	-	-	95%	88%
Surgical Care Improvement Project				
Appropriate Beta Blocker Usage[2,7]	-	-	75%	98%
Appropriate VTP Within 24 Hours[2]	98	4%	90%	98%
Controlled Postoperative Blood Glucose[2,7]	-	-	81%	97%
Perioperative Temperature Management[2]	104	99%	98%	100%
Prophylactic Antibiotic Selection[2]	92	87%	96%	99%
Prophylactic Antibiotic Selection (Outpatient)	-	-	-	98%
Prophylactic Antibiotic Stopped[2]	92	97%	83%	98%
Prophylactic Antibiotic Timing[2]	106	61%	89%	99%
Prophylactic Antibiotic Timing (Outpatient)	-	-	-	98%
Urinary Catheter Removal[2]	20	100%	91%	97%
Survey of Patients' Hospital Experiences				
Area Around Room 'Always' Quiet at Night[5]	-	-	-	61%
Doctors 'Always' Communicated Well[5]	-	-	-	82%
Home Recovery Information Given[5]	-	-	-	85%
Hospital Given 9 or 10 on 10 Point Scale[5]	-	-	-	71%
Meds 'Always' Explained Before Given[5]	-	-	-	64%
Nurses 'Always' Communicated Well[5]	-	-	-	79%
Pain 'Always' Well Controlled[5]	-	-	-	71%
Room and Bathroom 'Always' Clean[5]	-	-	-	73%
Timely Help 'Always' Received[5]	-	-	-	68%
Would Definitely Recommend Hospital[5]	-	-	-	71%
Use of Medical Imaging				
Cardiac Imaging Stress Test before Surgery	-	-	4.5%	5.3%
Combination Abdominal CT Scan	-	-	7.4%	10.5%
Combination Brain/Sinus CT Scan	-	-	0.8%	2.7%
Combination Chest CT Scan	-	-	6.1%	2.7%
Follow-up Mammogram/Ultrasound	-	-	43.2%	8.8%
Lumbar Spine MRI for Low Back Pain	-	-	44.3%	37.2%

Lafayette Hospital

Carr.753 Km.0.1 - Sector Cuatro Calles — Phone: 787-839-3232
Arroyo, PR 714 — Fax: 787-839-4330
Type: Acute Care Hospitals — Emergency Services: Yes
Ownership: Voluntary non-profit - Private — Beds: 38

Key Personnel:
Emergency Room . . . . Jofe Rivira
Chief of Medical Staff. . . . . Jorge Rodles, MD
CEO/President. . . . . Francisco A Vazquez

Measure	Cases	This Hosp.	State Avg.	U.S. Avg.
Blood Clot Prevention and Treatment				
Anticoagulation Overlap Therapy[5]	-	-	50%	93%
ICU Venous Thromboembolism Prophylaxis[5]	-	-	-	92%
Incidence of Potentially Preventable VTE[5]	-	-	-	10%
UFH with Dosages/Platelet Monitoring[5]	-	-	100%	97%
Venous Thromboembolism Prophylaxis[5]	-	-	98%	85%
Warfarin Therapy Discharge Instructions[5]	-	-	92%	75%
Chest Pain/Possible Heart Attack Care				
Aspirin Given Within 24 Hours of Arrival	-	-	-	96%
Fibrinolytic Meds Within 30 Min. of Arrival	-	-	-	58%
Average Time to ECG (minutes)	-	-	-	7
Average Time to Transfer (minutes)	-	-	-	60
Children's Asthma Care				
Received Home Management Plan of Care	-	-	-	88%
Received Reliever Medication	-	-	-	100%
Received Systemic Corticosteroids	-	-	-	100%
Emergency Department				
Admittance Decision Time (minutes)[5]	-	-	190	98
Head CT Results Within 45 Min. of Arrival	-	-	-	57%
Patients Who Left ER Before Being Seen	-	-	-	2%
Time from ER Arrival to Admit. (minutes)[5]	-	-	635	274
Time from ER Arrival to Discharge (minutes)	-	-	-	134
Time in ER Before Being Evaluated (minutes)	-	-	-	26
Time to Pain Meds for Fractures (minutes)	-	-	-	57
Heart Attack Care				
Aspirin Given at Discharge[1,2]	-	-	94%	99%
Fibrinolytic Meds Within 30 Min. of Arrival[2,3]	-	-	47%	54%
PCI Within 90 Minutes of Arrival[2,3]	-	-	53%	96%
Statin Prescribed at Discharge[1,2]	-	-	89%	98%
Heart Failure Care				
ACE Inhibitor or ARB for LVSD[1,2]	-	-	92%	97%
Discharge Instructions Given[2,3]	14	100%	87%	94%
Evaluation of LVS Function[2,3]	14	86%	94%	99%
Medicare Spending				
Medicare Spending per Patient (ratio)	-	-	-	0.98
Pneumonia Care				
Appropriate Initial Antibiotic Given[2,3]	11	45%	82%	95%
Blood Culture Timing[2,3]	11	64%	82%	98%
Pregnancy and Delivery Care				
Newborn Deliveries Scheduled Early[5]	-	-	-	6%
Preventive Care				
Immunization for Influenza[2]	18	17%	42%	90%
Immunization for Pneumonia[2,3]	16	50%	29%	92%
Stroke Care				
Anticoagulation Therapy for Atrial Fibrillation[5]	-	-	60%	95%
Antithrombotic Therapy Timing[5]	-	-	77%	98%
Assessed for Rehabilitation[5]	-	-	59%	97%
Discharged on Antithrombotic Therapy[5]	-	-	63%	99%
Discharged on Statin Medication[5]	-	-	90%	94%
Thrombolytic Therapy Timing[5]	-	-	-	66%
Venous Thromboembolism Prophylaxis[5]	-	-	52%	94%
Written Stroke Educational Materials Given[5]	-	-	95%	88%
Surgical Care Improvement Project				
Appropriate Beta Blocker Usage[5]	-	-	75%	98%
Appropriate VTP Within 24 Hours[5]	-	-	90%	98%
Controlled Postoperative Blood Glucose[5]	-	-	81%	97%

NOTE: Hospital profiles are in alphabetical order by state, then city, then hospital within the city; Rankings exclude hospitals with less than 25 cases except for patient surveys which excludes hospitals with less than 100 cases; (a) 100-299 cases; (1) The number of cases/patients is too few to report; (2) Data submitted were based on a sample of cases/patients; (3) Results are based on a shorter time period than required; (4) Data suppressed by CMS for one or more quarters; (5) Results are not available for this reporting period; (6) Fewer than 100 patients completed the HCAHPS survey; (7) No cases met the criteria for this measure; (8) The lower limit of the confidence interval cannot be calculated if the number of observed infections equals zero; (9) No data are available from the state/territory for this reporting period; (10) The scores shown reflect fewer than 50 completed surveys; (11) There were discrepancies in the data collection process; (12) This measure does not apply to this hospital for this reporting period; (13) Results cannot be calculated for this reporting period; (14) The results for this state are combined with nearby states to protect confidentiality; Please refer to the User's Guide for a full explanation of data.

Measure	Cases	This Hosp.	State Avg.	U.S. Avg.
Perioperative Temperature Management[5]	-	-	98%	100%
Prophylactic Antibiotic Selection[5]	-	-	96%	99%
Prophylactic Antibiotic Selection (Outpatient)	-	-	-	98%
Prophylactic Antibiotic Stopped[5]	-	-	83%	98%
Prophylactic Antibiotic Timing[5]	-	-	89%	99%
Prophylactic Antibiotic Timing (Outpatient)	-	-	-	98%
Urinary Catheter Removal[5]	-	-	91%	97%
Survey of Patients' Hospital Experiences				
Area Around Room 'Always' Quiet at Night[5]	-	-	-	61%
Doctors 'Always' Communicated Well[5]	-	-	-	82%
Home Recovery Information Given[5]	-	-	-	85%
Hospital Given 9 or 10 on 10 Point Scale[5]	-	-	-	71%
Meds 'Always' Explained Before Given[5]	-	-	-	64%
Nurses 'Always' Communicated Well[5]	-	-	-	79%
Pain 'Always' Well Controlled[5]	-	-	-	71%
Room and Bathroom 'Always' Clean[5]	-	-	-	73%
Timely Help 'Always' Received[5]	-	-	-	68%
Would Definitely Recommend Hospital[5]	-	-	-	71%
Use of Medical Imaging				
Cardiac Imaging Stress Test before Surgery	-	-	4.5%	5.3%
Combination Abdominal CT Scan	-	-	7.4%	10.5%
Combination Brain/Sinus CT Scan	-	-	0.8%	2.7%
Combination Chest CT Scan	-	-	6.1%	2.7%
Follow-up Mammogram/Ultrasound	-	-	43.2%	8.8%
Lumbar Spine MRI for Low Back Pain	-	-	44.3%	37.2%

Doctors Center Hospital Bayamon

9 J Street Ext Hermanas Davila
Bayamon, PR 959
Phone: 787-622-5420
Fax: 787-622-5432
Type: Acute Care Hospitals
Emergency Services: Yes
Ownership: Proprietary
Beds: 106

Measure	Cases	This Hosp.	State Avg.	U.S. Avg.
Blood Clot Prevention and Treatment				
Anticoagulation Overlap Therapy[5]	-	-	50%	93%
ICU Venous Thromboembolism Prophylaxis[5]	-	-	-	92%
Incidence of Potentially Preventable VTE[5]	-	-	-	10%
UFH with Dosages/Platelet Monitoring[5]	-	-	100%	97%
Venous Thromboembolism Prophylaxis[5]	-	-	98%	85%
Warfarin Therapy Discharge Instructions[5]	-	-	92%	75%
Chest Pain/Possible Heart Attack Care				
Aspirin Given Within 24 Hours of Arrival	-	-	-	96%
Fibrinolytic Meds Within 30 Min. of Arrival	-	-	-	58%
Average Time to ECG (minutes)	-	-	-	7
Average Time to Transfer (minutes)	-	-	-	60
Children's Asthma Care				
Received Home Management Plan of Care	-	-	-	88%
Received Reliever Medication	-	-	-	100%
Received Systemic Corticosteroids	-	-	-	100%
Emergency Department				
Admittance Decision Time (minutes)[5]	-	-	190	98
Head CT Results Within 45 Min. of Arrival	-	-	-	57%
Patients Who Left ER Before Being Seen	-	-	-	2%
Time from ER Arrival to Admit. (minutes)[5]	-	-	635	274
Time from ER Arrival to Discharge (minutes)	-	-	-	134
Time in ER Before Being Evaluated (minutes)	-	-	-	26
Time to Pain Meds for Fractures (minutes)	-	-	-	57
Heart Attack Care				
Aspirin Given at Discharge[2]	16	81%	94%	99%
Fibrinolytic Meds Within 30 Min. of Arrival[2,7]	-	-	47%	54%
PCI Within 90 Minutes of Arrival[2,7]	-	-	53%	96%
Statin Prescribed at Discharge[2]	23	61%	89%	98%
Heart Failure Care				
ACE Inhibitor or ARB for LVSD[2]	21	95%	92%	97%
Discharge Instructions Given[2]	84	67%	87%	94%
Evaluation of LVS Function[2]	84	83%	94%	99%
Medicare Spending				
Medicare Spending per Patient (ratio)	-	-	-	0.98
Pneumonia Care				
Appropriate Initial Antibiotic Given[2]	46	80%	82%	95%
Blood Culture Timing[2]	26	65%	82%	98%
Pregnancy and Delivery Care				
Newborn Deliveries Scheduled Early[5]	-	-	-	6%
Preventive Care				
Immunization for Influenza[5]	-	-	42%	90%
Immunization for Pneumonia[5]	-	-	29%	92%
Stroke Care				
Anticoagulation Therapy for Atrial Fibrillation[5]	-	-	60%	95%
Antithrombotic Therapy Timing[5]	-	-	77%	98%
Assessed for Rehabilitation[5]	-	-	59%	97%
Discharged on Antithrombotic Therapy[5]	-	-	63%	99%
Discharged on Statin Medication[5]	-	-	90%	94%
Thrombolytic Therapy Timing[5]	-	-	-	66%
Venous Thromboembolism Prophylaxis[5]	-	-	52%	94%
Written Stroke Educational Materials Given[5]	-	-	95%	88%
Surgical Care Improvement Project				
Appropriate Beta Blocker Usage[1,2]	-	-	75%	98%
Appropriate VTP Within 24 Hours[2]	95	98%	90%	98%
Controlled Postoperative Blood Glucose[2,7]	-	-	81%	97%
Perioperative Temperature Management[2]	100	100%	98%	100%
Prophylactic Antibiotic Selection[2]	90	92%	96%	99%
Prophylactic Antibiotic Selection (Outpatient)	-	-	-	98%
Prophylactic Antibiotic Stopped[2]	84	98%	83%	98%
Prophylactic Antibiotic Timing[2]	91	82%	89%	99%
Prophylactic Antibiotic Timing (Outpatient)	-	-	-	98%
Urinary Catheter Removal[1,2]	-	-	91%	97%
Survey of Patients' Hospital Experiences				
Area Around Room 'Always' Quiet at Night[5]	-	-	-	61%
Doctors 'Always' Communicated Well[5]	-	-	-	82%
Home Recovery Information Given[5]	-	-	-	85%
Hospital Given 9 or 10 on 10 Point Scale[5]	-	-	-	71%
Meds 'Always' Explained Before Given[5]	-	-	-	64%
Nurses 'Always' Communicated Well[5]	-	-	-	79%
Pain 'Always' Well Controlled[5]	-	-	-	71%
Room and Bathroom 'Always' Clean[5]	-	-	-	73%
Timely Help 'Always' Received[5]	-	-	-	68%
Would Definitely Recommend Hospital[5]	-	-	-	71%
Use of Medical Imaging				
Cardiac Imaging Stress Test before Surgery	-	-	4.5%	5.3%
Combination Abdominal CT Scan	-	-	7.4%	10.5%
Combination Brain/Sinus CT Scan	-	-	0.8%	2.7%
Combination Chest CT Scan	-	-	6.1%	2.7%
Follow-up Mammogram/Ultrasound	-	-	43.2%	8.8%
Lumbar Spine MRI for Low Back Pain	-	-	44.3%	37.2%

Hospital Hermanos Melendez

Carretera #2 Km 11 7
Bayamon, PR 960
Phone: 787-620-8181
Fax: 787-269-0085
URL: www.hospitalhermanosmelendez.net
Type: Acute Care Hospitals
Emergency Services: Yes
Ownership: Proprietary
Beds: 270

Key Personnel:

Operating Room. . . . . Neysis Alejandro
Quality Assurance . . . . Dennise J Javierre
Emergency Room . . . . Gary Labadie, MD
Pediatric In-Patient Care . . . . Evelyn Lopez, MD
Anesthesiology. . . . . Carlos Munoz, MD
Chief of Medical Staff . . . . Antonio Reyes-Beltran, MD

Measure	Cases	This Hosp.	State Avg.	U.S. Avg.
Blood Clot Prevention and Treatment				
Anticoagulation Overlap Therapy[1,2]	-	-	50%	93%
ICU Venous Thromboembolism Prophylaxis[2,3]	-	-	-	92%
Incidence of Potentially Preventable VTE[2,3]	-	-	-	10%
UFH with Dosages/Platelet Monitoring[1,2]	-	-	100%	97%
Venous Thromboembolism Prophylaxis[2,3]	36	100%	98%	85%
Warfarin Therapy Discharge Instructions[1,2]	-	-	92%	75%
Chest Pain/Possible Heart Attack Care				
Aspirin Given Within 24 Hours of Arrival	-	-	-	96%
Fibrinolytic Meds Within 30 Min. of Arrival	-	-	-	58%
Average Time to ECG (minutes)	-	-	-	7
Average Time to Transfer (minutes)	-	-	-	60
Children's Asthma Care				
Received Home Management Plan of Care	-	-	-	88%
Received Reliever Medication	-	-	-	100%
Received Systemic Corticosteroids	-	-	-	100%
Emergency Department				
Admittance Decision Time (minutes)[2]	513	190	190	98
Head CT Results Within 45 Min. of Arrival	-	-	-	57%
Patients Who Left ER Before Being Seen	-	-	-	2%
Time from ER Arrival to Admit. (minutes)[2]	513	645	635	274
Time from ER Arrival to Discharge (minutes)	-	-	-	134
Time in ER Before Being Evaluated (minutes)	-	-	-	26
Time to Pain Meds for Fractures (minutes)	-	-	-	57
Heart Attack Care				
Aspirin Given at Discharge	77	97%	94%	99%
Fibrinolytic Meds Within 30 Min. of Arrival[7]	-	-	47%	54%
PCI Within 90 Minutes of Arrival[7]	-	-	53%	96%
Statin Prescribed at Discharge	85	100%	89%	98%
Heart Failure Care				
ACE Inhibitor or ARB for LVSD	58	100%	92%	97%
Discharge Instructions Given	273	100%	87%	94%
Evaluation of LVS Function	274	97%	94%	99%
Medicare Spending				
Medicare Spending per Patient (ratio)	-	-	-	0.98
Pneumonia Care				
Appropriate Initial Antibiotic Given	116	93%	82%	95%
Blood Culture Timing	106	94%	82%	98%
Pregnancy and Delivery Care				
Newborn Deliveries Scheduled Early[5]	-	-	-	6%
Preventive Care				
Immunization for Influenza[2]	283	44%	42%	90%
Immunization for Pneumonia[2]	461	28%	29%	92%
Stroke Care				
Anticoagulation Therapy for Atrial Fibrillation[2,3]	-	-	60%	95%
Antithrombotic Therapy Timing[2,3]	-	-	77%	98%
Assessed for Rehabilitation[1,2]	-	-	59%	97%
Discharged on Antithrombotic Therapy[1,2]	-	-	63%	99%
Discharged on Statin Medication[1,2]	-	-	90%	94%
Thrombolytic Therapy Timing[1,2]	-	-	-	66%
Venous Thromboembolism Prophylaxis[2,3]	11	100%	52%	94%
Written Stroke Educational Materials Given[1,2]	-	-	95%	88%
Surgical Care Improvement Project				
Appropriate Beta Blocker Usage[1]	-	-	75%	98%
Appropriate VTP Within 24 Hours	57	100%	90%	98%
Controlled Postoperative Blood Glucose[1]	-	-	81%	97%
Perioperative Temperature Management	66	100%	98%	100%
Prophylactic Antibiotic Selection	78	96%	96%	99%
Prophylactic Antibiotic Selection (Outpatient)	-	-	-	98%
Prophylactic Antibiotic Stopped	78	100%	83%	98%
Prophylactic Antibiotic Timing	79	94%	89%	99%
Prophylactic Antibiotic Timing (Outpatient)	-	-	-	98%
Urinary Catheter Removal[1]	-	-	91%	97%
Survey of Patients' Hospital Experiences				
Area Around Room 'Always' Quiet at Night[5]	-	-	-	61%
Doctors 'Always' Communicated Well[5]	-	-	-	82%
Home Recovery Information Given[5]	-	-	-	85%
Hospital Given 9 or 10 on 10 Point Scale[5]	-	-	-	71%
Meds 'Always' Explained Before Given[5]	-	-	-	64%
Nurses 'Always' Communicated Well[5]	-	-	-	79%
Pain 'Always' Well Controlled[5]	-	-	-	71%
Room and Bathroom 'Always' Clean[5]	-	-	-	73%
Timely Help 'Always' Received[5]	-	-	-	68%
Would Definitely Recommend Hospital[5]	-	-	-	71%
Use of Medical Imaging				
Cardiac Imaging Stress Test before Surgery	-	-	4.5%	5.3%
Combination Abdominal CT Scan	-	-	7.4%	10.5%
Combination Brain/Sinus CT Scan	-	-	0.8%	2.7%
Combination Chest CT Scan	-	-	6.1%	2.7%
Follow-up Mammogram/Ultrasound	-	-	43.2%	8.8%
Lumbar Spine MRI for Low Back Pain	-	-	44.3%	37.2%

Hospital Hima - San Pablo Bayamon

Calle Santa Cruz Numero 70 Urb Santa Cruz
Phone: 787-620-4747
Bayamon, PR 960
Fax: 787-798-5495
Type: Acute Care Hospitals
Emergency Services: Yes
Ownership: Proprietary
Beds: 395

Key Personnel:

Quality Assurance . . . . Silva Cortes
Operating Room. . . . . Gloria Cruz
Administrator . . . . Anabel Irizarry, MHSA

NOTE: Hospital profiles are in alphabetical order by state, then city, then hospital within the city; Rankings exclude hospitals with less than 25 cases except for patient surveys which excludes hospitals with less than 100 cases; (a) 100-299 cases; (1) The number of cases/patients is too few to report; (2) Data submitted were based on a sample of cases/patients; (3) Results are based on a shorter time period than required; (4) Data suppressed by CMS for one or more quarters; (5) Results are not available for this reporting period; (6) Fewer than 100 patients completed the HCAHPS survey; (7) No cases met the criteria for this measure; (8) The lower limit of the confidence interval cannot be calculated if the number of observed infections equals zero; (9) No data are available from the state/territory for this reporting period; (10) The scores shown reflect fewer than 50 completed surveys; (11) There were discrepancies in the data collection process; (12) This measure does not apply to this hospital for this reporting period; (13) Results cannot be calculated for this reporting period; (14) The results for this state are combined with nearby states to protect confidentiality; Please refer to the User's Guide for a full explanation of data.

Chief of Medical Staff.......... Jaime Rivera, MD
Chairman/CEO .... Joaquin Rodriguez, Sr., JD

Measure	Cases	This Hosp.	State Avg.	U.S. Avg.
Blood Clot Prevention and Treatment				
Anticoagulation Overlap Therapy[5]	-	-	50%	93%
ICU Venous Thromboembolism Prophylaxis[5]	-		-	92%
Incidence of Potentially Preventable VTE[5]	-	-	-	10%
UFH with Dosages/Platelet Monitoring[5]	-	-	100%	97%
Venous Thromboembolism Prophylaxis[5]	-	-	98%	85%
Warfarin Therapy Discharge Instructions[5]	-	-	92%	75%
Chest Pain/Possible Heart Attack Care				
Aspirin Given Within 24 Hours of Arrival	-	-	-	96%
Fibrinolytic Meds Within 30 Min. of Arrival	-	-	-	58%
Average Time to ECG (minutes)	-	-	-	7
Average Time to Transfer (minutes)	-	-	-	60
Children's Asthma Care				
Received Home Management Plan of Care	-	-	-	88%
Received Reliever Medication	-	-	-	100%
Received Systemic Corticosteroids	-	-	-	100%
Emergency Department				
Admittance Decision Time (minutes)[5]	-	-	190	98
Head CT Results Within 45 Min. of Arrival	-	-	-	57%
Patients Who Left ER Before Being Seen	-	-	-	2%
Time from ER Arrival to Admit. (minutes)[5]	-	-	635	274
Time from ER Arrival to Discharge (minutes)	-	-	-	134
Time in ER Before Being Evaluated (minutes)	-	-	-	26
Time to Pain Meds for Fractures (minutes)	-	-	-	57
Heart Attack Care				
Aspirin Given at Discharge	342	97%	94%	99%
Fibrinolytic Meds Within 30 Min. of Arrival[5]	-	-	47%	54%
PCI Within 90 Minutes of Arrival[5]	-	-	53%	96%
Statin Prescribed at Discharge	390	96%	89%	98%
Heart Failure Care				
ACE Inhibitor or ARB for LVSD[2]	130	95%	92%	97%
Discharge Instructions Given[2]	300	99%	87%	94%
Evaluation of LVS Function[2]	302	100%	94%	99%
Medicare Spending				
Medicare Spending per Patient (ratio)	-	-	-	0.98
Pneumonia Care				
Appropriate Initial Antibiotic Given[2]	135	84%	82%	95%
Blood Culture Timing[2]	166	89%	82%	98%
Pregnancy and Delivery Care				
Newborn Deliveries Scheduled Early[5]	-	-	-	6%
Preventive Care				
Immunization for Influenza[5]	-	-	42%	90%
Immunization for Pneumonia[5]	-	-	29%	92%
Stroke Care				
Anticoagulation Therapy for Atrial Fibrillation[5]	-	-	60%	95%
Antithrombotic Therapy Timing[5]	-	-	77%	98%
Assessed for Rehabilitation[5]	-	-	59%	97%
Discharged on Antithrombotic Therapy[5]	-	-	63%	99%
Discharged on Statin Medication[5]	-	-	90%	94%
Thrombolytic Therapy Timing[5]	-	-	-	66%
Venous Thromboembolism Prophylaxis[5]	-	-	52%	94%
Written Stroke Educational Materials Given[5]	-	-	95%	88%
Surgical Care Improvement Project				
Appropriate Beta Blocker Usage[5]	-	-	75%	98%
Appropriate VTP Within 24 Hours[2]	351	95%	90%	98%
Controlled Postoperative Blood Glucose[2]	129	97%	81%	97%
Perioperative Temperature Management[2]	391	100%	98%	100%
Prophylactic Antibiotic Selection[2]	437	98%	96%	99%
Prophylactic Antibiotic Selection (Outpatient)	-	-	-	98%
Prophylactic Antibiotic Stopped[2]	421	87%	83%	98%
Prophylactic Antibiotic Timing[2]	438	97%	89%	99%
Prophylactic Antibiotic Timing (Outpatient)	-	-	-	98%
Urinary Catheter Removal[5]	-	-	91%	97%
Survey of Patients' Hospital Experiences				
Area Around Room 'Always' Quiet at Night[5]	-	-	-	61%
Doctors 'Always' Communicated Well[5]	-	-	-	82%
Home Recovery Information Given[5]	-	-	-	85%
Hospital Given 9 or 10 on 10 Point Scale[5]	-	-	-	71%
Meds 'Always' Explained Before Given[5]	-	-	-	64%
Nurses 'Always' Communicated Well[5]	-	-	-	79%
Pain 'Always' Well Controlled[5]	-	-	-	71%
Room and Bathroom 'Always' Clean[5]	-	-	-	73%
Timely Help 'Always' Received[5]	-	-	-	68%
Would Definitely Recommend Hospital[5]	-	-	-	71%
Use of Medical Imaging				
Cardiac Imaging Stress Test before Surgery	-	-	4.5%	5.3%
Combination Abdominal CT Scan	-	-	7.4%	10.5%
Combination Brain/Sinus CT Scan	-	-	0.8%	2.7%
Combination Chest CT Scan	-	-	6.1%	2.7%
Follow-up Mammogram/Ultrasound	-	-	43.2%	8.8%
Lumbar Spine MRI for Low Back Pain	-	-	44.3%	37.2%

Hospital Universitario Doctor Ruiz Arnau

Laurel Ave Santa Juanita #100 Phone: 787-787-5151
Bayamon, PR 956 Fax: 787-787-7979
E-mail: rafgarcia@salud.gov.pr
Type: Acute Care Hospitals Emergency Services: Yes
Ownership: Government - State Beds: 415

Key Personnel:
CEO/President................ Rafael Garcia Alvarez
Emergency Room .... Eva Y Calderon, MD
Quality Assurance .... A Julia Fernandez, MD
Pediatric In-Patient Care .... Frances Garcia, MD
Radiology.................. Aida Gonzalez
Chief of Medical Staff.......... Robert Hunter
Operating Room.............. Maria Nunez
Intensive Care Unit........... Maria Torres Davilla

Measure	Cases	This Hosp.	State Avg.	U.S. Avg.
Blood Clot Prevention and Treatment				
Anticoagulation Overlap Therapy[5]	-	-	50%	93%
ICU Venous Thromboembolism Prophylaxis[5]	-	-	-	92%
Incidence of Potentially Preventable VTE[5]	-			10%
UFH with Dosages/Platelet Monitoring[5]	-	-	100%	97%
Venous Thromboembolism Prophylaxis[5]	-	-	98%	85%
Warfarin Therapy Discharge Instructions[5]	-	-	92%	75%
Chest Pain/Possible Heart Attack Care				
Aspirin Given Within 24 Hours of Arrival	-	-	-	96%
Fibrinolytic Meds Within 30 Min. of Arrival	-	-	-	58%
Average Time to ECG (minutes)	-	-	-	7
Average Time to Transfer (minutes)	-	-	-	60
Children's Asthma Care				
Received Home Management Plan of Care	-	-	-	88%
Received Reliever Medication	-	-	-	100%
Received Systemic Corticosteroids	-	-	-	100%
Emergency Department				
Admittance Decision Time (minutes)[5]	-	-	190	98
Head CT Results Within 45 Min. of Arrival	-	-	-	57%
Patients Who Left ER Before Being Seen	-	-	-	2%
Time from ER Arrival to Admit. (minutes)[5]	-	-	635	274
Time from ER Arrival to Discharge (minutes)	-	-	-	134
Time in ER Before Being Evaluated (minutes)	-	-	-	26
Time to Pain Meds for Fractures (minutes)	-	-	-	57
Heart Attack Care				
Aspirin Given at Discharge	24	79%	94%	99%
Fibrinolytic Meds Within 30 Min. of Arrival[1]	-	-	47%	54%
PCI Within 90 Minutes of Arrival[7]	-	-	53%	96%
Statin Prescribed at Discharge	20	80%	89%	98%
Heart Failure Care				
ACE Inhibitor or ARB for LVSD	20	85%	92%	97%
Discharge Instructions Given	42	90%	87%	94%
Evaluation of LVS Function	53	96%	94%	99%
Medicare Spending				
Medicare Spending per Patient (ratio)	-	-	-	0.98
Pneumonia Care				
Appropriate Initial Antibiotic Given	93	72%	82%	95%
Blood Culture Timing	97	71%	82%	98%
Pregnancy and Delivery Care				
Newborn Deliveries Scheduled Early[5]	-	-	-	6%
Preventive Care				
Immunization for Influenza[5]	-	-	42%	90%
Immunization for Pneumonia[5]	-	-	29%	92%
Stroke Care				
Anticoagulation Therapy for Atrial Fibrillation[5]	-	-	60%	95%
Antithrombotic Therapy Timing[5]	-	-	77%	98%
Assessed for Rehabilitation[5]	-	-	59%	97%
Discharged on Antithrombotic Therapy[5]	-	-	63%	99%
Discharged on Statin Medication[5]	-	-	90%	94%
Thrombolytic Therapy Timing[5]	-	-	-	66%
Venous Thromboembolism Prophylaxis[5]	-	-	52%	94%
Written Stroke Educational Materials Given[5]	-	-	95%	88%
Surgical Care Improvement Project				
Appropriate Beta Blocker Usage[1]	-	-	75%	98%
Appropriate VTP Within 24 Hours	124	99%	90%	98%
Controlled Postoperative Blood Glucose[7]	-	-	81%	97%
Perioperative Temperature Management	149	74%	98%	100%
Prophylactic Antibiotic Selection	134	96%	96%	99%
Prophylactic Antibiotic Selection (Outpatient)	-	-	-	98%
Prophylactic Antibiotic Stopped	134	100%	83%	98%
Prophylactic Antibiotic Timing	135	92%	89%	99%
Prophylactic Antibiotic Timing (Outpatient)	-	-	-	98%
Urinary Catheter Removal	39	90%	91%	97%
Survey of Patients' Hospital Experiences				
Area Around Room 'Always' Quiet at Night[5]	-	-	-	61%
Doctors 'Always' Communicated Well[5]	-	-	-	82%
Home Recovery Information Given[5]	-	-	-	85%
Hospital Given 9 or 10 on 10 Point Scale[5]	-	-	-	71%
Meds 'Always' Explained Before Given[5]	-	-	-	64%
Nurses 'Always' Communicated Well[5]	-	-	-	79%
Pain 'Always' Well Controlled[5]	-	-	-	71%
Room and Bathroom 'Always' Clean[5]	-	-	-	73%
Timely Help 'Always' Received[5]	-	-	-	68%
Would Definitely Recommend Hospital[5]	-	-	-	71%
Use of Medical Imaging				
Cardiac Imaging Stress Test before Surgery	-	-	4.5%	5.3%
Combination Abdominal CT Scan	-	-	7.4%	10.5%
Combination Brain/Sinus CT Scan	-	-	0.8%	2.7%
Combination Chest CT Scan	-	-	6.1%	2.7%
Follow-up Mammogram/Ultrasound	-	-	43.2%	8.8%
Lumbar Spine MRI for Low Back Pain	-	-	44.3%	37.2%

Hospital Metropolitano De La Montana

Calle Isaac Gonzalez Esquina Ledesma Phone: 787-933-1100
Bda Nueva, PR 641
Type: Acute Care Hospitals Emergency Services: Yes
Ownership: Proprietary

Measure	Cases	This Hosp.	State Avg.	U.S. Avg.
Blood Clot Prevention and Treatment				
Anticoagulation Overlap Therapy[5]	-	-	50%	93%
ICU Venous Thromboembolism Prophylaxis[5]	-	-	-	92%
Incidence of Potentially Preventable VTE[5]	-	-	-	10%
UFH with Dosages/Platelet Monitoring[5]	-	-	100%	97%
Venous Thromboembolism Prophylaxis[5]	-	-	98%	85%
Warfarin Therapy Discharge Instructions[5]	-	-	92%	75%
Chest Pain/Possible Heart Attack Care				
Aspirin Given Within 24 Hours of Arrival	-	-	-	96%
Fibrinolytic Meds Within 30 Min. of Arrival	-	-	-	58%
Average Time to ECG (minutes)	-	-	-	7
Average Time to Transfer (minutes)	-	-	-	60
Children's Asthma Care				
Received Home Management Plan of Care	-	-	-	88%
Received Reliever Medication	-	-	-	100%
Received Systemic Corticosteroids	-	-	-	100%
Emergency Department				
Admittance Decision Time (minutes)[5]	-	-	190	98
Head CT Results Within 45 Min. of Arrival	-	-	-	57%
Patients Who Left ER Before Being Seen	-	-	-	2%
Time from ER Arrival to Admit. (minutes)[5]	-	-	635	274
Time from ER Arrival to Discharge (minutes)	-	-	-	134
Time in ER Before Being Evaluated (minutes)	-	-	-	26
Time to Pain Meds for Fractures (minutes)	-	-	-	57
Heart Attack Care				
Aspirin Given at Discharge[5]	-	-	94%	99%
Fibrinolytic Meds Within 30 Min. of Arrival[5]	-	-	47%	54%
PCI Within 90 Minutes of Arrival[5]	-	-	53%	96%
Statin Prescribed at Discharge[5]	-	-	89%	98%

NOTE: Hospital profiles are in alphabetical order by state, then city, then hospital within the city; Rankings exclude hospitals with less than 25 cases except for patient surveys which excludes hospitals with less than 100 cases; (a) 100-299 cases; (1) The number of cases/patients is too few to report; (2) Data submitted were based on a sample of cases/patients; (3) Results are based on a shorter time period than required; (4) Data suppressed by CMS for one or more quarters; (5) Results are not available for this reporting period; (6) Fewer than 100 patients completed the HCAHPS survey; (7) No cases met the criteria for this measure; (8) The lower limit of the confidence interval cannot be calculated if the number of observed infections equals zero; (9) No data are available from the state/territory for this reporting period; (10) The scores shown reflect fewer than 50 completed surveys; (11) There were discrepancies in the data collection process; (12) This measure does not apply to this hospital for this reporting period; (13) Results cannot be calculated for this reporting period; (14) The results for this state are combined with nearby states to protect confidentiality; Please refer to the User's Guide for a full explanation of data.

Measure	Cases	This Hosp.	State Avg.	U.S. Avg.
Heart Failure Care				
ACE Inhibitor or ARB for LVSD[5]	-	-	92%	97%
Discharge Instructions Given[5]	-	-	87%	94%
Evaluation of LVS Function[5]	-	-	94%	99%
Medicare Spending				
Medicare Spending per Patient (ratio)	-	-	-	0.98
Pneumonia Care				
Appropriate Initial Antibiotic Given[5]	-	-	82%	95%
Blood Culture Timing[5]	-	-	82%	98%
Pregnancy and Delivery Care				
Newborn Deliveries Scheduled Early[5]	-	-	-	6%
Preventive Care				
Immunization for Influenza[5]	-	-	42%	90%
Immunization for Pneumonia[5]	-	-	29%	92%
Stroke Care				
Anticoagulation Therapy for Atrial Fibrillation[5]	-	-	60%	95%
Antithrombotic Therapy Timing[5]	-	-	77%	98%
Assessed for Rehabilitation[5]	-	-	59%	97%
Discharged on Antithrombotic Therapy[5]	-	-	63%	99%
Discharged on Statin Medication[5]	-	-	90%	94%
Thrombolytic Therapy Timing[5]	-	-	-	66%
Venous Thromboembolism Prophylaxis[5]	-	-	52%	94%
Written Stroke Educational Materials Given[5]	-	-	95%	88%
Surgical Care Improvement Project				
Appropriate Beta Blocker Usage[5]	-	-	75%	98%
Appropriate VTP Within 24 Hours[5]	-	-	90%	98%
Controlled Postoperative Blood Glucose[5]	-	-	81%	97%
Perioperative Temperature Management[5]	-	-	98%	100%
Prophylactic Antibiotic Selection[5]	-	-	96%	99%
Prophylactic Antibiotic Selection (Outpatient)	-	-	-	98%
Prophylactic Antibiotic Stopped[5]	-	-	83%	98%
Prophylactic Antibiotic Timing[5]	-	-	89%	99%
Prophylactic Antibiotic Timing (Outpatient)	-	-	-	98%
Urinary Catheter Removal[5]	-	-	91%	97%
Survey of Patients' Hospital Experiences				
Area Around Room 'Always' Quiet at Night[5]	-	-	-	61%
Doctors 'Always' Communicated Well[5]	-	-	-	82%
Home Recovery Information Given[5]	-	-	-	85%
Hospital Given 9 or 10 on 10 Point Scale[5]	-	-	-	71%
Meds 'Always' Explained Before Given[5]	-	-	-	64%
Nurses 'Always' Communicated Well[5]	-	-	-	79%
Pain 'Always' Well Controlled[5]	-	-	-	71%
Room and Bathroom 'Always' Clean[5]	-	-	-	73%
Timely Help 'Always' Received[5]	-	-	-	68%
Would Definitely Recommend Hospital[5]	-	-	-	71%
Use of Medical Imaging				
Cardiac Imaging Stress Test before Surgery	-	-	4.5%	5.3%
Combination Abdominal CT Scan	-	-	7.4%	10.5%
Combination Brain/Sinus CT Scan	-	-	0.8%	2.7%
Combination Chest CT Scan	-	-	6.1%	2.7%
Follow-up Mammogram/Ultrasound	-	-	43.2%	8.8%
Lumbar Spine MRI for Low Back Pain	-	-	44.3%	37.2%

Hima San Pablo - Caguas

Ave Luis Munoz Marin | Phone: 787-653-3434
Caguas, PR 725
Type: Acute Care Hospitals | Emergency Services: Yes
Ownership: Proprietary

Measure	Cases	This Hosp.	State Avg.	U.S. Avg.
Blood Clot Prevention and Treatment				
Anticoagulation Overlap Therapy[5]	-	-	50%	93%
ICU Venous Thromboembolism Prophylaxis[5]	-	-	-	92%
Incidence of Potentially Preventable VTE[5]	-	-	-	10%
UFH with Dosages/Platelet Monitoring[5]	-	-	100%	97%
Venous Thromboembolism Prophylaxis[5]	-	-	98%	85%
Warfarin Therapy Discharge Instructions[5]	-	-	92%	75%
Chest Pain/Possible Heart Attack Care				
Aspirin Given Within 24 Hours of Arrival	-	-	-	96%
Fibrinolytic Meds Within 30 Min. of Arrival	-	-	-	58%
Average Time to ECG (minutes)	-	-	-	7
Average Time to Transfer (minutes)	-	-	-	60
Children's Asthma Care				
Received Home Management Plan of Care	-	-	-	88%
Received Reliever Medication	-	-	-	100%
Received Systemic Corticosteroids	-	-	-	100%
Emergency Department				
Admittance Decision Time (minutes)[5]	-	-	190	98
Head CT Results Within 45 Min. of Arrival	-	-	-	57%
Patients Who Left ER Before Being Seen	-	-	-	2%
Time from ER Arrival to Admit. (minutes)[5]	-	-	635	274
Time from ER Arrival to Discharge (minutes)	-	-	-	134
Time in ER Before Being Evaluated (minutes)	-	-	-	26
Time to Pain Meds for Fractures (minutes)	-	-	-	57
Heart Attack Care				
Aspirin Given at Discharge	64	95%	94%	99%
Fibrinolytic Meds Within 30 Min. of Arrival[7]	-	-	47%	54%
PCI Within 90 Minutes of Arrival[7]	-	-	53%	96%
Statin Prescribed at Discharge	73	99%	89%	98%
Heart Failure Care				
ACE Inhibitor or ARB for LVSD	94	100%	92%	97%
Discharge Instructions Given	201	100%	87%	94%
Evaluation of LVS Function	204	99%	94%	99%
Medicare Spending				
Medicare Spending per Patient (ratio)	-	-	-	0.98
Pneumonia Care				
Appropriate Initial Antibiotic Given[2]	111	81%	82%	95%
Blood Culture Timing[2]	146	84%	82%	98%
Pregnancy and Delivery Care				
Newborn Deliveries Scheduled Early[5]	-	-	-	6%
Preventive Care				
Immunization for Influenza[5]	-	-	42%	90%
Immunization for Pneumonia[5]	-	-	29%	92%
Stroke Care				
Anticoagulation Therapy for Atrial Fibrillation[5]	-	-	60%	95%
Antithrombotic Therapy Timing[5]	-	-	77%	98%
Assessed for Rehabilitation[5]	-	-	59%	97%
Discharged on Antithrombotic Therapy[5]	-	-	63%	99%
Discharged on Statin Medication[5]	-	-	90%	94%
Thrombolytic Therapy Timing[5]	-	-	-	66%
Venous Thromboembolism Prophylaxis[5]	-	-	52%	94%
Written Stroke Educational Materials Given[5]	-	-	95%	88%
Surgical Care Improvement Project				
Appropriate Beta Blocker Usage[2]	12	8%	75%	98%
Appropriate VTP Within 24 Hours[2]	301	95%	90%	98%
Controlled Postoperative Blood Glucose[2,7]	-	-	81%	97%
Perioperative Temperature Management[2]	314	100%	98%	100%
Prophylactic Antibiotic Selection[2]	301	97%	96%	99%
Prophylactic Antibiotic Selection (Outpatient)	-	-	-	98%
Prophylactic Antibiotic Stopped[2]	296	97%	83%	98%
Prophylactic Antibiotic Timing[2]	302	89%	89%	99%
Prophylactic Antibiotic Timing (Outpatient)	-	-	-	98%
Urinary Catheter Removal[2]	42	93%	91%	97%
Survey of Patients' Hospital Experiences				
Area Around Room 'Always' Quiet at Night[5]	-	-	-	61%
Doctors 'Always' Communicated Well[5]	-	-	-	82%
Home Recovery Information Given[5]	-	-	-	85%
Hospital Given 9 or 10 on 10 Point Scale[5]	-	-	-	71%
Meds 'Always' Explained Before Given[5]	-	-	-	64%
Nurses 'Always' Communicated Well[5]	-	-	-	79%
Pain 'Always' Well Controlled[5]	-	-	-	71%
Room and Bathroom 'Always' Clean[5]	-	-	-	73%
Timely Help 'Always' Received[5]	-	-	-	68%
Would Definitely Recommend Hospital[5]	-	-	-	71%
Use of Medical Imaging				
Cardiac Imaging Stress Test before Surgery	-	-	4.5%	5.3%
Combination Abdominal CT Scan	-	-	7.4%	10.5%
Combination Brain/Sinus CT Scan	-	-	0.8%	2.7%
Combination Chest CT Scan	-	-	6.1%	2.7%
Follow-up Mammogram/Ultrasound	-	-	43.2%	8.8%
Lumbar Spine MRI for Low Back Pain	-	-	44.3%	37.2%

Hospital Menonita Caguas

Carr 172 Exit 21 Urb Turabo Gardens | Phone: 787-744-3141
Caguas, PR 725
Type: Acute Care Hospitals | Emergency Services: Yes
Ownership: Voluntary non-profit - Private | Beds: 373

Measure	Cases	This Hosp.	State Avg.	U.S. Avg.
Blood Clot Prevention and Treatment				
Anticoagulation Overlap Therapy[5]	-	-	50%	93%
ICU Venous Thromboembolism Prophylaxis[5]	-	-	-	92%
Incidence of Potentially Preventable VTE[5]	-	-	-	10%
UFH with Dosages/Platelet Monitoring[5]	-	-	100%	97%
Venous Thromboembolism Prophylaxis[5]	-	-	98%	85%
Warfarin Therapy Discharge Instructions[5]	-	-	92%	75%
Chest Pain/Possible Heart Attack Care				
Aspirin Given Within 24 Hours of Arrival	-	-	-	96%
Fibrinolytic Meds Within 30 Min. of Arrival	-	-	-	58%
Average Time to ECG (minutes)	-	-	-	7
Average Time to Transfer (minutes)	-	-	-	60
Children's Asthma Care				
Received Home Management Plan of Care	-	-	-	88%
Received Reliever Medication	-	-	-	100%
Received Systemic Corticosteroids	-	-	-	100%
Emergency Department				
Admittance Decision Time (minutes)[5]	-	-	190	98
Head CT Results Within 45 Min. of Arrival	-	-	-	57%
Patients Who Left ER Before Being Seen	-	-	-	2%
Time from ER Arrival to Admit. (minutes)[5]	-	-	635	274
Time from ER Arrival to Discharge (minutes)	-	-	-	134
Time in ER Before Being Evaluated (minutes)	-	-	-	26
Time to Pain Meds for Fractures (minutes)	-	-	-	57
Heart Attack Care				
Aspirin Given at Discharge	147	94%	94%	99%
Fibrinolytic Meds Within 30 Min. of Arrival[7]	-	-	47%	54%
PCI Within 90 Minutes of Arrival[7]	-	-	53%	96%
Statin Prescribed at Discharge	143	92%	89%	98%
Heart Failure Care				
ACE Inhibitor or ARB for LVSD[1,3]	-	-	92%	97%
Discharge Instructions Given[1,3]	-	-	87%	94%
Evaluation of LVS Function[1,3]	-	-	94%	99%
Medicare Spending				
Medicare Spending per Patient (ratio)	-	-	-	0.98
Pneumonia Care				
Appropriate Initial Antibiotic Given	37	46%	82%	95%
Blood Culture Timing	24	62%	82%	98%
Pregnancy and Delivery Care				
Newborn Deliveries Scheduled Early[5]	-	-	-	6%
Preventive Care				
Immunization for Influenza[5]	-	-	42%	90%
Immunization for Pneumonia[5]	-	-	29%	92%
Stroke Care				
Anticoagulation Therapy for Atrial Fibrillation[5]	-	-	60%	95%
Antithrombotic Therapy Timing[5]	-	-	77%	98%
Assessed for Rehabilitation[5]	-	-	59%	97%
Discharged on Antithrombotic Therapy[5]	-	-	63%	99%
Discharged on Statin Medication[5]	-	-	90%	94%
Thrombolytic Therapy Timing[5]	-	-	-	66%
Venous Thromboembolism Prophylaxis[5]	-	-	52%	94%
Written Stroke Educational Materials Given[5]	-	-	95%	88%
Surgical Care Improvement Project				
Appropriate Beta Blocker Usage[5]	-	-	75%	98%
Appropriate VTP Within 24 Hours[5]	-	-	90%	98%
Controlled Postoperative Blood Glucose[5]	-	-	81%	97%
Perioperative Temperature Management[5]	-	-	98%	100%
Prophylactic Antibiotic Selection[5]	-	-	96%	99%
Prophylactic Antibiotic Selection (Outpatient)	-	-	-	98%
Prophylactic Antibiotic Stopped[5]	-	-	83%	98%
Prophylactic Antibiotic Timing[5]	-	-	89%	99%
Prophylactic Antibiotic Timing (Outpatient)	-	-	-	98%
Urinary Catheter Removal[5]	-	-	91%	97%
Survey of Patients' Hospital Experiences				
Area Around Room 'Always' Quiet at Night[5]	-	-	-	61%
Doctors 'Always' Communicated Well[5]	-	-	-	82%

NOTE: Hospital profiles are in alphabetical order by state, then city, then hospital within the city; Rankings exclude hospitals with less than 25 cases except for patient surveys which excludes hospitals with less than 100 cases; (a) 100-299 cases; (1) The number of cases/patients is too few to report; (2) Data submitted were based on a sample of cases/patients; (3) Results are based on a shorter time period than required; (4) Data suppressed by CMS for one or more quarters; (5) Results are not available for this reporting period; (6) Fewer than 100 patients completed the HCAHPS survey; (7) No cases met the criteria for this measure; (8) The lower limit of the confidence interval cannot be calculated if the number of observed infections equals zero; (9) No data are available from the state/territory for this reporting period; (10) The scores shown reflect fewer than 50 completed surveys; (11) There were discrepancies in the data collection process; (12) This measure does not apply to this hospital for this reporting period; (13) Results cannot be calculated for this reporting period; (14) The results for this state are combined with nearby states to protect confidentiality; Please refer to the User's Guide for a full explanation of data.

Measure	Cases	This Hosp.	State Avg.	U.S. Avg.
Home Recovery Information Given[5]	-	-	-	85%
Hospital Given 9 or 10 on 10 Point Scale[5]	-	-	-	71%
Meds 'Always' Explained Before Given[5]	-	-	-	64%
Nurses 'Always' Communicated Well[5]	-	-	-	79%
Pain 'Always' Well Controlled[5]	-	-	-	71%
Room and Bathroom 'Always' Clean[5]	-	-	-	73%
Timely Help 'Always' Received[5]	-	-	-	68%
Would Definitely Recommend Hospital[5]	-	-	-	71%
Use of Medical Imaging				
Cardiac Imaging Stress Test before Surgery	-	-	4.5%	5.3%
Combination Abdominal CT Scan	-	-	7.4%	10.5%
Combination Brain/Sinus CT Scan	-	-	0.8%	2.7%
Combination Chest CT Scan	-	-	6.1%	2.7%
Follow-up Mammogram/Ultrasound	-	-	43.2%	8.8%
Lumbar Spine MRI for Low Back Pain	-	-	44.3%	37.2%

Hospital UPR - Doctor Federico Trilla

Carr 3 Km 8 3 Ave 65th Infanteria, Box 6021
Phone: 787-757-1800
Carolina, PR 984
Type: Acute Care Hospitals — Emergency Services: No
Ownership: Proprietary

Measure	Cases	This Hosp.	State Avg.	U.S. Avg.
Blood Clot Prevention and Treatment				
Anticoagulation Overlap Therapy[5]	-	-	50%	93%
ICU Venous Thromboembolism Prophylaxis[5]	-	-	-	92%
Incidence of Potentially Preventable VTE[5]	-	-	-	10%
UFH with Dosages/Platelet Monitoring[5]	-	-	100%	97%
Venous Thromboembolism Prophylaxis[5]	-	-	98%	85%
Warfarin Therapy Discharge Instructions[5]	-	-	92%	75%
Chest Pain/Possible Heart Attack Care				
Aspirin Given Within 24 Hours of Arrival	-	-	-	96%
Fibrinolytic Meds Within 30 Min. of Arrival	-	-	-	58%
Average Time to ECG (minutes)	-	-	-	7
Average Time to Transfer (minutes)	-	-	-	60
Children's Asthma Care				
Received Home Management Plan of Care	-	-	-	88%
Received Reliever Medication	-	-	-	100%
Received Systemic Corticosteroids	-	-	-	100%
Emergency Department				
Admittance Decision Time (minutes)[5]	-	-	190	98
Head CT Results Within 45 Min. of Arrival	-	-	-	57%
Patients Who Left ER Before Being Seen	-	-	-	2%
Time from ER Arrival to Admit. (minutes)[5]	-	-	635	274
Time from ER Arrival to Discharge (minutes)	-	-	-	134
Time in ER Before Being Evaluated (minutes)	-	-	-	26
Time to Pain Meds for Fractures (minutes)	-	-	-	57
Heart Attack Care				
Aspirin Given at Discharge	108	99%	94%	99%
Fibrinolytic Meds Within 30 Min. of Arrival[1]	-	-	47%	54%
PCI Within 90 Minutes of Arrival[7]	-	-	53%	96%
Statin Prescribed at Discharge	114	99%	89%	98%
Heart Failure Care				
ACE Inhibitor or ARB for LVSD	96	100%	92%	97%
Discharge Instructions Given	211	96%	87%	94%
Evaluation of LVS Function	211	100%	94%	99%
Medicare Spending				
Medicare Spending per Patient (ratio)	-	-	-	0.98
Pneumonia Care				
Appropriate Initial Antibiotic Given	142	89%	82%	95%
Blood Culture Timing	145	80%	82%	98%
Pregnancy and Delivery Care				
Newborn Deliveries Scheduled Early[5]	-	-	-	6%
Preventive Care				
Immunization for Influenza[5]	-	-	42%	90%
Immunization for Pneumonia[5]	-	-	29%	92%
Stroke Care				
Anticoagulation Therapy for Atrial Fibrillation[5]	-	-	60%	95%
Antithrombotic Therapy Timing[5]	-	-	77%	98%
Assessed for Rehabilitation[5]	-	-	59%	97%
Discharged on Antithrombotic Therapy[5]	-	-	63%	99%
Discharged on Statin Medication[5]	-	-	90%	94%
Thrombolytic Therapy Timing[5]	-	-	-	66%
Venous Thromboembolism Prophylaxis[5]	-	-	52%	94%
Written Stroke Educational Materials Given[5]	-	-	95%	88%
Surgical Care Improvement Project				
Appropriate Beta Blocker Usage	12	100%	75%	98%
Appropriate VTP Within 24 Hours	106	95%	90%	98%
Controlled Postoperative Blood Glucose[3,7]	-	-	81%	97%
Perioperative Temperature Management	122	100%	98%	100%
Prophylactic Antibiotic Selection	111	95%	96%	99%
Prophylactic Antibiotic Selection (Outpatient)	-	-	-	98%
Prophylactic Antibiotic Stopped	110	85%	83%	98%
Prophylactic Antibiotic Timing	113	89%	89%	99%
Prophylactic Antibiotic Timing (Outpatient)	-	-	-	98%
Urinary Catheter Removal	22	100%	91%	97%
Survey of Patients' Hospital Experiences				
Area Around Room 'Always' Quiet at Night[5]	-	-	-	61%
Doctors 'Always' Communicated Well[5]	-	-	-	82%
Home Recovery Information Given[5]	-	-	-	85%
Hospital Given 9 or 10 on 10 Point Scale[5]	-	-	-	71%
Meds 'Always' Explained Before Given[5]	-	-	-	64%
Nurses 'Always' Communicated Well[5]	-	-	-	79%
Pain 'Always' Well Controlled[5]	-	-	-	71%
Room and Bathroom 'Always' Clean[5]	-	-	-	73%
Timely Help 'Always' Received[5]	-	-	-	68%
Would Definitely Recommend Hospital[5]	-	-	-	71%
Use of Medical Imaging				
Cardiac Imaging Stress Test before Surgery	-	-	4.5%	5.3%
Combination Abdominal CT Scan	-	-	7.4%	10.5%
Combination Brain/Sinus CT Scan	-	-	0.8%	2.7%
Combination Chest CT Scan	-	-	6.1%	2.7%
Follow-up Mammogram/Ultrasound	-	-	43.2%	8.8%
Lumbar Spine MRI for Low Back Pain	-	-	44.3%	37.2%

Castaner General Hospital

Saint 135 Km 64 2 — Phone: 787-829-5010
Castaner, PR 631
Type: Acute Care Hospitals — Emergency Services: Yes
Ownership: Government - Local

Key Personnel:
Operating Room. . . . . Analiz Acosta
CEO/President. . . . . Domingo Monroig
Radiology. . . . . Aida Quinonez
Emergency Room . . . . Margarita Rentas

Measure	Cases	This Hosp.	State Avg.	U.S. Avg.
Blood Clot Prevention and Treatment				
Anticoagulation Overlap Therapy[5]	-	-	50%	93%
ICU Venous Thromboembolism Prophylaxis[5]	-	-	-	92%
Incidence of Potentially Preventable VTE[5]	-	-	-	10%
UFH with Dosages/Platelet Monitoring[5]	-	-	100%	97%
Venous Thromboembolism Prophylaxis[5]	-	-	98%	85%
Warfarin Therapy Discharge Instructions[5]	-	-	92%	75%
Chest Pain/Possible Heart Attack Care				
Aspirin Given Within 24 Hours of Arrival	-	-	-	96%
Fibrinolytic Meds Within 30 Min. of Arrival	-	-	-	58%
Average Time to ECG (minutes)	-	-	-	7
Average Time to Transfer (minutes)	-	-	-	60
Children's Asthma Care				
Received Home Management Plan of Care	-	-	-	88%
Received Reliever Medication	-	-	-	100%
Received Systemic Corticosteroids	-	-	-	100%
Emergency Department				
Admittance Decision Time (minutes)[5]	-	-	190	98
Head CT Results Within 45 Min. of Arrival	-	-	-	57%
Patients Who Left ER Before Being Seen	-	-	-	2%
Time from ER Arrival to Admit. (minutes)[5]	-	-	635	274
Time from ER Arrival to Discharge (minutes)	-	-	-	134
Time in ER Before Being Evaluated (minutes)	-	-	-	26
Time to Pain Meds for Fractures (minutes)	-	-	-	57
Heart Attack Care				
Aspirin Given at Discharge[5]	-	-	94%	99%
Fibrinolytic Meds Within 30 Min. of Arrival[5]	-	-	47%	54%
PCI Within 90 Minutes of Arrival[5]	-	-	53%	96%
Statin Prescribed at Discharge[5]	-	-	89%	98%
Heart Failure Care				
ACE Inhibitor or ARB for LVSD[2,3]	-	-	92%	97%
Discharge Instructions Given[1,2]	-	-	87%	94%
Evaluation of LVS Function[1,2]	-	-	94%	99%
Medicare Spending				
Medicare Spending per Patient (ratio)	-	-	-	0.98
Pneumonia Care				
Appropriate Initial Antibiotic Given[1,2]	-	-	82%	95%
Blood Culture Timing[2,3]	-	-	82%	98%
Pregnancy and Delivery Care				
Newborn Deliveries Scheduled Early[5]	-	-	-	6%
Preventive Care				
Immunization for Influenza[5]	-	-	42%	90%
Immunization for Pneumonia[5]	-	-	29%	92%
Stroke Care				
Anticoagulation Therapy for Atrial Fibrillation[5]	-	-	60%	95%
Antithrombotic Therapy Timing[5]	-	-	77%	98%
Assessed for Rehabilitation[5]	-	-	59%	97%
Discharged on Antithrombotic Therapy[5]	-	-	63%	99%
Discharged on Statin Medication[5]	-	-	90%	94%
Thrombolytic Therapy Timing[5]	-	-	-	66%
Venous Thromboembolism Prophylaxis[5]	-	-	52%	94%
Written Stroke Educational Materials Given[5]	-	-	95%	88%
Surgical Care Improvement Project				
Appropriate Beta Blocker Usage[5]	-	-	75%	98%
Appropriate VTP Within 24 Hours[5]	-	-	90%	98%
Controlled Postoperative Blood Glucose[5]	-	-	81%	97%
Perioperative Temperature Management[5]	-	-	98%	100%
Prophylactic Antibiotic Selection[5]	-	-	96%	99%
Prophylactic Antibiotic Selection (Outpatient)	-	-	-	98%
Prophylactic Antibiotic Stopped[5]	-	-	83%	98%
Prophylactic Antibiotic Timing[5]	-	-	89%	99%
Prophylactic Antibiotic Timing (Outpatient)	-	-	-	98%
Urinary Catheter Removal[5]	-	-	91%	97%
Survey of Patients' Hospital Experiences				
Area Around Room 'Always' Quiet at Night[5]	-	-	-	61%
Doctors 'Always' Communicated Well[5]	-	-	-	82%
Home Recovery Information Given[5]	-	-	-	85%
Hospital Given 9 or 10 on 10 Point Scale[5]	-	-	-	71%
Meds 'Always' Explained Before Given[5]	-	-	-	64%
Nurses 'Always' Communicated Well[5]	-	-	-	79%
Pain 'Always' Well Controlled[5]	-	-	-	71%
Room and Bathroom 'Always' Clean[5]	-	-	-	73%
Timely Help 'Always' Received[5]	-	-	-	68%
Would Definitely Recommend Hospital[5]	-	-	-	71%
Use of Medical Imaging				
Cardiac Imaging Stress Test before Surgery	-	-	4.5%	5.3%
Combination Abdominal CT Scan	-	-	7.4%	10.5%
Combination Brain/Sinus CT Scan	-	-	0.8%	2.7%
Combination Chest CT Scan	-	-	6.1%	2.7%
Follow-up Mammogram/Ultrasound	-	-	43.2%	8.8%
Lumbar Spine MRI for Low Back Pain	-	-	44.3%	37.2%

Hospital Menonita De Cayey

Bo. Rincon Sector Las Lomas Km.3.1 Carr 14
Phone: 787-535-1001
Cayey, PR 737 — Fax: 787-535-1034
Type: Acute Care Hospitals — Emergency Services: Yes
Ownership: Voluntary non-profit - Private — Beds: 118

Key Personnel:
Infection Control. . . . . Carmen E Flores, RN
Emergency Room . . . . Ruben Mendez, MD
Intensive Care Unit. . . . . Eric Ramirez, MD
Pediatric Ambulatory Care . . . . . . Idalia Rivera, MD
Pediatric In-Patient Care . . . . Idalia Rivera, MD
Quality Assurance . . . . Lisbeth Rodriguez
Anesthesiology. . . . . Jose A Rodriguez Colom, MD
Chief of Medical Staff. . . . . Sandra Vazquez

Measure	Cases	This Hosp.	State Avg.	U.S. Avg.
Blood Clot Prevention and Treatment				
Anticoagulation Overlap Therapy[5]	-	-	50%	93%
ICU Venous Thromboembolism Prophylaxis[5]	-	-	-	92%
Incidence of Potentially Preventable VTE[5]	-	-	-	10%
UFH with Dosages/Platelet Monitoring[5]	-	-	100%	97%

NOTE: Hospital profiles are in alphabetical order by state, then city, then hospital within the city; Rankings exclude hospitals with less than 25 cases except for patient surveys which excludes hospitals with less than 100 cases; (a) 100-299 cases; (1) The number of cases/patients is too few to report; (2) Data submitted were based on a sample of cases/patients; (3) Results are based on a shorter time period than required; (4) Data suppressed by CMS for one or more quarters; (5) Results are not available for this reporting period; (6) Fewer than 100 patients completed the HCAHPS survey; (7) No cases met the criteria for this measure; (8) The lower limit of the confidence interval cannot be calculated if the number of observed infections equals zero; (9) No data are available from the state/territory for this reporting period; (10) The scores shown reflect fewer than 50 completed surveys; (11) There were discrepancies in the data collection process; (12) This measure does not apply to this hospital for this reporting period; (13) Results cannot be calculated for this reporting period; (14) The results for this state are combined with nearby states to protect confidentiality; Please refer to the User's Guide for a full explanation of data.

Measure	Cases	This Hosp.	State Avg.	U.S. Avg.
Venous Thromboembolism Prophylaxis[5]	-	-	98%	85%
Warfarin Therapy Discharge Instructions[5]	-	-	92%	75%
Chest Pain/Possible Heart Attack Care				
Aspirin Given Within 24 Hours of Arrival	-	-	-	96%
Fibrinolytic Meds Within 30 Min. of Arrival	-	-	-	58%
Average Time to ECG (minutes)	-	-	-	7
Average Time to Transfer (minutes)	-	-	-	60
Children's Asthma Care				
Received Home Management Plan of Care	-	-	-	88%
Received Reliever Medication	-	-	-	100%
Received Systemic Corticosteroids	-	-	-	100%
Emergency Department				
Admittance Decision Time (minutes)[5]	-	-	190	98
Head CT Results Within 45 Min. of Arrival	-	-	-	57%
Patients Who Left ER Before Being Seen	-	-	-	2%
Time from ER Arrival to Admit. (minutes)[5]	-	-	635	274
Time from ER Arrival to Discharge (minutes)	-	-	-	134
Time in ER Before Being Evaluated (minutes)	-	-	-	26
Time to Pain Meds for Fractures (minutes)	-	-	-	57
Heart Attack Care				
Aspirin Given at Discharge	133	85%	94%	99%
Fibrinolytic Meds Within 30 Min. of Arrival[1]	-	-	47%	54%
PCI Within 90 Minutes of Arrival[3,7]	-	-	53%	96%
Statin Prescribed at Discharge	150	81%	89%	98%
Heart Failure Care				
ACE Inhibitor or ARB for LVSD	45	100%	92%	97%
Discharge Instructions Given	170	93%	87%	94%
Evaluation of LVS Function	172	98%	94%	99%
Medicare Spending				
Medicare Spending per Patient (ratio)	-	-	-	0.98
Pneumonia Care				
Appropriate Initial Antibiotic Given	93	87%	82%	95%
Blood Culture Timing	128	90%	82%	98%
Pregnancy and Delivery Care				
Newborn Deliveries Scheduled Early[5]	-	-	-	6%
Preventive Care				
Immunization for Influenza[5]	-	-	42%	90%
Immunization for Pneumonia[5]	-	-	29%	92%
Stroke Care				
Anticoagulation Therapy for Atrial Fibrillation[5]	-	-	60%	95%
Antithrombotic Therapy Timing[5]	-	-	77%	98%
Assessed for Rehabilitation[5]	-	-	59%	97%
Discharged on Antithrombotic Therapy[5]	-	-	63%	99%
Discharged on Statin Medication[5]	-	-	90%	94%
Thrombolytic Therapy Timing[5]	-	-	-	66%
Venous Thromboembolism Prophylaxis[5]	-	-	52%	94%
Written Stroke Educational Materials Given[5]	-	-	95%	88%
Surgical Care Improvement Project				
Appropriate Beta Blocker Usage[2]	18	100%	75%	98%
Appropriate VTP Within 24 Hours[2]	255	97%	90%	98%
Controlled Postoperative Blood Glucose[2,7]	-	-	81%	97%
Perioperative Temperature Management[2]	286	100%	98%	100%
Prophylactic Antibiotic Selection[2]	154	96%	96%	99%
Prophylactic Antibiotic Selection (Outpatient)	-	-	-	98%
Prophylactic Antibiotic Stopped[2]	153	95%	83%	98%
Prophylactic Antibiotic Timing[2]	154	90%	89%	99%
Prophylactic Antibiotic Timing (Outpatient)	-	-	-	98%
Urinary Catheter Removal[2]	140	97%	91%	97%
Survey of Patients' Hospital Experiences				
Area Around Room 'Always' Quiet at Night[5]	-	-	-	61%
Doctors 'Always' Communicated Well[5]	-	-	-	82%
Home Recovery Information Given[5]	-	-	-	85%
Hospital Given 9 or 10 on 10 Point Scale[5]	-	-	-	71%
Meds 'Always' Explained Before Given[5]	-	-	-	64%
Nurses 'Always' Communicated Well[5]	-	-	-	79%
Pain 'Always' Well Controlled[5]	-	-	-	71%
Room and Bathroom 'Always' Clean[5]	-	-	-	73%
Timely Help 'Always' Received[5]	-	-	-	68%
Would Definitely Recommend Hospital[5]	-	-	-	71%
Use of Medical Imaging				
Cardiac Imaging Stress Test before Surgery	-	-	4.5%	5.3%
Combination Abdominal CT Scan	-	-	7.4%	10.5%
Combination Brain/Sinus CT Scan	-	-	0.8%	2.7%
Combination Chest CT Scan	-	-	6.1%	2.7%
Follow-up Mammogram/Ultrasound	-	-	43.2%	8.8%
Lumbar Spine MRI for Low Back Pain	-	-	44.3%	37.2%

Hospital San Cristobal

Carr 506 Km 1 0 Phone: 787-848-2100
Coto Laurel, PR 780
Type: Acute Care Hospitals Emergency Services: Yes
Ownership: Voluntary non-profit - Private
Key Personnel:
CEO/President. . . . . Edwin R Marques

Measure	Cases	This Hosp.	State Avg.	U.S. Avg.
Blood Clot Prevention and Treatment				
Anticoagulation Overlap Therapy[1]	-	-	50%	93%
ICU Venous Thromboembolism Prophylaxis[7]	-	-	-	92%
Incidence of Potentially Preventable VTE[7]	-	-	-	10%
UFH with Dosages/Platelet Monitoring[1]	-	-	100%	97%
Venous Thromboembolism Prophylaxis[1]	-	-	98%	85%
Warfarin Therapy Discharge Instructions	13	100%	92%	75%
Chest Pain/Possible Heart Attack Care				
Aspirin Given Within 24 Hours of Arrival	-	-	-	96%
Fibrinolytic Meds Within 30 Min. of Arrival	-	-	-	58%
Average Time to ECG (minutes)	-	-	-	7
Average Time to Transfer (minutes)	-	-	-	60
Children's Asthma Care				
Received Home Management Plan of Care	-	-	-	88%
Received Reliever Medication	-	-	-	100%
Received Systemic Corticosteroids	-	-	-	100%
Emergency Department				
Admittance Decision Time (minutes)[7]	-	-	190	98
Head CT Results Within 45 Min. of Arrival	-	-	-	57%
Patients Who Left ER Before Being Seen	-	-	-	2%
Time from ER Arrival to Admit. (minutes)[1]	-	-	635	274
Time from ER Arrival to Discharge (minutes)	-	-	-	134
Time in ER Before Being Evaluated (minutes)	-	-	-	26
Time to Pain Meds for Fractures (minutes)	-	-	-	57
Heart Attack Care				
Aspirin Given at Discharge[2]	79	100%	94%	99%
Fibrinolytic Meds Within 30 Min. of Arrival[1,2]	-	-	47%	54%
PCI Within 90 Minutes of Arrival[2,7]	-	-	53%	96%
Statin Prescribed at Discharge[2]	76	100%	89%	98%
Heart Failure Care				
ACE Inhibitor or ARB for LVSD[2]	58	100%	92%	97%
Discharge Instructions Given[2]	75	99%	87%	94%
Evaluation of LVS Function[2]	76	93%	94%	99%
Medicare Spending				
Medicare Spending per Patient (ratio)	-	-	-	0.98
Pneumonia Care				
Appropriate Initial Antibiotic Given[1,2]	-	-	82%	95%
Blood Culture Timing[2]	16	56%	82%	98%
Pregnancy and Delivery Care				
Newborn Deliveries Scheduled Early[5]	-	-	-	6%
Preventive Care				
Immunization for Influenza[5]	-	-	42%	90%
Immunization for Pneumonia[5]	-	-	29%	92%
Stroke Care				
Anticoagulation Therapy for Atrial Fibrillation[1]	-	-	60%	95%
Antithrombotic Therapy Timing	14	50%	77%	98%
Assessed for Rehabilitation	13	0%	59%	97%
Discharged on Antithrombotic Therapy	13	62%	63%	99%
Discharged on Statin Medication	13	85%	90%	94%
Thrombolytic Therapy Timing[1]	-	-	-	66%
Venous Thromboembolism Prophylaxis	14	79%	52%	94%
Written Stroke Educational Materials Given	11	73%	95%	88%
Surgical Care Improvement Project				
Appropriate Beta Blocker Usage[1,2]	-	-	75%	98%
Appropriate VTP Within 24 Hours[2]	42	29%	90%	98%
Controlled Postoperative Blood Glucose[2,7]	-	-	81%	97%
Perioperative Temperature Management[2]	59	97%	98%	100%
Prophylactic Antibiotic Selection[2]	59	100%	96%	99%
Prophylactic Antibiotic Selection (Outpatient)	-	-	-	98%
Prophylactic Antibiotic Stopped[2]	59	85%	83%	98%
Prophylactic Antibiotic Timing[2]	60	62%	89%	99%
Prophylactic Antibiotic Timing (Outpatient)	-	-	-	98%
Urinary Catheter Removal[1,2]	-	-	91%	97%
Survey of Patients' Hospital Experiences				
Area Around Room 'Always' Quiet at Night[5]	-	-	-	61%
Doctors 'Always' Communicated Well[5]	-	-	-	82%
Home Recovery Information Given[5]	-	-	-	85%
Hospital Given 9 or 10 on 10 Point Scale[5]	-	-	-	71%
Meds 'Always' Explained Before Given[5]	-	-	-	64%
Nurses 'Always' Communicated Well[5]	-	-	-	79%
Pain 'Always' Well Controlled[5]	-	-	-	71%
Room and Bathroom 'Always' Clean[5]	-	-	-	73%
Timely Help 'Always' Received[5]	-	-	-	68%
Would Definitely Recommend Hospital[5]	-	-	-	71%
Use of Medical Imaging				
Cardiac Imaging Stress Test before Surgery	-	-	4.5%	5.3%
Combination Abdominal CT Scan	-	-	7.4%	10.5%
Combination Brain/Sinus CT Scan	-	-	0.8%	2.7%
Combination Chest CT Scan	-	-	6.1%	2.7%
Follow-up Mammogram/Ultrasound	-	-	43.2%	8.8%
Lumbar Spine MRI for Low Back Pain	-	-	44.3%	37.2%

Hima - San Pablo Fajardo

General Valero Ave#404 Phone: 787-655-0505
Fajardo, PR 738
Type: Acute Care Hospitals Emergency Services: Yes
Ownership: Proprietary

Measure	Cases	This Hosp.	State Avg.	U.S. Avg.
Blood Clot Prevention and Treatment				
Anticoagulation Overlap Therapy[5]	-	-	50%	93%
ICU Venous Thromboembolism Prophylaxis[5]	-	-	-	92%
Incidence of Potentially Preventable VTE[5]	-	-	-	10%
UFH with Dosages/Platelet Monitoring[5]	-	-	100%	97%
Venous Thromboembolism Prophylaxis[5]	-	-	98%	85%
Warfarin Therapy Discharge Instructions[5]	-	-	92%	75%
Chest Pain/Possible Heart Attack Care				
Aspirin Given Within 24 Hours of Arrival	-	-	-	96%
Fibrinolytic Meds Within 30 Min. of Arrival	-	-	-	58%
Average Time to ECG (minutes)	-	-	-	7
Average Time to Transfer (minutes)	-	-	-	60
Children's Asthma Care				
Received Home Management Plan of Care	-	-	-	88%
Received Reliever Medication	-	-	-	100%
Received Systemic Corticosteroids	-	-	-	100%
Emergency Department				
Admittance Decision Time (minutes)[5]	-	-	190	98
Head CT Results Within 45 Min. of Arrival	-	-	-	57%
Patients Who Left ER Before Being Seen	-	-	-	2%
Time from ER Arrival to Admit. (minutes)[5]	-	-	635	274
Time from ER Arrival to Discharge (minutes)	-	-	-	134
Time in ER Before Being Evaluated (minutes)	-	-	-	26
Time to Pain Meds for Fractures (minutes)	-	-	-	57
Heart Attack Care				
Aspirin Given at Discharge	32	88%	94%	99%
Fibrinolytic Meds Within 30 Min. of Arrival[1]	-	-	47%	54%
PCI Within 90 Minutes of Arrival[7]	-	-	53%	96%
Statin Prescribed at Discharge	40	60%	89%	98%
Heart Failure Care				
ACE Inhibitor or ARB for LVSD	50	94%	92%	97%
Discharge Instructions Given	160	84%	87%	94%
Evaluation of LVS Function	160	92%	94%	99%
Medicare Spending				
Medicare Spending per Patient (ratio)	-	-	-	0.98
Pneumonia Care				
Appropriate Initial Antibiotic Given	57	67%	82%	95%
Blood Culture Timing	59	78%	82%	98%
Pregnancy and Delivery Care				
Newborn Deliveries Scheduled Early[5]	-	-	-	6%
Preventive Care				
Immunization for Influenza[5]	-	-	42%	90%
Immunization for Pneumonia[5]	-	-	29%	92%
Stroke Care				

NOTE: Hospital profiles are in alphabetical order by state, then city, then hospital within the city; Rankings exclude hospitals with less than 25 cases except for patient surveys which excludes hospitals with less than 100 cases; (a) 100-299 cases; (1) The number of cases/patients is too few to report; (2) Data submitted were based on a sample of cases/patients; (3) Results are based on a shorter time period than required; (4) Data suppressed by CMS for one or more quarters; (5) Results are not available for this reporting period; (6) Fewer than 100 patients completed the HCAHPS survey; (7) No cases met the criteria for this measure; (8) The lower limit of the confidence interval cannot be calculated if the number of observed infections equals zero; (9) No data are available from the state/territory for this reporting period; (10) The scores shown reflect fewer than 50 completed surveys; (11) There were discrepancies in the data collection process; (12) This measure does not apply to this hospital for this reporting period; (13) Results cannot be calculated for this reporting period; (14) The results for this state are combined with nearby states to protect confidentiality; Please refer to the User's Guide for a full explanation of data.

Measure	Cases	This Hosp.	State Avg.	U.S. Avg.
Anticoagulation Therapy for Atrial Fibrillation[5]	-	-	60%	95%
Antithrombotic Therapy Timing[5]	-	-	77%	98%
Assessed for Rehabilitation[5]	-	-	59%	97%
Discharged on Antithrombotic Therapy[5]	-	-	63%	99%
Discharged on Statin Medication[5]	-	-	90%	94%
Thrombolytic Therapy Timing[5]	-	-	-	66%
Venous Thromboembolism Prophylaxis[5]	-	-	52%	94%
Written Stroke Educational Materials Given[5]	-	-	95%	88%
Surgical Care Improvement Project				
Appropriate Beta Blocker Usage	28	54%	75%	98%
Appropriate VTP Within 24 Hours	225	79%	90%	98%
Controlled Postoperative Blood Glucose[7]	-	-	81%	97%
Perioperative Temperature Management	220	100%	98%	100%
Prophylactic Antibiotic Selection	213	98%	96%	99%
Prophylactic Antibiotic Selection (Outpatient)	-	-	-	98%
Prophylactic Antibiotic Stopped	211	52%	83%	98%
Prophylactic Antibiotic Timing	213	75%	89%	99%
Prophylactic Antibiotic Timing (Outpatient)	-	-	-	98%
Urinary Catheter Removal	41	63%	91%	97%
Survey of Patients' Hospital Experiences				
Area Around Room 'Always' Quiet at Night[5]	-	-	-	61%
Doctors 'Always' Communicated Well[5]	-	-	-	82%
Home Recovery Information Given[5]	-	-	-	85%
Hospital Given 9 or 10 on 10 Point Scale[5]	-	-	-	71%
Meds 'Always' Explained Before Given[5]	-	-	-	64%
Nurses 'Always' Communicated Well[5]	-	-	-	79%
Pain 'Always' Well Controlled[5]	-	-	-	71%
Room and Bathroom 'Always' Clean[5]	-	-	-	73%
Timely Help 'Always' Received[5]	-	-	-	68%
Would Definitely Recommend Hospital[5]	-	-	-	71%
Use of Medical Imaging				
Cardiac Imaging Stress Test before Surgery	-	-	4.5%	5.3%
Combination Abdominal CT Scan	-	-	7.4%	10.5%
Combination Brain/Sinus CT Scan	-	-	0.8%	2.7%
Combination Chest CT Scan	-	-	6.1%	2.7%
Follow-up Mammogram/Ultrasound	-	-	43.2%	8.8%
Lumbar Spine MRI for Low Back Pain	-	-	44.3%	37.2%

Doctors' Center Hospital San Juan

Pda. 20 C/ San Rafael # 1395
Fernandez Juncos, PR 909
Phone: 787-723-2950
Fax: 787-725-2124
Type: Acute Care Hospitals
Emergency Services: Yes
Ownership: Proprietary
Beds: 132

Key Personnel:
Quality Assurance . . . . Carmen Alvarado
Chair/CEO . . . . Walter D. Bristol
Chief of Medical Staff . . . . Anarda Gonzalez
CEO/President . . . . James A. Guest
Infection Control . . . . Madeline Vargas

Measure	Cases	This Hosp.	State Avg.	U.S. Avg.
Blood Clot Prevention and Treatment				
Anticoagulation Overlap Therapy[1,2]	-	-	50%	93%
ICU Venous Thromboembolism Prophylaxis[2,3]	-	-	-	92%
Incidence of Potentially Preventable VTE[2,3]	-	-	-	10%
UFH with Dosages/Platelet Monitoring[2,3]	-	-	100%	97%
Venous Thromboembolism Prophylaxis[1,2]	-	-	98%	85%
Warfarin Therapy Discharge Instructions[1,2]	-	-	92%	75%
Chest Pain/Possible Heart Attack Care				
Aspirin Given Within 24 Hours of Arrival	-	-	-	96%
Fibrinolytic Meds Within 30 Min. of Arrival	-	-	-	58%
Average Time to ECG (minutes)	-	-	-	7
Average Time to Transfer (minutes)	-	-	-	60
Children's Asthma Care				
Received Home Management Plan of Care	-	-	-	88%
Received Reliever Medication	-	-	-	100%
Received Systemic Corticosteroids	-	-	-	100%
Emergency Department				
Admittance Decision Time (minutes)[5]	-	-	190	98
Head CT Results Within 45 Min. of Arrival	-	-	-	57%
Patients Who Left ER Before Being Seen	-	-	-	2%
Time from ER Arrival to Admit. (minutes)[5]	-	-	635	274
Time from ER Arrival to Discharge (minutes)	-	-	-	134
Time in ER Before Being Evaluated (minutes)	-	-	-	26
Time to Pain Meds for Fractures (minutes)	-	-	-	57
Heart Attack Care				
Aspirin Given at Discharge[1,2]	-	-	94%	99%
Fibrinolytic Meds Within 30 Min. of Arrival[2,7]	-	-	47%	54%
PCI Within 90 Minutes of Arrival[2,7]	-	-	53%	96%
Statin Prescribed at Discharge[1,2]	-	-	89%	98%
Heart Failure Care				
ACE Inhibitor or ARB for LVSD[2]	22	27%	92%	97%
Discharge Instructions Given[2]	75	47%	87%	94%
Evaluation of LVS Function[2]	50	68%	94%	99%
Medicare Spending				
Medicare Spending per Patient (ratio)	-	-	-	0.98
Pneumonia Care				
Appropriate Initial Antibiotic Given[1,2]	-	-	82%	95%
Blood Culture Timing[1,2]	-	-	82%	98%
Pregnancy and Delivery Care				
Newborn Deliveries Scheduled Early[5]	-	-	-	6%
Preventive Care				
Immunization for Influenza[5]	-	-	42%	90%
Immunization for Pneumonia[5]	-	-	29%	92%
Stroke Care				
Anticoagulation Therapy for Atrial Fibrillation[1,2]	-	-	60%	95%
Antithrombotic Therapy Timing[1,2]	-	-	77%	98%
Assessed for Rehabilitation[1,2]	-	-	59%	97%
Discharged on Antithrombotic Therapy[1,2]	-	-	63%	99%
Discharged on Statin Medication[1,2]	-	-	90%	94%
Thrombolytic Therapy Timing[2,3]	-	-	-	66%
Venous Thromboembolism Prophylaxis[1,2]	-	-	52%	94%
Written Stroke Educational Materials Given[1,2]	-	-	95%	88%
Surgical Care Improvement Project				
Appropriate Beta Blocker Usage[5]	-	-	75%	98%
Appropriate VTP Within 24 Hours[5]	-	-	90%	98%
Controlled Postoperative Blood Glucose[5]	-	-	81%	97%
Perioperative Temperature Management[5]	-	-	98%	100%
Prophylactic Antibiotic Selection[5]	-	-	96%	99%
Prophylactic Antibiotic Selection (Outpatient)	-	-	-	98%
Prophylactic Antibiotic Stopped[5]	-	-	83%	98%
Prophylactic Antibiotic Timing[5]	-	-	89%	99%
Prophylactic Antibiotic Timing (Outpatient)	-	-	-	98%
Urinary Catheter Removal[5]	-	-	91%	97%
Survey of Patients' Hospital Experiences				
Area Around Room 'Always' Quiet at Night[5]	-	-	-	61%
Doctors 'Always' Communicated Well[5]	-	-	-	82%
Home Recovery Information Given[5]	-	-	-	85%
Hospital Given 9 or 10 on 10 Point Scale[5]	-	-	-	71%
Meds 'Always' Explained Before Given[5]	-	-	-	64%
Nurses 'Always' Communicated Well[5]	-	-	-	79%
Pain 'Always' Well Controlled[5]	-	-	-	71%
Room and Bathroom 'Always' Clean[5]	-	-	-	73%
Timely Help 'Always' Received[5]	-	-	-	68%
Would Definitely Recommend Hospital[5]	-	-	-	71%
Use of Medical Imaging				
Cardiac Imaging Stress Test before Surgery	-	-	4.5%	5.3%
Combination Abdominal CT Scan	-	-	7.4%	10.5%
Combination Brain/Sinus CT Scan	-	-	0.8%	2.7%
Combination Chest CT Scan	-	-	6.1%	2.7%
Follow-up Mammogram/Ultrasound	-	-	43.2%	8.8%
Lumbar Spine MRI for Low Back Pain	-	-	44.3%	37.2%

Hospital Pavia Santurce

Calle Profesor Augusto Rodriguez #1462
Fernandez Juncos, PR 910
Phone: 787-727-6060
Fax: 787-727-7500
URL: www.paviahospitalsanturce.com
Type: Acute Care Hospitals
Emergency Services: Yes
Ownership: Voluntary non-profit - Private
Beds: 193

Key Personnel:
Chief of Medical Staff . . . . Roberto Munoz Marin, MD
Intensive Care Unit . . . . Manuel Quiles, MD
Operating Room . . . . Maria Salva
Emergency Room . . . . Joaquin Vargas, MD
Infection Control . . . . Guillermo Vazquez, MD
Quality Assurance . . . . Nancy Velasquez
Anesthesiology . . . . Raul Porro Vizcarra, MD

Measure	Cases	This Hosp.	State Avg.	U.S. Avg.
Blood Clot Prevention and Treatment				
Anticoagulation Overlap Therapy[5]	-	-	50%	93%
ICU Venous Thromboembolism Prophylaxis[5]	-	-	-	92%
Incidence of Potentially Preventable VTE[5]	-	-	-	10%
UFH with Dosages/Platelet Monitoring[5]	-	-	100%	97%
Venous Thromboembolism Prophylaxis[5]	-	-	98%	85%
Warfarin Therapy Discharge Instructions[5]	-	-	92%	75%
Chest Pain/Possible Heart Attack Care				
Aspirin Given Within 24 Hours of Arrival	-	-	-	96%
Fibrinolytic Meds Within 30 Min. of Arrival	-	-	-	58%
Average Time to ECG (minutes)	-	-	-	7
Average Time to Transfer (minutes)	-	-	-	60
Children's Asthma Care				
Received Home Management Plan of Care	-	-	-	88%
Received Reliever Medication	-	-	-	100%
Received Systemic Corticosteroids	-	-	-	100%
Emergency Department				
Admittance Decision Time (minutes)[5]	-	-	190	98
Head CT Results Within 45 Min. of Arrival	-	-	-	57%
Patients Who Left ER Before Being Seen	-	-	-	2%
Time from ER Arrival to Admit. (minutes)[5]	-	-	635	274
Time from ER Arrival to Discharge (minutes)	-	-	-	134
Time in ER Before Being Evaluated (minutes)	-	-	-	26
Time to Pain Meds for Fractures (minutes)	-	-	-	57
Heart Attack Care				
Aspirin Given at Discharge	232	98%	94%	99%
Fibrinolytic Meds Within 30 Min. of Arrival[7]	-	-	47%	54%
PCI Within 90 Minutes of Arrival[1]	-	-	53%	96%
Statin Prescribed at Discharge	237	96%	89%	98%
Heart Failure Care				
ACE Inhibitor or ARB for LVSD	98	100%	92%	97%
Discharge Instructions Given	260	100%	87%	94%
Evaluation of LVS Function	260	100%	94%	99%
Medicare Spending				
Medicare Spending per Patient (ratio)	-	-	-	0.98
Pneumonia Care				
Appropriate Initial Antibiotic Given	63	100%	82%	95%
Blood Culture Timing	69	100%	82%	98%
Pregnancy and Delivery Care				
Newborn Deliveries Scheduled Early[5]	-	-	-	6%
Preventive Care				
Immunization for Influenza[5]	-	-	42%	90%
Immunization for Pneumonia[5]	-	-	29%	92%
Stroke Care				
Anticoagulation Therapy for Atrial Fibrillation[5]	-	-	60%	95%
Antithrombotic Therapy Timing[5]	-	-	77%	98%
Assessed for Rehabilitation[5]	-	-	59%	97%
Discharged on Antithrombotic Therapy[5]	-	-	63%	99%
Discharged on Statin Medication[5]	-	-	90%	94%
Thrombolytic Therapy Timing[5]	-	-	-	66%
Venous Thromboembolism Prophylaxis[5]	-	-	52%	94%
Written Stroke Educational Materials Given[5]	-	-	95%	88%
Surgical Care Improvement Project				
Appropriate Beta Blocker Usage	110	65%	75%	98%
Appropriate VTP Within 24 Hours	303	89%	90%	98%
Controlled Postoperative Blood Glucose	196	71%	81%	97%
Perioperative Temperature Management	375	100%	98%	100%
Prophylactic Antibiotic Selection	388	94%	96%	99%
Prophylactic Antibiotic Selection (Outpatient)	-	-	-	98%
Prophylactic Antibiotic Stopped	355	75%	83%	98%
Prophylactic Antibiotic Timing	392	92%	89%	99%
Prophylactic Antibiotic Timing (Outpatient)	-	-	-	98%
Urinary Catheter Removal	201	99%	91%	97%
Survey of Patients' Hospital Experiences				
Area Around Room 'Always' Quiet at Night[5]	-	-	-	61%
Doctors 'Always' Communicated Well[5]	-	-	-	82%
Home Recovery Information Given[5]	-	-	-	85%
Hospital Given 9 or 10 on 10 Point Scale[5]	-	-	-	71%
Meds 'Always' Explained Before Given[5]	-	-	-	64%
Nurses 'Always' Communicated Well[5]	-	-	-	79%
Pain 'Always' Well Controlled[5]	-	-	-	71%
Room and Bathroom 'Always' Clean[5]	-	-	-	73%

NOTE: Hospital profiles are in alphabetical order by state, then city, then hospital within the city; Rankings exclude hospitals with less than 25 cases except for patient surveys which excludes hospitals with less than 100 cases; (a) 100-299 cases; (1) The number of cases/patients is too few to report; (2) Data submitted were based on a sample of cases/patients; (3) Results are based on a shorter time period than required; (4) Data suppressed by CMS for one or more quarters; (5) Results are not available for this reporting period; (6) Fewer than 100 patients completed the HCAHPS survey; (7) No cases met the criteria for this measure; (8) The lower limit of the confidence interval cannot be calculated if the number of observed infections equals zero; (9) No data are available from the state/territory for this reporting period; (10) The scores shown reflect fewer than 50 completed surveys; (11) There were discrepancies in the data collection process; (12) This measure does not apply to this hospital for this reporting period; (13) Results cannot be calculated for this reporting period; (14) The results for this state are combined with nearby states to protect confidentiality; Please refer to the User's Guide for a full explanation of data.

Timely Help 'Always' Received[5]	-	-	-	68%
Would Definitely Recommend Hospital[5]	-	-	-	71%
Use of Medical Imaging				
Cardiac Imaging Stress Test before Surgery	-	-	4.5%	5.3%
Combination Abdominal CT Scan	-	-	7.4%	10.5%
Combination Brain/Sinus CT Scan	-	-	0.8%	2.7%
Combination Chest CT Scan	-	-	6.1%	2.7%
Follow-up Mammogram/Ultrasound	-	-	43.2%	8.8%
Lumbar Spine MRI for Low Back Pain	-	-	44.3%	37.2%

Hospital Episcopal San Lucas Guayama

Ave. Pedro Albizu Campos Urb. La Hacienda
Phone: 787-864-4300
Guayama, PR 785 Fax: 787-864-4466
URL: www.ssepr.com/cr_bienvenido.htm
Type: Acute Care Hospitals Emergency Services: Yes
Ownership: Proprietary Beds: 115

Key Personnel:
Emergency Room . . . . Jose Anglero Ramos
Intensive Care Unit. . . . . Jozita Carrasquillo
Chief of Medical Staff. . . . . Jorge Del Pozo
Anesthesiology. . . . . Miguel Fonpanos
Operating Room. . . . . Evangelina Laboy
Quality Assurance . . . . Pedro Rosario
Pediatric In-Patient Care . . . . Hiram Sosa
Infection Control. . . . . Carlos Leon Valiente

Measure	Cases	This Hosp.	State Avg.	U.S. Avg.
Blood Clot Prevention and Treatment				
Anticoagulation Overlap Therapy[5]	-	-	50%	93%
ICU Venous Thromboembolism Prophylaxis[5]	-	-	-	92%
Incidence of Potentially Preventable VTE[5]	-	-	-	10%
UFH with Dosages/Platelet Monitoring[5]	-	-	100%	97%
Venous Thromboembolism Prophylaxis[5]	-	-	98%	85%
Warfarin Therapy Discharge Instructions[5]	-	-	92%	75%
Chest Pain/Possible Heart Attack Care				
Aspirin Given Within 24 Hours of Arrival	-	-	-	96%
Fibrinolytic Meds Within 30 Min. of Arrival	-	-	-	58%
Average Time to ECG (minutes)	-	-	-	7
Average Time to Transfer (minutes)	-	-	-	60
Children's Asthma Care				
Received Home Management Plan of Care	-	-	-	88%
Received Reliever Medication	-	-	-	100%
Received Systemic Corticosteroids	-	-	-	100%
Emergency Department				
Admittance Decision Time (minutes)[5]	-	-	190	98
Head CT Results Within 45 Min. of Arrival	-	-	-	57%
Patients Who Left ER Before Being Seen	-	-	-	2%
Time from ER Arrival to Admit. (minutes)[5]	-	-	635	274
Time from ER Arrival to Discharge (minutes)	-	-	-	134
Time in ER Before Being Evaluated (minutes)	-	-	-	26
Time to Pain Meds for Fractures (minutes)	-	-	-	57
Heart Attack Care				
Aspirin Given at Discharge	37	100%	94%	99%
Fibrinolytic Meds Within 30 Min. of Arrival[7]	-	-	47%	54%
PCI Within 90 Minutes of Arrival[3,7]	-	-	53%	96%
Statin Prescribed at Discharge	44	100%	89%	98%
Heart Failure Care				
ACE Inhibitor or ARB for LVSD	17	100%	92%	97%
Discharge Instructions Given	67	100%	87%	94%
Evaluation of LVS Function	66	98%	94%	99%
Medicare Spending				
Medicare Spending per Patient (ratio)	-	-	-	0.98
Pneumonia Care				
Appropriate Initial Antibiotic Given	51	88%	82%	95%
Blood Culture Timing	34	88%	82%	98%
Pregnancy and Delivery Care				
Newborn Deliveries Scheduled Early[5]	-	-	-	6%
Preventive Care				
Immunization for Influenza[5]	-	-	42%	90%
Immunization for Pneumonia[5]	-	-	29%	92%
Stroke Care				
Anticoagulation Therapy for Atrial Fibrillation[5]	-	-	60%	95%
Antithrombotic Therapy Timing[5]	-	-	77%	98%
Assessed for Rehabilitation[5]	-	-	59%	97%
Discharged on Antithrombotic Therapy[5]	-	-	63%	99%
Discharged on Statin Medication[5]	-	-	90%	94%
Thrombolytic Therapy Timing[5]	-	-	-	66%
Venous Thromboembolism Prophylaxis[5]	-	-	52%	94%
Written Stroke Educational Materials Given[5]	-	-	95%	88%
Surgical Care Improvement Project				
Appropriate Beta Blocker Usage	16	94%	75%	98%
Appropriate VTP Within 24 Hours	162	96%	90%	98%
Controlled Postoperative Blood Glucose[7]	-	-	81%	97%
Perioperative Temperature Management	165	100%	98%	100%
Prophylactic Antibiotic Selection	163	98%	96%	99%
Prophylactic Antibiotic Selection (Outpatient)	-	-	-	98%
Prophylactic Antibiotic Stopped	151	99%	83%	98%
Prophylactic Antibiotic Timing	164	98%	89%	99%
Prophylactic Antibiotic Timing (Outpatient)	-	-	-	98%
Urinary Catheter Removal[7]	-	-	91%	97%
Survey of Patients' Hospital Experiences				
Area Around Room 'Always' Quiet at Night[5]	-	-	-	61%
Doctors 'Always' Communicated Well[5]	-	-	-	82%
Home Recovery Information Given[5]	-	-	-	85%
Hospital Given 9 or 10 on 10 Point Scale[5]	-	-	-	71%
Meds 'Always' Explained Before Given[5]	-	-	-	64%
Nurses 'Always' Communicated Well[5]	-	-	-	79%
Pain 'Always' Well Controlled[5]	-	-	-	71%
Room and Bathroom 'Always' Clean[5]	-	-	-	73%
Timely Help 'Always' Received[5]	-	-	-	68%
Would Definitely Recommend Hospital[5]	-	-	-	71%
Use of Medical Imaging				
Cardiac Imaging Stress Test before Surgery	-	-	4.5%	5.3%
Combination Abdominal CT Scan	-	-	7.4%	10.5%
Combination Brain/Sinus CT Scan	-	-	0.8%	2.7%
Combination Chest CT Scan	-	-	6.1%	2.7%
Follow-up Mammogram/Ultrasound	-	-	43.2%	8.8%
Lumbar Spine MRI for Low Back Pain	-	-	44.3%	37.2%

Santa Rosa Clinic

Ave. Los Veteranos #3 Km 135 7 Exit To Arroyo
Phone: 787-864-0101
Guayama, PR 785 Fax: 787-866-0489
Type: Acute Care Hospitals Emergency Services: Yes
Ownership: Voluntary non-profit - Private Beds: 89

Key Personnel:
CEO/President. . . . . Herson Lomorales

Measure	Cases	This Hosp.	State Avg.	U.S. Avg.
Blood Clot Prevention and Treatment				
Anticoagulation Overlap Therapy[5]	-	-	50%	93%
ICU Venous Thromboembolism Prophylaxis[5]	-	-	-	92%
Incidence of Potentially Preventable VTE[5]	-	-	-	10%
UFH with Dosages/Platelet Monitoring[5]	-	-	100%	97%
Venous Thromboembolism Prophylaxis[5]	-	-	98%	85%
Warfarin Therapy Discharge Instructions[5]	-	-	92%	75%
Chest Pain/Possible Heart Attack Care				
Aspirin Given Within 24 Hours of Arrival	-	-	-	96%
Fibrinolytic Meds Within 30 Min. of Arrival	-	-	-	58%
Average Time to ECG (minutes)	-	-	-	7
Average Time to Transfer (minutes)	-	-	-	60
Children's Asthma Care				
Received Home Management Plan of Care	-	-	-	88%
Received Reliever Medication	-	-	-	100%
Received Systemic Corticosteroids	-	-	-	100%
Emergency Department				
Admittance Decision Time (minutes)[5]	-	-	190	98
Head CT Results Within 45 Min. of Arrival	-	-	-	57%
Patients Who Left ER Before Being Seen	-	-	-	2%
Time from ER Arrival to Admit. (minutes)[5]	-	-	635	274
Time from ER Arrival to Discharge (minutes)	-	-	-	134
Time in ER Before Being Evaluated (minutes)	-	-	-	26
Time to Pain Meds for Fractures (minutes)	-	-	-	57
Heart Attack Care				
Aspirin Given at Discharge	22	100%	94%	99%
Fibrinolytic Meds Within 30 Min. of Arrival[7]	-	-	47%	54%
PCI Within 90 Minutes of Arrival[7]	-	-	53%	96%
Statin Prescribed at Discharge	21	76%	89%	98%
Heart Failure Care				
ACE Inhibitor or ARB for LVSD[1,3]	-	-	92%	97%
Discharge Instructions Given[3]	28	71%	87%	94%
Evaluation of LVS Function[3]	28	96%	94%	99%
Medicare Spending				
Medicare Spending per Patient (ratio)	-	-	-	0.98
Pneumonia Care				
Appropriate Initial Antibiotic Given	25	56%	82%	95%
Blood Culture Timing[7]	-	-	82%	98%
Pregnancy and Delivery Care				
Newborn Deliveries Scheduled Early[5]	-	-	-	6%
Preventive Care				
Immunization for Influenza[5]	-	-	42%	90%
Immunization for Pneumonia[5]	-	-	29%	92%
Stroke Care				
Anticoagulation Therapy for Atrial Fibrillation[5]	-	-	60%	95%
Antithrombotic Therapy Timing[5]	-	-	77%	98%
Assessed for Rehabilitation[5]	-	-	59%	97%
Discharged on Antithrombotic Therapy[5]	-	-	63%	99%
Discharged on Statin Medication[5]	-	-	90%	94%
Thrombolytic Therapy Timing[5]	-	-	-	66%
Venous Thromboembolism Prophylaxis[5]	-	-	52%	94%
Written Stroke Educational Materials Given[5]	-	-	95%	88%
Surgical Care Improvement Project				
Appropriate Beta Blocker Usage[1,3]	-	-	75%	98%
Appropriate VTP Within 24 Hours[1,3]	-	-	90%	98%
Controlled Postoperative Blood Glucose[3,7]	-	-	81%	97%
Perioperative Temperature Management[1,3]	-	-	98%	100%
Prophylactic Antibiotic Selection[1,3]	-	-	96%	99%
Prophylactic Antibiotic Selection (Outpatient)	-	-	-	98%
Prophylactic Antibiotic Stopped[1,3]	-	-	83%	98%
Prophylactic Antibiotic Timing[1,3]	-	-	89%	99%
Prophylactic Antibiotic Timing (Outpatient)	-	-	-	98%
Urinary Catheter Removal[1,3]	-	-	91%	97%
Survey of Patients' Hospital Experiences				
Area Around Room 'Always' Quiet at Night[5]	-	-	-	61%
Doctors 'Always' Communicated Well[5]	-	-	-	82%
Home Recovery Information Given[5]	-	-	-	85%
Hospital Given 9 or 10 on 10 Point Scale[5]	-	-	-	71%
Meds 'Always' Explained Before Given[5]	-	-	-	64%
Nurses 'Always' Communicated Well[5]	-	-	-	79%
Pain 'Always' Well Controlled[5]	-	-	-	71%
Room and Bathroom 'Always' Clean[5]	-	-	-	73%
Timely Help 'Always' Received[5]	-	-	-	68%
Would Definitely Recommend Hospital[5]	-	-	-	71%
Use of Medical Imaging				
Cardiac Imaging Stress Test before Surgery	-	-	4.5%	5.3%
Combination Abdominal CT Scan	-	-	7.4%	10.5%
Combination Brain/Sinus CT Scan	-	-	0.8%	2.7%
Combination Chest CT Scan	-	-	6.1%	2.7%
Follow-up Mammogram/Ultrasound	-	-	43.2%	8.8%
Lumbar Spine MRI for Low Back Pain	-	-	44.3%	37.2%

Auxilio Mutuo Hospital

Ponce De Leon Avenue Stop 36 1/2 #735 Phone: 787-758-2000
Hato Rey, PR 918 Fax: 787-771-7951
E-mail: jgalarce@auxilio.com
URL: www.auxiliopr.com
Type: Acute Care Hospitals Emergency Services: Yes
Ownership: Voluntary non-profit - Private Beds: 510

Key Personnel:
Infection Control. . . . . Quirico Canario-Brea, MD
Operating Room. . . . . Celia Cuadrado
CEO/President. . . . . Enrique Fierres
Pediatric Ambulatory Care . . . . . . Hector Fontanet, MD
Pediatric In-Patient Care . . . . Hector Fontanet, MD
Quality Assurance . . . . Sonia Jimenez
Chief of Medical Staff . . . . Angel Rodriguez
Radiology. . . . . Fernando Salduondo, MD

Measure	Cases	This Hosp.	State Avg.	U.S. Avg.
Blood Clot Prevention and Treatment				
Anticoagulation Overlap Therapy[5]	-	-	50%	93%
ICU Venous Thromboembolism Prophylaxis[5]	-	-	-	92%
Incidence of Potentially Preventable VTE[5]	-	-	-	10%

NOTE: Hospital profiles are in alphabetical order by state, then city, then hospital within the city; Rankings exclude hospitals with less than 25 cases except for patient surveys which excludes hospitals with less than 100 cases; (a) 100-299 cases; (1) The number of cases/patients is too few to report; (2) Data submitted were based on a sample of cases/patients; (3) Results are based on a shorter time period than required; (4) Data suppressed by CMS for one or more quarters; (5) Results are not available for this reporting period; (6) Fewer than 100 patients completed the HCAHPS survey; (7) No cases met the criteria for this measure; (8) The lower limit of the confidence interval cannot be calculated if the number of observed infections equals zero; (9) No data are available from the state/territory for this reporting period; (10) The scores shown reflect fewer than 50 completed surveys; (11) There were discrepancies in the data collection process; (12) This measure does not apply to this hospital for this reporting period; (13) Results cannot be calculated for this reporting period; (14) The results for this state are combined with nearby states to protect confidentiality; Please refer to the User's Guide for a full explanation of data.

Measure	Cases	This Hosp.	State Avg.	U.S. Avg.
UFH with Dosages/Platelet Monitoring[5]	-	-	100%	97%
Venous Thromboembolism Prophylaxis[5]	-	-	98%	85%
Warfarin Therapy Discharge Instructions[5]	-	-	92%	75%
Chest Pain/Possible Heart Attack Care				
Aspirin Given Within 24 Hours of Arrival	-	-	-	96%
Fibrinolytic Meds Within 30 Min. of Arrival	-	-	-	58%
Average Time to ECG (minutes)	-	-	-	7
Average Time to Transfer (minutes)	-	-	-	60
Children's Asthma Care				
Received Home Management Plan of Care	-	-	-	88%
Received Reliever Medication	-	-	-	100%
Received Systemic Corticosteroids	-	-	-	100%
Emergency Department				
Admittance Decision Time (minutes)[5]	-	-	190	98
Head CT Results Within 45 Min. of Arrival	-	-	-	57%
Patients Who Left ER Before Being Seen	-	-	-	2%
Time from ER Arrival to Admit. (minutes)[5]	-	-	635	274
Time from ER Arrival to Discharge (minutes)	-	-	-	134
Time in ER Before Being Evaluated (minutes)	-	-	-	26
Time to Pain Meds for Fractures (minutes)	-	-	-	57
Heart Attack Care				
Aspirin Given at Discharge	114	89%	94%	99%
Fibrinolytic Meds Within 30 Min. of Arrival[7]	-	-	47%	54%
PCI Within 90 Minutes of Arrival	13	15%	53%	96%
Statin Prescribed at Discharge	115	63%	89%	98%
Heart Failure Care				
ACE Inhibitor or ARB for LVSD	107	68%	92%	97%
Discharge Instructions Given	395	59%	87%	94%
Evaluation of LVS Function	399	87%	94%	99%
Medicare Spending				
Medicare Spending per Patient (ratio)	-	-	-	0.98
Pneumonia Care				
Appropriate Initial Antibiotic Given	88	76%	82%	95%
Blood Culture Timing	128	73%	82%	98%
Pregnancy and Delivery Care				
Newborn Deliveries Scheduled Early[5]	-	-	-	6%
Preventive Care				
Immunization for Influenza[5]	-	-	42%	90%
Immunization for Pneumonia[5]	-	-	29%	92%
Stroke Care				
Anticoagulation Therapy for Atrial Fibrillation[5]	-	-	60%	95%
Antithrombotic Therapy Timing[5]	-	-	77%	98%
Assessed for Rehabilitation[5]	-	-	59%	97%
Discharged on Antithrombotic Therapy[5]	-	-	63%	99%
Discharged on Statin Medication[5]	-	-	90%	94%
Thrombolytic Therapy Timing[5]	-	-	-	66%
Venous Thromboembolism Prophylaxis[5]	-	-	52%	94%
Written Stroke Educational Materials Given[5]	-	-	95%	88%
Surgical Care Improvement Project				
Appropriate Beta Blocker Usage[2]	203	84%	75%	98%
Appropriate VTP Within 24 Hours[2]	689	92%	90%	98%
Controlled Postoperative Blood Glucose[2]	103	70%	81%	97%
Perioperative Temperature Management[2]	729	100%	98%	100%
Prophylactic Antibiotic Selection[2]	738	97%	96%	99%
Prophylactic Antibiotic Selection (Outpatient)	-	-	-	98%
Prophylactic Antibiotic Stopped[2]	723	83%	83%	98%
Prophylactic Antibiotic Timing[2]	740	88%	89%	99%
Prophylactic Antibiotic Timing (Outpatient)	-	-	-	98%
Urinary Catheter Removal[2]	157	77%	91%	97%
Survey of Patients' Hospital Experiences				
Area Around Room 'Always' Quiet at Night[5]	-	-	-	61%
Doctors 'Always' Communicated Well[5]	-	-	-	82%
Home Recovery Information Given[5]	-	-	-	85%
Hospital Given 9 or 10 on 10 Point Scale[5]	-	-	-	71%
Meds 'Always' Explained Before Given[5]	-	-	-	64%
Nurses 'Always' Communicated Well[5]	-	-	-	79%
Pain 'Always' Well Controlled[5]	-	-	-	71%
Room and Bathroom 'Always' Clean[5]	-	-	-	73%
Timely Help 'Always' Received[5]	-	-	-	68%
Would Definitely Recommend Hospital[5]	-	-	-	71%
Use of Medical Imaging				
Cardiac Imaging Stress Test before Surgery	-	-	4.5%	5.3%
Combination Abdominal CT Scan	-	-	7.4%	10.5%
Combination Brain/Sinus CT Scan	-	-	0.8%	2.7%
Combination Chest CT Scan	-	-	6.1%	2.7%
Follow-up Mammogram/Ultrasound	-	-	43.2%	8.8%
Lumbar Spine MRI for Low Back Pain	-	-	44.3%	37.2%

Hospital Pavia Hato Rey

Ave Ponce De Leon 435 Phone: 787-754-0909
Hato Rey, PR 919
Type: Acute Care Hospitals Emergency Services: Yes
Ownership: Voluntary non-profit - Private
Key Personnel:
CEO/President. . . . . Jose Luis Rodriguez

Measure	Cases	This Hosp.	State Avg.	U.S. Avg.
Blood Clot Prevention and Treatment				
Anticoagulation Overlap Therapy[5]	-	-	50%	93%
ICU Venous Thromboembolism Prophylaxis[5]	-	-	-	92%
Incidence of Potentially Preventable VTE[5]	-	-	-	10%
UFH with Dosages/Platelet Monitoring[5]	-	-	100%	97%
Venous Thromboembolism Prophylaxis[5]	-	-	98%	85%
Warfarin Therapy Discharge Instructions[5]	-	-	92%	75%
Chest Pain/Possible Heart Attack Care				
Aspirin Given Within 24 Hours of Arrival	-	-	-	96%
Fibrinolytic Meds Within 30 Min. of Arrival	-	-	-	58%
Average Time to ECG (minutes)	-	-	-	7
Average Time to Transfer (minutes)	-	-	-	60
Children's Asthma Care				
Received Home Management Plan of Care	-	-	-	88%
Received Reliever Medication	-	-	-	100%
Received Systemic Corticosteroids	-	-	-	100%
Emergency Department				
Admittance Decision Time (minutes)[5]	-	-	190	98
Head CT Results Within 45 Min. of Arrival	-	-	-	57%
Patients Who Left ER Before Being Seen	-	-	-	2%
Time from ER Arrival to Admit. (minutes)[5]	-	-	635	274
Time from ER Arrival to Discharge (minutes)	-	-	-	134
Time in ER Before Being Evaluated (minutes)	-	-	-	26
Time to Pain Meds for Fractures (minutes)	-	-	-	57
Heart Attack Care				
Aspirin Given at Discharge	28	93%	94%	99%
Fibrinolytic Meds Within 30 Min. of Arrival[7]	-	-	47%	54%
PCI Within 90 Minutes of Arrival[7]	-	-	53%	96%
Statin Prescribed at Discharge	26	100%	89%	98%
Heart Failure Care				
ACE Inhibitor or ARB for LVSD	25	96%	92%	97%
Discharge Instructions Given	57	96%	87%	94%
Evaluation of LVS Function	63	98%	94%	99%
Medicare Spending				
Medicare Spending per Patient (ratio)	-	-	-	0.98
Pneumonia Care				
Appropriate Initial Antibiotic Given	80	81%	82%	95%
Blood Culture Timing	48	98%	82%	98%
Pregnancy and Delivery Care				
Newborn Deliveries Scheduled Early[5]	-	-	-	6%
Preventive Care				
Immunization for Influenza[5]	-	-	42%	90%
Immunization for Pneumonia[5]	-	-	29%	92%
Stroke Care				
Anticoagulation Therapy for Atrial Fibrillation[5]	-	-	60%	95%
Antithrombotic Therapy Timing[5]	-	-	77%	98%
Assessed for Rehabilitation[5]	-	-	59%	97%
Discharged on Antithrombotic Therapy[5]	-	-	63%	99%
Discharged on Statin Medication[5]	-	-	90%	94%
Thrombolytic Therapy Timing[5]	-	-	-	66%
Venous Thromboembolism Prophylaxis[5]	-	-	52%	94%
Written Stroke Educational Materials Given[5]	-	-	95%	88%
Surgical Care Improvement Project				
Appropriate Beta Blocker Usage[1]	-	-	75%	98%
Appropriate VTP Within 24 Hours	88	90%	90%	98%
Controlled Postoperative Blood Glucose[7]	-	-	81%	97%
Perioperative Temperature Management	90	100%	98%	100%
Prophylactic Antibiotic Selection	82	93%	96%	99%
Prophylactic Antibiotic Selection (Outpatient)	-	-	-	98%
Prophylactic Antibiotic Stopped	82	99%	83%	98%
Prophylactic Antibiotic Timing	82	83%	89%	99%
Prophylactic Antibiotic Timing (Outpatient)	-	-	-	98%
Urinary Catheter Removal[1]	-	-	91%	97%
Survey of Patients' Hospital Experiences				
Area Around Room 'Always' Quiet at Night[5]	-	-	-	61%
Doctors 'Always' Communicated Well[5]	-	-	-	82%
Home Recovery Information Given[5]	-	-	-	85%
Hospital Given 9 or 10 on 10 Point Scale[5]	-	-	-	71%
Meds 'Always' Explained Before Given[5]	-	-	-	64%
Nurses 'Always' Communicated Well[5]	-	-	-	79%
Pain 'Always' Well Controlled[5]	-	-	-	71%
Room and Bathroom 'Always' Clean[5]	-	-	-	73%
Timely Help 'Always' Received[5]	-	-	-	68%
Would Definitely Recommend Hospital[5]	-	-	-	71%
Use of Medical Imaging				
Cardiac Imaging Stress Test before Surgery	-	-	4.5%	5.3%
Combination Abdominal CT Scan	-	-	7.4%	10.5%
Combination Brain/Sinus CT Scan	-	-	0.8%	2.7%
Combination Chest CT Scan	-	-	6.1%	2.7%
Follow-up Mammogram/Ultrasound	-	-	43.2%	8.8%
Lumbar Spine MRI for Low Back Pain	-	-	44.3%	37.2%

Hima San Pablo Humacao

Calle Font Martelo #3 Phone: 787-852-2424
Humacao, PR 791
Type: Acute Care Hospitals Emergency Services: Yes
Ownership: Proprietary

Measure	Cases	This Hosp.	State Avg.	U.S. Avg.
Blood Clot Prevention and Treatment				
Anticoagulation Overlap Therapy[5]	-	-	50%	93%
ICU Venous Thromboembolism Prophylaxis[5]	-	-	-	92%
Incidence of Potentially Preventable VTE[5]	-	-	-	10%
UFH with Dosages/Platelet Monitoring[5]	-	-	100%	97%
Venous Thromboembolism Prophylaxis[5]	-	-	98%	85%
Warfarin Therapy Discharge Instructions[5]	-	-	92%	75%
Chest Pain/Possible Heart Attack Care				
Aspirin Given Within 24 Hours of Arrival	-	-	-	96%
Fibrinolytic Meds Within 30 Min. of Arrival	-	-	-	58%
Average Time to ECG (minutes)	-	-	-	7
Average Time to Transfer (minutes)	-	-	-	60
Children's Asthma Care				
Received Home Management Plan of Care	-	-	-	88%
Received Reliever Medication	-	-	-	100%
Received Systemic Corticosteroids	-	-	-	100%
Emergency Department				
Admittance Decision Time (minutes)[5]	-	-	190	98
Head CT Results Within 45 Min. of Arrival	-	-	-	57%
Patients Who Left ER Before Being Seen	-	-	-	2%
Time from ER Arrival to Admit. (minutes)[5]	-	-	635	274
Time from ER Arrival to Discharge (minutes)	-	-	-	134
Time in ER Before Being Evaluated (minutes)	-	-	-	26
Time to Pain Meds for Fractures (minutes)	-	-	-	57
Heart Attack Care				
Aspirin Given at Discharge	40	98%	94%	99%
Fibrinolytic Meds Within 30 Min. of Arrival[7]	-	-	47%	54%
PCI Within 90 Minutes of Arrival[7]	-	-	53%	96%
Statin Prescribed at Discharge	48	90%	89%	98%
Heart Failure Care				
ACE Inhibitor or ARB for LVSD	18	89%	92%	97%
Discharge Instructions Given	64	100%	87%	94%
Evaluation of LVS Function	65	89%	94%	99%
Medicare Spending				
Medicare Spending per Patient (ratio)	-	-	-	0.98
Pneumonia Care				
Appropriate Initial Antibiotic Given	74	95%	82%	95%
Blood Culture Timing	82	82%	82%	98%
Pregnancy and Delivery Care				
Newborn Deliveries Scheduled Early[5]	-	-	-	6%
Preventive Care				
Immunization for Influenza[5]	-	-	42%	90%
Immunization for Pneumonia[5]	-	-	29%	92%

NOTE: Hospital profiles are in alphabetical order by state, then city, then hospital within the city; Rankings exclude hospitals with less than 25 cases except for patient surveys which excludes hospitals with less than 100 cases; (a) 100-299 cases; (1) The number of cases/patients is too few to report; (2) Data submitted were based on a sample of cases/patients; (3) Results are based on a shorter time period than required; (4) Data suppressed by CMS for one or more quarters; (5) Results are not available for this reporting period; (6) Fewer than 100 patients completed the HCAHPS survey; (7) No cases met the criteria for this measure; (8) The lower limit of the confidence interval cannot be calculated if the number of observed infections equals zero; (9) No data are available from the state/territory for this reporting period; (10) The scores shown reflect fewer than 50 completed surveys; (11) There were discrepancies in the data collection process; (12) This measure does not apply to this hospital for this reporting period; (13) Results cannot be calculated for this reporting period; (14) The results for this state are combined with nearby states to protect confidentiality; Please refer to the User's Guide for a full explanation of data.

Stroke Care				
Anticoagulation Therapy for Atrial Fibrillation[5]	-	-	60%	95%
Antithrombotic Therapy Timing[5]	-	-	77%	98%
Assessed for Rehabilitation[5]	-	-	59%	97%
Discharged on Antithrombotic Therapy[5]	-	-	63%	99%
Discharged on Statin Medication[5]	-	-	90%	94%
Thrombolytic Therapy Timing[5]	-	-	-	66%
Venous Thromboembolism Prophylaxis[5]	-	-	52%	94%
Written Stroke Educational Materials Given[5]	-	-	95%	88%
Surgical Care Improvement Project				
Appropriate Beta Blocker Usage	11	91%	75%	98%
Appropriate VTP Within 24 Hours	79	91%	90%	98%
Controlled Postoperative Blood Glucose[7]	-	-	81%	97%
Perioperative Temperature Management	84	100%	98%	100%
Prophylactic Antibiotic Selection	73	88%	96%	99%
Prophylactic Antibiotic Selection (Outpatient)	-	-	-	98%
Prophylactic Antibiotic Stopped	72	26%	83%	98%
Prophylactic Antibiotic Timing	73	85%	89%	99%
Prophylactic Antibiotic Timing (Outpatient)	-	-	-	98%
Urinary Catheter Removal	16	88%	91%	97%
Survey of Patients' Hospital Experiences				
Area Around Room 'Always' Quiet at Night[5]	-	-	-	61%
Doctors 'Always' Communicated Well[5]	-	-	-	82%
Home Recovery Information Given[5]	-	-	-	85%
Hospital Given 9 or 10 on 10 Point Scale[5]	-	-	-	71%
Meds 'Always' Explained Before Given[5]	-	-	-	64%
Nurses 'Always' Communicated Well[5]	-	-	-	79%
Pain 'Always' Well Controlled[5]	-	-	-	71%
Room and Bathroom 'Always' Clean[5]	-	-	-	73%
Timely Help 'Always' Received[5]	-	-	-	68%
Would Definitely Recommend Hospital[5]	-	-	-	71%
Use of Medical Imaging				
Cardiac Imaging Stress Test before Surgery	-	-	4.5%	5.3%
Combination Abdominal CT Scan	-	-	7.4%	10.5%
Combination Brain/Sinus CT Scan	-	-	0.8%	2.7%
Combination Chest CT Scan	-	-	6.1%	2.7%
Follow-up Mammogram/Ultrasound	-	-	43.2%	8.8%
Lumbar Spine MRI for Low Back Pain	-	-	44.3%	37.2%

Hospital Oriente

300 Font Martello Street
Humacao, PR 792
Type: Acute Care Hospitals
Ownership: Proprietary

Phone: 787-852-0505
Fax: 787-850-4230
Emergency Services: Yes
Beds: 60

Key Personnel:
Anesthesiology. . . . . Ahmed Bajandad, MD
Intensive Care Unit. . . . . Osvaldo Figueroa, MD
Chief of Medical Staff . . . . Carmelo Herrero, MD
Infection Control. . . . . Agripino Lugo, MD
Operating Room. . . . . Wauda Morell
Pediatric In-Patient Care . . . . Ruddy Oquendo, MD

Measure	Cases	This Hosp.	State Avg.	U.S. Avg.
Blood Clot Prevention and Treatment				
Anticoagulation Overlap Therapy[5]	-	-	50%	93%
ICU Venous Thromboembolism Prophylaxis[5]	-	-	-	92%
Incidence of Potentially Preventable VTE[5]	-	-	-	10%
UFH with Dosages/Platelet Monitoring[5]	-	-	100%	97%
Venous Thromboembolism Prophylaxis[5]	-	-	98%	85%
Warfarin Therapy Discharge Instructions[5]	-	-	92%	75%
Chest Pain/Possible Heart Attack Care				
Aspirin Given Within 24 Hours of Arrival	-	-	-	96%
Fibrinolytic Meds Within 30 Min. of Arrival	-	-	-	58%
Average Time to ECG (minutes)	-	-	-	7
Average Time to Transfer (minutes)	-	-	-	60
Children's Asthma Care				
Received Home Management Plan of Care	-	-	-	88%
Received Reliever Medication	-	-	-	100%
Received Systemic Corticosteroids	-	-	-	100%
Emergency Department				
Admittance Decision Time (minutes)[5]	-	-	190	98
Head CT Results Within 45 Min. of Arrival	-	-	-	57%
Patients Who Left ER Before Being Seen	-	-	-	2%
Time from ER Arrival to Admit. (minutes)[5]	-	-	635	274
Time from ER Arrival to Discharge (minutes)	-	-	-	134
Time in ER Before Being Evaluated (minutes)	-	-	-	26
Time to Pain Meds for Fractures (minutes)	-	-	-	57
Heart Attack Care				
Aspirin Given at Discharge[1]	-	-	94%	99%
Fibrinolytic Meds Within 30 Min. of Arrival[7]	-	-	47%	54%
PCI Within 90 Minutes of Arrival[3,7]	-	-	53%	96%
Statin Prescribed at Discharge[1]	-	-	89%	98%
Heart Failure Care				
ACE Inhibitor or ARB for LVSD[1]	-	-	92%	97%
Discharge Instructions Given	28	89%	87%	94%
Evaluation of LVS Function	28	100%	94%	99%
Medicare Spending				
Medicare Spending per Patient (ratio)	-	-	-	0.98
Pneumonia Care				
Appropriate Initial Antibiotic Given	19	79%	82%	95%
Blood Culture Timing[1]	-	-	82%	98%
Pregnancy and Delivery Care				
Newborn Deliveries Scheduled Early[5]	-	-	-	6%
Preventive Care				
Immunization for Influenza[5]	-	-	42%	90%
Immunization for Pneumonia[5]	-	-	29%	92%
Stroke Care				
Anticoagulation Therapy for Atrial Fibrillation[5]	-	-	60%	95%
Antithrombotic Therapy Timing[5]	-	-	77%	98%
Assessed for Rehabilitation[5]	-	-	59%	97%
Discharged on Antithrombotic Therapy[5]	-	-	63%	99%
Discharged on Statin Medication[5]	-	-	90%	94%
Thrombolytic Therapy Timing[5]	-	-	-	66%
Venous Thromboembolism Prophylaxis[5]	-	-	52%	94%
Written Stroke Educational Materials Given[5]	-	-	95%	88%
Surgical Care Improvement Project				
Appropriate Beta Blocker Usage[5]	-	-	75%	98%
Appropriate VTP Within 24 Hours[5]	-	-	90%	98%
Controlled Postoperative Blood Glucose[5]	-	-	81%	97%
Perioperative Temperature Management[5]	-	-	98%	100%
Prophylactic Antibiotic Selection[5]	-	-	96%	99%
Prophylactic Antibiotic Selection (Outpatient)	-	-	-	98%
Prophylactic Antibiotic Stopped[5]	-	-	83%	98%
Prophylactic Antibiotic Timing[5]	-	-	89%	99%
Prophylactic Antibiotic Timing (Outpatient)	-	-	-	98%
Urinary Catheter Removal[5]	-	-	91%	97%
Survey of Patients' Hospital Experiences				
Area Around Room 'Always' Quiet at Night[5]	-	-	-	61%
Doctors 'Always' Communicated Well[5]	-	-	-	82%
Home Recovery Information Given[5]	-	-	-	85%
Hospital Given 9 or 10 on 10 Point Scale[5]	-	-	-	71%
Meds 'Always' Explained Before Given[5]	-	-	-	64%
Nurses 'Always' Communicated Well[5]	-	-	-	79%
Pain 'Always' Well Controlled[5]	-	-	-	71%
Room and Bathroom 'Always' Clean[5]	-	-	-	73%
Timely Help 'Always' Received[5]	-	-	-	68%
Would Definitely Recommend Hospital[5]	-	-	-	71%
Use of Medical Imaging				
Cardiac Imaging Stress Test before Surgery	-	-	4.5%	5.3%
Combination Abdominal CT Scan	-	-	7.4%	10.5%
Combination Brain/Sinus CT Scan	-	-	0.8%	2.7%
Combination Chest CT Scan	-	-	6.1%	2.7%
Follow-up Mammogram/Ultrasound	-	-	43.2%	8.8%
Lumbar Spine MRI for Low Back Pain	-	-	44.3%	37.2%

Ryder Memorial Hospital

355 Ave Font Martelo
Humacao, PR 791
Type: Acute Care Hospitals
Ownership: Voluntary non-profit - Private

Phone: 787-852-0768
Fax: 787-656-0737
Emergency Services: Yes
Beds: 227

Key Personnel:
CEO/President. . . . . Nemuel Artiles
Cardiac Laboratory. . . . . Wistremondo Dones, MD
Chief of Medical Staff . . . . Juan Gonsalez, MD
Emergency Room . . . . Juan Hernandez

Measure	Cases	This Hosp.	State Avg.	U.S. Avg.
Blood Clot Prevention and Treatment				
Anticoagulation Overlap Therapy[5]	-	-	50%	93%
ICU Venous Thromboembolism Prophylaxis[5]	-	-	-	92%
Incidence of Potentially Preventable VTE[5]	-	-	-	10%
UFH with Dosages/Platelet Monitoring[5]	-	-	100%	97%
Venous Thromboembolism Prophylaxis[5]	-	-	98%	85%
Warfarin Therapy Discharge Instructions[5]	-	-	92%	75%
Chest Pain/Possible Heart Attack Care				
Aspirin Given Within 24 Hours of Arrival	-	-	-	96%
Fibrinolytic Meds Within 30 Min. of Arrival	-	-	-	58%
Average Time to ECG (minutes)	-	-	-	7
Average Time to Transfer (minutes)	-	-	-	60
Children's Asthma Care				
Received Home Management Plan of Care	-	-	-	88%
Received Reliever Medication	-	-	-	100%
Received Systemic Corticosteroids	-	-	-	100%
Emergency Department				
Admittance Decision Time (minutes)[5]	-	-	190	98
Head CT Results Within 45 Min. of Arrival	-	-	-	57%
Patients Who Left ER Before Being Seen	-	-	-	2%
Time from ER Arrival to Admit. (minutes)[5]	-	-	635	274
Time from ER Arrival to Discharge (minutes)	-	-	-	134
Time in ER Before Being Evaluated (minutes)	-	-	-	26
Time to Pain Meds for Fractures (minutes)	-	-	-	57
Heart Attack Care				
Aspirin Given at Discharge[3]	61	69%	94%	99%
Fibrinolytic Meds Within 30 Min. of Arrival[1,3]	-	-	47%	54%
PCI Within 90 Minutes of Arrival[5]	-	-	53%	96%
Statin Prescribed at Discharge[3]	57	25%	89%	98%
Heart Failure Care				
ACE Inhibitor or ARB for LVSD[3]	42	69%	92%	97%
Discharge Instructions Given[3]	110	8%	87%	94%
Evaluation of LVS Function[3]	101	90%	94%	99%
Medicare Spending				
Medicare Spending per Patient (ratio)	-	-	-	0.98
Pneumonia Care				
Appropriate Initial Antibiotic Given[1,3]	-	-	82%	95%
Blood Culture Timing[5]	-	-	82%	98%
Pregnancy and Delivery Care				
Newborn Deliveries Scheduled Early[5]	-	-	-	6%
Preventive Care				
Immunization for Influenza[5]	-	-	42%	90%
Immunization for Pneumonia[5]	-	-	29%	92%
Stroke Care				
Anticoagulation Therapy for Atrial Fibrillation[5]	-	-	60%	95%
Antithrombotic Therapy Timing[5]	-	-	77%	98%
Assessed for Rehabilitation[5]	-	-	59%	97%
Discharged on Antithrombotic Therapy[5]	-	-	63%	99%
Discharged on Statin Medication[5]	-	-	90%	94%
Thrombolytic Therapy Timing[5]	-	-	-	66%
Venous Thromboembolism Prophylaxis[5]	-	-	52%	94%
Written Stroke Educational Materials Given[5]	-	-	95%	88%
Surgical Care Improvement Project				
Appropriate Beta Blocker Usage[5]	-	-	75%	98%
Appropriate VTP Within 24 Hours[5]	-	-	90%	98%
Controlled Postoperative Blood Glucose[5]	-	-	81%	97%
Perioperative Temperature Management[3]	82	15%	98%	100%
Prophylactic Antibiotic Selection[3]	52	38%	96%	99%
Prophylactic Antibiotic Selection (Outpatient)	-	-	-	98%
Prophylactic Antibiotic Stopped[3]	52	38%	83%	98%
Prophylactic Antibiotic Timing[3]	54	33%	89%	99%
Prophylactic Antibiotic Timing (Outpatient)	-	-	-	98%
Urinary Catheter Removal[3]	25	4%	91%	97%
Survey of Patients' Hospital Experiences				
Area Around Room 'Always' Quiet at Night[5]	-	-	-	61%
Doctors 'Always' Communicated Well[5]	-	-	-	82%
Home Recovery Information Given[5]	-	-	-	85%
Hospital Given 9 or 10 on 10 Point Scale[5]	-	-	-	71%
Meds 'Always' Explained Before Given[5]	-	-	-	64%
Nurses 'Always' Communicated Well[5]	-	-	-	79%
Pain 'Always' Well Controlled[5]	-	-	-	71%
Room and Bathroom 'Always' Clean[5]	-	-	-	73%
Timely Help 'Always' Received[5]	-	-	-	68%

NOTE: Hospital profiles are in alphabetical order by state, then city, then hospital within the city; Rankings exclude hospitals with less than 25 cases except for patient surveys which excludes hospitals with less than 100 cases; (a) 100-299 cases; (1) The number of cases/patients is too few to report; (2) Data submitted were based on a sample of cases/patients; (3) Results are based on a shorter time period than required; (4) Data suppressed by CMS for one or more quarters; (5) Results are not available for this reporting period; (6) Fewer than 100 patients completed the HCAHPS survey; (7) No cases met the criteria for this measure; (8) The lower limit of the confidence interval cannot be calculated if the number of observed infections equals zero; (9) No data are available from the state/territory for this reporting period; (10) The scores shown reflect fewer than 50 completed surveys; (11) There were discrepancies in the data collection process; (12) This measure does not apply to this hospital for this reporting period; (13) Results cannot be calculated for this reporting period; (14) The results for this state are combined with nearby states to protect confidentiality; Please refer to the User's Guide for a full explanation of data.

Measure	Cases	This Hosp.	State Avg.	U.S. Avg.
Would Definitely Recommend Hospital[5]	-	-	-	71%
Use of Medical Imaging				
Cardiac Imaging Stress Test before Surgery	-	-	4.5%	5.3%
Combination Abdominal CT Scan	-	-	7.4%	10.5%
Combination Brain/Sinus CT Scan	-	-	0.8%	2.7%
Combination Chest CT Scan	-	-	6.1%	2.7%
Follow-up Mammogram/Ultrasound	-	-	43.2%	8.8%
Lumbar Spine MRI for Low Back Pain	-	-	44.3%	37.2%

Doctors' Center Hospital

Marginal Carretera No 2, Km 47 7 Phone: 787-854-3322
Manati, PR 674
Type: Acute Care Hospitals Emergency Services: Yes
Ownership: Proprietary

Measure	Cases	This Hosp.	State Avg.	U.S. Avg.
Blood Clot Prevention and Treatment				
Anticoagulation Overlap Therapy[5]	-	-	50%	93%
ICU Venous Thromboembolism Prophylaxis[5]	-	-	-	92%
Incidence of Potentially Preventable VTE[5]	-	-	-	10%
UFH with Dosages/Platelet Monitoring[5]	-	-	100%	97%
Venous Thromboembolism Prophylaxis[5]	-	-	98%	85%
Warfarin Therapy Discharge Instructions[5]	-	-	92%	75%
Chest Pain/Possible Heart Attack Care				
Aspirin Given Within 24 Hours of Arrival	-	-	-	96%
Fibrinolytic Meds Within 30 Min. of Arrival	-	-	-	58%
Average Time to ECG (minutes)	-	-	-	7
Average Time to Transfer (minutes)	-	-	-	60
Children's Asthma Care				
Received Home Management Plan of Care	-	-	-	88%
Received Reliever Medication	-	-	-	100%
Received Systemic Corticosteroids	-	-	-	100%
Emergency Department				
Admittance Decision Time (minutes)[5]	-	-	190	98
Head CT Results Within 45 Min. of Arrival	-	-	-	57%
Patients Who Left ER Before Being Seen	-	-	-	2%
Time from ER Arrival to Admit. (minutes)[5]	-	-	635	274
Time from ER Arrival to Discharge (minutes)	-	-	-	134
Time in ER Before Being Evaluated (minutes)	-	-	-	26
Time to Pain Meds for Fractures (minutes)	-	-	-	57
Heart Attack Care				
Aspirin Given at Discharge	63	100%	94%	99%
Fibrinolytic Meds Within 30 Min. of Arrival[1]	-	-	47%	54%
PCI Within 90 Minutes of Arrival[7]	-	-	53%	96%
Statin Prescribed at Discharge	70	100%	89%	98%
Heart Failure Care				
ACE Inhibitor or ARB for LVSD	85	100%	92%	97%
Discharge Instructions Given	147	100%	87%	94%
Evaluation of LVS Function	150	99%	94%	99%
Medicare Spending				
Medicare Spending per Patient (ratio)	-	-	-	0.98
Pneumonia Care				
Appropriate Initial Antibiotic Given	74	95%	82%	95%
Blood Culture Timing	37	100%	82%	98%
Pregnancy and Delivery Care				
Newborn Deliveries Scheduled Early[5]	-	-	-	6%
Preventive Care				
Immunization for Influenza[5]	-	-	42%	90%
Immunization for Pneumonia[5]	-	-	29%	92%
Stroke Care				
Anticoagulation Therapy for Atrial Fibrillation[5]	-	-	60%	95%
Antithrombotic Therapy Timing[5]	-	-	77%	98%
Assessed for Rehabilitation[5]	-	-	59%	97%
Discharged on Antithrombotic Therapy[5]	-	-	63%	99%
Discharged on Statin Medication[5]	-	-	90%	94%
Thrombolytic Therapy Timing[5]	-	-	-	66%
Venous Thromboembolism Prophylaxis[5]	-	-	52%	94%
Written Stroke Educational Materials Given[5]	-	-	95%	88%
Surgical Care Improvement Project				
Appropriate Beta Blocker Usage[1]	-	-	75%	98%
Appropriate VTP Within 24 Hours	170	100%	90%	98%
Controlled Postoperative Blood Glucose[7]	-	-	81%	97%
Perioperative Temperature Management	175	100%	98%	100%
Prophylactic Antibiotic Selection	154	97%	96%	99%
Prophylactic Antibiotic Selection (Outpatient)	-	-	-	98%
Prophylactic Antibiotic Stopped	154	98%	83%	98%
Prophylactic Antibiotic Timing	154	100%	89%	99%
Prophylactic Antibiotic Timing (Outpatient)	-	-	-	98%
Urinary Catheter Removal	54	100%	91%	97%
Survey of Patients' Hospital Experiences				
Area Around Room 'Always' Quiet at Night[5]	-	-	-	61%
Doctors 'Always' Communicated Well[5]	-	-	-	82%
Home Recovery Information Given[5]	-	-	-	85%
Hospital Given 9 or 10 on 10 Point Scale[5]	-	-	-	71%
Meds 'Always' Explained Before Given[5]	-	-	-	64%
Nurses 'Always' Communicated Well[5]	-	-	-	79%
Pain 'Always' Well Controlled[5]	-	-	-	71%
Room and Bathroom 'Always' Clean[5]	-	-	-	73%
Timely Help 'Always' Received[5]	-	-	-	68%
Would Definitely Recommend Hospital[5]	-	-	-	71%
Use of Medical Imaging				
Cardiac Imaging Stress Test before Surgery	-	-	4.5%	5.3%
Combination Abdominal CT Scan	-	-	7.4%	10.5%
Combination Brain/Sinus CT Scan	-	-	0.8%	2.7%
Combination Chest CT Scan	-	-	6.1%	2.7%
Follow-up Mammogram/Ultrasound	-	-	43.2%	8.8%
Lumbar Spine MRI for Low Back Pain	-	-	44.3%	37.2%

Manati Medical Center Doctor Otero Lopez

Calle Hernandez Carrion Urb Atenas Phone: 787-621-3700
Manati, PR 674 Fax: 787-621-3710
URL: www.mmcaol.com
Type: Acute Care Hospitals Emergency Services: Yes
Ownership: Proprietary

Measure	Cases	This Hosp.	State Avg.	U.S. Avg.
Blood Clot Prevention and Treatment				
Anticoagulation Overlap Therapy[5]	-	-	50%	93%
ICU Venous Thromboembolism Prophylaxis[5]	-	-	-	92%
Incidence of Potentially Preventable VTE[5]	-	-	-	10%
UFH with Dosages/Platelet Monitoring[5]	-	-	100%	97%
Venous Thromboembolism Prophylaxis[5]	-	-	98%	85%
Warfarin Therapy Discharge Instructions[5]	-	-	92%	75%
Chest Pain/Possible Heart Attack Care				
Aspirin Given Within 24 Hours of Arrival	-	-	-	96%
Fibrinolytic Meds Within 30 Min. of Arrival	-	-	-	58%
Average Time to ECG (minutes)	-	-	-	7
Average Time to Transfer (minutes)	-	-	-	60
Children's Asthma Care				
Received Home Management Plan of Care	-	-	-	88%
Received Reliever Medication	-	-	-	100%
Received Systemic Corticosteroids	-	-	-	100%
Emergency Department				
Admittance Decision Time (minutes)[5]	-	-	190	98
Head CT Results Within 45 Min. of Arrival	-	-	-	57%
Patients Who Left ER Before Being Seen	-	-	-	2%
Time from ER Arrival to Admit. (minutes)[5]	-	-	635	274
Time from ER Arrival to Discharge (minutes)	-	-	-	134
Time in ER Before Being Evaluated (minutes)	-	-	-	26
Time to Pain Meds for Fractures (minutes)	-	-	-	57
Heart Attack Care				
Aspirin Given at Discharge[3]	57	100%	94%	99%
Fibrinolytic Meds Within 30 Min. of Arrival[1,3]	-	-	47%	54%
PCI Within 90 Minutes of Arrival[3,7]	-	-	53%	96%
Statin Prescribed at Discharge[3]	47	100%	89%	98%
Heart Failure Care				
ACE Inhibitor or ARB for LVSD[3]	45	100%	92%	97%
Discharge Instructions Given[3]	146	100%	87%	94%
Evaluation of LVS Function[3]	149	99%	94%	99%
Medicare Spending				
Medicare Spending per Patient (ratio)	-	-	-	0.98
Pneumonia Care				
Appropriate Initial Antibiotic Given[3]	139	91%	82%	95%
Blood Culture Timing[3]	115	87%	82%	98%
Pregnancy and Delivery Care				
Newborn Deliveries Scheduled Early[5]	-	-	-	6%
Preventive Care				
Immunization for Influenza[5]	-	-	42%	90%
Immunization for Pneumonia[5]	-	-	29%	92%
Stroke Care				
Anticoagulation Therapy for Atrial Fibrillation[1,3]	-	-	60%	95%
Antithrombotic Therapy Timing[3]	44	89%	77%	98%
Assessed for Rehabilitation[3]	62	39%	59%	97%
Discharged on Antithrombotic Therapy[3]	59	44%	63%	99%
Discharged on Statin Medication[3]	59	100%	90%	94%
Thrombolytic Therapy Timing[3,7]	-	-	-	66%
Venous Thromboembolism Prophylaxis[3]	60	82%	52%	94%
Written Stroke Educational Materials Given[3]	62	100%	95%	88%
Surgical Care Improvement Project				
Appropriate Beta Blocker Usage[3]	27	100%	75%	98%
Appropriate VTP Within 24 Hours[3]	90	100%	90%	98%
Controlled Postoperative Blood Glucose[3,7]	-	-	81%	97%
Perioperative Temperature Management[3]	90	100%	98%	100%
Prophylactic Antibiotic Selection[3]	94	93%	96%	99%
Prophylactic Antibiotic Selection (Outpatient)	-	-	-	98%
Prophylactic Antibiotic Stopped[3]	93	99%	83%	98%
Prophylactic Antibiotic Timing[3]	94	86%	89%	99%
Prophylactic Antibiotic Timing (Outpatient)	-	-	-	98%
Urinary Catheter Removal[3]	22	100%	91%	97%
Survey of Patients' Hospital Experiences				
Area Around Room 'Always' Quiet at Night[5]	-	-	-	61%
Doctors 'Always' Communicated Well[5]	-	-	-	82%
Home Recovery Information Given[5]	-	-	-	85%
Hospital Given 9 or 10 on 10 Point Scale[5]	-	-	-	71%
Meds 'Always' Explained Before Given[5]	-	-	-	64%
Nurses 'Always' Communicated Well[5]	-	-	-	79%
Pain 'Always' Well Controlled[5]	-	-	-	71%
Room and Bathroom 'Always' Clean[5]	-	-	-	73%
Timely Help 'Always' Received[5]	-	-	-	68%
Would Definitely Recommend Hospital[5]	-	-	-	71%
Use of Medical Imaging				
Cardiac Imaging Stress Test before Surgery	-	-	4.5%	5.3%
Combination Abdominal CT Scan	-	-	7.4%	10.5%
Combination Brain/Sinus CT Scan	-	-	0.8%	2.7%
Combination Chest CT Scan	-	-	6.1%	2.7%
Follow-up Mammogram/Ultrasound	-	-	43.2%	8.8%
Lumbar Spine MRI for Low Back Pain	-	-	44.3%	37.2%

Bella Vista Hospital

Carr 349 Km 2 7 Cerro Las Mesas Phone: 787-652-6045
Mayaguez, PR 681 Fax: 787-831-6315
Type: Acute Care Hospitals Emergency Services: Yes
Ownership: Voluntary non-profit - Church Beds: 199

Measure	Cases	This Hosp.	State Avg.	U.S. Avg.
Blood Clot Prevention and Treatment				
Anticoagulation Overlap Therapy[5]	-	-	50%	93%
ICU Venous Thromboembolism Prophylaxis[5]	-	-	-	92%
Incidence of Potentially Preventable VTE[5]	-	-	-	10%
UFH with Dosages/Platelet Monitoring[5]	-	-	100%	97%
Venous Thromboembolism Prophylaxis[5]	-	-	98%	85%
Warfarin Therapy Discharge Instructions[5]	-	-	92%	75%
Chest Pain/Possible Heart Attack Care				
Aspirin Given Within 24 Hours of Arrival	-	-	-	96%
Fibrinolytic Meds Within 30 Min. of Arrival	-	-	-	58%
Average Time to ECG (minutes)	-	-	-	7
Average Time to Transfer (minutes)	-	-	-	60
Children's Asthma Care				
Received Home Management Plan of Care	-	-	-	88%
Received Reliever Medication	-	-	-	100%
Received Systemic Corticosteroids	-	-	-	100%
Emergency Department				
Admittance Decision Time (minutes)[5]	-	-	190	98
Head CT Results Within 45 Min. of Arrival	-	-	-	57%
Patients Who Left ER Before Being Seen	-	-	-	2%
Time from ER Arrival to Admit. (minutes)[5]	-	-	635	274
Time from ER Arrival to Discharge (minutes)	-	-	-	134
Time in ER Before Being Evaluated (minutes)	-	-	-	26
Time to Pain Meds for Fractures (minutes)	-	-	-	57

NOTE: Hospital profiles are in alphabetical order by state, then city, then hospital within the city; Rankings exclude hospitals with less than 25 cases except for patient surveys which excludes hospitals with less than 100 cases; (a) 100-299 cases; (1) The number of cases/patients is too few to report; (2) Data submitted were based on a sample of cases/patients; (3) Results are based on a shorter time period than required; (4) Data suppressed by CMS for one or more quarters; (5) Results are not available for this reporting period; (6) Fewer than 100 patients completed the HCAHPS survey; (7) No cases met the criteria for this measure; (8) The lower limit of the confidence interval cannot be calculated if the number of observed infections equals zero; (9) No data are available from the state/territory for this reporting period; (10) The scores shown reflect fewer than 50 completed surveys; (11) There were discrepancies in the data collection process; (12) This measure does not apply to this hospital for this reporting period; (13) Results cannot be calculated for this reporting period; (14) The results for this state are combined with nearby states to protect confidentiality; Please refer to the User's Guide for a full explanation of data.

Measure	Cases	This Hosp.	State Avg.	U.S. Avg.
Heart Attack Care				
Aspirin Given at Discharge	39	90%	94%	99%
Fibrinolytic Meds Within 30 Min. of Arrival[1]	-	-	47%	54%
PCI Within 90 Minutes of Arrival[7]	-	-	53%	96%
Statin Prescribed at Discharge	46	76%	89%	98%
Heart Failure Care				
ACE Inhibitor or ARB for LVSD	43	84%	92%	97%
Discharge Instructions Given	136	94%	87%	94%
Evaluation of LVS Function	139	92%	94%	99%
Medicare Spending				
Medicare Spending per Patient (ratio)	-	-	-	0.98
Pneumonia Care				
Appropriate Initial Antibiotic Given	107	80%	82%	95%
Blood Culture Timing	123	61%	82%	98%
Pregnancy and Delivery Care				
Newborn Deliveries Scheduled Early[5]	-	-	-	6%
Preventive Care				
Immunization for Influenza[5]	-	-	42%	90%
Immunization for Pneumonia[5]	-	-	29%	92%
Stroke Care				
Anticoagulation Therapy for Atrial Fibrillation[5]	-	-	60%	95%
Antithrombotic Therapy Timing[5]	-	-	77%	98%
Assessed for Rehabilitation[5]	-	-	59%	97%
Discharged on Antithrombotic Therapy[5]	-	-	63%	99%
Discharged on Statin Medication[5]	-	-	90%	94%
Thrombolytic Therapy Timing[5]	-	-	-	66%
Venous Thromboembolism Prophylaxis[5]	-	-	52%	94%
Written Stroke Educational Materials Given[5]	-	-	95%	88%
Surgical Care Improvement Project				
Appropriate Beta Blocker Usage	192	85%	75%	98%
Appropriate VTP Within 24 Hours	864	88%	90%	98%
Controlled Postoperative Blood Glucose[7]	-	-	81%	97%
Perioperative Temperature Management	893	100%	98%	100%
Prophylactic Antibiotic Selection	727	98%	96%	99%
Prophylactic Antibiotic Selection (Outpatient)	-	-	-	98%
Prophylactic Antibiotic Stopped	719	50%	83%	98%
Prophylactic Antibiotic Timing	729	95%	89%	99%
Prophylactic Antibiotic Timing (Outpatient)	-	-	-	98%
Urinary Catheter Removal	334	69%	91%	97%
Survey of Patients' Hospital Experiences				
Area Around Room 'Always' Quiet at Night[5]	-	-	-	61%
Doctors 'Always' Communicated Well[5]	-	-	-	82%
Home Recovery Information Given[5]	-	-	-	85%
Hospital Given 9 or 10 on 10 Point Scale[5]	-	-	-	71%
Meds 'Always' Explained Before Given[5]	-	-	-	64%
Nurses 'Always' Communicated Well[5]	-	-	-	79%
Pain 'Always' Well Controlled[5]	-	-	-	71%
Room and Bathroom 'Always' Clean[5]	-	-	-	73%
Timely Help 'Always' Received[5]	-	-	-	68%
Would Definitely Recommend Hospital[5]	-	-	-	71%
Use of Medical Imaging				
Cardiac Imaging Stress Test before Surgery	-	-	4.5%	5.3%
Combination Abdominal CT Scan	-	-	7.4%	10.5%
Combination Brain/Sinus CT Scan	-	-	0.8%	2.7%
Combination Chest CT Scan	-	-	6.1%	2.7%
Follow-up Mammogram/Ultrasound	-	-	43.2%	8.8%
Lumbar Spine MRI for Low Back Pain	-	-	44.3%	37.2%

Hospital Perea

15 Dr Basora Street
Mayaguez, PR 681
Type: Acute Care Hospitals
Ownership: Voluntary non-profit - Private
Phone: 787-834-0101
Fax: 787-265-2455
Emergency Services: Yes
Beds: 103

Key Personnel:
CEO/President. . . . . Rafael Alvarado, MHSA
Anesthesiology. . . . . Jesus Becerea
Intensive Care Unit. . . . . Janet Crespo, RN
Chief of Medical Staff. . . . . Humberto Olivencia
Emergency Room . . . . Zoe Pizarro
Quality Assurance . . . . Carmen Rivera
Operating Room. . . . . Elida Soto, RN
Infection Control. . . . . Carmen Tomassini, RN

Measure	Cases	This Hosp.	State Avg.	U.S. Avg.
Blood Clot Prevention and Treatment				
Anticoagulation Overlap Therapy[5]	-	-	50%	93%
ICU Venous Thromboembolism Prophylaxis[5]	-	-	-	92%
Incidence of Potentially Preventable VTE[5]	-	-	-	10%
UFH with Dosages/Platelet Monitoring[5]	-	-	100%	97%
Venous Thromboembolism Prophylaxis[5]	-	-	98%	85%
Warfarin Therapy Discharge Instructions[5]	-	-	92%	75%
Chest Pain/Possible Heart Attack Care				
Aspirin Given Within 24 Hours of Arrival	-	-	-	96%
Fibrinolytic Meds Within 30 Min. of Arrival	-	-	-	58%
Average Time to ECG (minutes)	-	-	-	7
Average Time to Transfer (minutes)	-	-	-	60
Children's Asthma Care				
Received Home Management Plan of Care	-	-	-	88%
Received Reliever Medication	-	-	-	100%
Received Systemic Corticosteroids	-	-	-	100%
Emergency Department				
Admittance Decision Time (minutes)[5]	-	-	190	98
Head CT Results Within 45 Min. of Arrival	-	-	-	57%
Patients Who Left ER Before Being Seen	-	-	-	2%
Time from ER Arrival to Admit. (minutes)[5]	-	-	635	274
Time from ER Arrival to Discharge (minutes)	-	-	-	134
Time in ER Before Being Evaluated (minutes)	-	-	-	26
Time to Pain Meds for Fractures (minutes)	-	-	-	57
Heart Attack Care				
Aspirin Given at Discharge[2]	21	81%	94%	99%
Fibrinolytic Meds Within 30 Min. of Arrival[1,2]	-	-	47%	54%
PCI Within 90 Minutes of Arrival[2,3]	-	-	53%	96%
Statin Prescribed at Discharge[2]	20	70%	89%	98%
Heart Failure Care				
ACE Inhibitor or ARB for LVSD[2]	13	85%	92%	97%
Discharge Instructions Given[2]	35	100%	87%	94%
Evaluation of LVS Function[2]	35	100%	94%	99%
Medicare Spending				
Medicare Spending per Patient (ratio)	-	-	-	0.98
Pneumonia Care				
Appropriate Initial Antibiotic Given[2]	99	70%	82%	95%
Blood Culture Timing[2]	29	45%	82%	98%
Pregnancy and Delivery Care				
Newborn Deliveries Scheduled Early[5]	-	-	-	6%
Preventive Care				
Immunization for Influenza[5]	-	-	42%	90%
Immunization for Pneumonia[5]	-	-	29%	92%
Stroke Care				
Anticoagulation Therapy for Atrial Fibrillation[5]	-	-	60%	95%
Antithrombotic Therapy Timing[5]	-	-	77%	98%
Assessed for Rehabilitation[5]	-	-	59%	97%
Discharged on Antithrombotic Therapy[5]	-	-	63%	99%
Discharged on Statin Medication[5]	-	-	90%	94%
Thrombolytic Therapy Timing[5]	-	-	-	66%
Venous Thromboembolism Prophylaxis[5]	-	-	52%	94%
Written Stroke Educational Materials Given[5]	-	-	95%	88%
Surgical Care Improvement Project				
Appropriate Beta Blocker Usage[2,7]	-	-	75%	98%
Appropriate VTP Within 24 Hours[1,2]	-	-	90%	98%
Controlled Postoperative Blood Glucose[2,7]	-	-	81%	97%
Perioperative Temperature Management[2]	13	77%	98%	100%
Prophylactic Antibiotic Selection[2]	13	85%	96%	99%
Prophylactic Antibiotic Selection (Outpatient)	-	-	-	98%
Prophylactic Antibiotic Stopped[2]	13	92%	83%	98%
Prophylactic Antibiotic Timing[2]	13	85%	89%	99%
Prophylactic Antibiotic Timing (Outpatient)	-	-	-	98%
Urinary Catheter Removal[2,7]	-	-	91%	97%
Survey of Patients' Hospital Experiences				
Area Around Room 'Always' Quiet at Night[5]	-	-	-	61%
Doctors 'Always' Communicated Well[5]	-	-	-	82%
Home Recovery Information Given[5]	-	-	-	85%
Hospital Given 9 or 10 on 10 Point Scale[5]	-	-	-	71%
Meds 'Always' Explained Before Given[5]	-	-	-	64%
Nurses 'Always' Communicated Well[5]	-	-	-	79%
Pain 'Always' Well Controlled[5]	-	-	-	71%
Room and Bathroom 'Always' Clean[5]	-	-	-	73%
Timely Help 'Always' Received[5]	-	-	-	68%
Would Definitely Recommend Hospital[5]	-	-	-	71%
Use of Medical Imaging				
Cardiac Imaging Stress Test before Surgery	-	-	4.5%	5.3%
Combination Abdominal CT Scan	-	-	7.4%	10.5%
Combination Brain/Sinus CT Scan	-	-	0.8%	2.7%
Combination Chest CT Scan	-	-	6.1%	2.7%
Follow-up Mammogram/Ultrasound	-	-	43.2%	8.8%
Lumbar Spine MRI for Low Back Pain	-	-	44.3%	37.2%

Sistema Integrados De Salud Del Sur Oeste

Ave Hostos 410
Mayaguez, PR 681
Type: Acute Care Hospitals
Ownership: Proprietary
Phone: 787-652-9200
Fax: 787-834-3010
Emergency Services: Yes
Beds: 120

Key Personnel:
Emergency Room . . . . Virgilio Cora, MD
Pediatric In-Patient Care . . . . Arturo Lopez, MD
Chief of Medical Staff. . . . . Franklyn Plaguez, MD
Intensive Care Unit. . . . . Jessie Romeu, MD
Anesthesiology. . . . . Ivan Suarez, MD
CEO/President. . . . . Maria del Pilar Rodri

Measure	Cases	This Hosp.	State Avg.	U.S. Avg.
Blood Clot Prevention and Treatment				
Anticoagulation Overlap Therapy[5]	-	-	50%	93%
ICU Venous Thromboembolism Prophylaxis[5]	-	-	-	92%
Incidence of Potentially Preventable VTE[5]	-	-	-	10%
UFH with Dosages/Platelet Monitoring[5]	-	-	100%	97%
Venous Thromboembolism Prophylaxis[5]	-	-	98%	85%
Warfarin Therapy Discharge Instructions[5]	-	-	92%	75%
Chest Pain/Possible Heart Attack Care				
Aspirin Given Within 24 Hours of Arrival	-	-	-	96%
Fibrinolytic Meds Within 30 Min. of Arrival	-	-	-	58%
Average Time to ECG (minutes)	-	-	-	7
Average Time to Transfer (minutes)	-	-	-	60
Children's Asthma Care				
Received Home Management Plan of Care	-	-	-	88%
Received Reliever Medication	-	-	-	100%
Received Systemic Corticosteroids	-	-	-	100%
Emergency Department				
Admittance Decision Time (minutes)[5]	-	-	190	98
Head CT Results Within 45 Min. of Arrival	-	-	-	57%
Patients Who Left ER Before Being Seen	-	-	-	2%
Time from ER Arrival to Admit. (minutes)[5]	-	-	635	274
Time from ER Arrival to Discharge (minutes)	-	-	-	134
Time in ER Before Being Evaluated (minutes)	-	-	-	26
Time to Pain Meds for Fractures (minutes)	-	-	-	57
Heart Attack Care				
Aspirin Given at Discharge	212	100%	94%	99%
Fibrinolytic Meds Within 30 Min. of Arrival[1]	-	-	47%	54%
PCI Within 90 Minutes of Arrival[1]	-	-	53%	96%
Statin Prescribed at Discharge	224	100%	89%	98%
Heart Failure Care				
ACE Inhibitor or ARB for LVSD	63	100%	92%	97%
Discharge Instructions Given	170	100%	87%	94%
Evaluation of LVS Function	171	100%	94%	99%
Medicare Spending				
Medicare Spending per Patient (ratio)	-	-	-	0.98
Pneumonia Care				
Appropriate Initial Antibiotic Given	94	69%	82%	95%
Blood Culture Timing	178	80%	82%	98%
Pregnancy and Delivery Care				
Newborn Deliveries Scheduled Early[5]	-	-	-	6%
Preventive Care				
Immunization for Influenza[5]	-	-	42%	90%
Immunization for Pneumonia[5]	-	-	29%	92%
Stroke Care				
Anticoagulation Therapy for Atrial Fibrillation[5]	-	-	60%	95%
Antithrombotic Therapy Timing[5]	-	-	77%	98%
Assessed for Rehabilitation[5]	-	-	59%	97%
Discharged on Antithrombotic Therapy[5]	-	-	63%	99%
Discharged on Statin Medication[5]	-	-	90%	94%
Thrombolytic Therapy Timing[5]	-	-	-	66%
Venous Thromboembolism Prophylaxis[5]	-	-	52%	94%
Written Stroke Educational Materials Given[5]	-	-	95%	88%

NOTE: Hospital profiles are in alphabetical order by state, then city, then hospital within the city; Rankings exclude hospitals with less than 25 cases except for patient surveys which excludes hospitals with less than 100 cases; (a) 100-299 cases; (1) The number of cases/patients is too few to report; (2) Data submitted were based on a sample of cases/patients; (3) Results are based on a shorter time period than required; (4) Data suppressed by CMS for one or more quarters; (5) Results are not available for this reporting period; (6) Fewer than 100 patients completed the HCAHPS survey; (7) No cases met the criteria for this measure; (8) The lower limit of the confidence interval cannot be calculated if the number of observed infections equals zero; (9) No data are available from the state/territory for this reporting period; (10) The scores shown reflect fewer than 50 completed surveys; (11) There were discrepancies in the data collection process; (12) This measure does not apply to this hospital for this reporting period; (13) Results cannot be calculated for this reporting period; (14) The results for this state are combined with nearby states to protect confidentiality; Please refer to the User's Guide for a full explanation of data.

Surgical Care Improvement Project				
Appropriate Beta Blocker Usage	113	94%	75%	98%
Appropriate VTP Within 24 Hours	37	86%	90%	98%
Controlled Postoperative Blood Glucose	144	60%	81%	97%
Perioperative Temperature Management	262	100%	98%	100%
Prophylactic Antibiotic Selection	214	97%	96%	99%
Prophylactic Antibiotic Selection (Outpatient)	-	-	-	98%
Prophylactic Antibiotic Stopped	210	81%	83%	98%
Prophylactic Antibiotic Timing	222	63%	89%	99%
Prophylactic Antibiotic Timing (Outpatient)	-	-	-	98%
Urinary Catheter Removal	66	100%	91%	97%
Survey of Patients' Hospital Experiences				
Area Around Room 'Always' Quiet at Night[5]	-	-	-	61%
Doctors 'Always' Communicated Well[5]	-	-	-	82%
Home Recovery Information Given[5]	-	-	-	85%
Hospital Given 9 or 10 on 10 Point Scale[5]	-	-	-	71%
Meds 'Always' Explained Before Given[5]	-	-	-	64%
Nurses 'Always' Communicated Well[5]	-	-	-	79%
Pain 'Always' Well Controlled[5]	-	-	-	71%
Room and Bathroom 'Always' Clean[5]	-	-	-	73%
Timely Help 'Always' Received[5]	-	-	-	68%
Would Definitely Recommend Hospital[5]	-	-	-	71%
Use of Medical Imaging				
Cardiac Imaging Stress Test before Surgery	-	-	4.5%	5.3%
Combination Abdominal CT Scan	-	-	7.4%	10.5%
Combination Brain/Sinus CT Scan	-	-	0.8%	2.7%
Combination Chest CT Scan	-	-	6.1%	2.7%
Follow-up Mammogram/Ultrasound	-	-	43.2%	8.8%
Lumbar Spine MRI for Low Back Pain	-	-	44.3%	37.2%

Hospital San Carlos Borromeo

Calle Concepcion Vera Ayala #550 S Phone: 787-877-8000
Moca, PR 676
Type: Acute Care Hospitals Emergency Services: Yes
Ownership: Voluntary non-profit - Private

Measure	Cases	This Hosp.	State Avg.	U.S. Avg.
Blood Clot Prevention and Treatment				
Anticoagulation Overlap Therapy[5]	-	-	50%	93%
ICU Venous Thromboembolism Prophylaxis[5]	-	-	-	92%
Incidence of Potentially Preventable VTE[5]	-	-	-	10%
UFH with Dosages/Platelet Monitoring[5]	-	-	100%	97%
Venous Thromboembolism Prophylaxis[5]	-	-	98%	85%
Warfarin Therapy Discharge Instructions[5]	-	-	92%	75%
Chest Pain/Possible Heart Attack Care				
Aspirin Given Within 24 Hours of Arrival	-	-	-	96%
Fibrinolytic Meds Within 30 Min. of Arrival	-	-	-	58%
Average Time to ECG (minutes)	-	-	-	7
Average Time to Transfer (minutes)	-	-	-	60
Children's Asthma Care				
Received Home Management Plan of Care	-	-	-	88%
Received Reliever Medication	-	-	-	100%
Received Systemic Corticosteroids	-	-	-	100%
Emergency Department				
Admittance Decision Time (minutes)[5]	-	-	190	98
Head CT Results Within 45 Min. of Arrival	-	-	-	57%
Patients Who Left ER Before Being Seen	-	-	-	2%
Time from ER Arrival to Admit. (minutes)[5]	-	-	635	274
Time from ER Arrival to Discharge (minutes)	-	-	-	134
Time in ER Before Being Evaluated (minutes)	-	-	-	26
Time to Pain Meds for Fractures (minutes)	-	-	-	57
Heart Attack Care				
Aspirin Given at Discharge	52	96%	94%	99%
Fibrinolytic Meds Within 30 Min. of Arrival[1]	-	-	47%	54%
PCI Within 90 Minutes of Arrival[7]	-	-	53%	96%
Statin Prescribed at Discharge	60	92%	89%	98%
Heart Failure Care				
ACE Inhibitor or ARB for LVSD[2]	35	100%	92%	97%
Discharge Instructions Given[2]	81	96%	87%	94%
Evaluation of LVS Function[2]	81	80%	94%	99%
Medicare Spending				
Medicare Spending per Patient (ratio)	-	-	-	0.98
Pneumonia Care				
Appropriate Initial Antibiotic Given[2]	37	51%	82%	95%
Blood Culture Timing[2]	35	71%	82%	98%
Pregnancy and Delivery Care				
Newborn Deliveries Scheduled Early[5]	-	-	-	6%
Preventive Care				
Immunization for Influenza[5]	-	-	42%	90%
Immunization for Pneumonia[5]	-	-	29%	92%
Stroke Care				
Anticoagulation Therapy for Atrial Fibrillation[5]	-	-	60%	95%
Antithrombotic Therapy Timing[5]	-	-	77%	98%
Assessed for Rehabilitation[5]	-	-	59%	97%
Discharged on Antithrombotic Therapy[5]	-	-	63%	99%
Discharged on Statin Medication[5]	-	-	90%	94%
Thrombolytic Therapy Timing[5]	-	-	-	66%
Venous Thromboembolism Prophylaxis[5]	-	-	52%	94%
Written Stroke Educational Materials Given[5]	-	-	95%	88%
Surgical Care Improvement Project				
Appropriate Beta Blocker Usage[5]	-	-	75%	98%
Appropriate VTP Within 24 Hours[5]	-	-	90%	98%
Controlled Postoperative Blood Glucose[5]	-	-	81%	97%
Perioperative Temperature Management[5]	-	-	98%	100%
Prophylactic Antibiotic Selection[5]	-	-	96%	99%
Prophylactic Antibiotic Selection (Outpatient)	-	-	-	98%
Prophylactic Antibiotic Stopped[5]	-	-	83%	98%
Prophylactic Antibiotic Timing[5]	-	-	89%	99%
Prophylactic Antibiotic Timing (Outpatient)	-	-	-	98%
Urinary Catheter Removal[5]	-	-	91%	97%
Survey of Patients' Hospital Experiences				
Area Around Room 'Always' Quiet at Night[5]	-	-	-	61%
Doctors 'Always' Communicated Well[5]	-	-	-	82%
Home Recovery Information Given[5]	-	-	-	85%
Hospital Given 9 or 10 on 10 Point Scale[5]	-	-	-	71%
Meds 'Always' Explained Before Given[5]	-	-	-	64%
Nurses 'Always' Communicated Well[5]	-	-	-	79%
Pain 'Always' Well Controlled[5]	-	-	-	71%
Room and Bathroom 'Always' Clean[5]	-	-	-	73%
Timely Help 'Always' Received[5]	-	-	-	68%
Would Definitely Recommend Hospital[5]	-	-	-	71%
Use of Medical Imaging				
Cardiac Imaging Stress Test before Surgery	-	-	4.5%	5.3%
Combination Abdominal CT Scan	-	-	7.4%	10.5%
Combination Brain/Sinus CT Scan	-	-	0.8%	2.7%
Combination Chest CT Scan	-	-	6.1%	2.7%
Follow-up Mammogram/Ultrasound	-	-	43.2%	8.8%
Lumbar Spine MRI for Low Back Pain	-	-	44.3%	37.2%

Hospital Damas

Ponce By Pass #2213 Phone: 787-840-8460
Ponce, PR 717 Fax: 787-813-0592
E-mail: recursoshumanos@hospitaldamas.com
Type: Acute Care Hospitals Emergency Services: Yes
Ownership: Voluntary non-profit - Private Beds: 306

Key Personnel:

Chief of Medical Staff.......... Pedro Benitz, MD
Radiology................... German Chavez, MD
Operating Room............. Sharleen Irizarry
CEO/President.............. Mariano McConnie
Infection Control............. Ivetle Rodriquez
Pediatric Ambulatory Care ...... Francisco Torres, MD
Pediatric In-Patient Care .... Francisco Torres, MD
Quality Assurance .... Maria Torres

Measure	Cases	This Hosp.	State Avg.	U.S. Avg.
Blood Clot Prevention and Treatment				
Anticoagulation Overlap Therapy[5]	-	-	50%	93%
ICU Venous Thromboembolism Prophylaxis[5]	-	-	-	92%
Incidence of Potentially Preventable VTE[5]	-	-	-	10%
UFH with Dosages/Platelet Monitoring[5]	-	-	100%	97%
Venous Thromboembolism Prophylaxis[5]	-	-	98%	85%
Warfarin Therapy Discharge Instructions[5]	-	-	92%	75%
Chest Pain/Possible Heart Attack Care				
Aspirin Given Within 24 Hours of Arrival	-	-	-	96%
Fibrinolytic Meds Within 30 Min. of Arrival	-	-	-	58%
Average Time to ECG (minutes)	-	-	-	7
Average Time to Transfer (minutes)	-	-	-	60
Children's Asthma Care				
Received Home Management Plan of Care	-	-	-	88%
Received Reliever Medication	-	-	-	100%
Received Systemic Corticosteroids	-	-	-	100%
Emergency Department				
Admittance Decision Time (minutes)[5]	-	-	190	98
Head CT Results Within 45 Min. of Arrival	-	-	-	57%
Patients Who Left ER Before Being Seen	-	-	-	2%
Time from ER Arrival to Admit. (minutes)[5]	-	-	635	274
Time from ER Arrival to Discharge (minutes)	-	-	-	134
Time in ER Before Being Evaluated (minutes)	-	-	-	26
Time to Pain Meds for Fractures (minutes)	-	-	-	57
Heart Attack Care				
Aspirin Given at Discharge	66	98%	94%	99%
Fibrinolytic Meds Within 30 Min. of Arrival[1]	-	-	47%	54%
PCI Within 90 Minutes of Arrival[1]	-	-	53%	96%
Statin Prescribed at Discharge	68	94%	89%	98%
Heart Failure Care				
ACE Inhibitor or ARB for LVSD	51	98%	92%	97%
Discharge Instructions Given	125	86%	87%	94%
Evaluation of LVS Function	118	100%	94%	99%
Medicare Spending				
Medicare Spending per Patient (ratio)	-	-	-	0.98
Pneumonia Care				
Appropriate Initial Antibiotic Given	21	90%	82%	95%
Blood Culture Timing	26	92%	82%	98%
Pregnancy and Delivery Care				
Newborn Deliveries Scheduled Early[5]	-	-	-	6%
Preventive Care				
Immunization for Influenza[5]	-	-	42%	90%
Immunization for Pneumonia[5]	-	-	29%	92%
Stroke Care				
Anticoagulation Therapy for Atrial Fibrillation[5]	-	-	60%	95%
Antithrombotic Therapy Timing[5]	-	-	77%	98%
Assessed for Rehabilitation[5]	-	-	59%	97%
Discharged on Antithrombotic Therapy[5]	-	-	63%	99%
Discharged on Statin Medication[5]	-	-	90%	94%
Thrombolytic Therapy Timing[5]	-	-	-	66%
Venous Thromboembolism Prophylaxis[5]	-	-	52%	94%
Written Stroke Educational Materials Given[5]	-	-	95%	88%
Surgical Care Improvement Project				
Appropriate Beta Blocker Usage	36	100%	75%	98%
Appropriate VTP Within 24 Hours	265	99%	90%	98%
Controlled Postoperative Blood Glucose	69	97%	81%	97%
Perioperative Temperature Management	276	89%	98%	100%
Prophylactic Antibiotic Selection	341	99%	96%	99%
Prophylactic Antibiotic Selection (Outpatient)	-	-	-	98%
Prophylactic Antibiotic Stopped	338	91%	83%	98%
Prophylactic Antibiotic Timing	341	97%	89%	99%
Prophylactic Antibiotic Timing (Outpatient)	-	-	-	98%
Urinary Catheter Removal	18	100%	91%	97%
Survey of Patients' Hospital Experiences				
Area Around Room 'Always' Quiet at Night[5]	-	-	-	61%
Doctors 'Always' Communicated Well[5]	-	-	-	82%
Home Recovery Information Given[5]	-	-	-	85%
Hospital Given 9 or 10 on 10 Point Scale[5]	-	-	-	71%
Meds 'Always' Explained Before Given[5]	-	-	-	64%
Nurses 'Always' Communicated Well[5]	-	-	-	79%
Pain 'Always' Well Controlled[5]	-	-	-	71%
Room and Bathroom 'Always' Clean[5]	-	-	-	73%
Timely Help 'Always' Received[5]	-	-	-	68%
Would Definitely Recommend Hospital[5]	-	-	-	71%
Use of Medical Imaging				
Cardiac Imaging Stress Test before Surgery	-	-	4.5%	5.3%
Combination Abdominal CT Scan	-	-	7.4%	10.5%
Combination Brain/Sinus CT Scan	-	-	0.8%	2.7%
Combination Chest CT Scan	-	-	6.1%	2.7%
Follow-up Mammogram/Ultrasound	-	-	43.2%	8.8%
Lumbar Spine MRI for Low Back Pain	-	-	44.3%	37.2%

NOTE: Hospital profiles are in alphabetical order by state, then city, then hospital within the city; Rankings exclude hospitals with less than 25 cases except for patient surveys which excludes hospitals with less than 100 cases; (a) 100-299 cases; (1) The number of cases/patients is too few to report; (2) Data submitted were based on a sample of cases/patients; (3) Results are based on a shorter time period than required; (4) Data suppressed by CMS for one or more quarters; (5) Results are not available for this reporting period; (6) Fewer than 100 patients completed the HCAHPS survey; (7) No cases met the criteria for this measure; (8) The lower limit of the confidence interval cannot be calculated if the number of observed infections equals zero; (9) No data are available from the state/territory for this reporting period; (10) The scores shown reflect fewer than 50 completed surveys; (11) There were discrepancies in the data collection process; (12) This measure does not apply to this hospital for this reporting period; (13) Results cannot be calculated for this reporting period; (14) The results for this state are combined with nearby states to protect confidentiality; Please refer to the User's Guide for a full explanation of data.

Hospital Metropolitano Doctor Pila

2435 Las Americas Ave
Ponce, PR 733
Phone: 787-848-5600
Fax: 787-841-3454
Type: Acute Care Hospitals
Emergency Services: Yes
Ownership: Voluntary non-profit - Private
Beds: 183

Key Personnel:

Radiology. Adrian A Alvarez de la C
CEO/President. . . . . Lcda. Karen Z. Artau Feliciano, MHSA
Infection Control. . . . . Ana Cintron
Quality Assurance . . . . Ana Cintron
Operating Room. . . . . Melba Febus
Chief of Medical Staff. . . . . Thomas Hernand_z
Pediatric Ambulatory Care . . . . . . Jose Lisazoain
Pediatric In-Patient Care . . . . Jose Lisazoain

Measure	Cases	This Hosp.	State Avg.	U.S. Avg.
Blood Clot Prevention and Treatment				
Anticoagulation Overlap Therapy[5]	-	-	50%	93%
ICU Venous Thromboembolism Prophylaxis[5]	-	-	-	92%
Incidence of Potentially Preventable VTE[5]	-	-	-	10%
UFH with Dosages/Platelet Monitoring[5]	-	-	100%	97%
Venous Thromboembolism Prophylaxis[5]	-	-	98%	85%
Warfarin Therapy Discharge Instructions[5]	-	-	92%	75%
Chest Pain/Possible Heart Attack Care				
Aspirin Given Within 24 Hours of Arrival	-	-	-	96%
Fibrinolytic Meds Within 30 Min. of Arrival	-	-	-	58%
Average Time to ECG (minutes)	-	-	-	7
Average Time to Transfer (minutes)	-	-	-	60
Children's Asthma Care				
Received Home Management Plan of Care	-	-	-	88%
Received Reliever Medication	-	-	-	100%
Received Systemic Corticosteroids	-	-	-	100%
Emergency Department				
Admittance Decision Time (minutes)[5]	-	-	190	98
Head CT Results Within 45 Min. of Arrival	-	-	-	57%
Patients Who Left ER Before Being Seen	-	-	-	2%
Time from ER Arrival to Admit. (minutes)[5]	-	-	635	274
Time from ER Arrival to Discharge (minutes)	-	-	-	134
Time in ER Before Being Evaluated (minutes)	-	-	-	26
Time to Pain Meds for Fractures (minutes)	-	-	-	57
Heart Attack Care				
Aspirin Given at Discharge	36	92%	94%	99%
Fibrinolytic Meds Within 30 Min. of Arrival[7]	-	-	47%	54%
PCI Within 90 Minutes of Arrival[3,7]	-	-	53%	96%
Statin Prescribed at Discharge	33	73%	89%	98%
Heart Failure Care				
ACE Inhibitor or ARB for LVSD	50	70%	92%	97%
Discharge Instructions Given	116	61%	87%	94%
Evaluation of LVS Function	120	92%	94%	99%
Medicare Spending				
Medicare Spending per Patient (ratio)	-	-	-	0.98
Pneumonia Care				
Appropriate Initial Antibiotic Given	106	73%	82%	95%
Blood Culture Timing	77	84%	82%	98%
Pregnancy and Delivery Care				
Newborn Deliveries Scheduled Early[5]	-	-	-	6%
Preventive Care				
Immunization for Influenza[5]	-	-	42%	90%
Immunization for Pneumonia[5]	-	-	29%	92%
Stroke Care				
Anticoagulation Therapy for Atrial Fibrillation[5]	-	-	60%	95%
Antithrombotic Therapy Timing[5]	-	-	77%	98%
Assessed for Rehabilitation[5]	-	-	59%	97%
Discharged on Antithrombotic Therapy[5]	-	-	63%	99%
Discharged on Statin Medication[5]	-	-	90%	94%
Thrombolytic Therapy Timing[5]	-	-	-	66%
Venous Thromboembolism Prophylaxis[5]	-	-	52%	94%
Written Stroke Educational Materials Given[5]	-	-	95%	88%
Surgical Care Improvement Project				
Appropriate Beta Blocker Usage	25	100%	75%	98%
Appropriate VTP Within 24 Hours	129	91%	90%	98%
Controlled Postoperative Blood Glucose[3,7]	-	-	81%	97%
Perioperative Temperature Management	138	100%	98%	100%
Prophylactic Antibiotic Selection	136	96%	96%	99%
Prophylactic Antibiotic Selection (Outpatient)	-	-	-	98%
Prophylactic Antibiotic Stopped	130	95%	83%	98%
Prophylactic Antibiotic Timing	136	92%	89%	99%
Prophylactic Antibiotic Timing (Outpatient)	-	-	-	98%
Urinary Catheter Removal	49	96%	91%	97%
Survey of Patients' Hospital Experiences				
Area Around Room 'Always' Quiet at Night[5]	-	-	-	61%
Doctors 'Always' Communicated Well[5]	-	-	-	82%
Home Recovery Information Given[5]	-	-	-	85%
Hospital Given 9 or 10 on 10 Point Scale[5]	-	-	-	71%
Meds 'Always' Explained Before Given[5]	-	-	-	64%
Nurses 'Always' Communicated Well[5]	-	-	-	79%
Pain 'Always' Well Controlled[5]	-	-	-	71%
Room and Bathroom 'Always' Clean[5]	-	-	-	73%
Timely Help 'Always' Received[5]	-	-	-	68%
Would Definitely Recommend Hospital[5]	-	-	-	71%
Use of Medical Imaging				
Cardiac Imaging Stress Test before Surgery	-	-	4.5%	5.3%
Combination Abdominal CT Scan	-	-	7.4%	10.5%
Combination Brain/Sinus CT Scan	-	-	0.8%	2.7%
Combination Chest CT Scan	-	-	6.1%	2.7%
Follow-up Mammogram/Ultrasound	-	-	43.2%	8.8%
Lumbar Spine MRI for Low Back Pain	-	-	44.3%	37.2%

San Luke's Memorial Hospital

Tito Castro Ave #917
Ponce, PR 733
Phone: 787-844-2080
Fax: 787-841-3454
URL: www.ssepr.com/hospital_sanlucas.html
Type: Acute Care Hospitals
Emergency Services: Yes
Ownership: Voluntary non-profit - Church

Key Personnel:

Emergency Room . . . . Antonio Albite Vélez
CEO/President. . . . . Guillermo J Martin
Chief of Medical Staff. . . . . Jenaro Scarano

Measure	Cases	This Hosp.	State Avg.	U.S. Avg.
Blood Clot Prevention and Treatment				
Anticoagulation Overlap Therapy[5]	-	-	50%	93%
ICU Venous Thromboembolism Prophylaxis[5]	-	-	-	92%
Incidence of Potentially Preventable VTE[5]	-	-	-	10%
UFH with Dosages/Platelet Monitoring[5]	-	-	100%	97%
Venous Thromboembolism Prophylaxis[5]	-	-	98%	85%
Warfarin Therapy Discharge Instructions[5]	-	-	92%	75%
Chest Pain/Possible Heart Attack Care				
Aspirin Given Within 24 Hours of Arrival	-	-	-	96%
Fibrinolytic Meds Within 30 Min. of Arrival	-	-	-	58%
Average Time to ECG (minutes)	-	-	-	7
Average Time to Transfer (minutes)	-	-	-	60
Children's Asthma Care				
Received Home Management Plan of Care	-	-	-	88%
Received Reliever Medication	-	-	-	100%
Received Systemic Corticosteroids	-	-	-	100%
Emergency Department				
Admittance Decision Time (minutes)[5]	-	-	190	98
Head CT Results Within 45 Min. of Arrival	-	-	-	57%
Patients Who Left ER Before Being Seen	-	-	-	2%
Time from ER Arrival to Admit. (minutes)[5]	-	-	635	274
Time from ER Arrival to Discharge (minutes)	-	-	-	134
Time in ER Before Being Evaluated (minutes)	-	-	-	26
Time to Pain Meds for Fractures (minutes)	-	-	-	57
Heart Attack Care				
Aspirin Given at Discharge	655	99%	94%	99%
Fibrinolytic Meds Within 30 Min. of Arrival[7]	-	-	47%	54%
PCI Within 90 Minutes of Arrival	36	58%	53%	96%
Statin Prescribed at Discharge	621	86%	89%	98%
Heart Failure Care				
ACE Inhibitor or ARB for LVSD	112	97%	92%	97%
Discharge Instructions Given	401	100%	87%	94%
Evaluation of LVS Function	401	95%	94%	99%
Medicare Spending				
Medicare Spending per Patient (ratio)	-	-	-	0.98
Pneumonia Care				
Appropriate Initial Antibiotic Given	144	82%	82%	95%
Blood Culture Timing	77	88%	82%	98%
Pregnancy and Delivery Care				
Newborn Deliveries Scheduled Early[5]	-	-	-	6%
Preventive Care				
Immunization for Influenza[5]	-	-	42%	90%
Immunization for Pneumonia[5]	-	-	29%	92%
Stroke Care				
Anticoagulation Therapy for Atrial Fibrillation[5]	-	-	60%	95%
Antithrombotic Therapy Timing[5]	-	-	77%	98%
Assessed for Rehabilitation[5]	-	-	59%	97%
Discharged on Antithrombotic Therapy[5]	-	-	63%	99%
Discharged on Statin Medication[5]	-	-	90%	94%
Thrombolytic Therapy Timing[5]	-	-	-	66%
Venous Thromboembolism Prophylaxis[5]	-	-	52%	94%
Written Stroke Educational Materials Given[5]	-	-	95%	88%
Surgical Care Improvement Project				
Appropriate Beta Blocker Usage	42	81%	75%	98%
Appropriate VTP Within 24 Hours	214	98%	90%	98%
Controlled Postoperative Blood Glucose	79	81%	81%	97%
Perioperative Temperature Management	300	100%	98%	100%
Prophylactic Antibiotic Selection	291	91%	96%	99%
Prophylactic Antibiotic Selection (Outpatient)	-	-	-	98%
Prophylactic Antibiotic Stopped	287	80%	83%	98%
Prophylactic Antibiotic Timing	292	91%	89%	99%
Prophylactic Antibiotic Timing (Outpatient)	-	-	-	98%
Urinary Catheter Removal	65	97%	91%	97%
Survey of Patients' Hospital Experiences				
Area Around Room 'Always' Quiet at Night[5]	-	-	-	61%
Doctors 'Always' Communicated Well[5]	-	-	-	82%
Home Recovery Information Given[5]	-	-	-	85%
Hospital Given 9 or 10 on 10 Point Scale[5]	-	-	-	71%
Meds 'Always' Explained Before Given[5]	-	-	-	64%
Nurses 'Always' Communicated Well[5]	-	-	-	79%
Pain 'Always' Well Controlled[5]	-	-	-	71%
Room and Bathroom 'Always' Clean[5]	-	-	-	73%
Timely Help 'Always' Received[5]	-	-	-	68%
Would Definitely Recommend Hospital[5]	-	-	-	71%
Use of Medical Imaging				
Cardiac Imaging Stress Test before Surgery	-	-	4.5%	5.3%
Combination Abdominal CT Scan	-	-	7.4%	10.5%
Combination Brain/Sinus CT Scan	-	-	0.8%	2.7%
Combination Chest CT Scan	-	-	6.1%	2.7%
Follow-up Mammogram/Ultrasound	-	-	43.2%	8.8%
Lumbar Spine MRI for Low Back Pain	-	-	44.3%	37.2%

Centro Cardiovascular

Avenida Americo Miranda, Entrada Principal Cm
Phone: 787-754-8500
Rio Piedras, PR 936
Fax: 787-999-0860
URL: www.cardiovascular.gobierno.pr
Type: Acute Care Hospitals
Emergency Services: Yes
Ownership: Government - State
Beds: 122

Measure	Cases	This Hosp.	State Avg.	U.S. Avg.
Blood Clot Prevention and Treatment				
Anticoagulation Overlap Therapy[5]	-	-	50%	93%
ICU Venous Thromboembolism Prophylaxis[5]	-	-	-	92%
Incidence of Potentially Preventable VTE[5]	-	-	-	10%
UFH with Dosages/Platelet Monitoring[5]	-	-	100%	97%
Venous Thromboembolism Prophylaxis[5]	-	-	98%	85%
Warfarin Therapy Discharge Instructions[5]	-	-	92%	75%
Chest Pain/Possible Heart Attack Care				
Aspirin Given Within 24 Hours of Arrival	-	-	-	96%
Fibrinolytic Meds Within 30 Min. of Arrival	-	-	-	58%
Average Time to ECG (minutes)	-	-	-	7
Average Time to Transfer (minutes)	-	-	-	60
Children's Asthma Care				
Received Home Management Plan of Care	-	-	-	88%
Received Reliever Medication	-	-	-	100%
Received Systemic Corticosteroids	-	-	-	100%
Emergency Department				
Admittance Decision Time (minutes)[5]	-	-	190	98
Head CT Results Within 45 Min. of Arrival	-	-	-	57%
Patients Who Left ER Before Being Seen	-	-	-	2%

NOTE: Hospital profiles are in alphabetical order by state, then city, then hospital within the city; Rankings exclude hospitals with less than 25 cases except for patient surveys which excludes hospitals with less than 100 cases; (a) 100-299 cases; (1) The number of cases/patients is too few to report; (2) Data submitted were based on a sample of cases/patients; (3) Results are based on a shorter time period than required; (4) Data suppressed by CMS for one or more quarters; (5) Results are not available for this reporting period; (6) Fewer than 100 patients completed the HCAHPS survey; (7) No cases met the criteria for this measure; (8) The lower limit of the confidence interval cannot be calculated if the number of observed infections equals zero; (9) No data are available from the state/territory for this reporting period; (10) The scores shown reflect fewer than 50 completed surveys; (11) There were discrepancies in the data collection process; (12) This measure does not apply to this hospital for this reporting period; (13) Results cannot be calculated for this reporting period; (14) The results for this state are combined with nearby states to protect confidentiality; Please refer to the User's Guide for a full explanation of data.

Time from ER Arrival to Admit. (minutes)[5]	-	-	635	274
Time from ER Arrival to Discharge (minutes)	-	-	-	134
Time in ER Before Being Evaluated (minutes)	-	-	-	26
Time to Pain Meds for Fractures (minutes)	-	-	-	57
Heart Attack Care				
Aspirin Given at Discharge	383	89%	94%	99%
Fibrinolytic Meds Within 30 Min. of Arrival[7]	-	-	47%	54%
PCI Within 90 Minutes of Arrival	16	31%	53%	96%
Statin Prescribed at Discharge	415	89%	89%	98%
Heart Failure Care				
ACE Inhibitor or ARB for LVSD	227	95%	92%	97%
Discharge Instructions Given	388	97%	87%	94%
Evaluation of LVS Function	389	95%	94%	99%
Medicare Spending				
Medicare Spending per Patient (ratio)	-	-	-	0.98
Pneumonia Care				
Appropriate Initial Antibiotic Given[5]	-	-	82%	95%
Blood Culture Timing[5]	-	-	82%	98%
Pregnancy and Delivery Care				
Newborn Deliveries Scheduled Early[5]	-	-	-	6%
Preventive Care				
Immunization for Influenza[5]	-	-	42%	90%
Immunization for Pneumonia[5]	-	-	29%	92%
Stroke Care				
Anticoagulation Therapy for Atrial Fibrillation[5]	-	-	60%	95%
Antithrombotic Therapy Timing[5]	-	-	77%	98%
Assessed for Rehabilitation[5]	-	-	59%	97%
Discharged on Antithrombotic Therapy[5]	-	-	63%	99%
Discharged on Statin Medication[5]	-	-	90%	94%
Thrombolytic Therapy Timing[5]	-	-	-	66%
Venous Thromboembolism Prophylaxis[5]	-	-	52%	94%
Written Stroke Educational Materials Given[5]	-	-	95%	88%
Surgical Care Improvement Project				
Appropriate Beta Blocker Usage[2]	298	79%	75%	98%
Appropriate VTP Within 24 Hours[2,7]	-	-	90%	98%
Controlled Postoperative Blood Glucose[2]	928	83%	81%	97%
Perioperative Temperature Management[2,7]	-	-	98%	100%
Prophylactic Antibiotic Selection[2]	938	100%	96%	99%
Prophylactic Antibiotic Selection (Outpatient)	-	-	-	98%
Prophylactic Antibiotic Stopped[2]	934	92%	83%	98%
Prophylactic Antibiotic Timing[2]	947	92%	89%	99%
Prophylactic Antibiotic Timing (Outpatient)	-	-	-	98%
Urinary Catheter Removal[2]	650	100%	91%	97%
Survey of Patients' Hospital Experiences				
Area Around Room 'Always' Quiet at Night[5]	-	-	-	61%
Doctors 'Always' Communicated Well[5]	-	-	-	82%
Home Recovery Information Given[5]	-	-	-	85%
Hospital Given 9 or 10 on 10 Point Scale[5]	-	-	-	71%
Meds 'Always' Explained Before Given[5]	-	-	-	64%
Nurses 'Always' Communicated Well[5]	-	-	-	79%
Pain 'Always' Well Controlled[5]	-	-	-	71%
Room and Bathroom 'Always' Clean[5]	-	-	-	73%
Timely Help 'Always' Received[5]	-	-	-	68%
Would Definitely Recommend Hospital[5]	-	-	-	71%
Use of Medical Imaging				
Cardiac Imaging Stress Test before Surgery	-	-	4.5%	5.3%
Combination Abdominal CT Scan	-	-	7.4%	10.5%
Combination Brain/Sinus CT Scan	-	-	0.8%	2.7%
Combination Chest CT Scan	-	-	6.1%	2.7%
Follow-up Mammogram/Ultrasound	-	-	43.2%	8.8%
Lumbar Spine MRI for Low Back Pain	-	-	44.3%	37.2%

Hospital San Gerardo

Road No 844 Km 0 5 PO Cupey Bajo
Rio Piedras, PR 928
Type: Acute Care Hospitals
Ownership: Voluntary non-profit - Private
Phone: 787-761-8383
Emergency Services: Yes
Beds: 60

Measure	Cases	This Hosp.	State Avg.	U.S. Avg.
Blood Clot Prevention and Treatment				
Anticoagulation Overlap Therapy[5]	-	-	50%	93%
ICU Venous Thromboembolism Prophylaxis[5]	-	-	-	92%
Incidence of Potentially Preventable VTE[5]	-	-	-	10%
UFH with Dosages/Platelet Monitoring[5]	-	-	100%	97%
Venous Thromboembolism Prophylaxis[5]	-	-	98%	85%
Warfarin Therapy Discharge Instructions[5]	-	-	92%	75%
Chest Pain/Possible Heart Attack Care				
Aspirin Given Within 24 Hours of Arrival	-	-	-	96%
Fibrinolytic Meds Within 30 Min. of Arrival	-	-	-	58%
Average Time to ECG (minutes)	-	-	-	7
Average Time to Transfer (minutes)	-	-	-	60
Children's Asthma Care				
Received Home Management Plan of Care	-	-	-	88%
Received Reliever Medication	-	-	-	100%
Received Systemic Corticosteroids	-	-	-	100%
Emergency Department				
Admittance Decision Time (minutes)[5]	-	-	190	98
Head CT Results Within 45 Min. of Arrival	-	-	-	57%
Patients Who Left ER Before Being Seen	-	-	-	2%
Time from ER Arrival to Admit. (minutes)[5]	-	-	635	274
Time from ER Arrival to Discharge (minutes)	-	-	-	134
Time in ER Before Being Evaluated (minutes)	-	-	-	26
Time to Pain Meds for Fractures (minutes)	-	-	-	57
Heart Attack Care				
Aspirin Given at Discharge[2,3]	-	-	94%	99%
Fibrinolytic Meds Within 30 Min. of Arrival[1,2]	-	-	47%	54%
PCI Within 90 Minutes of Arrival[2,3]	-	-	53%	96%
Statin Prescribed at Discharge[2,3]	-	-	89%	98%
Heart Failure Care				
ACE Inhibitor or ARB for LVSD[2,3]	-	-	92%	97%
Discharge Instructions Given[1,2]	-	-	87%	94%
Evaluation of LVS Function[1,2]	-	-	94%	99%
Medicare Spending				
Medicare Spending per Patient (ratio)	-	-	-	0.98
Pneumonia Care				
Appropriate Initial Antibiotic Given[2,3]	-	-	82%	95%
Blood Culture Timing[2,3]	-	-	82%	98%
Pregnancy and Delivery Care				
Newborn Deliveries Scheduled Early[5]	-	-	-	6%
Preventive Care				
Immunization for Influenza[5]	-	-	42%	90%
Immunization for Pneumonia[5]	-	-	29%	92%
Stroke Care				
Anticoagulation Therapy for Atrial Fibrillation[5]	-	-	60%	95%
Antithrombotic Therapy Timing[5]	-	-	77%	98%
Assessed for Rehabilitation[5]	-	-	59%	97%
Discharged on Antithrombotic Therapy[5]	-	-	63%	99%
Discharged on Statin Medication[5]	-	-	90%	94%
Thrombolytic Therapy Timing[5]	-	-	-	66%
Venous Thromboembolism Prophylaxis[5]	-	-	52%	94%
Written Stroke Educational Materials Given[5]	-	-	95%	88%
Surgical Care Improvement Project				
Appropriate Beta Blocker Usage[5]	-	-	75%	98%
Appropriate VTP Within 24 Hours[5]	-	-	90%	98%
Controlled Postoperative Blood Glucose[5]	-	-	81%	97%
Perioperative Temperature Management[5]	-	-	98%	100%
Prophylactic Antibiotic Selection[5]	-	-	96%	99%
Prophylactic Antibiotic Selection (Outpatient)	-	-	-	98%
Prophylactic Antibiotic Stopped[5]	-	-	83%	98%
Prophylactic Antibiotic Timing[5]	-	-	89%	99%
Prophylactic Antibiotic Timing (Outpatient)	-	-	-	98%
Urinary Catheter Removal[5]	-	-	91%	97%
Survey of Patients' Hospital Experiences				
Area Around Room 'Always' Quiet at Night[5]	-	-	-	61%
Doctors 'Always' Communicated Well[5]	-	-	-	82%
Home Recovery Information Given[5]	-	-	-	85%
Hospital Given 9 or 10 on 10 Point Scale[5]	-	-	-	71%
Meds 'Always' Explained Before Given[5]	-	-	-	64%
Nurses 'Always' Communicated Well[5]	-	-	-	79%
Pain 'Always' Well Controlled[5]	-	-	-	71%
Room and Bathroom 'Always' Clean[5]	-	-	-	73%
Timely Help 'Always' Received[5]	-	-	-	68%
Would Definitely Recommend Hospital[5]	-	-	-	71%
Use of Medical Imaging				
Cardiac Imaging Stress Test before Surgery	-	-	4.5%	5.3%
Combination Abdominal CT Scan	-	-	7.4%	10.5%
Combination Brain/Sinus CT Scan	-	-	0.8%	2.7%
Combination Chest CT Scan	-	-	6.1%	2.7%
Follow-up Mammogram/Ultrasound	-	-	43.2%	8.8%
Lumbar Spine MRI for Low Back Pain	-	-	44.3%	37.2%

Hospital Universitario De Adulto

Barrio Monacillos Centromedico
Rio Piedras, PR 927
Type: Acute Care Hospitals
Ownership: Government - State
Phone: 787-754-0101
Fax: 787-294-3703
Emergency Services: Yes
Beds: 390

Measure	Cases	This Hosp.	State Avg.	U.S. Avg.
Blood Clot Prevention and Treatment				
Anticoagulation Overlap Therapy[5]	-	-	50%	93%
ICU Venous Thromboembolism Prophylaxis[5]	-	-	-	92%
Incidence of Potentially Preventable VTE[5]	-	-	-	10%
UFH with Dosages/Platelet Monitoring[5]	-	-	100%	97%
Venous Thromboembolism Prophylaxis[5]	-	-	98%	85%
Warfarin Therapy Discharge Instructions[5]	-	-	92%	75%
Chest Pain/Possible Heart Attack Care				
Aspirin Given Within 24 Hours of Arrival	-	-	-	96%
Fibrinolytic Meds Within 30 Min. of Arrival	-	-	-	58%
Average Time to ECG (minutes)	-	-	-	7
Average Time to Transfer (minutes)	-	-	-	60
Children's Asthma Care				
Received Home Management Plan of Care	-	-	-	88%
Received Reliever Medication	-	-	-	100%
Received Systemic Corticosteroids	-	-	-	100%
Emergency Department				
Admittance Decision Time (minutes)[5]	-	-	190	98
Head CT Results Within 45 Min. of Arrival	-	-	-	57%
Patients Who Left ER Before Being Seen	-	-	-	2%
Time from ER Arrival to Admit. (minutes)[5]	-	-	635	274
Time from ER Arrival to Discharge (minutes)	-	-	-	134
Time in ER Before Being Evaluated (minutes)	-	-	-	26
Time to Pain Meds for Fractures (minutes)	-	-	-	57
Heart Attack Care				
Aspirin Given at Discharge[1,3]	-	-	94%	99%
Fibrinolytic Meds Within 30 Min. of Arrival[3,7]	-	-	47%	54%
PCI Within 90 Minutes of Arrival[3,7]	-	-	53%	96%
Statin Prescribed at Discharge[1,3]	-	-	89%	98%
Heart Failure Care				
ACE Inhibitor or ARB for LVSD[1]	-	-	92%	97%
Discharge Instructions Given	18	0%	87%	94%
Evaluation of LVS Function	23	78%	94%	99%
Medicare Spending				
Medicare Spending per Patient (ratio)	-	-	-	0.98
Pneumonia Care				
Appropriate Initial Antibiotic Given[1]	-	-	82%	95%
Blood Culture Timing[1]	-	-	82%	98%
Pregnancy and Delivery Care				
Newborn Deliveries Scheduled Early[5]	-	-	-	6%
Preventive Care				
Immunization for Influenza[5]	-	-	42%	90%
Immunization for Pneumonia[5]	-	-	29%	92%
Stroke Care				
Anticoagulation Therapy for Atrial Fibrillation[1]	-	-	60%	95%
Antithrombotic Therapy Timing	66	80%	77%	98%
Assessed for Rehabilitation	125	80%	59%	97%
Discharged on Antithrombotic Therapy	55	82%	63%	99%
Discharged on Statin Medication	51	84%	90%	94%
Thrombolytic Therapy Timing	64	0%	-	66%
Venous Thromboembolism Prophylaxis	150	34%	52%	94%
Written Stroke Educational Materials Given	99	94%	95%	88%
Surgical Care Improvement Project				
Appropriate Beta Blocker Usage	22	18%	75%	98%
Appropriate VTP Within 24 Hours	189	89%	90%	98%
Controlled Postoperative Blood Glucose[7]	-	-	81%	97%
Perioperative Temperature Management	205	93%	98%	100%
Prophylactic Antibiotic Selection	149	88%	96%	99%
Prophylactic Antibiotic Selection (Outpatient)	-	-	-	98%
Prophylactic Antibiotic Stopped	149	61%	83%	98%

NOTE: Hospital profiles are in alphabetical order by state, then city, then hospital within the city; Rankings exclude hospitals with less than 25 cases except for patient surveys which excludes hospitals with less than 100 cases; (a) 100-299 cases; (1) The number of cases/patients is too few to report; (2) Data submitted were based on a sample of cases/patients; (3) Results are based on a shorter time period than required; (4) Data suppressed by CMS for one or more quarters; (5) Results are not available for this reporting period; (6) Fewer than 100 patients completed the HCAHPS survey; (7) No cases met the criteria for this measure; (8) The lower limit of the confidence interval cannot be calculated if the number of observed infections equals zero; (9) No data are available from the state/territory for this reporting period; (10) The scores shown reflect fewer than 50 completed surveys; (11) There were discrepancies in the data collection process; (12) This measure does not apply to this hospital for this reporting period; (13) Results cannot be calculated for this reporting period; (14) The results for this state are combined with nearby states to protect confidentiality; Please refer to the User's Guide for a full explanation of data.

Measure	Cases	This Hosp.	State Avg.	U.S. Avg.
Prophylactic Antibiotic Timing	151	79%	89%	99%
Prophylactic Antibiotic Timing (Outpatient)	-	-	-	98%
Urinary Catheter Removal	74	74%	91%	97%
Survey of Patients' Hospital Experiences				
Area Around Room 'Always' Quiet at Night[5]	-	-	-	61%
Doctors 'Always' Communicated Well[5]	-	-	-	82%
Home Recovery Information Given[5]	-	-	-	85%
Hospital Given 9 or 10 on 10 Point Scale[5]	-	-	-	71%
Meds 'Always' Explained Before Given[5]	-	-	-	64%
Nurses 'Always' Communicated Well[5]	-	-	-	79%
Pain 'Always' Well Controlled[5]	-	-	-	71%
Room and Bathroom 'Always' Clean[5]	-	-	-	73%
Timely Help 'Always' Received[5]	-	-	-	68%
Would Definitely Recommend Hospital[5]	-	-	-	71%
Use of Medical Imaging				
Cardiac Imaging Stress Test before Surgery	-	-	4.5%	5.3%
Combination Abdominal CT Scan	-	-	7.4%	10.5%
Combination Brain/Sinus CT Scan	-	-	0.8%	2.7%
Combination Chest CT Scan	-	-	6.1%	2.7%
Follow-up Mammogram/Ultrasound	-	-	43.2%	8.8%
Lumbar Spine MRI for Low Back Pain	-	-	44.3%	37.2%

San Juan Municipal Hospital

Barrio Monacillos,centro Medico
Rio Piedras, PR 936
Phone: 787-756-8535
Type: Acute Care Hospitals
Emergency Services: Yes
Ownership: Voluntary non-profit - Other

Measure	Cases	This Hosp.	State Avg.	U.S. Avg.
Blood Clot Prevention and Treatment				
Anticoagulation Overlap Therapy[5]	-	-	50%	93%
ICU Venous Thromboembolism Prophylaxis[5]	-	-	-	92%
Incidence of Potentially Preventable VTE[5]	-	-	-	10%
UFH with Dosages/Platelet Monitoring[5]	-	-	100%	97%
Venous Thromboembolism Prophylaxis[5]	-	-	98%	85%
Warfarin Therapy Discharge Instructions[5]	-	-	92%	75%
Chest Pain/Possible Heart Attack Care				
Aspirin Given Within 24 Hours of Arrival	-	-	-	96%
Fibrinolytic Meds Within 30 Min. of Arrival	-	-	-	58%
Average Time to ECG (minutes)	-	-	-	7
Average Time to Transfer (minutes)	-	-	-	60
Children's Asthma Care				
Received Home Management Plan of Care	-	-	-	88%
Received Reliever Medication	-	-	-	100%
Received Systemic Corticosteroids	-	-	-	100%
Emergency Department				
Admittance Decision Time (minutes)[5]	-	-	190	98
Head CT Results Within 45 Min. of Arrival	-	-	-	57%
Patients Who Left ER Before Being Seen	-	-	-	2%
Time from ER Arrival to Admit. (minutes)[5]	-	-	635	274
Time from ER Arrival to Discharge (minutes)	-	-	-	134
Time in ER Before Being Evaluated (minutes)	-	-	-	26
Time to Pain Meds for Fractures (minutes)	-	-	-	57
Heart Attack Care				
Aspirin Given at Discharge[3]	14	100%	94%	99%
Fibrinolytic Meds Within 30 Min. of Arrival[3,7]	-	-	47%	54%
PCI Within 90 Minutes of Arrival[3,7]	-	-	53%	96%
Statin Prescribed at Discharge[3]	13	100%	89%	98%
Heart Failure Care				
ACE Inhibitor or ARB for LVSD	49	100%	92%	97%
Discharge Instructions Given	49	100%	87%	94%
Evaluation of LVS Function	49	100%	94%	99%
Medicare Spending				
Medicare Spending per Patient (ratio)	-	-	-	0.98
Pneumonia Care				
Appropriate Initial Antibiotic Given	22	95%	82%	95%
Blood Culture Timing	27	100%	82%	98%
Pregnancy and Delivery Care				
Newborn Deliveries Scheduled Early[5]	-	-	-	6%
Preventive Care				
Immunization for Influenza[5]	-	-	42%	90%
Immunization for Pneumonia[5]	-	-	29%	92%
Stroke Care				
Anticoagulation Therapy for Atrial Fibrillation[5]	-	-	60%	95%
Antithrombotic Therapy Timing[5]	-	-	77%	98%
Assessed for Rehabilitation[5]	-	-	59%	97%
Discharged on Antithrombotic Therapy[5]	-	-	63%	99%
Discharged on Statin Medication[5]	-	-	90%	94%
Thrombolytic Therapy Timing[5]	-	-	-	66%
Venous Thromboembolism Prophylaxis[5]	-	-	52%	94%
Written Stroke Educational Materials Given[5]	-	-	95%	88%
Surgical Care Improvement Project				
Appropriate Beta Blocker Usage[7]	-	-	75%	98%
Appropriate VTP Within 24 Hours	107	93%	90%	98%
Controlled Postoperative Blood Glucose[7]	-	-	81%	97%
Perioperative Temperature Management	112	100%	98%	100%
Prophylactic Antibiotic Selection	109	98%	96%	99%
Prophylactic Antibiotic Selection (Outpatient)	-	-	-	98%
Prophylactic Antibiotic Stopped	109	100%	83%	98%
Prophylactic Antibiotic Timing	109	95%	89%	99%
Prophylactic Antibiotic Timing (Outpatient)	-	-	-	98%
Urinary Catheter Removal	43	100%	91%	97%
Survey of Patients' Hospital Experiences				
Area Around Room 'Always' Quiet at Night[5]	-	-	-	61%
Doctors 'Always' Communicated Well[5]	-	-	-	82%
Home Recovery Information Given[5]	-	-	-	85%
Hospital Given 9 or 10 on 10 Point Scale[5]	-	-	-	71%
Meds 'Always' Explained Before Given[5]	-	-	-	64%
Nurses 'Always' Communicated Well[5]	-	-	-	79%
Pain 'Always' Well Controlled[5]	-	-	-	71%
Room and Bathroom 'Always' Clean[5]	-	-	-	73%
Timely Help 'Always' Received[5]	-	-	-	68%
Would Definitely Recommend Hospital[5]	-	-	-	71%
Use of Medical Imaging				
Cardiac Imaging Stress Test before Surgery	-	-	4.5%	5.3%
Combination Abdominal CT Scan	-	-	7.4%	10.5%
Combination Brain/Sinus CT Scan	-	-	0.8%	2.7%
Combination Chest CT Scan	-	-	6.1%	2.7%
Follow-up Mammogram/Ultrasound	-	-	43.2%	8.8%
Lumbar Spine MRI for Low Back Pain	-	-	44.3%	37.2%

Hospital De La Concepcion

Road Number 2 Km 173.4
San German, PR 683
URL: www.hospitalconcepcion.org
Phone: 787-892-1860
Fax: 787-892-6465
Type: Acute Care Hospitals
Emergency Services: Yes
Ownership: Voluntary non-profit - Church
Beds: 155

Key Personnel:

Radiology. . . . . Wanda I Benitez Lopez
Quality Assurance . . . . Felicita Bonilla
Chief of Medical Staff. . . . . Francisco Jaume
Coronary Care . . . . Maria L Lebron
CEO/President. . . . . Jaime F Maestre Grau
Pediatric In-Patient Care . . . . Rosa Tones

Measure	Cases	This Hosp.	State Avg.	U.S. Avg.
Blood Clot Prevention and Treatment				
Anticoagulation Overlap Therapy[5]	-	-	50%	93%
ICU Venous Thromboembolism Prophylaxis[5]	-	-	-	92%
Incidence of Potentially Preventable VTE[5]	-	-	-	10%
UFH with Dosages/Platelet Monitoring[5]	-	-	100%	97%
Venous Thromboembolism Prophylaxis[5]	-	-	98%	85%
Warfarin Therapy Discharge Instructions[5]	-	-	92%	75%
Chest Pain/Possible Heart Attack Care				
Aspirin Given Within 24 Hours of Arrival	-	-	-	96%
Fibrinolytic Meds Within 30 Min. of Arrival	-	-	-	58%
Average Time to ECG (minutes)	-	-	-	7
Average Time to Transfer (minutes)	-	-	-	60
Children's Asthma Care				
Received Home Management Plan of Care	-	-	-	88%
Received Reliever Medication	-	-	-	100%
Received Systemic Corticosteroids	-	-	-	100%
Emergency Department				
Admittance Decision Time (minutes)[5]	-	-	190	98
Head CT Results Within 45 Min. of Arrival	-	-	-	57%
Patients Who Left ER Before Being Seen	-	-	-	2%
Time from ER Arrival to Admit. (minutes)[5]	-	-	635	274
Time from ER Arrival to Discharge (minutes)	-	-	-	134
Time in ER Before Being Evaluated (minutes)	-	-	-	26
Time to Pain Meds for Fractures (minutes)	-	-	-	57
Heart Attack Care				
Aspirin Given at Discharge	147	100%	94%	99%
Fibrinolytic Meds Within 30 Min. of Arrival[5]	-	-	47%	54%
PCI Within 90 Minutes of Arrival[7]	-	-	53%	96%
Statin Prescribed at Discharge	163	100%	89%	98%
Heart Failure Care				
ACE Inhibitor or ARB for LVSD	84	100%	92%	97%
Discharge Instructions Given	151	100%	87%	94%
Evaluation of LVS Function	150	100%	94%	99%
Medicare Spending				
Medicare Spending per Patient (ratio)	-	-	-	0.98
Pneumonia Care				
Appropriate Initial Antibiotic Given	46	93%	82%	95%
Blood Culture Timing[1]	-	-	82%	98%
Pregnancy and Delivery Care				
Newborn Deliveries Scheduled Early[5]	-	-	-	6%
Preventive Care				
Immunization for Influenza[5]	-	-	42%	90%
Immunization for Pneumonia[5]	-	-	29%	92%
Stroke Care				
Anticoagulation Therapy for Atrial Fibrillation[5]	-	-	60%	95%
Antithrombotic Therapy Timing[5]	-	-	77%	98%
Assessed for Rehabilitation[5]	-	-	59%	97%
Discharged on Antithrombotic Therapy[5]	-	-	63%	99%
Discharged on Statin Medication[5]	-	-	90%	94%
Thrombolytic Therapy Timing[5]	-	-	-	66%
Venous Thromboembolism Prophylaxis[5]	-	-	52%	94%
Written Stroke Educational Materials Given[5]	-	-	95%	88%
Surgical Care Improvement Project				
Appropriate Beta Blocker Usage	19	89%	75%	98%
Appropriate VTP Within 24 Hours	132	100%	90%	98%
Controlled Postoperative Blood Glucose[3,7]	-	-	81%	97%
Perioperative Temperature Management[3]	27	96%	98%	100%
Prophylactic Antibiotic Selection	130	98%	96%	99%
Prophylactic Antibiotic Selection (Outpatient)	-	-	-	98%
Prophylactic Antibiotic Stopped[5]	-	-	83%	98%
Prophylactic Antibiotic Timing	130	87%	89%	99%
Prophylactic Antibiotic Timing (Outpatient)	-	-	-	98%
Urinary Catheter Removal[5]	-	-	91%	97%
Survey of Patients' Hospital Experiences				
Area Around Room 'Always' Quiet at Night[5]	-	-	-	61%
Doctors 'Always' Communicated Well[5]	-	-	-	82%
Home Recovery Information Given[5]	-	-	-	85%
Hospital Given 9 or 10 on 10 Point Scale[5]	-	-	-	71%
Meds 'Always' Explained Before Given[5]	-	-	-	64%
Nurses 'Always' Communicated Well[5]	-	-	-	79%
Pain 'Always' Well Controlled[5]	-	-	-	71%
Room and Bathroom 'Always' Clean[5]	-	-	-	73%
Timely Help 'Always' Received[5]	-	-	-	68%
Would Definitely Recommend Hospital[5]	-	-	-	71%
Use of Medical Imaging				
Cardiac Imaging Stress Test before Surgery	-	-	4.5%	5.3%
Combination Abdominal CT Scan	-	-	7.4%	10.5%
Combination Brain/Sinus CT Scan	-	-	0.8%	2.7%
Combination Chest CT Scan	-	-	6.1%	2.7%
Follow-up Mammogram/Ultrasound	-	-	43.2%	8.8%
Lumbar Spine MRI for Low Back Pain	-	-	44.3%	37.2%

Hospital Metropolitano San German

Calle Javilla #8 Al Costado Parque De Bombas
Phone: 787-892-5300
San German, PR 683
Type: Acute Care Hospitals
Emergency Services: Yes
Ownership: Voluntary non-profit - Private

Measure	Cases	This Hosp.	State Avg.	U.S. Avg.
Blood Clot Prevention and Treatment				
Anticoagulation Overlap Therapy[5]	-	-	50%	93%
ICU Venous Thromboembolism Prophylaxis[5]	-	-	-	92%
Incidence of Potentially Preventable VTE[5]	-	-	-	10%
UFH with Dosages/Platelet Monitoring[5]	-	-	100%	97%

NOTE: Hospital profiles are in alphabetical order by state, then city, then hospital within the city; Rankings exclude hospitals with less than 25 cases except for patient surveys which excludes hospitals with less than 100 cases; (a) 100-299 cases; (1) The number of cases/patients is too few to report; (2) Data submitted were based on a sample of cases/patients; (3) Results are based on a shorter time period than required; (4) Data suppressed by CMS for one or more quarters; (5) Results are not available for this reporting period; (6) Fewer than 100 patients completed the HCAHPS survey; (7) No cases met the criteria for this measure; (8) The lower limit of the confidence interval cannot be calculated if the number of observed infections equals zero; (9) No data are available from the state/territory for this reporting period; (10) The scores shown reflect fewer than 50 completed surveys; (11) There were discrepancies in the data collection process; (12) This measure does not apply to this hospital for this reporting period; (13) Results cannot be calculated for this reporting period; (14) The results for this state are combined with nearby states to protect confidentiality; Please refer to the User's Guide for a full explanation of data.

Measure	Cases	This Hosp.	State Avg.	U.S. Avg.
Venous Thromboembolism Prophylaxis[5]	-	-	98%	85%
Warfarin Therapy Discharge Instructions[5]	-	-	92%	75%
Chest Pain/Possible Heart Attack Care				
Aspirin Given Within 24 Hours of Arrival	-	-	-	96%
Fibrinolytic Meds Within 30 Min. of Arrival	-	-	-	58%
Average Time to ECG (minutes)	-	-	-	7
Average Time to Transfer (minutes)	-	-	-	60
Children's Asthma Care				
Received Home Management Plan of Care	-	-	-	88%
Received Reliever Medication	-	-	-	100%
Received Systemic Corticosteroids	-	-	-	100%
Emergency Department				
Admittance Decision Time (minutes)[5]	-	-	190	98
Head CT Results Within 45 Min. of Arrival	-	-	-	57%
Patients Who Left ER Before Being Seen	-	-	-	2%
Time from ER Arrival to Admit. (minutes)[5]	-	-	635	274
Time from ER Arrival to Discharge (minutes)	-	-	-	134
Time in ER Before Being Evaluated (minutes)	-	-	-	26
Time to Pain Meds for Fractures (minutes)	-	-	-	57
Heart Attack Care				
Aspirin Given at Discharge[2]	63	89%	94%	99%
Fibrinolytic Meds Within 30 Min. of Arrival[1,2]	-	-	47%	54%
PCI Within 90 Minutes of Arrival[2,7]	-	-	53%	96%
Statin Prescribed at Discharge[2]	64	84%	89%	98%
Heart Failure Care				
ACE Inhibitor or ARB for LVSD[1,2]	-	-	92%	97%
Discharge Instructions Given[2]	45	60%	87%	94%
Evaluation of LVS Function[2]	46	80%	94%	99%
Medicare Spending				
Medicare Spending per Patient (ratio)	-	-	-	0.98
Pneumonia Care				
Appropriate Initial Antibiotic Given[1,2]	-	-	82%	95%
Blood Culture Timing[2]	12	67%	82%	98%
Pregnancy and Delivery Care				
Newborn Deliveries Scheduled Early[5]	-	-	-	6%
Preventive Care				
Immunization for Influenza[5]	-	-	42%	90%
Immunization for Pneumonia[5]	-	-	29%	92%
Stroke Care				
Anticoagulation Therapy for Atrial Fibrillation[5]	-	-	60%	95%
Antithrombotic Therapy Timing[5]	-	-	77%	98%
Assessed for Rehabilitation[5]	-	-	59%	97%
Discharged on Antithrombotic Therapy[5]	-	-	63%	99%
Discharged on Statin Medication[5]	-	-	90%	94%
Thrombolytic Therapy Timing[5]	-	-	-	66%
Venous Thromboembolism Prophylaxis[5]	-	-	52%	94%
Written Stroke Educational Materials Given[5]	-	-	95%	88%
Surgical Care Improvement Project				
Appropriate Beta Blocker Usage[1,2]	-	-	75%	98%
Appropriate VTP Within 24 Hours[2,3]	13	38%	90%	98%
Controlled Postoperative Blood Glucose[2,3]	-	-	81%	97%
Perioperative Temperature Management[2,3]	23	87%	98%	100%
Prophylactic Antibiotic Selection[1,2]	-	-	96%	99%
Prophylactic Antibiotic Selection (Outpatient)	-	-	-	98%
Prophylactic Antibiotic Stopped[1,2]	-	-	83%	98%
Prophylactic Antibiotic Timing[1,2]	-	-	89%	99%
Prophylactic Antibiotic Timing (Outpatient)	-	-	-	98%
Urinary Catheter Removal[1,2]	-	-	91%	97%
Survey of Patients' Hospital Experiences				
Area Around Room 'Always' Quiet at Night[5]	-	-	-	61%
Doctors 'Always' Communicated Well[5]	-	-	-	82%
Home Recovery Information Given[5]	-	-	-	85%
Hospital Given 9 or 10 on 10 Point Scale[5]	-	-	-	71%
Meds 'Always' Explained Before Given[5]	-	-	-	64%
Nurses 'Always' Communicated Well[5]	-	-	-	79%
Pain 'Always' Well Controlled[5]	-	-	-	71%
Room and Bathroom 'Always' Clean[5]	-	-	-	73%
Timely Help 'Always' Received[5]	-	-	-	68%
Would Definitely Recommend Hospital[5]	-	-	-	71%
Use of Medical Imaging				
Cardiac Imaging Stress Test before Surgery	-	-	4.5%	5.3%
Combination Abdominal CT Scan	-	-	7.4%	10.5%
Combination Brain/Sinus CT Scan	-	-	0.8%	2.7%
Combination Chest CT Scan	-	-	6.1%	2.7%
Follow-up Mammogram/Ultrasound	-	-	43.2%	8.8%
Lumbar Spine MRI for Low Back Pain	-	-	44.3%	37.2%

Admin de Servicios Medicos - Puerto Rico

Bo Monacillo Carr Num 22
San Juan, PR 935
Type: Acute Care Hospitals
Ownership: Government - Local
Phone: 787-777-3535
Fax: 787-777-3403
Emergency Services: Yes
Beds: 58

Measure	Cases	This Hosp.	State Avg.	U.S. Avg.
Blood Clot Prevention and Treatment				
Anticoagulation Overlap Therapy[5]	-	-	50%	93%
ICU Venous Thromboembolism Prophylaxis[5]	-	-	-	92%
Incidence of Potentially Preventable VTE[5]	-	-	-	10%
UFH with Dosages/Platelet Monitoring[5]	-	-	100%	97%
Venous Thromboembolism Prophylaxis[5]	-	-	98%	85%
Warfarin Therapy Discharge Instructions[5]	-	-	92%	75%
Chest Pain/Possible Heart Attack Care				
Aspirin Given Within 24 Hours of Arrival	-	-	-	96%
Fibrinolytic Meds Within 30 Min. of Arrival	-	-	-	58%
Average Time to ECG (minutes)	-	-	-	7
Average Time to Transfer (minutes)	-	-	-	60
Children's Asthma Care				
Received Home Management Plan of Care	-	-	-	88%
Received Reliever Medication	-	-	-	100%
Received Systemic Corticosteroids	-	-	-	100%
Emergency Department				
Admittance Decision Time (minutes)[5]	-	-	190	98
Head CT Results Within 45 Min. of Arrival	-	-	-	57%
Patients Who Left ER Before Being Seen	-	-	-	2%
Time from ER Arrival to Admit. (minutes)[5]	-	-	635	274
Time from ER Arrival to Discharge (minutes)	-	-	-	134
Time in ER Before Being Evaluated (minutes)	-	-	-	26
Time to Pain Meds for Fractures (minutes)	-	-	-	57
Heart Attack Care				
Aspirin Given at Discharge[5]	-	-	94%	99%
Fibrinolytic Meds Within 30 Min. of Arrival[5]	-	-	47%	54%
PCI Within 90 Minutes of Arrival[5]	-	-	53%	96%
Statin Prescribed at Discharge[5]	-	-	89%	98%
Heart Failure Care				
ACE Inhibitor or ARB for LVSD[5]	-	-	92%	97%
Discharge Instructions Given[5]	-	-	87%	94%
Evaluation of LVS Function[5]	-	-	94%	99%
Medicare Spending				
Medicare Spending per Patient (ratio)	-	-	-	0.98
Pneumonia Care				
Appropriate Initial Antibiotic Given[5]	-	-	82%	95%
Blood Culture Timing[5]	-	-	82%	98%
Pregnancy and Delivery Care				
Newborn Deliveries Scheduled Early[5]	-	-	-	6%
Preventive Care				
Immunization for Influenza[5]	-	-	42%	90%
Immunization for Pneumonia[5]	-	-	29%	92%
Stroke Care				
Anticoagulation Therapy for Atrial Fibrillation[5]	-	-	60%	95%
Antithrombotic Therapy Timing[5]	-	-	77%	98%
Assessed for Rehabilitation[5]	-	-	59%	97%
Discharged on Antithrombotic Therapy[5]	-	-	63%	99%
Discharged on Statin Medication[5]	-	-	90%	94%
Thrombolytic Therapy Timing[5]	-	-	-	66%
Venous Thromboembolism Prophylaxis[5]	-	-	52%	94%
Written Stroke Educational Materials Given[5]	-	-	95%	88%
Surgical Care Improvement Project				
Appropriate Beta Blocker Usage[1,3]	-	-	75%	98%
Appropriate VTP Within 24 Hours[1,3]	-	-	90%	98%
Controlled Postoperative Blood Glucose[3,7]	-	-	81%	97%
Perioperative Temperature Management[1,3]	-	-	98%	100%
Prophylactic Antibiotic Selection[3,7]	-	-	96%	99%
Prophylactic Antibiotic Selection (Outpatient)	-	-	-	98%
Prophylactic Antibiotic Stopped[3,7]	-	-	83%	98%
Prophylactic Antibiotic Timing[3,7]	-	-	89%	99%
Prophylactic Antibiotic Timing (Outpatient)	-	-	-	98%
Urinary Catheter Removal[3,7]	-	-	91%	97%
Survey of Patients' Hospital Experiences				
Area Around Room 'Always' Quiet at Night[5]	-	-	-	61%
Doctors 'Always' Communicated Well[5]	-	-	-	82%
Home Recovery Information Given[5]	-	-	-	85%
Hospital Given 9 or 10 on 10 Point Scale[5]	-	-	-	71%
Meds 'Always' Explained Before Given[5]	-	-	-	64%
Nurses 'Always' Communicated Well[5]	-	-	-	79%
Pain 'Always' Well Controlled[5]	-	-	-	71%
Room and Bathroom 'Always' Clean[5]	-	-	-	73%
Timely Help 'Always' Received[5]	-	-	-	68%
Would Definitely Recommend Hospital[5]	-	-	-	71%
Use of Medical Imaging				
Cardiac Imaging Stress Test before Surgery	-	-	4.5%	5.3%
Combination Abdominal CT Scan	-	-	7.4%	10.5%
Combination Brain/Sinus CT Scan	-	-	0.8%	2.7%
Combination Chest CT Scan	-	-	6.1%	2.7%
Follow-up Mammogram/Ultrasound	-	-	43.2%	8.8%
Lumbar Spine MRI for Low Back Pain	-	-	44.3%	37.2%

Asociacion Hospital Del Maestro

Sergio Cuevas Bustamante Street 550
San Juan, PR 936
E-mail: info@maestrofacmed.com
URL: www.maestrofacmed.com
Type: Acute Care Hospitals
Ownership: Voluntary non-profit - Other
Phone: 787-758-6420
Fax: 787-758-0105
Emergency Services: Yes
Beds: 216

Key Personnel:
CEO/President. . . . . Milton Maldonado
Chief of Medical Staff. . . . . Jose Montalvo
Operating Room. . . . . Carmen Perez, RN
Quality Assurance . . . . Ruth Plata
Pediatric In-Patient Care . . . . Mario Ramirez, MD
Hemotology Center . . . . Rafael Rizek
Emergency Room . . . . Luis Sarzalejo, MD
Infection Control. . . . . Carlos Leon Valiente, MD

Measure	Cases	This Hosp.	State Avg.	U.S. Avg.
Blood Clot Prevention and Treatment				
Anticoagulation Overlap Therapy[5]	-	-	50%	93%
ICU Venous Thromboembolism Prophylaxis[5]	-	-	-	92%
Incidence of Potentially Preventable VTE[5]	-	-	-	10%
UFH with Dosages/Platelet Monitoring[5]	-	-	100%	97%
Venous Thromboembolism Prophylaxis[5]	-	-	98%	85%
Warfarin Therapy Discharge Instructions[5]	-	-	92%	75%
Chest Pain/Possible Heart Attack Care				
Aspirin Given Within 24 Hours of Arrival	-	-	-	96%
Fibrinolytic Meds Within 30 Min. of Arrival	-	-	-	58%
Average Time to ECG (minutes)	-	-	-	7
Average Time to Transfer (minutes)	-	-	-	60
Children's Asthma Care				
Received Home Management Plan of Care	-	-	-	88%
Received Reliever Medication	-	-	-	100%
Received Systemic Corticosteroids	-	-	-	100%
Emergency Department				
Admittance Decision Time (minutes)[5]	-	-	190	98
Head CT Results Within 45 Min. of Arrival	-	-	-	57%
Patients Who Left ER Before Being Seen	-	-	-	2%
Time from ER Arrival to Admit. (minutes)[5]	-	-	635	274
Time from ER Arrival to Discharge (minutes)	-	-	-	134
Time in ER Before Being Evaluated (minutes)	-	-	-	26
Time to Pain Meds for Fractures (minutes)	-	-	-	57
Heart Attack Care				
Aspirin Given at Discharge	12	100%	94%	99%
Fibrinolytic Meds Within 30 Min. of Arrival[3,7]	-	-	47%	54%
PCI Within 90 Minutes of Arrival[3,7]	-	-	53%	96%
Statin Prescribed at Discharge	21	90%	89%	98%
Heart Failure Care				
ACE Inhibitor or ARB for LVSD	33	100%	92%	97%
Discharge Instructions Given	147	99%	87%	94%
Evaluation of LVS Function	149	100%	94%	99%
Medicare Spending				
Medicare Spending per Patient (ratio)	-	-	-	0.98
Pneumonia Care				

NOTE: Hospital profiles are in alphabetical order by state, then city, then hospital within the city; Rankings exclude hospitals with less than 25 cases except for patient surveys which excludes hospitals with less than 100 cases; (a) 100-299 cases; (1) The number of cases/patients is too few to report; (2) Data submitted were based on a sample of cases/patients; (3) Results are based on a shorter time period than required; (4) Data suppressed by CMS for one or more quarters; (5) Results are not available for this reporting period; (6) Fewer than 100 patients completed the HCAHPS survey; (7) No cases met the criteria for this measure; (8) The lower limit of the confidence interval cannot be calculated if the number of observed infections equals zero; (9) No data are available from the state/territory for this reporting period; (10) The scores shown reflect fewer than 50 completed surveys; (11) There were discrepancies in the data collection process; (12) This measure does not apply to this hospital for this reporting period; (13) Results cannot be calculated for this reporting period; (14) The results for this state are combined with nearby states to protect confidentiality; Please refer to the User's Guide for a full explanation of data.

Measure	Cases	This Hosp.	State Avg.	U.S. Avg.
Appropriate Initial Antibiotic Given	88	78%	82%	95%
Blood Culture Timing	81	79%	82%	98%
Pregnancy and Delivery Care				
Newborn Deliveries Scheduled Early[5]	-	-	-	6%
Preventive Care				
Immunization for Influenza[5]	-	-	42%	90%
Immunization for Pneumonia[5]	-	-	29%	92%
Stroke Care				
Anticoagulation Therapy for Atrial Fibrillation[5]	-	-	60%	95%
Antithrombotic Therapy Timing[5]	-	-	77%	98%
Assessed for Rehabilitation[5]	-	-	59%	97%
Discharged on Antithrombotic Therapy[5]	-	-	63%	99%
Discharged on Statin Medication[5]	-	-	90%	94%
Thrombolytic Therapy Timing[5]	-	-	-	66%
Venous Thromboembolism Prophylaxis[5]	-	-	52%	94%
Written Stroke Educational Materials Given[5]	-	-	95%	88%
Surgical Care Improvement Project				
Appropriate Beta Blocker Usage[1]	-	-	75%	98%
Appropriate VTP Within 24 Hours	145	98%	90%	98%
Controlled Postoperative Blood Glucose[7]	-	-	81%	97%
Perioperative Temperature Management	148	100%	98%	100%
Prophylactic Antibiotic Selection	125	87%	96%	99%
Prophylactic Antibiotic Selection (Outpatient)	-	-	-	98%
Prophylactic Antibiotic Stopped	125	100%	83%	98%
Prophylactic Antibiotic Timing	127	93%	89%	99%
Prophylactic Antibiotic Timing (Outpatient)	-	-	-	98%
Urinary Catheter Removal[7]	-	-	91%	97%
Survey of Patients' Hospital Experiences				
Area Around Room 'Always' Quiet at Night[5]	-	-	-	61%
Doctors 'Always' Communicated Well[5]	-	-	-	82%
Home Recovery Information Given[5]	-	-	-	85%
Hospital Given 9 or 10 on 10 Point Scale[5]	-	-	-	71%
Meds 'Always' Explained Before Given[5]	-	-	-	64%
Nurses 'Always' Communicated Well[5]	-	-	-	79%
Pain 'Always' Well Controlled[5]	-	-	-	71%
Room and Bathroom 'Always' Clean[5]	-	-	-	73%
Timely Help 'Always' Received[5]	-	-	-	68%
Would Definitely Recommend Hospital[5]	-	-	-	71%
Use of Medical Imaging				
Cardiac Imaging Stress Test before Surgery	-	-	4.5%	5.3%
Combination Abdominal CT Scan	-	-	7.4%	10.5%
Combination Brain/Sinus CT Scan	-	-	0.8%	2.7%
Combination Chest CT Scan	-	-	6.1%	2.7%
Follow-up Mammogram/Ultrasound	-	-	43.2%	8.8%
Lumbar Spine MRI for Low Back Pain	-	-	44.3%	37.2%

Doctor I Gonzalez Martinez Oncology Hospital

Bo. Monacillos Centro Medico Phone: 787-763-4149
San Juan, PR 919 Fax: 787-751-7940
Type: Acute Care Hospitals Emergency Services: No
Ownership: Voluntary non-profit - Private Beds: 143

Key Personnel:
CEO/President. . . . . Milagros Bargas
Chief of Medical Staff . . . . Carlos Chevere
Intensive Care Unit. . . . . Elizabeth De Jesus, RN
Infection Control. . . . . Francisca Marin, RN
Anesthesiology. . . . . Lourdes Medina, MD
Operating Room. . . . . Sylvia Quiles
Radiology. . . . . Jose Riviera, MD
Quality Assurance . . . . Milagros Vargas

Measure	Cases	This Hosp.	State Avg.	U.S. Avg.
Blood Clot Prevention and Treatment				
Anticoagulation Overlap Therapy[1]	-	-	50%	93%
ICU Venous Thromboembolism Prophylaxis[1]	-	-	-	92%
Incidence of Potentially Preventable VTE[7]	-	-	-	10%
UFH with Dosages/Platelet Monitoring[7]	-	-	100%	97%
Venous Thromboembolism Prophylaxis[1]	-	-	98%	85%
Warfarin Therapy Discharge Instructions[1]	-	-	92%	75%
Chest Pain/Possible Heart Attack Care				
Aspirin Given Within 24 Hours of Arrival	-	-	-	96%
Fibrinolytic Meds Within 30 Min. of Arrival	-	-	-	58%
Average Time to ECG (minutes)	-	-	-	7
Average Time to Transfer (minutes)	-	-	-	60
Children's Asthma Care				
Received Home Management Plan of Care	-	-	-	88%
Received Reliever Medication	-	-	-	100%
Received Systemic Corticosteroids	-	-	-	100%
Emergency Department				
Admittance Decision Time (minutes)[5]	-	-	190	98
Head CT Results Within 45 Min. of Arrival	-	-	-	57%
Patients Who Left ER Before Being Seen	-	-	-	2%
Time from ER Arrival to Admit. (minutes)[5]	-	-	635	274
Time from ER Arrival to Discharge (minutes)	-	-	-	134
Time in ER Before Being Evaluated (minutes)	-	-	-	26
Time to Pain Meds for Fractures (minutes)	-	-	-	57
Heart Attack Care				
Aspirin Given at Discharge[5]	-	-	94%	99%
Fibrinolytic Meds Within 30 Min. of Arrival[5]	-	-	47%	54%
PCI Within 90 Minutes of Arrival[5]	-	-	53%	96%
Statin Prescribed at Discharge[5]	-	-	89%	98%
Heart Failure Care				
ACE Inhibitor or ARB for LVSD[5]	-	-	92%	97%
Discharge Instructions Given[5]	-	-	87%	94%
Evaluation of LVS Function[5]	-	-	94%	99%
Medicare Spending				
Medicare Spending per Patient (ratio)	-	-	-	0.98
Pneumonia Care				
Appropriate Initial Antibiotic Given[5]	-	-	82%	95%
Blood Culture Timing[5]	-	-	82%	98%
Pregnancy and Delivery Care				
Newborn Deliveries Scheduled Early[5]	-	-	-	6%
Preventive Care				
Immunization for Influenza[5]	-	-	42%	90%
Immunization for Pneumonia[5]	-	-	29%	92%
Stroke Care				
Anticoagulation Therapy for Atrial Fibrillation[5]	-	-	60%	95%
Antithrombotic Therapy Timing[5]	-	-	77%	98%
Assessed for Rehabilitation[5]	-	-	59%	97%
Discharged on Antithrombotic Therapy[5]	-	-	63%	99%
Discharged on Statin Medication[5]	-	-	90%	94%
Thrombolytic Therapy Timing[5]	-	-	-	66%
Venous Thromboembolism Prophylaxis[5]	-	-	52%	94%
Written Stroke Educational Materials Given[5]	-	-	95%	88%
Surgical Care Improvement Project				
Appropriate Beta Blocker Usage[1,2]	-	-	75%	98%
Appropriate VTP Within 24 Hours[2,3]	138	98%	90%	98%
Controlled Postoperative Blood Glucose[2,3]	-	-	81%	97%
Perioperative Temperature Management[2,3]	205	100%	98%	100%
Prophylactic Antibiotic Selection[2,3]	184	98%	96%	99%
Prophylactic Antibiotic Selection (Outpatient)	-	-	-	98%
Prophylactic Antibiotic Stopped[2,3]	180	82%	83%	98%
Prophylactic Antibiotic Timing[2,3]	186	75%	89%	99%
Prophylactic Antibiotic Timing (Outpatient)	-	-	-	98%
Urinary Catheter Removal[2,3]	101	95%	91%	97%
Survey of Patients' Hospital Experiences				
Area Around Room 'Always' Quiet at Night[5]	-	-	-	61%
Doctors 'Always' Communicated Well[5]	-	-	-	82%
Home Recovery Information Given[5]	-	-	-	85%
Hospital Given 9 or 10 on 10 Point Scale[5]	-	-	-	71%
Meds 'Always' Explained Before Given[5]	-	-	-	64%
Nurses 'Always' Communicated Well[5]	-	-	-	79%
Pain 'Always' Well Controlled[5]	-	-	-	71%
Room and Bathroom 'Always' Clean[5]	-	-	-	73%
Timely Help 'Always' Received[5]	-	-	-	68%
Would Definitely Recommend Hospital[5]	-	-	-	71%
Use of Medical Imaging				
Cardiac Imaging Stress Test before Surgery	-	-	4.5%	5.3%
Combination Abdominal CT Scan	-	-	7.4%	10.5%
Combination Brain/Sinus CT Scan	-	-	0.8%	2.7%
Combination Chest CT Scan	-	-	6.1%	2.7%
Follow-up Mammogram/Ultrasound	-	-	43.2%	8.8%
Lumbar Spine MRI for Low Back Pain	-	-	44.3%	37.2%

Hospital San Francisco

371 De Diego Ave Phone: 787-767-5100
San Juan, PR 923
Type: Acute Care Hospitals Emergency Services: Yes
Ownership: Proprietary

Measure	Cases	This Hosp.	State Avg.	U.S. Avg.
Blood Clot Prevention and Treatment				
Anticoagulation Overlap Therapy[5]	-	-	50%	93%
ICU Venous Thromboembolism Prophylaxis[5]	-	-	-	92%
Incidence of Potentially Preventable VTE[5]	-	-	-	10%
UFH with Dosages/Platelet Monitoring[5]	-	-	100%	97%
Venous Thromboembolism Prophylaxis[5]	-	-	98%	85%
Warfarin Therapy Discharge Instructions[5]	-	-	92%	75%
Chest Pain/Possible Heart Attack Care				
Aspirin Given Within 24 Hours of Arrival	-	-	-	96%
Fibrinolytic Meds Within 30 Min. of Arrival	-	-	-	58%
Average Time to ECG (minutes)	-	-	-	7
Average Time to Transfer (minutes)	-	-	-	60
Children's Asthma Care				
Received Home Management Plan of Care	-	-	-	88%
Received Reliever Medication	-	-	-	100%
Received Systemic Corticosteroids	-	-	-	100%
Emergency Department				
Admittance Decision Time (minutes)[5]	-	-	190	98
Head CT Results Within 45 Min. of Arrival	-	-	-	57%
Patients Who Left ER Before Being Seen	-	-	-	2%
Time from ER Arrival to Admit. (minutes)[5]	-	-	635	274
Time from ER Arrival to Discharge (minutes)	-	-	-	134
Time in ER Before Being Evaluated (minutes)	-	-	-	26
Time to Pain Meds for Fractures (minutes)	-	-	-	57
Heart Attack Care				
Aspirin Given at Discharge	24	92%	94%	99%
Fibrinolytic Meds Within 30 Min. of Arrival[7]	-	-	47%	54%
PCI Within 90 Minutes of Arrival[7]	-	-	53%	96%
Statin Prescribed at Discharge	33	52%	89%	98%
Heart Failure Care				
ACE Inhibitor or ARB for LVSD	19	74%	92%	97%
Discharge Instructions Given	49	37%	87%	94%
Evaluation of LVS Function	50	96%	94%	99%
Medicare Spending				
Medicare Spending per Patient (ratio)	-	-	-	0.98
Pneumonia Care				
Appropriate Initial Antibiotic Given	39	54%	82%	95%
Blood Culture Timing	106	54%	82%	98%
Pregnancy and Delivery Care				
Newborn Deliveries Scheduled Early[5]	-	-	-	6%
Preventive Care				
Immunization for Influenza[5]	-	-	42%	90%
Immunization for Pneumonia[5]	-	-	29%	92%
Stroke Care				
Anticoagulation Therapy for Atrial Fibrillation[5]	-	-	60%	95%
Antithrombotic Therapy Timing[5]	-	-	77%	98%
Assessed for Rehabilitation[5]	-	-	59%	97%
Discharged on Antithrombotic Therapy[5]	-	-	63%	99%
Discharged on Statin Medication[5]	-	-	90%	94%
Thrombolytic Therapy Timing[5]	-	-	-	66%
Venous Thromboembolism Prophylaxis[5]	-	-	52%	94%
Written Stroke Educational Materials Given[5]	-	-	95%	88%
Surgical Care Improvement Project				
Appropriate Beta Blocker Usage	31	35%	75%	98%
Appropriate VTP Within 24 Hours	137	78%	90%	98%
Controlled Postoperative Blood Glucose[7]	-	-	81%	97%
Perioperative Temperature Management	141	100%	98%	100%
Prophylactic Antibiotic Selection	110	88%	96%	99%
Prophylactic Antibiotic Selection (Outpatient)	-	-	-	98%
Prophylactic Antibiotic Stopped	109	54%	83%	98%
Prophylactic Antibiotic Timing	110	75%	89%	99%
Prophylactic Antibiotic Timing (Outpatient)	-	-	-	98%
Urinary Catheter Removal	61	93%	91%	97%
Survey of Patients' Hospital Experiences				
Area Around Room 'Always' Quiet at Night[5]	-	-	-	61%
Doctors 'Always' Communicated Well[5]	-	-	-	82%

NOTE: Hospital profiles are in alphabetical order by state, then city, then hospital within the city; Rankings exclude hospitals with less than 25 cases except for patient surveys which excludes hospitals with less than 100 cases; (a) 100-299 cases; (1) The number of cases/patients is too few to report; (2) Data submitted were based on a sample of cases/patients; (3) Results are based on a shorter time period than required; (4) Data suppressed by CMS for one or more quarters; (5) Results are not available for this reporting period; (6) Fewer than 100 patients completed the HCAHPS survey; (7) No cases met the criteria for this measure; (8) The lower limit of the confidence interval cannot be calculated if the number of observed infections equals zero; (9) No data are available from the state/territory for this reporting period; (10) The scores shown reflect fewer than 50 completed surveys; (11) There were discrepancies in the data collection process; (12) This measure does not apply to this hospital for this reporting period; (13) Results cannot be calculated for this reporting period; (14) The results for this state are combined with nearby states to protect confidentiality; Please refer to the User's Guide for a full explanation of data.

Measure	Cases	This Hosp.	State Avg.	U.S. Avg.
Home Recovery Information Given[5]	-	-	-	85%
Hospital Given 9 or 10 on 10 Point Scale[5]	-	-	-	71%
Meds 'Always' Explained Before Given[5]	-	-	-	64%
Nurses 'Always' Communicated Well[5]	-	-	-	79%
Pain 'Always' Well Controlled[5]	-	-	-	71%
Room and Bathroom 'Always' Clean[5]	-	-	-	73%
Timely Help 'Always' Received[5]	-	-	-	68%
Would Definitely Recommend Hospital[5]	-	-	-	71%
Use of Medical Imaging				
Cardiac Imaging Stress Test before Surgery	-	-	4.5%	5.3%
Combination Abdominal CT Scan	-	-	7.4%	10.5%
Combination Brain/Sinus CT Scan	-	-	0.8%	2.7%
Combination Chest CT Scan	-	-	6.1%	2.7%
Follow-up Mammogram/Ultrasound	-	-	43.2%	8.8%
Lumbar Spine MRI for Low Back Pain	-	-	44.3%	37.2%

Metropolitan Hospital

Carretera 21 1785 Urb Las Lomas
San Juan, PR 915
Phone: 787-782-9999
Type: Acute Care Hospitals
Emergency Services: Yes
Ownership: Proprietary

Measure	Cases	This Hosp.	State Avg.	U.S. Avg.
Blood Clot Prevention and Treatment				
Anticoagulation Overlap Therapy[5]	-	-	50%	93%
ICU Venous Thromboembolism Prophylaxis[5]	-	-	-	92%
Incidence of Potentially Preventable VTE[5]	-	-	-	10%
UFH with Dosages/Platelet Monitoring[5]	-	-	100%	97%
Venous Thromboembolism Prophylaxis[5]	-	-	98%	85%
Warfarin Therapy Discharge Instructions[5]	-	-	92%	75%
Chest Pain/Possible Heart Attack Care				
Aspirin Given Within 24 Hours of Arrival	-	-	-	96%
Fibrinolytic Meds Within 30 Min. of Arrival	-	-	-	58%
Average Time to ECG (minutes)	-	-	-	7
Average Time to Transfer (minutes)	-	-	-	60
Children's Asthma Care				
Received Home Management Plan of Care	-	-	-	88%
Received Reliever Medication	-	-	-	100%
Received Systemic Corticosteroids	-	-	-	100%
Emergency Department				
Admittance Decision Time (minutes)[5]	-	-	190	98
Head CT Results Within 45 Min. of Arrival	-	-	-	57%
Patients Who Left ER Before Being Seen	-	-	-	2%
Time from ER Arrival to Admit. (minutes)[5]	-	-	635	274
Time from ER Arrival to Discharge (minutes)	-	-	-	134
Time in ER Before Being Evaluated (minutes)	-	-	-	26
Time to Pain Meds for Fractures (minutes)	-	-	-	57
Heart Attack Care				
Aspirin Given at Discharge	23	100%	94%	99%
Fibrinolytic Meds Within 30 Min. of Arrival[7]	-	-	47%	54%
PCI Within 90 Minutes of Arrival[7]	-	-	53%	96%
Statin Prescribed at Discharge	26	92%	89%	98%
Heart Failure Care				
ACE Inhibitor or ARB for LVSD	55	98%	92%	97%
Discharge Instructions Given	113	90%	87%	94%
Evaluation of LVS Function	112	99%	94%	99%
Medicare Spending				
Medicare Spending per Patient (ratio)	-	-	-	0.98
Pneumonia Care				
Appropriate Initial Antibiotic Given	158	93%	82%	95%
Blood Culture Timing	186	89%	82%	98%
Pregnancy and Delivery Care				
Newborn Deliveries Scheduled Early[5]	-	-	-	6%
Preventive Care				
Immunization for Influenza[5]	-	-	42%	90%
Immunization for Pneumonia[5]	-	-	29%	92%
Stroke Care				
Anticoagulation Therapy for Atrial Fibrillation[5]	-	-	60%	95%
Antithrombotic Therapy Timing[5]	-	-	77%	98%
Assessed for Rehabilitation[5]	-	-	59%	97%
Discharged on Antithrombotic Therapy[5]	-	-	63%	99%
Discharged on Statin Medication[5]	-	-	90%	94%
Thrombolytic Therapy Timing[5]	-	-	-	66%
Venous Thromboembolism Prophylaxis[5]	-	-	52%	94%
Written Stroke Educational Materials Given[5]	-	-	95%	88%
Surgical Care Improvement Project				
Appropriate Beta Blocker Usage[7]	-	-	75%	98%
Appropriate VTP Within 24 Hours	57	98%	90%	98%
Controlled Postoperative Blood Glucose[7]	-	-	81%	97%
Perioperative Temperature Management	64	98%	98%	100%
Prophylactic Antibiotic Selection	61	98%	96%	99%
Prophylactic Antibiotic Selection (Outpatient)	-	-	-	98%
Prophylactic Antibiotic Stopped	59	98%	83%	98%
Prophylactic Antibiotic Timing	61	90%	89%	99%
Prophylactic Antibiotic Timing (Outpatient)	-	-	-	98%
Urinary Catheter Removal	12	100%	91%	97%
Survey of Patients' Hospital Experiences				
Area Around Room 'Always' Quiet at Night[5]	-	-	-	61%
Doctors 'Always' Communicated Well[5]	-	-	-	82%
Home Recovery Information Given[5]	-	-	-	85%
Hospital Given 9 or 10 on 10 Point Scale[5]	-	-	-	71%
Meds 'Always' Explained Before Given[5]	-	-	-	64%
Nurses 'Always' Communicated Well[5]	-	-	-	79%
Pain 'Always' Well Controlled[5]	-	-	-	71%
Room and Bathroom 'Always' Clean[5]	-	-	-	73%
Timely Help 'Always' Received[5]	-	-	-	68%
Would Definitely Recommend Hospital[5]	-	-	-	71%
Use of Medical Imaging				
Cardiac Imaging Stress Test before Surgery	-	-	4.5%	5.3%
Combination Abdominal CT Scan	-	-	7.4%	10.5%
Combination Brain/Sinus CT Scan	-	-	0.8%	2.7%
Combination Chest CT Scan	-	-	6.1%	2.7%
Follow-up Mammogram/Ultrasound	-	-	43.2%	8.8%
Lumbar Spine MRI for Low Back Pain	-	-	44.3%	37.2%

Presbyterian Community Hospital

1451 Ashford Avenue
San Juan, PR 907
Phone: 787-721-2160
Fax: 787-723-3797
URL: www.presbypr.com
Type: Acute Care Hospitals
Emergency Services: Yes
Ownership: Voluntary non-profit - Other
Beds: 207

Key Personnel:

Infection Control. . . . . Hilda Aleman, BSN
Operating Room. . . . . Nancy Casares
CEO/President. . . . . Pedro J Gonzales, MHSH
Cardiac Laboratory. . . . . Josue Mercado, MD
Chief of Medical Staff. . . . . Josue Mercado
Radiology. . . . . Frances Aulet Morales
Quality Assurance . . . . Janet Perez
Pediatric Ambulatory Care . . . . . . Humberto Vozques, MD

Measure	Cases	This Hosp.	State Avg.	U.S. Avg.
Blood Clot Prevention and Treatment				
Anticoagulation Overlap Therapy[5]	-	-	50%	93%
ICU Venous Thromboembolism Prophylaxis[5]	-	-	-	92%
Incidence of Potentially Preventable VTE[5]	-	-	-	10%
UFH with Dosages/Platelet Monitoring[5]	-	-	100%	97%
Venous Thromboembolism Prophylaxis[5]	-	-	98%	85%
Warfarin Therapy Discharge Instructions[5]	-	-	92%	75%
Chest Pain/Possible Heart Attack Care				
Aspirin Given Within 24 Hours of Arrival	-	-	-	96%
Fibrinolytic Meds Within 30 Min. of Arrival	-	-	-	58%
Average Time to ECG (minutes)	-	-	-	7
Average Time to Transfer (minutes)	-	-	-	60
Children's Asthma Care				
Received Home Management Plan of Care	-	-	-	88%
Received Reliever Medication	-	-	-	100%
Received Systemic Corticosteroids	-	-	-	100%
Emergency Department				
Admittance Decision Time (minutes)[5]	-	-	190	98
Head CT Results Within 45 Min. of Arrival	-	-	-	57%
Patients Who Left ER Before Being Seen	-	-	-	2%
Time from ER Arrival to Admit. (minutes)[5]	-	-	635	274
Time from ER Arrival to Discharge (minutes)	-	-	-	134
Time in ER Before Being Evaluated (minutes)	-	-	-	26
Time to Pain Meds for Fractures (minutes)	-	-	-	57
Heart Attack Care				
Aspirin Given at Discharge	55	100%	94%	99%
Fibrinolytic Meds Within 30 Min. of Arrival[3,7]	-	-	47%	54%
PCI Within 90 Minutes of Arrival[3,7]	-	-	53%	96%
Statin Prescribed at Discharge	51	100%	89%	98%
Heart Failure Care				
ACE Inhibitor or ARB for LVSD	27	100%	92%	97%
Discharge Instructions Given	94	100%	87%	94%
Evaluation of LVS Function	33	100%	94%	99%
Medicare Spending				
Medicare Spending per Patient (ratio)	-	-	-	0.98
Pneumonia Care				
Appropriate Initial Antibiotic Given[1]	-	-	82%	95%
Blood Culture Timing	23	100%	82%	98%
Pregnancy and Delivery Care				
Newborn Deliveries Scheduled Early[5]	-	-	-	6%
Preventive Care				
Immunization for Influenza[5]	-	-	42%	90%
Immunization for Pneumonia[5]	-	-	29%	92%
Stroke Care				
Anticoagulation Therapy for Atrial Fibrillation[5]	-	-	60%	95%
Antithrombotic Therapy Timing[5]	-	-	77%	98%
Assessed for Rehabilitation[5]	-	-	59%	97%
Discharged on Antithrombotic Therapy[5]	-	-	63%	99%
Discharged on Statin Medication[5]	-	-	90%	94%
Thrombolytic Therapy Timing[5]	-	-	-	66%
Venous Thromboembolism Prophylaxis[5]	-	-	52%	94%
Written Stroke Educational Materials Given[5]	-	-	95%	88%
Surgical Care Improvement Project				
Appropriate Beta Blocker Usage	17	100%	75%	98%
Appropriate VTP Within 24 Hours	796	99%	90%	98%
Controlled Postoperative Blood Glucose[3,7]	-	-	81%	97%
Perioperative Temperature Management	846	100%	98%	100%
Prophylactic Antibiotic Selection	615	99%	96%	99%
Prophylactic Antibiotic Selection (Outpatient)	-	-	-	98%
Prophylactic Antibiotic Stopped	615	100%	83%	98%
Prophylactic Antibiotic Timing	615	99%	89%	99%
Prophylactic Antibiotic Timing (Outpatient)	-	-	-	98%
Urinary Catheter Removal	452	100%	91%	97%
Survey of Patients' Hospital Experiences				
Area Around Room 'Always' Quiet at Night[5]	-	-	-	61%
Doctors 'Always' Communicated Well[5]	-	-	-	82%
Home Recovery Information Given[5]	-	-	-	85%
Hospital Given 9 or 10 on 10 Point Scale[5]	-	-	-	71%
Meds 'Always' Explained Before Given[5]	-	-	-	64%
Nurses 'Always' Communicated Well[5]	-	-	-	79%
Pain 'Always' Well Controlled[5]	-	-	-	71%
Room and Bathroom 'Always' Clean[5]	-	-	-	73%
Timely Help 'Always' Received[5]	-	-	-	68%
Would Definitely Recommend Hospital[5]	-	-	-	71%
Use of Medical Imaging				
Cardiac Imaging Stress Test before Surgery	-	-	4.5%	5.3%
Combination Abdominal CT Scan	-	-	7.4%	10.5%
Combination Brain/Sinus CT Scan	-	-	0.8%	2.7%
Combination Chest CT Scan	-	-	6.1%	2.7%
Follow-up Mammogram/Ultrasound	-	-	43.2%	8.8%
Lumbar Spine MRI for Low Back Pain	-	-	44.3%	37.2%

San Juan VA Medical Center

10 Calle Casia
San Juan, PR 921
Phone: 800-449-8729
Fax: 787-641-4557
URL: www.visn8.med.va.gov/caribbean
Type: Acute Care - VA
Emergency Services: No
Ownership: Government Federal
Beds: 348

Key Personnel:

Hemotology Center . . . . Luis Baez, MD
Patient Relations . . . . Rafael Cuevas
Ambulatory Care . . . . Geraldo Franceshi, MD
Emergency Room . . . . Armaldo Martinez, MD
Radiology. . . . . Edda Quintero, MD
Infection Control. . . . . Sonia Saavedra, MD

Measure	Cases	This Hosp.	State Avg.	U.S. Avg.
Blood Clot Prevention and Treatment				
Anticoagulation Overlap Therapy	-	-	50%	93%
ICU Venous Thromboembolism Prophylaxis	-	-	-	92%
Incidence of Potentially Preventable VTE	-	-	-	10%

NOTE: Hospital profiles are in alphabetical order by state, then city, then hospital within the city; Rankings exclude hospitals with less than 25 cases except for patient surveys which excludes hospitals with less than 100 cases; (a) 100-299 cases; (1) The number of cases/patients is too few to report; (2) Data submitted were based on a sample of cases/patients; (3) Results are based on a shorter time period than required; (4) Data suppressed by CMS for one or more quarters; (5) Results are not available for this reporting period; (6) Fewer than 100 patients completed the HCAHPS survey; (7) No cases met the criteria for this measure; (8) The lower limit of the confidence interval cannot be calculated if the number of observed infections equals zero; (9) No data are available from the state/territory for this reporting period; (10) The scores shown reflect fewer than 50 completed surveys; (11) There were discrepancies in the data collection process; (12) This measure does not apply to this hospital for this reporting period; (13) Results cannot be calculated for this reporting period; (14) The results for this state are combined with nearby states to protect confidentiality; Please refer to the User's Guide for a full explanation of data.

Measure	Cases	This Hosp.	State Avg.	U.S. Avg.
UFH with Dosages/Platelet Monitoring	-	-	100%	97%
Venous Thromboembolism Prophylaxis	-	-	98%	85%
Warfarin Therapy Discharge Instructions	-	-	92%	75%
Chest Pain/Possible Heart Attack Care				
Aspirin Given Within 24 Hours of Arrival	-	-	-	96%
Fibrinolytic Meds Within 30 Min. of Arrival	-	-	-	58%
Average Time to ECG (minutes)	-	-	-	7
Average Time to Transfer (minutes)	-	-	-	60
Children's Asthma Care				
Received Home Management Plan of Care	-	-	-	88%
Received Reliever Medication	-	-	-	100%
Received Systemic Corticosteroids	-	-	-	100%
Emergency Department				
Admittance Decision Time (minutes)	-	-	190	98
Head CT Results Within 45 Min. of Arrival	-	-	-	57%
Patients Who Left ER Before Being Seen	-	-	-	2%
Time from ER Arrival to Admit. (minutes)	-	-	635	274
Time from ER Arrival to Discharge (minutes)	-	-	-	134
Time in ER Before Being Evaluated (minutes)	-	-	-	26
Time to Pain Meds for Fractures (minutes)	-	-	-	57
Heart Attack Care				
Aspirin Given at Discharge	119	100%	94%	99%
Fibrinolytic Meds Within 30 Min. of Arrival[1]	-	-	47%	54%
PCI Within 90 Minutes of Arrival[1]	-	-	53%	96%
Statin Prescribed at Discharge	128	98%	89%	98%
Heart Failure Care				
ACE Inhibitor or ARB for LVSD	95	100%	92%	97%
Discharge Instructions Given	256	100%	87%	94%
Evaluation of LVS Function	268	100%	94%	99%
Medicare Spending				
Medicare Spending per Patient (ratio)	-	-	-	0.98
Pneumonia Care				
Appropriate Initial Antibiotic Given	79	97%	82%	95%
Blood Culture Timing	291	99%	82%	98%
Pregnancy and Delivery Care				
Newborn Deliveries Scheduled Early	-	-	-	6%
Preventive Care				
Immunization for Influenza[5]	-	-	42%	90%
Immunization for Pneumonia[5]	-	-	29%	92%
Stroke Care				
Anticoagulation Therapy for Atrial Fibrillation	-	-	60%	95%
Antithrombotic Therapy Timing	-	-	77%	98%
Assessed for Rehabilitation	-	-	59%	97%
Discharged on Antithrombotic Therapy	-	-	63%	99%
Discharged on Statin Medication	-	-	90%	94%
Thrombolytic Therapy Timing	-	-	-	66%
Venous Thromboembolism Prophylaxis	-	-	52%	94%
Written Stroke Educational Materials Given	-	-	95%	88%
Surgical Care Improvement Project				
Appropriate Beta Blocker Usage[2]	66	94%	75%	98%
Appropriate VTP Within 24 Hours[2]	161	99%	90%	98%
Controlled Postoperative Blood Glucose[2]	57	98%	81%	97%
Perioperative Temperature Management[2]	157	99%	98%	100%
Prophylactic Antibiotic Selection	105	100%	96%	99%
Prophylactic Antibiotic Selection (Outpatient)	-	-	-	98%
Prophylactic Antibiotic Stopped	100	97%	83%	98%
Prophylactic Antibiotic Timing	105	99%	89%	99%
Prophylactic Antibiotic Timing (Outpatient)	-	-	-	98%
Urinary Catheter Removal[2]	116	97%	91%	97%
Survey of Patients' Hospital Experiences				
Area Around Room 'Always' Quiet at Night	-	-	-	61%
Doctors 'Always' Communicated Well	-	-	-	82%
Home Recovery Information Given	-	-	-	85%
Hospital Given 9 or 10 on 10 Point Scale	-	-	-	71%
Meds 'Always' Explained Before Given	-	-	-	64%
Nurses 'Always' Communicated Well	-	-	-	79%
Pain 'Always' Well Controlled	-	-	-	71%
Room and Bathroom 'Always' Clean	-	-	-	73%
Timely Help 'Always' Received	-	-	-	68%
Would Definitely Recommend Hospital	-	-	-	71%
Use of Medical Imaging				
Cardiac Imaging Stress Test before Surgery	-	-	4.5%	5.3%
Combination Abdominal CT Scan	-	-	7.4%	10.5%
Combination Brain/Sinus CT Scan	-	-	0.8%	2.7%
Combination Chest CT Scan	-	-	6.1%	2.7%
Follow-up Mammogram/Ultrasound	-	-	43.2%	8.8%
Lumbar Spine MRI for Low Back Pain	-	-	44.3%	37.2%

Centro Medico Wilma N Vazquez

Carr. 2 Km 39.5, Road Number 2 Bo Algarrobo
Phone: 787-858-1580
Vega Baja, PR 693
Type: Acute Care Hospitals Emergency Services: Yes
Ownership: Proprietary

Measure	Cases	This Hosp.	State Avg.	U.S. Avg.
Blood Clot Prevention and Treatment				
Anticoagulation Overlap Therapy[5]	-	-	50%	93%
ICU Venous Thromboembolism Prophylaxis[5]	-	-	-	92%
Incidence of Potentially Preventable VTE[5]	-	-	-	10%
UFH with Dosages/Platelet Monitoring[5]	-	-	100%	97%
Venous Thromboembolism Prophylaxis[5]	-	-	98%	85%
Warfarin Therapy Discharge Instructions[5]	-	-	92%	75%
Chest Pain/Possible Heart Attack Care				
Aspirin Given Within 24 Hours of Arrival	-	-	-	96%
Fibrinolytic Meds Within 30 Min. of Arrival	-	-	-	58%
Average Time to ECG (minutes)	-	-	-	7
Average Time to Transfer (minutes)	-	-	-	60
Children's Asthma Care				
Received Home Management Plan of Care	-	-	-	88%
Received Reliever Medication	-	-	-	100%
Received Systemic Corticosteroids	-	-	-	100%
Emergency Department				
Admittance Decision Time (minutes)[5]	-	-	190	98
Head CT Results Within 45 Min. of Arrival	-	-	-	57%
Patients Who Left ER Before Being Seen	-	-	-	2%
Time from ER Arrival to Admit. (minutes)[5]	-	-	635	274
Time from ER Arrival to Discharge (minutes)	-	-	-	134
Time in ER Before Being Evaluated (minutes)	-	-	-	26
Time to Pain Meds for Fractures (minutes)	-	-	-	57
Heart Attack Care				
Aspirin Given at Discharge[2,3]	11	100%	94%	99%
Fibrinolytic Meds Within 30 Min. of Arrival[1,2]	-	-	47%	54%
PCI Within 90 Minutes of Arrival[2,3]	-	-	53%	96%
Statin Prescribed at Discharge[2,3]	11	100%	89%	98%
Heart Failure Care				
ACE Inhibitor or ARB for LVSD[1,2]	-	-	92%	97%
Discharge Instructions Given[2,3]	29	97%	87%	94%
Evaluation of LVS Function[2,3]	30	100%	94%	99%
Medicare Spending				
Medicare Spending per Patient (ratio)	-	-	-	0.98
Pneumonia Care				
Appropriate Initial Antibiotic Given[1,2]	-	-	82%	95%
Blood Culture Timing[1,2]	-	-	82%	98%
Pregnancy and Delivery Care				
Newborn Deliveries Scheduled Early[5]	-	-	-	6%
Preventive Care				
Immunization for Influenza[5]	-	-	42%	90%
Immunization for Pneumonia[5]	-	-	29%	92%
Stroke Care				
Anticoagulation Therapy for Atrial Fibrillation[5]	-	-	60%	95%
Antithrombotic Therapy Timing[5]	-	-	77%	98%
Assessed for Rehabilitation[5]	-	-	59%	97%
Discharged on Antithrombotic Therapy[5]	-	-	63%	99%
Discharged on Statin Medication[5]	-	-	90%	94%
Thrombolytic Therapy Timing[5]	-	-	-	66%
Venous Thromboembolism Prophylaxis[5]	-	-	52%	94%
Written Stroke Educational Materials Given[5]	-	-	95%	88%
Surgical Care Improvement Project				
Appropriate Beta Blocker Usage[5]	-	-	75%	98%
Appropriate VTP Within 24 Hours[5]	-	-	90%	98%
Controlled Postoperative Blood Glucose[5]	-	-	81%	97%
Perioperative Temperature Management[5]	-	-	98%	100%
Prophylactic Antibiotic Selection[5]	-	-	96%	99%
Prophylactic Antibiotic Selection (Outpatient)	-	-	-	98%
Prophylactic Antibiotic Stopped[5]	-	-	83%	98%
Prophylactic Antibiotic Timing[5]	-	-	89%	99%
Prophylactic Antibiotic Timing (Outpatient)	-	-	-	98%
Urinary Catheter Removal[5]	-	-	91%	97%
Survey of Patients' Hospital Experiences				
Area Around Room 'Always' Quiet at Night[5]	-	-	-	61%
Doctors 'Always' Communicated Well[5]	-	-	-	82%
Home Recovery Information Given[5]	-	-	-	85%
Hospital Given 9 or 10 on 10 Point Scale[5]	-	-	-	71%
Meds 'Always' Explained Before Given[5]	-	-	-	64%
Nurses 'Always' Communicated Well[5]	-	-	-	79%
Pain 'Always' Well Controlled[5]	-	-	-	71%
Room and Bathroom 'Always' Clean[5]	-	-	-	73%
Timely Help 'Always' Received[5]	-	-	-	68%
Would Definitely Recommend Hospital[5]	-	-	-	71%
Use of Medical Imaging				
Cardiac Imaging Stress Test before Surgery	-	-	4.5%	5.3%
Combination Abdominal CT Scan	-	-	7.4%	10.5%
Combination Brain/Sinus CT Scan	-	-	0.8%	2.7%
Combination Chest CT Scan	-	-	6.1%	2.7%
Follow-up Mammogram/Ultrasound	-	-	43.2%	8.8%
Lumbar Spine MRI for Low Back Pain	-	-	44.3%	37.2%

Hospital Metropolitano Doctor Tito Mattei

Road 128 Km 1.0 Phone: 787-856-1000
Yauco, PR 698
Type: Acute Care Hospitals Emergency Services: Yes
Ownership: Proprietary

Measure	Cases	This Hosp.	State Avg.	U.S. Avg.
Blood Clot Prevention and Treatment				
Anticoagulation Overlap Therapy[5]	-	-	50%	93%
ICU Venous Thromboembolism Prophylaxis[5]	-	-	-	92%
Incidence of Potentially Preventable VTE[5]	-	-	-	10%
UFH with Dosages/Platelet Monitoring[5]	-	-	100%	97%
Venous Thromboembolism Prophylaxis[5]	-	-	98%	85%
Warfarin Therapy Discharge Instructions[5]	-	-	92%	75%
Chest Pain/Possible Heart Attack Care				
Aspirin Given Within 24 Hours of Arrival	-	-	-	96%
Fibrinolytic Meds Within 30 Min. of Arrival	-	-	-	58%
Average Time to ECG (minutes)	-	-	-	7
Average Time to Transfer (minutes)	-	-	-	60
Children's Asthma Care				
Received Home Management Plan of Care	-	-	-	88%
Received Reliever Medication	-	-	-	100%
Received Systemic Corticosteroids	-	-	-	100%
Emergency Department				
Admittance Decision Time (minutes)[5]	-	-	190	98
Head CT Results Within 45 Min. of Arrival	-	-	-	57%
Patients Who Left ER Before Being Seen	-	-	-	2%
Time from ER Arrival to Admit. (minutes)[5]	-	-	635	274
Time from ER Arrival to Discharge (minutes)	-	-	-	134
Time in ER Before Being Evaluated (minutes)	-	-	-	26
Time to Pain Meds for Fractures (minutes)	-	-	-	57
Heart Attack Care				
Aspirin Given at Discharge	128	92%	94%	99%
Fibrinolytic Meds Within 30 Min. of Arrival[1]	-	-	47%	54%
PCI Within 90 Minutes of Arrival[7]	-	-	53%	96%
Statin Prescribed at Discharge	140	88%	89%	98%
Heart Failure Care				
ACE Inhibitor or ARB for LVSD	76	86%	92%	97%
Discharge Instructions Given	184	82%	87%	94%
Evaluation of LVS Function	184	88%	94%	99%
Medicare Spending				
Medicare Spending per Patient (ratio)	-	-	-	0.98
Pneumonia Care				
Appropriate Initial Antibiotic Given	24	67%	82%	95%
Blood Culture Timing	11	64%	82%	98%
Pregnancy and Delivery Care				
Newborn Deliveries Scheduled Early[5]	-	-	-	6%
Preventive Care				
Immunization for Influenza[5]	-	-	42%	90%
Immunization for Pneumonia[5]	-	-	29%	92%

NOTE: Hospital profiles are in alphabetical order by state, then city, then hospital within the city; Rankings exclude hospitals with less than 25 cases except for patient surveys which excludes hospitals with less than 100 cases; (a) 100-299 cases; (1) The number of cases/patients is too few to report; (2) Data submitted were based on a sample of cases/patients; (3) Results are based on a shorter time period than required; (4) Data suppressed by CMS for one or more quarters; (5) Results are not available for this reporting period; (6) Fewer than 100 patients completed the HCAHPS survey; (7) No cases met the criteria for this measure; (8) The lower limit of the confidence interval cannot be calculated if the number of observed infections equals zero; (9) No data are available from the state/territory for this reporting period; (10) The scores shown reflect fewer than 50 completed surveys; (11) There were discrepancies in the data collection process; (12) This measure does not apply to this hospital for this reporting period; (13) Results cannot be calculated for this reporting period; (14) The results for this state are combined with nearby states to protect confidentiality; Please refer to the User's Guide for a full explanation of data.

Stroke Care				
Anticoagulation Therapy for Atrial Fibrillation[5]	-	-	60%	95%
Antithrombotic Therapy Timing[5]	-	-	77%	98%
Assessed for Rehabilitation[5]	-	-	59%	97%
Discharged on Antithrombotic Therapy[5]	-	-	63%	99%
Discharged on Statin Medication[5]	-	-	90%	94%
Thrombolytic Therapy Timing[5]	-	-	-	66%
Venous Thromboembolism Prophylaxis[5]	-	-	52%	94%
Written Stroke Educational Materials Given[5]	-	-	95%	88%
Surgical Care Improvement Project				
Appropriate Beta Blocker Usage	22	86%	75%	98%
Appropriate VTP Within 24 Hours	40	82%	90%	98%
Controlled Postoperative Blood Glucose[7]	-	-	81%	97%
Perioperative Temperature Management	75	100%	98%	100%
Prophylactic Antibiotic Selection	28	96%	96%	99%
Prophylactic Antibiotic Selection (Outpatient)	-	-	-	98%
Prophylactic Antibiotic Stopped	28	71%	83%	98%
Prophylactic Antibiotic Timing	28	75%	89%	99%
Prophylactic Antibiotic Timing (Outpatient)	-	-	-	98%
Urinary Catheter Removal	36	92%	91%	97%
Survey of Patients' Hospital Experiences				
Area Around Room 'Always' Quiet at Night[5]	-	-	-	61%
Doctors 'Always' Communicated Well[5]	-	-	-	82%
Home Recovery Information Given[5]	-	-	-	85%
Hospital Given 9 or 10 on 10 Point Scale[5]	-	-	-	71%
Meds 'Always' Explained Before Given[5]	-	-	-	64%
Nurses 'Always' Communicated Well[5]	-	-	-	79%
Pain 'Always' Well Controlled[5]	-	-	-	71%
Room and Bathroom 'Always' Clean[5]	-	-	-	73%
Timely Help 'Always' Received[5]	-	-	-	68%
Would Definitely Recommend Hospital[5]	-	-	-	71%
Use of Medical Imaging				
Cardiac Imaging Stress Test before Surgery	-	-	4.5%	5.3%
Combination Abdominal CT Scan	-	-	7.4%	10.5%
Combination Brain/Sinus CT Scan	-	-	0.8%	2.7%
Combination Chest CT Scan	-	-	6.1%	2.7%
Follow-up Mammogram/Ultrasound	-	-	43.2%	8.8%
Lumbar Spine MRI for Low Back Pain	-	-	44.3%	37.2%

NOTE: Hospital profiles are in alphabetical order by state, then city, then hospital within the city; Rankings exclude hospitals with less than 25 cases except for patient surveys which excludes hospitals with less than 100 cases; (a) 100-299 cases; (1) The number of cases/patients is too few to report; (2) Data submitted were based on a sample of cases/patients; (3) Results are based on a shorter time period than required; (4) Data suppressed by CMS for one or more quarters; (5) Results are not available for this reporting period; (6) Fewer than 100 patients completed the HCAHPS survey; (7) No cases met the criteria for this measure; (8) The lower limit of the confidence interval cannot be calculated if the number of observed infections equals zero; (9) No data are available from the state/territory for this reporting period; (10) The scores shown reflect fewer than 50 completed surveys; (11) There were discrepancies in the data collection process; (12) This measure does not apply to this hospital for this reporting period; (13) Results cannot be calculated for this reporting period; (14) The results for this state are combined with nearby states to protect confidentiality; Please refer to the User's Guide for a full explanation of data.

Blood Clot Prevention and Treatment

Anticoagulation Overlap Therapy

Hospital Name	City	Rate	Cases
Beaufort County Memorial Hospital[2]	Beaufort	100%	63
Carolina Pines Regional Medical Center[2]	Hartsville	100%	25
Grand Strand Regional Medical Center[2]	Myrtle Beach	100%	91
Self Regional Healthcare[2]	Greenwood	100%	130
Trident Medical Center[2]	Charleston	100%	150
Musc Medical Center[2]	Charleston	98%	133
Roper Hospital[2]	Charleston	98%	84
Saint Francis - Downtown[2]	Greenville	98%	88
Springs Memorial Hospital[2]	Lancaster	98%	51
Baptist Easley Hospital[2]	Easley	97%	29
Hilton Head Regional Medical Center[2]	Hilton Head Isl	97%	62
Tuomey Healthcare System[2]	Sumter	97%	76
Bon Secours-St Francis Xavier Hosp[2]	Charleston	96%	57
Mary Black Memorial Hospital[2]	Spartanburg	96%	45
Waccamaw Community Hospital[2]	Murrells Inlet	96%	26
Mcleod Regional Medical Center - Pee Dee[2]	Florence	95%	103
Sisters of Charity Providence Hospitals[2]	Columbia	95%	108
GHS Greenville Memorial Medical Center[2]	Greenville	93%	180
Carolinas Hospital System[2]	Florence	92%	79
Colleton Medical Center[2]	Walterboro	92%	40
Lexington Medical Center[2]	West Columbia	92%	199
Palmetto Health Richland[2]	Columbia	92%	178
Aiken Regional Medical Center[2]	Aiken	91%	55
Palmetto Health Baptist[2]	Columbia	91%	95
Trmc of Orangeburg & Calhoun[2]	Orangeburg	90%	84
Anmed Health[2]	Anderson	88%	151
Piedmont Medical Center[2]	Rock Hill	88%	141
Oconee Medical Center[2]	Seneca	82%	34
Spartanburg Regional Medical Center[2]	Spartanburg	80%	172
Mcleod Loris Seacoast Hospital[2]	Loris	79%	42
Coastal Carolina Hospital[2]	Hardeeville	74%	43
Kershaw Health[2]	Camden	67%	36
Wallace Thomson Hospital[2]	Union	67%	27

ICU Venous Thromboembolism Prophylaxis

Hospital Name	City	Rate	Cases
Baptist Easley Hospital[2]	Easley	100%	105
Bon Secours-St Francis Xavier Hosp[2]	Charleston	100%	57
Chesterfield General Hospital[2]	Cheraw	100%	102
Coastal Carolina Hospital[2]	Hardeeville	100%	25
Marlboro Park Hospital[2]	Bennettsville	100%	35
Springs Memorial Hospital[2]	Lancaster	100%	107
Village Hospital[2]	Greer	100%	31
GHS Greer Memorial Hospital[2]	Greer	99%	74
Mcleod Regional Medical Center - Pee Dee[2]	Florence	99%	127
Roper Hospital[2]	Charleston	99%	97
Anmed Health[2]	Anderson	98%	98
Beaufort County Memorial Hospital[2]	Beaufort	98%	54
Conway Medical Center[2]	Conway	98%	47
Grand Strand Regional Medical Center[2]	Myrtle Beach	98%	107
Hilton Head Regional Medical Center[2]	Hilton Head Isl	98%	60
Trident Medical Center[2]	Charleston	98%	114
Cannon Memorial Hospital[2]	Pickens	97%	33
Palmetto Health Richland[2]	Columbia	97%	86
Saint Francis - Downtown[2]	Greenville	97%	219
Mary Black Memorial Hospital[2]	Spartanburg	96%	82
Mcleod Medical Center - Dillon[2]	Dillon	96%	73
Newberry County Memorial Hospital[2]	Newberry	96%	54
Novant Health Gaffney Medical Center[2]	Gaffney	96%	100
Carolinas Hospital System[2]	Florence	95%	130
GHS Laurens County Memorial Hospital[2]	Clinton	95%	60
Georgetown Memorial Hospital[2]	Georgetown	94%	49
GHS - Hillcrest Memorial Hospital[2]	Simpsonville	94%	51
Self Regional Healthcare[2]	Greenwood	94%	109
Trmc of Orangeburg & Calhoun[2]	Orangeburg	94%	65
Waccamaw Community Hospital[2]	Murrells Inlet	94%	32
East Cooper Medical Center[2]	Mount Pleasant	93%	43
Musc Medical Center[2]	Charleston	93%	95
Sisters of Charity Providence Hospitals[2]	Columbia	93%	124
Kershaw Health[2]	Camden	92%	71
Wallace Thomson Hospital[2]	Union	92%	64
GHS Greenville Memorial Medical Center[2]	Greenville	91%	127
Palmetto Health Baptist[2]	Columbia	91%	47
Carolina Pines Regional Medical Center[2]	Hartsville	90%	98
Mcleod Loris Seacoast Hospital[2]	Loris	90%	115
Lexington Medical Center[2]	West Columbia	89%	70
Spartanburg Regional Medical Center[2]	Spartanburg	89%	114
Aiken Regional Medical Center[2]	Aiken	87%	86
Tuomey Healthcare System[2]	Sumter	87%	69
Carolinas Hospital System Marion[2]	Mullins	86%	96
Piedmont Medical Center[2]	Rock Hill	86%	78
Colleton Medical Center[2]	Walterboro	85%	203
Oconee Medical Center[2]	Seneca	85%	48
Clarendon Memorial Hospital[2]	Manning	81%	37
Chester Regional Medical Center[2]	Chester	80%	50

Incidence of Potentially Preventable VTE

Hospital Name	City	Rate	Cases
Spartanburg Regional Medical Center[2]	Spartanburg	0%	32
Grand Strand Regional Medical Center[2]	Myrtle Beach	3%	30
Mcleod Regional Medical Center - Pee Dee[2]	Florence	3%	31
Musc Medical Center[2]	Charleston	3%	98
Trident Medical Center[2]	Charleston	3%	34
GHS Greenville Memorial Medical Center[2]	Greenville	8%	61
Self Regional Healthcare[2]	Greenwood	8%	26
Palmetto Health Richland[2]	Columbia	18%	56
Lexington Medical Center[2]	West Columbia	20%	30

UFH with Dosages/Platelet Count Monitoring

Hospital Name	City	Rate	Cases
Anmed Health[2]	Anderson	100%	42
Beaufort County Memorial Hospital[2]	Beaufort	100%	48
Bon Secours-St Francis Xavier Hosp[2]	Charleston	100%	25
GHS Greenville Memorial Medical Center[2]	Greenville	100%	156
Grand Strand Regional Medical Center[2]	Myrtle Beach	100%	74
Lexington Medical Center[2]	West Columbia	100%	78
Mary Black Memorial Hospital[2]	Spartanburg	100%	46
Mcleod Regional Medical Center - Pee Dee[2]	Florence	100%	47
Palmetto Health Baptist[2]	Columbia	100%	44
Palmetto Health Richland[2]	Columbia	100%	103
Piedmont Medical Center[2]	Rock Hill	100%	57
Roper Hospital[2]	Charleston	100%	81
Self Regional Healthcare[2]	Greenwood	100%	44
Sisters of Charity Providence Hospitals[2]	Columbia	100%	55
Springs Memorial Hospital[2]	Lancaster	100%	35
Trident Medical Center[2]	Charleston	100%	41
Musc Medical Center[2]	Charleston	99%	92
Spartanburg Regional Medical Center[2]	Spartanburg	99%	148
Saint Francis - Downtown[2]	Greenville	98%	55
Trmc of Orangeburg & Calhoun[2]	Orangeburg	73%	51

Venous Thromboembolism Prophylaxis

Hospital Name	City	Rate	Cases
Newberry County Memorial Hospital[2]	Newberry	100%	128
Springs Memorial Hospital[2]	Lancaster	100%	378
Chesterfield General Hospital[2]	Cheraw	99%	359
Marlboro Park Hospital[2]	Bennettsville	99%	314
Mount Pleasant Hospital[2]	Mount Pleasant	99%	91
Anmed Health[2]	Anderson	98%	347
Bon Secours-St Francis Xavier Hosp[2]	Charleston	98%	347
GHS - Hillcrest Memorial Hospital[2]	Simpsonville	98%	178
Mcleod Regional Medical Center - Pee Dee[2]	Florence	98%	291
Village Hospital[2]	Greer	98%	150
GHS Greer Memorial Hospital[2]	Greer	97%	206
Hilton Head Regional Medical Center[2]	Hilton Head Isl	97%	352
Mary Black Memorial Hospital[2]	Spartanburg	97%	348
Baptist Easley Hospital[2]	Easley	96%	384
Roper Hospital[2]	Charleston	96%	284
Trident Medical Center[2]	Charleston	96%	362
Coastal Carolina Hospital[2]	Hardeeville	95%	197
Mcleod Medical Center - Dillon[2]	Dillon	95%	151
Novant Health Gaffney Medical Center[2]	Gaffney	94%	179
Cannon Memorial Hospital[2]	Pickens	93%	72
East Cooper Medical Center[2]	Mount Pleasant	93%	266
Spartanburg Regional Medical Center[2]	Spartanburg	93%	347
Waccamaw Community Hospital[2]	Murrells Inlet	93%	323
Wallace Thomson Hospital[2]	Union	93%	187
Grand Strand Regional Medical Center[2]	Myrtle Beach	92%	343
Palmetto Health Baptist[2]	Columbia	92%	409
Saint Francis - Downtown[2]	Greenville	92%	724
Aiken Regional Medical Center[2]	Aiken	91%	350
Beaufort County Memorial Hospital[2]	Beaufort	91%	386
Conway Medical Center[2]	Conway	89%	324
Self Regional Healthcare[2]	Greenwood	89%	271
Georgetown Memorial Hospital[2]	Georgetown	88%	352
Kershaw Health[2]	Camden	88%	368
Carolinas Hospital System[2]	Florence	87%	484
Mcleod Medical Center - Darlington	Darlington	87%	91
GHS Greenville Memorial Medical Center[2]	Greenville	86%	315
Mcleod Loris Seacoast Hospital[2]	Loris	86%	259
Colleton Medical Center[2]	Walterboro	85%	771
Lexington Medical Center[2]	West Columbia	84%	350
Piedmont Medical Center[2]	Rock Hill	83%	368
Sisters of Charity Providence Hospitals[2]	Columbia	81%	300
Musc Medical Center[2]	Charleston	80%	306
Carolinas Hospital System Marion[2]	Mullins	78%	237
GHS Laurens County Memorial Hospital[2]	Clinton	78%	216
Palmetto Health Richland[2]	Columbia	77%	391
Trmc of Orangeburg & Calhoun[2]	Orangeburg	77%	363
Oconee Medical Center[2]	Seneca	75%	329
Chester Regional Medical Center[2]	Chester	74%	144
Hampton Regional Medical Center[2]	Varnville	73%	112
Tuomey Healthcare System[2]	Sumter	69%	368
Carolina Pines Regional Medical Center[2]	Hartsville	66%	317
Clarendon Memorial Hospital[2]	Manning	65%	165
Lake City Community Hospital[2]	Lake City	54%	109
Barnwell County Hospital[2]	Barnwell	52%	114

Warfarin Therapy Discharge Instructions

Hospital Name	City	Rate	Cases
Colleton Medical Center[2]	Walterboro	100%	36
Saint Francis - Downtown[2]	Greenville	100%	59
Springs Memorial Hospital[2]	Lancaster	100%	44
Anmed Health[2]	Anderson	99%	104
Trident Medical Center[2]	Charleston	99%	109
Aiken Regional Medical Center[2]	Aiken	97%	36
Grand Strand Regional Medical Center[2]	Myrtle Beach	97%	70
Carolinas Hospital System[2]	Florence	96%	53
Lexington Medical Center[2]	West Columbia	96%	152
Sisters of Charity Providence Hospitals[2]	Columbia	93%	71
Beaufort County Memorial Hospital[2]	Beaufort	92%	49
Hilton Head Regional Medical Center[2]	Hilton Head Isl	92%	49
Bon Secours-St Francis Xavier Hosp[2]	Charleston	89%	44
Mary Black Memorial Hospital[2]	Spartanburg	88%	26
Roper Hospital[2]	Charleston	88%	64
Palmetto Health Baptist[2]	Columbia	86%	72
Mcleod Regional Medical Center - Pee Dee[2]	Florence	85%	65
Self Regional Healthcare[2]	Greenwood	75%	103
Tuomey Healthcare System[2]	Sumter	74%	70
Mcleod Loris Seacoast Hospital[2]	Loris	72%	29
Piedmont Medical Center[2]	Rock Hill	70%	103
Musc Medical Center[2]	Charleston	67%	103
Trmc of Orangeburg & Calhoun[2]	Orangeburg	67%	70
Coastal Carolina Hospital[2]	Hardeeville	53%	36
Palmetto Health Richland[2]	Columbia	49%	133
GHS Greenville Memorial Medical Center[2]	Greenville	4%	138
Spartanburg Regional Medical Center[2]	Spartanburg	0%	140

Chest Pain/Possible Heart Attack Care

Aspirin Given Within 24 Hours of Arrival

Hospital Name	City	Rate	Cases
Baptist Easley Hospital	Easley	100%	96
Beaufort County Memorial Hospital	Beaufort	100%	55
Cannon Memorial Hospital	Pickens	100%	38
Chester Regional Medical Center	Chester	100%	60
Colleton Medical Center	Walterboro	100%	45
Conway Medical Center	Conway	100%	76
GHS Greer Memorial Hospital	Greer	100%	94
Kershaw Health	Camden	100%	43
Mount Pleasant Hospital	Mount Pleasant	100%	26
Oconee Medical Center	Seneca	100%	73
Springs Memorial Hospital	Lancaster	100%	67
Wallace Thomson Hospital	Union	100%	33
Bon Secours-St Francis Xavier Hosp	Charleston	99%	75
GHS - Hillcrest Memorial Hospital	Simpsonville	99%	82
GHS Laurens County Memorial Hospital	Clinton	99%	69
Mcleod Medical Center - Dillon	Dillon	99%	94
Trmc of Orangeburg & Calhoun	Orangeburg	99%	99
Carolina Pines Regional Medical Center	Hartsville	98%	95
Chesterfield General Hospital	Cheraw	97%	37
East Cooper Medical Center	Mount Pleasant	97%	39
Novant Health Gaffney Medical Center	Gaffney	97%	61
Waccamaw Community Hospital	Murrells Inlet	97%	32
Tuomey Healthcare System	Sumter	96%	150
Carolinas Hospital System Marion	Mullins	95%	74
Newberry County Memorial Hospital	Newberry	95%	38
Mary Black Memorial Hospital	Spartanburg	94%	36
Mcleod Loris Seacoast Hospital	Loris	93%	86
Barnwell County Hospital	Barnwell	92%	36
Hampton Regional Medical Center	Varnville	89%	45
Clarendon Memorial Hospital	Manning	82%	91

Average Time to ECG (minutes)

Hospital Name	City	Min.	Cases
Baptist Easley Hospital	Easley	1	97
Chesterfield General Hospital	Cheraw	1	39
Conway Medical Center	Conway	1	76
GHS - Hillcrest Memorial Hospital	Simpsonville	1	83
Springs Memorial Hospital	Lancaster	1	69
Trmc of Orangeburg & Calhoun	Orangeburg	1	101
Carolina Pines Regional Medical Center	Hartsville	2	102
Novant Health Gaffney Medical Center	Gaffney	2	68
Beaufort County Memorial Hospital	Beaufort	3	55
Chester Regional Medical Center	Chester	3	64
East Cooper Medical Center	Mount Pleasant	3	40
GHS Greer Memorial Hospital	Greer	3	95
Cannon Memorial Hospital	Pickens	4	38
Mary Black Memorial Hospital	Spartanburg	4	35
Mcleod Medical Center - Dillon	Dillon	4	93
Mount Pleasant Hospital	Mount Pleasant	4	29
Colleton Medical Center	Walterboro	5	47
Newberry County Memorial Hospital	Newberry	5	37
Kershaw Health	Camden	6	44

NOTE: Hospital profiles are in alphabetical order by state, then city, then hospital within the city; Rankings exclude hospitals with less than 25 cases except for patient surveys which excludes hospitals with less than 100 cases; (a) 100-299 cases; (1) The number of cases/patients is too few to report; (2) Data submitted were based on a sample of cases/patients; (3) Results are based on a shorter time period than required; (4) Data suppressed by CMS for one or more quarters; (5) Results are not available for this reporting period; (6) Fewer than 100 patients completed the HCAHPS survey; (7) No cases met the criteria for this measure; (8) The lower limit of the confidence interval cannot be calculated if the number of observed infections equals zero; (9) No data are available from the state/territory for this reporting period; (10) The scores shown reflect fewer than 50 completed surveys; (11) There were discrepancies in the data collection process; (12) This measure does not apply to this hospital for this reporting period; (13) Results cannot be calculated for this reporting period; (14) The results for this state are combined with nearby states to protect confidentiality; Please refer to the User's Guide for a full explanation of data.

Hospital Name	City	Min.	Cases
Waccamaw Community Hospital	Murrells Inlet	7	33
Abbeville Area Medical Center	Abbeville	8	25
Bon Secours-St Francis Xavier Hosp	Charleston	8	79
Tuomey Healthcare System	Sumter	9	156
Hampton Regional Medical Center	Varnville	10	47
Mcleod Loris Seacoast Hospital	Loris	10	87
Oconee Medical Center	Seneca	10	73
Clarendon Memorial Hospital	Manning	17	91
GHS Laurens County Memorial Hospital	Clinton	18	68
Wallace Thomson Hospital	Union	23	37
Carolinas Hospital System Marion	Mullins	26	76
Barnwell County Hospital	Barnwell	36	33

Average Time to Transfer (minutes)

Hospital Name	City	Min.	Cases
Novant Health Gaffney Medical Center	Gaffney	44	27

Children's Asthma Care

Received Home Management Plan of Care

Hospital Name	City	Rate	Cases
Musc Medical Center	Charleston	97%	173

Received Reliever Medication

Hospital Name	City	Rate	Cases
Musc Medical Center	Charleston	100%	173

Received Systemic Corticosteroids

Hospital Name	City	Rate	Cases
Musc Medical Center	Charleston	99%	171

Emergency Department

Admittance Decision Time (minutes)

Hospital Name	City	Min.	Cases
Mcleod Medical Center - Dillon[2]	Dillon	36	258
Abbeville Area Medical Center[2]	Abbeville	45	245
Baptist Easley Hospital[2]	Easley	49	552
Barnwell County Hospital[2]	Barnwell	50	320
Chesterfield General Hospital[2]	Cheraw	51	674
Colleton Medical Center[2]	Walterboro	52	599
Marlboro Park Hospital[2]	Bennettsville	54	574
Hampton Regional Medical Center	Varnville	55	371
East Cooper Medical Center[2]	Mount Pleasant	56	263
Mcleod Loris Seacoast Hospital[2]	Loris	56	610
Springs Memorial Hospital[2]	Lancaster	56	828
Chester Regional Medical Center[2]	Chester	63	525
Lake City Community Hospital[2]	Lake City	70	304
Newberry County Memorial Hospital[2]	Newberry	73	272
Mount Pleasant Hospital[2]	Mount Pleasant	76	227
Waccamaw Community Hospital[2]	Murrells Inlet	76	592
Oconee Medical Center[2]	Seneca	77	782
Wallace Thomson Hospital[2]	Union	77	362
Cannon Memorial Hospital[2]	Pickens	78	398
Roper Hospital[2]	Charleston	82	539
Trmc of Orangeburg & Calhoun[2]	Orangeburg	83	747
Georgetown Memorial Hospital[2]	Georgetown	85	641
Palmetto Health Baptist[2]	Columbia	85	325
Tuomey Healthcare System[2]	Sumter	85	537
Anmed Health[2]	Anderson	88	687
Clarendon Memorial Hospital[2]	Manning	95	269
Conway Medical Center[2]	Conway	96	581
Carolina Pines Regional Medical Center[2]	Hartsville	97	555
Bon Secours-St Francis Xavier Hosp[2]	Charleston	98	412
Kershaw Health[2]	Camden	98	566
Carolinas Hospital System Marion[2]	Mullins	100	406
Novant Health Gaffney Medical Center[2]	Gaffney	100	481
GHS Greer Memorial Hospital[2]	Greer	102	368
Saint Francis - Downtown[2]	Greenville	103	549
Trident Medical Center[2]	Charleston	107	750
Musc Medical Center[2]	Charleston	108	358
GHS - Hillcrest Memorial Hospital[2]	Simpsonville	111	312
Carolinas Hospital System[2]	Florence	112	592
Self Regional Healthcare[2]	Greenwood	116	575
GHS Laurens County Memorial Hospital[2]	Clinton	120	278
Palmetto Health Richland[2]	Columbia	120	559
Grand Strand Regional Medical Center[2]	Myrtle Beach	121	881
Village Hospital[2]	Greer	125	463
Coastal Carolina Hospital[2]	Hardeeville	128	647
Aiken Regional Medical Center[2]	Aiken	134	508
Beaufort County Memorial Hospital[2]	Beaufort	144	675
Mary Black Memorial Hospital[2]	Spartanburg	149	625
Mcleod Regional Medical Center - Pee Dee[2]	Florence	162	526
Piedmont Medical Center[2]	Rock Hill	163	646
GHS Greenville Memorial Medical Center[2]	Greenville	165	401
Sisters of Charity Providence Hospitals[2]	Columbia	165	479
Hilton Head Regional Medical Center[2]	Hilton Head Isl	166	662
Lexington Medical Center[2]	West Columbia	174	365
Spartanburg Regional Medical Center[2]	Spartanburg	196	648

Head CT Results Within 45 Minutes of Arrival

Hospital Name	City	Rate	Cases
Sisters of Charity Providence Hospitals	Columbia	54%	28
Tuomey Healthcare System	Sumter	42%	26
Self Regional Healthcare	Greenwood	24%	34

Patients Who Left ER Before Being Seen

Hospital Name	City	Rate	Cases
Bon Secours-St Francis Xavier Hosp	Charleston	0%	45604
East Cooper Medical Center	Mount Pleasant	0%	15261
Mount Pleasant Hospital	Mount Pleasant	0%	11528
Abbeville Area Medical Center	Abbeville	1%	11897
Coastal Carolina Hospital	Hardeeville	1%	19382
Colleton Medical Center	Walterboro	1%	26681
Conway Medical Center	Conway	1%	48961
Grand Strand Regional Medical Center	Myrtle Beach	1%	78289
Hilton Head Regional Medical Center	Hilton Head Isl	1%	22912
Marlboro Park Hospital	Bennettsville	1%	13912
Roper Hospital	Charleston	1%	70083
Trident Medical Center	Charleston	1%	108047
Baptist Easley Hospital	Easley	2%	45690
Beaufort County Memorial Hospital	Beaufort	2%	41919
Cannon Memorial Hospital	Pickens	2%	20792
Carolina Pines Regional Medical Center	Hartsville	2%	32757
Carolinas Hospital System	Florence	2%	39471
Carolinas Hospital System Marion	Mullins	2%	21089
Chesterfield General Hospital	Cheraw	2%	12814
GHS - Hillcrest Memorial Hospital	Simpsonville	2%	30710
GHS Greer Memorial Hospital	Greer	2%	33606
Hampton Regional Medical Center	Varnville	2%	12215
Kershaw Health	Camden	2%	28467
Lexington Medical Center	West Columbia	2%	109559
Mcleod Medical Center - Dillon	Dillon	2%	28657
Novant Health Gaffney Medical Center	Gaffney	2%	36468
Oconee Medical Center	Seneca	2%	40285
Saint Francis - Downtown	Greenville	2%	80204
Trmc of Orangeburg & Calhoun	Orangeburg	2%	60567
Waccamaw Community Hospital	Murrells Inlet	2%	30738
Chester Regional Medical Center	Chester	3%	19449
GHS Greenville Memorial Medical Center	Greenville	3%	100766
GHS Laurens County Memorial Hospital	Clinton	3%	29443
Lake City Community Hospital	Lake City	3%	16814
Musc Medical Center	Charleston	3%	51739
Newberry County Memorial Hospital	Newberry	3%	21750
Piedmont Medical Center	Rock Hill	3%	67661
Springs Memorial Hospital	Lancaster	3%	36613
Tuomey Healthcare System	Sumter	3%	63090
Wallace Thomson Hospital	Union	3%	17546
Aiken Regional Medical Center	Aiken	4%	51471
Georgetown Memorial Hospital	Georgetown	4%	30890
Mary Black Memorial Hospital	Spartanburg	4%	39090
Palmetto Health Baptist	Columbia	4%	46648
Self Regional Healthcare	Greenwood	4%	48915
Village Hospital	Greer	4%	21260
Anmed Health	Anderson	5%	94610
Barnwell County Hospital	Barnwell	5%	12062
Mcleod Loris Seacoast Hospital	Loris	5%	45632
Mcleod Regional Medical Center - Pee Dee	Florence	5%	61428
Sisters of Charity Providence Hospitals	Columbia	5%	64608
Clarendon Memorial Hospital	Manning	6%	19353
Palmetto Health Richland	Columbia	9%	89440
Spartanburg Regional Medical Center	Spartanburg	9%	103738

Time from ER Arrival to Being Admitted (minutes)

Hospital Name	City	Min.	Cases
Mount Pleasant Hospital[2]	Mount Pleasant	196	230
Chesterfield General Hospital[2]	Cheraw	199	677
Marlboro Park Hospital[2]	Bennettsville	203	592
Roper Hospital[2]	Charleston	203	556
Abbeville Area Medical Center[2]	Abbeville	208	245
East Cooper Medical Center[2]	Mount Pleasant	215	263
Springs Memorial Hospital[2]	Lancaster	215	838
Wallace Thomson Hospital[2]	Union	216	374
Mcleod Loris Seacoast Hospital[2]	Loris	222	610
Chester Regional Medical Center[2]	Chester	223	529
Cannon Memorial Hospital[2]	Pickens	224	400
Conway Medical Center[2]	Conway	229	581
Oconee Medical Center[2]	Seneca	233	783
Mcleod Medical Center - Dillon[2]	Dillon	236	276
Waccamaw Community Hospital[2]	Murrells Inlet	242	606
Carolina Pines Regional Medical Center[2]	Hartsville	246	556
Colleton Medical Center[2]	Walterboro	248	599
Baptist Easley Hospital[2]	Easley	250	618
Newberry County Memorial Hospital[2]	Newberry	254	285
Lake City Community Hospital[2]	Lake City	255	305
Trmc of Orangeburg & Calhoun[2]	Orangeburg	256	756
Georgetown Memorial Hospital[2]	Georgetown	258	657
Hampton Regional Medical Center	Varnville	259	391
Kershaw Health[2]	Camden	261	566
Trident Medical Center[2]	Charleston	272	750
Musc Medical Center[2]	Charleston	273	375
Saint Francis - Downtown[2]	Greenville	273	565
Grand Strand Regional Medical Center[2]	Myrtle Beach	277	881
Carolinas Hospital System Marion[2]	Mullins	282	414
Bon Secours-St Francis Xavier Hosp[2]	Charleston	284	430
Carolinas Hospital System[2]	Florence	286	611
Tuomey Healthcare System[2]	Sumter	286	546
Self Regional Healthcare[2]	Greenwood	288	578
Coastal Carolina Hospital[2]	Hardeeville	300	660
Novant Health Gaffney Medical Center[2]	Gaffney	300	481
Village Hospital[2]	Greer	305	467
GHS Laurens County Memorial Hospital[2]	Clinton	306	323
Clarendon Memorial Hospital[2]	Manning	309	281
Barnwell County Hospital[2]	Barnwell	310	324
GHS - Hillcrest Memorial Hospital[2]	Simpsonville	316	316
Sisters of Charity Providence Hospitals[2]	Columbia	317	495
GHS Greer Memorial Hospital[2]	Greer	322	370
Piedmont Medical Center[2]	Rock Hill	324	651
Anmed Health[2]	Anderson	332	696
Hilton Head Regional Medical Center[2]	Hilton Head Isl	341	677
Aiken Regional Medical Center[2]	Aiken	342	527
Beaufort County Memorial Hospital[2]	Beaufort	344	676
Lexington Medical Center[2]	West Columbia	347	380
Mary Black Memorial Hospital[2]	Spartanburg	356	635
GHS Greenville Memorial Medical Center[2]	Greenville	357	411
Palmetto Health Baptist[2]	Columbia	366	352
Mcleod Regional Medical Center - Pee Dee[2]	Florence	376	535
Spartanburg Regional Medical Center[2]	Spartanburg	382	653
Palmetto Health Richland[2]	Columbia	422	586

Time from ER Arrival to Discharge (minutes)

Hospital Name	City	Min.	Cases
Lake City Community Hospital	Lake City	84	383
Cannon Memorial Hospital	Pickens	88	375
Chesterfield General Hospital	Cheraw	88	418
Wallace Thomson Hospital	Union	92	370
Mount Pleasant Hospital	Mount Pleasant	94	393
East Cooper Medical Center	Mount Pleasant	95	359
Marlboro Park Hospital	Bennettsville	95	410
Newberry County Memorial Hospital	Newberry	99	360
Roper Hospital	Charleston	99	389
Chester Regional Medical Center	Chester	105	589
Novant Health Gaffney Medical Center	Gaffney	113	456
Abbeville Area Medical Center	Abbeville	118	160
Colleton Medical Center	Walterboro	120	437
Grand Strand Regional Medical Center	Myrtle Beach	122	436
Coastal Carolina Hospital	Hardeeville	123	415
GHS Laurens County Memorial Hospital	Clinton	124	363
Mcleod Loris Seacoast Hospital	Loris	125	367
Trident Medical Center	Charleston	126	459
Village Hospital	Greer	126	441
Carolina Pines Regional Medical Center	Hartsville	128	423
Conway Medical Center	Conway	129	381
Baptist Easley Hospital	Easley	133	365
GHS - Hillcrest Memorial Hospital	Simpsonville	134	372
Aiken Regional Medical Center	Aiken	135	403
Carolinas Hospital System	Florence	135	371
Carolinas Hospital System Marion	Mullins	135	377
Oconee Medical Center	Seneca	138	343
Sisters of Charity Providence Hospitals	Columbia	138	395
Hampton Regional Medical Center	Varnville	140	368
Hilton Head Regional Medical Center	Hilton Head Isl	140	450
Mcleod Medical Center - Dillon	Dillon	142	307
Mary Black Memorial Hospital	Spartanburg	144	403
Kershaw Health	Camden	146	382
Springs Memorial Hospital	Lancaster	146	381
Trmc of Orangeburg & Calhoun	Orangeburg	150	448
Beaufort County Memorial Hospital	Beaufort	152	436
Tuomey Healthcare System	Sumter	153	369
Waccamaw Community Hospital	Murrells Inlet	154	376
Barnwell County Hospital	Barnwell	155	321
Georgetown Memorial Hospital	Georgetown	155	383
Saint Francis - Downtown	Greenville	155	1286
GHS Greer Memorial Hospital	Greer	158	376
Bon Secours-St Francis Xavier Hosp	Charleston	160	396
Musc Medical Center	Charleston	165	504
Palmetto Health Baptist	Columbia	165	409
Lexington Medical Center	West Columbia	168	332
Piedmont Medical Center	Rock Hill	175	331
Spartanburg Regional Medical Center	Spartanburg	178	377
GHS Greenville Memorial Medical Center	Greenville	188	345
Palmetto Health Richland	Columbia	189	384
Clarendon Memorial Hospital	Manning	192	411
Mcleod Regional Medical Center - Pee Dee	Florence	192	328
Self Regional Healthcare	Greenwood	195	360
Anmed Health	Anderson	244	351

NOTE: Hospital profiles are in alphabetical order by state, then city, then hospital within the city; Rankings exclude hospitals with less than 25 cases except for patient surveys which excludes hospitals with less than 100 cases; (a) 100-299 cases; (1) The number of cases/patients is too few to report; (2) Data submitted were based on a sample of cases/patients; (3) Results are based on a shorter time period than required; (4) Data suppressed by CMS for one or more quarters; (5) Results are not available for this reporting period; (6) Fewer than 100 patients completed the HCAHPS survey; (7) No cases met the criteria for this measure; (8) The lower limit of the confidence interval cannot be calculated if the number of observed infections equals zero; (9) No data are available from the state/territory for this reporting period; (10) The scores shown reflect fewer than 50 completed surveys; (11) There were discrepancies in the data collection process; (12) This measure does not apply to this hospital for this reporting period; (13) Results cannot be calculated for this reporting period; (14) The results for this state are combined with nearby states to protect confidentiality; Please refer to the User's Guide for a full explanation of data.

Time in ER Before Being Evaluated (minutes)

Hospital Name	City	Min.	Cases
Chesterfield General Hospital	Cheraw	6	511
Mount Pleasant Hospital	Mount Pleasant	10	413
East Cooper Medical Center	Mount Pleasant	12	380
Colleton Medical Center	Walterboro	13	515
Grand Strand Regional Medical Center	Myrtle Beach	16	486
Trident Medical Center	Charleston	16	521
Roper Hospital	Charleston	18	383
Beaufort County Memorial Hospital	Beaufort	19	506
Marlboro Park Hospital	Bennettsville	19	464
Palmetto Health Richland	Columbia	20	400
Hilton Head Regional Medical Center	Hilton Head Isl	23	472
Novant Health Gaffney Medical Center	Gaffney	23	473
Conway Medical Center	Conway	24	417
Wallace Thomson Hospital	Union	24	393
Newberry County Memorial Hospital	Newberry	25	336
Abbeville Area Medical Center	Abbeville	26	193
Springs Memorial Hospital	Lancaster	26	417
Coastal Carolina Hospital	Hardeeville	27	435
Baptist Easley Hospital	Easley	28	384
Mcleod Loris Seacoast Hospital	Loris	29	384
Lexington Medical Center	West Columbia	30	334
Hampton Regional Medical Center	Varnville	31	359
Saint Francis - Downtown	Greenville	33	1326
Palmetto Health Baptist	Columbia	34	357
Cannon Memorial Hospital	Pickens	35	409
Georgetown Memorial Hospital	Georgetown	36	349
Musc Medical Center	Charleston	36	487
Piedmont Medical Center	Rock Hill	36	365
Carolinas Hospital System	Florence	37	402
Carolina Pines Regional Medical Center	Hartsville	39	454
Carolinas Hospital System Marion	Mullins	39	413
Sisters of Charity Providence Hospitals	Columbia	39	419
Waccamaw Community Hospital	Murrells Inlet	39	379
Barnwell County Hospital	Barnwell	40	366
Bon Secours-St Francis Xavier Hosp	Charleston	40	406
Lake City Community Hospital	Lake City	40	385
Village Hospital	Greer	42	438
Mcleod Medical Center - Dillon	Dillon	43	375
Kershaw Health	Camden	44	404
Mary Black Memorial Hospital	Spartanburg	45	418
Chester Regional Medical Center	Chester	47	641
Trmc of Orangeburg & Calhoun	Orangeburg	48	304
GHS Laurens County Memorial Hospital	Clinton	49	387
Aiken Regional Medical Center	Aiken	58	416
GHS Greer Memorial Hospital	Greer	66	380
Self Regional Healthcare	Greenwood	66	398
Clarendon Memorial Hospital	Manning	68	440
Oconee Medical Center	Seneca	68	344
GHS - Hillcrest Memorial Hospital	Simpsonville	69	353
Spartanburg Regional Medical Center	Spartanburg	72	410
Mcleod Regional Medical Center - Pee Dee	Florence	76	367
GHS Greenville Memorial Medical Center	Greenville	79	357
Anmed Health	Anderson	88	362

Time to Pain Meds for Bone Fractures (minutes)

Hospital Name	City	Min.	Cases
East Cooper Medical Center	Mount Pleasant	26	64
GHS Greenville Memorial Medical Center	Greenville	28	341
Mount Pleasant Hospital	Mount Pleasant	36	31
Coastal Carolina Hospital	Hardeeville	42	68
Marlboro Park Hospital	Bennettsville	47	52
Baptist Easley Hospital	Easley	48	128
Newberry County Memorial Hospital	Newberry	48	87
Beaufort County Memorial Hospital	Beaufort	50	122
Carolinas Hospital System	Florence	50	73
Mcleod Loris Seacoast Hospital	Loris	50	142
Colleton Medical Center	Walterboro	52	59
Lexington Medical Center	West Columbia	53	247
Sisters of Charity Providence Hospitals	Columbia	53	131
GHS Greer Memorial Hospital	Greer	54	131
Hilton Head Regional Medical Center	Hilton Head Isl	54	81
Oconee Medical Center	Seneca	54	150
Conway Medical Center	Conway	55	162
Roper Hospital	Charleston	55	78
Village Hospital	Greer	55	114
Waccamaw Community Hospital	Murrells Inlet	57	56
Springs Memorial Hospital	Lancaster	58	155
Novant Health Gaffney Medical Center	Gaffney	59	91
Hampton Regional Medical Center	Varnville	60	36
Trident Medical Center	Charleston	60	219
Lake City Community Hospital	Lake City	61	34
Mcleod Medical Center - Dillon	Dillon	61	91
Palmetto Health Baptist	Columbia	61	38
Spartanburg Regional Medical Center	Spartanburg	61	205
Chester Regional Medical Center	Chester	63	61
Grand Strand Regional Medical Center	Myrtle Beach	63	197
Saint Francis - Downtown	Greenville	63	155
Carolina Pines Regional Medical Center	Hartsville	64	65
Carolinas Hospital System Marion	Mullins	64	69
GHS - Hillcrest Memorial Hospital	Simpsonville	64	105
Bon Secours-St Francis Xavier Hosp	Charleston	66	86
Wallace Thomson Hospital	Union	66	71
Trmc of Orangeburg & Calhoun	Orangeburg	67	119
Cannon Memorial Hospital	Pickens	69	55
Musc Medical Center	Charleston	70	237
Palmetto Health Richland	Columbia	73	249
Chesterfield General Hospital	Cheraw	74	60
Kershaw Health	Camden	75	112
Piedmont Medical Center	Rock Hill	76	214
Georgetown Memorial Hospital	Georgetown	77	47
Aiken Regional Medical Center	Aiken	78	110
Mary Black Memorial Hospital	Spartanburg	79	91
Anmed Health	Anderson	80	43
Mcleod Regional Medical Center - Pee Dee	Florence	81	147
GHS Laurens County Memorial Hospital	Clinton	82	78
Self Regional Healthcare	Greenwood	92	164
Tuomey Healthcare System	Sumter	92	70
Clarendon Memorial Hospital	Manning	103	74
Barnwell County Hospital	Barnwell	110	42

Heart Attack Care

Aspirin Given at Discharge

Hospital Name	City	Rate	Cases
Anmed Health	Anderson	100%	259
Beaufort County Memorial Hospital	Beaufort	100%	32
Carolinas Hospital System	Florence	100%	220
Charleston VA Medical Center	Charleston	100%	49
Georgetown Memorial Hospital[2]	Georgetown	100%	86
GHS Greenville Memorial Medical Center	Greenville	100%	750
Grand Strand Regional Medical Center[2]	Myrtle Beach	100%	299
Hilton Head Regional Medical Center	Hilton Head Isl	100%	118
Lexington Medical Center[2]	West Columbia	100%	270
Mcleod Regional Medical Center - Pee Dee	Florence	100%	615
Oconee Medical Center	Seneca	100%	32
Roper Hospital	Charleston	100%	334
Saint Francis - Downtown[2]	Greenville	100%	334
Sisters of Charity Providence Hospitals[2]	Columbia	100%	317
Spartanburg Regional Medical Center	Spartanburg	100%	653
Springs Memorial Hospital	Lancaster	100%	25
Trident Medical Center	Charleston	100%	379
Tuomey Healthcare System	Sumter	100%	43
Waccamaw Community Hospital[2]	Murrells Inlet	100%	35
Aiken Regional Medical Center	Aiken	99%	156
Musc Medical Center	Charleston	99%	368
Palmetto Health Richland	Columbia	99%	489
Piedmont Medical Center	Rock Hill	99%	412
Self Regional Healthcare	Greenwood	99%	290
Kershaw Health	Camden	98%	43
Trmc of Orangeburg & Calhoun	Orangeburg	97%	60
Mcleod Medical Center - Dillon	Dillon	96%	25
Carolinas Hospital System Marion	Mullins	95%	74
Mcleod Loris Seacoast Hospital	Loris	86%	37

PCI Within 90 Minutes of Arrival

Hospital Name	City	Rate	Cases
Anmed Health	Anderson	100%	88
GHS Greenville Memorial Medical Center	Greenville	100%	146
Grand Strand Regional Medical Center[2]	Myrtle Beach	100%	72
Roper Hospital	Charleston	100%	36
Saint Francis - Downtown[2]	Greenville	100%	56
Trident Medical Center	Charleston	99%	81
Musc Medical Center	Charleston	98%	42
Hilton Head Regional Medical Center	Hilton Head Isl	97%	35
Self Regional Healthcare	Greenwood	97%	36
Palmetto Health Richland	Columbia	96%	89
Spartanburg Regional Medical Center	Spartanburg	96%	142
Piedmont Medical Center	Rock Hill	95%	63
Aiken Regional Medical Center	Aiken	94%	33
Mcleod Regional Medical Center - Pee Dee	Florence	93%	45
Sisters of Charity Providence Hospitals[2]	Columbia	90%	29
Lexington Medical Center[2]	West Columbia	81%	63

Statin Prescribed at Discharge

Hospital Name	City	Rate	Cases
Anmed Health	Anderson	100%	254
Beaufort County Memorial Hospital	Beaufort	100%	36
Carolinas Hospital System	Florence	100%	219
Charleston VA Medical Center	Charleston	100%	49
Georgetown Memorial Hospital[2]	Georgetown	100%	82
Hilton Head Regional Medical Center	Hilton Head Isl	100%	116
Lexington Medical Center[2]	West Columbia	100%	261
Mcleod Loris Seacoast Hospital	Loris	100%	35
Piedmont Medical Center	Rock Hill	100%	400
Roper Hospital	Charleston	100%	330
Saint Francis - Downtown[2]	Greenville	100%	320
Sisters of Charity Providence Hospitals[2]	Columbia	100%	285
Trident Medical Center	Charleston	100%	371
GHS Greenville Memorial Medical Center	Greenville	99%	743
Grand Strand Regional Medical Center[2]	Myrtle Beach	99%	288
Mcleod Regional Medical Center - Pee Dee	Florence	99%	576
Musc Medical Center	Charleston	99%	363
Palmetto Health Richland	Columbia	99%	476
Spartanburg Regional Medical Center	Spartanburg	99%	641
Trmc of Orangeburg & Calhoun	Orangeburg	97%	60
Carolinas Hospital System Marion	Mullins	96%	70
Aiken Regional Medical Center	Aiken	95%	141
Self Regional Healthcare	Greenwood	95%	285
Waccamaw Community Hospital[2]	Murrells Inlet	94%	35
Kershaw Health	Camden	93%	45
Mcleod Medical Center - Dillon	Dillon	92%	26
Oconee Medical Center	Seneca	90%	29
Tuomey Healthcare System	Sumter	83%	48

Heart Failure Care

ACE Inhibitor or ARB for LVSD

Hospital Name	City	Rate	Cases
Baptist Easley Hospital	Easley	100%	42
Bon Secours-St Francis Xavier Hosp	Charleston	100%	49
Carolina Pines Regional Medical Center	Hartsville	100%	46
Carolinas Hospital System	Florence	100%	154
Charleston VA Medical Center	Charleston	100%	64
Colleton Medical Center	Walterboro	100%	61
Conway Medical Center[2]	Conway	100%	71
Georgetown Memorial Hospital[2]	Georgetown	100%	67
GHS Greer Memorial Hospital	Greer	100%	30
Grand Strand Regional Medical Center[2]	Myrtle Beach	100%	84
Lexington Medical Center[2]	West Columbia	100%	94
Mary Black Memorial Hospital	Spartanburg	100%	26
Novant Health Gaffney Medical Center	Gaffney	100%	29
Palmetto Health Baptist	Columbia	100%	77
Piedmont Medical Center	Rock Hill	100%	117
Roper Hospital	Charleston	100%	154
Saint Francis - Downtown[2]	Greenville	100%	107
Springs Memorial Hospital	Lancaster	100%	71
Trident Medical Center	Charleston	100%	194
Anmed Health	Anderson	99%	188
Columbia SC VA Medical Center	Columbia	99%	78
Mcleod Regional Medical Center - Pee Dee	Florence	99%	283
Palmetto Health Richland	Columbia	99%	355
Self Regional Healthcare	Greenwood	99%	104
GHS Greenville Memorial Medical Center	Greenville	98%	206
Musc Medical Center	Charleston	98%	254
Sisters of Charity Providence Hospitals[2]	Columbia	98%	100
Waccamaw Community Hospital[2]	Murrells Inlet	98%	62
Mcleod Medical Center - Dillon	Dillon	97%	32
Spartanburg Regional Medical Center	Spartanburg	97%	243
Trmc of Orangeburg & Calhoun	Orangeburg	97%	104
Aiken Regional Medical Center[2]	Aiken	96%	105
Carolinas Hospital System Marion	Mullins	96%	45
Mcleod Loris Seacoast Hospital	Loris	96%	57
Hilton Head Regional Medical Center	Hilton Head Isl	95%	40
Beaufort County Memorial Hospital	Beaufort	94%	94
Oconee Medical Center	Seneca	94%	51
Tuomey Healthcare System	Sumter	93%	192
Chester Regional Medical Center	Chester	92%	26
Kershaw Health[2]	Camden	89%	64
GHS Laurens County Memorial Hospital	Clinton	87%	31
Clarendon Memorial Hospital	Manning	66%	41

Discharge Instructions Given

Hospital Name	City	Rate	Cases
Anmed Health	Anderson	100%	462
Bon Secours-St Francis Xavier Hosp	Charleston	100%	116
Clarendon Memorial Hospital	Manning	100%	85
Colleton Medical Center	Walterboro	100%	229
Columbia SC VA Medical Center	Columbia	100%	226
East Cooper Medical Center	Mount Pleasant	100%	25
GHS Greer Memorial Hospital	Greer	100%	70
Hilton Head Regional Medical Center	Hilton Head Isl	100%	139
Marlboro Park Hospital	Bennettsville	100%	50
Mount Pleasant Hospital	Mount Pleasant	100%	30
Newberry County Memorial Hospital[2]	Newberry	100%	42
Roper Hospital	Charleston	100%	430
Springs Memorial Hospital	Lancaster	100%	176
Beaufort County Memorial Hospital	Beaufort	99%	230
Carolina Pines Regional Medical Center	Hartsville	99%	147
Palmetto Health Baptist	Columbia	99%	137
Self Regional Healthcare	Greenwood	99%	229
Trident Medical Center	Charleston	99%	531
Baptist Easley Hospital	Easley	98%	179
Chesterfield General Hospital	Cheraw	98%	51
Mcleod Regional Medical Center - Pee Dee	Florence	98%	616
Piedmont Medical Center	Rock Hill	98%	328
Charleston VA Medical Center	Charleston	97%	159
GHS - Hillcrest Memorial Hospital	Simpsonville	97%	33

NOTE: Hospital profiles are in alphabetical order by state, then city, then hospital within the city; Rankings exclude hospitals with less than 25 cases except for patient surveys which excludes hospitals with less than 100 cases; (a) 100-299 cases; (1) The number of cases/patients is too few to report; (2) Data submitted were based on a sample of cases/patients; (3) Results are based on a shorter time period than required; (4) Data suppressed by CMS for one or more quarters; (5) Results are not available for this reporting period; (6) Fewer than 100 patients completed the HCAHPS survey; (7) No cases met the criteria for this measure; (8) The lower limit of the confidence interval cannot be calculated if the number of observed infections equals zero; (9) No data are available from the state/territory for this reporting period; (10) The scores shown reflect fewer than 50 completed surveys; (11) There were discrepancies in the data collection process; (12) This measure does not apply to this hospital for this reporting period; (13) Results cannot be calculated for this reporting period; (14) The results for this state are combined with nearby states to protect confidentiality; Please refer to the User's Guide for a full explanation of data.

Hospital Name	City	Rate	Cases
Grand Strand Regional Medical Center[2]	Myrtle Beach	97%	262
Waccamaw Community Hospital[2]	Murrells Inlet	97%	146
Palmetto Health Richland	Columbia	96%	627
Village Hospital	Greer	96%	48
GHS Greenville Memorial Medical Center	Greenville	95%	543
Novant Health Gaffney Medical Center	Gaffney	95%	92
Saint Francis - Downtown[2]	Greenville	95%	253
Chester Regional Medical Center	Chester	94%	63
Kershaw Health[2]	Camden	94%	203
Aiken Regional Medical Center[2]	Aiken	93%	257
Mary Black Memorial Hospital	Spartanburg	93%	90
Trmc of Orangeburg & Calhoun	Orangeburg	93%	335
Wallace Thomson Hospital	Union	93%	85
Carolinas Hospital System	Florence	92%	431
Coastal Carolina Hospital	Hardeeville	92%	60
Mcleod Medical Center - Dillon	Dillon	92%	96
Musc Medical Center	Charleston	92%	518
Lexington Medical Center[2]	West Columbia	90%	228
Mcleod Loris Seacoast Hospital	Loris	90%	187
Spartanburg Regional Medical Center	Spartanburg	90%	706
Barnwell County Hospital	Barnwell	88%	25
Hampton Regional Medical Center	Varnville	88%	43
Tuomey Healthcare System	Sumter	88%	459
Conway Medical Center[2]	Conway	87%	178
Georgetown Memorial Hospital[2]	Georgetown	87%	133
GHS Laurens County Memorial Hospital	Clinton	87%	79
Oconee Medical Center	Seneca	83%	145
Carolinas Hospital System Marion	Mullins	81%	96
Sisters of Charity Providence Hospitals[2]	Columbia	77%	271
Williamsburg Regional Hospital	Kingstree	42%	40

Evaluation of LVS Function

Hospital Name	City	Rate	Cases
Anmed Health	Anderson	100%	595
Baptist Easley Hospital	Easley	100%	215
Beaufort County Memorial Hospital	Beaufort	100%	245
Bon Secours-St Francis Xavier Hosp	Charleston	100%	135
Carolinas Hospital System	Florence	100%	502
Carolinas Hospital System Marion	Mullins	100%	119
Charleston VA Medical Center	Charleston	100%	171
Chester Regional Medical Center	Chester	100%	76
Chesterfield General Hospital	Cheraw	100%	59
Coastal Carolina Hospital	Hardeeville	100%	71
Colleton Medical Center	Walterboro	100%	268
Columbia SC VA Medical Center	Columbia	100%	232
Conway Medical Center[2]	Conway	100%	206
East Cooper Medical Center	Mount Pleasant	100%	48
Georgetown Memorial Hospital[2]	Georgetown	100%	157
GHS - Hillcrest Memorial Hospital	Simpsonville	100%	41
GHS Greenville Memorial Medical Center	Greenville	100%	668
GHS Greer Memorial Hospital	Greer	100%	89
Grand Strand Regional Medical Center[2]	Myrtle Beach	100%	315
Hilton Head Regional Medical Center	Hilton Head Isl	100%	178
Lake City Community Hospital	Lake City	100%	25
Lexington Medical Center[2]	West Columbia	100%	272
Marlboro Park Hospital	Bennettsville	100%	57
Mcleod Medical Center - Dillon	Dillon	100%	105
Mcleod Regional Medical Center - Pee Dee	Florence	100%	723
Mount Pleasant Hospital	Mount Pleasant	100%	35
Musc Medical Center	Charleston	100%	548
Newberry County Memorial Hospital[2]	Newberry	100%	60
Novant Health Gaffney Medical Center	Gaffney	100%	116
Oconee Medical Center	Seneca	100%	173
Palmetto Health Baptist	Columbia	100%	178
Palmetto Health Richland	Columbia	100%	724
Roper Hospital	Charleston	100%	496
Saint Francis - Downtown[2]	Greenville	100%	300
Self Regional Healthcare	Greenwood	100%	274
Sisters of Charity Providence Hospitals[2]	Columbia	100%	313
Spartanburg Regional Medical Center	Spartanburg	100%	812
Springs Memorial Hospital	Lancaster	100%	204
Trident Medical Center	Charleston	100%	616
Trmc of Orangeburg & Calhoun	Orangeburg	100%	383
Village Hospital	Greer	100%	55
Waccamaw Community Hospital[2]	Murrells Inlet	100%	171
Aiken Regional Medical Center[2]	Aiken	99%	302
Carolina Pines Regional Medical Center	Hartsville	99%	164
Kershaw Health[2]	Camden	99%	245
Mary Black Memorial Hospital	Spartanburg	99%	107
Piedmont Medical Center	Rock Hill	99%	384
Tuomey Healthcare System	Sumter	99%	513
Cannon Memorial Hospital	Pickens	97%	31
Mcleod Loris Seacoast Hospital	Loris	97%	204
Hampton Regional Medical Center	Varnville	96%	48
Wallace Thomson Hospital	Union	96%	94
GHS Laurens County Memorial Hospital	Clinton	95%	105
Clarendon Memorial Hospital	Manning	93%	101
Williamsburg Regional Hospital	Kingstree	86%	49
Abbeville Area Medical Center	Abbeville	81%	26
Barnwell County Hospital	Barnwell	50%	32

Medicare Spending

Medicare Spending per Patient (ratio)

Hospital Name	City	Ratio	Cases
Chesterfield General Hospital	Cheraw	0.82	-
Mcleod Medical Center - Darlington	Darlington	0.86	-
GHS Patewood Memorial Hospital	Greenville	0.89	-
Hampton Regional Medical Center	Varnville	0.90	-
GHS - Hillcrest Memorial Hospital	Simpsonville	0.91	-
Marlboro Park Hospital	Bennettsville	0.91	-
Novant Health Gaffney Medical Center	Gaffney	0.91	-
GHS Greer Memorial Hospital	Greer	0.93	-
Mcleod Medical Center - Dillon	Dillon	0.93	-
Mcleod Loris Seacoast Hospital	Loris	0.94	-
Baptist Easley Hospital	Easley	0.95	-
Beaufort County Memorial Hospital	Beaufort	0.96	-
Carolinas Hospital System Marion	Mullins	0.96	-
Clarendon Memorial Hospital	Manning	0.96	-
Conway Medical Center	Conway	0.96	-
Georgetown Memorial Hospital	Georgetown	0.96	-
Mcleod Regional Medical Center - Pee Dee	Florence	0.96	-
Oconee Medical Center	Seneca	0.96	-
Spartanburg Regional Medical Center	Spartanburg	0.96	-
Tuomey Healthcare System	Sumter	0.96	-
Carolina Pines Regional Medical Center	Hartsville	0.97	-
Springs Memorial Hospital	Lancaster	0.97	-
Trmc of Orangeburg & Calhoun	Orangeburg	0.97	-
Bon Secours-St Francis Xavier Hosp	Charleston	0.98	-
Chester Regional Medical Center	Chester	0.98	-
Colleton Medical Center	Walterboro	0.98	-
GHS Greenville Memorial Medical Center	Greenville	0.98	-
Grand Strand Regional Medical Center	Myrtle Beach	0.98	-
Mount Pleasant Hospital	Mount Pleasant	0.98	-
Waccamaw Community Hospital	Murrells Inlet	0.98	-
Cannon Memorial Hospital	Pickens	0.99	-
Carolinas Hospital System	Florence	0.99	-
Musc Medical Center	Charleston	0.99	-
Palmetto Health Richland	Columbia	0.99	-
Sisters of Charity Providence Hospitals	Columbia	0.99	-
Coastal Carolina Hospital	Hardeeville	1.00	-
Kershaw Health	Camden	1.00	-
Newberry County Memorial Hospital	Newberry	1.00	-
Lexington Medical Center	West Columbia	1.01	-
Palmetto Health Baptist	Columbia	1.01	-
Trident Medical Center	Charleston	1.01	-
Village Hospital	Greer	1.01	-
Aiken Regional Medical Center	Aiken	1.02	-
Mary Black Memorial Hospital	Spartanburg	1.02	-
Roper Hospital	Charleston	1.02	-
Saint Francis - Downtown	Greenville	1.02	-
Self Regional Healthcare	Greenwood	1.02	-
Wallace Thomson Hospital	Union	1.02	-
GHS Laurens County Memorial Hospital	Clinton	1.03	-
Hilton Head Regional Medical Center	Hilton Head Isl	1.04	-
Piedmont Medical Center	Rock Hill	1.05	-
Anmed Health	Anderson	1.08	-
East Cooper Medical Center	Mount Pleasant	1.08	-
Lake City Community Hospital	Lake City	1.09	-
Barnwell County Hospital	Barnwell	1.16	-

Pneumonia Care

Appropriate Initial Antibiotic Given

Hospital Name	City	Rate	Cases
Aiken Regional Medical Center[2]	Aiken	100%	101
Anmed Health	Anderson	100%	348
Cannon Memorial Hospital	Pickens	100%	55
Carolinas Hospital System	Florence	100%	135
Chester Regional Medical Center	Chester	100%	50
Chesterfield General Hospital	Cheraw	100%	78
Georgetown Memorial Hospital[2]	Georgetown	100%	68
Mount Pleasant Hospital	Mount Pleasant	100%	25
Roper Hospital	Charleston	100%	98
Saint Francis - Downtown[2]	Greenville	100%	95
Springs Memorial Hospital	Lancaster	100%	74
Baptist Easley Hospital	Easley	99%	149
Bon Secours-St Francis Xavier Hosp	Charleston	99%	142
Carolina Pines Regional Medical Center	Hartsville	99%	128
Conway Medical Center[2]	Conway	99%	141
GHS - Hillcrest Memorial Hospital	Simpsonville	99%	91
Grand Strand Regional Medical Center[2]	Myrtle Beach	99%	80
Mcleod Medical Center - Dillon	Dillon	99%	90
Self Regional Healthcare	Greenwood	99%	173
Spartanburg Regional Medical Center	Spartanburg	99%	351
Village Hospital	Greer	99%	73
Columbia SC VA Medical Center	Columbia	98%	53
East Cooper Medical Center	Mount Pleasant	98%	48
GHS Greer Memorial Hospital	Greer	98%	121
Lexington Medical Center[2]	West Columbia	98%	80
Marlboro Park Hospital	Bennettsville	98%	46
Sisters of Charity Providence Hospitals[2]	Columbia	98%	83
Trident Medical Center	Charleston	98%	311
Trmc of Orangeburg & Calhoun	Orangeburg	98%	126
Coastal Carolina Hospital	Hardeeville	97%	69
Colleton Medical Center	Walterboro	97%	74
GHS Greenville Memorial Medical Center	Greenville	97%	263
Mary Black Memorial Hospital	Spartanburg	97%	148
Novant Health Gaffney Medical Center	Gaffney	97%	64
Beaufort County Memorial Hospital	Beaufort	96%	83
Carolinas Hospital System Marion	Mullins	96%	45
Hampton Regional Medical Center	Varnville	96%	28
Hilton Head Regional Medical Center	Hilton Head Isl	96%	111
Mcleod Loris Seacoast Hospital	Loris	96%	140
Musc Medical Center	Charleston	96%	69
Newberry County Memorial Hospital[2]	Newberry	96%	69
Oconee Medical Center	Seneca	96%	265
Waccamaw Community Hospital[2]	Murrells Inlet	96%	91
Mcleod Regional Medical Center - Pee Dee	Florence	95%	218
Palmetto Health Baptist	Columbia	95%	100
Kershaw Health[2]	Camden	94%	127
Tuomey Healthcare System	Sumter	94%	148
Piedmont Medical Center[2]	Rock Hill	93%	118
Lake City Community Hospital	Lake City	92%	48
Palmetto Health Richland	Columbia	92%	127
GHS Laurens County Memorial Hospital	Clinton	90%	67
Abbeville Area Medical Center	Abbeville	88%	41
Wallace Thomson Hospital	Union	81%	72
Clarendon Memorial Hospital	Manning	71%	56
Barnwell County Hospital	Barnwell	64%	44

Blood Culture Timing

Hospital Name	City	Rate	Cases
Baptist Easley Hospital	Easley	100%	248
Bon Secours-St Francis Xavier Hosp	Charleston	100%	220
Carolinas Hospital System	Florence	100%	205
Coastal Carolina Hospital	Hardeeville	100%	85
Colleton Medical Center	Walterboro	100%	127
Columbia SC VA Medical Center	Columbia	100%	84
Conway Medical Center[2]	Conway	100%	245
East Cooper Medical Center	Mount Pleasant	100%	70
Georgetown Memorial Hospital[2]	Georgetown	100%	140
Grand Strand Regional Medical Center[2]	Myrtle Beach	100%	118
Marlboro Park Hospital	Bennettsville	100%	73
Mcleod Medical Center - Dillon	Dillon	100%	107
Mount Pleasant Hospital	Mount Pleasant	100%	35
Roper Hospital	Charleston	100%	197
Trident Medical Center	Charleston	100%	611
Village Hospital	Greer	100%	85
Anmed Health	Anderson	99%	649
Cannon Memorial Hospital	Pickens	99%	68
Carolinas Hospital System Marion	Mullins	99%	85
Charleston VA Medical Center	Charleston	99%	75
Chester Regional Medical Center	Chester	99%	74
Chesterfield General Hospital	Cheraw	99%	132
GHS - Hillcrest Memorial Hospital	Simpsonville	99%	118
GHS Greer Memorial Hospital	Greer	99%	168
Hilton Head Regional Medical Center	Hilton Head Isl	99%	164
Mary Black Memorial Hospital	Spartanburg	99%	275
Mcleod Regional Medical Center - Pee Dee	Florence	99%	414
Newberry County Memorial Hospital[2]	Newberry	99%	92
Novant Health Gaffney Medical Center	Gaffney	99%	109
Self Regional Healthcare	Greenwood	99%	337
Spartanburg Regional Medical Center	Spartanburg	99%	617
Springs Memorial Hospital	Lancaster	99%	151
Waccamaw Community Hospital[2]	Murrells Inlet	99%	160
Carolina Pines Regional Medical Center	Hartsville	98%	151
GHS Greenville Memorial Medical Center	Greenville	98%	511
Lexington Medical Center[2]	West Columbia	98%	128
Palmetto Health Richland	Columbia	98%	211
Piedmont Medical Center[2]	Rock Hill	98%	129
Tuomey Healthcare System	Sumter	98%	232
Abbeville Area Medical Center	Abbeville	97%	34
Beaufort County Memorial Hospital	Beaufort	97%	99
Hampton Regional Medical Center	Varnville	97%	32
Mcleod Loris Seacoast Hospital	Loris	97%	194
Trmc of Orangeburg & Calhoun	Orangeburg	97%	226
Aiken Regional Medical Center[2]	Aiken	96%	151
Kershaw Health[2]	Camden	96%	136
Musc Medical Center	Charleston	96%	255
Oconee Medical Center	Seneca	96%	308
Palmetto Health Baptist	Columbia	96%	167
Saint Francis - Downtown[2]	Greenville	95%	174
GHS Laurens County Memorial Hospital	Clinton	94%	95
Sisters of Charity Providence Hospitals[2]	Columbia	94%	110
Allendale County Hospital[2]	Fairfax	93%	27
Clarendon Memorial Hospital	Manning	93%	61
Lake City Community Hospital	Lake City	88%	32
Wallace Thomson Hospital	Union	77%	65
Barnwell County Hospital	Barnwell	69%	62

NOTE: Hospital profiles are in alphabetical order by state, then city, then hospital within the city; Rankings exclude hospitals with less than 25 cases except for patient surveys which excludes hospitals with less than 100 cases; (a) 100-299 cases; (1) The number of cases/patients is too few to report; (2) Data submitted were based on a sample of cases/patients; (3) Results are based on a shorter time period than required; (4) Data suppressed by CMS for one or more quarters; (5) Results are not available for this reporting period; (6) Fewer than 100 patients completed the HCAHPS survey; (7) No cases met the criteria for this measure; (8) The lower limit of the confidence interval cannot be calculated if the number of observed infections equals zero; (9) No data are available from the state/territory for this reporting period; (10) The scores shown reflect fewer than 50 completed surveys; (11) There were discrepancies in the data collection process; (12) This measure does not apply to this hospital for this reporting period; (13) Results cannot be calculated for this reporting period; (14) The results for this state are combined with nearby states to protect confidentiality; Please refer to the User's Guide for a full explanation of data.

Pregnancy and Delivery Care

Newborns whose Deliveries were Scheduled Early

Hospital Name	City	Rate	Cases
Carolinas Hospital System Marion[2]	Mullins	0%	31
Colleton Medical Center[2]	Walterboro	0%	30
Georgetown Memorial Hospital[2]	Georgetown	0%	25
GHS Greer Memorial Hospital[2]	Greer	0%	25
Grand Strand Regional Medical Center[2]	Myrtle Beach	0%	29
Mary Black Memorial Hospital[2]	Spartanburg	0%	31
Mcleod Loris Seacoast Hospital[2]	Loris	0%	44
Mcleod Medical Center - Dillon[2]	Dillon	0%	41
Novant Health Gaffney Medical Center[2]	Gaffney	0%	37
Oconee Medical Center	Seneca	0%	36
Saint Francis - Downtown[2]	Greenville	0%	44
Trident Medical Center[2]	Charleston	0%	63
Anmed Health	Anderson	1%	334
Bon Secours-St Francis Xavier Hosp	Charleston	1%	233
GHS Greenville Memorial Medical Center[2]	Greenville	1%	67
Hilton Head Regional Medical Center[2]	Hilton Head Isl	1%	105
Palmetto Health Baptist[2]	Columbia	1%	286
Musc Medical Center[2]	Charleston	2%	110
Trmc of Orangeburg & Calhoun[2]	Orangeburg	2%	45
East Cooper Medical Center[2]	Mount Pleasant	3%	30
Mount Pleasant Hospital	Mount Pleasant	3%	32
Palmetto Health Richland[2]	Columbia	3%	180
Tuomey Healthcare System[2]	Sumter	3%	32
Aiken Regional Medical Center[2]	Aiken	4%	25
Carolina Pines Regional Medical Center	Hartsville	4%	54
GHS Laurens County Memorial Hospital	Clinton	4%	28
Newberry County Memorial Hospital[2]	Newberry	4%	49
Baptist Easley Hospital	Easley	5%	43
Clarendon Memorial Hospital[2]	Manning	5%	38
Piedmont Medical Center[2]	Rock Hill	5%	41
Spartanburg Regional Medical Center[2]	Spartanburg	5%	58
Conway Medical Center[2]	Conway	7%	28
Lexington Medical Center[2]	West Columbia	8%	62
Self Regional Healthcare	Greenwood	8%	120
Beaufort County Memorial Hospital[2]	Beaufort	15%	78

Preventive Care

Immunization for Influenza

Hospital Name	City	Rate	Cases
Chesterfield General Hospital[2]	Cheraw	100%	538
Newberry County Memorial Hospital[2]	Newberry	100%	246
Baptist Easley Hospital[2]	Easley	99%	406
Bon Secours-St Francis Xavier Hosp[2]	Charleston	99%	508
Cannon Memorial Hospital[2]	Pickens	99%	287
Conway Medical Center[2]	Conway	99%	528
GHS Patewood Memorial Hospital[2]	Greenville	99%	319
Grand Strand Regional Medical Center[2]	Myrtle Beach	99%	620
Marlboro Park Hospital[2]	Bennettsville	99%	380
Mcleod Regional Medical Center - Pee Dee[2]	Florence	99%	543
Oconee Medical Center[2]	Seneca	99%	547
Springs Memorial Hospital[2]	Lancaster	99%	580
Trident Medical Center[2]	Charleston	99%	651
Beaufort County Memorial Hospital[2]	Beaufort	98%	530
Colleton Medical Center[2]	Walterboro	98%	464
East Cooper Medical Center[2]	Mount Pleasant	98%	510
Mount Pleasant Hospital[2]	Mount Pleasant	98%	249
Roper Hospital[2]	Charleston	98%	607
Tuomey Healthcare System[2]	Sumter	98%	507
Village Hospital[2]	Greer	98%	318
Carolina Pines Regional Medical Center[2]	Hartsville	97%	495
Chester Regional Medical Center[2]	Chester	97%	374
GHS - Hillcrest Memorial Hospital[2]	Simpsonville	97%	310
GHS Greer Memorial Hospital[2]	Greer	97%	372
Hilton Head Regional Medical Center[2]	Hilton Head Isl	97%	521
Mary Black Memorial Hospital[2]	Spartanburg	97%	578
Mcleod Medical Center - Dillon[2]	Dillon	97%	276
Palmetto Health Baptist[2]	Columbia	97%	529
Waccamaw Community Hospital[2]	Murrells Inlet	97%	551
Anmed Health[2]	Anderson	96%	528
Carolinas Hospital System[2]	Florence	96%	629
Georgetown Memorial Hospital[2]	Georgetown	96%	444
Mcleod Loris Seacoast Hospital[2]	Loris	95%	398
Coastal Carolina Hospital[2]	Hardeeville	94%	352
Kershaw Health[2]	Camden	94%	487
Novant Health Gaffney Medical Center[2]	Gaffney	94%	309
Saint Francis - Downtown[2]	Greenville	94%	859
Aiken Regional Medical Center[2]	Aiken	93%	559
Carolinas Hospital System Marion[2]	Mullins	93%	329
GHS Greenville Memorial Medical Center[2]	Greenville	93%	546
Spartanburg Regional Medical Center[2]	Spartanburg	93%	558
Trmc of Orangeburg & Calhoun[2]	Orangeburg	93%	527
Mcleod Medical Center - Darlington	Darlington	92%	66
Musc Medical Center[2]	Charleston	91%	545
Self Regional Healthcare[2]	Greenwood	91%	560
Piedmont Medical Center[2]	Rock Hill	90%	545
Sisters of Charity Providence Hospitals[2]	Columbia	90%	627
Clarendon Memorial Hospital[2]	Manning	89%	267
Hampton Regional Medical Center[2]	Varnville	87%	314
Palmetto Health Richland[2]	Columbia	84%	616
Lake City Community Hospital[2]	Lake City	83%	288
GHS Laurens County Memorial Hospital[2]	Clinton	82%	258
Lexington Medical Center[2]	West Columbia	81%	493
Abbeville Area Medical Center[2]	Abbeville	74%	269
Wallace Thomson Hospital[2]	Union	71%	288
Barnwell County Hospital[2]	Barnwell	70%	285

Immunization for Pneumonia

Hospital Name	City	Rate	Cases
Bon Secours-St Francis Xavier Hosp[2]	Charleston	100%	506
Chesterfield General Hospital[2]	Cheraw	100%	636
Marlboro Park Hospital[2]	Bennettsville	100%	481
Newberry County Memorial Hospital[2]	Newberry	100%	275
Springs Memorial Hospital[2]	Lancaster	100%	703
Baptist Easley Hospital[2]	Easley	99%	579
Conway Medical Center[2]	Conway	99%	604
GHS Patewood Memorial Hospital[2]	Greenville	99%	367
Mary Black Memorial Hospital[2]	Spartanburg	99%	740
Mcleod Medical Center - Dillon[2]	Dillon	99%	318
Mcleod Regional Medical Center - Pee Dee[2]	Florence	99%	653
Novant Health Gaffney Medical Center[2]	Gaffney	99%	383
Oconee Medical Center[2]	Seneca	99%	735
Roper Hospital[2]	Charleston	99%	914
Trident Medical Center[2]	Charleston	99%	800
Anmed Health[2]	Anderson	98%	739
Beaufort County Memorial Hospital[2]	Beaufort	98%	606
Cannon Memorial Hospital[2]	Pickens	98%	432
GHS Greer Memorial Hospital[2]	Greer	98%	408
Hilton Head Regional Medical Center[2]	Hilton Head Isl	98%	703
Mcleod Medical Center - Darlington[2]	Darlington	98%	119
Mount Pleasant Hospital[2]	Mount Pleasant	98%	239
Village Hospital[2]	Greer	98%	446
Waccamaw Community Hospital[2]	Murrells Inlet	98%	728
Carolinas Hospital System[2]	Florence	97%	909
Chester Regional Medical Center[2]	Chester	97%	457
Colleton Medical Center[2]	Walterboro	97%	607
East Cooper Medical Center[2]	Mount Pleasant	97%	462
Georgetown Memorial Hospital[2]	Georgetown	97%	572
GHS - Hillcrest Memorial Hospital[2]	Simpsonville	97%	396
Mcleod Loris Seacoast Hospital[2]	Loris	97%	530
Tuomey Healthcare System[2]	Sumter	97%	623
Carolina Pines Regional Medical Center[2]	Hartsville	96%	558
Coastal Carolina Hospital[2]	Hardeeville	96%	554
Grand Strand Regional Medical Center[2]	Myrtle Beach	96%	832
Palmetto Health Baptist[2]	Columbia	96%	492
Spartanburg Regional Medical Center[2]	Spartanburg	96%	723
Saint Francis - Downtown[2]	Greenville	95%	1242
Trmc of Orangeburg & Calhoun[2]	Orangeburg	95%	688
Carolinas Hospital System Marion[2]	Mullins	94%	389
Kershaw Health[2]	Camden	93%	634
Piedmont Medical Center[2]	Rock Hill	93%	679
Aiken Regional Medical Center[2]	Aiken	92%	720
GHS Greenville Memorial Medical Center[2]	Greenville	92%	530
Hampton Regional Medical Center[2]	Varnville	92%	489
Sisters of Charity Providence Hospitals[2]	Columbia	92%	967
Musc Medical Center[2]	Charleston	90%	490
Palmetto Health Richland[2]	Columbia	90%	637
Self Regional Healthcare[2]	Greenwood	89%	827
Clarendon Memorial Hospital[2]	Manning	87%	297
GHS Laurens County Memorial Hospital[2]	Clinton	85%	342
Abbeville Area Medical Center[2]	Abbeville	82%	400
Lexington Medical Center[2]	West Columbia	80%	583
Lake City Community Hospital[2]	Lake City	79%	389
Wallace Thomson Hospital[2]	Union	76%	412
Barnwell County Hospital[2]	Barnwell	69%	401

Stroke Care

Anticoagulation Therapy for Atrial Fibrillation

Hospital Name	City	Rate	Cases
Anmed Health	Anderson	100%	33
Musc Medical Center	Charleston	96%	50
Spartanburg Regional Medical Center	Spartanburg	96%	54
Palmetto Health Richland	Columbia	95%	44

Antithrombotic Therapy Timing

Hospital Name	City	Rate	Cases
Aiken Regional Medical Center[2]	Aiken	100%	91
Anmed Health	Anderson	100%	214
Bon Secours-St Francis Xavier Hosp	Charleston	100%	76
Chesterfield General Hospital	Cheraw	100%	36
Coastal Carolina Hospital	Hardeeville	100%	35
Colleton Medical Center	Walterboro	100%	44
Conway Medical Center[2]	Conway	100%	81
Georgetown Memorial Hospital[2]	Georgetown	100%	50
GHS Laurens County Memorial Hospital	Clinton	100%	34
Grand Strand Regional Medical Center[2]	Myrtle Beach	100%	87
Kershaw Health	Camden	100%	72
Mcleod Medical Center - Dillon[2]	Dillon	100%	38
Piedmont Medical Center	Rock Hill	100%	175
Roper Hospital	Charleston	100%	107
Sisters of Charity Providence Hospitals[2]	Columbia	100%	71
Springs Memorial Hospital	Lancaster	100%	96
Trident Medical Center[2]	Charleston	100%	100
Lexington Medical Center[2]	West Columbia	99%	77
Mary Black Memorial Hospital	Spartanburg	99%	68
Saint Francis - Downtown	Greenville	99%	163
Spartanburg Regional Medical Center	Spartanburg	99%	343
Mcleod Loris Seacoast Hospital[2]	Loris	98%	59
Oconee Medical Center	Seneca	98%	54
Trmc of Orangeburg & Calhoun	Orangeburg	98%	146
Waccamaw Community Hospital[2]	Murrells Inlet	98%	64
Baptist Easley Hospital	Easley	97%	29
Beaufort County Memorial Hospital	Beaufort	97%	59
Carolinas Hospital System Marion	Mullins	97%	36
Palmetto Health Baptist	Columbia	97%	71
Hilton Head Regional Medical Center	Hilton Head Isl	96%	50
Mcleod Regional Medical Center - Pee Dee[2]	Florence	96%	77
Musc Medical Center	Charleston	96%	214
Palmetto Health Richland	Columbia	96%	295
Self Regional Healthcare	Greenwood	96%	129
Tuomey Healthcare System[2]	Sumter	95%	120
GHS Greenville Memorial Medical Center[2]	Greenville	94%	79
Carolinas Hospital System	Florence	93%	134
Carolina Pines Regional Medical Center	Hartsville	91%	34
Clarendon Memorial Hospital	Manning	71%	34

Assessed for Rehabilitation

Hospital Name	City	Rate	Cases
Baptist Easley Hospital	Easley	100%	29
Chesterfield General Hospital	Cheraw	100%	42
Colleton Medical Center	Walterboro	100%	47
East Cooper Medical Center	Mount Pleasant	100%	25
Georgetown Memorial Hospital[2]	Georgetown	100%	51
Saint Francis - Downtown	Greenville	100%	199
Springs Memorial Hospital	Lancaster	100%	95
Waccamaw Community Hospital[2]	Murrells Inlet	100%	71
Grand Strand Regional Medical Center[2]	Myrtle Beach	99%	104
Palmetto Health Richland	Columbia	99%	458
Piedmont Medical Center	Rock Hill	99%	182
Roper Hospital	Charleston	99%	145
Self Regional Healthcare	Greenwood	99%	162
Sisters of Charity Providence Hospitals[2]	Columbia	99%	74
Trident Medical Center[2]	Charleston	99%	114
Trmc of Orangeburg & Calhoun	Orangeburg	99%	151
Anmed Health	Anderson	98%	235
Carolinas Hospital System	Florence	98%	150
Mcleod Loris Seacoast Hospital[2]	Loris	98%	54
Palmetto Health Baptist	Columbia	98%	85
Bon Secours-St Francis Xavier Hosp	Charleston	97%	105
GHS Greenville Memorial Medical Center[2]	Greenville	97%	110
Lexington Medical Center[2]	West Columbia	97%	92
Musc Medical Center	Charleston	97%	548
Tuomey Healthcare System[2]	Sumter	97%	121
Carolina Pines Regional Medical Center	Hartsville	95%	42
Conway Medical Center[2]	Conway	95%	82
Hilton Head Regional Medical Center	Hilton Head Isl	95%	58
Oconee Medical Center	Seneca	95%	56
Spartanburg Regional Medical Center	Spartanburg	95%	394
Beaufort County Memorial Hospital	Beaufort	94%	68
Carolinas Hospital System Marion	Mullins	94%	36
Aiken Regional Medical Center[2]	Aiken	93%	111
Clarendon Memorial Hospital	Manning	93%	28
Mary Black Memorial Hospital	Spartanburg	93%	74
Mcleod Medical Center - Dillon[2]	Dillon	93%	42
Mcleod Regional Medical Center - Pee Dee[2]	Florence	92%	90
Coastal Carolina Hospital	Hardeeville	91%	34
GHS Laurens County Memorial Hospital	Clinton	91%	35
Kershaw Health	Camden	90%	73

Discharged on Antithrombotic Therapy

Hospital Name	City	Rate	Cases
Anmed Health	Anderson	100%	208
Baptist Easley Hospital	Easley	100%	28
Bon Secours-St Francis Xavier Hosp	Charleston	100%	95
Carolinas Hospital System Marion	Mullins	100%	36
Coastal Carolina Hospital	Hardeeville	100%	34
Colleton Medical Center	Walterboro	100%	46
Georgetown Memorial Hospital[2]	Georgetown	100%	49
Grand Strand Regional Medical Center[2]	Myrtle Beach	100%	92
Hilton Head Regional Medical Center	Hilton Head Isl	100%	56
Lexington Medical Center[2]	West Columbia	100%	81
Mary Black Memorial Hospital	Spartanburg	100%	68
Oconee Medical Center	Seneca	100%	52
Palmetto Health Baptist	Columbia	100%	75

NOTE: Hospital profiles are in alphabetical order by state, then city, then hospital within the city; Rankings exclude hospitals with less than 25 cases except for patient surveys which excludes hospitals with less than 100 cases; (a) 100-299 cases; (1) The number of cases/patients is too few to report; (2) Data submitted were based on a sample of cases/patients; (3) Results are based on a shorter time period than required; (4) Data suppressed by CMS for one or more quarters; (5) Results are not available for this reporting period; (6) Fewer than 100 patients completed the HCAHPS survey; (7) No cases met the criteria for this measure; (8) The lower limit of the confidence interval cannot be calculated if the number of observed infections equals zero; (9) No data are available from the state/territory for this reporting period; (10) The scores shown reflect fewer than 50 completed surveys; (11) There were discrepancies in the data collection process; (12) This measure does not apply to this hospital for this reporting period; (13) Results cannot be calculated for this reporting period; (14) The results for this state are combined with nearby states to protect confidentiality; Please refer to the User's Guide for a full explanation of data.

Hospital Name	City	Rate	Cases
Piedmont Medical Center	Rock Hill	100%	175
Roper Hospital	Charleston	100%	124
Saint Francis - Downtown	Greenville	100%	167
Sisters of Charity Providence Hospitals[2]	Columbia	100%	67
Springs Memorial Hospital	Lancaster	100%	92
Waccamaw Community Hospital[2]	Murrells Inlet	100%	71
Beaufort County Memorial Hospital	Beaufort	99%	62
Carolinas Hospital System	Florence	99%	122
Conway Medical Center[2]	Conway	99%	80
Kershaw Health	Camden	99%	68
Mcleod Regional Medical Center - Pee Dee[2]	Florence	99%	78
Palmetto Health Richland	Columbia	99%	337
Self Regional Healthcare	Greenwood	99%	146
Spartanburg Regional Medical Center	Spartanburg	99%	349
Trident Medical Center[2]	Charleston	99%	104
Trmc of Orangeburg & Calhoun	Orangeburg	99%	144
Aiken Regional Medical Center[2]	Aiken	98%	93
Carolina Pines Regional Medical Center	Hartsville	98%	40
Chesterfield General Hospital	Cheraw	98%	40
GHS Greenville Memorial Medical Center[2]	Greenville	98%	92
Mcleod Medical Center - Dillon[2]	Dillon	98%	41
Musc Medical Center	Charleston	98%	376
Tuomey Healthcare System[2]	Sumter	97%	116
Mcleod Loris Seacoast Hospital[2]	Loris	96%	51
GHS Laurens County Memorial Hospital	Clinton	88%	32
Clarendon Memorial Hospital	Manning	85%	27

Discharged on Statin Medication

Hospital Name	City	Rate	Cases
Bon Secours-St Francis Xavier Hosp	Charleston	100%	76
Chesterfield General Hospital	Cheraw	100%	31
Colleton Medical Center	Walterboro	100%	40
Georgetown Memorial Hospital[2]	Georgetown	100%	38
Springs Memorial Hospital	Lancaster	100%	85
Trident Medical Center[2]	Charleston	100%	86
Palmetto Health Richland	Columbia	99%	271
Roper Hospital	Charleston	99%	95
Anmed Health	Anderson	98%	162
Musc Medical Center	Charleston	98%	306
Piedmont Medical Center	Rock Hill	98%	139
Spartanburg Regional Medical Center	Spartanburg	98%	270
Waccamaw Community Hospital[2]	Murrells Inlet	98%	50
Carolinas Hospital System	Florence	97%	107
Trmc of Orangeburg & Calhoun	Orangeburg	96%	122
Grand Strand Regional Medical Center[2]	Myrtle Beach	95%	79
Lexington Medical Center[2]	West Columbia	95%	65
Mcleod Medical Center - Dillon[2]	Dillon	95%	39
Sisters of Charity Providence Hospitals[2]	Columbia	95%	55
Mary Black Memorial Hospital	Spartanburg	94%	50
Mcleod Regional Medical Center - Pee Dee[2]	Florence	94%	62
Palmetto Health Baptist	Columbia	94%	66
Self Regional Healthcare	Greenwood	94%	119
Mcleod Loris Seacoast Hospital[2]	Loris	93%	45
Saint Francis - Downtown	Greenville	93%	123
Carolina Pines Regional Medical Center	Hartsville	92%	36
GHS Greenville Memorial Medical Center[2]	Greenville	92%	79
GHS Laurens County Memorial Hospital	Clinton	92%	25
Coastal Carolina Hospital	Hardeeville	89%	27
Kershaw Health	Camden	88%	58
Conway Medical Center[2]	Conway	86%	64
Beaufort County Memorial Hospital	Beaufort	85%	59
Carolinas Hospital System Marion	Mullins	84%	31
Aiken Regional Medical Center[2]	Aiken	82%	77
Hilton Head Regional Medical Center	Hilton Head Isl	81%	47
Tuomey Healthcare System[2]	Sumter	77%	92
Oconee Medical Center	Seneca	67%	45

Thrombolytic Therapy Timing

Hospital Name	City	Rate	Cases
Palmetto Health Richland	Columbia	89%	28
Musc Medical Center	Charleston	85%	26
Spartanburg Regional Medical Center	Spartanburg	82%	28
Saint Francis - Downtown	Greenville	30%	37

Venous Thromboembolism (VTE) Prophylaxis

Hospital Name	City	Rate	Cases
Anmed Health	Anderson	100%	251
Baptist Easley Hospital	Easley	100%	30
Chesterfield General Hospital	Cheraw	100%	36
Coastal Carolina Hospital	Hardeeville	100%	32
Grand Strand Regional Medical Center[2]	Myrtle Beach	100%	110
Mcleod Medical Center - Dillon[2]	Dillon	100%	35
Spartanburg Regional Medical Center	Spartanburg	100%	406
Springs Memorial Hospital	Lancaster	100%	93
Trident Medical Center[2]	Charleston	100%	116
Waccamaw Community Hospital[2]	Murrells Inlet	100%	61
Bon Secours-St Francis Xavier Hosp	Charleston	99%	82
Mcleod Regional Medical Center - Pee Dee[2]	Florence	99%	99
Georgetown Memorial Hospital[2]	Georgetown	98%	50
Roper Hospital	Charleston	98%	134
GHS Greenville Memorial Medical Center[2]	Greenville	97%	118
Mary Black Memorial Hospital	Spartanburg	97%	75
Musc Medical Center	Charleston	97%	545
Piedmont Medical Center	Rock Hill	97%	180
Conway Medical Center[2]	Conway	96%	84
Colleton Medical Center	Walterboro	95%	39
Saint Francis - Downtown	Greenville	95%	202
Trmc of Orangeburg & Calhoun	Orangeburg	95%	152
Carolinas Hospital System	Florence	94%	165
Lexington Medical Center[2]	West Columbia	93%	98
Palmetto Health Richland	Columbia	93%	510
Mcleod Loris Seacoast Hospital[2]	Loris	92%	60
Palmetto Health Baptist	Columbia	92%	91
Wallace Thomson Hospital	Union	92%	25
Hilton Head Regional Medical Center	Hilton Head Isl	91%	55
Kershaw Health	Camden	91%	79
Beaufort County Memorial Hospital	Beaufort	90%	61
East Cooper Medical Center	Mount Pleasant	89%	28
Aiken Regional Medical Center[2]	Aiken	87%	116
Carolina Pines Regional Medical Center	Hartsville	87%	38
Carolinas Hospital System Marion	Mullins	86%	37
Tuomey Healthcare System[2]	Sumter	84%	128
GHS Laurens County Memorial Hospital	Clinton	83%	41
Sisters of Charity Providence Hospitals[2]	Columbia	81%	80
Self Regional Healthcare	Greenwood	80%	158
Oconee Medical Center	Seneca	75%	56
Clarendon Memorial Hospital	Manning	70%	33

Written Stroke Educational Materials Given

Hospital Name	City	Rate	Cases
Bon Secours-St Francis Xavier Hosp	Charleston	100%	73
Colleton Medical Center	Walterboro	100%	29
Springs Memorial Hospital	Lancaster	100%	61
Trident Medical Center[2]	Charleston	99%	69
Grand Strand Regional Medical Center[2]	Myrtle Beach	98%	64
Mary Black Memorial Hospital	Spartanburg	98%	41
Palmetto Health Baptist	Columbia	98%	49
Piedmont Medical Center	Rock Hill	98%	109
Anmed Health	Anderson	97%	147
Georgetown Memorial Hospital[2]	Georgetown	97%	37
Musc Medical Center	Charleston	97%	348
Palmetto Health Richland	Columbia	97%	292
Chesterfield General Hospital	Cheraw	96%	26
Saint Francis - Downtown	Greenville	96%	115
Aiken Regional Medical Center[2]	Aiken	95%	64
Self Regional Healthcare	Greenwood	94%	95
Tuomey Healthcare System[2]	Sumter	94%	63
Spartanburg Regional Medical Center	Spartanburg	93%	268
Trmc of Orangeburg & Calhoun	Orangeburg	93%	81
Waccamaw Community Hospital[2]	Murrells Inlet	93%	42
Roper Hospital	Charleston	88%	65
Mcleod Regional Medical Center - Pee Dee[2]	Florence	87%	55
Lexington Medical Center[2]	West Columbia	86%	49
Mcleod Loris Seacoast Hospital[2]	Loris	86%	29
Carolinas Hospital System	Florence	85%	95
Conway Medical Center[2]	Conway	84%	56
GHS Greenville Memorial Medical Center[2]	Greenville	83%	58
Kershaw Health	Camden	82%	39
Mcleod Medical Center - Dillon[2]	Dillon	79%	34
Hilton Head Regional Medical Center	Hilton Head Isl	71%	38
Beaufort County Memorial Hospital	Beaufort	65%	40
Sisters of Charity Providence Hospitals[2]	Columbia	63%	43
Oconee Medical Center	Seneca	18%	28

Surgical Care Improvement Project

Appropriate Beta Blocker Usage

Hospital Name	City	Rate	Cases
Baptist Easley Hospital	Easley	100%	63
Colleton Medical Center	Walterboro	100%	26
Columbia SC VA Medical Center[2]	Columbia	100%	25
East Cooper Medical Center	Mount Pleasant	100%	72
Grand Strand Regional Medical Center[2]	Myrtle Beach	100%	266
Hilton Head Regional Medical Center	Hilton Head Isl	100%	126
Mary Black Memorial Hospital	Spartanburg	100%	157
Musc Medical Center[2]	Charleston	100%	228
Spartanburg Regional Medical Center[2]	Spartanburg	100%	588
Springs Memorial Hospital	Lancaster	100%	31
Trident Medical Center[2]	Charleston	100%	269
Waccamaw Community Hospital[2]	Murrells Inlet	100%	105
Beaufort County Memorial Hospital	Beaufort	99%	155
Carolinas Hospital System	Florence	99%	234
GHS - Hillcrest Memorial Hospital[2]	Simpsonville	99%	67
GHS Patewood Memorial Hospital[2]	Greenville	99%	227
Mcleod Regional Medical Center - Pee Dee[2]	Florence	99%	206
Saint Francis - Downtown[2]	Greenville	99%	210
Self Regional Healthcare[2]	Greenwood	99%	302
Aiken Regional Medical Center[2]	Aiken	98%	127
Anmed Health[2]	Anderson	98%	288
Bon Secours-St Francis Xavier Hosp[2]	Charleston	98%	43
Charleston VA Medical Center[2]	Charleston	98%	92
Conway Medical Center[2]	Conway	98%	80
GHS Greenville Memorial Medical Center[2]	Greenville	98%	364
GHS Greer Memorial Hospital[2]	Greer	98%	134
Newberry County Memorial Hospital[2]	Newberry	98%	40
Roper Hospital[2]	Charleston	98%	248
Georgetown Memorial Hospital[2]	Georgetown	97%	64
Lexington Medical Center[2]	West Columbia	97%	148
Palmetto Health Richland	Columbia	97%	550
Sisters of Charity Providence Hospitals[2]	Columbia	97%	218
Tuomey Healthcare System[2]	Sumter	97%	152
Palmetto Health Baptist	Columbia	96%	314
Kershaw Health	Camden	95%	75
GHS Laurens County Memorial Hospital	Clinton	94%	62
Mcleod Loris Seacoast Hospital	Loris	94%	94
Trmc of Orangeburg & Calhoun[2]	Orangeburg	94%	72
Village Hospital	Greer	94%	48
Carolinas Hospital System Marion	Mullins	93%	29
Oconee Medical Center[2]	Seneca	93%	71
Piedmont Medical Center[2]	Rock Hill	93%	249
Carolina Pines Regional Medical Center	Hartsville	92%	49
Clarendon Memorial Hospital	Manning	85%	27

Appropriate VTP Within 24 Hours

Hospital Name	City	Rate	Cases
Abbeville Area Medical Center	Abbeville	100%	42
Anmed Health[2]	Anderson	100%	711
Carolina Pines Regional Medical Center	Hartsville	100%	205
Charleston VA Medical Center[2]	Charleston	100%	144
Chesterfield General Hospital	Cheraw	100%	34
Colleton Medical Center	Walterboro	100%	118
GHS Patewood Memorial Hospital[2]	Greenville	100%	644
Grand Strand Regional Medical Center[2]	Myrtle Beach	100%	414
Mount Pleasant Hospital	Mount Pleasant	100%	68
Musc Medical Center[2]	Charleston	100%	523
Novant Health Gaffney Medical Center	Gaffney	100%	65
Roper Hospital[2]	Charleston	100%	469
Springs Memorial Hospital	Lancaster	100%	156
Aiken Regional Medical Center[2]	Aiken	99%	421
Baptist Easley Hospital	Easley	99%	200
Beaufort County Memorial Hospital	Beaufort	99%	551
Bon Secours-St Francis Xavier Hosp[2]	Charleston	99%	237
Carolinas Hospital System	Florence	99%	509
Columbia SC VA Medical Center[2]	Columbia	99%	123
GHS - Hillcrest Memorial Hospital[2]	Simpsonville	99%	236
GHS Greer Memorial Hospital[2]	Greer	99%	490
Hilton Head Regional Medical Center	Hilton Head Isl	99%	267
Mcleod Medical Center - Dillon	Dillon	99%	76
Mcleod Regional Medical Center - Pee Dee[2]	Florence	99%	296
Newberry County Memorial Hospital[2]	Newberry	99%	135
Oconee Medical Center[2]	Seneca	99%	242
Palmetto Health Baptist	Columbia	99%	1033
Saint Francis - Downtown[2]	Greenville	99%	439
Sisters of Charity Providence Hospitals[2]	Columbia	99%	398
Trident Medical Center[2]	Charleston	99%	482
Tuomey Healthcare System[2]	Sumter	99%	436
Village Hospital	Greer	99%	189
Waccamaw Community Hospital[2]	Murrells Inlet	99%	376
Cannon Memorial Hospital	Pickens	98%	46
Conway Medical Center[2]	Conway	98%	300
East Cooper Medical Center	Mount Pleasant	98%	338
GHS Greenville Memorial Medical Center[2]	Greenville	98%	350
Kershaw Health	Camden	98%	178
Lexington Medical Center[2]	West Columbia	98%	293
Mary Black Memorial Hospital	Spartanburg	98%	471
Piedmont Medical Center[2]	Rock Hill	98%	484
Self Regional Healthcare[2]	Greenwood	98%	628
Spartanburg Regional Medical Center[2]	Spartanburg	98%	946
Chester Regional Medical Center	Chester	97%	67
Coastal Carolina Hospital	Hardeeville	97%	64
Georgetown Memorial Hospital[2]	Georgetown	97%	232
Hampton Regional Medical Center	Varnville	97%	31
Trmc of Orangeburg & Calhoun[2]	Orangeburg	97%	239
Clarendon Memorial Hospital	Manning	96%	124
GHS Laurens County Memorial Hospital	Clinton	96%	163
Palmetto Health Richland	Columbia	96%	1164
Carolinas Hospital System Marion	Mullins	95%	106
Mcleod Loris Seacoast Hospital	Loris	95%	301
Wallace Thomson Hospital	Union	63%	35

Controlled Postoperative Blood Glucose

Hospital Name	City	Rate	Cases
Lexington Medical Center[2]	West Columbia	100%	98
Roper Hospital[2]	Charleston	100%	198
Self Regional Healthcare[2]	Greenwood	100%	100
Spartanburg Regional Medical Center[2]	Spartanburg	100%	343
GHS Greenville Memorial Medical Center[2]	Greenville	99%	349
Grand Strand Regional Medical Center[2]	Myrtle Beach	99%	188
Mcleod Regional Medical Center - Pee Dee[2]	Florence	99%	97
Palmetto Health Richland	Columbia	99%	295

NOTE: Hospital profiles are in alphabetical order by state, then city, then hospital within the city; Rankings exclude hospitals with less than 25 cases except for patient surveys which excludes hospitals with less than 100 cases; (a) 100-299 cases; (1) The number of cases/patients is too few to report; (2) Data submitted were based on a sample of cases/patients; (3) Results are based on a shorter time period than required; (4) Data suppressed by CMS for one or more quarters; (5) Results are not available for this reporting period; (6) Fewer than 100 patients completed the HCAHPS survey; (7) No cases met the criteria for this measure; (8) The lower limit of the confidence interval cannot be calculated if the number of observed infections equals zero; (9) No data are available from the state/territory for this reporting period; (10) The scores shown reflect fewer than 50 completed surveys; (11) There were discrepancies in the data collection process; (12) This measure does not apply to this hospital for this reporting period; (13) Results cannot be calculated for this reporting period; (14) The results for this state are combined with nearby states to protect confidentiality; Please refer to the User's Guide for a full explanation of data.

Saint Francis - Downtown[2]	Greenville	99%	151
Sisters of Charity Providence Hospitals[2]	Columbia	99%	182
Trident Medical Center[2]	Charleston	99%	146
Anmed Health[2]	Anderson	97%	181
Carolinas Hospital System	Florence	97%	102
Charleston VA Medical Center[2]	Charleston	97%	62
Musc Medical Center[2]	Charleston	96%	130
Piedmont Medical Center[2]	Rock Hill	96%	101
Hilton Head Regional Medical Center	Hilton Head Isl	94%	63
Aiken Regional Medical Center[2]	Aiken	87%	30

Perioperative Temperature Management

Hospital Name	City	Rate	Cases
Abbeville Area Medical Center	Abbeville	100%	41
Aiken Regional Medical Center[2]	Aiken	100%	482
Anmed Health[2]	Anderson	100%	792
Baptist Easley Hospital	Easley	100%	213
Beaufort County Memorial Hospital	Beaufort	100%	597
Bon Secours-St Francis Xavier Hosp[2]	Charleston	100%	271
Cannon Memorial Hospital	Pickens	100%	49
Carolina Pines Regional Medical Center	Hartsville	100%	222
Charleston VA Medical Center[2]	Charleston	100%	168
Chester Regional Medical Center	Chester	100%	70
Chesterfield General Hospital	Cheraw	100%	39
Coastal Carolina Hospital	Hardeeville	100%	72
Colleton Medical Center	Walterboro	100%	134
Columbia SC VA Medical Center[2]	Columbia	100%	120
Conway Medical Center[2]	Conway	100%	397
East Cooper Medical Center	Mount Pleasant	100%	452
Georgetown Memorial Hospital[2]	Georgetown	100%	260
GHS - Hillcrest Memorial Hospital[2]	Simpsonville	100%	243
GHS Greenville Memorial Medical Center[2]	Greenville	100%	515
GHS Greer Memorial Hospital[2]	Greer	100%	553
GHS Laurens County Memorial Hospital	Clinton	100%	192
GHS Patewood Memorial Hospital[2]	Greenville	100%	824
Grand Strand Regional Medical Center[2]	Myrtle Beach	100%	494
Hilton Head Regional Medical Center	Hilton Head Isl	100%	357
Kershaw Health	Camden	100%	207
Lexington Medical Center[2]	West Columbia	100%	414
Mary Black Memorial Hospital	Spartanburg	100%	535
Mcleod Loris Seacoast Hospital	Loris	100%	324
Mcleod Medical Center - Dillon	Dillon	100%	81
Mcleod Regional Medical Center - Pee Dee[2]	Florence	100%	423
Mount Pleasant Hospital	Mount Pleasant	100%	94
Musc Medical Center[2]	Charleston	100%	689
Palmetto Health Baptist	Columbia	100%	1258
Palmetto Health Richland	Columbia	100%	1558
Piedmont Medical Center[2]	Rock Hill	100%	550
Roper Hospital[2]	Charleston	100%	596
Saint Francis - Downtown[2]	Greenville	100%	492
Self Regional Healthcare[2]	Greenwood	100%	738
Sisters of Charity Providence Hospitals[2]	Columbia	100%	561
Spartanburg Regional Medical Center[2]	Spartanburg	100%	1148
Springs Memorial Hospital	Lancaster	100%	166
Trident Medical Center[2]	Charleston	100%	638
Trmc of Orangeburg & Calhoun[2]	Orangeburg	100%	299
Tuomey Healthcare System[2]	Sumter	100%	481
Village Hospital	Greer	100%	195
Waccamaw Community Hospital[2]	Murrells Inlet	100%	447
Wallace Thomson Hospital	Union	100%	43
Carolinas Hospital System	Florence	99%	594
Carolinas Hospital System Marion	Mullins	99%	118
Newberry County Memorial Hospital[2]	Newberry	99%	154
Novant Health Gaffney Medical Center	Gaffney	99%	76
Oconee Medical Center[2]	Seneca	99%	274
Clarendon Memorial Hospital	Manning	96%	136
Hampton Regional Medical Center	Varnville	70%	33

Prophylactic Antibiotic Selection

Hospital Name	City	Rate	Cases
Aiken Regional Medical Center[2]	Aiken	100%	356
Beaufort County Memorial Hospital	Beaufort	100%	457
Cannon Memorial Hospital	Pickens	100%	33
Carolina Pines Regional Medical Center	Hartsville	100%	143
Carolinas Hospital System	Florence	100%	387
Carolinas Hospital System Marion	Mullins	100%	68
Charleston VA Medical Center	Charleston	100%	135
Chester Regional Medical Center	Chester	100%	49
Coastal Carolina Hospital	Hardeeville	100%	39
Colleton Medical Center	Walterboro	100%	96
Columbia SC VA Medical Center	Columbia	100%	85
Conway Medical Center[2]	Conway	100%	274
East Cooper Medical Center	Mount Pleasant	100%	303
Georgetown Memorial Hospital[2]	Georgetown	100%	153
GHS Greenville Memorial Medical Center[2]	Greenville	100%	587
GHS Greer Memorial Hospital[2]	Greer	100%	397
GHS Patewood Memorial Hospital[2]	Greenville	100%	684
Grand Strand Regional Medical Center[2]	Myrtle Beach	100%	474
Hilton Head Regional Medical Center	Hilton Head Isl	100%	292
Mary Black Memorial Hospital	Spartanburg	100%	387
Mount Pleasant Hospital	Mount Pleasant	100%	55
Palmetto Health Baptist	Columbia	100%	650
Palmetto Health Richland	Columbia	100%	1072
Roper Hospital[2]	Charleston	100%	575
Saint Francis - Downtown[2]	Greenville	100%	467
Spartanburg Regional Medical Center[2]	Spartanburg	100%	1158
Anmed Health[2]	Anderson	99%	767
Baptist Easley Hospital	Easley	99%	153
Bon Secours-St Francis Xavier Hosp[2]	Charleston	99%	125
GHS - Hillcrest Memorial Hospital[2]	Simpsonville	99%	172
Kershaw Health	Camden	99%	136
Lexington Medical Center[2]	West Columbia	99%	368
Mcleod Loris Seacoast Hospital	Loris	99%	201
Mcleod Regional Medical Center - Pee Dee[2]	Florence	99%	370
Musc Medical Center[2]	Charleston	99%	515
Oconee Medical Center[2]	Seneca	99%	175
Piedmont Medical Center[2]	Rock Hill	99%	498
Self Regional Healthcare[2]	Greenwood	99%	645
Sisters of Charity Providence Hospitals[2]	Columbia	99%	443
Springs Memorial Hospital	Lancaster	99%	91
Trident Medical Center[2]	Charleston	99%	563
Trmc of Orangeburg & Calhoun[2]	Orangeburg	99%	175
Tuomey Healthcare System[2]	Sumter	99%	318
Village Hospital	Greer	99%	151
Waccamaw Community Hospital[2]	Murrells Inlet	99%	304
GHS Laurens County Memorial Hospital	Clinton	98%	149
Mcleod Medical Center - Dillon	Dillon	98%	54
Newberry County Memorial Hospital[2]	Newberry	98%	117
Novant Health Gaffney Medical Center	Gaffney	98%	50
Clarendon Memorial Hospital	Manning	96%	85

Prophylactic Antibiotic Selection (Outpatient)

Hospital Name	City	Rate	Cases
Bon Secours-St Francis Xavier Hosp	Charleston	100%	407
Carolina Pines Regional Medical Center	Hartsville	100%	76
Clarendon Memorial Hospital	Manning	100%	31
Coastal Carolina Hospital	Hardeeville	100%	53
Colleton Medical Center	Walterboro	100%	25
GHS Greer Memorial Hospital	Greer	100%	46
Mcleod Medical Center - Darlington	Darlington	100%	34
Saint Francis - Downtown	Greenville	100%	923
Sisters of Charity Providence Hospitals	Columbia	100%	513
Springs Memorial Hospital	Lancaster	100%	70
Tuomey Healthcare System	Sumter	100%	110
Aiken Regional Medical Center	Aiken	99%	255
Anmed Health	Anderson	99%	513
Baptist Easley Hospital	Easley	99%	91
Carolinas Hospital System	Florence	99%	277
East Cooper Medical Center	Mount Pleasant	99%	181
Georgetown Memorial Hospital	Georgetown	99%	146
GHS Greenville Memorial Medical Center	Greenville	99%	765
GHS Patewood Memorial Hospital	Greenville	99%	157
Hilton Head Regional Medical Center	Hilton Head Isl	99%	289
Kershaw Health	Camden	99%	141
Lexington Medical Center	West Columbia	99%	681
Mary Black Memorial Hospital	Spartanburg	99%	233
Mount Pleasant Hospital	Mount Pleasant	99%	91
Musc Medical Center	Charleston	99%	824
Oconee Medical Center	Seneca	99%	94
Roper Hospital	Charleston	99%	681
Trident Medical Center	Charleston	99%	580
Conway Medical Center	Conway	98%	252
Grand Strand Regional Medical Center	Myrtle Beach	98%	329
Palmetto Health Baptist	Columbia	98%	430
Piedmont Medical Center	Rock Hill	98%	461
Self Regional Healthcare	Greenwood	98%	443
Spartanburg Regional Medical Center	Spartanburg	98%	927
Trmc of Orangeburg & Calhoun	Orangeburg	98%	275
Village Hospital	Greer	98%	122
Beaufort County Memorial Hospital	Beaufort	97%	216
Palmetto Health Richland	Columbia	97%	545
Waccamaw Community Hospital	Murrells Inlet	97%	64
Mcleod Regional Medical Center - Pee Dee	Florence	96%	565
Mcleod Loris Seacoast Hospital	Loris	95%	111

Prophylactic Antibiotic Stopped

Hospital Name	City	Rate	Cases
Anmed Health[2]	Anderson	100%	738
Charleston VA Medical Center	Charleston	100%	132
Chester Regional Medical Center	Chester	100%	47
Colleton Medical Center	Walterboro	100%	96
Columbia SC VA Medical Center	Columbia	100%	83
GHS - Hillcrest Memorial Hospital[2]	Simpsonville	100%	165
GHS Patewood Memorial Hospital[2]	Greenville	100%	682
Musc Medical Center[2]	Charleston	100%	487
Waccamaw Community Hospital[2]	Murrells Inlet	100%	299
Baptist Easley Hospital	Easley	99%	144
Carolinas Hospital System	Florence	99%	365
Conway Medical Center[2]	Conway	99%	269
GHS Greer Memorial Hospital[2]	Greer	99%	391
Grand Strand Regional Medical Center[2]	Myrtle Beach	99%	448
Newberry County Memorial Hospital[2]	Newberry	99%	113
Oconee Medical Center[2]	Seneca	99%	166
Palmetto Health Baptist	Columbia	99%	647
Roper Hospital[2]	Charleston	99%	566
Springs Memorial Hospital	Lancaster	99%	88
Trident Medical Center[2]	Charleston	99%	542
Village Hospital	Greer	99%	148
Beaufort County Memorial Hospital	Beaufort	98%	441
Carolina Pines Regional Medical Center	Hartsville	98%	131
GHS Greenville Memorial Medical Center[2]	Greenville	98%	563
Kershaw Health	Camden	98%	133
Lexington Medical Center[2]	West Columbia	98%	364
Mary Black Memorial Hospital	Spartanburg	98%	368
Mcleod Loris Seacoast Hospital	Loris	98%	199
Mcleod Regional Medical Center - Pee Dee[2]	Florence	98%	356
Novant Health Gaffney Medical Center	Gaffney	98%	47
Palmetto Health Richland	Columbia	98%	1048
Saint Francis - Downtown[2]	Greenville	98%	457
Spartanburg Regional Medical Center[2]	Spartanburg	98%	1120
Aiken Regional Medical Center[2]	Aiken	97%	339
Bon Secours-St Francis Xavier Hosp[2]	Charleston	97%	119
East Cooper Medical Center	Mount Pleasant	97%	301
Hilton Head Regional Medical Center	Hilton Head Isl	97%	286
Sisters of Charity Providence Hospitals[2]	Columbia	97%	440
Tuomey Healthcare System[2]	Sumter	97%	310
Georgetown Memorial Hospital[2]	Georgetown	96%	148
Mount Pleasant Hospital	Mount Pleasant	96%	50
Piedmont Medical Center[2]	Rock Hill	96%	485
Self Regional Healthcare[2]	Greenwood	96%	638
Coastal Carolina Hospital	Hardeeville	95%	37
GHS Laurens County Memorial Hospital	Clinton	95%	146
Trmc of Orangeburg & Calhoun[2]	Orangeburg	95%	173
Cannon Memorial Hospital	Pickens	94%	33
Mcleod Medical Center - Dillon	Dillon	94%	49
Carolinas Hospital System Marion	Mullins	90%	63
Clarendon Memorial Hospital	Manning	88%	85

Prophylactic Antibiotic Timing

Hospital Name	City	Rate	Cases
Aiken Regional Medical Center[2]	Aiken	100%	356
Anmed Health[2]	Anderson	100%	769
Beaufort County Memorial Hospital	Beaufort	100%	458
Cannon Memorial Hospital	Pickens	100%	33
Carolinas Hospital System	Florence	100%	387
Carolinas Hospital System Marion	Mullins	100%	68
Coastal Carolina Hospital	Hardeeville	100%	39
Colleton Medical Center	Walterboro	100%	96
Columbia SC VA Medical Center	Columbia	100%	85
Georgetown Memorial Hospital[2]	Georgetown	100%	153
GHS Greer Memorial Hospital[2]	Greer	100%	397
GHS Patewood Memorial Hospital[2]	Greenville	100%	684
Grand Strand Regional Medical Center[2]	Myrtle Beach	100%	474
Hilton Head Regional Medical Center	Hilton Head Isl	100%	294
Kershaw Health	Camden	100%	136
Mcleod Medical Center - Dillon	Dillon	100%	54
Mcleod Regional Medical Center - Pee Dee[2]	Florence	100%	379
Mount Pleasant Hospital	Mount Pleasant	100%	55
Newberry County Memorial Hospital[2]	Newberry	100%	117
Novant Health Gaffney Medical Center	Gaffney	100%	50
Palmetto Health Baptist	Columbia	100%	649
Palmetto Health Richland	Columbia	100%	1075
Roper Hospital[2]	Charleston	100%	575
Saint Francis - Downtown[2]	Greenville	100%	467
Sisters of Charity Providence Hospitals[2]	Columbia	100%	443
Springs Memorial Hospital	Lancaster	100%	91
Trident Medical Center[2]	Charleston	100%	563
Baptist Easley Hospital	Easley	99%	153
Bon Secours-St Francis Xavier Hosp[2]	Charleston	99%	125
Carolina Pines Regional Medical Center	Hartsville	99%	143
Charleston VA Medical Center	Charleston	99%	135
Conway Medical Center[2]	Conway	99%	276
East Cooper Medical Center	Mount Pleasant	99%	303
GHS - Hillcrest Memorial Hospital[2]	Simpsonville	99%	172
GHS Greenville Memorial Medical Center[2]	Greenville	99%	587
GHS Laurens County Memorial Hospital	Clinton	99%	149
Lexington Medical Center[2]	West Columbia	99%	369
Mary Black Memorial Hospital	Spartanburg	99%	387
Musc Medical Center[2]	Charleston	99%	518
Oconee Medical Center[2]	Seneca	99%	175
Piedmont Medical Center[2]	Rock Hill	99%	498
Self Regional Healthcare[2]	Greenwood	99%	646
Spartanburg Regional Medical Center[2]	Spartanburg	99%	1158
Trmc of Orangeburg & Calhoun[2]	Orangeburg	99%	178
Village Hospital	Greer	99%	151
Waccamaw Community Hospital[2]	Murrells Inlet	99%	304
Chester Regional Medical Center	Chester	98%	49
Mcleod Loris Seacoast Hospital	Loris	97%	201
Tuomey Healthcare System[2]	Sumter	97%	318
Clarendon Memorial Hospital	Manning	93%	85

NOTE: Hospital profiles are in alphabetical order by state, then city, then hospital within the city; Rankings exclude hospitals with less than 25 cases except for patient surveys which excludes hospitals with less than 100 cases; (a) 100-299 cases; (1) The number of cases/patients is too few to report; (2) Data submitted were based on a sample of cases/patients; (3) Results are based on a shorter time period than required; (4) Data suppressed by CMS for one or more quarters; (5) Results are not available for this reporting period; (6) Fewer than 100 patients completed the HCAHPS survey; (7) No cases met the criteria for this measure; (8) The lower limit of the confidence interval cannot be calculated if the number of observed infections equals zero; (9) No data are available from the state/territory for this reporting period; (10) The scores shown reflect fewer than 50 completed surveys; (11) There were discrepancies in the data collection process; (12) This measure does not apply to this hospital for this reporting period; (13) Results cannot be calculated for this reporting period; (14) The results for this state are combined with nearby states to protect confidentiality; Please refer to the User's Guide for a full explanation of data.

Prophylactic Antibiotic Timing (Outpatient)

Hospital Name	City	Rate	Cases
Aiken Regional Medical Center	Aiken	100%	255
Baptist Easley Hospital	Easley	100%	91
Bon Secours-St Francis Xavier Hosp	Charleston	100%	407
Carolina Pines Regional Medical Center	Hartsville	100%	76
East Cooper Medical Center	Mount Pleasant	100%	181
GHS Greer Memorial Hospital	Greer	100%	46
GHS Patewood Memorial Hospital	Greenville	100%	157
Hilton Head Regional Medical Center	Hilton Head Isl	100%	289
Mcleod Medical Center - Darlington	Darlington	100%	34
Mount Pleasant Hospital	Mount Pleasant	100%	91
Saint Francis - Downtown	Greenville	100%	923
Springs Memorial Hospital	Lancaster	100%	70
Trident Medical Center	Charleston	100%	580
Beaufort County Memorial Hospital	Beaufort	99%	216
GHS Greenville Memorial Medical Center	Greenville	99%	770
Mcleod Regional Medical Center - Pee Dee	Florence	99%	566
Musc Medical Center	Charleston	99%	715
Roper Hospital	Charleston	99%	674
Sisters of Charity Providence Hospitals	Columbia	99%	513
Trmc of Orangeburg & Calhoun	Orangeburg	99%	273
Village Hospital	Greer	99%	122
Carolinas Hospital System	Florence	98%	277
Conway Medical Center	Conway	98%	252
Grand Strand Regional Medical Center	Myrtle Beach	98%	330
Kershaw Health	Camden	98%	139
Lexington Medical Center	West Columbia	98%	682
Mary Black Memorial Hospital	Spartanburg	98%	233
Piedmont Medical Center	Rock Hill	98%	465
Spartanburg Regional Medical Center	Spartanburg	98%	934
Clarendon Memorial Hospital	Manning	97%	32
Georgetown Memorial Hospital	Georgetown	97%	146
Oconee Medical Center	Seneca	97%	96
Anmed Health	Anderson	96%	523
Coastal Carolina Hospital	Hardeeville	96%	54
Palmetto Health Richland	Columbia	96%	551
Self Regional Healthcare	Greenwood	96%	447
Mcleod Loris Seacoast Hospital	Loris	95%	112
Tuomey Healthcare System	Sumter	95%	114
Waccamaw Community Hospital	Murrells Inlet	95%	66
Palmetto Health Baptist	Columbia	94%	445
Colleton Medical Center	Walterboro	92%	26

Urinary Catheter Removal

Hospital Name	City	Rate	Cases
Aiken Regional Medical Center[2]	Aiken	100%	234
Beaufort County Memorial Hospital	Beaufort	100%	362
Cannon Memorial Hospital	Pickens	100%	37
GHS Patewood Memorial Hospital[2]	Greenville	100%	657
Mcleod Medical Center - Dillon	Dillon	100%	58
Newberry County Memorial Hospital[2]	Newberry	100%	106
Springs Memorial Hospital	Lancaster	100%	32
Anmed Health[2]	Anderson	99%	549
Baptist Easley Hospital	Easley	99%	162
Bon Secours-St Francis Xavier Hosp[2]	Charleston	99%	135
Carolinas Hospital System	Florence	99%	307
Columbia SC VA Medical Center[2]	Columbia	99%	87
East Cooper Medical Center	Mount Pleasant	99%	264
GHS Greer Memorial Hospital[2]	Greer	99%	468
Grand Strand Regional Medical Center[2]	Myrtle Beach	99%	427
Mcleod Regional Medical Center - Pee Dee[2]	Florence	99%	264
Musc Medical Center[2]	Charleston	99%	325
Roper Hospital[2]	Charleston	99%	270
Sisters of Charity Providence Hospitals[2]	Columbia	99%	540
Village Hospital	Greer	99%	173
Charleston VA Medical Center[2]	Charleston	98%	50
Conway Medical Center[2]	Conway	98%	191
Hilton Head Regional Medical Center	Hilton Head Isl	98%	101
Saint Francis - Downtown[2]	Greenville	98%	479
Spartanburg Regional Medical Center[2]	Spartanburg	98%	971
Trident Medical Center[2]	Charleston	98%	250
Tuomey Healthcare System[2]	Sumter	98%	341
Waccamaw Community Hospital[2]	Murrells Inlet	98%	298
GHS - Hillcrest Memorial Hospital[2]	Simpsonville	97%	226
Kershaw Health	Camden	97%	76
Lexington Medical Center[2]	West Columbia	97%	269
Palmetto Health Baptist	Columbia	97%	544
Palmetto Health Richland	Columbia	97%	1089
Piedmont Medical Center[2]	Rock Hill	97%	476
Mary Black Memorial Hospital	Spartanburg	96%	338
Carolina Pines Regional Medical Center	Hartsville	95%	111
Coastal Carolina Hospital	Hardeeville	95%	37
GHS Laurens County Memorial Hospital	Clinton	95%	157
Oconee Medical Center[2]	Seneca	95%	190
Georgetown Memorial Hospital[2]	Georgetown	94%	183
Mcleod Loris Seacoast Hospital	Loris	93%	188
GHS Greenville Memorial Medical Center[2]	Greenville	91%	473
Self Regional Healthcare[2]	Greenwood	90%	220
Clarendon Memorial Hospital	Manning	89%	88
Trmc of Orangeburg & Calhoun[2]	Orangeburg	87%	95

Survey of Patients' Hospital Experiences

Area Around Room 'Always' Quiet at Night

Hospital Name	City	Rate	Cases
GHS Patewood Memorial Hospital	Greenville	90%	300+
Village Hospital	Greer	77%	300+
Marlboro Park Hospital	Bennettsville	76%	(a)
East Cooper Medical Center	Mount Pleasant	74%	300+
Mount Pleasant Hospital	Mount Pleasant	74%	(a)
Abbeville Area Medical Center	Abbeville	73%	(a)
Mary Black Memorial Hospital	Spartanburg	73%	300+
Baptist Easley Hospital	Easley	72%	300+
Mcleod Medical Center - Dillon	Dillon	72%	300+
Williamsburg Regional Hospital	Kingstree	72%	(a)
Barnwell County Hospital	Barnwell	71%	(a)
Carolinas Hospital System	Florence	71%	300+
GHS - Hillcrest Memorial Hospital	Simpsonville	71%	300+
Carolinas Hospital System Marion	Mullins	70%	300+
Hampton Regional Medical Center	Varnville	70%	(a)
Mcleod Loris Seacoast Hospital	Loris	70%	300+
Saint Francis - Downtown	Greenville	70%	300+
Clarendon Memorial Hospital	Manning	69%	(a)
Georgetown Memorial Hospital	Georgetown	69%	300+
GHS Greer Memorial Hospital	Greer	69%	300+
Oconee Medical Center	Seneca	69%	300+
Self Regional Healthcare	Greenwood	69%	300+
Spartanburg Regional Medical Center	Spartanburg	69%	300+
Colleton Medical Center	Walterboro	68%	300+
Conway Medical Center	Conway	68%	300+
Palmetto Health Baptist	Columbia	68%	300+
Sisters of Charity Providence Hospitals	Columbia	68%	300+
Trmc of Orangeburg & Calhoun	Orangeburg	68%	300+
Anmed Health[11]	Anderson	67%	300+
Bon Secours-St Francis Xavier Hosp	Charleston	67%	300+
Carolina Pines Regional Medical Center	Hartsville	67%	300+
Lake City Community Hospital	Lake City	67%	(a)
Mcleod Regional Medical Center - Pee Dee	Florence	67%	300+
Springs Memorial Hospital	Lancaster	67%	300+
Wallace Thomson Hospital	Union	67%	300+
Chesterfield General Hospital	Cheraw	66%	300+
Musc Medical Center	Charleston	66%	300+
Roper Hospital	Charleston	66%	300+
Tuomey Healthcare System	Sumter	66%	300+
GHS Laurens County Memorial Hospital	Clinton	65%	300+
Kershaw Health	Camden	65%	300+
Palmetto Health Richland	Columbia	65%	300+
Beaufort County Memorial Hospital	Beaufort	64%	300+
Chester Regional Medical Center	Chester	63%	(a)
Coastal Carolina Hospital	Hardeeville	63%	300+
GHS Greenville Memorial Medical Center	Greenville	63%	300+
Aiken Regional Medical Center	Aiken	62%	300+
Cannon Memorial Hospital	Pickens	62%	(a)
Lexington Medical Center	West Columbia	62%	300+
Grand Strand Regional Medical Center	Myrtle Beach	60%	300+
Newberry County Memorial Hospital	Newberry	60%	300+
Novant Health Gaffney Medical Center	Gaffney	60%	(a)
Piedmont Medical Center	Rock Hill	59%	300+
Trident Medical Center	Charleston	59%	300+
Waccamaw Community Hospital	Murrells Inlet	57%	300+
Hilton Head Regional Medical Center	Hilton Head Isl	49%	300+

Doctors 'Always' Communicated Well

Hospital Name	City	Rate	Cases
Abbeville Area Medical Center	Abbeville	96%	(a)
Lake City Community Hospital	Lake City	92%	(a)
Wallace Thomson Hospital	Union	90%	300+
GHS Patewood Memorial Hospital	Greenville	89%	300+
Mcleod Medical Center - Dillon	Dillon	89%	300+
Mount Pleasant Hospital	Mount Pleasant	89%	(a)
Williamsburg Regional Hospital	Kingstree	88%	(a)
Palmetto Health Richland	Columbia	87%	300+
Village Hospital	Greer	87%	300+
East Cooper Medical Center	Mount Pleasant	86%	300+
GHS - Hillcrest Memorial Hospital	Simpsonville	86%	300+
GHS Greer Memorial Hospital	Greer	86%	300+
Newberry County Memorial Hospital	Newberry	86%	300+
Baptist Easley Hospital	Easley	85%	300+
Bon Secours-St Francis Xavier Hosp	Charleston	85%	300+
Carolina Pines Regional Medical Center	Hartsville	85%	300+
Carolinas Hospital System Marion	Mullins	85%	300+
Chesterfield General Hospital	Cheraw	85%	300+
Clarendon Memorial Hospital	Manning	85%	(a)
Marlboro Park Hospital	Bennettsville	85%	(a)
Self Regional Healthcare	Greenwood	85%	300+
Beaufort County Memorial Hospital	Beaufort	84%	300+
Hampton Regional Medical Center	Varnville	84%	(a)
Lexington Medical Center	West Columbia	84%	300+
Mary Black Memorial Hospital	Spartanburg	84%	300+
Mcleod Regional Medical Center - Pee Dee	Florence	84%	300+
Roper Hospital	Charleston	84%	300+
Springs Memorial Hospital	Lancaster	84%	300+
Trmc of Orangeburg & Calhoun	Orangeburg	84%	300+
Tuomey Healthcare System	Sumter	84%	300+
Cannon Memorial Hospital	Pickens	83%	(a)
Carolinas Hospital System	Florence	83%	300+
Mcleod Loris Seacoast Hospital	Loris	83%	300+
Oconee Medical Center	Seneca	83%	300+
Palmetto Health Baptist	Columbia	83%	300+
Sisters of Charity Providence Hospitals	Columbia	83%	300+
Anmed Health[11]	Anderson	82%	300+
Chester Regional Medical Center	Chester	82%	(a)
Georgetown Memorial Hospital	Georgetown	82%	300+
Kershaw Health	Camden	82%	300+
Musc Medical Center	Charleston	82%	300+
Saint Francis - Downtown	Greenville	82%	300+
Spartanburg Regional Medical Center	Spartanburg	82%	300+
Waccamaw Community Hospital	Murrells Inlet	82%	300+
Conway Medical Center	Conway	81%	300+
GHS Laurens County Memorial Hospital	Clinton	81%	300+
Hilton Head Regional Medical Center	Hilton Head Isl	81%	300+
Piedmont Medical Center	Rock Hill	81%	300+
Aiken Regional Medical Center	Aiken	80%	300+
Barnwell County Hospital	Barnwell	80%	(a)
Coastal Carolina Hospital	Hardeeville	80%	300+
Colleton Medical Center	Walterboro	80%	300+
Grand Strand Regional Medical Center	Myrtle Beach	79%	300+
Trident Medical Center	Charleston	79%	300+
GHS Greenville Memorial Medical Center	Greenville	78%	300+
Novant Health Gaffney Medical Center	Gaffney	76%	(a)

Home Recovery Information Given

Hospital Name	City	Rate	Cases
GHS Patewood Memorial Hospital	Greenville	93%	300+
Chester Regional Medical Center	Chester	92%	(a)
Village Hospital	Greer	91%	300+
Abbeville Area Medical Center	Abbeville	90%	(a)
Baptist Easley Hospital	Easley	90%	300+
GHS Greer Memorial Hospital	Greer	90%	300+
Springs Memorial Hospital	Lancaster	90%	300+
GHS - Hillcrest Memorial Hospital	Simpsonville	89%	300+
Hampton Regional Medical Center	Varnville	89%	(a)
Mount Pleasant Hospital	Mount Pleasant	89%	(a)
Spartanburg Regional Medical Center	Spartanburg	89%	300+
Williamsburg Regional Hospital	Kingstree	89%	(a)
Beaufort County Memorial Hospital	Beaufort	88%	300+
Bon Secours-St Francis Xavier Hosp	Charleston	88%	300+
East Cooper Medical Center	Mount Pleasant	88%	300+
Mary Black Memorial Hospital	Spartanburg	88%	300+
Roper Hospital	Charleston	88%	300+
Saint Francis - Downtown	Greenville	88%	300+
Marlboro Park Hospital	Bennettsville	87%	(a)
Mcleod Medical Center - Dillon	Dillon	87%	300+
Mcleod Regional Medical Center - Pee Dee	Florence	87%	300+
Palmetto Health Richland	Columbia	87%	300+
Self Regional Healthcare	Greenwood	87%	300+
Wallace Thomson Hospital	Union	87%	300+
Cannon Memorial Hospital	Pickens	86%	(a)
Hilton Head Regional Medical Center	Hilton Head Isl	86%	300+
Musc Medical Center	Charleston	86%	300+
Newberry County Memorial Hospital	Newberry	86%	300+
Sisters of Charity Providence Hospitals	Columbia	86%	300+
Aiken Regional Medical Center	Aiken	85%	300+
Anmed Health[11]	Anderson	85%	300+
Carolinas Hospital System	Florence	85%	300+
Clarendon Memorial Hospital	Manning	85%	(a)
Coastal Carolina Hospital	Hardeeville	85%	300+
GHS Laurens County Memorial Hospital	Clinton	85%	300+
Mcleod Loris Seacoast Hospital	Loris	85%	300+
Oconee Medical Center	Seneca	85%	300+
Piedmont Medical Center	Rock Hill	85%	300+
Tuomey Healthcare System	Sumter	85%	300+
Carolinas Hospital System Marion	Mullins	84%	300+
GHS Greenville Memorial Medical Center	Greenville	84%	300+
Kershaw Health	Camden	84%	300+
Lexington Medical Center	West Columbia	84%	300+
Novant Health Gaffney Medical Center	Gaffney	84%	(a)
Trident Medical Center	Charleston	84%	300+
Waccamaw Community Hospital	Murrells Inlet	84%	300+
Grand Strand Regional Medical Center	Myrtle Beach	83%	300+
Palmetto Health Baptist	Columbia	83%	300+
Carolina Pines Regional Medical Center	Hartsville	82%	300+
Colleton Medical Center	Walterboro	82%	300+
Conway Medical Center	Conway	82%	300+
Georgetown Memorial Hospital	Georgetown	82%	300+
Trmc of Orangeburg & Calhoun	Orangeburg	82%	300+
Chesterfield General Hospital	Cheraw	81%	300+
Barnwell County Hospital	Barnwell	80%	(a)
Lake City Community Hospital	Lake City	77%	(a)

NOTE: Hospital profiles are in alphabetical order by state, then city, then hospital within the city; Rankings exclude hospitals with less than 25 cases except for patient surveys which excludes hospitals with less than 100 cases; (a) 100-299 cases; (1) The number of cases/patients is too few to report; (2) Data submitted were based on a sample of cases/patients; (3) Results are based on a shorter time period than required; (4) Data suppressed by CMS for one or more quarters; (5) Results are not available for this reporting period; (6) Fewer than 100 patients completed the HCAHPS survey; (7) No cases met the criteria for this measure; (8) The lower limit of the confidence interval cannot be calculated if the number of observed infections equals zero; (9) No data are available from the state/territory for this reporting period; (10) The scores shown reflect fewer than 50 completed surveys; (11) There were discrepancies in the data collection process; (12) This measure does not apply to this hospital for this reporting period; (13) Results cannot be calculated for this reporting period; (14) The results for this state are combined with nearby states to protect confidentiality; Please refer to the User's Guide for a full explanation of data.

Hospital Given 9 or 10 on 10 Point Scale

Hospital Name	City	Rate	Cases
GHS Patewood Memorial Hospital	Greenville	91%	300+
GHS Greer Memorial Hospital	Greer	85%	300+
Abbeville Area Medical Center	Abbeville	81%	(a)
Mcleod Regional Medical Center - Pee Dee	Florence	81%	300+
Mount Pleasant Hospital	Mount Pleasant	81%	(a)
Village Hospital	Greer	81%	300+
Bon Secours-St Francis Xavier Hosp	Charleston	80%	300+
East Cooper Medical Center	Mount Pleasant	80%	300+
Musc Medical Center	Charleston	80%	300+
Hampton Regional Medical Center	Varnville	79%	(a)
Waccamaw Community Hospital	Murrells Inlet	79%	300+
Baptist Easley Hospital	Easley	78%	300+
Mary Black Memorial Hospital	Spartanburg	78%	300+
Roper Hospital	Charleston	78%	300+
Sisters of Charity Providence Hospitals	Columbia	78%	300+
GHS - Hillcrest Memorial Hospital	Simpsonville	77%	300+
Saint Francis - Downtown	Greenville	77%	300+
Lexington Medical Center	West Columbia	76%	300+
Palmetto Health Richland	Columbia	76%	300+
Carolinas Hospital System	Florence	75%	300+
Newberry County Memorial Hospital	Newberry	74%	300+
Self Regional Healthcare	Greenwood	74%	300+
Mcleod Loris Seacoast Hospital	Loris	73%	300+
Mcleod Medical Center - Dillon	Dillon	73%	300+
Anmed Health[11]	Anderson	72%	300+
Beaufort County Memorial Hospital	Beaufort	72%	300+
Clarendon Memorial Hospital	Manning	72%	(a)
Palmetto Health Baptist	Columbia	72%	300+
Spartanburg Regional Medical Center	Spartanburg	72%	300+
Conway Medical Center	Conway	71%	300+
GHS Greenville Memorial Medical Center	Greenville	71%	300+
Springs Memorial Hospital	Lancaster	71%	300+
Oconee Medical Center	Seneca	70%	300+
Williamsburg Regional Hospital	Kingstree	70%	(a)
Cannon Memorial Hospital	Pickens	69%	(a)
Coastal Carolina Hospital	Hardeeville	69%	300+
Georgetown Memorial Hospital	Georgetown	69%	300+
Wallace Thomson Hospital	Union	68%	300+
Chesterfield General Hospital	Cheraw	67%	300+
Hilton Head Regional Medical Center	Hilton Head Isl	67%	300+
Marlboro Park Hospital	Bennettsville	67%	(a)
Aiken Regional Medical Center	Aiken	66%	300+
Grand Strand Regional Medical Center	Myrtle Beach	66%	300+
Kershaw Health	Camden	66%	300+
Carolina Pines Regional Medical Center	Hartsville	65%	300+
Carolinas Hospital System Marion	Mullins	65%	300+
Colleton Medical Center	Walterboro	65%	300+
Piedmont Medical Center	Rock Hill	65%	300+
Trmc of Orangeburg & Calhoun	Orangeburg	64%	300+
Trident Medical Center	Charleston	63%	300+
Lake City Community Hospital	Lake City	62%	(a)
Chester Regional Medical Center	Chester	61%	(a)
GHS Laurens County Memorial Hospital	Clinton	61%	300+
Barnwell County Hospital	Barnwell	60%	(a)
Tuomey Healthcare System	Sumter	59%	300+
Novant Health Gaffney Medical Center	Gaffney	55%	(a)

Meds 'Always' Explained Before Given

Hospital Name	City	Rate	Cases
Abbeville Area Medical Center	Abbeville	78%	(a)
Mcleod Medical Center - Dillon	Dillon	72%	300+
Mount Pleasant Hospital	Mount Pleasant	72%	(a)
Williamsburg Regional Hospital	Kingstree	72%	(a)
Baptist Easley Hospital	Easley	71%	300+
GHS Patewood Memorial Hospital	Greenville	71%	300+
Hampton Regional Medical Center	Varnville	71%	(a)
Mcleod Loris Seacoast Hospital	Loris	71%	300+
Palmetto Health Richland	Columbia	70%	300+
GHS Greer Memorial Hospital	Greer	69%	300+
Marlboro Park Hospital	Bennettsville	69%	(a)
Mary Black Memorial Hospital	Spartanburg	69%	300+
Mcleod Regional Medical Center - Pee Dee	Florence	69%	300+
Village Hospital	Greer	69%	300+
Roper Hospital	Charleston	68%	300+
Springs Memorial Hospital	Lancaster	68%	300+
Bon Secours-St Francis Xavier Hosp	Charleston	67%	300+
Clarendon Memorial Hospital	Manning	67%	(a)
Self Regional Healthcare	Greenwood	67%	300+
Trmc of Orangeburg & Calhoun	Orangeburg	67%	300+
Wallace Thomson Hospital	Union	67%	300+
Beaufort County Memorial Hospital	Beaufort	66%	300+
Carolinas Hospital System	Florence	66%	300+
Kershaw Health	Camden	66%	300+
Musc Medical Center	Charleston	66%	300+
Newberry County Memorial Hospital	Newberry	66%	300+
Palmetto Health Baptist	Columbia	66%	300+
Carolinas Hospital System Marion	Mullins	65%	300+
Chesterfield General Hospital	Cheraw	65%	300+
East Cooper Medical Center	Mount Pleasant	65%	300+
Georgetown Memorial Hospital	Georgetown	65%	300+
Hilton Head Regional Medical Center	Hilton Head Isl	65%	300+
Spartanburg Regional Medical Center	Spartanburg	65%	300+
Waccamaw Community Hospital	Murrells Inlet	65%	300+
Anmed Health[11]	Anderson	64%	300+
GHS - Hillcrest Memorial Hospital	Simpsonville	64%	300+
Oconee Medical Center	Seneca	64%	300+
Sisters of Charity Providence Hospitals	Columbia	64%	300+
Cannon Memorial Hospital	Pickens	63%	(a)
Conway Medical Center	Conway	63%	300+
GHS Laurens County Memorial Hospital	Clinton	63%	300+
Saint Francis - Downtown	Greenville	63%	300+
Barnwell County Hospital	Barnwell	62%	(a)
Carolina Pines Regional Medical Center	Hartsville	62%	300+
Chester Regional Medical Center	Chester	62%	(a)
Coastal Carolina Hospital	Hardeeville	62%	300+
GHS Greenville Memorial Medical Center	Greenville	62%	300+
Lake City Community Hospital	Lake City	62%	(a)
Tuomey Healthcare System	Sumter	62%	300+
Colleton Medical Center	Walterboro	61%	300+
Piedmont Medical Center	Rock Hill	61%	300+
Lexington Medical Center	West Columbia	60%	300+
Trident Medical Center	Charleston	60%	300+
Grand Strand Regional Medical Center	Myrtle Beach	57%	300+
Aiken Regional Medical Center	Aiken	56%	300+
Novant Health Gaffney Medical Center	Gaffney	55%	(a)

Nurses 'Always' Communicated Well

Hospital Name	City	Rate	Cases
Abbeville Area Medical Center	Abbeville	92%	(a)
GHS Patewood Memorial Hospital	Greenville	90%	300+
Mount Pleasant Hospital	Mount Pleasant	86%	(a)
GHS Greer Memorial Hospital	Greer	85%	300+
Baptist Easley Hospital	Easley	84%	300+
Palmetto Health Richland	Columbia	84%	300+
Self Regional Healthcare	Greenwood	84%	300+
Mcleod Loris Seacoast Hospital	Loris	83%	300+
Mcleod Medical Center - Dillon	Dillon	83%	300+
Springs Memorial Hospital	Lancaster	83%	300+
Waccamaw Community Hospital	Murrells Inlet	83%	300+
Williamsburg Regional Hospital	Kingstree	83%	(a)
Bon Secours-St Francis Xavier Hosp	Charleston	82%	300+
GHS - Hillcrest Memorial Hospital	Simpsonville	82%	300+
Mary Black Memorial Hospital	Spartanburg	82%	300+
Mcleod Regional Medical Center - Pee Dee	Florence	82%	300+
Newberry County Memorial Hospital	Newberry	82%	300+
Roper Hospital	Charleston	82%	300+
Tuomey Healthcare System	Sumter	82%	300+
Village Hospital	Greer	82%	300+
Anmed Health[11]	Anderson	81%	300+
Barnwell County Hospital	Barnwell	81%	(a)
Cannon Memorial Hospital	Pickens	81%	(a)
Georgetown Memorial Hospital	Georgetown	81%	300+
Lake City Community Hospital	Lake City	81%	(a)
Marlboro Park Hospital	Bennettsville	81%	(a)
Musc Medical Center	Charleston	81%	300+
Spartanburg Regional Medical Center	Spartanburg	81%	300+
Beaufort County Memorial Hospital	Beaufort	80%	300+
Carolina Pines Regional Medical Center	Hartsville	80%	300+
Clarendon Memorial Hospital	Manning	80%	(a)
Conway Medical Center	Conway	80%	300+
East Cooper Medical Center	Mount Pleasant	80%	300+
Kershaw Health	Camden	80%	300+
Oconee Medical Center	Seneca	80%	300+
Palmetto Health Baptist	Columbia	80%	300+
Saint Francis - Downtown	Greenville	80%	300+
Trmc of Orangeburg & Calhoun	Orangeburg	80%	300+
Hampton Regional Medical Center	Varnville	79%	(a)
Lexington Medical Center	West Columbia	79%	300+
Wallace Thomson Hospital	Union	79%	300+
Carolinas Hospital System	Florence	78%	300+
Carolinas Hospital System Marion	Mullins	78%	300+
Chester Regional Medical Center	Chester	78%	(a)
Chesterfield General Hospital	Cheraw	78%	300+
Coastal Carolina Hospital	Hardeeville	78%	300+
GHS Greenville Memorial Medical Center	Greenville	78%	300+
GHS Laurens County Memorial Hospital	Clinton	78%	300+
Piedmont Medical Center	Rock Hill	78%	300+
Sisters of Charity Providence Hospitals	Columbia	78%	300+
Colleton Medical Center	Walterboro	77%	300+
Hilton Head Regional Medical Center	Hilton Head Isl	77%	300+
Aiken Regional Medical Center	Aiken	74%	300+
Grand Strand Regional Medical Center	Myrtle Beach	73%	300+
Trident Medical Center	Charleston	73%	300+
Novant Health Gaffney Medical Center	Gaffney	70%	(a)

Pain 'Always' Well Controlled

Hospital Name	City	Rate	Cases
Abbeville Area Medical Center	Abbeville	82%	(a)
GHS Patewood Memorial Hospital	Greenville	80%	300+
Mcleod Medical Center - Dillon	Dillon	77%	300+
Baptist Easley Hospital	Easley	76%	300+
Marlboro Park Hospital	Bennettsville	76%	(a)
Tuomey Healthcare System	Sumter	76%	300+
Waccamaw Community Hospital	Murrells Inlet	76%	300+
GHS Greer Memorial Hospital	Greer	75%	300+
Kershaw Health	Camden	75%	300+
Newberry County Memorial Hospital	Newberry	75%	300+
Palmetto Health Richland	Columbia	75%	300+
Coastal Carolina Hospital	Hardeeville	74%	300+
Mary Black Memorial Hospital	Spartanburg	74%	300+
Mcleod Loris Seacoast Hospital	Loris	74%	300+
Mcleod Regional Medical Center - Pee Dee	Florence	74%	300+
Mount Pleasant Hospital	Mount Pleasant	74%	(a)
Roper Hospital	Charleston	74%	300+
Self Regional Healthcare	Greenwood	74%	300+
Sisters of Charity Providence Hospitals	Columbia	74%	300+
Springs Memorial Hospital	Lancaster	74%	300+
Bon Secours-St Francis Xavier Hosp	Charleston	73%	300+
East Cooper Medical Center	Mount Pleasant	73%	300+
GHS - Hillcrest Memorial Hospital	Simpsonville	73%	300+
GHS Laurens County Memorial Hospital	Clinton	73%	300+
Lake City Community Hospital	Lake City	73%	(a)
Oconee Medical Center	Seneca	73%	300+
Saint Francis - Downtown	Greenville	73%	300+
Carolinas Hospital System	Florence	72%	300+
Chester Regional Medical Center	Chester	72%	(a)
Musc Medical Center	Charleston	72%	300+
Palmetto Health Baptist	Columbia	72%	300+
Spartanburg Regional Medical Center	Spartanburg	72%	300+
Wallace Thomson Hospital	Union	72%	300+
Anmed Health[11]	Anderson	71%	300+
Beaufort County Memorial Hospital	Beaufort	71%	300+
Chesterfield General Hospital	Cheraw	71%	300+
Hilton Head Regional Medical Center	Hilton Head Isl	71%	300+
Lexington Medical Center	West Columbia	71%	300+
Trmc of Orangeburg & Calhoun	Orangeburg	71%	300+
Village Hospital	Greer	71%	300+
Aiken Regional Medical Center	Aiken	70%	300+
Clarendon Memorial Hospital	Manning	70%	(a)
Georgetown Memorial Hospital	Georgetown	70%	300+
GHS Greenville Memorial Medical Center	Greenville	70%	300+
Williamsburg Regional Hospital	Kingstree	70%	(a)
Carolinas Hospital System Marion	Mullins	69%	300+
Colleton Medical Center	Walterboro	69%	300+
Hampton Regional Medical Center	Varnville	69%	(a)
Piedmont Medical Center	Rock Hill	69%	300+
Cannon Memorial Hospital	Pickens	68%	(a)
Carolina Pines Regional Medical Center	Hartsville	68%	300+
Conway Medical Center	Conway	68%	300+
Trident Medical Center	Charleston	68%	300+
Grand Strand Regional Medical Center	Myrtle Beach	66%	300+
Barnwell County Hospital	Barnwell	65%	(a)
Novant Health Gaffney Medical Center	Gaffney	62%	(a)

Room and Bathroom 'Always' Clean

Hospital Name	City	Rate	Cases
GHS Patewood Memorial Hospital	Greenville	90%	300+
Abbeville Area Medical Center	Abbeville	89%	(a)
Williamsburg Regional Hospital	Kingstree	82%	(a)
Baptist Easley Hospital	Easley	81%	300+
Self Regional Healthcare	Greenwood	81%	300+
Village Hospital	Greer	80%	300+
GHS Greer Memorial Hospital	Greer	79%	300+
Hampton Regional Medical Center	Varnville	79%	(a)
Newberry County Memorial Hospital	Newberry	79%	300+
Cannon Memorial Hospital	Pickens	78%	(a)
Mcleod Medical Center - Dillon	Dillon	78%	300+
Springs Memorial Hospital	Lancaster	78%	300+
Chester Regional Medical Center	Chester	76%	(a)
Clarendon Memorial Hospital	Manning	76%	(a)
Colleton Medical Center	Walterboro	76%	300+
Conway Medical Center	Conway	76%	300+
East Cooper Medical Center	Mount Pleasant	76%	300+
GHS - Hillcrest Memorial Hospital	Simpsonville	75%	300+
Anmed Health[11]	Anderson	74%	300+
Coastal Carolina Hospital	Hardeeville	73%	300+
Lexington Medical Center	West Columbia	73%	300+
Bon Secours-St Francis Xavier Hosp	Charleston	72%	300+
Mary Black Memorial Hospital	Spartanburg	72%	300+
Mcleod Regional Medical Center - Pee Dee	Florence	72%	300+
Trmc of Orangeburg & Calhoun	Orangeburg	72%	300+
Georgetown Memorial Hospital	Georgetown	71%	300+
Kershaw Health	Camden	71%	300+
Musc Medical Center	Charleston	71%	300+
Palmetto Health Richland	Columbia	71%	300+
Sisters of Charity Providence Hospitals	Columbia	71%	300+
Spartanburg Regional Medical Center	Spartanburg	71%	300+
Waccamaw Community Hospital	Murrells Inlet	71%	300+
Carolina Pines Regional Medical Center	Hartsville	70%	300+

NOTE: Hospital profiles are in alphabetical order by state, then city, then hospital within the city; Rankings exclude hospitals with less than 25 cases except for patient surveys which excludes hospitals with less than 100 cases; (a) 100-299 cases; (1) The number of cases/patients is too few to report; (2) Data submitted were based on a sample of cases/patients; (3) Results are based on a shorter time period than required; (4) Data suppressed by CMS for one or more quarters; (5) Results are not available for this reporting period; (6) Fewer than 100 patients completed the HCAHPS survey; (7) No cases met the criteria for this measure; (8) The lower limit of the confidence interval cannot be calculated if the number of observed infections equals zero; (9) No data are available from the state/territory for this reporting period; (10) The scores shown reflect fewer than 50 completed surveys; (11) There were discrepancies in the data collection process; (12) This measure does not apply to this hospital for this reporting period; (13) Results cannot be calculated for this reporting period; (14) The results for this state are combined with nearby states to protect confidentiality; Please refer to the User's Guide for a full explanation of data.

Carolinas Hospital System	Florence	70%	300+
Carolinas Hospital System Marion	Mullins	70%	300+
GHS Greenville Memorial Medical Center	Greenville	70%	300+
Roper Hospital	Charleston	70%	300+
Marlboro Park Hospital	Bennettsville	69%	(a)
Mcleod Loris Seacoast Hospital	Loris	69%	300+
Oconee Medical Center	Seneca	69%	300+
Palmetto Health Baptist	Columbia	69%	300+
Tuomey Healthcare System	Sumter	69%	300+
Beaufort County Memorial Hospital	Beaufort	68%	300+
Mount Pleasant Hospital	Mount Pleasant	68%	(a)
Novant Health Gaffney Medical Center	Gaffney	68%	(a)
Chesterfield General Hospital	Cheraw	67%	300+
Hilton Head Regional Medical Center	Hilton Head Isl	67%	300+
Barnwell County Hospital	Barnwell	66%	(a)
Grand Strand Regional Medical Center	Myrtle Beach	66%	300+
Saint Francis - Downtown	Greenville	66%	300+
Wallace Thomson Hospital	Union	66%	300+
Piedmont Medical Center	Rock Hill	65%	300+
Trident Medical Center	Charleston	65%	300+
GHS Laurens County Memorial Hospital	Clinton	62%	300+
Lake City Community Hospital	Lake City	62%	(a)
Aiken Regional Medical Center	Aiken	61%	300+

Timely Help 'Always' Received

Hospital Name	City	Rate	Cases
Abbeville Area Medical Center	Abbeville	85%	(a)
GHS Patewood Memorial Hospital	Greenville	84%	300+
Williamsburg Regional Hospital	Kingstree	77%	(a)
GHS Greer Memorial Hospital	Greer	75%	300+
Lake City Community Hospital	Lake City	74%	(a)
Marlboro Park Hospital	Bennettsville	74%	(a)
Mcleod Medical Center - Dillon	Dillon	73%	300+
Barnwell County Hospital	Barnwell	72%	(a)
Hampton Regional Medical Center	Varnville	72%	(a)
Mary Black Memorial Hospital	Spartanburg	72%	300+
Mcleod Regional Medical Center - Pee Dee	Florence	72%	300+
Mount Pleasant Hospital	Mount Pleasant	72%	(a)
Waccamaw Community Hospital	Murrells Inlet	72%	300+
Bon Secours-St Francis Xavier Hosp	Charleston	71%	300+
Springs Memorial Hospital	Lancaster	71%	300+
Wallace Thomson Hospital	Union	71%	300+
East Cooper Medical Center	Mount Pleasant	70%	300+
Village Hospital	Greer	70%	300+
Anmed Health[11]	Anderson	69%	300+
Carolina Pines Regional Medical Center	Hartsville	69%	300+
Chesterfield General Hospital	Cheraw	69%	300+
Georgetown Memorial Hospital	Georgetown	69%	300+
Mcleod Loris Seacoast Hospital	Loris	69%	300+
Musc Medical Center	Charleston	69%	300+
Newberry County Memorial Hospital	Newberry	69%	300+
Saint Francis - Downtown	Greenville	69%	300+
GHS - Hillcrest Memorial Hospital	Simpsonville	68%	300+
Kershaw Health	Camden	68%	300+
Palmetto Health Richland	Columbia	68%	300+
Roper Hospital	Charleston	68%	300+
Beaufort County Memorial Hospital	Beaufort	67%	300+
Cannon Memorial Hospital	Pickens	67%	(a)
Self Regional Healthcare	Greenwood	67%	300+
Chester Regional Medical Center	Chester	66%	(a)
Coastal Carolina Hospital	Hardeeville	66%	300+
Oconee Medical Center	Seneca	66%	300+
Spartanburg Regional Medical Center	Spartanburg	66%	300+
Baptist Easley Hospital	Easley	65%	300+
Carolinas Hospital System	Florence	65%	300+
Conway Medical Center	Conway	65%	300+
GHS Greenville Memorial Medical Center	Greenville	65%	300+
GHS Laurens County Memorial Hospital	Clinton	65%	300+
Lexington Medical Center	West Columbia	65%	300+
Carolinas Hospital System Marion	Mullins	64%	300+
Clarendon Memorial Hospital	Manning	64%	(a)
Piedmont Medical Center	Rock Hill	64%	300+
Trmc of Orangeburg & Calhoun	Orangeburg	64%	300+
Tuomey Healthcare System	Sumter	64%	300+
Hilton Head Regional Medical Center	Hilton Head Isl	63%	300+
Colleton Medical Center	Walterboro	62%	300+
Palmetto Health Baptist	Columbia	61%	300+
Aiken Regional Medical Center	Aiken	60%	300+
Sisters of Charity Providence Hospitals	Columbia	60%	300+
Trident Medical Center	Charleston	60%	300+
Grand Strand Regional Medical Center	Myrtle Beach	58%	300+
Novant Health Gaffney Medical Center	Gaffney	54%	(a)

Would Definitely Recommend Hospital

Hospital Name	City	Rate	Cases
GHS Patewood Memorial Hospital	Greenville	92%	300+
GHS Greer Memorial Hospital	Greer	87%	300+
Musc Medical Center	Charleston	85%	300+
Mcleod Regional Medical Center - Pee Dee	Florence	84%	300+
Village Hospital	Greer	84%	300+
Waccamaw Community Hospital	Murrells Inlet	83%	300+
Abbeville Area Medical Center	Abbeville	82%	(a)
Mount Pleasant Hospital	Mount Pleasant	82%	(a)
Roper Hospital	Charleston	82%	300+
Sisters of Charity Providence Hospitals	Columbia	82%	300+
Bon Secours-St Francis Xavier Hosp	Charleston	81%	300+
Saint Francis - Downtown	Greenville	81%	300+
East Cooper Medical Center	Mount Pleasant	80%	300+
Palmetto Health Richland	Columbia	80%	300+
GHS - Hillcrest Memorial Hospital	Simpsonville	79%	300+
Mary Black Memorial Hospital	Spartanburg	78%	300+
Baptist Easley Hospital	Easley	77%	300+
Spartanburg Regional Medical Center	Spartanburg	77%	300+
Carolinas Hospital System	Florence	76%	300+
Lexington Medical Center	West Columbia	76%	300+
Hampton Regional Medical Center	Varnville	75%	(a)
Palmetto Health Baptist	Columbia	75%	300+
Self Regional Healthcare	Greenwood	75%	300+
Beaufort County Memorial Hospital	Beaufort	73%	300+
GHS Greenville Memorial Medical Center	Greenville	73%	300+
Anmed Health[11]	Anderson	72%	300+
Conway Medical Center	Conway	71%	300+
Mcleod Loris Seacoast Hospital	Loris	71%	300+
Newberry County Memorial Hospital	Newberry	71%	300+
Grand Strand Regional Medical Center	Myrtle Beach	70%	300+
Mcleod Medical Center - Dillon	Dillon	70%	300+
Clarendon Memorial Hospital	Manning	68%	(a)
Coastal Carolina Hospital	Hardeeville	68%	300+
Hilton Head Regional Medical Center	Hilton Head Isl	68%	300+
Cannon Memorial Hospital	Pickens	67%	(a)
Oconee Medical Center	Seneca	67%	300+
Aiken Regional Medical Center	Aiken	66%	300+
Kershaw Health	Camden	66%	300+
Georgetown Memorial Hospital	Georgetown	65%	300+
Wallace Thomson Hospital	Union	65%	300+
Marlboro Park Hospital	Bennettsville	64%	(a)
Springs Memorial Hospital	Lancaster	64%	300+
Barnwell County Hospital	Barnwell	63%	(a)
Chesterfield General Hospital	Cheraw	63%	300+
Piedmont Medical Center	Rock Hill	63%	300+
Trident Medical Center	Charleston	63%	300+
Williamsburg Regional Hospital	Kingstree	61%	(a)
Carolina Pines Regional Medical Center	Hartsville	60%	300+
Carolinas Hospital System Marion	Mullins	59%	300+
Colleton Medical Center	Walterboro	59%	300+
Lake City Community Hospital	Lake City	59%	(a)
Trmc of Orangeburg & Calhoun	Orangeburg	59%	300+
Tuomey Healthcare System	Sumter	58%	300+
Chester Regional Medical Center	Chester	57%	(a)
GHS Laurens County Memorial Hospital	Clinton	57%	300+
Novant Health Gaffney Medical Center	Gaffney	50%	(a)

Use of Medical Imaging

Cardiac Imaging Stress Test before OP Surgery

Hospital Name	City	Rate	Cases
GHS Patewood Memorial Hospital	Greenville	0.7%	146
Lake City Community Hospital	Lake City	1.2%	82
Colleton Medical Center	Walterboro	2.1%	146
Newberry County Memorial Hospital	Newberry	2.4%	82
Abbeville Area Medical Center	Abbeville	2.9%	70
Georgetown Memorial Hospital	Georgetown	3.1%	259
Clarendon Memorial Hospital	Manning	3.2%	189
Mary Black Memorial Hospital	Spartanburg	3.3%	91
Oconee Medical Center	Seneca	3.5%	685
Anmed Health	Anderson	3.6%	1505
Kershaw Health	Camden	3.6%	387
Baptist Easley Hospital	Easley	3.8%	132
Carolina Pines Regional Medical Center	Hartsville	4.1%	267
Chester Regional Medical Center	Chester	4.2%	72
GHS - Hillcrest Memorial Hospital	Simpsonville	4.2%	312
Carolinas Hospital System Marion	Mullins	4.3%	141
Sisters of Charity Providence Hospitals	Columbia	4.4%	1658
Carolinas Hospital System	Florence	4.7%	299
Mount Pleasant Hospital	Mount Pleasant	4.7%	128
Palmetto Health Richland	Columbia	4.7%	1035
Hampton Regional Medical Center	Varnville	4.8%	83
GHS Greenville Memorial Medical Center	Greenville	4.9%	1164
Beaufort County Memorial Hospital	Beaufort	5.0%	441
Palmetto Health Baptist	Columbia	5.0%	323
Grand Strand Regional Medical Center	Myrtle Beach	5.4%	740
Musc Medical Center	Charleston	5.4%	644
GHS Greer Memorial Hospital	Greer	5.7%	386
Trmc of Orangeburg & Calhoun	Orangeburg	6.0%	151
Wallace Thomson Hospital	Union	6.0%	67
Spartanburg Regional Medical Center	Spartanburg	6.1%	477
Conway Medical Center	Conway	6.3%	317
Mcleod Loris Seacoast Hospital	Loris	6.3%	239
Mcleod Regional Medical Center - Pee Dee	Florence	6.6%	594
GHS Laurens County Memorial Hospital	Clinton	6.7%	89
Village Hospital	Greer	6.9%	87
Lexington Medical Center	West Columbia	7.0%	370
Chesterfield General Hospital	Cheraw	7.1%	99
Roper Hospital	Charleston	7.2%	488
Self Regional Healthcare	Greenwood	7.7%	416
Trident Medical Center	Charleston	8.0%	502
Waccamaw Community Hospital	Murrells Inlet	8.5%	212
Saint Francis - Downtown	Greenville	9.1%	66
Novant Health Gaffney Medical Center	Gaffney	10.8%	130

Combination Abdominal CT Scan

Hospital Name	City	Rate	Cases
Springs Memorial Hospital	Lancaster	0.3%	394
Carolinas Hospital System Marion	Mullins	0.7%	411
Novant Health Gaffney Medical Center	Gaffney	1.1%	281
Village Hospital	Greer	1.7%	301
Lexington Medical Center	West Columbia	1.8%	1947
Marlboro Park Hospital	Bennettsville	1.8%	113
Carolina Pines Regional Medical Center	Hartsville	2.0%	595
Palmetto Health Richland	Columbia	2.5%	649
Chester Regional Medical Center	Chester	2.6%	227
Mcleod Medical Center - Darlington	Darlington	2.8%	71
Aiken Regional Medical Center	Aiken	2.9%	1079
Beaufort County Memorial Hospital	Beaufort	3.1%	1045
Piedmont Medical Center	Rock Hill	3.2%	1223
Spartanburg Regional Medical Center	Spartanburg	3.2%	1709
Grand Strand Regional Medical Center	Myrtle Beach	3.6%	1546
Mcleod Medical Center - Dillon	Dillon	3.7%	401
Mcleod Regional Medical Center - Pee Dee	Florence	3.9%	2066
Saint Francis - Downtown	Greenville	4.2%	1609
Chesterfield General Hospital	Cheraw	4.3%	328
Mary Black Memorial Hospital	Spartanburg	4.3%	557
Palmetto Health Baptist	Columbia	4.5%	798
Newberry County Memorial Hospital	Newberry	4.6%	435
Baptist Easley Hospital	Easley	5.0%	436
Colleton Medical Center	Walterboro	5.3%	435
GHS - Hillcrest Memorial Hospital	Simpsonville	5.5%	474
GHS Laurens County Memorial Hospital	Clinton	5.5%	292
Mcleod Loris Seacoast Hospital	Loris	5.8%	1066
Hampton Regional Medical Center	Varnville	5.9%	169
Conway Medical Center	Conway	6.2%	881
Oconee Medical Center	Seneca	6.5%	818
Cannon Memorial Hospital	Pickens	6.8%	146
GHS Greer Memorial Hospital	Greer	6.8%	663
Coastal Carolina Hospital	Hardeeville	7.1%	482
Musc Medical Center	Charleston	7.4%	1661
Trmc of Orangeburg & Calhoun	Orangeburg	7.7%	832
East Cooper Medical Center	Mount Pleasant	8.0%	201
Mount Pleasant Hospital	Mount Pleasant	8.1%	455
Bon Secours-St Francis Xavier Hosp	Charleston	8.2%	1285
Sisters of Charity Providence Hospitals	Columbia	8.3%	1302
Trident Medical Center	Charleston	8.3%	1572
GHS Greenville Memorial Medical Center	Greenville	9.2%	1872
Barnwell County Hospital	Barnwell	9.3%	172
Carolinas Hospital System	Florence	9.7%	945
Hilton Head Regional Medical Center	Hilton Head Isl	9.7%	589
Roper Hospital	Charleston	9.7%	1525
Lake City Community Hospital	Lake City	10.1%	307
Self Regional Healthcare	Greenwood	10.1%	1183
GHS Patewood Memorial Hospital	Greenville	18.5%	509
Tuomey Healthcare System	Sumter	20.8%	929
Clarendon Memorial Hospital	Manning	21.0%	443
Wallace Thomson Hospital	Union	25.1%	231
Georgetown Memorial Hospital	Georgetown	28.5%	534
Kershaw Health	Camden	30.4%	451
Waccamaw Community Hospital	Murrells Inlet	34.3%	995
Abbeville Area Medical Center	Abbeville	36.9%	195
Anmed Health	Anderson	61.8%	1702

Combination Brain/Sinus CT Scan

Hospital Name	City	Rate	Cases
Baptist Easley Hospital	Easley	0.2%	592
Kershaw Health	Camden	0.6%	642
Hilton Head Regional Medical Center	Hilton Head Isl	0.8%	472
Village Hospital	Greer	0.8%	266
Conway Medical Center	Conway	0.9%	782
Roper Hospital	Charleston	1.1%	1234
Bon Secours-St Francis Xavier Hosp	Charleston	1.2%	1108
Piedmont Medical Center	Rock Hill	1.2%	1047
Mcleod Loris Seacoast Hospital	Loris	1.3%	1058
Oconee Medical Center	Seneca	1.5%	794
GHS Laurens County Memorial Hospital	Clinton	1.8%	443
Georgetown Memorial Hospital	Georgetown	1.9%	701
Musc Medical Center	Charleston	1.9%	896
Spartanburg Regional Medical Center	Spartanburg	1.9%	1398
Trmc of Orangeburg & Calhoun	Orangeburg	1.9%	847
Newberry County Memorial Hospital	Newberry	2.0%	410
Carolina Pines Regional Medical Center	Hartsville	2.1%	612
GHS Greer Memorial Hospital	Greer	2.1%	520
Lexington Medical Center	West Columbia	2.1%	1781

NOTE: Hospital profiles are in alphabetical order by state, then city, then hospital within the city; Rankings exclude hospitals with less than 25 cases except for patient surveys which excludes hospitals with less than 100 cases; (a) 100-299 cases; (1) The number of cases/patients is too few to report; (2) Data submitted were based on a sample of cases/patients; (3) Results are based on a shorter time period than required; (4) Data suppressed by CMS for one or more quarters; (5) Results are not available for this reporting period; (6) Fewer than 100 patients completed the HCAHPS survey; (7) No cases met the criteria for this measure; (8) The lower limit of the confidence interval cannot be calculated if the number of observed infections equals zero; (9) No data are available from the state/territory for this reporting period; (10) The scores shown reflect fewer than 50 completed surveys; (11) There were discrepancies in the data collection process; (12) This measure does not apply to this hospital for this reporting period; (13) Results cannot be calculated for this reporting period; (14) The results for this state are combined with nearby states to protect confidentiality; Please refer to the User's Guide for a full explanation of data.

Trident Medical Center	Charleston	2.1%	1634
Sisters of Charity Providence Hospitals	Columbia	2.3%	1392
Anmed Health	Anderson	2.4%	1508
GHS Greenville Memorial Medical Center	Greenville	2.5%	1691
Self Regional Healthcare	Greenwood	2.7%	1132
Aiken Regional Medical Center	Aiken	2.9%	816
Palmetto Health Richland	Columbia	2.9%	903
Saint Francis - Downtown	Greenville	2.9%	1609
Grand Strand Regional Medical Center	Myrtle Beach	3.0%	1465
Tuomey Healthcare System	Sumter	3.1%	1080
Mcleod Regional Medical Center - Pee Dee	Florence	3.7%	1506
Waccamaw Community Hospital	Murrells Inlet	4.3%	951
Coastal Carolina Hospital	Hardeeville	4.4%	564
Novant Health Gaffney Medical Center	Gaffney	4.4%	472
Springs Memorial Hospital	Lancaster	4.4%	796
Carolinas Hospital System	Florence	4.7%	773
Mary Black Memorial Hospital	Spartanburg	4.7%	594
Beaufort County Memorial Hospital	Beaufort	5.3%	795
Hampton Regional Medical Center	Varnville	6.4%	280
Marlboro Park Hospital	Bennettsville	6.9%	204

Combination Chest CT Scan

Hospital Name	City	Rate	Cases
Anmed Health	Anderson	0.0%	1047
Baptist Easley Hospital	Easley	0.0%	321
Cannon Memorial Hospital	Pickens	0.0%	101
Carolinas Hospital System Marion	Mullins	0.0%	95
GHS - Hillcrest Memorial Hospital	Simpsonville	0.0%	331
GHS Patewood Memorial Hospital	Greenville	0.0%	443
Mcleod Medical Center - Darlington	Darlington	0.0%	47
Mount Pleasant Hospital	Mount Pleasant	0.0%	396
Piedmont Medical Center	Rock Hill	0.0%	643
Spartanburg Regional Medical Center	Spartanburg	0.0%	1803
Village Hospital	Greer	0.0%	150
Bon Secours-St Francis Xavier Hosp	Charleston	0.1%	949
GHS Greenville Memorial Medical Center	Greenville	0.1%	1560
Beaufort County Memorial Hospital	Beaufort	0.2%	611
Musc Medical Center	Charleston	0.2%	2534
Roper Hospital	Charleston	0.2%	965
Aiken Regional Medical Center	Aiken	0.3%	639
GHS Greer Memorial Hospital	Greer	0.3%	368
Palmetto Health Richland	Columbia	0.3%	652
Trmc of Orangeburg & Calhoun	Orangeburg	0.4%	537
Carolina Pines Regional Medical Center	Hartsville	0.5%	391
Lexington Medical Center	West Columbia	0.5%	1083
Mcleod Regional Medical Center - Pee Dee	Florence	0.5%	1669
Mcleod Medical Center - Dillon	Dillon	0.6%	317
Novant Health Gaffney Medical Center	Gaffney	0.6%	156
GHS Laurens County Memorial Hospital	Clinton	0.7%	143
Grand Strand Regional Medical Center	Myrtle Beach	0.9%	855
Mary Black Memorial Hospital	Spartanburg	0.9%	235
Saint Francis - Downtown	Greenville	0.9%	1529
Springs Memorial Hospital	Lancaster	1.0%	208
Coastal Carolina Hospital	Hardeeville	1.1%	186
Colleton Medical Center	Walterboro	1.2%	162
Sisters of Charity Providence Hospitals	Columbia	1.2%	889
Palmetto Health Baptist	Columbia	1.3%	302
Mcleod Loris Seacoast Hospital	Loris	1.5%	599
Clarendon Memorial Hospital	Manning	1.6%	188
Oconee Medical Center	Seneca	1.9%	413
Conway Medical Center	Conway	2.3%	556
Kershaw Health	Camden	2.4%	411
Carolinas Hospital System	Florence	2.6%	832
Newberry County Memorial Hospital	Newberry	2.8%	246
Trident Medical Center	Charleston	2.8%	708
Chester Regional Medical Center	Chester	3.1%	97
Self Regional Healthcare	Greenwood	3.3%	639
Chesterfield General Hospital	Cheraw	3.6%	112
Hilton Head Regional Medical Center	Hilton Head Isl	4.5%	337
Tuomey Healthcare System	Sumter	4.6%	563
Barnwell County Hospital	Barnwell	5.4%	56
Waccamaw Community Hospital	Murrells Inlet	5.5%	669
East Cooper Medical Center	Mount Pleasant	7.4%	81
Hampton Regional Medical Center	Varnville	7.6%	66
Georgetown Memorial Hospital	Georgetown	7.8%	255
Lake City Community Hospital	Lake City	10.5%	114
Wallace Thomson Hospital	Union	11.9%	159
Abbeville Area Medical Center	Abbeville	13.2%	68

Follow-up Mammogram/Ultrasound

A follow-up rate near zero may indicate missed cancer; a rate higher than 14% may mean there is unnecessary follow up.

Hospital Name	City	Rate	Cases
Palmetto Health Baptist	Columbia	3.3%	6264
Hampton Regional Medical Center	Varnville	3.6%	447
Aiken Regional Medical Center	Aiken	3.7%	2123
Palmetto Health Richland	Columbia	3.7%	2451
Carolinas Hospital System Marion	Mullins	4.4%	956
Lexington Medical Center	West Columbia	4.4%	2435
Wallace Thomson Hospital	Union	4.7%	422
Grand Strand Regional Medical Center	Myrtle Beach	5.1%	3875
Bon Secours-St Francis Xavier Hosp	Charleston	5.2%	3530
Springs Memorial Hospital	Lancaster	5.3%	187
Conway Medical Center	Conway	5.6%	1592
Kershaw Health	Camden	6.0%	1748
Mount Pleasant Hospital	Mount Pleasant	6.0%	695
Carolina Pines Regional Medical Center	Hartsville	6.1%	804
Trident Medical Center	Charleston	6.1%	5968
Roper Hospital	Charleston	6.3%	1775
Coastal Carolina Hospital	Hardeeville	6.4%	267
Beaufort County Memorial Hospital	Beaufort	6.5%	2176
Mcleod Regional Medical Center - Pee Dee	Florence	6.8%	3733
Mary Black Memorial Hospital	Spartanburg	6.9%	1660
Mcleod Loris Seacoast Hospital	Loris	6.9%	2177
Mcleod Medical Center - Darlington	Darlington	7.1%	703
Village Hospital	Greer	7.4%	462
Colleton Medical Center	Walterboro	7.5%	764
Abbeville Area Medical Center	Abbeville	7.8%	357
Mcleod Medical Center - Dillon	Dillon	7.8%	309
Self Regional Healthcare	Greenwood	8.0%	3474
Clarendon Memorial Hospital	Manning	8.5%	576
Newberry County Memorial Hospital	Newberry	8.6%	776
Spartanburg Regional Medical Center	Spartanburg	8.9%	4585
GHS - Hillcrest Memorial Hospital	Simpsonville	9.0%	767
GHS Greer Memorial Hospital	Greer	9.4%	868
Lake City Community Hospital	Lake City	9.5%	571
Carolinas Hospital System	Florence	9.7%	1386
Chester Regional Medical Center	Chester	9.8%	440
Chesterfield General Hospital	Cheraw	10.1%	426
GHS Patewood Memorial Hospital	Greenville	10.3%	2633
Piedmont Medical Center	Rock Hill	10.4%	2179
Tuomey Healthcare System	Sumter	10.4%	3068
GHS Greenville Memorial Medical Center	Greenville	10.7%	2650
Saint Francis - Downtown	Greenville	11.0%	3028
Novant Health Gaffney Medical Center	Gaffney	11.1%	687
Waccamaw Community Hospital	Murrells Inlet	11.1%	2078
Baptist Easley Hospital	Easley	11.2%	1420
East Cooper Medical Center	Mount Pleasant	11.3%	1543
Hilton Head Regional Medical Center	Hilton Head Isl	11.4%	2593
Anmed Health	Anderson	12.1%	2294
Trmc of Orangeburg & Calhoun	Orangeburg	12.2%	789
GHS Laurens County Memorial Hospital	Clinton	12.6%	795
Musc Medical Center	Charleston	13.5%	1626
Oconee Medical Center	Seneca	13.9%	1016
Barnwell County Hospital	Barnwell	14.4%	222
Cannon Memorial Hospital	Pickens	14.7%	463
Georgetown Memorial Hospital	Georgetown	14.7%	865
Marlboro Park Hospital	Bennettsville	15.6%	314

Lumbar Spine MRI for Low Back Pain

Hospital Name	City	Rate	Cases
Trmc of Orangeburg & Calhoun	Orangeburg	29.5%	78
Trident Medical Center	Charleston	31.0%	129
GHS Patewood Memorial Hospital	Greenville	31.3%	224
Sisters of Charity Providence Hospitals	Columbia	31.3%	80
Piedmont Medical Center	Rock Hill	31.4%	102
Springs Memorial Hospital	Lancaster	31.4%	51
Palmetto Health Richland	Columbia	32.5%	169
Saint Francis - Downtown	Greenville	34.1%	276
Village Hospital	Greer	34.2%	117
Mcleod Loris Seacoast Hospital	Loris	34.3%	134
Aiken Regional Medical Center	Aiken	35.7%	154
GHS Greer Memorial Hospital	Greer	35.9%	117
Self Regional Healthcare	Greenwood	36.5%	304
Kershaw Health	Camden	36.7%	98
Lexington Medical Center	West Columbia	37.1%	124
Palmetto Health Baptist	Columbia	37.4%	190
Conway Medical Center	Conway	37.5%	104
Georgetown Memorial Hospital	Georgetown	38.0%	71
GHS Greenville Memorial Medical Center	Greenville	38.1%	194
Roper Hospital	Charleston	38.5%	327
Newberry County Memorial Hospital	Newberry	38.8%	80
Hilton Head Regional Medical Center	Hilton Head Isl	39.1%	46
GHS - Hillcrest Memorial Hospital	Simpsonville	39.2%	102
Bon Secours-St Francis Xavier Hosp	Charleston	39.3%	405
Mary Black Memorial Hospital	Spartanburg	40.0%	80
Carolina Pines Regional Medical Center	Hartsville	40.5%	153
Waccamaw Community Hospital	Murrells Inlet	40.7%	226
Grand Strand Regional Medical Center	Myrtle Beach	40.8%	130
Anmed Health	Anderson	41.0%	183
Mount Pleasant Hospital	Mount Pleasant	41.1%	168
Beaufort County Memorial Hospital	Beaufort	41.7%	211
Mcleod Medical Center - Dillon	Dillon	41.7%	84
Spartanburg Regional Medical Center	Spartanburg	42.0%	188
Tuomey Healthcare System	Sumter	42.1%	195
GHS Laurens County Memorial Hospital	Clinton	42.2%	45
Baptist Easley Hospital	Easley	42.5%	113
Musc Medical Center	Charleston	42.9%	163
Oconee Medical Center	Seneca	44.1%	93
Clarendon Memorial Hospital	Manning	45.0%	60
Colleton Medical Center	Walterboro	45.3%	75
Carolinas Hospital System Marion	Mullins	46.7%	45
Mcleod Regional Medical Center - Pee Dee	Florence	47.4%	293
Carolinas Hospital System	Florence	51.7%	89
Wallace Thomson Hospital	Union	56.3%	48

NOTE: Hospital profiles are in alphabetical order by state, then city, then hospital within the city; Rankings exclude hospitals with less than 25 cases except for patient surveys which excludes hospitals with less than 100 cases; (a) 100-299 cases; (1) The number of cases/patients is too few to report; (2) Data submitted were based on a sample of cases/patients; (3) Results are based on a shorter time period than required; (4) Data suppressed by CMS for one or more quarters; (5) Results are not available for this reporting period; (6) Fewer than 100 patients completed the HCAHPS survey; (7) No cases met the criteria for this measure; (8) The lower limit of the confidence interval cannot be calculated if the number of observed infections equals zero; (9) No data are available from the state/territory for this reporting period; (10) The scores shown reflect fewer than 50 completed surveys; (11) There were discrepancies in the data collection process; (12) This measure does not apply to this hospital for this reporting period; (13) Results cannot be calculated for this reporting period; (14) The results for this state are combined with nearby states to protect confidentiality; Please refer to the User's Guide for a full explanation of data.

Abbeville Area Medical Center

420 Thomson Circle
Abbeville, SC 29620
URL: www.abbevilleareamc.com
Type: Critical Access Hospitals
Ownership: Government - Local

Phone: 864-366-5011
Fax: 864-366-3317
Emergency Services: Yes
Beds: 25

Key Personnel:

Radiology. . . . . Kinchen W Ballentine, MD
Emergency Room . . . . Debbie Erwin
Anesthesiology. . . . . Doug Fuller
Chief of Medical Staff . . . . Loren Helmuth
Cardiac Laboratory. . . . . Brenda Holtzclaw
Intensive Care Unit. . . . . Angie Miller
CEO . . . . Rich Osmus
Operating Room. . . . . Lisa Ravencraft

Measure	Cases	This Hosp.	State Avg.	U.S. Avg.
Blood Clot Prevention and Treatment				
Anticoagulation Overlap Therapy[5]	-	-	92%	93%
ICU Venous Thromboembolism Prophylaxis[5]	-	-	94%	92%
Incidence of Potentially Preventable VTE[5]	-	-	8%	10%
UFH with Dosages/Platelet Monitoring[5]	-	-	98%	97%
Venous Thromboembolism Prophylaxis[5]	-	-	88%	85%
Warfarin Therapy Discharge Instructions[5]	-	-	72%	75%
Chest Pain/Possible Heart Attack Care				
Aspirin Given Within 24 Hours of Arrival	23	96%	97%	96%
Fibrinolytic Meds Within 30 Min. of Arrival[7]	-	-	68%	58%
Average Time to ECG (minutes)	25	8	5	7
Average Time to Transfer (minutes)[7]	-	-	43	60
Children's Asthma Care				
Received Home Management Plan of Care	-	-	-	88%
Received Reliever Medication	-	-	-	100%
Received Systemic Corticosteroids	-	-	-	100%
Emergency Department				
Admittance Decision Time (minutes)[2]	245	45	94	98
Head CT Results Within 45 Min. of Arrival[3,7]	-	-	61%	57%
Patients Who Left ER Before Being Seen	11,897	1%	3%	2%
Time from ER Arrival to Admit. (minutes)[2]	245	208	274	274
Time from ER Arrival to Discharge (minutes)	160	118	136	134
Time in ER Before Being Evaluated (minutes)	193	26	33	26
Time to Pain Meds for Fractures (minutes)[3]	11	58	61	57
Heart Attack Care				
Aspirin Given at Discharge[3,7]	-	-	99%	99%
Fibrinolytic Meds Within 30 Min. of Arrival[3,7]	-	-	50%	54%
PCI Within 90 Minutes of Arrival[3,7]	-	-	97%	96%
Statin Prescribed at Discharge[3,7]	-	-	99%	98%
Heart Failure Care				
ACE Inhibitor or ARB for LVSD[1]	-	-	98%	97%
Discharge Instructions Given	22	91%	94%	94%
Evaluation of LVS Function	26	81%	99%	99%
Medicare Spending				
Medicare Spending per Patient (ratio)	-	-	0.98	0.98
Pneumonia Care				
Appropriate Initial Antibiotic Given	41	88%	97%	95%
Blood Culture Timing	34	97%	98%	98%
Pregnancy and Delivery Care				
Newborn Deliveries Scheduled Early[3,7]	-	-	3%	6%
Preventive Care				
Immunization for Influenza[2]	269	74%	94%	90%
Immunization for Pneumonia[2]	400	82%	95%	92%
Stroke Care				
Anticoagulation Therapy for Atrial Fibrillation[5]	-	-	95%	95%
Antithrombotic Therapy Timing[5]	-	-	98%	98%
Assessed for Rehabilitation[5]	-	-	97%	97%
Discharged on Antithrombotic Therapy[5]	-	-	99%	99%
Discharged on Statin Medication[5]	-	-	94%	94%
Thrombolytic Therapy Timing[5]	-	-	58%	66%
Venous Thromboembolism Prophylaxis[5]	-	-	94%	94%
Written Stroke Educational Materials Given[5]	-	-	91%	88%
Surgical Care Improvement Project				
Appropriate Beta Blocker Usage	12	92%	98%	98%
Appropriate VTP Within 24 Hours	42	100%	98%	98%
Controlled Postoperative Blood Glucose[3,7]	-	-	99%	97%
Perioperative Temperature Management	41	100%	100%	100%
Prophylactic Antibiotic Selection[1]	-	-	99%	99%
Prophylactic Antibiotic Selection (Outpatient)[1,3]	-	-	99%	98%
Prophylactic Antibiotic Stopped[1]	-	-	98%	98%
Prophylactic Antibiotic Timing[1]	-	-	99%	99%
Prophylactic Antibiotic Timing (Outpatient)[1,3]	-	-	98%	98%
Urinary Catheter Removal[1]	-	-	97%	97%
Survey of Patients' Hospital Experiences				
Area Around Room 'Always' Quiet at Night		(a)	73% 67%	61%
Doctors 'Always' Communicated Well		(a)	96% 84%	82%
Home Recovery Information Given		(a)	90% 86%	85%
Hospital Given 9 or 10 on 10 Point Scale		(a)	81% 72%	71%
Meds 'Always' Explained Before Given		(a)	78% 66%	64%
Nurses 'Always' Communicated Well		(a)	92% 81%	79%
Pain 'Always' Well Controlled		(a)	82% 72%	71%
Room and Bathroom 'Always' Clean		(a)	89% 72%	73%
Timely Help 'Always' Received		(a)	85% 68%	68%
Would Definitely Recommend Hospital		(a)	82% 71%	71%
Use of Medical Imaging				
Cardiac Imaging Stress Test before Surgery	70	2.9%	5.1%	5.3%
Combination Abdominal CT Scan	195	36.9%	10.1%	10.5%
Combination Brain/Sinus CT Scan[1]	-	-	2.5%	2.7%
Combination Chest CT Scan	68	13.2%	1.3%	2.7%
Follow-up Mammogram/Ultrasound	357	7.8%	8%	8.8%
Lumbar Spine MRI for Low Back Pain[1]	-	-	39%	37.2%

Aiken Regional Medical Center

302 University Parkway
Aiken, SC 29801
URL: www.aikenregional.com
Type: Acute Care Hospitals
Ownership: Proprietary

Phone: 803-641-5900
Fax: 803-641-5179
Emergency Services: Yes
Beds: 230

Key Personnel:

Emergency Room . . . . John Arnold
Cardiology . . . . Gregory Eave, MD
Quality Assurance . . . . Lois Ell, RN
Chief of Medical Staff . . . . Donald McCartney
CEO . . . . Carlos Milanes
Radiology. . . . . Bob Queen

Measure	Cases	This Hosp.	State Avg.	U.S. Avg.
Blood Clot Prevention and Treatment				
Anticoagulation Overlap Therapy[2]	55	91%	92%	93%
ICU Venous Thromboembolism Prophylaxis[2]	86	87%	94%	92%
Incidence of Potentially Preventable VTE[1,2]	-	-	8%	10%
UFH with Dosages/Platelet Monitoring[1,2]	-	-	98%	97%
Venous Thromboembolism Prophylaxis[2]	350	91%	88%	85%
Warfarin Therapy Discharge Instructions[2]	36	97%	72%	75%
Chest Pain/Possible Heart Attack Care				
Aspirin Given Within 24 Hours of Arrival[1,3]	-	-	97%	96%
Fibrinolytic Meds Within 30 Min. of Arrival[3,7]	-	-	68%	58%
Average Time to ECG (minutes)[1,3]	-	-	5	7
Average Time to Transfer (minutes)[3,7]	-	-	43	60
Children's Asthma Care				
Received Home Management Plan of Care	-	-	-	88%
Received Reliever Medication	-	-	-	100%
Received Systemic Corticosteroids	-	-	-	100%
Emergency Department				
Admittance Decision Time (minutes)[2]	508	134	94	98
Head CT Results Within 45 Min. of Arrival	14	64%	61%	57%
Patients Who Left ER Before Being Seen	51,471	4%	3%	2%
Time from ER Arrival to Admit. (minutes)[2]	527	342	274	274
Time from ER Arrival to Discharge (minutes)	403	135	136	134
Time in ER Before Being Evaluated (minutes)	416	58	33	26
Time to Pain Meds for Fractures (minutes)	110	78	61	57
Heart Attack Care				
Aspirin Given at Discharge	156	99%	99%	99%
Fibrinolytic Meds Within 30 Min. of Arrival[7]	-	-	50%	54%
PCI Within 90 Minutes of Arrival	33	94%	97%	96%
Statin Prescribed at Discharge	141	95%	99%	98%
Heart Failure Care				
ACE Inhibitor or ARB for LVSD[2]	105	96%	98%	97%
Discharge Instructions Given[2]	257	93%	94%	94%
Evaluation of LVS Function[2]	302	99%	99%	99%
Medicare Spending				
Medicare Spending per Patient (ratio)	-	1.02	0.98	0.98
Pneumonia Care				
Appropriate Initial Antibiotic Given[2]	101	100%	97%	95%
Blood Culture Timing[2]	151	96%	98%	98%
Pregnancy and Delivery Care				
Newborn Deliveries Scheduled Early[2]	25	4%	3%	6%
Preventive Care				
Immunization for Influenza[2]	559	93%	94%	90%
Immunization for Pneumonia[2]	720	92%	95%	92%
Stroke Care				
Anticoagulation Therapy for Atrial Fibrillation[1,2]	-	-	95%	95%
Antithrombotic Therapy Timing[2]	91	100%	98%	98%
Assessed for Rehabilitation[2]	111	93%	97%	97%
Discharged on Antithrombotic Therapy[2]	93	98%	99%	99%
Discharged on Statin Medication[2]	77	82%	94%	94%
Thrombolytic Therapy Timing[2]	14	43%	58%	66%
Venous Thromboembolism Prophylaxis[2]	116	87%	94%	94%
Written Stroke Educational Materials Given[2]	64	95%	91%	88%
Surgical Care Improvement Project				
Appropriate Beta Blocker Usage[2]	127	98%	98%	98%
Appropriate VTP Within 24 Hours[2]	421	99%	98%	98%
Controlled Postoperative Blood Glucose[2]	30	87%	99%	97%
Perioperative Temperature Management[2]	482	100%	100%	100%
Prophylactic Antibiotic Selection[2]	356	100%	99%	99%
Prophylactic Antibiotic Selection (Outpatient)	255	99%	99%	98%
Prophylactic Antibiotic Stopped[2]	339	97%	98%	98%
Prophylactic Antibiotic Timing[2]	356	100%	99%	99%
Prophylactic Antibiotic Timing (Outpatient)	255	100%	98%	98%
Urinary Catheter Removal[2]	234	100%	97%	97%
Survey of Patients' Hospital Experiences				
Area Around Room 'Always' Quiet at Night	300+	62%	67%	61%
Doctors 'Always' Communicated Well	300+	80%	84%	82%
Home Recovery Information Given	300+	85%	86%	85%
Hospital Given 9 or 10 on 10 Point Scale	300+	66%	72%	71%
Meds 'Always' Explained Before Given	300+	56%	66%	64%
Nurses 'Always' Communicated Well	300+	74%	81%	79%
Pain 'Always' Well Controlled	300+	70%	72%	71%
Room and Bathroom 'Always' Clean	300+	61%	72%	73%
Timely Help 'Always' Received	300+	60%	68%	68%
Would Definitely Recommend Hospital	300+	66%	71%	71%
Use of Medical Imaging				
Cardiac Imaging Stress Test before Surgery[1]	-	-	5.1%	5.3%
Combination Abdominal CT Scan	1,079	2.9%	10.1%	10.5%
Combination Brain/Sinus CT Scan	816	2.9%	2.5%	2.7%
Combination Chest CT Scan	639	0.3%	1.3%	2.7%
Follow-up Mammogram/Ultrasound	2,123	3.7%	8%	8.8%
Lumbar Spine MRI for Low Back Pain	154	35.7%	39%	37.2%

Anmed Health

800 N Fant St
Anderson, SC 29621
URL: www.anmed.com
Type: Acute Care Hospitals
Ownership: Voluntary non-profit - Private

Phone: 864-261-1109
Fax: 864-512-1952
Emergency Services: Yes
Beds: 461

Key Personnel:

Pediatric Ambulatory Care . . . . . . James Carson, MD
Pediatric In-Patient Care . . . . James Carson, MD
Infection Control. . . . . Thomas Crocker, MD
Radiology. . . . . Carl Geier, MD
Operating Room. . . . . Mae Madden, RN
Chief of Medical Staff . . . . Harold Morse, MD
Quality Assurance . . . . Robert Pierce

Measure	Cases	This Hosp.	State Avg.	U.S. Avg.
Blood Clot Prevention and Treatment				
Anticoagulation Overlap Therapy[2]	151	88%	92%	93%
ICU Venous Thromboembolism Prophylaxis[2]	98	98%	94%	92%
Incidence of Potentially Preventable VTE[2]	18	0%	8%	10%
UFH with Dosages/Platelet Monitoring[2]	42	100%	98%	97%
Venous Thromboembolism Prophylaxis[2]	347	98%	88%	85%
Warfarin Therapy Discharge Instructions[2]	104	99%	72%	75%
Chest Pain/Possible Heart Attack Care				
Aspirin Given Within 24 Hours of Arrival[5]	-	-	97%	96%
Fibrinolytic Meds Within 30 Min. of Arrival[5]	-	-	68%	58%
Average Time to ECG (minutes)[5]	-	-	5	7
Average Time to Transfer (minutes)[5]	-	-	43	60
Children's Asthma Care				

NOTE: Hospital profiles are in alphabetical order by state, then city, then hospital within the city; Rankings exclude hospitals with less than 25 cases except for patient surveys which excludes hospitals with less than 100 cases; (a) 100-299 cases; (1) The number of cases/patients is too few to report; (2) Data submitted were based on a sample of cases/patients; (3) Results are based on a shorter time period than required; (4) Data suppressed by CMS for one or more quarters; (5) Results are not available for this reporting period; (6) Fewer than 100 patients completed the HCAHPS survey; (7) No cases met the criteria for this measure; (8) The lower limit of the confidence interval cannot be calculated if the number of observed infections equals zero; (9) No data are available from the state/territory for this reporting period; (10) The scores shown reflect fewer than 50 completed surveys; (11) There were discrepancies in the data collection process; (12) This measure does not apply to this hospital for this reporting period; (13) Results cannot be calculated for this reporting period; (14) The results for this state are combined with nearby states to protect confidentiality; Please refer to the User's Guide for a full explanation of data.

Measure	Cases	This Hosp.	State Avg.	U.S. Avg.
Received Home Management Plan of Care	-	-	-	88%
Received Reliever Medication	-	-	-	100%
Received Systemic Corticosteroids	-	-	-	100%
Emergency Department				
Admittance Decision Time (minutes)[2]	687	88	94	98
Head CT Results Within 45 Min. of Arrival[1]	-	-	61%	57%
Patients Who Left ER Before Being Seen	94,610	5%	3%	2%
Time from ER Arrival to Admit. (minutes)[2]	696	332	274	274
Time from ER Arrival to Discharge (minutes)	351	244	136	134
Time in ER Before Being Evaluated (minutes)	362	88	33	26
Time to Pain Meds for Fractures (minutes)	43	80	61	57
Heart Attack Care				
Aspirin Given at Discharge	259	100%	99%	99%
Fibrinolytic Meds Within 30 Min. of Arrival[7]	-	-	50%	54%
PCI Within 90 Minutes of Arrival	88	100%	97%	96%
Statin Prescribed at Discharge	254	100%	99%	98%
Heart Failure Care				
ACE Inhibitor or ARB for LVSD	188	99%	98%	97%
Discharge Instructions Given	462	100%	94%	94%
Evaluation of LVS Function	595	100%	99%	99%
Medicare Spending				
Medicare Spending per Patient (ratio)	-	1.08	0.98	0.98
Pneumonia Care				
Appropriate Initial Antibiotic Given	348	100%	97%	95%
Blood Culture Timing	649	99%	98%	98%
Pregnancy and Delivery Care				
Newborn Deliveries Scheduled Early	334	1%	3%	6%
Preventive Care				
Immunization for Influenza[2]	528	96%	94%	90%
Immunization for Pneumonia[2]	739	98%	95%	92%
Stroke Care				
Anticoagulation Therapy for Atrial Fibrillation	33	100%	95%	95%
Antithrombotic Therapy Timing	214	100%	98%	98%
Assessed for Rehabilitation	235	98%	97%	97%
Discharged on Antithrombotic Therapy	208	100%	99%	99%
Discharged on Statin Medication	162	98%	94%	94%
Thrombolytic Therapy Timing	11	91%	58%	66%
Venous Thromboembolism Prophylaxis	251	100%	94%	94%
Written Stroke Educational Materials Given	147	97%	91%	88%
Surgical Care Improvement Project				
Appropriate Beta Blocker Usage[2]	288	98%	98%	98%
Appropriate VTP Within 24 Hours[2]	711	100%	98%	98%
Controlled Postoperative Blood Glucose[2]	181	97%	99%	97%
Perioperative Temperature Management[2]	792	100%	100%	100%
Prophylactic Antibiotic Selection[2]	767	99%	99%	99%
Prophylactic Antibiotic Selection (Outpatient)	513	99%	99%	98%
Prophylactic Antibiotic Stopped[2]	738	100%	98%	98%
Prophylactic Antibiotic Timing[2]	769	100%	99%	99%
Prophylactic Antibiotic Timing (Outpatient)	523	96%	98%	98%
Urinary Catheter Removal[2]	549	99%	97%	97%
Survey of Patients' Hospital Experiences				
Area Around Room 'Always' Quiet at Night[11]	300+	67%	67%	61%
Doctors 'Always' Communicated Well[11]	300+	82%	84%	82%
Home Recovery Information Given[11]	300+	85%	86%	85%
Hospital Given 9 or 10 on 10 Point Scale[11]	300+	72%	72%	71%
Meds 'Always' Explained Before Given[11]	300+	64%	66%	64%
Nurses 'Always' Communicated Well[11]	300+	81%	81%	79%
Pain 'Always' Well Controlled[11]	300+	71%	72%	71%
Room and Bathroom 'Always' Clean[11]	300+	74%	72%	73%
Timely Help 'Always' Received[11]	300+	69%	68%	68%
Would Definitely Recommend Hospital[11]	300+	72%	71%	71%
Use of Medical Imaging				
Cardiac Imaging Stress Test before Surgery	1,505	3.6%	5.1%	5.3%
Combination Abdominal CT Scan	1,702	61.8%	10.1%	10.5%
Combination Brain/Sinus CT Scan	1,508	2.4%	2.5%	2.7%
Combination Chest CT Scan	1,047	0.0%	1.3%	2.7%
Follow-up Mammogram/Ultrasound	2,294	12.1%	8%	8.8%
Lumbar Spine MRI for Low Back Pain	183	41.0%	39%	37.2%

Barnwell County Hospital

PO Box 588 811 Reynolds Road
Barnwell, SC 29812
Phone: 803-259-1000
Fax: 803-541-4387
URL: www.barnwellcountysc.com/healthcare
Type: Acute Care Hospitals
Emergency Services: Yes
Ownership: Proprietary
Beds: 56

Key Personnel:

Quality Assurance . . . . Sherry Donaldson
Operating Room. . . . . Fran Kinard
Pediatric In-Patient Care . . . . Abe H Moskow, MD
Chief of Medical Staff . . . . S Richard, MD
Intensive Care Unit. . . . . Syed Shamsi
Infection Control. . . . . Allene Townes, RN
CEO/President. . . . . Robert Walters
Emergency Room . . . . Afsar Waraich, MD

Measure	Cases	This Hosp.	State Avg.	U.S. Avg.
Blood Clot Prevention and Treatment				
Anticoagulation Overlap Therapy[1,2]	-	-	92%	93%
ICU Venous Thromboembolism Prophylaxis[2,7]	-	-	94%	92%
Incidence of Potentially Preventable VTE[2,7]	-	-	8%	10%
UFH with Dosages/Platelet Monitoring[2,7]	-	-	98%	97%
Venous Thromboembolism Prophylaxis[2]	114	52%	88%	85%
Warfarin Therapy Discharge Instructions[1,2]	-	-	72%	75%
Chest Pain/Possible Heart Attack Care				
Aspirin Given Within 24 Hours of Arrival	36	92%	97%	96%
Fibrinolytic Meds Within 30 Min. of Arrival[7]	-	-	68%	58%
Average Time to ECG (minutes)	33	36	5	7
Average Time to Transfer (minutes)[1]	-	-	43	60
Children's Asthma Care				
Received Home Management Plan of Care	-	-	-	88%
Received Reliever Medication	-	-	-	100%
Received Systemic Corticosteroids	-	-	-	100%
Emergency Department				
Admittance Decision Time (minutes)[2]	320	50	94	98
Head CT Results Within 45 Min. of Arrival[1]	-	-	61%	57%
Patients Who Left ER Before Being Seen	12,062	5%	3%	2%
Time from ER Arrival to Admit. (minutes)[2]	324	310	274	274
Time from ER Arrival to Discharge (minutes)	321	155	136	134
Time in ER Before Being Evaluated (minutes)	366	40	33	26
Time to Pain Meds for Fractures (minutes)	42	110	61	57
Heart Attack Care				
Aspirin Given at Discharge[3,7]	-	-	99%	99%
Fibrinolytic Meds Within 30 Min. of Arrival[3,7]	-	-	50%	54%
PCI Within 90 Minutes of Arrival[3,7]	-	-	97%	96%
Statin Prescribed at Discharge[3,7]	-	-	99%	98%
Heart Failure Care				
ACE Inhibitor or ARB for LVSD[1]	-	-	98%	97%
Discharge Instructions Given	25	88%	94%	94%
Evaluation of LVS Function	32	50%	99%	99%
Medicare Spending				
Medicare Spending per Patient (ratio)	-	1.16	0.98	0.98
Pneumonia Care				
Appropriate Initial Antibiotic Given	44	64%	97%	95%
Blood Culture Timing	62	69%	98%	98%
Pregnancy and Delivery Care				
Newborn Deliveries Scheduled Early[7]	-	-	3%	6%
Preventive Care				
Immunization for Influenza[2]	285	70%	94%	90%
Immunization for Pneumonia[2]	401	69%	95%	92%
Stroke Care				
Anticoagulation Therapy for Atrial Fibrillation[1]	-	-	95%	95%
Antithrombotic Therapy Timing[1]	-	-	98%	98%
Assessed for Rehabilitation[1]	-	-	97%	97%
Discharged on Antithrombotic Therapy[1]	-	-	99%	99%
Discharged on Statin Medication[1]	-	-	94%	94%
Thrombolytic Therapy Timing[1]	-	-	58%	66%
Venous Thromboembolism Prophylaxis[1]	-	-	94%	94%
Written Stroke Educational Materials Given[1]	-	-	91%	88%
Surgical Care Improvement Project				
Appropriate Beta Blocker Usage[3,7]	-	-	98%	98%
Appropriate VTP Within 24 Hours[1,3]	-	-	98%	98%
Controlled Postoperative Blood Glucose[3,7]	-	-	99%	97%
Perioperative Temperature Management[1,3]	-	-	100%	100%
Prophylactic Antibiotic Selection[1,3]	-	-	99%	99%
Prophylactic Antibiotic Selection (Outpatient)[3,7]	-	-	99%	98%
Prophylactic Antibiotic Stopped[1,3]	-	-	98%	98%
Prophylactic Antibiotic Timing[1,3]	-	-	99%	99%
Prophylactic Antibiotic Timing (Outpatient)[1,3]	-	-	98%	98%
Urinary Catheter Removal[3,7]	-	-	97%	97%
Survey of Patients' Hospital Experiences				
Area Around Room 'Always' Quiet at Night	(a)	71%	67%	61%
Doctors 'Always' Communicated Well	(a)	80%	84%	82%
Home Recovery Information Given	(a)	80%	86%	85%
Hospital Given 9 or 10 on 10 Point Scale	(a)	60%	72%	71%
Meds 'Always' Explained Before Given	(a)	62%	66%	64%
Nurses 'Always' Communicated Well	(a)	81%	81%	79%
Pain 'Always' Well Controlled	(a)	65%	72%	71%
Room and Bathroom 'Always' Clean	(a)	66%	72%	73%
Timely Help 'Always' Received	(a)	72%	68%	68%
Would Definitely Recommend Hospital	(a)	63%	71%	71%
Use of Medical Imaging				
Cardiac Imaging Stress Test before Surgery[7]	-	-	5.1%	5.3%
Combination Abdominal CT Scan	172	9.3%	10.1%	10.5%
Combination Brain/Sinus CT Scan[1]	-	-	2.5%	2.7%
Combination Chest CT Scan	56	5.4%	1.3%	2.7%
Follow-up Mammogram/Ultrasound	222	14.4%	8%	8.8%
Lumbar Spine MRI for Low Back Pain[1]	-	-	39%	37.2%

Beaufort County Memorial Hospital

955 Ribaut Rd
Beaufort, SC 29902
Phone: 843-522-5200
Fax: 843-522-5671
URL: www.bmhsc.org
Type: Acute Care Hospitals
Emergency Services: Yes
Ownership: Government - Local
Beds: 197

Key Personnel:

CEO/President. . . . . David E Brown
Quality Assurance . . . . Pat Foulger
Chief of Medical Staff . . . . Curt Gambla
Emergency Room . . . . Connie Gowdowns, RN
Radiology. . . . . William A Jackson
Cardiac Laboratory. . . . . Daniel Mark

Measure	Cases	This Hosp.	State Avg.	U.S. Avg.
Blood Clot Prevention and Treatment				
Anticoagulation Overlap Therapy[2]	63	100%	92%	93%
ICU Venous Thromboembolism Prophylaxis[2]	54	98%	94%	92%
Incidence of Potentially Preventable VTE[1,2]	-	-	8%	10%
UFH with Dosages/Platelet Monitoring[2]	48	100%	98%	97%
Venous Thromboembolism Prophylaxis[2]	386	91%	88%	85%
Warfarin Therapy Discharge Instructions[2]	49	92%	72%	75%
Chest Pain/Possible Heart Attack Care				
Aspirin Given Within 24 Hours of Arrival	55	100%	97%	96%
Fibrinolytic Meds Within 30 Min. of Arrival	15	87%	68%	58%
Average Time to ECG (minutes)	55	3	5	7
Average Time to Transfer (minutes)[7]	-	-	43	60
Children's Asthma Care				
Received Home Management Plan of Care	-	-	-	88%
Received Reliever Medication	-	-	-	100%
Received Systemic Corticosteroids	-	-	-	100%
Emergency Department				
Admittance Decision Time (minutes)[2]	675	144	94	98
Head CT Results Within 45 Min. of Arrival[1]	-	-	61%	57%
Patients Who Left ER Before Being Seen	41,919	2%	3%	2%
Time from ER Arrival to Admit. (minutes)[2]	676	344	274	274
Time from ER Arrival to Discharge (minutes)	436	152	136	134
Time in ER Before Being Evaluated (minutes)	506	19	33	26
Time to Pain Meds for Fractures (minutes)	122	50	61	57
Heart Attack Care				
Aspirin Given at Discharge	32	100%	99%	99%
Fibrinolytic Meds Within 30 Min. of Arrival[7]	-	-	50%	54%
PCI Within 90 Minutes of Arrival[1]	-	-	97%	96%
Statin Prescribed at Discharge	36	100%	99%	98%
Heart Failure Care				
ACE Inhibitor or ARB for LVSD	94	94%	98%	97%
Discharge Instructions Given	230	99%	94%	94%
Evaluation of LVS Function	245	100%	99%	99%
Medicare Spending				
Medicare Spending per Patient (ratio)	-	0.96	0.98	0.98
Pneumonia Care				

NOTE: Hospital profiles are in alphabetical order by state, then city, then hospital within the city; Rankings exclude hospitals with less than 25 cases except for patient surveys which excludes hospitals with less than 100 cases; (a) 100-299 cases; (1) The number of cases/patients is too few to report; (2) Data submitted were based on a sample of cases/patients; (3) Results are based on a shorter time period than required; (4) Data suppressed by CMS for one or more quarters; (5) Results are not available for this reporting period; (6) Fewer than 100 patients completed the HCAHPS survey; (7) No cases met the criteria for this measure; (8) The lower limit of the confidence interval cannot be calculated if the number of observed infections equals zero; (9) No data are available from the state/territory for this reporting period; (10) The scores shown reflect fewer than 50 completed surveys; (11) There were discrepancies in the data collection process; (12) This measure does not apply to this hospital for this reporting period; (13) Results cannot be calculated for this reporting period; (14) The results for this state are combined with nearby states to protect confidentiality; Please refer to the User's Guide for a full explanation of data.

Appropriate Initial Antibiotic Given	83	96%	97%	95%
Blood Culture Timing	99	97%	98%	98%
Pregnancy and Delivery Care				
Newborn Deliveries Scheduled Early[2]	78	15%	3%	6%
Preventive Care				
Immunization for Influenza[2]	530	98%	94%	90%
Immunization for Pneumonia[2]	606	98%	95%	92%
Stroke Care				
Anticoagulation Therapy for Atrial Fibrillation[1]	-	-	95%	95%
Antithrombotic Therapy Timing	59	97%	98%	98%
Assessed for Rehabilitation	68	94%	97%	97%
Discharged on Antithrombotic Therapy	67	99%	99%	99%
Discharged on Statin Medication	59	85%	94%	94%
Thrombolytic Therapy Timing[1]	-	-	58%	66%
Venous Thromboembolism Prophylaxis	61	90%	94%	94%
Written Stroke Educational Materials Given	40	65%	91%	88%
Surgical Care Improvement Project				
Appropriate Beta Blocker Usage	155	99%	98%	98%
Appropriate VTP Within 24 Hours	551	99%	98%	98%
Controlled Postoperative Blood Glucose[7]	-	-	99%	97%
Perioperative Temperature Management	597	100%	100%	100%
Prophylactic Antibiotic Selection	457	100%	99%	99%
Prophylactic Antibiotic Selection (Outpatient)	216	97%	99%	98%
Prophylactic Antibiotic Stopped	441	98%	98%	98%
Prophylactic Antibiotic Timing	458	100%	99%	99%
Prophylactic Antibiotic Timing (Outpatient)	216	99%	98%	98%
Urinary Catheter Removal	362	100%	97%	97%
Survey of Patients' Hospital Experiences				
Area Around Room 'Always' Quiet at Night	300+	64%	67%	61%
Doctors 'Always' Communicated Well	300+	84%	84%	82%
Home Recovery Information Given	300+	88%	86%	85%
Hospital Given 9 or 10 on 10 Point Scale	300+	72%	72%	71%
Meds 'Always' Explained Before Given	300+	66%	66%	64%
Nurses 'Always' Communicated Well	300+	80%	81%	79%
Pain 'Always' Well Controlled	300+	71%	72%	71%
Room and Bathroom 'Always' Clean	300+	68%	72%	73%
Timely Help 'Always' Received	300+	67%	68%	68%
Would Definitely Recommend Hospital	300+	73%	71%	71%
Use of Medical Imaging				
Cardiac Imaging Stress Test before Surgery	441	5.0%	5.1%	5.3%
Combination Abdominal CT Scan	1,045	3.1%	10.1%	10.5%
Combination Brain/Sinus CT Scan	795	5.3%	2.5%	2.7%
Combination Chest CT Scan	611	0.2%	1.3%	2.7%
Follow-up Mammogram/Ultrasound	2,176	6.5%	8%	8.8%
Lumbar Spine MRI for Low Back Pain	211	41.7%	39%	37.2%

Marlboro Park Hospital

1138 Cheraw Highway
Bennettsville, SC 29512
Phone: 843-479-2881
Fax: 843-479-5860
URL: www.marlboroparkhospital.com
Type: Acute Care Hospitals
Emergency Services: Yes
Ownership: Proprietary
Beds: 102

Key Personnel:
CEO/President. . . . . Mark W Caton
Chief of Medical Staff . . . . Dell A Dembosky, MD
Intensive Care Unit. . . . . Jane Hodkin
Radiology. . . . . Misha Lee
Quality Assurance . . . . Ann Trotter

Measure	Cases	This Hosp.	State Avg.	U.S. Avg.
Blood Clot Prevention and Treatment				
Anticoagulation Overlap Therapy[1,2]	-	-	92%	93%
ICU Venous Thromboembolism Prophylaxis[2]	35	100%	94%	92%
Incidence of Potentially Preventable VTE[1,2]	-	-	8%	10%
UFH with Dosages/Platelet Monitoring[2,7]	-	-	98%	97%
Venous Thromboembolism Prophylaxis[2]	314	99%	88%	85%
Warfarin Therapy Discharge Instructions[1,2]	-	-	72%	75%
Chest Pain/Possible Heart Attack Care				
Aspirin Given Within 24 Hours of Arrival	15	100%	97%	96%
Fibrinolytic Meds Within 30 Min. of Arrival[3,7]	-	-	68%	58%
Average Time to ECG (minutes)	16	7	5	7
Average Time to Transfer (minutes)[3,7]	-	-	43	60
Children's Asthma Care				
Received Home Management Plan of Care	-	-	-	88%
Received Reliever Medication	-	-	-	100%
Received Systemic Corticosteroids	-	-	-	100%
Emergency Department				
Admittance Decision Time (minutes)[2]	574	54	94	98
Head CT Results Within 45 Min. of Arrival[3,7]	-	-	61%	57%
Patients Who Left ER Before Being Seen	13,912	1%	3%	2%
Time from ER Arrival to Admit. (minutes)[2]	592	203	274	274
Time from ER Arrival to Discharge (minutes)	410	95	136	134
Time in ER Before Being Evaluated (minutes)	464	19	33	26
Time to Pain Meds for Fractures (minutes)	52	47	61	57
Heart Attack Care				
Aspirin Given at Discharge[1]	-	-	99%	99%
Fibrinolytic Meds Within 30 Min. of Arrival[7]	-	-	50%	54%
PCI Within 90 Minutes of Arrival[7]	-	-	97%	96%
Statin Prescribed at Discharge[1]	-	-	99%	98%
Heart Failure Care				
ACE Inhibitor or ARB for LVSD	18	100%	98%	97%
Discharge Instructions Given	50	100%	94%	94%
Evaluation of LVS Function	57	100%	99%	99%
Medicare Spending				
Medicare Spending per Patient (ratio)	-	0.91	0.98	0.98
Pneumonia Care				
Appropriate Initial Antibiotic Given	46	98%	97%	95%
Blood Culture Timing	73	100%	98%	98%
Pregnancy and Delivery Care				
Newborn Deliveries Scheduled Early[1,2]	-	-	3%	6%
Preventive Care				
Immunization for Influenza[2]	380	99%	94%	90%
Immunization for Pneumonia[2]	481	100%	95%	92%
Stroke Care				
Anticoagulation Therapy for Atrial Fibrillation[1]	-	-	95%	95%
Antithrombotic Therapy Timing[1]	-	-	98%	98%
Assessed for Rehabilitation[1]	-	-	97%	97%
Discharged on Antithrombotic Therapy[1]	-	-	99%	99%
Discharged on Statin Medication[1]	-	-	94%	94%
Thrombolytic Therapy Timing[7]	-	-	58%	66%
Venous Thromboembolism Prophylaxis[1]	-	-	94%	94%
Written Stroke Educational Materials Given[1]	-	-	91%	88%
Surgical Care Improvement Project				
Appropriate Beta Blocker Usage[7]	-	-	98%	98%
Appropriate VTP Within 24 Hours[1]	-	-	98%	98%
Controlled Postoperative Blood Glucose[7]	-	-	99%	97%
Perioperative Temperature Management	11	100%	100%	100%
Prophylactic Antibiotic Selection[1]	-	-	99%	99%
Prophylactic Antibiotic Selection (Outpatient)[1,3]	-	-	99%	98%
Prophylactic Antibiotic Stopped[1]	-	-	98%	98%
Prophylactic Antibiotic Timing[1]	-	-	99%	99%
Prophylactic Antibiotic Timing (Outpatient)[1,3]	-	-	98%	98%
Urinary Catheter Removal[1]	-	-	97%	97%
Survey of Patients' Hospital Experiences				
Area Around Room 'Always' Quiet at Night	(a)	76%	67%	61%
Doctors 'Always' Communicated Well	(a)	85%	84%	82%
Home Recovery Information Given	(a)	87%	86%	85%
Hospital Given 9 or 10 on 10 Point Scale	(a)	67%	72%	71%
Meds 'Always' Explained Before Given	(a)	69%	66%	64%
Nurses 'Always' Communicated Well	(a)	81%	81%	79%
Pain 'Always' Well Controlled	(a)	76%	72%	71%
Room and Bathroom 'Always' Clean	(a)	69%	72%	73%
Timely Help 'Always' Received	(a)	74%	68%	68%
Would Definitely Recommend Hospital	(a)	64%	71%	71%
Use of Medical Imaging				
Cardiac Imaging Stress Test before Surgery[1]	-	-	5.1%	5.3%
Combination Abdominal CT Scan	113	1.8%	10.1%	10.5%
Combination Brain/Sinus CT Scan	204	6.9%	2.5%	2.7%
Combination Chest CT Scan[1]	-	-	1.3%	2.7%
Follow-up Mammogram/Ultrasound	314	15.6%	8%	8.8%
Lumbar Spine MRI for Low Back Pain[1]	-	-	39%	37.2%

Kershaw Health

Haile & Roberts Streets, Box 7003
Camden, SC 29020
Phone: 803-432-4311
Fax: 803-713-6369
E-mail: info@kcmc.org
URL: www.kcmc.org
Type: Acute Care Hospitals
Emergency Services: Yes
Ownership: Voluntary non-profit - Other
Beds: 201

Key Personnel:
Chief of Medical Staff . . . . M Todd Alderson, MD
Anesthesiology. . . . . Dan Brown, MD
Radiology. . . . . Donald J Copley, MD
CEO . . . . Terry J. Gunn, FACHE
Pediatric In-Patient Care . . . . Thomas Joseph, MD
Surgery . . . . Michael Nienhuis, MD
Emergency Room . . . . Tommy Norris, MD
Operating Room. . . . . Robert Puchalski, MD

Measure	Cases	This Hosp.	State Avg.	U.S. Avg.
Blood Clot Prevention and Treatment				
Anticoagulation Overlap Therapy[2]	36	67%	92%	93%
ICU Venous Thromboembolism Prophylaxis[2]	71	92%	94%	92%
Incidence of Potentially Preventable VTE[1,2]	-	-	8%	10%
UFH with Dosages/Platelet Monitoring[2]	14	100%	98%	97%
Venous Thromboembolism Prophylaxis[2]	368	88%	88%	85%
Warfarin Therapy Discharge Instructions[2]	24	83%	72%	75%
Chest Pain/Possible Heart Attack Care				
Aspirin Given Within 24 Hours of Arrival	43	100%	97%	96%
Fibrinolytic Meds Within 30 Min. of Arrival[7]	-	-	68%	58%
Average Time to ECG (minutes)	44	6	5	7
Average Time to Transfer (minutes)	15	41	43	60
Children's Asthma Care				
Received Home Management Plan of Care	-	-	-	88%
Received Reliever Medication	-	-	-	100%
Received Systemic Corticosteroids	-	-	-	100%
Emergency Department				
Admittance Decision Time (minutes)[2]	566	98	94	98
Head CT Results Within 45 Min. of Arrival	11	91%	61%	57%
Patients Who Left ER Before Being Seen	28,467	2%	3%	2%
Time from ER Arrival to Admit. (minutes)[2]	566	261	274	274
Time from ER Arrival to Discharge (minutes)	382	146	136	134
Time in ER Before Being Evaluated (minutes)	404	44	33	26
Time to Pain Meds for Fractures (minutes)	112	75	61	57
Heart Attack Care				
Aspirin Given at Discharge	43	98%	99%	99%
Fibrinolytic Meds Within 30 Min. of Arrival[7]	-	-	50%	54%
PCI Within 90 Minutes of Arrival[7]	-	-	97%	96%
Statin Prescribed at Discharge	45	93%	99%	98%
Heart Failure Care				
ACE Inhibitor or ARB for LVSD[2]	64	89%	98%	97%
Discharge Instructions Given[2]	203	94%	94%	94%
Evaluation of LVS Function[2]	245	99%	99%	99%
Medicare Spending				
Medicare Spending per Patient (ratio)	-	1.00	0.98	0.98
Pneumonia Care				
Appropriate Initial Antibiotic Given[2]	127	94%	97%	95%
Blood Culture Timing[2]	136	96%	98%	98%
Pregnancy and Delivery Care				
Newborn Deliveries Scheduled Early	21	5%	3%	6%
Preventive Care				
Immunization for Influenza[2]	487	94%	94%	90%
Immunization for Pneumonia[2]	634	93%	95%	92%
Stroke Care				
Anticoagulation Therapy for Atrial Fibrillation[1]	-	-	95%	95%
Antithrombotic Therapy Timing	72	100%	98%	98%
Assessed for Rehabilitation	73	90%	97%	97%
Discharged on Antithrombotic Therapy	68	99%	99%	99%
Discharged on Statin Medication	58	88%	94%	94%
Thrombolytic Therapy Timing[1]	-	-	58%	66%
Venous Thromboembolism Prophylaxis	79	91%	94%	94%
Written Stroke Educational Materials Given	39	82%	91%	88%
Surgical Care Improvement Project				
Appropriate Beta Blocker Usage	75	95%	98%	98%
Appropriate VTP Within 24 Hours	178	98%	98%	98%
Controlled Postoperative Blood Glucose[7]	-	-	99%	97%
Perioperative Temperature Management	207	100%	100%	100%

NOTE: Hospital profiles are in alphabetical order by state, then city, then hospital within the city; Rankings exclude hospitals with less than 25 cases except for patient surveys which excludes hospitals with less than 100 cases; (a) 100-299 cases; (1) The number of cases/patients is too few to report; (2) Data submitted were based on a sample of cases/patients; (3) Results are based on a shorter time period than required; (4) Data suppressed by CMS for one or more quarters; (5) Results are not available for this reporting period; (6) Fewer than 100 patients completed the HCAHPS survey; (7) No cases met the criteria for this measure; (8) The lower limit of the confidence interval cannot be calculated if the number of observed infections equals zero; (9) No data are available from the state/territory for this reporting period; (10) The scores shown reflect fewer than 50 completed surveys; (11) There were discrepancies in the data collection process; (12) This measure does not apply to this hospital for this reporting period; (13) Results cannot be calculated for this reporting period; (14) The results for this state are combined with nearby states to protect confidentiality; Please refer to the User's Guide for a full explanation of data.

Prophylactic Antibiotic Selection	136	99%	99%	99%
Prophylactic Antibiotic Selection (Outpatient)	141	99%	99%	98%
Prophylactic Antibiotic Stopped	133	98%	98%	98%
Prophylactic Antibiotic Timing	136	100%	99%	99%
Prophylactic Antibiotic Timing (Outpatient)	139	98%	98%	98%
Urinary Catheter Removal	76	97%	97%	97%
Survey of Patients' Hospital Experiences				
Area Around Room 'Always' Quiet at Night	300+	65%	67%	61%
Doctors 'Always' Communicated Well	300+	82%	84%	82%
Home Recovery Information Given	300+	84%	86%	85%
Hospital Given 9 or 10 on 10 Point Scale	300+	66%	72%	71%
Meds 'Always' Explained Before Given	300+	66%	66%	64%
Nurses 'Always' Communicated Well	300+	80%	81%	79%
Pain 'Always' Well Controlled	300+	75%	72%	71%
Room and Bathroom 'Always' Clean	300+	71%	72%	73%
Timely Help 'Always' Received	300+	68%	68%	68%
Would Definitely Recommend Hospital	300+	66%	71%	71%
Use of Medical Imaging				
Cardiac Imaging Stress Test before Surgery	387	3.6%	5.1%	5.3%
Combination Abdominal CT Scan	451	30.4%	10.1%	10.5%
Combination Brain/Sinus CT Scan	642	0.6%	2.5%	2.7%
Combination Chest CT Scan	411	2.4%	1.3%	2.7%
Follow-up Mammogram/Ultrasound	1,748	6.0%	8%	8.8%
Lumbar Spine MRI for Low Back Pain	98	36.7%	39%	37.2%

Bon Secours - Saint Francis Xavier Hospital

2095 Henry Tecklenburg Drive
Charleston, SC 29414
Phone: 843-402-1006
Fax: 843-720-5761
URL: www.stfrancishealth.org
Type: Acute Care Hospitals
Emergency Services: Yes
Ownership: Voluntary non-profit - Private
Beds: 141

Key Personnel:
Quality Assurance . . . . Lee Budd, RN
CEO/President. . . . . David L. Dunlap, FACHE
Cardiac Laboratory. . . . . James J Morris, MD
Pediatric Ambulatory Care . . . . . . Stephen Shapiro, MD
Pediatric In-Patient Care . . . . Stephen Shapiro, MD
Chief of Medical Staff. . . . . Steven Shapiro, MD
Operating Room. . . . . Allison Walters, RN
Infection Control. . . . . Timothy West, MD

Measure	Cases	This Hosp.	State Avg.	U.S. Avg.
Blood Clot Prevention and Treatment				
Anticoagulation Overlap Therapy[2]	57	96%	92%	93%
ICU Venous Thromboembolism Prophylaxis[2]	57	100%	94%	92%
Incidence of Potentially Preventable VTE[1,2]	-	-	8%	10%
UFH with Dosages/Platelet Monitoring[2]	25	100%	98%	97%
Venous Thromboembolism Prophylaxis[2]	347	98%	88%	85%
Warfarin Therapy Discharge Instructions[2]	44	89%	72%	75%
Chest Pain/Possible Heart Attack Care				
Aspirin Given Within 24 Hours of Arrival	75	99%	97%	96%
Fibrinolytic Meds Within 30 Min. of Arrival[7]	-	-	68%	58%
Average Time to ECG (minutes)	79	8	5	7
Average Time to Transfer (minutes)[1]	-	-	43	60
Children's Asthma Care				
Received Home Management Plan of Care	-	-	-	88%
Received Reliever Medication	-	-	-	100%
Received Systemic Corticosteroids	-	-	-	100%
Emergency Department				
Admittance Decision Time (minutes)[2]	412	98	94	98
Head CT Results Within 45 Min. of Arrival	12	75%	61%	57%
Patients Who Left ER Before Being Seen	45,604	0%	3%	2%
Time from ER Arrival to Admit. (minutes)[2]	430	284	274	274
Time from ER Arrival to Discharge (minutes)	396	160	136	134
Time in ER Before Being Evaluated (minutes)	406	40	33	26
Time to Pain Meds for Fractures (minutes)	86	66	61	57
Heart Attack Care				
Aspirin Given at Discharge[1]	-	-	99%	99%
Fibrinolytic Meds Within 30 Min. of Arrival[7]	-	-	50%	54%
PCI Within 90 Minutes of Arrival[7]	-	-	97%	96%
Statin Prescribed at Discharge[1]	-	-	99%	98%
Heart Failure Care				
ACE Inhibitor or ARB for LVSD	49	100%	98%	97%
Discharge Instructions Given	116	100%	94%	94%
Evaluation of LVS Function	135	100%	99%	99%
Medicare Spending				
Medicare Spending per Patient (ratio)	-	0.98	0.98	0.98
Pneumonia Care				
Appropriate Initial Antibiotic Given	142	99%	97%	95%
Blood Culture Timing	220	100%	98%	98%
Pregnancy and Delivery Care				
Newborn Deliveries Scheduled Early	233	1%	3%	6%
Preventive Care				
Immunization for Influenza[2]	508	99%	94%	90%
Immunization for Pneumonia[2]	506	100%	95%	92%
Stroke Care				
Anticoagulation Therapy for Atrial Fibrillation	12	100%	95%	95%
Antithrombotic Therapy Timing	76	100%	98%	98%
Assessed for Rehabilitation	105	97%	97%	97%
Discharged on Antithrombotic Therapy	95	100%	99%	99%
Discharged on Statin Medication	76	100%	94%	94%
Thrombolytic Therapy Timing[1]	-	-	58%	66%
Venous Thromboembolism Prophylaxis	82	99%	94%	94%
Written Stroke Educational Materials Given	73	100%	91%	88%
Surgical Care Improvement Project				
Appropriate Beta Blocker Usage[2]	43	98%	98%	98%
Appropriate VTP Within 24 Hours[2]	237	99%	98%	98%
Controlled Postoperative Blood Glucose[2,7]	-	-	99%	97%
Perioperative Temperature Management[2]	271	100%	100%	100%
Prophylactic Antibiotic Selection[2]	125	99%	99%	99%
Prophylactic Antibiotic Selection (Outpatient)	407	100%	99%	98%
Prophylactic Antibiotic Stopped[2]	119	97%	98%	98%
Prophylactic Antibiotic Timing[2]	125	99%	99%	99%
Prophylactic Antibiotic Timing (Outpatient)	407	100%	98%	98%
Urinary Catheter Removal[2]	135	99%	97%	97%
Survey of Patients' Hospital Experiences				
Area Around Room 'Always' Quiet at Night	300+	67%	67%	61%
Doctors 'Always' Communicated Well	300+	85%	84%	82%
Home Recovery Information Given	300+	88%	86%	85%
Hospital Given 9 or 10 on 10 Point Scale	300+	80%	72%	71%
Meds 'Always' Explained Before Given	300+	67%	66%	64%
Nurses 'Always' Communicated Well	300+	82%	81%	79%
Pain 'Always' Well Controlled	300+	73%	72%	71%
Room and Bathroom 'Always' Clean	300+	72%	72%	73%
Timely Help 'Always' Received	300+	71%	68%	68%
Would Definitely Recommend Hospital	300+	81%	71%	71%
Use of Medical Imaging				
Cardiac Imaging Stress Test before Surgery[1]	-	-	5.1%	5.3%
Combination Abdominal CT Scan	1,285	8.2%	10.1%	10.5%
Combination Brain/Sinus CT Scan	1,108	1.2%	2.5%	2.7%
Combination Chest CT Scan	949	0.1%	1.3%	2.7%
Follow-up Mammogram/Ultrasound	3,530	5.2%	8%	8.8%
Lumbar Spine MRI for Low Back Pain	405	39.3%	39%	37.2%

Charleston VA Medical Center

109 Bee Street
Charleston, SC 29401
Phone: 843-577-5011
Fax: 843-937-6100
URL: www1.va.gov/directory/guide/facility.asp?id=28
Type: Acute Care - VA
Emergency Services: No
Ownership: Government Federal
Beds: 145

Key Personnel:
CEO/President. . . . . John E Barilich
Quality Assurance . . . . Shirley Cooper, RN
Operating Room. . . . . Michael Denny
Radiology. . . . . Philip Freedland, MD
Chief of Medical Staff . . . . Florence N Hutchinson

Measure	Cases	This Hosp.	State Avg.	U.S. Avg.
Blood Clot Prevention and Treatment				
Anticoagulation Overlap Therapy	-	-	92%	93%
ICU Venous Thromboembolism Prophylaxis	-	-	94%	92%
Incidence of Potentially Preventable VTE	-	-	8%	10%
UFH with Dosages/Platelet Monitoring	-	-	98%	97%
Venous Thromboembolism Prophylaxis	-	-	88%	85%
Warfarin Therapy Discharge Instructions	-	-	72%	75%
Chest Pain/Possible Heart Attack Care				
Aspirin Given Within 24 Hours of Arrival	-	-	97%	96%
Fibrinolytic Meds Within 30 Min. of Arrival	-	-	68%	58%
Average Time to ECG (minutes)	-	-	5	7
Average Time to Transfer (minutes)	-	-	43	60
Children's Asthma Care				
Received Home Management Plan of Care	-	-	-	88%
Received Reliever Medication	-	-	-	100%
Received Systemic Corticosteroids	-	-	-	100%
Emergency Department				
Admittance Decision Time (minutes)	-	-	94	98
Head CT Results Within 45 Min. of Arrival	-	-	61%	57%
Patients Who Left ER Before Being Seen	-	-	3%	2%
Time from ER Arrival to Admit. (minutes)	-	-	274	274
Time from ER Arrival to Discharge (minutes)	-	-	136	134
Time in ER Before Being Evaluated (minutes)	-	-	33	26
Time to Pain Meds for Fractures (minutes)	-	-	61	57
Heart Attack Care				
Aspirin Given at Discharge	49	100%	99%	99%
Fibrinolytic Meds Within 30 Min. of Arrival[5]	-	-	50%	54%
PCI Within 90 Minutes of Arrival[1]	-	-	97%	96%
Statin Prescribed at Discharge	49	100%	99%	98%
Heart Failure Care				
ACE Inhibitor or ARB for LVSD	64	100%	98%	97%
Discharge Instructions Given	159	97%	94%	94%
Evaluation of LVS Function	171	100%	99%	99%
Medicare Spending				
Medicare Spending per Patient (ratio)	-	-	0.98	0.98
Pneumonia Care				
Appropriate Initial Antibiotic Given[1]	21	100%	97%	95%
Blood Culture Timing	75	99%	98%	98%
Pregnancy and Delivery Care				
Newborn Deliveries Scheduled Early	-	-	3%	6%
Preventive Care				
Immunization for Influenza[5]	-	-	94%	90%
Immunization for Pneumonia[5]	-	-	95%	92%
Stroke Care				
Anticoagulation Therapy for Atrial Fibrillation	-	-	95%	95%
Antithrombotic Therapy Timing	-	-	98%	98%
Assessed for Rehabilitation	-	-	97%	97%
Discharged on Antithrombotic Therapy	-	-	99%	99%
Discharged on Statin Medication	-	-	94%	94%
Thrombolytic Therapy Timing	-	-	58%	66%
Venous Thromboembolism Prophylaxis	-	-	94%	94%
Written Stroke Educational Materials Given	-	-	91%	88%
Surgical Care Improvement Project				
Appropriate Beta Blocker Usage[2]	92	98%	98%	98%
Appropriate VTP Within 24 Hours[2]	144	100%	98%	98%
Controlled Postoperative Blood Glucose[2]	62	97%	99%	97%
Perioperative Temperature Management[2]	168	100%	100%	100%
Prophylactic Antibiotic Selection	135	100%	99%	99%
Prophylactic Antibiotic Selection (Outpatient)	-	-	99%	98%
Prophylactic Antibiotic Stopped	132	100%	98%	98%
Prophylactic Antibiotic Timing	135	99%	99%	99%
Prophylactic Antibiotic Timing (Outpatient)	-	-	98%	98%
Urinary Catheter Removal[2]	50	98%	97%	97%
Survey of Patients' Hospital Experiences				
Area Around Room 'Always' Quiet at Night	-	-	67%	61%
Doctors 'Always' Communicated Well	-	-	84%	82%
Home Recovery Information Given	-	-	86%	85%
Hospital Given 9 or 10 on 10 Point Scale	-	-	72%	71%
Meds 'Always' Explained Before Given	-	-	66%	64%
Nurses 'Always' Communicated Well	-	-	81%	79%
Pain 'Always' Well Controlled	-	-	72%	71%
Room and Bathroom 'Always' Clean	-	-	72%	73%
Timely Help 'Always' Received	-	-	68%	68%
Would Definitely Recommend Hospital	-	-	71%	71%
Use of Medical Imaging				
Cardiac Imaging Stress Test before Surgery	-	-	5.1%	5.3%
Combination Abdominal CT Scan	-	-	10.1%	10.5%
Combination Brain/Sinus CT Scan	-	-	2.5%	2.7%
Combination Chest CT Scan	-	-	1.3%	2.7%
Follow-up Mammogram/Ultrasound	-	-	8%	8.8%
Lumbar Spine MRI for Low Back Pain	-	-	39%	37.2%

NOTE: Hospital profiles are in alphabetical order by state, then city, then hospital within the city; Rankings exclude hospitals with less than 25 cases except for patient surveys which excludes hospitals with less than 100 cases; (a) 100-299 cases; (1) The number of cases/patients is too few to report; (2) Data submitted were based on a sample of cases/patients; (3) Results are based on a shorter time period than required; (4) Data suppressed by CMS for one or more quarters; (5) Results are not available for this reporting period; (6) Fewer than 100 patients completed the HCAHPS survey; (7) No cases met the criteria for this measure; (8) The lower limit of the confidence interval cannot be calculated if the number of observed infections equals zero; (9) No data are available from the state/territory for this reporting period; (10) The scores shown reflect fewer than 50 completed surveys; (11) There were discrepancies in the data collection process; (12) This measure does not apply to this hospital for this reporting period; (13) Results cannot be calculated for this reporting period; (14) The results for this state are combined with nearby states to protect confidentiality; Please refer to the User's Guide for a full explanation of data.

Musc Medical Center

169 Ashley Ave Phone: 843-792-2300
Charleston, SC 29425 Fax: 843-792-6682
URL: www.musc.edu
Type: Acute Care Hospitals Emergency Services: Yes
Ownership: Government - State Beds: 596

Key Personnel:
Chief of Medical Staff. . . . . Patrick Cawley
CEO/President. . . . . Dr. David J. Cole
Pediatric Ambulatory Care . . . . . . Charles Darby, MD
Pediatric In-Patient Care . . . . Charles Darby, MD
Infection Control. . . . . Linda Formby
Quality Assurance . . . . Karen Pellegrin
Operating Room. . . . . Karen Weaver
Radiology. . . . . Jeremy Young, MD

Measure	Cases	This Hosp.	State Avg.	U.S. Avg.
Blood Clot Prevention and Treatment				
Anticoagulation Overlap Therapy[2]	133	98%	92%	93%
ICU Venous Thromboembolism Prophylaxis[2]	95	93%	94%	92%
Incidence of Potentially Preventable VTE[2]	98	3%	8%	10%
UFH with Dosages/Platelet Monitoring[2]	92	99%	98%	97%
Venous Thromboembolism Prophylaxis[2]	306	80%	88%	85%
Warfarin Therapy Discharge Instructions[2]	103	67%	72%	75%
Chest Pain/Possible Heart Attack Care				
Aspirin Given Within 24 Hours of Arrival	16	75%	97%	96%
Fibrinolytic Meds Within 30 Min. of Arrival[5]	-	-	68%	58%
Average Time to ECG (minutes)	17	3	5	7
Average Time to Transfer (minutes)[5]	-	-	43	60
Children's Asthma Care				
Received Home Management Plan of Care	173	97%	-	88%
Received Reliever Medication	173	100%	-	100%
Received Systemic Corticosteroids	171	99%	-	100%
Emergency Department				
Admittance Decision Time (minutes)[2]	358	108	94	98
Head CT Results Within 45 Min. of Arrival[1]	-	-	61%	57%
Patients Who Left ER Before Being Seen	51,739	3%	3%	2%
Time from ER Arrival to Admit. (minutes)[2]	375	273	274	274
Time from ER Arrival to Discharge (minutes)	504	165	136	134
Time in ER Before Being Evaluated (minutes)	487	36	33	26
Time to Pain Meds for Fractures (minutes)	237	70	61	57
Heart Attack Care				
Aspirin Given at Discharge	368	99%	99%	99%
Fibrinolytic Meds Within 30 Min. of Arrival[7]	-	-	50%	54%
PCI Within 90 Minutes of Arrival	42	98%	97%	96%
Statin Prescribed at Discharge	363	99%	99%	98%
Heart Failure Care				
ACE Inhibitor or ARB for LVSD	254	98%	98%	97%
Discharge Instructions Given	518	92%	94%	94%
Evaluation of LVS Function	548	100%	99%	99%
Medicare Spending				
Medicare Spending per Patient (ratio)	-	0.99	0.98	0.98
Pneumonia Care				
Appropriate Initial Antibiotic Given	69	96%	97%	95%
Blood Culture Timing	255	96%	98%	98%
Pregnancy and Delivery Care				
Newborn Deliveries Scheduled Early[2]	110	2%	3%	6%
Preventive Care				
Immunization for Influenza[2]	545	91%	94%	90%
Immunization for Pneumonia[2]	490	90%	95%	92%
Stroke Care				
Anticoagulation Therapy for Atrial Fibrillation	50	96%	95%	95%
Antithrombotic Therapy Timing	214	96%	98%	98%
Assessed for Rehabilitation	548	97%	97%	97%
Discharged on Antithrombotic Therapy	376	98%	99%	99%
Discharged on Statin Medication	306	98%	94%	94%
Thrombolytic Therapy Timing	26	85%	58%	66%
Venous Thromboembolism Prophylaxis	545	97%	94%	94%
Written Stroke Educational Materials Given	348	97%	91%	88%
Surgical Care Improvement Project				
Appropriate Beta Blocker Usage[2]	228	100%	98%	98%
Appropriate VTP Within 24 Hours[2]	523	100%	98%	98%
Controlled Postoperative Blood Glucose[2]	130	96%	99%	97%
Perioperative Temperature Management[2]	689	100%	100%	100%
Prophylactic Antibiotic Selection[2]	515	99%	99%	99%
Prophylactic Antibiotic Selection (Outpatient)	824	99%	99%	98%
Prophylactic Antibiotic Stopped[2]	487	100%	98%	98%
Prophylactic Antibiotic Timing[2]	518	99%	99%	99%
Prophylactic Antibiotic Timing (Outpatient)	715	99%	98%	98%
Urinary Catheter Removal[2]	325	99%	97%	97%
Survey of Patients' Hospital Experiences				
Area Around Room 'Always' Quiet at Night	300+	66%	67%	61%
Doctors 'Always' Communicated Well	300+	82%	84%	82%
Home Recovery Information Given	300+	86%	86%	85%
Hospital Given 9 or 10 on 10 Point Scale	300+	80%	72%	71%
Meds 'Always' Explained Before Given	300+	66%	66%	64%
Nurses 'Always' Communicated Well	300+	81%	81%	79%
Pain 'Always' Well Controlled	300+	72%	72%	71%
Room and Bathroom 'Always' Clean	300+	71%	72%	73%
Timely Help 'Always' Received	300+	69%	68%	68%
Would Definitely Recommend Hospital	300+	85%	71%	71%
Use of Medical Imaging				
Cardiac Imaging Stress Test before Surgery	644	5.4%	5.1%	5.3%
Combination Abdominal CT Scan	1,661	7.4%	10.1%	10.5%
Combination Brain/Sinus CT Scan	896	1.9%	2.5%	2.7%
Combination Chest CT Scan	2,534	0.2%	1.3%	2.7%
Follow-up Mammogram/Ultrasound	1,626	13.5%	8%	8.8%
Lumbar Spine MRI for Low Back Pain	163	42.9%	39%	37.2%

Roper Hospital

316 Calhoun St Phone: 843-724-2800
Charleston, SC 29401 Fax: 843-724-1987
URL: www.ropersaintfrancis.com
Type: Acute Care Hospitals Emergency Services: Yes
Ownership: Voluntary non-profit - Private Beds: 453

Key Personnel:
CEO/President. . . . . David L. Dunlap

Measure	Cases	This Hosp.	State Avg.	U.S. Avg.
Blood Clot Prevention and Treatment				
Anticoagulation Overlap Therapy[2]	84	98%	92%	93%
ICU Venous Thromboembolism Prophylaxis[2]	97	99%	94%	92%
Incidence of Potentially Preventable VTE[1,2]	-	-	8%	10%
UFH with Dosages/Platelet Monitoring[2]	81	100%	98%	97%
Venous Thromboembolism Prophylaxis[2]	284	96%	88%	85%
Warfarin Therapy Discharge Instructions[2]	64	88%	72%	75%
Chest Pain/Possible Heart Attack Care				
Aspirin Given Within 24 Hours of Arrival[1]	-	-	97%	96%
Fibrinolytic Meds Within 30 Min. of Arrival[3,7]	-	-	68%	58%
Average Time to ECG (minutes)[1]	-	-	5	7
Average Time to Transfer (minutes)[1,3]	-	-	43	60
Children's Asthma Care				
Received Home Management Plan of Care	-	-	-	88%
Received Reliever Medication	-	-	-	100%
Received Systemic Corticosteroids	-	-	-	100%
Emergency Department				
Admittance Decision Time (minutes)[2]	539	82	94	98
Head CT Results Within 45 Min. of Arrival	11	73%	61%	57%
Patients Who Left ER Before Being Seen	70,083	1%	3%	2%
Time from ER Arrival to Admit. (minutes)[2]	556	203	274	274
Time from ER Arrival to Discharge (minutes)	389	99	136	134
Time in ER Before Being Evaluated (minutes)	383	18	33	26
Time to Pain Meds for Fractures (minutes)	78	55	61	57
Heart Attack Care				
Aspirin Given at Discharge	334	100%	99%	99%
Fibrinolytic Meds Within 30 Min. of Arrival[7]	-	-	50%	54%
PCI Within 90 Minutes of Arrival	36	100%	97%	96%
Statin Prescribed at Discharge	330	100%	99%	98%
Heart Failure Care				
ACE Inhibitor or ARB for LVSD	154	100%	98%	97%
Discharge Instructions Given	430	100%	94%	94%
Evaluation of LVS Function	496	100%	99%	99%
Medicare Spending				
Medicare Spending per Patient (ratio)	-	1.02	0.98	0.98
Pneumonia Care				
Appropriate Initial Antibiotic Given	98	100%	97%	95%
Blood Culture Timing	197	100%	98%	98%
Pregnancy and Delivery Care				
Newborn Deliveries Scheduled Early[7]	-	-	3%	6%
Preventive Care				
Immunization for Influenza[2]	607	98%	94%	90%
Immunization for Pneumonia[2]	914	99%	95%	92%
Stroke Care				
Anticoagulation Therapy for Atrial Fibrillation	14	100%	95%	95%
Antithrombotic Therapy Timing	107	100%	98%	98%
Assessed for Rehabilitation	145	99%	97%	97%
Discharged on Antithrombotic Therapy	124	100%	99%	99%
Discharged on Statin Medication	95	99%	94%	94%
Thrombolytic Therapy Timing[1]	-	-	58%	66%
Venous Thromboembolism Prophylaxis	134	98%	94%	94%
Written Stroke Educational Materials Given	65	88%	91%	88%
Surgical Care Improvement Project				
Appropriate Beta Blocker Usage[2]	248	98%	98%	98%
Appropriate VTP Within 24 Hours[2]	469	100%	98%	98%
Controlled Postoperative Blood Glucose[2]	198	100%	99%	97%
Perioperative Temperature Management[2]	596	100%	100%	100%
Prophylactic Antibiotic Selection[2]	575	100%	99%	99%
Prophylactic Antibiotic Selection (Outpatient)	681	99%	99%	98%
Prophylactic Antibiotic Stopped[2]	566	99%	98%	98%
Prophylactic Antibiotic Timing[2]	575	100%	99%	99%
Prophylactic Antibiotic Timing (Outpatient)	674	99%	98%	98%
Urinary Catheter Removal[2]	270	99%	97%	97%
Survey of Patients' Hospital Experiences				
Area Around Room 'Always' Quiet at Night	300+	66%	67%	61%
Doctors 'Always' Communicated Well	300+	84%	84%	82%
Home Recovery Information Given	300+	88%	86%	85%
Hospital Given 9 or 10 on 10 Point Scale	300+	78%	72%	71%
Meds 'Always' Explained Before Given	300+	68%	66%	64%
Nurses 'Always' Communicated Well	300+	82%	81%	79%
Pain 'Always' Well Controlled	300+	74%	72%	71%
Room and Bathroom 'Always' Clean	300+	70%	72%	73%
Timely Help 'Always' Received	300+	68%	68%	68%
Would Definitely Recommend Hospital	300+	82%	71%	71%
Use of Medical Imaging				
Cardiac Imaging Stress Test before Surgery	488	7.2%	5.1%	5.3%
Combination Abdominal CT Scan	1,525	9.7%	10.1%	10.5%
Combination Brain/Sinus CT Scan	1,234	1.1%	2.5%	2.7%
Combination Chest CT Scan	965	0.2%	1.3%	2.7%
Follow-up Mammogram/Ultrasound	1,775	6.3%	8%	8.8%
Lumbar Spine MRI for Low Back Pain	327	38.5%	39%	37.2%

Trident Medical Center

9330 Medical Plaza Dr Phone: 843-797-8800
Charleston, SC 29406 Fax: 843-797-4958
URL: www.tridenthealthsystem.com
Type: Acute Care Hospitals Emergency Services: Yes
Ownership: Proprietary Beds: 296

Key Personnel:
Quality Assurance . . . . Toni Bunch
CEO/President. . . . . Todd Gallati
Infection Control. . . . . Dale Haselden
Pediatric Ambulatory Care . . . . . John Howe, MD
Pediatric In-Patient Care . . . . . . John Howe, MD
Operating Room. . . . . Dawn Jackson
Chief of Medical Staff. . . . . Lloyd Mandell, MD
Radiology. . . . . Al Wilson, MD

Measure	Cases	This Hosp.	State Avg.	U.S. Avg.
Blood Clot Prevention and Treatment				
Anticoagulation Overlap Therapy[2]	150	100%	92%	93%
ICU Venous Thromboembolism Prophylaxis[2]	114	98%	94%	92%
Incidence of Potentially Preventable VTE[2]	34	3%	8%	10%
UFH with Dosages/Platelet Monitoring[2]	41	100%	98%	97%
Venous Thromboembolism Prophylaxis[2]	362	96%	88%	85%
Warfarin Therapy Discharge Instructions[2]	109	99%	72%	75%
Chest Pain/Possible Heart Attack Care				
Aspirin Given Within 24 Hours of Arrival	20	100%	97%	96%
Fibrinolytic Meds Within 30 Min. of Arrival[3,7]	-	-	68%	58%
Average Time to ECG (minutes)	22	1	5	7
Average Time to Transfer (minutes)[3,7]	-	-	43	60
Children's Asthma Care				
Received Home Management Plan of Care	-	-	-	88%
Received Reliever Medication	-	-	-	100%
Received Systemic Corticosteroids	-	-	-	100%

NOTE: Hospital profiles are in alphabetical order by state, then city, then hospital within the city; Rankings exclude hospitals with less than 25 cases except for patient surveys which excludes hospitals with less than 100 cases; (a) 100-299 cases; (1) The number of cases/patients is too few to report; (2) Data submitted were based on a sample of cases/patients; (3) Results are based on a shorter time period than required; (4) Data suppressed by CMS for one or more quarters; (5) Results are not available for this reporting period; (6) Fewer than 100 patients completed the HCAHPS survey; (7) No cases met the criteria for this measure; (8) The lower limit of the confidence interval cannot be calculated if the number of observed infections equals zero; (9) No data are available from the state/territory for this reporting period; (10) The scores shown reflect fewer than 50 completed surveys; (11) There were discrepancies in the data collection process; (12) This measure does not apply to this hospital for this reporting period; (13) Results cannot be calculated for this reporting period; (14) The results for this state are combined with nearby states to protect confidentiality; Please refer to the User's Guide for a full explanation of data.

Measure	Cases	This Hosp.	State Avg.	U.S. Avg.
Emergency Department				
Admittance Decision Time (minutes)[2]	750	107	94	98
Head CT Results Within 45 Min. of Arrival	19	84%	61%	57%
Patients Who Left ER Before Being Seen	>100k	1%	3%	2%
Time from ER Arrival to Admit. (minutes)[2]	750	272	274	274
Time from ER Arrival to Discharge (minutes)	459	126	136	134
Time in ER Before Being Evaluated (minutes)	521	16	33	26
Time to Pain Meds for Fractures (minutes)	219	60	61	57
Heart Attack Care				
Aspirin Given at Discharge	379	100%	99%	99%
Fibrinolytic Meds Within 30 Min. of Arrival[7]	-	-	50%	54%
PCI Within 90 Minutes of Arrival	81	99%	97%	96%
Statin Prescribed at Discharge	371	100%	99%	98%
Heart Failure Care				
ACE Inhibitor or ARB for LVSD	194	100%	98%	97%
Discharge Instructions Given	531	99%	94%	94%
Evaluation of LVS Function	616	100%	99%	99%
Medicare Spending				
Medicare Spending per Patient (ratio)	-	1.01	0.98	0.98
Pneumonia Care				
Appropriate Initial Antibiotic Given	311	98%	97%	95%
Blood Culture Timing	611	100%	98%	98%
Pregnancy and Delivery Care				
Newborn Deliveries Scheduled Early[2]	63	0%	3%	6%
Preventive Care				
Immunization for Influenza[2]	651	99%	94%	90%
Immunization for Pneumonia[2]	800	99%	95%	92%
Stroke Care				
Anticoagulation Therapy for Atrial Fibrillation[2]	13	100%	95%	95%
Antithrombotic Therapy Timing[2]	100	100%	98%	98%
Assessed for Rehabilitation[2]	114	99%	97%	97%
Discharged on Antithrombotic Therapy[2]	104	99%	99%	99%
Discharged on Statin Medication[2]	86	100%	94%	94%
Thrombolytic Therapy Timing[1,2]	-	-	58%	66%
Venous Thromboembolism Prophylaxis[2]	116	100%	94%	94%
Written Stroke Educational Materials Given[2]	69	99%	91%	88%
Surgical Care Improvement Project				
Appropriate Beta Blocker Usage[2]	269	100%	98%	98%
Appropriate VTP Within 24 Hours[2]	482	99%	98%	98%
Controlled Postoperative Blood Glucose[2]	146	99%	99%	97%
Perioperative Temperature Management[2]	638	100%	100%	100%
Prophylactic Antibiotic Selection[2]	563	99%	99%	99%
Prophylactic Antibiotic Selection (Outpatient)	580	99%	99%	98%
Prophylactic Antibiotic Stopped[2]	542	99%	98%	98%
Prophylactic Antibiotic Timing[2]	563	100%	99%	99%
Prophylactic Antibiotic Timing (Outpatient)	580	100%	98%	98%
Urinary Catheter Removal[2]	250	98%	97%	97%
Survey of Patients' Hospital Experiences				
Area Around Room 'Always' Quiet at Night	300+	59%	67%	61%
Doctors 'Always' Communicated Well	300+	79%	84%	82%
Home Recovery Information Given	300+	84%	86%	85%
Hospital Given 9 or 10 on 10 Point Scale	300+	63%	72%	71%
Meds 'Always' Explained Before Given	300+	60%	66%	64%
Nurses 'Always' Communicated Well	300+	73%	81%	79%
Pain 'Always' Well Controlled	300+	68%	72%	71%
Room and Bathroom 'Always' Clean	300+	65%	72%	73%
Timely Help 'Always' Received	300+	60%	68%	68%
Would Definitely Recommend Hospital	300+	63%	71%	71%
Use of Medical Imaging				
Cardiac Imaging Stress Test before Surgery	502	8.0%	5.1%	5.3%
Combination Abdominal CT Scan	1,572	8.3%	10.1%	10.5%
Combination Brain/Sinus CT Scan	1,634	2.1%	2.5%	2.7%
Combination Chest CT Scan	708	2.8%	1.3%	2.7%
Follow-up Mammogram/Ultrasound	5,968	6.1%	8%	8.8%
Lumbar Spine MRI for Low Back Pain	129	31.0%	39%	37.2%

Chesterfield General Hospital

711 Chesterfield Highway
Cheraw, SC 29520
URL: www.chesterfieldgeneral.com
Type: Acute Care Hospitals
Ownership: Voluntary non-profit - Private
Phone: 843-537-7881
Fax: 843-320-3491
Emergency Services: Yes
Beds: 59

Key Personnel:
Radiology. . . . . Sharon Kimrey
CEO/President. . . . . Vance Reynolds

Measure	Cases	This Hosp.	State Avg.	U.S. Avg.
Blood Clot Prevention and Treatment				
Anticoagulation Overlap Therapy[2]	17	100%	92%	93%
ICU Venous Thromboembolism Prophylaxis[2]	102	100%	94%	92%
Incidence of Potentially Preventable VTE[1,2]	-	-	8%	10%
UFH with Dosages/Platelet Monitoring[2,7]	-	-	98%	97%
Venous Thromboembolism Prophylaxis[2]	359	99%	88%	85%
Warfarin Therapy Discharge Instructions[1,2]	-	-	72%	75%
Chest Pain/Possible Heart Attack Care				
Aspirin Given Within 24 Hours of Arrival	37	97%	97%	96%
Fibrinolytic Meds Within 30 Min. of Arrival[1]	-	-	68%	58%
Average Time to ECG (minutes)	39	1	5	7
Average Time to Transfer (minutes)[1]	-	-	43	60
Children's Asthma Care				
Received Home Management Plan of Care	-	-	-	88%
Received Reliever Medication	-	-	-	100%
Received Systemic Corticosteroids	-	-	-	100%
Emergency Department				
Admittance Decision Time (minutes)[2]	674	51	94	98
Head CT Results Within 45 Min. of Arrival[1]	-	-	61%	57%
Patients Who Left ER Before Being Seen	12,814	2%	3%	2%
Time from ER Arrival to Admit. (minutes)[2]	677	199	274	274
Time from ER Arrival to Discharge (minutes)	418	88	136	134
Time in ER Before Being Evaluated (minutes)	511	6	33	26
Time to Pain Meds for Fractures (minutes)	60	74	61	57
Heart Attack Care				
Aspirin Given at Discharge[1]	-	-	99%	99%
Fibrinolytic Meds Within 30 Min. of Arrival[7]	-	-	50%	54%
PCI Within 90 Minutes of Arrival[7]	-	-	97%	96%
Statin Prescribed at Discharge[1]	-	-	99%	98%
Heart Failure Care				
ACE Inhibitor or ARB for LVSD	24	100%	98%	97%
Discharge Instructions Given	51	98%	94%	94%
Evaluation of LVS Function	59	100%	99%	99%
Medicare Spending				
Medicare Spending per Patient (ratio)	-	0.82	0.98	0.98
Pneumonia Care				
Appropriate Initial Antibiotic Given	78	100%	97%	95%
Blood Culture Timing	132	99%	98%	98%
Pregnancy and Delivery Care				
Newborn Deliveries Scheduled Early[2]	11	0%	3%	6%
Preventive Care				
Immunization for Influenza[2]	538	100%	94%	90%
Immunization for Pneumonia[2]	636	100%	95%	92%
Stroke Care				
Anticoagulation Therapy for Atrial Fibrillation[1]	-	-	95%	95%
Antithrombotic Therapy Timing	36	100%	98%	98%
Assessed for Rehabilitation	42	100%	97%	97%
Discharged on Antithrombotic Therapy	40	98%	99%	99%
Discharged on Statin Medication	31	100%	94%	94%
Thrombolytic Therapy Timing[7]	-	-	58%	66%
Venous Thromboembolism Prophylaxis	36	100%	94%	94%
Written Stroke Educational Materials Given	26	96%	91%	88%
Surgical Care Improvement Project				
Appropriate Beta Blocker Usage[1]	-	-	98%	98%
Appropriate VTP Within 24 Hours	34	100%	98%	98%
Controlled Postoperative Blood Glucose[7]	-	-	99%	97%
Perioperative Temperature Management	39	100%	100%	100%
Prophylactic Antibiotic Selection	14	100%	99%	99%
Prophylactic Antibiotic Selection (Outpatient)[1]	-	-	99%	98%
Prophylactic Antibiotic Stopped	13	100%	98%	98%
Prophylactic Antibiotic Timing	14	100%	99%	99%
Prophylactic Antibiotic Timing (Outpatient)[1]	-	-	98%	98%
Urinary Catheter Removal[1]	-	-	97%	97%
Survey of Patients' Hospital Experiences				
Area Around Room 'Always' Quiet at Night	300+	66%	67%	61%
Doctors 'Always' Communicated Well	300+	85%	84%	82%
Home Recovery Information Given	300+	81%	86%	85%
Hospital Given 9 or 10 on 10 Point Scale	300+	67%	72%	71%
Meds 'Always' Explained Before Given	300+	65%	66%	64%
Nurses 'Always' Communicated Well	300+	78%	81%	79%
Pain 'Always' Well Controlled	300+	71%	72%	71%
Room and Bathroom 'Always' Clean	300+	67%	72%	73%
Timely Help 'Always' Received	300+	69%	68%	68%
Would Definitely Recommend Hospital	300+	63%	71%	71%
Use of Medical Imaging				
Cardiac Imaging Stress Test before Surgery	99	7.1%	5.1%	5.3%
Combination Abdominal CT Scan	328	4.3%	10.1%	10.5%
Combination Brain/Sinus CT Scan[1]	-	-	2.5%	2.7%
Combination Chest CT Scan	112	3.6%	1.3%	2.7%
Follow-up Mammogram/Ultrasound	426	10.1%	8%	8.8%
Lumbar Spine MRI for Low Back Pain[1]	-	-	39%	37.2%

Chester Regional Medical Center

1 Medical Park Drive
Chester, SC 29706
E-mail: whbundy@infoave.net
URL: www.chospital.org
Type: Acute Care Hospitals
Ownership: Proprietary
Phone: 803-581-3151
Fax: 803-581-2565
Emergency Services: Yes
Beds: 182

Key Personnel:
Quality Assurance . . . . Angie Bagley
Emergency Room . . . . Daniel R Crow
Chief of Medical Staff. . . . . Jennifer Edwards
Patient Relations . . . . Linda Fairfax
Radiology. . . . . Geoffrey T Gilleland
Operating Room. . . . . Joseph Rondina
Infection Control. . . . . Amy Shehane
CEO . . . . Page Vaughan

Measure	Cases	This Hosp.	State Avg.	U.S. Avg.
Blood Clot Prevention and Treatment				
Anticoagulation Overlap Therapy[1,2]	-	-	92%	93%
ICU Venous Thromboembolism Prophylaxis[2]	50	80%	94%	92%
Incidence of Potentially Preventable VTE[1,2]	-	-	8%	10%
UFH with Dosages/Platelet Monitoring[1,2]	-	-	98%	97%
Venous Thromboembolism Prophylaxis[2]	144	74%	88%	85%
Warfarin Therapy Discharge Instructions[1,2]	-	-	72%	75%
Chest Pain/Possible Heart Attack Care				
Aspirin Given Within 24 Hours of Arrival	60	100%	97%	96%
Fibrinolytic Meds Within 30 Min. of Arrival[1]	-	-	68%	58%
Average Time to ECG (minutes)	64	3	5	7
Average Time to Transfer (minutes)[1]	-	-	43	60
Children's Asthma Care				
Received Home Management Plan of Care	-	-	-	88%
Received Reliever Medication	-	-	-	100%
Received Systemic Corticosteroids	-	-	-	100%
Emergency Department				
Admittance Decision Time (minutes)[2]	525	63	94	98
Head CT Results Within 45 Min. of Arrival	11	9%	61%	57%
Patients Who Left ER Before Being Seen	19,449	3%	3%	2%
Time from ER Arrival to Admit. (minutes)[2]	529	223	274	274
Time from ER Arrival to Discharge (minutes)	589	105	136	134
Time in ER Before Being Evaluated (minutes)	641	47	33	26
Time to Pain Meds for Fractures (minutes)	61	63	61	57
Heart Attack Care				
Aspirin Given at Discharge	12	100%	99%	99%
Fibrinolytic Meds Within 30 Min. of Arrival[7]	-	-	50%	54%
PCI Within 90 Minutes of Arrival[7]	-	-	97%	96%
Statin Prescribed at Discharge	12	75%	99%	98%
Heart Failure Care				
ACE Inhibitor or ARB for LVSD	26	92%	98%	97%
Discharge Instructions Given	63	94%	94%	94%
Evaluation of LVS Function	76	100%	99%	99%
Medicare Spending				
Medicare Spending per Patient (ratio)	-	0.98	0.98	0.98
Pneumonia Care				
Appropriate Initial Antibiotic Given	50	100%	97%	95%
Blood Culture Timing	74	99%	98%	98%
Pregnancy and Delivery Care				
Newborn Deliveries Scheduled Early[7]	-	-	3%	6%
Preventive Care				
Immunization for Influenza[2]	374	97%	94%	90%
Immunization for Pneumonia[2]	457	97%	95%	92%
Stroke Care				

NOTE: Hospital profiles are in alphabetical order by state, then city, then hospital within the city; Rankings exclude hospitals with less than 25 cases except for patient surveys which excludes hospitals with less than 100 cases; (a) 100-299 cases; (1) The number of cases/patients is too few to report; (2) Data submitted were based on a sample of cases/patients; (3) Results are based on a shorter time period than required; (4) Data suppressed by CMS for one or more quarters; (5) Results are not available for this reporting period; (6) Fewer than 100 patients completed the HCAHPS survey; (7) No cases met the criteria for this measure; (8) The lower limit of the confidence interval cannot be calculated if the number of observed infections equals zero; (9) No data are available from the state/territory for this reporting period; (10) The scores shown reflect fewer than 50 completed surveys; (11) There were discrepancies in the data collection process; (12) This measure does not apply to this hospital for this reporting period; (13) Results cannot be calculated for this reporting period; (14) The results for this state are combined with nearby states to protect confidentiality; Please refer to the User's Guide for a full explanation of data.

Measure	Cases	This Hosp.	State Avg.	U.S. Avg.
Anticoagulation Therapy for Atrial Fibrillation[1,2]	-	-	95%	95%
Antithrombotic Therapy Timing[2]	16	100%	98%	98%
Assessed for Rehabilitation[2]	18	78%	97%	97%
Discharged on Antithrombotic Therapy[2]	18	100%	99%	99%
Discharged on Statin Medication[2]	14	93%	94%	94%
Thrombolytic Therapy Timing[1,2]	-	-	58%	66%
Venous Thromboembolism Prophylaxis[2]	16	94%	94%	94%
Written Stroke Educational Materials Given[2]	14	86%	91%	88%
Surgical Care Improvement Project				
Appropriate Beta Blocker Usage	15	100%	98%	98%
Appropriate VTP Within 24 Hours	67	97%	98%	98%
Controlled Postoperative Blood Glucose[7]	-	-	99%	97%
Perioperative Temperature Management	70	100%	100%	100%
Prophylactic Antibiotic Selection	49	100%	99%	99%
Prophylactic Antibiotic Selection (Outpatient)	18	94%	99%	98%
Prophylactic Antibiotic Stopped	47	100%	98%	98%
Prophylactic Antibiotic Timing	49	98%	99%	99%
Prophylactic Antibiotic Timing (Outpatient)	18	100%	98%	98%
Urinary Catheter Removal	23	96%	97%	97%
Survey of Patients' Hospital Experiences				
Area Around Room 'Always' Quiet at Night	(a)	63%	67%	61%
Doctors 'Always' Communicated Well	(a)	82%	84%	82%
Home Recovery Information Given	(a)	92%	86%	85%
Hospital Given 9 or 10 on 10 Point Scale	(a)	61%	72%	71%
Meds 'Always' Explained Before Given	(a)	62%	66%	64%
Nurses 'Always' Communicated Well	(a)	78%	81%	79%
Pain 'Always' Well Controlled	(a)	72%	72%	71%
Room and Bathroom 'Always' Clean	(a)	76%	72%	73%
Timely Help 'Always' Received	(a)	66%	68%	68%
Would Definitely Recommend Hospital	(a)	57%	71%	71%
Use of Medical Imaging				
Cardiac Imaging Stress Test before Surgery	72	4.2%	5.1%	5.3%
Combination Abdominal CT Scan	227	2.6%	10.1%	10.5%
Combination Brain/Sinus CT Scan[1]	-	-	2.5%	2.7%
Combination Chest CT Scan	97	3.1%	1.3%	2.7%
Follow-up Mammogram/Ultrasound	440	9.8%	8%	8.8%
Lumbar Spine MRI for Low Back Pain[1]	-	-	39%	37.2%

GHS Laurens County Memorial Hospital

22725 Highway 76 East
Clinton, SC 29325
Phone: 864-833-9100
Fax: 863-833-9471
E-mail: lroper@lchcs.org
URL: www.lchcs.org
Type: Acute Care Hospitals
Emergency Services: Yes
Ownership: Govt - Hospital Dist/Auth
Beds: 90
Key Personnel:
Radiology.................... Michael Evert

Measure	Cases	This Hosp.	State Avg.	U.S. Avg.
Blood Clot Prevention and Treatment				
Anticoagulation Overlap Therapy[1,2]	-	-	92%	93%
ICU Venous Thromboembolism Prophylaxis[2]	60	95%	94%	92%
Incidence of Potentially Preventable VTE[1,2]	-	-	8%	10%
UFH with Dosages/Platelet Monitoring[1,2]	-	-	98%	97%
Venous Thromboembolism Prophylaxis[2]	216	78%	88%	85%
Warfarin Therapy Discharge Instructions[1,2]	-	-	72%	75%
Chest Pain/Possible Heart Attack Care				
Aspirin Given Within 24 Hours of Arrival	69	99%	97%	96%
Fibrinolytic Meds Within 30 Min. of Arrival[7]	-	-	68%	58%
Average Time to ECG (minutes)	68	18	5	7
Average Time to Transfer (minutes)[1]	-	-	43	60
Children's Asthma Care				
Received Home Management Plan of Care	-	-	-	88%
Received Reliever Medication	-	-	-	100%
Received Systemic Corticosteroids	-	-	-	100%
Emergency Department				
Admittance Decision Time (minutes)[2]	278	120	94	98
Head CT Results Within 45 Min. of Arrival[1]	-	-	61%	57%
Patients Who Left ER Before Being Seen	29,443	3%	3%	2%
Time from ER Arrival to Admit. (minutes)[2]	323	306	274	274
Time from ER Arrival to Discharge (minutes)	363	124	136	134
Time in ER Before Being Evaluated (minutes)	387	49	33	26
Time to Pain Meds for Fractures (minutes)	78	82	61	57
Heart Attack Care				
Aspirin Given at Discharge[1]	-	-	99%	99%
Fibrinolytic Meds Within 30 Min. of Arrival[7]	-	-	50%	54%
PCI Within 90 Minutes of Arrival[7]	-	-	97%	96%
Statin Prescribed at Discharge[1]	-	-	99%	98%
Heart Failure Care				
ACE Inhibitor or ARB for LVSD	31	87%	98%	97%
Discharge Instructions Given	79	87%	94%	94%
Evaluation of LVS Function	105	95%	99%	99%
Medicare Spending				
Medicare Spending per Patient (ratio)	-	1.03	0.98	0.98
Pneumonia Care				
Appropriate Initial Antibiotic Given	67	90%	97%	95%
Blood Culture Timing	95	94%	98%	98%
Pregnancy and Delivery Care				
Newborn Deliveries Scheduled Early	28	4%	3%	6%
Preventive Care				
Immunization for Influenza[2]	258	82%	94%	90%
Immunization for Pneumonia[2]	342	85%	95%	92%
Stroke Care				
Anticoagulation Therapy for Atrial Fibrillation[1]	-	-	95%	95%
Antithrombotic Therapy Timing	34	100%	98%	98%
Assessed for Rehabilitation	35	91%	97%	97%
Discharged on Antithrombotic Therapy	32	88%	99%	99%
Discharged on Statin Medication	25	92%	94%	94%
Thrombolytic Therapy Timing[1]	-	-	58%	66%
Venous Thromboembolism Prophylaxis	41	83%	94%	94%
Written Stroke Educational Materials Given	17	88%	91%	88%
Surgical Care Improvement Project				
Appropriate Beta Blocker Usage	62	94%	98%	98%
Appropriate VTP Within 24 Hours	163	96%	98%	98%
Controlled Postoperative Blood Glucose[7]	-	-	99%	97%
Perioperative Temperature Management	192	100%	100%	100%
Prophylactic Antibiotic Selection	149	98%	99%	99%
Prophylactic Antibiotic Selection (Outpatient)[3]	12	100%	99%	98%
Prophylactic Antibiotic Stopped	146	95%	98%	98%
Prophylactic Antibiotic Timing	149	99%	99%	99%
Prophylactic Antibiotic Timing (Outpatient)[3]	12	100%	98%	98%
Urinary Catheter Removal	157	95%	97%	97%
Survey of Patients' Hospital Experiences				
Area Around Room 'Always' Quiet at Night	300+	65%	67%	61%
Doctors 'Always' Communicated Well	300+	81%	84%	82%
Home Recovery Information Given	300+	85%	86%	85%
Hospital Given 9 or 10 on 10 Point Scale	300+	61%	72%	71%
Meds 'Always' Explained Before Given	300+	63%	66%	64%
Nurses 'Always' Communicated Well	300+	78%	81%	79%
Pain 'Always' Well Controlled	300+	73%	72%	71%
Room and Bathroom 'Always' Clean	300+	62%	72%	73%
Timely Help 'Always' Received	300+	65%	68%	68%
Would Definitely Recommend Hospital	300+	57%	71%	71%
Use of Medical Imaging				
Cardiac Imaging Stress Test before Surgery	89	6.7%	5.1%	5.3%
Combination Abdominal CT Scan	292	5.5%	10.1%	10.5%
Combination Brain/Sinus CT Scan	443	1.8%	2.5%	2.7%
Combination Chest CT Scan	143	0.7%	1.3%	2.7%
Follow-up Mammogram/Ultrasound	795	12.6%	8%	8.8%
Lumbar Spine MRI for Low Back Pain	45	42.2%	39%	37.2%

Columbia SC VA Medical Center

6439 Garners Ferry Road
Columbia, SC 29209
Phone: 803-695-7980
Fax: 803-695-6739
URL: www.va.gov/columbiasc
Type: Acute Care - VA
Emergency Services: No
Ownership: Government Federal
Beds: 216
Key Personnel:
Chief of Medical Staff.......... Brian Heckert
Quality Assurance .... Carol Truslow, RN

Measure	Cases	This Hosp.	State Avg.	U.S. Avg.
Blood Clot Prevention and Treatment				
Anticoagulation Overlap Therapy	-	-	92%	93%
ICU Venous Thromboembolism Prophylaxis	-	-	94%	92%
Incidence of Potentially Preventable VTE	-	-	8%	10%
UFH with Dosages/Platelet Monitoring	-	-	98%	97%
Venous Thromboembolism Prophylaxis	-	-	88%	85%
Warfarin Therapy Discharge Instructions	-	-	72%	75%
Chest Pain/Possible Heart Attack Care				
Aspirin Given Within 24 Hours of Arrival	-	-	97%	96%
Fibrinolytic Meds Within 30 Min. of Arrival	-	-	68%	58%
Average Time to ECG (minutes)	-	-	5	7
Average Time to Transfer (minutes)	-	-	43	60
Children's Asthma Care				
Received Home Management Plan of Care	-	-	-	88%
Received Reliever Medication	-	-	-	100%
Received Systemic Corticosteroids	-	-	-	100%
Emergency Department				
Admittance Decision Time (minutes)	-	-	94	98
Head CT Results Within 45 Min. of Arrival	-	-	61%	57%
Patients Who Left ER Before Being Seen	-	-	3%	2%
Time from ER Arrival to Admit. (minutes)	-	-	274	274
Time from ER Arrival to Discharge (minutes)	-	-	136	134
Time in ER Before Being Evaluated (minutes)	-	-	33	26
Time to Pain Meds for Fractures (minutes)	-	-	61	57
Heart Attack Care				
Aspirin Given at Discharge[1]	-	-	99%	99%
Fibrinolytic Meds Within 30 Min. of Arrival[5]	-	-	50%	54%
PCI Within 90 Minutes of Arrival[5]	-	-	97%	96%
Statin Prescribed at Discharge[1]	-	-	99%	98%
Heart Failure Care				
ACE Inhibitor or ARB for LVSD	78	99%	98%	97%
Discharge Instructions Given	226	100%	94%	94%
Evaluation of LVS Function	232	100%	99%	99%
Medicare Spending				
Medicare Spending per Patient (ratio)	-	-	0.98	0.98
Pneumonia Care				
Appropriate Initial Antibiotic Given	53	98%	97%	95%
Blood Culture Timing	84	100%	98%	98%
Pregnancy and Delivery Care				
Newborn Deliveries Scheduled Early	-	-	3%	6%
Preventive Care				
Immunization for Influenza[5]	-	-	94%	90%
Immunization for Pneumonia[5]	-	-	95%	92%
Stroke Care				
Anticoagulation Therapy for Atrial Fibrillation	-	-	95%	95%
Antithrombotic Therapy Timing	-	-	98%	98%
Assessed for Rehabilitation	-	-	97%	97%
Discharged on Antithrombotic Therapy	-	-	99%	99%
Discharged on Statin Medication	-	-	94%	94%
Thrombolytic Therapy Timing	-	-	58%	66%
Venous Thromboembolism Prophylaxis	-	-	94%	94%
Written Stroke Educational Materials Given	-	-	91%	88%
Surgical Care Improvement Project				
Appropriate Beta Blocker Usage[2]	25	100%	98%	98%
Appropriate VTP Within 24 Hours[2]	123	99%	98%	98%
Controlled Postoperative Blood Glucose[5]	-	-	99%	97%
Perioperative Temperature Management[2]	120	100%	100%	100%
Prophylactic Antibiotic Selection	85	100%	99%	99%
Prophylactic Antibiotic Selection (Outpatient)	-	-	99%	98%
Prophylactic Antibiotic Stopped	83	100%	98%	98%
Prophylactic Antibiotic Timing	85	100%	99%	99%
Prophylactic Antibiotic Timing (Outpatient)	-	-	98%	98%
Urinary Catheter Removal[2]	87	99%	97%	97%
Survey of Patients' Hospital Experiences				
Area Around Room 'Always' Quiet at Night	-	-	67%	61%
Doctors 'Always' Communicated Well	-	-	84%	82%
Home Recovery Information Given	-	-	86%	85%
Hospital Given 9 or 10 on 10 Point Scale	-	-	72%	71%
Meds 'Always' Explained Before Given	-	-	66%	64%
Nurses 'Always' Communicated Well	-	-	81%	79%
Pain 'Always' Well Controlled	-	-	72%	71%
Room and Bathroom 'Always' Clean	-	-	72%	73%
Timely Help 'Always' Received	-	-	68%	68%
Would Definitely Recommend Hospital	-	-	71%	71%
Use of Medical Imaging				
Cardiac Imaging Stress Test before Surgery	-	-	5.1%	5.3%
Combination Abdominal CT Scan	-	-	10.1%	10.5%
Combination Brain/Sinus CT Scan	-	-	2.5%	2.7%

NOTE: Hospital profiles are in alphabetical order by state, then city, then hospital within the city; Rankings exclude hospitals with less than 25 cases except for patient surveys which excludes hospitals with less than 100 cases; (a) 100-299 cases; (1) The number of cases/patients is too few to report; (2) Data submitted were based on a sample of cases/patients; (3) Results are based on a shorter time period than required; (4) Data suppressed by CMS for one or more quarters; (5) Results are not available for this reporting period; (6) Fewer than 100 patients completed the HCAHPS survey; (7) No cases met the criteria for this measure; (8) The lower limit of the confidence interval cannot be calculated if the number of observed infections equals zero; (9) No data are available from the state/territory for this reporting period; (10) The scores shown reflect fewer than 50 completed surveys; (11) There were discrepancies in the data collection process; (12) This measure does not apply to this hospital for this reporting period; (13) Results cannot be calculated for this reporting period; (14) The results for this state are combined with nearby states to protect confidentiality; Please refer to the User's Guide for a full explanation of data.

Combination Chest CT Scan	-	-	1.3%	2.7%
Follow-up Mammogram/Ultrasound	-	-	8%	8.8%
Lumbar Spine MRI for Low Back Pain	-	-	39%	37.2%

Palmetto Health Baptist

Taylor at Marion St Phone: 803-296-5678
Columbia, SC 29220 Fax: 205-783-7076
URL: www.palmettohealth.org
Type: Acute Care Hospitals Emergency Services: Yes
Ownership: Voluntary non-profit - Private Beds: 489

Key Personnel:
CEO/President.............. Charles D Beaman, Jr
Infection Control.............. Gwen Floyd
Quality Assurance .... Kathleen Kelly
Radiology.................. Mark A Lovern, MD
Pediatric Ambulatory Care ...... Philip Mubarak, MD
Pediatric In-Patient Care .... Philip Mubarak, MD
Chief of Medical Staff.......... Dr William J Savoca
Operating Room.............. Lynn Wythe, RN

Measure	Cases	This Hosp.	State Avg.	U.S. Avg.
Blood Clot Prevention and Treatment				
Anticoagulation Overlap Therapy[2]	95	91%	92%	93%
ICU Venous Thromboembolism Prophylaxis[2]	47	91%	94%	92%
Incidence of Potentially Preventable VTE[2]	14	7%	8%	10%
UFH with Dosages/Platelet Monitoring[2]	44	100%	98%	97%
Venous Thromboembolism Prophylaxis[2]	409	92%	88%	85%
Warfarin Therapy Discharge Instructions[2]	72	86%	72%	75%
Chest Pain/Possible Heart Attack Care				
Aspirin Given Within 24 Hours of Arrival	15	100%	97%	96%
Fibrinolytic Meds Within 30 Min. of Arrival[7]	-	-	68%	58%
Average Time to ECG (minutes)	15	19	5	7
Average Time to Transfer (minutes)[1]	-	-	43	60
Children's Asthma Care				
Received Home Management Plan of Care	-	-	-	88%
Received Reliever Medication	-	-	-	100%
Received Systemic Corticosteroids	-	-	-	100%
Emergency Department				
Admittance Decision Time (minutes)[2]	325	85	94	98
Head CT Results Within 45 Min. of Arrival[1,3]	-	-	61%	57%
Patients Who Left ER Before Being Seen	46,648	4%	3%	2%
Time from ER Arrival to Admit. (minutes)[2]	352	366	274	274
Time from ER Arrival to Discharge (minutes)	409	165	136	134
Time in ER Before Being Evaluated (minutes)	357	34	33	26
Time to Pain Meds for Fractures (minutes)	38	61	61	57
Heart Attack Care				
Aspirin Given at Discharge	12	100%	99%	99%
Fibrinolytic Meds Within 30 Min. of Arrival[7]	-	-	50%	54%
PCI Within 90 Minutes of Arrival[7]	-	-	97%	96%
Statin Prescribed at Discharge	12	100%	99%	98%
Heart Failure Care				
ACE Inhibitor or ARB for LVSD	77	100%	98%	97%
Discharge Instructions Given	137	99%	94%	94%
Evaluation of LVS Function	178	100%	99%	99%
Medicare Spending				
Medicare Spending per Patient (ratio)	-	1.01	0.98	0.98
Pneumonia Care				
Appropriate Initial Antibiotic Given	100	95%	97%	95%
Blood Culture Timing	167	96%	98%	98%
Pregnancy and Delivery Care				
Newborn Deliveries Scheduled Early[2]	286	1%	3%	6%
Preventive Care				
Immunization for Influenza[2]	529	97%	94%	90%
Immunization for Pneumonia[2]	492	96%	95%	92%
Stroke Care				
Anticoagulation Therapy for Atrial Fibrillation[1]	-	-	95%	95%
Antithrombotic Therapy Timing	71	97%	98%	98%
Assessed for Rehabilitation	85	98%	97%	97%
Discharged on Antithrombotic Therapy	75	100%	99%	99%
Discharged on Statin Medication	66	94%	94%	94%
Thrombolytic Therapy Timing[1]	-	-	58%	66%
Venous Thromboembolism Prophylaxis	91	92%	94%	94%
Written Stroke Educational Materials Given	49	98%	91%	88%
Surgical Care Improvement Project				
Appropriate Beta Blocker Usage	314	96%	98%	98%
Appropriate VTP Within 24 Hours	1,033	99%	98%	98%
Controlled Postoperative Blood Glucose[7]	-	-	99%	97%
Perioperative Temperature Management	1,258	100%	100%	100%
Prophylactic Antibiotic Selection	650	100%	99%	99%
Prophylactic Antibiotic Selection (Outpatient)	430	98%	99%	98%
Prophylactic Antibiotic Stopped	647	99%	98%	98%
Prophylactic Antibiotic Timing	649	100%	99%	99%
Prophylactic Antibiotic Timing (Outpatient)	445	94%	98%	98%
Urinary Catheter Removal	544	97%	97%	97%
Survey of Patients' Hospital Experiences				
Area Around Room 'Always' Quiet at Night	300+	68%	67%	61%
Doctors 'Always' Communicated Well	300+	83%	84%	82%
Home Recovery Information Given	300+	83%	86%	85%
Hospital Given 9 or 10 on 10 Point Scale	300+	72%	72%	71%
Meds 'Always' Explained Before Given	300+	66%	66%	64%
Nurses 'Always' Communicated Well	300+	80%	81%	79%
Pain 'Always' Well Controlled	300+	72%	72%	71%
Room and Bathroom 'Always' Clean	300+	69%	72%	73%
Timely Help 'Always' Received	300+	61%	68%	68%
Would Definitely Recommend Hospital	300+	75%	71%	71%
Use of Medical Imaging				
Cardiac Imaging Stress Test before Surgery	323	5.0%	5.1%	5.3%
Combination Abdominal CT Scan	798	4.5%	10.1%	10.5%
Combination Brain/Sinus CT Scan[1]	-	-	2.5%	2.7%
Combination Chest CT Scan	302	1.3%	1.3%	2.7%
Follow-up Mammogram/Ultrasound	6,264	3.3%	8%	8.8%
Lumbar Spine MRI for Low Back Pain	190	37.4%	39%	37.2%

Palmetto Health Richland

5 Richland Medical Park Phone: 803-296-5678
Columbia, SC 29203 Fax: 803-434-2885
URL: www.palmettohealth.org
Type: Acute Care Hospitals Emergency Services: Yes
Ownership: Voluntary non-profit - Private Beds: 649

Key Personnel:
CEO/President.............. Charles D Beaman, Jr
Infection Control.............. Charles S Bryan, MD
Quality Assurance .... Fran King
Chief of Medical Staff.......... James I Raymond, MD
President.................. John J. Singerling, III
Intensive Care Unit............ Saundra Swygert

Measure	Cases	This Hosp.	State Avg.	U.S. Avg.
Blood Clot Prevention and Treatment				
Anticoagulation Overlap Therapy[2]	178	92%	92%	93%
ICU Venous Thromboembolism Prophylaxis[2]	86	97%	94%	92%
Incidence of Potentially Preventable VTE[2]	56	18%	8%	10%
UFH with Dosages/Platelet Monitoring[2]	103	100%	98%	97%
Venous Thromboembolism Prophylaxis[2]	391	77%	88%	85%
Warfarin Therapy Discharge Instructions[2]	133	49%	72%	75%
Chest Pain/Possible Heart Attack Care				
Aspirin Given Within 24 Hours of Arrival[3,7]	-	-	97%	96%
Fibrinolytic Meds Within 30 Min. of Arrival[5]	-	-	68%	58%
Average Time to ECG (minutes)[3,7]	-	-	5	7
Average Time to Transfer (minutes)[5]	-	-	43	60
Children's Asthma Care				
Received Home Management Plan of Care	-	-	-	88%
Received Reliever Medication	-	-	-	100%
Received Systemic Corticosteroids	-	-	-	100%
Emergency Department				
Admittance Decision Time (minutes)[2]	559	120	94	98
Head CT Results Within 45 Min. of Arrival[1]	-	-	61%	57%
Patients Who Left ER Before Being Seen	89,440	9%	3%	2%
Time from ER Arrival to Admit. (minutes)[2]	586	422	274	274
Time from ER Arrival to Discharge (minutes)	384	189	136	134
Time in ER Before Being Evaluated (minutes)	400	20	33	26
Time to Pain Meds for Fractures (minutes)	249	73	61	57
Heart Attack Care				
Aspirin Given at Discharge	489	99%	99%	99%
Fibrinolytic Meds Within 30 Min. of Arrival[7]	-	-	50%	54%
PCI Within 90 Minutes of Arrival	89	96%	97%	96%
Statin Prescribed at Discharge	476	99%	99%	98%
Heart Failure Care				
ACE Inhibitor or ARB for LVSD	355	99%	98%	97%
Discharge Instructions Given	627	96%	94%	94%
Evaluation of LVS Function	724	100%	99%	99%
Medicare Spending				
Medicare Spending per Patient (ratio)	-	0.99	0.98	0.98
Pneumonia Care				
Appropriate Initial Antibiotic Given	127	92%	97%	95%
Blood Culture Timing	211	98%	98%	98%
Pregnancy and Delivery Care				
Newborn Deliveries Scheduled Early[2]	180	3%	3%	6%
Preventive Care				
Immunization for Influenza[2]	616	84%	94%	90%
Immunization for Pneumonia[2]	637	90%	95%	92%
Stroke Care				
Anticoagulation Therapy for Atrial Fibrillation	44	95%	95%	95%
Antithrombotic Therapy Timing	295	96%	98%	98%
Assessed for Rehabilitation	458	99%	97%	97%
Discharged on Antithrombotic Therapy	337	99%	99%	99%
Discharged on Statin Medication	271	99%	94%	94%
Thrombolytic Therapy Timing	28	89%	58%	66%
Venous Thromboembolism Prophylaxis	510	93%	94%	94%
Written Stroke Educational Materials Given	292	97%	91%	88%
Surgical Care Improvement Project				
Appropriate Beta Blocker Usage	550	97%	98%	98%
Appropriate VTP Within 24 Hours	1,164	96%	98%	98%
Controlled Postoperative Blood Glucose	295	99%	99%	97%
Perioperative Temperature Management	1,558	100%	100%	100%
Prophylactic Antibiotic Selection	1,072	100%	99%	99%
Prophylactic Antibiotic Selection (Outpatient)	545	97%	99%	98%
Prophylactic Antibiotic Stopped	1,048	98%	98%	98%
Prophylactic Antibiotic Timing	1,075	100%	99%	99%
Prophylactic Antibiotic Timing (Outpatient)	551	96%	98%	98%
Urinary Catheter Removal	1,089	97%	97%	97%
Survey of Patients' Hospital Experiences				
Area Around Room 'Always' Quiet at Night	300+	65%	67%	61%
Doctors 'Always' Communicated Well	300+	87%	84%	82%
Home Recovery Information Given	300+	87%	86%	85%
Hospital Given 9 or 10 on 10 Point Scale	300+	76%	72%	71%
Meds 'Always' Explained Before Given	300+	70%	66%	64%
Nurses 'Always' Communicated Well	300+	84%	81%	79%
Pain 'Always' Well Controlled	300+	75%	72%	71%
Room and Bathroom 'Always' Clean	300+	71%	72%	73%
Timely Help 'Always' Received	300+	68%	68%	68%
Would Definitely Recommend Hospital	300+	80%	71%	71%
Use of Medical Imaging				
Cardiac Imaging Stress Test before Surgery	1,035	4.7%	5.1%	5.3%
Combination Abdominal CT Scan	649	2.5%	10.1%	10.5%
Combination Brain/Sinus CT Scan	903	2.9%	2.5%	2.7%
Combination Chest CT Scan	652	0.3%	1.3%	2.7%
Follow-up Mammogram/Ultrasound	2,451	3.7%	8%	8.8%
Lumbar Spine MRI for Low Back Pain	169	32.5%	39%	37.2%

Sisters of Charity Providence Hospitals

2435 Forest Dr Phone: 803-256-5300
Columbia, SC 29204 Fax: 803-256-5935
E-mail: info@provhosp.com
URL: www.providencehospitals.com
Type: Acute Care Hospitals Emergency Services: Yes
Ownership: Voluntary non-profit - Private Beds: 239

Key Personnel:
Chief of Medical Staff.......... Daniel Bouknight, MD
Radiology.................. Douglas Bull
Quality Assurance .... Linda Flemming
Emergency Room .... Diane Kerenick
CEO/President.............. George A Zara, CSA

Measure	Cases	This Hosp.	State Avg.	U.S. Avg.
Blood Clot Prevention and Treatment				
Anticoagulation Overlap Therapy[2]	108	95%	92%	93%
ICU Venous Thromboembolism Prophylaxis[2]	124	93%	94%	92%
Incidence of Potentially Preventable VTE[2]	15	20%	8%	10%
UFH with Dosages/Platelet Monitoring[2]	55	100%	98%	97%
Venous Thromboembolism Prophylaxis[2]	300	81%	88%	85%
Warfarin Therapy Discharge Instructions[2]	71	93%	72%	75%
Chest Pain/Possible Heart Attack Care				
Aspirin Given Within 24 Hours of Arrival[1,3]	-	-	97%	96%
Fibrinolytic Meds Within 30 Min. of Arrival[3,7]	-	-	68%	58%

NOTE: Hospital profiles are in alphabetical order by state, then city, then hospital within the city; Rankings exclude hospitals with less than 25 cases except for patient surveys which excludes hospitals with less than 100 cases; (a) 100-299 cases; (1) The number of cases/patients is too few to report; (2) Data submitted were based on a sample of cases/patients; (3) Results are based on a shorter time period than required; (4) Data suppressed by CMS for one or more quarters; (5) Results are not available for this reporting period; (6) Fewer than 100 patients completed the HCAHPS survey; (7) No cases met the criteria for this measure; (8) The lower limit of the confidence interval cannot be calculated if the number of observed infections equals zero; (9) No data are available from the state/territory for this reporting period; (10) The scores shown reflect fewer than 50 completed surveys; (11) There were discrepancies in the data collection process; (12) This measure does not apply to this hospital for this reporting period; (13) Results cannot be calculated for this reporting period; (14) The results for this state are combined with nearby states to protect confidentiality; Please refer to the User's Guide for a full explanation of data.

Average Time to ECG (minutes)[1,3]	-	-	5	7
Average Time to Transfer (minutes)[3,7]	-	-	43	60
Children's Asthma Care				
Received Home Management Plan of Care	-	-	-	88%
Received Reliever Medication	-	-	-	100%
Received Systemic Corticosteroids	-	-	-	100%
Emergency Department				
Admittance Decision Time (minutes)[2]	479	165	94	98
Head CT Results Within 45 Min. of Arrival	28	54%	61%	57%
Patients Who Left ER Before Being Seen	64,608	5%	3%	2%
Time from ER Arrival to Admit. (minutes)[2]	495	317	274	274
Time from ER Arrival to Discharge (minutes)	395	138	136	134
Time in ER Before Being Evaluated (minutes)	419	39	33	26
Time to Pain Meds for Fractures (minutes)	131	53	61	57
Heart Attack Care				
Aspirin Given at Discharge[2]	317	100%	99%	99%
Fibrinolytic Meds Within 30 Min. of Arrival[2,7]	-	-	50%	54%
PCI Within 90 Minutes of Arrival[2]	29	90%	97%	96%
Statin Prescribed at Discharge[2]	285	100%	99%	98%
Heart Failure Care				
ACE Inhibitor or ARB for LVSD[2]	100	98%	98%	97%
Discharge Instructions Given[2]	271	77%	94%	94%
Evaluation of LVS Function[2]	313	100%	99%	99%
Medicare Spending				
Medicare Spending per Patient (ratio)	-	0.99	0.98	0.98
Pneumonia Care				
Appropriate Initial Antibiotic Given[2]	83	98%	97%	95%
Blood Culture Timing[2]	110	94%	98%	98%
Pregnancy and Delivery Care				
Newborn Deliveries Scheduled Early[7]	-	-	3%	6%
Preventive Care				
Immunization for Influenza[2]	627	90%	94%	90%
Immunization for Pneumonia[2]	967	92%	95%	92%
Stroke Care				
Anticoagulation Therapy for Atrial Fibrillation[1,2]	-	-	95%	95%
Antithrombotic Therapy Timing[2]	71	100%	98%	98%
Assessed for Rehabilitation[2]	74	99%	97%	97%
Discharged on Antithrombotic Therapy[2]	67	100%	99%	99%
Discharged on Statin Medication[2]	55	95%	94%	94%
Thrombolytic Therapy Timing[1,2]	-	-	58%	66%
Venous Thromboembolism Prophylaxis[2]	80	81%	94%	94%
Written Stroke Educational Materials Given[2]	43	63%	91%	88%
Surgical Care Improvement Project				
Appropriate Beta Blocker Usage[2]	218	97%	98%	98%
Appropriate VTP Within 24 Hours[2]	398	99%	98%	98%
Controlled Postoperative Blood Glucose[2]	182	99%	99%	97%
Perioperative Temperature Management[2]	561	100%	100%	100%
Prophylactic Antibiotic Selection[2]	443	99%	99%	99%
Prophylactic Antibiotic Selection (Outpatient)	513	100%	99%	98%
Prophylactic Antibiotic Stopped[2]	440	97%	98%	98%
Prophylactic Antibiotic Timing[2]	443	100%	99%	99%
Prophylactic Antibiotic Timing (Outpatient)	513	99%	98%	98%
Urinary Catheter Removal[2]	540	99%	97%	97%
Survey of Patients' Hospital Experiences				
Area Around Room 'Always' Quiet at Night	300+	68%	67%	61%
Doctors 'Always' Communicated Well	300+	83%	84%	82%
Home Recovery Information Given	300+	86%	86%	85%
Hospital Given 9 or 10 on 10 Point Scale	300+	78%	72%	71%
Meds 'Always' Explained Before Given	300+	64%	66%	64%
Nurses 'Always' Communicated Well	300+	78%	81%	79%
Pain 'Always' Well Controlled	300+	74%	72%	71%
Room and Bathroom 'Always' Clean	300+	71%	72%	73%
Timely Help 'Always' Received	300+	60%	68%	68%
Would Definitely Recommend Hospital	300+	82%	71%	71%
Use of Medical Imaging				
Cardiac Imaging Stress Test before Surgery	1,658	4.4%	5.1%	5.3%
Combination Abdominal CT Scan	1,302	8.3%	10.1%	10.5%
Combination Brain/Sinus CT Scan	1,392	2.3%	2.5%	2.7%
Combination Chest CT Scan	889	1.2%	1.3%	2.7%
Follow-up Mammogram/Ultrasound[7]	-	-	8%	8.8%
Lumbar Spine MRI for Low Back Pain	80	31.3%	39%	37.2%

Conway Medical Center

300 Singleton Ridge Road
Conway, SC 29526
Phone: 843-347-8037
Fax: 843-347-8056
E-mail: jsnowden@conwaymedicalcenter.com
URL: www.conwayhospital.com
Type: Acute Care Hospitals
Emergency Services: Yes
Ownership: Voluntary non-profit - Private
Beds: 248

Key Personnel:
Radiology. . . . . Michael Brown
Emergency Room . . . . Barbara Bryant, RN
CEO/President. . . . . Philip A Clayton
Quality Assurance . . . . Angela Willisord

Measure	Cases	This Hosp.	State Avg.	U.S. Avg.
Blood Clot Prevention and Treatment				
Anticoagulation Overlap Therapy[2]	24	83%	92%	93%
ICU Venous Thromboembolism Prophylaxis[2]	47	98%	94%	92%
Incidence of Potentially Preventable VTE[1,2]	-	-	8%	10%
UFH with Dosages/Platelet Monitoring[1,2]	-	-	98%	97%
Venous Thromboembolism Prophylaxis[2]	324	89%	88%	85%
Warfarin Therapy Discharge Instructions[2]	19	74%	72%	75%
Chest Pain/Possible Heart Attack Care				
Aspirin Given Within 24 Hours of Arrival	76	100%	97%	96%
Fibrinolytic Meds Within 30 Min. of Arrival[7]	-	-	68%	58%
Average Time to ECG (minutes)	76	1	5	7
Average Time to Transfer (minutes)	19	40	43	60
Children's Asthma Care				
Received Home Management Plan of Care	-	-	-	88%
Received Reliever Medication	-	-	-	100%
Received Systemic Corticosteroids	-	-	-	100%
Emergency Department				
Admittance Decision Time (minutes)[2]	581	96	94	98
Head CT Results Within 45 Min. of Arrival[1]	-	-	61%	57%
Patients Who Left ER Before Being Seen	48,961	1%	3%	2%
Time from ER Arrival to Admit. (minutes)[2]	581	229	274	274
Time from ER Arrival to Discharge (minutes)	381	129	136	134
Time in ER Before Being Evaluated (minutes)	417	24	33	26
Time to Pain Meds for Fractures (minutes)	162	55	61	57
Heart Attack Care				
Aspirin Given at Discharge[2]	20	100%	99%	99%
Fibrinolytic Meds Within 30 Min. of Arrival[2,7]	-	-	50%	54%
PCI Within 90 Minutes of Arrival[2,7]	-	-	97%	96%
Statin Prescribed at Discharge[2]	18	100%	99%	98%
Heart Failure Care				
ACE Inhibitor or ARB for LVSD[2]	71	100%	98%	97%
Discharge Instructions Given[2]	178	87%	94%	94%
Evaluation of LVS Function[2]	206	100%	99%	99%
Medicare Spending				
Medicare Spending per Patient (ratio)	-	0.96	0.98	0.98
Pneumonia Care				
Appropriate Initial Antibiotic Given[2]	141	99%	97%	95%
Blood Culture Timing[2]	245	100%	98%	98%
Pregnancy and Delivery Care				
Newborn Deliveries Scheduled Early[2]	28	7%	3%	6%
Preventive Care				
Immunization for Influenza[2]	528	99%	94%	90%
Immunization for Pneumonia[2]	604	99%	95%	92%
Stroke Care				
Anticoagulation Therapy for Atrial Fibrillation[2]	14	86%	95%	95%
Antithrombotic Therapy Timing[2]	81	100%	98%	98%
Assessed for Rehabilitation[2]	82	95%	97%	97%
Discharged on Antithrombotic Therapy[2]	80	99%	99%	99%
Discharged on Statin Medication[2]	64	86%	94%	94%
Thrombolytic Therapy Timing[1,2]	-	-	58%	66%
Venous Thromboembolism Prophylaxis[2]	84	96%	94%	94%
Written Stroke Educational Materials Given[2]	56	84%	91%	88%
Surgical Care Improvement Project				
Appropriate Beta Blocker Usage[2]	80	98%	98%	98%
Appropriate VTP Within 24 Hours[2]	300	98%	98%	98%
Controlled Postoperative Blood Glucose[2,7]	-	-	99%	97%
Perioperative Temperature Management[2]	397	100%	100%	100%
Prophylactic Antibiotic Selection[2]	274	100%	99%	99%
Prophylactic Antibiotic Selection (Outpatient)	252	98%	99%	98%
Prophylactic Antibiotic Stopped[2]	269	99%	98%	98%
Prophylactic Antibiotic Timing[2]	276	99%	99%	99%
Prophylactic Antibiotic Timing (Outpatient)	252	98%	98%	98%
Urinary Catheter Removal[2]	191	98%	97%	97%
Survey of Patients' Hospital Experiences				
Area Around Room 'Always' Quiet at Night	300+	68%	67%	61%
Doctors 'Always' Communicated Well	300+	81%	84%	82%
Home Recovery Information Given	300+	82%	86%	85%
Hospital Given 9 or 10 on 10 Point Scale	300+	71%	72%	71%
Meds 'Always' Explained Before Given	300+	63%	66%	64%
Nurses 'Always' Communicated Well	300+	80%	81%	79%
Pain 'Always' Well Controlled	300+	68%	72%	71%
Room and Bathroom 'Always' Clean	300+	76%	72%	73%
Timely Help 'Always' Received	300+	65%	68%	68%
Would Definitely Recommend Hospital	300+	71%	71%	71%
Use of Medical Imaging				
Cardiac Imaging Stress Test before Surgery	317	6.3%	5.1%	5.3%
Combination Abdominal CT Scan	881	6.2%	10.1%	10.5%
Combination Brain/Sinus CT Scan	782	0.9%	2.5%	2.7%
Combination Chest CT Scan	556	2.3%	1.3%	2.7%
Follow-up Mammogram/Ultrasound	1,592	5.6%	8%	8.8%
Lumbar Spine MRI for Low Back Pain	104	37.5%	39%	37.2%

Mcleod Medical Center - Darlington

701 Cashua Ferry Road
Darlington, SC 29540
Phone: 843-395-1100
Fax: 843-777-1146
URL: www.mcleodhealth.org/facilities
Type: Acute Care Hospitals
Emergency Services: No
Ownership: Voluntary non-profit - Private
Beds: 49

Key Personnel:
Quality Assurance . . . . Johnna Black
Chief of Medical Staff. . . . . Tom Dickinson, MD
Emergency Room . . . . Richard Rogers
Infection Control. . . . . Nancy Vivian

Measure	Cases	This Hosp.	State Avg.	U.S. Avg.
Blood Clot Prevention and Treatment				
Anticoagulation Overlap Therapy[7]	-	-	92%	93%
ICU Venous Thromboembolism Prophylaxis[7]	-	-	94%	92%
Incidence of Potentially Preventable VTE[7]	-	-	8%	10%
UFH with Dosages/Platelet Monitoring[7]	-	-	98%	97%
Venous Thromboembolism Prophylaxis	91	87%	88%	85%
Warfarin Therapy Discharge Instructions[7]	-	-	72%	75%
Chest Pain/Possible Heart Attack Care				
Aspirin Given Within 24 Hours of Arrival[5]	-	-	97%	96%
Fibrinolytic Meds Within 30 Min. of Arrival[5]	-	-	68%	58%
Average Time to ECG (minutes)[5]	-	-	5	7
Average Time to Transfer (minutes)[5]	-	-	43	60
Children's Asthma Care				
Received Home Management Plan of Care	-	-	-	88%
Received Reliever Medication	-	-	-	100%
Received Systemic Corticosteroids	-	-	-	100%
Emergency Department				
Admittance Decision Time (minutes)[7]	-	-	94	98
Head CT Results Within 45 Min. of Arrival[5]	-	-	61%	57%
Patients Who Left ER Before Being Seen[5]	-	-	3%	2%
Time from ER Arrival to Admit. (minutes)[7]	-	-	274	274
Time from ER Arrival to Discharge (minutes)[5]	-	-	136	134
Time in ER Before Being Evaluated (minutes)[5]	-	-	33	26
Time to Pain Meds for Fractures (minutes)[5]	-	-	61	57
Heart Attack Care				
Aspirin Given at Discharge[3,7]	-	-	99%	99%
Fibrinolytic Meds Within 30 Min. of Arrival[3,7]	-	-	50%	54%
PCI Within 90 Minutes of Arrival[3,7]	-	-	97%	96%
Statin Prescribed at Discharge[3,7]	-	-	99%	98%
Heart Failure Care				
ACE Inhibitor or ARB for LVSD[1,3]	-	-	98%	97%
Discharge Instructions Given[1,3]	-	-	94%	94%
Evaluation of LVS Function[1,3]	-	-	99%	99%
Medicare Spending				
Medicare Spending per Patient (ratio)	-	0.86	0.98	0.98
Pneumonia Care				
Appropriate Initial Antibiotic Given[1]	-	-	97%	95%
Blood Culture Timing[7]	-	-	98%	98%
Pregnancy and Delivery Care				

NOTE: Hospital profiles are in alphabetical order by state, then city, then hospital within the city; Rankings exclude hospitals with less than 25 cases except for patient surveys which excludes hospitals with less than 100 cases; (a) 100-299 cases; (1) The number of cases/patients is too few to report; (2) Data submitted were based on a sample of cases/patients; (3) Results are based on a shorter time period than required; (4) Data suppressed by CMS for one or more quarters; (5) Results are not available for this reporting period; (6) Fewer than 100 patients completed the HCAHPS survey; (7) No cases met the criteria for this measure; (8) The lower limit of the confidence interval cannot be calculated if the number of observed infections equals zero; (9) No data are available from the state/territory for this reporting period; (10) The scores shown reflect fewer than 50 completed surveys; (11) There were discrepancies in the data collection process; (12) This measure does not apply to this hospital for this reporting period; (13) Results cannot be calculated for this reporting period; (14) The results for this state are combined with nearby states to protect confidentiality; Please refer to the User's Guide for a full explanation of data.

Measure	Cases	This Hosp.	State Avg.	U.S. Avg.
Newborn Deliveries Scheduled Early[2,7]	-	-	3%	6%
Preventive Care				
Immunization for Influenza	66	92%	94%	90%
Immunization for Pneumonia[2]	119	98%	95%	92%
Stroke Care				
Anticoagulation Therapy for Atrial Fibrillation[1,3]	-	-	95%	95%
Antithrombotic Therapy Timing[1,3]	-	-	98%	98%
Assessed for Rehabilitation[1,3]	-	-	97%	97%
Discharged on Antithrombotic Therapy[1,3]	-	-	99%	99%
Discharged on Statin Medication[1,3]	-	-	94%	94%
Thrombolytic Therapy Timing[3,7]	-	-	58%	66%
Venous Thromboembolism Prophylaxis[1,3]	-	-	94%	94%
Written Stroke Educational Materials Given[1,3]	-	-	91%	88%
Surgical Care Improvement Project				
Appropriate Beta Blocker Usage[5]	-	-	98%	98%
Appropriate VTP Within 24 Hours[5]	-	-	98%	98%
Controlled Postoperative Blood Glucose[5]	-	-	99%	97%
Perioperative Temperature Management[5]	-	-	100%	100%
Prophylactic Antibiotic Selection[5]	-	-	99%	99%
Prophylactic Antibiotic Selection (Outpatient)	34	100%	99%	98%
Prophylactic Antibiotic Stopped[5]	-	-	98%	98%
Prophylactic Antibiotic Timing[5]	-	-	99%	99%
Prophylactic Antibiotic Timing (Outpatient)	34	100%	98%	98%
Urinary Catheter Removal[5]	-	-	97%	97%
Survey of Patients' Hospital Experiences				
Area Around Room 'Always' Quiet at Night[10]	<100	63%	67%	61%
Doctors 'Always' Communicated Well[10]	<100	96%	84%	82%
Home Recovery Information Given[10]	<100	89%	86%	85%
Hospital Given 9 or 10 on 10 Point Scale[10]	<100	80%	72%	71%
Meds 'Always' Explained Before Given[10]	<100	79%	66%	64%
Nurses 'Always' Communicated Well[10]	<100	86%	81%	79%
Pain 'Always' Well Controlled[10]	<100	73%	72%	71%
Room and Bathroom 'Always' Clean[10]	<100	73%	72%	73%
Timely Help 'Always' Received[10]	<100	77%	68%	68%
Would Definitely Recommend Hospital[10]	<100	82%	71%	71%
Use of Medical Imaging				
Cardiac Imaging Stress Test before Surgery[7]	-	-	5.1%	5.3%
Combination Abdominal CT Scan	71	2.8%	10.1%	10.5%
Combination Brain/Sinus CT Scan[1]	-	-	2.5%	2.7%
Combination Chest CT Scan	47	0.0%	1.3%	2.7%
Follow-up Mammogram/Ultrasound	703	7.1%	8%	8.8%
Lumbar Spine MRI for Low Back Pain[1]	-	-	39%	37.2%

Mcleod Medical Center - Dillon

301 E Jackson St
Dillon, SC 29536
Phone: 843-774-4111
Fax: 843-774-1563
URL: www.mcleodhealth.org/facilities
Type: Acute Care Hospitals
Emergency Services: Yes
Ownership: Voluntary non-profit - Private
Beds: 79

Key Personnel:

Infection Control. . . . . Mary Kay Bagnal
Operating Room. . . . . Walter B Blum
Quality Assurance . . . . Celeste Campbell
Radiology. . . . . Matthew John Cerny, Jr, MD
Emergency Room . . . . Lance Davis, MD
Intensive Care Unit. . . . . James J Kelly, MD
Chief of Medical Staff. . . . . Yvonne Ramirez-Welden, MD
Pediatric In-Patient Care . . . . Feliciano B Yu, MD

Measure	Cases	This Hosp.	State Avg.	U.S. Avg.
Blood Clot Prevention and Treatment				
Anticoagulation Overlap Therapy[1,2]	-	-	92%	93%
ICU Venous Thromboembolism Prophylaxis[2]	73	96%	94%	92%
Incidence of Potentially Preventable VTE[2,7]	-	-	8%	10%
UFH with Dosages/Platelet Monitoring[2,7]	-	-	98%	97%
Venous Thromboembolism Prophylaxis[2]	151	95%	88%	85%
Warfarin Therapy Discharge Instructions[1,2]	-	-	72%	75%
Chest Pain/Possible Heart Attack Care				
Aspirin Given Within 24 Hours of Arrival	94	99%	97%	96%
Fibrinolytic Meds Within 30 Min. of Arrival[1]	-	-	68%	58%
Average Time to ECG (minutes)	93	4	5	7
Average Time to Transfer (minutes)[1]	-	-	43	60
Children's Asthma Care				
Received Home Management Plan of Care	-	-	-	88%
Received Reliever Medication	-	-	-	100%
Received Systemic Corticosteroids	-	-	-	100%
Emergency Department				
Admittance Decision Time (minutes)[2]	258	36	94	98
Head CT Results Within 45 Min. of Arrival	24	67%	61%	57%
Patients Who Left ER Before Being Seen	28,657	2%	3%	2%
Time from ER Arrival to Admit. (minutes)[2]	276	236	274	274
Time from ER Arrival to Discharge (minutes)	307	142	136	134
Time in ER Before Being Evaluated (minutes)	375	43	33	26
Time to Pain Meds for Fractures (minutes)	91	61	61	57
Heart Attack Care				
Aspirin Given at Discharge	25	96%	99%	99%
Fibrinolytic Meds Within 30 Min. of Arrival[7]	-	-	50%	54%
PCI Within 90 Minutes of Arrival[7]	-	-	97%	96%
Statin Prescribed at Discharge	26	92%	99%	98%
Heart Failure Care				
ACE Inhibitor or ARB for LVSD	32	97%	98%	97%
Discharge Instructions Given	96	92%	94%	94%
Evaluation of LVS Function	105	100%	99%	99%
Medicare Spending				
Medicare Spending per Patient (ratio)	-	0.93	0.98	0.98
Pneumonia Care				
Appropriate Initial Antibiotic Given	90	99%	97%	95%
Blood Culture Timing	107	100%	98%	98%
Pregnancy and Delivery Care				
Newborn Deliveries Scheduled Early[2]	41	0%	3%	6%
Preventive Care				
Immunization for Influenza[2]	276	97%	94%	90%
Immunization for Pneumonia[2]	318	99%	95%	92%
Stroke Care				
Anticoagulation Therapy for Atrial Fibrillation[1,2]	-	-	95%	95%
Antithrombotic Therapy Timing[2]	38	100%	98%	98%
Assessed for Rehabilitation[2]	42	93%	97%	97%
Discharged on Antithrombotic Therapy[2]	41	98%	99%	99%
Discharged on Statin Medication[2]	39	95%	94%	94%
Thrombolytic Therapy Timing[1,2]	-	-	58%	66%
Venous Thromboembolism Prophylaxis[2]	35	100%	94%	94%
Written Stroke Educational Materials Given[2]	34	79%	91%	88%
Surgical Care Improvement Project				
Appropriate Beta Blocker Usage	13	92%	98%	98%
Appropriate VTP Within 24 Hours	76	99%	98%	98%
Controlled Postoperative Blood Glucose[7]	-	-	99%	97%
Perioperative Temperature Management	81	100%	100%	100%
Prophylactic Antibiotic Selection	54	98%	99%	99%
Prophylactic Antibiotic Selection (Outpatient)	17	94%	99%	98%
Prophylactic Antibiotic Stopped	49	94%	98%	98%
Prophylactic Antibiotic Timing	54	100%	99%	99%
Prophylactic Antibiotic Timing (Outpatient)	17	88%	98%	98%
Urinary Catheter Removal	58	100%	97%	97%
Survey of Patients' Hospital Experiences				
Area Around Room 'Always' Quiet at Night	300+	72%	67%	61%
Doctors 'Always' Communicated Well	300+	89%	84%	82%
Home Recovery Information Given	300+	87%	86%	85%
Hospital Given 9 or 10 on 10 Point Scale	300+	73%	72%	71%
Meds 'Always' Explained Before Given	300+	72%	66%	64%
Nurses 'Always' Communicated Well	300+	83%	81%	79%
Pain 'Always' Well Controlled	300+	77%	72%	71%
Room and Bathroom 'Always' Clean	300+	78%	72%	73%
Timely Help 'Always' Received	300+	73%	68%	68%
Would Definitely Recommend Hospital	300+	70%	71%	71%
Use of Medical Imaging				
Cardiac Imaging Stress Test before Surgery[1]	-	-	5.1%	5.3%
Combination Abdominal CT Scan	401	3.7%	10.1%	10.5%
Combination Brain/Sinus CT Scan[1]	-	-	2.5%	2.7%
Combination Chest CT Scan	317	0.6%	1.3%	2.7%
Follow-up Mammogram/Ultrasound	309	7.8%	8%	8.8%
Lumbar Spine MRI for Low Back Pain	84	41.7%	39%	37.2%

Baptist Easley Hospital

200 Fleetwood Drive
Easley, SC 29640
Phone: 864-442-7200
Fax: 864-442-7890
URL: www.palmettohealth.org
Type: Acute Care Hospitals
Emergency Services: Yes
Ownership: Voluntary non-profit - Private
Beds: 109

Key Personnel:

Chief of Medical Staff . . . . Collis Barksdale, MD
CEO . . . . Charles D. Beaman, Jr
Radiology. . . . . Matthew D Carson
Infection Control. . . . . Julie Chastain
Emergency Room . . . . Brad Howard, MD
Intensive Care Unit. . . . . Sandy Myers
Quality Assurance . . . . Dale Powell
Operating Room. . . . . Robert Waters, MD

Measure	Cases	This Hosp.	State Avg.	U.S. Avg.
Blood Clot Prevention and Treatment				
Anticoagulation Overlap Therapy[2]	29	97%	92%	93%
ICU Venous Thromboembolism Prophylaxis[2]	105	100%	94%	92%
Incidence of Potentially Preventable VTE[1,2]	-	-	8%	10%
UFH with Dosages/Platelet Monitoring[1,2]	-	-	98%	97%
Venous Thromboembolism Prophylaxis[2]	384	96%	88%	85%
Warfarin Therapy Discharge Instructions[2]	24	92%	72%	75%
Chest Pain/Possible Heart Attack Care				
Aspirin Given Within 24 Hours of Arrival	96	100%	97%	96%
Fibrinolytic Meds Within 30 Min. of Arrival[7]	-	-	68%	58%
Average Time to ECG (minutes)	97	1	5	7
Average Time to Transfer (minutes)	13	19	43	60
Children's Asthma Care				
Received Home Management Plan of Care	-	-	-	88%
Received Reliever Medication	-	-	-	100%
Received Systemic Corticosteroids	-	-	-	100%
Emergency Department				
Admittance Decision Time (minutes)[2]	552	49	94	98
Head CT Results Within 45 Min. of Arrival[1]	-	-	61%	57%
Patients Who Left ER Before Being Seen	45,690	2%	3%	2%
Time from ER Arrival to Admit. (minutes)[2]	618	250	274	274
Time from ER Arrival to Discharge (minutes)	365	133	136	134
Time in ER Before Being Evaluated (minutes)	384	28	33	26
Time to Pain Meds for Fractures (minutes)	128	48	61	57
Heart Attack Care				
Aspirin Given at Discharge	15	100%	99%	99%
Fibrinolytic Meds Within 30 Min. of Arrival[7]	-	-	50%	54%
PCI Within 90 Minutes of Arrival[7]	-	-	97%	96%
Statin Prescribed at Discharge	12	100%	99%	98%
Heart Failure Care				
ACE Inhibitor or ARB for LVSD	42	100%	98%	97%
Discharge Instructions Given	179	98%	94%	94%
Evaluation of LVS Function	215	100%	99%	99%
Medicare Spending				
Medicare Spending per Patient (ratio)	-	0.95	0.98	0.98
Pneumonia Care				
Appropriate Initial Antibiotic Given	149	99%	97%	95%
Blood Culture Timing	248	100%	98%	98%
Pregnancy and Delivery Care				
Newborn Deliveries Scheduled Early	43	5%	3%	6%
Preventive Care				
Immunization for Influenza[2]	406	99%	94%	90%
Immunization for Pneumonia[2]	579	99%	95%	92%
Stroke Care				
Anticoagulation Therapy for Atrial Fibrillation[1]	-	-	95%	95%
Antithrombotic Therapy Timing	29	97%	98%	98%
Assessed for Rehabilitation	29	100%	97%	97%
Discharged on Antithrombotic Therapy	28	100%	99%	99%
Discharged on Statin Medication	17	100%	94%	94%
Thrombolytic Therapy Timing[7]	-	-	58%	66%
Venous Thromboembolism Prophylaxis	30	100%	94%	94%
Written Stroke Educational Materials Given	19	100%	91%	88%
Surgical Care Improvement Project				
Appropriate Beta Blocker Usage	63	100%	98%	98%
Appropriate VTP Within 24 Hours	200	99%	98%	98%
Controlled Postoperative Blood Glucose[7]	-	-	99%	97%
Perioperative Temperature Management	213	100%	100%	100%
Prophylactic Antibiotic Selection	153	99%	99%	99%

NOTE: Hospital profiles are in alphabetical order by state, then city, then hospital within the city; Rankings exclude hospitals with less than 25 cases except for patient surveys which excludes hospitals with less than 100 cases; (a) 100-299 cases; (1) The number of cases/patients is too few to report; (2) Data submitted were based on a sample of cases/patients; (3) Results are based on a shorter time period than required; (4) Data suppressed by CMS for one or more quarters; (5) Results are not available for this reporting period; (6) Fewer than 100 patients completed the HCAHPS survey; (7) No cases met the criteria for this measure; (8) The lower limit of the confidence interval cannot be calculated if the number of observed infections equals zero; (9) No data are available from the state/territory for this reporting period; (10) The scores shown reflect fewer than 50 completed surveys; (11) There were discrepancies in the data collection process; (12) This measure does not apply to this hospital for this reporting period; (13) Results cannot be calculated for this reporting period; (14) The results for this state are combined with nearby states to protect confidentiality; Please refer to the User's Guide for a full explanation of data.

Measure	Cases	This Hosp.	State Avg.	U.S. Avg.
Prophylactic Antibiotic Selection (Outpatient)	91	99%	99%	98%
Prophylactic Antibiotic Stopped	144	99%	98%	98%
Prophylactic Antibiotic Timing	153	99%	99%	99%
Prophylactic Antibiotic Timing (Outpatient)	91	100%	98%	98%
Urinary Catheter Removal	162	99%	97%	97%
Survey of Patients' Hospital Experiences				
Area Around Room 'Always' Quiet at Night	300+	72%	67%	61%
Doctors 'Always' Communicated Well	300+	85%	84%	82%
Home Recovery Information Given	300+	90%	86%	85%
Hospital Given 9 or 10 on 10 Point Scale	300+	78%	72%	71%
Meds 'Always' Explained Before Given	300+	71%	66%	64%
Nurses 'Always' Communicated Well	300+	84%	81%	79%
Pain 'Always' Well Controlled	300+	76%	72%	71%
Room and Bathroom 'Always' Clean	300+	81%	72%	73%
Timely Help 'Always' Received	300+	65%	68%	68%
Would Definitely Recommend Hospital	300+	77%	71%	71%
Use of Medical Imaging				
Cardiac Imaging Stress Test before Surgery	132	3.8%	5.1%	5.3%
Combination Abdominal CT Scan	436	5.0%	10.1%	10.5%
Combination Brain/Sinus CT Scan	592	0.2%	2.5%	2.7%
Combination Chest CT Scan	321	0.0%	1.3%	2.7%
Follow-up Mammogram/Ultrasound	1,420	11.2%	8%	8.8%
Lumbar Spine MRI for Low Back Pain	113	42.5%	39%	37.2%

Edgefield County Hospital

300 Ridge Medical Plaza — Phone: 803-637-1193
Edgefield, SC 29824 — Fax: 803-637-3174
E-mail: leslie.seigler@edgefieldcohospital.org
URL: www.edgefieldcohospital.org
Type: Critical Access Hospitals — Emergency Services: Yes
Ownership: Government - Local — Beds: 20

Key Personnel:
Emergency Room . . . . Paul Espinoza
CEO/President. . . . . Ray J Price
Chief of Medical Staff . . . . George Rainsord

Measure	Cases	This Hosp.	State Avg.	U.S. Avg.
Blood Clot Prevention and Treatment				
Anticoagulation Overlap Therapy[5]	-	-	92%	93%
ICU Venous Thromboembolism Prophylaxis[5]	-	-	94%	92%
Incidence of Potentially Preventable VTE[5]	-	-	8%	10%
UFH with Dosages/Platelet Monitoring[5]	-	-	98%	97%
Venous Thromboembolism Prophylaxis[5]	-	-	88%	85%
Warfarin Therapy Discharge Instructions[5]	-	-	72%	75%
Chest Pain/Possible Heart Attack Care				
Aspirin Given Within 24 Hours of Arrival	-	-	97%	96%
Fibrinolytic Meds Within 30 Min. of Arrival	-	-	68%	58%
Average Time to ECG (minutes)	-	-	5	7
Average Time to Transfer (minutes)	-	-	43	60
Children's Asthma Care				
Received Home Management Plan of Care	-	-	-	88%
Received Reliever Medication	-	-	-	100%
Received Systemic Corticosteroids	-	-	-	100%
Emergency Department				
Admittance Decision Time (minutes)[5]	-	-	94	98
Head CT Results Within 45 Min. of Arrival	-	-	61%	57%
Patients Who Left ER Before Being Seen	-	-	3%	2%
Time from ER Arrival to Admit. (minutes)[5]	-	-	274	274
Time from ER Arrival to Discharge (minutes)	-	-	136	134
Time in ER Before Being Evaluated (minutes)	-	-	33	26
Time to Pain Meds for Fractures (minutes)	-	-	61	57
Heart Attack Care				
Aspirin Given at Discharge[5]	-	-	99%	99%
Fibrinolytic Meds Within 30 Min. of Arrival[5]	-	-	50%	54%
PCI Within 90 Minutes of Arrival[5]	-	-	97%	96%
Statin Prescribed at Discharge[5]	-	-	99%	98%
Heart Failure Care				
ACE Inhibitor or ARB for LVSD[1,3]	-	-	98%	97%
Discharge Instructions Given[1,3]	-	-	94%	94%
Evaluation of LVS Function[3]	11	73%	99%	99%
Medicare Spending				
Medicare Spending per Patient (ratio)	-	-	0.98	0.98
Pneumonia Care				
Appropriate Initial Antibiotic Given[1,3]	-	-	97%	95%
Blood Culture Timing[3,7]	-	-	98%	98%
Pregnancy and Delivery Care				
Newborn Deliveries Scheduled Early[5]	-	-	3%	6%
Preventive Care				
Immunization for Influenza[5]	-	-	94%	90%
Immunization for Pneumonia[5]	-	-	95%	92%
Stroke Care				
Anticoagulation Therapy for Atrial Fibrillation[5]	-	-	95%	95%
Antithrombotic Therapy Timing[5]	-	-	98%	98%
Assessed for Rehabilitation[5]	-	-	97%	97%
Discharged on Antithrombotic Therapy[5]	-	-	99%	99%
Discharged on Statin Medication[5]	-	-	94%	94%
Thrombolytic Therapy Timing[5]	-	-	58%	66%
Venous Thromboembolism Prophylaxis[5]	-	-	94%	94%
Written Stroke Educational Materials Given[5]	-	-	91%	88%
Surgical Care Improvement Project				
Appropriate Beta Blocker Usage[5]	-	-	98%	98%
Appropriate VTP Within 24 Hours[5]	-	-	98%	98%
Controlled Postoperative Blood Glucose[5]	-	-	99%	97%
Perioperative Temperature Management[5]	-	-	100%	100%
Prophylactic Antibiotic Selection[5]	-	-	99%	99%
Prophylactic Antibiotic Selection (Outpatient)	-	-	99%	98%
Prophylactic Antibiotic Stopped[5]	-	-	98%	98%
Prophylactic Antibiotic Timing[5]	-	-	99%	99%
Prophylactic Antibiotic Timing (Outpatient)	-	-	98%	98%
Urinary Catheter Removal[5]	-	-	97%	97%
Survey of Patients' Hospital Experiences				
Area Around Room 'Always' Quiet at Night[5]	-	-	67%	61%
Doctors 'Always' Communicated Well[5]	-	-	84%	82%
Home Recovery Information Given[5]	-	-	86%	85%
Hospital Given 9 or 10 on 10 Point Scale[5]	-	-	72%	71%
Meds 'Always' Explained Before Given[5]	-	-	66%	64%
Nurses 'Always' Communicated Well[5]	-	-	81%	79%
Pain 'Always' Well Controlled[5]	-	-	72%	71%
Room and Bathroom 'Always' Clean[5]	-	-	72%	73%
Timely Help 'Always' Received[5]	-	-	68%	68%
Would Definitely Recommend Hospital[5]	-	-	71%	71%
Use of Medical Imaging				
Cardiac Imaging Stress Test before Surgery	-	-	5.1%	5.3%
Combination Abdominal CT Scan	-	-	10.1%	10.5%
Combination Brain/Sinus CT Scan	-	-	2.5%	2.7%
Combination Chest CT Scan	-	-	1.3%	2.7%
Follow-up Mammogram/Ultrasound	-	-	8%	8.8%
Lumbar Spine MRI for Low Back Pain	-	-	39%	37.2%

Allendale County Hospital

1787 Allendale Fairfax Rd — Phone: 803-632-3311
Fairfax, SC 29827
Type: Critical Access Hospitals — Emergency Services: Yes
Ownership: Government - Local

Measure	Cases	This Hosp.	State Avg.	U.S. Avg.
Blood Clot Prevention and Treatment				
Anticoagulation Overlap Therapy[5]	-	-	92%	93%
ICU Venous Thromboembolism Prophylaxis[5]	-	-	94%	92%
Incidence of Potentially Preventable VTE[5]	-	-	8%	10%
UFH with Dosages/Platelet Monitoring[5]	-	-	98%	97%
Venous Thromboembolism Prophylaxis[5]	-	-	88%	85%
Warfarin Therapy Discharge Instructions[5]	-	-	72%	75%
Chest Pain/Possible Heart Attack Care				
Aspirin Given Within 24 Hours of Arrival	-	-	97%	96%
Fibrinolytic Meds Within 30 Min. of Arrival	-	-	68%	58%
Average Time to ECG (minutes)	-	-	5	7
Average Time to Transfer (minutes)	-	-	43	60
Children's Asthma Care				
Received Home Management Plan of Care	-	-	-	88%
Received Reliever Medication	-	-	-	100%
Received Systemic Corticosteroids	-	-	-	100%
Emergency Department				
Admittance Decision Time (minutes)[5]	-	-	94	98
Head CT Results Within 45 Min. of Arrival	-	-	61%	57%
Patients Who Left ER Before Being Seen	-	-	3%	2%
Time from ER Arrival to Admit. (minutes)[5]	-	-	274	274
Time from ER Arrival to Discharge (minutes)	-	-	136	134
Time in ER Before Being Evaluated (minutes)	-	-	33	26
Time to Pain Meds for Fractures (minutes)	-	-	61	57
Heart Attack Care				
Aspirin Given at Discharge[5]	-	-	99%	99%
Fibrinolytic Meds Within 30 Min. of Arrival[5]	-	-	50%	54%
PCI Within 90 Minutes of Arrival[5]	-	-	97%	96%
Statin Prescribed at Discharge[5]	-	-	99%	98%
Heart Failure Care				
ACE Inhibitor or ARB for LVSD[5]	-	-	98%	97%
Discharge Instructions Given[5]	-	-	94%	94%
Evaluation of LVS Function[5]	-	-	99%	99%
Medicare Spending				
Medicare Spending per Patient (ratio)	-	-	0.98	0.98
Pneumonia Care				
Appropriate Initial Antibiotic Given[2]	21	90%	97%	95%
Blood Culture Timing[2]	27	93%	98%	98%
Pregnancy and Delivery Care				
Newborn Deliveries Scheduled Early[5]	-	-	3%	6%
Preventive Care				
Immunization for Influenza[5]	-	-	94%	90%
Immunization for Pneumonia[5]	-	-	95%	92%
Stroke Care				
Anticoagulation Therapy for Atrial Fibrillation[5]	-	-	95%	95%
Antithrombotic Therapy Timing[5]	-	-	98%	98%
Assessed for Rehabilitation[5]	-	-	97%	97%
Discharged on Antithrombotic Therapy[5]	-	-	99%	99%
Discharged on Statin Medication[5]	-	-	94%	94%
Thrombolytic Therapy Timing[5]	-	-	58%	66%
Venous Thromboembolism Prophylaxis[5]	-	-	94%	94%
Written Stroke Educational Materials Given[5]	-	-	91%	88%
Surgical Care Improvement Project				
Appropriate Beta Blocker Usage[5]	-	-	98%	98%
Appropriate VTP Within 24 Hours[5]	-	-	98%	98%
Controlled Postoperative Blood Glucose[5]	-	-	99%	97%
Perioperative Temperature Management[5]	-	-	100%	100%
Prophylactic Antibiotic Selection[5]	-	-	99%	99%
Prophylactic Antibiotic Selection (Outpatient)	-	-	99%	98%
Prophylactic Antibiotic Stopped[5]	-	-	98%	98%
Prophylactic Antibiotic Timing[5]	-	-	99%	99%
Prophylactic Antibiotic Timing (Outpatient)	-	-	98%	98%
Urinary Catheter Removal[5]	-	-	97%	97%
Survey of Patients' Hospital Experiences				
Area Around Room 'Always' Quiet at Night[5]	-	-	67%	61%
Doctors 'Always' Communicated Well[5]	-	-	84%	82%
Home Recovery Information Given[5]	-	-	86%	85%
Hospital Given 9 or 10 on 10 Point Scale[5]	-	-	72%	71%
Meds 'Always' Explained Before Given[5]	-	-	66%	64%
Nurses 'Always' Communicated Well[5]	-	-	81%	79%
Pain 'Always' Well Controlled[5]	-	-	72%	71%
Room and Bathroom 'Always' Clean[5]	-	-	72%	73%
Timely Help 'Always' Received[5]	-	-	68%	68%
Would Definitely Recommend Hospital[5]	-	-	71%	71%
Use of Medical Imaging				
Cardiac Imaging Stress Test before Surgery	-	-	5.1%	5.3%
Combination Abdominal CT Scan	-	-	10.1%	10.5%
Combination Brain/Sinus CT Scan	-	-	2.5%	2.7%
Combination Chest CT Scan	-	-	1.3%	2.7%
Follow-up Mammogram/Ultrasound	-	-	8%	8.8%
Lumbar Spine MRI for Low Back Pain	-	-	39%	37.2%

Carolinas Hospital System

805 Pamplico Hwy Box 100550 — Phone: 843-674-2500
Florence, SC 29505 — Fax: 843-674-2647
E-mail: info@carolinashospital.com
URL: www.carolinashospital.com
Type: Acute Care Hospitals — Emergency Services: Yes
Ownership: Voluntary non-profit - Other — Beds: 420

Key Personnel:
Infection Control. . . . . Sue Ann Avin, RN
Emergency Room . . . . William Cauthen, MD
Pediatric Ambulatory Care . . . . . . Thomas Cox Jr, MD
Cardiac Laboratory. . . . . Rilla Hemmingsen, RN
Radiology. . . . . Carey Hindman
CEO/President. . . . . James O'Loughlin

NOTE: Hospital profiles are in alphabetical order by state, then city, then hospital within the city; Rankings exclude hospitals with less than 25 cases except for patient surveys which excludes hospitals with less than 100 cases; (a) 100-299 cases; (1) The number of cases/patients is too few to report; (2) Data submitted were based on a sample of cases/patients; (3) Results are based on a shorter time period than required; (4) Data suppressed by CMS for one or more quarters; (5) Results are not available for this reporting period; (6) Fewer than 100 patients completed the HCAHPS survey; (7) No cases met the criteria for this measure; (8) The lower limit of the confidence interval cannot be calculated if the number of observed infections equals zero; (9) No data are available from the state/territory for this reporting period; (10) The scores shown reflect fewer than 50 completed surveys; (11) There were discrepancies in the data collection process; (12) This measure does not apply to this hospital for this reporting period; (13) Results cannot be calculated for this reporting period; (14) The results for this state are combined with nearby states to protect confidentiality; Please refer to the User's Guide for a full explanation of data.

Chief of Medical Staff.......... Kevin W Shea, MD
Intensive Care Unit............ Beverly Shields, RN

Measure	Cases	This Hosp.	State Avg.	U.S. Avg.
Blood Clot Prevention and Treatment				
Anticoagulation Overlap Therapy[2]	79	92%	92%	93%
ICU Venous Thromboembolism Prophylaxis[2]	130	95%	94%	92%
Incidence of Potentially Preventable VTE[2]	19	11%	8%	10%
UFH with Dosages/Platelet Monitoring[2]	19	100%	98%	97%
Venous Thromboembolism Prophylaxis[2]	484	87%	88%	85%
Warfarin Therapy Discharge Instructions[2]	53	96%	72%	75%
Chest Pain/Possible Heart Attack Care				
Aspirin Given Within 24 Hours of Arrival[1,3]	-	-	97%	96%
Fibrinolytic Meds Within 30 Min. of Arrival[5]	-	-	68%	58%
Average Time to ECG (minutes)[1,3]	-	-	5	7
Average Time to Transfer (minutes)[5]	-	-	43	60
Children's Asthma Care				
Received Home Management Plan of Care	-	-	-	88%
Received Reliever Medication	-	-	-	100%
Received Systemic Corticosteroids	-	-	-	100%
Emergency Department				
Admittance Decision Time (minutes)[2]	592	112	94	98
Head CT Results Within 45 Min. of Arrival[3,7]	-	-	61%	57%
Patients Who Left ER Before Being Seen	39,471	2%	3%	2%
Time from ER Arrival to Admit. (minutes)[2]	611	286	274	274
Time from ER Arrival to Discharge (minutes)	371	135	136	134
Time in ER Before Being Evaluated (minutes)	402	37	33	26
Time to Pain Meds for Fractures (minutes)	73	50	61	57
Heart Attack Care				
Aspirin Given at Discharge	220	100%	99%	99%
Fibrinolytic Meds Within 30 Min. of Arrival[7]	-	-	50%	54%
PCI Within 90 Minutes of Arrival[1]	-	-	97%	96%
Statin Prescribed at Discharge	219	100%	99%	98%
Heart Failure Care				
ACE Inhibitor or ARB for LVSD	154	100%	98%	97%
Discharge Instructions Given	431	92%	94%	94%
Evaluation of LVS Function	502	100%	99%	99%
Medicare Spending				
Medicare Spending per Patient (ratio)	-	0.99	0.98	0.98
Pneumonia Care				
Appropriate Initial Antibiotic Given	135	100%	97%	95%
Blood Culture Timing	205	100%	98%	98%
Pregnancy and Delivery Care				
Newborn Deliveries Scheduled Early[2]	19	0%	3%	6%
Preventive Care				
Immunization for Influenza[2]	629	96%	94%	90%
Immunization for Pneumonia[2]	909	97%	95%	92%
Stroke Care				
Anticoagulation Therapy for Atrial Fibrillation	11	100%	95%	95%
Antithrombotic Therapy Timing	134	93%	98%	98%
Assessed for Rehabilitation	150	98%	97%	97%
Discharged on Antithrombotic Therapy	122	99%	99%	99%
Discharged on Statin Medication	107	97%	94%	94%
Thrombolytic Therapy Timing[1]	-	-	58%	66%
Venous Thromboembolism Prophylaxis	165	94%	94%	94%
Written Stroke Educational Materials Given	95	85%	91%	88%
Surgical Care Improvement Project				
Appropriate Beta Blocker Usage	234	99%	98%	98%
Appropriate VTP Within 24 Hours	509	99%	98%	98%
Controlled Postoperative Blood Glucose	102	97%	99%	97%
Perioperative Temperature Management	594	99%	100%	100%
Prophylactic Antibiotic Selection	387	100%	99%	99%
Prophylactic Antibiotic Selection (Outpatient)	277	99%	99%	98%
Prophylactic Antibiotic Stopped	365	99%	98%	98%
Prophylactic Antibiotic Timing	387	100%	99%	99%
Prophylactic Antibiotic Timing (Outpatient)	277	98%	98%	98%
Urinary Catheter Removal	307	99%	97%	97%
Survey of Patients' Hospital Experiences				
Area Around Room 'Always' Quiet at Night	300+	71%	67%	61%
Doctors 'Always' Communicated Well	300+	83%	84%	82%
Home Recovery Information Given	300+	85%	86%	85%
Hospital Given 9 or 10 on 10 Point Scale	300+	75%	72%	71%
Meds 'Always' Explained Before Given	300+	66%	66%	64%
Nurses 'Always' Communicated Well	300+	78%	81%	79%
Pain 'Always' Well Controlled	300+	72%	72%	71%
Room and Bathroom 'Always' Clean	300+	70%	72%	73%
Timely Help 'Always' Received	300+	65%	68%	68%
Would Definitely Recommend Hospital	300+	76%	71%	71%
Use of Medical Imaging				
Cardiac Imaging Stress Test before Surgery	299	4.7%	5.1%	5.3%
Combination Abdominal CT Scan	945	9.7%	10.1%	10.5%
Combination Brain/Sinus CT Scan	773	4.7%	2.5%	2.7%
Combination Chest CT Scan	832	2.6%	1.3%	2.7%
Follow-up Mammogram/Ultrasound	1,386	9.7%	8%	8.8%
Lumbar Spine MRI for Low Back Pain	89	51.7%	39%	37.2%

Mcleod Regional Medical Center - Pee Dee

555 E Cheves Saint Box 8700
Florence, SC 29506
Phone: 843-777-2900
Fax: 843-777-2810
URL: www.mcleodhealth.org
Type: Acute Care Hospitals
Emergency Services: Yes
Ownership: Voluntary non-profit - Private
Beds: 371

Key Personnel:
Operating Room.............. Judy D Brown, RN
Pediatric Ambulatory Care ...... Michael Collins, MD
Pediatric In-Patient Care .... Michael Collins, MD
CEO/President............... Robert Colones
Quality Assurance .... Carole Davis, RN
Chief of Medical Staff.......... Richard Ervin, MD
Radiology.................... Raymond L Thomas
Infection Control.............. Vicky Zelenka, RN

Measure	Cases	This Hosp.	State Avg.	U.S. Avg.
Blood Clot Prevention and Treatment				
Anticoagulation Overlap Therapy[2]	103	95%	92%	93%
ICU Venous Thromboembolism Prophylaxis[2]	127	99%	94%	92%
Incidence of Potentially Preventable VTE[2]	31	3%	8%	10%
UFH with Dosages/Platelet Monitoring[2]	47	100%	98%	97%
Venous Thromboembolism Prophylaxis[2]	291	98%	88%	85%
Warfarin Therapy Discharge Instructions[2]	65	85%	72%	75%
Chest Pain/Possible Heart Attack Care				
Aspirin Given Within 24 Hours of Arrival[1,3]	-	-	97%	96%
Fibrinolytic Meds Within 30 Min. of Arrival[5]	-	-	68%	58%
Average Time to ECG (minutes)[1,3]	-	-	5	7
Average Time to Transfer (minutes)[5]	-	-	43	60
Children's Asthma Care				
Received Home Management Plan of Care	-	-	-	88%
Received Reliever Medication	-	-	-	100%
Received Systemic Corticosteroids	-	-	-	100%
Emergency Department				
Admittance Decision Time (minutes)[2]	526	162	94	98
Head CT Results Within 45 Min. of Arrival	13	85%	61%	57%
Patients Who Left ER Before Being Seen	61,428	5%	3%	2%
Time from ER Arrival to Admit. (minutes)[2]	535	376	274	274
Time from ER Arrival to Discharge (minutes)	328	192	136	134
Time in ER Before Being Evaluated (minutes)	367	76	33	26
Time to Pain Meds for Fractures (minutes)	147	81	61	57
Heart Attack Care				
Aspirin Given at Discharge	615	100%	99%	99%
Fibrinolytic Meds Within 30 Min. of Arrival[7]	-	-	50%	54%
PCI Within 90 Minutes of Arrival	45	93%	97%	96%
Statin Prescribed at Discharge	576	99%	99%	98%
Heart Failure Care				
ACE Inhibitor or ARB for LVSD	283	99%	98%	97%
Discharge Instructions Given	616	98%	94%	94%
Evaluation of LVS Function	723	100%	99%	99%
Medicare Spending				
Medicare Spending per Patient (ratio)	-	0.96	0.98	0.98
Pneumonia Care				
Appropriate Initial Antibiotic Given	218	95%	97%	95%
Blood Culture Timing	414	99%	98%	98%
Pregnancy and Delivery Care				
Newborn Deliveries Scheduled Early[2]	20	0%	3%	6%
Preventive Care				
Immunization for Influenza[2]	543	99%	94%	90%
Immunization for Pneumonia[2]	653	99%	95%	92%
Stroke Care				
Anticoagulation Therapy for Atrial Fibrillation[1,2]	-	-	95%	95%
Antithrombotic Therapy Timing[2]	77	96%	98%	98%
Assessed for Rehabilitation[2]	90	92%	97%	97%
Discharged on Antithrombotic Therapy[2]	78	99%	99%	99%
Discharged on Statin Medication[2]	62	94%	94%	94%
Thrombolytic Therapy Timing[1,2]	-	-	58%	66%
Venous Thromboembolism Prophylaxis[2]	99	99%	94%	94%
Written Stroke Educational Materials Given[2]	55	87%	91%	88%
Surgical Care Improvement Project				
Appropriate Beta Blocker Usage[2]	206	99%	98%	98%
Appropriate VTP Within 24 Hours[2]	296	99%	98%	98%
Controlled Postoperative Blood Glucose[2]	97	99%	99%	97%
Perioperative Temperature Management[2]	423	100%	100%	100%
Prophylactic Antibiotic Selection[2]	370	99%	99%	99%
Prophylactic Antibiotic Selection (Outpatient)	565	96%	99%	98%
Prophylactic Antibiotic Stopped[2]	356	98%	98%	98%
Prophylactic Antibiotic Timing[2]	379	100%	99%	99%
Prophylactic Antibiotic Timing (Outpatient)	566	99%	98%	98%
Urinary Catheter Removal[2]	264	99%	97%	97%
Survey of Patients' Hospital Experiences				
Area Around Room 'Always' Quiet at Night	300+	67%	67%	61%
Doctors 'Always' Communicated Well	300+	84%	84%	82%
Home Recovery Information Given	300+	87%	86%	85%
Hospital Given 9 or 10 on 10 Point Scale	300+	81%	72%	71%
Meds 'Always' Explained Before Given	300+	69%	66%	64%
Nurses 'Always' Communicated Well	300+	82%	81%	79%
Pain 'Always' Well Controlled	300+	74%	72%	71%
Room and Bathroom 'Always' Clean	300+	72%	72%	73%
Timely Help 'Always' Received	300+	72%	68%	68%
Would Definitely Recommend Hospital	300+	84%	71%	71%
Use of Medical Imaging				
Cardiac Imaging Stress Test before Surgery	594	6.6%	5.1%	5.3%
Combination Abdominal CT Scan	2,066	3.9%	10.1%	10.5%
Combination Brain/Sinus CT Scan	1,506	3.7%	2.5%	2.7%
Combination Chest CT Scan	1,669	0.5%	1.3%	2.7%
Follow-up Mammogram/Ultrasound	3,733	6.8%	8%	8.8%
Lumbar Spine MRI for Low Back Pain	293	47.4%	39%	37.2%

Novant Health Gaffney Medical Center

1530 N Limestone St
Gaffney, SC 29340
Phone: 864-487-4271
Fax: 864-489-0585
Type: Acute Care Hospitals
Emergency Services: Yes
Ownership: Proprietary
Beds: 125

Key Personnel:
Infection Control.............. Sherri Almond
Radiology.................... Kay Brown
Operating Room.............. Todd Hamrick
CEO/President............... Jo Howell
Quality Assurance .... Alice Jackson
Emergency Room .... Dan Kams, MD
Chief of Medical Staff.......... Donald McIntosh, MD
Intensive Care Unit............ Gerry Wicklund

Measure	Cases	This Hosp.	State Avg.	U.S. Avg.
Blood Clot Prevention and Treatment				
Anticoagulation Overlap Therapy[2]	22	100%	92%	93%
ICU Venous Thromboembolism Prophylaxis[2]	100	96%	94%	92%
Incidence of Potentially Preventable VTE[1,2]	-	-	8%	10%
UFH with Dosages/Platelet Monitoring[2]	15	100%	98%	97%
Venous Thromboembolism Prophylaxis[2]	179	94%	88%	85%
Warfarin Therapy Discharge Instructions[2]	20	85%	72%	75%
Chest Pain/Possible Heart Attack Care				
Aspirin Given Within 24 Hours of Arrival	61	97%	97%	96%
Fibrinolytic Meds Within 30 Min. of Arrival[7]	-	-	68%	58%
Average Time to ECG (minutes)	68	2	5	7
Average Time to Transfer (minutes)	27	44	43	60
Children's Asthma Care				
Received Home Management Plan of Care	17	88%	-	88%
Received Reliever Medication	18	100%	-	100%
Received Systemic Corticosteroids	16	100%	-	100%
Emergency Department				
Admittance Decision Time (minutes)[2]	481	100	94	98
Head CT Results Within 45 Min. of Arrival[1]	-	-	61%	57%
Patients Who Left ER Before Being Seen	36,468	2%	3%	2%
Time from ER Arrival to Admit. (minutes)[2]	481	300	274	274
Time from ER Arrival to Discharge (minutes)	456	113	136	134

NOTE: Hospital profiles are in alphabetical order by state, then city, then hospital within the city; Rankings exclude hospitals with less than 25 cases except for patient surveys which excludes hospitals with less than 100 cases; (a) 100-299 cases; (1) The number of cases/patients is too few to report; (2) Data submitted were based on a sample of cases/patients; (3) Results are based on a shorter time period than required; (4) Data suppressed by CMS for one or more quarters; (5) Results are not available for this reporting period; (6) Fewer than 100 patients completed the HCAHPS survey; (7) No cases met the criteria for this measure; (8) The lower limit of the confidence interval cannot be calculated if the number of observed infections equals zero; (9) No data are available from the state/territory for this reporting period; (10) The scores shown reflect fewer than 50 completed surveys; (11) There were discrepancies in the data collection process; (12) This measure does not apply to this hospital for this reporting period; (13) Results cannot be calculated for this reporting period; (14) The results for this state are combined with nearby states to protect confidentiality; Please refer to the User's Guide for a full explanation of data.

Measure	Cases	This Hosp.	State Avg.	U.S. Avg.
Time in ER Before Being Evaluated (minutes)	473	23	33	26
Time to Pain Meds for Fractures (minutes)	91	59	61	57
Heart Attack Care				
Aspirin Given at Discharge[1]	-	-	99%	99%
Fibrinolytic Meds Within 30 Min. of Arrival[7]	-	-	50%	54%
PCI Within 90 Minutes of Arrival[7]	-	-	97%	96%
Statin Prescribed at Discharge[1]	-	-	99%	98%
Heart Failure Care				
ACE Inhibitor or ARB for LVSD	29	100%	98%	97%
Discharge Instructions Given	92	95%	94%	94%
Evaluation of LVS Function	116	100%	99%	99%
Medicare Spending				
Medicare Spending per Patient (ratio)	-	0.91	0.98	0.98
Pneumonia Care				
Appropriate Initial Antibiotic Given	64	97%	97%	95%
Blood Culture Timing	109	99%	98%	98%
Pregnancy and Delivery Care				
Newborn Deliveries Scheduled Early[2]	37	0%	3%	6%
Preventive Care				
Immunization for Influenza[2]	309	94%	94%	90%
Immunization for Pneumonia[2]	383	99%	95%	92%
Stroke Care				
Anticoagulation Therapy for Atrial Fibrillation[1]	-	-	95%	95%
Antithrombotic Therapy Timing	16	100%	98%	98%
Assessed for Rehabilitation	19	95%	97%	97%
Discharged on Antithrombotic Therapy	17	100%	99%	99%
Discharged on Statin Medication	14	86%	94%	94%
Thrombolytic Therapy Timing[1]	-	-	58%	66%
Venous Thromboembolism Prophylaxis	18	100%	94%	94%
Written Stroke Educational Materials Given	13	69%	91%	88%
Surgical Care Improvement Project				
Appropriate Beta Blocker Usage	20	90%	98%	98%
Appropriate VTP Within 24 Hours	65	100%	98%	98%
Controlled Postoperative Blood Glucose[7]	-	-	99%	97%
Perioperative Temperature Management	76	99%	100%	100%
Prophylactic Antibiotic Selection	50	98%	99%	99%
Prophylactic Antibiotic Selection (Outpatient)[1,3]	-	-	99%	98%
Prophylactic Antibiotic Stopped	47	98%	98%	98%
Prophylactic Antibiotic Timing	50	100%	99%	99%
Prophylactic Antibiotic Timing (Outpatient)[1,3]	-	-	98%	98%
Urinary Catheter Removal	18	83%	97%	97%
Survey of Patients' Hospital Experiences				
Area Around Room 'Always' Quiet at Night	(a)	60%	67%	61%
Doctors 'Always' Communicated Well	(a)	76%	84%	82%
Home Recovery Information Given	(a)	84%	86%	85%
Hospital Given 9 or 10 on 10 Point Scale	(a)	55%	72%	71%
Meds 'Always' Explained Before Given	(a)	55%	66%	64%
Nurses 'Always' Communicated Well	(a)	70%	81%	79%
Pain 'Always' Well Controlled	(a)	62%	72%	71%
Room and Bathroom 'Always' Clean	(a)	68%	72%	73%
Timely Help 'Always' Received	(a)	54%	68%	68%
Would Definitely Recommend Hospital	(a)	50%	71%	71%
Use of Medical Imaging				
Cardiac Imaging Stress Test before Surgery	130	10.8%	5.1%	5.3%
Combination Abdominal CT Scan	281	1.1%	10.1%	10.5%
Combination Brain/Sinus CT Scan	472	4.4%	2.5%	2.7%
Combination Chest CT Scan	156	0.6%	1.3%	2.7%
Follow-up Mammogram/Ultrasound	687	11.1%	8%	8.8%
Lumbar Spine MRI for Low Back Pain[1]	-	-	39%	37.2%

Georgetown Memorial Hospital

606 Black River Rd Drawer 1718
Georgetown, SC 29440
Phone: 843-527-7000
Fax: 843-520-7887
E-mail: georgettem@gmhsc.com
URL: www.gmhsc.com
Type: Acute Care Hospitals
Emergency Services: Yes
Ownership: Voluntary non-profit - Private
Beds: 131

Key Personnel:

Radiology. . . . . David R Anderson, MD
CEO/President. . . . . Bruce P Bailey
Quality Assurance . . . . Bruce P Bailey
Infection Control. . . . . Erma Miller, RN
Operating Room. . . . . Dianne Rainwater
Chairman/CEO . . . . H. McRoy Skipper, MD
Chief of Medical Staff. . . . . Mark E Triana, DO

Measure	Cases	This Hosp.	State Avg.	U.S. Avg.
Blood Clot Prevention and Treatment				
Anticoagulation Overlap Therapy[2]	14	93%	92%	93%
ICU Venous Thromboembolism Prophylaxis[2]	49	94%	94%	92%
Incidence of Potentially Preventable VTE[1,2]	-	-	8%	10%
UFH with Dosages/Platelet Monitoring[1,2]	-	-	98%	97%
Venous Thromboembolism Prophylaxis[2]	352	88%	88%	85%
Warfarin Therapy Discharge Instructions[1,2]	-	-	72%	75%
Chest Pain/Possible Heart Attack Care				
Aspirin Given Within 24 Hours of Arrival[1]	-	-	97%	96%
Fibrinolytic Meds Within 30 Min. of Arrival[3,7]	-	-	68%	58%
Average Time to ECG (minutes)[1]	-	-	5	7
Average Time to Transfer (minutes)[3,7]	-	-	43	60
Children's Asthma Care				
Received Home Management Plan of Care	-	-	-	88%
Received Reliever Medication	-	-	-	100%
Received Systemic Corticosteroids	-	-	-	100%
Emergency Department				
Admittance Decision Time (minutes)[2]	641	85	94	98
Head CT Results Within 45 Min. of Arrival	14	93%	61%	57%
Patients Who Left ER Before Being Seen	30,890	4%	3%	2%
Time from ER Arrival to Admit. (minutes)[2]	657	258	274	274
Time from ER Arrival to Discharge (minutes)	383	155	136	134
Time in ER Before Being Evaluated (minutes)	349	36	33	26
Time to Pain Meds for Fractures (minutes)	47	77	61	57
Heart Attack Care				
Aspirin Given at Discharge[2]	86	100%	99%	99%
Fibrinolytic Meds Within 30 Min. of Arrival[2,7]	-	-	50%	54%
PCI Within 90 Minutes of Arrival[2]	17	94%	97%	96%
Statin Prescribed at Discharge[2]	82	100%	99%	98%
Heart Failure Care				
ACE Inhibitor or ARB for LVSD[2]	67	100%	98%	97%
Discharge Instructions Given[2]	133	87%	94%	94%
Evaluation of LVS Function[2]	157	100%	99%	99%
Medicare Spending				
Medicare Spending per Patient (ratio)	-	0.96	0.98	0.98
Pneumonia Care				
Appropriate Initial Antibiotic Given[2]	68	100%	97%	95%
Blood Culture Timing[2]	140	100%	98%	98%
Pregnancy and Delivery Care				
Newborn Deliveries Scheduled Early[2]	25	0%	3%	6%
Preventive Care				
Immunization for Influenza[2]	444	96%	94%	90%
Immunization for Pneumonia[2]	572	97%	95%	92%
Stroke Care				
Anticoagulation Therapy for Atrial Fibrillation[1,2]	-	-	95%	95%
Antithrombotic Therapy Timing[2]	50	100%	98%	98%
Assessed for Rehabilitation[2]	51	100%	97%	97%
Discharged on Antithrombotic Therapy[2]	49	100%	99%	99%
Discharged on Statin Medication[2]	38	100%	94%	94%
Thrombolytic Therapy Timing[1,2]	-	-	58%	66%
Venous Thromboembolism Prophylaxis[2]	50	98%	94%	94%
Written Stroke Educational Materials Given[2]	37	97%	91%	88%
Surgical Care Improvement Project				
Appropriate Beta Blocker Usage[2]	64	97%	98%	98%
Appropriate VTP Within 24 Hours[2]	232	97%	98%	98%
Controlled Postoperative Blood Glucose[2,7]	-	-	99%	97%
Perioperative Temperature Management[2]	260	100%	100%	100%
Prophylactic Antibiotic Selection[2]	153	100%	99%	99%
Prophylactic Antibiotic Selection (Outpatient)	146	99%	99%	98%
Prophylactic Antibiotic Stopped[2]	148	96%	98%	98%
Prophylactic Antibiotic Timing[2]	153	100%	99%	99%
Prophylactic Antibiotic Timing (Outpatient)	146	97%	98%	98%
Urinary Catheter Removal[2]	183	94%	97%	97%
Survey of Patients' Hospital Experiences				
Area Around Room 'Always' Quiet at Night	300+	69%	67%	61%
Doctors 'Always' Communicated Well	300+	82%	84%	82%
Home Recovery Information Given	300+	82%	86%	85%
Hospital Given 9 or 10 on 10 Point Scale	300+	69%	72%	71%
Meds 'Always' Explained Before Given	300+	65%	66%	64%
Nurses 'Always' Communicated Well	300+	81%	81%	79%
Pain 'Always' Well Controlled	300+	70%	72%	71%
Room and Bathroom 'Always' Clean	300+	71%	72%	73%
Timely Help 'Always' Received	300+	69%	68%	68%
Would Definitely Recommend Hospital	300+	65%	71%	71%
Use of Medical Imaging				
Cardiac Imaging Stress Test before Surgery	259	3.1%	5.1%	5.3%
Combination Abdominal CT Scan	534	28.5%	10.1%	10.5%
Combination Brain/Sinus CT Scan	701	1.9%	2.5%	2.7%
Combination Chest CT Scan	255	7.8%	1.3%	2.7%
Follow-up Mammogram/Ultrasound	865	14.7%	8%	8.8%
Lumbar Spine MRI for Low Back Pain	71	38.0%	39%	37.2%

GHS Greenville Memorial Medical Center

701 Grove Rd
Greenville, SC 29605
Phone: 864-455-7000
Fax: 864-455-6218
URL: www.ghs.org
Type: Acute Care Hospitals
Emergency Services: Yes
Ownership: Government - State
Beds: 710

Key Personnel:

Radiology. . . . . Michael Brannon
CEO/President. . . . . Michael C Riordan

Measure	Cases	This Hosp.	State Avg.	U.S. Avg.
Blood Clot Prevention and Treatment				
Anticoagulation Overlap Therapy[2]	180	93%	92%	93%
ICU Venous Thromboembolism Prophylaxis[2]	127	91%	94%	92%
Incidence of Potentially Preventable VTE[2]	61	8%	8%	10%
UFH with Dosages/Platelet Monitoring[2]	156	100%	98%	97%
Venous Thromboembolism Prophylaxis[2]	315	86%	88%	85%
Warfarin Therapy Discharge Instructions[2]	138	4%	72%	75%
Chest Pain/Possible Heart Attack Care				
Aspirin Given Within 24 Hours of Arrival[3,7]	-	-	97%	96%
Fibrinolytic Meds Within 30 Min. of Arrival[5]	-	-	68%	58%
Average Time to ECG (minutes)[3,7]	-	-	5	7
Average Time to Transfer (minutes)[5]	-	-	43	60
Children's Asthma Care				
Received Home Management Plan of Care	-	-	-	88%
Received Reliever Medication	-	-	-	100%
Received Systemic Corticosteroids	-	-	-	100%
Emergency Department				
Admittance Decision Time (minutes)[2]	401	165	94	98
Head CT Results Within 45 Min. of Arrival	14	79%	61%	57%
Patients Who Left ER Before Being Seen	>100k	3%	3%	2%
Time from ER Arrival to Admit. (minutes)[2]	411	357	274	274
Time from ER Arrival to Discharge (minutes)	345	188	136	134
Time in ER Before Being Evaluated (minutes)	357	79	33	26
Time to Pain Meds for Fractures (minutes)	341	28	61	57
Heart Attack Care				
Aspirin Given at Discharge	750	100%	99%	99%
Fibrinolytic Meds Within 30 Min. of Arrival[7]	-	-	50%	54%
PCI Within 90 Minutes of Arrival	146	100%	97%	96%
Statin Prescribed at Discharge	743	99%	99%	98%
Heart Failure Care				
ACE Inhibitor or ARB for LVSD	206	98%	98%	97%
Discharge Instructions Given	543	95%	94%	94%
Evaluation of LVS Function	668	100%	99%	99%
Medicare Spending				
Medicare Spending per Patient (ratio)	-	0.98	0.98	0.98
Pneumonia Care				
Appropriate Initial Antibiotic Given	263	97%	97%	95%
Blood Culture Timing	511	98%	98%	98%
Pregnancy and Delivery Care				
Newborn Deliveries Scheduled Early[2]	67	1%	3%	6%
Preventive Care				
Immunization for Influenza[2]	546	93%	94%	90%
Immunization for Pneumonia[2]	530	92%	95%	92%
Stroke Care				
Anticoagulation Therapy for Atrial Fibrillation[1,2]	-	-	95%	95%
Antithrombotic Therapy Timing[2]	79	94%	98%	98%
Assessed for Rehabilitation[2]	110	97%	97%	97%
Discharged on Antithrombotic Therapy[2]	92	98%	99%	99%
Discharged on Statin Medication[2]	79	92%	94%	94%
Thrombolytic Therapy Timing[1,2]	-	-	58%	66%
Venous Thromboembolism Prophylaxis[2]	118	97%	94%	94%
Written Stroke Educational Materials Given[2]	58	83%	91%	88%

NOTE: Hospital profiles are in alphabetical order by state, then city, then hospital within the city; Rankings exclude hospitals with less than 25 cases except for patient surveys which excludes hospitals with less than 100 cases; (a) 100-299 cases; (1) The number of cases/patients is too few to report; (2) Data submitted were based on a sample of cases/patients; (3) Results are based on a shorter time period than required; (4) Data suppressed by CMS for one or more quarters; (5) Results are not available for this reporting period; (6) Fewer than 100 patients completed the HCAHPS survey; (7) No cases met the criteria for this measure; (8) The lower limit of the confidence interval cannot be calculated if the number of observed infections equals zero; (9) No data are available from the state/territory for this reporting period; (10) The scores shown reflect fewer than 50 completed surveys; (11) There were discrepancies in the data collection process; (12) This measure does not apply to this hospital for this reporting period; (13) Results cannot be calculated for this reporting period; (14) The results for this state are combined with nearby states to protect confidentiality; Please refer to the User's Guide for a full explanation of data.

Measure	Cases	This Hosp.	State Avg.	U.S. Avg.
Surgical Care Improvement Project				
Appropriate Beta Blocker Usage[2]	364	98%	98%	98%
Appropriate VTP Within 24 Hours[2]	350	98%	98%	98%
Controlled Postoperative Blood Glucose[2]	349	99%	99%	97%
Perioperative Temperature Management[2]	515	100%	100%	100%
Prophylactic Antibiotic Selection[2]	587	100%	99%	99%
Prophylactic Antibiotic Selection (Outpatient)	765	99%	99%	98%
Prophylactic Antibiotic Stopped[2]	563	98%	98%	98%
Prophylactic Antibiotic Timing[2]	587	99%	99%	99%
Prophylactic Antibiotic Timing (Outpatient)	770	99%	98%	98%
Urinary Catheter Removal[2]	473	91%	97%	97%
Survey of Patients' Hospital Experiences				
Area Around Room 'Always' Quiet at Night	300+	63%	67%	61%
Doctors 'Always' Communicated Well	300+	78%	84%	82%
Home Recovery Information Given	300+	84%	86%	85%
Hospital Given 9 or 10 on 10 Point Scale	300+	71%	72%	71%
Meds 'Always' Explained Before Given	300+	62%	66%	64%
Nurses 'Always' Communicated Well	300+	78%	81%	79%
Pain 'Always' Well Controlled	300+	70%	72%	71%
Room and Bathroom 'Always' Clean	300+	70%	72%	73%
Timely Help 'Always' Received	300+	65%	68%	68%
Would Definitely Recommend Hospital	300+	73%	71%	71%
Use of Medical Imaging				
Cardiac Imaging Stress Test before Surgery	1,164	4.9%	5.1%	5.3%
Combination Abdominal CT Scan	1,872	9.2%	10.1%	10.5%
Combination Brain/Sinus CT Scan	1,691	2.5%	2.5%	2.7%
Combination Chest CT Scan	1,560	0.1%	1.3%	2.7%
Follow-up Mammogram/Ultrasound	2,650	10.7%	8%	8.8%
Lumbar Spine MRI for Low Back Pain	194	38.1%	39%	37.2%

GHS Patewood Memorial Hospital

175 Patewood Drive Phone: 864-797-1000
Greenville, SC 29615
URL: www.ghs.org
Type: Acute Care Hospitals Emergency Services: No
Ownership: Govt - Hospital Dist/Auth

Measure	Cases	This Hosp.	State Avg.	U.S. Avg.
Blood Clot Prevention and Treatment				
Anticoagulation Overlap Therapy[1,2]	-	-	92%	93%
ICU Venous Thromboembolism Prophylaxis[2,7]	-	-	94%	92%
Incidence of Potentially Preventable VTE[1,2]	-	-	8%	10%
UFH with Dosages/Platelet Monitoring[2,7]	-	-	98%	97%
Venous Thromboembolism Prophylaxis[2]	21	100%	88%	85%
Warfarin Therapy Discharge Instructions[1,2]	-	-	72%	75%
Chest Pain/Possible Heart Attack Care				
Aspirin Given Within 24 Hours of Arrival[5]	-	-	97%	96%
Fibrinolytic Meds Within 30 Min. of Arrival[5]	-	-	68%	58%
Average Time to ECG (minutes)[5]	-	-	5	7
Average Time to Transfer (minutes)[5]	-	-	43	60
Children's Asthma Care				
Received Home Management Plan of Care	-	-	-	88%
Received Reliever Medication	-	-	-	100%
Received Systemic Corticosteroids	-	-	-	100%
Emergency Department				
Admittance Decision Time (minutes)[2,7]	-	-	94	98
Head CT Results Within 45 Min. of Arrival[5]	-	-	61%	57%
Patients Who Left ER Before Being Seen[5]	-	-	3%	2%
Time from ER Arrival to Admit. (minutes)[2,7]	-	-	274	274
Time from ER Arrival to Discharge (minutes)[5]	-	-	136	134
Time in ER Before Being Evaluated (minutes)[5]	-	-	33	26
Time to Pain Meds for Fractures (minutes)[5]	-	-	61	57
Heart Attack Care				
Aspirin Given at Discharge[5]	-	-	99%	99%
Fibrinolytic Meds Within 30 Min. of Arrival[5]	-	-	50%	54%
PCI Within 90 Minutes of Arrival[5]	-	-	97%	96%
Statin Prescribed at Discharge[5]	-	-	99%	98%
Heart Failure Care				
ACE Inhibitor or ARB for LVSD[5]	-	-	98%	97%
Discharge Instructions Given[5]	-	-	94%	94%
Evaluation of LVS Function[5]	-	-	99%	99%
Medicare Spending				
Medicare Spending per Patient (ratio)	-	0.89	0.98	0.98
Pneumonia Care				
Appropriate Initial Antibiotic Given[5]	-	-	97%	95%
Blood Culture Timing[5]	-	-	98%	98%
Pregnancy and Delivery Care				
Newborn Deliveries Scheduled Early[2,7]	-	-	3%	6%
Preventive Care				
Immunization for Influenza[2]	319	99%	94%	90%
Immunization for Pneumonia[2]	367	99%	95%	92%
Stroke Care				
Anticoagulation Therapy for Atrial Fibrillation[5]	-	-	95%	95%
Antithrombotic Therapy Timing[5]	-	-	98%	98%
Assessed for Rehabilitation[5]	-	-	97%	97%
Discharged on Antithrombotic Therapy[5]	-	-	99%	99%
Discharged on Statin Medication[5]	-	-	94%	94%
Thrombolytic Therapy Timing[5]	-	-	58%	66%
Venous Thromboembolism Prophylaxis[5]	-	-	94%	94%
Written Stroke Educational Materials Given[5]	-	-	91%	88%
Surgical Care Improvement Project				
Appropriate Beta Blocker Usage[2]	227	99%	98%	98%
Appropriate VTP Within 24 Hours[2]	644	100%	98%	98%
Controlled Postoperative Blood Glucose[2,7]	-	-	99%	97%
Perioperative Temperature Management[2]	824	100%	100%	100%
Prophylactic Antibiotic Selection[2]	684	100%	99%	99%
Prophylactic Antibiotic Selection (Outpatient)	157	99%	99%	98%
Prophylactic Antibiotic Stopped[2]	682	100%	98%	98%
Prophylactic Antibiotic Timing[2]	684	100%	99%	99%
Prophylactic Antibiotic Timing (Outpatient)	157	100%	98%	98%
Urinary Catheter Removal[2]	657	100%	97%	97%
Survey of Patients' Hospital Experiences				
Area Around Room 'Always' Quiet at Night	300+	90%	67%	61%
Doctors 'Always' Communicated Well	300+	89%	84%	82%
Home Recovery Information Given	300+	93%	86%	85%
Hospital Given 9 or 10 on 10 Point Scale	300+	91%	72%	71%
Meds 'Always' Explained Before Given	300+	71%	66%	64%
Nurses 'Always' Communicated Well	300+	90%	81%	79%
Pain 'Always' Well Controlled	300+	80%	72%	71%
Room and Bathroom 'Always' Clean	300+	90%	72%	73%
Timely Help 'Always' Received	300+	84%	68%	68%
Would Definitely Recommend Hospital	300+	92%	71%	71%
Use of Medical Imaging				
Cardiac Imaging Stress Test before Surgery	146	0.7%	5.1%	5.3%
Combination Abdominal CT Scan	509	18.5%	10.1%	10.5%
Combination Brain/Sinus CT Scan[1]	-	-	2.5%	2.7%
Combination Chest CT Scan	443	0.0%	1.3%	2.7%
Follow-up Mammogram/Ultrasound	2,633	10.3%	8%	8.8%
Lumbar Spine MRI for Low Back Pain	224	31.3%	39%	37.2%

Saint Francis - Downtown

One Saint Francis Dr Phone: 864-255-1000
Greenville, SC 29601 Fax: 864-255-1013
E-mail: stfrancisfoundation@stfrancishealth.org
URL: www.stfrancishealth.org
Type: Acute Care Hospitals Emergency Services: Yes
Ownership: Voluntary non-profit - Church Beds: 257

Key Personnel:

Hemotology Center . . . . Michelle Abascal
Patient Relations . . . . Mina Bagwell
Radiology. . . . . Jeff Hamlin
Infection Control. . . . . Patricia McGauly
Chief of Medical Staff. . . . . Robert Mobley, MD
Quality Assurance . . . . Judy Pew
CEO/President. . . . . Valinda Rutledge
Coronary Care . . . . Carol Winckler

Measure	Cases	This Hosp.	State Avg.	U.S. Avg.
Blood Clot Prevention and Treatment				
Anticoagulation Overlap Therapy[2]	88	98%	92%	93%
ICU Venous Thromboembolism Prophylaxis[2]	219	97%	94%	92%
Incidence of Potentially Preventable VTE[1,2]	-	-	8%	10%
UFH with Dosages/Platelet Monitoring[2]	55	98%	98%	97%
Venous Thromboembolism Prophylaxis[2]	724	92%	88%	85%
Warfarin Therapy Discharge Instructions[2]	59	100%	72%	75%
Chest Pain/Possible Heart Attack Care				
Aspirin Given Within 24 Hours of Arrival[1,3]	-	-	97%	96%
Fibrinolytic Meds Within 30 Min. of Arrival[3,7]	-	-	68%	58%
Average Time to ECG (minutes)[1,3]	-	-	5	7
Average Time to Transfer (minutes)[3,7]	-	-	43	60
Children's Asthma Care				
Received Home Management Plan of Care	-	-	-	88%
Received Reliever Medication	-	-	-	100%
Received Systemic Corticosteroids	-	-	-	100%
Emergency Department				
Admittance Decision Time (minutes)[2]	549	103	94	98
Head CT Results Within 45 Min. of Arrival[1]	-	-	61%	57%
Patients Who Left ER Before Being Seen	80,204	2%	3%	2%
Time from ER Arrival to Admit. (minutes)[2]	565	273	274	274
Time from ER Arrival to Discharge (minutes)	1,286	155	136	134
Time in ER Before Being Evaluated (minutes)	1,326	33	33	26
Time to Pain Meds for Fractures (minutes)	155	63	61	57
Heart Attack Care				
Aspirin Given at Discharge[2]	334	100%	99%	99%
Fibrinolytic Meds Within 30 Min. of Arrival[2,7]	-	-	50%	54%
PCI Within 90 Minutes of Arrival[2]	56	100%	97%	96%
Statin Prescribed at Discharge[2]	320	100%	99%	98%
Heart Failure Care				
ACE Inhibitor or ARB for LVSD[2]	107	100%	98%	97%
Discharge Instructions Given[2]	253	95%	94%	94%
Evaluation of LVS Function[2]	300	100%	99%	99%
Medicare Spending				
Medicare Spending per Patient (ratio)	-	1.02	0.98	0.98
Pneumonia Care				
Appropriate Initial Antibiotic Given[2]	95	100%	97%	95%
Blood Culture Timing[2]	174	95%	98%	98%
Pregnancy and Delivery Care				
Newborn Deliveries Scheduled Early[2]	44	0%	3%	6%
Preventive Care				
Immunization for Influenza[2]	859	94%	94%	90%
Immunization for Pneumonia[2]	1,242	95%	95%	92%
Stroke Care				
Anticoagulation Therapy for Atrial Fibrillation	17	100%	95%	95%
Antithrombotic Therapy Timing	163	99%	98%	98%
Assessed for Rehabilitation	199	100%	97%	97%
Discharged on Antithrombotic Therapy	167	100%	99%	99%
Discharged on Statin Medication	123	93%	94%	94%
Thrombolytic Therapy Timing	37	30%	58%	66%
Venous Thromboembolism Prophylaxis	202	95%	94%	94%
Written Stroke Educational Materials Given	115	96%	91%	88%
Surgical Care Improvement Project				
Appropriate Beta Blocker Usage[2]	210	99%	98%	98%
Appropriate VTP Within 24 Hours[2]	439	99%	98%	98%
Controlled Postoperative Blood Glucose[2]	151	99%	99%	97%
Perioperative Temperature Management[2]	492	100%	100%	100%
Prophylactic Antibiotic Selection[2]	467	100%	99%	99%
Prophylactic Antibiotic Selection (Outpatient)	923	100%	99%	98%
Prophylactic Antibiotic Stopped[2]	457	98%	98%	98%
Prophylactic Antibiotic Timing[2]	467	100%	99%	99%
Prophylactic Antibiotic Timing (Outpatient)	923	100%	98%	98%
Urinary Catheter Removal[2]	479	98%	97%	97%
Survey of Patients' Hospital Experiences				
Area Around Room 'Always' Quiet at Night	300+	70%	67%	61%
Doctors 'Always' Communicated Well	300+	82%	84%	82%
Home Recovery Information Given	300+	88%	86%	85%
Hospital Given 9 or 10 on 10 Point Scale	300+	77%	72%	71%
Meds 'Always' Explained Before Given	300+	63%	66%	64%
Nurses 'Always' Communicated Well	300+	80%	81%	79%
Pain 'Always' Well Controlled	300+	73%	72%	71%
Room and Bathroom 'Always' Clean	300+	66%	72%	73%
Timely Help 'Always' Received	300+	69%	68%	68%
Would Definitely Recommend Hospital	300+	81%	71%	71%
Use of Medical Imaging				
Cardiac Imaging Stress Test before Surgery	66	9.1%	5.1%	5.3%
Combination Abdominal CT Scan	1,609	4.2%	10.1%	10.5%
Combination Brain/Sinus CT Scan	1,609	2.9%	2.5%	2.7%
Combination Chest CT Scan	1,529	0.9%	1.3%	2.7%
Follow-up Mammogram/Ultrasound	3,028	11.0%	8%	8.8%
Lumbar Spine MRI for Low Back Pain	276	34.1%	39%	37.2%

NOTE: Hospital profiles are in alphabetical order by state, then city, then hospital within the city; Rankings exclude hospitals with less than 25 cases except for patient surveys which excludes hospitals with less than 100 cases; (a) 100-299 cases; (1) The number of cases/patients is too few to report; (2) Data submitted were based on a sample of cases/patients; (3) Results are based on a shorter time period than required; (4) Data suppressed by CMS for one or more quarters; (5) Results are not available for this reporting period; (6) Fewer than 100 patients completed the HCAHPS survey; (7) No cases met the criteria for this measure; (8) The lower limit of the confidence interval cannot be calculated if the number of observed infections equals zero; (9) No data are available from the state/territory for this reporting period; (10) The scores shown reflect fewer than 50 completed surveys; (11) There were discrepancies in the data collection process; (12) This measure does not apply to this hospital for this reporting period; (13) Results cannot be calculated for this reporting period; (14) The results for this state are combined with nearby states to protect confidentiality; Please refer to the User's Guide for a full explanation of data.

Self Regional Healthcare

1325 Spring Street | Phone: 864-227-4111
Greenwood, SC 29646 | Fax: 864-725-4711
URL: www.selfregional.org
Type: Acute Care Hospitals | Emergency Services: Yes
Ownership: Voluntary non-profit - Private | Beds: 421

Key Personnel:
Infection Control. . . . . Dorrell Antley
CEO/President. . . . . M John Heydel
Quality Assurance . . . . Mary Margaret Jackson
Chief of Medical Staff . . . . Julius Leary, MD
Pediatric In-Patient Care . . . . Margaret Quarles, RN
Radiology. . . . . Jerry Ryans
Operating Room. . . . . Debbie Strickland, RN
Coronary Care . . . . Jackie Thornton

Measure	Cases	This Hosp.	State Avg.	U.S. Avg.
Blood Clot Prevention and Treatment				
Anticoagulation Overlap Therapy[2]	130	100%	92%	93%
ICU Venous Thromboembolism Prophylaxis[2]	109	94%	94%	92%
Incidence of Potentially Preventable VTE[2]	26	8%	8%	10%
UFH with Dosages/Platelet Monitoring[2]	44	100%	98%	97%
Venous Thromboembolism Prophylaxis[2]	271	89%	88%	85%
Warfarin Therapy Discharge Instructions[2]	103	75%	72%	75%
Chest Pain/Possible Heart Attack Care				
Aspirin Given Within 24 Hours of Arrival[5]	-	-	97%	96%
Fibrinolytic Meds Within 30 Min. of Arrival[5]	-	-	68%	58%
Average Time to ECG (minutes)[5]	-	-	5	7
Average Time to Transfer (minutes)[5]	-	-	43	60
Children's Asthma Care				
Received Home Management Plan of Care	-	-	-	88%
Received Reliever Medication	-	-	-	100%
Received Systemic Corticosteroids	-	-	-	100%
Emergency Department				
Admittance Decision Time (minutes)[2]	575	116	94	98
Head CT Results Within 45 Min. of Arrival	34	24%	61%	57%
Patients Who Left ER Before Being Seen	48,915	4%	3%	2%
Time from ER Arrival to Admit. (minutes)[2]	578	288	274	274
Time from ER Arrival to Discharge (minutes)	360	195	136	134
Time in ER Before Being Evaluated (minutes)	398	66	33	26
Time to Pain Meds for Fractures (minutes)	164	92	61	57
Heart Attack Care				
Aspirin Given at Discharge	290	99%	99%	99%
Fibrinolytic Meds Within 30 Min. of Arrival[1]	-	-	50%	54%
PCI Within 90 Minutes of Arrival	36	97%	97%	96%
Statin Prescribed at Discharge	285	95%	99%	98%
Heart Failure Care				
ACE Inhibitor or ARB for LVSD	104	99%	98%	97%
Discharge Instructions Given	229	99%	94%	94%
Evaluation of LVS Function	274	100%	99%	99%
Medicare Spending				
Medicare Spending per Patient (ratio)	-	1.02	0.98	0.98
Pneumonia Care				
Appropriate Initial Antibiotic Given	173	99%	97%	95%
Blood Culture Timing	337	99%	98%	98%
Pregnancy and Delivery Care				
Newborn Deliveries Scheduled Early	120	8%	3%	6%
Preventive Care				
Immunization for Influenza[2]	560	91%	94%	90%
Immunization for Pneumonia[2]	827	89%	95%	92%
Stroke Care				
Anticoagulation Therapy for Atrial Fibrillation	22	100%	95%	95%
Antithrombotic Therapy Timing	129	96%	98%	98%
Assessed for Rehabilitation	162	99%	97%	97%
Discharged on Antithrombotic Therapy	146	99%	99%	99%
Discharged on Statin Medication	119	94%	94%	94%
Thrombolytic Therapy Timing[1]	-	-	58%	66%
Venous Thromboembolism Prophylaxis	158	80%	94%	94%
Written Stroke Educational Materials Given	95	94%	91%	88%
Surgical Care Improvement Project				
Appropriate Beta Blocker Usage[2]	302	99%	98%	98%
Appropriate VTP Within 24 Hours[2]	628	98%	98%	98%
Controlled Postoperative Blood Glucose[2]	100	100%	99%	97%
Perioperative Temperature Management[2]	738	100%	100%	100%
Prophylactic Antibiotic Selection[2]	645	99%	99%	99%
Prophylactic Antibiotic Selection (Outpatient)	443	98%	99%	98%
Prophylactic Antibiotic Stopped[2]	638	96%	98%	98%
Prophylactic Antibiotic Timing[2]	646	99%	99%	99%
Prophylactic Antibiotic Timing (Outpatient)	447	96%	98%	98%
Urinary Catheter Removal[2]	220	90%	97%	97%
Survey of Patients' Hospital Experiences				
Area Around Room 'Always' Quiet at Night	300+	69%	67%	61%
Doctors 'Always' Communicated Well	300+	85%	84%	82%
Home Recovery Information Given	300+	87%	86%	85%
Hospital Given 9 or 10 on 10 Point Scale	300+	74%	72%	71%
Meds 'Always' Explained Before Given	300+	67%	66%	64%
Nurses 'Always' Communicated Well	300+	84%	81%	79%
Pain 'Always' Well Controlled	300+	74%	72%	71%
Room and Bathroom 'Always' Clean	300+	81%	72%	73%
Timely Help 'Always' Received	300+	67%	68%	68%
Would Definitely Recommend Hospital	300+	75%	71%	71%
Use of Medical Imaging				
Cardiac Imaging Stress Test before Surgery	416	7.7%	5.1%	5.3%
Combination Abdominal CT Scan	1,183	10.1%	10.1%	10.5%
Combination Brain/Sinus CT Scan	1,132	2.7%	2.5%	2.7%
Combination Chest CT Scan	639	3.3%	1.3%	2.7%
Follow-up Mammogram/Ultrasound	3,474	8.0%	8%	8.8%
Lumbar Spine MRI for Low Back Pain	304	36.5%	39%	37.2%

GHS Greer Memorial Hospital

830 South Buncombe Road | Phone: 864-848-8200
Greer, SC 29650
Type: Acute Care Hospitals | Emergency Services: Yes
Ownership: Voluntary non-profit - Private

Measure	Cases	This Hosp.	State Avg.	U.S. Avg.
Blood Clot Prevention and Treatment				
Anticoagulation Overlap Therapy[2]	21	100%	92%	93%
ICU Venous Thromboembolism Prophylaxis[2]	74	99%	94%	92%
Incidence of Potentially Preventable VTE[2,7]	-	-	8%	10%
UFH with Dosages/Platelet Monitoring[1,2]	-	-	98%	97%
Venous Thromboembolism Prophylaxis[2]	206	97%	88%	85%
Warfarin Therapy Discharge Instructions[2]	18	28%	72%	75%
Chest Pain/Possible Heart Attack Care				
Aspirin Given Within 24 Hours of Arrival	94	100%	97%	96%
Fibrinolytic Meds Within 30 Min. of Arrival[7]	-	-	68%	58%
Average Time to ECG (minutes)	95	3	5	7
Average Time to Transfer (minutes)[1]	-	-	43	60
Children's Asthma Care				
Received Home Management Plan of Care	-	-	-	88%
Received Reliever Medication	-	-	-	100%
Received Systemic Corticosteroids	-	-	-	100%
Emergency Department				
Admittance Decision Time (minutes)[2]	368	102	94	98
Head CT Results Within 45 Min. of Arrival[1]	-	-	61%	57%
Patients Who Left ER Before Being Seen	33,606	2%	3%	2%
Time from ER Arrival to Admit. (minutes)[2]	370	322	274	274
Time from ER Arrival to Discharge (minutes)	376	158	136	134
Time in ER Before Being Evaluated (minutes)	380	66	33	26
Time to Pain Meds for Fractures (minutes)	131	54	61	57
Heart Attack Care				
Aspirin Given at Discharge[1]	-	-	99%	99%
Fibrinolytic Meds Within 30 Min. of Arrival[7]	-	-	50%	54%
PCI Within 90 Minutes of Arrival[7]	-	-	97%	96%
Statin Prescribed at Discharge[1]	-	-	99%	98%
Heart Failure Care				
ACE Inhibitor or ARB for LVSD	30	100%	98%	97%
Discharge Instructions Given	70	100%	94%	94%
Evaluation of LVS Function	89	100%	99%	99%
Medicare Spending				
Medicare Spending per Patient (ratio)	-	0.93	0.98	0.98
Pneumonia Care				
Appropriate Initial Antibiotic Given	121	98%	97%	95%
Blood Culture Timing	168	99%	98%	98%
Pregnancy and Delivery Care				
Newborn Deliveries Scheduled Early[2]	25	0%	3%	6%
Preventive Care				
Immunization for Influenza[2]	372	97%	94%	90%
Immunization for Pneumonia[2]	408	98%	95%	92%
Stroke Care				
Anticoagulation Therapy for Atrial Fibrillation[2,7]	-	-	95%	95%
Antithrombotic Therapy Timing[1,2]	-	-	98%	98%
Assessed for Rehabilitation[1,2]	-	-	97%	97%
Discharged on Antithrombotic Therapy[1,2]	-	-	99%	99%
Discharged on Statin Medication[1,2]	-	-	94%	94%
Thrombolytic Therapy Timing[2,7]	-	-	58%	66%
Venous Thromboembolism Prophylaxis[1,2]	-	-	94%	94%
Written Stroke Educational Materials Given[1,2]	-	-	91%	88%
Surgical Care Improvement Project				
Appropriate Beta Blocker Usage[2]	134	98%	98%	98%
Appropriate VTP Within 24 Hours[2]	490	99%	98%	98%
Controlled Postoperative Blood Glucose[2,7]	-	-	99%	97%
Perioperative Temperature Management[2]	553	100%	100%	100%
Prophylactic Antibiotic Selection[2]	397	100%	99%	99%
Prophylactic Antibiotic Selection (Outpatient)	46	100%	99%	98%
Prophylactic Antibiotic Stopped[2]	391	99%	98%	98%
Prophylactic Antibiotic Timing[2]	397	100%	99%	99%
Prophylactic Antibiotic Timing (Outpatient)	46	100%	98%	98%
Urinary Catheter Removal[2]	468	99%	97%	97%
Survey of Patients' Hospital Experiences				
Area Around Room 'Always' Quiet at Night	300+	69%	67%	61%
Doctors 'Always' Communicated Well	300+	86%	84%	82%
Home Recovery Information Given	300+	90%	86%	85%
Hospital Given 9 or 10 on 10 Point Scale	300+	85%	72%	71%
Meds 'Always' Explained Before Given	300+	69%	66%	64%
Nurses 'Always' Communicated Well	300+	85%	81%	79%
Pain 'Always' Well Controlled	300+	75%	72%	71%
Room and Bathroom 'Always' Clean	300+	79%	72%	73%
Timely Help 'Always' Received	300+	75%	68%	68%
Would Definitely Recommend Hospital	300+	87%	71%	71%
Use of Medical Imaging				
Cardiac Imaging Stress Test before Surgery	386	5.7%	5.1%	5.3%
Combination Abdominal CT Scan	663	6.8%	10.1%	10.5%
Combination Brain/Sinus CT Scan	520	2.1%	2.5%	2.7%
Combination Chest CT Scan	368	0.3%	1.3%	2.7%
Follow-up Mammogram/Ultrasound	868	9.4%	8%	8.8%
Lumbar Spine MRI for Low Back Pain	117	35.9%	39%	37.2%

Village Hospital

250 Westmoreland Road | Phone: 864-530-6000
Greer, SC 29651
URL: www.villageatpelham.com
Type: Acute Care Hospitals | Emergency Services: Yes
Ownership: Govt - Hospital Dist/Auth | Beds: 48

Key Personnel:
President . . . . David H Parks

Measure	Cases	This Hosp.	State Avg.	U.S. Avg.
Blood Clot Prevention and Treatment				
Anticoagulation Overlap Therapy[2]	23	83%	92%	93%
ICU Venous Thromboembolism Prophylaxis[2]	31	100%	94%	92%
Incidence of Potentially Preventable VTE[1,2]	-	-	8%	10%
UFH with Dosages/Platelet Monitoring[2]	17	100%	98%	97%
Venous Thromboembolism Prophylaxis[2]	150	98%	88%	85%
Warfarin Therapy Discharge Instructions[2]	20	0%	72%	75%
Chest Pain/Possible Heart Attack Care				
Aspirin Given Within 24 Hours of Arrival[5]	-	-	97%	96%
Fibrinolytic Meds Within 30 Min. of Arrival[5]	-	-	68%	58%
Average Time to ECG (minutes)[5]	-	-	5	7
Average Time to Transfer (minutes)[5]	-	-	43	60
Children's Asthma Care				
Received Home Management Plan of Care	-	-	-	88%
Received Reliever Medication	-	-	-	100%
Received Systemic Corticosteroids	-	-	-	100%
Emergency Department				
Admittance Decision Time (minutes)[2]	463	125	94	98
Head CT Results Within 45 Min. of Arrival[1,3]	-	-	61%	57%
Patients Who Left ER Before Being Seen	21,260	4%	3%	2%
Time from ER Arrival to Admit. (minutes)[2]	467	305	274	274
Time from ER Arrival to Discharge (minutes)	441	126	136	134
Time in ER Before Being Evaluated (minutes)	438	42	33	26
Time to Pain Meds for Fractures (minutes)	114	55	61	57

NOTE: Hospital profiles are in alphabetical order by state, then city, then hospital within the city; Rankings exclude hospitals with less than 25 cases except for patient surveys which excludes hospitals with less than 100 cases; (a) 100-299 cases; (1) The number of cases/patients is too few to report; (2) Data submitted were based on a sample of cases/patients; (3) Results are based on a shorter time period than required; (4) Data suppressed by CMS for one or more quarters; (5) Results are not available for this reporting period; (6) Fewer than 100 patients completed the HCAHPS survey; (7) No cases met the criteria for this measure; (8) The lower limit of the confidence interval cannot be calculated if the number of observed infections equals zero; (9) No data are available from the state/territory for this reporting period; (10) The scores shown reflect fewer than 50 completed surveys; (11) There were discrepancies in the data collection process; (12) This measure does not apply to this hospital for this reporting period; (13) Results cannot be calculated for this reporting period; (14) The results for this state are combined with nearby states to protect confidentiality; Please refer to the User's Guide for a full explanation of data.

Heart Attack Care				
Aspirin Given at Discharge[7]	-	-	99%	99%
Fibrinolytic Meds Within 30 Min. of Arrival[7]	-	-	50%	54%
PCI Within 90 Minutes of Arrival[7]	-	-	97%	96%
Statin Prescribed at Discharge[7]	-	-	99%	98%
Heart Failure Care				
ACE Inhibitor or ARB for LVSD	14	100%	98%	97%
Discharge Instructions Given	48	96%	94%	94%
Evaluation of LVS Function	55	100%	99%	99%
Medicare Spending				
Medicare Spending per Patient (ratio)	-	1.01	0.98	0.98
Pneumonia Care				
Appropriate Initial Antibiotic Given	73	99%	97%	95%
Blood Culture Timing	85	100%	98%	98%
Pregnancy and Delivery Care				
Newborn Deliveries Scheduled Early[7]	-	-	3%	6%
Preventive Care				
Immunization for Influenza[2]	318	98%	94%	90%
Immunization for Pneumonia[2]	446	98%	95%	92%
Stroke Care				
Anticoagulation Therapy for Atrial Fibrillation[7]	-	-	95%	95%
Antithrombotic Therapy Timing	18	100%	98%	98%
Assessed for Rehabilitation	19	100%	97%	97%
Discharged on Antithrombotic Therapy	18	100%	99%	99%
Discharged on Statin Medication	12	100%	94%	94%
Thrombolytic Therapy Timing[7]	-	-	58%	66%
Venous Thromboembolism Prophylaxis	16	100%	94%	94%
Written Stroke Educational Materials Given[1]	-	-	91%	88%
Surgical Care Improvement Project				
Appropriate Beta Blocker Usage	48	94%	98%	98%
Appropriate VTP Within 24 Hours	189	99%	98%	98%
Controlled Postoperative Blood Glucose[7]	-	-	99%	97%
Perioperative Temperature Management	195	100%	100%	100%
Prophylactic Antibiotic Selection	151	99%	99%	99%
Prophylactic Antibiotic Selection (Outpatient)	122	98%	99%	98%
Prophylactic Antibiotic Stopped	148	99%	98%	98%
Prophylactic Antibiotic Timing	151	99%	99%	99%
Prophylactic Antibiotic Timing (Outpatient)	122	99%	98%	98%
Urinary Catheter Removal	173	99%	97%	97%
Survey of Patients' Hospital Experiences				
Area Around Room 'Always' Quiet at Night	300+	77%	67%	61%
Doctors 'Always' Communicated Well	300+	87%	84%	82%
Home Recovery Information Given	300+	91%	86%	85%
Hospital Given 9 or 10 on 10 Point Scale	300+	81%	72%	71%
Meds 'Always' Explained Before Given	300+	69%	66%	64%
Nurses 'Always' Communicated Well	300+	82%	81%	79%
Pain 'Always' Well Controlled	300+	71%	72%	71%
Room and Bathroom 'Always' Clean	300+	80%	72%	73%
Timely Help 'Always' Received	300+	70%	68%	68%
Would Definitely Recommend Hospital	300+	84%	71%	71%
Use of Medical Imaging				
Cardiac Imaging Stress Test before Surgery	87	6.9%	5.1%	5.3%
Combination Abdominal CT Scan	301	1.7%	10.1%	10.5%
Combination Brain/Sinus CT Scan	266	0.8%	2.5%	2.7%
Combination Chest CT Scan	150	0.0%	1.3%	2.7%
Follow-up Mammogram/Ultrasound	462	7.4%	8%	8.8%
Lumbar Spine MRI for Low Back Pain	117	34.2%	39%	37.2%

Coastal Carolina Hospital

1000 Medical Center Drive
Hardeeville, SC 29927
Phone: 843-784-8000
Type: Acute Care Hospitals
Emergency Services: Yes
Ownership: Proprietary

Key Personnel:
Operating Room. . . . . Dr Brendan Smith
CEO . . . . Bradley S. Talbert, FACHE
Chief of Medical Staff . . . . Peter White, MD

Measure	Cases	This Hosp.	State Avg.	U.S. Avg.
Blood Clot Prevention and Treatment				
Anticoagulation Overlap Therapy[2]	43	74%	92%	93%
ICU Venous Thromboembolism Prophylaxis[2]	25	100%	94%	92%
Incidence of Potentially Preventable VTE[1,2]	-	-	8%	10%
UFH with Dosages/Platelet Monitoring[1,2]	-	-	98%	97%
Venous Thromboembolism Prophylaxis[2]	197	95%	88%	85%
Warfarin Therapy Discharge Instructions[2]	36	53%	72%	75%
Chest Pain/Possible Heart Attack Care				
Aspirin Given Within 24 Hours of Arrival	23	100%	97%	96%
Fibrinolytic Meds Within 30 Min. of Arrival[7]	-	-	68%	58%
Average Time to ECG (minutes)	20	4	5	7
Average Time to Transfer (minutes)[1]	-	-	43	60
Children's Asthma Care				
Received Home Management Plan of Care	-	-	-	88%
Received Reliever Medication	-	-	-	100%
Received Systemic Corticosteroids	-	-	-	100%
Emergency Department				
Admittance Decision Time (minutes)[2]	647	128	94	98
Head CT Results Within 45 Min. of Arrival	20	90%	61%	57%
Patients Who Left ER Before Being Seen	19,382	1%	3%	2%
Time from ER Arrival to Admit. (minutes)[2]	660	300	274	274
Time from ER Arrival to Discharge (minutes)	415	123	136	134
Time in ER Before Being Evaluated (minutes)	435	27	33	26
Time to Pain Meds for Fractures (minutes)	68	42	61	57
Heart Attack Care				
Aspirin Given at Discharge[1]	-	-	99%	99%
Fibrinolytic Meds Within 30 Min. of Arrival[7]	-	-	50%	54%
PCI Within 90 Minutes of Arrival[7]	-	-	97%	96%
Statin Prescribed at Discharge[1]	-	-	99%	98%
Heart Failure Care				
ACE Inhibitor or ARB for LVSD	18	94%	98%	97%
Discharge Instructions Given	60	92%	94%	94%
Evaluation of LVS Function	71	100%	99%	99%
Medicare Spending				
Medicare Spending per Patient (ratio)	-	1.00	0.98	0.98
Pneumonia Care				
Appropriate Initial Antibiotic Given	69	97%	97%	95%
Blood Culture Timing	85	100%	98%	98%
Pregnancy and Delivery Care				
Newborn Deliveries Scheduled Early[7]	-	-	3%	6%
Preventive Care				
Immunization for Influenza[2]	352	94%	94%	90%
Immunization for Pneumonia[2]	554	96%	95%	92%
Stroke Care				
Anticoagulation Therapy for Atrial Fibrillation[1]	-	-	95%	95%
Antithrombotic Therapy Timing	35	100%	98%	98%
Assessed for Rehabilitation	34	91%	97%	97%
Discharged on Antithrombotic Therapy	34	100%	99%	99%
Discharged on Statin Medication	27	89%	94%	94%
Thrombolytic Therapy Timing[1]	-	-	58%	66%
Venous Thromboembolism Prophylaxis	32	100%	94%	94%
Written Stroke Educational Materials Given	21	57%	91%	88%
Surgical Care Improvement Project				
Appropriate Beta Blocker Usage	20	95%	98%	98%
Appropriate VTP Within 24 Hours	64	97%	98%	98%
Controlled Postoperative Blood Glucose[7]	-	-	99%	97%
Perioperative Temperature Management	72	100%	100%	100%
Prophylactic Antibiotic Selection	39	100%	99%	99%
Prophylactic Antibiotic Selection (Outpatient)	53	100%	99%	98%
Prophylactic Antibiotic Stopped	37	95%	98%	98%
Prophylactic Antibiotic Timing	39	100%	99%	99%
Prophylactic Antibiotic Timing (Outpatient)	54	96%	98%	98%
Urinary Catheter Removal	37	95%	97%	97%
Survey of Patients' Hospital Experiences				
Area Around Room 'Always' Quiet at Night	300+	63%	67%	61%
Doctors 'Always' Communicated Well	300+	80%	84%	82%
Home Recovery Information Given	300+	85%	86%	85%
Hospital Given 9 or 10 on 10 Point Scale	300+	69%	72%	71%
Meds 'Always' Explained Before Given	300+	62%	66%	64%
Nurses 'Always' Communicated Well	300+	78%	81%	79%
Pain 'Always' Well Controlled	300+	74%	72%	71%
Room and Bathroom 'Always' Clean	300+	73%	72%	73%
Timely Help 'Always' Received	300+	66%	68%	68%
Would Definitely Recommend Hospital	300+	68%	71%	71%
Use of Medical Imaging				
Cardiac Imaging Stress Test before Surgery[1]	-	-	5.1%	5.3%
Combination Abdominal CT Scan	482	7.1%	10.1%	10.5%
Combination Brain/Sinus CT Scan	564	4.4%	2.5%	2.7%
Combination Chest CT Scan	186	1.1%	1.3%	2.7%
Follow-up Mammogram/Ultrasound	267	6.4%	8%	8.8%
Lumbar Spine MRI for Low Back Pain[1]	-	-	39%	37.2%

Carolina Pines Regional Medical Center

1304 W Bobo Newsom Hwy
Hartsville, SC 29550
Phone: 864-339-2100
Fax: 843-339-4116
E-mail: tiletha.lane@cprmc.hma-corp.com
URL: www.cprmc.com
Type: Acute Care Hospitals
Emergency Services: Yes
Ownership: Proprietary
Beds: 116

Key Personnel:
Emergency Room . . . . James Balvich, MD
Chief of Medical Staff. . . . . Gary A Barker, MD
Infection Control. . . . . Shari Carter, RN
CEO/President. . . . . David Castleberry
Intensive Care Unit. . . . . Sherry Hudson
Patient Relations . . . . Janice Hutson
Quality Assurance . . . . Barbara Kelly, RN
Pediatric In-Patient Care . . . . JO Morphis, MD

Measure	Cases	This Hosp.	State Avg.	U.S. Avg.
Blood Clot Prevention and Treatment				
Anticoagulation Overlap Therapy[2]	25	100%	92%	93%
ICU Venous Thromboembolism Prophylaxis[2]	98	90%	94%	92%
Incidence of Potentially Preventable VTE[1,2]	-	-	8%	10%
UFH with Dosages/Platelet Monitoring[2]	14	100%	98%	97%
Venous Thromboembolism Prophylaxis[2]	317	66%	88%	85%
Warfarin Therapy Discharge Instructions[2]	19	100%	72%	75%
Chest Pain/Possible Heart Attack Care				
Aspirin Given Within 24 Hours of Arrival	95	98%	97%	96%
Fibrinolytic Meds Within 30 Min. of Arrival[7]	-	-	68%	58%
Average Time to ECG (minutes)	102	2	5	7
Average Time to Transfer (minutes)[1]	-	-	43	60
Children's Asthma Care				
Received Home Management Plan of Care	-	-	-	88%
Received Reliever Medication	-	-	-	100%
Received Systemic Corticosteroids	-	-	-	100%
Emergency Department				
Admittance Decision Time (minutes)[2]	555	97	94	98
Head CT Results Within 45 Min. of Arrival	17	94%	61%	57%
Patients Who Left ER Before Being Seen	32,757	2%	3%	2%
Time from ER Arrival to Admit. (minutes)[2]	556	246	274	274
Time from ER Arrival to Discharge (minutes)	423	128	136	134
Time in ER Before Being Evaluated (minutes)	454	39	33	26
Time to Pain Meds for Fractures (minutes)	65	64	61	57
Heart Attack Care				
Aspirin Given at Discharge[1]	-	-	99%	99%
Fibrinolytic Meds Within 30 Min. of Arrival[7]	-	-	50%	54%
PCI Within 90 Minutes of Arrival[7]	-	-	97%	96%
Statin Prescribed at Discharge[1]	-	-	99%	98%
Heart Failure Care				
ACE Inhibitor or ARB for LVSD	46	100%	98%	97%
Discharge Instructions Given	147	99%	94%	94%
Evaluation of LVS Function	164	99%	99%	99%
Medicare Spending				
Medicare Spending per Patient (ratio)	-	0.97	0.98	0.98
Pneumonia Care				
Appropriate Initial Antibiotic Given	128	99%	97%	95%
Blood Culture Timing	151	98%	98%	98%
Pregnancy and Delivery Care				
Newborn Deliveries Scheduled Early	54	4%	3%	6%
Preventive Care				
Immunization for Influenza[2]	495	97%	94%	90%
Immunization for Pneumonia[2]	558	96%	95%	92%
Stroke Care				
Anticoagulation Therapy for Atrial Fibrillation[1]	-	-	95%	95%
Antithrombotic Therapy Timing	34	91%	98%	98%
Assessed for Rehabilitation	42	95%	97%	97%
Discharged on Antithrombotic Therapy	40	98%	99%	99%
Discharged on Statin Medication	36	92%	94%	94%
Thrombolytic Therapy Timing[1]	-	-	58%	66%
Venous Thromboembolism Prophylaxis	38	87%	94%	94%
Written Stroke Educational Materials Given	24	75%	91%	88%

NOTE: Hospital profiles are in alphabetical order by state, then city, then hospital within the city; Rankings exclude hospitals with less than 25 cases except for patient surveys which excludes hospitals with less than 100 cases; (a) 100-299 cases; (1) The number of cases/patients is too few to report; (2) Data submitted were based on a sample of cases/patients; (3) Results are based on a shorter time period than required; (4) Data suppressed by CMS for one or more quarters; (5) Results are not available for this reporting period; (6) Fewer than 100 patients completed the HCAHPS survey; (7) No cases met the criteria for this measure; (8) The lower limit of the confidence interval cannot be calculated if the number of observed infections equals zero; (9) No data are available from the state/territory for this reporting period; (10) The scores shown reflect fewer than 50 completed surveys; (11) There were discrepancies in the data collection process; (12) This measure does not apply to this hospital for this reporting period; (13) Results cannot be calculated for this reporting period; (14) The results for this state are combined with nearby states to protect confidentiality; Please refer to the User's Guide for a full explanation of data.

Surgical Care Improvement Project				
Appropriate Beta Blocker Usage	49	92%	98%	98%
Appropriate VTP Within 24 Hours	205	100%	98%	98%
Controlled Postoperative Blood Glucose[7]	-	-	99%	97%
Perioperative Temperature Management	222	100%	100%	100%
Prophylactic Antibiotic Selection	143	100%	99%	99%
Prophylactic Antibiotic Selection (Outpatient)	76	100%	99%	98%
Prophylactic Antibiotic Stopped	131	98%	98%	98%
Prophylactic Antibiotic Timing	143	99%	99%	99%
Prophylactic Antibiotic Timing (Outpatient)	76	100%	98%	98%
Urinary Catheter Removal	111	95%	97%	97%
Survey of Patients' Hospital Experiences				
Area Around Room 'Always' Quiet at Night	300+	67%	67%	61%
Doctors 'Always' Communicated Well	300+	85%	84%	82%
Home Recovery Information Given	300+	82%	86%	85%
Hospital Given 9 or 10 on 10 Point Scale	300+	65%	72%	71%
Meds 'Always' Explained Before Given	300+	62%	66%	64%
Nurses 'Always' Communicated Well	300+	80%	81%	79%
Pain 'Always' Well Controlled	300+	68%	72%	71%
Room and Bathroom 'Always' Clean	300+	70%	72%	73%
Timely Help 'Always' Received	300+	69%	68%	68%
Would Definitely Recommend Hospital	300+	60%	71%	71%
Use of Medical Imaging				
Cardiac Imaging Stress Test before Surgery	267	4.1%	5.1%	5.3%
Combination Abdominal CT Scan	595	2.0%	10.1%	10.5%
Combination Brain/Sinus CT Scan	612	2.1%	2.5%	2.7%
Combination Chest CT Scan	391	0.5%	1.3%	2.7%
Follow-up Mammogram/Ultrasound	804	6.1%	8%	8.8%
Lumbar Spine MRI for Low Back Pain	153	40.5%	39%	37.2%

Hilton Head Regional Medical Center

25 Hospital Center Blvd — Phone: 843-681-6122
Hilton Head Island, SC 29925 — Fax: 843-689-3670
URL: www.hiltonheadmedctr.com
Type: Acute Care Hospitals — Emergency Services: Yes
Ownership: Proprietary — Beds: 93
Key Personnel:
CEO/President. . . . . Todd Lockcuff
Operating Room. . . . . Thomas Rzeczycki, MD
Chief of Medical Staff . . . . George W Warner, MD

Measure	Cases	This Hosp.	State Avg.	U.S. Avg.
Blood Clot Prevention and Treatment				
Anticoagulation Overlap Therapy[2]	62	97%	92%	93%
ICU Venous Thromboembolism Prophylaxis[2]	60	98%	94%	92%
Incidence of Potentially Preventable VTE[2]	16	0%	8%	10%
UFH with Dosages/Platelet Monitoring[1,2]	-	-	98%	97%
Venous Thromboembolism Prophylaxis[2]	352	97%	88%	85%
Warfarin Therapy Discharge Instructions[2]	49	92%	72%	75%
Chest Pain/Possible Heart Attack Care				
Aspirin Given Within 24 Hours of Arrival[1,3]	-	-	97%	96%
Fibrinolytic Meds Within 30 Min. of Arrival[5]	-	-	68%	58%
Average Time to ECG (minutes)[1,3]	-	-	5	7
Average Time to Transfer (minutes)[5]	-	-	43	60
Children's Asthma Care				
Received Home Management Plan of Care	-	-	-	88%
Received Reliever Medication	-	-	-	100%
Received Systemic Corticosteroids	-	-	-	100%
Emergency Department				
Admittance Decision Time (minutes)[2]	662	166	94	98
Head CT Results Within 45 Min. of Arrival[1]	-	-	61%	57%
Patients Who Left ER Before Being Seen	22,912	1%	3%	2%
Time from ER Arrival to Admit. (minutes)[2]	677	341	274	274
Time from ER Arrival to Discharge (minutes)	450	140	136	134
Time in ER Before Being Evaluated (minutes)	472	23	33	26
Time to Pain Meds for Fractures (minutes)	81	54	61	57
Heart Attack Care				
Aspirin Given at Discharge	118	100%	99%	99%
Fibrinolytic Meds Within 30 Min. of Arrival[7]	-	-	50%	54%
PCI Within 90 Minutes of Arrival	35	97%	97%	96%
Statin Prescribed at Discharge	116	100%	99%	98%
Heart Failure Care				
ACE Inhibitor or ARB for LVSD	40	95%	98%	97%
Discharge Instructions Given	139	100%	94%	94%
Evaluation of LVS Function	178	100%	99%	99%
Medicare Spending				
Medicare Spending per Patient (ratio)	-	1.04	0.98	0.98
Pneumonia Care				
Appropriate Initial Antibiotic Given	111	96%	97%	95%
Blood Culture Timing	164	99%	98%	98%
Pregnancy and Delivery Care				
Newborn Deliveries Scheduled Early[2]	105	1%	3%	6%
Preventive Care				
Immunization for Influenza[2]	521	97%	94%	90%
Immunization for Pneumonia[2]	703	98%	95%	92%
Stroke Care				
Anticoagulation Therapy for Atrial Fibrillation	14	86%	95%	95%
Antithrombotic Therapy Timing	50	96%	98%	98%
Assessed for Rehabilitation	58	95%	97%	97%
Discharged on Antithrombotic Therapy	56	100%	99%	99%
Discharged on Statin Medication	47	81%	94%	94%
Thrombolytic Therapy Timing[1]	-	-	58%	66%
Venous Thromboembolism Prophylaxis	55	91%	94%	94%
Written Stroke Educational Materials Given	38	71%	91%	88%
Surgical Care Improvement Project				
Appropriate Beta Blocker Usage	126	100%	98%	98%
Appropriate VTP Within 24 Hours	267	99%	98%	98%
Controlled Postoperative Blood Glucose	63	94%	99%	97%
Perioperative Temperature Management	357	100%	100%	100%
Prophylactic Antibiotic Selection	292	100%	99%	99%
Prophylactic Antibiotic Selection (Outpatient)	289	99%	99%	98%
Prophylactic Antibiotic Stopped	286	97%	98%	98%
Prophylactic Antibiotic Timing	294	100%	99%	99%
Prophylactic Antibiotic Timing (Outpatient)	289	100%	98%	98%
Urinary Catheter Removal	101	98%	97%	97%
Survey of Patients' Hospital Experiences				
Area Around Room 'Always' Quiet at Night	300+	49%	67%	61%
Doctors 'Always' Communicated Well	300+	81%	84%	82%
Home Recovery Information Given	300+	86%	86%	85%
Hospital Given 9 or 10 on 10 Point Scale	300+	67%	72%	71%
Meds 'Always' Explained Before Given	300+	65%	66%	64%
Nurses 'Always' Communicated Well	300+	77%	81%	79%
Pain 'Always' Well Controlled	300+	71%	72%	71%
Room and Bathroom 'Always' Clean	300+	67%	72%	73%
Timely Help 'Always' Received	300+	63%	68%	68%
Would Definitely Recommend Hospital	300+	68%	71%	71%
Use of Medical Imaging				
Cardiac Imaging Stress Test before Surgery[1]	-	-	5.1%	5.3%
Combination Abdominal CT Scan	589	9.7%	10.1%	10.5%
Combination Brain/Sinus CT Scan	472	0.8%	2.5%	2.7%
Combination Chest CT Scan	337	4.5%	1.3%	2.7%
Follow-up Mammogram/Ultrasound	2,593	11.4%	8%	8.8%
Lumbar Spine MRI for Low Back Pain	46	39.1%	39%	37.2%

Williamsburg Regional Hospital

500 Nelson Boulevard — Phone: 843-355-8888
Kingstree, SC 29556 — Fax: 843-355-0128
URL: www.w-rh.org
Type: Critical Access Hospitals — Emergency Services: Yes
Ownership: Voluntary non-profit - Private — Beds: 25
Key Personnel:
Emergency Room . . . . Chris Davis, RN
Quality Assurance . . . . Mary Lois Huggins, RN
CEO/President. . . . . Mitch Monsour
Chief of Medical Staff . . . . Frank Trefny

Measure	Cases	This Hosp.	State Avg.	U.S. Avg.
Blood Clot Prevention and Treatment				
Anticoagulation Overlap Therapy[5]	-	-	92%	93%
ICU Venous Thromboembolism Prophylaxis[5]	-	-	94%	92%
Incidence of Potentially Preventable VTE[5]	-	-	8%	10%
UFH with Dosages/Platelet Monitoring[5]	-	-	98%	97%
Venous Thromboembolism Prophylaxis[5]	-	-	88%	85%
Warfarin Therapy Discharge Instructions[5]	-	-	72%	75%
Chest Pain/Possible Heart Attack Care				
Aspirin Given Within 24 Hours of Arrival	-	-	97%	96%
Fibrinolytic Meds Within 30 Min. of Arrival	-	-	68%	58%
Average Time to ECG (minutes)	-	-	5	7
Average Time to Transfer (minutes)	-	-	43	60
Children's Asthma Care				
Received Home Management Plan of Care	-	-	-	88%
Received Reliever Medication	-	-	-	100%
Received Systemic Corticosteroids	-	-	-	100%
Emergency Department				
Admittance Decision Time (minutes)[5]	-	-	94	98
Head CT Results Within 45 Min. of Arrival	-	-	61%	57%
Patients Who Left ER Before Being Seen	-	-	3%	2%
Time from ER Arrival to Admit. (minutes)[5]	-	-	274	274
Time from ER Arrival to Discharge (minutes)	-	-	136	134
Time in ER Before Being Evaluated (minutes)	-	-	33	26
Time to Pain Meds for Fractures (minutes)	-	-	61	57
Heart Attack Care				
Aspirin Given at Discharge[1]	-	-	99%	99%
Fibrinolytic Meds Within 30 Min. of Arrival[7]	-	-	50%	54%
PCI Within 90 Minutes of Arrival[7]	-	-	97%	96%
Statin Prescribed at Discharge[1]	-	-	99%	98%
Heart Failure Care				
ACE Inhibitor or ARB for LVSD	16	88%	98%	97%
Discharge Instructions Given	40	42%	94%	94%
Evaluation of LVS Function	49	86%	99%	99%
Medicare Spending				
Medicare Spending per Patient (ratio)	-	-	0.98	0.98
Pneumonia Care				
Appropriate Initial Antibiotic Given	24	96%	97%	95%
Blood Culture Timing	21	86%	98%	98%
Pregnancy and Delivery Care				
Newborn Deliveries Scheduled Early[5]	-	-	3%	6%
Preventive Care				
Immunization for Influenza[5]	-	-	94%	90%
Immunization for Pneumonia[5]	-	-	95%	92%
Stroke Care				
Anticoagulation Therapy for Atrial Fibrillation[5]	-	-	95%	95%
Antithrombotic Therapy Timing[5]	-	-	98%	98%
Assessed for Rehabilitation[5]	-	-	97%	97%
Discharged on Antithrombotic Therapy[5]	-	-	99%	99%
Discharged on Statin Medication[5]	-	-	94%	94%
Thrombolytic Therapy Timing[5]	-	-	58%	66%
Venous Thromboembolism Prophylaxis[5]	-	-	94%	94%
Written Stroke Educational Materials Given[5]	-	-	91%	88%
Surgical Care Improvement Project				
Appropriate Beta Blocker Usage[1]	-	-	98%	98%
Appropriate VTP Within 24 Hours	12	100%	98%	98%
Controlled Postoperative Blood Glucose[7]	-	-	99%	97%
Perioperative Temperature Management	14	93%	100%	100%
Prophylactic Antibiotic Selection[1]	-	-	99%	99%
Prophylactic Antibiotic Selection (Outpatient)	-	-	99%	98%
Prophylactic Antibiotic Stopped[1]	-	-	98%	98%
Prophylactic Antibiotic Timing[1]	-	-	99%	99%
Prophylactic Antibiotic Timing (Outpatient)	-	-	98%	98%
Urinary Catheter Removal	15	100%	97%	97%
Survey of Patients' Hospital Experiences				
Area Around Room 'Always' Quiet at Night	(a)	72%	67%	61%
Doctors 'Always' Communicated Well	(a)	88%	84%	82%
Home Recovery Information Given	(a)	89%	86%	85%
Hospital Given 9 or 10 on 10 Point Scale	(a)	70%	72%	71%
Meds 'Always' Explained Before Given	(a)	72%	66%	64%
Nurses 'Always' Communicated Well	(a)	83%	81%	79%
Pain 'Always' Well Controlled	(a)	70%	72%	71%
Room and Bathroom 'Always' Clean	(a)	82%	72%	73%
Timely Help 'Always' Received	(a)	77%	68%	68%
Would Definitely Recommend Hospital	(a)	61%	71%	71%
Use of Medical Imaging				
Cardiac Imaging Stress Test before Surgery	-	-	5.1%	5.3%
Combination Abdominal CT Scan	-	-	10.1%	10.5%
Combination Brain/Sinus CT Scan	-	-	2.5%	2.7%
Combination Chest CT Scan	-	-	1.3%	2.7%
Follow-up Mammogram/Ultrasound	-	-	8%	8.8%
Lumbar Spine MRI for Low Back Pain	-	-	39%	37.2%

NOTE: Hospital profiles are in alphabetical order by state, then city, then hospital within the city; Rankings exclude hospitals with less than 25 cases except for patient surveys which excludes hospitals with less than 100 cases; (a) 100-299 cases; (1) The number of cases/patients is too few to report; (2) Data submitted were based on a sample of cases/patients; (3) Results are based on a shorter time period than required; (4) Data suppressed by CMS for one or more quarters; (5) Results are not available for this reporting period; (6) Fewer than 100 patients completed the HCAHPS survey; (7) No cases met the criteria for this measure; (8) The lower limit of the confidence interval cannot be calculated if the number of observed infections equals zero; (9) No data are available from the state/territory for this reporting period; (10) The scores shown reflect fewer than 50 completed surveys; (11) There were discrepancies in the data collection process; (12) This measure does not apply to this hospital for this reporting period; (13) Results cannot be calculated for this reporting period; (14) The results for this state are combined with nearby states to protect confidentiality; Please refer to the User's Guide for a full explanation of data.

Lake City Community Hospital

258 N Ron Mcnair Blvd Phone: 843-374-2036
Lake City, SC 29560 Fax: 843-374-5675
E-mail: leesa@lcchospital.org
URL: www.lcchospital.org
Type: Acute Care Hospitals Emergency Services: Yes
Ownership: Govt - Hospital Dist/Auth Beds: 48

Key Personnel:
CEO/President. . . . . Clarence Bowman
Radiology. . . . . Michael H Brown
Emergency Room . . . . Randall Davis
Quality Assurance . . . . Teresa Dullaghan
Chief of Medical Staff. . . . . Iris Hanna
Infection Control. . . . . Cindy Moon
Operating Room. . . . . Sherry Parrot

Measure	Cases	This Hosp.	State Avg.	U.S. Avg.
Blood Clot Prevention and Treatment				
Anticoagulation Overlap Therapy[2]	11	91%	92%	93%
ICU Venous Thromboembolism Prophylaxis[2,7]	-	-	94%	92%
Incidence of Potentially Preventable VTE[2,7]	-	-	8%	10%
UFH with Dosages/Platelet Monitoring[2,7]	-	-	98%	97%
Venous Thromboembolism Prophylaxis[2]	109	54%	88%	85%
Warfarin Therapy Discharge Instructions[1,2]	-	-	72%	75%
Chest Pain/Possible Heart Attack Care				
Aspirin Given Within 24 Hours of Arrival[3]	14	86%	97%	96%
Fibrinolytic Meds Within 30 Min. of Arrival[1,3]	-	-	68%	58%
Average Time to ECG (minutes)[3]	13	12	5	7
Average Time to Transfer (minutes)[3,7]	-	-	43	60
Children's Asthma Care				
Received Home Management Plan of Care	-	-	-	88%
Received Reliever Medication	-	-	-	100%
Received Systemic Corticosteroids	-	-	-	100%
Emergency Department				
Admittance Decision Time (minutes)[2]	304	70	94	98
Head CT Results Within 45 Min. of Arrival[1,3]	-	-	61%	57%
Patients Who Left ER Before Being Seen	16,814	3%	3%	2%
Time from ER Arrival to Admit. (minutes)[2]	305	255	274	274
Time from ER Arrival to Discharge (minutes)	383	84	136	134
Time in ER Before Being Evaluated (minutes)	385	40	33	26
Time to Pain Meds for Fractures (minutes)	34	61	61	57
Heart Attack Care				
Aspirin Given at Discharge[1]	-	-	99%	99%
Fibrinolytic Meds Within 30 Min. of Arrival[7]	-	-	50%	54%
PCI Within 90 Minutes of Arrival[7]	-	-	97%	96%
Statin Prescribed at Discharge[1]	-	-	99%	98%
Heart Failure Care				
ACE Inhibitor or ARB for LVSD[1]	-	-	98%	97%
Discharge Instructions Given	24	100%	94%	94%
Evaluation of LVS Function	25	100%	99%	99%
Medicare Spending				
Medicare Spending per Patient (ratio)	-	1.09	0.98	0.98
Pneumonia Care				
Appropriate Initial Antibiotic Given	48	92%	97%	95%
Blood Culture Timing	32	88%	98%	98%
Pregnancy and Delivery Care				
Newborn Deliveries Scheduled Early[7]	-	-	3%	6%
Preventive Care				
Immunization for Influenza[2]	288	83%	94%	90%
Immunization for Pneumonia[2]	389	79%	95%	92%
Stroke Care				
Anticoagulation Therapy for Atrial Fibrillation[1]	-	-	95%	95%
Antithrombotic Therapy Timing[1]	-	-	98%	98%
Assessed for Rehabilitation[1]	-	-	97%	97%
Discharged on Antithrombotic Therapy[1]	-	-	99%	99%
Discharged on Statin Medication[1]	-	-	94%	94%
Thrombolytic Therapy Timing[1]	-	-	58%	66%
Venous Thromboembolism Prophylaxis	12	67%	94%	94%
Written Stroke Educational Materials Given[1]	-	-	91%	88%
Surgical Care Improvement Project				
Appropriate Beta Blocker Usage[7]	-	-	98%	98%
Appropriate VTP Within 24 Hours[1]	-	-	98%	98%
Controlled Postoperative Blood Glucose[7]	-	-	99%	97%
Perioperative Temperature Management	11	82%	100%	100%
Prophylactic Antibiotic Selection[1]	-	-	99%	99%
Prophylactic Antibiotic Selection (Outpatient)[5]	-	-	99%	98%
Prophylactic Antibiotic Stopped[1]	-	-	98%	98%
Prophylactic Antibiotic Timing[1]	-	-	99%	99%
Prophylactic Antibiotic Timing (Outpatient)[5]	-	-	98%	98%
Urinary Catheter Removal[1]	-	-	97%	97%
Survey of Patients' Hospital Experiences				
Area Around Room 'Always' Quiet at Night	(a)	67%	67%	61%
Doctors 'Always' Communicated Well	(a)	92%	84%	82%
Home Recovery Information Given	(a)	77%	86%	85%
Hospital Given 9 or 10 on 10 Point Scale	(a)	62%	72%	71%
Meds 'Always' Explained Before Given	(a)	62%	66%	64%
Nurses 'Always' Communicated Well	(a)	81%	81%	79%
Pain 'Always' Well Controlled	(a)	73%	72%	71%
Room and Bathroom 'Always' Clean	(a)	62%	72%	73%
Timely Help 'Always' Received	(a)	74%	68%	68%
Would Definitely Recommend Hospital	(a)	59%	71%	71%
Use of Medical Imaging				
Cardiac Imaging Stress Test before Surgery	82	1.2%	5.1%	5.3%
Combination Abdominal CT Scan	307	10.1%	10.1%	10.5%
Combination Brain/Sinus CT Scan[1]	-	-	2.5%	2.7%
Combination Chest CT Scan	114	10.5%	1.3%	2.7%
Follow-up Mammogram/Ultrasound	571	9.5%	8%	8.8%
Lumbar Spine MRI for Low Back Pain[1]	-	-	39%	37.2%

Springs Memorial Hospital

800 W Meeting St Phone: 803-286-1481
Lancaster, SC 29720 Fax: 803-286-1367
URL: www.springsmemorial.com
Type: Acute Care Hospitals Emergency Services: Yes
Ownership: Proprietary Beds: 200

Key Personnel:
Radiology. . . . . Gautam Agrawal, MD
CEO . . . . Janice Dabney, FACHE
Coronary Care . . . . Annie Fongheiser
Chief of Medical Staff. . . . . RS Glickenberger, MD
Infection Control. . . . . Sharon Jowers
Pediatric In-Patient Care . . . . A Morris, MD
Quality Assurance . . . . Judy Robinson
Operating Room. . . . . Barbara Smith, RN

Measure	Cases	This Hosp.	State Avg.	U.S. Avg.
Blood Clot Prevention and Treatment				
Anticoagulation Overlap Therapy[2]	51	98%	92%	93%
ICU Venous Thromboembolism Prophylaxis[2]	107	100%	94%	92%
Incidence of Potentially Preventable VTE[1,2]	-	-	8%	10%
UFH with Dosages/Platelet Monitoring[2]	35	100%	98%	97%
Venous Thromboembolism Prophylaxis[2]	378	100%	88%	85%
Warfarin Therapy Discharge Instructions[2]	44	100%	72%	75%
Chest Pain/Possible Heart Attack Care				
Aspirin Given Within 24 Hours of Arrival	67	100%	97%	96%
Fibrinolytic Meds Within 30 Min. of Arrival[7]	-	-	68%	58%
Average Time to ECG (minutes)	69	1	5	7
Average Time to Transfer (minutes)	20	54	43	60
Children's Asthma Care				
Received Home Management Plan of Care	-	-	-	88%
Received Reliever Medication	-	-	-	100%
Received Systemic Corticosteroids	-	-	-	100%
Emergency Department				
Admittance Decision Time (minutes)[2]	828	56	94	98
Head CT Results Within 45 Min. of Arrival	16	94%	61%	57%
Patients Who Left ER Before Being Seen	36,613	3%	3%	2%
Time from ER Arrival to Admit. (minutes)[2]	838	215	274	274
Time from ER Arrival to Discharge (minutes)	381	146	136	134
Time in ER Before Being Evaluated (minutes)	417	26	33	26
Time to Pain Meds for Fractures (minutes)	155	58	61	57
Heart Attack Care				
Aspirin Given at Discharge	25	100%	99%	99%
Fibrinolytic Meds Within 30 Min. of Arrival[7]	-	-	50%	54%
PCI Within 90 Minutes of Arrival[7]	-	-	97%	96%
Statin Prescribed at Discharge	24	100%	99%	98%
Heart Failure Care				
ACE Inhibitor or ARB for LVSD	71	100%	98%	97%
Discharge Instructions Given	176	100%	94%	94%
Evaluation of LVS Function	204	100%	99%	99%
Medicare Spending				
Medicare Spending per Patient (ratio)	-	0.97	0.98	0.98
Pneumonia Care				
Appropriate Initial Antibiotic Given	74	100%	97%	95%
Blood Culture Timing	151	99%	98%	98%
Pregnancy and Delivery Care				
Newborn Deliveries Scheduled Early[2]	24	0%	3%	6%
Preventive Care				
Immunization for Influenza[2]	580	99%	94%	90%
Immunization for Pneumonia[2]	703	100%	95%	92%
Stroke Care				
Anticoagulation Therapy for Atrial Fibrillation	12	100%	95%	95%
Antithrombotic Therapy Timing	96	100%	98%	98%
Assessed for Rehabilitation	95	100%	97%	97%
Discharged on Antithrombotic Therapy	92	100%	99%	99%
Discharged on Statin Medication	85	100%	94%	94%
Thrombolytic Therapy Timing[7]	-	-	58%	66%
Venous Thromboembolism Prophylaxis	93	100%	94%	94%
Written Stroke Educational Materials Given	61	100%	91%	88%
Surgical Care Improvement Project				
Appropriate Beta Blocker Usage	31	100%	98%	98%
Appropriate VTP Within 24 Hours	156	100%	98%	98%
Controlled Postoperative Blood Glucose[7]	-	-	99%	97%
Perioperative Temperature Management	166	100%	100%	100%
Prophylactic Antibiotic Selection	91	99%	99%	99%
Prophylactic Antibiotic Selection (Outpatient)	70	100%	99%	98%
Prophylactic Antibiotic Stopped	88	99%	98%	98%
Prophylactic Antibiotic Timing	91	100%	99%	99%
Prophylactic Antibiotic Timing (Outpatient)	70	100%	98%	98%
Urinary Catheter Removal	32	100%	97%	97%
Survey of Patients' Hospital Experiences				
Area Around Room 'Always' Quiet at Night	300+	67%	67%	61%
Doctors 'Always' Communicated Well	300+	84%	84%	82%
Home Recovery Information Given	300+	90%	86%	85%
Hospital Given 9 or 10 on 10 Point Scale	300+	71%	72%	71%
Meds 'Always' Explained Before Given	300+	68%	66%	64%
Nurses 'Always' Communicated Well	300+	83%	81%	79%
Pain 'Always' Well Controlled	300+	74%	72%	71%
Room and Bathroom 'Always' Clean	300+	78%	72%	73%
Timely Help 'Always' Received	300+	71%	68%	68%
Would Definitely Recommend Hospital	300+	64%	71%	71%
Use of Medical Imaging				
Cardiac Imaging Stress Test before Surgery[1]	-	-	5.1%	5.3%
Combination Abdominal CT Scan	394	0.3%	10.1%	10.5%
Combination Brain/Sinus CT Scan	796	4.4%	2.5%	2.7%
Combination Chest CT Scan	208	1.0%	1.3%	2.7%
Follow-up Mammogram/Ultrasound	187	5.3%	8%	8.8%
Lumbar Spine MRI for Low Back Pain	51	31.4%	39%	37.2%

Mcleod Loris Seacoast Hospital

3655 Mitchell Street Phone: 843-716-7000
Loris, SC 29569
Type: Acute Care Hospitals Emergency Services: Yes
Ownership: Voluntary non-profit - Private

Measure	Cases	This Hosp.	State Avg.	U.S. Avg.
Blood Clot Prevention and Treatment				
Anticoagulation Overlap Therapy[2]	42	79%	92%	93%
ICU Venous Thromboembolism Prophylaxis[2]	115	90%	94%	92%
Incidence of Potentially Preventable VTE[1,2]	-	-	8%	10%
UFH with Dosages/Platelet Monitoring[1,2]	-	-	98%	97%
Venous Thromboembolism Prophylaxis[2]	259	86%	88%	85%
Warfarin Therapy Discharge Instructions[2]	29	72%	72%	75%
Chest Pain/Possible Heart Attack Care				
Aspirin Given Within 24 Hours of Arrival	86	93%	97%	96%
Fibrinolytic Meds Within 30 Min. of Arrival[7]	-	-	68%	58%
Average Time to ECG (minutes)	87	10	5	7
Average Time to Transfer (minutes)[1]	-	-	43	60
Children's Asthma Care				
Received Home Management Plan of Care	-	-	-	88%
Received Reliever Medication	-	-	-	100%
Received Systemic Corticosteroids	-	-	-	100%
Emergency Department				
Admittance Decision Time (minutes)[2]	610	56	94	98

NOTE: Hospital profiles are in alphabetical order by state, then city, then hospital within the city; Rankings exclude hospitals with less than 25 cases except for patient surveys which excludes hospitals with less than 100 cases; (a) 100-299 cases; (1) The number of cases/patients is too few to report; (2) Data submitted were based on a sample of cases/patients; (3) Results are based on a shorter time period than required; (4) Data suppressed by CMS for one or more quarters; (5) Results are not available for this reporting period; (6) Fewer than 100 patients completed the HCAHPS survey; (7) No cases met the criteria for this measure; (8) The lower limit of the confidence interval cannot be calculated if the number of observed infections equals zero; (9) No data are available from the state/territory for this reporting period; (10) The scores shown reflect fewer than 50 completed surveys; (11) There were discrepancies in the data collection process; (12) This measure does not apply to this hospital for this reporting period; (13) Results cannot be calculated for this reporting period; (14) The results for this state are combined with nearby states to protect confidentiality; Please refer to the User's Guide for a full explanation of data.

Measure	Cases	This Hosp.	State Avg.	U.S. Avg.
Head CT Results Within 45 Min. of Arrival	17	24%	61%	57%
Patients Who Left ER Before Being Seen	45,632	5%	3%	2%
Time from ER Arrival to Admit. (minutes)[2]	610	222	274	274
Time from ER Arrival to Discharge (minutes)	367	125	136	134
Time in ER Before Being Evaluated (minutes)	384	29	33	26
Time to Pain Meds for Fractures (minutes)	142	50	61	57
Heart Attack Care				
Aspirin Given at Discharge	37	86%	99%	99%
Fibrinolytic Meds Within 30 Min. of Arrival[7]	-	-	50%	54%
PCI Within 90 Minutes of Arrival[7]	-	-	97%	96%
Statin Prescribed at Discharge	35	100%	99%	98%
Heart Failure Care				
ACE Inhibitor or ARB for LVSD	57	96%	98%	97%
Discharge Instructions Given	187	90%	94%	94%
Evaluation of LVS Function	204	97%	99%	99%
Medicare Spending				
Medicare Spending per Patient (ratio)	-	0.94	0.98	0.98
Pneumonia Care				
Appropriate Initial Antibiotic Given	140	96%	97%	95%
Blood Culture Timing	194	97%	98%	98%
Pregnancy and Delivery Care				
Newborn Deliveries Scheduled Early[2]	44	0%	3%	6%
Preventive Care				
Immunization for Influenza[2]	398	95%	94%	90%
Immunization for Pneumonia[2]	530	97%	95%	92%
Stroke Care				
Anticoagulation Therapy for Atrial Fibrillation[1,2]	-	-	95%	95%
Antithrombotic Therapy Timing[2]	59	98%	98%	98%
Assessed for Rehabilitation[2]	54	98%	97%	97%
Discharged on Antithrombotic Therapy[2]	51	96%	99%	99%
Discharged on Statin Medication[2]	45	93%	94%	94%
Thrombolytic Therapy Timing[2,7]	-	-	58%	66%
Venous Thromboembolism Prophylaxis[2]	60	92%	94%	94%
Written Stroke Educational Materials Given[2]	29	86%	91%	88%
Surgical Care Improvement Project				
Appropriate Beta Blocker Usage	94	94%	98%	98%
Appropriate VTP Within 24 Hours	301	95%	98%	98%
Controlled Postoperative Blood Glucose[7]	-	-	99%	97%
Perioperative Temperature Management	324	100%	100%	100%
Prophylactic Antibiotic Selection	201	99%	99%	99%
Prophylactic Antibiotic Selection (Outpatient)	111	95%	99%	98%
Prophylactic Antibiotic Stopped	199	98%	98%	98%
Prophylactic Antibiotic Timing	201	97%	99%	99%
Prophylactic Antibiotic Timing (Outpatient)	112	95%	98%	98%
Urinary Catheter Removal	188	93%	97%	97%
Survey of Patients' Hospital Experiences				
Area Around Room 'Always' Quiet at Night	300+	70%	67%	61%
Doctors 'Always' Communicated Well	300+	83%	84%	82%
Home Recovery Information Given	300+	85%	86%	85%
Hospital Given 9 or 10 on 10 Point Scale	300+	73%	72%	71%
Meds 'Always' Explained Before Given	300+	71%	66%	64%
Nurses 'Always' Communicated Well	300+	83%	81%	79%
Pain 'Always' Well Controlled	300+	74%	72%	71%
Room and Bathroom 'Always' Clean	300+	69%	72%	73%
Timely Help 'Always' Received	300+	69%	68%	68%
Would Definitely Recommend Hospital	300+	71%	71%	71%
Use of Medical Imaging				
Cardiac Imaging Stress Test before Surgery	239	6.3%	5.1%	5.3%
Combination Abdominal CT Scan	1,066	5.8%	10.1%	10.5%
Combination Brain/Sinus CT Scan	1,058	1.3%	2.5%	2.7%
Combination Chest CT Scan	599	1.5%	1.3%	2.7%
Follow-up Mammogram/Ultrasound	2,177	6.9%	8%	8.8%
Lumbar Spine MRI for Low Back Pain	134	34.3%	39%	37.2%

Clarendon Memorial Hospital

10 Hospital Saint Box 550
Manning, SC 29102
Phone: 803-435-8463
Fax: 803-435-3256
URL: www.clarendonhealth.com
Type: Acute Care Hospitals
Emergency Services: Yes
Ownership: Govt - Hospital Dist/Auth
Beds: 56

Key Personnel:
Pediatric Ambulatory Care . . . . . . Beryl Bachus-Keith, MD
Operating Room. . . . . Karen eth Baxley, RN
Chief of Medical Staff. . . . . Beryl Bchus-Keith, MD
Radiology. . . . . Steve Davis, MD
CEO/President. . . . . Edward R Frye, Jr
Infection Control. . . . . Vicki Myers
Quality Assurance . . . . Lin Rainey

Measure	Cases	This Hosp.	State Avg.	U.S. Avg.
Blood Clot Prevention and Treatment				
Anticoagulation Overlap Therapy[2]	21	62%	92%	93%
ICU Venous Thromboembolism Prophylaxis[2]	37	81%	94%	92%
Incidence of Potentially Preventable VTE[1,2]	-	-	8%	10%
UFH with Dosages/Platelet Monitoring[2,7]	-	-	98%	97%
Venous Thromboembolism Prophylaxis[2]	165	65%	88%	85%
Warfarin Therapy Discharge Instructions[2]	16	100%	72%	75%
Chest Pain/Possible Heart Attack Care				
Aspirin Given Within 24 Hours of Arrival	91	82%	97%	96%
Fibrinolytic Meds Within 30 Min. of Arrival[1]	-	-	68%	58%
Average Time to ECG (minutes)	91	17	5	7
Average Time to Transfer (minutes)[1]	-	-	43	60
Children's Asthma Care				
Received Home Management Plan of Care	-	-	-	88%
Received Reliever Medication	-	-	-	100%
Received Systemic Corticosteroids	-	-	-	100%
Emergency Department				
Admittance Decision Time (minutes)[2]	269	95	94	98
Head CT Results Within 45 Min. of Arrival[1]	-	-	61%	57%
Patients Who Left ER Before Being Seen	19,353	6%	3%	2%
Time from ER Arrival to Admit. (minutes)[2]	281	309	274	274
Time from ER Arrival to Discharge (minutes)	411	192	136	134
Time in ER Before Being Evaluated (minutes)	440	68	33	26
Time to Pain Meds for Fractures (minutes)	74	103	61	57
Heart Attack Care				
Aspirin Given at Discharge[1]	-	-	99%	99%
Fibrinolytic Meds Within 30 Min. of Arrival[7]	-	-	50%	54%
PCI Within 90 Minutes of Arrival[7]	-	-	97%	96%
Statin Prescribed at Discharge[1]	-	-	99%	98%
Heart Failure Care				
ACE Inhibitor or ARB for LVSD	41	66%	98%	97%
Discharge Instructions Given	85	100%	94%	94%
Evaluation of LVS Function	101	93%	99%	99%
Medicare Spending				
Medicare Spending per Patient (ratio)	-	0.96	0.98	0.98
Pneumonia Care				
Appropriate Initial Antibiotic Given	56	71%	97%	95%
Blood Culture Timing	61	93%	98%	98%
Pregnancy and Delivery Care				
Newborn Deliveries Scheduled Early[2]	38	5%	3%	6%
Preventive Care				
Immunization for Influenza[2]	267	89%	94%	90%
Immunization for Pneumonia[2]	297	87%	95%	92%
Stroke Care				
Anticoagulation Therapy for Atrial Fibrillation[1]	-	-	95%	95%
Antithrombotic Therapy Timing	34	71%	98%	98%
Assessed for Rehabilitation	28	93%	97%	97%
Discharged on Antithrombotic Therapy	27	85%	99%	99%
Discharged on Statin Medication	21	33%	94%	94%
Thrombolytic Therapy Timing[1]	-	-	58%	66%
Venous Thromboembolism Prophylaxis	33	70%	94%	94%
Written Stroke Educational Materials Given	12	100%	91%	88%
Surgical Care Improvement Project				
Appropriate Beta Blocker Usage	27	85%	98%	98%
Appropriate VTP Within 24 Hours	124	96%	98%	98%
Controlled Postoperative Blood Glucose[7]	-	-	99%	97%
Perioperative Temperature Management	136	96%	100%	100%
Prophylactic Antibiotic Selection	85	96%	99%	99%
Prophylactic Antibiotic Selection (Outpatient)	31	100%	99%	98%
Prophylactic Antibiotic Stopped	85	88%	98%	98%
Prophylactic Antibiotic Timing	85	93%	99%	99%
Prophylactic Antibiotic Timing (Outpatient)	32	97%	98%	98%
Urinary Catheter Removal	88	89%	97%	97%
Survey of Patients' Hospital Experiences				
Area Around Room 'Always' Quiet at Night	(a)	69%	67%	61%
Doctors 'Always' Communicated Well	(a)	85%	84%	82%
Home Recovery Information Given	(a)	85%	86%	85%
Hospital Given 9 or 10 on 10 Point Scale	(a)	72%	72%	71%
Meds 'Always' Explained Before Given	(a)	67%	66%	64%
Nurses 'Always' Communicated Well	(a)	80%	81%	79%
Pain 'Always' Well Controlled	(a)	70%	72%	71%
Room and Bathroom 'Always' Clean	(a)	76%	72%	73%
Timely Help 'Always' Received	(a)	64%	68%	68%
Would Definitely Recommend Hospital	(a)	68%	71%	71%
Use of Medical Imaging				
Cardiac Imaging Stress Test before Surgery	189	3.2%	5.1%	5.3%
Combination Abdominal CT Scan	443	21.0%	10.1%	10.5%
Combination Brain/Sinus CT Scan[1]	-	-	2.5%	2.7%
Combination Chest CT Scan	188	1.6%	1.3%	2.7%
Follow-up Mammogram/Ultrasound	576	8.5%	8%	8.8%
Lumbar Spine MRI for Low Back Pain	60	45.0%	39%	37.2%

East Cooper Medical Center

2000 Hospital Dr
Mount Pleasant, SC 29464
Phone: 843-881-0100
Fax: 843-881-4396
URL: www.eastcoopermedctr.com
Type: Acute Care Hospitals
Emergency Services: Yes
Ownership: Proprietary
Beds: 100

Key Personnel:
CEO/President. . . . . Jack Dusenbery
Quality Assurance . . . . Levvy Hutchinson
Emergency Room . . . . Zack Phillips
Chief of Medical Staff. . . . . William Wilson

Measure	Cases	This Hosp.	State Avg.	U.S. Avg.
Blood Clot Prevention and Treatment				
Anticoagulation Overlap Therapy[2]	15	100%	92%	93%
ICU Venous Thromboembolism Prophylaxis[2]	43	93%	94%	92%
Incidence of Potentially Preventable VTE[1,2]	-	-	8%	10%
UFH with Dosages/Platelet Monitoring[1,2]	-	-	98%	97%
Venous Thromboembolism Prophylaxis[2]	266	93%	88%	85%
Warfarin Therapy Discharge Instructions[1,2]	-	-	72%	75%
Chest Pain/Possible Heart Attack Care				
Aspirin Given Within 24 Hours of Arrival	39	97%	97%	96%
Fibrinolytic Meds Within 30 Min. of Arrival[3,7]	-	-	68%	58%
Average Time to ECG (minutes)	40	3	5	7
Average Time to Transfer (minutes)[1,3]	-	-	43	60
Children's Asthma Care				
Received Home Management Plan of Care	-	-	-	88%
Received Reliever Medication	-	-	-	100%
Received Systemic Corticosteroids	-	-	-	100%
Emergency Department				
Admittance Decision Time (minutes)[2]	263	56	94	98
Head CT Results Within 45 Min. of Arrival[1]	-	-	61%	57%
Patients Who Left ER Before Being Seen	15,261	0%	3%	2%
Time from ER Arrival to Admit. (minutes)[2]	263	215	274	274
Time from ER Arrival to Discharge (minutes)	359	95	136	134
Time in ER Before Being Evaluated (minutes)	380	12	33	26
Time to Pain Meds for Fractures (minutes)	64	26	61	57
Heart Attack Care				
Aspirin Given at Discharge[1,3]	-	-	99%	99%
Fibrinolytic Meds Within 30 Min. of Arrival[3,7]	-	-	50%	54%
PCI Within 90 Minutes of Arrival[3,7]	-	-	97%	96%
Statin Prescribed at Discharge[1,3]	-	-	99%	98%
Heart Failure Care				
ACE Inhibitor or ARB for LVSD[1]	-	-	98%	97%
Discharge Instructions Given	25	100%	94%	94%
Evaluation of LVS Function	48	100%	99%	99%
Medicare Spending				
Medicare Spending per Patient (ratio)	-	1.08	0.98	0.98
Pneumonia Care				
Appropriate Initial Antibiotic Given	48	98%	97%	95%
Blood Culture Timing	70	100%	98%	98%
Pregnancy and Delivery Care				
Newborn Deliveries Scheduled Early[2]	30	3%	3%	6%
Preventive Care				
Immunization for Influenza[2]	510	98%	94%	90%
Immunization for Pneumonia[2]	462	97%	95%	92%
Stroke Care				
Anticoagulation Therapy for Atrial Fibrillation[1]	-	-	95%	95%
Antithrombotic Therapy Timing	14	93%	98%	98%

NOTE: Hospital profiles are in alphabetical order by state, then city, then hospital within the city; Rankings exclude hospitals with less than 25 cases except for patient surveys which excludes hospitals with less than 100 cases; (a) 100-299 cases; (1) The number of cases/patients is too few to report; (2) Data submitted were based on a sample of cases/patients; (3) Results are based on a shorter time period than required; (4) Data suppressed by CMS for one or more quarters; (5) Results are not available for this reporting period; (6) Fewer than 100 patients completed the HCAHPS survey; (7) No cases met the criteria for this measure; (8) The lower limit of the confidence interval cannot be calculated if the number of observed infections equals zero; (9) No data are available from the state/territory for this reporting period; (10) The scores shown reflect fewer than 50 completed surveys; (11) There were discrepancies in the data collection process; (12) This measure does not apply to this hospital for this reporting period; (13) Results cannot be calculated for this reporting period; (14) The results for this state are combined with nearby states to protect confidentiality; Please refer to the User's Guide for a full explanation of data.

Measure	Cases	This Hosp.	State Avg.	U.S. Avg.
Assessed for Rehabilitation	25	100%	97%	97%
Discharged on Antithrombotic Therapy	24	96%	99%	99%
Discharged on Statin Medication[1]	-	-	94%	94%
Thrombolytic Therapy Timing[1]	-	-	58%	66%
Venous Thromboembolism Prophylaxis	28	89%	94%	94%
Written Stroke Educational Materials Given	13	77%	91%	88%
Surgical Care Improvement Project				
Appropriate Beta Blocker Usage	72	100%	98%	98%
Appropriate VTP Within 24 Hours	338	98%	98%	98%
Controlled Postoperative Blood Glucose[7]	-	-	99%	97%
Perioperative Temperature Management	452	100%	100%	100%
Prophylactic Antibiotic Selection	303	100%	99%	99%
Prophylactic Antibiotic Selection (Outpatient)	181	99%	99%	98%
Prophylactic Antibiotic Stopped	301	97%	98%	98%
Prophylactic Antibiotic Timing	303	99%	99%	99%
Prophylactic Antibiotic Timing (Outpatient)	181	100%	98%	98%
Urinary Catheter Removal	264	99%	97%	97%
Survey of Patients' Hospital Experiences				
Area Around Room 'Always' Quiet at Night	300+	74%	67%	61%
Doctors 'Always' Communicated Well	300+	86%	84%	82%
Home Recovery Information Given	300+	88%	86%	85%
Hospital Given 9 or 10 on 10 Point Scale	300+	80%	72%	71%
Meds 'Always' Explained Before Given	300+	65%	66%	64%
Nurses 'Always' Communicated Well	300+	80%	81%	79%
Pain 'Always' Well Controlled	300+	73%	72%	71%
Room and Bathroom 'Always' Clean	300+	76%	72%	73%
Timely Help 'Always' Received	300+	70%	68%	68%
Would Definitely Recommend Hospital	300+	80%	71%	71%
Use of Medical Imaging				
Cardiac Imaging Stress Test before Surgery[1]	-	-	5.1%	5.3%
Combination Abdominal CT Scan	201	8.0%	10.1%	10.5%
Combination Brain/Sinus CT Scan[1]	-	-	2.5%	2.7%
Combination Chest CT Scan	81	7.4%	1.3%	2.7%
Follow-up Mammogram/Ultrasound	1,543	11.3%	8%	8.8%
Lumbar Spine MRI for Low Back Pain[1]	-	-	39%	37.2%

Mount Pleasant Hospital

3500 Highway 17 North
Mount Pleasant, SC 29466
URL: www.rsfh.com
Type: Acute Care Hospitals
Ownership: Voluntary non-profit - Private
Phone: 843-724-2954
Emergency Services: Yes

Measure	Cases	This Hosp.	State Avg.	U.S. Avg.
Blood Clot Prevention and Treatment				
Anticoagulation Overlap Therapy[1,2]	-	-	92%	93%
ICU Venous Thromboembolism Prophylaxis[2]	23	100%	94%	92%
Incidence of Potentially Preventable VTE[1,2]	-	-	8%	10%
UFH with Dosages/Platelet Monitoring[1,2]	-	-	98%	97%
Venous Thromboembolism Prophylaxis[2]	91	99%	88%	85%
Warfarin Therapy Discharge Instructions[1,2]	-	-	72%	75%
Chest Pain/Possible Heart Attack Care				
Aspirin Given Within 24 Hours of Arrival	26	100%	97%	96%
Fibrinolytic Meds Within 30 Min. of Arrival[3,7]	-	-	68%	58%
Average Time to ECG (minutes)	29	4	5	7
Average Time to Transfer (minutes)[1,3]	-	-	43	60
Children's Asthma Care				
Received Home Management Plan of Care	-	-	-	88%
Received Reliever Medication	-	-	-	100%
Received Systemic Corticosteroids	-	-	-	100%
Emergency Department				
Admittance Decision Time (minutes)[2]	227	76	94	98
Head CT Results Within 45 Min. of Arrival[1]	-	-	61%	57%
Patients Who Left ER Before Being Seen	11,528	0%	3%	2%
Time from ER Arrival to Admit. (minutes)[2]	230	196	274	274
Time from ER Arrival to Discharge (minutes)	393	94	136	134
Time in ER Before Being Evaluated (minutes)	413	10	33	26
Time to Pain Meds for Fractures (minutes)	31	36	61	57
Heart Attack Care				
Aspirin Given at Discharge[1,3]	-	-	99%	99%
Fibrinolytic Meds Within 30 Min. of Arrival[3,7]	-	-	50%	54%
PCI Within 90 Minutes of Arrival[3,7]	-	-	97%	96%
Statin Prescribed at Discharge[1,3]	-	-	99%	98%
Heart Failure Care				
ACE Inhibitor or ARB for LVSD[1]	-	-	98%	97%
Discharge Instructions Given	30	100%	94%	94%
Evaluation of LVS Function	35	100%	99%	99%
Medicare Spending				
Medicare Spending per Patient (ratio)	-	0.98	0.98	0.98
Pneumonia Care				
Appropriate Initial Antibiotic Given	25	100%	97%	95%
Blood Culture Timing	35	100%	98%	98%
Pregnancy and Delivery Care				
Newborn Deliveries Scheduled Early	32	3%	3%	6%
Preventive Care				
Immunization for Influenza[2]	249	98%	94%	90%
Immunization for Pneumonia[2]	239	98%	95%	92%
Stroke Care				
Anticoagulation Therapy for Atrial Fibrillation[1]	-	-	95%	95%
Antithrombotic Therapy Timing[1]	-	-	98%	98%
Assessed for Rehabilitation[1]	-	-	97%	97%
Discharged on Antithrombotic Therapy[1]	-	-	99%	99%
Discharged on Statin Medication[1]	-	-	94%	94%
Thrombolytic Therapy Timing[7]	-	-	58%	66%
Venous Thromboembolism Prophylaxis[1]	-	-	94%	94%
Written Stroke Educational Materials Given[1]	-	-	91%	88%
Surgical Care Improvement Project				
Appropriate Beta Blocker Usage[1]	-	-	98%	98%
Appropriate VTP Within 24 Hours	68	100%	98%	98%
Controlled Postoperative Blood Glucose[7]	-	-	99%	97%
Perioperative Temperature Management	94	100%	100%	100%
Prophylactic Antibiotic Selection	55	100%	99%	99%
Prophylactic Antibiotic Selection (Outpatient)	91	99%	99%	98%
Prophylactic Antibiotic Stopped	50	96%	98%	98%
Prophylactic Antibiotic Timing	55	100%	99%	99%
Prophylactic Antibiotic Timing (Outpatient)	91	100%	98%	98%
Urinary Catheter Removal	21	100%	97%	97%
Survey of Patients' Hospital Experiences				
Area Around Room 'Always' Quiet at Night	(a)	74%	67%	61%
Doctors 'Always' Communicated Well	(a)	89%	84%	82%
Home Recovery Information Given	(a)	89%	86%	85%
Hospital Given 9 or 10 on 10 Point Scale	(a)	81%	72%	71%
Meds 'Always' Explained Before Given	(a)	72%	66%	64%
Nurses 'Always' Communicated Well	(a)	86%	81%	79%
Pain 'Always' Well Controlled	(a)	74%	72%	71%
Room and Bathroom 'Always' Clean	(a)	68%	72%	73%
Timely Help 'Always' Received	(a)	72%	68%	68%
Would Definitely Recommend Hospital	(a)	82%	71%	71%
Use of Medical Imaging				
Cardiac Imaging Stress Test before Surgery	128	4.7%	5.1%	5.3%
Combination Abdominal CT Scan	455	8.1%	10.1%	10.5%
Combination Brain/Sinus CT Scan[1]	-	-	2.5%	2.7%
Combination Chest CT Scan	396	0.0%	1.3%	2.7%
Follow-up Mammogram/Ultrasound	695	6.0%	8%	8.8%
Lumbar Spine MRI for Low Back Pain	168	41.1%	39%	37.2%

Carolinas Hospital System Marion

2829 E Hwy 76
Mullins, SC 29574
Type: Acute Care Hospitals
Ownership: Proprietary
Phone: 843-431-2000
Fax: 843-431-2414
Emergency Services: Yes
Beds: 124

Key Personnel:

Chief of Medical Staff.......... Marc G Bahan, Jr, DM
Infection Control............. Sharon Elvington, MD
Quality Assurance .... Gena Jones, RN
Radiology.................... Thomas O Klauber, MD
Pediatric Ambulatory Care ...... Vege R Rao, MD
Pediatric In-Patient Care .... Vege R Rao, MD
Operating Room............. Stephen P Regec, RN
CEO/President............... Gene Tucker

Measure	Cases	This Hosp.	State Avg.	U.S. Avg.
Blood Clot Prevention and Treatment				
Anticoagulation Overlap Therapy[2]	18	67%	92%	93%
ICU Venous Thromboembolism Prophylaxis[2]	96	86%	94%	92%
Incidence of Potentially Preventable VTE[2,7]	-	-	8%	10%
UFH with Dosages/Platelet Monitoring[2,7]	-	-	98%	97%
Venous Thromboembolism Prophylaxis[2]	237	78%	88%	85%
Warfarin Therapy Discharge Instructions[2]	11	82%	72%	75%
Chest Pain/Possible Heart Attack Care				
Aspirin Given Within 24 Hours of Arrival	74	95%	97%	96%
Fibrinolytic Meds Within 30 Min. of Arrival[1]	-	-	68%	58%
Average Time to ECG (minutes)	76	26	5	7
Average Time to Transfer (minutes)[7]	-	-	43	60
Children's Asthma Care				
Received Home Management Plan of Care	-	-	-	88%
Received Reliever Medication	-	-	-	100%
Received Systemic Corticosteroids	-	-	-	100%
Emergency Department				
Admittance Decision Time (minutes)[2]	406	100	94	98
Head CT Results Within 45 Min. of Arrival	13	38%	61%	57%
Patients Who Left ER Before Being Seen	21,089	2%	3%	2%
Time from ER Arrival to Admit. (minutes)[2]	414	282	274	274
Time from ER Arrival to Discharge (minutes)	377	135	136	134
Time in ER Before Being Evaluated (minutes)	413	39	33	26
Time to Pain Meds for Fractures (minutes)	69	64	61	57
Heart Attack Care				
Aspirin Given at Discharge	74	95%	99%	99%
Fibrinolytic Meds Within 30 Min. of Arrival[7]	-	-	50%	54%
PCI Within 90 Minutes of Arrival[7]	-	-	97%	96%
Statin Prescribed at Discharge	70	96%	99%	98%
Heart Failure Care				
ACE Inhibitor or ARB for LVSD	45	96%	98%	97%
Discharge Instructions Given	96	81%	94%	94%
Evaluation of LVS Function	119	100%	99%	99%
Medicare Spending				
Medicare Spending per Patient (ratio)	-	0.96	0.98	0.98
Pneumonia Care				
Appropriate Initial Antibiotic Given	45	96%	97%	95%
Blood Culture Timing	85	99%	98%	98%
Pregnancy and Delivery Care				
Newborn Deliveries Scheduled Early[2]	31	0%	3%	6%
Preventive Care				
Immunization for Influenza[2]	329	93%	94%	90%
Immunization for Pneumonia[2]	389	94%	95%	92%
Stroke Care				
Anticoagulation Therapy for Atrial Fibrillation[1]	-	-	95%	95%
Antithrombotic Therapy Timing	36	97%	98%	98%
Assessed for Rehabilitation	36	94%	97%	97%
Discharged on Antithrombotic Therapy	36	100%	99%	99%
Discharged on Statin Medication	31	84%	94%	94%
Thrombolytic Therapy Timing[7]	-	-	58%	66%
Venous Thromboembolism Prophylaxis	37	86%	94%	94%
Written Stroke Educational Materials Given	21	86%	91%	88%
Surgical Care Improvement Project				
Appropriate Beta Blocker Usage	29	93%	98%	98%
Appropriate VTP Within 24 Hours	106	95%	98%	98%
Controlled Postoperative Blood Glucose[7]	-	-	99%	97%
Perioperative Temperature Management	118	99%	100%	100%
Prophylactic Antibiotic Selection	68	100%	99%	99%
Prophylactic Antibiotic Selection (Outpatient)	12	92%	99%	98%
Prophylactic Antibiotic Stopped	63	90%	98%	98%
Prophylactic Antibiotic Timing	68	100%	99%	99%
Prophylactic Antibiotic Timing (Outpatient)	13	92%	98%	98%
Urinary Catheter Removal	16	88%	97%	97%
Survey of Patients' Hospital Experiences				
Area Around Room 'Always' Quiet at Night	300+	70%	67%	61%
Doctors 'Always' Communicated Well	300+	85%	84%	82%
Home Recovery Information Given	300+	84%	86%	85%
Hospital Given 9 or 10 on 10 Point Scale	300+	65%	72%	71%
Meds 'Always' Explained Before Given	300+	65%	66%	64%
Nurses 'Always' Communicated Well	300+	78%	81%	79%
Pain 'Always' Well Controlled	300+	69%	72%	71%
Room and Bathroom 'Always' Clean	300+	70%	72%	73%
Timely Help 'Always' Received	300+	64%	68%	68%
Would Definitely Recommend Hospital	300+	59%	71%	71%
Use of Medical Imaging				
Cardiac Imaging Stress Test before Surgery	141	4.3%	5.1%	5.3%
Combination Abdominal CT Scan	411	0.7%	10.1%	10.5%
Combination Brain/Sinus CT Scan[1]	-	-	2.5%	2.7%

NOTE: Hospital profiles are in alphabetical order by state, then city, then hospital within the city; Rankings exclude hospitals with less than 25 cases except for patient surveys which excludes hospitals with less than 100 cases; (a) 100-299 cases; (1) The number of cases/patients is too few to report; (2) Data submitted were based on a sample of cases/patients; (3) Results are based on a shorter time period than required; (4) Data suppressed by CMS for one or more quarters; (5) Results are not available for this reporting period; (6) Fewer than 100 patients completed the HCAHPS survey; (7) No cases met the criteria for this measure; (8) The lower limit of the confidence interval cannot be calculated if the number of observed infections equals zero; (9) No data are available from the state/territory for this reporting period; (10) The scores shown reflect fewer than 50 completed surveys; (11) There were discrepancies in the data collection process; (12) This measure does not apply to this hospital for this reporting period; (13) Results cannot be calculated for this reporting period; (14) The results for this state are combined with nearby states to protect confidentiality; Please refer to the User's Guide for a full explanation of data.

Combination Chest CT Scan	95	0.0%	1.3%	2.7%
Follow-up Mammogram/Ultrasound	956	4.4%	8%	8.8%
Lumbar Spine MRI for Low Back Pain	45	46.7%	39%	37.2%

Waccamaw Community Hospital

4070 Highway 17 Bypass — Phone: 843-652-1000
Murrells Inlet, SC 29576 — Fax: 843-652-1700
URL: www.gmhsc.com
Type: Acute Care Hospitals — Emergency Services: Yes
Ownership: Voluntary non-profit - Private — Beds: 111

Key Personnel:
Radiology. . . . . David R Anderson
President/CEO. . . . . Bruce P Bailey
Operating Room. . . . . N Craig Brackett, MD
Emergency Room . . . . Scott Burns
Chief of Medical Staff . . . . Gerald E Harmon, MD
Patient Relations . . . . Pam Maxwell, BSN RN
Cardiac Laboratory. . . . . Robert Pugh
Surgery . . . . David G. Thomas, MD

Measure	Cases	This Hosp.	State Avg.	U.S. Avg.
Blood Clot Prevention and Treatment				
Anticoagulation Overlap Therapy[2]	26	96%	92%	93%
ICU Venous Thromboembolism Prophylaxis[2]	32	94%	94%	92%
Incidence of Potentially Preventable VTE[1,2]	-	-	8%	10%
UFH with Dosages/Platelet Monitoring[2]	12	100%	98%	97%
Venous Thromboembolism Prophylaxis[2]	323	93%	88%	85%
Warfarin Therapy Discharge Instructions[2]	23	91%	72%	75%
Chest Pain/Possible Heart Attack Care				
Aspirin Given Within 24 Hours of Arrival	32	97%	97%	96%
Fibrinolytic Meds Within 30 Min. of Arrival[7]	-	-	68%	58%
Average Time to ECG (minutes)	33	7	5	7
Average Time to Transfer (minutes)[1]	-	-	43	60
Children's Asthma Care				
Received Home Management Plan of Care	-	-	-	88%
Received Reliever Medication	-	-	-	100%
Received Systemic Corticosteroids	-	-	-	100%
Emergency Department				
Admittance Decision Time (minutes)[2]	592	76	94	98
Head CT Results Within 45 Min. of Arrival	17	94%	61%	57%
Patients Who Left ER Before Being Seen	30,738	2%	3%	2%
Time from ER Arrival to Admit. (minutes)[2]	606	242	274	274
Time from ER Arrival to Discharge (minutes)	376	154	136	134
Time in ER Before Being Evaluated (minutes)	379	39	33	26
Time to Pain Meds for Fractures (minutes)	56	57	61	57
Heart Attack Care				
Aspirin Given at Discharge[2]	35	100%	99%	99%
Fibrinolytic Meds Within 30 Min. of Arrival[2,7]	-	-	50%	54%
PCI Within 90 Minutes of Arrival[2,7]	-	-	97%	96%
Statin Prescribed at Discharge[2]	35	94%	99%	98%
Heart Failure Care				
ACE Inhibitor or ARB for LVSD[2]	62	98%	98%	97%
Discharge Instructions Given[2]	146	97%	94%	94%
Evaluation of LVS Function[2]	171	100%	99%	99%
Medicare Spending				
Medicare Spending per Patient (ratio)	-	0.98	0.98	0.98
Pneumonia Care				
Appropriate Initial Antibiotic Given[2]	91	96%	97%	95%
Blood Culture Timing[2]	160	99%	98%	98%
Pregnancy and Delivery Care				
Newborn Deliveries Scheduled Early[2]	23	0%	3%	6%
Preventive Care				
Immunization for Influenza[2]	551	97%	94%	90%
Immunization for Pneumonia[2]	728	98%	95%	92%
Stroke Care				
Anticoagulation Therapy for Atrial Fibrillation[2]	11	91%	95%	95%
Antithrombotic Therapy Timing[2]	64	98%	98%	98%
Assessed for Rehabilitation[2]	71	100%	97%	97%
Discharged on Antithrombotic Therapy[2]	71	100%	99%	99%
Discharged on Statin Medication[2]	50	98%	94%	94%
Thrombolytic Therapy Timing[1,2]	-	-	58%	66%
Venous Thromboembolism Prophylaxis[2]	61	100%	94%	94%
Written Stroke Educational Materials Given[2]	42	93%	91%	88%
Surgical Care Improvement Project				
Appropriate Beta Blocker Usage[2]	105	100%	98%	98%
Appropriate VTP Within 24 Hours[2]	376	99%	98%	98%
Controlled Postoperative Blood Glucose[2,7]	-	-	99%	97%
Perioperative Temperature Management[2]	447	100%	100%	100%
Prophylactic Antibiotic Selection[2]	304	99%	99%	99%
Prophylactic Antibiotic Selection (Outpatient)	64	97%	99%	98%
Prophylactic Antibiotic Stopped[2]	299	100%	98%	98%
Prophylactic Antibiotic Timing[2]	304	99%	99%	99%
Prophylactic Antibiotic Timing (Outpatient)	66	95%	98%	98%
Urinary Catheter Removal[2]	298	98%	97%	97%
Survey of Patients' Hospital Experiences				
Area Around Room 'Always' Quiet at Night	300+	57%	67%	61%
Doctors 'Always' Communicated Well	300+	82%	84%	82%
Home Recovery Information Given	300+	84%	86%	85%
Hospital Given 9 or 10 on 10 Point Scale	300+	79%	72%	71%
Meds 'Always' Explained Before Given	300+	65%	66%	64%
Nurses 'Always' Communicated Well	300+	83%	81%	79%
Pain 'Always' Well Controlled	300+	76%	72%	71%
Room and Bathroom 'Always' Clean	300+	71%	72%	73%
Timely Help 'Always' Received	300+	72%	68%	68%
Would Definitely Recommend Hospital	300+	83%	71%	71%
Use of Medical Imaging				
Cardiac Imaging Stress Test before Surgery	212	8.5%	5.1%	5.3%
Combination Abdominal CT Scan	995	34.3%	10.1%	10.5%
Combination Brain/Sinus CT Scan	951	4.3%	2.5%	2.7%
Combination Chest CT Scan	669	5.5%	1.3%	2.7%
Follow-up Mammogram/Ultrasound	2,078	11.1%	8%	8.8%
Lumbar Spine MRI for Low Back Pain	226	40.7%	39%	37.2%

Grand Strand Regional Medical Center

809 82nd Parkway — Phone: 843-692-1000
Myrtle Beach, SC 29572 — Fax: 843-692-1109
URL: www.grandstrandmed.com
Type: Acute Care Hospitals — Emergency Services: Yes
Ownership: Proprietary — Beds: 219

Key Personnel:
Anesthesiology. . . . . Frederick Bellamy, MD
Emergency Room . . . . Jim Hunter, MD
Infection Control. . . . . Winona McLamb
Intensive Care Unit. . . . . Cheryl Paul
Chief of Medical Staff. . . . . Lyle Shelver, MD
CEO/President. . . . . Doug White

Measure	Cases	This Hosp.	State Avg.	U.S. Avg.
Blood Clot Prevention and Treatment				
Anticoagulation Overlap Therapy[2]	91	100%	92%	93%
ICU Venous Thromboembolism Prophylaxis[2]	107	98%	94%	92%
Incidence of Potentially Preventable VTE[2]	30	3%	8%	10%
UFH with Dosages/Platelet Monitoring[2]	74	100%	98%	97%
Venous Thromboembolism Prophylaxis[2]	343	92%	88%	85%
Warfarin Therapy Discharge Instructions[2]	70	97%	72%	75%
Chest Pain/Possible Heart Attack Care				
Aspirin Given Within 24 Hours of Arrival[3,7]	-	-	97%	96%
Fibrinolytic Meds Within 30 Min. of Arrival[5]	-	-	68%	58%
Average Time to ECG (minutes)[3,7]	-	-	5	7
Average Time to Transfer (minutes)[5]	-	-	43	60
Children's Asthma Care				
Received Home Management Plan of Care	-	-	-	88%
Received Reliever Medication	-	-	-	100%
Received Systemic Corticosteroids	-	-	-	100%
Emergency Department				
Admittance Decision Time (minutes)[2]	881	121	94	98
Head CT Results Within 45 Min. of Arrival	12	83%	61%	57%
Patients Who Left ER Before Being Seen	78,289	1%	3%	2%
Time from ER Arrival to Admit. (minutes)[2]	881	277	274	274
Time from ER Arrival to Discharge (minutes)	436	122	136	134
Time in ER Before Being Evaluated (minutes)	486	16	33	26
Time to Pain Meds for Fractures (minutes)	197	63	61	57
Heart Attack Care				
Aspirin Given at Discharge[2]	299	100%	99%	99%
Fibrinolytic Meds Within 30 Min. of Arrival[2,7]	-	-	50%	54%
PCI Within 90 Minutes of Arrival[2]	72	100%	97%	96%
Statin Prescribed at Discharge[2]	288	99%	99%	98%
Heart Failure Care				
ACE Inhibitor or ARB for LVSD[2]	84	100%	98%	97%
Discharge Instructions Given[2]	262	97%	94%	94%
Evaluation of LVS Function[2]	315	100%	99%	99%
Medicare Spending				
Medicare Spending per Patient (ratio)	-	0.98	0.98	0.98
Pneumonia Care				
Appropriate Initial Antibiotic Given[2]	80	99%	97%	95%
Blood Culture Timing[2]	118	100%	98%	98%
Pregnancy and Delivery Care				
Newborn Deliveries Scheduled Early[2]	29	0%	3%	6%
Preventive Care				
Immunization for Influenza[2]	620	99%	94%	90%
Immunization for Pneumonia[2]	832	96%	95%	92%
Stroke Care				
Anticoagulation Therapy for Atrial Fibrillation[2]	14	93%	95%	95%
Antithrombotic Therapy Timing[2]	87	100%	98%	98%
Assessed for Rehabilitation[2]	104	99%	97%	97%
Discharged on Antithrombotic Therapy[2]	92	100%	99%	99%
Discharged on Statin Medication[2]	79	95%	94%	94%
Thrombolytic Therapy Timing[1,2]	-	-	58%	66%
Venous Thromboembolism Prophylaxis[2]	110	100%	94%	94%
Written Stroke Educational Materials Given[2]	64	98%	91%	88%
Surgical Care Improvement Project				
Appropriate Beta Blocker Usage[2]	266	100%	98%	98%
Appropriate VTP Within 24 Hours[2]	414	100%	98%	98%
Controlled Postoperative Blood Glucose[2]	188	99%	99%	97%
Perioperative Temperature Management[2]	494	100%	100%	100%
Prophylactic Antibiotic Selection[2]	474	100%	99%	99%
Prophylactic Antibiotic Selection (Outpatient)	329	98%	99%	98%
Prophylactic Antibiotic Stopped[2]	448	99%	98%	98%
Prophylactic Antibiotic Timing[2]	474	100%	99%	99%
Prophylactic Antibiotic Timing (Outpatient)	330	98%	98%	98%
Urinary Catheter Removal[2]	427	99%	97%	97%
Survey of Patients' Hospital Experiences				
Area Around Room 'Always' Quiet at Night	300+	60%	67%	61%
Doctors 'Always' Communicated Well	300+	79%	84%	82%
Home Recovery Information Given	300+	83%	86%	85%
Hospital Given 9 or 10 on 10 Point Scale	300+	66%	72%	71%
Meds 'Always' Explained Before Given	300+	57%	66%	64%
Nurses 'Always' Communicated Well	300+	73%	81%	79%
Pain 'Always' Well Controlled	300+	66%	72%	71%
Room and Bathroom 'Always' Clean	300+	66%	72%	73%
Timely Help 'Always' Received	300+	58%	68%	68%
Would Definitely Recommend Hospital	300+	70%	71%	71%
Use of Medical Imaging				
Cardiac Imaging Stress Test before Surgery	740	5.4%	5.1%	5.3%
Combination Abdominal CT Scan	1,546	3.6%	10.1%	10.5%
Combination Brain/Sinus CT Scan	1,465	3.0%	2.5%	2.7%
Combination Chest CT Scan	855	0.9%	1.3%	2.7%
Follow-up Mammogram/Ultrasound	3,875	5.1%	8%	8.8%
Lumbar Spine MRI for Low Back Pain	130	40.8%	39%	37.2%

Newberry County Memorial Hospital

2669 Kinard Saint PO Box 497 — Phone: 803-405-7145
Newberry, SC 29108 — Fax: 803-276-6885
URL: www.newberryhospital.org
Type: Acute Care Hospitals — Emergency Services: Yes
Ownership: Government - Local — Beds: 102

Key Personnel:
CEO/President. . . . . Lynn W Beasley
Infection Control. . . . . Lindy Beaver, RN
Radiology. . . . . Lawrence Lough, MD
Patient Relations . . . . Debra G Roberts
Pediatric Ambulatory Care . . . . . . Tanya Russo, DO
Operating Room. . . . . Kathy Stroud
Coronary Care . . . . Kay Traylor
Intensive Care Unit. . . . . Kay Traylor

Measure	Cases	This Hosp.	State Avg.	U.S. Avg.
Blood Clot Prevention and Treatment				
Anticoagulation Overlap Therapy[1,2]	-	-	92%	93%
ICU Venous Thromboembolism Prophylaxis[2]	54	96%	94%	92%
Incidence of Potentially Preventable VTE[2,7]	-	-	8%	10%
UFH with Dosages/Platelet Monitoring[2,7]	-	-	98%	97%
Venous Thromboembolism Prophylaxis[2]	128	100%	88%	85%
Warfarin Therapy Discharge Instructions[1,2]	-	-	72%	75%
Chest Pain/Possible Heart Attack Care				

NOTE: Hospital profiles are in alphabetical order by state, then city, then hospital within the city; Rankings exclude hospitals with less than 25 cases except for patient surveys which excludes hospitals with less than 100 cases; (a) 100-299 cases; (1) The number of cases/patients is too few to report; (2) Data submitted were based on a sample of cases/patients; (3) Results are based on a shorter time period than required; (4) Data suppressed by CMS for one or more quarters; (5) Results are not available for this reporting period; (6) Fewer than 100 patients completed the HCAHPS survey; (7) No cases met the criteria for this measure; (8) The lower limit of the confidence interval cannot be calculated if the number of observed infections equals zero; (9) No data are available from the state/territory for this reporting period; (10) The scores shown reflect fewer than 50 completed surveys; (11) There were discrepancies in the data collection process; (12) This measure does not apply to this hospital for this reporting period; (13) Results cannot be calculated for this reporting period; (14) The results for this state are combined with nearby states to protect confidentiality; Please refer to the User's Guide for a full explanation of data.

Measure	Cases	This Hosp.	State Avg.	U.S. Avg.
Aspirin Given Within 24 Hours of Arrival	38	95%	97%	96%
Fibrinolytic Meds Within 30 Min. of Arrival[7]	-	-	68%	58%
Average Time to ECG (minutes)	37	5	5	7
Average Time to Transfer (minutes)[7]	-	-	43	60
Children's Asthma Care				
Received Home Management Plan of Care	-	-	-	88%
Received Reliever Medication	-	-	-	100%
Received Systemic Corticosteroids	-	-	-	100%
Emergency Department				
Admittance Decision Time (minutes)[2]	272	73	94	98
Head CT Results Within 45 Min. of Arrival	11	55%	61%	57%
Patients Who Left ER Before Being Seen	21,750	3%	3%	2%
Time from ER Arrival to Admit. (minutes)[2]	285	254	274	274
Time from ER Arrival to Discharge (minutes)	360	99	136	134
Time in ER Before Being Evaluated (minutes)	336	25	33	26
Time to Pain Meds for Fractures (minutes)	87	48	61	57
Heart Attack Care				
Aspirin Given at Discharge[5]	-	-	99%	99%
Fibrinolytic Meds Within 30 Min. of Arrival[5]	-	-	50%	54%
PCI Within 90 Minutes of Arrival[5]	-	-	97%	96%
Statin Prescribed at Discharge[5]	-	-	99%	98%
Heart Failure Care				
ACE Inhibitor or ARB for LVSD[2]	16	100%	98%	97%
Discharge Instructions Given[2]	42	100%	94%	94%
Evaluation of LVS Function[2]	60	100%	99%	99%
Medicare Spending				
Medicare Spending per Patient (ratio)	-	1.00	0.98	0.98
Pneumonia Care				
Appropriate Initial Antibiotic Given[2]	69	96%	97%	95%
Blood Culture Timing[2]	92	99%	98%	98%
Pregnancy and Delivery Care				
Newborn Deliveries Scheduled Early[2]	49	4%	3%	6%
Preventive Care				
Immunization for Influenza[2]	246	100%	94%	90%
Immunization for Pneumonia[2]	275	100%	95%	92%
Stroke Care				
Anticoagulation Therapy for Atrial Fibrillation[2,7]	-	-	95%	95%
Antithrombotic Therapy Timing[2]	17	94%	98%	98%
Assessed for Rehabilitation[2]	17	88%	97%	97%
Discharged on Antithrombotic Therapy[2]	15	100%	99%	99%
Discharged on Statin Medication[1,2]	-	-	94%	94%
Thrombolytic Therapy Timing[1,2]	-	-	58%	66%
Venous Thromboembolism Prophylaxis[2]	18	100%	94%	94%
Written Stroke Educational Materials Given[1,2]	-	-	91%	88%
Surgical Care Improvement Project				
Appropriate Beta Blocker Usage[2]	40	98%	98%	98%
Appropriate VTP Within 24 Hours[2]	135	99%	98%	98%
Controlled Postoperative Blood Glucose[2,7]	-	-	99%	97%
Perioperative Temperature Management[2]	154	99%	100%	100%
Prophylactic Antibiotic Selection[2]	117	98%	99%	99%
Prophylactic Antibiotic Selection (Outpatient)[1]	-	-	99%	98%
Prophylactic Antibiotic Stopped[2]	113	99%	98%	98%
Prophylactic Antibiotic Timing[2]	117	100%	99%	99%
Prophylactic Antibiotic Timing (Outpatient)[1]	-	-	98%	98%
Urinary Catheter Removal[2]	106	100%	97%	97%
Survey of Patients' Hospital Experiences				
Area Around Room 'Always' Quiet at Night	300+	60%	67%	61%
Doctors 'Always' Communicated Well	300+	86%	84%	82%
Home Recovery Information Given	300+	86%	86%	85%
Hospital Given 9 or 10 on 10 Point Scale	300+	74%	72%	71%
Meds 'Always' Explained Before Given	300+	66%	66%	64%
Nurses 'Always' Communicated Well	300+	82%	81%	79%
Pain 'Always' Well Controlled	300+	75%	72%	71%
Room and Bathroom 'Always' Clean	300+	79%	72%	73%
Timely Help 'Always' Received	300+	69%	68%	68%
Would Definitely Recommend Hospital	300+	71%	71%	71%
Use of Medical Imaging				
Cardiac Imaging Stress Test before Surgery	82	2.4%	5.1%	5.3%
Combination Abdominal CT Scan	435	4.6%	10.1%	10.5%
Combination Brain/Sinus CT Scan	410	2.0%	2.5%	2.7%
Combination Chest CT Scan	246	2.8%	1.3%	2.7%
Follow-up Mammogram/Ultrasound	776	8.6%	8%	8.8%
Lumbar Spine MRI for Low Back Pain	80	38.8%	39%	37.2%

Trmc of Orangeburg & Calhoun

3000 Saint Matthews Rd Box 1806
Orangeburg, SC 29115
Phone: 803-533-2460
Fax: 803-395-2304
E-mail: contactus@trmchealth.org
URL: www.trmchealth.org
Type: Acute Care Hospitals
Emergency Services: Yes
Ownership: Government - Local
Beds: 286

Key Personnel:

Radiology. . . . . Sandra Connor
CEO/President. . . . . Thomas C Dandridge, FACHE
Infection Control. . . . . Sonya Ehrnhardt
Chief of Medical Staff. . . . . M Said Nassri, MD
Patient Relations . . . . Sandra Perry
Operating Room. . . . . Martha Plant
Emergency Room . . . . Robert Swetnam, MD
Quality Assurance . . . . Charlie Thiret

Measure	Cases	This Hosp.	State Avg.	U.S. Avg.
Blood Clot Prevention and Treatment				
Anticoagulation Overlap Therapy[2]	84	90%	92%	93%
ICU Venous Thromboembolism Prophylaxis[2]	65	94%	94%	92%
Incidence of Potentially Preventable VTE[2]	15	20%	8%	10%
UFH with Dosages/Platelet Monitoring[2]	51	73%	98%	97%
Venous Thromboembolism Prophylaxis[2]	363	77%	88%	85%
Warfarin Therapy Discharge Instructions[2]	70	67%	72%	75%
Chest Pain/Possible Heart Attack Care				
Aspirin Given Within 24 Hours of Arrival	99	99%	97%	96%
Fibrinolytic Meds Within 30 Min. of Arrival[7]	-	-	68%	58%
Average Time to ECG (minutes)	101	1	5	7
Average Time to Transfer (minutes)	19	50	43	60
Children's Asthma Care				
Received Home Management Plan of Care	-	-	-	88%
Received Reliever Medication	-	-	-	100%
Received Systemic Corticosteroids	-	-	-	100%
Emergency Department				
Admittance Decision Time (minutes)[2]	747	83	94	98
Head CT Results Within 45 Min. of Arrival[1]	-	-	61%	57%
Patients Who Left ER Before Being Seen	60,567	2%	3%	2%
Time from ER Arrival to Admit. (minutes)[2]	756	256	274	274
Time from ER Arrival to Discharge (minutes)	448	150	136	134
Time in ER Before Being Evaluated (minutes)	304	48	33	26
Time to Pain Meds for Fractures (minutes)	119	67	61	57
Heart Attack Care				
Aspirin Given at Discharge	60	97%	99%	99%
Fibrinolytic Meds Within 30 Min. of Arrival[7]	-	-	50%	54%
PCI Within 90 Minutes of Arrival[7]	-	-	97%	96%
Statin Prescribed at Discharge	60	97%	99%	98%
Heart Failure Care				
ACE Inhibitor or ARB for LVSD	104	97%	98%	97%
Discharge Instructions Given	335	93%	94%	94%
Evaluation of LVS Function	383	100%	99%	99%
Medicare Spending				
Medicare Spending per Patient (ratio)	-	0.97	0.98	0.98
Pneumonia Care				
Appropriate Initial Antibiotic Given	126	98%	97%	95%
Blood Culture Timing	226	97%	98%	98%
Pregnancy and Delivery Care				
Newborn Deliveries Scheduled Early[2]	45	2%	3%	6%
Preventive Care				
Immunization for Influenza[2]	527	93%	94%	90%
Immunization for Pneumonia[2]	688	95%	95%	92%
Stroke Care				
Anticoagulation Therapy for Atrial Fibrillation	11	100%	95%	95%
Antithrombotic Therapy Timing	146	98%	98%	98%
Assessed for Rehabilitation	151	99%	97%	97%
Discharged on Antithrombotic Therapy	144	99%	99%	99%
Discharged on Statin Medication	122	96%	94%	94%
Thrombolytic Therapy Timing[1]	-	-	58%	66%
Venous Thromboembolism Prophylaxis	152	95%	94%	94%
Written Stroke Educational Materials Given	81	93%	91%	88%
Surgical Care Improvement Project				
Appropriate Beta Blocker Usage[2]	72	94%	98%	98%
Appropriate VTP Within 24 Hours[2]	239	97%	98%	98%
Controlled Postoperative Blood Glucose[2,7]	-	-	99%	97%
Perioperative Temperature Management[2]	299	100%	100%	100%
Prophylactic Antibiotic Selection[2]	175	99%	99%	99%
Prophylactic Antibiotic Selection (Outpatient)	275	98%	99%	98%
Prophylactic Antibiotic Stopped[2]	173	95%	98%	98%
Prophylactic Antibiotic Timing[2]	178	99%	99%	99%
Prophylactic Antibiotic Timing (Outpatient)	273	99%	98%	98%
Urinary Catheter Removal[2]	95	87%	97%	97%
Survey of Patients' Hospital Experiences				
Area Around Room 'Always' Quiet at Night	300+	68%	67%	61%
Doctors 'Always' Communicated Well	300+	84%	84%	82%
Home Recovery Information Given	300+	82%	86%	85%
Hospital Given 9 or 10 on 10 Point Scale	300+	64%	72%	71%
Meds 'Always' Explained Before Given	300+	67%	66%	64%
Nurses 'Always' Communicated Well	300+	80%	81%	79%
Pain 'Always' Well Controlled	300+	71%	72%	71%
Room and Bathroom 'Always' Clean	300+	72%	72%	73%
Timely Help 'Always' Received	300+	64%	68%	68%
Would Definitely Recommend Hospital	300+	59%	71%	71%
Use of Medical Imaging				
Cardiac Imaging Stress Test before Surgery	151	6.0%	5.1%	5.3%
Combination Abdominal CT Scan	832	7.7%	10.1%	10.5%
Combination Brain/Sinus CT Scan	847	1.9%	2.5%	2.7%
Combination Chest CT Scan	537	0.4%	1.3%	2.7%
Follow-up Mammogram/Ultrasound	789	12.2%	8%	8.8%
Lumbar Spine MRI for Low Back Pain	78	29.5%	39%	37.2%

Cannon Memorial Hospital

123 Medical Park Drive PO Box 188
Pickens, SC 29671
Phone: 864-878-4791
Fax: 864-878-8354
URL: www.cannonhospital.org
Type: Acute Care Hospitals
Emergency Services: Yes
Ownership: Voluntary non-profit - Private
Beds: 55

Key Personnel:

Infection Control. . . . . Donna Anderson, RN
Emergency Room . . . . Michael L Dillard, MD
Quality Assurance . . . . Vicki Livingston, MT
CEO/President. . . . . Norman G Rentz
Operating Room. . . . . Peter Schriver, RN
Chief of Medical Staff. . . . . Martha Seaborn
Intensive Care Unit. . . . . Jean Watson, RN

Measure	Cases	This Hosp.	State Avg.	U.S. Avg.
Blood Clot Prevention and Treatment				
Anticoagulation Overlap Therapy[1,2]	-	-	92%	93%
ICU Venous Thromboembolism Prophylaxis[2]	33	97%	94%	92%
Incidence of Potentially Preventable VTE[2,7]	-	-	8%	10%
UFH with Dosages/Platelet Monitoring[2,7]	-	-	98%	97%
Venous Thromboembolism Prophylaxis[2]	72	93%	88%	85%
Warfarin Therapy Discharge Instructions[1,2]	-	-	72%	75%
Chest Pain/Possible Heart Attack Care				
Aspirin Given Within 24 Hours of Arrival	38	100%	97%	96%
Fibrinolytic Meds Within 30 Min. of Arrival[7]	-	-	68%	58%
Average Time to ECG (minutes)	38	4	5	7
Average Time to Transfer (minutes)	11	44	43	60
Children's Asthma Care				
Received Home Management Plan of Care	-	-	-	88%
Received Reliever Medication	-	-	-	100%
Received Systemic Corticosteroids	-	-	-	100%
Emergency Department				
Admittance Decision Time (minutes)[2]	398	78	94	98
Head CT Results Within 45 Min. of Arrival[1]	-	-	61%	57%
Patients Who Left ER Before Being Seen	20,792	2%	3%	2%
Time from ER Arrival to Admit. (minutes)[2]	400	224	274	274
Time from ER Arrival to Discharge (minutes)	375	88	136	134
Time in ER Before Being Evaluated (minutes)	409	35	33	26
Time to Pain Meds for Fractures (minutes)	55	69	61	57
Heart Attack Care				
Aspirin Given at Discharge[1]	-	-	99%	99%
Fibrinolytic Meds Within 30 Min. of Arrival[7]	-	-	50%	54%
PCI Within 90 Minutes of Arrival[7]	-	-	97%	96%
Statin Prescribed at Discharge[1]	-	-	99%	98%
Heart Failure Care				
ACE Inhibitor or ARB for LVSD[1]	-	-	98%	97%
Discharge Instructions Given	22	100%	94%	94%

NOTE: Hospital profiles are in alphabetical order by state, then city, then hospital within the city; Rankings exclude hospitals with less than 25 cases except for patient surveys which excludes hospitals with less than 100 cases; (a) 100-299 cases; (1) The number of cases/patients is too few to report; (2) Data submitted were based on a sample of cases/patients; (3) Results are based on a shorter time period than required; (4) Data suppressed by CMS for one or more quarters; (5) Results are not available for this reporting period; (6) Fewer than 100 patients completed the HCAHPS survey; (7) No cases met the criteria for this measure; (8) The lower limit of the confidence interval cannot be calculated if the number of observed infections equals zero; (9) No data are available from the state/territory for this reporting period; (10) The scores shown reflect fewer than 50 completed surveys; (11) There were discrepancies in the data collection process; (12) This measure does not apply to this hospital for this reporting period; (13) Results cannot be calculated for this reporting period; (14) The results for this state are combined with nearby states to protect confidentiality; Please refer to the User's Guide for a full explanation of data.

Evaluation of LVS Function	31	97%	99%	99%
Medicare Spending				
Medicare Spending per Patient (ratio)	-	0.99	0.98	0.98
Pneumonia Care				
Appropriate Initial Antibiotic Given	55	100%	97%	95%
Blood Culture Timing	68	99%	98%	98%
Pregnancy and Delivery Care				
Newborn Deliveries Scheduled Early[7]	-	-	3%	6%
Preventive Care				
Immunization for Influenza[2]	287	99%	94%	90%
Immunization for Pneumonia[2]	432	98%	95%	92%
Stroke Care				
Anticoagulation Therapy for Atrial Fibrillation[1,3]	-	-	95%	95%
Antithrombotic Therapy Timing[1,3]	-	-	98%	98%
Assessed for Rehabilitation[1,3]	-	-	97%	97%
Discharged on Antithrombotic Therapy[1,3]	-	-	99%	99%
Discharged on Statin Medication[1,3]	-	-	94%	94%
Thrombolytic Therapy Timing[3,7]	-	-	58%	66%
Venous Thromboembolism Prophylaxis[1,3]	-	-	94%	94%
Written Stroke Educational Materials Given[1,3]	-	-	91%	88%
Surgical Care Improvement Project				
Appropriate Beta Blocker Usage	15	87%	98%	98%
Appropriate VTP Within 24 Hours	46	98%	98%	98%
Controlled Postoperative Blood Glucose[7]	-	-	99%	97%
Perioperative Temperature Management	49	100%	100%	100%
Prophylactic Antibiotic Selection	33	100%	99%	99%
Prophylactic Antibiotic Selection (Outpatient)[1,3]	-	-	99%	98%
Prophylactic Antibiotic Stopped	33	94%	98%	98%
Prophylactic Antibiotic Timing	33	100%	99%	99%
Prophylactic Antibiotic Timing (Outpatient)[1,3]	-	-	98%	98%
Urinary Catheter Removal	37	100%	97%	97%
Survey of Patients' Hospital Experiences				
Area Around Room 'Always' Quiet at Night	(a)	62%	67%	61%
Doctors 'Always' Communicated Well	(a)	83%	84%	82%
Home Recovery Information Given	(a)	86%	86%	85%
Hospital Given 9 or 10 on 10 Point Scale	(a)	69%	72%	71%
Meds 'Always' Explained Before Given	(a)	63%	66%	64%
Nurses 'Always' Communicated Well	(a)	81%	81%	79%
Pain 'Always' Well Controlled	(a)	68%	72%	71%
Room and Bathroom 'Always' Clean	(a)	78%	72%	73%
Timely Help 'Always' Received	(a)	67%	68%	68%
Would Definitely Recommend Hospital	(a)	67%	71%	71%
Use of Medical Imaging				
Cardiac Imaging Stress Test before Surgery[1]	-	-	5.1%	5.3%
Combination Abdominal CT Scan	146	6.8%	10.1%	10.5%
Combination Brain/Sinus CT Scan[1]	-	-	2.5%	2.7%
Combination Chest CT Scan	101	0.0%	1.3%	2.7%
Follow-up Mammogram/Ultrasound	463	14.7%	8%	8.8%
Lumbar Spine MRI for Low Back Pain[1]	-	-	39%	37.2%

Piedmont Medical Center

222 S Herlong Ave
Rock Hill, SC 29730
Phone: 803-329-1234
Fax: 803-329-0979
URL: www.piedmontmedicalcenter.com
Type: Acute Care Hospitals
Emergency Services: Yes
Ownership: Proprietary
Beds: 268

Key Personnel:

Pediatric Ambulatory Care . . . . . . Dexter Cook, MD
Pediatric In-Patient Care . . . . . . Dexter Cook, MD
Operating Room. . . . . Gary Fillers
Quality Assurance . . . . Janet Griewe
Emergency Room . . . . Wilma Jenkins
CEO/President. . . . . Bill Masterton
Radiology. . . . . Howard Snider, MD
Chief of Medical Staff . . . . James Wood, MD

Measure	Cases	This Hosp.	State Avg.	U.S. Avg.
Blood Clot Prevention and Treatment				
Anticoagulation Overlap Therapy[2]	141	88%	92%	93%
ICU Venous Thromboembolism Prophylaxis[2]	78	86%	94%	92%
Incidence of Potentially Preventable VTE[2]	13	15%	8%	10%
UFH with Dosages/Platelet Monitoring[2]	57	100%	98%	97%
Venous Thromboembolism Prophylaxis[2]	368	83%	88%	85%
Warfarin Therapy Discharge Instructions[2]	103	70%	72%	75%
Chest Pain/Possible Heart Attack Care				
Aspirin Given Within 24 Hours of Arrival[1]	-	-	97%	96%
Fibrinolytic Meds Within 30 Min. of Arrival[3,7]	-	-	68%	58%
Average Time to ECG (minutes)[1]	-	-	5	7
Average Time to Transfer (minutes)[3,7]	-	-	43	60
Children's Asthma Care				
Received Home Management Plan of Care	-	-	-	88%
Received Reliever Medication	-	-	-	100%
Received Systemic Corticosteroids	-	-	-	100%
Emergency Department				
Admittance Decision Time (minutes)[2]	646	163	94	98
Head CT Results Within 45 Min. of Arrival	13	69%	61%	57%
Patients Who Left ER Before Being Seen	67,661	3%	3%	2%
Time from ER Arrival to Admit. (minutes)[2]	651	324	274	274
Time from ER Arrival to Discharge (minutes)	331	175	136	134
Time in ER Before Being Evaluated (minutes)	365	36	33	26
Time to Pain Meds for Fractures (minutes)	214	76	61	57
Heart Attack Care				
Aspirin Given at Discharge	412	99%	99%	99%
Fibrinolytic Meds Within 30 Min. of Arrival[1]	-	-	50%	54%
PCI Within 90 Minutes of Arrival	63	95%	97%	96%
Statin Prescribed at Discharge	400	100%	99%	98%
Heart Failure Care				
ACE Inhibitor or ARB for LVSD	117	100%	98%	97%
Discharge Instructions Given	328	98%	94%	94%
Evaluation of LVS Function	384	99%	99%	99%
Medicare Spending				
Medicare Spending per Patient (ratio)	-	1.05	0.98	0.98
Pneumonia Care				
Appropriate Initial Antibiotic Given[2]	118	93%	97%	95%
Blood Culture Timing[2]	129	98%	98%	98%
Pregnancy and Delivery Care				
Newborn Deliveries Scheduled Early[2]	41	5%	3%	6%
Preventive Care				
Immunization for Influenza[2]	545	90%	94%	90%
Immunization for Pneumonia[2]	679	93%	95%	92%
Stroke Care				
Anticoagulation Therapy for Atrial Fibrillation	18	94%	95%	95%
Antithrombotic Therapy Timing	175	100%	98%	98%
Assessed for Rehabilitation	182	99%	97%	97%
Discharged on Antithrombotic Therapy	175	100%	99%	99%
Discharged on Statin Medication	139	98%	94%	94%
Thrombolytic Therapy Timing[1]	-	-	58%	66%
Venous Thromboembolism Prophylaxis	180	97%	94%	94%
Written Stroke Educational Materials Given	109	98%	91%	88%
Surgical Care Improvement Project				
Appropriate Beta Blocker Usage[2]	249	93%	98%	98%
Appropriate VTP Within 24 Hours[2]	484	98%	98%	98%
Controlled Postoperative Blood Glucose[2]	101	96%	99%	97%
Perioperative Temperature Management[2]	550	100%	100%	100%
Prophylactic Antibiotic Selection[2]	498	99%	99%	99%
Prophylactic Antibiotic Selection (Outpatient)	461	98%	99%	98%
Prophylactic Antibiotic Stopped[2]	485	96%	98%	98%
Prophylactic Antibiotic Timing[2]	498	99%	99%	99%
Prophylactic Antibiotic Timing (Outpatient)	465	98%	98%	98%
Urinary Catheter Removal[2]	476	97%	97%	97%
Survey of Patients' Hospital Experiences				
Area Around Room 'Always' Quiet at Night	300+	59%	67%	61%
Doctors 'Always' Communicated Well	300+	81%	84%	82%
Home Recovery Information Given	300+	85%	86%	85%
Hospital Given 9 or 10 on 10 Point Scale	300+	65%	72%	71%
Meds 'Always' Explained Before Given	300+	61%	66%	64%
Nurses 'Always' Communicated Well	300+	78%	81%	79%
Pain 'Always' Well Controlled	300+	69%	72%	71%
Room and Bathroom 'Always' Clean	300+	65%	72%	73%
Timely Help 'Always' Received	300+	64%	68%	68%
Would Definitely Recommend Hospital	300+	63%	71%	71%
Use of Medical Imaging				
Cardiac Imaging Stress Test before Surgery[1]	-	-	5.1%	5.3%
Combination Abdominal CT Scan	1,223	3.2%	10.1%	10.5%
Combination Brain/Sinus CT Scan	1,047	1.2%	2.5%	2.7%
Combination Chest CT Scan	643	0.0%	1.3%	2.7%
Follow-up Mammogram/Ultrasound	2,179	10.4%	8%	8.8%
Lumbar Spine MRI for Low Back Pain	102	31.4%	39%	37.2%

Oconee Medical Center

298 Memorial Drive
Seneca, SC 29672
Phone: 864-882-3351
Fax: 864-885-7391
URL: www.oconeememorial.org
Type: Acute Care Hospitals
Emergency Services: Yes
Ownership: Voluntary non-profit - Private
Beds: 160

Key Personnel:

Radiology. . . . . Bonnie Anderson
Quality Assurance . . . . Jane Bryant
Chief of Medical Staff . . . . Raza Hassan, MD
Emergency Room . . . . Patrick Johannes
Chairman/CEO . . . . Rick Phillips
CEO/President. . . . . Jeanne L Ward

Measure	Cases	This Hosp.	State Avg.	U.S. Avg.
Blood Clot Prevention and Treatment				
Anticoagulation Overlap Therapy[2]	34	82%	92%	93%
ICU Venous Thromboembolism Prophylaxis[2]	48	85%	94%	92%
Incidence of Potentially Preventable VTE[2]	12	0%	8%	10%
UFH with Dosages/Platelet Monitoring[1,2]	-	-	98%	97%
Venous Thromboembolism Prophylaxis[2]	329	75%	88%	85%
Warfarin Therapy Discharge Instructions[2]	19	5%	72%	75%
Chest Pain/Possible Heart Attack Care				
Aspirin Given Within 24 Hours of Arrival	73	100%	97%	96%
Fibrinolytic Meds Within 30 Min. of Arrival[7]	-	-	68%	58%
Average Time to ECG (minutes)	73	10	5	7
Average Time to Transfer (minutes)	18	44	43	60
Children's Asthma Care				
Received Home Management Plan of Care	-	-	-	88%
Received Reliever Medication	-	-	-	100%
Received Systemic Corticosteroids	-	-	-	100%
Emergency Department				
Admittance Decision Time (minutes)[2]	782	77	94	98
Head CT Results Within 45 Min. of Arrival	15	33%	61%	57%
Patients Who Left ER Before Being Seen	40,285	2%	3%	2%
Time from ER Arrival to Admit. (minutes)[2]	783	233	274	274
Time from ER Arrival to Discharge (minutes)	343	138	136	134
Time in ER Before Being Evaluated (minutes)	344	68	33	26
Time to Pain Meds for Fractures (minutes)	150	54	61	57
Heart Attack Care				
Aspirin Given at Discharge	32	100%	99%	99%
Fibrinolytic Meds Within 30 Min. of Arrival[7]	-	-	50%	54%
PCI Within 90 Minutes of Arrival[7]	-	-	97%	96%
Statin Prescribed at Discharge	29	90%	99%	98%
Heart Failure Care				
ACE Inhibitor or ARB for LVSD	51	94%	98%	97%
Discharge Instructions Given	145	83%	94%	94%
Evaluation of LVS Function	173	100%	99%	99%
Medicare Spending				
Medicare Spending per Patient (ratio)	-	0.96	0.98	0.98
Pneumonia Care				
Appropriate Initial Antibiotic Given	265	96%	97%	95%
Blood Culture Timing	308	96%	98%	98%
Pregnancy and Delivery Care				
Newborn Deliveries Scheduled Early	36	0%	3%	6%
Preventive Care				
Immunization for Influenza[2]	547	99%	94%	90%
Immunization for Pneumonia[2]	735	99%	95%	92%
Stroke Care				
Anticoagulation Therapy for Atrial Fibrillation[1]	-	-	95%	95%
Antithrombotic Therapy Timing	54	98%	98%	98%
Assessed for Rehabilitation	56	95%	97%	97%
Discharged on Antithrombotic Therapy	52	100%	99%	99%
Discharged on Statin Medication	45	67%	94%	94%
Thrombolytic Therapy Timing[1]	-	-	58%	66%
Venous Thromboembolism Prophylaxis	56	75%	94%	94%
Written Stroke Educational Materials Given	28	18%	91%	88%
Surgical Care Improvement Project				
Appropriate Beta Blocker Usage[2]	71	93%	98%	98%
Appropriate VTP Within 24 Hours[2]	242	99%	98%	98%
Controlled Postoperative Blood Glucose[2,7]	-	-	99%	97%
Perioperative Temperature Management[2]	274	99%	100%	100%
Prophylactic Antibiotic Selection[2]	175	99%	99%	99%

NOTE: Hospital profiles are in alphabetical order by state, then city, then hospital within the city; Rankings exclude hospitals with less than 25 cases except for patient surveys which excludes hospitals with less than 100 cases; (a) 100-299 cases; (1) The number of cases/patients is too few to report; (2) Data submitted were based on a sample of cases/patients; (3) Results are based on a shorter time period than required; (4) Data suppressed by CMS for one or more quarters; (5) Results are not available for this reporting period; (6) Fewer than 100 patients completed the HCAHPS survey; (7) No cases met the criteria for this measure; (8) The lower limit of the confidence interval cannot be calculated if the number of observed infections equals zero; (9) No data are available from the state/territory for this reporting period; (10) The scores shown reflect fewer than 50 completed surveys; (11) There were discrepancies in the data collection process; (12) This measure does not apply to this hospital for this reporting period; (13) Results cannot be calculated for this reporting period; (14) The results for this state are combined with nearby states to protect confidentiality; Please refer to the User's Guide for a full explanation of data.

Measure	Cases	This Hosp.	State Avg.	U.S. Avg.
Prophylactic Antibiotic Selection (Outpatient)	94	99%	99%	98%
Prophylactic Antibiotic Stopped[2]	166	99%	98%	98%
Prophylactic Antibiotic Timing[2]	175	99%	99%	99%
Prophylactic Antibiotic Timing (Outpatient)	96	97%	98%	98%
Urinary Catheter Removal[2]	190	95%	97%	97%
Survey of Patients' Hospital Experiences				
Area Around Room 'Always' Quiet at Night	300+	69%	67%	61%
Doctors 'Always' Communicated Well	300+	83%	84%	82%
Home Recovery Information Given	300+	85%	86%	85%
Hospital Given 9 or 10 on 10 Point Scale	300+	70%	72%	71%
Meds 'Always' Explained Before Given	300+	64%	66%	64%
Nurses 'Always' Communicated Well	300+	80%	81%	79%
Pain 'Always' Well Controlled	300+	73%	72%	71%
Room and Bathroom 'Always' Clean	300+	69%	72%	73%
Timely Help 'Always' Received	300+	66%	68%	68%
Would Definitely Recommend Hospital	300+	67%	71%	71%
Use of Medical Imaging				
Cardiac Imaging Stress Test before Surgery	685	3.5%	5.1%	5.3%
Combination Abdominal CT Scan	818	6.5%	10.1%	10.5%
Combination Brain/Sinus CT Scan	794	1.5%	2.5%	2.7%
Combination Chest CT Scan	413	1.9%	1.3%	2.7%
Follow-up Mammogram/Ultrasound	1,016	13.9%	8%	8.8%
Lumbar Spine MRI for Low Back Pain	93	44.1%	39%	37.2%

GHS - Hillcrest Memorial Hospital

729 South East Main Street
Simpsonville, SC 29681
Phone: 864-454-6151
Fax: 864-967-6147
URL: www.ghs.org
Type: Acute Care Hospitals
Emergency Services: Yes
Ownership: Govt - Hospital Dist/Auth
Beds: 43

Key Personnel:

Quality Assurance . . . . Lynette Ali
Operating Room. . . . . Alice Bagley
Anesthesiology. . . . . Thomas Helm
Infection Control . . . . Judy Major
Chief of Medical Staff . . . . David C Silkiner, MD

Measure	Cases	This Hosp.	State Avg.	U.S. Avg.
Blood Clot Prevention and Treatment				
Anticoagulation Overlap Therapy[2]	19	89%	92%	93%
ICU Venous Thromboembolism Prophylaxis[2]	51	94%	94%	92%
Incidence of Potentially Preventable VTE[1,2]	-	-	8%	10%
UFH with Dosages/Platelet Monitoring[1,2]	-	-	98%	97%
Venous Thromboembolism Prophylaxis[2]	178	98%	88%	85%
Warfarin Therapy Discharge Instructions[2]	17	0%	72%	75%
Chest Pain/Possible Heart Attack Care				
Aspirin Given Within 24 Hours of Arrival	82	99%	97%	96%
Fibrinolytic Meds Within 30 Min. of Arrival[7]	-	-	68%	58%
Average Time to ECG (minutes)	83	1	5	7
Average Time to Transfer (minutes)	13	21	43	60
Children's Asthma Care				
Received Home Management Plan of Care	-	-	-	88%
Received Reliever Medication	-	-	-	100%
Received Systemic Corticosteroids	-	-	-	100%
Emergency Department				
Admittance Decision Time (minutes)[2]	312	111	94	98
Head CT Results Within 45 Min. of Arrival[1]	-	-	61%	57%
Patients Who Left ER Before Being Seen	30,710	2%	3%	2%
Time from ER Arrival to Admit. (minutes)[2]	316	316	274	274
Time from ER Arrival to Discharge (minutes)	372	134	136	134
Time in ER Before Being Evaluated (minutes)	353	69	33	26
Time to Pain Meds for Fractures (minutes)	105	64	61	57
Heart Attack Care				
Aspirin Given at Discharge[3,7]	-	-	99%	99%
Fibrinolytic Meds Within 30 Min. of Arrival[3,7]	-	-	50%	54%
PCI Within 90 Minutes of Arrival[3,7]	-	-	97%	96%
Statin Prescribed at Discharge[3,7]	-	-	99%	98%
Heart Failure Care				
ACE Inhibitor or ARB for LVSD[1]	-	-	98%	97%
Discharge Instructions Given	33	97%	94%	94%
Evaluation of LVS Function	41	100%	99%	99%
Medicare Spending				
Medicare Spending per Patient (ratio)	-	0.91	0.98	0.98
Pneumonia Care				
Appropriate Initial Antibiotic Given	91	99%	97%	95%
Blood Culture Timing	118	99%	98%	98%
Pregnancy and Delivery Care				
Newborn Deliveries Scheduled Early[2,7]	-	-	3%	6%
Preventive Care				
Immunization for Influenza[2]	310	97%	94%	90%
Immunization for Pneumonia[2]	396	97%	95%	92%
Stroke Care				
Anticoagulation Therapy for Atrial Fibrillation[2,7]	-	-	95%	95%
Antithrombotic Therapy Timing[1,2]	-	-	98%	98%
Assessed for Rehabilitation[1,2]	-	-	97%	97%
Discharged on Antithrombotic Therapy[1,2]	-	-	99%	99%
Discharged on Statin Medication[1,2]	-	-	94%	94%
Thrombolytic Therapy Timing[2,7]	-	-	58%	66%
Venous Thromboembolism Prophylaxis[1,2]	-	-	94%	94%
Written Stroke Educational Materials Given[1,2]	-	-	91%	88%
Surgical Care Improvement Project				
Appropriate Beta Blocker Usage[2]	67	99%	98%	98%
Appropriate VTP Within 24 Hours[2]	236	99%	98%	98%
Controlled Postoperative Blood Glucose[2,7]	-	-	99%	97%
Perioperative Temperature Management[2]	243	100%	100%	100%
Prophylactic Antibiotic Selection[2]	172	99%	99%	99%
Prophylactic Antibiotic Selection (Outpatient)[1]	-	-	99%	98%
Prophylactic Antibiotic Stopped[2]	165	100%	98%	98%
Prophylactic Antibiotic Timing[2]	172	99%	99%	99%
Prophylactic Antibiotic Timing (Outpatient)[1]	-	-	98%	98%
Urinary Catheter Removal[2]	226	97%	97%	97%
Survey of Patients' Hospital Experiences				
Area Around Room 'Always' Quiet at Night	300+	71%	67%	61%
Doctors 'Always' Communicated Well	300+	86%	84%	82%
Home Recovery Information Given	300+	89%	86%	85%
Hospital Given 9 or 10 on 10 Point Scale	300+	77%	72%	71%
Meds 'Always' Explained Before Given	300+	64%	66%	64%
Nurses 'Always' Communicated Well	300+	82%	81%	79%
Pain 'Always' Well Controlled	300+	73%	72%	71%
Room and Bathroom 'Always' Clean	300+	75%	72%	73%
Timely Help 'Always' Received	300+	68%	68%	68%
Would Definitely Recommend Hospital	300+	79%	71%	71%
Use of Medical Imaging				
Cardiac Imaging Stress Test before Surgery	312	4.2%	5.1%	5.3%
Combination Abdominal CT Scan	474	5.5%	10.1%	10.5%
Combination Brain/Sinus CT Scan[1]	-	-	2.5%	2.7%
Combination Chest CT Scan	331	0.0%	1.3%	2.7%
Follow-up Mammogram/Ultrasound	767	9.0%	8%	8.8%
Lumbar Spine MRI for Low Back Pain	102	39.2%	39%	37.2%

Mary Black Memorial Hospital

1700 Skylyn Dr Box 3217
Spartanburg, SC 29307
Phone: 864-573-3000
Fax: 864-573-3454
E-mail: webmaster@maryblack.org
URL: www.maryblackhealthsystem.com
Type: Acute Care Hospitals
Emergency Services: Yes
Ownership: Proprietary
Beds: 226

Key Personnel:

Pediatric Ambulatory Care . . . . . . William Burns, MD
Pediatric In-Patient Care . . . . William Burns, MD
Operating Room. . . . . Ernest Camp
Emergency Room . . . . Deepak Malhan
Quality Assurance . . . . Diane Parker, RN
Chief of Medical Staff . . . . Vickie Shehan
CEO/President. . . . . Phillip L Wright

Measure	Cases	This Hosp.	State Avg.	U.S. Avg.
Blood Clot Prevention and Treatment				
Anticoagulation Overlap Therapy[2]	45	96%	92%	93%
ICU Venous Thromboembolism Prophylaxis[2]	82	96%	94%	92%
Incidence of Potentially Preventable VTE[2]	11	0%	8%	10%
UFH with Dosages/Platelet Monitoring[2]	46	100%	98%	97%
Venous Thromboembolism Prophylaxis[2]	348	97%	88%	85%
Warfarin Therapy Discharge Instructions[2]	26	88%	72%	75%
Chest Pain/Possible Heart Attack Care				
Aspirin Given Within 24 Hours of Arrival	36	94%	97%	96%
Fibrinolytic Meds Within 30 Min. of Arrival[7]	-	-	68%	58%
Average Time to ECG (minutes)	35	4	5	7
Average Time to Transfer (minutes)[1]	-	-	43	60
Children's Asthma Care				
Received Home Management Plan of Care	-	-	-	88%
Received Reliever Medication	-	-	-	100%
Received Systemic Corticosteroids	-	-	-	100%
Emergency Department				
Admittance Decision Time (minutes)[2]	625	149	94	98
Head CT Results Within 45 Min. of Arrival[1]	-	-	61%	57%
Patients Who Left ER Before Being Seen	39,090	4%	3%	2%
Time from ER Arrival to Admit. (minutes)[2]	635	356	274	274
Time from ER Arrival to Discharge (minutes)	403	144	136	134
Time in ER Before Being Evaluated (minutes)	418	45	33	26
Time to Pain Meds for Fractures (minutes)	91	79	61	57
Heart Attack Care				
Aspirin Given at Discharge[1]	-	-	99%	99%
Fibrinolytic Meds Within 30 Min. of Arrival[7]	-	-	50%	54%
PCI Within 90 Minutes of Arrival[7]	-	-	97%	96%
Statin Prescribed at Discharge[1]	-	-	99%	98%
Heart Failure Care				
ACE Inhibitor or ARB for LVSD	26	100%	98%	97%
Discharge Instructions Given	90	93%	94%	94%
Evaluation of LVS Function	107	99%	99%	99%
Medicare Spending				
Medicare Spending per Patient (ratio)	-	1.02	0.98	0.98
Pneumonia Care				
Appropriate Initial Antibiotic Given	148	97%	97%	95%
Blood Culture Timing	275	99%	98%	98%
Pregnancy and Delivery Care				
Newborn Deliveries Scheduled Early[2]	31	0%	3%	6%
Preventive Care				
Immunization for Influenza[2]	578	97%	94%	90%
Immunization for Pneumonia[2]	740	99%	95%	92%
Stroke Care				
Anticoagulation Therapy for Atrial Fibrillation[1]	-	-	95%	95%
Antithrombotic Therapy Timing	68	99%	98%	98%
Assessed for Rehabilitation	74	93%	97%	97%
Discharged on Antithrombotic Therapy	68	100%	99%	99%
Discharged on Statin Medication	50	94%	94%	94%
Thrombolytic Therapy Timing[1]	-	-	58%	66%
Venous Thromboembolism Prophylaxis	75	97%	94%	94%
Written Stroke Educational Materials Given	41	98%	91%	88%
Surgical Care Improvement Project				
Appropriate Beta Blocker Usage	157	100%	98%	98%
Appropriate VTP Within 24 Hours	471	98%	98%	98%
Controlled Postoperative Blood Glucose[7]	-	-	99%	97%
Perioperative Temperature Management	535	100%	100%	100%
Prophylactic Antibiotic Selection	387	100%	99%	99%
Prophylactic Antibiotic Selection (Outpatient)	233	99%	99%	98%
Prophylactic Antibiotic Stopped	368	98%	98%	98%
Prophylactic Antibiotic Timing	387	99%	99%	99%
Prophylactic Antibiotic Timing (Outpatient)	233	98%	98%	98%
Urinary Catheter Removal	338	96%	97%	97%
Survey of Patients' Hospital Experiences				
Area Around Room 'Always' Quiet at Night	300+	73%	67%	61%
Doctors 'Always' Communicated Well	300+	84%	84%	82%
Home Recovery Information Given	300+	88%	86%	85%
Hospital Given 9 or 10 on 10 Point Scale	300+	78%	72%	71%
Meds 'Always' Explained Before Given	300+	69%	66%	64%
Nurses 'Always' Communicated Well	300+	82%	81%	79%
Pain 'Always' Well Controlled	300+	74%	72%	71%
Room and Bathroom 'Always' Clean	300+	72%	72%	73%
Timely Help 'Always' Received	300+	72%	68%	68%
Would Definitely Recommend Hospital	300+	78%	71%	71%
Use of Medical Imaging				
Cardiac Imaging Stress Test before Surgery	91	3.3%	5.1%	5.3%
Combination Abdominal CT Scan	557	4.3%	10.1%	10.5%
Combination Brain/Sinus CT Scan	594	4.7%	2.5%	2.7%
Combination Chest CT Scan	235	0.9%	1.3%	2.7%
Follow-up Mammogram/Ultrasound	1,660	6.9%	8%	8.8%
Lumbar Spine MRI for Low Back Pain	80	40.0%	39%	37.2%

NOTE: Hospital profiles are in alphabetical order by state, then city, then hospital within the city; Rankings exclude hospitals with less than 25 cases except for patient surveys which excludes hospitals with less than 100 cases; (a) 100-299 cases; (1) The number of cases/patients is too few to report; (2) Data submitted were based on a sample of cases/patients; (3) Results are based on a shorter time period than required; (4) Data suppressed by CMS for one or more quarters; (5) Results are not available for this reporting period; (6) Fewer than 100 patients completed the HCAHPS survey; (7) No cases met the criteria for this measure; (8) The lower limit of the confidence interval cannot be calculated if the number of observed infections equals zero; (9) No data are available from the state/territory for this reporting period; (10) The scores shown reflect fewer than 50 completed surveys; (11) There were discrepancies in the data collection process; (12) This measure does not apply to this hospital for this reporting period; (13) Results cannot be calculated for this reporting period; (14) The results for this state are combined with nearby states to protect confidentiality; Please refer to the User's Guide for a full explanation of data.

Spartanburg Regional Medical Center

101 E Wood St | Phone: 864-560-6000
Spartanburg, SC 29303 | Fax: 864-560-6001
URL: www.srhs.com
Type: Acute Care Hospitals | Emergency Services: Yes
Ownership: Government - Local | Beds: 588

Key Personnel:
CEO/President. . . . . Ingo Angermeier
Infection Control. . . . . Lynn Cromer
Operating Room. . . . . Tonie Edwards
Pediatric Ambulatory Care . . . . . . Dennis Jurs, MD
Pediatric In-Patient Care . . . . Dennis Jurs, MD
Radiology. . . . . Noel Rhodes
Chief of Medical Staff. . . . . Robert Riehle, MD
Quality Assurance . . . . Cindy Shifflett

Measure	Cases	This Hosp.	State Avg.	U.S. Avg.
Blood Clot Prevention and Treatment				
Anticoagulation Overlap Therapy[2]	172	80%	92%	93%
ICU Venous Thromboembolism Prophylaxis[2]	114	89%	94%	92%
Incidence of Potentially Preventable VTE[2]	32	0%	8%	10%
UFH with Dosages/Platelet Monitoring[2]	148	99%	98%	97%
Venous Thromboembolism Prophylaxis[2]	347	93%	88%	85%
Warfarin Therapy Discharge Instructions[2]	140	0%	72%	75%
Chest Pain/Possible Heart Attack Care				
Aspirin Given Within 24 Hours of Arrival[5]	-	-	97%	96%
Fibrinolytic Meds Within 30 Min. of Arrival[5]	-	-	68%	58%
Average Time to ECG (minutes)[5]	-	-	5	7
Average Time to Transfer (minutes)[5]	-	-	43	60
Children's Asthma Care				
Received Home Management Plan of Care	-	-	-	88%
Received Reliever Medication	-	-	-	100%
Received Systemic Corticosteroids	-	-	-	100%
Emergency Department				
Admittance Decision Time (minutes)[2]	648	196	94	98
Head CT Results Within 45 Min. of Arrival	14	71%	61%	57%
Patients Who Left ER Before Being Seen	>100k	9%	3%	2%
Time from ER Arrival to Admit. (minutes)[2]	653	382	274	274
Time from ER Arrival to Discharge (minutes)	377	178	136	134
Time in ER Before Being Evaluated (minutes)	410	72	33	26
Time to Pain Meds for Fractures (minutes)	205	61	61	57
Heart Attack Care				
Aspirin Given at Discharge	653	100%	99%	99%
Fibrinolytic Meds Within 30 Min. of Arrival[7]	-	-	50%	54%
PCI Within 90 Minutes of Arrival	142	96%	97%	96%
Statin Prescribed at Discharge	641	99%	99%	98%
Heart Failure Care				
ACE Inhibitor or ARB for LVSD	243	97%	98%	97%
Discharge Instructions Given	706	90%	94%	94%
Evaluation of LVS Function	812	100%	99%	99%
Medicare Spending				
Medicare Spending per Patient (ratio)	-	0.96	0.98	0.98
Pneumonia Care				
Appropriate Initial Antibiotic Given	351	99%	97%	95%
Blood Culture Timing	617	99%	98%	98%
Pregnancy and Delivery Care				
Newborn Deliveries Scheduled Early[2]	58	5%	3%	6%
Preventive Care				
Immunization for Influenza[2]	558	93%	94%	90%
Immunization for Pneumonia[2]	723	96%	95%	92%
Stroke Care				
Anticoagulation Therapy for Atrial Fibrillation	54	96%	95%	95%
Antithrombotic Therapy Timing	343	99%	98%	98%
Assessed for Rehabilitation	394	95%	97%	97%
Discharged on Antithrombotic Therapy	349	99%	99%	99%
Discharged on Statin Medication	270	98%	94%	94%
Thrombolytic Therapy Timing	28	82%	58%	66%
Venous Thromboembolism Prophylaxis	406	100%	94%	94%
Written Stroke Educational Materials Given	268	93%	91%	88%
Surgical Care Improvement Project				
Appropriate Beta Blocker Usage[2]	588	100%	98%	98%
Appropriate VTP Within 24 Hours[2]	946	98%	98%	98%
Controlled Postoperative Blood Glucose[2]	343	100%	99%	97%
Perioperative Temperature Management[2]	1,148	100%	100%	100%
Prophylactic Antibiotic Selection[2]	1,158	100%	99%	99%
Prophylactic Antibiotic Selection (Outpatient)	927	98%	99%	98%
Prophylactic Antibiotic Stopped[2]	1,120	98%	98%	98%
Prophylactic Antibiotic Timing[2]	1,158	99%	99%	99%
Prophylactic Antibiotic Timing (Outpatient)	934	98%	98%	98%
Urinary Catheter Removal[2]	971	98%	97%	97%
Survey of Patients' Hospital Experiences				
Area Around Room 'Always' Quiet at Night	300+	69%	67%	61%
Doctors 'Always' Communicated Well	300+	82%	84%	82%
Home Recovery Information Given	300+	89%	86%	85%
Hospital Given 9 or 10 on 10 Point Scale	300+	72%	72%	71%
Meds 'Always' Explained Before Given	300+	65%	66%	64%
Nurses 'Always' Communicated Well	300+	81%	81%	79%
Pain 'Always' Well Controlled	300+	72%	72%	71%
Room and Bathroom 'Always' Clean	300+	71%	72%	73%
Timely Help 'Always' Received	300+	66%	68%	68%
Would Definitely Recommend Hospital	300+	77%	71%	71%
Use of Medical Imaging				
Cardiac Imaging Stress Test before Surgery	477	6.1%	5.1%	5.3%
Combination Abdominal CT Scan	1,709	3.2%	10.1%	10.5%
Combination Brain/Sinus CT Scan	1,398	1.9%	2.5%	2.7%
Combination Chest CT Scan	1,803	0.0%	1.3%	2.7%
Follow-up Mammogram/Ultrasound	4,585	8.9%	8%	8.8%
Lumbar Spine MRI for Low Back Pain	188	42.0%	39%	37.2%

Tuomey Healthcare System

129 N Washington St | Phone: 803-774-8900
Sumter, SC 29150 | Fax: 803-774-9494
URL: www.tuomey.com
Type: Acute Care Hospitals | Emergency Services: Yes
Ownership: Voluntary non-profit - Private | Beds: 266

Key Personnel:
Cardiac Laboratory. . . . . Dale J. Cannon, Jr., MD
CEO/President. . . . . Jay Cox
Chief of Medical Staff. . . . . Mark Crabbe
Emergency Room . . . . Scot Dilts, MD
Pediatric In-Patient Care . . . . James DuRant, MD
Anesthesiology. . . . . Carlos Lecca, MD
Radiology. . . . . Michael Mease, MD
Surgery . . . . Henry Moses, MD

Measure	Cases	This Hosp.	State Avg.	U.S. Avg.
Blood Clot Prevention and Treatment				
Anticoagulation Overlap Therapy[2]	76	97%	92%	93%
ICU Venous Thromboembolism Prophylaxis[2]	69	87%	94%	92%
Incidence of Potentially Preventable VTE[1,2]	-	-	8%	10%
UFH with Dosages/Platelet Monitoring[1,2]	-	-	98%	97%
Venous Thromboembolism Prophylaxis[2]	368	69%	88%	85%
Warfarin Therapy Discharge Instructions[2]	70	74%	72%	75%
Chest Pain/Possible Heart Attack Care				
Aspirin Given Within 24 Hours of Arrival	150	96%	97%	96%
Fibrinolytic Meds Within 30 Min. of Arrival[1]	-	-	68%	58%
Average Time to ECG (minutes)	156	9	5	7
Average Time to Transfer (minutes)	21	24	43	60
Children's Asthma Care				
Received Home Management Plan of Care	-	-	-	88%
Received Reliever Medication	-	-	-	100%
Received Systemic Corticosteroids	-	-	-	100%
Emergency Department				
Admittance Decision Time (minutes)[2]	537	85	94	98
Head CT Results Within 45 Min. of Arrival	26	42%	61%	57%
Patients Who Left ER Before Being Seen	63,090	3%	3%	2%
Time from ER Arrival to Admit. (minutes)[2]	546	286	274	274
Time from ER Arrival to Discharge (minutes)	369	153	136	134
Time in ER Before Being Evaluated (minutes)[7]	-	-	33	26
Time to Pain Meds for Fractures (minutes)	70	92	61	57
Heart Attack Care				
Aspirin Given at Discharge	43	100%	99%	99%
Fibrinolytic Meds Within 30 Min. of Arrival[7]	-	-	50%	54%
PCI Within 90 Minutes of Arrival[7]	-	-	97%	96%
Statin Prescribed at Discharge	48	83%	99%	98%
Heart Failure Care				
ACE Inhibitor or ARB for LVSD	192	93%	98%	97%
Discharge Instructions Given	459	88%	94%	94%
Evaluation of LVS Function	513	99%	99%	99%
Medicare Spending				
Medicare Spending per Patient (ratio)	-	0.96	0.98	0.98
Pneumonia Care				
Appropriate Initial Antibiotic Given	148	94%	97%	95%
Blood Culture Timing	232	98%	98%	98%
Pregnancy and Delivery Care				
Newborn Deliveries Scheduled Early[2]	32	3%	3%	6%
Preventive Care				
Immunization for Influenza[2]	507	98%	94%	90%
Immunization for Pneumonia[2]	623	97%	95%	92%
Stroke Care				
Anticoagulation Therapy for Atrial Fibrillation[1,2]	-	-	95%	95%
Antithrombotic Therapy Timing[2]	120	95%	98%	98%
Assessed for Rehabilitation[2]	121	97%	97%	97%
Discharged on Antithrombotic Therapy[2]	116	97%	99%	99%
Discharged on Statin Medication[2]	92	77%	94%	94%
Thrombolytic Therapy Timing[1,2]	-	-	58%	66%
Venous Thromboembolism Prophylaxis[2]	128	84%	94%	94%
Written Stroke Educational Materials Given[2]	63	94%	91%	88%
Surgical Care Improvement Project				
Appropriate Beta Blocker Usage[2]	152	97%	98%	98%
Appropriate VTP Within 24 Hours[2]	436	99%	98%	98%
Controlled Postoperative Blood Glucose[2,7]	-	-	99%	97%
Perioperative Temperature Management[2]	481	100%	100%	100%
Prophylactic Antibiotic Selection[2]	318	99%	99%	99%
Prophylactic Antibiotic Selection (Outpatient)	110	100%	99%	98%
Prophylactic Antibiotic Stopped[2]	310	97%	98%	98%
Prophylactic Antibiotic Timing[2]	318	97%	99%	99%
Prophylactic Antibiotic Timing (Outpatient)	114	95%	98%	98%
Urinary Catheter Removal[2]	341	98%	97%	97%
Survey of Patients' Hospital Experiences				
Area Around Room 'Always' Quiet at Night	300+	66%	67%	61%
Doctors 'Always' Communicated Well	300+	84%	84%	82%
Home Recovery Information Given	300+	85%	86%	85%
Hospital Given 9 or 10 on 10 Point Scale	300+	59%	72%	71%
Meds 'Always' Explained Before Given	300+	62%	66%	64%
Nurses 'Always' Communicated Well	300+	82%	81%	79%
Pain 'Always' Well Controlled	300+	76%	72%	71%
Room and Bathroom 'Always' Clean	300+	69%	72%	73%
Timely Help 'Always' Received	300+	64%	68%	68%
Would Definitely Recommend Hospital	300+	58%	71%	71%
Use of Medical Imaging				
Cardiac Imaging Stress Test before Surgery[1]	-	-	5.1%	5.3%
Combination Abdominal CT Scan	929	20.8%	10.1%	10.5%
Combination Brain/Sinus CT Scan	1,080	3.1%	2.5%	2.7%
Combination Chest CT Scan	563	4.6%	1.3%	2.7%
Follow-up Mammogram/Ultrasound	3,068	10.4%	8%	8.8%
Lumbar Spine MRI for Low Back Pain	195	42.1%	39%	37.2%

Wallace Thomson Hospital

322 W South Saint PO Box 789 | Phone: 864-427-0351
Union, SC 29379 | Fax: 864-429-2524
E-mail: nbrown@wallacethomson.com
URL: www.wallacethomson.com
Type: Acute Care Hospitals | Emergency Services: Yes
Ownership: Govt - Hospital Dist/Auth | Beds: 143

Key Personnel:
Quality Assurance . . . . Paul C Akers, MD
Infection Control. . . . . J Louis Becton, MD
Pediatric In-Patient Care . . . . J Louis Becton, Jr, MD
Chief of Medical Staff . . . . M. John Flood, MD
Chairman/CEO . . . . Rhonda C. Ingle, MBA
Radiology. . . . . Stephen Muehlen, RT

Measure	Cases	This Hosp.	State Avg.	U.S. Avg.
Blood Clot Prevention and Treatment				
Anticoagulation Overlap Therapy[2]	27	67%	92%	93%
ICU Venous Thromboembolism Prophylaxis[2]	64	92%	94%	92%
Incidence of Potentially Preventable VTE[1,2]	-	-	8%	10%
UFH with Dosages/Platelet Monitoring[1,2]	-	-	98%	97%
Venous Thromboembolism Prophylaxis[2]	187	93%	88%	85%
Warfarin Therapy Discharge Instructions[2]	18	72%	72%	75%
Chest Pain/Possible Heart Attack Care				
Aspirin Given Within 24 Hours of Arrival	33	100%	97%	96%
Fibrinolytic Meds Within 30 Min. of Arrival[7]	-	-	68%	58%
Average Time to ECG (minutes)	37	23	5	7

NOTE: Hospital profiles are in alphabetical order by state, then city, then hospital within the city; Rankings exclude hospitals with less than 25 cases except for patient surveys which excludes hospitals with less than 100 cases; (a) 100-299 cases; (1) The number of cases/patients is too few to report; (2) Data submitted were based on a sample of cases/patients; (3) Results are based on a shorter time period than required; (4) Data suppressed by CMS for one or more quarters; (5) Results are not available for this reporting period; (6) Fewer than 100 patients completed the HCAHPS survey; (7) No cases met the criteria for this measure; (8) The lower limit of the confidence interval cannot be calculated if the number of observed infections equals zero; (9) No data are available from the state/territory for this reporting period; (10) The scores shown reflect fewer than 50 completed surveys; (11) There were discrepancies in the data collection process; (12) This measure does not apply to this hospital for this reporting period; (13) Results cannot be calculated for this reporting period; (14) The results for this state are combined with nearby states to protect confidentiality; Please refer to the User's Guide for a full explanation of data.

Measure	Cases	This Hosp.	State Avg.	U.S. Avg.
Average Time to Transfer (minutes)[7]	-	-	43	60
Children's Asthma Care				
Received Home Management Plan of Care	-	-	-	88%
Received Reliever Medication	-	-	-	100%
Received Systemic Corticosteroids	-	-	-	100%
Emergency Department				
Admittance Decision Time (minutes)[2]	362	77	94	98
Head CT Results Within 45 Min. of Arrival[1]	-	-	61%	57%
Patients Who Left ER Before Being Seen	17,546	3%	3%	2%
Time from ER Arrival to Admit. (minutes)[2]	374	216	274	274
Time from ER Arrival to Discharge (minutes)	370	92	136	134
Time in ER Before Being Evaluated (minutes)	393	24	33	26
Time to Pain Meds for Fractures (minutes)	71	66	61	57
Heart Attack Care				
Aspirin Given at Discharge[1]	-	-	99%	99%
Fibrinolytic Meds Within 30 Min. of Arrival[7]	-	-	50%	54%
PCI Within 90 Minutes of Arrival[7]	-	-	97%	96%
Statin Prescribed at Discharge[1]	-	-	99%	98%
Heart Failure Care				
ACE Inhibitor or ARB for LVSD	19	84%	98%	97%
Discharge Instructions Given	85	93%	94%	94%
Evaluation of LVS Function	94	96%	99%	99%
Medicare Spending				
Medicare Spending per Patient (ratio)	-	1.02	0.98	0.98
Pneumonia Care				
Appropriate Initial Antibiotic Given	72	81%	97%	95%
Blood Culture Timing	65	77%	98%	98%
Pregnancy and Delivery Care				
Newborn Deliveries Scheduled Early	14	0%	3%	6%
Preventive Care				
Immunization for Influenza[2]	288	71%	94%	90%
Immunization for Pneumonia[2]	412	76%	95%	92%
Stroke Care				
Anticoagulation Therapy for Atrial Fibrillation[1]	-	-	95%	95%
Antithrombotic Therapy Timing	20	95%	98%	98%
Assessed for Rehabilitation	22	91%	97%	97%
Discharged on Antithrombotic Therapy	17	100%	99%	99%
Discharged on Statin Medication	19	89%	94%	94%
Thrombolytic Therapy Timing[1]	-	-	58%	66%
Venous Thromboembolism Prophylaxis	25	92%	94%	94%
Written Stroke Educational Materials Given	14	86%	91%	88%
Surgical Care Improvement Project				
Appropriate Beta Blocker Usage[1]	-	-	98%	98%
Appropriate VTP Within 24 Hours	35	63%	98%	98%
Controlled Postoperative Blood Glucose[7]	-	-	99%	97%
Perioperative Temperature Management	43	100%	100%	100%
Prophylactic Antibiotic Selection[7]	-	-	99%	99%
Prophylactic Antibiotic Selection (Outpatient)[1,3]	-	-	99%	98%
Prophylactic Antibiotic Stopped[7]	-	-	98%	98%
Prophylactic Antibiotic Timing[7]	-	-	99%	99%
Prophylactic Antibiotic Timing (Outpatient)[1,3]	-	-	98%	98%
Urinary Catheter Removal	16	81%	97%	97%
Survey of Patients' Hospital Experiences				
Area Around Room 'Always' Quiet at Night	300+	67%	67%	61%
Doctors 'Always' Communicated Well	300+	90%	84%	82%
Home Recovery Information Given	300+	87%	86%	85%
Hospital Given 9 or 10 on 10 Point Scale	300+	68%	72%	71%
Meds 'Always' Explained Before Given	300+	67%	66%	64%
Nurses 'Always' Communicated Well	300+	79%	81%	79%
Pain 'Always' Well Controlled	300+	72%	72%	71%
Room and Bathroom 'Always' Clean	300+	66%	72%	73%
Timely Help 'Always' Received	300+	71%	68%	68%
Would Definitely Recommend Hospital	300+	65%	71%	71%
Use of Medical Imaging				
Cardiac Imaging Stress Test before Surgery	67	6.0%	5.1%	5.3%
Combination Abdominal CT Scan	231	25.1%	10.1%	10.5%
Combination Brain/Sinus CT Scan[1]	-	-	2.5%	2.7%
Combination Chest CT Scan	159	11.9%	1.3%	2.7%
Follow-up Mammogram/Ultrasound	422	4.7%	8%	8.8%
Lumbar Spine MRI for Low Back Pain	48	56.3%	39%	37.2%

Hampton Regional Medical Center

595 West Carolina Avenue
Varnville, SC 29944
Phone: 803-943-2771
Fax: 803-943-1241
Type: Acute Care Hospitals
Emergency Services: Yes
Ownership: Voluntary non-profit - Private
Beds: 68

Key Personnel:
Operating Room. . . . . Mario Cerame
Infection Control. . . . . Lauren Ginn
CEO/President. . . . . Dave H Hamill
Anesthesiology. . . . . H Roman, MD
Radiology. . . . . Edward Warren
Chief of Medical Staff. . . . . Glenn W Welcker, MD

Measure	Cases	This Hosp.	State Avg.	U.S. Avg.
Blood Clot Prevention and Treatment				
Anticoagulation Overlap Therapy[2]	22	73%	92%	93%
ICU Venous Thromboembolism Prophylaxis[2,7]	-	-	94%	92%
Incidence of Potentially Preventable VTE[1,2]	-	-	8%	10%
UFH with Dosages/Platelet Monitoring[1,2]	-	-	98%	97%
Venous Thromboembolism Prophylaxis[2]	112	73%	88%	85%
Warfarin Therapy Discharge Instructions[2]	20	75%	72%	75%
Chest Pain/Possible Heart Attack Care				
Aspirin Given Within 24 Hours of Arrival	45	89%	97%	96%
Fibrinolytic Meds Within 30 Min. of Arrival[1]	-	-	68%	58%
Average Time to ECG (minutes)	47	10	5	7
Average Time to Transfer (minutes)[7]	-	-	43	60
Children's Asthma Care				
Received Home Management Plan of Care	-	-	-	88%
Received Reliever Medication	-	-	-	100%
Received Systemic Corticosteroids	-	-	-	100%
Emergency Department				
Admittance Decision Time (minutes)	371	55	94	98
Head CT Results Within 45 Min. of Arrival[1]	-	-	61%	57%
Patients Who Left ER Before Being Seen	12,215	2%	3%	2%
Time from ER Arrival to Admit. (minutes)	391	259	274	274
Time from ER Arrival to Discharge (minutes)	368	140	136	134
Time in ER Before Being Evaluated (minutes)	359	31	33	26
Time to Pain Meds for Fractures (minutes)	36	60	61	57
Heart Attack Care				
Aspirin Given at Discharge[3,7]	-	-	99%	99%
Fibrinolytic Meds Within 30 Min. of Arrival[3,7]	-	-	50%	54%
PCI Within 90 Minutes of Arrival[3,7]	-	-	97%	96%
Statin Prescribed at Discharge[1,3]	-	-	99%	98%
Heart Failure Care				
ACE Inhibitor or ARB for LVSD	16	69%	98%	97%
Discharge Instructions Given	43	88%	94%	94%
Evaluation of LVS Function	48	96%	99%	99%
Medicare Spending				
Medicare Spending per Patient (ratio)	-	0.90	0.98	0.98
Pneumonia Care				
Appropriate Initial Antibiotic Given	28	96%	97%	95%
Blood Culture Timing	32	97%	98%	98%
Pregnancy and Delivery Care				
Newborn Deliveries Scheduled Early[7]	-	-	3%	6%
Preventive Care				
Immunization for Influenza[2]	314	87%	94%	90%
Immunization for Pneumonia[2]	489	92%	95%	92%
Stroke Care				
Anticoagulation Therapy for Atrial Fibrillation[3,7]	-	-	95%	95%
Antithrombotic Therapy Timing[1,3]	-	-	98%	98%
Assessed for Rehabilitation[1,3]	-	-	97%	97%
Discharged on Antithrombotic Therapy[1,3]	-	-	99%	99%
Discharged on Statin Medication[1,3]	-	-	94%	94%
Thrombolytic Therapy Timing[3,7]	-	-	58%	66%
Venous Thromboembolism Prophylaxis[1,3]	-	-	94%	94%
Written Stroke Educational Materials Given[1,3]	-	-	91%	88%
Surgical Care Improvement Project				
Appropriate Beta Blocker Usage[1]	-	-	98%	98%
Appropriate VTP Within 24 Hours	31	97%	98%	98%
Controlled Postoperative Blood Glucose[7]	-	-	99%	97%
Perioperative Temperature Management	33	70%	100%	100%
Prophylactic Antibiotic Selection	22	100%	99%	99%
Prophylactic Antibiotic Selection (Outpatient)[1,3]	-	-	99%	98%
Prophylactic Antibiotic Stopped	22	100%	98%	98%
Prophylactic Antibiotic Timing	23	91%	99%	99%
Prophylactic Antibiotic Timing (Outpatient)[1,3]	-	-	98%	98%
Urinary Catheter Removal[1]	-	-	97%	97%
Survey of Patients' Hospital Experiences				
Area Around Room 'Always' Quiet at Night	(a)	70%	67%	61%
Doctors 'Always' Communicated Well	(a)	84%	84%	82%
Home Recovery Information Given	(a)	89%	86%	85%
Hospital Given 9 or 10 on 10 Point Scale	(a)	79%	72%	71%
Meds 'Always' Explained Before Given	(a)	71%	66%	64%
Nurses 'Always' Communicated Well	(a)	79%	81%	79%
Pain 'Always' Well Controlled	(a)	69%	72%	71%
Room and Bathroom 'Always' Clean	(a)	79%	72%	73%
Timely Help 'Always' Received	(a)	72%	68%	68%
Would Definitely Recommend Hospital	(a)	75%	71%	71%
Use of Medical Imaging				
Cardiac Imaging Stress Test before Surgery	83	4.8%	5.1%	5.3%
Combination Abdominal CT Scan	169	5.9%	10.1%	10.5%
Combination Brain/Sinus CT Scan	280	6.4%	2.5%	2.7%
Combination Chest CT Scan	66	7.6%	1.3%	2.7%
Follow-up Mammogram/Ultrasound	447	3.6%	8%	8.8%
Lumbar Spine MRI for Low Back Pain[1]	-	-	39%	37.2%

Colleton Medical Center

501 Robertson Boulevard
Walterboro, SC 29488
Phone: 843-782-2000
Fax: 843-549-0246
URL: www.colletonmedical.com
Type: Acute Care Hospitals
Emergency Services: Yes
Ownership: Proprietary
Beds: 131

Key Personnel:
CEO/President. . . . . Rebecca Brewer
CEO . . . . Jeffrey A. Cook
Quality Assurance . . . . Debbie Drew
Emergency Room . . . . D Meacher, MD
Chief of Medical Staff. . . . . Kim Rakes-Stephens, MD
Operating Room. . . . . Dusty Rhoades
Infection Control. . . . . Gail Sartain

Measure	Cases	This Hosp.	State Avg.	U.S. Avg.
Blood Clot Prevention and Treatment				
Anticoagulation Overlap Therapy[2]	40	92%	92%	93%
ICU Venous Thromboembolism Prophylaxis[2]	203	85%	94%	92%
Incidence of Potentially Preventable VTE[2,7]	-	-	8%	10%
UFH with Dosages/Platelet Monitoring[1,2]	-	-	98%	97%
Venous Thromboembolism Prophylaxis[2]	771	85%	88%	85%
Warfarin Therapy Discharge Instructions[2]	36	100%	72%	75%
Chest Pain/Possible Heart Attack Care				
Aspirin Given Within 24 Hours of Arrival	45	100%	97%	96%
Fibrinolytic Meds Within 30 Min. of Arrival[7]	-	-	68%	58%
Average Time to ECG (minutes)	47	5	5	7
Average Time to Transfer (minutes)[1]	-	-	43	60
Children's Asthma Care				
Received Home Management Plan of Care	-	-	-	88%
Received Reliever Medication	-	-	-	100%
Received Systemic Corticosteroids	-	-	-	100%
Emergency Department				
Admittance Decision Time (minutes)[2]	599	52	94	98
Head CT Results Within 45 Min. of Arrival	22	55%	61%	57%
Patients Who Left ER Before Being Seen	26,681	1%	3%	2%
Time from ER Arrival to Admit. (minutes)[2]	599	248	274	274
Time from ER Arrival to Discharge (minutes)	437	120	136	134
Time in ER Before Being Evaluated (minutes)	515	13	33	26
Time to Pain Meds for Fractures (minutes)	59	52	61	57
Heart Attack Care				
Aspirin Given at Discharge[1]	-	-	99%	99%
Fibrinolytic Meds Within 30 Min. of Arrival[7]	-	-	50%	54%
PCI Within 90 Minutes of Arrival[7]	-	-	97%	96%
Statin Prescribed at Discharge[1]	-	-	99%	98%
Heart Failure Care				
ACE Inhibitor or ARB for LVSD	61	100%	98%	97%
Discharge Instructions Given	229	100%	94%	94%
Evaluation of LVS Function	268	100%	99%	99%
Medicare Spending				
Medicare Spending per Patient (ratio)	-	0.98	0.98	0.98
Pneumonia Care				
Appropriate Initial Antibiotic Given	74	97%	97%	95%

NOTE: Hospital profiles are in alphabetical order by state, then city, then hospital within the city; Rankings exclude hospitals with less than 25 cases except for patient surveys which excludes hospitals with less than 100 cases; (a) 100-299 cases; (1) The number of cases/patients is too few to report; (2) Data submitted were based on a sample of cases/patients; (3) Results are based on a shorter time period than required; (4) Data suppressed by CMS for one or more quarters; (5) Results are not available for this reporting period; (6) Fewer than 100 patients completed the HCAHPS survey; (7) No cases met the criteria for this measure; (8) The lower limit of the confidence interval cannot be calculated if the number of observed infections equals zero; (9) No data are available from the state/territory for this reporting period; (10) The scores shown reflect fewer than 50 completed surveys; (11) There were discrepancies in the data collection process; (12) This measure does not apply to this hospital for this reporting period; (13) Results cannot be calculated for this reporting period; (14) The results for this state are combined with nearby states to protect confidentiality; Please refer to the User's Guide for a full explanation of data.

Measure	Cases	This Hosp.	State Avg.	U.S. Avg.
Blood Culture Timing	127	100%	98%	98%
Pregnancy and Delivery Care				
Newborn Deliveries Scheduled Early[2]	30	0%	3%	6%
Preventive Care				
Immunization for Influenza[2]	464	98%	94%	90%
Immunization for Pneumonia[2]	607	97%	95%	92%
Stroke Care				
Anticoagulation Therapy for Atrial Fibrillation[1]	-	-	95%	95%
Antithrombotic Therapy Timing	44	100%	98%	98%
Assessed for Rehabilitation	47	100%	97%	97%
Discharged on Antithrombotic Therapy	46	100%	99%	99%
Discharged on Statin Medication	40	100%	94%	94%
Thrombolytic Therapy Timing[7]	-	-	58%	66%
Venous Thromboembolism Prophylaxis	39	95%	94%	94%
Written Stroke Educational Materials Given	29	100%	91%	88%
Surgical Care Improvement Project				
Appropriate Beta Blocker Usage	26	100%	98%	98%
Appropriate VTP Within 24 Hours	118	100%	98%	98%
Controlled Postoperative Blood Glucose[7]	-	-	99%	97%
Perioperative Temperature Management	134	100%	100%	100%
Prophylactic Antibiotic Selection	96	100%	99%	99%
Prophylactic Antibiotic Selection (Outpatient)	25	100%	99%	98%
Prophylactic Antibiotic Stopped	96	100%	98%	98%
Prophylactic Antibiotic Timing	96	100%	99%	99%
Prophylactic Antibiotic Timing (Outpatient)	26	92%	98%	98%
Urinary Catheter Removal	20	100%	97%	97%
Survey of Patients' Hospital Experiences				
Area Around Room 'Always' Quiet at Night	300+	68%	67%	61%
Doctors 'Always' Communicated Well	300+	80%	84%	82%
Home Recovery Information Given	300+	82%	86%	85%
Hospital Given 9 or 10 on 10 Point Scale	300+	65%	72%	71%
Meds 'Always' Explained Before Given	300+	61%	66%	64%
Nurses 'Always' Communicated Well	300+	77%	81%	79%
Pain 'Always' Well Controlled	300+	69%	72%	71%
Room and Bathroom 'Always' Clean	300+	76%	72%	73%
Timely Help 'Always' Received	300+	62%	68%	68%
Would Definitely Recommend Hospital	300+	59%	71%	71%
Use of Medical Imaging				
Cardiac Imaging Stress Test before Surgery	146	2.1%	5.1%	5.3%
Combination Abdominal CT Scan	435	5.3%	10.1%	10.5%
Combination Brain/Sinus CT Scan[1]	-	-	2.5%	2.7%
Combination Chest CT Scan	162	1.2%	1.3%	2.7%
Follow-up Mammogram/Ultrasound	764	7.5%	8%	8.8%
Lumbar Spine MRI for Low Back Pain	75	45.3%	39%	37.2%

Lexington Medical Center

2720 Sunset Blvd
West Columbia, SC 29169
Phone: 803-791-2000
Fax: 803-791-2660
E-mail: magregory@lexhealth.org
URL: www.lexmed.com
Type: Acute Care Hospitals
Emergency Services: No
Ownership: Govt - Hospital Dist/Auth
Beds: 380

Key Personnel:
CEO/President . . . . Michael J Biediger
Operating Room . . . . Sharon Hickman, RN
Radiology . . . . Charles Hood
Chief of Medical Staff . . . . Steven A Madden, MD
Pediatric Ambulatory Care . . . . . . Dwight Reynolds, MD
Pediatric In-Patient Care . . . . Dwight Reynolds, MD
Quality Assurance . . . . Barbara Warren

Measure	Cases	This Hosp.	State Avg.	U.S. Avg.
Blood Clot Prevention and Treatment				
Anticoagulation Overlap Therapy[2]	199	92%	92%	93%
ICU Venous Thromboembolism Prophylaxis[2]	70	89%	94%	92%
Incidence of Potentially Preventable VTE[2]	30	20%	8%	10%
UFH with Dosages/Platelet Monitoring[2]	78	100%	98%	97%
Venous Thromboembolism Prophylaxis[2]	350	84%	88%	85%
Warfarin Therapy Discharge Instructions[2]	152	96%	72%	75%
Chest Pain/Possible Heart Attack Care				
Aspirin Given Within 24 Hours of Arrival[5]	-	-	97%	96%
Fibrinolytic Meds Within 30 Min. of Arrival[5]	-	-	68%	58%
Average Time to ECG (minutes)[5]	-	-	5	7
Average Time to Transfer (minutes)[5]	-	-	43	60
Children's Asthma Care				
Received Home Management Plan of Care	-	-	-	88%
Received Reliever Medication	-	-	-	100%
Received Systemic Corticosteroids	-	-	-	100%
Emergency Department				
Admittance Decision Time (minutes)[2]	365	174	94	98
Head CT Results Within 45 Min. of Arrival[1]	-	-	61%	57%
Patients Who Left ER Before Being Seen	>100k	2%	3%	2%
Time from ER Arrival to Admit. (minutes)[2]	380	347	274	274
Time from ER Arrival to Discharge (minutes)	332	168	136	134
Time in ER Before Being Evaluated (minutes)	334	30	33	26
Time to Pain Meds for Fractures (minutes)	247	53	61	57
Heart Attack Care				
Aspirin Given at Discharge[2]	270	100%	99%	99%
Fibrinolytic Meds Within 30 Min. of Arrival[2,7]	-	-	50%	54%
PCI Within 90 Minutes of Arrival[2]	63	81%	97%	96%
Statin Prescribed at Discharge[2]	261	100%	99%	98%
Heart Failure Care				
ACE Inhibitor or ARB for LVSD[2]	94	100%	98%	97%
Discharge Instructions Given[2]	228	90%	94%	94%
Evaluation of LVS Function[2]	272	100%	99%	99%
Medicare Spending				
Medicare Spending per Patient (ratio)	-	1.01	0.98	0.98
Pneumonia Care				
Appropriate Initial Antibiotic Given[2]	80	98%	97%	95%
Blood Culture Timing[2]	128	98%	98%	98%
Pregnancy and Delivery Care				
Newborn Deliveries Scheduled Early[2]	62	8%	3%	6%
Preventive Care				
Immunization for Influenza[2]	493	81%	94%	90%
Immunization for Pneumonia[2]	583	80%	95%	92%
Stroke Care				
Anticoagulation Therapy for Atrial Fibrillation[1,2]	-	-	95%	95%
Antithrombotic Therapy Timing[2]	77	99%	98%	98%
Assessed for Rehabilitation[2]	92	97%	97%	97%
Discharged on Antithrombotic Therapy[2]	81	100%	99%	99%
Discharged on Statin Medication[2]	65	95%	94%	94%
Thrombolytic Therapy Timing[1,2]	-	-	58%	66%
Venous Thromboembolism Prophylaxis[2]	98	93%	94%	94%
Written Stroke Educational Materials Given[2]	49	86%	91%	88%
Surgical Care Improvement Project				
Appropriate Beta Blocker Usage[2]	148	97%	98%	98%
Appropriate VTP Within 24 Hours[2]	293	98%	98%	98%
Controlled Postoperative Blood Glucose[2]	98	100%	99%	97%
Perioperative Temperature Management[2]	414	100%	100%	100%
Prophylactic Antibiotic Selection[2]	368	99%	99%	99%
Prophylactic Antibiotic Selection (Outpatient)	681	99%	99%	98%
Prophylactic Antibiotic Stopped[2]	364	98%	98%	98%
Prophylactic Antibiotic Timing[2]	369	99%	99%	99%
Prophylactic Antibiotic Timing (Outpatient)	682	98%	98%	98%
Urinary Catheter Removal[2]	269	97%	97%	97%
Survey of Patients' Hospital Experiences				
Area Around Room 'Always' Quiet at Night	300+	62%	67%	61%
Doctors 'Always' Communicated Well	300+	84%	84%	82%
Home Recovery Information Given	300+	84%	86%	85%
Hospital Given 9 or 10 on 10 Point Scale	300+	76%	72%	71%
Meds 'Always' Explained Before Given	300+	60%	66%	64%
Nurses 'Always' Communicated Well	300+	79%	81%	79%
Pain 'Always' Well Controlled	300+	71%	72%	71%
Room and Bathroom 'Always' Clean	300+	73%	72%	73%
Timely Help 'Always' Received	300+	65%	68%	68%
Would Definitely Recommend Hospital	300+	76%	71%	71%
Use of Medical Imaging				
Cardiac Imaging Stress Test before Surgery	370	7.0%	5.1%	5.3%
Combination Abdominal CT Scan	1,947	1.8%	10.1%	10.5%
Combination Brain/Sinus CT Scan	1,781	2.1%	2.5%	2.7%
Combination Chest CT Scan	1,083	0.5%	1.3%	2.7%
Follow-up Mammogram/Ultrasound	2,435	4.4%	8%	8.8%
Lumbar Spine MRI for Low Back Pain	124	37.1%	39%	37.2%

Fairfield Memorial Hospital

321 Bypass PO Box 620
Winnsboro, SC 29180
Phone: 803-635-0233
Fax: 803-635-5612
URL: www.fairfieldmemorial.com
Type: Critical Access Hospitals
Emergency Services: Yes
Ownership: Government - Local
Beds: 25

Key Personnel:
Hemotology Center . . . . Cheryl Baxter
Chief of Medical Staff . . . . Dr Larry Cantey
Radiology . . . . Chris Carlton
Infection Control . . . . Shirley Hall, RN
Quality Assurance . . . . Shirley Hall
Patient Relations . . . . Mary Lynn Kinley
Emergency Room . . . . Mary Sas, RN
CEO . . . . Michael L Wiliams

Measure	Cases	This Hosp.	State Avg.	U.S. Avg.
Blood Clot Prevention and Treatment				
Anticoagulation Overlap Therapy[5]	-	-	92%	93%
ICU Venous Thromboembolism Prophylaxis[5]	-	-	94%	92%
Incidence of Potentially Preventable VTE[5]	-	-	8%	10%
UFH with Dosages/Platelet Monitoring[5]	-	-	98%	97%
Venous Thromboembolism Prophylaxis[5]	-	-	88%	85%
Warfarin Therapy Discharge Instructions[5]	-	-	72%	75%
Chest Pain/Possible Heart Attack Care				
Aspirin Given Within 24 Hours of Arrival	-	-	97%	96%
Fibrinolytic Meds Within 30 Min. of Arrival	-	-	68%	58%
Average Time to ECG (minutes)	-	-	5	7
Average Time to Transfer (minutes)	-	-	43	60
Children's Asthma Care				
Received Home Management Plan of Care	-	-	-	88%
Received Reliever Medication	-	-	-	100%
Received Systemic Corticosteroids	-	-	-	100%
Emergency Department				
Admittance Decision Time (minutes)[5]	-	-	94	98
Head CT Results Within 45 Min. of Arrival	-	-	61%	57%
Patients Who Left ER Before Being Seen	-	-	3%	2%
Time from ER Arrival to Admit. (minutes)[5]	-	-	274	274
Time from ER Arrival to Discharge (minutes)	-	-	136	134
Time in ER Before Being Evaluated (minutes)	-	-	33	26
Time to Pain Meds for Fractures (minutes)	-	-	61	57
Heart Attack Care				
Aspirin Given at Discharge[5]	-	-	99%	99%
Fibrinolytic Meds Within 30 Min. of Arrival[5]	-	-	50%	54%
PCI Within 90 Minutes of Arrival[5]	-	-	97%	96%
Statin Prescribed at Discharge[5]	-	-	99%	98%
Heart Failure Care				
ACE Inhibitor or ARB for LVSD[7]	-	-	98%	97%
Discharge Instructions Given	11	27%	94%	94%
Evaluation of LVS Function	11	55%	99%	99%
Medicare Spending				
Medicare Spending per Patient (ratio)	-	-	0.98	0.98
Pneumonia Care				
Appropriate Initial Antibiotic Given	20	70%	97%	95%
Blood Culture Timing	21	81%	98%	98%
Pregnancy and Delivery Care				
Newborn Deliveries Scheduled Early[5]	-	-	3%	6%
Preventive Care				
Immunization for Influenza[5]	-	-	94%	90%
Immunization for Pneumonia[5]	-	-	95%	92%
Stroke Care				
Anticoagulation Therapy for Atrial Fibrillation[5]	-	-	95%	95%
Antithrombotic Therapy Timing[5]	-	-	98%	98%
Assessed for Rehabilitation[5]	-	-	97%	97%
Discharged on Antithrombotic Therapy[5]	-	-	99%	99%
Discharged on Statin Medication[5]	-	-	94%	94%
Thrombolytic Therapy Timing[5]	-	-	58%	66%
Venous Thromboembolism Prophylaxis[5]	-	-	94%	94%
Written Stroke Educational Materials Given[5]	-	-	91%	88%
Surgical Care Improvement Project				
Appropriate Beta Blocker Usage[5]	-	-	98%	98%
Appropriate VTP Within 24 Hours[5]	-	-	98%	98%
Controlled Postoperative Blood Glucose[5]	-	-	99%	97%
Perioperative Temperature Management[5]	-	-	100%	100%
Prophylactic Antibiotic Selection[5]	-	-	99%	99%

NOTE: Hospital profiles are in alphabetical order by state, then city, then hospital within the city; Rankings exclude hospitals with less than 25 cases except for patient surveys which excludes hospitals with less than 100 cases; (a) 100-299 cases; (1) The number of cases/patients is too few to report; (2) Data submitted were based on a sample of cases/patients; (3) Results are based on a shorter time period than required; (4) Data suppressed by CMS for one or more quarters; (5) Results are not available for this reporting period; (6) Fewer than 100 patients completed the HCAHPS survey; (7) No cases met the criteria for this measure; (8) The lower limit of the confidence interval cannot be calculated if the number of observed infections equals zero; (9) No data are available from the state/territory for this reporting period; (10) The scores shown reflect fewer than 50 completed surveys; (11) There were discrepancies in the data collection process; (12) This measure does not apply to this hospital for this reporting period; (13) Results cannot be calculated for this reporting period; (14) The results for this state are combined with nearby states to protect confidentiality; Please refer to the User's Guide for a full explanation of data.

Prophylactic Antibiotic Selection (Outpatient)	-	-	99%	98%
Prophylactic Antibiotic Stopped[5]	-	-	98%	98%
Prophylactic Antibiotic Timing[5]	-	-	99%	99%
Prophylactic Antibiotic Timing (Outpatient)	-	-	98%	98%
Urinary Catheter Removal[5]	-	-	97%	97%
Survey of Patients' Hospital Experiences				
Area Around Room 'Always' Quiet at Night[5]	-	-	67%	61%
Doctors 'Always' Communicated Well[5]	-	-	84%	82%
Home Recovery Information Given[5]	-	-	86%	85%
Hospital Given 9 or 10 on 10 Point Scale[5]	-	-	72%	71%
Meds 'Always' Explained Before Given[5]	-	-	66%	64%
Nurses 'Always' Communicated Well[5]	-	-	81%	79%
Pain 'Always' Well Controlled[5]	-	-	72%	71%
Room and Bathroom 'Always' Clean[5]	-	-	72%	73%
Timely Help 'Always' Received[5]	-	-	68%	68%
Would Definitely Recommend Hospital[5]	-	-	71%	71%
Use of Medical Imaging				
Cardiac Imaging Stress Test before Surgery	-	-	5.1%	5.3%
Combination Abdominal CT Scan	-	-	10.1%	10.5%
Combination Brain/Sinus CT Scan	-	-	2.5%	2.7%
Combination Chest CT Scan	-	-	1.3%	2.7%
Follow-up Mammogram/Ultrasound	-	-	8%	8.8%
Lumbar Spine MRI for Low Back Pain	-	-	39%	37.2%

NOTE: Hospital profiles are in alphabetical order by state, then city, then hospital within the city; Rankings exclude hospitals with less than 25 cases except for patient surveys which excludes hospitals with less than 100 cases; (a) 100-299 cases; (1) The number of cases/patients is too few to report; (2) Data submitted were based on a sample of cases/patients; (3) Results are based on a shorter time period than required; (4) Data suppressed by CMS for one or more quarters; (5) Results are not available for this reporting period; (6) Fewer than 100 patients completed the HCAHPS survey; (7) No cases met the criteria for this measure; (8) The lower limit of the confidence interval cannot be calculated if the number of observed infections equals zero; (9) No data are available from the state/territory for this reporting period; (10) The scores shown reflect fewer than 50 completed surveys; (11) There were discrepancies in the data collection process; (12) This measure does not apply to this hospital for this reporting period; (13) Results cannot be calculated for this reporting period; (14) The results for this state are combined with nearby states to protect confidentiality; Please refer to the User's Guide for a full explanation of data.

Blood Clot Prevention and Treatment

Anticoagulation Overlap Therapy

Hospital Name	City	Rate	Cases
Baylor Medical Center at Mckinney[2]	Mc Kinney	100%	55
Baylor Regional Medical Center at Plano[2]	Plano	100%	73
Bayshore Medical Center[2]	Pasadena	100%	96
College Station Medical Center[2]	College Station	100%	32
Conroe Regional Medical Center[2]	Conroe	100%	106
Cypress Fairbanks Medical Center[2]	Houston	100%	39
Detar Hospital Navarro[2]	Victoria	100%	25
Huntsville Memorial Hospital[2]	Huntsville	100%	35
Longview Regional Medical Center[2]	Longview	100%	49
Medical Center of Plano[2]	Plano	100%	135
Medical City Dallas Hospital[2]	Dallas	100%	83
Memorial Hermann Sugar Land Hospital[2]	Sugar Land	100%	34
Methodist Dallas Medical Center[2]	Dallas	100%	100
Methodist Mansfield Medical Center[2]	Mansfield	100%	85
Methodist Richardson Medical Center[2]	Richardson	100%	35
Methodist Stone Oak Hospital[2]	San Antonio	100%	41
Methodist Sugar Land Hospital[2]	Sugar Land	100%	95
North Hills Hospital[2]	N Richland Hls	100%	83
Plaza Medical Center of Fort Worth[2]	Fort Worth	100%	82
Rio Grande Regional Hospital[2]	Mcallen	100%	47
Round Rock Medical Center[2]	Round Rock	100%	48
Saint Joseph Medical Center[2]	Houston	100%	67
Seton Medical Center Hays[2]	Kyle	100%	36
Texas Health Presbyterian Hospital - WNJ[2]	Sherman	100%	41
Texas Reg Med Ctr at Sunnyvale[2]	Sunnyvale	100%	30
Texoma Medical Center[2]	Denison	100%	64
University Medical Center[2]	Lubbock	100%	82
University Medical Center of El Paso[2]	El Paso	100%	99
Wadley Regional Medical Center[2]	Texarkana	100%	48
Weatherford Regional Medical Center[2]	Weatherford	100%	35
West Houston Medical Center[2]	Houston	100%	59
Woodland Heights Medical Center[2]	Lufkin	100%	30
Baylor Reg Med Ctr at Grapevine[2]	Grapevine	99%	85
Clear Lake Regional Medical Center[2]	Webster	99%	153
Good Shepherd Medical Center[2]	Longview	99%	93
Methodist Charlton Medical Center[2]	Dallas	99%	131
North Austin Medical Center[2]	Austin	99%	109
Saint David's Medical Center[2]	Austin	99%	83
Scott & White Memorial Hospital[2]	Temple	99%	192
South Texas Health System[2]	Edinburg	99%	77
The Corpus Christi Medical Center[2]	Corpus Christi	98%	64
Harris Health System[2]	Houston	98%	166
JPS Health Network[2]	Fort Worth	98%	165
Medical Center of Mckinney[2]	Mckinney	98%	65
Memorial Hermann Northeast[2]	Humble	98%	98
Memorial Hermann Texas Medical Center[2]	Houston	98%	175
Methodist West Houston Hospital[2]	Houston	98%	46
Methodist Willowbrook Hospital[2]	Houston	98%	82
Midland Memorial Hospital[2]	Midland	98%	64
Saint David's South Austin Medical Center[2]	Austin	98%	105
Saint Luke's Hospital at the Vintage[2]	Houston	98%	43
University Health System[2]	San Antonio	98%	87
Valley Regional Medical Center[2]	Brownsville	98%	41
Baylor Medical Center at Irving[2]	Irving	97%	69
Baylor University Medical Center[2]	Dallas	97%	174
Las Colinas Medical Center[2]	Irving	97%	36
Memorial Hermann Hospital System[2]	Houston	97%	434
Methodist Hospital[2]	San Antonio	97%	310
Parkland Health & Hospital System[2]	Dallas	97%	155
Texas Health Presbyterian Hospital Denton[2]	Denton	97%	60
TX Health Presbyterian Hosp Rockwall[2]	Rockwall	97%	36
United Regional Health Care System[2]	Wichita Falls	97%	118
Baptist Medical Center[2]	San Antonio	96%	217
Dallas Regional Medical Center[2]	Mesquite	96%	27
Doctors Hospital[2]	Dallas	96%	28
Heart Hospital Baylor Plano[2]	Plano	96%	26
Hunt Regional Medical Center[2]	Greenville	96%	46
Medical Center of Arlington[2]	Arlington	96%	75
Medical Center of Lewisville[2]	Lewisville	96%	51
Memorial Hermann Katy Hospital[2]	Katy	96%	52
Memorial Medical Center of East Texas[2]	Lufkin	96%	47
Mother Frances Hospital[2]	Tyler	96%	134
Palestine Regional Medical Center[2]	Palestine	96%	28
Scott & White Hospital - Round Rock[2]	Round Rock	96%	52
Seton Medical Center Williamson[2]	Round Rock	96%	45
UT Southwestern University Hospital[2]	Dallas	96%	119
Citizens Medical Center[2]	Victoria	95%	37
Lake Pointe Medical Center[2]	Rowlett	95%	44
Saint Luke's Episcopal Hospital[2]	Houston	95%	211
Texas Health Arlington Memorial Hospital[2]	Arlington	95%	106
TX Hlth Harris Meth Hosp SW Ft Worth[2]	Fort Worth	95%	58
TX Hlth Presbyterian Hosp-Flower Mound[2]	Flower Mound	95%	37
Baylor Medical Center at Garland[2]	Garland	94%	77
Baylor Medical Center at Waxahachie[2]	Waxahachie	94%	34
Cedar Park Regional Medical Center[2]	Cedar Park	94%	32
Christus Saint Michael Health System[2]	Texarkana	94%	111
Covenant Medical Center[2]	Lubbock	94%	164
Hillcrest Baptist Medical Center[2]	Waco	94%	34
Houston Northwest Medical Center[2]	Houston	94%	93
Paris Regional Medical Center[2]	Paris	94%	48
Park Plaza Hospital[2]	Houston	94%	36
Providence Health Center[2]	Waco	94%	123
Seton Medical Center Austin[2]	Austin	94%	82
University Medical Center at Brackenridge[2]	Austin	94%	49
Baptist Saint Anthony's Hospital[2]	Amarillo	93%	144
Mem Hermann Mem City Med Ctr[2]	Houston	93%	116
Northwest Texas Hospital[2]	Amarillo	93%	45
Saint Luke's Sugar Land Hospital[2]	Sugar Land	93%	28
Abilene Regional Medical Center[2]	Abilene	92%	26
Centennial Medical Center[2]	Frisco	92%	51
Denton Regional Medical Center[2]	Denton	92%	89
Doctors Hospital at Renaissance[2]	Edinburg	92%	73
Kingwood Medical Center[2]	Kingwood	92%	96
Medical Center Hospital[2]	Odessa	92%	124
The Methodist Hospital[2]	Houston	92%	200
Metroplex Hospital[2]	Killeen	92%	38
TX Hlth Harris Meth Hosp-Alliance[2]	Fort Worth	92%	26
Univ of Texas Med Branch Galveston[2]	Galveston	92%	85
Baptist Beaumont Hospital[2]	Beaumont	91%	78
Sierra Providence East Medical Center[2]	El Paso	91%	46
Providence Memorial Hospital[2]	El Paso	90%	61
Texas Health Harris Methodist[2]	Bedford	90%	115
Baylor All Saints Medical Center at FW[2]	Fort Worth	89%	65
Hendrick Medical Center[2]	Abilene	89%	82
San Jacinto Methodist Hospital[2]	Baytown	89%	75
Sierra Medical Center[2]	El Paso	89%	61
Texas Health Harris Methodist Fort Worth[2]	Fort Worth	89%	219
Central Texas Medical Center[2]	San Marcos	88%	25
Christus Saint John Hospital[2]	Nassau Bay	88%	33
Saint Joseph Regional Health Center[2]	Bryan	87%	116
Christus Santa Rosa Hospital[2]	San Antonio	86%	110
North Cypress Medical Center[2]	Cypress	86%	78
Texas Health Presbyterian Hospital Plano[2]	Plano	86%	101
TX Hlth Harris Meth Hosp-Cleburne[2]	Cleburne	84%	44
Texas Health Presbyterian Hospital Dallas[2]	Dallas	83%	100
East Texas Medical Center[2]	Tyler	82%	137
The Medical Center of Southeast Texas[2]	Port Arthur	80%	59
Shannon Medical Center[2]	San Angelo	80%	64
Tomball Regional Medical Center[2]	Tomball	80%	46
Las Palmas Medical Center[2]	El Paso	79%	109
Christus Hospital[2]	Beaumont	75%	48
Saint Luke's the Woodlands Hospital[2]	The Woodlands	75%	67
Christus Spohn Hospital Corpus Christi[2]	Corpus Christi	73%	147
Laredo Medical Center[2]	Laredo	71%	34
Oakbend Medical Center[2]	Richmond	71%	28
Huguley Memorial Medical Center[2]	Burleson	70%	77
Saint Luke's Patients Medical Center[2]	Pasadena	68%	40
VHS Harlingen Hospital Company[2]	Harlingen	66%	62
Memorial Hospital[2]	Nacogdoches	59%	32
Nacogdoches Medical Center[2]	Nacogdoches	55%	38
Lubbock Heart Hospital[2]	Lubbock	45%	29

ICU Venous Thromboembolism Prophylaxis

Hospital Name	City	Rate	Cases
Baylor Medical Center at Mckinney[2]	Mc Kinney	100%	69
Baylor University Medical Center[2]	Dallas	100%	101
Brazosport Regional Health System[2]	Lake Jackson	100%	49
The Corpus Christi Medical Center[2]	Corpus Christi	100%	115
Cuero Community Hospital[2]	Cuero	100%	26
Detar Hospital Navarro[2]	Victoria	100%	113
Good Shepherd Medical Center[2]	Longview	100%	61
Heart Hospital Baylor Plano[2]	Plano	100%	254
JPS Health Network[2]	Fort Worth	100%	91
Lake Granbury Medical Center[2]	Granbury	100%	67
Lake Pointe Medical Center[2]	Rowlett	100%	41
Longview Regional Medical Center[2]	Longview	100%	91
Medical Center of Plano[2]	Plano	100%	117
Medical City Dallas Hospital[2]	Dallas	100%	96
Memorial Hermann Northeast[2]	Humble	100%	68
Methodist Dallas Medical Center[2]	Dallas	100%	126
Methodist Richardson Medical Center[2]	Richardson	100%	66
Methodist Stone Oak Hospital[2]	San Antonio	100%	93
Methodist Sugar Land Hospital[2]	Sugar Land	100%	102
Moore County Hospital District[2]	Dumas	100%	31
Parkland Health & Hospital System[2]	Dallas	100%	109
Scenic Mountain Medical Center[2]	Big Spring	100%	54
Sierra Providence East Medical Center[2]	El Paso	100%	72
South Texas Regional Medical Center[2]	Jourdanton	100%	45
TX Hlth Harris Meth Hosp SW Ft Worth[2]	Fort Worth	100%	41
Texas Health Presbyterian Hospital Allen[2]	Allen	100%	36
TX Hlth Presbyterian Hosp-Kaufman[2]	Kaufman	100%	29
Texas Health Presbyterian Hospital Plano[2]	Plano	100%	109
Texoma Medical Center[2]	Denison	100%	90
University Medical Center of El Paso[2]	El Paso	100%	130
Univ of TX Health Science Ctr-Tyler[2]	Tyler	100%	56
Weatherford Regional Medical Center[2]	Weatherford	100%	100
Woodland Heights Medical Center[2]	Lufkin	100%	98
Abilene Regional Medical Center[2]	Abilene	99%	106
Baptist Medical Center[2]	San Antonio	99%	258
Baylor Heart & Vascular Hospital[2]	Dallas	99%	76
Baylor Regional Medical Center at Plano[2]	Plano	99%	100
Bayshore Medical Center[2]	Pasadena	99%	121
Kingwood Medical Center[2]	Kingwood	99%	110
Memorial Hermann Katy Hospital[2]	Katy	99%	81
Methodist Hospital[2]	San Antonio	99%	126
Metroplex Hospital[2]	Killeen	99%	103
North Hills Hospital[2]	N Richland Hls	99%	80
Palestine Regional Medical Center[2]	Palestine	99%	86
Peterson Regional Medical Center[2]	Kerrville	99%	93
Providence Memorial Hospital[2]	El Paso	99%	77
Rio Grande Regional Hospital[2]	Mcallen	99%	97
Saint Joseph Regional Health Center[2]	Bryan	99%	75
Scott & White Memorial Hospital[2]	Temple	99%	85
Sierra Medical Center[2]	El Paso	99%	113
South Texas Health System[2]	Edinburg	99%	103
Texas Health Presbyterian Hospital Denton[2]	Denton	99%	78
Univ of Texas Med Branch Galveston[2]	Galveston	99%	97
West Houston Medical Center[2]	Houston	99%	116
Baylor Reg Med Ctr at Grapevine[2]	Grapevine	98%	60
Clear Lake Regional Medical Center[2]	Webster	98%	146
Doctors Hospital[2]	Dallas	98%	63
Hill Country Memorial Hospital[2]	Fredericksburg	98%	50
Knapp Medical Center[2]	Weslaco	98%	92
Laredo Medical Center[2]	Laredo	98%	62
Las Colinas Medical Center[2]	Irving	98%	61
Memorial Hermann Hospital System[2]	Houston	98%	338
Mem Hermann Mem City Med Ctr[2]	Houston	98%	89
Memorial Hermann Texas Medical Center[2]	Houston	98%	143
Methodist Charlton Medical Center[2]	Dallas	98%	84
Methodist West Houston Hospital[2]	Houston	98%	88
Mother Frances Hospital[2]	Tyler	98%	90
Round Rock Medical Center[2]	Round Rock	98%	53
Saint David's Medical Center[2]	Austin	98%	90
Seton Medical Center Williamson[2]	Round Rock	98%	134
Texas Health Arlington Memorial Hospital[2]	Arlington	98%	85
TX Hlth Harris Meth Hosp-Cleburne[2]	Cleburne	98%	55
Texas Health Harris Methodist[2]	Bedford	98%	63
TX Hlth Heart & Vasc Hosp-Arlington[2]	Arlington	98%	86
Texas Health Presbyterian Hospital Dallas[2]	Dallas	98%	59
UT SW Univ Hosp-Zale Lipshy[2]	Dallas	98%	110
Wadley Regional Medical Center[2]	Texarkana	98%	111
Baptist Beaumont Hospital[2]	Beaumont	97%	95
Baylor Medical Center at Irving[2]	Irving	97%	119
College Station Medical Center[2]	College Station	97%	110
Conroe Regional Medical Center[2]	Conroe	97%	130
Covenant Hospital Plainview[2]	Plainview	97%	34
Cypress Fairbanks Medical Center[2]	Houston	97%	113
Medical Center of Arlington[2]	Arlington	97%	89
Medical Center of Lewisville[2]	Lewisville	97%	38
North Austin Medical Center[2]	Austin	97%	77
TX Hlth Harris Meth Hosp-Stephenville[2]	Stephenville	97%	33
University Medical Center at Brackenridge[2]	Austin	97%	71
Baylor Medical Center at Garland[2]	Garland	96%	102
Cleveland Regional Medical Center[2]	Cleveland	96%	47
Methodist Willowbrook Hospital[2]	Houston	96%	96
TX Hlth Harris Methodist Hosp-Azle[2]	Azle	96%	48
UT Southwestern University Hospital[2]	Dallas	96%	124
Baylor Medical Center at Waxahachie[2]	Waxahachie	95%	73
Cedar Park Regional Medical Center[2]	Cedar Park	95%	41
Central Texas Medical Center[2]	San Marcos	95%	63
Matagorda Regional Medical Center[2]	Bay City	95%	61
Memorial Hermann Sugar Land Hospital[2]	Sugar Land	95%	66
Methodist Mansfield Medical Center[2]	Mansfield	95%	81
Midland Memorial Hospital[2]	Midland	95%	87
North Texas Medical Center[2]	Gainesville	95%	42
Seton Northwest Hospital[2]	Austin	95%	62
Texas Health Harris Methodist Fort Worth[2]	Fort Worth	95%	135
United Regional Health Care System[2]	Wichita Falls	95%	66
University Medical Center[2]	Lubbock	95%	147
Angleton - Danbury Medical Center[2]	Angleton	94%	36
Denton Regional Medical Center[2]	Denton	94%	108
Doctors Hospital at Renaissance[2]	Edinburg	94%	48
Harris Health System[2]	Houston	94%	124
Medical Center of Mckinney[2]	Mckinney	94%	80
Odessa Regional Hospital[2]	Odessa	94%	99
Paris Regional Medical Center[2]	Paris	94%	72
Saint David's South Austin Medical Center[2]	Austin	94%	80
San Angelo Community Medical Center[2]	San Angelo	94%	89
University Health System[2]	San Antonio	94%	81
VHS Harlingen Hospital Company[2]	Harlingen	94%	71
Christus Saint John Hospital[2]	Nassau Bay	93%	71
Mission Regional Medical Center[2]	Mission	93%	131
Seton Medical Center Harker Heights[2]	Harker Heights	93%	90
Seton Medical Center Hays[2]	Kyle	93%	68
Texas Reg Med Ctr at Sunnyvale[2]	Sunnyvale	93%	60
Tomball Regional Medical Center[2]	Tomball	93%	107
Brownwood Regional Medical Center[2]	Brownwood	92%	52
Houston Northwest Medical Center[2]	Houston	92%	119

NOTE: Hospital profiles are in alphabetical order by state, then city, then hospital within the city; Rankings exclude hospitals with less than 25 cases except for patient surveys which excludes hospitals with less than 100 cases; (a) 100-299 cases; (1) The number of cases/patients is too few to report; (2) Data submitted were based on a sample of cases/patients; (3) Results are based on a shorter time period than required; (4) Data suppressed by CMS for one or more quarters; (5) Results are not available for this reporting period; (6) Fewer than 100 patients completed the HCAHPS survey; (7) No cases met the criteria for this measure; (8) The lower limit of the confidence interval cannot be calculated if the number of observed infections equals zero; (9) No data are available from the state/territory for this reporting period; (10) The scores shown reflect fewer than 50 completed surveys; (11) There were discrepancies in the data collection process; (12) This measure does not apply to this hospital for this reporting period; (13) Results cannot be calculated for this reporting period; (14) The results for this state are combined with nearby states to protect confidentiality; Please refer to the User's Guide for a full explanation of data.

The Methodist Hospital[2]	Houston	92%	134
Northwest Texas Hospital[2]	Amarillo	92%	186
Oakbend Medical Center[2]	Richmond	92%	92
Pampa Regional Medical Center[2]	Pampa	92%	49
Plaza Medical Center of Fort Worth[2]	Fort Worth	92%	104
Saint Joseph Medical Center[2]	Houston	92%	108
Texas General Hospital[3]	Grand Prairie	92%	25
East Texas Medical Center[2]	Tyler	91%	102
Las Palmas Medical Center[2]	El Paso	91%	117
North Cypress Medical Center[2]	Cypress	91%	69
Park Plaza Hospital[2]	Houston	91%	65
TX Hlth Harris Meth Hosp-Alliance[2]	Fort Worth	91%	57
Dallas Regional Medical Center[2]	Mesquite	90%	94
Hendrick Medical Center[2]	Abilene	90%	71
Medical Center Hospital[2]	Odessa	90%	132
Memorial Medical Center of East Texas[2]	Lufkin	90%	93
Nacogdoches Medical Center[2]	Nacogdoches	90%	90
San Jacinto Methodist Hospital[2]	Baytown	90%	121
Uvalde Memorial Hospital[2]	Uvalde	90%	186
Baylor Medical Center at Carrollton[2]	Carrollton	89%	88
Centennial Medical Center[2]	Frisco	89%	65
Rolling Plains Memorial Hospital[2]	Sweetwater	89%	53
Southwest General Hospital[2]	San Antonio	89%	71
Valley Regional Medical Center[2]	Brownsville	89%	73
Baylor All Saints Medical Center at FW[2]	Fort Worth	88%	84
Citizens Medical Center[2]	Victoria	88%	72
Doctors Hospital of Laredo[2]	Laredo	88%	102
Hillcrest Baptist Medical Center[2]	Waco	88%	112
Scott & White Hospital - Round Rock[2]	Round Rock	88%	41
Shannon Medical Center[2]	San Angelo	88%	66
Texas Health Presbyterian Hospital - WNJ[2]	Sherman	88%	113
Saint Luke's the Woodlands Hospital[2]	The Woodlands	87%	79
TX Hlth Presbyterian Hosp-Flower Mound[2]	Flower Mound	87%	39
TX Health Presbyterian Hosp Rockwall[2]	Rockwall	87%	103
Wise Regional Health System[2]	Decatur	87%	145
Gulf Coast Medical Center[2]	Wharton	86%	49
Seton Medical Center Austin[2]	Austin	86%	71
Huguley Memorial Medical Center[2]	Burleson	85%	87
Huntsville Memorial Hospital[2]	Huntsville	85%	47
Lakeway Regional Medical Center[2]	Lakeway	84%	49
Memorial Medical Center Livingston[2]	Livingston	84%	45
Providence Health Center[2]	Waco	84%	100
VHS Brownsville Hospital Company[2]	Brownsville	84%	69
Baptist Saint Anthony's Hospital[2]	Amarillo	83%	153
Guadalupe Regional Medical Center[2]	Seguin	83%	59
Fort Duncan Medical Center[2]	Eagle Pass	82%	102
Harlingen Medical Center[2]	Harlingen	82%	71
Hunt Regional Medical Center[2]	Greenville	82%	124
Memorial Hermann Baptist Orange Hospital[2]	Orange	82%	38
Saint Luke's Sugar Land Hospital[2]	Sugar Land	81%	75
Titus Regional Medical Center[2]	Mount Pleasant	81%	42
Christus Spohn Hospital Corpus Christi[2]	Corpus Christi	80%	94
Saint Luke's Patients Medical Center[2]	Pasadena	80%	61
Christus Spohn Hospital Beeville[2]	Beeville	79%	57
Covenant Medical Center[2]	Lubbock	79%	103
Care Regional Medical Center[2]	Aransas Pass	78%	93
Saint Luke's Episcopal Hospital[2]	Houston	77%	108
Navarro Regional Hospital[2]	Corsicana	76%	63
University General Hospital[2]	Houston	76%	49
The Medical Center of Southeast Texas[2]	Port Arthur	75%	127
Nix Health Care System[2]	San Antonio	75%	60
Christus Saint Michael Health System[2]	Texarkana	74%	97
Saint Luke's Hospital at the Vintage[2]	Houston	74%	61
Lubbock Heart Hospital[2]	Lubbock	73%	79
Val Verde Regional Medical Center[2]	Del Rio	73%	51
Christus Hospital[2]	Beaumont	69%	72
Christus Saint Catherine Hospital[2]	Katy	69%	67
Christus Santa Rosa Hospital[2]	San Antonio	69%	149
East Texas Medical Center Jacksonville[2]	Jacksonville	69%	26
Christus Spohn Hospital Alice[2]	Alice	68%	94
Hopkins County Memorial Hospital[2]	Sulphur Springs	68%	40
Christus Spohn Hospital Kleberg[2]	Kingsville	67%	89
Palo Pinto General Hospital[2]	Mineral Wells	67%	39
Dallas Medical Center[2]	Dallas	63%	38
Starr County Memorial Hospital[2]	Rio Grande City	63%	84
El Campo Memorial Hospital[2]	El Campo	62%	26
Doctors Hospital Tidwell[2]	Houston	60%	80
Saint Anthony's Hospital[2]	Houston	60%	86
East Texas Medical Center Athens[2]	Athens	59%	49
Memorial Hospital[2]	Nacogdoches	53%	131
University General Hospital Dallas[2]	Dallas	42%	53
Christus Jasper Memorial Hospital[2]	Jasper	36%	47

Incidence of Potentially Preventable VTE

Hospital Name	City	Rate	Cases
JPS Health Network[2]	Fort Worth	0%	57
Medical Center of Plano[2]	Plano	0%	47
University Medical Center of El Paso[2]	El Paso	0%	33
Univ of Texas Med Branch Galveston[2]	Galveston	0%	27
Harris Health System[2]	Houston	2%	53
Memorial Hermann Texas Medical Center[2]	Houston	2%	109
Methodist Hospital[2]	San Antonio	3%	86
UT Southwestern University Hospital[2]	Dallas	3%	35
East Texas Medical Center[2]	Tyler	4%	25
Baylor University Medical Center[2]	Dallas	5%	56
University Health System[2]	San Antonio	5%	42
Memorial Hermann Hospital System[2]	Houston	6%	85
Saint Luke's Episcopal Hospital[2]	Houston	6%	62
Texas Health Harris Methodist Fort Worth[2]	Fort Worth	6%	71
Baptist Medical Center[2]	San Antonio	7%	46
Medical Center of Arlington[2]	Arlington	7%	27
Scott & White Memorial Hospital[2]	Temple	8%	38
Seton Medical Center Austin[2]	Austin	8%	25
Doctors Hospital at Renaissance[2]	Edinburg	10%	30
Christus Saint Michael Health System[2]	Texarkana	15%	26
Covenant Medical Center[2]	Lubbock	19%	48
Parkland Health & Hospital System[2]	Dallas	19%	67
Las Palmas Medical Center[2]	El Paso	20%	30
The Methodist Hospital[2]	Houston	20%	87
Christus Spohn Hospital Corpus Christi[2]	Corpus Christi	25%	61

UFH with Dosages/Platelet Count Monitoring

Hospital Name	City	Rate	Cases
Baylor All Saints Medical Center at FW[2]	Fort Worth	100%	29
Baylor Medical Center at Irving[2]	Irving	100%	68
Baylor University Medical Center[2]	Dallas	100%	131
Bayshore Medical Center[2]	Pasadena	100%	42
Christus Spohn Hospital Corpus Christi[2]	Corpus Christi	100%	33
Clear Lake Regional Medical Center[2]	Webster	100%	38
Conroe Regional Medical Center[2]	Conroe	100%	38
Harris Health System[2]	Houston	100%	138
JPS Health Network[2]	Fort Worth	100%	68
Kingwood Medical Center[2]	Kingwood	100%	46
Medical Center of Mckinney[2]	Mckinney	100%	29
Medical Center of Plano[2]	Plano	100%	44
Mem Hermann Mem City Med Ctr[2]	Houston	100%	46
Memorial Hermann Northeast[2]	Humble	100%	37
Memorial Hermann Texas Medical Center[2]	Houston	100%	177
Memorial Medical Center of East Texas[2]	Lufkin	100%	52
Methodist Charlton Medical Center[2]	Dallas	100%	76
Methodist Dallas Medical Center[2]	Dallas	100%	72
Methodist Hospital[2]	San Antonio	100%	126
Methodist Mansfield Medical Center[2]	Mansfield	100%	27
Methodist Willowbrook Hospital[2]	Houston	100%	44
Mother Frances Hospital[2]	Tyler	100%	43
North Cypress Medical Center[2]	Cypress	100%	41
Northwest Texas Hospital[2]	Amarillo	100%	43
Park Plaza Hospital[2]	Houston	100%	26
Parkland Health & Hospital System[2]	Dallas	100%	140
Saint Luke's Episcopal Hospital[2]	Houston	100%	179
San Jacinto Methodist Hospital[2]	Baytown	100%	57
Scott & White Memorial Hospital[2]	Temple	100%	144
Seton Medical Center Austin[2]	Austin	100%	27
South Texas Health System[2]	Edinburg	100%	42
Texas Health Presbyterian Hospital - WNJ[2]	Sherman	100%	31
Texas Health Presbyterian Hospital Plano[2]	Plano	100%	32
Texoma Medical Center[2]	Denison	100%	25
Tomball Regional Medical Center[2]	Tomball	100%	42
United Regional Health Care System[2]	Wichita Falls	100%	42
University Health System[2]	San Antonio	100%	56
University Medical Center[2]	Lubbock	100%	29
Univ of Texas Med Branch Galveston[2]	Galveston	100%	89
UT Southwestern University Hospital[2]	Dallas	100%	115
Baptist Saint Anthony's Hospital[2]	Amarillo	99%	74
Memorial Hermann Hospital System[2]	Houston	99%	105
The Methodist Hospital[2]	Houston	99%	179
Texas Health Harris Methodist Fort Worth[2]	Fort Worth	99%	73
Baptist Medical Center[2]	San Antonio	98%	96
Plaza Medical Center of Fort Worth[2]	Fort Worth	97%	38
Saint Luke's the Woodlands Hospital[2]	The Woodlands	96%	27
Christus Santa Rosa Hospital[2]	San Antonio	92%	40
Texas Health Presbyterian Hospital Dallas[2]	Dallas	88%	40
East Texas Medical Center[2]	Tyler	84%	31
Medical Center Hospital[2]	Odessa	74%	27
Doctors Hospital at Renaissance[2]	Edinburg	26%	135

Venous Thromboembolism Prophylaxis

Hospital Name	City	Rate	Cases
Baylor Medical Center at Mckinney[2]	Mc Kinney	100%	327
Baylor Surgical Hospital at Fort Worth[2]	Fort Worth	100%	61
Fdn Surgical Hosp of San Antonio[2]	San Antonio	100%	100
Houston Physicians' Hospital	Webster	100%	94
Medical Center of Plano[2]	Plano	100%	341
Methodist Ambulatory Surgery Hospital NW[2]	San Antonio	100%	43
Methodist Dallas Medical Center[2]	Dallas	100%	350
Methodist Hospital For Surgery[2]	Addison	100%	94
Methodist Stone Oak Hospital[2]	San Antonio	100%	331
North Hills Hospital[2]	N Richland Hls	100%	340
Peterson Regional Medical Center[2]	Kerrville	100%	342
Sugar Land Surgical Hospital[2]	Sugar Land	100%	30
TX Health Ctr for Diag & Surgery	Plano	100%	306
TX Hlth Harris Meth Hosp-Southlake	Southlake	100%	117
Texoma Medical Center[2]	Denison	100%	362
Tops Surgical Specialty Hospital[2]	Houston	100%	30
University Medical Center of El Paso[2]	El Paso	100%	330
Woodland Heights Medical Center[2]	Lufkin	100%	322
Abilene Regional Medical Center[2]	Abilene	99%	343
Baylor Heart & Vascular Hospital[2]	Dallas	99%	201
Baylor Medical Center at Frisco[2]	Frisco	99%	110
Baylor Medical Center at Trophy Club[2]	Trophy Club	99%	70
Baylor Medical Center at Uptown[2]	Dallas	99%	69
College Station Medical Center[2]	College Station	99%	346
The Corpus Christi Medical Center[2]	Corpus Christi	99%	326
Detar Hospital Navarro[2]	Victoria	99%	371
El Paso Specialty Hospital[2]	El Paso	99%	234
Hill Country Memorial Hospital[2]	Fredericksburg	99%	190
The Hospital at Westlake Medical Center[2]	Austin	99%	155
Houston Orthopedic & Spine Hospital[2]	Bellaire	99%	112
Lake Granbury Medical Center[2]	Granbury	99%	195
Memorial Hermann Sugar Land Hospital[2]	Sugar Land	99%	311
Palestine Regional Medical Center[2]	Palestine	99%	234
Quail Creek Surgical Hospital	Amarillo	99%	227
Rio Grande Regional Hospital[2]	Mcallen	99%	400
Saint Marks Medical Center[2]	La Grange	99%	188
Texas Orthopedic Hospital[2]	Houston	99%	144
Baylor Regional Medical Center at Plano[2]	Plano	98%	364
Baylor Surgical Hospital at Las Colinas[2]	Irving	98%	45
Big Bend Regional Medical Center[2]	Alpine	98%	187
Cedar Park Regional Medical Center[2]	Cedar Park	98%	249
First Surgical Hospital	Bellaire	98%	122
Lake Pointe Medical Center[2]	Rowlett	98%	347
Northwest Hills Surgical Hospital	Austin	98%	43
Saint Luke's Lakeside Hospital[2]	The Woodlands	98%	51
Seton Smithville Regional Hospital[2]	Smithville	98%	130
South Texas Spine & Surgical Hospital	San Antonio	98%	422
Texas Health Harris Methodist[2]	Bedford	98%	312
Texas Health Presbyterian Hospital Denton[2]	Denton	98%	416
Tyler County Hospital[2]	Woodville	98%	352
USMD Hospital at Fort Worth	Fort Worth	98%	57
Weatherford Regional Medical Center[2]	Weatherford	98%	359
Baylor Medical Center at Irving[2]	Irving	97%	347
Baylor Ortho & Spine Hosp-Arlington[2]	Arlington	97%	36
Brownwood Regional Medical Center[2]	Brownwood	97%	304
Kingwood Medical Center[2]	Kingwood	97%	403
Memorial Hermann Katy Hospital[2]	Katy	97%	322
Methodist Sugar Land Hospital[2]	Sugar Land	97%	345
Metroplex Hospital[2]	Killeen	97%	305
North Austin Medical Center[2]	Austin	97%	394
Round Rock Medical Center[2]	Round Rock	97%	357
Seton Medical Center Williamson[2]	Round Rock	97%	307
TX Hlth Presbyterian Hosp-Kaufman[2]	Kaufman	97%	180
Univ of Texas Med Branch Galveston[2]	Galveston	97%	316
UT SW Univ Hosp-Zale Lipshy[2]	Dallas	97%	205
Baylor Medical Center at Garland[2]	Garland	96%	364
Bayshore Medical Center[2]	Pasadena	96%	395
Brazosport Regional Health System[2]	Lake Jackson	96%	392
Longview Regional Medical Center[2]	Longview	96%	428
Methodist Charlton Medical Center[2]	Dallas	96%	376
Pine Creek Medical Center[2]	Dallas	96%	110
Providence Memorial Hospital[2]	El Paso	96%	373
Saint David's Medical Center[2]	Austin	96%	337
San Angelo Community Medical Center[2]	San Angelo	96%	339
TX Hlth Harris Methodist Hosp-Azle[2]	Azle	96%	211
TX Hlth Harris Meth Hosp-Cleburne[2]	Cleburne	96%	369
Texas Health Presbyterian Hospital Allen[2]	Allen	96%	283
United Regional Health Care System[2]	Wichita Falls	96%	369
Baylor Reg Med Ctr at Grapevine[2]	Grapevine	95%	357
Central Texas Medical Center[2]	San Marcos	95%	303
Doctors Hospital at Renaissance[2]	Edinburg	95%	307
Heart Hospital Baylor Plano[2]	Plano	95%	291
Laredo Medical Center[2]	Laredo	95%	451
Las Colinas Medical Center[2]	Irving	95%	279
Matagorda Regional Medical Center[2]	Bay City	95%	202
Medical Center of Lewisville[2]	Lewisville	95%	382
Memorial Hermann Texas Medical Center[2]	Houston	95%	286
Saint David's South Austin Medical Center[2]	Austin	95%	380
Sierra Providence East Medical Center[2]	El Paso	95%	399
Univ of TX Health Science Ctr-Tyler[2]	Tyler	95%	140
Baylor Medical Center at Waxahachie[2]	Waxahachie	94%	262
Grace Medical Center	Lubbock	94%	232
Mem Hermann Mem City Med Ctr[2]	Houston	94%	319
Methodist Hospital[2]	San Antonio	94%	438
North Central Surgical Center[2]	Dallas	94%	62
Odessa Regional Hospital[2]	Odessa	94%	190
Rolling Plains Memorial Hospital[2]	Sweetwater	94%	127
South Texas Regional Medical Center[2]	Jourdanton	94%	197
TX Hlth Harris Meth Hosp-Alliance[2]	Fort Worth	94%	126
TX Hlth Presbyterian Hosp-Flower Mound[2]	Flower Mound	94%	314
University Health System[2]	San Antonio	94%	285
Clear Lake Regional Medical Center[2]	Webster	93%	364
Cleveland Regional Medical Center[2]	Cleveland	93%	227
Ennis Regional Medical Center[2]	Ennis	93%	175

NOTE: Hospital profiles are in alphabetical order by state, then city, then hospital within the city; Rankings exclude hospitals with less than 25 cases except for patient surveys which excludes hospitals with less than 100 cases; (a) 100-299 cases; (1) The number of cases/patients is too few to report; (2) Data submitted were based on a sample of cases/patients; (3) Results are based on a shorter time period than required; (4) Data suppressed by CMS for one or more quarters; (5) Results are not available for this reporting period; (6) Fewer than 100 patients completed the HCAHPS survey; (7) No cases met the criteria for this measure; (8) The lower limit of the confidence interval cannot be calculated if the number of observed infections equals zero; (9) No data are available from the state/territory for this reporting period; (10) The scores shown reflect fewer than 50 completed surveys; (11) There were discrepancies in the data collection process; (12) This measure does not apply to this hospital for this reporting period; (13) Results cannot be calculated for this reporting period; (14) The results for this state are combined with nearby states to protect confidentiality; Please refer to the User's Guide for a full explanation of data.

Hillcrest Baptist Medical Center[2]	Waco	93%	285
Medical City Dallas Hospital[2]	Dallas	93%	371
Methodist Richardson Medical Center[2]	Richardson	93%	341
Scenic Mountain Medical Center[2]	Big Spring	93%	235
Scott & White Hospital - Round Rock[2]	Round Rock	93%	335
Baylor University Medical Center[2]	Dallas	92%	355
Connally Memorial Medical Center[2]	Floresville	92%	145
JPS Health Network[2]	Fort Worth	92%	401
Lakeway Regional Medical Center[2]	Lakeway	92%	87
Memorial Hermann Hospital System[2]	Houston	92%	1432
Angleton - Danbury Medical Center[2]	Angleton	91%	111
Covenant Hospital Plainview[2]	Plainview	91%	170
Memorial Hermann Northeast[2]	Humble	91%	385
Methodist Mansfield Medical Center[2]	Mansfield	91%	401
North Cypress Medical Center[2]	Cypress	91%	371
Saint Joseph Regional Health Center[2]	Bryan	91%	342
Sierra Medical Center[2]	El Paso	91%	358
TX Hlth Harris Meth Hosp SW Ft Worth[2]	Fort Worth	91%	400
TX Inst for Surgery at Presby Hosp	Dallas	91%	57
UT Southwestern University Hospital[2]	Dallas	91%	383
Wadley Regional Medical Center[2]	Texarkana	91%	405
West Houston Medical Center[2]	Houston	91%	370
The Womans Hospital of Texas[2]	Houston	91%	105
Baylor Medical Center at Carrollton[2]	Carrollton	90%	335
Conroe Regional Medical Center[2]	Conroe	90%	364
Huguley Memorial Medical Center[2]	Burleson	90%	356
Kell West Regional Hospital	Wichita Falls	90%	344
Knapp Medical Center[2]	Weslaco	90%	301
Seton Northwest Hospital[2]	Austin	90%	300
South Texas Surgical Hospital	Corpus Christi	90%	262
Texas General Hospital[3]	Grand Prairie	90%	116
TX Hlth Heart & Vasc Hosp-Arlington[2]	Arlington	90%	71
University Medical Center[2]	Lubbock	90%	294
Denton Regional Medical Center[2]	Denton	89%	326
Medical Center of Mckinney[2]	Mckinney	89%	362
Shannon Medical Center[2]	San Angelo	89%	340
South Texas Health System[2]	Edinburg	89%	334
Texas Health Harris Methodist Fort Worth[2]	Fort Worth	89%	355
TX Hlth Harris Meth Hosp-Stephenville[2]	Stephenville	89%	132
Good Shepherd Medical Center Marshall[2]	Marshall	88%	281
Mission Regional Medical Center[2]	Mission	88%	339
Mother Frances Hospital[2]	Tyler	88%	336
Parkview Regional Hospital[2]	Mexia	88%	112
Valley Regional Medical Center[2]	Brownsville	88%	388
Cypress Fairbanks Medical Center[2]	Houston	87%	335
Doctors Hospital[2]	Dallas	87%	369
East Texas Medical Center - Gilmer[2]	Gilmer	87%	117
Houston Hospital for Specialized Surgery	Houston	87%	30
Pampa Regional Medical Center[2]	Pampa	87%	90
Rollins Brook Community Hospital[2]	Lampasas	87%	87
Seton Medical Center Harker Heights[2]	Harker Heights	87%	282
Texas Health Arlington Memorial Hospital[2]	Arlington	87%	443
University Medical Center at Brackenridge[2]	Austin	87%	313
Seton Medical Center Hays[2]	Kyle	86%	348
Texas Health Presbyterian Hospital Plano[2]	Plano	86%	283
Titus Regional Medical Center[2]	Mount Pleasant	86%	118
Arise Austin Medical Center[2]	Austin	85%	27
Centennial Medical Center[2]	Frisco	85%	341
Graham Regional Medical Center[2]	Graham	85%	113
Midland Memorial Hospital[2]	Midland	85%	356
Park Plaza Hospital[2]	Houston	85%	386
Scott & White Memorial Hospital[2]	Temple	85%	326
Texas Health Presbyterian Hospital Dallas[2]	Dallas	85%	376
Texas Reg Med Ctr at Sunnyvale[2]	Sunnyvale	85%	358
Baptist Saint Anthony's Hospital[2]	Amarillo	84%	316
Baylor All Saints Medical Center at FW[2]	Fort Worth	84%	331
Medical Center of Arlington[2]	Arlington	84%	433
Moore County Hospital District[2]	Dumas	84%	57
Northwest Texas Hospital[2]	Amarillo	84%	227
Parkland Health & Hospital System[2]	Dallas	84%	292
Plaza Medical Center of Fort Worth[2]	Fort Worth	84%	313
Seton Medical Center Austin[2]	Austin	84%	329
East Texas Medical Center[2]	Tyler	83%	271
Houston Northwest Medical Center[2]	Houston	83%	350
Methodist Mckinney Hospital[2]	Mc Kinney	83%	30
Nacogdoches Medical Center[2]	Nacogdoches	83%	255
Medical Arts Hospital[2]	Lamesa	82%	142
Methodist Willowbrook Hospital[2]	Houston	82%	347
The Physicians Centre	Bryan	82%	50
Christus Spohn Hospital Beeville[2]	Beeville	81%	151
Hendrick Medical Center[2]	Abilene	81%	367
Hill Regional Hospital[2]	Hillsboro	81%	221
Hunt Regional Medical Center[2]	Greenville	81%	291
Medical Center Hospital[2]	Odessa	81%	291
Memorial Medical Center Livingston[2]	Livingston	81%	204
Permian Regional Medical Center	Andrews	81%	166
Saint Luke's Hospital at the Vintage[2]	Houston	81%	268
Saint Luke's Patients Medical Center[2]	Pasadena	81%	392
San Jacinto Methodist Hospital[2]	Baytown	81%	352
Scott & White Hospital Brenham[2]	Brenham	81%	93
Foundation Surgical Hospital of El Paso[2]	El Paso	80%	35
Uvalde Memorial Hospital[2]	Uvalde	80%	441
Wise Regional Health System[2]	Decatur	80%	269
Fort Duncan Medical Center[2]	Eagle Pass	79%	307
Methodist West Houston Hospital[2]	Houston	79%	339
Seymour Hospital[2]	Seymour	79%	211
Anson General Hospital	Anson	78%	185
Cuero Community Hospital[2]	Cuero	78%	105
Guadalupe Regional Medical Center[2]	Seguin	78%	261
Saint Joseph Medical Center[2]	Houston	78%	340
Baptist Medical Center[2]	San Antonio	77%	908
Dallas Regional Medical Center[2]	Mesquite	77%	295
North Texas Medical Center[2]	Gainesville	77%	79
Paris Regional Medical Center[2]	Paris	77%	426
Saint Luke's Sugar Land Hospital[2]	Sugar Land	77%	312
USMD Hospital at Arlington[2]	Arlington	77%	115
Saint Luke's Episcopal Hospital[2]	Houston	76%	357
Seton Southwest Hospital[2]	Austin	76%	85
TX Health Presbyterian Hosp Rockwall[2]	Rockwall	76%	703
Christus Spohn Hospital Corpus Christi[2]	Corpus Christi	75%	334
Harlingen Medical Center[2]	Harlingen	75%	323
Huntsville Memorial Hospital[2]	Huntsville	75%	378
Southwest General Hospital[2]	San Antonio	75%	409
Harris Health System[2]	Houston	74%	673
Memorial Hermann Baptist Orange Hospital[2]	Orange	74%	129
Oakbend Medical Center[2]	Richmond	74%	294
Providence Health Center[2]	Waco	74%	308
Doctors Hospital of Laredo[2]	Laredo	73%	400
Gulf Coast Medical Center[2]	Wharton	73%	55
Memorial Medical Center of East Texas[2]	Lufkin	73%	340
Saint Luke's the Woodlands Hospital[2]	The Woodlands	73%	330
Christus Saint John Hospital[2]	Nassau Bay	72%	330
Christus Saint Michael Health System[2]	Texarkana	72%	380
Good Shepherd Medical Center[2]	Longview	72%	359
Las Palmas Medical Center[2]	El Paso	72%	409
Citizens Medical Center[2]	Victoria	71%	345
Covenant Medical Center[2]	Lubbock	71%	307
Hereford Regional Medical Center[2]	Hereford	71%	129
Nix Health Care System[2]	San Antonio	70%	258
Cogdell Memorial Hospital	Snyder	67%	220
Texas Health Presbyterian Hospital - WNJ[2]	Sherman	67%	321
Tomball Regional Medical Center[2]	Tomball	67%	416
Stamford Memorial Hospital[2]	Stamford	66%	148
Christus Spohn Hospital Kleberg[2]	Kingsville	65%	361
Etmc Carthage[2]	Carthage	65%	106
The Methodist Hospital[2]	Houston	65%	298
Baptist Beaumont Hospital[2]	Beaumont	64%	389
Care Regional Medical Center[2]	Aransas Pass	64%	70
Scott & White Hospital - Llano[2]	Llano	64%	132
Childress Regional Medical Center	Childress	63%	224
East Texas Medical Center Pittsburg[2]	Pittsburg	63%	131
Christus Hospital[2]	Beaumont	60%	368
Dallas Medical Center[2]	Dallas	59%	235
Val Verde Regional Medical Center[2]	Del Rio	59%	239
Lubbock Heart Hospital[2]	Lubbock	58%	224
Navarro Regional Hospital[2]	Corsicana	58%	224
Christus Spohn Hospital Alice[2]	Alice	57%	215
Glen Rose Medical Center	Glen Rose	57%	367
Christus Saint Catherine Hospital[2]	Katy	56%	225
Good Shephard Medical Center - Linden[2]	Linden	56%	114
Etmc Henderson[2]	Henderson	55%	148
Hopkins County Memorial Hospital[2]	Sulphur Springs	55%	230
The Medical Center of Southeast Texas[2]	Port Arthur	55%	325
Christus Santa Rosa Hospital[2]	San Antonio	54%	712
Palo Pinto General Hospital[2]	Mineral Wells	54%	160
VHS Harlingen Hospital Company[2]	Harlingen	54%	336
East Texas Medical Center Crockett[2]	Crockett	52%	104
VHS Brownsville Hospital Company[2]	Brownsville	52%	330
University General Hospital Dallas[2]	Dallas	51%	249
East Texas Medical Center Jacksonville[2]	Jacksonville	50%	96
El Campo Memorial Hospital[2]	El Campo	50%	127
Memorial Hospital[2]	Nacogdoches	50%	323
Starr County Memorial Hospital[2]	Rio Grande City	50%	131
Frio Regional Hospital[2]	Pearsall	49%	95
Heritage Park Surgical Hospital	Sherman	49%	77
Wilbarger General Hospital[2]	Vernon	49%	137
Covenant Hospital Levelland	Levelland	48%	296
Doctors Diagnostic Hospital[2]	Cleveland	48%	83
Goodall Witcher Hospital[2]	Clifton	48%	117
Stephens Memorial Hospital[2]	Breckenridge	47%	258
East Texas Medical Center - Fairfield	Fairfield	45%	266
Hamilton General Hospital[2]	Hamilton	43%	170
Saint Anthony's Hospital[2]	Houston	42%	293
Memorial Hospital[2]	Gonzales	41%	320
Doctors Hospital Tidwell[2]	Houston	40%	125
University General Hospital[2]	Houston	40%	224
Columbus Community Hospital[2]	Columbus	37%	158
Pecos County Memorial Hospital[2]	Fort Stockton	37%	172
East Texas Medical Center Athens[2]	Athens	35%	407
Bowie Memorial Hospital[2]	Bowie	33%	153
Etmc Clarksville[2]	Clarksville	33%	137
Trustpoint Hospital	Lubbock	29%	184
East Texas Medical Center Quitman[2]	Quitman	28%	124
East Texas Medical Center Trinity[2]	Trinity	27%	266
Eastland Memorial Hospital[2]	Eastland	26%	133
Allegiance Specialty Hospital of Kilgore[2]	Kilgore	24%	76
East Texas Medical Center Mount Vernon[2]	Mount Vernon	24%	120
Nocona General Hospital[2]	Nocona	22%	140
Christus Jasper Memorial Hospital[2]	Jasper	21%	114
Brownfield Regional Medical Center[2]	Brownfield	19%	125
Basin Healthcare Center	Odessa	18%	66
Knox County Hospital	Knox City	18%	60
Hamlin Memorial Hospital[2]	Hamlin	13%	98
Hemphill County Hospital[2]	Canadian	12%	81
Lake Whitney Medical Center[2]	Whitney	12%	98
Faith Community Hospital[2]	Jacksboro	11%	102
Dimmit Regional Hospital[2]	Carrizo Springs	7%	94
Lamb Healthcare Center	Littlefield	5%	120
Bellville General Hospital[2]	Bellville	0%	98
Falls Community Hospital & Clinic[2]	Marlin	0%	123

Warfarin Therapy Discharge Instructions

Hospital Name	City	Rate	Cases
Baylor Medical Center at Mckinney[2]	Mc Kinney	100%	45
Baylor Medical Center at Waxahachie[2]	Waxahachie	100%	30
Baylor Reg Med Ctr at Grapevine[2]	Grapevine	100%	68
Baylor Regional Medical Center at Plano[2]	Plano	100%	59
The Corpus Christi Medical Center[2]	Corpus Christi	100%	42
Good Shepherd Medical Center[2]	Longview	100%	79
Good Shepherd Medical Center Marshall[2]	Marshall	100%	26
Houston Northwest Medical Center[2]	Houston	100%	66
Huguley Memorial Medical Center[2]	Burleson	100%	52
Hunt Regional Medical Center[2]	Greenville	100%	40
Lake Pointe Medical Center[2]	Rowlett	100%	28
Laredo Medical Center[2]	Laredo	100%	26
Las Colinas Medical Center[2]	Irving	100%	34
Longview Regional Medical Center[2]	Longview	100%	32
Medical Center of Plano[2]	Plano	100%	102
Methodist Stone Oak Hospital[2]	San Antonio	100%	34
Methodist Sugar Land Hospital[2]	Sugar Land	100%	68
Mother Frances Hospital[2]	Tyler	100%	87
North Hills Hospital[2]	N Richland Hls	100%	62
Providence Memorial Hospital[2]	El Paso	100%	44
Round Rock Medical Center[2]	Round Rock	100%	38
Saint David's Medical Center[2]	Austin	100%	72
Saint David's South Austin Medical Center[2]	Austin	100%	79
Saint Joseph Regional Health Center[2]	Bryan	100%	85
Sierra Medical Center[2]	El Paso	100%	44
Sierra Providence East Medical Center[2]	El Paso	100%	37
TX Hlth Presbyterian Hosp-Flower Mound[2]	Flower Mound	100%	32
United Regional Health Care System[2]	Wichita Falls	100%	78
Valley Regional Medical Center[2]	Brownsville	100%	29
Wadley Regional Medical Center[2]	Texarkana	100%	36
Weatherford Regional Medical Center[2]	Weatherford	100%	27
West Houston Medical Center[2]	Houston	100%	46
Baylor University Medical Center[2]	Dallas	99%	123
Bayshore Medical Center[2]	Pasadena	99%	75
Clear Lake Regional Medical Center[2]	Webster	99%	102
Methodist Charlton Medical Center[2]	Dallas	99%	90
Methodist Dallas Medical Center[2]	Dallas	99%	76
North Austin Medical Center[2]	Austin	99%	75
Baptist Beaumont Hospital[2]	Beaumont	98%	63
Baylor All Saints Medical Center at FW[2]	Fort Worth	98%	46
Kingwood Medical Center[2]	Kingwood	98%	56
Saint Joseph Medical Center[2]	Houston	98%	47
University Medical Center of El Paso[2]	El Paso	98%	81
Medical Center of Arlington[2]	Arlington	97%	60
Medical City Dallas Hospital[2]	Dallas	97%	62
Methodist Hospital[2]	San Antonio	97%	230
Methodist Mansfield Medical Center[2]	Mansfield	97%	69
Metroplex Hospital[2]	Killeen	97%	31
Nacogdoches Medical Center[2]	Nacogdoches	97%	31
Rio Grande Regional Hospital[2]	Mcallen	97%	37
Saint Luke's Hospital at the Vintage[2]	Houston	97%	31
TX Hlth Harris Meth Hosp-Cleburne[2]	Cleburne	97%	35
Baylor Medical Center at Irving[2]	Irving	96%	56
Cedar Park Regional Medical Center[2]	Cedar Park	96%	25
Methodist Richardson Medical Center[2]	Richardson	96%	26
South Texas Health System[2]	Edinburg	96%	49
Texoma Medical Center[2]	Denison	96%	46
The Medical Center of Southeast Texas[2]	Port Arthur	95%	42
TX Hlth Harris Meth Hosp SW Ft Worth[2]	Fort Worth	95%	43
Methodist Willowbrook Hospital[2]	Houston	94%	65
University Medical Center[2]	Lubbock	94%	63
Conroe Regional Medical Center[2]	Conroe	93%	70
Methodist West Houston Hospital[2]	Houston	93%	28
Centennial Medical Center[2]	Frisco	92%	37
Doctors Hospital at Renaissance[2]	Edinburg	92%	38
Hendrick Medical Center[2]	Abilene	92%	64
Midland Memorial Hospital[2]	Midland	92%	50
Baptist Medical Center[2]	San Antonio	91%	150
Denton Regional Medical Center[2]	Denton	91%	75
Harris Health System[2]	Houston	91%	138

NOTE: Hospital profiles are in alphabetical order by state, then city, then hospital within the city; Rankings exclude hospitals with less than 25 cases except for patient surveys which excludes hospitals with less than 100 cases; (a) 100-299 cases; (1) The number of cases/patients is too few to report; (2) Data submitted were based on a sample of cases/patients; (3) Results are based on a shorter time period than required; (4) Data suppressed by CMS for one or more quarters; (5) Results are not available for this reporting period; (6) Fewer than 100 patients completed the HCAHPS survey; (7) No cases met the criteria for this measure; (8) The lower limit of the confidence interval cannot be calculated if the number of observed infections equals zero; (9) No data are available from the state/territory for this reporting period; (10) The scores shown reflect fewer than 50 completed surveys; (11) There were discrepancies in the data collection process; (12) This measure does not apply to this hospital for this reporting period; (13) Results cannot be calculated for this reporting period; (14) The results for this state are combined with nearby states to protect confidentiality; Please refer to the User's Guide for a full explanation of data.

Hospital Name	City	Rate	Cases
Tomball Regional Medical Center[2]	Tomball	91%	32
VHS Harlingen Hospital Company[2]	Harlingen	91%	46
Texas Health Presbyterian Hospital - WNJ[2]	Sherman	90%	30
UT Southwestern University Hospital[2]	Dallas	90%	88
Covenant Medical Center[2]	Lubbock	89%	113
Medical Center of Lewisville[2]	Lewisville	89%	37
Texas Health Arlington Memorial Hospital[2]	Arlington	89%	83
University Health System[2]	San Antonio	89%	66
Memorial Medical Center of East Texas[2]	Lufkin	88%	34
Mem Hermann Mem City Med Ctr[2]	Houston	87%	85
Texas Health Harris Methodist[2]	Bedford	87%	95
Cypress Fairbanks Medical Center[2]	Houston	86%	28
Medical Center of Mckinney[2]	Mckinney	85%	53
Baptist Saint Anthony's Hospital[2]	Amarillo	84%	104
JPS Health Network[2]	Fort Worth	84%	126
Baylor Medical Center at Garland[2]	Garland	83%	54
Memorial Hermann Hospital System[2]	Houston	81%	335
Paris Regional Medical Center[2]	Paris	81%	42
Saint Luke's Patients Medical Center[2]	Pasadena	81%	26
Christus Spohn Hospital Corpus Christi[2]	Corpus Christi	80%	98
The Methodist Hospital[2]	Houston	80%	155
Memorial Hermann Sugar Land Hospital[2]	Sugar Land	79%	29
Scott & White Hospital - Round Rock[2]	Round Rock	78%	40
East Texas Medical Center[2]	Tyler	76%	105
Memorial Hermann Northeast[2]	Humble	76%	82
Northwest Texas Hospital[2]	Amarillo	76%	38
Providence Health Center[2]	Waco	76%	94
Shannon Medical Center[2]	San Angelo	76%	51
Las Palmas Medical Center[2]	El Paso	75%	71
Plaza Medical Center of Fort Worth[2]	Fort Worth	73%	48
Saint Luke's Sugar Land Hospital[2]	Sugar Land	72%	25
North Cypress Medical Center[2]	Cypress	71%	55
Medical Center Hospital[2]	Odessa	70%	93
University Medical Center at Brackenridge[2]	Austin	70%	44
Saint Luke's Episcopal Hospital[2]	Houston	69%	143
San Jacinto Methodist Hospital[2]	Baytown	69%	58
Memorial Hermann Katy Hospital[2]	Katy	68%	31
Texas Health Presbyterian Hospital Plano[2]	Plano	68%	80
Christus Hospital[2]	Beaumont	67%	42
Memorial Hermann Texas Medical Center[2]	Houston	67%	111
Texas Health Harris Methodist Fort Worth[2]	Fort Worth	62%	133
Christus Santa Rosa Hospital[2]	San Antonio	61%	69
Seton Medical Center Williamson[2]	Round Rock	61%	36
Christus Saint Michael Health System[2]	Texarkana	55%	76
Texas Health Presbyterian Hospital Denton[2]	Denton	49%	51
Univ of Texas Med Branch Galveston[2]	Galveston	48%	75
Saint Luke's the Woodlands Hospital[2]	The Woodlands	47%	45
Scott & White Memorial Hospital[2]	Temple	43%	152
Seton Medical Center Austin[2]	Austin	36%	66
Texas Health Presbyterian Hospital Dallas[2]	Dallas	31%	67
Parkland Health & Hospital System[2]	Dallas	1%	144

Chest Pain/Possible Heart Attack Care

Aspirin Given Within 24 Hours of Arrival

Hospital Name	City	Rate	Cases
Baylor Regional Medical Center at Plano	Plano	100%	33
Brazosport Regional Health System	Lake Jackson	100%	34
Brownwood Regional Medical Center	Brownwood	100%	171
Care Regional Medical Center	Aransas Pass	100%	29
Cedar Park Regional Medical Center	Cedar Park	100%	29
Central Texas Medical Center	San Marcos	100%	31
Covenant Hospital Plainview	Plainview	100%	39
East Texas Medical Center - Fairfield	Fairfield	100%	64
Gulf Coast Medical Center	Wharton	100%	27
Hopkins County Memorial Hospital	Sulphur Springs	100%	41
Lake Pointe Medical Center	Rowlett	100%	30
Memorial Hermann Sugar Land Hospital	Sugar Land	100%	55
Permian Regional Medical Center	Andrews	100%	28
Peterson Regional Medical Center	Kerrville	100%	90
Saint David's Medical Center	Austin	100%	49
Saint Marks Medical Center	La Grange	100%	72
South Texas Regional Medical Center	Jourdanton	100%	93
Stephens Memorial Hospital	Breckenridge	100%	32
TX Hlth Harris Meth Hosp SW Ft Worth	Fort Worth	100%	50
Weatherford Regional Medical Center	Weatherford	100%	48
Memorial Hermann Katy Hospital	Katy	99%	67
Rolling Plains Memorial Hospital	Sweetwater	99%	76
TX Hlth Harris Methodist Hosp-Azle	Azle	99%	118
Baylor Medical Center at Waxahachie	Waxahachie	98%	63
Baylor University Medical Center	Dallas	98%	477
Columbus Community Hospital	Columbus	98%	54
Coryell Memorial Healthcare System	Gatesville	98%	59
East Texas Medical Center - Gilmer	Gilmer	98%	42
Good Shepherd Medical Center Marshall	Marshall	98%	105
Hill Country Memorial Hospital	Fredericksburg	98%	48
Hunt Regional Medical Center	Greenville	98%	97
Methodist Hospital	San Antonio	98%	40
Navarro Regional Hospital	Corsicana	98%	41
North Texas Medical Center	Gainesville	98%	58
Seton Northwest Hospital	Austin	98%	52
Texas Health Presbyterian Hospital Allen	Allen	98%	62
Uvalde Memorial Hospital	Uvalde	98%	115
Angleton - Danbury Medical Center	Angleton	97%	67
Cuero Community Hospital	Cuero	97%	29
East Texas Medical Center Athens	Athens	97%	168
Good Shepherd Medical Center - Linden	Linden	97%	31
Hill Regional Hospital	Hillsboro	97%	31
Hillcrest Baptist Medical Center[3]	Waco	97%	31
Huntsville Memorial Hospital	Huntsville	97%	118
Memorial Hermann Baptist Orange Hospital	Orange	97%	38
Oakbend Medical Center	Richmond	97%	32
Saint Joseph Regional Health Center	Bryan	97%	36
TX Hlth Presbyterian Hosp-Kaufman	Kaufman	97%	71
Big Bend Regional Medical Center	Alpine	96%	28
Christus Jasper Memorial Hospital	Jasper	96%	110
Christus Spohn Hospital Kleberg	Kingsville	96%	97
Connally Memorial Medical Center	Floresville	96%	56
East Texas Medical Center Jacksonville	Jacksonville	96%	26
Ennis Regional Medical Center	Ennis	96%	48
Palo Pinto General Hospital[3]	Mineral Wells	96%	49
Scott & White Hospital - Llano	Llano	96%	51
Seton Southwest Hospital	Austin	96%	257
TX Hlth Harris Meth Hosp-Alliance[3]	Fort Worth	96%	27
TX Health Presbyterian Hosp Rockwall	Rockwall	96%	68
Moore County Hospital District	Dumas	95%	43
Scenic Mountain Medical Center	Big Spring	95%	80
Scott & White Hospital Brenham	Brenham	95%	78
TX Hlth Harris Meth Hosp-Cleburne	Cleburne	95%	169
Guadalupe Regional Medical Center	Seguin	94%	102
Palestine Regional Medical Center	Palestine	94%	95
Titus Regional Medical Center	Mount Pleasant	94%	77
Etmc Henderson	Henderson	93%	42
Fort Duncan Medical Center	Eagle Pass	93%	74
Knapp Medical Center	Weslaco	93%	29
Parkview Regional Hospital	Mexia	93%	89
Rollins Brook Community Hospital	Lampasas	93%	41
Texas Health Arlington Memorial Hospital	Arlington	93%	315
East Texas Medical Center Crockett	Crockett	92%	40
East Texas Medical Center Quitman	Quitman	92%	52
Medical Arts Hospital	Lamesa	92%	38
Seton Smithville Regional Hospital	Smithville	92%	37
Brownfield Regional Medical Center	Brownfield	91%	70
TX Hlth Harris Meth Hosp-Stephenville	Stephenville	90%	105
USMD Hospital at Arlington	Arlington	90%	39
Val Verde Regional Medical Center	Del Rio	90%	102
Christus Spohn Hospital Beeville	Beeville	89%	80
Cleveland Regional Medical Center	Cleveland	89%	27
Etmc Carthage	Carthage	89%	36
Memorial Hospital	Gonzales	89%	27
Cogdell Memorial Hospital	Snyder	88%	42
Graham Regional Medical Center	Graham	88%	76
Kell West Regional Hospital	Wichita Falls	88%	26
Memorial Medical Center Livingston	Livingston	88%	160
Wilbarger General Hospital	Vernon	88%	25
Bowie Memorial Hospital	Bowie	86%	28
Eastland Memorial Hospital	Eastland	86%	28
Dimmit Regional Hospital	Carrizo Springs	83%	110
Christus Santa Rosa Hospital	San Antonio	82%	57
Tyler County Hospital	Woodville	80%	49
Christus Spohn Hospital Alice	Alice	79%	119
Glen Rose Medical Center	Glen Rose	78%	27
Starr County Memorial Hospital	Rio Grande City	74%	69

Fibrinolytic Meds Within 30 Minutes of Arrival

Hospital Name	City	Rate	Cases
Memorial Medical Center Livingston	Livingston	17%	59

Average Time to ECG (minutes)

Hospital Name	City	Min.	Cases
Eastland Memorial Hospital	Eastland	0	30
Peterson Regional Medical Center	Kerrville	0	92
East Texas Medical Center Quitman	Quitman	2	54
Good Shepherd Medical Center Marshall	Marshall	2	112
Palestine Regional Medical Center	Palestine	2	96
Palo Pinto General Hospital[3]	Mineral Wells	2	50
Baylor University Medical Center	Dallas	3	480
Cuero Community Hospital	Cuero	3	30
Scott & White Hospital - Llano	Llano	3	50
TX Hlth Harris Meth Hosp-Stephenville	Stephenville	3	111
Big Bend Regional Medical Center	Alpine	4	29
Cedar Park Regional Medical Center	Cedar Park	4	29
Central Texas Medical Center	San Marcos	4	30
East Texas Medical Center - Fairfield	Fairfield	4	65
Etmc Carthage	Carthage	4	36
Memorial Hermann Sugar Land Hospital	Sugar Land	4	58
Methodist Hospital	San Antonio	4	40
Oakbend Medical Center	Richmond	4	31
Saint David's Medical Center	Austin	4	51
Scenic Mountain Medical Center	Big Spring	4	88
Stephens Memorial Hospital	Breckenridge	4	33
Bowie Memorial Hospital	Bowie	5	30
East Texas Medical Center Crockett	Crockett	5	40
Fort Duncan Medical Center	Eagle Pass	5	76
Hill Regional Hospital	Hillsboro	5	35
Hopkins County Memorial Hospital	Sulphur Springs	5	43
Memorial Hospital	Gonzales	5	27
Cleveland Regional Medical Center	Cleveland	6	27
East Texas Medical Center Athens	Athens	6	174
East Texas Medical Center Jacksonville	Jacksonville	6	26
Ennis Regional Medical Center	Ennis	6	50
Gulf Coast Medical Center	Wharton	6	28
Hill Country Memorial Hospital	Fredericksburg	6	50
Lake Pointe Medical Center	Rowlett	6	33
Texas Health Presbyterian Hospital Allen	Allen	6	63
TX Hlth Presbyterian Hosp-Kaufman	Kaufman	6	72
TX Health Presbyterian Hosp Rockwall	Rockwall	6	73
Val Verde Regional Medical Center	Del Rio	6	107
Weatherford Regional Medical Center	Weatherford	6	49
Baylor Medical Center at Waxahachie	Waxahachie	7	64
Columbus Community Hospital	Columbus	7	55
Etmc Henderson	Henderson	7	49
Hunt Regional Medical Center	Greenville	7	103
Memorial Hermann Katy Hospital	Katy	7	69
Seton Southwest Hospital	Austin	7	263
TX Hlth Harris Meth Hosp-Alliance[3]	Fort Worth	7	29
Angleton - Danbury Medical Center	Angleton	8	76
Baylor Regional Medical Center at Plano	Plano	8	33
Brazosport Regional Health System	Lake Jackson	8	34
Brownwood Regional Medical Center	Brownwood	8	180
Connally Memorial Medical Center	Floresville	8	57
Covenant Hospital Plainview	Plainview	8	42
East Texas Medical Center - Gilmer	Gilmer	8	44
Good Shephard Medical Center - Linden	Linden	8	34
Moore County Hospital District	Dumas	8	44
Navarro Regional Hospital	Corsicana	8	42
Parkview Regional Hospital	Mexia	8	94
Permian Regional Medical Center	Andrews	8	28
Saint Joseph Regional Health Center	Bryan	8	37
Seton Northwest Hospital	Austin	8	52
TX Hlth Harris Methodist Hosp-Azle	Azle	8	123
TX Hlth Harris Meth Hosp SW Ft Worth	Fort Worth	8	52
Uvalde Memorial Hospital	Uvalde	8	123
Guadalupe Regional Medical Center	Seguin	9	105
Scott & White Hospital Brenham	Brenham	9	77
Seton Smithville Regional Hospital	Smithville	9	37
South Texas Regional Medical Center	Jourdanton	9	95
TX Hlth Harris Meth Hosp-Cleburne	Cleburne	9	175
Christus Jasper Memorial Hospital	Jasper	10	115
Cogdell Memorial Hospital	Snyder	10	41
Matagorda Regional Medical Center	Bay City	10	26
Medical Arts Hospital	Lamesa	10	39
North Texas Medical Center	Gainesville	10	60
Rollins Brook Community Hospital	Lampasas	10	46
Saint Marks Medical Center	La Grange	10	74
Texas Health Arlington Memorial Hospital	Arlington	10	334
USMD Hospital at Arlington	Arlington	10	39
Coryell Memorial Healthcare System	Gatesville	11	64
Huntsville Memorial Hospital	Huntsville	11	126
Memorial Hermann Baptist Orange Hospital	Orange	11	37
El Campo Memorial Hospital	El Campo	12	27
Brownfield Regional Medical Center	Brownfield	14	77
Care Regional Medical Center	Aransas Pass	14	29
Christus Santa Rosa Hospital	San Antonio	14	55
Hillcrest Baptist Medical Center[3]	Waco	14	30
Titus Regional Medical Center	Mount Pleasant	14	82
Wilbarger General Hospital	Vernon	14	26
Graham Regional Medical Center	Graham	15	79
Knapp Medical Center	Weslaco	15	29
Rolling Plains Memorial Hospital	Sweetwater	15	84
Christus Spohn Hospital Kleberg	Kingsville	16	107
Dimmit Regional Hospital	Carrizo Springs	18	110
Tyler County Hospital	Woodville	18	50
Christus Spohn Hospital Beeville	Beeville	22	84
Memorial Medical Center Livingston	Livingston	22	158
Starr County Memorial Hospital	Rio Grande City	23	78
Christus Spohn Hospital Alice	Alice	24	119
Kell West Regional Hospital	Wichita Falls	32	26

Average Time to Transfer (minutes)

Hospital Name	City	Min.	Cases
Baylor University Medical Center	Dallas	43	95
Memorial Hermann Katy Hospital	Katy	46	29
TX Hlth Harris Meth Hosp-Cleburne	Cleburne	46	26
Texas Health Arlington Memorial Hospital	Arlington	48	49
Good Shepherd Medical Center Marshall	Marshall	129	59

NOTE: Hospital profiles are in alphabetical order by state, then city, then hospital within the city; Rankings exclude hospitals with less than 25 cases except for patient surveys which excludes hospitals with less than 100 cases; (a) 100-299 cases; (1) The number of cases/patients is too few to report; (2) Data submitted were based on a sample of cases/patients; (3) Results are based on a shorter time period than required; (4) Data suppressed by CMS for one or more quarters; (5) Results are not available for this reporting period; (6) Fewer than 100 patients completed the HCAHPS survey; (7) No cases met the criteria for this measure; (8) The lower limit of the confidence interval cannot be calculated if the number of observed infections equals zero; (9) No data are available from the state/territory for this reporting period; (10) The scores shown reflect fewer than 50 completed surveys; (11) There were discrepancies in the data collection process; (12) This measure does not apply to this hospital for this reporting period; (13) Results cannot be calculated for this reporting period; (14) The results for this state are combined with nearby states to protect confidentiality; Please refer to the User's Guide for a full explanation of data.

Children's Asthma Care

Received Home Management Plan of Care

Hospital Name	City	Rate	Cases
Methodist Hospital	San Antonio	98%	523
Baptist Medical Center	San Antonio	91%	268
Christus Santa Rosa Hospital	San Antonio	91%	147
Cook Childrens Medical Center[2]	Fort Worth	90%	284
Driscoll Childrens Hospital	Corpus Christi	81%	141

Received Reliever Medication

Hospital Name	City	Rate	Cases
Baptist Medical Center	San Antonio	100%	269
Christus Santa Rosa Hospital	San Antonio	100%	148
Cook Childrens Medical Center[2]	Fort Worth	100%	284
Driscoll Childrens Hospital	Corpus Christi	100%	141
Methodist Hospital	San Antonio	100%	523

Received Systemic Corticosteroids

Hospital Name	City	Rate	Cases
Baptist Medical Center	San Antonio	100%	269
Cook Childrens Medical Center[2]	Fort Worth	100%	284
Methodist Hospital	San Antonio	100%	522
Christus Santa Rosa Hospital	San Antonio	99%	148
Driscoll Childrens Hospital	Corpus Christi	99%	141

Emergency Department

Admittance Decision Time (minutes)

Hospital Name	City	Min.	Cases
Hamlin Memorial Hospital[2]	Hamlin	0	89
Seymour Hospital	Seymour	0	173
The Womans Hospital of Texas[2]	Houston	0	311
Faith Community Hospital[2]	Jacksboro	3	65
Hemphill County Hospital[2]	Canadian	10	68
Plains Memorial Hospital	Dimmitt	10	66
Electra Memorial Hospital	Electra	14	40
Stamford Memorial Hospital	Stamford	15	107
Lamb Healthcare Center	Littlefield	20	86
Nocona General Hospital[2]	Nocona	20	302
Anson General Hospital	Anson	22	49
El Paso Specialty Hospital[2]	El Paso	26	43
Medical Arts Hospital[2]	Lamesa	27	249
Childress Regional Medical Center[2]	Childress	28	94
Moore County Hospital District[2]	Dumas	29	144
Good Shephard Medical Center - Linden[2]	Linden	30	199
Stephens Memorial Hospital[2]	Breckenridge	30	165
Goodall Witcher Hospital[2]	Clifton	32	105
Otto Kaiser Memorial Hospital[2]	Kenedy	32	165
Permian Regional Medical Center[2]	Andrews	34	83
Brownfield Regional Medical Center[2]	Brownfield	35	146
Cogdell Memorial Hospital	Snyder	40	198
East Texas Medical Center Mount Vernon[2]	Mount Vernon	40	130
Memorial Hospital[2]	Gonzales	40	283
Scott & White Hospital - Llano	Llano	40	248
Uvalde Memorial Hospital[2]	Uvalde	41	613
Hill Regional Hospital[2]	Hillsboro	43	280
Val Verde Regional Medical Center[2]	Del Rio	43	327
East Texas Medical Center Pittsburg[2]	Pittsburg	45	303
Etmc Clarksville[2]	Clarksville	45	255
Houston Orthopedic & Spine Hospital	Bellaire	45	36
Lake Whitney Medical Center[2]	Whitney	45	289
Methodist Mckinney Hospital[2]	Mc Kinney	45	32
Tyler County Hospital[2]	Woodville	45	455
Glen Rose Medical Center	Glen Rose	47	466
Saint Marks Medical Center[2]	La Grange	47	393
Baylor Medical Center at Trophy Club[2]	Trophy Club	48	32
Frio Regional Hospital[2]	Pearsall	48	44
El Campo Memorial Hospital	El Campo	49	117
Hamilton General Hospital[2]	Hamilton	49	437
TX Hlth Harris Meth Hosp-Stephenville[2]	Stephenville	49	299
East Texas Medical Center - Fairfield	Fairfield	50	381
Covenant Hospital Plainview[2]	Plainview	54	102
Lubbock Heart Hospital[2]	Lubbock	54	100
Rolling Plains Memorial Hospital[2]	Sweetwater	54	236
Central Texas Hospital[2,3]	Cameron	55	103
Cuero Community Hospital[2]	Cuero	55	309
Grace Medical Center	Lubbock	55	115
Longview Regional Medical Center[2]	Longview	55	465
Texas General Hospital[3]	Grand Prairie	55	79
Hopkins County Memorial Hospital[2]	Sulphur Springs	56	322
Graham Regional Medical Center[2]	Graham	57	362
Gulf Coast Medical Center[2]	Wharton	58	293
Golden Plains Community Hospital[2]	Borger	59	255
Rollins Brook Community Hospital[2]	Lampasas	59	234
University Medical Center[2]	Lubbock	59	546
Detar Hospital Navarro[2]	Victoria	60	489
Doctors Diagnostic Hospital[2]	Cleveland	60	88
East Texas Medical Center - Gilmer[2]	Gilmer	60	243
Good Shepherd Medical Center[2]	Longview	60	624
Lavaca Medical Center[2]	Hallettsville	60	342
Palestine Regional Medical Center[2]	Palestine	60	372
Citizens Medical Center[2]	Victoria	61	377
Seton Smithville Regional Hospital[2]	Smithville	61	306
Starr County Memorial Hospital[2]	Rio Grande City	62	431
Titus Regional Medical Center[2]	Mount Pleasant	62	111
Baylor Regional Medical Center at Plano[2]	Plano	63	494
Big Bend Regional Medical Center[2]	Alpine	64	318
Dallas Regional Medical Center[2]	Mesquite	64	1321
East Texas Medical Center Crockett[2]	Crockett	65	226
East Texas Medical Center Jacksonville[2]	Jacksonville	65	150
Valley Regional Medical Center[2]	Brownsville	65	592
Good Shepherd Medical Center Marshall[2]	Marshall	66	506
Scott & White Hospital Brenham[2]	Brenham	66	228
Seton Medical Center Harker Heights[2]	Harker Heights	66	370
Covenant Hospital Levelland[2]	Levelland	68	163
Nix Health Care System[2]	San Antonio	68	60
Woodland Heights Medical Center[2]	Lufkin	68	498
Metroplex Hospital[2]	Killeen	69	459
Huntsville Memorial Hospital[2]	Huntsville	70	461
Mitchell County Hospital District	Colorado City	70	247
North Texas Medical Center[2]	Gainesville	70	185
Univ of TX Health Science Ctr-Tyler[2]	Tyler	70	352
Memorial Hospital[2]	Nacogdoches	71	296
Navarro Regional Hospital[2]	Corsicana	71	435
Pampa Regional Medical Center[2]	Pampa	71	394
TX Hlth Harris Meth Hosp SW Ft Worth[2]	Fort Worth	71	603
Weatherford Regional Medical Center[2]	Weatherford	71	640
Etmc Henderson[2]	Henderson	72	296
Saint Luke's Lakeside Hospital[2]	The Woodlands	72	29
Wilbarger General Hospital[2]	Vernon	72	210
Hill Country Memorial Hospital[2]	Fredericksburg	73	223
Memorial Hermann Katy Hospital[2]	Katy	73	460
Scott & White Hospital - Round Rock[2]	Round Rock	73	493
College Station Medical Center[2]	College Station	74	569
East Texas Medical Center Quitman[2]	Quitman	74	231
Memorial Hermann Sugar Land Hospital[2]	Sugar Land	74	431
Nacogdoches Medical Center[2]	Nacogdoches	74	471
San Angelo Community Medical Center[2]	San Angelo	74	476
TX Health Presbyterian Hosp Rockwall[2]	Rockwall	74	438
Dimmit Regional Hospital[2]	Carrizo Springs	75	157
East Texas Medical Center Trinity[2]	Trinity	75	248
Hereford Regional Medical Center[2]	Hereford	75	140
University General Hospital Dallas[2]	Dallas	75	217
Scenic Mountain Medical Center[2]	Big Spring	76	344
Lake Pointe Medical Center[2]	Rowlett	77	657
TX Hlth Harris Methodist Hosp-Azle[2]	Azle	77	699
Cedar Park Regional Medical Center[2]	Cedar Park	78	539
Ennis Regional Medical Center[2]	Ennis	78	296
Etmc Carthage[2]	Carthage	78	387
Lake Granbury Medical Center[2]	Granbury	78	387
Methodist Stone Oak Hospital[2]	San Antonio	78	412
University General Hospital[2]	Houston	79	925
Baylor Medical Center at Garland[2]	Garland	80	447
Bowie Memorial Hospital[2]	Bowie	80	284
Brownwood Regional Medical Center[2]	Brownwood	80	522
Knapp Medical Center[2]	Weslaco	80	347
Medina Regional Hospital[3]	Hondo	80	272
Palo Pinto General Hospital[2]	Mineral Wells	80	257
Shannon Medical Center[2]	San Angelo	80	582
Texas Reg Med Ctr at Sunnyvale[2]	Sunnyvale	80	514
East Texas Medical Center Athens[2]	Athens	81	556
Lakeway Regional Medical Center[2,3]	Lakeway	81	245
TX Hlth Presbyterian Hosp-Flower Mound[2]	Flower Mound	81	317
Baylor Medical Center at Waxahachie[2]	Waxahachie	82	310
Dallas Medical Center[2]	Dallas	82	287
Sierra Medical Center[2]	El Paso	83	591
Baylor Medical Center at Mckinney[2]	Mc Kinney	84	607
Scott & White Memorial Hospital[2]	Temple	84	575
Wise Regional Health System[2]	Decatur	84	511
Baylor Medical Center at Irving[2]	Irving	85	672
Columbus Community Hospital[2]	Columbus	85	183
Connally Memorial Medical Center[2]	Floresville	85	391
Eastland Memorial Hospital[2]	Eastland	85	112
Matagorda Regional Medical Center[2]	Bay City	85	243
Parkview Regional Hospital[2]	Mexia	85	445
Texas Health Arlington Memorial Hospital[2]	Arlington	85	693
VHS Brownsville Hospital Company[2]	Brownsville	85	534
Cleveland Regional Medical Center[2]	Cleveland	86	268
Heart Hospital Baylor Plano[2]	Plano	86	189
Sierra Providence East Medical Center[2]	El Paso	86	658
The Corpus Christi Medical Center[2]	Corpus Christi	87	589
Mem Hermann Mem City Med Ctr[2]	Houston	87	487
Paris Regional Medical Center[2]	Paris	88	558
Saint Anthony's Hospital[2,3]	Houston	88	205
TX Hlth Harris Meth Hosp-Cleburne[2]	Cleburne	88	502
Texas Health Presbyterian Hospital - WNJ[2]	Sherman	89	672
Care Regional Medical Center[2]	Aransas Pass	90	408
TX Hlth Presbyterian Hosp-Kaufman[2]	Kaufman	90	298
Harlingen Medical Center[2]	Harlingen	91	613
Memorial Medical Center Livingston[2]	Livingston	91	268
TX Hlth Harris Meth Hosp-Alliance[2,3]	Fort Worth	91	263
Texas Health Presbyterian Hospital Plano[2]	Plano	92	274
Baylor Reg Med Ctr at Grapevine[2]	Grapevine	93	531
Mission Regional Medical Center[2]	Mission	93	344
Texas Health Harris Methodist[2]	Bedford	93	521
Park Plaza Hospital[2]	Houston	94	431
Tomball Regional Medical Center[2]	Tomball	94	719
USMD Hospital at Arlington[2]	Arlington	94	108
The Hospital at Westlake Medical Center[2]	Austin	95	292
Hunt Regional Medical Center[2]	Greenville	95	549
Kell West Regional Hospital	Wichita Falls	95	195
Oakbend Medical Center[2]	Richmond	96	421
Saint Joseph Medical Center[2]	Houston	97	588
Texas Health Presbyterian Hospital Allen[2]	Allen	97	463
Abilene Regional Medical Center[2]	Abilene	98	412
Baylor Medical Center at Carrollton[2]	Carrollton	98	613
South Texas Regional Medical Center[2]	Jourdanton	98	351
Doctors Hospital Tidwell[2]	Houston	99	270
Methodist Richardson Medical Center[2]	Richardson	100	522
VHS Harlingen Hospital Company[2]	Harlingen	100	565
Doctors Hospital at Renaissance[2]	Edinburg	101	291
Methodist Hospital[2]	San Antonio	103	585
Providence Memorial Hospital[2]	El Paso	103	441
Covenant Medical Center[2]	Lubbock	104	586
Methodist Sugar Land Hospital[2]	Sugar Land	104	330
Central Texas Medical Center[2]	San Marcos	105	540
Pecos County Memorial Hospital[2]	Fort Stockton	105	257
Christus Jasper Memorial Hospital[2]	Jasper	106	374
Hillcrest Baptist Medical Center[2]	Waco	106	445
Clear Lake Regional Medical Center[2]	Webster	107	850
Doctors Hospital[2]	Dallas	108	698
Saint Joseph Regional Health Center[2]	Bryan	108	688
Memorial Hermann Baptist Orange Hospital[2]	Orange	110	337
Texas Health Harris Methodist Fort Worth[2]	Fort Worth	111	827
Memorial Hermann Texas Medical Center[2]	Houston	112	508
Las Colinas Medical Center[2]	Irving	113	609
Texas Health Presbyterian Hospital Denton[2]	Denton	113	650
Baptist Saint Anthony's Hospital[2]	Amarillo	114	677
Las Palmas Medical Center[2]	El Paso	115	778
Angleton - Danbury Medical Center[2]	Angleton	116	230
Baylor All Saints Medical Center at FW[2]	Fort Worth	118	376
The Medical Center of Southeast Texas[2]	Port Arthur	119	704
Memorial Medical Center of East Texas[2]	Lufkin	119	387
United Regional Health Care System[2]	Wichita Falls	120	531
Centennial Medical Center[2]	Frisco	122	427
Medical Center of Lewisville[2]	Lewisville	122	722
North Hills Hospital[2]	N Richland Hls	122	750
UT Southwestern University Hospital[2]	Dallas	122	436
Guadalupe Regional Medical Center[2]	Seguin	123	371
Mother Frances Hospital[2]	Tyler	125	476
Cypress Fairbanks Medical Center[2]	Houston	126	546
Saint Luke's the Woodlands Hospital[2]	The Woodlands	126	371
Medical Center of Plano[2]	Plano	127	804
Methodist Willowbrook Hospital[2]	Houston	127	551
Odessa Regional Hospital[2]	Odessa	127	275
Saint David's South Austin Medical Center[2]	Austin	127	784
Medical Center Hospital[2]	Odessa	128	826
West Houston Medical Center[2]	Houston	128	614
Midland Memorial Hospital[2]	Midland	129	1431
Christus Santa Rosa Hospital[2]	San Antonio	130	648
Christus Spohn Hospital Beeville[2]	Beeville	130	379
Medical City Dallas Hospital[2]	Dallas	130	671
North Cypress Medical Center[2]	Cypress	130	625
Bayshore Medical Center[2]	Pasadena	131	540
Hendrick Medical Center[2]	Abilene	131	591
Christus Hospital[2]	Beaumont	132	654
Methodist West Houston Hospital[2]	Houston	132	561
Peterson Regional Medical Center[2]	Kerrville	132	559
Providence Health Center[2]	Waco	132	671
Christus Saint Catherine Hospital[2]	Katy	135	415
JPS Health Network[2]	Fort Worth	136	704
Memorial Hermann Hospital System[2]	Houston	137	2033
Doctors Hospital of Laredo[2]	Laredo	138	361
Round Rock Medical Center[2]	Round Rock	138	621
Christus Spohn Hospital Alice[2]	Alice	140	450
East Texas Medical Center[2]	Tyler	140	274
Denton Regional Medical Center[2]	Denton	142	768
Saint Luke's Episcopal Hospital[2]	Houston	142	573
The Methodist Hospital[2]	Houston	144	438
Christus Saint Michael Health System[2]	Texarkana	146	669
University Medical Center of El Paso[2]	El Paso	146	672
Medical Center of Mckinney[2]	Mckinney	147	812
Methodist Mansfield Medical Center[2]	Mansfield	150	232
North Austin Medical Center[2]	Austin	150	502
Texoma Medical Center[2]	Denison	150	497
Baptist Medical Center[2]	San Antonio	151	2184
Wadley Regional Medical Center[2]	Texarkana	151	573
Conroe Regional Medical Center[2]	Conroe	153	659
Northwest Texas Hospital[2]	Amarillo	153	511
Fort Duncan Medical Center[2]	Eagle Pass	154	233

NOTE: Hospital profiles are in alphabetical order by state, then city, then hospital within the city; Rankings exclude hospitals with less than 25 cases except for patient surveys which excludes hospitals with less than 100 cases; (a) 100-299 cases; (1) The number of cases/patients is too few to report; (2) Data submitted were based on a sample of cases/patients; (3) Results are based on a shorter time period than required; (4) Data suppressed by CMS for one or more quarters; (5) Results are not available for this reporting period; (6) Fewer than 100 patients completed the HCAHPS survey; (7) No cases met the criteria for this measure; (8) The lower limit of the confidence interval cannot be calculated if the number of observed infections equals zero; (9) No data are available from the state/territory for this reporting period; (10) The scores shown reflect fewer than 50 completed surveys; (11) There were discrepancies in the data collection process; (12) This measure does not apply to this hospital for this reporting period; (13) Results cannot be calculated for this reporting period; (14) The results for this state are combined with nearby states to protect confidentiality; Please refer to the User's Guide for a full explanation of data.

Hospital Name	City	Rate	Cases
Houston Northwest Medical Center[2]	Houston	155	683
Medical Center of Arlington[2]	Arlington	158	724
Baylor University Medical Center[2]	Dallas	159	503
South Texas Health System[2]	Edinburg	159	625
Rio Grande Regional Hospital[2]	Mcallen	160	568
Saint David's Medical Center[2]	Austin	162	532
Huguley Memorial Medical Center[2]	Burleson	164	573
Baptist Beaumont Hospital[2]	Beaumont	167	777
Brazosport Regional Health System[2]	Lake Jackson	168	523
Texas Health Presbyterian Hospital Dallas[2]	Dallas	170	432
Christus Saint John Hospital[2]	Nassau Bay	174	827
Methodist Charlton Medical Center[2]	Dallas	178	507
Saint Luke's Patients Medical Center[2]	Pasadena	180	393
San Jacinto Methodist Hospital[2]	Baytown	180	682
Plaza Medical Center of Fort Worth[2]	Fort Worth	182	712
Saint Luke's Hospital at the Vintage[2]	Houston	184	310
Methodist Dallas Medical Center[2]	Dallas	189	477
Saint Luke's Sugar Land Hospital[2]	Sugar Land	189	479
Christus Spohn Hospital Kleberg[2]	Kingsville	208	412
Southwest General Hospital[2]	San Antonio	208	636
Christus Spohn Hospital Corpus Christi[2]	Corpus Christi	214	876
Memorial Hermann Northeast[2]	Humble	214	656
University Health System[2]	San Antonio	228	429
Univ of Texas Med Branch Galveston[2]	Galveston	238	221
Laredo Medical Center[2]	Laredo	240	584
Parkland Health & Hospital System[2]	Dallas	243	515
Kingwood Medical Center[2]	Kingwood	290	588
Harris Health System[2]	Houston	332	1076
Falls Community Hospital & Clinic[2]	Marlin	1026	246

Head CT Results Within 45 Minutes of Arrival

Hospital Name	City	Rate	Cases
Baptist Beaumont Hospital	Beaumont	97%	34
The Corpus Christi Medical Center	Corpus Christi	90%	30
Methodist Hospital	San Antonio	87%	39
Medical Center of Lewisville	Lewisville	81%	26
Christus Saint John Hospital	Nassau Bay	78%	41
Texoma Medical Center	Denison	66%	32
UT Southwestern University Hospital	Dallas	66%	41
Christus Hospital	Beaumont	65%	34
Good Shepherd Medical Center Marshall	Marshall	50%	36
Memorial Hermann Hospital System	Houston	48%	48
Knapp Medical Center	Weslaco	41%	29
Val Verde Regional Medical Center	Del Rio	27%	26
Guadalupe Regional Medical Center	Seguin	24%	33
Christus Santa Rosa Hospital	San Antonio	22%	40
Covenant Hospital Plainview	Plainview	21%	29
Starr County Memorial Hospital	Rio Grande City	15%	27

Patients Who Left ER Before Being Seen

Hospital Name	City	Rate	Cases
Anson General Hospital	Anson	0%	2711
Arise Austin Medical Center	Austin	0%	414
Basin Healthcare Center	Odessa	0%	2131
Baylor Emergency Medical Center	Aubrey	0%	7897
Baylor Surgical Hospital at Fort Worth	Fort Worth	0%	400
Big Bend Regional Medical Center	Alpine	0%	4509
East Texas Medical Center Trinity	Trinity	0%	7293
Eastland Memorial Hospital	Eastland	0%	8882
El Paso Specialty Hospital	El Paso	0%	2200
Faith Community Hospital	Jacksboro	0%	2081
Frio Regional Hospital	Pearsall	0%	8384
Heart Hospital Baylor Plano	Plano	0%	4023
Heritage Park Surgical Hospital	Sherman	0%	622
Hill Country Memorial Hospital	Fredericksburg	0%	14228
The Hospital at Westlake Medical Center	Austin	0%	4762
Houston Hospital for Specialized Surgery	Houston	0%	36
Houston Orthopedic & Spine Hospital	Bellaire	0%	422
Jackson Healthcare Center	Edna	0%	4358
Knox County Hospital	Knox City	0%	1476
Lakeway Regional Medical Center	Lakeway	0%	5068
Methodist Mckinney Hospital	Mc Kinney	0%	3480
North Central Surgical Center	Dallas	0%	1423
North Cypress Medical Center	Cypress	0%	14719
Northwest Hills Surgical Hospital	Austin	0%	71
Saint Anthony's Hospital	Houston	0%	11963
Saint Luke's Lakeside Hospital	The Woodlands	0%	2332
Seymour Hospital	Seymour	0%	1945
South Texas Spine & Surgical Hospital	San Antonio	0%	166
Surgery Specialty Hosps of America	Pasadena	0%	333
Texas General Hospital	Grand Prairie	0%	4176
TX Hlth Presbyterian Hosp-Flower Mound	Flower Mound	0%	14068
TX Inst for Surgery at Presby Hosp	Dallas	0%	46
Texas Orthopedic Hospital	Houston	0%	575
Tops Surgical Specialty Hospital	Houston	0%	525
Univ of Texas Med Branch Galveston	Galveston	0%	39423
The Womans Hospital of Texas	Houston	0%	3886
Baptist Emergency Hospital	San Antonio	1%	14272
Baylor Medical Center at Mckinney	Mc Kinney	1%	10169
Baylor Medical Center at Trophy Club	Trophy Club	1%	2613
Baylor Medical Center at Uptown	Dallas	1%	1782
Baylor Reg Med Ctr at Grapevine	Grapevine	1%	46129
Baylor Surgical Hospital at Las Colinas	Irving	1%	2374
Bellville General Hospital	Bellville	1%	5218
Bowie Memorial Hospital	Bowie	1%	4952
Brownwood Regional Medical Center	Brownwood	1%	22713
Centennial Medical Center	Frisco	1%	21988
Christus Saint Catherine Hospital	Katy	1%	23960
Citizens Medical Center	Victoria	1%	33747
Clear Lake Regional Medical Center	Webster	1%	76822
Cogdell Memorial Hospital	Snyder	1%	8651
College Station Medical Center	College Station	1%	31071
Connally Memorial Medical Center	Floresville	1%	13088
Conroe Regional Medical Center	Conroe	1%	50349
Cook Childrens Northeast Hospital	Hurst	1%	3055
The Corpus Christi Medical Center	Corpus Christi	1%	71892
East Texas Medical Center - Fairfield	Fairfield	1%	9698
East Texas Medical Center Athens	Athens	1%	61171
East Texas Medical Center Crockett	Crockett	1%	14134
East Texas Medical Center Mount Vernon	Mount Vernon	1%	3146
East Texas Medical Center Quitman	Quitman	1%	9219
Emerus Hospital	Sugar Land	1%	7914
Fort Duncan Medical Center	Eagle Pass	1%	19162
Foundation Surgical Hospital of El Paso	El Paso	1%	10736
Fdn Surgical Hosp of San Antonio	San Antonio	1%	186
Glen Rose Medical Center	Glen Rose	1%	7703
Good Shepherd Medical Center Marshall	Marshall	1%	30727
Goodall Witcher Hospital	Clifton	1%	4448
Graham Regional Medical Center	Graham	1%	9491
Guadalupe Regional Medical Center	Seguin	1%	36470
Hamilton General Hospital	Hamilton	1%	6075
Harlingen Medical Center	Harlingen	1%	29594
Heart Hospital Baylor Denton	Denton	1%	283
Hereford Regional Medical Center	Hereford	1%	7761
Hill Regional Hospital	Hillsboro	1%	11387
Houston Physicians' Hospital	Webster	1%	298
Lake Granbury Medical Center	Granbury	1%	20193
Lake Pointe Medical Center	Rowlett	1%	29195
Lamb Healthcare Center	Littlefield	1%	3592
Las Colinas Medical Center	Irving	1%	26547
Longview Regional Medical Center	Longview	1%	31728
Lubbock Heart Hospital	Lubbock	1%	4597
Lynn County Hospital District	Tahoka	1%	2190
Medical Center of Lewisville	Lewisville	1%	45113
Memorial Hermann Sugar Land Hospital	Sugar Land	1%	25892
Memorial Medical Center	Port Lavaca	1%	38604
Methodist Ambulatory Surgery Hospital NW	San Antonio	1%	858
Methodist Hospital	San Antonio	1%	275021
Methodist Hospital For Surgery	Addison	1%	1268
Methodist Richardson Medical Center	Richardson	1%	34693
Methodist Stone Oak Hospital	San Antonio	1%	22998
Mission Regional Medical Center	Mission	1%	37723
Moore County Hospital District	Dumas	1%	9031
Oakbend Medical Center	Richmond	1%	28946
Otto Kaiser Memorial Hospital	Kenedy	1%	9111
Pampa Regional Medical Center	Pampa	1%	12671
Park Plaza Hospital	Houston	1%	10381
Parkview Regional Hospital	Mexia	1%	9505
Peterson Regional Medical Center	Kerrville	1%	30534
The Physicians Centre	Bryan	1%	1110
Plains Memorial Hospital	Dimmitt	1%	2869
Rio Grande Regional Hospital	Mcallen	1%	35920
Rolling Plains Memorial Hospital	Sweetwater	1%	12002
Round Rock Medical Center	Round Rock	1%	41385
Saint David's Medical Center	Austin	1%	53708
Saint David's South Austin Medical Center	Austin	1%	103143
Saint Luke's Episcopal Hospital	Houston	1%	84705
Saint Luke's Hospital at the Vintage	Houston	1%	17173
Saint Luke's Sugar Land Hospital	Sugar Land	1%	18633
Saint Marks Medical Center	La Grange	1%	10595
Scott & White Hospital - Llano	Llano	1%	7005
Scott & White Hospital - Round Rock	Round Rock	1%	23016
Scott & White Memorial Hospital	Temple	1%	78537
Seton Medical Center Austin	Austin	1%	38221
Seton Medical Center Williamson	Round Rock	1%	30755
Seton Northwest Hospital	Austin	1%	35588
Seton Smithville Regional Hospital	Smithville	1%	10758
Seton Southwest Hospital	Austin	1%	38221
South Texas Regional Medical Center	Jourdanton	1%	19758
Stamford Memorial Hospital	Stamford	1%	2427
Texas Health Harris Methodist Fort Worth	Fort Worth	1%	133512
TX Hlth Harris Meth Hosp-Alliance	Fort Worth	1%	5851
TX Hlth Harris Meth Hosp-Cleburne	Cleburne	1%	35652
TX Hlth Harris Meth Hosp-Southlake	Southlake	1%	1943
TX Hlth Harris Meth Hosp SW Ft Worth	Fort Worth	1%	59141
Texas Health Presbyterian Hospital Dallas	Dallas	1%	84477
Texas Spine & Joint Hospital	Tyler	1%	399
Titus Regional Medical Center	Mount Pleasant	1%	21681
Tomball Regional Medical Center	Tomball	1%	33869
Tyler County Hospital	Woodville	1%	10455
University General Hospital	Houston	1%	2914
University Medical Center	Lubbock	1%	773959
Univ of TX Health Science Ctr-Tyler	Tyler	1%	14853
USMD Hospital at Fort Worth	Fort Worth	1%	728
VHS Harlingen Hospital Company	Harlingen	1%	56970
Wise Regional Health System	Decatur	1%	25611
Woodland Heights Medical Center	Lufkin	1%	17231
Baptist Beaumont Hospital	Beaumont	2%	75401
Baylor All Saints Medical Center at FW	Fort Worth	2%	48539
Baylor Medical Center at Carrollton	Carrollton	2%	35987
Baylor Medical Center at Frisco	Frisco	2%	2682
Baylor Medical Center at Garland	Garland	2%	66900
Baylor Medical Center at Waxahachie	Waxahachie	2%	43318
Baylor Ortho & Spine Hosp-Arlington	Arlington	2%	953
Baylor Regional Medical Center at Plano	Plano	2%	24455
Bayshore Medical Center	Pasadena	2%	115478
Cedar Park Regional Medical Center	Cedar Park	2%	28927
Central Texas Medical Center	San Marcos	2%	38953
Childress Regional Medical Center	Childress	2%	5051
Columbus Community Hospital	Columbus	2%	6152
Dallas Medical Center	Dallas	2%	11335
Denton Regional Medical Center	Denton	2%	44917
Doctors Diagnostic Hospital	Cleveland	2%	542
Doctors Hospital of Laredo	Laredo	2%	29386
East Texas Medical Center - Gilmer	Gilmer	2%	11532
East Texas Medical Center Jacksonville	Jacksonville	2%	14801
El Campo Memorial Hospital	El Campo	2%	5984
Etmc Carthage	Carthage	2%	14446
Etmc Clarksville	Clarksville	2%	5428
Etmc Henderson	Henderson	2%	14008
First Surgical Hospital	Bellaire	2%	262
Gulf Coast Medical Center	Wharton	2%	11481
Hamlin Memorial Hospital	Hamlin	2%	1218
Hunt Regional Medical Center	Greenville	2%	47992
Las Palmas Medical Center	El Paso	2%	43553
Medical Center of Arlington	Arlington	2%	69263
Medical Center of Mckinney	Mckinney	2%	32478
Medical Center of Plano	Plano	2%	40849
Medical City Dallas Hospital	Dallas	2%	76716
Memorial Hermann Katy Hospital	Katy	2%	36447
Memorial Hermann Northeast	Humble	2%	58680
Mem Hermann Surgical Hosp Kingwood	Kingwood	2%	162
Memorial Hospital	Gonzales	2%	9620
The Methodist Hospital	Houston	2%	54453
Navarro Regional Hospital	Corsicana	2%	26127
North Austin Medical Center	Austin	2%	63017
North Hills Hospital	N Richland Hls	2%	67164
North Texas Medical Center	Gainesville	2%	17441
Palo Pinto General Hospital	Mineral Wells	2%	22304
Paris Regional Medical Center	Paris	2%	35322
Pecos County Memorial Hospital	Fort Stockton	2%	7013
Plaza Medical Center of Fort Worth	Fort Worth	2%	18118
Providence Memorial Hospital	El Paso	2%	47232
Saint Joseph Regional Health Center	Bryan	2%	56221
San Angelo Community Medical Center	San Angelo	2%	26203
Scott & White Hospital Brenham	Brenham	2%	15881
Shannon Medical Center	San Angelo	2%	55207
Sugar Land Surgical Hospital	Sugar Land	2%	297
TX Hlth Harris Meth Hosp-Stephenville	Stephenville	2%	18340
Texas Health Presbyterian Hospital - WNJ	Sherman	2%	29700
Texas Health Presbyterian Hospital Allen	Allen	2%	30030
Texas Health Presbyterian Hospital Denton	Denton	2%	43158
TX Hlth Presbyterian Hosp-Kaufman	Kaufman	2%	27890
Texas Health Presbyterian Hospital Plano	Plano	2%	45716
TX Health Presbyterian Hosp Rockwall	Rockwall	2%	25529
Texoma Medical Center	Denison	2%	44225
Val Verde Regional Medical Center	Del Rio	2%	25335
Valley Regional Medical Center	Brownsville	2%	32770
VHS Brownsville Hospital Company	Brownsville	2%	32439
Weatherford Regional Medical Center	Weatherford	2%	26270
West Houston Medical Center	Houston	2%	51437
Wilbarger General Hospital	Vernon	2%	7344
Baptist Saint Anthony's Hospital	Amarillo	3%	62217
Baylor Medical Center at Irving	Irving	3%	73987
Christus Santa Rosa Hospital	San Antonio	3%	238530
Cornerstone Regional Hospital	Edinburg	3%	38
Covenant Medical Center	Lubbock	3%	64104
Cuero Community Hospital	Cuero	3%	8815
Detar Hospital Navarro	Victoria	3%	23684
Doctors Hospital at Renaissance	Edinburg	3%	33853
Ennis Regional Medical Center	Ennis	3%	16845
Falls Community Hospital & Clinic	Marlin	3%	7605
Good Shepherd Medical Center	Longview	3%	81537
Grace Medical Center	Lubbock	3%	11305
Huguley Memorial Medical Center	Burleson	3%	47555
Kell West Regional Hospital	Wichita Falls	3%	12886
Kingwood Medical Center	Kingwood	3%	57791
Lake Whitney Medical Center	Whitney	3%	3621
Medical Arts Hospital	Lamesa	3%	6798
The Medical Center of Southeast Texas	Port Arthur	3%	32006
Memorial Hermann Hospital System	Houston	3%	229088
Methodist Mansfield Medical Center	Mansfield	3%	52769

NOTE: Hospital profiles are in alphabetical order by state, then city, then hospital within the city; Rankings exclude hospitals with less than 25 cases except for patient surveys which excludes hospitals with less than 100 cases; (a) 100-299 cases; (1) The number of cases/patients is too few to report; (2) Data submitted were based on a sample of cases/patients; (3) Results are based on a shorter time period than required; (4) Data suppressed by CMS for one or more quarters; (5) Results are not available for this reporting period; (6) Fewer than 100 patients completed the HCAHPS survey; (7) No cases met the criteria for this measure; (8) The lower limit of the confidence interval cannot be calculated if the number of observed infections equals zero; (9) No data are available from the state/territory for this reporting period; (10) The scores shown reflect fewer than 50 completed surveys; (11) There were discrepancies in the data collection process; (12) This measure does not apply to this hospital for this reporting period; (13) Results cannot be calculated for this reporting period; (14) The results for this state are combined with nearby states to protect confidentiality; Please refer to the User's Guide for a full explanation of data.

Methodist West Houston Hospital	Houston	3%	23095
Mother Frances Hospital	Tyler	3%	69804
Odessa Regional Hospital	Odessa	3%	27035
Permian Regional Medical Center	Andrews	3%	8536
Providence Health Center	Waco	3%	86396
Seton Medical Center Harker Heights	Harker Heights	3%	17819
Seton Medical Center Hays	Kyle	3%	32850
Sierra Providence East Medical Center	El Paso	3%	51708
South Texas Health System	Edinburg	3%	74555
South Texas Surgical Hospital	Corpus Christi	3%	1090
Southwest General Hospital	San Antonio	3%	48609
Stephens Memorial Hospital	Breckenridge	3%	5679
TX Hlth Harris Methodist Hosp-Azle	Azle	3%	27241
USMD Hospital at Arlington	Arlington	3%	22604
Wadley Regional Medical Center	Texarkana	3%	44596
Baptist Medical Center	San Antonio	4%	23304
Baylor University Medical Center	Dallas	4%	117265
Christus Hospital	Beaumont	4%	53806
Christus Saint Michael Health System	Texarkana	4%	66047
Hillcrest Baptist Medical Center	Waco	4%	56609
Hopkins County Memorial Hospital	Sulphur Springs	4%	17631
Matagorda Regional Medical Center	Bay City	4%	18863
Medical Center Hospital	Odessa	4%	53180
Memorial Hospital	Nacogdoches	4%	26845
Memorial Medical Center Livingston	Livingston	4%	23617
Methodist Sugar Land Hospital	Sugar Land	4%	38524
Methodist Willowbrook Hospital	Houston	4%	54403
Midland Memorial Hospital	Midland	4%	63743
Northwest Texas Hospital	Amarillo	4%	50021
Palestine Regional Medical Center	Palestine	4%	31689
Scenic Mountain Medical Center	Big Spring	4%	17518
Texas Health Harris Methodist	Bedford	4%	61881
United Regional Health Care System	Wichita Falls	4%	81450
UT Southwestern University Hospital	Dallas	4%	37102
Abilene Regional Medical Center	Abilene	5%	25892
Angleton - Danbury Medical Center	Angleton	5%	17591
Christus Saint John Hospital	Nassau Bay	5%	25910
Christus Spohn Hospital Corpus Christi	Corpus Christi	5%	122277
Cleveland Regional Medical Center	Cleveland	5%	2777
Covenant Hospital Levelland	Levelland	5%	6780
Cypress Fairbanks Medical Center	Houston	5%	34807
Dimmit Regional Hospital	Carrizo Springs	5%	5083
Huntsville Memorial Hospital	Huntsville	5%	22385
JPS Health Network	Fort Worth	5%	108335
Knapp Medical Center	Weslaco	5%	39196
Mem Hermann Mem City Med Ctr	Houston	5%	58239
Memorial Medical Center of East Texas	Lufkin	5%	38783
Methodist Dallas Medical Center	Dallas	5%	63702
Metroplex Hospital	Killeen	5%	51746
Saint Joseph Medical Center	Houston	5%	32034
Saint Luke's Patients Medical Center	Pasadena	5%	15237
Saint Luke's the Woodlands Hospital	The Woodlands	5%	37967
San Jacinto Methodist Hospital	Baytown	5%	54340
Sierra Medical Center	El Paso	5%	27050
Texas Health Arlington Memorial Hospital	Arlington	5%	75924
Uvalde Memorial Hospital	Uvalde	5%	18378
Brownfield Regional Medical Center	Brownfield	6%	5335
Christus Spohn Hospital Alice	Alice	6%	29341
Christus Spohn Hospital Beeville	Beeville	6%	20594
Covenant Hospital Plainview	Plainview	6%	13838
Hendrick Medical Center	Abilene	6%	62307
University Medical Center at Brackenridge	Austin	6%	71280
University Medical Center of El Paso	El Paso	6%	54863
Christus Jasper Memorial Hospital	Jasper	7%	24159
Christus Spohn Hospital Kleberg	Kingsville	7%	19773
East Texas Medical Center	Tyler	7%	66359
Houston Northwest Medical Center	Houston	7%	78889
Laredo Medical Center	Laredo	7%	58248
University General Hospital Dallas	Dallas	7%	12576
Memorial Hermann Baptist Orange Hospital	Orange	8%	18697
Memorial Hermann Texas Medical Center	Houston	8%	61592
Parkland Health & Hospital System	Dallas	8%	218047
University Health System	San Antonio	8%	66831
Care Regional Medical Center	Aransas Pass	9%	10699
Methodist Charlton Medical Center	Dallas	9%	72069
Brazosport Regional Health System	Lake Jackson	10%	29238
Hemphill County Hospital	Canadian	10%	2017
Texas Reg Med Ctr at Sunnyvale	Sunnyvale	10%	30374
TX Health Ctr for Diag & Surgery	Plano	13%	92
Harris Health System	Houston	14%	173681
Nocona General Hospital	Nocona	14%	2866
Starr County Memorial Hospital	Rio Grande City	15%	11761
Doctors Hospital Tidwell	Houston	16%	16721
Dallas Regional Medical Center	Mesquite	17%	1861
Doctors Hospital	Dallas	18%	5818
Pine Creek Medical Center	Dallas	20%	80
Nacogdoches Medical Center	Nacogdoches	86%	790

Time from ER Arrival to Being Admitted (minutes)

Hospital Name	City	Min.	Cases
The Womans Hospital of Texas[2]	Houston	52	311
Nocona General Hospital[2]	Nocona	86	320
Hamlin Memorial Hospital[2]	Hamlin	88	92
Knox County Hospital[2]	Knox City	89	55
Electra Memorial Hospital	Electra	95	40
Seymour Hospital	Seymour	95	180
Stephens Memorial Hospital[2]	Breckenridge	113	165
Houston Orthopedic & Spine Hospital	Bellaire	114	38
Hemphill County Hospital[2]	Canadian	120	87
Stamford Memorial Hospital	Stamford	120	134
Lamb Healthcare Center	Littlefield	122	132
Childress Regional Medical Center[2]	Childress	126	136
Anson General Hospital	Anson	130	61
Lubbock Heart Hospital[2]	Lubbock	134	202
Faith Community Hospital[2]	Jacksboro	141	65
Hamilton General Hospital[2]	Hamilton	145	440
Plains Memorial Hospital	Dimmitt	145	69
Central Texas Hospital[2,3]	Cameron	150	103
Mitchell County Hospital District	Colorado City	150	252
Good Shephard Medical Center - Linden[2]	Linden	155	213
East Texas Medical Center Mount Vernon[2]	Mount Vernon	158	148
Lake Whitney Medical Center[2]	Whitney	159	325
Hill Regional Hospital[2]	Hillsboro	160	280
Brownfield Regional Medical Center[2]	Brownfield	163	173
Otto Kaiser Memorial Hospital[2]	Kenedy	172	200
El Paso Specialty Hospital[2]	El Paso	175	43
Goodall Witcher Hospital[2]	Clifton	176	164
TX Hlth Harris Meth Hosp-Stephenville[2]	Stephenville	176	300
Cogdell Memorial Hospital	Snyder	178	202
Scott & White Hospital - Llano	Llano	183	258
Seton Smithville Regional Hospital[2]	Smithville	183	307
Doctors Diagnostic Hospital[2]	Cleveland	185	88
Medical Arts Hospital[2]	Lamesa	186	249
Methodist Mckinney Hospital[2]	Mc Kinney	186	41
Moore County Hospital District[2]	Dumas	186	151
Big Bend Regional Medical Center[2]	Alpine	190	318
Etmc Clarksville[2]	Clarksville	190	278
Citizens Medical Center[2]	Victoria	193	581
Palestine Regional Medical Center[2]	Palestine	193	380
Glen Rose Medical Center	Glen Rose	194	466
Memorial Hospital[2]	Gonzales	194	283
Seton Medical Center Williamson[2]	Round Rock	194	648
Rolling Plains Memorial Hospital[2]	Sweetwater	195	236
Tyler County Hospital[2]	Woodville	195	480
Hopkins County Memorial Hospital[2]	Sulphur Springs	196	331
Detar Hospital Navarro[2]	Victoria	197	489
Medical Center of Lewisville[2]	Lewisville	198	722
Palo Pinto General Hospital[2]	Mineral Wells	198	268
Scott & White Hospital - Round Rock[2]	Round Rock	198	494
Cuero Community Hospital[2]	Cuero	199	309
Frio Regional Hospital[2]	Pearsall	200	78
Saint Luke's Lakeside Hospital[2]	The Woodlands	200	33
East Texas Medical Center Pittsburg[2]	Pittsburg	202	356
El Campo Memorial Hospital	El Campo	203	208
Lavaca Medical Center[2]	Hallettsville	203	342
Permian Regional Medical Center[2]	Andrews	204	138
Saint Marks Medical Center[2]	La Grange	205	398
East Texas Medical Center Crockett[2]	Crockett	206	228
Covenant Hospital Plainview[2]	Plainview	208	115
Rollins Brook Community Hospital[2]	Lampasas	209	319
TX Hlth Harris Methodist Hosp-Azle[2]	Azle	209	699
Baylor Regional Medical Center at Plano[2]	Plano	210	594
East Texas Medical Center Trinity[2]	Trinity	210	248
Golden Plains Community Hospital[2]	Borger	210	289
Lake Pointe Medical Center[2]	Rowlett	210	671
Las Colinas Medical Center[2]	Irving	210	610
Bowie Memorial Hospital[2]	Bowie	211	311
The Hospital at Westlake Medical Center[2]	Austin	211	293
Brownwood Regional Medical Center[2]	Brownwood	212	523
Methodist Richardson Medical Center[2]	Richardson	212	563
Nix Health Care System[2]	San Antonio	212	110
Val Verde Regional Medical Center[2]	Del Rio	213	343
Scenic Mountain Medical Center[2]	Big Spring	214	368
Graham Regional Medical Center[2]	Graham	215	362
TX Hlth Presbyterian Hosp-Flower Mound[2]	Flower Mound	215	317
East Texas Medical Center - Gilmer[2]	Gilmer	216	291
Medical Center of Plano[2]	Plano	216	804
Hereford Regional Medical Center[2]	Hereford	217	261
Wilbarger General Hospital[2]	Vernon	217	246
Navarro Regional Hospital[2]	Corsicana	218	436
Conroe Regional Medical Center[2]	Conroe	219	659
San Angelo Community Medical Center[2]	San Angelo	219	503
University General Hospital[2]	Houston	220	1122
Pampa Regional Medical Center[2]	Pampa	222	424
Uvalde Memorial Hospital[2]	Uvalde	222	614
Medical Center of Mckinney[2]	Mckinney	223	817
North Texas Medical Center[2]	Gainesville	223	190
College Station Medical Center[2]	College Station	224	578
Lakeway Regional Medical Center[2,3]	Lakeway	225	247
Univ of TX Health Science Ctr-Tyler[2]	Tyler	225	353
East Texas Medical Center Quitman[2]	Quitman	226	332
Lake Granbury Medical Center[2]	Granbury	226	392
Shannon Medical Center[2]	San Angelo	226	703
Titus Regional Medical Center[2]	Mount Pleasant	226	148
Covenant Hospital Levelland[2]	Levelland	228	169
Woodland Heights Medical Center[2]	Lufkin	228	508
TX Hlth Harris Meth Hosp SW Ft Worth[2]	Fort Worth	229	603
Good Shepherd Medical Center Marshall[2]	Marshall	230	508
Texas Health Presbyterian Hospital Allen[2]	Allen	230	462
East Texas Medical Center Jacksonville[2]	Jacksonville	231	167
Grace Medical Center	Lubbock	232	120
Etmc Carthage[2]	Carthage	233	414
Rio Grande Regional Hospital[2]	Mcallen	233	575
Longview Regional Medical Center[2]	Longview	234	493
TX Health Presbyterian Hosp Rockwall[2]	Rockwall	234	449
Baylor Medical Center at Garland[2]	Garland	235	461
Heart Hospital Baylor Plano[2]	Plano	235	190
TX Hlth Presbyterian Hosp-Kaufman[2]	Kaufman	235	314
Good Shepherd Medical Center[2]	Longview	236	627
Gulf Coast Medical Center[2]	Wharton	236	315
Parkview Regional Hospital[2]	Mexia	236	445
Pecos County Memorial Hospital[2]	Fort Stockton	236	298
Wise Regional Health System[2]	Decatur	237	511
Connally Memorial Medical Center[2]	Floresville	238	437
Saint Joseph Regional Health Center[2]	Bryan	238	688
Scott & White Hospital Brenham[2]	Brenham	238	239
Valley Regional Medical Center[2]	Brownsville	240	600
Weatherford Regional Medical Center[2]	Weatherford	240	640
Baylor Medical Center at Trophy Club[2]	Trophy Club	241	33
Etmc Henderson[2]	Henderson	241	313
Eastland Memorial Hospital[2]	Eastland	243	156
Hunt Regional Medical Center[2]	Greenville	245	576
Baylor Reg Med Ctr at Grapevine[2]	Grapevine	246	536
Dallas Regional Medical Center[2]	Mesquite	246	1323
Saint Anthony's Hospital[2,3]	Houston	248	210
Harlingen Medical Center[2]	Harlingen	249	616
East Texas Medical Center - Fairfield	Fairfield	251	401
North Hills Hospital[2]	N Richland Hls	251	759
Cedar Park Regional Medical Center[2]	Cedar Park	252	548
Methodist Stone Oak Hospital[2]	San Antonio	252	413
United Regional Health Care System[2]	Wichita Falls	252	536
Hill Country Memorial Hospital[2]	Fredericksburg	253	224
Plaza Medical Center of Fort Worth[2]	Fort Worth	254	714
Seton Medical Center Harker Heights[2]	Harker Heights	254	371
Seton Southwest Hospital[2]	Austin	254	46
Kell West Regional Hospital	Wichita Falls	255	196
Baylor Medical Center at Waxahachie[2]	Waxahachie	256	336
Nacogdoches Medical Center[2]	Nacogdoches	256	471
Baylor Medical Center at Mckinney[2]	Mc Kinney	257	607
University Medical Center[2]	Lubbock	258	557
Memorial Hermann Katy Hospital[2]	Katy	259	487
TX Hlth Harris Meth Hosp-Cleburne[2]	Cleburne	259	503
Texas Health Presbyterian Hospital Plano[2]	Plano	260	275
Columbus Community Hospital[2]	Columbus	261	184
Providence Memorial Hospital[2]	El Paso	261	443
Texas Health Harris Methodist[2]	Bedford	261	523
Texas Health Presbyterian Hospital - WNJ[2]	Sherman	262	674
Doctors Hospital at Renaissance[2]	Edinburg	263	292
Matagorda Regional Medical Center[2]	Bay City	263	317
Memorial Hermann Sugar Land Hospital[2]	Sugar Land	263	453
Guadalupe Regional Medical Center[2]	Seguin	264	379
Saint David's South Austin Medical Center[2]	Austin	264	785
Memorial Hospital[2]	Nacogdoches	265	398
Centennial Medical Center[2]	Frisco	266	428
The Corpus Christi Medical Center[2]	Corpus Christi	266	589
Oakbend Medical Center[2]	Richmond	266	428
Peterson Regional Medical Center[2]	Kerrville	266	578
Saint Joseph Medical Center[2]	Houston	266	590
Seton Medical Center Austin[2]	Austin	266	467
Texas Health Harris Methodist Fort Worth[2]	Fort Worth	266	827
TX Hlth Harris Meth Hosp-Alliance[2,3]	Fort Worth	267	265
Dallas Medical Center[2]	Dallas	268	322
North Cypress Medical Center[2]	Cypress	268	625
Texas Reg Med Ctr at Sunnyvale[2]	Sunnyvale	268	514
Texas Health Presbyterian Hospital Denton[2]	Denton	269	649
Medical City Dallas Hospital[2]	Dallas	270	671
Knapp Medical Center[2]	Weslaco	271	518
Round Rock Medical Center[2]	Round Rock	273	621
Tomball Regional Medical Center[2]	Tomball	273	728
Cleveland Regional Medical Center[2]	Cleveland	275	270
Dimmit Regional Hospital[2]	Carrizo Springs	275	161
University General Hospital Dallas[2]	Dallas	275	216
Baylor Medical Center at Carrollton[2]	Carrollton	276	616
Covenant Medical Center[2]	Lubbock	278	610
Seton Medical Center Hays[2]	Kyle	278	778
Denton Regional Medical Center[2]	Denton	280	768
Medina Regional Hospital[3]	Hondo	280	273
Scott & White Memorial Hospital[2]	Temple	280	580
South Texas Regional Medical Center[2]	Jourdanton	280	355
Clear Lake Regional Medical Center[2]	Webster	282	859
Ennis Regional Medical Center[2]	Ennis	282	299
VHS Brownsville Hospital Company[2]	Brownsville	282	534
Doctors Hospital[2]	Dallas	283	698

NOTE: Hospital profiles are in alphabetical order by state, then city, then hospital within the city; Rankings exclude hospitals with less than 25 cases except for patient surveys which excludes hospitals with less than 100 cases; (a) 100-299 cases; (1) The number of cases/patients is too few to report; (2) Data submitted were based on a sample of cases/patients; (3) Results are based on a shorter time period than required; (4) Data suppressed by CMS for one or more quarters; (5) Results are not available for this reporting period; (6) Fewer than 100 patients completed the HCAHPS survey; (7) No cases met the criteria for this measure; (8) The lower limit of the confidence interval cannot be calculated if the number of observed infections equals zero; (9) No data are available from the state/territory for this reporting period; (10) The scores shown reflect fewer than 50 completed surveys; (11) There were discrepancies in the data collection process; (12) This measure does not apply to this hospital for this reporting period; (13) Results cannot be calculated for this reporting period; (14) The results for this state are combined with nearby states to protect confidentiality; Please refer to the User's Guide for a full explanation of data.

VHS Harlingen Hospital Company[2]	Harlingen	283	566
Saint David's Medical Center[2]	Austin	284	532
Sierra Medical Center[2]	El Paso	284	595
Texas Health Arlington Memorial Hospital[2]	Arlington	284	693
Park Plaza Hospital[2]	Houston	286	431
Metroplex Hospital[2]	Killeen	287	461
Paris Regional Medical Center[2]	Paris	287	573
East Texas Medical Center Athens[2]	Athens	288	605
Mem Hermann Mem City Med Ctr[2]	Houston	288	520
Methodist Hospital[2]	San Antonio	291	595
USMD Hospital at Arlington[2]	Arlington	291	106
Huntsville Memorial Hospital[2]	Huntsville	292	495
Medical Center of Arlington[2]	Arlington	292	727
Midland Memorial Hospital[2]	Midland	293	1438
Seton Northwest Hospital[2]	Austin	293	597
Mission Regional Medical Center[2]	Mission	294	360
Methodist Sugar Land Hospital[2]	Sugar Land	301	397
Abilene Regional Medical Center[2]	Abilene	302	415
Christus Jasper Memorial Hospital[2]	Jasper	302	403
Baylor Medical Center at Irving[2]	Irving	304	674
Methodist Mansfield Medical Center[2]	Mansfield	304	239
Texoma Medical Center[2]	Denison	304	552
North Austin Medical Center[2]	Austin	305	503
Saint Luke's Episcopal Hospital[2]	Houston	307	606
Bayshore Medical Center[2]	Pasadena	308	551
Central Texas Medical Center[2]	San Marcos	308	541
Las Palmas Medical Center[2]	El Paso	308	778
Medical Center Hospital[2]	Odessa	309	834
Cypress Fairbanks Medical Center[2]	Houston	313	553
Mother Frances Hospital[2]	Tyler	313	490
Odessa Regional Hospital[2]	Odessa	318	275
Providence Health Center[2]	Waco	318	683
Methodist West Houston Hospital[2]	Houston	319	614
Christus Santa Rosa Hospital[2]	San Antonio	320	648
Methodist Willowbrook Hospital[2]	Houston	320	634
Hillcrest Baptist Medical Center[2]	Waco	324	456
The Methodist Hospital[2]	Houston	324	440
Memorial Medical Center Livingston[2]	Livingston	325	301
Wadley Regional Medical Center[2]	Texarkana	325	597
Baptist Saint Anthony's Hospital[2]	Amarillo	328	680
Sierra Providence East Medical Center[2]	El Paso	328	670
Baptist Medical Center[2]	San Antonio	330	2272
Baylor All Saints Medical Center at FW[2]	Fort Worth	330	382
Christus Saint Catherine Hospital[2]	Katy	331	416
West Houston Medical Center[2]	Houston	332	618
Huguley Memorial Medical Center[2]	Burleson	335	593
Christus Saint Michael Health System[2]	Texarkana	336	696
Hendrick Medical Center[2]	Abilene	338	597
Baptist Beaumont Hospital[2]	Beaumont	340	781
Memorial Hermann Texas Medical Center[2]	Houston	340	528
Christus Saint John Hospital[2]	Nassau Bay	341	827
Christus Hospital[2]	Beaumont	347	667
Texas General Hospital[3]	Grand Prairie	348	80
Brazosport Regional Health System[2]	Lake Jackson	349	529
Memorial Hermann Baptist Orange Hospital[2]	Orange	350	377
Univ of Texas Med Branch Galveston[2]	Galveston	350	222
Houston Northwest Medical Center[2]	Houston	351	684
East Texas Medical Center[2]	Tyler	352	288
Texas Health Presbyterian Hospital Dallas[2]	Dallas	352	432
Angleton - Danbury Medical Center[2]	Angleton	354	231
The Medical Center of Southeast Texas[2]	Port Arthur	354	718
Saint Luke's Sugar Land Hospital[2]	Sugar Land	357	486
University Medical Center at Brackenridge[2]	Austin	357	698
South Texas Health System[2]	Edinburg	358	668
Christus Spohn Hospital Beeville[2]	Beeville	360	380
Memorial Hermann Hospital System[2]	Houston	360	2182
Saint Luke's Hospital at the Vintage[2]	Houston	360	314
Care Regional Medical Center[2]	Aransas Pass	365	422
Saint Luke's the Woodlands Hospital[2]	The Woodlands	365	403
Doctors Hospital Tidwell[2]	Houston	366	286
Fort Duncan Medical Center[2]	Eagle Pass	368	239
Methodist Dallas Medical Center[2]	Dallas	368	476
UT Southwestern University Hospital[2]	Dallas	374	447
Christus Spohn Hospital Alice[2]	Alice	378	450
JPS Health Network[2]	Fort Worth	384	722
Starr County Memorial Hospital[2]	Rio Grande City	384	542
Memorial Medical Center of East Texas[2]	Lufkin	387	415
Northwest Texas Hospital[2]	Amarillo	387	528
San Jacinto Methodist Hospital[2]	Baytown	388	697
Saint Luke's Patients Medical Center[2]	Pasadena	389	441
Christus Spohn Hospital Kleberg[2]	Kingsville	395	412
Southwest General Hospital[2]	San Antonio	395	653
Doctors Hospital of Laredo[2]	Laredo	400	370
Baylor University Medical Center[2]	Dallas	405	505
Methodist Charlton Medical Center[2]	Dallas	416	506
Christus Spohn Hospital Corpus Christi[2]	Corpus Christi	417	879
Kingwood Medical Center[2]	Kingwood	420	611
University Health System[2]	San Antonio	438	448
Laredo Medical Center[2]	Laredo	439	593
Parkland Health & Hospital System[2]	Dallas	442	538
Memorial Hermann Northeast[2]	Humble	454	713
University Medical Center of El Paso[2]	El Paso	504	672
Harris Health System[2]	Houston	786	1081
Falls Community Hospital & Clinic[2]	Marlin	926	280

Time from ER Arrival to Discharge (minutes)

Hospital Name	City	Min.	Cases
Methodist Ambulatory Surgery Hospital NW	San Antonio	57	252
Anson General Hospital	Anson	60	348
Northwest Hills Surgical Hospital	Austin	60	53
Surgery Specialty Hosps of America[3]	Pasadena	60	222
Nocona General Hospital	Nocona	64	298
Hill Regional Hospital	Hillsboro	70	390
Hamlin Memorial Hospital	Hamlin	71	250
Lamb Healthcare Center	Littlefield	71	223
Mitchell County Hospital District	Colorado City	71	392
Knox County Hospital	Knox City	74	228
Tops Surgical Specialty Hospital	Houston	74	272
Basin Healthcare Center	Odessa	75	387
Jackson Healthcare Center[3]	Edna	75	79
The Physicians Centre	Bryan	75	465
USMD Hospital at Fort Worth	Fort Worth	75	237
Moore County Hospital District	Dumas	76	349
Palo Pinto General Hospital	Mineral Wells	76	384
Stamford Memorial Hospital	Stamford	76	285
Good Shephard Medical Center - Linden	Linden	79	357
Baylor Surgical Hospital at Las Colinas	Irving	80	279
Bayside Community Hospital	Anahuac	80	264
Methodist Mckinney Hospital	Mc Kinney	80	249
Seymour Hospital	Seymour	80	328
Baylor Ortho & Spine Hosp-Arlington	Arlington	82	272
North Central Surgical Center	Dallas	82	289
Baylor Medical Center at Uptown	Dallas	83	286
Bowie Memorial Hospital	Bowie	83	618
Cogdell Memorial Hospital	Snyder	83	319
El Paso Specialty Hospital	El Paso	83	325
Lake Whitney Medical Center	Whitney	84	214
First Surgical Hospital	Bellaire	85	264
The Hospital at Westlake Medical Center	Austin	86	395
Sugar Land Surgical Hospital	Sugar Land	87	253
Heart Hospital Baylor Denton	Denton	88	46
Methodist Hospital For Surgery	Addison	88	267
TX Hlth Harris Meth Hosp-Southlake	Southlake	88	250
Baylor Medical Center at Trophy Club	Trophy Club	89	258
Scott & White Hospital - Round Rock	Round Rock	90	428
Eastland Memorial Hospital	Eastland	91	360
Goodall Witcher Hospital	Clifton	91	324
Baylor Medical Center at Frisco[3]	Frisco	92	448
East Texas Medical Center Mount Vernon	Mount Vernon	92	266
Grace Medical Center	Lubbock	92	10336
Nix Health Care System[3]	San Antonio	92	544
Parkview Regional Hospital	Mexia	92	347
Houston Physicians' Hospital	Webster	93	219
Lakeway Regional Medical Center[3]	Lakeway	93	247
Cypress Fairbanks Medical Center	Houston	94	471
Heritage Park Surgical Hospital	Sherman	94	239
Oakbend Medical Center	Richmond	94	357
Seton Smithville Regional Hospital	Smithville	94	356
Big Bend Regional Medical Center	Alpine	95	352
Fdn Surgical Hosp of San Antonio	San Antonio	95	230
Hemphill County Hospital	Canadian	95	366
South Texas Spine & Surgical Hospital	San Antonio	95	159
South Texas Surgical Hospital	Corpus Christi	95	448
Stephens Memorial Hospital	Breckenridge	95	2588
Faith Community Hospital	Jacksboro	96	292
Scenic Mountain Medical Center	Big Spring	96	375
Childress Regional Medical Center	Childress	97	384
Hamilton General Hospital	Hamilton	97	394
Arise Austin Medical Center	Austin	98	212
Scott & White Memorial Hospital	Temple	98	417
Mem Hermann Surgical Hosp Kingwood	Kingwood	99	129
North Texas Medical Center	Gainesville	99	354
Saint Luke's Lakeside Hospital	The Woodlands	99	248
Bellville General Hospital	Bellville	100	365
Cook Childrens Northeast Hospital	Hurst	100	248
Tyler County Hospital	Woodville	100	343
El Campo Memorial Hospital	El Campo	101	388
East Texas Medical Center Crockett	Crockett	102	413
Memorial Hospital	Gonzales	102	350
Permian Regional Medical Center	Andrews	102	358
Detar Hospital Navarro	Victoria	103	397
Saint Luke's Episcopal Hospital	Houston	103	427
Texas Orthopedic Hospital	Houston	103	261
Wadley Regional Medical Center	Texarkana	103	461
Cuero Community Hospital	Cuero	104	434
Etmc Carthage	Carthage	104	355
Frio Regional Hospital	Pearsall	104	350
Medical Arts Hospital	Lamesa	104	339
Baylor Surgical Hospital at Fort Worth	Fort Worth	105	291
Pampa Regional Medical Center	Pampa	105	887
Pine Creek Medical Center	Dallas	105	45
TX Hlth Harris Meth Hosp-Stephenville	Stephenville	105	414
Titus Regional Medical Center	Mount Pleasant	105	380
Medical Center of Lewisville	Lewisville	106	440
Rolling Plains Memorial Hospital	Sweetwater	106	324
Saint Joseph Regional Health Center	Bryan	106	396
Scott & White Hospital - Llano	Llano	106	374
Etmc Clarksville	Clarksville	107	607
Rollins Brook Community Hospital	Lampasas	107	341
Christus Saint Catherine Hospital	Katy	108	379
Kell West Regional Hospital	Wichita Falls	108	915
Palestine Regional Medical Center	Palestine	108	421
Hereford Regional Medical Center	Hereford	109	344
Dallas Regional Medical Center	Mesquite	110	1479
Falls Community Hospital & Clinic	Marlin	110	381
Foundation Surgical Hospital of El Paso	El Paso	110	546
Houston Orthopedic & Spine Hospital	Bellaire	110	402
Baylor Medical Center at Waxahachie	Waxahachie	111	392
Dallas Medical Center	Dallas	111	481
East Texas Medical Center - Gilmer	Gilmer	112	666
Centennial Medical Center	Frisco	113	458
Glen Rose Medical Center	Glen Rose	113	220
Lake Granbury Medical Center	Granbury	113	391
North Hills Hospital	N Richland Hls	113	472
San Angelo Community Medical Center	San Angelo	113	383
College Station Medical Center	College Station	114	400
Doctors Diagnostic Hospital	Cleveland	114	306
Navarro Regional Hospital	Corsicana	114	390
Connally Memorial Medical Center	Floresville	115	391
Good Shepherd Medical Center Marshall	Marshall	115	363
Hansford County Hospital[3]	Spearman	115	136
Univ of TX Health Science Ctr-Tyler	Tyler	115	385
Val Verde Regional Medical Center	Del Rio	115	1430
Brownwood Regional Medical Center	Brownwood	116	373
Gulf Coast Medical Center	Wharton	116	426
Hopkins County Memorial Hospital	Sulphur Springs	116	478
TX Hlth Presbyterian Hosp-Flower Mound	Flower Mound	116	448
Wilbarger General Hospital	Vernon	116	494
Brownfield Regional Medical Center	Brownfield	117	252
Harlingen Medical Center	Harlingen	118	371
North Cypress Medical Center	Cypress	118	367
South Texas Regional Medical Center	Jourdanton	118	370
East Texas Medical Center Trinity	Trinity	119	273
Lake Pointe Medical Center	Rowlett	119	443
Lubbock Heart Hospital	Lubbock	119	223
Providence Memorial Hospital	El Paso	119	397
Rio Grande Regional Hospital	Mcallen	119	473
Shannon Medical Center	San Angelo	119	417
Citizens Medical Center	Victoria	120	353
East Texas Medical Center - Fairfield	Fairfield	120	382
Saint Marks Medical Center	La Grange	120	460
Columbus Community Hospital	Columbus	121	385
Graham Regional Medical Center	Graham	121	329
Texas Health Presbyterian Hospital - WNJ	Sherman	121	415
Texas Spine & Joint Hospital	Tyler	121	238
University General Hospital Dallas[3]	Dallas	121	244
Methodist Richardson Medical Center	Richardson	122	389
TX Health Ctr for Diag & Surgery	Plano	122	85
Texas Health Presbyterian Hospital Allen	Allen	122	413
Wise Regional Health System	Decatur	123	546
Covenant Hospital Levelland	Levelland	124	371
Ennis Regional Medical Center	Ennis	124	384
Hill Country Memorial Hospital	Fredericksburg	124	487
Pecos County Memorial Hospital	Fort Stockton	124	374
Doctors Hospital	Dallas	125	445
Medical Center of Mckinney	Mckinney	126	406
TX Hlth Harris Methodist Hosp-Azle	Azle	126	435
East Texas Medical Center Jacksonville	Jacksonville	127	331
Abilene Regional Medical Center	Abilene	128	392
Good Shepherd Medical Center	Longview	128	394
TX Hlth Harris Meth Hosp-Cleburne	Cleburne	128	409
Saint David's South Austin Medical Center	Austin	129	509
Medical Center of Arlington	Arlington	130	490
TX Hlth Harris Meth Hosp SW Ft Worth	Fort Worth	130	423
Texas Reg Med Ctr at Sunnyvale	Sunnyvale	130	337
Matagorda Regional Medical Center	Bay City	132	426
Christus Santa Rosa Hospital	San Antonio	134	1305
The Methodist Hospital	Houston	134	404
Texoma Medical Center	Denison	134	396
USMD Hospital at Arlington	Arlington	134	360
Clear Lake Regional Medical Center	Webster	135	499
Covenant Hospital Plainview	Plainview	135	345
Dimmit Regional Hospital	Carrizo Springs	135	129
Las Colinas Medical Center	Irving	135	416
Peterson Regional Medical Center	Kerrville	135	471
Scott & White Hospital Brenham	Brenham	135	351
Central Texas Medical Center	San Marcos	136	367
Guadalupe Regional Medical Center	Seguin	136	345
Texas General Hospital[3]	Grand Prairie	136	258
United Regional Health Care System	Wichita Falls	137	463
Cleveland Regional Medical Center	Cleveland	138	855
Conroe Regional Medical Center	Conroe	138	447
Houston Northwest Medical Center	Houston	138	511

NOTE: Hospital profiles are in alphabetical order by state, then city, then hospital within the city; Rankings exclude hospitals with less than 25 cases except for patient surveys which excludes hospitals with less than 100 cases; (a) 100-299 cases; (1) The number of cases/patients is too few to report; (2) Data submitted were based on a sample of cases/patients; (3) Results are based on a shorter time period than required; (4) Data suppressed by CMS for one or more quarters; (5) Results are not available for this reporting period; (6) Fewer than 100 patients completed the HCAHPS survey; (7) No cases met the criteria for this measure; (8) The lower limit of the confidence interval cannot be calculated if the number of observed infections equals zero; (9) No data are available from the state/territory for this reporting period; (10) The scores shown reflect fewer than 50 completed surveys; (11) There were discrepancies in the data collection process; (12) This measure does not apply to this hospital for this reporting period; (13) Results cannot be calculated for this reporting period; (14) The results for this state are combined with nearby states to protect confidentiality; Please refer to the User's Guide for a full explanation of data.

Hospital Name	City	Min.	Cases
Hunt Regional Medical Center	Greenville	138	369
Methodist Hospital	San Antonio	138	500
Saint Anthony's Hospital	Houston	138	315
Weatherford Regional Medical Center	Weatherford	138	374
Baylor Medical Center at Garland	Garland	139	379
Christus Jasper Memorial Hospital	Jasper	140	386
Seton Medical Center Harker Heights	Harker Heights	140	762
Coryell Memorial Healthcare System	Gatesville	141	846
East Texas Medical Center Quitman	Quitman	141	347
Longview Regional Medical Center	Longview	141	393
Mother Frances Hospital	Tyler	141	406
Doctors Hospital of Laredo	Laredo	142	363
East Texas Medical Center	Tyler	142	351
Etmc Henderson	Henderson	142	358
Medical City Dallas Hospital	Dallas	142	444
North Austin Medical Center	Austin	142	515
The Corpus Christi Medical Center	Corpus Christi	143	517
Las Palmas Medical Center	El Paso	143	527
Nacogdoches Medical Center	Nacogdoches	143	371
Medical Center of Plano	Plano	144	438
TX Health Presbyterian Hosp Rockwall	Rockwall	144	443
Baylor Reg Med Ctr at Grapevine	Grapevine	145	378
Cedar Park Regional Medical Center	Cedar Park	145	394
TX Hlth Presbyterian Hosp-Kaufman	Kaufman	145	400
Denton Regional Medical Center	Denton	146	414
Bayshore Medical Center	Pasadena	148	441
Plaza Medical Center of Fort Worth	Fort Worth	148	438
Texas Health Presbyterian Hospital Denton	Denton	148	414
Christus Spohn Hospital Beeville	Beeville	149	399
Memorial Medical Center Livingston	Livingston	149	330
Midland Memorial Hospital	Midland	149	429
Southwest General Hospital	San Antonio	149	673
Sierra Providence East Medical Center	El Paso	150	457
Tomball Regional Medical Center	Tomball	150	489
VHS Brownsville Hospital Company	Brownsville	150	530
Woodland Heights Medical Center	Lufkin	150	381
Seton Southwest Hospital	Austin	151	330
Uvalde Memorial Hospital	Uvalde	151	742
Baylor Regional Medical Center at Plano	Plano	152	395
Heart Hospital Baylor Plano	Plano	152	374
Round Rock Medical Center	Round Rock	153	497
TX Hlth Harris Meth Hosp-Alliance[3]	Fort Worth	153	316
Park Plaza Hospital	Houston	154	426
Seton Medical Center Williamson	Round Rock	154	371
Texas Health Harris Methodist Fort Worth	Fort Worth	155	409
Baylor Medical Center at Carrollton	Carrollton	156	388
Baylor Medical Center at Mckinney	Mc Kinney	156	431
Saint David's Medical Center	Austin	156	503
Texas Health Presbyterian Hospital Plano	Plano	156	399
Care Regional Medical Center	Aransas Pass	157	488
Memorial Hermann Sugar Land Hospital	Sugar Land	157	371
Baptist Medical Center	San Antonio	158	392
East Texas Medical Center Athens	Athens	158	394
Hillcrest Baptist Medical Center	Waco	158	360
Paris Regional Medical Center	Paris	158	448
Saint Luke's Patients Medical Center	Pasadena	158	443
Sierra Medical Center	El Paso	158	390
Covenant Medical Center	Lubbock	159	539
Huntsville Memorial Hospital	Huntsville	159	349
Memorial Hermann Baptist Orange Hospital	Orange	159	364
Memorial Hospital	Nacogdoches	160	354
Methodist Mansfield Medical Center	Mansfield	162	385
Saint Luke's Hospital at the Vintage	Houston	162	369
Christus Saint Michael Health System	Texarkana	163	460
Odessa Regional Hospital	Odessa	163	296
Mission Regional Medical Center	Mission	164	356
Saint Joseph Medical Center	Houston	164	577
Huguley Memorial Medical Center	Burleson	165	350
San Jacinto Methodist Hospital	Baytown	165	415
The Womans Hospital of Texas	Houston	165	437
Christus Saint John Hospital	Nassau Bay	166	372
Texas Health Harris Methodist	Bedford	168	398
Seton Medical Center Austin	Austin	170	330
Methodist Willowbrook Hospital	Houston	171	396
Baptist Beaumont Hospital	Beaumont	172	426
University General Hospital	Houston	173	1037
Christus Hospital	Beaumont	174	382
Medical Center Hospital	Odessa	174	943
Seton Medical Center Hays	Kyle	175	373
Methodist Stone Oak Hospital	San Antonio	176	446
Seton Northwest Hospital	Austin	176	362
South Texas Health System	Edinburg	176	403
Univ of Texas Med Branch Galveston	Galveston	176	337
Valley Regional Medical Center	Brownsville	176	461
Baptist Saint Anthony's Hospital	Amarillo	177	441
Saint Luke's Sugar Land Hospital	Sugar Land	177	386
West Houston Medical Center	Houston	177	475
Memorial Medical Center of East Texas	Lufkin	178	362
Doctors Hospital at Renaissance	Edinburg	179	583
Hendrick Medical Center	Abilene	179	398
Fort Duncan Medical Center	Eagle Pass	180	379
University Medical Center	Lubbock	180	380
Knapp Medical Center	Weslaco	181	348
Texas Health Arlington Memorial Hospital	Arlington	181	415
Angleton - Danbury Medical Center	Angleton	182	358
Metroplex Hospital	Killeen	182	346
Northwest Texas Hospital	Amarillo	182	400
Christus Spohn Hospital Kleberg	Kingsville	185	471
Christus Spohn Hospital Corpus Christi	Corpus Christi	186	379
Memorial Hermann Katy Hospital	Katy	188	342
VHS Harlingen Hospital Company	Harlingen	189	342
Brazosport Regional Health System	Lake Jackson	190	361
Christus Spohn Hospital Alice	Alice	192	391
Saint Luke's the Woodlands Hospital	The Woodlands	192	385
The Medical Center of Southeast Texas	Port Arthur	193	713
Methodist West Houston Hospital	Houston	195	381
Texas Health Presbyterian Hospital Dallas	Dallas	200	394
Methodist Sugar Land Hospital	Sugar Land	202	353
Baylor All Saints Medical Center at FW	Fort Worth	203	401
Baylor Medical Center at Irving	Irving	203	377
Memorial Hermann Hospital System	Houston	204	1486
Mem Hermann Mem City Med Ctr	Houston	205	360
Laredo Medical Center	Laredo	207	355
Methodist Dallas Medical Center	Dallas	212	360
Providence Health Center	Waco	212	362
University Medical Center at Brackenridge	Austin	214	327
Kingwood Medical Center	Kingwood	215	414
Memorial Hermann Northeast	Humble	217	368
UT Southwestern University Hospital	Dallas	219	444
Doctors Hospital Tidwell	Houston	228	338
Methodist Charlton Medical Center	Dallas	228	364
Baylor University Medical Center	Dallas	239	363
Memorial Hermann Texas Medical Center	Houston	243	351
JPS Health Network	Fort Worth	245	731
Starr County Memorial Hospital	Rio Grande City	280	393
University Medical Center of El Paso	El Paso	336	397
Parkland Health & Hospital System	Dallas	356	355
University Health System	San Antonio	383	177
Harris Health System	Houston	441	716

Time in ER Before Being Evaluated (minutes)

Hospital Name	City	Min.	Cases
Bayside Community Hospital	Anahuac	0	296
Care Regional Medical Center	Aransas Pass	0	628
Pine Creek Medical Center	Dallas	0	82
Doctors Hospital of Laredo	Laredo	4	397
Northwest Hills Surgical Hospital	Austin	5	56
Mem Hermann Surgical Hosp Kingwood	Kingwood	6	237
Stephens Memorial Hospital	Breckenridge	6	3042
Sugar Land Surgical Hospital	Sugar Land	6	278
The Hospital at Westlake Medical Center	Austin	7	407
Baylor Ortho & Spine Hosp-Arlington	Arlington	8	271
Hill Regional Hospital	Hillsboro	9	419
Lakeway Regional Medical Center[3]	Lakeway	9	270
The Womans Hospital of Texas	Houston	9	456
Basin Healthcare Center	Odessa	10	403
Baylor Surgical Hospital at Fort Worth	Fort Worth	10	264
First Surgical Hospital	Bellaire	10	307
Medical Center of Lewisville	Lewisville	10	457
Methodist Ambulatory Surgery Hospital NW	San Antonio	10	264
North Central Surgical Center	Dallas	10	300
Baylor Medical Center at Uptown	Dallas	11	293
Good Shephard Medical Center - Linden	Linden	11	424
Laredo Medical Center	Laredo	11	396
Methodist Mckinney Hospital	Mc Kinney	11	169
Scott & White Hospital - Llano	Llano	11	342
Seton Medical Center Williamson	Round Rock	11	404
TX Hlth Presbyterian Hosp-Flower Mound	Flower Mound	11	502
Big Bend Regional Medical Center	Alpine	12	463
Brownwood Regional Medical Center	Brownwood	12	424
Central Texas Medical Center	San Marcos	12	383
El Paso Specialty Hospital	El Paso	12	330
Heart Hospital Baylor Plano	Plano	12	324
Jackson Healthcare Center[3]	Edna	12	73
Rio Grande Regional Hospital	Mcallen	12	531
TX Hlth Harris Meth Hosp-Southlake	Southlake	12	275
Abilene Regional Medical Center	Abilene	13	404
Baylor Medical Center at Frisco[3]	Frisco	13	468
Baylor Medical Center at Trophy Club	Trophy Club	13	267
Las Colinas Medical Center	Irving	13	449
Medical Center of Mckinney	Mckinney	13	460
Methodist Hospital	San Antonio	13	523
Methodist Stone Oak Hospital	San Antonio	13	487
Nix Health Care System[3]	San Antonio	13	511
North Hills Hospital	N Richland Hls	13	501
Centennial Medical Center	Frisco	14	501
East Texas Medical Center Quitman	Quitman	14	376
Knox County Hospital	Knox City	14	258
Methodist Richardson Medical Center	Richardson	14	409
Plaza Medical Center of Fort Worth	Fort Worth	14	474
Saint Joseph Regional Health Center	Bryan	14	406
Baylor Surgical Hospital at Las Colinas	Irving	15	292
Bayshore Medical Center	Pasadena	15	495
Christus Saint Catherine Hospital	Katy	15	399
Detar Hospital Navarro	Victoria	15	430
Doctors Diagnostic Hospital	Cleveland	15	321
Eastland Memorial Hospital	Eastland	15	344
Glen Rose Medical Center	Glen Rose	15	462
Lamb Healthcare Center	Littlefield	15	230
Longview Regional Medical Center	Longview	15	407
Medical Center of Arlington	Arlington	15	520
Nocona General Hospital	Nocona	15	277
North Cypress Medical Center	Cypress	15	430
Oakbend Medical Center	Richmond	15	336
The Physicians Centre	Bryan	15	482
South Texas Spine & Surgical Hospital	San Antonio	15	179
Tops Surgical Specialty Hospital	Houston	15	294
Baylor Medical Center at Irving	Irving	16	327
Bellville General Hospital	Bellville	16	384
Clear Lake Regional Medical Center	Webster	16	545
Cogdell Memorial Hospital	Snyder	16	400
College Station Medical Center	College Station	16	423
The Corpus Christi Medical Center	Corpus Christi	16	545
East Texas Medical Center Trinity	Trinity	16	352
Faith Community Hospital	Jacksboro	16	416
Lubbock Heart Hospital	Lubbock	16	283
Mitchell County Hospital District	Colorado City	16	413
Moore County Hospital District	Dumas	16	341
Palo Pinto General Hospital	Mineral Wells	16	344
San Angelo Community Medical Center	San Angelo	16	413
East Texas Medical Center Mount Vernon	Mount Vernon	17	322
Hansford County Hospital[3]	Spearman	17	149
Seton Southwest Hospital	Austin	17	342
Texas Health Presbyterian Hospital Allen	Allen	17	441
Cedar Park Regional Medical Center	Cedar Park	18	418
Cuero Community Hospital	Cuero	18	476
Dallas Regional Medical Center	Mesquite	18	1548
East Texas Medical Center - Fairfield	Fairfield	18	496
East Texas Medical Center Crockett	Crockett	18	407
Houston Physicians' Hospital	Webster	18	231
Medical Center of Plano	Plano	18	489
Palestine Regional Medical Center	Palestine	18	491
Parkview Regional Hospital	Mexia	18	408
Peterson Regional Medical Center	Kerrville	18	527
Rollins Brook Community Hospital	Lampasas	18	299
Anson General Hospital	Anson	19	312
Denton Regional Medical Center	Denton	19	479
East Texas Medical Center - Gilmer	Gilmer	19	667
Medical City Dallas Hospital	Dallas	19	520
Memorial Hospital	Gonzales	19	428
Scott & White Hospital - Round Rock	Round Rock	19	440
Seton Medical Center Hays	Kyle	19	388
USMD Hospital at Fort Worth	Fort Worth	19	256
VHS Brownsville Hospital Company	Brownsville	19	590
Wise Regional Health System	Decatur	19	597
Bowie Memorial Hospital	Bowie	20	452
Christus Jasper Memorial Hospital	Jasper	20	421
El Campo Memorial Hospital	El Campo	20	357
Harlingen Medical Center	Harlingen	20	392
Heart Hospital Baylor Denton	Denton	20	125
Hill Country Memorial Hospital	Fredericksburg	20	529
Houston Orthopedic & Spine Hospital	Bellaire	20	424
Methodist Hospital For Surgery	Addison	20	287
Rolling Plains Memorial Hospital	Sweetwater	20	375
Round Rock Medical Center	Round Rock	20	510
Saint David's South Austin Medical Center	Austin	20	549
South Texas Surgical Hospital	Corpus Christi	20	438
Stamford Memorial Hospital	Stamford	20	257
TX Health Ctr for Diag & Surgery	Plano	20	108
Texas Health Harris Methodist Fort Worth	Fort Worth	20	443
TX Hlth Harris Meth Hosp-Alliance[3]	Fort Worth	20	339
Conroe Regional Medical Center	Conroe	21	523
Good Shepherd Medical Center Marshall	Marshall	21	405
North Texas Medical Center	Gainesville	21	364
Seton Smithville Regional Hospital	Smithville	21	385
Texas Health Harris Methodist	Bedford	21	442
Val Verde Regional Medical Center	Del Rio	21	1492
Dimmit Regional Hospital	Carrizo Springs	22	404
Etmc Clarksville	Clarksville	22	485
Foundation Surgical Hospital of El Paso	El Paso	22	569
Lake Pointe Medical Center	Rowlett	22	460
Saint David's Medical Center	Austin	22	527
Baylor Reg Med Ctr at Grapevine	Grapevine	23	376
Cypress Fairbanks Medical Center	Houston	23	37
East Texas Medical Center Athens	Athens	23	418
Ennis Regional Medical Center	Ennis	23	427
Etmc Henderson	Henderson	23	390
Fort Duncan Medical Center	Eagle Pass	23	423
Navarro Regional Hospital	Corsicana	23	417
TX Hlth Harris Meth Hosp-Cleburne	Cleburne	23	445
TX Hlth Harris Meth Hosp-Stephenville	Stephenville	23	442
Christus Saint John Hospital	Nassau Bay	24	404
Citizens Medical Center	Victoria	24	370

NOTE: Hospital profiles are in alphabetical order by state, then city, then hospital within the city; Rankings exclude hospitals with less than 25 cases except for patient surveys which excludes hospitals with less than 100 cases; (a) 100-299 cases; (1) The number of cases/patients is too few to report; (2) Data submitted were based on a sample of cases/patients; (3) Results are based on a shorter time period than required; (4) Data suppressed by CMS for one or more quarters; (5) Results are not available for this reporting period; (6) Fewer than 100 patients completed the HCAHPS survey; (7) No cases met the criteria for this measure; (8) The lower limit of the confidence interval cannot be calculated if the number of observed infections equals zero; (9) No data are available from the state/territory for this reporting period; (10) The scores shown reflect fewer than 50 completed surveys; (11) There were discrepancies in the data collection process; (12) This measure does not apply to this hospital for this reporting period; (13) Results cannot be calculated for this reporting period; (14) The results for this state are combined with nearby states to protect confidentiality; Please refer to the User's Guide for a full explanation of data.

Falls Community Hospital & Clinic	Marlin	24	353
Gulf Coast Medical Center	Wharton	24	485
Hamilton General Hospital	Hamilton	24	484
Heritage Park Surgical Hospital	Sherman	24	255
Lake Granbury Medical Center	Granbury	24	415
Las Palmas Medical Center	El Paso	24	548
Pampa Regional Medical Center	Pampa	24	814
Park Plaza Hospital	Houston	24	486
Shannon Medical Center	San Angelo	24	432
Texas Health Presbyterian Hospital Plano	Plano	24	440
Valley Regional Medical Center	Brownsville	24	513
Cook Childrens Northeast Hospital	Hurst	25	247
Etmc Carthage	Carthage	25	299
Hopkins County Memorial Hospital	Sulphur Springs	25	514
Paris Regional Medical Center	Paris	25	465
Providence Memorial Hospital	El Paso	25	410
South Texas Regional Medical Center	Jourdanton	25	408
Texas General Hospital[3]	Grand Prairie	25	274
Univ of TX Health Science Ctr-Tyler	Tyler	25	401
Woodland Heights Medical Center	Lufkin	25	403
Christus Santa Rosa Hospital	San Antonio	26	1385
Seton Medical Center Austin	Austin	26	357
Starr County Memorial Hospital	Rio Grande City	26	602
Surgery Specialty Hosps of America[3]	Pasadena	26	227
Texas Health Presbyterian Hospital Denton	Denton	26	440
Titus Regional Medical Center	Mount Pleasant	26	352
Tyler County Hospital	Woodville	26	380
Weatherford Regional Medical Center	Weatherford	26	422
Wilbarger General Hospital	Vernon	26	504
Baylor Medical Center at Waxahachie	Waxahachie	27	103
Columbus Community Hospital	Columbus	27	422
Covenant Medical Center	Lubbock	27	568
East Texas Medical Center Jacksonville	Jacksonville	27	325
Goodall Witcher Hospital	Clifton	27	187
Memorial Hermann Sugar Land Hospital	Sugar Land	27	419
North Austin Medical Center	Austin	27	538
Scenic Mountain Medical Center	Big Spring	27	413
Seton Medical Center Harker Heights	Harker Heights	27	821
Childress Regional Medical Center	Childress	28	316
Midland Memorial Hospital	Midland	28	436
Providence Health Center	Waco	28	353
Saint Luke's Lakeside Hospital	The Woodlands	28	270
Saint Marks Medical Center	La Grange	28	514
Scott & White Hospital Brenham	Brenham	28	366
Univ of Texas Med Branch Galveston	Galveston	28	385
Baylor Medical Center at Carrollton	Carrollton	29	135
Doctors Hospital	Dallas	29	491
Nacogdoches Medical Center	Nacogdoches	29	381
Pecos County Memorial Hospital	Fort Stockton	29	396
Seton Northwest Hospital	Austin	29	381
Texoma Medical Center	Denison	29	418
University Medical Center at Brackenridge	Austin	29	391
Uvalde Memorial Hospital	Uvalde	29	824
Arise Austin Medical Center	Austin	30	238
Doctors Hospital at Renaissance	Edinburg	30	706
Fdn Surgical Hosp of San Antonio	San Antonio	30	200
Frio Regional Hospital	Pearsall	30	294
Graham Regional Medical Center	Graham	30	369
Hamlin Memorial Hospital	Hamlin	30	269
Hereford Regional Medical Center	Hereford	30	367
Houston Northwest Medical Center	Houston	30	552
Lake Whitney Medical Center	Whitney	30	191
Memorial Hermann Katy Hospital	Katy	30	408
The Methodist Hospital	Houston	30	448
Seymour Hospital	Seymour	30	311
South Texas Health System	Edinburg	30	426
West Houston Medical Center	Houston	30	531
Connally Memorial Medical Center	Floresville	31	416
Covenant Hospital Levelland	Levelland	31	391
Huntsville Memorial Hospital	Huntsville	31	397
Methodist Mansfield Medical Center	Mansfield	31	405
Mission Regional Medical Center	Mission	31	265
Saint Luke's Episcopal Hospital	Houston	31	374
TX Hlth Harris Meth Hosp SW Ft Worth	Fort Worth	31	444
Texas Health Presbyterian Hospital - WNJ	Sherman	31	443
Matagorda Regional Medical Center	Bay City	32	451
Methodist West Houston Hospital	Houston	32	421
TX Health Presbyterian Hosp Rockwall	Rockwall	32	455
Good Shepherd Medical Center	Longview	33	410
Hunt Regional Medical Center	Greenville	33	407
Saint Joseph Medical Center	Houston	33	665
Baylor Medical Center at Mckinney	Mc Kinney	34	443
Sierra Medical Center	El Paso	34	411
TX Hlth Presbyterian Hosp-Kaufman	Kaufman	34	442
Sierra Providence East Medical Center	El Paso	35	479
East Texas Medical Center	Tyler	36	368
Guadalupe Regional Medical Center	Seguin	36	382
Covenant Hospital Plainview	Plainview	37	387
Memorial Medical Center Livingston	Livingston	37	343
Texas Orthopedic Hospital	Houston	37	270
Christus Hospital	Beaumont	38	418
Memorial Hermann Hospital System	Houston	38	1664
Scott & White Memorial Hospital	Temple	38	429
United Regional Health Care System	Wichita Falls	38	491
University General Hospital Dallas[3]	Dallas	38	248
Christus Spohn Hospital Beeville	Beeville	39	404
Medical Arts Hospital	Lamesa	39	384
Permian Regional Medical Center	Andrews	39	361
Grace Medical Center	Lubbock	40	10588
Hemphill County Hospital	Canadian	40	356
Kingwood Medical Center	Kingwood	40	515
Saint Anthony's Hospital	Houston	40	357
TX Hlth Harris Methodist Hosp-Azle	Azle	40	501
Kell West Regional Hospital	Wichita Falls	41	959
Memorial Hermann Northeast	Humble	41	411
University Medical Center	Lubbock	41	405
Dallas Medical Center	Dallas	42	490
Hillcrest Baptist Medical Center	Waco	42	355
Mem Hermann Mem City Med Ctr	Houston	42	410
Texas Spine & Joint Hospital	Tyler	42	249
Wadley Regional Medical Center	Texarkana	42	474
Baptist Beaumont Hospital	Beaumont	43	438
Christus Saint Michael Health System	Texarkana	43	474
Methodist Dallas Medical Center	Dallas	43	403
UT Southwestern University Hospital	Dallas	43	477
Baptist Saint Anthony's Hospital	Amarillo	44	456
Coryell Memorial Healthcare System	Gatesville	44	897
Memorial Hermann Texas Medical Center	Houston	44	403
Baptist Medical Center	San Antonio	45	408
Cleveland Regional Medical Center	Cleveland	45	923
Knapp Medical Center	Weslaco	45	364
Medical Center Hospital	Odessa	45	991
Saint Luke's Patients Medical Center	Pasadena	45	419
Huguley Memorial Medical Center	Burleson	46	379
University General Hospital	Houston	46	991
USMD Hospital at Arlington	Arlington	49	364
Baylor Medical Center at Garland	Garland	50	57
Baylor University Medical Center	Dallas	50	418
Hendrick Medical Center	Abilene	51	422
Memorial Hermann Baptist Orange Hospital	Orange	52	359
Mother Frances Hospital	Tyler	52	424
Texas Health Arlington Memorial Hospital	Arlington	52	444
Texas Health Presbyterian Hospital Dallas	Dallas	52	362
Christus Spohn Hospital Kleberg	Kingsville	53	503
Methodist Willowbrook Hospital	Houston	53	417
Saint Luke's Hospital at the Vintage	Houston	54	274
Memorial Medical Center of East Texas	Lufkin	55	343
Angleton - Danbury Medical Center	Angleton	56	404
Baylor All Saints Medical Center at FW	Fort Worth	56	399
JPS Health Network	Fort Worth	56	868
Christus Spohn Hospital Alice	Alice	57	427
Christus Spohn Hospital Corpus Christi	Corpus Christi	58	405
Metroplex Hospital	Killeen	60	383
Odessa Regional Hospital	Odessa	60	311
Texas Reg Med Ctr at Sunnyvale	Sunnyvale	60	381
Southwest General Hospital	San Antonio	62	754
San Jacinto Methodist Hospital	Baytown	63	454
Brownfield Regional Medical Center	Brownfield	64	418
The Medical Center of Southeast Texas	Port Arthur	64	743
Brazosport Regional Health System	Lake Jackson	65	387
VHS Harlingen Hospital Company	Harlingen	67	369
Methodist Sugar Land Hospital	Sugar Land	70	424
Tomball Regional Medical Center	Tomball	71	441
Memorial Hospital	Nacogdoches	73	352
Northwest Texas Hospital	Amarillo	73	382
Saint Luke's Sugar Land Hospital	Sugar Land	73	364
Methodist Charlton Medical Center	Dallas	74	401
University Health System	San Antonio	80	176
Saint Luke's the Woodlands Hospital	The Woodlands	84	366
Doctors Hospital Tidwell	Houston	95	363
Parkland Health & Hospital System	Dallas	106	228
University Medical Center of El Paso	El Paso	115	415
Harris Health System	Houston	130	800

Time to Pain Meds for Bone Fractures (minutes)

Hospital Name	City	Min.	Cases
Doctors Hospital of Laredo	Laredo	20	158
Seton Medical Center Williamson	Round Rock	22	36
Baptist Saint Anthony's Hospital	Amarillo	23	180
The Hospital at Westlake Medical Center	Austin	25	56
El Paso Specialty Hospital	El Paso	28	84
Medical Center of Lewisville	Lewisville	28	269
Seton Smithville Regional Hospital	Smithville	29	41
Bellville General Hospital	Bellville	30	31
Centennial Medical Center	Frisco	30	98
Good Shephard Medical Center - Linden	Linden	31	35
Christus Saint Catherine Hospital	Katy	32	121
Las Colinas Medical Center	Irving	32	86
TX Hlth Presbyterian Hosp-Flower Mound	Flower Mound	32	104
Cypress Fairbanks Medical Center	Houston	33	175
Memorial Medical Center[3]	Port Lavaca	33	25
Moore County Hospital District	Dumas	34	36
Hill Regional Hospital	Hillsboro	35	50
Medical Center of Arlington	Arlington	35	237
Medical Center of Mckinney	Mckinney	35	102
Eastland Memorial Hospital	Eastland	36	36
Hamilton General Hospital	Hamilton	36	36
Seton Southwest Hospital	Austin	36	43
Lake Pointe Medical Center	Rowlett	37	156
North Texas Medical Center	Gainesville	37	74
Saint Luke's Episcopal Hospital	Houston	37	189
Baylor Medical Center at Irving	Irving	38	197
Methodist Richardson Medical Center	Richardson	38	123
Medical Center Hospital	Odessa	39	141
VHS Brownsville Hospital Company	Brownsville	39	155
Bowie Memorial Hospital	Bowie	40	43
North Central Surgical Center	Dallas	40	31
Pecos County Memorial Hospital	Fort Stockton	40	45
Scott & White Hospital Brenham	Brenham	40	88
Baylor Medical Center at Waxahachie	Waxahachie	41	169
Baylor Reg Med Ctr at Grapevine	Grapevine	41	151
Providence Memorial Hospital	El Paso	41	277
Rolling Plains Memorial Hospital	Sweetwater	41	43
Oakbend Medical Center	Richmond	42	102
Good Shepherd Medical Center	Longview	43	279
Harlingen Medical Center	Harlingen	43	155
The Methodist Hospital	Houston	43	99
Baylor Regional Medical Center at Plano	Plano	44	90
College Station Medical Center	College Station	44	159
Medical City Dallas Hospital	Dallas	44	292
Parkview Regional Hospital	Mexia	44	44
Round Rock Medical Center	Round Rock	44	152
Saint David's South Austin Medical Center	Austin	44	194
Baylor Medical Center at Mckinney	Mc Kinney	45	121
Cogdell Memorial Hospital	Snyder	45	35
Columbus Community Hospital	Columbus	45	44
Rio Grande Regional Hospital	Mcallen	45	197
Saint David's Medical Center	Austin	45	129
Conroe Regional Medical Center	Conroe	46	206
Graham Regional Medical Center	Graham	46	56
North Cypress Medical Center	Cypress	46	250
Seton Medical Center Austin	Austin	46	27
TX Hlth Harris Meth Hosp-Stephenville	Stephenville	46	52
Univ of TX Health Science Ctr-Tyler	Tyler	46	32
Clear Lake Regional Medical Center	Webster	47	459
Detar Hospital Navarro	Victoria	47	108
North Hills Hospital	N Richland Hls	47	166
San Angelo Community Medical Center	San Angelo	47	81
Cedar Park Regional Medical Center	Cedar Park	48	239
Childress Regional Medical Center	Childress	48	33
The Corpus Christi Medical Center	Corpus Christi	48	198
Dallas Regional Medical Center	Mesquite	48	162
East Texas Medical Center - Fairfield	Fairfield	48	52
Glen Rose Medical Center	Glen Rose	48	47
Good Shepherd Medical Center Marshall	Marshall	48	131
Memorial Hospital	Gonzales	48	46
North Austin Medical Center	Austin	48	174
TX Hlth Harris Meth Hosp-Alliance[3]	Fort Worth	48	108
Tomball Regional Medical Center	Tomball	48	122
El Campo Memorial Hospital	El Campo	49	27
Ennis Regional Medical Center	Ennis	49	90
Frio Regional Hospital	Pearsall	49	59
Sierra Medical Center	El Paso	49	84
TX Health Presbyterian Hosp Rockwall	Rockwall	49	164
Baptist Medical Center	San Antonio	50	466
Baylor Medical Center at Carrollton	Carrollton	50	136
Brownwood Regional Medical Center	Brownwood	50	160
Connally Memorial Medical Center	Floresville	50	80
Guadalupe Regional Medical Center	Seguin	50	86
Medical Center of Plano	Plano	50	124
Memorial Hermann Sugar Land Hospital	Sugar Land	50	141
Methodist Hospital	San Antonio	50	502
Rollins Brook Community Hospital	Lampasas	50	63
Shannon Medical Center	San Angelo	50	150
University Medical Center at Brackenridge	Austin	50	56
Etmc Henderson	Henderson	51	77
Las Palmas Medical Center	El Paso	51	381
Mission Regional Medical Center	Mission	51	100
Scott & White Hospital - Llano	Llano	51	55
Central Texas Medical Center	San Marcos	52	206
Falls Community Hospital & Clinic	Marlin	52	35
Palestine Regional Medical Center	Palestine	52	108
Texas Health Presbyterian Hospital Allen	Allen	52	122
TX Hlth Presbyterian Hosp-Kaufman	Kaufman	52	105
Christus Jasper Memorial Hospital	Jasper	53	130
Christus Santa Rosa Hospital	San Antonio	53	533
Cleveland Regional Medical Center	Cleveland	53	76
Scenic Mountain Medical Center	Big Spring	53	89
Foundation Surgical Hospital of El Paso	El Paso	54	41
Matagorda Regional Medical Center	Bay City	54	75
Texas Health Presbyterian Hospital Denton	Denton	54	173
Bayshore Medical Center	Pasadena	55	284
Gulf Coast Medical Center	Wharton	55	58

NOTE: Hospital profiles are in alphabetical order by state, then city, then hospital within the city; Rankings exclude hospitals with less than 25 cases except for patient surveys which excludes hospitals with less than 100 cases; (a) 100-299 cases; (1) The number of cases/patients is too few to report; (2) Data submitted were based on a sample of cases/patients; (3) Results are based on a shorter time period than required; (4) Data suppressed by CMS for one or more quarters; (5) Results are not available for this reporting period; (6) Fewer than 100 patients completed the HCAHPS survey; (7) No cases met the criteria for this measure; (8) The lower limit of the confidence interval cannot be calculated if the number of observed infections equals zero; (9) No data are available from the state/territory for this reporting period; (10) The scores shown reflect fewer than 50 completed surveys; (11) There were discrepancies in the data collection process; (12) This measure does not apply to this hospital for this reporting period; (13) Results cannot be calculated for this reporting period; (14) The results for this state are combined with nearby states to protect confidentiality; Please refer to the User's Guide for a full explanation of data.

Knapp Medical Center	Weslaco	55	149
Lake Granbury Medical Center	Granbury	55	87
Navarro Regional Hospital	Corsicana	55	130
Scott & White Memorial Hospital	Temple	55	142
Texoma Medical Center	Denison	55	191
Baylor Medical Center at Garland	Garland	56	233
Big Bend Regional Medical Center	Alpine	56	47
Christus Spohn Hospital Kleberg	Kingsville	56	88
Hopkins County Memorial Hospital	Sulphur Springs	56	73
Longview Regional Medical Center	Longview	56	96
Methodist Stone Oak Hospital	San Antonio	56	110
TX Hlth Harris Meth Hosp-Cleburne	Cleburne	56	128
West Houston Medical Center	Houston	56	165
Midland Memorial Hospital	Midland	57	262
Permian Regional Medical Center	Andrews	57	29
Saint Joseph Regional Health Center	Bryan	57	144
Saint Marks Medical Center	La Grange	57	50
Titus Regional Medical Center	Mount Pleasant	57	137
Denton Regional Medical Center	Denton	58	210
Doctors Hospital	Dallas	58	106
Methodist Mansfield Medical Center	Mansfield	58	251
Saint Luke's Hospital at the Vintage	Houston	58	73
South Texas Regional Medical Center	Jourdanton	58	119
VHS Harlingen Hospital Company	Harlingen	58	225
Baylor University Medical Center	Dallas	59	187
Pampa Regional Medical Center	Pampa	59	46
Plaza Medical Center of Fort Worth	Fort Worth	59	25
Stephens Memorial Hospital	Breckenridge	59	27
Val Verde Regional Medical Center	Del Rio	59	144
East Texas Medical Center Athens	Athens	60	156
Fort Duncan Medical Center	Eagle Pass	60	104
Huguley Memorial Medical Center	Burleson	60	169
Huntsville Memorial Hospital	Huntsville	60	133
Kell West Regional Hospital	Wichita Falls	60	88
Saint Luke's the Woodlands Hospital	The Woodlands	60	225
South Texas Health System	Edinburg	60	368
Texas Health Harris Methodist Fort Worth	Fort Worth	60	342
Tyler County Hospital	Woodville	60	49
Valley Regional Medical Center	Brownsville	60	212
Wise Regional Health System	Decatur	60	123
Baptist Beaumont Hospital	Beaumont	61	174
East Texas Medical Center - Gilmer	Gilmer	61	37
Peterson Regional Medical Center	Kerrville	61	142
TX Hlth Harris Meth Hosp SW Ft Worth	Fort Worth	61	244
Covenant Hospital Levelland	Levelland	62	34
Saint Luke's Sugar Land Hospital	Sugar Land	62	84
Scott & White Hospital - Round Rock	Round Rock	62	69
TX Hlth Harris Methodist Hosp-Azle	Azle	62	100
Texas Health Presbyterian Hospital Plano	Plano	62	165
East Texas Medical Center Quitman	Quitman	63	65
Memorial Medical Center Livingston	Livingston	63	112
Univ of Texas Med Branch Galveston	Galveston	63	124
Christus Saint John Hospital	Nassau Bay	64	115
Covenant Hospital Plainview	Plainview	64	81
Palo Pinto General Hospital	Mineral Wells	64	43
Seton Northwest Hospital	Austin	64	26
Texas Reg Med Ctr at Sunnyvale	Sunnyvale	64	182
Wadley Regional Medical Center	Texarkana	64	115
Christus Spohn Hospital Beeville	Beeville	65	72
Coryell Memorial Healthcare System	Gatesville	65	53
Methodist West Houston Hospital	Houston	65	99
Citizens Medical Center	Victoria	66	103
Hill Country Memorial Hospital	Fredericksburg	66	72
Hillcrest Baptist Medical Center	Waco	66	317
Hunt Regional Medical Center	Greenville	66	192
Memorial Hermann Hospital System	Houston	66	944
Seton Medical Center Harker Heights	Harker Heights	66	139
Doctors Hospital at Renaissance	Edinburg	67	126
East Texas Medical Center Jacksonville	Jacksonville	67	45
Seton Medical Center Hays	Kyle	67	46
United Regional Health Care System	Wichita Falls	67	292
Mem Hermann Mem City Med Ctr	Houston	68	206
University Medical Center	Lubbock	68	274
Wilbarger General Hospital	Vernon	68	26
Abilene Regional Medical Center	Abilene	69	95
Texas Health Presbyterian Hospital Dallas	Dallas	69	103
Brazosport Regional Health System	Lake Jackson	71	184
Sierra Providence East Medical Center	El Paso	71	248
Angleton - Danbury Medical Center	Angleton	72	80
Baylor All Saints Medical Center at FW	Fort Worth	72	70
Houston Northwest Medical Center	Houston	72	203
Methodist Sugar Land Hospital	Sugar Land	72	144
Mother Frances Hospital	Tyler	72	231
Southwest General Hospital	San Antonio	72	153
Christus Saint Michael Health System	Texarkana	73	262
Memorial Hermann Katy Hospital	Katy	73	175
Dallas Medical Center	Dallas	74	37
Memorial Hermann Northeast	Humble	74	224
Methodist Willowbrook Hospital	Houston	74	193
Providence Health Center	Waco	74	31
Care Regional Medical Center	Aransas Pass	75	58
Memorial Hermann Baptist Orange Hospital	Orange	75	70
Starr County Memorial Hospital	Rio Grande City	75	60
Etmc Carthage	Carthage	76	37
Nacogdoches Medical Center	Nacogdoches	76	74
Christus Hospital	Beaumont	77	285
JPS Health Network	Fort Worth	77	245
Texas Health Arlington Memorial Hospital	Arlington	77	194
Texas Health Harris Methodist	Bedford	79	172
Texas Health Presbyterian Hospital - WNJ	Sherman	79	117
Saint Joseph Medical Center	Houston	80	96
Uvalde Memorial Hospital	Uvalde	81	129
Metroplex Hospital	Killeen	82	191
Saint Luke's Patients Medical Center	Pasadena	82	54
USMD Hospital at Arlington	Arlington	82	75
Methodist Dallas Medical Center	Dallas	83	197
Christus Spohn Hospital Alice	Alice	84	172
Weatherford Regional Medical Center	Weatherford	84	106
Christus Spohn Hospital Corpus Christi	Corpus Christi	86	154
San Jacinto Methodist Hospital	Baytown	86	171
Woodland Heights Medical Center	Lufkin	86	80
Paris Regional Medical Center	Paris	87	94
UT Southwestern University Hospital	Dallas	87	61
East Texas Medical Center	Tyler	88	218
The Medical Center of Southeast Texas	Port Arthur	88	90
Memorial Medical Center of East Texas	Lufkin	88	110
Odessa Regional Hospital	Odessa	89	57
Parkland Health & Hospital System	Dallas	90	51
Covenant Medical Center	Lubbock	91	111
Hendrick Medical Center	Abilene	91	181
Memorial Hermann Texas Medical Center	Houston	92	256
Kingwood Medical Center	Kingwood	96	150
Laredo Medical Center	Laredo	97	327
Methodist Charlton Medical Center	Dallas	97	181
University Medical Center of El Paso	El Paso	99	257
Northwest Texas Hospital	Amarillo	102	155
Memorial Hospital	Nacogdoches	125	62
Doctors Hospital Tidwell	Houston	126	58
University Health System	San Antonio	130	144
Harris Health System	Houston	202	386

Heart Attack Care

Aspirin Given at Discharge

Hospital Name	City	Rate	Cases
Abilene Regional Medical Center	Abilene	100%	142
Baptist Medical Center	San Antonio	100%	1141
Baylor Heart & Vascular Hospital	Dallas	100%	457
Baylor Medical Center at Carrollton	Carrollton	100%	80
Baylor Medical Center at Mckinney	Mc Kinney	100%	83
Bayshore Medical Center	Pasadena	100%	324
Brazosport Regional Health System	Lake Jackson	100%	46
Cedar Park Regional Medical Center	Cedar Park	100%	41
Citizens Medical Center	Victoria	100%	205
Clear Lake Regional Medical Center[2]	Webster	100%	431
College Station Medical Center	College Station	100%	88
Conroe Regional Medical Center	Conroe	100%	332
The Corpus Christi Medical Center	Corpus Christi	100%	257
Dallas Regional Medical Center	Mesquite	100%	110
Denton Regional Medical Center	Denton	100%	251
Detar Hospital Navarro	Victoria	100%	144
Doctors Hospital	Dallas	100%	119
Doctors Hospital at Renaissance[2]	Edinburg	100%	234
East Texas Medical Center[2]	Tyler	100%	271
Hendrick Medical Center	Abilene	100%	375
Hopkins County Memorial Hospital	Sulphur Springs	100%	50
Houston Northwest Medical Center	Houston	100%	274
Huguley Memorial Medical Center	Burleson	100%	265
JPS Health Network	Fort Worth	100%	295
Kingwood Medical Center[2]	Kingwood	100%	271
Knapp Medical Center	Weslaco	100%	29
Lake Granbury Medical Center	Granbury	100%	35
Lake Pointe Medical Center	Rowlett	100%	83
Lakeway Regional Medical Center[3]	Lakeway	100%	34
Laredo Medical Center	Laredo	100%	149
Las Colinas Medical Center	Irving	100%	87
Las Palmas Medical Center	El Paso	100%	308
Longview Regional Medical Center	Longview	100%	130
Lubbock Heart Hospital[2]	Lubbock	100%	176
Medical Center of Arlington	Arlington	100%	210
Medical Center of Lewisville	Lewisville	100%	143
Medical Center of Mckinney	Mckinney	100%	144
Medical Center of Plano[2]	Plano	100%	203
Medical City Dallas Hospital	Dallas	100%	161
Memorial Hermann Hospital System[2]	Houston	100%	945
Memorial Hermann Katy Hospital	Katy	100%	28
Memorial Hermann Texas Medical Center[2]	Houston	100%	282
Methodist Charlton Medical Center	Dallas	100%	300
Methodist Dallas Medical Center	Dallas	100%	264
Methodist Hospital	San Antonio	100%	1317
Methodist Mansfield Medical Center	Mansfield	100%	214
Methodist Richardson Medical Center	Richardson	100%	117
Methodist Stone Oak Hospital[2]	San Antonio	100%	142
Methodist Sugar Land Hospital[2]	Sugar Land	100%	232
Methodist West Houston Hospital[2]	Houston	100%	230
Methodist Willowbrook Hospital[2]	Houston	100%	271
Midland Memorial Hospital	Midland	100%	223
Nacogdoches Medical Center	Nacogdoches	100%	41
Nix Health Care System	San Antonio	100%	37
North Austin Medical Center	Austin	100%	169
North Cypress Medical Center	Cypress	100%	207
North Hills Hospital	N Richland Hls	100%	201
Northwest Texas Hospital[2]	Amarillo	100%	257
Paris Regional Medical Center	Paris	100%	151
Parkland Health & Hospital System[2]	Dallas	100%	253
Plaza Medical Center of Fort Worth[2]	Fort Worth	100%	265
Providence Memorial Hospital	El Paso	100%	116
Rio Grande Regional Hospital[2]	Mcallen	100%	158
Round Rock Medical Center	Round Rock	100%	171
Saint David's Medical Center	Austin	100%	414
Saint David's South Austin Medical Center[2]	Austin	100%	311
Saint Joseph Regional Health Center	Bryan	100%	245
Saint Luke's the Woodlands Hospital	The Woodlands	100%	153
San Angelo Community Medical Center	San Angelo	100%	90
San Antonio VA Medical Center	San Antonio	100%	71
San Jacinto Methodist Hospital	Baytown	100%	209
Scott & White Memorial Hospital[2]	Temple	100%	301
Seton Medical Center Harker Heights	Harker Heights	100%	46
Seton Medical Center Williamson	Round Rock	100%	148
Shannon Medical Center	San Angelo	100%	234
Sierra Medical Center	El Paso	100%	95
Sierra Providence East Medical Center	El Paso	100%	78
South Texas Health System[2]	Edinburg	100%	281
Temple VA Med Ctr-VA Central Texas	Temple	100%	41
Texas Health Harris Methodist	Bedford	100%	219
TX Hlth Heart & Vasc Hosp-Arlington	Arlington	100%	183
Texas Health Presbyterian Hospital Dallas	Dallas	100%	432
Texoma Medical Center[2]	Denison	100%	271
United Regional Health Care System	Wichita Falls	100%	319
University Medical Center	Lubbock	100%	262
University Medical Center at Brackenridge	Austin	100%	86
University Medical Center of El Paso	El Paso	100%	156
Wadley Regional Medical Center	Texarkana	100%	152
Weatherford Regional Medical Center	Weatherford	100%	27
West Houston Medical Center	Houston	100%	174
Woodland Heights Medical Center	Lufkin	100%	83
Baptist Beaumont Hospital	Beaumont	99%	295
Baylor All Saints Medical Center at FW	Fort Worth	99%	165
Baylor Medical Center at Garland	Garland	99%	216
Baylor Medical Center at Irving	Irving	99%	195
Baylor Reg Med Ctr at Grapevine	Grapevine	99%	196
Baylor University Medical Center	Dallas	99%	139
Centennial Medical Center	Frisco	99%	101
Christus Hospital[2]	Beaumont	99%	320
Covenant Medical Center	Lubbock	99%	654
Cypress Fairbanks Medical Center	Houston	99%	128
Dallas VA Medical Center - VA North Texas	Dallas	99%	102
Good Shepherd Medical Center[2]	Longview	99%	298
Harlingen Medical Center	Harlingen	99%	119
Heart Hospital Baylor Plano	Plano	99%	324
The Medical Center of Southeast Texas	Port Arthur	99%	83
Mem Hermann Mem City Med Ctr[2]	Houston	99%	279
Memorial Hospital	Nacogdoches	99%	78
The Methodist Hospital	Houston	99%	552
Metroplex Hospital[2]	Killeen	99%	91
Mother Frances Hospital	Tyler	99%	691
Providence Health Center	Waco	99%	313
Scott & White Hospital - Round Rock	Round Rock	99%	109
Seton Medical Center Austin	Austin	99%	186
Seton Medical Center Hays	Kyle	99%	146
Texas Health Harris Methodist Fort Worth	Fort Worth	99%	902
Texas Health Presbyterian Hospital Denton	Denton	99%	126
Texas Health Presbyterian Hospital Plano	Plano	99%	179
Texas Reg Med Ctr at Sunnyvale	Sunnyvale	99%	112
Univ of Texas Med Branch Galveston[2]	Galveston	99%	231
Valley Regional Medical Center	Brownsville	99%	236
VHS Brownsville Hospital Company	Brownsville	99%	211
Christus Saint Michael Health System	Texarkana	98%	315
Christus Santa Rosa Hospital	San Antonio	98%	419
Christus Spohn Hospital Corpus Christi	Corpus Christi	98%	529
Harris Health System	Houston	98%	387
Medical Center Hospital	Odessa	98%	313
Memorial Hermann Northeast[2]	Humble	98%	210
Memorial Medical Center of East Texas[2]	Lufkin	98%	243
Odessa Regional Hospital	Odessa	98%	172
Palestine Regional Medical Center	Palestine	98%	52
Saint Luke's Episcopal Hospital[2]	Houston	98%	303
Saint Luke's Hospital at the Vintage	Houston	98%	48
Saint Luke's Sugar Land Hospital	Sugar Land	98%	86
TX Hlth Harris Meth Hosp SW Ft Worth	Fort Worth	98%	44
Texas Health Presbyterian Hospital - WNJ	Sherman	98%	135
University Health System	San Antonio	98%	168

NOTE: Hospital profiles are in alphabetical order by state, then city, then hospital within the city; Rankings exclude hospitals with less than 25 cases except for patient surveys which excludes hospitals with less than 100 cases; (a) 100-299 cases; (1) The number of cases/patients is too few to report; (2) Data submitted were based on a sample of cases/patients; (3) Results are based on a shorter time period than required; (4) Data suppressed by CMS for one or more quarters; (5) Results are not available for this reporting period; (6) Fewer than 100 patients completed the HCAHPS survey; (7) No cases met the criteria for this measure; (8) The lower limit of the confidence interval cannot be calculated if the number of observed infections equals zero; (9) No data are available from the state/territory for this reporting period; (10) The scores shown reflect fewer than 50 completed surveys; (11) There were discrepancies in the data collection process; (12) This measure does not apply to this hospital for this reporting period; (13) Results cannot be calculated for this reporting period; (14) The results for this state are combined with nearby states to protect confidentiality; Please refer to the User's Guide for a full explanation of data.

Hospital Name	City	Rate	Cases
UT Southwestern University Hospital	Dallas	98%	109
Christus Saint John Hospital	Nassau Bay	97%	93
Houston VA Medical Center	Houston	97%	136
Saint Joseph Medical Center	Houston	97%	108
VHS Harlingen Hospital Company	Harlingen	97%	197
Baptist Saint Anthony's Hospital[2]	Amarillo	96%	316
Park Plaza Hospital	Houston	96%	25
Wise Regional Health System	Decatur	96%	150
Saint Luke's Patients Medical Center	Pasadena	95%	56
Hillcrest Baptist Medical Center	Waco	94%	200
Matagorda Regional Medical Center	Bay City	94%	36
Mission Regional Medical Center	Mission	94%	107
Tomball Regional Medical Center	Tomball	94%	145
Doctors Hospital of Laredo	Laredo	93%	44
Oakbend Medical Center	Richmond	93%	76
Southwest General Hospital	San Antonio	92%	216
Doctors Hospital Tidwell	Houston	64%	33
Starr County Memorial Hospital	Rio Grande City	54%	37

PCI Within 90 Minutes of Arrival

Hospital Name	City	Rate	Cases
Baylor Medical Center at Garland	Garland	100%	58
Bayshore Medical Center	Pasadena	100%	50
Christus Saint Michael Health System	Texarkana	100%	31
Conroe Regional Medical Center	Conroe	100%	46
The Corpus Christi Medical Center	Corpus Christi	100%	30
Denton Regional Medical Center	Denton	100%	33
Detar Hospital Navarro	Victoria	100%	25
Good Shepherd Medical Center[2]	Longview	100%	50
Hendrick Medical Center	Abilene	100%	41
Houston Northwest Medical Center	Houston	100%	51
Laredo Medical Center	Laredo	100%	25
Medical Center of Arlington	Arlington	100%	31
Medical Center of Lewisville	Lewisville	100%	35
Medical Center of Mckinney	Mckinney	100%	36
Memorial Hermann Northeast[2]	Humble	100%	33
The Methodist Hospital	Houston	100%	34
Methodist Sugar Land Hospital[2]	Sugar Land	100%	52
North Austin Medical Center	Austin	100%	57
North Cypress Medical Center	Cypress	100%	27
North Hills Hospital	N Richland Hls	100%	59
Providence Memorial Hospital	El Paso	100%	28
Round Rock Medical Center	Round Rock	100%	39
Saint David's Medical Center	Austin	100%	59
Saint David's South Austin Medical Center[2]	Austin	100%	68
Saint Joseph Regional Health Center	Bryan	100%	25
Saint Luke's Episcopal Hospital[2]	Houston	100%	35
Texas Health Harris Methodist Fort Worth	Fort Worth	100%	87
Texas Health Harris Methodist	Bedford	100%	54
Texoma Medical Center[2]	Denison	100%	52
Valley Regional Medical Center	Brownsville	100%	27
Covenant Medical Center	Lubbock	98%	48
Medical Center of Plano[2]	Plano	98%	46
Methodist West Houston Hospital[2]	Houston	98%	40
University Medical Center	Lubbock	98%	59
Baylor Medical Center at Irving	Irving	97%	39
Harris Health System	Houston	97%	30
Memorial Hermann Texas Medical Center[2]	Houston	97%	39
Methodist Dallas Medical Center	Dallas	97%	33
Methodist Willowbrook Hospital[2]	Houston	97%	33
Midland Memorial Hospital	Midland	97%	62
Northwest Texas Hospital[2]	Amarillo	97%	39
Seton Medical Center Hays	Kyle	97%	31
Shannon Medical Center	San Angelo	97%	32
Sierra Providence East Medical Center	El Paso	97%	31
West Houston Medical Center	Houston	97%	30
Baylor Reg Med Ctr at Grapevine	Grapevine	96%	53
Clear Lake Regional Medical Center[2]	Webster	96%	75
Huguley Memorial Medical Center	Burleson	96%	46
Las Palmas Medical Center	El Paso	96%	45
Methodist Hospital	San Antonio	96%	182
Saint Luke's the Woodlands Hospital	The Woodlands	96%	27
Baptist Medical Center	San Antonio	95%	143
JPS Health Network	Fort Worth	95%	60
Kingwood Medical Center[2]	Kingwood	95%	42
Methodist Charlton Medical Center	Dallas	95%	55
Texas Health Presbyterian Hospital Dallas	Dallas	95%	39
Christus Hospital[2]	Beaumont	94%	32
Christus Spohn Hospital Corpus Christi	Corpus Christi	94%	53
Mother Frances Hospital	Tyler	94%	82
Texas Health Presbyterian Hospital Plano	Plano	94%	32
Providence Health Center	Waco	93%	60
San Jacinto Methodist Hospital	Baytown	93%	29
Memorial Hermann Hospital System[2]	Houston	92%	147
University Medical Center of El Paso	El Paso	92%	26
Christus Santa Rosa Hospital	San Antonio	91%	64
Medical City Dallas Hospital	Dallas	91%	35
Scott & White Memorial Hospital[2]	Temple	91%	34
Baptist Saint Anthony's Hospital[2]	Amarillo	90%	42
United Regional Health Care System	Wichita Falls	89%	35
Mem Hermann Mem City Med Ctr[2]	Houston	88%	43
Seton Medical Center Williamson	Round Rock	88%	25
Baptist Beaumont Hospital	Beaumont	86%	44
Memorial Medical Center of East Texas[2]	Lufkin	86%	29
VHS Harlingen Hospital Company	Harlingen	85%	26
Parkland Health & Hospital System[2]	Dallas	84%	31
Wadley Regional Medical Center	Texarkana	84%	35
Medical Center Hospital	Odessa	83%	35
Tomball Regional Medical Center	Tomball	73%	30

Statin Prescribed at Discharge

Hospital Name	City	Rate	Cases
Baptist Beaumont Hospital	Beaumont	100%	281
Baylor Heart & Vascular Hospital	Dallas	100%	447
Baylor Medical Center at Carrollton	Carrollton	100%	84
Baylor Medical Center at Garland	Garland	100%	203
Bayshore Medical Center	Pasadena	100%	328
Brazosport Regional Health System	Lake Jackson	100%	47
Cedar Park Regional Medical Center	Cedar Park	100%	41
Clear Lake Regional Medical Center[2]	Webster	100%	405
College Station Medical Center	College Station	100%	85
Conroe Regional Medical Center	Conroe	100%	311
The Corpus Christi Medical Center	Corpus Christi	100%	248
Dallas VA Medical Center - VA North Texas	Dallas	100%	102
Denton Regional Medical Center	Denton	100%	241
Doctors Hospital of Laredo	Laredo	100%	45
East Texas Medical Center[2]	Tyler	100%	252
Hendrick Medical Center	Abilene	100%	346
Houston Northwest Medical Center	Houston	100%	271
Huguley Memorial Medical Center	Burleson	100%	248
JPS Health Network	Fort Worth	100%	285
Kingwood Medical Center[2]	Kingwood	100%	249
Lake Granbury Medical Center	Granbury	100%	29
Lake Pointe Medical Center	Rowlett	100%	80
Laredo Medical Center	Laredo	100%	145
Las Colinas Medical Center	Irving	100%	76
Las Palmas Medical Center	El Paso	100%	298
Medical Center of Arlington	Arlington	100%	202
Medical Center of Lewisville	Lewisville	100%	140
Medical Center of Plano[2]	Plano	100%	197
Medical City Dallas Hospital	Dallas	100%	152
Methodist Charlton Medical Center	Dallas	100%	297
Methodist Dallas Medical Center	Dallas	100%	252
Methodist Hospital	San Antonio	100%	1307
Methodist Mansfield Medical Center	Mansfield	100%	219
Methodist Stone Oak Hospital[2]	San Antonio	100%	136
Methodist Sugar Land Hospital[2]	Sugar Land	100%	216
Methodist Willowbrook Hospital[2]	Houston	100%	250
Metroplex Hospital[2]	Killeen	100%	85
Nix Health Care System	San Antonio	100%	35
North Austin Medical Center	Austin	100%	164
North Cypress Medical Center	Cypress	100%	203
North Hills Hospital	N Richland Hls	100%	199
Northwest Texas Hospital[2]	Amarillo	100%	246
Palestine Regional Medical Center	Palestine	100%	52
Plaza Medical Center of Fort Worth[2]	Fort Worth	100%	258
Providence Memorial Hospital	El Paso	100%	116
Round Rock Medical Center	Round Rock	100%	163
Saint David's Medical Center	Austin	100%	395
Saint David's South Austin Medical Center[2]	Austin	100%	299
Saint Joseph Regional Health Center	Bryan	100%	241
Saint Luke's Sugar Land Hospital	Sugar Land	100%	83
Saint Luke's the Woodlands Hospital	The Woodlands	100%	147
San Angelo Community Medical Center	San Angelo	100%	86
San Antonio VA Medical Center	San Antonio	100%	69
Scott & White Memorial Hospital[2]	Temple	100%	287
Sierra Providence East Medical Center	El Paso	100%	82
South Texas Health System[2]	Edinburg	100%	268
Temple VA Med Ctr-VA Central Texas	Temple	100%	43
Texas Health Arlington Memorial Hospital	Arlington	100%	25
Texas Health Harris Methodist	Bedford	100%	214
Texas Health Presbyterian Hospital Denton	Denton	100%	125
Texas Health Presbyterian Hospital Plano	Plano	100%	174
Texoma Medical Center[2]	Denison	100%	248
United Regional Health Care System	Wichita Falls	100%	319
UT Southwestern University Hospital	Dallas	100%	105
Wadley Regional Medical Center	Texarkana	100%	149
West Houston Medical Center	Houston	100%	161
Woodland Heights Medical Center	Lufkin	100%	76
Abilene Regional Medical Center	Abilene	99%	133
Baptist Medical Center	San Antonio	99%	1127
Baylor Medical Center at Irving	Irving	99%	188
Baylor University Medical Center	Dallas	99%	135
Centennial Medical Center	Frisco	99%	94
Covenant Medical Center	Lubbock	99%	613
Cypress Fairbanks Medical Center	Houston	99%	123
Dallas Regional Medical Center	Mesquite	99%	111
Detar Hospital Navarro	Victoria	99%	132
Doctors Hospital	Dallas	99%	124
Good Shepherd Medical Center[2]	Longview	99%	292
Harlingen Medical Center	Harlingen	99%	113
Harris Health System	Houston	99%	377
Houston VA Medical Center	Houston	99%	134
Longview Regional Medical Center	Longview	99%	120
Medical Center of Mckinney	Mckinney	99%	138
The Medical Center of Southeast Texas	Port Arthur	99%	81
Memorial Hermann Hospital System[2]	Houston	99%	900
Memorial Hermann Northeast[2]	Humble	99%	207
Memorial Hermann Texas Medical Center[2]	Houston	99%	269
The Methodist Hospital	Houston	99%	523
Methodist Richardson Medical Center	Richardson	99%	119
Methodist West Houston Hospital[2]	Houston	99%	217
Paris Regional Medical Center	Paris	99%	146
Parkland Health & Hospital System[2]	Dallas	99%	252
Providence Health Center	Waco	99%	303
Rio Grande Regional Hospital[2]	Mcallen	99%	150
Saint Luke's Episcopal Hospital[2]	Houston	99%	293
San Jacinto Methodist Hospital	Baytown	99%	213
Scott & White Hospital - Round Rock	Round Rock	99%	108
Seton Medical Center Hays	Kyle	99%	142
Seton Medical Center Williamson	Round Rock	99%	144
Texas Health Harris Methodist Fort Worth	Fort Worth	99%	879
TX Hlth Heart & Vasc Hosp-Arlington	Arlington	99%	190
Texas Health Presbyterian Hospital Dallas	Dallas	99%	417
University Medical Center	Lubbock	99%	269
University Medical Center at Brackenridge	Austin	99%	79
University Medical Center of El Paso	El Paso	99%	158
Univ of Texas Med Branch Galveston[2]	Galveston	99%	217
Valley Regional Medical Center	Brownsville	99%	236
Baptist Saint Anthony's Hospital[2]	Amarillo	98%	291
Baylor All Saints Medical Center at FW	Fort Worth	98%	157
Baylor Medical Center at Mckinney	Mc Kinney	98%	82
Baylor Reg Med Ctr at Grapevine	Grapevine	98%	189
Christus Hospital[2]	Beaumont	98%	314
Christus Saint Michael Health System	Texarkana	98%	300
Christus Santa Rosa Hospital	San Antonio	98%	400
Doctors Hospital at Renaissance[2]	Edinburg	98%	221
Heart Hospital Baylor Plano	Plano	98%	316
Hopkins County Memorial Hospital	Sulphur Springs	98%	48
Medical Center Hospital	Odessa	98%	317
Nacogdoches Medical Center	Nacogdoches	98%	41
Seton Medical Center Austin	Austin	98%	176
Seton Medical Center Harker Heights	Harker Heights	98%	44
Shannon Medical Center	San Angelo	98%	231
Sierra Medical Center	El Paso	98%	103
TX Hlth Harris Meth Hosp SW Ft Worth	Fort Worth	98%	47
Citizens Medical Center	Victoria	97%	208
Mem Hermann Mem City Med Ctr[2]	Houston	97%	272
Memorial Hospital	Nacogdoches	97%	76
Midland Memorial Hospital	Midland	97%	227
Mother Frances Hospital	Tyler	97%	672
Oakbend Medical Center	Richmond	97%	76
Saint Luke's Patients Medical Center	Pasadena	97%	62
Texas Health Presbyterian Hospital - WNJ	Sherman	97%	127
University Health System	San Antonio	97%	165
VHS Harlingen Hospital Company	Harlingen	97%	183
Christus Saint John Hospital	Nassau Bay	96%	82
Memorial Medical Center of East Texas[2]	Lufkin	96%	237
Saint Luke's Hospital at the Vintage	Houston	96%	47
Southwest General Hospital	San Antonio	96%	196
VHS Brownsville Hospital Company	Brownsville	96%	197
Wise Regional Health System	Decatur	96%	148
Christus Spohn Hospital Corpus Christi	Corpus Christi	95%	519
Texas Reg Med Ctr at Sunnyvale	Sunnyvale	95%	102
Hillcrest Baptist Medical Center	Waco	94%	187
Saint Joseph Medical Center	Houston	94%	103
Odessa Regional Hospital	Odessa	93%	148
Matagorda Regional Medical Center	Bay City	91%	34
Tomball Regional Medical Center	Tomball	91%	140
Mission Regional Medical Center	Mission	90%	105
Knapp Medical Center	Weslaco	89%	28
Lakeway Regional Medical Center[3]	Lakeway	88%	34
Lubbock Heart Hospital[2]	Lubbock	86%	147
Doctors Hospital Tidwell	Houston	75%	32
Starr County Memorial Hospital	Rio Grande City	43%	30

Heart Failure Care

ACE Inhibitor or ARB for LVSD

Hospital Name	City	Rate	Cases
Baptist Medical Center	San Antonio	100%	417
Baylor Heart & Vascular Hospital	Dallas	100%	58
Baylor Medical Center at Carrollton	Carrollton	100%	42
Baylor Medical Center at Mckinney	Mc Kinney	100%	39
Bayshore Medical Center	Pasadena	100%	174
Central Texas Medical Center	San Marcos	100%	28
Christus Saint Catherine Hospital	Katy	100%	30
Clear Lake Regional Medical Center[2]	Webster	100%	92
College Station Medical Center	College Station	100%	104
Conroe Regional Medical Center	Conroe	100%	137
The Corpus Christi Medical Center	Corpus Christi	100%	109
Cuero Community Hospital	Cuero	100%	34

NOTE: Hospital profiles are in alphabetical order by state, then city, then hospital within the city; Rankings exclude hospitals with less than 25 cases except for patient surveys which excludes hospitals with less than 100 cases; (a) 100-299 cases; (1) The number of cases/patients is too few to report; (2) Data submitted were based on a sample of cases/patients; (3) Results are based on a shorter time period than required; (4) Data suppressed by CMS for one or more quarters; (5) Results are not available for this reporting period; (6) Fewer than 100 patients completed the HCAHPS survey; (7) No cases met the criteria for this measure; (8) The lower limit of the confidence interval cannot be calculated if the number of observed infections equals zero; (9) No data are available from the state/territory for this reporting period; (10) The scores shown reflect fewer than 50 completed surveys; (11) There were discrepancies in the data collection process; (12) This measure does not apply to this hospital for this reporting period; (13) Results cannot be calculated for this reporting period; (14) The results for this state are combined with nearby states to protect confidentiality; Please refer to the User's Guide for a full explanation of data.

Hospital Name	City	Rate	Cases
Denton Regional Medical Center	Denton	100%	88
Detar Hospital Navarro	Victoria	100%	75
Doctors Hospital	Dallas	100%	108
Harlingen Medical Center	Harlingen	100%	37
Hopkins County Memorial Hospital	Sulphur Springs	100%	29
Houston Northwest Medical Center	Houston	100%	158
Huguley Memorial Medical Center	Burleson	100%	89
Hunt Regional Medical Center	Greenville	100%	46
Lake Pointe Medical Center	Rowlett	100%	43
Laredo Medical Center	Laredo	100%	117
Las Colinas Medical Center	Irving	100%	36
Las Palmas Medical Center	El Paso	100%	221
Longview Regional Medical Center	Longview	100%	41
Medical Center of Arlington	Arlington	100%	95
Medical Center of Lewisville	Lewisville	100%	57
Medical Center of Plano[2]	Plano	100%	80
Medical City Dallas Hospital	Dallas	100%	148
Memorial Hermann Northeast[2]	Humble	100%	116
Memorial Hermann Sugar Land Hospital	Sugar Land	100%	32
Methodist Charlton Medical Center	Dallas	100%	225
Methodist Dallas Medical Center	Dallas	100%	173
Methodist Mansfield Medical Center	Mansfield	100%	90
Methodist Richardson Medical Center	Richardson	100%	38
Methodist Sugar Land Hospital[2]	Sugar Land	100%	105
Methodist Willowbrook Hospital[2]	Houston	100%	113
Metroplex Hospital[2]	Killeen	100%	73
Nacogdoches Medical Center	Nacogdoches	100%	31
North Austin Medical Center	Austin	100%	63
North Cypress Medical Center	Cypress	100%	68
North Hills Hospital	N Richland Hls	100%	84
Pampa Regional Medical Center	Pampa	100%	34
Park Plaza Hospital	Houston	100%	43
Plaza Medical Center of Fort Worth[2]	Fort Worth	100%	80
Providence Memorial Hospital	El Paso	100%	84
Red River Regional Hospital	Bonham	100%	27
Round Rock Medical Center	Round Rock	100%	47
Saint David's Medical Center	Austin	100%	203
Saint David's South Austin Medical Center[2]	Austin	100%	92
San Angelo Community Medical Center	San Angelo	100%	25
Seton Medical Center Austin[2]	Austin	100%	79
Seton Medical Center Hays	Kyle	100%	46
Sierra Medical Center	El Paso	100%	81
Sierra Providence East Medical Center	El Paso	100%	75
South Texas Health System[2]	Edinburg	100%	88
Texas Health Arlington Memorial Hospital	Arlington	100%	57
TX Hlth Harris Meth Hosp-Cleburne	Cleburne	100%	31
TX Hlth Heart & Vasc Hosp-Arlington	Arlington	100%	92
Texas Health Presbyterian Hospital Dallas	Dallas	100%	200
Texas Health Presbyterian Hospital Denton	Denton	100%	75
Texas Health Presbyterian Hospital Plano	Plano	100%	56
UT Southwestern University Hospital	Dallas	100%	225
Val Verde Regional Medical Center	Del Rio	100%	36
Valley Regional Medical Center	Brownsville	100%	98
Weatherford Regional Medical Center	Weatherford	100%	30
West Houston Medical Center	Houston	100%	96
Woodland Heights Medical Center	Lufkin	100%	53
Baylor University Medical Center	Dallas	99%	391
Christus Saint Michael Health System	Texarkana	99%	186
Christus Santa Rosa Hospital	San Antonio	99%	178
Hendrick Medical Center	Abilene	99%	142
Mem Hermann Mem City Med Ctr[2]	Houston	99%	101
Memorial Hermann Texas Medical Center[2]	Houston	99%	131
Methodist Hospital	San Antonio	99%	522
Northwest Texas Hospital[2]	Amarillo	99%	96
Parkland Health & Hospital System[2]	Dallas	99%	153
Saint Joseph Regional Health Center	Bryan	99%	189
Texas Health Presbyterian Hospital - WNJ	Sherman	99%	73
Texoma Medical Center[2]	Denison	99%	99
University Medical Center at Brackenridge	Austin	99%	84
University Medical Center of El Paso	El Paso	99%	107
Wadley Regional Medical Center	Texarkana	99%	89
Baptist Beaumont Hospital[2]	Beaumont	98%	121
Baylor Medical Center at Garland	Garland	98%	121
Baylor Medical Center at Waxahachie	Waxahachie	98%	66
Baylor Reg Med Ctr at Grapevine	Grapevine	98%	49
Christus Saint John Hospital	Nassau Bay	98%	58
Covenant Medical Center	Lubbock	98%	161
Dallas Regional Medical Center	Mesquite	98%	64
Doctors Hospital at Renaissance[2]	Edinburg	98%	119
Fort Duncan Medical Center	Eagle Pass	98%	47
Good Shepherd Medical Center Marshall	Marshall	98%	55
Hillcrest Baptist Medical Center	Waco	98%	66
JPS Health Network	Fort Worth	98%	259
Kingwood Medical Center	Kingwood	98%	121
Knapp Medical Center	Weslaco	98%	47
The Medical Center of Southeast Texas	Port Arthur	98%	81
Memorial Hermann Hospital System[2]	Houston	98%	439
Seton Medical Center Williamson	Round Rock	98%	52
Shannon Medical Center	San Angelo	98%	92
Texas Health Harris Methodist	Bedford	98%	110
Texas Reg Med Ctr at Sunnyvale[2]	Sunnyvale	98%	57
Univ of Texas Med Branch Galveston[2]	Galveston	98%	117
VHS Harlingen Hospital Company	Harlingen	98%	121
Abilene Regional Medical Center	Abilene	97%	69
Cedar Park Regional Medical Center	Cedar Park	97%	33
Christus Hospital[2]	Beaumont	97%	106
Dallas VA Medical Center - VA North Texas	Dallas	97%	237
Memorial Hermann Katy Hospital	Katy	97%	68
The Methodist Hospital	Houston	97%	319
Methodist West Houston Hospital[2]	Houston	97%	113
Mother Frances Hospital[2]	Tyler	97%	182
Odessa Regional Hospital	Odessa	97%	37
Rio Grande Regional Hospital	Mcallen	97%	95
Saint Joseph Medical Center	Houston	97%	162
Saint Luke's the Woodlands Hospital	The Woodlands	97%	125
San Antonio VA Medical Center	San Antonio	97%	101
San Jacinto Methodist Hospital	Baytown	97%	134
Southwest General Hospital	San Antonio	97%	63
Texas Health Harris Methodist Fort Worth	Fort Worth	97%	266
United Regional Health Care System	Wichita Falls	97%	155
Baylor All Saints Medical Center at FW	Fort Worth	96%	77
Baylor Medical Center at Irving	Irving	96%	82
East Texas Medical Center[2]	Tyler	96%	104
Harris Health System[2]	Houston	96%	318
Heart Hospital Baylor Plano	Plano	96%	106
Houston VA Medical Center	Houston	96%	253
Medical Center of Mckinney	Mckinney	96%	52
Saint Luke's Episcopal Hospital[2]	Houston	96%	112
Temple VA Med Ctr-VA Central Texas	Temple	96%	105
TX Hlth Harris Meth Hosp SW Ft Worth	Fort Worth	96%	78
TX Health Presbyterian Hosp Rockwall	Rockwall	96%	26
University Health System	San Antonio	96%	131
VA Amarillo Healthcare System	Amarillo	96%	27
Brazosport Regional Health System	Lake Jackson	95%	44
Christus Spohn Hospital Beeville	Beeville	95%	40
Cypress Fairbanks Medical Center	Houston	95%	44
Huntsville Memorial Hospital	Huntsville	95%	43
Palestine Regional Medical Center	Palestine	95%	65
Scenic Mountain Medical Center	Big Spring	95%	42
Scott & White Hospital - Round Rock	Round Rock	95%	39
University Medical Center[2]	Lubbock	95%	105
Saint Luke's Sugar Land Hospital	Sugar Land	94%	31
Scott & White Memorial Hospital[2]	Temple	94%	105
Medical Center Hospital	Odessa	93%	125
Memorial Medical Center of East Texas[2]	Lufkin	93%	92
Midland Memorial Hospital	Midland	93%	113
Peterson Regional Medical Center	Kerrville	93%	41
Seton Medical Center Harker Heights	Harker Heights	93%	42
Christus Spohn Hospital Corpus Christi	Corpus Christi	92%	307
Doctors Hospital of Laredo	Laredo	92%	78
Good Shepherd Medical Center[2]	Longview	92%	115
Wise Regional Health System	Decatur	92%	53
Baptist Saint Anthony's Hospital[2]	Amarillo	91%	97
Citizens Medical Center	Victoria	91%	96
Oakbend Medical Center	Richmond	91%	33
Providence Health Center	Waco	91%	151
Saint Luke's Hospital at the Vintage	Houston	91%	34
Tomball Regional Medical Center	Tomball	91%	88
Guadalupe Regional Medical Center	Seguin	89%	35
VHS Brownsville Hospital Company	Brownsville	88%	69
Christus Spohn Hospital Alice	Alice	87%	39
Memorial Hospital	Nacogdoches	87%	47
Pecos County Memorial Hospital[2]	Fort Stockton	87%	47
Saint Luke's Patients Medical Center	Pasadena	87%	61
Mission Regional Medical Center	Mission	86%	57
Paris Regional Medical Center[2]	Paris	85%	73
Christus Jasper Memorial Hospital	Jasper	84%	25
Doctors Hospital Tidwell	Houston	83%	54
Navarro Regional Hospital	Corsicana	83%	42
Lubbock Heart Hospital[2]	Lubbock	79%	81
East Texas Medical Center Athens	Athens	78%	60
Christus Spohn Hospital Kleberg	Kingsville	68%	44

Discharge Instructions Given

Hospital Name	City	Rate	Cases
Baylor Heart & Vascular Hospital	Dallas	100%	95
Baylor Medical Center at Mckinney	Mc Kinney	100%	113
Baylor Regional Medical Center at Plano	Plano	100%	57
Brownwood Regional Medical Center	Brownwood	100%	67
Central Texas Medical Center	San Marcos	100%	115
Christus Saint Catherine Hospital	Katy	100%	85
Christus Spohn Hospital Alice	Alice	100%	107
Citizens Medical Center	Victoria	100%	229
Connally Memorial Medical Center	Floresville	100%	29
Cuero Community Hospital	Cuero	100%	55
Detar Hospital Navarro	Victoria	100%	183
Doctors Hospital	Dallas	100%	223
Doctors Hospital at Renaissance[2]	Edinburg	100%	300
Graham Regional Medical Center[2]	Graham	100%	44
Harlingen Medical Center	Harlingen	100%	123
Hill Country Memorial Hospital	Fredericksburg	100%	52
Laredo Medical Center	Laredo	100%	348
Las Colinas Medical Center	Irving	100%	102
Las Palmas Medical Center	El Paso	100%	565
Longview Regional Medical Center	Longview	100%	117
Medical Center of Arlington	Arlington	100%	282
Memorial Medical Center	Port Lavaca	100%	26
Methodist Mansfield Medical Center	Mansfield	100%	266
Methodist Richardson Medical Center	Richardson	100%	88
Methodist Sugar Land Hospital[2]	Sugar Land	100%	253
Methodist West Houston Hospital[2]	Houston	100%	216
Metroplex Hospital[2]	Killeen	100%	196
North Hills Hospital	N Richland Hls	100%	222
Palo Pinto General Hospital	Mineral Wells	100%	38
Pampa Regional Medical Center	Pampa	100%	54
Plaza Medical Center of Fort Worth[2]	Fort Worth	100%	234
Providence Memorial Hospital	El Paso	100%	227
Rolling Plains Memorial Hospital	Sweetwater	100%	42
Round Rock Medical Center	Round Rock	100%	120
Saint Marks Medical Center	La Grange	100%	30
San Antonio VA Medical Center	San Antonio	100%	236
San Jacinto Methodist Hospital	Baytown	100%	268
Scott & White Hospital - Round Rock	Round Rock	100%	92
Scott & White Memorial Hospital[2]	Temple	100%	258
Seton Edgar B Davis Hospital	Luling	100%	30
Seton Highland Lakes	Burnet	100%	28
Seton Medical Center Williamson	Round Rock	100%	137
Sierra Providence East Medical Center	El Paso	100%	156
Temple VA Med Ctr-VA Central Texas	Temple	100%	204
Texas Health Harris Methodist Fort Worth	Fort Worth	100%	671
TX Hlth Harris Methodist Hosp-Azle	Azle	100%	68
TX Hlth Harris Meth Hosp-Cleburne	Cleburne	100%	134
Valley Regional Medical Center	Brownsville	100%	229
Weatherford Regional Medical Center	Weatherford	100%	88
Baylor Medical Center at Carrollton	Carrollton	99%	104
Baylor Medical Center at Garland	Garland	99%	244
Baylor Medical Center at Irving	Irving	99%	218
Baylor Medical Center at Waxahachie	Waxahachie	99%	144
Baylor Reg Med Ctr at Grapevine	Grapevine	99%	124
Brazosport Regional Health System	Lake Jackson	99%	141
Christus Hospital[2]	Beaumont	99%	270
Christus Spohn Hospital Corpus Christi	Corpus Christi	99%	794
Conroe Regional Medical Center	Conroe	99%	361
The Corpus Christi Medical Center	Corpus Christi	99%	372
Cypress Fairbanks Medical Center	Houston	99%	102
Doctors Hospital Tidwell	Houston	99%	84
Heart Hospital Baylor Plano	Plano	99%	219
Hunt Regional Medical Center	Greenville	99%	101
Kingwood Medical Center	Kingwood	99%	370
Medical Center of Lewisville	Lewisville	99%	129
Medical City Dallas Hospital	Dallas	99%	402
Methodist Dallas Medical Center	Dallas	99%	417
Methodist Stone Oak Hospital[2]	San Antonio	99%	83
Mother Frances Hospital[2]	Tyler	99%	492
North Austin Medical Center	Austin	99%	197
Parkland Health & Hospital System[2]	Dallas	99%	283
Saint Joseph Regional Health Center	Bryan	99%	472
TX Hlth Harris Meth Hosp SW Ft Worth	Fort Worth	99%	228
Texas Health Harris Methodist	Bedford	99%	266
Texas Health Presbyterian Hospital - WNJ	Sherman	99%	175
Texas Health Presbyterian Hospital Denton	Denton	99%	165
TX Hlth Presbyterian Hosp-Kaufman	Kaufman	99%	71
University Medical Center[2]	Lubbock	99%	220
Univ of TX Health Science Ctr-Tyler	Tyler	99%	87
Univ of Texas Med Branch Galveston[2]	Galveston	99%	272
Val Verde Regional Medical Center	Del Rio	99%	122
VHS Harlingen Hospital Company	Harlingen	99%	370
West Houston Medical Center	Houston	99%	225
Abilene Regional Medical Center	Abilene	98%	113
Bayshore Medical Center	Pasadena	98%	441
Christus Saint John Hospital	Nassau Bay	98%	119
Christus Santa Rosa Hospital	San Antonio	98%	421
Clear Lake Regional Medical Center[2]	Webster	98%	245
Denton Regional Medical Center	Denton	98%	182
Hill Regional Hospital	Hillsboro	98%	40
Hopkins County Memorial Hospital	Sulphur Springs	98%	60
Knapp Medical Center	Weslaco	98%	201
Lake Pointe Medical Center	Rowlett	98%	126
Medical Center of Plano[2]	Plano	98%	187
Midland Memorial Hospital	Midland	98%	316
Mother Frances Hospital Jacksonville	Jacksonville	98%	57
North Cypress Medical Center	Cypress	98%	204
Saint David's South Austin Medical Center[2]	Austin	98%	296
Saint Luke's Hospital at the Vintage	Houston	98%	89
San Angelo Community Medical Center	San Angelo	98%	113
Scott & White Hospital Brenham	Brenham	98%	43
Texas Health Arlington Memorial Hospital	Arlington	98%	192
Texas Health Presbyterian Hospital Dallas	Dallas	98%	389
United Regional Health Care System	Wichita Falls	98%	327
Woodland Heights Medical Center	Lufkin	98%	113
Christus Jasper Memorial Hospital	Jasper	97%	59
Covenant Medical Center	Lubbock	97%	468
Huntsville Memorial Hospital	Huntsville	97%	125

NOTE: Hospital profiles are in alphabetical order by state, then city, then hospital within the city; Rankings exclude hospitals with less than 25 cases except for patient surveys which excludes hospitals with less than 100 cases; (a) 100-299 cases; (1) The number of cases/patients is too few to report; (2) Data submitted were based on a sample of cases/patients; (3) Results are based on a shorter time period than required; (4) Data suppressed by CMS for one or more quarters; (5) Results are not available for this reporting period; (6) Fewer than 100 patients completed the HCAHPS survey; (7) No cases met the criteria for this measure; (8) The lower limit of the confidence interval cannot be calculated if the number of observed infections equals zero; (9) No data are available from the state/territory for this reporting period; (10) The scores shown reflect fewer than 50 completed surveys; (11) There were discrepancies in the data collection process; (12) This measure does not apply to this hospital for this reporting period; (13) Results cannot be calculated for this reporting period; (14) The results for this state are combined with nearby states to protect confidentiality; Please refer to the User's Guide for a full explanation of data.

JPS Health Network	Fort Worth	97%	445
Memorial Hospital	Gonzales	97%	30
Methodist Charlton Medical Center	Dallas	97%	465
Rio Grande Regional Hospital	Mcallen	97%	325
Saint David's Medical Center	Austin	97%	587
Saint Luke's Episcopal Hospital[2]	Houston	97%	293
Saint Luke's Sugar Land Hospital	Sugar Land	97%	88
Saint Luke's the Woodlands Hospital	The Woodlands	97%	253
Seton Northwest Hospital	Austin	97%	78
Shannon Medical Center	San Angelo	97%	215
Southwest General Hospital	San Antonio	97%	177
TX Hlth Heart & Vasc Hosp-Arlington	Arlington	97%	183
Texoma Medical Center[2]	Denison	97%	219
University Medical Center of El Paso	El Paso	97%	232
Baylor All Saints Medical Center at FW	Fort Worth	96%	194
Baylor University Medical Center	Dallas	96%	770
Christus Spohn Hospital Kleberg	Kingsville	96%	160
Cleveland Regional Medical Center	Cleveland	96%	26
Dallas Regional Medical Center	Mesquite	96%	162
Lake Granbury Medical Center	Granbury	96%	69
Matagorda Regional Medical Center	Bay City	96%	69
Medical Center of Mckinney	Mckinney	96%	177
Memorial Hermann Northeast[2]	Humble	96%	283
Memorial Hermann Sugar Land Hospital	Sugar Land	96%	98
Memorial Medical Center of East Texas[2]	Lufkin	96%	185
Methodist Hospital	San Antonio	96%	1250
Palestine Regional Medical Center	Palestine	96%	112
Texas Health Presbyterian Hospital Allen	Allen	96%	48
VHS Brownsville Hospital Company	Brownsville	96%	184
Wadley Regional Medical Center	Texarkana	96%	159
Baptist Medical Center	San Antonio	95%	1111
College Station Medical Center	College Station	95%	173
Dallas VA Medical Center - VA North Texas	Dallas	95%	552
East Texas Medical Center[2]	Tyler	95%	225
Hamilton General Hospital	Hamilton	95%	59
Hendrick Medical Center	Abilene	95%	266
Huguley Memorial Medical Center	Burleson	95%	288
Memorial Hermann Hospital System[2]	Houston	95%	979
Memorial Medical Center Livingston[2]	Livingston	95%	56
Mission Regional Medical Center	Mission	95%	174
Paris Regional Medical Center[2]	Paris	95%	188
Peterson Regional Medical Center	Kerrville	95%	104
Seton Medical Center Austin[2]	Austin	95%	247
Sierra Medical Center	El Paso	95%	169
TX Hlth Harris Meth Hosp-Stephenville	Stephenville	95%	41
Texas Reg Med Ctr at Sunnyvale[2]	Sunnyvale	95%	152
Titus Regional Medical Center	Mount Pleasant	95%	44
Good Shepherd Medical Center[2]	Longview	94%	262
Good Shepherd Medical Center Marshall	Marshall	94%	97
Houston Northwest Medical Center	Houston	94%	382
Memorial Hermann Katy Hospital	Katy	94%	139
Northwest Texas Hospital[2]	Amarillo	94%	221
Parkview Regional Hospital	Mexia	94%	31
Red River Regional Hospital	Bonham	94%	34
Saint Luke's Patients Medical Center	Pasadena	94%	140
South Texas Health System[2]	Edinburg	94%	268
Texas Health Presbyterian Hospital Plano	Plano	94%	161
University Medical Center at Brackenridge	Austin	94%	220
UT Southwestern University Hospital	Dallas	94%	502
Wise Regional Health System	Decatur	94%	114
Yoakum Community Hospital	Yoakum	94%	35
Columbus Community Hospital	Columbus	93%	29
Eastland Memorial Hospital	Eastland	93%	28
Fort Duncan Medical Center	Eagle Pass	93%	98
Methodist Willowbrook Hospital[2]	Houston	93%	244
Seton Medical Center Hays	Kyle	93%	91
Uvalde Memorial Hospital	Uvalde	93%	44
VA Amarillo Healthcare System	Amarillo	93%	72
Baptist Beaumont Hospital[2]	Beaumont	92%	272
Christus Saint Michael Health System	Texarkana	92%	451
Lubbock Heart Hospital[2]	Lubbock	92%	252
North Texas Medical Center	Gainesville	92%	26
Park Plaza Hospital	Houston	92%	145
Medical Center Hospital	Odessa	91%	273
Mem Hermann Mem City Med Ctr[2]	Houston	91%	232
Nacogdoches Medical Center	Nacogdoches	91%	66
South Texas Regional Medical Center	Jourdanton	91%	43
Etmc Henderson	Henderson	90%	40
Harris Health System[2]	Houston	90%	633
Nix Health Care System	San Antonio	90%	71
Saint Joseph Medical Center	Houston	90%	374
Scenic Mountain Medical Center	Big Spring	90%	60
TX Health Presbyterian Hosp Rockwall	Rockwall	90%	103
University Health System	San Antonio	90%	303
Ennis Regional Medical Center	Ennis	88%	51
Guadalupe Regional Medical Center	Seguin	88%	86
The Methodist Hospital	Houston	88%	826
Providence Health Center	Waco	88%	320
Cedar Park Regional Medical Center	Cedar Park	87%	84
Centennial Medical Center	Frisco	87%	38
Dallas Medical Center	Dallas	87%	39
Houston VA Medical Center	Houston	87%	530
Memorial Hermann Texas Medical Center[2]	Houston	87%	285
Tomball Regional Medical Center	Tomball	87%	244
Care Regional Medical Center[2]	Aransas Pass	86%	44
East Texas Medical Center Jacksonville	Jacksonville	86%	35
Memorial Hermann Baptist Orange Hospital	Orange	86%	42
Odessa Regional Hospital	Odessa	86%	94
Baptist Saint Anthony's Hospital[2]	Amarillo	84%	255
Christus Spohn Hospital Beeville	Beeville	84%	95
Saint Anthony's Hospital[2,3]	Houston	83%	60
Angleton - Danbury Medical Center	Angleton	82%	57
Hillcrest Baptist Medical Center	Waco	82%	143
Oakbend Medical Center	Richmond	82%	85
Navarro Regional Hospital	Corsicana	81%	104
The Medical Center of Southeast Texas	Port Arthur	80%	236
Memorial Hospital	Nacogdoches	80%	84
Seton Medical Center Harker Heights	Harker Heights	80%	110
East Texas Medical Center Quitman[2]	Quitman	79%	28
East Texas Medical Center Mount Vernon	Mount Vernon	78%	27
Doctors Hospital of Laredo	Laredo	77%	178
TX Hlth Presbyterian Hosp-Flower Mound	Flower Mound	75%	56
Etmc Clarksville	Clarksville	74%	31
Pecos County Memorial Hospital[2]	Fort Stockton	70%	63
East Texas Medical Center Crockett	Crockett	60%	57
Etmc Carthage	Carthage	57%	30
East Texas Medical Center Athens	Athens	56%	152
Lakeway Regional Medical Center[3]	Lakeway	56%	25
East Texas Medical Center Pittsburg[2]	Pittsburg	52%	54
University General Hospital	Houston	50%	36
University General Hospital Dallas[2]	Dallas	5%	42

Evaluation of LVS Function

Hospital Name	City	Rate	Cases
Abilene Regional Medical Center	Abilene	100%	141
Baptist Medical Center	San Antonio	100%	1323
Baylor All Saints Medical Center at FW	Fort Worth	100%	234
Baylor Heart & Vascular Hospital	Dallas	100%	106
Baylor Medical Center at Carrollton	Carrollton	100%	136
Baylor Medical Center at Garland	Garland	100%	308
Baylor Medical Center at Irving	Irving	100%	243
Baylor Medical Center at Mckinney	Mc Kinney	100%	108
Baylor Reg Med Ctr at Grapevine	Grapevine	100%	166
Baylor Regional Medical Center at Plano	Plano	100%	84
Baylor University Medical Center	Dallas	100%	867
Bayshore Medical Center	Pasadena	100%	513
Big Bend Regional Medical Center	Alpine	100%	26
Brazosport Regional Health System	Lake Jackson	100%	173
Cedar Park Regional Medical Center	Cedar Park	100%	99
Centennial Medical Center	Frisco	100%	56
Central Texas Medical Center	San Marcos	100%	154
Christus Saint Catherine Hospital	Katy	100%	96
Christus Saint John Hospital	Nassau Bay	100%	141
Christus Saint Michael Health System	Texarkana	100%	565
Christus Spohn Hospital Alice	Alice	100%	125
College Station Medical Center	College Station	100%	200
Connally Memorial Medical Center	Floresville	100%	42
Conroe Regional Medical Center	Conroe	100%	451
The Corpus Christi Medical Center	Corpus Christi	100%	434
Covenant Hospital Plainview	Plainview	100%	25
Cuero Community Hospital	Cuero	100%	84
Dallas Medical Center	Dallas	100%	56
Dallas Regional Medical Center	Mesquite	100%	197
Denton Regional Medical Center	Denton	100%	232
Detar Hospital Navarro	Victoria	100%	228
Doctors Hospital	Dallas	100%	285
Doctors Hospital at Renaissance[2]	Edinburg	100%	360
East Texas Medical Center[2]	Tyler	100%	296
Good Shepherd Medical Center[2]	Longview	100%	316
Harlingen Medical Center	Harlingen	100%	138
Harris Health System[2]	Houston	100%	648
Heart Hospital Baylor Plano	Plano	100%	272
Hendrick Medical Center	Abilene	100%	316
Hill Country Memorial Hospital	Fredericksburg	100%	67
Hill Regional Hospital	Hillsboro	100%	55
Houston Northwest Medical Center	Houston	100%	453
Houston VA Medical Center	Houston	100%	553
Huguley Memorial Medical Center	Burleson	100%	398
Hunt Regional Medical Center	Greenville	100%	135
JPS Health Network	Fort Worth	100%	480
Kingwood Medical Center	Kingwood	100%	461
Lake Granbury Medical Center	Granbury	100%	99
Lakeway Regional Medical Center[3]	Lakeway	100%	29
Laredo Medical Center	Laredo	100%	384
Las Colinas Medical Center	Irving	100%	118
Las Palmas Medical Center	El Paso	100%	647
Longview Regional Medical Center	Longview	100%	147
Matagorda Regional Medical Center	Bay City	100%	94
Medical Center of Arlington	Arlington	100%	357
Medical Center of Lewisville	Lewisville	100%	161
Medical Center of Mckinney	Mckinney	100%	236
Medical Center of Plano[2]	Plano	100%	262
The Medical Center of Southeast Texas	Port Arthur	100%	284
Medical City Dallas Hospital	Dallas	100%	489
Memorial Hermann Hospital System[2]	Houston	100%	1205
Memorial Hermann Katy Hospital	Katy	100%	177
Mem Hermann Mem City Med Ctr[2]	Houston	100%	308
Memorial Hermann Northeast[2]	Humble	100%	321
Memorial Hermann Sugar Land Hospital	Sugar Land	100%	114
Memorial Hermann Texas Medical Center[2]	Houston	100%	307
Memorial Medical Center	Port Lavaca	100%	31
Memorial Medical Center of East Texas[2]	Lufkin	100%	230
Methodist Charlton Medical Center	Dallas	100%	549
Methodist Dallas Medical Center	Dallas	100%	455
Methodist Hospital	San Antonio	100%	1537
The Methodist Hospital	Houston	100%	960
Methodist Mansfield Medical Center	Mansfield	100%	311
Methodist Richardson Medical Center	Richardson	100%	114
Methodist Stone Oak Hospital[2]	San Antonio	100%	109
Methodist Sugar Land Hospital[2]	Sugar Land	100%	325
Methodist West Houston Hospital[2]	Houston	100%	261
Methodist Willowbrook Hospital[2]	Houston	100%	304
Metroplex Hospital[2]	Killeen	100%	230
Midland Memorial Hospital	Midland	100%	377
Mother Frances Hospital[2]	Tyler	100%	625
Mother Frances Hospital Jacksonville	Jacksonville	100%	64
Nacogdoches Medical Center	Nacogdoches	100%	84
North Austin Medical Center	Austin	100%	233
North Cypress Medical Center	Cypress	100%	257
North Hills Hospital	N Richland Hls	100%	278
Northwest Texas Hospital[2]	Amarillo	100%	260
Odessa Regional Hospital	Odessa	100%	109
Palestine Regional Medical Center	Palestine	100%	144
Palo Pinto General Hospital	Mineral Wells	100%	47
Pampa Regional Medical Center	Pampa	100%	71
Paris Regional Medical Center[2]	Paris	100%	240
Park Plaza Hospital	Houston	100%	165
Parkland Health & Hospital System[2]	Dallas	100%	294
Plaza Medical Center of Fort Worth[2]	Fort Worth	100%	285
Providence Memorial Hospital	El Paso	100%	247
Red River Regional Hospital	Bonham	100%	70
Rolling Plains Memorial Hospital	Sweetwater	100%	61
Round Rock Medical Center	Round Rock	100%	147
Saint David's Medical Center	Austin	100%	675
Saint David's South Austin Medical Center[2]	Austin	100%	360
Saint Joseph Regional Health Center	Bryan	100%	566
Saint Luke's Episcopal Hospital[2]	Houston	100%	329
Saint Luke's Patients Medical Center	Pasadena	100%	186
Saint Luke's the Woodlands Hospital	The Woodlands	100%	318
Saint Marks Medical Center	La Grange	100%	45
San Angelo Community Medical Center	San Angelo	100%	149
San Antonio VA Medical Center	San Antonio	100%	263
San Jacinto Methodist Hospital	Baytown	100%	344
Scenic Mountain Medical Center	Big Spring	100%	90
Scott & White Hospital - Round Rock	Round Rock	100%	122
Scott & White Hospital Brenham	Brenham	100%	57
Scott & White Memorial Hospital[2]	Temple	100%	324
Seton Edgar B Davis Hospital	Luling	100%	37
Seton Medical Center Austin[2]	Austin	100%	285
Seton Medical Center Hays	Kyle	100%	110
Seton Medical Center Williamson	Round Rock	100%	162
Seton Northwest Hospital	Austin	100%	91
Shannon Medical Center	San Angelo	100%	256
Sierra Medical Center	El Paso	100%	199
Sierra Providence East Medical Center	El Paso	100%	174
South Texas Health System[2]	Edinburg	100%	310
South Texas Regional Medical Center	Jourdanton	100%	51
Southwest General Hospital	San Antonio	100%	200
Temple VA Med Ctr-VA Central Texas	Temple	100%	222
Texas Health Arlington Memorial Hospital	Arlington	100%	260
Texas Health Harris Methodist Fort Worth	Fort Worth	100%	826
TX Hlth Harris Meth Hosp-Alliance[3]	Fort Worth	100%	32
TX Hlth Harris Methodist Hosp-Azle	Azle	100%	96
TX Hlth Harris Meth Hosp-Cleburne	Cleburne	100%	161
TX Hlth Harris Meth Hosp-Stephenville	Stephenville	100%	51
TX Hlth Harris Meth Hosp SW Ft Worth	Fort Worth	100%	291
Texas Health Harris Methodist	Bedford	100%	367
TX Hlth Heart & Vasc Hosp-Arlington	Arlington	100%	202
Texas Health Presbyterian Hospital Allen	Allen	100%	61
Texas Health Presbyterian Hospital Dallas	Dallas	100%	566
Texas Health Presbyterian Hospital Denton	Denton	100%	213
TX Hlth Presbyterian Hosp-Flower Mound	Flower Mound	100%	67
TX Hlth Presbyterian Hosp-Kaufman	Kaufman	100%	79
Texas Health Presbyterian Hospital Plano	Plano	100%	195
Texoma Medical Center[2]	Denison	100%	267
Titus Regional Medical Center	Mount Pleasant	100%	63
Tyler County Hospital	Woodville	100%	29
United Regional Health Care System	Wichita Falls	100%	394
University Medical Center[2]	Lubbock	100%	262
University Medical Center at Brackenridge	Austin	100%	241
University Medical Center of El Paso	El Paso	100%	244
Univ of Texas Med Branch Galveston[2]	Galveston	100%	298
UT Southwestern University Hospital	Dallas	100%	566

NOTE: Hospital profiles are in alphabetical order by state, then city, then hospital within the city; Rankings exclude hospitals with less than 25 cases except for patient surveys which excludes hospitals with less than 100 cases; (a) 100-299 cases; (1) The number of cases/patients is too few to report; (2) Data submitted were based on a sample of cases/patients; (3) Results are based on a shorter time period than required; (4) Data suppressed by CMS for one or more quarters; (5) Results are not available for this reporting period; (6) Fewer than 100 patients completed the HCAHPS survey; (7) No cases met the criteria for this measure; (8) The lower limit of the confidence interval cannot be calculated if the number of observed infections equals zero; (9) No data are available from the state/territory for this reporting period; (10) The scores shown reflect fewer than 50 completed surveys; (11) There were discrepancies in the data collection process; (12) This measure does not apply to this hospital for this reporting period; (13) Results cannot be calculated for this reporting period; (14) The results for this state are combined with nearby states to protect confidentiality; Please refer to the User's Guide for a full explanation of data.

VA Amarillo Healthcare System	Amarillo	100%	95
Val Verde Regional Medical Center	Del Rio	100%	136
Valley Regional Medical Center	Brownsville	100%	261
Wadley Regional Medical Center	Texarkana	100%	204
Weatherford Regional Medical Center	Weatherford	100%	115
West Houston Medical Center	Houston	100%	274
Woodland Heights Medical Center	Lufkin	100%	160
Baptist Beaumont Hospital[2]	Beaumont	99%	309
Baptist Saint Anthony's Hospital[2]	Amarillo	99%	315
Baylor Medical Center at Waxahachie	Waxahachie	99%	166
Brownwood Regional Medical Center	Brownwood	99%	91
Christus Hospital[2]	Beaumont	99%	331
Christus Santa Rosa Hospital	San Antonio	99%	524
Clear Lake Regional Medical Center[2]	Webster	99%	310
Covenant Medical Center	Lubbock	99%	587
Cypress Fairbanks Medical Center	Houston	99%	131
Dallas VA Medical Center - VA North Texas	Dallas	99%	589
Doctors Hospital of Laredo	Laredo	99%	194
Fort Duncan Medical Center	Eagle Pass	99%	146
Good Shepherd Medical Center Marshall	Marshall	99%	109
Hamilton General Hospital	Hamilton	99%	94
Hillcrest Baptist Medical Center	Waco	99%	190
Hopkins County Memorial Hospital	Sulphur Springs	99%	85
Lake Pointe Medical Center	Rowlett	99%	146
Memorial Hospital	Nacogdoches	99%	110
Navarro Regional Hospital	Corsicana	99%	139
Nix Health Care System	San Antonio	99%	100
Pecos County Memorial Hospital[2]	Fort Stockton	99%	68
Peterson Regional Medical Center	Kerrville	99%	152
Providence Health Center	Waco	99%	411
Rio Grande Regional Hospital	Mcallen	99%	385
Saint Joseph Medical Center	Houston	99%	424
Saint Luke's Hospital at the Vintage	Houston	99%	119
Saint Luke's Sugar Land Hospital	Sugar Land	99%	107
Seton Medical Center Harker Heights	Harker Heights	99%	120
Texas Health Presbyterian Hospital - WNJ	Sherman	99%	217
TX Health Presbyterian Hosp Rockwall	Rockwall	99%	132
University Health System	San Antonio	99%	308
Univ of TX Health Science Ctr-Tyler	Tyler	99%	107
VHS Harlingen Hospital Company	Harlingen	99%	423
Wise Regional Health System	Decatur	99%	145
Christus Spohn Hospital Beeville	Beeville	98%	115
Columbus Community Hospital	Columbus	98%	57
East Texas Medical Center Jacksonville	Jacksonville	98%	51
Memorial Hermann Baptist Orange Hospital	Orange	98%	48
Texas Reg Med Ctr at Sunnyvale[2]	Sunnyvale	98%	193
Tomball Regional Medical Center	Tomball	98%	311
VHS Brownsville Hospital Company	Brownsville	98%	220
Bowie Memorial Hospital[2]	Bowie	97%	34
Christus Jasper Memorial Hospital	Jasper	97%	74
Christus Spohn Hospital Corpus Christi	Corpus Christi	97%	937
Citizens Medical Center	Victoria	97%	274
Cleveland Regional Medical Center	Cleveland	97%	36
Medical Center Hospital	Odessa	97%	298
Memorial Medical Center Livingston[2]	Livingston	97%	79
Mission Regional Medical Center	Mission	97%	218
Doctors Hospital Tidwell	Houston	96%	101
Guadalupe Regional Medical Center	Seguin	96%	113
Lubbock Heart Hospital[2]	Lubbock	96%	275
Rollins Brook Community Hospital[2]	Lampasas	96%	25
University General Hospital	Houston	96%	47
Uvalde Memorial Hospital	Uvalde	96%	57
Angleton - Danbury Medical Center	Angleton	95%	64
Eastland Memorial Hospital	Eastland	95%	44
Ennis Regional Medical Center	Ennis	95%	65
Graham Regional Medical Center[2]	Graham	95%	59
Oakbend Medical Center	Richmond	95%	119
Care Regional Medical Center[2]	Aransas Pass	94%	54
Christus Spohn Hospital Kleberg	Kingsville	93%	192
Knapp Medical Center	Weslaco	93%	234
Parkview Regional Hospital	Mexia	93%	41
Huntsville Memorial Hospital	Huntsville	92%	143
Yoakum Community Hospital	Yoakum	92%	61
North Texas Medical Center	Gainesville	91%	35
East Texas Medical Center Athens	Athens	90%	193
Lavaca Medical Center	Hallettsville	89%	28
Memorial Hospital	Gonzales	89%	38
East Texas Medical Center - Gilmer	Gilmer	88%	26
Glen Rose Medical Center	Glen Rose	87%	31
Etmc Clarksville	Clarksville	86%	44
Covenant Hospital Levelland	Levelland	85%	26
Etmc Carthage	Carthage	85%	40
Etmc Henderson	Henderson	84%	51
East Texas Medical Center Pittsburg[2]	Pittsburg	82%	68
East Texas Medical Center Quitman[2]	Quitman	82%	39
East Texas Medical Center Trinity[2]	Trinity	78%	40
University General Hospital Dallas[2]	Dallas	71%	51
East Texas Medical Center Crockett	Crockett	61%	96
East Texas Medical Center Mount Vernon	Mount Vernon	60%	42
Golden Plains Community Hospital	Borger	59%	27
Saint Anthony's Hospital[2,3]	Houston	31%	67

Medicare Spending

Medicare Spending per Patient (ratio)

Hospital Name	City	Ratio	Cases
Basin Healthcare Center	Odessa	0.71	-
Lake Whitney Medical Center	Whitney	0.80	-
Moore County Hospital District	Dumas	0.80	-
Anson General Hospital	Anson	0.81	-
Hemphill County Hospital	Canadian	0.81	-
Lamb Healthcare Center	Littlefield	0.82	-
Pecos County Memorial Hospital	Fort Stockton	0.82	-
Hamlin Memorial Hospital	Hamlin	0.83	-
First Surgical Hospital	Bellaire	0.85	-
Seton Smithville Regional Hospital	Smithville	0.85	-
Central Texas Hospital	Cameron	0.86	-
Hill Regional Hospital	Hillsboro	0.86	-
Knox County Hospital	Knox City	0.86	-
Frio Regional Hospital	Pearsall	0.88	-
Glen Rose Medical Center	Glen Rose	0.88	-
Permian Regional Medical Center	Andrews	0.88	-
Riverside General Hospital	Houston	0.88	-
Scott & White Hospital Brenham	Brenham	0.88	-
Starr County Memorial Hospital	Rio Grande City	0.88	-
Texas Orthopedic Hospital	Houston	0.88	-
Val Verde Regional Medical Center	Del Rio	0.88	-
Graham Regional Medical Center	Graham	0.89	-
Brownfield Regional Medical Center	Brownfield	0.91	-
El Campo Memorial Hospital	El Campo	0.91	-
Parkland Health & Hospital System	Dallas	0.91	-
Quail Creek Surgical Hospital	Amarillo	0.91	-
Shannon Medical Center	San Angelo	0.91	-
Bowie Memorial Hospital	Bowie	0.92	-
East Texas Medical Center Mount Vernon	Mount Vernon	0.92	-
Etmc Carthage	Carthage	0.92	-
Hamilton General Hospital	Hamilton	0.92	-
Scott & White Memorial Hospital	Temple	0.92	-
Covenant Hospital Levelland	Levelland	0.93	-
Rolling Plains Memorial Hospital	Sweetwater	0.93	-
Seymour Hospital	Seymour	0.93	-
Stamford Memorial Hospital	Stamford	0.93	-
TX Health Ctr for Diag & Surgery	Plano	0.93	-
Cogdell Memorial Hospital	Snyder	0.94	-
Faith Community Hospital	Jacksboro	0.94	-
Hill Country Memorial Hospital	Fredericksburg	0.94	-
Medical Arts Hospital	Lamesa	0.94	-
Memorial Hospital	Gonzales	0.94	-
Scott & White Hospital - Llano	Llano	0.94	-
Scott & White Hospital - Round Rock	Round Rock	0.94	-
Stephens Memorial Hospital	Breckenridge	0.94	-
University Health System	San Antonio	0.94	-
UT SW Univ Hosp-Zale Lipshy	Dallas	0.94	-
Covenant Hospital Plainview	Plainview	0.95	-
East Texas Medical Center - Fairfield	Fairfield	0.95	-
Parkview Regional Hospital	Mexia	0.95	-
Sugar Land Surgical Hospital	Sugar Land	0.95	-
Arise Austin Medical Center	Austin	0.96	-
Brazosport Regional Health System	Lake Jackson	0.96	-
The Corpus Christi Medical Center	Corpus Christi	0.96	-
Goodall Witcher Hospital	Clifton	0.96	-
Harris Health System	Houston	0.96	-
Metroplex Hospital	Killeen	0.96	-
Nocona General Hospital	Nocona	0.96	-
Pampa Regional Medical Center	Pampa	0.96	-
Scenic Mountain Medical Center	Big Spring	0.96	-
Seton Medical Center Harker Heights	Harker Heights	0.96	-
South Texas Spine & Surgical Hospital	San Antonio	0.96	-
Wilbarger General Hospital	Vernon	0.96	-
Baylor Heart & Vascular Hospital	Dallas	0.97	-
Lubbock Heart Hospital	Lubbock	0.97	-
Providence Health Center	Waco	0.97	-
Tops Surgical Specialty Hospital	Houston	0.97	-
The Womans Hospital of Texas	Houston	0.97	-
Woodland Heights Medical Center	Lufkin	0.97	-
Christus Spohn Hospital Beeville	Beeville	0.98	-
College Station Medical Center	College Station	0.98	-
Connally Memorial Medical Center	Floresville	0.98	-
Knapp Medical Center	Weslaco	0.98	-
Methodist Dallas Medical Center	Dallas	0.98	-
The Methodist Hospital	Houston	0.98	-
Seton Northwest Hospital	Austin	0.98	-
Seton Southwest Hospital	Austin	0.98	-
Texas Spine & Joint Hospital	Tyler	0.98	-
Abilene Regional Medical Center	Abilene	0.99	-
Baptist Saint Anthony's Hospital	Amarillo	0.99	-
Childress Regional Medical Center	Childress	0.99	-
Christus Jasper Memorial Hospital	Jasper	0.99	-
Citizens Medical Center	Victoria	0.99	-
Columbus Community Hospital	Columbus	0.99	-
Dimmit Regional Hospital	Carrizo Springs	0.99	-
East Texas Medical Center Crockett	Crockett	0.99	-
Hendrick Medical Center	Abilene	0.99	-
Laredo Medical Center	Laredo	0.99	-
Longview Regional Medical Center	Longview	0.99	-
Memorial Hermann Texas Medical Center	Houston	0.99	-
Saint Joseph Regional Health Center	Bryan	0.99	-
TX Hlth Harris Meth Hosp-Cleburne	Cleburne	0.99	-
University Medical Center of El Paso	El Paso	0.99	-
Univ of TX Health Science Ctr-Tyler	Tyler	0.99	-
Univ of Texas Med Branch Galveston	Galveston	0.99	-
USMD Hospital at Arlington	Arlington	0.99	-
Brownwood Regional Medical Center	Brownwood	1.00	-
Christus Spohn Hospital Kleberg	Kingsville	1.00	-
Cornerstone Regional Hospital	Edinburg	1.00	-
Doctors Hospital of Laredo	Laredo	1.00	-
East Texas Medical Center Athens	Athens	1.00	-
Good Shepherd Medical Center	Longview	1.00	-
Las Colinas Medical Center	Irving	1.00	-
Odessa Regional Hospital	Odessa	1.00	-
Providence Memorial Hospital	El Paso	1.00	-
Saint Luke's Episcopal Hospital	Houston	1.00	-
Tyler County Hospital	Woodville	1.00	-
Uvalde Memorial Hospital	Uvalde	1.00	-
Covenant Medical Center	Lubbock	1.01	-
Detar Hospital Navarro	Victoria	1.01	-
Doctors Diagnostic Hospital	Cleveland	1.01	-
El Paso Specialty Hospital	El Paso	1.01	-
Good Shepherd Medical Center Marshall	Marshall	1.01	-
Grace Medical Center	Lubbock	1.01	-
Harlingen Medical Center	Harlingen	1.01	-
Heart Hospital Baylor Plano	Plano	1.01	-
Hillcrest Baptist Medical Center	Waco	1.01	-
The Hospital at Westlake Medical Center	Austin	1.01	-
Houston Orthopedic & Spine Hospital	Bellaire	1.01	-
Las Palmas Medical Center	El Paso	1.01	-
Methodist Ambulatory Surgery Hospital NW	San Antonio	1.01	-
Methodist Hospital For Surgery	Addison	1.01	-
Mission Regional Medical Center	Mission	1.01	-
Nix Health Care System	San Antonio	1.01	-
The Physicians Centre	Bryan	1.01	-
Rio Grande Regional Hospital	Mcallen	1.01	-
San Angelo Community Medical Center	San Angelo	1.01	-
San Jacinto Methodist Hospital	Baytown	1.01	-
Sierra Medical Center	El Paso	1.01	-
South Texas Surgical Hospital	Corpus Christi	1.01	-
TX Hlth Harris Meth Hosp-Stephenville	Stephenville	1.01	-
Texas Health Presbyterian Hospital - WNJ	Sherman	1.01	-
VHS Harlingen Hospital Company	Harlingen	1.01	-
Baylor Medical Center at Mckinney	Mc Kinney	1.02	-
Christus Spohn Hospital Corpus Christi	Corpus Christi	1.02	-
Eastland Memorial Hospital	Eastland	1.02	-
Fort Duncan Medical Center	Eagle Pass	1.02	-
Medical Center Hospital	Odessa	1.02	-
Memorial Hermann Baptist Orange Hospital	Orange	1.02	-
Memorial Medical Center of East Texas	Lufkin	1.02	-
Methodist Mckinney Hospital	Mc Kinney	1.02	-
Palestine Regional Medical Center	Palestine	1.02	-
Sierra Providence East Medical Center	El Paso	1.02	-
TX Hlth Harris Meth Hosp SW Ft Worth	Fort Worth	1.02	-
Angleton - Danbury Medical Center	Angleton	1.03	-
Baptist Beaumont Hospital	Beaumont	1.03	-
Baylor Medical Center at Irving	Irving	1.03	-
Bellville General Hospital	Bellville	1.03	-
Christus Hospital	Beaumont	1.03	-
Christus Saint Catherine Hospital	Katy	1.03	-
Christus Saint Michael Health System	Texarkana	1.03	-
Doctors Hospital at Renaissance	Edinburg	1.03	-
East Texas Medical Center - Gilmer	Gilmer	1.03	-
Foundation Surgical Hospital of El Paso	El Paso	1.03	-
Hereford Regional Medical Center	Hereford	1.03	-
Lake Granbury Medical Center	Granbury	1.03	-
Mother Frances Hospital	Tyler	1.03	-
Nacogdoches Medical Center	Nacogdoches	1.03	-
Navarro Regional Hospital	Corsicana	1.03	-
Northwest Texas Hospital	Amarillo	1.03	-
Saint David's Medical Center	Austin	1.03	-
Saint David's South Austin Medical Center	Austin	1.03	-
South Texas Regional Medical Center	Jourdanton	1.03	-
UT Southwestern University Hospital	Dallas	1.03	-
Valley Regional Medical Center	Brownsville	1.03	-
Baptist Medical Center	San Antonio	1.04	-
Baylor All Saints Medical Center at FW	Fort Worth	1.04	-
Baylor Medical Center at Waxahachie	Waxahachie	1.04	-
Baylor University Medical Center	Dallas	1.04	-
Central Texas Medical Center	San Marcos	1.04	-
Christus Spohn Hospital Alice	Alice	1.04	-
Guadalupe Regional Medical Center	Seguin	1.04	-
Huntsville Memorial Hospital	Huntsville	1.04	-
Medical Center of Lewisville	Lewisville	1.04	-
Memorial Hermann Katy Hospital	Katy	1.04	-
Methodist Hospital	San Antonio	1.04	-
Seton Medical Center Austin	Austin	1.04	-
South Texas Health System	Edinburg	1.04	-

NOTE: Hospital profiles are in alphabetical order by state, then city, then hospital within the city; Rankings exclude hospitals with less than 25 cases except for patient surveys which excludes hospitals with less than 100 cases; (a) 100-299 cases; (1) The number of cases/patients is too few to report; (2) Data submitted were based on a sample of cases/patients; (3) Results are based on a shorter time period than required; (4) Data suppressed by CMS for one or more quarters; (5) Results are not available for this reporting period; (6) Fewer than 100 patients completed the HCAHPS survey; (7) No cases met the criteria for this measure; (8) The lower limit of the confidence interval cannot be calculated if the number of observed infections equals zero; (9) No data are available from the state/territory for this reporting period; (10) The scores shown reflect fewer than 50 completed surveys; (11) There were discrepancies in the data collection process; (12) This measure does not apply to this hospital for this reporting period; (13) Results cannot be calculated for this reporting period; (14) The results for this state are combined with nearby states to protect confidentiality; Please refer to the User's Guide for a full explanation of data.

Southwest General Hospital	San Antonio	1.04	-
Titus Regional Medical Center	Mount Pleasant	1.04	-
University Medical Center	Lubbock	1.04	-
Care Regional Medical Center	Aransas Pass	1.05	-
Cedar Park Regional Medical Center	Cedar Park	1.05	-
Etmc Clarksville	Clarksville	1.05	-
Etmc Henderson	Henderson	1.05	-
JPS Health Network	Fort Worth	1.05	-
Medical City Dallas Hospital	Dallas	1.05	-
Memorial Medical Center Livingston	Livingston	1.05	-
North Austin Medical Center	Austin	1.05	-
North Texas Medical Center	Gainesville	1.05	-
Peterson Regional Medical Center	Kerrville	1.05	-
Round Rock Medical Center	Round Rock	1.05	-
TX Hlth Presbyterian Hosp-Flower Mound	Flower Mound	1.05	-
United Regional Health Care System	Wichita Falls	1.05	-
University Medical Center at Brackenridge	Austin	1.05	-
VHS Brownsville Hospital Company	Brownsville	1.05	-
Dallas Regional Medical Center	Mesquite	1.06	-
Gulf Coast Medical Center	Wharton	1.06	-
Hopkins County Memorial Hospital	Sulphur Springs	1.06	-
North Central Surgical Center	Dallas	1.06	-
North Hills Hospital	N Richland Hls	1.06	-
Palo Pinto General Hospital	Mineral Wells	1.06	-
Park Plaza Hospital	Houston	1.06	-
Saint Joseph Medical Center	Houston	1.06	-
Saint Marks Medical Center	La Grange	1.06	-
Texas Health Harris Methodist	Bedford	1.06	-
TX Hlth Presbyterian Hosp-Kaufman	Kaufman	1.06	-
TX Health Presbyterian Hosp Rockwall	Rockwall	1.06	-
Weatherford Regional Medical Center	Weatherford	1.06	-
Baylor Medical Center at Uptown	Dallas	1.07	-
Christus Santa Rosa Hospital	San Antonio	1.07	-
Conroe Regional Medical Center	Conroe	1.07	-
East Texas Medical Center	Tyler	1.07	-
East Texas Medical Center Jacksonville	Jacksonville	1.07	-
Falls Community Hospital & Clinic	Marlin	1.07	-
Heart Hospital Baylor Denton	Denton	1.07	-
Houston Physicians' Hospital	Webster	1.07	-
Kell West Regional Hospital	Wichita Falls	1.07	-
Kingwood Medical Center	Kingwood	1.07	-
Lakeway Regional Medical Center	Lakeway	1.07	-
Methodist Stone Oak Hospital	San Antonio	1.07	-
Pine Creek Medical Center	Dallas	1.07	-
Plaza Medical Center of Fort Worth	Fort Worth	1.07	-
Seton Medical Center Hays	Kyle	1.07	-
Texas Health Presbyterian Hospital Plano	Plano	1.07	-
Wise Regional Health System	Decatur	1.07	-
Baylor Medical Center at Garland	Garland	1.08	-
Baylor Reg Med Ctr at Grapevine	Grapevine	1.08	-
Ennis Regional Medical Center	Ennis	1.08	-
Heritage Park Surgical Hospital	Sherman	1.08	-
Hunt Regional Medical Center	Greenville	1.08	-
Medical Center of Arlington	Arlington	1.08	-
Methodist Mansfield Medical Center	Mansfield	1.08	-
Methodist West Houston Hospital	Houston	1.08	-
Midland Memorial Hospital	Midland	1.08	-
Paris Regional Medical Center	Paris	1.08	-
Texas Health Harris Methodist Fort Worth	Fort Worth	1.08	-
Texas Health Presbyterian Hospital Dallas	Dallas	1.08	-
Texoma Medical Center	Denison	1.08	-
Wadley Regional Medical Center	Texarkana	1.08	-
Baylor Ortho & Spine Hosp-Arlington	Arlington	1.09	-
Baylor Regional Medical Center at Plano	Plano	1.09	-
Clear Lake Regional Medical Center	Webster	1.09	-
Doctors Hospital	Dallas	1.09	-
Matagorda Regional Medical Center	Bay City	1.09	-
Memorial Hermann Northeast	Humble	1.09	-
Methodist Sugar Land Hospital	Sugar Land	1.09	-
Seton Medical Center Williamson	Round Rock	1.09	-
Tomball Regional Medical Center	Tomball	1.09	-
Medical Center of Mckinney	Mckinney	1.10	-
Mem Hermann Mem City Med Ctr	Houston	1.10	-
Memorial Hermann Sugar Land Hospital	Sugar Land	1.10	-
Methodist Charlton Medical Center	Dallas	1.10	-
Northwest Hills Surgical Hospital	Austin	1.10	-
USMD Hospital at Fort Worth	Fort Worth	1.10	-
Baylor Medical Center at Frisco	Frisco	1.11	-
The Medical Center of Southeast Texas	Port Arthur	1.11	-
Saint Luke's Lakeside Hospital	The Woodlands	1.11	-
TX Hlth Heart & Vasc Hosp-Arlington	Arlington	1.11	-
Baylor Medical Center at Carrollton	Carrollton	1.12	-
Christus Saint John Hospital	Nassau Bay	1.12	-
Houston Northwest Medical Center	Houston	1.12	-
Huguley Memorial Medical Center	Burleson	1.12	-
Methodist Willowbrook Hospital	Houston	1.12	-
Bayshore Medical Center	Pasadena	1.13	-
Denton Regional Medical Center	Denton	1.13	-
Lake Pointe Medical Center	Rowlett	1.13	-
Medical Center of Plano	Plano	1.13	-
Memorial Hospital	Nacogdoches	1.13	-
Saint Luke's the Woodlands Hospital	The Woodlands	1.13	-
Texas Health Arlington Memorial Hospital	Arlington	1.13	-
Texas Health Presbyterian Hospital Denton	Denton	1.13	-
Allegiance Specialty Hospital of Kilgore	Kilgore	1.14	-
Cypress Fairbanks Medical Center	Houston	1.14	-
Memorial Hermann Hospital System	Houston	1.14	-
North Cypress Medical Center	Cypress	1.14	-
Centennial Medical Center	Frisco	1.15	-
Cuero Community Hospital	Cuero	1.15	-
Mem Hermann Surgical Hosp Kingwood	Kingwood	1.15	-
Northwest Texas Surgery Center	Amarillo	1.15	-
Texas Health Presbyterian Hospital Allen	Allen	1.16	-
Texas Reg Med Ctr at Sunnyvale	Sunnyvale	1.16	-
West Houston Medical Center	Houston	1.16	-
Baylor Surgical Hospital at Fort Worth	Fort Worth	1.17	-
Oakbend Medical Center	Richmond	1.17	-
Saint Luke's Sugar Land Hospital	Sugar Land	1.17	-
Cleveland Regional Medical Center	Cleveland	1.19	-
Fdn Surgical Hosp of San Antonio	San Antonio	1.19	-
Methodist Richardson Medical Center	Richardson	1.19	-
TX Hlth Harris Meth Hosp-Southlake	Southlake	1.19	-
TX Hlth Harris Methodist Hosp-Azle	Azle	1.20	-
Baylor Surgical Hospital at Las Colinas	Irving	1.22	-
Dallas Medical Center	Dallas	1.22	-
Saint Luke's Hospital at the Vintage	Houston	1.22	-
Doctors Hospital Tidwell	Houston	1.23	-
East Texas Medical Center Trinity	Trinity	1.26	-
Saint Luke's Patients Medical Center	Pasadena	1.26	-
University General Hospital	Houston	1.29	-
University General Hospital Dallas	Dallas	1.29	-
Saint Anthony's Hospital	Houston	1.31	-
Baylor Medical Center at Trophy Club	Trophy Club	1.45	-
TX Inst for Surgery at Presby Hosp	Dallas	1.65	-

Pneumonia Care

Appropriate Initial Antibiotic Given

Hospital Name	City	Rate	Cases
Abilene Regional Medical Center	Abilene	100%	53
Baylor Medical Center at Mckinney	Mc Kinney	100%	99
Big Bend Regional Medical Center	Alpine	100%	25
Clear Lake Regional Medical Center[2]	Webster	100%	87
Conroe Regional Medical Center	Conroe	100%	140
The Corpus Christi Medical Center	Corpus Christi	100%	139
Detar Hospital Navarro	Victoria	100%	80
East Texas Medical Center - Fairfield	Fairfield	100%	38
East Texas Medical Center - Gilmer	Gilmer	100%	25
Electra Memorial Hospital	Electra	100%	33
Good Shepherd Medical Center[2]	Longview	100%	106
Harlingen Medical Center	Harlingen	100%	85
Houston Northwest Medical Center	Houston	100%	173
Laredo Medical Center	Laredo	100%	152
Las Colinas Medical Center	Irving	100%	56
Medical Center of Arlington[2]	Arlington	100%	75
Medical City Dallas Hospital	Dallas	100%	104
Methodist Mansfield Medical Center	Mansfield	100%	155
Methodist Richardson Medical Center[2]	Richardson	100%	80
Methodist Willowbrook Hospital[2]	Houston	100%	95
Metroplex Hospital[2]	Killeen	100%	56
North Austin Medical Center	Austin	100%	128
Northwest Texas Hospital[2]	Amarillo	100%	79
Paris Regional Medical Center[2]	Paris	100%	72
Rolling Plains Memorial Hospital	Sweetwater	100%	52
San Angelo Community Medical Center	San Angelo	100%	77
Scott & White Hospital - Llano	Llano	100%	27
Seton Edgar B Davis Hospital	Luling	100%	38
Seton Highland Lakes	Burnet	100%	51
South Texas Health System[2]	Edinburg	100%	77
Texas Health Arlington Memorial Hospital	Arlington	100%	270
TX Hlth Harris Meth Hosp-Alliance[3]	Fort Worth	100%	49
TX Hlth Presbyterian Hosp-Kaufman	Kaufman	100%	74
Texoma Medical Center[2]	Denison	100%	82
University Medical Center of El Paso	El Paso	100%	120
UT Southwestern University Hospital	Dallas	100%	87
VA Amarillo Healthcare System	Amarillo	100%	35
Weatherford Regional Medical Center	Weatherford	100%	105
Woodland Heights Medical Center	Lufkin	100%	57
Baptist Beaumont Hospital[2]	Beaumont	99%	130
Baylor Medical Center at Garland	Garland	99%	184
Baylor University Medical Center[2]	Dallas	99%	69
Bayshore Medical Center	Pasadena	99%	270
Brazosport Regional Health System[2]	Lake Jackson	99%	71
Central Texas Medical Center	San Marcos	99%	86
College Station Medical Center	College Station	99%	70
Denton Regional Medical Center[2]	Denton	99%	110
Lake Granbury Medical Center	Granbury	99%	85
Las Palmas Medical Center	El Paso	99%	298
Medical Center of Lewisville	Lewisville	99%	93
Mem Hermann Mem City Med Ctr[2]	Houston	99%	72
Methodist Charlton Medical Center	Dallas	99%	156
Methodist Sugar Land Hospital[2]	Sugar Land	99%	68
Round Rock Medical Center	Round Rock	99%	93
Scott & White Memorial Hospital[2]	Temple	99%	71
Seton Northwest Hospital	Austin	99%	94
Shannon Medical Center	San Angelo	99%	146
TX Hlth Harris Meth Hosp-Cleburne	Cleburne	99%	144
TX Health Presbyterian Hosp Rockwall	Rockwall	99%	137
Baptist Medical Center	San Antonio	98%	592
Baylor Medical Center at Irving[2]	Irving	98%	120
Baylor Regional Medical Center at Plano	Plano	98%	107
Christus Saint Catherine Hospital	Katy	98%	50
Doctors Hospital	Dallas	98%	122
East Texas Medical Center[2]	Tyler	98%	49
Good Shepherd Medical Center Marshall	Marshall	98%	109
Harris Health System[2]	Houston	98%	153
Hill Regional Hospital	Hillsboro	98%	47
Hillcrest Baptist Medical Center[2]	Waco	98%	80
Huguley Memorial Medical Center	Burleson	98%	180
Methodist Dallas Medical Center	Dallas	98%	101
Methodist Hospital	San Antonio	98%	673
Methodist Stone Oak Hospital[2]	San Antonio	98%	65
North Cypress Medical Center	Cypress	98%	149
North Hills Hospital[2]	N Richland Hls	98%	91
Pampa Regional Medical Center	Pampa	98%	41
Parkview Regional Hospital	Mexia	98%	59
Providence Memorial Hospital[2]	El Paso	98%	121
Rio Grande Regional Hospital	Mcallen	98%	188
Saint David's Medical Center	Austin	98%	188
Saint Luke's Hospital at the Vintage	Houston	98%	102
Saint Luke's Patients Medical Center[2]	Pasadena	98%	92
Saint Luke's Sugar Land Hospital	Sugar Land	98%	85
Sierra Providence East Medical Center[2]	El Paso	98%	111
South Texas Regional Medical Center	Jourdanton	98%	50
Southwest General Hospital	San Antonio	98%	91
Texas Health Presbyterian Hospital Dallas	Dallas	98%	181
Texas Health Presbyterian Hospital Denton	Denton	98%	169
Texas Health Presbyterian Hospital Plano	Plano	98%	151
Texas Reg Med Ctr at Sunnyvale	Sunnyvale	98%	65
Univ of TX Health Science Ctr-Tyler[2]	Tyler	98%	66
Valley Regional Medical Center	Brownsville	98%	89
West Houston Medical Center	Houston	98%	81
Baylor All Saints Medical Center at FW	Fort Worth	97%	184
Baylor Medical Center at Carrollton	Carrollton	97%	106
Baylor Medical Center at Waxahachie	Waxahachie	97%	116
Baylor Reg Med Ctr at Grapevine	Grapevine	97%	154
Brownfield Regional Medical Center	Brownfield	97%	29
Christus Saint Michael Health System	Texarkana	97%	269
Christus Santa Rosa Hospital	San Antonio	97%	369
Citizens Medical Center	Victoria	97%	96
Cypress Fairbanks Medical Center	Houston	97%	118
Dallas Medical Center[2]	Dallas	97%	33
Doctors Hospital of Laredo[2]	Laredo	97%	69
Fort Duncan Medical Center[2]	Eagle Pass	97%	72
Good Shephard Medical Center - Linden	Linden	97%	37
JPS Health Network	Fort Worth	97%	217
Longview Regional Medical Center	Longview	97%	99
Medical Center Hospital	Odessa	97%	147
Medical Center of Plano[2]	Plano	97%	75
Memorial Hermann Hospital System[2]	Houston	97%	298
Memorial Hermann Sugar Land Hospital[2]	Sugar Land	97%	73
Memorial Medical Center	Port Lavaca	97%	58
Methodist West Houston Hospital[2]	Houston	97%	118
Mother Frances Hospital[2]	Tyler	97%	235
Nacogdoches Medical Center	Nacogdoches	97%	59
Parkland Health & Hospital System[2]	Dallas	97%	67
Peterson Regional Medical Center	Kerrville	97%	136
Saint David's South Austin Medical Center[2]	Austin	97%	98
San Antonio VA Medical Center	San Antonio	97%	72
Seton Medical Center Austin	Austin	97%	162
Seton Medical Center Harker Heights	Harker Heights	97%	70
TX Hlth Harris Methodist Hosp-Azle	Azle	97%	103
TX Hlth Harris Meth Hosp SW Ft Worth	Fort Worth	97%	237
Uvalde Memorial Hospital	Uvalde	97%	62
Wise Regional Health System	Decatur	97%	96
Baptist Saint Anthony's Hospital[2]	Amarillo	96%	93
Cedar Park Regional Medical Center	Cedar Park	96%	89
Centennial Medical Center	Frisco	96%	53
Christus Spohn Hospital Kleberg[2]	Kingsville	96%	90
Doctors Hospital at Renaissance[2]	Edinburg	96%	137
East Texas Medical Center Crockett	Crockett	96%	25
Hill Country Memorial Hospital	Fredericksburg	96%	55
Huntsville Memorial Hospital	Huntsville	96%	101
Kingwood Medical Center	Kingwood	96%	194
Knapp Medical Center	Weslaco	96%	112
Lake Pointe Medical Center	Rowlett	96%	105
Memorial Hermann Baptist Orange Hospital	Orange	96%	76
Memorial Hermann Northeast[2]	Humble	96%	69
Memorial Medical Center of East Texas[2]	Lufkin	96%	71
Mission Regional Medical Center	Mission	96%	163
Providence Health Center	Waco	96%	267
Saint Joseph Medical Center	Houston	96%	108

NOTE: Hospital profiles are in alphabetical order by state, then city, then hospital within the city; Rankings exclude hospitals with less than 25 cases except for patient surveys which excludes hospitals with less than 100 cases; (a) 100-299 cases; (1) The number of cases/patients is too few to report; (2) Data submitted were based on a sample of cases/patients; (3) Results are based on a shorter time period than required; (4) Data suppressed by CMS for one or more quarters; (5) Results are not available for this reporting period; (6) Fewer than 100 patients completed the HCAHPS survey; (7) No cases met the criteria for this measure; (8) The lower limit of the confidence interval cannot be calculated if the number of observed infections equals zero; (9) No data are available from the state/territory for this reporting period; (10) The scores shown reflect fewer than 50 completed surveys; (11) There were discrepancies in the data collection process; (12) This measure does not apply to this hospital for this reporting period; (13) Results cannot be calculated for this reporting period; (14) The results for this state are combined with nearby states to protect confidentiality; Please refer to the User's Guide for a full explanation of data.

Saint Luke's Episcopal Hospital[2]	Houston	96%	79
Saint Marks Medical Center	La Grange	96%	52
San Jacinto Methodist Hospital	Baytown	96%	162
Sierra Medical Center[2]	El Paso	96%	106
Texas Health Harris Methodist	Bedford	96%	250
Texas Health Presbyterian Hospital Allen	Allen	96%	84
United Regional Health Care System	Wichita Falls	96%	243
University Medical Center[2]	Lubbock	96%	49
Wadley Regional Medical Center	Texarkana	96%	96
Covenant Medical Center	Lubbock	95%	314
Ennis Regional Medical Center	Ennis	95%	75
Hunt Regional Medical Center	Greenville	95%	168
Medical Center of Mckinney	Mckinney	95%	109
The Methodist Hospital[2]	Houston	95%	168
Park Plaza Hospital	Houston	95%	38
Scott & White Hospital - Round Rock[2]	Round Rock	95%	84
Scott & White Hospital Brenham	Brenham	95%	41
Seton Medical Center Williamson	Round Rock	95%	98
Temple VA Med Ctr-VA Central Texas	Temple	95%	64
Texas Health Harris Methodist Fort Worth	Fort Worth	95%	350
Texas Health Presbyterian Hospital - WNJ	Sherman	95%	86
Titus Regional Medical Center	Mount Pleasant	95%	95
Val Verde Regional Medical Center	Del Rio	95%	42
VHS Harlingen Hospital Company	Harlingen	95%	241
Angleton - Danbury Medical Center	Angleton	94%	31
Brownwood Regional Medical Center	Brownwood	94%	82
Dallas Regional Medical Center	Mesquite	94%	69
Memorial Hermann Katy Hospital[2]	Katy	94%	89
North Texas Medical Center	Gainesville	94%	53
Palestine Regional Medical Center	Palestine	94%	110
Saint Joseph Regional Health Center	Bryan	94%	162
Bowie Memorial Hospital[2]	Bowie	93%	29
Christus Saint John Hospital	Nassau Bay	93%	117
Connally Memorial Medical Center	Floresville	93%	45
Covenant Hospital Plainview	Plainview	93%	46
Hopkins County Memorial Hospital	Sulphur Springs	93%	121
Matagorda Regional Medical Center	Bay City	93%	44
TX Hlth Harris Meth Hosp-Stephenville	Stephenville	93%	45
University Medical Center at Brackenridge	Austin	93%	74
Univ of Texas Med Branch Galveston[2]	Galveston	93%	41
Christus Hospital[2]	Beaumont	92%	119
Christus Spohn Hospital Alice	Alice	92%	59
Christus Spohn Hospital Beeville	Beeville	92%	50
East Texas Medical Center Jacksonville	Jacksonville	92%	40
Graham Regional Medical Center[2]	Graham	92%	39
Hendrick Medical Center	Abilene	92%	202
Houston VA Medical Center	Houston	92%	75
Lavaca Medical Center	Hallettsville	92%	37
Tomball Regional Medical Center	Tomball	92%	156
Etmc Henderson	Henderson	91%	44
The Medical Center of Southeast Texas	Port Arthur	91%	117
Mother Frances Hospital Jacksonville	Jacksonville	91%	35
Plaza Medical Center of Fort Worth[2]	Fort Worth	91%	54
Seton Medical Center Hays	Kyle	91%	108
Columbus Community Hospital	Columbus	90%	29
Dallas VA Medical Center - VA North Texas	Dallas	90%	96
East Texas Medical Center Quitman	Quitman	90%	42
Etmc Carthage	Carthage	90%	42
Memorial Hospital	Nacogdoches	90%	61
Nix Health Care System	San Antonio	90%	42
Palo Pinto General Hospital	Mineral Wells	90%	67
Christus Jasper Memorial Hospital	Jasper	89%	61
Christus Spohn Hospital Corpus Christi	Corpus Christi	89%	347
Hamilton General Hospital	Hamilton	89%	47
Memorial Medical Center Livingston[2]	Livingston	89%	95
Nocona General Hospital[2]	Nocona	89%	35
Saint Luke's the Woodlands Hospital[2]	The Woodlands	89%	111
Starr County Memorial Hospital	Rio Grande City	89%	103
TX Hlth Presbyterian Hosp-Flower Mound	Flower Mound	89%	84
VHS Brownsville Hospital Company[2]	Brownsville	89%	103
Guadalupe Regional Medical Center	Seguin	88%	64
Memorial Hermann Texas Medical Center[2]	Houston	88%	66
Odessa Regional Hospital	Odessa	88%	57
W J Mangold Memorial Hospital	Lockney	88%	40
Midland Memorial Hospital	Midland	87%	135
Cuero Community Hospital	Cuero	86%	36
East Texas Medical Center Athens[2]	Athens	86%	155
Goodall Witcher Hospital[2]	Clifton	86%	28
Navarro Regional Hospital	Corsicana	86%	58
Tyler County Hospital	Woodville	86%	28
Oakbend Medical Center	Richmond	84%	58
Seymour Hospital	Seymour	84%	43
University Health System[2]	San Antonio	81%	53
East Texas Medical Center Pittsburg	Pittsburg	80%	49
Coryell Memorial Healthcare System	Gatesville	77%	35
Doctors Hospital Tidwell	Houston	76%	45
Lake Whitney Medical Center[2]	Whitney	75%	36
Etmc Clarksville	Clarksville	73%	82
Glen Rose Medical Center	Glen Rose	71%	35
Care Regional Medical Center[2]	Aransas Pass	70%	30
Wilbarger General Hospital[2]	Vernon	70%	30
Sabine County Hospital	Hemphill	68%	34
Covenant Hospital Levelland	Levelland	62%	29
Permian Regional Medical Center	Andrews	55%	40
Falls Community Hospital & Clinic[2]	Marlin	44%	77

Blood Culture Timing

Hospital Name	City	Rate	Cases
Abilene Regional Medical Center	Abilene	100%	88
Baptist Beaumont Hospital[2]	Beaumont	100%	225
Baylor Medical Center at Carrollton	Carrollton	100%	163
Baylor Medical Center at Garland	Garland	100%	283
Baylor Medical Center at Waxahachie	Waxahachie	100%	151
Bayshore Medical Center	Pasadena	100%	425
Big Bend Regional Medical Center	Alpine	100%	33
Christus Saint John Hospital	Nassau Bay	100%	148
Cleveland Regional Medical Center	Cleveland	100%	48
Cogdell Memorial Hospital	Snyder	100%	26
College Station Medical Center	College Station	100%	124
Columbus Community Hospital	Columbus	100%	35
Conroe Regional Medical Center	Conroe	100%	222
The Corpus Christi Medical Center	Corpus Christi	100%	294
Cuero Community Hospital	Cuero	100%	49
Denton Regional Medical Center[2]	Denton	100%	235
Detar Hospital Navarro	Victoria	100%	144
Doctors Hospital of Laredo[2]	Laredo	100%	71
East Texas Medical Center - Gilmer	Gilmer	100%	36
Good Shephard Medical Center - Linden	Linden	100%	45
Harlingen Medical Center	Harlingen	100%	124
Laredo Medical Center	Laredo	100%	341
Las Colinas Medical Center	Irving	100%	101
Las Palmas Medical Center	El Paso	100%	546
Medical Center of Arlington[2]	Arlington	100%	136
Medical Center of Mckinney	Mckinney	100%	215
Medical Center of Plano[2]	Plano	100%	118
Medical City Dallas Hospital	Dallas	100%	203
Memorial Hermann Hospital System[2]	Houston	100%	567
Memorial Hermann Northeast[2]	Humble	100%	110
Memorial Hermann Sugar Land Hospital[2]	Sugar Land	100%	127
Memorial Medical Center	Port Lavaca	100%	50
Methodist Richardson Medical Center[2]	Richardson	100%	130
Methodist Stone Oak Hospital[2]	San Antonio	100%	92
Methodist Sugar Land Hospital[2]	Sugar Land	100%	106
Metroplex Hospital[2]	Killeen	100%	101
Mother Frances Hospital Jacksonville	Jacksonville	100%	47
Nacogdoches Medical Center	Nacogdoches	100%	92
North Austin Medical Center	Austin	100%	278
North Cypress Medical Center	Cypress	100%	302
North Texas Medical Center	Gainesville	100%	76
Peterson Regional Medical Center	Kerrville	100%	224
Plaza Medical Center of Fort Worth[2]	Fort Worth	100%	53
Providence Memorial Hospital[2]	El Paso	100%	143
Round Rock Medical Center	Round Rock	100%	201
Saint Marks Medical Center	La Grange	100%	79
San Angelo Community Medical Center	San Angelo	100%	110
San Jacinto Methodist Hospital	Baytown	100%	261
Scott & White Memorial Hospital[2]	Temple	100%	222
Seton Highland Lakes	Burnet	100%	71
Seton Smithville Regional Hospital	Smithville	100%	38
Sierra Providence East Medical Center[2]	El Paso	100%	123
Texas Health Arlington Memorial Hospital	Arlington	100%	407
TX Hlth Harris Meth Hosp-Alliance[3]	Fort Worth	100%	53
TX Hlth Harris Methodist Hosp-Azle	Azle	100%	156
TX Hlth Harris Meth Hosp-Cleburne	Cleburne	100%	205
Texas Health Presbyterian Hospital - WNJ	Sherman	100%	228
Texas Health Presbyterian Hospital Denton	Denton	100%	270
Texoma Medical Center[2]	Denison	100%	162
United Regional Health Care System	Wichita Falls	100%	329
Val Verde Regional Medical Center	Del Rio	100%	83
Weatherford Regional Medical Center	Weatherford	100%	213
West Houston Medical Center	Houston	100%	200
Baptist Medical Center	San Antonio	99%	1129
Baylor All Saints Medical Center at FW	Fort Worth	99%	358
Baylor Medical Center at Mckinney	Mc Kinney	99%	183
Baylor Regional Medical Center at Plano	Plano	99%	219
Baylor University Medical Center[2]	Dallas	99%	152
Brownwood Regional Medical Center	Brownwood	99%	141
Centennial Medical Center	Frisco	99%	84
Central Texas Medical Center	San Marcos	99%	166
Clear Lake Regional Medical Center[2]	Webster	99%	169
Cypress Fairbanks Medical Center	Houston	99%	204
Dallas Regional Medical Center	Mesquite	99%	144
Dallas VA Medical Center - VA North Texas	Dallas	99%	175
Doctors Hospital	Dallas	99%	198
Doctors Hospital at Renaissance[2]	Edinburg	99%	199
East Texas Medical Center[2]	Tyler	99%	103
Fort Duncan Medical Center[2]	Eagle Pass	99%	115
Good Shepherd Medical Center[2]	Longview	99%	195
Guadalupe Regional Medical Center	Seguin	99%	103
Houston Northwest Medical Center	Houston	99%	197
Lake Granbury Medical Center	Granbury	99%	154
Lake Pointe Medical Center	Rowlett	99%	138
Medical Center of Lewisville	Lewisville	99%	197
The Medical Center of Southeast Texas	Port Arthur	99%	173
Memorial Hermann Katy Hospital[2]	Katy	99%	168
Mem Hermann Mem City Med Ctr[2]	Houston	99%	145
Memorial Hermann Texas Medical Center[2]	Houston	99%	104
Methodist Dallas Medical Center	Dallas	99%	254
Methodist Hospital	San Antonio	99%	1244
Methodist Mansfield Medical Center	Mansfield	99%	226
Methodist Willowbrook Hospital[2]	Houston	99%	180
Midland Memorial Hospital	Midland	99%	202
Mother Frances Hospital[2]	Tyler	99%	360
North Hills Hospital[2]	N Richland Hls	99%	188
Palestine Regional Medical Center	Palestine	99%	161
Parkland Health & Hospital System[2]	Dallas	99%	137
Red River Regional Hospital	Bonham	99%	76
Rio Grande Regional Hospital	Mcallen	99%	239
Saint David's Medical Center	Austin	99%	366
Saint David's South Austin Medical Center[2]	Austin	99%	159
Saint Joseph Regional Health Center	Bryan	99%	304
Saint Luke's Episcopal Hospital[2]	Houston	99%	147
Saint Luke's Hospital at the Vintage	Houston	99%	128
Saint Luke's Patients Medical Center[2]	Pasadena	99%	109
Saint Luke's the Woodlands Hospital[2]	The Woodlands	99%	142
Scott & White Hospital - Round Rock[2]	Round Rock	99%	146
Scott & White Hospital Brenham	Brenham	99%	67
Shannon Medical Center	San Angelo	99%	363
Sierra Medical Center[2]	El Paso	99%	152
Southwest General Hospital	San Antonio	99%	157
Temple VA Med Ctr-VA Central Texas	Temple	99%	135
Texas Health Harris Methodist Fort Worth	Fort Worth	99%	691
TX Hlth Harris Meth Hosp-Stephenville	Stephenville	99%	86
TX Hlth Harris Meth Hosp SW Ft Worth	Fort Worth	99%	413
Texas Health Harris Methodist	Bedford	99%	375
Texas Health Presbyterian Hospital Allen	Allen	99%	124
Texas Health Presbyterian Hospital Dallas	Dallas	99%	198
TX Hlth Presbyterian Hosp-Kaufman	Kaufman	99%	123
TX Health Presbyterian Hosp Rockwall	Rockwall	99%	207
Tomball Regional Medical Center	Tomball	99%	225
University Medical Center[2]	Lubbock	99%	125
University Medical Center of El Paso	El Paso	99%	159
UT Southwestern University Hospital	Dallas	99%	241
Valley Regional Medical Center	Brownsville	99%	167
VHS Harlingen Hospital Company	Harlingen	99%	441
Wise Regional Health System	Decatur	99%	167
Woodland Heights Medical Center	Lufkin	99%	92
Baptist Saint Anthony's Hospital[2]	Amarillo	98%	196
Baylor Medical Center at Irving[2]	Irving	98%	190
Baylor Reg Med Ctr at Grapevine	Grapevine	98%	284
Cedar Park Regional Medical Center	Cedar Park	98%	133
Christus Santa Rosa Hospital	San Antonio	98%	541
Citizens Medical Center	Victoria	98%	174
Coleman County Medical Center Company	Coleman	98%	40
Connally Memorial Medical Center	Floresville	98%	47
Dallas Medical Center[2]	Dallas	98%	42
East Texas Medical Center Jacksonville	Jacksonville	98%	56
Good Shepherd Medical Center Marshall	Marshall	98%	190
Hill Country Memorial Hospital	Fredericksburg	98%	61
Hill Regional Hospital	Hillsboro	98%	60
Kingwood Medical Center	Kingwood	98%	250
Lavaca Medical Center	Hallettsville	98%	41
Medical Center Hospital	Odessa	98%	234
Memorial Hermann Baptist Orange Hospital	Orange	98%	97
The Methodist Hospital[2]	Houston	98%	340
Navarro Regional Hospital	Corsicana	98%	94
Nix Health Care System	San Antonio	98%	43
Oakbend Medical Center	Richmond	98%	145
Palo Pinto General Hospital	Mineral Wells	98%	96
Park Plaza Hospital	Houston	98%	90
Providence Health Center	Waco	98%	542
Rolling Plains Memorial Hospital	Sweetwater	98%	50
Saint Joseph Medical Center	Houston	98%	196
Saint Luke's Sugar Land Hospital	Sugar Land	98%	122
San Antonio VA Medical Center	San Antonio	98%	165
Scenic Mountain Medical Center	Big Spring	98%	50
Scott & White Hospital - Llano	Llano	98%	53
Seton Edgar B Davis Hospital	Luling	98%	52
Seton Medical Center Austin	Austin	98%	276
Seton Medical Center Williamson	Round Rock	98%	194
Seton Northwest Hospital	Austin	98%	145
South Texas Health System[2]	Edinburg	98%	131
South Texas Regional Medical Center	Jourdanton	98%	87
TX Hlth Presbyterian Hosp-Flower Mound	Flower Mound	98%	122
Texas Health Presbyterian Hospital Plano	Plano	98%	247
Texas Reg Med Ctr at Sunnyvale	Sunnyvale	98%	125
Titus Regional Medical Center	Mount Pleasant	98%	81
University Medical Center at Brackenridge	Austin	98%	143
Univ of TX Health Science Ctr-Tyler[2]	Tyler	98%	109
Univ of Texas Med Branch Galveston[2]	Galveston	98%	84
VA Amarillo Healthcare System	Amarillo	98%	66
Wadley Regional Medical Center	Texarkana	98%	182
Christus Hospital[2]	Beaumont	97%	149

NOTE: Hospital profiles are in alphabetical order by state, then city, then hospital within the city; Rankings exclude hospitals with less than 25 cases except for patient surveys which excludes hospitals with less than 100 cases; (a) 100-299 cases; (1) The number of cases/patients is too few to report; (2) Data submitted were based on a sample of cases/patients; (3) Results are based on a shorter time period than required; (4) Data suppressed by CMS for one or more quarters; (5) Results are not available for this reporting period; (6) Fewer than 100 patients completed the HCAHPS survey; (7) No cases met the criteria for this measure; (8) The lower limit of the confidence interval cannot be calculated if the number of observed infections equals zero; (9) No data are available from the state/territory for this reporting period; (10) The scores shown reflect fewer than 50 completed surveys; (11) There were discrepancies in the data collection process; (12) This measure does not apply to this hospital for this reporting period; (13) Results cannot be calculated for this reporting period; (14) The results for this state are combined with nearby states to protect confidentiality; Please refer to the User's Guide for a full explanation of data.

Christus Saint Michael Health System	Texarkana	97%	383
Christus Spohn Hospital Kleberg[2]	Kingsville	97%	92
Covenant Medical Center	Lubbock	97%	499
Glen Rose Medical Center	Glen Rose	97%	39
Harris Health System[2]	Houston	97%	313
The Hospital at Westlake Medical Center	Austin	97%	33
Houston VA Medical Center	Houston	97%	158
Huguley Memorial Medical Center	Burleson	97%	311
Hunt Regional Medical Center	Greenville	97%	307
Longview Regional Medical Center	Longview	97%	155
Lubbock Heart Hospital[2]	Lubbock	97%	34
Memorial Hospital	Nacogdoches	97%	100
Memorial Medical Center Livingston[2]	Livingston	97%	129
Memorial Medical Center of East Texas[2]	Lufkin	97%	100
Methodist Charlton Medical Center	Dallas	97%	212
Methodist West Houston Hospital[2]	Houston	97%	206
Mission Regional Medical Center	Mission	97%	302
Pampa Regional Medical Center	Pampa	97%	58
Seton Medical Center Harker Heights	Harker Heights	97%	92
Seton Medical Center Hays	Kyle	97%	219
Tyler County Hospital	Woodville	97%	29
Brazosport Regional Health System[2]	Lake Jackson	96%	164
Christus Saint Catherine Hospital	Katy	96%	80
Christus Spohn Hospital Alice	Alice	96%	84
Christus Spohn Hospital Beeville	Beeville	96%	81
East Texas Medical Center - Fairfield	Fairfield	96%	57
East Texas Medical Center Athens[2]	Athens	96%	297
Etmc Henderson	Henderson	96%	76
Graham Regional Medical Center[2]	Graham	96%	47
Hendrick Medical Center	Abilene	96%	313
Huntsville Memorial Hospital	Huntsville	96%	160
JPS Health Network	Fort Worth	96%	308
Medina Regional Hospital[3]	Hondo	96%	28
Northwest Texas Hospital[2]	Amarillo	96%	110
Seymour Hospital	Seymour	96%	25
VHS Brownsville Hospital Company[2]	Brownsville	96%	262
Doctors Hospital Tidwell	Houston	95%	56
Hamilton General Hospital	Hamilton	95%	102
Hillcrest Baptist Medical Center[2]	Waco	95%	162
Knapp Medical Center	Weslaco	95%	190
Odessa Regional Hospital	Odessa	95%	80
Ennis Regional Medical Center	Ennis	94%	122
Gulf Coast Medical Center[2]	Wharton	94%	34
Uvalde Memorial Hospital	Uvalde	94%	90
Covenant Hospital Plainview	Plainview	93%	45
Etmc Carthage	Carthage	93%	54
Golden Plains Community Hospital	Borger	93%	30
Hopkins County Memorial Hospital	Sulphur Springs	93%	132
Christus Jasper Memorial Hospital	Jasper	92%	86
Christus Spohn Hospital Corpus Christi	Corpus Christi	92%	814
El Campo Memorial Hospital	El Campo	92%	25
Frio Regional Hospital	Pearsall	92%	26
East Texas Medical Center Quitman	Quitman	91%	32
Paris Regional Medical Center[2]	Paris	91%	133
Parkview Regional Hospital	Mexia	91%	66
Etmc Clarksville	Clarksville	90%	62
Angleton - Danbury Medical Center	Angleton	89%	37
East Texas Medical Center Trinity[2]	Trinity	89%	35
Goodall Witcher Hospital[2]	Clifton	89%	27
Matagorda Regional Medical Center	Bay City	89%	64
East Texas Medical Center Pittsburg	Pittsburg	88%	57
Pecos County Memorial Hospital[2]	Fort Stockton	87%	31
Starr County Memorial Hospital	Rio Grande City	87%	143
Coryell Memorial Healthcare System	Gatesville	84%	51
Bowie Memorial Hospital[2]	Bowie	82%	33
Eastland Memorial Hospital[2]	Eastland	81%	26
Care Regional Medical Center[2]	Aransas Pass	80%	70
Falls Community Hospital & Clinic[2]	Marlin	78%	27
Permian Regional Medical Center	Andrews	75%	32
University Health System[2]	San Antonio	74%	85
Wilbarger General Hospital[2]	Vernon	68%	25

Pregnancy and Delivery Care

Newborns whose Deliveries were Scheduled Early

Hospital Name	City	Rate	Cases
Baptist Saint Anthony's Hospital[2]	Amarillo	0%	42
Cedar Park Regional Medical Center[2]	Cedar Park	0%	28
Centennial Medical Center[2]	Frisco	0%	47
Christus Spohn Hospital Beeville[2]	Beeville	0%	34
Clear Lake Regional Medical Center[2]	Webster	0%	82
Dimmit Regional Hospital[2]	Carrizo Springs	0%	43
Good Shepherd Medical Center Marshall	Marshall	0%	25
Houston Northwest Medical Center[2]	Houston	0%	68
Kingwood Medical Center[2]	Kingwood	0%	54
Laredo Medical Center[2]	Laredo	0%	167
Las Colinas Medical Center[2]	Irving	0%	44
Memorial Hermann Northeast[2]	Humble	0%	38
The Methodist Hospital	Houston	0%	97
Methodist Willowbrook Hospital[2]	Houston	0%	84
Nacogdoches Medical Center[2]	Nacogdoches	0%	32
Navarro Regional Hospital[2]	Corsicana	0%	46
North Texas Medical Center[2]	Gainesville	0%	29
Northwest Texas Hospital[2]	Amarillo	0%	40
Pampa Regional Medical Center	Pampa	0%	28
Rio Grande Regional Hospital[2]	Mcallen	0%	79
Rolling Plains Memorial Hospital	Sweetwater	0%	31
Saint David's South Austin Medical Center[2]	Austin	0%	47
Seton Medical Center Austin	Austin	0%	227
Seton Medical Center Hays	Kyle	0%	60
Seton Medical Center Williamson	Round Rock	0%	72
Seton Northwest Hospital	Austin	0%	77
Seton Southwest Hospital	Austin	0%	49
South Texas Regional Medical Center[2]	Jourdanton	0%	42
Texas Reg Med Ctr at Sunnyvale[2]	Sunnyvale	0%	31
University Medical Center[2]	Lubbock	0%	60
University Medical Center at Brackenridge	Austin	0%	97
UT Southwestern University Hospital[2]	Dallas	0%	42
Valley Regional Medical Center[2]	Brownsville	0%	71
Wadley Regional Medical Center[2]	Texarkana	0%	26
West Houston Medical Center[2]	Houston	0%	61
Woodland Heights Medical Center[2]	Lufkin	0%	47
JPS Health Network[2]	Fort Worth	1%	68
Memorial Hospital	Nacogdoches	1%	102
Methodist Hospital[2]	San Antonio	1%	144
North Austin Medical Center[2]	Austin	1%	96
Saint David's Medical Center[2]	Austin	1%	94
Scott & White Memorial Hospital[2]	Temple	1%	75
Shannon Medical Center	San Angelo	1%	119
University Medical Center of El Paso[2]	El Paso	1%	77
Baylor Medical Center at Frisco	Frisco	2%	235
Baylor Medical Center at Irving	Irving	2%	211
Bayshore Medical Center[2]	Pasadena	2%	115
East Texas Medical Center Jacksonville	Jacksonville	2%	45
Good Shepherd Medical Center[2]	Longview	2%	56
Hopkins County Memorial Hospital[2]	Sulphur Springs	2%	44
Knapp Medical Center[2]	Weslaco	2%	47
Medical Center of Plano[2]	Plano	2%	43
Methodist Charlton Medical Center[2]	Dallas	2%	257
Methodist Dallas Medical Center[2]	Dallas	2%	316
Methodist Stone Oak Hospital[2]	San Antonio	2%	43
Peterson Regional Medical Center	Kerrville	2%	51
Texas Health Arlington Memorial Hospital	Arlington	2%	214
Texoma Medical Center[2]	Denison	2%	42
Val Verde Regional Medical Center	Del Rio	2%	133
VHS Brownsville Hospital Company	Brownsville	2%	217
The Womans Hospital of Texas[2]	Houston	2%	122
Baptist Beaumont Hospital[2]	Beaumont	3%	31
Baptist Medical Center[2]	San Antonio	3%	138
Baylor All Saints Medical Center at FW	Fort Worth	3%	510
Baylor University Medical Center	Dallas	3%	354
The Corpus Christi Medical Center[2]	Corpus Christi	3%	60
Denton Regional Medical Center[2]	Denton	3%	34
Doctors Hospital of Laredo[2]	Laredo	3%	63
Ennis Regional Medical Center[2]	Ennis	3%	39
Hill Country Memorial Hospital	Fredericksburg	3%	29
Hunt Regional Medical Center[2]	Greenville	3%	35
Las Palmas Medical Center[2]	El Paso	3%	115
North Hills Hospital[2]	N Richland Hls	3%	32
Parkland Health & Hospital System[2]	Dallas	3%	78
Sierra Medical Center[2]	El Paso	3%	62
South Texas Health System[2]	Edinburg	3%	35
Texas Health Presbyterian Hospital - WNJ	Sherman	3%	34
University Health System[2]	San Antonio	3%	30
Baylor Medical Center at Carrollton	Carrollton	4%	126
Columbus Community Hospital	Columbus	4%	25
Detar Hospital Navarro[2]	Victoria	4%	56
Harlingen Medical Center	Harlingen	4%	105
Huntsville Memorial Hospital	Huntsville	4%	45
Medical Center Hospital[2]	Odessa	4%	48
Medical Center of Mckinney[2]	Mckinney	4%	51
Medical City Dallas Hospital[2]	Dallas	4%	57
Methodist Sugar Land Hospital[2]	Sugar Land	4%	56
Paris Regional Medical Center	Paris	4%	120
Providence Memorial Hospital[2]	El Paso	4%	95
San Angelo Community Medical Center[2]	San Angelo	4%	57
TX Hlth Harris Meth Hosp SW Ft Worth	Fort Worth	4%	315
Uvalde Memorial Hospital	Uvalde	4%	25
Covenant Hospital Levelland[2]	Levelland	5%	39
Memorial Hermann Hospital System[2]	Houston	5%	299
Memorial Hospital[2]	Gonzales	5%	61
San Jacinto Methodist Hospital	Baytown	5%	142
Seton Medical Center Harker Heights	Harker Heights	5%	87
Sierra Providence East Medical Center[2]	El Paso	5%	66
Weatherford Regional Medical Center[2]	Weatherford	5%	38
Baylor Medical Center at Garland	Garland	6%	151
Doctors Hospital at Renaissance[2,3]	Edinburg	6%	1288
Harris Health System	Houston	6%	425
Hendrick Medical Center[2]	Abilene	6%	31
TX Hlth Harris Meth Hosp-Stephenville	Stephenville	6%	31
Titus Regional Medical Center	Mount Pleasant	6%	135
Tomball Regional Medical Center[2]	Tomball	6%	34
Brazosport Regional Health System[2]	Lake Jackson	7%	27
Brownwood Regional Medical Center[2]	Brownwood	7%	44
Citizens Medical Center[2]	Victoria	7%	45
Doctors Hospital[2]	Dallas	7%	45
Guadalupe Regional Medical Center	Seguin	7%	103
Lake Pointe Medical Center[2]	Rowlett	7%	41
Medical Center of Arlington[2]	Arlington	7%	82
Medical Center of Lewisville[2]	Lewisville	7%	28
Methodist Mansfield Medical Center[2]	Mansfield	7%	188
Saint Joseph Medical Center[2]	Houston	7%	83
Southwest General Hospital[2]	San Antonio	7%	56
Texas Health Harris Methodist	Bedford	7%	227
TX Hlth Presbyterian Hosp-Flower Mound[2]	Flower Mound	7%	29
TX Health Presbyterian Hosp Rockwall	Rockwall	7%	85
College Station Medical Center[2]	College Station	8%	61
Cypress Fairbanks Medical Center[2]	Houston	8%	71
Hereford Regional Medical Center	Hereford	8%	51
Matagorda Regional Medical Center	Bay City	8%	66
TX Hlth Harris Meth Hosp-Cleburne	Cleburne	8%	65
Texas Health Presbyterian Hospital Dallas	Dallas	8%	575
Baylor Medical Center at Mckinney	Mc Kinney	9%	124
Christus Saint Catherine Hospital[2]	Katy	9%	32
Hillcrest Baptist Medical Center[2]	Waco	9%	85
Huguley Memorial Medical Center[2]	Burleson	9%	44
Mem Hermann Mem City Med Ctr[2]	Houston	9%	68
Saint Luke's Hospital at the Vintage	Houston	9%	47
Texas Health Harris Methodist Fort Worth	Fort Worth	9%	249
Abilene Regional Medical Center[2]	Abilene	10%	42
Christus Saint Michael Health System[2]	Texarkana	10%	31
East Texas Medical Center Athens	Athens	10%	83
Mother Frances Hospital	Tyler	10%	207
Round Rock Medical Center[2]	Round Rock	10%	31
Texas Health Presbyterian Hospital Allen	Allen	10%	59
Univ of Texas Med Branch Galveston[2]	Galveston	10%	73
Oakbend Medical Center	Richmond	11%	148
Saint Joseph Regional Health Center[2]	Bryan	11%	73
TX Hlth Harris Meth Hosp-Alliance	Fort Worth	11%	81
Texas Health Presbyterian Hospital Denton	Denton	11%	188
Mission Regional Medical Center[2]	Mission	12%	73
VHS Harlingen Hospital Company[2]	Harlingen	12%	83
Christus Santa Rosa Hospital	San Antonio	13%	216
Methodist West Houston Hospital[2]	Houston	13%	52
Midland Memorial Hospital[2]	Midland	13%	237
United Regional Health Care System	Wichita Falls	13%	186
Memorial Hermann Texas Medical Center[2]	Houston	14%	107
Methodist Richardson Medical Center	Richardson	15%	34
Covenant Hospital Plainview[2]	Plainview	16%	49
Baylor Reg Med Ctr at Grapevine	Grapevine	17%	230
Christus Saint John Hospital	Nassau Bay	17%	69
Park Plaza Hospital[2]	Houston	18%	28
Saint Luke's the Woodlands Hospital	The Woodlands	18%	146
Texas Health Presbyterian Hospital Plano	Plano	18%	369
Angleton - Danbury Medical Center	Angleton	19%	54
The Medical Center of Southeast Texas[2]	Port Arthur	19%	48
Odessa Regional Hospital[2]	Odessa	19%	43
Palo Pinto General Hospital[2]	Mineral Wells	19%	27
Wise Regional Health System	Decatur	20%	70
Memorial Hermann Katy Hospital[2]	Katy	22%	65
Christus Spohn Hospital Kleberg[2]	Kingsville	23%	30
Fort Duncan Medical Center[2]	Eagle Pass	23%	53
Memorial Medical Center of East Texas[2]	Lufkin	23%	112
Doctors Hospital Tidwell	Houston	24%	186
Palestine Regional Medical Center[2]	Palestine	26%	27
Central Texas Medical Center[2]	San Marcos	28%	40
Christus Spohn Hospital Alice[2]	Alice	28%	32
Covenant Medical Center[2]	Lubbock	31%	55
Memorial Medical Center Livingston[2]	Livingston	37%	49
Christus Hospital[2]	Beaumont	55%	76
Permian Regional Medical Center	Andrews	55%	58

Preventive Care

Immunization for Influenza

Hospital Name	City	Rate	Cases
Abilene Regional Medical Center[2]	Abilene	100%	548
Baylor Medical Center at Trophy Club[2]	Trophy Club	100%	400
Baylor Regional Medical Center at Plano[2]	Plano	100%	597
Conroe Regional Medical Center[2]	Conroe	100%	625
The Corpus Christi Medical Center[2]	Corpus Christi	100%	549
Detar Hospital Navarro[2]	Victoria	100%	552
Electra Memorial Hospital	Electra	100%	28
Heart Hospital Baylor Plano[2]	Plano	100%	395
The Hospital at Westlake Medical Center[2]	Austin	100%	495
Huntsville Memorial Hospital[2]	Huntsville	100%	415
Laredo Medical Center[2]	Laredo	100%	547
Las Colinas Medical Center[2]	Irving	100%	460
Longview Regional Medical Center[2]	Longview	100%	579
Medical Center of Plano[2]	Plano	100%	622
Methodist Stone Oak Hospital[2]	San Antonio	100%	524

NOTE: Hospital profiles are in alphabetical order by state, then city, then hospital within the city; Rankings exclude hospitals with less than 25 cases except for patient surveys which excludes hospitals with less than 100 cases; (a) 100-299 cases; (1) The number of cases/patients is too few to report; (2) Data submitted were based on a sample of cases/patients; (3) Results are based on a shorter time period than required; (4) Data suppressed by CMS for one or more quarters; (5) Results are not available for this reporting period; (6) Fewer than 100 patients completed the HCAHPS survey; (7) No cases met the criteria for this measure; (8) The lower limit of the confidence interval cannot be calculated if the number of observed infections equals zero; (9) No data are available from the state/territory for this reporting period; (10) The scores shown reflect fewer than 50 completed surveys; (11) There were discrepancies in the data collection process; (12) This measure does not apply to this hospital for this reporting period; (13) Results cannot be calculated for this reporting period; (14) The results for this state are combined with nearby states to protect confidentiality; Please refer to the User's Guide for a full explanation of data.

Pampa Regional Medical Center[2]	Pampa	100%	443
Rio Grande Regional Hospital[2]	Mcallen	100%	554
Rolling Plains Memorial Hospital[2]	Sweetwater	100%	279
Southwest General Hospital[2]	San Antonio	100%	601
TX Hlth Harris Methodist Hosp-Azle[2]	Azle	100%	361
TX Hlth Harris Meth Hosp-Cleburne[2]	Cleburne	100%	401
Texoma Medical Center[2]	Denison	100%	563
Weatherford Regional Medical Center[2]	Weatherford	100%	527
Woodland Heights Medical Center[2]	Lufkin	100%	526
Baylor Heart & Vascular Hospital[2]	Dallas	99%	298
Baylor Medical Center at Frisco[2]	Frisco	99%	414
Baylor Medical Center at Mckinney[2]	Mc Kinney	99%	451
Brownwood Regional Medical Center[2]	Brownwood	99%	483
Cornerstone Regional Hospital[2]	Edinburg	99%	247
Cuero Community Hospital[2]	Cuero	99%	276
El Campo Memorial Hospital	El Campo	99%	169
Graham Regional Medical Center[2]	Graham	99%	283
Harlingen Medical Center[2]	Harlingen	99%	533
Heart Hospital Baylor Denton	Denton	99%	109
Kingwood Medical Center[2]	Kingwood	99%	572
Lake Granbury Medical Center[2]	Granbury	99%	299
Lake Pointe Medical Center[2]	Rowlett	99%	541
Medical Center of Lewisville[2]	Lewisville	99%	496
Mem Hermann Surgical Hosp Kingwood	Kingwood	99%	83
Methodist Ambulatory Surgery Hospital NW[2]	San Antonio	99%	303
Methodist Dallas Medical Center[2]	Dallas	99%	483
Methodist Sugar Land Hospital[2]	Sugar Land	99%	528
North Cypress Medical Center[2]	Cypress	99%	674
The Physicians Centre	Bryan	99%	195
Providence Memorial Hospital[2]	El Paso	99%	498
Saint David's Medical Center[2]	Austin	99%	532
Saint David's South Austin Medical Center[2]	Austin	99%	575
Saint Luke's Patients Medical Center[2]	Pasadena	99%	356
Sierra Providence East Medical Center[2]	El Paso	99%	539
Texas Health Arlington Memorial Hospital[2]	Arlington	99%	585
TX Hlth Harris Meth Hosp-Alliance[2,3]	Fort Worth	99%	138
TX Hlth Harris Meth Hosp-Stephenville[2]	Stephenville	99%	285
Texas Health Harris Methodist[2]	Bedford	99%	631
TX Hlth Heart & Vasc Hosp-Arlington[2]	Arlington	99%	293
Texas Health Presbyterian Hospital Dallas[2]	Dallas	99%	560
Texas Orthopedic Hospital[2]	Houston	99%	361
University Medical Center of El Paso[2]	El Paso	99%	518
Valley Regional Medical Center[2]	Brownsville	99%	487
Baylor Medical Center at Carrollton[2]	Carrollton	98%	509
Big Bend Regional Medical Center[2]	Alpine	98%	323
Cedar Park Regional Medical Center[2]	Cedar Park	98%	500
Christus Saint John Hospital[2]	Nassau Bay	98%	551
Clear Lake Regional Medical Center[2]	Webster	98%	629
Connally Memorial Medical Center[2]	Floresville	98%	312
Dallas Regional Medical Center[2]	Mesquite	98%	1108
Mem Hermann Mem City Med Ctr[2]	Houston	98%	530
Memorial Hermann Northeast[2]	Humble	98%	561
Memorial Hermann Sugar Land Hospital[2]	Sugar Land	98%	482
Memorial Hospital[2]	Gonzales	98%	307
Methodist Charlton Medical Center[2]	Dallas	98%	523
Methodist Hospital[2]	San Antonio	98%	631
Methodist Willowbrook Hospital[2]	Houston	98%	497
Midland Memorial Hospital[2]	Midland	98%	1259
North Hills Hospital[2]	N Richland Hls	98%	553
Odessa Regional Hospital[2]	Odessa	98%	548
Round Rock Medical Center[2]	Round Rock	98%	475
San Jacinto Methodist Hospital[2]	Baytown	98%	676
Seton Medical Center Williamson[2]	Round Rock	98%	543
South Texas Regional Medical Center[2]	Jourdanton	98%	272
Surgery Specialty Hosps of America[2]	Pasadena	98%	51
TX Hlth Harris Meth Hosp SW Ft Worth[2]	Fort Worth	98%	556
Texas Health Presbyterian Hospital Allen[2]	Allen	98%	459
Texas Health Presbyterian Hospital Denton[2]	Denton	98%	581
Baptist Saint Anthony's Hospital[2]	Amarillo	97%	618
Baylor All Saints Medical Center at FW[2]	Fort Worth	97%	461
Baylor Medical Center at Garland[2]	Garland	97%	555
Baylor Medical Center at Irving[2]	Irving	97%	521
Bayshore Medical Center[2]	Pasadena	97%	541
Centennial Medical Center[2]	Frisco	97%	471
Christus Saint Catherine Hospital[2]	Katy	97%	354
Columbus Community Hospital[2]	Columbus	97%	291
Hill Country Memorial Hospital[2]	Fredericksburg	97%	316
Lavaca Medical Center	Hallettsville	97%	259
Medical Center Hospital[2]	Odessa	97%	748
Medical Center of Mckinney[2]	Mckinney	97%	585
Medical City Dallas Hospital[2]	Dallas	97%	640
Memorial Hermann Katy Hospital[2]	Katy	97%	493
Methodist Mansfield Medical Center[2]	Mansfield	97%	497
Methodist Richardson Medical Center[2]	Richardson	97%	452
Navarro Regional Hospital[2]	Corsicana	97%	371
North Austin Medical Center[2]	Austin	97%	532
Peterson Regional Medical Center[2]	Kerrville	97%	442
Quail Creek Surgical Hospital	Amarillo	97%	715
Saint Joseph Regional Health Center[2]	Bryan	97%	571
San Angelo Community Medical Center[2]	San Angelo	97%	559
Scenic Mountain Medical Center[2]	Big Spring	97%	316

Scott & White Hospital Brenham[2]	Brenham	97%	244
Sierra Medical Center[2]	El Paso	97%	555
South Texas Spine & Surgical Hospital	San Antonio	97%	526
Texas Health Harris Methodist Fort Worth[2]	Fort Worth	97%	627
TX Hlth Presbyterian Hosp-Flower Mound[2]	Flower Mound	97%	463
TX Hlth Presbyterian Hosp-Kaufman[2]	Kaufman	97%	317
TX Health Presbyterian Hosp Rockwall[2]	Rockwall	97%	426
United Regional Health Care System[2]	Wichita Falls	97%	496
Baptist Beaumont Hospital[2]	Beaumont	96%	555
Baptist Medical Center[2]	San Antonio	96%	2241
Baylor Ortho & Spine Hosp-Arlington[2]	Arlington	96%	331
Baylor Surgical Hospital at Las Colinas[2]	Irving	96%	232
Baylor University Medical Center[2]	Dallas	96%	547
Cleveland Regional Medical Center[2]	Cleveland	96%	396
Doctors Hospital at Renaissance[2]	Edinburg	96%	439
Houston Northwest Medical Center[2]	Houston	96%	527
Hunt Regional Medical Center[2]	Greenville	96%	505
Matagorda Regional Medical Center[2]	Bay City	96%	254
Memorial Hermann Hospital System[2]	Houston	96%	2066
The Methodist Hospital[2]	Houston	96%	602
Methodist West Houston Hospital[2]	Houston	96%	562
Palestine Regional Medical Center[2]	Palestine	96%	426
Parkview Regional Hospital[2]	Mexia	96%	297
Saint Marks Medical Center[2]	La Grange	96%	304
Seton Southwest Hospital[2]	Austin	96%	186
Sugar Land Surgical Hospital	Sugar Land	96%	137
Texas Health Presbyterian Hospital - WNJ[2]	Sherman	96%	576
Tops Surgical Specialty Hospital[2]	Houston	96%	315
UT Southwestern University Hospital[2]	Dallas	96%	545
UT SW Univ Hosp-Zale Lipshy[2]	Dallas	96%	607
West Houston Medical Center[2]	Houston	96%	539
Baylor Medical Center at Waxahachie[2]	Waxahachie	95%	331
Covenant Medical Center[2]	Lubbock	95%	601
Cypress Fairbanks Medical Center[2]	Houston	95%	493
Denton Regional Medical Center[2]	Denton	95%	621
East Texas Medical Center[2]	Tyler	95%	555
Grace Medical Center	Lubbock	95%	456
Kell West Regional Hospital	Wichita Falls	95%	458
Medical Center of Arlington[2]	Arlington	95%	531
Memorial Hermann Baptist Orange Hospital[2]	Orange	95%	257
Nix Health Care System[2]	San Antonio	95%	788
Paris Regional Medical Center[2]	Paris	95%	524
Plaza Medical Center of Fort Worth[2]	Fort Worth	95%	663
Seton Smithville Regional Hospital[2]	Smithville	95%	222
South Texas Health System[2]	Edinburg	95%	551
TX Hlth Harris Meth Hosp-Southlake[2]	Southlake	95%	354
Angleton - Danbury Medical Center[2]	Angleton	94%	251
Christus Saint Michael Health System[2]	Texarkana	94%	556
Citizens Medical Center[2]	Victoria	94%	553
College Station Medical Center[2]	College Station	94%	600
Good Shepherd Medical Center[2]	Longview	94%	553
Guadalupe Regional Medical Center[2]	Seguin	94%	370
Metroplex Hospital[2]	Killeen	94%	462
Nacogdoches Medical Center[2]	Nacogdoches	94%	428
Rollins Brook Community Hospital[2]	Lampasas	94%	281
Saint Luke's the Woodlands Hospital[2]	The Woodlands	94%	526
Seton Medical Center Hays[2]	Kyle	94%	541
Basin Healthcare Center	Odessa	93%	73
Central Texas Medical Center[2]	San Marcos	93%	442
Gulf Coast Medical Center[2]	Wharton	93%	245
JPS Health Network[2]	Fort Worth	93%	645
Memorial Medical Center of East Texas[2]	Lufkin	93%	548
Moore County Hospital District[2]	Dumas	93%	211
Scott & White Hospital - Round Rock[2]	Round Rock	93%	487
Stephens Memorial Hospital[2]	Breckenridge	93%	229
Texas Health Presbyterian Hospital Plano[2]	Plano	93%	537
VHS Brownsville Hospital Company[2]	Brownsville	93%	525
East Texas Medical Center Jacksonville[2]	Jacksonville	92%	227
Hillcrest Baptist Medical Center[2]	Waco	92%	476
Houston Physicians' Hospital	Webster	92%	264
North Texas Medical Center[2]	Gainesville	92%	231
Park Plaza Hospital[2]	Houston	92%	531
Saint Luke's Episcopal Hospital[2]	Houston	92%	639
Saint Luke's Sugar Land Hospital[2]	Sugar Land	92%	341
TX Health Ctr for Diag & Surgery	Plano	92%	311
Wise Regional Health System[2]	Decatur	92%	501
Christus Spohn Hospital Corpus Christi[2]	Corpus Christi	91%	601
Christus Spohn Hospital Kleberg[2]	Kingsville	91%	371
East Texas Medical Center - Fairfield	Fairfield	91%	231
Ennis Regional Medical Center[2]	Ennis	91%	319
Hendrick Medical Center[2]	Abilene	91%	563
Saint Joseph Medical Center[2]	Houston	91%	609
Saint Luke's Hospital at the Vintage[2]	Houston	91%	346
Saint Luke's Lakeside Hospital[2]	The Woodlands	91%	326
Seton Northwest Hospital[2]	Austin	91%	480
University Medical Center at Brackenridge[2]	Austin	91%	532
Val Verde Regional Medical Center[2]	Del Rio	91%	298
VHS Harlingen Hospital Company[2]	Harlingen	91%	497
Hamilton General Hospital[2]	Hamilton	90%	336
Hill Regional Hospital[2]	Hillsboro	90%	285
Hopkins County Memorial Hospital[2]	Sulphur Springs	90%	344

The Medical Center of Southeast Texas[2]	Port Arthur	90%	688
Otto Kaiser Memorial Hospital	Kenedy	90%	88
Shannon Medical Center[2]	San Angelo	90%	667
Wadley Regional Medical Center[2]	Texarkana	90%	557
Christus Santa Rosa Hospital[2]	San Antonio	89%	637
Christus Spohn Hospital Beeville[2]	Beeville	89%	277
Doctors Hospital[2]	Dallas	89%	565
East Texas Medical Center - Gilmer[2]	Gilmer	89%	226
El Paso Specialty Hospital[2]	El Paso	89%	329
Etmc Carthage[2]	Carthage	89%	312
Falls Community Hospital & Clinic[2]	Marlin	89%	197
Memorial Medical Center Livingston[2]	Livingston	89%	261
Northwest Texas Hospital[2]	Amarillo	89%	527
Pecos County Memorial Hospital[2]	Fort Stockton	89%	235
Brazosport Regional Health System[2]	Lake Jackson	88%	494
Dallas Medical Center[2]	Dallas	88%	310
Doctors Hospital of Laredo[2]	Laredo	88%	431
Foundation Surgical Hospital of El Paso[2]	El Paso	88%	304
Frio Regional Hospital	Pearsall	88%	167
Harris Health System[2]	Houston	88%	966
Huguley Memorial Medical Center[2]	Burleson	88%	540
Knapp Medical Center[2]	Weslaco	88%	411
Allegiance Specialty Hospital of Kilgore[2]	Kilgore	87%	336
Baylor Medical Center at Uptown[2]	Dallas	87%	316
Doctors Diagnostic Hospital[2]	Cleveland	87%	244
East Texas Medical Center Quitman[2]	Quitman	87%	292
Mission Regional Medical Center[2]	Mission	87%	436
Scott & White Hospital - Llano	Llano	87%	314
Scott & White Memorial Hospital[2]	Temple	87%	563
Seton Medical Center Austin[2]	Austin	87%	517
Childress Regional Medical Center[2]	Childress	86%	237
Memorial Hermann Texas Medical Center[2]	Houston	86%	520
Memorial Hospital[2]	Nacogdoches	86%	418
Parkland Health & Hospital System[2]	Dallas	86%	479
Saint Anthony's Hospital[2,3]	Houston	86%	153
Seymour Hospital	Seymour	86%	199
Univ of TX Health Science Ctr-Tyler[2]	Tyler	86%	326
USMD Hospital at Fort Worth	Fort Worth	86%	236
Doctors Hospital Tidwell[2]	Houston	85%	339
Glen Rose Medical Center	Glen Rose	85%	265
Providence Health Center[2]	Waco	85%	537
Baylor Reg Med Ctr at Grapevine[2]	Grapevine	84%	516
East Texas Medical Center Trinity[2]	Trinity	84%	281
Good Shepherd Medical Center Marshall[2]	Marshall	84%	409
Lubbock Heart Hospital[2]	Lubbock	84%	347
Nocona General Hospital[2]	Nocona	84%	207
Oakbend Medical Center[2]	Richmond	84%	463
Stamford Memorial Hospital	Stamford	84%	135
Tomball Regional Medical Center[2]	Tomball	84%	619
USMD Hospital at Arlington[2]	Arlington	84%	306
Central Texas Hospital[2,3]	Cameron	83%	104
South Texas Surgical Hospital[2]	Corpus Christi	83%	367
Univ of Texas Med Branch Galveston[2]	Galveston	83%	462
Eastland Memorial Hospital[2]	Eastland	82%	295
Faith Community Hospital[2]	Jacksboro	82%	83
Heritage Park Surgical Hospital	Sherman	82%	139
Las Palmas Medical Center[2]	El Paso	82%	661
University Medical Center[2]	Lubbock	82%	524
Titus Regional Medical Center[2]	Mount Pleasant	81%	298
Covenant Hospital Plainview[2]	Plainview	80%	244
Palo Pinto General Hospital[2]	Mineral Wells	80%	253
Texas Reg Med Ctr at Sunnyvale[2]	Sunnyvale	80%	443
University Health System[2]	San Antonio	80%	530
Methodist Hospital For Surgery[2]	Addison	79%	339
Christus Jasper Memorial Hospital[2]	Jasper	77%	258
Goodall Witcher Hospital[2]	Clifton	77%	226
Baylor Surgical Hospital at Fort Worth[2]	Fort Worth	76%	476
Christus Spohn Hospital Alice[2]	Alice	76%	342
Cogdell Memorial Hospital	Snyder	76%	247
Mother Frances Hospital[2]	Tyler	76%	564
Wilbarger General Hospital[2]	Vernon	76%	231
First Surgical Hospital[2]	Bellaire	75%	248
Starr County Memorial Hospital[2]	Rio Grande City	75%	432
Texas Spine & Joint Hospital[2]	Tyler	75%	345
Bowie Memorial Hospital[2]	Bowie	74%	277
East Texas Medical Center Pittsburg[2]	Pittsburg	74%	299
Good Shephard Medical Center - Linden[2]	Linden	74%	205
East Texas Medical Center Mount Vernon[2]	Mount Vernon	73%	241
Plains Memorial Hospital	Dimmitt	73%	49
Lamb Healthcare Center	Littlefield	72%	148
Golden Plains Community Hospital[2]	Borger	71%	382
Mayhill Hospital[2]	Denton	71%	296
Anson General Hospital	Anson	70%	148
Northwest Texas Surgery Center	Amarillo	70%	93
Bellville General Hospital[2]	Bellville	69%	158
Christus Hospital[2]	Beaumont	68%	535
Knox County Hospital[2]	Knox City	68%	53
Uvalde Memorial Hospital[2]	Uvalde	68%	518
Etmc Clarksville[2]	Clarksville	67%	286
Hamlin Memorial Hospital[2]	Hamlin	66%	65
Mitchell County Hospital District	Colorado City	66%	164

NOTE: Hospital profiles are in alphabetical order by state, then city, then hospital within the city; Rankings exclude hospitals with less than 25 cases except for patient surveys which excludes hospitals with less than 100 cases; (a) 100-299 cases; (1) The number of cases/patients is too few to report; (2) Data submitted were based on a sample of cases/patients; (3) Results are based on a shorter time period than required; (4) Data suppressed by CMS for one or more quarters; (5) Results are not available for this reporting period; (6) Fewer than 100 patients completed the HCAHPS survey; (7) No cases met the criteria for this measure; (8) The lower limit of the confidence interval cannot be calculated if the number of observed infections equals zero; (9) No data are available from the state/territory for this reporting period; (10) The scores shown reflect fewer than 50 completed surveys; (11) There were discrepancies in the data collection process; (12) This measure does not apply to this hospital for this reporting period; (13) Results cannot be calculated for this reporting period; (14) The results for this state are combined with nearby states to protect confidentiality; Please refer to the User's Guide for a full explanation of data.

The Womans Hospital of Texas[2]	Houston	66%	352
Fort Duncan Medical Center[2]	Eagle Pass	65%	446
North Central Surgical Center[2]	Dallas	64%	323
Etmc Henderson[2]	Henderson	63%	261
Fdn Surgical Hosp of San Antonio[2]	San Antonio	63%	305
Houston Orthopedic & Spine Hospital[2]	Bellaire	63%	1090
East Texas Medical Center Athens[2]	Athens	62%	574
Arise Austin Medical Center[2]	Austin	60%	315
Care Regional Medical Center[2]	Aransas Pass	59%	306
TX Inst for Surgery at Presby Hosp	Dallas	59%	135
Tyler County Hospital[2]	Woodville	57%	359
Brownfield Regional Medical Center[2]	Brownfield	56%	285
Covenant Hospital Levelland[2]	Levelland	55%	225
Houston Hospital for Specialized Surgery	Houston	55%	114
East Texas Medical Center Crockett[2]	Crockett	53%	244
Methodist Mckinney Hospital[2]	Mc Kinney	48%	241
Medical Arts Hospital	Lamesa	46%	215
Northwest Hills Surgical Hospital	Austin	43%	217
University General Hospital Dallas[2]	Dallas	43%	266
Dimmit Regional Hospital[2]	Carrizo Springs	42%	151
Hemphill County Hospital[2]	Canadian	41%	74
University General Hospital[2]	Houston	41%	1025
Pine Creek Medical Center[2]	Dallas	37%	302
Trustpoint Hospital	Lubbock	36%	114
Seton Medical Center Harker Heights[2]	Harker Heights	32%	287
Lakeway Regional Medical Center[2,3]	Lakeway	29%	132
Lake Whitney Medical Center[2]	Whitney	23%	288
Permian Regional Medical Center[2]	Andrews	21%	174
Hereford Regional Medical Center[2]	Hereford	17%	254
Emerus Hospital[3]	Sugar Land	0%	34
Riverside General Hospital[2]	Houston	0%	254

Immunization for Pneumonia

Hospital Name	City	Rate	Cases
Abilene Regional Medical Center[2]	Abilene	100%	642
The Corpus Christi Medical Center[2]	Corpus Christi	100%	590
Detar Hospital Navarro[2]	Victoria	100%	628
El Campo Memorial Hospital	El Campo	100%	245
The Hospital at Westlake Medical Center[2]	Austin	100%	504
Laredo Medical Center[2]	Laredo	100%	557
Medical Center of Plano[2]	Plano	100%	649
Methodist Stone Oak Hospital[2]	San Antonio	100%	528
Pampa Regional Medical Center[2]	Pampa	100%	480
Providence Memorial Hospital[2]	El Paso	100%	407
Rolling Plains Memorial Hospital[2]	Sweetwater	100%	371
Sierra Providence East Medical Center[2]	El Paso	100%	561
Southwest General Hospital[2]	San Antonio	100%	602
TX Hlth Harris Methodist Hosp-Azle[2]	Azle	100%	570
Valley Regional Medical Center[2]	Brownsville	100%	449
Weatherford Regional Medical Center[2]	Weatherford	100%	647
Woodland Heights Medical Center[2]	Lufkin	100%	666
Baylor Medical Center at Mckinney[2]	Mc Kinney	99%	463
Baylor Regional Medical Center at Plano[2]	Plano	99%	841
Brownwood Regional Medical Center[2]	Brownwood	99%	580
Central Texas Medical Center[2]	San Marcos	99%	507
Clear Lake Regional Medical Center[2]	Webster	99%	732
Conroe Regional Medical Center[2]	Conroe	99%	844
Cuero Community Hospital[2]	Cuero	99%	407
Graham Regional Medical Center[2]	Graham	99%	399
Heart Hospital Baylor Plano[2]	Plano	99%	672
Hunt Regional Medical Center[2]	Greenville	99%	575
Lake Granbury Medical Center[2]	Granbury	99%	386
Lake Pointe Medical Center[2]	Rowlett	99%	537
Las Colinas Medical Center[2]	Irving	99%	407
Longview Regional Medical Center[2]	Longview	99%	674
Medical Center of Lewisville[2]	Lewisville	99%	542
Memorial Hermann Baptist Orange Hospital[2]	Orange	99%	327
Methodist Ambulatory Surgery Hospital NW[2]	San Antonio	99%	342
Methodist Hospital[2]	San Antonio	99%	671
Nacogdoches Medical Center[2]	Nacogdoches	99%	477
North Cypress Medical Center[2]	Cypress	99%	893
North Hills Hospital[2]	N Richland Hls	99%	718
Rio Grande Regional Hospital[2]	Mcallen	99%	556
Saint David's Medical Center[2]	Austin	99%	625
Saint Joseph Regional Health Center[2]	Bryan	99%	723
San Angelo Community Medical Center[2]	San Angelo	99%	592
San Jacinto Methodist Hospital[2]	Baytown	99%	812
Seton Medical Center Williamson[2]	Round Rock	99%	622
South Texas Regional Medical Center[2]	Jourdanton	99%	336
TX Hlth Harris Meth Hosp-Cleburne[2]	Cleburne	99%	551
TX Hlth Heart & Vasc Hosp-Arlington[2]	Arlington	99%	488
Texas Health Presbyterian Hospital - WNJ[2]	Sherman	99%	815
Texas Health Presbyterian Hospital Dallas[2]	Dallas	99%	602
TX Hlth Presbyterian Hosp-Flower Mound[2]	Flower Mound	99%	437
Texoma Medical Center[2]	Denison	99%	723
University Medical Center of El Paso[2]	El Paso	99%	383
Baptist Beaumont Hospital[2]	Beaumont	98%	713
Baylor Heart & Vascular Hospital[2]	Dallas	98%	443
Baylor Medical Center at Garland[2]	Garland	98%	717
Big Bend Regional Medical Center[2]	Alpine	98%	294
Christus Saint John Hospital[2]	Nassau Bay	98%	686
Columbus Community Hospital[2]	Columbus	98%	338
Connally Memorial Medical Center[2]	Floresville	98%	507
Dallas Regional Medical Center[2]	Mesquite	98%	1091
Medical Center of Mckinney[2]	Mckinney	98%	787
Memorial Hermann Sugar Land Hospital[2]	Sugar Land	98%	447
Methodist Charlton Medical Center[2]	Dallas	98%	705
Methodist Dallas Medical Center[2]	Dallas	98%	569
Methodist Richardson Medical Center[2]	Richardson	98%	562
Methodist Sugar Land Hospital[2]	Sugar Land	98%	566
Methodist West Houston Hospital[2]	Houston	98%	580
North Austin Medical Center[2]	Austin	98%	506
Peterson Regional Medical Center[2]	Kerrville	98%	632
Quail Creek Surgical Hospital	Amarillo	98%	730
Saint David's South Austin Medical Center[2]	Austin	98%	730
Saint Luke's Patients Medical Center[2]	Pasadena	98%	541
Saint Marks Medical Center[2]	La Grange	98%	398
Scenic Mountain Medical Center[2]	Big Spring	98%	380
TX Hlth Harris Meth Hosp-Stephenville[2]	Stephenville	98%	354
UT Southwestern University Hospital[2]	Dallas	98%	652
Baptist Saint Anthony's Hospital[2]	Amarillo	97%	710
Baylor Medical Center at Irving[2]	Irving	97%	597
Bayshore Medical Center[2]	Pasadena	97%	567
Cedar Park Regional Medical Center[2]	Cedar Park	97%	465
Centennial Medical Center[2]	Frisco	97%	437
Cleveland Regional Medical Center[2]	Cleveland	97%	342
Doctors Hospital[2]	Dallas	97%	772
Doctors Hospital at Renaissance[2]	Edinburg	97%	316
East Texas Medical Center[2]	Tyler	97%	683
Grace Medical Center	Lubbock	97%	577
Harlingen Medical Center[2]	Harlingen	97%	654
Heart Hospital Baylor Denton[3]	Denton	97%	31
Kingwood Medical Center[2]	Kingwood	97%	669
Medical Center Hospital[2]	Odessa	97%	886
Medical City Dallas Hospital[2]	Dallas	97%	568
Mem Hermann Mem City Med Ctr[2]	Houston	97%	595
Memorial Hermann Northeast[2]	Humble	97%	754
The Methodist Hospital[2]	Houston	97%	799
Methodist Willowbrook Hospital[2]	Houston	97%	534
Navarro Regional Hospital[2]	Corsicana	97%	440
Odessa Regional Hospital[2]	Odessa	97%	374
Plaza Medical Center of Fort Worth[2]	Fort Worth	97%	1013
Round Rock Medical Center[2]	Round Rock	97%	521
Saint Luke's the Woodlands Hospital[2]	The Woodlands	97%	602
Seton Smithville Regional Hospital[2]	Smithville	97%	301
Sierra Medical Center[2]	El Paso	97%	696
South Texas Spine & Surgical Hospital	San Antonio	97%	546
TX Hlth Harris Meth Hosp SW Ft Worth[2]	Fort Worth	97%	632
Texas Health Harris Methodist[2]	Bedford	97%	768
Texas Health Presbyterian Hospital Allen[2]	Allen	97%	444
Texas Health Presbyterian Hospital Denton[2]	Denton	97%	700
TX Hlth Presbyterian Hosp-Kaufman[2]	Kaufman	97%	417
Texas Orthopedic Hospital[2]	Houston	97%	392
UT SW Univ Hosp-Zale Lipshy[2]	Dallas	97%	639
Baptist Medical Center[2]	San Antonio	96%	2607
Baylor All Saints Medical Center at FW[2]	Fort Worth	96%	411
Baylor Medical Center at Carrollton[2]	Carrollton	96%	525
Baylor Medical Center at Frisco[2]	Frisco	96%	196
Baylor Medical Center at Trophy Club[2]	Trophy Club	96%	170
Baylor Surgical Hospital at Las Colinas[2]	Irving	96%	156
Baylor University Medical Center[2]	Dallas	96%	594
Christus Spohn Hospital Beeville[2]	Beeville	96%	354
College Station Medical Center[2]	College Station	96%	742
Cypress Fairbanks Medical Center[2]	Houston	96%	339
Heritage Park Surgical Hospital	Sherman	96%	121
Hill Country Memorial Hospital[2]	Fredericksburg	96%	383
Hill Regional Hospital[2]	Hillsboro	96%	341
Huntsville Memorial Hospital[2]	Huntsville	96%	483
Kell West Regional Hospital	Wichita Falls	96%	567
Lavaca Medical Center	Hallettsville	96%	391
Matagorda Regional Medical Center[2]	Bay City	96%	313
Memorial Hermann Hospital System[2]	Houston	96%	2213
Memorial Hermann Katy Hospital[2]	Katy	96%	452
Metroplex Hospital[2]	Killeen	96%	450
Midland Memorial Hospital[2]	Midland	96%	1854
Palestine Regional Medical Center[2]	Palestine	96%	410
Paris Regional Medical Center[2]	Paris	96%	816
South Texas Health System[2]	Edinburg	96%	664
Sugar Land Surgical Hospital	Sugar Land	96%	152
Texas Health Arlington Memorial Hospital[2]	Arlington	96%	723
TX Hlth Harris Meth Hosp-Southlake[2]	Southlake	96%	454
TX Health Presbyterian Hosp Rockwall[2]	Rockwall	96%	437
West Houston Medical Center[2]	Houston	96%	562
Childress Regional Medical Center[2]	Childress	95%	249
Christus Saint Michael Health System[2]	Texarkana	95%	709
Christus Spohn Hospital Kleberg[2]	Kingsville	95%	487
Cornerstone Regional Hospital[2]	Edinburg	95%	382
East Texas Medical Center - Gilmer[2]	Gilmer	95%	354
Electra Memorial Hospital	Electra	95%	40
Glen Rose Medical Center	Glen Rose	95%	449
Good Shepherd Medical Center Marshall[2]	Marshall	95%	450
Guadalupe Regional Medical Center[2]	Seguin	95%	386
Memorial Hospital[2]	Gonzales	95%	350
Nix Health Care System[2]	San Antonio	95%	660
Park Plaza Hospital[2]	Houston	95%	641
Rollins Brook Community Hospital[2]	Lampasas	95%	461
Saint Luke's Hospital at the Vintage[2]	Houston	95%	371
Surgery Specialty Hosps of America[2]	Pasadena	95%	38
TX Health Ctr for Diag & Surgery	Plano	95%	191
Texas Health Harris Methodist Fort Worth[2]	Fort Worth	95%	841
Texas Reg Med Ctr at Sunnyvale[2]	Sunnyvale	95%	501
USMD Hospital at Fort Worth	Fort Worth	95%	227
VHS Harlingen Hospital Company[2]	Harlingen	95%	589
Wadley Regional Medical Center[2]	Texarkana	95%	666
Faith Community Hospital[2]	Jacksboro	94%	109
Hopkins County Memorial Hospital[2]	Sulphur Springs	94%	312
Houston Northwest Medical Center[2]	Houston	94%	573
Mem Hermann Surgical Hosp Kingwood	Kingwood	94%	80
Methodist Mansfield Medical Center[2]	Mansfield	94%	526
Mission Regional Medical Center[2]	Mission	94%	465
Nocona General Hospital[2]	Nocona	94%	265
Scott & White Hospital Brenham[2]	Brenham	94%	275
Seton Northwest Hospital[2]	Austin	94%	419
VHS Brownsville Hospital Company[2]	Brownsville	94%	521
Wise Regional Health System[2]	Decatur	94%	643
Baylor Medical Center at Waxahachie[2]	Waxahachie	93%	472
Baylor Ortho & Spine Hosp-Arlington[2]	Arlington	93%	383
Brazosport Regional Health System[2]	Lake Jackson	93%	550
Denton Regional Medical Center[2]	Denton	93%	770
Good Shepherd Medical Center[2]	Longview	93%	691
Hillcrest Baptist Medical Center[2]	Waco	93%	447
Medical Center of Arlington[2]	Arlington	93%	511
Parkview Regional Hospital[2]	Mexia	93%	460
Saint Luke's Sugar Land Hospital[2]	Sugar Land	93%	420
Seton Medical Center Hays[2]	Kyle	93%	648
Seymour Hospital	Seymour	93%	250
TX Hlth Harris Meth Hosp-Alliance[2,3]	Fort Worth	93%	183
Titus Regional Medical Center[2]	Mount Pleasant	93%	241
United Regional Health Care System[2]	Wichita Falls	93%	611
Val Verde Regional Medical Center[2]	Del Rio	93%	301
Citizens Medical Center[2]	Victoria	92%	715
Etmc Carthage[2]	Carthage	92%	451
Frio Regional Hospital[2]	Pearsall	92%	132
Hamilton General Hospital[2]	Hamilton	92%	539
Huguley Memorial Medical Center[2]	Burleson	92%	722
Knapp Medical Center[2]	Weslaco	92%	491
The Medical Center of Southeast Texas[2]	Port Arthur	92%	816
Moore County Hospital District[2]	Dumas	92%	162
The Physicians Centre	Bryan	92%	167
Saint Luke's Lakeside Hospital[2]	The Woodlands	92%	386
Scott & White Hospital - Round Rock[2]	Round Rock	92%	677
Stephens Memorial Hospital[2]	Breckenridge	92%	314
Texas Health Presbyterian Hospital Plano[2]	Plano	92%	480
Univ of TX Health Science Ctr-Tyler[2]	Tyler	92%	475
Christus Saint Catherine Hospital[2]	Katy	91%	329
Covenant Medical Center[2]	Lubbock	91%	786
East Texas Medical Center Quitman[2]	Quitman	91%	411
Fort Duncan Medical Center[2]	Eagle Pass	91%	445
Gulf Coast Medical Center[2]	Wharton	91%	342
Harris Health System[2]	Houston	91%	817
Hendrick Medical Center[2]	Abilene	91%	686
Baylor Medical Center at Uptown[2]	Dallas	90%	292
Houston Orthopedic & Spine Hospital[2]	Bellaire	90%	1141
JPS Health Network[2]	Fort Worth	90%	491
Memorial Hospital[2]	Nacogdoches	90%	479
North Texas Medical Center[2]	Gainesville	90%	233
Scott & White Memorial Hospital[2]	Temple	90%	643
Tops Surgical Specialty Hospital[2]	Houston	90%	391
University Medical Center at Brackenridge[2]	Austin	90%	425
Allegiance Specialty Hospital of Kilgore[2]	Kilgore	89%	598
Angleton - Danbury Medical Center[2]	Angleton	89%	250
Basin Healthcare Center[2]	Odessa	89%	36
Covenant Hospital Plainview[2]	Plainview	89%	257
East Texas Medical Center Jacksonville[2]	Jacksonville	89%	223
El Paso Specialty Hospital[2]	El Paso	89%	377
Houston Physicians' Hospital	Webster	89%	262
Pecos County Memorial Hospital[2]	Fort Stockton	89%	313
Providence Health Center[2]	Waco	89%	721
Shannon Medical Center[2]	San Angelo	89%	746
Christus Jasper Memorial Hospital[2]	Jasper	88%	367
Christus Santa Rosa Hospital[2]	San Antonio	88%	864
Covenant Hospital Levelland[2]	Levelland	88%	204
East Texas Medical Center - Fairfield	Fairfield	88%	367
Ennis Regional Medical Center[2]	Ennis	88%	268
Etmc Henderson[2]	Henderson	88%	305
Las Palmas Medical Center[2]	El Paso	88%	762
Memorial Medical Center of East Texas[2]	Lufkin	88%	773
Saint Joseph Medical Center[2]	Houston	88%	564
Saint Luke's Episcopal Hospital[2]	Houston	88%	902
Tomball Regional Medical Center[2]	Tomball	88%	819
Baylor Reg Med Ctr at Grapevine[2]	Grapevine	87%	485
Bowie Memorial Hospital[2]	Bowie	87%	431
East Texas Medical Center Trinity[2]	Trinity	87%	345

NOTE: Hospital profiles are in alphabetical order by state, then city, then hospital within the city; Rankings exclude hospitals with less than 25 cases except for patient surveys which excludes hospitals with less than 100 cases; (a) 100-299 cases; (1) The number of cases/patients is too few to report; (2) Data submitted were based on a sample of cases/patients; (3) Results are based on a shorter time period than required; (4) Data suppressed by CMS for one or more quarters; (5) Results are not available for this reporting period; (6) Fewer than 100 patients completed the HCAHPS survey; (7) No cases met the criteria for this measure; (8) The lower limit of the confidence interval cannot be calculated if the number of observed infections equals zero; (9) No data are available from the state/territory for this reporting period; (10) The scores shown reflect fewer than 50 completed surveys; (11) There were discrepancies in the data collection process; (12) This measure does not apply to this hospital for this reporting period; (13) Results cannot be calculated for this reporting period; (14) The results for this state are combined with nearby states to protect confidentiality; Please refer to the User's Guide for a full explanation of data.

Hospital Name	City	Rate	Cases
Memorial Medical Center Livingston[2]	Livingston	87%	323
Plains Memorial Hospital	Dimmitt	87%	91
Christus Spohn Hospital Corpus Christi[2]	Corpus Christi	86%	828
Oakbend Medical Center[2]	Richmond	86%	427
Palo Pinto General Hospital[2]	Mineral Wells	86%	323
Parkland Health & Hospital System[2]	Dallas	86%	380
Seton Medical Center Austin[2]	Austin	86%	614
South Texas Surgical Hospital[2]	Corpus Christi	86%	601
University Medical Center[2]	Lubbock	86%	534
Doctors Diagnostic Hospital[2]	Cleveland	85%	236
East Texas Medical Center Pittsburg[2]	Pittsburg	85%	386
Foundation Surgical Hospital of El Paso[2]	El Paso	85%	362
Seton Southwest Hospital[2]	Austin	85%	27
Doctors Hospital of Laredo[2]	Laredo	84%	328
Doctors Hospital Tidwell[2]	Houston	84%	261
Eastland Memorial Hospital[2]	Eastland	84%	468
Lubbock Heart Hospital[2]	Lubbock	84%	553
Memorial Hermann Texas Medical Center[2]	Houston	84%	419
Scott & White Hospital - Llano	Llano	84%	346
Wilbarger General Hospital[2]	Vernon	84%	308
Central Texas Hospital[2,3]	Cameron	83%	48
Good Shephard Medical Center - Linden[2]	Linden	83%	269
Goodall Witcher Hospital[2]	Clifton	83%	265
Starr County Memorial Hospital[2]	Rio Grande City	83%	525
USMD Hospital at Arlington[2]	Arlington	83%	332
Mother Frances Hospital[2]	Tyler	82%	679
Northwest Texas Hospital[2]	Amarillo	82%	480
Uvalde Memorial Hospital[2]	Uvalde	82%	542
East Texas Medical Center Mount Vernon[2]	Mount Vernon	81%	360
Otto Kaiser Memorial Hospital[2]	Kenedy	81%	202
Univ of Texas Med Branch Galveston[2]	Galveston	81%	396
Christus Spohn Hospital Alice[2]	Alice	80%	392
Dallas Medical Center[2]	Dallas	79%	380
University Health System[2]	San Antonio	79%	405
East Texas Medical Center Crockett[2]	Crockett	78%	310
Stamford Memorial Hospital	Stamford	78%	184
Baylor Surgical Hospital at Fort Worth[2]	Fort Worth	77%	387
Mitchell County Hospital District	Colorado City	76%	221
Etmc Clarksville[2]	Clarksville	75%	422
Lamb Healthcare Center[2]	Littlefield	75%	182
Medical Arts Hospital	Lamesa	75%	134
Texas General Hospital[3]	Grand Prairie	75%	61
East Texas Medical Center Athens[2]	Athens	74%	680
Fdn Surgical Hosp of San Antonio[2]	San Antonio	74%	121
Golden Plains Community Hospital[2]	Borger	74%	351
Arise Austin Medical Center[2]	Austin	72%	368
Care Regional Medical Center[2]	Aransas Pass	72%	489
Cogdell Memorial Hospital	Snyder	72%	262
Knox County Hospital[2]	Knox City	72%	86
Christus Hospital[2]	Beaumont	71%	598
Methodist Hospital For Surgery[2]	Addison	71%	336
First Surgical Hospital[2]	Bellaire	69%	147
Mayhill Hospital[2]	Denton	69%	327
North Central Surgical Center[2]	Dallas	69%	283
Northwest Texas Surgery Center[2]	Amarillo	69%	71
Houston Hospital for Specialized Surgery	Houston	65%	40
Trustpoint Hospital[2]	Lubbock	65%	221
Saint Anthony's Hospital[2,3]	Houston	64%	170
Anson General Hospital	Anson	62%	212
Texas Spine & Joint Hospital[2]	Tyler	61%	494
Tyler County Hospital[2]	Woodville	59%	508
The Womans Hospital of Texas[2]	Houston	59%	44
Northwest Hills Surgical Hospital	Austin	57%	160
University General Hospital[2]	Houston	57%	1511
Bellville General Hospital[2]	Bellville	56%	216
Falls Community Hospital & Clinic[2]	Marlin	55%	286
Methodist Mckinney Hospital[2]	Mc Kinney	55%	268
Brownfield Regional Medical Center[2]	Brownfield	53%	332
Hamlin Memorial Hospital[2]	Hamlin	53%	113
TX Inst for Surgery at Presby Hosp	Dallas	51%	83
Lakeway Regional Medical Center[2,3]	Lakeway	50%	226
University General Hospital Dallas[2]	Dallas	48%	335
Permian Regional Medical Center[2]	Andrews	46%	103
Hemphill County Hospital[2]	Canadian	43%	88
Dimmit Regional Hospital[2]	Carrizo Springs	42%	118
Seton Medical Center Harker Heights[2]	Harker Heights	37%	325
Lake Whitney Medical Center[2]	Whitney	34%	387
Pine Creek Medical Center[2]	Dallas	32%	171
Hereford Regional Medical Center[2]	Hereford	29%	186

Stroke Care

Anticoagulation Therapy for Atrial Fibrillation

Hospital Name	City	Rate	Cases
East Texas Medical Center	Tyler	100%	34
Medical Center Hospital	Odessa	100%	28
Medical City Dallas Hospital	Dallas	100%	36
Memorial Hermann Texas Medical Center	Houston	100%	80
Methodist Sugar Land Hospital	Sugar Land	100%	27
Methodist Willowbrook Hospital	Houston	100%	25
United Regional Health Care System	Wichita Falls	100%	27
VHS Harlingen Hospital Company	Harlingen	100%	25
Memorial Hermann Hospital System	Houston	99%	74
Methodist Hospital	San Antonio	99%	107
Mem Hermann Mem City Med Ctr	Houston	98%	44
The Methodist Hospital	Houston	98%	104
Seton Medical Center Austin	Austin	98%	40
Good Shepherd Medical Center	Longview	96%	49
Mother Frances Hospital	Tyler	95%	37
Baptist Medical Center	San Antonio	94%	111
Wadley Regional Medical Center	Texarkana	94%	32
Christus Spohn Hospital Corpus Christi[2]	Corpus Christi	88%	51
Providence Health Center	Waco	69%	26

Antithrombotic Therapy Timing

Hospital Name	City	Rate	Cases
Abilene Regional Medical Center	Abilene	100%	50
Baylor All Saints Medical Center at FW[2]	Fort Worth	100%	71
Baylor Medical Center at Carrollton	Carrollton	100%	27
Baylor Medical Center at Irving[2]	Irving	100%	83
Baylor Medical Center at Mckinney	Mc Kinney	100%	40
Baylor Reg Med Ctr at Grapevine	Grapevine	100%	60
Bayshore Medical Center	Pasadena	100%	194
Brazosport Regional Health System	Lake Jackson	100%	33
Brownwood Regional Medical Center	Brownwood	100%	25
Centennial Medical Center	Frisco	100%	28
Clear Lake Regional Medical Center[2]	Webster	100%	102
The Corpus Christi Medical Center[2]	Corpus Christi	100%	65
Cypress Fairbanks Medical Center	Houston	100%	50
Dallas Regional Medical Center	Mesquite	100%	40
Detar Hospital Navarro	Victoria	100%	79
East Texas Medical Center	Tyler	100%	255
Good Shepherd Medical Center	Longview	100%	287
Harlingen Medical Center	Harlingen	100%	31
Hendrick Medical Center	Abilene	100%	116
Hillcrest Baptist Medical Center	Waco	100%	110
Huguley Memorial Medical Center	Burleson	100%	79
Hunt Regional Medical Center[2]	Greenville	100%	76
JPS Health Network	Fort Worth	100%	210
Knapp Medical Center[2]	Weslaco	100%	71
Lake Pointe Medical Center	Rowlett	100%	54
Longview Regional Medical Center	Longview	100%	44
Medical Center of Arlington[2]	Arlington	100%	102
Memorial Medical Center Livingston[2]	Livingston	100%	28
Methodist Dallas Medical Center[2]	Dallas	100%	153
Methodist Mansfield Medical Center[2]	Mansfield	100%	77
Methodist Richardson Medical Center	Richardson	100%	37
Methodist Sugar Land Hospital	Sugar Land	100%	170
Methodist West Houston Hospital	Houston	100%	79
Metroplex Hospital[2]	Killeen	100%	47
Navarro Regional Hospital	Corsicana	100%	28
North Austin Medical Center[2]	Austin	100%	69
North Cypress Medical Center	Cypress	100%	117
North Hills Hospital	N Richland Hls	100%	108
Oakbend Medical Center[2]	Richmond	100%	46
Odessa Regional Hospital	Odessa	100%	32
Park Plaza Hospital	Houston	100%	28
Plaza Medical Center of Fort Worth[2]	Fort Worth	100%	76
Providence Health Center	Waco	100%	213
Round Rock Medical Center	Round Rock	100%	73
Saint Joseph Medical Center	Houston	100%	73
Saint Luke's Hospital at the Vintage	Houston	100%	27
Saint Luke's Sugar Land Hospital	Sugar Land	100%	30
San Angelo Community Medical Center	San Angelo	100%	32
Scott & White Hospital - Round Rock	Round Rock	100%	50
South Texas Health System[2]	Edinburg	100%	93
Southwest General Hospital	San Antonio	100%	53
TX Hlth Harris Meth Hosp SW Ft Worth[2]	Fort Worth	100%	59
Texas Health Harris Methodist[2]	Bedford	100%	104
Texas Health Presbyterian Hospital - WNJ	Sherman	100%	49
Texas Health Presbyterian Hospital Dallas[2]	Dallas	100%	81
TX Hlth Presbyterian Hosp-Kaufman[2]	Kaufman	100%	25
Texas Health Presbyterian Hospital Plano[2]	Plano	100%	80
TX Health Presbyterian Hosp Rockwall	Rockwall	100%	25
Texas Reg Med Ctr at Sunnyvale	Sunnyvale	100%	46
Texoma Medical Center[2]	Denison	100%	95
University Medical Center of El Paso	El Paso	100%	82
Univ of Texas Med Branch Galveston[2]	Galveston	100%	60
Valley Regional Medical Center[2]	Brownsville	100%	48
VHS Brownsville Hospital Company	Brownsville	100%	76
West Houston Medical Center	Houston	100%	99
Woodland Heights Medical Center	Lufkin	100%	39
Baptist Saint Anthony's Hospital[2]	Amarillo	99%	95
Baylor University Medical Center[2]	Dallas	99%	105
Conroe Regional Medical Center	Conroe	99%	136
Doctors Hospital	Dallas	99%	72
Doctors Hospital at Renaissance	Edinburg	99%	127
Kingwood Medical Center[2]	Kingwood	99%	102
Las Palmas Medical Center[2]	El Paso	99%	95
Medical Center of Mckinney[2]	Mckinney	99%	67
Medical City Dallas Hospital	Dallas	99%	164
Memorial Hermann Katy Hospital	Katy	99%	80
Mem Hermann Mem City Med Ctr	Houston	99%	237
Memorial Hermann Northeast	Humble	99%	173
Methodist Stone Oak Hospital[2]	San Antonio	99%	98
Parkland Health & Hospital System[2]	Dallas	99%	82
Saint David's Medical Center[2]	Austin	99%	77
Saint David's South Austin Medical Center[2]	Austin	99%	67
Saint Luke's the Woodlands Hospital	The Woodlands	99%	112
Scott & White Memorial Hospital[2]	Temple	99%	92
Shannon Medical Center	San Angelo	99%	140
Texas Health Arlington Memorial Hospital[2]	Arlington	99%	112
Texas Health Harris Methodist Fort Worth[2]	Fort Worth	99%	173
Texas Health Presbyterian Hospital Denton[2]	Denton	99%	81
United Regional Health Care System	Wichita Falls	99%	194
UT SW Univ Hosp-Zale Lipshy[2]	Dallas	99%	80
VHS Harlingen Hospital Company	Harlingen	99%	164
Baylor Medical Center at Garland[2]	Garland	98%	107
Baylor Regional Medical Center at Plano	Plano	98%	66
Central Texas Medical Center	San Marcos	98%	45
Christus Saint Michael Health System	Texarkana	98%	163
Christus Spohn Hospital Corpus Christi[2]	Corpus Christi	98%	303
College Station Medical Center	College Station	98%	48
Medical Center Hospital	Odessa	98%	178
Medical Center of Lewisville	Lewisville	98%	51
Medical Center of Plano[2]	Plano	98%	89
Memorial Hermann Hospital System	Houston	98%	601
Methodist Charlton Medical Center[2]	Dallas	98%	180
Methodist Hospital	San Antonio	98%	640
Methodist Willowbrook Hospital	Houston	98%	149
Mission Regional Medical Center	Mission	98%	56
Mother Frances Hospital	Tyler	98%	344
Paris Regional Medical Center	Paris	98%	50
Peterson Regional Medical Center	Kerrville	98%	52
Saint Joseph Regional Health Center[2]	Bryan	98%	110
Saint Luke's Episcopal Hospital[2]	Houston	98%	90
San Jacinto Methodist Hospital	Baytown	98%	166
Tomball Regional Medical Center	Tomball	98%	95
Baptist Beaumont Hospital[2]	Beaumont	97%	129
Baptist Medical Center	San Antonio	97%	629
Baylor Medical Center at Waxahachie	Waxahachie	97%	33
Covenant Medical Center	Lubbock	97%	184
Denton Regional Medical Center[2]	Denton	97%	73
Harris Health System	Houston	97%	196
Houston Northwest Medical Center	Houston	97%	160
Huntsville Memorial Hospital	Huntsville	97%	31
Memorial Hermann Sugar Land Hospital	Sugar Land	97%	38
The Methodist Hospital	Houston	97%	351
Northwest Texas Hospital[2]	Amarillo	97%	89
Providence Memorial Hospital	El Paso	97%	70
Seton Northwest Hospital	Austin	97%	30
Wise Regional Health System	Decatur	97%	38
Christus Saint John Hospital	Nassau Bay	96%	28
Memorial Hermann Texas Medical Center	Houston	96%	374
Memorial Hospital	Nacogdoches	96%	46
Nix Health Care System	San Antonio	96%	25
Rio Grande Regional Hospital[2]	Mcallen	96%	73
Saint Luke's Patients Medical Center	Pasadena	96%	28
Seton Medical Center Austin	Austin	96%	165
Sierra Providence East Medical Center	El Paso	96%	84
University Health System[2]	San Antonio	96%	110
University Medical Center	Lubbock	96%	135
UT Southwestern University Hospital	Dallas	96%	26
Wadley Regional Medical Center	Texarkana	96%	140
Christus Santa Rosa Hospital	San Antonio	95%	129
Citizens Medical Center	Victoria	95%	60
Nacogdoches Medical Center	Nacogdoches	95%	44
Seton Medical Center Hays	Kyle	95%	63
Sierra Medical Center	El Paso	95%	77
Christus Hospital[2]	Beaumont	94%	96
The Medical Center of Southeast Texas	Port Arthur	94%	78
Memorial Medical Center of East Texas	Lufkin	94%	116
Midland Memorial Hospital	Midland	94%	111
Seton Medical Center Williamson	Round Rock	93%	71
University Medical Center at Brackenridge	Austin	93%	116
Hopkins County Memorial Hospital	Sulphur Springs	92%	26
Palestine Regional Medical Center	Palestine	92%	40
East Texas Medical Center Athens	Athens	89%	80
Doctors Hospital of Laredo	Laredo	85%	48
Laredo Medical Center	Laredo	85%	198

Assessed for Rehabilitation

Hospital Name	City	Rate	Cases
Abilene Regional Medical Center	Abilene	100%	55
Baylor Medical Center at Mckinney	Mc Kinney	100%	49
Baylor Medical Center at Waxahachie	Waxahachie	100%	29
Baylor Reg Med Ctr at Grapevine	Grapevine	100%	80
Baylor University Medical Center[2]	Dallas	100%	157
Bayshore Medical Center	Pasadena	100%	211
Brownwood Regional Medical Center	Brownwood	100%	35
Central Texas Medical Center	San Marcos	100%	47
College Station Medical Center	College Station	100%	69

NOTE: Hospital profiles are in alphabetical order by state, then city, then hospital within the city; Rankings exclude hospitals with less than 25 cases except for patient surveys which excludes hospitals with less than 100 cases; (a) 100-299 cases; (1) The number of cases/patients is too few to report; (2) Data submitted were based on a sample of cases/patients; (3) Results are based on a shorter time period than required; (4) Data suppressed by CMS for one or more quarters; (5) Results are not available for this reporting period; (6) Fewer than 100 patients completed the HCAHPS survey; (7) No cases met the criteria for this measure; (8) The lower limit of the confidence interval cannot be calculated if the number of observed infections equals zero; (9) No data are available from the state/territory for this reporting period; (10) The scores shown reflect fewer than 50 completed surveys; (11) There were discrepancies in the data collection process; (12) This measure does not apply to this hospital for this reporting period; (13) Results cannot be calculated for this reporting period; (14) The results for this state are combined with nearby states to protect confidentiality; Please refer to the User's Guide for a full explanation of data.

Conroe Regional Medical Center	Conroe	100%	183
The Corpus Christi Medical Center[2]	Corpus Christi	100%	83
Cypress Fairbanks Medical Center	Houston	100%	52
Denton Regional Medical Center[2]	Denton	100%	87
Detar Hospital Navarro	Victoria	100%	78
East Texas Medical Center	Tyler	100%	339
Hendrick Medical Center	Abilene	100%	128
Hillcrest Baptist Medical Center	Waco	100%	128
Houston Northwest Medical Center	Houston	100%	193
Kingwood Medical Center[2]	Kingwood	100%	118
Knapp Medical Center[2]	Weslaco	100%	81
Lake Pointe Medical Center	Rowlett	100%	72
Longview Regional Medical Center	Longview	100%	50
Medical Center of Lewisville	Lewisville	100%	46
Medical City Dallas Hospital	Dallas	100%	220
Memorial Hermann Hospital System	Houston	100%	664
Memorial Hermann Katy Hospital	Katy	100%	86
Mem Hermann Mem City Med Ctr	Houston	100%	300
Memorial Hermann Northeast	Humble	100%	180
Memorial Hermann Sugar Land Hospital	Sugar Land	100%	46
Memorial Hermann Texas Medical Center	Houston	100%	855
Memorial Hospital	Nacogdoches	100%	52
Memorial Medical Center of East Texas	Lufkin	100%	143
Methodist Dallas Medical Center[2]	Dallas	100%	209
Methodist Hospital	San Antonio	100%	835
Methodist Mansfield Medical Center[2]	Mansfield	100%	79
Methodist Richardson Medical Center	Richardson	100%	53
Methodist Stone Oak Hospital[2]	San Antonio	100%	121
Metroplex Hospital[2]	Killeen	100%	46
Midland Memorial Hospital	Midland	100%	133
North Austin Medical Center[2]	Austin	100%	79
North Hills Hospital	N Richland Hls	100%	108
Oakbend Medical Center[2]	Richmond	100%	45
Paris Regional Medical Center	Paris	100%	50
Parkland Health & Hospital System[2]	Dallas	100%	131
Providence Memorial Hospital	El Paso	100%	100
Saint David's South Austin Medical Center[2]	Austin	100%	75
San Angelo Community Medical Center	San Angelo	100%	34
Scott & White Hospital - Round Rock	Round Rock	100%	64
Shannon Medical Center	San Angelo	100%	160
Sierra Providence East Medical Center	El Paso	100%	96
Texas Health Harris Methodist[2]	Bedford	100%	110
Texas Health Presbyterian Hospital - WNJ	Sherman	100%	59
TX Hlth Presbyterian Hosp-Kaufman[2]	Kaufman	100%	25
Texas Health Presbyterian Hospital Plano[2]	Plano	100%	94
TX Health Presbyterian Hosp Rockwall	Rockwall	100%	29
Texas Reg Med Ctr at Sunnyvale	Sunnyvale	100%	43
Texoma Medical Center[2]	Denison	100%	107
University Medical Center of El Paso	El Paso	100%	132
UT Southwestern University Hospital	Dallas	100%	35
Valley Regional Medical Center[2]	Brownsville	100%	58
VHS Brownsville Hospital Company	Brownsville	100%	99
VHS Harlingen Hospital Company	Harlingen	100%	270
West Houston Medical Center	Houston	100%	124
Wise Regional Health System	Decatur	100%	57
Woodland Heights Medical Center	Lufkin	100%	44
Baptist Medical Center	San Antonio	99%	866
Baylor All Saints Medical Center at FW[2]	Fort Worth	99%	78
Baylor Medical Center at Garland[2]	Garland	99%	123
Baylor Medical Center at Irving[2]	Irving	99%	94
Doctors Hospital at Renaissance	Edinburg	99%	162
Las Palmas Medical Center[2]	El Paso	99%	123
Medical Center of Arlington[2]	Arlington	99%	119
Medical Center of Plano[2]	Plano	99%	135
Methodist Charlton Medical Center[2]	Dallas	99%	183
The Methodist Hospital	Houston	99%	533
Methodist Sugar Land Hospital	Sugar Land	99%	195
North Cypress Medical Center	Cypress	99%	146
Round Rock Medical Center	Round Rock	99%	76
Saint David's Medical Center[2]	Austin	99%	119
Scott & White Memorial Hospital[2]	Temple	99%	154
South Texas Health System[2]	Edinburg	99%	125
Texas Health Arlington Memorial Hospital[2]	Arlington	99%	134
Tomball Regional Medical Center	Tomball	99%	105
United Regional Health Care System	Wichita Falls	99%	249
UT SW Univ Hosp-Zale Lipshy[2]	Dallas	99%	153
Wadley Regional Medical Center	Texarkana	99%	196
Baptist Beaumont Hospital[2]	Beaumont	98%	157
Baylor Regional Medical Center at Plano	Plano	98%	89
Christus Saint Michael Health System	Texarkana	98%	182
Dallas Regional Medical Center	Mesquite	98%	40
Harris Health System	Houston	98%	284
JPS Health Network	Fort Worth	98%	269
Medical Center Hospital	Odessa	98%	185
Medical Center of Mckinney[2]	Mckinney	98%	81
Methodist Willowbrook Hospital	Houston	98%	179
Mother Frances Hospital	Tyler	98%	393
Peterson Regional Medical Center	Kerrville	98%	50
Rio Grande Regional Hospital[2]	Mcallen	98%	95
Saint Joseph Regional Health Center[2]	Bryan	98%	121
Seton Northwest Hospital	Austin	98%	40
Sierra Medical Center	El Paso	98%	111
Southwest General Hospital	San Antonio	98%	56
Texas Health Presbyterian Hospital Denton[2]	Denton	98%	89
University Health System[2]	San Antonio	98%	172
University Medical Center at Brackenridge	Austin	98%	188
Univ of Texas Med Branch Galveston[2]	Galveston	98%	104
Brazosport Regional Health System	Lake Jackson	97%	37
Centennial Medical Center	Frisco	97%	37
Clear Lake Regional Medical Center[2]	Webster	97%	112
Covenant Medical Center	Lubbock	97%	281
Good Shepherd Medical Center	Longview	97%	359
Providence Health Center	Waco	97%	247
Seton Medical Center Williamson	Round Rock	97%	103
Texas Health Harris Methodist Fort Worth[2]	Fort Worth	97%	228
Christus Saint John Hospital	Nassau Bay	96%	25
Christus Spohn Hospital Corpus Christi[2]	Corpus Christi	96%	446
Citizens Medical Center	Victoria	96%	67
Huguley Memorial Medical Center	Burleson	96%	81
Hunt Regional Medical Center[2]	Greenville	96%	77
Saint Luke's Patients Medical Center	Pasadena	96%	28
San Jacinto Methodist Hospital	Baytown	96%	166
Seton Medical Center Austin	Austin	96%	223
Texas Health Presbyterian Hospital Dallas[2]	Dallas	96%	115
University Medical Center	Lubbock	96%	187
Baptist Saint Anthony's Hospital[2]	Amarillo	95%	110
Baylor Medical Center at Carrollton	Carrollton	95%	39
Palestine Regional Medical Center	Palestine	95%	37
Plaza Medical Center of Fort Worth[2]	Fort Worth	95%	108
Saint Joseph Medical Center	Houston	95%	88
Saint Luke's Sugar Land Hospital	Sugar Land	95%	37
Huntsville Memorial Hospital	Huntsville	94%	31
Methodist West Houston Hospital	Houston	94%	96
Nacogdoches Medical Center	Nacogdoches	94%	52
Saint Luke's Hospital at the Vintage	Houston	94%	36
Northwest Texas Hospital[2]	Amarillo	93%	114
TX Hlth Harris Meth Hosp SW Ft Worth[2]	Fort Worth	93%	74
Doctors Hospital	Dallas	92%	79
Mission Regional Medical Center	Mission	92%	77
Seton Medical Center Hays	Kyle	92%	74
Christus Santa Rosa Hospital	San Antonio	91%	142
Doctors Hospital of Laredo	Laredo	91%	47
Laredo Medical Center	Laredo	91%	209
The Medical Center of Southeast Texas	Port Arthur	91%	81
Saint Luke's Episcopal Hospital[2]	Houston	90%	136
Saint Luke's the Woodlands Hospital	The Woodlands	90%	163
Odessa Regional Hospital	Odessa	89%	28
Park Plaza Hospital	Houston	88%	26
Harlingen Medical Center	Harlingen	85%	33
Christus Hospital[2]	Beaumont	82%	120
Memorial Medical Center Livingston[2]	Livingston	81%	26
Hopkins County Memorial Hospital	Sulphur Springs	78%	27
East Texas Medical Center Athens	Athens	71%	79
Navarro Regional Hospital	Corsicana	70%	27

Discharged on Antithrombotic Therapy

Hospital Name	City	Rate	Cases
Abilene Regional Medical Center	Abilene	100%	52
Baptist Medical Center	San Antonio	100%	709
Baylor All Saints Medical Center at FW[2]	Fort Worth	100%	70
Baylor Medical Center at Carrollton	Carrollton	100%	29
Baylor Medical Center at Garland[2]	Garland	100%	122
Baylor Medical Center at Mckinney	Mc Kinney	100%	42
Baylor Medical Center at Waxahachie	Waxahachie	100%	29
Baylor Reg Med Ctr at Grapevine	Grapevine	100%	79
Baylor University Medical Center[2]	Dallas	100%	123
Bayshore Medical Center	Pasadena	100%	195
Brazosport Regional Health System	Lake Jackson	100%	32
Brownwood Regional Medical Center	Brownwood	100%	35
Centennial Medical Center	Frisco	100%	28
Clear Lake Regional Medical Center[2]	Webster	100%	103
College Station Medical Center	College Station	100%	62
Conroe Regional Medical Center	Conroe	100%	156
Cypress Fairbanks Medical Center	Houston	100%	50
Dallas Regional Medical Center	Mesquite	100%	39
Denton Regional Medical Center[2]	Denton	100%	79
Detar Hospital Navarro	Victoria	100%	75
Doctors Hospital	Dallas	100%	74
East Texas Medical Center	Tyler	100%	291
Harlingen Medical Center	Harlingen	100%	29
Harris Health System	Houston	100%	216
Hendrick Medical Center	Abilene	100%	110
Hillcrest Baptist Medical Center	Waco	100%	112
Houston Northwest Medical Center	Houston	100%	164
Huguley Memorial Medical Center	Burleson	100%	81
Hunt Regional Medical Center[2]	Greenville	100%	73
Kingwood Medical Center[2]	Kingwood	100%	99
Lake Pointe Medical Center	Rowlett	100%	72
Longview Regional Medical Center	Longview	100%	47
Medical Center of Arlington[2]	Arlington	100%	110
Medical Center of Lewisville	Lewisville	100%	46
Medical Center of Mckinney[2]	Mckinney	100%	68
Medical Center of Plano[2]	Plano	100%	110
Medical City Dallas Hospital	Dallas	100%	180
Memorial Hermann Hospital System	Houston	100%	636
Memorial Hermann Katy Hospital	Katy	100%	84
Mem Hermann Mem City Med Ctr	Houston	100%	261
Memorial Hermann Sugar Land Hospital	Sugar Land	100%	46
Methodist Charlton Medical Center[2]	Dallas	100%	179
Methodist Dallas Medical Center[2]	Dallas	100%	160
Methodist Hospital	San Antonio	100%	666
The Methodist Hospital	Houston	100%	413
Methodist Mansfield Medical Center[2]	Mansfield	100%	77
Methodist Richardson Medical Center	Richardson	100%	45
Methodist Stone Oak Hospital[2]	San Antonio	100%	107
Methodist West Houston Hospital	Houston	100%	93
Methodist Willowbrook Hospital	Houston	100%	158
Metroplex Hospital[2]	Killeen	100%	46
North Austin Medical Center[2]	Austin	100%	68
North Cypress Medical Center	Cypress	100%	119
North Hills Hospital	N Richland Hls	100%	105
Oakbend Medical Center[2]	Richmond	100%	44
Paris Regional Medical Center	Paris	100%	47
Parkland Health & Hospital System[2]	Dallas	100%	107
Peterson Regional Medical Center	Kerrville	100%	50
Plaza Medical Center of Fort Worth[2]	Fort Worth	100%	87
Providence Health Center	Waco	100%	213
Rio Grande Regional Hospital[2]	Mcallen	100%	70
Round Rock Medical Center	Round Rock	100%	74
Saint David's Medical Center[2]	Austin	100%	89
Saint David's South Austin Medical Center[2]	Austin	100%	71
Saint Joseph Regional Health Center[2]	Bryan	100%	103
Saint Luke's Hospital at the Vintage	Houston	100%	33
Saint Luke's Sugar Land Hospital	Sugar Land	100%	33
Saint Luke's the Woodlands Hospital	The Woodlands	100%	133
San Angelo Community Medical Center	San Angelo	100%	33
San Jacinto Methodist Hospital	Baytown	100%	158
Scott & White Hospital - Round Rock	Round Rock	100%	63
Scott & White Memorial Hospital[2]	Temple	100%	114
Seton Medical Center Austin	Austin	100%	201
Seton Medical Center Hays	Kyle	100%	71
Shannon Medical Center	San Angelo	100%	140
Sierra Medical Center	El Paso	100%	83
Sierra Providence East Medical Center	El Paso	100%	84
South Texas Health System[2]	Edinburg	100%	95
Texas Health Arlington Memorial Hospital[2]	Arlington	100%	115
TX Hlth Harris Meth Hosp SW Ft Worth[2]	Fort Worth	100%	71
Texas Health Harris Methodist[2]	Bedford	100%	108
Texas Health Presbyterian Hospital - WNJ	Sherman	100%	49
Texas Health Presbyterian Hospital Dallas[2]	Dallas	100%	97
Texas Health Presbyterian Hospital Denton[2]	Denton	100%	88
TX Hlth Presbyterian Hosp-Kaufman[2]	Kaufman	100%	25
Texas Health Presbyterian Hospital Plano[2]	Plano	100%	89
TX Health Presbyterian Hosp Rockwall	Rockwall	100%	29
Texoma Medical Center[2]	Denison	100%	100
Univ of Texas Med Branch Galveston[2]	Galveston	100%	80
UT Southwestern University Hospital	Dallas	100%	32
Valley Regional Medical Center[2]	Brownsville	100%	50
VHS Brownsville Hospital Company	Brownsville	100%	80
VHS Harlingen Hospital Company	Harlingen	100%	213
Woodland Heights Medical Center	Lufkin	100%	41
Baptist Beaumont Hospital[2]	Beaumont	99%	134
Baylor Medical Center at Irving[2]	Irving	99%	84
Baylor Regional Medical Center at Plano	Plano	99%	80
Christus Saint Michael Health System	Texarkana	99%	171
Christus Santa Rosa Hospital	San Antonio	99%	127
The Corpus Christi Medical Center[2]	Corpus Christi	99%	68
Doctors Hospital at Renaissance	Edinburg	99%	135
Good Shepherd Medical Center	Longview	99%	326
Knapp Medical Center[2]	Weslaco	99%	71
Las Palmas Medical Center[2]	El Paso	99%	105
Medical Center Hospital	Odessa	99%	166
Memorial Hermann Northeast	Humble	99%	176
Memorial Hermann Texas Medical Center	Houston	99%	528
Memorial Medical Center of East Texas	Lufkin	99%	130
Methodist Sugar Land Hospital	Sugar Land	99%	174
Providence Memorial Hospital	El Paso	99%	70
Saint Joseph Medical Center	Houston	99%	77
Texas Health Harris Methodist Fort Worth[2]	Fort Worth	99%	180
United Regional Health Care System	Wichita Falls	99%	222
University Health System[2]	San Antonio	99%	146
University Medical Center at Brackenridge	Austin	99%	138
University Medical Center of El Paso	El Paso	99%	97
UT SW Univ Hosp-Zale Lipshy[2]	Dallas	99%	92
Wadley Regional Medical Center	Texarkana	99%	181
West Houston Medical Center	Houston	99%	99
Baptist Saint Anthony's Hospital[2]	Amarillo	98%	96
Central Texas Medical Center	San Marcos	98%	45
Christus Spohn Hospital Corpus Christi[2]	Corpus Christi	98%	356
JPS Health Network	Fort Worth	98%	223
Memorial Hospital	Nacogdoches	98%	44
Midland Memorial Hospital	Midland	98%	127
Mother Frances Hospital	Tyler	98%	357

NOTE: Hospital profiles are in alphabetical order by state, then city, then hospital within the city; Rankings exclude hospitals with less than 25 cases except for patient surveys which excludes hospitals with less than 100 cases; (a) 100-299 cases; (1) The number of cases/patients is too few to report; (2) Data submitted were based on a sample of cases/patients; (3) Results are based on a shorter time period than required; (4) Data suppressed by CMS for one or more quarters; (5) Results are not available for this reporting period; (6) Fewer than 100 patients completed the HCAHPS survey; (7) No cases met the criteria for this measure; (8) The lower limit of the confidence interval cannot be calculated if the number of observed infections equals zero; (9) No data are available from the state/territory for this reporting period; (10) The scores shown reflect fewer than 50 completed surveys; (11) There were discrepancies in the data collection process; (12) This measure does not apply to this hospital for this reporting period; (13) Results cannot be calculated for this reporting period; (14) The results for this state are combined with nearby states to protect confidentiality; Please refer to the User's Guide for a full explanation of data.

Hospital Name	City	Rate	Cases
Nacogdoches Medical Center	Nacogdoches	98%	48
Seton Medical Center Williamson	Round Rock	98%	89
Texas Reg Med Ctr at Sunnyvale	Sunnyvale	98%	43
Wise Regional Health System	Decatur	98%	55
Northwest Texas Hospital[2]	Amarillo	97%	93
Palestine Regional Medical Center	Palestine	97%	36
Saint Luke's Episcopal Hospital[2]	Houston	97%	109
University Medical Center	Lubbock	97%	156
Huntsville Memorial Hospital	Huntsville	96%	26
The Medical Center of Southeast Texas	Port Arthur	96%	78
Odessa Regional Hospital	Odessa	96%	28
Park Plaza Hospital	Houston	96%	25
Mission Regional Medical Center	Mission	95%	58
Seton Northwest Hospital	Austin	95%	40
Tomball Regional Medical Center	Tomball	95%	101
Covenant Medical Center	Lubbock	94%	217
Laredo Medical Center	Laredo	94%	190
Saint Luke's Patients Medical Center	Pasadena	93%	27
Christus Hospital[2]	Beaumont	91%	91
Citizens Medical Center	Victoria	91%	65
Doctors Hospital of Laredo	Laredo	91%	47
Southwest General Hospital	San Antonio	89%	54
East Texas Medical Center Athens	Athens	87%	78
Hopkins County Memorial Hospital	Sulphur Springs	85%	26
Memorial Medical Center Livingston[2]	Livingston	85%	26

Discharged on Statin Medication

Hospital Name	City	Rate	Cases
Bayshore Medical Center	Pasadena	100%	158
Conroe Regional Medical Center	Conroe	100%	117
The Corpus Christi Medical Center[2]	Corpus Christi	100%	52
Detar Hospital Navarro	Victoria	100%	59
Houston Northwest Medical Center	Houston	100%	138
Lake Pointe Medical Center	Rowlett	100%	60
Medical Center of Lewisville	Lewisville	100%	34
Memorial Hermann Hospital System	Houston	100%	483
Memorial Hermann Sugar Land Hospital	Sugar Land	100%	36
Memorial Hermann Texas Medical Center	Houston	100%	382
Methodist Mansfield Medical Center[2]	Mansfield	100%	62
Methodist Richardson Medical Center	Richardson	100%	41
Methodist Stone Oak Hospital[2]	San Antonio	100%	82
Methodist Willowbrook Hospital	Houston	100%	125
Metroplex Hospital[2]	Killeen	100%	34
Midland Memorial Hospital	Midland	100%	94
North Austin Medical Center[2]	Austin	100%	55
North Cypress Medical Center	Cypress	100%	101
North Hills Hospital	N Richland Hls	100%	81
Parkland Health & Hospital System[2]	Dallas	100%	77
Providence Memorial Hospital	El Paso	100%	52
Saint David's Medical Center[2]	Austin	100%	69
Saint David's South Austin Medical Center[2]	Austin	100%	52
San Angelo Community Medical Center	San Angelo	100%	29
Scott & White Hospital - Round Rock	Round Rock	100%	46
Scott & White Memorial Hospital[2]	Temple	100%	88
Sierra Medical Center	El Paso	100%	54
Texas Health Arlington Memorial Hospital[2]	Arlington	100%	88
Texas Health Presbyterian Hospital Dallas[2]	Dallas	100%	80
Texas Health Presbyterian Hospital Denton[2]	Denton	100%	67
Texas Health Presbyterian Hospital Plano[2]	Plano	100%	63
Texoma Medical Center[2]	Denison	100%	67
University Medical Center of El Paso	El Paso	100%	71
West Houston Medical Center	Houston	100%	71
Woodland Heights Medical Center	Lufkin	100%	31
Kingwood Medical Center[2]	Kingwood	99%	69
Las Palmas Medical Center[2]	El Paso	99%	80
Medical Center of Arlington[2]	Arlington	99%	88
Medical Center of Plano[2]	Plano	99%	85
Medical City Dallas Hospital	Dallas	99%	122
Mem Hermann Mem City Med Ctr	Houston	99%	171
Methodist Charlton Medical Center[2]	Dallas	99%	136
Methodist Dallas Medical Center[2]	Dallas	99%	110
Methodist Hospital	San Antonio	99%	514
Seton Medical Center Austin	Austin	99%	158
South Texas Health System[2]	Edinburg	99%	69
Texas Health Harris Methodist[2]	Bedford	99%	87
United Regional Health Care System	Wichita Falls	99%	169
Baptist Beaumont Hospital[2]	Beaumont	98%	106
Baptist Medical Center	San Antonio	98%	552
Baylor Medical Center at Irving[2]	Irving	98%	62
Baylor Reg Med Ctr at Grapevine	Grapevine	98%	62
Clear Lake Regional Medical Center[2]	Webster	98%	81
College Station Medical Center	College Station	98%	46
Harris Health System	Houston	98%	169
Medical Center of Mckinney[2]	Mckinney	98%	61
Memorial Hermann Katy Hospital	Katy	98%	55
Memorial Hermann Northeast	Humble	98%	129
San Jacinto Methodist Hospital	Baytown	98%	124
Seton Medical Center Hays	Kyle	98%	55
Sierra Providence East Medical Center	El Paso	98%	54
Texas Health Harris Methodist Fort Worth[2]	Fort Worth	98%	140
University Health System[2]	San Antonio	98%	113
Univ of Texas Med Branch Galveston[2]	Galveston	98%	50
Valley Regional Medical Center[2]	Brownsville	98%	43
Abilene Regional Medical Center	Abilene	97%	38
Baylor University Medical Center[2]	Dallas	97%	98
Central Texas Medical Center	San Marcos	97%	39
Dallas Regional Medical Center	Mesquite	97%	29
Hendrick Medical Center	Abilene	97%	74
Medical Center Hospital	Odessa	97%	119
Methodist Sugar Land Hospital	Sugar Land	97%	136
Methodist West Houston Hospital	Houston	97%	74
Oakbend Medical Center[2]	Richmond	97%	33
Peterson Regional Medical Center	Kerrville	97%	36
Plaza Medical Center of Fort Worth[2]	Fort Worth	97%	64
TX Hlth Harris Meth Hosp SW Ft Worth[2]	Fort Worth	97%	62
University Medical Center at Brackenridge	Austin	97%	96
UT SW Univ Hosp-Zale Lipshy[2]	Dallas	97%	62
VHS Harlingen Hospital Company	Harlingen	97%	152
Doctors Hospital	Dallas	96%	56
Hillcrest Baptist Medical Center	Waco	96%	93
JPS Health Network	Fort Worth	96%	199
Knapp Medical Center[2]	Weslaco	96%	53
Memorial Medical Center of East Texas	Lufkin	96%	96
The Methodist Hospital	Houston	96%	313
Round Rock Medical Center	Round Rock	96%	55
Saint Joseph Regional Health Center[2]	Bryan	96%	84
Seton Medical Center Williamson	Round Rock	96%	57
Shannon Medical Center	San Angelo	96%	112
Baylor Medical Center at Garland[2]	Garland	95%	94
Denton Regional Medical Center[2]	Denton	95%	58
Doctors Hospital at Renaissance	Edinburg	95%	95
Huguley Memorial Medical Center	Burleson	95%	61
Saint Luke's the Woodlands Hospital	The Woodlands	95%	104
VHS Brownsville Hospital Company	Brownsville	95%	44
Wadley Regional Medical Center	Texarkana	95%	143
Baylor Medical Center at Mckinney	Mc Kinney	94%	36
Baylor Regional Medical Center at Plano	Plano	94%	62
Mother Frances Hospital	Tyler	94%	289
Providence Health Center	Waco	94%	168
Christus Saint Michael Health System	Texarkana	93%	130
Longview Regional Medical Center	Longview	93%	29
Rio Grande Regional Hospital[2]	Mcallen	93%	44
Cypress Fairbanks Medical Center	Houston	92%	39
Good Shepherd Medical Center	Longview	92%	257
Harlingen Medical Center	Harlingen	92%	26
University Medical Center	Lubbock	92%	132
UT Southwestern University Hospital	Dallas	92%	26
Christus Santa Rosa Hospital	San Antonio	91%	105
East Texas Medical Center	Tyler	91%	214
Northwest Texas Hospital[2]	Amarillo	90%	70
Paris Regional Medical Center	Paris	90%	39
Saint Luke's Episcopal Hospital[2]	Houston	90%	93
Saint Luke's Hospital at the Vintage	Houston	90%	30
Baylor All Saints Medical Center at FW[2]	Fort Worth	89%	55
Tomball Regional Medical Center	Tomball	89%	80
Brazosport Regional Health System	Lake Jackson	88%	26
Covenant Medical Center	Lubbock	88%	171
Saint Luke's Sugar Land Hospital	Sugar Land	88%	26
Seton Northwest Hospital	Austin	88%	34
Texas Health Presbyterian Hospital - WNJ	Sherman	88%	40
Texas Reg Med Ctr at Sunnyvale	Sunnyvale	88%	34
Wise Regional Health System	Decatur	88%	34
Baptist Saint Anthony's Hospital[2]	Amarillo	87%	79
Christus Spohn Hospital Corpus Christi[2]	Corpus Christi	87%	284
Doctors Hospital of Laredo	Laredo	86%	37
Saint Joseph Medical Center	Houston	86%	65
Mission Regional Medical Center	Mission	85%	46
Palestine Regional Medical Center	Palestine	85%	26
Citizens Medical Center	Victoria	83%	54
Laredo Medical Center	Laredo	83%	138
Southwest General Hospital	San Antonio	83%	41
Nacogdoches Medical Center	Nacogdoches	82%	39
Hunt Regional Medical Center[2]	Greenville	81%	58
Christus Hospital[2]	Beaumont	74%	88
The Medical Center of Southeast Texas	Port Arthur	74%	61
Memorial Hospital	Nacogdoches	74%	39
Hopkins County Memorial Hospital	Sulphur Springs	72%	25
Huntsville Memorial Hospital	Huntsville	64%	25
East Texas Medical Center Athens	Athens	52%	65

Thrombolytic Therapy Timing

Hospital Name	City	Rate	Cases
The Methodist Hospital	Houston	98%	43
Methodist Hospital	San Antonio	97%	32
VHS Harlingen Hospital Company	Harlingen	97%	30
Memorial Hermann Texas Medical Center	Houston	95%	65
Baptist Medical Center	San Antonio	94%	83
University Health System[2]	San Antonio	88%	25
JPS Health Network	Fort Worth	83%	30
Memorial Hermann Hospital System	Houston	77%	43
Christus Spohn Hospital Corpus Christi[2]	Corpus Christi	76%	41
Mem Hermann Mem City Med Ctr	Houston	73%	33
Seton Medical Center Austin	Austin	67%	30
Northwest Texas Hospital[2]	Amarillo	11%	36

Venous Thromboembolism (VTE) Prophylaxis

Hospital Name	City	Rate	Cases
Baylor Regional Medical Center at Plano	Plano	100%	74
Baylor University Medical Center[2]	Dallas	100%	163
Central Texas Medical Center	San Marcos	100%	45
College Station Medical Center	College Station	100%	60
The Corpus Christi Medical Center[2]	Corpus Christi	100%	79
Detar Hospital Navarro	Victoria	100%	84
Lake Pointe Medical Center	Rowlett	100%	62
Medical Center of Arlington[2]	Arlington	100%	129
Medical Center of Lewisville	Lewisville	100%	51
Medical Center of Plano[2]	Plano	100%	152
Mem Hermann Mem City Med Ctr	Houston	100%	300
Memorial Hermann Sugar Land Hospital	Sugar Land	100%	37
Memorial Hermann Texas Medical Center	Houston	100%	939
Methodist Dallas Medical Center[2]	Dallas	100%	236
Methodist Hospital	San Antonio	100%	889
Methodist Mansfield Medical Center[2]	Mansfield	100%	72
Methodist Richardson Medical Center	Richardson	100%	44
Methodist Stone Oak Hospital[2]	San Antonio	100%	118
Methodist Sugar Land Hospital	Sugar Land	100%	181
Metroplex Hospital[2]	Killeen	100%	47
North Austin Medical Center[2]	Austin	100%	76
North Hills Hospital	N Richland Hls	100%	112
Peterson Regional Medical Center	Kerrville	100%	52
San Angelo Community Medical Center	San Angelo	100%	36
Sierra Providence East Medical Center	El Paso	100%	106
TX Health Presbyterian Hosp Rockwall	Rockwall	100%	25
Texas Reg Med Ctr at Sunnyvale	Sunnyvale	100%	47
Texoma Medical Center[2]	Denison	100%	104
West Houston Medical Center	Houston	100%	142
Woodland Heights Medical Center	Lufkin	100%	43
Baylor Reg Med Ctr at Grapevine	Grapevine	99%	75
Bayshore Medical Center	Pasadena	99%	215
Conroe Regional Medical Center	Conroe	99%	177
Hendrick Medical Center	Abilene	99%	135
Kingwood Medical Center[2]	Kingwood	99%	126
Knapp Medical Center[2]	Weslaco	99%	91
Las Palmas Medical Center[2]	El Paso	99%	134
Memorial Hermann Hospital System	Houston	99%	636
Memorial Hermann Katy Hospital	Katy	99%	77
North Cypress Medical Center	Cypress	99%	146
Parkland Health & Hospital System[2]	Dallas	99%	129
Rio Grande Regional Hospital[2]	Mcallen	99%	107
Round Rock Medical Center	Round Rock	99%	76
Saint David's South Austin Medical Center[2]	Austin	99%	70
Scott & White Memorial Hospital[2]	Temple	99%	151
Shannon Medical Center	San Angelo	99%	178
Texas Health Harris Methodist[2]	Bedford	99%	108
Texas Health Presbyterian Hospital Dallas[2]	Dallas	99%	115
Texas Health Presbyterian Hospital Denton[2]	Denton	99%	85
United Regional Health Care System	Wichita Falls	99%	251
University Health System[2]	San Antonio	99%	166
University Medical Center of El Paso	El Paso	99%	143
Univ of Texas Med Branch Galveston[2]	Galveston	99%	111
UT SW Univ Hosp-Zale Lipshy[2]	Dallas	99%	165
Baylor Medical Center at Irving[2]	Irving	98%	97
Baylor Medical Center at Mckinney	Mc Kinney	98%	43
Good Shepherd Medical Center	Longview	98%	350
Medical Center Hospital	Odessa	98%	206
Medical City Dallas Hospital	Dallas	98%	225
Memorial Hermann Northeast	Humble	98%	179
Methodist Charlton Medical Center[2]	Dallas	98%	182
Oakbend Medical Center[2]	Richmond	98%	48
Palestine Regional Medical Center	Palestine	98%	41
Providence Memorial Hospital	El Paso	98%	122
Saint David's Medical Center[2]	Austin	98%	125
Saint Joseph Regional Health Center[2]	Bryan	98%	128
Seton Medical Center Williamson	Round Rock	98%	105
Sierra Medical Center	El Paso	98%	131
South Texas Health System[2]	Edinburg	98%	137
Texas Health Harris Methodist Fort Worth[2]	Fort Worth	98%	254
Texas Health Presbyterian Hospital Plano[2]	Plano	98%	84
Valley Regional Medical Center[2]	Brownsville	98%	57
Wadley Regional Medical Center	Texarkana	98%	195
Baylor Medical Center at Garland[2]	Garland	97%	115
Brazosport Regional Health System	Lake Jackson	97%	32
Brownwood Regional Medical Center	Brownwood	97%	34
Hillcrest Baptist Medical Center	Waco	97%	131
Memorial Medical Center of East Texas	Lufkin	97%	149
Methodist Willowbrook Hospital	Houston	97%	179
Seton Northwest Hospital	Austin	97%	30
Texas Health Arlington Memorial Hospital[2]	Arlington	97%	118
Denton Regional Medical Center[2]	Denton	96%	84
JPS Health Network	Fort Worth	96%	306
Longview Regional Medical Center	Longview	96%	50
Medical Center of Mckinney[2]	Mckinney	96%	85
The Methodist Hospital	Houston	96%	560

NOTE: Hospital profiles are in alphabetical order by state, then city, then hospital within the city; Rankings exclude hospitals with less than 25 cases except for patient surveys which excludes hospitals with less than 100 cases; (a) 100-299 cases; (1) The number of cases/patients is too few to report; (2) Data submitted were based on a sample of cases/patients; (3) Results are based on a shorter time period than required; (4) Data suppressed by CMS for one or more quarters; (5) Results are not available for this reporting period; (6) Fewer than 100 patients completed the HCAHPS survey; (7) No cases met the criteria for this measure; (8) The lower limit of the confidence interval cannot be calculated if the number of observed infections equals zero; (9) No data are available from the state/territory for this reporting period; (10) The scores shown reflect fewer than 50 completed surveys; (11) There were discrepancies in the data collection process; (12) This measure does not apply to this hospital for this reporting period; (13) Results cannot be calculated for this reporting period; (14) The results for this state are combined with nearby states to protect confidentiality; Please refer to the User's Guide for a full explanation of data.

Midland Memorial Hospital	Midland	96%	136
Mother Frances Hospital	Tyler	96%	400
Northwest Texas Hospital[2]	Amarillo	96%	126
Scott & White Hospital - Round Rock	Round Rock	96%	54
VHS Harlingen Hospital Company	Harlingen	96%	289
Wise Regional Health System	Decatur	96%	48
Abilene Regional Medical Center	Abilene	95%	55
Baptist Medical Center	San Antonio	95%	897
Christus Saint Michael Health System	Texarkana	95%	186
Doctors Hospital at Renaissance	Edinburg	95%	171
Houston Northwest Medical Center	Houston	95%	209
Laredo Medical Center	Laredo	95%	217
Seton Medical Center Austin	Austin	95%	220
VHS Brownsville Hospital Company	Brownsville	95%	111
Baptist Beaumont Hospital[2]	Beaumont	94%	162
Clear Lake Regional Medical Center[2]	Webster	94%	107
East Texas Medical Center	Tyler	94%	348
Plaza Medical Center of Fort Worth[2]	Fort Worth	94%	121
Saint Luke's Sugar Land Hospital	Sugar Land	94%	36
University Medical Center at Brackenridge	Austin	94%	195
Harris Health System	Houston	93%	274
San Jacinto Methodist Hospital	Baytown	93%	173
Centennial Medical Center	Frisco	92%	40
Citizens Medical Center	Victoria	92%	65
Mission Regional Medical Center	Mission	92%	87
Providence Health Center	Waco	92%	254
Baylor Medical Center at Waxahachie	Waxahachie	91%	34
Covenant Medical Center	Lubbock	91%	297
Dallas Regional Medical Center	Mesquite	91%	43
Huguley Memorial Medical Center	Burleson	91%	75
Seton Medical Center Hays	Kyle	91%	68
Southwest General Hospital	San Antonio	91%	55
Baptist Saint Anthony's Hospital[2]	Amarillo	90%	115
Christus Spohn Hospital Corpus Christi[2]	Corpus Christi	90%	459
Doctors Hospital	Dallas	90%	77
Saint Luke's the Woodlands Hospital	The Woodlands	90%	154
Texas Health Presbyterian Hospital - WNJ	Sherman	90%	61
Cypress Fairbanks Medical Center	Houston	89%	53
Doctors Hospital of Laredo	Laredo	89%	54
Saint Luke's Patients Medical Center	Pasadena	89%	27
Baylor Medical Center at Carrollton	Carrollton	86%	42
Saint Luke's Hospital at the Vintage	Houston	86%	36
Tomball Regional Medical Center	Tomball	86%	108
Methodist West Houston Hospital	Houston	85%	86
Nacogdoches Medical Center	Nacogdoches	84%	49
Saint Joseph Medical Center	Houston	84%	94
Saint Luke's Episcopal Hospital[2]	Houston	84%	142
Baylor All Saints Medical Center at FW[2]	Fort Worth	83%	82
Hunt Regional Medical Center[2]	Greenville	82%	66
TX Hlth Harris Meth Hosp SW Ft Worth[2]	Fort Worth	82%	57
Fort Duncan Medical Center	Eagle Pass	81%	26
University Medical Center	Lubbock	80%	208
UT Southwestern University Hospital	Dallas	80%	35
Nix Health Care System	San Antonio	79%	28
Odessa Regional Hospital	Odessa	77%	30
Memorial Medical Center Livingston[2]	Livingston	76%	29
Paris Regional Medical Center	Paris	76%	50
Park Plaza Hospital	Houston	76%	29
Christus Hospital[2]	Beaumont	70%	124
Huntsville Memorial Hospital	Huntsville	70%	33
Christus Saint John Hospital	Nassau Bay	69%	29
The Medical Center of Southeast Texas	Port Arthur	68%	84
Harlingen Medical Center	Harlingen	64%	36
Memorial Hospital	Nacogdoches	61%	57
Christus Santa Rosa Hospital	San Antonio	58%	135
Navarro Regional Hospital	Corsicana	48%	31
East Texas Medical Center Athens	Athens	42%	81
Hopkins County Memorial Hospital	Sulphur Springs	35%	26

Written Stroke Educational Materials Given

Hospital Name	City	Rate	Cases
Baylor Medical Center at Garland[2]	Garland	100%	76
Baylor Medical Center at Mckinney	Mc Kinney	100%	26
Baylor University Medical Center[2]	Dallas	100%	88
Detar Hospital Navarro	Victoria	100%	41
Doctors Hospital	Dallas	100%	44
Kingwood Medical Center[2]	Kingwood	100%	69
Knapp Medical Center[2]	Weslaco	100%	41
Lake Pointe Medical Center	Rowlett	100%	38
Methodist Mansfield Medical Center[2]	Mansfield	100%	53
Methodist Richardson Medical Center	Richardson	100%	27
Metroplex Hospital[2]	Killeen	100%	26
Mission Regional Medical Center	Mission	100%	43
North Austin Medical Center[2]	Austin	100%	56
North Cypress Medical Center	Cypress	100%	81
North Hills Hospital	N Richland Hls	100%	58
Providence Memorial Hospital	El Paso	100%	55
Sierra Providence East Medical Center	El Paso	100%	61
Southwest General Hospital	San Antonio	100%	32
Texas Health Harris Methodist[2]	Bedford	100%	62
Texas Health Presbyterian Hospital Plano[2]	Plano	100%	52
Texoma Medical Center[2]	Denison	100%	60
West Houston Medical Center	Houston	100%	69
Covenant Medical Center	Lubbock	99%	141
Methodist Dallas Medical Center[2]	Dallas	99%	115
Methodist Stone Oak Hospital[2]	San Antonio	99%	70
Mother Frances Hospital	Tyler	99%	201
Parkland Health & Hospital System[2]	Dallas	99%	92
Saint David's Medical Center[2]	Austin	99%	67
South Texas Health System[2]	Edinburg	99%	81
UT SW Univ Hosp-Zale Lipshy[2]	Dallas	99%	77
Wadley Regional Medical Center	Texarkana	99%	94
Baylor Reg Med Ctr at Grapevine	Grapevine	98%	53
Las Palmas Medical Center[2]	El Paso	98%	80
Medical Center of Mckinney[2]	Mckinney	98%	49
Memorial Hermann Hospital System	Houston	98%	415
Memorial Medical Center of East Texas	Lufkin	98%	63
Methodist Charlton Medical Center[2]	Dallas	98%	95
Methodist Hospital	San Antonio	98%	412
Shannon Medical Center	San Angelo	98%	91
TX Hlth Harris Meth Hosp SW Ft Worth[2]	Fort Worth	98%	48
Texas Health Presbyterian Hospital Dallas[2]	Dallas	98%	66
Texas Health Presbyterian Hospital Denton[2]	Denton	98%	58
United Regional Health Care System	Wichita Falls	98%	126
VHS Harlingen Hospital Company	Harlingen	98%	147
Baylor Medical Center at Irving[2]	Irving	97%	60
Bayshore Medical Center	Pasadena	97%	138
Brazosport Regional Health System	Lake Jackson	97%	30
Conroe Regional Medical Center	Conroe	97%	106
Cypress Fairbanks Medical Center	Houston	97%	34
Doctors Hospital at Renaissance	Edinburg	97%	90
Longview Regional Medical Center	Longview	97%	30
Medical Center of Arlington[2]	Arlington	97%	58
Medical Center of Lewisville	Lewisville	97%	32
Mem Hermann Mem City Med Ctr	Houston	97%	184
San Jacinto Methodist Hospital	Baytown	97%	106
Texas Health Presbyterian Hospital - WNJ	Sherman	97%	33
VHS Brownsville Hospital Company	Brownsville	97%	39
Wise Regional Health System	Decatur	97%	29
The Corpus Christi Medical Center[2]	Corpus Christi	96%	53
Good Shepherd Medical Center	Longview	96%	193
Hendrick Medical Center	Abilene	96%	78
Hillcrest Baptist Medical Center	Waco	96%	69
Huguley Memorial Medical Center	Burleson	96%	53
JPS Health Network	Fort Worth	96%	202
Medical Center of Plano[2]	Plano	96%	70
Memorial Hermann Texas Medical Center	Houston	96%	500
Methodist Willowbrook Hospital	Houston	96%	109
Midland Memorial Hospital	Midland	96%	73
Peterson Regional Medical Center	Kerrville	96%	28
Saint Joseph Regional Health Center[2]	Bryan	96%	67
Scott & White Hospital - Round Rock	Round Rock	96%	27
Woodland Heights Medical Center	Lufkin	96%	25
Citizens Medical Center	Victoria	95%	38
Denton Regional Medical Center[2]	Denton	95%	56
Laredo Medical Center	Laredo	95%	132
Medical City Dallas Hospital	Dallas	95%	114
Methodist Sugar Land Hospital	Sugar Land	95%	108
Scott & White Memorial Hospital[2]	Temple	95%	80
University Health System[2]	San Antonio	95%	130
Baptist Beaumont Hospital[2]	Beaumont	94%	80
Clear Lake Regional Medical Center[2]	Webster	94%	72
Memorial Hermann Northeast	Humble	94%	113
Seton Medical Center Austin	Austin	94%	124
Texas Health Arlington Memorial Hospital[2]	Arlington	94%	82
University Medical Center of El Paso	El Paso	94%	105
Baylor All Saints Medical Center at FW[2]	Fort Worth	93%	30
College Station Medical Center	College Station	93%	45
Houston Northwest Medical Center	Houston	93%	119
Memorial Hermann Katy Hospital	Katy	93%	54
The Methodist Hospital	Houston	93%	299
Round Rock Medical Center	Round Rock	93%	45
University Medical Center	Lubbock	93%	109
Baptist Medical Center	San Antonio	92%	433
Memorial Hermann Sugar Land Hospital	Sugar Land	92%	36
Texas Health Harris Methodist Fort Worth[2]	Fort Worth	92%	127
Christus Spohn Hospital Corpus Christi[2]	Corpus Christi	91%	227
Methodist West Houston Hospital	Houston	91%	66
Plaza Medical Center of Fort Worth[2]	Fort Worth	91%	55
Harris Health System	Houston	90%	209
Baylor Regional Medical Center at Plano	Plano	89%	55
Sierra Medical Center	El Paso	89%	63
Dallas Regional Medical Center	Mesquite	88%	25
Providence Health Center	Waco	88%	130
Seton Medical Center Williamson	Round Rock	88%	60
Medical Center Hospital	Odessa	87%	122
Rio Grande Regional Hospital[2]	Mcallen	87%	70
East Texas Medical Center	Tyler	86%	160
Texas Reg Med Ctr at Sunnyvale	Sunnyvale	86%	28
Saint Joseph Medical Center	Houston	85%	55
Saint Luke's the Woodlands Hospital	The Woodlands	85%	104
Harlingen Medical Center	Harlingen	84%	25
East Texas Medical Center Athens	Athens	83%	42
Nacogdoches Medical Center	Nacogdoches	83%	30
Northwest Texas Hospital[2]	Amarillo	83%	70
Saint David's South Austin Medical Center[2]	Austin	83%	42
Christus Saint Michael Health System	Texarkana	81%	78
Hunt Regional Medical Center[2]	Greenville	81%	36
Univ of Texas Med Branch Galveston[2]	Galveston	78%	64
Tomball Regional Medical Center	Tomball	77%	66
Saint Luke's Episcopal Hospital[2]	Houston	75%	81
University Medical Center at Brackenridge	Austin	75%	125
Valley Regional Medical Center[2]	Brownsville	74%	31
The Medical Center of Southeast Texas	Port Arthur	70%	44
Seton Medical Center Hays	Kyle	70%	47
Baptist Saint Anthony's Hospital[2]	Amarillo	68%	57
Doctors Hospital of Laredo	Laredo	56%	25
Christus Hospital[2]	Beaumont	55%	65
Seton Northwest Hospital	Austin	39%	33
Christus Santa Rosa Hospital	San Antonio	27%	74
Memorial Hospital	Nacogdoches	4%	27

Surgical Care Improvement Project

Appropriate Beta Blocker Usage

Hospital Name	City	Rate	Cases
Baylor Heart & Vascular Hospital	Dallas	100%	68
Baylor Medical Center at Mckinney[2]	Mc Kinney	100%	64
Baylor Medical Center at Uptown	Dallas	100%	99
Bayshore Medical Center[2]	Pasadena	100%	119
Brownwood Regional Medical Center	Brownwood	100%	65
Centennial Medical Center	Frisco	100%	58
Central Texas Medical Center	San Marcos	100%	38
Christus Saint Catherine Hospital	Katy	100%	31
Conroe Regional Medical Center[2]	Conroe	100%	199
Cornerstone Regional Hospital[2]	Edinburg	100%	50
Dallas Regional Medical Center	Mesquite	100%	65
Denton Regional Medical Center[2]	Denton	100%	266
Good Shepherd Medical Center Marshall	Marshall	100%	67
Heart Hospital Baylor Plano	Plano	100%	746
Heritage Park Surgical Hospital	Sherman	100%	46
Hill Country Memorial Hospital[2]	Fredericksburg	100%	157
The Hospital at Westlake Medical Center	Austin	100%	57
Huguley Memorial Medical Center	Burleson	100%	230
Kingwood Medical Center[2]	Kingwood	100%	164
Medical Center of Arlington[2]	Arlington	100%	114
Medical Center of Lewisville[2]	Lewisville	100%	102
Medical City Dallas Hospital[2]	Dallas	100%	253
Memorial Hermann Katy Hospital[2]	Katy	100%	100
Methodist Dallas Medical Center	Dallas	100%	319
Methodist Mansfield Medical Center	Mansfield	100%	98
Methodist Mckinney Hospital[2]	Mc Kinney	100%	69
Methodist Richardson Medical Center[2]	Richardson	100%	80
Navarro Regional Hospital	Corsicana	100%	36
North Austin Medical Center[2]	Austin	100%	165
North Central Surgical Center	Dallas	100%	48
North Cypress Medical Center	Cypress	100%	201
Odessa Regional Hospital	Odessa	100%	72
Parkland Health & Hospital System[2]	Dallas	100%	72
Quail Creek Surgical Hospital	Amarillo	100%	232
Round Rock Medical Center[2]	Round Rock	100%	119
Saint David's Medical Center[2]	Austin	100%	236
Saint Luke's the Woodlands Hospital[2]	The Woodlands	100%	232
San Angelo Community Medical Center	San Angelo	100%	139
Scott & White Hospital Brenham	Brenham	100%	31
Seton Highland Lakes	Burnet	100%	30
South Texas Spine & Surgical Hospital	San Antonio	100%	49
Texas Health Arlington Memorial Hospital[2]	Arlington	100%	110
Texas Health Harris Methodist Fort Worth[2]	Fort Worth	100%	445
TX Hlth Harris Meth Hosp-Southlake	Southlake	100%	154
TX Hlth Harris Meth Hosp SW Ft Worth[2]	Fort Worth	100%	101
TX Hlth Heart & Vasc Hosp-Arlington	Arlington	100%	64
Texas Health Presbyterian Hospital - WNJ	Sherman	100%	135
Texas Health Presbyterian Hospital Allen[2]	Allen	100%	34
TX Hlth Presbyterian Hosp-Flower Mound	Flower Mound	100%	93
TX Hlth Presbyterian Hosp-Kaufman[2]	Kaufman	100%	32
TX Health Presbyterian Hosp Rockwall	Rockwall	100%	96
Texas Orthopedic Hospital[2]	Houston	100%	77
Texas Reg Med Ctr at Sunnyvale[2]	Sunnyvale	100%	71
Texoma Medical Center[2]	Denison	100%	221
Titus Regional Medical Center	Mount Pleasant	100%	39
University Medical Center[2]	Lubbock	100%	206
University Medical Center at Brackenridge[2]	Austin	100%	58
University Medical Center of El Paso[2]	El Paso	100%	66
UT SW Univ Hosp-Zale Lipshy[2]	Dallas	100%	29
Val Verde Regional Medical Center	Del Rio	100%	28
Weatherford Regional Medical Center	Weatherford	100%	110
West Houston Medical Center[2]	Houston	100%	147
Woodland Heights Medical Center	Lufkin	100%	195
Abilene Regional Medical Center	Abilene	99%	217
Baptist Medical Center[2]	San Antonio	99%	1097
Baylor Medical Center at Carrollton	Carrollton	99%	86

NOTE: Hospital profiles are in alphabetical order by state, then city, then hospital within the city; Rankings exclude hospitals with less than 25 cases except for patient surveys which excludes hospitals with less than 100 cases; (a) 100-299 cases; (1) The number of cases/patients is too few to report; (2) Data submitted were based on a sample of cases/patients; (3) Results are based on a shorter time period than required; (4) Data suppressed by CMS for one or more quarters; (5) Results are not available for this reporting period; (6) Fewer than 100 patients completed the HCAHPS survey; (7) No cases met the criteria for this measure; (8) The lower limit of the confidence interval cannot be calculated if the number of observed infections equals zero; (9) No data are available from the state/territory for this reporting period; (10) The scores shown reflect fewer than 50 completed surveys; (11) There were discrepancies in the data collection process; (12) This measure does not apply to this hospital for this reporting period; (13) Results cannot be calculated for this reporting period; (14) The results for this state are combined with nearby states to protect confidentiality; Please refer to the User's Guide for a full explanation of data.

Baylor Medical Center at Frisco	Frisco	99%	179
Baylor Medical Center at Garland[2]	Garland	99%	103
Baylor Ortho & Spine Hosp-Arlington	Arlington	99%	165
Baylor Regional Medical Center at Plano[2]	Plano	99%	136
Baylor Surgical Hospital at Fort Worth	Fort Worth	99%	122
Baylor University Medical Center[2]	Dallas	99%	776
College Station Medical Center	College Station	99%	209
The Corpus Christi Medical Center[2]	Corpus Christi	99%	223
Dallas VA Medical Center - VA North Texas[2]	Dallas	99%	130
Detar Hospital Navarro	Victoria	99%	141
Doctors Hospital at Renaissance[2]	Edinburg	99%	260
East Texas Medical Center[2]	Tyler	99%	215
JPS Health Network[2]	Fort Worth	99%	198
Las Palmas Medical Center[2]	El Paso	99%	188
Longview Regional Medical Center	Longview	99%	259
Methodist Charlton Medical Center	Dallas	99%	189
Methodist Hospital[2]	San Antonio	99%	393
Methodist Sugar Land Hospital[2]	Sugar Land	99%	203
Methodist West Houston Hospital[2]	Houston	99%	165
Methodist Willowbrook Hospital[2]	Houston	99%	141
North Hills Hospital[2]	N Richland Hls	99%	152
Northwest Texas Hospital[2]	Amarillo	99%	138
Palestine Regional Medical Center	Palestine	99%	73
Plaza Medical Center of Fort Worth[2]	Fort Worth	99%	284
Providence Memorial Hospital[2]	El Paso	99%	115
Saint David's South Austin Medical Center[2]	Austin	99%	188
Saint Luke's Lakeside Hospital	The Woodlands	99%	138
San Jacinto Methodist Hospital[2]	Baytown	99%	126
Seton Medical Center Williamson	Round Rock	99%	87
Shannon Medical Center	San Angelo	99%	351
Southwest General Hospital	San Antonio	99%	69
Texas Health Harris Methodist[2]	Bedford	99%	165
Texas Health Presbyterian Hospital Dallas[2]	Dallas	99%	203
Texas Health Presbyterian Hospital Plano[2]	Plano	99%	457
Texas Spine & Joint Hospital[2]	Tyler	99%	72
United Regional Health Care System	Wichita Falls	99%	282
UT Southwestern University Hospital[2]	Dallas	99%	267
Angleton - Danbury Medical Center[2]	Angleton	98%	44
Baptist Beaumont Hospital[2]	Beaumont	98%	184
Baylor Medical Center at Irving[2]	Irving	98%	131
Baylor Reg Med Ctr at Grapevine[2]	Grapevine	98%	160
Christus Hospital[2]	Beaumont	98%	355
Christus Saint Michael Health System[2]	Texarkana	98%	354
Christus Santa Rosa Hospital	San Antonio	98%	350
Cypress Fairbanks Medical Center[2]	Houston	98%	50
Doctors Hospital[2]	Dallas	98%	103
Good Shepherd Medical Center[2]	Longview	98%	183
Harlingen Medical Center[2]	Harlingen	98%	187
Harris Health System[2]	Houston	98%	120
Hendrick Medical Center[2]	Abilene	98%	200
Houston Northwest Medical Center[2]	Houston	98%	181
Houston Physicians' Hospital	Webster	98%	62
Houston VA Medical Center[2]	Houston	98%	332
Huntsville Memorial Hospital	Huntsville	98%	57
Kell West Regional Hospital	Wichita Falls	98%	98
Knapp Medical Center	Weslaco	98%	88
Lake Granbury Medical Center	Granbury	98%	59
Lake Pointe Medical Center	Rowlett	98%	82
Laredo Medical Center	Laredo	98%	122
Las Colinas Medical Center[2]	Irving	98%	55
Medical Center Hospital[2]	Odessa	98%	188
Medical Center of Plano[2]	Plano	98%	195
Memorial Hermann Sugar Land Hospital[2]	Sugar Land	98%	94
Memorial Hermann Texas Medical Center[2]	Houston	98%	243
Memorial Medical Center Livingston[2]	Livingston	98%	40
Memorial Medical Center of East Texas[2]	Lufkin	98%	136
Methodist Stone Oak Hospital[2]	San Antonio	98%	189
Mother Frances Hospital[2]	Tyler	98%	312
Rio Grande Regional Hospital[2]	Mcallen	98%	119
Saint Luke's Episcopal Hospital[2]	Houston	98%	359
Scott & White Memorial Hospital[2]	Temple	98%	312
Seton Medical Center Austin[2]	Austin	98%	204
Sierra Providence East Medical Center[2]	El Paso	98%	43
South Texas Health System[2]	Edinburg	98%	168
Sugar Land Surgical Hospital	Sugar Land	98%	45
TX Hlth Harris Meth Hosp-Cleburne[2]	Cleburne	98%	82
USMD Hospital at Fort Worth	Fort Worth	98%	49
Baptist Saint Anthony's Hospital[2]	Amarillo	97%	302
Baylor All Saints Medical Center at FW[2]	Fort Worth	97%	169
Clear Lake Regional Medical Center[2]	Webster	97%	235
Hillcrest Baptist Medical Center[2]	Waco	97%	199
Medical Center of Mckinney[2]	Mckinney	97%	158
Memorial Hermann Hospital System[2]	Houston	97%	663
Mem Hermann Mem City Med Ctr[2]	Houston	97%	205
Memorial Hermann Northeast[2]	Humble	97%	76
Mem Hermann Surgical Hosp Kingwood	Kingwood	97%	35
Methodist Ambulatory Surgery Hospital NW[2]	San Antonio	97%	38
Methodist Hospital For Surgery[2]	Addison	97%	159
The Methodist Hospital[2]	Houston	97%	384
Paris Regional Medical Center[2]	Paris	97%	183
The Physicians Centre	Bryan	97%	32
Saint Joseph Medical Center	Houston	97%	144
Saint Joseph Regional Health Center[2]	Bryan	97%	149
Scott & White Hospital - Round Rock[2]	Round Rock	97%	154
Seton Medical Center Hays	Kyle	97%	71
Seton Northwest Hospital	Austin	97%	59
South Texas Surgical Hospital	Corpus Christi	97%	120
TX Hlth Harris Meth Hosp-Stephenville[2]	Stephenville	97%	31
Tops Surgical Specialty Hospital	Houston	97%	75
Univ of Texas Med Branch Galveston[2]	Galveston	97%	156
Valley Regional Medical Center	Brownsville	97%	96
Cedar Park Regional Medical Center	Cedar Park	96%	92
Christus Saint John Hospital	Nassau Bay	96%	125
Covenant Medical Center	Lubbock	96%	890
First Surgical Hospital	Bellaire	96%	25
The Medical Center of Southeast Texas	Port Arthur	96%	156
Nix Health Care System	San Antonio	96%	85
Pampa Regional Medical Center	Pampa	96%	51
San Antonio VA Medical Center[2]	San Antonio	96%	182
Sierra Medical Center[2]	El Paso	96%	182
University Health System[2]	San Antonio	96%	158
Univ of TX Health Science Ctr-Tyler	Tyler	96%	28
VHS Brownsville Hospital Company[2]	Brownsville	96%	73
Wadley Regional Medical Center	Texarkana	96%	192
Wise Regional Health System[2]	Decatur	96%	112
Baylor Medical Center at Waxahachie[2]	Waxahachie	95%	86
Brazosport Regional Health System	Lake Jackson	95%	42
Christus Spohn Hospital Corpus Christi	Corpus Christi	95%	516
Dallas Medical Center[2]	Dallas	95%	38
Midland Memorial Hospital	Midland	95%	279
Park Plaza Hospital[2]	Houston	95%	92
Peterson Regional Medical Center	Kerrville	95%	164
Texas Health Presbyterian Hospital Denton[2]	Denton	95%	108
USMD Hospital at Arlington[2]	Arlington	95%	43
VHS Harlingen Hospital Company[2]	Harlingen	95%	338
Citizens Medical Center	Victoria	94%	179
Doctors Hospital of Laredo[2]	Laredo	94%	31
Grace Medical Center	Lubbock	94%	77
Guadalupe Regional Medical Center	Seguin	94%	67
Metroplex Hospital[2]	Killeen	94%	65
Mission Regional Medical Center	Mission	94%	80
El Paso Specialty Hospital	El Paso	93%	101
Nacogdoches Medical Center[2]	Nacogdoches	93%	57
Northwest Texas Surgery Center	Amarillo	93%	30
Temple VA Med Ctr-VA Central Texas[2]	Temple	93%	91
East Texas Medical Center Athens[2]	Athens	91%	57
Lubbock Heart Hospital[2]	Lubbock	91%	146
Saint Luke's Patients Medical Center[2]	Pasadena	91%	104
Foundation Surgical Hospital of El Paso[2]	El Paso	90%	30
Hunt Regional Medical Center	Greenville	89%	54
Providence Health Center[2]	Waco	88%	185
Saint Luke's Hospital at the Vintage	Houston	88%	32
Houston Orthopedic & Spine Hospital	Bellaire	87%	210
Tomball Regional Medical Center	Tomball	87%	137
Hopkins County Memorial Hospital	Sulphur Springs	86%	28
East Texas Medical Center Jacksonville	Jacksonville	85%	33
Seton Medical Center Harker Heights	Harker Heights	85%	27
Memorial Hospital	Nacogdoches	83%	77
VA Amarillo Healthcare System[2]	Amarillo	82%	33
Arise Austin Medical Center[2]	Austin	71%	45
University General Hospital	Houston	63%	38
Pine Creek Medical Center[2]	Dallas	49%	41

Appropriate VTP Within 24 Hours

Hospital Name	City	Rate	Cases
Baylor Medical Center at Frisco	Frisco	100%	880
Baylor Medical Center at Trophy Club	Trophy Club	100%	67
Baylor Medical Center at Uptown	Dallas	100%	373
Baylor Regional Medical Center at Plano[2]	Plano	100%	447
Baylor Surgical Hospital at Fort Worth	Fort Worth	100%	443
Bayshore Medical Center[2]	Pasadena	100%	314
Brownwood Regional Medical Center	Brownwood	100%	210
Cleveland Regional Medical Center	Cleveland	100%	31
Columbus Community Hospital	Columbus	100%	38
Conroe Regional Medical Center[2]	Conroe	100%	358
Cornerstone Regional Hospital[2]	Edinburg	100%	339
The Corpus Christi Medical Center[2]	Corpus Christi	100%	435
Dallas Regional Medical Center	Mesquite	100%	207
East Texas Medical Center[2]	Tyler	100%	299
El Paso Specialty Hospital	El Paso	100%	422
Fdn Surgical Hosp of San Antonio[2]	San Antonio	100%	119
Harlingen Medical Center[2]	Harlingen	100%	323
Houston Orthopedic & Spine Hospital	Bellaire	100%	846
Houston Physicians' Hospital	Webster	100%	217
Kingwood Medical Center[2]	Kingwood	100%	355
Lake Granbury Medical Center	Granbury	100%	230
Lake Pointe Medical Center	Rowlett	100%	176
Laredo Medical Center	Laredo	100%	502
Las Colinas Medical Center[2]	Irving	100%	211
Las Palmas Medical Center[2]	El Paso	100%	453
Matagorda Regional Medical Center	Bay City	100%	38
Medical Center of Plano[2]	Plano	100%	449
Medical City Dallas Hospital[2]	Dallas	100%	525
Methodist Ambulatory Surgery Hospital NW[2]	San Antonio	100%	197
Methodist Charlton Medical Center	Dallas	100%	527
Methodist Dallas Medical Center	Dallas	100%	1047
Methodist Hospital For Surgery[2]	Addison	100%	688
Methodist Mansfield Medical Center	Mansfield	100%	205
Methodist Mckinney Hospital[2]	Mc Kinney	100%	277
Methodist Richardson Medical Center[2]	Richardson	100%	255
Methodist Stone Oak Hospital[2]	San Antonio	100%	381
Methodist Sugar Land Hospital[2]	Sugar Land	100%	463
Methodist Willowbrook Hospital[2]	Houston	100%	294
Metroplex Hospital[2]	Killeen	100%	220
Palestine Regional Medical Center	Palestine	100%	226
The Physicians Centre	Bryan	100%	96
Quail Creek Surgical Hospital	Amarillo	100%	777
Rio Grande Regional Hospital[2]	Mcallen	100%	231
Round Rock Medical Center[2]	Round Rock	100%	339
Saint David's Medical Center[2]	Austin	100%	484
Saint David's South Austin Medical Center[2]	Austin	100%	407
Saint Luke's Lakeside Hospital	The Woodlands	100%	361
Saint Luke's Sugar Land Hospital	Sugar Land	100%	83
Saint Marks Medical Center	La Grange	100%	72
San Angelo Community Medical Center	San Angelo	100%	332
San Jacinto Methodist Hospital[2]	Baytown	100%	409
Scenic Mountain Medical Center	Big Spring	100%	64
Scott & White Memorial Hospital[2]	Temple	100%	464
South Texas Spine & Surgical Hospital	San Antonio	100%	149
Sugar Land Surgical Hospital	Sugar Land	100%	175
Temple VA Med Ctr-VA Central Texas[2]	Temple	100%	240
TX Health Ctr for Diag & Surgery	Plano	100%	60
Texas Health Presbyterian Hospital Allen[2]	Allen	100%	156
Texas Health Presbyterian Hospital Plano[2]	Plano	100%	1643
TX Inst for Surgery at Presby Hosp[3]	Dallas	100%	152
Texas Orthopedic Hospital[2]	Houston	100%	357
Texas Spine & Joint Hospital[2]	Tyler	100%	212
Texoma Medical Center[2]	Denison	100%	393
UT SW Univ Hosp-Zale Lipshy[2]	Dallas	100%	96
Val Verde Regional Medical Center	Del Rio	100%	115
Weatherford Regional Medical Center	Weatherford	100%	344
West Houston Medical Center[2]	Houston	100%	305
Woodland Heights Medical Center	Lufkin	100%	371
Abilene Regional Medical Center	Abilene	99%	429
Baptist Medical Center[2]	San Antonio	99%	2615
Baylor Medical Center at Carrollton	Carrollton	99%	408
Baylor Medical Center at Irving[2]	Irving	99%	404
Baylor Medical Center at Mckinney[2]	Mc Kinney	99%	170
Baylor Medical Center at Waxahachie[2]	Waxahachie	99%	282
Baylor Ortho & Spine Hosp-Arlington	Arlington	99%	742
Baylor Reg Med Ctr at Grapevine[2]	Grapevine	99%	595
Baylor Surgical Hospital at Las Colinas	Irving	99%	134
Baylor University Medical Center[2]	Dallas	99%	1719
Cedar Park Regional Medical Center	Cedar Park	99%	308
Christus Hospital[2]	Beaumont	99%	769
Christus Saint Michael Health System[2]	Texarkana	99%	795
Clear Lake Regional Medical Center[2]	Webster	99%	471
Detar Hospital Navarro	Victoria	99%	380
Doctors Hospital at Renaissance[2]	Edinburg	99%	710
East Texas Medical Center Jacksonville	Jacksonville	99%	84
Fort Duncan Medical Center[2]	Eagle Pass	99%	93
Good Shepherd Medical Center[2]	Longview	99%	404
Grace Medical Center	Lubbock	99%	309
Guadalupe Regional Medical Center	Seguin	99%	310
Harris Health System[2]	Houston	99%	628
Hill Country Memorial Hospital[2]	Fredericksburg	99%	446
Hillcrest Baptist Medical Center[2]	Waco	99%	514
The Hospital at Westlake Medical Center	Austin	99%	290
Houston Northwest Medical Center[2]	Houston	99%	418
Huguley Memorial Medical Center	Burleson	99%	366
JPS Health Network[2]	Fort Worth	99%	576
Kell West Regional Hospital	Wichita Falls	99%	317
Longview Regional Medical Center	Longview	99%	526
Medical Center Hospital[2]	Odessa	99%	419
Medical Center of Arlington[2]	Arlington	99%	268
Medical Center of Lewisville[2]	Lewisville	99%	190
Medical Center of Mckinney[2]	Mckinney	99%	282
The Medical Center of Southeast Texas	Port Arthur	99%	390
Memorial Hermann Hospital System[2]	Houston	99%	1550
Mem Hermann Surgical Hosp Kingwood	Kingwood	99%	116
Memorial Hermann Texas Medical Center[2]	Houston	99%	444
Midland Memorial Hospital	Midland	99%	776
Navarro Regional Hospital	Corsicana	99%	141
North Austin Medical Center[2]	Austin	99%	448
North Central Surgical Center	Dallas	99%	507
North Cypress Medical Center	Cypress	99%	550
North Hills Hospital[2]	N Richland Hls	99%	296
Northwest Texas Surgery Center	Amarillo	99%	112
Odessa Regional Hospital	Odessa	99%	217
Providence Memorial Hospital[2]	El Paso	99%	348
Saint Joseph Regional Health Center[2]	Bryan	99%	320
Saint Luke's the Woodlands Hospital[2]	The Woodlands	99%	423
Scott & White Hospital Brenham	Brenham	99%	107

NOTE: Hospital profiles are in alphabetical order by state, then city, then hospital within the city; Rankings exclude hospitals with less than 25 cases except for patient surveys which excludes hospitals with less than 100 cases; (a) 100-299 cases; (1) The number of cases/patients is too few to report; (2) Data submitted were based on a sample of cases/patients; (3) Results are based on a shorter time period than required; (4) Data suppressed by CMS for one or more quarters; (5) Results are not available for this reporting period; (6) Fewer than 100 patients completed the HCAHPS survey; (7) No cases met the criteria for this measure; (8) The lower limit of the confidence interval cannot be calculated if the number of observed infections equals zero; (9) No data are available from the state/territory for this reporting period; (10) The scores shown reflect fewer than 50 completed surveys; (11) There were discrepancies in the data collection process; (12) This measure does not apply to this hospital for this reporting period; (13) Results cannot be calculated for this reporting period; (14) The results for this state are combined with nearby states to protect confidentiality; Please refer to the User's Guide for a full explanation of data.

Seton Highland Lakes	Burnet	99%	90
Seton Northwest Hospital	Austin	99%	271
Shannon Medical Center	San Angelo	99%	713
South Texas Health System[2]	Edinburg	99%	370
Southwest General Hospital	San Antonio	99%	210
Texas Health Arlington Memorial Hospital[2]	Arlington	99%	305
Texas Health Harris Methodist Fort Worth[2]	Fort Worth	99%	812
TX Hlth Harris Meth Hosp-Southlake	Southlake	99%	495
Texas Health Presbyterian Hospital - WNJ	Sherman	99%	191
Texas Health Presbyterian Hospital Dallas[2]	Dallas	99%	478
TX Hlth Presbyterian Hosp-Kaufman[2]	Kaufman	99%	105
Tops Surgical Specialty Hospital	Houston	99%	355
United Regional Health Care System	Wichita Falls	99%	718
University Medical Center[2]	Lubbock	99%	381
University Medical Center of El Paso[2]	El Paso	99%	342
Univ of Texas Med Branch Galveston[2]	Galveston	99%	263
UT Southwestern University Hospital[2]	Dallas	99%	487
Valley Regional Medical Center	Brownsville	99%	274
The Womans Hospital of Texas[2]	Houston	99%	182
Baylor All Saints Medical Center at FW[2]	Fort Worth	98%	588
Baylor Medical Center at Garland[2]	Garland	98%	214
Central Texas Medical Center	San Marcos	98%	167
Christus Saint Catherine Hospital	Katy	98%	146
College Station Medical Center	College Station	98%	465
Covenant Medical Center	Lubbock	98%	2285
Cypress Fairbanks Medical Center[2]	Houston	98%	176
Denton Regional Medical Center[2]	Denton	98%	338
Doctors Hospital[2]	Dallas	98%	276
Etmc Henderson	Henderson	98%	59
Graham Regional Medical Center[2]	Graham	98%	50
Houston VA Medical Center[2]	Houston	98%	382
Huntsville Memorial Hospital	Huntsville	98%	229
Memorial Hermann Baptist Orange Hospital	Orange	98%	44
Memorial Hermann Katy Hospital[2]	Katy	98%	405
Memorial Hermann Sugar Land Hospital[2]	Sugar Land	98%	313
Methodist Hospital[2]	San Antonio	98%	684
Park Plaza Hospital[2]	Houston	98%	357
Peterson Regional Medical Center	Kerrville	98%	432
Plaza Medical Center of Fort Worth[2]	Fort Worth	98%	467
Saint Joseph Medical Center	Houston	98%	563
Seton Medical Center Austin[2]	Austin	98%	489
Seton Medical Center Hays	Kyle	98%	184
Seton Medical Center Williamson	Round Rock	98%	231
Sierra Providence East Medical Center[2]	El Paso	98%	187
South Texas Regional Medical Center	Jourdanton	98%	57
TX Hlth Harris Meth Hosp-Stephenville[2]	Stephenville	98%	150
Texas Health Harris Methodist[2]	Bedford	98%	327
Texas Health Presbyterian Hospital Denton[2]	Denton	98%	247
TX Health Presbyterian Hosp Rockwall	Rockwall	98%	408
Texas Reg Med Ctr at Sunnyvale[2]	Sunnyvale	98%	156
Wise Regional Health System[2]	Decatur	98%	226
Angleton - Danbury Medical Center[2]	Angleton	97%	156
Baptist Saint Anthony's Hospital[2]	Amarillo	97%	457
Christus Santa Rosa Hospital	San Antonio	97%	999
Covenant Hospital Plainview	Plainview	97%	155
Eastland Memorial Hospital[2]	Eastland	97%	29
Heritage Park Surgical Hospital	Sherman	97%	142
Hunt Regional Medical Center	Greenville	97%	236
Knapp Medical Center	Weslaco	97%	369
Lubbock Heart Hospital[2]	Lubbock	97%	192
Memorial Hermann Northeast[2]	Humble	97%	229
The Methodist Hospital[2]	Houston	97%	592
Methodist West Houston Hospital[2]	Houston	97%	210
Northwest Texas Hospital[2]	Amarillo	97%	317
Paris Regional Medical Center[2]	Paris	97%	357
Saint Luke's Patients Medical Center[2]	Pasadena	97%	335
Scott & White Hospital - Round Rock[2]	Round Rock	97%	317
Sierra Medical Center[2]	El Paso	97%	412
TX Hlth Harris Methodist Hosp-Azle[2]	Azle	97%	31
TX Hlth Harris Meth Hosp-Cleburne[2]	Cleburne	97%	245
TX Hlth Harris Meth Hosp SW Ft Worth[2]	Fort Worth	97%	395
University Medical Center at Brackenridge[2]	Austin	97%	298
USMD Hospital at Fort Worth	Fort Worth	97%	152
Baptist Beaumont Hospital[2]	Beaumont	96%	385
Brazosport Regional Health System	Lake Jackson	96%	138
Centennial Medical Center	Frisco	96%	143
Christus Spohn Hospital Beeville	Beeville	96%	26
Christus Spohn Hospital Kleberg	Kingsville	96%	70
Dallas VA Medical Center - VA North Texas[2]	Dallas	96%	218
East Texas Medical Center Crockett	Crockett	96%	26
Foundation Surgical Hospital of El Paso[2]	El Paso	96%	148
Good Shepherd Medical Center Marshall	Marshall	96%	205
Hendrick Medical Center[2]	Abilene	96%	376
Lakeway Regional Medical Center[3]	Lakeway	96%	28
Mem Hermann Mem City Med Ctr[2]	Houston	96%	427
Mother Frances Hospital[2]	Tyler	96%	420
Nix Health Care System	San Antonio	96%	293
Pampa Regional Medical Center	Pampa	96%	137
Providence Health Center[2]	Waco	96%	362
Saint Luke's Episcopal Hospital[2]	Houston	96%	484
Saint Luke's Hospital at the Vintage	Houston	96%	121
San Antonio VA Medical Center[2]	San Antonio	96%	296
University General Hospital Dallas[2]	Dallas	96%	25
Wadley Regional Medical Center	Texarkana	96%	422
Arise Austin Medical Center[2]	Austin	95%	350
Christus Saint John Hospital	Nassau Bay	95%	462
Dallas Medical Center[2]	Dallas	95%	154
Ennis Regional Medical Center	Ennis	95%	40
First Surgical Hospital	Bellaire	95%	95
Mission Regional Medical Center	Mission	95%	273
Seton Medical Center Harker Heights	Harker Heights	95%	114
South Texas Surgical Hospital	Corpus Christi	95%	530
TX Hlth Presbyterian Hosp-Flower Mound	Flower Mound	95%	383
Tomball Regional Medical Center	Tomball	95%	374
University Health System[2]	San Antonio	95%	440
East Texas Medical Center Athens[2]	Athens	94%	217
Memorial Medical Center of East Texas[2]	Lufkin	94%	220
Nacogdoches Medical Center[2]	Nacogdoches	94%	158
North Texas Medical Center	Gainesville	94%	72
Univ of TX Health Science Ctr-Tyler	Tyler	94%	85
USMD Hospital at Arlington[2]	Arlington	94%	125
VHS Harlingen Hospital Company[2]	Harlingen	94%	886
Doctors Hospital of Laredo[2]	Laredo	93%	182
Hill Regional Hospital	Hillsboro	93%	55
Palo Pinto General Hospital	Mineral Wells	93%	75
Parkland Health & Hospital System[2]	Dallas	93%	359
Doctors Hospital Tidwell	Houston	92%	62
Titus Regional Medical Center	Mount Pleasant	92%	156
Christus Spohn Hospital Corpus Christi	Corpus Christi	91%	1316
Citizens Medical Center	Victoria	91%	476
Golden Plains Community Hospital	Borger	91%	34
TX Hlth Harris Meth Hosp-Alliance[2,3]	Fort Worth	91%	33
VA Amarillo Healthcare System[2]	Amarillo	91%	94
Uvalde Memorial Hospital	Uvalde	90%	42
VHS Brownsville Hospital Company[2]	Brownsville	90%	210
Oakbend Medical Center[2]	Richmond	89%	128
Pine Creek Medical Center[2]	Dallas	89%	248
University General Hospital	Houston	89%	134
Hopkins County Memorial Hospital	Sulphur Springs	88%	120
Memorial Hospital	Nacogdoches	87%	191
Christus Spohn Hospital Alice	Alice	86%	37
Memorial Medical Center Livingston[2]	Livingston	84%	134

Controlled Postoperative Blood Glucose

Hospital Name	City	Rate	Cases
Baylor Medical Center at Garland[2]	Garland	100%	27
College Station Medical Center	College Station	100%	63
Detar Hospital Navarro	Victoria	100%	27
Doctors Hospital[2]	Dallas	100%	32
East Texas Medical Center[2]	Tyler	100%	113
Houston Northwest Medical Center[2]	Houston	100%	71
Las Palmas Medical Center[2]	El Paso	100%	104
Medical Center Hospital[2]	Odessa	100%	76
Medical Center of Arlington[2]	Arlington	100%	61
Medical Center of Mckinney[2]	Mckinney	100%	25
Methodist Charlton Medical Center	Dallas	100%	55
Methodist Dallas Medical Center	Dallas	100%	97
San Angelo Community Medical Center	San Angelo	100%	30
Southwest General Hospital	San Antonio	100%	27
United Regional Health Care System	Wichita Falls	100%	133
University Medical Center[2]	Lubbock	100%	114
Valley Regional Medical Center	Brownsville	100%	41
VHS Brownsville Hospital Company[2]	Brownsville	100%	41
West Houston Medical Center[2]	Houston	100%	78
Conroe Regional Medical Center[2]	Conroe	99%	101
Doctors Hospital at Renaissance[2]	Edinburg	99%	198
Harlingen Medical Center[2]	Harlingen	99%	127
Heart Hospital Baylor Plano	Plano	99%	1053
JPS Health Network[2]	Fort Worth	99%	115
Longview Regional Medical Center	Longview	99%	111
Medical City Dallas Hospital[2]	Dallas	99%	105
Mem Hermann Mem City Med Ctr[2]	Houston	99%	137
Methodist Mansfield Medical Center	Mansfield	99%	92
North Austin Medical Center[2]	Austin	99%	95
Rio Grande Regional Hospital[2]	Mcallen	99%	87
South Texas Health System[2]	Edinburg	99%	121
Texas Health Harris Methodist Fort Worth[2]	Fort Worth	99%	240
Texas Health Presbyterian Hospital Dallas[2]	Dallas	99%	145
Baylor Reg Med Ctr at Grapevine[2]	Grapevine	98%	66
Baylor University Medical Center[2]	Dallas	98%	405
Christus Hospital[2]	Beaumont	98%	126
Houston VA Medical Center[2]	Houston	98%	248
Memorial Hermann Hospital System[2]	Houston	98%	234
Methodist Hospital[2]	San Antonio	98%	212
Methodist Sugar Land Hospital[2]	Sugar Land	98%	105
Methodist West Houston Hospital[2]	Houston	98%	122
Providence Health Center[2]	Waco	98%	110
Saint David's South Austin Medical Center[2]	Austin	98%	124
Seton Medical Center Hays	Kyle	98%	45
Seton Medical Center Williamson	Round Rock	98%	59
TX Hlth Heart & Vasc Hosp-Arlington	Arlington	98%	157
University Medical Center of El Paso[2]	El Paso	98%	42
Bayshore Medical Center[2]	Pasadena	97%	34
Citizens Medical Center	Victoria	97%	31
Covenant Medical Center	Lubbock	97%	255
Hendrick Medical Center[2]	Abilene	97%	107
Laredo Medical Center	Laredo	97%	78
Medical Center of Plano[2]	Plano	97%	92
Methodist Willowbrook Hospital[2]	Houston	97%	67
Midland Memorial Hospital	Midland	97%	74
Mother Frances Hospital[2]	Tyler	97%	196
North Hills Hospital[2]	N Richland Hls	97%	62
Northwest Texas Hospital[2]	Amarillo	97%	98
Plaza Medical Center of Fort Worth[2]	Fort Worth	97%	139
Saint David's Medical Center[2]	Austin	97%	216
San Antonio VA Medical Center[2]	San Antonio	97%	93
San Jacinto Methodist Hospital[2]	Baytown	97%	65
Scott & White Memorial Hospital[2]	Temple	97%	148
Shannon Medical Center	San Angelo	97%	117
Sierra Medical Center[2]	El Paso	97%	89
UT Southwestern University Hospital[2]	Dallas	97%	185
Baptist Beaumont Hospital[2]	Beaumont	96%	76
Baptist Medical Center[2]	San Antonio	96%	488
Baylor All Saints Medical Center at FW[2]	Fort Worth	96%	28
Christus Saint Michael Health System[2]	Texarkana	96%	132
The Corpus Christi Medical Center[2]	Corpus Christi	96%	122
Hillcrest Baptist Medical Center[2]	Waco	96%	68
The Medical Center of Southeast Texas	Port Arthur	96%	67
Memorial Hermann Texas Medical Center[2]	Houston	96%	135
Providence Memorial Hospital[2]	El Paso	96%	49
Round Rock Medical Center[2]	Round Rock	96%	28
Saint Joseph Regional Health Center[2]	Bryan	96%	90
Saint Luke's the Woodlands Hospital[2]	The Woodlands	96%	118
Texas Health Harris Methodist[2]	Bedford	96%	50
Texas Health Presbyterian Hospital - WNJ	Sherman	96%	56
Baptist Saint Anthony's Hospital[2]	Amarillo	95%	141
Clear Lake Regional Medical Center[2]	Webster	95%	118
Kingwood Medical Center[2]	Kingwood	95%	95
Methodist Stone Oak Hospital[2]	San Antonio	95%	83
Saint Luke's Episcopal Hospital[2]	Houston	95%	195
Seton Medical Center Austin[2]	Austin	95%	134
Texoma Medical Center[2]	Denison	95%	98
Univ of Texas Med Branch Galveston[2]	Galveston	95%	86
Harris Health System[2]	Houston	94%	110
Huguley Memorial Medical Center	Burleson	94%	86
Medical Center of Lewisville[2]	Lewisville	94%	50
Odessa Regional Hospital	Odessa	94%	52
Scott & White Hospital - Round Rock[2]	Round Rock	94%	63
Texas Health Presbyterian Hospital Denton[2]	Denton	94%	62
Wadley Regional Medical Center	Texarkana	94%	68
Wise Regional Health System[2]	Decatur	94%	48
Baylor Medical Center at Irving[2]	Irving	93%	29
Christus Santa Rosa Hospital	San Antonio	93%	188
Dallas VA Medical Center - VA North Texas[2]	Dallas	93%	74
Good Shepherd Medical Center[2]	Longview	93%	113
The Methodist Hospital[2]	Houston	93%	191
University Health System[2]	San Antonio	93%	138
Denton Regional Medical Center[2]	Denton	92%	106
North Cypress Medical Center	Cypress	92%	50
Abilene Regional Medical Center	Abilene	91%	133
Texas Health Presbyterian Hospital Plano[2]	Plano	91%	92
VHS Harlingen Hospital Company[2]	Harlingen	91%	97
Woodland Heights Medical Center	Lufkin	91%	57
Memorial Medical Center of East Texas[2]	Lufkin	90%	60
Paris Regional Medical Center[2]	Paris	90%	115
Christus Spohn Hospital Corpus Christi	Corpus Christi	89%	360
Lubbock Heart Hospital[2]	Lubbock	86%	105
Tomball Regional Medical Center	Tomball	86%	51
Saint Joseph Medical Center	Houston	84%	63

Perioperative Temperature Management

Hospital Name	City	Rate	Cases
Abilene Regional Medical Center	Abilene	100%	520
Angleton - Danbury Medical Center[2]	Angleton	100%	174
Baptist Beaumont Hospital[2]	Beaumont	100%	501
Baptist Medical Center[2]	San Antonio	100%	3017
Baptist Saint Anthony's Hospital[2]	Amarillo	100%	580
Basin Healthcare Center[2]	Odessa	100%	25
Baylor All Saints Medical Center at FW[2]	Fort Worth	100%	701
Baylor Heart & Vascular Hospital	Dallas	100%	130
Baylor Medical Center at Carrollton	Carrollton	100%	457
Baylor Medical Center at Frisco	Frisco	100%	906
Baylor Medical Center at Garland[2]	Garland	100%	284
Baylor Medical Center at Irving[2]	Irving	100%	436
Baylor Medical Center at Mckinney[2]	Mc Kinney	100%	198
Baylor Medical Center at Trophy Club	Trophy Club	100%	68
Baylor Medical Center at Uptown	Dallas	100%	415
Baylor Medical Center at Waxahachie[2]	Waxahachie	100%	294
Baylor Ortho & Spine Hosp-Arlington	Arlington	100%	750
Baylor Reg Med Ctr at Grapevine[2]	Grapevine	100%	680
Baylor Regional Medical Center at Plano[2]	Plano	100%	498
Baylor Surgical Hospital at Fort Worth	Fort Worth	100%	446
Baylor Surgical Hospital at Las Colinas	Irving	100%	139

NOTE: Hospital profiles are in alphabetical order by state, then city, then hospital within the city; Rankings exclude hospitals with less than 25 cases except for patient surveys which excludes hospitals with less than 100 cases; (a) 100-299 cases; (1) The number of cases/patients is too few to report; (2) Data submitted were based on a sample of cases/patients; (3) Results are based on a shorter time period than required; (4) Data suppressed by CMS for one or more quarters; (5) Results are not available for this reporting period; (6) Fewer than 100 patients completed the HCAHPS survey; (7) No cases met the criteria for this measure; (8) The lower limit of the confidence interval cannot be calculated if the number of observed infections equals zero; (9) No data are available from the state/territory for this reporting period; (10) The scores shown reflect fewer than 50 completed surveys; (11) There were discrepancies in the data collection process; (12) This measure does not apply to this hospital for this reporting period; (13) Results cannot be calculated for this reporting period; (14) The results for this state are combined with nearby states to protect confidentiality; Please refer to the User's Guide for a full explanation of data.

Hospital Name	City	Rate	Cases
Baylor University Medical Center[2]	Dallas	100%	2005
Bayshore Medical Center[2]	Pasadena	100%	424
Brazosport Regional Health System	Lake Jackson	100%	155
Brownwood Regional Medical Center	Brownwood	100%	261
Cedar Park Regional Medical Center	Cedar Park	100%	381
Central Texas Medical Center	San Marcos	100%	183
Christus Hospital[2]	Beaumont	100%	907
Christus Saint Catherine Hospital	Katy	100%	174
Christus Saint John Hospital	Nassau Bay	100%	518
Christus Saint Michael Health System[2]	Texarkana	100%	1042
Christus Santa Rosa Hospital	San Antonio	100%	1270
Christus Spohn Hospital Alice	Alice	100%	40
Christus Spohn Hospital Beeville	Beeville	100%	28
Christus Spohn Hospital Corpus Christi	Corpus Christi	100%	1632
Christus Spohn Hospital Kleberg	Kingsville	100%	85
Citizens Medical Center	Victoria	100%	548
Clear Lake Regional Medical Center[2]	Webster	100%	602
Cleveland Regional Medical Center	Cleveland	100%	42
College Station Medical Center	College Station	100%	646
Columbus Community Hospital	Columbus	100%	44
Conroe Regional Medical Center[2]	Conroe	100%	480
Cornerstone Regional Hospital[2]	Edinburg	100%	383
The Corpus Christi Medical Center[2]	Corpus Christi	100%	657
Covenant Hospital Plainview	Plainview	100%	178
Covenant Medical Center	Lubbock	100%	2760
Cypress Fairbanks Medical Center[2]	Houston	100%	213
Dallas Regional Medical Center	Mesquite	100%	251
Denton Regional Medical Center[2]	Denton	100%	515
Detar Hospital Navarro	Victoria	100%	417
Doctors Hospital at Renaissance[2]	Edinburg	100%	895
Doctors Hospital of Laredo[2]	Laredo	100%	219
Doctors Hospital Tidwell	Houston	100%	52
East Texas Medical Center[2]	Tyler	100%	417
East Texas Medical Center Athens[2]	Athens	100%	269
East Texas Medical Center Crockett	Crockett	100%	32
East Texas Medical Center Jacksonville	Jacksonville	100%	94
Eastland Memorial Hospital[2]	Eastland	100%	33
El Paso Specialty Hospital	El Paso	100%	433
Ennis Regional Medical Center	Ennis	100%	46
Etmc Henderson	Henderson	100%	75
First Surgical Hospital	Bellaire	100%	147
Fort Duncan Medical Center[2]	Eagle Pass	100%	109
Foundation Surgical Hospital of El Paso[2]	El Paso	100%	192
Fdn Surgical Hosp of San Antonio[2]	San Antonio	100%	123
Golden Plains Community Hospital	Borger	100%	39
Good Shepherd Medical Center[2]	Longview	100%	499
Good Shepherd Medical Center Marshall	Marshall	100%	261
Grace Medical Center	Lubbock	100%	326
Graham Regional Medical Center[2]	Graham	100%	62
Guadalupe Regional Medical Center	Seguin	100%	353
Gulf Coast Medical Center	Wharton	100%	29
Harlingen Medical Center[2]	Harlingen	100%	380
Harris Health System[2]	Houston	100%	714
Heart Hospital Baylor Plano	Plano	100%	287
Heritage Park Surgical Hospital	Sherman	100%	152
Hill Country Memorial Hospital[2]	Fredericksburg	100%	507
Hill Regional Hospital	Hillsboro	100%	61
Hillcrest Baptist Medical Center[2]	Waco	100%	572
Hopkins County Memorial Hospital	Sulphur Springs	100%	146
The Hospital at Westlake Medical Center	Austin	100%	308
Houston Northwest Medical Center[2]	Houston	100%	510
Houston Orthopedic & Spine Hospital	Bellaire	100%	924
Houston Physicians' Hospital	Webster	100%	229
Houston VA Medical Center[2]	Houston	100%	531
Huguley Memorial Medical Center	Burleson	100%	427
Hunt Regional Medical Center	Greenville	100%	271
Huntsville Memorial Hospital	Huntsville	100%	235
JPS Health Network[2]	Fort Worth	100%	796
Kingwood Medical Center[2]	Kingwood	100%	460
Knapp Medical Center	Weslaco	100%	418
Lake Granbury Medical Center	Granbury	100%	248
Lake Pointe Medical Center	Rowlett	100%	217
Lakeway Regional Medical Center[3]	Lakeway	100%	36
Laredo Medical Center	Laredo	100%	579
Las Colinas Medical Center[2]	Irving	100%	240
Las Palmas Medical Center[2]	El Paso	100%	549
Longview Regional Medical Center	Longview	100%	750
Matagorda Regional Medical Center	Bay City	100%	42
Medical Center Hospital[2]	Odessa	100%	559
Medical Center of Arlington[2]	Arlington	100%	378
Medical Center of Lewisville[2]	Lewisville	100%	290
Medical Center of Mckinney[2]	Mckinney	100%	353
Medical Center of Plano[2]	Plano	100%	517
The Medical Center of Southeast Texas	Port Arthur	100%	424
Medical City Dallas Hospital[2]	Dallas	100%	681
Memorial Hermann Baptist Orange Hospital	Orange	100%	50
Memorial Hermann Hospital System[2]	Houston	100%	1953
Memorial Hermann Katy Hospital[2]	Katy	100%	435
Mem Hermann Mem City Med Ctr[2]	Houston	100%	619
Memorial Hermann Northeast[2]	Humble	100%	280
Memorial Hermann Sugar Land Hospital[2]	Sugar Land	100%	350
Mem Hermann Surgical Hosp Kingwood	Kingwood	100%	128
Memorial Hermann Texas Medical Center[2]	Houston	100%	634
Memorial Hospital	Nacogdoches	100%	246
Memorial Medical Center Livingston[2]	Livingston	100%	153
Memorial Medical Center of East Texas[2]	Lufkin	100%	295
Methodist Ambulatory Surgery Hospital NW[2]	San Antonio	100%	207
Methodist Charlton Medical Center	Dallas	100%	579
Methodist Dallas Medical Center	Dallas	100%	1298
Methodist Hospital[2]	San Antonio	100%	907
Methodist Hospital For Surgery[2]	Addison	100%	724
The Methodist Hospital[2]	Houston	100%	827
Methodist Mansfield Medical Center	Mansfield	100%	341
Methodist Mckinney Hospital[2]	Mc Kinney	100%	314
Methodist Richardson Medical Center[2]	Richardson	100%	286
Methodist Stone Oak Hospital[2]	San Antonio	100%	514
Methodist Sugar Land Hospital[2]	Sugar Land	100%	584
Methodist West Houston Hospital[2]	Houston	100%	318
Methodist Willowbrook Hospital[2]	Houston	100%	346
Metroplex Hospital[2]	Killeen	100%	249
Midland Memorial Hospital	Midland	100%	968
Mission Regional Medical Center	Mission	100%	304
Mother Frances Hospital[2]	Tyler	100%	638
Nacogdoches Medical Center[2]	Nacogdoches	100%	188
Nix Health Care System	San Antonio	100%	311
North Austin Medical Center[2]	Austin	100%	508
North Central Surgical Center	Dallas	100%	510
North Cypress Medical Center	Cypress	100%	701
North Hills Hospital[2]	N Richland Hls	100%	437
North Texas Medical Center	Gainesville	100%	75
Oakbend Medical Center[2]	Richmond	100%	153
Odessa Regional Hospital	Odessa	100%	268
Palestine Regional Medical Center	Palestine	100%	271
Palo Pinto General Hospital	Mineral Wells	100%	96
Pampa Regional Medical Center	Pampa	100%	168
Paris Regional Medical Center[2]	Paris	100%	410
Park Plaza Hospital[2]	Houston	100%	396
Parkland Health & Hospital System[2]	Dallas	100%	423
Peterson Regional Medical Center	Kerrville	100%	498
The Physicians Centre	Bryan	100%	150
Plaza Medical Center of Fort Worth[2]	Fort Worth	100%	681
Providence Memorial Hospital[2]	El Paso	100%	393
Quail Creek Surgical Hospital	Amarillo	100%	834
Rio Grande Regional Hospital[2]	Mcallen	100%	312
Round Rock Medical Center[2]	Round Rock	100%	358
Saint David's Medical Center[2]	Austin	100%	596
Saint David's South Austin Medical Center[2]	Austin	100%	473
Saint Joseph Medical Center	Houston	100%	648
Saint Joseph Regional Health Center[2]	Bryan	100%	406
Saint Luke's Episcopal Hospital[2]	Houston	100%	629
Saint Luke's Hospital at the Vintage	Houston	100%	135
Saint Luke's Lakeside Hospital	The Woodlands	100%	367
Saint Luke's Patients Medical Center[2]	Pasadena	100%	378
Saint Luke's Sugar Land Hospital	Sugar Land	100%	92
Saint Luke's the Woodlands Hospital[2]	The Woodlands	100%	531
Saint Marks Medical Center	La Grange	100%	78
San Angelo Community Medical Center	San Angelo	100%	458
San Antonio VA Medical Center[2]	San Antonio	100%	314
San Jacinto Methodist Hospital[2]	Baytown	100%	480
Scenic Mountain Medical Center	Big Spring	100%	79
Scott & White Hospital Brenham	Brenham	100%	125
Scott & White Memorial Hospital[2]	Temple	100%	601
Seton Highland Lakes	Burnet	100%	100
Seton Medical Center Austin[2]	Austin	100%	581
Seton Medical Center Harker Heights	Harker Heights	100%	150
Seton Medical Center Hays	Kyle	100%	215
Seton Medical Center Williamson	Round Rock	100%	268
Seton Northwest Hospital	Austin	100%	289
Seton Southwest Hospital[3]	Austin	100%	26
Shannon Medical Center	San Angelo	100%	903
Sierra Medical Center[2]	El Paso	100%	466
Sierra Providence East Medical Center[2]	El Paso	100%	219
South Texas Health System[2]	Edinburg	100%	419
South Texas Regional Medical Center	Jourdanton	100%	43
South Texas Spine & Surgical Hospital	San Antonio	100%	271
South Texas Surgical Hospital	Corpus Christi	100%	552
Southwest General Hospital	San Antonio	100%	272
Sugar Land Surgical Hospital	Sugar Land	100%	185
Temple VA Med Ctr-VA Central Texas[2]	Temple	100%	287
Texas Health Arlington Memorial Hospital[2]	Arlington	100%	406
TX Health Ctr for Diag & Surgery	Plano	100%	61
Texas Health Harris Methodist Fort Worth[2]	Fort Worth	100%	972
TX Hlth Harris Meth Hosp-Alliance[2,3]	Fort Worth	100%	43
TX Hlth Harris Meth Hosp-Cleburne[2]	Cleburne	100%	259
TX Hlth Harris Meth Hosp-Southlake	Southlake	100%	546
TX Hlth Harris Meth Hosp-Stephenville[2]	Stephenville	100%	166
TX Hlth Harris Meth Hosp SW Ft Worth[2]	Fort Worth	100%	445
TX Hlth Heart & Vasc Hosp-Arlington	Arlington	100%	66
Texas Health Presbyterian Hospital - WNJ	Sherman	100%	225
Texas Health Presbyterian Hospital Allen[2]	Allen	100%	195
Texas Health Presbyterian Hospital Dallas[2]	Dallas	100%	591
Texas Health Presbyterian Hospital Denton[2]	Denton	100%	337
TX Hlth Presbyterian Hosp-Flower Mound	Flower Mound	100%	416
TX Hlth Presbyterian Hosp-Kaufman[2]	Kaufman	100%	115
Texas Health Presbyterian Hospital Plano[2]	Plano	100%	1912
TX Health Presbyterian Hosp Rockwall	Rockwall	100%	422
Texas Orthopedic Hospital[2]	Houston	100%	381
Texas Reg Med Ctr at Sunnyvale[2]	Sunnyvale	100%	190
Texas Spine & Joint Hospital[2]	Tyler	100%	236
Texoma Medical Center[2]	Denison	100%	480
Titus Regional Medical Center	Mount Pleasant	100%	166
Tops Surgical Specialty Hospital	Houston	100%	369
United Regional Health Care System	Wichita Falls	100%	806
University Health System[2]	San Antonio	100%	510
University Medical Center[2]	Lubbock	100%	519
University Medical Center at Brackenridge[2]	Austin	100%	347
University Medical Center of El Paso[2]	El Paso	100%	392
Univ of TX Health Science Ctr-Tyler	Tyler	100%	99
Univ of Texas Med Branch Galveston[2]	Galveston	100%	353
USMD Hospital at Arlington[2]	Arlington	100%	213
USMD Hospital at Fort Worth	Fort Worth	100%	213
UT Southwestern University Hospital[2]	Dallas	100%	576
Uvalde Memorial Hospital	Uvalde	100%	44
VA Amarillo Healthcare System[2]	Amarillo	100%	98
Val Verde Regional Medical Center	Del Rio	100%	121
VHS Brownsville Hospital Company[2]	Brownsville	100%	238
VHS Harlingen Hospital Company[2]	Harlingen	100%	965
Wadley Regional Medical Center	Texarkana	100%	524
Weatherford Regional Medical Center	Weatherford	100%	367
West Houston Medical Center[2]	Houston	100%	370
Wise Regional Health System[2]	Decatur	100%	290
The Womans Hospital of Texas[2]	Houston	100%	223
Woodland Heights Medical Center	Lufkin	100%	438
Arise Austin Medical Center[2]	Austin	99%	373
Centennial Medical Center	Frisco	99%	181
Dallas Medical Center[2]	Dallas	99%	167
Dallas VA Medical Center - VA North Texas[2]	Dallas	99%	247
Doctors Hospital[2]	Dallas	99%	230
Hendrick Medical Center[2]	Abilene	99%	466
Kell West Regional Hospital	Wichita Falls	99%	345
Navarro Regional Hospital	Corsicana	99%	156
Northwest Texas Hospital[2]	Amarillo	99%	387
Providence Health Center[2]	Waco	99%	428
Texas Health Harris Methodist[2]	Bedford	99%	437
TX Inst for Surgery at Presby Hosp[3]	Dallas	99%	146
Tomball Regional Medical Center	Tomball	99%	452
UT SW Univ Hosp-Zale Lipshy[2]	Dallas	99%	127
Valley Regional Medical Center	Brownsville	99%	312
Northwest Texas Surgery Center	Amarillo	97%	126
Pine Creek Medical Center[2]	Dallas	97%	287
Scott & White Hospital - Round Rock[2]	Round Rock	97%	418
TX Hlth Harris Methodist Hosp-Azle[2]	Azle	97%	32
Covenant Hospital Levelland	Levelland	96%	27
Memorial Hospital[2]	Gonzales	96%	25
Lubbock Heart Hospital[2]	Lubbock	95%	241
University General Hospital	Houston	95%	167
University General Hospital Dallas[2]	Dallas	57%	30

Prophylactic Antibiotic Selection

Hospital Name	City	Rate	Cases
Abilene Regional Medical Center	Abilene	100%	500
Baptist Medical Center[2]	San Antonio	100%	2970
Baylor Heart & Vascular Hospital	Dallas	100%	88
Baylor Medical Center at Carrollton	Carrollton	100%	327
Baylor Medical Center at Garland[2]	Garland	100%	152
Baylor Medical Center at Irving[2]	Irving	100%	298
Baylor Medical Center at Mckinney[2]	Mc Kinney	100%	82
Baylor Medical Center at Trophy Club	Trophy Club	100%	52
Baylor Medical Center at Uptown	Dallas	100%	409
Baylor Medical Center at Waxahachie[2]	Waxahachie	100%	201
Baylor Ortho & Spine Hosp-Arlington	Arlington	100%	677
Baylor Reg Med Ctr at Grapevine[2]	Grapevine	100%	455
Baylor Regional Medical Center at Plano[2]	Plano	100%	300
Baylor Surgical Hospital at Fort Worth	Fort Worth	100%	423
Baylor Surgical Hospital at Las Colinas	Irving	100%	122
Baylor University Medical Center[2]	Dallas	100%	1850
Christus Hospital[2]	Beaumont	100%	664
Christus Saint Catherine Hospital	Katy	100%	98
Clear Lake Regional Medical Center[2]	Webster	100%	429
Cleveland Regional Medical Center	Cleveland	100%	25
Conroe Regional Medical Center[2]	Conroe	100%	328
The Corpus Christi Medical Center[2]	Corpus Christi	100%	428
Denton Regional Medical Center[2]	Denton	100%	352
Detar Hospital Navarro	Victoria	100%	271
Doctors Hospital[2]	Dallas	100%	252
Doctors Hospital at Renaissance[2]	Edinburg	100%	654
Fort Duncan Medical Center[2]	Eagle Pass	100%	57
Fdn Surgical Hosp of San Antonio[2]	San Antonio	100%	37
Golden Plains Community Hospital	Borger	100%	31
Graham Regional Medical Center[2]	Graham	100%	40
Guadalupe Regional Medical Center	Seguin	100%	268
Harlingen Medical Center[2]	Harlingen	100%	401
Heart Hospital Baylor Plano	Plano	100%	1058

NOTE: Hospital profiles are in alphabetical order by state, then city, then hospital within the city; Rankings exclude hospitals with less than 25 cases except for patient surveys which excludes hospitals with less than 100 cases; (a) 100-299 cases; (1) The number of cases/patients is too few to report; (2) Data submitted were based on a sample of cases/patients; (3) Results are based on a shorter time period than required; (4) Data suppressed by CMS for one or more quarters; (5) Results are not available for this reporting period; (6) Fewer than 100 patients completed the HCAHPS survey; (7) No cases met the criteria for this measure; (8) The lower limit of the confidence interval cannot be calculated if the number of observed infections equals zero; (9) No data are available from the state/territory for this reporting period; (10) The scores shown reflect fewer than 50 completed surveys; (11) There were discrepancies in the data collection process; (12) This measure does not apply to this hospital for this reporting period; (13) Results cannot be calculated for this reporting period; (14) The results for this state are combined with nearby states to protect confidentiality; Please refer to the User's Guide for a full explanation of data.

Hill Country Memorial Hospital[2]	Fredericksburg	100%	391
The Hospital at Westlake Medical Center	Austin	100%	281
Houston Orthopedic & Spine Hospital	Bellaire	100%	756
Huguley Memorial Medical Center	Burleson	100%	320
Kell West Regional Hospital	Wichita Falls	100%	266
Kingwood Medical Center[2]	Kingwood	100%	302
Lake Pointe Medical Center	Rowlett	100%	118
Lakeway Regional Medical Center[3]	Lakeway	100%	25
Laredo Medical Center	Laredo	100%	397
Las Colinas Medical Center[2]	Irving	100%	139
Las Palmas Medical Center[2]	El Paso	100%	435
Medical Center of Arlington[2]	Arlington	100%	208
Medical Center of Mckinney[2]	Mckinney	100%	217
Medical Center of Plano[2]	Plano	100%	355
Memorial Hermann Baptist Orange Hospital	Orange	100%	25
Memorial Hermann Katy Hospital[2]	Katy	100%	280
Memorial Hermann Northeast[2]	Humble	100%	129
Methodist Ambulatory Surgery Hospital NW[2]	San Antonio	100%	161
Methodist Charlton Medical Center	Dallas	100%	432
Methodist Dallas Medical Center	Dallas	100%	543
Methodist Hospital For Surgery[2]	Addison	100%	695
Methodist Mansfield Medical Center	Mansfield	100%	218
Methodist Richardson Medical Center[2]	Richardson	100%	198
Methodist Willowbrook Hospital[2]	Houston	100%	244
Mother Frances Hospital[2]	Tyler	100%	559
Nacogdoches Medical Center[2]	Nacogdoches	100%	108
Navarro Regional Hospital	Corsicana	100%	70
North Austin Medical Center[2]	Austin	100%	396
North Central Surgical Center	Dallas	100%	491
North Cypress Medical Center	Cypress	100%	425
North Hills Hospital[2]	N Richland Hls	100%	271
Pampa Regional Medical Center	Pampa	100%	138
The Physicians Centre	Bryan	100%	85
Plaza Medical Center of Fort Worth[2]	Fort Worth	100%	516
Quail Creek Surgical Hospital	Amarillo	100%	719
Rio Grande Regional Hospital[2]	Mcallen	100%	216
Round Rock Medical Center[2]	Round Rock	100%	249
Saint David's Medical Center[2]	Austin	100%	586
Saint David's South Austin Medical Center[2]	Austin	100%	381
Saint Joseph Regional Health Center[2]	Bryan	100%	346
Saint Luke's Lakeside Hospital	The Woodlands	100%	349
Saint Luke's the Woodlands Hospital[2]	The Woodlands	100%	436
Saint Marks Medical Center	La Grange	100%	45
San Angelo Community Medical Center	San Angelo	100%	382
San Antonio VA Medical Center	San Antonio	100%	258
Seton Highland Lakes	Burnet	100%	77
Shannon Medical Center	San Angelo	100%	638
Sierra Providence East Medical Center[2]	El Paso	100%	126
South Texas Health System[2]	Edinburg	100%	318
South Texas Regional Medical Center	Jourdanton	100%	29
South Texas Spine & Surgical Hospital	San Antonio	100%	231
Sugar Land Surgical Hospital	Sugar Land	100%	170
Texas Health Arlington Memorial Hospital[2]	Arlington	100%	232
TX Hlth Harris Meth Hosp-Cleburne[2]	Cleburne	100%	172
TX Hlth Harris Meth Hosp-Southlake	Southlake	100%	468
TX Hlth Harris Meth Hosp-Stephenville[2]	Stephenville	100%	131
TX Hlth Heart & Vasc Hosp-Arlington	Arlington	100%	154
Texas Health Presbyterian Hospital Allen[2]	Allen	100%	117
Texas Health Presbyterian Hospital Dallas[2]	Dallas	100%	486
TX Health Presbyterian Hosp Rockwall	Rockwall	100%	286
Texas Orthopedic Hospital[2]	Houston	100%	258
Texas Reg Med Ctr at Sunnyvale[2]	Sunnyvale	100%	168
Texas Spine & Joint Hospital[2]	Tyler	100%	213
Texoma Medical Center[2]	Denison	100%	379
Tops Surgical Specialty Hospital	Houston	100%	348
United Regional Health Care System	Wichita Falls	100%	526
Univ of TX Health Science Ctr-Tyler	Tyler	100%	51
USMD Hospital at Arlington[2]	Arlington	100%	51
USMD Hospital at Fort Worth	Fort Worth	100%	189
Uvalde Memorial Hospital	Uvalde	100%	28
VA Amarillo Healthcare System	Amarillo	100%	56
Valley Regional Medical Center	Brownsville	100%	221
West Houston Medical Center[2]	Houston	100%	289
Woodland Heights Medical Center	Lufkin	100%	245
Baptist Beaumont Hospital[2]	Beaumont	99%	386
Baptist Saint Anthony's Hospital[2]	Amarillo	99%	491
Baylor All Saints Medical Center at FW[2]	Fort Worth	99%	521
Baylor Medical Center at Frisco	Frisco	99%	793
Bayshore Medical Center[2]	Pasadena	99%	263
Brownwood Regional Medical Center	Brownwood	99%	170
Central Texas Medical Center	San Marcos	99%	77
Christus Saint Michael Health System[2]	Texarkana	99%	794
Christus Santa Rosa Hospital	San Antonio	99%	702
Citizens Medical Center	Victoria	99%	358
College Station Medical Center	College Station	99%	440
Cornerstone Regional Hospital[2]	Edinburg	99%	355
Covenant Hospital Plainview	Plainview	99%	72
Cypress Fairbanks Medical Center[2]	Houston	99%	122
Dallas VA Medical Center - VA North Texas	Dallas	99%	231
Doctors Hospital of Laredo[2]	Laredo	99%	116
East Texas Medical Center[2]	Tyler	99%	398
El Paso Specialty Hospital	El Paso	99%	417
Foundation Surgical Hospital of El Paso[2]	El Paso	99%	148
Good Shepherd Medical Center[2]	Longview	99%	399
Good Shepherd Medical Center Marshall	Marshall	99%	154
Grace Medical Center	Lubbock	99%	268
Harris Health System[2]	Houston	99%	475
Hendrick Medical Center[2]	Abilene	99%	401
Hillcrest Baptist Medical Center[2]	Waco	99%	497
Houston Northwest Medical Center[2]	Houston	99%	388
Houston Physicians' Hospital	Webster	99%	214
Houston VA Medical Center	Houston	99%	515
Huntsville Memorial Hospital	Huntsville	99%	167
JPS Health Network[2]	Fort Worth	99%	557
Medical Center Hospital[2]	Odessa	99%	426
Medical Center of Lewisville[2]	Lewisville	99%	198
The Medical Center of Southeast Texas	Port Arthur	99%	350
Medical City Dallas Hospital[2]	Dallas	99%	517
Memorial Hermann Hospital System[2]	Houston	99%	1410
Mem Hermann Mem City Med Ctr[2]	Houston	99%	481
Memorial Hermann Sugar Land Hospital[2]	Sugar Land	99%	235
Mem Hermann Surgical Hosp Kingwood	Kingwood	99%	117
Memorial Hospital	Nacogdoches	99%	134
Methodist Hospital[2]	San Antonio	99%	704
The Methodist Hospital[2]	Houston	99%	592
Methodist Mckinney Hospital[2]	Mc Kinney	99%	268
Methodist Stone Oak Hospital[2]	San Antonio	99%	380
Methodist Sugar Land Hospital[2]	Sugar Land	99%	470
Midland Memorial Hospital	Midland	99%	590
Odessa Regional Hospital	Odessa	99%	211
Paris Regional Medical Center[2]	Paris	99%	387
Peterson Regional Medical Center	Kerrville	99%	378
Providence Memorial Hospital[2]	El Paso	99%	312
Saint Luke's Episcopal Hospital[2]	Houston	99%	559
Scott & White Hospital - Round Rock[2]	Round Rock	99%	303
Scott & White Hospital Brenham	Brenham	99%	91
Scott & White Memorial Hospital[2]	Temple	99%	506
Seton Medical Center Austin[2]	Austin	99%	559
Sierra Medical Center[2]	El Paso	99%	402
South Texas Surgical Hospital	Corpus Christi	99%	467
Southwest General Hospital	San Antonio	99%	78
Texas Health Harris Methodist Fort Worth[2]	Fort Worth	99%	947
Texas Health Presbyterian Hospital - WNJ	Sherman	99%	162
Texas Health Presbyterian Hospital Denton[2]	Denton	99%	216
TX Hlth Presbyterian Hosp-Kaufman[2]	Kaufman	99%	69
Texas Health Presbyterian Hospital Plano[2]	Plano	99%	1503
TX Inst for Surgery at Presby Hosp[3]	Dallas	99%	155
University Medical Center[2]	Lubbock	99%	400
University Medical Center at Brackenridge[2]	Austin	99%	224
Univ of Texas Med Branch Galveston[2]	Galveston	99%	300
Val Verde Regional Medical Center	Del Rio	99%	78
Wadley Regional Medical Center	Texarkana	99%	336
Weatherford Regional Medical Center	Weatherford	99%	254
The Womans Hospital of Texas[2]	Houston	99%	117
Brazosport Regional Health System	Lake Jackson	98%	94
Cedar Park Regional Medical Center	Cedar Park	98%	225
Christus Saint John Hospital	Nassau Bay	98%	383
Christus Spohn Hospital Corpus Christi	Corpus Christi	98%	1118
Covenant Medical Center	Lubbock	98%	1786
Dallas Medical Center[2]	Dallas	98%	98
Dallas Regional Medical Center	Mesquite	98%	210
East Texas Medical Center Athens[2]	Athens	98%	177
East Texas Medical Center Jacksonville	Jacksonville	98%	65
Lake Granbury Medical Center	Granbury	98%	193
Longview Regional Medical Center	Longview	98%	559
Lubbock Heart Hospital[2]	Lubbock	98%	284
Memorial Hermann Texas Medical Center[2]	Houston	98%	406
Methodist West Houston Hospital[2]	Houston	98%	249
Metroplex Hospital[2]	Killeen	98%	166
Mission Regional Medical Center	Mission	98%	161
Nix Health Care System	San Antonio	98%	186
North Texas Medical Center	Gainesville	98%	51
Northwest Texas Hospital[2]	Amarillo	98%	314
Parkland Health & Hospital System[2]	Dallas	98%	270
Saint Luke's Hospital at the Vintage	Houston	98%	55
Saint Luke's Patients Medical Center[2]	Pasadena	98%	258
San Jacinto Methodist Hospital[2]	Baytown	98%	335
Seton Medical Center Harker Heights	Harker Heights	98%	95
Seton Medical Center Hays	Kyle	98%	149
Seton Medical Center Williamson	Round Rock	98%	134
TX Hlth Harris Meth Hosp SW Ft Worth[2]	Fort Worth	98%	289
Texas Health Harris Methodist[2]	Bedford	98%	255
TX Hlth Presbyterian Hosp-Flower Mound	Flower Mound	98%	323
Tomball Regional Medical Center	Tomball	98%	260
University Health System[2]	San Antonio	98%	467
University Medical Center of El Paso[2]	El Paso	98%	253
UT Southwestern University Hospital[2]	Dallas	98%	560
Angleton - Danbury Medical Center[2]	Angleton	97%	140
Centennial Medical Center	Frisco	97%	92
Doctors Hospital Tidwell	Houston	97%	35
First Surgical Hospital	Bellaire	97%	127
Heritage Park Surgical Hospital	Sherman	97%	139
Knapp Medical Center	Weslaco	97%	294
Memorial Medical Center Livingston[2]	Livingston	97%	107
Oakbend Medical Center[2]	Richmond	97%	89
Palestine Regional Medical Center	Palestine	97%	37
Park Plaza Hospital[2]	Houston	97%	282
Providence Health Center[2]	Waco	97%	379
Saint Joseph Medical Center	Houston	97%	407
Saint Luke's Sugar Land Hospital	Sugar Land	97%	35
Seton Northwest Hospital	Austin	97%	188
VHS Harlingen Hospital Company[2]	Harlingen	97%	887
Arise Austin Medical Center[2]	Austin	96%	316
Etmc Henderson	Henderson	96%	46
Hunt Regional Medical Center	Greenville	96%	197
Temple VA Med Ctr-VA Central Texas	Temple	96%	194
TX Health Ctr for Diag & Surgery	Plano	96%	51
Titus Regional Medical Center	Mount Pleasant	96%	78
Memorial Medical Center of East Texas[2]	Lufkin	95%	238
Palo Pinto General Hospital	Mineral Wells	95%	65
Pine Creek Medical Center[2]	Dallas	95%	64
University General Hospital	Houston	94%	70
Christus Spohn Hospital Kleberg	Kingsville	93%	45
Northwest Texas Surgery Center	Amarillo	93%	116
Hopkins County Memorial Hospital	Sulphur Springs	92%	84
VHS Brownsville Hospital Company[2]	Brownsville	92%	53
Scenic Mountain Medical Center	Big Spring	91%	44
Wise Regional Health System[2]	Decatur	91%	223
Hill Regional Hospital	Hillsboro	83%	41

Prophylactic Antibiotic Selection (Outpatient)

Hospital Name	City	Rate	Cases
Baylor Reg Med Ctr at Grapevine	Grapevine	100%	474
Baylor Regional Medical Center at Plano	Plano	100%	259
Baylor Surgical Hospital at Fort Worth	Fort Worth	100%	239
Clear Lake Regional Medical Center	Webster	100%	572
Dallas Medical Center	Dallas	100%	37
Detar Hospital Navarro	Victoria	100%	421
El Paso Specialty Hospital	El Paso	100%	45
Graham Regional Medical Center	Graham	100%	32
Hendrick Medical Center	Abilene	100%	375
Kingwood Medical Center	Kingwood	100%	259
Lake Granbury Medical Center	Granbury	100%	154
Medical Center of Arlington	Arlington	100%	322
Medical City Dallas Hospital	Dallas	100%	620
Memorial Hermann Northeast	Humble	100%	117
Methodist Ambulatory Surgery Hospital NW	San Antonio	100%	40
Methodist Hospital	San Antonio	100%	1068
Navarro Regional Hospital	Corsicana	100%	41
North Central Surgical Center	Dallas	100%	364
North Hills Hospital	N Richland Hls	100%	253
Northwest Hills Surgical Hospital	Austin	100%	201
Northwest Texas Hospital	Amarillo	100%	222
Palestine Regional Medical Center	Palestine	100%	68
The Physicians Centre	Bryan	100%	35
Plaza Medical Center of Fort Worth	Fort Worth	100%	320
Providence Memorial Hospital	El Paso	100%	444
Quail Creek Surgical Hospital	Amarillo	100%	200
Saint David's Medical Center	Austin	100%	724
Saint Luke's Lakeside Hospital	The Woodlands	100%	320
San Angelo Community Medical Center	San Angelo	100%	151
Scott & White Hospital Brenham	Brenham	100%	45
Seton Medical Center Hays	Kyle	100%	55
Seton Northwest Hospital	Austin	100%	43
Sierra Medical Center	El Paso	100%	487
South Texas Regional Medical Center	Jourdanton	100%	33
TX Hlth Heart & Vasc Hosp-Arlington	Arlington	100%	365
TX Inst for Surgery at Presby Hosp	Dallas	100%	258
Texas Orthopedic Hospital	Houston	100%	428
Tops Surgical Specialty Hospital	Houston	100%	50
Valley Regional Medical Center	Brownsville	100%	189
Weatherford Regional Medical Center	Weatherford	100%	51
Woodland Heights Medical Center	Lufkin	100%	152
Abilene Regional Medical Center	Abilene	99%	300
Baylor Heart & Vascular Hospital	Dallas	99%	734
Baylor Medical Center at Carrollton	Carrollton	99%	67
Baylor Medical Center at Irving	Irving	99%	271
Baylor Medical Center at Trophy Club	Trophy Club	99%	105
Baylor Medical Center at Uptown	Dallas	99%	185
Baylor Ortho & Spine Hosp-Arlington	Arlington	99%	149
Bayshore Medical Center	Pasadena	99%	138
Cedar Park Regional Medical Center	Cedar Park	99%	161
Central Texas Medical Center	San Marcos	99%	154
Citizens Medical Center	Victoria	99%	274
College Station Medical Center	College Station	99%	316
The Corpus Christi Medical Center	Corpus Christi	99%	536
Dallas Regional Medical Center	Mesquite	99%	88
Doctors Hospital	Dallas	99%	193
Good Shepherd Medical Center	Longview	99%	466
Harris Health System	Houston	99%	625
The Hospital at Westlake Medical Center	Austin	99%	166
Houston Physicians' Hospital	Webster	99%	266
JPS Health Network	Fort Worth	99%	392

NOTE: Hospital profiles are in alphabetical order by state, then city, then hospital within the city; Rankings exclude hospitals with less than 25 cases except for patient surveys which excludes hospitals with less than 100 cases; (a) 100-299 cases; (1) The number of cases/patients is too few to report; (2) Data submitted were based on a sample of cases/patients; (3) Results are based on a shorter time period than required; (4) Data suppressed by CMS for one or more quarters; (5) Results are not available for this reporting period; (6) Fewer than 100 patients completed the HCAHPS survey; (7) No cases met the criteria for this measure; (8) The lower limit of the confidence interval cannot be calculated if the number of observed infections equals zero; (9) No data are available from the state/territory for this reporting period; (10) The scores shown reflect fewer than 50 completed surveys; (11) There were discrepancies in the data collection process; (12) This measure does not apply to this hospital for this reporting period; (13) Results cannot be calculated for this reporting period; (14) The results for this state are combined with nearby states to protect confidentiality; Please refer to the User's Guide for a full explanation of data.

Lake Pointe Medical Center	Rowlett	99%	200
Laredo Medical Center	Laredo	99%	262
Las Colinas Medical Center	Irving	99%	158
Las Palmas Medical Center	El Paso	99%	828
Longview Regional Medical Center	Longview	99%	386
Medical Center Hospital	Odessa	99%	289
Memorial Hermann Katy Hospital	Katy	99%	254
Mem Hermann Mem City Med Ctr	Houston	99%	526
Memorial Hermann Sugar Land Hospital	Sugar Land	99%	118
Memorial Hermann Texas Medical Center	Houston	99%	480
Methodist Charlton Medical Center	Dallas	99%	136
Methodist Dallas Medical Center	Dallas	99%	739
Methodist Hospital For Surgery	Addison	99%	477
The Methodist Hospital	Houston	99%	1265
Methodist Mansfield Medical Center	Mansfield	99%	193
Methodist Stone Oak Hospital	San Antonio	99%	593
Methodist Willowbrook Hospital	Houston	99%	343
Nacogdoches Medical Center	Nacogdoches	99%	192
Nix Health Care System	San Antonio	99%	108
North Austin Medical Center	Austin	99%	593
Odessa Regional Hospital	Odessa	99%	123
Parkland Health & Hospital System	Dallas	99%	400
Round Rock Medical Center	Round Rock	99%	242
Saint David's South Austin Medical Center	Austin	99%	449
Saint Joseph Regional Health Center	Bryan	99%	348
Saint Luke's the Woodlands Hospital	The Woodlands	99%	310
Seton Medical Center Austin	Austin	99%	578
Seton Medical Center Harker Heights	Harker Heights	99%	120
Seton Medical Center Williamson	Round Rock	99%	184
Shannon Medical Center	San Angelo	99%	457
South Texas Health System	Edinburg	99%	283
South Texas Spine & Surgical Hospital	San Antonio	99%	360
Southwest General Hospital	San Antonio	99%	149
Sugar Land Surgical Hospital	Sugar Land	99%	133
TX Health Ctr for Diag & Surgery	Plano	99%	436
TX Hlth Harris Meth Hosp-Southlake	Southlake	99%	317
Texas Health Presbyterian Hospital - WNJ	Sherman	99%	146
Texas Health Presbyterian Hospital Denton	Denton	99%	308
Texas Spine & Joint Hospital	Tyler	99%	396
Texoma Medical Center	Denison	99%	400
United Regional Health Care System	Wichita Falls	99%	582
University Medical Center	Lubbock	99%	176
University Medical Center at Brackenridge	Austin	99%	270
University Medical Center of El Paso	El Paso	99%	222
UT Southwestern University Hospital	Dallas	99%	248
UT SW Univ Hosp-Zale Lipshy	Dallas	99%	237
The Womans Hospital of Texas	Houston	99%	1064
Baptist Medical Center	San Antonio	98%	1533
Baptist Saint Anthony's Hospital	Amarillo	98%	599
Baylor Medical Center at Frisco	Frisco	98%	528
Baylor Medical Center at Garland	Garland	98%	170
Baylor Medical Center at Mckinney	Mc Kinney	98%	165
Baylor University Medical Center	Dallas	98%	571
Centennial Medical Center	Frisco	98%	60
Christus Saint Michael Health System	Texarkana	98%	492
Conroe Regional Medical Center	Conroe	98%	263
Covenant Medical Center	Lubbock	98%	744
Doctors Hospital at Renaissance	Edinburg	98%	817
Foundation Surgical Hospital of El Paso	El Paso	98%	99
Grace Medical Center	Lubbock	98%	264
Guadalupe Regional Medical Center	Seguin	98%	92
Harlingen Medical Center	Harlingen	98%	107
Hill Country Memorial Hospital	Fredericksburg	98%	63
Houston Northwest Medical Center	Houston	98%	194
Hunt Regional Medical Center	Greenville	98%	98
Kell West Regional Hospital	Wichita Falls	98%	291
Lubbock Heart Hospital	Lubbock	98%	273
Matagorda Regional Medical Center	Bay City	98%	115
Medical Center of Lewisville	Lewisville	98%	43
Memorial Hermann Baptist Orange Hospital	Orange	98%	47
Memorial Hermann Hospital System	Houston	98%	1335
Mem Hermann Surgical Hosp Kingwood	Kingwood	98%	179
Mother Frances Hospital	Tyler	98%	1220
Saint Luke's Hospital at the Vintage	Houston	98%	43
San Jacinto Methodist Hospital	Baytown	98%	160
Scott & White Hospital - Round Rock	Round Rock	98%	196
Scott & White Memorial Hospital	Temple	98%	743
Texas Health Harris Methodist	Bedford	98%	425
Texas Health Presbyterian Hospital Allen	Allen	98%	92
TX Health Presbyterian Hosp Rockwall	Rockwall	98%	413
Univ of Texas Med Branch Galveston	Galveston	98%	352
VHS Brownsville Hospital Company	Brownsville	98%	180
West Houston Medical Center	Houston	98%	176
Wise Regional Health System	Decatur	98%	166
Baptist Beaumont Hospital	Beaumont	97%	277
Baylor Surgical Hospital at Las Colinas	Irving	97%	73
Brownwood Regional Medical Center	Brownwood	97%	109
Christus Saint John Hospital	Nassau Bay	97%	165
Columbus Community Hospital	Columbus	97%	33
East Texas Medical Center	Tyler	97%	399
Huntsville Memorial Hospital	Huntsville	97%	98
Medical Center of Plano	Plano	97%	277
Methodist Richardson Medical Center	Richardson	97%	229
Palo Pinto General Hospital	Mineral Wells	97%	32
Paris Regional Medical Center	Paris	97%	232
Park Plaza Hospital	Houston	97%	267
Peterson Regional Medical Center	Kerrville	97%	157
Providence Health Center	Waco	97%	261
Saint Luke's Episcopal Hospital	Houston	97%	715
Texas Health Arlington Memorial Hospital	Arlington	97%	218
Texas Health Harris Methodist Fort Worth	Fort Worth	97%	745
TX Hlth Harris Meth Hosp-Cleburne	Cleburne	97%	36
Texas Health Presbyterian Hospital Dallas	Dallas	97%	667
Titus Regional Medical Center	Mount Pleasant	97%	97
USMD Hospital at Arlington	Arlington	97%	593
Baylor All Saints Medical Center at FW	Fort Worth	96%	524
Covenant Hospital Plainview	Plainview	96%	46
Good Shepherd Medical Center Marshall	Marshall	96%	27
Heart Hospital Baylor Denton[3]	Denton	96%	89
Heart Hospital Baylor Plano	Plano	96%	622
Heritage Park Surgical Hospital	Sherman	96%	159
Houston Orthopedic & Spine Hospital	Bellaire	96%	357
Knapp Medical Center	Weslaco	96%	26
Methodist Sugar Land Hospital	Sugar Land	96%	493
Midland Memorial Hospital	Midland	96%	255
North Cypress Medical Center	Cypress	96%	189
Northwest Texas Surgery Center	Amarillo	96%	46
Sierra Providence East Medical Center	El Paso	96%	79
TX Hlth Presbyterian Hosp-Flower Mound	Flower Mound	96%	322
Tomball Regional Medical Center	Tomball	96%	186
University Health System	San Antonio	96%	387
Brazosport Regional Health System	Lake Jackson	95%	41
Christus Hospital	Beaumont	95%	597
Christus Spohn Hospital Corpus Christi	Corpus Christi	95%	532
Huguley Memorial Medical Center	Burleson	95%	256
Memorial Hospital	Nacogdoches	95%	175
Rio Grande Regional Hospital	Mcallen	95%	95
Saint Luke's Patients Medical Center	Pasadena	95%	218
Wadley Regional Medical Center	Texarkana	95%	347
Cornerstone Regional Hospital[3]	Edinburg	94%	31
Cypress Fairbanks Medical Center	Houston	94%	100
Hillcrest Baptist Medical Center	Waco	94%	141
Medical Center of Mckinney	Mckinney	94%	109
Methodist West Houston Hospital	Houston	94%	291
Denton Regional Medical Center	Denton	93%	295
Doctors Hospital of Laredo	Laredo	93%	119
East Texas Medical Center Athens	Athens	93%	41
Saint Joseph Medical Center	Houston	93%	285
Seton Highland Lakes[3]	Burnet	93%	44
TX Hlth Harris Meth Hosp SW Ft Worth	Fort Worth	93%	355
University General Hospital	Houston	93%	116
University General Hospital Dallas	Dallas	93%	46
Val Verde Regional Medical Center	Del Rio	93%	30
Christus Santa Rosa Hospital	San Antonio	92%	463
The Medical Center of Southeast Texas	Port Arthur	92%	145
Memorial Medical Center of East Texas	Lufkin	92%	219
Texas Reg Med Ctr at Sunnyvale	Sunnyvale	92%	52
Basin Healthcare Center	Odessa	91%	277
Pine Creek Medical Center	Dallas	90%	249
USMD Hospital at Fort Worth	Fort Worth	90%	299
Hopkins County Memorial Hospital	Sulphur Springs	89%	132
Metroplex Hospital	Killeen	89%	130
Texas Health Presbyterian Hospital Plano	Plano	89%	338
VHS Harlingen Hospital Company	Harlingen	89%	280
First Surgical Hospital	Bellaire	88%	130
Methodist Mckinney Hospital	Mc Kinney	85%	111
Mission Regional Medical Center	Mission	85%	27
South Texas Surgical Hospital	Corpus Christi	85%	129
Christus Spohn Hospital Alice	Alice	59%	54

Prophylactic Antibiotic Stopped

Hospital Name	City	Rate	Cases
Baylor Medical Center at Carrollton	Carrollton	100%	312
Baylor Medical Center at Irving[2]	Irving	100%	292
Baylor Medical Center at Uptown	Dallas	100%	408
Baylor Regional Medical Center at Plano[2]	Plano	100%	277
Central Texas Medical Center	San Marcos	100%	64
Christus Spohn Hospital Kleberg	Kingsville	100%	44
Conroe Regional Medical Center[2]	Conroe	100%	304
Covenant Hospital Plainview	Plainview	100%	72
Dallas Regional Medical Center	Mesquite	100%	209
Etmc Henderson	Henderson	100%	44
The Hospital at Westlake Medical Center	Austin	100%	280
Lake Granbury Medical Center	Granbury	100%	192
Lakeway Regional Medical Center[3]	Lakeway	100%	25
Medical Center of Lewisville[2]	Lewisville	100%	193
Memorial Hermann Sugar Land Hospital[2]	Sugar Land	100%	225
Methodist Dallas Medical Center	Dallas	100%	538
Methodist Hospital For Surgery[2]	Addison	100%	695
Methodist Mansfield Medical Center	Mansfield	100%	209
Methodist Stone Oak Hospital[2]	San Antonio	100%	361
Methodist Willowbrook Hospital[2]	Houston	100%	222
North Austin Medical Center[2]	Austin	100%	394
North Central Surgical Center	Dallas	100%	491
North Cypress Medical Center	Cypress	100%	409
North Hills Hospital[2]	N Richland Hls	100%	258
Palestine Regional Medical Center	Palestine	100%	35
Palo Pinto General Hospital	Mineral Wells	100%	63
Peterson Regional Medical Center	Kerrville	100%	373
The Physicians Centre	Bryan	100%	85
Quail Creek Surgical Hospital	Amarillo	100%	719
Round Rock Medical Center[2]	Round Rock	100%	246
Saint David's Medical Center[2]	Austin	100%	574
Saint Luke's Lakeside Hospital	The Woodlands	100%	345
Saint Marks Medical Center	La Grange	100%	41
San Angelo Community Medical Center	San Angelo	100%	378
TX Hlth Harris Meth Hosp-Southlake	Southlake	100%	468
TX Hlth Heart & Vasc Hosp-Arlington	Arlington	100%	149
Texas Health Presbyterian Hospital - WNJ	Sherman	100%	152
Texas Health Presbyterian Hospital Denton[2]	Denton	100%	211
Texas Health Presbyterian Hospital Plano[2]	Plano	100%	1494
TX Inst for Surgery at Presby Hosp[3]	Dallas	100%	155
Texoma Medical Center[2]	Denison	100%	338
Titus Regional Medical Center	Mount Pleasant	100%	77
University Medical Center at Brackenridge[2]	Austin	100%	220
Univ of TX Health Science Ctr-Tyler	Tyler	100%	47
Valley Regional Medical Center	Brownsville	100%	212
West Houston Medical Center[2]	Houston	100%	267
The Womans Hospital of Texas[2]	Houston	100%	109
Woodland Heights Medical Center	Lufkin	100%	224
Abilene Regional Medical Center	Abilene	99%	475
Baptist Beaumont Hospital[2]	Beaumont	99%	363
Baptist Medical Center[2]	San Antonio	99%	2868
Baylor All Saints Medical Center at FW[2]	Fort Worth	99%	492
Baylor Heart & Vascular Hospital	Dallas	99%	82
Baylor Medical Center at Frisco	Frisco	99%	789
Baylor Medical Center at Waxahachie[2]	Waxahachie	99%	190
Baylor Ortho & Spine Hosp-Arlington	Arlington	99%	677
Baylor Reg Med Ctr at Grapevine[2]	Grapevine	99%	446
Bayshore Medical Center[2]	Pasadena	99%	242
Brazosport Regional Health System	Lake Jackson	99%	91
Cedar Park Regional Medical Center	Cedar Park	99%	222
Christus Hospital[2]	Beaumont	99%	639
Christus Saint John Hospital	Nassau Bay	99%	374
Christus Santa Rosa Hospital	San Antonio	99%	691
Cornerstone Regional Hospital[2]	Edinburg	99%	351
Denton Regional Medical Center[2]	Denton	99%	343
Detar Hospital Navarro	Victoria	99%	262
Foundation Surgical Hospital of El Paso[2]	El Paso	99%	143
Good Shepherd Medical Center Marshall	Marshall	99%	152
Heart Hospital Baylor Plano	Plano	99%	1007
Hendrick Medical Center[2]	Abilene	99%	390
Heritage Park Surgical Hospital	Sherman	99%	139
Hill Country Memorial Hospital[2]	Fredericksburg	99%	387
Hillcrest Baptist Medical Center[2]	Waco	99%	482
Huntsville Memorial Hospital	Huntsville	99%	165
JPS Health Network[2]	Fort Worth	99%	547
Kingwood Medical Center[2]	Kingwood	99%	286
Knapp Medical Center	Weslaco	99%	289
Lake Pointe Medical Center	Rowlett	99%	110
Laredo Medical Center	Laredo	99%	364
Las Colinas Medical Center[2]	Irving	99%	133
Las Palmas Medical Center[2]	El Paso	99%	426
Longview Regional Medical Center	Longview	99%	536
Medical Center of Mckinney[2]	Mckinney	99%	203
Medical Center of Plano[2]	Plano	99%	338
Medical City Dallas Hospital[2]	Dallas	99%	481
Memorial Hermann Katy Hospital[2]	Katy	99%	273
Methodist Charlton Medical Center	Dallas	99%	422
Methodist Hospital[2]	San Antonio	99%	679
Methodist Sugar Land Hospital[2]	Sugar Land	99%	417
Methodist West Houston Hospital[2]	Houston	99%	241
Metroplex Hospital[2]	Killeen	99%	166
Nacogdoches Medical Center[2]	Nacogdoches	99%	101
Nix Health Care System	San Antonio	99%	185
Park Plaza Hospital[2]	Houston	99%	274
Providence Memorial Hospital[2]	El Paso	99%	294
Saint Joseph Regional Health Center[2]	Bryan	99%	338
Scott & White Hospital Brenham	Brenham	99%	91
Scott & White Memorial Hospital[2]	Temple	99%	486
Seton Highland Lakes	Burnet	99%	77
Seton Medical Center Williamson	Round Rock	99%	128
Seton Northwest Hospital	Austin	99%	178
Sierra Providence East Medical Center[2]	El Paso	99%	114
South Texas Spine & Surgical Hospital	San Antonio	99%	231
Sugar Land Surgical Hospital	Sugar Land	99%	169
Texas Health Arlington Memorial Hospital[2]	Arlington	99%	218
TX Hlth Harris Meth Hosp SW Ft Worth[2]	Fort Worth	99%	288
Texas Health Presbyterian Hospital Dallas[2]	Dallas	99%	479
TX Hlth Presbyterian Hosp-Kaufman[2]	Kaufman	99%	68
Texas Orthopedic Hospital[2]	Houston	99%	255
United Regional Health Care System	Wichita Falls	99%	510
University Medical Center of El Paso[2]	El Paso	99%	241

NOTE: Hospital profiles are in alphabetical order by state, then city, then hospital within the city; Rankings exclude hospitals with less than 25 cases except for patient surveys which excludes hospitals with less than 100 cases; (a) 100-299 cases; (1) The number of cases/patients is too few to report; (2) Data submitted were based on a sample of cases/patients; (3) Results are based on a shorter time period than required; (4) Data suppressed by CMS for one or more quarters; (5) Results are not available for this reporting period; (6) Fewer than 100 patients completed the HCAHPS survey; (7) No cases met the criteria for this measure; (8) The lower limit of the confidence interval cannot be calculated if the number of observed infections equals zero; (9) No data are available from the state/territory for this reporting period; (10) The scores shown reflect fewer than 50 completed surveys; (11) There were discrepancies in the data collection process; (12) This measure does not apply to this hospital for this reporting period; (13) Results cannot be calculated for this reporting period; (14) The results for this state are combined with nearby states to protect confidentiality; Please refer to the User's Guide for a full explanation of data.

USMD Hospital at Fort Worth	Fort Worth	99%	187
Baylor Medical Center at Mckinney[2]	Mc Kinney	98%	82
Baylor Surgical Hospital at Las Colinas	Irving	98%	121
Baylor University Medical Center[2]	Dallas	98%	1803
College Station Medical Center	College Station	98%	435
Doctors Hospital at Renaissance[2]	Edinburg	98%	615
East Texas Medical Center[2]	Tyler	98%	392
El Paso Specialty Hospital	El Paso	98%	417
Good Shepherd Medical Center[2]	Longview	98%	393
Guadalupe Regional Medical Center	Seguin	98%	266
Harlingen Medical Center[2]	Harlingen	98%	390
Medical Center of Arlington[2]	Arlington	98%	194
Memorial Hermann Hospital System[2]	Houston	98%	1344
Memorial Hermann Northeast[2]	Humble	98%	128
Methodist Mckinney Hospital[2]	Mc Kinney	98%	267
Methodist Richardson Medical Center[2]	Richardson	98%	196
Midland Memorial Hospital	Midland	98%	581
Mother Frances Hospital[2]	Tyler	98%	543
Paris Regional Medical Center[2]	Paris	98%	370
Rio Grande Regional Hospital[2]	Mcallen	98%	205
Saint David's South Austin Medical Center[2]	Austin	98%	364
Saint Luke's the Woodlands Hospital[2]	The Woodlands	98%	416
San Antonio VA Medical Center	San Antonio	98%	249
San Jacinto Methodist Hospital[2]	Baytown	98%	319
Scenic Mountain Medical Center	Big Spring	98%	41
Scott & White Hospital - Round Rock[2]	Round Rock	98%	292
Seton Medical Center Austin[2]	Austin	98%	546
Shannon Medical Center	San Angelo	98%	622
Temple VA Med Ctr-VA Central Texas	Temple	98%	191
Texas Health Harris Methodist Fort Worth[2]	Fort Worth	98%	923
TX Health Presbyterian Hosp Rockwall	Rockwall	98%	281
Texas Reg Med Ctr at Sunnyvale[2]	Sunnyvale	98%	167
University Medical Center[2]	Lubbock	98%	381
Univ of Texas Med Branch Galveston[2]	Galveston	98%	295
USMD Hospital at Arlington[2]	Arlington	98%	50
UT Southwestern University Hospital[2]	Dallas	98%	555
VHS Harlingen Hospital Company[2]	Harlingen	98%	876
Arise Austin Medical Center[2]	Austin	97%	316
Baylor Surgical Hospital at Fort Worth	Fort Worth	97%	420
Centennial Medical Center	Frisco	97%	79
Christus Saint Catherine Hospital	Katy	97%	98
Christus Saint Michael Health System[2]	Texarkana	97%	759
Citizens Medical Center	Victoria	97%	354
Clear Lake Regional Medical Center[2]	Webster	97%	414
The Corpus Christi Medical Center[2]	Corpus Christi	97%	391
Cypress Fairbanks Medical Center[2]	Houston	97%	113
Doctors Hospital[2]	Dallas	97%	246
Doctors Hospital Tidwell	Houston	97%	34
East Texas Medical Center Jacksonville	Jacksonville	97%	64
Golden Plains Community Hospital	Borger	97%	31
Grace Medical Center	Lubbock	97%	267
Harris Health System[2]	Houston	97%	444
Houston Northwest Medical Center[2]	Houston	97%	367
Houston VA Medical Center	Houston	97%	483
Huguley Memorial Medical Center	Burleson	97%	290
Hunt Regional Medical Center	Greenville	97%	188
Kell West Regional Hospital	Wichita Falls	97%	262
The Medical Center of Southeast Texas	Port Arthur	97%	325
Mem Hermann Surgical Hosp Kingwood	Kingwood	97%	117
Methodist Ambulatory Surgery Hospital NW[2]	San Antonio	97%	157
Mission Regional Medical Center	Mission	97%	141
Navarro Regional Hospital	Corsicana	97%	68
Northwest Texas Hospital[2]	Amarillo	97%	305
Odessa Regional Hospital	Odessa	97%	188
Pampa Regional Medical Center	Pampa	97%	131
Pine Creek Medical Center[2]	Dallas	97%	64
Providence Health Center[2]	Waco	97%	366
Saint Joseph Medical Center	Houston	97%	387
Seton Medical Center Hays	Kyle	97%	142
South Texas Health System[2]	Edinburg	97%	297
South Texas Regional Medical Center	Jourdanton	97%	29
Southwest General Hospital	San Antonio	97%	73
TX Hlth Harris Meth Hosp-Cleburne[2]	Cleburne	97%	171
Texas Health Harris Methodist[2]	Bedford	97%	248
Texas Health Presbyterian Hospital Allen[2]	Allen	97%	111
TX Hlth Presbyterian Hosp-Flower Mound	Flower Mound	97%	315
Texas Spine & Joint Hospital[2]	Tyler	97%	213
Tops Surgical Specialty Hospital	Houston	97%	348
Wadley Regional Medical Center	Texarkana	97%	325
Baptist Saint Anthony's Hospital[2]	Amarillo	96%	470
Baylor Medical Center at Garland[2]	Garland	96%	138
Baylor Medical Center at Trophy Club	Trophy Club	96%	52
Christus Spohn Hospital Corpus Christi	Corpus Christi	96%	1078
Dallas VA Medical Center - VA North Texas	Dallas	96%	188
Medical Center Hospital[2]	Odessa	96%	402
Memorial Hermann Baptist Orange Hospital	Orange	96%	25
Mem Hermann Mem City Med Ctr[2]	Houston	96%	467
Memorial Hermann Texas Medical Center[2]	Houston	96%	387
Parkland Health & Hospital System[2]	Dallas	96%	266
Plaza Medical Center of Fort Worth[2]	Fort Worth	96%	510
Saint Luke's Episcopal Hospital[2]	Houston	96%	531
Saint Luke's Hospital at the Vintage	Houston	96%	54
Saint Luke's Patients Medical Center[2]	Pasadena	96%	253
Sierra Medical Center[2]	El Paso	96%	391
TX Health Ctr for Diag & Surgery	Plano	96%	49
Uvalde Memorial Hospital	Uvalde	96%	27
Val Verde Regional Medical Center	Del Rio	96%	76
VHS Brownsville Hospital Company[2]	Brownsville	96%	48
Weatherford Regional Medical Center	Weatherford	96%	248
Brownwood Regional Medical Center	Brownwood	95%	155
Covenant Medical Center	Lubbock	95%	1754
Doctors Hospital of Laredo[2]	Laredo	95%	108
Fort Duncan Medical Center[2]	Eagle Pass	95%	56
Graham Regional Medical Center[2]	Graham	95%	40
Houston Orthopedic & Spine Hospital	Bellaire	95%	744
Memorial Medical Center Livingston[2]	Livingston	95%	99
The Methodist Hospital[2]	Houston	95%	578
Northwest Texas Surgery Center	Amarillo	95%	116
South Texas Surgical Hospital	Corpus Christi	95%	465
University Health System[2]	San Antonio	95%	453
Fdn Surgical Hosp of San Antonio[2]	San Antonio	94%	36
Houston Physicians' Hospital	Webster	94%	211
Memorial Hospital	Nacogdoches	94%	129
Memorial Medical Center of East Texas[2]	Lufkin	94%	226
North Texas Medical Center	Gainesville	94%	51
Oakbend Medical Center[2]	Richmond	94%	86
Angleton - Danbury Medical Center[2]	Angleton	93%	140
VA Amarillo Healthcare System	Amarillo	93%	56
TX Hlth Harris Meth Hosp-Stephenville[2]	Stephenville	92%	126
Tomball Regional Medical Center	Tomball	91%	246
Seton Medical Center Harker Heights	Harker Heights	90%	89
Hopkins County Memorial Hospital	Sulphur Springs	88%	83
University General Hospital	Houston	88%	64
Saint Luke's Sugar Land Hospital	Sugar Land	85%	34
Dallas Medical Center[2]	Dallas	84%	93
Lubbock Heart Hospital[2]	Lubbock	84%	281
Wise Regional Health System[2]	Decatur	83%	210
East Texas Medical Center Athens[2]	Athens	82%	175
Hill Regional Hospital	Hillsboro	80%	40
First Surgical Hospital	Bellaire	72%	127

Prophylactic Antibiotic Timing

Hospital Name	City	Rate	Cases
Baylor All Saints Medical Center at FW[2]	Fort Worth	100%	521
Baylor Heart & Vascular Hospital	Dallas	100%	88
Baylor Medical Center at Carrollton	Carrollton	100%	327
Baylor Medical Center at Irving[2]	Irving	100%	299
Baylor Medical Center at Mckinney[2]	Mc Kinney	100%	83
Baylor Medical Center at Trophy Club	Trophy Club	100%	52
Baylor Medical Center at Uptown	Dallas	100%	410
Baylor Medical Center at Waxahachie[2]	Waxahachie	100%	201
Baylor Reg Med Ctr at Grapevine[2]	Grapevine	100%	453
Baylor Regional Medical Center at Plano[2]	Plano	100%	300
Bayshore Medical Center[2]	Pasadena	100%	264
Christus Hospital[2]	Beaumont	100%	664
Clear Lake Regional Medical Center[2]	Webster	100%	429
Cleveland Regional Medical Center	Cleveland	100%	25
Conroe Regional Medical Center[2]	Conroe	100%	328
The Corpus Christi Medical Center[2]	Corpus Christi	100%	428
Dallas Regional Medical Center	Mesquite	100%	211
Doctors Hospital at Renaissance[2]	Edinburg	100%	660
El Paso Specialty Hospital	El Paso	100%	417
Foundation Surgical Hospital of El Paso[2]	El Paso	100%	149
Good Shepherd Medical Center Marshall	Marshall	100%	154
Harlingen Medical Center[2]	Harlingen	100%	401
Heart Hospital Baylor Plano	Plano	100%	1058
Hendrick Medical Center[2]	Abilene	100%	403
The Hospital at Westlake Medical Center	Austin	100%	281
Houston Physicians' Hospital	Webster	100%	214
Hunt Regional Medical Center	Greenville	100%	196
JPS Health Network[2]	Fort Worth	100%	559
Kingwood Medical Center[2]	Kingwood	100%	302
Knapp Medical Center	Weslaco	100%	297
Lake Pointe Medical Center	Rowlett	100%	118
Lakeway Regional Medical Center[3]	Lakeway	100%	25
Laredo Medical Center	Laredo	100%	397
Las Colinas Medical Center[2]	Irving	100%	139
Las Palmas Medical Center[2]	El Paso	100%	436
Medical Center of Arlington[2]	Arlington	100%	208
Medical Center of Mckinney[2]	Mckinney	100%	217
The Medical Center of Southeast Texas	Port Arthur	100%	353
Medical City Dallas Hospital[2]	Dallas	100%	517
Memorial Hermann Baptist Orange Hospital	Orange	100%	25
Memorial Hermann Katy Hospital[2]	Katy	100%	280
Memorial Hermann Northeast[2]	Humble	100%	129
Memorial Hermann Sugar Land Hospital[2]	Sugar Land	100%	235
Mem Hermann Surgical Hosp Kingwood	Kingwood	100%	117
Memorial Medical Center of East Texas[2]	Lufkin	100%	238
Methodist Ambulatory Surgery Hospital NW[2]	San Antonio	100%	161
Methodist Charlton Medical Center	Dallas	100%	432
Methodist Dallas Medical Center	Dallas	100%	544
Methodist Hospital For Surgery[2]	Addison	100%	696
The Methodist Hospital[2]	Houston	100%	592
Methodist Mansfield Medical Center	Mansfield	100%	219
Methodist Sugar Land Hospital[2]	Sugar Land	100%	470
Methodist Willowbrook Hospital[2]	Houston	100%	245
Nacogdoches Medical Center[2]	Nacogdoches	100%	108
Navarro Regional Hospital	Corsicana	100%	71
North Central Surgical Center	Dallas	100%	491
North Cypress Medical Center	Cypress	100%	425
North Hills Hospital[2]	N Richland Hls	100%	271
North Texas Medical Center	Gainesville	100%	51
Palestine Regional Medical Center	Palestine	100%	37
Pampa Regional Medical Center	Pampa	100%	138
Providence Memorial Hospital[2]	El Paso	100%	312
Round Rock Medical Center[2]	Round Rock	100%	249
Saint David's South Austin Medical Center[2]	Austin	100%	381
Saint Luke's Lakeside Hospital	The Woodlands	100%	349
Saint Luke's the Woodlands Hospital[2]	The Woodlands	100%	436
Saint Marks Medical Center	La Grange	100%	45
Scenic Mountain Medical Center	Big Spring	100%	44
Seton Medical Center Harker Heights	Harker Heights	100%	96
Seton Northwest Hospital	Austin	100%	188
Shannon Medical Center	San Angelo	100%	640
Sierra Medical Center[2]	El Paso	100%	402
Sierra Providence East Medical Center[2]	El Paso	100%	126
South Texas Regional Medical Center	Jourdanton	100%	29
Texas Health Arlington Memorial Hospital[2]	Arlington	100%	232
TX Hlth Harris Meth Hosp-Southlake	Southlake	100%	468
TX Hlth Heart & Vasc Hosp-Arlington	Arlington	100%	154
TX Hlth Presbyterian Hosp-Flower Mound	Flower Mound	100%	323
TX Hlth Presbyterian Hosp-Kaufman[2]	Kaufman	100%	69
TX Health Presbyterian Hosp Rockwall	Rockwall	100%	287
Texas Orthopedic Hospital[2]	Houston	100%	258
Texas Reg Med Ctr at Sunnyvale[2]	Sunnyvale	100%	167
Texas Spine & Joint Hospital[2]	Tyler	100%	213
Texoma Medical Center[2]	Denison	100%	380
United Regional Health Care System	Wichita Falls	100%	532
University Medical Center[2]	Lubbock	100%	400
University Medical Center of El Paso[2]	El Paso	100%	253
Val Verde Regional Medical Center	Del Rio	100%	79
Valley Regional Medical Center	Brownsville	100%	221
Weatherford Regional Medical Center	Weatherford	100%	254
West Houston Medical Center[2]	Houston	100%	289
The Womans Hospital of Texas[2]	Houston	100%	116
Woodland Heights Medical Center	Lufkin	100%	246
Abilene Regional Medical Center	Abilene	99%	500
Baptist Beaumont Hospital[2]	Beaumont	99%	386
Baptist Medical Center[2]	San Antonio	99%	2971
Baptist Saint Anthony's Hospital[2]	Amarillo	99%	492
Baylor Medical Center at Frisco	Frisco	99%	793
Baylor Medical Center at Garland[2]	Garland	99%	152
Baylor Ortho & Spine Hosp-Arlington	Arlington	99%	677
Baylor University Medical Center[2]	Dallas	99%	1855
Brazosport Regional Health System	Lake Jackson	99%	94
Brownwood Regional Medical Center	Brownwood	99%	170
Cedar Park Regional Medical Center	Cedar Park	99%	226
Centennial Medical Center	Frisco	99%	92
Central Texas Medical Center	San Marcos	99%	77
Christus Saint Catherine Hospital	Katy	99%	98
Christus Saint Michael Health System[2]	Texarkana	99%	794
Christus Santa Rosa Hospital	San Antonio	99%	702
Cornerstone Regional Hospital[2]	Edinburg	99%	355
Covenant Hospital Plainview	Plainview	99%	72
Detar Hospital Navarro	Victoria	99%	271
Doctors Hospital[2]	Dallas	99%	253
Doctors Hospital of Laredo[2]	Laredo	99%	116
East Texas Medical Center Athens[2]	Athens	99%	177
Good Shepherd Medical Center[2]	Longview	99%	402
Harris Health System[2]	Houston	99%	476
Hill Country Memorial Hospital[2]	Fredericksburg	99%	392
Hillcrest Baptist Medical Center[2]	Waco	99%	498
Houston Northwest Medical Center[2]	Houston	99%	388
Houston VA Medical Center	Houston	99%	515
Huguley Memorial Medical Center	Burleson	99%	320
Kell West Regional Hospital	Wichita Falls	99%	266
Lake Granbury Medical Center	Granbury	99%	194
Longview Regional Medical Center	Longview	99%	559
Medical Center of Lewisville[2]	Lewisville	99%	199
Medical Center of Plano[2]	Plano	99%	356
Memorial Hermann Hospital System[2]	Houston	99%	1412
Mem Hermann Mem City Med Ctr[2]	Houston	99%	481
Memorial Hermann Texas Medical Center[2]	Houston	99%	406
Memorial Hospital	Nacogdoches	99%	134
Methodist Hospital[2]	San Antonio	99%	708
Methodist Richardson Medical Center[2]	Richardson	99%	198
Methodist Stone Oak Hospital[2]	San Antonio	99%	380
Methodist West Houston Hospital[2]	Houston	99%	250
Metroplex Hospital[2]	Killeen	99%	167
Midland Memorial Hospital	Midland	99%	590
Mother Frances Hospital[2]	Tyler	99%	559
Nix Health Care System	San Antonio	99%	186
North Austin Medical Center[2]	Austin	99%	396

NOTE: Hospital profiles are in alphabetical order by state, then city, then hospital within the city; Rankings exclude hospitals with less than 25 cases except for patient surveys which excludes hospitals with less than 100 cases; (a) 100-299 cases; (1) The number of cases/patients is too few to report; (2) Data submitted were based on a sample of cases/patients; (3) Results are based on a shorter time period than required; (4) Data suppressed by CMS for one or more quarters; (5) Results are not available for this reporting period; (6) Fewer than 100 patients completed the HCAHPS survey; (7) No cases met the criteria for this measure; (8) The lower limit of the confidence interval cannot be calculated if the number of observed infections equals zero; (9) No data are available from the state/territory for this reporting period; (10) The scores shown reflect fewer than 50 completed surveys; (11) There were discrepancies in the data collection process; (12) This measure does not apply to this hospital for this reporting period; (13) Results cannot be calculated for this reporting period; (14) The results for this state are combined with nearby states to protect confidentiality; Please refer to the User's Guide for a full explanation of data.

Northwest Texas Hospital[2]	Amarillo	99%	316
Odessa Regional Hospital	Odessa	99%	211
Park Plaza Hospital[2]	Houston	99%	282
Peterson Regional Medical Center	Kerrville	99%	379
Plaza Medical Center of Fort Worth[2]	Fort Worth	99%	517
Providence Health Center[2]	Waco	99%	381
Quail Creek Surgical Hospital	Amarillo	99%	719
Rio Grande Regional Hospital[2]	Mcallen	99%	216
Saint David's Medical Center[2]	Austin	99%	588
Saint Joseph Regional Health Center[2]	Bryan	99%	347
Saint Luke's Episcopal Hospital[2]	Houston	99%	560
Saint Luke's Patients Medical Center[2]	Pasadena	99%	258
San Angelo Community Medical Center	San Angelo	99%	383
San Jacinto Methodist Hospital[2]	Baytown	99%	335
Scott & White Hospital - Round Rock[2]	Round Rock	99%	304
Scott & White Memorial Hospital[2]	Temple	99%	508
Seton Medical Center Austin[2]	Austin	99%	560
Seton Medical Center Hays	Kyle	99%	149
Seton Medical Center Williamson	Round Rock	99%	135
South Texas Spine & Surgical Hospital	San Antonio	99%	231
South Texas Surgical Hospital	Corpus Christi	99%	467
Southwest General Hospital	San Antonio	99%	80
Sugar Land Surgical Hospital	Sugar Land	99%	170
Texas Health Harris Methodist Fort Worth[2]	Fort Worth	99%	950
TX Hlth Harris Meth Hosp-Stephenville[2]	Stephenville	99%	131
Texas Health Presbyterian Hospital - WNJ	Sherman	99%	162
Texas Health Presbyterian Hospital Allen[2]	Allen	99%	116
Texas Health Presbyterian Hospital Dallas[2]	Dallas	99%	489
Texas Health Presbyterian Hospital Denton[2]	Denton	99%	216
Titus Regional Medical Center	Mount Pleasant	99%	78
Tomball Regional Medical Center	Tomball	99%	262
University Medical Center at Brackenridge[2]	Austin	99%	224
Univ of Texas Med Branch Galveston[2]	Galveston	99%	302
VHS Harlingen Hospital Company[2]	Harlingen	99%	888
Wadley Regional Medical Center	Texarkana	99%	337
Baylor Surgical Hospital at Fort Worth	Fort Worth	98%	423
Baylor Surgical Hospital at Las Colinas	Irving	98%	123
Christus Saint John Hospital	Nassau Bay	98%	383
Citizens Medical Center	Victoria	98%	368
College Station Medical Center	College Station	98%	440
Covenant Medical Center	Lubbock	98%	1788
Cypress Fairbanks Medical Center[2]	Houston	98%	122
Denton Regional Medical Center[2]	Denton	98%	352
East Texas Medical Center[2]	Tyler	98%	398
Fort Duncan Medical Center[2]	Eagle Pass	98%	57
Houston Orthopedic & Spine Hospital	Bellaire	98%	757
Medical Center Hospital[2]	Odessa	98%	426
Methodist Mckinney Hospital[2]	Mc Kinney	98%	268
Mission Regional Medical Center	Mission	98%	161
Palo Pinto General Hospital	Mineral Wells	98%	66
Paris Regional Medical Center[2]	Paris	98%	387
Parkland Health & Hospital System[2]	Dallas	98%	271
The Physicians Centre	Bryan	98%	85
Saint Luke's Hospital at the Vintage	Houston	98%	55
San Antonio VA Medical Center	San Antonio	98%	259
Scott & White Hospital Brenham	Brenham	98%	91
South Texas Health System[2]	Edinburg	98%	318
Temple VA Med Ctr-VA Central Texas	Temple	98%	195
TX Health Ctr for Diag & Surgery	Plano	98%	51
TX Hlth Harris Meth Hosp-Cleburne[2]	Cleburne	98%	174
TX Hlth Harris Meth Hosp SW Ft Worth[2]	Fort Worth	98%	292
Texas Health Harris Methodist[2]	Bedford	98%	256
Texas Health Presbyterian Hospital Plano[2]	Plano	98%	1506
Tops Surgical Specialty Hospital	Houston	98%	348
University Health System[2]	San Antonio	98%	468
USMD Hospital at Arlington[2]	Arlington	98%	51
USMD Hospital at Fort Worth	Fort Worth	98%	189
UT Southwestern University Hospital[2]	Dallas	98%	565
VHS Brownsville Hospital Company[2]	Brownsville	98%	53
Wise Regional Health System[2]	Decatur	98%	224
Angleton - Danbury Medical Center[2]	Angleton	97%	140
Arise Austin Medical Center[2]	Austin	97%	316
Christus Spohn Hospital Corpus Christi	Corpus Christi	97%	1121
Dallas Medical Center[2]	Dallas	97%	98
Dallas VA Medical Center - VA North Texas	Dallas	97%	194
East Texas Medical Center Jacksonville	Jacksonville	97%	65
Fdn Surgical Hosp of San Antonio[2]	San Antonio	97%	37
Guadalupe Regional Medical Center	Seguin	97%	269
Heritage Park Surgical Hospital	Sherman	97%	139
Saint Luke's Sugar Land Hospital	Sugar Land	97%	35
TX Inst for Surgery at Presby Hosp[3]	Dallas	97%	156
Christus Spohn Hospital Kleberg	Kingsville	96%	45
Grace Medical Center	Lubbock	96%	270
Huntsville Memorial Hospital	Huntsville	96%	167
Lubbock Heart Hospital[2]	Lubbock	96%	284
Oakbend Medical Center[2]	Richmond	96%	89
Saint Joseph Medical Center	Houston	96%	412
Seton Highland Lakes	Burnet	96%	77
Univ of TX Health Science Ctr-Tyler	Tyler	96%	51
VA Amarillo Healthcare System	Amarillo	96%	56
Hill Regional Hospital	Hillsboro	95%	41
Northwest Texas Surgery Center	Amarillo	95%	116
Doctors Hospital Tidwell	Houston	94%	35
Etmc Henderson	Henderson	93%	46
Hopkins County Memorial Hospital	Sulphur Springs	93%	84
Graham Regional Medical Center[2]	Graham	92%	40
Memorial Medical Center Livingston[2]	Livingston	91%	107
Pine Creek Medical Center[2]	Dallas	89%	64
Uvalde Memorial Hospital	Uvalde	89%	28
Golden Plains Community Hospital	Borger	87%	31
University General Hospital	Houston	84%	74
First Surgical Hospital	Bellaire	73%	129

Prophylactic Antibiotic Timing (Outpatient)

Hospital Name	City	Rate	Cases
Abilene Regional Medical Center	Abilene	100%	300
Baylor Heart & Vascular Hospital	Dallas	100%	734
Baylor Medical Center at Uptown	Dallas	100%	185
Baylor Ortho & Spine Hosp-Arlington	Arlington	100%	149
Baylor Reg Med Ctr at Grapevine	Grapevine	100%	474
Baylor Regional Medical Center at Plano	Plano	100%	259
Baylor Surgical Hospital at Las Colinas	Irving	100%	73
Cedar Park Regional Medical Center	Cedar Park	100%	161
Centennial Medical Center	Frisco	100%	60
Central Texas Medical Center	San Marcos	100%	154
Clear Lake Regional Medical Center	Webster	100%	572
College Station Medical Center	College Station	100%	269
Columbus Community Hospital	Columbus	100%	33
The Corpus Christi Medical Center	Corpus Christi	100%	536
Covenant Hospital Plainview	Plainview	100%	46
Detar Hospital Navarro	Victoria	100%	421
El Paso Specialty Hospital	El Paso	100%	45
Foundation Surgical Hospital of El Paso	El Paso	100%	99
Graham Regional Medical Center	Graham	100%	32
Harlingen Medical Center	Harlingen	100%	107
Hendrick Medical Center	Abilene	100%	376
Hill Country Memorial Hospital	Fredericksburg	100%	62
Houston Northwest Medical Center	Houston	100%	194
Houston Physicians' Hospital	Webster	100%	266
Lake Pointe Medical Center	Rowlett	100%	200
Laredo Medical Center	Laredo	100%	262
Las Colinas Medical Center	Irving	100%	158
Las Palmas Medical Center	El Paso	100%	828
Medical Center of Arlington	Arlington	100%	322
Medical Center of Mckinney	Mckinney	100%	109
Medical City Dallas Hospital	Dallas	100%	620
Memorial Hermann Katy Hospital	Katy	100%	255
Memorial Hermann Sugar Land Hospital	Sugar Land	100%	118
Mem Hermann Surgical Hosp Kingwood	Kingwood	100%	179
Methodist Ambulatory Surgery Hospital NW	San Antonio	100%	40
Methodist Dallas Medical Center	Dallas	100%	738
Methodist Hospital	San Antonio	100%	1068
Methodist Hospital For Surgery	Addison	100%	477
Methodist Stone Oak Hospital	San Antonio	100%	593
Methodist Willowbrook Hospital	Houston	100%	343
North Austin Medical Center	Austin	100%	594
North Central Surgical Center	Dallas	100%	364
Palestine Regional Medical Center	Palestine	100%	68
Palo Pinto General Hospital	Mineral Wells	100%	32
The Physicians Centre	Bryan	100%	35
Plaza Medical Center of Fort Worth	Fort Worth	100%	320
Providence Memorial Hospital	El Paso	100%	428
Quail Creek Surgical Hospital	Amarillo	100%	200
Round Rock Medical Center	Round Rock	100%	242
Saint David's South Austin Medical Center	Austin	100%	449
Saint Joseph Regional Health Center	Bryan	100%	347
Saint Luke's Hospital at the Vintage	Houston	100%	43
Saint Luke's Lakeside Hospital	The Woodlands	100%	321
Saint Luke's the Woodlands Hospital	The Woodlands	100%	310
San Angelo Community Medical Center	San Angelo	100%	151
Sierra Medical Center	El Paso	100%	487
South Texas Regional Medical Center	Jourdanton	100%	33
South Texas Spine & Surgical Hospital	San Antonio	100%	360
Southwest General Hospital	San Antonio	100%	149
TX Health Ctr for Diag & Surgery	Plano	100%	436
TX Hlth Harris Meth Hosp-Southlake	Southlake	100%	317
TX Hlth Heart & Vasc Hosp-Arlington	Arlington	100%	365
TX Health Presbyterian Hosp Rockwall	Rockwall	100%	413
Texas Orthopedic Hospital	Houston	100%	428
Texoma Medical Center	Denison	100%	400
Tops Surgical Specialty Hospital	Houston	100%	50
University Medical Center	Lubbock	100%	176
University Medical Center of El Paso	El Paso	100%	223
USMD Hospital at Fort Worth	Fort Worth	100%	300
Valley Regional Medical Center	Brownsville	100%	189
Weatherford Regional Medical Center	Weatherford	100%	51
The Womans Hospital of Texas	Houston	100%	1064
Woodland Heights Medical Center	Lufkin	100%	152
Baptist Beaumont Hospital	Beaumont	99%	279
Basin Healthcare Center	Odessa	99%	279
Baylor All Saints Medical Center at FW	Fort Worth	99%	524
Baylor Medical Center at Frisco	Frisco	99%	528
Baylor Medical Center at Garland	Garland	99%	170
Baylor Medical Center at Irving	Irving	99%	271
Baylor Medical Center at Mckinney	Mc Kinney	99%	165
Baylor Surgical Hospital at Fort Worth	Fort Worth	99%	241
Bayshore Medical Center	Pasadena	99%	139
Brownwood Regional Medical Center	Brownwood	99%	110
Christus Saint Michael Health System	Texarkana	99%	494
Citizens Medical Center	Victoria	99%	276
Conroe Regional Medical Center	Conroe	99%	265
Denton Regional Medical Center	Denton	99%	295
Doctors Hospital	Dallas	99%	195
Good Shepherd Medical Center	Longview	99%	467
Heart Hospital Baylor Denton[3]	Denton	99%	90
Heart Hospital Baylor Plano	Plano	99%	623
Houston Orthopedic & Spine Hospital	Bellaire	99%	357
Huntsville Memorial Hospital	Huntsville	99%	98
Kell West Regional Hospital	Wichita Falls	99%	290
Kingwood Medical Center	Kingwood	99%	259
Longview Regional Medical Center	Longview	99%	387
Lubbock Heart Hospital	Lubbock	99%	274
Medical Center Hospital	Odessa	99%	290
Medical Center of Plano	Plano	99%	277
Memorial Hermann Hospital System	Houston	99%	1336
Methodist Charlton Medical Center	Dallas	99%	137
The Methodist Hospital	Houston	99%	1266
Methodist Mansfield Medical Center	Mansfield	99%	194
Metroplex Hospital	Killeen	99%	130
Mother Frances Hospital	Tyler	99%	1223
Nacogdoches Medical Center	Nacogdoches	99%	192
North Cypress Medical Center	Cypress	99%	190
North Hills Hospital	N Richland Hls	99%	253
Northwest Hills Surgical Hospital	Austin	99%	203
Northwest Texas Hospital	Amarillo	99%	224
Odessa Regional Hospital	Odessa	99%	123
Peterson Regional Medical Center	Kerrville	99%	157
Saint David's Medical Center	Austin	99%	725
Saint Luke's Patients Medical Center	Pasadena	99%	218
San Jacinto Methodist Hospital	Baytown	99%	161
Seton Medical Center Williamson	Round Rock	99%	184
Shannon Medical Center	San Angelo	99%	460
Sierra Providence East Medical Center	El Paso	99%	80
Texas Health Harris Methodist Fort Worth	Fort Worth	99%	752
TX Hlth Harris Meth Hosp SW Ft Worth	Fort Worth	99%	356
Texas Health Harris Methodist	Bedford	99%	426
Texas Health Presbyterian Hospital - WNJ	Sherman	99%	146
TX Hlth Presbyterian Hosp-Flower Mound	Flower Mound	99%	323
Texas Spine & Joint Hospital	Tyler	99%	396
University Medical Center at Brackenridge	Austin	99%	270
Univ of Texas Med Branch Galveston	Galveston	99%	280
USMD Hospital at Arlington	Arlington	99%	591
UT SW Univ Hosp-Zale Lipshy	Dallas	99%	237
Wadley Regional Medical Center	Texarkana	99%	349
Baptist Saint Anthony's Hospital	Amarillo	98%	600
Baylor University Medical Center	Dallas	98%	573
Christus Hospital	Beaumont	98%	597
Dallas Regional Medical Center	Mesquite	98%	88
Doctors Hospital at Renaissance	Edinburg	98%	824
Grace Medical Center	Lubbock	98%	267
Harris Health System	Houston	98%	633
The Hospital at Westlake Medical Center	Austin	98%	168
Mem Hermann Mem City Med Ctr	Houston	98%	528
Memorial Hermann Texas Medical Center	Houston	98%	482
Memorial Medical Center of East Texas	Lufkin	98%	219
Methodist Mckinney Hospital	Mc Kinney	98%	113
Methodist Richardson Medical Center	Richardson	98%	232
Methodist Sugar Land Hospital	Sugar Land	98%	494
Methodist West Houston Hospital	Houston	98%	293
Midland Memorial Hospital	Midland	98%	257
Paris Regional Medical Center	Paris	98%	234
Park Plaza Hospital	Houston	98%	229
Rio Grande Regional Hospital	Mcallen	98%	96
Saint Luke's Episcopal Hospital	Houston	98%	718
Scott & White Memorial Hospital	Temple	98%	565
Seton Medical Center Austin	Austin	98%	582
Seton Medical Center Hays	Kyle	98%	56
Seton Northwest Hospital	Austin	98%	44
South Texas Health System	Edinburg	98%	287
United Regional Health Care System	Wichita Falls	98%	586
UT Southwestern University Hospital	Dallas	98%	248
Wise Regional Health System	Decatur	98%	168
Baptist Medical Center	San Antonio	97%	1543
Christus Saint John Hospital	Nassau Bay	97%	166
Christus Santa Rosa Hospital	San Antonio	97%	469
Cornerstone Regional Hospital[3]	Edinburg	97%	31
Covenant Medical Center	Lubbock	97%	754
Cypress Fairbanks Medical Center	Houston	97%	101
Heritage Park Surgical Hospital	Sherman	97%	164
Huguley Memorial Medical Center	Burleson	97%	259
Lake Granbury Medical Center	Granbury	97%	158
Texas Health Arlington Memorial Hospital	Arlington	97%	220
Texas Health Presbyterian Hospital Allen	Allen	97%	93

NOTE: Hospital profiles are in alphabetical order by state, then city, then hospital within the city; Rankings exclude hospitals with less than 25 cases except for patient surveys which excludes hospitals with less than 100 cases; (a) 100-299 cases; (1) The number of cases/patients is too few to report; (2) Data submitted were based on a sample of cases/patients; (3) Results are based on a shorter time period than required; (4) Data suppressed by CMS for one or more quarters; (5) Results are not available for this reporting period; (6) Fewer than 100 patients completed the HCAHPS survey; (7) No cases met the criteria for this measure; (8) The lower limit of the confidence interval cannot be calculated if the number of observed infections equals zero; (9) No data are available from the state/territory for this reporting period; (10) The scores shown reflect fewer than 50 completed surveys; (11) There were discrepancies in the data collection process; (12) This measure does not apply to this hospital for this reporting period; (13) Results cannot be calculated for this reporting period; (14) The results for this state are combined with nearby states to protect confidentiality; Please refer to the User's Guide for a full explanation of data.

Texas Health Presbyterian Hospital Dallas	Dallas	97%	659
Texas Health Presbyterian Hospital Denton	Denton	97%	310
Titus Regional Medical Center	Mount Pleasant	97%	97
West Houston Medical Center	Houston	97%	177
Baylor Medical Center at Carrollton	Carrollton	96%	67
Good Shepherd Medical Center Marshall	Marshall	96%	28
Hillcrest Baptist Medical Center	Waco	96%	146
JPS Health Network	Fort Worth	96%	368
Matagorda Regional Medical Center	Bay City	96%	119
Memorial Hermann Baptist Orange Hospital	Orange	96%	48
Memorial Hermann Northeast	Humble	96%	118
Nix Health Care System	San Antonio	96%	108
Northwest Texas Surgery Center	Amarillo	96%	48
Scott & White Hospital - Round Rock	Round Rock	96%	140
Seton Medical Center Harker Heights	Harker Heights	96%	122
Sugar Land Surgical Hospital	Sugar Land	96%	133
TX Inst for Surgery at Presby Hosp	Dallas	96%	258
University Health System	San Antonio	96%	390
Baylor Medical Center at Trophy Club	Trophy Club	95%	106
East Texas Medical Center	Tyler	95%	402
Medical Center of Lewisville	Lewisville	95%	43
TX Hlth Harris Meth Hosp-Cleburne	Cleburne	95%	37
Christus Spohn Hospital Corpus Christi	Corpus Christi	94%	546
Parkland Health & Hospital System	Dallas	94%	356
Providence Health Center	Waco	94%	264
Hopkins County Memorial Hospital	Sulphur Springs	93%	134
Memorial Hospital	Nacogdoches	93%	177
Saint Joseph Medical Center	Houston	93%	297
Texas Health Presbyterian Hospital Plano	Plano	93%	349
VHS Harlingen Hospital Company	Harlingen	93%	292
Guadalupe Regional Medical Center	Seguin	92%	93
Hunt Regional Medical Center	Greenville	92%	105
Navarro Regional Hospital	Corsicana	92%	39
Brazosport Regional Health System	Lake Jackson	91%	44
Doctors Hospital of Laredo	Laredo	91%	129
East Texas Medical Center Athens	Athens	91%	44
The Medical Center of Southeast Texas	Port Arthur	91%	157
Pine Creek Medical Center	Dallas	90%	252
Tomball Regional Medical Center	Tomball	90%	198
Texas Reg Med Ctr at Sunnyvale	Sunnyvale	88%	56
Val Verde Regional Medical Center	Del Rio	88%	32
Seton Highland Lakes[3]	Burnet	87%	46
Christus Spohn Hospital Alice	Alice	86%	58
Knapp Medical Center	Weslaco	85%	26
South Texas Surgical Hospital	Corpus Christi	85%	130
Mission Regional Medical Center	Mission	84%	31
University General Hospital Dallas	Dallas	83%	54
VHS Brownsville Hospital Company	Brownsville	83%	200
First Surgical Hospital	Bellaire	81%	136
Dallas Medical Center	Dallas	75%	48
University General Hospital	Houston	74%	143

Urinary Catheter Removal

Hospital Name	City	Rate	Cases
Abilene Regional Medical Center	Abilene	100%	356
Baylor Heart & Vascular Hospital	Dallas	100%	99
Baylor Medical Center at Carrollton	Carrollton	100%	235
Baylor Medical Center at Trophy Club	Trophy Club	100%	61
Baylor Medical Center at Uptown	Dallas	100%	261
Baylor Medical Center at Waxahachie[2]	Waxahachie	100%	227
Baylor Regional Medical Center at Plano[2]	Plano	100%	258
Baylor Surgical Hospital at Fort Worth	Fort Worth	100%	435
Baylor Surgical Hospital at Las Colinas	Irving	100%	115
College Station Medical Center	College Station	100%	322
Conroe Regional Medical Center[2]	Conroe	100%	293
The Corpus Christi Medical Center[2]	Corpus Christi	100%	426
Dallas Regional Medical Center	Mesquite	100%	196
Doctors Hospital Tidwell	Houston	100%	28
El Paso Specialty Hospital	El Paso	100%	27
First Surgical Hospital	Bellaire	100%	45
Heart Hospital Baylor Plano	Plano	100%	802
Hendrick Medical Center[2]	Abilene	100%	325
Hill Country Memorial Hospital[2]	Fredericksburg	100%	424
The Hospital at Westlake Medical Center	Austin	100%	89
Houston Orthopedic & Spine Hospital	Bellaire	100%	428
Knapp Medical Center	Weslaco	100%	229
Lake Granbury Medical Center	Granbury	100%	166
Laredo Medical Center	Laredo	100%	404
Las Colinas Medical Center[2]	Irving	100%	117
Medical Center of Lewisville[2]	Lewisville	100%	192
Medical Center of Mckinney[2]	Mckinney	100%	238
Medical Center of Plano[2]	Plano	100%	339
Memorial Hermann Katy Hospital[2]	Katy	100%	259
Memorial Hermann Sugar Land Hospital[2]	Sugar Land	100%	168
Methodist Ambulatory Surgery Hospital NW[2]	San Antonio	100%	59
Methodist Charlton Medical Center	Dallas	100%	391
Methodist Dallas Medical Center	Dallas	100%	720
Methodist Mansfield Medical Center	Mansfield	100%	182
Methodist Richardson Medical Center[2]	Richardson	100%	166
Methodist Stone Oak Hospital[2]	San Antonio	100%	334
Methodist Sugar Land Hospital[2]	Sugar Land	100%	339
Methodist Willowbrook Hospital[2]	Houston	100%	205
Metroplex Hospital[2]	Killeen	100%	116
North Austin Medical Center[2]	Austin	100%	330
North Central Surgical Center	Dallas	100%	458
North Cypress Medical Center	Cypress	100%	173
North Texas Medical Center	Gainesville	100%	37
Northwest Texas Surgery Center	Amarillo	100%	115
Palestine Regional Medical Center	Palestine	100%	144
The Physicians Centre	Bryan	100%	87
Quail Creek Surgical Hospital	Amarillo	100%	743
Rio Grande Regional Hospital[2]	Mcallen	100%	190
San Antonio VA Medical Center[2]	San Antonio	100%	219
San Jacinto Methodist Hospital[2]	Baytown	100%	316
Scott & White Hospital Brenham	Brenham	100%	78
Seton Highland Lakes	Burnet	100%	82
Texas Health Harris Methodist Fort Worth[2]	Fort Worth	100%	927
TX Hlth Harris Meth Hosp-Southlake	Southlake	100%	422
Texas Health Presbyterian Hospital Plano[2]	Plano	100%	1426
TX Inst for Surgery at Presby Hosp[3]	Dallas	100%	151
Texoma Medical Center[2]	Denison	100%	265
University Medical Center of El Paso[2]	El Paso	100%	153
Valley Regional Medical Center	Brownsville	100%	136
West Houston Medical Center[2]	Houston	100%	237
Woodland Heights Medical Center	Lufkin	100%	331
Baylor Medical Center at Frisco	Frisco	99%	695
Baylor Medical Center at Garland[2]	Garland	99%	204
Baylor Medical Center at Mckinney[2]	Mc Kinney	99%	83
Baylor Ortho & Spine Hosp-Arlington	Arlington	99%	348
Baylor University Medical Center[2]	Dallas	99%	1322
Bayshore Medical Center[2]	Pasadena	99%	138
Clear Lake Regional Medical Center[2]	Webster	99%	377
Cypress Fairbanks Medical Center[2]	Houston	99%	83
Denton Regional Medical Center[2]	Denton	99%	264
Detar Hospital Navarro	Victoria	99%	128
Doctors Hospital[2]	Dallas	99%	256
Doctors Hospital at Renaissance[2]	Edinburg	99%	467
East Texas Medical Center[2]	Tyler	99%	336
Good Shepherd Medical Center Marshall	Marshall	99%	130
Harlingen Medical Center[2]	Harlingen	99%	374
Huguley Memorial Medical Center	Burleson	99%	268
Kell West Regional Hospital	Wichita Falls	99%	162
Lake Pointe Medical Center	Rowlett	99%	139
Longview Regional Medical Center	Longview	99%	375
Medical Center Hospital[2]	Odessa	99%	433
Medical Center of Arlington[2]	Arlington	99%	176
The Medical Center of Southeast Texas	Port Arthur	99%	302
Medical City Dallas Hospital[2]	Dallas	99%	365
Memorial Hermann Hospital System[2]	Houston	99%	1136
Memorial Hermann Northeast[2]	Humble	99%	134
Methodist West Houston Hospital[2]	Houston	99%	239
North Hills Hospital[2]	N Richland Hls	99%	283
Pampa Regional Medical Center	Pampa	99%	102
Providence Memorial Hospital[2]	El Paso	99%	96
Round Rock Medical Center[2]	Round Rock	99%	293
Saint David's Medical Center[2]	Austin	99%	458
Saint David's South Austin Medical Center[2]	Austin	99%	246
Saint Luke's Lakeside Hospital	The Woodlands	99%	352
San Angelo Community Medical Center	San Angelo	99%	109
Seton Medical Center Williamson	Round Rock	99%	190
Seton Northwest Hospital	Austin	99%	130
South Texas Spine & Surgical Hospital	San Antonio	99%	124
Sugar Land Surgical Hospital	Sugar Land	99%	122
Texas Health Arlington Memorial Hospital[2]	Arlington	99%	213
TX Hlth Harris Meth Hosp-Cleburne[2]	Cleburne	99%	189
Texas Health Harris Methodist[2]	Bedford	99%	300
TX Hlth Heart & Vasc Hosp-Arlington	Arlington	99%	113
Texas Health Presbyterian Hospital Allen[2]	Allen	99%	105
Texas Health Presbyterian Hospital Dallas[2]	Dallas	99%	496
Texas Health Presbyterian Hospital Denton[2]	Denton	99%	202
Texas Orthopedic Hospital[2]	Houston	99%	138
Texas Spine & Joint Hospital[2]	Tyler	99%	170
United Regional Health Care System	Wichita Falls	99%	578
University Medical Center[2]	Lubbock	99%	336
Univ of Texas Med Branch Galveston[2]	Galveston	99%	271
USMD Hospital at Fort Worth	Fort Worth	99%	180
UT Southwestern University Hospital[2]	Dallas	99%	526
Weatherford Regional Medical Center	Weatherford	99%	301
Baptist Medical Center[2]	San Antonio	98%	1685
Baylor Medical Center at Irving[2]	Irving	98%	346
Baylor Reg Med Ctr at Grapevine[2]	Grapevine	98%	424
Centennial Medical Center	Frisco	98%	98
Central Texas Medical Center	San Marcos	98%	101
Christus Saint Michael Health System[2]	Texarkana	98%	710
Christus Santa Rosa Hospital	San Antonio	98%	639
Covenant Hospital Plainview	Plainview	98%	98
Dallas VA Medical Center - VA North Texas[2]	Dallas	98%	214
Fort Duncan Medical Center[2]	Eagle Pass	98%	44
Hill Regional Hospital	Hillsboro	98%	43
Hillcrest Baptist Medical Center[2]	Waco	98%	356
Houston Physicians' Hospital	Webster	98%	176
Houston VA Medical Center[2]	Houston	98%	439
Kingwood Medical Center[2]	Kingwood	98%	226
Las Palmas Medical Center[2]	El Paso	98%	184
Methodist Hospital[2]	San Antonio	98%	399
The Methodist Hospital[2]	Houston	98%	515
Methodist Mckinney Hospital[2]	Mc Kinney	98%	266
Midland Memorial Hospital	Midland	98%	561
Nacogdoches Medical Center[2]	Nacogdoches	98%	94
Park Plaza Hospital[2]	Houston	98%	261
Plaza Medical Center of Fort Worth[2]	Fort Worth	98%	573
Saint Joseph Regional Health Center[2]	Bryan	98%	300
Saint Luke's Episcopal Hospital[2]	Houston	98%	482
Saint Luke's Patients Medical Center[2]	Pasadena	98%	173
Saint Luke's the Woodlands Hospital[2]	The Woodlands	98%	397
Shannon Medical Center	San Angelo	98%	531
Sierra Providence East Medical Center[2]	El Paso	98%	59
South Texas Regional Medical Center	Jourdanton	98%	40
TX Hlth Harris Meth Hosp-Stephenville[2]	Stephenville	98%	107
TX Hlth Presbyterian Hosp-Flower Mound	Flower Mound	98%	300
TX Hlth Presbyterian Hosp-Kaufman[2]	Kaufman	98%	55
TX Health Presbyterian Hosp Rockwall	Rockwall	98%	289
Tops Surgical Specialty Hospital	Houston	98%	202
Univ of TX Health Science Ctr-Tyler	Tyler	98%	63
USMD Hospital at Arlington[2]	Arlington	98%	55
VHS Brownsville Hospital Company[2]	Brownsville	98%	100
Arise Austin Medical Center[2]	Austin	97%	37
Baptist Saint Anthony's Hospital[2]	Amarillo	97%	507
Brownwood Regional Medical Center	Brownwood	97%	89
Christus Hospital[2]	Beaumont	97%	493
Columbus Community Hospital	Columbus	97%	31
Good Shepherd Medical Center[2]	Longview	97%	335
JPS Health Network[2]	Fort Worth	97%	468
Mem Hermann Mem City Med Ctr[2]	Houston	97%	275
Memorial Hermann Texas Medical Center[2]	Houston	97%	347
Northwest Texas Hospital[2]	Amarillo	97%	259
Palo Pinto General Hospital	Mineral Wells	97%	36
Scott & White Hospital - Round Rock[2]	Round Rock	97%	267
Scott & White Memorial Hospital[2]	Temple	97%	263
Sierra Medical Center[2]	El Paso	97%	150
South Texas Health System[2]	Edinburg	97%	270
Southwest General Hospital	San Antonio	97%	151
TX Hlth Harris Meth Hosp SW Ft Worth[2]	Fort Worth	97%	257
University Medical Center at Brackenridge[2]	Austin	97%	114
Uvalde Memorial Hospital	Uvalde	97%	29
Baylor All Saints Medical Center at FW[2]	Fort Worth	96%	256
Christus Saint Catherine Hospital	Katy	96%	81
Covenant Medical Center	Lubbock	96%	1520
Harris Health System[2]	Houston	96%	286
Houston Northwest Medical Center[2]	Houston	96%	257
Hunt Regional Medical Center	Greenville	96%	189
Memorial Medical Center Livingston[2]	Livingston	96%	93
Mission Regional Medical Center	Mission	96%	70
Nix Health Care System	San Antonio	96%	180
Odessa Regional Hospital	Odessa	96%	133
Paris Regional Medical Center[2]	Paris	96%	313
Parkland Health & Hospital System[2]	Dallas	96%	244
Peterson Regional Medical Center	Kerrville	96%	392
Temple VA Med Ctr-VA Central Texas[2]	Temple	96%	180
Titus Regional Medical Center	Mount Pleasant	96%	113
UT SW Univ Hosp-Zale Lipshy[2]	Dallas	96%	26
VA Amarillo Healthcare System[2]	Amarillo	96%	67
Foundation Surgical Hospital of El Paso[2]	El Paso	95%	59
Guadalupe Regional Medical Center	Seguin	95%	58
Methodist Hospital For Surgery[2]	Addison	95%	624
Seton Medical Center Austin[2]	Austin	95%	262
Seton Medical Center Hays	Kyle	95%	148
Val Verde Regional Medical Center	Del Rio	95%	62
Wadley Regional Medical Center	Texarkana	95%	364
Baptist Beaumont Hospital[2]	Beaumont	94%	232
Cedar Park Regional Medical Center	Cedar Park	94%	102
Doctors Hospital of Laredo[2]	Laredo	94%	85
Huntsville Memorial Hospital	Huntsville	94%	175
Lubbock Heart Hospital[2]	Lubbock	94%	221
Saint Joseph Medical Center	Houston	94%	248
Saint Luke's Hospital at the Vintage	Houston	94%	64
Seton Medical Center Harker Heights	Harker Heights	94%	63
South Texas Surgical Hospital	Corpus Christi	94%	138
Texas Reg Med Ctr at Sunnyvale[2]	Sunnyvale	94%	126
VHS Harlingen Hospital Company[2]	Harlingen	94%	869
Dallas Medical Center[2]	Dallas	93%	101
Navarro Regional Hospital	Corsicana	93%	101
Pine Creek Medical Center[2]	Dallas	93%	202
Texas Health Presbyterian Hospital - WNJ	Sherman	93%	149
Wise Regional Health System[2]	Decatur	93%	202
Memorial Medical Center of East Texas[2]	Lufkin	92%	243
Mother Frances Hospital[2]	Tyler	92%	466
Christus Saint John Hospital	Nassau Bay	91%	317
East Texas Medical Center Jacksonville	Jacksonville	91%	58
Hopkins County Memorial Hospital	Sulphur Springs	91%	44
Lakeway Regional Medical Center[3]	Lakeway	91%	32
Providence Health Center[2]	Waco	91%	221
Christus Spohn Hospital Corpus Christi	Corpus Christi	90%	740

NOTE: Hospital profiles are in alphabetical order by state, then city, then hospital within the city; Rankings exclude hospitals with less than 25 cases except for patient surveys which excludes hospitals with less than 100 cases; (a) 100-299 cases; (1) The number of cases/patients is too few to report; (2) Data submitted were based on a sample of cases/patients; (3) Results are based on a shorter time period than required; (4) Data suppressed by CMS for one or more quarters; (5) Results are not available for this reporting period; (6) Fewer than 100 patients completed the HCAHPS survey; (7) No cases met the criteria for this measure; (8) The lower limit of the confidence interval cannot be calculated if the number of observed infections equals zero; (9) No data are available from the state/territory for this reporting period; (10) The scores shown reflect fewer than 50 completed surveys; (11) There were discrepancies in the data collection process; (12) This measure does not apply to this hospital for this reporting period; (13) Results cannot be calculated for this reporting period; (14) The results for this state are combined with nearby states to protect confidentiality; Please refer to the User's Guide for a full explanation of data.

Memorial Hospital	Nacogdoches	89%	122
Citizens Medical Center	Victoria	88%	167
Etmc Henderson	Henderson	88%	41
TX Hlth Harris Methodist Hosp-Azle[2]	Azle	88%	25
Saint Luke's Sugar Land Hospital	Sugar Land	87%	60
Brazosport Regional Health System	Lake Jackson	85%	47
University Health System[2]	San Antonio	85%	261
Ennis Regional Medical Center	Ennis	82%	28
Graham Regional Medical Center[2]	Graham	81%	52
Scenic Mountain Medical Center	Big Spring	81%	32
Tomball Regional Medical Center	Tomball	81%	262
Fdn Surgical Hosp of San Antonio[2]	San Antonio	80%	41
University General Hospital	Houston	77%	113
East Texas Medical Center Athens[2]	Athens	73%	102
Oakbend Medical Center[2]	Richmond	71%	38
Christus Spohn Hospital Kleberg	Kingsville	68%	40

Survey of Patients' Hospital Experiences

Area Around Room 'Always' Quiet at Night

Hospital Name	City	Rate	Cases
The Physicians Centre	Bryan	93%	(a)
Baptist Emergency Hospital	San Antonio	92%	(a)
Northwest Hills Surgical Hospital	Austin	91%	(a)
Sugar Land Surgical Hospital	Sugar Land	89%	(a)
TX Hlth Harris Meth Hosp-Southlake	Southlake	89%	300+
USMD Hospital at Fort Worth	Fort Worth	88%	(a)
Baylor Medical Center at Uptown	Dallas	87%	300+
Saint Luke's Lakeside Hospital	The Woodlands	87%	300+
Houston Orthopedic & Spine Hospital	Bellaire	86%	300+
South Texas Spine & Surgical Hospital	San Antonio	86%	300+
Tops Surgical Specialty Hospital	Houston	86%	(a)
First Surgical Hospital	Bellaire	85%	(a)
Fdn Surgical Hosp of San Antonio	San Antonio	85%	300+
Methodist Mckinney Hospital	Mc Kinney	85%	(a)
Arise Austin Medical Center[3]	Austin	84%	(a)
Heritage Park Surgical Hospital	Sherman	84%	(a)
Quail Creek Surgical Hospital	Amarillo	84%	300+
TX Health Ctr for Diag & Surgery	Plano	84%	(a)
USMD Hospital at Arlington	Arlington	84%	300+
Basin Healthcare Center	Odessa	82%	(a)
Baylor Medical Center at Trophy Club	Trophy Club	82%	(a)
Baylor Ortho & Spine Hosp-Arlington	Arlington	82%	300+
Baylor Surgical Hospital at Las Colinas	Irving	82%	(a)
Houston Physicians' Hospital	Webster	82%	(a)
Methodist Hospital For Surgery	Addison	82%	300+
North Central Surgical Center	Dallas	82%	300+
Methodist Ambulatory Surgery Hospital NW	San Antonio	81%	(a)
South Texas Surgical Hospital	Corpus Christi	81%	300+
Heart Hospital Baylor Plano	Plano	80%	300+
Baylor Medical Center at Frisco	Frisco	79%	300+
Good Shephard Medical Center - Linden	Linden	79%	(a)
East Texas Medical Center Pittsburg	Pittsburg	78%	(a)
Pine Creek Medical Center	Dallas	77%	300+
Baylor Heart & Vascular Hospital	Dallas	76%	300+
East Texas Medical Center - Gilmer	Gilmer	76%	(a)
Electra Memorial Hospital	Electra	76%	(a)
Graham Regional Medical Center	Graham	76%	(a)
Hill Country Memorial Hospital	Fredericksburg	76%	300+
Memorial Hermann Baptist Orange Hospital	Orange	76%	300+
Cornerstone Regional Hospital	Edinburg	75%	(a)
Etmc Carthage	Carthage	75%	(a)
Guadalupe Regional Medical Center	Seguin	75%	300+
Kell West Regional Hospital	Wichita Falls	75%	(a)
Parkview Regional Hospital	Mexia	75%	(a)
TX Hlth Presbyterian Hosp-Kaufman	Kaufman	75%	300+
Tyler County Hospital	Woodville	75%	(a)
Yoakum Community Hospital	Yoakum	75%	(a)
Baylor Regional Medical Center at Plano	Plano	74%	300+
The Hospital at Westlake Medical Center	Austin	74%	300+
The Medical Center of Southeast Texas	Port Arthur	74%	300+
Seton Medical Center Harker Heights	Harker Heights	74%	300+
Eastland Memorial Hospital	Eastland	73%	(a)
Falls Community Hospital & Clinic	Marlin	73%	(a)
Glen Rose Medical Center	Glen Rose	73%	(a)
North Cypress Medical Center	Cypress	73%	300+
Texas Spine & Joint Hospital	Tyler	73%	300+
University General Hospital Dallas	Dallas	73%	(a)
UT SW Univ Hosp-Zale Lipshy	Dallas	73%	300+
W J Mangold Memorial Hospital	Lockney	73%	(a)
Childress Regional Medical Center	Childress	72%	(a)
Christus Saint Catherine Hospital	Katy	72%	300+
Christus Spohn Hospital Alice	Alice	72%	300+
Citizens Medical Center	Victoria	72%	300+
Cuero Community Hospital	Cuero	72%	(a)
Etmc Henderson	Henderson	72%	300+
TX Inst for Surgery at Presby Hosp	Dallas	72%	(a)
Titus Regional Medical Center	Mount Pleasant	72%	300+
Baylor Medical Center at Waxahachie	Waxahachie	71%	300+
Big Bend Regional Medical Center	Alpine	71%	(a)
Brownfield Regional Medical Center	Brownfield	71%	(a)
Care Regional Medical Center	Aransas Pass	71%	(a)
El Paso Specialty Hospital	El Paso	71%	(a)
Hill Regional Hospital	Hillsboro	71%	300+
Medical City Dallas Hospital	Dallas	71%	300+
Park Plaza Hospital	Houston	71%	300+
Permian Regional Medical Center	Andrews	71%	(a)
Saint Anthony's Hospital	Houston	71%	(a)
Seton Edgar B Davis Hospital	Luling	71%	(a)
TX Hlth Presbyterian Hosp-Flower Mound	Flower Mound	71%	300+
Weatherford Regional Medical Center	Weatherford	71%	300+
Foundation Surgical Hospital of El Paso	El Paso	70%	300+
Good Shepherd Medical Center	Longview	70%	300+
Grace Medical Center	Lubbock	70%	300+
Hendrick Medical Center	Abilene	70%	300+
Medina Regional Hospital	Hondo	70%	(a)
Methodist West Houston Hospital	Houston	70%	300+
Pecos County Memorial Hospital	Fort Stockton	70%	(a)
Rollins Brook Community Hospital[11]	Lampasas	70%	(a)
Saint Luke's Sugar Land Hospital	Sugar Land	70%	300+
Seton Southwest Hospital	Austin	70%	(a)
Texas Health Presbyterian Hospital Plano	Plano	70%	300+
University General Hospital	Houston	70%	300+
Woodland Heights Medical Center	Lufkin	70%	300+
Baptist Beaumont Hospital	Beaumont	69%	300+
Covenant Hospital Plainview	Plainview	69%	300+
Medical Center of Mckinney	Mckinney	69%	300+
Memorial Hermann Sugar Land Hospital	Sugar Land	69%	300+
Memorial Medical Center Livingston	Livingston	69%	300+
Memorial Medical Center of East Texas	Lufkin	69%	300+
Methodist Charlton Medical Center	Dallas	69%	300+
Methodist Willowbrook Hospital	Houston	69%	300+
Saint Joseph Regional Health Center	Bryan	69%	300+
Centennial Medical Center	Frisco	68%	300+
Detar Hospital Navarro	Victoria	68%	300+
Lubbock Heart Hospital	Lubbock	68%	300+
Matagorda Regional Medical Center	Bay City	68%	(a)
Methodist Stone Oak Hospital	San Antonio	68%	300+
Metroplex Hospital[11]	Killeen	68%	300+
Nacogdoches Medical Center	Nacogdoches	68%	300+
Saint David's Medical Center	Austin	68%	300+
Shannon Medical Center	San Angelo	68%	300+
TX Hlth Harris Meth Hosp-Stephenville	Stephenville	68%	300+
TX Hlth Harris Meth Hosp SW Ft Worth	Fort Worth	68%	300+
United Regional Health Care System	Wichita Falls	68%	300+
Baylor Medical Center at Garland	Garland	67%	300+
Christus Hospital	Beaumont	67%	300+
College Station Medical Center	College Station	67%	300+
Coryell Memorial Healthcare System	Gatesville	67%	(a)
Doctors Hospital of Laredo	Laredo	67%	300+
Harlingen Medical Center[11]	Harlingen	67%	300+
Hereford Regional Medical Center	Hereford	67%	(a)
Memorial Medical Center	Port Lavaca	67%	(a)
Methodist Mansfield Medical Center	Mansfield	67%	300+
Plaza Medical Center of Fort Worth	Fort Worth	67%	300+
Providence Health Center	Waco	67%	300+
Saint Luke's Hospital at the Vintage	Houston	67%	300+
San Jacinto Methodist Hospital	Baytown	67%	300+
University Medical Center	Lubbock	67%	300+
Abilene Regional Medical Center	Abilene	66%	300+
Christus Saint Michael Health System	Texarkana	66%	300+
Columbus Community Hospital	Columbus	66%	(a)
Covenant Hospital Levelland	Levelland	66%	(a)
Doctors Hospital	Dallas	66%	300+
Doctors Hospital at Renaissance	Edinburg	66%	300+
East Texas Medical Center Crockett	Crockett	66%	(a)
East Texas Medical Center Quitman	Quitman	66%	(a)
Hillcrest Baptist Medical Center	Waco	66%	300+
Hopkins County Memorial Hospital	Sulphur Springs	66%	300+
Hunt Regional Medical Center	Greenville	66%	300+
Huntsville Memorial Hospital	Huntsville	66%	(a)
Longview Regional Medical Center	Longview	66%	300+
Medical Center Hospital	Odessa	66%	300+
Memorial Hermann Katy Hospital	Katy	66%	300+
Methodist Sugar Land Hospital	Sugar Land	66%	300+
Scott & White Hospital - Round Rock	Round Rock	66%	300+
Seton Medical Center Williamson	Round Rock	66%	300+
TX Hlth Harris Meth Hosp-Cleburne	Cleburne	66%	300+
Texas Health Presbyterian Hospital Allen	Allen	66%	300+
Texas Orthopedic Hospital	Houston	66%	300+
Texoma Medical Center	Denison	66%	300+
UT Southwestern University Hospital	Dallas	66%	300+
Angleton - Danbury Medical Center	Angleton	65%	300+
Baylor University Medical Center	Dallas	65%	300+
Central Texas Medical Center[11]	San Marcos	65%	300+
Christus Spohn Hospital Beeville	Beeville	65%	(a)
Methodist Richardson Medical Center	Richardson	65%	300+
Northwest Texas Hospital	Amarillo	65%	300+
Saint Luke's Episcopal Hospital	Houston	65%	300+
San Angelo Community Medical Center	San Angelo	65%	300+
Scott & White Hospital - Llano	Llano	65%	(a)
Seton Medical Center Hays	Kyle	65%	300+
South Texas Health System	Edinburg	65%	300+
TX Hlth Heart & Vasc Hosp-Arlington	Arlington	65%	300+
TX Health Presbyterian Hosp Rockwall	Rockwall	65%	300+
Tomball Regional Medical Center	Tomball	65%	300+
The Womans Hospital of Texas	Houston	65%	300+
Baylor Medical Center at Mckinney	Mc Kinney	64%	300+
Christus Spohn Hospital Kleberg	Kingsville	64%	300+
Clear Lake Regional Medical Center	Webster	64%	300+
Covenant Medical Center	Lubbock	64%	300+
East Texas Medical Center Jacksonville	Jacksonville	64%	300+
Good Shepherd Medical Center Marshall	Marshall	64%	300+
Las Colinas Medical Center	Irving	64%	300+
Memorial Hermann Northeast	Humble	64%	300+
North Hills Hospital	N Richland Hls	64%	300+
Saint David's South Austin Medical Center	Austin	64%	300+
Scenic Mountain Medical Center	Big Spring	64%	300+
Scott & White Hospital Brenham	Brenham	64%	300+
South Texas Regional Medical Center	Jourdanton	64%	(a)
TX Hlth Harris Methodist Hosp-Azle	Azle	64%	300+
Texas Health Presbyterian Hospital - WNJ	Sherman	64%	300+
University Medical Center of El Paso	El Paso	64%	300+
Wadley Regional Medical Center	Texarkana	64%	300+
Wise Regional Health System	Decatur	64%	300+
Baylor All Saints Medical Center at FW	Fort Worth	63%	300+
Baylor Reg Med Ctr at Grapevine	Grapevine	63%	300+
Etmc Clarksville	Clarksville	63%	(a)
Hamilton General Hospital	Hamilton	63%	(a)
Huguley Memorial Medical Center[11]	Burleson	63%	300+
Lake Granbury Medical Center	Granbury	63%	300+
Lake Pointe Medical Center	Rowlett	63%	300+
Medical Center of Lewisville	Lewisville	63%	300+
Mem Hermann Mem City Med Ctr	Houston	63%	300+
Methodist Dallas Medical Center	Dallas	63%	300+
The Methodist Hospital	Houston	63%	300+
Moore County Hospital District	Dumas	63%	(a)
Mother Frances Hospital	Tyler	63%	300+
Odessa Regional Hospital	Odessa	63%	300+
Palestine Regional Medical Center	Palestine	63%	300+
Pampa Regional Medical Center	Pampa	63%	300+
Rio Grande Regional Hospital	Mcallen	63%	300+
Saint Joseph Medical Center	Houston	63%	300+
Saint Marks Medical Center	La Grange	63%	(a)
Seton Highland Lakes	Burnet	63%	300+
Southwest General Hospital	San Antonio	63%	300+
Texas Health Arlington Memorial Hospital	Arlington	63%	300+
Baptist Saint Anthony's Hospital	Amarillo	62%	300+
Baylor Surgical Hospital at Fort Worth	Fort Worth	62%	300+
Christus Santa Rosa Hospital	San Antonio	62%	300+
The Corpus Christi Medical Center	Corpus Christi	62%	300+
Ennis Regional Medical Center	Ennis	62%	300+
Las Palmas Medical Center	El Paso	62%	300+
Memorial Hermann Hospital System	Houston	62%	300+
Memorial Hospital	Nacogdoches	62%	300+
North Austin Medical Center	Austin	62%	300+
Rolling Plains Memorial Hospital	Sweetwater	62%	(a)
Round Rock Medical Center	Round Rock	62%	300+
Scott & White Memorial Hospital[11]	Temple	62%	300+
Sierra Providence East Medical Center	El Paso	62%	300+
Starr County Memorial Hospital	Rio Grande City	62%	(a)
Texas Health Presbyterian Hospital Dallas	Dallas	62%	300+
Uvalde Memorial Hospital[11]	Uvalde	62%	(a)
Baptist Medical Center[11]	San Antonio	61%	300+
Brownwood Regional Medical Center	Brownwood	61%	300+
Christus Jasper Memorial Hospital	Jasper	61%	(a)
Conroe Regional Medical Center	Conroe	61%	300+
Dallas Regional Medical Center	Mesquite	61%	300+
East Texas Medical Center Athens	Athens	61%	300+
Medical Center of Arlington	Arlington	61%	300+
Medical Center of Plano	Plano	61%	300+
Methodist Hospital	San Antonio	61%	300+
Navarro Regional Hospital	Corsicana	61%	300+
Nix Health Care System	San Antonio	61%	300+
Oakbend Medical Center	Richmond	61%	300+
Palo Pinto General Hospital	Mineral Wells	61%	300+
Saint Luke's the Woodlands Hospital	The Woodlands	61%	300+
Univ of TX Health Science Ctr-Tyler	Tyler	61%	(a)
Val Verde Regional Medical Center	Del Rio	61%	300+
Baylor Medical Center at Carrollton	Carrollton	60%	300+
Christus Spohn Hospital Corpus Christi	Corpus Christi	60%	300+
Dallas Medical Center	Dallas	60%	300+
Fort Duncan Medical Center	Eagle Pass	60%	300+
Houston Northwest Medical Center	Houston	60%	300+
Lake Whitney Medical Center[11]	Whitney	60%	(a)
Laredo Medical Center	Laredo	60%	300+
Memorial Hermann Texas Medical Center	Houston	60%	300+
Midland Memorial Hospital	Midland	60%	300+
Seton Northwest Hospital	Austin	60%	300+
Texas Health Harris Methodist	Bedford	60%	300+
Texas Health Presbyterian Hospital Denton	Denton	60%	300+
Texas Reg Med Ctr at Sunnyvale	Sunnyvale	60%	300+

NOTE: Hospital profiles are in alphabetical order by state, then city, then hospital within the city; Rankings exclude hospitals with less than 25 cases except for patient surveys which excludes hospitals with less than 100 cases; (a) 100-299 cases; (1) The number of cases/patients is too few to report; (2) Data submitted were based on a sample of cases/patients; (3) Results are based on a shorter time period than required; (4) Data suppressed by CMS for one or more quarters; (5) Results are not available for this reporting period; (6) Fewer than 100 patients completed the HCAHPS survey; (7) No cases met the criteria for this measure; (8) The lower limit of the confidence interval cannot be calculated if the number of observed infections equals zero; (9) No data are available from the state/territory for this reporting period; (10) The scores shown reflect fewer than 50 completed surveys; (11) There were discrepancies in the data collection process; (12) This measure does not apply to this hospital for this reporting period; (13) Results cannot be calculated for this reporting period; (14) The results for this state are combined with nearby states to protect confidentiality; Please refer to the User's Guide for a full explanation of data.

University Medical Center at Brackenridge	Austin	60%	300+
Univ of Texas Med Branch Galveston	Galveston	60%	300+
VHS Brownsville Hospital Company[11]	Brownsville	60%	300+
West Houston Medical Center	Houston	60%	300+
Brazosport Regional Health System	Lake Jackson	59%	300+
Cedar Park Regional Medical Center	Cedar Park	59%	300+
Kingwood Medical Center	Kingwood	59%	300+
Knapp Medical Center	Weslaco	59%	300+
Mission Regional Medical Center	Mission	59%	300+
North Texas Medical Center	Gainesville	59%	(a)
Providence Memorial Hospital	El Paso	59%	300+
Texas Health Harris Methodist Fort Worth	Fort Worth	59%	300+
VHS Harlingen Hospital Company[11]	Harlingen	59%	300+
Bayshore Medical Center	Pasadena	58%	300+
Christus Saint John Hospital	Nassau Bay	58%	300+
Connally Memorial Medical Center	Floresville	58%	(a)
Denton Regional Medical Center	Denton	58%	300+
East Texas Medical Center	Tyler	58%	300+
JPS Health Network	Fort Worth	58%	300+
Saint Luke's Patients Medical Center	Pasadena	58%	300+
Baylor Medical Center at Irving	Irving	57%	300+
Cypress Fairbanks Medical Center	Houston	56%	300+
Doctors Hospital Tidwell	Houston	56%	300+
Paris Regional Medical Center	Paris	56%	300+
Seton Medical Center Austin	Austin	56%	300+
Valley Regional Medical Center	Brownsville	55%	300+
Peterson Regional Medical Center	Kerrville	54%	300+
Sierra Medical Center	El Paso	53%	300+
Harris Health System	Houston	52%	300+
Parkland Health & Hospital System	Dallas	52%	300+
University Health System	San Antonio	52%	300+

Doctors 'Always' Communicated Well

Hospital Name	City	Rate	Cases
W J Mangold Memorial Hospital	Lockney	99%	(a)
East Texas Medical Center - Gilmer	Gilmer	97%	(a)
Falls Community Hospital & Clinic	Marlin	96%	(a)
Tyler County Hospital	Woodville	96%	(a)
Baptist Emergency Hospital	San Antonio	93%	(a)
Electra Memorial Hospital	Electra	93%	(a)
Glen Rose Medical Center	Glen Rose	93%	(a)
Eastland Memorial Hospital	Eastland	92%	(a)
Hamilton General Hospital	Hamilton	92%	(a)
Pecos County Memorial Hospital	Fort Stockton	92%	(a)
Rollins Brook Community Hospital[11]	Lampasas	92%	(a)
Yoakum Community Hospital	Yoakum	92%	(a)
East Texas Medical Center Pittsburg	Pittsburg	91%	(a)
East Texas Medical Center Quitman	Quitman	91%	(a)
Graham Regional Medical Center	Graham	91%	(a)
Quail Creek Surgical Hospital	Amarillo	91%	300+
Baylor Medical Center at Uptown	Dallas	90%	300+
Childress Regional Medical Center	Childress	90%	(a)
Hill Regional Hospital	Hillsboro	90%	300+
Nacogdoches Medical Center	Nacogdoches	90%	300+
Park Plaza Hospital	Houston	90%	300+
South Texas Spine & Surgical Hospital	San Antonio	90%	300+
TX Inst for Surgery at Presby Hosp	Dallas	90%	(a)
Tops Surgical Specialty Hospital	Houston	90%	(a)
Baylor Ortho & Spine Hosp-Arlington	Arlington	89%	300+
Covenant Hospital Levelland	Levelland	89%	(a)
Hill Country Memorial Hospital	Fredericksburg	89%	300+
Medina Regional Hospital	Hondo	89%	(a)
Memorial Hermann Baptist Orange Hospital	Orange	89%	300+
North Central Surgical Center	Dallas	89%	300+
The Physicians Centre	Bryan	89%	(a)
Seton Edgar B Davis Hospital	Luling	89%	(a)
TX Hlth Harris Meth Hosp-Southlake	Southlake	89%	300+
TX Hlth Harris Meth Hosp-Stephenville	Stephenville	89%	300+
Baylor Heart & Vascular Hospital	Dallas	88%	300+
Heritage Park Surgical Hospital	Sherman	88%	(a)
Kell West Regional Hospital	Wichita Falls	88%	(a)
Memorial Medical Center	Port Lavaca	88%	(a)
Rolling Plains Memorial Hospital	Sweetwater	88%	(a)
South Texas Surgical Hospital	Corpus Christi	88%	300+
Sugar Land Surgical Hospital	Sugar Land	88%	(a)
Texas Spine & Joint Hospital	Tyler	88%	300+
Univ of TX Health Science Ctr-Tyler	Tyler	88%	(a)
USMD Hospital at Fort Worth	Fort Worth	88%	(a)
Baylor Medical Center at Frisco	Frisco	87%	300+
Baylor Surgical Hospital at Las Colinas	Irving	87%	(a)
Christus Spohn Hospital Kleberg	Kingsville	87%	300+
Covenant Hospital Plainview	Plainview	87%	300+
East Texas Medical Center Crockett	Crockett	87%	(a)
Etmc Carthage	Carthage	87%	(a)
Grace Medical Center	Lubbock	87%	300+
Heart Hospital Baylor Plano	Plano	87%	300+
Houston Physicians' Hospital	Webster	87%	(a)
Saint Luke's Lakeside Hospital	The Woodlands	87%	300+
Starr County Memorial Hospital	Rio Grande City	87%	(a)
Brownfield Regional Medical Center	Brownfield	86%	(a)
Christus Jasper Memorial Hospital	Jasper	86%	(a)
Columbus Community Hospital	Columbus	86%	(a)
Coryell Memorial Healthcare System	Gatesville	86%	(a)
Fdn Surgical Hosp of San Antonio	San Antonio	86%	300+
Huntsville Memorial Hospital	Huntsville	86%	(a)
Methodist Mckinney Hospital	Mc Kinney	86%	(a)
Saint Marks Medical Center	La Grange	86%	(a)
Scott & White Hospital - Llano	Llano	86%	(a)
Seton Medical Center Harker Heights	Harker Heights	86%	300+
UT Southwestern University Hospital	Dallas	86%	300+
Uvalde Memorial Hospital[11]	Uvalde	86%	(a)
Baylor Medical Center at Trophy Club	Trophy Club	85%	(a)
Big Bend Regional Medical Center	Alpine	85%	(a)
College Station Medical Center	College Station	85%	300+
Doctors Hospital	Dallas	85%	300+
First Surgical Hospital	Bellaire	85%	(a)
Good Shephard Medical Center - Linden	Linden	85%	(a)
Parkview Regional Hospital	Mexia	85%	(a)
Scott & White Hospital - Round Rock	Round Rock	85%	300+
TX Health Ctr for Diag & Surgery	Plano	85%	(a)
TX Hlth Presbyterian Hosp-Flower Mound	Flower Mound	85%	300+
Texas Orthopedic Hospital	Houston	85%	300+
USMD Hospital at Arlington	Arlington	85%	300+
UT SW Univ Hosp-Zale Lipshy	Dallas	85%	300+
Arise Austin Medical Center[3]	Austin	84%	(a)
Baptist Beaumont Hospital	Beaumont	84%	300+
Basin Healthcare Center	Odessa	84%	(a)
Baylor Reg Med Ctr at Grapevine	Grapevine	84%	300+
Citizens Medical Center	Victoria	84%	300+
East Texas Medical Center Jacksonville	Jacksonville	84%	300+
Guadalupe Regional Medical Center	Seguin	84%	300+
Methodist Hospital For Surgery	Addison	84%	300+
Saint Anthony's Hospital	Houston	84%	(a)
Seton Highland Lakes	Burnet	84%	300+
Shannon Medical Center	San Angelo	84%	300+
TX Hlth Presbyterian Hosp-Kaufman	Kaufman	84%	300+
Baylor University Medical Center	Dallas	83%	300+
Brownwood Regional Medical Center	Brownwood	83%	300+
Christus Hospital	Beaumont	83%	300+
Christus Saint Catherine Hospital	Katy	83%	300+
El Paso Specialty Hospital	El Paso	83%	(a)
Etmc Clarksville	Clarksville	83%	(a)
Etmc Henderson	Henderson	83%	300+
Hendrick Medical Center	Abilene	83%	300+
Hereford Regional Medical Center	Hereford	83%	(a)
Houston Orthopedic & Spine Hospital	Bellaire	83%	300+
Longview Regional Medical Center	Longview	83%	300+
Lubbock Heart Hospital	Lubbock	83%	300+
Medical City Dallas Hospital	Dallas	83%	300+
Methodist Ambulatory Surgery Hospital NW	San Antonio	83%	(a)
Mission Regional Medical Center	Mission	83%	300+
Moore County Hospital District	Dumas	83%	(a)
Northwest Hills Surgical Hospital	Austin	83%	(a)
Pine Creek Medical Center	Dallas	83%	300+
Providence Memorial Hospital	El Paso	83%	300+
Saint David's Medical Center	Austin	83%	300+
Saint Luke's Episcopal Hospital	Houston	83%	300+
San Angelo Community Medical Center	San Angelo	83%	300+
Scott & White Hospital Brenham	Brenham	83%	300+
TX Hlth Harris Methodist Hosp-Azle	Azle	83%	300+
TX Hlth Harris Meth Hosp SW Ft Worth	Fort Worth	83%	300+
Texas Health Presbyterian Hospital Allen	Allen	83%	300+
Titus Regional Medical Center	Mount Pleasant	83%	300+
Woodland Heights Medical Center	Lufkin	83%	300+
Abilene Regional Medical Center	Abilene	82%	300+
Baylor Surgical Hospital at Fort Worth	Fort Worth	82%	300+
Centennial Medical Center	Frisco	82%	300+
Christus Saint Michael Health System	Texarkana	82%	300+
Christus Spohn Hospital Alice	Alice	82%	300+
The Corpus Christi Medical Center	Corpus Christi	82%	300+
Covenant Medical Center	Lubbock	82%	300+
Cuero Community Hospital	Cuero	82%	(a)
Detar Hospital Navarro	Victoria	82%	300+
Doctors Hospital of Laredo	Laredo	82%	300+
East Texas Medical Center Athens	Athens	82%	300+
Foundation Surgical Hospital of El Paso	El Paso	82%	300+
Good Shepherd Medical Center	Longview	82%	300+
The Hospital at Westlake Medical Center	Austin	82%	300+
Knapp Medical Center	Weslaco	82%	300+
Lake Pointe Medical Center	Rowlett	82%	300+
Memorial Hermann Katy Hospital	Katy	82%	300+
Memorial Hermann Sugar Land Hospital	Sugar Land	82%	300+
Memorial Medical Center of East Texas	Lufkin	82%	300+
The Methodist Hospital	Houston	82%	300+
Metroplex Hospital[11]	Killeen	82%	300+
North Texas Medical Center	Gainesville	82%	(a)
Palo Pinto General Hospital	Mineral Wells	82%	300+
Saint Joseph Regional Health Center	Bryan	82%	300+
Scott & White Memorial Hospital[11]	Temple	82%	300+
Seton Medical Center Austin	Austin	82%	300+
Seton Southwest Hospital	Austin	82%	(a)
TX Hlth Harris Meth Hosp-Cleburne	Cleburne	82%	300+
Texas Health Presbyterian Hospital Plano	Plano	82%	300+
University Medical Center	Lubbock	82%	300+
Wise Regional Health System	Decatur	82%	300+
The Womans Hospital of Texas	Houston	82%	300+
Baptist Medical Center[11]	San Antonio	81%	300+
Baptist Saint Anthony's Hospital	Amarillo	81%	300+
Baylor Medical Center at Garland	Garland	81%	300+
Baylor Medical Center at Mckinney	Mc Kinney	81%	300+
Baylor Regional Medical Center at Plano	Plano	81%	300+
Care Regional Medical Center	Aransas Pass	81%	(a)
Christus Santa Rosa Hospital	San Antonio	81%	300+
Fort Duncan Medical Center	Eagle Pass	81%	300+
Hillcrest Baptist Medical Center	Waco	81%	300+
Houston Northwest Medical Center	Houston	81%	300+
Lake Granbury Medical Center	Granbury	81%	300+
Matagorda Regional Medical Center	Bay City	81%	(a)
The Medical Center of Southeast Texas	Port Arthur	81%	300+
Memorial Hospital	Nacogdoches	81%	300+
Navarro Regional Hospital	Corsicana	81%	300+
Nix Health Care System	San Antonio	81%	300+
Providence Health Center	Waco	81%	300+
Scenic Mountain Medical Center	Big Spring	81%	300+
Sierra Medical Center	El Paso	81%	300+
Texas Health Harris Methodist	Bedford	81%	300+
Texas Health Presbyterian Hospital Dallas	Dallas	81%	300+
Texoma Medical Center	Denison	81%	300+
Val Verde Regional Medical Center	Del Rio	81%	300+
VHS Brownsville Hospital Company[11]	Brownsville	81%	300+
VHS Harlingen Hospital Company[11]	Harlingen	81%	300+
Angleton - Danbury Medical Center	Angleton	80%	300+
Baylor All Saints Medical Center at FW	Fort Worth	80%	300+
Brazosport Regional Health System	Lake Jackson	80%	300+
Cedar Park Regional Medical Center	Cedar Park	80%	300+
Central Texas Medical Center[11]	San Marcos	80%	300+
Christus Spohn Hospital Beeville	Beeville	80%	(a)
Cypress Fairbanks Medical Center	Houston	80%	300+
Huguley Memorial Medical Center[11]	Burleson	80%	300+
Medical Center of Mckinney	Mckinney	80%	300+
Mem Hermann Mem City Med Ctr	Houston	80%	300+
Memorial Hermann Texas Medical Center	Houston	80%	300+
Methodist Dallas Medical Center	Dallas	80%	300+
Methodist Hospital	San Antonio	80%	300+
Methodist Mansfield Medical Center	Mansfield	80%	300+
Methodist Richardson Medical Center	Richardson	80%	300+
Methodist Sugar Land Hospital	Sugar Land	80%	300+
Methodist West Houston Hospital	Houston	80%	300+
Mother Frances Hospital	Tyler	80%	300+
North Austin Medical Center	Austin	80%	300+
North Cypress Medical Center	Cypress	80%	300+
Oakbend Medical Center	Richmond	80%	300+
Odessa Regional Hospital	Odessa	80%	300+
Pampa Regional Medical Center	Pampa	80%	300+
Permian Regional Medical Center	Andrews	80%	(a)
Peterson Regional Medical Center	Kerrville	80%	300+
Plaza Medical Center of Fort Worth	Fort Worth	80%	300+
Saint Joseph Medical Center	Houston	80%	300+
Saint Luke's Patients Medical Center	Pasadena	80%	300+
Saint Luke's Sugar Land Hospital	Sugar Land	80%	300+
San Jacinto Methodist Hospital	Baytown	80%	300+
Seton Medical Center Hays	Kyle	80%	300+
Seton Northwest Hospital	Austin	80%	300+
Texas Health Harris Methodist Fort Worth	Fort Worth	80%	300+
TX Hlth Heart & Vasc Hosp-Arlington	Arlington	80%	300+
United Regional Health Care System	Wichita Falls	80%	300+
University General Hospital Dallas	Dallas	80%	(a)
Valley Regional Medical Center	Brownsville	80%	300+
Wadley Regional Medical Center	Texarkana	80%	300+
Clear Lake Regional Medical Center	Webster	79%	300+
Doctors Hospital at Renaissance	Edinburg	79%	300+
Ennis Regional Medical Center	Ennis	79%	300+
Harris Health System	Houston	79%	300+
Laredo Medical Center	Laredo	79%	300+
Las Colinas Medical Center	Irving	79%	300+
Medical Center Hospital	Odessa	79%	300+
Medical Center of Lewisville	Lewisville	79%	300+
Memorial Hermann Hospital System	Houston	79%	300+
Methodist Stone Oak Hospital	San Antonio	79%	300+
Paris Regional Medical Center	Paris	79%	300+
Rio Grande Regional Hospital	Mcallen	79%	300+
Saint David's South Austin Medical Center	Austin	79%	300+
Saint Luke's the Woodlands Hospital	The Woodlands	79%	300+
Seton Medical Center Williamson	Round Rock	79%	300+
Sierra Providence East Medical Center	El Paso	79%	300+
South Texas Regional Medical Center	Jourdanton	79%	(a)
Texas Health Presbyterian Hospital - WNJ	Sherman	79%	300+
Texas Health Presbyterian Hospital Denton	Denton	79%	300+
Tomball Regional Medical Center	Tomball	79%	300+
University Medical Center of El Paso	El Paso	79%	300+
Weatherford Regional Medical Center	Weatherford	79%	300+
Baylor Medical Center at Irving	Irving	78%	300+
Christus Spohn Hospital Corpus Christi	Corpus Christi	78%	300+

NOTE: Hospital profiles are in alphabetical order by state, then city, then hospital within the city; Rankings exclude hospitals with less than 25 cases except for patient surveys which excludes hospitals with less than 100 cases; (a) 100-299 cases; (1) The number of cases/patients is too few to report; (2) Data submitted were based on a sample of cases/patients; (3) Results are based on a shorter time period than required; (4) Data suppressed by CMS for one or more quarters; (5) Results are not available for this reporting period; (6) Fewer than 100 patients completed the HCAHPS survey; (7) No cases met the criteria for this measure; (8) The lower limit of the confidence interval cannot be calculated if the number of observed infections equals zero; (9) No data are available from the state/territory for this reporting period; (10) The scores shown reflect fewer than 50 completed surveys; (11) There were discrepancies in the data collection process; (12) This measure does not apply to this hospital for this reporting period; (13) Results cannot be calculated for this reporting period; (14) The results for this state are combined with nearby states to protect confidentiality; Please refer to the User's Guide for a full explanation of data.

Connally Memorial Medical Center	Floresville	78%	(a)
Denton Regional Medical Center	Denton	78%	300+
Doctors Hospital Tidwell	Houston	78%	300+
East Texas Medical Center	Tyler	78%	300+
Harlingen Medical Center[11]	Harlingen	78%	300+
Hopkins County Memorial Hospital	Sulphur Springs	78%	300+
Hunt Regional Medical Center	Greenville	78%	300+
JPS Health Network	Fort Worth	78%	300+
Lake Whitney Medical Center[11]	Whitney	78%	(a)
Medical Center of Plano	Plano	78%	300+
Memorial Hermann Northeast	Humble	78%	300+
Memorial Medical Center Livingston	Livingston	78%	300+
Northwest Texas Hospital	Amarillo	78%	300+
Parkland Health & Hospital System	Dallas	78%	300+
Round Rock Medical Center	Round Rock	78%	300+
South Texas Health System	Edinburg	78%	300+
TX Health Presbyterian Hosp Rockwall	Rockwall	78%	300+
University General Hospital	Houston	78%	300+
University Health System	San Antonio	78%	300+
Univ of Texas Med Branch Galveston	Galveston	78%	300+
Conroe Regional Medical Center	Conroe	77%	300+
Cornerstone Regional Hospital	Edinburg	77%	(a)
Good Shepherd Medical Center Marshall	Marshall	77%	300+
Kingwood Medical Center	Kingwood	77%	300+
Las Palmas Medical Center	El Paso	77%	300+
Medical Center of Arlington	Arlington	77%	300+
Midland Memorial Hospital	Midland	77%	300+
North Hills Hospital	N Richland Hls	77%	300+
Palestine Regional Medical Center	Palestine	77%	300+
Southwest General Hospital	San Antonio	77%	300+
Texas Health Arlington Memorial Hospital	Arlington	77%	300+
Texas Reg Med Ctr at Sunnyvale	Sunnyvale	77%	300+
University Medical Center at Brackenridge	Austin	77%	300+
Baylor Medical Center at Carrollton	Carrollton	76%	300+
Baylor Medical Center at Waxahachie	Waxahachie	76%	300+
Bayshore Medical Center	Pasadena	76%	300+
Methodist Charlton Medical Center	Dallas	76%	300+
Methodist Willowbrook Hospital	Houston	76%	300+
West Houston Medical Center	Houston	75%	300+
Christus Saint John Hospital	Nassau Bay	74%	300+
Dallas Regional Medical Center	Mesquite	74%	300+
Saint Luke's Hospital at the Vintage	Houston	74%	300+
Dallas Medical Center	Dallas	71%	300+

Home Recovery Information Given

Hospital Name	City	Rate	Cases
TX Inst for Surgery at Presby Hosp	Dallas	97%	(a)
Electra Memorial Hospital	Electra	95%	(a)
Heritage Park Surgical Hospital	Sherman	94%	(a)
Eastland Memorial Hospital	Eastland	93%	(a)
Houston Orthopedic & Spine Hospital	Bellaire	93%	300+
North Central Surgical Center	Dallas	93%	300+
TX Hlth Harris Meth Hosp-Southlake	Southlake	93%	300+
Arise Austin Medical Center[3]	Austin	92%	(a)
Baylor Medical Center at Uptown	Dallas	92%	300+
Baylor Ortho & Spine Hosp-Arlington	Arlington	92%	300+
Big Bend Regional Medical Center	Alpine	91%	(a)
East Texas Medical Center Quitman	Quitman	91%	(a)
Hill Country Memorial Hospital	Fredericksburg	91%	300+
Northwest Hills Surgical Hospital	Austin	91%	(a)
Quail Creek Surgical Hospital	Amarillo	91%	300+
Rollins Brook Community Hospital[11]	Lampasas	91%	(a)
Sugar Land Surgical Hospital	Sugar Land	91%	(a)
TX Health Ctr for Diag & Surgery	Plano	91%	(a)
TX Hlth Harris Methodist Hosp-Azle	Azle	91%	300+
Univ of TX Health Science Ctr-Tyler	Tyler	91%	(a)
Uvalde Memorial Hospital[11]	Uvalde	91%	(a)
Childress Regional Medical Center	Childress	90%	(a)
East Texas Medical Center - Gilmer	Gilmer	90%	(a)
Methodist Hospital For Surgery	Addison	90%	300+
Moore County Hospital District	Dumas	90%	(a)
North Texas Medical Center	Gainesville	90%	(a)
The Physicians Centre	Bryan	90%	(a)
South Texas Regional Medical Center	Jourdanton	90%	(a)
Texas Spine & Joint Hospital	Tyler	90%	300+
Baylor Surgical Hospital at Las Colinas	Irving	89%	(a)
East Texas Medical Center Pittsburg	Pittsburg	89%	(a)
The Hospital at Westlake Medical Center	Austin	89%	300+
Mem Hermann Mem City Med Ctr	Houston	89%	300+
Memorial Medical Center	Port Lavaca	89%	(a)
Palo Pinto General Hospital	Mineral Wells	89%	300+
Parkview Regional Hospital	Mexia	89%	(a)
Providence Health Center	Waco	89%	300+
Seton Southwest Hospital	Austin	89%	(a)
South Texas Spine & Surgical Hospital	San Antonio	89%	300+
TX Hlth Harris Meth Hosp-Stephenville	Stephenville	89%	300+
Texas Orthopedic Hospital	Houston	89%	300+
Tops Surgical Specialty Hospital	Houston	89%	(a)
USMD Hospital at Fort Worth	Fort Worth	89%	(a)
Baylor Medical Center at Frisco	Frisco	88%	300+
Baylor Medical Center at Trophy Club	Trophy Club	88%	(a)
Brownfield Regional Medical Center	Brownfield	88%	(a)
Brownwood Regional Medical Center	Brownwood	88%	300+
El Paso Specialty Hospital	El Paso	88%	(a)
Grace Medical Center	Lubbock	88%	300+
Heart Hospital Baylor Plano	Plano	88%	300+
Houston Physicians' Hospital	Webster	88%	(a)
Kell West Regional Hospital	Wichita Falls	88%	(a)
Longview Regional Medical Center	Longview	88%	300+
Methodist Ambulatory Surgery Hospital NW	San Antonio	88%	(a)
Methodist Mckinney Hospital	Mc Kinney	88%	(a)
Metroplex Hospital[11]	Killeen	88%	300+
North Austin Medical Center	Austin	88%	300+
Round Rock Medical Center	Round Rock	88%	300+
Saint David's Medical Center	Austin	88%	300+
Saint Luke's Lakeside Hospital	The Woodlands	88%	300+
Seton Medical Center Harker Heights	Harker Heights	88%	300+
Starr County Memorial Hospital	Rio Grande City	88%	(a)
TX Hlth Harris Meth Hosp-Cleburne	Cleburne	88%	300+
Univ of Texas Med Branch Galveston	Galveston	88%	300+
UT Southwestern University Hospital	Dallas	88%	300+
VHS Harlingen Hospital Company[11]	Harlingen	88%	300+
Wadley Regional Medical Center	Texarkana	88%	300+
Baptist Beaumont Hospital	Beaumont	87%	300+
Baylor Surgical Hospital at Fort Worth	Fort Worth	87%	300+
Covenant Medical Center	Lubbock	87%	300+
East Texas Medical Center Jacksonville	Jacksonville	87%	300+
Fdn Surgical Hosp of San Antonio	San Antonio	87%	300+
Good Shepherd Medical Center	Longview	87%	300+
Graham Regional Medical Center	Graham	87%	(a)
Harlingen Medical Center[11]	Harlingen	87%	300+
Matagorda Regional Medical Center	Bay City	87%	(a)
Memorial Hermann Texas Medical Center	Houston	87%	300+
Memorial Medical Center Livingston	Livingston	87%	300+
Nacogdoches Medical Center	Nacogdoches	87%	300+
San Angelo Community Medical Center	San Angelo	87%	300+
Seton Edgar B Davis Hospital	Luling	87%	(a)
Seton Medical Center Austin	Austin	87%	300+
South Texas Surgical Hospital	Corpus Christi	87%	300+
Texas Health Harris Methodist Fort Worth	Fort Worth	87%	300+
Texas Health Harris Methodist	Bedford	87%	300+
Texas Health Presbyterian Hospital Plano	Plano	87%	300+
United Regional Health Care System	Wichita Falls	87%	300+
UT SW Univ Hosp-Zale Lipshy	Dallas	87%	300+
Woodland Heights Medical Center	Lufkin	87%	300+
Abilene Regional Medical Center	Abilene	86%	300+
Angleton - Danbury Medical Center	Angleton	86%	300+
Baptist Medical Center[11]	San Antonio	86%	300+
Baylor Regional Medical Center at Plano	Plano	86%	300+
Cedar Park Regional Medical Center	Cedar Park	86%	300+
Central Texas Medical Center[11]	San Marcos	86%	300+
College Station Medical Center	College Station	86%	300+
The Corpus Christi Medical Center	Corpus Christi	86%	300+
Covenant Hospital Levelland	Levelland	86%	(a)
Denton Regional Medical Center	Denton	86%	300+
Detar Hospital Navarro	Victoria	86%	300+
Doctors Hospital of Laredo	Laredo	86%	300+
First Surgical Hospital	Bellaire	86%	(a)
Hamilton General Hospital	Hamilton	86%	(a)
Hendrick Medical Center	Abilene	86%	300+
Huguley Memorial Medical Center[11]	Burleson	86%	300+
Hunt Regional Medical Center	Greenville	86%	300+
Las Colinas Medical Center	Irving	86%	300+
Medical Center of Mckinney	Mckinney	86%	300+
Medical City Dallas Hospital	Dallas	86%	300+
Memorial Hermann Katy Hospital	Katy	86%	300+
Memorial Hermann Northeast	Humble	86%	300+
Memorial Hermann Sugar Land Hospital	Sugar Land	86%	300+
Memorial Medical Center of East Texas	Lufkin	86%	300+
The Methodist Hospital	Houston	86%	300+
Methodist West Houston Hospital	Houston	86%	300+
Odessa Regional Hospital	Odessa	86%	300+
Pecos County Memorial Hospital	Fort Stockton	86%	(a)
Pine Creek Medical Center	Dallas	86%	300+
Rolling Plains Memorial Hospital	Sweetwater	86%	(a)
Saint David's South Austin Medical Center	Austin	86%	300+
Saint Joseph Regional Health Center	Bryan	86%	300+
Scott & White Hospital - Llano	Llano	86%	(a)
Scott & White Hospital - Round Rock	Round Rock	86%	300+
Seton Highland Lakes	Burnet	86%	300+
Seton Medical Center Hays	Kyle	86%	300+
TX Hlth Harris Meth Hosp SW Ft Worth	Fort Worth	86%	300+
TX Hlth Heart & Vasc Hosp-Arlington	Arlington	86%	300+
Texas Health Presbyterian Hospital Allen	Allen	86%	300+
Texas Health Presbyterian Hospital Denton	Denton	86%	300+
TX Hlth Presbyterian Hosp-Flower Mound	Flower Mound	86%	300+
Texoma Medical Center	Denison	86%	300+
University Medical Center at Brackenridge	Austin	86%	300+
University Medical Center of El Paso	El Paso	86%	300+
VHS Brownsville Hospital Company[11]	Brownsville	86%	300+
Weatherford Regional Medical Center	Weatherford	86%	300+
Wise Regional Health System	Decatur	86%	300+
Basin Healthcare Center	Odessa	85%	(a)
Baylor Heart & Vascular Hospital	Dallas	85%	300+
Baylor Medical Center at Mckinney	Mc Kinney	85%	300+
Baylor Reg Med Ctr at Grapevine	Grapevine	85%	300+
Baylor University Medical Center	Dallas	85%	300+
Care Regional Medical Center	Aransas Pass	85%	(a)
Centennial Medical Center	Frisco	85%	300+
Christus Saint Catherine Hospital	Katy	85%	300+
Christus Saint Michael Health System	Texarkana	85%	300+
Christus Santa Rosa Hospital	San Antonio	85%	300+
Christus Spohn Hospital Alice	Alice	85%	300+
Christus Spohn Hospital Beeville	Beeville	85%	(a)
Connally Memorial Medical Center	Floresville	85%	(a)
Covenant Hospital Plainview	Plainview	85%	300+
Cypress Fairbanks Medical Center	Houston	85%	300+
Ennis Regional Medical Center	Ennis	85%	300+
Hill Regional Hospital	Hillsboro	85%	300+
Hopkins County Memorial Hospital	Sulphur Springs	85%	300+
Lubbock Heart Hospital	Lubbock	85%	300+
Medical Center of Lewisville	Lewisville	85%	300+
The Medical Center of Southeast Texas	Port Arthur	85%	300+
Memorial Hermann Baptist Orange Hospital	Orange	85%	300+
Memorial Hermann Hospital System	Houston	85%	300+
Methodist Hospital	San Antonio	85%	300+
Methodist Stone Oak Hospital	San Antonio	85%	300+
Methodist Sugar Land Hospital	Sugar Land	85%	300+
Mission Regional Medical Center	Mission	85%	300+
Navarro Regional Hospital	Corsicana	85%	300+
North Hills Hospital	N Richland Hls	85%	300+
Northwest Texas Hospital	Amarillo	85%	300+
Parkland Health & Hospital System	Dallas	85%	300+
Peterson Regional Medical Center	Kerrville	85%	300+
Plaza Medical Center of Fort Worth	Fort Worth	85%	300+
Scott & White Hospital Brenham	Brenham	85%	300+
Scott & White Memorial Hospital[11]	Temple	85%	300+
Seton Medical Center Williamson	Round Rock	85%	300+
Seton Northwest Hospital	Austin	85%	300+
TX Hlth Presbyterian Hosp-Kaufman	Kaufman	85%	300+
TX Health Presbyterian Hosp Rockwall	Rockwall	85%	300+
University Health System	San Antonio	85%	300+
USMD Hospital at Arlington	Arlington	85%	300+
The Womans Hospital of Texas	Houston	85%	300+
Baylor Medical Center at Garland	Garland	84%	300+
Baylor Medical Center at Waxahachie	Waxahachie	84%	300+
Christus Spohn Hospital Kleberg	Kingsville	84%	300+
Clear Lake Regional Medical Center	Webster	84%	300+
Conroe Regional Medical Center	Conroe	84%	300+
Cuero Community Hospital	Cuero	84%	(a)
Falls Community Hospital & Clinic	Marlin	84%	(a)
Foundation Surgical Hospital of El Paso	El Paso	84%	300+
Guadalupe Regional Medical Center	Seguin	84%	300+
Knapp Medical Center	Weslaco	84%	300+
Lake Granbury Medical Center	Granbury	84%	300+
Las Palmas Medical Center	El Paso	84%	300+
Medical Center of Plano	Plano	84%	300+
Medina Regional Hospital	Hondo	84%	(a)
Methodist Willowbrook Hospital	Houston	84%	300+
Mother Frances Hospital	Tyler	84%	300+
North Cypress Medical Center	Cypress	84%	300+
Providence Memorial Hospital	El Paso	84%	300+
Saint Marks Medical Center	La Grange	84%	(a)
San Jacinto Methodist Hospital	Baytown	84%	300+
Shannon Medical Center	San Angelo	84%	300+
Texas Health Arlington Memorial Hospital	Arlington	84%	300+
Texas Health Presbyterian Hospital Dallas	Dallas	84%	300+
Titus Regional Medical Center	Mount Pleasant	84%	300+
University Medical Center	Lubbock	84%	300+
Valley Regional Medical Center	Brownsville	84%	300+
Yoakum Community Hospital	Yoakum	84%	(a)
Baptist Saint Anthony's Hospital	Amarillo	83%	300+
Baylor All Saints Medical Center at FW	Fort Worth	83%	300+
Baylor Medical Center at Irving	Irving	83%	300+
Brazosport Regional Health System	Lake Jackson	83%	300+
Christus Jasper Memorial Hospital	Jasper	83%	(a)
Christus Saint John Hospital	Nassau Bay	83%	300+
Doctors Hospital	Dallas	83%	300+
East Texas Medical Center Crockett	Crockett	83%	(a)
Etmc Carthage	Carthage	83%	(a)
Etmc Henderson	Henderson	83%	300+
Fort Duncan Medical Center	Eagle Pass	83%	300+
JPS Health Network	Fort Worth	83%	300+
Kingwood Medical Center	Kingwood	83%	300+
Lake Pointe Medical Center	Rowlett	83%	300+
Medical Center of Arlington	Arlington	83%	300+
Memorial Hospital	Nacogdoches	83%	300+
Methodist Mansfield Medical Center	Mansfield	83%	300+
Methodist Richardson Medical Center	Richardson	83%	300+
Oakbend Medical Center	Richmond	83%	300+
Palestine Regional Medical Center	Palestine	83%	300+
Saint Joseph Medical Center	Houston	83%	300+
Saint Luke's Hospital at the Vintage	Houston	83%	300+

NOTE: Hospital profiles are in alphabetical order by state, then city, then hospital within the city; Rankings exclude hospitals with less than 25 cases except for patient surveys which excludes hospitals with less than 100 cases; (a) 100-299 cases; (1) The number of cases/patients is too few to report; (2) Data submitted were based on a sample of cases/patients; (3) Results are based on a shorter time period than required; (4) Data suppressed by CMS for one or more quarters; (5) Results are not available for this reporting period; (6) Fewer than 100 patients completed the HCAHPS survey; (7) No cases met the criteria for this measure; (8) The lower limit of the confidence interval cannot be calculated if the number of observed infections equals zero; (9) No data are available from the state/territory for this reporting period; (10) The scores shown reflect fewer than 50 completed surveys; (11) There were discrepancies in the data collection process; (12) This measure does not apply to this hospital for this reporting period; (13) Results cannot be calculated for this reporting period; (14) The results for this state are combined with nearby states to protect confidentiality; Please refer to the User's Guide for a full explanation of data.

Sierra Medical Center	El Paso	83%	300+
Sierra Providence East Medical Center	El Paso	83%	300+
Southwest General Hospital	San Antonio	83%	300+
Texas Health Presbyterian Hospital - WNJ	Sherman	83%	300+
Tomball Regional Medical Center	Tomball	83%	300+
Val Verde Regional Medical Center	Del Rio	83%	300+
Christus Spohn Hospital Corpus Christi	Corpus Christi	82%	300+
Cornerstone Regional Hospital	Edinburg	82%	(a)
Doctors Hospital at Renaissance	Edinburg	82%	300+
East Texas Medical Center	Tyler	82%	300+
East Texas Medical Center Athens	Athens	82%	300+
Etmc Clarksville	Clarksville	82%	(a)
Good Shepherd Medical Center Marshall	Marshall	82%	300+
Hillcrest Baptist Medical Center	Waco	82%	300+
Midland Memorial Hospital	Midland	82%	300+
Pampa Regional Medical Center	Pampa	82%	300+
Scenic Mountain Medical Center	Big Spring	82%	300+
South Texas Health System	Edinburg	82%	300+
University General Hospital	Houston	82%	300+
Baptist Emergency Hospital	San Antonio	81%	(a)
Baylor Medical Center at Carrollton	Carrollton	81%	300+
Bayshore Medical Center	Pasadena	81%	300+
Christus Hospital	Beaumont	81%	300+
Coryell Memorial Healthcare System	Gatesville	81%	(a)
Harris Health System	Houston	81%	300+
Laredo Medical Center	Laredo	81%	300+
Medical Center Hospital	Odessa	81%	300+
Methodist Dallas Medical Center	Dallas	81%	300+
Nix Health Care System	San Antonio	81%	300+
Rio Grande Regional Hospital	Mcallen	81%	300+
Saint Anthony's Hospital	Houston	81%	(a)
Saint Luke's Episcopal Hospital	Houston	81%	300+
Saint Luke's Patients Medical Center	Pasadena	81%	300+
University General Hospital Dallas	Dallas	81%	(a)
West Houston Medical Center	Houston	81%	300+
Citizens Medical Center	Victoria	80%	300+
Columbus Community Hospital	Columbus	80%	(a)
Houston Northwest Medical Center	Houston	80%	300+
Huntsville Memorial Hospital	Huntsville	80%	(a)
Methodist Charlton Medical Center	Dallas	80%	300+
Park Plaza Hospital	Houston	80%	300+
Saint Luke's Sugar Land Hospital	Sugar Land	80%	300+
Good Shephard Medical Center - Linden	Linden	79%	(a)
Glen Rose Medical Center	Glen Rose	78%	(a)
Saint Luke's the Woodlands Hospital	The Woodlands	78%	300+
Hereford Regional Medical Center	Hereford	77%	(a)
Texas Reg Med Ctr at Sunnyvale	Sunnyvale	77%	(a)
Dallas Medical Center	Dallas	76%	300+
Paris Regional Medical Center	Paris	76%	300+
Dallas Regional Medical Center	Mesquite	75%	300+
Permian Regional Medical Center	Andrews	75%	(a)
Tyler County Hospital	Woodville	75%	(a)
W J Mangold Memorial Hospital	Lockney	75%	(a)
Doctors Hospital Tidwell	Houston	73%	300+
Lake Whitney Medical Center[11]	Whitney	72%	(a)

Hospital Given 9 or 10 on 10 Point Scale

Hospital Name	City	Rate	Cases
The Physicians Centre	Bryan	92%	(a)
Hill Country Memorial Hospital	Fredericksburg	91%	300+
Quail Creek Surgical Hospital	Amarillo	91%	300+
Heart Hospital Baylor Plano	Plano	90%	300+
North Central Surgical Center	Dallas	90%	300+
Sugar Land Surgical Hospital	Sugar Land	90%	(a)
TX Hlth Harris Meth Hosp-Southlake	Southlake	90%	300+
TX Inst for Surgery at Presby Hosp	Dallas	90%	(a)
Baylor Medical Center at Frisco	Frisco	89%	300+
Heritage Park Surgical Hospital	Sherman	89%	(a)
Houston Orthopedic & Spine Hospital	Bellaire	89%	300+
TX Health Ctr for Diag & Surgery	Plano	89%	(a)
Baylor Heart & Vascular Hospital	Dallas	88%	300+
Baylor Medical Center at Uptown	Dallas	88%	300+
Baylor Ortho & Spine Hosp-Arlington	Arlington	88%	300+
USMD Hospital at Fort Worth	Fort Worth	88%	(a)
Electra Memorial Hospital	Electra	87%	(a)
Rollins Brook Community Hospital[11]	Lampasas	87%	(a)
Saint Luke's Lakeside Hospital	The Woodlands	87%	300+
East Texas Medical Center - Gilmer	Gilmer	86%	(a)
Northwest Hills Surgical Hospital	Austin	86%	(a)
Texas Spine & Joint Hospital	Tyler	86%	300+
Baylor Medical Center at Mckinney	Mc Kinney	85%	300+
Fdn Surgical Hosp of San Antonio	San Antonio	85%	300+
Houston Physicians' Hospital	Webster	85%	(a)
UT SW Univ Hosp-Zale Lipshy	Dallas	85%	300+
Baylor Medical Center at Trophy Club	Trophy Club	84%	(a)
South Texas Spine & Surgical Hospital	San Antonio	84%	300+
South Texas Surgical Hospital	Corpus Christi	84%	300+
USMD Hospital at Arlington	Arlington	84%	300+
W J Mangold Memorial Hospital	Lockney	84%	(a)
Baptist Emergency Hospital	San Antonio	83%	(a)
Hamilton General Hospital	Hamilton	82%	(a)
Lubbock Heart Hospital	Lubbock	82%	300+
Methodist Hospital For Surgery	Addison	82%	300+
Tops Surgical Specialty Hospital	Houston	82%	(a)
Baylor Surgical Hospital at Las Colinas	Irving	81%	(a)
East Texas Medical Center Pittsburg	Pittsburg	81%	(a)
Seton Edgar B Davis Hospital	Luling	81%	(a)
Seton Southwest Hospital	Austin	81%	(a)
Texas Health Presbyterian Hospital Plano	Plano	81%	300+
Baylor Regional Medical Center at Plano	Plano	80%	300+
The Hospital at Westlake Medical Center	Austin	80%	300+
Methodist Ambulatory Surgery Hospital NW	San Antonio	80%	(a)
Methodist Mansfield Medical Center	Mansfield	80%	300+
Univ of TX Health Science Ctr-Tyler	Tyler	80%	(a)
Childress Regional Medical Center	Childress	79%	(a)
East Texas Medical Center Quitman	Quitman	79%	(a)
Methodist West Houston Hospital	Houston	79%	300+
Saint David's Medical Center	Austin	79%	300+
Seton Medical Center Harker Heights	Harker Heights	79%	300+
TX Hlth Heart & Vasc Hosp-Arlington	Arlington	79%	300+
TX Hlth Presbyterian Hosp-Flower Mound	Flower Mound	79%	300+
University Medical Center	Lubbock	79%	300+
Baylor Reg Med Ctr at Grapevine	Grapevine	78%	300+
Eastland Memorial Hospital	Eastland	78%	(a)
Kell West Regional Hospital	Wichita Falls	78%	(a)
The Methodist Hospital	Houston	78%	300+
Methodist Sugar Land Hospital	Sugar Land	78%	300+
TX Hlth Harris Meth Hosp SW Ft Worth	Fort Worth	78%	300+
TX Hlth Presbyterian Hosp-Kaufman	Kaufman	78%	(a)
United Regional Health Care System	Wichita Falls	78%	300+
Woodland Heights Medical Center	Lufkin	78%	300+
Covenant Medical Center	Lubbock	77%	300+
Glen Rose Medical Center	Glen Rose	77%	(a)
Medina Regional Hospital	Hondo	77%	(a)
Mem Hermann Mem City Med Ctr	Houston	77%	300+
Methodist Mckinney Hospital	Mc Kinney	77%	(a)
Mission Regional Medical Center	Mission	77%	300+
Parkview Regional Hospital	Mexia	77%	(a)
Pecos County Memorial Hospital	Fort Stockton	77%	(a)
Providence Health Center	Waco	77%	300+
Seton Highland Lakes	Burnet	77%	(a)
Texoma Medical Center	Denison	77%	300+
UT Southwestern University Hospital	Dallas	77%	300+
Uvalde Memorial Hospital[11]	Uvalde	77%	(a)
Arise Austin Medical Center[3]	Austin	76%	(a)
Baptist Saint Anthony's Hospital	Amarillo	76%	300+
Baylor All Saints Medical Center at FW	Fort Worth	76%	300+
Doctors Hospital at Renaissance	Edinburg	76%	300+
Hendrick Medical Center	Abilene	76%	300+
Medical City Dallas Hospital	Dallas	76%	300+
Memorial Hermann Katy Hospital	Katy	76%	300+
Memorial Hermann Sugar Land Hospital	Sugar Land	76%	300+
Saint Joseph Regional Health Center	Bryan	76%	300+
Saint Luke's the Woodlands Hospital	The Woodlands	76%	300+
San Angelo Community Medical Center	San Angelo	76%	300+
Texas Health Harris Methodist Fort Worth	Fort Worth	76%	300+
TX Hlth Harris Meth Hosp-Stephenville	Stephenville	76%	300+
Texas Health Harris Methodist	Bedford	76%	300+
Texas Health Presbyterian Hospital Allen	Allen	76%	300+
TX Health Presbyterian Hosp Rockwall	Rockwall	76%	300+
Texas Orthopedic Hospital	Houston	76%	300+
Big Bend Regional Medical Center	Alpine	75%	(a)
Christus Saint Catherine Hospital	Katy	75%	300+
Covenant Hospital Levelland	Levelland	75%	(a)
Detar Hospital Navarro	Victoria	75%	300+
Memorial Hermann Hospital System	Houston	75%	300+
Methodist Willowbrook Hospital	Houston	75%	300+
North Austin Medical Center	Austin	75%	300+
Pine Creek Medical Center	Dallas	75%	300+
Round Rock Medical Center	Round Rock	75%	300+
Saint Luke's Episcopal Hospital	Houston	75%	300+
Seton Medical Center Williamson	Round Rock	75%	300+
Shannon Medical Center	San Angelo	75%	300+
VHS Brownsville Hospital Company[11]	Brownsville	75%	300+
Yoakum Community Hospital	Yoakum	75%	(a)
Basin Healthcare Center	Odessa	74%	(a)
Baylor University Medical Center	Dallas	74%	300+
Christus Saint Michael Health System	Texarkana	74%	300+
East Texas Medical Center Jacksonville	Jacksonville	74%	300+
First Surgical Hospital	Bellaire	74%	(a)
Graham Regional Medical Center	Graham	74%	(a)
Medical Center of Lewisville	Lewisville	74%	300+
Mother Frances Hospital	Tyler	74%	300+
Rolling Plains Memorial Hospital	Sweetwater	74%	(a)
Saint David's South Austin Medical Center	Austin	74%	300+
Saint Luke's Hospital at the Vintage	Houston	74%	300+
San Jacinto Methodist Hospital	Baytown	74%	300+
Scott & White Hospital - Round Rock	Round Rock	74%	300+
Seton Medical Center Hays	Kyle	74%	300+
Texas Health Presbyterian Hospital Dallas	Dallas	74%	300+
University Medical Center of El Paso	El Paso	74%	300+
Wise Regional Health System	Decatur	74%	300+
Baptist Beaumont Hospital	Beaumont	73%	300+
Baylor Medical Center at Waxahachie	Waxahachie	73%	300+
Central Texas Medical Center[11]	San Marcos	73%	300+
Christus Saint John Hospital	Nassau Bay	73%	300+
Cuero Community Hospital	Cuero	73%	(a)
Foundation Surgical Hospital of El Paso	El Paso	73%	300+
Grace Medical Center	Lubbock	73%	300+
Guadalupe Regional Medical Center	Seguin	73%	300+
JPS Health Network	Fort Worth	73%	300+
Longview Regional Medical Center	Longview	73%	300+
Memorial Hermann Baptist Orange Hospital	Orange	73%	300+
Memorial Hermann Texas Medical Center	Houston	73%	300+
Memorial Medical Center of East Texas	Lufkin	73%	300+
Methodist Dallas Medical Center	Dallas	73%	300+
Methodist Stone Oak Hospital	San Antonio	73%	300+
Moore County Hospital District	Dumas	73%	(a)
North Cypress Medical Center	Cypress	73%	300+
Sierra Providence East Medical Center	El Paso	73%	300+
TX Hlth Harris Meth Hosp-Cleburne	Cleburne	73%	300+
University Medical Center at Brackenridge	Austin	73%	300+
The Womans Hospital of Texas	Houston	73%	300+
Baptist Medical Center[11]	San Antonio	72%	300+
College Station Medical Center	College Station	72%	300+
Doctors Hospital of Laredo	Laredo	72%	300+
El Paso Specialty Hospital	El Paso	72%	(a)
Harlingen Medical Center[11]	Harlingen	72%	300+
Park Plaza Hospital	Houston	72%	300+
Rio Grande Regional Hospital	Mcallen	72%	300+
Saint Luke's Sugar Land Hospital	Sugar Land	72%	300+
Seton Medical Center Austin	Austin	72%	300+
TX Hlth Harris Methodist Hosp-Azle	Azle	72%	300+
Texas Health Presbyterian Hospital Denton	Denton	72%	300+
Baylor Medical Center at Irving	Irving	71%	300+
Christus Santa Rosa Hospital	San Antonio	71%	300+
Christus Spohn Hospital Alice	Alice	71%	300+
The Corpus Christi Medical Center	Corpus Christi	71%	300+
Falls Community Hospital & Clinic	Marlin	71%	(a)
Good Shepherd Medical Center	Longview	71%	300+
Hill Regional Hospital	Hillsboro	71%	300+
Hillcrest Baptist Medical Center	Waco	71%	300+
Hopkins County Memorial Hospital	Sulphur Springs	71%	300+
Lake Pointe Medical Center	Rowlett	71%	300+
Matagorda Regional Medical Center	Bay City	71%	(a)
Medical Center of Mckinney	Mckinney	71%	300+
Memorial Hermann Northeast	Humble	71%	300+
Nacogdoches Medical Center	Nacogdoches	71%	300+
Nix Health Care System	San Antonio	71%	300+
North Texas Medical Center	Gainesville	71%	(a)
Saint Luke's Patients Medical Center	Pasadena	71%	300+
Saint Marks Medical Center	La Grange	71%	(a)
Scott & White Memorial Hospital[11]	Temple	71%	300+
Texas Reg Med Ctr at Sunnyvale	Sunnyvale	71%	300+
Univ of Texas Med Branch Galveston	Galveston	71%	300+
Centennial Medical Center	Frisco	70%	300+
Citizens Medical Center	Victoria	70%	300+
Columbus Community Hospital	Columbus	70%	(a)
Cornerstone Regional Hospital	Edinburg	70%	(a)
Good Shepherd Medical Center - Linden	Linden	70%	(a)
Medical Center Hospital	Odessa	70%	300+
Metroplex Hospital[11]	Killeen	70%	300+
Odessa Regional Hospital	Odessa	70%	300+
Plaza Medical Center of Fort Worth	Fort Worth	70%	300+
Texas Health Arlington Memorial Hospital	Arlington	70%	300+
University Health System	San Antonio	70%	300+
VHS Harlingen Hospital Company[11]	Harlingen	70%	300+
Weatherford Regional Medical Center	Weatherford	70%	300+
Angleton - Danbury Medical Center	Angleton	69%	300+
Baylor Medical Center at Garland	Garland	69%	300+
Christus Hospital	Beaumont	69%	300+
Christus Spohn Hospital Corpus Christi	Corpus Christi	69%	300+
Connally Memorial Medical Center	Floresville	69%	(a)
Cypress Fairbanks Medical Center	Houston	69%	300+
Etmc Henderson	Henderson	69%	300+
Harris Health System	Houston	69%	300+
Laredo Medical Center	Laredo	69%	300+
Medical Center of Plano	Plano	69%	300+
Methodist Charlton Medical Center	Dallas	69%	300+
Methodist Hospital	San Antonio	69%	300+
North Hills Hospital	N Richland Hls	69%	300+
Northwest Texas Hospital	Amarillo	69%	300+
Peterson Regional Medical Center	Kerrville	69%	300+
Seton Northwest Hospital	Austin	69%	300+
South Texas Health System	Edinburg	69%	300+
Wadley Regional Medical Center	Texarkana	69%	300+
Baylor Surgical Hospital at Fort Worth	Fort Worth	68%	300+
Covenant Hospital Plainview	Plainview	68%	300+
Denton Regional Medical Center	Denton	68%	300+
East Texas Medical Center	Tyler	68%	300+
Las Colinas Medical Center	Irving	68%	300+
The Medical Center of Southeast Texas	Port Arthur	68%	300+
Methodist Richardson Medical Center	Richardson	68%	300+

NOTE: Hospital profiles are in alphabetical order by state, then city, then hospital within the city; Rankings exclude hospitals with less than 25 cases except for patient surveys which excludes hospitals with less than 100 cases; (a) 100-299 cases; (1) The number of cases/patients is too few to report; (2) Data submitted were based on a sample of cases/patients; (3) Results are based on a shorter time period than required; (4) Data suppressed by CMS for one or more quarters; (5) Results are not available for this reporting period; (6) Fewer than 100 patients completed the HCAHPS survey; (7) No cases met the criteria for this measure; (8) The lower limit of the confidence interval cannot be calculated if the number of observed infections equals zero; (9) No data are available from the state/territory for this reporting period; (10) The scores shown reflect fewer than 50 completed surveys; (11) There were discrepancies in the data collection process; (12) This measure does not apply to this hospital for this reporting period; (13) Results cannot be calculated for this reporting period; (14) The results for this state are combined with nearby states to protect confidentiality; Please refer to the User's Guide for a full explanation of data.

Oakbend Medical Center	Richmond	68%	300+
Palo Pinto General Hospital	Mineral Wells	68%	300+
Providence Memorial Hospital	El Paso	68%	300+
Scott & White Hospital Brenham	Brenham	68%	300+
Titus Regional Medical Center	Mount Pleasant	68%	300+
Valley Regional Medical Center	Brownsville	68%	300+
Abilene Regional Medical Center	Abilene	67%	300+
Baylor Medical Center at Carrollton	Carrollton	67%	300+
Coryell Memorial Healthcare System	Gatesville	67%	(a)
Doctors Hospital	Dallas	67%	300+
Good Shepherd Medical Center Marshall	Marshall	67%	300+
Huguley Memorial Medical Center[11]	Burleson	67%	300+
Las Palmas Medical Center	El Paso	67%	300+
Medical Center of Arlington	Arlington	67%	300+
Parkland Health & Hospital System	Dallas	67%	300+
Saint Anthony's Hospital	Houston	67%	(a)
Tyler County Hospital	Woodville	67%	(a)
University General Hospital	Houston	67%	300+
Clear Lake Regional Medical Center	Webster	66%	300+
Conroe Regional Medical Center	Conroe	66%	300+
Knapp Medical Center	Weslaco	66%	300+
Memorial Medical Center Livingston	Livingston	66%	300+
South Texas Regional Medical Center	Jourdanton	66%	(a)
Tomball Regional Medical Center	Tomball	66%	300+
Cedar Park Regional Medical Center	Cedar Park	65%	300+
Christus Spohn Hospital Beeville	Beeville	65%	(a)
East Texas Medical Center Athens	Athens	65%	300+
Ennis Regional Medical Center	Ennis	65%	(a)
Hunt Regional Medical Center	Greenville	65%	300+
Lake Granbury Medical Center	Granbury	65%	300+
Memorial Hospital	Nacogdoches	65%	300+
Starr County Memorial Hospital	Rio Grande City	65%	(a)
Care Regional Medical Center	Aransas Pass	64%	(a)
East Texas Medical Center Crockett	Crockett	64%	(a)
Fort Duncan Medical Center	Eagle Pass	64%	300+
Hereford Regional Medical Center	Hereford	64%	(a)
Houston Northwest Medical Center	Houston	64%	300+
Kingwood Medical Center	Kingwood	64%	300+
Midland Memorial Hospital	Midland	64%	300+
Pampa Regional Medical Center	Pampa	64%	300+
Saint Joseph Medical Center	Houston	64%	300+
Scott & White Hospital - Llano	Llano	64%	(a)
Texas Health Presbyterian Hospital - WNJ	Sherman	64%	300+
Brownfield Regional Medical Center	Brownfield	63%	(a)
Brownwood Regional Medical Center	Brownwood	63%	300+
Doctors Hospital Tidwell	Houston	63%	300+
Etmc Carthage	Carthage	63%	(a)
Memorial Medical Center	Port Lavaca	63%	(a)
Sierra Medical Center	El Paso	63%	300+
Bayshore Medical Center	Pasadena	62%	300+
Christus Spohn Hospital Kleberg	Kingsville	62%	300+
Etmc Clarksville	Clarksville	62%	(a)
Navarro Regional Hospital	Corsicana	62%	300+
Permian Regional Medical Center	Andrews	62%	(a)
West Houston Medical Center	Houston	62%	300+
Christus Jasper Memorial Hospital	Jasper	60%	(a)
Huntsville Memorial Hospital	Huntsville	60%	(a)
Palestine Regional Medical Center	Palestine	60%	300+
Southwest General Hospital	San Antonio	60%	300+
Scenic Mountain Medical Center	Big Spring	59%	300+
Brazosport Regional Health System	Lake Jackson	58%	300+
Val Verde Regional Medical Center	Del Rio	58%	300+
University General Hospital Dallas	Dallas	57%	(a)
Lake Whitney Medical Center[11]	Whitney	55%	(a)
Dallas Regional Medical Center	Mesquite	52%	300+
Paris Regional Medical Center	Paris	50%	300+
Dallas Medical Center	Dallas	45%	300+

Meds 'Always' Explained Before Given

Hospital Name	City	Rate	Cases
Heritage Park Surgical Hospital	Sherman	86%	(a)
Sugar Land Surgical Hospital	Sugar Land	85%	(a)
East Texas Medical Center - Gilmer	Gilmer	83%	(a)
The Physicians Centre	Bryan	83%	(a)
Tyler County Hospital	Woodville	82%	(a)
Parkview Regional Hospital	Mexia	80%	(a)
Rollins Brook Community Hospital[11]	Lampasas	80%	(a)
TX Hlth Harris Meth Hosp-Southlake	Southlake	79%	300+
USMD Hospital at Fort Worth	Fort Worth	79%	(a)
Falls Community Hospital & Clinic	Marlin	78%	(a)
Hill Country Memorial Hospital	Fredericksburg	78%	300+
Quail Creek Surgical Hospital	Amarillo	78%	300+
Texas Spine & Joint Hospital	Tyler	78%	300+
Baylor Medical Center at Uptown	Dallas	77%	300+
Seton Edgar B Davis Hospital	Luling	76%	(a)
South Texas Spine & Surgical Hospital	San Antonio	76%	300+
W J Mangold Memorial Hospital	Lockney	76%	(a)
Big Bend Regional Medical Center	Alpine	75%	(a)
Childress Regional Medical Center	Childress	75%	(a)
North Central Surgical Center	Dallas	75%	300+
Northwest Hills Surgical Hospital	Austin	75%	(a)
South Texas Surgical Hospital	Corpus Christi	75%	300+
TX Hlth Presbyterian Hosp-Kaufman	Kaufman	75%	300+
East Texas Medical Center Pittsburg	Pittsburg	74%	(a)
Eastland Memorial Hospital	Eastland	74%	(a)
Kell West Regional Hospital	Wichita Falls	74%	(a)
Memorial Hermann Baptist Orange Hospital	Orange	74%	300+
TX Hlth Harris Meth Hosp-Stephenville	Stephenville	74%	300+
Baylor Ortho & Spine Hosp-Arlington	Arlington	73%	300+
Hamilton General Hospital	Hamilton	73%	(a)
Rolling Plains Memorial Hospital	Sweetwater	73%	(a)
TX Health Ctr for Diag & Surgery	Plano	73%	(a)
University Medical Center	Lubbock	73%	300+
Baylor Heart & Vascular Hospital	Dallas	72%	300+
East Texas Medical Center Quitman	Quitman	72%	(a)
Fdn Surgical Hosp of San Antonio	San Antonio	72%	300+
Houston Physicians' Hospital	Webster	72%	(a)
Uvalde Memorial Hospital[11]	Uvalde	72%	(a)
Electra Memorial Hospital	Electra	71%	(a)
Glen Rose Medical Center	Glen Rose	71%	(a)
Heart Hospital Baylor Plano	Plano	71%	300+
Scott & White Hospital - Llano	Llano	71%	(a)
TX Inst for Surgery at Presby Hosp	Dallas	71%	(a)
Tops Surgical Specialty Hospital	Houston	71%	(a)
USMD Hospital at Arlington	Arlington	71%	300+
UT SW Univ Hosp-Zale Lipshy	Dallas	71%	300+
Baylor Surgical Hospital at Las Colinas	Irving	70%	(a)
Good Shephard Medical Center - Linden	Linden	70%	(a)
Memorial Medical Center	Port Lavaca	70%	(a)
Methodist Ambulatory Surgery Hospital NW	San Antonio	70%	(a)
Saint Anthony's Hospital	Houston	70%	(a)
Saint Luke's Lakeside Hospital	The Woodlands	70%	300+
Baptist Beaumont Hospital	Beaumont	69%	300+
Baylor Medical Center at Frisco	Frisco	69%	300+
Baylor Medical Center at Trophy Club	Trophy Club	69%	(a)
Hill Regional Hospital	Hillsboro	69%	300+
The Hospital at Westlake Medical Center	Austin	69%	(a)
Methodist Richardson Medical Center	Richardson	69%	300+
North Texas Medical Center	Gainesville	69%	(a)
Saint Marks Medical Center	La Grange	69%	(a)
Starr County Memorial Hospital	Rio Grande City	69%	(a)
Univ of TX Health Science Ctr-Tyler	Tyler	69%	(a)
Baylor Medical Center at Waxahachie	Waxahachie	68%	300+
Care Regional Medical Center	Aransas Pass	68%	(a)
Covenant Hospital Plainview	Plainview	68%	300+
East Texas Medical Center Jacksonville	Jacksonville	68%	300+
Houston Orthopedic & Spine Hospital	Bellaire	68%	300+
Mem Hermann Mem City Med Ctr	Houston	68%	300+
Moore County Hospital District	Dumas	68%	(a)
Nacogdoches Medical Center	Nacogdoches	68%	300+
Odessa Regional Hospital	Odessa	68%	300+
Park Plaza Hospital	Houston	68%	300+
Saint David's South Austin Medical Center	Austin	68%	300+
Saint Joseph Regional Health Center	Bryan	68%	300+
Seton Highland Lakes	Burnet	68%	300+
TX Hlth Harris Meth Hosp-Cleburne	Cleburne	68%	300+
University General Hospital Dallas	Dallas	68%	(a)
Baylor University Medical Center	Dallas	67%	300+
Brownwood Regional Medical Center	Brownwood	67%	300+
Christus Saint Michael Health System	Texarkana	67%	300+
Christus Spohn Hospital Alice	Alice	67%	300+
Christus Spohn Hospital Beeville	Beeville	67%	(a)
Coryell Memorial Healthcare System	Gatesville	67%	(a)
Covenant Medical Center	Lubbock	67%	300+
Etmc Carthage	Carthage	67%	(a)
Etmc Henderson	Henderson	67%	300+
Medina Regional Hospital	Hondo	67%	(a)
Methodist Hospital For Surgery	Addison	67%	300+
Methodist Mckinney Hospital	Mc Kinney	67%	(a)
Pine Creek Medical Center	Dallas	67%	300+
Round Rock Medical Center	Round Rock	67%	300+
San Angelo Community Medical Center	San Angelo	67%	300+
Scott & White Hospital Brenham	Brenham	67%	300+
Shannon Medical Center	San Angelo	67%	300+
Texas Health Harris Methodist	Bedford	67%	300+
Woodland Heights Medical Center	Lufkin	67%	300+
Abilene Regional Medical Center	Abilene	66%	300+
Angleton - Danbury Medical Center	Angleton	66%	300+
Arise Austin Medical Center[3]	Austin	66%	(a)
Baylor Medical Center at Garland	Garland	66%	300+
Baylor Surgical Hospital at Fort Worth	Fort Worth	66%	300+
College Station Medical Center	College Station	66%	300+
Fort Duncan Medical Center	Eagle Pass	66%	300+
Good Shepherd Medical Center	Longview	66%	300+
Graham Regional Medical Center	Graham	66%	(a)
Hereford Regional Medical Center	Hereford	66%	(a)
Hopkins County Memorial Hospital	Sulphur Springs	66%	300+
Methodist Dallas Medical Center	Dallas	66%	300+
Methodist Sugar Land Hospital	Sugar Land	66%	300+
Metroplex Hospital[11]	Killeen	66%	300+
Northwest Texas Hospital	Amarillo	66%	300+
Pecos County Memorial Hospital	Fort Stockton	66%	(a)
Providence Memorial Hospital	El Paso	66%	300+
Saint David's Medical Center	Austin	66%	300+
Seton Medical Center Harker Heights	Harker Heights	66%	300+
Seton Medical Center Williamson	Round Rock	66%	300+
TX Hlth Harris Methodist Hosp-Azle	Azle	66%	300+
TX Hlth Presbyterian Hosp-Flower Mound	Flower Mound	66%	300+
Texas Health Presbyterian Hospital Plano	Plano	66%	300+
Titus Regional Medical Center	Mount Pleasant	66%	300+
Univ of Texas Med Branch Galveston	Galveston	66%	300+
UT Southwestern University Hospital	Dallas	66%	300+
Basin Healthcare Center	Odessa	65%	(a)
Baylor Reg Med Ctr at Grapevine	Grapevine	65%	300+
Christus Hospital	Beaumont	65%	300+
Christus Jasper Memorial Hospital	Jasper	65%	(a)
Christus Spohn Hospital Kleberg	Kingsville	65%	300+
Detar Hospital Navarro	Victoria	65%	300+
First Surgical Hospital	Bellaire	65%	(a)
Grace Medical Center	Lubbock	65%	300+
Lubbock Heart Hospital	Lubbock	65%	300+
Medical Center of Lewisville	Lewisville	65%	300+
Medical Center of Mckinney	Mckinney	65%	300+
Mission Regional Medical Center	Mission	65%	300+
North Austin Medical Center	Austin	65%	300+
Providence Health Center	Waco	65%	300+
San Jacinto Methodist Hospital	Baytown	65%	300+
Scott & White Hospital - Round Rock	Round Rock	65%	300+
Seton Medical Center Hays	Kyle	65%	300+
Texas Health Harris Methodist Fort Worth	Fort Worth	65%	300+
TX Hlth Harris Meth Hosp SW Ft Worth	Fort Worth	65%	300+
Texas Health Presbyterian Hospital Allen	Allen	65%	300+
Texoma Medical Center	Denison	65%	300+
University Medical Center of El Paso	El Paso	65%	300+
Brownfield Regional Medical Center	Brownfield	64%	(a)
Central Texas Medical Center[11]	San Marcos	64%	300+
Conroe Regional Medical Center	Conroe	64%	300+
Covenant Hospital Levelland	Levelland	64%	(a)
Doctors Hospital of Laredo	Laredo	64%	300+
Ennis Regional Medical Center	Ennis	64%	300+
Harlingen Medical Center[11]	Harlingen	64%	300+
Hendrick Medical Center	Abilene	64%	300+
Hunt Regional Medical Center	Greenville	64%	300+
Huntsville Memorial Hospital	Huntsville	64%	(a)
Knapp Medical Center	Weslaco	64%	300+
Longview Regional Medical Center	Longview	64%	300+
Memorial Hermann Katy Hospital	Katy	64%	300+
Memorial Medical Center Livingston	Livingston	64%	300+
Memorial Medical Center of East Texas	Lufkin	64%	300+
The Methodist Hospital	Houston	64%	300+
Methodist Mansfield Medical Center	Mansfield	64%	300+
Navarro Regional Hospital	Corsicana	64%	300+
Seton Medical Center Austin	Austin	64%	300+
Sierra Providence East Medical Center	El Paso	64%	300+
Texas Health Presbyterian Hospital Denton	Denton	64%	300+
TX Health Presbyterian Hosp Rockwall	Rockwall	64%	300+
University Medical Center at Brackenridge	Austin	64%	300+
VHS Brownsville Hospital Company[11]	Brownsville	64%	300+
VHS Harlingen Hospital Company[11]	Harlingen	64%	300+
Wise Regional Health System	Decatur	64%	300+
Baptist Emergency Hospital	San Antonio	63%	(a)
Baptist Saint Anthony's Hospital	Amarillo	63%	300+
Baylor All Saints Medical Center at FW	Fort Worth	63%	300+
Baylor Medical Center at Mckinney	Mc Kinney	63%	300+
Brazosport Regional Health System	Lake Jackson	63%	300+
Christus Saint Catherine Hospital	Katy	63%	300+
Cornerstone Regional Hospital	Edinburg	63%	(a)
Cuero Community Hospital	Cuero	63%	(a)
Doctors Hospital at Renaissance	Edinburg	63%	300+
Guadalupe Regional Medical Center	Seguin	63%	300+
Harris Health System	Houston	63%	300+
Las Palmas Medical Center	El Paso	63%	300+
Matagorda Regional Medical Center	Bay City	63%	(a)
Memorial Hermann Northeast	Humble	63%	300+
Memorial Hermann Texas Medical Center	Houston	63%	300+
Methodist West Houston Hospital	Houston	63%	300+
Mother Frances Hospital	Tyler	63%	300+
Nix Health Care System	San Antonio	63%	300+
Plaza Medical Center of Fort Worth	Fort Worth	63%	300+
Saint Luke's Episcopal Hospital	Houston	63%	300+
Saint Luke's Sugar Land Hospital	Sugar Land	63%	300+
Scott & White Memorial Hospital[11]	Temple	63%	300+
Seton Southwest Hospital	Austin	63%	(a)
South Texas Regional Medical Center	Jourdanton	63%	(a)
TX Hlth Heart & Vasc Hosp-Arlington	Arlington	63%	300+
United Regional Health Care System	Wichita Falls	63%	300+
Val Verde Regional Medical Center	Del Rio	63%	300+
Wadley Regional Medical Center	Texarkana	63%	300+
Baylor Regional Medical Center at Plano	Plano	62%	300+
Christus Spohn Hospital Corpus Christi	Corpus Christi	62%	300+
Citizens Medical Center	Victoria	62%	300+
Clear Lake Regional Medical Center	Webster	62%	300+
East Texas Medical Center Crockett	Crockett	62%	(a)

NOTE: Hospital profiles are in alphabetical order by state, then city, then hospital within the city; Rankings exclude hospitals with less than 25 cases except for patient surveys which excludes hospitals with less than 100 cases; (a) 100-299 cases; (1) The number of cases/patients is too few to report; (2) Data submitted were based on a sample of cases/patients; (3) Results are based on a shorter time period than required; (4) Data suppressed by CMS for one or more quarters; (5) Results are not available for this reporting period; (6) Fewer than 100 patients completed the HCAHPS survey; (7) No cases met the criteria for this measure; (8) The lower limit of the confidence interval cannot be calculated if the number of observed infections equals zero; (9) No data are available from the state/territory for this reporting period; (10) The scores shown reflect fewer than 50 completed surveys; (11) There were discrepancies in the data collection process; (12) This measure does not apply to this hospital for this reporting period; (13) Results cannot be calculated for this reporting period; (14) The results for this state are combined with nearby states to protect confidentiality; Please refer to the User's Guide for a full explanation of data.

Lake Pointe Medical Center	Rowlett	62%	300+
Medical City Dallas Hospital	Dallas	62%	300+
Memorial Hermann Sugar Land Hospital	Sugar Land	62%	300+
Memorial Hospital	Nacogdoches	62%	300+
Methodist Hospital	San Antonio	62%	300+
Methodist Willowbrook Hospital	Houston	62%	300+
North Cypress Medical Center	Cypress	62%	300+
Parkland Health & Hospital System	Dallas	62%	300+
Peterson Regional Medical Center	Kerrville	62%	300+
Texas Reg Med Ctr at Sunnyvale	Sunnyvale	62%	300+
University Health System	San Antonio	62%	300+
Weatherford Regional Medical Center	Weatherford	62%	300+
The Womans Hospital of Texas	Houston	62%	300+
Baptist Medical Center[11]	San Antonio	61%	300+
Christus Santa Rosa Hospital	San Antonio	61%	300+
Columbus Community Hospital	Columbus	61%	(a)
Connally Memorial Medical Center	Floresville	61%	(a)
The Corpus Christi Medical Center	Corpus Christi	61%	300+
Denton Regional Medical Center	Denton	61%	300+
East Texas Medical Center	Tyler	61%	300+
East Texas Medical Center Athens	Athens	61%	300+
Hillcrest Baptist Medical Center	Waco	61%	300+
Huguley Memorial Medical Center[11]	Burleson	61%	300+
JPS Health Network	Fort Worth	61%	300+
Las Colinas Medical Center	Irving	61%	300+
The Medical Center of Southeast Texas	Port Arthur	61%	300+
Memorial Hermann Hospital System	Houston	61%	300+
Permian Regional Medical Center	Andrews	61%	(a)
Rio Grande Regional Hospital	Mcallen	61%	300+
South Texas Health System	Edinburg	61%	300+
Texas Health Arlington Memorial Hospital	Arlington	61%	300+
Texas Health Presbyterian Hospital Dallas	Dallas	61%	300+
Texas Orthopedic Hospital	Houston	61%	300+
Valley Regional Medical Center	Brownsville	61%	300+
Yoakum Community Hospital	Yoakum	61%	(a)
Baylor Medical Center at Irving	Irving	60%	300+
Cedar Park Regional Medical Center	Cedar Park	60%	300+
Doctors Hospital	Dallas	60%	300+
El Paso Specialty Hospital	El Paso	60%	(a)
Etmc Clarksville	Clarksville	60%	(a)
Foundation Surgical Hospital of El Paso	El Paso	60%	300+
Lake Granbury Medical Center	Granbury	60%	300+
Laredo Medical Center	Laredo	60%	300+
Medical Center Hospital	Odessa	60%	300+
Medical Center of Plano	Plano	60%	300+
Methodist Charlton Medical Center	Dallas	60%	300+
Oakbend Medical Center	Richmond	60%	300+
Saint Joseph Medical Center	Houston	60%	300+
Seton Northwest Hospital	Austin	60%	300+
Centennial Medical Center	Frisco	59%	300+
Cypress Fairbanks Medical Center	Houston	59%	300+
Medical Center of Arlington	Arlington	59%	300+
Methodist Stone Oak Hospital	San Antonio	59%	300+
Saint Luke's the Woodlands Hospital	The Woodlands	59%	300+
Tomball Regional Medical Center	Tomball	59%	300+
Baylor Medical Center at Carrollton	Carrollton	58%	300+
Christus Saint John Hospital	Nassau Bay	58%	300+
Lake Whitney Medical Center[11]	Whitney	58%	(a)
Palo Pinto General Hospital	Mineral Wells	58%	300+
Saint Luke's Patients Medical Center	Pasadena	58%	300+
Scenic Mountain Medical Center	Big Spring	58%	300+
Sierra Medical Center	El Paso	58%	300+
Southwest General Hospital	San Antonio	58%	300+
Doctors Hospital Tidwell	Houston	57%	300+
Houston Northwest Medical Center	Houston	57%	300+
Kingwood Medical Center	Kingwood	57%	300+
Palestine Regional Medical Center	Palestine	57%	300+
Saint Luke's Hospital at the Vintage	Houston	57%	300+
Texas Health Presbyterian Hospital - WNJ	Sherman	57%	300+
Bayshore Medical Center	Pasadena	56%	300+
North Hills Hospital	N Richland Hls	56%	300+
Paris Regional Medical Center	Paris	56%	300+
Good Shepherd Medical Center Marshall	Marshall	55%	300+
University General Hospital	Houston	55%	300+
Midland Memorial Hospital	Midland	54%	300+
West Houston Medical Center	Houston	54%	300+
Pampa Regional Medical Center	Pampa	53%	300+
Dallas Regional Medical Center	Mesquite	47%	300+
Dallas Medical Center	Dallas	43%	300+

Nurses 'Always' Communicated Well

Hospital Name	City	Rate	Cases
Sugar Land Surgical Hospital	Sugar Land	95%	(a)
The Physicians Centre	Bryan	94%	(a)
Heritage Park Surgical Hospital	Sherman	93%	(a)
Quail Creek Surgical Hospital	Amarillo	93%	300+
W J Mangold Memorial Hospital	Lockney	92%	(a)
Tyler County Hospital	Woodville	91%	(a)
Baylor Medical Center at Uptown	Dallas	90%	300+
USMD Hospital at Fort Worth	Fort Worth	90%	(a)
Hill Country Memorial Hospital	Fredericksburg	89%	300+
Northwest Hills Surgical Hospital	Austin	89%	(a)
Rollins Brook Community Hospital[11]	Lampasas	89%	(a)
TX Health Ctr for Diag & Surgery	Plano	89%	(a)
Baylor Ortho & Spine Hosp-Arlington	Arlington	88%	300+
East Texas Medical Center - Gilmer	Gilmer	88%	(a)
North Central Surgical Center	Dallas	88%	300+
TX Hlth Harris Meth Hosp-Southlake	Southlake	88%	300+
Baptist Emergency Hospital	San Antonio	87%	(a)
Baylor Heart & Vascular Hospital	Dallas	87%	300+
Baylor Medical Center at Frisco	Frisco	87%	300+
Electra Memorial Hospital	Electra	87%	(a)
South Texas Surgical Hospital	Corpus Christi	87%	300+
Texas Spine & Joint Hospital	Tyler	87%	300+
Baylor Medical Center at Trophy Club	Trophy Club	86%	(a)
East Texas Medical Center Pittsburg	Pittsburg	86%	(a)
East Texas Medical Center Quitman	Quitman	86%	(a)
Falls Community Hospital & Clinic	Marlin	86%	(a)
Heart Hospital Baylor Plano	Plano	86%	300+
Houston Physicians' Hospital	Webster	86%	(a)
South Texas Spine & Surgical Hospital	San Antonio	86%	300+
Tops Surgical Specialty Hospital	Houston	86%	(a)
Yoakum Community Hospital	Yoakum	86%	(a)
Childress Regional Medical Center	Childress	85%	(a)
Fdn Surgical Hosp of San Antonio	San Antonio	85%	300+
Glen Rose Medical Center	Glen Rose	85%	(a)
Parkview Regional Hospital	Mexia	85%	(a)
Seton Edgar B Davis Hospital	Luling	85%	(a)
TX Hlth Presbyterian Hosp-Kaufman	Kaufman	85%	300+
Big Bend Regional Medical Center	Alpine	84%	(a)
Memorial Hermann Baptist Orange Hospital	Orange	84%	300+
Rolling Plains Memorial Hospital	Sweetwater	84%	(a)
Saint Luke's Lakeside Hospital	The Woodlands	84%	300+
TX Hlth Harris Meth Hosp-Cleburne	Cleburne	84%	300+
TX Hlth Harris Meth Hosp-Stephenville	Stephenville	84%	300+
USMD Hospital at Arlington	Arlington	84%	300+
UT SW Univ Hosp-Zale Lipshy	Dallas	84%	300+
Eastland Memorial Hospital	Eastland	83%	(a)
First Surgical Hospital	Bellaire	83%	(a)
Hendrick Medical Center	Abilene	83%	300+
Houston Orthopedic & Spine Hospital	Bellaire	83%	300+
Kell West Regional Hospital	Wichita Falls	83%	(a)
Methodist Ambulatory Surgery Hospital NW	San Antonio	83%	(a)
TX Inst for Surgery at Presby Hosp	Dallas	83%	(a)
United Regional Health Care System	Wichita Falls	83%	300+
Uvalde Memorial Hospital[11]	Uvalde	83%	(a)
Baylor Medical Center at Waxahachie	Waxahachie	82%	300+
Baylor Surgical Hospital at Las Colinas	Irving	82%	(a)
Cornerstone Regional Hospital	Edinburg	82%	(a)
Covenant Hospital Levelland	Levelland	82%	(a)
Hopkins County Memorial Hospital	Sulphur Springs	82%	300+
Lubbock Heart Hospital	Lubbock	82%	300+
Memorial Medical Center	Port Lavaca	82%	(a)
Pecos County Memorial Hospital	Fort Stockton	82%	(a)
Starr County Memorial Hospital	Rio Grande City	82%	(a)
University Medical Center	Lubbock	82%	300+
UT Southwestern University Hospital	Dallas	82%	300+
Brownfield Regional Medical Center	Brownfield	81%	(a)
Christus Hospital	Beaumont	81%	300+
Christus Saint Michael Health System	Texarkana	81%	300+
Christus Spohn Hospital Alice	Alice	81%	300+
Coryell Memorial Healthcare System	Gatesville	81%	(a)
East Texas Medical Center Crockett	Crockett	81%	(a)
East Texas Medical Center Jacksonville	Jacksonville	81%	300+
Medina Regional Hospital	Hondo	81%	(a)
Methodist Mansfield Medical Center	Mansfield	81%	300+
Methodist Mckinney Hospital	Mc Kinney	81%	(a)
Moore County Hospital District	Dumas	81%	(a)
Nacogdoches Medical Center	Nacogdoches	81%	300+
Saint Joseph Regional Health Center	Bryan	81%	300+
San Jacinto Methodist Hospital	Baytown	81%	300+
Seton Highland Lakes	Burnet	81%	300+
Seton Medical Center Harker Heights	Harker Heights	81%	300+
Seton Southwest Hospital	Austin	81%	(a)
Shannon Medical Center	San Angelo	81%	300+
TX Hlth Heart & Vasc Hosp-Arlington	Arlington	81%	300+
TX Hlth Presbyterian Hosp-Flower Mound	Flower Mound	81%	300+
Texas Health Presbyterian Hospital Plano	Plano	81%	300+
Titus Regional Medical Center	Mount Pleasant	81%	300+
Woodland Heights Medical Center	Lufkin	81%	300+
Baptist Beaumont Hospital	Beaumont	80%	300+
Basin Healthcare Center	Odessa	80%	(a)
Baylor Medical Center at Mckinney	Mc Kinney	80%	300+
Central Texas Medical Center[11]	San Marcos	80%	300+
Columbus Community Hospital	Columbus	80%	(a)
Connally Memorial Medical Center	Floresville	80%	(a)
Covenant Medical Center	Lubbock	80%	300+
Good Shephard Medical Center - Linden	Linden	80%	(a)
Graham Regional Medical Center	Graham	80%	(a)
Guadalupe Regional Medical Center	Seguin	80%	300+
Hamilton General Hospital	Hamilton	80%	(a)
Hunt Regional Medical Center	Greenville	80%	300+
Lake Pointe Medical Center	Rowlett	80%	300+
Matagorda Regional Medical Center	Bay City	80%	(a)
Memorial Hermann Northeast	Humble	80%	300+
Methodist Hospital For Surgery	Addison	80%	300+
Metroplex Hospital[11]	Killeen	80%	300+
Saint David's Medical Center	Austin	80%	300+
Saint David's South Austin Medical Center	Austin	80%	300+
Saint Marks Medical Center	La Grange	80%	(a)
San Angelo Community Medical Center	San Angelo	80%	300+
Texas Health Harris Methodist Fort Worth	Fort Worth	80%	300+
TX Hlth Harris Methodist Hosp-Azle	Azle	80%	300+
TX Hlth Harris Meth Hosp SW Ft Worth	Fort Worth	80%	300+
TX Health Presbyterian Hosp Rockwall	Rockwall	80%	300+
Wadley Regional Medical Center	Texarkana	80%	300+
Baylor All Saints Medical Center at FW	Fort Worth	79%	300+
Baylor Reg Med Ctr at Grapevine	Grapevine	79%	300+
Baylor Regional Medical Center at Plano	Plano	79%	300+
Christus Spohn Hospital Beeville	Beeville	79%	(a)
Etmc Clarksville	Clarksville	79%	(a)
Etmc Henderson	Henderson	79%	300+
Hill Regional Hospital	Hillsboro	79%	300+
Medical Center of Mckinney	Mckinney	79%	300+
Memorial Hermann Hospital System	Houston	79%	300+
Methodist West Houston Hospital	Houston	79%	300+
Mission Regional Medical Center	Mission	79%	300+
North Texas Medical Center	Gainesville	79%	(a)
Palo Pinto General Hospital	Mineral Wells	79%	300+
Providence Health Center	Waco	79%	300+
Texas Health Harris Methodist	Bedford	79%	300+
Texas Health Presbyterian Hospital Allen	Allen	79%	300+
Wise Regional Health System	Decatur	79%	300+
Angleton - Danbury Medical Center	Angleton	78%	300+
Baptist Saint Anthony's Hospital	Amarillo	78%	300+
Baylor Medical Center at Garland	Garland	78%	300+
Baylor University Medical Center	Dallas	78%	300+
Care Regional Medical Center	Aransas Pass	78%	(a)
Christus Santa Rosa Hospital	San Antonio	78%	300+
Christus Spohn Hospital Kleberg	Kingsville	78%	300+
Citizens Medical Center	Victoria	78%	300+
College Station Medical Center	College Station	78%	300+
Covenant Hospital Plainview	Plainview	78%	300+
Detar Hospital Navarro	Victoria	78%	300+
Good Shepherd Medical Center	Longview	78%	300+
The Hospital at Westlake Medical Center	Austin	78%	300+
Huguley Memorial Medical Center[11]	Burleson	78%	300+
Longview Regional Medical Center	Longview	78%	300+
Memorial Hermann Katy Hospital	Katy	78%	300+
Methodist Dallas Medical Center	Dallas	78%	300+
Methodist Sugar Land Hospital	Sugar Land	78%	300+
Park Plaza Hospital	Houston	78%	300+
Round Rock Medical Center	Round Rock	78%	300+
Saint Anthony's Hospital	Houston	78%	(a)
Saint Luke's the Woodlands Hospital	The Woodlands	78%	300+
Scott & White Hospital - Llano	Llano	78%	(a)
Scott & White Hospital - Round Rock	Round Rock	78%	300+
Texoma Medical Center	Denison	78%	300+
Univ of Texas Med Branch Galveston	Galveston	78%	300+
Weatherford Regional Medical Center	Weatherford	78%	300+
Arise Austin Medical Center[3]	Austin	77%	(a)
Baptist Medical Center[11]	San Antonio	77%	300+
Baylor Medical Center at Irving	Irving	77%	300+
Brownwood Regional Medical Center	Brownwood	77%	300+
Christus Saint Catherine Hospital	Katy	77%	300+
Cuero Community Hospital	Cuero	77%	(a)
Doctors Hospital of Laredo	Laredo	77%	300+
Foundation Surgical Hospital of El Paso	El Paso	77%	300+
Huntsville Memorial Hospital	Huntsville	77%	(a)
JPS Health Network	Fort Worth	77%	300+
Medical Center of Lewisville	Lewisville	77%	300+
Medical City Dallas Hospital	Dallas	77%	300+
Mem Hermann Mem City Med Ctr	Houston	77%	300+
Memorial Hermann Sugar Land Hospital	Sugar Land	77%	300+
Memorial Hermann Texas Medical Center	Houston	77%	300+
Memorial Hospital	Nacogdoches	77%	300+
Memorial Medical Center Livingston	Livingston	77%	300+
Memorial Medical Center of East Texas	Lufkin	77%	300+
The Methodist Hospital	Houston	77%	300+
Methodist Willowbrook Hospital	Houston	77%	300+
Mother Frances Hospital	Tyler	77%	300+
North Austin Medical Center	Austin	77%	300+
Northwest Texas Hospital	Amarillo	77%	300+
Permian Regional Medical Center	Andrews	77%	(a)
Pine Creek Medical Center	Dallas	77%	300+
Scott & White Hospital Brenham	Brenham	77%	300+
Scott & White Memorial Hospital[11]	Temple	77%	300+
Seton Medical Center Hays	Kyle	77%	300+
Seton Medical Center Williamson	Round Rock	77%	300+
Sierra Providence East Medical Center	El Paso	77%	300+
Texas Health Presbyterian Hospital Dallas	Dallas	77%	300+
Texas Health Presbyterian Hospital Denton	Denton	77%	300+
Texas Reg Med Ctr at Sunnyvale	Sunnyvale	77%	300+

NOTE: Hospital profiles are in alphabetical order by state, then city, then hospital within the city; Rankings exclude hospitals with less than 25 cases except for patient surveys which excludes hospitals with less than 100 cases; (a) 100-299 cases; (1) The number of cases/patients is too few to report; (2) Data submitted were based on a sample of cases/patients; (3) Results are based on a shorter time period than required; (4) Data suppressed by CMS for one or more quarters; (5) Results are not available for this reporting period; (6) Fewer than 100 patients completed the HCAHPS survey; (7) No cases met the criteria for this measure; (8) The lower limit of the confidence interval cannot be calculated if the number of observed infections equals zero; (9) No data are available from the state/territory for this reporting period; (10) The scores shown reflect fewer than 50 completed surveys; (11) There were discrepancies in the data collection process; (12) This measure does not apply to this hospital for this reporting period; (13) Results cannot be calculated for this reporting period; (14) The results for this state are combined with nearby states to protect confidentiality; Please refer to the User's Guide for a full explanation of data.

Hospital Name	City	Rate	Cases
University Medical Center of El Paso	El Paso	77%	300+
Univ of TX Health Science Ctr-Tyler	Tyler	77%	(a)
Val Verde Regional Medical Center	Del Rio	77%	300+
VHS Brownsville Hospital Company[11]	Brownsville	77%	300+
VHS Harlingen Hospital Company[11]	Harlingen	77%	300+
Abilene Regional Medical Center	Abilene	76%	300+
Baylor Surgical Hospital at Fort Worth	Fort Worth	76%	300+
Brazosport Regional Health System	Lake Jackson	76%	300+
Centennial Medical Center	Frisco	76%	300+
Christus Jasper Memorial Hospital	Jasper	76%	(a)
Christus Spohn Hospital Corpus Christi	Corpus Christi	76%	300+
Clear Lake Regional Medical Center	Webster	76%	300+
The Corpus Christi Medical Center	Corpus Christi	76%	300+
Doctors Hospital	Dallas	76%	300+
Doctors Hospital at Renaissance	Edinburg	76%	300+
East Texas Medical Center	Tyler	76%	300+
East Texas Medical Center Athens	Athens	76%	300+
Etmc Carthage	Carthage	76%	(a)
Grace Medical Center	Lubbock	76%	300+
Harlingen Medical Center[11]	Harlingen	76%	300+
Hillcrest Baptist Medical Center	Waco	76%	300+
Medical Center Hospital	Odessa	76%	300+
Methodist Charlton Medical Center	Dallas	76%	300+
Navarro Regional Hospital	Corsicana	76%	300+
Rio Grande Regional Hospital	Mcallen	76%	300+
Saint Luke's Episcopal Hospital	Houston	76%	300+
Seton Medical Center Austin	Austin	76%	300+
Seton Northwest Hospital	Austin	76%	300+
South Texas Regional Medical Center	Jourdanton	76%	(a)
Texas Health Arlington Memorial Hospital	Arlington	76%	300+
Texas Orthopedic Hospital	Houston	76%	300+
Christus Saint John Hospital	Nassau Bay	75%	300+
Denton Regional Medical Center	Denton	75%	300+
El Paso Specialty Hospital	El Paso	75%	(a)
Good Shepherd Medical Center Marshall	Marshall	75%	300+
Hereford Regional Medical Center	Hereford	75%	(a)
Knapp Medical Center	Weslaco	75%	300+
Las Colinas Medical Center	Irving	75%	300+
Las Palmas Medical Center	El Paso	75%	300+
Medical Center of Arlington	Arlington	75%	300+
Medical Center of Plano	Plano	75%	300+
The Medical Center of Southeast Texas	Port Arthur	75%	300+
Methodist Hospital	San Antonio	75%	300+
Methodist Richardson Medical Center	Richardson	75%	300+
North Cypress Medical Center	Cypress	75%	300+
Odessa Regional Hospital	Odessa	75%	300+
Peterson Regional Medical Center	Kerrville	75%	300+
Saint Joseph Medical Center	Houston	75%	300+
Saint Luke's Hospital at the Vintage	Houston	75%	300+
Saint Luke's Sugar Land Hospital	Sugar Land	75%	300+
Scenic Mountain Medical Center	Big Spring	75%	300+
Texas Health Presbyterian Hospital - WNJ	Sherman	75%	300+
Tomball Regional Medical Center	Tomball	75%	300+
University Medical Center at Brackenridge	Austin	75%	300+
Conroe Regional Medical Center	Conroe	74%	300+
Cypress Fairbanks Medical Center	Houston	74%	300+
Fort Duncan Medical Center	Eagle Pass	74%	300+
Harris Health System	Houston	74%	300+
Houston Northwest Medical Center	Houston	74%	300+
Lake Granbury Medical Center	Granbury	74%	300+
Methodist Stone Oak Hospital	San Antonio	74%	300+
Nix Health Care System	San Antonio	74%	300+
North Hills Hospital	N Richland Hls	74%	300+
Palestine Regional Medical Center	Palestine	74%	300+
Plaza Medical Center of Fort Worth	Fort Worth	74%	300+
Providence Memorial Hospital	El Paso	74%	300+
Saint Luke's Patients Medical Center	Pasadena	74%	300+
University General Hospital Dallas	Dallas	74%	(a)
Laredo Medical Center	Laredo	73%	300+
Pampa Regional Medical Center	Pampa	73%	300+
Sierra Medical Center	El Paso	73%	300+
South Texas Health System	Edinburg	73%	300+
Valley Regional Medical Center	Brownsville	73%	300+
The Womans Hospital of Texas	Houston	73%	300+
Baylor Medical Center at Carrollton	Carrollton	72%	300+
Bayshore Medical Center	Pasadena	72%	300+
Cedar Park Regional Medical Center	Cedar Park	72%	300+
Ennis Regional Medical Center	Ennis	72%	300+
Kingwood Medical Center	Kingwood	72%	300+
Midland Memorial Hospital	Midland	72%	300+
Oakbend Medical Center	Richmond	72%	300+
Paris Regional Medical Center	Paris	72%	300+
Parkland Health & Hospital System	Dallas	72%	300+
Southwest General Hospital	San Antonio	71%	300+
University Health System	San Antonio	71%	300+
West Houston Medical Center	Houston	71%	300+
Doctors Hospital Tidwell	Houston	70%	300+
Lake Whitney Medical Center[11]	Whitney	70%	(a)
University General Hospital	Houston	68%	300+
Dallas Regional Medical Center	Mesquite	66%	300+
Dallas Medical Center	Dallas	59%	300+

Pain 'Always' Well Controlled

Hospital Name	City	Rate	Cases
The Physicians Centre	Bryan	85%	(a)
Yoakum Community Hospital	Yoakum	84%	(a)
Falls Community Hospital & Clinic	Marlin	83%	(a)
Rollins Brook Community Hospital[11]	Lampasas	83%	(a)
Sugar Land Surgical Hospital	Sugar Land	83%	(a)
Baylor Medical Center at Trophy Club	Trophy Club	82%	(a)
Heritage Park Surgical Hospital	Sherman	82%	(a)
Quail Creek Surgical Hospital	Amarillo	82%	300+
Basin Healthcare Center	Odessa	81%	(a)
Eastland Memorial Hospital	Eastland	81%	(a)
Hill Country Memorial Hospital	Fredericksburg	81%	300+
USMD Hospital at Fort Worth	Fort Worth	81%	(a)
Baptist Emergency Hospital	San Antonio	80%	(a)
Baylor Medical Center at Frisco	Frisco	80%	300+
Baylor Ortho & Spine Hosp-Arlington	Arlington	80%	300+
Glen Rose Medical Center	Glen Rose	80%	(a)
Graham Regional Medical Center	Graham	80%	(a)
Heart Hospital Baylor Plano	Plano	80%	300+
Northwest Hills Surgical Hospital	Austin	80%	(a)
Pecos County Memorial Hospital	Fort Stockton	80%	(a)
South Texas Spine & Surgical Hospital	San Antonio	80%	300+
TX Hlth Harris Meth Hosp-Southlake	Southlake	80%	300+
Tops Surgical Specialty Hospital	Houston	80%	(a)
W J Mangold Memorial Hospital	Lockney	80%	(a)
Baylor Medical Center at Uptown	Dallas	79%	300+
Cuero Community Hospital	Cuero	79%	(a)
East Texas Medical Center - Gilmer	Gilmer	79%	(a)
East Texas Medical Center Quitman	Quitman	79%	(a)
Parkview Regional Hospital	Mexia	79%	(a)
South Texas Surgical Hospital	Corpus Christi	79%	300+
TX Hlth Harris Meth Hosp-Cleburne	Cleburne	79%	300+
Big Bend Regional Medical Center	Alpine	78%	(a)
Brownfield Regional Medical Center	Brownfield	78%	(a)
Electra Memorial Hospital	Electra	78%	(a)
Houston Physicians' Hospital	Webster	78%	(a)
North Central Surgical Center	Dallas	78%	300+
TX Hlth Presbyterian Hosp-Kaufman	Kaufman	78%	300+
Texas Spine & Joint Hospital	Tyler	78%	300+
UT SW Univ Hosp-Zale Lipshy	Dallas	78%	300+
Uvalde Memorial Hospital[11]	Uvalde	78%	(a)
Baylor Heart & Vascular Hospital	Dallas	77%	300+
Baylor Surgical Hospital at Las Colinas	Irving	77%	(a)
East Texas Medical Center Pittsburg	Pittsburg	77%	(a)
First Surgical Hospital	Bellaire	77%	(a)
Fdn Surgical Hosp of San Antonio	San Antonio	77%	300+
Childress Regional Medical Center	Childress	76%	(a)
Christus Hospital	Beaumont	76%	300+
Connally Memorial Medical Center	Floresville	76%	(a)
Lake Pointe Medical Center	Rowlett	76%	300+
Saint Luke's Lakeside Hospital	The Woodlands	76%	300+
San Jacinto Methodist Hospital	Baytown	76%	300+
Scott & White Hospital - Llano	Llano	76%	(a)
Seton Edgar B Davis Hospital	Luling	76%	(a)
TX Health Ctr for Diag & Surgery	Plano	76%	(a)
TX Hlth Harris Meth Hosp-Stephenville	Stephenville	76%	300+
TX Hlth Heart & Vasc Hosp-Arlington	Arlington	76%	300+
Titus Regional Medical Center	Mount Pleasant	76%	300+
Christus Spohn Hospital Alice	Alice	75%	300+
Covenant Hospital Levelland	Levelland	75%	(a)
East Texas Medical Center Crockett	Crockett	75%	(a)
Guadalupe Regional Medical Center	Seguin	75%	300+
Houston Orthopedic & Spine Hospital	Bellaire	75%	300+
Medical Center of Mckinney	Mckinney	75%	300+
Methodist Mansfield Medical Center	Mansfield	75%	300+
TX Hlth Presbyterian Hosp-Flower Mound	Flower Mound	75%	300+
Texas Health Presbyterian Hospital Plano	Plano	75%	300+
USMD Hospital at Arlington	Arlington	75%	300+
Baptist Beaumont Hospital	Beaumont	74%	300+
Baylor Medical Center at Mckinney	Mc Kinney	74%	300+
Baylor Medical Center at Waxahachie	Waxahachie	74%	300+
Baylor Regional Medical Center at Plano	Plano	74%	300+
Coryell Memorial Healthcare System	Gatesville	74%	(a)
Matagorda Regional Medical Center	Bay City	74%	(a)
Medical City Dallas Hospital	Dallas	74%	300+
Memorial Hermann Baptist Orange Hospital	Orange	74%	300+
Methodist Hospital For Surgery	Addison	74%	300+
Methodist Mckinney Hospital	Mc Kinney	74%	(a)
Nacogdoches Medical Center	Nacogdoches	74%	300+
North Austin Medical Center	Austin	74%	300+
North Texas Medical Center	Gainesville	74%	(a)
Park Plaza Hospital	Houston	74%	300+
Saint David's Medical Center	Austin	74%	300+
Saint David's South Austin Medical Center	Austin	74%	300+
Saint Marks Medical Center	La Grange	74%	(a)
Seton Highland Lakes	Burnet	74%	300+
Texas Reg Med Ctr at Sunnyvale	Sunnyvale	74%	300+
United Regional Health Care System	Wichita Falls	74%	300+
Baylor All Saints Medical Center at FW	Fort Worth	73%	300+
Baylor Reg Med Ctr at Grapevine	Grapevine	73%	300+
Centennial Medical Center	Frisco	73%	300+
Central Texas Medical Center[11]	San Marcos	73%	300+
Christus Saint Catherine Hospital	Katy	73%	300+
Christus Saint Michael Health System	Texarkana	73%	300+
Christus Spohn Hospital Beeville	Beeville	73%	(a)
College Station Medical Center	College Station	73%	300+
Covenant Medical Center	Lubbock	73%	300+
Detar Hospital Navarro	Victoria	73%	300+
East Texas Medical Center Jacksonville	Jacksonville	73%	300+
Hendrick Medical Center	Abilene	73%	300+
Huntsville Memorial Hospital	Huntsville	73%	(a)
Kell West Regional Hospital	Wichita Falls	73%	(a)
Lake Granbury Medical Center	Granbury	73%	300+
Medina Regional Hospital	Hondo	73%	(a)
Memorial Hermann Northeast	Humble	73%	300+
Methodist Ambulatory Surgery Hospital NW	San Antonio	73%	(a)
Mission Regional Medical Center	Mission	73%	300+
Moore County Hospital District	Dumas	73%	(a)
Palo Pinto General Hospital	Mineral Wells	73%	300+
Providence Health Center	Waco	73%	300+
San Angelo Community Medical Center	San Angelo	73%	300+
Starr County Memorial Hospital	Rio Grande City	73%	(a)
TX Hlth Harris Meth Hosp SW Ft Worth	Fort Worth	73%	300+
Texas Health Harris Methodist	Bedford	73%	300+
TX Inst for Surgery at Presby Hosp	Dallas	73%	(a)
University General Hospital Dallas	Dallas	73%	(a)
University Medical Center	Lubbock	73%	300+
Weatherford Regional Medical Center	Weatherford	73%	300+
Woodland Heights Medical Center	Lufkin	73%	300+
Angleton - Danbury Medical Center	Angleton	72%	300+
Baylor University Medical Center	Dallas	72%	300+
Brownwood Regional Medical Center	Brownwood	72%	300+
Christus Saint John Hospital	Nassau Bay	72%	300+
Christus Spohn Hospital Kleberg	Kingsville	72%	300+
Covenant Hospital Plainview	Plainview	72%	300+
Doctors Hospital of Laredo	Laredo	72%	300+
Fort Duncan Medical Center	Eagle Pass	72%	300+
Foundation Surgical Hospital of El Paso	El Paso	72%	300+
Hopkins County Memorial Hospital	Sulphur Springs	72%	300+
Huguley Memorial Medical Center[11]	Burleson	72%	300+
Knapp Medical Center	Weslaco	72%	300+
Las Colinas Medical Center	Irving	72%	300+
Memorial Hermann Hospital System	Houston	72%	300+
Memorial Hermann Sugar Land Hospital	Sugar Land	72%	300+
Memorial Medical Center Livingston	Livingston	72%	300+
Methodist Dallas Medical Center	Dallas	72%	300+
Methodist Richardson Medical Center	Richardson	72%	300+
Metroplex Hospital[11]	Killeen	72%	300+
Navarro Regional Hospital	Corsicana	72%	300+
Pine Creek Medical Center	Dallas	72%	300+
Rolling Plains Memorial Hospital	Sweetwater	72%	(a)
Round Rock Medical Center	Round Rock	72%	300+
Saint Luke's Episcopal Hospital	Houston	72%	300+
Scott & White Hospital Brenham	Brenham	72%	300+
Seton Southwest Hospital	Austin	72%	(a)
Shannon Medical Center	San Angelo	72%	300+
Sierra Providence East Medical Center	El Paso	72%	300+
Texas Health Harris Methodist Fort Worth	Fort Worth	72%	300+
UT Southwestern University Hospital	Dallas	72%	300+
Val Verde Regional Medical Center	Del Rio	72%	300+
Baylor Medical Center at Garland	Garland	71%	300+
Care Regional Medical Center	Aransas Pass	71%	(a)
Columbus Community Hospital	Columbus	71%	(a)
Cornerstone Regional Hospital	Edinburg	71%	(a)
The Corpus Christi Medical Center	Corpus Christi	71%	300+
Cypress Fairbanks Medical Center	Houston	71%	300+
Denton Regional Medical Center	Denton	71%	300+
Doctors Hospital	Dallas	71%	300+
Doctors Hospital at Renaissance	Edinburg	71%	300+
Lubbock Heart Hospital	Lubbock	71%	300+
Medical Center Hospital	Odessa	71%	300+
Memorial Hermann Katy Hospital	Katy	71%	300+
Mem Hermann Mem City Med Ctr	Houston	71%	300+
The Methodist Hospital	Houston	71%	300+
Methodist Sugar Land Hospital	Sugar Land	71%	300+
North Cypress Medical Center	Cypress	71%	300+
Northwest Texas Hospital	Amarillo	71%	300+
Permian Regional Medical Center	Andrews	71%	(a)
Peterson Regional Medical Center	Kerrville	71%	300+
Saint Anthony's Hospital	Houston	71%	(a)
Saint Joseph Regional Health Center	Bryan	71%	300+
Scenic Mountain Medical Center	Big Spring	71%	300+
Seton Medical Center Harker Heights	Harker Heights	71%	300+
Seton Medical Center Hays	Kyle	71%	300+
Texas Health Arlington Memorial Hospital	Arlington	71%	300+
Texas Health Presbyterian Hospital Dallas	Dallas	71%	300+
TX Health Presbyterian Hosp Rockwall	Rockwall	71%	300+
Texas Orthopedic Hospital	Houston	71%	300+
Texoma Medical Center	Denison	71%	300+
VHS Brownsville Hospital Company[11]	Brownsville	71%	300+

NOTE: Hospital profiles are in alphabetical order by state, then city, then hospital within the city; Rankings exclude hospitals with less than 25 cases except for patient surveys which excludes hospitals with less than 100 cases; (a) 100-299 cases; (1) The number of cases/patients is too few to report; (2) Data submitted were based on a sample of cases/patients; (3) Results are based on a shorter time period than required; (4) Data suppressed by CMS for one or more quarters; (5) Results are not available for this reporting period; (6) Fewer than 100 patients completed the HCAHPS survey; (7) No cases met the criteria for this measure; (8) The lower limit of the confidence interval cannot be calculated if the number of observed infections equals zero; (9) No data are available from the state/territory for this reporting period; (10) The scores shown reflect fewer than 50 completed surveys; (11) There were discrepancies in the data collection process; (12) This measure does not apply to this hospital for this reporting period; (13) Results cannot be calculated for this reporting period; (14) The results for this state are combined with nearby states to protect confidentiality; Please refer to the User's Guide for a full explanation of data.

Wise Regional Health System	Decatur	71%	300+
Baptist Medical Center[11]	San Antonio	70%	300+
Baptist Saint Anthony's Hospital	Amarillo	70%	300+
Baylor Medical Center at Irving	Irving	70%	300+
Christus Jasper Memorial Hospital	Jasper	70%	(a)
Christus Santa Rosa Hospital	San Antonio	70%	300+
Christus Spohn Hospital Corpus Christi	Corpus Christi	70%	300+
Citizens Medical Center	Victoria	70%	300+
Clear Lake Regional Medical Center	Webster	70%	300+
East Texas Medical Center	Tyler	70%	300+
Etmc Henderson	Henderson	70%	300+
Good Shepherd Medical Center	Longview	70%	300+
Hillcrest Baptist Medical Center	Waco	70%	300+
Houston Northwest Medical Center	Houston	70%	300+
Longview Regional Medical Center	Longview	70%	300+
Medical Center of Arlington	Arlington	70%	300+
Medical Center of Lewisville	Lewisville	70%	300+
Memorial Medical Center of East Texas	Lufkin	70%	300+
Methodist Charlton Medical Center	Dallas	70%	300+
Methodist Hospital	San Antonio	70%	300+
Methodist West Houston Hospital	Houston	70%	300+
Methodist Willowbrook Hospital	Houston	70%	300+
Rio Grande Regional Hospital	Mcallen	70%	300+
Scott & White Hospital - Round Rock	Round Rock	70%	300+
Seton Medical Center Austin	Austin	70%	300+
TX Hlth Harris Methodist Hosp-Azle	Azle	70%	300+
Texas Health Presbyterian Hospital Allen	Allen	70%	300+
Tyler County Hospital	Woodville	70%	(a)
Univ of TX Health Science Ctr-Tyler	Tyler	70%	(a)
VHS Harlingen Hospital Company[11]	Harlingen	70%	300+
Wadley Regional Medical Center	Texarkana	70%	300+
The Womans Hospital of Texas	Houston	70%	300+
Arise Austin Medical Center[3]	Austin	69%	(a)
Conroe Regional Medical Center	Conroe	69%	300+
El Paso Specialty Hospital	El Paso	69%	(a)
Grace Medical Center	Lubbock	69%	300+
Hamilton General Hospital	Hamilton	69%	(a)
Harlingen Medical Center[11]	Harlingen	69%	300+
Harris Health System	Houston	69%	300+
Hereford Regional Medical Center	Hereford	69%	(a)
The Hospital at Westlake Medical Center	Austin	69%	300+
Hunt Regional Medical Center	Greenville	69%	300+
Las Palmas Medical Center	El Paso	69%	300+
Memorial Hermann Texas Medical Center	Houston	69%	300+
Memorial Medical Center	Port Lavaca	69%	(a)
Nix Health Care System	San Antonio	69%	300+
Oakbend Medical Center	Richmond	69%	300+
Odessa Regional Hospital	Odessa	69%	300+
Providence Memorial Hospital	El Paso	69%	300+
Saint Joseph Medical Center	Houston	69%	300+
Seton Medical Center Williamson	Round Rock	69%	300+
Seton Northwest Hospital	Austin	69%	300+
South Texas Health System	Edinburg	69%	300+
Texas Health Presbyterian Hospital Denton	Denton	69%	300+
University Medical Center of El Paso	El Paso	69%	300+
Etmc Clarksville	Clarksville	68%	(a)
Hill Regional Hospital	Hillsboro	68%	300+
Medical Center of Plano	Plano	68%	300+
Methodist Stone Oak Hospital	San Antonio	68%	300+
Midland Memorial Hospital	Midland	68%	300+
Mother Frances Hospital	Tyler	68%	300+
North Hills Hospital	N Richland Hls	68%	300+
Pampa Regional Medical Center	Pampa	68%	300+
Saint Luke's the Woodlands Hospital	The Woodlands	68%	300+
Scott & White Memorial Hospital[11]	Temple	68%	300+
South Texas Regional Medical Center	Jourdanton	68%	(a)
Tomball Regional Medical Center	Tomball	68%	300+
University Health System	San Antonio	68%	300+
University Medical Center at Brackenridge	Austin	68%	300+
Univ of Texas Med Branch Galveston	Galveston	68%	300+
Baylor Surgical Hospital at Fort Worth	Fort Worth	67%	300+
Bayshore Medical Center	Pasadena	67%	300+
Doctors Hospital Tidwell	Houston	67%	300+
East Texas Medical Center Athens	Athens	67%	300+
JPS Health Network	Fort Worth	67%	300+
Laredo Medical Center	Laredo	67%	300+
The Medical Center of Southeast Texas	Port Arthur	67%	300+
Parkland Health & Hospital System	Dallas	67%	300+
Plaza Medical Center of Fort Worth	Fort Worth	67%	300+
Saint Luke's Sugar Land Hospital	Sugar Land	67%	300+
Texas Health Presbyterian Hospital - WNJ	Sherman	67%	300+
West Houston Medical Center	Houston	67%	300+
Abilene Regional Medical Center	Abilene	66%	300+
Baylor Medical Center at Carrollton	Carrollton	66%	300+
Cedar Park Regional Medical Center	Cedar Park	66%	300+
Ennis Regional Medical Center	Ennis	66%	300+
Etmc Carthage	Carthage	66%	(a)
Kingwood Medical Center	Kingwood	66%	300+
Southwest General Hospital	San Antonio	66%	300+
Valley Regional Medical Center	Brownsville	66%	300+
Brazosport Regional Health System	Lake Jackson	65%	300+
Dallas Regional Medical Center	Mesquite	65%	300+
Good Shepherd Medical Center - Linden	Linden	65%	(a)
Good Shepherd Medical Center Marshall	Marshall	65%	300+
Memorial Hospital	Nacogdoches	64%	300+
Palestine Regional Medical Center	Palestine	64%	300+
Paris Regional Medical Center	Paris	64%	300+
Saint Luke's Hospital at the Vintage	Houston	64%	300+
University General Hospital	Houston	64%	300+
Saint Luke's Patients Medical Center	Pasadena	63%	300+
Sierra Medical Center	El Paso	63%	300+
Dallas Medical Center	Dallas	59%	300+
Lake Whitney Medical Center[11]	Whitney	57%	(a)

Room and Bathroom 'Always' Clean

Hospital Name	City	Rate	Cases
Baylor Medical Center at Frisco	Frisco	91%	300+
North Central Surgical Center	Dallas	91%	300+
Electra Memorial Hospital	Electra	89%	(a)
Sugar Land Surgical Hospital	Sugar Land	89%	(a)
Baylor Surgical Hospital at Las Colinas	Irving	88%	(a)
East Texas Medical Center - Gilmer	Gilmer	88%	(a)
Falls Community Hospital & Clinic	Marlin	88%	(a)
Quail Creek Surgical Hospital	Amarillo	88%	300+
TX Inst for Surgery at Presby Hosp	Dallas	88%	(a)
USMD Hospital at Arlington	Arlington	88%	300+
TX Hlth Harris Meth Hosp-Stephenville	Stephenville	87%	300+
USMD Hospital at Fort Worth	Fort Worth	87%	(a)
Baylor Medical Center at Uptown	Dallas	86%	300+
Baylor Ortho & Spine Hosp-Arlington	Arlington	86%	300+
Northwest Hills Surgical Hospital	Austin	86%	(a)
The Physicians Centre	Bryan	86%	(a)
TX Hlth Harris Meth Hosp-Southlake	Southlake	86%	300+
Houston Orthopedic & Spine Hospital	Bellaire	85%	300+
TX Health Ctr for Diag & Surgery	Plano	85%	(a)
Baylor Medical Center at Trophy Club	Trophy Club	84%	(a)
East Texas Medical Center Pittsburg	Pittsburg	84%	(a)
Methodist Hospital For Surgery	Addison	84%	300+
Rolling Plains Memorial Hospital	Sweetwater	84%	(a)
Starr County Memorial Hospital	Rio Grande City	84%	(a)
Tyler County Hospital	Woodville	84%	(a)
W J Mangold Memorial Hospital	Lockney	84%	(a)
Hill Country Memorial Hospital	Fredericksburg	83%	300+
Saint Luke's Lakeside Hospital	The Woodlands	83%	300+
TX Hlth Harris Methodist Hosp-Azle	Azle	83%	300+
TX Health Presbyterian Hosp Rockwall	Rockwall	83%	300+
Tops Surgical Specialty Hospital	Houston	83%	(a)
East Texas Medical Center Quitman	Quitman	82%	(a)
Heart Hospital Baylor Plano	Plano	82%	300+
Heritage Park Surgical Hospital	Sherman	82%	(a)
Kell West Regional Hospital	Wichita Falls	82%	(a)
Parkview Regional Hospital	Mexia	82%	(a)
South Texas Surgical Hospital	Corpus Christi	82%	300+
Guadalupe Regional Medical Center	Seguin	81%	300+
Rollins Brook Community Hospital[11]	Lampasas	81%	(a)
TX Hlth Heart & Vasc Hosp-Arlington	Arlington	81%	300+
Baylor Heart & Vascular Hospital	Dallas	80%	300+
Cuero Community Hospital	Cuero	80%	(a)
First Surgical Hospital	Bellaire	80%	(a)
Hamilton General Hospital	Hamilton	80%	(a)
Hereford Regional Medical Center	Hereford	80%	(a)
Memorial Medical Center	Port Lavaca	80%	(a)
Methodist West Houston Hospital	Houston	80%	300+
Pecos County Memorial Hospital	Fort Stockton	80%	(a)
South Texas Spine & Surgical Hospital	San Antonio	80%	300+
United Regional Health Care System	Wichita Falls	80%	300+
Yoakum Community Hospital	Yoakum	80%	(a)
Baylor Reg Med Ctr at Grapevine	Grapevine	79%	300+
Christus Spohn Hospital Beeville	Beeville	79%	(a)
Connally Memorial Medical Center	Floresville	79%	(a)
Cornerstone Regional Hospital	Edinburg	79%	(a)
Doctors Hospital of Laredo	Laredo	79%	300+
The Hospital at Westlake Medical Center	Austin	79%	300+
Methodist Ambulatory Surgery Hospital NW	San Antonio	79%	(a)
Methodist Mckinney Hospital	Mc Kinney	79%	(a)
Moore County Hospital District	Dumas	79%	(a)
North Austin Medical Center	Austin	79%	300+
Seton Edgar B Davis Hospital	Luling	79%	(a)
Texas Health Presbyterian Hospital Plano	Plano	79%	300+
Texas Spine & Joint Hospital	Tyler	79%	300+
Baylor Regional Medical Center at Plano	Plano	78%	300+
Coryell Memorial Healthcare System	Gatesville	78%	(a)
Fdn Surgical Hosp of San Antonio	San Antonio	78%	300+
Glen Rose Medical Center	Glen Rose	78%	(a)
Good Shephard Medical Center - Linden	Linden	78%	(a)
Houston Physicians' Hospital	Webster	78%	(a)
Knapp Medical Center	Weslaco	78%	300+
Matagorda Regional Medical Center	Bay City	78%	(a)
Medina Regional Hospital	Hondo	78%	(a)
Memorial Medical Center Livingston	Livingston	78%	300+
TX Hlth Harris Meth Hosp-Cleburne	Cleburne	78%	300+
Baptist Saint Anthony's Hospital	Amarillo	77%	300+
Baylor Medical Center at Mckinney	Mc Kinney	77%	300+
Christus Saint Catherine Hospital	Katy	77%	300+
East Texas Medical Center Jacksonville	Jacksonville	77%	300+
Etmc Clarksville	Clarksville	77%	(a)
Hopkins County Memorial Hospital	Sulphur Springs	77%	300+
Longview Regional Medical Center	Longview	77%	300+
Metroplex Hospital[11]	Killeen	77%	300+
Saint Luke's Sugar Land Hospital	Sugar Land	77%	300+
Scott & White Hospital - Round Rock	Round Rock	77%	300+
Texas Health Presbyterian Hospital Allen	Allen	77%	300+
TX Hlth Presbyterian Hosp-Kaufman	Kaufman	77%	300+
Titus Regional Medical Center	Mount Pleasant	77%	300+
Val Verde Regional Medical Center	Del Rio	77%	300+
Abilene Regional Medical Center	Abilene	76%	300+
Angleton - Danbury Medical Center	Angleton	76%	300+
Arise Austin Medical Center[3]	Austin	76%	(a)
Baylor Medical Center at Waxahachie	Waxahachie	76%	300+
Christus Spohn Hospital Alice	Alice	76%	300+
Doctors Hospital at Renaissance	Edinburg	76%	300+
El Paso Specialty Hospital	El Paso	76%	(a)
Etmc Henderson	Henderson	76%	300+
Hendrick Medical Center	Abilene	76%	300+
Hill Regional Hospital	Hillsboro	76%	300+
Methodist Mansfield Medical Center	Mansfield	76%	300+
Methodist Richardson Medical Center	Richardson	76%	300+
Nix Health Care System	San Antonio	76%	300+
Saint Luke's Hospital at the Vintage	Houston	76%	300+
Saint Marks Medical Center	La Grange	76%	(a)
San Jacinto Methodist Hospital	Baytown	76%	300+
Seton Southwest Hospital	Austin	76%	(a)
Sierra Providence East Medical Center	El Paso	76%	300+
Texas Health Arlington Memorial Hospital	Arlington	76%	300+
Texas Health Harris Methodist Fort Worth	Fort Worth	76%	300+
TX Hlth Presbyterian Hosp-Flower Mound	Flower Mound	76%	300+
Univ of TX Health Science Ctr-Tyler	Tyler	76%	(a)
Baptist Emergency Hospital	San Antonio	75%	(a)
Basin Healthcare Center	Odessa	75%	(a)
Baylor Medical Center at Garland	Garland	75%	300+
Childress Regional Medical Center	Childress	75%	(a)
Christus Saint Michael Health System	Texarkana	75%	300+
Columbus Community Hospital	Columbus	75%	(a)
Covenant Hospital Plainview	Plainview	75%	300+
Fort Duncan Medical Center	Eagle Pass	75%	300+
Harlingen Medical Center[11]	Harlingen	75%	300+
Medical City Dallas Hospital	Dallas	75%	300+
Memorial Hermann Katy Hospital	Katy	75%	300+
Memorial Hermann Sugar Land Hospital	Sugar Land	75%	300+
Methodist Charlton Medical Center	Dallas	75%	300+
Methodist Stone Oak Hospital	San Antonio	75%	300+
North Texas Medical Center	Gainesville	75%	(a)
Seton Highland Lakes	Burnet	75%	300+
Shannon Medical Center	San Angelo	75%	300+
UT SW Univ Hosp-Zale Lipshy	Dallas	75%	300+
VHS Brownsville Hospital Company[11]	Brownsville	75%	300+
Woodland Heights Medical Center	Lufkin	75%	300+
Big Bend Regional Medical Center	Alpine	74%	(a)
Brownfield Regional Medical Center	Brownfield	74%	(a)
Christus Saint John Hospital	Nassau Bay	74%	300+
Citizens Medical Center	Victoria	74%	300+
Covenant Hospital Levelland	Levelland	74%	(a)
Ennis Regional Medical Center	Ennis	74%	300+
Memorial Hermann Hospital System	Houston	74%	300+
Saint David's South Austin Medical Center	Austin	74%	300+
University Medical Center	Lubbock	74%	300+
Wise Regional Health System	Decatur	74%	300+
Central Texas Medical Center[11]	San Marcos	73%	300+
Christus Spohn Hospital Kleberg	Kingsville	73%	300+
Eastland Memorial Hospital	Eastland	73%	(a)
Huntsville Memorial Hospital	Huntsville	73%	(a)
Medical Center of Lewisville	Lewisville	73%	300+
Medical Center of Mckinney	Mckinney	73%	300+
Mem Hermann Mem City Med Ctr	Houston	73%	300+
Mission Regional Medical Center	Mission	73%	300+
Navarro Regional Hospital	Corsicana	73%	300+
North Hills Hospital	N Richland Hls	73%	300+
Pine Creek Medical Center	Dallas	73%	300+
Round Rock Medical Center	Round Rock	73%	300+
Saint David's Medical Center	Austin	73%	300+
Saint Joseph Regional Health Center	Bryan	73%	300+
Seton Medical Center Harker Heights	Harker Heights	73%	300+
Texas Health Presbyterian Hospital Denton	Denton	73%	300+
Texas Reg Med Ctr at Sunnyvale	Sunnyvale	73%	300+
University Medical Center of El Paso	El Paso	73%	300+
Uvalde Memorial Hospital[11]	Uvalde	73%	(a)
Christus Hospital	Beaumont	72%	300+
Christus Jasper Memorial Hospital	Jasper	72%	(a)
Foundation Surgical Hospital of El Paso	El Paso	72%	300+
Hunt Regional Medical Center	Greenville	72%	300+
Lubbock Heart Hospital	Lubbock	72%	300+
Memorial Hermann Baptist Orange Hospital	Orange	72%	300+
Methodist Sugar Land Hospital	Sugar Land	72%	300+

NOTE: Hospital profiles are in alphabetical order by state, then city, then hospital within the city; Rankings exclude hospitals with less than 25 cases except for patient surveys which excludes hospitals with less than 100 cases; (a) 100-299 cases; (1) The number of cases/patients is too few to report; (2) Data submitted were based on a sample of cases/patients; (3) Results are based on a shorter time period than required; (4) Data suppressed by CMS for one or more quarters; (5) Results are not available for this reporting period; (6) Fewer than 100 patients completed the HCAHPS survey; (7) No cases met the criteria for this measure; (8) The lower limit of the confidence interval cannot be calculated if the number of observed infections equals zero; (9) No data are available from the state/territory for this reporting period; (10) The scores shown reflect fewer than 50 completed surveys; (11) There were discrepancies in the data collection process; (12) This measure does not apply to this hospital for this reporting period; (13) Results cannot be calculated for this reporting period; (14) The results for this state are combined with nearby states to protect confidentiality; Please refer to the User's Guide for a full explanation of data.

Park Plaza Hospital	Houston	72%	300+
South Texas Regional Medical Center	Jourdanton	72%	(a)
Texas Health Presbyterian Hospital Dallas	Dallas	72%	300+
Valley Regional Medical Center	Brownsville	72%	300+
Baylor Medical Center at Irving	Irving	71%	300+
Brazosport Regional Health System	Lake Jackson	71%	300+
Good Shepherd Medical Center	Longview	71%	300+
Good Shepherd Medical Center Marshall	Marshall	71%	300+
JPS Health Network	Fort Worth	71%	300+
Las Colinas Medical Center	Irving	71%	300+
Medical Center of Plano	Plano	71%	300+
Memorial Hermann Texas Medical Center	Houston	71%	300+
Memorial Medical Center of East Texas	Lufkin	71%	300+
Methodist Dallas Medical Center	Dallas	71%	300+
The Methodist Hospital	Houston	71%	300+
Permian Regional Medical Center	Andrews	71%	(a)
Plaza Medical Center of Fort Worth	Fort Worth	71%	300+
Providence Health Center	Waco	71%	300+
Rio Grande Regional Hospital	Mcallen	71%	300+
Saint Luke's the Woodlands Hospital	The Woodlands	71%	300+
Baylor Surgical Hospital at Fort Worth	Fort Worth	70%	300+
Baylor University Medical Center	Dallas	70%	300+
Cedar Park Regional Medical Center	Cedar Park	70%	300+
Christus Santa Rosa Hospital	San Antonio	70%	300+
Clear Lake Regional Medical Center	Webster	70%	300+
Covenant Medical Center	Lubbock	70%	300+
Denton Regional Medical Center	Denton	70%	300+
Detar Hospital Navarro	Victoria	70%	300+
Hillcrest Baptist Medical Center	Waco	70%	300+
Laredo Medical Center	Laredo	70%	300+
Las Palmas Medical Center	El Paso	70%	300+
Mother Frances Hospital	Tyler	70%	300+
Saint Anthony's Hospital	Houston	70%	(a)
Saint Luke's Episcopal Hospital	Houston	70%	300+
Scenic Mountain Medical Center	Big Spring	70%	300+
Scott & White Hospital - Llano	Llano	70%	(a)
Seton Medical Center Williamson	Round Rock	70%	300+
Texas Orthopedic Hospital	Houston	70%	300+
Texoma Medical Center	Denison	70%	300+
UT Southwestern University Hospital	Dallas	70%	300+
VHS Harlingen Hospital Company[11]	Harlingen	70%	300+
Wadley Regional Medical Center	Texarkana	70%	300+
Baptist Beaumont Hospital	Beaumont	69%	300+
Baylor All Saints Medical Center at FW	Fort Worth	69%	300+
Bayshore Medical Center	Pasadena	69%	300+
Christus Spohn Hospital Corpus Christi	Corpus Christi	69%	300+
College Station Medical Center	College Station	69%	300+
The Corpus Christi Medical Center	Corpus Christi	69%	300+
East Texas Medical Center	Tyler	69%	300+
Huguley Memorial Medical Center[11]	Burleson	69%	300+
Methodist Hospital	San Antonio	69%	300+
North Cypress Medical Center	Cypress	69%	300+
Peterson Regional Medical Center	Kerrville	69%	300+
San Angelo Community Medical Center	San Angelo	69%	300+
Scott & White Hospital Brenham	Brenham	69%	300+
Texas Health Harris Methodist	Bedford	69%	300+
University General Hospital Dallas	Dallas	69%	(a)
Univ of Texas Med Branch Galveston	Galveston	69%	300+
West Houston Medical Center	Houston	69%	300+
Baylor Medical Center at Carrollton	Carrollton	68%	300+
Dallas Regional Medical Center	Mesquite	68%	300+
Doctors Hospital Tidwell	Houston	68%	300+
Grace Medical Center	Lubbock	68%	300+
Lake Pointe Medical Center	Rowlett	68%	300+
Memorial Hermann Northeast	Humble	68%	300+
Methodist Willowbrook Hospital	Houston	68%	300+
Odessa Regional Hospital	Odessa	68%	300+
Providence Memorial Hospital	El Paso	68%	300+
Saint Luke's Patients Medical Center	Pasadena	68%	300+
Seton Northwest Hospital	Austin	68%	300+
South Texas Health System	Edinburg	68%	300+
The Womans Hospital of Texas	Houston	68%	300+
Brownwood Regional Medical Center	Brownwood	67%	300+
Care Regional Medical Center	Aransas Pass	67%	(a)
Centennial Medical Center	Frisco	67%	300+
Kingwood Medical Center	Kingwood	67%	300+
Medical Center of Arlington	Arlington	67%	300+
Palo Pinto General Hospital	Mineral Wells	67%	300+
Parkland Health & Hospital System	Dallas	67%	300+
Seton Medical Center Hays	Kyle	67%	300+
University General Hospital	Houston	67%	300+
University Health System	San Antonio	67%	300+
Conroe Regional Medical Center	Conroe	66%	300+
Doctors Hospital	Dallas	66%	300+
Houston Northwest Medical Center	Houston	66%	300+
Palestine Regional Medical Center	Palestine	66%	300+
TX Hlth Harris Meth Hosp SW Ft Worth	Fort Worth	66%	300+
Baptist Medical Center[11]	San Antonio	65%	300+
East Texas Medical Center Athens	Athens	65%	300+
East Texas Medical Center Crockett	Crockett	65%	(a)
Etmc Carthage	Carthage	65%	(a)
Scott & White Memorial Hospital[11]	Temple	65%	300+
Seton Medical Center Austin	Austin	65%	300+
Sierra Medical Center	El Paso	65%	300+
Tomball Regional Medical Center	Tomball	65%	300+
University Medical Center at Brackenridge	Austin	65%	300+
Weatherford Regional Medical Center	Weatherford	65%	300+
Harris Health System	Houston	64%	300+
Lake Granbury Medical Center	Granbury	64%	300+
The Medical Center of Southeast Texas	Port Arthur	64%	300+
Northwest Texas Hospital	Amarillo	64%	300+
Paris Regional Medical Center	Paris	64%	300+
Saint Joseph Medical Center	Houston	64%	300+
Cypress Fairbanks Medical Center	Houston	63%	300+
Graham Regional Medical Center	Graham	63%	(a)
Medical Center Hospital	Odessa	63%	300+
Memorial Hospital	Nacogdoches	63%	300+
Nacogdoches Medical Center	Nacogdoches	63%	300+
Pampa Regional Medical Center	Pampa	63%	300+
Oakbend Medical Center	Richmond	62%	300+
Southwest General Hospital	San Antonio	62%	300+
Midland Memorial Hospital	Midland	61%	300+
Texas Health Presbyterian Hospital - WNJ	Sherman	61%	300+
Dallas Medical Center	Dallas	58%	300+
Lake Whitney Medical Center[11]	Whitney	53%	(a)

Timely Help 'Always' Received

Hospital Name	City	Rate	Cases
Sugar Land Surgical Hospital	Sugar Land	94%	(a)
Quail Creek Surgical Hospital	Amarillo	93%	300+
Heritage Park Surgical Hospital	Sherman	90%	(a)
Northwest Hills Surgical Hospital	Austin	90%	(a)
Baylor Medical Center at Uptown	Dallas	89%	300+
TX Inst for Surgery at Presby Hosp	Dallas	87%	(a)
East Texas Medical Center - Gilmer	Gilmer	86%	(a)
TX Health Ctr for Diag & Surgery	Plano	86%	(a)
TX Hlth Harris Meth Hosp-Southlake	Southlake	86%	300+
USMD Hospital at Fort Worth	Fort Worth	86%	(a)
North Central Surgical Center	Dallas	85%	300+
The Physicians Centre	Bryan	85%	(a)
W J Mangold Memorial Hospital	Lockney	85%	(a)
Baylor Surgical Hospital at Las Colinas	Irving	84%	(a)
Tops Surgical Specialty Hospital	Houston	84%	(a)
Baylor Ortho & Spine Hosp-Arlington	Arlington	83%	300+
Electra Memorial Hospital	Electra	83%	(a)
Texas Spine & Joint Hospital	Tyler	83%	300+
Tyler County Hospital	Woodville	83%	(a)
Yoakum Community Hospital	Yoakum	83%	(a)
South Texas Spine & Surgical Hospital	San Antonio	82%	300+
Fdn Surgical Hosp of San Antonio	San Antonio	81%	300+
Saint Luke's Lakeside Hospital	The Woodlands	81%	300+
Baylor Medical Center at Trophy Club	Trophy Club	80%	(a)
Childress Regional Medical Center	Childress	80%	(a)
Hill Country Memorial Hospital	Fredericksburg	80%	300+
Parkview Regional Hospital	Mexia	80%	(a)
Baptist Emergency Hospital	San Antonio	79%	(a)
East Texas Medical Center Pittsburg	Pittsburg	79%	(a)
First Surgical Hospital	Bellaire	79%	(a)
Glen Rose Medical Center	Glen Rose	79%	(a)
Heart Hospital Baylor Plano	Plano	79%	300+
Basin Healthcare Center	Odessa	78%	(a)
Baylor Heart & Vascular Hospital	Dallas	78%	300+
Big Bend Regional Medical Center	Alpine	78%	(a)
Houston Orthopedic & Spine Hospital	Bellaire	78%	300+
Houston Physicians' Hospital	Webster	78%	(a)
Kell West Regional Hospital	Wichita Falls	78%	(a)
Rollins Brook Community Hospital[11]	Lampasas	78%	(a)
USMD Hospital at Arlington	Arlington	78%	300+
Good Shephard Medical Center - Linden	Linden	77%	(a)
Methodist Mckinney Hospital	Mc Kinney	77%	(a)
North Texas Medical Center	Gainesville	77%	(a)
Rolling Plains Memorial Hospital	Sweetwater	77%	(a)
Eastland Memorial Hospital	Eastland	76%	(a)
Saint Marks Medical Center	La Grange	76%	(a)
TX Hlth Harris Methodist Hosp-Azle	Azle	76%	300+
TX Hlth Harris Meth Hosp-Stephenville	Stephenville	76%	300+
Baylor Medical Center at Frisco	Frisco	75%	300+
South Texas Surgical Hospital	Corpus Christi	75%	300+
Cornerstone Regional Hospital	Edinburg	74%	(a)
Coryell Memorial Healthcare System	Gatesville	74%	(a)
East Texas Medical Center Crockett	Crockett	74%	(a)
Graham Regional Medical Center	Graham	74%	(a)
The Hospital at Westlake Medical Center	Austin	74%	(a)
Memorial Hermann Baptist Orange Hospital	Orange	74%	300+
Methodist Hospital For Surgery	Addison	74%	300+
TX Hlth Heart & Vasc Hosp-Arlington	Arlington	74%	300+
TX Hlth Presbyterian Hosp-Kaufman	Kaufman	74%	300+
Uvalde Memorial Hospital[11]	Uvalde	74%	(a)
Woodland Heights Medical Center	Lufkin	74%	300+
Covenant Hospital Levelland	Levelland	73%	(a)
Falls Community Hospital & Clinic	Marlin	73%	(a)
Lubbock Heart Hospital	Lubbock	73%	300+
Methodist Ambulatory Surgery Hospital NW	San Antonio	73%	(a)
Pecos County Memorial Hospital	Fort Stockton	73%	(a)
Pine Creek Medical Center	Dallas	73%	300+
San Jacinto Methodist Hospital	Baytown	73%	300+
Scott & White Hospital - Llano	Llano	73%	(a)
TX Hlth Presbyterian Hosp-Flower Mound	Flower Mound	73%	300+
United Regional Health Care System	Wichita Falls	73%	300+
Cuero Community Hospital	Cuero	72%	(a)
East Texas Medical Center Quitman	Quitman	72%	(a)
Foundation Surgical Hospital of El Paso	El Paso	72%	300+
Hill Regional Hospital	Hillsboro	72%	300+
Palo Pinto General Hospital	Mineral Wells	72%	300+
Seton Highland Lakes	Burnet	72%	300+
Seton Southwest Hospital	Austin	72%	(a)
Titus Regional Medical Center	Mount Pleasant	72%	300+
Christus Spohn Hospital Alice	Alice	71%	300+
Christus Spohn Hospital Beeville	Beeville	71%	(a)
Memorial Medical Center	Port Lavaca	71%	(a)
UT SW Univ Hosp-Zale Lipshy	Dallas	71%	300+
Angleton - Danbury Medical Center	Angleton	70%	300+
Brownfield Regional Medical Center	Brownfield	70%	(a)
Christus Saint Michael Health System	Texarkana	70%	300+
Etmc Clarksville	Clarksville	70%	(a)
Nacogdoches Medical Center	Nacogdoches	70%	300+
Seton Edgar B Davis Hospital	Luling	70%	(a)
Seton Medical Center Harker Heights	Harker Heights	70%	300+
Texas Health Harris Methodist Fort Worth	Fort Worth	70%	300+
Texas Reg Med Ctr at Sunnyvale	Sunnyvale	70%	300+
University Medical Center	Lubbock	70%	300+
Baptist Beaumont Hospital	Beaumont	69%	300+
Christus Jasper Memorial Hospital	Jasper	69%	(a)
Covenant Hospital Plainview	Plainview	69%	300+
East Texas Medical Center Jacksonville	Jacksonville	69%	300+
Guadalupe Regional Medical Center	Seguin	69%	300+
Hereford Regional Medical Center	Hereford	69%	(a)
Medical Center of Mckinney	Mckinney	69%	300+
San Angelo Community Medical Center	San Angelo	69%	300+
TX Hlth Harris Meth Hosp-Cleburne	Cleburne	69%	300+
Texas Health Presbyterian Hospital Allen	Allen	69%	300+
TX Health Presbyterian Hosp Rockwall	Rockwall	69%	300+
Baylor Medical Center at Waxahachie	Waxahachie	68%	300+
Central Texas Medical Center[11]	San Marcos	68%	300+
Covenant Medical Center	Lubbock	68%	300+
El Paso Specialty Hospital	El Paso	68%	(a)
Grace Medical Center	Lubbock	68%	300+
Hendrick Medical Center	Abilene	68%	300+
Matagorda Regional Medical Center	Bay City	68%	(a)
Mission Regional Medical Center	Mission	68%	300+
Moore County Hospital District	Dumas	68%	(a)
Park Plaza Hospital	Houston	68%	300+
Round Rock Medical Center	Round Rock	68%	300+
Saint Joseph Regional Health Center	Bryan	68%	300+
Shannon Medical Center	San Angelo	68%	300+
Sierra Providence East Medical Center	El Paso	68%	300+
Starr County Memorial Hospital	Rio Grande City	68%	(a)
Wadley Regional Medical Center	Texarkana	68%	300+
Wise Regional Health System	Decatur	68%	300+
Baylor Medical Center at Mckinney	Mc Kinney	67%	300+
Baylor Regional Medical Center at Plano	Plano	67%	300+
Care Regional Medical Center	Aransas Pass	67%	(a)
Connally Memorial Medical Center	Floresville	67%	(a)
Etmc Carthage	Carthage	67%	(a)
Etmc Henderson	Henderson	67%	300+
Hamilton General Hospital	Hamilton	67%	(a)
Hopkins County Memorial Hospital	Sulphur Springs	67%	300+
Huguley Memorial Medical Center[11]	Burleson	67%	300+
Hunt Regional Medical Center	Greenville	67%	300+
Medina Regional Hospital	Hondo	67%	(a)
Mem Hermann Mem City Med Ctr	Houston	67%	300+
Memorial Hospital	Nacogdoches	67%	300+
Northwest Texas Hospital	Amarillo	67%	300+
Saint Anthony's Hospital	Houston	67%	(a)
Saint David's Medical Center	Austin	67%	300+
Texas Health Presbyterian Hospital Plano	Plano	67%	300+
Univ of Texas Med Branch Galveston	Galveston	67%	300+
Arise Austin Medical Center[3]	Austin	66%	(a)
Christus Hospital	Beaumont	66%	300+
Detar Hospital Navarro	Victoria	66%	300+
Lake Pointe Medical Center	Rowlett	66%	300+
Longview Regional Medical Center	Longview	66%	300+
Memorial Hermann Katy Hospital	Katy	66%	300+
Methodist Sugar Land Hospital	Sugar Land	66%	300+
Texas Health Arlington Memorial Hospital	Arlington	66%	300+
Texas Health Harris Methodist	Bedford	66%	300+
Val Verde Regional Medical Center	Del Rio	66%	300+
Weatherford Regional Medical Center	Weatherford	66%	300+
Baylor Medical Center at Garland	Garland	65%	300+
Centennial Medical Center	Frisco	65%	300+
Christus Saint John Hospital	Nassau Bay	65%	300+
Citizens Medical Center	Victoria	65%	300+
Denton Regional Medical Center	Denton	65%	300+

NOTE: Hospital profiles are in alphabetical order by state, then city, then hospital within the city; Rankings exclude hospitals with less than 25 cases except for patient surveys which excludes hospitals with less than 100 cases; (a) 100-299 cases; (1) The number of cases/patients is too few to report; (2) Data submitted were based on a sample of cases/patients; (3) Results are based on a shorter time period than required; (4) Data suppressed by CMS for one or more quarters; (5) Results are not available for this reporting period; (6) Fewer than 100 patients completed the HCAHPS survey; (7) No cases met the criteria for this measure; (8) The lower limit of the confidence interval cannot be calculated if the number of observed infections equals zero; (9) No data are available from the state/territory for this reporting period; (10) The scores shown reflect fewer than 50 completed surveys; (11) There were discrepancies in the data collection process; (12) This measure does not apply to this hospital for this reporting period; (13) Results cannot be calculated for this reporting period; (14) The results for this state are combined with nearby states to protect confidentiality; Please refer to the User's Guide for a full explanation of data.

Doctors Hospital of Laredo	Laredo	65%	300+
Good Shepherd Medical Center	Longview	65%	300+
Lake Whitney Medical Center[11]	Whitney	65%	(a)
Methodist Mansfield Medical Center	Mansfield	65%	300+
Methodist Richardson Medical Center	Richardson	65%	300+
Methodist West Houston Hospital	Houston	65%	300+
Pampa Regional Medical Center	Pampa	65%	300+
Saint David's South Austin Medical Center	Austin	65%	300+
Saint Luke's Episcopal Hospital	Houston	65%	300+
Scenic Mountain Medical Center	Big Spring	65%	300+
Scott & White Hospital - Round Rock	Round Rock	65%	300+
Scott & White Hospital Brenham	Brenham	65%	300+
TX Hlth Harris Meth Hosp SW Ft Worth	Fort Worth	65%	300+
Texas Health Presbyterian Hospital Denton	Denton	65%	300+
UT Southwestern University Hospital	Dallas	65%	300+
Baptist Saint Anthony's Hospital	Amarillo	64%	300+
Baylor Surgical Hospital at Fort Worth	Fort Worth	64%	300+
Christus Saint Catherine Hospital	Katy	64%	300+
Christus Santa Rosa Hospital	San Antonio	64%	300+
Christus Spohn Hospital Kleberg	Kingsville	64%	300+
College Station Medical Center	College Station	64%	300+
Columbus Community Hospital	Columbus	64%	(a)
Doctors Hospital	Dallas	64%	300+
Harlingen Medical Center[11]	Harlingen	64%	300+
Huntsville Memorial Hospital	Huntsville	64%	(a)
Medical Center of Lewisville	Lewisville	64%	300+
Memorial Hermann Hospital System	Houston	64%	300+
Memorial Hermann Northeast	Humble	64%	300+
Memorial Medical Center Livingston	Livingston	64%	300+
Metroplex Hospital[11]	Killeen	64%	300+
North Austin Medical Center	Austin	64%	300+
North Cypress Medical Center	Cypress	64%	300+
Permian Regional Medical Center	Andrews	64%	(a)
Peterson Regional Medical Center	Kerrville	64%	300+
Providence Health Center	Waco	64%	300+
Saint Luke's Patients Medical Center	Pasadena	64%	300+
Seton Medical Center Williamson	Round Rock	64%	300+
Texas Orthopedic Hospital	Houston	64%	300+
Baylor All Saints Medical Center at FW	Fort Worth	63%	300+
Baylor Reg Med Ctr at Grapevine	Grapevine	63%	300+
Cedar Park Regional Medical Center	Cedar Park	63%	300+
Memorial Hermann Texas Medical Center	Houston	63%	300+
The Methodist Hospital	Houston	63%	300+
Methodist Willowbrook Hospital	Houston	63%	300+
North Hills Hospital	N Richland Hls	63%	300+
Oakbend Medical Center	Richmond	63%	300+
Seton Medical Center Hays	Kyle	63%	300+
Seton Northwest Hospital	Austin	63%	300+
Texas Health Presbyterian Hospital - WNJ	Sherman	63%	300+
University Medical Center of El Paso	El Paso	63%	300+
Univ of TX Health Science Ctr-Tyler	Tyler	63%	(a)
Abilene Regional Medical Center	Abilene	62%	300+
Baylor University Medical Center	Dallas	62%	300+
Brownwood Regional Medical Center	Brownwood	62%	300+
Conroe Regional Medical Center	Conroe	62%	300+
The Corpus Christi Medical Center	Corpus Christi	62%	300+
Cypress Fairbanks Medical Center	Houston	62%	300+
Doctors Hospital at Renaissance	Edinburg	62%	300+
Harris Health System	Houston	62%	300+
Houston Northwest Medical Center	Houston	62%	300+
JPS Health Network	Fort Worth	62%	300+
Knapp Medical Center	Weslaco	62%	300+
Medical City Dallas Hospital	Dallas	62%	300+
Memorial Medical Center of East Texas	Lufkin	62%	300+
Navarro Regional Hospital	Corsicana	62%	300+
Odessa Regional Hospital	Odessa	62%	300+
Plaza Medical Center of Fort Worth	Fort Worth	62%	300+
Providence Memorial Hospital	El Paso	62%	300+
Saint Luke's Hospital at the Vintage	Houston	62%	300+
Texas Health Presbyterian Hospital Dallas	Dallas	62%	300+
Texoma Medical Center	Denison	62%	300+
VHS Brownsville Hospital Company[11]	Brownsville	62%	300+
Baptist Medical Center[11]	San Antonio	61%	300+
Baylor Medical Center at Carrollton	Carrollton	61%	300+
Baylor Medical Center at Irving	Irving	61%	300+
Brazosport Regional Health System	Lake Jackson	61%	300+
East Texas Medical Center	Tyler	61%	300+
East Texas Medical Center Athens	Athens	61%	300+
Las Palmas Medical Center	El Paso	61%	300+
Medical Center Hospital	Odessa	61%	300+
The Medical Center of Southeast Texas	Port Arthur	61%	300+
Seton Medical Center Austin	Austin	61%	300+
Sierra Medical Center	El Paso	61%	300+
Christus Spohn Hospital Corpus Christi	Corpus Christi	60%	300+
Clear Lake Regional Medical Center	Webster	60%	300+
Hillcrest Baptist Medical Center	Waco	60%	300+
Methodist Dallas Medical Center	Dallas	60%	300+
Saint Luke's The Woodlands Hospital	The Woodlands	60%	300+
South Texas Health System	Edinburg	60%	300+
Tomball Regional Medical Center	Tomball	60%	300+
University General Hospital Dallas	Dallas	60%	(a)
University Medical Center at Brackenridge	Austin	60%	300+
VHS Harlingen Hospital Company[11]	Harlingen	60%	300+
Fort Duncan Medical Center	Eagle Pass	59%	300+
Lake Granbury Medical Center	Granbury	59%	300+
Las Colinas Medical Center	Irving	59%	300+
Memorial Hermann Sugar Land Hospital	Sugar Land	59%	300+
Methodist Hospital	San Antonio	59%	300+
Mother Frances Hospital	Tyler	59%	300+
Saint Joseph Medical Center	Houston	59%	300+
Scott & White Memorial Hospital[11]	Temple	59%	300+
South Texas Regional Medical Center	Jourdanton	59%	(a)
Medical Center of Arlington	Arlington	58%	300+
Methodist Charlton Medical Center	Dallas	58%	300+
Midland Memorial Hospital	Midland	58%	300+
Palestine Regional Medical Center	Palestine	58%	300+
Paris Regional Medical Center	Paris	58%	300+
Parkland Health & Hospital System	Dallas	58%	300+
Rio Grande Regional Hospital	Mcallen	58%	300+
Bayshore Medical Center	Pasadena	57%	300+
Doctors Hospital Tidwell	Houston	57%	300+
Ennis Regional Medical Center	Ennis	57%	300+
Good Shepherd Medical Center Marshall	Marshall	57%	300+
Kingwood Medical Center	Kingwood	57%	300+
Medical Center of Plano	Plano	57%	300+
Methodist Stone Oak Hospital	San Antonio	57%	300+
Saint Luke's Sugar Land Hospital	Sugar Land	57%	300+
University Health System	San Antonio	57%	300+
Dallas Regional Medical Center	Mesquite	56%	300+
The Womans Hospital of Texas	Houston	56%	300+
Laredo Medical Center	Laredo	55%	300+
Valley Regional Medical Center	Brownsville	55%	300+
Nix Health Care System	San Antonio	54%	300+
West Houston Medical Center	Houston	53%	300+
Southwest General Hospital	San Antonio	52%	300+
University General Hospital	Houston	52%	300+
Dallas Medical Center	Dallas	48%	300+

Would Definitely Recommend Hospital

Hospital Name	City	Rate	Cases
The Physicians Centre	Bryan	95%	(a)
Heart Hospital Baylor Plano	Plano	93%	300+
Heritage Park Surgical Hospital	Sherman	92%	(a)
Hill Country Memorial Hospital	Fredericksburg	92%	300+
North Central Surgical Center	Dallas	92%	300+
Quail Creek Surgical Hospital	Amarillo	92%	300+
Sugar Land Surgical Hospital	Sugar Land	92%	(a)
Baylor Heart & Vascular Hospital	Dallas	91%	300+
TX Hlth Harris Meth Hosp-Southlake	Southlake	91%	300+
TX Inst for Surgery at Presby Hosp	Dallas	91%	(a)
USMD Hospital at Fort Worth	Fort Worth	91%	(a)
Baylor Ortho & Spine Hosp-Arlington	Arlington	90%	300+
TX Health Ctr for Diag & Surgery	Plano	90%	(a)
Texas Spine & Joint Hospital	Tyler	90%	300+
Baylor Medical Center at Frisco	Frisco	89%	300+
Baylor Medical Center at Uptown	Dallas	89%	300+
Electra Memorial Hospital	Electra	89%	(a)
UT SW Univ Hosp-Zale Lipshy	Dallas	89%	300+
Houston Orthopedic & Spine Hospital	Bellaire	88%	300+
Saint Luke's Lakeside Hospital	The Woodlands	88%	300+
Baptist Emergency Hospital	San Antonio	87%	(a)
Baylor Medical Center at Mckinney	Mc Kinney	87%	300+
South Texas Spine & Surgical Hospital	San Antonio	87%	300+
South Texas Surgical Hospital	Corpus Christi	87%	300+
Fdn Surgical Hosp of San Antonio	San Antonio	86%	300+
Tops Surgical Specialty Hospital	Houston	86%	(a)
USMD Hospital at Arlington	Arlington	86%	300+
Baylor Regional Medical Center at Plano	Plano	85%	300+
Houston Physicians' Hospital	Webster	85%	(a)
Kell West Regional Hospital	Wichita Falls	85%	(a)
Lubbock Heart Hospital	Lubbock	85%	300+
East Texas Medical Center Pittsburg	Pittsburg	84%	(a)
Methodist Mansfield Medical Center	Mansfield	84%	300+
Texas Health Presbyterian Hospital Plano	Plano	84%	300+
Univ of TX Health Science Ctr-Tyler	Tyler	84%	(a)
Baylor Medical Center at Trophy Club	Trophy Club	83%	(a)
Glen Rose Medical Center	Glen Rose	83%	(a)
Methodist Hospital For Surgery	Addison	83%	300+
Northwest Hills Surgical Hospital	Austin	83%	(a)
TX Hlth Heart & Vasc Hosp-Arlington	Arlington	83%	300+
University Medical Center	Lubbock	83%	300+
W J Mangold Memorial Hospital	Lockney	83%	(a)
Baylor Reg Med Ctr at Grapevine	Grapevine	82%	300+
Childress Regional Medical Center	Childress	82%	(a)
East Texas Medical Center - Gilmer	Gilmer	82%	(a)
The Methodist Hospital	Houston	82%	300+
Hendrick Medical Center	Abilene	81%	300+
Mem Hermann Mem City Med Ctr	Houston	81%	300+
Methodist Ambulatory Surgery Hospital NW	San Antonio	81%	(a)
Providence Health Center	Waco	81%	300+
Seton Edgar B Davis Hospital	Luling	81%	(a)
Texas Orthopedic Hospital	Houston	81%	300+
UT Southwestern University Hospital	Dallas	81%	300+
Baptist Saint Anthony's Hospital	Amarillo	80%	300+
Baylor Surgical Hospital at Las Colinas	Irving	80%	(a)
Graham Regional Medical Center	Graham	80%	(a)
Methodist West Houston Hospital	Houston	80%	300+
Rollins Brook Community Hospital[11]	Lampasas	80%	(a)
Saint David's Medical Center	Austin	80%	300+
Seton Medical Center Harker Heights	Harker Heights	80%	300+
Seton Southwest Hospital	Austin	80%	(a)
Texas Health Harris Methodist Fort Worth	Fort Worth	80%	300+
TX Hlth Harris Meth Hosp SW Ft Worth	Fort Worth	80%	300+
TX Health Presbyterian Hosp Rockwall	Rockwall	80%	300+
Texoma Medical Center	Denison	80%	300+
Arise Austin Medical Center[3]	Austin	79%	(a)
Baylor All Saints Medical Center at FW	Fort Worth	79%	300+
Baylor University Medical Center	Dallas	79%	300+
Christus Saint John Hospital	Nassau Bay	79%	300+
Hamilton General Hospital	Hamilton	79%	(a)
The Hospital at Westlake Medical Center	Austin	79%	300+
Medical City Dallas Hospital	Dallas	79%	300+
Memorial Hermann Katy Hospital	Katy	79%	300+
Methodist Sugar Land Hospital	Sugar Land	79%	300+
Mother Frances Hospital	Tyler	79%	300+
North Austin Medical Center	Austin	79%	300+
Saint Luke's the Woodlands Hospital	The Woodlands	79%	300+
Scott & White Hospital - Round Rock	Round Rock	79%	300+
Seton Medical Center Williamson	Round Rock	79%	300+
Texas Health Harris Methodist	Bedford	79%	300+
Texas Health Presbyterian Hospital Dallas	Dallas	79%	300+
Woodland Heights Medical Center	Lufkin	79%	300+
Baptist Beaumont Hospital	Beaumont	78%	300+
Cornerstone Regional Hospital	Edinburg	78%	(a)
East Texas Medical Center Quitman	Quitman	78%	(a)
Saint Joseph Regional Health Center	Bryan	78%	300+
Saint Luke's Patients Medical Center	Pasadena	78%	300+
Seton Medical Center Hays	Kyle	78%	300+
Shannon Medical Center	San Angelo	78%	300+
TX Hlth Presbyterian Hosp-Flower Mound	Flower Mound	78%	300+
United Regional Health Care System	Wichita Falls	78%	300+
Wise Regional Health System	Decatur	78%	300+
Christus Saint Catherine Hospital	Katy	77%	300+
Christus Saint Michael Health System	Texarkana	77%	300+
Covenant Medical Center	Lubbock	77%	300+
Doctors Hospital at Renaissance	Edinburg	77%	300+
First Surgical Hospital	Bellaire	77%	(a)
Harlingen Medical Center[11]	Harlingen	77%	300+
Memorial Hermann Sugar Land Hospital	Sugar Land	77%	300+
Methodist Willowbrook Hospital	Houston	77%	300+
Saint Luke's Hospital at the Vintage	Houston	77%	300+
San Angelo Community Medical Center	San Angelo	77%	300+
TX Hlth Harris Meth Hosp-Stephenville	Stephenville	77%	300+
Texas Health Presbyterian Hospital Allen	Allen	77%	300+
Big Bend Regional Medical Center	Alpine	76%	(a)
Citizens Medical Center	Victoria	76%	300+
Columbus Community Hospital	Columbus	76%	(a)
El Paso Specialty Hospital	El Paso	76%	(a)
JPS Health Network	Fort Worth	76%	300+
Memorial Hermann Hospital System	Houston	76%	300+
Methodist Mckinney Hospital	Mc Kinney	76%	(a)
Round Rock Medical Center	Round Rock	76%	300+
Saint David's South Austin Medical Center	Austin	76%	300+
Saint Luke's Episcopal Hospital	Houston	76%	300+
Saint Marks Medical Center	La Grange	76%	(a)
Scott & White Memorial Hospital[11]	Temple	76%	300+
Sierra Providence East Medical Center	El Paso	76%	300+
Texas Health Presbyterian Hospital Denton	Denton	76%	300+
Good Shephard Medical Center - Linden	Linden	75%	(a)
Good Shepherd Medical Center	Longview	75%	300+
Grace Medical Center	Lubbock	75%	300+
Longview Regional Medical Center	Longview	75%	300+
Memorial Hermann Texas Medical Center	Houston	75%	300+
Memorial Medical Center of East Texas	Lufkin	75%	300+
Mission Regional Medical Center	Mission	75%	300+
North Cypress Medical Center	Cypress	75%	300+
Parkview Regional Hospital	Mexia	75%	(a)
Rolling Plains Memorial Hospital	Sweetwater	75%	(a)
Saint Luke's Sugar Land Hospital	Sugar Land	75%	300+
Seton Highland Lakes	Burnet	75%	300+
Seton Medical Center Austin	Austin	75%	300+
University Medical Center of El Paso	El Paso	75%	300+
The Womans Hospital of Texas	Houston	75%	300+
College Station Medical Center	College Station	74%	300+
Covenant Hospital Levelland	Levelland	74%	(a)
Detar Hospital Navarro	Victoria	74%	300+
Falls Community Hospital & Clinic	Marlin	74%	(a)
Foundation Surgical Hospital of El Paso	El Paso	74%	(a)
Hillcrest Baptist Medical Center	Waco	74%	300+
Medical Center of Lewisville	Lewisville	74%	300+
Memorial Medical Center	Port Lavaca	74%	(a)
Methodist Stone Oak Hospital	San Antonio	74%	300+
Nacogdoches Medical Center	Nacogdoches	74%	300+

NOTE: Hospital profiles are in alphabetical order by state, then city, then hospital within the city; Rankings exclude hospitals with less than 25 cases except for patient surveys which excludes hospitals with less than 100 cases; (a) 100-299 cases; (1) The number of cases/patients is too few to report; (2) Data submitted were based on a sample of cases/patients; (3) Results are based on a shorter time period than required; (4) Data suppressed by CMS for one or more quarters; (5) Results are not available for this reporting period; (6) Fewer than 100 patients completed the HCAHPS survey; (7) No cases met the criteria for this measure; (8) The lower limit of the confidence interval cannot be calculated if the number of observed infections equals zero; (9) No data are available from the state/territory for this reporting period; (10) The scores shown reflect fewer than 50 completed surveys; (11) There were discrepancies in the data collection process; (12) This measure does not apply to this hospital for this reporting period; (13) Results cannot be calculated for this reporting period; (14) The results for this state are combined with nearby states to protect confidentiality; Please refer to the User's Guide for a full explanation of data.

Odessa Regional Hospital	Odessa	74%	300+
Pecos County Memorial Hospital	Fort Stockton	74%	(a)
Plaza Medical Center of Fort Worth	Fort Worth	74%	300+
Seton Northwest Hospital	Austin	74%	300+
TX Hlth Presbyterian Hosp-Kaufman	Kaufman	74%	300+
Texas Reg Med Ctr at Sunnyvale	Sunnyvale	74%	300+
Tyler County Hospital	Woodville	74%	(a)
Baptist Medical Center[11]	San Antonio	73%	300+
Basin Healthcare Center	Odessa	73%	(a)
Baylor Medical Center at Garland	Garland	73%	300+
Baylor Medical Center at Waxahachie	Waxahachie	73%	300+
Centennial Medical Center	Frisco	73%	300+
Central Texas Medical Center[11]	San Marcos	73%	300+
Christus Hospital	Beaumont	73%	300+
Christus Santa Rosa Hospital	San Antonio	73%	300+
The Corpus Christi Medical Center	Corpus Christi	73%	300+
Doctors Hospital of Laredo	Laredo	73%	300+
Guadalupe Regional Medical Center	Seguin	73%	300+
Medina Regional Hospital	Hondo	73%	(a)
Memorial Hermann Northeast	Humble	73%	300+
Methodist Dallas Medical Center	Dallas	73%	300+
Pine Creek Medical Center	Dallas	73%	300+
San Jacinto Methodist Hospital	Baytown	73%	300+
Texas Health Arlington Memorial Hospital	Arlington	73%	300+
Baylor Medical Center at Irving	Irving	72%	300+
Christus Spohn Hospital Corpus Christi	Corpus Christi	72%	300+
Cypress Fairbanks Medical Center	Houston	72%	300+
East Texas Medical Center Jacksonville	Jacksonville	72%	300+
Eastland Memorial Hospital	Eastland	72%	(a)
Park Plaza Hospital	Houston	72%	300+
TX Hlth Harris Meth Hosp-Cleburne	Cleburne	72%	300+
Univ of Texas Med Branch Galveston	Galveston	72%	300+
Uvalde Memorial Hospital[11]	Uvalde	72%	(a)
VHS Harlingen Hospital Company[11]	Harlingen	72%	300+
Yoakum Community Hospital	Yoakum	72%	(a)
Abilene Regional Medical Center	Abilene	71%	300+
Baylor Surgical Hospital at Fort Worth	Fort Worth	71%	300+
Denton Regional Medical Center	Denton	71%	300+
East Texas Medical Center	Tyler	71%	300+
Las Colinas Medical Center	Irving	71%	300+
Medical Center Hospital	Odessa	71%	300+
Medical Center of Mckinney	Mckinney	71%	300+
Methodist Hospital	San Antonio	71%	300+
Northwest Texas Hospital	Amarillo	71%	300+
VHS Brownsville Hospital Company[11]	Brownsville	71%	300+
Doctors Hospital	Dallas	70%	300+
Medical Center of Plano	Plano	70%	300+
Nix Health Care System	San Antonio	70%	300+
North Hills Hospital	N Richland Hls	70%	300+
Peterson Regional Medical Center	Kerrville	70%	300+
Rio Grande Regional Hospital	Mcallen	70%	300+
TX Hlth Harris Methodist Hosp-Azle	Azle	70%	300+
University Medical Center at Brackenridge	Austin	70%	300+
Angleton - Danbury Medical Center	Angleton	69%	300+
Cedar Park Regional Medical Center	Cedar Park	69%	300+
Cuero Community Hospital	Cuero	69%	(a)
Harris Health System	Houston	69%	300+
Hill Regional Hospital	Hillsboro	69%	300+
Lake Pointe Medical Center	Rowlett	69%	300+
The Medical Center of Southeast Texas	Port Arthur	69%	300+
Memorial Hermann Baptist Orange Hospital	Orange	69%	300+
Moore County Hospital District	Dumas	69%	(a)
Providence Memorial Hospital	El Paso	69%	300+
South Texas Health System	Edinburg	69%	300+
University Health System	San Antonio	69%	300+
Baylor Medical Center at Carrollton	Carrollton	68%	300+
Covenant Hospital Plainview	Plainview	68%	300+
Hopkins County Memorial Hospital	Sulphur Springs	68%	300+
Matagorda Regional Medical Center	Bay City	68%	(a)
Methodist Richardson Medical Center	Richardson	68%	300+
Parkland Health & Hospital System	Dallas	68%	300+
Sierra Medical Center	El Paso	68%	300+
Tomball Regional Medical Center	Tomball	68%	300+
Valley Regional Medical Center	Brownsville	68%	300+
Christus Spohn Hospital Alice	Alice	67%	300+
Clear Lake Regional Medical Center	Webster	67%	300+
Etmc Henderson	Henderson	67%	300+
Houston Northwest Medical Center	Houston	67%	300+
Huguley Memorial Medical Center[11]	Burleson	67%	300+
Kingwood Medical Center	Kingwood	67%	300+
Las Palmas Medical Center	El Paso	67%	300+
Memorial Hospital	Nacogdoches	67%	300+
Saint Joseph Medical Center	Houston	67%	300+
University General Hospital	Houston	67%	300+
Wadley Regional Medical Center	Texarkana	67%	300+
Weatherford Regional Medical Center	Weatherford	67%	300+
Laredo Medical Center	Laredo	66%	300+
Medical Center of Arlington	Arlington	66%	300+
Methodist Charlton Medical Center	Dallas	66%	300+
Metroplex Hospital[11]	Killeen	66%	300+
Saint Anthony's Hospital	Houston	66%	(a)
Titus Regional Medical Center	Mount Pleasant	66%	300+
Care Regional Medical Center	Aransas Pass	65%	(a)
Connally Memorial Medical Center	Floresville	65%	(a)
East Texas Medical Center Athens	Athens	65%	300+
Etmc Clarksville	Clarksville	65%	(a)
Lake Granbury Medical Center	Granbury	65%	300+
West Houston Medical Center	Houston	65%	300+
Brownfield Regional Medical Center	Brownfield	64%	(a)
Conroe Regional Medical Center	Conroe	64%	300+
Oakbend Medical Center	Richmond	64%	300+
Palo Pinto General Hospital	Mineral Wells	64%	300+
Texas Health Presbyterian Hospital - WNJ	Sherman	64%	300+
Hunt Regional Medical Center	Greenville	63%	300+
Knapp Medical Center	Weslaco	63%	300+
Midland Memorial Hospital	Midland	63%	300+
North Texas Medical Center	Gainesville	63%	(a)
South Texas Regional Medical Center	Jourdanton	63%	(a)
Starr County Memorial Hospital	Rio Grande City	63%	(a)
Fort Duncan Medical Center	Eagle Pass	62%	300+
Good Shepherd Medical Center Marshall	Marshall	62%	300+
Scott & White Hospital Brenham	Brenham	62%	300+
Christus Spohn Hospital Beeville	Beeville	61%	(a)
Hereford Regional Medical Center	Hereford	61%	(a)
Memorial Medical Center Livingston	Livingston	61%	300+
Val Verde Regional Medical Center	Del Rio	61%	300+
East Texas Medical Center Crockett	Crockett	60%	(a)
Ennis Regional Medical Center	Ennis	60%	300+
Pampa Regional Medical Center	Pampa	60%	300+
Scott & White Hospital - Llano	Llano	60%	(a)
Bayshore Medical Center	Pasadena	59%	300+
Brownwood Regional Medical Center	Brownwood	59%	300+
Coryell Memorial Healthcare System	Gatesville	59%	(a)
Southwest General Hospital	San Antonio	59%	300+
Christus Spohn Hospital Kleberg	Kingsville	58%	300+
Navarro Regional Hospital	Corsicana	58%	300+
Permian Regional Medical Center	Andrews	58%	(a)
Huntsville Memorial Hospital	Huntsville	57%	(a)
University General Hospital Dallas	Dallas	57%	(a)
Brazosport Regional Health System	Lake Jackson	56%	300+
Christus Jasper Memorial Hospital	Jasper	56%	(a)
Doctors Hospital Tidwell	Houston	54%	300+
Etmc Carthage	Carthage	54%	(a)
Scenic Mountain Medical Center	Big Spring	54%	300+
Palestine Regional Medical Center	Palestine	52%	300+
Lake Whitney Medical Center[11]	Whitney	51%	(a)
Paris Regional Medical Center	Paris	50%	300+
Dallas Regional Medical Center	Mesquite	49%	300+
Dallas Medical Center	Dallas	39%	300+

Use of Medical Imaging

Cardiac Imaging Stress Test before OP Surgery

Hospital Name	City	Rate	Cases
Christus Hospital	Beaumont	0.0%	62
Christus Spohn Hospital Corpus Christi	Corpus Christi	0.0%	59
Odessa Regional Hospital	Odessa	0.0%	47
Val Verde Regional Medical Center	Del Rio	0.0%	67
Cogdell Memorial Hospital	Snyder	1.2%	85
Texas Health Harris Methodist Fort Worth	Fort Worth	1.4%	70
Cuero Community Hospital	Cuero	1.6%	64
Christus Saint Catherine Hospital	Katy	1.8%	56
Etmc Carthage	Carthage	1.8%	55
Hendrick Medical Center	Abilene	1.8%	1169
Medical Center of Arlington	Arlington	1.9%	106
Nacogdoches Medical Center	Nacogdoches	1.9%	54
Huguley Memorial Medical Center	Burleson	2.0%	150
Detar Hospital Navarro	Victoria	2.2%	93
Medical Arts Hospital	Lamesa	2.2%	45
Midland Memorial Hospital	Midland	2.2%	316
South Texas Health System	Edinburg	2.3%	88
Texas Health Presbyterian Hospital Dallas	Dallas	2.4%	249
Methodist Willowbrook Hospital	Houston	2.5%	79
Scott & White Hospital - Llano	Llano	2.6%	77
Cedar Park Regional Medical Center	Cedar Park	2.7%	185
Sierra Providence East Medical Center	El Paso	2.9%	105
TX Hlth Presbyterian Hosp-Kaufman	Kaufman	3.0%	200
Etmc Clarksville	Clarksville	3.1%	98
Harris Health System	Houston	3.1%	324
University Medical Center	Lubbock	3.2%	529
JPS Health Network	Fort Worth	3.3%	397
Parkland Health & Hospital System	Dallas	3.4%	411
Providence Health Center	Waco	3.4%	179
Paris Regional Medical Center	Paris	3.5%	85
Baylor Medical Center at Waxahachie	Waxahachie	3.6%	137
Baylor Reg Med Ctr at Grapevine	Grapevine	3.6%	194
Kingwood Medical Center	Kingwood	3.6%	55
University Medical Center of El Paso	El Paso	3.6%	83
Christus Saint Michael Health System	Texarkana	3.8%	260
Hill Regional Hospital	Hillsboro	3.8%	52
Hillcrest Baptist Medical Center	Waco	3.8%	264
Lake Granbury Medical Center	Granbury	3.8%	368
Good Shepherd Medical Center	Longview	3.9%	483
Hopkins County Memorial Hospital	Sulphur Springs	3.9%	414
Saint Joseph Regional Health Center	Bryan	3.9%	308
Tomball Regional Medical Center	Tomball	3.9%	129
University Medical Center at Brackenridge	Austin	3.9%	51
Northwest Texas Hospital	Amarillo	4.0%	126
Good Shepherd Medical Center Marshall	Marshall	4.1%	121
Memorial Medical Center of East Texas	Lufkin	4.1%	344
Metroplex Hospital	Killeen	4.1%	196
Texas Health Presbyterian Hospital Plano	Plano	4.1%	74
United Regional Health Care System	Wichita Falls	4.1%	242
Baptist Saint Anthony's Hospital	Amarillo	4.2%	331
Baylor University Medical Center	Dallas	4.2%	71
Cypress Fairbanks Medical Center	Houston	4.2%	48
Hill Country Memorial Hospital	Fredericksburg	4.3%	116
Saint David's Medical Center	Austin	4.3%	4459
Seton Medical Center Williamson	Round Rock	4.4%	158
Seton Southwest Hospital	Austin	4.4%	45
Round Rock Medical Center	Round Rock	4.5%	247
Seton Northwest Hospital	Austin	4.5%	110
Texas Reg Med Ctr at Sunnyvale	Sunnyvale	4.5%	88
University Health System	San Antonio	4.5%	336
Guadalupe Regional Medical Center	Seguin	4.6%	151
Mother Frances Hospital	Tyler	4.6%	2196
Uvalde Memorial Hospital	Uvalde	4.6%	65
Knapp Medical Center	Weslaco	4.7%	192
Medical Center of Mckinney	Mckinney	4.7%	64
South Texas Regional Medical Center	Jourdanton	4.7%	64
Baylor Medical Center at Carrollton	Carrollton	4.8%	145
Brownwood Regional Medical Center	Brownwood	4.8%	357
Citizens Medical Center	Victoria	4.8%	437
Conroe Regional Medical Center	Conroe	4.8%	789
Methodist Charlton Medical Center	Dallas	4.8%	227
Navarro Regional Hospital	Corsicana	4.8%	145
Shannon Medical Center	San Angelo	4.8%	229
VHS Harlingen Hospital Company	Harlingen	4.8%	433
Medical City Dallas Hospital	Dallas	4.9%	528
Texas Health Presbyterian Hospital - WNJ	Sherman	4.9%	512
East Texas Medical Center Athens	Athens	5.0%	202
Lakeway Regional Medical Center	Lakeway	5.0%	199
Scott & White Hospital - Round Rock	Round Rock	5.0%	420
Univ of Texas Med Branch Galveston	Galveston	5.0%	663
Seton Medical Center Hays	Kyle	5.1%	195
Abilene Regional Medical Center	Abilene	5.2%	363
Baptist Medical Center	San Antonio	5.2%	726
Glen Rose Medical Center	Glen Rose	5.2%	97
Saint David's South Austin Medical Center	Austin	5.2%	288
Saint Luke's Episcopal Hospital	Houston	5.2%	504
Connally Memorial Medical Center	Floresville	5.3%	57
Methodist Hospital	San Antonio	5.4%	3598
Clear Lake Regional Medical Center	Webster	5.5%	436
Rolling Plains Memorial Hospital	Sweetwater	5.5%	73
Seton Medical Center Austin	Austin	5.6%	640
West Houston Medical Center	Houston	5.6%	126
Covenant Medical Center	Lubbock	5.8%	225
East Texas Medical Center	Tyler	5.8%	362
Seton Highland Lakes	Burnet	5.8%	154
Texas Health Harris Methodist	Bedford	5.8%	104
Titus Regional Medical Center	Mount Pleasant	5.8%	104
Doctors Hospital	Dallas	6.0%	248
Huntsville Memorial Hospital	Huntsville	6.0%	150
North Austin Medical Center	Austin	6.0%	217
Longview Regional Medical Center	Longview	6.1%	114
East Texas Medical Center Jacksonville	Jacksonville	6.3%	95
Hunt Regional Medical Center	Greenville	6.3%	238
Palestine Regional Medical Center	Palestine	6.3%	63
San Jacinto Methodist Hospital	Baytown	6.3%	95
Baylor Medical Center at Mckinney	Mc Kinney	6.4%	110
The Methodist Hospital	Houston	6.4%	566
Park Plaza Hospital	Houston	6.4%	171
Rio Grande Regional Hospital	Mcallen	6.4%	281
Scott & White Memorial Hospital	Temple	6.5%	902
Palo Pinto General Hospital	Mineral Wells	6.7%	210
Univ of TX Health Science Ctr-Tyler	Tyler	6.7%	179
San Angelo Community Medical Center	San Angelo	6.8%	530
Methodist Mansfield Medical Center	Mansfield	6.9%	174
Baylor Medical Center at Garland	Garland	7.0%	300
Baylor Medical Center at Irving	Irving	7.0%	257
Heart Hospital Baylor Plano	Plano	7.0%	527
Seton Medical Center Harker Heights	Harker Heights	7.0%	86
Texoma Medical Center	Denison	7.1%	156
Houston Northwest Medical Center	Houston	7.2%	320
The Hospital at Westlake Medical Center	Austin	7.3%	124
Las Palmas Medical Center	El Paso	7.3%	109
Saint Luke's the Woodlands Hospital	The Woodlands	7.4%	176
Wadley Regional Medical Center	Texarkana	7.4%	122
Memorial Hermann Hospital System	Houston	7.5%	843
Memorial Hospital	Nacogdoches	7.5%	93
Methodist Stone Oak Hospital	San Antonio	7.5%	174
Peterson Regional Medical Center	Kerrville	7.5%	252

NOTE: Hospital profiles are in alphabetical order by state, then city, then hospital within the city; Rankings exclude hospitals with less than 25 cases except for patient surveys which excludes hospitals with less than 100 cases; (a) 100-299 cases; (1) The number of cases/patients is too few to report; (2) Data submitted were based on a sample of cases/patients; (3) Results are based on a shorter time period than required; (4) Data suppressed by CMS for one or more quarters; (5) Results are not available for this reporting period; (6) Fewer than 100 patients completed the HCAHPS survey; (7) No cases met the criteria for this measure; (8) The lower limit of the confidence interval cannot be calculated if the number of observed infections equals zero; (9) No data are available from the state/territory for this reporting period; (10) The scores shown reflect fewer than 50 completed surveys; (11) There were discrepancies in the data collection process; (12) This measure does not apply to this hospital for this reporting period; (13) Results cannot be calculated for this reporting period; (14) The results for this state are combined with nearby states to protect confidentiality; Please refer to the User's Guide for a full explanation of data.

Hospital Name	City	Rate	Cases
Saint Joseph Medical Center	Houston	7.6%	119
Central Texas Medical Center	San Marcos	7.8%	102
Memorial Hermann Texas Medical Center	Houston	7.8%	180
Methodist Dallas Medical Center	Dallas	7.8%	141
Plaza Medical Center of Fort Worth	Fort Worth	7.8%	129
Texas Health Presbyterian Hospital Allen	Allen	7.8%	64
Christus Santa Rosa Hospital	San Antonio	7.9%	305
Methodist Sugar Land Hospital	Sugar Land	8.0%	212
Baptist Beaumont Hospital	Beaumont	8.1%	149
Nix Health Care System	San Antonio	8.1%	185
Texas Health Arlington Memorial Hospital	Arlington	8.6%	139
UT Southwestern University Hospital	Dallas	8.6%	290
Bayshore Medical Center	Pasadena	8.9%	315
Mem Hermann Mem City Med Ctr	Houston	9.9%	141
Covenant Hospital Plainview	Plainview	10.0%	80
Lubbock Heart Hospital	Lubbock	10.0%	230
North Cypress Medical Center	Cypress	11.0%	146

Combination Abdominal CT Scan

Hospital Name	City	Rate	Cases
East Texas Medical Center Mount Vernon	Mount Vernon	0.0%	50
Hansford County Hospital	Spearman	0.0%	70
Rolling Plains Memorial Hospital	Sweetwater	0.0%	133
Baptist Saint Anthony's Hospital	Amarillo	0.6%	1499
Methodist Stone Oak Hospital	San Antonio	0.6%	352
Texas Health Harris Methodist Fort Worth	Fort Worth	0.9%	1068
Baptist Emergency Hospital	San Antonio	1.1%	184
Baptist Medical Center	San Antonio	1.1%	1839
Round Rock Medical Center	Round Rock	1.1%	359
Saint David's South Austin Medical Center	Austin	1.1%	627
East Texas Medical Center - Gilmer	Gilmer	1.3%	149
Medical Center of Arlington	Arlington	1.3%	394
TX Hlth Harris Meth Hosp-Alliance	Fort Worth	1.3%	75
East Texas Medical Center Trinity	Trinity	1.4%	70
North Austin Medical Center	Austin	1.4%	567
Seton Medical Center Williamson	Round Rock	1.5%	264
Southwest General Hospital	San Antonio	1.5%	196
Cedar Park Regional Medical Center	Cedar Park	1.7%	359
Methodist Richardson Medical Center	Richardson	1.7%	634
Fort Duncan Medical Center	Eagle Pass	1.8%	509
Seton Southwest Hospital	Austin	1.8%	167
Texas Health Harris Methodist	Bedford	1.8%	615
Emerus Hospital	Sugar Land	1.9%	54
Seymour Hospital	Seymour	1.9%	54
Seton Northwest Hospital	Austin	2.0%	254
Texas Health Presbyterian Hospital Dallas	Dallas	2.0%	555
Falls Community Hospital & Clinic	Marlin	2.1%	96
University Medical Center at Brackenridge	Austin	2.1%	240
Heart Hospital Baylor Plano	Plano	2.2%	93
Hereford Regional Medical Center	Hereford	2.2%	92
Paris Regional Medical Center	Paris	2.3%	398
Seton Medical Center Harker Heights	Harker Heights	2.3%	218
Seton Medical Center Austin	Austin	2.5%	404
Seton Medical Center Hays	Kyle	2.5%	363
Etmc Carthage	Carthage	2.6%	191
Brownfield Regional Medical Center	Brownfield	2.7%	74
Sierra Providence East Medical Center	El Paso	2.9%	339
North Hills Hospital	N Richland Hls	3.0%	502
College Station Medical Center	College Station	3.1%	321
Saint David's Medical Center	Austin	3.2%	759
The Corpus Christi Medical Center	Corpus Christi	3.4%	502
Nacogdoches Medical Center	Nacogdoches	3.4%	406
Parkview Regional Hospital	Mexia	3.4%	145
Rio Grande Regional Hospital	Mcallen	3.5%	396
Plains Memorial Hospital	Dimmitt	3.6%	56
San Angelo Community Medical Center	San Angelo	3.7%	301
Texas Health Arlington Memorial Hospital	Arlington	3.7%	595
Baylor Medical Center at Waxahachie	Waxahachie	3.8%	660
Citizens Medical Center	Victoria	3.8%	1020
Cuero Community Hospital	Cuero	3.8%	235
Pecos County Memorial Hospital	Fort Stockton	3.8%	132
Shannon Medical Center	San Angelo	4.2%	523
Baylor Medical Center at Irving	Irving	4.3%	726
Brazosport Regional Health System	Lake Jackson	4.4%	771
Peterson Regional Medical Center	Kerrville	4.4%	902
University Medical Center of El Paso	El Paso	4.5%	440
South Texas Regional Medical Center	Jourdanton	4.6%	324
Good Shephard Medical Center - Linden	Linden	4.8%	126
Medical Center of Lewisville	Lewisville	4.8%	271
Baylor University Medical Center	Dallas	5.0%	2199
Saint Luke's Patients Medical Center	Pasadena	5.1%	455
Seton Highland Lakes	Burnet	5.1%	693
Clear Lake Regional Medical Center	Webster	5.2%	1395
Central Texas Hospital	Cameron	5.3%	57
Medical Center of Mckinney	Mckinney	5.4%	465
Christus Santa Rosa Hospital	San Antonio	5.5%	1596
East Texas Medical Center Crockett	Crockett	5.5%	163
Las Palmas Medical Center	El Paso	5.6%	1006
Hillcrest Baptist Medical Center	Waco	5.8%	1017
Seton Edgar B Davis Hospital	Luling	5.8%	311
East Texas Medical Center Quitman	Quitman	6.0%	200
Saint Joseph Regional Health Center	Bryan	6.1%	822
Texas Health Presbyterian Hospital Allen	Allen	6.1%	214
East Texas Medical Center	Tyler	6.2%	1430
Goodall Witcher Hospital	Clifton	6.2%	81
Baylor Medical Center at Mckinney	Mc Kinney	6.4%	497
Baylor Reg Med Ctr at Grapevine	Grapevine	6.4%	547
Baptist Beaumont Hospital	Beaumont	6.5%	721
Matagorda Regional Medical Center	Bay City	6.5%	214
Saint Joseph Medical Center	Houston	6.5%	369
Hendrick Medical Center	Abilene	6.6%	1053
Otto Kaiser Memorial Hospital	Kenedy	6.6%	183
Methodist Hospital	San Antonio	6.7%	2332
Scott & White Hospital - Llano	Llano	6.7%	255
TX Hlth Harris Meth Hosp-Cleburne	Cleburne	6.7%	419
Lakeway Regional Medical Center	Lakeway	6.8%	176
Sweeny Community Hospital	Sweeny	6.9%	72
USMD Hospital at Arlington	Arlington	6.9%	259
Parkland Health & Hospital System	Dallas	7.0%	1153
East Texas Medical Center - Fairfield	Fairfield	7.1%	113
Centennial Medical Center	Frisco	7.3%	232
Doctors Hospital	Dallas	7.3%	424
Scott & White Hospital - Round Rock	Round Rock	7.3%	896
Stephens Memorial Hospital	Breckenridge	7.4%	68
Medical City Dallas Hospital	Dallas	7.5%	616
Methodist Mansfield Medical Center	Mansfield	7.6%	543
Christus Saint John Hospital	Nassau Bay	7.7%	378
Saint Luke's Sugar Land Hospital	Sugar Land	7.7%	246
Navarro Regional Hospital	Corsicana	7.9%	316
Plaza Medical Center of Fort Worth	Fort Worth	7.9%	216
Providence Health Center	Waco	7.9%	1206
Sierra Medical Center	El Paso	8.0%	614
Reeves County Hospital District	Pecos	8.2%	110
Woodland Heights Medical Center	Lufkin	8.2%	353
Covenant Hospital Plainview	Plainview	8.3%	192
Baylor Medical Center at Carrollton	Carrollton	8.4%	380
Laredo Medical Center	Laredo	8.5%	1065
Scott & White Memorial Hospital	Temple	8.5%	2428
Harris Health System	Houston	8.6%	910
Moore County Hospital District	Dumas	8.6%	105
Baylor Regional Medical Center at Plano	Plano	8.7%	643
Memorial Hospital	Gonzales	8.8%	125
Uvalde Memorial Hospital	Uvalde	8.8%	443
Lake Pointe Medical Center	Rowlett	8.9%	576
Baylor Medical Center at Frisco	Frisco	9.1%	99
Longview Regional Medical Center	Longview	9.1%	584
Rollins Brook Community Hospital	Lampasas	9.1%	175
Denton Regional Medical Center	Denton	9.2%	369
Las Colinas Medical Center	Irving	9.2%	206
Methodist Charlton Medical Center	Dallas	9.3%	851
Coryell Memorial Healthcare System	Gatesville	9.4%	96
United Regional Health Care System	Wichita Falls	9.5%	833
Weatherford Regional Medical Center	Weatherford	9.5%	419
Good Shepherd Medical Center Marshall	Marshall	9.8%	457
Ennis Regional Medical Center	Ennis	9.9%	151
Stamford Memorial Hospital	Stamford	9.9%	71
TX Hlth Harris Meth Hosp SW Ft Worth	Fort Worth	9.9%	770
Texas Reg Med Ctr at Sunnyvale	Sunnyvale	10.1%	278
Bayshore Medical Center	Pasadena	10.2%	688
Connally Memorial Medical Center	Floresville	10.2%	186
Dallas Regional Medical Center	Mesquite	10.2%	274
JPS Health Network	Fort Worth	10.3%	1008
Memorial Hermann Sugar Land Hospital	Sugar Land	10.3%	380
Central Texas Medical Center	San Marcos	10.5%	467
Hamilton General Hospital	Hamilton	10.5%	124
TX Hlth Harris Methodist Hosp-Azle	Azle	10.6%	360
Texas Health Presbyterian Hospital Plano	Plano	10.7%	542
Baylor All Saints Medical Center at FW	Fort Worth	10.9%	707
Guadalupe Regional Medical Center	Seguin	10.9%	726
Good Shepherd Medical Center	Longview	11.0%	1299
Memorial Hospital	Nacogdoches	11.1%	405
Midland Memorial Hospital	Midland	11.1%	970
Metroplex Hospital	Killeen	11.7%	606
Seton Smithville Regional Hospital	Smithville	11.7%	266
East Texas Medical Center Athens	Athens	11.8%	825
Houston Northwest Medical Center	Houston	11.8%	595
Texas Health Presbyterian Hospital Denton	Denton	11.8%	448
Medical Arts Hospital	Lamesa	11.9%	134
Wise Regional Health System	Decatur	11.9%	605
Baylor Medical Center at Garland	Garland	12.4%	1028
The Physicians Centre	Bryan	12.4%	113
Texas Health Presbyterian Hospital - WNJ	Sherman	12.4%	364
TX Health Presbyterian Hosp Rockwall	Rockwall	12.6%	413
Huntsville Memorial Hospital	Huntsville	12.7%	536
Scott & White Hospital Brenham	Brenham	12.7%	228
Frio Regional Hospital	Pearsall	13.2%	91
Gulf Coast Medical Center	Wharton	13.3%	105
Medical Center Hospital	Odessa	13.4%	791
Mission Regional Medical Center	Mission	13.4%	253
Etmc Henderson	Henderson	13.8%	240
East Texas Medical Center Jacksonville	Jacksonville	13.9%	287
North Texas Medical Center	Gainesville	14.0%	221
Memorial Hermann Northeast	Humble	14.1%	625
Nix Health Care System	San Antonio	14.1%	227
Providence Memorial Hospital	El Paso	14.1%	547
Univ of TX Health Science Ctr-Tyler	Tyler	14.1%	433
UT Southwestern University Hospital	Dallas	14.1%	1423
VHS Brownsville Hospital Company	Brownsville	14.1%	552
Val Verde Regional Medical Center	Del Rio	14.3%	442
Christus Jasper Memorial Hospital	Jasper	14.5%	373
Dimmit Regional Hospital	Carrizo Springs	14.6%	82
West Houston Medical Center	Houston	14.7%	339
South Texas Health System	Edinburg	15.3%	588
TX Hlth Presbyterian Hosp-Flower Mound	Flower Mound	15.3%	288
Doctors Hospital of Laredo	Laredo	15.6%	359
Detar Hospital Navarro	Victoria	15.9%	508
Lake Granbury Medical Center	Granbury	16.2%	543
Saint Marks Medical Center	La Grange	16.2%	315
Cypress Fairbanks Medical Center	Houston	16.3%	215
Scenic Mountain Medical Center	Big Spring	16.4%	238
Memorial Hermann Hospital System	Houston	16.7%	3617
Saint Luke's Hospital at the Vintage	Houston	16.7%	228
VHS Harlingen Hospital Company	Harlingen	16.7%	893
Huguley Memorial Medical Center	Burleson	16.8%	743
Wadley Regional Medical Center	Texarkana	17.1%	387
Odessa Regional Hospital	Odessa	17.2%	174
Medical Center of Plano	Plano	17.3%	693
Saint Luke's the Woodlands Hospital	The Woodlands	17.5%	775
Cleveland Regional Medical Center	Cleveland	17.7%	113
Methodist Willowbrook Hospital	Houston	17.7%	566
Big Bend Regional Medical Center	Alpine	17.8%	118
Christus Saint Catherine Hospital	Katy	17.8%	253
Conroe Regional Medical Center	Conroe	17.8%	675
University General Hospital Dallas	Dallas	17.9%	67
Christus Saint Michael Health System	Texarkana	18.1%	1115
Tyler County Hospital	Woodville	18.3%	131
Foundation Surgical Hospital of El Paso	El Paso	18.4%	316
Northwest Texas Hospital	Amarillo	18.6%	388
Permian Regional Medical Center	Andrews	18.6%	86
Glen Rose Medical Center	Glen Rose	18.7%	155
Saint Luke's Episcopal Hospital	Houston	18.8%	1312
Kingwood Medical Center	Kingwood	19.1%	571
University Health System	San Antonio	19.1%	618
Bellville General Hospital	Bellville	19.6%	112
Palestine Regional Medical Center	Palestine	19.6%	317
TX Hlth Presbyterian Hosp-Kaufman	Kaufman	20.6%	247
Univ of Texas Med Branch Galveston	Galveston	21.1%	1104
Dallas Medical Center	Dallas	21.2%	104
Jackson Healthcare Center	Edna	21.6%	74
Starr County Memorial Hospital	Rio Grande City	21.8%	78
Memorial Medical Center Livingston	Livingston	22.0%	323
Park Plaza Hospital	Houston	22.3%	309
Hill Regional Hospital	Hillsboro	22.6%	168
Methodist Sugar Land Hospital	Sugar Land	22.8%	851
Tomball Regional Medical Center	Tomball	23.0%	718
Methodist West Houston Hospital	Houston	23.1%	324
TX Hlth Harris Meth Hosp-Stephenville	Stephenville	23.4%	273
Memorial Hermann Katy Hospital	Katy	23.6%	788
University Medical Center	Lubbock	23.8%	1236
Etmc Clarksville	Clarksville	24.0%	129
Harlingen Medical Center	Harlingen	24.1%	340
Mitchell County Hospital District	Colorado City	24.2%	66
Christus Spohn Hospital Beeville	Beeville	24.5%	163
Methodist Dallas Medical Center	Dallas	24.5%	1017
Valley Regional Medical Center	Brownsville	24.5%	445
Mother Frances Hospital	Tyler	24.8%	1640
San Jacinto Methodist Hospital	Baytown	25.1%	514
Abilene Regional Medical Center	Abilene	25.7%	428
Memorial Hermann Texas Medical Center	Houston	25.8%	809
Kell West Regional Hospital	Wichita Falls	26.0%	327
Wilbarger General Hospital	Vernon	26.8%	179
Oakbend Medical Center	Richmond	27.6%	381
Childress Regional Medical Center	Childress	28.1%	121
Doctors Hospital Tidwell	Houston	28.3%	60
Texoma Medical Center	Denison	28.5%	1203
Hill Country Memorial Hospital	Fredericksburg	29.0%	613
Pampa Regional Medical Center	Pampa	29.4%	180
Basin Healthcare Center	Odessa	29.5%	129
Christus Hospital	Beaumont	30.7%	1209
Palo Pinto General Hospital	Mineral Wells	31.1%	283
The Medical Center of Southeast Texas	Port Arthur	31.2%	446
Covenant Medical Center	Lubbock	31.3%	1279
UT SW Univ Hosp-Zale Lipshy	Dallas	31.9%	552
Angleton - Danbury Medical Center	Angleton	32.7%	171
Covenant Hospital Levelland	Levelland	33.3%	51
The Methodist Hospital	Houston	33.4%	2000
Graham Regional Medical Center	Graham	33.5%	284
Hamilton Hospital	Olney	34.4%	93
Lubbock Heart Hospital	Lubbock	34.7%	75
Cogdell Memorial Hospital	Snyder	35.0%	103
Mem Hermann Mem City Med Ctr	Houston	35.4%	1365
Hopkins County Memorial Hospital	Sulphur Springs	38.5%	449
Memorial Hermann Baptist Orange Hospital	Orange	38.5%	377

NOTE: Hospital profiles are in alphabetical order by state, then city, then hospital within the city; Rankings exclude hospitals with less than 25 cases except for patient surveys which excludes hospitals with less than 100 cases; (a) 100-299 cases; (1) The number of cases/patients is too few to report; (2) Data submitted were based on a sample of cases/patients; (3) Results are based on a shorter time period than required; (4) Data suppressed by CMS for one or more quarters; (5) Results are not available for this reporting period; (6) Fewer than 100 patients completed the HCAHPS survey; (7) No cases met the criteria for this measure; (8) The lower limit of the confidence interval cannot be calculated if the number of observed infections equals zero; (9) No data are available from the state/territory for this reporting period; (10) The scores shown reflect fewer than 50 completed surveys; (11) There were discrepancies in the data collection process; (12) This measure does not apply to this hospital for this reporting period; (13) Results cannot be calculated for this reporting period; (14) The results for this state are combined with nearby states to protect confidentiality; Please refer to the User's Guide for a full explanation of data.

Hospital Name	City	Rate	Cases
Christus Spohn Hospital Corpus Christi	Corpus Christi	40.3%	553
Hunt Regional Medical Center	Greenville	40.5%	1062
Brownwood Regional Medical Center	Brownwood	43.0%	551
Grace Medical Center	Lubbock	43.3%	353
El Campo Memorial Hospital	El Campo	44.6%	112
Titus Regional Medical Center	Mount Pleasant	45.2%	473
Eastland Memorial Hospital	Eastland	45.9%	133
Memorial Medical Center	Port Lavaca	46.2%	199
Doctors Hospital at Renaissance	Edinburg	46.4%	2163
Saint Luke's Lakeside Hospital	The Woodlands	46.8%	94
Heart Hospital Baylor Denton	Denton	48.8%	41
Bowie Memorial Hospital	Bowie	52.1%	94
Christus Spohn Hospital Alice	Alice	52.1%	257
Knapp Medical Center	Weslaco	52.1%	630
University General Hospital	Houston	52.8%	231
TX Health Ctr for Diag & Surgery	Plano	54.7%	75
Columbus Community Hospital	Columbus	55.5%	290
Care Regional Medical Center	Aransas Pass	55.8%	181
Christus Spohn Hospital Kleberg	Kingsville	56.0%	257
Memorial Medical Center of East Texas	Lufkin	59.1%	606
Houston Physicians' Hospital	Webster	59.5%	126
Doctors Diagnostic Hospital	Cleveland	62.0%	142
North Cypress Medical Center	Cypress	65.9%	936
Heritage Park Surgical Hospital	Sherman	75.0%	196

Combination Brain/Sinus CT Scan

Hospital Name	City	Rate	Cases
Basin Healthcare Center	Odessa	0.0%	35
Baylor Emergency Medical Center	Aubrey	0.0%	31
Baylor Surgical Hospital at Fort Worth	Fort Worth	0.0%	34
Bayside Community Hospital	Anahuac	0.0%	51
Electra Memorial Hospital	Electra	0.0%	44
Hamilton Hospital	Olney	0.0%	127
Lake Whitney Medical Center	Whitney	0.0%	72
Medical Arts Hospital	Lamesa	0.0%	115
Mitchell County Hospital District	Colorado City	0.0%	68
Nocona General Hospital	Nocona	0.0%	39
Saint Anthony's Hospital	Houston	0.0%	46
Stamford Memorial Hospital	Stamford	0.0%	76
Texas Spine & Joint Hospital	Tyler	0.0%	97
UT SW Univ Hosp-Zale Lipshy	Dallas	0.0%	56
Columbus Community Hospital	Columbus	0.4%	242
Guadalupe Regional Medical Center	Seguin	0.4%	550
Longview Regional Medical Center	Longview	0.4%	720
Cuero Community Hospital	Cuero	0.5%	215
Good Shepherd Medical Center Marshall	Marshall	0.6%	495
Heart Hospital Baylor Plano	Plano	0.6%	162
Mission Regional Medical Center	Mission	0.6%	522
Providence Health Center	Waco	0.6%	1159
Tyler County Hospital	Woodville	0.6%	178
Bellville General Hospital	Bellville	0.7%	135
Christus Jasper Memorial Hospital	Jasper	0.7%	595
Coryell Memorial Healthcare System	Gatesville	0.7%	150
Saint Luke's Lakeside Hospital	The Woodlands	0.7%	135
Hill Country Memorial Hospital	Fredericksburg	0.8%	356
Brownwood Regional Medical Center	Brownwood	0.9%	555
Lubbock Heart Hospital	Lubbock	0.9%	225
Methodist Dallas Medical Center	Dallas	0.9%	774
Palo Pinto General Hospital	Mineral Wells	0.9%	340
Kell West Regional Hospital	Wichita Falls	1.0%	202
Dallas Regional Medical Center	Mesquite	1.1%	350
Good Shepherd Medical Center	Longview	1.1%	1309
Hill Regional Hospital	Hillsboro	1.1%	188
UT Southwestern University Hospital	Dallas	1.1%	791
Baylor University Medical Center	Dallas	1.2%	1989
Memorial Hermann Sugar Land Hospital	Sugar Land	1.2%	335
Navarro Regional Hospital	Corsicana	1.2%	497
Univ of TX Health Science Ctr-Tyler	Tyler	1.2%	242
Wadley Regional Medical Center	Texarkana	1.2%	573
Baptist Medical Center	San Antonio	1.3%	1930
Medical Center Hospital	Odessa	1.3%	718
Saint Luke's the Woodlands Hospital	The Woodlands	1.4%	586
Citizens Medical Center	Victoria	1.5%	729
Memorial Hermann Northeast	Humble	1.5%	743
Nacogdoches Medical Center	Nacogdoches	1.5%	336
Baylor Medical Center at Waxahachie	Waxahachie	1.6%	699
Christus Saint Michael Health System	Texarkana	1.6%	1265
Hendrick Medical Center	Abilene	1.6%	935
Mem Hermann Mem City Med Ctr	Houston	1.6%	1466
Scott & White Memorial Hospital	Temple	1.6%	1282
Univ of Texas Med Branch Galveston	Galveston	1.6%	828
Baylor Medical Center at Irving	Irving	1.7%	888
Houston Northwest Medical Center	Houston	1.7%	522
Paris Regional Medical Center	Paris	1.7%	638
Saint Luke's Episcopal Hospital	Houston	1.7%	1050
San Angelo Community Medical Center	San Angelo	1.7%	401
San Jacinto Methodist Hospital	Baytown	1.7%	769
Scott & White Hospital - Round Rock	Round Rock	1.7%	577
Uvalde Memorial Hospital	Uvalde	1.7%	350
Brazosport Regional Health System	Lake Jackson	1.8%	731
Christus Hospital	Beaumont	1.8%	1172
Hunt Regional Medical Center	Greenville	1.8%	1007
Memorial Hermann Texas Medical Center	Houston	1.8%	758
North Austin Medical Center	Austin	1.8%	605
Texas Health Presbyterian Hospital Dallas	Dallas	1.8%	881
United Regional Health Care System	Wichita Falls	1.8%	1182
Memorial Hermann Hospital System	Houston	1.9%	3649
Mother Frances Hospital	Tyler	1.9%	1406
Peterson Regional Medical Center	Kerrville	1.9%	751
TX Health Presbyterian Hosp Rockwall	Rockwall	1.9%	426
Valley Regional Medical Center	Brownsville	1.9%	486
Doctors Hospital at Renaissance	Edinburg	2.0%	1624
Methodist Mansfield Medical Center	Mansfield	2.0%	500
TX Hlth Presbyterian Hosp-Kaufman	Kaufman	2.0%	403
Memorial Hospital	Nacogdoches	2.1%	473
Methodist West Houston Hospital	Houston	2.1%	481
Midland Memorial Hospital	Midland	2.1%	605
Providence Memorial Hospital	El Paso	2.1%	513
Saint David's South Austin Medical Center	Austin	2.1%	874
Texas Health Arlington Memorial Hospital	Arlington	2.1%	878
Harlingen Medical Center	Harlingen	2.2%	412
Metroplex Hospital	Killeen	2.2%	627
Parkland Health & Hospital System	Dallas	2.2%	810
Texoma Medical Center	Denison	2.2%	1230
Medical City Dallas Hospital	Dallas	2.3%	562
Methodist Charlton Medical Center	Dallas	2.3%	1063
Saint Joseph Regional Health Center	Bryan	2.3%	945
TX Hlth Harris Meth Hosp SW Ft Worth	Fort Worth	2.3%	730
Baptist Saint Anthony's Hospital	Amarillo	2.4%	1241
Bayshore Medical Center	Pasadena	2.4%	746
Methodist Sugar Land Hospital	Sugar Land	2.4%	1100
Sierra Medical Center	El Paso	2.4%	588
Palestine Regional Medical Center	Palestine	2.5%	516
Shannon Medical Center	San Angelo	2.5%	650
Texas Health Harris Methodist	Bedford	2.5%	911
East Texas Medical Center Athens	Athens	2.6%	802
Titus Regional Medical Center	Mount Pleasant	2.6%	507
Tomball Regional Medical Center	Tomball	2.6%	732
Baylor All Saints Medical Center at FW	Fort Worth	2.7%	624
Christus Santa Rosa Hospital	San Antonio	2.7%	1684
The Medical Center of Southeast Texas	Port Arthur	2.7%	600
The Methodist Hospital	Houston	2.7%	1620
Saint David's Medical Center	Austin	2.7%	997
Seton Highland Lakes	Burnet	2.7%	639
Baylor Reg Med Ctr at Grapevine	Grapevine	2.8%	618
Knapp Medical Center	Weslaco	2.8%	985
Hillcrest Baptist Medical Center	Waco	2.9%	833
Methodist Willowbrook Hospital	Houston	2.9%	664
The Corpus Christi Medical Center	Corpus Christi	3.0%	1002
Texas Health Presbyterian Hospital Plano	Plano	3.0%	643
Baptist Beaumont Hospital	Beaumont	3.2%	1024
Baylor Medical Center at Garland	Garland	3.3%	1230
Covenant Medical Center	Lubbock	3.3%	1080
Las Palmas Medical Center	El Paso	3.3%	1120
Texas Health Harris Methodist Fort Worth	Fort Worth	3.3%	2097
East Texas Medical Center	Tyler	3.4%	1133
South Texas Health System	Edinburg	3.4%	860
Clear Lake Regional Medical Center	Webster	3.5%	1587
Conroe Regional Medical Center	Conroe	3.5%	789
Methodist Hospital	San Antonio	3.7%	2853
Medical Center of Mckinney	Mckinney	3.8%	448
North Cypress Medical Center	Cypress	3.8%	978
VHS Harlingen Hospital Company	Harlingen	4.0%	902
Central Texas Medical Center	San Marcos	4.1%	515
Detar Hospital Navarro	Victoria	4.2%	527
Harris Health System	Houston	4.2%	669
Texas Health Presbyterian Hospital - WNJ	Sherman	4.2%	620
Baylor Regional Medical Center at Plano	Plano	4.3%	904
Huntsville Memorial Hospital	Huntsville	4.3%	646
Lake Granbury Medical Center	Granbury	4.3%	585
Southwest General Hospital	San Antonio	4.3%	374
Laredo Medical Center	Laredo	4.4%	1171
Weatherford Regional Medical Center	Weatherford	4.4%	526
Woodland Heights Medical Center	Lufkin	4.5%	465
JPS Health Network	Fort Worth	4.6%	1003
Covenant Hospital Plainview	Plainview	4.8%	290
Oakbend Medical Center	Richmond	4.8%	418
University Medical Center at Brackenridge	Austin	4.8%	395
College Station Medical Center	College Station	4.9%	410
Huguley Memorial Medical Center	Burleson	5.0%	719
Memorial Medical Center of East Texas	Lufkin	5.0%	760
University Medical Center of El Paso	El Paso	5.0%	339
Val Verde Regional Medical Center	Del Rio	5.0%	439
Christus Spohn Hospital Alice	Alice	5.1%	514
Christus Spohn Hospital Corpus Christi	Corpus Christi	5.1%	1025
Etmc Carthage	Carthage	5.1%	236
East Texas Medical Center Jacksonville	Jacksonville	5.2%	248
University Medical Center	Lubbock	5.4%	1156
Etmc Clarksville	Clarksville	5.7%	176
Medical Center of Plano	Plano	6.1%	578
Pampa Regional Medical Center	Pampa	6.1%	244
Glen Rose Medical Center	Glen Rose	6.2%	226
North Hills Hospital	N Richland Hls	6.2%	617
Texas Health Presbyterian Hospital Allen	Allen	6.3%	255
Memorial Hermann Baptist Orange Hospital	Orange	6.6%	438
Grace Medical Center	Lubbock	7.0%	128
Scenic Mountain Medical Center	Big Spring	7.1%	239
Central Texas Hospital	Cameron	16.3%	43

Combination Chest CT Scan

Hospital Name	City	Rate	Cases
Abilene Regional Medical Center	Abilene	0.0%	241
Baptist Emergency Hospital	San Antonio	0.0%	56
Christus Saint John Hospital	Nassau Bay	0.0%	238
Denton Regional Medical Center	Denton	0.0%	215
East Texas Medical Center - Fairfield	Fairfield	0.0%	50
East Texas Medical Center - Gilmer	Gilmer	0.0%	63
Eastland Memorial Hospital	Eastland	0.0%	70
Etmc Carthage	Carthage	0.0%	101
Fort Duncan Medical Center	Eagle Pass	0.0%	131
Goodall Witcher Hospital	Clifton	0.0%	52
Graham Regional Medical Center	Graham	0.0%	208
Hendrick Medical Center	Abilene	0.0%	827
Hill Country Memorial Hospital	Fredericksburg	0.0%	322
Kingwood Medical Center	Kingwood	0.0%	324
Medical Center of Arlington	Arlington	0.0%	47
Methodist Stone Oak Hospital	San Antonio	0.0%	56
Methodist Willowbrook Hospital	Houston	0.0%	375
Nacogdoches Medical Center	Nacogdoches	0.0%	270
North Texas Medical Center	Gainesville	0.0%	97
Oakbend Medical Center	Richmond	0.0%	178
Parkview Regional Hospital	Mexia	0.0%	82
The Physicians Centre	Bryan	0.0%	47
Providence Memorial Hospital	El Paso	0.0%	243
Rolling Plains Memorial Hospital	Sweetwater	0.0%	70
Round Rock Medical Center	Round Rock	0.0%	144
Saint Luke's Sugar Land Hospital	Sugar Land	0.0%	215
San Angelo Community Medical Center	San Angelo	0.0%	212
Seton Medical Center Harker Heights	Harker Heights	0.0%	82
Seton Medical Center Hays	Kyle	0.0%	217
Seton Northwest Hospital	Austin	0.0%	58
Seymour Hospital	Seymour	0.0%	46
Sierra Providence East Medical Center	El Paso	0.0%	107
South Texas Regional Medical Center	Jourdanton	0.0%	218
Sweeny Community Hospital	Sweeny	0.0%	52
University Medical Center at Brackenridge	Austin	0.0%	143
UT Southwestern University Hospital	Dallas	0.0%	2053
Harris Health System	Houston	0.1%	819
Mother Frances Hospital	Tyler	0.1%	1396
Scott & White Memorial Hospital	Temple	0.1%	2047
Clear Lake Regional Medical Center	Webster	0.2%	628
East Texas Medical Center	Tyler	0.2%	1004
Parkland Health & Hospital System	Dallas	0.2%	1204
Memorial Medical Center of East Texas	Lufkin	0.3%	375
Peterson Regional Medical Center	Kerrville	0.3%	673
Providence Health Center	Waco	0.3%	736
Texas Health Harris Methodist Fort Worth	Fort Worth	0.3%	346
Baylor Reg Med Ctr at Grapevine	Grapevine	0.4%	232
Huntsville Memorial Hospital	Huntsville	0.4%	496
Methodist West Houston Hospital	Houston	0.4%	229
Saint Luke's Patients Medical Center	Pasadena	0.4%	239
Seton Edgar B Davis Hospital	Luling	0.4%	228
University Health System	San Antonio	0.4%	484
University Medical Center of El Paso	El Paso	0.4%	231
UT SW Univ Hosp-Zale Lipshy	Dallas	0.4%	471
Baptist Saint Anthony's Hospital	Amarillo	0.5%	597
Citizens Medical Center	Victoria	0.5%	824
Doctors Hospital	Dallas	0.5%	202
Baptist Beaumont Hospital	Beaumont	0.6%	321
Christus Spohn Hospital Corpus Christi	Corpus Christi	0.6%	178
Longview Regional Medical Center	Longview	0.6%	664
Methodist Hospital	San Antonio	0.6%	880
The Methodist Hospital	Houston	0.7%	1831
Texas Health Presbyterian Hospital Dallas	Dallas	0.7%	143
Univ of TX Health Science Ctr-Tyler	Tyler	0.7%	840
Lake Pointe Medical Center	Rowlett	0.8%	263
Seton Highland Lakes	Burnet	0.8%	385
Woodland Heights Medical Center	Lufkin	0.8%	256
Heart Hospital Baylor Plano	Plano	0.9%	112
Park Plaza Hospital	Houston	0.9%	117
Saint Joseph Regional Health Center	Bryan	0.9%	344
Baylor All Saints Medical Center at FW	Fort Worth	1.0%	298
East Texas Medical Center Crockett	Crockett	1.0%	100
Saint David's Medical Center	Austin	1.0%	209
Scott & White Hospital - Llano	Llano	1.0%	201
West Houston Medical Center	Houston	1.0%	102
College Station Medical Center	College Station	1.1%	174
Hillcrest Baptist Medical Center	Waco	1.1%	641
Medical City Dallas Hospital	Dallas	1.1%	356
Cypress Fairbanks Medical Center	Houston	1.2%	85
East Texas Medical Center Quitman	Quitman	1.2%	86
Paris Regional Medical Center	Paris	1.2%	85
Baylor Medical Center at Mckinney	Mc Kinney	1.3%	158

NOTE: Hospital profiles are in alphabetical order by state, then city, then hospital within the city; Rankings exclude hospitals with less than 25 cases except for patient surveys which excludes hospitals with less than 100 cases; (a) 100-299 cases; (1) The number of cases/patients is too few to report; (2) Data submitted were based on a sample of cases/patients; (3) Results are based on a shorter time period than required; (4) Data suppressed by CMS for one or more quarters; (5) Results are not available for this reporting period; (6) Fewer than 100 patients completed the HCAHPS survey; (7) No cases met the criteria for this measure; (8) The lower limit of the confidence interval cannot be calculated if the number of observed infections equals zero; (9) No data are available from the state/territory for this reporting period; (10) The scores shown reflect fewer than 50 completed surveys; (11) There were discrepancies in the data collection process; (12) This measure does not apply to this hospital for this reporting period; (13) Results cannot be calculated for this reporting period; (14) The results for this state are combined with nearby states to protect confidentiality; Please refer to the User's Guide for a full explanation of data.

Baylor University Medical Center	Dallas	1.3%	1352
Methodist Richardson Medical Center	Richardson	1.3%	478
Scott & White Hospital - Round Rock	Round Rock	1.3%	521
TX Hlth Harris Meth Hosp SW Ft Worth	Fort Worth	1.3%	313
Wise Regional Health System	Decatur	1.3%	391
Bayshore Medical Center	Pasadena	1.5%	274
Cleveland Regional Medical Center	Cleveland	1.5%	65
Memorial Hermann Baptist Orange Hospital	Orange	1.6%	129
North Hills Hospital	N Richland Hls	1.6%	126
Seton Medical Center Williamson	Round Rock	1.8%	110
Sierra Medical Center	El Paso	1.8%	325
Medical Center of Lewisville	Lewisville	1.9%	105
Shannon Medical Center	San Angelo	1.9%	261
Cuero Community Hospital	Cuero	2.0%	100
The Hospital at Westlake Medical Center	Austin	2.1%	48
Christus Spohn Hospital Alice	Alice	2.2%	92
Baylor Medical Center at Irving	Irving	2.3%	519
Seton Medical Center Austin	Austin	2.3%	88
Texas Health Harris Methodist	Bedford	2.3%	261
Baylor Medical Center at Waxahachie	Waxahachie	2.4%	381
Hamilton General Hospital	Hamilton	2.4%	84
Tomball Regional Medical Center	Tomball	2.4%	581
Univ of Texas Med Branch Galveston	Galveston	2.4%	781
Medical Center of Mckinney	Mckinney	2.5%	321
Covenant Medical Center	Lubbock	2.6%	1088
North Austin Medical Center	Austin	2.6%	114
Saint Luke's Episcopal Hospital	Houston	2.6%	1340
Methodist Sugar Land Hospital	Sugar Land	2.7%	843
Christus Santa Rosa Hospital	San Antonio	2.8%	424
Gulf Coast Medical Center	Wharton	2.8%	71
Memorial Hermann Hospital System	Houston	2.9%	2413
North Cypress Medical Center	Cypress	3.0%	760
Covenant Hospital Plainview	Plainview	3.1%	129
Rio Grande Regional Hospital	Mcallen	3.1%	65
Saint Joseph Medical Center	Houston	3.1%	130
JPS Health Network	Fort Worth	3.2%	822
Brazosport Regional Health System	Lake Jackson	3.4%	494
Centennial Medical Center	Frisco	3.6%	168
Christus Spohn Hospital Kleberg	Kingsville	3.7%	82
Coryell Memorial Healthcare System	Gatesville	4.1%	49
Baylor Medical Center at Frisco	Frisco	4.2%	48
TX Hlth Presbyterian Hosp-Flower Mound	Flower Mound	4.2%	120
Medical Arts Hospital	Lamesa	4.5%	66
Baylor Medical Center at Garland	Garland	4.7%	426
Baptist Medical Center	San Antonio	4.8%	273
Mission Regional Medical Center	Mission	4.8%	105
Southwest General Hospital	San Antonio	4.8%	63
Kell West Regional Hospital	Wichita Falls	5.0%	120
TX Health Presbyterian Hosp Rockwall	Rockwall	5.0%	219
United Regional Health Care System	Wichita Falls	5.2%	382
Las Palmas Medical Center	El Paso	5.3%	133
Nix Health Care System	San Antonio	5.3%	76
Saint David's South Austin Medical Center	Austin	5.3%	131
Weatherford Regional Medical Center	Weatherford	5.3%	360
Laredo Medical Center	Laredo	5.6%	445
Las Colinas Medical Center	Irving	5.6%	71
Midland Memorial Hospital	Midland	5.6%	726
Texas Health Arlington Memorial Hospital	Arlington	5.6%	126
Care Regional Medical Center	Aransas Pass	5.7%	123
Memorial Hermann Northeast	Humble	5.7%	420
Plaza Medical Center of Fort Worth	Fort Worth	5.7%	70
Dallas Regional Medical Center	Mesquite	5.8%	104
Memorial Hermann Sugar Land Hospital	Sugar Land	5.8%	208
Houston Northwest Medical Center	Houston	5.9%	437
The Corpus Christi Medical Center	Corpus Christi	6.1%	66
Starr County Memorial Hospital	Rio Grande City	6.1%	147
VHS Brownsville Hospital Company	Brownsville	6.2%	145
Memorial Hermann Texas Medical Center	Houston	6.4%	685
Central Texas Medical Center	San Marcos	6.6%	182
Good Shepherd Medical Center	Longview	6.6%	641
Angleton - Danbury Medical Center	Angleton	6.7%	105
Christus Spohn Hospital Beeville	Beeville	6.7%	75
Lakeway Regional Medical Center	Lakeway	6.7%	89
Lubbock Heart Hospital	Lubbock	6.7%	282
Saint Luke's the Woodlands Hospital	The Woodlands	7.0%	612
Memorial Hermann Katy Hospital	Katy	7.2%	306
Medical Center of Plano	Plano	7.4%	434
Good Shephard Medical Center - Linden	Linden	7.6%	66
Methodist Charlton Medical Center	Dallas	7.6%	197
TX Hlth Harris Meth Hosp-Cleburne	Cleburne	7.6%	197
Hill Regional Hospital	Hillsboro	7.7%	65
Palo Pinto General Hospital	Mineral Wells	7.8%	153
South Texas Health System	Edinburg	7.8%	206
Christus Saint Catherine Hospital	Katy	7.9%	126
Cedar Park Regional Medical Center	Cedar Park	8.0%	138
Guadalupe Regional Medical Center	Seguin	8.0%	325
Metroplex Hospital	Killeen	8.1%	469
Saint Luke's Hospital at the Vintage	Houston	8.1%	148
Scott & White Hospital Brenham	Brenham	8.2%	159
Texas Health Presbyterian Hospital Plano	Plano	8.5%	247
Scenic Mountain Medical Center	Big Spring	8.7%	92
Val Verde Regional Medical Center	Del Rio	9.2%	173
Huguley Memorial Medical Center	Burleson	9.3%	462
Lake Granbury Medical Center	Granbury	9.3%	441
Mem Hermann Mem City Med Ctr	Houston	9.3%	907
Conroe Regional Medical Center	Conroe	9.5%	317
Memorial Hospital	Nacogdoches	9.5%	284
Seton Smithville Regional Hospital	Smithville	9.5%	179
Baylor Regional Medical Center at Plano	Plano	9.7%	145
Matagorda Regional Medical Center	Bay City	10.2%	98
Etmc Henderson	Henderson	10.3%	97
Connally Memorial Medical Center	Floresville	10.6%	132
Uvalde Memorial Hospital	Uvalde	10.9%	192
Rollins Brook Community Hospital	Lampasas	11.1%	108
TX Hlth Harris Methodist Hosp-Azle	Azle	11.3%	97
Good Shepherd Medical Center Marshall	Marshall	11.6%	267
Saint Marks Medical Center	La Grange	11.6%	173
Navarro Regional Hospital	Corsicana	11.8%	153
Texas Reg Med Ctr at Sunnyvale	Sunnyvale	11.9%	67
Etmc Clarksville	Clarksville	12.0%	92
Baylor Medical Center at Carrollton	Carrollton	13.1%	221
East Texas Medical Center Jacksonville	Jacksonville	13.1%	206
Methodist Mansfield Medical Center	Mansfield	13.6%	132
Harlingen Medical Center	Harlingen	13.9%	194
Saint Luke's Lakeside Hospital	The Woodlands	14.4%	90
Texas Health Presbyterian Hospital Denton	Denton	14.6%	213
Texas Health Presbyterian Hospital - WNJ	Sherman	14.9%	377
East Texas Medical Center Athens	Athens	15.1%	530
Memorial Hospital	Gonzales	15.2%	79
Doctors Hospital of Laredo	Laredo	15.8%	184
Christus Jasper Memorial Hospital	Jasper	16.3%	209
Columbus Community Hospital	Columbus	17.0%	159
Christus Saint Michael Health System	Texarkana	19.5%	514
Valley Regional Medical Center	Brownsville	19.6%	240
Hopkins County Memorial Hospital	Sulphur Springs	21.4%	220
Foundation Surgical Hospital of El Paso	El Paso	21.6%	74
University Medical Center	Lubbock	21.6%	633
VHS Harlingen Hospital Company	Harlingen	22.5%	307
Medical Center Hospital	Odessa	23.2%	341
Detar Hospital Navarro	Victoria	24.3%	239
Wadley Regional Medical Center	Texarkana	24.7%	174
Northwest Texas Hospital	Amarillo	25.1%	199
Brownwood Regional Medical Center	Brownwood	25.6%	215
Grace Medical Center	Lubbock	25.7%	113
Memorial Medical Center Livingston	Livingston	28.6%	189
Methodist Dallas Medical Center	Dallas	29.1%	683
Texoma Medical Center	Denison	29.9%	772
San Jacinto Methodist Hospital	Baytown	30.5%	220
Wilbarger General Hospital	Vernon	31.3%	96
Glen Rose Medical Center	Glen Rose	31.4%	105
Titus Regional Medical Center	Mount Pleasant	31.4%	398
University General Hospital	Houston	31.9%	135
TX Hlth Harris Meth Hosp-Stephenville	Stephenville	32.4%	170
Doctors Hospital at Renaissance	Edinburg	33.8%	1602
Christus Hospital	Beaumont	34.0%	533
Palestine Regional Medical Center	Palestine	34.4%	93
The Medical Center of Southeast Texas	Port Arthur	35.6%	163
Pampa Regional Medical Center	Pampa	37.7%	61
Hunt Regional Medical Center	Greenville	38.4%	1040
TX Hlth Presbyterian Hosp-Kaufman	Kaufman	39.3%	117
Knapp Medical Center	Weslaco	40.2%	373
Memorial Medical Center	Port Lavaca	57.6%	99

Follow-up Mammogram/Ultrasound

A follow-up rate near zero may indicate missed cancer; a rate higher than 14% may mean there is unnecessary follow up.

Hospital Name	City	Rate	Cases
El Campo Memorial Hospital	El Campo	0.0%	241
Central Texas Medical Center	San Marcos	0.9%	668
Matagorda Regional Medical Center	Bay City	1.1%	280
Hopkins County Memorial Hospital	Sulphur Springs	1.7%	360
Sweeny Community Hospital	Sweeny	2.2%	91
Rollins Brook Community Hospital	Lampasas	2.3%	349
Knapp Medical Center	Weslaco	2.4%	1313
North Hills Hospital	N Richland Hls	2.6%	534
Providence Health Center	Waco	2.6%	2407
Harlingen Medical Center	Harlingen	2.9%	342
Christus Santa Rosa Hospital	San Antonio	3.2%	1931
Parkland Health & Hospital System	Dallas	3.4%	2134
Saint Marks Medical Center	La Grange	3.4%	557
Hunt Regional Medical Center	Greenville	3.5%	1749
Texas Health Harris Methodist Fort Worth	Fort Worth	3.5%	805
Palestine Regional Medical Center	Palestine	3.6%	449
Las Palmas Medical Center	El Paso	3.7%	819
Saint Joseph Medical Center	Houston	3.9%	826
Saint Luke's Patients Medical Center	Pasadena	3.9%	128
VHS Harlingen Hospital Company	Harlingen	3.9%	1553
Methodist Mansfield Medical Center	Mansfield	4.0%	580
Columbus Community Hospital	Columbus	4.3%	374
Bowie Memorial Hospital	Bowie	4.4%	68
Stephens Memorial Hospital	Breckenridge	4.4%	45
Odessa Regional Hospital	Odessa	4.5%	912
Texas Health Presbyterian Hospital Denton	Denton	4.5%	1106
San Angelo Community Medical Center	San Angelo	4.6%	1021
Seton Northwest Hospital	Austin	4.6%	260
Shannon Medical Center	San Angelo	4.6%	2113
Tops Surgical Specialty Hospital	Houston	4.8%	2482
Val Verde Regional Medical Center	Del Rio	4.8%	460
Uvalde Memorial Hospital	Uvalde	4.9%	370
East Texas Medical Center Quitman	Quitman	5.0%	222
Ennis Regional Medical Center	Ennis	5.0%	403
Hill Regional Hospital	Hillsboro	5.1%	513
United Regional Health Care System	Wichita Falls	5.1%	1462
University Health System	San Antonio	5.2%	1581
The Corpus Christi Medical Center	Corpus Christi	5.4%	504
East Texas Medical Center	Tyler	5.4%	3066
TX Hlth Presbyterian Hosp-Flower Mound	Flower Mound	5.4%	166
Texas Health Presbyterian Hospital Plano	Plano	5.4%	994
East Texas Medical Center - Fairfield	Fairfield	5.5%	128
Grace Medical Center	Lubbock	5.5%	688
Kingwood Medical Center	Kingwood	5.5%	346
Medical City Dallas Hospital	Dallas	5.5%	1202
Childress Regional Medical Center	Childress	5.6%	214
Memorial Hermann Baptist Orange Hospital	Orange	5.6%	576
Round Rock Medical Center	Round Rock	5.6%	355
Saint Joseph Regional Health Center	Bryan	5.6%	568
East Texas Medical Center Jacksonville	Jacksonville	5.7%	282
Fort Duncan Medical Center	Eagle Pass	5.7%	557
The Medical Center of Southeast Texas	Port Arthur	5.7%	421
Methodist Richardson Medical Center	Richardson	5.7%	1254
TX Hlth Harris Meth Hosp-Cleburne	Cleburne	5.7%	441
Christus Spohn Hospital Beeville	Beeville	5.8%	329
Cleveland Regional Medical Center	Cleveland	5.8%	120
Mission Regional Medical Center	Mission	5.8%	1285
Harris Health System	Houston	5.9%	1200
Dallas Regional Medical Center	Mesquite	6.0%	448
Etmc Carthage	Carthage	6.0%	248
North Austin Medical Center	Austin	6.0%	251
Baptist Beaumont Hospital	Beaumont	6.1%	955
Texas Health Arlington Memorial Hospital	Arlington	6.1%	1321
Baylor Medical Center at Garland	Garland	6.2%	2456
Memorial Hermann Hospital System	Houston	6.2%	6651
Saint Luke's Episcopal Hospital	Houston	6.3%	1109
Bellville General Hospital	Bellville	6.4%	265
East Texas Medical Center Athens	Athens	6.4%	606
Eastland Memorial Hospital	Eastland	6.4%	140
Good Shepherd Medical Center Marshall	Marshall	6.4%	733
Saint David's Medical Center	Austin	6.4%	1863
Christus Saint Catherine Hospital	Katy	6.6%	483
East Texas Medical Center Crockett	Crockett	6.6%	271
Glen Rose Medical Center	Glen Rose	6.6%	378
Memorial Hermann Sugar Land Hospital	Sugar Land	6.7%	853
TX Hlth Harris Meth Hosp SW Ft Worth	Fort Worth	6.7%	1654
Citizens Medical Center	Victoria	6.8%	1121
Medical Center Hospital	Odessa	6.8%	1611
Christus Spohn Hospital Kleberg	Kingsville	6.9%	346
Connally Memorial Medical Center	Floresville	6.9%	202
Park Plaza Hospital	Houston	6.9%	576
Christus Saint Michael Health System	Texarkana	7.0%	1606
Memorial Medical Center of East Texas	Lufkin	7.0%	1700
Mother Frances Hospital	Tyler	7.0%	6818
Mem Hermann Mem City Med Ctr	Houston	7.1%	4518
Scott & White Hospital - Llano	Llano	7.1%	326
Laredo Medical Center	Laredo	7.2%	1246
Saint David's South Austin Medical Center	Austin	7.2%	97
Texas Health Presbyterian Hospital Dallas	Dallas	7.2%	2714
Etmc Henderson	Henderson	7.3%	330
Good Shepherd Medical Center	Longview	7.3%	2278
Guadalupe Regional Medical Center	Seguin	7.3%	716
Methodist Sugar Land Hospital	Sugar Land	7.3%	841
Oakbend Medical Center	Richmond	7.3%	521
Hamilton General Hospital	Hamilton	7.4%	190
San Jacinto Methodist Hospital	Baytown	7.4%	1014
Seton Highland Lakes	Burnet	7.4%	1032
Graham Regional Medical Center	Graham	7.5%	494
Memorial Medical Center	Port Lavaca	7.5%	292
Memorial Hermann Texas Medical Center	Houston	7.6%	397
Metroplex Hospital	Killeen	7.6%	1063
Permian Regional Medical Center	Andrews	7.6%	251
Texas Health Presbyterian Hospital - WNJ	Sherman	7.6%	2021
Univ of Texas Med Branch Galveston	Galveston	7.6%	2073
Valley Regional Medical Center	Brownsville	7.6%	970
Baylor Medical Center at Carrollton	Carrollton	7.7%	1058
The Physicians Centre	Bryan	7.7%	491
Baylor Medical Center at Irving	Irving	7.8%	1914
Scott & White Hospital - Round Rock	Round Rock	7.8%	1609
Doctors Hospital at Renaissance	Edinburg	7.9%	3174
Nix Health Care System	San Antonio	7.9%	887
TX Hlth Presbyterian Hosp-Kaufman	Kaufman	7.9%	343
The Womans Hospital of Texas	Houston	7.9%	1081
College Station Medical Center	College Station	8.0%	627
Detar Hospital Navarro	Victoria	8.0%	672
Methodist Dallas Medical Center	Dallas	8.0%	1070

NOTE: Hospital profiles are in alphabetical order by state, then city, then hospital within the city; Rankings exclude hospitals with less than 25 cases except for patient surveys which excludes hospitals with less than 100 cases; (a) 100-299 cases; (1) The number of cases/patients is too few to report; (2) Data submitted were based on a sample of cases/patients; (3) Results are based on a shorter time period than required; (4) Data suppressed by CMS for one or more quarters; (5) Results are not available for this reporting period; (6) Fewer than 100 patients completed the HCAHPS survey; (7) No cases met the criteria for this measure; (8) The lower limit of the confidence interval cannot be calculated if the number of observed infections equals zero; (9) No data are available from the state/territory for this reporting period; (10) The scores shown reflect fewer than 50 completed surveys; (11) There were discrepancies in the data collection process; (12) This measure does not apply to this hospital for this reporting period; (13) Results cannot be calculated for this reporting period; (14) The results for this state are combined with nearby states to protect confidentiality; Please refer to the User's Guide for a full explanation of data.

Midland Memorial Hospital	Midland	8.0%	2468
Providence Memorial Hospital	El Paso	8.0%	1055
Memorial Hermann Northeast	Humble	8.1%	824
Scott & White Hospital Brenham	Brenham	8.1%	185
Covenant Medical Center	Lubbock	8.2%	2412
University Medical Center of El Paso	El Paso	8.2%	911
Bayshore Medical Center	Pasadena	8.3%	517
Lake Pointe Medical Center	Rowlett	8.3%	1154
Baylor University Medical Center	Dallas	8.4%	4921
Seton Edgar B Davis Hospital	Luling	8.4%	286
Starr County Memorial Hospital	Rio Grande City	8.4%	214
Centennial Medical Center	Frisco	8.5%	331
Conroe Regional Medical Center	Conroe	8.5%	1762
Hillcrest Baptist Medical Center	Waco	8.5%	1880
JPS Health Network	Fort Worth	8.5%	1416
Baylor Medical Center at Waxahachie	Waxahachie	8.6%	1226
Baylor Reg Med Ctr at Grapevine	Grapevine	8.6%	1300
Scott & White Memorial Hospital	Temple	8.6%	3688
Huntsville Memorial Hospital	Huntsville	8.7%	715
University Medical Center at Brackenridge	Austin	8.8%	102
Wilbarger General Hospital	Vernon	8.8%	194
Christus Spohn Hospital Alice	Alice	8.9%	214
Hendrick Medical Center	Abilene	8.9%	3327
Christus Hospital	Beaumont	9.0%	3100
Saint Luke's the Woodlands Hospital	The Woodlands	9.0%	634
Brazosport Regional Health System	Lake Jackson	9.1%	853
Cuero Community Hospital	Cuero	9.1%	340
Methodist Charlton Medical Center	Dallas	9.1%	2286
Seton Medical Center Hays	Kyle	9.1%	88
Sierra Providence East Medical Center	El Paso	9.2%	141
Abilene Regional Medical Center	Abilene	9.3%	634
Baylor Regional Medical Center at Plano	Plano	9.3%	2359
Dallas Medical Center	Dallas	9.3%	182
Rio Grande Regional Hospital	Mcallen	9.3%	568
Seton Southwest Hospital	Austin	9.3%	108
South Texas Health System	Edinburg	9.3%	549
Angleton - Danbury Medical Center	Angleton	9.4%	298
Medical Center of Mckinney	Mckinney	9.4%	1092
Memorial Hermann Katy Hospital	Katy	9.4%	1289
Wadley Regional Medical Center	Texarkana	9.5%	970
Seton Medical Center Williamson	Round Rock	9.7%	93
Wise Regional Health System	Decatur	9.7%	486
Goodall Witcher Hospital	Clifton	9.8%	296
Huguley Memorial Medical Center	Burleson	9.8%	795
Sierra Medical Center	El Paso	9.8%	1783
Navarro Regional Hospital	Corsicana	9.9%	736
VHS Brownsville Hospital Company	Brownsville	10.0%	782
Clear Lake Regional Medical Center	Webster	10.1%	2599
North Texas Medical Center	Gainesville	10.1%	515
Texoma Medical Center	Denison	10.2%	1571
Houston Northwest Medical Center	Houston	10.3%	1336
Parkview Regional Hospital	Mexia	10.3%	261
UT Southwestern University Hospital	Dallas	10.3%	2792
Woodland Heights Medical Center	Lufkin	10.3%	631
Doctors Hospital of Laredo	Laredo	10.4%	443
Care Regional Medical Center	Aransas Pass	10.5%	162
Doctors Hospital	Dallas	10.6%	1052
TX Hlth Harris Methodist Hosp-Azle	Azle	10.7%	475
Peterson Regional Medical Center	Kerrville	10.8%	1560
Memorial Hospital	Gonzales	10.9%	165
Nacogdoches Medical Center	Nacogdoches	10.9%	855
Medical Center of Plano	Plano	11.0%	584
Las Colinas Medical Center	Irving	11.1%	324
Medical Center of Lewisville	Lewisville	11.2%	1100
Texas Health Presbyterian Hospital Allen	Allen	11.2%	662
West Houston Medical Center	Houston	11.4%	808
Palo Pinto General Hospital	Mineral Wells	11.7%	298
Seton Smithville Regional Hospital	Smithville	11.8%	626
Brownwood Regional Medical Center	Brownwood	11.9%	859
Lakeway Regional Medical Center	Lakeway	11.9%	67
Covenant Hospital Levelland	Levelland	12.0%	209
Scenic Mountain Medical Center	Big Spring	12.0%	234
University Medical Center	Lubbock	12.2%	1155
Christus Jasper Memorial Hospital	Jasper	12.7%	639
Baylor Medical Center at Mckinney	Mc Kinney	12.9%	325
Memorial Medical Center Livingston	Livingston	12.9%	865
North Cypress Medical Center	Cypress	12.9%	742
Northwest Texas Hospital	Amarillo	12.9%	510
Pampa Regional Medical Center	Pampa	12.9%	155
Rolling Plains Memorial Hospital	Sweetwater	13.0%	146
Christus Spohn Hospital Corpus Christi	Corpus Christi	13.1%	398
Lake Granbury Medical Center	Granbury	13.1%	1027
Hill Country Memorial Hospital	Fredericksburg	13.2%	1649
South Texas Regional Medical Center	Jourdanton	13.5%	349
TX Hlth Harris Meth Hosp-Stephenville	Stephenville	13.6%	110
Univ of TX Health Science Ctr-Tyler	Tyler	13.7%	665
Christus Saint John Hospital	Nassau Bay	13.9%	281
The Methodist Hospital	Houston	13.9%	1140
University General Hospital	Houston	13.9%	395
Paris Regional Medical Center	Paris	14.0%	272
Saint Luke's Hospital at the Vintage	Houston	14.1%	71
Cogdell Memorial Hospital	Snyder	14.4%	167
Methodist Willowbrook Hospital	Houston	14.4%	418
TX Health Presbyterian Hosp Rockwall	Rockwall	14.5%	331
Cypress Fairbanks Medical Center	Houston	14.6%	742
Jackson Healthcare Center	Edna	14.7%	68
Tomball Regional Medical Center	Tomball	14.9%	850
Saint Luke's Sugar Land Hospital	Sugar Land	15.5%	84
Coryell Memorial Healthcare System	Gatesville	15.9%	251
Frio Regional Hospital	Pearsall	16.8%	119
Methodist West Houston Hospital	Houston	17.0%	165
Texas Reg Med Ctr at Sunnyvale	Sunnyvale	17.1%	117
Memorial Hospital	Nacogdoches	18.0%	957
Otto Kaiser Memorial Hospital	Kenedy	19.4%	67
Moore County Hospital District	Dumas	21.6%	125
Titus Regional Medical Center	Mount Pleasant	21.8%	629
Seton Medical Center Harker Heights	Harker Heights	27.8%	54
Cedar Park Regional Medical Center	Cedar Park	32.2%	326

Lumbar Spine MRI for Low Back Pain

Hospital Name	City	Rate	Cases
Harlingen Medical Center	Harlingen	23.1%	117
Knapp Medical Center	Weslaco	26.0%	104
Christus Jasper Memorial Hospital	Jasper	26.8%	82
Good Shepherd Medical Center Marshall	Marshall	28.3%	60
Basin Healthcare Center	Odessa	29.1%	55
The Medical Center of Southeast Texas	Port Arthur	29.5%	61
Christus Saint John Hospital	Nassau Bay	30.8%	78
TX Hlth Presbyterian Hosp-Flower Mound	Flower Mound	30.8%	78
Medical Center of Plano	Plano	31.5%	54
Heart Hospital Baylor Denton	Denton	31.8%	66
Tomball Regional Medical Center	Tomball	31.9%	91
Doctors Hospital at Renaissance	Edinburg	32.3%	533
Navarro Regional Hospital	Corsicana	32.7%	49
Saint Luke's Episcopal Hospital	Houston	32.7%	98
Texas Health Harris Methodist Fort Worth	Fort Worth	32.7%	150
VHS Harlingen Hospital Company	Harlingen	32.8%	116
Baylor Medical Center at Garland	Garland	33.3%	162
Methodist Sugar Land Hospital	Sugar Land	33.5%	245
Citizens Medical Center	Victoria	33.7%	86
Medical Center Hospital	Odessa	33.8%	154
Methodist Dallas Medical Center	Dallas	33.8%	80
North Central Surgical Center	Dallas	33.9%	280
Sierra Medical Center	El Paso	34.1%	82
Huguley Memorial Medical Center	Burleson	34.2%	73
Doctors Hospital of Laredo	Laredo	34.3%	70
Saint Luke's Lakeside Hospital	The Woodlands	34.5%	87
Scott & White Hospital - Round Rock	Round Rock	34.5%	110
Christus Santa Rosa Hospital	San Antonio	34.6%	182
Memorial Hermann Hospital System	Houston	34.6%	382
TX Health Ctr for Diag & Surgery	Plano	34.6%	179
Memorial Hospital	Nacogdoches	34.9%	86
Wise Regional Health System	Decatur	34.9%	292
Methodist Willowbrook Hospital	Houston	35.0%	100
Texas Spine & Joint Hospital	Tyler	35.0%	900
North Cypress Medical Center	Cypress	35.1%	228
Saint Joseph Regional Health Center	Bryan	35.3%	173
Heritage Park Surgical Hospital	Sherman	35.4%	113
Harris Health System	Houston	35.6%	59
Baylor Reg Med Ctr at Grapevine	Grapevine	35.7%	115
Fort Duncan Medical Center	Eagle Pass	35.8%	67
Baylor Medical Center at Uptown	Dallas	36.0%	50
Parkland Health & Hospital System	Dallas	36.3%	171
Baylor Regional Medical Center at Plano	Plano	36.5%	74
TX Health Presbyterian Hosp Rockwall	Rockwall	36.5%	159
Christus Hospital	Beaumont	36.8%	209
Clear Lake Regional Medical Center	Webster	36.8%	125
Baylor Medical Center at Waxahachie	Waxahachie	37.0%	100
Shannon Medical Center	San Angelo	37.0%	316
Mem Hermann Mem City Med Ctr	Houston	37.1%	377
Huntsville Memorial Hospital	Huntsville	37.2%	86
Memorial Hermann Northeast	Humble	37.3%	59
Baylor Medical Center at Carrollton	Carrollton	37.8%	45
Midland Memorial Hospital	Midland	37.8%	233
Texas Health Presbyterian Hospital - WNJ	Sherman	38.0%	71
VHS Brownsville Hospital Company	Brownsville	38.0%	71
Metroplex Hospital	Killeen	38.2%	241
Peterson Regional Medical Center	Kerrville	38.2%	246
Brownwood Regional Medical Center	Brownwood	38.6%	158
Memorial Hermann Sugar Land Hospital	Sugar Land	38.8%	178
Univ of Texas Med Branch Galveston	Galveston	38.8%	245
UT Southwestern University Hospital	Dallas	38.9%	244
Baylor University Medical Center	Dallas	39.3%	272
Abilene Regional Medical Center	Abilene	39.5%	114
JPS Health Network	Fort Worth	39.5%	81
Texas Health Presbyterian Hospital Denton	Denton	39.5%	76
Baylor Surgical Hospital at Fort Worth	Fort Worth	39.6%	53
TX Hlth Harris Meth Hosp-Southlake	Southlake	39.6%	217
University Health System	San Antonio	39.7%	63
University General Hospital	Houston	39.8%	123
Mother Frances Hospital	Tyler	40.0%	445
Texas Health Arlington Memorial Hospital	Arlington	40.0%	55
TX Hlth Presbyterian Hosp-Kaufman	Kaufman	40.0%	40
Hendrick Medical Center	Abilene	40.1%	309
Texas Orthopedic Hospital	Houston	40.1%	172
Hill Country Memorial Hospital	Fredericksburg	40.3%	139
Longview Regional Medical Center	Longview	40.3%	201
Texoma Medical Center	Denison	40.4%	151
Graham Regional Medical Center	Graham	40.6%	96
Providence Memorial Hospital	El Paso	40.7%	150
Detar Hospital Navarro	Victoria	40.8%	71
Hunt Regional Medical Center	Greenville	40.9%	137
Memorial Hermann Texas Medical Center	Houston	40.9%	110
Houston Orthopedic & Spine Hospital	Bellaire	41.0%	188
Scott & White Memorial Hospital	Temple	41.0%	427
Cuero Community Hospital	Cuero	41.2%	68
East Texas Medical Center Athens	Athens	41.4%	152
Memorial Medical Center Livingston	Livingston	41.5%	41
Saint Luke's Patients Medical Center	Pasadena	41.5%	53
United Regional Health Care System	Wichita Falls	41.6%	101
Good Shepherd Medical Center	Longview	41.9%	136
Conroe Regional Medical Center	Conroe	42.0%	81
Columbus Community Hospital	Columbus	42.1%	38
Memorial Medical Center of East Texas	Lufkin	42.1%	221
Saint Marks Medical Center	La Grange	42.1%	57
Baptist Beaumont Hospital	Beaumont	42.3%	71
Laredo Medical Center	Laredo	42.6%	101
Houston Physicians' Hospital	Webster	42.9%	182
East Texas Medical Center	Tyler	43.1%	202
Starr County Memorial Hospital	Rio Grande City	43.1%	51
Doctors Hospital	Dallas	43.2%	37
Baylor Medical Center at Irving	Irving	43.4%	83
Medical Center of Mckinney	Mckinney	43.5%	46
San Angelo Community Medical Center	San Angelo	43.8%	64
Christus Saint Michael Health System	Texarkana	44.1%	261
Brazosport Regional Health System	Lake Jackson	44.4%	117
Methodist Charlton Medical Center	Dallas	44.4%	63
Baptist Saint Anthony's Hospital	Amarillo	44.5%	227
Lake Granbury Medical Center	Granbury	44.5%	137
The Methodist Hospital	Houston	44.6%	417
Grace Medical Center	Lubbock	44.8%	105
Palo Pinto General Hospital	Mineral Wells	44.9%	69
Methodist Richardson Medical Center	Richardson	45.2%	62
TX Hlth Harris Meth Hosp-Stephenville	Stephenville	45.2%	62
Val Verde Regional Medical Center	Del Rio	45.3%	53
Guadalupe Regional Medical Center	Seguin	45.7%	81
The Physicians Centre	Bryan	45.7%	94
Providence Health Center	Waco	45.9%	133
Nix Health Care System	San Antonio	46.2%	52
Memorial Hermann Baptist Orange Hospital	Orange	46.3%	41
Foundation Surgical Hospital of El Paso	El Paso	46.8%	47
College Station Medical Center	College Station	46.9%	49
Hill Regional Hospital	Hillsboro	47.1%	34
Wadley Regional Medical Center	Texarkana	47.2%	108
Hillcrest Baptist Medical Center	Waco	47.3%	91
Woodland Heights Medical Center	Lufkin	47.3%	91
Memorial Hermann Katy Hospital	Katy	48.0%	75
West Houston Medical Center	Houston	48.5%	33
Weatherford Regional Medical Center	Weatherford	48.8%	41
TX Hlth Harris Meth Hosp SW Ft Worth	Fort Worth	49.1%	53
Nacogdoches Medical Center	Nacogdoches	49.5%	105
East Texas Medical Center Jacksonville	Jacksonville	50.0%	36
Methodist Hospital For Surgery	Addison	50.0%	34
Centennial Medical Center	Frisco	51.5%	33
Lake Pointe Medical Center	Rowlett	51.5%	134
University Medical Center	Lubbock	51.7%	176
Wilbarger General Hospital	Vernon	52.6%	57
Etmc Carthage	Carthage	52.8%	36
Las Palmas Medical Center	El Paso	52.8%	36
Northwest Texas Hospital	Amarillo	53.4%	58
Titus Regional Medical Center	Mount Pleasant	55.4%	121
Hopkins County Memorial Hospital	Sulphur Springs	56.7%	67
Memorial Medical Center	Port Lavaca	56.9%	72
North Texas Medical Center	Gainesville	57.4%	47
San Jacinto Methodist Hospital	Baytown	58.0%	50
East Texas Medical Center Crockett	Crockett	58.2%	55

NOTE: Hospital profiles are in alphabetical order by state, then city, then hospital within the city; Rankings exclude hospitals with less than 25 cases except for patient surveys which excludes hospitals with less than 100 cases; (a) 100-299 cases; (1) The number of cases/patients is too few to report; (2) Data submitted were based on a sample of cases/patients; (3) Results are based on a shorter time period than required; (4) Data suppressed by CMS for one or more quarters; (5) Results are not available for this reporting period; (6) Fewer than 100 patients completed the HCAHPS survey; (7) No cases met the criteria for this measure; (8) The lower limit of the confidence interval cannot be calculated if the number of observed infections equals zero; (9) No data are available from the state/territory for this reporting period; (10) The scores shown reflect fewer than 50 completed surveys; (11) There were discrepancies in the data collection process; (12) This measure does not apply to this hospital for this reporting period; (13) Results cannot be calculated for this reporting period; (14) The results for this state are combined with nearby states to protect confidentiality; Please refer to the User's Guide for a full explanation of data.

Abilene Regional Medical Center

6250 Hwy 83/84 Phone: 325-428-1000
Abilene, TX 79606 Fax: 325-428-1029
E-mail: debbie_mcclure@armc.net
URL: www.abileneregional.com
Type: Acute Care Hospitals Emergency Services: Yes
Ownership: Proprietary Beds: 187

Key Personnel:
Radiology. . . . . Johnny Bliznak
Chief of Medical Staff. . . . . Glennon Einspanier
CEO/President. . . . . Michael Murphy
Emergency Room . . . . Chrie Six, RN

Measure	Cases	This Hosp.	State Avg.	U.S. Avg.
Blood Clot Prevention and Treatment				
Anticoagulation Overlap Therapy[2]	26	92%	93%	93%
ICU Venous Thromboembolism Prophylaxis[2]	106	99%	92%	92%
Incidence of Potentially Preventable VTE[1,2]	-	-	9%	10%
UFH with Dosages/Platelet Monitoring[1,2]	-	-	96%	97%
Venous Thromboembolism Prophylaxis[2]	343	99%	82%	85%
Warfarin Therapy Discharge Instructions[2]	16	94%	84%	75%
Chest Pain/Possible Heart Attack Care				
Aspirin Given Within 24 Hours of Arrival[1,3]	-	-	94%	96%
Fibrinolytic Meds Within 30 Min. of Arrival[5]	-	-	47%	58%
Average Time to ECG (minutes)[1,3]	-	-	8	7
Average Time to Transfer (minutes)[5]	-	-	62	60
Children's Asthma Care				
Received Home Management Plan of Care	-	-	93%	88%
Received Reliever Medication	-	-	100%	100%
Received Systemic Corticosteroids	-	-	100%	100%
Emergency Department				
Admittance Decision Time (minutes)[2]	412	98	99	98
Head CT Results Within 45 Min. of Arrival[1]	-	-	54%	57%
Patients Who Left ER Before Being Seen	25,892	5%	3%	2%
Time from ER Arrival to Admit. (minutes)[2]	415	302	270	274
Time from ER Arrival to Discharge (minutes)	392	128	127	134
Time in ER Before Being Evaluated (minutes)	404	13	26	26
Time to Pain Meds for Fractures (minutes)	95	69	57	57
Heart Attack Care				
Aspirin Given at Discharge	142	100%	99%	99%
Fibrinolytic Meds Within 30 Min. of Arrival[7]	-	-	49%	54%
PCI Within 90 Minutes of Arrival	20	100%	95%	96%
Statin Prescribed at Discharge	133	99%	98%	98%
Heart Failure Care				
ACE Inhibitor or ARB for LVSD	69	97%	97%	97%
Discharge Instructions Given	113	98%	95%	94%
Evaluation of LVS Function	141	100%	99%	99%
Medicare Spending				
Medicare Spending per Patient (ratio)	-	0.99	1.03	0.98
Pneumonia Care				
Appropriate Initial Antibiotic Given	53	100%	95%	95%
Blood Culture Timing	88	100%	98%	98%
Pregnancy and Delivery Care				
Newborn Deliveries Scheduled Early[2]	42	10%	7%	6%
Preventive Care				
Immunization for Influenza[2]	548	100%	90%	90%
Immunization for Pneumonia[2]	642	100%	92%	92%
Stroke Care				
Anticoagulation Therapy for Atrial Fibrillation	11	100%	96%	95%
Antithrombotic Therapy Timing	50	100%	98%	98%
Assessed for Rehabilitation	55	100%	98%	97%
Discharged on Antithrombotic Therapy	52	100%	99%	99%
Discharged on Statin Medication	38	97%	95%	94%
Thrombolytic Therapy Timing[7]	-	-	68%	66%
Venous Thromboembolism Prophylaxis	55	95%	94%	94%
Written Stroke Educational Materials Given	18	94%	92%	88%
Surgical Care Improvement Project				
Appropriate Beta Blocker Usage	217	99%	98%	98%
Appropriate VTP Within 24 Hours	429	99%	98%	98%
Controlled Postoperative Blood Glucose	133	91%	96%	97%
Perioperative Temperature Management	520	100%	100%	100%
Prophylactic Antibiotic Selection	500	100%	99%	99%
Prophylactic Antibiotic Selection (Outpatient)	300	99%	98%	98%
Prophylactic Antibiotic Stopped	475	99%	98%	98%
Prophylactic Antibiotic Timing	500	99%	99%	99%
Prophylactic Antibiotic Timing (Outpatient)	300	100%	98%	98%
Urinary Catheter Removal	356	100%	98%	97%
Survey of Patients' Hospital Experiences				
Area Around Room 'Always' Quiet at Night	300+	66%	68%	61%
Doctors 'Always' Communicated Well	300+	82%	83%	82%
Home Recovery Information Given	300+	86%	85%	85%
Hospital Given 9 or 10 on 10 Point Scale	300+	67%	73%	71%
Meds 'Always' Explained Before Given	300+	66%	66%	64%
Nurses 'Always' Communicated Well	300+	76%	80%	79%
Pain 'Always' Well Controlled	300+	66%	72%	71%
Room and Bathroom 'Always' Clean	300+	76%	75%	73%
Timely Help 'Always' Received	300+	62%	69%	68%
Would Definitely Recommend Hospital	300+	71%	73%	71%
Use of Medical Imaging				
Cardiac Imaging Stress Test before Surgery	363	5.2%	5.3%	5.3%
Combination Abdominal CT Scan	428	25.7%	16.4%	10.5%
Combination Brain/Sinus CT Scan[1]	-	-	2.7%	2.7%
Combination Chest CT Scan	241	0.0%	5.6%	2.7%
Follow-up Mammogram/Ultrasound	634	9.3%	7.9%	8.8%
Lumbar Spine MRI for Low Back Pain	114	39.5%	39.6%	37.2%

Hendrick Medical Center

1900 Pine Phone: 325-670-2000
Abilene, TX 79601 Fax: 325-670-2293
URL: www.ehendrick.org
Type: Acute Care Hospitals Emergency Services: Yes
Ownership: Voluntary non-profit - Private Beds: 522

Key Personnel:
Cardiac Laboratory. . . . . Steve Albrient
Infection Control. . . . . Patty Bull
Quality Assurance . . . . Patt Bunorant
Pediatric Ambulatory Care . . . . . . Beth Jointer
CEO/President. . . . . Tim Lancaster
Hemotology Center . . . . Sandi Saringer
Radiology. . . . . Richard Snelburn, MD
Chief of Medical Staff. . . . . Jerry Strader, DDS

Measure	Cases	This Hosp.	State Avg.	U.S. Avg.
Blood Clot Prevention and Treatment				
Anticoagulation Overlap Therapy[2]	82	89%	93%	93%
ICU Venous Thromboembolism Prophylaxis[2]	71	90%	92%	92%
Incidence of Potentially Preventable VTE[2]	16	19%	9%	10%
UFH with Dosages/Platelet Monitoring[2]	19	100%	96%	97%
Venous Thromboembolism Prophylaxis[2]	367	81%	82%	85%
Warfarin Therapy Discharge Instructions[2]	64	92%	84%	75%
Chest Pain/Possible Heart Attack Care				
Aspirin Given Within 24 Hours of Arrival[5]	-	-	94%	96%
Fibrinolytic Meds Within 30 Min. of Arrival[5]	-	-	47%	58%
Average Time to ECG (minutes)[5]	-	-	8	7
Average Time to Transfer (minutes)[5]	-	-	62	60
Children's Asthma Care				
Received Home Management Plan of Care	-	-	93%	88%
Received Reliever Medication	-	-	100%	100%
Received Systemic Corticosteroids	-	-	100%	100%
Emergency Department				
Admittance Decision Time (minutes)[2]	591	131	99	98
Head CT Results Within 45 Min. of Arrival	21	86%	54%	57%
Patients Who Left ER Before Being Seen	62,307	6%	3%	2%
Time from ER Arrival to Admit. (minutes)[2]	597	338	270	274
Time from ER Arrival to Discharge (minutes)	398	179	127	134
Time in ER Before Being Evaluated (minutes)	422	51	26	26
Time to Pain Meds for Fractures (minutes)	181	91	57	57
Heart Attack Care				
Aspirin Given at Discharge	375	100%	99%	99%
Fibrinolytic Meds Within 30 Min. of Arrival[7]	-	-	49%	54%
PCI Within 90 Minutes of Arrival	41	100%	95%	96%
Statin Prescribed at Discharge	346	100%	98%	98%
Heart Failure Care				
ACE Inhibitor or ARB for LVSD	142	99%	97%	97%
Discharge Instructions Given	266	95%	95%	94%
Evaluation of LVS Function	316	100%	99%	99%
Medicare Spending				
Medicare Spending per Patient (ratio)	-	0.99	1.03	0.98
Pneumonia Care				
Appropriate Initial Antibiotic Given	202	92%	95%	95%
Blood Culture Timing	313	96%	98%	98%
Pregnancy and Delivery Care				
Newborn Deliveries Scheduled Early[2]	31	6%	7%	6%
Preventive Care				
Immunization for Influenza[2]	563	91%	90%	90%
Immunization for Pneumonia[2]	686	91%	92%	92%
Stroke Care				
Anticoagulation Therapy for Atrial Fibrillation	15	100%	96%	95%
Antithrombotic Therapy Timing	116	100%	98%	98%
Assessed for Rehabilitation	128	100%	98%	97%
Discharged on Antithrombotic Therapy	110	100%	99%	99%
Discharged on Statin Medication	74	97%	95%	94%
Thrombolytic Therapy Timing[1]	-	-	68%	66%
Venous Thromboembolism Prophylaxis	135	99%	94%	94%
Written Stroke Educational Materials Given	78	96%	92%	88%
Surgical Care Improvement Project				
Appropriate Beta Blocker Usage[2]	200	98%	98%	98%
Appropriate VTP Within 24 Hours[2]	376	96%	98%	98%
Controlled Postoperative Blood Glucose[2]	107	97%	96%	97%
Perioperative Temperature Management[2]	466	99%	100%	100%
Prophylactic Antibiotic Selection[2]	401	99%	99%	99%
Prophylactic Antibiotic Selection (Outpatient)	375	100%	98%	98%
Prophylactic Antibiotic Stopped[2]	390	99%	98%	98%
Prophylactic Antibiotic Timing[2]	403	100%	99%	99%
Prophylactic Antibiotic Timing (Outpatient)	376	100%	98%	98%
Urinary Catheter Removal[2]	325	100%	98%	97%
Survey of Patients' Hospital Experiences				
Area Around Room 'Always' Quiet at Night	300+	70%	68%	61%
Doctors 'Always' Communicated Well	300+	83%	83%	82%
Home Recovery Information Given	300+	86%	85%	85%
Hospital Given 9 or 10 on 10 Point Scale	300+	76%	73%	71%
Meds 'Always' Explained Before Given	300+	64%	66%	64%
Nurses 'Always' Communicated Well	300+	83%	80%	79%
Pain 'Always' Well Controlled	300+	73%	72%	71%
Room and Bathroom 'Always' Clean	300+	76%	75%	73%
Timely Help 'Always' Received	300+	68%	69%	68%
Would Definitely Recommend Hospital	300+	81%	73%	71%
Use of Medical Imaging				
Cardiac Imaging Stress Test before Surgery	1,169	1.8%	5.3%	5.3%
Combination Abdominal CT Scan	1,053	6.6%	16.4%	10.5%
Combination Brain/Sinus CT Scan	935	1.6%	2.7%	2.7%
Combination Chest CT Scan	827	0.0%	5.6%	2.7%
Follow-up Mammogram/Ultrasound	3,327	8.9%	7.9%	8.8%
Lumbar Spine MRI for Low Back Pain	309	40.1%	39.6%	37.2%

Methodist Hospital For Surgery

17101 Dallas Parkway Phone: 469-248-3900
Addison, TX 75001
Type: Acute Care Hospitals Emergency Services: Yes
Ownership: Proprietary

Measure	Cases	This Hosp.	State Avg.	U.S. Avg.
Blood Clot Prevention and Treatment				
Anticoagulation Overlap Therapy[1,2]	-	-	93%	93%
ICU Venous Thromboembolism Prophylaxis[1,2]	-	-	92%	92%
Incidence of Potentially Preventable VTE[1,2]	-	-	9%	10%
UFH with Dosages/Platelet Monitoring[2,7]	-	-	96%	97%
Venous Thromboembolism Prophylaxis[2]	94	100%	82%	85%
Warfarin Therapy Discharge Instructions[1,2]	-	-	84%	75%
Chest Pain/Possible Heart Attack Care				
Aspirin Given Within 24 Hours of Arrival[5]	-	-	94%	96%
Fibrinolytic Meds Within 30 Min. of Arrival[5]	-	-	47%	58%
Average Time to ECG (minutes)[5]	-	-	8	7
Average Time to Transfer (minutes)[5]	-	-	62	60
Children's Asthma Care				
Received Home Management Plan of Care	-	-	93%	88%
Received Reliever Medication	-	-	100%	100%
Received Systemic Corticosteroids	-	-	100%	100%
Emergency Department				
Admittance Decision Time (minutes)[1,2]	-	-	99	98
Head CT Results Within 45 Min. of Arrival[5]	-	-	54%	57%
Patients Who Left ER Before Being Seen	1,268	1%	3%	2%

NOTE: Hospital profiles are in alphabetical order by state, then city, then hospital within the city; Rankings exclude hospitals with less than 25 cases except for patient surveys which excludes hospitals with less than 100 cases; (a) 100-299 cases; (1) The number of cases/patients is too few to report; (2) Data submitted were based on a sample of cases/patients; (3) Results are based on a shorter time period than required; (4) Data suppressed by CMS for one or more quarters; (5) Results are not available for this reporting period; (6) Fewer than 100 patients completed the HCAHPS survey; (7) No cases met the criteria for this measure; (8) The lower limit of the confidence interval cannot be calculated if the number of observed infections equals zero; (9) No data are available from the state/territory for this reporting period; (10) The scores shown reflect fewer than 50 completed surveys; (11) There were discrepancies in the data collection process; (12) This measure does not apply to this hospital for this reporting period; (13) Results cannot be calculated for this reporting period; (14) The results for this state are combined with nearby states to protect confidentiality; Please refer to the User's Guide for a full explanation of data.

Measure	Cases	This Hosp.	State Avg.	U.S. Avg.
Time from ER Arrival to Admit. (minutes)[1,2]	-	-	270	274
Time from ER Arrival to Discharge (minutes)	267	88	127	134
Time in ER Before Being Evaluated (minutes)	287	20	26	26
Time to Pain Meds for Fractures (minutes)[5]	-	-	57	57
Heart Attack Care				
Aspirin Given at Discharge[5]	-	-	99%	99%
Fibrinolytic Meds Within 30 Min. of Arrival[5]	-	-	49%	54%
PCI Within 90 Minutes of Arrival[5]	-	-	95%	96%
Statin Prescribed at Discharge[5]	-	-	98%	98%
Heart Failure Care				
ACE Inhibitor or ARB for LVSD[5]	-	-	97%	97%
Discharge Instructions Given[5]	-	-	95%	94%
Evaluation of LVS Function[5]	-	-	99%	99%
Medicare Spending				
Medicare Spending per Patient (ratio)	-	1.01	1.03	0.98
Pneumonia Care				
Appropriate Initial Antibiotic Given[5]	-	-	95%	95%
Blood Culture Timing[5]	-	-	98%	98%
Pregnancy and Delivery Care				
Newborn Deliveries Scheduled Early[7]	-	-	7%	6%
Preventive Care				
Immunization for Influenza[2]	339	79%	90%	90%
Immunization for Pneumonia[2]	336	71%	92%	92%
Stroke Care				
Anticoagulation Therapy for Atrial Fibrillation[5]	-	-	96%	95%
Antithrombotic Therapy Timing[5]	-	-	98%	98%
Assessed for Rehabilitation[5]	-	-	98%	97%
Discharged on Antithrombotic Therapy[5]	-	-	99%	99%
Discharged on Statin Medication[5]	-	-	95%	94%
Thrombolytic Therapy Timing[5]	-	-	68%	66%
Venous Thromboembolism Prophylaxis[5]	-	-	94%	94%
Written Stroke Educational Materials Given[5]	-	-	92%	88%
Surgical Care Improvement Project				
Appropriate Beta Blocker Usage[2]	159	97%	98%	98%
Appropriate VTP Within 24 Hours[2]	688	100%	98%	98%
Controlled Postoperative Blood Glucose[2,7]	-	-	96%	97%
Perioperative Temperature Management[2]	724	100%	100%	100%
Prophylactic Antibiotic Selection[2]	695	100%	99%	99%
Prophylactic Antibiotic Selection (Outpatient)	477	99%	98%	98%
Prophylactic Antibiotic Stopped[2]	695	100%	98%	98%
Prophylactic Antibiotic Timing[2]	696	100%	99%	99%
Prophylactic Antibiotic Timing (Outpatient)	477	100%	98%	98%
Urinary Catheter Removal[2]	624	95%	98%	97%
Survey of Patients' Hospital Experiences				
Area Around Room 'Always' Quiet at Night	300+	82%	68%	61%
Doctors 'Always' Communicated Well	300+	84%	83%	82%
Home Recovery Information Given	300+	90%	85%	85%
Hospital Given 9 or 10 on 10 Point Scale	300+	82%	73%	71%
Meds 'Always' Explained Before Given	300+	67%	66%	64%
Nurses 'Always' Communicated Well	300+	80%	80%	79%
Pain 'Always' Well Controlled	300+	74%	72%	71%
Room and Bathroom 'Always' Clean	300+	84%	75%	73%
Timely Help 'Always' Received	300+	74%	69%	68%
Would Definitely Recommend Hospital	300+	83%	73%	71%
Use of Medical Imaging				
Cardiac Imaging Stress Test before Surgery[7]	-	-	5.3%	5.3%
Combination Abdominal CT Scan[1]	-	-	16.4%	10.5%
Combination Brain/Sinus CT Scan[1]	-	-	2.7%	2.7%
Combination Chest CT Scan[1]	-	-	5.6%	2.7%
Follow-up Mammogram/Ultrasound[7]	-	-	7.9%	8.8%
Lumbar Spine MRI for Low Back Pain	34	50.0%	39.6%	37.2%

Christus Spohn Hospital Alice

2500 E Main Street Phone: 361-661-8016
Alice, TX 78332 Fax: 361-883-6478
URL: www.christusspohn.org
Type: Acute Care Hospitals Emergency Services: Yes
Ownership: Voluntary non-profit - Private Beds: 148

Key Personnel:

Radiology. . . . . Larry H Adams
Cardiac Laboratory. . . . . Jennifer Anbmendi
Operating Room. . . . . Alberto Belalcazar
Intensive Care Unit. . . . . Elvira DeTorres
Quality Assurance . . . . Brenda Garett
Emergency Room . . . . Larry Johnson
Hemotology Center . . . . Martha Siemonsma
Chief of Medical Staff. . . . . Charles T. Volk, MD

Measure	Cases	This Hosp.	State Avg.	U.S. Avg.
Blood Clot Prevention and Treatment				
Anticoagulation Overlap Therapy[1,2]	-	-	93%	93%
ICU Venous Thromboembolism Prophylaxis[2]	94	68%	92%	92%
Incidence of Potentially Preventable VTE[1,2]	-	-	9%	10%
UFH with Dosages/Platelet Monitoring[1,2]	-	-	96%	97%
Venous Thromboembolism Prophylaxis[2]	215	57%	82%	85%
Warfarin Therapy Discharge Instructions[1,2]	-	-	84%	75%
Chest Pain/Possible Heart Attack Care				
Aspirin Given Within 24 Hours of Arrival	119	79%	94%	96%
Fibrinolytic Meds Within 30 Min. of Arrival	11	27%	47%	58%
Average Time to ECG (minutes)	119	24	8	7
Average Time to Transfer (minutes)[1]	-	-	62	60
Children's Asthma Care				
Received Home Management Plan of Care	-	-	93%	88%
Received Reliever Medication	-	-	100%	100%
Received Systemic Corticosteroids	-	-	100%	100%
Emergency Department				
Admittance Decision Time (minutes)[2]	450	140	99	98
Head CT Results Within 45 Min. of Arrival	22	36%	54%	57%
Patients Who Left ER Before Being Seen	29,341	6%	3%	2%
Time from ER Arrival to Admit. (minutes)[2]	450	378	270	274
Time from ER Arrival to Discharge (minutes)	391	192	127	134
Time in ER Before Being Evaluated (minutes)	427	57	26	26
Time to Pain Meds for Fractures (minutes)	172	84	57	57
Heart Attack Care				
Aspirin Given at Discharge	20	100%	99%	99%
Fibrinolytic Meds Within 30 Min. of Arrival[7]	-	-	49%	54%
PCI Within 90 Minutes of Arrival[7]	-	-	95%	96%
Statin Prescribed at Discharge	20	80%	98%	98%
Heart Failure Care				
ACE Inhibitor or ARB for LVSD	39	87%	97%	97%
Discharge Instructions Given	107	100%	95%	94%
Evaluation of LVS Function	125	100%	99%	99%
Medicare Spending				
Medicare Spending per Patient (ratio)	-	1.04	1.03	0.98
Pneumonia Care				
Appropriate Initial Antibiotic Given	59	92%	95%	95%
Blood Culture Timing	84	96%	98%	98%
Pregnancy and Delivery Care				
Newborn Deliveries Scheduled Early[2]	32	28%	7%	6%
Preventive Care				
Immunization for Influenza[2]	342	76%	90%	90%
Immunization for Pneumonia[2]	392	80%	92%	92%
Stroke Care				
Anticoagulation Therapy for Atrial Fibrillation[1]	-	-	96%	95%
Antithrombotic Therapy Timing[1]	-	-	98%	98%
Assessed for Rehabilitation[1]	-	-	98%	97%
Discharged on Antithrombotic Therapy[1]	-	-	99%	99%
Discharged on Statin Medication[1]	-	-	95%	94%
Thrombolytic Therapy Timing[1]	-	-	68%	66%
Venous Thromboembolism Prophylaxis[1]	-	-	94%	94%
Written Stroke Educational Materials Given[1]	-	-	92%	88%
Surgical Care Improvement Project				
Appropriate Beta Blocker Usage[1]	-	-	98%	98%
Appropriate VTP Within 24 Hours	37	86%	98%	98%
Controlled Postoperative Blood Glucose[7]	-	-	96%	97%
Perioperative Temperature Management	40	100%	100%	100%
Prophylactic Antibiotic Selection	11	100%	99%	99%
Prophylactic Antibiotic Selection (Outpatient)	54	59%	98%	98%
Prophylactic Antibiotic Stopped[1]	-	-	98%	98%
Prophylactic Antibiotic Timing	12	83%	99%	99%
Prophylactic Antibiotic Timing (Outpatient)	58	86%	98%	98%
Urinary Catheter Removal	23	91%	98%	97%
Survey of Patients' Hospital Experiences				
Area Around Room 'Always' Quiet at Night	300+	72%	68%	61%
Doctors 'Always' Communicated Well	300+	82%	83%	82%
Home Recovery Information Given	300+	85%	85%	85%
Hospital Given 9 or 10 on 10 Point Scale	300+	71%	73%	71%
Meds 'Always' Explained Before Given	300+	67%	66%	64%
Nurses 'Always' Communicated Well	300+	81%	80%	79%
Pain 'Always' Well Controlled	300+	75%	72%	71%
Room and Bathroom 'Always' Clean	300+	76%	75%	73%
Timely Help 'Always' Received	300+	71%	69%	68%
Would Definitely Recommend Hospital	300+	67%	73%	71%
Use of Medical Imaging				
Cardiac Imaging Stress Test before Surgery[1]	-	-	5.3%	5.3%
Combination Abdominal CT Scan	257	52.1%	16.4%	10.5%
Combination Brain/Sinus CT Scan	514	5.1%	2.7%	2.7%
Combination Chest CT Scan	92	2.2%	5.6%	2.7%
Follow-up Mammogram/Ultrasound	214	8.9%	7.9%	8.8%
Lumbar Spine MRI for Low Back Pain[1]	-	-	39.6%	37.2%

Texas Health Presbyterian Hospital Allen

1105 Central Expressway North Phone: 972-747-6197
Allen, TX 75013
URL: www.texashealth.org/pha
Type: Acute Care Hospitals Emergency Services: Yes
Ownership: Government - Federal Beds: 73

Key Personnel:

CEO/President. . . . . Jeff Reecer
Chief of Medical Staff . . . . Robert Schwab, MD

Measure	Cases	This Hosp.	State Avg.	U.S. Avg.
Blood Clot Prevention and Treatment				
Anticoagulation Overlap Therapy[2]	21	100%	93%	93%
ICU Venous Thromboembolism Prophylaxis[2]	36	100%	92%	92%
Incidence of Potentially Preventable VTE[1,2]	-	-	9%	10%
UFH with Dosages/Platelet Monitoring[1,2]	-	-	96%	97%
Venous Thromboembolism Prophylaxis[2]	283	96%	82%	85%
Warfarin Therapy Discharge Instructions[2]	17	53%	84%	75%
Chest Pain/Possible Heart Attack Care				
Aspirin Given Within 24 Hours of Arrival	62	98%	94%	96%
Fibrinolytic Meds Within 30 Min. of Arrival[7]	-	-	47%	58%
Average Time to ECG (minutes)	63	6	8	7
Average Time to Transfer (minutes)[1]	-	-	62	60
Children's Asthma Care				
Received Home Management Plan of Care	-	-	93%	88%
Received Reliever Medication	-	-	100%	100%
Received Systemic Corticosteroids	-	-	100%	100%
Emergency Department				
Admittance Decision Time (minutes)[2]	463	97	99	98
Head CT Results Within 45 Min. of Arrival[1]	-	-	54%	57%
Patients Who Left ER Before Being Seen	30,030	2%	3%	2%
Time from ER Arrival to Admit. (minutes)[2]	462	230	270	274
Time from ER Arrival to Discharge (minutes)	413	122	127	134
Time in ER Before Being Evaluated (minutes)	441	17	26	26
Time to Pain Meds for Fractures (minutes)	122	52	57	57
Heart Attack Care				
Aspirin Given at Discharge[1,3]	-	-	99%	99%
Fibrinolytic Meds Within 30 Min. of Arrival[3,7]	-	-	49%	54%
PCI Within 90 Minutes of Arrival[3,7]	-	-	95%	96%
Statin Prescribed at Discharge[1,3]	-	-	98%	98%
Heart Failure Care				
ACE Inhibitor or ARB for LVSD	12	100%	97%	97%
Discharge Instructions Given	48	96%	95%	94%
Evaluation of LVS Function	61	100%	99%	99%
Medicare Spending				
Medicare Spending per Patient (ratio)	-	1.16	1.03	0.98
Pneumonia Care				
Appropriate Initial Antibiotic Given	84	96%	95%	95%
Blood Culture Timing	124	99%	98%	98%
Pregnancy and Delivery Care				
Newborn Deliveries Scheduled Early	59	10%	7%	6%
Preventive Care				
Immunization for Influenza[2]	459	98%	90%	90%
Immunization for Pneumonia[2]	444	97%	92%	92%
Stroke Care				
Anticoagulation Therapy for Atrial Fibrillation[1,2]	-	-	96%	95%
Antithrombotic Therapy Timing[1,2]	-	-	98%	98%
Assessed for Rehabilitation[1,2]	-	-	98%	97%
Discharged on Antithrombotic Therapy[1,2]	-	-	99%	99%
Discharged on Statin Medication[1,2]	-	-	95%	94%
Thrombolytic Therapy Timing[2,7]	-	-	68%	66%

NOTE: Hospital profiles are in alphabetical order by state, then city, then hospital within the city; Rankings exclude hospitals with less than 25 cases except for patient surveys which excludes hospitals with less than 100 cases; (a) 100-299 cases; (1) The number of cases/patients is too few to report; (2) Data submitted were based on a sample of cases/patients; (3) Results are based on a shorter time period than required; (4) Data suppressed by CMS for one or more quarters; (5) Results are not available for this reporting period; (6) Fewer than 100 patients completed the HCAHPS survey; (7) No cases met the criteria for this measure; (8) The lower limit of the confidence interval cannot be calculated if the number of observed infections equals zero; (9) No data are available from the state/territory for this reporting period; (10) The scores shown reflect fewer than 50 completed surveys; (11) There were discrepancies in the data collection process; (12) This measure does not apply to this hospital for this reporting period; (13) Results cannot be calculated for this reporting period; (14) The results for this state are combined with nearby states to protect confidentiality; Please refer to the User's Guide for a full explanation of data.

Measure	Cases	This Hosp.	State Avg.	U.S. Avg.
Venous Thromboembolism Prophylaxis[1,2]	-	-	94%	94%
Written Stroke Educational Materials Given[1,2]	-	-	92%	88%
Surgical Care Improvement Project				
Appropriate Beta Blocker Usage[2]	34	100%	98%	98%
Appropriate VTP Within 24 Hours[2]	156	100%	98%	98%
Controlled Postoperative Blood Glucose[2,7]	-	-	96%	97%
Perioperative Temperature Management[2]	195	100%	100%	100%
Prophylactic Antibiotic Selection[2]	117	100%	99%	99%
Prophylactic Antibiotic Selection (Outpatient)	92	98%	98%	98%
Prophylactic Antibiotic Stopped[2]	111	97%	98%	98%
Prophylactic Antibiotic Timing[2]	116	99%	99%	99%
Prophylactic Antibiotic Timing (Outpatient)	93	97%	98%	98%
Urinary Catheter Removal[2]	105	99%	98%	97%
Survey of Patients' Hospital Experiences				
Area Around Room 'Always' Quiet at Night	300+	66%	68%	61%
Doctors 'Always' Communicated Well	300+	83%	83%	82%
Home Recovery Information Given	300+	86%	85%	85%
Hospital Given 9 or 10 on 10 Point Scale	300+	76%	73%	71%
Meds 'Always' Explained Before Given	300+	65%	66%	64%
Nurses 'Always' Communicated Well	300+	79%	80%	79%
Pain 'Always' Well Controlled	300+	70%	72%	71%
Room and Bathroom 'Always' Clean	300+	77%	75%	73%
Timely Help 'Always' Received	300+	69%	69%	68%
Would Definitely Recommend Hospital	300+	77%	73%	71%
Use of Medical Imaging				
Cardiac Imaging Stress Test before Surgery	64	7.8%	5.3%	5.3%
Combination Abdominal CT Scan	214	6.1%	16.4%	10.5%
Combination Brain/Sinus CT Scan	255	6.3%	2.7%	2.7%
Combination Chest CT Scan[1]	-	-	5.6%	2.7%
Follow-up Mammogram/Ultrasound	662	11.2%	7.9%	8.8%
Lumbar Spine MRI for Low Back Pain[1]	-	-	39.6%	37.2%

Big Bend Regional Medical Center

2600 Highway 118 North
Alpine, TX 79830
Phone: 432-837-3447
Fax: 915-837-0255
URL: www.bigbendhealthcare.com
Type: Critical Access Hospitals
Emergency Services: Yes
Ownership: Proprietary
Beds: 40

Key Personnel:
Operating Room. . . . . George Alsop, RN
Quality Assurance . . . . Karen Davidson
Anesthesiology. . . . . Vicki Friddell
Chief of Medical Staff . . . . David Sanchez, MD
Patient Relations . . . . Heidi Wolf
CEO/President. . . . . Fred Woody

Measure	Cases	This Hosp.	State Avg.	U.S. Avg.
Blood Clot Prevention and Treatment				
Anticoagulation Overlap Therapy[2,7]	-	-	93%	93%
ICU Venous Thromboembolism Prophylaxis[2]	14	86%	92%	92%
Incidence of Potentially Preventable VTE[1,2]	-	-	9%	10%
UFH with Dosages/Platelet Monitoring[1,2]	-	-	96%	97%
Venous Thromboembolism Prophylaxis[2]	187	98%	82%	85%
Warfarin Therapy Discharge Instructions[2,7]	-	-	84%	75%
Chest Pain/Possible Heart Attack Care				
Aspirin Given Within 24 Hours of Arrival	28	96%	94%	96%
Fibrinolytic Meds Within 30 Min. of Arrival[1,3]	-	-	47%	58%
Average Time to ECG (minutes)	29	4	8	7
Average Time to Transfer (minutes)[3,7]	-	-	62	60
Children's Asthma Care				
Received Home Management Plan of Care	-	-	93%	88%
Received Reliever Medication	-	-	100%	100%
Received Systemic Corticosteroids	-	-	100%	100%
Emergency Department				
Admittance Decision Time (minutes)[2]	318	64	99	98
Head CT Results Within 45 Min. of Arrival[1]	-	-	54%	57%
Patients Who Left ER Before Being Seen	4,509	0%	3%	2%
Time from ER Arrival to Admit. (minutes)[2]	318	190	270	274
Time from ER Arrival to Discharge (minutes)	352	95	127	134
Time in ER Before Being Evaluated (minutes)	463	12	26	26
Time to Pain Meds for Fractures (minutes)	47	56	57	57
Heart Attack Care				
Aspirin Given at Discharge[3,7]	-	-	99%	99%
Fibrinolytic Meds Within 30 Min. of Arrival[3,7]	-	-	49%	54%
PCI Within 90 Minutes of Arrival[3,7]	-	-	95%	96%
Statin Prescribed at Discharge[1,3]	-	-	98%	98%
Heart Failure Care				
ACE Inhibitor or ARB for LVSD[1]	-	-	97%	97%
Discharge Instructions Given	22	100%	95%	94%
Evaluation of LVS Function	26	100%	99%	99%
Medicare Spending				
Medicare Spending per Patient (ratio)	-	-	1.03	0.98
Pneumonia Care				
Appropriate Initial Antibiotic Given	25	100%	95%	95%
Blood Culture Timing	33	100%	98%	98%
Pregnancy and Delivery Care				
Newborn Deliveries Scheduled Early[1,2]	-	-	7%	6%
Preventive Care				
Immunization for Influenza[2]	323	98%	90%	90%
Immunization for Pneumonia[2]	294	98%	92%	92%
Stroke Care				
Anticoagulation Therapy for Atrial Fibrillation[1]	-	-	96%	95%
Antithrombotic Therapy Timing[7]	-	-	98%	98%
Assessed for Rehabilitation[1]	-	-	98%	97%
Discharged on Antithrombotic Therapy[1]	-	-	99%	99%
Discharged on Statin Medication[1]	-	-	95%	94%
Thrombolytic Therapy Timing[7]	-	-	68%	66%
Venous Thromboembolism Prophylaxis[1]	-	-	94%	94%
Written Stroke Educational Materials Given[1]	-	-	92%	88%
Surgical Care Improvement Project				
Appropriate Beta Blocker Usage[1]	-	-	98%	98%
Appropriate VTP Within 24 Hours	14	100%	98%	98%
Controlled Postoperative Blood Glucose[7]	-	-	96%	97%
Perioperative Temperature Management	16	100%	100%	100%
Prophylactic Antibiotic Selection[1]	-	-	99%	99%
Prophylactic Antibiotic Selection (Outpatient)[1,3]	-	-	98%	98%
Prophylactic Antibiotic Stopped[1]	-	-	98%	98%
Prophylactic Antibiotic Timing[1]	-	-	99%	99%
Prophylactic Antibiotic Timing (Outpatient)[1,3]	-	-	98%	98%
Urinary Catheter Removal[1]	-	-	98%	97%
Survey of Patients' Hospital Experiences				
Area Around Room 'Always' Quiet at Night	(a)	71%	68%	61%
Doctors 'Always' Communicated Well	(a)	85%	83%	82%
Home Recovery Information Given	(a)	91%	85%	85%
Hospital Given 9 or 10 on 10 Point Scale	(a)	75%	73%	71%
Meds 'Always' Explained Before Given	(a)	75%	66%	64%
Nurses 'Always' Communicated Well	(a)	84%	80%	79%
Pain 'Always' Well Controlled	(a)	78%	72%	71%
Room and Bathroom 'Always' Clean	(a)	74%	75%	73%
Timely Help 'Always' Received	(a)	78%	69%	68%
Would Definitely Recommend Hospital	(a)	76%	73%	71%
Use of Medical Imaging				
Cardiac Imaging Stress Test before Surgery[7]	-	-	5.3%	5.3%
Combination Abdominal CT Scan	118	17.8%	16.4%	10.5%
Combination Brain/Sinus CT Scan[1]	-	-	2.7%	2.7%
Combination Chest CT Scan[1]	-	-	5.6%	2.7%
Follow-up Mammogram/Ultrasound[7]	-	-	7.9%	8.8%
Lumbar Spine MRI for Low Back Pain[1]	-	-	39.6%	37.2%

Baptist Saint Anthony's Hospital

1600 Wallace Blvd
Amarillo, TX 79106
Phone: 806-212-2000
Fax: 806-212-2853
URL: www.bsahs.com
Type: Acute Care Hospitals
Emergency Services: Yes
Ownership: Government - Federal
Beds: 451

Key Personnel:
Radiology. . . . . Shay Christian
Operating Room. . . . . Lanell Clayton
Coronary Care . . . . Kelly Fuller
CEO/President. . . . . John Hicks
Chief of Medical Staff . . . . Kenneth Johnston, MD
Quality Assurance . . . . Terry Long
Pediatric Ambulatory Care . . . . . . Teri Skelton
Infection Control. . . . . Charlotte Wheeler

Measure	Cases	This Hosp.	State Avg.	U.S. Avg.
Blood Clot Prevention and Treatment				
Anticoagulation Overlap Therapy[2]	144	93%	93%	93%
ICU Venous Thromboembolism Prophylaxis[2]	153	83%	92%	92%
Incidence of Potentially Preventable VTE[2]	20	15%	9%	10%
UFH with Dosages/Platelet Monitoring[2]	74	99%	96%	97%
Venous Thromboembolism Prophylaxis[2]	316	84%	82%	85%
Warfarin Therapy Discharge Instructions[2]	104	84%	84%	75%
Chest Pain/Possible Heart Attack Care				
Aspirin Given Within 24 Hours of Arrival[1,3]	-	-	94%	96%
Fibrinolytic Meds Within 30 Min. of Arrival[5]	-	-	47%	58%
Average Time to ECG (minutes)[1,3]	-	-	8	7
Average Time to Transfer (minutes)[5]	-	-	62	60
Children's Asthma Care				
Received Home Management Plan of Care	-	-	93%	88%
Received Reliever Medication	-	-	100%	100%
Received Systemic Corticosteroids	-	-	100%	100%
Emergency Department				
Admittance Decision Time (minutes)[2]	677	114	99	98
Head CT Results Within 45 Min. of Arrival[1]	-	-	54%	57%
Patients Who Left ER Before Being Seen	62,217	3%	3%	2%
Time from ER Arrival to Admit. (minutes)[2]	680	328	270	274
Time from ER Arrival to Discharge (minutes)	441	177	127	134
Time in ER Before Being Evaluated (minutes)	456	44	26	26
Time to Pain Meds for Fractures (minutes)	180	23	57	57
Heart Attack Care				
Aspirin Given at Discharge[2]	316	96%	99%	99%
Fibrinolytic Meds Within 30 Min. of Arrival[2,7]	-	-	49%	54%
PCI Within 90 Minutes of Arrival[2]	42	90%	95%	96%
Statin Prescribed at Discharge[2]	291	98%	98%	98%
Heart Failure Care				
ACE Inhibitor or ARB for LVSD[2]	97	91%	97%	97%
Discharge Instructions Given[2]	255	84%	95%	94%
Evaluation of LVS Function[2]	315	99%	99%	99%
Medicare Spending				
Medicare Spending per Patient (ratio)	-	0.99	1.03	0.98
Pneumonia Care				
Appropriate Initial Antibiotic Given[2]	93	96%	95%	95%
Blood Culture Timing[2]	196	98%	98%	98%
Pregnancy and Delivery Care				
Newborn Deliveries Scheduled Early[2]	42	0%	7%	6%
Preventive Care				
Immunization for Influenza[2]	618	97%	90%	90%
Immunization for Pneumonia[2]	710	97%	92%	92%
Stroke Care				
Anticoagulation Therapy for Atrial Fibrillation[2]	13	92%	96%	95%
Antithrombotic Therapy Timing[2]	95	99%	98%	98%
Assessed for Rehabilitation[2]	110	95%	98%	97%
Discharged on Antithrombotic Therapy[2]	96	98%	99%	99%
Discharged on Statin Medication[2]	79	87%	95%	94%
Thrombolytic Therapy Timing[1,2]	-	-	68%	66%
Venous Thromboembolism Prophylaxis[2]	115	90%	94%	94%
Written Stroke Educational Materials Given[2]	57	68%	92%	88%
Surgical Care Improvement Project				
Appropriate Beta Blocker Usage[2]	302	97%	98%	98%
Appropriate VTP Within 24 Hours[2]	457	97%	98%	98%
Controlled Postoperative Blood Glucose[2]	141	95%	96%	97%
Perioperative Temperature Management[2]	580	100%	100%	100%
Prophylactic Antibiotic Selection[2]	491	99%	99%	99%
Prophylactic Antibiotic Selection (Outpatient)	599	98%	98%	98%
Prophylactic Antibiotic Stopped[2]	470	96%	98%	98%
Prophylactic Antibiotic Timing[2]	492	99%	99%	99%
Prophylactic Antibiotic Timing (Outpatient)	600	98%	98%	98%
Urinary Catheter Removal[2]	507	97%	98%	97%
Survey of Patients' Hospital Experiences				
Area Around Room 'Always' Quiet at Night	300+	62%	68%	61%
Doctors 'Always' Communicated Well	300+	81%	83%	82%
Home Recovery Information Given	300+	83%	85%	85%
Hospital Given 9 or 10 on 10 Point Scale	300+	76%	73%	71%
Meds 'Always' Explained Before Given	300+	63%	66%	64%
Nurses 'Always' Communicated Well	300+	78%	80%	79%
Pain 'Always' Well Controlled	300+	70%	72%	71%
Room and Bathroom 'Always' Clean	300+	77%	75%	73%
Timely Help 'Always' Received	300+	64%	69%	68%
Would Definitely Recommend Hospital	300+	80%	73%	71%
Use of Medical Imaging				
Cardiac Imaging Stress Test before Surgery	331	4.2%	5.3%	5.3%

NOTE: Hospital profiles are in alphabetical order by state, then city, then hospital within the city; Rankings exclude hospitals with less than 25 cases except for patient surveys which excludes hospitals with less than 100 cases; (a) 100-299 cases; (1) The number of cases/patients is too few to report; (2) Data submitted were based on a sample of cases/patients; (3) Results are based on a shorter time period than required; (4) Data suppressed by CMS for one or more quarters; (5) Results are not available for this reporting period; (6) Fewer than 100 patients completed the HCAHPS survey; (7) No cases met the criteria for this measure; (8) The lower limit of the confidence interval cannot be calculated if the number of observed infections equals zero; (9) No data are available from the state/territory for this reporting period; (10) The scores shown reflect fewer than 50 completed surveys; (11) There were discrepancies in the data collection process; (12) This measure does not apply to this hospital for this reporting period; (13) Results cannot be calculated for this reporting period; (14) The results for this state are combined with nearby states to protect confidentiality; Please refer to the User's Guide for a full explanation of data.

Combination Abdominal CT Scan	1,499	0.6%	16.4%	10.5%
Combination Brain/Sinus CT Scan	1,241	2.4%	2.7%	2.7%
Combination Chest CT Scan	597	0.5%	5.6%	2.7%
Follow-up Mammogram/Ultrasound[7]	-	-	7.9%	8.8%
Lumbar Spine MRI for Low Back Pain	227	44.5%	39.6%	37.2%

Northwest Texas Hospital

1501 Coulter Road
Amarillo, TX 79106
URL: www.nxtexashealthcare.com
Type: Acute Care Hospitals
Ownership: Proprietary
Phone: 806-354-1110
Fax: 806-354-1109
Emergency Services: Yes
Beds: 489
Key Personnel:
CEO/President. . . . . Mark Crawford

Measure	Cases	This Hosp.	State Avg.	U.S. Avg.
Blood Clot Prevention and Treatment				
Anticoagulation Overlap Therapy[2]	45	93%	93%	93%
ICU Venous Thromboembolism Prophylaxis[2]	186	92%	92%	92%
Incidence of Potentially Preventable VTE[2]	21	5%	9%	10%
UFH with Dosages/Platelet Monitoring[2]	43	100%	96%	97%
Venous Thromboembolism Prophylaxis[2]	227	84%	82%	85%
Warfarin Therapy Discharge Instructions[2]	38	76%	84%	75%
Chest Pain/Possible Heart Attack Care				
Aspirin Given Within 24 Hours of Arrival[1]	-	-	94%	96%
Fibrinolytic Meds Within 30 Min. of Arrival[5]	-	-	47%	58%
Average Time to ECG (minutes)[1]	-	-	8	7
Average Time to Transfer (minutes)[5]	-	-	62	60
Children's Asthma Care				
Received Home Management Plan of Care	-	-	93%	88%
Received Reliever Medication	-	-	100%	100%
Received Systemic Corticosteroids	-	-	100%	100%
Emergency Department				
Admittance Decision Time (minutes)[2]	511	153	99	98
Head CT Results Within 45 Min. of Arrival[1]	-	-	54%	57%
Patients Who Left ER Before Being Seen	50,021	4%	3%	2%
Time from ER Arrival to Admit. (minutes)[2]	528	387	270	274
Time from ER Arrival to Discharge (minutes)	400	182	127	134
Time in ER Before Being Evaluated (minutes)	382	73	26	26
Time to Pain Meds for Fractures (minutes)	155	102	57	57
Heart Attack Care				
Aspirin Given at Discharge[2]	257	100%	99%	99%
Fibrinolytic Meds Within 30 Min. of Arrival[2,7]	-	-	49%	54%
PCI Within 90 Minutes of Arrival[2]	39	97%	95%	96%
Statin Prescribed at Discharge[2]	246	100%	98%	98%
Heart Failure Care				
ACE Inhibitor or ARB for LVSD[2]	96	99%	97%	97%
Discharge Instructions Given[2]	221	94%	95%	94%
Evaluation of LVS Function[2]	260	100%	99%	99%
Medicare Spending				
Medicare Spending per Patient (ratio)	-	1.03	1.03	0.98
Pneumonia Care				
Appropriate Initial Antibiotic Given[2]	79	100%	95%	95%
Blood Culture Timing[2]	110	96%	98%	98%
Pregnancy and Delivery Care				
Newborn Deliveries Scheduled Early[2]	40	0%	7%	6%
Preventive Care				
Immunization for Influenza[2]	527	89%	90%	90%
Immunization for Pneumonia[2]	480	82%	92%	92%
Stroke Care				
Anticoagulation Therapy for Atrial Fibrillation[2]	14	100%	96%	95%
Antithrombotic Therapy Timing[2]	89	97%	98%	98%
Assessed for Rehabilitation[2]	114	93%	98%	97%
Discharged on Antithrombotic Therapy[2]	93	97%	99%	99%
Discharged on Statin Medication[2]	70	90%	95%	94%
Thrombolytic Therapy Timing[2]	36	11%	68%	66%
Venous Thromboembolism Prophylaxis[2]	126	96%	94%	94%
Written Stroke Educational Materials Given[2]	70	83%	92%	88%
Surgical Care Improvement Project				
Appropriate Beta Blocker Usage[2]	138	99%	98%	98%
Appropriate VTP Within 24 Hours[2]	317	97%	98%	98%
Controlled Postoperative Blood Glucose[2]	98	97%	96%	97%
Perioperative Temperature Management[2]	387	99%	100%	100%
Prophylactic Antibiotic Selection[2]	314	98%	99%	99%
Prophylactic Antibiotic Selection (Outpatient)	222	100%	98%	98%
Prophylactic Antibiotic Stopped[2]	305	97%	98%	98%
Prophylactic Antibiotic Timing[2]	316	99%	99%	99%
Prophylactic Antibiotic Timing (Outpatient)	224	99%	98%	98%
Urinary Catheter Removal[2]	259	97%	98%	97%
Survey of Patients' Hospital Experiences				
Area Around Room 'Always' Quiet at Night	300+	65%	68%	61%
Doctors 'Always' Communicated Well	300+	78%	83%	82%
Home Recovery Information Given	300+	85%	85%	85%
Hospital Given 9 or 10 on 10 Point Scale	300+	69%	73%	71%
Meds 'Always' Explained Before Given	300+	66%	66%	64%
Nurses 'Always' Communicated Well	300+	77%	80%	79%
Pain 'Always' Well Controlled	300+	71%	72%	71%
Room and Bathroom 'Always' Clean	300+	64%	75%	73%
Timely Help 'Always' Received	300+	67%	69%	68%
Would Definitely Recommend Hospital	300+	71%	73%	71%
Use of Medical Imaging				
Cardiac Imaging Stress Test before Surgery	126	4.0%	5.3%	5.3%
Combination Abdominal CT Scan	388	18.6%	16.4%	10.5%
Combination Brain/Sinus CT Scan[1]	-	-	2.7%	2.7%
Combination Chest CT Scan	199	25.1%	5.6%	2.7%
Follow-up Mammogram/Ultrasound	510	12.9%	7.9%	8.8%
Lumbar Spine MRI for Low Back Pain	58	53.4%	39.6%	37.2%

Northwest Texas Surgery Center

3501 Soncy Rd Suite 118
Amarillo, TX 79109
Type: Acute Care Hospitals
Ownership: Proprietary
Phone: 806-359-7999
Emergency Services: Yes
Beds: 6
Key Personnel:
Anesthesiology. . . . . Scott Bass
CEO/President. . . . . Dave Clark
Cardiology . . . . Suresh Neelagaru

Measure	Cases	This Hosp.	State Avg.	U.S. Avg.
Blood Clot Prevention and Treatment				
Anticoagulation Overlap Therapy[7]	-	-	93%	93%
ICU Venous Thromboembolism Prophylaxis[7]	-	-	92%	92%
Incidence of Potentially Preventable VTE[7]	-	-	9%	10%
UFH with Dosages/Platelet Monitoring[7]	-	-	96%	97%
Venous Thromboembolism Prophylaxis[1]	-	-	82%	85%
Warfarin Therapy Discharge Instructions[7]	-	-	84%	75%
Chest Pain/Possible Heart Attack Care				
Aspirin Given Within 24 Hours of Arrival[5]	-	-	94%	96%
Fibrinolytic Meds Within 30 Min. of Arrival[5]	-	-	47%	58%
Average Time to ECG (minutes)[5]	-	-	8	7
Average Time to Transfer (minutes)[5]	-	-	62	60
Children's Asthma Care				
Received Home Management Plan of Care	-	-	93%	88%
Received Reliever Medication	-	-	100%	100%
Received Systemic Corticosteroids	-	-	100%	100%
Emergency Department				
Admittance Decision Time (minutes)[2,7]	-	-	99	98
Head CT Results Within 45 Min. of Arrival[5]	-	-	54%	57%
Patients Who Left ER Before Being Seen[5]	-	-	3%	2%
Time from ER Arrival to Admit. (minutes)[2,7]	-	-	270	274
Time from ER Arrival to Discharge (minutes)[5]	-	-	127	134
Time in ER Before Being Evaluated (minutes)[5]	-	-	26	26
Time to Pain Meds for Fractures (minutes)[5]	-	-	57	57
Heart Attack Care				
Aspirin Given at Discharge[5]	-	-	99%	99%
Fibrinolytic Meds Within 30 Min. of Arrival[5]	-	-	49%	54%
PCI Within 90 Minutes of Arrival[5]	-	-	95%	96%
Statin Prescribed at Discharge[5]	-	-	98%	98%
Heart Failure Care				
ACE Inhibitor or ARB for LVSD[5]	-	-	97%	97%
Discharge Instructions Given[5]	-	-	95%	94%
Evaluation of LVS Function[5]	-	-	99%	99%
Medicare Spending				
Medicare Spending per Patient (ratio)	-	1.15	1.03	0.98
Pneumonia Care				
Appropriate Initial Antibiotic Given[5]	-	-	95%	95%
Blood Culture Timing[5]	-	-	98%	98%
Pregnancy and Delivery Care				
Newborn Deliveries Scheduled Early[7]	-	-	7%	6%
Preventive Care				
Immunization for Influenza	93	70%	90%	90%
Immunization for Pneumonia[2]	71	69%	92%	92%
Stroke Care				
Anticoagulation Therapy for Atrial Fibrillation[5]	-	-	96%	95%
Antithrombotic Therapy Timing[5]	-	-	98%	98%
Assessed for Rehabilitation[5]	-	-	98%	97%
Discharged on Antithrombotic Therapy[5]	-	-	99%	99%
Discharged on Statin Medication[5]	-	-	95%	94%
Thrombolytic Therapy Timing[5]	-	-	68%	66%
Venous Thromboembolism Prophylaxis[5]	-	-	94%	94%
Written Stroke Educational Materials Given[5]	-	-	92%	88%
Surgical Care Improvement Project				
Appropriate Beta Blocker Usage	30	93%	98%	98%
Appropriate VTP Within 24 Hours	112	99%	98%	98%
Controlled Postoperative Blood Glucose[7]	-	-	96%	97%
Perioperative Temperature Management	126	97%	100%	100%
Prophylactic Antibiotic Selection	116	93%	99%	99%
Prophylactic Antibiotic Selection (Outpatient)	46	96%	98%	98%
Prophylactic Antibiotic Stopped	116	95%	98%	98%
Prophylactic Antibiotic Timing	116	95%	99%	99%
Prophylactic Antibiotic Timing (Outpatient)	48	96%	98%	98%
Urinary Catheter Removal	115	100%	98%	97%
Survey of Patients' Hospital Experiences				
Area Around Room 'Always' Quiet at Night[6]	<100	85%	68%	61%
Doctors 'Always' Communicated Well[6]	<100	91%	83%	82%
Home Recovery Information Given[6]	<100	93%	85%	85%
Hospital Given 9 or 10 on 10 Point Scale[6]	<100	84%	73%	71%
Meds 'Always' Explained Before Given[6]	<100	82%	66%	64%
Nurses 'Always' Communicated Well[6]	<100	87%	80%	79%
Pain 'Always' Well Controlled[6]	<100	80%	72%	71%
Room and Bathroom 'Always' Clean[6]	<100	86%	75%	73%
Timely Help 'Always' Received[6]	<100	89%	69%	68%
Would Definitely Recommend Hospital[6]	<100	83%	73%	71%
Use of Medical Imaging				
Cardiac Imaging Stress Test before Surgery[7]	-	-	5.3%	5.3%
Combination Abdominal CT Scan[7]	-	-	16.4%	10.5%
Combination Brain/Sinus CT Scan[7]	-	-	2.7%	2.7%
Combination Chest CT Scan[7]	-	-	5.6%	2.7%
Follow-up Mammogram/Ultrasound[7]	-	-	7.9%	8.8%
Lumbar Spine MRI for Low Back Pain[7]	-	-	39.6%	37.2%

Quail Creek Surgical Hospital

6819 Plum Creek
Amarillo, TX 79124
URL: www.physurg.com
Type: Acute Care Hospitals
Ownership: Proprietary
Phone: 806-354-6100
Emergency Services: Yes
Beds: 32

Measure	Cases	This Hosp.	State Avg.	U.S. Avg.
Blood Clot Prevention and Treatment				
Anticoagulation Overlap Therapy[7]	-	-	93%	93%
ICU Venous Thromboembolism Prophylaxis[7]	-	-	92%	92%
Incidence of Potentially Preventable VTE[7]	-	-	9%	10%
UFH with Dosages/Platelet Monitoring[7]	-	-	96%	97%
Venous Thromboembolism Prophylaxis	227	99%	82%	85%
Warfarin Therapy Discharge Instructions[7]	-	-	84%	75%
Chest Pain/Possible Heart Attack Care				
Aspirin Given Within 24 Hours of Arrival[5]	-	-	94%	96%
Fibrinolytic Meds Within 30 Min. of Arrival[5]	-	-	47%	58%
Average Time to ECG (minutes)[5]	-	-	8	7
Average Time to Transfer (minutes)[5]	-	-	62	60
Children's Asthma Care				
Received Home Management Plan of Care	-	-	93%	88%
Received Reliever Medication	-	-	100%	100%
Received Systemic Corticosteroids	-	-	100%	100%
Emergency Department				
Admittance Decision Time (minutes)[7]	-	-	99	98
Head CT Results Within 45 Min. of Arrival[5]	-	-	54%	57%
Patients Who Left ER Before Being Seen[5]	-	-	3%	2%
Time from ER Arrival to Admit. (minutes)[7]	-	-	270	274
Time from ER Arrival to Discharge (minutes)[5]	-	-	127	134

NOTE: Hospital profiles are in alphabetical order by state, then city, then hospital within the city; Rankings exclude hospitals with less than 25 cases except for patient surveys which excludes hospitals with less than 100 cases; (a) 100-299 cases; (1) The number of cases/patients is too few to report; (2) Data submitted were based on a sample of cases/patients; (3) Results are based on a shorter time period than required; (4) Data suppressed by CMS for one or more quarters; (5) Results are not available for this reporting period; (6) Fewer than 100 patients completed the HCAHPS survey; (7) No cases met the criteria for this measure; (8) The lower limit of the confidence interval cannot be calculated if the number of observed infections equals zero; (9) No data are available from the state/territory for this reporting period; (10) The scores shown reflect fewer than 50 completed surveys; (11) There were discrepancies in the data collection process; (12) This measure does not apply to this hospital for this reporting period; (13) Results cannot be calculated for this reporting period; (14) The results for this state are combined with nearby states to protect confidentiality; Please refer to the User's Guide for a full explanation of data.

Measure	Cases	This Hosp.	State Avg.	U.S. Avg.
Time in ER Before Being Evaluated (minutes)[5]	-	-	26	26
Time to Pain Meds for Fractures (minutes)[5]	-	-	57	57
Heart Attack Care				
Aspirin Given at Discharge[5]	-	-	99%	99%
Fibrinolytic Meds Within 30 Min. of Arrival[5]	-	-	49%	54%
PCI Within 90 Minutes of Arrival[5]	-	-	95%	96%
Statin Prescribed at Discharge[5]	-	-	98%	98%
Heart Failure Care				
ACE Inhibitor or ARB for LVSD[5]	-	-	97%	97%
Discharge Instructions Given[5]	-	-	95%	94%
Evaluation of LVS Function[5]	-	-	99%	99%
Medicare Spending				
Medicare Spending per Patient (ratio)	-	0.91	1.03	0.98
Pneumonia Care				
Appropriate Initial Antibiotic Given[5]	-	-	95%	95%
Blood Culture Timing[5]	-	-	98%	98%
Pregnancy and Delivery Care				
Newborn Deliveries Scheduled Early[7]	-	-	7%	6%
Preventive Care				
Immunization for Influenza	715	97%	90%	90%
Immunization for Pneumonia	730	98%	92%	92%
Stroke Care				
Anticoagulation Therapy for Atrial Fibrillation[5]	-	-	96%	95%
Antithrombotic Therapy Timing[5]	-	-	98%	98%
Assessed for Rehabilitation[5]	-	-	98%	97%
Discharged on Antithrombotic Therapy[5]	-	-	99%	99%
Discharged on Statin Medication[5]	-	-	95%	94%
Thrombolytic Therapy Timing[5]	-	-	68%	66%
Venous Thromboembolism Prophylaxis[5]	-	-	94%	94%
Written Stroke Educational Materials Given[5]	-	-	92%	88%
Surgical Care Improvement Project				
Appropriate Beta Blocker Usage	232	100%	98%	98%
Appropriate VTP Within 24 Hours	777	100%	98%	98%
Controlled Postoperative Blood Glucose[7]	-	-	96%	97%
Perioperative Temperature Management	834	100%	100%	100%
Prophylactic Antibiotic Selection	719	100%	99%	99%
Prophylactic Antibiotic Selection (Outpatient)	200	100%	98%	98%
Prophylactic Antibiotic Stopped	719	100%	98%	98%
Prophylactic Antibiotic Timing	719	99%	99%	99%
Prophylactic Antibiotic Timing (Outpatient)	200	100%	98%	98%
Urinary Catheter Removal	743	100%	98%	97%
Survey of Patients' Hospital Experiences				
Area Around Room 'Always' Quiet at Night	300+	84%	68%	61%
Doctors 'Always' Communicated Well	300+	91%	83%	82%
Home Recovery Information Given	300+	91%	85%	85%
Hospital Given 9 or 10 on 10 Point Scale	300+	91%	73%	71%
Meds 'Always' Explained Before Given	300+	78%	66%	64%
Nurses 'Always' Communicated Well	300+	93%	80%	79%
Pain 'Always' Well Controlled	300+	82%	72%	71%
Room and Bathroom 'Always' Clean	300+	88%	75%	73%
Timely Help 'Always' Received	300+	93%	69%	68%
Would Definitely Recommend Hospital	300+	92%	73%	71%
Use of Medical Imaging				
Cardiac Imaging Stress Test before Surgery[7]	-	-	5.3%	5.3%
Combination Abdominal CT Scan[7]	-	-	16.4%	10.5%
Combination Brain/Sinus CT Scan[7]	-	-	2.7%	2.7%
Combination Chest CT Scan[7]	-	-	5.6%	2.7%
Follow-up Mammogram/Ultrasound[7]	-	-	7.9%	8.8%
Lumbar Spine MRI for Low Back Pain[7]	-	-	39.6%	37.2%

VA Amarillo Healthcare System

6010 Amarillo Blvd. West
Amarillo, TX 79106
Type: Acute Care - VA
Ownership: Government Federal
Phone: 806-355-9703
Fax: 806-354-7860
Emergency Services: No
Beds: 290

Key Personnel:
Operating Room. . . . . Linda Brattin
Chief of Medical Staff. . . . . Dennis A. Ice
Infection Control. . . . . Ona Mountgonery
Quality Assurance . . . . Colleen Sloan
Emergency Room . . . . Thomas Turner, MD
CEO/President. . . . . Andrew M Welch MHA FACHE

Measure	Cases	This Hosp.	State Avg.	U.S. Avg.
Blood Clot Prevention and Treatment				
Anticoagulation Overlap Therapy	-	-	93%	93%
ICU Venous Thromboembolism Prophylaxis	-	-	92%	92%
Incidence of Potentially Preventable VTE	-	-	9%	10%
UFH with Dosages/Platelet Monitoring	-	-	96%	97%
Venous Thromboembolism Prophylaxis	-	-	82%	85%
Warfarin Therapy Discharge Instructions	-	-	84%	75%
Chest Pain/Possible Heart Attack Care				
Aspirin Given Within 24 Hours of Arrival	-	-	94%	96%
Fibrinolytic Meds Within 30 Min. of Arrival	-	-	47%	58%
Average Time to ECG (minutes)	-	-	8	7
Average Time to Transfer (minutes)	-	-	62	60
Children's Asthma Care				
Received Home Management Plan of Care	-	-	93%	88%
Received Reliever Medication	-	-	100%	100%
Received Systemic Corticosteroids	-	-	100%	100%
Emergency Department				
Admittance Decision Time (minutes)	-	-	99	98
Head CT Results Within 45 Min. of Arrival	-	-	54%	57%
Patients Who Left ER Before Being Seen	-	-	3%	2%
Time from ER Arrival to Admit. (minutes)	-	-	270	274
Time from ER Arrival to Discharge (minutes)	-	-	127	134
Time in ER Before Being Evaluated (minutes)	-	-	26	26
Time to Pain Meds for Fractures (minutes)	-	-	57	57
Heart Attack Care				
Aspirin Given at Discharge[1]	-	-	99%	99%
Fibrinolytic Meds Within 30 Min. of Arrival[5]	-	-	49%	54%
PCI Within 90 Minutes of Arrival[5]	-	-	95%	96%
Statin Prescribed at Discharge[1]	-	-	98%	98%
Heart Failure Care				
ACE Inhibitor or ARB for LVSD	27	96%	97%	97%
Discharge Instructions Given	72	93%	95%	94%
Evaluation of LVS Function	95	100%	99%	99%
Medicare Spending				
Medicare Spending per Patient (ratio)	-	-	1.03	0.98
Pneumonia Care				
Appropriate Initial Antibiotic Given	35	100%	95%	95%
Blood Culture Timing	66	98%	98%	98%
Pregnancy and Delivery Care				
Newborn Deliveries Scheduled Early	-	-	7%	6%
Preventive Care				
Immunization for Influenza[5]	-	-	90%	90%
Immunization for Pneumonia[5]	-	-	92%	92%
Stroke Care				
Anticoagulation Therapy for Atrial Fibrillation	-	-	96%	95%
Antithrombotic Therapy Timing	-	-	98%	98%
Assessed for Rehabilitation	-	-	98%	97%
Discharged on Antithrombotic Therapy	-	-	99%	99%
Discharged on Statin Medication	-	-	95%	94%
Thrombolytic Therapy Timing	-	-	68%	66%
Venous Thromboembolism Prophylaxis	-	-	94%	94%
Written Stroke Educational Materials Given	-	-	92%	88%
Surgical Care Improvement Project				
Appropriate Beta Blocker Usage[2]	33	82%	98%	98%
Appropriate VTP Within 24 Hours[2]	94	91%	98%	98%
Controlled Postoperative Blood Glucose[5]	-	-	96%	97%
Perioperative Temperature Management[2]	98	100%	100%	100%
Prophylactic Antibiotic Selection	56	100%	99%	99%
Prophylactic Antibiotic Selection (Outpatient)	-	-	98%	98%
Prophylactic Antibiotic Stopped	56	93%	98%	98%
Prophylactic Antibiotic Timing	56	96%	99%	99%
Prophylactic Antibiotic Timing (Outpatient)	-	-	98%	98%
Urinary Catheter Removal[2]	67	96%	98%	97%
Survey of Patients' Hospital Experiences				
Area Around Room 'Always' Quiet at Night	-	-	68%	61%
Doctors 'Always' Communicated Well	-	-	83%	82%
Home Recovery Information Given	-	-	85%	85%
Hospital Given 9 or 10 on 10 Point Scale	-	-	73%	71%
Meds 'Always' Explained Before Given	-	-	66%	64%
Nurses 'Always' Communicated Well	-	-	80%	79%
Pain 'Always' Well Controlled	-	-	72%	71%
Room and Bathroom 'Always' Clean	-	-	75%	73%
Timely Help 'Always' Received	-	-	69%	68%
Would Definitely Recommend Hospital	-	-	73%	71%
Use of Medical Imaging				
Cardiac Imaging Stress Test before Surgery	-	-	5.3%	5.3%
Combination Abdominal CT Scan	-	-	16.4%	10.5%
Combination Brain/Sinus CT Scan	-	-	2.7%	2.7%
Combination Chest CT Scan	-	-	5.6%	2.7%
Follow-up Mammogram/Ultrasound	-	-	7.9%	8.8%
Lumbar Spine MRI for Low Back Pain	-	-	39.6%	37.2%

Bayside Community Hospital

200 Hospital Drive
Anahuac, TX 77514
Type: Critical Access Hospitals
Ownership: Government - Local
Phone: 409-267-3143
Fax: 409-267-3608
Emergency Services: Yes
Beds: 30

Key Personnel:
Chief of Medical Staff. . . . . Leonidas Andres, MD
Emergency Room . . . . Leonidas S Andres, MD
Infection Control. . . . . Donna Bruce
Quality Assurance . . . . Donna Bruce
Radiology. . . . . Rajendrakumar Desai
Operating Room. . . . . Cathy Muscat, RN
CEO/President. . . . . Robert Pascasio

Measure	Cases	This Hosp.	State Avg.	U.S. Avg.
Blood Clot Prevention and Treatment				
Anticoagulation Overlap Therapy[5]	-	-	93%	93%
ICU Venous Thromboembolism Prophylaxis[5]	-	-	92%	92%
Incidence of Potentially Preventable VTE[5]	-	-	9%	10%
UFH with Dosages/Platelet Monitoring[5]	-	-	96%	97%
Venous Thromboembolism Prophylaxis[5]	-	-	82%	85%
Warfarin Therapy Discharge Instructions[5]	-	-	84%	75%
Chest Pain/Possible Heart Attack Care				
Aspirin Given Within 24 Hours of Arrival[5]	-	-	94%	96%
Fibrinolytic Meds Within 30 Min. of Arrival[5]	-	-	47%	58%
Average Time to ECG (minutes)[5]	-	-	8	7
Average Time to Transfer (minutes)[5]	-	-	62	60
Children's Asthma Care				
Received Home Management Plan of Care	-	-	93%	88%
Received Reliever Medication	-	-	100%	100%
Received Systemic Corticosteroids	-	-	100%	100%
Emergency Department				
Admittance Decision Time (minutes)[5]	-	-	99	98
Head CT Results Within 45 Min. of Arrival[5]	-	-	54%	57%
Patients Who Left ER Before Being Seen[5]	-	-	3%	2%
Time from ER Arrival to Admit. (minutes)[5]	-	-	270	274
Time from ER Arrival to Discharge (minutes)	264	80	127	134
Time in ER Before Being Evaluated (minutes)	296	0	26	26
Time to Pain Meds for Fractures (minutes)[5]	-	-	57	57
Heart Attack Care				
Aspirin Given at Discharge[5]	-	-	99%	99%
Fibrinolytic Meds Within 30 Min. of Arrival[5]	-	-	49%	54%
PCI Within 90 Minutes of Arrival[5]	-	-	95%	96%
Statin Prescribed at Discharge[5]	-	-	98%	98%
Heart Failure Care				
ACE Inhibitor or ARB for LVSD[3,7]	-	-	97%	97%
Discharge Instructions Given[1,3]	-	-	95%	94%
Evaluation of LVS Function[1,3]	-	-	99%	99%
Medicare Spending				
Medicare Spending per Patient (ratio)	-	-	1.03	0.98
Pneumonia Care				
Appropriate Initial Antibiotic Given[1]	-	-	95%	95%
Blood Culture Timing[1]	-	-	98%	98%
Pregnancy and Delivery Care				
Newborn Deliveries Scheduled Early[5]	-	-	7%	6%
Preventive Care				
Immunization for Influenza[5]	-	-	90%	90%
Immunization for Pneumonia[5]	-	-	92%	92%
Stroke Care				
Anticoagulation Therapy for Atrial Fibrillation[5]	-	-	96%	95%
Antithrombotic Therapy Timing[5]	-	-	98%	98%
Assessed for Rehabilitation[5]	-	-	98%	97%
Discharged on Antithrombotic Therapy[5]	-	-	99%	99%
Discharged on Statin Medication[5]	-	-	95%	94%
Thrombolytic Therapy Timing[5]	-	-	68%	66%
Venous Thromboembolism Prophylaxis[5]	-	-	94%	94%

NOTE: Hospital profiles are in alphabetical order by state, then city, then hospital within the city; Rankings exclude hospitals with less than 25 cases except for patient surveys which excludes hospitals with less than 100 cases; (a) 100-299 cases; (1) The number of cases/patients is too few to report; (2) Data submitted were based on a sample of cases/patients; (3) Results are based on a shorter time period than required; (4) Data suppressed by CMS for one or more quarters; (5) Results are not available for this reporting period; (6) Fewer than 100 patients completed the HCAHPS survey; (7) No cases met the criteria for this measure; (8) The lower limit of the confidence interval cannot be calculated if the number of observed infections equals zero; (9) No data are available from the state/territory for this reporting period; (10) The scores shown reflect fewer than 50 completed surveys; (11) There were discrepancies in the data collection process; (12) This measure does not apply to this hospital for this reporting period; (13) Results cannot be calculated for this reporting period; (14) The results for this state are combined with nearby states to protect confidentiality; Please refer to the User's Guide for a full explanation of data.

Measure	Cases	This Hosp.	State Avg.	U.S. Avg.
Written Stroke Educational Materials Given[5]	-	-	92%	88%
Surgical Care Improvement Project				
Appropriate Beta Blocker Usage[5]	-	-	98%	98%
Appropriate VTP Within 24 Hours[5]	-	-	98%	98%
Controlled Postoperative Blood Glucose[5]	-	-	96%	97%
Perioperative Temperature Management[5]	-	-	100%	100%
Prophylactic Antibiotic Selection[5]	-	-	99%	99%
Prophylactic Antibiotic Selection (Outpatient)[5]	-	-	98%	98%
Prophylactic Antibiotic Stopped[5]	-	-	98%	98%
Prophylactic Antibiotic Timing[5]	-	-	99%	99%
Prophylactic Antibiotic Timing (Outpatient)[5]	-	-	98%	98%
Urinary Catheter Removal[5]	-	-	98%	97%
Survey of Patients' Hospital Experiences				
Area Around Room 'Always' Quiet at Night[10]	<100	90%	68%	61%
Doctors 'Always' Communicated Well[10]	<100	97%	83%	82%
Home Recovery Information Given[10]	<100	83%	85%	85%
Hospital Given 9 or 10 on 10 Point Scale[10]	<100	73%	73%	71%
Meds 'Always' Explained Before Given[10]	<100	73%	66%	64%
Nurses 'Always' Communicated Well[10]	<100	89%	80%	79%
Pain 'Always' Well Controlled[10]	<100	79%	72%	71%
Room and Bathroom 'Always' Clean[10]	<100	85%	75%	73%
Timely Help 'Always' Received[10]	<100	82%	69%	68%
Would Definitely Recommend Hospital[10]	<100	75%	73%	71%
Use of Medical Imaging				
Cardiac Imaging Stress Test before Surgery[7]	-	-	5.3%	5.3%
Combination Abdominal CT Scan[1]	-	-	16.4%	10.5%
Combination Brain/Sinus CT Scan	51	0.0%	2.7%	2.7%
Combination Chest CT Scan[1]	-	-	5.6%	2.7%
Follow-up Mammogram/Ultrasound[7]	-	-	7.9%	8.8%
Lumbar Spine MRI for Low Back Pain[1]	-	-	39.6%	37.2%

Permian Regional Medical Center

720 Hospital Drive
Andrews, TX 79714
Phone: 432-523-2200
Fax: 423-464-2180
E-mail: rrichards@permianregional.com
URL: www.permianregional.com
Type: Acute Care Hospitals
Emergency Services: Yes
Ownership: Govt - Hospital Dist/Auth
Beds: 175

Key Personnel:
Pediatric Ambulatory Care . . . . . . Sylvia Cala, MD
Pediatric In-Patient Care . . . . Sylvia Cala, MD
Radiology. . . . . Ken Cox, RT, MBA
Chief of Medical Staff. . . . . Natver Jariwala, MD
Infection Control. . . . . Lynn Mock
Quality Assurance . . . . Lynn Mock
Operating Room. . . . . Doytt Redmond, RN
CEO . . . . Russell Tippin

Measure	Cases	This Hosp.	State Avg.	U.S. Avg.
Blood Clot Prevention and Treatment				
Anticoagulation Overlap Therapy[1]	-	-	93%	93%
ICU Venous Thromboembolism Prophylaxis[1]	-	-	92%	92%
Incidence of Potentially Preventable VTE[7]	-	-	9%	10%
UFH with Dosages/Platelet Monitoring[7]	-	-	96%	97%
Venous Thromboembolism Prophylaxis	166	81%	82%	85%
Warfarin Therapy Discharge Instructions[1]	-	-	84%	75%
Chest Pain/Possible Heart Attack Care				
Aspirin Given Within 24 Hours of Arrival	28	100%	94%	96%
Fibrinolytic Meds Within 30 Min. of Arrival[7]	-	-	47%	58%
Average Time to ECG (minutes)	28	8	8	7
Average Time to Transfer (minutes)[1]	-	-	62	60
Children's Asthma Care				
Received Home Management Plan of Care	-	-	93%	88%
Received Reliever Medication	-	-	100%	100%
Received Systemic Corticosteroids	-	-	100%	100%
Emergency Department				
Admittance Decision Time (minutes)[2]	83	34	99	98
Head CT Results Within 45 Min. of Arrival[1,3]	-	-	54%	57%
Patients Who Left ER Before Being Seen	8,536	3%	3%	2%
Time from ER Arrival to Admit. (minutes)[2]	138	204	270	274
Time from ER Arrival to Discharge (minutes)	358	102	127	134
Time in ER Before Being Evaluated (minutes)	361	39	26	26
Time to Pain Meds for Fractures (minutes)	29	57	57	57
Heart Attack Care				
Aspirin Given at Discharge[3,7]	-	-	99%	99%
Fibrinolytic Meds Within 30 Min. of Arrival[3,7]	-	-	49%	54%
PCI Within 90 Minutes of Arrival[3,7]	-	-	95%	96%
Statin Prescribed at Discharge[3,7]	-	-	98%	98%
Heart Failure Care				
ACE Inhibitor or ARB for LVSD[3,7]	-	-	97%	97%
Discharge Instructions Given[1,3]	-	-	95%	94%
Evaluation of LVS Function[1,3]	-	-	99%	99%
Medicare Spending				
Medicare Spending per Patient (ratio)	-	0.88	1.03	0.98
Pneumonia Care				
Appropriate Initial Antibiotic Given	40	55%	95%	95%
Blood Culture Timing	32	75%	98%	98%
Pregnancy and Delivery Care				
Newborn Deliveries Scheduled Early	58	55%	7%	6%
Preventive Care				
Immunization for Influenza[2]	174	21%	90%	90%
Immunization for Pneumonia[2]	103	46%	92%	92%
Stroke Care				
Anticoagulation Therapy for Atrial Fibrillation[3,7]	-	-	96%	95%
Antithrombotic Therapy Timing[1,3]	-	-	98%	98%
Assessed for Rehabilitation[1,3]	-	-	98%	97%
Discharged on Antithrombotic Therapy[1,3]	-	-	99%	99%
Discharged on Statin Medication[1,3]	-	-	95%	94%
Thrombolytic Therapy Timing[3,7]	-	-	68%	66%
Venous Thromboembolism Prophylaxis[1,3]	-	-	94%	94%
Written Stroke Educational Materials Given[3,7]	-	-	92%	88%
Surgical Care Improvement Project				
Appropriate Beta Blocker Usage[7]	-	-	98%	98%
Appropriate VTP Within 24 Hours[1]	-	-	98%	98%
Controlled Postoperative Blood Glucose[7]	-	-	96%	97%
Perioperative Temperature Management	19	89%	100%	100%
Prophylactic Antibiotic Selection	11	45%	99%	99%
Prophylactic Antibiotic Selection (Outpatient)	13	69%	98%	98%
Prophylactic Antibiotic Stopped	11	91%	98%	98%
Prophylactic Antibiotic Timing	12	75%	99%	99%
Prophylactic Antibiotic Timing (Outpatient)	11	73%	98%	98%
Urinary Catheter Removal[1]	-	-	98%	97%
Survey of Patients' Hospital Experiences				
Area Around Room 'Always' Quiet at Night	(a)	71%	68%	61%
Doctors 'Always' Communicated Well	(a)	80%	83%	82%
Home Recovery Information Given	(a)	75%	85%	85%
Hospital Given 9 or 10 on 10 Point Scale	(a)	62%	73%	71%
Meds 'Always' Explained Before Given	(a)	61%	66%	64%
Nurses 'Always' Communicated Well	(a)	77%	80%	79%
Pain 'Always' Well Controlled	(a)	71%	72%	71%
Room and Bathroom 'Always' Clean	(a)	71%	75%	73%
Timely Help 'Always' Received	(a)	64%	69%	68%
Would Definitely Recommend Hospital	(a)	58%	73%	71%
Use of Medical Imaging				
Cardiac Imaging Stress Test before Surgery[1]	-	-	5.3%	5.3%
Combination Abdominal CT Scan	86	18.6%	16.4%	10.5%
Combination Brain/Sinus CT Scan[1]	-	-	2.7%	2.7%
Combination Chest CT Scan[1]	-	-	5.6%	2.7%
Follow-up Mammogram/Ultrasound	251	7.6%	7.9%	8.8%
Lumbar Spine MRI for Low Back Pain[1]	-	-	39.6%	37.2%

Angleton - Danbury Medical Center

132 Hospital Dr
Angleton, TX 77515
Phone: 979-849-7721
Fax: 979-849-0581
URL: www.admc.org
Type: Acute Care Hospitals
Emergency Services: Yes
Ownership: Govt - Hospital Dist/Auth
Beds: 62

Key Personnel:
Quality Assurance . . . . Sara Allen
Chief of Medical Staff. . . . . Marcia Filipp
Pediatric In-Patient Care . . . . Hubert Lu, MD
Operating Room. . . . . James P Maguire
Infection Control. . . . . Loretta Miles
Emergency Room . . . . Sheraz Pirali, MD
Anesthesiology. . . . . Manjit Randhawa, D.O.
CEO/President. . . . . Donna K. Sollenberger, MA

Measure	Cases	This Hosp.	State Avg.	U.S. Avg.
Blood Clot Prevention and Treatment				
Anticoagulation Overlap Therapy[2]	13	85%	93%	93%
ICU Venous Thromboembolism Prophylaxis[2]	36	94%	92%	92%
Incidence of Potentially Preventable VTE[1,2]	-	-	9%	10%
UFH with Dosages/Platelet Monitoring[1,2]	-	-	96%	97%
Venous Thromboembolism Prophylaxis[2]	111	91%	82%	85%
Warfarin Therapy Discharge Instructions[1,2]	-	-	84%	75%
Chest Pain/Possible Heart Attack Care				
Aspirin Given Within 24 Hours of Arrival	67	97%	94%	96%
Fibrinolytic Meds Within 30 Min. of Arrival[1]	-	-	47%	58%
Average Time to ECG (minutes)	76	8	8	7
Average Time to Transfer (minutes)	12	273	62	60
Children's Asthma Care				
Received Home Management Plan of Care	-	-	93%	88%
Received Reliever Medication	-	-	100%	100%
Received Systemic Corticosteroids	-	-	100%	100%
Emergency Department				
Admittance Decision Time (minutes)[2]	230	116	99	98
Head CT Results Within 45 Min. of Arrival[1]	-	-	54%	57%
Patients Who Left ER Before Being Seen	17,591	5%	3%	2%
Time from ER Arrival to Admit. (minutes)[2]	231	354	270	274
Time from ER Arrival to Discharge (minutes)	358	182	127	134
Time in ER Before Being Evaluated (minutes)	404	56	26	26
Time to Pain Meds for Fractures (minutes)	80	72	57	57
Heart Attack Care				
Aspirin Given at Discharge[1,3]	-	-	99%	99%
Fibrinolytic Meds Within 30 Min. of Arrival[3,7]	-	-	49%	54%
PCI Within 90 Minutes of Arrival[3,7]	-	-	95%	96%
Statin Prescribed at Discharge[1,3]	-	-	98%	98%
Heart Failure Care				
ACE Inhibitor or ARB for LVSD	21	95%	97%	97%
Discharge Instructions Given	57	82%	95%	94%
Evaluation of LVS Function	64	95%	99%	99%
Medicare Spending				
Medicare Spending per Patient (ratio)	-	1.03	1.03	0.98
Pneumonia Care				
Appropriate Initial Antibiotic Given	31	94%	95%	95%
Blood Culture Timing	37	89%	98%	98%
Pregnancy and Delivery Care				
Newborn Deliveries Scheduled Early	54	19%	7%	6%
Preventive Care				
Immunization for Influenza[2]	251	94%	90%	90%
Immunization for Pneumonia[2]	250	89%	92%	92%
Stroke Care				
Anticoagulation Therapy for Atrial Fibrillation[1,3]	-	-	96%	95%
Antithrombotic Therapy Timing[1,3]	-	-	98%	98%
Assessed for Rehabilitation[1,3]	-	-	98%	97%
Discharged on Antithrombotic Therapy[1,3]	-	-	99%	99%
Discharged on Statin Medication[1,3]	-	-	95%	94%
Thrombolytic Therapy Timing[3,7]	-	-	68%	66%
Venous Thromboembolism Prophylaxis[1,3]	-	-	94%	94%
Written Stroke Educational Materials Given[1,3]	-	-	92%	88%
Surgical Care Improvement Project				
Appropriate Beta Blocker Usage[2]	44	98%	98%	98%
Appropriate VTP Within 24 Hours[2]	156	97%	98%	98%
Controlled Postoperative Blood Glucose[2,7]	-	-	96%	97%
Perioperative Temperature Management[2]	174	100%	100%	100%
Prophylactic Antibiotic Selection[2]	140	97%	99%	99%
Prophylactic Antibiotic Selection (Outpatient)	11	91%	98%	98%
Prophylactic Antibiotic Stopped[2]	140	93%	98%	98%
Prophylactic Antibiotic Timing[2]	140	97%	99%	99%
Prophylactic Antibiotic Timing (Outpatient)	11	100%	98%	98%
Urinary Catheter Removal[2]	17	59%	98%	97%
Survey of Patients' Hospital Experiences				
Area Around Room 'Always' Quiet at Night	300+	65%	68%	61%
Doctors 'Always' Communicated Well	300+	80%	83%	82%
Home Recovery Information Given	300+	86%	85%	85%
Hospital Given 9 or 10 on 10 Point Scale	300+	69%	73%	71%
Meds 'Always' Explained Before Given	300+	66%	66%	64%
Nurses 'Always' Communicated Well	300+	78%	80%	79%
Pain 'Always' Well Controlled	300+	72%	72%	71%
Room and Bathroom 'Always' Clean	300+	76%	75%	73%
Timely Help 'Always' Received	300+	70%	69%	68%
Would Definitely Recommend Hospital	300+	69%	73%	71%

NOTE: Hospital profiles are in alphabetical order by state, then city, then hospital within the city; Rankings exclude hospitals with less than 25 cases except for patient surveys which excludes hospitals with less than 100 cases; (a) 100-299 cases; (1) The number of cases/patients is too few to report; (2) Data submitted were based on a sample of cases/patients; (3) Results are based on a shorter time period than required; (4) Data suppressed by CMS for one or more quarters; (5) Results are not available for this reporting period; (6) Fewer than 100 patients completed the HCAHPS survey; (7) No cases met the criteria for this measure; (8) The lower limit of the confidence interval cannot be calculated if the number of observed infections equals zero; (9) No data are available from the state/territory for this reporting period; (10) The scores shown reflect fewer than 50 completed surveys; (11) There were discrepancies in the data collection process; (12) This measure does not apply to this hospital for this reporting period; (13) Results cannot be calculated for this reporting period; (14) The results for this state are combined with nearby states to protect confidentiality; Please refer to the User's Guide for a full explanation of data.

Use of Medical Imaging				
Cardiac Imaging Stress Test before Surgery[1]	-	-	5.3%	5.3%
Combination Abdominal CT Scan	171	32.7%	16.4%	10.5%
Combination Brain/Sinus CT Scan[1]	-	-	2.7%	2.7%
Combination Chest CT Scan	105	6.7%	5.6%	2.7%
Follow-up Mammogram/Ultrasound	298	9.4%	7.9%	8.8%
Lumbar Spine MRI for Low Back Pain[1]	-	-	39.6%	37.2%

Anson General Hospital

101 Avenue J
Anson, TX 79501
Phone: 325-823-3231
Fax: 325-823-3098
Type: Acute Care Hospitals
Emergency Services: Yes
Ownership: Voluntary non-profit - Other
Beds: 45

Key Personnel:
Chair/CEO . . . . Yves Carrière
CEO . . . . Paul Chatelain
Chief of Medical Staff . . . . Stephen Chiang, MD
Infection Control . . . . Margaret Gates
Quality Assurance . . . . Margaret Gates, RN
Operating Room . . . . Sheila A Layne, RN
CEO/President . . . . Ted D Matthews
Emergency Room . . . . Sal Torres, MD

Measure	Cases	This Hosp.	State Avg.	U.S. Avg.
Blood Clot Prevention and Treatment				
Anticoagulation Overlap Therapy[1]	-	-	93%	93%
ICU Venous Thromboembolism Prophylaxis[7]	-	-	92%	92%
Incidence of Potentially Preventable VTE[7]	-	-	9%	10%
UFH with Dosages/Platelet Monitoring[7]	-	-	96%	97%
Venous Thromboembolism Prophylaxis	185	78%	82%	85%
Warfarin Therapy Discharge Instructions[1]	-	-	84%	75%
Chest Pain/Possible Heart Attack Care				
Aspirin Given Within 24 Hours of Arrival[5]	-	-	94%	96%
Fibrinolytic Meds Within 30 Min. of Arrival[5]	-	-	47%	58%
Average Time to ECG (minutes)[5]	-	-	8	7
Average Time to Transfer (minutes)[5]	-	-	62	60
Children's Asthma Care				
Received Home Management Plan of Care	-	-	93%	88%
Received Reliever Medication	-	-	100%	100%
Received Systemic Corticosteroids	-	-	100%	100%
Emergency Department				
Admittance Decision Time (minutes)	49	22	99	98
Head CT Results Within 45 Min. of Arrival[5]	-	-	54%	57%
Patients Who Left ER Before Being Seen	2,711	0%	3%	2%
Time from ER Arrival to Admit. (minutes)	61	130	270	274
Time from ER Arrival to Discharge (minutes)	348	60	127	134
Time in ER Before Being Evaluated (minutes)	312	19	26	26
Time to Pain Meds for Fractures (minutes)[1,3]	-	-	57	57
Heart Attack Care				
Aspirin Given at Discharge[5]	-	-	99%	99%
Fibrinolytic Meds Within 30 Min. of Arrival[5]	-	-	49%	54%
PCI Within 90 Minutes of Arrival[5]	-	-	95%	96%
Statin Prescribed at Discharge[5]	-	-	98%	98%
Heart Failure Care				
ACE Inhibitor or ARB for LVSD[5]	-	-	97%	97%
Discharge Instructions Given[5]	-	-	95%	94%
Evaluation of LVS Function[5]	-	-	99%	99%
Medicare Spending				
Medicare Spending per Patient (ratio)	-	0.81	1.03	0.98
Pneumonia Care				
Appropriate Initial Antibiotic Given[5]	-	-	95%	95%
Blood Culture Timing[5]	-	-	98%	98%
Pregnancy and Delivery Care				
Newborn Deliveries Scheduled Early[7]	-	-	7%	6%
Preventive Care				
Immunization for Influenza	148	70%	90%	90%
Immunization for Pneumonia	212	62%	92%	92%
Stroke Care				
Anticoagulation Therapy for Atrial Fibrillation[5]	-	-	96%	95%
Antithrombotic Therapy Timing[5]	-	-	98%	98%
Assessed for Rehabilitation[5]	-	-	98%	97%
Discharged on Antithrombotic Therapy[5]	-	-	99%	99%
Discharged on Statin Medication[5]	-	-	95%	94%
Thrombolytic Therapy Timing[5]	-	-	68%	66%
Venous Thromboembolism Prophylaxis[5]	-	-	94%	94%
Written Stroke Educational Materials Given[5]	-	-	92%	88%
Surgical Care Improvement Project				
Appropriate Beta Blocker Usage[5]	-	-	98%	98%
Appropriate VTP Within 24 Hours[5]	-	-	98%	98%
Controlled Postoperative Blood Glucose[5]	-	-	96%	97%
Perioperative Temperature Management[5]	-	-	100%	100%
Prophylactic Antibiotic Selection[5]	-	-	99%	99%
Prophylactic Antibiotic Selection (Outpatient)[5]	-	-	98%	98%
Prophylactic Antibiotic Stopped[5]	-	-	98%	98%
Prophylactic Antibiotic Timing[5]	-	-	99%	99%
Prophylactic Antibiotic Timing (Outpatient)[5]	-	-	98%	98%
Urinary Catheter Removal[5]	-	-	98%	97%
Survey of Patients' Hospital Experiences				
Area Around Room 'Always' Quiet at Night[6]	<100	75%	68%	61%
Doctors 'Always' Communicated Well[6]	<100	91%	83%	82%
Home Recovery Information Given[6]	<100	86%	85%	85%
Hospital Given 9 or 10 on 10 Point Scale[6]	<100	82%	73%	71%
Meds 'Always' Explained Before Given[6]	<100	82%	66%	64%
Nurses 'Always' Communicated Well[6]	<100	86%	80%	79%
Pain 'Always' Well Controlled[6]	<100	85%	72%	71%
Room and Bathroom 'Always' Clean[6]	<100	89%	75%	73%
Timely Help 'Always' Received[6]	<100	84%	69%	68%
Would Definitely Recommend Hospital[6]	<100	81%	73%	71%
Use of Medical Imaging				
Cardiac Imaging Stress Test before Surgery[7]	-	-	5.3%	5.3%
Combination Abdominal CT Scan[1]	-	-	16.4%	10.5%
Combination Brain/Sinus CT Scan[1]	-	-	2.7%	2.7%
Combination Chest CT Scan[1]	-	-	5.6%	2.7%
Follow-up Mammogram/Ultrasound[7]	-	-	7.9%	8.8%
Lumbar Spine MRI for Low Back Pain[1]	-	-	39.6%	37.2%

Care Regional Medical Center

1711 W Wheeler Avenue
Aransas Pass, TX 78336
Phone: 361-758-8585
Fax: 361-758-3476
URL: www.nbhtx.com
Type: Acute Care Hospitals
Emergency Services: Yes
Ownership: Proprietary
Beds: 75

Key Personnel:
CEO/President . . . . Christopher W Dux

Measure	Cases	This Hosp.	State Avg.	U.S. Avg.
Blood Clot Prevention and Treatment				
Anticoagulation Overlap Therapy[2]	11	73%	93%	93%
ICU Venous Thromboembolism Prophylaxis[2]	93	78%	92%	92%
Incidence of Potentially Preventable VTE[1,2]	-	-	9%	10%
UFH with Dosages/Platelet Monitoring[2,7]	-	-	96%	97%
Venous Thromboembolism Prophylaxis[2]	70	64%	82%	85%
Warfarin Therapy Discharge Instructions[1,2]	-	-	84%	75%
Chest Pain/Possible Heart Attack Care				
Aspirin Given Within 24 Hours of Arrival	29	100%	94%	96%
Fibrinolytic Meds Within 30 Min. of Arrival[1,3]	-	-	47%	58%
Average Time to ECG (minutes)	29	14	8	7
Average Time to Transfer (minutes)[1,3]	-	-	62	60
Children's Asthma Care				
Received Home Management Plan of Care	-	-	93%	88%
Received Reliever Medication	-	-	100%	100%
Received Systemic Corticosteroids	-	-	100%	100%
Emergency Department				
Admittance Decision Time (minutes)[2]	408	90	99	98
Head CT Results Within 45 Min. of Arrival[1]	-	-	54%	57%
Patients Who Left ER Before Being Seen	10,699	9%	3%	2%
Time from ER Arrival to Admit. (minutes)[2]	422	365	270	274
Time from ER Arrival to Discharge (minutes)	488	157	127	134
Time in ER Before Being Evaluated (minutes)	628	0	26	26
Time to Pain Meds for Fractures (minutes)	58	75	57	57
Heart Attack Care				
Aspirin Given at Discharge[1]	-	-	99%	99%
Fibrinolytic Meds Within 30 Min. of Arrival[7]	-	-	49%	54%
PCI Within 90 Minutes of Arrival[7]	-	-	95%	96%
Statin Prescribed at Discharge[1]	-	-	98%	98%
Heart Failure Care				
ACE Inhibitor or ARB for LVSD[2]	18	94%	97%	97%
Discharge Instructions Given[2]	44	86%	95%	94%
Evaluation of LVS Function[2]	54	94%	99%	99%
Medicare Spending				
Medicare Spending per Patient (ratio)	-	1.05	1.03	0.98
Pneumonia Care				
Appropriate Initial Antibiotic Given[2]	30	70%	95%	95%
Blood Culture Timing[2]	70	80%	98%	98%
Pregnancy and Delivery Care				
Newborn Deliveries Scheduled Early[7]	-	-	7%	6%
Preventive Care				
Immunization for Influenza[2]	306	59%	90%	90%
Immunization for Pneumonia[2]	489	72%	92%	92%
Stroke Care				
Anticoagulation Therapy for Atrial Fibrillation[5]	-	-	96%	95%
Antithrombotic Therapy Timing[5]	-	-	98%	98%
Assessed for Rehabilitation[5]	-	-	98%	97%
Discharged on Antithrombotic Therapy[5]	-	-	99%	99%
Discharged on Statin Medication[5]	-	-	95%	94%
Thrombolytic Therapy Timing[5]	-	-	68%	66%
Venous Thromboembolism Prophylaxis[5]	-	-	94%	94%
Written Stroke Educational Materials Given[5]	-	-	92%	88%
Surgical Care Improvement Project				
Appropriate Beta Blocker Usage[1]	-	-	98%	98%
Appropriate VTP Within 24 Hours	16	38%	98%	98%
Controlled Postoperative Blood Glucose[7]	-	-	96%	97%
Perioperative Temperature Management	19	95%	100%	100%
Prophylactic Antibiotic Selection[1]	-	-	99%	99%
Prophylactic Antibiotic Selection (Outpatient)[5]	-	-	98%	98%
Prophylactic Antibiotic Stopped[1]	-	-	98%	98%
Prophylactic Antibiotic Timing[1]	-	-	99%	99%
Prophylactic Antibiotic Timing (Outpatient)[5]	-	-	98%	98%
Urinary Catheter Removal	13	62%	98%	97%
Survey of Patients' Hospital Experiences				
Area Around Room 'Always' Quiet at Night	(a)	71%	68%	61%
Doctors 'Always' Communicated Well	(a)	81%	83%	82%
Home Recovery Information Given	(a)	85%	85%	85%
Hospital Given 9 or 10 on 10 Point Scale	(a)	64%	73%	71%
Meds 'Always' Explained Before Given	(a)	68%	66%	64%
Nurses 'Always' Communicated Well	(a)	78%	80%	79%
Pain 'Always' Well Controlled	(a)	71%	72%	71%
Room and Bathroom 'Always' Clean	(a)	67%	75%	73%
Timely Help 'Always' Received	(a)	67%	69%	68%
Would Definitely Recommend Hospital	(a)	65%	73%	71%
Use of Medical Imaging				
Cardiac Imaging Stress Test before Surgery[1]	-	-	5.3%	5.3%
Combination Abdominal CT Scan	181	55.8%	16.4%	10.5%
Combination Brain/Sinus CT Scan[1]	-	-	2.7%	2.7%
Combination Chest CT Scan	123	5.7%	5.6%	2.7%
Follow-up Mammogram/Ultrasound	162	10.5%	7.9%	8.8%
Lumbar Spine MRI for Low Back Pain[1]	-	-	39.6%	37.2%

Baylor Orthopedic & Spine Hospital at Arlington

707 Highlander Blvd
Arlington, TX 76015
Phone: 817-549-2364
URL: www.baylorarlington.com
Type: Acute Care Hospitals
Emergency Services: Yes
Ownership: Proprietary

Key Personnel:
CEO . . . . Allen Beck
Radiology . . . . Charlene Kirby

Measure	Cases	This Hosp.	State Avg.	U.S. Avg.
Blood Clot Prevention and Treatment				
Anticoagulation Overlap Therapy[2,7]	-	-	93%	93%
ICU Venous Thromboembolism Prophylaxis[2,7]	-	-	92%	92%
Incidence of Potentially Preventable VTE[2,7]	-	-	9%	10%
UFH with Dosages/Platelet Monitoring[2,7]	-	-	96%	97%
Venous Thromboembolism Prophylaxis[2]	36	97%	82%	85%
Warfarin Therapy Discharge Instructions[2,7]	-	-	84%	75%
Chest Pain/Possible Heart Attack Care				
Aspirin Given Within 24 Hours of Arrival[5]	-	-	94%	96%
Fibrinolytic Meds Within 30 Min. of Arrival[5]	-	-	47%	58%
Average Time to ECG (minutes)[5]	-	-	8	7
Average Time to Transfer (minutes)[5]	-	-	62	60
Children's Asthma Care				
Received Home Management Plan of Care	-	-	93%	88%

NOTE: Hospital profiles are in alphabetical order by state, then city, then hospital within the city; Rankings exclude hospitals with less than 25 cases except for patient surveys which excludes hospitals with less than 100 cases; (a) 100-299 cases; (1) The number of cases/patients is too few to report; (2) Data submitted were based on a sample of cases/patients; (3) Results are based on a shorter time period than required; (4) Data suppressed by CMS for one or more quarters; (5) Results are not available for this reporting period; (6) Fewer than 100 patients completed the HCAHPS survey; (7) No cases met the criteria for this measure; (8) The lower limit of the confidence interval cannot be calculated if the number of observed infections equals zero; (9) No data are available from the state/territory for this reporting period; (10) The scores shown reflect fewer than 50 completed surveys; (11) There were discrepancies in the data collection process; (12) This measure does not apply to this hospital for this reporting period; (13) Results cannot be calculated for this reporting period; (14) The results for this state are combined with nearby states to protect confidentiality; Please refer to the User's Guide for a full explanation of data.

Measure	Cases	This Hosp.	State Avg.	U.S. Avg.
Received Reliever Medication	-	-	100%	100%
Received Systemic Corticosteroids	-	-	100%	100%
Emergency Department				
Admittance Decision Time (minutes)[1,2]	-	-	99	98
Head CT Results Within 45 Min. of Arrival[5]	-	-	54%	57%
Patients Who Left ER Before Being Seen	953	2%	3%	2%
Time from ER Arrival to Admit. (minutes)[1,2]	-	-	270	274
Time from ER Arrival to Discharge (minutes)	272	82	127	134
Time in ER Before Being Evaluated (minutes)	271	8	26	26
Time to Pain Meds for Fractures (minutes)[1]	-	-	57	57
Heart Attack Care				
Aspirin Given at Discharge[5]	-	-	99%	99%
Fibrinolytic Meds Within 30 Min. of Arrival[5]	-	-	49%	54%
PCI Within 90 Minutes of Arrival[5]	-	-	95%	96%
Statin Prescribed at Discharge[5]	-	-	98%	98%
Heart Failure Care				
ACE Inhibitor or ARB for LVSD[5]	-	-	97%	97%
Discharge Instructions Given[5]	-	-	95%	94%
Evaluation of LVS Function[5]	-	-	99%	99%
Medicare Spending				
Medicare Spending per Patient (ratio)	-	1.09	1.03	0.98
Pneumonia Care				
Appropriate Initial Antibiotic Given[5]	-	-	95%	95%
Blood Culture Timing[5]	-	-	98%	98%
Pregnancy and Delivery Care				
Newborn Deliveries Scheduled Early[7]	-	-	7%	6%
Preventive Care				
Immunization for Influenza[2]	331	96%	90%	90%
Immunization for Pneumonia[2]	383	93%	92%	92%
Stroke Care				
Anticoagulation Therapy for Atrial Fibrillation[5]	-	-	96%	95%
Antithrombotic Therapy Timing[5]	-	-	98%	98%
Assessed for Rehabilitation[5]	-	-	98%	97%
Discharged on Antithrombotic Therapy[5]	-	-	99%	99%
Discharged on Statin Medication[5]	-	-	95%	94%
Thrombolytic Therapy Timing[5]	-	-	68%	66%
Venous Thromboembolism Prophylaxis[5]	-	-	94%	94%
Written Stroke Educational Materials Given[5]	-	-	92%	88%
Surgical Care Improvement Project				
Appropriate Beta Blocker Usage	165	99%	98%	98%
Appropriate VTP Within 24 Hours	742	99%	98%	98%
Controlled Postoperative Blood Glucose[7]	-	-	96%	97%
Perioperative Temperature Management	750	100%	100%	100%
Prophylactic Antibiotic Selection	677	100%	99%	99%
Prophylactic Antibiotic Selection (Outpatient)	149	99%	98%	98%
Prophylactic Antibiotic Stopped	677	99%	98%	98%
Prophylactic Antibiotic Timing	677	99%	99%	99%
Prophylactic Antibiotic Timing (Outpatient)	149	100%	98%	98%
Urinary Catheter Removal	348	99%	98%	97%
Survey of Patients' Hospital Experiences				
Area Around Room 'Always' Quiet at Night	300+	82%	68%	61%
Doctors 'Always' Communicated Well	300+	89%	83%	82%
Home Recovery Information Given	300+	92%	85%	85%
Hospital Given 9 or 10 on 10 Point Scale	300+	88%	73%	71%
Meds 'Always' Explained Before Given	300+	73%	66%	64%
Nurses 'Always' Communicated Well	300+	88%	80%	79%
Pain 'Always' Well Controlled	300+	80%	72%	71%
Room and Bathroom 'Always' Clean	300+	86%	75%	73%
Timely Help 'Always' Received	300+	83%	69%	68%
Would Definitely Recommend Hospital	300+	90%	73%	71%
Use of Medical Imaging				
Cardiac Imaging Stress Test before Surgery[7]	-	-	5.3%	5.3%
Combination Abdominal CT Scan[1]	-	-	16.4%	10.5%
Combination Brain/Sinus CT Scan[1]	-	-	2.7%	2.7%
Combination Chest CT Scan[1]	-	-	5.6%	2.7%
Follow-up Mammogram/Ultrasound[7]	-	-	7.9%	8.8%
Lumbar Spine MRI for Low Back Pain[1]	-	-	39.6%	37.2%

Medical Center of Arlington

3301 Matlock Road
Arlington, TX 76015
Phone: 817-465-3241
Fax: 817-472-4878
URL: www.medicalcenterarlington.com
Type: Acute Care Hospitals
Emergency Services: Yes
Ownership: Proprietary
Beds: 298

Key Personnel:

Patient Relations . . . . Kay Adams
CEO/President. . . . . Patrick D Brilliant
Emergency Room . . . . Bill Crawley, RN
Radiology. . . . . Terry Doyle
Infection Control. . . . . Carol Hill, RN
Intensive Care Unit. . . . . Kathy Srokosz, RN
Quality Assurance . . . . Emelda Valcarcel
Chief of Medical Staff. . . . . Richard Wray, MD

Measure	Cases	This Hosp.	State Avg.	U.S. Avg.
Blood Clot Prevention and Treatment				
Anticoagulation Overlap Therapy[2]	75	96%	93%	93%
ICU Venous Thromboembolism Prophylaxis[2]	89	97%	92%	92%
Incidence of Potentially Preventable VTE[2]	27	7%	9%	10%
UFH with Dosages/Platelet Monitoring[2]	14	100%	96%	97%
Venous Thromboembolism Prophylaxis[2]	433	84%	82%	85%
Warfarin Therapy Discharge Instructions[2]	60	97%	84%	75%
Chest Pain/Possible Heart Attack Care				
Aspirin Given Within 24 Hours of Arrival[1,3]	-	-	94%	96%
Fibrinolytic Meds Within 30 Min. of Arrival[5]	-	-	47%	58%
Average Time to ECG (minutes)[1,3]	-	-	8	7
Average Time to Transfer (minutes)[5]	-	-	62	60
Children's Asthma Care				
Received Home Management Plan of Care	-	-	93%	88%
Received Reliever Medication	-	-	100%	100%
Received Systemic Corticosteroids	-	-	100%	100%
Emergency Department				
Admittance Decision Time (minutes)[2]	724	158	99	98
Head CT Results Within 45 Min. of Arrival	17	82%	54%	57%
Patients Who Left ER Before Being Seen	69,263	2%	3%	2%
Time from ER Arrival to Admit. (minutes)[2]	727	292	270	274
Time from ER Arrival to Discharge (minutes)	490	130	127	134
Time in ER Before Being Evaluated (minutes)	520	15	26	26
Time to Pain Meds for Fractures (minutes)	237	35	57	57
Heart Attack Care				
Aspirin Given at Discharge	210	100%	99%	99%
Fibrinolytic Meds Within 30 Min. of Arrival[7]	-	-	49%	54%
PCI Within 90 Minutes of Arrival	31	100%	95%	96%
Statin Prescribed at Discharge	202	100%	98%	98%
Heart Failure Care				
ACE Inhibitor or ARB for LVSD	95	100%	97%	97%
Discharge Instructions Given	282	100%	95%	94%
Evaluation of LVS Function	357	100%	99%	99%
Medicare Spending				
Medicare Spending per Patient (ratio)	-	1.08	1.03	0.98
Pneumonia Care				
Appropriate Initial Antibiotic Given[2]	75	100%	95%	95%
Blood Culture Timing[2]	136	100%	98%	98%
Pregnancy and Delivery Care				
Newborn Deliveries Scheduled Early[2]	82	7%	7%	6%
Preventive Care				
Immunization for Influenza[2]	531	95%	90%	90%
Immunization for Pneumonia[2]	511	93%	92%	92%
Stroke Care				
Anticoagulation Therapy for Atrial Fibrillation[2]	12	100%	96%	95%
Antithrombotic Therapy Timing[2]	102	100%	98%	98%
Assessed for Rehabilitation[2]	119	99%	98%	97%
Discharged on Antithrombotic Therapy[2]	110	100%	99%	99%
Discharged on Statin Medication[2]	88	99%	95%	94%
Thrombolytic Therapy Timing[2]	12	100%	68%	66%
Venous Thromboembolism Prophylaxis[2]	129	100%	94%	94%
Written Stroke Educational Materials Given[2]	58	97%	92%	88%
Surgical Care Improvement Project				
Appropriate Beta Blocker Usage[2]	114	100%	98%	98%
Appropriate VTP Within 24 Hours[2]	268	99%	98%	98%
Controlled Postoperative Blood Glucose[2]	61	100%	96%	97%
Perioperative Temperature Management[2]	378	100%	100%	100%
Prophylactic Antibiotic Selection[2]	208	100%	99%	99%
Prophylactic Antibiotic Selection (Outpatient)	322	100%	98%	98%
Prophylactic Antibiotic Stopped[2]	194	98%	98%	98%
Prophylactic Antibiotic Timing[2]	208	100%	99%	99%
Prophylactic Antibiotic Timing (Outpatient)	322	100%	98%	98%
Urinary Catheter Removal[2]	176	99%	98%	97%
Survey of Patients' Hospital Experiences				
Area Around Room 'Always' Quiet at Night	300+	61%	68%	61%
Doctors 'Always' Communicated Well	300+	77%	83%	82%
Home Recovery Information Given	300+	83%	85%	85%
Hospital Given 9 or 10 on 10 Point Scale	300+	67%	73%	71%
Meds 'Always' Explained Before Given	300+	59%	66%	64%
Nurses 'Always' Communicated Well	300+	75%	80%	79%
Pain 'Always' Well Controlled	300+	70%	72%	71%
Room and Bathroom 'Always' Clean	300+	67%	75%	73%
Timely Help 'Always' Received	300+	58%	69%	68%
Would Definitely Recommend Hospital	300+	66%	73%	71%
Use of Medical Imaging				
Cardiac Imaging Stress Test before Surgery	106	1.9%	5.3%	5.3%
Combination Abdominal CT Scan	394	1.3%	16.4%	10.5%
Combination Brain/Sinus CT Scan[1]	-	-	2.7%	2.7%
Combination Chest CT Scan	47	0.0%	5.6%	2.7%
Follow-up Mammogram/Ultrasound[1]	-	-	7.9%	8.8%
Lumbar Spine MRI for Low Back Pain[1]	-	-	39.6%	37.2%

Texas Health Arlington Memorial Hospital

800 W Randol Mill Rd
Arlington, TX 76012
Phone: 817-548-6100
URL: www.texashealth.org
Type: Acute Care Hospitals
Emergency Services: Yes
Ownership: Voluntary non-profit - Private
Beds: 417

Key Personnel:

CEO/President. . . . . Douglas D. Hawthorne

Measure	Cases	This Hosp.	State Avg.	U.S. Avg.
Blood Clot Prevention and Treatment				
Anticoagulation Overlap Therapy[2]	106	95%	93%	93%
ICU Venous Thromboembolism Prophylaxis[2]	85	98%	92%	92%
Incidence of Potentially Preventable VTE[2]	13	15%	9%	10%
UFH with Dosages/Platelet Monitoring[2]	22	95%	96%	97%
Venous Thromboembolism Prophylaxis[2]	443	87%	82%	85%
Warfarin Therapy Discharge Instructions[2]	83	89%	84%	75%
Chest Pain/Possible Heart Attack Care				
Aspirin Given Within 24 Hours of Arrival	315	93%	94%	96%
Fibrinolytic Meds Within 30 Min. of Arrival[7]	-	-	47%	58%
Average Time to ECG (minutes)	334	10	8	7
Average Time to Transfer (minutes)	49	48	62	60
Children's Asthma Care				
Received Home Management Plan of Care	-	-	93%	88%
Received Reliever Medication	-	-	100%	100%
Received Systemic Corticosteroids	-	-	100%	100%
Emergency Department				
Admittance Decision Time (minutes)[2]	693	85	99	98
Head CT Results Within 45 Min. of Arrival[1]	-	-	54%	57%
Patients Who Left ER Before Being Seen	75,924	5%	3%	2%
Time from ER Arrival to Admit. (minutes)[2]	693	284	270	274
Time from ER Arrival to Discharge (minutes)	415	181	127	134
Time in ER Before Being Evaluated (minutes)	444	52	26	26
Time to Pain Meds for Fractures (minutes)	194	77	57	57
Heart Attack Care				
Aspirin Given at Discharge	24	100%	99%	99%
Fibrinolytic Meds Within 30 Min. of Arrival[7]	-	-	49%	54%
PCI Within 90 Minutes of Arrival[7]	-	-	95%	96%
Statin Prescribed at Discharge	25	100%	98%	98%
Heart Failure Care				
ACE Inhibitor or ARB for LVSD	57	100%	97%	97%
Discharge Instructions Given	192	98%	95%	94%
Evaluation of LVS Function	260	100%	99%	99%
Medicare Spending				
Medicare Spending per Patient (ratio)	-	1.13	1.03	0.98
Pneumonia Care				
Appropriate Initial Antibiotic Given	270	100%	95%	95%
Blood Culture Timing	407	100%	98%	98%
Pregnancy and Delivery Care				
Newborn Deliveries Scheduled Early	214	2%	7%	6%

NOTE: Hospital profiles are in alphabetical order by state, then city, then hospital within the city; Rankings exclude hospitals with less than 25 cases except for patient surveys which excludes hospitals with less than 100 cases; (a) 100-299 cases; (1) The number of cases/patients is too few to report; (2) Data submitted were based on a sample of cases/patients; (3) Results are based on a shorter time period than required; (4) Data suppressed by CMS for one or more quarters; (5) Results are not available for this reporting period; (6) Fewer than 100 patients completed the HCAHPS survey; (7) No cases met the criteria for this measure; (8) The lower limit of the confidence interval cannot be calculated if the number of observed infections equals zero; (9) No data are available from the state/territory for this reporting period; (10) The scores shown reflect fewer than 50 completed surveys; (11) There were discrepancies in the data collection process; (12) This measure does not apply to this hospital for this reporting period; (13) Results cannot be calculated for this reporting period; (14) The results for this state are combined with nearby states to protect confidentiality; Please refer to the User's Guide for a full explanation of data.

Preventive Care				
Immunization for Influenza[2]	585	99%	90%	90%
Immunization for Pneumonia[2]	723	96%	92%	92%
Stroke Care				
Anticoagulation Therapy for Atrial Fibrillation[2]	12	100%	96%	95%
Antithrombotic Therapy Timing[2]	112	99%	98%	98%
Assessed for Rehabilitation[2]	134	99%	98%	97%
Discharged on Antithrombotic Therapy[2]	115	100%	99%	99%
Discharged on Statin Medication[2]	88	100%	95%	94%
Thrombolytic Therapy Timing[1,2]	-	-	68%	66%
Venous Thromboembolism Prophylaxis[2]	118	97%	94%	94%
Written Stroke Educational Materials Given[2]	82	94%	92%	88%
Surgical Care Improvement Project				
Appropriate Beta Blocker Usage[2]	110	100%	98%	98%
Appropriate VTP Within 24 Hours[2]	305	99%	98%	98%
Controlled Postoperative Blood Glucose[2,7]	-	-	96%	97%
Perioperative Temperature Management[2]	406	100%	100%	100%
Prophylactic Antibiotic Selection[2]	232	100%	99%	99%
Prophylactic Antibiotic Selection (Outpatient)	218	97%	98%	98%
Prophylactic Antibiotic Stopped[2]	218	99%	98%	98%
Prophylactic Antibiotic Timing[2]	232	100%	99%	99%
Prophylactic Antibiotic Timing (Outpatient)	220	97%	98%	98%
Urinary Catheter Removal[2]	213	99%	98%	97%
Survey of Patients' Hospital Experiences				
Area Around Room 'Always' Quiet at Night	300+	63%	68%	61%
Doctors 'Always' Communicated Well	300+	77%	83%	82%
Home Recovery Information Given	300+	84%	85%	85%
Hospital Given 9 or 10 on 10 Point Scale	300+	70%	73%	71%
Meds 'Always' Explained Before Given	300+	61%	66%	64%
Nurses 'Always' Communicated Well	300+	76%	80%	79%
Pain 'Always' Well Controlled	300+	71%	72%	71%
Room and Bathroom 'Always' Clean	300+	76%	75%	73%
Timely Help 'Always' Received	300+	66%	69%	68%
Would Definitely Recommend Hospital	300+	73%	73%	71%
Use of Medical Imaging				
Cardiac Imaging Stress Test before Surgery	139	8.6%	5.3%	5.3%
Combination Abdominal CT Scan	595	3.7%	16.4%	10.5%
Combination Brain/Sinus CT Scan	878	2.1%	2.7%	2.7%
Combination Chest CT Scan	126	5.6%	5.6%	2.7%
Follow-up Mammogram/Ultrasound	1,321	6.1%	7.9%	8.8%
Lumbar Spine MRI for Low Back Pain	55	40.0%	39.6%	37.2%

Texas Health Heart & Vascular Hospital Arlington

811 Wright Street Phone: 817-960-3500
Arlington, TX 76012
Type: Acute Care Hospitals Emergency Services: No
Ownership: Proprietary

Measure	Cases	This Hosp.	State Avg.	U.S. Avg.
Blood Clot Prevention and Treatment				
Anticoagulation Overlap Therapy[1,2]	-	-	93%	93%
ICU Venous Thromboembolism Prophylaxis[2]	86	98%	92%	92%
Incidence of Potentially Preventable VTE[1,2]	-	-	9%	10%
UFH with Dosages/Platelet Monitoring[1,2]	-	-	96%	97%
Venous Thromboembolism Prophylaxis[2]	71	90%	82%	85%
Warfarin Therapy Discharge Instructions[1,2]	-	-	84%	75%
Chest Pain/Possible Heart Attack Care				
Aspirin Given Within 24 Hours of Arrival[5]	-	-	94%	96%
Fibrinolytic Meds Within 30 Min. of Arrival[5]	-	-	47%	58%
Average Time to ECG (minutes)[5]	-	-	8	7
Average Time to Transfer (minutes)[5]	-	-	62	60
Children's Asthma Care				
Received Home Management Plan of Care	-	-	93%	88%
Received Reliever Medication	-	-	100%	100%
Received Systemic Corticosteroids	-	-	100%	100%
Emergency Department				
Admittance Decision Time (minutes)[2,7]	-	-	99	98
Head CT Results Within 45 Min. of Arrival[5]	-	-	54%	57%
Patients Who Left ER Before Being Seen[5]	-	-	3%	2%
Time from ER Arrival to Admit. (minutes)[2,7]	-	-	270	274
Time from ER Arrival to Discharge (minutes)[5]	-	-	127	134
Time in ER Before Being Evaluated (minutes)[5]	-	-	26	26
Time to Pain Meds for Fractures (minutes)[5]	-	-	57	57
Heart Attack Care				
Aspirin Given at Discharge	183	100%	99%	99%
Fibrinolytic Meds Within 30 Min. of Arrival[7]	-	-	49%	54%
PCI Within 90 Minutes of Arrival[7]	-	-	95%	96%
Statin Prescribed at Discharge	190	99%	98%	98%
Heart Failure Care				
ACE Inhibitor or ARB for LVSD	92	100%	97%	97%
Discharge Instructions Given	183	97%	95%	94%
Evaluation of LVS Function	202	100%	99%	99%
Medicare Spending				
Medicare Spending per Patient (ratio)	-	1.11	1.03	0.98
Pneumonia Care				
Appropriate Initial Antibiotic Given[7]	-	-	95%	95%
Blood Culture Timing[1]	-	-	98%	98%
Pregnancy and Delivery Care				
Newborn Deliveries Scheduled Early[7]	-	-	7%	6%
Preventive Care				
Immunization for Influenza[2]	293	99%	90%	90%
Immunization for Pneumonia[2]	488	99%	92%	92%
Stroke Care				
Anticoagulation Therapy for Atrial Fibrillation[7]	-	-	96%	95%
Antithrombotic Therapy Timing[7]	-	-	98%	98%
Assessed for Rehabilitation[7]	-	-	98%	97%
Discharged on Antithrombotic Therapy[7]	-	-	99%	99%
Discharged on Statin Medication[7]	-	-	95%	94%
Thrombolytic Therapy Timing[7]	-	-	68%	66%
Venous Thromboembolism Prophylaxis[7]	-	-	94%	94%
Written Stroke Educational Materials Given[7]	-	-	92%	88%
Surgical Care Improvement Project				
Appropriate Beta Blocker Usage	64	100%	98%	98%
Appropriate VTP Within 24 Hours[1]	-	-	98%	98%
Controlled Postoperative Blood Glucose	157	98%	96%	97%
Perioperative Temperature Management	66	100%	100%	100%
Prophylactic Antibiotic Selection	154	100%	99%	99%
Prophylactic Antibiotic Selection (Outpatient)	365	100%	98%	98%
Prophylactic Antibiotic Stopped	149	100%	98%	98%
Prophylactic Antibiotic Timing	154	100%	99%	99%
Prophylactic Antibiotic Timing (Outpatient)	365	100%	98%	98%
Urinary Catheter Removal	113	99%	98%	97%
Survey of Patients' Hospital Experiences				
Area Around Room 'Always' Quiet at Night	300+	65%	68%	61%
Doctors 'Always' Communicated Well	300+	80%	83%	82%
Home Recovery Information Given	300+	86%	85%	85%
Hospital Given 9 or 10 on 10 Point Scale	300+	79%	73%	71%
Meds 'Always' Explained Before Given	300+	63%	66%	64%
Nurses 'Always' Communicated Well	300+	81%	80%	79%
Pain 'Always' Well Controlled	300+	76%	72%	71%
Room and Bathroom 'Always' Clean	300+	81%	75%	73%
Timely Help 'Always' Received	300+	74%	69%	68%
Would Definitely Recommend Hospital	300+	83%	73%	71%
Use of Medical Imaging				
Cardiac Imaging Stress Test before Surgery[1]	-	-	5.3%	5.3%
Combination Abdominal CT Scan[1]	-	-	16.4%	10.5%
Combination Brain/Sinus CT Scan[1]	-	-	2.7%	2.7%
Combination Chest CT Scan[1]	-	-	5.6%	2.7%
Follow-up Mammogram/Ultrasound[7]	-	-	7.9%	8.8%
Lumbar Spine MRI for Low Back Pain[7]	-	-	39.6%	37.2%

USMD Hospital at Arlington

801 W Interstate 20 Phone: 817-472-3400
Arlington, TX 76017 Fax: 817-472-3090
URL: www.usmdhospital.com
Type: Acute Care Hospitals Emergency Services: Yes
Ownership: Physician Beds: 18
Key Personnel:
Radiology. Stuart Aronson
CEO/President. . . . . Gordon Davis

Measure	Cases	This Hosp.	State Avg.	U.S. Avg.
Blood Clot Prevention and Treatment				
Anticoagulation Overlap Therapy[2]	11	73%	93%	93%
ICU Venous Thromboembolism Prophylaxis[1,2]	-	-	92%	92%
Incidence of Potentially Preventable VTE[1,2]	-	-	9%	10%
UFH with Dosages/Platelet Monitoring[1,2]	-	-	96%	97%
Venous Thromboembolism Prophylaxis[2]	115	77%	82%	85%
Warfarin Therapy Discharge Instructions[2]	12	83%	84%	75%
Chest Pain/Possible Heart Attack Care				
Aspirin Given Within 24 Hours of Arrival	39	90%	94%	96%
Fibrinolytic Meds Within 30 Min. of Arrival[7]	-	-	47%	58%
Average Time to ECG (minutes)	39	10	8	7
Average Time to Transfer (minutes)[1]	-	-	62	60
Children's Asthma Care				
Received Home Management Plan of Care	-	-	93%	88%
Received Reliever Medication	-	-	100%	100%
Received Systemic Corticosteroids	-	-	100%	100%
Emergency Department				
Admittance Decision Time (minutes)[2]	108	94	99	98
Head CT Results Within 45 Min. of Arrival[1]	-	-	54%	57%
Patients Who Left ER Before Being Seen	22,604	3%	3%	2%
Time from ER Arrival to Admit. (minutes)[2]	106	291	270	274
Time from ER Arrival to Discharge (minutes)	360	134	127	134
Time in ER Before Being Evaluated (minutes)	364	49	26	26
Time to Pain Meds for Fractures (minutes)	75	82	57	57
Heart Attack Care				
Aspirin Given at Discharge[5]	-	-	99%	99%
Fibrinolytic Meds Within 30 Min. of Arrival[5]	-	-	49%	54%
PCI Within 90 Minutes of Arrival[5]	-	-	95%	96%
Statin Prescribed at Discharge[5]	-	-	98%	98%
Heart Failure Care				
ACE Inhibitor or ARB for LVSD[5]	-	-	97%	97%
Discharge Instructions Given[5]	-	-	95%	94%
Evaluation of LVS Function[5]	-	-	99%	99%
Medicare Spending				
Medicare Spending per Patient (ratio)	-	0.99	1.03	0.98
Pneumonia Care				
Appropriate Initial Antibiotic Given[2]	15	87%	95%	95%
Blood Culture Timing[2]	15	93%	98%	98%
Pregnancy and Delivery Care				
Newborn Deliveries Scheduled Early[7]	-	-	7%	6%
Preventive Care				
Immunization for Influenza[2]	306	84%	90%	90%
Immunization for Pneumonia[2]	332	83%	92%	92%
Stroke Care				
Anticoagulation Therapy for Atrial Fibrillation[5]	-	-	96%	95%
Antithrombotic Therapy Timing[5]	-	-	98%	98%
Assessed for Rehabilitation[5]	-	-	98%	97%
Discharged on Antithrombotic Therapy[5]	-	-	99%	99%
Discharged on Statin Medication[5]	-	-	95%	94%
Thrombolytic Therapy Timing[5]	-	-	68%	66%
Venous Thromboembolism Prophylaxis[5]	-	-	94%	94%
Written Stroke Educational Materials Given[5]	-	-	92%	88%
Surgical Care Improvement Project				
Appropriate Beta Blocker Usage[2]	43	95%	98%	98%
Appropriate VTP Within 24 Hours[2]	125	94%	98%	98%
Controlled Postoperative Blood Glucose[2,7]	-	-	96%	97%
Perioperative Temperature Management[2]	213	100%	100%	100%
Prophylactic Antibiotic Selection[2]	51	100%	99%	99%
Prophylactic Antibiotic Selection (Outpatient)	593	97%	98%	98%
Prophylactic Antibiotic Stopped[2]	50	98%	98%	98%
Prophylactic Antibiotic Timing[2]	51	98%	99%	99%
Prophylactic Antibiotic Timing (Outpatient)	591	99%	98%	98%
Urinary Catheter Removal[2]	55	98%	98%	97%
Survey of Patients' Hospital Experiences				
Area Around Room 'Always' Quiet at Night	300+	84%	68%	61%
Doctors 'Always' Communicated Well	300+	85%	83%	82%
Home Recovery Information Given	300+	85%	85%	85%
Hospital Given 9 or 10 on 10 Point Scale	300+	84%	73%	71%
Meds 'Always' Explained Before Given	300+	71%	66%	64%
Nurses 'Always' Communicated Well	300+	84%	80%	79%
Pain 'Always' Well Controlled	300+	75%	72%	71%
Room and Bathroom 'Always' Clean	300+	88%	75%	73%
Timely Help 'Always' Received	300+	78%	69%	68%
Would Definitely Recommend Hospital	300+	86%	73%	71%
Use of Medical Imaging				
Cardiac Imaging Stress Test before Surgery[7]	-	-	5.3%	5.3%
Combination Abdominal CT Scan	259	6.9%	16.4%	10.5%

NOTE: Hospital profiles are in alphabetical order by state, then city, then hospital within the city; Rankings exclude hospitals with less than 25 cases except for patient surveys which excludes hospitals with less than 100 cases; (a) 100-299 cases; (1) The number of cases/patients is too few to report; (2) Data submitted were based on a sample of cases/patients; (3) Results are based on a shorter time period than required; (4) Data suppressed by CMS for one or more quarters; (5) Results are not available for this reporting period; (6) Fewer than 100 patients completed the HCAHPS survey; (7) No cases met the criteria for this measure; (8) The lower limit of the confidence interval cannot be calculated if the number of observed infections equals zero; (9) No data are available from the state/territory for this reporting period; (10) The scores shown reflect fewer than 50 completed surveys; (11) There were discrepancies in the data collection process; (12) This measure does not apply to this hospital for this reporting period; (13) Results cannot be calculated for this reporting period; (14) The results for this state are combined with nearby states to protect confidentiality; Please refer to the User's Guide for a full explanation of data.

Measure	Cases	This Hosp.	State Avg.	U.S. Avg.
Combination Brain/Sinus CT Scan[1]	-	-	2.7%	2.7%
Combination Chest CT Scan[1]	-	-	5.6%	2.7%
Follow-up Mammogram/Ultrasound[7]	-	-	7.9%	8.8%
Lumbar Spine MRI for Low Back Pain[1]	-	-	39.6%	37.2%

East Texas Medical Center Athens

2000 South Palestine
Athens, TX 75751
Phone: 903-676-1000
Fax: 903-676-3153
E-mail: info@etmc.org
URL: www.etmc.org/athens
Type: Acute Care Hospitals
Emergency Services: Yes
Ownership: Voluntary non-profit - Private
Beds: 117

Key Personnel:
Chief of Medical Staff . . . . Marcus G Abadie
Radiology. E Maxey Abernathy
CEO/President. . . . . Patrick L Wallace

Measure	Cases	This Hosp.	State Avg.	U.S. Avg.
Blood Clot Prevention and Treatment				
Anticoagulation Overlap Therapy[2]	24	79%	93%	93%
ICU Venous Thromboembolism Prophylaxis[2]	49	59%	92%	92%
Incidence of Potentially Preventable VTE[1,2]	-	-	9%	10%
UFH with Dosages/Platelet Monitoring[1,2]	-	-	96%	97%
Venous Thromboembolism Prophylaxis[2]	407	35%	82%	85%
Warfarin Therapy Discharge Instructions[2]	20	100%	84%	75%
Chest Pain/Possible Heart Attack Care				
Aspirin Given Within 24 Hours of Arrival	168	97%	94%	96%
Fibrinolytic Meds Within 30 Min. of Arrival	20	70%	47%	58%
Average Time to ECG (minutes)	174	6	8	7
Average Time to Transfer (minutes)[1]	-	-	62	60
Children's Asthma Care				
Received Home Management Plan of Care	-	-	93%	88%
Received Reliever Medication	-	-	100%	100%
Received Systemic Corticosteroids	-	-	100%	100%
Emergency Department				
Admittance Decision Time (minutes)[2]	556	81	99	98
Head CT Results Within 45 Min. of Arrival	16	50%	54%	57%
Patients Who Left ER Before Being Seen	61,171	1%	3%	2%
Time from ER Arrival to Admit. (minutes)[2]	605	288	270	274
Time from ER Arrival to Discharge (minutes)	394	158	127	134
Time in ER Before Being Evaluated (minutes)	418	23	26	26
Time to Pain Meds for Fractures (minutes)	156	60	57	57
Heart Attack Care				
Aspirin Given at Discharge	16	75%	99%	99%
Fibrinolytic Meds Within 30 Min. of Arrival[7]	-	-	49%	54%
PCI Within 90 Minutes of Arrival[7]	-	-	95%	96%
Statin Prescribed at Discharge	15	80%	98%	98%
Heart Failure Care				
ACE Inhibitor or ARB for LVSD	60	78%	97%	97%
Discharge Instructions Given	152	56%	95%	94%
Evaluation of LVS Function	193	90%	99%	99%
Medicare Spending				
Medicare Spending per Patient (ratio)	-	1.00	1.03	0.98
Pneumonia Care				
Appropriate Initial Antibiotic Given[2]	155	86%	95%	95%
Blood Culture Timing[2]	297	96%	98%	98%
Pregnancy and Delivery Care				
Newborn Deliveries Scheduled Early	83	10%	7%	6%
Preventive Care				
Immunization for Influenza[2]	574	62%	90%	90%
Immunization for Pneumonia[2]	680	74%	92%	92%
Stroke Care				
Anticoagulation Therapy for Atrial Fibrillation	13	62%	96%	95%
Antithrombotic Therapy Timing	80	89%	98%	98%
Assessed for Rehabilitation	79	71%	98%	97%
Discharged on Antithrombotic Therapy	78	87%	99%	99%
Discharged on Statin Medication	65	52%	95%	94%
Thrombolytic Therapy Timing	16	6%	68%	66%
Venous Thromboembolism Prophylaxis	81	42%	94%	94%
Written Stroke Educational Materials Given	42	83%	92%	88%
Surgical Care Improvement Project				
Appropriate Beta Blocker Usage[2]	57	91%	98%	98%
Appropriate VTP Within 24 Hours[2]	217	94%	98%	98%
Controlled Postoperative Blood Glucose[2,7]	-	-	96%	97%
Perioperative Temperature Management[2]	269	100%	100%	100%
Prophylactic Antibiotic Selection[2]	177	98%	99%	99%
Prophylactic Antibiotic Selection (Outpatient)	41	93%	98%	98%
Prophylactic Antibiotic Stopped[2]	175	82%	98%	98%
Prophylactic Antibiotic Timing[2]	177	99%	99%	99%
Prophylactic Antibiotic Timing (Outpatient)	44	91%	98%	98%
Urinary Catheter Removal[2]	102	73%	98%	97%
Survey of Patients' Hospital Experiences				
Area Around Room 'Always' Quiet at Night	300+	61%	68%	61%
Doctors 'Always' Communicated Well	300+	82%	83%	82%
Home Recovery Information Given	300+	82%	85%	85%
Hospital Given 9 or 10 on 10 Point Scale	300+	65%	73%	71%
Meds 'Always' Explained Before Given	300+	61%	66%	64%
Nurses 'Always' Communicated Well	300+	76%	80%	79%
Pain 'Always' Well Controlled	300+	67%	72%	71%
Room and Bathroom 'Always' Clean	300+	65%	75%	73%
Timely Help 'Always' Received	300+	61%	69%	68%
Would Definitely Recommend Hospital	300+	65%	73%	71%
Use of Medical Imaging				
Cardiac Imaging Stress Test before Surgery	202	5.0%	5.3%	5.3%
Combination Abdominal CT Scan	825	11.8%	16.4%	10.5%
Combination Brain/Sinus CT Scan	802	2.6%	2.7%	2.7%
Combination Chest CT Scan	530	15.1%	5.6%	2.7%
Follow-up Mammogram/Ultrasound	606	6.4%	7.9%	8.8%
Lumbar Spine MRI for Low Back Pain	152	41.4%	39.6%	37.2%

Baylor Emergency Medical Center

26791 Highway 380
Aubrey, TX 76227
Phone: 972-347-2525
Type: Acute Care Hospitals
Emergency Services: Yes
Ownership: Proprietary

Measure	Cases	This Hosp.	State Avg.	U.S. Avg.
Blood Clot Prevention and Treatment				
Anticoagulation Overlap Therapy[5]	-	-	93%	93%
ICU Venous Thromboembolism Prophylaxis[5]	-	-	92%	92%
Incidence of Potentially Preventable VTE[5]	-	-	9%	10%
UFH with Dosages/Platelet Monitoring[5]	-	-	96%	97%
Venous Thromboembolism Prophylaxis[5]	-	-	82%	85%
Warfarin Therapy Discharge Instructions[5]	-	-	84%	75%
Chest Pain/Possible Heart Attack Care				
Aspirin Given Within 24 Hours of Arrival[5]	-	-	94%	96%
Fibrinolytic Meds Within 30 Min. of Arrival[5]	-	-	47%	58%
Average Time to ECG (minutes)[5]	-	-	8	7
Average Time to Transfer (minutes)[5]	-	-	62	60
Children's Asthma Care				
Received Home Management Plan of Care	-	-	93%	88%
Received Reliever Medication	-	-	100%	100%
Received Systemic Corticosteroids	-	-	100%	100%
Emergency Department				
Admittance Decision Time (minutes)[5]	-	-	99	98
Head CT Results Within 45 Min. of Arrival[5]	-	-	54%	57%
Patients Who Left ER Before Being Seen	7,897	0%	3%	2%
Time from ER Arrival to Admit. (minutes)[5]	-	-	270	274
Time from ER Arrival to Discharge (minutes)[5]	-	-	127	134
Time in ER Before Being Evaluated (minutes)[5]	-	-	26	26
Time to Pain Meds for Fractures (minutes)[5]	-	-	57	57
Heart Attack Care				
Aspirin Given at Discharge[5]	-	-	99%	99%
Fibrinolytic Meds Within 30 Min. of Arrival[5]	-	-	49%	54%
PCI Within 90 Minutes of Arrival[5]	-	-	95%	96%
Statin Prescribed at Discharge[5]	-	-	98%	98%
Heart Failure Care				
ACE Inhibitor or ARB for LVSD[5]	-	-	97%	97%
Discharge Instructions Given[5]	-	-	95%	94%
Evaluation of LVS Function[5]	-	-	99%	99%
Medicare Spending				
Medicare Spending per Patient (ratio)[1]	-	-	1.03	0.98
Pneumonia Care				
Appropriate Initial Antibiotic Given[5]	-	-	95%	95%
Blood Culture Timing[5]	-	-	98%	98%
Pregnancy and Delivery Care				
Newborn Deliveries Scheduled Early[7]	-	-	7%	6%
Preventive Care				
Immunization for Influenza[5]	-	-	90%	90%
Immunization for Pneumonia[5]	-	-	92%	92%
Stroke Care				
Anticoagulation Therapy for Atrial Fibrillation[5]	-	-	96%	95%
Antithrombotic Therapy Timing[5]	-	-	98%	98%
Assessed for Rehabilitation[5]	-	-	98%	97%
Discharged on Antithrombotic Therapy[5]	-	-	99%	99%
Discharged on Statin Medication[5]	-	-	95%	94%
Thrombolytic Therapy Timing[5]	-	-	68%	66%
Venous Thromboembolism Prophylaxis[5]	-	-	94%	94%
Written Stroke Educational Materials Given[5]	-	-	92%	88%
Surgical Care Improvement Project				
Appropriate Beta Blocker Usage[5]	-	-	98%	98%
Appropriate VTP Within 24 Hours[5]	-	-	98%	98%
Controlled Postoperative Blood Glucose[5]	-	-	96%	97%
Perioperative Temperature Management[5]	-	-	100%	100%
Prophylactic Antibiotic Selection[5]	-	-	99%	99%
Prophylactic Antibiotic Selection (Outpatient)[5]	-	-	98%	98%
Prophylactic Antibiotic Stopped[5]	-	-	98%	98%
Prophylactic Antibiotic Timing[5]	-	-	99%	99%
Prophylactic Antibiotic Timing (Outpatient)[5]	-	-	98%	98%
Urinary Catheter Removal[5]	-	-	98%	97%
Survey of Patients' Hospital Experiences				
Area Around Room 'Always' Quiet at Night[10]	<100	90%	68%	61%
Doctors 'Always' Communicated Well[10]	<100	94%	83%	82%
Home Recovery Information Given[10]	<100	77%	85%	85%
Hospital Given 9 or 10 on 10 Point Scale[10]	<100	91%	73%	71%
Meds 'Always' Explained Before Given[10]	<100	91%	66%	64%
Nurses 'Always' Communicated Well[10]	<100	100%	80%	79%
Pain 'Always' Well Controlled[10]	<100	98%	72%	71%
Room and Bathroom 'Always' Clean[10]	<100	90%	75%	73%
Timely Help 'Always' Received[10]	<100	100%	69%	68%
Would Definitely Recommend Hospital[10]	<100	100%	73%	71%
Use of Medical Imaging				
Cardiac Imaging Stress Test before Surgery[7]	-	-	5.3%	5.3%
Combination Abdominal CT Scan[1]	-	-	16.4%	10.5%
Combination Brain/Sinus CT Scan	31	0.0%	2.7%	2.7%
Combination Chest CT Scan[1]	-	-	5.6%	2.7%
Follow-up Mammogram/Ultrasound[7]	-	-	7.9%	8.8%
Lumbar Spine MRI for Low Back Pain[7]	-	-	39.6%	37.2%

Arise Austin Medical Center

3003 Bee Caves Road
Austin, TX 78746
Phone: 512-347-9888
Type: Acute Care Hospitals
Emergency Services: Yes
Ownership: Physician

Key Personnel:
Chief of Medical Staff . . . . Robert Wills, MD
CEO . . . . Diana Zamora Magallan

Measure	Cases	This Hosp.	State Avg.	U.S. Avg.
Blood Clot Prevention and Treatment				
Anticoagulation Overlap Therapy[2,7]	-	-	93%	93%
ICU Venous Thromboembolism Prophylaxis[2,7]	-	-	92%	92%
Incidence of Potentially Preventable VTE[2,7]	-	-	9%	10%
UFH with Dosages/Platelet Monitoring[2,7]	-	-	96%	97%
Venous Thromboembolism Prophylaxis[2]	27	85%	82%	85%
Warfarin Therapy Discharge Instructions[2,7]	-	-	84%	75%
Chest Pain/Possible Heart Attack Care				
Aspirin Given Within 24 Hours of Arrival[5]	-	-	94%	96%
Fibrinolytic Meds Within 30 Min. of Arrival[5]	-	-	47%	58%
Average Time to ECG (minutes)[5]	-	-	8	7
Average Time to Transfer (minutes)[5]	-	-	62	60
Children's Asthma Care				
Received Home Management Plan of Care	-	-	93%	88%
Received Reliever Medication	-	-	100%	100%
Received Systemic Corticosteroids	-	-	100%	100%
Emergency Department				
Admittance Decision Time (minutes)[1,2]	-	-	99	98
Head CT Results Within 45 Min. of Arrival[5]	-	-	54%	57%
Patients Who Left ER Before Being Seen	414	0%	3%	2%
Time from ER Arrival to Admit. (minutes)[1,2]	-	-	270	274
Time from ER Arrival to Discharge (minutes)	212	98	127	134

NOTE: Hospital profiles are in alphabetical order by state, then city, then hospital within the city; Rankings exclude hospitals with less than 25 cases except for patient surveys which excludes hospitals with less than 100 cases; (a) 100-299 cases; (1) The number of cases/patients is too few to report; (2) Data submitted were based on a sample of cases/patients; (3) Results are based on a shorter time period than required; (4) Data suppressed by CMS for one or more quarters; (5) Results are not available for this reporting period; (6) Fewer than 100 patients completed the HCAHPS survey; (7) No cases met the criteria for this measure; (8) The lower limit of the confidence interval cannot be calculated if the number of observed infections equals zero; (9) No data are available from the state/territory for this reporting period; (10) The scores shown reflect fewer than 50 completed surveys; (11) There were discrepancies in the data collection process; (12) This measure does not apply to this hospital for this reporting period; (13) Results cannot be calculated for this reporting period; (14) The results for this state are combined with nearby states to protect confidentiality; Please refer to the User's Guide for a full explanation of data.

Measure	Cases	This Hosp.	State Avg.	U.S. Avg.
Time in ER Before Being Evaluated (minutes)	238	30	26	26
Time to Pain Meds for Fractures (minutes)[5]	-	-	57	57
Heart Attack Care				
Aspirin Given at Discharge[5]	-	-	99%	99%
Fibrinolytic Meds Within 30 Min. of Arrival[5]	-	-	49%	54%
PCI Within 90 Minutes of Arrival[5]	-	-	95%	96%
Statin Prescribed at Discharge[5]	-	-	98%	98%
Heart Failure Care				
ACE Inhibitor or ARB for LVSD[5]	-	-	97%	97%
Discharge Instructions Given[5]	-	-	95%	94%
Evaluation of LVS Function[5]	-	-	99%	99%
Medicare Spending				
Medicare Spending per Patient (ratio)	-	0.96	1.03	0.98
Pneumonia Care				
Appropriate Initial Antibiotic Given[5]	-	-	95%	95%
Blood Culture Timing[5]	-	-	98%	98%
Pregnancy and Delivery Care				
Newborn Deliveries Scheduled Early[7]	-	-	7%	6%
Preventive Care				
Immunization for Influenza[2]	315	60%	90%	90%
Immunization for Pneumonia[2]	368	72%	92%	92%
Stroke Care				
Anticoagulation Therapy for Atrial Fibrillation[5]	-	-	96%	95%
Antithrombotic Therapy Timing[5]	-	-	98%	98%
Assessed for Rehabilitation[5]	-	-	98%	97%
Discharged on Antithrombotic Therapy[5]	-	-	99%	99%
Discharged on Statin Medication[5]	-	-	95%	94%
Thrombolytic Therapy Timing[5]	-	-	68%	66%
Venous Thromboembolism Prophylaxis[5]	-	-	94%	94%
Written Stroke Educational Materials Given[5]	-	-	92%	88%
Surgical Care Improvement Project				
Appropriate Beta Blocker Usage[2]	45	71%	98%	98%
Appropriate VTP Within 24 Hours[2]	350	95%	98%	98%
Controlled Postoperative Blood Glucose[2,7]	-	-	96%	97%
Perioperative Temperature Management[2]	373	99%	100%	100%
Prophylactic Antibiotic Selection[2]	316	96%	99%	99%
Prophylactic Antibiotic Selection (Outpatient)[5]	-	-	98%	98%
Prophylactic Antibiotic Stopped[2]	316	97%	98%	98%
Prophylactic Antibiotic Timing[2]	316	97%	99%	99%
Prophylactic Antibiotic Timing (Outpatient)[5]	-	-	98%	98%
Urinary Catheter Removal[2]	37	97%	98%	97%
Survey of Patients' Hospital Experiences				
Area Around Room 'Always' Quiet at Night[3]	(a)	84%	68%	61%
Doctors 'Always' Communicated Well[3]	(a)	84%	83%	82%
Home Recovery Information Given[3]	(a)	92%	85%	85%
Hospital Given 9 or 10 on 10 Point Scale[3]	(a)	76%	73%	71%
Meds 'Always' Explained Before Given[3]	(a)	66%	66%	64%
Nurses 'Always' Communicated Well[3]	(a)	77%	80%	79%
Pain 'Always' Well Controlled[3]	(a)	69%	72%	71%
Room and Bathroom 'Always' Clean[3]	(a)	76%	75%	73%
Timely Help 'Always' Received[3]	(a)	66%	69%	68%
Would Definitely Recommend Hospital[3]	(a)	79%	73%	71%
Use of Medical Imaging				
Cardiac Imaging Stress Test before Surgery[7]	-	-	5.3%	5.3%
Combination Abdominal CT Scan[1]	-	-	16.4%	10.5%
Combination Brain/Sinus CT Scan[1]	-	-	2.7%	2.7%
Combination Chest CT Scan[1]	-	-	5.6%	2.7%
Follow-up Mammogram/Ultrasound[7]	-	-	7.9%	8.8%
Lumbar Spine MRI for Low Back Pain[1]	-	-	39.6%	37.2%

Dell Children's Medical Center of Central Texas

4900 Mueller Blvd
Austin, TX 78723
Phone: 512-324-0000
Type: Childrens
Emergency Services: Yes
Ownership: Voluntary non-profit - Private

Measure	Cases	This Hosp.	State Avg.	U.S. Avg.
Blood Clot Prevention and Treatment				
Anticoagulation Overlap Therapy[5]	-	-	93%	93%
ICU Venous Thromboembolism Prophylaxis[5]	-	-	92%	92%
Incidence of Potentially Preventable VTE[5]	-	-	9%	10%
UFH with Dosages/Platelet Monitoring[5]	-	-	96%	97%
Venous Thromboembolism Prophylaxis[5]	-	-	82%	85%
Warfarin Therapy Discharge Instructions[5]	-	-	84%	75%
Chest Pain/Possible Heart Attack Care				
Aspirin Given Within 24 Hours of Arrival	-	-	94%	96%
Fibrinolytic Meds Within 30 Min. of Arrival	-	-	47%	58%
Average Time to ECG (minutes)	-	-	8	7
Average Time to Transfer (minutes)	-	-	62	60
Children's Asthma Care				
Received Home Management Plan of Care	-	-	93%	88%
Received Reliever Medication	-	-	100%	100%
Received Systemic Corticosteroids	-	-	100%	100%
Emergency Department				
Admittance Decision Time (minutes)[5]	-	-	99	98
Head CT Results Within 45 Min. of Arrival	-	-	54%	57%
Patients Who Left ER Before Being Seen	-	-	3%	2%
Time from ER Arrival to Admit. (minutes)[5]	-	-	270	274
Time from ER Arrival to Discharge (minutes)	-	-	127	134
Time in ER Before Being Evaluated (minutes)	-	-	26	26
Time to Pain Meds for Fractures (minutes)	-	-	57	57
Heart Attack Care				
Aspirin Given at Discharge[5]	-	-	99%	99%
Fibrinolytic Meds Within 30 Min. of Arrival[5]	-	-	49%	54%
PCI Within 90 Minutes of Arrival[5]	-	-	95%	96%
Statin Prescribed at Discharge[5]	-	-	98%	98%
Heart Failure Care				
ACE Inhibitor or ARB for LVSD[5]	-	-	97%	97%
Discharge Instructions Given[5]	-	-	95%	94%
Evaluation of LVS Function[5]	-	-	99%	99%
Medicare Spending				
Medicare Spending per Patient (ratio)	-	-	1.03	0.98
Pneumonia Care				
Appropriate Initial Antibiotic Given[5]	-	-	95%	95%
Blood Culture Timing[5]	-	-	98%	98%
Pregnancy and Delivery Care				
Newborn Deliveries Scheduled Early[5]	-	-	7%	6%
Preventive Care				
Immunization for Influenza[5]	-	-	90%	90%
Immunization for Pneumonia[5]	-	-	92%	92%
Stroke Care				
Anticoagulation Therapy for Atrial Fibrillation[5]	-	-	96%	95%
Antithrombotic Therapy Timing[5]	-	-	98%	98%
Assessed for Rehabilitation[5]	-	-	98%	97%
Discharged on Antithrombotic Therapy[5]	-	-	99%	99%
Discharged on Statin Medication[5]	-	-	95%	94%
Thrombolytic Therapy Timing[5]	-	-	68%	66%
Venous Thromboembolism Prophylaxis[5]	-	-	94%	94%
Written Stroke Educational Materials Given[5]	-	-	92%	88%
Surgical Care Improvement Project				
Appropriate Beta Blocker Usage[5]	-	-	98%	98%
Appropriate VTP Within 24 Hours[5]	-	-	98%	98%
Controlled Postoperative Blood Glucose[5]	-	-	96%	97%
Perioperative Temperature Management[5]	-	-	100%	100%
Prophylactic Antibiotic Selection[5]	-	-	99%	99%
Prophylactic Antibiotic Selection (Outpatient)	-	-	98%	98%
Prophylactic Antibiotic Stopped[5]	-	-	98%	98%
Prophylactic Antibiotic Timing[5]	-	-	99%	99%
Prophylactic Antibiotic Timing (Outpatient)	-	-	98%	98%
Urinary Catheter Removal[5]	-	-	98%	97%
Survey of Patients' Hospital Experiences				
Area Around Room 'Always' Quiet at Night[5]	-	-	68%	61%
Doctors 'Always' Communicated Well[5]	-	-	83%	82%
Home Recovery Information Given[5]	-	-	85%	85%
Hospital Given 9 or 10 on 10 Point Scale[5]	-	-	73%	71%
Meds 'Always' Explained Before Given[5]	-	-	66%	64%
Nurses 'Always' Communicated Well[5]	-	-	80%	79%
Pain 'Always' Well Controlled[5]	-	-	72%	71%
Room and Bathroom 'Always' Clean[5]	-	-	75%	73%
Timely Help 'Always' Received[5]	-	-	69%	68%
Would Definitely Recommend Hospital[5]	-	-	73%	71%
Use of Medical Imaging				
Cardiac Imaging Stress Test before Surgery	-	-	5.3%	5.3%
Combination Abdominal CT Scan	-	-	16.4%	10.5%
Combination Brain/Sinus CT Scan	-	-	2.7%	2.7%
Combination Chest CT Scan	-	-	5.6%	2.7%
Follow-up Mammogram/Ultrasound	-	-	7.9%	8.8%
Lumbar Spine MRI for Low Back Pain	-	-	39.6%	37.2%

The Hospital at Westlake Medical Center

5656 Bee Caves Road, Suite M-302
Austin, TX 78746
Phone: 512-327-0000
URL: www.westlakemedical.com
Type: Acute Care Hospitals
Emergency Services: Yes
Ownership: Proprietary
Beds: 21

Key Personnel:
CEO/President. . . . . Rip Miller

Measure	Cases	This Hosp.	State Avg.	U.S. Avg.
Blood Clot Prevention and Treatment				
Anticoagulation Overlap Therapy[2]	11	100%	93%	93%
ICU Venous Thromboembolism Prophylaxis[2]	18	100%	92%	92%
Incidence of Potentially Preventable VTE[2,7]	-	-	9%	10%
UFH with Dosages/Platelet Monitoring[2,7]	-	-	96%	97%
Venous Thromboembolism Prophylaxis[2]	155	99%	82%	85%
Warfarin Therapy Discharge Instructions[1,2]	-	-	84%	75%
Chest Pain/Possible Heart Attack Care				
Aspirin Given Within 24 Hours of Arrival[5]	-	-	94%	96%
Fibrinolytic Meds Within 30 Min. of Arrival[5]	-	-	47%	58%
Average Time to ECG (minutes)[5]	-	-	8	7
Average Time to Transfer (minutes)[5]	-	-	62	60
Children's Asthma Care				
Received Home Management Plan of Care	-	-	93%	88%
Received Reliever Medication	-	-	100%	100%
Received Systemic Corticosteroids	-	-	100%	100%
Emergency Department				
Admittance Decision Time (minutes)[2]	292	95	99	98
Head CT Results Within 45 Min. of Arrival[1,3]	-	-	54%	57%
Patients Who Left ER Before Being Seen	4,762	0%	3%	2%
Time from ER Arrival to Admit. (minutes)[2]	293	211	270	274
Time from ER Arrival to Discharge (minutes)	395	86	127	134
Time in ER Before Being Evaluated (minutes)	407	7	26	26
Time to Pain Meds for Fractures (minutes)	56	25	57	57
Heart Attack Care				
Aspirin Given at Discharge	11	100%	99%	99%
Fibrinolytic Meds Within 30 Min. of Arrival[7]	-	-	49%	54%
PCI Within 90 Minutes of Arrival[1]	-	-	95%	96%
Statin Prescribed at Discharge	12	100%	98%	98%
Heart Failure Care				
ACE Inhibitor or ARB for LVSD[1]	-	-	97%	97%
Discharge Instructions Given[1]	-	-	95%	94%
Evaluation of LVS Function	14	100%	99%	99%
Medicare Spending				
Medicare Spending per Patient (ratio)	-	1.01	1.03	0.98
Pneumonia Care				
Appropriate Initial Antibiotic Given	18	100%	95%	95%
Blood Culture Timing	33	97%	98%	98%
Pregnancy and Delivery Care				
Newborn Deliveries Scheduled Early[7]	-	-	7%	6%
Preventive Care				
Immunization for Influenza[2]	495	100%	90%	90%
Immunization for Pneumonia[2]	504	100%	92%	92%
Stroke Care				
Anticoagulation Therapy for Atrial Fibrillation[3,7]	-	-	96%	95%
Antithrombotic Therapy Timing[1,3]	-	-	98%	98%
Assessed for Rehabilitation[1,3]	-	-	98%	97%
Discharged on Antithrombotic Therapy[1,3]	-	-	99%	99%
Discharged on Statin Medication[1,3]	-	-	95%	94%
Thrombolytic Therapy Timing[3,7]	-	-	68%	66%
Venous Thromboembolism Prophylaxis[1,3]	-	-	94%	94%
Written Stroke Educational Materials Given[3,7]	-	-	92%	88%
Surgical Care Improvement Project				
Appropriate Beta Blocker Usage	57	100%	98%	98%
Appropriate VTP Within 24 Hours	290	99%	98%	98%
Controlled Postoperative Blood Glucose	15	87%	96%	97%
Perioperative Temperature Management	308	100%	100%	100%
Prophylactic Antibiotic Selection	281	100%	99%	99%
Prophylactic Antibiotic Selection (Outpatient)	166	99%	98%	98%
Prophylactic Antibiotic Stopped	280	100%	98%	98%

NOTE: Hospital profiles are in alphabetical order by state, then city, then hospital within the city; Rankings exclude hospitals with less than 25 cases except for patient surveys which excludes hospitals with less than 100 cases; (a) 100-299 cases; (1) The number of cases/patients is too few to report; (2) Data submitted were based on a sample of cases/patients; (3) Results are based on a shorter time period than required; (4) Data suppressed by CMS for one or more quarters; (5) Results are not available for this reporting period; (6) Fewer than 100 patients completed the HCAHPS survey; (7) No cases met the criteria for this measure; (8) The lower limit of the confidence interval cannot be calculated if the number of observed infections equals zero; (9) No data are available from the state/territory for this reporting period; (10) The scores shown reflect fewer than 50 completed surveys; (11) There were discrepancies in the data collection process; (12) This measure does not apply to this hospital for this reporting period; (13) Results cannot be calculated for this reporting period; (14) The results for this state are combined with nearby states to protect confidentiality; Please refer to the User's Guide for a full explanation of data.

Measure	Cases	This Hosp.	State Avg.	U.S. Avg.
Prophylactic Antibiotic Timing	281	100%	99%	99%
Prophylactic Antibiotic Timing (Outpatient)	168	98%	98%	98%
Urinary Catheter Removal	89	100%	98%	97%
Survey of Patients' Hospital Experiences				
Area Around Room 'Always' Quiet at Night	300+	74%	68%	61%
Doctors 'Always' Communicated Well	300+	82%	83%	82%
Home Recovery Information Given	300+	89%	85%	85%
Hospital Given 9 or 10 on 10 Point Scale	300+	80%	73%	71%
Meds 'Always' Explained Before Given	300+	69%	66%	64%
Nurses 'Always' Communicated Well	300+	78%	80%	79%
Pain 'Always' Well Controlled	300+	69%	72%	71%
Room and Bathroom 'Always' Clean	300+	79%	75%	73%
Timely Help 'Always' Received	300+	74%	69%	68%
Would Definitely Recommend Hospital	300+	79%	73%	71%
Use of Medical Imaging				
Cardiac Imaging Stress Test before Surgery	124	7.3%	5.3%	5.3%
Combination Abdominal CT Scan[1]	-	-	16.4%	10.5%
Combination Brain/Sinus CT Scan[1]	-	-	2.7%	2.7%
Combination Chest CT Scan	48	2.1%	5.6%	2.7%
Follow-up Mammogram/Ultrasound[7]	-	-	7.9%	8.8%
Lumbar Spine MRI for Low Back Pain[1]	-	-	39.6%	37.2%

North Austin Medical Center

12221 Mopac Expressway North
Austin, TX 78758
Phone: 512-901-1000
Fax: 512-901-1871
URL: www.cornerstonehealthcaregroup.com
Type: Acute Care Hospitals
Emergency Services: Yes
Ownership: Voluntary non-profit - Other
Beds: 133
Key Personnel:
CEO/President. . . . . C. David Huffstutler
Chief of Medical Staff. . . . . Thomas W. Knight, MD
Emergency Room . . . . Robert Mills

Measure	Cases	This Hosp.	State Avg.	U.S. Avg.
Blood Clot Prevention and Treatment				
Anticoagulation Overlap Therapy[2]	109	99%	93%	93%
ICU Venous Thromboembolism Prophylaxis[2]	77	97%	92%	92%
Incidence of Potentially Preventable VTE[2]	17	0%	9%	10%
UFH with Dosages/Platelet Monitoring[1,2]	-	-	96%	97%
Venous Thromboembolism Prophylaxis[2]	394	97%	82%	85%
Warfarin Therapy Discharge Instructions[2]	75	99%	84%	75%
Chest Pain/Possible Heart Attack Care				
Aspirin Given Within 24 Hours of Arrival[1,3]	-	-	94%	96%
Fibrinolytic Meds Within 30 Min. of Arrival[3,7]	-	-	47%	58%
Average Time to ECG (minutes)[1,3]	-	-	8	7
Average Time to Transfer (minutes)[3,7]	-	-	62	60
Children's Asthma Care				
Received Home Management Plan of Care	-	-	93%	88%
Received Reliever Medication	-	-	100%	100%
Received Systemic Corticosteroids	-	-	100%	100%
Emergency Department				
Admittance Decision Time (minutes)[2]	502	150	99	98
Head CT Results Within 45 Min. of Arrival[1,3]	-	-	54%	57%
Patients Who Left ER Before Being Seen	63,017	2%	3%	2%
Time from ER Arrival to Admit. (minutes)[2]	503	305	270	274
Time from ER Arrival to Discharge (minutes)	515	142	127	134
Time in ER Before Being Evaluated (minutes)	538	27	26	26
Time to Pain Meds for Fractures (minutes)	174	48	57	57
Heart Attack Care				
Aspirin Given at Discharge	169	100%	99%	99%
Fibrinolytic Meds Within 30 Min. of Arrival[7]	-	-	49%	54%
PCI Within 90 Minutes of Arrival	57	100%	95%	96%
Statin Prescribed at Discharge	164	100%	98%	98%
Heart Failure Care				
ACE Inhibitor or ARB for LVSD	63	100%	97%	97%
Discharge Instructions Given	197	99%	95%	94%
Evaluation of LVS Function	233	100%	99%	99%
Medicare Spending				
Medicare Spending per Patient (ratio)	-	1.05	1.03	0.98
Pneumonia Care				
Appropriate Initial Antibiotic Given	128	100%	95%	95%
Blood Culture Timing	278	100%	98%	98%
Pregnancy and Delivery Care				
Newborn Deliveries Scheduled Early[2]	96	1%	7%	6%
Preventive Care				
Immunization for Influenza[2]	532	97%	90%	90%
Immunization for Pneumonia[2]	506	98%	92%	92%
Stroke Care				
Anticoagulation Therapy for Atrial Fibrillation[1,2]	-	-	96%	95%
Antithrombotic Therapy Timing[2]	69	100%	98%	98%
Assessed for Rehabilitation[2]	79	100%	98%	97%
Discharged on Antithrombotic Therapy[2]	68	100%	99%	99%
Discharged on Statin Medication[2]	55	100%	95%	94%
Thrombolytic Therapy Timing[1,2]	-	-	68%	66%
Venous Thromboembolism Prophylaxis[2]	76	100%	94%	94%
Written Stroke Educational Materials Given[2]	56	100%	92%	88%
Surgical Care Improvement Project				
Appropriate Beta Blocker Usage[2]	165	100%	98%	98%
Appropriate VTP Within 24 Hours[2]	448	99%	98%	98%
Controlled Postoperative Blood Glucose[2]	95	99%	96%	97%
Perioperative Temperature Management[2]	508	100%	100%	100%
Prophylactic Antibiotic Selection[2]	396	100%	99%	99%
Prophylactic Antibiotic Selection (Outpatient)	593	99%	98%	98%
Prophylactic Antibiotic Stopped[2]	394	100%	98%	98%
Prophylactic Antibiotic Timing[2]	396	99%	99%	99%
Prophylactic Antibiotic Timing (Outpatient)	594	100%	98%	98%
Urinary Catheter Removal[2]	330	100%	98%	97%
Survey of Patients' Hospital Experiences				
Area Around Room 'Always' Quiet at Night	300+	62%	68%	61%
Doctors 'Always' Communicated Well	300+	80%	83%	82%
Home Recovery Information Given	300+	88%	85%	85%
Hospital Given 9 or 10 on 10 Point Scale	300+	75%	73%	71%
Meds 'Always' Explained Before Given	300+	65%	66%	64%
Nurses 'Always' Communicated Well	300+	77%	80%	79%
Pain 'Always' Well Controlled	300+	74%	72%	71%
Room and Bathroom 'Always' Clean	300+	79%	75%	73%
Timely Help 'Always' Received	300+	64%	69%	68%
Would Definitely Recommend Hospital	300+	79%	73%	71%
Use of Medical Imaging				
Cardiac Imaging Stress Test before Surgery	217	6.0%	5.3%	5.3%
Combination Abdominal CT Scan	567	1.4%	16.4%	10.5%
Combination Brain/Sinus CT Scan	605	1.8%	2.7%	2.7%
Combination Chest CT Scan	114	2.6%	5.6%	2.7%
Follow-up Mammogram/Ultrasound	251	6.0%	7.9%	8.8%
Lumbar Spine MRI for Low Back Pain[1]	-	-	39.6%	37.2%

Northwest Hills Surgical Hospital

6818 Austin Center Blvd Suite 100
Austin, TX 78731
Phone: 512-346-1994
URL: www.scasurgery.com
Type: Acute Care Hospitals
Emergency Services: Yes
Ownership: Proprietary
Key Personnel:
CEO/President. . . . . Andrew Hayek

Measure	Cases	This Hosp.	State Avg.	U.S. Avg.
Blood Clot Prevention and Treatment				
Anticoagulation Overlap Therapy[7]	-	-	93%	93%
ICU Venous Thromboembolism Prophylaxis[7]	-	-	92%	92%
Incidence of Potentially Preventable VTE[7]	-	-	9%	10%
UFH with Dosages/Platelet Monitoring[7]	-	-	96%	97%
Venous Thromboembolism Prophylaxis	43	98%	82%	85%
Warfarin Therapy Discharge Instructions[7]	-	-	84%	75%
Chest Pain/Possible Heart Attack Care				
Aspirin Given Within 24 Hours of Arrival[5]	-	-	94%	96%
Fibrinolytic Meds Within 30 Min. of Arrival[5]	-	-	47%	58%
Average Time to ECG (minutes)[5]	-	-	8	7
Average Time to Transfer (minutes)[5]	-	-	62	60
Children's Asthma Care				
Received Home Management Plan of Care	-	-	93%	88%
Received Reliever Medication	-	-	100%	100%
Received Systemic Corticosteroids	-	-	100%	100%
Emergency Department				
Admittance Decision Time (minutes)[7]	-	-	99	98
Head CT Results Within 45 Min. of Arrival[5]	-	-	54%	57%
Patients Who Left ER Before Being Seen	71	0%	3%	2%
Time from ER Arrival to Admit. (minutes)[7]	-	-	270	274
Time from ER Arrival to Discharge (minutes)	53	60	127	134
Time in ER Before Being Evaluated (minutes)	56	5	26	26
Time to Pain Meds for Fractures (minutes)[5]	-	-	57	57
Heart Attack Care				
Aspirin Given at Discharge[5]	-	-	99%	99%
Fibrinolytic Meds Within 30 Min. of Arrival[5]	-	-	49%	54%
PCI Within 90 Minutes of Arrival[5]	-	-	95%	96%
Statin Prescribed at Discharge[5]	-	-	98%	98%
Heart Failure Care				
ACE Inhibitor or ARB for LVSD[5]	-	-	97%	97%
Discharge Instructions Given[5]	-	-	95%	94%
Evaluation of LVS Function[5]	-	-	99%	99%
Medicare Spending				
Medicare Spending per Patient (ratio)	-	1.10	1.03	0.98
Pneumonia Care				
Appropriate Initial Antibiotic Given[5]	-	-	95%	95%
Blood Culture Timing[5]	-	-	98%	98%
Pregnancy and Delivery Care				
Newborn Deliveries Scheduled Early[7]	-	-	7%	6%
Preventive Care				
Immunization for Influenza	217	43%	90%	90%
Immunization for Pneumonia	160	57%	92%	92%
Stroke Care				
Anticoagulation Therapy for Atrial Fibrillation[5]	-	-	96%	95%
Antithrombotic Therapy Timing[5]	-	-	98%	98%
Assessed for Rehabilitation[5]	-	-	98%	97%
Discharged on Antithrombotic Therapy[5]	-	-	99%	99%
Discharged on Statin Medication[5]	-	-	95%	94%
Thrombolytic Therapy Timing[5]	-	-	68%	66%
Venous Thromboembolism Prophylaxis[5]	-	-	94%	94%
Written Stroke Educational Materials Given[5]	-	-	92%	88%
Surgical Care Improvement Project				
Appropriate Beta Blocker Usage[1]	-	-	98%	98%
Appropriate VTP Within 24 Hours	16	100%	98%	98%
Controlled Postoperative Blood Glucose[7]	-	-	96%	97%
Perioperative Temperature Management	17	59%	100%	100%
Prophylactic Antibiotic Selection[1]	-	-	99%	99%
Prophylactic Antibiotic Selection (Outpatient)	201	100%	98%	98%
Prophylactic Antibiotic Stopped[1]	-	-	98%	98%
Prophylactic Antibiotic Timing[1]	-	-	99%	99%
Prophylactic Antibiotic Timing (Outpatient)	203	99%	98%	98%
Urinary Catheter Removal[7]	-	-	98%	97%
Survey of Patients' Hospital Experiences				
Area Around Room 'Always' Quiet at Night	(a)	91%	68%	61%
Doctors 'Always' Communicated Well	(a)	83%	83%	82%
Home Recovery Information Given	(a)	91%	85%	85%
Hospital Given 9 or 10 on 10 Point Scale	(a)	86%	73%	71%
Meds 'Always' Explained Before Given	(a)	75%	66%	64%
Nurses 'Always' Communicated Well	(a)	89%	80%	79%
Pain 'Always' Well Controlled	(a)	80%	72%	71%
Room and Bathroom 'Always' Clean	(a)	86%	75%	73%
Timely Help 'Always' Received	(a)	90%	69%	68%
Would Definitely Recommend Hospital	(a)	83%	73%	71%
Use of Medical Imaging				
Cardiac Imaging Stress Test before Surgery[7]	-	-	5.3%	5.3%
Combination Abdominal CT Scan[7]	-	-	16.4%	10.5%
Combination Brain/Sinus CT Scan[7]	-	-	2.7%	2.7%
Combination Chest CT Scan[7]	-	-	5.6%	2.7%
Follow-up Mammogram/Ultrasound[7]	-	-	7.9%	8.8%
Lumbar Spine MRI for Low Back Pain[7]	-	-	39.6%	37.2%

Saint David's Medical Center

919 E 32nd St
Austin, TX 78705
Phone: 512-476-7111
Fax: 512-867-5831
URL: www.stdavidsrehab.com
Type: Acute Care Hospitals
Emergency Services: Yes
Ownership: Voluntary non-profit - Private
Beds: 107
Key Personnel:
Quality Assurance . . . . Cynthia Duggins
CEO/President. . . . . Cole Eslyn
Chief of Medical Staff. . . . . Cioo Race, MD

Measure	Cases	This Hosp.	State Avg.	U.S. Avg.
Blood Clot Prevention and Treatment				
Anticoagulation Overlap Therapy[2]	83	99%	93%	93%

NOTE: Hospital profiles are in alphabetical order by state, then city, then hospital within the city; Rankings exclude hospitals with less than 25 cases except for patient surveys which excludes hospitals with less than 100 cases; (a) 100-299 cases; (1) The number of cases/patients is too few to report; (2) Data submitted were based on a sample of cases/patients; (3) Results are based on a shorter time period than required; (4) Data suppressed by CMS for one or more quarters; (5) Results are not available for this reporting period; (6) Fewer than 100 patients completed the HCAHPS survey; (7) No cases met the criteria for this measure; (8) The lower limit of the confidence interval cannot be calculated if the number of observed infections equals zero; (9) No data are available from the state/territory for this reporting period; (10) The scores shown reflect fewer than 50 completed surveys; (11) There were discrepancies in the data collection process; (12) This measure does not apply to this hospital for this reporting period; (13) Results cannot be calculated for this reporting period; (14) The results for this state are combined with nearby states to protect confidentiality; Please refer to the User's Guide for a full explanation of data.

Measure	Cases	This Hosp.	State Avg.	U.S. Avg.
ICU Venous Thromboembolism Prophylaxis[2]	90	98%	92%	92%
Incidence of Potentially Preventable VTE[1,2]	-	-	9%	10%
UFH with Dosages/Platelet Monitoring[2]	24	100%	96%	97%
Venous Thromboembolism Prophylaxis[2]	337	96%	82%	85%
Warfarin Therapy Discharge Instructions[2]	72	100%	84%	75%
Chest Pain/Possible Heart Attack Care				
Aspirin Given Within 24 Hours of Arrival	49	100%	94%	96%
Fibrinolytic Meds Within 30 Min. of Arrival[7]	-	-	47%	58%
Average Time to ECG (minutes)	51	4	8	7
Average Time to Transfer (minutes)[1]	-	-	62	60
Children's Asthma Care				
Received Home Management Plan of Care	-	-	93%	88%
Received Reliever Medication	-	-	100%	100%
Received Systemic Corticosteroids	-	-	100%	100%
Emergency Department				
Admittance Decision Time (minutes)[2]	532	162	99	98
Head CT Results Within 45 Min. of Arrival[1]	-	-	54%	57%
Patients Who Left ER Before Being Seen	53,708	1%	3%	2%
Time from ER Arrival to Admit. (minutes)[2]	532	284	270	274
Time from ER Arrival to Discharge (minutes)	503	156	127	134
Time in ER Before Being Evaluated (minutes)	527	22	26	26
Time to Pain Meds for Fractures (minutes)	129	45	57	57
Heart Attack Care				
Aspirin Given at Discharge	414	100%	99%	99%
Fibrinolytic Meds Within 30 Min. of Arrival[7]	-	-	49%	54%
PCI Within 90 Minutes of Arrival	59	100%	95%	96%
Statin Prescribed at Discharge	395	100%	98%	98%
Heart Failure Care				
ACE Inhibitor or ARB for LVSD	203	100%	97%	97%
Discharge Instructions Given	587	97%	95%	94%
Evaluation of LVS Function	675	100%	99%	99%
Medicare Spending				
Medicare Spending per Patient (ratio)	-	1.03	1.03	0.98
Pneumonia Care				
Appropriate Initial Antibiotic Given	188	98%	95%	95%
Blood Culture Timing	366	99%	98%	98%
Pregnancy and Delivery Care				
Newborn Deliveries Scheduled Early[2]	94	1%	7%	6%
Preventive Care				
Immunization for Influenza[2]	532	99%	90%	90%
Immunization for Pneumonia[2]	625	99%	92%	92%
Stroke Care				
Anticoagulation Therapy for Atrial Fibrillation[2]	11	100%	96%	95%
Antithrombotic Therapy Timing[2]	77	99%	98%	98%
Assessed for Rehabilitation[2]	119	99%	98%	97%
Discharged on Antithrombotic Therapy[2]	89	100%	99%	99%
Discharged on Statin Medication[2]	69	100%	95%	94%
Thrombolytic Therapy Timing[1,2]	-	-	68%	66%
Venous Thromboembolism Prophylaxis[2]	125	98%	94%	94%
Written Stroke Educational Materials Given[2]	67	99%	92%	88%
Surgical Care Improvement Project				
Appropriate Beta Blocker Usage[2]	236	100%	98%	98%
Appropriate VTP Within 24 Hours[2]	484	100%	98%	98%
Controlled Postoperative Blood Glucose[2]	216	97%	96%	97%
Perioperative Temperature Management[2]	596	100%	100%	100%
Prophylactic Antibiotic Selection[2]	586	100%	99%	99%
Prophylactic Antibiotic Selection (Outpatient)	724	100%	98%	98%
Prophylactic Antibiotic Stopped[2]	574	100%	98%	98%
Prophylactic Antibiotic Timing[2]	588	99%	99%	99%
Prophylactic Antibiotic Timing (Outpatient)	725	99%	98%	98%
Urinary Catheter Removal[2]	458	99%	98%	97%
Survey of Patients' Hospital Experiences				
Area Around Room 'Always' Quiet at Night	300+	68%	68%	61%
Doctors 'Always' Communicated Well	300+	83%	83%	82%
Home Recovery Information Given	300+	88%	85%	85%
Hospital Given 9 or 10 on 10 Point Scale	300+	79%	73%	71%
Meds 'Always' Explained Before Given	300+	66%	66%	64%
Nurses 'Always' Communicated Well	300+	80%	80%	79%
Pain 'Always' Well Controlled	300+	74%	72%	71%
Room and Bathroom 'Always' Clean	300+	73%	75%	73%
Timely Help 'Always' Received	300+	67%	69%	68%
Would Definitely Recommend Hospital	300+	80%	73%	71%
Use of Medical Imaging				
Cardiac Imaging Stress Test before Surgery	4,459	4.3%	5.3%	5.3%
Combination Abdominal CT Scan	759	3.2%	16.4%	10.5%
Combination Brain/Sinus CT Scan	997	2.7%	2.7%	2.7%
Combination Chest CT Scan	209	1.0%	5.6%	2.7%
Follow-up Mammogram/Ultrasound	1,863	6.4%	7.9%	8.8%
Lumbar Spine MRI for Low Back Pain[1]	-	-	39.6%	37.2%

Saint David's South Austin Medical Center

901 West Ben White Blvd
Austin, TX 78704
Phone: 512-448-7107
Fax: 512-416-6213
URL: www.southaustinhospital.com
Type: Acute Care Hospitals
Emergency Services: Yes
Ownership: Proprietary
Beds: 252

Key Personnel:
Emergency Room . . . . Jerry Anderson
President/CEO. . . . . C. David Huffstutler
Chief of Medical Staff. . . . . Thomas W. Knight, MD
Ambulatory Care . . . . Phillip Neeley
Quality Assurance . . . . Dave Thomsen

Measure	Cases	This Hosp.	State Avg.	U.S. Avg.
Blood Clot Prevention and Treatment				
Anticoagulation Overlap Therapy[2]	105	98%	93%	93%
ICU Venous Thromboembolism Prophylaxis[2]	80	94%	92%	92%
Incidence of Potentially Preventable VTE[2]	22	0%	9%	10%
UFH with Dosages/Platelet Monitoring[2]	19	95%	96%	97%
Venous Thromboembolism Prophylaxis[2]	380	95%	82%	85%
Warfarin Therapy Discharge Instructions[2]	79	100%	84%	75%
Chest Pain/Possible Heart Attack Care				
Aspirin Given Within 24 Hours of Arrival	12	100%	94%	96%
Fibrinolytic Meds Within 30 Min. of Arrival[3,7]	-	-	47%	58%
Average Time to ECG (minutes)	12	10	8	7
Average Time to Transfer (minutes)[3,7]	-	-	62	60
Children's Asthma Care				
Received Home Management Plan of Care	-	-	93%	88%
Received Reliever Medication	-	-	100%	100%
Received Systemic Corticosteroids	-	-	100%	100%
Emergency Department				
Admittance Decision Time (minutes)[2]	784	127	99	98
Head CT Results Within 45 Min. of Arrival	17	41%	54%	57%
Patients Who Left ER Before Being Seen	>100k	1%	3%	2%
Time from ER Arrival to Admit. (minutes)[2]	785	264	270	274
Time from ER Arrival to Discharge (minutes)	509	129	127	134
Time in ER Before Being Evaluated (minutes)	549	20	26	26
Time to Pain Meds for Fractures (minutes)	194	44	57	57
Heart Attack Care				
Aspirin Given at Discharge[2]	311	100%	99%	99%
Fibrinolytic Meds Within 30 Min. of Arrival[2,7]	-	-	49%	54%
PCI Within 90 Minutes of Arrival[2]	68	100%	95%	96%
Statin Prescribed at Discharge[2]	299	100%	98%	98%
Heart Failure Care				
ACE Inhibitor or ARB for LVSD[2]	92	100%	97%	97%
Discharge Instructions Given[2]	296	98%	95%	94%
Evaluation of LVS Function[2]	360	100%	99%	99%
Medicare Spending				
Medicare Spending per Patient (ratio)	-	1.03	1.03	0.98
Pneumonia Care				
Appropriate Initial Antibiotic Given[2]	98	97%	95%	95%
Blood Culture Timing[2]	159	99%	98%	98%
Pregnancy and Delivery Care				
Newborn Deliveries Scheduled Early[2]	47	0%	7%	6%
Preventive Care				
Immunization for Influenza[2]	575	99%	90%	90%
Immunization for Pneumonia[2]	730	98%	92%	92%
Stroke Care				
Anticoagulation Therapy for Atrial Fibrillation[1,2]	-	-	96%	95%
Antithrombotic Therapy Timing[2]	67	99%	98%	98%
Assessed for Rehabilitation[2]	75	100%	98%	97%
Discharged on Antithrombotic Therapy[2]	71	100%	99%	99%
Discharged on Statin Medication[2]	52	100%	95%	94%
Thrombolytic Therapy Timing[1,2]	-	-	68%	66%
Venous Thromboembolism Prophylaxis[2]	70	99%	94%	94%
Written Stroke Educational Materials Given[2]	42	83%	92%	88%
Surgical Care Improvement Project				
Appropriate Beta Blocker Usage[2]	188	99%	98%	98%
Appropriate VTP Within 24 Hours[2]	407	100%	98%	98%
Controlled Postoperative Blood Glucose[2]	124	98%	96%	97%
Perioperative Temperature Management[2]	473	100%	100%	100%
Prophylactic Antibiotic Selection[2]	381	100%	99%	99%
Prophylactic Antibiotic Selection (Outpatient)	449	99%	98%	98%
Prophylactic Antibiotic Stopped[2]	364	98%	98%	98%
Prophylactic Antibiotic Timing[2]	381	100%	99%	99%
Prophylactic Antibiotic Timing (Outpatient)	449	100%	98%	98%
Urinary Catheter Removal[2]	246	99%	98%	97%
Survey of Patients' Hospital Experiences				
Area Around Room 'Always' Quiet at Night	300+	64%	68%	61%
Doctors 'Always' Communicated Well	300+	79%	83%	82%
Home Recovery Information Given	300+	86%	85%	85%
Hospital Given 9 or 10 on 10 Point Scale	300+	74%	73%	71%
Meds 'Always' Explained Before Given	300+	68%	66%	64%
Nurses 'Always' Communicated Well	300+	80%	80%	79%
Pain 'Always' Well Controlled	300+	74%	72%	71%
Room and Bathroom 'Always' Clean	300+	74%	75%	73%
Timely Help 'Always' Received	300+	65%	69%	68%
Would Definitely Recommend Hospital	300+	76%	73%	71%
Use of Medical Imaging				
Cardiac Imaging Stress Test before Surgery	288	5.2%	5.3%	5.3%
Combination Abdominal CT Scan	627	1.1%	16.4%	10.5%
Combination Brain/Sinus CT Scan	874	2.1%	2.7%	2.7%
Combination Chest CT Scan	131	5.3%	5.6%	2.7%
Follow-up Mammogram/Ultrasound	97	7.2%	7.9%	8.8%
Lumbar Spine MRI for Low Back Pain[1]	-	-	39.6%	37.2%

Seton Medical Center Austin

1201 W 38th St
Austin, TX 78705
Phone: 512-324-1000
Fax: 512-380-7527
URL: www.seton.net
Type: Acute Care Hospitals
Emergency Services: Yes
Ownership: Voluntary non-profit - Private
Beds: 471

Key Personnel:
CEO/President. . . . . John Brindley
Chief of Medical Staff. . . . . Phillip Church
Cardiac Laboratory. . . . . Joseph Gallinger
Emergency Room . . . . Mark Vassallo

Measure	Cases	This Hosp.	State Avg.	U.S. Avg.
Blood Clot Prevention and Treatment				
Anticoagulation Overlap Therapy[2]	82	94%	93%	93%
ICU Venous Thromboembolism Prophylaxis[2]	71	86%	92%	92%
Incidence of Potentially Preventable VTE[2]	25	8%	9%	10%
UFH with Dosages/Platelet Monitoring[2]	27	100%	96%	97%
Venous Thromboembolism Prophylaxis[2]	329	84%	82%	85%
Warfarin Therapy Discharge Instructions[2]	66	36%	84%	75%
Chest Pain/Possible Heart Attack Care				
Aspirin Given Within 24 Hours of Arrival[1]	-	-	94%	96%
Fibrinolytic Meds Within 30 Min. of Arrival[3,7]	-	-	47%	58%
Average Time to ECG (minutes)[1]	-	-	8	7
Average Time to Transfer (minutes)[3,7]	-	-	62	60
Children's Asthma Care				
Received Home Management Plan of Care	-	-	93%	88%
Received Reliever Medication	-	-	100%	100%
Received Systemic Corticosteroids	-	-	100%	100%
Emergency Department				
Admittance Decision Time (minutes)[2,7]	-	-	99	98
Head CT Results Within 45 Min. of Arrival[1]	-	-	54%	57%
Patients Who Left ER Before Being Seen	38,221	1%	3%	2%
Time from ER Arrival to Admit. (minutes)[2]	467	266	270	274
Time from ER Arrival to Discharge (minutes)	330	170	127	134
Time in ER Before Being Evaluated (minutes)	357	26	26	26
Time to Pain Meds for Fractures (minutes)	27	46	57	57
Heart Attack Care				
Aspirin Given at Discharge	186	99%	99%	99%
Fibrinolytic Meds Within 30 Min. of Arrival[7]	-	-	49%	54%
PCI Within 90 Minutes of Arrival	22	100%	95%	96%
Statin Prescribed at Discharge	176	98%	98%	98%
Heart Failure Care				
ACE Inhibitor or ARB for LVSD[2]	79	100%	97%	97%
Discharge Instructions Given[2]	247	95%	95%	94%

NOTE: Hospital profiles are in alphabetical order by state, then city, then hospital within the city; Rankings exclude hospitals with less than 25 cases except for patient surveys which excludes hospitals with less than 100 cases; (a) 100-299 cases; (1) The number of cases/patients is too few to report; (2) Data submitted were based on a sample of cases/patients; (3) Results are based on a shorter time period than required; (4) Data suppressed by CMS for one or more quarters; (5) Results are not available for this reporting period; (6) Fewer than 100 patients completed the HCAHPS survey; (7) No cases met the criteria for this measure; (8) The lower limit of the confidence interval cannot be calculated if the number of observed infections equals zero; (9) No data are available from the state/territory for this reporting period; (10) The scores shown reflect fewer than 50 completed surveys; (11) There were discrepancies in the data collection process; (12) This measure does not apply to this hospital for this reporting period; (13) Results cannot be calculated for this reporting period; (14) The results for this state are combined with nearby states to protect confidentiality; Please refer to the User's Guide for a full explanation of data.

Measure	Cases	This Hosp.	State Avg.	U.S. Avg.
Evaluation of LVS Function[2]	285	100%	99%	99%
Medicare Spending				
Medicare Spending per Patient (ratio)	-	1.04	1.03	0.98
Pneumonia Care				
Appropriate Initial Antibiotic Given	162	97%	95%	95%
Blood Culture Timing	276	98%	98%	98%
Pregnancy and Delivery Care				
Newborn Deliveries Scheduled Early	227	0%	7%	6%
Preventive Care				
Immunization for Influenza[2]	517	87%	90%	90%
Immunization for Pneumonia[2]	614	86%	92%	92%
Stroke Care				
Anticoagulation Therapy for Atrial Fibrillation	40	98%	96%	95%
Antithrombotic Therapy Timing	165	96%	98%	98%
Assessed for Rehabilitation	223	96%	98%	97%
Discharged on Antithrombotic Therapy	201	100%	99%	99%
Discharged on Statin Medication	158	99%	95%	94%
Thrombolytic Therapy Timing	30	67%	68%	66%
Venous Thromboembolism Prophylaxis	220	95%	94%	94%
Written Stroke Educational Materials Given	124	94%	92%	88%
Surgical Care Improvement Project				
Appropriate Beta Blocker Usage[2]	204	98%	98%	98%
Appropriate VTP Within 24 Hours[2]	489	98%	98%	98%
Controlled Postoperative Blood Glucose[2]	134	95%	96%	97%
Perioperative Temperature Management[2]	581	100%	100%	100%
Prophylactic Antibiotic Selection[2]	559	99%	99%	99%
Prophylactic Antibiotic Selection (Outpatient)	578	99%	98%	98%
Prophylactic Antibiotic Stopped[2]	546	98%	98%	98%
Prophylactic Antibiotic Timing[2]	560	99%	99%	99%
Prophylactic Antibiotic Timing (Outpatient)	582	98%	98%	98%
Urinary Catheter Removal[2]	262	95%	98%	97%
Survey of Patients' Hospital Experiences				
Area Around Room 'Always' Quiet at Night	300+	56%	68%	61%
Doctors 'Always' Communicated Well	300+	82%	83%	82%
Home Recovery Information Given	300+	87%	85%	85%
Hospital Given 9 or 10 on 10 Point Scale	300+	72%	73%	71%
Meds 'Always' Explained Before Given	300+	64%	66%	64%
Nurses 'Always' Communicated Well	300+	76%	80%	79%
Pain 'Always' Well Controlled	300+	70%	72%	71%
Room and Bathroom 'Always' Clean	300+	65%	75%	73%
Timely Help 'Always' Received	300+	61%	69%	68%
Would Definitely Recommend Hospital	300+	75%	73%	71%
Use of Medical Imaging				
Cardiac Imaging Stress Test before Surgery	640	5.6%	5.3%	5.3%
Combination Abdominal CT Scan	404	2.5%	16.4%	10.5%
Combination Brain/Sinus CT Scan[1]	-	-	2.7%	2.7%
Combination Chest CT Scan	88	2.3%	5.6%	2.7%
Follow-up Mammogram/Ultrasound[1]	-	-	7.9%	8.8%
Lumbar Spine MRI for Low Back Pain[1]	-	-	39.6%	37.2%

Seton Northwest Hospital

11113 Research Boulevard Phone: 512-324-6000
Austin, TX 78759 Fax: 512-324-6123
URL: www.seton.net
Type: Acute Care Hospitals Emergency Services: Yes
Ownership: Voluntary non-profit - Private Beds: 103

Key Personnel:
Radiology. . . . . George R Brown
President/CEO. . . . . Jeff Cook
President/CEO. . . . . Ken Galadish
President/CEO. . . . . Jesus Garza
President . . . . Greg W. Hartman
President/CEO. . . . . Prathibha Varkey, MD, MPH, MBA
Quality Assurance . . . . Carol Wratten, MD, MBA, FACOG

Measure	Cases	This Hosp.	State Avg.	U.S. Avg.
Blood Clot Prevention and Treatment				
Anticoagulation Overlap Therapy[2]	22	100%	93%	93%
ICU Venous Thromboembolism Prophylaxis[2]	62	95%	92%	92%
Incidence of Potentially Preventable VTE[1,2]	-	-	9%	10%
UFH with Dosages/Platelet Monitoring[1,2]	-	-	96%	97%
Venous Thromboembolism Prophylaxis[2]	300	90%	82%	85%
Warfarin Therapy Discharge Instructions[2]	20	75%	84%	75%
Chest Pain/Possible Heart Attack Care				
Aspirin Given Within 24 Hours of Arrival	52	98%	94%	96%
Fibrinolytic Meds Within 30 Min. of Arrival[7]	-	-	47%	58%
Average Time to ECG (minutes)	52	8	8	7
Average Time to Transfer (minutes)	14	30	62	60
Children's Asthma Care				
Received Home Management Plan of Care	-	-	93%	88%
Received Reliever Medication	-	-	100%	100%
Received Systemic Corticosteroids	-	-	100%	100%
Emergency Department				
Admittance Decision Time (minutes)[2,7]	-	-	99	98
Head CT Results Within 45 Min. of Arrival[1]	-	-	54%	57%
Patients Who Left ER Before Being Seen	35,588	1%	3%	2%
Time from ER Arrival to Admit. (minutes)[2]	597	293	270	274
Time from ER Arrival to Discharge (minutes)	362	176	127	134
Time in ER Before Being Evaluated (minutes)	381	29	26	26
Time to Pain Meds for Fractures (minutes)	26	64	57	57
Heart Attack Care				
Aspirin Given at Discharge[1,3]	-	-	99%	99%
Fibrinolytic Meds Within 30 Min. of Arrival[3,7]	-	-	49%	54%
PCI Within 90 Minutes of Arrival[3,7]	-	-	95%	96%
Statin Prescribed at Discharge[1,3]	-	-	98%	98%
Heart Failure Care				
ACE Inhibitor or ARB for LVSD	15	93%	97%	97%
Discharge Instructions Given	78	97%	95%	94%
Evaluation of LVS Function	91	100%	99%	99%
Medicare Spending				
Medicare Spending per Patient (ratio)	-	0.98	1.03	0.98
Pneumonia Care				
Appropriate Initial Antibiotic Given	94	99%	95%	95%
Blood Culture Timing	145	98%	98%	98%
Pregnancy and Delivery Care				
Newborn Deliveries Scheduled Early	77	0%	7%	6%
Preventive Care				
Immunization for Influenza[2]	480	91%	90%	90%
Immunization for Pneumonia[2]	419	94%	92%	92%
Stroke Care				
Anticoagulation Therapy for Atrial Fibrillation[1]	-	-	96%	95%
Antithrombotic Therapy Timing	30	97%	98%	98%
Assessed for Rehabilitation	40	98%	98%	97%
Discharged on Antithrombotic Therapy	40	95%	99%	99%
Discharged on Statin Medication	34	88%	95%	94%
Thrombolytic Therapy Timing[1]	-	-	68%	66%
Venous Thromboembolism Prophylaxis	30	97%	94%	94%
Written Stroke Educational Materials Given	33	39%	92%	88%
Surgical Care Improvement Project				
Appropriate Beta Blocker Usage	59	97%	98%	98%
Appropriate VTP Within 24 Hours	271	99%	98%	98%
Controlled Postoperative Blood Glucose[7]	-	-	96%	97%
Perioperative Temperature Management	289	100%	100%	100%
Prophylactic Antibiotic Selection	188	97%	99%	99%
Prophylactic Antibiotic Selection (Outpatient)	43	100%	98%	98%
Prophylactic Antibiotic Stopped	178	99%	98%	98%
Prophylactic Antibiotic Timing	188	100%	99%	99%
Prophylactic Antibiotic Timing (Outpatient)	44	98%	98%	98%
Urinary Catheter Removal	130	99%	98%	97%
Survey of Patients' Hospital Experiences				
Area Around Room 'Always' Quiet at Night	300+	60%	68%	61%
Doctors 'Always' Communicated Well	300+	80%	83%	82%
Home Recovery Information Given	300+	85%	85%	85%
Hospital Given 9 or 10 on 10 Point Scale	300+	69%	73%	71%
Meds 'Always' Explained Before Given	300+	60%	66%	64%
Nurses 'Always' Communicated Well	300+	76%	80%	79%
Pain 'Always' Well Controlled	300+	69%	72%	71%
Room and Bathroom 'Always' Clean	300+	68%	75%	73%
Timely Help 'Always' Received	300+	63%	69%	68%
Would Definitely Recommend Hospital	300+	74%	73%	71%
Use of Medical Imaging				
Cardiac Imaging Stress Test before Surgery	110	4.5%	5.3%	5.3%
Combination Abdominal CT Scan	254	2.0%	16.4%	10.5%
Combination Brain/Sinus CT Scan[1]	-	-	2.7%	2.7%
Combination Chest CT Scan	58	0.0%	5.6%	2.7%
Follow-up Mammogram/Ultrasound	260	4.6%	7.9%	8.8%
Lumbar Spine MRI for Low Back Pain[1]	-	-	39.6%	37.2%

Seton Southwest Hospital

7900 Fm 1826 Phone: 512-324-9000
Austin, TX 78737 Fax: 512-324-9040
URL: www.seton.net
Type: Acute Care Hospitals Emergency Services: Yes
Ownership: Voluntary non-profit - Private Beds: 17

Key Personnel:
Radiology. . . . . Scott E Campbell
CEO/President. . . . . Jesus Garza
Quality Assurance . . . . Carol Wratten, MD, MBA, FACOG

Measure	Cases	This Hosp.	State Avg.	U.S. Avg.
Blood Clot Prevention and Treatment				
Anticoagulation Overlap Therapy[2,7]	-	-	93%	93%
ICU Venous Thromboembolism Prophylaxis[2,7]	-	-	92%	92%
Incidence of Potentially Preventable VTE[2,7]	-	-	9%	10%
UFH with Dosages/Platelet Monitoring[2,7]	-	-	96%	97%
Venous Thromboembolism Prophylaxis[2]	85	76%	82%	85%
Warfarin Therapy Discharge Instructions[2,7]	-	-	84%	75%
Chest Pain/Possible Heart Attack Care				
Aspirin Given Within 24 Hours of Arrival	257	96%	94%	96%
Fibrinolytic Meds Within 30 Min. of Arrival[7]	-	-	47%	58%
Average Time to ECG (minutes)	263	7	8	7
Average Time to Transfer (minutes)[1]	-	-	62	60
Children's Asthma Care				
Received Home Management Plan of Care	-	-	93%	88%
Received Reliever Medication	-	-	100%	100%
Received Systemic Corticosteroids	-	-	100%	100%
Emergency Department				
Admittance Decision Time (minutes)[2,7]	-	-	99	98
Head CT Results Within 45 Min. of Arrival[1]	-	-	54%	57%
Patients Who Left ER Before Being Seen	38,221	1%	3%	2%
Time from ER Arrival to Admit. (minutes)[2]	46	254	270	274
Time from ER Arrival to Discharge (minutes)	330	151	127	134
Time in ER Before Being Evaluated (minutes)	342	17	26	26
Time to Pain Meds for Fractures (minutes)	43	36	57	57
Heart Attack Care				
Aspirin Given at Discharge[5]	-	-	99%	99%
Fibrinolytic Meds Within 30 Min. of Arrival[5]	-	-	49%	54%
PCI Within 90 Minutes of Arrival[5]	-	-	95%	96%
Statin Prescribed at Discharge[5]	-	-	98%	98%
Heart Failure Care				
ACE Inhibitor or ARB for LVSD[5]	-	-	97%	97%
Discharge Instructions Given[5]	-	-	95%	94%
Evaluation of LVS Function[5]	-	-	99%	99%
Medicare Spending				
Medicare Spending per Patient (ratio)	-	0.98	1.03	0.98
Pneumonia Care				
Appropriate Initial Antibiotic Given[5]	-	-	95%	95%
Blood Culture Timing[5]	-	-	98%	98%
Pregnancy and Delivery Care				
Newborn Deliveries Scheduled Early	49	0%	7%	6%
Preventive Care				
Immunization for Influenza[2]	186	96%	90%	90%
Immunization for Pneumonia[2]	27	85%	92%	92%
Stroke Care				
Anticoagulation Therapy for Atrial Fibrillation[5]	-	-	96%	95%
Antithrombotic Therapy Timing[5]	-	-	98%	98%
Assessed for Rehabilitation[5]	-	-	98%	97%
Discharged on Antithrombotic Therapy[5]	-	-	99%	99%
Discharged on Statin Medication[5]	-	-	95%	94%
Thrombolytic Therapy Timing[5]	-	-	68%	66%
Venous Thromboembolism Prophylaxis[5]	-	-	94%	94%
Written Stroke Educational Materials Given[5]	-	-	92%	88%
Surgical Care Improvement Project				
Appropriate Beta Blocker Usage[1,3]	-	-	98%	98%
Appropriate VTP Within 24 Hours[3]	16	100%	98%	98%
Controlled Postoperative Blood Glucose[3,7]	-	-	96%	97%
Perioperative Temperature Management[3]	26	100%	100%	100%
Prophylactic Antibiotic Selection[3]	13	92%	99%	99%
Prophylactic Antibiotic Selection (Outpatient)[1]	-	-	98%	98%
Prophylactic Antibiotic Stopped[3]	13	100%	98%	98%
Prophylactic Antibiotic Timing[3]	13	100%	99%	99%
Prophylactic Antibiotic Timing (Outpatient)[1]	-	-	98%	98%

NOTE: Hospital profiles are in alphabetical order by state, then city, then hospital within the city; Rankings exclude hospitals with less than 25 cases except for patient surveys which excludes hospitals with less than 100 cases; (a) 100-299 cases; (1) The number of cases/patients is too few to report; (2) Data submitted were based on a sample of cases/patients; (3) Results are based on a shorter time period than required; (4) Data suppressed by CMS for one or more quarters; (5) Results are not available for this reporting period; (6) Fewer than 100 patients completed the HCAHPS survey; (7) No cases met the criteria for this measure; (8) The lower limit of the confidence interval cannot be calculated if the number of observed infections equals zero; (9) No data are available from the state/territory for this reporting period; (10) The scores shown reflect fewer than 50 completed surveys; (11) There were discrepancies in the data collection process; (12) This measure does not apply to this hospital for this reporting period; (13) Results cannot be calculated for this reporting period; (14) The results for this state are combined with nearby states to protect confidentiality; Please refer to the User's Guide for a full explanation of data.

Measure	Cases	This Hosp.	State Avg.	U.S. Avg.
Urinary Catheter Removal[3]	15	100%	98%	97%
Survey of Patients' Hospital Experiences				
Area Around Room 'Always' Quiet at Night	(a)	70%	68%	61%
Doctors 'Always' Communicated Well	(a)	82%	83%	82%
Home Recovery Information Given	(a)	89%	85%	85%
Hospital Given 9 or 10 on 10 Point Scale	(a)	81%	73%	71%
Meds 'Always' Explained Before Given	(a)	63%	66%	64%
Nurses 'Always' Communicated Well	(a)	81%	80%	79%
Pain 'Always' Well Controlled	(a)	72%	72%	71%
Room and Bathroom 'Always' Clean	(a)	76%	75%	73%
Timely Help 'Always' Received	(a)	72%	69%	68%
Would Definitely Recommend Hospital	(a)	80%	73%	71%
Use of Medical Imaging				
Cardiac Imaging Stress Test before Surgery	45	4.4%	5.3%	5.3%
Combination Abdominal CT Scan	167	1.8%	16.4%	10.5%
Combination Brain/Sinus CT Scan[1]	-	-	2.7%	2.7%
Combination Chest CT Scan[1]	-	-	5.6%	2.7%
Follow-up Mammogram/Ultrasound	108	9.3%	7.9%	8.8%
Lumbar Spine MRI for Low Back Pain[1]	-	-	39.6%	37.2%

University Medical Center at Brackenridge

601 E 15th Street Phone: 512-324-7000
Austin, TX 78701
URL: www.seton.net/locations/brackenridge
Type: Acute Care Hospitals Emergency Services: Yes
Ownership: Voluntary non-profit - Private
Key Personnel:
Chief of Medical Staff.......... Dr Tom Caven
CEO/President............... Jesus Garza
Emergency Room .... Cindy Joy-McCoy, RN
Quality Assurance .... Carol Wratten, MD, MBA, FACOG

Measure	Cases	This Hosp.	State Avg.	U.S. Avg.
Blood Clot Prevention and Treatment				
Anticoagulation Overlap Therapy[2]	49	94%	93%	93%
ICU Venous Thromboembolism Prophylaxis[2]	71	97%	92%	92%
Incidence of Potentially Preventable VTE[2]	23	4%	9%	10%
UFH with Dosages/Platelet Monitoring[2]	17	100%	96%	97%
Venous Thromboembolism Prophylaxis[2]	313	87%	82%	85%
Warfarin Therapy Discharge Instructions[2]	44	70%	84%	75%
Chest Pain/Possible Heart Attack Care				
Aspirin Given Within 24 Hours of Arrival[1,3]	-	-	94%	96%
Fibrinolytic Meds Within 30 Min. of Arrival[5]	-	-	47%	58%
Average Time to ECG (minutes)[1,3]	-	-	8	7
Average Time to Transfer (minutes)[5]	-	-	62	60
Children's Asthma Care				
Received Home Management Plan of Care	-	-	93%	88%
Received Reliever Medication	-	-	100%	100%
Received Systemic Corticosteroids	-	-	100%	100%
Emergency Department				
Admittance Decision Time (minutes)[2,7]	-	-	99	98
Head CT Results Within 45 Min. of Arrival[3,7]	-	-	54%	57%
Patients Who Left ER Before Being Seen	71,280	6%	3%	2%
Time from ER Arrival to Admit. (minutes)[2]	698	357	270	274
Time from ER Arrival to Discharge (minutes)	327	214	127	134
Time in ER Before Being Evaluated (minutes)	391	29	26	26
Time to Pain Meds for Fractures (minutes)	56	50	57	57
Heart Attack Care				
Aspirin Given at Discharge	86	100%	99%	99%
Fibrinolytic Meds Within 30 Min. of Arrival[7]	-	-	49%	54%
PCI Within 90 Minutes of Arrival	24	92%	95%	96%
Statin Prescribed at Discharge	79	99%	98%	98%
Heart Failure Care				
ACE Inhibitor or ARB for LVSD	84	99%	97%	97%
Discharge Instructions Given	220	94%	95%	94%
Evaluation of LVS Function	241	100%	99%	99%
Medicare Spending				
Medicare Spending per Patient (ratio)	-	1.05	1.03	0.98
Pneumonia Care				
Appropriate Initial Antibiotic Given	74	93%	95%	95%
Blood Culture Timing	143	98%	98%	98%
Pregnancy and Delivery Care				
Newborn Deliveries Scheduled Early	97	0%	7%	6%
Preventive Care				
Immunization for Influenza[2]	532	91%	90%	90%
Immunization for Pneumonia[2]	425	90%	92%	92%
Stroke Care				
Anticoagulation Therapy for Atrial Fibrillation	14	100%	96%	95%
Antithrombotic Therapy Timing	116	93%	98%	98%
Assessed for Rehabilitation	188	98%	98%	97%
Discharged on Antithrombotic Therapy	138	99%	99%	99%
Discharged on Statin Medication	96	97%	95%	94%
Thrombolytic Therapy Timing	16	75%	68%	66%
Venous Thromboembolism Prophylaxis	195	94%	94%	94%
Written Stroke Educational Materials Given	125	75%	92%	88%
Surgical Care Improvement Project				
Appropriate Beta Blocker Usage[2]	58	100%	98%	98%
Appropriate VTP Within 24 Hours[2]	298	97%	98%	98%
Controlled Postoperative Blood Glucose[1,2]	-	-	96%	97%
Perioperative Temperature Management[2]	347	100%	100%	100%
Prophylactic Antibiotic Selection[2]	224	99%	99%	99%
Prophylactic Antibiotic Selection (Outpatient)	270	99%	98%	98%
Prophylactic Antibiotic Stopped[2]	220	100%	98%	98%
Prophylactic Antibiotic Timing[2]	224	99%	99%	99%
Prophylactic Antibiotic Timing (Outpatient)	270	99%	98%	98%
Urinary Catheter Removal[2]	114	97%	98%	97%
Survey of Patients' Hospital Experiences				
Area Around Room 'Always' Quiet at Night	300+	60%	68%	61%
Doctors 'Always' Communicated Well	300+	77%	83%	82%
Home Recovery Information Given	300+	86%	85%	85%
Hospital Given 9 or 10 on 10 Point Scale	300+	73%	73%	71%
Meds 'Always' Explained Before Given	300+	64%	66%	64%
Nurses 'Always' Communicated Well	300+	75%	80%	79%
Pain 'Always' Well Controlled	300+	68%	72%	71%
Room and Bathroom 'Always' Clean	300+	65%	75%	73%
Timely Help 'Always' Received	300+	60%	69%	68%
Would Definitely Recommend Hospital	300+	70%	73%	71%
Use of Medical Imaging				
Cardiac Imaging Stress Test before Surgery	51	3.9%	5.3%	5.3%
Combination Abdominal CT Scan	240	2.1%	16.4%	10.5%
Combination Brain/Sinus CT Scan	395	4.8%	2.7%	2.7%
Combination Chest CT Scan	143	0.0%	5.6%	2.7%
Follow-up Mammogram/Ultrasound	102	8.8%	7.9%	8.8%
Lumbar Spine MRI for Low Back Pain[1]	-	-	39.6%	37.2%

Texas Health Harris Methodist Hospital Azle

108 Denver Trail Phone: 817-444-8700
Azle, TX 76020 Fax: 817-882-2553
URL: www.hmhs.org
Type: Acute Care Hospitals Emergency Services: Yes
Ownership: Voluntary non-profit - Church Beds: 44
Key Personnel:
Infection Control............. Jean Earls
CEO/President............... Bob Ellzey, FACHE
Quality Assurance .... Monica Goth
Chief of Medical Staff.......... Judy Laviolette, MD
Anesthesiology............... William Sanders, D.O.

Measure	Cases	This Hosp.	State Avg.	U.S. Avg.
Blood Clot Prevention and Treatment				
Anticoagulation Overlap Therapy[2]	17	82%	93%	93%
ICU Venous Thromboembolism Prophylaxis[2]	48	96%	92%	92%
Incidence of Potentially Preventable VTE[1,2]	-	-	9%	10%
UFH with Dosages/Platelet Monitoring[2,7]	-	-	96%	97%
Venous Thromboembolism Prophylaxis[2]	211	96%	82%	85%
Warfarin Therapy Discharge Instructions[2]	11	82%	84%	75%
Chest Pain/Possible Heart Attack Care				
Aspirin Given Within 24 Hours of Arrival	118	99%	94%	96%
Fibrinolytic Meds Within 30 Min. of Arrival[1]	-	-	47%	58%
Average Time to ECG (minutes)	123	8	8	7
Average Time to Transfer (minutes)	19	81	62	60
Children's Asthma Care				
Received Home Management Plan of Care	-	-	93%	88%
Received Reliever Medication	-	-	100%	100%
Received Systemic Corticosteroids	-	-	100%	100%
Emergency Department				
Admittance Decision Time (minutes)[2]	699	77	99	98
Head CT Results Within 45 Min. of Arrival[1]	-	-	54%	57%
Patients Who Left ER Before Being Seen	27,241	3%	3%	2%
Time from ER Arrival to Admit. (minutes)[2]	699	209	270	274
Time from ER Arrival to Discharge (minutes)	435	126	127	134
Time in ER Before Being Evaluated (minutes)	501	40	26	26
Time to Pain Meds for Fractures (minutes)	100	62	57	57
Heart Attack Care				
Aspirin Given at Discharge[1]	-	-	99%	99%
Fibrinolytic Meds Within 30 Min. of Arrival[7]	-	-	49%	54%
PCI Within 90 Minutes of Arrival[7]	-	-	95%	96%
Statin Prescribed at Discharge[1]	-	-	98%	98%
Heart Failure Care				
ACE Inhibitor or ARB for LVSD	18	100%	97%	97%
Discharge Instructions Given	68	100%	95%	94%
Evaluation of LVS Function	96	100%	99%	99%
Medicare Spending				
Medicare Spending per Patient (ratio)	-	1.20	1.03	0.98
Pneumonia Care				
Appropriate Initial Antibiotic Given	103	97%	95%	95%
Blood Culture Timing	156	100%	98%	98%
Pregnancy and Delivery Care				
Newborn Deliveries Scheduled Early[7]	-	-	7%	6%
Preventive Care				
Immunization for Influenza[2]	361	100%	90%	90%
Immunization for Pneumonia[2]	570	100%	92%	92%
Stroke Care				
Anticoagulation Therapy for Atrial Fibrillation[1,2]	-	-	96%	95%
Antithrombotic Therapy Timing[1,2]	-	-	98%	98%
Assessed for Rehabilitation[1,2]	-	-	98%	97%
Discharged on Antithrombotic Therapy[1,2]	-	-	99%	99%
Discharged on Statin Medication[1,2]	-	-	95%	94%
Thrombolytic Therapy Timing[2,7]	-	-	68%	66%
Venous Thromboembolism Prophylaxis[1,2]	-	-	94%	94%
Written Stroke Educational Materials Given[1,2]	-	-	92%	88%
Surgical Care Improvement Project				
Appropriate Beta Blocker Usage[1,2]	-	-	98%	98%
Appropriate VTP Within 24 Hours[2]	31	97%	98%	98%
Controlled Postoperative Blood Glucose[2,7]	-	-	96%	97%
Perioperative Temperature Management[2]	32	97%	100%	100%
Prophylactic Antibiotic Selection[2]	23	100%	99%	99%
Prophylactic Antibiotic Selection (Outpatient)[1,3]	-	-	98%	98%
Prophylactic Antibiotic Stopped[2]	21	95%	98%	98%
Prophylactic Antibiotic Timing[2]	23	96%	99%	99%
Prophylactic Antibiotic Timing (Outpatient)[1,3]	-	-	98%	98%
Urinary Catheter Removal[2]	25	88%	98%	97%
Survey of Patients' Hospital Experiences				
Area Around Room 'Always' Quiet at Night	300+	64%	68%	61%
Doctors 'Always' Communicated Well	300+	83%	83%	82%
Home Recovery Information Given	300+	91%	85%	85%
Hospital Given 9 or 10 on 10 Point Scale	300+	72%	73%	71%
Meds 'Always' Explained Before Given	300+	66%	66%	64%
Nurses 'Always' Communicated Well	300+	80%	80%	79%
Pain 'Always' Well Controlled	300+	70%	72%	71%
Room and Bathroom 'Always' Clean	300+	83%	75%	73%
Timely Help 'Always' Received	300+	76%	69%	68%
Would Definitely Recommend Hospital	300+	70%	73%	71%
Use of Medical Imaging				
Cardiac Imaging Stress Test before Surgery[1]	-	-	5.3%	5.3%
Combination Abdominal CT Scan	360	10.6%	16.4%	10.5%
Combination Brain/Sinus CT Scan[1]	-	-	2.7%	2.7%
Combination Chest CT Scan	97	11.3%	5.6%	2.7%
Follow-up Mammogram/Ultrasound	475	10.7%	7.9%	8.8%
Lumbar Spine MRI for Low Back Pain[1]	-	-	39.6%	37.2%

Ballinger Memorial Hospital

608 Avenue B Phone: 325-365-2531
Ballinger, TX 76821
Type: Critical Access Hospitals Emergency Services: Yes
Ownership: Govt - Hospital Dist/Auth

Measure	Cases	This Hosp.	State Avg.	U.S. Avg.
Blood Clot Prevention and Treatment				
Anticoagulation Overlap Therapy[5]	-	-	93%	93%
ICU Venous Thromboembolism Prophylaxis[5]	-	-	92%	92%

NOTE: Hospital profiles are in alphabetical order by state, then city, then hospital within the city; Rankings exclude hospitals with less than 25 cases except for patient surveys which excludes hospitals with less than 100 cases; (a) 100-299 cases; (1) The number of cases/patients is too few to report; (2) Data submitted were based on a sample of cases/patients; (3) Results are based on a shorter time period than required; (4) Data suppressed by CMS for one or more quarters; (5) Results are not available for this reporting period; (6) Fewer than 100 patients completed the HCAHPS survey; (7) No cases met the criteria for this measure; (8) The lower limit of the confidence interval cannot be calculated if the number of observed infections equals zero; (9) No data are available from the state/territory for this reporting period; (10) The scores shown reflect fewer than 50 completed surveys; (11) There were discrepancies in the data collection process; (12) This measure does not apply to this hospital for this reporting period; (13) Results cannot be calculated for this reporting period; (14) The results for this state are combined with nearby states to protect confidentiality; Please refer to the User's Guide for a full explanation of data.

Measure	Cases	This Hosp.	State Avg.	U.S. Avg.
Incidence of Potentially Preventable VTE[5]	-	-	9%	10%
UFH with Dosages/Platelet Monitoring[5]	-	-	96%	97%
Venous Thromboembolism Prophylaxis[5]	-	-	82%	85%
Warfarin Therapy Discharge Instructions[5]	-	-	84%	75%
Chest Pain/Possible Heart Attack Care				
Aspirin Given Within 24 Hours of Arrival	-	-	94%	96%
Fibrinolytic Meds Within 30 Min. of Arrival	-	-	47%	58%
Average Time to ECG (minutes)	-	-	8	7
Average Time to Transfer (minutes)	-	-	62	60
Children's Asthma Care				
Received Home Management Plan of Care	-	-	93%	88%
Received Reliever Medication	-	-	100%	100%
Received Systemic Corticosteroids	-	-	100%	100%
Emergency Department				
Admittance Decision Time (minutes)[5]	-	-	99	98
Head CT Results Within 45 Min. of Arrival	-	-	54%	57%
Patients Who Left ER Before Being Seen	-	-	3%	2%
Time from ER Arrival to Admit. (minutes)[5]	-	-	270	274
Time from ER Arrival to Discharge (minutes)	-	-	127	134
Time in ER Before Being Evaluated (minutes)	-	-	26	26
Time to Pain Meds for Fractures (minutes)	-	-	57	57
Heart Attack Care				
Aspirin Given at Discharge[3,7]	-	-	99%	99%
Fibrinolytic Meds Within 30 Min. of Arrival[3,7]	-	-	49%	54%
PCI Within 90 Minutes of Arrival[3,7]	-	-	95%	96%
Statin Prescribed at Discharge[3,7]	-	-	98%	98%
Heart Failure Care				
ACE Inhibitor or ARB for LVSD[1]	-	-	97%	97%
Discharge Instructions Given[1]	-	-	95%	94%
Evaluation of LVS Function	11	100%	99%	99%
Medicare Spending				
Medicare Spending per Patient (ratio)	-	-	1.03	0.98
Pneumonia Care				
Appropriate Initial Antibiotic Given[1]	-	-	95%	95%
Blood Culture Timing[1]	-	-	98%	98%
Pregnancy and Delivery Care				
Newborn Deliveries Scheduled Early[5]	-	-	7%	6%
Preventive Care				
Immunization for Influenza[5]	-	-	90%	90%
Immunization for Pneumonia[5]	-	-	92%	92%
Stroke Care				
Anticoagulation Therapy for Atrial Fibrillation[5]	-	-	96%	95%
Antithrombotic Therapy Timing[5]	-	-	98%	98%
Assessed for Rehabilitation[5]	-	-	98%	97%
Discharged on Antithrombotic Therapy[5]	-	-	99%	99%
Discharged on Statin Medication[5]	-	-	95%	94%
Thrombolytic Therapy Timing[5]	-	-	68%	66%
Venous Thromboembolism Prophylaxis[5]	-	-	94%	94%
Written Stroke Educational Materials Given[5]	-	-	92%	88%
Surgical Care Improvement Project				
Appropriate Beta Blocker Usage[5]	-	-	98%	98%
Appropriate VTP Within 24 Hours[5]	-	-	98%	98%
Controlled Postoperative Blood Glucose[5]	-	-	96%	97%
Perioperative Temperature Management[5]	-	-	100%	100%
Prophylactic Antibiotic Selection[5]	-	-	99%	99%
Prophylactic Antibiotic Selection (Outpatient)	-	-	98%	98%
Prophylactic Antibiotic Stopped[5]	-	-	98%	98%
Prophylactic Antibiotic Timing[5]	-	-	99%	99%
Prophylactic Antibiotic Timing (Outpatient)	-	-	98%	98%
Urinary Catheter Removal[5]	-	-	98%	97%
Survey of Patients' Hospital Experiences				
Area Around Room 'Always' Quiet at Night[10]	<100	68%	68%	61%
Doctors 'Always' Communicated Well[10]	<100	85%	83%	82%
Home Recovery Information Given[10]	<100	83%	85%	85%
Hospital Given 9 or 10 on 10 Point Scale[10]	<100	64%	73%	71%
Meds 'Always' Explained Before Given[10]	<100	65%	66%	64%
Nurses 'Always' Communicated Well[10]	<100	85%	80%	79%
Pain 'Always' Well Controlled[10]	<100	36%	72%	71%
Room and Bathroom 'Always' Clean[10]	<100	73%	75%	73%
Timely Help 'Always' Received[10]	<100	84%	69%	68%
Would Definitely Recommend Hospital[10]	<100	54%	73%	71%
Use of Medical Imaging				
Cardiac Imaging Stress Test before Surgery	-	-	5.3%	5.3%
Combination Abdominal CT Scan	-	-	16.4%	10.5%
Combination Brain/Sinus CT Scan	-	-	2.7%	2.7%
Combination Chest CT Scan	-	-	5.6%	2.7%
Follow-up Mammogram/Ultrasound	-	-	7.9%	8.8%
Lumbar Spine MRI for Low Back Pain	-	-	39.6%	37.2%

Matagorda Regional Medical Center

104 7th Street
Bay City, TX 77414
URL: www.matagordageneral.org
Type: Acute Care Hospitals
Ownership: Govt - Hospital Dist/Auth
Phone: 979-245-6383
Fax: 979-245-1525
Emergency Services: Yes
Beds: 66

Key Personnel:
Chief of Medical Staff.......... Alan Barker
Radiology.................... Bob Maxcey

Measure	Cases	This Hosp.	State Avg.	U.S. Avg.
Blood Clot Prevention and Treatment				
Anticoagulation Overlap Therapy[2]	11	91%	93%	93%
ICU Venous Thromboembolism Prophylaxis[2]	61	95%	92%	92%
Incidence of Potentially Preventable VTE[1,2]	-	-	9%	10%
UFH with Dosages/Platelet Monitoring[1,2]	-	-	96%	97%
Venous Thromboembolism Prophylaxis[2]	202	95%	82%	85%
Warfarin Therapy Discharge Instructions[1,2]	-	-	84%	75%
Chest Pain/Possible Heart Attack Care				
Aspirin Given Within 24 Hours of Arrival	24	88%	94%	96%
Fibrinolytic Meds Within 30 Min. of Arrival[1,3]	-	-	47%	58%
Average Time to ECG (minutes)	26	10	8	7
Average Time to Transfer (minutes)[1,3]	-	-	62	60
Children's Asthma Care				
Received Home Management Plan of Care	-	-	93%	88%
Received Reliever Medication	-	-	100%	100%
Received Systemic Corticosteroids	-	-	100%	100%
Emergency Department				
Admittance Decision Time (minutes)[2]	243	85	99	98
Head CT Results Within 45 Min. of Arrival	15	40%	54%	57%
Patients Who Left ER Before Being Seen	18,863	4%	3%	2%
Time from ER Arrival to Admit. (minutes)[2]	317	263	270	274
Time from ER Arrival to Discharge (minutes)	426	132	127	134
Time in ER Before Being Evaluated (minutes)	451	32	26	26
Time to Pain Meds for Fractures (minutes)	75	54	57	57
Heart Attack Care				
Aspirin Given at Discharge	36	94%	99%	99%
Fibrinolytic Meds Within 30 Min. of Arrival[7]	-	-	49%	54%
PCI Within 90 Minutes of Arrival[7]	-	-	95%	96%
Statin Prescribed at Discharge	34	91%	98%	98%
Heart Failure Care				
ACE Inhibitor or ARB for LVSD	22	91%	97%	97%
Discharge Instructions Given	69	96%	95%	94%
Evaluation of LVS Function	94	100%	99%	99%
Medicare Spending				
Medicare Spending per Patient (ratio)	-	1.09	1.03	0.98
Pneumonia Care				
Appropriate Initial Antibiotic Given	44	93%	95%	95%
Blood Culture Timing	64	89%	98%	98%
Pregnancy and Delivery Care				
Newborn Deliveries Scheduled Early	66	8%	7%	6%
Preventive Care				
Immunization for Influenza[2]	254	96%	90%	90%
Immunization for Pneumonia[2]	313	96%	92%	92%
Stroke Care				
Anticoagulation Therapy for Atrial Fibrillation[1]	-	-	96%	95%
Antithrombotic Therapy Timing[1]	-	-	98%	98%
Assessed for Rehabilitation[1]	-	-	98%	97%
Discharged on Antithrombotic Therapy[1]	-	-	99%	99%
Discharged on Statin Medication[1]	-	-	95%	94%
Thrombolytic Therapy Timing[1]	-	-	68%	66%
Venous Thromboembolism Prophylaxis[1]	-	-	94%	94%
Written Stroke Educational Materials Given[1]	-	-	92%	88%
Surgical Care Improvement Project				
Appropriate Beta Blocker Usage	11	100%	98%	98%
Appropriate VTP Within 24 Hours	38	100%	98%	98%
Controlled Postoperative Blood Glucose[7]	-	-	96%	97%
Perioperative Temperature Management	42	100%	100%	100%
Prophylactic Antibiotic Selection	15	100%	99%	99%
Prophylactic Antibiotic Selection (Outpatient)	115	98%	98%	98%
Prophylactic Antibiotic Stopped	13	77%	98%	98%
Prophylactic Antibiotic Timing	15	100%	99%	99%
Prophylactic Antibiotic Timing (Outpatient)	119	96%	98%	98%
Urinary Catheter Removal	21	95%	98%	97%
Survey of Patients' Hospital Experiences				
Area Around Room 'Always' Quiet at Night	(a)	68%	68%	61%
Doctors 'Always' Communicated Well	(a)	81%	83%	82%
Home Recovery Information Given	(a)	87%	85%	85%
Hospital Given 9 or 10 on 10 Point Scale	(a)	71%	73%	71%
Meds 'Always' Explained Before Given	(a)	63%	66%	64%
Nurses 'Always' Communicated Well	(a)	80%	80%	79%
Pain 'Always' Well Controlled	(a)	74%	72%	71%
Room and Bathroom 'Always' Clean	(a)	78%	75%	73%
Timely Help 'Always' Received	(a)	68%	69%	68%
Would Definitely Recommend Hospital	(a)	68%	73%	71%
Use of Medical Imaging				
Cardiac Imaging Stress Test before Surgery[1]	-	-	5.3%	5.3%
Combination Abdominal CT Scan	214	6.5%	16.4%	10.5%
Combination Brain/Sinus CT Scan[1]	-	-	2.7%	2.7%
Combination Chest CT Scan	98	10.2%	5.6%	2.7%
Follow-up Mammogram/Ultrasound	280	1.1%	7.9%	8.8%
Lumbar Spine MRI for Low Back Pain[1]	-	-	39.6%	37.2%

San Jacinto Methodist Hospital

4401 Garth Road
Baytown, TX 77521
URL: www.methodisthealth.com/sanjacinto
Type: Acute Care Hospitals
Ownership: Voluntary non-profit - Private
Phone: 281-420-8600
Fax: 281-420-8852
Emergency Services: No
Beds: 335

Key Personnel:
Quality Assurance .... Robert Bains
CEO/President.............. Donna A. Gares
Infection Control.............. Barbara Gils
Intensive Care Unit............ Denise Hopper
Chief of Medical Staff.......... Bruce Kennedy, MD
Operating Room............. Nancy Vespa

Measure	Cases	This Hosp.	State Avg.	U.S. Avg.
Blood Clot Prevention and Treatment				
Anticoagulation Overlap Therapy[2]	75	89%	93%	93%
ICU Venous Thromboembolism Prophylaxis[2]	121	90%	92%	92%
Incidence of Potentially Preventable VTE[2]	20	20%	9%	10%
UFH with Dosages/Platelet Monitoring[2]	57	100%	96%	97%
Venous Thromboembolism Prophylaxis[2]	352	81%	82%	85%
Warfarin Therapy Discharge Instructions[2]	58	69%	84%	75%
Chest Pain/Possible Heart Attack Care				
Aspirin Given Within 24 Hours of Arrival[1,3]	-	-	94%	96%
Fibrinolytic Meds Within 30 Min. of Arrival[3,7]	-	-	47%	58%
Average Time to ECG (minutes)[1,3]	-	-	8	7
Average Time to Transfer (minutes)[3,7]	-	-	62	60
Children's Asthma Care				
Received Home Management Plan of Care	-	-	93%	88%
Received Reliever Medication	-	-	100%	100%
Received Systemic Corticosteroids	-	-	100%	100%
Emergency Department				
Admittance Decision Time (minutes)[2]	682	180	99	98
Head CT Results Within 45 Min. of Arrival[1]	-	-	54%	57%
Patients Who Left ER Before Being Seen	54,340	5%	3%	2%
Time from ER Arrival to Admit. (minutes)[2]	697	388	270	274
Time from ER Arrival to Discharge (minutes)	415	165	127	134
Time in ER Before Being Evaluated (minutes)	454	63	26	26
Time to Pain Meds for Fractures (minutes)	171	86	57	57
Heart Attack Care				
Aspirin Given at Discharge	209	100%	99%	99%
Fibrinolytic Meds Within 30 Min. of Arrival[7]	-	-	49%	54%
PCI Within 90 Minutes of Arrival	29	93%	95%	96%
Statin Prescribed at Discharge	213	99%	98%	98%
Heart Failure Care				
ACE Inhibitor or ARB for LVSD	134	97%	97%	97%
Discharge Instructions Given	268	100%	95%	94%
Evaluation of LVS Function	344	100%	99%	99%
Medicare Spending				

NOTE: Hospital profiles are in alphabetical order by state, then city, then hospital within the city; Rankings exclude hospitals with less than 25 cases except for patient surveys which excludes hospitals with less than 100 cases; (a) 100-299 cases; (1) The number of cases/patients is too few to report; (2) Data submitted were based on a sample of cases/patients; (3) Results are based on a shorter time period than required; (4) Data suppressed by CMS for one or more quarters; (5) Results are not available for this reporting period; (6) Fewer than 100 patients completed the HCAHPS survey; (7) No cases met the criteria for this measure; (8) The lower limit of the confidence interval cannot be calculated if the number of observed infections equals zero; (9) No data are available from the state/territory for this reporting period; (10) The scores shown reflect fewer than 50 completed surveys; (11) There were discrepancies in the data collection process; (12) This measure does not apply to this hospital for this reporting period; (13) Results cannot be calculated for this reporting period; (14) The results for this state are combined with nearby states to protect confidentiality; Please refer to the User's Guide for a full explanation of data.

Medicare Spending per Patient (ratio)	-	1.01	1.03	0.98
Pneumonia Care				
Appropriate Initial Antibiotic Given	162	96%	95%	95%
Blood Culture Timing	261	100%	98%	98%
Pregnancy and Delivery Care				
Newborn Deliveries Scheduled Early	142	5%	7%	6%
Preventive Care				
Immunization for Influenza[2]	676	98%	90%	90%
Immunization for Pneumonia[2]	812	99%	92%	92%
Stroke Care				
Anticoagulation Therapy for Atrial Fibrillation	17	94%	96%	95%
Antithrombotic Therapy Timing	166	98%	98%	98%
Assessed for Rehabilitation	166	96%	98%	97%
Discharged on Antithrombotic Therapy	158	100%	99%	99%
Discharged on Statin Medication	124	98%	95%	94%
Thrombolytic Therapy Timing[1]	-	-	68%	66%
Venous Thromboembolism Prophylaxis	173	93%	94%	94%
Written Stroke Educational Materials Given	106	97%	92%	88%
Surgical Care Improvement Project				
Appropriate Beta Blocker Usage[2]	126	99%	98%	98%
Appropriate VTP Within 24 Hours[2]	409	100%	98%	98%
Controlled Postoperative Blood Glucose[2]	65	97%	96%	97%
Perioperative Temperature Management[2]	480	100%	100%	100%
Prophylactic Antibiotic Selection[2]	335	98%	99%	99%
Prophylactic Antibiotic Selection (Outpatient)	160	98%	98%	98%
Prophylactic Antibiotic Stopped[2]	319	98%	98%	98%
Prophylactic Antibiotic Timing[2]	335	99%	99%	99%
Prophylactic Antibiotic Timing (Outpatient)	161	99%	98%	98%
Urinary Catheter Removal[2]	316	100%	98%	97%
Survey of Patients' Hospital Experiences				
Area Around Room 'Always' Quiet at Night	300+	67%	68%	61%
Doctors 'Always' Communicated Well	300+	80%	83%	82%
Home Recovery Information Given	300+	84%	85%	85%
Hospital Given 9 or 10 on 10 Point Scale	300+	74%	73%	71%
Meds 'Always' Explained Before Given	300+	65%	66%	64%
Nurses 'Always' Communicated Well	300+	81%	80%	79%
Pain 'Always' Well Controlled	300+	76%	72%	71%
Room and Bathroom 'Always' Clean	300+	76%	75%	73%
Timely Help 'Always' Received	300+	73%	69%	68%
Would Definitely Recommend Hospital	300+	73%	73%	71%
Use of Medical Imaging				
Cardiac Imaging Stress Test before Surgery	95	6.3%	5.3%	5.3%
Combination Abdominal CT Scan	514	25.1%	16.4%	10.5%
Combination Brain/Sinus CT Scan	769	1.7%	2.7%	2.7%
Combination Chest CT Scan	220	30.5%	5.6%	2.7%
Follow-up Mammogram/Ultrasound	1,014	7.4%	7.9%	8.8%
Lumbar Spine MRI for Low Back Pain	50	58.0%	39.6%	37.2%

Baptist Beaumont Hospital

3080 College Street — Phone: 409-212-5012
Beaumont, TX 77701 — Fax: 409-212-6016
URL: www.mhbh.org
Type: Acute Care Hospitals — Emergency Services: Yes
Ownership: Voluntary non-profit - Private — Beds: 22

Key Personnel:
Hemotology Center . . . . Gay-Lynne Jones
Operating Room. . . . . Miriam Kay
Emergency Room . . . . Connie Raymond
CEO/President. . . . . Louis Silva
Anesthesiology. . . . . Howard Sperling
Quality Assurance . . . . Maureen Thompson

Measure	Cases	This Hosp.	State Avg.	U.S. Avg.
Blood Clot Prevention and Treatment				
Anticoagulation Overlap Therapy[2]	78	91%	93%	93%
ICU Venous Thromboembolism Prophylaxis[2]	95	97%	92%	92%
Incidence of Potentially Preventable VTE[1,2]	-	-	9%	10%
UFH with Dosages/Platelet Monitoring[1,2]	-	-	96%	97%
Venous Thromboembolism Prophylaxis[2]	389	64%	82%	85%
Warfarin Therapy Discharge Instructions[2]	63	98%	84%	75%
Chest Pain/Possible Heart Attack Care				
Aspirin Given Within 24 Hours of Arrival[1]	-	-	94%	96%
Fibrinolytic Meds Within 30 Min. of Arrival[5]	-	-	47%	58%
Average Time to ECG (minutes)[1]	-	-	8	7
Average Time to Transfer (minutes)[5]	-	-	62	60
Children's Asthma Care				
Received Home Management Plan of Care	-	-	93%	88%
Received Reliever Medication	-	-	100%	100%
Received Systemic Corticosteroids	-	-	100%	100%
Emergency Department				
Admittance Decision Time (minutes)[2]	777	167	99	98
Head CT Results Within 45 Min. of Arrival	34	97%	54%	57%
Patients Who Left ER Before Being Seen	75,401	2%	3%	2%
Time from ER Arrival to Admit. (minutes)[2]	781	340	270	274
Time from ER Arrival to Discharge (minutes)	426	172	127	134
Time in ER Before Being Evaluated (minutes)	438	43	26	26
Time to Pain Meds for Fractures (minutes)	174	61	57	57
Heart Attack Care				
Aspirin Given at Discharge	295	99%	99%	99%
Fibrinolytic Meds Within 30 Min. of Arrival[7]	-	-	49%	54%
PCI Within 90 Minutes of Arrival	44	86%	95%	96%
Statin Prescribed at Discharge	281	100%	98%	98%
Heart Failure Care				
ACE Inhibitor or ARB for LVSD[2]	121	98%	97%	97%
Discharge Instructions Given[2]	272	92%	95%	94%
Evaluation of LVS Function[2]	309	99%	99%	99%
Medicare Spending				
Medicare Spending per Patient (ratio)	-	1.03	1.03	0.98
Pneumonia Care				
Appropriate Initial Antibiotic Given[2]	130	99%	95%	95%
Blood Culture Timing[2]	225	100%	98%	98%
Pregnancy and Delivery Care				
Newborn Deliveries Scheduled Early[2]	31	3%	7%	6%
Preventive Care				
Immunization for Influenza[2]	555	96%	90%	90%
Immunization for Pneumonia[2]	713	98%	92%	92%
Stroke Care				
Anticoagulation Therapy for Atrial Fibrillation[2]	19	100%	96%	95%
Antithrombotic Therapy Timing[2]	129	97%	98%	98%
Assessed for Rehabilitation[2]	157	98%	98%	97%
Discharged on Antithrombotic Therapy[2]	134	99%	99%	99%
Discharged on Statin Medication[2]	106	98%	95%	94%
Thrombolytic Therapy Timing[2]	12	83%	68%	66%
Venous Thromboembolism Prophylaxis[2]	162	94%	94%	94%
Written Stroke Educational Materials Given[2]	80	94%	92%	88%
Surgical Care Improvement Project				
Appropriate Beta Blocker Usage[2]	184	98%	98%	98%
Appropriate VTP Within 24 Hours[2]	385	96%	98%	98%
Controlled Postoperative Blood Glucose[2]	76	96%	96%	97%
Perioperative Temperature Management[2]	501	100%	100%	100%
Prophylactic Antibiotic Selection[2]	386	99%	99%	99%
Prophylactic Antibiotic Selection (Outpatient)	277	97%	98%	98%
Prophylactic Antibiotic Stopped[2]	363	99%	98%	98%
Prophylactic Antibiotic Timing[2]	386	99%	99%	99%
Prophylactic Antibiotic Timing (Outpatient)	279	99%	98%	98%
Urinary Catheter Removal[2]	232	94%	98%	97%
Survey of Patients' Hospital Experiences				
Area Around Room 'Always' Quiet at Night	300+	69%	68%	61%
Doctors 'Always' Communicated Well	300+	84%	83%	82%
Home Recovery Information Given	300+	87%	85%	85%
Hospital Given 9 or 10 on 10 Point Scale	300+	73%	73%	71%
Meds 'Always' Explained Before Given	300+	69%	66%	64%
Nurses 'Always' Communicated Well	300+	80%	80%	79%
Pain 'Always' Well Controlled	300+	74%	72%	71%
Room and Bathroom 'Always' Clean	300+	69%	75%	73%
Timely Help 'Always' Received	300+	69%	69%	68%
Would Definitely Recommend Hospital	300+	78%	73%	71%
Use of Medical Imaging				
Cardiac Imaging Stress Test before Surgery	149	8.1%	5.3%	5.3%
Combination Abdominal CT Scan	721	6.5%	16.4%	10.5%
Combination Brain/Sinus CT Scan	1,024	3.2%	2.7%	2.7%
Combination Chest CT Scan	321	0.6%	5.6%	2.7%
Follow-up Mammogram/Ultrasound	955	6.1%	7.9%	8.8%
Lumbar Spine MRI for Low Back Pain	71	42.3%	39.6%	37.2%

Christus Hospital

2830 Calder Avenue — Phone: 409-892-7171
Beaumont, TX 77702 — Fax: 409-899-8191
E-mail: communications@christushealth.org
URL: www.christushealth.org
Type: Acute Care Hospitals — Emergency Services: Yes
Ownership: Voluntary non-profit - Church — Beds: 461

Key Personnel:
Radiology. . . . . Douglas C Connor
President/CEO. . . . . Ellen Jones
Infection Control. . . . . Cindy Powell
Chief of Medical Staff . . . . Herman William, MD

Measure	Cases	This Hosp.	State Avg.	U.S. Avg.
Blood Clot Prevention and Treatment				
Anticoagulation Overlap Therapy[2]	48	75%	93%	93%
ICU Venous Thromboembolism Prophylaxis[2]	72	69%	92%	92%
Incidence of Potentially Preventable VTE[2]	12	17%	9%	10%
UFH with Dosages/Platelet Monitoring[1,2]	-	-	96%	97%
Venous Thromboembolism Prophylaxis[2]	368	60%	82%	85%
Warfarin Therapy Discharge Instructions[2]	42	67%	84%	75%
Chest Pain/Possible Heart Attack Care				
Aspirin Given Within 24 Hours of Arrival	12	100%	94%	96%
Fibrinolytic Meds Within 30 Min. of Arrival[3,7]	-	-	47%	58%
Average Time to ECG (minutes)	12	14	8	7
Average Time to Transfer (minutes)[3,7]	-	-	62	60
Children's Asthma Care				
Received Home Management Plan of Care	-	-	93%	88%
Received Reliever Medication	-	-	100%	100%
Received Systemic Corticosteroids	-	-	100%	100%
Emergency Department				
Admittance Decision Time (minutes)[2]	654	132	99	98
Head CT Results Within 45 Min. of Arrival	34	65%	54%	57%
Patients Who Left ER Before Being Seen	53,806	4%	3%	2%
Time from ER Arrival to Admit. (minutes)[2]	667	347	270	274
Time from ER Arrival to Discharge (minutes)	382	174	127	134
Time in ER Before Being Evaluated (minutes)	418	38	26	26
Time to Pain Meds for Fractures (minutes)	285	77	57	57
Heart Attack Care				
Aspirin Given at Discharge[2]	320	99%	99%	99%
Fibrinolytic Meds Within 30 Min. of Arrival[2,7]	-	-	49%	54%
PCI Within 90 Minutes of Arrival[2]	32	94%	95%	96%
Statin Prescribed at Discharge[2]	314	98%	98%	98%
Heart Failure Care				
ACE Inhibitor or ARB for LVSD[2]	106	97%	97%	97%
Discharge Instructions Given[2]	270	99%	95%	94%
Evaluation of LVS Function[2]	331	99%	99%	99%
Medicare Spending				
Medicare Spending per Patient (ratio)	-	1.03	1.03	0.98
Pneumonia Care				
Appropriate Initial Antibiotic Given[2]	119	92%	95%	95%
Blood Culture Timing[2]	149	97%	98%	98%
Pregnancy and Delivery Care				
Newborn Deliveries Scheduled Early[2]	76	55%	7%	6%
Preventive Care				
Immunization for Influenza[2]	535	68%	90%	90%
Immunization for Pneumonia[2]	598	71%	92%	92%
Stroke Care				
Anticoagulation Therapy for Atrial Fibrillation[2]	11	82%	96%	95%
Antithrombotic Therapy Timing[2]	96	94%	98%	98%
Assessed for Rehabilitation[2]	120	82%	98%	97%
Discharged on Antithrombotic Therapy[2]	91	91%	99%	99%
Discharged on Statin Medication[2]	88	74%	95%	94%
Thrombolytic Therapy Timing[1,2]	-	-	68%	66%
Venous Thromboembolism Prophylaxis[2]	124	70%	94%	94%
Written Stroke Educational Materials Given[2]	65	55%	92%	88%
Surgical Care Improvement Project				
Appropriate Beta Blocker Usage[2]	355	98%	98%	98%
Appropriate VTP Within 24 Hours[2]	769	99%	98%	98%
Controlled Postoperative Blood Glucose[2]	126	98%	96%	97%
Perioperative Temperature Management[2]	907	100%	100%	100%
Prophylactic Antibiotic Selection[2]	664	100%	99%	99%
Prophylactic Antibiotic Selection (Outpatient)	597	95%	98%	98%
Prophylactic Antibiotic Stopped[2]	639	99%	98%	98%

NOTE: Hospital profiles are in alphabetical order by state, then city, then hospital within the city; Rankings exclude hospitals with less than 25 cases except for patient surveys which excludes hospitals with less than 100 cases; (a) 100-299 cases; (1) The number of cases/patients is too few to report; (2) Data submitted were based on a sample of cases/patients; (3) Results are based on a shorter time period than required; (4) Data suppressed by CMS for one or more quarters; (5) Results are not available for this reporting period; (6) Fewer than 100 patients completed the HCAHPS survey; (7) No cases met the criteria for this measure; (8) The lower limit of the confidence interval cannot be calculated if the number of observed infections equals zero; (9) No data are available from the state/territory for this reporting period; (10) The scores shown reflect fewer than 50 completed surveys; (11) There were discrepancies in the data collection process; (12) This measure does not apply to this hospital for this reporting period; (13) Results cannot be calculated for this reporting period; (14) The results for this state are combined with nearby states to protect confidentiality; Please refer to the User's Guide for a full explanation of data.

Measure	Cases	This Hosp.	State Avg.	U.S. Avg.
Prophylactic Antibiotic Timing[2]	664	100%	99%	99%
Prophylactic Antibiotic Timing (Outpatient)	597	98%	98%	98%
Urinary Catheter Removal[2]	493	97%	98%	97%
Survey of Patients' Hospital Experiences				
Area Around Room 'Always' Quiet at Night	300+	67%	68%	61%
Doctors 'Always' Communicated Well	300+	83%	83%	82%
Home Recovery Information Given	300+	81%	85%	85%
Hospital Given 9 or 10 on 10 Point Scale	300+	69%	73%	71%
Meds 'Always' Explained Before Given	300+	65%	66%	64%
Nurses 'Always' Communicated Well	300+	81%	80%	79%
Pain 'Always' Well Controlled	300+	76%	72%	71%
Room and Bathroom 'Always' Clean	300+	72%	75%	73%
Timely Help 'Always' Received	300+	66%	69%	68%
Would Definitely Recommend Hospital	300+	73%	73%	71%
Use of Medical Imaging				
Cardiac Imaging Stress Test before Surgery	62	0.0%	5.3%	5.3%
Combination Abdominal CT Scan	1,209	30.7%	16.4%	10.5%
Combination Brain/Sinus CT Scan	1,172	1.8%	2.7%	2.7%
Combination Chest CT Scan	533	34.0%	5.6%	2.7%
Follow-up Mammogram/Ultrasound	3,100	9.0%	7.9%	8.8%
Lumbar Spine MRI for Low Back Pain	209	36.8%	39.6%	37.2%

Texas Health Harris Methodist Hurst - Euless - Bedford

1600 Hospital Parkway Phone: 817-848-4000
Bedford, TX 76022 Fax: 817-685-4890
URL: www.texashealth.org
Type: Acute Care Hospitals Emergency Services: Yes
Ownership: Voluntary non-profit - Private Beds: 300

Key Personnel:

Quality Assurance . . . . Dorothy Bartz, RN
Pediatric Ambulatory Care . . . . . . Marsha Blackman
Pediatric In-Patient Care . . . . Marsha Blackman
Radiology. . . . . Stanley Cook, MD
CEO/President. . . . . Deborah Paganelli, FACHE
Infection Control. . . . . Rama Stevens
Chief of Medical Staff. . . . . Gregory A. Tichenor, MD
Coronary Care . . . . Gary Wallace

Measure	Cases	This Hosp.	State Avg.	U.S. Avg.
Blood Clot Prevention and Treatment				
Anticoagulation Overlap Therapy[2]	115	90%	93%	93%
ICU Venous Thromboembolism Prophylaxis[2]	63	98%	92%	92%
Incidence of Potentially Preventable VTE[1,2]	-	-	9%	10%
UFH with Dosages/Platelet Monitoring[2]	15	100%	96%	97%
Venous Thromboembolism Prophylaxis[2]	312	98%	82%	85%
Warfarin Therapy Discharge Instructions[2]	95	87%	84%	75%
Chest Pain/Possible Heart Attack Care				
Aspirin Given Within 24 Hours of Arrival[1,3]	-	-	94%	96%
Fibrinolytic Meds Within 30 Min. of Arrival[3,7]	-	-	47%	58%
Average Time to ECG (minutes)[1,3]	-	-	8	7
Average Time to Transfer (minutes)[3,7]	-	-	62	60
Children's Asthma Care				
Received Home Management Plan of Care	-	-	93%	88%
Received Reliever Medication	-	-	100%	100%
Received Systemic Corticosteroids	-	-	100%	100%
Emergency Department				
Admittance Decision Time (minutes)[2]	521	93	99	98
Head CT Results Within 45 Min. of Arrival	15	47%	54%	57%
Patients Who Left ER Before Being Seen	61,881	4%	3%	2%
Time from ER Arrival to Admit. (minutes)[2]	523	261	270	274
Time from ER Arrival to Discharge (minutes)	398	168	127	134
Time in ER Before Being Evaluated (minutes)	442	21	26	26
Time to Pain Meds for Fractures (minutes)	172	79	57	57
Heart Attack Care				
Aspirin Given at Discharge	219	100%	99%	99%
Fibrinolytic Meds Within 30 Min. of Arrival[1]	-	-	49%	54%
PCI Within 90 Minutes of Arrival	54	100%	95%	96%
Statin Prescribed at Discharge	214	100%	98%	98%
Heart Failure Care				
ACE Inhibitor or ARB for LVSD	110	98%	97%	97%
Discharge Instructions Given	266	99%	95%	94%
Evaluation of LVS Function	367	100%	99%	99%
Medicare Spending				
Medicare Spending per Patient (ratio)	-	1.06	1.03	0.98
Pneumonia Care				
Appropriate Initial Antibiotic Given	250	96%	95%	95%
Blood Culture Timing	375	99%	98%	98%
Pregnancy and Delivery Care				
Newborn Deliveries Scheduled Early	227	7%	7%	6%
Preventive Care				
Immunization for Influenza[2]	631	99%	90%	90%
Immunization for Pneumonia[2]	768	97%	92%	92%
Stroke Care				
Anticoagulation Therapy for Atrial Fibrillation[2]	14	100%	96%	95%
Antithrombotic Therapy Timing[2]	104	100%	98%	98%
Assessed for Rehabilitation[2]	110	100%	98%	97%
Discharged on Antithrombotic Therapy[2]	108	100%	99%	99%
Discharged on Statin Medication[2]	87	99%	95%	94%
Thrombolytic Therapy Timing[1,2]	-	-	68%	66%
Venous Thromboembolism Prophylaxis[2]	108	99%	94%	94%
Written Stroke Educational Materials Given[2]	62	100%	92%	88%
Surgical Care Improvement Project				
Appropriate Beta Blocker Usage[2]	165	99%	98%	98%
Appropriate VTP Within 24 Hours[2]	327	98%	98%	98%
Controlled Postoperative Blood Glucose[2]	50	96%	96%	97%
Perioperative Temperature Management[2]	437	99%	100%	100%
Prophylactic Antibiotic Selection[2]	255	98%	99%	99%
Prophylactic Antibiotic Selection (Outpatient)	425	98%	98%	98%
Prophylactic Antibiotic Stopped[2]	248	97%	98%	98%
Prophylactic Antibiotic Timing[2]	256	98%	99%	99%
Prophylactic Antibiotic Timing (Outpatient)	426	99%	98%	98%
Urinary Catheter Removal[2]	300	99%	98%	97%
Survey of Patients' Hospital Experiences				
Area Around Room 'Always' Quiet at Night	300+	60%	68%	61%
Doctors 'Always' Communicated Well	300+	81%	83%	82%
Home Recovery Information Given	300+	87%	85%	85%
Hospital Given 9 or 10 on 10 Point Scale	300+	76%	73%	71%
Meds 'Always' Explained Before Given	300+	67%	66%	64%
Nurses 'Always' Communicated Well	300+	79%	80%	79%
Pain 'Always' Well Controlled	300+	73%	72%	71%
Room and Bathroom 'Always' Clean	300+	69%	75%	73%
Timely Help 'Always' Received	300+	66%	69%	68%
Would Definitely Recommend Hospital	300+	79%	73%	71%
Use of Medical Imaging				
Cardiac Imaging Stress Test before Surgery	104	5.8%	5.3%	5.3%
Combination Abdominal CT Scan	615	1.8%	16.4%	10.5%
Combination Brain/Sinus CT Scan	911	2.5%	2.7%	2.7%
Combination Chest CT Scan	261	2.3%	5.6%	2.7%
Follow-up Mammogram/Ultrasound[7]	-	-	7.9%	8.8%
Lumbar Spine MRI for Low Back Pain[1]	-	-	39.6%	37.2%

Christus Spohn Hospital Beeville

1500 E Houston Hwy Phone: 361-354-2000
Beeville, TX 78102 Fax: 361-358-9322
URL: www.christushealth.org
Type: Acute Care Hospitals Emergency Services: Yes
Ownership: Voluntary non-profit - Church Beds: 69

Key Personnel:

Infection Control. . . . . Michael G Bullen, MD
CEO/President. . . . . Kathy J McDonagh

Measure	Cases	This Hosp.	State Avg.	U.S. Avg.
Blood Clot Prevention and Treatment				
Anticoagulation Overlap Therapy[1,2]	-	-	93%	93%
ICU Venous Thromboembolism Prophylaxis[2]	57	79%	92%	92%
Incidence of Potentially Preventable VTE[2,7]	-	-	9%	10%
UFH with Dosages/Platelet Monitoring[2,7]	-	-	96%	97%
Venous Thromboembolism Prophylaxis[2]	151	81%	82%	85%
Warfarin Therapy Discharge Instructions[1,2]	-	-	84%	75%
Chest Pain/Possible Heart Attack Care				
Aspirin Given Within 24 Hours of Arrival	80	89%	94%	96%
Fibrinolytic Meds Within 30 Min. of Arrival[1]	-	-	47%	58%
Average Time to ECG (minutes)	84	22	8	7
Average Time to Transfer (minutes)[7]	-	-	62	60
Children's Asthma Care				
Received Home Management Plan of Care	-	-	93%	88%
Received Reliever Medication	-	-	100%	100%
Received Systemic Corticosteroids	-	-	100%	100%
Emergency Department				
Admittance Decision Time (minutes)[2]	379	130	99	98
Head CT Results Within 45 Min. of Arrival	16	50%	54%	57%
Patients Who Left ER Before Being Seen	20,594	6%	3%	2%
Time from ER Arrival to Admit. (minutes)[2]	380	360	270	274
Time from ER Arrival to Discharge (minutes)	399	149	127	134
Time in ER Before Being Evaluated (minutes)	404	39	26	26
Time to Pain Meds for Fractures (minutes)	72	65	57	57
Heart Attack Care				
Aspirin Given at Discharge[1]	-	-	99%	99%
Fibrinolytic Meds Within 30 Min. of Arrival[7]	-	-	49%	54%
PCI Within 90 Minutes of Arrival[7]	-	-	95%	96%
Statin Prescribed at Discharge[1]	-	-	98%	98%
Heart Failure Care				
ACE Inhibitor or ARB for LVSD	40	95%	97%	97%
Discharge Instructions Given	95	84%	95%	94%
Evaluation of LVS Function	115	98%	99%	99%
Medicare Spending				
Medicare Spending per Patient (ratio)	-	0.98	1.03	0.98
Pneumonia Care				
Appropriate Initial Antibiotic Given	50	92%	95%	95%
Blood Culture Timing	81	96%	98%	98%
Pregnancy and Delivery Care				
Newborn Deliveries Scheduled Early[2]	34	0%	7%	6%
Preventive Care				
Immunization for Influenza[2]	277	89%	90%	90%
Immunization for Pneumonia[2]	354	96%	92%	92%
Stroke Care				
Anticoagulation Therapy for Atrial Fibrillation[7]	-	-	96%	95%
Antithrombotic Therapy Timing	12	83%	98%	98%
Assessed for Rehabilitation[1]	-	-	98%	97%
Discharged on Antithrombotic Therapy[1]	-	-	99%	99%
Discharged on Statin Medication[1]	-	-	95%	94%
Thrombolytic Therapy Timing[1]	-	-	68%	66%
Venous Thromboembolism Prophylaxis	12	67%	94%	94%
Written Stroke Educational Materials Given[1]	-	-	92%	88%
Surgical Care Improvement Project				
Appropriate Beta Blocker Usage[1]	-	-	98%	98%
Appropriate VTP Within 24 Hours	26	96%	98%	98%
Controlled Postoperative Blood Glucose[7]	-	-	96%	97%
Perioperative Temperature Management	28	100%	100%	100%
Prophylactic Antibiotic Selection	16	94%	99%	99%
Prophylactic Antibiotic Selection (Outpatient)[1,3]	-	-	98%	98%
Prophylactic Antibiotic Stopped	16	81%	98%	98%
Prophylactic Antibiotic Timing	16	100%	99%	99%
Prophylactic Antibiotic Timing (Outpatient)[1,3]	-	-	98%	98%
Urinary Catheter Removal[1]	-	-	98%	97%
Survey of Patients' Hospital Experiences				
Area Around Room 'Always' Quiet at Night	(a)	65%	68%	61%
Doctors 'Always' Communicated Well	(a)	80%	83%	82%
Home Recovery Information Given	(a)	85%	85%	85%
Hospital Given 9 or 10 on 10 Point Scale	(a)	65%	73%	71%
Meds 'Always' Explained Before Given	(a)	67%	66%	64%
Nurses 'Always' Communicated Well	(a)	79%	80%	79%
Pain 'Always' Well Controlled	(a)	73%	72%	71%
Room and Bathroom 'Always' Clean	(a)	79%	75%	73%
Timely Help 'Always' Received	(a)	71%	69%	68%
Would Definitely Recommend Hospital	(a)	61%	73%	71%
Use of Medical Imaging				
Cardiac Imaging Stress Test before Surgery[1]	-	-	5.3%	5.3%
Combination Abdominal CT Scan	163	24.5%	16.4%	10.5%
Combination Brain/Sinus CT Scan[1]	-	-	2.7%	2.7%
Combination Chest CT Scan	75	6.7%	5.6%	2.7%
Follow-up Mammogram/Ultrasound	329	5.8%	7.9%	8.8%
Lumbar Spine MRI for Low Back Pain[1]	-	-	39.6%	37.2%

First Surgical Hospital

4801 Bissonnet Blvd Phone: 713-713-7133
Bellaire, TX 77401
URL: www.firststreethospital.com
Type: Acute Care Hospitals Emergency Services: Yes
Ownership: Proprietary

Key Personnel:

CEO . . . . Walter Leleux

NOTE: Hospital profiles are in alphabetical order by state, then city, then hospital within the city; Rankings exclude hospitals with less than 25 cases except for patient surveys which excludes hospitals with less than 100 cases; (a) 100-299 cases; (1) The number of cases/patients is too few to report; (2) Data submitted were based on a sample of cases/patients; (3) Results are based on a shorter time period than required; (4) Data suppressed by CMS for one or more quarters; (5) Results are not available for this reporting period; (6) Fewer than 100 patients completed the HCAHPS survey; (7) No cases met the criteria for this measure; (8) The lower limit of the confidence interval cannot be calculated if the number of observed infections equals zero; (9) No data are available from the state/territory for this reporting period; (10) The scores shown reflect fewer than 50 completed surveys; (11) There were discrepancies in the data collection process; (12) This measure does not apply to this hospital for this reporting period; (13) Results cannot be calculated for this reporting period; (14) The results for this state are combined with nearby states to protect confidentiality; Please refer to the User's Guide for a full explanation of data.

Measure	Cases	This Hosp.	State Avg.	U.S. Avg.
Blood Clot Prevention and Treatment				
Anticoagulation Overlap Therapy[7]	-	-	93%	93%
ICU Venous Thromboembolism Prophylaxis[7]	-	-	92%	92%
Incidence of Potentially Preventable VTE[7]	-	-	9%	10%
UFH with Dosages/Platelet Monitoring[7]	-	-	96%	97%
Venous Thromboembolism Prophylaxis	122	98%	82%	85%
Warfarin Therapy Discharge Instructions[7]	-	-	84%	75%
Chest Pain/Possible Heart Attack Care				
Aspirin Given Within 24 Hours of Arrival[1,3]	-	-	94%	96%
Fibrinolytic Meds Within 30 Min. of Arrival[5]	-	-	47%	58%
Average Time to ECG (minutes)[1,3]	-	-	8	7
Average Time to Transfer (minutes)[5]	-	-	62	60
Children's Asthma Care				
Received Home Management Plan of Care	-	-	93%	88%
Received Reliever Medication	-	-	100%	100%
Received Systemic Corticosteroids	-	-	100%	100%
Emergency Department				
Admittance Decision Time (minutes)	12	34	99	98
Head CT Results Within 45 Min. of Arrival[3,7]	-	-	54%	57%
Patients Who Left ER Before Being Seen	262	2%	3%	2%
Time from ER Arrival to Admit. (minutes)	12	175	270	274
Time from ER Arrival to Discharge (minutes)	264	85	127	134
Time in ER Before Being Evaluated (minutes)	307	10	26	26
Time to Pain Meds for Fractures (minutes)[1,3]	-	-	57	57
Heart Attack Care				
Aspirin Given at Discharge[5]	-	-	99%	99%
Fibrinolytic Meds Within 30 Min. of Arrival[5]	-	-	49%	54%
PCI Within 90 Minutes of Arrival[5]	-	-	95%	96%
Statin Prescribed at Discharge[5]	-	-	98%	98%
Heart Failure Care				
ACE Inhibitor or ARB for LVSD[5]	-	-	97%	97%
Discharge Instructions Given[5]	-	-	95%	94%
Evaluation of LVS Function[5]	-	-	99%	99%
Medicare Spending				
Medicare Spending per Patient (ratio)	-	0.85	1.03	0.98
Pneumonia Care				
Appropriate Initial Antibiotic Given[5]	-	-	95%	95%
Blood Culture Timing[5]	-	-	98%	98%
Pregnancy and Delivery Care				
Newborn Deliveries Scheduled Early[7]	-	-	7%	6%
Preventive Care				
Immunization for Influenza[2]	248	75%	90%	90%
Immunization for Pneumonia[2]	147	69%	92%	92%
Stroke Care				
Anticoagulation Therapy for Atrial Fibrillation[5]	-	-	96%	95%
Antithrombotic Therapy Timing[5]	-	-	98%	98%
Assessed for Rehabilitation[5]	-	-	98%	97%
Discharged on Antithrombotic Therapy[5]	-	-	99%	99%
Discharged on Statin Medication[5]	-	-	95%	94%
Thrombolytic Therapy Timing[5]	-	-	68%	66%
Venous Thromboembolism Prophylaxis[5]	-	-	94%	94%
Written Stroke Educational Materials Given[5]	-	-	92%	88%
Surgical Care Improvement Project				
Appropriate Beta Blocker Usage	25	96%	98%	98%
Appropriate VTP Within 24 Hours	95	95%	98%	98%
Controlled Postoperative Blood Glucose[7]	-	-	96%	97%
Perioperative Temperature Management	147	100%	100%	100%
Prophylactic Antibiotic Selection	127	97%	99%	99%
Prophylactic Antibiotic Selection (Outpatient)	130	88%	98%	98%
Prophylactic Antibiotic Stopped	127	72%	98%	98%
Prophylactic Antibiotic Timing	129	73%	99%	99%
Prophylactic Antibiotic Timing (Outpatient)	136	81%	98%	98%
Urinary Catheter Removal	45	100%	98%	97%
Survey of Patients' Hospital Experiences				
Area Around Room 'Always' Quiet at Night	(a)	85%	68%	61%
Doctors 'Always' Communicated Well	(a)	85%	83%	82%
Home Recovery Information Given	(a)	86%	85%	85%
Hospital Given 9 or 10 on 10 Point Scale	(a)	74%	73%	71%
Meds 'Always' Explained Before Given	(a)	65%	66%	64%
Nurses 'Always' Communicated Well	(a)	83%	80%	79%
Pain 'Always' Well Controlled	(a)	77%	72%	71%
Room and Bathroom 'Always' Clean	(a)	80%	75%	73%
Timely Help 'Always' Received	(a)	79%	69%	68%
Would Definitely Recommend Hospital	(a)	77%	73%	71%
Use of Medical Imaging				
Cardiac Imaging Stress Test before Surgery[7]	-	-	5.3%	5.3%
Combination Abdominal CT Scan[1]	-	-	16.4%	10.5%
Combination Brain/Sinus CT Scan[1]	-	-	2.7%	2.7%
Combination Chest CT Scan[1]	-	-	5.6%	2.7%
Follow-up Mammogram/Ultrasound[7]	-	-	7.9%	8.8%
Lumbar Spine MRI for Low Back Pain[7]	-	-	39.6%	37.2%

Houston Orthopedic & Spine Hospital

5410 West Loop South
Bellaire, TX 77401
Phone: 713-622-2262
URL: www.foundationsurgicalhospital.com
Type: Acute Care Hospitals
Emergency Services: Yes
Ownership: Proprietary
Beds: 64

Key Personnel:
Surgery . . . . Lee Ansell, MD
CEO . . . . Andrew Knizley
Radiology. . . . . David Nunez

Measure	Cases	This Hosp.	State Avg.	U.S. Avg.
Blood Clot Prevention and Treatment				
Anticoagulation Overlap Therapy[1,2]	-	-	93%	93%
ICU Venous Thromboembolism Prophylaxis[2,7]	-	-	92%	92%
Incidence of Potentially Preventable VTE[2,7]	-	-	9%	10%
UFH with Dosages/Platelet Monitoring[2,7]	-	-	96%	97%
Venous Thromboembolism Prophylaxis[2]	112	99%	82%	85%
Warfarin Therapy Discharge Instructions[2,7]	-	-	84%	75%
Chest Pain/Possible Heart Attack Care				
Aspirin Given Within 24 Hours of Arrival[3,7]	-	-	94%	96%
Fibrinolytic Meds Within 30 Min. of Arrival[5]	-	-	47%	58%
Average Time to ECG (minutes)[3,7]	-	-	8	7
Average Time to Transfer (minutes)[5]	-	-	62	60
Children's Asthma Care				
Received Home Management Plan of Care	-	-	93%	88%
Received Reliever Medication	-	-	100%	100%
Received Systemic Corticosteroids	-	-	100%	100%
Emergency Department				
Admittance Decision Time (minutes)	36	45	99	98
Head CT Results Within 45 Min. of Arrival[5]	-	-	54%	57%
Patients Who Left ER Before Being Seen	422	0%	3%	2%
Time from ER Arrival to Admit. (minutes)	38	114	270	274
Time from ER Arrival to Discharge (minutes)	402	110	127	134
Time in ER Before Being Evaluated (minutes)	424	20	26	26
Time to Pain Meds for Fractures (minutes)[1]	-	-	57	57
Heart Attack Care				
Aspirin Given at Discharge[5]	-	-	99%	99%
Fibrinolytic Meds Within 30 Min. of Arrival[5]	-	-	49%	54%
PCI Within 90 Minutes of Arrival[5]	-	-	95%	96%
Statin Prescribed at Discharge[5]	-	-	98%	98%
Heart Failure Care				
ACE Inhibitor or ARB for LVSD[5]	-	-	97%	97%
Discharge Instructions Given[5]	-	-	95%	94%
Evaluation of LVS Function[5]	-	-	99%	99%
Medicare Spending				
Medicare Spending per Patient (ratio)	-	1.01	1.03	0.98
Pneumonia Care				
Appropriate Initial Antibiotic Given[5]	-	-	95%	95%
Blood Culture Timing[5]	-	-	98%	98%
Pregnancy and Delivery Care				
Newborn Deliveries Scheduled Early[7]	-	-	7%	6%
Preventive Care				
Immunization for Influenza[2]	1,090	63%	90%	90%
Immunization for Pneumonia[2]	1,141	90%	92%	92%
Stroke Care				
Anticoagulation Therapy for Atrial Fibrillation[5]	-	-	96%	95%
Antithrombotic Therapy Timing[5]	-	-	98%	98%
Assessed for Rehabilitation[5]	-	-	98%	97%
Discharged on Antithrombotic Therapy[5]	-	-	99%	99%
Discharged on Statin Medication[5]	-	-	95%	94%
Thrombolytic Therapy Timing[5]	-	-	68%	66%
Venous Thromboembolism Prophylaxis[5]	-	-	94%	94%
Written Stroke Educational Materials Given[5]	-	-	92%	88%
Surgical Care Improvement Project				
Appropriate Beta Blocker Usage	210	87%	98%	98%
Appropriate VTP Within 24 Hours	846	100%	98%	98%
Controlled Postoperative Blood Glucose[7]	-	-	96%	97%
Perioperative Temperature Management	924	100%	100%	100%
Prophylactic Antibiotic Selection	756	100%	99%	99%
Prophylactic Antibiotic Selection (Outpatient)	357	96%	98%	98%
Prophylactic Antibiotic Stopped	744	95%	98%	98%
Prophylactic Antibiotic Timing	757	98%	99%	99%
Prophylactic Antibiotic Timing (Outpatient)	357	99%	98%	98%
Urinary Catheter Removal	428	100%	98%	97%
Survey of Patients' Hospital Experiences				
Area Around Room 'Always' Quiet at Night	300+	86%	68%	61%
Doctors 'Always' Communicated Well	300+	83%	83%	82%
Home Recovery Information Given	300+	93%	85%	85%
Hospital Given 9 or 10 on 10 Point Scale	300+	89%	73%	71%
Meds 'Always' Explained Before Given	300+	68%	66%	64%
Nurses 'Always' Communicated Well	300+	83%	80%	79%
Pain 'Always' Well Controlled	300+	75%	72%	71%
Room and Bathroom 'Always' Clean	300+	85%	75%	73%
Timely Help 'Always' Received	300+	78%	69%	68%
Would Definitely Recommend Hospital	300+	88%	73%	71%
Use of Medical Imaging				
Cardiac Imaging Stress Test before Surgery[7]	-	-	5.3%	5.3%
Combination Abdominal CT Scan[1]	-	-	16.4%	10.5%
Combination Brain/Sinus CT Scan[1]	-	-	2.7%	2.7%
Combination Chest CT Scan[1]	-	-	5.6%	2.7%
Follow-up Mammogram/Ultrasound[7]	-	-	7.9%	8.8%
Lumbar Spine MRI for Low Back Pain	188	41.0%	39.6%	37.2%

Bellville General Hospital

44 N Cummings
Bellville, TX 77418
Phone: 979-865-3141
Fax: 979-865-9631
URL: www.bellvillehospital.com
Type: Acute Care Hospitals
Emergency Services: Yes
Ownership: Voluntary non-profit - Private
Beds: 32

Key Personnel:
Radiology. . . . . Mir Zulfiqua Alikhan
CEO/President. . . . . Michael J. Spicer

Measure	Cases	This Hosp.	State Avg.	U.S. Avg.
Blood Clot Prevention and Treatment				
Anticoagulation Overlap Therapy[2,7]	-	-	93%	93%
ICU Venous Thromboembolism Prophylaxis[2,7]	-	-	92%	92%
Incidence of Potentially Preventable VTE[2,7]	-	-	9%	10%
UFH with Dosages/Platelet Monitoring[2,7]	-	-	96%	97%
Venous Thromboembolism Prophylaxis[2]	98	0%	82%	85%
Warfarin Therapy Discharge Instructions[2,7]	-	-	84%	75%
Chest Pain/Possible Heart Attack Care				
Aspirin Given Within 24 Hours of Arrival[5]	-	-	94%	96%
Fibrinolytic Meds Within 30 Min. of Arrival[5]	-	-	47%	58%
Average Time to ECG (minutes)[5]	-	-	8	7
Average Time to Transfer (minutes)[5]	-	-	62	60
Children's Asthma Care				
Received Home Management Plan of Care	-	-	93%	88%
Received Reliever Medication	-	-	100%	100%
Received Systemic Corticosteroids	-	-	100%	100%
Emergency Department				
Admittance Decision Time (minutes)[1,2]	-	-	99	98
Head CT Results Within 45 Min. of Arrival[5]	-	-	54%	57%
Patients Who Left ER Before Being Seen	5,218	1%	3%	2%
Time from ER Arrival to Admit. (minutes)[1,2]	-	-	270	274
Time from ER Arrival to Discharge (minutes)	365	100	127	134
Time in ER Before Being Evaluated (minutes)	384	16	26	26
Time to Pain Meds for Fractures (minutes)	31	30	57	57
Heart Attack Care				
Aspirin Given at Discharge[5]	-	-	99%	99%
Fibrinolytic Meds Within 30 Min. of Arrival[5]	-	-	49%	54%
PCI Within 90 Minutes of Arrival[5]	-	-	95%	96%
Statin Prescribed at Discharge[5]	-	-	98%	98%
Heart Failure Care				
ACE Inhibitor or ARB for LVSD[1,3]	-	-	97%	97%
Discharge Instructions Given[1,3]	-	-	95%	94%

NOTE: Hospital profiles are in alphabetical order by state, then city, then hospital within the city; Rankings exclude hospitals with less than 25 cases except for patient surveys which excludes hospitals with less than 100 cases; (a) 100-299 cases; (1) The number of cases/patients is too few to report; (2) Data submitted were based on a sample of cases/patients; (3) Results are based on a shorter time period than required; (4) Data suppressed by CMS for one or more quarters; (5) Results are not available for this reporting period; (6) Fewer than 100 patients completed the HCAHPS survey; (7) No cases met the criteria for this measure; (8) The lower limit of the confidence interval cannot be calculated if the number of observed infections equals zero; (9) No data are available from the state/territory for this reporting period; (10) The scores shown reflect fewer than 50 completed surveys; (11) There were discrepancies in the data collection process; (12) This measure does not apply to this hospital for this reporting period; (13) Results cannot be calculated for this reporting period; (14) The results for this state are combined with nearby states to protect confidentiality; Please refer to the User's Guide for a full explanation of data.

Measure	Cases	This Hosp.	State Avg.	U.S. Avg.
Evaluation of LVS Function[1,3]	-	-	99%	99%
Medicare Spending				
Medicare Spending per Patient (ratio)	-	1.03	1.03	0.98
Pneumonia Care				
Appropriate Initial Antibiotic Given[1,3]	-	-	95%	95%
Blood Culture Timing[1,3]	-	-	98%	98%
Pregnancy and Delivery Care				
Newborn Deliveries Scheduled Early[7]	-	-	7%	6%
Preventive Care				
Immunization for Influenza[2]	158	69%	90%	90%
Immunization for Pneumonia[2]	216	56%	92%	92%
Stroke Care				
Anticoagulation Therapy for Atrial Fibrillation[5]	-	-	96%	95%
Antithrombotic Therapy Timing[5]	-	-	98%	98%
Assessed for Rehabilitation[5]	-	-	98%	97%
Discharged on Antithrombotic Therapy[5]	-	-	99%	99%
Discharged on Statin Medication[5]	-	-	95%	94%
Thrombolytic Therapy Timing[5]	-	-	68%	66%
Venous Thromboembolism Prophylaxis[5]	-	-	94%	94%
Written Stroke Educational Materials Given[5]	-	-	92%	88%
Surgical Care Improvement Project				
Appropriate Beta Blocker Usage[5]	-	-	98%	98%
Appropriate VTP Within 24 Hours[5]	-	-	98%	98%
Controlled Postoperative Blood Glucose[5]	-	-	96%	97%
Perioperative Temperature Management[5]	-	-	100%	100%
Prophylactic Antibiotic Selection[5]	-	-	99%	99%
Prophylactic Antibiotic Selection (Outpatient)[5]	-	-	98%	98%
Prophylactic Antibiotic Stopped[5]	-	-	98%	98%
Prophylactic Antibiotic Timing[5]	-	-	99%	99%
Prophylactic Antibiotic Timing (Outpatient)[5]	-	-	98%	98%
Urinary Catheter Removal[5]	-	-	98%	97%
Survey of Patients' Hospital Experiences				
Area Around Room 'Always' Quiet at Night[6]	<100	86%	68%	61%
Doctors 'Always' Communicated Well[6]	<100	90%	83%	82%
Home Recovery Information Given[6]	<100	84%	85%	85%
Hospital Given 9 or 10 on 10 Point Scale[6]	<100	84%	73%	71%
Meds 'Always' Explained Before Given[6]	<100	59%	66%	64%
Nurses 'Always' Communicated Well[6]	<100	84%	80%	79%
Pain 'Always' Well Controlled[6]	<100	70%	72%	71%
Room and Bathroom 'Always' Clean[6]	<100	88%	75%	73%
Timely Help 'Always' Received[6]	<100	90%	69%	68%
Would Definitely Recommend Hospital[6]	<100	79%	73%	71%
Use of Medical Imaging				
Cardiac Imaging Stress Test before Surgery[7]	-	-	5.3%	5.3%
Combination Abdominal CT Scan	112	19.6%	16.4%	10.5%
Combination Brain/Sinus CT Scan	135	0.7%	2.7%	2.7%
Combination Chest CT Scan[1]	-	-	5.6%	2.7%
Follow-up Mammogram/Ultrasound	265	6.4%	7.9%	8.8%
Lumbar Spine MRI for Low Back Pain[1]	-	-	39.6%	37.2%

Reagan Memorial Hospital

805 North Main
Big Lake, TX 76932
Phone: 325-844-2561
Fax: 325-884-2891
Type: Critical Access Hospitals
Emergency Services: Yes
Ownership: Govt - Hospital Dist/Auth
Beds: 14

Key Personnel:
Infection Control . . . . Karen Gore, RN
Chief of Medical Staff . . . . Joseph Sudokan, MD
Emergency Room . . . . Joseph Sudokan, MD

Measure	Cases	This Hosp.	State Avg.	U.S. Avg.
Blood Clot Prevention and Treatment				
Anticoagulation Overlap Therapy[5]	-	-	93%	93%
ICU Venous Thromboembolism Prophylaxis[5]	-	-	92%	92%
Incidence of Potentially Preventable VTE[5]	-	-	9%	10%
UFH with Dosages/Platelet Monitoring[5]	-	-	96%	97%
Venous Thromboembolism Prophylaxis[5]	-	-	82%	85%
Warfarin Therapy Discharge Instructions[5]	-	-	84%	75%
Chest Pain/Possible Heart Attack Care				
Aspirin Given Within 24 Hours of Arrival[1,3]	-	-	94%	96%
Fibrinolytic Meds Within 30 Min. of Arrival[1,3]	-	-	47%	58%
Average Time to ECG (minutes)[1,3]	-	-	8	7
Average Time to Transfer (minutes)[3,7]	-	-	62	60
Children's Asthma Care				
Received Home Management Plan of Care	-	-	93%	88%
Received Reliever Medication	-	-	100%	100%
Received Systemic Corticosteroids	-	-	100%	100%
Emergency Department				
Admittance Decision Time (minutes)[5]	-	-	99	98
Head CT Results Within 45 Min. of Arrival[5]	-	-	54%	57%
Patients Who Left ER Before Being Seen[5]	-	-	3%	2%
Time from ER Arrival to Admit. (minutes)[5]	-	-	270	274
Time from ER Arrival to Discharge (minutes)[5]	-	-	127	134
Time in ER Before Being Evaluated (minutes)[5]	-	-	26	26
Time to Pain Meds for Fractures (minutes)[5]	-	-	57	57
Heart Attack Care				
Aspirin Given at Discharge[5]	-	-	99%	99%
Fibrinolytic Meds Within 30 Min. of Arrival[5]	-	-	49%	54%
PCI Within 90 Minutes of Arrival[5]	-	-	95%	96%
Statin Prescribed at Discharge[5]	-	-	98%	98%
Heart Failure Care				
ACE Inhibitor or ARB for LVSD[5]	-	-	97%	97%
Discharge Instructions Given[5]	-	-	95%	94%
Evaluation of LVS Function[5]	-	-	99%	99%
Medicare Spending				
Medicare Spending per Patient (ratio)	-	-	1.03	0.98
Pneumonia Care				
Appropriate Initial Antibiotic Given[3,7]	-	-	95%	95%
Blood Culture Timing[3,7]	-	-	98%	98%
Pregnancy and Delivery Care				
Newborn Deliveries Scheduled Early[5]	-	-	7%	6%
Preventive Care				
Immunization for Influenza[5]	-	-	90%	90%
Immunization for Pneumonia[5]	-	-	92%	92%
Stroke Care				
Anticoagulation Therapy for Atrial Fibrillation[5]	-	-	96%	95%
Antithrombotic Therapy Timing[5]	-	-	98%	98%
Assessed for Rehabilitation[5]	-	-	98%	97%
Discharged on Antithrombotic Therapy[5]	-	-	99%	99%
Discharged on Statin Medication[5]	-	-	95%	94%
Thrombolytic Therapy Timing[5]	-	-	68%	66%
Venous Thromboembolism Prophylaxis[5]	-	-	94%	94%
Written Stroke Educational Materials Given[5]	-	-	92%	88%
Surgical Care Improvement Project				
Appropriate Beta Blocker Usage[5]	-	-	98%	98%
Appropriate VTP Within 24 Hours[5]	-	-	98%	98%
Controlled Postoperative Blood Glucose[5]	-	-	96%	97%
Perioperative Temperature Management[5]	-	-	100%	100%
Prophylactic Antibiotic Selection[5]	-	-	99%	99%
Prophylactic Antibiotic Selection (Outpatient)[5]	-	-	98%	98%
Prophylactic Antibiotic Stopped[5]	-	-	98%	98%
Prophylactic Antibiotic Timing[5]	-	-	99%	99%
Prophylactic Antibiotic Timing (Outpatient)[5]	-	-	98%	98%
Urinary Catheter Removal[5]	-	-	98%	97%
Survey of Patients' Hospital Experiences				
Area Around Room 'Always' Quiet at Night[10]	<100	49%	68%	61%
Doctors 'Always' Communicated Well[10]	<100	100%	83%	82%
Home Recovery Information Given[10]	<100	100%	85%	85%
Hospital Given 9 or 10 on 10 Point Scale[10]	<100	52%	73%	71%
Meds 'Always' Explained Before Given[10]	<100	98%	66%	64%
Nurses 'Always' Communicated Well[10]	<100	100%	80%	79%
Pain 'Always' Well Controlled[10]	<100	-	72%	71%
Room and Bathroom 'Always' Clean[10]	<100	99%	75%	73%
Timely Help 'Always' Received[10]	<100	100%	69%	68%
Would Definitely Recommend Hospital[10]	<100	54%	73%	71%
Use of Medical Imaging				
Cardiac Imaging Stress Test before Surgery[7]	-	-	5.3%	5.3%
Combination Abdominal CT Scan[1]	-	-	16.4%	10.5%
Combination Brain/Sinus CT Scan[1]	-	-	2.7%	2.7%
Combination Chest CT Scan[1]	-	-	5.6%	2.7%
Follow-up Mammogram/Ultrasound[7]	-	-	7.9%	8.8%
Lumbar Spine MRI for Low Back Pain[7]	-	-	39.6%	37.2%

Scenic Mountain Medical Center

1601 W 11th Place
Big Spring, TX 79720
URL: www.smmccares.com
Phone: 432-263-1211
Fax: 432-268-4962
Type: Acute Care Hospitals
Emergency Services: Yes
Ownership: Proprietary
Beds: 150

Key Personnel:
Pediatric Ambulatory Care . . . . . . Steve Ahmed, MD
Pediatric In-Patient Care . . . . Steve Ahmed, MD
Radiology. . . . . Rajesh Bhojwani
Chief of Medical Staff . . . . James Huston, MD
CEO/President. . . . . George N Parsley
Quality Assurance . . . . Pat Timpe, RN

Measure	Cases	This Hosp.	State Avg.	U.S. Avg.
Blood Clot Prevention and Treatment				
Anticoagulation Overlap Therapy[2]	16	94%	93%	93%
ICU Venous Thromboembolism Prophylaxis[2]	54	100%	92%	92%
Incidence of Potentially Preventable VTE[1,2]	-	-	9%	10%
UFH with Dosages/Platelet Monitoring[2,7]	-	-	96%	97%
Venous Thromboembolism Prophylaxis[2]	235	93%	82%	85%
Warfarin Therapy Discharge Instructions[2]	12	100%	84%	75%
Chest Pain/Possible Heart Attack Care				
Aspirin Given Within 24 Hours of Arrival	80	95%	94%	96%
Fibrinolytic Meds Within 30 Min. of Arrival	12	75%	47%	58%
Average Time to ECG (minutes)	88	4	8	7
Average Time to Transfer (minutes)[1]	-	-	62	60
Children's Asthma Care				
Received Home Management Plan of Care	-	-	93%	88%
Received Reliever Medication	-	-	100%	100%
Received Systemic Corticosteroids	-	-	100%	100%
Emergency Department				
Admittance Decision Time (minutes)[2]	344	76	99	98
Head CT Results Within 45 Min. of Arrival[1]	-	-	54%	57%
Patients Who Left ER Before Being Seen	17,518	4%	3%	2%
Time from ER Arrival to Admit. (minutes)[2]	368	214	270	274
Time from ER Arrival to Discharge (minutes)	375	96	127	134
Time in ER Before Being Evaluated (minutes)	413	27	26	26
Time to Pain Meds for Fractures (minutes)	89	53	57	57
Heart Attack Care				
Aspirin Given at Discharge	13	100%	99%	99%
Fibrinolytic Meds Within 30 Min. of Arrival[1]	-	-	49%	54%
PCI Within 90 Minutes of Arrival[7]	-	-	95%	96%
Statin Prescribed at Discharge	14	86%	98%	98%
Heart Failure Care				
ACE Inhibitor or ARB for LVSD	42	95%	97%	97%
Discharge Instructions Given	60	90%	95%	94%
Evaluation of LVS Function	90	100%	99%	99%
Medicare Spending				
Medicare Spending per Patient (ratio)	-	0.96	1.03	0.98
Pneumonia Care				
Appropriate Initial Antibiotic Given	22	95%	95%	95%
Blood Culture Timing	50	98%	98%	98%
Pregnancy and Delivery Care				
Newborn Deliveries Scheduled Early[2]	19	0%	7%	6%
Preventive Care				
Immunization for Influenza[2]	316	97%	90%	90%
Immunization for Pneumonia[2]	380	98%	92%	92%
Stroke Care				
Anticoagulation Therapy for Atrial Fibrillation[1]	-	-	96%	95%
Antithrombotic Therapy Timing[1]	-	-	98%	98%
Assessed for Rehabilitation[1]	-	-	98%	97%
Discharged on Antithrombotic Therapy[1]	-	-	99%	99%
Discharged on Statin Medication[1]	-	-	95%	94%
Thrombolytic Therapy Timing[7]	-	-	68%	66%
Venous Thromboembolism Prophylaxis[1]	-	-	94%	94%
Written Stroke Educational Materials Given[1]	-	-	92%	88%
Surgical Care Improvement Project				
Appropriate Beta Blocker Usage	18	100%	98%	98%
Appropriate VTP Within 24 Hours	64	100%	98%	98%
Controlled Postoperative Blood Glucose[7]	-	-	96%	97%
Perioperative Temperature Management	79	100%	100%	100%
Prophylactic Antibiotic Selection	44	91%	99%	99%
Prophylactic Antibiotic Selection (Outpatient)	15	100%	98%	98%
Prophylactic Antibiotic Stopped	41	98%	98%	98%

NOTE: Hospital profiles are in alphabetical order by state, then city, then hospital within the city; Rankings exclude hospitals with less than 25 cases except for patient surveys which excludes hospitals with less than 100 cases; (a) 100-299 cases; (1) The number of cases/patients is too few to report; (2) Data submitted were based on a sample of cases/patients; (3) Results are based on a shorter time period than required; (4) Data suppressed by CMS for one or more quarters; (5) Results are not available for this reporting period; (6) Fewer than 100 patients completed the HCAHPS survey; (7) No cases met the criteria for this measure; (8) The lower limit of the confidence interval cannot be calculated if the number of observed infections equals zero; (9) No data are available from the state/territory for this reporting period; (10) The scores shown reflect fewer than 50 completed surveys; (11) There were discrepancies in the data collection process; (12) This measure does not apply to this hospital for this reporting period; (13) Results cannot be calculated for this reporting period; (14) The results for this state are combined with nearby states to protect confidentiality; Please refer to the User's Guide for a full explanation of data.

Measure	Cases	This Hosp.	State Avg.	U.S. Avg.
Prophylactic Antibiotic Timing	44	100%	99%	99%
Prophylactic Antibiotic Timing (Outpatient)	15	100%	98%	98%
Urinary Catheter Removal	32	81%	98%	97%
Survey of Patients' Hospital Experiences				
Area Around Room 'Always' Quiet at Night	300+	64%	68%	61%
Doctors 'Always' Communicated Well	300+	81%	83%	82%
Home Recovery Information Given	300+	82%	85%	85%
Hospital Given 9 or 10 on 10 Point Scale	300+	59%	73%	71%
Meds 'Always' Explained Before Given	300+	58%	66%	64%
Nurses 'Always' Communicated Well	300+	75%	80%	79%
Pain 'Always' Well Controlled	300+	71%	72%	71%
Room and Bathroom 'Always' Clean	300+	70%	75%	73%
Timely Help 'Always' Received	300+	65%	69%	68%
Would Definitely Recommend Hospital	300+	54%	73%	71%
Use of Medical Imaging				
Cardiac Imaging Stress Test before Surgery[1]	-	-	5.3%	5.3%
Combination Abdominal CT Scan	238	16.4%	16.4%	10.5%
Combination Brain/Sinus CT Scan	239	7.1%	2.7%	2.7%
Combination Chest CT Scan	92	8.7%	5.6%	2.7%
Follow-up Mammogram/Ultrasound	234	12.0%	7.9%	8.8%
Lumbar Spine MRI for Low Back Pain[1]	-	-	39.6%	37.2%

VA West Texas Healthcare System

300 Veterans Blvd.
Big Spring, TX 79720
Phone: 432-263-7361
Fax: 432-264-4834
URL: www1.va.gov/directory/guide/facilities
Type: Acute Care - VA
Emergency Services: No
Ownership: Government Federal
Beds: 95

Key Personnel:
Chief of Medical Staff . . . . Martin S Schnier, MD
Quality Assurance . . . . Debra Wallace, RN

Measure	Cases	This Hosp.	State Avg.	U.S. Avg.
Blood Clot Prevention and Treatment				
Anticoagulation Overlap Therapy	-	-	93%	93%
ICU Venous Thromboembolism Prophylaxis	-	-	92%	92%
Incidence of Potentially Preventable VTE	-	-	9%	10%
UFH with Dosages/Platelet Monitoring	-	-	96%	97%
Venous Thromboembolism Prophylaxis	-	-	82%	85%
Warfarin Therapy Discharge Instructions	-	-	84%	75%
Chest Pain/Possible Heart Attack Care				
Aspirin Given Within 24 Hours of Arrival	-	-	94%	96%
Fibrinolytic Meds Within 30 Min. of Arrival	-	-	47%	58%
Average Time to ECG (minutes)	-	-	8	7
Average Time to Transfer (minutes)	-	-	62	60
Children's Asthma Care				
Received Home Management Plan of Care	-	-	93%	88%
Received Reliever Medication	-	-	100%	100%
Received Systemic Corticosteroids	-	-	100%	100%
Emergency Department				
Admittance Decision Time (minutes)	-	-	99	98
Head CT Results Within 45 Min. of Arrival	-	-	54%	57%
Patients Who Left ER Before Being Seen	-	-	3%	2%
Time from ER Arrival to Admit. (minutes)	-	-	270	274
Time from ER Arrival to Discharge (minutes)	-	-	127	134
Time in ER Before Being Evaluated (minutes)	-	-	26	26
Time to Pain Meds for Fractures (minutes)	-	-	57	57
Heart Attack Care				
Aspirin Given at Discharge[5]	-	-	99%	99%
Fibrinolytic Meds Within 30 Min. of Arrival[5]	-	-	49%	54%
PCI Within 90 Minutes of Arrival[5]	-	-	95%	96%
Statin Prescribed at Discharge[5]	-	-	98%	98%
Heart Failure Care				
ACE Inhibitor or ARB for LVSD[5]	-	-	97%	97%
Discharge Instructions Given[5]	-	-	95%	94%
Evaluation of LVS Function[5]	-	-	99%	99%
Medicare Spending				
Medicare Spending per Patient (ratio)	-	-	1.03	0.98
Pneumonia Care				
Appropriate Initial Antibiotic Given[5]	-	-	95%	95%
Blood Culture Timing[5]	-	-	98%	98%
Pregnancy and Delivery Care				
Newborn Deliveries Scheduled Early	-	-	7%	6%
Preventive Care				
Immunization for Influenza[5]	-	-	90%	90%
Immunization for Pneumonia[5]	-	-	92%	92%
Stroke Care				
Anticoagulation Therapy for Atrial Fibrillation	-	-	96%	95%
Antithrombotic Therapy Timing	-	-	98%	98%
Assessed for Rehabilitation	-	-	98%	97%
Discharged on Antithrombotic Therapy	-	-	99%	99%
Discharged on Statin Medication	-	-	95%	94%
Thrombolytic Therapy Timing	-	-	68%	66%
Venous Thromboembolism Prophylaxis	-	-	94%	94%
Written Stroke Educational Materials Given	-	-	92%	88%
Surgical Care Improvement Project				
Appropriate Beta Blocker Usage[5]	-	-	98%	98%
Appropriate VTP Within 24 Hours[5]	-	-	98%	98%
Controlled Postoperative Blood Glucose[5]	-	-	96%	97%
Perioperative Temperature Management[5]	-	-	100%	100%
Prophylactic Antibiotic Selection[5]	-	-	99%	99%
Prophylactic Antibiotic Selection (Outpatient)	-	-	98%	98%
Prophylactic Antibiotic Stopped[5]	-	-	98%	98%
Prophylactic Antibiotic Timing[5]	-	-	99%	99%
Prophylactic Antibiotic Timing (Outpatient)	-	-	98%	98%
Urinary Catheter Removal[5]	-	-	98%	97%
Survey of Patients' Hospital Experiences				
Area Around Room 'Always' Quiet at Night	-	-	68%	61%
Doctors 'Always' Communicated Well	-	-	83%	82%
Home Recovery Information Given	-	-	85%	85%
Hospital Given 9 or 10 on 10 Point Scale	-	-	73%	71%
Meds 'Always' Explained Before Given	-	-	66%	64%
Nurses 'Always' Communicated Well	-	-	80%	79%
Pain 'Always' Well Controlled	-	-	72%	71%
Room and Bathroom 'Always' Clean	-	-	75%	73%
Timely Help 'Always' Received	-	-	69%	68%
Would Definitely Recommend Hospital	-	-	73%	71%
Use of Medical Imaging				
Cardiac Imaging Stress Test before Surgery	-	-	5.3%	5.3%
Combination Abdominal CT Scan	-	-	16.4%	10.5%
Combination Brain/Sinus CT Scan	-	-	2.7%	2.7%
Combination Chest CT Scan	-	-	5.6%	2.7%
Follow-up Mammogram/Ultrasound	-	-	7.9%	8.8%
Lumbar Spine MRI for Low Back Pain	-	-	39.6%	37.2%

Red River Regional Hospital

504 Lipscomb Street
Bonham, TX 75418
Phone: 903-640-7311
Fax: 903-640-7601
Type: Critical Access Hospitals
Emergency Services: Yes
Ownership: Proprietary
Beds: 75

Key Personnel:
Radiology. . . . . Scott M Baker
CEO . . . . David Conejo
Emergency Room . . . . Tina Elliotte
Chief of Medical Staff . . . . George George
Quality Assurance . . . . Clarissa McCollun

Measure	Cases	This Hosp.	State Avg.	U.S. Avg.
Blood Clot Prevention and Treatment				
Anticoagulation Overlap Therapy[5]	-	-	93%	93%
ICU Venous Thromboembolism Prophylaxis[5]	-	-	92%	92%
Incidence of Potentially Preventable VTE[5]	-	-	9%	10%
UFH with Dosages/Platelet Monitoring[5]	-	-	96%	97%
Venous Thromboembolism Prophylaxis[5]	-	-	82%	85%
Warfarin Therapy Discharge Instructions[5]	-	-	84%	75%
Chest Pain/Possible Heart Attack Care				
Aspirin Given Within 24 Hours of Arrival	-	-	94%	96%
Fibrinolytic Meds Within 30 Min. of Arrival	-	-	47%	58%
Average Time to ECG (minutes)	-	-	8	7
Average Time to Transfer (minutes)	-	-	62	60
Children's Asthma Care				
Received Home Management Plan of Care	-	-	93%	88%
Received Reliever Medication	-	-	100%	100%
Received Systemic Corticosteroids	-	-	100%	100%
Emergency Department				
Admittance Decision Time (minutes)[5]	-	-	99	98
Head CT Results Within 45 Min. of Arrival	-	-	54%	57%
Patients Who Left ER Before Being Seen	-	-	3%	2%
Time from ER Arrival to Admit. (minutes)[5]	-	-	270	274
Time from ER Arrival to Discharge (minutes)	-	-	127	134
Time in ER Before Being Evaluated (minutes)	-	-	26	26
Time to Pain Meds for Fractures (minutes)	-	-	57	57
Heart Attack Care				
Aspirin Given at Discharge[1,3]	-	-	99%	99%
Fibrinolytic Meds Within 30 Min. of Arrival[1,3]	-	-	49%	54%
PCI Within 90 Minutes of Arrival[3,7]	-	-	95%	96%
Statin Prescribed at Discharge[1,3]	-	-	98%	98%
Heart Failure Care				
ACE Inhibitor or ARB for LVSD	27	100%	97%	97%
Discharge Instructions Given	34	94%	95%	94%
Evaluation of LVS Function	70	100%	99%	99%
Medicare Spending				
Medicare Spending per Patient (ratio)	-	-	1.03	0.98
Pneumonia Care				
Appropriate Initial Antibiotic Given	20	95%	95%	95%
Blood Culture Timing	76	99%	98%	98%
Pregnancy and Delivery Care				
Newborn Deliveries Scheduled Early[5]	-	-	7%	6%
Preventive Care				
Immunization for Influenza[5]	-	-	90%	90%
Immunization for Pneumonia[5]	-	-	92%	92%
Stroke Care				
Anticoagulation Therapy for Atrial Fibrillation[3,7]	-	-	96%	95%
Antithrombotic Therapy Timing[3,7]	-	-	98%	98%
Assessed for Rehabilitation[1,3]	-	-	98%	97%
Discharged on Antithrombotic Therapy[3,7]	-	-	99%	99%
Discharged on Statin Medication[1,3]	-	-	95%	94%
Thrombolytic Therapy Timing[3,7]	-	-	68%	66%
Venous Thromboembolism Prophylaxis[1,3]	-	-	94%	94%
Written Stroke Educational Materials Given[3,7]	-	-	92%	88%
Surgical Care Improvement Project				
Appropriate Beta Blocker Usage[3,7]	-	-	98%	98%
Appropriate VTP Within 24 Hours[5]	-	-	98%	98%
Controlled Postoperative Blood Glucose[3,7]	-	-	96%	97%
Perioperative Temperature Management[1,3]	-	-	100%	100%
Prophylactic Antibiotic Selection[5]	-	-	99%	99%
Prophylactic Antibiotic Selection (Outpatient)	-	-	98%	98%
Prophylactic Antibiotic Stopped[5]	-	-	98%	98%
Prophylactic Antibiotic Timing[5]	-	-	99%	99%
Prophylactic Antibiotic Timing (Outpatient)	-	-	98%	98%
Urinary Catheter Removal[3,7]	-	-	98%	97%
Survey of Patients' Hospital Experiences				
Area Around Room 'Always' Quiet at Night[5]	-	-	68%	61%
Doctors 'Always' Communicated Well[5]	-	-	83%	82%
Home Recovery Information Given[5]	-	-	85%	85%
Hospital Given 9 or 10 on 10 Point Scale[5]	-	-	73%	71%
Meds 'Always' Explained Before Given[5]	-	-	66%	64%
Nurses 'Always' Communicated Well[5]	-	-	80%	79%
Pain 'Always' Well Controlled[5]	-	-	72%	71%
Room and Bathroom 'Always' Clean[5]	-	-	75%	73%
Timely Help 'Always' Received[5]	-	-	69%	68%
Would Definitely Recommend Hospital[5]	-	-	73%	71%
Use of Medical Imaging				
Cardiac Imaging Stress Test before Surgery	-	-	5.3%	5.3%
Combination Abdominal CT Scan	-	-	16.4%	10.5%
Combination Brain/Sinus CT Scan	-	-	2.7%	2.7%
Combination Chest CT Scan	-	-	5.6%	2.7%
Follow-up Mammogram/Ultrasound	-	-	7.9%	8.8%
Lumbar Spine MRI for Low Back Pain	-	-	39.6%	37.2%

Golden Plains Community Hospital

100 Medical Drive
Borger, TX 79007
Phone: 806-273-1100
Fax: 806-273-1104
E-mail: ceogpch@goldenplains.org
URL: www.goldenplains.org
Type: Critical Access Hospitals
Emergency Services: Yes
Ownership: Government - Federal
Beds: 25

Key Personnel:
Pediatric In-Patient Care . . . . Vicky Cato, RN
Quality Assurance . . . . Melody Henderson
Radiology. . . . . Cyndey Hester
Operating Room. . . . . Sherry Kramer, RN
Chief of Medical Staff . . . . Hank Landers, MD

NOTE: Hospital profiles are in alphabetical order by state, then city, then hospital within the city; Rankings exclude hospitals with less than 25 cases except for patient surveys which excludes hospitals with less than 100 cases; (a) 100-299 cases; (1) The number of cases/patients is too few to report; (2) Data submitted were based on a sample of cases/patients; (3) Results are based on a shorter time period than required; (4) Data suppressed by CMS for one or more quarters; (5) Results are not available for this reporting period; (6) Fewer than 100 patients completed the HCAHPS survey; (7) No cases met the criteria for this measure; (8) The lower limit of the confidence interval cannot be calculated if the number of observed infections equals zero; (9) No data are available from the state/territory for this reporting period; (10) The scores shown reflect fewer than 50 completed surveys; (11) There were discrepancies in the data collection process; (12) This measure does not apply to this hospital for this reporting period; (13) Results cannot be calculated for this reporting period; (14) The results for this state are combined with nearby states to protect confidentiality; Please refer to the User's Guide for a full explanation of data.

Infection Control. . . . . Becky Peery, RN
CEO . . . . Kevin Storey

Measure	Cases	This Hosp.	State Avg.	U.S. Avg.
Blood Clot Prevention and Treatment				
Anticoagulation Overlap Therapy[5]	-	-	93%	93%
ICU Venous Thromboembolism Prophylaxis[5]	-	-	92%	92%
Incidence of Potentially Preventable VTE[5]	-	-	9%	10%
UFH with Dosages/Platelet Monitoring[5]	-	-	96%	97%
Venous Thromboembolism Prophylaxis[5]	-	-	82%	85%
Warfarin Therapy Discharge Instructions[5]	-	-	84%	75%
Chest Pain/Possible Heart Attack Care				
Aspirin Given Within 24 Hours of Arrival	-	-	94%	96%
Fibrinolytic Meds Within 30 Min. of Arrival	-	-	47%	58%
Average Time to ECG (minutes)	-	-	8	7
Average Time to Transfer (minutes)	-	-	62	60
Children's Asthma Care				
Received Home Management Plan of Care	-	-	93%	88%
Received Reliever Medication	-	-	100%	100%
Received Systemic Corticosteroids	-	-	100%	100%
Emergency Department				
Admittance Decision Time (minutes)[2]	255	59	99	98
Head CT Results Within 45 Min. of Arrival	-	-	54%	57%
Patients Who Left ER Before Being Seen	-	-	3%	2%
Time from ER Arrival to Admit. (minutes)[2]	289	210	270	274
Time from ER Arrival to Discharge (minutes)	-	-	127	134
Time in ER Before Being Evaluated (minutes)	-	-	26	26
Time to Pain Meds for Fractures (minutes)	-	-	57	57
Heart Attack Care				
Aspirin Given at Discharge[1]	-	-	99%	99%
Fibrinolytic Meds Within 30 Min. of Arrival[7]	-	-	49%	54%
PCI Within 90 Minutes of Arrival[7]	-	-	95%	96%
Statin Prescribed at Discharge[1]	-	-	98%	98%
Heart Failure Care				
ACE Inhibitor or ARB for LVSD[7]	-	-	97%	97%
Discharge Instructions Given	24	67%	95%	94%
Evaluation of LVS Function	27	59%	99%	99%
Medicare Spending				
Medicare Spending per Patient (ratio)	-	-	1.03	0.98
Pneumonia Care				
Appropriate Initial Antibiotic Given	16	69%	95%	95%
Blood Culture Timing	30	93%	98%	98%
Pregnancy and Delivery Care				
Newborn Deliveries Scheduled Early[5]	-	-	7%	6%
Preventive Care				
Immunization for Influenza[2]	382	71%	90%	90%
Immunization for Pneumonia[2]	351	74%	92%	92%
Stroke Care				
Anticoagulation Therapy for Atrial Fibrillation[5]	-	-	96%	95%
Antithrombotic Therapy Timing[5]	-	-	98%	98%
Assessed for Rehabilitation[5]	-	-	98%	97%
Discharged on Antithrombotic Therapy[5]	-	-	99%	99%
Discharged on Statin Medication[5]	-	-	95%	94%
Thrombolytic Therapy Timing[5]	-	-	68%	66%
Venous Thromboembolism Prophylaxis[5]	-	-	94%	94%
Written Stroke Educational Materials Given[5]	-	-	92%	88%
Surgical Care Improvement Project				
Appropriate Beta Blocker Usage[1]	-	-	98%	98%
Appropriate VTP Within 24 Hours	34	91%	98%	98%
Controlled Postoperative Blood Glucose[7]	-	-	96%	97%
Perioperative Temperature Management	39	100%	100%	100%
Prophylactic Antibiotic Selection	31	100%	99%	99%
Prophylactic Antibiotic Selection (Outpatient)	-	-	98%	98%
Prophylactic Antibiotic Stopped	31	97%	98%	98%
Prophylactic Antibiotic Timing	31	87%	99%	99%
Prophylactic Antibiotic Timing (Outpatient)	-	-	98%	98%
Urinary Catheter Removal	21	86%	98%	97%
Survey of Patients' Hospital Experiences				
Area Around Room 'Always' Quiet at Night[5]	-	-	68%	61%
Doctors 'Always' Communicated Well[5]	-	-	83%	82%
Home Recovery Information Given[5]	-	-	85%	85%
Hospital Given 9 or 10 on 10 Point Scale[5]	-	-	73%	71%
Meds 'Always' Explained Before Given[5]	-	-	66%	64%
Nurses 'Always' Communicated Well[5]	-	-	80%	79%
Pain 'Always' Well Controlled[5]	-	-	72%	71%
Room and Bathroom 'Always' Clean[5]	-	-	75%	73%
Timely Help 'Always' Received[5]	-	-	69%	68%
Would Definitely Recommend Hospital[5]	-	-	73%	71%
Use of Medical Imaging				
Cardiac Imaging Stress Test before Surgery	-	-	5.3%	5.3%
Combination Abdominal CT Scan	-	-	16.4%	10.5%
Combination Brain/Sinus CT Scan	-	-	2.7%	2.7%
Combination Chest CT Scan	-	-	5.6%	2.7%
Follow-up Mammogram/Ultrasound	-	-	7.9%	8.8%
Lumbar Spine MRI for Low Back Pain	-	-	39.6%	37.2%

Bowie Memorial Hospital

705 East Greenwood Av
Bowie, TX 76230
Phone: 940-872-1126
Fax: 940-872-1561
Type: Acute Care Hospitals
Emergency Services: Yes
Ownership: Govt - Hospital Dist/Auth
Beds: 49

Key Personnel:
Anesthesiology. . . . . Andy Crawford, CRNA
Chief of Medical Staff. . . . . Gary Evans, MD
CEO/President. . . . . Kim Lee
Emergency Room . . . . Diane Neu, DON, RN
Infection Control. . . . . Peggy Raley, LVN
Quality Assurance . . . . Peggy Raley, LVN

Measure	Cases	This Hosp.	State Avg.	U.S. Avg.
Blood Clot Prevention and Treatment				
Anticoagulation Overlap Therapy[1,2]	-	-	93%	93%
ICU Venous Thromboembolism Prophylaxis[2,7]	-	-	92%	92%
Incidence of Potentially Preventable VTE[2,7]	-	-	9%	10%
UFH with Dosages/Platelet Monitoring[1,2]	-	-	96%	97%
Venous Thromboembolism Prophylaxis[2]	153	33%	82%	85%
Warfarin Therapy Discharge Instructions[1,2]	-	-	84%	75%
Chest Pain/Possible Heart Attack Care				
Aspirin Given Within 24 Hours of Arrival	28	86%	94%	96%
Fibrinolytic Meds Within 30 Min. of Arrival[1]	-	-	47%	58%
Average Time to ECG (minutes)	30	5	8	7
Average Time to Transfer (minutes)[1]	-	-	62	60
Children's Asthma Care				
Received Home Management Plan of Care	-	-	93%	88%
Received Reliever Medication	-	-	100%	100%
Received Systemic Corticosteroids	-	-	100%	100%
Emergency Department				
Admittance Decision Time (minutes)[2]	284	80	99	98
Head CT Results Within 45 Min. of Arrival[1,3]	-	-	54%	57%
Patients Who Left ER Before Being Seen	4,952	1%	3%	2%
Time from ER Arrival to Admit. (minutes)[2]	311	211	270	274
Time from ER Arrival to Discharge (minutes)	618	83	127	134
Time in ER Before Being Evaluated (minutes)	452	20	26	26
Time to Pain Meds for Fractures (minutes)	43	40	57	57
Heart Attack Care				
Aspirin Given at Discharge[1,3]	-	-	99%	99%
Fibrinolytic Meds Within 30 Min. of Arrival[1,3]	-	-	49%	54%
PCI Within 90 Minutes of Arrival[3,7]	-	-	95%	96%
Statin Prescribed at Discharge[1,3]	-	-	98%	98%
Heart Failure Care				
ACE Inhibitor or ARB for LVSD[2]	22	100%	97%	97%
Discharge Instructions Given[2]	15	100%	95%	94%
Evaluation of LVS Function[2]	34	97%	99%	99%
Medicare Spending				
Medicare Spending per Patient (ratio)	-	0.92	1.03	0.98
Pneumonia Care				
Appropriate Initial Antibiotic Given[2]	29	93%	95%	95%
Blood Culture Timing[2]	33	82%	98%	98%
Pregnancy and Delivery Care				
Newborn Deliveries Scheduled Early[7]	-	-	7%	6%
Preventive Care				
Immunization for Influenza[2]	277	74%	90%	90%
Immunization for Pneumonia[2]	431	87%	92%	92%
Stroke Care				
Anticoagulation Therapy for Atrial Fibrillation[3,7]	-	-	96%	95%
Antithrombotic Therapy Timing[1,3]	-	-	98%	98%
Assessed for Rehabilitation[1,3]	-	-	98%	97%
Discharged on Antithrombotic Therapy[1,3]	-	-	99%	99%
Discharged on Statin Medication[1,3]	-	-	95%	94%
Thrombolytic Therapy Timing[1,3]	-	-	68%	66%
Venous Thromboembolism Prophylaxis[1,3]	-	-	94%	94%
Written Stroke Educational Materials Given[3,7]	-	-	92%	88%
Surgical Care Improvement Project				
Appropriate Beta Blocker Usage[5]	-	-	98%	98%
Appropriate VTP Within 24 Hours[5]	-	-	98%	98%
Controlled Postoperative Blood Glucose[5]	-	-	96%	97%
Perioperative Temperature Management[5]	-	-	100%	100%
Prophylactic Antibiotic Selection[5]	-	-	99%	99%
Prophylactic Antibiotic Selection (Outpatient)[1,3]	-	-	98%	98%
Prophylactic Antibiotic Stopped[5]	-	-	98%	98%
Prophylactic Antibiotic Timing[5]	-	-	99%	99%
Prophylactic Antibiotic Timing (Outpatient)[1,3]	-	-	98%	98%
Urinary Catheter Removal[5]	-	-	98%	97%
Survey of Patients' Hospital Experiences				
Area Around Room 'Always' Quiet at Night[6]	<100	64%	68%	61%
Doctors 'Always' Communicated Well[6]	<100	94%	83%	82%
Home Recovery Information Given[6]	<100	86%	85%	85%
Hospital Given 9 or 10 on 10 Point Scale[6]	<100	74%	73%	71%
Meds 'Always' Explained Before Given[6]	<100	61%	66%	64%
Nurses 'Always' Communicated Well[6]	<100	83%	80%	79%
Pain 'Always' Well Controlled[6]	<100	76%	72%	71%
Room and Bathroom 'Always' Clean[6]	<100	76%	75%	73%
Timely Help 'Always' Received[6]	<100	80%	69%	68%
Would Definitely Recommend Hospital[6]	<100	70%	73%	71%
Use of Medical Imaging				
Cardiac Imaging Stress Test before Surgery[7]	-	-	5.3%	5.3%
Combination Abdominal CT Scan	94	52.1%	16.4%	10.5%
Combination Brain/Sinus CT Scan[1]	-	-	2.7%	2.7%
Combination Chest CT Scan[1]	-	-	5.6%	2.7%
Follow-up Mammogram/Ultrasound	68	4.4%	7.9%	8.8%
Lumbar Spine MRI for Low Back Pain[1]	-	-	39.6%	37.2%

Stephens Memorial Hospital

200 South Geneva Street
Breckenridge, TX 76424
Phone: 254-559-2241
Fax: 254-559-9000
URL: www.smhtx.com
Type: Acute Care Hospitals
Emergency Services: Yes
Ownership: Government - Local
Beds: 40

Key Personnel:
Radiology. . . . . Jim Andrus, RT
CEO/President. . . . . Robbie Dewberry
Chief of Medical Staff . . . . Matthew T Proctor
Infection Control. . . . . Alicia Whitt, RN, ACNO

Measure	Cases	This Hosp.	State Avg.	U.S. Avg.
Blood Clot Prevention and Treatment				
Anticoagulation Overlap Therapy[1,2]	-	-	93%	93%
ICU Venous Thromboembolism Prophylaxis[2,7]	-	-	92%	92%
Incidence of Potentially Preventable VTE[2,7]	-	-	9%	10%
UFH with Dosages/Platelet Monitoring[2,7]	-	-	96%	97%
Venous Thromboembolism Prophylaxis[2]	258	47%	82%	85%
Warfarin Therapy Discharge Instructions[1,2]	-	-	84%	75%
Chest Pain/Possible Heart Attack Care				
Aspirin Given Within 24 Hours of Arrival	32	100%	94%	96%
Fibrinolytic Meds Within 30 Min. of Arrival[1]	-	-	47%	58%
Average Time to ECG (minutes)	33	4	8	7
Average Time to Transfer (minutes)[7]	-	-	62	60
Children's Asthma Care				
Received Home Management Plan of Care	-	-	93%	88%
Received Reliever Medication	-	-	100%	100%
Received Systemic Corticosteroids	-	-	100%	100%
Emergency Department				
Admittance Decision Time (minutes)[2]	165	30	99	98
Head CT Results Within 45 Min. of Arrival[3,7]	-	-	54%	57%
Patients Who Left ER Before Being Seen	5,679	3%	3%	2%
Time from ER Arrival to Admit. (minutes)[2]	165	113	270	274
Time from ER Arrival to Discharge (minutes)	2,588	95	127	134
Time in ER Before Being Evaluated (minutes)	3,042	6	26	26
Time to Pain Meds for Fractures (minutes)	27	59	57	57
Heart Attack Care				
Aspirin Given at Discharge[1,3]	-	-	99%	99%
Fibrinolytic Meds Within 30 Min. of Arrival[3,7]	-	-	49%	54%

NOTE: Hospital profiles are in alphabetical order by state, then city, then hospital within the city; Rankings exclude hospitals with less than 25 cases except for patient surveys which excludes hospitals with less than 100 cases; (a) 100-299 cases; (1) The number of cases/patients is too few to report; (2) Data submitted were based on a sample of cases/patients; (3) Results are based on a shorter time period than required; (4) Data suppressed by CMS for one or more quarters; (5) Results are not available for this reporting period; (6) Fewer than 100 patients completed the HCAHPS survey; (7) No cases met the criteria for this measure; (8) The lower limit of the confidence interval cannot be calculated if the number of observed infections equals zero; (9) No data are available from the state/territory for this reporting period; (10) The scores shown reflect fewer than 50 completed surveys; (11) There were discrepancies in the data collection process; (12) This measure does not apply to this hospital for this reporting period; (13) Results cannot be calculated for this reporting period; (14) The results for this state are combined with nearby states to protect confidentiality; Please refer to the User's Guide for a full explanation of data.

Measure	Cases	This Hosp.	State Avg.	U.S. Avg.
PCI Within 90 Minutes of Arrival[3,7]	-	-	95%	96%
Statin Prescribed at Discharge[1,3]	-	-	98%	98%
Heart Failure Care				
ACE Inhibitor or ARB for LVSD[1]	-	-	97%	97%
Discharge Instructions Given	18	94%	95%	94%
Evaluation of LVS Function	19	63%	99%	99%
Medicare Spending				
Medicare Spending per Patient (ratio)	-	0.94	1.03	0.98
Pneumonia Care				
Appropriate Initial Antibiotic Given	18	89%	95%	95%
Blood Culture Timing	20	80%	98%	98%
Pregnancy and Delivery Care				
Newborn Deliveries Scheduled Early[7]	-	-	7%	6%
Preventive Care				
Immunization for Influenza[2]	229	93%	90%	90%
Immunization for Pneumonia[2]	314	92%	92%	92%
Stroke Care				
Anticoagulation Therapy for Atrial Fibrillation[7]	-	-	96%	95%
Antithrombotic Therapy Timing[1]	-	-	98%	98%
Assessed for Rehabilitation[1]	-	-	98%	97%
Discharged on Antithrombotic Therapy[1]	-	-	99%	99%
Discharged on Statin Medication[1]	-	-	95%	94%
Thrombolytic Therapy Timing[1]	-	-	68%	66%
Venous Thromboembolism Prophylaxis[1]	-	-	94%	94%
Written Stroke Educational Materials Given[1]	-	-	92%	88%
Surgical Care Improvement Project				
Appropriate Beta Blocker Usage[5]	-	-	98%	98%
Appropriate VTP Within 24 Hours[5]	-	-	98%	98%
Controlled Postoperative Blood Glucose[5]	-	-	96%	97%
Perioperative Temperature Management[5]	-	-	100%	100%
Prophylactic Antibiotic Selection[5]	-	-	99%	99%
Prophylactic Antibiotic Selection (Outpatient)[5]	-	-	98%	98%
Prophylactic Antibiotic Stopped[5]	-	-	98%	98%
Prophylactic Antibiotic Timing[5]	-	-	99%	99%
Prophylactic Antibiotic Timing (Outpatient)[5]	-	-	98%	98%
Urinary Catheter Removal[5]	-	-	98%	97%
Survey of Patients' Hospital Experiences				
Area Around Room 'Always' Quiet at Night[6]	<100	71%	68%	61%
Doctors 'Always' Communicated Well[6]	<100	85%	83%	82%
Home Recovery Information Given[6]	<100	74%	85%	85%
Hospital Given 9 or 10 on 10 Point Scale[6]	<100	68%	73%	71%
Meds 'Always' Explained Before Given[6]	<100	46%	66%	64%
Nurses 'Always' Communicated Well[6]	<100	85%	80%	79%
Pain 'Always' Well Controlled[6]	<100	75%	72%	71%
Room and Bathroom 'Always' Clean[6]	<100	68%	75%	73%
Timely Help 'Always' Received[6]	<100	81%	69%	68%
Would Definitely Recommend Hospital[6]	<100	78%	73%	71%
Use of Medical Imaging				
Cardiac Imaging Stress Test before Surgery[7]	-	-	5.3%	5.3%
Combination Abdominal CT Scan	68	7.4%	16.4%	10.5%
Combination Brain/Sinus CT Scan[1]	-	-	2.7%	2.7%
Combination Chest CT Scan[1]	-	-	5.6%	2.7%
Follow-up Mammogram/Ultrasound	45	4.4%	7.9%	8.8%
Lumbar Spine MRI for Low Back Pain[1]	-	-	39.6%	37.2%

Scott & White Hospital Brenham

700 Medical Parkway		Phone: 979-836-6173
Brenham, TX 77833		Fax: 979-830-2277
URL: www.trinitymed.com
Type: Acute Care Hospitals		Emergency Services: Yes
Ownership: Voluntary non-profit - Private		Beds: 60

Key Personnel:
Cardiac Laboratory............ Lynn Boeaer
Quality Assurance .... Teresa Gabriel
Emergency Room .... Garry L. Gore, MD, FACEP
Radiology.................... Ian Hamilton, PhD, CHP, DABR(
Chair/CEO.................... Tommy Ladewig
Administrator .... Michael Pittman, FACHE, RN
Chief of Medical Staff.......... Michael Schlabach, MD, MPPH
CEO/President................ John Simms

Measure	Cases	This Hosp.	State Avg.	U.S. Avg.
Blood Clot Prevention and Treatment				
Anticoagulation Overlap Therapy[1,2]	-	-	93%	93%
ICU Venous Thromboembolism Prophylaxis[2]	21	86%	92%	92%
Incidence of Potentially Preventable VTE[2,7]	-	-	9%	10%
UFH with Dosages/Platelet Monitoring[2,7]	-	-	96%	97%
Venous Thromboembolism Prophylaxis[2]	93	81%	82%	85%
Warfarin Therapy Discharge Instructions[1,2]	-	-	84%	75%
Chest Pain/Possible Heart Attack Care				
Aspirin Given Within 24 Hours of Arrival	78	95%	94%	96%
Fibrinolytic Meds Within 30 Min. of Arrival[1]	-	-	47%	58%
Average Time to ECG (minutes)	77	9	8	7
Average Time to Transfer (minutes)[1]	-	-	62	60
Children's Asthma Care				
Received Home Management Plan of Care	-	-	93%	88%
Received Reliever Medication	-	-	100%	100%
Received Systemic Corticosteroids	-	-	100%	100%
Emergency Department				
Admittance Decision Time (minutes)[2]	228	66	99	98
Head CT Results Within 45 Min. of Arrival	11	91%	54%	57%
Patients Who Left ER Before Being Seen	15,881	2%	3%	2%
Time from ER Arrival to Admit. (minutes)[2]	239	238	270	274
Time from ER Arrival to Discharge (minutes)	351	135	127	134
Time in ER Before Being Evaluated (minutes)	366	28	26	26
Time to Pain Meds for Fractures (minutes)	88	40	57	57
Heart Attack Care				
Aspirin Given at Discharge[1]	-	-	99%	99%
Fibrinolytic Meds Within 30 Min. of Arrival[7]	-	-	49%	54%
PCI Within 90 Minutes of Arrival[7]	-	-	95%	96%
Statin Prescribed at Discharge[1]	-	-	98%	98%
Heart Failure Care				
ACE Inhibitor or ARB for LVSD	17	94%	97%	97%
Discharge Instructions Given	43	98%	95%	94%
Evaluation of LVS Function	57	100%	99%	99%
Medicare Spending				
Medicare Spending per Patient (ratio)	-	0.88	1.03	0.98
Pneumonia Care				
Appropriate Initial Antibiotic Given	41	95%	95%	95%
Blood Culture Timing	67	99%	98%	98%
Pregnancy and Delivery Care				
Newborn Deliveries Scheduled Early	23	9%	7%	6%
Preventive Care				
Immunization for Influenza[2]	244	97%	90%	90%
Immunization for Pneumonia[2]	275	94%	92%	92%
Stroke Care				
Anticoagulation Therapy for Atrial Fibrillation[1]	-	-	96%	95%
Antithrombotic Therapy Timing[1]	-	-	98%	98%
Assessed for Rehabilitation[1]	-	-	98%	97%
Discharged on Antithrombotic Therapy[1]	-	-	99%	99%
Discharged on Statin Medication[1]	-	-	95%	94%
Thrombolytic Therapy Timing[7]	-	-	68%	66%
Venous Thromboembolism Prophylaxis[1]	-	-	94%	94%
Written Stroke Educational Materials Given[1]	-	-	92%	88%
Surgical Care Improvement Project				
Appropriate Beta Blocker Usage	31	100%	98%	98%
Appropriate VTP Within 24 Hours	107	99%	98%	98%
Controlled Postoperative Blood Glucose[7]	-	-	96%	97%
Perioperative Temperature Management	125	100%	100%	100%
Prophylactic Antibiotic Selection	91	99%	99%	99%
Prophylactic Antibiotic Selection (Outpatient)	45	100%	98%	98%
Prophylactic Antibiotic Stopped	91	99%	98%	98%
Prophylactic Antibiotic Timing	91	98%	99%	99%
Prophylactic Antibiotic Timing (Outpatient)	16	100%	98%	98%
Urinary Catheter Removal	78	100%	98%	97%
Survey of Patients' Hospital Experiences				
Area Around Room 'Always' Quiet at Night	300+	64%	68%	61%
Doctors 'Always' Communicated Well	300+	83%	83%	82%
Home Recovery Information Given	300+	85%	85%	85%
Hospital Given 9 or 10 on 10 Point Scale	300+	68%	73%	71%
Meds 'Always' Explained Before Given	300+	67%	66%	64%
Nurses 'Always' Communicated Well	300+	77%	80%	79%
Pain 'Always' Well Controlled	300+	72%	72%	71%
Room and Bathroom 'Always' Clean	300+	69%	75%	73%
Timely Help 'Always' Received	300+	65%	69%	68%
Would Definitely Recommend Hospital	300+	62%	73%	71%
Use of Medical Imaging				
Cardiac Imaging Stress Test before Surgery[1]	-	-	5.3%	5.3%
Combination Abdominal CT Scan	228	12.7%	16.4%	10.5%
Combination Brain/Sinus CT Scan[1]	-	-	2.7%	2.7%
Combination Chest CT Scan	159	8.2%	5.6%	2.7%
Follow-up Mammogram/Ultrasound	185	8.1%	7.9%	8.8%
Lumbar Spine MRI for Low Back Pain[1]	-	-	39.6%	37.2%

Brownfield Regional Medical Center

705 East Felt Street		Phone: 806-637-3551
Brownfield, TX 79316		Fax: 806-637-9083
E-mail: webmaster@brownfield-rmc.org
URL: www.brownfield-rmc.org
Type: Acute Care Hospitals		Emergency Services: Yes
Ownership: Govt - Hospital Dist/Auth		Beds: 71

Key Personnel:
Chief of Medical Staff.......... Paul Chebib, MD
CEO/President................ Mike Click, RN
Operating Room............. Nell Coder, RN
Infection Control............. Michelle McElly, RN

Measure	Cases	This Hosp.	State Avg.	U.S. Avg.
Blood Clot Prevention and Treatment				
Anticoagulation Overlap Therapy[2,7]	-	-	93%	93%
ICU Venous Thromboembolism Prophylaxis[2,7]	-	-	92%	92%
Incidence of Potentially Preventable VTE[2,7]	-	-	9%	10%
UFH with Dosages/Platelet Monitoring[2,7]	-	-	96%	97%
Venous Thromboembolism Prophylaxis[2]	125	19%	82%	85%
Warfarin Therapy Discharge Instructions[2,7]	-	-	84%	75%
Chest Pain/Possible Heart Attack Care				
Aspirin Given Within 24 Hours of Arrival	70	91%	94%	96%
Fibrinolytic Meds Within 30 Min. of Arrival[3,7]	-	-	47%	58%
Average Time to ECG (minutes)	77	14	8	7
Average Time to Transfer (minutes)[1,3]	-	-	62	60
Children's Asthma Care				
Received Home Management Plan of Care	-	-	93%	88%
Received Reliever Medication	-	-	100%	100%
Received Systemic Corticosteroids	-	-	100%	100%
Emergency Department				
Admittance Decision Time (minutes)[2]	146	35	99	98
Head CT Results Within 45 Min. of Arrival[7]	-	-	54%	57%
Patients Who Left ER Before Being Seen	5,335	6%	3%	2%
Time from ER Arrival to Admit. (minutes)[2]	173	163	270	274
Time from ER Arrival to Discharge (minutes)	252	117	127	134
Time in ER Before Being Evaluated (minutes)	418	64	26	26
Time to Pain Meds for Fractures (minutes)	20	81	57	57
Heart Attack Care				
Aspirin Given at Discharge[1]	-	-	99%	99%
Fibrinolytic Meds Within 30 Min. of Arrival[1]	-	-	49%	54%
PCI Within 90 Minutes of Arrival[7]	-	-	95%	96%
Statin Prescribed at Discharge[1]	-	-	98%	98%
Heart Failure Care				
ACE Inhibitor or ARB for LVSD[1]	-	-	97%	97%
Discharge Instructions Given	21	29%	95%	94%
Evaluation of LVS Function	21	43%	99%	99%
Medicare Spending				
Medicare Spending per Patient (ratio)	-	0.91	1.03	0.98
Pneumonia Care				
Appropriate Initial Antibiotic Given	29	97%	95%	95%
Blood Culture Timing[1]	-	-	98%	98%
Pregnancy and Delivery Care				
Newborn Deliveries Scheduled Early	21	5%	7%	6%
Preventive Care				
Immunization for Influenza[2]	285	56%	90%	90%
Immunization for Pneumonia[2]	332	53%	92%	92%
Stroke Care				
Anticoagulation Therapy for Atrial Fibrillation[7]	-	-	96%	95%
Antithrombotic Therapy Timing[1]	-	-	98%	98%
Assessed for Rehabilitation[1]	-	-	98%	97%
Discharged on Antithrombotic Therapy[1]	-	-	99%	99%
Discharged on Statin Medication[1]	-	-	95%	94%
Thrombolytic Therapy Timing[7]	-	-	68%	66%
Venous Thromboembolism Prophylaxis[1]	-	-	94%	94%
Written Stroke Educational Materials Given[1]	-	-	92%	88%
Surgical Care Improvement Project				
Appropriate Beta Blocker Usage[5]	-	-	98%	98%

NOTE: Hospital profiles are in alphabetical order by state, then city, then hospital within the city; Rankings exclude hospitals with less than 25 cases except for patient surveys which excludes hospitals with less than 100 cases; (a) 100-299 cases; (1) The number of cases/patients is too few to report; (2) Data submitted were based on a sample of cases/patients; (3) Results are based on a shorter time period than required; (4) Data suppressed by CMS for one or more quarters; (5) Results are not available for this reporting period; (6) Fewer than 100 patients completed the HCAHPS survey; (7) No cases met the criteria for this measure; (8) The lower limit of the confidence interval cannot be calculated if the number of observed infections equals zero; (9) No data are available from the state/territory for this reporting period; (10) The scores shown reflect fewer than 50 completed surveys; (11) There were discrepancies in the data collection process; (12) This measure does not apply to this hospital for this reporting period; (13) Results cannot be calculated for this reporting period; (14) The results for this state are combined with nearby states to protect confidentiality; Please refer to the User's Guide for a full explanation of data.

Measure	Cases	This Hosp.	State Avg.	U.S. Avg.
Appropriate VTP Within 24 Hours[5]	-	-	98%	98%
Controlled Postoperative Blood Glucose[5]	-	-	96%	97%
Perioperative Temperature Management[5]	-	-	100%	100%
Prophylactic Antibiotic Selection[5]	-	-	99%	99%
Prophylactic Antibiotic Selection (Outpatient)[5]	-	-	98%	98%
Prophylactic Antibiotic Stopped[5]	-	-	98%	98%
Prophylactic Antibiotic Timing[5]	-	-	99%	99%
Prophylactic Antibiotic Timing (Outpatient)[5]	-	-	98%	98%
Urinary Catheter Removal[5]	-	-	98%	97%
Survey of Patients' Hospital Experiences				
Area Around Room 'Always' Quiet at Night	(a)	71%	68%	61%
Doctors 'Always' Communicated Well	(a)	86%	83%	82%
Home Recovery Information Given	(a)	88%	85%	85%
Hospital Given 9 or 10 on 10 Point Scale	(a)	63%	73%	71%
Meds 'Always' Explained Before Given	(a)	64%	66%	64%
Nurses 'Always' Communicated Well	(a)	81%	80%	79%
Pain 'Always' Well Controlled	(a)	78%	72%	71%
Room and Bathroom 'Always' Clean	(a)	74%	75%	73%
Timely Help 'Always' Received	(a)	70%	69%	68%
Would Definitely Recommend Hospital	(a)	64%	73%	71%
Use of Medical Imaging				
Cardiac Imaging Stress Test before Surgery[7]	-	-	5.3%	5.3%
Combination Abdominal CT Scan	74	2.7%	16.4%	10.5%
Combination Brain/Sinus CT Scan[1]	-	-	2.7%	2.7%
Combination Chest CT Scan[1]	-	-	5.6%	2.7%
Follow-up Mammogram/Ultrasound[7]	-	-	7.9%	8.8%
Lumbar Spine MRI for Low Back Pain[1]	-	-	39.6%	37.2%

Valley Regional Medical Center

100 A Alton Gloor
Brownsville, TX 78526
Phone: 956-350-7000
Fax: 956-350-7191
URL: www.valleyregionalmedicalcenter.com
Type: Acute Care Hospitals
Emergency Services: Yes
Ownership: Proprietary
Beds: 214

Key Personnel:

CEO . . . . Susan Andrews
Surgery . . . . Kwang Lee
Chief of Medical Staff . . . . Juan F. Rodriguez
Pediatrics . . . . Asim Zamir

Measure	Cases	This Hosp.	State Avg.	U.S. Avg.
Blood Clot Prevention and Treatment				
Anticoagulation Overlap Therapy[2]	41	98%	93%	93%
ICU Venous Thromboembolism Prophylaxis[2]	73	89%	92%	92%
Incidence of Potentially Preventable VTE[2]	12	0%	9%	10%
UFH with Dosages/Platelet Monitoring[1,2]	-	-	96%	97%
Venous Thromboembolism Prophylaxis[2]	388	88%	82%	85%
Warfarin Therapy Discharge Instructions[2]	29	100%	84%	75%
Chest Pain/Possible Heart Attack Care				
Aspirin Given Within 24 Hours of Arrival[5]	-	-	94%	96%
Fibrinolytic Meds Within 30 Min. of Arrival[5]	-	-	47%	58%
Average Time to ECG (minutes)[5]	-	-	8	7
Average Time to Transfer (minutes)[5]	-	-	62	60
Children's Asthma Care				
Received Home Management Plan of Care	-	-	93%	88%
Received Reliever Medication	-	-	100%	100%
Received Systemic Corticosteroids	-	-	100%	100%
Emergency Department				
Admittance Decision Time (minutes)[2]	592	65	99	98
Head CT Results Within 45 Min. of Arrival[1]	-	-	54%	57%
Patients Who Left ER Before Being Seen	32,770	2%	3%	2%
Time from ER Arrival to Admit. (minutes)[2]	600	240	270	274
Time from ER Arrival to Discharge (minutes)	461	176	127	134
Time in ER Before Being Evaluated (minutes)	513	24	26	26
Time to Pain Meds for Fractures (minutes)	212	60	57	57
Heart Attack Care				
Aspirin Given at Discharge	236	99%	99%	99%
Fibrinolytic Meds Within 30 Min. of Arrival[7]	-	-	49%	54%
PCI Within 90 Minutes of Arrival	27	100%	95%	96%
Statin Prescribed at Discharge	236	99%	98%	98%
Heart Failure Care				
ACE Inhibitor or ARB for LVSD	98	100%	97%	97%
Discharge Instructions Given	229	100%	95%	94%
Evaluation of LVS Function	261	100%	99%	99%
Medicare Spending				
Medicare Spending per Patient (ratio)	-	1.03	1.03	0.98
Pneumonia Care				
Appropriate Initial Antibiotic Given	89	98%	95%	95%
Blood Culture Timing	167	99%	98%	98%
Pregnancy and Delivery Care				
Newborn Deliveries Scheduled Early[2]	71	0%	7%	6%
Preventive Care				
Immunization for Influenza[2]	487	99%	90%	90%
Immunization for Pneumonia[2]	449	100%	92%	92%
Stroke Care				
Anticoagulation Therapy for Atrial Fibrillation[1,2]	-	-	96%	95%
Antithrombotic Therapy Timing[2]	48	100%	98%	98%
Assessed for Rehabilitation[2]	58	100%	98%	97%
Discharged on Antithrombotic Therapy[2]	50	100%	99%	99%
Discharged on Statin Medication[2]	43	98%	95%	94%
Thrombolytic Therapy Timing[1,2]	-	-	68%	66%
Venous Thromboembolism Prophylaxis[2]	57	98%	94%	94%
Written Stroke Educational Materials Given[2]	31	74%	92%	88%
Surgical Care Improvement Project				
Appropriate Beta Blocker Usage	96	97%	98%	98%
Appropriate VTP Within 24 Hours	274	99%	98%	98%
Controlled Postoperative Blood Glucose	41	100%	96%	97%
Perioperative Temperature Management	312	99%	100%	100%
Prophylactic Antibiotic Selection	221	100%	99%	99%
Prophylactic Antibiotic Selection (Outpatient)	189	100%	98%	98%
Prophylactic Antibiotic Stopped	212	100%	98%	98%
Prophylactic Antibiotic Timing	221	100%	99%	99%
Prophylactic Antibiotic Timing (Outpatient)	189	100%	98%	98%
Urinary Catheter Removal	136	100%	98%	97%
Survey of Patients' Hospital Experiences				
Area Around Room 'Always' Quiet at Night	300+	55%	68%	61%
Doctors 'Always' Communicated Well	300+	80%	83%	82%
Home Recovery Information Given	300+	84%	85%	85%
Hospital Given 9 or 10 on 10 Point Scale	300+	68%	73%	71%
Meds 'Always' Explained Before Given	300+	61%	66%	64%
Nurses 'Always' Communicated Well	300+	73%	80%	79%
Pain 'Always' Well Controlled	300+	66%	72%	71%
Room and Bathroom 'Always' Clean	300+	72%	75%	73%
Timely Help 'Always' Received	300+	55%	69%	68%
Would Definitely Recommend Hospital	300+	68%	73%	71%
Use of Medical Imaging				
Cardiac Imaging Stress Test before Surgery[1]	-	-	5.3%	5.3%
Combination Abdominal CT Scan	445	24.5%	16.4%	10.5%
Combination Brain/Sinus CT Scan	486	1.9%	2.7%	2.7%
Combination Chest CT Scan	240	19.6%	5.6%	2.7%
Follow-up Mammogram/Ultrasound	970	7.6%	7.9%	8.8%
Lumbar Spine MRI for Low Back Pain[1]	-	-	39.6%	37.2%

VHS Brownsville Hospital Company

1040 W Jefferson St
Brownsville, TX 78520
Phone: 956-544-1400
Fax: 956-698-5712
URL: www.brownsvillemedical.com
Type: Acute Care Hospitals
Emergency Services: Yes
Ownership: Proprietary
Beds: 243

Key Personnel:

Radiology . . . . Mark Boykin, MD
Quality Assurance . . . . Julie Cass, RN
Anesthesiology . . . . John Wells, MD
CEO/President . . . . Jim Wesson

Measure	Cases	This Hosp.	State Avg.	U.S. Avg.
Blood Clot Prevention and Treatment				
Anticoagulation Overlap Therapy[2]	21	67%	93%	93%
ICU Venous Thromboembolism Prophylaxis[2]	69	84%	92%	92%
Incidence of Potentially Preventable VTE[2]	17	29%	9%	10%
UFH with Dosages/Platelet Monitoring[1,2]	-	-	96%	97%
Venous Thromboembolism Prophylaxis[2]	330	52%	82%	85%
Warfarin Therapy Discharge Instructions[2]	16	94%	84%	75%
Chest Pain/Possible Heart Attack Care				
Aspirin Given Within 24 Hours of Arrival[1,3]	-	-	94%	96%
Fibrinolytic Meds Within 30 Min. of Arrival[5]	-	-	47%	58%
Average Time to ECG (minutes)[1,3]	-	-	8	7
Average Time to Transfer (minutes)[5]	-	-	62	60
Children's Asthma Care				
Received Home Management Plan of Care	-	-	93%	88%
Received Reliever Medication	-	-	100%	100%
Received Systemic Corticosteroids	-	-	100%	100%
Emergency Department				
Admittance Decision Time (minutes)[2]	534	85	99	98
Head CT Results Within 45 Min. of Arrival[1]	-	-	54%	57%
Patients Who Left ER Before Being Seen	32,439	2%	3%	2%
Time from ER Arrival to Admit. (minutes)[2]	534	282	270	274
Time from ER Arrival to Discharge (minutes)	530	150	127	134
Time in ER Before Being Evaluated (minutes)	590	19	26	26
Time to Pain Meds for Fractures (minutes)	155	39	57	57
Heart Attack Care				
Aspirin Given at Discharge	211	99%	99%	99%
Fibrinolytic Meds Within 30 Min. of Arrival[7]	-	-	49%	54%
PCI Within 90 Minutes of Arrival	21	95%	95%	96%
Statin Prescribed at Discharge	197	96%	98%	98%
Heart Failure Care				
ACE Inhibitor or ARB for LVSD	69	88%	97%	97%
Discharge Instructions Given	184	96%	95%	94%
Evaluation of LVS Function	220	98%	99%	99%
Medicare Spending				
Medicare Spending per Patient (ratio)	-	1.05	1.03	0.98
Pneumonia Care				
Appropriate Initial Antibiotic Given[2]	103	89%	95%	95%
Blood Culture Timing[2]	262	96%	98%	98%
Pregnancy and Delivery Care				
Newborn Deliveries Scheduled Early	217	2%	7%	6%
Preventive Care				
Immunization for Influenza[2]	525	93%	90%	90%
Immunization for Pneumonia[2]	521	94%	92%	92%
Stroke Care				
Anticoagulation Therapy for Atrial Fibrillation[1]	-	-	96%	95%
Antithrombotic Therapy Timing	76	100%	98%	98%
Assessed for Rehabilitation	99	100%	98%	97%
Discharged on Antithrombotic Therapy	80	100%	99%	99%
Discharged on Statin Medication	44	95%	95%	94%
Thrombolytic Therapy Timing[1]	-	-	68%	66%
Venous Thromboembolism Prophylaxis	111	95%	94%	94%
Written Stroke Educational Materials Given	39	97%	92%	88%
Surgical Care Improvement Project				
Appropriate Beta Blocker Usage[2]	73	96%	98%	98%
Appropriate VTP Within 24 Hours[2]	210	90%	98%	98%
Controlled Postoperative Blood Glucose[2]	41	100%	96%	97%
Perioperative Temperature Management[2]	238	100%	100%	100%
Prophylactic Antibiotic Selection[2]	53	92%	99%	99%
Prophylactic Antibiotic Selection (Outpatient)	180	98%	98%	98%
Prophylactic Antibiotic Stopped[2]	48	96%	98%	98%
Prophylactic Antibiotic Timing[2]	53	98%	99%	99%
Prophylactic Antibiotic Timing (Outpatient)	200	83%	98%	98%
Urinary Catheter Removal[2]	100	98%	98%	97%
Survey of Patients' Hospital Experiences				
Area Around Room 'Always' Quiet at Night[11]	300+	60%	68%	61%
Doctors 'Always' Communicated Well[11]	300+	81%	83%	82%
Home Recovery Information Given[11]	300+	86%	85%	85%
Hospital Given 9 or 10 on 10 Point Scale[11]	300+	75%	73%	71%
Meds 'Always' Explained Before Given[11]	300+	64%	66%	64%
Nurses 'Always' Communicated Well[11]	300+	77%	80%	79%
Pain 'Always' Well Controlled[11]	300+	71%	72%	71%
Room and Bathroom 'Always' Clean[11]	300+	75%	75%	73%
Timely Help 'Always' Received[11]	300+	62%	69%	68%
Would Definitely Recommend Hospital[11]	300+	71%	73%	71%
Use of Medical Imaging				
Cardiac Imaging Stress Test before Surgery[1]	-	-	5.3%	5.3%
Combination Abdominal CT Scan	552	14.1%	16.4%	10.5%
Combination Brain/Sinus CT Scan[1]	-	-	2.7%	2.7%
Combination Chest CT Scan	145	6.2%	5.6%	2.7%
Follow-up Mammogram/Ultrasound	782	10.0%	7.9%	8.8%
Lumbar Spine MRI for Low Back Pain	71	38.0%	39.6%	37.2%

NOTE: Hospital profiles are in alphabetical order by state, then city, then hospital within the city; Rankings exclude hospitals with less than 25 cases except for patient surveys which excludes hospitals with less than 100 cases; (a) 100-299 cases; (1) The number of cases/patients is too few to report; (2) Data submitted were based on a sample of cases/patients; (3) Results are based on a shorter time period than required; (4) Data suppressed by CMS for one or more quarters; (5) Results are not available for this reporting period; (6) Fewer than 100 patients completed the HCAHPS survey; (7) No cases met the criteria for this measure; (8) The lower limit of the confidence interval cannot be calculated if the number of observed infections equals zero; (9) No data are available from the state/territory for this reporting period; (10) The scores shown reflect fewer than 50 completed surveys; (11) There were discrepancies in the data collection process; (12) This measure does not apply to this hospital for this reporting period; (13) Results cannot be calculated for this reporting period; (14) The results for this state are combined with nearby states to protect confidentiality; Please refer to the User's Guide for a full explanation of data.

Brownwood Regional Medical Center

1501 Burnet Dr
Brownwood, TX 76801
Phone: 325-646-8541
Fax: 325-649-3434
URL: www.brmc-cares.com
Type: Acute Care Hospitals
Emergency Services: Yes
Ownership: Proprietary
Beds: 196

Key Personnel:

Coronary Care . . . . Kasey Bonnema, RN
Pediatric In-Patient Care . . . . Cindy Ferguson, RN
Radiology. Rick Jennings
Operating Room. . . . . Dan Locker, RN
CEO/President. . . . . Matt T Maxfield
Chief of Medical Staff. . . . . David Morales, MD
Quality Assurance . . . . Cindy Orr, RN
Infection Control. . . . . Sandy Porter, RN

Measure	Cases	This Hosp.	State Avg.	U.S. Avg.
Blood Clot Prevention and Treatment				
Anticoagulation Overlap Therapy[2]	14	100%	93%	93%
ICU Venous Thromboembolism Prophylaxis[2]	52	92%	92%	92%
Incidence of Potentially Preventable VTE[1,2]	-	-	9%	10%
UFH with Dosages/Platelet Monitoring[1,2]	-	-	96%	97%
Venous Thromboembolism Prophylaxis[2]	304	97%	82%	85%
Warfarin Therapy Discharge Instructions[2]	13	100%	84%	75%
Chest Pain/Possible Heart Attack Care				
Aspirin Given Within 24 Hours of Arrival	171	100%	94%	96%
Fibrinolytic Meds Within 30 Min. of Arrival	19	84%	47%	58%
Average Time to ECG (minutes)	180	8	8	7
Average Time to Transfer (minutes)[7]	-	-	62	60
Children's Asthma Care				
Received Home Management Plan of Care	-	-	93%	88%
Received Reliever Medication	-	-	100%	100%
Received Systemic Corticosteroids	-	-	100%	100%
Emergency Department				
Admittance Decision Time (minutes)[2]	522	80	99	98
Head CT Results Within 45 Min. of Arrival[7]	-	-	54%	57%
Patients Who Left ER Before Being Seen	22,713	1%	3%	2%
Time from ER Arrival to Admit. (minutes)[2]	523	212	270	274
Time from ER Arrival to Discharge (minutes)	373	116	127	134
Time in ER Before Being Evaluated (minutes)	424	12	26	26
Time to Pain Meds for Fractures (minutes)	160	50	57	57
Heart Attack Care				
Aspirin Given at Discharge[1]	-	-	99%	99%
Fibrinolytic Meds Within 30 Min. of Arrival[1]	-	-	49%	54%
PCI Within 90 Minutes of Arrival[7]	-	-	95%	96%
Statin Prescribed at Discharge[1]	-	-	98%	98%
Heart Failure Care				
ACE Inhibitor or ARB for LVSD	24	100%	97%	97%
Discharge Instructions Given	67	100%	95%	94%
Evaluation of LVS Function	91	99%	99%	99%
Medicare Spending				
Medicare Spending per Patient (ratio)	-	1.00	1.03	0.98
Pneumonia Care				
Appropriate Initial Antibiotic Given	82	94%	95%	95%
Blood Culture Timing	141	99%	98%	98%
Pregnancy and Delivery Care				
Newborn Deliveries Scheduled Early[2]	44	7%	7%	6%
Preventive Care				
Immunization for Influenza[2]	483	99%	90%	90%
Immunization for Pneumonia[2]	580	99%	92%	92%
Stroke Care				
Anticoagulation Therapy for Atrial Fibrillation[1]	-	-	96%	95%
Antithrombotic Therapy Timing	25	100%	98%	98%
Assessed for Rehabilitation	35	100%	98%	97%
Discharged on Antithrombotic Therapy	35	100%	99%	99%
Discharged on Statin Medication	17	88%	95%	94%
Thrombolytic Therapy Timing[1]	-	-	68%	66%
Venous Thromboembolism Prophylaxis	34	97%	94%	94%
Written Stroke Educational Materials Given	20	90%	92%	88%
Surgical Care Improvement Project				
Appropriate Beta Blocker Usage	65	100%	98%	98%
Appropriate VTP Within 24 Hours	210	100%	98%	98%
Controlled Postoperative Blood Glucose[7]	-	-	96%	97%
Perioperative Temperature Management	261	100%	100%	100%
Prophylactic Antibiotic Selection	170	99%	99%	99%
Prophylactic Antibiotic Selection (Outpatient)	109	97%	98%	98%
Prophylactic Antibiotic Stopped	155	95%	98%	98%
Prophylactic Antibiotic Timing	170	99%	99%	99%
Prophylactic Antibiotic Timing (Outpatient)	110	99%	98%	98%
Urinary Catheter Removal	89	97%	98%	97%
Survey of Patients' Hospital Experiences				
Area Around Room 'Always' Quiet at Night	300+	61%	68%	61%
Doctors 'Always' Communicated Well	300+	83%	83%	82%
Home Recovery Information Given	300+	88%	85%	85%
Hospital Given 9 or 10 on 10 Point Scale	300+	63%	73%	71%
Meds 'Always' Explained Before Given	300+	67%	66%	64%
Nurses 'Always' Communicated Well	300+	77%	80%	79%
Pain 'Always' Well Controlled	300+	72%	72%	71%
Room and Bathroom 'Always' Clean	300+	67%	75%	73%
Timely Help 'Always' Received	300+	62%	69%	68%
Would Definitely Recommend Hospital	300+	59%	73%	71%
Use of Medical Imaging				
Cardiac Imaging Stress Test before Surgery	357	4.8%	5.3%	5.3%
Combination Abdominal CT Scan	551	43.0%	16.4%	10.5%
Combination Brain/Sinus CT Scan	555	0.9%	2.7%	2.7%
Combination Chest CT Scan	215	25.6%	5.6%	2.7%
Follow-up Mammogram/Ultrasound	859	11.9%	7.9%	8.8%
Lumbar Spine MRI for Low Back Pain	158	38.6%	39.6%	37.2%

The Physicians Centre

3131 University Drive East
Bryan, TX 77802
Phone: 979-731-3100
Fax: 979-731-3957
URL: www.thephysicianscentre.com
Type: Acute Care Hospitals
Emergency Services: Yes
Ownership: Proprietary

Key Personnel:

Radiology. . . . . LeeAnn Ford
CEO . . . . Kori Rich

Measure	Cases	This Hosp.	State Avg.	U.S. Avg.
Blood Clot Prevention and Treatment				
Anticoagulation Overlap Therapy[7]	-	-	93%	93%
ICU Venous Thromboembolism Prophylaxis[7]	-	-	92%	92%
Incidence of Potentially Preventable VTE[7]	-	-	9%	10%
UFH with Dosages/Platelet Monitoring[7]	-	-	96%	97%
Venous Thromboembolism Prophylaxis	50	82%	82%	85%
Warfarin Therapy Discharge Instructions[7]	-	-	84%	75%
Chest Pain/Possible Heart Attack Care				
Aspirin Given Within 24 Hours of Arrival[1,3]	-	-	94%	96%
Fibrinolytic Meds Within 30 Min. of Arrival[5]	-	-	47%	58%
Average Time to ECG (minutes)[1,3]	-	-	8	7
Average Time to Transfer (minutes)[5]	-	-	62	60
Children's Asthma Care				
Received Home Management Plan of Care	-	-	93%	88%
Received Reliever Medication	-	-	100%	100%
Received Systemic Corticosteroids	-	-	100%	100%
Emergency Department				
Admittance Decision Time (minutes)	12	58	99	98
Head CT Results Within 45 Min. of Arrival[3,7]	-	-	54%	57%
Patients Who Left ER Before Being Seen	1,110	1%	3%	2%
Time from ER Arrival to Admit. (minutes)	12	213	270	274
Time from ER Arrival to Discharge (minutes)	465	75	127	134
Time in ER Before Being Evaluated (minutes)	482	15	26	26
Time to Pain Meds for Fractures (minutes)[1,3]	-	-	57	57
Heart Attack Care				
Aspirin Given at Discharge[5]	-	-	99%	99%
Fibrinolytic Meds Within 30 Min. of Arrival[5]	-	-	49%	54%
PCI Within 90 Minutes of Arrival[5]	-	-	95%	96%
Statin Prescribed at Discharge[5]	-	-	98%	98%
Heart Failure Care				
ACE Inhibitor or ARB for LVSD[5]	-	-	97%	97%
Discharge Instructions Given[5]	-	-	95%	94%
Evaluation of LVS Function[5]	-	-	99%	99%
Medicare Spending				
Medicare Spending per Patient (ratio)	-	1.01	1.03	0.98
Pneumonia Care				
Appropriate Initial Antibiotic Given[5]	-	-	95%	95%
Blood Culture Timing[5]	-	-	98%	98%
Pregnancy and Delivery Care				
Newborn Deliveries Scheduled Early[7]	-	-	7%	6%
Preventive Care				
Immunization for Influenza	195	99%	90%	90%
Immunization for Pneumonia	167	92%	92%	92%
Stroke Care				
Anticoagulation Therapy for Atrial Fibrillation[5]	-	-	96%	95%
Antithrombotic Therapy Timing[5]	-	-	98%	98%
Assessed for Rehabilitation[5]	-	-	98%	97%
Discharged on Antithrombotic Therapy[5]	-	-	99%	99%
Discharged on Statin Medication[5]	-	-	95%	94%
Thrombolytic Therapy Timing[5]	-	-	68%	66%
Venous Thromboembolism Prophylaxis[5]	-	-	94%	94%
Written Stroke Educational Materials Given[5]	-	-	92%	88%
Surgical Care Improvement Project				
Appropriate Beta Blocker Usage	32	97%	98%	98%
Appropriate VTP Within 24 Hours	96	100%	98%	98%
Controlled Postoperative Blood Glucose[7]	-	-	96%	97%
Perioperative Temperature Management	150	100%	100%	100%
Prophylactic Antibiotic Selection	85	100%	99%	99%
Prophylactic Antibiotic Selection (Outpatient)	35	100%	98%	98%
Prophylactic Antibiotic Stopped	85	100%	98%	98%
Prophylactic Antibiotic Timing	85	98%	99%	99%
Prophylactic Antibiotic Timing (Outpatient)	35	100%	98%	98%
Urinary Catheter Removal	87	100%	98%	97%
Survey of Patients' Hospital Experiences				
Area Around Room 'Always' Quiet at Night	(a)	93%	68%	61%
Doctors 'Always' Communicated Well	(a)	89%	83%	82%
Home Recovery Information Given	(a)	90%	85%	85%
Hospital Given 9 or 10 on 10 Point Scale	(a)	92%	73%	71%
Meds 'Always' Explained Before Given	(a)	83%	66%	64%
Nurses 'Always' Communicated Well	(a)	94%	80%	79%
Pain 'Always' Well Controlled	(a)	85%	72%	71%
Room and Bathroom 'Always' Clean	(a)	86%	75%	73%
Timely Help 'Always' Received	(a)	85%	69%	68%
Would Definitely Recommend Hospital	(a)	95%	73%	71%
Use of Medical Imaging				
Cardiac Imaging Stress Test before Surgery[7]	-	-	5.3%	5.3%
Combination Abdominal CT Scan	113	12.4%	16.4%	10.5%
Combination Brain/Sinus CT Scan[1]	-	-	2.7%	2.7%
Combination Chest CT Scan	47	0.0%	5.6%	2.7%
Follow-up Mammogram/Ultrasound	491	7.7%	7.9%	8.8%
Lumbar Spine MRI for Low Back Pain	94	45.7%	39.6%	37.2%

Saint Joseph Regional Health Center

2801 Franciscan Dr
Bryan, TX 77802
Phone: 979-776-3912
URL: www.st-joseph.org/sjrhc
Type: Acute Care Hospitals
Emergency Services: Yes
Ownership: Voluntary non-profit - Church
Beds: 210

Key Personnel:

Radiology. . . . . Mir Zulfiquar Alikhan
Emergency Room . . . . Anthony David Amoroso
Intensive Care Unit. . . . . Stephanie Cumpton
Chief of Medical Staff. . . . . Robert Emmick, MD
Chief of Medical Staff . . . . Garth Morgan
President/CEO. . . . . James W. Pope, MHHA, FACHE
Infection Control. . . . . Jan Shay
Operating Room. . . . . Steve Thomas

Measure	Cases	This Hosp.	State Avg.	U.S. Avg.
Blood Clot Prevention and Treatment				
Anticoagulation Overlap Therapy[2]	116	87%	93%	93%
ICU Venous Thromboembolism Prophylaxis[2]	75	99%	92%	92%
Incidence of Potentially Preventable VTE[2]	20	5%	9%	10%
UFH with Dosages/Platelet Monitoring[1,2]	-	-	96%	97%
Venous Thromboembolism Prophylaxis[2]	342	91%	82%	85%
Warfarin Therapy Discharge Instructions[2]	85	100%	84%	75%
Chest Pain/Possible Heart Attack Care				
Aspirin Given Within 24 Hours of Arrival	36	97%	94%	96%
Fibrinolytic Meds Within 30 Min. of Arrival[3,7]	-	-	47%	58%
Average Time to ECG (minutes)	37	8	8	7
Average Time to Transfer (minutes)[3,7]	-	-	62	60
Children's Asthma Care				
Received Home Management Plan of Care	-	-	93%	88%
Received Reliever Medication	-	-	100%	100%

NOTE: Hospital profiles are in alphabetical order by state, then city, then hospital within the city; Rankings exclude hospitals with less than 25 cases except for patient surveys which excludes hospitals with less than 100 cases; (a) 100-299 cases; (1) The number of cases/patients is too few to report; (2) Data submitted were based on a sample of cases/patients; (3) Results are based on a shorter time period than required; (4) Data suppressed by CMS for one or more quarters; (5) Results are not available for this reporting period; (6) Fewer than 100 patients completed the HCAHPS survey; (7) No cases met the criteria for this measure; (8) The lower limit of the confidence interval cannot be calculated if the number of observed infections equals zero; (9) No data are available from the state/territory for this reporting period; (10) The scores shown reflect fewer than 50 completed surveys; (11) There were discrepancies in the data collection process; (12) This measure does not apply to this hospital for this reporting period; (13) Results cannot be calculated for this reporting period; (14) The results for this state are combined with nearby states to protect confidentiality; Please refer to the User's Guide for a full explanation of data.

Measure	Cases	This Hosp.	State Avg.	U.S. Avg.
Received Systemic Corticosteroids	-	-	100%	100%
Emergency Department				
Admittance Decision Time (minutes)[2]	688	108	99	98
Head CT Results Within 45 Min. of Arrival[1]	-	-	54%	57%
Patients Who Left ER Before Being Seen	56,221	2%	3%	2%
Time from ER Arrival to Admit. (minutes)[2]	688	238	270	274
Time from ER Arrival to Discharge (minutes)	396	106	127	134
Time in ER Before Being Evaluated (minutes)	406	14	26	26
Time to Pain Meds for Fractures (minutes)	144	57	57	57
Heart Attack Care				
Aspirin Given at Discharge	245	100%	99%	99%
Fibrinolytic Meds Within 30 Min. of Arrival[7]	-	-	49%	54%
PCI Within 90 Minutes of Arrival	25	100%	95%	96%
Statin Prescribed at Discharge	241	100%	98%	98%
Heart Failure Care				
ACE Inhibitor or ARB for LVSD	189	99%	97%	97%
Discharge Instructions Given	472	99%	95%	94%
Evaluation of LVS Function	566	100%	99%	99%
Medicare Spending				
Medicare Spending per Patient (ratio)	-	0.99	1.03	0.98
Pneumonia Care				
Appropriate Initial Antibiotic Given	162	94%	95%	95%
Blood Culture Timing	304	99%	98%	98%
Pregnancy and Delivery Care				
Newborn Deliveries Scheduled Early[2]	73	11%	7%	6%
Preventive Care				
Immunization for Influenza[2]	571	97%	90%	90%
Immunization for Pneumonia[2]	723	99%	92%	92%
Stroke Care				
Anticoagulation Therapy for Atrial Fibrillation[1,2]	-	-	96%	95%
Antithrombotic Therapy Timing[2]	110	98%	98%	98%
Assessed for Rehabilitation[2]	121	98%	98%	97%
Discharged on Antithrombotic Therapy[2]	103	100%	99%	99%
Discharged on Statin Medication[2]	84	96%	95%	94%
Thrombolytic Therapy Timing[1,2]	-	-	68%	66%
Venous Thromboembolism Prophylaxis[2]	128	98%	94%	94%
Written Stroke Educational Materials Given[2]	67	96%	92%	88%
Surgical Care Improvement Project				
Appropriate Beta Blocker Usage[2]	149	97%	98%	98%
Appropriate VTP Within 24 Hours[2]	320	99%	98%	98%
Controlled Postoperative Blood Glucose[2]	90	96%	96%	97%
Perioperative Temperature Management[2]	406	100%	100%	100%
Prophylactic Antibiotic Selection[2]	346	100%	99%	99%
Prophylactic Antibiotic Selection (Outpatient)	348	99%	98%	98%
Prophylactic Antibiotic Stopped[2]	338	99%	98%	98%
Prophylactic Antibiotic Timing[2]	347	99%	99%	99%
Prophylactic Antibiotic Timing (Outpatient)	347	100%	98%	98%
Urinary Catheter Removal[2]	300	98%	98%	97%
Survey of Patients' Hospital Experiences				
Area Around Room 'Always' Quiet at Night	300+	69%	68%	61%
Doctors 'Always' Communicated Well	300+	82%	83%	82%
Home Recovery Information Given	300+	86%	85%	85%
Hospital Given 9 or 10 on 10 Point Scale	300+	76%	73%	71%
Meds 'Always' Explained Before Given	300+	68%	66%	64%
Nurses 'Always' Communicated Well	300+	81%	80%	79%
Pain 'Always' Well Controlled	300+	71%	72%	71%
Room and Bathroom 'Always' Clean	300+	73%	75%	73%
Timely Help 'Always' Received	300+	68%	69%	68%
Would Definitely Recommend Hospital	300+	78%	73%	71%
Use of Medical Imaging				
Cardiac Imaging Stress Test before Surgery	308	3.9%	5.3%	5.3%
Combination Abdominal CT Scan	822	6.1%	16.4%	10.5%
Combination Brain/Sinus CT Scan	945	2.3%	2.7%	2.7%
Combination Chest CT Scan	344	0.9%	5.6%	2.7%
Follow-up Mammogram/Ultrasound	568	5.6%	7.9%	8.8%
Lumbar Spine MRI for Low Back Pain	173	35.3%	39.6%	37.2%

Huguley Memorial Medical Center

11801 South Freeway Phone: 817-568-5317
Burleson, TX 76028 Fax: 817-568-1296
E-mail: huguley-admin@ahss.org
URL: www.huguley.org
Type: Acute Care Hospitals Emergency Services: Yes
Ownership: Voluntary non-profit - Church Beds: 213

Key Personnel:
Operating Room. . . . . Barry Bass, RN
President/CEO. . . . . Ken Finch
Emergency Room . . . . John K Griswell, MD
Quality Assurance . . . . Valerie Hunt
Chief of Medical Staff. . . . . Edward Laue, MD
Pediatric Ambulatory Care . . . . . . Ylicia Richards, MD
Pediatric In-Patient Care . . . . Ylicia Richards, MD
Infection Control. . . . . Linda Stair, RN

Measure	Cases	This Hosp.	State Avg.	U.S. Avg.
Blood Clot Prevention and Treatment				
Anticoagulation Overlap Therapy[2]	77	70%	93%	93%
ICU Venous Thromboembolism Prophylaxis[2]	87	85%	92%	92%
Incidence of Potentially Preventable VTE[2]	16	6%	9%	10%
UFH with Dosages/Platelet Monitoring[2]	19	95%	96%	97%
Venous Thromboembolism Prophylaxis[2]	356	90%	82%	85%
Warfarin Therapy Discharge Instructions[2]	52	100%	84%	75%
Chest Pain/Possible Heart Attack Care				
Aspirin Given Within 24 Hours of Arrival[1]	-	-	94%	96%
Fibrinolytic Meds Within 30 Min. of Arrival[5]	-	-	47%	58%
Average Time to ECG (minutes)[1]	-	-	8	7
Average Time to Transfer (minutes)[5]	-	-	62	60
Children's Asthma Care				
Received Home Management Plan of Care	-	-	93%	88%
Received Reliever Medication	-	-	100%	100%
Received Systemic Corticosteroids	-	-	100%	100%
Emergency Department				
Admittance Decision Time (minutes)[2]	573	164	99	98
Head CT Results Within 45 Min. of Arrival[1]	-	-	54%	57%
Patients Who Left ER Before Being Seen	47,555	3%	3%	2%
Time from ER Arrival to Admit. (minutes)[2]	593	335	270	274
Time from ER Arrival to Discharge (minutes)	350	165	127	134
Time in ER Before Being Evaluated (minutes)	379	46	26	26
Time to Pain Meds for Fractures (minutes)	169	60	57	57
Heart Attack Care				
Aspirin Given at Discharge	265	100%	99%	99%
Fibrinolytic Meds Within 30 Min. of Arrival[7]	-	-	49%	54%
PCI Within 90 Minutes of Arrival	46	96%	95%	96%
Statin Prescribed at Discharge	248	100%	98%	98%
Heart Failure Care				
ACE Inhibitor or ARB for LVSD	89	100%	97%	97%
Discharge Instructions Given	288	95%	95%	94%
Evaluation of LVS Function	398	100%	99%	99%
Medicare Spending				
Medicare Spending per Patient (ratio)	-	1.12	1.03	0.98
Pneumonia Care				
Appropriate Initial Antibiotic Given	180	98%	95%	95%
Blood Culture Timing	311	97%	98%	98%
Pregnancy and Delivery Care				
Newborn Deliveries Scheduled Early[2]	44	9%	7%	6%
Preventive Care				
Immunization for Influenza[2]	540	88%	90%	90%
Immunization for Pneumonia[2]	722	92%	92%	92%
Stroke Care				
Anticoagulation Therapy for Atrial Fibrillation[1]	-	-	96%	95%
Antithrombotic Therapy Timing	79	100%	98%	98%
Assessed for Rehabilitation	81	96%	98%	97%
Discharged on Antithrombotic Therapy	81	100%	99%	99%
Discharged on Statin Medication	61	95%	95%	94%
Thrombolytic Therapy Timing	13	8%	68%	66%
Venous Thromboembolism Prophylaxis	75	91%	94%	94%
Written Stroke Educational Materials Given	53	96%	92%	88%
Surgical Care Improvement Project				
Appropriate Beta Blocker Usage	230	100%	98%	98%
Appropriate VTP Within 24 Hours	366	99%	98%	98%
Controlled Postoperative Blood Glucose	86	94%	96%	97%
Perioperative Temperature Management	427	100%	100%	100%
Prophylactic Antibiotic Selection	320	100%	99%	99%
Prophylactic Antibiotic Selection (Outpatient)	256	95%	98%	98%
Prophylactic Antibiotic Stopped	290	97%	98%	98%
Prophylactic Antibiotic Timing	320	99%	99%	99%
Prophylactic Antibiotic Timing (Outpatient)	259	97%	98%	98%
Urinary Catheter Removal	268	99%	98%	97%
Survey of Patients' Hospital Experiences				
Area Around Room 'Always' Quiet at Night[11]	300+	63%	68%	61%
Doctors 'Always' Communicated Well[11]	300+	80%	83%	82%
Home Recovery Information Given[11]	300+	86%	85%	85%
Hospital Given 9 or 10 on 10 Point Scale[11]	300+	67%	73%	71%
Meds 'Always' Explained Before Given[11]	300+	61%	66%	64%
Nurses 'Always' Communicated Well[11]	300+	78%	80%	79%
Pain 'Always' Well Controlled[11]	300+	72%	72%	71%
Room and Bathroom 'Always' Clean[11]	300+	69%	75%	73%
Timely Help 'Always' Received[11]	300+	67%	69%	68%
Would Definitely Recommend Hospital[11]	300+	67%	73%	71%
Use of Medical Imaging				
Cardiac Imaging Stress Test before Surgery	150	2.0%	5.3%	5.3%
Combination Abdominal CT Scan	743	16.8%	16.4%	10.5%
Combination Brain/Sinus CT Scan	719	5.0%	2.7%	2.7%
Combination Chest CT Scan	462	9.3%	5.6%	2.7%
Follow-up Mammogram/Ultrasound	795	9.8%	7.9%	8.8%
Lumbar Spine MRI for Low Back Pain	73	34.2%	39.6%	37.2%

Seton Highland Lakes

Highway 281 South Phone: 512-715-3000
Burnet, TX 78611 Fax: 512-756-6405
URL: www.seton.net
Type: Critical Access Hospitals Emergency Services: Yes
Ownership: Voluntary non-profit - Private Beds: 25

Key Personnel:
CEO/President. . . . . Dr. Robert I. Bonar, Jr., HA
Chief of Medical Staff. . . . . Scott Liggett
Emergency Room . . . . Elizabeth Stevenson

Measure	Cases	This Hosp.	State Avg.	U.S. Avg.
Blood Clot Prevention and Treatment				
Anticoagulation Overlap Therapy[5]	-	-	93%	93%
ICU Venous Thromboembolism Prophylaxis[5]	-	-	92%	92%
Incidence of Potentially Preventable VTE[5]	-	-	9%	10%
UFH with Dosages/Platelet Monitoring[5]	-	-	96%	97%
Venous Thromboembolism Prophylaxis[5]	-	-	82%	85%
Warfarin Therapy Discharge Instructions[5]	-	-	84%	75%
Chest Pain/Possible Heart Attack Care				
Aspirin Given Within 24 Hours of Arrival[5]	-	-	94%	96%
Fibrinolytic Meds Within 30 Min. of Arrival[5]	-	-	47%	58%
Average Time to ECG (minutes)[5]	-	-	8	7
Average Time to Transfer (minutes)[5]	-	-	62	60
Children's Asthma Care				
Received Home Management Plan of Care	-	-	93%	88%
Received Reliever Medication	-	-	100%	100%
Received Systemic Corticosteroids	-	-	100%	100%
Emergency Department				
Admittance Decision Time (minutes)[5]	-	-	99	98
Head CT Results Within 45 Min. of Arrival[5]	-	-	54%	57%
Patients Who Left ER Before Being Seen[5]	-	-	3%	2%
Time from ER Arrival to Admit. (minutes)[5]	-	-	270	274
Time from ER Arrival to Discharge (minutes)[5]	-	-	127	134
Time in ER Before Being Evaluated (minutes)[5]	-	-	26	26
Time to Pain Meds for Fractures (minutes)[5]	-	-	57	57
Heart Attack Care				
Aspirin Given at Discharge[3,7]	-	-	99%	99%
Fibrinolytic Meds Within 30 Min. of Arrival[3,7]	-	-	49%	54%
PCI Within 90 Minutes of Arrival[3,7]	-	-	95%	96%
Statin Prescribed at Discharge[3,7]	-	-	98%	98%
Heart Failure Care				
ACE Inhibitor or ARB for LVSD	14	93%	97%	97%
Discharge Instructions Given	28	100%	95%	94%
Evaluation of LVS Function	22	100%	99%	99%
Medicare Spending				
Medicare Spending per Patient (ratio)	-	-	1.03	0.98
Pneumonia Care				
Appropriate Initial Antibiotic Given	51	100%	95%	95%

NOTE: Hospital profiles are in alphabetical order by state, then city, then hospital within the city; Rankings exclude hospitals with less than 25 cases except for patient surveys which excludes hospitals with less than 100 cases; (a) 100-299 cases; (1) The number of cases/patients is too few to report; (2) Data submitted were based on a sample of cases/patients; (3) Results are based on a shorter time period than required; (4) Data suppressed by CMS for one or more quarters; (5) Results are not available for this reporting period; (6) Fewer than 100 patients completed the HCAHPS survey; (7) No cases met the criteria for this measure; (8) The lower limit of the confidence interval cannot be calculated if the number of observed infections equals zero; (9) No data are available from the state/territory for this reporting period; (10) The scores shown reflect fewer than 50 completed surveys; (11) There were discrepancies in the data collection process; (12) This measure does not apply to this hospital for this reporting period; (13) Results cannot be calculated for this reporting period; (14) The results for this state are combined with nearby states to protect confidentiality; Please refer to the User's Guide for a full explanation of data.

Measure	Cases	This Hosp.	State Avg.	U.S. Avg.
Blood Culture Timing	71	100%	98%	98%
Pregnancy and Delivery Care				
Newborn Deliveries Scheduled Early[5]	-	-	7%	6%
Preventive Care				
Immunization for Influenza[5]	-	-	90%	90%
Immunization for Pneumonia[5]	-	-	92%	92%
Stroke Care				
Anticoagulation Therapy for Atrial Fibrillation[5]	-	-	96%	95%
Antithrombotic Therapy Timing[5]	-	-	98%	98%
Assessed for Rehabilitation[5]	-	-	98%	97%
Discharged on Antithrombotic Therapy[5]	-	-	99%	99%
Discharged on Statin Medication[5]	-	-	95%	94%
Thrombolytic Therapy Timing[5]	-	-	68%	66%
Venous Thromboembolism Prophylaxis[5]	-	-	94%	94%
Written Stroke Educational Materials Given[5]	-	-	92%	88%
Surgical Care Improvement Project				
Appropriate Beta Blocker Usage	30	100%	98%	98%
Appropriate VTP Within 24 Hours	90	99%	98%	98%
Controlled Postoperative Blood Glucose[3,7]	-	-	96%	97%
Perioperative Temperature Management	100	100%	100%	100%
Prophylactic Antibiotic Selection	77	100%	99%	99%
Prophylactic Antibiotic Selection (Outpatient)[3]	44	93%	98%	98%
Prophylactic Antibiotic Stopped	77	99%	98%	98%
Prophylactic Antibiotic Timing	77	96%	99%	99%
Prophylactic Antibiotic Timing (Outpatient)[3]	46	87%	98%	98%
Urinary Catheter Removal	82	100%	98%	97%
Survey of Patients' Hospital Experiences				
Area Around Room 'Always' Quiet at Night	300+	63%	68%	61%
Doctors 'Always' Communicated Well	300+	84%	83%	82%
Home Recovery Information Given	300+	86%	85%	85%
Hospital Given 9 or 10 on 10 Point Scale	300+	77%	73%	71%
Meds 'Always' Explained Before Given	300+	68%	66%	64%
Nurses 'Always' Communicated Well	300+	81%	80%	79%
Pain 'Always' Well Controlled	300+	74%	72%	71%
Room and Bathroom 'Always' Clean	300+	75%	75%	73%
Timely Help 'Always' Received	300+	72%	69%	68%
Would Definitely Recommend Hospital	300+	75%	73%	71%
Use of Medical Imaging				
Cardiac Imaging Stress Test before Surgery	154	5.8%	5.3%	5.3%
Combination Abdominal CT Scan	693	5.1%	16.4%	10.5%
Combination Brain/Sinus CT Scan	639	2.7%	2.7%	2.7%
Combination Chest CT Scan	385	0.8%	5.6%	2.7%
Follow-up Mammogram/Ultrasound	1,032	7.4%	7.9%	8.8%
Lumbar Spine MRI for Low Back Pain[1]	-	-	39.6%	37.2%

Burleson Saint Joseph Health Center

1101 Woodson Drive
Caldwell, TX 77836
URL: www.st-joseph.org/burleson
Phone: 979-567-3245
Fax: 979-567-0616
Type: Critical Access Hospitals
Emergency Services: Yes
Ownership: Voluntary non-profit - Church
Beds: 15

Measure	Cases	This Hosp.	State Avg.	U.S. Avg.
Blood Clot Prevention and Treatment				
Anticoagulation Overlap Therapy[5]	-	-	93%	93%
ICU Venous Thromboembolism Prophylaxis[5]	-	-	92%	92%
Incidence of Potentially Preventable VTE[5]	-	-	9%	10%
UFH with Dosages/Platelet Monitoring[5]	-	-	96%	97%
Venous Thromboembolism Prophylaxis[5]	-	-	82%	85%
Warfarin Therapy Discharge Instructions[5]	-	-	84%	75%
Chest Pain/Possible Heart Attack Care				
Aspirin Given Within 24 Hours of Arrival	-	-	94%	96%
Fibrinolytic Meds Within 30 Min. of Arrival	-	-	47%	58%
Average Time to ECG (minutes)	-	-	8	7
Average Time to Transfer (minutes)	-	-	62	60
Children's Asthma Care				
Received Home Management Plan of Care	-	-	93%	88%
Received Reliever Medication	-	-	100%	100%
Received Systemic Corticosteroids	-	-	100%	100%
Emergency Department				
Admittance Decision Time (minutes)[5]	-	-	99	98
Head CT Results Within 45 Min. of Arrival	-	-	54%	57%
Patients Who Left ER Before Being Seen	-	-	3%	2%
Time from ER Arrival to Admit. (minutes)[5]	-	-	270	274
Time from ER Arrival to Discharge (minutes)	-	-	127	134
Time in ER Before Being Evaluated (minutes)	-	-	26	26
Time to Pain Meds for Fractures (minutes)	-	-	57	57
Heart Attack Care				
Aspirin Given at Discharge[5]	-	-	99%	99%
Fibrinolytic Meds Within 30 Min. of Arrival[5]	-	-	49%	54%
PCI Within 90 Minutes of Arrival[5]	-	-	95%	96%
Statin Prescribed at Discharge[5]	-	-	98%	98%
Heart Failure Care				
ACE Inhibitor or ARB for LVSD[1]	-	-	97%	97%
Discharge Instructions Given[1]	-	-	95%	94%
Evaluation of LVS Function[1]	-	-	99%	99%
Medicare Spending				
Medicare Spending per Patient (ratio)	-	-	1.03	0.98
Pneumonia Care				
Appropriate Initial Antibiotic Given[7]	-	-	95%	95%
Blood Culture Timing[7]	-	-	98%	98%
Pregnancy and Delivery Care				
Newborn Deliveries Scheduled Early[5]	-	-	7%	6%
Preventive Care				
Immunization for Influenza[5]	-	-	90%	90%
Immunization for Pneumonia[5]	-	-	92%	92%
Stroke Care				
Anticoagulation Therapy for Atrial Fibrillation[5]	-	-	96%	95%
Antithrombotic Therapy Timing[5]	-	-	98%	98%
Assessed for Rehabilitation[5]	-	-	98%	97%
Discharged on Antithrombotic Therapy[5]	-	-	99%	99%
Discharged on Statin Medication[5]	-	-	95%	94%
Thrombolytic Therapy Timing[5]	-	-	68%	66%
Venous Thromboembolism Prophylaxis[5]	-	-	94%	94%
Written Stroke Educational Materials Given[5]	-	-	92%	88%
Surgical Care Improvement Project				
Appropriate Beta Blocker Usage[5]	-	-	98%	98%
Appropriate VTP Within 24 Hours[5]	-	-	98%	98%
Controlled Postoperative Blood Glucose[5]	-	-	96%	97%
Perioperative Temperature Management[5]	-	-	100%	100%
Prophylactic Antibiotic Selection[5]	-	-	99%	99%
Prophylactic Antibiotic Selection (Outpatient)	-	-	98%	98%
Prophylactic Antibiotic Stopped[5]	-	-	98%	98%
Prophylactic Antibiotic Timing[5]	-	-	99%	99%
Prophylactic Antibiotic Timing (Outpatient)	-	-	98%	98%
Urinary Catheter Removal[5]	-	-	98%	97%
Survey of Patients' Hospital Experiences				
Area Around Room 'Always' Quiet at Night[5]	-	-	68%	61%
Doctors 'Always' Communicated Well[5]	-	-	83%	82%
Home Recovery Information Given[5]	-	-	85%	85%
Hospital Given 9 or 10 on 10 Point Scale[5]	-	-	73%	71%
Meds 'Always' Explained Before Given[5]	-	-	66%	64%
Nurses 'Always' Communicated Well[5]	-	-	80%	79%
Pain 'Always' Well Controlled[5]	-	-	72%	71%
Room and Bathroom 'Always' Clean[5]	-	-	75%	73%
Timely Help 'Always' Received[5]	-	-	69%	68%
Would Definitely Recommend Hospital[5]	-	-	73%	71%
Use of Medical Imaging				
Cardiac Imaging Stress Test before Surgery	-	-	5.3%	5.3%
Combination Abdominal CT Scan	-	-	16.4%	10.5%
Combination Brain/Sinus CT Scan	-	-	2.7%	2.7%
Combination Chest CT Scan	-	-	5.6%	2.7%
Follow-up Mammogram/Ultrasound	-	-	7.9%	8.8%
Lumbar Spine MRI for Low Back Pain	-	-	39.6%	37.2%

Central Texas Hospital

806 N Crockett
Cameron, TX 76520
Phone: 254-697-6591
Type: Acute Care Hospitals
Emergency Services: Yes
Ownership: Proprietary
Key Personnel:
CEO/President. . . . . Tariq Mahmood

Measure	Cases	This Hosp.	State Avg.	U.S. Avg.
Blood Clot Prevention and Treatment				
Anticoagulation Overlap Therapy[5]	-	-	93%	93%
ICU Venous Thromboembolism Prophylaxis[5]	-	-	92%	92%
Incidence of Potentially Preventable VTE[5]	-	-	9%	10%
UFH with Dosages/Platelet Monitoring[5]	-	-	96%	97%
Venous Thromboembolism Prophylaxis[5]	-	-	82%	85%
Warfarin Therapy Discharge Instructions[5]	-	-	84%	75%
Chest Pain/Possible Heart Attack Care				
Aspirin Given Within 24 Hours of Arrival[5]	-	-	94%	96%
Fibrinolytic Meds Within 30 Min. of Arrival[5]	-	-	47%	58%
Average Time to ECG (minutes)[5]	-	-	8	7
Average Time to Transfer (minutes)[5]	-	-	62	60
Children's Asthma Care				
Received Home Management Plan of Care	-	-	93%	88%
Received Reliever Medication	-	-	100%	100%
Received Systemic Corticosteroids	-	-	100%	100%
Emergency Department				
Admittance Decision Time (minutes)[2,3]	103	55	99	98
Head CT Results Within 45 Min. of Arrival[5]	-	-	54%	57%
Patients Who Left ER Before Being Seen[5]	-	-	3%	2%
Time from ER Arrival to Admit. (minutes)[2,3]	103	150	270	274
Time from ER Arrival to Discharge (minutes)[5]	-	-	127	134
Time in ER Before Being Evaluated (minutes)[5]	-	-	26	26
Time to Pain Meds for Fractures (minutes)[5]	-	-	57	57
Heart Attack Care				
Aspirin Given at Discharge[5]	-	-	99%	99%
Fibrinolytic Meds Within 30 Min. of Arrival[5]	-	-	49%	54%
PCI Within 90 Minutes of Arrival[5]	-	-	95%	96%
Statin Prescribed at Discharge[5]	-	-	98%	98%
Heart Failure Care				
ACE Inhibitor or ARB for LVSD[5]	-	-	97%	97%
Discharge Instructions Given[5]	-	-	95%	94%
Evaluation of LVS Function[5]	-	-	99%	99%
Medicare Spending				
Medicare Spending per Patient (ratio)	-	0.86	1.03	0.98
Pneumonia Care				
Appropriate Initial Antibiotic Given[1,3]	-	-	95%	95%
Blood Culture Timing[1,3]	-	-	98%	98%
Pregnancy and Delivery Care				
Newborn Deliveries Scheduled Early[5]	-	-	7%	6%
Preventive Care				
Immunization for Influenza[2,3]	104	83%	90%	90%
Immunization for Pneumonia[2,3]	48	83%	92%	92%
Stroke Care				
Anticoagulation Therapy for Atrial Fibrillation[5]	-	-	96%	95%
Antithrombotic Therapy Timing[5]	-	-	98%	98%
Assessed for Rehabilitation[5]	-	-	98%	97%
Discharged on Antithrombotic Therapy[5]	-	-	99%	99%
Discharged on Statin Medication[5]	-	-	95%	94%
Thrombolytic Therapy Timing[5]	-	-	68%	66%
Venous Thromboembolism Prophylaxis[5]	-	-	94%	94%
Written Stroke Educational Materials Given[5]	-	-	92%	88%
Surgical Care Improvement Project				
Appropriate Beta Blocker Usage[5]	-	-	98%	98%
Appropriate VTP Within 24 Hours[5]	-	-	98%	98%
Controlled Postoperative Blood Glucose[5]	-	-	96%	97%
Perioperative Temperature Management[5]	-	-	100%	100%
Prophylactic Antibiotic Selection[5]	-	-	99%	99%
Prophylactic Antibiotic Selection (Outpatient)[5]	-	-	98%	98%
Prophylactic Antibiotic Stopped[5]	-	-	98%	98%
Prophylactic Antibiotic Timing[5]	-	-	99%	99%
Prophylactic Antibiotic Timing (Outpatient)[5]	-	-	98%	98%
Urinary Catheter Removal[5]	-	-	98%	97%
Survey of Patients' Hospital Experiences				
Area Around Room 'Always' Quiet at Night[5]	-	-	68%	61%
Doctors 'Always' Communicated Well[5]	-	-	83%	82%
Home Recovery Information Given[5]	-	-	85%	85%
Hospital Given 9 or 10 on 10 Point Scale[5]	-	-	73%	71%
Meds 'Always' Explained Before Given[5]	-	-	66%	64%
Nurses 'Always' Communicated Well[5]	-	-	80%	79%
Pain 'Always' Well Controlled[5]	-	-	72%	71%
Room and Bathroom 'Always' Clean[5]	-	-	75%	73%
Timely Help 'Always' Received[5]	-	-	69%	68%
Would Definitely Recommend Hospital[5]	-	-	73%	71%

NOTE: Hospital profiles are in alphabetical order by state, then city, then hospital within the city; Rankings exclude hospitals with less than 25 cases except for patient surveys which excludes hospitals with less than 100 cases; (a) 100-299 cases; (1) The number of cases/patients is too few to report; (2) Data submitted were based on a sample of cases/patients; (3) Results are based on a shorter time period than required; (4) Data suppressed by CMS for one or more quarters; (5) Results are not available for this reporting period; (6) Fewer than 100 patients completed the HCAHPS survey; (7) No cases met the criteria for this measure; (8) The lower limit of the confidence interval cannot be calculated if the number of observed infections equals zero; (9) No data are available from the state/territory for this reporting period; (10) The scores shown reflect fewer than 50 completed surveys; (11) There were discrepancies in the data collection process; (12) This measure does not apply to this hospital for this reporting period; (13) Results cannot be calculated for this reporting period; (14) The results for this state are combined with nearby states to protect confidentiality; Please refer to the User's Guide for a full explanation of data.

Measure	Cases	This Hosp.	State Avg.	U.S. Avg.
Use of Medical Imaging				
Cardiac Imaging Stress Test before Surgery[7]	-	-	5.3%	5.3%
Combination Abdominal CT Scan	57	5.3%	16.4%	10.5%
Combination Brain/Sinus CT Scan	43	16.3%	2.7%	2.7%
Combination Chest CT Scan[1]	-	-	5.6%	2.7%
Follow-up Mammogram/Ultrasound[7]	-	-	7.9%	8.8%
Lumbar Spine MRI for Low Back Pain[7]	-	-	39.6%	37.2%

Hemphill County Hospital

1020 S 4th St
Canadian, TX 79014
Phone: 806-323-6622
Fax: 806-323-8061
URL: www.hch.dst.ts.us
Type: Acute Care Hospitals
Emergency Services: Yes
Ownership: Govt - Hospital Dist/Auth
Beds: 26

Key Personnel:

Quality Assurance . . . . David Albin
CEO . . . . Christy Francis
Infection Control. . . . . Cary George
Chief of Medical Staff. . . . . Valerie Verbi, MD
Emergency Room . . . . Valerie Verbi, MD

Measure	Cases	This Hosp.	State Avg.	U.S. Avg.
Blood Clot Prevention and Treatment				
Anticoagulation Overlap Therapy[1,2]	-	-	93%	93%
ICU Venous Thromboembolism Prophylaxis[2,7]	-	-	92%	92%
Incidence of Potentially Preventable VTE[2,7]	-	-	9%	10%
UFH with Dosages/Platelet Monitoring[2,7]	-	-	96%	97%
Venous Thromboembolism Prophylaxis[2]	81	12%	82%	85%
Warfarin Therapy Discharge Instructions[1,2]	-	-	84%	75%
Chest Pain/Possible Heart Attack Care				
Aspirin Given Within 24 Hours of Arrival[1,3]	-	-	94%	96%
Fibrinolytic Meds Within 30 Min. of Arrival[5]	-	-	47%	58%
Average Time to ECG (minutes)[3,7]	-	-	8	7
Average Time to Transfer (minutes)[5]	-	-	62	60
Children's Asthma Care				
Received Home Management Plan of Care	-	-	93%	88%
Received Reliever Medication	-	-	100%	100%
Received Systemic Corticosteroids	-	-	100%	100%
Emergency Department				
Admittance Decision Time (minutes)[2]	68	10	99	98
Head CT Results Within 45 Min. of Arrival[5]	-	-	54%	57%
Patients Who Left ER Before Being Seen	2,017	10%	3%	2%
Time from ER Arrival to Admit. (minutes)[2]	87	120	270	274
Time from ER Arrival to Discharge (minutes)	366	95	127	134
Time in ER Before Being Evaluated (minutes)	356	40	26	26
Time to Pain Meds for Fractures (minutes)[1,3]	-	-	57	57
Heart Attack Care				
Aspirin Given at Discharge[5]	-	-	99%	99%
Fibrinolytic Meds Within 30 Min. of Arrival[5]	-	-	49%	54%
PCI Within 90 Minutes of Arrival[5]	-	-	95%	96%
Statin Prescribed at Discharge[5]	-	-	98%	98%
Heart Failure Care				
ACE Inhibitor or ARB for LVSD[2,3]	-	-	97%	97%
Discharge Instructions Given[1,2]	-	-	95%	94%
Evaluation of LVS Function[1,2]	-	-	99%	99%
Medicare Spending				
Medicare Spending per Patient (ratio)	-	0.81	1.03	0.98
Pneumonia Care				
Appropriate Initial Antibiotic Given[1,2]	-	-	95%	95%
Blood Culture Timing[1,2]	-	-	98%	98%
Pregnancy and Delivery Care				
Newborn Deliveries Scheduled Early[7]	-	-	7%	6%
Preventive Care				
Immunization for Influenza[2]	74	41%	90%	90%
Immunization for Pneumonia[2]	88	43%	92%	92%
Stroke Care				
Anticoagulation Therapy for Atrial Fibrillation[5]	-	-	96%	95%
Antithrombotic Therapy Timing[5]	-	-	98%	98%
Assessed for Rehabilitation[5]	-	-	98%	97%
Discharged on Antithrombotic Therapy[5]	-	-	99%	99%
Discharged on Statin Medication[5]	-	-	95%	94%
Thrombolytic Therapy Timing[5]	-	-	68%	66%
Venous Thromboembolism Prophylaxis[5]	-	-	94%	94%
Written Stroke Educational Materials Given[5]	-	-	92%	88%
Surgical Care Improvement Project				
Appropriate Beta Blocker Usage[5]	-	-	98%	98%
Appropriate VTP Within 24 Hours[5]	-	-	98%	98%
Controlled Postoperative Blood Glucose[5]	-	-	96%	97%
Perioperative Temperature Management[5]	-	-	100%	100%
Prophylactic Antibiotic Selection[5]	-	-	99%	99%
Prophylactic Antibiotic Selection (Outpatient)[5]	-	-	98%	98%
Prophylactic Antibiotic Stopped[5]	-	-	98%	98%
Prophylactic Antibiotic Timing[5]	-	-	99%	99%
Prophylactic Antibiotic Timing (Outpatient)[5]	-	-	98%	98%
Urinary Catheter Removal[5]	-	-	98%	97%
Survey of Patients' Hospital Experiences				
Area Around Room 'Always' Quiet at Night[10]	<100	83%	68%	61%
Doctors 'Always' Communicated Well[10]	<100	94%	83%	82%
Home Recovery Information Given[10]	<100	91%	85%	85%
Hospital Given 9 or 10 on 10 Point Scale[10]	<100	81%	73%	71%
Meds 'Always' Explained Before Given[10]	<100	66%	66%	64%
Nurses 'Always' Communicated Well[10]	<100	95%	80%	79%
Pain 'Always' Well Controlled[10]	<100	79%	72%	71%
Room and Bathroom 'Always' Clean[10]	<100	84%	75%	73%
Timely Help 'Always' Received[10]	<100	83%	69%	68%
Would Definitely Recommend Hospital[10]	<100	72%	73%	71%
Use of Medical Imaging				
Cardiac Imaging Stress Test before Surgery[7]	-	-	5.3%	5.3%
Combination Abdominal CT Scan[1]	-	-	16.4%	10.5%
Combination Brain/Sinus CT Scan[1]	-	-	2.7%	2.7%
Combination Chest CT Scan[1]	-	-	5.6%	2.7%
Follow-up Mammogram/Ultrasound[7]	-	-	7.9%	8.8%
Lumbar Spine MRI for Low Back Pain[7]	-	-	39.6%	37.2%

Dimmit Regional Hospital

704 Hospital Drive
Carrizo Springs, TX 78834
Phone: 830-876-2424
Fax: 830-876-3099
URL: www.dcmhospital.org
Type: Acute Care Hospitals
Emergency Services: Yes
Ownership: Govt - Hospital Dist/Auth
Beds: 35

Key Personnel:

CEO/President. . . . . Ernest Flores Jr
Chief of Medical Staff. . . . . Carlos Salazer

Measure	Cases	This Hosp.	State Avg.	U.S. Avg.
Blood Clot Prevention and Treatment				
Anticoagulation Overlap Therapy[1,2]	-	-	93%	93%
ICU Venous Thromboembolism Prophylaxis[2,7]	-	-	92%	92%
Incidence of Potentially Preventable VTE[2,7]	-	-	9%	10%
UFH with Dosages/Platelet Monitoring[1,2]	-	-	96%	97%
Venous Thromboembolism Prophylaxis[2]	94	7%	82%	85%
Warfarin Therapy Discharge Instructions[1,2]	-	-	84%	75%
Chest Pain/Possible Heart Attack Care				
Aspirin Given Within 24 Hours of Arrival	110	83%	94%	96%
Fibrinolytic Meds Within 30 Min. of Arrival[1]	-	-	47%	58%
Average Time to ECG (minutes)	110	18	8	7
Average Time to Transfer (minutes)[1]	-	-	62	60
Children's Asthma Care				
Received Home Management Plan of Care	-	-	93%	88%
Received Reliever Medication	-	-	100%	100%
Received Systemic Corticosteroids	-	-	100%	100%
Emergency Department				
Admittance Decision Time (minutes)[2]	157	75	99	98
Head CT Results Within 45 Min. of Arrival	16	12%	54%	57%
Patients Who Left ER Before Being Seen	5,083	5%	3%	2%
Time from ER Arrival to Admit. (minutes)[2]	161	275	270	274
Time from ER Arrival to Discharge (minutes)	129	135	127	134
Time in ER Before Being Evaluated (minutes)	404	22	26	26
Time to Pain Meds for Fractures (minutes)[5]	-	-	57	57
Heart Attack Care				
Aspirin Given at Discharge[2,3]	-	-	99%	99%
Fibrinolytic Meds Within 30 Min. of Arrival[2,3]	-	-	49%	54%
PCI Within 90 Minutes of Arrival[2,3]	-	-	95%	96%
Statin Prescribed at Discharge[2,3]	-	-	98%	98%
Heart Failure Care				
ACE Inhibitor or ARB for LVSD[1,2]	-	-	97%	97%
Discharge Instructions Given[2]	14	71%	95%	94%
Evaluation of LVS Function[2]	13	15%	99%	99%
Medicare Spending				
Medicare Spending per Patient (ratio)	-	0.99	1.03	0.98
Pneumonia Care				
Appropriate Initial Antibiotic Given[1,2]	-	-	95%	95%
Blood Culture Timing[1,2]	-	-	98%	98%
Pregnancy and Delivery Care				
Newborn Deliveries Scheduled Early[2]	43	0%	7%	6%
Preventive Care				
Immunization for Influenza[2]	151	42%	90%	90%
Immunization for Pneumonia[2]	118	42%	92%	92%
Stroke Care				
Anticoagulation Therapy for Atrial Fibrillation[2,3]	-	-	96%	95%
Antithrombotic Therapy Timing[1,2]	-	-	98%	98%
Assessed for Rehabilitation[1,2]	-	-	98%	97%
Discharged on Antithrombotic Therapy[1,2]	-	-	99%	99%
Discharged on Statin Medication[1,2]	-	-	95%	94%
Thrombolytic Therapy Timing[1,2]	-	-	68%	66%
Venous Thromboembolism Prophylaxis[1,2]	-	-	94%	94%
Written Stroke Educational Materials Given[1,2]	-	-	92%	88%
Surgical Care Improvement Project				
Appropriate Beta Blocker Usage[2,7]	-	-	98%	98%
Appropriate VTP Within 24 Hours[1,2]	-	-	98%	98%
Controlled Postoperative Blood Glucose[2,7]	-	-	96%	97%
Perioperative Temperature Management[1,2]	-	-	100%	100%
Prophylactic Antibiotic Selection[1,2]	-	-	99%	99%
Prophylactic Antibiotic Selection (Outpatient)[5]	-	-	98%	98%
Prophylactic Antibiotic Stopped[1,2]	-	-	98%	98%
Prophylactic Antibiotic Timing[1,2]	-	-	99%	99%
Prophylactic Antibiotic Timing (Outpatient)[5]	-	-	98%	98%
Urinary Catheter Removal[2,7]	-	-	98%	97%
Survey of Patients' Hospital Experiences				
Area Around Room 'Always' Quiet at Night[6]	<100	45%	68%	61%
Doctors 'Always' Communicated Well[6]	<100	80%	83%	82%
Home Recovery Information Given[6]	<100	77%	85%	85%
Hospital Given 9 or 10 on 10 Point Scale[6]	<100	33%	73%	71%
Meds 'Always' Explained Before Given[6]	<100	43%	66%	64%
Nurses 'Always' Communicated Well[6]	<100	59%	80%	79%
Pain 'Always' Well Controlled[6]	<100	58%	72%	71%
Room and Bathroom 'Always' Clean[6]	<100	69%	75%	73%
Timely Help 'Always' Received[6]	<100	59%	69%	68%
Would Definitely Recommend Hospital[6]	<100	39%	73%	71%
Use of Medical Imaging				
Cardiac Imaging Stress Test before Surgery[7]	-	-	5.3%	5.3%
Combination Abdominal CT Scan	82	14.6%	16.4%	10.5%
Combination Brain/Sinus CT Scan[1]	-	-	2.7%	2.7%
Combination Chest CT Scan[1]	-	-	5.6%	2.7%
Follow-up Mammogram/Ultrasound[7]	-	-	7.9%	8.8%
Lumbar Spine MRI for Low Back Pain[7]	-	-	39.6%	37.2%

Baylor Medical Center at Carrollton

4343 North Josey Lane
Carrollton, TX 75010
Phone: 972-492-1010
Fax: 972-394-4783
URL: www.trinitymedicalcenter.com
Type: Acute Care Hospitals
Emergency Services: Yes
Ownership: Proprietary
Beds: 149

Key Personnel:

Operating Room. . . . . Diana Beck
Radiology. . . . . Joseph Chan
Pediatric Ambulatory Care . . . . . . Eitel Colberg
Pediatric In-Patient Care . . . . Eitel Colberg
Chief of Medical Staff. . . . . Farrah Hamid
Infection Control. . . . . Denise Lavacak
Quality Assurance . . . . Jack Peterson
CEO/President. . . . . Craig Sims

Measure	Cases	This Hosp.	State Avg.	U.S. Avg.
Blood Clot Prevention and Treatment				
Anticoagulation Overlap Therapy[2]	16	100%	93%	93%
ICU Venous Thromboembolism Prophylaxis[2]	88	89%	92%	92%
Incidence of Potentially Preventable VTE[1,2]	-	-	9%	10%
UFH with Dosages/Platelet Monitoring[1,2]	-	-	96%	97%
Venous Thromboembolism Prophylaxis[2]	335	90%	82%	85%
Warfarin Therapy Discharge Instructions[2]	15	100%	84%	75%
Chest Pain/Possible Heart Attack Care				
Aspirin Given Within 24 Hours of Arrival[3]	14	100%	94%	96%
Fibrinolytic Meds Within 30 Min. of Arrival[3,7]	-	-	47%	58%

NOTE: Hospital profiles are in alphabetical order by state, then city, then hospital within the city; Rankings exclude hospitals with less than 25 cases except for patient surveys which excludes hospitals with less than 100 cases; (a) 100-299 cases; (1) The number of cases/patients is too few to report; (2) Data submitted were based on a sample of cases/patients; (3) Results are based on a shorter time period than required; (4) Data suppressed by CMS for one or more quarters; (5) Results are not available for this reporting period; (6) Fewer than 100 patients completed the HCAHPS survey; (7) No cases met the criteria for this measure; (8) The lower limit of the confidence interval cannot be calculated if the number of observed infections equals zero; (9) No data are available from the state/territory for this reporting period; (10) The scores shown reflect fewer than 50 completed surveys; (11) There were discrepancies in the data collection process; (12) This measure does not apply to this hospital for this reporting period; (13) Results cannot be calculated for this reporting period; (14) The results for this state are combined with nearby states to protect confidentiality; Please refer to the User's Guide for a full explanation of data.

Measure	Cases	This Hosp.	State Avg.	U.S. Avg.
Average Time to ECG (minutes)[3]	14	1	8	7
Average Time to Transfer (minutes)[1,3]	-	-	62	60
Children's Asthma Care				
Received Home Management Plan of Care	-	-	93%	88%
Received Reliever Medication	-	-	100%	100%
Received Systemic Corticosteroids	-	-	100%	100%
Emergency Department				
Admittance Decision Time (minutes)[2]	613	98	99	98
Head CT Results Within 45 Min. of Arrival[1]	-	-	54%	57%
Patients Who Left ER Before Being Seen	35,987	2%	3%	2%
Time from ER Arrival to Admit. (minutes)[2]	616	276	270	274
Time from ER Arrival to Discharge (minutes)	388	156	127	134
Time in ER Before Being Evaluated (minutes)	135	29	26	26
Time to Pain Meds for Fractures (minutes)	136	50	57	57
Heart Attack Care				
Aspirin Given at Discharge	80	100%	99%	99%
Fibrinolytic Meds Within 30 Min. of Arrival[7]	-	-	49%	54%
PCI Within 90 Minutes of Arrival	16	100%	95%	96%
Statin Prescribed at Discharge	84	100%	98%	98%
Heart Failure Care				
ACE Inhibitor or ARB for LVSD	42	100%	97%	97%
Discharge Instructions Given	104	99%	95%	94%
Evaluation of LVS Function	136	100%	99%	99%
Medicare Spending				
Medicare Spending per Patient (ratio)	-	1.12	1.03	0.98
Pneumonia Care				
Appropriate Initial Antibiotic Given	106	97%	95%	95%
Blood Culture Timing	163	100%	98%	98%
Pregnancy and Delivery Care				
Newborn Deliveries Scheduled Early	126	4%	7%	6%
Preventive Care				
Immunization for Influenza[2]	509	98%	90%	90%
Immunization for Pneumonia[2]	525	96%	92%	92%
Stroke Care				
Anticoagulation Therapy for Atrial Fibrillation[1]	-	-	96%	95%
Antithrombotic Therapy Timing	27	100%	98%	98%
Assessed for Rehabilitation	39	95%	98%	97%
Discharged on Antithrombotic Therapy	29	100%	99%	99%
Discharged on Statin Medication	24	79%	95%	94%
Thrombolytic Therapy Timing[1]	-	-	68%	66%
Venous Thromboembolism Prophylaxis	42	86%	94%	94%
Written Stroke Educational Materials Given	15	87%	92%	88%
Surgical Care Improvement Project				
Appropriate Beta Blocker Usage	86	99%	98%	98%
Appropriate VTP Within 24 Hours	408	99%	98%	98%
Controlled Postoperative Blood Glucose[7]	-	-	96%	97%
Perioperative Temperature Management	457	100%	100%	100%
Prophylactic Antibiotic Selection	327	100%	99%	99%
Prophylactic Antibiotic Selection (Outpatient)	67	99%	98%	98%
Prophylactic Antibiotic Stopped	312	100%	98%	98%
Prophylactic Antibiotic Timing	327	100%	99%	99%
Prophylactic Antibiotic Timing (Outpatient)	67	96%	98%	98%
Urinary Catheter Removal	235	100%	98%	97%
Survey of Patients' Hospital Experiences				
Area Around Room 'Always' Quiet at Night	300+	60%	68%	61%
Doctors 'Always' Communicated Well	300+	76%	83%	82%
Home Recovery Information Given	300+	81%	85%	85%
Hospital Given 9 or 10 on 10 Point Scale	300+	67%	73%	71%
Meds 'Always' Explained Before Given	300+	58%	66%	64%
Nurses 'Always' Communicated Well	300+	72%	80%	79%
Pain 'Always' Well Controlled	300+	66%	72%	71%
Room and Bathroom 'Always' Clean	300+	68%	75%	73%
Timely Help 'Always' Received	300+	61%	69%	68%
Would Definitely Recommend Hospital	300+	68%	73%	71%
Use of Medical Imaging				
Cardiac Imaging Stress Test before Surgery	145	4.8%	5.3%	5.3%
Combination Abdominal CT Scan	380	8.4%	16.4%	10.5%
Combination Brain/Sinus CT Scan[1]	-	-	2.7%	2.7%
Combination Chest CT Scan	221	13.1%	5.6%	2.7%
Follow-up Mammogram/Ultrasound	1,058	7.7%	7.9%	8.8%
Lumbar Spine MRI for Low Back Pain	45	37.8%	39.6%	37.2%

Etmc Carthage

409 West Cottage
Carthage, TX 75633
E-mail: info@etmc.org
URL: www.etmc.org
Phone: 936933841
Fax: 903-694-4625
Type: Acute Care Hospitals
Ownership: Voluntary non-profit - Private
Emergency Services: Yes
Beds: 49

Key Personnel:
Operating Room. . . . . Robert Callahan, RN
Anesthesiology. . . . . John Hernandez, CRNA
Infection Control. . . . . Royce Hill, MD
Chief of Medical Staff. . . . . Linda Nagle
Emergency Room . . . . Gary Sweek, DO
Quality Assurance . . . . Jay Wright

Measure	Cases	This Hosp.	State Avg.	U.S. Avg.
Blood Clot Prevention and Treatment				
Anticoagulation Overlap Therapy[1,2]	-	-	93%	93%
ICU Venous Thromboembolism Prophylaxis[2,7]	-	-	92%	92%
Incidence of Potentially Preventable VTE[2,7]	-	-	9%	10%
UFH with Dosages/Platelet Monitoring[2,7]	-	-	96%	97%
Venous Thromboembolism Prophylaxis[2]	106	65%	82%	85%
Warfarin Therapy Discharge Instructions[1,2]	-	-	84%	75%
Chest Pain/Possible Heart Attack Care				
Aspirin Given Within 24 Hours of Arrival	36	89%	94%	96%
Fibrinolytic Meds Within 30 Min. of Arrival[1]	-	-	47%	58%
Average Time to ECG (minutes)	36	4	8	7
Average Time to Transfer (minutes)[1]	-	-	62	60
Children's Asthma Care				
Received Home Management Plan of Care	-	-	93%	88%
Received Reliever Medication	-	-	100%	100%
Received Systemic Corticosteroids	-	-	100%	100%
Emergency Department				
Admittance Decision Time (minutes)[2]	387	78	99	98
Head CT Results Within 45 Min. of Arrival[1]	-	-	54%	57%
Patients Who Left ER Before Being Seen	14,446	2%	3%	2%
Time from ER Arrival to Admit. (minutes)[2]	414	233	270	274
Time from ER Arrival to Discharge (minutes)	355	104	127	134
Time in ER Before Being Evaluated (minutes)	299	25	26	26
Time to Pain Meds for Fractures (minutes)	37	76	57	57
Heart Attack Care				
Aspirin Given at Discharge[1]	-	-	99%	99%
Fibrinolytic Meds Within 30 Min. of Arrival[7]	-	-	49%	54%
PCI Within 90 Minutes of Arrival[7]	-	-	95%	96%
Statin Prescribed at Discharge[1]	-	-	98%	98%
Heart Failure Care				
ACE Inhibitor or ARB for LVSD	13	100%	97%	97%
Discharge Instructions Given	30	57%	95%	94%
Evaluation of LVS Function	40	85%	99%	99%
Medicare Spending				
Medicare Spending per Patient (ratio)	-	0.92	1.03	0.98
Pneumonia Care				
Appropriate Initial Antibiotic Given	42	90%	95%	95%
Blood Culture Timing	54	93%	98%	98%
Pregnancy and Delivery Care				
Newborn Deliveries Scheduled Early[7]	-	-	7%	6%
Preventive Care				
Immunization for Influenza[2]	312	89%	90%	90%
Immunization for Pneumonia[2]	451	92%	92%	92%
Stroke Care				
Anticoagulation Therapy for Atrial Fibrillation[1]	-	-	96%	95%
Antithrombotic Therapy Timing	12	100%	98%	98%
Assessed for Rehabilitation	13	85%	98%	97%
Discharged on Antithrombotic Therapy	12	100%	99%	99%
Discharged on Statin Medication[1]	-	-	95%	94%
Thrombolytic Therapy Timing[7]	-	-	68%	66%
Venous Thromboembolism Prophylaxis	12	75%	94%	94%
Written Stroke Educational Materials Given[1]	-	-	92%	88%
Surgical Care Improvement Project				
Appropriate Beta Blocker Usage[1,3]	-	-	98%	98%
Appropriate VTP Within 24 Hours[1,3]	-	-	98%	98%
Controlled Postoperative Blood Glucose[3,7]	-	-	96%	97%
Perioperative Temperature Management[1,3]	-	-	100%	100%
Prophylactic Antibiotic Selection[1,3]	-	-	99%	99%
Prophylactic Antibiotic Selection (Outpatient)[1,3]	-	-	98%	98%
Prophylactic Antibiotic Stopped[1,3]	-	-	98%	98%
Prophylactic Antibiotic Timing[1,3]	-	-	99%	99%
Prophylactic Antibiotic Timing (Outpatient)[1,3]	-	-	98%	98%
Urinary Catheter Removal[1,3]	-	-	98%	97%
Survey of Patients' Hospital Experiences				
Area Around Room 'Always' Quiet at Night	(a)	75%	68%	61%
Doctors 'Always' Communicated Well	(a)	87%	83%	82%
Home Recovery Information Given	(a)	83%	85%	85%
Hospital Given 9 or 10 on 10 Point Scale	(a)	63%	73%	71%
Meds 'Always' Explained Before Given	(a)	67%	66%	64%
Nurses 'Always' Communicated Well	(a)	76%	80%	79%
Pain 'Always' Well Controlled	(a)	66%	72%	71%
Room and Bathroom 'Always' Clean	(a)	65%	75%	73%
Timely Help 'Always' Received	(a)	67%	69%	68%
Would Definitely Recommend Hospital	(a)	54%	73%	71%
Use of Medical Imaging				
Cardiac Imaging Stress Test before Surgery	55	1.8%	5.3%	5.3%
Combination Abdominal CT Scan	191	2.6%	16.4%	10.5%
Combination Brain/Sinus CT Scan	236	5.1%	2.7%	2.7%
Combination Chest CT Scan	101	0.0%	5.6%	2.7%
Follow-up Mammogram/Ultrasound	248	6.0%	7.9%	8.8%
Lumbar Spine MRI for Low Back Pain	36	52.8%	39.6%	37.2%

Cedar Park Regional Medical Center

1401 Medical Parkway
Cedar Park, TX 78613
URL: www.cedarparkregional.com
Phone: 512-528-7000
Type: Acute Care Hospitals
Ownership: Proprietary
Emergency Services: Yes
Beds: 150

Key Personnel:
President . . . . Jonathan B Buten
Radiology. Bill Cummings

Measure	Cases	This Hosp.	State Avg.	U.S. Avg.
Blood Clot Prevention and Treatment				
Anticoagulation Overlap Therapy[2]	32	94%	93%	93%
ICU Venous Thromboembolism Prophylaxis[2]	41	95%	92%	92%
Incidence of Potentially Preventable VTE[1,2]	-	-	9%	10%
UFH with Dosages/Platelet Monitoring[1,2]	-	-	96%	97%
Venous Thromboembolism Prophylaxis[2]	249	98%	82%	85%
Warfarin Therapy Discharge Instructions[2]	25	96%	84%	75%
Chest Pain/Possible Heart Attack Care				
Aspirin Given Within 24 Hours of Arrival	29	100%	94%	96%
Fibrinolytic Meds Within 30 Min. of Arrival[3,7]	-	-	47%	58%
Average Time to ECG (minutes)	29	4	8	7
Average Time to Transfer (minutes)[1,3]	-	-	62	60
Children's Asthma Care				
Received Home Management Plan of Care	-	-	93%	88%
Received Reliever Medication	-	-	100%	100%
Received Systemic Corticosteroids	-	-	100%	100%
Emergency Department				
Admittance Decision Time (minutes)[2]	539	78	99	98
Head CT Results Within 45 Min. of Arrival[1]	-	-	54%	57%
Patients Who Left ER Before Being Seen	28,927	2%	3%	2%
Time from ER Arrival to Admit. (minutes)[2]	548	252	270	274
Time from ER Arrival to Discharge (minutes)	394	145	127	134
Time in ER Before Being Evaluated (minutes)	418	18	26	26
Time to Pain Meds for Fractures (minutes)	239	48	57	57
Heart Attack Care				
Aspirin Given at Discharge	41	100%	99%	99%
Fibrinolytic Meds Within 30 Min. of Arrival[7]	-	-	49%	54%
PCI Within 90 Minutes of Arrival	12	100%	95%	96%
Statin Prescribed at Discharge	41	100%	98%	98%
Heart Failure Care				
ACE Inhibitor or ARB for LVSD	33	97%	97%	97%
Discharge Instructions Given	84	87%	95%	94%
Evaluation of LVS Function	99	100%	99%	99%
Medicare Spending				
Medicare Spending per Patient (ratio)	-	1.05	1.03	0.98
Pneumonia Care				
Appropriate Initial Antibiotic Given	89	96%	95%	95%
Blood Culture Timing	133	98%	98%	98%
Pregnancy and Delivery Care				
Newborn Deliveries Scheduled Early[2]	28	0%	7%	6%

NOTE: Hospital profiles are in alphabetical order by state, then city, then hospital within the city; Rankings exclude hospitals with less than 25 cases except for patient surveys which excludes hospitals with less than 100 cases; (a) 100-299 cases; (1) The number of cases/patients is too few to report; (2) Data submitted were based on a sample of cases/patients; (3) Results are based on a shorter time period than required; (4) Data suppressed by CMS for one or more quarters; (5) Results are not available for this reporting period; (6) Fewer than 100 patients completed the HCAHPS survey; (7) No cases met the criteria for this measure; (8) The lower limit of the confidence interval cannot be calculated if the number of observed infections equals zero; (9) No data are available from the state/territory for this reporting period; (10) The scores shown reflect fewer than 50 completed surveys; (11) There were discrepancies in the data collection process; (12) This measure does not apply to this hospital for this reporting period; (13) Results cannot be calculated for this reporting period; (14) The results for this state are combined with nearby states to protect confidentiality; Please refer to the User's Guide for a full explanation of data.

Measure	Cases	This Hosp.	State Avg.	U.S. Avg.
Preventive Care				
Immunization for Influenza[2]	500	98%	90%	90%
Immunization for Pneumonia[2]	465	97%	92%	92%
Stroke Care				
Anticoagulation Therapy for Atrial Fibrillation[1]	-	-	96%	95%
Antithrombotic Therapy Timing	20	100%	98%	98%
Assessed for Rehabilitation	24	100%	98%	97%
Discharged on Antithrombotic Therapy	24	100%	99%	99%
Discharged on Statin Medication	12	100%	95%	94%
Thrombolytic Therapy Timing[1]	-	-	68%	66%
Venous Thromboembolism Prophylaxis	18	94%	94%	94%
Written Stroke Educational Materials Given	12	100%	92%	88%
Surgical Care Improvement Project				
Appropriate Beta Blocker Usage	92	96%	98%	98%
Appropriate VTP Within 24 Hours	308	99%	98%	98%
Controlled Postoperative Blood Glucose[7]	-	-	96%	97%
Perioperative Temperature Management	381	100%	100%	100%
Prophylactic Antibiotic Selection	225	98%	99%	99%
Prophylactic Antibiotic Selection (Outpatient)	161	99%	98%	98%
Prophylactic Antibiotic Stopped	222	99%	98%	98%
Prophylactic Antibiotic Timing	226	99%	99%	99%
Prophylactic Antibiotic Timing (Outpatient)	161	100%	98%	98%
Urinary Catheter Removal	102	94%	98%	97%
Survey of Patients' Hospital Experiences				
Area Around Room 'Always' Quiet at Night	300+	59%	68%	61%
Doctors 'Always' Communicated Well	300+	80%	83%	82%
Home Recovery Information Given	300+	86%	85%	85%
Hospital Given 9 or 10 on 10 Point Scale	300+	65%	73%	71%
Meds 'Always' Explained Before Given	300+	60%	66%	64%
Nurses 'Always' Communicated Well	300+	72%	80%	79%
Pain 'Always' Well Controlled	300+	66%	72%	71%
Room and Bathroom 'Always' Clean	300+	70%	75%	73%
Timely Help 'Always' Received	300+	63%	69%	68%
Would Definitely Recommend Hospital	300+	69%	73%	71%
Use of Medical Imaging				
Cardiac Imaging Stress Test before Surgery	185	2.7%	5.3%	5.3%
Combination Abdominal CT Scan	359	1.7%	16.4%	10.5%
Combination Brain/Sinus CT Scan[1]	-	-	2.7%	2.7%
Combination Chest CT Scan	138	8.0%	5.6%	2.7%
Follow-up Mammogram/Ultrasound	326	32.2%	7.9%	8.8%
Lumbar Spine MRI for Low Back Pain[1]	-	-	39.6%	37.2%

Scott & White Emergency Hospital at Cedar Park

900 East Whitestone Blvd
Cedar Park, TX 78613
Phone: 512-684-4911
Type: Acute Care Hospitals
Emergency Services: Yes
Ownership: Proprietary

Measure	Cases	This Hosp.	State Avg.	U.S. Avg.
Blood Clot Prevention and Treatment				
Anticoagulation Overlap Therapy[5]	-	-	93%	93%
ICU Venous Thromboembolism Prophylaxis[5]	-	-	92%	92%
Incidence of Potentially Preventable VTE[5]	-	-	9%	10%
UFH with Dosages/Platelet Monitoring[5]	-	-	96%	97%
Venous Thromboembolism Prophylaxis[5]	-	-	82%	85%
Warfarin Therapy Discharge Instructions[5]	-	-	84%	75%
Chest Pain/Possible Heart Attack Care				
Aspirin Given Within 24 Hours of Arrival[5]	-	-	94%	96%
Fibrinolytic Meds Within 30 Min. of Arrival[5]	-	-	47%	58%
Average Time to ECG (minutes)[5]	-	-	8	7
Average Time to Transfer (minutes)[5]	-	-	62	60
Children's Asthma Care				
Received Home Management Plan of Care	-	-	93%	88%
Received Reliever Medication	-	-	100%	100%
Received Systemic Corticosteroids	-	-	100%	100%
Emergency Department				
Admittance Decision Time (minutes)[5]	-	-	99	98
Head CT Results Within 45 Min. of Arrival[5]	-	-	54%	57%
Patients Who Left ER Before Being Seen[5]	-	-	3%	2%
Time from ER Arrival to Admit. (minutes)[5]	-	-	270	274
Time from ER Arrival to Discharge (minutes)[5]	-	-	127	134
Time in ER Before Being Evaluated (minutes)[5]	-	-	26	26
Time to Pain Meds for Fractures (minutes)[5]	-	-	57	57
Heart Attack Care				
Aspirin Given at Discharge[5]	-	-	99%	99%
Fibrinolytic Meds Within 30 Min. of Arrival[5]	-	-	49%	54%
PCI Within 90 Minutes of Arrival[5]	-	-	95%	96%
Statin Prescribed at Discharge[5]	-	-	98%	98%
Heart Failure Care				
ACE Inhibitor or ARB for LVSD[5]	-	-	97%	97%
Discharge Instructions Given[5]	-	-	95%	94%
Evaluation of LVS Function[5]	-	-	99%	99%
Medicare Spending				
Medicare Spending per Patient (ratio)	-	-	1.03	0.98
Pneumonia Care				
Appropriate Initial Antibiotic Given[5]	-	-	95%	95%
Blood Culture Timing[5]	-	-	98%	98%
Pregnancy and Delivery Care				
Newborn Deliveries Scheduled Early[3,7]	-	-	7%	6%
Preventive Care				
Immunization for Influenza[5]	-	-	90%	90%
Immunization for Pneumonia[5]	-	-	92%	92%
Stroke Care				
Anticoagulation Therapy for Atrial Fibrillation[5]	-	-	96%	95%
Antithrombotic Therapy Timing[5]	-	-	98%	98%
Assessed for Rehabilitation[5]	-	-	98%	97%
Discharged on Antithrombotic Therapy[5]	-	-	99%	99%
Discharged on Statin Medication[5]	-	-	95%	94%
Thrombolytic Therapy Timing[5]	-	-	68%	66%
Venous Thromboembolism Prophylaxis[5]	-	-	94%	94%
Written Stroke Educational Materials Given[5]	-	-	92%	88%
Surgical Care Improvement Project				
Appropriate Beta Blocker Usage[5]	-	-	98%	98%
Appropriate VTP Within 24 Hours[5]	-	-	98%	98%
Controlled Postoperative Blood Glucose[5]	-	-	96%	97%
Perioperative Temperature Management[5]	-	-	100%	100%
Prophylactic Antibiotic Selection[5]	-	-	99%	99%
Prophylactic Antibiotic Selection (Outpatient)[5]	-	-	98%	98%
Prophylactic Antibiotic Stopped[5]	-	-	98%	98%
Prophylactic Antibiotic Timing[5]	-	-	99%	99%
Prophylactic Antibiotic Timing (Outpatient)[5]	-	-	98%	98%
Urinary Catheter Removal[5]	-	-	98%	97%
Survey of Patients' Hospital Experiences				
Area Around Room 'Always' Quiet at Night[5]	-	-	68%	61%
Doctors 'Always' Communicated Well[5]	-	-	83%	82%
Home Recovery Information Given[5]	-	-	85%	85%
Hospital Given 9 or 10 on 10 Point Scale[5]	-	-	73%	71%
Meds 'Always' Explained Before Given[5]	-	-	66%	64%
Nurses 'Always' Communicated Well[5]	-	-	80%	79%
Pain 'Always' Well Controlled[5]	-	-	72%	71%
Room and Bathroom 'Always' Clean[5]	-	-	75%	73%
Timely Help 'Always' Received[5]	-	-	69%	68%
Would Definitely Recommend Hospital[5]	-	-	73%	71%
Use of Medical Imaging				
Cardiac Imaging Stress Test before Surgery[5]	-	-	5.3%	5.3%
Combination Abdominal CT Scan[5]	-	-	16.4%	10.5%
Combination Brain/Sinus CT Scan[5]	-	-	2.7%	2.7%
Combination Chest CT Scan[5]	-	-	5.6%	2.7%
Follow-up Mammogram/Ultrasound[5]	-	-	7.9%	8.8%
Lumbar Spine MRI for Low Back Pain[5]	-	-	39.6%	37.2%

Childress Regional Medical Center

Hwy 83 North
Childress, TX 79201
Phone: 940-937-6371
Fax: 940-937-9133
E-mail: crmc11@chipshot.net
URL: www.childresshospital.com
Type: Acute Care Hospitals
Emergency Services: Yes
Ownership: Govt - Hospital Dist/Auth
Beds: 60

Key Personnel:

Quality Assurance . . . . Sue Allen
Emergency Room . . . . T. Stephen Carter, MD
Surgery . . . . Richard A. Katseres, MD
Operating Room. . . . . Betty Seagroves

Measure	Cases	This Hosp.	State Avg.	U.S. Avg.
Blood Clot Prevention and Treatment				
Anticoagulation Overlap Therapy[1]	-	-	93%	93%
ICU Venous Thromboembolism Prophylaxis[7]	-	-	92%	92%
Incidence of Potentially Preventable VTE[7]	-	-	9%	10%
UFH with Dosages/Platelet Monitoring[7]	-	-	96%	97%
Venous Thromboembolism Prophylaxis	224	63%	82%	85%
Warfarin Therapy Discharge Instructions[1]	-	-	84%	75%
Chest Pain/Possible Heart Attack Care				
Aspirin Given Within 24 Hours of Arrival	23	100%	94%	96%
Fibrinolytic Meds Within 30 Min. of Arrival[1]	-	-	47%	58%
Average Time to ECG (minutes)	23	4	8	7
Average Time to Transfer (minutes)[7]	-	-	62	60
Children's Asthma Care				
Received Home Management Plan of Care	-	-	93%	88%
Received Reliever Medication	-	-	100%	100%
Received Systemic Corticosteroids	-	-	100%	100%
Emergency Department				
Admittance Decision Time (minutes)[2]	94	28	99	98
Head CT Results Within 45 Min. of Arrival[1]	-	-	54%	57%
Patients Who Left ER Before Being Seen	5,051	2%	3%	2%
Time from ER Arrival to Admit. (minutes)[2]	136	126	270	274
Time from ER Arrival to Discharge (minutes)	384	97	127	134
Time in ER Before Being Evaluated (minutes)	316	28	26	26
Time to Pain Meds for Fractures (minutes)	33	48	57	57
Heart Attack Care				
Aspirin Given at Discharge[3,7]	-	-	99%	99%
Fibrinolytic Meds Within 30 Min. of Arrival[3,7]	-	-	49%	54%
PCI Within 90 Minutes of Arrival[3,7]	-	-	95%	96%
Statin Prescribed at Discharge[3,7]	-	-	98%	98%
Heart Failure Care				
ACE Inhibitor or ARB for LVSD[1,3]	-	-	97%	97%
Discharge Instructions Given[1,3]	-	-	95%	94%
Evaluation of LVS Function[1,3]	-	-	99%	99%
Medicare Spending				
Medicare Spending per Patient (ratio)	-	0.99	1.03	0.98
Pneumonia Care				
Appropriate Initial Antibiotic Given	22	100%	95%	95%
Blood Culture Timing	15	100%	98%	98%
Pregnancy and Delivery Care				
Newborn Deliveries Scheduled Early	19	0%	7%	6%
Preventive Care				
Immunization for Influenza[2]	237	86%	90%	90%
Immunization for Pneumonia[2]	249	95%	92%	92%
Stroke Care				
Anticoagulation Therapy for Atrial Fibrillation[1]	-	-	96%	95%
Antithrombotic Therapy Timing[1]	-	-	98%	98%
Assessed for Rehabilitation[1]	-	-	98%	97%
Discharged on Antithrombotic Therapy[1]	-	-	99%	99%
Discharged on Statin Medication[1]	-	-	95%	94%
Thrombolytic Therapy Timing[7]	-	-	68%	66%
Venous Thromboembolism Prophylaxis[1]	-	-	94%	94%
Written Stroke Educational Materials Given[1]	-	-	92%	88%
Surgical Care Improvement Project				
Appropriate Beta Blocker Usage[1]	-	-	98%	98%
Appropriate VTP Within 24 Hours	21	100%	98%	98%
Controlled Postoperative Blood Glucose[7]	-	-	96%	97%
Perioperative Temperature Management	22	100%	100%	100%
Prophylactic Antibiotic Selection	22	100%	99%	99%
Prophylactic Antibiotic Selection (Outpatient)[1,3]	-	-	98%	98%
Prophylactic Antibiotic Stopped	22	100%	98%	98%
Prophylactic Antibiotic Timing	22	95%	99%	99%
Prophylactic Antibiotic Timing (Outpatient)[1,3]	-	-	98%	98%
Urinary Catheter Removal[1]	-	-	98%	97%
Survey of Patients' Hospital Experiences				
Area Around Room 'Always' Quiet at Night	(a)	72%	68%	61%
Doctors 'Always' Communicated Well	(a)	90%	83%	82%
Home Recovery Information Given	(a)	90%	85%	85%
Hospital Given 9 or 10 on 10 Point Scale	(a)	79%	73%	71%
Meds 'Always' Explained Before Given	(a)	75%	66%	64%
Nurses 'Always' Communicated Well	(a)	85%	80%	79%
Pain 'Always' Well Controlled	(a)	76%	72%	71%
Room and Bathroom 'Always' Clean	(a)	75%	75%	73%
Timely Help 'Always' Received	(a)	80%	69%	68%
Would Definitely Recommend Hospital	(a)	82%	73%	71%
Use of Medical Imaging				

NOTE: Hospital profiles are in alphabetical order by state, then city, then hospital within the city; Rankings exclude hospitals with less than 25 cases except for patient surveys which excludes hospitals with less than 100 cases; (a) 100-299 cases; (1) The number of cases/patients is too few to report; (2) Data submitted were based on a sample of cases/patients; (3) Results are based on a shorter time period than required; (4) Data suppressed by CMS for one or more quarters; (5) Results are not available for this reporting period; (6) Fewer than 100 patients completed the HCAHPS survey; (7) No cases met the criteria for this measure; (8) The lower limit of the confidence interval cannot be calculated if the number of observed infections equals zero; (9) No data are available from the state/territory for this reporting period; (10) The scores shown reflect fewer than 50 completed surveys; (11) There were discrepancies in the data collection process; (12) This measure does not apply to this hospital for this reporting period; (13) Results cannot be calculated for this reporting period; (14) The results for this state are combined with nearby states to protect confidentiality; Please refer to the User's Guide for a full explanation of data.

Cardiac Imaging Stress Test before Surgery[1]	-	-	5.3%	5.3%
Combination Abdominal CT Scan	121	28.1%	16.4%	10.5%
Combination Brain/Sinus CT Scan[1]	-	-	2.7%	2.7%
Combination Chest CT Scan[1]	-	-	5.6%	2.7%
Follow-up Mammogram/Ultrasound	214	5.6%	7.9%	8.8%
Lumbar Spine MRI for Low Back Pain[1]	-	-	39.6%	37.2%

Chillicothe Hospital District

303 Avenue I
Chillicothe, TX 79225
Phone: 940-852-5131
Type: Critical Access Hospitals
Emergency Services: Yes
Ownership: Govt - Hospital Dist/Auth

Measure	Cases	This Hosp.	State Avg.	U.S. Avg.
Blood Clot Prevention and Treatment				
Anticoagulation Overlap Therapy[5]	-	-	93%	93%
ICU Venous Thromboembolism Prophylaxis[5]	-	-	92%	92%
Incidence of Potentially Preventable VTE[5]	-	-	9%	10%
UFH with Dosages/Platelet Monitoring[5]	-	-	96%	97%
Venous Thromboembolism Prophylaxis[5]	-	-	82%	85%
Warfarin Therapy Discharge Instructions[5]	-	-	84%	75%
Chest Pain/Possible Heart Attack Care				
Aspirin Given Within 24 Hours of Arrival	-	-	94%	96%
Fibrinolytic Meds Within 30 Min. of Arrival	-	-	47%	58%
Average Time to ECG (minutes)	-	-	8	7
Average Time to Transfer (minutes)	-	-	62	60
Children's Asthma Care				
Received Home Management Plan of Care	-	-	93%	88%
Received Reliever Medication	-	-	100%	100%
Received Systemic Corticosteroids	-	-	100%	100%
Emergency Department				
Admittance Decision Time (minutes)[5]	-	-	99	98
Head CT Results Within 45 Min. of Arrival	-	-	54%	57%
Patients Who Left ER Before Being Seen	-	-	3%	2%
Time from ER Arrival to Admit. (minutes)[5]	-	-	270	274
Time from ER Arrival to Discharge (minutes)	-	-	127	134
Time in ER Before Being Evaluated (minutes)	-	-	26	26
Time to Pain Meds for Fractures (minutes)	-	-	57	57
Heart Attack Care				
Aspirin Given at Discharge[5]	-	-	99%	99%
Fibrinolytic Meds Within 30 Min. of Arrival[5]	-	-	49%	54%
PCI Within 90 Minutes of Arrival[5]	-	-	95%	96%
Statin Prescribed at Discharge[5]	-	-	98%	98%
Heart Failure Care				
ACE Inhibitor or ARB for LVSD[3,7]	-	-	97%	97%
Discharge Instructions Given[3,7]	-	-	95%	94%
Evaluation of LVS Function[3,7]	-	-	99%	99%
Medicare Spending				
Medicare Spending per Patient (ratio)	-	-	1.03	0.98
Pneumonia Care				
Appropriate Initial Antibiotic Given[5]	-	-	95%	95%
Blood Culture Timing[5]	-	-	98%	98%
Pregnancy and Delivery Care				
Newborn Deliveries Scheduled Early[5]	-	-	7%	6%
Preventive Care				
Immunization for Influenza[5]	-	-	90%	90%
Immunization for Pneumonia[5]	-	-	92%	92%
Stroke Care				
Anticoagulation Therapy for Atrial Fibrillation[5]	-	-	96%	95%
Antithrombotic Therapy Timing[5]	-	-	98%	98%
Assessed for Rehabilitation[5]	-	-	98%	97%
Discharged on Antithrombotic Therapy[5]	-	-	99%	99%
Discharged on Statin Medication[5]	-	-	95%	94%
Thrombolytic Therapy Timing[5]	-	-	68%	66%
Venous Thromboembolism Prophylaxis[5]	-	-	94%	94%
Written Stroke Educational Materials Given[5]	-	-	92%	88%
Surgical Care Improvement Project				
Appropriate Beta Blocker Usage[5]	-	-	98%	98%
Appropriate VTP Within 24 Hours[5]	-	-	98%	98%
Controlled Postoperative Blood Glucose[5]	-	-	96%	97%
Perioperative Temperature Management[5]	-	-	100%	100%
Prophylactic Antibiotic Selection[5]	-	-	99%	99%
Prophylactic Antibiotic Selection (Outpatient)	-	-	98%	98%
Prophylactic Antibiotic Stopped[5]	-	-	98%	98%
Prophylactic Antibiotic Timing[5]	-	-	99%	99%
Prophylactic Antibiotic Timing (Outpatient)	-	-	98%	98%
Urinary Catheter Removal[5]	-	-	98%	97%
Survey of Patients' Hospital Experiences				
Area Around Room 'Always' Quiet at Night[5]	-	-	68%	61%
Doctors 'Always' Communicated Well[5]	-	-	83%	82%
Home Recovery Information Given[5]	-	-	85%	85%
Hospital Given 9 or 10 on 10 Point Scale[5]	-	-	73%	71%
Meds 'Always' Explained Before Given[5]	-	-	66%	64%
Nurses 'Always' Communicated Well[5]	-	-	80%	79%
Pain 'Always' Well Controlled[5]	-	-	72%	71%
Room and Bathroom 'Always' Clean[5]	-	-	75%	73%
Timely Help 'Always' Received[5]	-	-	69%	68%
Would Definitely Recommend Hospital[5]	-	-	73%	71%
Use of Medical Imaging				
Cardiac Imaging Stress Test before Surgery	-	-	5.3%	5.3%
Combination Abdominal CT Scan	-	-	16.4%	10.5%
Combination Brain/Sinus CT Scan	-	-	2.7%	2.7%
Combination Chest CT Scan	-	-	5.6%	2.7%
Follow-up Mammogram/Ultrasound	-	-	7.9%	8.8%
Lumbar Spine MRI for Low Back Pain	-	-	39.6%	37.2%

Etmc Clarksville

3000 W Main St
Clarksville, TX 75426
Phone: 903-427-3851
Fax: 903-427-2719
URL: www.etmc.org
Type: Acute Care Hospitals
Emergency Services: Yes
Ownership: Voluntary non-profit - Other
Beds: 36

Key Personnel:

Patient Relations . . . . Irene Bryant, RN
CEO/President. . . . . Elmer Ellis
Quality Assurance . . . . Carolyn Jones
Coronary Care . . . . Sharla McCulloch, RN
Intensive Care Unit. . . . . Sharla McCulloch, RN
Operating Room. . . . . BC Muthappa, RN
Infection Control. . . . . Amber Sims, RN
Emergency Room . . . . Linda Tabb, RN

Measure	Cases	This Hosp.	State Avg.	U.S. Avg.
Blood Clot Prevention and Treatment				
Anticoagulation Overlap Therapy[1,2]	-	-	93%	93%
ICU Venous Thromboembolism Prophylaxis[2,7]	-	-	92%	92%
Incidence of Potentially Preventable VTE[2,7]	-	-	9%	10%
UFH with Dosages/Platelet Monitoring[2,7]	-	-	96%	97%
Venous Thromboembolism Prophylaxis[2]	137	33%	82%	85%
Warfarin Therapy Discharge Instructions[1,2]	-	-	84%	75%
Chest Pain/Possible Heart Attack Care				
Aspirin Given Within 24 Hours of Arrival	17	100%	94%	96%
Fibrinolytic Meds Within 30 Min. of Arrival[3,7]	-	-	47%	58%
Average Time to ECG (minutes)	18	10	8	7
Average Time to Transfer (minutes)[3,7]	-	-	62	60
Children's Asthma Care				
Received Home Management Plan of Care	-	-	93%	88%
Received Reliever Medication	-	-	100%	100%
Received Systemic Corticosteroids	-	-	100%	100%
Emergency Department				
Admittance Decision Time (minutes)[2]	255	45	99	98
Head CT Results Within 45 Min. of Arrival[3,7]	-	-	54%	57%
Patients Who Left ER Before Being Seen	5,428	2%	3%	2%
Time from ER Arrival to Admit. (minutes)[2]	278	190	270	274
Time from ER Arrival to Discharge (minutes)	607	107	127	134
Time in ER Before Being Evaluated (minutes)	485	22	26	26
Time to Pain Meds for Fractures (minutes)	16	62	57	57
Heart Attack Care				
Aspirin Given at Discharge[1]	-	-	99%	99%
Fibrinolytic Meds Within 30 Min. of Arrival[7]	-	-	49%	54%
PCI Within 90 Minutes of Arrival[7]	-	-	95%	96%
Statin Prescribed at Discharge[1]	-	-	98%	98%
Heart Failure Care				
ACE Inhibitor or ARB for LVSD[1]	-	-	97%	97%
Discharge Instructions Given	31	74%	95%	94%
Evaluation of LVS Function	44	86%	99%	99%
Medicare Spending				
Medicare Spending per Patient (ratio)	-	1.05	1.03	0.98
Pneumonia Care				
Appropriate Initial Antibiotic Given	82	73%	95%	95%
Blood Culture Timing	62	90%	98%	98%
Pregnancy and Delivery Care				
Newborn Deliveries Scheduled Early[7]	-	-	7%	6%
Preventive Care				
Immunization for Influenza[2]	286	67%	90%	90%
Immunization for Pneumonia[2]	422	75%	92%	92%
Stroke Care				
Anticoagulation Therapy for Atrial Fibrillation[7]	-	-	96%	95%
Antithrombotic Therapy Timing[1]	-	-	98%	98%
Assessed for Rehabilitation[1]	-	-	98%	97%
Discharged on Antithrombotic Therapy[1]	-	-	99%	99%
Discharged on Statin Medication[1]	-	-	95%	94%
Thrombolytic Therapy Timing[7]	-	-	68%	66%
Venous Thromboembolism Prophylaxis[1]	-	-	94%	94%
Written Stroke Educational Materials Given[1]	-	-	92%	88%
Surgical Care Improvement Project				
Appropriate Beta Blocker Usage[5]	-	-	98%	98%
Appropriate VTP Within 24 Hours[5]	-	-	98%	98%
Controlled Postoperative Blood Glucose[5]	-	-	96%	97%
Perioperative Temperature Management[5]	-	-	100%	100%
Prophylactic Antibiotic Selection[5]	-	-	99%	99%
Prophylactic Antibiotic Selection (Outpatient)[3,7]	-	-	98%	98%
Prophylactic Antibiotic Stopped[5]	-	-	98%	98%
Prophylactic Antibiotic Timing[5]	-	-	99%	99%
Prophylactic Antibiotic Timing (Outpatient)[1,3]	-	-	98%	98%
Urinary Catheter Removal[5]	-	-	98%	97%
Survey of Patients' Hospital Experiences				
Area Around Room 'Always' Quiet at Night	(a)	63%	68%	61%
Doctors 'Always' Communicated Well	(a)	83%	83%	82%
Home Recovery Information Given	(a)	82%	85%	85%
Hospital Given 9 or 10 on 10 Point Scale	(a)	62%	73%	71%
Meds 'Always' Explained Before Given	(a)	60%	66%	64%
Nurses 'Always' Communicated Well	(a)	79%	80%	79%
Pain 'Always' Well Controlled	(a)	68%	72%	71%
Room and Bathroom 'Always' Clean	(a)	77%	75%	73%
Timely Help 'Always' Received	(a)	70%	69%	68%
Would Definitely Recommend Hospital	(a)	65%	73%	71%
Use of Medical Imaging				
Cardiac Imaging Stress Test before Surgery	98	3.1%	5.3%	5.3%
Combination Abdominal CT Scan	129	24.0%	16.4%	10.5%
Combination Brain/Sinus CT Scan	176	5.7%	2.7%	2.7%
Combination Chest CT Scan	92	12.0%	5.6%	2.7%
Follow-up Mammogram/Ultrasound[7]	-	-	7.9%	8.8%
Lumbar Spine MRI for Low Back Pain[1]	-	-	39.6%	37.2%

Texas Health Harris Methodist Hospital Cleburne

201 Walls Drive
Cleburne, TX 76033
Phone: 817-641-2551
Fax: 817-641-4346
URL: www.texashealth.org
Type: Acute Care Hospitals
Emergency Services: Yes
Ownership: Voluntary non-profit - Church
Beds: 137

Key Personnel:

Emergency Room . . . . Nettie Davis
CEO . . . . Douglas D. Hawthorne
Quality Assurance . . . . Beth Herrick, RN
Chief of Medical Staff. . . . . Barney Maddox, MD
CEO/President. . . . . Brent D Magers
President . . . . Shawn D. Parsley, DO

Measure	Cases	This Hosp.	State Avg.	U.S. Avg.
Blood Clot Prevention and Treatment				
Anticoagulation Overlap Therapy[2]	44	84%	93%	93%
ICU Venous Thromboembolism Prophylaxis[2]	55	98%	92%	92%
Incidence of Potentially Preventable VTE[1,2]	-	-	9%	10%
UFH with Dosages/Platelet Monitoring[1,2]	-	-	96%	97%
Venous Thromboembolism Prophylaxis[2]	369	96%	82%	85%
Warfarin Therapy Discharge Instructions[2]	35	97%	84%	75%
Chest Pain/Possible Heart Attack Care				
Aspirin Given Within 24 Hours of Arrival	169	95%	94%	96%
Fibrinolytic Meds Within 30 Min. of Arrival[7]	-	-	47%	58%
Average Time to ECG (minutes)	175	9	8	7
Average Time to Transfer (minutes)	26	46	62	60
Children's Asthma Care				

NOTE: Hospital profiles are in alphabetical order by state, then city, then hospital within the city; Rankings exclude hospitals with less than 25 cases except for patient surveys which excludes hospitals with less than 100 cases; (a) 100-299 cases; (1) The number of cases/patients is too few to report; (2) Data submitted were based on a sample of cases/patients; (3) Results are based on a shorter time period than required; (4) Data suppressed by CMS for one or more quarters; (5) Results are not available for this reporting period; (6) Fewer than 100 patients completed the HCAHPS survey; (7) No cases met the criteria for this measure; (8) The lower limit of the confidence interval cannot be calculated if the number of observed infections equals zero; (9) No data are available from the state/territory for this reporting period; (10) The scores shown reflect fewer than 50 completed surveys; (11) There were discrepancies in the data collection process; (12) This measure does not apply to this hospital for this reporting period; (13) Results cannot be calculated for this reporting period; (14) The results for this state are combined with nearby states to protect confidentiality; Please refer to the User's Guide for a full explanation of data.

Measure	Cases	This Hosp.	State Avg.	U.S. Avg.
Received Home Management Plan of Care	-	-	93%	88%
Received Reliever Medication	-	-	100%	100%
Received Systemic Corticosteroids	-	-	100%	100%
Emergency Department				
Admittance Decision Time (minutes)[2]	502	88	99	98
Head CT Results Within 45 Min. of Arrival	12	67%	54%	57%
Patients Who Left ER Before Being Seen	35,652	1%	3%	2%
Time from ER Arrival to Admit. (minutes)[2]	503	259	270	274
Time from ER Arrival to Discharge (minutes)	409	128	127	134
Time in ER Before Being Evaluated (minutes)	445	23	26	26
Time to Pain Meds for Fractures (minutes)	128	56	57	57
Heart Attack Care				
Aspirin Given at Discharge[1,3]	-	-	99%	99%
Fibrinolytic Meds Within 30 Min. of Arrival[3,7]	-	-	49%	54%
PCI Within 90 Minutes of Arrival[3,7]	-	-	95%	96%
Statin Prescribed at Discharge[1,3]	-	-	98%	98%
Heart Failure Care				
ACE Inhibitor or ARB for LVSD	31	100%	97%	97%
Discharge Instructions Given	134	100%	95%	94%
Evaluation of LVS Function	161	100%	99%	99%
Medicare Spending				
Medicare Spending per Patient (ratio)	-	0.99	1.03	0.98
Pneumonia Care				
Appropriate Initial Antibiotic Given	144	99%	95%	95%
Blood Culture Timing	205	100%	98%	98%
Pregnancy and Delivery Care				
Newborn Deliveries Scheduled Early	65	8%	7%	6%
Preventive Care				
Immunization for Influenza[2]	401	100%	90%	90%
Immunization for Pneumonia[2]	551	99%	92%	92%
Stroke Care				
Anticoagulation Therapy for Atrial Fibrillation[2,7]	-	-	96%	95%
Antithrombotic Therapy Timing[1,2]	-	-	98%	98%
Assessed for Rehabilitation[1,2]	-	-	98%	97%
Discharged on Antithrombotic Therapy[1,2]	-	-	99%	99%
Discharged on Statin Medication[1,2]	-	-	95%	94%
Thrombolytic Therapy Timing[2,7]	-	-	68%	66%
Venous Thromboembolism Prophylaxis[1,2]	-	-	94%	94%
Written Stroke Educational Materials Given[1,2]	-	-	92%	88%
Surgical Care Improvement Project				
Appropriate Beta Blocker Usage[2]	82	98%	98%	98%
Appropriate VTP Within 24 Hours[2]	245	97%	98%	98%
Controlled Postoperative Blood Glucose[2,7]	-	-	96%	97%
Perioperative Temperature Management[2]	259	100%	100%	100%
Prophylactic Antibiotic Selection[2]	172	100%	99%	99%
Prophylactic Antibiotic Selection (Outpatient)	36	97%	98%	98%
Prophylactic Antibiotic Stopped[2]	171	97%	98%	98%
Prophylactic Antibiotic Timing[2]	174	98%	99%	99%
Prophylactic Antibiotic Timing (Outpatient)	37	95%	98%	98%
Urinary Catheter Removal[2]	189	99%	98%	97%
Survey of Patients' Hospital Experiences				
Area Around Room 'Always' Quiet at Night	300+	66%	68%	61%
Doctors 'Always' Communicated Well	300+	82%	83%	82%
Home Recovery Information Given	300+	88%	85%	85%
Hospital Given 9 or 10 on 10 Point Scale	300+	73%	73%	71%
Meds 'Always' Explained Before Given	300+	68%	66%	64%
Nurses 'Always' Communicated Well	300+	84%	80%	79%
Pain 'Always' Well Controlled	300+	79%	72%	71%
Room and Bathroom 'Always' Clean	300+	78%	75%	73%
Timely Help 'Always' Received	300+	69%	69%	68%
Would Definitely Recommend Hospital	300+	72%	73%	71%
Use of Medical Imaging				
Cardiac Imaging Stress Test before Surgery[1]	-	-	5.3%	5.3%
Combination Abdominal CT Scan	419	6.7%	16.4%	10.5%
Combination Brain/Sinus CT Scan[1]	-	-	2.7%	2.7%
Combination Chest CT Scan	197	7.6%	5.6%	2.7%
Follow-up Mammogram/Ultrasound	441	5.7%	7.9%	8.8%
Lumbar Spine MRI for Low Back Pain[1]	-	-	39.6%	37.2%

Cleveland Regional Medical Center

300 E Crockett
Cleveland, TX 77327
Phone: 281-593-1811
Fax: 281-432-4369
URL: www.clevelandregionalmedical.com
Type: Acute Care Hospitals
Emergency Services: Yes
Ownership: Proprietary
Beds: 107
Key Personnel:
Quality Assurance . . . . Julie Darbonne
Operating Room. . . . . James Fleming

Measure	Cases	This Hosp.	State Avg.	U.S. Avg.
Blood Clot Prevention and Treatment				
Anticoagulation Overlap Therapy[1,2]	-	-	93%	93%
ICU Venous Thromboembolism Prophylaxis[2]	47	96%	92%	92%
Incidence of Potentially Preventable VTE[2,7]	-	-	9%	10%
UFH with Dosages/Platelet Monitoring[2,7]	-	-	96%	97%
Venous Thromboembolism Prophylaxis[2]	227	93%	82%	85%
Warfarin Therapy Discharge Instructions[1,2]	-	-	84%	75%
Chest Pain/Possible Heart Attack Care				
Aspirin Given Within 24 Hours of Arrival	27	89%	94%	96%
Fibrinolytic Meds Within 30 Min. of Arrival[1]	-	-	47%	58%
Average Time to ECG (minutes)	27	6	8	7
Average Time to Transfer (minutes)[1]	-	-	62	60
Children's Asthma Care				
Received Home Management Plan of Care	-	-	93%	88%
Received Reliever Medication	-	-	100%	100%
Received Systemic Corticosteroids	-	-	100%	100%
Emergency Department				
Admittance Decision Time (minutes)[2]	268	86	99	98
Head CT Results Within 45 Min. of Arrival[1]	-	-	54%	57%
Patients Who Left ER Before Being Seen	2,777	5%	3%	2%
Time from ER Arrival to Admit. (minutes)[2]	270	275	270	274
Time from ER Arrival to Discharge (minutes)	855	138	127	134
Time in ER Before Being Evaluated (minutes)	923	45	26	26
Time to Pain Meds for Fractures (minutes)	76	53	57	57
Heart Attack Care				
Aspirin Given at Discharge[3]	13	100%	99%	99%
Fibrinolytic Meds Within 30 Min. of Arrival[3,7]	-	-	49%	54%
PCI Within 90 Minutes of Arrival[3,7]	-	-	95%	96%
Statin Prescribed at Discharge[3]	12	83%	98%	98%
Heart Failure Care				
ACE Inhibitor or ARB for LVSD[1]	-	-	97%	97%
Discharge Instructions Given	26	96%	95%	94%
Evaluation of LVS Function	36	97%	99%	99%
Medicare Spending				
Medicare Spending per Patient (ratio)	-	1.19	1.03	0.98
Pneumonia Care				
Appropriate Initial Antibiotic Given	24	88%	95%	95%
Blood Culture Timing	48	100%	98%	98%
Pregnancy and Delivery Care				
Newborn Deliveries Scheduled Early[1,2]	-	-	7%	6%
Preventive Care				
Immunization for Influenza[2]	396	96%	90%	90%
Immunization for Pneumonia[2]	342	97%	92%	92%
Stroke Care				
Anticoagulation Therapy for Atrial Fibrillation[5]	-	-	96%	95%
Antithrombotic Therapy Timing[5]	-	-	98%	98%
Assessed for Rehabilitation[5]	-	-	98%	97%
Discharged on Antithrombotic Therapy[5]	-	-	99%	99%
Discharged on Statin Medication[5]	-	-	95%	94%
Thrombolytic Therapy Timing[5]	-	-	68%	66%
Venous Thromboembolism Prophylaxis[5]	-	-	94%	94%
Written Stroke Educational Materials Given[5]	-	-	92%	88%
Surgical Care Improvement Project				
Appropriate Beta Blocker Usage[1]	-	-	98%	98%
Appropriate VTP Within 24 Hours	31	100%	98%	98%
Controlled Postoperative Blood Glucose[7]	-	-	96%	97%
Perioperative Temperature Management	42	100%	100%	100%
Prophylactic Antibiotic Selection	25	100%	99%	99%
Prophylactic Antibiotic Selection (Outpatient)[3]	11	100%	98%	98%
Prophylactic Antibiotic Stopped	24	100%	98%	98%
Prophylactic Antibiotic Timing	25	100%	99%	99%
Prophylactic Antibiotic Timing (Outpatient)[3]	11	100%	98%	98%
Urinary Catheter Removal[1]	-	-	98%	97%
Survey of Patients' Hospital Experiences				
Area Around Room 'Always' Quiet at Night[5]	-	-	68%	61%
Doctors 'Always' Communicated Well[5]	-	-	83%	82%
Home Recovery Information Given[5]	-	-	85%	85%
Hospital Given 9 or 10 on 10 Point Scale[5]	-	-	73%	71%
Meds 'Always' Explained Before Given[5]	-	-	66%	64%
Nurses 'Always' Communicated Well[5]	-	-	80%	79%
Pain 'Always' Well Controlled[5]	-	-	72%	71%
Room and Bathroom 'Always' Clean[5]	-	-	75%	73%
Timely Help 'Always' Received[5]	-	-	69%	68%
Would Definitely Recommend Hospital[5]	-	-	73%	71%
Use of Medical Imaging				
Cardiac Imaging Stress Test before Surgery[7]	-	-	5.3%	5.3%
Combination Abdominal CT Scan	113	17.7%	16.4%	10.5%
Combination Brain/Sinus CT Scan[1]	-	-	2.7%	2.7%
Combination Chest CT Scan	65	1.5%	5.6%	2.7%
Follow-up Mammogram/Ultrasound	120	5.8%	7.9%	8.8%
Lumbar Spine MRI for Low Back Pain[1]	-	-	39.6%	37.2%

Doctors Diagnostic Hospital

1017 South Travis
Cleveland, TX 77328
Phone: 281-622-2900
URL: www.doctorsdiagnostichospital.com
Type: Acute Care Hospitals
Emergency Services: Yes
Ownership: Physician
Key Personnel:
Administrator . . . . Jeff Ackerman, MD
Radiology. . . . . Belinda Valdez

Measure	Cases	This Hosp.	State Avg.	U.S. Avg.
Blood Clot Prevention and Treatment				
Anticoagulation Overlap Therapy[2,7]	-	-	93%	93%
ICU Venous Thromboembolism Prophylaxis[2,7]	-	-	92%	92%
Incidence of Potentially Preventable VTE[2,7]	-	-	9%	10%
UFH with Dosages/Platelet Monitoring[2,7]	-	-	96%	97%
Venous Thromboembolism Prophylaxis[2]	83	48%	82%	85%
Warfarin Therapy Discharge Instructions[2,7]	-	-	84%	75%
Chest Pain/Possible Heart Attack Care				
Aspirin Given Within 24 Hours of Arrival[5]	-	-	94%	96%
Fibrinolytic Meds Within 30 Min. of Arrival[5]	-	-	47%	58%
Average Time to ECG (minutes)[5]	-	-	8	7
Average Time to Transfer (minutes)[5]	-	-	62	60
Children's Asthma Care				
Received Home Management Plan of Care	-	-	93%	88%
Received Reliever Medication	-	-	100%	100%
Received Systemic Corticosteroids	-	-	100%	100%
Emergency Department				
Admittance Decision Time (minutes)[2]	88	60	99	98
Head CT Results Within 45 Min. of Arrival[5]	-	-	54%	57%
Patients Who Left ER Before Being Seen	542	2%	3%	2%
Time from ER Arrival to Admit. (minutes)[2]	88	185	270	274
Time from ER Arrival to Discharge (minutes)	306	114	127	134
Time in ER Before Being Evaluated (minutes)	321	15	26	26
Time to Pain Meds for Fractures (minutes)[5]	-	-	57	57
Heart Attack Care				
Aspirin Given at Discharge[5]	-	-	99%	99%
Fibrinolytic Meds Within 30 Min. of Arrival[5]	-	-	49%	54%
PCI Within 90 Minutes of Arrival[5]	-	-	95%	96%
Statin Prescribed at Discharge[5]	-	-	98%	98%
Heart Failure Care				
ACE Inhibitor or ARB for LVSD[5]	-	-	97%	97%
Discharge Instructions Given[5]	-	-	95%	94%
Evaluation of LVS Function[5]	-	-	99%	99%
Medicare Spending				
Medicare Spending per Patient (ratio)	-	1.01	1.03	0.98
Pneumonia Care				
Appropriate Initial Antibiotic Given[5]	-	-	95%	95%
Blood Culture Timing[5]	-	-	98%	98%
Pregnancy and Delivery Care				
Newborn Deliveries Scheduled Early[7]	-	-	7%	6%
Preventive Care				
Immunization for Influenza[2]	244	87%	90%	90%
Immunization for Pneumonia[2]	236	85%	92%	92%
Stroke Care				

NOTE: Hospital profiles are in alphabetical order by state, then city, then hospital within the city; Rankings exclude hospitals with less than 25 cases except for patient surveys which excludes hospitals with less than 100 cases; (a) 100-299 cases; (1) The number of cases/patients is too few to report; (2) Data submitted were based on a sample of cases/patients; (3) Results are based on a shorter time period than required; (4) Data suppressed by CMS for one or more quarters; (5) Results are not available for this reporting period; (6) Fewer than 100 patients completed the HCAHPS survey; (7) No cases met the criteria for this measure; (8) The lower limit of the confidence interval cannot be calculated if the number of observed infections equals zero; (9) No data are available from the state/territory for this reporting period; (10) The scores shown reflect fewer than 50 completed surveys; (11) There were discrepancies in the data collection process; (12) This measure does not apply to this hospital for this reporting period; (13) Results cannot be calculated for this reporting period; (14) The results for this state are combined with nearby states to protect confidentiality; Please refer to the User's Guide for a full explanation of data.

Measure	Cases	This Hosp.	State Avg.	U.S. Avg.
Anticoagulation Therapy for Atrial Fibrillation[5]	-	-	96%	95%
Antithrombotic Therapy Timing[5]	-	-	98%	98%
Assessed for Rehabilitation[5]	-	-	98%	97%
Discharged on Antithrombotic Therapy[5]	-	-	99%	99%
Discharged on Statin Medication[5]	-	-	95%	94%
Thrombolytic Therapy Timing[5]	-	-	68%	66%
Venous Thromboembolism Prophylaxis[5]	-	-	94%	94%
Written Stroke Educational Materials Given[5]	-	-	92%	88%
Surgical Care Improvement Project				
Appropriate Beta Blocker Usage[1,3]	-	-	98%	98%
Appropriate VTP Within 24 Hours[1,3]	-	-	98%	98%
Controlled Postoperative Blood Glucose[3,7]	-	-	96%	97%
Perioperative Temperature Management[1,3]	-	-	100%	100%
Prophylactic Antibiotic Selection[1,3]	-	-	99%	99%
Prophylactic Antibiotic Selection (Outpatient)[5]	-	-	98%	98%
Prophylactic Antibiotic Stopped[1,3]	-	-	98%	98%
Prophylactic Antibiotic Timing[1,3]	-	-	99%	99%
Prophylactic Antibiotic Timing (Outpatient)[5]	-	-	98%	98%
Urinary Catheter Removal[3,7]	-	-	98%	97%
Survey of Patients' Hospital Experiences				
Area Around Room 'Always' Quiet at Night[6]	<100	86%	68%	61%
Doctors 'Always' Communicated Well[6]	<100	83%	83%	82%
Home Recovery Information Given[6]	<100	83%	85%	85%
Hospital Given 9 or 10 on 10 Point Scale[6]	<100	59%	73%	71%
Meds 'Always' Explained Before Given[6]	<100	54%	66%	64%
Nurses 'Always' Communicated Well[6]	<100	79%	80%	79%
Pain 'Always' Well Controlled[6]	<100	71%	72%	71%
Room and Bathroom 'Always' Clean[6]	<100	66%	75%	73%
Timely Help 'Always' Received[6]	<100	63%	69%	68%
Would Definitely Recommend Hospital[6]	<100	65%	73%	71%
Use of Medical Imaging				
Cardiac Imaging Stress Test before Surgery[1]	-	-	5.3%	5.3%
Combination Abdominal CT Scan	142	62.0%	16.4%	10.5%
Combination Brain/Sinus CT Scan[1]	-	-	2.7%	2.7%
Combination Chest CT Scan[1]	-	-	5.6%	2.7%
Follow-up Mammogram/Ultrasound[7]	-	-	7.9%	8.8%
Lumbar Spine MRI for Low Back Pain[1]	-	-	39.6%	37.2%

Goodall Witcher Hospital

101 Posey Avenue
Clifton, TX 76634
URL: www.gwhf.org
Type: Acute Care Hospitals
Ownership: Govt - Hospital Dist/Auth

Phone: 254-675-8322
Fax: 254-675-2246
Emergency Services: Yes
Beds: 72

Key Personnel:
Operating Room. . . . . L Cotten
Chief of Medical Staff . . . . Leon Cotten, MD
Radiology. . . . . Deborah Davis
Quality Assurance . . . . Anita Diebenow
CEO/President. . . . . Clarence Fields, Jr
Patient Relations . . . . Kenneth Lowrance, RN, FNP-C
Infection Control. . . . . Pat Massingill, RN
Emergency Room . . . . Joyce McDowell, RN

Measure	Cases	This Hosp.	State Avg.	U.S. Avg.
Blood Clot Prevention and Treatment				
Anticoagulation Overlap Therapy[1,2]	-	-	93%	93%
ICU Venous Thromboembolism Prophylaxis[2,7]	-	-	92%	92%
Incidence of Potentially Preventable VTE[1,2]	-	-	9%	10%
UFH with Dosages/Platelet Monitoring[2,7]	-	-	96%	97%
Venous Thromboembolism Prophylaxis[2]	117	48%	82%	85%
Warfarin Therapy Discharge Instructions[1,2]	-	-	84%	75%
Chest Pain/Possible Heart Attack Care				
Aspirin Given Within 24 Hours of Arrival[1,3]	-	-	94%	96%
Fibrinolytic Meds Within 30 Min. of Arrival[3,7]	-	-	47%	58%
Average Time to ECG (minutes)[1,3]	-	-	8	7
Average Time to Transfer (minutes)[3,7]	-	-	62	60
Children's Asthma Care				
Received Home Management Plan of Care	-	-	93%	88%
Received Reliever Medication	-	-	100%	100%
Received Systemic Corticosteroids	-	-	100%	100%
Emergency Department				
Admittance Decision Time (minutes)[2]	105	32	99	98
Head CT Results Within 45 Min. of Arrival[1,3]	-	-	54%	57%
Patients Who Left ER Before Being Seen	4,448	1%	3%	2%
Time from ER Arrival to Admit. (minutes)[2]	164	176	270	274
Time from ER Arrival to Discharge (minutes)	324	91	127	134
Time in ER Before Being Evaluated (minutes)	187	27	26	26
Time to Pain Meds for Fractures (minutes)	24	34	57	57
Heart Attack Care				
Aspirin Given at Discharge[5]	-	-	99%	99%
Fibrinolytic Meds Within 30 Min. of Arrival[5]	-	-	49%	54%
PCI Within 90 Minutes of Arrival[5]	-	-	95%	96%
Statin Prescribed at Discharge[5]	-	-	98%	98%
Heart Failure Care				
ACE Inhibitor or ARB for LVSD[1,2]	-	-	97%	97%
Discharge Instructions Given[1,2]	-	-	95%	94%
Evaluation of LVS Function[2]	11	82%	99%	99%
Medicare Spending				
Medicare Spending per Patient (ratio)	-	0.96	1.03	0.98
Pneumonia Care				
Appropriate Initial Antibiotic Given[2]	28	86%	95%	95%
Blood Culture Timing[2]	27	89%	98%	98%
Pregnancy and Delivery Care				
Newborn Deliveries Scheduled Early	19	0%	7%	6%
Preventive Care				
Immunization for Influenza[2]	226	77%	90%	90%
Immunization for Pneumonia[2]	265	83%	92%	92%
Stroke Care				
Anticoagulation Therapy for Atrial Fibrillation[5]	-	-	96%	95%
Antithrombotic Therapy Timing[5]	-	-	98%	98%
Assessed for Rehabilitation[5]	-	-	98%	97%
Discharged on Antithrombotic Therapy[5]	-	-	99%	99%
Discharged on Statin Medication[5]	-	-	95%	94%
Thrombolytic Therapy Timing[5]	-	-	68%	66%
Venous Thromboembolism Prophylaxis[5]	-	-	94%	94%
Written Stroke Educational Materials Given[5]	-	-	92%	88%
Surgical Care Improvement Project				
Appropriate Beta Blocker Usage[1,2]	-	-	98%	98%
Appropriate VTP Within 24 Hours[1,2]	-	-	98%	98%
Controlled Postoperative Blood Glucose[2,7]	-	-	96%	97%
Perioperative Temperature Management[1,2]	-	-	100%	100%
Prophylactic Antibiotic Selection[1,2]	-	-	99%	99%
Prophylactic Antibiotic Selection (Outpatient)[5]	-	-	98%	98%
Prophylactic Antibiotic Stopped[1,2]	-	-	98%	98%
Prophylactic Antibiotic Timing[1,2]	-	-	99%	99%
Prophylactic Antibiotic Timing (Outpatient)[5]	-	-	98%	98%
Urinary Catheter Removal[1,2]	-	-	98%	97%
Survey of Patients' Hospital Experiences				
Area Around Room 'Always' Quiet at Night[6]	<100	66%	68%	61%
Doctors 'Always' Communicated Well[6]	<100	81%	83%	82%
Home Recovery Information Given[6]	<100	91%	85%	85%
Hospital Given 9 or 10 on 10 Point Scale[6]	<100	70%	73%	71%
Meds 'Always' Explained Before Given[6]	<100	53%	66%	64%
Nurses 'Always' Communicated Well[6]	<100	77%	80%	79%
Pain 'Always' Well Controlled[6]	<100	68%	72%	71%
Room and Bathroom 'Always' Clean[6]	<100	72%	75%	73%
Timely Help 'Always' Received[6]	<100	63%	69%	68%
Would Definitely Recommend Hospital[6]	<100	66%	73%	71%
Use of Medical Imaging				
Cardiac Imaging Stress Test before Surgery[7]	-	-	5.3%	5.3%
Combination Abdominal CT Scan	81	6.2%	16.4%	10.5%
Combination Brain/Sinus CT Scan[1]	-	-	2.7%	2.7%
Combination Chest CT Scan	52	0.0%	5.6%	2.7%
Follow-up Mammogram/Ultrasound	296	9.8%	7.9%	8.8%
Lumbar Spine MRI for Low Back Pain[1]	-	-	39.6%	37.2%

Coleman County Medical Center Company

310 South Pecos Street
Coleman, TX 76834
Type: Critical Access Hospitals
Ownership: Govt - Hospital Dist/Auth

Phone: 325-625-2135
Fax: 325-625-5730
Emergency Services: Yes
Beds: 46

Key Personnel:
Chief of Medical Staff . . . . Michael Bailey, DO
Infection Control. . . . . Lynn Corbelt
Pediatric In-Patient Care . . . . Bobbie Jones
CEO/President. . . . . Douglas Langley
Operating Room. . . . . Becky Matthews, RN
Anesthesiology. . . . . Ed Pi Neiro, CRNA
Administrator . . . . Mike Pruitt

Measure	Cases	This Hosp.	State Avg.	U.S. Avg.
Blood Clot Prevention and Treatment				
Anticoagulation Overlap Therapy[5]	-	-	93%	93%
ICU Venous Thromboembolism Prophylaxis[5]	-	-	92%	92%
Incidence of Potentially Preventable VTE[5]	-	-	9%	10%
UFH with Dosages/Platelet Monitoring[5]	-	-	96%	97%
Venous Thromboembolism Prophylaxis[5]	-	-	82%	85%
Warfarin Therapy Discharge Instructions[5]	-	-	84%	75%
Chest Pain/Possible Heart Attack Care				
Aspirin Given Within 24 Hours of Arrival	-	-	94%	96%
Fibrinolytic Meds Within 30 Min. of Arrival	-	-	47%	58%
Average Time to ECG (minutes)	-	-	8	7
Average Time to Transfer (minutes)	-	-	62	60
Children's Asthma Care				
Received Home Management Plan of Care	-	-	93%	88%
Received Reliever Medication	-	-	100%	100%
Received Systemic Corticosteroids	-	-	100%	100%
Emergency Department				
Admittance Decision Time (minutes)[5]	-	-	99	98
Head CT Results Within 45 Min. of Arrival	-	-	54%	57%
Patients Who Left ER Before Being Seen	-	-	3%	2%
Time from ER Arrival to Admit. (minutes)[5]	-	-	270	274
Time from ER Arrival to Discharge (minutes)	-	-	127	134
Time in ER Before Being Evaluated (minutes)	-	-	26	26
Time to Pain Meds for Fractures (minutes)	-	-	57	57
Heart Attack Care				
Aspirin Given at Discharge[5]	-	-	99%	99%
Fibrinolytic Meds Within 30 Min. of Arrival[5]	-	-	49%	54%
PCI Within 90 Minutes of Arrival[5]	-	-	95%	96%
Statin Prescribed at Discharge[5]	-	-	98%	98%
Heart Failure Care				
ACE Inhibitor or ARB for LVSD[1]	-	-	97%	97%
Discharge Instructions Given	13	85%	95%	94%
Evaluation of LVS Function	20	90%	99%	99%
Medicare Spending				
Medicare Spending per Patient (ratio)	-	-	1.03	0.98
Pneumonia Care				
Appropriate Initial Antibiotic Given	22	91%	95%	95%
Blood Culture Timing	40	98%	98%	98%
Pregnancy and Delivery Care				
Newborn Deliveries Scheduled Early[5]	-	-	7%	6%
Preventive Care				
Immunization for Influenza[5]	-	-	90%	90%
Immunization for Pneumonia[5]	-	-	92%	92%
Stroke Care				
Anticoagulation Therapy for Atrial Fibrillation[5]	-	-	96%	95%
Antithrombotic Therapy Timing[5]	-	-	98%	98%
Assessed for Rehabilitation[5]	-	-	98%	97%
Discharged on Antithrombotic Therapy[5]	-	-	99%	99%
Discharged on Statin Medication[5]	-	-	95%	94%
Thrombolytic Therapy Timing[5]	-	-	68%	66%
Venous Thromboembolism Prophylaxis[5]	-	-	94%	94%
Written Stroke Educational Materials Given[5]	-	-	92%	88%
Surgical Care Improvement Project				
Appropriate Beta Blocker Usage[5]	-	-	98%	98%
Appropriate VTP Within 24 Hours[5]	-	-	98%	98%
Controlled Postoperative Blood Glucose[5]	-	-	96%	97%
Perioperative Temperature Management[5]	-	-	100%	100%
Prophylactic Antibiotic Selection[5]	-	-	99%	99%
Prophylactic Antibiotic Selection (Outpatient)	-	-	98%	98%
Prophylactic Antibiotic Stopped[5]	-	-	98%	98%
Prophylactic Antibiotic Timing[5]	-	-	99%	99%
Prophylactic Antibiotic Timing (Outpatient)	-	-	98%	98%
Urinary Catheter Removal[5]	-	-	98%	97%
Survey of Patients' Hospital Experiences				
Area Around Room 'Always' Quiet at Night[5]	-	-	68%	61%
Doctors 'Always' Communicated Well[5]	-	-	83%	82%
Home Recovery Information Given[5]	-	-	85%	85%
Hospital Given 9 or 10 on 10 Point Scale[5]	-	-	73%	71%
Meds 'Always' Explained Before Given[5]	-	-	66%	64%
Nurses 'Always' Communicated Well[5]	-	-	80%	79%
Pain 'Always' Well Controlled[5]	-	-	72%	71%

NOTE: Hospital profiles are in alphabetical order by state, then city, then hospital within the city; Rankings exclude hospitals with less than 25 cases except for patient surveys which excludes hospitals with less than 100 cases; (a) 100-299 cases; (1) The number of cases/patients is too few to report; (2) Data submitted were based on a sample of cases/patients; (3) Results are based on a shorter time period than required; (4) Data suppressed by CMS for one or more quarters; (5) Results are not available for this reporting period; (6) Fewer than 100 patients completed the HCAHPS survey; (7) No cases met the criteria for this measure; (8) The lower limit of the confidence interval cannot be calculated if the number of observed infections equals zero; (9) No data are available from the state/territory for this reporting period; (10) The scores shown reflect fewer than 50 completed surveys; (11) There were discrepancies in the data collection process; (12) This measure does not apply to this hospital for this reporting period; (13) Results cannot be calculated for this reporting period; (14) The results for this state are combined with nearby states to protect confidentiality; Please refer to the User's Guide for a full explanation of data.

Measure	Cases	This Hosp.	State Avg.	U.S. Avg.
Room and Bathroom 'Always' Clean[5]	-	-	75%	73%
Timely Help 'Always' Received[5]	-	-	69%	68%
Would Definitely Recommend Hospital[5]	-	-	73%	71%
Use of Medical Imaging				
Cardiac Imaging Stress Test before Surgery	-	-	5.3%	5.3%
Combination Abdominal CT Scan	-	-	16.4%	10.5%
Combination Brain/Sinus CT Scan	-	-	2.7%	2.7%
Combination Chest CT Scan	-	-	5.6%	2.7%
Follow-up Mammogram/Ultrasound	-	-	7.9%	8.8%
Lumbar Spine MRI for Low Back Pain	-	-	39.6%	37.2%

College Station Medical Center

1604 Rock Prairie Road
College Station, TX 77842
Phone: 979-764-5151
Fax: 979-693-3294
URL: www.csmedcenter.com
Type: Acute Care Hospitals
Emergency Services: Yes
Ownership: Proprietary
Beds: 119

Key Personnel:

Radiology. . . . . Mir Zulfiquar Alikhan, MD
CEO/President. . . . . Thomas W Jackson
Emergency Room . . . . Joe Jones, MD
Pediatric Ambulatory Care . . . . . . Terri Tomlin, MD
Pediatric In-Patient Care . . . . . . Terri Tomlin, MD
Chief of Medical Staff. . . . . Usha Venkatraj
Patient Relations . . . . Sherri Welch
Infection Control. . . . . Yeojin Zee

Measure	Cases	This Hosp.	State Avg.	U.S. Avg.
Blood Clot Prevention and Treatment				
Anticoagulation Overlap Therapy[2]	32	100%	93%	93%
ICU Venous Thromboembolism Prophylaxis[2]	110	97%	92%	92%
Incidence of Potentially Preventable VTE[1,2]	-	-	9%	10%
UFH with Dosages/Platelet Monitoring[1,2]	-	-	96%	97%
Venous Thromboembolism Prophylaxis[2]	346	99%	82%	85%
Warfarin Therapy Discharge Instructions[2]	20	90%	84%	75%
Chest Pain/Possible Heart Attack Care				
Aspirin Given Within 24 Hours of Arrival	12	100%	94%	96%
Fibrinolytic Meds Within 30 Min. of Arrival[5]	-	-	47%	58%
Average Time to ECG (minutes)	12	4	8	7
Average Time to Transfer (minutes)[5]	-	-	62	60
Children's Asthma Care				
Received Home Management Plan of Care	-	-	93%	88%
Received Reliever Medication	-	-	100%	100%
Received Systemic Corticosteroids	-	-	100%	100%
Emergency Department				
Admittance Decision Time (minutes)[2]	569	74	99	98
Head CT Results Within 45 Min. of Arrival[1]	-	-	54%	57%
Patients Who Left ER Before Being Seen	31,071	1%	3%	2%
Time from ER Arrival to Admit. (minutes)[2]	578	224	270	274
Time from ER Arrival to Discharge (minutes)	400	114	127	134
Time in ER Before Being Evaluated (minutes)	423	16	26	26
Time to Pain Meds for Fractures (minutes)	159	44	57	57
Heart Attack Care				
Aspirin Given at Discharge	88	100%	99%	99%
Fibrinolytic Meds Within 30 Min. of Arrival[7]	-	-	49%	54%
PCI Within 90 Minutes of Arrival[1]	-	-	95%	96%
Statin Prescribed at Discharge	85	100%	98%	98%
Heart Failure Care				
ACE Inhibitor or ARB for LVSD	104	100%	97%	97%
Discharge Instructions Given	173	95%	95%	94%
Evaluation of LVS Function	200	100%	99%	99%
Medicare Spending				
Medicare Spending per Patient (ratio)	-	0.98	1.03	0.98
Pneumonia Care				
Appropriate Initial Antibiotic Given	70	99%	95%	95%
Blood Culture Timing	124	100%	98%	98%
Pregnancy and Delivery Care				
Newborn Deliveries Scheduled Early[2]	61	8%	7%	6%
Preventive Care				
Immunization for Influenza[2]	600	94%	90%	90%
Immunization for Pneumonia[2]	742	96%	92%	92%
Stroke Care				
Anticoagulation Therapy for Atrial Fibrillation[1]	-	-	96%	95%
Antithrombotic Therapy Timing	48	98%	98%	98%
Assessed for Rehabilitation	69	100%	98%	97%
Discharged on Antithrombotic Therapy	62	100%	99%	99%
Discharged on Statin Medication	46	98%	95%	94%
Thrombolytic Therapy Timing[1]	-	-	68%	66%
Venous Thromboembolism Prophylaxis	60	100%	94%	94%
Written Stroke Educational Materials Given	45	93%	92%	88%
Surgical Care Improvement Project				
Appropriate Beta Blocker Usage	209	99%	98%	98%
Appropriate VTP Within 24 Hours	465	98%	98%	98%
Controlled Postoperative Blood Glucose	63	100%	96%	97%
Perioperative Temperature Management	646	100%	100%	100%
Prophylactic Antibiotic Selection	440	99%	99%	99%
Prophylactic Antibiotic Selection (Outpatient)	316	99%	98%	98%
Prophylactic Antibiotic Stopped	435	98%	98%	98%
Prophylactic Antibiotic Timing	440	98%	99%	99%
Prophylactic Antibiotic Timing (Outpatient)	269	100%	98%	98%
Urinary Catheter Removal	322	100%	98%	97%
Survey of Patients' Hospital Experiences				
Area Around Room 'Always' Quiet at Night	300+	67%	68%	61%
Doctors 'Always' Communicated Well	300+	85%	83%	82%
Home Recovery Information Given	300+	86%	85%	85%
Hospital Given 9 or 10 on 10 Point Scale	300+	72%	73%	71%
Meds 'Always' Explained Before Given	300+	66%	66%	64%
Nurses 'Always' Communicated Well	300+	78%	80%	79%
Pain 'Always' Well Controlled	300+	73%	72%	71%
Room and Bathroom 'Always' Clean	300+	69%	75%	73%
Timely Help 'Always' Received	300+	64%	69%	68%
Would Definitely Recommend Hospital	300+	74%	73%	71%
Use of Medical Imaging				
Cardiac Imaging Stress Test before Surgery[1]	-	-	5.3%	5.3%
Combination Abdominal CT Scan	321	3.1%	16.4%	10.5%
Combination Brain/Sinus CT Scan	410	4.9%	2.7%	2.7%
Combination Chest CT Scan	174	1.1%	5.6%	2.7%
Follow-up Mammogram/Ultrasound	627	8.0%	7.9%	8.8%
Lumbar Spine MRI for Low Back Pain	49	46.9%	39.6%	37.2%

Scott & White Hospital- College Station

700 Scott & White Drive
College Station, TX 77845
Phone: 979-691-3701
Type: Acute Care Hospitals
Emergency Services: Yes
Ownership: Voluntary non-profit - Private

Measure	Cases	This Hosp.	State Avg.	U.S. Avg.
Blood Clot Prevention and Treatment				
Anticoagulation Overlap Therapy[5]	-	-	93%	93%
ICU Venous Thromboembolism Prophylaxis[5]	-	-	92%	92%
Incidence of Potentially Preventable VTE[5]	-	-	9%	10%
UFH with Dosages/Platelet Monitoring[5]	-	-	96%	97%
Venous Thromboembolism Prophylaxis[5]	-	-	82%	85%
Warfarin Therapy Discharge Instructions[5]	-	-	84%	75%
Chest Pain/Possible Heart Attack Care				
Aspirin Given Within 24 Hours of Arrival[5]	-	-	94%	96%
Fibrinolytic Meds Within 30 Min. of Arrival[5]	-	-	47%	58%
Average Time to ECG (minutes)[5]	-	-	8	7
Average Time to Transfer (minutes)[5]	-	-	62	60
Children's Asthma Care				
Received Home Management Plan of Care	-	-	93%	88%
Received Reliever Medication	-	-	100%	100%
Received Systemic Corticosteroids	-	-	100%	100%
Emergency Department				
Admittance Decision Time (minutes)[5]	-	-	99	98
Head CT Results Within 45 Min. of Arrival[5]	-	-	54%	57%
Patients Who Left ER Before Being Seen[5]	-	-	3%	2%
Time from ER Arrival to Admit. (minutes)[5]	-	-	270	274
Time from ER Arrival to Discharge (minutes)[5]	-	-	127	134
Time in ER Before Being Evaluated (minutes)[5]	-	-	26	26
Time to Pain Meds for Fractures (minutes)[5]	-	-	57	57
Heart Attack Care				
Aspirin Given at Discharge[5]	-	-	99%	99%
Fibrinolytic Meds Within 30 Min. of Arrival[5]	-	-	49%	54%
PCI Within 90 Minutes of Arrival[5]	-	-	95%	96%
Statin Prescribed at Discharge[5]	-	-	98%	98%
Heart Failure Care				
ACE Inhibitor or ARB for LVSD[5]	-	-	97%	97%
Discharge Instructions Given[5]	-	-	95%	94%
Evaluation of LVS Function[5]	-	-	99%	99%
Medicare Spending				
Medicare Spending per Patient (ratio)	-	-	1.03	0.98
Pneumonia Care				
Appropriate Initial Antibiotic Given[5]	-	-	95%	95%
Blood Culture Timing[5]	-	-	98%	98%
Pregnancy and Delivery Care				
Newborn Deliveries Scheduled Early[5]	-	-	7%	6%
Preventive Care				
Immunization for Influenza[5]	-	-	90%	90%
Immunization for Pneumonia[5]	-	-	92%	92%
Stroke Care				
Anticoagulation Therapy for Atrial Fibrillation[5]	-	-	96%	95%
Antithrombotic Therapy Timing[5]	-	-	98%	98%
Assessed for Rehabilitation[5]	-	-	98%	97%
Discharged on Antithrombotic Therapy[5]	-	-	99%	99%
Discharged on Statin Medication[5]	-	-	95%	94%
Thrombolytic Therapy Timing[5]	-	-	68%	66%
Venous Thromboembolism Prophylaxis[5]	-	-	94%	94%
Written Stroke Educational Materials Given[5]	-	-	92%	88%
Surgical Care Improvement Project				
Appropriate Beta Blocker Usage[5]	-	-	98%	98%
Appropriate VTP Within 24 Hours[5]	-	-	98%	98%
Controlled Postoperative Blood Glucose[5]	-	-	96%	97%
Perioperative Temperature Management[5]	-	-	100%	100%
Prophylactic Antibiotic Selection[5]	-	-	99%	99%
Prophylactic Antibiotic Selection (Outpatient)[5]	-	-	98%	98%
Prophylactic Antibiotic Stopped[5]	-	-	98%	98%
Prophylactic Antibiotic Timing[5]	-	-	99%	99%
Prophylactic Antibiotic Timing (Outpatient)[5]	-	-	98%	98%
Urinary Catheter Removal[5]	-	-	98%	97%
Survey of Patients' Hospital Experiences				
Area Around Room 'Always' Quiet at Night[5]	-	-	68%	61%
Doctors 'Always' Communicated Well[5]	-	-	83%	82%
Home Recovery Information Given[5]	-	-	85%	85%
Hospital Given 9 or 10 on 10 Point Scale[5]	-	-	73%	71%
Meds 'Always' Explained Before Given[5]	-	-	66%	64%
Nurses 'Always' Communicated Well[5]	-	-	80%	79%
Pain 'Always' Well Controlled[5]	-	-	72%	71%
Room and Bathroom 'Always' Clean[5]	-	-	75%	73%
Timely Help 'Always' Received[5]	-	-	69%	68%
Would Definitely Recommend Hospital[5]	-	-	73%	71%
Use of Medical Imaging				
Cardiac Imaging Stress Test before Surgery[5]	-	-	5.3%	5.3%
Combination Abdominal CT Scan[5]	-	-	16.4%	10.5%
Combination Brain/Sinus CT Scan[5]	-	-	2.7%	2.7%
Combination Chest CT Scan[5]	-	-	5.6%	2.7%
Follow-up Mammogram/Ultrasound[5]	-	-	7.9%	8.8%
Lumbar Spine MRI for Low Back Pain[5]	-	-	39.6%	37.2%

Mitchell County Hospital District

997 West I-20
Colorado City, TX 79512
Phone: 325-728-3431
Fax: 325-728-8974
URL: www.mitchellcountyhospital.com
Type: Critical Access Hospitals
Emergency Services: Yes
Ownership: Govt - Hospital Dist/Auth
Beds: 39

Key Personnel:

CEO/President. . . . . Robbie Dewberry
Emergency Room . . . . Cindy Hale, RN
Surgery . . . . Lufkin Moses, DO
Chief of Medical Staff. . . . . Dee A Raach, MD

Measure	Cases	This Hosp.	State Avg.	U.S. Avg.
Blood Clot Prevention and Treatment				
Anticoagulation Overlap Therapy[5]	-	-	93%	93%
ICU Venous Thromboembolism Prophylaxis[5]	-	-	92%	92%
Incidence of Potentially Preventable VTE[5]	-	-	9%	10%
UFH with Dosages/Platelet Monitoring[5]	-	-	96%	97%
Venous Thromboembolism Prophylaxis[5]	-	-	82%	85%
Warfarin Therapy Discharge Instructions[5]	-	-	84%	75%
Chest Pain/Possible Heart Attack Care				
Aspirin Given Within 24 Hours of Arrival[5]	-	-	94%	96%
Fibrinolytic Meds Within 30 Min. of Arrival[5]	-	-	47%	58%

NOTE: Hospital profiles are in alphabetical order by state, then city, then hospital within the city; Rankings exclude hospitals with less than 25 cases except for patient surveys which excludes hospitals with less than 100 cases; (a) 100-299 cases; (1) The number of cases/patients is too few to report; (2) Data submitted were based on a sample of cases/patients; (3) Results are based on a shorter time period than required; (4) Data suppressed by CMS for one or more quarters; (5) Results are not available for this reporting period; (6) Fewer than 100 patients completed the HCAHPS survey; (7) No cases met the criteria for this measure; (8) The lower limit of the confidence interval cannot be calculated if the number of observed infections equals zero; (9) No data are available from the state/territory for this reporting period; (10) The scores shown reflect fewer than 50 completed surveys; (11) There were discrepancies in the data collection process; (12) This measure does not apply to this hospital for this reporting period; (13) Results cannot be calculated for this reporting period; (14) The results for this state are combined with nearby states to protect confidentiality; Please refer to the User's Guide for a full explanation of data.

Measure	Cases	This Hosp.	State Avg.	U.S. Avg.
Average Time to ECG (minutes)[5]	-	-	8	7
Average Time to Transfer (minutes)[5]	-	-	62	60
Children's Asthma Care				
Received Home Management Plan of Care	-	-	93%	88%
Received Reliever Medication	-	-	100%	100%
Received Systemic Corticosteroids	-	-	100%	100%
Emergency Department				
Admittance Decision Time (minutes)	247	70	99	98
Head CT Results Within 45 Min. of Arrival[5]	-	-	54%	57%
Patients Who Left ER Before Being Seen[5]	-	-	3%	2%
Time from ER Arrival to Admit. (minutes)	252	150	270	274
Time from ER Arrival to Discharge (minutes)	392	71	127	134
Time in ER Before Being Evaluated (minutes)	413	16	26	26
Time to Pain Meds for Fractures (minutes)	13	83	57	57
Heart Attack Care				
Aspirin Given at Discharge[5]	-	-	99%	99%
Fibrinolytic Meds Within 30 Min. of Arrival[5]	-	-	49%	54%
PCI Within 90 Minutes of Arrival[5]	-	-	95%	96%
Statin Prescribed at Discharge[5]	-	-	98%	98%
Heart Failure Care				
ACE Inhibitor or ARB for LVSD[1]	-	-	97%	97%
Discharge Instructions Given[1]	-	-	95%	94%
Evaluation of LVS Function[1]	-	-	99%	99%
Medicare Spending				
Medicare Spending per Patient (ratio)	-	-	1.03	0.98
Pneumonia Care				
Appropriate Initial Antibiotic Given	24	92%	95%	95%
Blood Culture Timing	16	94%	98%	98%
Pregnancy and Delivery Care				
Newborn Deliveries Scheduled Early[5]	-	-	7%	6%
Preventive Care				
Immunization for Influenza	164	66%	90%	90%
Immunization for Pneumonia	221	76%	92%	92%
Stroke Care				
Anticoagulation Therapy for Atrial Fibrillation[5]	-	-	96%	95%
Antithrombotic Therapy Timing[5]	-	-	98%	98%
Assessed for Rehabilitation[5]	-	-	98%	97%
Discharged on Antithrombotic Therapy[5]	-	-	99%	99%
Discharged on Statin Medication[5]	-	-	95%	94%
Thrombolytic Therapy Timing[5]	-	-	68%	66%
Venous Thromboembolism Prophylaxis[5]	-	-	94%	94%
Written Stroke Educational Materials Given[5]	-	-	92%	88%
Surgical Care Improvement Project				
Appropriate Beta Blocker Usage[5]	-	-	98%	98%
Appropriate VTP Within 24 Hours[5]	-	-	98%	98%
Controlled Postoperative Blood Glucose[5]	-	-	96%	97%
Perioperative Temperature Management[5]	-	-	100%	100%
Prophylactic Antibiotic Selection[5]	-	-	99%	99%
Prophylactic Antibiotic Selection (Outpatient)[5]	-	-	98%	98%
Prophylactic Antibiotic Stopped[5]	-	-	98%	98%
Prophylactic Antibiotic Timing[5]	-	-	99%	99%
Prophylactic Antibiotic Timing (Outpatient)[5]	-	-	98%	98%
Urinary Catheter Removal[5]	-	-	98%	97%
Survey of Patients' Hospital Experiences				
Area Around Room 'Always' Quiet at Night[5]	-	-	68%	61%
Doctors 'Always' Communicated Well[5]	-	-	83%	82%
Home Recovery Information Given[5]	-	-	85%	85%
Hospital Given 9 or 10 on 10 Point Scale[5]	-	-	73%	71%
Meds 'Always' Explained Before Given[5]	-	-	66%	64%
Nurses 'Always' Communicated Well[5]	-	-	80%	79%
Pain 'Always' Well Controlled[5]	-	-	72%	71%
Room and Bathroom 'Always' Clean[5]	-	-	75%	73%
Timely Help 'Always' Received[5]	-	-	69%	68%
Would Definitely Recommend Hospital[5]	-	-	73%	71%
Use of Medical Imaging				
Cardiac Imaging Stress Test before Surgery[7]	-	-	5.3%	5.3%
Combination Abdominal CT Scan	66	24.2%	16.4%	10.5%
Combination Brain/Sinus CT Scan	68	0.0%	2.7%	2.7%
Combination Chest CT Scan[1]	-	-	5.6%	2.7%
Follow-up Mammogram/Ultrasound[7]	-	-	7.9%	8.8%
Lumbar Spine MRI for Low Back Pain[1]	-	-	39.6%	37.2%

Columbus Community Hospital

110 Shult Dr Phone: 979-732-2371
Columbus, TX 78934 Fax: 979-732-9242
URL: www.columbusch.com
Type: Acute Care Hospitals Emergency Services: Yes
Ownership: Voluntary non-profit - Private Beds: 40

Key Personnel:
Operating Room. . . . . Lynn Butler, RN
Radiology. . . . . Stanley Faldyn
Emergency Room . . . . Jeno Hargrove, RN
Anesthesiology. . . . . Scott Huffman, MD
Quality Assurance . . . . Tracy Lilie, RHIT
Infection Control. . . . . Carol Rooks, RN
CEO . . . . Rob Thomas
Chief of Medical Staff. . . . . David Wilkinson, MD

Measure	Cases	This Hosp.	State Avg.	U.S. Avg.
Blood Clot Prevention and Treatment				
Anticoagulation Overlap Therapy[2]	12	75%	93%	93%
ICU Venous Thromboembolism Prophylaxis[2,7]	-	-	92%	92%
Incidence of Potentially Preventable VTE[1,2]	-	-	9%	10%
UFH with Dosages/Platelet Monitoring[1,2]	-	-	96%	97%
Venous Thromboembolism Prophylaxis[2]	158	37%	82%	85%
Warfarin Therapy Discharge Instructions[1,2]	-	-	84%	75%
Chest Pain/Possible Heart Attack Care				
Aspirin Given Within 24 Hours of Arrival	54	98%	94%	96%
Fibrinolytic Meds Within 30 Min. of Arrival[1]	-	-	47%	58%
Average Time to ECG (minutes)	55	7	8	7
Average Time to Transfer (minutes)[1]	-	-	62	60
Children's Asthma Care				
Received Home Management Plan of Care	-	-	93%	88%
Received Reliever Medication	-	-	100%	100%
Received Systemic Corticosteroids	-	-	100%	100%
Emergency Department				
Admittance Decision Time (minutes)[2]	183	85	99	98
Head CT Results Within 45 Min. of Arrival	13	15%	54%	57%
Patients Who Left ER Before Being Seen	6,152	2%	3%	2%
Time from ER Arrival to Admit. (minutes)[2]	184	261	270	274
Time from ER Arrival to Discharge (minutes)	385	121	127	134
Time in ER Before Being Evaluated (minutes)	422	27	26	26
Time to Pain Meds for Fractures (minutes)	44	45	57	57
Heart Attack Care				
Aspirin Given at Discharge[1]	-	-	99%	99%
Fibrinolytic Meds Within 30 Min. of Arrival[7]	-	-	49%	54%
PCI Within 90 Minutes of Arrival[7]	-	-	95%	96%
Statin Prescribed at Discharge[1]	-	-	98%	98%
Heart Failure Care				
ACE Inhibitor or ARB for LVSD[1]	-	-	97%	97%
Discharge Instructions Given	29	93%	95%	94%
Evaluation of LVS Function	57	98%	99%	99%
Medicare Spending				
Medicare Spending per Patient (ratio)	-	0.99	1.03	0.98
Pneumonia Care				
Appropriate Initial Antibiotic Given	29	90%	95%	95%
Blood Culture Timing	35	100%	98%	98%
Pregnancy and Delivery Care				
Newborn Deliveries Scheduled Early	25	4%	7%	6%
Preventive Care				
Immunization for Influenza[2]	291	97%	90%	90%
Immunization for Pneumonia[2]	338	98%	92%	92%
Stroke Care				
Anticoagulation Therapy for Atrial Fibrillation[3,7]	-	-	96%	95%
Antithrombotic Therapy Timing[1,3]	-	-	98%	98%
Assessed for Rehabilitation[1,3]	-	-	98%	97%
Discharged on Antithrombotic Therapy[1,3]	-	-	99%	99%
Discharged on Statin Medication[1,3]	-	-	95%	94%
Thrombolytic Therapy Timing[1,3]	-	-	68%	66%
Venous Thromboembolism Prophylaxis[1,3]	-	-	94%	94%
Written Stroke Educational Materials Given[1,3]	-	-	92%	88%
Surgical Care Improvement Project				
Appropriate Beta Blocker Usage	14	100%	98%	98%
Appropriate VTP Within 24 Hours	38	100%	98%	98%
Controlled Postoperative Blood Glucose[7]	-	-	96%	97%
Perioperative Temperature Management	44	100%	100%	100%
Prophylactic Antibiotic Selection	17	100%	99%	99%
Prophylactic Antibiotic Selection (Outpatient)	33	97%	98%	98%
Prophylactic Antibiotic Stopped	17	88%	98%	98%
Prophylactic Antibiotic Timing	17	100%	99%	99%
Prophylactic Antibiotic Timing (Outpatient)	33	100%	98%	98%
Urinary Catheter Removal	31	97%	98%	97%
Survey of Patients' Hospital Experiences				
Area Around Room 'Always' Quiet at Night	(a)	66%	68%	61%
Doctors 'Always' Communicated Well	(a)	86%	83%	82%
Home Recovery Information Given	(a)	80%	85%	85%
Hospital Given 9 or 10 on 10 Point Scale	(a)	70%	73%	71%
Meds 'Always' Explained Before Given	(a)	61%	66%	64%
Nurses 'Always' Communicated Well	(a)	80%	80%	79%
Pain 'Always' Well Controlled	(a)	71%	72%	71%
Room and Bathroom 'Always' Clean	(a)	75%	75%	73%
Timely Help 'Always' Received	(a)	64%	69%	68%
Would Definitely Recommend Hospital	(a)	76%	73%	71%
Use of Medical Imaging				
Cardiac Imaging Stress Test before Surgery[1]	-	-	5.3%	5.3%
Combination Abdominal CT Scan	290	55.5%	16.4%	10.5%
Combination Brain/Sinus CT Scan	242	0.4%	2.7%	2.7%
Combination Chest CT Scan	159	17.0%	5.6%	2.7%
Follow-up Mammogram/Ultrasound	374	4.3%	7.9%	8.8%
Lumbar Spine MRI for Low Back Pain	38	42.1%	39.6%	37.2%

Hunt Regional Community Hospital

2900 Sterling Hart Drive Phone: 903-408-1881
Commerce, TX 75428
URL: www.hmhd.org
Type: Critical Access Hospitals Emergency Services: Yes
Ownership: Govt - Hospital Dist/Auth

Key Personnel:
CEO . . . . Richard Carter

Measure	Cases	This Hosp.	State Avg.	U.S. Avg.
Blood Clot Prevention and Treatment				
Anticoagulation Overlap Therapy[5]	-	-	93%	93%
ICU Venous Thromboembolism Prophylaxis[5]	-	-	92%	92%
Incidence of Potentially Preventable VTE[5]	-	-	9%	10%
UFH with Dosages/Platelet Monitoring[5]	-	-	96%	97%
Venous Thromboembolism Prophylaxis[5]	-	-	82%	85%
Warfarin Therapy Discharge Instructions[5]	-	-	84%	75%
Chest Pain/Possible Heart Attack Care				
Aspirin Given Within 24 Hours of Arrival	-	-	94%	96%
Fibrinolytic Meds Within 30 Min. of Arrival	-	-	47%	58%
Average Time to ECG (minutes)	-	-	8	7
Average Time to Transfer (minutes)	-	-	62	60
Children's Asthma Care				
Received Home Management Plan of Care	-	-	93%	88%
Received Reliever Medication	-	-	100%	100%
Received Systemic Corticosteroids	-	-	100%	100%
Emergency Department				
Admittance Decision Time (minutes)[5]	-	-	99	98
Head CT Results Within 45 Min. of Arrival	-	-	54%	57%
Patients Who Left ER Before Being Seen	-	-	3%	2%
Time from ER Arrival to Admit. (minutes)[5]	-	-	270	274
Time from ER Arrival to Discharge (minutes)	-	-	127	134
Time in ER Before Being Evaluated (minutes)	-	-	26	26
Time to Pain Meds for Fractures (minutes)	-	-	57	57
Heart Attack Care				
Aspirin Given at Discharge[5]	-	-	99%	99%
Fibrinolytic Meds Within 30 Min. of Arrival[5]	-	-	49%	54%
PCI Within 90 Minutes of Arrival[5]	-	-	95%	96%
Statin Prescribed at Discharge[5]	-	-	98%	98%
Heart Failure Care				
ACE Inhibitor or ARB for LVSD[5]	-	-	97%	97%
Discharge Instructions Given[5]	-	-	95%	94%
Evaluation of LVS Function[5]	-	-	99%	99%
Medicare Spending				
Medicare Spending per Patient (ratio)	-	-	1.03	0.98
Pneumonia Care				
Appropriate Initial Antibiotic Given[3]	12	92%	95%	95%
Blood Culture Timing[3]	15	100%	98%	98%
Pregnancy and Delivery Care				
Newborn Deliveries Scheduled Early[5]	-	-	7%	6%

NOTE: Hospital profiles are in alphabetical order by state, then city, then hospital within the city; Rankings exclude hospitals with less than 25 cases except for patient surveys which excludes hospitals with less than 100 cases; (a) 100-299 cases; (1) The number of cases/patients is too few to report; (2) Data submitted were based on a sample of cases/patients; (3) Results are based on a shorter time period than required; (4) Data suppressed by CMS for one or more quarters; (5) Results are not available for this reporting period; (6) Fewer than 100 patients completed the HCAHPS survey; (7) No cases met the criteria for this measure; (8) The lower limit of the confidence interval cannot be calculated if the number of observed infections equals zero; (9) No data are available from the state/territory for this reporting period; (10) The scores shown reflect fewer than 50 completed surveys; (11) There were discrepancies in the data collection process; (12) This measure does not apply to this hospital for this reporting period; (13) Results cannot be calculated for this reporting period; (14) The results for this state are combined with nearby states to protect confidentiality; Please refer to the User's Guide for a full explanation of data.

Measure	Cases	This Hosp.	State Avg.	U.S. Avg.
Preventive Care				
Immunization for Influenza[5]	-	-	90%	90%
Immunization for Pneumonia[5]	-	-	92%	92%
Stroke Care				
Anticoagulation Therapy for Atrial Fibrillation[5]	-	-	96%	95%
Antithrombotic Therapy Timing[5]	-	-	98%	98%
Assessed for Rehabilitation[5]	-	-	98%	97%
Discharged on Antithrombotic Therapy[5]	-	-	99%	99%
Discharged on Statin Medication[5]	-	-	95%	94%
Thrombolytic Therapy Timing[5]	-	-	68%	66%
Venous Thromboembolism Prophylaxis[5]	-	-	94%	94%
Written Stroke Educational Materials Given[5]	-	-	92%	88%
Surgical Care Improvement Project				
Appropriate Beta Blocker Usage[5]	-	-	98%	98%
Appropriate VTP Within 24 Hours[5]	-	-	98%	98%
Controlled Postoperative Blood Glucose[5]	-	-	96%	97%
Perioperative Temperature Management[5]	-	-	100%	100%
Prophylactic Antibiotic Selection[5]	-	-	99%	99%
Prophylactic Antibiotic Selection (Outpatient)	-	-	98%	98%
Prophylactic Antibiotic Stopped[5]	-	-	98%	98%
Prophylactic Antibiotic Timing[5]	-	-	99%	99%
Prophylactic Antibiotic Timing (Outpatient)	-	-	98%	98%
Urinary Catheter Removal[5]	-	-	98%	97%
Survey of Patients' Hospital Experiences				
Area Around Room 'Always' Quiet at Night[5]	-	-	68%	61%
Doctors 'Always' Communicated Well[5]	-	-	83%	82%
Home Recovery Information Given[5]	-	-	85%	85%
Hospital Given 9 or 10 on 10 Point Scale[5]	-	-	73%	71%
Meds 'Always' Explained Before Given[5]	-	-	66%	64%
Nurses 'Always' Communicated Well[5]	-	-	80%	79%
Pain 'Always' Well Controlled[5]	-	-	72%	71%
Room and Bathroom 'Always' Clean[5]	-	-	75%	73%
Timely Help 'Always' Received[5]	-	-	69%	68%
Would Definitely Recommend Hospital[5]	-	-	73%	71%
Use of Medical Imaging				
Cardiac Imaging Stress Test before Surgery	-	-	5.3%	5.3%
Combination Abdominal CT Scan	-	-	16.4%	10.5%
Combination Brain/Sinus CT Scan	-	-	2.7%	2.7%
Combination Chest CT Scan	-	-	5.6%	2.7%
Follow-up Mammogram/Ultrasound	-	-	7.9%	8.8%
Lumbar Spine MRI for Low Back Pain	-	-	39.6%	37.2%

Conroe Regional Medical Center

504 Medical Center Blvd
Conroe, TX 77304
Phone: 936-539-1111
Fax: 936-539-7059
URL: www.conroeregional.com
Type: Acute Care Hospitals
Emergency Services: Yes
Ownership: Proprietary
Beds: 342

Key Personnel:

Quality Assurance . . . . Linda Chapman
CEO/President. . . . . Matt Davis, FACHE
Chief of Medical Staff. . . . . Rochelle Evans, DO
Operating Room. . . . . Judith Gerst, RN
Pediatric Ambulatory Care . . . . . . Jayne Schulte
Pediatric In-Patient Care . . . . . . Jayne Schulte
Intensive Care Unit. . . . . Sharla Shumaker, RN
Infection Control. . . . . Elaine Whaley, RN

Measure	Cases	This Hosp.	State Avg.	U.S. Avg.
Blood Clot Prevention and Treatment				
Anticoagulation Overlap Therapy[2]	106	100%	93%	93%
ICU Venous Thromboembolism Prophylaxis[2]	130	97%	92%	92%
Incidence of Potentially Preventable VTE[2]	11	0%	9%	10%
UFH with Dosages/Platelet Monitoring[2]	38	100%	96%	97%
Venous Thromboembolism Prophylaxis[2]	364	90%	82%	85%
Warfarin Therapy Discharge Instructions[2]	70	93%	84%	75%
Chest Pain/Possible Heart Attack Care				
Aspirin Given Within 24 Hours of Arrival[1,3]	-	-	94%	96%
Fibrinolytic Meds Within 30 Min. of Arrival[5]	-	-	47%	58%
Average Time to ECG (minutes)[1,3]	-	-	8	7
Average Time to Transfer (minutes)[5]	-	-	62	60
Children's Asthma Care				
Received Home Management Plan of Care	-	-	93%	88%
Received Reliever Medication	-	-	100%	100%
Received Systemic Corticosteroids	-	-	100%	100%
Emergency Department				
Admittance Decision Time (minutes)[2]	659	153	99	98
Head CT Results Within 45 Min. of Arrival[1]	-	-	54%	57%
Patients Who Left ER Before Being Seen	50,349	1%	3%	2%
Time from ER Arrival to Admit. (minutes)[2]	659	219	270	274
Time from ER Arrival to Discharge (minutes)	447	138	127	134
Time in ER Before Being Evaluated (minutes)	523	21	26	26
Time to Pain Meds for Fractures (minutes)	206	46	57	57
Heart Attack Care				
Aspirin Given at Discharge	332	100%	99%	99%
Fibrinolytic Meds Within 30 Min. of Arrival[7]	-	-	49%	54%
PCI Within 90 Minutes of Arrival	46	100%	95%	96%
Statin Prescribed at Discharge	311	100%	98%	98%
Heart Failure Care				
ACE Inhibitor or ARB for LVSD	137	100%	97%	97%
Discharge Instructions Given	361	99%	95%	94%
Evaluation of LVS Function	451	100%	99%	99%
Medicare Spending				
Medicare Spending per Patient (ratio)	-	1.07	1.03	0.98
Pneumonia Care				
Appropriate Initial Antibiotic Given	140	100%	95%	95%
Blood Culture Timing	222	100%	98%	98%
Pregnancy and Delivery Care				
Newborn Deliveries Scheduled Early[2]	21	0%	7%	6%
Preventive Care				
Immunization for Influenza[2]	625	100%	90%	90%
Immunization for Pneumonia[2]	844	99%	92%	92%
Stroke Care				
Anticoagulation Therapy for Atrial Fibrillation	15	100%	96%	95%
Antithrombotic Therapy Timing	136	99%	98%	98%
Assessed for Rehabilitation	183	100%	98%	97%
Discharged on Antithrombotic Therapy	156	100%	99%	99%
Discharged on Statin Medication	117	100%	95%	94%
Thrombolytic Therapy Timing	13	92%	68%	66%
Venous Thromboembolism Prophylaxis	177	99%	94%	94%
Written Stroke Educational Materials Given	106	97%	92%	88%
Surgical Care Improvement Project				
Appropriate Beta Blocker Usage[2]	199	100%	98%	98%
Appropriate VTP Within 24 Hours[2]	358	100%	98%	98%
Controlled Postoperative Blood Glucose[2]	101	99%	96%	97%
Perioperative Temperature Management[2]	480	100%	100%	100%
Prophylactic Antibiotic Selection[2]	328	100%	99%	99%
Prophylactic Antibiotic Selection (Outpatient)	263	98%	98%	98%
Prophylactic Antibiotic Stopped[2]	304	100%	98%	98%
Prophylactic Antibiotic Timing[2]	328	100%	99%	99%
Prophylactic Antibiotic Timing (Outpatient)	265	99%	98%	98%
Urinary Catheter Removal[2]	293	100%	98%	97%
Survey of Patients' Hospital Experiences				
Area Around Room 'Always' Quiet at Night	300+	61%	68%	61%
Doctors 'Always' Communicated Well	300+	77%	83%	82%
Home Recovery Information Given	300+	84%	85%	85%
Hospital Given 9 or 10 on 10 Point Scale	300+	66%	73%	71%
Meds 'Always' Explained Before Given	300+	64%	66%	64%
Nurses 'Always' Communicated Well	300+	74%	80%	79%
Pain 'Always' Well Controlled	300+	69%	72%	71%
Room and Bathroom 'Always' Clean	300+	66%	75%	73%
Timely Help 'Always' Received	300+	62%	69%	68%
Would Definitely Recommend Hospital	300+	64%	73%	71%
Use of Medical Imaging				
Cardiac Imaging Stress Test before Surgery	789	4.8%	5.3%	5.3%
Combination Abdominal CT Scan	675	17.8%	16.4%	10.5%
Combination Brain/Sinus CT Scan	789	3.5%	2.7%	2.7%
Combination Chest CT Scan	317	9.5%	5.6%	2.7%
Follow-up Mammogram/Ultrasound	1,762	8.5%	7.9%	8.8%
Lumbar Spine MRI for Low Back Pain	81	42.0%	39.6%	37.2%

Christus Spohn Hospital Corpus Christi

600 Elizabeth Street
Corpus Christi, TX 78404
Phone: 361-902-4103
Fax: 361-881-1427
E-mail: spohn@christushealth.org
URL: www.christusspohn.org
Type: Acute Care Hospitals
Emergency Services: Yes
Ownership: Voluntary non-profit - Church
Beds: 397

Key Personnel:

Intensive Care Unit. . . . . Brian Grant, RN
CEO/President. . . . . Bruce Holstein
Emergency Room . . . . Melanie Kasper
Operating Room. . . . . Melanie Kasper
Infection Control. . . . . Leona Kocinek
Chief of Medical Staff. . . . . John McKeever
Radiology. . . . . Dale Obermueller

Measure	Cases	This Hosp.	State Avg.	U.S. Avg.
Blood Clot Prevention and Treatment				
Anticoagulation Overlap Therapy[2]	147	73%	93%	93%
ICU Venous Thromboembolism Prophylaxis[2]	94	80%	92%	92%
Incidence of Potentially Preventable VTE[2]	61	25%	9%	10%
UFH with Dosages/Platelet Monitoring[2]	33	100%	96%	97%
Venous Thromboembolism Prophylaxis[2]	334	75%	82%	85%
Warfarin Therapy Discharge Instructions[2]	98	80%	84%	75%
Chest Pain/Possible Heart Attack Care				
Aspirin Given Within 24 Hours of Arrival[1]	-	-	94%	96%
Fibrinolytic Meds Within 30 Min. of Arrival[3,7]	-	-	47%	58%
Average Time to ECG (minutes)[1]	-	-	8	7
Average Time to Transfer (minutes)[1,3]	-	-	62	60
Children's Asthma Care				
Received Home Management Plan of Care	-	-	93%	88%
Received Reliever Medication	-	-	100%	100%
Received Systemic Corticosteroids	-	-	100%	100%
Emergency Department				
Admittance Decision Time (minutes)[2]	876	214	99	98
Head CT Results Within 45 Min. of Arrival	11	55%	54%	57%
Patients Who Left ER Before Being Seen	>100k	5%	3%	2%
Time from ER Arrival to Admit. (minutes)[2]	879	417	270	274
Time from ER Arrival to Discharge (minutes)	379	186	127	134
Time in ER Before Being Evaluated (minutes)	405	58	26	26
Time to Pain Meds for Fractures (minutes)	154	86	57	57
Heart Attack Care				
Aspirin Given at Discharge	529	98%	99%	99%
Fibrinolytic Meds Within 30 Min. of Arrival[1]	-	-	49%	54%
PCI Within 90 Minutes of Arrival	53	94%	95%	96%
Statin Prescribed at Discharge	519	95%	98%	98%
Heart Failure Care				
ACE Inhibitor or ARB for LVSD	307	92%	97%	97%
Discharge Instructions Given	794	99%	95%	94%
Evaluation of LVS Function	937	97%	99%	99%
Medicare Spending				
Medicare Spending per Patient (ratio)	-	1.02	1.03	0.98
Pneumonia Care				
Appropriate Initial Antibiotic Given	347	89%	95%	95%
Blood Culture Timing	814	92%	98%	98%
Pregnancy and Delivery Care				
Newborn Deliveries Scheduled Early[2]	16	6%	7%	6%
Preventive Care				
Immunization for Influenza[2]	601	91%	90%	90%
Immunization for Pneumonia[2]	828	86%	92%	92%
Stroke Care				
Anticoagulation Therapy for Atrial Fibrillation[2]	51	88%	96%	95%
Antithrombotic Therapy Timing[2]	303	98%	98%	98%
Assessed for Rehabilitation[2]	446	96%	98%	97%
Discharged on Antithrombotic Therapy[2]	356	98%	99%	99%
Discharged on Statin Medication[2]	284	87%	95%	94%
Thrombolytic Therapy Timing[2]	41	76%	68%	66%
Venous Thromboembolism Prophylaxis[2]	459	90%	94%	94%
Written Stroke Educational Materials Given[2]	227	91%	92%	88%
Surgical Care Improvement Project				
Appropriate Beta Blocker Usage	516	95%	98%	98%
Appropriate VTP Within 24 Hours	1,316	91%	98%	98%
Controlled Postoperative Blood Glucose	360	89%	96%	97%
Perioperative Temperature Management	1,632	100%	100%	100%
Prophylactic Antibiotic Selection	1,118	98%	99%	99%

NOTE: Hospital profiles are in alphabetical order by state, then city, then hospital within the city; Rankings exclude hospitals with less than 25 cases except for patient surveys which excludes hospitals with less than 100 cases; (a) 100-299 cases; (1) The number of cases/patients is too few to report; (2) Data submitted were based on a sample of cases/patients; (3) Results are based on a shorter time period than required; (4) Data suppressed by CMS for one or more quarters; (5) Results are not available for this reporting period; (6) Fewer than 100 patients completed the HCAHPS survey; (7) No cases met the criteria for this measure; (8) The lower limit of the confidence interval cannot be calculated if the number of observed infections equals zero; (9) No data are available from the state/territory for this reporting period; (10) The scores shown reflect fewer than 50 completed surveys; (11) There were discrepancies in the data collection process; (12) This measure does not apply to this hospital for this reporting period; (13) Results cannot be calculated for this reporting period; (14) The results for this state are combined with nearby states to protect confidentiality; Please refer to the User's Guide for a full explanation of data.

Measure	Cases	This Hosp.	State Avg.	U.S. Avg.
Prophylactic Antibiotic Selection (Outpatient)	532	95%	98%	98%
Prophylactic Antibiotic Stopped	1,078	96%	98%	98%
Prophylactic Antibiotic Timing	1,121	97%	99%	99%
Prophylactic Antibiotic Timing (Outpatient)	546	94%	98%	98%
Urinary Catheter Removal	740	90%	98%	97%
Survey of Patients' Hospital Experiences				
Area Around Room 'Always' Quiet at Night	300+	60%	68%	61%
Doctors 'Always' Communicated Well	300+	78%	83%	82%
Home Recovery Information Given	300+	82%	85%	85%
Hospital Given 9 or 10 on 10 Point Scale	300+	69%	73%	71%
Meds 'Always' Explained Before Given	300+	62%	66%	64%
Nurses 'Always' Communicated Well	300+	76%	80%	79%
Pain 'Always' Well Controlled	300+	70%	72%	71%
Room and Bathroom 'Always' Clean	300+	69%	75%	73%
Timely Help 'Always' Received	300+	60%	69%	68%
Would Definitely Recommend Hospital	300+	72%	73%	71%
Use of Medical Imaging				
Cardiac Imaging Stress Test before Surgery	59	0.0%	5.3%	5.3%
Combination Abdominal CT Scan	553	40.3%	16.4%	10.5%
Combination Brain/Sinus CT Scan	1,025	5.1%	2.7%	2.7%
Combination Chest CT Scan	178	0.6%	5.6%	2.7%
Follow-up Mammogram/Ultrasound	398	13.1%	7.9%	8.8%
Lumbar Spine MRI for Low Back Pain[1]	-	-	39.6%	37.2%

The Corpus Christi Medical Center

7101 S Padre Island Dr
Corpus Christi, TX 78412
Phone: 361-761-1501
URL: www.ccmedicalcenter.com
Type: Acute Care Hospitals
Emergency Services: Yes
Ownership: Proprietary

Measure	Cases	This Hosp.	State Avg.	U.S. Avg.
Blood Clot Prevention and Treatment				
Anticoagulation Overlap Therapy[2]	64	98%	93%	93%
ICU Venous Thromboembolism Prophylaxis[2]	115	100%	92%	92%
Incidence of Potentially Preventable VTE[1,2]	-	-	9%	10%
UFH with Dosages/Platelet Monitoring[2]	17	100%	96%	97%
Venous Thromboembolism Prophylaxis[2]	326	99%	82%	85%
Warfarin Therapy Discharge Instructions[2]	42	100%	84%	75%
Chest Pain/Possible Heart Attack Care				
Aspirin Given Within 24 Hours of Arrival[1]	-	-	94%	96%
Fibrinolytic Meds Within 30 Min. of Arrival[7]	-	-	47%	58%
Average Time to ECG (minutes)[1]	-	-	8	7
Average Time to Transfer (minutes)[7]	-	-	62	60
Children's Asthma Care				
Received Home Management Plan of Care	-	-	93%	88%
Received Reliever Medication	-	-	100%	100%
Received Systemic Corticosteroids	-	-	100%	100%
Emergency Department				
Admittance Decision Time (minutes)[2]	589	87	99	98
Head CT Results Within 45 Min. of Arrival	30	90%	54%	57%
Patients Who Left ER Before Being Seen	71,892	1%	3%	2%
Time from ER Arrival to Admit. (minutes)[2]	589	266	270	274
Time from ER Arrival to Discharge (minutes)	517	143	127	134
Time in ER Before Being Evaluated (minutes)	545	16	26	26
Time to Pain Meds for Fractures (minutes)	198	48	57	57
Heart Attack Care				
Aspirin Given at Discharge	257	100%	99%	99%
Fibrinolytic Meds Within 30 Min. of Arrival[7]	-	-	49%	54%
PCI Within 90 Minutes of Arrival	30	100%	95%	96%
Statin Prescribed at Discharge	248	100%	98%	98%
Heart Failure Care				
ACE Inhibitor or ARB for LVSD	109	100%	97%	97%
Discharge Instructions Given	372	99%	95%	94%
Evaluation of LVS Function	434	100%	99%	99%
Medicare Spending				
Medicare Spending per Patient (ratio)	-	0.96	1.03	0.98
Pneumonia Care				
Appropriate Initial Antibiotic Given	139	100%	95%	95%
Blood Culture Timing	294	100%	98%	98%
Pregnancy and Delivery Care				
Newborn Deliveries Scheduled Early[2]	60	3%	7%	6%
Preventive Care				
Immunization for Influenza[2]	549	100%	90%	90%
Immunization for Pneumonia[2]	590	100%	92%	92%
Stroke Care				
Anticoagulation Therapy for Atrial Fibrillation[1,2]	-	-	96%	95%
Antithrombotic Therapy Timing[2]	65	100%	98%	98%
Assessed for Rehabilitation[2]	83	100%	98%	97%
Discharged on Antithrombotic Therapy[2]	68	99%	99%	99%
Discharged on Statin Medication[2]	52	100%	95%	94%
Thrombolytic Therapy Timing[1,2]	-	-	68%	66%
Venous Thromboembolism Prophylaxis[2]	79	100%	94%	94%
Written Stroke Educational Materials Given[2]	53	96%	92%	88%
Surgical Care Improvement Project				
Appropriate Beta Blocker Usage[2]	223	99%	98%	98%
Appropriate VTP Within 24 Hours[2]	435	100%	98%	98%
Controlled Postoperative Blood Glucose[2]	122	96%	96%	97%
Perioperative Temperature Management[2]	657	100%	100%	100%
Prophylactic Antibiotic Selection[2]	428	100%	99%	99%
Prophylactic Antibiotic Selection (Outpatient)	536	99%	98%	98%
Prophylactic Antibiotic Stopped[2]	391	97%	98%	98%
Prophylactic Antibiotic Timing[2]	428	100%	99%	99%
Prophylactic Antibiotic Timing (Outpatient)	536	100%	98%	98%
Urinary Catheter Removal[2]	426	100%	98%	97%
Survey of Patients' Hospital Experiences				
Area Around Room 'Always' Quiet at Night	300+	62%	68%	61%
Doctors 'Always' Communicated Well	300+	82%	83%	82%
Home Recovery Information Given	300+	86%	85%	85%
Hospital Given 9 or 10 on 10 Point Scale	300+	71%	73%	71%
Meds 'Always' Explained Before Given	300+	61%	66%	64%
Nurses 'Always' Communicated Well	300+	76%	80%	79%
Pain 'Always' Well Controlled	300+	71%	72%	71%
Room and Bathroom 'Always' Clean	300+	69%	75%	73%
Timely Help 'Always' Received	300+	62%	69%	68%
Would Definitely Recommend Hospital	300+	73%	73%	71%
Use of Medical Imaging				
Cardiac Imaging Stress Test before Surgery[1]	-	-	5.3%	5.3%
Combination Abdominal CT Scan	502	3.4%	16.4%	10.5%
Combination Brain/Sinus CT Scan	1,002	3.0%	2.7%	2.7%
Combination Chest CT Scan	66	6.1%	5.6%	2.7%
Follow-up Mammogram/Ultrasound	504	5.4%	7.9%	8.8%
Lumbar Spine MRI for Low Back Pain[1]	-	-	39.6%	37.2%

Driscoll Childrens Hospital

3533 S Alameda Box 6530
Corpus Christi, TX 78411
Phone: 512-850-5000
Fax: 361-694-5317
URL: www.driscollchildrens.org
Type: Childrens
Emergency Services: Yes
Ownership: Voluntary non-profit - Other
Beds: 188

Key Personnel:
Chief of Medical Staff. . . . . Fae Bryan
Anesthesiology. . . . . Guy Giesecke
Quality Assurance . . . . Judy Hayden
Emergency Room . . . . Lois Koester
CEO/President. . . . . Rick W Merrill

Measure	Cases	This Hosp.	State Avg.	U.S. Avg.
Blood Clot Prevention and Treatment				
Anticoagulation Overlap Therapy[5]	-	-	93%	93%
ICU Venous Thromboembolism Prophylaxis[5]	-	-	92%	92%
Incidence of Potentially Preventable VTE[5]	-	-	9%	10%
UFH with Dosages/Platelet Monitoring[5]	-	-	96%	97%
Venous Thromboembolism Prophylaxis[5]	-	-	82%	85%
Warfarin Therapy Discharge Instructions[5]	-	-	84%	75%
Chest Pain/Possible Heart Attack Care				
Aspirin Given Within 24 Hours of Arrival	-	-	94%	96%
Fibrinolytic Meds Within 30 Min. of Arrival	-	-	47%	58%
Average Time to ECG (minutes)	-	-	8	7
Average Time to Transfer (minutes)	-	-	62	60
Children's Asthma Care				
Received Home Management Plan of Care	141	81%	93%	88%
Received Reliever Medication	141	100%	100%	100%
Received Systemic Corticosteroids	141	99%	100%	100%
Emergency Department				
Admittance Decision Time (minutes)[5]	-	-	99	98
Head CT Results Within 45 Min. of Arrival	-	-	54%	57%
Patients Who Left ER Before Being Seen	-	-	3%	2%
Time from ER Arrival to Admit. (minutes)[5]	-	-	270	274
Time from ER Arrival to Discharge (minutes)	-	-	127	134
Time in ER Before Being Evaluated (minutes)	-	-	26	26
Time to Pain Meds for Fractures (minutes)	-	-	57	57
Heart Attack Care				
Aspirin Given at Discharge[5]	-	-	99%	99%
Fibrinolytic Meds Within 30 Min. of Arrival[5]	-	-	49%	54%
PCI Within 90 Minutes of Arrival[5]	-	-	95%	96%
Statin Prescribed at Discharge[5]	-	-	98%	98%
Heart Failure Care				
ACE Inhibitor or ARB for LVSD[5]	-	-	97%	97%
Discharge Instructions Given[5]	-	-	95%	94%
Evaluation of LVS Function[5]	-	-	99%	99%
Medicare Spending				
Medicare Spending per Patient (ratio)	-	-	1.03	0.98
Pneumonia Care				
Appropriate Initial Antibiotic Given[5]	-	-	95%	95%
Blood Culture Timing[5]	-	-	98%	98%
Pregnancy and Delivery Care				
Newborn Deliveries Scheduled Early[5]	-	-	7%	6%
Preventive Care				
Immunization for Influenza[5]	-	-	90%	90%
Immunization for Pneumonia[5]	-	-	92%	92%
Stroke Care				
Anticoagulation Therapy for Atrial Fibrillation[5]	-	-	96%	95%
Antithrombotic Therapy Timing[5]	-	-	98%	98%
Assessed for Rehabilitation[5]	-	-	98%	97%
Discharged on Antithrombotic Therapy[5]	-	-	99%	99%
Discharged on Statin Medication[5]	-	-	95%	94%
Thrombolytic Therapy Timing[5]	-	-	68%	66%
Venous Thromboembolism Prophylaxis[5]	-	-	94%	94%
Written Stroke Educational Materials Given[5]	-	-	92%	88%
Surgical Care Improvement Project				
Appropriate Beta Blocker Usage[5]	-	-	98%	98%
Appropriate VTP Within 24 Hours[5]	-	-	98%	98%
Controlled Postoperative Blood Glucose[5]	-	-	96%	97%
Perioperative Temperature Management[5]	-	-	100%	100%
Prophylactic Antibiotic Selection[5]	-	-	99%	99%
Prophylactic Antibiotic Selection (Outpatient)	-	-	98%	98%
Prophylactic Antibiotic Stopped[5]	-	-	98%	98%
Prophylactic Antibiotic Timing[5]	-	-	99%	99%
Prophylactic Antibiotic Timing (Outpatient)	-	-	98%	98%
Urinary Catheter Removal[5]	-	-	98%	97%
Survey of Patients' Hospital Experiences				
Area Around Room 'Always' Quiet at Night[5]	-	-	68%	61%
Doctors 'Always' Communicated Well[5]	-	-	83%	82%
Home Recovery Information Given[5]	-	-	85%	85%
Hospital Given 9 or 10 on 10 Point Scale[5]	-	-	73%	71%
Meds 'Always' Explained Before Given[5]	-	-	66%	64%
Nurses 'Always' Communicated Well[5]	-	-	80%	79%
Pain 'Always' Well Controlled[5]	-	-	72%	71%
Room and Bathroom 'Always' Clean[5]	-	-	75%	73%
Timely Help 'Always' Received[5]	-	-	69%	68%
Would Definitely Recommend Hospital[5]	-	-	73%	71%
Use of Medical Imaging				
Cardiac Imaging Stress Test before Surgery	-	-	5.3%	5.3%
Combination Abdominal CT Scan	-	-	16.4%	10.5%
Combination Brain/Sinus CT Scan	-	-	2.7%	2.7%
Combination Chest CT Scan	-	-	5.6%	2.7%
Follow-up Mammogram/Ultrasound	-	-	7.9%	8.8%
Lumbar Spine MRI for Low Back Pain	-	-	39.6%	37.2%

South Texas Surgical Hospital

6130 Parkway Drive
Corpus Christi, TX 78414
Phone: 361-993-2000
URL: www.nshinc.com
Type: Acute Care Hospitals
Emergency Services: Yes
Ownership: Proprietary

Measure	Cases	This Hosp.	State Avg.	U.S. Avg.
Blood Clot Prevention and Treatment				
Anticoagulation Overlap Therapy[7]	-	-	93%	93%

NOTE: Hospital profiles are in alphabetical order by state, then city, then hospital within the city; Rankings exclude hospitals with less than 25 cases except for patient surveys which excludes hospitals with less than 100 cases; (a) 100-299 cases; (1) The number of cases/patients is too few to report; (2) Data submitted were based on a sample of cases/patients; (3) Results are based on a shorter time period than required; (4) Data suppressed by CMS for one or more quarters; (5) Results are not available for this reporting period; (6) Fewer than 100 patients completed the HCAHPS survey; (7) No cases met the criteria for this measure; (8) The lower limit of the confidence interval cannot be calculated if the number of observed infections equals zero; (9) No data are available from the state/territory for this reporting period; (10) The scores shown reflect fewer than 50 completed surveys; (11) There were discrepancies in the data collection process; (12) This measure does not apply to this hospital for this reporting period; (13) Results cannot be calculated for this reporting period; (14) The results for this state are combined with nearby states to protect confidentiality; Please refer to the User's Guide for a full explanation of data.

ICU Venous Thromboembolism Prophylaxis[7]	-	-	92%	92%
Incidence of Potentially Preventable VTE[7]	-	-	9%	10%
UFH with Dosages/Platelet Monitoring[7]	-	-	96%	97%
Venous Thromboembolism Prophylaxis	262	90%	82%	85%
Warfarin Therapy Discharge Instructions[7]	-	-	84%	75%
Chest Pain/Possible Heart Attack Care				
Aspirin Given Within 24 Hours of Arrival[5]	-	-	94%	96%
Fibrinolytic Meds Within 30 Min. of Arrival[5]	-	-	47%	58%
Average Time to ECG (minutes)[5]	-	-	8	7
Average Time to Transfer (minutes)[5]	-	-	62	60
Children's Asthma Care				
Received Home Management Plan of Care	-	-	93%	88%
Received Reliever Medication	-	-	100%	100%
Received Systemic Corticosteroids	-	-	100%	100%
Emergency Department				
Admittance Decision Time (minutes)[2]	24	70	99	98
Head CT Results Within 45 Min. of Arrival[5]	-	-	54%	57%
Patients Who Left ER Before Being Seen	1,090	3%	3%	2%
Time from ER Arrival to Admit. (minutes)[2]	24	195	270	274
Time from ER Arrival to Discharge (minutes)	448	95	127	134
Time in ER Before Being Evaluated (minutes)	438	20	26	26
Time to Pain Meds for Fractures (minutes)[5]	-	-	57	57
Heart Attack Care				
Aspirin Given at Discharge[5]	-	-	99%	99%
Fibrinolytic Meds Within 30 Min. of Arrival[5]	-	-	49%	54%
PCI Within 90 Minutes of Arrival[5]	-	-	95%	96%
Statin Prescribed at Discharge[5]	-	-	98%	98%
Heart Failure Care				
ACE Inhibitor or ARB for LVSD[5]	-	-	97%	97%
Discharge Instructions Given[5]	-	-	95%	94%
Evaluation of LVS Function[5]	-	-	99%	99%
Medicare Spending				
Medicare Spending per Patient (ratio)	-	1.01	1.03	0.98
Pneumonia Care				
Appropriate Initial Antibiotic Given[5]	-	-	95%	95%
Blood Culture Timing[5]	-	-	98%	98%
Pregnancy and Delivery Care				
Newborn Deliveries Scheduled Early[7]	-	-	7%	6%
Preventive Care				
Immunization for Influenza[2]	367	83%	90%	90%
Immunization for Pneumonia[2]	601	86%	92%	92%
Stroke Care				
Anticoagulation Therapy for Atrial Fibrillation[5]	-	-	96%	95%
Antithrombotic Therapy Timing[5]	-	-	98%	98%
Assessed for Rehabilitation[5]	-	-	98%	97%
Discharged on Antithrombotic Therapy[5]	-	-	99%	99%
Discharged on Statin Medication[5]	-	-	95%	94%
Thrombolytic Therapy Timing[5]	-	-	68%	66%
Venous Thromboembolism Prophylaxis[5]	-	-	94%	94%
Written Stroke Educational Materials Given[5]	-	-	92%	88%
Surgical Care Improvement Project				
Appropriate Beta Blocker Usage	120	97%	98%	98%
Appropriate VTP Within 24 Hours	530	95%	98%	98%
Controlled Postoperative Blood Glucose[7]	-	-	96%	97%
Perioperative Temperature Management	552	100%	100%	100%
Prophylactic Antibiotic Selection	467	99%	99%	99%
Prophylactic Antibiotic Selection (Outpatient)	129	85%	98%	98%
Prophylactic Antibiotic Stopped	465	95%	98%	98%
Prophylactic Antibiotic Timing	467	99%	99%	99%
Prophylactic Antibiotic Timing (Outpatient)	130	85%	98%	98%
Urinary Catheter Removal	138	94%	98%	97%
Survey of Patients' Hospital Experiences				
Area Around Room 'Always' Quiet at Night	300+	81%	68%	61%
Doctors 'Always' Communicated Well	300+	88%	83%	82%
Home Recovery Information Given	300+	87%	85%	85%
Hospital Given 9 or 10 on 10 Point Scale	300+	84%	73%	71%
Meds 'Always' Explained Before Given	300+	75%	66%	64%
Nurses 'Always' Communicated Well	300+	87%	80%	79%
Pain 'Always' Well Controlled	300+	79%	72%	71%
Room and Bathroom 'Always' Clean	300+	82%	75%	73%
Timely Help 'Always' Received	300+	75%	69%	68%
Would Definitely Recommend Hospital	300+	87%	73%	71%
Use of Medical Imaging				
Cardiac Imaging Stress Test before Surgery[7]	-	-	5.3%	5.3%
Combination Abdominal CT Scan[1]	-	-	16.4%	10.5%
Combination Brain/Sinus CT Scan[1]	-	-	2.7%	2.7%
Combination Chest CT Scan[7]	-	-	5.6%	2.7%
Follow-up Mammogram/Ultrasound[7]	-	-	7.9%	8.8%
Lumbar Spine MRI for Low Back Pain[7]	-	-	39.6%	37.2%

Navarro Regional Hospital

3201 West Highway 22
Corsicana, TX 75110
URL: www.navarrohospital.com
Type: Acute Care Hospitals
Ownership: Voluntary non-profit - Private
Phone: 903-654-6800
Fax: 903-654-6964
Emergency Services: Yes
Beds: 139

Key Personnel:
CEO/President. . . . . Fred Woody

Measure	Cases	This Hosp.	State Avg.	U.S. Avg.
Blood Clot Prevention and Treatment				
Anticoagulation Overlap Therapy[2]	12	92%	93%	93%
ICU Venous Thromboembolism Prophylaxis[2]	63	76%	92%	92%
Incidence of Potentially Preventable VTE[2,7]	-	-	9%	10%
UFH with Dosages/Platelet Monitoring[2,7]	-	-	96%	97%
Venous Thromboembolism Prophylaxis[2]	224	58%	82%	85%
Warfarin Therapy Discharge Instructions[2]	13	77%	84%	75%
Chest Pain/Possible Heart Attack Care				
Aspirin Given Within 24 Hours of Arrival	41	98%	94%	96%
Fibrinolytic Meds Within 30 Min. of Arrival[1]	-	-	47%	58%
Average Time to ECG (minutes)	42	8	8	7
Average Time to Transfer (minutes)[1]	-	-	62	60
Children's Asthma Care				
Received Home Management Plan of Care	-	-	93%	88%
Received Reliever Medication	-	-	100%	100%
Received Systemic Corticosteroids	-	-	100%	100%
Emergency Department				
Admittance Decision Time (minutes)[2]	435	71	99	98
Head CT Results Within 45 Min. of Arrival	11	55%	54%	57%
Patients Who Left ER Before Being Seen	26,127	2%	3%	2%
Time from ER Arrival to Admit. (minutes)[2]	436	218	270	274
Time from ER Arrival to Discharge (minutes)	390	114	127	134
Time in ER Before Being Evaluated (minutes)	417	23	26	26
Time to Pain Meds for Fractures (minutes)	130	55	57	57
Heart Attack Care				
Aspirin Given at Discharge[1]	-	-	99%	99%
Fibrinolytic Meds Within 30 Min. of Arrival[7]	-	-	49%	54%
PCI Within 90 Minutes of Arrival[7]	-	-	95%	96%
Statin Prescribed at Discharge[1]	-	-	98%	98%
Heart Failure Care				
ACE Inhibitor or ARB for LVSD	42	83%	97%	97%
Discharge Instructions Given	104	81%	95%	94%
Evaluation of LVS Function	139	99%	99%	99%
Medicare Spending				
Medicare Spending per Patient (ratio)	-	1.03	1.03	0.98
Pneumonia Care				
Appropriate Initial Antibiotic Given	58	86%	95%	95%
Blood Culture Timing	94	98%	98%	98%
Pregnancy and Delivery Care				
Newborn Deliveries Scheduled Early[2]	46	0%	7%	6%
Preventive Care				
Immunization for Influenza[2]	371	97%	90%	90%
Immunization for Pneumonia[2]	440	97%	92%	92%
Stroke Care				
Anticoagulation Therapy for Atrial Fibrillation[1]	-	-	96%	95%
Antithrombotic Therapy Timing	28	100%	98%	98%
Assessed for Rehabilitation	27	70%	98%	97%
Discharged on Antithrombotic Therapy	24	92%	99%	99%
Discharged on Statin Medication	23	70%	95%	94%
Thrombolytic Therapy Timing[1]	-	-	68%	66%
Venous Thromboembolism Prophylaxis	31	48%	94%	94%
Written Stroke Educational Materials Given	18	39%	92%	88%
Surgical Care Improvement Project				
Appropriate Beta Blocker Usage	36	100%	98%	98%
Appropriate VTP Within 24 Hours	141	99%	98%	98%
Controlled Postoperative Blood Glucose[7]	-	-	96%	97%
Perioperative Temperature Management	156	99%	100%	100%
Prophylactic Antibiotic Selection	70	100%	99%	99%
Prophylactic Antibiotic Selection (Outpatient)	41	100%	98%	98%
Prophylactic Antibiotic Stopped	68	97%	98%	98%
Prophylactic Antibiotic Timing	71	100%	99%	99%
Prophylactic Antibiotic Timing (Outpatient)	39	92%	98%	98%
Urinary Catheter Removal	101	93%	98%	97%
Survey of Patients' Hospital Experiences				
Area Around Room 'Always' Quiet at Night	300+	61%	68%	61%
Doctors 'Always' Communicated Well	300+	81%	83%	82%
Home Recovery Information Given	300+	85%	85%	85%
Hospital Given 9 or 10 on 10 Point Scale	300+	62%	73%	71%
Meds 'Always' Explained Before Given	300+	64%	66%	64%
Nurses 'Always' Communicated Well	300+	76%	80%	79%
Pain 'Always' Well Controlled	300+	72%	72%	71%
Room and Bathroom 'Always' Clean	300+	73%	75%	73%
Timely Help 'Always' Received	300+	62%	69%	68%
Would Definitely Recommend Hospital	300+	58%	73%	71%
Use of Medical Imaging				
Cardiac Imaging Stress Test before Surgery	145	4.8%	5.3%	5.3%
Combination Abdominal CT Scan	316	7.9%	16.4%	10.5%
Combination Brain/Sinus CT Scan	497	1.2%	2.7%	2.7%
Combination Chest CT Scan	153	11.8%	5.6%	2.7%
Follow-up Mammogram/Ultrasound	736	9.9%	7.9%	8.8%
Lumbar Spine MRI for Low Back Pain	49	32.7%	39.6%	37.2%

Crane County Hospital District

1310 S Alford St
Crane, TX 79731
Type: Critical Access Hospitals
Ownership: Govt - Hospital Dist/Auth
Phone: 432-558-3555
Emergency Services: Yes

Measure	Cases	This Hosp.	State Avg.	U.S. Avg.
Blood Clot Prevention and Treatment				
Anticoagulation Overlap Therapy[5]	-	-	93%	93%
ICU Venous Thromboembolism Prophylaxis[5]	-	-	92%	92%
Incidence of Potentially Preventable VTE[5]	-	-	9%	10%
UFH with Dosages/Platelet Monitoring[5]	-	-	96%	97%
Venous Thromboembolism Prophylaxis[5]	-	-	82%	85%
Warfarin Therapy Discharge Instructions[5]	-	-	84%	75%
Chest Pain/Possible Heart Attack Care				
Aspirin Given Within 24 Hours of Arrival	-	-	94%	96%
Fibrinolytic Meds Within 30 Min. of Arrival	-	-	47%	58%
Average Time to ECG (minutes)	-	-	8	7
Average Time to Transfer (minutes)	-	-	62	60
Children's Asthma Care				
Received Home Management Plan of Care	-	-	93%	88%
Received Reliever Medication	-	-	100%	100%
Received Systemic Corticosteroids	-	-	100%	100%
Emergency Department				
Admittance Decision Time (minutes)[5]	-	-	99	98
Head CT Results Within 45 Min. of Arrival	-	-	54%	57%
Patients Who Left ER Before Being Seen	-	-	3%	2%
Time from ER Arrival to Admit. (minutes)[5]	-	-	270	274
Time from ER Arrival to Discharge (minutes)	-	-	127	134
Time in ER Before Being Evaluated (minutes)	-	-	26	26
Time to Pain Meds for Fractures (minutes)	-	-	57	57
Heart Attack Care				
Aspirin Given at Discharge[5]	-	-	99%	99%
Fibrinolytic Meds Within 30 Min. of Arrival[5]	-	-	49%	54%
PCI Within 90 Minutes of Arrival[5]	-	-	95%	96%
Statin Prescribed at Discharge[5]	-	-	98%	98%
Heart Failure Care				
ACE Inhibitor or ARB for LVSD[3,7]	-	-	97%	97%
Discharge Instructions Given[1,3]	-	-	95%	94%
Evaluation of LVS Function[1,3]	-	-	99%	99%
Medicare Spending				
Medicare Spending per Patient (ratio)	-	-	1.03	0.98
Pneumonia Care				
Appropriate Initial Antibiotic Given[3,7]	-	-	95%	95%
Blood Culture Timing[3,7]	-	-	98%	98%
Pregnancy and Delivery Care				
Newborn Deliveries Scheduled Early[5]	-	-	7%	6%

NOTE: Hospital profiles are in alphabetical order by state, then city, then hospital within the city; Rankings exclude hospitals with less than 25 cases except for patient surveys which excludes hospitals with less than 100 cases; (a) 100-299 cases; (1) The number of cases/patients is too few to report; (2) Data submitted were based on a sample of cases/patients; (3) Results are based on a shorter time period than required; (4) Data suppressed by CMS for one or more quarters; (5) Results are not available for this reporting period; (6) Fewer than 100 patients completed the HCAHPS survey; (7) No cases met the criteria for this measure; (8) The lower limit of the confidence interval cannot be calculated if the number of observed infections equals zero; (9) No data are available from the state/territory for this reporting period; (10) The scores shown reflect fewer than 50 completed surveys; (11) There were discrepancies in the data collection process; (12) This measure does not apply to this hospital for this reporting period; (13) Results cannot be calculated for this reporting period; (14) The results for this state are combined with nearby states to protect confidentiality; Please refer to the User's Guide for a full explanation of data.

Measure	Cases	This Hosp.	State Avg.	U.S. Avg.
Preventive Care				
Immunization for Influenza[5]	-	-	90%	90%
Immunization for Pneumonia[3]	17	71%	92%	92%
Stroke Care				
Anticoagulation Therapy for Atrial Fibrillation[5]	-	-	96%	95%
Antithrombotic Therapy Timing[5]	-	-	98%	98%
Assessed for Rehabilitation[5]	-	-	98%	97%
Discharged on Antithrombotic Therapy[5]	-	-	99%	99%
Discharged on Statin Medication[5]	-	-	95%	94%
Thrombolytic Therapy Timing[5]	-	-	68%	66%
Venous Thromboembolism Prophylaxis[5]	-	-	94%	94%
Written Stroke Educational Materials Given[5]	-	-	92%	88%
Surgical Care Improvement Project				
Appropriate Beta Blocker Usage[5]	-	-	98%	98%
Appropriate VTP Within 24 Hours[5]	-	-	98%	98%
Controlled Postoperative Blood Glucose[5]	-	-	96%	97%
Perioperative Temperature Management[5]	-	-	100%	100%
Prophylactic Antibiotic Selection[5]	-	-	99%	99%
Prophylactic Antibiotic Selection (Outpatient)	-	-	98%	98%
Prophylactic Antibiotic Stopped[5]	-	-	98%	98%
Prophylactic Antibiotic Timing[5]	-	-	99%	99%
Prophylactic Antibiotic Timing (Outpatient)	-	-	98%	98%
Urinary Catheter Removal[5]	-	-	98%	97%
Survey of Patients' Hospital Experiences				
Area Around Room 'Always' Quiet at Night[5]	-	-	68%	61%
Doctors 'Always' Communicated Well[5]	-	-	83%	82%
Home Recovery Information Given[5]	-	-	85%	85%
Hospital Given 9 or 10 on 10 Point Scale[5]	-	-	73%	71%
Meds 'Always' Explained Before Given[5]	-	-	66%	64%
Nurses 'Always' Communicated Well[5]	-	-	80%	79%
Pain 'Always' Well Controlled[5]	-	-	72%	71%
Room and Bathroom 'Always' Clean[5]	-	-	75%	73%
Timely Help 'Always' Received[5]	-	-	69%	68%
Would Definitely Recommend Hospital[5]	-	-	73%	71%
Use of Medical Imaging				
Cardiac Imaging Stress Test before Surgery	-	-	5.3%	5.3%
Combination Abdominal CT Scan	-	-	16.4%	10.5%
Combination Brain/Sinus CT Scan	-	-	2.7%	2.7%
Combination Chest CT Scan	-	-	5.6%	2.7%
Follow-up Mammogram/Ultrasound	-	-	7.9%	8.8%
Lumbar Spine MRI for Low Back Pain	-	-	39.6%	37.2%

East Texas Medical Center Crockett

1100 Loop 304 East
Crockett, TX 75835
Phone: 936-546-3862
Fax: 936-546-3892
E-mail: info@etmc.org
URL: www.etmc.org/crockett
Type: Acute Care Hospitals
Emergency Services: Yes
Ownership: Voluntary non-profit - Private
Beds: 93

Key Personnel:

Chief of Medical Staff. . . . . Mike Cochran, MD
Emergency Room . . . . David Garner, RN
Quality Assurance . . . . Caroline Ramirez
CEO/President. . . . . Nelda Welch

Measure	Cases	This Hosp.	State Avg.	U.S. Avg.
Blood Clot Prevention and Treatment				
Anticoagulation Overlap Therapy[1,2]	-	-	93%	93%
ICU Venous Thromboembolism Prophylaxis[2]	21	57%	92%	92%
Incidence of Potentially Preventable VTE[2,7]	-	-	9%	10%
UFH with Dosages/Platelet Monitoring[2,7]	-	-	96%	97%
Venous Thromboembolism Prophylaxis[2]	104	52%	82%	85%
Warfarin Therapy Discharge Instructions[1,2]	-	-	84%	75%
Chest Pain/Possible Heart Attack Care				
Aspirin Given Within 24 Hours of Arrival	40	92%	94%	96%
Fibrinolytic Meds Within 30 Min. of Arrival[1]	-	-	47%	58%
Average Time to ECG (minutes)	40	5	8	7
Average Time to Transfer (minutes)[7]	-	-	62	60
Children's Asthma Care				
Received Home Management Plan of Care	-	-	93%	88%
Received Reliever Medication	-	-	100%	100%
Received Systemic Corticosteroids	-	-	100%	100%
Emergency Department				
Admittance Decision Time (minutes)[2]	226	65	99	98
Head CT Results Within 45 Min. of Arrival[1,3]	-	-	54%	57%
Patients Who Left ER Before Being Seen	14,134	1%	3%	2%
Time from ER Arrival to Admit. (minutes)[2]	228	206	270	274
Time from ER Arrival to Discharge (minutes)	413	102	127	134
Time in ER Before Being Evaluated (minutes)	407	18	26	26
Time to Pain Meds for Fractures (minutes)	15	71	57	57
Heart Attack Care				
Aspirin Given at Discharge[1,3]	-	-	99%	99%
Fibrinolytic Meds Within 30 Min. of Arrival[3,7]	-	-	49%	54%
PCI Within 90 Minutes of Arrival[3,7]	-	-	95%	96%
Statin Prescribed at Discharge[1,3]	-	-	98%	98%
Heart Failure Care				
ACE Inhibitor or ARB for LVSD	11	82%	97%	97%
Discharge Instructions Given	57	60%	95%	94%
Evaluation of LVS Function	96	61%	99%	99%
Medicare Spending				
Medicare Spending per Patient (ratio)	-	0.99	1.03	0.98
Pneumonia Care				
Appropriate Initial Antibiotic Given	25	96%	95%	95%
Blood Culture Timing	24	96%	98%	98%
Pregnancy and Delivery Care				
Newborn Deliveries Scheduled Early[2]	13	8%	7%	6%
Preventive Care				
Immunization for Influenza[2]	244	53%	90%	90%
Immunization for Pneumonia[2]	310	78%	92%	92%
Stroke Care				
Anticoagulation Therapy for Atrial Fibrillation[1]	-	-	96%	95%
Antithrombotic Therapy Timing[1]	-	-	98%	98%
Assessed for Rehabilitation[1]	-	-	98%	97%
Discharged on Antithrombotic Therapy[1]	-	-	99%	99%
Discharged on Statin Medication[1]	-	-	95%	94%
Thrombolytic Therapy Timing[7]	-	-	68%	66%
Venous Thromboembolism Prophylaxis[1]	-	-	94%	94%
Written Stroke Educational Materials Given[1]	-	-	92%	88%
Surgical Care Improvement Project				
Appropriate Beta Blocker Usage	11	91%	98%	98%
Appropriate VTP Within 24 Hours	26	96%	98%	98%
Controlled Postoperative Blood Glucose[7]	-	-	96%	97%
Perioperative Temperature Management	32	100%	100%	100%
Prophylactic Antibiotic Selection	15	100%	99%	99%
Prophylactic Antibiotic Selection (Outpatient)[1,3]	-	-	98%	98%
Prophylactic Antibiotic Stopped	13	92%	98%	98%
Prophylactic Antibiotic Timing	15	60%	99%	99%
Prophylactic Antibiotic Timing (Outpatient)[1,3]	-	-	98%	98%
Urinary Catheter Removal	17	76%	98%	97%
Survey of Patients' Hospital Experiences				
Area Around Room 'Always' Quiet at Night	(a)	66%	68%	61%
Doctors 'Always' Communicated Well	(a)	87%	83%	82%
Home Recovery Information Given	(a)	83%	85%	85%
Hospital Given 9 or 10 on 10 Point Scale	(a)	64%	73%	71%
Meds 'Always' Explained Before Given	(a)	62%	66%	64%
Nurses 'Always' Communicated Well	(a)	81%	80%	79%
Pain 'Always' Well Controlled	(a)	75%	72%	71%
Room and Bathroom 'Always' Clean	(a)	65%	75%	73%
Timely Help 'Always' Received	(a)	74%	69%	68%
Would Definitely Recommend Hospital	(a)	60%	73%	71%
Use of Medical Imaging				
Cardiac Imaging Stress Test before Surgery[1]	-	-	5.3%	5.3%
Combination Abdominal CT Scan	163	5.5%	16.4%	10.5%
Combination Brain/Sinus CT Scan[1]	-	-	2.7%	2.7%
Combination Chest CT Scan	100	1.0%	5.6%	2.7%
Follow-up Mammogram/Ultrasound	271	6.6%	7.9%	8.8%
Lumbar Spine MRI for Low Back Pain	55	58.2%	39.6%	37.2%

Cuero Community Hospital

2550 N Esplanade
Cuero, TX 77954
Phone: 361-275-6191
Fax: 361-275-3999
URL: www.cuerohosp.org
Type: Acute Care Hospitals
Emergency Services: Yes
Ownership: Govt - Hospital Dist/Auth
Beds: 60

Key Personnel:

Cardiology . . . . Harish Chandna, MD
Chair/CEO . . . . Amy Crain
Quality Assurance . . . . Carol Drozd
Infection Control. . . . . Debbie Irving, RN
Operating Room. . . . . Gale Jendrzey, RN
Emergency Room . . . . Patty Jetter
Chief of Medical Staff . . . . Ramond Ruise
Surgery . . . . William Wagner, MD

Measure	Cases	This Hosp.	State Avg.	U.S. Avg.
Blood Clot Prevention and Treatment				
Anticoagulation Overlap Therapy[1,2]	-	-	93%	93%
ICU Venous Thromboembolism Prophylaxis[2]	26	100%	92%	92%
Incidence of Potentially Preventable VTE[1,2]	-	-	9%	10%
UFH with Dosages/Platelet Monitoring[2,7]	-	-	96%	97%
Venous Thromboembolism Prophylaxis[2]	105	78%	82%	85%
Warfarin Therapy Discharge Instructions[1,2]	-	-	84%	75%
Chest Pain/Possible Heart Attack Care				
Aspirin Given Within 24 Hours of Arrival	29	97%	94%	96%
Fibrinolytic Meds Within 30 Min. of Arrival[1]	-	-	47%	58%
Average Time to ECG (minutes)	30	3	8	7
Average Time to Transfer (minutes)[7]	-	-	62	60
Children's Asthma Care				
Received Home Management Plan of Care	-	-	93%	88%
Received Reliever Medication	-	-	100%	100%
Received Systemic Corticosteroids	-	-	100%	100%
Emergency Department				
Admittance Decision Time (minutes)[2]	309	55	99	98
Head CT Results Within 45 Min. of Arrival[1]	-	-	54%	57%
Patients Who Left ER Before Being Seen	8,815	3%	3%	2%
Time from ER Arrival to Admit. (minutes)[2]	309	199	270	274
Time from ER Arrival to Discharge (minutes)	434	104	127	134
Time in ER Before Being Evaluated (minutes)	476	18	26	26
Time to Pain Meds for Fractures (minutes)	19	51	57	57
Heart Attack Care				
Aspirin Given at Discharge[1,3]	-	-	99%	99%
Fibrinolytic Meds Within 30 Min. of Arrival[3,7]	-	-	49%	54%
PCI Within 90 Minutes of Arrival[3,7]	-	-	95%	96%
Statin Prescribed at Discharge[1,3]	-	-	98%	98%
Heart Failure Care				
ACE Inhibitor or ARB for LVSD	34	100%	97%	97%
Discharge Instructions Given	55	100%	95%	94%
Evaluation of LVS Function	84	100%	99%	99%
Medicare Spending				
Medicare Spending per Patient (ratio)	-	1.15	1.03	0.98
Pneumonia Care				
Appropriate Initial Antibiotic Given	36	86%	95%	95%
Blood Culture Timing	49	100%	98%	98%
Pregnancy and Delivery Care				
Newborn Deliveries Scheduled Early[1]	-	-	7%	6%
Preventive Care				
Immunization for Influenza[2]	276	99%	90%	90%
Immunization for Pneumonia[2]	407	99%	92%	92%
Stroke Care				
Anticoagulation Therapy for Atrial Fibrillation[7]	-	-	96%	95%
Antithrombotic Therapy Timing[1]	-	-	98%	98%
Assessed for Rehabilitation[1]	-	-	98%	97%
Discharged on Antithrombotic Therapy[1]	-	-	99%	99%
Discharged on Statin Medication[1]	-	-	95%	94%
Thrombolytic Therapy Timing[7]	-	-	68%	66%
Venous Thromboembolism Prophylaxis	11	100%	94%	94%
Written Stroke Educational Materials Given[1]	-	-	92%	88%
Surgical Care Improvement Project				
Appropriate Beta Blocker Usage[1]	-	-	98%	98%
Appropriate VTP Within 24 Hours[1]	-	-	98%	98%
Controlled Postoperative Blood Glucose[7]	-	-	96%	97%
Perioperative Temperature Management[1]	-	-	100%	100%
Prophylactic Antibiotic Selection[1]	-	-	99%	99%
Prophylactic Antibiotic Selection (Outpatient)	12	92%	98%	98%
Prophylactic Antibiotic Stopped[1]	-	-	98%	98%
Prophylactic Antibiotic Timing[1]	-	-	99%	99%
Prophylactic Antibiotic Timing (Outpatient)[1]	-	-	98%	98%
Urinary Catheter Removal[1]	-	-	98%	97%
Survey of Patients' Hospital Experiences				
Area Around Room 'Always' Quiet at Night	(a)	72%	68%	61%
Doctors 'Always' Communicated Well	(a)	82%	83%	82%

NOTE: Hospital profiles are in alphabetical order by state, then city, then hospital within the city; Rankings exclude hospitals with less than 25 cases except for patient surveys which excludes hospitals with less than 100 cases; (a) 100-299 cases; (1) The number of cases/patients is too few to report; (2) Data submitted were based on a sample of cases/patients; (3) Results are based on a shorter time period than required; (4) Data suppressed by CMS for one or more quarters; (5) Results are not available for this reporting period; (6) Fewer than 100 patients completed the HCAHPS survey; (7) No cases met the criteria for this measure; (8) The lower limit of the confidence interval cannot be calculated if the number of observed infections equals zero; (9) No data are available from the state/territory for this reporting period; (10) The scores shown reflect fewer than 50 completed surveys; (11) There were discrepancies in the data collection process; (12) This measure does not apply to this hospital for this reporting period; (13) Results cannot be calculated for this reporting period; (14) The results for this state are combined with nearby states to protect confidentiality; Please refer to the User's Guide for a full explanation of data.

Measure	Cases	This Hosp.	State Avg.	U.S. Avg.
Home Recovery Information Given	(a)	84%	85%	85%
Hospital Given 9 or 10 on 10 Point Scale	(a)	73%	73%	71%
Meds 'Always' Explained Before Given	(a)	63%	66%	64%
Nurses 'Always' Communicated Well	(a)	77%	80%	79%
Pain 'Always' Well Controlled	(a)	79%	72%	71%
Room and Bathroom 'Always' Clean	(a)	80%	75%	73%
Timely Help 'Always' Received	(a)	72%	69%	68%
Would Definitely Recommend Hospital	(a)	69%	73%	71%
Use of Medical Imaging				
Cardiac Imaging Stress Test before Surgery	64	1.6%	5.3%	5.3%
Combination Abdominal CT Scan	235	3.8%	16.4%	10.5%
Combination Brain/Sinus CT Scan	215	0.5%	2.7%	2.7%
Combination Chest CT Scan	100	2.0%	5.6%	2.7%
Follow-up Mammogram/Ultrasound	340	9.1%	7.9%	8.8%
Lumbar Spine MRI for Low Back Pain	68	41.2%	39.6%	37.2%

North Cypress Medical Center

21214 Northwest Freeway Phone: 281-890-0203
Cypress, TX 77429
URL: www.ncmc-hospital.com
Type: Acute Care Hospitals Emergency Services: Yes
Ownership: Physician Beds: 175
Key Personnel:
Chairman/CEO .... Robert A Behar
Pediatrics.................... Neeta Bhardwaj, M.D.

Measure	Cases	This Hosp.	State Avg.	U.S. Avg.
Blood Clot Prevention and Treatment				
Anticoagulation Overlap Therapy[2]	78	86%	93%	93%
ICU Venous Thromboembolism Prophylaxis[2]	69	91%	92%	92%
Incidence of Potentially Preventable VTE[2]	20	0%	9%	10%
UFH with Dosages/Platelet Monitoring[2]	41	100%	96%	97%
Venous Thromboembolism Prophylaxis[2]	371	91%	82%	85%
Warfarin Therapy Discharge Instructions[2]	55	71%	84%	75%
Chest Pain/Possible Heart Attack Care				
Aspirin Given Within 24 Hours of Arrival[1,3]	-	-	94%	96%
Fibrinolytic Meds Within 30 Min. of Arrival[5]	-	-	47%	58%
Average Time to ECG (minutes)[1,3]	-	-	8	7
Average Time to Transfer (minutes)[5]	-	-	62	60
Children's Asthma Care				
Received Home Management Plan of Care	-	-	93%	88%
Received Reliever Medication	-	-	100%	100%
Received Systemic Corticosteroids	-	-	100%	100%
Emergency Department				
Admittance Decision Time (minutes)[2]	625	130	99	98
Head CT Results Within 45 Min. of Arrival[1]	-	-	54%	57%
Patients Who Left ER Before Being Seen	14,719	0%	3%	2%
Time from ER Arrival to Admit. (minutes)[2]	625	268	270	274
Time from ER Arrival to Discharge (minutes)	367	118	127	134
Time in ER Before Being Evaluated (minutes)	430	15	26	26
Time to Pain Meds for Fractures (minutes)	250	46	57	57
Heart Attack Care				
Aspirin Given at Discharge	207	100%	99%	99%
Fibrinolytic Meds Within 30 Min. of Arrival[7]	-	-	49%	54%
PCI Within 90 Minutes of Arrival	27	100%	95%	96%
Statin Prescribed at Discharge	203	100%	98%	98%
Heart Failure Care				
ACE Inhibitor or ARB for LVSD	68	100%	97%	97%
Discharge Instructions Given	204	98%	95%	94%
Evaluation of LVS Function	257	100%	99%	99%
Medicare Spending				
Medicare Spending per Patient (ratio)	-	1.14	1.03	0.98
Pneumonia Care				
Appropriate Initial Antibiotic Given	149	98%	95%	95%
Blood Culture Timing	302	100%	98%	98%
Pregnancy and Delivery Care				
Newborn Deliveries Scheduled Early[7]	-	-	7%	6%
Preventive Care				
Immunization for Influenza[2]	674	99%	90%	90%
Immunization for Pneumonia[2]	893	99%	92%	92%
Stroke Care				
Anticoagulation Therapy for Atrial Fibrillation	15	100%	96%	95%
Antithrombotic Therapy Timing	117	100%	98%	98%
Assessed for Rehabilitation	146	99%	98%	97%
Discharged on Antithrombotic Therapy	119	100%	99%	99%
Discharged on Statin Medication	101	100%	95%	94%
Thrombolytic Therapy Timing[1]	-	-	68%	66%
Venous Thromboembolism Prophylaxis	146	99%	94%	94%
Written Stroke Educational Materials Given	81	100%	92%	88%
Surgical Care Improvement Project				
Appropriate Beta Blocker Usage	201	100%	98%	98%
Appropriate VTP Within 24 Hours	550	99%	98%	98%
Controlled Postoperative Blood Glucose	50	92%	96%	97%
Perioperative Temperature Management	701	100%	100%	100%
Prophylactic Antibiotic Selection	425	100%	99%	99%
Prophylactic Antibiotic Selection (Outpatient)	189	96%	98%	98%
Prophylactic Antibiotic Stopped	409	100%	98%	98%
Prophylactic Antibiotic Timing	425	100%	99%	99%
Prophylactic Antibiotic Timing (Outpatient)	190	99%	98%	98%
Urinary Catheter Removal	173	100%	98%	97%
Survey of Patients' Hospital Experiences				
Area Around Room 'Always' Quiet at Night	300+	73%	68%	61%
Doctors 'Always' Communicated Well	300+	80%	83%	82%
Home Recovery Information Given	300+	84%	85%	85%
Hospital Given 9 or 10 on 10 Point Scale	300+	73%	73%	71%
Meds 'Always' Explained Before Given	300+	62%	66%	64%
Nurses 'Always' Communicated Well	300+	75%	80%	79%
Pain 'Always' Well Controlled	300+	71%	72%	71%
Room and Bathroom 'Always' Clean	300+	69%	75%	73%
Timely Help 'Always' Received	300+	64%	69%	68%
Would Definitely Recommend Hospital	300+	75%	73%	71%
Use of Medical Imaging				
Cardiac Imaging Stress Test before Surgery	146	11.0%	5.3%	5.3%
Combination Abdominal CT Scan	936	65.9%	16.4%	10.5%
Combination Brain/Sinus CT Scan	978	3.8%	2.7%	2.7%
Combination Chest CT Scan	760	3.0%	5.6%	2.7%
Follow-up Mammogram/Ultrasound	742	12.9%	7.9%	8.8%
Lumbar Spine MRI for Low Back Pain	228	35.1%	39.6%	37.2%

Coon Memorial Hospital

1411 Denver Avenue Phone: 806-244-4571
Dalhart, TX 79022 Fax: 806-244-5013
URL: www.coonmemorial.org
Type: Critical Access Hospitals Emergency Services: Yes
Ownership: Govt - Hospital Dist/Auth Beds: 23
Key Personnel:
CEO/President................ Sieto Mellema

Measure	Cases	This Hosp.	State Avg.	U.S. Avg.
Blood Clot Prevention and Treatment				
Anticoagulation Overlap Therapy[5]	-	-	93%	93%
ICU Venous Thromboembolism Prophylaxis[5]	-	-	92%	92%
Incidence of Potentially Preventable VTE[5]	-	-	9%	10%
UFH with Dosages/Platelet Monitoring[5]	-	-	96%	97%
Venous Thromboembolism Prophylaxis[5]	-	-	82%	85%
Warfarin Therapy Discharge Instructions[5]	-	-	84%	75%
Chest Pain/Possible Heart Attack Care				
Aspirin Given Within 24 Hours of Arrival	-	-	94%	96%
Fibrinolytic Meds Within 30 Min. of Arrival	-	-	47%	58%
Average Time to ECG (minutes)	-	-	8	7
Average Time to Transfer (minutes)	-	-	62	60
Children's Asthma Care				
Received Home Management Plan of Care	-	-	93%	88%
Received Reliever Medication	-	-	100%	100%
Received Systemic Corticosteroids	-	-	100%	100%
Emergency Department				
Admittance Decision Time (minutes)[5]	-	-	99	98
Head CT Results Within 45 Min. of Arrival	-	-	54%	57%
Patients Who Left ER Before Being Seen	-	-	3%	2%
Time from ER Arrival to Admit. (minutes)[5]	-	-	270	274
Time from ER Arrival to Discharge (minutes)	-	-	127	134
Time in ER Before Being Evaluated (minutes)	-	-	26	26
Time to Pain Meds for Fractures (minutes)	-	-	57	57
Heart Attack Care				
Aspirin Given at Discharge[5]	-	-	99%	99%
Fibrinolytic Meds Within 30 Min. of Arrival[5]	-	-	49%	54%
PCI Within 90 Minutes of Arrival[5]	-	-	95%	96%
Statin Prescribed at Discharge[5]	-	-	98%	98%
Heart Failure Care				
ACE Inhibitor or ARB for LVSD[3,7]	-	-	97%	97%
Discharge Instructions Given[1,3]	-	-	95%	94%
Evaluation of LVS Function[1,3]	-	-	99%	99%
Medicare Spending				
Medicare Spending per Patient (ratio)	-	-	1.03	0.98
Pneumonia Care				
Appropriate Initial Antibiotic Given	17	76%	95%	95%
Blood Culture Timing[1]	-	-	98%	98%
Pregnancy and Delivery Care				
Newborn Deliveries Scheduled Early[5]	-	-	7%	6%
Preventive Care				
Immunization for Influenza[5]	-	-	90%	90%
Immunization for Pneumonia[5]	-	-	92%	92%
Stroke Care				
Anticoagulation Therapy for Atrial Fibrillation[5]	-	-	96%	95%
Antithrombotic Therapy Timing[5]	-	-	98%	98%
Assessed for Rehabilitation[5]	-	-	98%	97%
Discharged on Antithrombotic Therapy[5]	-	-	99%	99%
Discharged on Statin Medication[5]	-	-	95%	94%
Thrombolytic Therapy Timing[5]	-	-	68%	66%
Venous Thromboembolism Prophylaxis[5]	-	-	94%	94%
Written Stroke Educational Materials Given[5]	-	-	92%	88%
Surgical Care Improvement Project				
Appropriate Beta Blocker Usage[1]	-	-	98%	98%
Appropriate VTP Within 24 Hours	16	100%	98%	98%
Controlled Postoperative Blood Glucose[7]	-	-	96%	97%
Perioperative Temperature Management	20	75%	100%	100%
Prophylactic Antibiotic Selection	20	90%	99%	99%
Prophylactic Antibiotic Selection (Outpatient)	-	-	98%	98%
Prophylactic Antibiotic Stopped	20	75%	98%	98%
Prophylactic Antibiotic Timing	20	40%	99%	99%
Prophylactic Antibiotic Timing (Outpatient)	-	-	98%	98%
Urinary Catheter Removal	12	83%	98%	97%
Survey of Patients' Hospital Experiences				
Area Around Room 'Always' Quiet at Night[6]	<100	62%	68%	61%
Doctors 'Always' Communicated Well[6]	<100	86%	83%	82%
Home Recovery Information Given[6]	<100	83%	85%	85%
Hospital Given 9 or 10 on 10 Point Scale[6]	<100	64%	73%	71%
Meds 'Always' Explained Before Given[6]	<100	64%	66%	64%
Nurses 'Always' Communicated Well[6]	<100	74%	80%	79%
Pain 'Always' Well Controlled[6]	<100	64%	72%	71%
Room and Bathroom 'Always' Clean[6]	<100	67%	75%	73%
Timely Help 'Always' Received[6]	<100	53%	69%	68%
Would Definitely Recommend Hospital[6]	<100	56%	73%	71%
Use of Medical Imaging				
Cardiac Imaging Stress Test before Surgery	-	-	5.3%	5.3%
Combination Abdominal CT Scan	-	-	16.4%	10.5%
Combination Brain/Sinus CT Scan	-	-	2.7%	2.7%
Combination Chest CT Scan	-	-	5.6%	2.7%
Follow-up Mammogram/Ultrasound	-	-	7.9%	8.8%
Lumbar Spine MRI for Low Back Pain	-	-	39.6%	37.2%

Baylor Heart & Vascular Hospital

621 North Hall Street Phone: 214-820-0670
Dallas, TX 75226
URL: www.baylorhearthospital.com
Type: Acute Care Hospitals Emergency Services: No
Ownership: Proprietary
Key Personnel:
CEO .... Joel T. Allison, FACHE
Chief of Medical Staff........... Irving Prengler, MD
Operating Room.............. Shirley Sample, RN

Measure	Cases	This Hosp.	State Avg.	U.S. Avg.
Blood Clot Prevention and Treatment				
Anticoagulation Overlap Therapy[2]	11	100%	93%	93%
ICU Venous Thromboembolism Prophylaxis[2]	76	99%	92%	92%
Incidence of Potentially Preventable VTE[1,2]	-	-	9%	10%
UFH with Dosages/Platelet Monitoring[2]	14	100%	96%	97%
Venous Thromboembolism Prophylaxis[2]	201	99%	82%	85%
Warfarin Therapy Discharge Instructions[1,2]	-	-	84%	75%
Chest Pain/Possible Heart Attack Care				
Aspirin Given Within 24 Hours of Arrival[5]	-	-	94%	96%

NOTE: Hospital profiles are in alphabetical order by state, then city, then hospital within the city; Rankings exclude hospitals with less than 25 cases except for patient surveys which excludes hospitals with less than 100 cases; (a) 100-299 cases; (1) The number of cases/patients is too few to report; (2) Data submitted were based on a sample of cases/patients; (3) Results are based on a shorter time period than required; (4) Data suppressed by CMS for one or more quarters; (5) Results are not available for this reporting period; (6) Fewer than 100 patients completed the HCAHPS survey; (7) No cases met the criteria for this measure; (8) The lower limit of the confidence interval cannot be calculated if the number of observed infections equals zero; (9) No data are available from the state/territory for this reporting period; (10) The scores shown reflect fewer than 50 completed surveys; (11) There were discrepancies in the data collection process; (12) This measure does not apply to this hospital for this reporting period; (13) Results cannot be calculated for this reporting period; (14) The results for this state are combined with nearby states to protect confidentiality; Please refer to the User's Guide for a full explanation of data.

Measure	Cases	This Hosp.	State Avg.	U.S. Avg.
Fibrinolytic Meds Within 30 Min. of Arrival[5]	-	-	47%	58%
Average Time to ECG (minutes)[5]	-	-	8	7
Average Time to Transfer (minutes)[5]	-	-	62	60
Children's Asthma Care				
Received Home Management Plan of Care	-	-	93%	88%
Received Reliever Medication	-	-	100%	100%
Received Systemic Corticosteroids	-	-	100%	100%
Emergency Department				
Admittance Decision Time (minutes)[2,7]	-	-	99	98
Head CT Results Within 45 Min. of Arrival[5]	-	-	54%	57%
Patients Who Left ER Before Being Seen[5]	-	-	3%	2%
Time from ER Arrival to Admit. (minutes)[2,7]	-	-	270	274
Time from ER Arrival to Discharge (minutes)[5]	-	-	127	134
Time in ER Before Being Evaluated (minutes)[5]	-	-	26	26
Time to Pain Meds for Fractures (minutes)[5]	-	-	57	57
Heart Attack Care				
Aspirin Given at Discharge	457	100%	99%	99%
Fibrinolytic Meds Within 30 Min. of Arrival[7]	-	-	49%	54%
PCI Within 90 Minutes of Arrival[7]	-	-	95%	96%
Statin Prescribed at Discharge	447	100%	98%	98%
Heart Failure Care				
ACE Inhibitor or ARB for LVSD	58	100%	97%	97%
Discharge Instructions Given	95	100%	95%	94%
Evaluation of LVS Function	106	100%	99%	99%
Medicare Spending				
Medicare Spending per Patient (ratio)	-	0.97	1.03	0.98
Pneumonia Care				
Appropriate Initial Antibiotic Given[3,7]	-	-	95%	95%
Blood Culture Timing[3,7]	-	-	98%	98%
Pregnancy and Delivery Care				
Newborn Deliveries Scheduled Early[7]	-	-	7%	6%
Preventive Care				
Immunization for Influenza[2]	298	99%	90%	90%
Immunization for Pneumonia[2]	443	98%	92%	92%
Stroke Care				
Anticoagulation Therapy for Atrial Fibrillation[7]	-	-	96%	95%
Antithrombotic Therapy Timing[1]	-	-	98%	98%
Assessed for Rehabilitation[7]	-	-	98%	97%
Discharged on Antithrombotic Therapy[7]	-	-	99%	99%
Discharged on Statin Medication[7]	-	-	95%	94%
Thrombolytic Therapy Timing[7]	-	-	68%	66%
Venous Thromboembolism Prophylaxis[1]	-	-	94%	94%
Written Stroke Educational Materials Given[7]	-	-	92%	88%
Surgical Care Improvement Project				
Appropriate Beta Blocker Usage	68	100%	98%	98%
Appropriate VTP Within 24 Hours[7]	-	-	98%	98%
Controlled Postoperative Blood Glucose[7]	-	-	96%	97%
Perioperative Temperature Management	130	100%	100%	100%
Prophylactic Antibiotic Selection	88	100%	99%	99%
Prophylactic Antibiotic Selection (Outpatient)	734	99%	98%	98%
Prophylactic Antibiotic Stopped	82	99%	98%	98%
Prophylactic Antibiotic Timing	88	100%	99%	99%
Prophylactic Antibiotic Timing (Outpatient)	734	100%	98%	98%
Urinary Catheter Removal	99	100%	98%	97%
Survey of Patients' Hospital Experiences				
Area Around Room 'Always' Quiet at Night	300+	76%	68%	61%
Doctors 'Always' Communicated Well	300+	88%	83%	82%
Home Recovery Information Given	300+	85%	85%	85%
Hospital Given 9 or 10 on 10 Point Scale	300+	88%	73%	71%
Meds 'Always' Explained Before Given	300+	72%	66%	64%
Nurses 'Always' Communicated Well	300+	87%	80%	79%
Pain 'Always' Well Controlled	300+	77%	72%	71%
Room and Bathroom 'Always' Clean	300+	80%	75%	73%
Timely Help 'Always' Received	300+	78%	69%	68%
Would Definitely Recommend Hospital	300+	91%	73%	71%
Use of Medical Imaging				
Cardiac Imaging Stress Test before Surgery[1]	-	-	5.3%	5.3%
Combination Abdominal CT Scan[1]	-	-	16.4%	10.5%
Combination Brain/Sinus CT Scan[1]	-	-	2.7%	2.7%
Combination Chest CT Scan[1]	-	-	5.6%	2.7%
Follow-up Mammogram/Ultrasound[7]	-	-	7.9%	8.8%
Lumbar Spine MRI for Low Back Pain[1]	-	-	39.6%	37.2%

Baylor Medical Center at Uptown

2727 East Lemmon Avenue Building I Phone: 214-443-3000
Dallas, TX 75204
URL: www.bmcuptown.com
Type: Acute Care Hospitals Emergency Services: Yes
Ownership: Voluntary non-profit - Private
Key Personnel:
Imaging . . . . Thomas Bosquet
Quality Assurance . . . . Linda Broome
CEO . . . . Matt Chance

Measure	Cases	This Hosp.	State Avg.	U.S. Avg.
Blood Clot Prevention and Treatment				
Anticoagulation Overlap Therapy[2,7]	-	-	93%	93%
ICU Venous Thromboembolism Prophylaxis[2,7]	-	-	92%	92%
Incidence of Potentially Preventable VTE[2,7]	-	-	9%	10%
UFH with Dosages/Platelet Monitoring[2,7]	-	-	96%	97%
Venous Thromboembolism Prophylaxis[2]	69	99%	82%	85%
Warfarin Therapy Discharge Instructions[2,7]	-	-	84%	75%
Chest Pain/Possible Heart Attack Care				
Aspirin Given Within 24 Hours of Arrival[1,3]	-	-	94%	96%
Fibrinolytic Meds Within 30 Min. of Arrival[5]	-	-	47%	58%
Average Time to ECG (minutes)[1,3]	-	-	8	7
Average Time to Transfer (minutes)[5]	-	-	62	60
Children's Asthma Care				
Received Home Management Plan of Care	-	-	93%	88%
Received Reliever Medication	-	-	100%	100%
Received Systemic Corticosteroids	-	-	100%	100%
Emergency Department				
Admittance Decision Time (minutes)[1,2]	-	-	99	98
Head CT Results Within 45 Min. of Arrival[1,3]	-	-	54%	57%
Patients Who Left ER Before Being Seen	1,782	1%	3%	2%
Time from ER Arrival to Admit. (minutes)[1,2]	-	-	270	274
Time from ER Arrival to Discharge (minutes)	286	83	127	134
Time in ER Before Being Evaluated (minutes)	293	11	26	26
Time to Pain Meds for Fractures (minutes)	12	46	57	57
Heart Attack Care				
Aspirin Given at Discharge[5]	-	-	99%	99%
Fibrinolytic Meds Within 30 Min. of Arrival[5]	-	-	49%	54%
PCI Within 90 Minutes of Arrival[5]	-	-	95%	96%
Statin Prescribed at Discharge[5]	-	-	98%	98%
Heart Failure Care				
ACE Inhibitor or ARB for LVSD[5]	-	-	97%	97%
Discharge Instructions Given[5]	-	-	95%	94%
Evaluation of LVS Function[5]	-	-	99%	99%
Medicare Spending				
Medicare Spending per Patient (ratio)	-	1.07	1.03	0.98
Pneumonia Care				
Appropriate Initial Antibiotic Given[5]	-	-	95%	95%
Blood Culture Timing[5]	-	-	98%	98%
Pregnancy and Delivery Care				
Newborn Deliveries Scheduled Early[7]	-	-	7%	6%
Preventive Care				
Immunization for Influenza[2]	316	87%	90%	90%
Immunization for Pneumonia[2]	292	90%	92%	92%
Stroke Care				
Anticoagulation Therapy for Atrial Fibrillation[5]	-	-	96%	95%
Antithrombotic Therapy Timing[5]	-	-	98%	98%
Assessed for Rehabilitation[5]	-	-	98%	97%
Discharged on Antithrombotic Therapy[5]	-	-	99%	99%
Discharged on Statin Medication[5]	-	-	95%	94%
Thrombolytic Therapy Timing[5]	-	-	68%	66%
Venous Thromboembolism Prophylaxis[5]	-	-	94%	94%
Written Stroke Educational Materials Given[5]	-	-	92%	88%
Surgical Care Improvement Project				
Appropriate Beta Blocker Usage	99	100%	98%	98%
Appropriate VTP Within 24 Hours	373	100%	98%	98%
Controlled Postoperative Blood Glucose[7]	-	-	96%	97%
Perioperative Temperature Management	415	100%	100%	100%
Prophylactic Antibiotic Selection	409	100%	99%	99%
Prophylactic Antibiotic Selection (Outpatient)	185	99%	98%	98%
Prophylactic Antibiotic Stopped	408	100%	98%	98%
Prophylactic Antibiotic Timing	410	100%	99%	99%
Prophylactic Antibiotic Timing (Outpatient)	185	100%	98%	98%
Urinary Catheter Removal	261	100%	98%	97%
Survey of Patients' Hospital Experiences				
Area Around Room 'Always' Quiet at Night	300+	87%	68%	61%
Doctors 'Always' Communicated Well	300+	90%	83%	82%
Home Recovery Information Given	300+	92%	85%	85%
Hospital Given 9 or 10 on 10 Point Scale	300+	88%	73%	71%
Meds 'Always' Explained Before Given	300+	77%	66%	64%
Nurses 'Always' Communicated Well	300+	90%	80%	79%
Pain 'Always' Well Controlled	300+	79%	72%	71%
Room and Bathroom 'Always' Clean	300+	86%	75%	73%
Timely Help 'Always' Received	300+	89%	69%	68%
Would Definitely Recommend Hospital	300+	89%	73%	71%
Use of Medical Imaging				
Cardiac Imaging Stress Test before Surgery[7]	-	-	5.3%	5.3%
Combination Abdominal CT Scan[1]	-	-	16.4%	10.5%
Combination Brain/Sinus CT Scan[1]	-	-	2.7%	2.7%
Combination Chest CT Scan[1]	-	-	5.6%	2.7%
Follow-up Mammogram/Ultrasound[7]	-	-	7.9%	8.8%
Lumbar Spine MRI for Low Back Pain	50	36.0%	39.6%	37.2%

Baylor University Medical Center

3500 Gaston Ave Phone: 214-820-0111
Dallas, TX 75246
URL: www.baylorhealth.com
Type: Acute Care Hospitals Emergency Services: Yes
Ownership: Voluntary non-profit - Church Beds: 1,025
Key Personnel:
CEO . . . . Joel T. Allison, FACHE
President . . . . John B McWhorter, III

Measure	Cases	This Hosp.	State Avg.	U.S. Avg.
Blood Clot Prevention and Treatment				
Anticoagulation Overlap Therapy[2]	174	97%	93%	93%
ICU Venous Thromboembolism Prophylaxis[2]	101	100%	92%	92%
Incidence of Potentially Preventable VTE[2]	56	5%	9%	10%
UFH with Dosages/Platelet Monitoring[2]	131	100%	96%	97%
Venous Thromboembolism Prophylaxis[2]	355	92%	82%	85%
Warfarin Therapy Discharge Instructions[2]	123	99%	84%	75%
Chest Pain/Possible Heart Attack Care				
Aspirin Given Within 24 Hours of Arrival	477	98%	94%	96%
Fibrinolytic Meds Within 30 Min. of Arrival[7]	-	-	47%	58%
Average Time to ECG (minutes)	480	3	8	7
Average Time to Transfer (minutes)	95	43	62	60
Children's Asthma Care				
Received Home Management Plan of Care	-	-	93%	88%
Received Reliever Medication	-	-	100%	100%
Received Systemic Corticosteroids	-	-	100%	100%
Emergency Department				
Admittance Decision Time (minutes)[2]	503	159	99	98
Head CT Results Within 45 Min. of Arrival[1]	-	-	54%	57%
Patients Who Left ER Before Being Seen	>100k	4%	3%	2%
Time from ER Arrival to Admit. (minutes)[2]	505	405	270	274
Time from ER Arrival to Discharge (minutes)	363	239	127	134
Time in ER Before Being Evaluated (minutes)	418	50	26	26
Time to Pain Meds for Fractures (minutes)	187	59	57	57
Heart Attack Care				
Aspirin Given at Discharge	139	99%	99%	99%
Fibrinolytic Meds Within 30 Min. of Arrival[7]	-	-	49%	54%
PCI Within 90 Minutes of Arrival[1]	-	-	95%	96%
Statin Prescribed at Discharge	135	99%	98%	98%
Heart Failure Care				
ACE Inhibitor or ARB for LVSD	391	99%	97%	97%
Discharge Instructions Given	770	96%	95%	94%
Evaluation of LVS Function	867	100%	99%	99%
Medicare Spending				
Medicare Spending per Patient (ratio)	-	1.04	1.03	0.98
Pneumonia Care				
Appropriate Initial Antibiotic Given[2]	69	99%	95%	95%
Blood Culture Timing[2]	152	99%	98%	98%
Pregnancy and Delivery Care				
Newborn Deliveries Scheduled Early	354	3%	7%	6%
Preventive Care				
Immunization for Influenza[2]	547	96%	90%	90%
Immunization for Pneumonia[2]	594	96%	92%	92%

NOTE: Hospital profiles are in alphabetical order by state, then city, then hospital within the city; Rankings exclude hospitals with less than 25 cases except for patient surveys which excludes hospitals with less than 100 cases; (a) 100-299 cases; (1) The number of cases/patients is too few to report; (2) Data submitted were based on a sample of cases/patients; (3) Results are based on a shorter time period than required; (4) Data suppressed by CMS for one or more quarters; (5) Results are not available for this reporting period; (6) Fewer than 100 patients completed the HCAHPS survey; (7) No cases met the criteria for this measure; (8) The lower limit of the confidence interval cannot be calculated if the number of observed infections equals zero; (9) No data are available from the state/territory for this reporting period; (10) The scores shown reflect fewer than 50 completed surveys; (11) There were discrepancies in the data collection process; (12) This measure does not apply to this hospital for this reporting period; (13) Results cannot be calculated for this reporting period; (14) The results for this state are combined with nearby states to protect confidentiality; Please refer to the User's Guide for a full explanation of data.

Measure	Cases	This Hosp.	State Avg.	U.S. Avg.
Stroke Care				
Anticoagulation Therapy for Atrial Fibrillation[2]	17	100%	96%	95%
Antithrombotic Therapy Timing[2]	105	99%	98%	98%
Assessed for Rehabilitation[2]	157	100%	98%	97%
Discharged on Antithrombotic Therapy[2]	123	100%	99%	99%
Discharged on Statin Medication[2]	98	97%	95%	94%
Thrombolytic Therapy Timing[2]	18	89%	68%	66%
Venous Thromboembolism Prophylaxis[2]	163	100%	94%	94%
Written Stroke Educational Materials Given[2]	88	100%	92%	88%
Surgical Care Improvement Project				
Appropriate Beta Blocker Usage[2]	776	99%	98%	98%
Appropriate VTP Within 24 Hours[2]	1,719	99%	98%	98%
Controlled Postoperative Blood Glucose[2]	405	98%	96%	97%
Perioperative Temperature Management[2]	2,005	100%	100%	100%
Prophylactic Antibiotic Selection[2]	1,850	100%	99%	99%
Prophylactic Antibiotic Selection (Outpatient)	571	98%	98%	98%
Prophylactic Antibiotic Stopped[2]	1,803	98%	98%	98%
Prophylactic Antibiotic Timing[2]	1,855	99%	99%	99%
Prophylactic Antibiotic Timing (Outpatient)	573	98%	98%	98%
Urinary Catheter Removal[2]	1,322	99%	98%	97%
Survey of Patients' Hospital Experiences				
Area Around Room 'Always' Quiet at Night	300+	65%	68%	61%
Doctors 'Always' Communicated Well	300+	83%	83%	82%
Home Recovery Information Given	300+	85%	85%	85%
Hospital Given 9 or 10 on 10 Point Scale	300+	74%	73%	71%
Meds 'Always' Explained Before Given	300+	67%	66%	64%
Nurses 'Always' Communicated Well	300+	78%	80%	79%
Pain 'Always' Well Controlled	300+	72%	72%	71%
Room and Bathroom 'Always' Clean	300+	70%	75%	73%
Timely Help 'Always' Received	300+	62%	69%	68%
Would Definitely Recommend Hospital	300+	79%	73%	71%
Use of Medical Imaging				
Cardiac Imaging Stress Test before Surgery	71	4.2%	5.3%	5.3%
Combination Abdominal CT Scan	2,199	5.0%	16.4%	10.5%
Combination Brain/Sinus CT Scan	1,989	1.2%	2.7%	2.7%
Combination Chest CT Scan	1,352	1.3%	5.6%	2.7%
Follow-up Mammogram/Ultrasound	4,921	8.4%	7.9%	8.8%
Lumbar Spine MRI for Low Back Pain	272	39.3%	39.6%	37.2%

Dallas Medical Center

7 Medical Parkway
Dallas, TX 75234
URL: www.rhdmemorial.com
Phone: 972-247-1000
Fax: 972-888-7090
Type: Acute Care Hospitals
Ownership: Proprietary
Emergency Services: Yes
Beds: 155

Key Personnel:

Operating Room. . . . . Tana Carpenter, RN
Radiology. . . . . Joseph Chan, MD
Pediatric Ambulatory Care . . . . . . Kimberly Chesshire, MD
Pediatric In-Patient Care . . . . Kimberly Chesshire, MD
Infection Control. . . . . Patti Grant, RN
Quality Assurance . . . . Priscila Miranda
Chief of Medical Staff. . . . . Chirag Patel, DO
CEO/President. . . . . Dr. Prem Reddy, MD, FACC, FCCP

Measure	Cases	This Hosp.	State Avg.	U.S. Avg.
Blood Clot Prevention and Treatment				
Anticoagulation Overlap Therapy[2]	11	64%	93%	93%
ICU Venous Thromboembolism Prophylaxis[2]	38	63%	92%	92%
Incidence of Potentially Preventable VTE[1,2]	-	-	9%	10%
UFH with Dosages/Platelet Monitoring[1,2]	-	-	96%	97%
Venous Thromboembolism Prophylaxis[2]	235	59%	82%	85%
Warfarin Therapy Discharge Instructions[1,2]	-	-	84%	75%
Chest Pain/Possible Heart Attack Care				
Aspirin Given Within 24 Hours of Arrival[5]	-	-	94%	96%
Fibrinolytic Meds Within 30 Min. of Arrival[5]	-	-	47%	58%
Average Time to ECG (minutes)[5]	-	-	8	7
Average Time to Transfer (minutes)[5]	-	-	62	60
Children's Asthma Care				
Received Home Management Plan of Care	-	-	93%	88%
Received Reliever Medication	-	-	100%	100%
Received Systemic Corticosteroids	-	-	100%	100%
Emergency Department				
Admittance Decision Time (minutes)[2]	287	82	99	98
Head CT Results Within 45 Min. of Arrival[3,7]	-	-	54%	57%
Patients Who Left ER Before Being Seen	11,335	2%	3%	2%
Time from ER Arrival to Admit. (minutes)[2]	322	268	270	274
Time from ER Arrival to Discharge (minutes)	481	111	127	134
Time in ER Before Being Evaluated (minutes)	490	42	26	26
Time to Pain Meds for Fractures (minutes)	37	74	57	57
Heart Attack Care				
Aspirin Given at Discharge	24	100%	99%	99%
Fibrinolytic Meds Within 30 Min. of Arrival[7]	-	-	49%	54%
PCI Within 90 Minutes of Arrival[1]	-	-	95%	96%
Statin Prescribed at Discharge	24	92%	98%	98%
Heart Failure Care				
ACE Inhibitor or ARB for LVSD	21	95%	97%	97%
Discharge Instructions Given	39	87%	95%	94%
Evaluation of LVS Function	56	100%	99%	99%
Medicare Spending				
Medicare Spending per Patient (ratio)	-	1.22	1.03	0.98
Pneumonia Care				
Appropriate Initial Antibiotic Given[2]	33	97%	95%	95%
Blood Culture Timing[2]	42	98%	98%	98%
Pregnancy and Delivery Care				
Newborn Deliveries Scheduled Early[7]	-	-	7%	6%
Preventive Care				
Immunization for Influenza[2]	310	88%	90%	90%
Immunization for Pneumonia[2]	380	79%	92%	92%
Stroke Care				
Anticoagulation Therapy for Atrial Fibrillation[1]	-	-	96%	95%
Antithrombotic Therapy Timing	18	89%	98%	98%
Assessed for Rehabilitation	20	80%	98%	97%
Discharged on Antithrombotic Therapy	18	94%	99%	99%
Discharged on Statin Medication	18	56%	95%	94%
Thrombolytic Therapy Timing[1]	-	-	68%	66%
Venous Thromboembolism Prophylaxis	20	65%	94%	94%
Written Stroke Educational Materials Given[1]	-	-	92%	88%
Surgical Care Improvement Project				
Appropriate Beta Blocker Usage[2]	38	95%	98%	98%
Appropriate VTP Within 24 Hours[2]	154	95%	98%	98%
Controlled Postoperative Blood Glucose[2,7]	-	-	96%	97%
Perioperative Temperature Management[2]	167	99%	100%	100%
Prophylactic Antibiotic Selection[2]	98	98%	99%	99%
Prophylactic Antibiotic Selection (Outpatient)	37	100%	98%	98%
Prophylactic Antibiotic Stopped[2]	93	84%	98%	98%
Prophylactic Antibiotic Timing[2]	98	97%	99%	99%
Prophylactic Antibiotic Timing (Outpatient)	48	75%	98%	98%
Urinary Catheter Removal[2]	101	93%	98%	97%
Survey of Patients' Hospital Experiences				
Area Around Room 'Always' Quiet at Night	300+	60%	68%	61%
Doctors 'Always' Communicated Well	300+	71%	83%	82%
Home Recovery Information Given	300+	76%	85%	85%
Hospital Given 9 or 10 on 10 Point Scale	300+	45%	73%	71%
Meds 'Always' Explained Before Given	300+	43%	66%	64%
Nurses 'Always' Communicated Well	300+	59%	80%	79%
Pain 'Always' Well Controlled	300+	59%	72%	71%
Room and Bathroom 'Always' Clean	300+	58%	75%	73%
Timely Help 'Always' Received	300+	48%	69%	68%
Would Definitely Recommend Hospital	300+	39%	73%	71%
Use of Medical Imaging				
Cardiac Imaging Stress Test before Surgery[1]	-	-	5.3%	5.3%
Combination Abdominal CT Scan	104	21.2%	16.4%	10.5%
Combination Brain/Sinus CT Scan[1]	-	-	2.7%	2.7%
Combination Chest CT Scan[1]	-	-	5.6%	2.7%
Follow-up Mammogram/Ultrasound	182	9.3%	7.9%	8.8%
Lumbar Spine MRI for Low Back Pain[1]	-	-	39.6%	37.2%

Dallas VA Medical Center - VA North Texas

4500 S. Lancaster Road
Dallas, TX 75216
Phone: 214-742-8387
Fax: 214-857-1678
E-mail: ntx_internet_information@med.va.gov
URL: www.north-texas.med.va.gov
Type: Acute Care - VA
Ownership: Government Federal
Emergency Services: No
Beds: 299

Key Personnel:

Radiology. Andre Duerinckx, MD
Quality Assurance . . . . Mike George
Infection Control. . . . . Beverly Gray, MD
Cardiac Laboratory. . . . . Paul Grayburn, MD
Chief of Medical Staff . . . . Clark R. Gregg, MD
CEO/President. . . . . Alan G Harper
Operating Room. . . . . Brenda Summers

Measure	Cases	This Hosp.	State Avg.	U.S. Avg.
Blood Clot Prevention and Treatment				
Anticoagulation Overlap Therapy	-	-	93%	93%
ICU Venous Thromboembolism Prophylaxis	-	-	92%	92%
Incidence of Potentially Preventable VTE	-	-	9%	10%
UFH with Dosages/Platelet Monitoring	-	-	96%	97%
Venous Thromboembolism Prophylaxis	-	-	82%	85%
Warfarin Therapy Discharge Instructions	-	-	84%	75%
Chest Pain/Possible Heart Attack Care				
Aspirin Given Within 24 Hours of Arrival	-	-	94%	96%
Fibrinolytic Meds Within 30 Min. of Arrival	-	-	47%	58%
Average Time to ECG (minutes)	-	-	8	7
Average Time to Transfer (minutes)	-	-	62	60
Children's Asthma Care				
Received Home Management Plan of Care	-	-	93%	88%
Received Reliever Medication	-	-	100%	100%
Received Systemic Corticosteroids	-	-	100%	100%
Emergency Department				
Admittance Decision Time (minutes)	-	-	99	98
Head CT Results Within 45 Min. of Arrival	-	-	54%	57%
Patients Who Left ER Before Being Seen	-	-	3%	2%
Time from ER Arrival to Admit. (minutes)	-	-	270	274
Time from ER Arrival to Discharge (minutes)	-	-	127	134
Time in ER Before Being Evaluated (minutes)	-	-	26	26
Time to Pain Meds for Fractures (minutes)	-	-	57	57
Heart Attack Care				
Aspirin Given at Discharge	102	99%	99%	99%
Fibrinolytic Meds Within 30 Min. of Arrival[5]	-	-	49%	54%
PCI Within 90 Minutes of Arrival[1]	-	-	95%	96%
Statin Prescribed at Discharge	102	100%	98%	98%
Heart Failure Care				
ACE Inhibitor or ARB for LVSD	237	97%	97%	97%
Discharge Instructions Given	552	95%	95%	94%
Evaluation of LVS Function	589	99%	99%	99%
Medicare Spending				
Medicare Spending per Patient (ratio)	-	-	1.03	0.98
Pneumonia Care				
Appropriate Initial Antibiotic Given	96	90%	95%	95%
Blood Culture Timing	175	99%	98%	98%
Pregnancy and Delivery Care				
Newborn Deliveries Scheduled Early	-	-	7%	6%
Preventive Care				
Immunization for Influenza[5]	-	-	90%	90%
Immunization for Pneumonia[5]	-	-	92%	92%
Stroke Care				
Anticoagulation Therapy for Atrial Fibrillation	-	-	96%	95%
Antithrombotic Therapy Timing	-	-	98%	98%
Assessed for Rehabilitation	-	-	98%	97%
Discharged on Antithrombotic Therapy	-	-	99%	99%
Discharged on Statin Medication	-	-	95%	94%
Thrombolytic Therapy Timing	-	-	68%	66%
Venous Thromboembolism Prophylaxis	-	-	94%	94%
Written Stroke Educational Materials Given	-	-	92%	88%
Surgical Care Improvement Project				
Appropriate Beta Blocker Usage[2]	130	99%	98%	98%
Appropriate VTP Within 24 Hours[2]	218	96%	98%	98%
Controlled Postoperative Blood Glucose[2]	74	93%	96%	97%
Perioperative Temperature Management[2]	247	99%	100%	100%
Prophylactic Antibiotic Selection	192	99%	99%	99%
Prophylactic Antibiotic Selection (Outpatient)	-	-	98%	98%
Prophylactic Antibiotic Stopped	188	96%	98%	98%
Prophylactic Antibiotic Timing	194	97%	99%	99%
Prophylactic Antibiotic Timing (Outpatient)	-	-	98%	98%
Urinary Catheter Removal[2]	214	98%	98%	97%
Survey of Patients' Hospital Experiences				
Area Around Room 'Always' Quiet at Night	-	-	68%	61%
Doctors 'Always' Communicated Well	-	-	83%	82%

NOTE: Hospital profiles are in alphabetical order by state, then city, then hospital within the city; Rankings exclude hospitals with less than 25 cases except for patient surveys which excludes hospitals with less than 100 cases; (a) 100-299 cases; (1) The number of cases/patients is too few to report; (2) Data submitted were based on a sample of cases/patients; (3) Results are based on a shorter time period than required; (4) Data suppressed by CMS for one or more quarters; (5) Results are not available for this reporting period; (6) Fewer than 100 patients completed the HCAHPS survey; (7) No cases met the criteria for this measure; (8) The lower limit of the confidence interval cannot be calculated if the number of observed infections equals zero; (9) No data are available from the state/territory for this reporting period; (10) The scores shown reflect fewer than 50 completed surveys; (11) There were discrepancies in the data collection process; (12) This measure does not apply to this hospital for this reporting period; (13) Results cannot be calculated for this reporting period; (14) The results for this state are combined with nearby states to protect confidentiality; Please refer to the User's Guide for a full explanation of data.

Measure	Cases	This Hosp.	State Avg.	U.S. Avg.
Home Recovery Information Given	-	-	85%	85%
Hospital Given 9 or 10 on 10 Point Scale	-	-	73%	71%
Meds 'Always' Explained Before Given	-	-	66%	64%
Nurses 'Always' Communicated Well	-	-	80%	79%
Pain 'Always' Well Controlled	-	-	72%	71%
Room and Bathroom 'Always' Clean	-	-	75%	73%
Timely Help 'Always' Received	-	-	69%	68%
Would Definitely Recommend Hospital	-	-	73%	71%
Use of Medical Imaging				
Cardiac Imaging Stress Test before Surgery	-	-	5.3%	5.3%
Combination Abdominal CT Scan	-	-	16.4%	10.5%
Combination Brain/Sinus CT Scan	-	-	2.7%	2.7%
Combination Chest CT Scan	-	-	5.6%	2.7%
Follow-up Mammogram/Ultrasound	-	-	7.9%	8.8%
Lumbar Spine MRI for Low Back Pain	-	-	39.6%	37.2%

Doctors Hospital

9440 Poppy Dr
Dallas, TX 75218
Phone: 214-324-6100
Fax: 214-324-0612
URL: www.doctorshospitaldallas.com
Type: Acute Care Hospitals
Emergency Services: Yes
Ownership: Proprietary
Beds: 222

Key Personnel:
Chief of Medical Staff . . . . Leonard Comia, MD
Radiology . . . . Dale Fisher, MD
CEO . . . . Jay Krishnaswamy
Pediatric In-Patient Care . . . . Karen Schaute, MD
Quality Assurance . . . . Linda Weld, RN

Measure	Cases	This Hosp.	State Avg.	U.S. Avg.
Blood Clot Prevention and Treatment				
Anticoagulation Overlap Therapy[2]	28	96%	93%	93%
ICU Venous Thromboembolism Prophylaxis[2]	63	98%	92%	92%
Incidence of Potentially Preventable VTE[2]	11	9%	9%	10%
UFH with Dosages/Platelet Monitoring[1,2]	-	-	96%	97%
Venous Thromboembolism Prophylaxis[2]	369	87%	82%	85%
Warfarin Therapy Discharge Instructions[2]	17	100%	84%	75%
Chest Pain/Possible Heart Attack Care				
Aspirin Given Within 24 Hours of Arrival[1,3]	-	-	94%	96%
Fibrinolytic Meds Within 30 Min. of Arrival[3,7]	-	-	47%	58%
Average Time to ECG (minutes)[1,3]	-	-	8	7
Average Time to Transfer (minutes)[3,7]	-	-	62	60
Children's Asthma Care				
Received Home Management Plan of Care	-	-	93%	88%
Received Reliever Medication	-	-	100%	100%
Received Systemic Corticosteroids	-	-	100%	100%
Emergency Department				
Admittance Decision Time (minutes)[2]	698	108	99	98
Head CT Results Within 45 Min. of Arrival[1]	-	-	54%	57%
Patients Who Left ER Before Being Seen	5,818	18%	3%	2%
Time from ER Arrival to Admit. (minutes)[2]	698	283	270	274
Time from ER Arrival to Discharge (minutes)	445	125	127	134
Time in ER Before Being Evaluated (minutes)	491	29	26	26
Time to Pain Meds for Fractures (minutes)	106	58	57	57
Heart Attack Care				
Aspirin Given at Discharge	119	100%	99%	99%
Fibrinolytic Meds Within 30 Min. of Arrival[7]	-	-	49%	54%
PCI Within 90 Minutes of Arrival	21	100%	95%	96%
Statin Prescribed at Discharge	124	99%	98%	98%
Heart Failure Care				
ACE Inhibitor or ARB for LVSD	108	100%	97%	97%
Discharge Instructions Given	223	100%	95%	94%
Evaluation of LVS Function	285	100%	99%	99%
Medicare Spending				
Medicare Spending per Patient (ratio)	-	1.09	1.03	0.98
Pneumonia Care				
Appropriate Initial Antibiotic Given	122	98%	95%	95%
Blood Culture Timing	198	99%	98%	98%
Pregnancy and Delivery Care				
Newborn Deliveries Scheduled Early[2]	45	7%	7%	6%
Preventive Care				
Immunization for Influenza[2]	565	89%	90%	90%
Immunization for Pneumonia[2]	772	97%	92%	92%
Stroke Care				
Anticoagulation Therapy for Atrial Fibrillation[1]	-	-	96%	95%
Antithrombotic Therapy Timing	72	99%	98%	98%
Assessed for Rehabilitation	79	92%	98%	97%
Discharged on Antithrombotic Therapy	74	100%	99%	99%
Discharged on Statin Medication	56	96%	95%	94%
Thrombolytic Therapy Timing[1]	-	-	68%	66%
Venous Thromboembolism Prophylaxis	77	90%	94%	94%
Written Stroke Educational Materials Given	44	100%	92%	88%
Surgical Care Improvement Project				
Appropriate Beta Blocker Usage[2]	103	98%	98%	98%
Appropriate VTP Within 24 Hours[2]	276	98%	98%	98%
Controlled Postoperative Blood Glucose[2]	32	100%	96%	97%
Perioperative Temperature Management[2]	230	99%	100%	100%
Prophylactic Antibiotic Selection[2]	252	100%	99%	99%
Prophylactic Antibiotic Selection (Outpatient)	193	99%	98%	98%
Prophylactic Antibiotic Stopped[2]	246	97%	98%	98%
Prophylactic Antibiotic Timing[2]	253	99%	99%	99%
Prophylactic Antibiotic Timing (Outpatient)	195	99%	98%	98%
Urinary Catheter Removal[2]	256	99%	98%	97%
Survey of Patients' Hospital Experiences				
Area Around Room 'Always' Quiet at Night	300+	66%	68%	61%
Doctors 'Always' Communicated Well	300+	85%	83%	82%
Home Recovery Information Given	300+	83%	85%	85%
Hospital Given 9 or 10 on 10 Point Scale	300+	67%	73%	71%
Meds 'Always' Explained Before Given	300+	60%	66%	64%
Nurses 'Always' Communicated Well	300+	76%	80%	79%
Pain 'Always' Well Controlled	300+	71%	72%	71%
Room and Bathroom 'Always' Clean	300+	66%	75%	73%
Timely Help 'Always' Received	300+	64%	69%	68%
Would Definitely Recommend Hospital	300+	70%	73%	71%
Use of Medical Imaging				
Cardiac Imaging Stress Test before Surgery	248	6.0%	5.3%	5.3%
Combination Abdominal CT Scan	424	7.3%	16.4%	10.5%
Combination Brain/Sinus CT Scan[1]	-	-	2.7%	2.7%
Combination Chest CT Scan	202	0.5%	5.6%	2.7%
Follow-up Mammogram/Ultrasound	1,052	10.6%	7.9%	8.8%
Lumbar Spine MRI for Low Back Pain	37	43.2%	39.6%	37.2%

Medical City Dallas Hospital

7777 Forest Lane
Dallas, TX 75230
Phone: 972-566-6222
Fax: 972-566-6248
E-mail: medcity.main@hcahealthcare.com
URL: www.medicalcityhospital.com
Type: Acute Care Hospitals
Emergency Services: Yes
Ownership: Proprietary
Beds: 598

Key Personnel:
Chief of Medical Staff . . . . Mark Hebert, MD
Quality Assurance . . . . Lisa Steele
CEO/President . . . . Troy A. Villarreal

Measure	Cases	This Hosp.	State Avg.	U.S. Avg.
Blood Clot Prevention and Treatment				
Anticoagulation Overlap Therapy[2]	83	100%	93%	93%
ICU Venous Thromboembolism Prophylaxis[2]	96	100%	92%	92%
Incidence of Potentially Preventable VTE[2]	21	0%	9%	10%
UFH with Dosages/Platelet Monitoring[2]	17	100%	96%	97%
Venous Thromboembolism Prophylaxis[2]	371	93%	82%	85%
Warfarin Therapy Discharge Instructions[2]	62	97%	84%	75%
Chest Pain/Possible Heart Attack Care				
Aspirin Given Within 24 Hours of Arrival[1,3]	-	-	94%	96%
Fibrinolytic Meds Within 30 Min. of Arrival[3,7]	-	-	47%	58%
Average Time to ECG (minutes)[1,3]	-	-	8	7
Average Time to Transfer (minutes)[3,7]	-	-	62	60
Children's Asthma Care				
Received Home Management Plan of Care	-	-	93%	88%
Received Reliever Medication	-	-	100%	100%
Received Systemic Corticosteroids	-	-	100%	100%
Emergency Department				
Admittance Decision Time (minutes)[2]	671	130	99	98
Head CT Results Within 45 Min. of Arrival[1]	-	-	54%	57%
Patients Who Left ER Before Being Seen	76,716	2%	3%	2%
Time from ER Arrival to Admit. (minutes)[2]	671	270	270	274
Time from ER Arrival to Discharge (minutes)	444	142	127	134
Time in ER Before Being Evaluated (minutes)	520	19	26	26
Time to Pain Meds for Fractures (minutes)	292	44	57	57
Heart Attack Care				
Aspirin Given at Discharge	161	100%	99%	99%
Fibrinolytic Meds Within 30 Min. of Arrival[7]	-	-	49%	54%
PCI Within 90 Minutes of Arrival	35	91%	95%	96%
Statin Prescribed at Discharge	152	100%	98%	98%
Heart Failure Care				
ACE Inhibitor or ARB for LVSD	148	100%	97%	97%
Discharge Instructions Given	402	99%	95%	94%
Evaluation of LVS Function	489	100%	99%	99%
Medicare Spending				
Medicare Spending per Patient (ratio)	-	1.05	1.03	0.98
Pneumonia Care				
Appropriate Initial Antibiotic Given	104	100%	95%	95%
Blood Culture Timing	203	100%	98%	98%
Pregnancy and Delivery Care				
Newborn Deliveries Scheduled Early[2]	57	4%	7%	6%
Preventive Care				
Immunization for Influenza[2]	640	97%	90%	90%
Immunization for Pneumonia[2]	568	97%	92%	92%
Stroke Care				
Anticoagulation Therapy for Atrial Fibrillation	36	100%	96%	95%
Antithrombotic Therapy Timing	164	99%	98%	98%
Assessed for Rehabilitation	220	100%	98%	97%
Discharged on Antithrombotic Therapy	180	100%	99%	99%
Discharged on Statin Medication	122	99%	95%	94%
Thrombolytic Therapy Timing[1]	-	-	68%	66%
Venous Thromboembolism Prophylaxis	225	98%	94%	94%
Written Stroke Educational Materials Given	114	95%	92%	88%
Surgical Care Improvement Project				
Appropriate Beta Blocker Usage[2]	253	100%	98%	98%
Appropriate VTP Within 24 Hours[2]	525	100%	98%	98%
Controlled Postoperative Blood Glucose[2]	105	99%	96%	97%
Perioperative Temperature Management[2]	681	100%	100%	100%
Prophylactic Antibiotic Selection[2]	517	99%	99%	99%
Prophylactic Antibiotic Selection (Outpatient)	620	100%	98%	98%
Prophylactic Antibiotic Stopped[2]	481	99%	98%	98%
Prophylactic Antibiotic Timing[2]	517	100%	99%	99%
Prophylactic Antibiotic Timing (Outpatient)	620	100%	98%	98%
Urinary Catheter Removal[2]	365	99%	98%	97%
Survey of Patients' Hospital Experiences				
Area Around Room 'Always' Quiet at Night	300+	71%	68%	61%
Doctors 'Always' Communicated Well	300+	83%	83%	82%
Home Recovery Information Given	300+	86%	85%	85%
Hospital Given 9 or 10 on 10 Point Scale	300+	76%	73%	71%
Meds 'Always' Explained Before Given	300+	62%	66%	64%
Nurses 'Always' Communicated Well	300+	77%	80%	79%
Pain 'Always' Well Controlled	300+	74%	72%	71%
Room and Bathroom 'Always' Clean	300+	75%	75%	73%
Timely Help 'Always' Received	300+	62%	69%	68%
Would Definitely Recommend Hospital	300+	79%	73%	71%
Use of Medical Imaging				
Cardiac Imaging Stress Test before Surgery	528	4.9%	5.3%	5.3%
Combination Abdominal CT Scan	616	7.5%	16.4%	10.5%
Combination Brain/Sinus CT Scan	562	2.3%	2.7%	2.7%
Combination Chest CT Scan	356	1.1%	5.6%	2.7%
Follow-up Mammogram/Ultrasound	1,202	5.5%	7.9%	8.8%
Lumbar Spine MRI for Low Back Pain[1]	-	-	39.6%	37.2%

Methodist Charlton Medical Center

3500 W Wheatland Road
Dallas, TX 75237
Phone: 214-947-7777
Fax: 214-947-7525
URL: www.methodisthealthsystem.org
Type: Acute Care Hospitals
Emergency Services: Yes
Ownership: Voluntary non-profit - Private
Beds: 245

Key Personnel:
Radiology . . . . Carla Anderson
Emergency Room . . . . Thomas Barrows
Operating Room . . . . Barry Bass
Cardiac Laboratory . . . . Kim Hollan
President/CEO . . . . Stephen L. Mansfield, PhD, FACHE

Measure	Cases	This Hosp.	State Avg.	U.S. Avg.
Blood Clot Prevention and Treatment				
Anticoagulation Overlap Therapy[2]	131	99%	93%	93%

NOTE: Hospital profiles are in alphabetical order by state, then city, then hospital within the city; Rankings exclude hospitals with less than 25 cases except for patient surveys which excludes hospitals with less than 100 cases; (a) 100-299 cases; (1) The number of cases/patients is too few to report; (2) Data submitted were based on a sample of cases/patients; (3) Results are based on a shorter time period than required; (4) Data suppressed by CMS for one or more quarters; (5) Results are not available for this reporting period; (6) Fewer than 100 patients completed the HCAHPS survey; (7) No cases met the criteria for this measure; (8) The lower limit of the confidence interval cannot be calculated if the number of observed infections equals zero; (9) No data are available from the state/territory for this reporting period; (10) The scores shown reflect fewer than 50 completed surveys; (11) There were discrepancies in the data collection process; (12) This measure does not apply to this hospital for this reporting period; (13) Results cannot be calculated for this reporting period; (14) The results for this state are combined with nearby states to protect confidentiality; Please refer to the User's Guide for a full explanation of data.

Measure	Cases	This Hosp.	State Avg.	U.S. Avg.
ICU Venous Thromboembolism Prophylaxis[2]	84	98%	92%	92%
Incidence of Potentially Preventable VTE[2]	23	0%	9%	10%
UFH with Dosages/Platelet Monitoring[2]	76	100%	96%	97%
Venous Thromboembolism Prophylaxis[2]	376	96%	82%	85%
Warfarin Therapy Discharge Instructions[2]	90	99%	84%	75%
Chest Pain/Possible Heart Attack Care				
Aspirin Given Within 24 Hours of Arrival	13	100%	94%	96%
Fibrinolytic Meds Within 30 Min. of Arrival[3,7]	-	-	47%	58%
Average Time to ECG (minutes)	13	11	8	7
Average Time to Transfer (minutes)[1,3]	-	-	62	60
Children's Asthma Care				
Received Home Management Plan of Care	-	-	93%	88%
Received Reliever Medication	-	-	100%	100%
Received Systemic Corticosteroids	-	-	100%	100%
Emergency Department				
Admittance Decision Time (minutes)[2]	507	178	99	98
Head CT Results Within 45 Min. of Arrival	20	75%	54%	57%
Patients Who Left ER Before Being Seen	72,069	9%	3%	2%
Time from ER Arrival to Admit. (minutes)[2]	506	416	270	274
Time from ER Arrival to Discharge (minutes)	364	228	127	134
Time in ER Before Being Evaluated (minutes)	401	74	26	26
Time to Pain Meds for Fractures (minutes)	181	97	57	57
Heart Attack Care				
Aspirin Given at Discharge	300	100%	99%	99%
Fibrinolytic Meds Within 30 Min. of Arrival[7]	-	-	49%	54%
PCI Within 90 Minutes of Arrival	55	95%	95%	96%
Statin Prescribed at Discharge	297	100%	98%	98%
Heart Failure Care				
ACE Inhibitor or ARB for LVSD	225	100%	97%	97%
Discharge Instructions Given	465	97%	95%	94%
Evaluation of LVS Function	549	100%	99%	99%
Medicare Spending				
Medicare Spending per Patient (ratio)	-	1.10	1.03	0.98
Pneumonia Care				
Appropriate Initial Antibiotic Given	156	99%	95%	95%
Blood Culture Timing	212	97%	98%	98%
Pregnancy and Delivery Care				
Newborn Deliveries Scheduled Early[2]	257	2%	7%	6%
Preventive Care				
Immunization for Influenza[2]	523	98%	90%	90%
Immunization for Pneumonia[2]	705	98%	92%	92%
Stroke Care				
Anticoagulation Therapy for Atrial Fibrillation[2]	21	100%	96%	95%
Antithrombotic Therapy Timing[2]	180	98%	98%	98%
Assessed for Rehabilitation[2]	183	99%	98%	97%
Discharged on Antithrombotic Therapy[2]	179	100%	99%	99%
Discharged on Statin Medication[2]	136	99%	95%	94%
Thrombolytic Therapy Timing[2]	11	55%	68%	66%
Venous Thromboembolism Prophylaxis[2]	182	98%	94%	94%
Written Stroke Educational Materials Given[2]	95	98%	92%	88%
Surgical Care Improvement Project				
Appropriate Beta Blocker Usage	189	99%	98%	98%
Appropriate VTP Within 24 Hours	527	100%	98%	98%
Controlled Postoperative Blood Glucose	55	100%	96%	97%
Perioperative Temperature Management	579	100%	100%	100%
Prophylactic Antibiotic Selection	432	100%	99%	99%
Prophylactic Antibiotic Selection (Outpatient)	136	99%	98%	98%
Prophylactic Antibiotic Stopped	422	99%	98%	98%
Prophylactic Antibiotic Timing	432	100%	99%	99%
Prophylactic Antibiotic Timing (Outpatient)	137	99%	98%	98%
Urinary Catheter Removal	391	100%	98%	97%
Survey of Patients' Hospital Experiences				
Area Around Room 'Always' Quiet at Night	300+	69%	68%	61%
Doctors 'Always' Communicated Well	300+	76%	83%	82%
Home Recovery Information Given	300+	80%	85%	85%
Hospital Given 9 or 10 on 10 Point Scale	300+	69%	73%	71%
Meds 'Always' Explained Before Given	300+	60%	66%	64%
Nurses 'Always' Communicated Well	300+	76%	80%	79%
Pain 'Always' Well Controlled	300+	70%	72%	71%
Room and Bathroom 'Always' Clean	300+	75%	75%	73%
Timely Help 'Always' Received	300+	58%	69%	68%
Would Definitely Recommend Hospital	300+	66%	73%	71%
Use of Medical Imaging				
Cardiac Imaging Stress Test before Surgery	227	4.8%	5.3%	5.3%
Combination Abdominal CT Scan	851	9.3%	16.4%	10.5%
Combination Brain/Sinus CT Scan	1,063	2.3%	2.7%	2.7%
Combination Chest CT Scan	197	7.6%	5.6%	2.7%
Follow-up Mammogram/Ultrasound	2,286	9.1%	7.9%	8.8%
Lumbar Spine MRI for Low Back Pain	63	44.4%	39.6%	37.2%

Methodist Dallas Medical Center

1441 North Beckley Avenue
Dallas, TX 75203
Phone: 214-947-2879
Fax: 214-947-2519
URL: www.mhd.com
Type: Acute Care Hospitals
Emergency Services: Yes
Ownership: Voluntary non-profit - Other
Beds: 478

Key Personnel:

Radiology. . . . . James Camak, MD
Operating Room. . . . . Larry Creech, RN
CEO/President. . . . . Stephen L Mansfield, FACHE, PhD
Pediatric Ambulatory Care . . . . . . Robert Nelson, MD
Pediatric In-Patient Care . . . . Robert Nelson, MD
Quality Assurance . . . . Sam Ruffing

Measure	Cases	This Hosp.	State Avg.	U.S. Avg.
Blood Clot Prevention and Treatment				
Anticoagulation Overlap Therapy[2]	100	100%	93%	93%
ICU Venous Thromboembolism Prophylaxis[2]	126	100%	92%	92%
Incidence of Potentially Preventable VTE[2]	15	7%	9%	10%
UFH with Dosages/Platelet Monitoring[2]	72	100%	96%	97%
Venous Thromboembolism Prophylaxis[2]	350	100%	82%	85%
Warfarin Therapy Discharge Instructions[2]	76	99%	84%	75%
Chest Pain/Possible Heart Attack Care				
Aspirin Given Within 24 Hours of Arrival[5]	-	-	94%	96%
Fibrinolytic Meds Within 30 Min. of Arrival[5]	-	-	47%	58%
Average Time to ECG (minutes)[5]	-	-	8	7
Average Time to Transfer (minutes)[5]	-	-	62	60
Children's Asthma Care				
Received Home Management Plan of Care	-	-	93%	88%
Received Reliever Medication	-	-	100%	100%
Received Systemic Corticosteroids	-	-	100%	100%
Emergency Department				
Admittance Decision Time (minutes)[2]	477	189	99	98
Head CT Results Within 45 Min. of Arrival[1]	-	-	54%	57%
Patients Who Left ER Before Being Seen	63,702	5%	3%	2%
Time from ER Arrival to Admit. (minutes)[2]	476	368	270	274
Time from ER Arrival to Discharge (minutes)	360	212	127	134
Time in ER Before Being Evaluated (minutes)	403	43	26	26
Time to Pain Meds for Fractures (minutes)	197	83	57	57
Heart Attack Care				
Aspirin Given at Discharge	264	100%	99%	99%
Fibrinolytic Meds Within 30 Min. of Arrival[7]	-	-	49%	54%
PCI Within 90 Minutes of Arrival	33	97%	95%	96%
Statin Prescribed at Discharge	252	100%	98%	98%
Heart Failure Care				
ACE Inhibitor or ARB for LVSD	173	100%	97%	97%
Discharge Instructions Given	417	99%	95%	94%
Evaluation of LVS Function	455	100%	99%	99%
Medicare Spending				
Medicare Spending per Patient (ratio)	-	0.98	1.03	0.98
Pneumonia Care				
Appropriate Initial Antibiotic Given	101	98%	95%	95%
Blood Culture Timing	254	99%	98%	98%
Pregnancy and Delivery Care				
Newborn Deliveries Scheduled Early[2]	316	2%	7%	6%
Preventive Care				
Immunization for Influenza[2]	483	99%	90%	90%
Immunization for Pneumonia[2]	569	98%	92%	92%
Stroke Care				
Anticoagulation Therapy for Atrial Fibrillation[2]	15	100%	96%	95%
Antithrombotic Therapy Timing[2]	153	100%	98%	98%
Assessed for Rehabilitation[2]	209	100%	98%	97%
Discharged on Antithrombotic Therapy[2]	160	100%	99%	99%
Discharged on Statin Medication[2]	110	99%	95%	94%
Thrombolytic Therapy Timing[2]	17	100%	68%	66%
Venous Thromboembolism Prophylaxis[2]	236	100%	94%	94%
Written Stroke Educational Materials Given[2]	115	99%	92%	88%
Surgical Care Improvement Project				
Appropriate Beta Blocker Usage	319	100%	98%	98%
Appropriate VTP Within 24 Hours	1,047	100%	98%	98%
Controlled Postoperative Blood Glucose	97	100%	96%	97%
Perioperative Temperature Management	1,298	100%	100%	100%
Prophylactic Antibiotic Selection	543	100%	99%	99%
Prophylactic Antibiotic Selection (Outpatient)	739	99%	98%	98%
Prophylactic Antibiotic Stopped	538	100%	98%	98%
Prophylactic Antibiotic Timing	544	100%	99%	99%
Prophylactic Antibiotic Timing (Outpatient)	738	100%	98%	98%
Urinary Catheter Removal	720	100%	98%	97%
Survey of Patients' Hospital Experiences				
Area Around Room 'Always' Quiet at Night	300+	63%	68%	61%
Doctors 'Always' Communicated Well	300+	80%	83%	82%
Home Recovery Information Given	300+	81%	85%	85%
Hospital Given 9 or 10 on 10 Point Scale	300+	73%	73%	71%
Meds 'Always' Explained Before Given	300+	66%	66%	64%
Nurses 'Always' Communicated Well	300+	78%	80%	79%
Pain 'Always' Well Controlled	300+	72%	72%	71%
Room and Bathroom 'Always' Clean	300+	71%	75%	73%
Timely Help 'Always' Received	300+	60%	69%	68%
Would Definitely Recommend Hospital	300+	73%	73%	71%
Use of Medical Imaging				
Cardiac Imaging Stress Test before Surgery	141	7.8%	5.3%	5.3%
Combination Abdominal CT Scan	1,017	24.5%	16.4%	10.5%
Combination Brain/Sinus CT Scan	774	0.9%	2.7%	2.7%
Combination Chest CT Scan	683	29.1%	5.6%	2.7%
Follow-up Mammogram/Ultrasound	1,070	8.0%	7.9%	8.8%
Lumbar Spine MRI for Low Back Pain	80	33.8%	39.6%	37.2%

North Central Surgical Center

9301 North Central Expressway Suite 100
Dallas, TX 75231
Phone: 214-265-2810
URL: www.northcentral-sc.com
Type: Acute Care Hospitals
Emergency Services: Yes
Ownership: Voluntary non-profit - Other
Beds: 25

Key Personnel:

Surgery . . . . Richard Anderson, MD
Administrator . . . . Suzanne Greever

Measure	Cases	This Hosp.	State Avg.	U.S. Avg.
Blood Clot Prevention and Treatment				
Anticoagulation Overlap Therapy[2,7]	-	-	93%	93%
ICU Venous Thromboembolism Prophylaxis[2,7]	-	-	92%	92%
Incidence of Potentially Preventable VTE[2,7]	-	-	9%	10%
UFH with Dosages/Platelet Monitoring[2,7]	-	-	96%	97%
Venous Thromboembolism Prophylaxis[2]	62	94%	82%	85%
Warfarin Therapy Discharge Instructions[2,7]	-	-	84%	75%
Chest Pain/Possible Heart Attack Care				
Aspirin Given Within 24 Hours of Arrival[1,3]	-	-	94%	96%
Fibrinolytic Meds Within 30 Min. of Arrival[5]	-	-	47%	58%
Average Time to ECG (minutes)[1,3]	-	-	8	7
Average Time to Transfer (minutes)[5]	-	-	62	60
Children's Asthma Care				
Received Home Management Plan of Care	-	-	93%	88%
Received Reliever Medication	-	-	100%	100%
Received Systemic Corticosteroids	-	-	100%	100%
Emergency Department				
Admittance Decision Time (minutes)[1,2]	-	-	99	98
Head CT Results Within 45 Min. of Arrival[3,7]	-	-	54%	57%
Patients Who Left ER Before Being Seen	1,423	0%	3%	2%
Time from ER Arrival to Admit. (minutes)[1,2]	-	-	270	274
Time from ER Arrival to Discharge (minutes)	289	82	127	134
Time in ER Before Being Evaluated (minutes)	300	10	26	26
Time to Pain Meds for Fractures (minutes)	31	40	57	57
Heart Attack Care				
Aspirin Given at Discharge[5]	-	-	99%	99%
Fibrinolytic Meds Within 30 Min. of Arrival[5]	-	-	49%	54%
PCI Within 90 Minutes of Arrival[5]	-	-	95%	96%
Statin Prescribed at Discharge[5]	-	-	98%	98%
Heart Failure Care				
ACE Inhibitor or ARB for LVSD[5]	-	-	97%	97%
Discharge Instructions Given[5]	-	-	95%	94%
Evaluation of LVS Function[5]	-	-	99%	99%

NOTE: Hospital profiles are in alphabetical order by state, then city, then hospital within the city; Rankings exclude hospitals with less than 25 cases except for patient surveys which excludes hospitals with less than 100 cases; (a) 100-299 cases; (1) The number of cases/patients is too few to report; (2) Data submitted were based on a sample of cases/patients; (3) Results are based on a shorter time period than required; (4) Data suppressed by CMS for one or more quarters; (5) Results are not available for this reporting period; (6) Fewer than 100 patients completed the HCAHPS survey; (7) No cases met the criteria for this measure; (8) The lower limit of the confidence interval cannot be calculated if the number of observed infections equals zero; (9) No data are available from the state/territory for this reporting period; (10) The scores shown reflect fewer than 50 completed surveys; (11) There were discrepancies in the data collection process; (12) This measure does not apply to this hospital for this reporting period; (13) Results cannot be calculated for this reporting period; (14) The results for this state are combined with nearby states to protect confidentiality; Please refer to the User's Guide for a full explanation of data.

Medicare Spending				
Medicare Spending per Patient (ratio)	-	1.06	1.03	0.98
Pneumonia Care				
Appropriate Initial Antibiotic Given[5]	-	-	95%	95%
Blood Culture Timing[5]	-	-	98%	98%
Pregnancy and Delivery Care				
Newborn Deliveries Scheduled Early[7]	-	-	7%	6%
Preventive Care				
Immunization for Influenza[2]	323	64%	90%	90%
Immunization for Pneumonia[2]	283	69%	92%	92%
Stroke Care				
Anticoagulation Therapy for Atrial Fibrillation[5]	-	-	96%	95%
Antithrombotic Therapy Timing[5]	-	-	98%	98%
Assessed for Rehabilitation[5]	-	-	98%	97%
Discharged on Antithrombotic Therapy[5]	-	-	99%	99%
Discharged on Statin Medication[5]	-	-	95%	94%
Thrombolytic Therapy Timing[5]	-	-	68%	66%
Venous Thromboembolism Prophylaxis[5]	-	-	94%	94%
Written Stroke Educational Materials Given[5]	-	-	92%	88%
Surgical Care Improvement Project				
Appropriate Beta Blocker Usage	48	100%	98%	98%
Appropriate VTP Within 24 Hours	507	99%	98%	98%
Controlled Postoperative Blood Glucose[7]	-	-	96%	97%
Perioperative Temperature Management	510	100%	100%	100%
Prophylactic Antibiotic Selection	491	100%	99%	99%
Prophylactic Antibiotic Selection (Outpatient)	364	100%	98%	98%
Prophylactic Antibiotic Stopped	491	100%	98%	98%
Prophylactic Antibiotic Timing	491	100%	99%	99%
Prophylactic Antibiotic Timing (Outpatient)	364	100%	98%	98%
Urinary Catheter Removal	458	100%	98%	97%
Survey of Patients' Hospital Experiences				
Area Around Room 'Always' Quiet at Night	300+	82%	68%	61%
Doctors 'Always' Communicated Well	300+	89%	83%	82%
Home Recovery Information Given	300+	93%	85%	85%
Hospital Given 9 or 10 on 10 Point Scale	300+	90%	73%	71%
Meds 'Always' Explained Before Given	300+	75%	66%	64%
Nurses 'Always' Communicated Well	300+	88%	80%	79%
Pain 'Always' Well Controlled	300+	78%	72%	71%
Room and Bathroom 'Always' Clean	300+	91%	75%	73%
Timely Help 'Always' Received	300+	85%	69%	68%
Would Definitely Recommend Hospital	300+	92%	73%	71%
Use of Medical Imaging				
Cardiac Imaging Stress Test before Surgery[7]	-	-	5.3%	5.3%
Combination Abdominal CT Scan[1]	-	-	16.4%	10.5%
Combination Brain/Sinus CT Scan[1]	-	-	2.7%	2.7%
Combination Chest CT Scan[1]	-	-	5.6%	2.7%
Follow-up Mammogram/Ultrasound[7]	-	-	7.9%	8.8%
Lumbar Spine MRI for Low Back Pain	280	33.9%	39.6%	37.2%

Parkland Health & Hospital System

5201 Harry Hines Blvd
Dallas, TX 75235
Phone: 214-590-8000
Fax: 214-590-8096
URL: www.parklandhospital.com
Type: Acute Care Hospitals
Emergency Services: Yes
Ownership: Govt - Hospital Dist/Auth
Beds: 997

Key Personnel:

CEO/President. . . . . Frederick P. Cerise, MD, MPH
Radiology. . . . . Julie Champine, MD, FACR
Coronary Care . . . . Annie Franklin
Chief of Medical Staff. . . . . Carlos E. Girod, MD, FCCP
Quality Assurance . . . . Terry L Jones
Surgery . . . . Joseph P. Minei, MD, MBA
Anesthesiology. . . . . Babatunde Ogunnaike, MD, MBBS
Pediatrics. . . . . Donna Persaud, MD

Measure	Cases	This Hosp.	State Avg.	U.S. Avg.
Blood Clot Prevention and Treatment				
Anticoagulation Overlap Therapy[2]	155	97%	93%	93%
ICU Venous Thromboembolism Prophylaxis[2]	109	100%	92%	92%
Incidence of Potentially Preventable VTE[2]	67	19%	9%	10%
UFH with Dosages/Platelet Monitoring[2]	140	100%	96%	97%
Venous Thromboembolism Prophylaxis[2]	292	84%	82%	85%
Warfarin Therapy Discharge Instructions[2]	144	1%	84%	75%
Chest Pain/Possible Heart Attack Care				
Aspirin Given Within 24 Hours of Arrival[5]	-	-	94%	96%
Fibrinolytic Meds Within 30 Min. of Arrival[5]	-	-	47%	58%
Average Time to ECG (minutes)[5]	-	-	8	7
Average Time to Transfer (minutes)[5]	-	-	62	60
Children's Asthma Care				
Received Home Management Plan of Care	-	-	93%	88%
Received Reliever Medication	-	-	100%	100%
Received Systemic Corticosteroids	-	-	100%	100%
Emergency Department				
Admittance Decision Time (minutes)[2]	515	243	99	98
Head CT Results Within 45 Min. of Arrival[3,7]	-	-	54%	57%
Patients Who Left ER Before Being Seen	>100k	8%	3%	2%
Time from ER Arrival to Admit. (minutes)[2]	538	442	270	274
Time from ER Arrival to Discharge (minutes)	355	356	127	134
Time in ER Before Being Evaluated (minutes)	228	106	26	26
Time to Pain Meds for Fractures (minutes)	51	90	57	57
Heart Attack Care				
Aspirin Given at Discharge[2]	253	100%	99%	99%
Fibrinolytic Meds Within 30 Min. of Arrival[2,7]	-	-	49%	54%
PCI Within 90 Minutes of Arrival[2]	31	84%	95%	96%
Statin Prescribed at Discharge[2]	252	99%	98%	98%
Heart Failure Care				
ACE Inhibitor or ARB for LVSD[2]	153	99%	97%	97%
Discharge Instructions Given[2]	283	99%	95%	94%
Evaluation of LVS Function[2]	294	100%	99%	99%
Medicare Spending				
Medicare Spending per Patient (ratio)	-	0.91	1.03	0.98
Pneumonia Care				
Appropriate Initial Antibiotic Given[2]	67	97%	95%	95%
Blood Culture Timing[2]	137	99%	98%	98%
Pregnancy and Delivery Care				
Newborn Deliveries Scheduled Early[2]	78	3%	7%	6%
Preventive Care				
Immunization for Influenza[2]	479	86%	90%	90%
Immunization for Pneumonia[2]	380	86%	92%	92%
Stroke Care				
Anticoagulation Therapy for Atrial Fibrillation[1,2]	-	-	96%	95%
Antithrombotic Therapy Timing[2]	82	99%	98%	98%
Assessed for Rehabilitation[2]	131	100%	98%	97%
Discharged on Antithrombotic Therapy[2]	107	100%	99%	99%
Discharged on Statin Medication[2]	77	100%	95%	94%
Thrombolytic Therapy Timing[2]	16	100%	68%	66%
Venous Thromboembolism Prophylaxis[2]	129	99%	94%	94%
Written Stroke Educational Materials Given[2]	92	99%	92%	88%
Surgical Care Improvement Project				
Appropriate Beta Blocker Usage[2]	72	100%	98%	98%
Appropriate VTP Within 24 Hours[2]	359	93%	98%	98%
Controlled Postoperative Blood Glucose[1,2]	-	-	96%	97%
Perioperative Temperature Management[2]	423	100%	100%	100%
Prophylactic Antibiotic Selection[2]	270	98%	99%	99%
Prophylactic Antibiotic Selection (Outpatient)	400	99%	98%	98%
Prophylactic Antibiotic Stopped[2]	266	96%	98%	98%
Prophylactic Antibiotic Timing[2]	271	98%	99%	99%
Prophylactic Antibiotic Timing (Outpatient)	356	94%	98%	98%
Urinary Catheter Removal[2]	244	96%	98%	97%
Survey of Patients' Hospital Experiences				
Area Around Room 'Always' Quiet at Night	300+	52%	68%	61%
Doctors 'Always' Communicated Well	300+	78%	83%	82%
Home Recovery Information Given	300+	85%	85%	85%
Hospital Given 9 or 10 on 10 Point Scale	300+	67%	73%	71%
Meds 'Always' Explained Before Given	300+	62%	66%	64%
Nurses 'Always' Communicated Well	300+	72%	80%	79%
Pain 'Always' Well Controlled	300+	67%	72%	71%
Room and Bathroom 'Always' Clean	300+	67%	75%	73%
Timely Help 'Always' Received	300+	58%	69%	68%
Would Definitely Recommend Hospital	300+	68%	73%	71%
Use of Medical Imaging				
Cardiac Imaging Stress Test before Surgery	411	3.4%	5.3%	5.3%
Combination Abdominal CT Scan	1,153	7.0%	16.4%	10.5%
Combination Brain/Sinus CT Scan	810	2.2%	2.7%	2.7%
Combination Chest CT Scan	1,204	0.2%	5.6%	2.7%
Follow-up Mammogram/Ultrasound	2,134	3.4%	7.9%	8.8%
Lumbar Spine MRI for Low Back Pain	171	36.3%	39.6%	37.2%

Pine Creek Medical Center

9032 Harry Hines Blvd
Dallas, TX 75235
Phone: 214-231-2273
Fax: 214-231-2271
URL: www.pinecreekmedicalcenter.com
Type: Acute Care Hospitals
Emergency Services: Yes
Ownership: Physician

Measure	Cases	This Hosp.	State Avg.	U.S. Avg.
Blood Clot Prevention and Treatment				
Anticoagulation Overlap Therapy[2,7]	-	-	93%	93%
ICU Venous Thromboembolism Prophylaxis[2,7]	-	-	92%	92%
Incidence of Potentially Preventable VTE[2,7]	-	-	9%	10%
UFH with Dosages/Platelet Monitoring[2,7]	-	-	96%	97%
Venous Thromboembolism Prophylaxis[2]	110	96%	82%	85%
Warfarin Therapy Discharge Instructions[2,7]	-	-	84%	75%
Chest Pain/Possible Heart Attack Care				
Aspirin Given Within 24 Hours of Arrival[5]	-	-	94%	96%
Fibrinolytic Meds Within 30 Min. of Arrival[5]	-	-	47%	58%
Average Time to ECG (minutes)[5]	-	-	8	7
Average Time to Transfer (minutes)[5]	-	-	62	60
Children's Asthma Care				
Received Home Management Plan of Care	-	-	93%	88%
Received Reliever Medication	-	-	100%	100%
Received Systemic Corticosteroids	-	-	100%	100%
Emergency Department				
Admittance Decision Time (minutes)[1,2]	-	-	99	98
Head CT Results Within 45 Min. of Arrival[5]	-	-	54%	57%
Patients Who Left ER Before Being Seen	80	20%	3%	2%
Time from ER Arrival to Admit. (minutes)[1,2]	-	-	270	274
Time from ER Arrival to Discharge (minutes)	45	105	127	134
Time in ER Before Being Evaluated (minutes)	82	0	26	26
Time to Pain Meds for Fractures (minutes)[5]	-	-	57	57
Heart Attack Care				
Aspirin Given at Discharge[5]	-	-	99%	99%
Fibrinolytic Meds Within 30 Min. of Arrival[5]	-	-	49%	54%
PCI Within 90 Minutes of Arrival[5]	-	-	95%	96%
Statin Prescribed at Discharge[5]	-	-	98%	98%
Heart Failure Care				
ACE Inhibitor or ARB for LVSD[5]	-	-	97%	97%
Discharge Instructions Given[5]	-	-	95%	94%
Evaluation of LVS Function[5]	-	-	99%	99%
Medicare Spending				
Medicare Spending per Patient (ratio)	-	1.07	1.03	0.98
Pneumonia Care				
Appropriate Initial Antibiotic Given[5]	-	-	95%	95%
Blood Culture Timing[5]	-	-	98%	98%
Pregnancy and Delivery Care				
Newborn Deliveries Scheduled Early[7]	-	-	7%	6%
Preventive Care				
Immunization for Influenza[2]	302	37%	90%	90%
Immunization for Pneumonia[2]	171	32%	92%	92%
Stroke Care				
Anticoagulation Therapy for Atrial Fibrillation[5]	-	-	96%	95%
Antithrombotic Therapy Timing[5]	-	-	98%	98%
Assessed for Rehabilitation[5]	-	-	98%	97%
Discharged on Antithrombotic Therapy[5]	-	-	99%	99%
Discharged on Statin Medication[5]	-	-	95%	94%
Thrombolytic Therapy Timing[5]	-	-	68%	66%
Venous Thromboembolism Prophylaxis[5]	-	-	94%	94%
Written Stroke Educational Materials Given[5]	-	-	92%	88%
Surgical Care Improvement Project				
Appropriate Beta Blocker Usage[2]	41	49%	98%	98%
Appropriate VTP Within 24 Hours[2]	248	89%	98%	98%
Controlled Postoperative Blood Glucose[2,7]	-	-	96%	97%
Perioperative Temperature Management[2]	287	97%	100%	100%
Prophylactic Antibiotic Selection[2]	64	95%	99%	99%
Prophylactic Antibiotic Selection (Outpatient)	249	90%	98%	98%
Prophylactic Antibiotic Stopped[2]	64	97%	98%	98%
Prophylactic Antibiotic Timing[2]	64	89%	99%	99%
Prophylactic Antibiotic Timing (Outpatient)	252	90%	98%	98%
Urinary Catheter Removal[2]	202	93%	98%	97%
Survey of Patients' Hospital Experiences				
Area Around Room 'Always' Quiet at Night	300+	77%	68%	61%

NOTE: Hospital profiles are in alphabetical order by state, then city, then hospital within the city; Rankings exclude hospitals with less than 25 cases except for patient surveys which excludes hospitals with less than 100 cases; (a) 100-299 cases; (1) The number of cases/patients is too few to report; (2) Data submitted were based on a sample of cases/patients; (3) Results are based on a shorter time period than required; (4) Data suppressed by CMS for one or more quarters; (5) Results are not available for this reporting period; (6) Fewer than 100 patients completed the HCAHPS survey; (7) No cases met the criteria for this measure; (8) The lower limit of the confidence interval cannot be calculated if the number of observed infections equals zero; (9) No data are available from the state/territory for this reporting period; (10) The scores shown reflect fewer than 50 completed surveys; (11) There were discrepancies in the data collection process; (12) This measure does not apply to this hospital for this reporting period; (13) Results cannot be calculated for this reporting period; (14) The results for this state are combined with nearby states to protect confidentiality; Please refer to the User's Guide for a full explanation of data.

Doctors 'Always' Communicated Well	300+	83%	83%	82%
Home Recovery Information Given	300+	86%	85%	85%
Hospital Given 9 or 10 on 10 Point Scale	300+	75%	73%	71%
Meds 'Always' Explained Before Given	300+	67%	66%	64%
Nurses 'Always' Communicated Well	300+	77%	80%	79%
Pain 'Always' Well Controlled	300+	72%	72%	71%
Room and Bathroom 'Always' Clean	300+	73%	75%	73%
Timely Help 'Always' Received	300+	73%	69%	68%
Would Definitely Recommend Hospital	300+	73%	73%	71%
Use of Medical Imaging				
Cardiac Imaging Stress Test before Surgery[7]	-	-	5.3%	5.3%
Combination Abdominal CT Scan[1]	-	-	16.4%	10.5%
Combination Brain/Sinus CT Scan[1]	-	-	2.7%	2.7%
Combination Chest CT Scan[1]	-	-	5.6%	2.7%
Follow-up Mammogram/Ultrasound[7]	-	-	7.9%	8.8%
Lumbar Spine MRI for Low Back Pain[1]	-	-	39.6%	37.2%

Texas Health Presbyterian Hospital Dallas

8200 Walnut Hill Lane
Dallas, TX 75231
Phone: 214-345-6789
Fax: 214-345-6093
URL: www.texashealth.org
Type: Acute Care Hospitals
Emergency Services: Yes
Ownership: Voluntary non-profit - Private
Beds: 866

Key Personnel:
Chief of Medical Staff.......... Bobby Abraham
Emergency Room .... A Compton Broders, MD
Operating Room.............. Fran Coch
Intensive Care Unit............ Bev Dorney, RN
CEO .... Douglas D. Hawthorne
CEO/President................ Shawn Parsley, D.O.
Quality Assurance .... Beth Peters
Anesthesiology................ Thomas Russell, MD

Measure	Cases	This Hosp.	State Avg.	U.S. Avg.
Blood Clot Prevention and Treatment				
Anticoagulation Overlap Therapy[2]	100	83%	93%	93%
ICU Venous Thromboembolism Prophylaxis[2]	59	98%	92%	92%
Incidence of Potentially Preventable VTE[2]	19	5%	9%	10%
UFH with Dosages/Platelet Monitoring[2]	40	88%	96%	97%
Venous Thromboembolism Prophylaxis[2]	376	85%	82%	85%
Warfarin Therapy Discharge Instructions[2]	67	31%	84%	75%
Chest Pain/Possible Heart Attack Care				
Aspirin Given Within 24 Hours of Arrival[3,7]	-	-	94%	96%
Fibrinolytic Meds Within 30 Min. of Arrival[5]	-	-	47%	58%
Average Time to ECG (minutes)[3,7]	-	-	8	7
Average Time to Transfer (minutes)[5]	-	-	62	60
Children's Asthma Care				
Received Home Management Plan of Care	-	-	93%	88%
Received Reliever Medication	-	-	100%	100%
Received Systemic Corticosteroids	-	-	100%	100%
Emergency Department				
Admittance Decision Time (minutes)[2]	432	170	99	98
Head CT Results Within 45 Min. of Arrival[1,3]	-	-	54%	57%
Patients Who Left ER Before Being Seen	84,477	1%	3%	2%
Time from ER Arrival to Admit. (minutes)[2]	432	352	270	274
Time from ER Arrival to Discharge (minutes)	394	200	127	134
Time in ER Before Being Evaluated (minutes)	362	52	26	26
Time to Pain Meds for Fractures (minutes)	103	69	57	57
Heart Attack Care				
Aspirin Given at Discharge	432	100%	99%	99%
Fibrinolytic Meds Within 30 Min. of Arrival[7]	-	-	49%	54%
PCI Within 90 Minutes of Arrival	39	95%	95%	96%
Statin Prescribed at Discharge	417	99%	98%	98%
Heart Failure Care				
ACE Inhibitor or ARB for LVSD	200	100%	97%	97%
Discharge Instructions Given	389	98%	95%	94%
Evaluation of LVS Function	566	100%	99%	99%
Medicare Spending				
Medicare Spending per Patient (ratio)	-	1.08	1.03	0.98
Pneumonia Care				
Appropriate Initial Antibiotic Given	181	98%	95%	95%
Blood Culture Timing	198	99%	98%	98%
Pregnancy and Delivery Care				
Newborn Deliveries Scheduled Early	575	8%	7%	6%
Preventive Care				
Immunization for Influenza[2]	560	99%	90%	90%
Immunization for Pneumonia[2]	602	99%	92%	92%
Stroke Care				
Anticoagulation Therapy for Atrial Fibrillation[2]	14	100%	96%	95%
Antithrombotic Therapy Timing[2]	81	100%	98%	98%
Assessed for Rehabilitation[2]	115	96%	98%	97%
Discharged on Antithrombotic Therapy[2]	97	100%	99%	99%
Discharged on Statin Medication[2]	80	100%	95%	94%
Thrombolytic Therapy Timing[1,2]	-	-	68%	66%
Venous Thromboembolism Prophylaxis[2]	115	99%	94%	94%
Written Stroke Educational Materials Given[2]	66	98%	92%	88%
Surgical Care Improvement Project				
Appropriate Beta Blocker Usage[2]	203	99%	98%	98%
Appropriate VTP Within 24 Hours[2]	478	99%	98%	98%
Controlled Postoperative Blood Glucose[2]	145	99%	96%	97%
Perioperative Temperature Management[2]	591	100%	100%	100%
Prophylactic Antibiotic Selection[2]	486	100%	99%	99%
Prophylactic Antibiotic Selection (Outpatient)	667	97%	98%	98%
Prophylactic Antibiotic Stopped[2]	479	99%	98%	98%
Prophylactic Antibiotic Timing[2]	489	99%	99%	99%
Prophylactic Antibiotic Timing (Outpatient)	659	97%	98%	98%
Urinary Catheter Removal[2]	496	99%	98%	97%
Survey of Patients' Hospital Experiences				
Area Around Room 'Always' Quiet at Night	300+	62%	68%	61%
Doctors 'Always' Communicated Well	300+	81%	83%	82%
Home Recovery Information Given	300+	84%	85%	85%
Hospital Given 9 or 10 on 10 Point Scale	300+	74%	73%	71%
Meds 'Always' Explained Before Given	300+	61%	66%	64%
Nurses 'Always' Communicated Well	300+	77%	80%	79%
Pain 'Always' Well Controlled	300+	71%	72%	71%
Room and Bathroom 'Always' Clean	300+	72%	75%	73%
Timely Help 'Always' Received	300+	62%	69%	68%
Would Definitely Recommend Hospital	300+	79%	73%	71%
Use of Medical Imaging				
Cardiac Imaging Stress Test before Surgery	249	2.4%	5.3%	5.3%
Combination Abdominal CT Scan	555	2.0%	16.4%	10.5%
Combination Brain/Sinus CT Scan	881	1.8%	2.7%	2.7%
Combination Chest CT Scan	143	0.7%	5.6%	2.7%
Follow-up Mammogram/Ultrasound	2,714	7.2%	7.9%	8.8%
Lumbar Spine MRI for Low Back Pain[1]	-	-	39.6%	37.2%

Texas Institute for Surgery at Presbyterian Hospital

7115 Greenville Avenue Suite 100
Dallas, TX 75231
Phone: 214-647-5300
Fax: 214-647-5301
URL: www.texasinstituteforsurgery.org
Type: Acute Care Hospitals
Emergency Services: Yes
Ownership: Proprietary

Key Personnel:
Operating Room.............. Rene Clark, RN
President.................... David Helfer
Chief of Medical Staff.......... Molly Hicks

Measure	Cases	This Hosp.	State Avg.	U.S. Avg.
Blood Clot Prevention and Treatment				
Anticoagulation Overlap Therapy[7]	-	-	93%	93%
ICU Venous Thromboembolism Prophylaxis[7]	-	-	92%	92%
Incidence of Potentially Preventable VTE[7]	-	-	9%	10%
UFH with Dosages/Platelet Monitoring[7]	-	-	96%	97%
Venous Thromboembolism Prophylaxis	57	91%	82%	85%
Warfarin Therapy Discharge Instructions[7]	-	-	84%	75%
Chest Pain/Possible Heart Attack Care				
Aspirin Given Within 24 Hours of Arrival[5]	-	-	94%	96%
Fibrinolytic Meds Within 30 Min. of Arrival[5]	-	-	47%	58%
Average Time to ECG (minutes)[5]	-	-	8	7
Average Time to Transfer (minutes)[5]	-	-	62	60
Children's Asthma Care				
Received Home Management Plan of Care	-	-	93%	88%
Received Reliever Medication	-	-	100%	100%
Received Systemic Corticosteroids	-	-	100%	100%
Emergency Department				
Admittance Decision Time (minutes)[7]	-	-	99	98
Head CT Results Within 45 Min. of Arrival[5]	-	-	54%	57%
Patients Who Left ER Before Being Seen	46	0%	3%	2%
Time from ER Arrival to Admit. (minutes)[7]	-	-	270	274
Time from ER Arrival to Discharge (minutes)[5]	-	-	127	134
Time in ER Before Being Evaluated (minutes)[5]	-	-	26	26
Time to Pain Meds for Fractures (minutes)[5]	-	-	57	57
Heart Attack Care				
Aspirin Given at Discharge[5]	-	-	99%	99%
Fibrinolytic Meds Within 30 Min. of Arrival[5]	-	-	49%	54%
PCI Within 90 Minutes of Arrival[5]	-	-	95%	96%
Statin Prescribed at Discharge[5]	-	-	98%	98%
Heart Failure Care				
ACE Inhibitor or ARB for LVSD[5]	-	-	97%	97%
Discharge Instructions Given[5]	-	-	95%	94%
Evaluation of LVS Function[5]	-	-	99%	99%
Medicare Spending				
Medicare Spending per Patient (ratio)	-	1.65	1.03	0.98
Pneumonia Care				
Appropriate Initial Antibiotic Given[5]	-	-	95%	95%
Blood Culture Timing[5]	-	-	98%	98%
Pregnancy and Delivery Care				
Newborn Deliveries Scheduled Early[7]	-	-	7%	6%
Preventive Care				
Immunization for Influenza	135	59%	90%	90%
Immunization for Pneumonia	83	51%	92%	92%
Stroke Care				
Anticoagulation Therapy for Atrial Fibrillation[5]	-	-	96%	95%
Antithrombotic Therapy Timing[5]	-	-	98%	98%
Assessed for Rehabilitation[5]	-	-	98%	97%
Discharged on Antithrombotic Therapy[5]	-	-	99%	99%
Discharged on Statin Medication[5]	-	-	95%	94%
Thrombolytic Therapy Timing[5]	-	-	68%	66%
Venous Thromboembolism Prophylaxis[5]	-	-	94%	94%
Written Stroke Educational Materials Given[5]	-	-	92%	88%
Surgical Care Improvement Project				
Appropriate Beta Blocker Usage[3,7]	-	-	98%	98%
Appropriate VTP Within 24 Hours[3]	152	100%	98%	98%
Controlled Postoperative Blood Glucose[3,7]	-	-	96%	97%
Perioperative Temperature Management[3]	146	99%	100%	100%
Prophylactic Antibiotic Selection[3]	155	99%	99%	99%
Prophylactic Antibiotic Selection (Outpatient)	258	100%	98%	98%
Prophylactic Antibiotic Stopped[3]	155	100%	98%	98%
Prophylactic Antibiotic Timing[3]	156	97%	99%	99%
Prophylactic Antibiotic Timing (Outpatient)	258	96%	98%	98%
Urinary Catheter Removal[3]	151	100%	98%	97%
Survey of Patients' Hospital Experiences				
Area Around Room 'Always' Quiet at Night	(a)	72%	68%	61%
Doctors 'Always' Communicated Well	(a)	90%	83%	82%
Home Recovery Information Given	(a)	97%	85%	85%
Hospital Given 9 or 10 on 10 Point Scale	(a)	90%	73%	71%
Meds 'Always' Explained Before Given	(a)	71%	66%	64%
Nurses 'Always' Communicated Well	(a)	83%	80%	79%
Pain 'Always' Well Controlled	(a)	73%	72%	71%
Room and Bathroom 'Always' Clean	(a)	88%	75%	73%
Timely Help 'Always' Received	(a)	87%	69%	68%
Would Definitely Recommend Hospital	(a)	91%	73%	71%
Use of Medical Imaging				
Cardiac Imaging Stress Test before Surgery[7]	-	-	5.3%	5.3%
Combination Abdominal CT Scan[7]	-	-	16.4%	10.5%
Combination Brain/Sinus CT Scan[7]	-	-	2.7%	2.7%
Combination Chest CT Scan[7]	-	-	5.6%	2.7%
Follow-up Mammogram/Ultrasound[7]	-	-	7.9%	8.8%
Lumbar Spine MRI for Low Back Pain[7]	-	-	39.6%	37.2%

University General Hospital Dallas

2929 South Hampton Road
Dallas, TX 75224
Phone: 214-623-4400
URL: www.shchospital.com
Type: Acute Care Hospitals
Emergency Services: Yes
Ownership: Proprietary
Beds: 111

Measure	Cases	This Hosp.	State Avg.	U.S. Avg.
Blood Clot Prevention and Treatment				
Anticoagulation Overlap Therapy[1,2]	-	-	93%	93%
ICU Venous Thromboembolism Prophylaxis[2]	53	42%	92%	92%
Incidence of Potentially Preventable VTE[2,7]	-	-	9%	10%

NOTE: Hospital profiles are in alphabetical order by state, then city, then hospital within the city; Rankings exclude hospitals with less than 25 cases except for patient surveys which excludes hospitals with less than 100 cases; (a) 100-299 cases; (1) The number of cases/patients is too few to report; (2) Data submitted were based on a sample of cases/patients; (3) Results are based on a shorter time period than required; (4) Data suppressed by CMS for one or more quarters; (5) Results are not available for this reporting period; (6) Fewer than 100 patients completed the HCAHPS survey; (7) No cases met the criteria for this measure; (8) The lower limit of the confidence interval cannot be calculated if the number of observed infections equals zero; (9) No data are available from the state/territory for this reporting period; (10) The scores shown reflect fewer than 50 completed surveys; (11) There were discrepancies in the data collection process; (12) This measure does not apply to this hospital for this reporting period; (13) Results cannot be calculated for this reporting period; (14) The results for this state are combined with nearby states to protect confidentiality; Please refer to the User's Guide for a full explanation of data.

Measure	Cases	This Hosp.	State Avg.	U.S. Avg.
UFH with Dosages/Platelet Monitoring[1,2]	-	-	96%	97%
Venous Thromboembolism Prophylaxis[2]	249	51%	82%	85%
Warfarin Therapy Discharge Instructions[1,2]	-	-	84%	75%
Chest Pain/Possible Heart Attack Care				
Aspirin Given Within 24 Hours of Arrival[1,3]	-	-	94%	96%
Fibrinolytic Meds Within 30 Min. of Arrival[3,7]	-	-	47%	58%
Average Time to ECG (minutes)[1,3]	-	-	8	7
Average Time to Transfer (minutes)[1,3]	-	-	62	60
Children's Asthma Care				
Received Home Management Plan of Care	-	-	93%	88%
Received Reliever Medication	-	-	100%	100%
Received Systemic Corticosteroids	-	-	100%	100%
Emergency Department				
Admittance Decision Time (minutes)[2]	217	75	99	98
Head CT Results Within 45 Min. of Arrival[3,7]	-	-	54%	57%
Patients Who Left ER Before Being Seen	12,576	7%	3%	2%
Time from ER Arrival to Admit. (minutes)[2]	216	275	270	274
Time from ER Arrival to Discharge (minutes)[3]	244	121	127	134
Time in ER Before Being Evaluated (minutes)[3]	248	38	26	26
Time to Pain Meds for Fractures (minutes)[3]	16	108	57	57
Heart Attack Care				
Aspirin Given at Discharge[5]	-	-	99%	99%
Fibrinolytic Meds Within 30 Min. of Arrival[5]	-	-	49%	54%
PCI Within 90 Minutes of Arrival[5]	-	-	95%	96%
Statin Prescribed at Discharge[5]	-	-	98%	98%
Heart Failure Care				
ACE Inhibitor or ARB for LVSD[2]	13	38%	97%	97%
Discharge Instructions Given[2]	42	5%	95%	94%
Evaluation of LVS Function[2]	51	71%	99%	99%
Medicare Spending				
Medicare Spending per Patient (ratio)	-	1.29	1.03	0.98
Pneumonia Care				
Appropriate Initial Antibiotic Given[1,2]	-	-	95%	95%
Blood Culture Timing[1,2]	-	-	98%	98%
Pregnancy and Delivery Care				
Newborn Deliveries Scheduled Early[2,7]	-	-	7%	6%
Preventive Care				
Immunization for Influenza[2]	266	43%	90%	90%
Immunization for Pneumonia[2]	335	48%	92%	92%
Stroke Care				
Anticoagulation Therapy for Atrial Fibrillation[3,7]	-	-	96%	95%
Antithrombotic Therapy Timing[1,3]	-	-	98%	98%
Assessed for Rehabilitation[1,3]	-	-	98%	97%
Discharged on Antithrombotic Therapy[1,3]	-	-	99%	99%
Discharged on Statin Medication[1,3]	-	-	95%	94%
Thrombolytic Therapy Timing[3,7]	-	-	68%	66%
Venous Thromboembolism Prophylaxis[1,3]	-	-	94%	94%
Written Stroke Educational Materials Given[1,3]	-	-	92%	88%
Surgical Care Improvement Project				
Appropriate Beta Blocker Usage[1,2]	-	-	98%	98%
Appropriate VTP Within 24 Hours[2]	25	96%	98%	98%
Controlled Postoperative Blood Glucose[2,7]	-	-	96%	97%
Perioperative Temperature Management[2]	30	57%	100%	100%
Prophylactic Antibiotic Selection[2]	13	100%	99%	99%
Prophylactic Antibiotic Selection (Outpatient)	46	93%	98%	98%
Prophylactic Antibiotic Stopped[2]	13	85%	98%	98%
Prophylactic Antibiotic Timing[2]	19	58%	99%	99%
Prophylactic Antibiotic Timing (Outpatient)	54	83%	98%	98%
Urinary Catheter Removal[2]	22	68%	98%	97%
Survey of Patients' Hospital Experiences				
Area Around Room 'Always' Quiet at Night	(a)	73%	68%	61%
Doctors 'Always' Communicated Well	(a)	80%	83%	82%
Home Recovery Information Given	(a)	81%	85%	85%
Hospital Given 9 or 10 on 10 Point Scale	(a)	57%	73%	71%
Meds 'Always' Explained Before Given	(a)	68%	66%	64%
Nurses 'Always' Communicated Well	(a)	74%	80%	79%
Pain 'Always' Well Controlled	(a)	73%	72%	71%
Room and Bathroom 'Always' Clean	(a)	69%	75%	73%
Timely Help 'Always' Received	(a)	60%	69%	68%
Would Definitely Recommend Hospital	(a)	57%	73%	71%
Use of Medical Imaging				
Cardiac Imaging Stress Test before Surgery[1]	-	-	5.3%	5.3%
Combination Abdominal CT Scan	67	17.9%	16.4%	10.5%
Combination Brain/Sinus CT Scan[1]	-	-	2.7%	2.7%
Combination Chest CT Scan[1]	-	-	5.6%	2.7%
Follow-up Mammogram/Ultrasound[7]	-	-	7.9%	8.8%
Lumbar Spine MRI for Low Back Pain[1]	-	-	39.6%	37.2%

UT Southwestern University Hospital

5909 Harry Hines Blvd
Dallas, TX 75390
Phone: 214-879-3758
URL: www.utsouthwestern.edu
Type: Acute Care Hospitals
Emergency Services: Yes
Ownership: Government - State
Beds: 271

Key Personnel:

Chief of Medical Staff.......... Patricia Bergen
Surgery.................... Michael Choti, MD
Patient Relations .... Carol Key
Ambulatory Care .... Bruce Meyer
Pediatrics................... Julio Perez Fontan, MD
CEO/President............... Daniel K. Podolsky, MD
Radiology................... Neil M. Rofsky, MD
Emergency Room .... Shannon Wentz

Measure	Cases	This Hosp.	State Avg.	U.S. Avg.
Blood Clot Prevention and Treatment				
Anticoagulation Overlap Therapy[2]	119	96%	93%	93%
ICU Venous Thromboembolism Prophylaxis[2]	124	96%	92%	92%
Incidence of Potentially Preventable VTE[2]	35	3%	9%	10%
UFH with Dosages/Platelet Monitoring[2]	115	100%	96%	97%
Venous Thromboembolism Prophylaxis[2]	383	91%	82%	85%
Warfarin Therapy Discharge Instructions[2]	88	90%	84%	75%
Chest Pain/Possible Heart Attack Care				
Aspirin Given Within 24 Hours of Arrival[5]	-	-	94%	96%
Fibrinolytic Meds Within 30 Min. of Arrival[5]	-	-	47%	58%
Average Time to ECG (minutes)[5]	-	-	8	7
Average Time to Transfer (minutes)[5]	-	-	62	60
Children's Asthma Care				
Received Home Management Plan of Care	-	-	93%	88%
Received Reliever Medication	-	-	100%	100%
Received Systemic Corticosteroids	-	-	100%	100%
Emergency Department				
Admittance Decision Time (minutes)[2]	436	122	99	98
Head CT Results Within 45 Min. of Arrival	41	66%	54%	57%
Patients Who Left ER Before Being Seen	37,102	4%	3%	2%
Time from ER Arrival to Admit. (minutes)[2]	447	374	270	274
Time from ER Arrival to Discharge (minutes)	444	219	127	134
Time in ER Before Being Evaluated (minutes)	477	43	26	26
Time to Pain Meds for Fractures (minutes)	61	87	57	57
Heart Attack Care				
Aspirin Given at Discharge	109	98%	99%	99%
Fibrinolytic Meds Within 30 Min. of Arrival[7]	-	-	49%	54%
PCI Within 90 Minutes of Arrival	14	100%	95%	96%
Statin Prescribed at Discharge	105	100%	98%	98%
Heart Failure Care				
ACE Inhibitor or ARB for LVSD	225	100%	97%	97%
Discharge Instructions Given	502	94%	95%	94%
Evaluation of LVS Function	566	100%	99%	99%
Medicare Spending				
Medicare Spending per Patient (ratio)	-	1.03	1.03	0.98
Pneumonia Care				
Appropriate Initial Antibiotic Given	87	100%	95%	95%
Blood Culture Timing	241	99%	98%	98%
Pregnancy and Delivery Care				
Newborn Deliveries Scheduled Early[2]	42	0%	7%	6%
Preventive Care				
Immunization for Influenza[2]	545	96%	90%	90%
Immunization for Pneumonia[2]	652	98%	92%	92%
Stroke Care				
Anticoagulation Therapy for Atrial Fibrillation[1]	-	-	96%	95%
Antithrombotic Therapy Timing	26	96%	98%	98%
Assessed for Rehabilitation	35	100%	98%	97%
Discharged on Antithrombotic Therapy	32	100%	99%	99%
Discharged on Statin Medication	26	92%	95%	94%
Thrombolytic Therapy Timing[7]	-	-	68%	66%
Venous Thromboembolism Prophylaxis	35	80%	94%	94%
Written Stroke Educational Materials Given	17	94%	92%	88%
Surgical Care Improvement Project				
Appropriate Beta Blocker Usage[2]	267	99%	98%	98%
Appropriate VTP Within 24 Hours[2]	487	99%	98%	98%
Controlled Postoperative Blood Glucose[2]	185	97%	96%	97%
Perioperative Temperature Management[2]	576	100%	100%	100%
Prophylactic Antibiotic Selection[2]	560	98%	99%	99%
Prophylactic Antibiotic Selection (Outpatient)	248	99%	98%	98%
Prophylactic Antibiotic Stopped[2]	555	98%	98%	98%
Prophylactic Antibiotic Timing[2]	565	98%	99%	99%
Prophylactic Antibiotic Timing (Outpatient)	248	98%	98%	98%
Urinary Catheter Removal[2]	526	99%	98%	97%
Survey of Patients' Hospital Experiences				
Area Around Room 'Always' Quiet at Night	300+	66%	68%	61%
Doctors 'Always' Communicated Well	300+	86%	83%	82%
Home Recovery Information Given	300+	88%	85%	85%
Hospital Given 9 or 10 on 10 Point Scale	300+	77%	73%	71%
Meds 'Always' Explained Before Given	300+	66%	66%	64%
Nurses 'Always' Communicated Well	300+	82%	80%	79%
Pain 'Always' Well Controlled	300+	72%	72%	71%
Room and Bathroom 'Always' Clean	300+	70%	75%	73%
Timely Help 'Always' Received	300+	65%	69%	68%
Would Definitely Recommend Hospital	300+	81%	73%	71%
Use of Medical Imaging				
Cardiac Imaging Stress Test before Surgery	290	8.6%	5.3%	5.3%
Combination Abdominal CT Scan	1,423	14.1%	16.4%	10.5%
Combination Brain/Sinus CT Scan	791	1.1%	2.7%	2.7%
Combination Chest CT Scan	2,053	0.0%	5.6%	2.7%
Follow-up Mammogram/Ultrasound	2,792	10.3%	7.9%	8.8%
Lumbar Spine MRI for Low Back Pain	244	38.9%	39.6%	37.2%

UT Southwestern University Hospital -Zale Lipshy

5151 Harry Hines Blvd
Dallas, TX 75390
Phone: 214-879-3758
Fax: 214-645-5663
URL: www.utsouthwestern.edu/utsw/home/pc/universityhospitals
Type: Acute Care Hospitals
Emergency Services: No
Ownership: Government - State
Beds: 151

Key Personnel:

Radiology.................. W Phil Evans
Chief of Medical Staff.......... Steven Leach, MD
Quality Assurance .... W. Gary Reed, MD
CEO/President................ Don Smithburg

Measure	Cases	This Hosp.	State Avg.	U.S. Avg.
Blood Clot Prevention and Treatment				
Anticoagulation Overlap Therapy[2]	12	100%	93%	93%
ICU Venous Thromboembolism Prophylaxis[2]	110	98%	92%	92%
Incidence of Potentially Preventable VTE[2]	18	6%	9%	10%
UFH with Dosages/Platelet Monitoring[1,2]	-	-	96%	97%
Venous Thromboembolism Prophylaxis[2]	205	97%	82%	85%
Warfarin Therapy Discharge Instructions[1,2]	-	-	84%	75%
Chest Pain/Possible Heart Attack Care				
Aspirin Given Within 24 Hours of Arrival[5]	-	-	94%	96%
Fibrinolytic Meds Within 30 Min. of Arrival[5]	-	-	47%	58%
Average Time to ECG (minutes)[5]	-	-	8	7
Average Time to Transfer (minutes)[5]	-	-	62	60
Children's Asthma Care				
Received Home Management Plan of Care	-	-	93%	88%
Received Reliever Medication	-	-	100%	100%
Received Systemic Corticosteroids	-	-	100%	100%
Emergency Department				
Admittance Decision Time (minutes)[2,7]	-	-	99	98
Head CT Results Within 45 Min. of Arrival[5]	-	-	54%	57%
Patients Who Left ER Before Being Seen[5]	-	-	3%	2%
Time from ER Arrival to Admit. (minutes)[2,7]	-	-	270	274
Time from ER Arrival to Discharge (minutes)[5]	-	-	127	134
Time in ER Before Being Evaluated (minutes)[5]	-	-	26	26
Time to Pain Meds for Fractures (minutes)[5]	-	-	57	57
Heart Attack Care				
Aspirin Given at Discharge[5]	-	-	99%	99%
Fibrinolytic Meds Within 30 Min. of Arrival[5]	-	-	49%	54%
PCI Within 90 Minutes of Arrival[5]	-	-	95%	96%
Statin Prescribed at Discharge[5]	-	-	98%	98%
Heart Failure Care				
ACE Inhibitor or ARB for LVSD[3,7]	-	-	97%	97%

NOTE: Hospital profiles are in alphabetical order by state, then city, then hospital within the city; Rankings exclude hospitals with less than 25 cases except for patient surveys which excludes hospitals with less than 100 cases; (a) 100-299 cases; (1) The number of cases/patients is too few to report; (2) Data submitted were based on a sample of cases/patients; (3) Results are based on a shorter time period than required; (4) Data suppressed by CMS for one or more quarters; (5) Results are not available for this reporting period; (6) Fewer than 100 patients completed the HCAHPS survey; (7) No cases met the criteria for this measure; (8) The lower limit of the confidence interval cannot be calculated if the number of observed infections equals zero; (9) No data are available from the state/territory for this reporting period; (10) The scores shown reflect fewer than 50 completed surveys; (11) There were discrepancies in the data collection process; (12) This measure does not apply to this hospital for this reporting period; (13) Results cannot be calculated for this reporting period; (14) The results for this state are combined with nearby states to protect confidentiality; Please refer to the User's Guide for a full explanation of data.

Measure	Cases	This Hosp.	State Avg.	U.S. Avg.
Discharge Instructions Given[3,7]	-	-	95%	94%
Evaluation of LVS Function[3,7]	-	-	99%	99%
Medicare Spending				
Medicare Spending per Patient (ratio)	-	0.94	1.03	0.98
Pneumonia Care				
Appropriate Initial Antibiotic Given[7]	-	-	95%	95%
Blood Culture Timing[7]	-	-	98%	98%
Pregnancy and Delivery Care				
Newborn Deliveries Scheduled Early[7]	-	-	7%	6%
Preventive Care				
Immunization for Influenza[2]	607	96%	90%	90%
Immunization for Pneumonia[2]	639	97%	92%	92%
Stroke Care				
Anticoagulation Therapy for Atrial Fibrillation[2]	15	100%	96%	95%
Antithrombotic Therapy Timing[2]	80	99%	98%	98%
Assessed for Rehabilitation[2]	153	99%	98%	97%
Discharged on Antithrombotic Therapy[2]	92	99%	99%	99%
Discharged on Statin Medication[2]	62	97%	95%	94%
Thrombolytic Therapy Timing[2,7]	-	-	68%	66%
Venous Thromboembolism Prophylaxis[2]	165	99%	94%	94%
Written Stroke Educational Materials Given[2]	77	99%	92%	88%
Surgical Care Improvement Project				
Appropriate Beta Blocker Usage[2]	29	100%	98%	98%
Appropriate VTP Within 24 Hours[2]	96	100%	98%	98%
Controlled Postoperative Blood Glucose[2,7]	-	-	96%	97%
Perioperative Temperature Management[2]	127	99%	100%	100%
Prophylactic Antibiotic Selection[1,2]	-	-	99%	99%
Prophylactic Antibiotic Selection (Outpatient)	237	99%	98%	98%
Prophylactic Antibiotic Stopped[1,2]	-	-	98%	98%
Prophylactic Antibiotic Timing[1,2]	-	-	99%	99%
Prophylactic Antibiotic Timing (Outpatient)	237	99%	98%	98%
Urinary Catheter Removal[2]	26	96%	98%	97%
Survey of Patients' Hospital Experiences				
Area Around Room 'Always' Quiet at Night	300+	73%	68%	61%
Doctors 'Always' Communicated Well	300+	85%	83%	82%
Home Recovery Information Given	300+	87%	85%	85%
Hospital Given 9 or 10 on 10 Point Scale	300+	85%	73%	71%
Meds 'Always' Explained Before Given	300+	71%	66%	64%
Nurses 'Always' Communicated Well	300+	84%	80%	79%
Pain 'Always' Well Controlled	300+	78%	72%	71%
Room and Bathroom 'Always' Clean	300+	75%	75%	73%
Timely Help 'Always' Received	300+	71%	69%	68%
Would Definitely Recommend Hospital	300+	89%	73%	71%
Use of Medical Imaging				
Cardiac Imaging Stress Test before Surgery[1]	-	-	5.3%	5.3%
Combination Abdominal CT Scan	552	31.9%	16.4%	10.5%
Combination Brain/Sinus CT Scan	56	0.0%	2.7%	2.7%
Combination Chest CT Scan	471	0.4%	5.6%	2.7%
Follow-up Mammogram/Ultrasound[7]	-	-	7.9%	8.8%
Lumbar Spine MRI for Low Back Pain[1]	-	-	39.6%	37.2%

Wise Regional Health System

609 Medical Center Drive
Decatur, TX 76234
Phone: 940-627-5921
Fax: 940-626-0119
URL: www.wiseregional.com
Type: Acute Care Hospitals
Emergency Services: Yes
Ownership: Govt - Hospital Dist/Auth
Beds: 99

Key Personnel:

Radiology. . . . . Douglas Beall
Anesthesiology. . . . . David Blaylock, MD
Operating Room. . . . . Mark Gross
Intensive Care Unit. . . . . Pam Martin
Emergency Room . . . . Tim McIntyre
Infection Control. . . . . Kay Pugsley
Pediatric In-Patient Care . . . . Ron Smith, MD
CEO/President. . . . . Steve Summers

Measure	Cases	This Hosp.	State Avg.	U.S. Avg.
Blood Clot Prevention and Treatment				
Anticoagulation Overlap Therapy[2]	24	100%	93%	93%
ICU Venous Thromboembolism Prophylaxis[2]	145	87%	92%	92%
Incidence of Potentially Preventable VTE[1,2]	-	-	9%	10%
UFH with Dosages/Platelet Monitoring[1,2]	-	-	96%	97%
Venous Thromboembolism Prophylaxis[2]	269	80%	82%	85%
Warfarin Therapy Discharge Instructions[2]	17	88%	84%	75%
Chest Pain/Possible Heart Attack Care				
Aspirin Given Within 24 Hours of Arrival[1,3]	-	-	94%	96%
Fibrinolytic Meds Within 30 Min. of Arrival[5]	-	-	47%	58%
Average Time to ECG (minutes)[1,3]	-	-	8	7
Average Time to Transfer (minutes)[5]	-	-	62	60
Children's Asthma Care				
Received Home Management Plan of Care	-	-	93%	88%
Received Reliever Medication	-	-	100%	100%
Received Systemic Corticosteroids	-	-	100%	100%
Emergency Department				
Admittance Decision Time (minutes)[2]	511	84	99	98
Head CT Results Within 45 Min. of Arrival	13	92%	54%	57%
Patients Who Left ER Before Being Seen	25,611	1%	3%	2%
Time from ER Arrival to Admit. (minutes)[2]	511	237	270	274
Time from ER Arrival to Discharge (minutes)	546	123	127	134
Time in ER Before Being Evaluated (minutes)	597	19	26	26
Time to Pain Meds for Fractures (minutes)	123	60	57	57
Heart Attack Care				
Aspirin Given at Discharge	150	96%	99%	99%
Fibrinolytic Meds Within 30 Min. of Arrival[7]	-	-	49%	54%
PCI Within 90 Minutes of Arrival	16	94%	95%	96%
Statin Prescribed at Discharge	148	96%	98%	98%
Heart Failure Care				
ACE Inhibitor or ARB for LVSD	53	92%	97%	97%
Discharge Instructions Given	114	94%	95%	94%
Evaluation of LVS Function	145	99%	99%	99%
Medicare Spending				
Medicare Spending per Patient (ratio)	-	1.07	1.03	0.98
Pneumonia Care				
Appropriate Initial Antibiotic Given	96	97%	95%	95%
Blood Culture Timing	167	99%	98%	98%
Pregnancy and Delivery Care				
Newborn Deliveries Scheduled Early	70	20%	7%	6%
Preventive Care				
Immunization for Influenza[2]	501	92%	90%	90%
Immunization for Pneumonia[2]	643	94%	92%	92%
Stroke Care				
Anticoagulation Therapy for Atrial Fibrillation[1]	-	-	96%	95%
Antithrombotic Therapy Timing	38	97%	98%	98%
Assessed for Rehabilitation	57	100%	98%	97%
Discharged on Antithrombotic Therapy	55	98%	99%	99%
Discharged on Statin Medication	34	88%	95%	94%
Thrombolytic Therapy Timing[1]	-	-	68%	66%
Venous Thromboembolism Prophylaxis	48	96%	94%	94%
Written Stroke Educational Materials Given	29	97%	92%	88%
Surgical Care Improvement Project				
Appropriate Beta Blocker Usage[2]	112	96%	98%	98%
Appropriate VTP Within 24 Hours[2]	226	98%	98%	98%
Controlled Postoperative Blood Glucose[2]	48	94%	96%	97%
Perioperative Temperature Management[2]	290	100%	100%	100%
Prophylactic Antibiotic Selection[2]	223	91%	99%	99%
Prophylactic Antibiotic Selection (Outpatient)	166	98%	98%	98%
Prophylactic Antibiotic Stopped[2]	210	83%	98%	98%
Prophylactic Antibiotic Timing[2]	224	98%	99%	99%
Prophylactic Antibiotic Timing (Outpatient)	168	98%	98%	98%
Urinary Catheter Removal[2]	202	93%	98%	97%
Survey of Patients' Hospital Experiences				
Area Around Room 'Always' Quiet at Night	300+	64%	68%	61%
Doctors 'Always' Communicated Well	300+	82%	83%	82%
Home Recovery Information Given	300+	86%	85%	85%
Hospital Given 9 or 10 on 10 Point Scale	300+	74%	73%	71%
Meds 'Always' Explained Before Given	300+	64%	66%	64%
Nurses 'Always' Communicated Well	300+	79%	80%	79%
Pain 'Always' Well Controlled	300+	71%	72%	71%
Room and Bathroom 'Always' Clean	300+	74%	75%	73%
Timely Help 'Always' Received	300+	68%	69%	68%
Would Definitely Recommend Hospital	300+	78%	73%	71%
Use of Medical Imaging				
Cardiac Imaging Stress Test before Surgery[1]	-	-	5.3%	5.3%
Combination Abdominal CT Scan	605	11.9%	16.4%	10.5%
Combination Brain/Sinus CT Scan[1]	-	-	2.7%	2.7%
Combination Chest CT Scan	391	1.3%	5.6%	2.7%
Follow-up Mammogram/Ultrasound	486	9.7%	7.9%	8.8%
Lumbar Spine MRI for Low Back Pain	292	34.9%	39.6%	37.2%

Val Verde Regional Medical Center

801 Bedell Ave
Del Rio, TX 78840
Phone: 830-775-8566
Fax: 830-768-2630
E-mail: info@vvrmc.org
URL: www.vvrmc.org
Type: Acute Care Hospitals
Emergency Services: Yes
Ownership: Govt - Hospital Dist/Auth
Beds: 93

Key Personnel:

Quality Assurance . . . . Kathy Fletcher
CEO/President. . . . . Jack Houghton
Operating Room. . . . . Terry Lindsey
Infection Control. . . . . Charlie Linebaugh
Emergency Room . . . . Marjorie Mellott
Radiology. . . . . Joe Sanders
Intensive Care Unit. . . . . Gloria Villegas, RN
Chief of Medical Staff . . . . Gloria Ziegler

Measure	Cases	This Hosp.	State Avg.	U.S. Avg.
Blood Clot Prevention and Treatment				
Anticoagulation Overlap Therapy[2]	16	100%	93%	93%
ICU Venous Thromboembolism Prophylaxis[2]	51	73%	92%	92%
Incidence of Potentially Preventable VTE[1,2]	-	-	9%	10%
UFH with Dosages/Platelet Monitoring[1,2]	-	-	96%	97%
Venous Thromboembolism Prophylaxis[2]	239	59%	82%	85%
Warfarin Therapy Discharge Instructions[2]	11	100%	84%	75%
Chest Pain/Possible Heart Attack Care				
Aspirin Given Within 24 Hours of Arrival	102	90%	94%	96%
Fibrinolytic Meds Within 30 Min. of Arrival[1]	-	-	47%	58%
Average Time to ECG (minutes)	107	6	8	7
Average Time to Transfer (minutes)[1]	-	-	62	60
Children's Asthma Care				
Received Home Management Plan of Care	-	-	93%	88%
Received Reliever Medication	-	-	100%	100%
Received Systemic Corticosteroids	-	-	100%	100%
Emergency Department				
Admittance Decision Time (minutes)[2]	327	43	99	98
Head CT Results Within 45 Min. of Arrival	26	27%	54%	57%
Patients Who Left ER Before Being Seen	25,335	2%	3%	2%
Time from ER Arrival to Admit. (minutes)[2]	343	213	270	274
Time from ER Arrival to Discharge (minutes)	1,430	115	127	134
Time in ER Before Being Evaluated (minutes)	1,492	21	26	26
Time to Pain Meds for Fractures (minutes)	144	59	57	57
Heart Attack Care				
Aspirin Given at Discharge	19	100%	99%	99%
Fibrinolytic Meds Within 30 Min. of Arrival[7]	-	-	49%	54%
PCI Within 90 Minutes of Arrival[7]	-	-	95%	96%
Statin Prescribed at Discharge	20	100%	98%	98%
Heart Failure Care				
ACE Inhibitor or ARB for LVSD	36	100%	97%	97%
Discharge Instructions Given	122	99%	95%	94%
Evaluation of LVS Function	136	100%	99%	99%
Medicare Spending				
Medicare Spending per Patient (ratio)	-	0.88	1.03	0.98
Pneumonia Care				
Appropriate Initial Antibiotic Given	42	95%	95%	95%
Blood Culture Timing	83	100%	98%	98%
Pregnancy and Delivery Care				
Newborn Deliveries Scheduled Early	133	2%	7%	6%
Preventive Care				
Immunization for Influenza[2]	298	91%	90%	90%
Immunization for Pneumonia[2]	301	93%	92%	92%
Stroke Care				
Anticoagulation Therapy for Atrial Fibrillation[1]	-	-	96%	95%
Antithrombotic Therapy Timing	13	100%	98%	98%
Assessed for Rehabilitation	13	77%	98%	97%
Discharged on Antithrombotic Therapy	12	100%	99%	99%
Discharged on Statin Medication[1]	-	-	95%	94%
Thrombolytic Therapy Timing[1]	-	-	68%	66%
Venous Thromboembolism Prophylaxis	19	63%	94%	94%
Written Stroke Educational Materials Given[1]	-	-	92%	88%
Surgical Care Improvement Project				
Appropriate Beta Blocker Usage	28	100%	98%	98%

NOTE: Hospital profiles are in alphabetical order by state, then city, then hospital within the city; Rankings exclude hospitals with less than 25 cases except for patient surveys which excludes hospitals with less than 100 cases; (a) 100-299 cases; (1) The number of cases/patients is too few to report; (2) Data submitted were based on a sample of cases/patients; (3) Results are based on a shorter time period than required; (4) Data suppressed by CMS for one or more quarters; (5) Results are not available for this reporting period; (6) Fewer than 100 patients completed the HCAHPS survey; (7) No cases met the criteria for this measure; (8) The lower limit of the confidence interval cannot be calculated if the number of observed infections equals zero; (9) No data are available from the state/territory for this reporting period; (10) The scores shown reflect fewer than 50 completed surveys; (11) There were discrepancies in the data collection process; (12) This measure does not apply to this hospital for this reporting period; (13) Results cannot be calculated for this reporting period; (14) The results for this state are combined with nearby states to protect confidentiality; Please refer to the User's Guide for a full explanation of data.

Appropriate VTP Within 24 Hours	115	100%	98%	98%
Controlled Postoperative Blood Glucose[7]	-	-	96%	97%
Perioperative Temperature Management	121	100%	100%	100%
Prophylactic Antibiotic Selection	78	99%	99%	99%
Prophylactic Antibiotic Selection (Outpatient)	30	93%	98%	98%
Prophylactic Antibiotic Stopped	76	96%	98%	98%
Prophylactic Antibiotic Timing	79	100%	99%	99%
Prophylactic Antibiotic Timing (Outpatient)	32	88%	98%	98%
Urinary Catheter Removal	62	95%	98%	97%
Survey of Patients' Hospital Experiences				
Area Around Room 'Always' Quiet at Night	300+	61%	68%	61%
Doctors 'Always' Communicated Well	300+	81%	83%	82%
Home Recovery Information Given	300+	83%	85%	85%
Hospital Given 9 or 10 on 10 Point Scale	300+	58%	73%	71%
Meds 'Always' Explained Before Given	300+	63%	66%	64%
Nurses 'Always' Communicated Well	300+	77%	80%	79%
Pain 'Always' Well Controlled	300+	72%	72%	71%
Room and Bathroom 'Always' Clean	300+	77%	75%	73%
Timely Help 'Always' Received	300+	66%	69%	68%
Would Definitely Recommend Hospital	300+	61%	73%	71%
Use of Medical Imaging				
Cardiac Imaging Stress Test before Surgery	67	0.0%	5.3%	5.3%
Combination Abdominal CT Scan	442	14.3%	16.4%	10.5%
Combination Brain/Sinus CT Scan	439	5.0%	2.7%	2.7%
Combination Chest CT Scan	173	9.2%	5.6%	2.7%
Follow-up Mammogram/Ultrasound	460	4.8%	7.9%	8.8%
Lumbar Spine MRI for Low Back Pain	53	45.3%	39.6%	37.2%

Texoma Medical Center

5016 S Us Highway 75
Denison, TX 75020
Phone: 903-416-4000
Fax: 903-416-4129
E-mail: contactus@thcs.org
URL: www.texomamedicalcenter.net
Type: Acute Care Hospitals
Emergency Services: Yes
Ownership: Proprietary
Beds: 246

Key Personnel:

Emergency Room . . . . Janet Baker, RN
Patient Relations . . . . Sheryl Bowen
Quality Assurance . . . . Minnie Burkhardt
Infection Control. . . . . Donna Glenn, RN
Radiology. . . . . Tom Jennings
CEO . . . . Ron Seal
Intensive Care Unit. . . . . Lana Snowden, RN
Operating Room. . . . . Angie Whitfield

Measure	Cases	This Hosp.	State Avg.	U.S. Avg.
Blood Clot Prevention and Treatment				
Anticoagulation Overlap Therapy[2]	64	100%	93%	93%
ICU Venous Thromboembolism Prophylaxis[2]	90	100%	92%	92%
Incidence of Potentially Preventable VTE[2]	13	0%	9%	10%
UFH with Dosages/Platelet Monitoring[2]	25	100%	96%	97%
Venous Thromboembolism Prophylaxis[2]	362	100%	82%	85%
Warfarin Therapy Discharge Instructions[2]	46	96%	84%	75%
Chest Pain/Possible Heart Attack Care				
Aspirin Given Within 24 Hours of Arrival[1,3]	-	-	94%	96%
Fibrinolytic Meds Within 30 Min. of Arrival[5]	-	-	47%	58%
Average Time to ECG (minutes)[1,3]	-	-	8	7
Average Time to Transfer (minutes)[5]	-	-	62	60
Children's Asthma Care				
Received Home Management Plan of Care	-	-	93%	88%
Received Reliever Medication	-	-	100%	100%
Received Systemic Corticosteroids	-	-	100%	100%
Emergency Department				
Admittance Decision Time (minutes)[2]	497	150	99	98
Head CT Results Within 45 Min. of Arrival	32	66%	54%	57%
Patients Who Left ER Before Being Seen	44,225	2%	3%	2%
Time from ER Arrival to Admit. (minutes)[2]	552	304	270	274
Time from ER Arrival to Discharge (minutes)	396	134	127	134
Time in ER Before Being Evaluated (minutes)	418	29	26	26
Time to Pain Meds for Fractures (minutes)	191	55	57	57
Heart Attack Care				
Aspirin Given at Discharge[2]	271	100%	99%	99%
Fibrinolytic Meds Within 30 Min. of Arrival[2,7]	-	-	49%	54%
PCI Within 90 Minutes of Arrival[2]	52	100%	95%	96%
Statin Prescribed at Discharge[2]	248	100%	98%	98%
Heart Failure Care				
ACE Inhibitor or ARB for LVSD[2]	99	99%	97%	97%
Discharge Instructions Given[2]	219	97%	95%	94%
Evaluation of LVS Function[2]	267	100%	99%	99%
Medicare Spending				
Medicare Spending per Patient (ratio)	-	1.08	1.03	0.98
Pneumonia Care				
Appropriate Initial Antibiotic Given[2]	82	100%	95%	95%
Blood Culture Timing[2]	162	100%	98%	98%
Pregnancy and Delivery Care				
Newborn Deliveries Scheduled Early[2]	42	2%	7%	6%
Preventive Care				
Immunization for Influenza[2]	563	100%	90%	90%
Immunization for Pneumonia[2]	723	99%	92%	92%
Stroke Care				
Anticoagulation Therapy for Atrial Fibrillation[1,2]	-	-	96%	95%
Antithrombotic Therapy Timing[2]	95	100%	98%	98%
Assessed for Rehabilitation[2]	107	100%	98%	97%
Discharged on Antithrombotic Therapy[2]	100	100%	99%	99%
Discharged on Statin Medication[2]	67	100%	95%	94%
Thrombolytic Therapy Timing[1,2]	-	-	68%	66%
Venous Thromboembolism Prophylaxis[2]	104	100%	94%	94%
Written Stroke Educational Materials Given[2]	60	100%	92%	88%
Surgical Care Improvement Project				
Appropriate Beta Blocker Usage[2]	221	100%	98%	98%
Appropriate VTP Within 24 Hours[2]	393	100%	98%	98%
Controlled Postoperative Blood Glucose[2]	98	95%	96%	97%
Perioperative Temperature Management[2]	480	100%	100%	100%
Prophylactic Antibiotic Selection[2]	379	100%	99%	99%
Prophylactic Antibiotic Selection (Outpatient)	400	99%	98%	98%
Prophylactic Antibiotic Stopped[2]	338	100%	98%	98%
Prophylactic Antibiotic Timing[2]	380	100%	99%	99%
Prophylactic Antibiotic Timing (Outpatient)	400	100%	98%	98%
Urinary Catheter Removal[2]	265	100%	98%	97%
Survey of Patients' Hospital Experiences				
Area Around Room 'Always' Quiet at Night	300+	66%	68%	61%
Doctors 'Always' Communicated Well	300+	81%	83%	82%
Home Recovery Information Given	300+	86%	85%	85%
Hospital Given 9 or 10 on 10 Point Scale	300+	77%	73%	71%
Meds 'Always' Explained Before Given	300+	65%	66%	64%
Nurses 'Always' Communicated Well	300+	78%	80%	79%
Pain 'Always' Well Controlled	300+	71%	72%	71%
Room and Bathroom 'Always' Clean	300+	70%	75%	73%
Timely Help 'Always' Received	300+	62%	69%	68%
Would Definitely Recommend Hospital	300+	80%	73%	71%
Use of Medical Imaging				
Cardiac Imaging Stress Test before Surgery	156	7.1%	5.3%	5.3%
Combination Abdominal CT Scan	1,203	28.5%	16.4%	10.5%
Combination Brain/Sinus CT Scan	1,230	2.2%	2.7%	2.7%
Combination Chest CT Scan	772	29.9%	5.6%	2.7%
Follow-up Mammogram/Ultrasound	1,571	10.2%	7.9%	8.8%
Lumbar Spine MRI for Low Back Pain	151	40.4%	39.6%	37.2%

Denton Regional Medical Center

3535 South I35 East
Denton, TX 76210
Phone: 940-384-3535
Fax: 940-384-4726
URL: www.dentonregional.com
Type: Acute Care Hospitals
Emergency Services: Yes
Ownership: Proprietary
Beds: 208

Key Personnel:

Chief of Medical Staff. . . . . Simon N Allo, MD
Infection Control. . . . . Janet Glowicz
Cardiac Laboratory. . . . . William T Gray
CEO/President. . . . . Robert Haley
Pediatric In-Patient Care . . . . Marilyn R Janke, MD
Radiology. . . . . Jason Ma, MD
Operating Room. . . . . Michelle Rainey, RN
Quality Assurance . . . . Sandra Smith

Measure	Cases	This Hosp.	State Avg.	U.S. Avg.
Blood Clot Prevention and Treatment				
Anticoagulation Overlap Therapy[2]	89	92%	93%	93%
ICU Venous Thromboembolism Prophylaxis[2]	108	94%	92%	92%
Incidence of Potentially Preventable VTE[1,2]	-	-	9%	10%
UFH with Dosages/Platelet Monitoring[1,2]	-	-	96%	97%
Venous Thromboembolism Prophylaxis[2]	326	89%	82%	85%
Warfarin Therapy Discharge Instructions[2]	75	91%	84%	75%
Chest Pain/Possible Heart Attack Care				
Aspirin Given Within 24 Hours of Arrival[1,3]	-	-	94%	96%
Fibrinolytic Meds Within 30 Min. of Arrival[5]	-	-	47%	58%
Average Time to ECG (minutes)[1,3]	-	-	8	7
Average Time to Transfer (minutes)[5]	-	-	62	60
Children's Asthma Care				
Received Home Management Plan of Care	-	-	93%	88%
Received Reliever Medication	-	-	100%	100%
Received Systemic Corticosteroids	-	-	100%	100%
Emergency Department				
Admittance Decision Time (minutes)[2]	768	142	99	98
Head CT Results Within 45 Min. of Arrival	19	89%	54%	57%
Patients Who Left ER Before Being Seen	44,917	2%	3%	2%
Time from ER Arrival to Admit. (minutes)[2]	768	280	270	274
Time from ER Arrival to Discharge (minutes)	414	146	127	134
Time in ER Before Being Evaluated (minutes)	479	19	26	26
Time to Pain Meds for Fractures (minutes)	210	58	57	57
Heart Attack Care				
Aspirin Given at Discharge	251	100%	99%	99%
Fibrinolytic Meds Within 30 Min. of Arrival[7]	-	-	49%	54%
PCI Within 90 Minutes of Arrival	33	100%	95%	96%
Statin Prescribed at Discharge	241	100%	98%	98%
Heart Failure Care				
ACE Inhibitor or ARB for LVSD	88	100%	97%	97%
Discharge Instructions Given	182	98%	95%	94%
Evaluation of LVS Function	232	100%	99%	99%
Medicare Spending				
Medicare Spending per Patient (ratio)	-	1.13	1.03	0.98
Pneumonia Care				
Appropriate Initial Antibiotic Given[2]	110	99%	95%	95%
Blood Culture Timing[2]	235	100%	98%	98%
Pregnancy and Delivery Care				
Newborn Deliveries Scheduled Early[2]	34	3%	7%	6%
Preventive Care				
Immunization for Influenza[2]	621	95%	90%	90%
Immunization for Pneumonia[2]	770	93%	92%	92%
Stroke Care				
Anticoagulation Therapy for Atrial Fibrillation[1,2]	-	-	96%	95%
Antithrombotic Therapy Timing[2]	73	97%	98%	98%
Assessed for Rehabilitation[2]	87	100%	98%	97%
Discharged on Antithrombotic Therapy[2]	79	100%	99%	99%
Discharged on Statin Medication[2]	58	95%	95%	94%
Thrombolytic Therapy Timing[2,7]	-	-	68%	66%
Venous Thromboembolism Prophylaxis[2]	84	96%	94%	94%
Written Stroke Educational Materials Given[2]	56	95%	92%	88%
Surgical Care Improvement Project				
Appropriate Beta Blocker Usage[2]	266	100%	98%	98%
Appropriate VTP Within 24 Hours[2]	338	98%	98%	98%
Controlled Postoperative Blood Glucose[2]	106	92%	96%	97%
Perioperative Temperature Management[2]	515	100%	100%	100%
Prophylactic Antibiotic Selection[2]	352	100%	99%	99%
Prophylactic Antibiotic Selection (Outpatient)	295	93%	98%	98%
Prophylactic Antibiotic Stopped[2]	343	99%	98%	98%
Prophylactic Antibiotic Timing[2]	352	98%	99%	99%
Prophylactic Antibiotic Timing (Outpatient)	295	99%	98%	98%
Urinary Catheter Removal[2]	264	99%	98%	97%
Survey of Patients' Hospital Experiences				
Area Around Room 'Always' Quiet at Night	300+	58%	68%	61%
Doctors 'Always' Communicated Well	300+	78%	83%	82%
Home Recovery Information Given	300+	86%	85%	85%
Hospital Given 9 or 10 on 10 Point Scale	300+	68%	73%	71%
Meds 'Always' Explained Before Given	300+	61%	66%	64%
Nurses 'Always' Communicated Well	300+	75%	80%	79%
Pain 'Always' Well Controlled	300+	71%	72%	71%
Room and Bathroom 'Always' Clean	300+	70%	75%	73%
Timely Help 'Always' Received	300+	65%	69%	68%
Would Definitely Recommend Hospital	300+	71%	73%	71%
Use of Medical Imaging				
Cardiac Imaging Stress Test before Surgery[1]	-	-	5.3%	5.3%
Combination Abdominal CT Scan	369	9.2%	16.4%	10.5%

NOTE: Hospital profiles are in alphabetical order by state, then city, then hospital within the city; Rankings exclude hospitals with less than 25 cases except for patient surveys which excludes hospitals with less than 100 cases; (a) 100-299 cases; (1) The number of cases/patients is too few to report; (2) Data submitted were based on a sample of cases/patients; (3) Results are based on a shorter time period than required; (4) Data suppressed by CMS for one or more quarters; (5) Results are not available for this reporting period; (6) Fewer than 100 patients completed the HCAHPS survey; (7) No cases met the criteria for this measure; (8) The lower limit of the confidence interval cannot be calculated if the number of observed infections equals zero; (9) No data are available from the state/territory for this reporting period; (10) The scores shown reflect fewer than 50 completed surveys; (11) There were discrepancies in the data collection process; (12) This measure does not apply to this hospital for this reporting period; (13) Results cannot be calculated for this reporting period; (14) The results for this state are combined with nearby states to protect confidentiality; Please refer to the User's Guide for a full explanation of data.

Measure	Cases	This Hosp.	State Avg.	U.S. Avg.
Combination Brain/Sinus CT Scan[1]	-	-	2.7%	2.7%
Combination Chest CT Scan	215	0.0%	5.6%	2.7%
Follow-up Mammogram/Ultrasound[7]	-	-	7.9%	8.8%
Lumbar Spine MRI for Low Back Pain[1]	-	-	39.6%	37.2%

Heart Hospital Baylor Denton

2801 South Mayhill Road Phone: 940-220-0600
Denton, TX 76208
URL: www.northtexashospital.com
Type: Acute Care Hospitals Emergency Services: Yes
Ownership: Physician
Key Personnel:
President . . . . Mark A. Valentine

Measure	Cases	This Hosp.	State Avg.	U.S. Avg.
Blood Clot Prevention and Treatment				
Anticoagulation Overlap Therapy[2,3]	-	-	93%	93%
ICU Venous Thromboembolism Prophylaxis[2,3]	-	-	92%	92%
Incidence of Potentially Preventable VTE[2,3]	-	-	9%	10%
UFH with Dosages/Platelet Monitoring[2,3]	-	-	96%	97%
Venous Thromboembolism Prophylaxis[1,2]	-	-	82%	85%
Warfarin Therapy Discharge Instructions[2,3]	-	-	84%	75%
Chest Pain/Possible Heart Attack Care				
Aspirin Given Within 24 Hours of Arrival[5]	-	-	94%	96%
Fibrinolytic Meds Within 30 Min. of Arrival[5]	-	-	47%	58%
Average Time to ECG (minutes)[5]	-	-	8	7
Average Time to Transfer (minutes)[5]	-	-	62	60
Children's Asthma Care				
Received Home Management Plan of Care	-	-	93%	88%
Received Reliever Medication	-	-	100%	100%
Received Systemic Corticosteroids	-	-	100%	100%
Emergency Department				
Admittance Decision Time (minutes)[3,7]	-	-	99	98
Head CT Results Within 45 Min. of Arrival[5]	-	-	54%	57%
Patients Who Left ER Before Being Seen	283	1%	3%	2%
Time from ER Arrival to Admit. (minutes)[3,7]	-	-	270	274
Time from ER Arrival to Discharge (minutes)	46	88	127	134
Time in ER Before Being Evaluated (minutes)	125	20	26	26
Time to Pain Meds for Fractures (minutes)[5]	-	-	57	57
Heart Attack Care				
Aspirin Given at Discharge[5]	-	-	99%	99%
Fibrinolytic Meds Within 30 Min. of Arrival[5]	-	-	49%	54%
PCI Within 90 Minutes of Arrival[5]	-	-	95%	96%
Statin Prescribed at Discharge[5]	-	-	98%	98%
Heart Failure Care				
ACE Inhibitor or ARB for LVSD[5]	-	-	97%	97%
Discharge Instructions Given[5]	-	-	95%	94%
Evaluation of LVS Function[5]	-	-	99%	99%
Medicare Spending				
Medicare Spending per Patient (ratio)	-	1.07	1.03	0.98
Pneumonia Care				
Appropriate Initial Antibiotic Given[5]	-	-	95%	95%
Blood Culture Timing[5]	-	-	98%	98%
Pregnancy and Delivery Care				
Newborn Deliveries Scheduled Early[7]	-	-	7%	6%
Preventive Care				
Immunization for Influenza	109	99%	90%	90%
Immunization for Pneumonia[3]	31	97%	92%	92%
Stroke Care				
Anticoagulation Therapy for Atrial Fibrillation[5]	-	-	96%	95%
Antithrombotic Therapy Timing[5]	-	-	98%	98%
Assessed for Rehabilitation[5]	-	-	98%	97%
Discharged on Antithrombotic Therapy[5]	-	-	99%	99%
Discharged on Statin Medication[5]	-	-	95%	94%
Thrombolytic Therapy Timing[5]	-	-	68%	66%
Venous Thromboembolism Prophylaxis[5]	-	-	94%	94%
Written Stroke Educational Materials Given[5]	-	-	92%	88%
Surgical Care Improvement Project				
Appropriate Beta Blocker Usage[1,3]	-	-	98%	98%
Appropriate VTP Within 24 Hours[3]	20	100%	98%	98%
Controlled Postoperative Blood Glucose[3,7]	-	-	96%	97%
Perioperative Temperature Management[3]	23	100%	100%	100%
Prophylactic Antibiotic Selection[3]	24	100%	99%	99%
Prophylactic Antibiotic Selection (Outpatient)[3]	89	96%	98%	98%
Prophylactic Antibiotic Stopped[3]	24	100%	98%	98%
Prophylactic Antibiotic Timing[3]	24	100%	99%	99%
Prophylactic Antibiotic Timing (Outpatient)[3]	90	99%	98%	98%
Urinary Catheter Removal[1,3]	-	-	98%	97%
Survey of Patients' Hospital Experiences				
Area Around Room 'Always' Quiet at Night[3,6]	<100	84%	68%	61%
Doctors 'Always' Communicated Well[3,6]	<100	89%	83%	82%
Home Recovery Information Given[3,6]	<100	91%	85%	85%
Hospital Given 9 or 10 on 10 Point Scale[3,6]	<100	82%	73%	71%
Meds 'Always' Explained Before Given[3,6]	<100	65%	66%	64%
Nurses 'Always' Communicated Well[3,6]	<100	90%	80%	79%
Pain 'Always' Well Controlled[3,6]	<100	69%	72%	71%
Room and Bathroom 'Always' Clean[3,6]	<100	85%	75%	73%
Timely Help 'Always' Received[3,6]	<100	85%	69%	68%
Would Definitely Recommend Hospital[3,6]	<100	86%	73%	71%
Use of Medical Imaging				
Cardiac Imaging Stress Test before Surgery[7]	-	-	5.3%	5.3%
Combination Abdominal CT Scan	41	48.8%	16.4%	10.5%
Combination Brain/Sinus CT Scan[1]	-	-	2.7%	2.7%
Combination Chest CT Scan[1]	-	-	5.6%	2.7%
Follow-up Mammogram/Ultrasound[7]	-	-	7.9%	8.8%
Lumbar Spine MRI for Low Back Pain	66	31.8%	39.6%	37.2%

Mayhill Hospital

2809 South Mayhill Road Phone: 940-239-3000
Denton, TX 76208
URL: www.mayhillhospital.com
Type: Acute Care Hospitals Emergency Services: No
Ownership: Proprietary
Key Personnel:
Administrator . . . . Dan Aller

Measure	Cases	This Hosp.	State Avg.	U.S. Avg.
Blood Clot Prevention and Treatment				
Anticoagulation Overlap Therapy[2,7]	-	-	93%	93%
ICU Venous Thromboembolism Prophylaxis[2,7]	-	-	92%	92%
Incidence of Potentially Preventable VTE[2,7]	-	-	9%	10%
UFH with Dosages/Platelet Monitoring[2,7]	-	-	96%	97%
Venous Thromboembolism Prophylaxis[2]	12	8%	82%	85%
Warfarin Therapy Discharge Instructions[2,7]	-	-	84%	75%
Chest Pain/Possible Heart Attack Care				
Aspirin Given Within 24 Hours of Arrival[5]	-	-	94%	96%
Fibrinolytic Meds Within 30 Min. of Arrival[5]	-	-	47%	58%
Average Time to ECG (minutes)[5]	-	-	8	7
Average Time to Transfer (minutes)[5]	-	-	62	60
Children's Asthma Care				
Received Home Management Plan of Care	-	-	93%	88%
Received Reliever Medication	-	-	100%	100%
Received Systemic Corticosteroids	-	-	100%	100%
Emergency Department				
Admittance Decision Time (minutes)[2,7]	-	-	99	98
Head CT Results Within 45 Min. of Arrival[5]	-	-	54%	57%
Patients Who Left ER Before Being Seen[5]	-	-	3%	2%
Time from ER Arrival to Admit. (minutes)[2,7]	-	-	270	274
Time from ER Arrival to Discharge (minutes)[5]	-	-	127	134
Time in ER Before Being Evaluated (minutes)[5]	-	-	26	26
Time to Pain Meds for Fractures (minutes)[5]	-	-	57	57
Heart Attack Care				
Aspirin Given at Discharge[5]	-	-	99%	99%
Fibrinolytic Meds Within 30 Min. of Arrival[5]	-	-	49%	54%
PCI Within 90 Minutes of Arrival[5]	-	-	95%	96%
Statin Prescribed at Discharge[5]	-	-	98%	98%
Heart Failure Care				
ACE Inhibitor or ARB for LVSD[5]	-	-	97%	97%
Discharge Instructions Given[5]	-	-	95%	94%
Evaluation of LVS Function[5]	-	-	99%	99%
Medicare Spending				
Medicare Spending per Patient (ratio)	-	-	1.03	0.98
Pneumonia Care				
Appropriate Initial Antibiotic Given[5]	-	-	95%	95%
Blood Culture Timing[5]	-	-	98%	98%
Pregnancy and Delivery Care				
Newborn Deliveries Scheduled Early[7]	-	-	7%	6%
Preventive Care				
Immunization for Influenza[2]	296	71%	90%	90%
Immunization for Pneumonia[2]	327	69%	92%	92%
Stroke Care				
Anticoagulation Therapy for Atrial Fibrillation[5]	-	-	96%	95%
Antithrombotic Therapy Timing[5]	-	-	98%	98%
Assessed for Rehabilitation[5]	-	-	98%	97%
Discharged on Antithrombotic Therapy[5]	-	-	99%	99%
Discharged on Statin Medication[5]	-	-	95%	94%
Thrombolytic Therapy Timing[5]	-	-	68%	66%
Venous Thromboembolism Prophylaxis[5]	-	-	94%	94%
Written Stroke Educational Materials Given[5]	-	-	92%	88%
Surgical Care Improvement Project				
Appropriate Beta Blocker Usage[5]	-	-	98%	98%
Appropriate VTP Within 24 Hours[5]	-	-	98%	98%
Controlled Postoperative Blood Glucose[5]	-	-	96%	97%
Perioperative Temperature Management[5]	-	-	100%	100%
Prophylactic Antibiotic Selection[5]	-	-	99%	99%
Prophylactic Antibiotic Selection (Outpatient)[5]	-	-	98%	98%
Prophylactic Antibiotic Stopped[5]	-	-	98%	98%
Prophylactic Antibiotic Timing[5]	-	-	99%	99%
Prophylactic Antibiotic Timing (Outpatient)[5]	-	-	98%	98%
Urinary Catheter Removal[5]	-	-	98%	97%
Survey of Patients' Hospital Experiences				
Area Around Room 'Always' Quiet at Night[5]	-	-	68%	61%
Doctors 'Always' Communicated Well[5]	-	-	83%	82%
Home Recovery Information Given[5]	-	-	85%	85%
Hospital Given 9 or 10 on 10 Point Scale[5]	-	-	73%	71%
Meds 'Always' Explained Before Given[5]	-	-	66%	64%
Nurses 'Always' Communicated Well[5]	-	-	80%	79%
Pain 'Always' Well Controlled[5]	-	-	72%	71%
Room and Bathroom 'Always' Clean[5]	-	-	75%	73%
Timely Help 'Always' Received[5]	-	-	69%	68%
Would Definitely Recommend Hospital[5]	-	-	73%	71%
Use of Medical Imaging				
Cardiac Imaging Stress Test before Surgery[7]	-	-	5.3%	5.3%
Combination Abdominal CT Scan[7]	-	-	16.4%	10.5%
Combination Brain/Sinus CT Scan[7]	-	-	2.7%	2.7%
Combination Chest CT Scan[7]	-	-	5.6%	2.7%
Follow-up Mammogram/Ultrasound[7]	-	-	7.9%	8.8%
Lumbar Spine MRI for Low Back Pain[7]	-	-	39.6%	37.2%

Texas Health Presbyterian Hospital Denton

3000 N I-35 Phone: 940-898-7000
Denton, TX 76201
URL: www.texashealth.org
Type: Acute Care Hospitals Emergency Services: Yes
Ownership: Voluntary non-profit - Private Beds: 255
Key Personnel:
CEO . . . . Barclay E. Berdan
Emergency Room . . . . Justin Miller, RN

Measure	Cases	This Hosp.	State Avg.	U.S. Avg.
Blood Clot Prevention and Treatment				
Anticoagulation Overlap Therapy[2]	60	97%	93%	93%
ICU Venous Thromboembolism Prophylaxis[2]	78	99%	92%	92%
Incidence of Potentially Preventable VTE[1,2]	-	-	9%	10%
UFH with Dosages/Platelet Monitoring[1,2]	-	-	96%	97%
Venous Thromboembolism Prophylaxis[2]	416	98%	82%	85%
Warfarin Therapy Discharge Instructions[2]	51	49%	84%	75%
Chest Pain/Possible Heart Attack Care				
Aspirin Given Within 24 Hours of Arrival[1,3]	-	-	94%	96%
Fibrinolytic Meds Within 30 Min. of Arrival[5]	-	-	47%	58%
Average Time to ECG (minutes)[1,3]	-	-	8	7
Average Time to Transfer (minutes)[5]	-	-	62	60
Children's Asthma Care				
Received Home Management Plan of Care	-	-	93%	88%
Received Reliever Medication	-	-	100%	100%
Received Systemic Corticosteroids	-	-	100%	100%
Emergency Department				
Admittance Decision Time (minutes)[2]	650	113	99	98
Head CT Results Within 45 Min. of Arrival[1]	-	-	54%	57%
Patients Who Left ER Before Being Seen	43,158	2%	3%	2%
Time from ER Arrival to Admit. (minutes)[2]	649	269	270	274
Time from ER Arrival to Discharge (minutes)	414	148	127	134

NOTE: Hospital profiles are in alphabetical order by state, then city, then hospital within the city; Rankings exclude hospitals with less than 25 cases except for patient surveys which excludes hospitals with less than 100 cases; (a) 100-299 cases; (1) The number of cases/patients is too few to report; (2) Data submitted were based on a sample of cases/patients; (3) Results are based on a shorter time period than required; (4) Data suppressed by CMS for one or more quarters; (5) Results are not available for this reporting period; (6) Fewer than 100 patients completed the HCAHPS survey; (7) No cases met the criteria for this measure; (8) The lower limit of the confidence interval cannot be calculated if the number of observed infections equals zero; (9) No data are available from the state/territory for this reporting period; (10) The scores shown reflect fewer than 50 completed surveys; (11) There were discrepancies in the data collection process; (12) This measure does not apply to this hospital for this reporting period; (13) Results cannot be calculated for this reporting period; (14) The results for this state are combined with nearby states to protect confidentiality; Please refer to the User's Guide for a full explanation of data.

Measure	Cases	This Hosp.	State Avg.	U.S. Avg.
Time in ER Before Being Evaluated (minutes)	440	26	26	26
Time to Pain Meds for Fractures (minutes)	173	54	57	57
Heart Attack Care				
Aspirin Given at Discharge	126	99%	99%	99%
Fibrinolytic Meds Within 30 Min. of Arrival[7]	-	-	49%	54%
PCI Within 90 Minutes of Arrival	18	89%	95%	96%
Statin Prescribed at Discharge	125	100%	98%	98%
Heart Failure Care				
ACE Inhibitor or ARB for LVSD	75	100%	97%	97%
Discharge Instructions Given	165	99%	95%	94%
Evaluation of LVS Function	213	100%	99%	99%
Medicare Spending				
Medicare Spending per Patient (ratio)	-	1.13	1.03	0.98
Pneumonia Care				
Appropriate Initial Antibiotic Given	169	98%	95%	95%
Blood Culture Timing	270	100%	98%	98%
Pregnancy and Delivery Care				
Newborn Deliveries Scheduled Early	188	11%	7%	6%
Preventive Care				
Immunization for Influenza[2]	581	98%	90%	90%
Immunization for Pneumonia[2]	700	97%	92%	92%
Stroke Care				
Anticoagulation Therapy for Atrial Fibrillation[2]	15	93%	96%	95%
Antithrombotic Therapy Timing[2]	81	99%	98%	98%
Assessed for Rehabilitation[2]	89	98%	98%	97%
Discharged on Antithrombotic Therapy[2]	88	100%	99%	99%
Discharged on Statin Medication[2]	67	100%	95%	94%
Thrombolytic Therapy Timing[1,2]	-	-	68%	66%
Venous Thromboembolism Prophylaxis[2]	85	99%	94%	94%
Written Stroke Educational Materials Given[2]	58	98%	92%	88%
Surgical Care Improvement Project				
Appropriate Beta Blocker Usage[2]	108	95%	98%	98%
Appropriate VTP Within 24 Hours[2]	247	98%	98%	98%
Controlled Postoperative Blood Glucose[2]	62	94%	96%	97%
Perioperative Temperature Management[2]	337	100%	100%	100%
Prophylactic Antibiotic Selection[2]	216	99%	99%	99%
Prophylactic Antibiotic Selection (Outpatient)	308	99%	98%	98%
Prophylactic Antibiotic Stopped[2]	211	100%	98%	98%
Prophylactic Antibiotic Timing[2]	216	99%	99%	99%
Prophylactic Antibiotic Timing (Outpatient)	310	97%	98%	98%
Urinary Catheter Removal[2]	202	99%	98%	97%
Survey of Patients' Hospital Experiences				
Area Around Room 'Always' Quiet at Night	300+	60%	68%	61%
Doctors 'Always' Communicated Well	300+	79%	83%	82%
Home Recovery Information Given	300+	86%	85%	85%
Hospital Given 9 or 10 on 10 Point Scale	300+	72%	73%	71%
Meds 'Always' Explained Before Given	300+	64%	66%	64%
Nurses 'Always' Communicated Well	300+	77%	80%	79%
Pain 'Always' Well Controlled	300+	69%	72%	71%
Room and Bathroom 'Always' Clean	300+	73%	75%	73%
Timely Help 'Always' Received	300+	65%	69%	68%
Would Definitely Recommend Hospital	300+	76%	73%	71%
Use of Medical Imaging				
Cardiac Imaging Stress Test before Surgery[1]	-	-	5.3%	5.3%
Combination Abdominal CT Scan	448	11.8%	16.4%	10.5%
Combination Brain/Sinus CT Scan[1]	-	-	2.7%	2.7%
Combination Chest CT Scan	213	14.6%	5.6%	2.7%
Follow-up Mammogram/Ultrasound	1,106	4.5%	7.9%	8.8%
Lumbar Spine MRI for Low Back Pain	76	39.5%	39.6%	37.2%

Yoakum County Hospital

412 Mustang Avenue Phone: 806-592-2121
Denver City, TX 79323
Type: Critical Access Hospitals Emergency Services: Yes
Ownership: Voluntary non-profit - Other

Measure	Cases	This Hosp.	State Avg.	U.S. Avg.
Blood Clot Prevention and Treatment				
Anticoagulation Overlap Therapy[5]	-	-	93%	93%
ICU Venous Thromboembolism Prophylaxis[5]	-	-	92%	92%
Incidence of Potentially Preventable VTE[5]	-	-	9%	10%
UFH with Dosages/Platelet Monitoring[5]	-	-	96%	97%
Venous Thromboembolism Prophylaxis[5]	-	-	82%	85%
Warfarin Therapy Discharge Instructions[5]	-	-	84%	75%
Chest Pain/Possible Heart Attack Care				
Aspirin Given Within 24 Hours of Arrival	-	-	94%	96%
Fibrinolytic Meds Within 30 Min. of Arrival	-	-	47%	58%
Average Time to ECG (minutes)	-	-	8	7
Average Time to Transfer (minutes)	-	-	62	60
Children's Asthma Care				
Received Home Management Plan of Care	-	-	93%	88%
Received Reliever Medication	-	-	100%	100%
Received Systemic Corticosteroids	-	-	100%	100%
Emergency Department				
Admittance Decision Time (minutes)[5]	-	-	99	98
Head CT Results Within 45 Min. of Arrival	-	-	54%	57%
Patients Who Left ER Before Being Seen	-	-	3%	2%
Time from ER Arrival to Admit. (minutes)[5]	-	-	270	274
Time from ER Arrival to Discharge (minutes)	-	-	127	134
Time in ER Before Being Evaluated (minutes)	-	-	26	26
Time to Pain Meds for Fractures (minutes)	-	-	57	57
Heart Attack Care				
Aspirin Given at Discharge[1,3]	-	-	99%	99%
Fibrinolytic Meds Within 30 Min. of Arrival[3,7]	-	-	49%	54%
PCI Within 90 Minutes of Arrival[3,7]	-	-	95%	96%
Statin Prescribed at Discharge[1,3]	-	-	98%	98%
Heart Failure Care				
ACE Inhibitor or ARB for LVSD[5]	-	-	97%	97%
Discharge Instructions Given[5]	-	-	95%	94%
Evaluation of LVS Function[5]	-	-	99%	99%
Medicare Spending				
Medicare Spending per Patient (ratio)	-	-	1.03	0.98
Pneumonia Care				
Appropriate Initial Antibiotic Given[3,7]	-	-	95%	95%
Blood Culture Timing[3,7]	-	-	98%	98%
Pregnancy and Delivery Care				
Newborn Deliveries Scheduled Early[5]	-	-	7%	6%
Preventive Care				
Immunization for Influenza[5]	-	-	90%	90%
Immunization for Pneumonia[5]	-	-	92%	92%
Stroke Care				
Anticoagulation Therapy for Atrial Fibrillation[5]	-	-	96%	95%
Antithrombotic Therapy Timing[5]	-	-	98%	98%
Assessed for Rehabilitation[5]	-	-	98%	97%
Discharged on Antithrombotic Therapy[5]	-	-	99%	99%
Discharged on Statin Medication[5]	-	-	95%	94%
Thrombolytic Therapy Timing[5]	-	-	68%	66%
Venous Thromboembolism Prophylaxis[5]	-	-	94%	94%
Written Stroke Educational Materials Given[5]	-	-	92%	88%
Surgical Care Improvement Project				
Appropriate Beta Blocker Usage[5]	-	-	98%	98%
Appropriate VTP Within 24 Hours[5]	-	-	98%	98%
Controlled Postoperative Blood Glucose[5]	-	-	96%	97%
Perioperative Temperature Management[5]	-	-	100%	100%
Prophylactic Antibiotic Selection[5]	-	-	99%	99%
Prophylactic Antibiotic Selection (Outpatient)	-	-	98%	98%
Prophylactic Antibiotic Stopped[5]	-	-	98%	98%
Prophylactic Antibiotic Timing[5]	-	-	99%	99%
Prophylactic Antibiotic Timing (Outpatient)	-	-	98%	98%
Urinary Catheter Removal[5]	-	-	98%	97%
Survey of Patients' Hospital Experiences				
Area Around Room 'Always' Quiet at Night[6]	<100	73%	68%	61%
Doctors 'Always' Communicated Well[6]	<100	91%	83%	82%
Home Recovery Information Given[6]	<100	82%	85%	85%
Hospital Given 9 or 10 on 10 Point Scale[6]	<100	84%	73%	71%
Meds 'Always' Explained Before Given[6]	<100	69%	66%	64%
Nurses 'Always' Communicated Well[6]	<100	85%	80%	79%
Pain 'Always' Well Controlled[6]	<100	72%	72%	71%
Room and Bathroom 'Always' Clean[6]	<100	86%	75%	73%
Timely Help 'Always' Received[6]	<100	79%	69%	68%
Would Definitely Recommend Hospital[6]	<100	77%	73%	71%
Use of Medical Imaging				
Cardiac Imaging Stress Test before Surgery	-	-	5.3%	5.3%
Combination Abdominal CT Scan	-	-	16.4%	10.5%
Combination Brain/Sinus CT Scan	-	-	2.7%	2.7%
Combination Chest CT Scan	-	-	5.6%	2.7%
Follow-up Mammogram/Ultrasound	-	-	7.9%	8.8%
Lumbar Spine MRI for Low Back Pain	-	-	39.6%	37.2%

Nix Community General Hospital

230 West Miller Street Phone: 210-271-2190
Dilley, TX 78017
Type: Acute Care Hospitals Emergency Services: Yes
Ownership: Voluntary non-profit - Private

Measure	Cases	This Hosp.	State Avg.	U.S. Avg.
Blood Clot Prevention and Treatment				
Anticoagulation Overlap Therapy[5]	-	-	93%	93%
ICU Venous Thromboembolism Prophylaxis[5]	-	-	92%	92%
Incidence of Potentially Preventable VTE[5]	-	-	9%	10%
UFH with Dosages/Platelet Monitoring[5]	-	-	96%	97%
Venous Thromboembolism Prophylaxis[5]	-	-	82%	85%
Warfarin Therapy Discharge Instructions[5]	-	-	84%	75%
Chest Pain/Possible Heart Attack Care				
Aspirin Given Within 24 Hours of Arrival[5]	-	-	94%	96%
Fibrinolytic Meds Within 30 Min. of Arrival[5]	-	-	47%	58%
Average Time to ECG (minutes)[5]	-	-	8	7
Average Time to Transfer (minutes)[5]	-	-	62	60
Children's Asthma Care				
Received Home Management Plan of Care	-	-	93%	88%
Received Reliever Medication	-	-	100%	100%
Received Systemic Corticosteroids	-	-	100%	100%
Emergency Department				
Admittance Decision Time (minutes)[5]	-	-	99	98
Head CT Results Within 45 Min. of Arrival[5]	-	-	54%	57%
Patients Who Left ER Before Being Seen[5]	-	-	3%	2%
Time from ER Arrival to Admit. (minutes)[5]	-	-	270	274
Time from ER Arrival to Discharge (minutes)[5]	-	-	127	134
Time in ER Before Being Evaluated (minutes)[5]	-	-	26	26
Time to Pain Meds for Fractures (minutes)[5]	-	-	57	57
Heart Attack Care				
Aspirin Given at Discharge[5]	-	-	99%	99%
Fibrinolytic Meds Within 30 Min. of Arrival[5]	-	-	49%	54%
PCI Within 90 Minutes of Arrival[5]	-	-	95%	96%
Statin Prescribed at Discharge[5]	-	-	98%	98%
Heart Failure Care				
ACE Inhibitor or ARB for LVSD[5]	-	-	97%	97%
Discharge Instructions Given[5]	-	-	95%	94%
Evaluation of LVS Function[5]	-	-	99%	99%
Medicare Spending				
Medicare Spending per Patient (ratio)	-	-	1.03	0.98
Pneumonia Care				
Appropriate Initial Antibiotic Given[5]	-	-	95%	95%
Blood Culture Timing[5]	-	-	98%	98%
Pregnancy and Delivery Care				
Newborn Deliveries Scheduled Early[5]	-	-	7%	6%
Preventive Care				
Immunization for Influenza[5]	-	-	90%	90%
Immunization for Pneumonia[5]	-	-	92%	92%
Stroke Care				
Anticoagulation Therapy for Atrial Fibrillation[5]	-	-	96%	95%
Antithrombotic Therapy Timing[5]	-	-	98%	98%
Assessed for Rehabilitation[5]	-	-	98%	97%
Discharged on Antithrombotic Therapy[5]	-	-	99%	99%
Discharged on Statin Medication[5]	-	-	95%	94%
Thrombolytic Therapy Timing[5]	-	-	68%	66%
Venous Thromboembolism Prophylaxis[5]	-	-	94%	94%
Written Stroke Educational Materials Given[5]	-	-	92%	88%
Surgical Care Improvement Project				
Appropriate Beta Blocker Usage[5]	-	-	98%	98%
Appropriate VTP Within 24 Hours[5]	-	-	98%	98%
Controlled Postoperative Blood Glucose[5]	-	-	96%	97%
Perioperative Temperature Management[5]	-	-	100%	100%
Prophylactic Antibiotic Selection[5]	-	-	99%	99%
Prophylactic Antibiotic Selection (Outpatient)[5]	-	-	98%	98%
Prophylactic Antibiotic Stopped[5]	-	-	98%	98%
Prophylactic Antibiotic Timing[5]	-	-	99%	99%
Prophylactic Antibiotic Timing (Outpatient)[5]	-	-	98%	98%

NOTE: Hospital profiles are in alphabetical order by state, then city, then hospital within the city; Rankings exclude hospitals with less than 25 cases except for patient surveys which excludes hospitals with less than 100 cases; (a) 100-299 cases; (1) The number of cases/patients is too few to report; (2) Data submitted were based on a sample of cases/patients; (3) Results are based on a shorter time period than required; (4) Data suppressed by CMS for one or more quarters; (5) Results are not available for this reporting period; (6) Fewer than 100 patients completed the HCAHPS survey; (7) No cases met the criteria for this measure; (8) The lower limit of the confidence interval cannot be calculated if the number of observed infections equals zero; (9) No data are available from the state/territory for this reporting period; (10) The scores shown reflect fewer than 50 completed surveys; (11) There were discrepancies in the data collection process; (12) This measure does not apply to this hospital for this reporting period; (13) Results cannot be calculated for this reporting period; (14) The results for this state are combined with nearby states to protect confidentiality; Please refer to the User's Guide for a full explanation of data.

Measure	Cases	This Hosp.	State Avg.	U.S. Avg.
Urinary Catheter Removal[5]	-	-	98%	97%
Survey of Patients' Hospital Experiences				
Area Around Room 'Always' Quiet at Night[5]	-	-	68%	61%
Doctors 'Always' Communicated Well[5]	-	-	83%	82%
Home Recovery Information Given[5]	-	-	85%	85%
Hospital Given 9 or 10 on 10 Point Scale[5]	-	-	73%	71%
Meds 'Always' Explained Before Given[5]	-	-	66%	64%
Nurses 'Always' Communicated Well[5]	-	-	80%	79%
Pain 'Always' Well Controlled[5]	-	-	72%	71%
Room and Bathroom 'Always' Clean[5]	-	-	75%	73%
Timely Help 'Always' Received[5]	-	-	69%	68%
Would Definitely Recommend Hospital[5]	-	-	73%	71%
Use of Medical Imaging				
Cardiac Imaging Stress Test before Surgery[5]	-	-	5.3%	5.3%
Combination Abdominal CT Scan[5]	-	-	16.4%	10.5%
Combination Brain/Sinus CT Scan[5]	-	-	2.7%	2.7%
Combination Chest CT Scan[5]	-	-	5.6%	2.7%
Follow-up Mammogram/Ultrasound[5]	-	-	7.9%	8.8%
Lumbar Spine MRI for Low Back Pain[5]	-	-	39.6%	37.2%

Plains Memorial Hospital

310 West Halsell Street
Dimmitt, TX 79027
Phone: 806-647-2191
Fax: 806-647-2407
URL: www.cchdonline.com
Type: Critical Access Hospitals
Emergency Services: No
Ownership: Govt - Hospital Dist/Auth
Beds: 25

Key Personnel:
Radiology. . . . . Deana Beames
Emergency Room . . . . Matt Clayton
Operating Room. . . . . Paula Proffitt, RN
CEO/President. . . . . Linda Rasor, RN, BSN
Anesthesiology. . . . . Joe Villeinueve
Quality Assurance . . . . Ruth Wayland, RN

Measure	Cases	This Hosp.	State Avg.	U.S. Avg.
Blood Clot Prevention and Treatment				
Anticoagulation Overlap Therapy[5]	-	-	93%	93%
ICU Venous Thromboembolism Prophylaxis[5]	-	-	92%	92%
Incidence of Potentially Preventable VTE[5]	-	-	9%	10%
UFH with Dosages/Platelet Monitoring[5]	-	-	96%	97%
Venous Thromboembolism Prophylaxis[5]	-	-	82%	85%
Warfarin Therapy Discharge Instructions[5]	-	-	84%	75%
Chest Pain/Possible Heart Attack Care				
Aspirin Given Within 24 Hours of Arrival[1,3]	-	-	94%	96%
Fibrinolytic Meds Within 30 Min. of Arrival[1,3]	-	-	47%	58%
Average Time to ECG (minutes)[1,3]	-	-	8	7
Average Time to Transfer (minutes)[3,7]	-	-	62	60
Children's Asthma Care				
Received Home Management Plan of Care	-	-	93%	88%
Received Reliever Medication	-	-	100%	100%
Received Systemic Corticosteroids	-	-	100%	100%
Emergency Department				
Admittance Decision Time (minutes)	66	10	99	98
Head CT Results Within 45 Min. of Arrival[5]	-	-	54%	57%
Patients Who Left ER Before Being Seen	2,869	1%	3%	2%
Time from ER Arrival to Admit. (minutes)	69	145	270	274
Time from ER Arrival to Discharge (minutes)[5]	-	-	127	134
Time in ER Before Being Evaluated (minutes)[5]	-	-	26	26
Time to Pain Meds for Fractures (minutes)[5]	-	-	57	57
Heart Attack Care				
Aspirin Given at Discharge[5]	-	-	99%	99%
Fibrinolytic Meds Within 30 Min. of Arrival[5]	-	-	49%	54%
PCI Within 90 Minutes of Arrival[5]	-	-	95%	96%
Statin Prescribed at Discharge[5]	-	-	98%	98%
Heart Failure Care				
ACE Inhibitor or ARB for LVSD[1]	-	-	97%	97%
Discharge Instructions Given[1]	-	-	95%	94%
Evaluation of LVS Function[1]	-	-	99%	99%
Medicare Spending				
Medicare Spending per Patient (ratio)	-	-	1.03	0.98
Pneumonia Care				
Appropriate Initial Antibiotic Given[1]	-	-	95%	95%
Blood Culture Timing[1]	-	-	98%	98%
Pregnancy and Delivery Care				
Newborn Deliveries Scheduled Early[5]	-	-	7%	6%
Preventive Care				
Immunization for Influenza	49	73%	90%	90%
Immunization for Pneumonia	91	87%	92%	92%
Stroke Care				
Anticoagulation Therapy for Atrial Fibrillation[5]	-	-	96%	95%
Antithrombotic Therapy Timing[5]	-	-	98%	98%
Assessed for Rehabilitation[5]	-	-	98%	97%
Discharged on Antithrombotic Therapy[5]	-	-	99%	99%
Discharged on Statin Medication[5]	-	-	95%	94%
Thrombolytic Therapy Timing[5]	-	-	68%	66%
Venous Thromboembolism Prophylaxis[5]	-	-	94%	94%
Written Stroke Educational Materials Given[5]	-	-	92%	88%
Surgical Care Improvement Project				
Appropriate Beta Blocker Usage[5]	-	-	98%	98%
Appropriate VTP Within 24 Hours[5]	-	-	98%	98%
Controlled Postoperative Blood Glucose[5]	-	-	96%	97%
Perioperative Temperature Management[5]	-	-	100%	100%
Prophylactic Antibiotic Selection[5]	-	-	99%	99%
Prophylactic Antibiotic Selection (Outpatient)[5]	-	-	98%	98%
Prophylactic Antibiotic Stopped[5]	-	-	98%	98%
Prophylactic Antibiotic Timing[5]	-	-	99%	99%
Prophylactic Antibiotic Timing (Outpatient)[5]	-	-	98%	98%
Urinary Catheter Removal[5]	-	-	98%	97%
Survey of Patients' Hospital Experiences				
Area Around Room 'Always' Quiet at Night[10]	<100	77%	68%	61%
Doctors 'Always' Communicated Well[10]	<100	82%	83%	82%
Home Recovery Information Given[10]	<100	84%	85%	85%
Hospital Given 9 or 10 on 10 Point Scale[10]	<100	71%	73%	71%
Meds 'Always' Explained Before Given[10]	<100	58%	66%	64%
Nurses 'Always' Communicated Well[10]	<100	76%	80%	79%
Pain 'Always' Well Controlled[10]	<100	80%	72%	71%
Room and Bathroom 'Always' Clean[10]	<100	82%	75%	73%
Timely Help 'Always' Received[10]	<100	71%	69%	68%
Would Definitely Recommend Hospital[10]	<100	64%	73%	71%
Use of Medical Imaging				
Cardiac Imaging Stress Test before Surgery[7]	-	-	5.3%	5.3%
Combination Abdominal CT Scan	56	3.6%	16.4%	10.5%
Combination Brain/Sinus CT Scan[1]	-	-	2.7%	2.7%
Combination Chest CT Scan[1]	-	-	5.6%	2.7%
Follow-up Mammogram/Ultrasound[7]	-	-	7.9%	8.8%
Lumbar Spine MRI for Low Back Pain[1]	-	-	39.6%	37.2%

Moore County Hospital District

224 E Second Street
Dumas, TX 79029
Phone: 806-935-7171
Fax: 806-934-7842
URL: www.mchd.net
Type: Acute Care Hospitals
Emergency Services: Yes
Ownership: Govt - Hospital Dist/Auth
Beds: 60

Key Personnel:
Intensive Care Unit. . . . . Anis Ansari, MD
Quality Assurance . . . . Yvonne Blue
Chairman/CEO . . . . Tom Ferguson
Emergency Room . . . . Mike Flores, MD
Operating Room. . . . . Hilliard Floyd, RN
Infection Control. . . . . Peggy Roberts, RN
Anesthesiology. . . . . Stella Tan, MD
CEO/President. . . . . Jeff Turner, FACHE

Measure	Cases	This Hosp.	State Avg.	U.S. Avg.
Blood Clot Prevention and Treatment				
Anticoagulation Overlap Therapy[1,2]	-	-	93%	93%
ICU Venous Thromboembolism Prophylaxis[2]	31	100%	92%	92%
Incidence of Potentially Preventable VTE[2,7]	-	-	9%	10%
UFH with Dosages/Platelet Monitoring[1,2]	-	-	96%	97%
Venous Thromboembolism Prophylaxis[2]	57	84%	82%	85%
Warfarin Therapy Discharge Instructions[1,2]	-	-	84%	75%
Chest Pain/Possible Heart Attack Care				
Aspirin Given Within 24 Hours of Arrival	43	95%	94%	96%
Fibrinolytic Meds Within 30 Min. of Arrival[1]	-	-	47%	58%
Average Time to ECG (minutes)	44	8	8	7
Average Time to Transfer (minutes)[1]	-	-	62	60
Children's Asthma Care				
Received Home Management Plan of Care	-	-	93%	88%
Received Reliever Medication	-	-	100%	100%
Received Systemic Corticosteroids	-	-	100%	100%
Emergency Department				
Admittance Decision Time (minutes)[2]	144	29	99	98
Head CT Results Within 45 Min. of Arrival[1]	-	-	54%	57%
Patients Who Left ER Before Being Seen	9,031	1%	3%	2%
Time from ER Arrival to Admit. (minutes)[2]	151	186	270	274
Time from ER Arrival to Discharge (minutes)	349	76	127	134
Time in ER Before Being Evaluated (minutes)	341	16	26	26
Time to Pain Meds for Fractures (minutes)	36	34	57	57
Heart Attack Care				
Aspirin Given at Discharge[1]	-	-	99%	99%
Fibrinolytic Meds Within 30 Min. of Arrival[7]	-	-	49%	54%
PCI Within 90 Minutes of Arrival[7]	-	-	95%	96%
Statin Prescribed at Discharge[1]	-	-	98%	98%
Heart Failure Care				
ACE Inhibitor or ARB for LVSD[7]	-	-	97%	97%
Discharge Instructions Given[1]	-	-	95%	94%
Evaluation of LVS Function	16	100%	99%	99%
Medicare Spending				
Medicare Spending per Patient (ratio)	-	0.80	1.03	0.98
Pneumonia Care				
Appropriate Initial Antibiotic Given[1]	-	-	95%	95%
Blood Culture Timing[1]	-	-	98%	98%
Pregnancy and Delivery Care				
Newborn Deliveries Scheduled Early[2]	17	12%	7%	6%
Preventive Care				
Immunization for Influenza[2]	211	93%	90%	90%
Immunization for Pneumonia[2]	162	92%	92%	92%
Stroke Care				
Anticoagulation Therapy for Atrial Fibrillation[7]	-	-	96%	95%
Antithrombotic Therapy Timing[1]	-	-	98%	98%
Assessed for Rehabilitation[1]	-	-	98%	97%
Discharged on Antithrombotic Therapy[1]	-	-	99%	99%
Discharged on Statin Medication[1]	-	-	95%	94%
Thrombolytic Therapy Timing[7]	-	-	68%	66%
Venous Thromboembolism Prophylaxis[1]	-	-	94%	94%
Written Stroke Educational Materials Given[1]	-	-	92%	88%
Surgical Care Improvement Project				
Appropriate Beta Blocker Usage[1]	-	-	98%	98%
Appropriate VTP Within 24 Hours	15	100%	98%	98%
Controlled Postoperative Blood Glucose[7]	-	-	96%	97%
Perioperative Temperature Management	13	100%	100%	100%
Prophylactic Antibiotic Selection[1]	-	-	99%	99%
Prophylactic Antibiotic Selection (Outpatient)[1,3]	-	-	98%	98%
Prophylactic Antibiotic Stopped[1]	-	-	98%	98%
Prophylactic Antibiotic Timing[1]	-	-	99%	99%
Prophylactic Antibiotic Timing (Outpatient)[1,3]	-	-	98%	98%
Urinary Catheter Removal[1]	-	-	98%	97%
Survey of Patients' Hospital Experiences				
Area Around Room 'Always' Quiet at Night	(a)	63%	68%	61%
Doctors 'Always' Communicated Well	(a)	83%	83%	82%
Home Recovery Information Given	(a)	90%	85%	85%
Hospital Given 9 or 10 on 10 Point Scale	(a)	73%	73%	71%
Meds 'Always' Explained Before Given	(a)	68%	66%	64%
Nurses 'Always' Communicated Well	(a)	81%	80%	79%
Pain 'Always' Well Controlled	(a)	73%	72%	71%
Room and Bathroom 'Always' Clean	(a)	79%	75%	73%
Timely Help 'Always' Received	(a)	68%	69%	68%
Would Definitely Recommend Hospital	(a)	69%	73%	71%
Use of Medical Imaging				
Cardiac Imaging Stress Test before Surgery[1]	-	-	5.3%	5.3%
Combination Abdominal CT Scan	105	8.6%	16.4%	10.5%
Combination Brain/Sinus CT Scan[1]	-	-	2.7%	2.7%
Combination Chest CT Scan[1]	-	-	5.6%	2.7%
Follow-up Mammogram/Ultrasound	125	21.6%	7.9%	8.8%
Lumbar Spine MRI for Low Back Pain[1]	-	-	39.6%	37.2%

Fort Duncan Medical Center

3333 N Foster Maldonado Blvd
Eagle Pass, TX 78852
Phone: 830-773-5321
Fax: 830-758-4851
URL: www.fortduncanmedicalcenter.com
Type: Acute Care Hospitals
Emergency Services: Yes
Ownership: Proprietary
Beds: 104

Key Personnel:
Intensive Care Unit. . . . . Wilma Carbonel, RN

NOTE: Hospital profiles are in alphabetical order by state, then city, then hospital within the city; Rankings exclude hospitals with less than 25 cases except for patient surveys which excludes hospitals with less than 100 cases; (a) 100-299 cases; (1) The number of cases/patients is too few to report; (2) Data submitted were based on a sample of cases/patients; (3) Results are based on a shorter time period than required; (4) Data suppressed by CMS for one or more quarters; (5) Results are not available for this reporting period; (6) Fewer than 100 patients completed the HCAHPS survey; (7) No cases met the criteria for this measure; (8) The lower limit of the confidence interval cannot be calculated if the number of observed infections equals zero; (9) No data are available from the state/territory for this reporting period; (10) The scores shown reflect fewer than 50 completed surveys; (11) There were discrepancies in the data collection process; (12) This measure does not apply to this hospital for this reporting period; (13) Results cannot be calculated for this reporting period; (14) The results for this state are combined with nearby states to protect confidentiality; Please refer to the User's Guide for a full explanation of data.

Pediatric In-Patient Care . . . . Ricardo De Los Santos, MD
Infection Control. . . . . Trinidad Justo, RN
Operating Room. . . . . Juliet Martinez, RN
CEO . . . . Richard Prati
Chief of Medical Staff. . . . . Carlos E Rodriguez, MD

Measure	Cases	This Hosp.	State Avg.	U.S. Avg.
Blood Clot Prevention and Treatment				
Anticoagulation Overlap Therapy[1,2]	-	-	93%	93%
ICU Venous Thromboembolism Prophylaxis[2]	102	82%	92%	92%
Incidence of Potentially Preventable VTE[1,2]	-	-	9%	10%
UFH with Dosages/Platelet Monitoring[1,2]	-	-	96%	97%
Venous Thromboembolism Prophylaxis[2]	307	79%	82%	85%
Warfarin Therapy Discharge Instructions[1,2]	-	-	84%	75%
Chest Pain/Possible Heart Attack Care				
Aspirin Given Within 24 Hours of Arrival	74	93%	94%	96%
Fibrinolytic Meds Within 30 Min. of Arrival[1]	-	-	47%	58%
Average Time to ECG (minutes)	76	5	8	7
Average Time to Transfer (minutes)[1]	-	-	62	60
Children's Asthma Care				
Received Home Management Plan of Care	-	-	93%	88%
Received Reliever Medication	-	-	100%	100%
Received Systemic Corticosteroids	-	-	100%	100%
Emergency Department				
Admittance Decision Time (minutes)[2]	233	154	99	98
Head CT Results Within 45 Min. of Arrival	18	22%	54%	57%
Patients Who Left ER Before Being Seen	19,162	1%	3%	2%
Time from ER Arrival to Admit. (minutes)[2]	239	368	270	274
Time from ER Arrival to Discharge (minutes)	379	180	127	134
Time in ER Before Being Evaluated (minutes)	423	23	26	26
Time to Pain Meds for Fractures (minutes)	104	60	57	57
Heart Attack Care				
Aspirin Given at Discharge	13	92%	99%	99%
Fibrinolytic Meds Within 30 Min. of Arrival[7]	-	-	49%	54%
PCI Within 90 Minutes of Arrival[7]	-	-	95%	96%
Statin Prescribed at Discharge	12	100%	98%	98%
Heart Failure Care				
ACE Inhibitor or ARB for LVSD	47	98%	97%	97%
Discharge Instructions Given	98	93%	95%	94%
Evaluation of LVS Function	146	99%	99%	99%
Medicare Spending				
Medicare Spending per Patient (ratio)	-	1.02	1.03	0.98
Pneumonia Care				
Appropriate Initial Antibiotic Given[2]	72	97%	95%	95%
Blood Culture Timing[2]	115	99%	98%	98%
Pregnancy and Delivery Care				
Newborn Deliveries Scheduled Early[2]	53	23%	7%	6%
Preventive Care				
Immunization for Influenza[2]	446	65%	90%	90%
Immunization for Pneumonia[2]	445	91%	92%	92%
Stroke Care				
Anticoagulation Therapy for Atrial Fibrillation[1]	-	-	96%	95%
Antithrombotic Therapy Timing	23	87%	98%	98%
Assessed for Rehabilitation	18	94%	98%	97%
Discharged on Antithrombotic Therapy	17	94%	99%	99%
Discharged on Statin Medication	12	75%	95%	94%
Thrombolytic Therapy Timing[7]	-	-	68%	66%
Venous Thromboembolism Prophylaxis	26	81%	94%	94%
Written Stroke Educational Materials Given[1]	-	-	92%	88%
Surgical Care Improvement Project				
Appropriate Beta Blocker Usage[2]	12	100%	98%	98%
Appropriate VTP Within 24 Hours[2]	93	99%	98%	98%
Controlled Postoperative Blood Glucose[2,7]	-	-	96%	97%
Perioperative Temperature Management[2]	109	100%	100%	100%
Prophylactic Antibiotic Selection[2]	57	100%	99%	99%
Prophylactic Antibiotic Selection (Outpatient)	17	88%	98%	98%
Prophylactic Antibiotic Stopped[2]	56	95%	98%	98%
Prophylactic Antibiotic Timing[2]	57	98%	99%	99%
Prophylactic Antibiotic Timing (Outpatient)	18	94%	98%	98%
Urinary Catheter Removal[2]	44	98%	98%	97%
Survey of Patients' Hospital Experiences				
Area Around Room 'Always' Quiet at Night	300+	60%	68%	61%
Doctors 'Always' Communicated Well	300+	81%	83%	82%
Home Recovery Information Given	300+	83%	85%	85%
Hospital Given 9 or 10 on 10 Point Scale	300+	64%	73%	71%
Meds 'Always' Explained Before Given	300+	66%	66%	64%
Nurses 'Always' Communicated Well	300+	74%	80%	79%
Pain 'Always' Well Controlled	300+	72%	72%	71%
Room and Bathroom 'Always' Clean	300+	75%	75%	73%
Timely Help 'Always' Received	300+	59%	69%	68%
Would Definitely Recommend Hospital	300+	62%	73%	71%
Use of Medical Imaging				
Cardiac Imaging Stress Test before Surgery[1]	-	-	5.3%	5.3%
Combination Abdominal CT Scan	509	1.8%	16.4%	10.5%
Combination Brain/Sinus CT Scan[1]	-	-	2.7%	2.7%
Combination Chest CT Scan	131	0.0%	5.6%	2.7%
Follow-up Mammogram/Ultrasound	557	5.7%	7.9%	8.8%
Lumbar Spine MRI for Low Back Pain	67	35.8%	39.6%	37.2%

Eastland Memorial Hospital

304 S Daugherty
Eastland, TX 76448
Phone: 254-629-2601
Fax: 254-629-8929
E-mail: rrm@eastland-mh.com
URL: www.eastlandmemorial.com
Type: Acute Care Hospitals
Emergency Services: Yes
Ownership: Govt - Hospital Dist/Auth
Beds: 83

Key Personnel:
Patient Relations . . . . Sherry L Clements, RN
CEO/President. . . . . Shane Kernell
Chief of Medical Staff. . . . . Alan Mickish
Radiology. . . . . Gorman Thorp
Infection Control. . . . . Sue Watkins

Measure	Cases	This Hosp.	State Avg.	U.S. Avg.
Blood Clot Prevention and Treatment				
Anticoagulation Overlap Therapy[1,2]	-	-	93%	93%
ICU Venous Thromboembolism Prophylaxis[2,7]	-	-	92%	92%
Incidence of Potentially Preventable VTE[1,2]	-	-	9%	10%
UFH with Dosages/Platelet Monitoring[2,7]	-	-	96%	97%
Venous Thromboembolism Prophylaxis[2]	133	26%	82%	85%
Warfarin Therapy Discharge Instructions[1,2]	-	-	84%	75%
Chest Pain/Possible Heart Attack Care				
Aspirin Given Within 24 Hours of Arrival	28	86%	94%	96%
Fibrinolytic Meds Within 30 Min. of Arrival[1]	-	-	47%	58%
Average Time to ECG (minutes)	30	0	8	7
Average Time to Transfer (minutes)[7]	-	-	62	60
Children's Asthma Care				
Received Home Management Plan of Care	-	-	93%	88%
Received Reliever Medication	-	-	100%	100%
Received Systemic Corticosteroids	-	-	100%	100%
Emergency Department				
Admittance Decision Time (minutes)[2]	112	85	99	98
Head CT Results Within 45 Min. of Arrival[1]	-	-	54%	57%
Patients Who Left ER Before Being Seen	8,882	0%	3%	2%
Time from ER Arrival to Admit. (minutes)[2]	156	243	270	274
Time from ER Arrival to Discharge (minutes)	360	91	127	134
Time in ER Before Being Evaluated (minutes)	344	15	26	26
Time to Pain Meds for Fractures (minutes)	36	36	57	57
Heart Attack Care				
Aspirin Given at Discharge[1,3]	-	-	99%	99%
Fibrinolytic Meds Within 30 Min. of Arrival[3,7]	-	-	49%	54%
PCI Within 90 Minutes of Arrival[3,7]	-	-	95%	96%
Statin Prescribed at Discharge[1,3]	-	-	98%	98%
Heart Failure Care				
ACE Inhibitor or ARB for LVSD[1]	-	-	97%	97%
Discharge Instructions Given	28	93%	95%	94%
Evaluation of LVS Function	44	95%	99%	99%
Medicare Spending				
Medicare Spending per Patient (ratio)	-	1.02	1.03	0.98
Pneumonia Care				
Appropriate Initial Antibiotic Given[2]	22	86%	95%	95%
Blood Culture Timing[2]	26	81%	98%	98%
Pregnancy and Delivery Care				
Newborn Deliveries Scheduled Early[7]	-	-	7%	6%
Preventive Care				
Immunization for Influenza[2]	295	82%	90%	90%
Immunization for Pneumonia[2]	468	84%	92%	92%
Stroke Care				
Anticoagulation Therapy for Atrial Fibrillation[1]	-	-	96%	95%
Antithrombotic Therapy Timing[1]	-	-	98%	98%
Assessed for Rehabilitation[1]	-	-	98%	97%
Discharged on Antithrombotic Therapy[1]	-	-	99%	99%
Discharged on Statin Medication[1]	-	-	95%	94%
Thrombolytic Therapy Timing[1]	-	-	68%	66%
Venous Thromboembolism Prophylaxis[1]	-	-	94%	94%
Written Stroke Educational Materials Given[1]	-	-	92%	88%
Surgical Care Improvement Project				
Appropriate Beta Blocker Usage[1,2]	-	-	98%	98%
Appropriate VTP Within 24 Hours[2]	29	97%	98%	98%
Controlled Postoperative Blood Glucose[2,7]	-	-	96%	97%
Perioperative Temperature Management[2]	33	100%	100%	100%
Prophylactic Antibiotic Selection[1,2]	-	-	99%	99%
Prophylactic Antibiotic Selection (Outpatient)[3,7]	-	-	98%	98%
Prophylactic Antibiotic Stopped[1,2]	-	-	98%	98%
Prophylactic Antibiotic Timing[1,2]	-	-	99%	99%
Prophylactic Antibiotic Timing (Outpatient)[3,7]	-	-	98%	98%
Urinary Catheter Removal[2]	11	55%	98%	97%
Survey of Patients' Hospital Experiences				
Area Around Room 'Always' Quiet at Night	(a)	73%	68%	61%
Doctors 'Always' Communicated Well	(a)	92%	83%	82%
Home Recovery Information Given	(a)	93%	85%	85%
Hospital Given 9 or 10 on 10 Point Scale	(a)	78%	73%	71%
Meds 'Always' Explained Before Given	(a)	74%	66%	64%
Nurses 'Always' Communicated Well	(a)	83%	80%	79%
Pain 'Always' Well Controlled	(a)	81%	72%	71%
Room and Bathroom 'Always' Clean	(a)	73%	75%	73%
Timely Help 'Always' Received	(a)	76%	69%	68%
Would Definitely Recommend Hospital	(a)	72%	73%	71%
Use of Medical Imaging				
Cardiac Imaging Stress Test before Surgery[7]	-	-	5.3%	5.3%
Combination Abdominal CT Scan	133	45.9%	16.4%	10.5%
Combination Brain/Sinus CT Scan[1]	-	-	2.7%	2.7%
Combination Chest CT Scan	70	0.0%	5.6%	2.7%
Follow-up Mammogram/Ultrasound	140	6.4%	7.9%	8.8%
Lumbar Spine MRI for Low Back Pain[1]	-	-	39.6%	37.2%

Cornerstone Regional Hospital

2302 Cornerstone Boulevard
Edinburg, TX 78539
Phone: 956-618-4444
URL: www.southtexashealthsystem.com
Type: Acute Care Hospitals
Emergency Services: Yes
Ownership: Proprietary

Key Personnel:
Operating Room. . . . . Raul Marquez, MD
CEO/President. . . . . Alma Medina
Chief of Medical Staff. . . . . John Orfanos, MD
Radiology. . . . . Rene Villarreal

Measure	Cases	This Hosp.	State Avg.	U.S. Avg.
Blood Clot Prevention and Treatment				
Anticoagulation Overlap Therapy[2,7]	-	-	93%	93%
ICU Venous Thromboembolism Prophylaxis[2,7]	-	-	92%	92%
Incidence of Potentially Preventable VTE[2,7]	-	-	9%	10%
UFH with Dosages/Platelet Monitoring[2,7]	-	-	96%	97%
Venous Thromboembolism Prophylaxis[2]	19	100%	82%	85%
Warfarin Therapy Discharge Instructions[2,7]	-	-	84%	75%
Chest Pain/Possible Heart Attack Care				
Aspirin Given Within 24 Hours of Arrival[5]	-	-	94%	96%
Fibrinolytic Meds Within 30 Min. of Arrival[5]	-	-	47%	58%
Average Time to ECG (minutes)[5]	-	-	8	7
Average Time to Transfer (minutes)[5]	-	-	62	60
Children's Asthma Care				
Received Home Management Plan of Care	-	-	93%	88%
Received Reliever Medication	-	-	100%	100%
Received Systemic Corticosteroids	-	-	100%	100%
Emergency Department				
Admittance Decision Time (minutes)[1,2]	-	-	99	98
Head CT Results Within 45 Min. of Arrival[5]	-	-	54%	57%
Patients Who Left ER Before Being Seen	38	3%	3%	2%
Time from ER Arrival to Admit. (minutes)[1,2]	-	-	270	274
Time from ER Arrival to Discharge (minutes)[3]	15	155	127	134
Time in ER Before Being Evaluated (minutes)[3]	24	98	26	26

NOTE: Hospital profiles are in alphabetical order by state, then city, then hospital within the city; Rankings exclude hospitals with less than 25 cases except for patient surveys which excludes hospitals with less than 100 cases; (a) 100-299 cases; (1) The number of cases/patients is too few to report; (2) Data submitted were based on a sample of cases/patients; (3) Results are based on a shorter time period than required; (4) Data suppressed by CMS for one or more quarters; (5) Results are not available for this reporting period; (6) Fewer than 100 patients completed the HCAHPS survey; (7) No cases met the criteria for this measure; (8) The lower limit of the confidence interval cannot be calculated if the number of observed infections equals zero; (9) No data are available from the state/territory for this reporting period; (10) The scores shown reflect fewer than 50 completed surveys; (11) There were discrepancies in the data collection process; (12) This measure does not apply to this hospital for this reporting period; (13) Results cannot be calculated for this reporting period; (14) The results for this state are combined with nearby states to protect confidentiality; Please refer to the User's Guide for a full explanation of data.

Measure	Cases	This Hosp.	State Avg.	U.S. Avg.
Time to Pain Meds for Fractures (minutes)[5]	-	-	57	57
Heart Attack Care				
Aspirin Given at Discharge[5]	-	-	99%	99%
Fibrinolytic Meds Within 30 Min. of Arrival[5]	-	-	49%	54%
PCI Within 90 Minutes of Arrival[5]	-	-	95%	96%
Statin Prescribed at Discharge[5]	-	-	98%	98%
Heart Failure Care				
ACE Inhibitor or ARB for LVSD[5]	-	-	97%	97%
Discharge Instructions Given[5]	-	-	95%	94%
Evaluation of LVS Function[5]	-	-	99%	99%
Medicare Spending				
Medicare Spending per Patient (ratio)	-	1.00	1.03	0.98
Pneumonia Care				
Appropriate Initial Antibiotic Given[2,3]	-	-	95%	95%
Blood Culture Timing[2,3]	-	-	98%	98%
Pregnancy and Delivery Care				
Newborn Deliveries Scheduled Early[2,7]	-	-	7%	6%
Preventive Care				
Immunization for Influenza[2]	247	99%	90%	90%
Immunization for Pneumonia[2]	382	95%	92%	92%
Stroke Care				
Anticoagulation Therapy for Atrial Fibrillation[5]	-	-	96%	95%
Antithrombotic Therapy Timing[5]	-	-	98%	98%
Assessed for Rehabilitation[5]	-	-	98%	97%
Discharged on Antithrombotic Therapy[5]	-	-	99%	99%
Discharged on Statin Medication[5]	-	-	95%	94%
Thrombolytic Therapy Timing[5]	-	-	68%	66%
Venous Thromboembolism Prophylaxis[5]	-	-	94%	94%
Written Stroke Educational Materials Given[5]	-	-	92%	88%
Surgical Care Improvement Project				
Appropriate Beta Blocker Usage[2]	50	100%	98%	98%
Appropriate VTP Within 24 Hours[2]	339	100%	98%	98%
Controlled Postoperative Blood Glucose[2,7]	-	-	96%	97%
Perioperative Temperature Management[2]	383	100%	100%	100%
Prophylactic Antibiotic Selection[2]	355	99%	99%	99%
Prophylactic Antibiotic Selection (Outpatient)[3]	31	94%	98%	98%
Prophylactic Antibiotic Stopped[2]	351	99%	98%	98%
Prophylactic Antibiotic Timing[2]	355	99%	99%	99%
Prophylactic Antibiotic Timing (Outpatient)[3]	31	97%	98%	98%
Urinary Catheter Removal[1,2]	-	-	98%	97%
Survey of Patients' Hospital Experiences				
Area Around Room 'Always' Quiet at Night	(a)	75%	68%	61%
Doctors 'Always' Communicated Well	(a)	77%	83%	82%
Home Recovery Information Given	(a)	82%	85%	85%
Hospital Given 9 or 10 on 10 Point Scale	(a)	70%	73%	71%
Meds 'Always' Explained Before Given	(a)	63%	66%	64%
Nurses 'Always' Communicated Well	(a)	82%	80%	79%
Pain 'Always' Well Controlled	(a)	71%	72%	71%
Room and Bathroom 'Always' Clean	(a)	79%	75%	73%
Timely Help 'Always' Received	(a)	74%	69%	68%
Would Definitely Recommend Hospital	(a)	78%	73%	71%
Use of Medical Imaging				
Cardiac Imaging Stress Test before Surgery[7]	-	-	5.3%	5.3%
Combination Abdominal CT Scan[1]	-	-	16.4%	10.5%
Combination Brain/Sinus CT Scan[1]	-	-	2.7%	2.7%
Combination Chest CT Scan[7]	-	-	5.6%	2.7%
Follow-up Mammogram/Ultrasound[7]	-	-	7.9%	8.8%
Lumbar Spine MRI for Low Back Pain[7]	-	-	39.6%	37.2%

Doctors Hospital at Renaissance

5501 South Mccoll
Edinburg, TX 78539
URL: www.dhr-rgv.com
Type: Acute Care Hospitals
Ownership: Proprietary
Phone: 956-362-8677
Fax: 956-661-7331
Emergency Services: Yes
Beds: 142
Key Personnel:
CEO/President. . . . . Joseph B Courtney

Measure	Cases	This Hosp.	State Avg.	U.S. Avg.
Blood Clot Prevention and Treatment				
Anticoagulation Overlap Therapy[2]	73	92%	93%	93%
ICU Venous Thromboembolism Prophylaxis[2]	48	94%	92%	92%
Incidence of Potentially Preventable VTE[2]	30	10%	9%	10%
UFH with Dosages/Platelet Monitoring[2]	135	26%	96%	97%
Venous Thromboembolism Prophylaxis[2]	307	95%	82%	85%
Warfarin Therapy Discharge Instructions[2]	38	92%	84%	75%
Chest Pain/Possible Heart Attack Care				
Aspirin Given Within 24 Hours of Arrival[5]	-	-	94%	96%
Fibrinolytic Meds Within 30 Min. of Arrival[5]	-	-	47%	58%
Average Time to ECG (minutes)[5]	-	-	8	7
Average Time to Transfer (minutes)[5]	-	-	62	60
Children's Asthma Care				
Received Home Management Plan of Care	-	-	93%	88%
Received Reliever Medication	-	-	100%	100%
Received Systemic Corticosteroids	-	-	100%	100%
Emergency Department				
Admittance Decision Time (minutes)[2]	291	101	99	98
Head CT Results Within 45 Min. of Arrival[5]	-	-	54%	57%
Patients Who Left ER Before Being Seen	33,853	3%	3%	2%
Time from ER Arrival to Admit. (minutes)[2]	292	263	270	274
Time from ER Arrival to Discharge (minutes)	583	179	127	134
Time in ER Before Being Evaluated (minutes)	706	30	26	26
Time to Pain Meds for Fractures (minutes)	126	67	57	57
Heart Attack Care				
Aspirin Given at Discharge[2]	234	100%	99%	99%
Fibrinolytic Meds Within 30 Min. of Arrival[2,7]	-	-	49%	54%
PCI Within 90 Minutes of Arrival[2]	23	100%	95%	96%
Statin Prescribed at Discharge[2]	221	98%	98%	98%
Heart Failure Care				
ACE Inhibitor or ARB for LVSD[2]	119	98%	97%	97%
Discharge Instructions Given[2]	300	100%	95%	94%
Evaluation of LVS Function[2]	360	100%	99%	99%
Medicare Spending				
Medicare Spending per Patient (ratio)	-	1.03	1.03	0.98
Pneumonia Care				
Appropriate Initial Antibiotic Given[2]	137	96%	95%	95%
Blood Culture Timing[2]	199	99%	98%	98%
Pregnancy and Delivery Care				
Newborn Deliveries Scheduled Early[2,3]	1,288	6%	7%	6%
Preventive Care				
Immunization for Influenza[2]	439	96%	90%	90%
Immunization for Pneumonia[2]	316	97%	92%	92%
Stroke Care				
Anticoagulation Therapy for Atrial Fibrillation[1]	-	-	96%	95%
Antithrombotic Therapy Timing	127	99%	98%	98%
Assessed for Rehabilitation	162	99%	98%	97%
Discharged on Antithrombotic Therapy	135	99%	99%	99%
Discharged on Statin Medication	95	95%	95%	94%
Thrombolytic Therapy Timing[1]	-	-	68%	66%
Venous Thromboembolism Prophylaxis	171	95%	94%	94%
Written Stroke Educational Materials Given	90	97%	92%	88%
Surgical Care Improvement Project				
Appropriate Beta Blocker Usage[2]	260	99%	98%	98%
Appropriate VTP Within 24 Hours[2]	710	99%	98%	98%
Controlled Postoperative Blood Glucose[2]	198	99%	96%	97%
Perioperative Temperature Management[2]	895	100%	100%	100%
Prophylactic Antibiotic Selection[2]	654	100%	99%	99%
Prophylactic Antibiotic Selection (Outpatient)	817	98%	98%	98%
Prophylactic Antibiotic Stopped[2]	615	98%	98%	98%
Prophylactic Antibiotic Timing[2]	660	100%	99%	99%
Prophylactic Antibiotic Timing (Outpatient)	824	98%	98%	98%
Urinary Catheter Removal[2]	467	99%	98%	97%
Survey of Patients' Hospital Experiences				
Area Around Room 'Always' Quiet at Night	300+	66%	68%	61%
Doctors 'Always' Communicated Well	300+	79%	83%	82%
Home Recovery Information Given	300+	82%	85%	85%
Hospital Given 9 or 10 on 10 Point Scale	300+	76%	73%	71%
Meds 'Always' Explained Before Given	300+	63%	66%	64%
Nurses 'Always' Communicated Well	300+	76%	80%	79%
Pain 'Always' Well Controlled	300+	71%	72%	71%
Room and Bathroom 'Always' Clean	300+	76%	75%	73%
Timely Help 'Always' Received	300+	62%	69%	68%
Would Definitely Recommend Hospital	300+	77%	73%	71%
Use of Medical Imaging				
Cardiac Imaging Stress Test before Surgery[1]	-	-	5.3%	5.3%
Combination Abdominal CT Scan	2,163	46.4%	16.4%	10.5%
Combination Brain/Sinus CT Scan	1,624	2.0%	2.7%	2.7%
Combination Chest CT Scan	1,602	33.8%	5.6%	2.7%
Follow-up Mammogram/Ultrasound	3,174	7.9%	7.9%	8.8%
Lumbar Spine MRI for Low Back Pain	533	32.3%	39.6%	37.2%

South Texas Health System

1102 W Trenton Road
Edinburg, TX 78539
URL: www.edinburgregional.com
Type: Acute Care Hospitals
Ownership: Proprietary
Phone: 956-632-4000
Fax: 956-388-6020
Emergency Services: Yes
Beds: 250
Key Personnel:
CEO/President. . . . . James Christian Smolik

Measure	Cases	This Hosp.	State Avg.	U.S. Avg.
Blood Clot Prevention and Treatment				
Anticoagulation Overlap Therapy[2]	77	99%	93%	93%
ICU Venous Thromboembolism Prophylaxis[2]	103	99%	92%	92%
Incidence of Potentially Preventable VTE[2]	22	0%	9%	10%
UFH with Dosages/Platelet Monitoring[2]	42	100%	96%	97%
Venous Thromboembolism Prophylaxis[2]	334	89%	82%	85%
Warfarin Therapy Discharge Instructions[2]	49	96%	84%	75%
Chest Pain/Possible Heart Attack Care				
Aspirin Given Within 24 Hours of Arrival[3,7]	-	-	94%	96%
Fibrinolytic Meds Within 30 Min. of Arrival[5]	-	-	47%	58%
Average Time to ECG (minutes)[3,7]	-	-	8	7
Average Time to Transfer (minutes)[5]	-	-	62	60
Children's Asthma Care				
Received Home Management Plan of Care	-	-	93%	88%
Received Reliever Medication	-	-	100%	100%
Received Systemic Corticosteroids	-	-	100%	100%
Emergency Department				
Admittance Decision Time (minutes)[2]	625	159	99	98
Head CT Results Within 45 Min. of Arrival[1]	-	-	54%	57%
Patients Who Left ER Before Being Seen	74,555	3%	3%	2%
Time from ER Arrival to Admit. (minutes)[2]	668	358	270	274
Time from ER Arrival to Discharge (minutes)	403	176	127	134
Time in ER Before Being Evaluated (minutes)	426	30	26	26
Time to Pain Meds for Fractures (minutes)	368	60	57	57
Heart Attack Care				
Aspirin Given at Discharge[2]	281	100%	99%	99%
Fibrinolytic Meds Within 30 Min. of Arrival[2,7]	-	-	49%	54%
PCI Within 90 Minutes of Arrival[2]	15	100%	95%	96%
Statin Prescribed at Discharge[2]	268	100%	98%	98%
Heart Failure Care				
ACE Inhibitor or ARB for LVSD[2]	88	100%	97%	97%
Discharge Instructions Given[2]	268	94%	95%	94%
Evaluation of LVS Function[2]	310	100%	99%	99%
Medicare Spending				
Medicare Spending per Patient (ratio)	-	1.04	1.03	0.98
Pneumonia Care				
Appropriate Initial Antibiotic Given[2]	77	100%	95%	95%
Blood Culture Timing[2]	131	98%	98%	98%
Pregnancy and Delivery Care				
Newborn Deliveries Scheduled Early[2]	35	3%	7%	6%
Preventive Care				
Immunization for Influenza[2]	551	95%	90%	90%
Immunization for Pneumonia[2]	664	96%	92%	92%
Stroke Care				
Anticoagulation Therapy for Atrial Fibrillation[1,2]	-	-	96%	95%
Antithrombotic Therapy Timing[2]	93	100%	98%	98%
Assessed for Rehabilitation[2]	125	99%	98%	97%
Discharged on Antithrombotic Therapy[2]	95	100%	99%	99%
Discharged on Statin Medication[2]	69	99%	95%	94%
Thrombolytic Therapy Timing[1,2]	-	-	68%	66%
Venous Thromboembolism Prophylaxis[2]	137	98%	94%	94%
Written Stroke Educational Materials Given[2]	81	99%	92%	88%
Surgical Care Improvement Project				
Appropriate Beta Blocker Usage[2]	168	98%	98%	98%
Appropriate VTP Within 24 Hours[2]	370	99%	98%	98%
Controlled Postoperative Blood Glucose[2]	121	99%	96%	97%
Perioperative Temperature Management[2]	419	100%	100%	100%
Prophylactic Antibiotic Selection[2]	318	100%	99%	99%
Prophylactic Antibiotic Selection (Outpatient)	283	99%	98%	98%

NOTE: Hospital profiles are in alphabetical order by state, then city, then hospital within the city; Rankings exclude hospitals with less than 25 cases except for patient surveys which excludes hospitals with less than 100 cases; (a) 100-299 cases; (1) The number of cases/patients is too few to report; (2) Data submitted were based on a sample of cases/patients; (3) Results are based on a shorter time period than required; (4) Data suppressed by CMS for one or more quarters; (5) Results are not available for this reporting period; (6) Fewer than 100 patients completed the HCAHPS survey; (7) No cases met the criteria for this measure; (8) The lower limit of the confidence interval cannot be calculated if the number of observed infections equals zero; (9) No data are available from the state/territory for this reporting period; (10) The scores shown reflect fewer than 50 completed surveys; (11) There were discrepancies in the data collection process; (12) This measure does not apply to this hospital for this reporting period; (13) Results cannot be calculated for this reporting period; (14) The results for this state are combined with nearby states to protect confidentiality; Please refer to the User's Guide for a full explanation of data.

Measure	Cases	This Hosp.	State Avg.	U.S. Avg.
Prophylactic Antibiotic Stopped[2]	297	97%	98%	98%
Prophylactic Antibiotic Timing[2]	318	98%	99%	99%
Prophylactic Antibiotic Timing (Outpatient)	287	98%	98%	98%
Urinary Catheter Removal[2]	270	97%	98%	97%
Survey of Patients' Hospital Experiences				
Area Around Room 'Always' Quiet at Night	300+	65%	68%	61%
Doctors 'Always' Communicated Well	300+	78%	83%	82%
Home Recovery Information Given	300+	82%	85%	85%
Hospital Given 9 or 10 on 10 Point Scale	300+	69%	73%	71%
Meds 'Always' Explained Before Given	300+	61%	66%	64%
Nurses 'Always' Communicated Well	300+	73%	80%	79%
Pain 'Always' Well Controlled	300+	69%	72%	71%
Room and Bathroom 'Always' Clean	300+	68%	75%	73%
Timely Help 'Always' Received	300+	60%	69%	68%
Would Definitely Recommend Hospital	300+	69%	73%	71%
Use of Medical Imaging				
Cardiac Imaging Stress Test before Surgery	88	2.3%	5.3%	5.3%
Combination Abdominal CT Scan	588	15.3%	16.4%	10.5%
Combination Brain/Sinus CT Scan	860	3.4%	2.7%	2.7%
Combination Chest CT Scan	206	7.8%	5.6%	2.7%
Follow-up Mammogram/Ultrasound	549	9.3%	7.9%	8.8%
Lumbar Spine MRI for Low Back Pain[1]	-	-	39.6%	37.2%

Jackson Healthcare Center

1013 S Wells
Edna, TX 77957
Phone: 361-782-7800
Type: Critical Access Hospitals
Emergency Services: Yes
Ownership: Govt - Hospital Dist/Auth

Measure	Cases	This Hosp.	State Avg.	U.S. Avg.
Blood Clot Prevention and Treatment				
Anticoagulation Overlap Therapy[2,3]	-	-	93%	93%
ICU Venous Thromboembolism Prophylaxis[2,3]	-	-	92%	92%
Incidence of Potentially Preventable VTE[2,3]	-	-	9%	10%
UFH with Dosages/Platelet Monitoring[2,3]	-	-	96%	97%
Venous Thromboembolism Prophylaxis[1,2]	-	-	82%	85%
Warfarin Therapy Discharge Instructions[2,3]	-	-	84%	75%
Chest Pain/Possible Heart Attack Care				
Aspirin Given Within 24 Hours of Arrival[1,3]	-	-	94%	96%
Fibrinolytic Meds Within 30 Min. of Arrival[5]	-	-	47%	58%
Average Time to ECG (minutes)[1,3]	-	-	8	7
Average Time to Transfer (minutes)[5]	-	-	62	60
Children's Asthma Care				
Received Home Management Plan of Care	-	-	93%	88%
Received Reliever Medication	-	-	100%	100%
Received Systemic Corticosteroids	-	-	100%	100%
Emergency Department				
Admittance Decision Time (minutes)[5]	-	-	99	98
Head CT Results Within 45 Min. of Arrival[5]	-	-	54%	57%
Patients Who Left ER Before Being Seen	4,358	0%	3%	2%
Time from ER Arrival to Admit. (minutes)[5]	-	-	270	274
Time from ER Arrival to Discharge (minutes)[3]	79	75	127	134
Time in ER Before Being Evaluated (minutes)[3]	73	12	26	26
Time to Pain Meds for Fractures (minutes)[5]	-	-	57	57
Heart Attack Care				
Aspirin Given at Discharge[5]	-	-	99%	99%
Fibrinolytic Meds Within 30 Min. of Arrival[5]	-	-	49%	54%
PCI Within 90 Minutes of Arrival[5]	-	-	95%	96%
Statin Prescribed at Discharge[5]	-	-	98%	98%
Heart Failure Care				
ACE Inhibitor or ARB for LVSD[2,3]	-	-	97%	97%
Discharge Instructions Given[2,3]	-	-	95%	94%
Evaluation of LVS Function[1,2]	-	-	99%	99%
Medicare Spending				
Medicare Spending per Patient (ratio)	-	-	1.03	0.98
Pneumonia Care				
Appropriate Initial Antibiotic Given[1,2]	-	-	95%	95%
Blood Culture Timing[1,2]	-	-	98%	98%
Pregnancy and Delivery Care				
Newborn Deliveries Scheduled Early[5]	-	-	7%	6%
Preventive Care				
Immunization for Influenza[5]	-	-	90%	90%
Immunization for Pneumonia[5]	-	-	92%	92%
Stroke Care				
Anticoagulation Therapy for Atrial Fibrillation[5]	-	-	96%	95%
Antithrombotic Therapy Timing[5]	-	-	98%	98%
Assessed for Rehabilitation[5]	-	-	98%	97%
Discharged on Antithrombotic Therapy[5]	-	-	99%	99%
Discharged on Statin Medication[5]	-	-	95%	94%
Thrombolytic Therapy Timing[5]	-	-	68%	66%
Venous Thromboembolism Prophylaxis[5]	-	-	94%	94%
Written Stroke Educational Materials Given[5]	-	-	92%	88%
Surgical Care Improvement Project				
Appropriate Beta Blocker Usage[5]	-	-	98%	98%
Appropriate VTP Within 24 Hours[5]	-	-	98%	98%
Controlled Postoperative Blood Glucose[5]	-	-	96%	97%
Perioperative Temperature Management[5]	-	-	100%	100%
Prophylactic Antibiotic Selection[5]	-	-	99%	99%
Prophylactic Antibiotic Selection (Outpatient)[5]	-	-	98%	98%
Prophylactic Antibiotic Stopped[5]	-	-	98%	98%
Prophylactic Antibiotic Timing[5]	-	-	99%	99%
Prophylactic Antibiotic Timing (Outpatient)[5]	-	-	98%	98%
Urinary Catheter Removal[5]	-	-	98%	97%
Survey of Patients' Hospital Experiences				
Area Around Room 'Always' Quiet at Night[5]	-	-	68%	61%
Doctors 'Always' Communicated Well[5]	-	-	83%	82%
Home Recovery Information Given[5]	-	-	85%	85%
Hospital Given 9 or 10 on 10 Point Scale[5]	-	-	73%	71%
Meds 'Always' Explained Before Given[5]	-	-	66%	64%
Nurses 'Always' Communicated Well[5]	-	-	80%	79%
Pain 'Always' Well Controlled[5]	-	-	72%	71%
Room and Bathroom 'Always' Clean[5]	-	-	75%	73%
Timely Help 'Always' Received[5]	-	-	69%	68%
Would Definitely Recommend Hospital[5]	-	-	73%	71%
Use of Medical Imaging				
Cardiac Imaging Stress Test before Surgery[7]	-	-	5.3%	5.3%
Combination Abdominal CT Scan	74	21.6%	16.4%	10.5%
Combination Brain/Sinus CT Scan[1]	-	-	2.7%	2.7%
Combination Chest CT Scan[1]	-	-	5.6%	2.7%
Follow-up Mammogram/Ultrasound	68	14.7%	7.9%	8.8%
Lumbar Spine MRI for Low Back Pain[1]	-	-	39.6%	37.2%

El Campo Memorial Hospital

303 Sandy Corner Rd
El Campo, TX 77437
Phone: 979-578-5251
Fax: 979-543-8420
E-mail: sgularte@ecmh.org
URL: www.ecmh.org
Type: Acute Care Hospitals
Emergency Services: Yes
Ownership: Voluntary non-profit - Other
Beds: 49

Key Personnel:
Emergency Room . . . . Carlos Duqua, MD
CEO/President. . . . . Steve Gularte
Infection Control. . . . . Sherrie Hardin, RN
Intensive Care Unit. . . . . Sherrie Hardin, RN
Quality Assurance . . . . Billie Jurasek, RN
Chief of Medical Staff. . . . . Ankus Sarkar
Anesthesiology. . . . . Pramodh Wadera, MD

Measure	Cases	This Hosp.	State Avg.	U.S. Avg.
Blood Clot Prevention and Treatment				
Anticoagulation Overlap Therapy[1,2]	-	-	93%	93%
ICU Venous Thromboembolism Prophylaxis[2]	26	62%	92%	92%
Incidence of Potentially Preventable VTE[2,7]	-	-	9%	10%
UFH with Dosages/Platelet Monitoring[1,2]	-	-	96%	97%
Venous Thromboembolism Prophylaxis[2]	127	50%	82%	85%
Warfarin Therapy Discharge Instructions[1,2]	-	-	84%	75%
Chest Pain/Possible Heart Attack Care				
Aspirin Given Within 24 Hours of Arrival	24	83%	94%	96%
Fibrinolytic Meds Within 30 Min. of Arrival[7]	-	-	47%	58%
Average Time to ECG (minutes)	27	12	8	7
Average Time to Transfer (minutes)[7]	-	-	62	60
Children's Asthma Care				
Received Home Management Plan of Care	-	-	93%	88%
Received Reliever Medication	-	-	100%	100%
Received Systemic Corticosteroids	-	-	100%	100%
Emergency Department				
Admittance Decision Time (minutes)	117	49	99	98
Head CT Results Within 45 Min. of Arrival[1]	-	-	54%	57%
Patients Who Left ER Before Being Seen	5,984	2%	3%	2%
Time from ER Arrival to Admit. (minutes)	208	203	270	274
Time from ER Arrival to Discharge (minutes)	388	101	127	134
Time in ER Before Being Evaluated (minutes)	357	20	26	26
Time to Pain Meds for Fractures (minutes)	27	49	57	57
Heart Attack Care				
Aspirin Given at Discharge[1]	-	-	99%	99%
Fibrinolytic Meds Within 30 Min. of Arrival[7]	-	-	49%	54%
PCI Within 90 Minutes of Arrival[7]	-	-	95%	96%
Statin Prescribed at Discharge[1]	-	-	98%	98%
Heart Failure Care				
ACE Inhibitor or ARB for LVSD[1]	-	-	97%	97%
Discharge Instructions Given	20	90%	95%	94%
Evaluation of LVS Function	22	95%	99%	99%
Medicare Spending				
Medicare Spending per Patient (ratio)	-	0.91	1.03	0.98
Pneumonia Care				
Appropriate Initial Antibiotic Given	18	78%	95%	95%
Blood Culture Timing	25	92%	98%	98%
Pregnancy and Delivery Care				
Newborn Deliveries Scheduled Early[7]	-	-	7%	6%
Preventive Care				
Immunization for Influenza	169	99%	90%	90%
Immunization for Pneumonia	245	100%	92%	92%
Stroke Care				
Anticoagulation Therapy for Atrial Fibrillation[7]	-	-	96%	95%
Antithrombotic Therapy Timing[1]	-	-	98%	98%
Assessed for Rehabilitation[1]	-	-	98%	97%
Discharged on Antithrombotic Therapy[1]	-	-	99%	99%
Discharged on Statin Medication[1]	-	-	95%	94%
Thrombolytic Therapy Timing[7]	-	-	68%	66%
Venous Thromboembolism Prophylaxis[1]	-	-	94%	94%
Written Stroke Educational Materials Given[1]	-	-	92%	88%
Surgical Care Improvement Project				
Appropriate Beta Blocker Usage[1,3]	-	-	98%	98%
Appropriate VTP Within 24 Hours[1,3]	-	-	98%	98%
Controlled Postoperative Blood Glucose[3,7]	-	-	96%	97%
Perioperative Temperature Management[1,3]	-	-	100%	100%
Prophylactic Antibiotic Selection[1,3]	-	-	99%	99%
Prophylactic Antibiotic Selection (Outpatient)[3,7]	-	-	98%	98%
Prophylactic Antibiotic Stopped[1,3]	-	-	98%	98%
Prophylactic Antibiotic Timing[1,3]	-	-	99%	99%
Prophylactic Antibiotic Timing (Outpatient)[3,7]	-	-	98%	98%
Urinary Catheter Removal[1,3]	-	-	98%	97%
Survey of Patients' Hospital Experiences				
Area Around Room 'Always' Quiet at Night[6]	<100	73%	68%	61%
Doctors 'Always' Communicated Well[6]	<100	85%	83%	82%
Home Recovery Information Given[6]	<100	85%	85%	85%
Hospital Given 9 or 10 on 10 Point Scale[6]	<100	67%	73%	71%
Meds 'Always' Explained Before Given[6]	<100	76%	66%	64%
Nurses 'Always' Communicated Well[6]	<100	89%	80%	79%
Pain 'Always' Well Controlled[6]	<100	89%	72%	71%
Room and Bathroom 'Always' Clean[6]	<100	82%	75%	73%
Timely Help 'Always' Received[6]	<100	80%	69%	68%
Would Definitely Recommend Hospital[6]	<100	67%	73%	71%
Use of Medical Imaging				
Cardiac Imaging Stress Test before Surgery[1]	-	-	5.3%	5.3%
Combination Abdominal CT Scan	112	44.6%	16.4%	10.5%
Combination Brain/Sinus CT Scan[1]	-	-	2.7%	2.7%
Combination Chest CT Scan[1]	-	-	5.6%	2.7%
Follow-up Mammogram/Ultrasound	241	0.0%	7.9%	8.8%
Lumbar Spine MRI for Low Back Pain[1]	-	-	39.6%	37.2%

El Paso Specialty Hospital

1755 Curie Suite A
El Paso, TX 79902
Phone: 915-544-3636
E-mail: vquiambao@nhsinc.com
URL: www.elpasospecialtyhospital.com
Type: Acute Care Hospitals
Emergency Services: Yes
Ownership: Proprietary
Beds: 31

Key Personnel:
CEO/President. . . . . Tom Meagher
Operating Room. . . . . Gloria Pena
Radiology. . . . . Richard Pena

NOTE: Hospital profiles are in alphabetical order by state, then city, then hospital within the city; Rankings exclude hospitals with less than 25 cases except for patient surveys which excludes hospitals with less than 100 cases; (a) 100-299 cases; (1) The number of cases/patients is too few to report; (2) Data submitted were based on a sample of cases/patients; (3) Results are based on a shorter time period than required; (4) Data suppressed by CMS for one or more quarters; (5) Results are not available for this reporting period; (6) Fewer than 100 patients completed the HCAHPS survey; (7) No cases met the criteria for this measure; (8) The lower limit of the confidence interval cannot be calculated if the number of observed infections equals zero; (9) No data are available from the state/territory for this reporting period; (10) The scores shown reflect fewer than 50 completed surveys; (11) There were discrepancies in the data collection process; (12) This measure does not apply to this hospital for this reporting period; (13) Results cannot be calculated for this reporting period; (14) The results for this state are combined with nearby states to protect confidentiality; Please refer to the User's Guide for a full explanation of data.

Measure	Cases	This Hosp.	State Avg.	U.S. Avg.
Blood Clot Prevention and Treatment				
Anticoagulation Overlap Therapy[1,2]	-	-	93%	93%
ICU Venous Thromboembolism Prophylaxis[2,7]	-	-	92%	92%
Incidence of Potentially Preventable VTE[1,2]	-	-	9%	10%
UFH with Dosages/Platelet Monitoring[2,7]	-	-	96%	97%
Venous Thromboembolism Prophylaxis[2]	234	99%	82%	85%
Warfarin Therapy Discharge Instructions[1,2]	-	-	84%	75%
Chest Pain/Possible Heart Attack Care				
Aspirin Given Within 24 Hours of Arrival[5]	-	-	94%	96%
Fibrinolytic Meds Within 30 Min. of Arrival[5]	-	-	47%	58%
Average Time to ECG (minutes)[5]	-	-	8	7
Average Time to Transfer (minutes)[5]	-	-	62	60
Children's Asthma Care				
Received Home Management Plan of Care	-	-	93%	88%
Received Reliever Medication	-	-	100%	100%
Received Systemic Corticosteroids	-	-	100%	100%
Emergency Department				
Admittance Decision Time (minutes)[2]	43	26	99	98
Head CT Results Within 45 Min. of Arrival[5]	-	-	54%	57%
Patients Who Left ER Before Being Seen	2,200	0%	3%	2%
Time from ER Arrival to Admit. (minutes)[2]	43	175	270	274
Time from ER Arrival to Discharge (minutes)	325	83	127	134
Time in ER Before Being Evaluated (minutes)	330	12	26	26
Time to Pain Meds for Fractures (minutes)	84	28	57	57
Heart Attack Care				
Aspirin Given at Discharge[5]	-	-	99%	99%
Fibrinolytic Meds Within 30 Min. of Arrival[5]	-	-	49%	54%
PCI Within 90 Minutes of Arrival[5]	-	-	95%	96%
Statin Prescribed at Discharge[5]	-	-	98%	98%
Heart Failure Care				
ACE Inhibitor or ARB for LVSD[5]	-	-	97%	97%
Discharge Instructions Given[5]	-	-	95%	94%
Evaluation of LVS Function[5]	-	-	99%	99%
Medicare Spending				
Medicare Spending per Patient (ratio)	-	1.01	1.03	0.98
Pneumonia Care				
Appropriate Initial Antibiotic Given[5]	-	-	95%	95%
Blood Culture Timing[5]	-	-	98%	98%
Pregnancy and Delivery Care				
Newborn Deliveries Scheduled Early[7]	-	-	7%	6%
Preventive Care				
Immunization for Influenza[2]	329	89%	90%	90%
Immunization for Pneumonia[2]	377	89%	92%	92%
Stroke Care				
Anticoagulation Therapy for Atrial Fibrillation[5]	-	-	96%	95%
Antithrombotic Therapy Timing[5]	-	-	98%	98%
Assessed for Rehabilitation[5]	-	-	98%	97%
Discharged on Antithrombotic Therapy[5]	-	-	99%	99%
Discharged on Statin Medication[5]	-	-	95%	94%
Thrombolytic Therapy Timing[5]	-	-	68%	66%
Venous Thromboembolism Prophylaxis[5]	-	-	94%	94%
Written Stroke Educational Materials Given[5]	-	-	92%	88%
Surgical Care Improvement Project				
Appropriate Beta Blocker Usage	101	93%	98%	98%
Appropriate VTP Within 24 Hours	422	100%	98%	98%
Controlled Postoperative Blood Glucose[7]	-	-	96%	97%
Perioperative Temperature Management	433	100%	100%	100%
Prophylactic Antibiotic Selection	417	99%	99%	99%
Prophylactic Antibiotic Selection (Outpatient)	45	100%	98%	98%
Prophylactic Antibiotic Stopped	417	98%	98%	98%
Prophylactic Antibiotic Timing	417	100%	99%	99%
Prophylactic Antibiotic Timing (Outpatient)	45	100%	98%	98%
Urinary Catheter Removal	27	100%	98%	97%
Survey of Patients' Hospital Experiences				
Area Around Room 'Always' Quiet at Night	(a)	71%	68%	61%
Doctors 'Always' Communicated Well	(a)	83%	83%	82%
Home Recovery Information Given	(a)	88%	85%	85%
Hospital Given 9 or 10 on 10 Point Scale	(a)	72%	73%	71%
Meds 'Always' Explained Before Given	(a)	60%	66%	64%
Nurses 'Always' Communicated Well	(a)	75%	80%	79%
Pain 'Always' Well Controlled	(a)	69%	72%	71%
Room and Bathroom 'Always' Clean	(a)	76%	75%	73%
Timely Help 'Always' Received	(a)	68%	69%	68%
Would Definitely Recommend Hospital	(a)	76%	73%	71%
Use of Medical Imaging				
Cardiac Imaging Stress Test before Surgery[7]	-	-	5.3%	5.3%
Combination Abdominal CT Scan[1]	-	-	16.4%	10.5%
Combination Brain/Sinus CT Scan[1]	-	-	2.7%	2.7%
Combination Chest CT Scan[7]	-	-	5.6%	2.7%
Follow-up Mammogram/Ultrasound[7]	-	-	7.9%	8.8%
Lumbar Spine MRI for Low Back Pain[7]	-	-	39.6%	37.2%

Foundation Surgical Hospital of El Paso

1416 George Dieter
El Paso, TX 79936
Phone: 915-598-4240
Fax: 9155984412
E-mail: info@physicianshospital.net
URL: www.physicianshospital.net
Type: Acute Care Hospitals
Emergency Services: Yes
Ownership: Physician

Measure	Cases	This Hosp.	State Avg.	U.S. Avg.
Blood Clot Prevention and Treatment				
Anticoagulation Overlap Therapy[1,2]	-	-	93%	93%
ICU Venous Thromboembolism Prophylaxis[1,2]	-	-	92%	92%
Incidence of Potentially Preventable VTE[2,7]	-	-	9%	10%
UFH with Dosages/Platelet Monitoring[1,2]	-	-	96%	97%
Venous Thromboembolism Prophylaxis[2]	35	80%	82%	85%
Warfarin Therapy Discharge Instructions[1,2]	-	-	84%	75%
Chest Pain/Possible Heart Attack Care				
Aspirin Given Within 24 Hours of Arrival[1,3]	-	-	94%	96%
Fibrinolytic Meds Within 30 Min. of Arrival[3,7]	-	-	47%	58%
Average Time to ECG (minutes)[1,3]	-	-	8	7
Average Time to Transfer (minutes)[3,7]	-	-	62	60
Children's Asthma Care				
Received Home Management Plan of Care	-	-	93%	88%
Received Reliever Medication	-	-	100%	100%
Received Systemic Corticosteroids	-	-	100%	100%
Emergency Department				
Admittance Decision Time (minutes)[1,2]	-	-	99	98
Head CT Results Within 45 Min. of Arrival[1,3]	-	-	54%	57%
Patients Who Left ER Before Being Seen	10,736	1%	3%	2%
Time from ER Arrival to Admit. (minutes)[1,2]	-	-	270	274
Time from ER Arrival to Discharge (minutes)	546	110	127	134
Time in ER Before Being Evaluated (minutes)	569	22	26	26
Time to Pain Meds for Fractures (minutes)	41	54	57	57
Heart Attack Care				
Aspirin Given at Discharge[5]	-	-	99%	99%
Fibrinolytic Meds Within 30 Min. of Arrival[5]	-	-	49%	54%
PCI Within 90 Minutes of Arrival[5]	-	-	95%	96%
Statin Prescribed at Discharge[5]	-	-	98%	98%
Heart Failure Care				
ACE Inhibitor or ARB for LVSD[5]	-	-	97%	97%
Discharge Instructions Given[5]	-	-	95%	94%
Evaluation of LVS Function[5]	-	-	99%	99%
Medicare Spending				
Medicare Spending per Patient (ratio)	-	1.03	1.03	0.98
Pneumonia Care				
Appropriate Initial Antibiotic Given[1,2]	-	-	95%	95%
Blood Culture Timing[1,2]	-	-	98%	98%
Pregnancy and Delivery Care				
Newborn Deliveries Scheduled Early[2,7]	-	-	7%	6%
Preventive Care				
Immunization for Influenza[2]	304	88%	90%	90%
Immunization for Pneumonia[2]	362	85%	92%	92%
Stroke Care				
Anticoagulation Therapy for Atrial Fibrillation[5]	-	-	96%	95%
Antithrombotic Therapy Timing[5]	-	-	98%	98%
Assessed for Rehabilitation[5]	-	-	98%	97%
Discharged on Antithrombotic Therapy[5]	-	-	99%	99%
Discharged on Statin Medication[5]	-	-	95%	94%
Thrombolytic Therapy Timing[5]	-	-	68%	66%
Venous Thromboembolism Prophylaxis[5]	-	-	94%	94%
Written Stroke Educational Materials Given[5]	-	-	92%	88%
Surgical Care Improvement Project				
Appropriate Beta Blocker Usage[2]	30	90%	98%	98%
Appropriate VTP Within 24 Hours[2]	148	96%	98%	98%
Controlled Postoperative Blood Glucose[2,7]	-	-	96%	97%
Perioperative Temperature Management[2]	192	100%	100%	100%
Prophylactic Antibiotic Selection[2]	148	99%	99%	99%
Prophylactic Antibiotic Selection (Outpatient)	99	98%	98%	98%
Prophylactic Antibiotic Stopped[2]	143	99%	98%	98%
Prophylactic Antibiotic Timing[2]	149	100%	99%	99%
Prophylactic Antibiotic Timing (Outpatient)	99	100%	98%	98%
Urinary Catheter Removal[2]	59	95%	98%	97%
Survey of Patients' Hospital Experiences				
Area Around Room 'Always' Quiet at Night	300+	70%	68%	61%
Doctors 'Always' Communicated Well	300+	82%	83%	82%
Home Recovery Information Given	300+	84%	85%	85%
Hospital Given 9 or 10 on 10 Point Scale	300+	73%	73%	71%
Meds 'Always' Explained Before Given	300+	60%	66%	64%
Nurses 'Always' Communicated Well	300+	77%	80%	79%
Pain 'Always' Well Controlled	300+	72%	72%	71%
Room and Bathroom 'Always' Clean	300+	72%	75%	73%
Timely Help 'Always' Received	300+	72%	69%	68%
Would Definitely Recommend Hospital	300+	74%	73%	71%
Use of Medical Imaging				
Cardiac Imaging Stress Test before Surgery[1]	-	-	5.3%	5.3%
Combination Abdominal CT Scan	316	18.4%	16.4%	10.5%
Combination Brain/Sinus CT Scan[1]	-	-	2.7%	2.7%
Combination Chest CT Scan	74	21.6%	5.6%	2.7%
Follow-up Mammogram/Ultrasound[7]	-	-	7.9%	8.8%
Lumbar Spine MRI for Low Back Pain	47	46.8%	39.6%	37.2%

Las Palmas Medical Center

1801 North Oregon Street
El Paso, TX 79902
Phone: 915-521-1200
Fax: 915-544-5203
Type: Acute Care Hospitals
Emergency Services: Yes
Ownership: Proprietary
Beds: 255

Key Personnel:

Pediatric In-Patient Care .... Eduardo Covarrubias, MD
Emergency Room .... Mitchell Farrell, MD
Chief of Medical Staff.......... Emilio Gonzalez-Ayala, MD
CEO .... Henry Hank Hernandez
Radiology.................. Hugo Isuani, MD
Quality Assurance .... Alan Napier
Intensive Care Unit........... Denise Porter
Operating Room............. Becky Van Haslen

Measure	Cases	This Hosp.	State Avg.	U.S. Avg.
Blood Clot Prevention and Treatment				
Anticoagulation Overlap Therapy[2]	109	79%	93%	93%
ICU Venous Thromboembolism Prophylaxis[2]	117	91%	92%	92%
Incidence of Potentially Preventable VTE[2]	30	20%	9%	10%
UFH with Dosages/Platelet Monitoring[2]	16	100%	96%	97%
Venous Thromboembolism Prophylaxis[2]	409	72%	82%	85%
Warfarin Therapy Discharge Instructions[2]	71	75%	84%	75%
Chest Pain/Possible Heart Attack Care				
Aspirin Given Within 24 Hours of Arrival[1,3]	-	-	94%	96%
Fibrinolytic Meds Within 30 Min. of Arrival[5]	-	-	47%	58%
Average Time to ECG (minutes)[1,3]	-	-	8	7
Average Time to Transfer (minutes)[5]	-	-	62	60
Children's Asthma Care				
Received Home Management Plan of Care	-	-	93%	88%
Received Reliever Medication	-	-	100%	100%
Received Systemic Corticosteroids	-	-	100%	100%
Emergency Department				
Admittance Decision Time (minutes)[2]	778	115	99	98
Head CT Results Within 45 Min. of Arrival[1]	-	-	54%	57%
Patients Who Left ER Before Being Seen	43,553	2%	3%	2%
Time from ER Arrival to Admit. (minutes)[2]	778	308	270	274
Time from ER Arrival to Discharge (minutes)	527	143	127	134
Time in ER Before Being Evaluated (minutes)	548	24	26	26
Time to Pain Meds for Fractures (minutes)	381	51	57	57
Heart Attack Care				
Aspirin Given at Discharge	308	100%	99%	99%
Fibrinolytic Meds Within 30 Min. of Arrival[1]	-	-	49%	54%
PCI Within 90 Minutes of Arrival	45	96%	95%	96%
Statin Prescribed at Discharge	298	100%	98%	98%
Heart Failure Care				
ACE Inhibitor or ARB for LVSD	221	100%	97%	97%

NOTE: Hospital profiles are in alphabetical order by state, then city, then hospital within the city; Rankings exclude hospitals with less than 25 cases except for patient surveys which excludes hospitals with less than 100 cases; (a) 100-299 cases; (1) The number of cases/patients is too few to report; (2) Data submitted were based on a sample of cases/patients; (3) Results are based on a shorter time period than required; (4) Data suppressed by CMS for one or more quarters; (5) Results are not available for this reporting period; (6) Fewer than 100 patients completed the HCAHPS survey; (7) No cases met the criteria for this measure; (8) The lower limit of the confidence interval cannot be calculated if the number of observed infections equals zero; (9) No data are available from the state/territory for this reporting period; (10) The scores shown reflect fewer than 50 completed surveys; (11) There were discrepancies in the data collection process; (12) This measure does not apply to this hospital for this reporting period; (13) Results cannot be calculated for this reporting period; (14) The results for this state are combined with nearby states to protect confidentiality; Please refer to the User's Guide for a full explanation of data.

Measure	Cases	This Hosp.	State Avg.	U.S. Avg.
Discharge Instructions Given	565	100%	95%	94%
Evaluation of LVS Function	647	100%	99%	99%
Medicare Spending				
Medicare Spending per Patient (ratio)	-	1.01	1.03	0.98
Pneumonia Care				
Appropriate Initial Antibiotic Given	298	99%	95%	95%
Blood Culture Timing	546	100%	98%	98%
Pregnancy and Delivery Care				
Newborn Deliveries Scheduled Early[2]	115	3%	7%	6%
Preventive Care				
Immunization for Influenza[2]	661	82%	90%	90%
Immunization for Pneumonia[2]	762	88%	92%	92%
Stroke Care				
Anticoagulation Therapy for Atrial Fibrillation[2]	12	100%	96%	95%
Antithrombotic Therapy Timing[2]	95	99%	98%	98%
Assessed for Rehabilitation[2]	123	99%	98%	97%
Discharged on Antithrombotic Therapy[2]	105	99%	99%	99%
Discharged on Statin Medication[2]	80	99%	95%	94%
Thrombolytic Therapy Timing[2]	19	95%	68%	66%
Venous Thromboembolism Prophylaxis[2]	134	99%	94%	94%
Written Stroke Educational Materials Given[2]	80	98%	92%	88%
Surgical Care Improvement Project				
Appropriate Beta Blocker Usage[2]	188	99%	98%	98%
Appropriate VTP Within 24 Hours[2]	453	100%	98%	98%
Controlled Postoperative Blood Glucose[2]	104	100%	96%	97%
Perioperative Temperature Management[2]	549	100%	100%	100%
Prophylactic Antibiotic Selection[2]	435	100%	99%	99%
Prophylactic Antibiotic Selection (Outpatient)	828	99%	98%	98%
Prophylactic Antibiotic Stopped[2]	426	99%	98%	98%
Prophylactic Antibiotic Timing[2]	436	100%	99%	99%
Prophylactic Antibiotic Timing (Outpatient)	828	100%	98%	98%
Urinary Catheter Removal[2]	184	98%	98%	97%
Survey of Patients' Hospital Experiences				
Area Around Room 'Always' Quiet at Night	300+	62%	68%	61%
Doctors 'Always' Communicated Well	300+	77%	83%	82%
Home Recovery Information Given	300+	84%	85%	85%
Hospital Given 9 or 10 on 10 Point Scale	300+	67%	73%	71%
Meds 'Always' Explained Before Given	300+	63%	66%	64%
Nurses 'Always' Communicated Well	300+	75%	80%	79%
Pain 'Always' Well Controlled	300+	69%	72%	71%
Room and Bathroom 'Always' Clean	300+	70%	75%	73%
Timely Help 'Always' Received	300+	61%	69%	68%
Would Definitely Recommend Hospital	300+	67%	73%	71%
Use of Medical Imaging				
Cardiac Imaging Stress Test before Surgery	109	7.3%	5.3%	5.3%
Combination Abdominal CT Scan	1,006	5.6%	16.4%	10.5%
Combination Brain/Sinus CT Scan	1,120	3.3%	2.7%	2.7%
Combination Chest CT Scan	133	5.3%	5.6%	2.7%
Follow-up Mammogram/Ultrasound	819	3.7%	7.9%	8.8%
Lumbar Spine MRI for Low Back Pain	36	52.8%	39.6%	37.2%

Providence Memorial Hospital

2001 N Oregon St
El Paso, TX 79902
URL: www.sphn.com
Phone: 915-577-6011
Fax: 915-577-6109
Type: Acute Care Hospitals
Ownership: Proprietary
Emergency Services: Yes
Beds: 508

Key Personnel:
CEO/President. . . . . John Harris
Cardiac Laboratory. . . . . Larry Lewis
Emergency Room . . . . Carl Templin

Measure	Cases	This Hosp.	State Avg.	U.S. Avg.
Blood Clot Prevention and Treatment				
Anticoagulation Overlap Therapy[2]	61	90%	93%	93%
ICU Venous Thromboembolism Prophylaxis[2]	77	99%	92%	92%
Incidence of Potentially Preventable VTE[2]	19	5%	9%	10%
UFH with Dosages/Platelet Monitoring[1,2]	-	-	96%	97%
Venous Thromboembolism Prophylaxis[2]	373	96%	82%	85%
Warfarin Therapy Discharge Instructions[2]	44	100%	84%	75%
Chest Pain/Possible Heart Attack Care				
Aspirin Given Within 24 Hours of Arrival[1,3]	-	-	94%	96%
Fibrinolytic Meds Within 30 Min. of Arrival[5]	-	-	47%	58%
Average Time to ECG (minutes)[1,3]	-	-	8	7
Average Time to Transfer (minutes)[5]	-	-	62	60
Children's Asthma Care				
Received Home Management Plan of Care	-	-	93%	88%
Received Reliever Medication	-	-	100%	100%
Received Systemic Corticosteroids	-	-	100%	100%
Emergency Department				
Admittance Decision Time (minutes)[2]	441	103	99	98
Head CT Results Within 45 Min. of Arrival[1,3]	-	-	54%	57%
Patients Who Left ER Before Being Seen	47,232	2%	3%	2%
Time from ER Arrival to Admit. (minutes)[2]	443	261	270	274
Time from ER Arrival to Discharge (minutes)	397	119	127	134
Time in ER Before Being Evaluated (minutes)	410	25	26	26
Time to Pain Meds for Fractures (minutes)	277	41	57	57
Heart Attack Care				
Aspirin Given at Discharge	116	100%	99%	99%
Fibrinolytic Meds Within 30 Min. of Arrival[1]	-	-	49%	54%
PCI Within 90 Minutes of Arrival	28	100%	95%	96%
Statin Prescribed at Discharge	116	100%	98%	98%
Heart Failure Care				
ACE Inhibitor or ARB for LVSD	84	100%	97%	97%
Discharge Instructions Given	227	100%	95%	94%
Evaluation of LVS Function	247	100%	99%	99%
Medicare Spending				
Medicare Spending per Patient (ratio)	-	1.00	1.03	0.98
Pneumonia Care				
Appropriate Initial Antibiotic Given[2]	121	98%	95%	95%
Blood Culture Timing[2]	143	100%	98%	98%
Pregnancy and Delivery Care				
Newborn Deliveries Scheduled Early[2]	95	4%	7%	6%
Preventive Care				
Immunization for Influenza[2]	498	99%	90%	90%
Immunization for Pneumonia[2]	407	100%	92%	92%
Stroke Care				
Anticoagulation Therapy for Atrial Fibrillation	12	100%	96%	95%
Antithrombotic Therapy Timing	70	97%	98%	98%
Assessed for Rehabilitation	100	100%	98%	97%
Discharged on Antithrombotic Therapy	70	99%	99%	99%
Discharged on Statin Medication	52	100%	95%	94%
Thrombolytic Therapy Timing	12	83%	68%	66%
Venous Thromboembolism Prophylaxis	122	98%	94%	94%
Written Stroke Educational Materials Given	55	100%	92%	88%
Surgical Care Improvement Project				
Appropriate Beta Blocker Usage[2]	115	99%	98%	98%
Appropriate VTP Within 24 Hours[2]	348	99%	98%	98%
Controlled Postoperative Blood Glucose[2]	49	96%	96%	97%
Perioperative Temperature Management[2]	393	100%	100%	100%
Prophylactic Antibiotic Selection[2]	312	99%	99%	99%
Prophylactic Antibiotic Selection (Outpatient)	444	100%	98%	98%
Prophylactic Antibiotic Stopped[2]	294	99%	98%	98%
Prophylactic Antibiotic Timing[2]	312	100%	99%	99%
Prophylactic Antibiotic Timing (Outpatient)	428	100%	98%	98%
Urinary Catheter Removal[2]	96	99%	98%	97%
Survey of Patients' Hospital Experiences				
Area Around Room 'Always' Quiet at Night	300+	59%	68%	61%
Doctors 'Always' Communicated Well	300+	83%	83%	82%
Home Recovery Information Given	300+	84%	85%	85%
Hospital Given 9 or 10 on 10 Point Scale	300+	68%	73%	71%
Meds 'Always' Explained Before Given	300+	66%	66%	64%
Nurses 'Always' Communicated Well	300+	74%	80%	79%
Pain 'Always' Well Controlled	300+	69%	72%	71%
Room and Bathroom 'Always' Clean	300+	68%	75%	73%
Timely Help 'Always' Received	300+	62%	69%	68%
Would Definitely Recommend Hospital	300+	69%	73%	71%
Use of Medical Imaging				
Cardiac Imaging Stress Test before Surgery[1]	-	-	5.3%	5.3%
Combination Abdominal CT Scan	547	14.1%	16.4%	10.5%
Combination Brain/Sinus CT Scan	513	2.1%	2.7%	2.7%
Combination Chest CT Scan	243	0.0%	5.6%	2.7%
Follow-up Mammogram/Ultrasound	1,055	8.0%	7.9%	8.8%
Lumbar Spine MRI for Low Back Pain	150	40.7%	39.6%	37.2%

Sierra Medical Center

1625 Medical Center Dr
El Paso, TX 79902
URL: www.sphn.com
Phone: 915-747-4000
Fax: 915-747-2550
Type: Acute Care Hospitals
Ownership: Proprietary
Emergency Services: Yes
Beds: 365

Key Personnel:
Operating Room. . . . . Paul Arellano
CEO/President. . . . . Thomas E Casaday
Quality Assurance . . . . Becky McDonald

Measure	Cases	This Hosp.	State Avg.	U.S. Avg.
Blood Clot Prevention and Treatment				
Anticoagulation Overlap Therapy[2]	61	89%	93%	93%
ICU Venous Thromboembolism Prophylaxis[2]	113	99%	92%	92%
Incidence of Potentially Preventable VTE[2]	22	0%	9%	10%
UFH with Dosages/Platelet Monitoring[2]	13	92%	96%	97%
Venous Thromboembolism Prophylaxis[2]	358	91%	82%	85%
Warfarin Therapy Discharge Instructions[2]	44	100%	84%	75%
Chest Pain/Possible Heart Attack Care				
Aspirin Given Within 24 Hours of Arrival[1,3]	-	-	94%	96%
Fibrinolytic Meds Within 30 Min. of Arrival[5]	-	-	47%	58%
Average Time to ECG (minutes)[1,3]	-	-	8	7
Average Time to Transfer (minutes)[5]	-	-	62	60
Children's Asthma Care				
Received Home Management Plan of Care	-	-	93%	88%
Received Reliever Medication	-	-	100%	100%
Received Systemic Corticosteroids	-	-	100%	100%
Emergency Department				
Admittance Decision Time (minutes)[2]	591	83	99	98
Head CT Results Within 45 Min. of Arrival[3,7]	-	-	54%	57%
Patients Who Left ER Before Being Seen	27,050	5%	3%	2%
Time from ER Arrival to Admit. (minutes)[2]	595	284	270	274
Time from ER Arrival to Discharge (minutes)	390	158	127	134
Time in ER Before Being Evaluated (minutes)	411	34	26	26
Time to Pain Meds for Fractures (minutes)	84	49	57	57
Heart Attack Care				
Aspirin Given at Discharge	95	100%	99%	99%
Fibrinolytic Meds Within 30 Min. of Arrival[7]	-	-	49%	54%
PCI Within 90 Minutes of Arrival	16	81%	95%	96%
Statin Prescribed at Discharge	103	98%	98%	98%
Heart Failure Care				
ACE Inhibitor or ARB for LVSD	81	100%	97%	97%
Discharge Instructions Given	169	95%	95%	94%
Evaluation of LVS Function	199	100%	99%	99%
Medicare Spending				
Medicare Spending per Patient (ratio)	-	1.01	1.03	0.98
Pneumonia Care				
Appropriate Initial Antibiotic Given[2]	106	96%	95%	95%
Blood Culture Timing[2]	152	99%	98%	98%
Pregnancy and Delivery Care				
Newborn Deliveries Scheduled Early[2]	62	3%	7%	6%
Preventive Care				
Immunization for Influenza[2]	555	97%	90%	90%
Immunization for Pneumonia[2]	696	97%	92%	92%
Stroke Care				
Anticoagulation Therapy for Atrial Fibrillation	14	100%	96%	95%
Antithrombotic Therapy Timing	77	95%	98%	98%
Assessed for Rehabilitation	111	98%	98%	97%
Discharged on Antithrombotic Therapy	83	100%	99%	99%
Discharged on Statin Medication	54	100%	95%	94%
Thrombolytic Therapy Timing	12	58%	68%	66%
Venous Thromboembolism Prophylaxis	131	98%	94%	94%
Written Stroke Educational Materials Given	63	89%	92%	88%
Surgical Care Improvement Project				
Appropriate Beta Blocker Usage[2]	182	96%	98%	98%
Appropriate VTP Within 24 Hours[2]	412	97%	98%	98%
Controlled Postoperative Blood Glucose[2]	89	97%	96%	97%
Perioperative Temperature Management[2]	466	100%	100%	100%
Prophylactic Antibiotic Selection[2]	402	99%	99%	99%
Prophylactic Antibiotic Selection (Outpatient)	487	100%	98%	98%
Prophylactic Antibiotic Stopped[2]	391	96%	98%	98%
Prophylactic Antibiotic Timing[2]	402	100%	99%	99%
Prophylactic Antibiotic Timing (Outpatient)	487	100%	98%	98%

NOTE: Hospital profiles are in alphabetical order by state, then city, then hospital within the city; Rankings exclude hospitals with less than 25 cases except for patient surveys which excludes hospitals with less than 100 cases; (a) 100-299 cases; (1) The number of cases/patients is too few to report; (2) Data submitted were based on a sample of cases/patients; (3) Results are based on a shorter time period than required; (4) Data suppressed by CMS for one or more quarters; (5) Results are not available for this reporting period; (6) Fewer than 100 patients completed the HCAHPS survey; (7) No cases met the criteria for this measure; (8) The lower limit of the confidence interval cannot be calculated if the number of observed infections equals zero; (9) No data are available from the state/territory for this reporting period; (10) The scores shown reflect fewer than 50 completed surveys; (11) There were discrepancies in the data collection process; (12) This measure does not apply to this hospital for this reporting period; (13) Results cannot be calculated for this reporting period; (14) The results for this state are combined with nearby states to protect confidentiality; Please refer to the User's Guide for a full explanation of data.

Urinary Catheter Removal[2]	150	97%	98%	97%
Survey of Patients' Hospital Experiences				
Area Around Room 'Always' Quiet at Night	300+	53%	68%	61%
Doctors 'Always' Communicated Well	300+	81%	83%	82%
Home Recovery Information Given	300+	83%	85%	85%
Hospital Given 9 or 10 on 10 Point Scale	300+	63%	73%	71%
Meds 'Always' Explained Before Given	300+	58%	66%	64%
Nurses 'Always' Communicated Well	300+	73%	80%	79%
Pain 'Always' Well Controlled	300+	63%	72%	71%
Room and Bathroom 'Always' Clean	300+	65%	75%	73%
Timely Help 'Always' Received	300+	61%	69%	68%
Would Definitely Recommend Hospital	300+	68%	73%	71%
Use of Medical Imaging				
Cardiac Imaging Stress Test before Surgery[1]	-	-	5.3%	5.3%
Combination Abdominal CT Scan	614	8.0%	16.4%	10.5%
Combination Brain/Sinus CT Scan	588	2.4%	2.7%	2.7%
Combination Chest CT Scan	325	1.8%	5.6%	2.7%
Follow-up Mammogram/Ultrasound	1,783	9.8%	7.9%	8.8%
Lumbar Spine MRI for Low Back Pain	82	34.1%	39.6%	37.2%

Sierra Providence East Medical Center

3280 Joe Battle Blvd
El Paso, TX 79938
Phone: 915-856-7349
URL: www.sphn.com
Type: Acute Care Hospitals
Emergency Services: Yes
Ownership: Proprietary
Beds: 110
Key Personnel:
CEO . . . . John Harris

Measure	Cases	This Hosp.	State Avg.	U.S. Avg.
Blood Clot Prevention and Treatment				
Anticoagulation Overlap Therapy[2]	46	91%	93%	93%
ICU Venous Thromboembolism Prophylaxis[2]	72	100%	92%	92%
Incidence of Potentially Preventable VTE[1,2]	-	-	9%	10%
UFH with Dosages/Platelet Monitoring[1,2]	-	-	96%	97%
Venous Thromboembolism Prophylaxis[2]	399	95%	82%	85%
Warfarin Therapy Discharge Instructions[2]	37	100%	84%	75%
Chest Pain/Possible Heart Attack Care				
Aspirin Given Within 24 Hours of Arrival[1]	-	-	94%	96%
Fibrinolytic Meds Within 30 Min. of Arrival[5]	-	-	47%	58%
Average Time to ECG (minutes)[1]	-	-	8	7
Average Time to Transfer (minutes)[5]	-	-	62	60
Children's Asthma Care				
Received Home Management Plan of Care	-	-	93%	88%
Received Reliever Medication	-	-	100%	100%
Received Systemic Corticosteroids	-	-	100%	100%
Emergency Department				
Admittance Decision Time (minutes)[2]	658	86	99	98
Head CT Results Within 45 Min. of Arrival[1]	-	-	54%	57%
Patients Who Left ER Before Being Seen	51,708	3%	3%	2%
Time from ER Arrival to Admit. (minutes)[2]	670	328	270	274
Time from ER Arrival to Discharge (minutes)	457	150	127	134
Time in ER Before Being Evaluated (minutes)	479	35	26	26
Time to Pain Meds for Fractures (minutes)	248	71	57	57
Heart Attack Care				
Aspirin Given at Discharge	78	100%	99%	99%
Fibrinolytic Meds Within 30 Min. of Arrival[7]	-	-	49%	54%
PCI Within 90 Minutes of Arrival	31	97%	95%	96%
Statin Prescribed at Discharge	82	100%	98%	98%
Heart Failure Care				
ACE Inhibitor or ARB for LVSD	75	100%	97%	97%
Discharge Instructions Given	156	100%	95%	94%
Evaluation of LVS Function	174	100%	99%	99%
Medicare Spending				
Medicare Spending per Patient (ratio)	-	1.02	1.03	0.98
Pneumonia Care				
Appropriate Initial Antibiotic Given[2]	111	98%	95%	95%
Blood Culture Timing[2]	123	100%	98%	98%
Pregnancy and Delivery Care				
Newborn Deliveries Scheduled Early[2]	66	5%	7%	6%
Preventive Care				
Immunization for Influenza[2]	539	99%	90%	90%
Immunization for Pneumonia[2]	561	100%	92%	92%
Stroke Care				
Anticoagulation Therapy for Atrial Fibrillation[1]	-	-	96%	95%
Antithrombotic Therapy Timing	84	96%	98%	98%
Assessed for Rehabilitation	96	100%	98%	97%
Discharged on Antithrombotic Therapy	84	100%	99%	99%
Discharged on Statin Medication	54	98%	95%	94%
Thrombolytic Therapy Timing[1]	-	-	68%	66%
Venous Thromboembolism Prophylaxis	106	100%	94%	94%
Written Stroke Educational Materials Given	61	100%	92%	88%
Surgical Care Improvement Project				
Appropriate Beta Blocker Usage[2]	43	98%	98%	98%
Appropriate VTP Within 24 Hours[2]	187	98%	98%	98%
Controlled Postoperative Blood Glucose[2,7]	-	-	96%	97%
Perioperative Temperature Management[2]	219	100%	100%	100%
Prophylactic Antibiotic Selection[2]	126	100%	99%	99%
Prophylactic Antibiotic Selection (Outpatient)	79	96%	98%	98%
Prophylactic Antibiotic Stopped[2]	114	99%	98%	98%
Prophylactic Antibiotic Timing[2]	126	100%	99%	99%
Prophylactic Antibiotic Timing (Outpatient)	80	99%	98%	98%
Urinary Catheter Removal[2]	59	98%	98%	97%
Survey of Patients' Hospital Experiences				
Area Around Room 'Always' Quiet at Night	300+	62%	68%	61%
Doctors 'Always' Communicated Well	300+	79%	83%	82%
Home Recovery Information Given	300+	83%	85%	85%
Hospital Given 9 or 10 on 10 Point Scale	300+	73%	73%	71%
Meds 'Always' Explained Before Given	300+	64%	66%	64%
Nurses 'Always' Communicated Well	300+	77%	80%	79%
Pain 'Always' Well Controlled	300+	72%	72%	71%
Room and Bathroom 'Always' Clean	300+	76%	75%	73%
Timely Help 'Always' Received	300+	68%	69%	68%
Would Definitely Recommend Hospital	300+	76%	73%	71%
Use of Medical Imaging				
Cardiac Imaging Stress Test before Surgery	105	2.9%	5.3%	5.3%
Combination Abdominal CT Scan	339	2.9%	16.4%	10.5%
Combination Brain/Sinus CT Scan[1]	-	-	2.7%	2.7%
Combination Chest CT Scan	107	0.0%	5.6%	2.7%
Follow-up Mammogram/Ultrasound	141	9.2%	7.9%	8.8%
Lumbar Spine MRI for Low Back Pain[1]	-	-	39.6%	37.2%

University Medical Center of El Paso

4815 Alameda Ave
El Paso, TX 79905
Phone: 915-521-7602
Fax: 915-521-7975
URL: www.thomasoncares.org
Type: Acute Care Hospitals
Emergency Services: Yes
Ownership: Govt - Hospital Dist/Auth
Beds: 346
Key Personnel:
Pediatric Ambulatory Care . . . . . . Gilbert A Handal, MD
Pediatric In-Patient Care . . . . Gilbert A Handal, MD
Chief of Medical Staff. . . . . Harold Hughes, MD
Quality Assurance . . . . Betty Johnson, RN
CEO/President. . . . . James N Valenti

Measure	Cases	This Hosp.	State Avg.	U.S. Avg.
Blood Clot Prevention and Treatment				
Anticoagulation Overlap Therapy[2]	99	100%	93%	93%
ICU Venous Thromboembolism Prophylaxis[2]	130	100%	92%	92%
Incidence of Potentially Preventable VTE[2]	33	0%	9%	10%
UFH with Dosages/Platelet Monitoring[2]	14	100%	96%	97%
Venous Thromboembolism Prophylaxis[2]	330	100%	82%	85%
Warfarin Therapy Discharge Instructions[2]	81	98%	84%	75%
Chest Pain/Possible Heart Attack Care				
Aspirin Given Within 24 Hours of Arrival[3,7]	-	-	94%	96%
Fibrinolytic Meds Within 30 Min. of Arrival[5]	-	-	47%	58%
Average Time to ECG (minutes)[3,7]	-	-	8	7
Average Time to Transfer (minutes)[5]	-	-	62	60
Children's Asthma Care				
Received Home Management Plan of Care	-	-	93%	88%
Received Reliever Medication	-	-	100%	100%
Received Systemic Corticosteroids	-	-	100%	100%
Emergency Department				
Admittance Decision Time (minutes)[2]	672	146	99	98
Head CT Results Within 45 Min. of Arrival[1]	-	-	54%	57%
Patients Who Left ER Before Being Seen	54,863	6%	3%	2%
Time from ER Arrival to Admit. (minutes)[2]	672	504	270	274
Time from ER Arrival to Discharge (minutes)	397	336	127	134
Time in ER Before Being Evaluated (minutes)	415	115	26	26
Time to Pain Meds for Fractures (minutes)	257	99	57	57
Heart Attack Care				
Aspirin Given at Discharge	156	100%	99%	99%
Fibrinolytic Meds Within 30 Min. of Arrival[1]	-	-	49%	54%
PCI Within 90 Minutes of Arrival	26	92%	95%	96%
Statin Prescribed at Discharge	158	99%	98%	98%
Heart Failure Care				
ACE Inhibitor or ARB for LVSD	107	99%	97%	97%
Discharge Instructions Given	232	97%	95%	94%
Evaluation of LVS Function	244	100%	99%	99%
Medicare Spending				
Medicare Spending per Patient (ratio)	-	0.99	1.03	0.98
Pneumonia Care				
Appropriate Initial Antibiotic Given	120	100%	95%	95%
Blood Culture Timing	159	99%	98%	98%
Pregnancy and Delivery Care				
Newborn Deliveries Scheduled Early[2]	77	1%	7%	6%
Preventive Care				
Immunization for Influenza[2]	518	99%	90%	90%
Immunization for Pneumonia[2]	383	99%	92%	92%
Stroke Care				
Anticoagulation Therapy for Atrial Fibrillation[1]	-	-	96%	95%
Antithrombotic Therapy Timing	82	100%	98%	98%
Assessed for Rehabilitation	132	100%	98%	97%
Discharged on Antithrombotic Therapy	97	99%	99%	99%
Discharged on Statin Medication	71	100%	95%	94%
Thrombolytic Therapy Timing[1]	-	-	68%	66%
Venous Thromboembolism Prophylaxis	143	99%	94%	94%
Written Stroke Educational Materials Given	105	94%	92%	88%
Surgical Care Improvement Project				
Appropriate Beta Blocker Usage[2]	66	100%	98%	98%
Appropriate VTP Within 24 Hours[2]	342	99%	98%	98%
Controlled Postoperative Blood Glucose[2]	42	98%	96%	97%
Perioperative Temperature Management[2]	392	100%	100%	100%
Prophylactic Antibiotic Selection[2]	253	98%	99%	99%
Prophylactic Antibiotic Selection (Outpatient)	222	99%	98%	98%
Prophylactic Antibiotic Stopped[2]	241	99%	98%	98%
Prophylactic Antibiotic Timing[2]	253	100%	99%	99%
Prophylactic Antibiotic Timing (Outpatient)	223	100%	98%	98%
Urinary Catheter Removal[2]	153	100%	98%	97%
Survey of Patients' Hospital Experiences				
Area Around Room 'Always' Quiet at Night	300+	64%	68%	61%
Doctors 'Always' Communicated Well	300+	79%	83%	82%
Home Recovery Information Given	300+	86%	85%	85%
Hospital Given 9 or 10 on 10 Point Scale	300+	74%	73%	71%
Meds 'Always' Explained Before Given	300+	65%	66%	64%
Nurses 'Always' Communicated Well	300+	77%	80%	79%
Pain 'Always' Well Controlled	300+	69%	72%	71%
Room and Bathroom 'Always' Clean	300+	73%	75%	73%
Timely Help 'Always' Received	300+	63%	69%	68%
Would Definitely Recommend Hospital	300+	75%	73%	71%
Use of Medical Imaging				
Cardiac Imaging Stress Test before Surgery	83	3.6%	5.3%	5.3%
Combination Abdominal CT Scan	440	4.5%	16.4%	10.5%
Combination Brain/Sinus CT Scan	339	5.0%	2.7%	2.7%
Combination Chest CT Scan	231	0.4%	5.6%	2.7%
Follow-up Mammogram/Ultrasound	911	8.2%	7.9%	8.8%
Lumbar Spine MRI for Low Back Pain[1]	-	-	39.6%	37.2%

Electra Memorial Hospital

1207 S Bailey Street
Electra, TX 76360
Phone: 940-495-3981
Fax: 940-495-4137
E-mail: emh@electrahospital.com
URL: www.electrahospital.com
Type: Critical Access Hospitals
Emergency Services: Yes
Ownership: Govt - Hospital Dist/Auth
Beds: 25
Key Personnel:
Chief of Medical Staff. . . . . Eloisa Banez, MD
CEO . . . . Jan A Reed
Emergency Room . . . . Ben Segler, RN
Infection Control. . . . . April Shelley

Measure	Cases	This Hosp.	State Avg.	U.S. Avg.
Blood Clot Prevention and Treatment				

NOTE: Hospital profiles are in alphabetical order by state, then city, then hospital within the city; Rankings exclude hospitals with less than 25 cases except for patient surveys which excludes hospitals with less than 100 cases; (a) 100-299 cases; (1) The number of cases/patients is too few to report; (2) Data submitted were based on a sample of cases/patients; (3) Results are based on a shorter time period than required; (4) Data suppressed by CMS for one or more quarters; (5) Results are not available for this reporting period; (6) Fewer than 100 patients completed the HCAHPS survey; (7) No cases met the criteria for this measure; (8) The lower limit of the confidence interval cannot be calculated if the number of observed infections equals zero; (9) No data are available from the state/territory for this reporting period; (10) The scores shown reflect fewer than 50 completed surveys; (11) There were discrepancies in the data collection process; (12) This measure does not apply to this hospital for this reporting period; (13) Results cannot be calculated for this reporting period; (14) The results for this state are combined with nearby states to protect confidentiality; Please refer to the User's Guide for a full explanation of data.

Anticoagulation Overlap Therapy[5]	-	-	93%	93%
ICU Venous Thromboembolism Prophylaxis[5]	-	-	92%	92%
Incidence of Potentially Preventable VTE[5]	-	-	9%	10%
UFH with Dosages/Platelet Monitoring[5]	-	-	96%	97%
Venous Thromboembolism Prophylaxis[5]	-	-	82%	85%
Warfarin Therapy Discharge Instructions[5]	-	-	84%	75%
Chest Pain/Possible Heart Attack Care				
Aspirin Given Within 24 Hours of Arrival[5]	-	-	94%	96%
Fibrinolytic Meds Within 30 Min. of Arrival[5]	-	-	47%	58%
Average Time to ECG (minutes)[5]	-	-	8	7
Average Time to Transfer (minutes)[5]	-	-	62	60
Children's Asthma Care				
Received Home Management Plan of Care	-	-	93%	88%
Received Reliever Medication	-	-	100%	100%
Received Systemic Corticosteroids	-	-	100%	100%
Emergency Department				
Admittance Decision Time (minutes)	40	14	99	98
Head CT Results Within 45 Min. of Arrival[5]	-	-	54%	57%
Patients Who Left ER Before Being Seen[5]	-	-	3%	2%
Time from ER Arrival to Admit. (minutes)	40	95	270	274
Time from ER Arrival to Discharge (minutes)[5]	-	-	127	134
Time in ER Before Being Evaluated (minutes)[5]	-	-	26	26
Time to Pain Meds for Fractures (minutes)[5]	-	-	57	57
Heart Attack Care				
Aspirin Given at Discharge[5]	-	-	99%	99%
Fibrinolytic Meds Within 30 Min. of Arrival[5]	-	-	49%	54%
PCI Within 90 Minutes of Arrival[5]	-	-	95%	96%
Statin Prescribed at Discharge[5]	-	-	98%	98%
Heart Failure Care				
ACE Inhibitor or ARB for LVSD[1]	-	-	97%	97%
Discharge Instructions Given[1]	-	-	95%	94%
Evaluation of LVS Function[1]	-	-	99%	99%
Medicare Spending				
Medicare Spending per Patient (ratio)	-	-	1.03	0.98
Pneumonia Care				
Appropriate Initial Antibiotic Given	33	100%	95%	95%
Blood Culture Timing	14	100%	98%	98%
Pregnancy and Delivery Care				
Newborn Deliveries Scheduled Early[5]	-	-	7%	6%
Preventive Care				
Immunization for Influenza	28	100%	90%	90%
Immunization for Pneumonia	40	95%	92%	92%
Stroke Care				
Anticoagulation Therapy for Atrial Fibrillation[5]	-	-	96%	95%
Antithrombotic Therapy Timing[5]	-	-	98%	98%
Assessed for Rehabilitation[5]	-	-	98%	97%
Discharged on Antithrombotic Therapy[5]	-	-	99%	99%
Discharged on Statin Medication[5]	-	-	95%	94%
Thrombolytic Therapy Timing[5]	-	-	68%	66%
Venous Thromboembolism Prophylaxis[5]	-	-	94%	94%
Written Stroke Educational Materials Given[5]	-	-	92%	88%
Surgical Care Improvement Project				
Appropriate Beta Blocker Usage[5]	-	-	98%	98%
Appropriate VTP Within 24 Hours[5]	-	-	98%	98%
Controlled Postoperative Blood Glucose[5]	-	-	96%	97%
Perioperative Temperature Management[5]	-	-	100%	100%
Prophylactic Antibiotic Selection[5]	-	-	99%	99%
Prophylactic Antibiotic Selection (Outpatient)[5]	-	-	98%	98%
Prophylactic Antibiotic Stopped[5]	-	-	98%	98%
Prophylactic Antibiotic Timing[5]	-	-	99%	99%
Prophylactic Antibiotic Timing (Outpatient)[5]	-	-	98%	98%
Urinary Catheter Removal[5]	-	-	98%	97%
Survey of Patients' Hospital Experiences				
Area Around Room 'Always' Quiet at Night	(a)	76%	68%	61%
Doctors 'Always' Communicated Well	(a)	93%	83%	82%
Home Recovery Information Given	(a)	95%	85%	85%
Hospital Given 9 or 10 on 10 Point Scale	(a)	87%	73%	71%
Meds 'Always' Explained Before Given	(a)	71%	66%	64%
Nurses 'Always' Communicated Well	(a)	87%	80%	79%
Pain 'Always' Well Controlled	(a)	78%	72%	71%
Room and Bathroom 'Always' Clean	(a)	89%	75%	73%
Timely Help 'Always' Received	(a)	83%	69%	68%
Would Definitely Recommend Hospital	(a)	89%	73%	71%
Use of Medical Imaging				
Cardiac Imaging Stress Test before Surgery[7]	-	-	5.3%	5.3%
Combination Abdominal CT Scan[1]	-	-	16.4%	10.5%
Combination Brain/Sinus CT Scan	44	0.0%	2.7%	2.7%
Combination Chest CT Scan[1]	-	-	5.6%	2.7%
Follow-up Mammogram/Ultrasound[7]	-	-	7.9%	8.8%
Lumbar Spine MRI for Low Back Pain[1]	-	-	39.6%	37.2%

Ennis Regional Medical Center

2201 West Lampasas Street
Ennis, TX 75119
Phone: 972-875-0900
Fax: 469-256-2154
E-mail: info@ennisregional.com
URL: www.ennisregional.com
Type: Acute Care Hospitals
Emergency Services: Yes
Ownership: Proprietary
Beds: 60

Key Personnel:
Surgery . . . . Alfonso Ballesteros, MD
Chief of Medical Staff. . . . . Raymond W. Blair, Jr., MD
Chairman/CEO . . . . Michael Montgomery
Radiology. . . . . Gary Waddell, MD
CEO/President. . . . . Kevin Zachary, MBA

Measure	Cases	This Hosp.	State Avg.	U.S. Avg.
Blood Clot Prevention and Treatment				
Anticoagulation Overlap Therapy[1,2]	-	-	93%	93%
ICU Venous Thromboembolism Prophylaxis[2]	20	100%	92%	92%
Incidence of Potentially Preventable VTE[2,7]	-	-	9%	10%
UFH with Dosages/Platelet Monitoring[1,2]	-	-	96%	97%
Venous Thromboembolism Prophylaxis[2]	175	93%	82%	85%
Warfarin Therapy Discharge Instructions[1,2]	-	-	84%	75%
Chest Pain/Possible Heart Attack Care				
Aspirin Given Within 24 Hours of Arrival	48	96%	94%	96%
Fibrinolytic Meds Within 30 Min. of Arrival[7]	-	-	47%	58%
Average Time to ECG (minutes)	50	6	8	7
Average Time to Transfer (minutes)[7]	-	-	62	60
Children's Asthma Care				
Received Home Management Plan of Care	-	-	93%	88%
Received Reliever Medication	-	-	100%	100%
Received Systemic Corticosteroids	-	-	100%	100%
Emergency Department				
Admittance Decision Time (minutes)[2]	296	78	99	98
Head CT Results Within 45 Min. of Arrival[1]	-	-	54%	57%
Patients Who Left ER Before Being Seen	16,845	3%	3%	2%
Time from ER Arrival to Admit. (minutes)[2]	299	282	270	274
Time from ER Arrival to Discharge (minutes)	384	124	127	134
Time in ER Before Being Evaluated (minutes)	427	23	26	26
Time to Pain Meds for Fractures (minutes)	90	49	57	57
Heart Attack Care				
Aspirin Given at Discharge[1,3]	-	-	99%	99%
Fibrinolytic Meds Within 30 Min. of Arrival[3,7]	-	-	49%	54%
PCI Within 90 Minutes of Arrival[3,7]	-	-	95%	96%
Statin Prescribed at Discharge[3,7]	-	-	98%	98%
Heart Failure Care				
ACE Inhibitor or ARB for LVSD	18	89%	97%	97%
Discharge Instructions Given	51	88%	95%	94%
Evaluation of LVS Function	65	95%	99%	99%
Medicare Spending				
Medicare Spending per Patient (ratio)	-	1.08	1.03	0.98
Pneumonia Care				
Appropriate Initial Antibiotic Given	75	95%	95%	95%
Blood Culture Timing	122	94%	98%	98%
Pregnancy and Delivery Care				
Newborn Deliveries Scheduled Early[2]	39	3%	7%	6%
Preventive Care				
Immunization for Influenza[2]	319	91%	90%	90%
Immunization for Pneumonia[2]	268	88%	92%	92%
Stroke Care				
Anticoagulation Therapy for Atrial Fibrillation[1]	-	-	96%	95%
Antithrombotic Therapy Timing	15	93%	98%	98%
Assessed for Rehabilitation	13	100%	98%	97%
Discharged on Antithrombotic Therapy	13	100%	99%	99%
Discharged on Statin Medication[1]	-	-	95%	94%
Thrombolytic Therapy Timing[1]	-	-	68%	66%
Venous Thromboembolism Prophylaxis	14	86%	94%	94%
Written Stroke Educational Materials Given[1]	-	-	92%	88%
Surgical Care Improvement Project				
Appropriate Beta Blocker Usage[1]	-	-	98%	98%
Appropriate VTP Within 24 Hours	40	95%	98%	98%
Controlled Postoperative Blood Glucose[7]	-	-	96%	97%
Perioperative Temperature Management	46	100%	100%	100%
Prophylactic Antibiotic Selection	21	100%	99%	99%
Prophylactic Antibiotic Selection (Outpatient)	23	100%	98%	98%
Prophylactic Antibiotic Stopped	21	95%	98%	98%
Prophylactic Antibiotic Timing	22	91%	99%	99%
Prophylactic Antibiotic Timing (Outpatient)	20	100%	98%	98%
Urinary Catheter Removal	28	82%	98%	97%
Survey of Patients' Hospital Experiences				
Area Around Room 'Always' Quiet at Night	300+	62%	68%	61%
Doctors 'Always' Communicated Well	300+	79%	83%	82%
Home Recovery Information Given	300+	85%	85%	85%
Hospital Given 9 or 10 on 10 Point Scale	300+	65%	73%	71%
Meds 'Always' Explained Before Given	300+	64%	66%	64%
Nurses 'Always' Communicated Well	300+	72%	80%	79%
Pain 'Always' Well Controlled	300+	66%	72%	71%
Room and Bathroom 'Always' Clean	300+	74%	75%	73%
Timely Help 'Always' Received	300+	57%	69%	68%
Would Definitely Recommend Hospital	300+	60%	73%	71%
Use of Medical Imaging				
Cardiac Imaging Stress Test before Surgery[7]	-	-	5.3%	5.3%
Combination Abdominal CT Scan	151	9.9%	16.4%	10.5%
Combination Brain/Sinus CT Scan[1]	-	-	2.7%	2.7%
Combination Chest CT Scan[1]	-	-	5.6%	2.7%
Follow-up Mammogram/Ultrasound	403	5.0%	7.9%	8.8%
Lumbar Spine MRI for Low Back Pain[1]	-	-	39.6%	37.2%

East Texas Medical Center - Fairfield

125 Newman St
Fairfield, TX 75840
Phone: 903-389-1612
Fax: 903-389-1601
URL: www.etmc.org
Type: Acute Care Hospitals
Emergency Services: Yes
Ownership: Voluntary non-profit - Private
Beds: 48

Key Personnel:
Chief of Medical Staff. . . . . Glenn Routhouska

Measure	Cases	This Hosp.	State Avg.	U.S. Avg.
Blood Clot Prevention and Treatment				
Anticoagulation Overlap Therapy[1]	-	-	93%	93%
ICU Venous Thromboembolism Prophylaxis[7]	-	-	92%	92%
Incidence of Potentially Preventable VTE[1]	-	-	9%	10%
UFH with Dosages/Platelet Monitoring[7]	-	-	96%	97%
Venous Thromboembolism Prophylaxis	266	45%	82%	85%
Warfarin Therapy Discharge Instructions[1]	-	-	84%	75%
Chest Pain/Possible Heart Attack Care				
Aspirin Given Within 24 Hours of Arrival	64	100%	94%	96%
Fibrinolytic Meds Within 30 Min. of Arrival[1]	-	-	47%	58%
Average Time to ECG (minutes)	65	4	8	7
Average Time to Transfer (minutes)[7]	-	-	62	60
Children's Asthma Care				
Received Home Management Plan of Care	-	-	93%	88%
Received Reliever Medication	-	-	100%	100%
Received Systemic Corticosteroids	-	-	100%	100%
Emergency Department				
Admittance Decision Time (minutes)	381	50	99	98
Head CT Results Within 45 Min. of Arrival[1,3]	-	-	54%	57%
Patients Who Left ER Before Being Seen	9,698	1%	3%	2%
Time from ER Arrival to Admit. (minutes)	401	251	270	274
Time from ER Arrival to Discharge (minutes)	382	120	127	134
Time in ER Before Being Evaluated (minutes)	496	18	26	26
Time to Pain Meds for Fractures (minutes)	52	48	57	57
Heart Attack Care				
Aspirin Given at Discharge[1,3]	-	-	99%	99%
Fibrinolytic Meds Within 30 Min. of Arrival[3,7]	-	-	49%	54%
PCI Within 90 Minutes of Arrival[3,7]	-	-	95%	96%
Statin Prescribed at Discharge[1,3]	-	-	98%	98%
Heart Failure Care				
ACE Inhibitor or ARB for LVSD[1]	-	-	97%	97%
Discharge Instructions Given	15	100%	95%	94%
Evaluation of LVS Function	20	90%	99%	99%

NOTE: Hospital profiles are in alphabetical order by state, then city, then hospital within the city; Rankings exclude hospitals with less than 25 cases except for patient surveys which excludes hospitals with less than 100 cases; (a) 100-299 cases; (1) The number of cases/patients is too few to report; (2) Data submitted were based on a sample of cases/patients; (3) Results are based on a shorter time period than required; (4) Data suppressed by CMS for one or more quarters; (5) Results are not available for this reporting period; (6) Fewer than 100 patients completed the HCAHPS survey; (7) No cases met the criteria for this measure; (8) The lower limit of the confidence interval cannot be calculated if the number of observed infections equals zero; (9) No data are available from the state/territory for this reporting period; (10) The scores shown reflect fewer than 50 completed surveys; (11) There were discrepancies in the data collection process; (12) This measure does not apply to this hospital for this reporting period; (13) Results cannot be calculated for this reporting period; (14) The results for this state are combined with nearby states to protect confidentiality; Please refer to the User's Guide for a full explanation of data.

Measure	Cases	This Hosp.	State Avg.	U.S. Avg.
Medicare Spending				
Medicare Spending per Patient (ratio)	-	0.95	1.03	0.98
Pneumonia Care				
Appropriate Initial Antibiotic Given	38	100%	95%	95%
Blood Culture Timing	57	96%	98%	98%
Pregnancy and Delivery Care				
Newborn Deliveries Scheduled Early[7]	-	-	7%	6%
Preventive Care				
Immunization for Influenza	231	91%	90%	90%
Immunization for Pneumonia	367	88%	92%	92%
Stroke Care				
Anticoagulation Therapy for Atrial Fibrillation[7]	-	-	96%	95%
Antithrombotic Therapy Timing[1]	-	-	98%	98%
Assessed for Rehabilitation[1]	-	-	98%	97%
Discharged on Antithrombotic Therapy[1]	-	-	99%	99%
Discharged on Statin Medication[1]	-	-	95%	94%
Thrombolytic Therapy Timing[7]	-	-	68%	66%
Venous Thromboembolism Prophylaxis[1]	-	-	94%	94%
Written Stroke Educational Materials Given[1]	-	-	92%	88%
Surgical Care Improvement Project				
Appropriate Beta Blocker Usage[5]	-	-	98%	98%
Appropriate VTP Within 24 Hours[5]	-	-	98%	98%
Controlled Postoperative Blood Glucose[5]	-	-	96%	97%
Perioperative Temperature Management[5]	-	-	100%	100%
Prophylactic Antibiotic Selection[5]	-	-	99%	99%
Prophylactic Antibiotic Selection (Outpatient)[3,7]	-	-	98%	98%
Prophylactic Antibiotic Stopped[5]	-	-	98%	98%
Prophylactic Antibiotic Timing[5]	-	-	99%	99%
Prophylactic Antibiotic Timing (Outpatient)[1,3]	-	-	98%	98%
Urinary Catheter Removal[5]	-	-	98%	97%
Survey of Patients' Hospital Experiences				
Area Around Room 'Always' Quiet at Night[6]	<100	73%	68%	61%
Doctors 'Always' Communicated Well[6]	<100	88%	83%	82%
Home Recovery Information Given[6]	<100	82%	85%	85%
Hospital Given 9 or 10 on 10 Point Scale[6]	<100	72%	73%	71%
Meds 'Always' Explained Before Given[6]	<100	73%	66%	64%
Nurses 'Always' Communicated Well[6]	<100	86%	80%	79%
Pain 'Always' Well Controlled[6]	<100	80%	72%	71%
Room and Bathroom 'Always' Clean[6]	<100	70%	75%	73%
Timely Help 'Always' Received[6]	<100	75%	69%	68%
Would Definitely Recommend Hospital[6]	<100	58%	73%	71%
Use of Medical Imaging				
Cardiac Imaging Stress Test before Surgery[1]	-	-	5.3%	5.3%
Combination Abdominal CT Scan	113	7.1%	16.4%	10.5%
Combination Brain/Sinus CT Scan[1]	-	-	2.7%	2.7%
Combination Chest CT Scan	50	0.0%	5.6%	2.7%
Follow-up Mammogram/Ultrasound	128	5.5%	7.9%	8.8%
Lumbar Spine MRI for Low Back Pain[1]	-	-	39.6%	37.2%

Connally Memorial Medical Center

499 10th Street Phone: 830-393-1300
Floresville, TX 78114
Type: Acute Care Hospitals Emergency Services: Yes
Ownership: Govt - Hospital Dist/Auth
Key Personnel:
CEO .... Brian Burnside, F.A.C.H.E.

Measure	Cases	This Hosp.	State Avg.	U.S. Avg.
Blood Clot Prevention and Treatment				
Anticoagulation Overlap Therapy[1,2]	-	-	93%	93%
ICU Venous Thromboembolism Prophylaxis[1,2]	-	-	92%	92%
Incidence of Potentially Preventable VTE[2,7]	-	-	9%	10%
UFH with Dosages/Platelet Monitoring[2,7]	-	-	96%	97%
Venous Thromboembolism Prophylaxis[2]	145	92%	82%	85%
Warfarin Therapy Discharge Instructions[1,2]	-	-	84%	75%
Chest Pain/Possible Heart Attack Care				
Aspirin Given Within 24 Hours of Arrival	56	96%	94%	96%
Fibrinolytic Meds Within 30 Min. of Arrival[1]	-	-	47%	58%
Average Time to ECG (minutes)	57	8	8	7
Average Time to Transfer (minutes)[1]	-	-	62	60
Children's Asthma Care				
Received Home Management Plan of Care	-	-	93%	88%
Received Reliever Medication	-	-	100%	100%
Received Systemic Corticosteroids	-	-	100%	100%
Emergency Department				
Admittance Decision Time (minutes)[2]	391	85	99	98
Head CT Results Within 45 Min. of Arrival[1]	-	-	54%	57%
Patients Who Left ER Before Being Seen	13,088	1%	3%	2%
Time from ER Arrival to Admit. (minutes)[2]	437	238	270	274
Time from ER Arrival to Discharge (minutes)	391	115	127	134
Time in ER Before Being Evaluated (minutes)	416	31	26	26
Time to Pain Meds for Fractures (minutes)	80	50	57	57
Heart Attack Care				
Aspirin Given at Discharge[1]	-	-	99%	99%
Fibrinolytic Meds Within 30 Min. of Arrival[7]	-	-	49%	54%
PCI Within 90 Minutes of Arrival[7]	-	-	95%	96%
Statin Prescribed at Discharge[1]	-	-	98%	98%
Heart Failure Care				
ACE Inhibitor or ARB for LVSD	18	100%	97%	97%
Discharge Instructions Given	29	100%	95%	94%
Evaluation of LVS Function	42	100%	99%	99%
Medicare Spending				
Medicare Spending per Patient (ratio)	-	0.98	1.03	0.98
Pneumonia Care				
Appropriate Initial Antibiotic Given	45	93%	95%	95%
Blood Culture Timing	47	98%	98%	98%
Pregnancy and Delivery Care				
Newborn Deliveries Scheduled Early[7]	-	-	7%	6%
Preventive Care				
Immunization for Influenza[2]	312	98%	90%	90%
Immunization for Pneumonia[2]	507	98%	92%	92%
Stroke Care				
Anticoagulation Therapy for Atrial Fibrillation[7]	-	-	96%	95%
Antithrombotic Therapy Timing[1]	-	-	98%	98%
Assessed for Rehabilitation[1]	-	-	98%	97%
Discharged on Antithrombotic Therapy[1]	-	-	99%	99%
Discharged on Statin Medication[1]	-	-	95%	94%
Thrombolytic Therapy Timing[7]	-	-	68%	66%
Venous Thromboembolism Prophylaxis[1]	-	-	94%	94%
Written Stroke Educational Materials Given[1]	-	-	92%	88%
Surgical Care Improvement Project				
Appropriate Beta Blocker Usage[1]	-	-	98%	98%
Appropriate VTP Within 24 Hours	18	100%	98%	98%
Controlled Postoperative Blood Glucose[7]	-	-	96%	97%
Perioperative Temperature Management	19	100%	100%	100%
Prophylactic Antibiotic Selection	16	94%	99%	99%
Prophylactic Antibiotic Selection (Outpatient)[1,3]	-	-	98%	98%
Prophylactic Antibiotic Stopped	15	100%	98%	98%
Prophylactic Antibiotic Timing	16	100%	99%	99%
Prophylactic Antibiotic Timing (Outpatient)[1,3]	-	-	98%	98%
Urinary Catheter Removal[1]	-	-	98%	97%
Survey of Patients' Hospital Experiences				
Area Around Room 'Always' Quiet at Night	(a)	58%	68%	61%
Doctors 'Always' Communicated Well	(a)	78%	83%	82%
Home Recovery Information Given	(a)	85%	85%	85%
Hospital Given 9 or 10 on 10 Point Scale	(a)	69%	73%	71%
Meds 'Always' Explained Before Given	(a)	61%	66%	64%
Nurses 'Always' Communicated Well	(a)	80%	80%	79%
Pain 'Always' Well Controlled	(a)	76%	72%	71%
Room and Bathroom 'Always' Clean	(a)	79%	75%	73%
Timely Help 'Always' Received	(a)	67%	69%	68%
Would Definitely Recommend Hospital	(a)	65%	73%	71%
Use of Medical Imaging				
Cardiac Imaging Stress Test before Surgery	57	5.3%	5.3%	5.3%
Combination Abdominal CT Scan	186	10.2%	16.4%	10.5%
Combination Brain/Sinus CT Scan[1]	-	-	2.7%	2.7%
Combination Chest CT Scan	132	10.6%	5.6%	2.7%
Follow-up Mammogram/Ultrasound	202	6.9%	7.9%	8.8%
Lumbar Spine MRI for Low Back Pain[1]	-	-	39.6%	37.2%

Texas Health Presbyterian Hospital Flower Mound

4400 Long Prairie Road Phone: 972-419-1530
Flower Mound, TX 75028
URL: www.phfmtexas.com
Type: Acute Care Hospitals Emergency Services: Yes
Ownership: Proprietary Beds: 103

Measure	Cases	This Hosp.	State Avg.	U.S. Avg.
Blood Clot Prevention and Treatment				
Anticoagulation Overlap Therapy[2]	37	95%	93%	93%
ICU Venous Thromboembolism Prophylaxis[2]	39	87%	92%	92%
Incidence of Potentially Preventable VTE[1,2]	-	-	9%	10%
UFH with Dosages/Platelet Monitoring[1,2]	-	-	96%	97%
Venous Thromboembolism Prophylaxis[2]	314	94%	82%	85%
Warfarin Therapy Discharge Instructions[2]	32	100%	84%	75%
Chest Pain/Possible Heart Attack Care				
Aspirin Given Within 24 Hours of Arrival	13	100%	94%	96%
Fibrinolytic Meds Within 30 Min. of Arrival[7]	-	-	47%	58%
Average Time to ECG (minutes)	14	8	8	7
Average Time to Transfer (minutes)[1]	-	-	62	60
Children's Asthma Care				
Received Home Management Plan of Care	-	-	93%	88%
Received Reliever Medication	-	-	100%	100%
Received Systemic Corticosteroids	-	-	100%	100%
Emergency Department				
Admittance Decision Time (minutes)[2]	317	81	99	98
Head CT Results Within 45 Min. of Arrival[1]	-	-	54%	57%
Patients Who Left ER Before Being Seen	14,068	0%	3%	2%
Time from ER Arrival to Admit. (minutes)[2]	317	215	270	274
Time from ER Arrival to Discharge (minutes)	448	116	127	134
Time in ER Before Being Evaluated (minutes)	502	11	26	26
Time to Pain Meds for Fractures (minutes)	104	32	57	57
Heart Attack Care				
Aspirin Given at Discharge	13	77%	99%	99%
Fibrinolytic Meds Within 30 Min. of Arrival[7]	-	-	49%	54%
PCI Within 90 Minutes of Arrival[7]	-	-	95%	96%
Statin Prescribed at Discharge	14	100%	98%	98%
Heart Failure Care				
ACE Inhibitor or ARB for LVSD	17	94%	97%	97%
Discharge Instructions Given	56	75%	95%	94%
Evaluation of LVS Function	67	100%	99%	99%
Medicare Spending				
Medicare Spending per Patient (ratio)	-	1.05	1.03	0.98
Pneumonia Care				
Appropriate Initial Antibiotic Given	84	89%	95%	95%
Blood Culture Timing	122	98%	98%	98%
Pregnancy and Delivery Care				
Newborn Deliveries Scheduled Early[2]	29	7%	7%	6%
Preventive Care				
Immunization for Influenza[2]	463	97%	90%	90%
Immunization for Pneumonia[2]	437	99%	92%	92%
Stroke Care				
Anticoagulation Therapy for Atrial Fibrillation[2,7]	-	-	96%	95%
Antithrombotic Therapy Timing[1,2]	-	-	98%	98%
Assessed for Rehabilitation[2]	11	91%	98%	97%
Discharged on Antithrombotic Therapy[2]	11	91%	99%	99%
Discharged on Statin Medication[1,2]	-	-	95%	94%
Thrombolytic Therapy Timing[1,2]	-	-	68%	66%
Venous Thromboembolism Prophylaxis[1,2]	-	-	94%	94%
Written Stroke Educational Materials Given[1,2]	-	-	92%	88%
Surgical Care Improvement Project				
Appropriate Beta Blocker Usage	93	100%	98%	98%
Appropriate VTP Within 24 Hours	383	95%	98%	98%
Controlled Postoperative Blood Glucose[7]	-	-	96%	97%
Perioperative Temperature Management	416	100%	100%	100%
Prophylactic Antibiotic Selection	323	98%	99%	99%
Prophylactic Antibiotic Selection (Outpatient)	322	96%	98%	98%
Prophylactic Antibiotic Stopped	315	97%	98%	98%
Prophylactic Antibiotic Timing	323	100%	99%	99%
Prophylactic Antibiotic Timing (Outpatient)	323	99%	98%	98%
Urinary Catheter Removal	300	98%	98%	97%
Survey of Patients' Hospital Experiences				
Area Around Room 'Always' Quiet at Night	300+	71%	68%	61%

NOTE: Hospital profiles are in alphabetical order by state, then city, then hospital within the city; Rankings exclude hospitals with less than 25 cases except for patient surveys which excludes hospitals with less than 100 cases; (a) 100-299 cases; (1) The number of cases/patients is too few to report; (2) Data submitted were based on a sample of cases/patients; (3) Results are based on a shorter time period than required; (4) Data suppressed by CMS for one or more quarters; (5) Results are not available for this reporting period; (6) Fewer than 100 patients completed the HCAHPS survey; (7) No cases met the criteria for this measure; (8) The lower limit of the confidence interval cannot be calculated if the number of observed infections equals zero; (9) No data are available from the state/territory for this reporting period; (10) The scores shown reflect fewer than 50 completed surveys; (11) There were discrepancies in the data collection process; (12) This measure does not apply to this hospital for this reporting period; (13) Results cannot be calculated for this reporting period; (14) The results for this state are combined with nearby states to protect confidentiality; Please refer to the User's Guide for a full explanation of data.

Measure	Cases	This Hosp.	State Avg.	U.S. Avg.
Doctors 'Always' Communicated Well	300+	85%	83%	82%
Home Recovery Information Given	300+	86%	85%	85%
Hospital Given 9 or 10 on 10 Point Scale	300+	79%	73%	71%
Meds 'Always' Explained Before Given	300+	66%	66%	64%
Nurses 'Always' Communicated Well	300+	81%	80%	79%
Pain 'Always' Well Controlled	300+	75%	72%	71%
Room and Bathroom 'Always' Clean	300+	76%	75%	73%
Timely Help 'Always' Received	300+	73%	69%	68%
Would Definitely Recommend Hospital	300+	78%	73%	71%
Use of Medical Imaging				
Cardiac Imaging Stress Test before Surgery[1]	-	-	5.3%	5.3%
Combination Abdominal CT Scan	288	15.3%	16.4%	10.5%
Combination Brain/Sinus CT Scan[1]	-	-	2.7%	2.7%
Combination Chest CT Scan	120	4.2%	5.6%	2.7%
Follow-up Mammogram/Ultrasound	166	5.4%	7.9%	8.8%
Lumbar Spine MRI for Low Back Pain	78	30.8%	39.6%	37.2%

Pecos County Memorial Hospital

387 West I 10
Fort Stockton, TX 79735
Phone: 432-336-4201
Fax: 432-336-4526
Type: Acute Care Hospitals
Emergency Services: Yes
Ownership: Government - Local
Beds: 37

Key Personnel:
Quality Assurance . . . . Linda Allen
Chief of Medical Staff . . . . Larry C. Boyd, Dr.
Anesthesiology. . . . . Mary Gonzales
CEO . . . . Jim Horton
Operating Room. . . . . Judy Minter, RN
Emergency Room . . . . Monica Sherwood
Infection Control. . . . . Kate Young

Measure	Cases	This Hosp.	State Avg.	U.S. Avg.
Blood Clot Prevention and Treatment				
Anticoagulation Overlap Therapy[2]	14	57%	93%	93%
ICU Venous Thromboembolism Prophylaxis[2,7]	-	-	92%	92%
Incidence of Potentially Preventable VTE[2,7]	-	-	9%	10%
UFH with Dosages/Platelet Monitoring[2,7]	-	-	96%	97%
Venous Thromboembolism Prophylaxis[2]	172	37%	82%	85%
Warfarin Therapy Discharge Instructions[2]	12	92%	84%	75%
Chest Pain/Possible Heart Attack Care				
Aspirin Given Within 24 Hours of Arrival[3]	14	93%	94%	96%
Fibrinolytic Meds Within 30 Min. of Arrival[1,3]	-	-	47%	58%
Average Time to ECG (minutes)[3]	14	12	8	7
Average Time to Transfer (minutes)[1,3]	-	-	62	60
Children's Asthma Care				
Received Home Management Plan of Care	-	-	93%	88%
Received Reliever Medication	-	-	100%	100%
Received Systemic Corticosteroids	-	-	100%	100%
Emergency Department				
Admittance Decision Time (minutes)[2]	257	105	99	98
Head CT Results Within 45 Min. of Arrival[1]	-	-	54%	57%
Patients Who Left ER Before Being Seen	7,013	2%	3%	2%
Time from ER Arrival to Admit. (minutes)[2]	298	236	270	274
Time from ER Arrival to Discharge (minutes)	374	124	127	134
Time in ER Before Being Evaluated (minutes)	396	29	26	26
Time to Pain Meds for Fractures (minutes)	45	40	57	57
Heart Attack Care				
Aspirin Given at Discharge[5]	-	-	99%	99%
Fibrinolytic Meds Within 30 Min. of Arrival[5]	-	-	49%	54%
PCI Within 90 Minutes of Arrival[5]	-	-	95%	96%
Statin Prescribed at Discharge[5]	-	-	98%	98%
Heart Failure Care				
ACE Inhibitor or ARB for LVSD[2]	47	87%	97%	97%
Discharge Instructions Given[2]	63	70%	95%	94%
Evaluation of LVS Function[2]	68	99%	99%	99%
Medicare Spending				
Medicare Spending per Patient (ratio)	-	0.82	1.03	0.98
Pneumonia Care				
Appropriate Initial Antibiotic Given[2]	24	79%	95%	95%
Blood Culture Timing[2]	31	87%	98%	98%
Pregnancy and Delivery Care				
Newborn Deliveries Scheduled Early	20	5%	7%	6%
Preventive Care				
Immunization for Influenza[2]	235	89%	90%	90%
Immunization for Pneumonia[2]	313	89%	92%	92%
Stroke Care				
Anticoagulation Therapy for Atrial Fibrillation[5]	-	-	96%	95%
Antithrombotic Therapy Timing[5]	-	-	98%	98%
Assessed for Rehabilitation[5]	-	-	98%	97%
Discharged on Antithrombotic Therapy[5]	-	-	99%	99%
Discharged on Statin Medication[5]	-	-	95%	94%
Thrombolytic Therapy Timing[5]	-	-	68%	66%
Venous Thromboembolism Prophylaxis[5]	-	-	94%	94%
Written Stroke Educational Materials Given[5]	-	-	92%	88%
Surgical Care Improvement Project				
Appropriate Beta Blocker Usage[3,7]	-	-	98%	98%
Appropriate VTP Within 24 Hours[1,3]	-	-	98%	98%
Controlled Postoperative Blood Glucose[3,7]	-	-	96%	97%
Perioperative Temperature Management[1,3]	-	-	100%	100%
Prophylactic Antibiotic Selection[1,3]	-	-	99%	99%
Prophylactic Antibiotic Selection (Outpatient)[5]	-	-	98%	98%
Prophylactic Antibiotic Stopped[1,3]	-	-	98%	98%
Prophylactic Antibiotic Timing[1,3]	-	-	99%	99%
Prophylactic Antibiotic Timing (Outpatient)[5]	-	-	98%	98%
Urinary Catheter Removal[3,7]	-	-	98%	97%
Survey of Patients' Hospital Experiences				
Area Around Room 'Always' Quiet at Night	(a)	70%	68%	61%
Doctors 'Always' Communicated Well	(a)	92%	83%	82%
Home Recovery Information Given	(a)	86%	85%	85%
Hospital Given 9 or 10 on 10 Point Scale	(a)	77%	73%	71%
Meds 'Always' Explained Before Given	(a)	66%	66%	64%
Nurses 'Always' Communicated Well	(a)	82%	80%	79%
Pain 'Always' Well Controlled	(a)	80%	72%	71%
Room and Bathroom 'Always' Clean	(a)	80%	75%	73%
Timely Help 'Always' Received	(a)	73%	69%	68%
Would Definitely Recommend Hospital	(a)	74%	73%	71%
Use of Medical Imaging				
Cardiac Imaging Stress Test before Surgery[7]	-	-	5.3%	5.3%
Combination Abdominal CT Scan	132	3.8%	16.4%	10.5%
Combination Brain/Sinus CT Scan[1]	-	-	2.7%	2.7%
Combination Chest CT Scan[1]	-	-	5.6%	2.7%
Follow-up Mammogram/Ultrasound[7]	-	-	7.9%	8.8%
Lumbar Spine MRI for Low Back Pain[1]	-	-	39.6%	37.2%

Baylor All Saints Medical Center at FW

1400 Eighth Ave
Fort Worth, TX 76104
Phone: 817-926-2544
Fax: 817-922-1593
URL: www.baylorhealth.com/locations/allsaints
Type: Acute Care Hospitals
Emergency Services: Yes
Ownership: Voluntary non-profit - Private
Beds: 275

Key Personnel:
CEO/President. . . . . David Klein, MD, MBA

Measure	Cases	This Hosp.	State Avg.	U.S. Avg.
Blood Clot Prevention and Treatment				
Anticoagulation Overlap Therapy[2]	65	89%	93%	93%
ICU Venous Thromboembolism Prophylaxis[2]	84	88%	92%	92%
Incidence of Potentially Preventable VTE[1,2]	-	-	9%	10%
UFH with Dosages/Platelet Monitoring[2]	29	100%	96%	97%
Venous Thromboembolism Prophylaxis[2]	331	84%	82%	85%
Warfarin Therapy Discharge Instructions[2]	46	98%	84%	75%
Chest Pain/Possible Heart Attack Care				
Aspirin Given Within 24 Hours of Arrival[1,3]	-	-	94%	96%
Fibrinolytic Meds Within 30 Min. of Arrival[5]	-	-	47%	58%
Average Time to ECG (minutes)[1,3]	-	-	8	7
Average Time to Transfer (minutes)[5]	-	-	62	60
Children's Asthma Care				
Received Home Management Plan of Care	-	-	93%	88%
Received Reliever Medication	-	-	100%	100%
Received Systemic Corticosteroids	-	-	100%	100%
Emergency Department				
Admittance Decision Time (minutes)[2]	376	118	99	98
Head CT Results Within 45 Min. of Arrival[1]	-	-	54%	57%
Patients Who Left ER Before Being Seen	48,539	2%	3%	2%
Time from ER Arrival to Admit. (minutes)[2]	382	330	270	274
Time from ER Arrival to Discharge (minutes)	401	203	127	134
Time in ER Before Being Evaluated (minutes)	399	56	26	26
Time to Pain Meds for Fractures (minutes)	70	72	57	57
Heart Attack Care				
Aspirin Given at Discharge	165	99%	99%	99%
Fibrinolytic Meds Within 30 Min. of Arrival[7]	-	-	49%	54%
PCI Within 90 Minutes of Arrival	15	87%	95%	96%
Statin Prescribed at Discharge	157	98%	98%	98%
Heart Failure Care				
ACE Inhibitor or ARB for LVSD	77	96%	97%	97%
Discharge Instructions Given	194	96%	95%	94%
Evaluation of LVS Function	234	100%	99%	99%
Medicare Spending				
Medicare Spending per Patient (ratio)	-	1.04	1.03	0.98
Pneumonia Care				
Appropriate Initial Antibiotic Given	184	97%	95%	95%
Blood Culture Timing	358	99%	98%	98%
Pregnancy and Delivery Care				
Newborn Deliveries Scheduled Early	510	3%	7%	6%
Preventive Care				
Immunization for Influenza[2]	461	97%	90%	90%
Immunization for Pneumonia[2]	411	96%	92%	92%
Stroke Care				
Anticoagulation Therapy for Atrial Fibrillation[1,2]	-	-	96%	95%
Antithrombotic Therapy Timing[2]	71	100%	98%	98%
Assessed for Rehabilitation[2]	78	99%	98%	97%
Discharged on Antithrombotic Therapy[2]	70	100%	99%	99%
Discharged on Statin Medication[2]	55	89%	95%	94%
Thrombolytic Therapy Timing[1,2]	-	-	68%	66%
Venous Thromboembolism Prophylaxis[2]	82	83%	94%	94%
Written Stroke Educational Materials Given[2]	30	93%	92%	88%
Surgical Care Improvement Project				
Appropriate Beta Blocker Usage[2]	169	97%	98%	98%
Appropriate VTP Within 24 Hours[2]	588	98%	98%	98%
Controlled Postoperative Blood Glucose[2]	28	96%	96%	97%
Perioperative Temperature Management[2]	701	100%	100%	100%
Prophylactic Antibiotic Selection[2]	521	99%	99%	99%
Prophylactic Antibiotic Selection (Outpatient)	524	96%	98%	98%
Prophylactic Antibiotic Stopped[2]	492	99%	98%	98%
Prophylactic Antibiotic Timing[2]	521	100%	99%	99%
Prophylactic Antibiotic Timing (Outpatient)	524	99%	98%	98%
Urinary Catheter Removal[2]	256	96%	98%	97%
Survey of Patients' Hospital Experiences				
Area Around Room 'Always' Quiet at Night	300+	63%	68%	61%
Doctors 'Always' Communicated Well	300+	80%	83%	82%
Home Recovery Information Given	300+	83%	85%	85%
Hospital Given 9 or 10 on 10 Point Scale	300+	76%	73%	71%
Meds 'Always' Explained Before Given	300+	63%	66%	64%
Nurses 'Always' Communicated Well	300+	79%	80%	79%
Pain 'Always' Well Controlled	300+	73%	72%	71%
Room and Bathroom 'Always' Clean	300+	69%	75%	73%
Timely Help 'Always' Received	300+	63%	69%	68%
Would Definitely Recommend Hospital	300+	79%	73%	71%
Use of Medical Imaging				
Cardiac Imaging Stress Test before Surgery[1]	-	-	5.3%	5.3%
Combination Abdominal CT Scan	707	10.9%	16.4%	10.5%
Combination Brain/Sinus CT Scan	624	2.7%	2.7%	2.7%
Combination Chest CT Scan	298	1.0%	5.6%	2.7%
Follow-up Mammogram/Ultrasound[7]	-	-	7.9%	8.8%
Lumbar Spine MRI for Low Back Pain[1]	-	-	39.6%	37.2%

Baylor Surgical Hospital at Fort Worth

750 12th Avenue
Fort Worth, TX 76104
Phone: 817-334-5050
URL: www.mcsh-hospital.com
Type: Acute Care Hospitals
Emergency Services: Yes
Ownership: Voluntary non-profit - Private

Key Personnel:
Quality Assurance . . . . Linda Leiwer
CEO . . . . Roger Rhodes

Measure	Cases	This Hosp.	State Avg.	U.S. Avg.
Blood Clot Prevention and Treatment				
Anticoagulation Overlap Therapy[1,2]	-	-	93%	93%
ICU Venous Thromboembolism Prophylaxis[2,7]	-	-	92%	92%
Incidence of Potentially Preventable VTE[2,7]	-	-	9%	10%
UFH with Dosages/Platelet Monitoring[1,2]	-	-	96%	97%
Venous Thromboembolism Prophylaxis[2]	61	100%	82%	85%

NOTE: Hospital profiles are in alphabetical order by state, then city, then hospital within the city; Rankings exclude hospitals with less than 25 cases except for patient surveys which excludes hospitals with less than 100 cases; (a) 100-299 cases; (1) The number of cases/patients is too few to report; (2) Data submitted were based on a sample of cases/patients; (3) Results are based on a shorter time period than required; (4) Data suppressed by CMS for one or more quarters; (5) Results are not available for this reporting period; (6) Fewer than 100 patients completed the HCAHPS survey; (7) No cases met the criteria for this measure; (8) The lower limit of the confidence interval cannot be calculated if the number of observed infections equals zero; (9) No data are available from the state/territory for this reporting period; (10) The scores shown reflect fewer than 50 completed surveys; (11) There were discrepancies in the data collection process; (12) This measure does not apply to this hospital for this reporting period; (13) Results cannot be calculated for this reporting period; (14) The results for this state are combined with nearby states to protect confidentiality; Please refer to the User's Guide for a full explanation of data.

Measure	Cases	This Hosp.	State Avg.	U.S. Avg.
Warfarin Therapy Discharge Instructions[1,2]	-	-	84%	75%
Chest Pain/Possible Heart Attack Care				
Aspirin Given Within 24 Hours of Arrival[5]	-	-	94%	96%
Fibrinolytic Meds Within 30 Min. of Arrival[5]	-	-	47%	58%
Average Time to ECG (minutes)[5]	-	-	8	7
Average Time to Transfer (minutes)[5]	-	-	62	60
Children's Asthma Care				
Received Home Management Plan of Care	-	-	93%	88%
Received Reliever Medication	-	-	100%	100%
Received Systemic Corticosteroids	-	-	100%	100%
Emergency Department				
Admittance Decision Time (minutes)[1,2]	-	-	99	98
Head CT Results Within 45 Min. of Arrival[5]	-	-	54%	57%
Patients Who Left ER Before Being Seen	400	0%	3%	2%
Time from ER Arrival to Admit. (minutes)[1,2]	-	-	270	274
Time from ER Arrival to Discharge (minutes)	291	105	127	134
Time in ER Before Being Evaluated (minutes)	264	10	26	26
Time to Pain Meds for Fractures (minutes)[1,3]	-	-	57	57
Heart Attack Care				
Aspirin Given at Discharge[5]	-	-	99%	99%
Fibrinolytic Meds Within 30 Min. of Arrival[5]	-	-	49%	54%
PCI Within 90 Minutes of Arrival[5]	-	-	95%	96%
Statin Prescribed at Discharge[5]	-	-	98%	98%
Heart Failure Care				
ACE Inhibitor or ARB for LVSD[5]	-	-	97%	97%
Discharge Instructions Given[5]	-	-	95%	94%
Evaluation of LVS Function[5]	-	-	99%	99%
Medicare Spending				
Medicare Spending per Patient (ratio)	-	1.17	1.03	0.98
Pneumonia Care				
Appropriate Initial Antibiotic Given[5]	-	-	95%	95%
Blood Culture Timing[5]	-	-	98%	98%
Pregnancy and Delivery Care				
Newborn Deliveries Scheduled Early[7]	-	-	7%	6%
Preventive Care				
Immunization for Influenza[2]	476	76%	90%	90%
Immunization for Pneumonia[2]	387	77%	92%	92%
Stroke Care				
Anticoagulation Therapy for Atrial Fibrillation[5]	-	-	96%	95%
Antithrombotic Therapy Timing[5]	-	-	98%	98%
Assessed for Rehabilitation[5]	-	-	98%	97%
Discharged on Antithrombotic Therapy[5]	-	-	99%	99%
Discharged on Statin Medication[5]	-	-	95%	94%
Thrombolytic Therapy Timing[5]	-	-	68%	66%
Venous Thromboembolism Prophylaxis[5]	-	-	94%	94%
Written Stroke Educational Materials Given[5]	-	-	92%	88%
Surgical Care Improvement Project				
Appropriate Beta Blocker Usage	122	99%	98%	98%
Appropriate VTP Within 24 Hours	443	100%	98%	98%
Controlled Postoperative Blood Glucose[7]	-	-	96%	97%
Perioperative Temperature Management	446	100%	100%	100%
Prophylactic Antibiotic Selection	423	100%	99%	99%
Prophylactic Antibiotic Selection (Outpatient)	239	100%	98%	98%
Prophylactic Antibiotic Stopped	420	97%	98%	98%
Prophylactic Antibiotic Timing	423	98%	99%	99%
Prophylactic Antibiotic Timing (Outpatient)	241	99%	98%	98%
Urinary Catheter Removal	435	100%	98%	97%
Survey of Patients' Hospital Experiences				
Area Around Room 'Always' Quiet at Night	300+	62%	68%	61%
Doctors 'Always' Communicated Well	300+	82%	83%	82%
Home Recovery Information Given	300+	87%	85%	85%
Hospital Given 9 or 10 on 10 Point Scale	300+	68%	73%	71%
Meds 'Always' Explained Before Given	300+	66%	66%	64%
Nurses 'Always' Communicated Well	300+	76%	80%	79%
Pain 'Always' Well Controlled	300+	67%	72%	71%
Room and Bathroom 'Always' Clean	300+	70%	75%	73%
Timely Help 'Always' Received	300+	64%	69%	68%
Would Definitely Recommend Hospital	300+	71%	73%	71%
Use of Medical Imaging				
Cardiac Imaging Stress Test before Surgery[7]	-	-	5.3%	5.3%
Combination Abdominal CT Scan[1]	-	-	16.4%	10.5%
Combination Brain/Sinus CT Scan	34	0.0%	2.7%	2.7%
Combination Chest CT Scan[1]	-	-	5.6%	2.7%
Follow-up Mammogram/Ultrasound[7]	-	-	7.9%	8.8%
Lumbar Spine MRI for Low Back Pain	53	39.6%	39.6%	37.2%

Cook Childrens Medical Center

801 Seventh Avenue
Fort Worth, TX 76104
URL: www.cookchildrens.org
Type: Childrens
Ownership: Voluntary non-profit - Private
Phone: 682-885-4000
Fax: 682-885-3947
Emergency Services: Yes
Beds: 282

Key Personnel:
Emergency Room . . . . Maggie Huey

Measure	Cases	This Hosp.	State Avg.	U.S. Avg.
Blood Clot Prevention and Treatment				
Anticoagulation Overlap Therapy[5]	-	-	93%	93%
ICU Venous Thromboembolism Prophylaxis[5]	-	-	92%	92%
Incidence of Potentially Preventable VTE[5]	-	-	9%	10%
UFH with Dosages/Platelet Monitoring[5]	-	-	96%	97%
Venous Thromboembolism Prophylaxis[5]	-	-	82%	85%
Warfarin Therapy Discharge Instructions[5]	-	-	84%	75%
Chest Pain/Possible Heart Attack Care				
Aspirin Given Within 24 Hours of Arrival	-	-	94%	96%
Fibrinolytic Meds Within 30 Min. of Arrival	-	-	47%	58%
Average Time to ECG (minutes)	-	-	8	7
Average Time to Transfer (minutes)	-	-	62	60
Children's Asthma Care				
Received Home Management Plan of Care[2]	284	90%	93%	88%
Received Reliever Medication[2]	284	100%	100%	100%
Received Systemic Corticosteroids[2]	284	100%	100%	100%
Emergency Department				
Admittance Decision Time (minutes)[5]	-	-	99	98
Head CT Results Within 45 Min. of Arrival	-	-	54%	57%
Patients Who Left ER Before Being Seen	-	-	3%	2%
Time from ER Arrival to Admit. (minutes)[5]	-	-	270	274
Time from ER Arrival to Discharge (minutes)	-	-	127	134
Time in ER Before Being Evaluated (minutes)	-	-	26	26
Time to Pain Meds for Fractures (minutes)	-	-	57	57
Heart Attack Care				
Aspirin Given at Discharge[5]	-	-	99%	99%
Fibrinolytic Meds Within 30 Min. of Arrival[5]	-	-	49%	54%
PCI Within 90 Minutes of Arrival[5]	-	-	95%	96%
Statin Prescribed at Discharge[5]	-	-	98%	98%
Heart Failure Care				
ACE Inhibitor or ARB for LVSD[5]	-	-	97%	97%
Discharge Instructions Given[5]	-	-	95%	94%
Evaluation of LVS Function[5]	-	-	99%	99%
Medicare Spending				
Medicare Spending per Patient (ratio)	-	-	1.03	0.98
Pneumonia Care				
Appropriate Initial Antibiotic Given[5]	-	-	95%	95%
Blood Culture Timing[5]	-	-	98%	98%
Pregnancy and Delivery Care				
Newborn Deliveries Scheduled Early[5]	-	-	7%	6%
Preventive Care				
Immunization for Influenza[5]	-	-	90%	90%
Immunization for Pneumonia[5]	-	-	92%	92%
Stroke Care				
Anticoagulation Therapy for Atrial Fibrillation[5]	-	-	96%	95%
Antithrombotic Therapy Timing[5]	-	-	98%	98%
Assessed for Rehabilitation[5]	-	-	98%	97%
Discharged on Antithrombotic Therapy[5]	-	-	99%	99%
Discharged on Statin Medication[5]	-	-	95%	94%
Thrombolytic Therapy Timing[5]	-	-	68%	66%
Venous Thromboembolism Prophylaxis[5]	-	-	94%	94%
Written Stroke Educational Materials Given[5]	-	-	92%	88%
Surgical Care Improvement Project				
Appropriate Beta Blocker Usage[5]	-	-	98%	98%
Appropriate VTP Within 24 Hours[5]	-	-	98%	98%
Controlled Postoperative Blood Glucose[5]	-	-	96%	97%
Perioperative Temperature Management[5]	-	-	100%	100%
Prophylactic Antibiotic Selection[5]	-	-	99%	99%
Prophylactic Antibiotic Selection (Outpatient)	-	-	98%	98%
Prophylactic Antibiotic Stopped[5]	-	-	98%	98%
Prophylactic Antibiotic Timing[5]	-	-	99%	99%
Prophylactic Antibiotic Timing (Outpatient)	-	-	98%	98%
Urinary Catheter Removal[5]	-	-	98%	97%
Survey of Patients' Hospital Experiences				
Area Around Room 'Always' Quiet at Night[5]	-	-	68%	61%
Doctors 'Always' Communicated Well[5]	-	-	83%	82%
Home Recovery Information Given[5]	-	-	85%	85%
Hospital Given 9 or 10 on 10 Point Scale[5]	-	-	73%	71%
Meds 'Always' Explained Before Given[5]	-	-	66%	64%
Nurses 'Always' Communicated Well[5]	-	-	80%	79%
Pain 'Always' Well Controlled[5]	-	-	72%	71%
Room and Bathroom 'Always' Clean[5]	-	-	75%	73%
Timely Help 'Always' Received[5]	-	-	69%	68%
Would Definitely Recommend Hospital[5]	-	-	73%	71%
Use of Medical Imaging				
Cardiac Imaging Stress Test before Surgery	-	-	5.3%	5.3%
Combination Abdominal CT Scan	-	-	16.4%	10.5%
Combination Brain/Sinus CT Scan	-	-	2.7%	2.7%
Combination Chest CT Scan	-	-	5.6%	2.7%
Follow-up Mammogram/Ultrasound	-	-	7.9%	8.8%
Lumbar Spine MRI for Low Back Pain	-	-	39.6%	37.2%

JPS Health Network

1500 S Main St
Fort Worth, TX 76104
URL: www.jpshealthnet.org
Type: Acute Care Hospitals
Ownership: Govt - Hospital Dist/Auth
Phone: 817-921-3431
Fax: 817-927-1664
Emergency Services: Yes
Beds: 459

Key Personnel:
Quality Assurance . . . . Carl Blumberg, RN
CEO/President. . . . . Robert Earley
Pediatric Ambulatory Care . . . . . . Janet Figueroa
Infection Control. . . . . Jan Hawley
Radiology. . . . . Mona Martinez
Chief of Medical Staff . . . . Robert Reddix, MD
Pediatric In-Patient Care . . . . . . Darryl Wilson
Operating Room. . . . . Pat Wright

Measure	Cases	This Hosp.	State Avg.	U.S. Avg.
Blood Clot Prevention and Treatment				
Anticoagulation Overlap Therapy[2]	165	98%	93%	93%
ICU Venous Thromboembolism Prophylaxis[2]	91	100%	92%	92%
Incidence of Potentially Preventable VTE[2]	57	0%	9%	10%
UFH with Dosages/Platelet Monitoring[2]	68	100%	96%	97%
Venous Thromboembolism Prophylaxis[2]	401	92%	82%	85%
Warfarin Therapy Discharge Instructions[2]	126	84%	84%	75%
Chest Pain/Possible Heart Attack Care				
Aspirin Given Within 24 Hours of Arrival[1]	-	-	94%	96%
Fibrinolytic Meds Within 30 Min. of Arrival[3,7]	-	-	47%	58%
Average Time to ECG (minutes)[1]	-	-	8	7
Average Time to Transfer (minutes)[1,3]	-	-	62	60
Children's Asthma Care				
Received Home Management Plan of Care	-	-	93%	88%
Received Reliever Medication	-	-	100%	100%
Received Systemic Corticosteroids	-	-	100%	100%
Emergency Department				
Admittance Decision Time (minutes)[2]	704	136	99	98
Head CT Results Within 45 Min. of Arrival[1]	-	-	54%	57%
Patients Who Left ER Before Being Seen	>100k	5%	3%	2%
Time from ER Arrival to Admit. (minutes)[2]	722	384	270	274
Time from ER Arrival to Discharge (minutes)	731	245	127	134
Time in ER Before Being Evaluated (minutes)	868	56	26	26
Time to Pain Meds for Fractures (minutes)	245	77	57	57
Heart Attack Care				
Aspirin Given at Discharge	295	100%	99%	99%
Fibrinolytic Meds Within 30 Min. of Arrival[7]	-	-	49%	54%
PCI Within 90 Minutes of Arrival	60	95%	95%	96%
Statin Prescribed at Discharge	285	100%	98%	98%
Heart Failure Care				
ACE Inhibitor or ARB for LVSD	259	98%	97%	97%
Discharge Instructions Given	445	97%	95%	94%
Evaluation of LVS Function	480	100%	99%	99%
Medicare Spending				
Medicare Spending per Patient (ratio)	-	1.05	1.03	0.98
Pneumonia Care				

NOTE: Hospital profiles are in alphabetical order by state, then city, then hospital within the city; Rankings exclude hospitals with less than 25 cases except for patient surveys which excludes hospitals with less than 100 cases; (a) 100-299 cases; (1) The number of cases/patients is too few to report; (2) Data submitted were based on a sample of cases/patients; (3) Results are based on a shorter time period than required; (4) Data suppressed by CMS for one or more quarters; (5) Results are not available for this reporting period; (6) Fewer than 100 patients completed the HCAHPS survey; (7) No cases met the criteria for this measure; (8) The lower limit of the confidence interval cannot be calculated if the number of observed infections equals zero; (9) No data are available from the state/territory for this reporting period; (10) The scores shown reflect fewer than 50 completed surveys; (11) There were discrepancies in the data collection process; (12) This measure does not apply to this hospital for this reporting period; (13) Results cannot be calculated for this reporting period; (14) The results for this state are combined with nearby states to protect confidentiality; Please refer to the User's Guide for a full explanation of data.

Measure	Cases	This Hosp.	State Avg.	U.S. Avg.
Appropriate Initial Antibiotic Given	217	97%	95%	95%
Blood Culture Timing	308	96%	98%	98%
Pregnancy and Delivery Care				
Newborn Deliveries Scheduled Early[2]	68	1%	7%	6%
Preventive Care				
Immunization for Influenza[2]	645	93%	90%	90%
Immunization for Pneumonia[2]	491	90%	92%	92%
Stroke Care				
Anticoagulation Therapy for Atrial Fibrillation	12	100%	96%	95%
Antithrombotic Therapy Timing	210	100%	98%	98%
Assessed for Rehabilitation	269	98%	98%	97%
Discharged on Antithrombotic Therapy	223	98%	99%	99%
Discharged on Statin Medication	199	96%	95%	94%
Thrombolytic Therapy Timing	30	83%	68%	66%
Venous Thromboembolism Prophylaxis	306	96%	94%	94%
Written Stroke Educational Materials Given	202	96%	92%	88%
Surgical Care Improvement Project				
Appropriate Beta Blocker Usage[2]	198	99%	98%	98%
Appropriate VTP Within 24 Hours[2]	576	99%	98%	98%
Controlled Postoperative Blood Glucose[2]	115	99%	96%	97%
Perioperative Temperature Management[2]	796	100%	100%	100%
Prophylactic Antibiotic Selection[2]	557	99%	99%	99%
Prophylactic Antibiotic Selection (Outpatient)	392	99%	98%	98%
Prophylactic Antibiotic Stopped[2]	547	99%	98%	98%
Prophylactic Antibiotic Timing[2]	559	100%	99%	99%
Prophylactic Antibiotic Timing (Outpatient)	368	96%	98%	98%
Urinary Catheter Removal[2]	468	97%	98%	97%
Survey of Patients' Hospital Experiences				
Area Around Room 'Always' Quiet at Night	300+	58%	68%	61%
Doctors 'Always' Communicated Well	300+	78%	83%	82%
Home Recovery Information Given	300+	83%	85%	85%
Hospital Given 9 or 10 on 10 Point Scale	300+	73%	73%	71%
Meds 'Always' Explained Before Given	300+	61%	66%	64%
Nurses 'Always' Communicated Well	300+	77%	80%	79%
Pain 'Always' Well Controlled	300+	67%	72%	71%
Room and Bathroom 'Always' Clean	300+	71%	75%	73%
Timely Help 'Always' Received	300+	62%	69%	68%
Would Definitely Recommend Hospital	300+	76%	73%	71%
Use of Medical Imaging				
Cardiac Imaging Stress Test before Surgery	397	3.3%	5.3%	5.3%
Combination Abdominal CT Scan	1,008	10.3%	16.4%	10.5%
Combination Brain/Sinus CT Scan	1,003	4.6%	2.7%	2.7%
Combination Chest CT Scan	822	3.2%	5.6%	2.7%
Follow-up Mammogram/Ultrasound	1,416	8.5%	7.9%	8.8%
Lumbar Spine MRI for Low Back Pain	81	39.5%	39.6%	37.2%

Plaza Medical Center of Fort Worth

900 Eighth Avenue
Fort Worth, TX 76104
URL: www.plazamedicalcenter.com
Type: Acute Care Hospitals
Ownership: Proprietary
Phone: 817-336-2100
Fax: 817-347-5796
Emergency Services: Yes
Beds: 320

Key Personnel:
Operating Room. . . . . Paula Barney
Chief of Medical Staff. . . . . MI Mughal
CEO/President. . . . . Tony Villarreal
Emergency Room . . . . Daniela Wallace, RN

Measure	Cases	This Hosp.	State Avg.	U.S. Avg.
Blood Clot Prevention and Treatment				
Anticoagulation Overlap Therapy[2]	82	100%	93%	93%
ICU Venous Thromboembolism Prophylaxis[2]	104	92%	92%	92%
Incidence of Potentially Preventable VTE[1,2]	-	-	9%	10%
UFH with Dosages/Platelet Monitoring[2]	38	97%	96%	97%
Venous Thromboembolism Prophylaxis[2]	313	84%	82%	85%
Warfarin Therapy Discharge Instructions[2]	48	73%	84%	75%
Chest Pain/Possible Heart Attack Care				
Aspirin Given Within 24 Hours of Arrival[1,3]	-	-	94%	96%
Fibrinolytic Meds Within 30 Min. of Arrival[5]	-	-	47%	58%
Average Time to ECG (minutes)[1,3]	-	-	8	7
Average Time to Transfer (minutes)[5]	-	-	62	60
Children's Asthma Care				
Received Home Management Plan of Care	-	-	93%	88%
Received Reliever Medication	-	-	100%	100%
Received Systemic Corticosteroids	-	-	100%	100%
Emergency Department				
Admittance Decision Time (minutes)[2]	712	182	99	98
Head CT Results Within 45 Min. of Arrival[3,7]	-	-	54%	57%
Patients Who Left ER Before Being Seen	18,118	2%	3%	2%
Time from ER Arrival to Admit. (minutes)[2]	714	254	270	274
Time from ER Arrival to Discharge (minutes)	438	148	127	134
Time in ER Before Being Evaluated (minutes)	474	14	26	26
Time to Pain Meds for Fractures (minutes)	25	59	57	57
Heart Attack Care				
Aspirin Given at Discharge[2]	265	100%	99%	99%
Fibrinolytic Meds Within 30 Min. of Arrival[2,7]	-	-	49%	54%
PCI Within 90 Minutes of Arrival[2]	14	100%	95%	96%
Statin Prescribed at Discharge[2]	258	100%	98%	98%
Heart Failure Care				
ACE Inhibitor or ARB for LVSD[2]	80	100%	97%	97%
Discharge Instructions Given[2]	234	100%	95%	94%
Evaluation of LVS Function[2]	285	100%	99%	99%
Medicare Spending				
Medicare Spending per Patient (ratio)	-	1.07	1.03	0.98
Pneumonia Care				
Appropriate Initial Antibiotic Given[2]	54	91%	95%	95%
Blood Culture Timing[2]	53	100%	98%	98%
Pregnancy and Delivery Care				
Newborn Deliveries Scheduled Early[2,7]	-	-	7%	6%
Preventive Care				
Immunization for Influenza[2]	663	95%	90%	90%
Immunization for Pneumonia[2]	1,013	97%	92%	92%
Stroke Care				
Anticoagulation Therapy for Atrial Fibrillation[2]	17	100%	96%	95%
Antithrombotic Therapy Timing[2]	76	100%	98%	98%
Assessed for Rehabilitation[2]	108	95%	98%	97%
Discharged on Antithrombotic Therapy[2]	87	100%	99%	99%
Discharged on Statin Medication[2]	64	97%	95%	94%
Thrombolytic Therapy Timing[1,2]	-	-	68%	66%
Venous Thromboembolism Prophylaxis[2]	121	94%	94%	94%
Written Stroke Educational Materials Given[2]	55	91%	92%	88%
Surgical Care Improvement Project				
Appropriate Beta Blocker Usage[2]	284	99%	98%	98%
Appropriate VTP Within 24 Hours[2]	467	98%	98%	98%
Controlled Postoperative Blood Glucose[2]	139	97%	96%	97%
Perioperative Temperature Management[2]	681	100%	100%	100%
Prophylactic Antibiotic Selection[2]	516	100%	99%	99%
Prophylactic Antibiotic Selection (Outpatient)	320	100%	98%	98%
Prophylactic Antibiotic Stopped[2]	510	96%	98%	98%
Prophylactic Antibiotic Timing[2]	517	99%	99%	99%
Prophylactic Antibiotic Timing (Outpatient)	320	100%	98%	98%
Urinary Catheter Removal[2]	573	98%	98%	97%
Survey of Patients' Hospital Experiences				
Area Around Room 'Always' Quiet at Night	300+	67%	68%	61%
Doctors 'Always' Communicated Well	300+	80%	83%	82%
Home Recovery Information Given	300+	85%	85%	85%
Hospital Given 9 or 10 on 10 Point Scale	300+	70%	73%	71%
Meds 'Always' Explained Before Given	300+	63%	66%	64%
Nurses 'Always' Communicated Well	300+	74%	80%	79%
Pain 'Always' Well Controlled	300+	67%	72%	71%
Room and Bathroom 'Always' Clean	300+	71%	75%	73%
Timely Help 'Always' Received	300+	62%	69%	68%
Would Definitely Recommend Hospital	300+	74%	73%	71%
Use of Medical Imaging				
Cardiac Imaging Stress Test before Surgery	129	7.8%	5.3%	5.3%
Combination Abdominal CT Scan	216	7.9%	16.4%	10.5%
Combination Brain/Sinus CT Scan[1]	-	-	2.7%	2.7%
Combination Chest CT Scan	70	5.7%	5.6%	2.7%
Follow-up Mammogram/Ultrasound[7]	-	-	7.9%	8.8%
Lumbar Spine MRI for Low Back Pain[1]	-	-	39.6%	37.2%

Texas Health Harris Methodist Fort Worth

1301 Pennsylvania Avenue
Fort Worth, TX 76104
URL: www.texashealth.org
Type: Acute Care Hospitals
Ownership: Voluntary non-profit - Church
Phone: 817-250-2100
Fax: 817-882-2865
Emergency Services: Yes
Beds: 628

Key Personnel:
Radiology. . . . . Ronald Alexander
Operating Room. . . . . Laura Barksdale
President . . . . Lillie Biggins, R.N., FACHE
Emergency Room . . . . John M Geesbreght, MD
CEO/President. . . . . Douglas D Hawthorne
Quality Assurance . . . . Margaret Proctor
Chief of Medical Staff. . . . . Joseph Prosser, M.D., M.B.A., C
Infection Control. . . . . Carol Trickey

Measure	Cases	This Hosp.	State Avg.	U.S. Avg.
Blood Clot Prevention and Treatment				
Anticoagulation Overlap Therapy[2]	219	89%	93%	93%
ICU Venous Thromboembolism Prophylaxis[2]	135	95%	92%	92%
Incidence of Potentially Preventable VTE[2]	71	6%	9%	10%
UFH with Dosages/Platelet Monitoring[2]	73	99%	96%	97%
Venous Thromboembolism Prophylaxis[2]	355	89%	82%	85%
Warfarin Therapy Discharge Instructions[2]	133	62%	84%	75%
Chest Pain/Possible Heart Attack Care				
Aspirin Given Within 24 Hours of Arrival	15	93%	94%	96%
Fibrinolytic Meds Within 30 Min. of Arrival[3,7]	-	-	47%	58%
Average Time to ECG (minutes)	17	7	8	7
Average Time to Transfer (minutes)[3,7]	-	-	62	60
Children's Asthma Care				
Received Home Management Plan of Care	-	-	93%	88%
Received Reliever Medication	-	-	100%	100%
Received Systemic Corticosteroids	-	-	100%	100%
Emergency Department				
Admittance Decision Time (minutes)[2]	827	111	99	98
Head CT Results Within 45 Min. of Arrival	20	45%	54%	57%
Patients Who Left ER Before Being Seen	>100k	1%	3%	2%
Time from ER Arrival to Admit. (minutes)[2]	827	266	270	274
Time from ER Arrival to Discharge (minutes)	409	155	127	134
Time in ER Before Being Evaluated (minutes)	443	20	26	26
Time to Pain Meds for Fractures (minutes)	342	60	57	57
Heart Attack Care				
Aspirin Given at Discharge	902	99%	99%	99%
Fibrinolytic Meds Within 30 Min. of Arrival[7]	-	-	49%	54%
PCI Within 90 Minutes of Arrival	87	100%	95%	96%
Statin Prescribed at Discharge	879	99%	98%	98%
Heart Failure Care				
ACE Inhibitor or ARB for LVSD	266	97%	97%	97%
Discharge Instructions Given	671	100%	95%	94%
Evaluation of LVS Function	826	100%	99%	99%
Medicare Spending				
Medicare Spending per Patient (ratio)	-	1.08	1.03	0.98
Pneumonia Care				
Appropriate Initial Antibiotic Given	350	95%	95%	95%
Blood Culture Timing	691	99%	98%	98%
Pregnancy and Delivery Care				
Newborn Deliveries Scheduled Early	249	9%	7%	6%
Preventive Care				
Immunization for Influenza[2]	627	97%	90%	90%
Immunization for Pneumonia[2]	841	95%	92%	92%
Stroke Care				
Anticoagulation Therapy for Atrial Fibrillation[2]	17	100%	96%	95%
Antithrombotic Therapy Timing[2]	173	99%	98%	98%
Assessed for Rehabilitation[2]	228	97%	98%	97%
Discharged on Antithrombotic Therapy[2]	180	99%	99%	99%
Discharged on Statin Medication[2]	140	98%	95%	94%
Thrombolytic Therapy Timing[2]	17	76%	68%	66%
Venous Thromboembolism Prophylaxis[2]	254	98%	94%	94%
Written Stroke Educational Materials Given[2]	127	92%	92%	88%
Surgical Care Improvement Project				
Appropriate Beta Blocker Usage[2]	445	100%	98%	98%
Appropriate VTP Within 24 Hours[2]	812	99%	98%	98%
Controlled Postoperative Blood Glucose[2]	240	99%	96%	97%
Perioperative Temperature Management[2]	972	100%	100%	100%
Prophylactic Antibiotic Selection[2]	947	99%	99%	99%

NOTE: Hospital profiles are in alphabetical order by state, then city, then hospital within the city; Rankings exclude hospitals with less than 25 cases except for patient surveys which excludes hospitals with less than 100 cases; (a) 100-299 cases; (1) The number of cases/patients is too few to report; (2) Data submitted were based on a sample of cases/patients; (3) Results are based on a shorter time period than required; (4) Data suppressed by CMS for one or more quarters; (5) Results are not available for this reporting period; (6) Fewer than 100 patients completed the HCAHPS survey; (7) No cases met the criteria for this measure; (8) The lower limit of the confidence interval cannot be calculated if the number of observed infections equals zero; (9) No data are available from the state/territory for this reporting period; (10) The scores shown reflect fewer than 50 completed surveys; (11) There were discrepancies in the data collection process; (12) This measure does not apply to this hospital for this reporting period; (13) Results cannot be calculated for this reporting period; (14) The results for this state are combined with nearby states to protect confidentiality; Please refer to the User's Guide for a full explanation of data.

Measure	Cases	This Hosp.	State Avg.	U.S. Avg.
Prophylactic Antibiotic Selection (Outpatient)	745	97%	98%	98%
Prophylactic Antibiotic Stopped[2]	923	98%	98%	98%
Prophylactic Antibiotic Timing[2]	950	99%	99%	99%
Prophylactic Antibiotic Timing (Outpatient)	752	99%	98%	98%
Urinary Catheter Removal[2]	927	100%	98%	97%
Survey of Patients' Hospital Experiences				
Area Around Room 'Always' Quiet at Night	300+	59%	68%	61%
Doctors 'Always' Communicated Well	300+	80%	83%	82%
Home Recovery Information Given	300+	87%	85%	85%
Hospital Given 9 or 10 on 10 Point Scale	300+	76%	73%	71%
Meds 'Always' Explained Before Given	300+	65%	66%	64%
Nurses 'Always' Communicated Well	300+	80%	80%	79%
Pain 'Always' Well Controlled	300+	72%	72%	71%
Room and Bathroom 'Always' Clean	300+	76%	75%	73%
Timely Help 'Always' Received	300+	70%	69%	68%
Would Definitely Recommend Hospital	300+	80%	73%	71%
Use of Medical Imaging				
Cardiac Imaging Stress Test before Surgery	70	1.4%	5.3%	5.3%
Combination Abdominal CT Scan	1,068	0.9%	16.4%	10.5%
Combination Brain/Sinus CT Scan	2,097	3.3%	2.7%	2.7%
Combination Chest CT Scan	346	0.3%	5.6%	2.7%
Follow-up Mammogram/Ultrasound	805	3.5%	7.9%	8.8%
Lumbar Spine MRI for Low Back Pain	150	32.7%	39.6%	37.2%

Texas Health Harris Methodist Hospital Alliance

10864 Texas Health Trail Phone: 682-212-2004
Fort Worth, TX 76244
URL: www.texashealth.org/alliance
Type: Acute Care Hospitals Emergency Services: Yes
Ownership: Voluntary non-profit - Private

Measure	Cases	This Hosp.	State Avg.	U.S. Avg.
Blood Clot Prevention and Treatment				
Anticoagulation Overlap Therapy[2]	26	92%	93%	93%
ICU Venous Thromboembolism Prophylaxis[2]	57	91%	92%	92%
Incidence of Potentially Preventable VTE[1,2]	-	-	9%	10%
UFH with Dosages/Platelet Monitoring[1,2]	-	-	96%	97%
Venous Thromboembolism Prophylaxis[2]	126	94%	82%	85%
Warfarin Therapy Discharge Instructions[2]	22	36%	84%	75%
Chest Pain/Possible Heart Attack Care				
Aspirin Given Within 24 Hours of Arrival[3]	27	96%	94%	96%
Fibrinolytic Meds Within 30 Min. of Arrival[3,7]	-	-	47%	58%
Average Time to ECG (minutes)[3]	29	7	8	7
Average Time to Transfer (minutes)[1,3]	-	-	62	60
Children's Asthma Care				
Received Home Management Plan of Care	-	-	93%	88%
Received Reliever Medication	-	-	100%	100%
Received Systemic Corticosteroids	-	-	100%	100%
Emergency Department				
Admittance Decision Time (minutes)[2,3]	263	91	99	98
Head CT Results Within 45 Min. of Arrival[1,3]	-	-	54%	57%
Patients Who Left ER Before Being Seen	5,851	1%	3%	2%
Time from ER Arrival to Admit. (minutes)[2,3]	265	267	270	274
Time from ER Arrival to Discharge (minutes)[3]	316	153	127	134
Time in ER Before Being Evaluated (minutes)[3]	339	20	26	26
Time to Pain Meds for Fractures (minutes)[3]	108	48	57	57
Heart Attack Care				
Aspirin Given at Discharge[1,3]	-	-	99%	99%
Fibrinolytic Meds Within 30 Min. of Arrival[3,7]	-	-	49%	54%
PCI Within 90 Minutes of Arrival[3,7]	-	-	95%	96%
Statin Prescribed at Discharge[1,3]	-	-	98%	98%
Heart Failure Care				
ACE Inhibitor or ARB for LVSD[1,3]	-	-	97%	97%
Discharge Instructions Given[3]	23	83%	95%	94%
Evaluation of LVS Function[3]	32	100%	99%	99%
Medicare Spending				
Medicare Spending per Patient (ratio)	-	-	1.03	0.98
Pneumonia Care				
Appropriate Initial Antibiotic Given[3]	49	100%	95%	95%
Blood Culture Timing[3]	53	100%	98%	98%
Pregnancy and Delivery Care				
Newborn Deliveries Scheduled Early	81	11%	7%	6%
Preventive Care				
Immunization for Influenza[2,3]	138	99%	90%	90%
Immunization for Pneumonia[2,3]	183	93%	92%	92%
Stroke Care				
Anticoagulation Therapy for Atrial Fibrillation[1,2]	-	-	96%	95%
Antithrombotic Therapy Timing[1,2]	-	-	98%	98%
Assessed for Rehabilitation[2]	14	100%	98%	97%
Discharged on Antithrombotic Therapy[2]	14	100%	99%	99%
Discharged on Statin Medication[2]	12	92%	95%	94%
Thrombolytic Therapy Timing[1,2]	-	-	68%	66%
Venous Thromboembolism Prophylaxis[1,2]	-	-	94%	94%
Written Stroke Educational Materials Given[1,2]	-	-	92%	88%
Surgical Care Improvement Project				
Appropriate Beta Blocker Usage[2,3]	11	100%	98%	98%
Appropriate VTP Within 24 Hours[2,3]	33	91%	98%	98%
Controlled Postoperative Blood Glucose[2,3]	-	-	96%	97%
Perioperative Temperature Management[2,3]	43	100%	100%	100%
Prophylactic Antibiotic Selection[2,3]	12	92%	99%	99%
Prophylactic Antibiotic Selection (Outpatient)[1,3]	-	-	98%	98%
Prophylactic Antibiotic Stopped[2,3]	11	100%	98%	98%
Prophylactic Antibiotic Timing[2,3]	12	75%	99%	99%
Prophylactic Antibiotic Timing (Outpatient)[1,3]	-	-	98%	98%
Urinary Catheter Removal[2,3]	23	91%	98%	97%
Survey of Patients' Hospital Experiences				
Area Around Room 'Always' Quiet at Night[5]	-	-	68%	61%
Doctors 'Always' Communicated Well[5]	-	-	83%	82%
Home Recovery Information Given[5]	-	-	85%	85%
Hospital Given 9 or 10 on 10 Point Scale[5]	-	-	73%	71%
Meds 'Always' Explained Before Given[5]	-	-	66%	64%
Nurses 'Always' Communicated Well[5]	-	-	80%	79%
Pain 'Always' Well Controlled[5]	-	-	72%	71%
Room and Bathroom 'Always' Clean[5]	-	-	75%	73%
Timely Help 'Always' Received[5]	-	-	69%	68%
Would Definitely Recommend Hospital[5]	-	-	73%	71%
Use of Medical Imaging				
Cardiac Imaging Stress Test before Surgery[1]	-	-	5.3%	5.3%
Combination Abdominal CT Scan	75	1.3%	16.4%	10.5%
Combination Brain/Sinus CT Scan[1]	-	-	2.7%	2.7%
Combination Chest CT Scan[1]	-	-	5.6%	2.7%
Follow-up Mammogram/Ultrasound[1]	-	-	7.9%	8.8%
Lumbar Spine MRI for Low Back Pain[1]	-	-	39.6%	37.2%

Texas Health Harris Methodist Hospital SW Fort Worth

6100 Harris Pkwy Phone: 817-433-5000
Fort Worth, TX 76132 Fax: 817-433-6099
URL: www.texahealth.org
Type: Acute Care Hospitals Emergency Services: Yes
Ownership: Voluntary non-profit - Private Beds: 85
Key Personnel:
Radiology. Frank Brown, MD
Intensive Care Unit. . . . . Jennifer Evans, RN
Emergency Room . . . . Sharon Gibson
Quality Assurance . . . . Barbara Hunt
Infection Control. . . . . Kim Strelczyk, RN
Chief of Medical Staff. . . . . Lynne R Tilkin, DO

Measure	Cases	This Hosp.	State Avg.	U.S. Avg.
Blood Clot Prevention and Treatment				
Anticoagulation Overlap Therapy[2]	58	95%	93%	93%
ICU Venous Thromboembolism Prophylaxis[2]	41	100%	92%	92%
Incidence of Potentially Preventable VTE[2]	18	0%	9%	10%
UFH with Dosages/Platelet Monitoring[1,2]	-	-	96%	97%
Venous Thromboembolism Prophylaxis[2]	400	91%	82%	85%
Warfarin Therapy Discharge Instructions[2]	43	95%	84%	75%
Chest Pain/Possible Heart Attack Care				
Aspirin Given Within 24 Hours of Arrival	50	100%	94%	96%
Fibrinolytic Meds Within 30 Min. of Arrival[7]	-	-	47%	58%
Average Time to ECG (minutes)	52	8	8	7
Average Time to Transfer (minutes)[7]	-	-	62	60
Children's Asthma Care				
Received Home Management Plan of Care	-	-	93%	88%
Received Reliever Medication	-	-	100%	100%
Received Systemic Corticosteroids	-	-	100%	100%
Emergency Department				
Admittance Decision Time (minutes)[2]	603	71	99	98
Head CT Results Within 45 Min. of Arrival	13	46%	54%	57%
Patients Who Left ER Before Being Seen	59,141	1%	3%	2%
Time from ER Arrival to Admit. (minutes)[2]	603	229	270	274
Time from ER Arrival to Discharge (minutes)	423	130	127	134
Time in ER Before Being Evaluated (minutes)	444	31	26	26
Time to Pain Meds for Fractures (minutes)	244	61	57	57
Heart Attack Care				
Aspirin Given at Discharge	44	98%	99%	99%
Fibrinolytic Meds Within 30 Min. of Arrival[7]	-	-	49%	54%
PCI Within 90 Minutes of Arrival[7]	-	-	95%	96%
Statin Prescribed at Discharge	47	98%	98%	98%
Heart Failure Care				
ACE Inhibitor or ARB for LVSD	78	96%	97%	97%
Discharge Instructions Given	228	99%	95%	94%
Evaluation of LVS Function	291	100%	99%	99%
Medicare Spending				
Medicare Spending per Patient (ratio)	-	1.02	1.03	0.98
Pneumonia Care				
Appropriate Initial Antibiotic Given	237	97%	95%	95%
Blood Culture Timing	413	99%	98%	98%
Pregnancy and Delivery Care				
Newborn Deliveries Scheduled Early	315	4%	7%	6%
Preventive Care				
Immunization for Influenza[2]	556	98%	90%	90%
Immunization for Pneumonia[2]	632	97%	92%	92%
Stroke Care				
Anticoagulation Therapy for Atrial Fibrillation[1,2]	-	-	96%	95%
Antithrombotic Therapy Timing[2]	59	100%	98%	98%
Assessed for Rehabilitation[2]	74	93%	98%	97%
Discharged on Antithrombotic Therapy[2]	71	100%	99%	99%
Discharged on Statin Medication[2]	62	97%	95%	94%
Thrombolytic Therapy Timing[2,7]	-	-	68%	66%
Venous Thromboembolism Prophylaxis[2]	57	82%	94%	94%
Written Stroke Educational Materials Given[2]	48	98%	92%	88%
Surgical Care Improvement Project				
Appropriate Beta Blocker Usage[2]	101	100%	98%	98%
Appropriate VTP Within 24 Hours[2]	395	97%	98%	98%
Controlled Postoperative Blood Glucose[2,7]	-	-	96%	97%
Perioperative Temperature Management[2]	445	100%	100%	100%
Prophylactic Antibiotic Selection[2]	289	98%	99%	99%
Prophylactic Antibiotic Selection (Outpatient)	355	93%	98%	98%
Prophylactic Antibiotic Stopped[2]	288	99%	98%	98%
Prophylactic Antibiotic Timing[2]	292	98%	99%	99%
Prophylactic Antibiotic Timing (Outpatient)	356	99%	98%	98%
Urinary Catheter Removal[2]	257	97%	98%	97%
Survey of Patients' Hospital Experiences				
Area Around Room 'Always' Quiet at Night	300+	68%	68%	61%
Doctors 'Always' Communicated Well	300+	83%	83%	82%
Home Recovery Information Given	300+	86%	85%	85%
Hospital Given 9 or 10 on 10 Point Scale	300+	78%	73%	71%
Meds 'Always' Explained Before Given	300+	65%	66%	64%
Nurses 'Always' Communicated Well	300+	80%	80%	79%
Pain 'Always' Well Controlled	300+	73%	72%	71%
Room and Bathroom 'Always' Clean	300+	66%	75%	73%
Timely Help 'Always' Received	300+	65%	69%	68%
Would Definitely Recommend Hospital	300+	80%	73%	71%
Use of Medical Imaging				
Cardiac Imaging Stress Test before Surgery[1]	-	-	5.3%	5.3%
Combination Abdominal CT Scan	770	9.9%	16.4%	10.5%
Combination Brain/Sinus CT Scan	730	2.3%	2.7%	2.7%
Combination Chest CT Scan	313	1.3%	5.6%	2.7%
Follow-up Mammogram/Ultrasound	1,654	6.7%	7.9%	8.8%
Lumbar Spine MRI for Low Back Pain	53	49.1%	39.6%	37.2%

USMD Hospital at Fort Worth

5900 Altamesa Blvd Phone: 817-433-9100
Fort Worth, TX 76132
URL: www.usmdfortworth.com
Type: Acute Care Hospitals Emergency Services: Yes
Ownership: Proprietary
Key Personnel:
Administrator . . . . Stephanie Atkins-Gudry

Measure	Cases	This Hosp.	State Avg.	U.S. Avg.

NOTE: Hospital profiles are in alphabetical order by state, then city, then hospital within the city; Rankings exclude hospitals with less than 25 cases except for patient surveys which excludes hospitals with less than 100 cases; (a) 100-299 cases; (1) The number of cases/patients is too few to report; (2) Data submitted were based on a sample of cases/patients; (3) Results are based on a shorter time period than required; (4) Data suppressed by CMS for one or more quarters; (5) Results are not available for this reporting period; (6) Fewer than 100 patients completed the HCAHPS survey; (7) No cases met the criteria for this measure; (8) The lower limit of the confidence interval cannot be calculated if the number of observed infections equals zero; (9) No data are available from the state/territory for this reporting period; (10) The scores shown reflect fewer than 50 completed surveys; (11) There were discrepancies in the data collection process; (12) This measure does not apply to this hospital for this reporting period; (13) Results cannot be calculated for this reporting period; (14) The results for this state are combined with nearby states to protect confidentiality; Please refer to the User's Guide for a full explanation of data.

Blood Clot Prevention and Treatment				
Anticoagulation Overlap Therapy[7]	-	-	93%	93%
ICU Venous Thromboembolism Prophylaxis[7]	-	-	92%	92%
Incidence of Potentially Preventable VTE[7]	-	-	9%	10%
UFH with Dosages/Platelet Monitoring[7]	-	-	96%	97%
Venous Thromboembolism Prophylaxis	57	98%	82%	85%
Warfarin Therapy Discharge Instructions[7]	-	-	84%	75%
Chest Pain/Possible Heart Attack Care				
Aspirin Given Within 24 Hours of Arrival[5]	-	-	94%	96%
Fibrinolytic Meds Within 30 Min. of Arrival[5]	-	-	47%	58%
Average Time to ECG (minutes)[5]	-	-	8	7
Average Time to Transfer (minutes)[5]	-	-	62	60
Children's Asthma Care				
Received Home Management Plan of Care	-	-	93%	88%
Received Reliever Medication	-	-	100%	100%
Received Systemic Corticosteroids	-	-	100%	100%
Emergency Department				
Admittance Decision Time (minutes)[7]	-	-	99	98
Head CT Results Within 45 Min. of Arrival[5]	-	-	54%	57%
Patients Who Left ER Before Being Seen	728	1%	3%	2%
Time from ER Arrival to Admit. (minutes)[7]	-	-	270	274
Time from ER Arrival to Discharge (minutes)	237	75	127	134
Time in ER Before Being Evaluated (minutes)	256	19	26	26
Time to Pain Meds for Fractures (minutes)[5]	-	-	57	57
Heart Attack Care				
Aspirin Given at Discharge[5]	-	-	99%	99%
Fibrinolytic Meds Within 30 Min. of Arrival[5]	-	-	49%	54%
PCI Within 90 Minutes of Arrival[5]	-	-	95%	96%
Statin Prescribed at Discharge[5]	-	-	98%	98%
Heart Failure Care				
ACE Inhibitor or ARB for LVSD[5]	-	-	97%	97%
Discharge Instructions Given[5]	-	-	95%	94%
Evaluation of LVS Function[5]	-	-	99%	99%
Medicare Spending				
Medicare Spending per Patient (ratio)	-	1.10	1.03	0.98
Pneumonia Care				
Appropriate Initial Antibiotic Given[5]	-	-	95%	95%
Blood Culture Timing[5]	-	-	98%	98%
Pregnancy and Delivery Care				
Newborn Deliveries Scheduled Early[7]	-	-	7%	6%
Preventive Care				
Immunization for Influenza	236	86%	90%	90%
Immunization for Pneumonia	227	95%	92%	92%
Stroke Care				
Anticoagulation Therapy for Atrial Fibrillation[5]	-	-	96%	95%
Antithrombotic Therapy Timing[5]	-	-	98%	98%
Assessed for Rehabilitation[5]	-	-	98%	97%
Discharged on Antithrombotic Therapy[5]	-	-	99%	99%
Discharged on Statin Medication[5]	-	-	95%	94%
Thrombolytic Therapy Timing[5]	-	-	68%	66%
Venous Thromboembolism Prophylaxis[5]	-	-	94%	94%
Written Stroke Educational Materials Given[5]	-	-	92%	88%
Surgical Care Improvement Project				
Appropriate Beta Blocker Usage	49	98%	98%	98%
Appropriate VTP Within 24 Hours	152	97%	98%	98%
Controlled Postoperative Blood Glucose[7]	-	-	96%	97%
Perioperative Temperature Management	213	100%	100%	100%
Prophylactic Antibiotic Selection	189	100%	99%	99%
Prophylactic Antibiotic Selection (Outpatient)	299	90%	98%	98%
Prophylactic Antibiotic Stopped	187	99%	98%	98%
Prophylactic Antibiotic Timing	189	98%	99%	99%
Prophylactic Antibiotic Timing (Outpatient)	300	100%	98%	98%
Urinary Catheter Removal	180	99%	98%	97%
Survey of Patients' Hospital Experiences				
Area Around Room 'Always' Quiet at Night	(a)	88%	68%	61%
Doctors 'Always' Communicated Well	(a)	88%	83%	82%
Home Recovery Information Given	(a)	89%	85%	85%
Hospital Given 9 or 10 on 10 Point Scale	(a)	88%	73%	71%
Meds 'Always' Explained Before Given	(a)	79%	66%	64%
Nurses 'Always' Communicated Well	(a)	90%	80%	79%
Pain 'Always' Well Controlled	(a)	81%	72%	71%
Room and Bathroom 'Always' Clean	(a)	87%	75%	73%
Timely Help 'Always' Received	(a)	86%	69%	68%
Would Definitely Recommend Hospital	(a)	91%	73%	71%
Use of Medical Imaging				
Cardiac Imaging Stress Test before Surgery[7]	-	-	5.3%	5.3%
Combination Abdominal CT Scan[1]	-	-	16.4%	10.5%
Combination Brain/Sinus CT Scan[1]	-	-	2.7%	2.7%
Combination Chest CT Scan[1]	-	-	5.6%	2.7%
Follow-up Mammogram/Ultrasound[7]	-	-	7.9%	8.8%
Lumbar Spine MRI for Low Back Pain[7]	-	-	39.6%	37.2%

Hill Country Memorial Hospital

1020 South State Highway 16
Fredericksburg, TX 78624
Phone: 830-997-4353
Fax: 830-997-1348
E-mail: jyoung@hcmbs.org
URL: www.hcmbs.org
Type: Acute Care Hospitals
Emergency Services: Yes
Ownership: Voluntary non-profit - Private
Beds: 84

Key Personnel:
Quality Assurance . . . . Bernice Basse
Radiology. . . . . W E Bishop
CEO/President. . . . . Jeff A Bourgeois
Infection Control . . . . Carl Evans, MD
Intensive Care Unit. . . . . Judy Frazier
Chief of Medical Staff . . . . Ottis Layne
Emergency Room . . . . Ottis Layne, MD
Anesthesiology. . . . . Michael Williams DO

Measure	Cases	This Hosp.	State Avg.	U.S. Avg.
Blood Clot Prevention and Treatment				
Anticoagulation Overlap Therapy[1,2]	-	-	93%	93%
ICU Venous Thromboembolism Prophylaxis[2]	50	98%	92%	92%
Incidence of Potentially Preventable VTE[2,7]	-	-	9%	10%
UFH with Dosages/Platelet Monitoring[1,2]	-	-	96%	97%
Venous Thromboembolism Prophylaxis[2]	190	99%	82%	85%
Warfarin Therapy Discharge Instructions[1,2]	-	-	84%	75%
Chest Pain/Possible Heart Attack Care				
Aspirin Given Within 24 Hours of Arrival	48	98%	94%	96%
Fibrinolytic Meds Within 30 Min. of Arrival[7]	-	-	47%	58%
Average Time to ECG (minutes)	50	6	8	7
Average Time to Transfer (minutes)[7]	-	-	62	60
Children's Asthma Care				
Received Home Management Plan of Care	-	-	93%	88%
Received Reliever Medication	-	-	100%	100%
Received Systemic Corticosteroids	-	-	100%	100%
Emergency Department				
Admittance Decision Time (minutes)[2]	223	73	99	98
Head CT Results Within 45 Min. of Arrival[1]	-	-	54%	57%
Patients Who Left ER Before Being Seen	14,228	0%	3%	2%
Time from ER Arrival to Admit. (minutes)[2]	224	253	270	274
Time from ER Arrival to Discharge (minutes)	487	124	127	134
Time in ER Before Being Evaluated (minutes)	529	20	26	26
Time to Pain Meds for Fractures (minutes)	72	66	57	57
Heart Attack Care				
Aspirin Given at Discharge[1,3]	-	-	99%	99%
Fibrinolytic Meds Within 30 Min. of Arrival[3,7]	-	-	49%	54%
PCI Within 90 Minutes of Arrival[3,7]	-	-	95%	96%
Statin Prescribed at Discharge[1,3]	-	-	98%	98%
Heart Failure Care				
ACE Inhibitor or ARB for LVSD	14	100%	97%	97%
Discharge Instructions Given	52	100%	95%	94%
Evaluation of LVS Function	67	100%	99%	99%
Medicare Spending				
Medicare Spending per Patient (ratio)	-	0.94	1.03	0.98
Pneumonia Care				
Appropriate Initial Antibiotic Given	55	96%	95%	95%
Blood Culture Timing	61	98%	98%	98%
Pregnancy and Delivery Care				
Newborn Deliveries Scheduled Early	29	3%	7%	6%
Preventive Care				
Immunization for Influenza[2]	316	97%	90%	90%
Immunization for Pneumonia[2]	383	96%	92%	92%
Stroke Care				
Anticoagulation Therapy for Atrial Fibrillation[1,2]	-	-	96%	95%
Antithrombotic Therapy Timing[2]	16	100%	98%	98%
Assessed for Rehabilitation[2]	19	100%	98%	97%
Discharged on Antithrombotic Therapy[2]	18	100%	99%	99%
Discharged on Statin Medication[2]	12	100%	95%	94%
Thrombolytic Therapy Timing[2,7]	-	-	68%	66%
Venous Thromboembolism Prophylaxis[2]	18	100%	94%	94%
Written Stroke Educational Materials Given[2]	12	92%	92%	88%
Surgical Care Improvement Project				
Appropriate Beta Blocker Usage[2]	157	100%	98%	98%
Appropriate VTP Within 24 Hours[2]	446	99%	98%	98%
Controlled Postoperative Blood Glucose[2,7]	-	-	96%	97%
Perioperative Temperature Management[2]	507	100%	100%	100%
Prophylactic Antibiotic Selection[2]	391	100%	99%	99%
Prophylactic Antibiotic Selection (Outpatient)	63	98%	98%	98%
Prophylactic Antibiotic Stopped[2]	387	99%	98%	98%
Prophylactic Antibiotic Timing[2]	392	99%	99%	99%
Prophylactic Antibiotic Timing (Outpatient)	62	100%	98%	98%
Urinary Catheter Removal[2]	424	100%	98%	97%
Survey of Patients' Hospital Experiences				
Area Around Room 'Always' Quiet at Night	300+	76%	68%	61%
Doctors 'Always' Communicated Well	300+	89%	83%	82%
Home Recovery Information Given	300+	91%	85%	85%
Hospital Given 9 or 10 on 10 Point Scale	300+	91%	73%	71%
Meds 'Always' Explained Before Given	300+	78%	66%	64%
Nurses 'Always' Communicated Well	300+	89%	80%	79%
Pain 'Always' Well Controlled	300+	81%	72%	71%
Room and Bathroom 'Always' Clean	300+	83%	75%	73%
Timely Help 'Always' Received	300+	80%	69%	68%
Would Definitely Recommend Hospital	300+	92%	73%	71%
Use of Medical Imaging				
Cardiac Imaging Stress Test before Surgery	116	4.3%	5.3%	5.3%
Combination Abdominal CT Scan	613	29.0%	16.4%	10.5%
Combination Brain/Sinus CT Scan	356	0.8%	2.7%	2.7%
Combination Chest CT Scan	322	0.0%	5.6%	2.7%
Follow-up Mammogram/Ultrasound	1,649	13.2%	7.9%	8.8%
Lumbar Spine MRI for Low Back Pain	139	40.3%	39.6%	37.2%

Baylor Medical Center at Frisco

5601 Warren Parkway
Phone: 214-618-2000
Frisco, TX 75034
URL: www.bmcf.com
Type: Acute Care Hospitals
Emergency Services: Yes
Ownership: Proprietary

Key Personnel:
President/CEO. . . . . William A Keaton
Imaging . . . . Kareith Ragan
Emergency . . . . Kenny Whirley

Measure	Cases	This Hosp.	State Avg.	U.S. Avg.
Blood Clot Prevention and Treatment				
Anticoagulation Overlap Therapy[1,2]	-	-	93%	93%
ICU Venous Thromboembolism Prophylaxis[2,7]	-	-	92%	92%
Incidence of Potentially Preventable VTE[1,2]	-	-	9%	10%
UFH with Dosages/Platelet Monitoring[2,7]	-	-	96%	97%
Venous Thromboembolism Prophylaxis[2]	110	99%	82%	85%
Warfarin Therapy Discharge Instructions[1,2]	-	-	84%	75%
Chest Pain/Possible Heart Attack Care				
Aspirin Given Within 24 Hours of Arrival[1,3]	-	-	94%	96%
Fibrinolytic Meds Within 30 Min. of Arrival[3,7]	-	-	47%	58%
Average Time to ECG (minutes)[1,3]	-	-	8	7
Average Time to Transfer (minutes)[1,3]	-	-	62	60
Children's Asthma Care				
Received Home Management Plan of Care	-	-	93%	88%
Received Reliever Medication	-	-	100%	100%
Received Systemic Corticosteroids	-	-	100%	100%
Emergency Department				
Admittance Decision Time (minutes)[1,2]	-	-	99	98
Head CT Results Within 45 Min. of Arrival[1,3]	-	-	54%	57%
Patients Who Left ER Before Being Seen	2,682	2%	3%	2%
Time from ER Arrival to Admit. (minutes)[1,2]	-	-	270	274
Time from ER Arrival to Discharge (minutes)[3]	448	92	127	134
Time in ER Before Being Evaluated (minutes)[3]	468	13	26	26
Time to Pain Meds for Fractures (minutes)[1,3]	-	-	57	57
Heart Attack Care				
Aspirin Given at Discharge[5]	-	-	99%	99%
Fibrinolytic Meds Within 30 Min. of Arrival[5]	-	-	49%	54%

NOTE: Hospital profiles are in alphabetical order by state, then city, then hospital within the city; Rankings exclude hospitals with less than 25 cases except for patient surveys which excludes hospitals with less than 100 cases; (a) 100-299 cases; (1) The number of cases/patients is too few to report; (2) Data submitted were based on a sample of cases/patients; (3) Results are based on a shorter time period than required; (4) Data suppressed by CMS for one or more quarters; (5) Results are not available for this reporting period; (6) Fewer than 100 patients completed the HCAHPS survey; (7) No cases met the criteria for this measure; (8) The lower limit of the confidence interval cannot be calculated if the number of observed infections equals zero; (9) No data are available from the state/territory for this reporting period; (10) The scores shown reflect fewer than 50 completed surveys; (11) There were discrepancies in the data collection process; (12) This measure does not apply to this hospital for this reporting period; (13) Results cannot be calculated for this reporting period; (14) The results for this state are combined with nearby states to protect confidentiality; Please refer to the User's Guide for a full explanation of data.

Measure	Cases	This Hosp.	State Avg.	U.S. Avg.
PCI Within 90 Minutes of Arrival[5]	-	-	95%	96%
Statin Prescribed at Discharge[5]	-	-	98%	98%
Heart Failure Care				
ACE Inhibitor or ARB for LVSD[5]	-	-	97%	97%
Discharge Instructions Given[5]	-	-	95%	94%
Evaluation of LVS Function[5]	-	-	99%	99%
Medicare Spending				
Medicare Spending per Patient (ratio)	-	1.11	1.03	0.98
Pneumonia Care				
Appropriate Initial Antibiotic Given[5]	-	-	95%	95%
Blood Culture Timing[5]	-	-	98%	98%
Pregnancy and Delivery Care				
Newborn Deliveries Scheduled Early	235	2%	7%	6%
Preventive Care				
Immunization for Influenza[2]	414	99%	90%	90%
Immunization for Pneumonia[2]	196	96%	92%	92%
Stroke Care				
Anticoagulation Therapy for Atrial Fibrillation[5]	-	-	96%	95%
Antithrombotic Therapy Timing[5]	-	-	98%	98%
Assessed for Rehabilitation[5]	-	-	98%	97%
Discharged on Antithrombotic Therapy[5]	-	-	99%	99%
Discharged on Statin Medication[5]	-	-	95%	94%
Thrombolytic Therapy Timing[5]	-	-	68%	66%
Venous Thromboembolism Prophylaxis[5]	-	-	94%	94%
Written Stroke Educational Materials Given[5]	-	-	92%	88%
Surgical Care Improvement Project				
Appropriate Beta Blocker Usage	179	99%	98%	98%
Appropriate VTP Within 24 Hours	880	100%	98%	98%
Controlled Postoperative Blood Glucose[7]	-	-	96%	97%
Perioperative Temperature Management	906	100%	100%	100%
Prophylactic Antibiotic Selection	793	99%	99%	99%
Prophylactic Antibiotic Selection (Outpatient)	528	98%	98%	98%
Prophylactic Antibiotic Stopped	789	99%	98%	98%
Prophylactic Antibiotic Timing	793	99%	99%	99%
Prophylactic Antibiotic Timing (Outpatient)	528	99%	98%	98%
Urinary Catheter Removal	695	99%	98%	97%
Survey of Patients' Hospital Experiences				
Area Around Room 'Always' Quiet at Night	300+	79%	68%	61%
Doctors 'Always' Communicated Well	300+	87%	83%	82%
Home Recovery Information Given	300+	88%	85%	85%
Hospital Given 9 or 10 on 10 Point Scale	300+	89%	73%	71%
Meds 'Always' Explained Before Given	300+	69%	66%	64%
Nurses 'Always' Communicated Well	300+	87%	80%	79%
Pain 'Always' Well Controlled	300+	80%	72%	71%
Room and Bathroom 'Always' Clean	300+	91%	75%	73%
Timely Help 'Always' Received	300+	75%	69%	68%
Would Definitely Recommend Hospital	300+	89%	73%	71%
Use of Medical Imaging				
Cardiac Imaging Stress Test before Surgery[7]	-	-	5.3%	5.3%
Combination Abdominal CT Scan	99	9.1%	16.4%	10.5%
Combination Brain/Sinus CT Scan[1]	-	-	2.7%	2.7%
Combination Chest CT Scan	48	4.2%	5.6%	2.7%
Follow-up Mammogram/Ultrasound[7]	-	-	7.9%	8.8%
Lumbar Spine MRI for Low Back Pain[1]	-	-	39.6%	37.2%

Centennial Medical Center

12505 Lebanon Road
Frisco, TX 75035
Phone: 972-963-3333
Fax: 972-963-3625
URL: www.centennialmedcenter.com
Type: Acute Care Hospitals
Emergency Services: Yes
Ownership: Proprietary
Beds: 165

Key Personnel:

CEO/President. . . . . William C Henning
Radiology. . . . . Subba Raju Kosuri
Chairman/CEO . . . . Rick Lewis
Pediatrics. . . . . Dr. Richard Nail
CEO . . . . Joe Thomason

Measure	Cases	This Hosp.	State Avg.	U.S. Avg.
Blood Clot Prevention and Treatment				
Anticoagulation Overlap Therapy[2]	51	92%	93%	93%
ICU Venous Thromboembolism Prophylaxis[2]	65	89%	92%	92%
Incidence of Potentially Preventable VTE[1,2]	-	-	9%	10%
UFH with Dosages/Platelet Monitoring[1,2]	-	-	96%	97%
Venous Thromboembolism Prophylaxis[2]	341	85%	82%	85%
Warfarin Therapy Discharge Instructions[2]	37	92%	84%	75%
Chest Pain/Possible Heart Attack Care				
Aspirin Given Within 24 Hours of Arrival[1,3]	-	-	94%	96%
Fibrinolytic Meds Within 30 Min. of Arrival[3,7]	-	-	47%	58%
Average Time to ECG (minutes)[1,3]	-	-	8	7
Average Time to Transfer (minutes)[3,7]	-	-	62	60
Children's Asthma Care				
Received Home Management Plan of Care	-	-	93%	88%
Received Reliever Medication	-	-	100%	100%
Received Systemic Corticosteroids	-	-	100%	100%
Emergency Department				
Admittance Decision Time (minutes)[2]	427	122	99	98
Head CT Results Within 45 Min. of Arrival[1]	-	-	54%	57%
Patients Who Left ER Before Being Seen	21,988	1%	3%	2%
Time from ER Arrival to Admit. (minutes)[2]	428	266	270	274
Time from ER Arrival to Discharge (minutes)	458	113	127	134
Time in ER Before Being Evaluated (minutes)	501	14	26	26
Time to Pain Meds for Fractures (minutes)	98	30	57	57
Heart Attack Care				
Aspirin Given at Discharge	101	99%	99%	99%
Fibrinolytic Meds Within 30 Min. of Arrival[7]	-	-	49%	54%
PCI Within 90 Minutes of Arrival	18	78%	95%	96%
Statin Prescribed at Discharge	94	99%	98%	98%
Heart Failure Care				
ACE Inhibitor or ARB for LVSD[1]	-	-	97%	97%
Discharge Instructions Given	38	87%	95%	94%
Evaluation of LVS Function	56	100%	99%	99%
Medicare Spending				
Medicare Spending per Patient (ratio)	-	1.15	1.03	0.98
Pneumonia Care				
Appropriate Initial Antibiotic Given	53	96%	95%	95%
Blood Culture Timing	84	99%	98%	98%
Pregnancy and Delivery Care				
Newborn Deliveries Scheduled Early[2]	47	0%	7%	6%
Preventive Care				
Immunization for Influenza[2]	471	97%	90%	90%
Immunization for Pneumonia[2]	437	97%	92%	92%
Stroke Care				
Anticoagulation Therapy for Atrial Fibrillation[7]	-	-	96%	95%
Antithrombotic Therapy Timing	28	100%	98%	98%
Assessed for Rehabilitation	37	97%	98%	97%
Discharged on Antithrombotic Therapy	28	100%	99%	99%
Discharged on Statin Medication	24	79%	95%	94%
Thrombolytic Therapy Timing[1]	-	-	68%	66%
Venous Thromboembolism Prophylaxis	40	92%	94%	94%
Written Stroke Educational Materials Given	22	77%	92%	88%
Surgical Care Improvement Project				
Appropriate Beta Blocker Usage	58	100%	98%	98%
Appropriate VTP Within 24 Hours	143	96%	98%	98%
Controlled Postoperative Blood Glucose	17	100%	96%	97%
Perioperative Temperature Management	181	99%	100%	100%
Prophylactic Antibiotic Selection	92	97%	99%	99%
Prophylactic Antibiotic Selection (Outpatient)	60	98%	98%	98%
Prophylactic Antibiotic Stopped	79	97%	98%	98%
Prophylactic Antibiotic Timing	92	99%	99%	99%
Prophylactic Antibiotic Timing (Outpatient)	60	100%	98%	98%
Urinary Catheter Removal	98	98%	98%	97%
Survey of Patients' Hospital Experiences				
Area Around Room 'Always' Quiet at Night	300+	68%	68%	61%
Doctors 'Always' Communicated Well	300+	82%	83%	82%
Home Recovery Information Given	300+	85%	85%	85%
Hospital Given 9 or 10 on 10 Point Scale	300+	70%	73%	71%
Meds 'Always' Explained Before Given	300+	59%	66%	64%
Nurses 'Always' Communicated Well	300+	76%	80%	79%
Pain 'Always' Well Controlled	300+	73%	72%	71%
Room and Bathroom 'Always' Clean	300+	67%	75%	73%
Timely Help 'Always' Received	300+	65%	69%	68%
Would Definitely Recommend Hospital	300+	73%	73%	71%
Use of Medical Imaging				
Cardiac Imaging Stress Test before Surgery[1]	-	-	5.3%	5.3%
Combination Abdominal CT Scan	232	7.3%	16.4%	10.5%
Combination Brain/Sinus CT Scan[1]	-	-	2.7%	2.7%
Combination Chest CT Scan	168	3.6%	5.6%	2.7%
Follow-up Mammogram/Ultrasound	331	8.5%	7.9%	8.8%
Lumbar Spine MRI for Low Back Pain	33	51.5%	39.6%	37.2%

North Texas Medical Center

1900 Hospital Blvd
Gainesville, TX 76240
Phone: 940-612-8600
Fax: 940-612-8612
URL: www.ntmconline.net
Type: Acute Care Hospitals
Emergency Services: Yes
Ownership: Govt - Hospital Dist/Auth
Beds: 60

Key Personnel:

Operating Room. . . . . Kerri Acuna
CEO/President. . . . . Randy Bacus, FACHE
Quality Assurance . . . . Robin Barton
Emergency Room . . . . Audie Hayes
Chief of Medical Staff. . . . . Mary Smith

Measure	Cases	This Hosp.	State Avg.	U.S. Avg.
Blood Clot Prevention and Treatment				
Anticoagulation Overlap Therapy[2]	13	77%	93%	93%
ICU Venous Thromboembolism Prophylaxis[2]	42	95%	92%	92%
Incidence of Potentially Preventable VTE[2,7]	-	-	9%	10%
UFH with Dosages/Platelet Monitoring[1,2]	-	-	96%	97%
Venous Thromboembolism Prophylaxis[2]	79	77%	82%	85%
Warfarin Therapy Discharge Instructions[2]	13	85%	84%	75%
Chest Pain/Possible Heart Attack Care				
Aspirin Given Within 24 Hours of Arrival	58	98%	94%	96%
Fibrinolytic Meds Within 30 Min. of Arrival[7]	-	-	47%	58%
Average Time to ECG (minutes)	60	10	8	7
Average Time to Transfer (minutes)[1]	-	-	62	60
Children's Asthma Care				
Received Home Management Plan of Care	-	-	93%	88%
Received Reliever Medication	-	-	100%	100%
Received Systemic Corticosteroids	-	-	100%	100%
Emergency Department				
Admittance Decision Time (minutes)[2]	185	70	99	98
Head CT Results Within 45 Min. of Arrival[1]	-	-	54%	57%
Patients Who Left ER Before Being Seen	17,441	2%	3%	2%
Time from ER Arrival to Admit. (minutes)[2]	190	223	270	274
Time from ER Arrival to Discharge (minutes)	354	99	127	134
Time in ER Before Being Evaluated (minutes)	364	21	26	26
Time to Pain Meds for Fractures (minutes)	74	37	57	57
Heart Attack Care				
Aspirin Given at Discharge[1]	-	-	99%	99%
Fibrinolytic Meds Within 30 Min. of Arrival[7]	-	-	49%	54%
PCI Within 90 Minutes of Arrival[7]	-	-	95%	96%
Statin Prescribed at Discharge[1]	-	-	98%	98%
Heart Failure Care				
ACE Inhibitor or ARB for LVSD[1]	-	-	97%	97%
Discharge Instructions Given	26	92%	95%	94%
Evaluation of LVS Function	35	91%	99%	99%
Medicare Spending				
Medicare Spending per Patient (ratio)	-	1.05	1.03	0.98
Pneumonia Care				
Appropriate Initial Antibiotic Given	53	94%	95%	95%
Blood Culture Timing	76	100%	98%	98%
Pregnancy and Delivery Care				
Newborn Deliveries Scheduled Early[2]	29	0%	7%	6%
Preventive Care				
Immunization for Influenza[2]	231	92%	90%	90%
Immunization for Pneumonia[2]	233	90%	92%	92%
Stroke Care				
Anticoagulation Therapy for Atrial Fibrillation[1]	-	-	96%	95%
Antithrombotic Therapy Timing[1]	-	-	98%	98%
Assessed for Rehabilitation[1]	-	-	98%	97%
Discharged on Antithrombotic Therapy[1]	-	-	99%	99%
Discharged on Statin Medication[1]	-	-	95%	94%
Thrombolytic Therapy Timing[1]	-	-	68%	66%
Venous Thromboembolism Prophylaxis[1]	-	-	94%	94%
Written Stroke Educational Materials Given[1]	-	-	92%	88%
Surgical Care Improvement Project				
Appropriate Beta Blocker Usage	22	86%	98%	98%
Appropriate VTP Within 24 Hours	72	94%	98%	98%
Controlled Postoperative Blood Glucose[7]	-	-	96%	97%

NOTE: Hospital profiles are in alphabetical order by state, then city, then hospital within the city; Rankings exclude hospitals with less than 25 cases except for patient surveys which excludes hospitals with less than 100 cases; (a) 100-299 cases; (1) The number of cases/patients is too few to report; (2) Data submitted were based on a sample of cases/patients; (3) Results are based on a shorter time period than required; (4) Data suppressed by CMS for one or more quarters; (5) Results are not available for this reporting period; (6) Fewer than 100 patients completed the HCAHPS survey; (7) No cases met the criteria for this measure; (8) The lower limit of the confidence interval cannot be calculated if the number of observed infections equals zero; (9) No data are available from the state/territory for this reporting period; (10) The scores shown reflect fewer than 50 completed surveys; (11) There were discrepancies in the data collection process; (12) This measure does not apply to this hospital for this reporting period; (13) Results cannot be calculated for this reporting period; (14) The results for this state are combined with nearby states to protect confidentiality; Please refer to the User's Guide for a full explanation of data.

Perioperative Temperature Management	75	100%	100%	100%
Prophylactic Antibiotic Selection	51	98%	99%	99%
Prophylactic Antibiotic Selection (Outpatient)[1,3]	-	-	98%	98%
Prophylactic Antibiotic Stopped	51	94%	98%	98%
Prophylactic Antibiotic Timing	51	100%	99%	99%
Prophylactic Antibiotic Timing (Outpatient)[1,3]	-	-	98%	98%
Urinary Catheter Removal	37	100%	98%	97%
Survey of Patients' Hospital Experiences				
Area Around Room 'Always' Quiet at Night	(a)	59%	68%	61%
Doctors 'Always' Communicated Well	(a)	82%	83%	82%
Home Recovery Information Given	(a)	90%	85%	85%
Hospital Given 9 or 10 on 10 Point Scale	(a)	71%	73%	71%
Meds 'Always' Explained Before Given	(a)	69%	66%	64%
Nurses 'Always' Communicated Well	(a)	79%	80%	79%
Pain 'Always' Well Controlled	(a)	74%	72%	71%
Room and Bathroom 'Always' Clean	(a)	75%	75%	73%
Timely Help 'Always' Received	(a)	77%	69%	68%
Would Definitely Recommend Hospital	(a)	63%	73%	71%
Use of Medical Imaging				
Cardiac Imaging Stress Test before Surgery[1]	-	-	5.3%	5.3%
Combination Abdominal CT Scan	221	14.0%	16.4%	10.5%
Combination Brain/Sinus CT Scan[1]	-	-	2.7%	2.7%
Combination Chest CT Scan	97	0.0%	5.6%	2.7%
Follow-up Mammogram/Ultrasound	515	10.1%	7.9%	8.8%
Lumbar Spine MRI for Low Back Pain	47	57.4%	39.6%	37.2%

University of Texas Medical Branch Galveston

301 University Boulevard
Galveston, TX 77555
Phone: 409-772-1011
Fax: 409-772-6216
E-mail: public.affairs@utmbhealth.com
URL: www.utmb.edu
Type: Acute Care Hospitals
Emergency Services: Yes
Ownership: Government - State

Key Personnel:

Quality Assurance .... Jennifer Baer
CEO/President............... David L Callendar, MD
Operating Room.............. Bud Cherry
Pediatric In-Patient Care .... Walter J Meyer, MD
Chief of Medical Staff.......... Don Powell, MD
Infection Control............. Norbert Roberts, MD
Pediatric Ambulatory Care ...... Patricia A Rogers, MD
Radiology.................. Leonard E Swischuk

Measure	Cases	This Hosp.	State Avg.	U.S. Avg.
Blood Clot Prevention and Treatment				
Anticoagulation Overlap Therapy[2]	85	92%	93%	93%
ICU Venous Thromboembolism Prophylaxis[2]	97	99%	92%	92%
Incidence of Potentially Preventable VTE[2]	27	0%	9%	10%
UFH with Dosages/Platelet Monitoring[2]	89	100%	96%	97%
Venous Thromboembolism Prophylaxis[2]	316	97%	82%	85%
Warfarin Therapy Discharge Instructions[2]	75	48%	84%	75%
Chest Pain/Possible Heart Attack Care				
Aspirin Given Within 24 Hours of Arrival[3,7]	-	-	94%	96%
Fibrinolytic Meds Within 30 Min. of Arrival[5]	-	-	47%	58%
Average Time to ECG (minutes)[3,7]	-	-	8	7
Average Time to Transfer (minutes)[5]	-	-	62	60
Children's Asthma Care				
Received Home Management Plan of Care	-	-	93%	88%
Received Reliever Medication	-	-	100%	100%
Received Systemic Corticosteroids	-	-	100%	100%
Emergency Department				
Admittance Decision Time (minutes)[2]	221	238	99	98
Head CT Results Within 45 Min. of Arrival[1]	-	-	54%	57%
Patients Who Left ER Before Being Seen	39,423	0%	3%	2%
Time from ER Arrival to Admit. (minutes)[2]	222	350	270	274
Time from ER Arrival to Discharge (minutes)	337	176	127	134
Time in ER Before Being Evaluated (minutes)	385	28	26	26
Time to Pain Meds for Fractures (minutes)	124	63	57	57
Heart Attack Care				
Aspirin Given at Discharge[2]	231	99%	99%	99%
Fibrinolytic Meds Within 30 Min. of Arrival[2,7]	-	-	49%	54%
PCI Within 90 Minutes of Arrival[2]	24	100%	95%	96%
Statin Prescribed at Discharge[2]	217	99%	98%	98%
Heart Failure Care				
ACE Inhibitor or ARB for LVSD[2]	117	98%	97%	97%
Discharge Instructions Given[2]	272	99%	95%	94%
Evaluation of LVS Function[2]	298	100%	99%	99%
Medicare Spending				
Medicare Spending per Patient (ratio)	-	0.99	1.03	0.98
Pneumonia Care				
Appropriate Initial Antibiotic Given[2]	41	93%	95%	95%
Blood Culture Timing[2]	84	98%	98%	98%
Pregnancy and Delivery Care				
Newborn Deliveries Scheduled Early[2]	73	10%	7%	6%
Preventive Care				
Immunization for Influenza[2]	462	83%	90%	90%
Immunization for Pneumonia[2]	396	81%	92%	92%
Stroke Care				
Anticoagulation Therapy for Atrial Fibrillation[1,2]	-	-	96%	95%
Antithrombotic Therapy Timing[2]	60	100%	98%	98%
Assessed for Rehabilitation[2]	104	98%	98%	97%
Discharged on Antithrombotic Therapy[2]	80	100%	99%	99%
Discharged on Statin Medication[2]	50	98%	95%	94%
Thrombolytic Therapy Timing[2]	17	71%	68%	66%
Venous Thromboembolism Prophylaxis[2]	111	99%	94%	94%
Written Stroke Educational Materials Given[2]	64	78%	92%	88%
Surgical Care Improvement Project				
Appropriate Beta Blocker Usage[2]	156	97%	98%	98%
Appropriate VTP Within 24 Hours[2]	263	99%	98%	98%
Controlled Postoperative Blood Glucose[2]	86	95%	96%	97%
Perioperative Temperature Management[2]	353	100%	100%	100%
Prophylactic Antibiotic Selection[2]	300	99%	99%	99%
Prophylactic Antibiotic Selection (Outpatient)	352	98%	98%	98%
Prophylactic Antibiotic Stopped[2]	295	98%	98%	98%
Prophylactic Antibiotic Timing[2]	302	99%	99%	99%
Prophylactic Antibiotic Timing (Outpatient)	280	99%	98%	98%
Urinary Catheter Removal[2]	271	99%	98%	97%
Survey of Patients' Hospital Experiences				
Area Around Room 'Always' Quiet at Night	300+	60%	68%	61%
Doctors 'Always' Communicated Well	300+	78%	83%	82%
Home Recovery Information Given	300+	88%	85%	85%
Hospital Given 9 or 10 on 10 Point Scale	300+	71%	73%	71%
Meds 'Always' Explained Before Given	300+	66%	66%	64%
Nurses 'Always' Communicated Well	300+	78%	80%	79%
Pain 'Always' Well Controlled	300+	68%	72%	71%
Room and Bathroom 'Always' Clean	300+	69%	75%	73%
Timely Help 'Always' Received	300+	67%	69%	68%
Would Definitely Recommend Hospital	300+	72%	73%	71%
Use of Medical Imaging				
Cardiac Imaging Stress Test before Surgery	663	5.0%	5.3%	5.3%
Combination Abdominal CT Scan	1,104	21.1%	16.4%	10.5%
Combination Brain/Sinus CT Scan	828	1.6%	2.7%	2.7%
Combination Chest CT Scan	781	2.4%	5.6%	2.7%
Follow-up Mammogram/Ultrasound	2,073	7.6%	7.9%	8.8%
Lumbar Spine MRI for Low Back Pain	245	38.8%	39.6%	37.2%

Baylor Medical Center at Garland

2300 Marie Curie Drive
Garland, TX 75042
Phone: 972-487-5000
Fax: 972-487-5005
URL: www.baylorhealth.com
Type: Acute Care Hospitals
Emergency Services: Yes
Ownership: Government - Federal
Beds: 223

Key Personnel:

CEO .... Joel Allison, FACHE
Emergency Room .... Tom Button, RN
Radiology.................. Patricia De Leon, MD
Chief of Medical Staff.......... Irving Prengler, MD
Pediatric In-Patient Care .... Vance Redfield, MD

Measure	Cases	This Hosp.	State Avg.	U.S. Avg.
Blood Clot Prevention and Treatment				
Anticoagulation Overlap Therapy[2]	77	94%	93%	93%
ICU Venous Thromboembolism Prophylaxis[2]	102	96%	92%	92%
Incidence of Potentially Preventable VTE[2]	14	0%	9%	10%
UFH with Dosages/Platelet Monitoring[1,2]	-	-	96%	97%
Venous Thromboembolism Prophylaxis[2]	364	96%	82%	85%
Warfarin Therapy Discharge Instructions[2]	54	83%	84%	75%
Chest Pain/Possible Heart Attack Care				
Aspirin Given Within 24 Hours of Arrival[1,3]	-	-	94%	96%
Fibrinolytic Meds Within 30 Min. of Arrival[3,7]	-	-	47%	58%
Average Time to ECG (minutes)[1,3]	-	-	8	7
Average Time to Transfer (minutes)[3,7]	-	-	62	60
Children's Asthma Care				
Received Home Management Plan of Care	-	-	93%	88%
Received Reliever Medication	-	-	100%	100%
Received Systemic Corticosteroids	-	-	100%	100%
Emergency Department				
Admittance Decision Time (minutes)[2]	447	80	99	98
Head CT Results Within 45 Min. of Arrival	19	79%	54%	57%
Patients Who Left ER Before Being Seen	66,900	2%	3%	2%
Time from ER Arrival to Admit. (minutes)[2]	461	235	270	274
Time from ER Arrival to Discharge (minutes)	379	139	127	134
Time in ER Before Being Evaluated (minutes)	57	50	26	26
Time to Pain Meds for Fractures (minutes)	233	56	57	57
Heart Attack Care				
Aspirin Given at Discharge	216	99%	99%	99%
Fibrinolytic Meds Within 30 Min. of Arrival[1]	-	-	49%	54%
PCI Within 90 Minutes of Arrival	58	100%	95%	96%
Statin Prescribed at Discharge	203	100%	98%	98%
Heart Failure Care				
ACE Inhibitor or ARB for LVSD	121	98%	97%	97%
Discharge Instructions Given	244	99%	95%	94%
Evaluation of LVS Function	308	100%	99%	99%
Medicare Spending				
Medicare Spending per Patient (ratio)	-	1.08	1.03	0.98
Pneumonia Care				
Appropriate Initial Antibiotic Given	184	99%	95%	95%
Blood Culture Timing	283	100%	98%	98%
Pregnancy and Delivery Care				
Newborn Deliveries Scheduled Early	151	6%	7%	6%
Preventive Care				
Immunization for Influenza[2]	555	97%	90%	90%
Immunization for Pneumonia[2]	717	98%	92%	92%
Stroke Care				
Anticoagulation Therapy for Atrial Fibrillation[2]	17	88%	96%	95%
Antithrombotic Therapy Timing[2]	107	98%	98%	98%
Assessed for Rehabilitation[2]	123	99%	98%	97%
Discharged on Antithrombotic Therapy[2]	122	100%	99%	99%
Discharged on Statin Medication[2]	94	95%	95%	94%
Thrombolytic Therapy Timing[2]	11	73%	68%	66%
Venous Thromboembolism Prophylaxis[2]	115	97%	94%	94%
Written Stroke Educational Materials Given[2]	76	100%	92%	88%
Surgical Care Improvement Project				
Appropriate Beta Blocker Usage[2]	103	99%	98%	98%
Appropriate VTP Within 24 Hours[2]	214	98%	98%	98%
Controlled Postoperative Blood Glucose[2]	27	100%	96%	97%
Perioperative Temperature Management[2]	284	100%	100%	100%
Prophylactic Antibiotic Selection[2]	152	100%	99%	99%
Prophylactic Antibiotic Selection (Outpatient)	170	98%	98%	98%
Prophylactic Antibiotic Stopped[2]	138	96%	98%	98%
Prophylactic Antibiotic Timing[2]	152	99%	99%	99%
Prophylactic Antibiotic Timing (Outpatient)	170	99%	98%	98%
Urinary Catheter Removal[2]	204	99%	98%	97%
Survey of Patients' Hospital Experiences				
Area Around Room 'Always' Quiet at Night	300+	67%	68%	61%
Doctors 'Always' Communicated Well	300+	81%	83%	82%
Home Recovery Information Given	300+	84%	85%	85%
Hospital Given 9 or 10 on 10 Point Scale	300+	69%	73%	71%
Meds 'Always' Explained Before Given	300+	66%	66%	64%
Nurses 'Always' Communicated Well	300+	78%	80%	79%
Pain 'Always' Well Controlled	300+	71%	72%	71%
Room and Bathroom 'Always' Clean	300+	75%	75%	73%
Timely Help 'Always' Received	300+	65%	69%	68%
Would Definitely Recommend Hospital	300+	73%	73%	71%
Use of Medical Imaging				
Cardiac Imaging Stress Test before Surgery	300	7.0%	5.3%	5.3%
Combination Abdominal CT Scan	1,028	12.4%	16.4%	10.5%
Combination Brain/Sinus CT Scan	1,230	3.3%	2.7%	2.7%
Combination Chest CT Scan	426	4.7%	5.6%	2.7%
Follow-up Mammogram/Ultrasound	2,456	6.2%	7.9%	8.8%
Lumbar Spine MRI for Low Back Pain	162	33.3%	39.6%	37.2%

NOTE: Hospital profiles are in alphabetical order by state, then city, then hospital within the city; Rankings exclude hospitals with less than 25 cases except for patient surveys which excludes hospitals with less than 100 cases; (a) 100-299 cases; (1) The number of cases/patients is too few to report; (2) Data submitted were based on a sample of cases/patients; (3) Results are based on a shorter time period than required; (4) Data suppressed by CMS for one or more quarters; (5) Results are not available for this reporting period; (6) Fewer than 100 patients completed the HCAHPS survey; (7) No cases met the criteria for this measure; (8) The lower limit of the confidence interval cannot be calculated if the number of observed infections equals zero; (9) No data are available from the state/territory for this reporting period; (10) The scores shown reflect fewer than 50 completed surveys; (11) There were discrepancies in the data collection process; (12) This measure does not apply to this hospital for this reporting period; (13) Results cannot be calculated for this reporting period; (14) The results for this state are combined with nearby states to protect confidentiality; Please refer to the User's Guide for a full explanation of data.

Coryell Memorial Healthcare System

1507 W Main Street
Gatesville, TX 76528
Phone: 254-865-8251
Fax: 254-248-6306
E-mail: adminsec@cmhos.org
URL: www.cmhos.org
Type: Critical Access Hospitals
Emergency Services: Yes
Ownership: Govt - Hospital Dist/Auth
Beds: 55
Key Personnel:
CEO/President. . . . . David K Byrom, CPA
Chief of Medical Staff. . . . . Regan Tipton

Measure	Cases	This Hosp.	State Avg.	U.S. Avg.
Blood Clot Prevention and Treatment				
Anticoagulation Overlap Therapy[5]	-	-	93%	93%
ICU Venous Thromboembolism Prophylaxis[5]	-	-	92%	92%
Incidence of Potentially Preventable VTE[5]	-	-	9%	10%
UFH with Dosages/Platelet Monitoring[5]	-	-	96%	97%
Venous Thromboembolism Prophylaxis[5]	-	-	82%	85%
Warfarin Therapy Discharge Instructions[5]	-	-	84%	75%
Chest Pain/Possible Heart Attack Care				
Aspirin Given Within 24 Hours of Arrival	59	98%	94%	96%
Fibrinolytic Meds Within 30 Min. of Arrival[7]	-	-	47%	58%
Average Time to ECG (minutes)	64	11	8	7
Average Time to Transfer (minutes)	11	115	62	60
Children's Asthma Care				
Received Home Management Plan of Care	-	-	93%	88%
Received Reliever Medication	-	-	100%	100%
Received Systemic Corticosteroids	-	-	100%	100%
Emergency Department				
Admittance Decision Time (minutes)[5]	-	-	99	98
Head CT Results Within 45 Min. of Arrival	14	21%	54%	57%
Patients Who Left ER Before Being Seen[5]	-	-	3%	2%
Time from ER Arrival to Admit. (minutes)[5]	-	-	270	274
Time from ER Arrival to Discharge (minutes)	846	141	127	134
Time in ER Before Being Evaluated (minutes)	897	44	26	26
Time to Pain Meds for Fractures (minutes)	53	65	57	57
Heart Attack Care				
Aspirin Given at Discharge[5]	-	-	99%	99%
Fibrinolytic Meds Within 30 Min. of Arrival[5]	-	-	49%	54%
PCI Within 90 Minutes of Arrival[5]	-	-	95%	96%
Statin Prescribed at Discharge[5]	-	-	98%	98%
Heart Failure Care				
ACE Inhibitor or ARB for LVSD[1]	-	-	97%	97%
Discharge Instructions Given[1]	-	-	95%	94%
Evaluation of LVS Function	16	94%	99%	99%
Medicare Spending				
Medicare Spending per Patient (ratio)	-	-	1.03	0.98
Pneumonia Care				
Appropriate Initial Antibiotic Given	35	77%	95%	95%
Blood Culture Timing	51	84%	98%	98%
Pregnancy and Delivery Care				
Newborn Deliveries Scheduled Early[5]	-	-	7%	6%
Preventive Care				
Immunization for Influenza[5]	-	-	90%	90%
Immunization for Pneumonia[5]	-	-	92%	92%
Stroke Care				
Anticoagulation Therapy for Atrial Fibrillation[5]	-	-	96%	95%
Antithrombotic Therapy Timing[5]	-	-	98%	98%
Assessed for Rehabilitation[5]	-	-	98%	97%
Discharged on Antithrombotic Therapy[5]	-	-	99%	99%
Discharged on Statin Medication[5]	-	-	95%	94%
Thrombolytic Therapy Timing[5]	-	-	68%	66%
Venous Thromboembolism Prophylaxis[5]	-	-	94%	94%
Written Stroke Educational Materials Given[5]	-	-	92%	88%
Surgical Care Improvement Project				
Appropriate Beta Blocker Usage[5]	-	-	98%	98%
Appropriate VTP Within 24 Hours[5]	-	-	98%	98%
Controlled Postoperative Blood Glucose[5]	-	-	96%	97%
Perioperative Temperature Management[5]	-	-	100%	100%
Prophylactic Antibiotic Selection[5]	-	-	99%	99%
Prophylactic Antibiotic Selection (Outpatient)[1,3]	-	-	98%	98%
Prophylactic Antibiotic Stopped[5]	-	-	98%	98%
Prophylactic Antibiotic Timing[5]	-	-	99%	99%
Prophylactic Antibiotic Timing (Outpatient)[1,3]	-	-	98%	98%
Urinary Catheter Removal[5]	-	-	98%	97%
Survey of Patients' Hospital Experiences				
Area Around Room 'Always' Quiet at Night	(a)	67%	68%	61%
Doctors 'Always' Communicated Well	(a)	86%	83%	82%
Home Recovery Information Given	(a)	81%	85%	85%
Hospital Given 9 or 10 on 10 Point Scale	(a)	67%	73%	71%
Meds 'Always' Explained Before Given	(a)	67%	66%	64%
Nurses 'Always' Communicated Well	(a)	81%	80%	79%
Pain 'Always' Well Controlled	(a)	74%	72%	71%
Room and Bathroom 'Always' Clean	(a)	78%	75%	73%
Timely Help 'Always' Received	(a)	74%	69%	68%
Would Definitely Recommend Hospital	(a)	59%	73%	71%
Use of Medical Imaging				
Cardiac Imaging Stress Test before Surgery[1]	-	-	5.3%	5.3%
Combination Abdominal CT Scan	96	9.4%	16.4%	10.5%
Combination Brain/Sinus CT Scan	150	0.7%	2.7%	2.7%
Combination Chest CT Scan	49	4.1%	5.6%	2.7%
Follow-up Mammogram/Ultrasound	251	15.9%	7.9%	8.8%
Lumbar Spine MRI for Low Back Pain[1]	-	-	39.6%	37.2%

East Texas Medical Center - Gilmer

712 North Wood
Gilmer, TX 75644
Phone: 903-841-7100
URL: www.etmc.org
Type: Acute Care Hospitals
Emergency Services: Yes
Ownership: Voluntary non-profit - Private
Key Personnel:
CEO/President. . . . . Elmer G Ellis

Measure	Cases	This Hosp.	State Avg.	U.S. Avg.
Blood Clot Prevention and Treatment				
Anticoagulation Overlap Therapy[1,2]	-	-	93%	93%
ICU Venous Thromboembolism Prophylaxis[2,7]	-	-	92%	92%
Incidence of Potentially Preventable VTE[1,2]	-	-	9%	10%
UFH with Dosages/Platelet Monitoring[2,7]	-	-	96%	97%
Venous Thromboembolism Prophylaxis[2]	117	87%	82%	85%
Warfarin Therapy Discharge Instructions[1,2]	-	-	84%	75%
Chest Pain/Possible Heart Attack Care				
Aspirin Given Within 24 Hours of Arrival	42	98%	94%	96%
Fibrinolytic Meds Within 30 Min. of Arrival[1]	-	-	47%	58%
Average Time to ECG (minutes)	44	8	8	7
Average Time to Transfer (minutes)[1]	-	-	62	60
Children's Asthma Care				
Received Home Management Plan of Care	-	-	93%	88%
Received Reliever Medication	-	-	100%	100%
Received Systemic Corticosteroids	-	-	100%	100%
Emergency Department				
Admittance Decision Time (minutes)[2]	243	60	99	98
Head CT Results Within 45 Min. of Arrival[1]	-	-	54%	57%
Patients Who Left ER Before Being Seen	11,532	2%	3%	2%
Time from ER Arrival to Admit. (minutes)[2]	291	216	270	274
Time from ER Arrival to Discharge (minutes)	666	112	127	134
Time in ER Before Being Evaluated (minutes)	667	19	26	26
Time to Pain Meds for Fractures (minutes)	37	61	57	57
Heart Attack Care				
Aspirin Given at Discharge[1]	-	-	99%	99%
Fibrinolytic Meds Within 30 Min. of Arrival[7]	-	-	49%	54%
PCI Within 90 Minutes of Arrival[7]	-	-	95%	96%
Statin Prescribed at Discharge[1]	-	-	98%	98%
Heart Failure Care				
ACE Inhibitor or ARB for LVSD[1]	-	-	97%	97%
Discharge Instructions Given	18	94%	95%	94%
Evaluation of LVS Function	26	88%	99%	99%
Medicare Spending				
Medicare Spending per Patient (ratio)	-	1.03	1.03	0.98
Pneumonia Care				
Appropriate Initial Antibiotic Given	25	100%	95%	95%
Blood Culture Timing	36	100%	98%	98%
Pregnancy and Delivery Care				
Newborn Deliveries Scheduled Early[7]	-	-	7%	6%
Preventive Care				
Immunization for Influenza[2]	226	89%	90%	90%
Immunization for Pneumonia[2]	354	95%	92%	92%
Stroke Care				
Anticoagulation Therapy for Atrial Fibrillation[7]	-	-	96%	95%
Antithrombotic Therapy Timing[1]	-	-	98%	98%
Assessed for Rehabilitation[1]	-	-	98%	97%
Discharged on Antithrombotic Therapy[1]	-	-	99%	99%
Discharged on Statin Medication[1]	-	-	95%	94%
Thrombolytic Therapy Timing[7]	-	-	68%	66%
Venous Thromboembolism Prophylaxis[1]	-	-	94%	94%
Written Stroke Educational Materials Given[1]	-	-	92%	88%
Surgical Care Improvement Project				
Appropriate Beta Blocker Usage[5]	-	-	98%	98%
Appropriate VTP Within 24 Hours[5]	-	-	98%	98%
Controlled Postoperative Blood Glucose[5]	-	-	96%	97%
Perioperative Temperature Management[5]	-	-	100%	100%
Prophylactic Antibiotic Selection[5]	-	-	99%	99%
Prophylactic Antibiotic Selection (Outpatient)[5]	-	-	98%	98%
Prophylactic Antibiotic Stopped[5]	-	-	98%	98%
Prophylactic Antibiotic Timing[5]	-	-	99%	99%
Prophylactic Antibiotic Timing (Outpatient)[5]	-	-	98%	98%
Urinary Catheter Removal[5]	-	-	98%	97%
Survey of Patients' Hospital Experiences				
Area Around Room 'Always' Quiet at Night	(a)	76%	68%	61%
Doctors 'Always' Communicated Well	(a)	97%	83%	82%
Home Recovery Information Given	(a)	90%	85%	85%
Hospital Given 9 or 10 on 10 Point Scale	(a)	86%	73%	71%
Meds 'Always' Explained Before Given	(a)	83%	66%	64%
Nurses 'Always' Communicated Well	(a)	88%	80%	79%
Pain 'Always' Well Controlled	(a)	79%	72%	71%
Room and Bathroom 'Always' Clean	(a)	88%	75%	73%
Timely Help 'Always' Received	(a)	86%	69%	68%
Would Definitely Recommend Hospital	(a)	82%	73%	71%
Use of Medical Imaging				
Cardiac Imaging Stress Test before Surgery[1]	-	-	5.3%	5.3%
Combination Abdominal CT Scan	149	1.3%	16.4%	10.5%
Combination Brain/Sinus CT Scan[1]	-	-	2.7%	2.7%
Combination Chest CT Scan	63	0.0%	5.6%	2.7%
Follow-up Mammogram/Ultrasound[7]	-	-	7.9%	8.8%
Lumbar Spine MRI for Low Back Pain[1]	-	-	39.6%	37.2%

Glen Rose Medical Center

1021 Holden Street
Glen Rose, TX 76043
Phone: 254-897-2215
Fax: 254-897-1427
Type: Acute Care Hospitals
Emergency Services: Yes
Ownership: Govt - Hospital Dist/Auth
Beds: 134
Key Personnel:
Chief of Medical Staff. . . . . Aimee Coker, MD
Operating Room. . . . . Nataline Fanning
CEO/President. . . . . Gary Marks
Infection Control. . . . . Jennifer Thrash
Radiology. . . . . D Matt Toups

Measure	Cases	This Hosp.	State Avg.	U.S. Avg.
Blood Clot Prevention and Treatment				
Anticoagulation Overlap Therapy[1]	-	-	93%	93%
ICU Venous Thromboembolism Prophylaxis[7]	-	-	92%	92%
Incidence of Potentially Preventable VTE[1]	-	-	9%	10%
UFH with Dosages/Platelet Monitoring[7]	-	-	96%	97%
Venous Thromboembolism Prophylaxis	367	57%	82%	85%
Warfarin Therapy Discharge Instructions[1]	-	-	84%	75%
Chest Pain/Possible Heart Attack Care				
Aspirin Given Within 24 Hours of Arrival	27	78%	94%	96%
Fibrinolytic Meds Within 30 Min. of Arrival[7]	-	-	47%	58%
Average Time to ECG (minutes)	20	8	8	7
Average Time to Transfer (minutes)[1]	-	-	62	60
Children's Asthma Care				
Received Home Management Plan of Care	-	-	93%	88%
Received Reliever Medication	-	-	100%	100%
Received Systemic Corticosteroids	-	-	100%	100%
Emergency Department				
Admittance Decision Time (minutes)	466	47	99	98
Head CT Results Within 45 Min. of Arrival[1]	-	-	54%	57%
Patients Who Left ER Before Being Seen	7,703	1%	3%	2%
Time from ER Arrival to Admit. (minutes)	466	194	270	274
Time from ER Arrival to Discharge (minutes)	220	113	127	134
Time in ER Before Being Evaluated (minutes)	462	15	26	26

NOTE: Hospital profiles are in alphabetical order by state, then city, then hospital within the city; Rankings exclude hospitals with less than 25 cases except for patient surveys which excludes hospitals with less than 100 cases; (a) 100-299 cases; (1) The number of cases/patients is too few to report; (2) Data submitted were based on a sample of cases/patients; (3) Results are based on a shorter time period than required; (4) Data suppressed by CMS for one or more quarters; (5) Results are not available for this reporting period; (6) Fewer than 100 patients completed the HCAHPS survey; (7) No cases met the criteria for this measure; (8) The lower limit of the confidence interval cannot be calculated if the number of observed infections equals zero; (9) No data are available from the state/territory for this reporting period; (10) The scores shown reflect fewer than 50 completed surveys; (11) There were discrepancies in the data collection process; (12) This measure does not apply to this hospital for this reporting period; (13) Results cannot be calculated for this reporting period; (14) The results for this state are combined with nearby states to protect confidentiality; Please refer to the User's Guide for a full explanation of data.

Time to Pain Meds for Fractures (minutes)	47	48	57	57
Heart Attack Care				
Aspirin Given at Discharge[1,3]	-	-	99%	99%
Fibrinolytic Meds Within 30 Min. of Arrival[3,7]	-	-	49%	54%
PCI Within 90 Minutes of Arrival[3,7]	-	-	95%	96%
Statin Prescribed at Discharge[1,3]	-	-	98%	98%
Heart Failure Care				
ACE Inhibitor or ARB for LVSD[1]	-	-	97%	97%
Discharge Instructions Given	20	35%	95%	94%
Evaluation of LVS Function	31	87%	99%	99%
Medicare Spending				
Medicare Spending per Patient (ratio)	-	0.88	1.03	0.98
Pneumonia Care				
Appropriate Initial Antibiotic Given	35	71%	95%	95%
Blood Culture Timing	39	97%	98%	98%
Pregnancy and Delivery Care				
Newborn Deliveries Scheduled Early[7]	-	-	7%	6%
Preventive Care				
Immunization for Influenza	265	85%	90%	90%
Immunization for Pneumonia	449	95%	92%	92%
Stroke Care				
Anticoagulation Therapy for Atrial Fibrillation[1,3]	-	-	96%	95%
Antithrombotic Therapy Timing[1,3]	-	-	98%	98%
Assessed for Rehabilitation[3]	13	46%	98%	97%
Discharged on Antithrombotic Therapy[3]	13	85%	99%	99%
Discharged on Statin Medication[3]	13	54%	95%	94%
Thrombolytic Therapy Timing[1,3]	-	-	68%	66%
Venous Thromboembolism Prophylaxis[1,3]	-	-	94%	94%
Written Stroke Educational Materials Given[1,3]	-	-	92%	88%
Surgical Care Improvement Project				
Appropriate Beta Blocker Usage[1]	-	-	98%	98%
Appropriate VTP Within 24 Hours[1]	-	-	98%	98%
Controlled Postoperative Blood Glucose[7]	-	-	96%	97%
Perioperative Temperature Management[1]	-	-	100%	100%
Prophylactic Antibiotic Selection[1]	-	-	99%	99%
Prophylactic Antibiotic Selection (Outpatient)[3]	11	55%	98%	98%
Prophylactic Antibiotic Stopped[1]	-	-	98%	98%
Prophylactic Antibiotic Timing[1]	-	-	99%	99%
Prophylactic Antibiotic Timing (Outpatient)[3]	11	100%	98%	98%
Urinary Catheter Removal[1]	-	-	98%	97%
Survey of Patients' Hospital Experiences				
Area Around Room 'Always' Quiet at Night	(a)	73%	68%	61%
Doctors 'Always' Communicated Well	(a)	93%	83%	82%
Home Recovery Information Given	(a)	78%	85%	85%
Hospital Given 9 or 10 on 10 Point Scale	(a)	77%	73%	71%
Meds 'Always' Explained Before Given	(a)	71%	66%	64%
Nurses 'Always' Communicated Well	(a)	85%	80%	79%
Pain 'Always' Well Controlled	(a)	80%	72%	71%
Room and Bathroom 'Always' Clean	(a)	78%	75%	73%
Timely Help 'Always' Received	(a)	79%	69%	68%
Would Definitely Recommend Hospital	(a)	83%	73%	71%
Use of Medical Imaging				
Cardiac Imaging Stress Test before Surgery	97	5.2%	5.3%	5.3%
Combination Abdominal CT Scan	155	18.7%	16.4%	10.5%
Combination Brain/Sinus CT Scan	226	6.2%	2.7%	2.7%
Combination Chest CT Scan	105	31.4%	5.6%	2.7%
Follow-up Mammogram/Ultrasound	378	6.6%	7.9%	8.8%
Lumbar Spine MRI for Low Back Pain[1]	-	-	39.6%	37.2%

Memorial Hospital

1110 North Sarah Dewitt Drive
Gonzales, TX 78629
Phone: 830-672-7581
Fax: 830-672-2401
E-mail: cnorris@gonzaleshealthcare.com
URL: www.gonzaleshealthcare.com
Type: Acute Care Hospitals
Emergency Services: Yes
Ownership: Govt - Hospital Dist/Auth
Beds: 35

Key Personnel:
President .... Lisa Gindler
Radiology..................... Charles Harvey
Chief of Medical Staff.......... Commie Hisey
Emergency Room .... Carl Jenkins, RN
CEO .... Chuck Norris
Operating Room.............. Phillip Sladek, RN

Measure	Cases	This Hosp.	State Avg.	U.S. Avg.
Blood Clot Prevention and Treatment				
Anticoagulation Overlap Therapy[1,2]	-	-	93%	93%
ICU Venous Thromboembolism Prophylaxis[2,7]	-	-	92%	92%
Incidence of Potentially Preventable VTE[2,7]	-	-	9%	10%
UFH with Dosages/Platelet Monitoring[1,2]	-	-	96%	97%
Venous Thromboembolism Prophylaxis[2]	320	41%	82%	85%
Warfarin Therapy Discharge Instructions[1,2]	-	-	84%	75%
Chest Pain/Possible Heart Attack Care				
Aspirin Given Within 24 Hours of Arrival	27	89%	94%	96%
Fibrinolytic Meds Within 30 Min. of Arrival[1,3]	-	-	47%	58%
Average Time to ECG (minutes)	27	5	8	7
Average Time to Transfer (minutes)[1,3]	-	-	62	60
Children's Asthma Care				
Received Home Management Plan of Care	-	-	93%	88%
Received Reliever Medication	-	-	100%	100%
Received Systemic Corticosteroids	-	-	100%	100%
Emergency Department				
Admittance Decision Time (minutes)[2]	283	40	99	98
Head CT Results Within 45 Min. of Arrival[1]	-	-	54%	57%
Patients Who Left ER Before Being Seen	9,620	2%	3%	2%
Time from ER Arrival to Admit. (minutes)[2]	283	194	270	274
Time from ER Arrival to Discharge (minutes)	350	102	127	134
Time in ER Before Being Evaluated (minutes)	428	19	26	26
Time to Pain Meds for Fractures (minutes)	46	48	57	57
Heart Attack Care				
Aspirin Given at Discharge[1,3]	-	-	99%	99%
Fibrinolytic Meds Within 30 Min. of Arrival[3,7]	-	-	49%	54%
PCI Within 90 Minutes of Arrival[3,7]	-	-	95%	96%
Statin Prescribed at Discharge[1,3]	-	-	98%	98%
Heart Failure Care				
ACE Inhibitor or ARB for LVSD	13	77%	97%	97%
Discharge Instructions Given	30	97%	95%	94%
Evaluation of LVS Function	38	89%	99%	99%
Medicare Spending				
Medicare Spending per Patient (ratio)	-	0.94	1.03	0.98
Pneumonia Care				
Appropriate Initial Antibiotic Given	23	91%	95%	95%
Blood Culture Timing	19	95%	98%	98%
Pregnancy and Delivery Care				
Newborn Deliveries Scheduled Early[2]	61	5%	7%	6%
Preventive Care				
Immunization for Influenza[2]	307	98%	90%	90%
Immunization for Pneumonia[2]	350	95%	92%	92%
Stroke Care				
Anticoagulation Therapy for Atrial Fibrillation[1,3]	-	-	96%	95%
Antithrombotic Therapy Timing[1,3]	-	-	98%	98%
Assessed for Rehabilitation[1,3]	-	-	98%	97%
Discharged on Antithrombotic Therapy[1,3]	-	-	99%	99%
Discharged on Statin Medication[1,3]	-	-	95%	94%
Thrombolytic Therapy Timing[1,3]	-	-	68%	66%
Venous Thromboembolism Prophylaxis[1,3]	-	-	94%	94%
Written Stroke Educational Materials Given[3,7]	-	-	92%	88%
Surgical Care Improvement Project				
Appropriate Beta Blocker Usage[1,2]	-	-	98%	98%
Appropriate VTP Within 24 Hours[2]	23	43%	98%	98%
Controlled Postoperative Blood Glucose[2,7]	-	-	96%	97%
Perioperative Temperature Management[2]	25	96%	100%	100%
Prophylactic Antibiotic Selection[1,2]	-	-	99%	99%
Prophylactic Antibiotic Selection (Outpatient)	24	92%	98%	98%
Prophylactic Antibiotic Stopped[1,2]	-	-	98%	98%
Prophylactic Antibiotic Timing[2]	11	73%	99%	99%
Prophylactic Antibiotic Timing (Outpatient)	13	85%	98%	98%
Urinary Catheter Removal[1,2]	-	-	98%	97%
Survey of Patients' Hospital Experiences				
Area Around Room 'Always' Quiet at Night[6]	<100	68%	68%	61%
Doctors 'Always' Communicated Well[6]	<100	89%	83%	82%
Home Recovery Information Given[6]	<100	89%	85%	85%
Hospital Given 9 or 10 on 10 Point Scale[6]	<100	77%	73%	71%
Meds 'Always' Explained Before Given[6]	<100	67%	66%	64%
Nurses 'Always' Communicated Well[6]	<100	83%	80%	79%
Pain 'Always' Well Controlled[6]	<100	69%	72%	71%
Room and Bathroom 'Always' Clean[6]	<100	80%	75%	73%
Timely Help 'Always' Received[6]	<100	79%	69%	68%
Would Definitely Recommend Hospital[6]	<100	70%	73%	71%
Use of Medical Imaging				
Cardiac Imaging Stress Test before Surgery[7]	-	-	5.3%	5.3%
Combination Abdominal CT Scan	125	8.8%	16.4%	10.5%
Combination Brain/Sinus CT Scan[1]	-	-	2.7%	2.7%
Combination Chest CT Scan	79	15.2%	5.6%	2.7%
Follow-up Mammogram/Ultrasound	165	10.9%	7.9%	8.8%
Lumbar Spine MRI for Low Back Pain[1]	-	-	39.6%	37.2%

Graham Regional Medical Center

1301 Montgomery Road
Graham, TX 76450
Phone: 940-549-3400
Fax: 940-521-5158
URL: www.grahamrmc.com
Type: Acute Care Hospitals
Emergency Services: Yes
Ownership: Government - Local
Beds: 37

Key Personnel:
Chief of Medical Staff.......... Pete Brown, MD
Quality Assurance .... Diane Grissom
Emergency Room .... Gerald Mitchell
President..................... Wyatt Pettus
Operating Room.............. Kim Steger

Measure	Cases	This Hosp.	State Avg.	U.S. Avg.
Blood Clot Prevention and Treatment				
Anticoagulation Overlap Therapy[1,2]	-	-	93%	93%
ICU Venous Thromboembolism Prophylaxis[2,7]	-	-	92%	92%
Incidence of Potentially Preventable VTE[2,7]	-	-	9%	10%
UFH with Dosages/Platelet Monitoring[2,7]	-	-	96%	97%
Venous Thromboembolism Prophylaxis[2]	113	85%	82%	85%
Warfarin Therapy Discharge Instructions[1,2]	-	-	84%	75%
Chest Pain/Possible Heart Attack Care				
Aspirin Given Within 24 Hours of Arrival	76	88%	94%	96%
Fibrinolytic Meds Within 30 Min. of Arrival[7]	-	-	47%	58%
Average Time to ECG (minutes)	79	15	8	7
Average Time to Transfer (minutes)[1]	-	-	62	60
Children's Asthma Care				
Received Home Management Plan of Care	-	-	93%	88%
Received Reliever Medication	-	-	100%	100%
Received Systemic Corticosteroids	-	-	100%	100%
Emergency Department				
Admittance Decision Time (minutes)[2]	362	57	99	98
Head CT Results Within 45 Min. of Arrival[1]	-	-	54%	57%
Patients Who Left ER Before Being Seen	9,491	1%	3%	2%
Time from ER Arrival to Admit. (minutes)[2]	362	215	270	274
Time from ER Arrival to Discharge (minutes)	329	121	127	134
Time in ER Before Being Evaluated (minutes)	369	30	26	26
Time to Pain Meds for Fractures (minutes)	56	46	57	57
Heart Attack Care				
Aspirin Given at Discharge[1,2]	-	-	99%	99%
Fibrinolytic Meds Within 30 Min. of Arrival[2,3]	-	-	49%	54%
PCI Within 90 Minutes of Arrival[2,3]	-	-	95%	96%
Statin Prescribed at Discharge[1,2]	-	-	98%	98%
Heart Failure Care				
ACE Inhibitor or ARB for LVSD[1,2]	-	-	97%	97%
Discharge Instructions Given[2]	44	100%	95%	94%
Evaluation of LVS Function[2]	59	95%	99%	99%
Medicare Spending				
Medicare Spending per Patient (ratio)	-	0.89	1.03	0.98
Pneumonia Care				
Appropriate Initial Antibiotic Given[2]	39	92%	95%	95%
Blood Culture Timing[2]	47	96%	98%	98%
Pregnancy and Delivery Care				
Newborn Deliveries Scheduled Early[7]	-	-	7%	6%
Preventive Care				
Immunization for Influenza[2]	283	99%	90%	90%
Immunization for Pneumonia[2]	399	99%	92%	92%
Stroke Care				
Anticoagulation Therapy for Atrial Fibrillation[2,7]	-	-	96%	95%
Antithrombotic Therapy Timing[1,2]	-	-	98%	98%
Assessed for Rehabilitation[1,2]	-	-	98%	97%
Discharged on Antithrombotic Therapy[1,2]	-	-	99%	99%
Discharged on Statin Medication[1,2]	-	-	95%	94%
Thrombolytic Therapy Timing[2,7]	-	-	68%	66%
Venous Thromboembolism Prophylaxis[1,2]	-	-	94%	94%

NOTE: Hospital profiles are in alphabetical order by state, then city, then hospital within the city; Rankings exclude hospitals with less than 25 cases except for patient surveys which excludes hospitals with less than 100 cases; (a) 100-299 cases; (1) The number of cases/patients is too few to report; (2) Data submitted were based on a sample of cases/patients; (3) Results are based on a shorter time period than required; (4) Data suppressed by CMS for one or more quarters; (5) Results are not available for this reporting period; (6) Fewer than 100 patients completed the HCAHPS survey; (7) No cases met the criteria for this measure; (8) The lower limit of the confidence interval cannot be calculated if the number of observed infections equals zero; (9) No data are available from the state/territory for this reporting period; (10) The scores shown reflect fewer than 50 completed surveys; (11) There were discrepancies in the data collection process; (12) This measure does not apply to this hospital for this reporting period; (13) Results cannot be calculated for this reporting period; (14) The results for this state are combined with nearby states to protect confidentiality; Please refer to the User's Guide for a full explanation of data.

Measure	Cases	This Hosp.	State Avg.	U.S. Avg.
Written Stroke Educational Materials Given[2,7]	-	-	92%	88%
Surgical Care Improvement Project				
Appropriate Beta Blocker Usage[2]	15	53%	98%	98%
Appropriate VTP Within 24 Hours[2]	50	98%	98%	98%
Controlled Postoperative Blood Glucose[2,7]	-	-	96%	97%
Perioperative Temperature Management[2]	62	100%	100%	100%
Prophylactic Antibiotic Selection[2]	40	100%	99%	99%
Prophylactic Antibiotic Selection (Outpatient)	32	100%	98%	98%
Prophylactic Antibiotic Stopped[2]	40	95%	98%	98%
Prophylactic Antibiotic Timing[2]	40	92%	99%	99%
Prophylactic Antibiotic Timing (Outpatient)	32	100%	98%	98%
Urinary Catheter Removal[2]	52	81%	98%	97%
Survey of Patients' Hospital Experiences				
Area Around Room 'Always' Quiet at Night	(a)	76%	68%	61%
Doctors 'Always' Communicated Well	(a)	91%	83%	82%
Home Recovery Information Given	(a)	87%	85%	85%
Hospital Given 9 or 10 on 10 Point Scale	(a)	74%	73%	71%
Meds 'Always' Explained Before Given	(a)	66%	66%	64%
Nurses 'Always' Communicated Well	(a)	80%	80%	79%
Pain 'Always' Well Controlled	(a)	80%	72%	71%
Room and Bathroom 'Always' Clean	(a)	63%	75%	73%
Timely Help 'Always' Received	(a)	74%	69%	68%
Would Definitely Recommend Hospital	(a)	80%	73%	71%
Use of Medical Imaging				
Cardiac Imaging Stress Test before Surgery[7]	-	-	5.3%	5.3%
Combination Abdominal CT Scan	284	33.5%	16.4%	10.5%
Combination Brain/Sinus CT Scan[1]	-	-	2.7%	2.7%
Combination Chest CT Scan	208	0.0%	5.6%	2.7%
Follow-up Mammogram/Ultrasound	494	7.5%	7.9%	8.8%
Lumbar Spine MRI for Low Back Pain	96	40.6%	39.6%	37.2%

Lake Granbury Medical Center

1310 Paluxy Rd
Granbury, TX 76048
URL: www.lakegranburymedicalcenter.com
Type: Acute Care Hospitals
Ownership: Proprietary
Phone: 817-573-2683
Fax: 817-408-3038
Emergency Services: Yes
Beds: 56

Key Personnel:
Intensive Care Unit. . . . . Gwen Aparicio
Radiology. . . . . Lillian Cavin, DO
Emergency Room . . . . Ken Filbeck, MD
Pediatric In-Patient Care . . . . . . Christy Massey, RN
Infection Control. . . . . Denise Pratz
CEO/President. . . . . Donnie L Romine
Operating Room. . . . . Joe Rudisaile, RN
Quality Assurance . . . . John Traly

Measure	Cases	This Hosp.	State Avg.	U.S. Avg.
Blood Clot Prevention and Treatment				
Anticoagulation Overlap Therapy[2]	15	100%	93%	93%
ICU Venous Thromboembolism Prophylaxis[2]	67	100%	92%	92%
Incidence of Potentially Preventable VTE[1,2]	-	-	9%	10%
UFH with Dosages/Platelet Monitoring[1,2]	-	-	96%	97%
Venous Thromboembolism Prophylaxis[2]	195	99%	82%	85%
Warfarin Therapy Discharge Instructions[2]	11	82%	84%	75%
Chest Pain/Possible Heart Attack Care				
Aspirin Given Within 24 Hours of Arrival	16	100%	94%	96%
Fibrinolytic Meds Within 30 Min. of Arrival[3,7]	-	-	47%	58%
Average Time to ECG (minutes)	17	8	8	7
Average Time to Transfer (minutes)[1,3]	-	-	62	60
Children's Asthma Care				
Received Home Management Plan of Care	-	-	93%	88%
Received Reliever Medication	-	-	100%	100%
Received Systemic Corticosteroids	-	-	100%	100%
Emergency Department				
Admittance Decision Time (minutes)[2]	387	78	99	98
Head CT Results Within 45 Min. of Arrival	15	80%	54%	57%
Patients Who Left ER Before Being Seen	20,193	1%	3%	2%
Time from ER Arrival to Admit. (minutes)[2]	392	226	270	274
Time from ER Arrival to Discharge (minutes)	391	113	127	134
Time in ER Before Being Evaluated (minutes)	415	24	26	26
Time to Pain Meds for Fractures (minutes)	87	55	57	57
Heart Attack Care				
Aspirin Given at Discharge	35	100%	99%	99%
Fibrinolytic Meds Within 30 Min. of Arrival[7]	-	-	49%	54%
PCI Within 90 Minutes of Arrival	14	100%	95%	96%
Statin Prescribed at Discharge	29	100%	98%	98%
Heart Failure Care				
ACE Inhibitor or ARB for LVSD	17	100%	97%	97%
Discharge Instructions Given	69	96%	95%	94%
Evaluation of LVS Function	99	100%	99%	99%
Medicare Spending				
Medicare Spending per Patient (ratio)	-	1.03	1.03	0.98
Pneumonia Care				
Appropriate Initial Antibiotic Given	85	99%	95%	95%
Blood Culture Timing	154	99%	98%	98%
Pregnancy and Delivery Care				
Newborn Deliveries Scheduled Early[2]	14	0%	7%	6%
Preventive Care				
Immunization for Influenza[2]	299	99%	90%	90%
Immunization for Pneumonia[2]	386	99%	92%	92%
Stroke Care				
Anticoagulation Therapy for Atrial Fibrillation[1]	-	-	96%	95%
Antithrombotic Therapy Timing[1]	-	-	98%	98%
Assessed for Rehabilitation	16	100%	98%	97%
Discharged on Antithrombotic Therapy	15	100%	99%	99%
Discharged on Statin Medication	11	91%	95%	94%
Thrombolytic Therapy Timing[7]	-	-	68%	66%
Venous Thromboembolism Prophylaxis	11	100%	94%	94%
Written Stroke Educational Materials Given[1]	-	-	92%	88%
Surgical Care Improvement Project				
Appropriate Beta Blocker Usage	59	98%	98%	98%
Appropriate VTP Within 24 Hours	230	100%	98%	98%
Controlled Postoperative Blood Glucose[7]	-	-	96%	97%
Perioperative Temperature Management	248	100%	100%	100%
Prophylactic Antibiotic Selection	193	98%	99%	99%
Prophylactic Antibiotic Selection (Outpatient)	154	100%	98%	98%
Prophylactic Antibiotic Stopped	192	100%	98%	98%
Prophylactic Antibiotic Timing	194	99%	99%	99%
Prophylactic Antibiotic Timing (Outpatient)	158	97%	98%	98%
Urinary Catheter Removal	166	100%	98%	97%
Survey of Patients' Hospital Experiences				
Area Around Room 'Always' Quiet at Night	300+	63%	68%	61%
Doctors 'Always' Communicated Well	300+	81%	83%	82%
Home Recovery Information Given	300+	84%	85%	85%
Hospital Given 9 or 10 on 10 Point Scale	300+	65%	73%	71%
Meds 'Always' Explained Before Given	300+	60%	66%	64%
Nurses 'Always' Communicated Well	300+	74%	80%	79%
Pain 'Always' Well Controlled	300+	73%	72%	71%
Room and Bathroom 'Always' Clean	300+	64%	75%	73%
Timely Help 'Always' Received	300+	59%	69%	68%
Would Definitely Recommend Hospital	300+	65%	73%	71%
Use of Medical Imaging				
Cardiac Imaging Stress Test before Surgery	368	3.8%	5.3%	5.3%
Combination Abdominal CT Scan	543	16.2%	16.4%	10.5%
Combination Brain/Sinus CT Scan	585	4.3%	2.7%	2.7%
Combination Chest CT Scan	441	9.3%	5.6%	2.7%
Follow-up Mammogram/Ultrasound	1,027	13.1%	7.9%	8.8%
Lumbar Spine MRI for Low Back Pain	137	44.5%	39.6%	37.2%

Texas General Hospital

2709 Hospital Blvd
Grand Prairie, TX 75051
Type: Acute Care Hospitals
Ownership: Proprietary
Phone: 469-635-2073
Emergency Services: Yes

Measure	Cases	This Hosp.	State Avg.	U.S. Avg.
Blood Clot Prevention and Treatment				
Anticoagulation Overlap Therapy[1,3]	-	-	93%	93%
ICU Venous Thromboembolism Prophylaxis[3]	25	92%	92%	92%
Incidence of Potentially Preventable VTE[3,7]	-	-	9%	10%
UFH with Dosages/Platelet Monitoring[3,7]	-	-	96%	97%
Venous Thromboembolism Prophylaxis[3]	116	90%	82%	85%
Warfarin Therapy Discharge Instructions[1,3]	-	-	84%	75%
Chest Pain/Possible Heart Attack Care				
Aspirin Given Within 24 Hours of Arrival[1,3]	-	-	94%	96%
Fibrinolytic Meds Within 30 Min. of Arrival[3,7]	-	-	47%	58%
Average Time to ECG (minutes)[1,3]	-	-	8	7
Average Time to Transfer (minutes)[3,7]	-	-	62	60
Children's Asthma Care				
Received Home Management Plan of Care	-	-	93%	88%
Received Reliever Medication	-	-	100%	100%
Received Systemic Corticosteroids	-	-	100%	100%
Emergency Department				
Admittance Decision Time (minutes)[3]	79	55	99	98
Head CT Results Within 45 Min. of Arrival[3,7]	-	-	54%	57%
Patients Who Left ER Before Being Seen	4,176	0%	3%	2%
Time from ER Arrival to Admit. (minutes)[3]	80	348	270	274
Time from ER Arrival to Discharge (minutes)[3]	258	136	127	134
Time in ER Before Being Evaluated (minutes)[3]	274	25	26	26
Time to Pain Meds for Fractures (minutes)[1,3]	-	-	57	57
Heart Attack Care				
Aspirin Given at Discharge[5]	-	-	99%	99%
Fibrinolytic Meds Within 30 Min. of Arrival[5]	-	-	49%	54%
PCI Within 90 Minutes of Arrival[5]	-	-	95%	96%
Statin Prescribed at Discharge[5]	-	-	98%	98%
Heart Failure Care				
ACE Inhibitor or ARB for LVSD[1,3]	-	-	97%	97%
Discharge Instructions Given[1,3]	-	-	95%	94%
Evaluation of LVS Function[1,3]	-	-	99%	99%
Medicare Spending				
Medicare Spending per Patient (ratio)[1]	-	-	1.03	0.98
Pneumonia Care				
Appropriate Initial Antibiotic Given[1,3]	-	-	95%	95%
Blood Culture Timing[1,3]	-	-	98%	98%
Pregnancy and Delivery Care				
Newborn Deliveries Scheduled Early[3,7]	-	-	7%	6%
Preventive Care				
Immunization for Influenza[5]	-	-	90%	90%
Immunization for Pneumonia[3]	61	75%	92%	92%
Stroke Care				
Anticoagulation Therapy for Atrial Fibrillation[1,3]	-	-	96%	95%
Antithrombotic Therapy Timing[1,3]	-	-	98%	98%
Assessed for Rehabilitation[1,3]	-	-	98%	97%
Discharged on Antithrombotic Therapy[1,3]	-	-	99%	99%
Discharged on Statin Medication[3,7]	-	-	95%	94%
Thrombolytic Therapy Timing[3,7]	-	-	68%	66%
Venous Thromboembolism Prophylaxis[1,3]	-	-	94%	94%
Written Stroke Educational Materials Given[3,7]	-	-	92%	88%
Surgical Care Improvement Project				
Appropriate Beta Blocker Usage[1,3]	-	-	98%	98%
Appropriate VTP Within 24 Hours[1,3]	-	-	98%	98%
Controlled Postoperative Blood Glucose[3,7]	-	-	96%	97%
Perioperative Temperature Management[1,3]	-	-	100%	100%
Prophylactic Antibiotic Selection[3,7]	-	-	99%	99%
Prophylactic Antibiotic Selection (Outpatient)[1,3]	-	-	98%	98%
Prophylactic Antibiotic Stopped[3,7]	-	-	98%	98%
Prophylactic Antibiotic Timing[3,7]	-	-	99%	99%
Prophylactic Antibiotic Timing (Outpatient)[1,3]	-	-	98%	98%
Urinary Catheter Removal[1,3]	-	-	98%	97%
Survey of Patients' Hospital Experiences				
Area Around Room 'Always' Quiet at Night[5]	-	-	68%	61%
Doctors 'Always' Communicated Well[5]	-	-	83%	82%
Home Recovery Information Given[5]	-	-	85%	85%
Hospital Given 9 or 10 on 10 Point Scale[5]	-	-	73%	71%
Meds 'Always' Explained Before Given[5]	-	-	66%	64%
Nurses 'Always' Communicated Well[5]	-	-	80%	79%
Pain 'Always' Well Controlled[5]	-	-	72%	71%
Room and Bathroom 'Always' Clean[5]	-	-	75%	73%
Timely Help 'Always' Received[5]	-	-	69%	68%
Would Definitely Recommend Hospital[5]	-	-	73%	71%
Use of Medical Imaging				
Cardiac Imaging Stress Test before Surgery[7]	-	-	5.3%	5.3%
Combination Abdominal CT Scan[1]	-	-	16.4%	10.5%
Combination Brain/Sinus CT Scan[1]	-	-	2.7%	2.7%
Combination Chest CT Scan[1]	-	-	5.6%	2.7%
Follow-up Mammogram/Ultrasound[7]	-	-	7.9%	8.8%
Lumbar Spine MRI for Low Back Pain[1]	-	-	39.6%	37.2%

NOTE: Hospital profiles are in alphabetical order by state, then city, then hospital within the city; Rankings exclude hospitals with less than 25 cases except for patient surveys which excludes hospitals with less than 100 cases; (a) 100-299 cases; (1) The number of cases/patients is too few to report; (2) Data submitted were based on a sample of cases/patients; (3) Results are based on a shorter time period than required; (4) Data suppressed by CMS for one or more quarters; (5) Results are not available for this reporting period; (6) Fewer than 100 patients completed the HCAHPS survey; (7) No cases met the criteria for this measure; (8) The lower limit of the confidence interval cannot be calculated if the number of observed infections equals zero; (9) No data are available from the state/territory for this reporting period; (10) The scores shown reflect fewer than 50 completed surveys; (11) There were discrepancies in the data collection process; (12) This measure does not apply to this hospital for this reporting period; (13) Results cannot be calculated for this reporting period; (14) The results for this state are combined with nearby states to protect confidentiality; Please refer to the User's Guide for a full explanation of data.

Baylor Regional Medical Center at Grapevine

1650 W College St — Phone: 817-481-1588
Grapevine, TX 76051 — Fax: 817-481-2962
URL: www.baylorhealth.com
Type: Acute Care Hospitals — Emergency Services: Yes
Ownership: Voluntary non-profit - Private — Beds: 190

Key Personnel:
CEO/President. . . . . Sandy Aaron
Infection Control. . . . . Brady Allen
Quality Assurance . . . . Julie Gunderson
Cardiac Laboratory. . . . . Phil Hecht, MD
Operating Room. . . . . Robbie Kreissler
Chief of Medical Staff. . . . . Stephen Lacey, MD
Radiology. . . . . Patricia De Leon
Emergency Room . . . . John Marcucci

Measure	Cases	This Hosp.	State Avg.	U.S. Avg.
Blood Clot Prevention and Treatment				
Anticoagulation Overlap Therapy[2]	85	99%	93%	93%
ICU Venous Thromboembolism Prophylaxis[2]	60	98%	92%	92%
Incidence of Potentially Preventable VTE[2]	16	12%	9%	10%
UFH with Dosages/Platelet Monitoring[2]	23	100%	96%	97%
Venous Thromboembolism Prophylaxis[2]	357	95%	82%	85%
Warfarin Therapy Discharge Instructions[2]	68	100%	84%	75%
Chest Pain/Possible Heart Attack Care				
Aspirin Given Within 24 Hours of Arrival[5]	-	-	94%	96%
Fibrinolytic Meds Within 30 Min. of Arrival[5]	-	-	47%	58%
Average Time to ECG (minutes)[5]	-	-	8	7
Average Time to Transfer (minutes)[5]	-	-	62	60
Children's Asthma Care				
Received Home Management Plan of Care	-	-	93%	88%
Received Reliever Medication	-	-	100%	100%
Received Systemic Corticosteroids	-	-	100%	100%
Emergency Department				
Admittance Decision Time (minutes)[2]	531	93	99	98
Head CT Results Within 45 Min. of Arrival	24	75%	54%	57%
Patients Who Left ER Before Being Seen	46,129	1%	3%	2%
Time from ER Arrival to Admit. (minutes)[2]	536	246	270	274
Time from ER Arrival to Discharge (minutes)	378	145	127	134
Time in ER Before Being Evaluated (minutes)	376	23	26	26
Time to Pain Meds for Fractures (minutes)	151	41	57	57
Heart Attack Care				
Aspirin Given at Discharge	196	99%	99%	99%
Fibrinolytic Meds Within 30 Min. of Arrival[7]	-	-	49%	54%
PCI Within 90 Minutes of Arrival	53	96%	95%	96%
Statin Prescribed at Discharge	189	98%	98%	98%
Heart Failure Care				
ACE Inhibitor or ARB for LVSD	49	98%	97%	97%
Discharge Instructions Given	124	99%	95%	94%
Evaluation of LVS Function	166	100%	99%	99%
Medicare Spending				
Medicare Spending per Patient (ratio)	-	1.08	1.03	0.98
Pneumonia Care				
Appropriate Initial Antibiotic Given	154	97%	95%	95%
Blood Culture Timing	284	98%	98%	98%
Pregnancy and Delivery Care				
Newborn Deliveries Scheduled Early	230	17%	7%	6%
Preventive Care				
Immunization for Influenza[2]	516	84%	90%	90%
Immunization for Pneumonia[2]	485	87%	92%	92%
Stroke Care				
Anticoagulation Therapy for Atrial Fibrillation	12	100%	96%	95%
Antithrombotic Therapy Timing	60	100%	98%	98%
Assessed for Rehabilitation	80	100%	98%	97%
Discharged on Antithrombotic Therapy	79	100%	99%	99%
Discharged on Statin Medication	62	98%	95%	94%
Thrombolytic Therapy Timing	11	100%	68%	66%
Venous Thromboembolism Prophylaxis	75	99%	94%	94%
Written Stroke Educational Materials Given	53	98%	92%	88%
Surgical Care Improvement Project				
Appropriate Beta Blocker Usage[2]	160	98%	98%	98%
Appropriate VTP Within 24 Hours[2]	595	99%	98%	98%
Controlled Postoperative Blood Glucose[2]	66	98%	96%	97%
Perioperative Temperature Management[2]	680	100%	100%	100%
Prophylactic Antibiotic Selection[2]	455	100%	99%	99%
Prophylactic Antibiotic Selection (Outpatient)	474	100%	98%	98%
Prophylactic Antibiotic Stopped[2]	446	99%	98%	98%
Prophylactic Antibiotic Timing[2]	453	100%	99%	99%
Prophylactic Antibiotic Timing (Outpatient)	474	100%	98%	98%
Urinary Catheter Removal[2]	424	98%	98%	97%
Survey of Patients' Hospital Experiences				
Area Around Room 'Always' Quiet at Night	300+	63%	68%	61%
Doctors 'Always' Communicated Well	300+	84%	83%	82%
Home Recovery Information Given	300+	85%	85%	85%
Hospital Given 9 or 10 on 10 Point Scale	300+	78%	73%	71%
Meds 'Always' Explained Before Given	300+	65%	66%	64%
Nurses 'Always' Communicated Well	300+	79%	80%	79%
Pain 'Always' Well Controlled	300+	73%	72%	71%
Room and Bathroom 'Always' Clean	300+	79%	75%	73%
Timely Help 'Always' Received	300+	63%	69%	68%
Would Definitely Recommend Hospital	300+	82%	73%	71%
Use of Medical Imaging				
Cardiac Imaging Stress Test before Surgery	194	3.6%	5.3%	5.3%
Combination Abdominal CT Scan	547	6.4%	16.4%	10.5%
Combination Brain/Sinus CT Scan	618	2.8%	2.7%	2.7%
Combination Chest CT Scan	232	0.4%	5.6%	2.7%
Follow-up Mammogram/Ultrasound	1,300	8.6%	7.9%	8.8%
Lumbar Spine MRI for Low Back Pain	115	35.7%	39.6%	37.2%

Hunt Regional Medical Center

4215 Joe Ramsey Blvd — Phone: 903-408-5000
Greenville, TX 75401 — Fax: 903-408-1609
E-mail: administration@hmhd.org
URL: www.hmhd.org
Type: Acute Care Hospitals — Emergency Services: Yes
Ownership: Govt - Hospital Dist/Auth — Beds: 139

Key Personnel:
CEO . . . . Richard Carter
Chief of Medical Staff. . . . . Syed Hamid, MD
Radiology. . . . . Lawrence W Kaler
Operating Room. . . . . Joseph Ronaghan, MD
Emergency Room . . . . Rick Selveggi, MD
Quality Assurance . . . . Betsy Sollenne
Chairman/CEO . . . . Ron Wensel

Measure	Cases	This Hosp.	State Avg.	U.S. Avg.
Blood Clot Prevention and Treatment				
Anticoagulation Overlap Therapy[2]	46	96%	93%	93%
ICU Venous Thromboembolism Prophylaxis[2]	124	82%	92%	92%
Incidence of Potentially Preventable VTE[1,2]	-	-	9%	10%
UFH with Dosages/Platelet Monitoring[1,2]	-	-	96%	97%
Venous Thromboembolism Prophylaxis[2]	291	81%	82%	85%
Warfarin Therapy Discharge Instructions[2]	40	100%	84%	75%
Chest Pain/Possible Heart Attack Care				
Aspirin Given Within 24 Hours of Arrival	97	98%	94%	96%
Fibrinolytic Meds Within 30 Min. of Arrival[1]	-	-	47%	58%
Average Time to ECG (minutes)	103	7	8	7
Average Time to Transfer (minutes)	15	44	62	60
Children's Asthma Care				
Received Home Management Plan of Care	-	-	93%	88%
Received Reliever Medication	-	-	100%	100%
Received Systemic Corticosteroids	-	-	100%	100%
Emergency Department				
Admittance Decision Time (minutes)[2]	549	95	99	98
Head CT Results Within 45 Min. of Arrival	13	46%	54%	57%
Patients Who Left ER Before Being Seen	47,992	2%	3%	2%
Time from ER Arrival to Admit. (minutes)[2]	576	245	270	274
Time from ER Arrival to Discharge (minutes)	369	138	127	134
Time in ER Before Being Evaluated (minutes)	407	33	26	26
Time to Pain Meds for Fractures (minutes)	192	66	57	57
Heart Attack Care				
Aspirin Given at Discharge[1]	-	-	99%	99%
Fibrinolytic Meds Within 30 Min. of Arrival[7]	-	-	49%	54%
PCI Within 90 Minutes of Arrival[7]	-	-	95%	96%
Statin Prescribed at Discharge[1]	-	-	98%	98%
Heart Failure Care				
ACE Inhibitor or ARB for LVSD	46	100%	97%	97%
Discharge Instructions Given	101	99%	95%	94%
Evaluation of LVS Function	135	100%	99%	99%
Medicare Spending				
Medicare Spending per Patient (ratio)	-	1.08	1.03	0.98
Pneumonia Care				
Appropriate Initial Antibiotic Given	168	95%	95%	95%
Blood Culture Timing	307	97%	98%	98%
Pregnancy and Delivery Care				
Newborn Deliveries Scheduled Early[2]	35	3%	7%	6%
Preventive Care				
Immunization for Influenza[2]	505	96%	90%	90%
Immunization for Pneumonia[2]	575	99%	92%	92%
Stroke Care				
Anticoagulation Therapy for Atrial Fibrillation[2]	11	91%	96%	95%
Antithrombotic Therapy Timing[2]	76	100%	98%	98%
Assessed for Rehabilitation[2]	77	96%	98%	97%
Discharged on Antithrombotic Therapy[2]	73	100%	99%	99%
Discharged on Statin Medication[2]	58	81%	95%	94%
Thrombolytic Therapy Timing[1,2]	-	-	68%	66%
Venous Thromboembolism Prophylaxis[2]	66	82%	94%	94%
Written Stroke Educational Materials Given[2]	36	81%	92%	88%
Surgical Care Improvement Project				
Appropriate Beta Blocker Usage	54	89%	98%	98%
Appropriate VTP Within 24 Hours	236	97%	98%	98%
Controlled Postoperative Blood Glucose[7]	-	-	96%	97%
Perioperative Temperature Management	271	100%	100%	100%
Prophylactic Antibiotic Selection	197	96%	99%	99%
Prophylactic Antibiotic Selection (Outpatient)	98	98%	98%	98%
Prophylactic Antibiotic Stopped	188	97%	98%	98%
Prophylactic Antibiotic Timing	196	100%	99%	99%
Prophylactic Antibiotic Timing (Outpatient)	105	92%	98%	98%
Urinary Catheter Removal	189	96%	98%	97%
Survey of Patients' Hospital Experiences				
Area Around Room 'Always' Quiet at Night	300+	66%	68%	61%
Doctors 'Always' Communicated Well	300+	78%	83%	82%
Home Recovery Information Given	300+	86%	85%	85%
Hospital Given 9 or 10 on 10 Point Scale	300+	65%	73%	71%
Meds 'Always' Explained Before Given	300+	64%	66%	64%
Nurses 'Always' Communicated Well	300+	80%	80%	79%
Pain 'Always' Well Controlled	300+	69%	72%	71%
Room and Bathroom 'Always' Clean	300+	72%	75%	73%
Timely Help 'Always' Received	300+	67%	69%	68%
Would Definitely Recommend Hospital	300+	63%	73%	71%
Use of Medical Imaging				
Cardiac Imaging Stress Test before Surgery	238	6.3%	5.3%	5.3%
Combination Abdominal CT Scan	1,062	40.5%	16.4%	10.5%
Combination Brain/Sinus CT Scan	1,007	1.8%	2.7%	2.7%
Combination Chest CT Scan	1,040	38.4%	5.6%	2.7%
Follow-up Mammogram/Ultrasound	1,749	3.5%	7.9%	8.8%
Lumbar Spine MRI for Low Back Pain	137	40.9%	39.6%	37.2%

Limestone Medical Center

701 Mcclintic Drive — Phone: 254-729-3281
Groesbeck, TX 76642 — Fax: 254-729-2689
E-mail: lmcadmin@lmchospital.com
URL: www.lmchospital.com
Type: Critical Access Hospitals — Emergency Services: Yes
Ownership: Govt - Hospital Dist/Auth — Beds: 20

Key Personnel:
Radiology. . . . . Jennifer Hixson
Chief of Medical Staff . . . . Larry Hughes
CEO . . . . Larry Price
Quality Assurance . . . . Larry Price
Patient Relations . . . . Sherald Wood
Emergency Room . . . . Jude Wright
Infection Control. . . . . Judy Wright, RN

Measure	Cases	This Hosp.	State Avg.	U.S. Avg.
Blood Clot Prevention and Treatment				
Anticoagulation Overlap Therapy[5]	-	-	93%	93%
ICU Venous Thromboembolism Prophylaxis[5]	-	-	92%	92%
Incidence of Potentially Preventable VTE[5]	-	-	9%	10%
UFH with Dosages/Platelet Monitoring[5]	-	-	96%	97%
Venous Thromboembolism Prophylaxis[5]	-	-	82%	85%
Warfarin Therapy Discharge Instructions[5]	-	-	84%	75%
Chest Pain/Possible Heart Attack Care				
Aspirin Given Within 24 Hours of Arrival	-	-	94%	96%
Fibrinolytic Meds Within 30 Min. of Arrival	-	-	47%	58%

NOTE: Hospital profiles are in alphabetical order by state, then city, then hospital within the city; Rankings exclude hospitals with less than 25 cases except for patient surveys which excludes hospitals with less than 100 cases; (a) 100-299 cases; (1) The number of cases/patients is too few to report; (2) Data submitted were based on a sample of cases/patients; (3) Results are based on a shorter time period than required; (4) Data suppressed by CMS for one or more quarters; (5) Results are not available for this reporting period; (6) Fewer than 100 patients completed the HCAHPS survey; (7) No cases met the criteria for this measure; (8) The lower limit of the confidence interval cannot be calculated if the number of observed infections equals zero; (9) No data are available from the state/territory for this reporting period; (10) The scores shown reflect fewer than 50 completed surveys; (11) There were discrepancies in the data collection process; (12) This measure does not apply to this hospital for this reporting period; (13) Results cannot be calculated for this reporting period; (14) The results for this state are combined with nearby states to protect confidentiality; Please refer to the User's Guide for a full explanation of data.

Average Time to ECG (minutes)	-	-	8	7
Average Time to Transfer (minutes)	-	-	62	60
Children's Asthma Care				
Received Home Management Plan of Care	-	-	93%	88%
Received Reliever Medication	-	-	100%	100%
Received Systemic Corticosteroids	-	-	100%	100%
Emergency Department				
Admittance Decision Time (minutes)[5]	-	-	99	98
Head CT Results Within 45 Min. of Arrival	-	-	54%	57%
Patients Who Left ER Before Being Seen	-	-	3%	2%
Time from ER Arrival to Admit. (minutes)[5]	-	-	270	274
Time from ER Arrival to Discharge (minutes)	-	-	127	134
Time in ER Before Being Evaluated (minutes)	-	-	26	26
Time to Pain Meds for Fractures (minutes)	-	-	57	57
Heart Attack Care				
Aspirin Given at Discharge[5]	-	-	99%	99%
Fibrinolytic Meds Within 30 Min. of Arrival[5]	-	-	49%	54%
PCI Within 90 Minutes of Arrival[5]	-	-	95%	96%
Statin Prescribed at Discharge[5]	-	-	98%	98%
Heart Failure Care				
ACE Inhibitor or ARB for LVSD[1,3]	-	-	97%	97%
Discharge Instructions Given[3,7]	-	-	95%	94%
Evaluation of LVS Function[1,3]	-	-	99%	99%
Medicare Spending				
Medicare Spending per Patient (ratio)	-	-	1.03	0.98
Pneumonia Care				
Appropriate Initial Antibiotic Given	12	83%	95%	95%
Blood Culture Timing[1]	-	-	98%	98%
Pregnancy and Delivery Care				
Newborn Deliveries Scheduled Early[5]	-	-	7%	6%
Preventive Care				
Immunization for Influenza[5]	-	-	90%	90%
Immunization for Pneumonia[5]	-	-	92%	92%
Stroke Care				
Anticoagulation Therapy for Atrial Fibrillation[5]	-	-	96%	95%
Antithrombotic Therapy Timing[5]	-	-	98%	98%
Assessed for Rehabilitation[5]	-	-	98%	97%
Discharged on Antithrombotic Therapy[5]	-	-	99%	99%
Discharged on Statin Medication[5]	-	-	95%	94%
Thrombolytic Therapy Timing[5]	-	-	68%	66%
Venous Thromboembolism Prophylaxis[5]	-	-	94%	94%
Written Stroke Educational Materials Given[5]	-	-	92%	88%
Surgical Care Improvement Project				
Appropriate Beta Blocker Usage[5]	-	-	98%	98%
Appropriate VTP Within 24 Hours[5]	-	-	98%	98%
Controlled Postoperative Blood Glucose[5]	-	-	96%	97%
Perioperative Temperature Management[5]	-	-	100%	100%
Prophylactic Antibiotic Selection[5]	-	-	99%	99%
Prophylactic Antibiotic Selection (Outpatient)	-	-	98%	98%
Prophylactic Antibiotic Stopped[5]	-	-	98%	98%
Prophylactic Antibiotic Timing[5]	-	-	99%	99%
Prophylactic Antibiotic Timing (Outpatient)	-	-	98%	98%
Urinary Catheter Removal[5]	-	-	98%	97%
Survey of Patients' Hospital Experiences				
Area Around Room 'Always' Quiet at Night[5]	-	-	68%	61%
Doctors 'Always' Communicated Well[5]	-	-	83%	82%
Home Recovery Information Given[5]	-	-	85%	85%
Hospital Given 9 or 10 on 10 Point Scale[5]	-	-	73%	71%
Meds 'Always' Explained Before Given[5]	-	-	66%	64%
Nurses 'Always' Communicated Well[5]	-	-	80%	79%
Pain 'Always' Well Controlled[5]	-	-	72%	71%
Room and Bathroom 'Always' Clean[5]	-	-	75%	73%
Timely Help 'Always' Received[5]	-	-	69%	68%
Would Definitely Recommend Hospital[5]	-	-	73%	71%
Use of Medical Imaging				
Cardiac Imaging Stress Test before Surgery	-	-	5.3%	5.3%
Combination Abdominal CT Scan	-	-	16.4%	10.5%
Combination Brain/Sinus CT Scan	-	-	2.7%	2.7%
Combination Chest CT Scan	-	-	5.6%	2.7%
Follow-up Mammogram/Ultrasound	-	-	7.9%	8.8%
Lumbar Spine MRI for Low Back Pain	-	-	39.6%	37.2%

Lavaca Medical Center

1400 North Texana Street
Hallettsville, TX 77964
Type: Critical Access Hospitals
Ownership: Govt - Hospital Dist/Auth
Phone: 361-798-3671
Fax: 361-798-2682
Emergency Services: Yes
Beds: 25

Key Personnel:
CEO/President. . . . . James E Vanek

Measure	Cases	This Hosp.	State Avg.	U.S. Avg.
Blood Clot Prevention and Treatment				
Anticoagulation Overlap Therapy[5]	-	-	93%	93%
ICU Venous Thromboembolism Prophylaxis[5]	-	-	92%	92%
Incidence of Potentially Preventable VTE[5]	-	-	9%	10%
UFH with Dosages/Platelet Monitoring[5]	-	-	96%	97%
Venous Thromboembolism Prophylaxis[5]	-	-	82%	85%
Warfarin Therapy Discharge Instructions[5]	-	-	84%	75%
Chest Pain/Possible Heart Attack Care				
Aspirin Given Within 24 Hours of Arrival	-	-	94%	96%
Fibrinolytic Meds Within 30 Min. of Arrival	-	-	47%	58%
Average Time to ECG (minutes)	-	-	8	7
Average Time to Transfer (minutes)	-	-	62	60
Children's Asthma Care				
Received Home Management Plan of Care	-	-	93%	88%
Received Reliever Medication	-	-	100%	100%
Received Systemic Corticosteroids	-	-	100%	100%
Emergency Department				
Admittance Decision Time (minutes)[2]	342	60	99	98
Head CT Results Within 45 Min. of Arrival	-	-	54%	57%
Patients Who Left ER Before Being Seen	-	-	3%	2%
Time from ER Arrival to Admit. (minutes)[2]	342	203	270	274
Time from ER Arrival to Discharge (minutes)	-	-	127	134
Time in ER Before Being Evaluated (minutes)	-	-	26	26
Time to Pain Meds for Fractures (minutes)	-	-	57	57
Heart Attack Care				
Aspirin Given at Discharge[3,7]	-	-	99%	99%
Fibrinolytic Meds Within 30 Min. of Arrival[3,7]	-	-	49%	54%
PCI Within 90 Minutes of Arrival[3,7]	-	-	95%	96%
Statin Prescribed at Discharge[3,7]	-	-	98%	98%
Heart Failure Care				
ACE Inhibitor or ARB for LVSD[1]	-	-	97%	97%
Discharge Instructions Given	13	100%	95%	94%
Evaluation of LVS Function	28	89%	99%	99%
Medicare Spending				
Medicare Spending per Patient (ratio)	-	-	1.03	0.98
Pneumonia Care				
Appropriate Initial Antibiotic Given	37	92%	95%	95%
Blood Culture Timing	41	98%	98%	98%
Pregnancy and Delivery Care				
Newborn Deliveries Scheduled Early[5]	-	-	7%	6%
Preventive Care				
Immunization for Influenza	259	97%	90%	90%
Immunization for Pneumonia	391	96%	92%	92%
Stroke Care				
Anticoagulation Therapy for Atrial Fibrillation[5]	-	-	96%	95%
Antithrombotic Therapy Timing[5]	-	-	98%	98%
Assessed for Rehabilitation[5]	-	-	98%	97%
Discharged on Antithrombotic Therapy[5]	-	-	99%	99%
Discharged on Statin Medication[5]	-	-	95%	94%
Thrombolytic Therapy Timing[5]	-	-	68%	66%
Venous Thromboembolism Prophylaxis[5]	-	-	94%	94%
Written Stroke Educational Materials Given[5]	-	-	92%	88%
Surgical Care Improvement Project				
Appropriate Beta Blocker Usage[5]	-	-	98%	98%
Appropriate VTP Within 24 Hours[5]	-	-	98%	98%
Controlled Postoperative Blood Glucose[5]	-	-	96%	97%
Perioperative Temperature Management[5]	-	-	100%	100%
Prophylactic Antibiotic Selection[5]	-	-	99%	99%
Prophylactic Antibiotic Selection (Outpatient)	-	-	98%	98%
Prophylactic Antibiotic Stopped[5]	-	-	98%	98%
Prophylactic Antibiotic Timing[5]	-	-	99%	99%
Prophylactic Antibiotic Timing (Outpatient)	-	-	98%	98%
Urinary Catheter Removal[5]	-	-	98%	97%
Survey of Patients' Hospital Experiences				
Area Around Room 'Always' Quiet at Night[5]	-	-	68%	61%
Doctors 'Always' Communicated Well[5]	-	-	83%	82%
Home Recovery Information Given[5]	-	-	85%	85%
Hospital Given 9 or 10 on 10 Point Scale[5]	-	-	73%	71%
Meds 'Always' Explained Before Given[5]	-	-	66%	64%
Nurses 'Always' Communicated Well[5]	-	-	80%	79%
Pain 'Always' Well Controlled[5]	-	-	72%	71%
Room and Bathroom 'Always' Clean[5]	-	-	75%	73%
Timely Help 'Always' Received[5]	-	-	69%	68%
Would Definitely Recommend Hospital[5]	-	-	73%	71%
Use of Medical Imaging				
Cardiac Imaging Stress Test before Surgery	-	-	5.3%	5.3%
Combination Abdominal CT Scan	-	-	16.4%	10.5%
Combination Brain/Sinus CT Scan	-	-	2.7%	2.7%
Combination Chest CT Scan	-	-	5.6%	2.7%
Follow-up Mammogram/Ultrasound	-	-	7.9%	8.8%
Lumbar Spine MRI for Low Back Pain	-	-	39.6%	37.2%

Hamilton General Hospital

400 N Brown
Hamilton, TX 76531
URL: www.hamiltonhospital.org
Type: Acute Care Hospitals
Ownership: Govt - Hospital Dist/Auth
Phone: 254-386-3151
Fax: 254-386-5173
Emergency Services: Yes

Key Personnel:
Quality Assurance . . . . Melissa DeLaGarza, RN BSN, CDE
Chief of Medical Staff. . . . . James R Lee, MD
CEO . . . . Brian Roland

Measure	Cases	This Hosp.	State Avg.	U.S. Avg.
Blood Clot Prevention and Treatment				
Anticoagulation Overlap Therapy[2]	14	100%	93%	93%
ICU Venous Thromboembolism Prophylaxis[2,7]	-	-	92%	92%
Incidence of Potentially Preventable VTE[2,7]	-	-	9%	10%
UFH with Dosages/Platelet Monitoring[2,7]	-	-	96%	97%
Venous Thromboembolism Prophylaxis[2]	170	43%	82%	85%
Warfarin Therapy Discharge Instructions[1,2]	-	-	84%	75%
Chest Pain/Possible Heart Attack Care				
Aspirin Given Within 24 Hours of Arrival[5]	-	-	94%	96%
Fibrinolytic Meds Within 30 Min. of Arrival[5]	-	-	47%	58%
Average Time to ECG (minutes)[5]	-	-	8	7
Average Time to Transfer (minutes)[5]	-	-	62	60
Children's Asthma Care				
Received Home Management Plan of Care	-	-	93%	88%
Received Reliever Medication	-	-	100%	100%
Received Systemic Corticosteroids	-	-	100%	100%
Emergency Department				
Admittance Decision Time (minutes)[2]	437	49	99	98
Head CT Results Within 45 Min. of Arrival[1,3]	-	-	54%	57%
Patients Who Left ER Before Being Seen	6,075	1%	3%	2%
Time from ER Arrival to Admit. (minutes)[2]	440	145	270	274
Time from ER Arrival to Discharge (minutes)	394	97	127	134
Time in ER Before Being Evaluated (minutes)	484	24	26	26
Time to Pain Meds for Fractures (minutes)	36	36	57	57
Heart Attack Care				
Aspirin Given at Discharge[1,3]	-	-	99%	99%
Fibrinolytic Meds Within 30 Min. of Arrival[3,7]	-	-	49%	54%
PCI Within 90 Minutes of Arrival[3,7]	-	-	95%	96%
Statin Prescribed at Discharge[1,3]	-	-	98%	98%
Heart Failure Care				
ACE Inhibitor or ARB for LVSD	21	95%	97%	97%
Discharge Instructions Given	59	95%	95%	94%
Evaluation of LVS Function	94	99%	99%	99%
Medicare Spending				
Medicare Spending per Patient (ratio)	-	0.92	1.03	0.98
Pneumonia Care				
Appropriate Initial Antibiotic Given	47	89%	95%	95%
Blood Culture Timing	102	95%	98%	98%
Pregnancy and Delivery Care				
Newborn Deliveries Scheduled Early[7]	-	-	7%	6%
Preventive Care				
Immunization for Influenza[2]	336	90%	90%	90%
Immunization for Pneumonia[2]	539	92%	92%	92%

NOTE: Hospital profiles are in alphabetical order by state, then city, then hospital within the city; Rankings exclude hospitals with less than 25 cases except for patient surveys which excludes hospitals with less than 100 cases; (a) 100-299 cases; (1) The number of cases/patients is too few to report; (2) Data submitted were based on a sample of cases/patients; (3) Results are based on a shorter time period than required; (4) Data suppressed by CMS for one or more quarters; (5) Results are not available for this reporting period; (6) Fewer than 100 patients completed the HCAHPS survey; (7) No cases met the criteria for this measure; (8) The lower limit of the confidence interval cannot be calculated if the number of observed infections equals zero; (9) No data are available from the state/territory for this reporting period; (10) The scores shown reflect fewer than 50 completed surveys; (11) There were discrepancies in the data collection process; (12) This measure does not apply to this hospital for this reporting period; (13) Results cannot be calculated for this reporting period; (14) The results for this state are combined with nearby states to protect confidentiality; Please refer to the User's Guide for a full explanation of data.

Measure	Cases	This Hosp.	State Avg.	U.S. Avg.
Stroke Care				
Anticoagulation Therapy for Atrial Fibrillation[3,7]	-	-	96%	95%
Antithrombotic Therapy Timing[1,3]	-	-	98%	98%
Assessed for Rehabilitation[1,3]	-	-	98%	97%
Discharged on Antithrombotic Therapy[1,3]	-	-	99%	99%
Discharged on Statin Medication[1,3]	-	-	95%	94%
Thrombolytic Therapy Timing[3,7]	-	-	68%	66%
Venous Thromboembolism Prophylaxis[1,3]	-	-	94%	94%
Written Stroke Educational Materials Given[3,7]	-	-	92%	88%
Surgical Care Improvement Project				
Appropriate Beta Blocker Usage[5]	-	-	98%	98%
Appropriate VTP Within 24 Hours[5]	-	-	98%	98%
Controlled Postoperative Blood Glucose[5]	-	-	96%	97%
Perioperative Temperature Management[5]	-	-	100%	100%
Prophylactic Antibiotic Selection[5]	-	-	99%	99%
Prophylactic Antibiotic Selection (Outpatient)[5]	-	-	98%	98%
Prophylactic Antibiotic Stopped[5]	-	-	98%	98%
Prophylactic Antibiotic Timing[5]	-	-	99%	99%
Prophylactic Antibiotic Timing (Outpatient)[5]	-	-	98%	98%
Urinary Catheter Removal[5]	-	-	98%	97%
Survey of Patients' Hospital Experiences				
Area Around Room 'Always' Quiet at Night	(a)	63%	68%	61%
Doctors 'Always' Communicated Well	(a)	92%	83%	82%
Home Recovery Information Given	(a)	86%	85%	85%
Hospital Given 9 or 10 on 10 Point Scale	(a)	82%	73%	71%
Meds 'Always' Explained Before Given	(a)	73%	66%	64%
Nurses 'Always' Communicated Well	(a)	80%	80%	79%
Pain 'Always' Well Controlled	(a)	69%	72%	71%
Room and Bathroom 'Always' Clean	(a)	80%	75%	73%
Timely Help 'Always' Received	(a)	67%	69%	68%
Would Definitely Recommend Hospital	(a)	79%	73%	71%
Use of Medical Imaging				
Cardiac Imaging Stress Test before Surgery[7]	-	-	5.3%	5.3%
Combination Abdominal CT Scan	124	10.5%	16.4%	10.5%
Combination Brain/Sinus CT Scan[1]	-	-	2.7%	2.7%
Combination Chest CT Scan	84	2.4%	5.6%	2.7%
Follow-up Mammogram/Ultrasound	190	7.4%	7.9%	8.8%
Lumbar Spine MRI for Low Back Pain[1]	-	-	39.6%	37.2%

Hamlin Memorial Hospital

632 N W Second Street
Hamlin, TX 79520
Type: Acute Care Hospitals
Ownership: Govt - Hospital Dist/Auth
Phone: 325-576-3646
Fax: 325-576-2922
Emergency Services: Yes
Beds: 25

Key Personnel:
CEO .... Keith L. Butler

Measure	Cases	This Hosp.	State Avg.	U.S. Avg.
Blood Clot Prevention and Treatment				
Anticoagulation Overlap Therapy[1,2]	-	-	93%	93%
ICU Venous Thromboembolism Prophylaxis[2,7]	-	-	92%	92%
Incidence of Potentially Preventable VTE[1,2]	-	-	9%	10%
UFH with Dosages/Platelet Monitoring[1,2]	-	-	96%	97%
Venous Thromboembolism Prophylaxis[2]	98	13%	82%	85%
Warfarin Therapy Discharge Instructions[1,2]	-	-	84%	75%
Chest Pain/Possible Heart Attack Care				
Aspirin Given Within 24 Hours of Arrival[5]	-	-	94%	96%
Fibrinolytic Meds Within 30 Min. of Arrival[5]	-	-	47%	58%
Average Time to ECG (minutes)[5]	-	-	8	7
Average Time to Transfer (minutes)[5]	-	-	62	60
Children's Asthma Care				
Received Home Management Plan of Care	-	-	93%	88%
Received Reliever Medication	-	-	100%	100%
Received Systemic Corticosteroids	-	-	100%	100%
Emergency Department				
Admittance Decision Time (minutes)[2]	89	0	99	98
Head CT Results Within 45 Min. of Arrival[3,7]	-	-	54%	57%
Patients Who Left ER Before Being Seen	1,218	2%	3%	2%
Time from ER Arrival to Admit. (minutes)[2]	92	88	270	274
Time from ER Arrival to Discharge (minutes)	250	71	127	134
Time in ER Before Being Evaluated (minutes)	269	30	26	26
Time to Pain Meds for Fractures (minutes)[1,3]	-	-	57	57
Heart Attack Care				
Aspirin Given at Discharge[5]	-	-	99%	99%
Fibrinolytic Meds Within 30 Min. of Arrival[5]	-	-	49%	54%
PCI Within 90 Minutes of Arrival[5]	-	-	95%	96%
Statin Prescribed at Discharge[5]	-	-	98%	98%
Heart Failure Care				
ACE Inhibitor or ARB for LVSD[2,3]	-	-	97%	97%
Discharge Instructions Given[1,2]	-	-	95%	94%
Evaluation of LVS Function[1,2]	-	-	99%	99%
Medicare Spending				
Medicare Spending per Patient (ratio)	-	0.83	1.03	0.98
Pneumonia Care				
Appropriate Initial Antibiotic Given[1,2]	-	-	95%	95%
Blood Culture Timing[1,2]	-	-	98%	98%
Pregnancy and Delivery Care				
Newborn Deliveries Scheduled Early[2,7]	-	-	7%	6%
Preventive Care				
Immunization for Influenza[2]	65	66%	90%	90%
Immunization for Pneumonia[2]	113	53%	92%	92%
Stroke Care				
Anticoagulation Therapy for Atrial Fibrillation[2,3]	-	-	96%	95%
Antithrombotic Therapy Timing[1,2]	-	-	98%	98%
Assessed for Rehabilitation[1,2]	-	-	98%	97%
Discharged on Antithrombotic Therapy[1,2]	-	-	99%	99%
Discharged on Statin Medication[1,2]	-	-	95%	94%
Thrombolytic Therapy Timing[2,3]	-	-	68%	66%
Venous Thromboembolism Prophylaxis[1,2]	-	-	94%	94%
Written Stroke Educational Materials Given[2,3]	-	-	92%	88%
Surgical Care Improvement Project				
Appropriate Beta Blocker Usage[5]	-	-	98%	98%
Appropriate VTP Within 24 Hours[5]	-	-	98%	98%
Controlled Postoperative Blood Glucose[5]	-	-	96%	97%
Perioperative Temperature Management[5]	-	-	100%	100%
Prophylactic Antibiotic Selection[5]	-	-	99%	99%
Prophylactic Antibiotic Selection (Outpatient)[3,7]	-	-	98%	98%
Prophylactic Antibiotic Stopped[5]	-	-	98%	98%
Prophylactic Antibiotic Timing[5]	-	-	99%	99%
Prophylactic Antibiotic Timing (Outpatient)[3,7]	-	-	98%	98%
Urinary Catheter Removal[5]	-	-	98%	97%
Survey of Patients' Hospital Experiences				
Area Around Room 'Always' Quiet at Night[10]	<100	90%	68%	61%
Doctors 'Always' Communicated Well[10]	<100	99%	83%	82%
Home Recovery Information Given[10]	<100	94%	85%	85%
Hospital Given 9 or 10 on 10 Point Scale[10]	<100	91%	73%	71%
Meds 'Always' Explained Before Given[10]	<100	94%	66%	64%
Nurses 'Always' Communicated Well[10]	<100	94%	80%	79%
Pain 'Always' Well Controlled[10]	<100	92%	72%	71%
Room and Bathroom 'Always' Clean[10]	<100	90%	75%	73%
Timely Help 'Always' Received[10]	<100	96%	69%	68%
Would Definitely Recommend Hospital[10]	<100	93%	73%	71%
Use of Medical Imaging				
Cardiac Imaging Stress Test before Surgery[7]	-	-	5.3%	5.3%
Combination Abdominal CT Scan[1]	-	-	16.4%	10.5%
Combination Brain/Sinus CT Scan[1]	-	-	2.7%	2.7%
Combination Chest CT Scan[1]	-	-	5.6%	2.7%
Follow-up Mammogram/Ultrasound[7]	-	-	7.9%	8.8%
Lumbar Spine MRI for Low Back Pain[1]	-	-	39.6%	37.2%

Seton Medical Center Harker Heights

850 W Central Texas Expressway
Harker Heights, TX 76548
Type: Acute Care Hospitals
Ownership: Proprietary
Phone: 254-953-8342
Emergency Services: Yes

Measure	Cases	This Hosp.	State Avg.	U.S. Avg.
Blood Clot Prevention and Treatment				
Anticoagulation Overlap Therapy[1,2]	-	-	93%	93%
ICU Venous Thromboembolism Prophylaxis[2]	90	93%	92%	92%
Incidence of Potentially Preventable VTE[1,2]	-	-	9%	10%
UFH with Dosages/Platelet Monitoring[1,2]	-	-	96%	97%
Venous Thromboembolism Prophylaxis[2]	282	87%	82%	85%
Warfarin Therapy Discharge Instructions[1,2]	-	-	84%	75%
Chest Pain/Possible Heart Attack Care				
Aspirin Given Within 24 Hours of Arrival	21	95%	94%	96%
Fibrinolytic Meds Within 30 Min. of Arrival[7]	-	-	47%	58%
Average Time to ECG (minutes)	20	15	8	7
Average Time to Transfer (minutes)[7]	-	-	62	60
Children's Asthma Care				
Received Home Management Plan of Care	-	-	93%	88%
Received Reliever Medication	-	-	100%	100%
Received Systemic Corticosteroids	-	-	100%	100%
Emergency Department				
Admittance Decision Time (minutes)[2]	370	66	99	98
Head CT Results Within 45 Min. of Arrival[1]	-	-	54%	57%
Patients Who Left ER Before Being Seen	17,819	3%	3%	2%
Time from ER Arrival to Admit. (minutes)[2]	371	254	270	274
Time from ER Arrival to Discharge (minutes)	762	140	127	134
Time in ER Before Being Evaluated (minutes)	821	27	26	26
Time to Pain Meds for Fractures (minutes)	139	66	57	57
Heart Attack Care				
Aspirin Given at Discharge	46	100%	99%	99%
Fibrinolytic Meds Within 30 Min. of Arrival[7]	-	-	49%	54%
PCI Within 90 Minutes of Arrival	12	92%	95%	96%
Statin Prescribed at Discharge	44	98%	98%	98%
Heart Failure Care				
ACE Inhibitor or ARB for LVSD	42	93%	97%	97%
Discharge Instructions Given	110	80%	95%	94%
Evaluation of LVS Function	120	99%	99%	99%
Medicare Spending				
Medicare Spending per Patient (ratio)	-	0.96	1.03	0.98
Pneumonia Care				
Appropriate Initial Antibiotic Given	70	97%	95%	95%
Blood Culture Timing	92	97%	98%	98%
Pregnancy and Delivery Care				
Newborn Deliveries Scheduled Early	87	5%	7%	6%
Preventive Care				
Immunization for Influenza[2]	287	32%	90%	90%
Immunization for Pneumonia[2]	325	37%	92%	92%
Stroke Care				
Anticoagulation Therapy for Atrial Fibrillation[1]	-	-	96%	95%
Antithrombotic Therapy Timing	23	100%	98%	98%
Assessed for Rehabilitation	21	95%	98%	97%
Discharged on Antithrombotic Therapy	20	100%	99%	99%
Discharged on Statin Medication	16	81%	95%	94%
Thrombolytic Therapy Timing[1]	-	-	68%	66%
Venous Thromboembolism Prophylaxis	24	92%	94%	94%
Written Stroke Educational Materials Given	15	20%	92%	88%
Surgical Care Improvement Project				
Appropriate Beta Blocker Usage	27	85%	98%	98%
Appropriate VTP Within 24 Hours	114	95%	98%	98%
Controlled Postoperative Blood Glucose[7]	-	-	96%	97%
Perioperative Temperature Management	150	100%	100%	100%
Prophylactic Antibiotic Selection	95	98%	99%	99%
Prophylactic Antibiotic Selection (Outpatient)	120	99%	98%	98%
Prophylactic Antibiotic Stopped	89	90%	98%	98%
Prophylactic Antibiotic Timing	96	100%	99%	99%
Prophylactic Antibiotic Timing (Outpatient)	122	96%	98%	98%
Urinary Catheter Removal	63	94%	98%	97%
Survey of Patients' Hospital Experiences				
Area Around Room 'Always' Quiet at Night	300+	74%	68%	61%
Doctors 'Always' Communicated Well	300+	86%	83%	82%
Home Recovery Information Given	300+	88%	85%	85%
Hospital Given 9 or 10 on 10 Point Scale	300+	79%	73%	71%
Meds 'Always' Explained Before Given	300+	66%	66%	64%
Nurses 'Always' Communicated Well	300+	81%	80%	79%
Pain 'Always' Well Controlled	300+	71%	72%	71%
Room and Bathroom 'Always' Clean	300+	73%	75%	73%
Timely Help 'Always' Received	300+	70%	69%	68%
Would Definitely Recommend Hospital	300+	80%	73%	71%
Use of Medical Imaging				
Cardiac Imaging Stress Test before Surgery	86	7.0%	5.3%	5.3%
Combination Abdominal CT Scan	218	2.3%	16.4%	10.5%
Combination Brain/Sinus CT Scan[1]	-	-	2.7%	2.7%
Combination Chest CT Scan	82	0.0%	5.6%	2.7%
Follow-up Mammogram/Ultrasound	54	27.8%	7.9%	8.8%
Lumbar Spine MRI for Low Back Pain[1]	-	-	39.6%	37.2%

NOTE: Hospital profiles are in alphabetical order by state, then city, then hospital within the city; Rankings exclude hospitals with less than 25 cases except for patient surveys which excludes hospitals with less than 100 cases; (a) 100-299 cases; (1) The number of cases/patients is too few to report; (2) Data submitted were based on a sample of cases/patients; (3) Results are based on a shorter time period than required; (4) Data suppressed by CMS for one or more quarters; (5) Results are not available for this reporting period; (6) Fewer than 100 patients completed the HCAHPS survey; (7) No cases met the criteria for this measure; (8) The lower limit of the confidence interval cannot be calculated if the number of observed infections equals zero; (9) No data are available from the state/territory for this reporting period; (10) The scores shown reflect fewer than 50 completed surveys; (11) There were discrepancies in the data collection process; (12) This measure does not apply to this hospital for this reporting period; (13) Results cannot be calculated for this reporting period; (14) The results for this state are combined with nearby states to protect confidentiality; Please refer to the User's Guide for a full explanation of data.

Harlingen Medical Center

5501 South Expressway 77
Harlingen, TX 78550
Phone: 956-365-1000
Fax: 956-365-1875
URL: www.harlingenmedicalcenter.com
Type: Acute Care Hospitals
Emergency Services: Yes
Ownership: Proprietary
Beds: 80

Key Personnel:
Chief of Medical Staff .... Ruby Byrd
CEO/President .... Brenda Ivory
Emergency Room .... Arturo Rodriguez

Measure	Cases	This Hosp.	State Avg.	U.S. Avg.
Blood Clot Prevention and Treatment				
Anticoagulation Overlap Therapy[2]	16	100%	93%	93%
ICU Venous Thromboembolism Prophylaxis[2]	71	82%	92%	92%
Incidence of Potentially Preventable VTE[1,2]	-	-	9%	10%
UFH with Dosages/Platelet Monitoring[1,2]	-	-	96%	97%
Venous Thromboembolism Prophylaxis[2]	323	75%	82%	85%
Warfarin Therapy Discharge Instructions[2]	12	92%	84%	75%
Chest Pain/Possible Heart Attack Care				
Aspirin Given Within 24 Hours of Arrival[5]	-	-	94%	96%
Fibrinolytic Meds Within 30 Min. of Arrival[5]	-	-	47%	58%
Average Time to ECG (minutes)[5]	-	-	8	7
Average Time to Transfer (minutes)[5]	-	-	62	60
Children's Asthma Care				
Received Home Management Plan of Care	-	-	93%	88%
Received Reliever Medication	-	-	100%	100%
Received Systemic Corticosteroids	-	-	100%	100%
Emergency Department				
Admittance Decision Time (minutes)[2]	613	91	99	98
Head CT Results Within 45 Min. of Arrival[1]	-	-	54%	57%
Patients Who Left ER Before Being Seen	29,594	1%	3%	2%
Time from ER Arrival to Admit. (minutes)[2]	616	249	270	274
Time from ER Arrival to Discharge (minutes)	371	118	127	134
Time in ER Before Being Evaluated (minutes)	392	20	26	26
Time to Pain Meds for Fractures (minutes)	155	43	57	57
Heart Attack Care				
Aspirin Given at Discharge	119	99%	99%	99%
Fibrinolytic Meds Within 30 Min. of Arrival[7]	-	-	49%	54%
PCI Within 90 Minutes of Arrival	14	86%	95%	96%
Statin Prescribed at Discharge	113	99%	98%	98%
Heart Failure Care				
ACE Inhibitor or ARB for LVSD	37	100%	97%	97%
Discharge Instructions Given	123	100%	95%	94%
Evaluation of LVS Function	138	100%	99%	99%
Medicare Spending				
Medicare Spending per Patient (ratio)	-	1.01	1.03	0.98
Pneumonia Care				
Appropriate Initial Antibiotic Given	85	100%	95%	95%
Blood Culture Timing	124	100%	98%	98%
Pregnancy and Delivery Care				
Newborn Deliveries Scheduled Early	105	4%	7%	6%
Preventive Care				
Immunization for Influenza[2]	533	99%	90%	90%
Immunization for Pneumonia[2]	654	97%	92%	92%
Stroke Care				
Anticoagulation Therapy for Atrial Fibrillation[1]	-	-	96%	95%
Antithrombotic Therapy Timing	31	100%	98%	98%
Assessed for Rehabilitation	33	85%	98%	97%
Discharged on Antithrombotic Therapy	29	100%	99%	99%
Discharged on Statin Medication	26	92%	95%	94%
Thrombolytic Therapy Timing[1]	-	-	68%	66%
Venous Thromboembolism Prophylaxis	36	64%	94%	94%
Written Stroke Educational Materials Given	25	84%	92%	88%
Surgical Care Improvement Project				
Appropriate Beta Blocker Usage[2]	187	98%	98%	98%
Appropriate VTP Within 24 Hours[2]	323	100%	98%	98%
Controlled Postoperative Blood Glucose[2]	127	99%	96%	97%
Perioperative Temperature Management[2]	380	100%	100%	100%
Prophylactic Antibiotic Selection[2]	401	100%	99%	99%
Prophylactic Antibiotic Selection (Outpatient)	107	98%	98%	98%
Prophylactic Antibiotic Stopped[2]	390	98%	98%	98%
Prophylactic Antibiotic Timing[2]	401	100%	99%	99%
Prophylactic Antibiotic Timing (Outpatient)	107	100%	98%	98%
Urinary Catheter Removal[2]	374	99%	98%	97%
Survey of Patients' Hospital Experiences				
Area Around Room 'Always' Quiet at Night[11]	300+	67%	68%	61%
Doctors 'Always' Communicated Well[11]	300+	78%	83%	82%
Home Recovery Information Given[11]	300+	87%	85%	85%
Hospital Given 9 or 10 on 10 Point Scale[11]	300+	72%	73%	71%
Meds 'Always' Explained Before Given[11]	300+	64%	66%	64%
Nurses 'Always' Communicated Well[11]	300+	76%	80%	79%
Pain 'Always' Well Controlled[11]	300+	69%	72%	71%
Room and Bathroom 'Always' Clean[11]	300+	75%	75%	73%
Timely Help 'Always' Received[11]	300+	64%	69%	68%
Would Definitely Recommend Hospital[11]	300+	77%	73%	71%
Use of Medical Imaging				
Cardiac Imaging Stress Test before Surgery[1]	-	-	5.3%	5.3%
Combination Abdominal CT Scan	340	24.1%	16.4%	10.5%
Combination Brain/Sinus CT Scan	412	2.2%	2.7%	2.7%
Combination Chest CT Scan	194	13.9%	5.6%	2.7%
Follow-up Mammogram/Ultrasound	342	2.9%	7.9%	8.8%
Lumbar Spine MRI for Low Back Pain	117	23.1%	39.6%	37.2%

VHS Harlingen Hospital Company

2101 Pease St
Harlingen, TX 78550
Phone: 956-389-1100
Fax: 956-389-1632
URL: www.vbmc.org
Type: Acute Care Hospitals
Emergency Services: Yes
Ownership: Proprietary
Beds: 588

Key Personnel:
Operating Room .... Patrick S Almond, RN
Radiology .... Robert S Andrews, MD
Infection Control .... Pat Brattin, RN
Quality Assurance .... Ward Cook
Chief of Medical Staff .... Robert Minor, MD
Pediatric Ambulatory Care ...... G Toland, MD
Pediatric In-Patient Care .... G Toland, MD

Measure	Cases	This Hosp.	State Avg.	U.S. Avg.
Blood Clot Prevention and Treatment				
Anticoagulation Overlap Therapy[2]	62	66%	93%	93%
ICU Venous Thromboembolism Prophylaxis[2]	71	94%	92%	92%
Incidence of Potentially Preventable VTE[2]	14	14%	9%	10%
UFH with Dosages/Platelet Monitoring[2]	15	93%	96%	97%
Venous Thromboembolism Prophylaxis[2]	336	54%	82%	85%
Warfarin Therapy Discharge Instructions[2]	46	91%	84%	75%
Chest Pain/Possible Heart Attack Care				
Aspirin Given Within 24 Hours of Arrival[1,3]	-	-	94%	96%
Fibrinolytic Meds Within 30 Min. of Arrival[5]	-	-	47%	58%
Average Time to ECG (minutes)[1,3]	-	-	8	7
Average Time to Transfer (minutes)[5]	-	-	62	60
Children's Asthma Care				
Received Home Management Plan of Care	-	-	93%	88%
Received Reliever Medication	-	-	100%	100%
Received Systemic Corticosteroids	-	-	100%	100%
Emergency Department				
Admittance Decision Time (minutes)[2]	565	100	99	98
Head CT Results Within 45 Min. of Arrival[1]	-	-	54%	57%
Patients Who Left ER Before Being Seen	56,970	1%	3%	2%
Time from ER Arrival to Admit. (minutes)[2]	566	283	270	274
Time from ER Arrival to Discharge (minutes)	342	189	127	134
Time in ER Before Being Evaluated (minutes)	369	67	26	26
Time to Pain Meds for Fractures (minutes)	225	58	57	57
Heart Attack Care				
Aspirin Given at Discharge	197	97%	99%	99%
Fibrinolytic Meds Within 30 Min. of Arrival[1]	-	-	49%	54%
PCI Within 90 Minutes of Arrival	26	85%	95%	96%
Statin Prescribed at Discharge	183	97%	98%	98%
Heart Failure Care				
ACE Inhibitor or ARB for LVSD	121	98%	97%	97%
Discharge Instructions Given	370	99%	95%	94%
Evaluation of LVS Function	423	99%	99%	99%
Medicare Spending				
Medicare Spending per Patient (ratio)	-	1.01	1.03	0.98
Pneumonia Care				
Appropriate Initial Antibiotic Given	241	95%	95%	95%
Blood Culture Timing	441	99%	98%	98%
Pregnancy and Delivery Care				
Newborn Deliveries Scheduled Early[2]	83	12%	7%	6%
Preventive Care				
Immunization for Influenza[2]	497	91%	90%	90%
Immunization for Pneumonia[2]	589	95%	92%	92%
Stroke Care				
Anticoagulation Therapy for Atrial Fibrillation	25	100%	96%	95%
Antithrombotic Therapy Timing	164	99%	98%	98%
Assessed for Rehabilitation	270	100%	98%	97%
Discharged on Antithrombotic Therapy	213	100%	99%	99%
Discharged on Statin Medication	152	97%	95%	94%
Thrombolytic Therapy Timing	30	97%	68%	66%
Venous Thromboembolism Prophylaxis	289	96%	94%	94%
Written Stroke Educational Materials Given	147	98%	92%	88%
Surgical Care Improvement Project				
Appropriate Beta Blocker Usage[2]	338	95%	98%	98%
Appropriate VTP Within 24 Hours[2]	886	94%	98%	98%
Controlled Postoperative Blood Glucose[2]	97	91%	96%	97%
Perioperative Temperature Management[2]	965	100%	100%	100%
Prophylactic Antibiotic Selection[2]	887	97%	99%	99%
Prophylactic Antibiotic Selection (Outpatient)	280	89%	98%	98%
Prophylactic Antibiotic Stopped[2]	876	98%	98%	98%
Prophylactic Antibiotic Timing[2]	888	99%	99%	99%
Prophylactic Antibiotic Timing (Outpatient)	292	93%	98%	98%
Urinary Catheter Removal[2]	869	94%	98%	97%
Survey of Patients' Hospital Experiences				
Area Around Room 'Always' Quiet at Night[11]	300+	59%	68%	61%
Doctors 'Always' Communicated Well[11]	300+	81%	83%	82%
Home Recovery Information Given[11]	300+	88%	85%	85%
Hospital Given 9 or 10 on 10 Point Scale[11]	300+	70%	73%	71%
Meds 'Always' Explained Before Given[11]	300+	64%	66%	64%
Nurses 'Always' Communicated Well[11]	300+	77%	80%	79%
Pain 'Always' Well Controlled[11]	300+	70%	72%	71%
Room and Bathroom 'Always' Clean[11]	300+	70%	75%	73%
Timely Help 'Always' Received[11]	300+	60%	69%	68%
Would Definitely Recommend Hospital[11]	300+	72%	73%	71%
Use of Medical Imaging				
Cardiac Imaging Stress Test before Surgery	433	4.8%	5.3%	5.3%
Combination Abdominal CT Scan	893	16.7%	16.4%	10.5%
Combination Brain/Sinus CT Scan	902	4.0%	2.7%	2.7%
Combination Chest CT Scan	307	22.5%	5.6%	2.7%
Follow-up Mammogram/Ultrasound	1,553	3.9%	7.9%	8.8%
Lumbar Spine MRI for Low Back Pain	116	32.8%	39.6%	37.2%

Haskell Memorial Hospital

1 North Avenue N PO Box 1117
Haskell, TX 79521
Phone: 940-864-2621
Type: Critical Access Hospitals
Emergency Services: Yes
Ownership: Govt - Hospital Dist/Auth

Measure	Cases	This Hosp.	State Avg.	U.S. Avg.
Blood Clot Prevention and Treatment				
Anticoagulation Overlap Therapy[5]	-	-	93%	93%
ICU Venous Thromboembolism Prophylaxis[5]	-	-	92%	92%
Incidence of Potentially Preventable VTE[5]	-	-	9%	10%
UFH with Dosages/Platelet Monitoring[5]	-	-	96%	97%
Venous Thromboembolism Prophylaxis[5]	-	-	82%	85%
Warfarin Therapy Discharge Instructions[5]	-	-	84%	75%
Chest Pain/Possible Heart Attack Care				
Aspirin Given Within 24 Hours of Arrival	-	-	94%	96%
Fibrinolytic Meds Within 30 Min. of Arrival	-	-	47%	58%
Average Time to ECG (minutes)	-	-	8	7
Average Time to Transfer (minutes)	-	-	62	60
Children's Asthma Care				
Received Home Management Plan of Care	-	-	93%	88%
Received Reliever Medication	-	-	100%	100%
Received Systemic Corticosteroids	-	-	100%	100%
Emergency Department				
Admittance Decision Time (minutes)[5]	-	-	99	98
Head CT Results Within 45 Min. of Arrival	-	-	54%	57%
Patients Who Left ER Before Being Seen	-	-	3%	2%
Time from ER Arrival to Admit. (minutes)[5]	-	-	270	274
Time from ER Arrival to Discharge (minutes)	-	-	127	134
Time in ER Before Being Evaluated (minutes)	-	-	26	26

NOTE: Hospital profiles are in alphabetical order by state, then city, then hospital within the city; Rankings exclude hospitals with less than 25 cases except for patient surveys which excludes hospitals with less than 100 cases; (a) 100-299 cases; (1) The number of cases/patients is too few to report; (2) Data submitted were based on a sample of cases/patients; (3) Results are based on a shorter time period than required; (4) Data suppressed by CMS for one or more quarters; (5) Results are not available for this reporting period; (6) Fewer than 100 patients completed the HCAHPS survey; (7) No cases met the criteria for this measure; (8) The lower limit of the confidence interval cannot be calculated if the number of observed infections equals zero; (9) No data are available from the state/territory for this reporting period; (10) The scores shown reflect fewer than 50 completed surveys; (11) There were discrepancies in the data collection process; (12) This measure does not apply to this hospital for this reporting period; (13) Results cannot be calculated for this reporting period; (14) The results for this state are combined with nearby states to protect confidentiality; Please refer to the User's Guide for a full explanation of data.

Time to Pain Meds for Fractures (minutes)	-	-	57	57
Heart Attack Care				
Aspirin Given at Discharge[5]	-	-	99%	99%
Fibrinolytic Meds Within 30 Min. of Arrival[5]	-	-	49%	54%
PCI Within 90 Minutes of Arrival[5]	-	-	95%	96%
Statin Prescribed at Discharge[5]	-	-	98%	98%
Heart Failure Care				
ACE Inhibitor or ARB for LVSD[5]	-	-	97%	97%
Discharge Instructions Given[5]	-	-	95%	94%
Evaluation of LVS Function[5]	-	-	99%	99%
Medicare Spending				
Medicare Spending per Patient (ratio)	-	-	1.03	0.98
Pneumonia Care				
Appropriate Initial Antibiotic Given[5]	-	-	95%	95%
Blood Culture Timing[5]	-	-	98%	98%
Pregnancy and Delivery Care				
Newborn Deliveries Scheduled Early[5]	-	-	7%	6%
Preventive Care				
Immunization for Influenza[5]	-	-	90%	90%
Immunization for Pneumonia[5]	-	-	92%	92%
Stroke Care				
Anticoagulation Therapy for Atrial Fibrillation[5]	-	-	96%	95%
Antithrombotic Therapy Timing[5]	-	-	98%	98%
Assessed for Rehabilitation[5]	-	-	98%	97%
Discharged on Antithrombotic Therapy[5]	-	-	99%	99%
Discharged on Statin Medication[5]	-	-	95%	94%
Thrombolytic Therapy Timing[5]	-	-	68%	66%
Venous Thromboembolism Prophylaxis[5]	-	-	94%	94%
Written Stroke Educational Materials Given[5]	-	-	92%	88%
Surgical Care Improvement Project				
Appropriate Beta Blocker Usage[5]	-	-	98%	98%
Appropriate VTP Within 24 Hours[5]	-	-	98%	98%
Controlled Postoperative Blood Glucose[5]	-	-	96%	97%
Perioperative Temperature Management[5]	-	-	100%	100%
Prophylactic Antibiotic Selection[5]	-	-	99%	99%
Prophylactic Antibiotic Selection (Outpatient)	-	-	98%	98%
Prophylactic Antibiotic Stopped[5]	-	-	98%	98%
Prophylactic Antibiotic Timing[5]	-	-	99%	99%
Prophylactic Antibiotic Timing (Outpatient)	-	-	98%	98%
Urinary Catheter Removal[5]	-	-	98%	97%
Survey of Patients' Hospital Experiences				
Area Around Room 'Always' Quiet at Night[5]	-	-	68%	61%
Doctors 'Always' Communicated Well[5]	-	-	83%	82%
Home Recovery Information Given[5]	-	-	85%	85%
Hospital Given 9 or 10 on 10 Point Scale[5]	-	-	73%	71%
Meds 'Always' Explained Before Given[5]	-	-	66%	64%
Nurses 'Always' Communicated Well[5]	-	-	80%	79%
Pain 'Always' Well Controlled[5]	-	-	72%	71%
Room and Bathroom 'Always' Clean[5]	-	-	75%	73%
Timely Help 'Always' Received[5]	-	-	69%	68%
Would Definitely Recommend Hospital[5]	-	-	73%	71%
Use of Medical Imaging				
Cardiac Imaging Stress Test before Surgery	-	-	5.3%	5.3%
Combination Abdominal CT Scan	-	-	16.4%	10.5%
Combination Brain/Sinus CT Scan	-	-	2.7%	2.7%
Combination Chest CT Scan	-	-	5.6%	2.7%
Follow-up Mammogram/Ultrasound	-	-	7.9%	8.8%
Lumbar Spine MRI for Low Back Pain	-	-	39.6%	37.2%

Sabine County Hospital

2301 Hwy 83 W — Phone: 409-787-3300
Hemphill, TX 75948
Type: Critical Access Hospitals — Emergency Services: Yes
Ownership: Govt - Hospital Dist/Auth

Measure	Cases	This Hosp.	State Avg.	U.S. Avg.
Blood Clot Prevention and Treatment				
Anticoagulation Overlap Therapy[5]	-	-	93%	93%
ICU Venous Thromboembolism Prophylaxis[5]	-	-	92%	92%
Incidence of Potentially Preventable VTE[5]	-	-	9%	10%
UFH with Dosages/Platelet Monitoring[5]	-	-	96%	97%
Venous Thromboembolism Prophylaxis[5]	-	-	82%	85%
Warfarin Therapy Discharge Instructions[5]	-	-	84%	75%
Chest Pain/Possible Heart Attack Care				
Aspirin Given Within 24 Hours of Arrival	-	-	94%	96%
Fibrinolytic Meds Within 30 Min. of Arrival	-	-	47%	58%
Average Time to ECG (minutes)	-	-	8	7
Average Time to Transfer (minutes)	-	-	62	60
Children's Asthma Care				
Received Home Management Plan of Care	-	-	93%	88%
Received Reliever Medication	-	-	100%	100%
Received Systemic Corticosteroids	-	-	100%	100%
Emergency Department				
Admittance Decision Time (minutes)[5]	-	-	99	98
Head CT Results Within 45 Min. of Arrival	-	-	54%	57%
Patients Who Left ER Before Being Seen	-	-	3%	2%
Time from ER Arrival to Admit. (minutes)[5]	-	-	270	274
Time from ER Arrival to Discharge (minutes)	-	-	127	134
Time in ER Before Being Evaluated (minutes)	-	-	26	26
Time to Pain Meds for Fractures (minutes)	-	-	57	57
Heart Attack Care				
Aspirin Given at Discharge[5]	-	-	99%	99%
Fibrinolytic Meds Within 30 Min. of Arrival[5]	-	-	49%	54%
PCI Within 90 Minutes of Arrival[5]	-	-	95%	96%
Statin Prescribed at Discharge[5]	-	-	98%	98%
Heart Failure Care				
ACE Inhibitor or ARB for LVSD[7]	-	-	97%	97%
Discharge Instructions Given[1]	-	-	95%	94%
Evaluation of LVS Function	11	18%	99%	99%
Medicare Spending				
Medicare Spending per Patient (ratio)	-	-	1.03	0.98
Pneumonia Care				
Appropriate Initial Antibiotic Given	34	68%	95%	95%
Blood Culture Timing	15	80%	98%	98%
Pregnancy and Delivery Care				
Newborn Deliveries Scheduled Early[5]	-	-	7%	6%
Preventive Care				
Immunization for Influenza[5]	-	-	90%	90%
Immunization for Pneumonia[5]	-	-	92%	92%
Stroke Care				
Anticoagulation Therapy for Atrial Fibrillation[5]	-	-	96%	95%
Antithrombotic Therapy Timing[5]	-	-	98%	98%
Assessed for Rehabilitation[5]	-	-	98%	97%
Discharged on Antithrombotic Therapy[5]	-	-	99%	99%
Discharged on Statin Medication[5]	-	-	95%	94%
Thrombolytic Therapy Timing[5]	-	-	68%	66%
Venous Thromboembolism Prophylaxis[5]	-	-	94%	94%
Written Stroke Educational Materials Given[5]	-	-	92%	88%
Surgical Care Improvement Project				
Appropriate Beta Blocker Usage[5]	-	-	98%	98%
Appropriate VTP Within 24 Hours[5]	-	-	98%	98%
Controlled Postoperative Blood Glucose[5]	-	-	96%	97%
Perioperative Temperature Management[5]	-	-	100%	100%
Prophylactic Antibiotic Selection[5]	-	-	99%	99%
Prophylactic Antibiotic Selection (Outpatient)	-	-	98%	98%
Prophylactic Antibiotic Stopped[5]	-	-	98%	98%
Prophylactic Antibiotic Timing[5]	-	-	99%	99%
Prophylactic Antibiotic Timing (Outpatient)	-	-	98%	98%
Urinary Catheter Removal[5]	-	-	98%	97%
Survey of Patients' Hospital Experiences				
Area Around Room 'Always' Quiet at Night[5]	-	-	68%	61%
Doctors 'Always' Communicated Well[5]	-	-	83%	82%
Home Recovery Information Given[5]	-	-	85%	85%
Hospital Given 9 or 10 on 10 Point Scale[5]	-	-	73%	71%
Meds 'Always' Explained Before Given[5]	-	-	66%	64%
Nurses 'Always' Communicated Well[5]	-	-	80%	79%
Pain 'Always' Well Controlled[5]	-	-	72%	71%
Room and Bathroom 'Always' Clean[5]	-	-	75%	73%
Timely Help 'Always' Received[5]	-	-	69%	68%
Would Definitely Recommend Hospital[5]	-	-	73%	71%
Use of Medical Imaging				
Cardiac Imaging Stress Test before Surgery	-	-	5.3%	5.3%
Combination Abdominal CT Scan	-	-	16.4%	10.5%
Combination Brain/Sinus CT Scan	-	-	2.7%	2.7%
Combination Chest CT Scan	-	-	5.6%	2.7%
Follow-up Mammogram/Ultrasound	-	-	7.9%	8.8%
Lumbar Spine MRI for Low Back Pain	-	-	39.6%	37.2%

Etmc Henderson

300 Wilson Street — Phone: 903-657-7541
Henderson, TX 75652 — Fax: 903-655-3661
URL: www.hmhtx.org
Type: Acute Care Hospitals — Emergency Services: Yes
Ownership: Voluntary non-profit - Private — Beds: 158

Key Personnel:
Intensive Care Unit. . . . . Dorothy Boone, RN
Operating Room. . . . . Brian Camazine, RN
Emergency Room . . . . Tom Curtis, MD
Infection Control. . . . . Tammy Koonce
CEO/President. . . . . Mark Leitner
Radiology. . . . . John Melvin, MD
Chief of Medical Staff . . . . Yogesh Pai, MD
Quality Assurance . . . . Chad Palmer

Measure	Cases	This Hosp.	State Avg.	U.S. Avg.
Blood Clot Prevention and Treatment				
Anticoagulation Overlap Therapy[1,2]	-	-	93%	93%
ICU Venous Thromboembolism Prophylaxis[1,2]	-	-	92%	92%
Incidence of Potentially Preventable VTE[2,7]	-	-	9%	10%
UFH with Dosages/Platelet Monitoring[1,2]	-	-	96%	97%
Venous Thromboembolism Prophylaxis[2]	148	55%	82%	85%
Warfarin Therapy Discharge Instructions[1,2]	-	-	84%	75%
Chest Pain/Possible Heart Attack Care				
Aspirin Given Within 24 Hours of Arrival	42	93%	94%	96%
Fibrinolytic Meds Within 30 Min. of Arrival[1]	-	-	47%	58%
Average Time to ECG (minutes)	49	7	8	7
Average Time to Transfer (minutes)[1]	-	-	62	60
Children's Asthma Care				
Received Home Management Plan of Care	-	-	93%	88%
Received Reliever Medication	-	-	100%	100%
Received Systemic Corticosteroids	-	-	100%	100%
Emergency Department				
Admittance Decision Time (minutes)[2]	296	72	99	98
Head CT Results Within 45 Min. of Arrival[1]	-	-	54%	57%
Patients Who Left ER Before Being Seen	14,008	2%	3%	2%
Time from ER Arrival to Admit. (minutes)[2]	313	241	270	274
Time from ER Arrival to Discharge (minutes)	358	142	127	134
Time in ER Before Being Evaluated (minutes)	390	23	26	26
Time to Pain Meds for Fractures (minutes)	77	51	57	57
Heart Attack Care				
Aspirin Given at Discharge[1]	-	-	99%	99%
Fibrinolytic Meds Within 30 Min. of Arrival[7]	-	-	49%	54%
PCI Within 90 Minutes of Arrival[7]	-	-	95%	96%
Statin Prescribed at Discharge[1]	-	-	98%	98%
Heart Failure Care				
ACE Inhibitor or ARB for LVSD[1]	-	-	97%	97%
Discharge Instructions Given	40	90%	95%	94%
Evaluation of LVS Function	51	84%	99%	99%
Medicare Spending				
Medicare Spending per Patient (ratio)	-	1.05	1.03	0.98
Pneumonia Care				
Appropriate Initial Antibiotic Given	44	91%	95%	95%
Blood Culture Timing	76	96%	98%	98%
Pregnancy and Delivery Care				
Newborn Deliveries Scheduled Early	24	17%	7%	6%
Preventive Care				
Immunization for Influenza[2]	261	63%	90%	90%
Immunization for Pneumonia[2]	305	88%	92%	92%
Stroke Care				
Anticoagulation Therapy for Atrial Fibrillation[1]	-	-	96%	95%
Antithrombotic Therapy Timing[1]	-	-	98%	98%
Assessed for Rehabilitation[1]	-	-	98%	97%
Discharged on Antithrombotic Therapy[1]	-	-	99%	99%
Discharged on Statin Medication[1]	-	-	95%	94%
Thrombolytic Therapy Timing[1]	-	-	68%	66%
Venous Thromboembolism Prophylaxis[1]	-	-	94%	94%
Written Stroke Educational Materials Given[1]	-	-	92%	88%
Surgical Care Improvement Project				
Appropriate Beta Blocker Usage	20	85%	98%	98%
Appropriate VTP Within 24 Hours	59	98%	98%	98%

NOTE: Hospital profiles are in alphabetical order by state, then city, then hospital within the city; Rankings exclude hospitals with less than 25 cases except for patient surveys which excludes hospitals with less than 100 cases; (a) 100-299 cases; (1) The number of cases/patients is too few to report; (2) Data submitted were based on a sample of cases/patients; (3) Results are based on a shorter time period than required; (4) Data suppressed by CMS for one or more quarters; (5) Results are not available for this reporting period; (6) Fewer than 100 patients completed the HCAHPS survey; (7) No cases met the criteria for this measure; (8) The lower limit of the confidence interval cannot be calculated if the number of observed infections equals zero; (9) No data are available from the state/territory for this reporting period; (10) The scores shown reflect fewer than 50 completed surveys; (11) There were discrepancies in the data collection process; (12) This measure does not apply to this hospital for this reporting period; (13) Results cannot be calculated for this reporting period; (14) The results for this state are combined with nearby states to protect confidentiality; Please refer to the User's Guide for a full explanation of data.

Measure	Cases	This Hosp.	State Avg.	U.S. Avg.
Controlled Postoperative Blood Glucose[7]	-	-	96%	97%
Perioperative Temperature Management	75	100%	100%	100%
Prophylactic Antibiotic Selection	46	96%	99%	99%
Prophylactic Antibiotic Selection (Outpatient)[1,3]	-	-	98%	98%
Prophylactic Antibiotic Stopped	44	100%	98%	98%
Prophylactic Antibiotic Timing	46	93%	99%	99%
Prophylactic Antibiotic Timing (Outpatient)[1,3]	-	-	98%	98%
Urinary Catheter Removal	41	88%	98%	97%
Survey of Patients' Hospital Experiences				
Area Around Room 'Always' Quiet at Night	300+	72%	68%	61%
Doctors 'Always' Communicated Well	300+	83%	83%	82%
Home Recovery Information Given	300+	83%	85%	85%
Hospital Given 9 or 10 on 10 Point Scale	300+	69%	73%	71%
Meds 'Always' Explained Before Given	300+	67%	66%	64%
Nurses 'Always' Communicated Well	300+	79%	80%	79%
Pain 'Always' Well Controlled	300+	70%	72%	71%
Room and Bathroom 'Always' Clean	300+	76%	75%	73%
Timely Help 'Always' Received	300+	67%	69%	68%
Would Definitely Recommend Hospital	300+	67%	73%	71%
Use of Medical Imaging				
Cardiac Imaging Stress Test before Surgery[1]	-	-	5.3%	5.3%
Combination Abdominal CT Scan	240	13.8%	16.4%	10.5%
Combination Brain/Sinus CT Scan[1]	-	-	2.7%	2.7%
Combination Chest CT Scan	97	10.3%	5.6%	2.7%
Follow-up Mammogram/Ultrasound	330	7.3%	7.9%	8.8%
Lumbar Spine MRI for Low Back Pain[1]	-	-	39.6%	37.2%

Hereford Regional Medical Center

801 East Third
Hereford, TX 79045
Phone: 806-364-2141
Fax: 806-349-9373
URL: www.herefordtx.org/deafsmithco/healthcare.htm
Type: Acute Care Hospitals
Emergency Services: Yes
Ownership: Govt - Hospital Dist/Auth
Beds: 40

Key Personnel:
Emergency Room . . . . Brinda Cozeby
Chief of Medical Staff. . . . . Nadir Khuri, MD
Quality Assurance . . . . Sheri Nedins
CEO/President. . . . . James Taylor

Measure	Cases	This Hosp.	State Avg.	U.S. Avg.
Blood Clot Prevention and Treatment				
Anticoagulation Overlap Therapy[1,2]	-	-	93%	93%
ICU Venous Thromboembolism Prophylaxis[1,2]	-	-	92%	92%
Incidence of Potentially Preventable VTE[2,7]	-	-	9%	10%
UFH with Dosages/Platelet Monitoring[1,2]	-	-	96%	97%
Venous Thromboembolism Prophylaxis[2]	129	71%	82%	85%
Warfarin Therapy Discharge Instructions[1,2]	-	-	84%	75%
Chest Pain/Possible Heart Attack Care				
Aspirin Given Within 24 Hours of Arrival	24	88%	94%	96%
Fibrinolytic Meds Within 30 Min. of Arrival[1]	-	-	47%	58%
Average Time to ECG (minutes)	24	7	8	7
Average Time to Transfer (minutes)[1]	-	-	62	60
Children's Asthma Care				
Received Home Management Plan of Care	-	-	93%	88%
Received Reliever Medication	-	-	100%	100%
Received Systemic Corticosteroids	-	-	100%	100%
Emergency Department				
Admittance Decision Time (minutes)[2]	140	75	99	98
Head CT Results Within 45 Min. of Arrival[1]	-	-	54%	57%
Patients Who Left ER Before Being Seen	7,761	1%	3%	2%
Time from ER Arrival to Admit. (minutes)[2]	261	217	270	274
Time from ER Arrival to Discharge (minutes)	344	109	127	134
Time in ER Before Being Evaluated (minutes)	367	30	26	26
Time to Pain Meds for Fractures (minutes)	24	48	57	57
Heart Attack Care				
Aspirin Given at Discharge[1,3]	-	-	99%	99%
Fibrinolytic Meds Within 30 Min. of Arrival[3,7]	-	-	49%	54%
PCI Within 90 Minutes of Arrival[3,7]	-	-	95%	96%
Statin Prescribed at Discharge[1,3]	-	-	98%	98%
Heart Failure Care				
ACE Inhibitor or ARB for LVSD[1]	-	-	97%	97%
Discharge Instructions Given	16	31%	95%	94%
Evaluation of LVS Function	20	90%	99%	99%
Medicare Spending				
Medicare Spending per Patient (ratio)	-	1.03	1.03	0.98
Pneumonia Care				
Appropriate Initial Antibiotic Given[1]	-	-	95%	95%
Blood Culture Timing	19	100%	98%	98%
Pregnancy and Delivery Care				
Newborn Deliveries Scheduled Early	51	8%	7%	6%
Preventive Care				
Immunization for Influenza[2]	254	17%	90%	90%
Immunization for Pneumonia[2]	186	29%	92%	92%
Stroke Care				
Anticoagulation Therapy for Atrial Fibrillation[1]	-	-	96%	95%
Antithrombotic Therapy Timing[1]	-	-	98%	98%
Assessed for Rehabilitation[1]	-	-	98%	97%
Discharged on Antithrombotic Therapy[1]	-	-	99%	99%
Discharged on Statin Medication[1]	-	-	95%	94%
Thrombolytic Therapy Timing[7]	-	-	68%	66%
Venous Thromboembolism Prophylaxis[1]	-	-	94%	94%
Written Stroke Educational Materials Given[7]	-	-	92%	88%
Surgical Care Improvement Project				
Appropriate Beta Blocker Usage[1]	-	-	98%	98%
Appropriate VTP Within 24 Hours	23	100%	98%	98%
Controlled Postoperative Blood Glucose[7]	-	-	96%	97%
Perioperative Temperature Management	24	100%	100%	100%
Prophylactic Antibiotic Selection	19	100%	99%	99%
Prophylactic Antibiotic Selection (Outpatient)[3,7]	-	-	98%	98%
Prophylactic Antibiotic Stopped	19	95%	98%	98%
Prophylactic Antibiotic Timing	19	68%	99%	99%
Prophylactic Antibiotic Timing (Outpatient)[3,7]	-	-	98%	98%
Urinary Catheter Removal	11	82%	98%	97%
Survey of Patients' Hospital Experiences				
Area Around Room 'Always' Quiet at Night	(a)	67%	68%	61%
Doctors 'Always' Communicated Well	(a)	83%	83%	82%
Home Recovery Information Given	(a)	77%	85%	85%
Hospital Given 9 or 10 on 10 Point Scale	(a)	64%	73%	71%
Meds 'Always' Explained Before Given	(a)	66%	66%	64%
Nurses 'Always' Communicated Well	(a)	75%	80%	79%
Pain 'Always' Well Controlled	(a)	69%	72%	71%
Room and Bathroom 'Always' Clean	(a)	80%	75%	73%
Timely Help 'Always' Received	(a)	69%	69%	68%
Would Definitely Recommend Hospital	(a)	61%	73%	71%
Use of Medical Imaging				
Cardiac Imaging Stress Test before Surgery[1]	-	-	5.3%	5.3%
Combination Abdominal CT Scan	92	2.2%	16.4%	10.5%
Combination Brain/Sinus CT Scan[1]	-	-	2.7%	2.7%
Combination Chest CT Scan[1]	-	-	5.6%	2.7%
Follow-up Mammogram/Ultrasound[1]	-	-	7.9%	8.8%
Lumbar Spine MRI for Low Back Pain[1]	-	-	39.6%	37.2%

Hill Regional Hospital

101 Circle Drive
Hillsboro, TX 76645
Phone: 254-580-8500
Fax: 254-582-2144
URL: www.hillregionalhospital.com
Type: Acute Care Hospitals
Emergency Services: Yes
Ownership: Voluntary non-profit - Private
Beds: 92

Key Personnel:
Radiology. . . . . Patricia Barnes
Pediatric In-Patient Care . . . . Carol Beyer, MD
Chief of Medical Staff. . . . . Paul Floy
Intensive Care Unit. . . . . Janice Markwardt
CEO/President. . . . . Jan McClure
Infection Control. . . . . Patricia Perez
Operating Room. . . . . Kay Wooten, RN

Measure	Cases	This Hosp.	State Avg.	U.S. Avg.
Blood Clot Prevention and Treatment				
Anticoagulation Overlap Therapy[2]	12	100%	93%	93%
ICU Venous Thromboembolism Prophylaxis[2]	17	88%	92%	92%
Incidence of Potentially Preventable VTE[1,2]	-	-	9%	10%
UFH with Dosages/Platelet Monitoring[2,7]	-	-	96%	97%
Venous Thromboembolism Prophylaxis[2]	221	81%	82%	85%
Warfarin Therapy Discharge Instructions[1,2]	-	-	84%	75%
Chest Pain/Possible Heart Attack Care				
Aspirin Given Within 24 Hours of Arrival	31	97%	94%	96%
Fibrinolytic Meds Within 30 Min. of Arrival[1]	-	-	47%	58%
Average Time to ECG (minutes)	35	5	8	7
Average Time to Transfer (minutes)[1]	-	-	62	60
Children's Asthma Care				
Received Home Management Plan of Care	-	-	93%	88%
Received Reliever Medication	-	-	100%	100%
Received Systemic Corticosteroids	-	-	100%	100%
Emergency Department				
Admittance Decision Time (minutes)[2]	280	43	99	98
Head CT Results Within 45 Min. of Arrival[1]	-	-	54%	57%
Patients Who Left ER Before Being Seen	11,387	1%	3%	2%
Time from ER Arrival to Admit. (minutes)[2]	280	160	270	274
Time from ER Arrival to Discharge (minutes)	390	70	127	134
Time in ER Before Being Evaluated (minutes)	419	9	26	26
Time to Pain Meds for Fractures (minutes)	50	35	57	57
Heart Attack Care				
Aspirin Given at Discharge[1]	-	-	99%	99%
Fibrinolytic Meds Within 30 Min. of Arrival[7]	-	-	49%	54%
PCI Within 90 Minutes of Arrival[7]	-	-	95%	96%
Statin Prescribed at Discharge	11	91%	98%	98%
Heart Failure Care				
ACE Inhibitor or ARB for LVSD[1]	-	-	97%	97%
Discharge Instructions Given	40	98%	95%	94%
Evaluation of LVS Function	55	100%	99%	99%
Medicare Spending				
Medicare Spending per Patient (ratio)	-	0.86	1.03	0.98
Pneumonia Care				
Appropriate Initial Antibiotic Given	47	98%	95%	95%
Blood Culture Timing	60	98%	98%	98%
Pregnancy and Delivery Care				
Newborn Deliveries Scheduled Early[2]	18	6%	7%	6%
Preventive Care				
Immunization for Influenza[2]	285	90%	90%	90%
Immunization for Pneumonia[2]	341	96%	92%	92%
Stroke Care				
Anticoagulation Therapy for Atrial Fibrillation[1]	-	-	96%	95%
Antithrombotic Therapy Timing[1]	-	-	98%	98%
Assessed for Rehabilitation	12	92%	98%	97%
Discharged on Antithrombotic Therapy[1]	-	-	99%	99%
Discharged on Statin Medication[1]	-	-	95%	94%
Thrombolytic Therapy Timing[7]	-	-	68%	66%
Venous Thromboembolism Prophylaxis	13	92%	94%	94%
Written Stroke Educational Materials Given[1]	-	-	92%	88%
Surgical Care Improvement Project				
Appropriate Beta Blocker Usage[1]	-	-	98%	98%
Appropriate VTP Within 24 Hours	55	93%	98%	98%
Controlled Postoperative Blood Glucose[7]	-	-	96%	97%
Perioperative Temperature Management	61	100%	100%	100%
Prophylactic Antibiotic Selection	41	83%	99%	99%
Prophylactic Antibiotic Selection (Outpatient)[1,3]	-	-	98%	98%
Prophylactic Antibiotic Stopped	40	80%	98%	98%
Prophylactic Antibiotic Timing	41	95%	99%	99%
Prophylactic Antibiotic Timing (Outpatient)[1,3]	-	-	98%	98%
Urinary Catheter Removal	43	98%	98%	97%
Survey of Patients' Hospital Experiences				
Area Around Room 'Always' Quiet at Night	300+	71%	68%	61%
Doctors 'Always' Communicated Well	300+	90%	83%	82%
Home Recovery Information Given	300+	85%	85%	85%
Hospital Given 9 or 10 on 10 Point Scale	300+	71%	73%	71%
Meds 'Always' Explained Before Given	300+	69%	66%	64%
Nurses 'Always' Communicated Well	300+	79%	80%	79%
Pain 'Always' Well Controlled	300+	68%	72%	71%
Room and Bathroom 'Always' Clean	300+	76%	75%	73%
Timely Help 'Always' Received	300+	72%	69%	68%
Would Definitely Recommend Hospital	300+	69%	73%	71%
Use of Medical Imaging				
Cardiac Imaging Stress Test before Surgery	52	3.8%	5.3%	5.3%
Combination Abdominal CT Scan	168	22.6%	16.4%	10.5%
Combination Brain/Sinus CT Scan	188	1.1%	2.7%	2.7%
Combination Chest CT Scan	65	7.7%	5.6%	2.7%
Follow-up Mammogram/Ultrasound	513	5.1%	7.9%	8.8%
Lumbar Spine MRI for Low Back Pain	34	47.1%	39.6%	37.2%

NOTE: Hospital profiles are in alphabetical order by state, then city, then hospital within the city; Rankings exclude hospitals with less than 25 cases except for patient surveys which excludes hospitals with less than 100 cases; (a) 100-299 cases; (1) The number of cases/patients is too few to report; (2) Data submitted were based on a sample of cases/patients; (3) Results are based on a shorter time period than required; (4) Data suppressed by CMS for one or more quarters; (5) Results are not available for this reporting period; (6) Fewer than 100 patients completed the HCAHPS survey; (7) No cases met the criteria for this measure; (8) The lower limit of the confidence interval cannot be calculated if the number of observed infections equals zero; (9) No data are available from the state/territory for this reporting period; (10) The scores shown reflect fewer than 50 completed surveys; (11) There were discrepancies in the data collection process; (12) This measure does not apply to this hospital for this reporting period; (13) Results cannot be calculated for this reporting period; (14) The results for this state are combined with nearby states to protect confidentiality; Please refer to the User's Guide for a full explanation of data.

Medina Regional Hospital

3100 Avenue E Phone: 830-426-7700
Hondo, TX 78861 Fax: 830-426-7479
E-mail: cgarcia@medinahospital.net
URL: www.medinahospital.net
Type: Critical Access Hospitals Emergency Services: Yes
Ownership: Voluntary non-profit - Other Beds: 25

Key Personnel:
Chief of Medical Staff. . . . . John Meyer
Emergency Room . . . . Kerry Porter, RN
Patient Relations . . . . Donna Sharp
Radiology. . . . . Stephanie Wanat

Measure	Cases	This Hosp.	State Avg.	U.S. Avg.
Blood Clot Prevention and Treatment				
Anticoagulation Overlap Therapy[5]	-	-	93%	93%
ICU Venous Thromboembolism Prophylaxis[5]	-	-	92%	92%
Incidence of Potentially Preventable VTE[5]	-	-	9%	10%
UFH with Dosages/Platelet Monitoring[5]	-	-	96%	97%
Venous Thromboembolism Prophylaxis[5]	-	-	82%	85%
Warfarin Therapy Discharge Instructions[5]	-	-	84%	75%
Chest Pain/Possible Heart Attack Care				
Aspirin Given Within 24 Hours of Arrival	-	-	94%	96%
Fibrinolytic Meds Within 30 Min. of Arrival	-	-	47%	58%
Average Time to ECG (minutes)	-	-	8	7
Average Time to Transfer (minutes)	-	-	62	60
Children's Asthma Care				
Received Home Management Plan of Care	-	-	93%	88%
Received Reliever Medication	-	-	100%	100%
Received Systemic Corticosteroids	-	-	100%	100%
Emergency Department				
Admittance Decision Time (minutes)[3]	272	80	99	98
Head CT Results Within 45 Min. of Arrival	-	-	54%	57%
Patients Who Left ER Before Being Seen	-	-	3%	2%
Time from ER Arrival to Admit. (minutes)[3]	273	280	270	274
Time from ER Arrival to Discharge (minutes)	-	-	127	134
Time in ER Before Being Evaluated (minutes)	-	-	26	26
Time to Pain Meds for Fractures (minutes)	-	-	57	57
Heart Attack Care				
Aspirin Given at Discharge[5]	-	-	99%	99%
Fibrinolytic Meds Within 30 Min. of Arrival[5]	-	-	49%	54%
PCI Within 90 Minutes of Arrival[5]	-	-	95%	96%
Statin Prescribed at Discharge[5]	-	-	98%	98%
Heart Failure Care				
ACE Inhibitor or ARB for LVSD[1,3]	-	-	97%	97%
Discharge Instructions Given[1,3]	-	-	95%	94%
Evaluation of LVS Function[3]	11	82%	99%	99%
Medicare Spending				
Medicare Spending per Patient (ratio)	-	-	1.03	0.98
Pneumonia Care				
Appropriate Initial Antibiotic Given[3]	24	100%	95%	95%
Blood Culture Timing[3]	28	96%	98%	98%
Pregnancy and Delivery Care				
Newborn Deliveries Scheduled Early[5]	-	-	7%	6%
Preventive Care				
Immunization for Influenza[5]	-	-	90%	90%
Immunization for Pneumonia[5]	-	-	92%	92%
Stroke Care				
Anticoagulation Therapy for Atrial Fibrillation[5]	-	-	96%	95%
Antithrombotic Therapy Timing[5]	-	-	98%	98%
Assessed for Rehabilitation[5]	-	-	98%	97%
Discharged on Antithrombotic Therapy[5]	-	-	99%	99%
Discharged on Statin Medication[5]	-	-	95%	94%
Thrombolytic Therapy Timing[5]	-	-	68%	66%
Venous Thromboembolism Prophylaxis[5]	-	-	94%	94%
Written Stroke Educational Materials Given[5]	-	-	92%	88%
Surgical Care Improvement Project				
Appropriate Beta Blocker Usage[5]	-	-	98%	98%
Appropriate VTP Within 24 Hours[5]	-	-	98%	98%
Controlled Postoperative Blood Glucose[5]	-	-	96%	97%
Perioperative Temperature Management[5]	-	-	100%	100%
Prophylactic Antibiotic Selection[5]	-	-	99%	99%
Prophylactic Antibiotic Selection (Outpatient)	-	-	98%	98%
Prophylactic Antibiotic Stopped[5]	-	-	98%	98%
Prophylactic Antibiotic Timing[5]	-	-	99%	99%
Prophylactic Antibiotic Timing (Outpatient)	-	-	98%	98%
Urinary Catheter Removal[5]	-	-	98%	97%
Survey of Patients' Hospital Experiences				
Area Around Room 'Always' Quiet at Night	(a)	70%	68%	61%
Doctors 'Always' Communicated Well	(a)	89%	83%	82%
Home Recovery Information Given	(a)	84%	85%	85%
Hospital Given 9 or 10 on 10 Point Scale	(a)	77%	73%	71%
Meds 'Always' Explained Before Given	(a)	67%	66%	64%
Nurses 'Always' Communicated Well	(a)	81%	80%	79%
Pain 'Always' Well Controlled	(a)	73%	72%	71%
Room and Bathroom 'Always' Clean	(a)	78%	75%	73%
Timely Help 'Always' Received	(a)	67%	69%	68%
Would Definitely Recommend Hospital	(a)	73%	73%	71%
Use of Medical Imaging				
Cardiac Imaging Stress Test before Surgery	-	-	5.3%	5.3%
Combination Abdominal CT Scan	-	-	16.4%	10.5%
Combination Brain/Sinus CT Scan	-	-	2.7%	2.7%
Combination Chest CT Scan	-	-	5.6%	2.7%
Follow-up Mammogram/Ultrasound	-	-	7.9%	8.8%
Lumbar Spine MRI for Low Back Pain	-	-	39.6%	37.2%

Cypress Fairbanks Medical Center

10655 Steepletop Drive Phone: 281-897-3100
Houston, TX 77065 Fax: 281-890-5341
URL: www.cyfairhospital.com
Type: Acute Care Hospitals Emergency Services: Yes
Ownership: Proprietary Beds: 160

Key Personnel:
Operating Room. . . . . Ziad Amr
Quality Assurance . . . . Mark Ayers
Infection Control. . . . . Cheryl Briggs, RN
Radiology. . . . . Danny Chow, MD
Chief of Medical Staff . . . . Dr Jennifer Daley
Emergency Room . . . . Bob Shepherd, MD
Anesthesiology. . . . . David Wagner, MD
CEO/President. . . . . James Wright

Measure	Cases	This Hosp.	State Avg.	U.S. Avg.
Blood Clot Prevention and Treatment				
Anticoagulation Overlap Therapy[2]	39	100%	93%	93%
ICU Venous Thromboembolism Prophylaxis[2]	113	97%	92%	92%
Incidence of Potentially Preventable VTE[1,2]	-	-	9%	10%
UFH with Dosages/Platelet Monitoring[2]	16	100%	96%	97%
Venous Thromboembolism Prophylaxis[2]	335	87%	82%	85%
Warfarin Therapy Discharge Instructions[2]	28	86%	84%	75%
Chest Pain/Possible Heart Attack Care				
Aspirin Given Within 24 Hours of Arrival[1,3]	-	-	94%	96%
Fibrinolytic Meds Within 30 Min. of Arrival[3,7]	-	-	47%	58%
Average Time to ECG (minutes)[1,3]	-	-	8	7
Average Time to Transfer (minutes)[3,7]	-	-	62	60
Children's Asthma Care				
Received Home Management Plan of Care	-	-	93%	88%
Received Reliever Medication	-	-	100%	100%
Received Systemic Corticosteroids	-	-	100%	100%
Emergency Department				
Admittance Decision Time (minutes)[2]	546	126	99	98
Head CT Results Within 45 Min. of Arrival[1]	-	-	54%	57%
Patients Who Left ER Before Being Seen	34,807	5%	3%	2%
Time from ER Arrival to Admit. (minutes)[2]	553	313	270	274
Time from ER Arrival to Discharge (minutes)	471	94	127	134
Time in ER Before Being Evaluated (minutes)	37	23	26	26
Time to Pain Meds for Fractures (minutes)	175	33	57	57
Heart Attack Care				
Aspirin Given at Discharge	128	99%	99%	99%
Fibrinolytic Meds Within 30 Min. of Arrival[7]	-	-	49%	54%
PCI Within 90 Minutes of Arrival	20	100%	95%	96%
Statin Prescribed at Discharge	123	99%	98%	98%
Heart Failure Care				
ACE Inhibitor or ARB for LVSD	44	95%	97%	97%
Discharge Instructions Given	102	99%	95%	94%
Evaluation of LVS Function	131	99%	99%	99%
Medicare Spending				
Medicare Spending per Patient (ratio)	-	1.14	1.03	0.98
Pneumonia Care				
Appropriate Initial Antibiotic Given	118	97%	95%	95%
Blood Culture Timing	204	99%	98%	98%
Pregnancy and Delivery Care				
Newborn Deliveries Scheduled Early[2]	71	8%	7%	6%
Preventive Care				
Immunization for Influenza[2]	493	95%	90%	90%
Immunization for Pneumonia[2]	339	96%	92%	92%
Stroke Care				
Anticoagulation Therapy for Atrial Fibrillation[1]	-	-	96%	95%
Antithrombotic Therapy Timing	50	100%	98%	98%
Assessed for Rehabilitation	52	100%	98%	97%
Discharged on Antithrombotic Therapy	50	100%	99%	99%
Discharged on Statin Medication	39	92%	95%	94%
Thrombolytic Therapy Timing[1]	-	-	68%	66%
Venous Thromboembolism Prophylaxis	53	89%	94%	94%
Written Stroke Educational Materials Given	34	97%	92%	88%
Surgical Care Improvement Project				
Appropriate Beta Blocker Usage[2]	50	98%	98%	98%
Appropriate VTP Within 24 Hours[2]	176	98%	98%	98%
Controlled Postoperative Blood Glucose[2]	16	100%	96%	97%
Perioperative Temperature Management[2]	213	100%	100%	100%
Prophylactic Antibiotic Selection[2]	122	99%	99%	99%
Prophylactic Antibiotic Selection (Outpatient)	100	94%	98%	98%
Prophylactic Antibiotic Stopped[2]	113	97%	98%	98%
Prophylactic Antibiotic Timing[2]	122	98%	99%	99%
Prophylactic Antibiotic Timing (Outpatient)	101	97%	98%	98%
Urinary Catheter Removal[2]	83	99%	98%	97%
Survey of Patients' Hospital Experiences				
Area Around Room 'Always' Quiet at Night	300+	56%	68%	61%
Doctors 'Always' Communicated Well	300+	80%	83%	82%
Home Recovery Information Given	300+	85%	85%	85%
Hospital Given 9 or 10 on 10 Point Scale	300+	69%	73%	71%
Meds 'Always' Explained Before Given	300+	59%	66%	64%
Nurses 'Always' Communicated Well	300+	74%	80%	79%
Pain 'Always' Well Controlled	300+	71%	72%	71%
Room and Bathroom 'Always' Clean	300+	63%	75%	73%
Timely Help 'Always' Received	300+	62%	69%	68%
Would Definitely Recommend Hospital	300+	72%	73%	71%
Use of Medical Imaging				
Cardiac Imaging Stress Test before Surgery	48	4.2%	5.3%	5.3%
Combination Abdominal CT Scan	215	16.3%	16.4%	10.5%
Combination Brain/Sinus CT Scan[1]	-	-	2.7%	2.7%
Combination Chest CT Scan	85	1.2%	5.6%	2.7%
Follow-up Mammogram/Ultrasound	742	14.6%	7.9%	8.8%
Lumbar Spine MRI for Low Back Pain[1]	-	-	39.6%	37.2%

Doctors Hospital Tidwell

510 W Tidwell Phone: 713-691-1111
Houston, TX 77091
URL: www.dhthou.com
Type: Acute Care Hospitals Emergency Services: Yes
Ownership: Physician Beds: 190

Key Personnel:
Quality Assurance . . . . Kathy Campbell
Coronary Care . . . . Kenneth Douglas
CEO/President. . . . . Max Ludeke, FACHE
Chief of Medical Staff . . . . Dr Carlos Palacios
Emergency Room . . . . Judy Reyes

Measure	Cases	This Hosp.	State Avg.	U.S. Avg.
Blood Clot Prevention and Treatment				
Anticoagulation Overlap Therapy[1,2]	-	-	93%	93%
ICU Venous Thromboembolism Prophylaxis[2]	80	60%	92%	92%
Incidence of Potentially Preventable VTE[1,2]	-	-	9%	10%
UFH with Dosages/Platelet Monitoring[2,7]	-	-	96%	97%
Venous Thromboembolism Prophylaxis[2]	125	40%	82%	85%
Warfarin Therapy Discharge Instructions[1,2]	-	-	84%	75%
Chest Pain/Possible Heart Attack Care				
Aspirin Given Within 24 Hours of Arrival[1,3]	-	-	94%	96%
Fibrinolytic Meds Within 30 Min. of Arrival[3,7]	-	-	47%	58%
Average Time to ECG (minutes)[1,3]	-	-	8	7
Average Time to Transfer (minutes)[1,3]	-	-	62	60
Children's Asthma Care				
Received Home Management Plan of Care	-	-	93%	88%

NOTE: Hospital profiles are in alphabetical order by state, then city, then hospital within the city; Rankings exclude hospitals with less than 25 cases except for patient surveys which excludes hospitals with less than 100 cases; (a) 100-299 cases; (1) The number of cases/patients is too few to report; (2) Data submitted were based on a sample of cases/patients; (3) Results are based on a shorter time period than required; (4) Data suppressed by CMS for one or more quarters; (5) Results are not available for this reporting period; (6) Fewer than 100 patients completed the HCAHPS survey; (7) No cases met the criteria for this measure; (8) The lower limit of the confidence interval cannot be calculated if the number of observed infections equals zero; (9) No data are available from the state/territory for this reporting period; (10) The scores shown reflect fewer than 50 completed surveys; (11) There were discrepancies in the data collection process; (12) This measure does not apply to this hospital for this reporting period; (13) Results cannot be calculated for this reporting period; (14) The results for this state are combined with nearby states to protect confidentiality; Please refer to the User's Guide for a full explanation of data.

Measure	Cases	This Hosp.	State Avg.	U.S. Avg.
Received Reliever Medication	-	-	100%	100%
Received Systemic Corticosteroids	-	-	100%	100%
Emergency Department				
Admittance Decision Time (minutes)[2]	270	99	99	98
Head CT Results Within 45 Min. of Arrival[1]	-	-	54%	57%
Patients Who Left ER Before Being Seen	16,721	16%	3%	2%
Time from ER Arrival to Admit. (minutes)[2]	286	366	270	274
Time from ER Arrival to Discharge (minutes)	338	228	127	134
Time in ER Before Being Evaluated (minutes)	363	95	26	26
Time to Pain Meds for Fractures (minutes)	58	126	57	57
Heart Attack Care				
Aspirin Given at Discharge	33	64%	99%	99%
Fibrinolytic Meds Within 30 Min. of Arrival[7]	-	-	49%	54%
PCI Within 90 Minutes of Arrival[7]	-	-	95%	96%
Statin Prescribed at Discharge	32	75%	98%	98%
Heart Failure Care				
ACE Inhibitor or ARB for LVSD	54	83%	97%	97%
Discharge Instructions Given	84	99%	95%	94%
Evaluation of LVS Function	101	96%	99%	99%
Medicare Spending				
Medicare Spending per Patient (ratio)	-	1.23	1.03	0.98
Pneumonia Care				
Appropriate Initial Antibiotic Given	45	76%	95%	95%
Blood Culture Timing	56	95%	98%	98%
Pregnancy and Delivery Care				
Newborn Deliveries Scheduled Early	186	24%	7%	6%
Preventive Care				
Immunization for Influenza[2]	339	85%	90%	90%
Immunization for Pneumonia[2]	261	84%	92%	92%
Stroke Care				
Anticoagulation Therapy for Atrial Fibrillation[1]	-	-	96%	95%
Antithrombotic Therapy Timing[1]	-	-	98%	98%
Assessed for Rehabilitation[1]	-	-	98%	97%
Discharged on Antithrombotic Therapy[1]	-	-	99%	99%
Discharged on Statin Medication[1]	-	-	95%	94%
Thrombolytic Therapy Timing[7]	-	-	68%	66%
Venous Thromboembolism Prophylaxis[1]	-	-	94%	94%
Written Stroke Educational Materials Given[1]	-	-	92%	88%
Surgical Care Improvement Project				
Appropriate Beta Blocker Usage[1]	-	-	98%	98%
Appropriate VTP Within 24 Hours	62	92%	98%	98%
Controlled Postoperative Blood Glucose[7]	-	-	96%	97%
Perioperative Temperature Management	52	100%	100%	100%
Prophylactic Antibiotic Selection	35	97%	99%	99%
Prophylactic Antibiotic Selection (Outpatient)[1]	-	-	98%	98%
Prophylactic Antibiotic Stopped	34	97%	98%	98%
Prophylactic Antibiotic Timing	35	94%	99%	99%
Prophylactic Antibiotic Timing (Outpatient)	11	82%	98%	98%
Urinary Catheter Removal	28	100%	98%	97%
Survey of Patients' Hospital Experiences				
Area Around Room 'Always' Quiet at Night	300+	56%	68%	61%
Doctors 'Always' Communicated Well	300+	78%	83%	82%
Home Recovery Information Given	300+	73%	85%	85%
Hospital Given 9 or 10 on 10 Point Scale	300+	63%	73%	71%
Meds 'Always' Explained Before Given	300+	57%	66%	64%
Nurses 'Always' Communicated Well	300+	70%	80%	79%
Pain 'Always' Well Controlled	300+	67%	72%	71%
Room and Bathroom 'Always' Clean	300+	68%	75%	73%
Timely Help 'Always' Received	300+	57%	69%	68%
Would Definitely Recommend Hospital	300+	54%	73%	71%
Use of Medical Imaging				
Cardiac Imaging Stress Test before Surgery[7]	-	-	5.3%	5.3%
Combination Abdominal CT Scan	60	28.3%	16.4%	10.5%
Combination Brain/Sinus CT Scan[1]	-	-	2.7%	2.7%
Combination Chest CT Scan[1]	-	-	5.6%	2.7%
Follow-up Mammogram/Ultrasound[7]	-	-	7.9%	8.8%
Lumbar Spine MRI for Low Back Pain[1]	-	-	39.6%	37.2%

Harris Health System

2525 Holly Hall
Houston, TX 77054
Phone: 713-566-6417
URL: www.hchdonline.com
Type: Acute Care Hospitals
Emergency Services: Yes
Ownership: Government - Local

Key Personnel:
Radiology. Cleveland Black
CEO . . . . Barbara Prince

Measure	Cases	This Hosp.	State Avg.	U.S. Avg.
Blood Clot Prevention and Treatment				
Anticoagulation Overlap Therapy[2]	166	98%	93%	93%
ICU Venous Thromboembolism Prophylaxis[2]	124	94%	92%	92%
Incidence of Potentially Preventable VTE[2]	53	2%	9%	10%
UFH with Dosages/Platelet Monitoring[2]	138	100%	96%	97%
Venous Thromboembolism Prophylaxis[2]	673	74%	82%	85%
Warfarin Therapy Discharge Instructions[2]	138	91%	84%	75%
Chest Pain/Possible Heart Attack Care				
Aspirin Given Within 24 Hours of Arrival[1,3]	-	-	94%	96%
Fibrinolytic Meds Within 30 Min. of Arrival[5]	-	-	47%	58%
Average Time to ECG (minutes)[1,3]	-	-	8	7
Average Time to Transfer (minutes)[5]	-	-	62	60
Children's Asthma Care				
Received Home Management Plan of Care	-	-	93%	88%
Received Reliever Medication	-	-	100%	100%
Received Systemic Corticosteroids	-	-	100%	100%
Emergency Department				
Admittance Decision Time (minutes)[2]	1,076	332	99	98
Head CT Results Within 45 Min. of Arrival[1]	-	-	54%	57%
Patients Who Left ER Before Being Seen	>100k	14%	3%	2%
Time from ER Arrival to Admit. (minutes)[2]	1,081	786	270	274
Time from ER Arrival to Discharge (minutes)	716	441	127	134
Time in ER Before Being Evaluated (minutes)	800	130	26	26
Time to Pain Meds for Fractures (minutes)	386	202	57	57
Heart Attack Care				
Aspirin Given at Discharge	387	98%	99%	99%
Fibrinolytic Meds Within 30 Min. of Arrival[7]	-	-	49%	54%
PCI Within 90 Minutes of Arrival	30	97%	95%	96%
Statin Prescribed at Discharge	377	99%	98%	98%
Heart Failure Care				
ACE Inhibitor or ARB for LVSD[2]	318	96%	97%	97%
Discharge Instructions Given[2]	633	90%	95%	94%
Evaluation of LVS Function[2]	648	100%	99%	99%
Medicare Spending				
Medicare Spending per Patient (ratio)	-	0.96	1.03	0.98
Pneumonia Care				
Appropriate Initial Antibiotic Given[2]	153	98%	95%	95%
Blood Culture Timing[2]	313	97%	98%	98%
Pregnancy and Delivery Care				
Newborn Deliveries Scheduled Early	425	6%	7%	6%
Preventive Care				
Immunization for Influenza[2]	966	88%	90%	90%
Immunization for Pneumonia[2]	817	91%	92%	92%
Stroke Care				
Anticoagulation Therapy for Atrial Fibrillation	16	100%	96%	95%
Antithrombotic Therapy Timing	196	97%	98%	98%
Assessed for Rehabilitation	284	98%	98%	97%
Discharged on Antithrombotic Therapy	216	100%	99%	99%
Discharged on Statin Medication	169	98%	95%	94%
Thrombolytic Therapy Timing[1]	-	-	68%	66%
Venous Thromboembolism Prophylaxis	274	93%	94%	94%
Written Stroke Educational Materials Given	209	90%	92%	88%
Surgical Care Improvement Project				
Appropriate Beta Blocker Usage[2]	120	98%	98%	98%
Appropriate VTP Within 24 Hours[2]	628	99%	98%	98%
Controlled Postoperative Blood Glucose[2]	110	94%	96%	97%
Perioperative Temperature Management[2]	714	100%	100%	100%
Prophylactic Antibiotic Selection[2]	475	99%	99%	99%
Prophylactic Antibiotic Selection (Outpatient)	625	99%	98%	98%
Prophylactic Antibiotic Stopped[2]	444	97%	98%	98%
Prophylactic Antibiotic Timing[2]	476	99%	99%	99%
Prophylactic Antibiotic Timing (Outpatient)	633	98%	98%	98%
Urinary Catheter Removal[2]	286	96%	98%	97%
Survey of Patients' Hospital Experiences				
Area Around Room 'Always' Quiet at Night	300+	52%	68%	61%
Doctors 'Always' Communicated Well	300+	79%	83%	82%
Home Recovery Information Given	300+	81%	85%	85%
Hospital Given 9 or 10 on 10 Point Scale	300+	69%	73%	71%
Meds 'Always' Explained Before Given	300+	63%	66%	64%
Nurses 'Always' Communicated Well	300+	74%	80%	79%
Pain 'Always' Well Controlled	300+	69%	72%	71%
Room and Bathroom 'Always' Clean	300+	64%	75%	73%
Timely Help 'Always' Received	300+	62%	69%	68%
Would Definitely Recommend Hospital	300+	69%	73%	71%
Use of Medical Imaging				
Cardiac Imaging Stress Test before Surgery	324	3.1%	5.3%	5.3%
Combination Abdominal CT Scan	910	8.6%	16.4%	10.5%
Combination Brain/Sinus CT Scan	669	4.2%	2.7%	2.7%
Combination Chest CT Scan	819	0.1%	5.6%	2.7%
Follow-up Mammogram/Ultrasound	1,200	5.9%	7.9%	8.8%
Lumbar Spine MRI for Low Back Pain	59	35.6%	39.6%	37.2%

Houston Hospital for Specialized Surgery

5445 Labranch Street
Houston, TX 77004
Phone: 713-528-6800
Type: Acute Care Hospitals
Emergency Services: No
Ownership: Proprietary

Measure	Cases	This Hosp.	State Avg.	U.S. Avg.
Blood Clot Prevention and Treatment				
Anticoagulation Overlap Therapy[7]	-	-	93%	93%
ICU Venous Thromboembolism Prophylaxis[7]	-	-	92%	92%
Incidence of Potentially Preventable VTE[7]	-	-	9%	10%
UFH with Dosages/Platelet Monitoring[7]	-	-	96%	97%
Venous Thromboembolism Prophylaxis	30	87%	82%	85%
Warfarin Therapy Discharge Instructions[7]	-	-	84%	75%
Chest Pain/Possible Heart Attack Care				
Aspirin Given Within 24 Hours of Arrival[5]	-	-	94%	96%
Fibrinolytic Meds Within 30 Min. of Arrival[5]	-	-	47%	58%
Average Time to ECG (minutes)[5]	-	-	8	7
Average Time to Transfer (minutes)[5]	-	-	62	60
Children's Asthma Care				
Received Home Management Plan of Care	-	-	93%	88%
Received Reliever Medication	-	-	100%	100%
Received Systemic Corticosteroids	-	-	100%	100%
Emergency Department				
Admittance Decision Time (minutes)[1]	-	-	99	98
Head CT Results Within 45 Min. of Arrival[5]	-	-	54%	57%
Patients Who Left ER Before Being Seen	36	0%	3%	2%
Time from ER Arrival to Admit. (minutes)[1]	-	-	270	274
Time from ER Arrival to Discharge (minutes)[1,3]	-	-	127	134
Time in ER Before Being Evaluated (minutes)[1,3]	-	-	26	26
Time to Pain Meds for Fractures (minutes)[5]	-	-	57	57
Heart Attack Care				
Aspirin Given at Discharge[5]	-	-	99%	99%
Fibrinolytic Meds Within 30 Min. of Arrival[5]	-	-	49%	54%
PCI Within 90 Minutes of Arrival[5]	-	-	95%	96%
Statin Prescribed at Discharge[5]	-	-	98%	98%
Heart Failure Care				
ACE Inhibitor or ARB for LVSD[5]	-	-	97%	97%
Discharge Instructions Given[5]	-	-	95%	94%
Evaluation of LVS Function[5]	-	-	99%	99%
Medicare Spending				
Medicare Spending per Patient (ratio)[1]	-	-	1.03	0.98
Pneumonia Care				
Appropriate Initial Antibiotic Given[5]	-	-	95%	95%
Blood Culture Timing[5]	-	-	98%	98%
Pregnancy and Delivery Care				
Newborn Deliveries Scheduled Early[7]	-	-	7%	6%
Preventive Care				
Immunization for Influenza	114	55%	90%	90%
Immunization for Pneumonia	40	65%	92%	92%
Stroke Care				
Anticoagulation Therapy for Atrial Fibrillation[5]	-	-	96%	95%
Antithrombotic Therapy Timing[5]	-	-	98%	98%

NOTE: Hospital profiles are in alphabetical order by state, then city, then hospital within the city; Rankings exclude hospitals with less than 25 cases except for patient surveys which excludes hospitals with less than 100 cases; (a) 100-299 cases; (1) The number of cases/patients is too few to report; (2) Data submitted were based on a sample of cases/patients; (3) Results are based on a shorter time period than required; (4) Data suppressed by CMS for one or more quarters; (5) Results are not available for this reporting period; (6) Fewer than 100 patients completed the HCAHPS survey; (7) No cases met the criteria for this measure; (8) The lower limit of the confidence interval cannot be calculated if the number of observed infections equals zero; (9) No data are available from the state/territory for this reporting period; (10) The scores shown reflect fewer than 50 completed surveys; (11) There were discrepancies in the data collection process; (12) This measure does not apply to this hospital for this reporting period; (13) Results cannot be calculated for this reporting period; (14) The results for this state are combined with nearby states to protect confidentiality; Please refer to the User's Guide for a full explanation of data.

Measure	Cases	This Hosp.	State Avg.	U.S. Avg.
Assessed for Rehabilitation[5]	-	-	98%	97%
Discharged on Antithrombotic Therapy[5]	-	-	99%	99%
Discharged on Statin Medication[5]	-	-	95%	94%
Thrombolytic Therapy Timing[5]	-	-	68%	66%
Venous Thromboembolism Prophylaxis[5]	-	-	94%	94%
Written Stroke Educational Materials Given[5]	-	-	92%	88%
Surgical Care Improvement Project				
Appropriate Beta Blocker Usage[3,7]	-	-	98%	98%
Appropriate VTP Within 24 Hours[1,3]	-	-	98%	98%
Controlled Postoperative Blood Glucose[3,7]	-	-	96%	97%
Perioperative Temperature Management[1,3]	-	-	100%	100%
Prophylactic Antibiotic Selection[1,3]	-	-	99%	99%
Prophylactic Antibiotic Selection (Outpatient)[1,3]	-	-	98%	98%
Prophylactic Antibiotic Stopped[1,3]	-	-	98%	98%
Prophylactic Antibiotic Timing[1,3]	-	-	99%	99%
Prophylactic Antibiotic Timing (Outpatient)[1,3]	-	-	98%	98%
Urinary Catheter Removal[3,7]	-	-	98%	97%
Survey of Patients' Hospital Experiences				
Area Around Room 'Always' Quiet at Night[6]	<100	84%	68%	61%
Doctors 'Always' Communicated Well[6]	<100	90%	83%	82%
Home Recovery Information Given[6]	<100	91%	85%	85%
Hospital Given 9 or 10 on 10 Point Scale[6]	<100	65%	73%	71%
Meds 'Always' Explained Before Given[6]	<100	67%	66%	64%
Nurses 'Always' Communicated Well[6]	<100	74%	80%	79%
Pain 'Always' Well Controlled[6]	<100	69%	72%	71%
Room and Bathroom 'Always' Clean[6]	<100	77%	75%	73%
Timely Help 'Always' Received[6]	<100	71%	69%	68%
Would Definitely Recommend Hospital[6]	<100	61%	73%	71%
Use of Medical Imaging				
Cardiac Imaging Stress Test before Surgery[7]	-	-	5.3%	5.3%
Combination Abdominal CT Scan[7]	-	-	16.4%	10.5%
Combination Brain/Sinus CT Scan[7]	-	-	2.7%	2.7%
Combination Chest CT Scan[7]	-	-	5.6%	2.7%
Follow-up Mammogram/Ultrasound[7]	-	-	7.9%	8.8%
Lumbar Spine MRI for Low Back Pain[7]	-	-	39.6%	37.2%

Houston Northwest Medical Center

710 Fm 1960 West
Houston, TX 77090
URL: www.hnmc.com
Phone: 281-440-1000
Fax: 281-440-2474
Type: Acute Care Hospitals
Ownership: Proprietary
Emergency Services: Yes
Beds: 494

Key Personnel:
Emergency Room . . . . David Arai, MD
Pediatric Ambulatory Care . . . . . . Susan Gardner
Pediatric In-Patient Care . . . . Susan Gardner
Intensive Care Unit. . . . . Grace Heffron, RN
Quality Assurance . . . . Melanie Lewis
CEO/President. . . . . Tim Puthoff
Radiology. . . . . M Elizabeth Sands, MD
Chief of Medical Staff . . . . Daniel Tuft

Measure	Cases	This Hosp.	State Avg.	U.S. Avg.
Blood Clot Prevention and Treatment				
Anticoagulation Overlap Therapy[2]	93	94%	93%	93%
ICU Venous Thromboembolism Prophylaxis[2]	119	92%	92%	92%
Incidence of Potentially Preventable VTE[2]	11	18%	9%	10%
UFH with Dosages/Platelet Monitoring[2]	23	100%	96%	97%
Venous Thromboembolism Prophylaxis[2]	350	83%	82%	85%
Warfarin Therapy Discharge Instructions[2]	66	100%	84%	75%
Chest Pain/Possible Heart Attack Care				
Aspirin Given Within 24 Hours of Arrival[3,7]	-	-	94%	96%
Fibrinolytic Meds Within 30 Min. of Arrival[5]	-	-	47%	58%
Average Time to ECG (minutes)[3,7]	-	-	8	7
Average Time to Transfer (minutes)[5]	-	-	62	60
Children's Asthma Care				
Received Home Management Plan of Care	-	-	93%	88%
Received Reliever Medication	-	-	100%	100%
Received Systemic Corticosteroids	-	-	100%	100%
Emergency Department				
Admittance Decision Time (minutes)[2]	683	155	99	98
Head CT Results Within 45 Min. of Arrival[1]	-	-	54%	57%
Patients Who Left ER Before Being Seen	78,889	7%	3%	2%
Time from ER Arrival to Admit. (minutes)[2]	684	351	270	274
Time from ER Arrival to Discharge (minutes)	511	138	127	134
Time in ER Before Being Evaluated (minutes)	552	30	26	26
Time to Pain Meds for Fractures (minutes)	203	72	57	57
Heart Attack Care				
Aspirin Given at Discharge	274	100%	99%	99%
Fibrinolytic Meds Within 30 Min. of Arrival[7]	-	-	49%	54%
PCI Within 90 Minutes of Arrival	51	100%	95%	96%
Statin Prescribed at Discharge	271	100%	98%	98%
Heart Failure Care				
ACE Inhibitor or ARB for LVSD	158	100%	97%	97%
Discharge Instructions Given	382	94%	95%	94%
Evaluation of LVS Function	453	100%	99%	99%
Medicare Spending				
Medicare Spending per Patient (ratio)	-	1.12	1.03	0.98
Pneumonia Care				
Appropriate Initial Antibiotic Given	173	100%	95%	95%
Blood Culture Timing	197	99%	98%	98%
Pregnancy and Delivery Care				
Newborn Deliveries Scheduled Early[2]	68	0%	7%	6%
Preventive Care				
Immunization for Influenza[2]	527	96%	90%	90%
Immunization for Pneumonia[2]	573	94%	92%	92%
Stroke Care				
Anticoagulation Therapy for Atrial Fibrillation	19	100%	96%	95%
Antithrombotic Therapy Timing	160	97%	98%	98%
Assessed for Rehabilitation	193	100%	98%	97%
Discharged on Antithrombotic Therapy	164	100%	99%	99%
Discharged on Statin Medication	138	100%	95%	94%
Thrombolytic Therapy Timing	17	94%	68%	66%
Venous Thromboembolism Prophylaxis	209	95%	94%	94%
Written Stroke Educational Materials Given	119	93%	92%	88%
Surgical Care Improvement Project				
Appropriate Beta Blocker Usage[2]	181	98%	98%	98%
Appropriate VTP Within 24 Hours[2]	418	99%	98%	98%
Controlled Postoperative Blood Glucose[2]	71	100%	96%	97%
Perioperative Temperature Management[2]	510	100%	100%	100%
Prophylactic Antibiotic Selection[2]	388	99%	99%	99%
Prophylactic Antibiotic Selection (Outpatient)	194	98%	98%	98%
Prophylactic Antibiotic Stopped[2]	367	97%	98%	98%
Prophylactic Antibiotic Timing[2]	388	99%	99%	99%
Prophylactic Antibiotic Timing (Outpatient)	194	100%	98%	98%
Urinary Catheter Removal[2]	257	96%	98%	97%
Survey of Patients' Hospital Experiences				
Area Around Room 'Always' Quiet at Night	300+	60%	68%	61%
Doctors 'Always' Communicated Well	300+	81%	83%	82%
Home Recovery Information Given	300+	80%	85%	85%
Hospital Given 9 or 10 on 10 Point Scale	300+	64%	73%	71%
Meds 'Always' Explained Before Given	300+	57%	66%	64%
Nurses 'Always' Communicated Well	300+	74%	80%	79%
Pain 'Always' Well Controlled	300+	70%	72%	71%
Room and Bathroom 'Always' Clean	300+	66%	75%	73%
Timely Help 'Always' Received	300+	62%	69%	68%
Would Definitely Recommend Hospital	300+	67%	73%	71%
Use of Medical Imaging				
Cardiac Imaging Stress Test before Surgery	320	7.2%	5.3%	5.3%
Combination Abdominal CT Scan	595	11.8%	16.4%	10.5%
Combination Brain/Sinus CT Scan	522	1.7%	2.7%	2.7%
Combination Chest CT Scan	437	5.9%	5.6%	2.7%
Follow-up Mammogram/Ultrasound	1,336	10.3%	7.9%	8.8%
Lumbar Spine MRI for Low Back Pain[1]	-	-	39.6%	37.2%

Houston VA Medical Center

2002 Holcombe Blvd.
Houston, TX 77030
URL: www.houston.med.va.gov
Phone: 713-794-7100
Fax: 713-794-7218
Type: Acute Care - VA
Ownership: Government Federal
Emergency Services: No
Beds: 343

Key Personnel:
Chief of Medical Staff . . . . J. Kalavar, MD
Hemotology Center . . . . Mike Kroll, MD
Operating Room. . . . . Nancy Napier, RN
Quality Assurance . . . . James Scheurich, MD
Intensive Care Unit. . . . . Loreta Tumangan
Emergency Room . . . . John L Urbanek, MD
Radiology. . . . . Meena Vig, MD
Infection Control. . . . . Ed Young, MD

Measure	Cases	This Hosp.	State Avg.	U.S. Avg.
Blood Clot Prevention and Treatment				
Anticoagulation Overlap Therapy	-	-	93%	93%
ICU Venous Thromboembolism Prophylaxis	-	-	92%	92%
Incidence of Potentially Preventable VTE	-	-	9%	10%
UFH with Dosages/Platelet Monitoring	-	-	96%	97%
Venous Thromboembolism Prophylaxis	-	-	82%	85%
Warfarin Therapy Discharge Instructions	-	-	84%	75%
Chest Pain/Possible Heart Attack Care				
Aspirin Given Within 24 Hours of Arrival	-	-	94%	96%
Fibrinolytic Meds Within 30 Min. of Arrival	-	-	47%	58%
Average Time to ECG (minutes)	-	-	8	7
Average Time to Transfer (minutes)	-	-	62	60
Children's Asthma Care				
Received Home Management Plan of Care	-	-	93%	88%
Received Reliever Medication	-	-	100%	100%
Received Systemic Corticosteroids	-	-	100%	100%
Emergency Department				
Admittance Decision Time (minutes)	-	-	99	98
Head CT Results Within 45 Min. of Arrival	-	-	54%	57%
Patients Who Left ER Before Being Seen	-	-	3%	2%
Time from ER Arrival to Admit. (minutes)	-	-	270	274
Time from ER Arrival to Discharge (minutes)	-	-	127	134
Time in ER Before Being Evaluated (minutes)	-	-	26	26
Time to Pain Meds for Fractures (minutes)	-	-	57	57
Heart Attack Care				
Aspirin Given at Discharge	136	97%	99%	99%
Fibrinolytic Meds Within 30 Min. of Arrival[5]	-	-	49%	54%
PCI Within 90 Minutes of Arrival[1]	11	82%	95%	96%
Statin Prescribed at Discharge	134	99%	98%	98%
Heart Failure Care				
ACE Inhibitor or ARB for LVSD	253	96%	97%	97%
Discharge Instructions Given	530	87%	95%	94%
Evaluation of LVS Function	553	100%	99%	99%
Medicare Spending				
Medicare Spending per Patient (ratio)	-	-	1.03	0.98
Pneumonia Care				
Appropriate Initial Antibiotic Given	75	92%	95%	95%
Blood Culture Timing	158	97%	98%	98%
Pregnancy and Delivery Care				
Newborn Deliveries Scheduled Early	-	-	7%	6%
Preventive Care				
Immunization for Influenza[5]	-	-	90%	90%
Immunization for Pneumonia[5]	-	-	92%	92%
Stroke Care				
Anticoagulation Therapy for Atrial Fibrillation	-	-	96%	95%
Antithrombotic Therapy Timing	-	-	98%	98%
Assessed for Rehabilitation	-	-	98%	97%
Discharged on Antithrombotic Therapy	-	-	99%	99%
Discharged on Statin Medication	-	-	95%	94%
Thrombolytic Therapy Timing	-	-	68%	66%
Venous Thromboembolism Prophylaxis	-	-	94%	94%
Written Stroke Educational Materials Given	-	-	92%	88%
Surgical Care Improvement Project				
Appropriate Beta Blocker Usage[2]	332	98%	98%	98%
Appropriate VTP Within 24 Hours[2]	382	98%	98%	98%
Controlled Postoperative Blood Glucose[2]	248	98%	96%	97%
Perioperative Temperature Management[2]	531	100%	100%	100%
Prophylactic Antibiotic Selection	515	99%	99%	99%
Prophylactic Antibiotic Selection (Outpatient)	-	-	98%	98%
Prophylactic Antibiotic Stopped	483	97%	98%	98%
Prophylactic Antibiotic Timing	515	99%	99%	99%
Prophylactic Antibiotic Timing (Outpatient)	-	-	98%	98%
Urinary Catheter Removal[2]	439	98%	98%	97%
Survey of Patients' Hospital Experiences				
Area Around Room 'Always' Quiet at Night	-	-	68%	61%
Doctors 'Always' Communicated Well	-	-	83%	82%
Home Recovery Information Given	-	-	85%	85%
Hospital Given 9 or 10 on 10 Point Scale	-	-	73%	71%
Meds 'Always' Explained Before Given	-	-	66%	64%
Nurses 'Always' Communicated Well	-	-	80%	79%
Pain 'Always' Well Controlled	-	-	72%	71%

NOTE: Hospital profiles are in alphabetical order by state, then city, then hospital within the city; Rankings exclude hospitals with less than 25 cases except for patient surveys which excludes hospitals with less than 100 cases; (a) 100-299 cases; (1) The number of cases/patients is too few to report; (2) Data submitted were based on a sample of cases/patients; (3) Results are based on a shorter time period than required; (4) Data suppressed by CMS for one or more quarters; (5) Results are not available for this reporting period; (6) Fewer than 100 patients completed the HCAHPS survey; (7) No cases met the criteria for this measure; (8) The lower limit of the confidence interval cannot be calculated if the number of observed infections equals zero; (9) No data are available from the state/territory for this reporting period; (10) The scores shown reflect fewer than 50 completed surveys; (11) There were discrepancies in the data collection process; (12) This measure does not apply to this hospital for this reporting period; (13) Results cannot be calculated for this reporting period; (14) The results for this state are combined with nearby states to protect confidentiality; Please refer to the User's Guide for a full explanation of data.

Measure	Cases	This Hosp.	State Avg.	U.S. Avg.
Room and Bathroom 'Always' Clean	-	-	75%	73%
Timely Help 'Always' Received	-	-	69%	68%
Would Definitely Recommend Hospital	-	-	73%	71%
Use of Medical Imaging				
Cardiac Imaging Stress Test before Surgery	-	-	5.3%	5.3%
Combination Abdominal CT Scan	-	-	16.4%	10.5%
Combination Brain/Sinus CT Scan	-	-	2.7%	2.7%
Combination Chest CT Scan	-	-	5.6%	2.7%
Follow-up Mammogram/Ultrasound	-	-	7.9%	8.8%
Lumbar Spine MRI for Low Back Pain	-	-	39.6%	37.2%

Memorial Hermann Hospital System

1635 North Loop West Phone: 713-448-6796
Houston, TX 77008
URL: www.memorialhermann.org
Type: Acute Care Hospitals Emergency Services: Yes
Ownership: Voluntary non-profit - Private Beds: 3,514

Measure	Cases	This Hosp.	State Avg.	U.S. Avg.
Blood Clot Prevention and Treatment				
Anticoagulation Overlap Therapy[2]	434	97%	93%	93%
ICU Venous Thromboembolism Prophylaxis[2]	338	98%	92%	92%
Incidence of Potentially Preventable VTE[2]	85	6%	9%	10%
UFH with Dosages/Platelet Monitoring[2]	105	99%	96%	97%
Venous Thromboembolism Prophylaxis[2]	1,432	92%	82%	85%
Warfarin Therapy Discharge Instructions[2]	335	81%	84%	75%
Chest Pain/Possible Heart Attack Care				
Aspirin Given Within 24 Hours of Arrival	14	100%	94%	96%
Fibrinolytic Meds Within 30 Min. of Arrival[7]	-	-	47%	58%
Average Time to ECG (minutes)	15	10	8	7
Average Time to Transfer (minutes)[1]	-	-	62	60
Children's Asthma Care				
Received Home Management Plan of Care	-	-	93%	88%
Received Reliever Medication	-	-	100%	100%
Received Systemic Corticosteroids	-	-	100%	100%
Emergency Department				
Admittance Decision Time (minutes)[2]	2,033	137	99	98
Head CT Results Within 45 Min. of Arrival	48	48%	54%	57%
Patients Who Left ER Before Being Seen	>100k	3%	3%	2%
Time from ER Arrival to Admit. (minutes)[2]	2,182	360	270	274
Time from ER Arrival to Discharge (minutes)	1,486	204	127	134
Time in ER Before Being Evaluated (minutes)	1,664	38	26	26
Time to Pain Meds for Fractures (minutes)	944	66	57	57
Heart Attack Care				
Aspirin Given at Discharge[2]	945	100%	99%	99%
Fibrinolytic Meds Within 30 Min. of Arrival[2,7]	-	-	49%	54%
PCI Within 90 Minutes of Arrival[2]	147	92%	95%	96%
Statin Prescribed at Discharge[2]	900	99%	98%	98%
Heart Failure Care				
ACE Inhibitor or ARB for LVSD[2]	439	98%	97%	97%
Discharge Instructions Given[2]	979	95%	95%	94%
Evaluation of LVS Function[2]	1,205	100%	99%	99%
Medicare Spending				
Medicare Spending per Patient (ratio)	-	1.14	1.03	0.98
Pneumonia Care				
Appropriate Initial Antibiotic Given[2]	298	97%	95%	95%
Blood Culture Timing[2]	567	100%	98%	98%
Pregnancy and Delivery Care				
Newborn Deliveries Scheduled Early[2]	299	5%	7%	6%
Preventive Care				
Immunization for Influenza[2]	2,066	96%	90%	90%
Immunization for Pneumonia[2]	2,213	96%	92%	92%
Stroke Care				
Anticoagulation Therapy for Atrial Fibrillation	74	99%	96%	95%
Antithrombotic Therapy Timing	601	98%	98%	98%
Assessed for Rehabilitation	664	100%	98%	97%
Discharged on Antithrombotic Therapy	636	100%	99%	99%
Discharged on Statin Medication	483	100%	95%	94%
Thrombolytic Therapy Timing	43	77%	68%	66%
Venous Thromboembolism Prophylaxis	636	99%	94%	94%
Written Stroke Educational Materials Given	415	98%	92%	88%
Surgical Care Improvement Project				
Appropriate Beta Blocker Usage[2]	663	97%	98%	98%
Appropriate VTP Within 24 Hours[2]	1,550	99%	98%	98%
Controlled Postoperative Blood Glucose[2]	234	98%	96%	97%
Perioperative Temperature Management[2]	1,953	100%	100%	100%
Prophylactic Antibiotic Selection[2]	1,410	99%	99%	99%
Prophylactic Antibiotic Selection (Outpatient)	1,335	98%	98%	98%
Prophylactic Antibiotic Stopped[2]	1,344	98%	98%	98%
Prophylactic Antibiotic Timing[2]	1,412	99%	99%	99%
Prophylactic Antibiotic Timing (Outpatient)	1,336	99%	98%	98%
Urinary Catheter Removal[2]	1,136	99%	98%	97%
Survey of Patients' Hospital Experiences				
Area Around Room 'Always' Quiet at Night	300+	62%	68%	61%
Doctors 'Always' Communicated Well	300+	79%	83%	82%
Home Recovery Information Given	300+	85%	85%	85%
Hospital Given 9 or 10 on 10 Point Scale	300+	75%	73%	71%
Meds 'Always' Explained Before Given	300+	61%	66%	64%
Nurses 'Always' Communicated Well	300+	79%	80%	79%
Pain 'Always' Well Controlled	300+	72%	72%	71%
Room and Bathroom 'Always' Clean	300+	74%	75%	73%
Timely Help 'Always' Received	300+	64%	69%	68%
Would Definitely Recommend Hospital	300+	76%	73%	71%
Use of Medical Imaging				
Cardiac Imaging Stress Test before Surgery	843	7.5%	5.3%	5.3%
Combination Abdominal CT Scan	3,617	16.7%	16.4%	10.5%
Combination Brain/Sinus CT Scan	3,649	1.9%	2.7%	2.7%
Combination Chest CT Scan	2,413	2.9%	5.6%	2.7%
Follow-up Mammogram/Ultrasound	6,651	6.2%	7.9%	8.8%
Lumbar Spine MRI for Low Back Pain	382	34.6%	39.6%	37.2%

Memorial Hermann Memorial City Medical Center

921 Gessner Phone: 713-242-3000
Houston, TX 77024 Fax: 713-827-4096
URL: www.mhhs.org
Type: Acute Care Hospitals Emergency Services: Yes
Ownership: Voluntary non-profit - Private Beds: 426

Key Personnel:
CEO/President. . . . . Keith Alexander
Infection Control. . . . . Christy Hodges
Operating Room. . . . . Elizabeth Jones
Quality Assurance . . . . Rhonda Kitieier
Pediatric In-Patient Care . . . . Elizabeth Lee
Radiology. . . . . Charles Mitchell
Chief of Medical Staff. . . . . Edward Rensimer, MD
Coronary Care. . . . . Suzy Robinson

Measure	Cases	This Hosp.	State Avg.	U.S. Avg.
Blood Clot Prevention and Treatment				
Anticoagulation Overlap Therapy[2]	116	93%	93%	93%
ICU Venous Thromboembolism Prophylaxis[2]	89	98%	92%	92%
Incidence of Potentially Preventable VTE[2]	19	16%	9%	10%
UFH with Dosages/Platelet Monitoring[2]	46	100%	96%	97%
Venous Thromboembolism Prophylaxis[2]	319	94%	82%	85%
Warfarin Therapy Discharge Instructions[2]	85	87%	84%	75%
Chest Pain/Possible Heart Attack Care				
Aspirin Given Within 24 Hours of Arrival[1,3]	-	-	94%	96%
Fibrinolytic Meds Within 30 Min. of Arrival[3,7]	-	-	47%	58%
Average Time to ECG (minutes)[1,3]	-	-	8	7
Average Time to Transfer (minutes)[3,7]	-	-	62	60
Children's Asthma Care				
Received Home Management Plan of Care	-	-	93%	88%
Received Reliever Medication	-	-	100%	100%
Received Systemic Corticosteroids	-	-	100%	100%
Emergency Department				
Admittance Decision Time (minutes)[2]	487	87	99	98
Head CT Results Within 45 Min. of Arrival[1]	-	-	54%	57%
Patients Who Left ER Before Being Seen	58,239	5%	3%	2%
Time from ER Arrival to Admit. (minutes)[2]	520	288	270	274
Time from ER Arrival to Discharge (minutes)	360	205	127	134
Time in ER Before Being Evaluated (minutes)	410	42	26	26
Time to Pain Meds for Fractures (minutes)	206	68	57	57
Heart Attack Care				
Aspirin Given at Discharge[2]	279	99%	99%	99%
Fibrinolytic Meds Within 30 Min. of Arrival[2,7]	-	-	49%	54%
PCI Within 90 Minutes of Arrival[2]	43	88%	95%	96%
Statin Prescribed at Discharge[2]	272	97%	98%	98%
Heart Failure Care				
ACE Inhibitor or ARB for LVSD[2]	101	99%	97%	97%
Discharge Instructions Given[2]	232	91%	95%	94%
Evaluation of LVS Function[2]	308	100%	99%	99%
Medicare Spending				
Medicare Spending per Patient (ratio)	-	1.10	1.03	0.98
Pneumonia Care				
Appropriate Initial Antibiotic Given[2]	72	99%	95%	95%
Blood Culture Timing[2]	145	99%	98%	98%
Pregnancy and Delivery Care				
Newborn Deliveries Scheduled Early[2]	68	9%	7%	6%
Preventive Care				
Immunization for Influenza[2]	530	98%	90%	90%
Immunization for Pneumonia[2]	595	97%	92%	92%
Stroke Care				
Anticoagulation Therapy for Atrial Fibrillation	44	98%	96%	95%
Antithrombotic Therapy Timing	237	99%	98%	98%
Assessed for Rehabilitation	300	100%	98%	97%
Discharged on Antithrombotic Therapy	261	100%	99%	99%
Discharged on Statin Medication	171	99%	95%	94%
Thrombolytic Therapy Timing	33	73%	68%	66%
Venous Thromboembolism Prophylaxis	300	100%	94%	94%
Written Stroke Educational Materials Given	184	97%	92%	88%
Surgical Care Improvement Project				
Appropriate Beta Blocker Usage[2]	205	97%	98%	98%
Appropriate VTP Within 24 Hours[2]	427	96%	98%	98%
Controlled Postoperative Blood Glucose[2]	137	99%	96%	97%
Perioperative Temperature Management[2]	619	100%	100%	100%
Prophylactic Antibiotic Selection[2]	481	99%	99%	99%
Prophylactic Antibiotic Selection (Outpatient)	526	99%	98%	98%
Prophylactic Antibiotic Stopped[2]	467	96%	98%	98%
Prophylactic Antibiotic Timing[2]	481	99%	99%	99%
Prophylactic Antibiotic Timing (Outpatient)	528	98%	98%	98%
Urinary Catheter Removal[2]	275	97%	98%	97%
Survey of Patients' Hospital Experiences				
Area Around Room 'Always' Quiet at Night	300+	63%	68%	61%
Doctors 'Always' Communicated Well	300+	80%	83%	82%
Home Recovery Information Given	300+	89%	85%	85%
Hospital Given 9 or 10 on 10 Point Scale	300+	77%	73%	71%
Meds 'Always' Explained Before Given	300+	68%	66%	64%
Nurses 'Always' Communicated Well	300+	77%	80%	79%
Pain 'Always' Well Controlled	300+	71%	72%	71%
Room and Bathroom 'Always' Clean	300+	73%	75%	73%
Timely Help 'Always' Received	300+	67%	69%	68%
Would Definitely Recommend Hospital	300+	81%	73%	71%
Use of Medical Imaging				
Cardiac Imaging Stress Test before Surgery	141	9.9%	5.3%	5.3%
Combination Abdominal CT Scan	1,365	35.4%	16.4%	10.5%
Combination Brain/Sinus CT Scan	1,466	1.6%	2.7%	2.7%
Combination Chest CT Scan	907	9.3%	5.6%	2.7%
Follow-up Mammogram/Ultrasound	4,518	7.1%	7.9%	8.8%
Lumbar Spine MRI for Low Back Pain	377	37.1%	39.6%	37.2%

Memorial Hermann Texas Medical Center

6411 Fannin Phone: 713-704-3700
Houston, TX 77030 Fax: 713-448-5665
URL: www.mhhs.org
Type: Acute Care Hospitals Emergency Services: Yes
Ownership: Voluntary non-profit - Private Beds: 908

Key Personnel:
CEO . . . . Craig Cordola
Radiology. . . . . Stanford Goldman, MD
Anesthesiology. . . . . Jeffrey Katz, MD
Quality Assurance . . . . Kathy Luther, RN
Intensive Care Unit. . . . . Lynn MaGuire
CEO/President. . . . . Juanita Romans
Chief of Medical Staff. . . . . David Taylor, MD

Measure	Cases	This Hosp.	State Avg.	U.S. Avg.
Blood Clot Prevention and Treatment				
Anticoagulation Overlap Therapy[2]	175	98%	93%	93%
ICU Venous Thromboembolism Prophylaxis[2]	143	98%	92%	92%
Incidence of Potentially Preventable VTE[2]	109	2%	9%	10%
UFH with Dosages/Platelet Monitoring[2]	177	100%	96%	97%
Venous Thromboembolism Prophylaxis[2]	286	95%	82%	85%
Warfarin Therapy Discharge Instructions[2]	111	67%	84%	75%

NOTE: Hospital profiles are in alphabetical order by state, then city, then hospital within the city; Rankings exclude hospitals with less than 25 cases except for patient surveys which excludes hospitals with less than 100 cases; (a) 100-299 cases; (1) The number of cases/patients is too few to report; (2) Data submitted were based on a sample of cases/patients; (3) Results are based on a shorter time period than required; (4) Data suppressed by CMS for one or more quarters; (5) Results are not available for this reporting period; (6) Fewer than 100 patients completed the HCAHPS survey; (7) No cases met the criteria for this measure; (8) The lower limit of the confidence interval cannot be calculated if the number of observed infections equals zero; (9) No data are available from the state/territory for this reporting period; (10) The scores shown reflect fewer than 50 completed surveys; (11) There were discrepancies in the data collection process; (12) This measure does not apply to this hospital for this reporting period; (13) Results cannot be calculated for this reporting period; (14) The results for this state are combined with nearby states to protect confidentiality; Please refer to the User's Guide for a full explanation of data.

Measure	Cases	This Hosp.	State Avg.	U.S. Avg.
Chest Pain/Possible Heart Attack Care				
Aspirin Given Within 24 Hours of Arrival[5]	-	-	94%	96%
Fibrinolytic Meds Within 30 Min. of Arrival[5]	-	-	47%	58%
Average Time to ECG (minutes)[5]	-	-	8	7
Average Time to Transfer (minutes)[5]	-	-	62	60
Children's Asthma Care				
Received Home Management Plan of Care	-	-	93%	88%
Received Reliever Medication	-	-	100%	100%
Received Systemic Corticosteroids	-	-	100%	100%
Emergency Department				
Admittance Decision Time (minutes)[2]	508	112	99	98
Head CT Results Within 45 Min. of Arrival[1]	-	-	54%	57%
Patients Who Left ER Before Being Seen	61,592	8%	3%	2%
Time from ER Arrival to Admit. (minutes)[2]	528	340	270	274
Time from ER Arrival to Discharge (minutes)	351	243	127	134
Time in ER Before Being Evaluated (minutes)	403	44	26	26
Time to Pain Meds for Fractures (minutes)	256	92	57	57
Heart Attack Care				
Aspirin Given at Discharge[2]	282	100%	99%	99%
Fibrinolytic Meds Within 30 Min. of Arrival[2,7]	-	-	49%	54%
PCI Within 90 Minutes of Arrival[2]	39	97%	95%	96%
Statin Prescribed at Discharge[2]	269	99%	98%	98%
Heart Failure Care				
ACE Inhibitor or ARB for LVSD[2]	131	99%	97%	97%
Discharge Instructions Given[2]	285	87%	95%	94%
Evaluation of LVS Function[2]	307	100%	99%	99%
Medicare Spending				
Medicare Spending per Patient (ratio)	-	0.99	1.03	0.98
Pneumonia Care				
Appropriate Initial Antibiotic Given[2]	33	88%	95%	95%
Blood Culture Timing[2]	104	99%	98%	98%
Pregnancy and Delivery Care				
Newborn Deliveries Scheduled Early[2]	107	14%	7%	6%
Preventive Care				
Immunization for Influenza[2]	520	86%	90%	90%
Immunization for Pneumonia[2]	419	84%	92%	92%
Stroke Care				
Anticoagulation Therapy for Atrial Fibrillation	80	100%	96%	95%
Antithrombotic Therapy Timing	374	96%	98%	98%
Assessed for Rehabilitation	855	100%	98%	97%
Discharged on Antithrombotic Therapy	528	99%	99%	99%
Discharged on Statin Medication	382	100%	95%	94%
Thrombolytic Therapy Timing	65	95%	68%	66%
Venous Thromboembolism Prophylaxis	939	100%	94%	94%
Written Stroke Educational Materials Given	500	96%	92%	88%
Surgical Care Improvement Project				
Appropriate Beta Blocker Usage[2]	243	98%	98%	98%
Appropriate VTP Within 24 Hours[2]	444	99%	98%	98%
Controlled Postoperative Blood Glucose[2]	135	96%	96%	97%
Perioperative Temperature Management[2]	634	100%	100%	100%
Prophylactic Antibiotic Selection[2]	406	98%	99%	99%
Prophylactic Antibiotic Selection (Outpatient)	480	99%	98%	98%
Prophylactic Antibiotic Stopped[2]	387	96%	98%	98%
Prophylactic Antibiotic Timing[2]	406	99%	99%	99%
Prophylactic Antibiotic Timing (Outpatient)	482	98%	98%	98%
Urinary Catheter Removal[2]	347	97%	98%	97%
Survey of Patients' Hospital Experiences				
Area Around Room 'Always' Quiet at Night	300+	60%	68%	61%
Doctors 'Always' Communicated Well	300+	80%	83%	82%
Home Recovery Information Given	300+	87%	85%	85%
Hospital Given 9 or 10 on 10 Point Scale	300+	73%	73%	71%
Meds 'Always' Explained Before Given	300+	63%	66%	64%
Nurses 'Always' Communicated Well	300+	77%	80%	79%
Pain 'Always' Well Controlled	300+	69%	72%	71%
Room and Bathroom 'Always' Clean	300+	71%	75%	73%
Timely Help 'Always' Received	300+	63%	69%	68%
Would Definitely Recommend Hospital	300+	75%	73%	71%
Use of Medical Imaging				
Cardiac Imaging Stress Test before Surgery	180	7.8%	5.3%	5.3%
Combination Abdominal CT Scan	809	25.8%	16.4%	10.5%
Combination Brain/Sinus CT Scan	758	1.8%	2.7%	2.7%
Combination Chest CT Scan	685	6.4%	5.6%	2.7%
Follow-up Mammogram/Ultrasound	397	7.6%	7.9%	8.8%
Lumbar Spine MRI for Low Back Pain	110	40.9%	39.6%	37.2%

The Methodist Hospital

6565 Fannin
Houston, TX 77030
URL: www.methodisthealth.com
Type: Acute Care Hospitals
Ownership: Voluntary non-profit - Private
Phone: 713-790-2221
Fax: 713-790-2605
Emergency Services: Yes
Beds: 1,299

Key Personnel:
Pediatric Ambulatory Care ...... Ralph D Feigin, MD
Pediatric In-Patient Care .... Ralph D Feigin, MD
Radiology.................... James Harrell, MD
Operating Room............. Jane Lee, RN
Infection Control............. Fran Slater
CEO/President............... Judy Spinella
Quality Assurance .... Connie Wallace
Chief of Medical Staff.......... Catherine Williams, MD

Measure	Cases	This Hosp.	State Avg.	U.S. Avg.
Blood Clot Prevention and Treatment				
Anticoagulation Overlap Therapy[2]	200	92%	93%	93%
ICU Venous Thromboembolism Prophylaxis[2]	134	92%	92%	92%
Incidence of Potentially Preventable VTE[2]	87	20%	9%	10%
UFH with Dosages/Platelet Monitoring[2]	179	99%	96%	97%
Venous Thromboembolism Prophylaxis[2]	298	65%	82%	85%
Warfarin Therapy Discharge Instructions[2]	155	80%	84%	75%
Chest Pain/Possible Heart Attack Care				
Aspirin Given Within 24 Hours of Arrival[5]	-	-	94%	96%
Fibrinolytic Meds Within 30 Min. of Arrival[5]	-	-	47%	58%
Average Time to ECG (minutes)[5]	-	-	8	7
Average Time to Transfer (minutes)[5]	-	-	62	60
Children's Asthma Care				
Received Home Management Plan of Care	-	-	93%	88%
Received Reliever Medication	-	-	100%	100%
Received Systemic Corticosteroids	-	-	100%	100%
Emergency Department				
Admittance Decision Time (minutes)[2]	438	144	99	98
Head CT Results Within 45 Min. of Arrival[1,3]	-	-	54%	57%
Patients Who Left ER Before Being Seen	54,453	2%	3%	2%
Time from ER Arrival to Admit. (minutes)[2]	440	324	270	274
Time from ER Arrival to Discharge (minutes)	404	134	127	134
Time in ER Before Being Evaluated (minutes)	448	30	26	26
Time to Pain Meds for Fractures (minutes)	99	43	57	57
Heart Attack Care				
Aspirin Given at Discharge	552	99%	99%	99%
Fibrinolytic Meds Within 30 Min. of Arrival[7]	-	-	49%	54%
PCI Within 90 Minutes of Arrival	34	100%	95%	96%
Statin Prescribed at Discharge	523	99%	98%	98%
Heart Failure Care				
ACE Inhibitor or ARB for LVSD	319	97%	97%	97%
Discharge Instructions Given	826	88%	95%	94%
Evaluation of LVS Function	960	100%	99%	99%
Medicare Spending				
Medicare Spending per Patient (ratio)	-	0.98	1.03	0.98
Pneumonia Care				
Appropriate Initial Antibiotic Given[2]	168	95%	95%	95%
Blood Culture Timing[2]	340	98%	98%	98%
Pregnancy and Delivery Care				
Newborn Deliveries Scheduled Early	97	0%	7%	6%
Preventive Care				
Immunization for Influenza[2]	602	96%	90%	90%
Immunization for Pneumonia[2]	799	97%	92%	92%
Stroke Care				
Anticoagulation Therapy for Atrial Fibrillation	104	98%	96%	95%
Antithrombotic Therapy Timing	351	97%	98%	98%
Assessed for Rehabilitation	533	99%	98%	97%
Discharged on Antithrombotic Therapy	413	100%	99%	99%
Discharged on Statin Medication	313	96%	95%	94%
Thrombolytic Therapy Timing	43	98%	68%	66%
Venous Thromboembolism Prophylaxis	560	96%	94%	94%
Written Stroke Educational Materials Given	299	93%	92%	88%
Surgical Care Improvement Project				
Appropriate Beta Blocker Usage[2]	384	97%	98%	98%
Appropriate VTP Within 24 Hours[2]	592	97%	98%	98%
Controlled Postoperative Blood Glucose[2]	191	93%	96%	97%
Perioperative Temperature Management[2]	827	100%	100%	100%
Prophylactic Antibiotic Selection[2]	592	99%	99%	99%
Prophylactic Antibiotic Selection (Outpatient)	1,265	99%	98%	98%
Prophylactic Antibiotic Stopped[2]	578	95%	98%	98%
Prophylactic Antibiotic Timing[2]	592	100%	99%	99%
Prophylactic Antibiotic Timing (Outpatient)	1,266	99%	98%	98%
Urinary Catheter Removal[2]	515	98%	98%	97%
Survey of Patients' Hospital Experiences				
Area Around Room 'Always' Quiet at Night	300+	63%	68%	61%
Doctors 'Always' Communicated Well	300+	82%	83%	82%
Home Recovery Information Given	300+	86%	85%	85%
Hospital Given 9 or 10 on 10 Point Scale	300+	78%	73%	71%
Meds 'Always' Explained Before Given	300+	64%	66%	64%
Nurses 'Always' Communicated Well	300+	77%	80%	79%
Pain 'Always' Well Controlled	300+	71%	72%	71%
Room and Bathroom 'Always' Clean	300+	71%	75%	73%
Timely Help 'Always' Received	300+	63%	69%	68%
Would Definitely Recommend Hospital	300+	82%	73%	71%
Use of Medical Imaging				
Cardiac Imaging Stress Test before Surgery	566	6.4%	5.3%	5.3%
Combination Abdominal CT Scan	2,000	33.4%	16.4%	10.5%
Combination Brain/Sinus CT Scan	1,620	2.7%	2.7%	2.7%
Combination Chest CT Scan	1,831	0.7%	5.6%	2.7%
Follow-up Mammogram/Ultrasound	1,140	13.9%	7.9%	8.8%
Lumbar Spine MRI for Low Back Pain	417	44.6%	39.6%	37.2%

Methodist West Houston Hospital

18500 Katy Freeway
Houston, TX 77094
Type: Acute Care Hospitals
Ownership: Voluntary non-profit - Private
Phone: 832-522-1000
Emergency Services: Yes

Measure	Cases	This Hosp.	State Avg.	U.S. Avg.
Blood Clot Prevention and Treatment				
Anticoagulation Overlap Therapy[2]	46	98%	93%	93%
ICU Venous Thromboembolism Prophylaxis[2]	88	98%	92%	92%
Incidence of Potentially Preventable VTE[1,2]	-	-	9%	10%
UFH with Dosages/Platelet Monitoring[2]	16	100%	96%	97%
Venous Thromboembolism Prophylaxis[2]	339	79%	82%	85%
Warfarin Therapy Discharge Instructions[2]	28	93%	84%	75%
Chest Pain/Possible Heart Attack Care				
Aspirin Given Within 24 Hours of Arrival[5]	-	-	94%	96%
Fibrinolytic Meds Within 30 Min. of Arrival[5]	-	-	47%	58%
Average Time to ECG (minutes)[5]	-	-	8	7
Average Time to Transfer (minutes)[5]	-	-	62	60
Children's Asthma Care				
Received Home Management Plan of Care	-	-	93%	88%
Received Reliever Medication	-	-	100%	100%
Received Systemic Corticosteroids	-	-	100%	100%
Emergency Department				
Admittance Decision Time (minutes)[2]	561	132	99	98
Head CT Results Within 45 Min. of Arrival[1,3]	-	-	54%	57%
Patients Who Left ER Before Being Seen	23,095	3%	3%	2%
Time from ER Arrival to Admit. (minutes)[2]	614	319	270	274
Time from ER Arrival to Discharge (minutes)	381	195	127	134
Time in ER Before Being Evaluated (minutes)	421	32	26	26
Time to Pain Meds for Fractures (minutes)	99	65	57	57
Heart Attack Care				
Aspirin Given at Discharge[2]	230	100%	99%	99%
Fibrinolytic Meds Within 30 Min. of Arrival[2,7]	-	-	49%	54%
PCI Within 90 Minutes of Arrival[2]	40	98%	95%	96%
Statin Prescribed at Discharge[2]	217	99%	98%	98%
Heart Failure Care				
ACE Inhibitor or ARB for LVSD[2]	113	97%	97%	97%
Discharge Instructions Given[2]	216	100%	95%	94%
Evaluation of LVS Function[2]	261	100%	99%	99%
Medicare Spending				
Medicare Spending per Patient (ratio)	-	1.08	1.03	0.98
Pneumonia Care				
Appropriate Initial Antibiotic Given[2]	118	97%	95%	95%
Blood Culture Timing[2]	206	97%	98%	98%
Pregnancy and Delivery Care				

NOTE: Hospital profiles are in alphabetical order by state, then city, then hospital within the city; Rankings exclude hospitals with less than 25 cases except for patient surveys which excludes hospitals with less than 100 cases; (a) 100-299 cases; (1) The number of cases/patients is too few to report; (2) Data submitted were based on a sample of cases/patients; (3) Results are based on a shorter time period than required; (4) Data suppressed by CMS for one or more quarters; (5) Results are not available for this reporting period; (6) Fewer than 100 patients completed the HCAHPS survey; (7) No cases met the criteria for this measure; (8) The lower limit of the confidence interval cannot be calculated if the number of observed infections equals zero; (9) No data are available from the state/territory for this reporting period; (10) The scores shown reflect fewer than 50 completed surveys; (11) There were discrepancies in the data collection process; (12) This measure does not apply to this hospital for this reporting period; (13) Results cannot be calculated for this reporting period; (14) The results for this state are combined with nearby states to protect confidentiality; Please refer to the User's Guide for a full explanation of data.

Measure	Cases	This Hosp.	State Avg.	U.S. Avg.
Newborn Deliveries Scheduled Early[2]	52	13%	7%	6%
Preventive Care				
Immunization for Influenza[2]	562	96%	90%	90%
Immunization for Pneumonia[2]	580	98%	92%	92%
Stroke Care				
Anticoagulation Therapy for Atrial Fibrillation	14	100%	96%	95%
Antithrombotic Therapy Timing	79	100%	98%	98%
Assessed for Rehabilitation	96	94%	98%	97%
Discharged on Antithrombotic Therapy	93	100%	99%	99%
Discharged on Statin Medication	74	97%	95%	94%
Thrombolytic Therapy Timing[1]	-	-	68%	66%
Venous Thromboembolism Prophylaxis	86	85%	94%	94%
Written Stroke Educational Materials Given	66	91%	92%	88%
Surgical Care Improvement Project				
Appropriate Beta Blocker Usage[2]	165	99%	98%	98%
Appropriate VTP Within 24 Hours[2]	210	97%	98%	98%
Controlled Postoperative Blood Glucose[2]	122	98%	96%	97%
Perioperative Temperature Management[2]	318	100%	100%	100%
Prophylactic Antibiotic Selection[2]	249	98%	99%	99%
Prophylactic Antibiotic Selection (Outpatient)	291	94%	98%	98%
Prophylactic Antibiotic Stopped[2]	241	99%	98%	98%
Prophylactic Antibiotic Timing[2]	250	99%	99%	99%
Prophylactic Antibiotic Timing (Outpatient)	293	98%	98%	98%
Urinary Catheter Removal[2]	239	99%	98%	97%
Survey of Patients' Hospital Experiences				
Area Around Room 'Always' Quiet at Night	300+	70%	68%	61%
Doctors 'Always' Communicated Well	300+	80%	83%	82%
Home Recovery Information Given	300+	86%	85%	85%
Hospital Given 9 or 10 on 10 Point Scale	300+	79%	73%	71%
Meds 'Always' Explained Before Given	300+	63%	66%	64%
Nurses 'Always' Communicated Well	300+	79%	80%	79%
Pain 'Always' Well Controlled	300+	70%	72%	71%
Room and Bathroom 'Always' Clean	300+	80%	75%	73%
Timely Help 'Always' Received	300+	65%	69%	68%
Would Definitely Recommend Hospital	300+	80%	73%	71%
Use of Medical Imaging				
Cardiac Imaging Stress Test before Surgery[1]	-	-	5.3%	5.3%
Combination Abdominal CT Scan	324	23.1%	16.4%	10.5%
Combination Brain/Sinus CT Scan	481	2.1%	2.7%	2.7%
Combination Chest CT Scan	229	0.4%	5.6%	2.7%
Follow-up Mammogram/Ultrasound	165	17.0%	7.9%	8.8%
Lumbar Spine MRI for Low Back Pain[1]	-	-	39.6%	37.2%

Methodist Willowbrook Hospital

18220 Tomball Parkway
Houston, TX 77070
Phone: 281-477-1000
URL: www.houstonmethodist.org/willowbrook-hospital
Type: Acute Care Hospitals
Emergency Services: Yes
Ownership: Voluntary non-profit - Church

Measure	Cases	This Hosp.	State Avg.	U.S. Avg.
Blood Clot Prevention and Treatment				
Anticoagulation Overlap Therapy[2]	82	98%	93%	93%
ICU Venous Thromboembolism Prophylaxis[2]	96	96%	92%	92%
Incidence of Potentially Preventable VTE[1,2]	-	-	9%	10%
UFH with Dosages/Platelet Monitoring[2]	44	100%	96%	97%
Venous Thromboembolism Prophylaxis[2]	347	82%	82%	85%
Warfarin Therapy Discharge Instructions[2]	65	94%	84%	75%
Chest Pain/Possible Heart Attack Care				
Aspirin Given Within 24 Hours of Arrival[5]	-	-	94%	96%
Fibrinolytic Meds Within 30 Min. of Arrival[5]	-	-	47%	58%
Average Time to ECG (minutes)[5]	-	-	8	7
Average Time to Transfer (minutes)[5]	-	-	62	60
Children's Asthma Care				
Received Home Management Plan of Care	-	-	93%	88%
Received Reliever Medication	-	-	100%	100%
Received Systemic Corticosteroids	-	-	100%	100%
Emergency Department				
Admittance Decision Time (minutes)[2]	551	127	99	98
Head CT Results Within 45 Min. of Arrival[1]	-	-	54%	57%
Patients Who Left ER Before Being Seen	54,403	4%	3%	2%
Time from ER Arrival to Admit. (minutes)[2]	634	320	270	274
Time from ER Arrival to Discharge (minutes)	396	171	127	134
Time in ER Before Being Evaluated (minutes)	417	53	26	26
Time to Pain Meds for Fractures (minutes)	193	74	57	57
Heart Attack Care				
Aspirin Given at Discharge[2]	271	100%	99%	99%
Fibrinolytic Meds Within 30 Min. of Arrival[2,7]	-	-	49%	54%
PCI Within 90 Minutes of Arrival[2]	33	97%	95%	96%
Statin Prescribed at Discharge[2]	250	100%	98%	98%
Heart Failure Care				
ACE Inhibitor or ARB for LVSD[2]	113	100%	97%	97%
Discharge Instructions Given[2]	244	93%	95%	94%
Evaluation of LVS Function[2]	304	100%	99%	99%
Medicare Spending				
Medicare Spending per Patient (ratio)	-	1.12	1.03	0.98
Pneumonia Care				
Appropriate Initial Antibiotic Given[2]	95	100%	95%	95%
Blood Culture Timing[2]	180	99%	98%	98%
Pregnancy and Delivery Care				
Newborn Deliveries Scheduled Early[2]	84	0%	7%	6%
Preventive Care				
Immunization for Influenza[2]	497	98%	90%	90%
Immunization for Pneumonia[2]	534	97%	92%	92%
Stroke Care				
Anticoagulation Therapy for Atrial Fibrillation	25	100%	96%	95%
Antithrombotic Therapy Timing	149	98%	98%	98%
Assessed for Rehabilitation	179	98%	98%	97%
Discharged on Antithrombotic Therapy	158	100%	99%	99%
Discharged on Statin Medication	125	100%	95%	94%
Thrombolytic Therapy Timing	11	91%	68%	66%
Venous Thromboembolism Prophylaxis	179	97%	94%	94%
Written Stroke Educational Materials Given	109	96%	92%	88%
Surgical Care Improvement Project				
Appropriate Beta Blocker Usage[2]	141	99%	98%	98%
Appropriate VTP Within 24 Hours[2]	294	100%	98%	98%
Controlled Postoperative Blood Glucose[2]	67	97%	96%	97%
Perioperative Temperature Management[2]	346	100%	100%	100%
Prophylactic Antibiotic Selection[2]	244	100%	99%	99%
Prophylactic Antibiotic Selection (Outpatient)	343	99%	98%	98%
Prophylactic Antibiotic Stopped[2]	222	100%	98%	98%
Prophylactic Antibiotic Timing[2]	245	100%	99%	99%
Prophylactic Antibiotic Timing (Outpatient)	343	100%	98%	98%
Urinary Catheter Removal[2]	205	100%	98%	97%
Survey of Patients' Hospital Experiences				
Area Around Room 'Always' Quiet at Night	300+	69%	68%	61%
Doctors 'Always' Communicated Well	300+	76%	83%	82%
Home Recovery Information Given	300+	84%	85%	85%
Hospital Given 9 or 10 on 10 Point Scale	300+	75%	73%	71%
Meds 'Always' Explained Before Given	300+	62%	66%	64%
Nurses 'Always' Communicated Well	300+	77%	80%	79%
Pain 'Always' Well Controlled	300+	70%	72%	71%
Room and Bathroom 'Always' Clean	300+	68%	75%	73%
Timely Help 'Always' Received	300+	63%	69%	68%
Would Definitely Recommend Hospital	300+	77%	73%	71%
Use of Medical Imaging				
Cardiac Imaging Stress Test before Surgery	79	2.5%	5.3%	5.3%
Combination Abdominal CT Scan	566	17.7%	16.4%	10.5%
Combination Brain/Sinus CT Scan	664	2.9%	2.7%	2.7%
Combination Chest CT Scan	375	0.0%	5.6%	2.7%
Follow-up Mammogram/Ultrasound	418	14.4%	7.9%	8.8%
Lumbar Spine MRI for Low Back Pain	100	35.0%	39.6%	37.2%

Park Plaza Hospital

1313 Hermann Dr
Houston, TX 77004
Phone: 713-527-5019
Fax: 713-527-5689
URL: www.parkplazahospital.com
Type: Acute Care Hospitals
Emergency Services: Yes
Ownership: Proprietary
Beds: 446

Key Personnel:

Chief of Medical Staff.......... Timothy Anderson, MD
Quality Assurance .... Mark Ayers
Patient Relations .... Gwen Banks
Emergency Room .... Mike Davis
Infection Control............. Pam Diffenbach
Radiology.................. Cathy Doughty
Operating Room............. Annie Moulder
CEO/President............... John Tressa, RN, MSN, MBA

Measure	Cases	This Hosp.	State Avg.	U.S. Avg.
Blood Clot Prevention and Treatment				
Anticoagulation Overlap Therapy[2]	36	94%	93%	93%
ICU Venous Thromboembolism Prophylaxis[2]	65	91%	92%	92%
Incidence of Potentially Preventable VTE[1,2]	-	-	9%	10%
UFH with Dosages/Platelet Monitoring[2]	26	100%	96%	97%
Venous Thromboembolism Prophylaxis[2]	386	85%	82%	85%
Warfarin Therapy Discharge Instructions[2]	21	95%	84%	75%
Chest Pain/Possible Heart Attack Care				
Aspirin Given Within 24 Hours of Arrival[1,3]	-	-	94%	96%
Fibrinolytic Meds Within 30 Min. of Arrival[3,7]	-	-	47%	58%
Average Time to ECG (minutes)[1,3]	-	-	8	7
Average Time to Transfer (minutes)[1,3]	-	-	62	60
Children's Asthma Care				
Received Home Management Plan of Care	-	-	93%	88%
Received Reliever Medication	-	-	100%	100%
Received Systemic Corticosteroids	-	-	100%	100%
Emergency Department				
Admittance Decision Time (minutes)[2]	431	94	99	98
Head CT Results Within 45 Min. of Arrival[1,3]	-	-	54%	57%
Patients Who Left ER Before Being Seen	10,381	1%	3%	2%
Time from ER Arrival to Admit. (minutes)[2]	431	286	270	274
Time from ER Arrival to Discharge (minutes)	426	154	127	134
Time in ER Before Being Evaluated (minutes)	486	24	26	26
Time to Pain Meds for Fractures (minutes)	11	40	57	57
Heart Attack Care				
Aspirin Given at Discharge	25	96%	99%	99%
Fibrinolytic Meds Within 30 Min. of Arrival[7]	-	-	49%	54%
PCI Within 90 Minutes of Arrival[1]	-	-	95%	96%
Statin Prescribed at Discharge	24	96%	98%	98%
Heart Failure Care				
ACE Inhibitor or ARB for LVSD	43	100%	97%	97%
Discharge Instructions Given	145	92%	95%	94%
Evaluation of LVS Function	165	100%	99%	99%
Medicare Spending				
Medicare Spending per Patient (ratio)	-	1.06	1.03	0.98
Pneumonia Care				
Appropriate Initial Antibiotic Given	38	95%	95%	95%
Blood Culture Timing	90	98%	98%	98%
Pregnancy and Delivery Care				
Newborn Deliveries Scheduled Early[2]	28	18%	7%	6%
Preventive Care				
Immunization for Influenza[2]	531	92%	90%	90%
Immunization for Pneumonia[2]	641	95%	92%	92%
Stroke Care				
Anticoagulation Therapy for Atrial Fibrillation[1]	-	-	96%	95%
Antithrombotic Therapy Timing	28	100%	98%	98%
Assessed for Rehabilitation	26	88%	98%	97%
Discharged on Antithrombotic Therapy	25	96%	99%	99%
Discharged on Statin Medication	22	91%	95%	94%
Thrombolytic Therapy Timing[1]	-	-	68%	66%
Venous Thromboembolism Prophylaxis	29	76%	94%	94%
Written Stroke Educational Materials Given	15	27%	92%	88%
Surgical Care Improvement Project				
Appropriate Beta Blocker Usage[2]	92	95%	98%	98%
Appropriate VTP Within 24 Hours[2]	357	98%	98%	98%
Controlled Postoperative Blood Glucose[2,7]	-	-	96%	97%
Perioperative Temperature Management[2]	396	100%	100%	100%
Prophylactic Antibiotic Selection[2]	282	97%	99%	99%
Prophylactic Antibiotic Selection (Outpatient)	267	97%	98%	98%
Prophylactic Antibiotic Stopped[2]	274	99%	98%	98%
Prophylactic Antibiotic Timing[2]	282	99%	99%	99%
Prophylactic Antibiotic Timing (Outpatient)	229	98%	98%	98%
Urinary Catheter Removal[2]	261	98%	98%	97%
Survey of Patients' Hospital Experiences				
Area Around Room 'Always' Quiet at Night	300+	71%	68%	61%
Doctors 'Always' Communicated Well	300+	90%	83%	82%
Home Recovery Information Given	300+	80%	85%	85%
Hospital Given 9 or 10 on 10 Point Scale	300+	72%	73%	71%
Meds 'Always' Explained Before Given	300+	68%	66%	64%
Nurses 'Always' Communicated Well	300+	78%	80%	79%
Pain 'Always' Well Controlled	300+	74%	72%	71%

NOTE: Hospital profiles are in alphabetical order by state, then city, then hospital within the city; Rankings exclude hospitals with less than 25 cases except for patient surveys which excludes hospitals with less than 100 cases; (a) 100-299 cases; (1) The number of cases/patients is too few to report; (2) Data submitted were based on a sample of cases/patients; (3) Results are based on a shorter time period than required; (4) Data suppressed by CMS for one or more quarters; (5) Results are not available for this reporting period; (6) Fewer than 100 patients completed the HCAHPS survey; (7) No cases met the criteria for this measure; (8) The lower limit of the confidence interval cannot be calculated if the number of observed infections equals zero; (9) No data are available from the state/territory for this reporting period; (10) The scores shown reflect fewer than 50 completed surveys; (11) There were discrepancies in the data collection process; (12) This measure does not apply to this hospital for this reporting period; (13) Results cannot be calculated for this reporting period; (14) The results for this state are combined with nearby states to protect confidentiality; Please refer to the User's Guide for a full explanation of data.

Measure	Cases	This Hosp.	State Avg.	U.S. Avg.
Room and Bathroom 'Always' Clean	300+	72%	75%	73%
Timely Help 'Always' Received	300+	68%	69%	68%
Would Definitely Recommend Hospital	300+	72%	73%	71%
Use of Medical Imaging				
Cardiac Imaging Stress Test before Surgery	171	6.4%	5.3%	5.3%
Combination Abdominal CT Scan	309	22.3%	16.4%	10.5%
Combination Brain/Sinus CT Scan[1]	-	-	2.7%	2.7%
Combination Chest CT Scan	117	0.9%	5.6%	2.7%
Follow-up Mammogram/Ultrasound	576	6.9%	7.9%	8.8%
Lumbar Spine MRI for Low Back Pain[1]	-	-	39.6%	37.2%

Riverside General Hospital

3204 Ennis St
Houston, TX 77004
Phone: 713-526-2441
Fax: 713-526-3554
URL: www.riversidegeneral.org
Type: Acute Care Hospitals
Emergency Services: Yes
Ownership: Voluntary non-profit - Private
Beds: 98
Key Personnel:
Chief of Medical Staff.......... Edith Jones

Measure	Cases	This Hosp.	State Avg.	U.S. Avg.
Blood Clot Prevention and Treatment				
Anticoagulation Overlap Therapy[2,3]	-	-	93%	93%
ICU Venous Thromboembolism Prophylaxis[2,3]	-	-	92%	92%
Incidence of Potentially Preventable VTE[2,3]	-	-	9%	10%
UFH with Dosages/Platelet Monitoring[2,3]	-	-	96%	97%
Venous Thromboembolism Prophylaxis[2,3]	-	-	82%	85%
Warfarin Therapy Discharge Instructions[2,3]	-	-	84%	75%
Chest Pain/Possible Heart Attack Care				
Aspirin Given Within 24 Hours of Arrival[5]	-	-	94%	96%
Fibrinolytic Meds Within 30 Min. of Arrival[5]	-	-	47%	58%
Average Time to ECG (minutes)[5]	-	-	8	7
Average Time to Transfer (minutes)[5]	-	-	62	60
Children's Asthma Care				
Received Home Management Plan of Care	-	-	93%	88%
Received Reliever Medication	-	-	100%	100%
Received Systemic Corticosteroids	-	-	100%	100%
Emergency Department				
Admittance Decision Time (minutes)[2,7]	-	-	99	98
Head CT Results Within 45 Min. of Arrival[5]	-	-	54%	57%
Patients Who Left ER Before Being Seen	19	16%	3%	2%
Time from ER Arrival to Admit. (minutes)[2,7]	-	-	270	274
Time from ER Arrival to Discharge (minutes)[5]	-	-	127	134
Time in ER Before Being Evaluated (minutes)[5]	-	-	26	26
Time to Pain Meds for Fractures (minutes)[5]	-	-	57	57
Heart Attack Care				
Aspirin Given at Discharge[5]	-	-	99%	99%
Fibrinolytic Meds Within 30 Min. of Arrival[5]	-	-	49%	54%
PCI Within 90 Minutes of Arrival[5]	-	-	95%	96%
Statin Prescribed at Discharge[5]	-	-	98%	98%
Heart Failure Care				
ACE Inhibitor or ARB for LVSD[5]	-	-	97%	97%
Discharge Instructions Given[5]	-	-	95%	94%
Evaluation of LVS Function[5]	-	-	99%	99%
Medicare Spending				
Medicare Spending per Patient (ratio)	-	0.88	1.03	0.98
Pneumonia Care				
Appropriate Initial Antibiotic Given[5]	-	-	95%	95%
Blood Culture Timing[5]	-	-	98%	98%
Pregnancy and Delivery Care				
Newborn Deliveries Scheduled Early[7]	-	-	7%	6%
Preventive Care				
Immunization for Influenza[2]	254	0%	90%	90%
Immunization for Pneumonia[2,7]	-	-	92%	92%
Stroke Care				
Anticoagulation Therapy for Atrial Fibrillation[5]	-	-	96%	95%
Antithrombotic Therapy Timing[5]	-	-	98%	98%
Assessed for Rehabilitation[5]	-	-	98%	97%
Discharged on Antithrombotic Therapy[5]	-	-	99%	99%
Discharged on Statin Medication[5]	-	-	95%	94%
Thrombolytic Therapy Timing[5]	-	-	68%	66%
Venous Thromboembolism Prophylaxis[5]	-	-	94%	94%
Written Stroke Educational Materials Given[5]	-	-	92%	88%
Surgical Care Improvement Project				
Appropriate Beta Blocker Usage[5]	-	-	98%	98%
Appropriate VTP Within 24 Hours[5]	-	-	98%	98%
Controlled Postoperative Blood Glucose[5]	-	-	96%	97%
Perioperative Temperature Management[5]	-	-	100%	100%
Prophylactic Antibiotic Selection[5]	-	-	99%	99%
Prophylactic Antibiotic Selection (Outpatient)[5]	-	-	98%	98%
Prophylactic Antibiotic Stopped[5]	-	-	98%	98%
Prophylactic Antibiotic Timing[5]	-	-	99%	99%
Prophylactic Antibiotic Timing (Outpatient)[5]	-	-	98%	98%
Urinary Catheter Removal[5]	-	-	98%	97%
Survey of Patients' Hospital Experiences				
Area Around Room 'Always' Quiet at Night[1]	-	-	68%	61%
Doctors 'Always' Communicated Well[1]	-	-	83%	82%
Home Recovery Information Given[1]	-	-	85%	85%
Hospital Given 9 or 10 on 10 Point Scale[1]	-	-	73%	71%
Meds 'Always' Explained Before Given[1]	-	-	66%	64%
Nurses 'Always' Communicated Well[1]	-	-	80%	79%
Pain 'Always' Well Controlled[1]	-	-	72%	71%
Room and Bathroom 'Always' Clean[1]	-	-	75%	73%
Timely Help 'Always' Received[1]	-	-	69%	68%
Would Definitely Recommend Hospital[1]	-	-	73%	71%
Use of Medical Imaging				
Cardiac Imaging Stress Test before Surgery[7]	-	-	5.3%	5.3%
Combination Abdominal CT Scan[7]	-	-	16.4%	10.5%
Combination Brain/Sinus CT Scan[7]	-	-	2.7%	2.7%
Combination Chest CT Scan[7]	-	-	5.6%	2.7%
Follow-up Mammogram/Ultrasound[7]	-	-	7.9%	8.8%
Lumbar Spine MRI for Low Back Pain[7]	-	-	39.6%	37.2%

Saint Anthony's Hospital

2807 Little York Rd
Houston, TX 77093
Phone: 713-697-2961
Fax: 713-696-4662
URL: www.renhealthcare.org/default.aspx
Type: Acute Care Hospitals
Emergency Services: Yes
Ownership: Proprietary
Beds: 39
Key Personnel:
Operating Room.............. Diane Conner
CEO/President.............. J Scott Douglass
Chief of Medical Staff.......... Annette Leonard
Emergency Room .... Kevin Pallesen
Quality Assurance .... Mickey Smensy

Measure	Cases	This Hosp.	State Avg.	U.S. Avg.
Blood Clot Prevention and Treatment				
Anticoagulation Overlap Therapy[1,2]	-	-	93%	93%
ICU Venous Thromboembolism Prophylaxis[2]	86	60%	92%	92%
Incidence of Potentially Preventable VTE[2,7]	-	-	9%	10%
UFH with Dosages/Platelet Monitoring[1,2]	-	-	96%	97%
Venous Thromboembolism Prophylaxis[2]	293	42%	82%	85%
Warfarin Therapy Discharge Instructions[1,2]	-	-	84%	75%
Chest Pain/Possible Heart Attack Care				
Aspirin Given Within 24 Hours of Arrival[5]	-	-	94%	96%
Fibrinolytic Meds Within 30 Min. of Arrival[5]	-	-	47%	58%
Average Time to ECG (minutes)[5]	-	-	8	7
Average Time to Transfer (minutes)[5]	-	-	62	60
Children's Asthma Care				
Received Home Management Plan of Care	-	-	93%	88%
Received Reliever Medication	-	-	100%	100%
Received Systemic Corticosteroids	-	-	100%	100%
Emergency Department				
Admittance Decision Time (minutes)[2,3]	205	88	99	98
Head CT Results Within 45 Min. of Arrival[5]	-	-	54%	57%
Patients Who Left ER Before Being Seen	11,963	0%	3%	2%
Time from ER Arrival to Admit. (minutes)[2,3]	210	248	270	274
Time from ER Arrival to Discharge (minutes)	315	138	127	134
Time in ER Before Being Evaluated (minutes)	357	40	26	26
Time to Pain Meds for Fractures (minutes)[5]	-	-	57	57
Heart Attack Care				
Aspirin Given at Discharge[1,2]	-	-	99%	99%
Fibrinolytic Meds Within 30 Min. of Arrival[2,3]	-	-	49%	54%
PCI Within 90 Minutes of Arrival[2,3]	-	-	95%	96%
Statin Prescribed at Discharge[1,2]	-	-	98%	98%
Heart Failure Care				
ACE Inhibitor or ARB for LVSD[2,3]	19	100%	97%	97%
Discharge Instructions Given[2,3]	60	83%	95%	94%
Evaluation of LVS Function[2,3]	67	31%	99%	99%
Medicare Spending				
Medicare Spending per Patient (ratio)	-	1.31	1.03	0.98
Pneumonia Care				
Appropriate Initial Antibiotic Given[2,3]	19	21%	95%	95%
Blood Culture Timing[2,3]	21	81%	98%	98%
Pregnancy and Delivery Care				
Newborn Deliveries Scheduled Early[2,7]	-	-	7%	6%
Preventive Care				
Immunization for Influenza[2,3]	153	86%	90%	90%
Immunization for Pneumonia[2,3]	170	64%	92%	92%
Stroke Care				
Anticoagulation Therapy for Atrial Fibrillation[2,3]	-	-	96%	95%
Antithrombotic Therapy Timing[1,2]	-	-	98%	98%
Assessed for Rehabilitation[1,2]	-	-	98%	97%
Discharged on Antithrombotic Therapy[1,2]	-	-	99%	99%
Discharged on Statin Medication[1,2]	-	-	95%	94%
Thrombolytic Therapy Timing[2,3]	-	-	68%	66%
Venous Thromboembolism Prophylaxis[1,2]	-	-	94%	94%
Written Stroke Educational Materials Given[1,2]	-	-	92%	88%
Surgical Care Improvement Project				
Appropriate Beta Blocker Usage[1,2]	-	-	98%	98%
Appropriate VTP Within 24 Hours[1,2]	-	-	98%	98%
Controlled Postoperative Blood Glucose[2,3]	-	-	96%	97%
Perioperative Temperature Management[1,2]	-	-	100%	100%
Prophylactic Antibiotic Selection[2,3]	-	-	99%	99%
Prophylactic Antibiotic Selection (Outpatient)[5]	-	-	98%	98%
Prophylactic Antibiotic Stopped[2,3]	-	-	98%	98%
Prophylactic Antibiotic Timing[2,3]	-	-	99%	99%
Prophylactic Antibiotic Timing (Outpatient)[5]	-	-	98%	98%
Urinary Catheter Removal[1,2]	-	-	98%	97%
Survey of Patients' Hospital Experiences				
Area Around Room 'Always' Quiet at Night	(a)	71%	68%	61%
Doctors 'Always' Communicated Well	(a)	84%	83%	82%
Home Recovery Information Given	(a)	81%	85%	85%
Hospital Given 9 or 10 on 10 Point Scale	(a)	67%	73%	71%
Meds 'Always' Explained Before Given	(a)	70%	66%	64%
Nurses 'Always' Communicated Well	(a)	78%	80%	79%
Pain 'Always' Well Controlled	(a)	71%	72%	71%
Room and Bathroom 'Always' Clean	(a)	70%	75%	73%
Timely Help 'Always' Received	(a)	67%	69%	68%
Would Definitely Recommend Hospital	(a)	66%	73%	71%
Use of Medical Imaging				
Cardiac Imaging Stress Test before Surgery[7]	-	-	5.3%	5.3%
Combination Abdominal CT Scan[1]	-	-	16.4%	10.5%
Combination Brain/Sinus CT Scan	46	0.0%	2.7%	2.7%
Combination Chest CT Scan[1]	-	-	5.6%	2.7%
Follow-up Mammogram/Ultrasound[7]	-	-	7.9%	8.8%
Lumbar Spine MRI for Low Back Pain[7]	-	-	39.6%	37.2%

Saint Joseph Medical Center

1401 Saint Joseph Parkway
Houston, TX 77002
Phone: 713-757-1000
Fax: 713-657-7123
E-mail: fritz.guthrie@sjmctx.com
URL: www.sjmctx.com
Type: Acute Care Hospitals
Emergency Services: Yes
Ownership: Government - Federal
Beds: 792
Key Personnel:
Quality Assurance .... Rhonda Delaney
CEO/President.............. Phillip D Robinson
Emergency Room .... Dori Upton

Measure	Cases	This Hosp.	State Avg.	U.S. Avg.
Blood Clot Prevention and Treatment				
Anticoagulation Overlap Therapy[2]	67	100%	93%	93%
ICU Venous Thromboembolism Prophylaxis[2]	108	92%	92%	92%
Incidence of Potentially Preventable VTE[2]	19	11%	9%	10%
UFH with Dosages/Platelet Monitoring[2]	11	100%	96%	97%
Venous Thromboembolism Prophylaxis[2]	340	78%	82%	85%
Warfarin Therapy Discharge Instructions[2]	47	98%	84%	75%
Chest Pain/Possible Heart Attack Care				
Aspirin Given Within 24 Hours of Arrival[3,7]	-	-	94%	96%
Fibrinolytic Meds Within 30 Min. of Arrival[5]	-	-	47%	58%

NOTE: Hospital profiles are in alphabetical order by state, then city, then hospital within the city; Rankings exclude hospitals with less than 25 cases except for patient surveys which excludes hospitals with less than 100 cases; (a) 100-299 cases; (1) The number of cases/patients is too few to report; (2) Data submitted were based on a sample of cases/patients; (3) Results are based on a shorter time period than required; (4) Data suppressed by CMS for one or more quarters; (5) Results are not available for this reporting period; (6) Fewer than 100 patients completed the HCAHPS survey; (7) No cases met the criteria for this measure; (8) The lower limit of the confidence interval cannot be calculated if the number of observed infections equals zero; (9) No data are available from the state/territory for this reporting period; (10) The scores shown reflect fewer than 50 completed surveys; (11) There were discrepancies in the data collection process; (12) This measure does not apply to this hospital for this reporting period; (13) Results cannot be calculated for this reporting period; (14) The results for this state are combined with nearby states to protect confidentiality; Please refer to the User's Guide for a full explanation of data.

Measure	Cases	This Hosp.	State Avg.	U.S. Avg.
Average Time to ECG (minutes)[3,7]	-	-	8	7
Average Time to Transfer (minutes)[5]	-	-	62	60
Children's Asthma Care				
Received Home Management Plan of Care	-	-	93%	88%
Received Reliever Medication	-	-	100%	100%
Received Systemic Corticosteroids	-	-	100%	100%
Emergency Department				
Admittance Decision Time (minutes)[2]	588	97	99	98
Head CT Results Within 45 Min. of Arrival[1]	-	-	54%	57%
Patients Who Left ER Before Being Seen	32,034	5%	3%	2%
Time from ER Arrival to Admit. (minutes)[2]	590	266	270	274
Time from ER Arrival to Discharge (minutes)	577	164	127	134
Time in ER Before Being Evaluated (minutes)	665	33	26	26
Time to Pain Meds for Fractures (minutes)	96	80	57	57
Heart Attack Care				
Aspirin Given at Discharge	108	97%	99%	99%
Fibrinolytic Meds Within 30 Min. of Arrival[7]	-	-	49%	54%
PCI Within 90 Minutes of Arrival[1]	-	-	95%	96%
Statin Prescribed at Discharge	103	94%	98%	98%
Heart Failure Care				
ACE Inhibitor or ARB for LVSD	162	97%	97%	97%
Discharge Instructions Given	374	90%	95%	94%
Evaluation of LVS Function	424	99%	99%	99%
Medicare Spending				
Medicare Spending per Patient (ratio)	-	1.06	1.03	0.98
Pneumonia Care				
Appropriate Initial Antibiotic Given	108	96%	95%	95%
Blood Culture Timing	196	98%	98%	98%
Pregnancy and Delivery Care				
Newborn Deliveries Scheduled Early[2]	83	7%	7%	6%
Preventive Care				
Immunization for Influenza[2]	609	91%	90%	90%
Immunization for Pneumonia[2]	564	88%	92%	92%
Stroke Care				
Anticoagulation Therapy for Atrial Fibrillation[1]	-	-	96%	95%
Antithrombotic Therapy Timing	73	100%	98%	98%
Assessed for Rehabilitation	88	95%	98%	97%
Discharged on Antithrombotic Therapy	77	99%	99%	99%
Discharged on Statin Medication	65	86%	95%	94%
Thrombolytic Therapy Timing[1]	-	-	68%	66%
Venous Thromboembolism Prophylaxis	94	84%	94%	94%
Written Stroke Educational Materials Given	55	85%	92%	88%
Surgical Care Improvement Project				
Appropriate Beta Blocker Usage	144	97%	98%	98%
Appropriate VTP Within 24 Hours	563	98%	98%	98%
Controlled Postoperative Blood Glucose	63	84%	96%	97%
Perioperative Temperature Management	648	100%	100%	100%
Prophylactic Antibiotic Selection	407	97%	99%	99%
Prophylactic Antibiotic Selection (Outpatient)	285	93%	98%	98%
Prophylactic Antibiotic Stopped	387	97%	98%	98%
Prophylactic Antibiotic Timing	412	96%	99%	99%
Prophylactic Antibiotic Timing (Outpatient)	297	93%	98%	98%
Urinary Catheter Removal	248	94%	98%	97%
Survey of Patients' Hospital Experiences				
Area Around Room 'Always' Quiet at Night	300+	63%	68%	61%
Doctors 'Always' Communicated Well	300+	80%	83%	82%
Home Recovery Information Given	300+	83%	85%	85%
Hospital Given 9 or 10 on 10 Point Scale	300+	64%	73%	71%
Meds 'Always' Explained Before Given	300+	60%	66%	64%
Nurses 'Always' Communicated Well	300+	75%	80%	79%
Pain 'Always' Well Controlled	300+	69%	72%	71%
Room and Bathroom 'Always' Clean	300+	64%	75%	73%
Timely Help 'Always' Received	300+	59%	69%	68%
Would Definitely Recommend Hospital	300+	67%	73%	71%
Use of Medical Imaging				
Cardiac Imaging Stress Test before Surgery	119	7.6%	5.3%	5.3%
Combination Abdominal CT Scan	369	6.5%	16.4%	10.5%
Combination Brain/Sinus CT Scan[1]	-	-	2.7%	2.7%
Combination Chest CT Scan	130	3.1%	5.6%	2.7%
Follow-up Mammogram/Ultrasound	826	3.9%	7.9%	8.8%
Lumbar Spine MRI for Low Back Pain[1]	-	-	39.6%	37.2%

Saint Luke's Episcopal Hospital

6720 Bertner Phone: 832-355-1000
Houston, TX 77030
URL: www.sleh.com
Type: Acute Care Hospitals Emergency Services: Yes
Ownership: Voluntary non-profit - Church Beds: 946

Key Personnel:
Quality Assurance .... Pat Crossman
Radiology.................... P Milton Gray, MD
Anesthesiology............... Tareq Khan, MD
Emergency Room .... Jacklincs Lynch
CEO/President............... David Pate, MD, JD
Chief of Medical Staff.......... Angela Shippy, MD

Measure	Cases	This Hosp.	State Avg.	U.S. Avg.
Blood Clot Prevention and Treatment				
Anticoagulation Overlap Therapy[2]	211	95%	93%	93%
ICU Venous Thromboembolism Prophylaxis[2]	108	77%	92%	92%
Incidence of Potentially Preventable VTE[2]	62	6%	9%	10%
UFH with Dosages/Platelet Monitoring[2]	179	100%	96%	97%
Venous Thromboembolism Prophylaxis[2]	357	76%	82%	85%
Warfarin Therapy Discharge Instructions[2]	143	69%	84%	75%
Chest Pain/Possible Heart Attack Care				
Aspirin Given Within 24 Hours of Arrival[1,3]	-	-	94%	96%
Fibrinolytic Meds Within 30 Min. of Arrival[3,7]	-	-	47%	58%
Average Time to ECG (minutes)[1,3]	-	-	8	7
Average Time to Transfer (minutes)[3,7]	-	-	62	60
Children's Asthma Care				
Received Home Management Plan of Care	-	-	93%	88%
Received Reliever Medication	-	-	100%	100%
Received Systemic Corticosteroids	-	-	100%	100%
Emergency Department				
Admittance Decision Time (minutes)[2]	573	142	99	98
Head CT Results Within 45 Min. of Arrival[1]	-	-	54%	57%
Patients Who Left ER Before Being Seen	84,705	1%	3%	2%
Time from ER Arrival to Admit. (minutes)[2]	606	307	270	274
Time from ER Arrival to Discharge (minutes)	427	103	127	134
Time in ER Before Being Evaluated (minutes)	374	31	26	26
Time to Pain Meds for Fractures (minutes)	189	37	57	57
Heart Attack Care				
Aspirin Given at Discharge[2]	303	98%	99%	99%
Fibrinolytic Meds Within 30 Min. of Arrival[2,7]	-	-	49%	54%
PCI Within 90 Minutes of Arrival[2]	35	100%	95%	96%
Statin Prescribed at Discharge[2]	293	99%	98%	98%
Heart Failure Care				
ACE Inhibitor or ARB for LVSD[2]	112	96%	97%	97%
Discharge Instructions Given[2]	293	97%	95%	94%
Evaluation of LVS Function[2]	329	100%	99%	99%
Medicare Spending				
Medicare Spending per Patient (ratio)	-	1.00	1.03	0.98
Pneumonia Care				
Appropriate Initial Antibiotic Given[2]	79	96%	95%	95%
Blood Culture Timing[2]	147	99%	98%	98%
Pregnancy and Delivery Care				
Newborn Deliveries Scheduled Early[7]	-	-	7%	6%
Preventive Care				
Immunization for Influenza[2]	639	92%	90%	90%
Immunization for Pneumonia[2]	902	88%	92%	92%
Stroke Care				
Anticoagulation Therapy for Atrial Fibrillation[2]	18	100%	96%	95%
Antithrombotic Therapy Timing[2]	90	98%	98%	98%
Assessed for Rehabilitation[2]	136	90%	98%	97%
Discharged on Antithrombotic Therapy[2]	109	97%	99%	99%
Discharged on Statin Medication[2]	93	90%	95%	94%
Thrombolytic Therapy Timing[1,2]	-	-	68%	66%
Venous Thromboembolism Prophylaxis[2]	142	84%	94%	94%
Written Stroke Educational Materials Given[2]	81	75%	92%	88%
Surgical Care Improvement Project				
Appropriate Beta Blocker Usage[2]	359	98%	98%	98%
Appropriate VTP Within 24 Hours[2]	484	96%	98%	98%
Controlled Postoperative Blood Glucose[2]	195	95%	96%	97%
Perioperative Temperature Management[2]	629	100%	100%	100%
Prophylactic Antibiotic Selection[2]	559	99%	99%	99%
Prophylactic Antibiotic Selection (Outpatient)	715	97%	98%	98%
Prophylactic Antibiotic Stopped[2]	531	96%	98%	98%
Prophylactic Antibiotic Timing[2]	560	99%	99%	99%
Prophylactic Antibiotic Timing (Outpatient)	718	98%	98%	98%
Urinary Catheter Removal[2]	482	98%	98%	97%
Survey of Patients' Hospital Experiences				
Area Around Room 'Always' Quiet at Night	300+	65%	68%	61%
Doctors 'Always' Communicated Well	300+	83%	83%	82%
Home Recovery Information Given	300+	81%	85%	85%
Hospital Given 9 or 10 on 10 Point Scale	300+	75%	73%	71%
Meds 'Always' Explained Before Given	300+	63%	66%	64%
Nurses 'Always' Communicated Well	300+	76%	80%	79%
Pain 'Always' Well Controlled	300+	72%	72%	71%
Room and Bathroom 'Always' Clean	300+	70%	75%	73%
Timely Help 'Always' Received	300+	65%	69%	68%
Would Definitely Recommend Hospital	300+	76%	73%	71%
Use of Medical Imaging				
Cardiac Imaging Stress Test before Surgery	504	5.2%	5.3%	5.3%
Combination Abdominal CT Scan	1,312	18.8%	16.4%	10.5%
Combination Brain/Sinus CT Scan	1,050	1.7%	2.7%	2.7%
Combination Chest CT Scan	1,340	2.6%	5.6%	2.7%
Follow-up Mammogram/Ultrasound	1,109	6.3%	7.9%	8.8%
Lumbar Spine MRI for Low Back Pain	98	32.7%	39.6%	37.2%

Saint Luke's Hospital at the Vintage

20171 Chasewood Park Drive Phone: 832-534-5000
Houston, TX 77070
Type: Acute Care Hospitals Emergency Services: Yes
Ownership: Proprietary

Measure	Cases	This Hosp.	State Avg.	U.S. Avg.
Blood Clot Prevention and Treatment				
Anticoagulation Overlap Therapy[2]	43	98%	93%	93%
ICU Venous Thromboembolism Prophylaxis[2]	61	74%	92%	92%
Incidence of Potentially Preventable VTE[1,2]	-	-	9%	10%
UFH with Dosages/Platelet Monitoring[1,2]	-	-	96%	97%
Venous Thromboembolism Prophylaxis[2]	268	81%	82%	85%
Warfarin Therapy Discharge Instructions[2]	31	97%	84%	75%
Chest Pain/Possible Heart Attack Care				
Aspirin Given Within 24 Hours of Arrival[1,3]	-	-	94%	96%
Fibrinolytic Meds Within 30 Min. of Arrival[3,7]	-	-	47%	58%
Average Time to ECG (minutes)[1,3]	-	-	8	7
Average Time to Transfer (minutes)[3,7]	-	-	62	60
Children's Asthma Care				
Received Home Management Plan of Care	-	-	93%	88%
Received Reliever Medication	-	-	100%	100%
Received Systemic Corticosteroids	-	-	100%	100%
Emergency Department				
Admittance Decision Time (minutes)[2]	310	184	99	98
Head CT Results Within 45 Min. of Arrival[1]	-	-	54%	57%
Patients Who Left ER Before Being Seen	17,173	1%	3%	2%
Time from ER Arrival to Admit. (minutes)[2]	314	360	270	274
Time from ER Arrival to Discharge (minutes)	369	162	127	134
Time in ER Before Being Evaluated (minutes)	274	54	26	26
Time to Pain Meds for Fractures (minutes)	73	58	57	57
Heart Attack Care				
Aspirin Given at Discharge	48	98%	99%	99%
Fibrinolytic Meds Within 30 Min. of Arrival[7]	-	-	49%	54%
PCI Within 90 Minutes of Arrival[1]	-	-	95%	96%
Statin Prescribed at Discharge	47	96%	98%	98%
Heart Failure Care				
ACE Inhibitor or ARB for LVSD	34	91%	97%	97%
Discharge Instructions Given	89	98%	95%	94%
Evaluation of LVS Function	119	99%	99%	99%
Medicare Spending				
Medicare Spending per Patient (ratio)	-	1.22	1.03	0.98
Pneumonia Care				
Appropriate Initial Antibiotic Given	102	98%	95%	95%
Blood Culture Timing	128	99%	98%	98%
Pregnancy and Delivery Care				
Newborn Deliveries Scheduled Early	47	9%	7%	6%
Preventive Care				
Immunization for Influenza[2]	346	91%	90%	90%
Immunization for Pneumonia[2]	371	95%	92%	92%
Stroke Care				

NOTE: Hospital profiles are in alphabetical order by state, then city, then hospital within the city; Rankings exclude hospitals with less than 25 cases except for patient surveys which excludes hospitals with less than 100 cases; (a) 100-299 cases; (1) The number of cases/patients is too few to report; (2) Data submitted were based on a sample of cases/patients; (3) Results are based on a shorter time period than required; (4) Data suppressed by CMS for one or more quarters; (5) Results are not available for this reporting period; (6) Fewer than 100 patients completed the HCAHPS survey; (7) No cases met the criteria for this measure; (8) The lower limit of the confidence interval cannot be calculated if the number of observed infections equals zero; (9) No data are available from the state/territory for this reporting period; (10) The scores shown reflect fewer than 50 completed surveys; (11) There were discrepancies in the data collection process; (12) This measure does not apply to this hospital for this reporting period; (13) Results cannot be calculated for this reporting period; (14) The results for this state are combined with nearby states to protect confidentiality; Please refer to the User's Guide for a full explanation of data.

Measure	Cases	This Hosp.	State Avg.	U.S. Avg.
Anticoagulation Therapy for Atrial Fibrillation[1]	-	-	96%	95%
Antithrombotic Therapy Timing	27	100%	98%	98%
Assessed for Rehabilitation	36	94%	98%	97%
Discharged on Antithrombotic Therapy	33	100%	99%	99%
Discharged on Statin Medication	30	90%	95%	94%
Thrombolytic Therapy Timing[1]	-	-	68%	66%
Venous Thromboembolism Prophylaxis	36	86%	94%	94%
Written Stroke Educational Materials Given	14	57%	92%	88%
Surgical Care Improvement Project				
Appropriate Beta Blocker Usage	32	88%	98%	98%
Appropriate VTP Within 24 Hours	121	96%	98%	98%
Controlled Postoperative Blood Glucose[7]	-	-	96%	97%
Perioperative Temperature Management	135	100%	100%	100%
Prophylactic Antibiotic Selection	55	98%	99%	99%
Prophylactic Antibiotic Selection (Outpatient)	43	98%	98%	98%
Prophylactic Antibiotic Stopped	54	96%	98%	98%
Prophylactic Antibiotic Timing	55	98%	99%	99%
Prophylactic Antibiotic Timing (Outpatient)	43	100%	98%	98%
Urinary Catheter Removal	64	94%	98%	97%
Survey of Patients' Hospital Experiences				
Area Around Room 'Always' Quiet at Night	300+	67%	68%	61%
Doctors 'Always' Communicated Well	300+	74%	83%	82%
Home Recovery Information Given	300+	83%	85%	85%
Hospital Given 9 or 10 on 10 Point Scale	300+	74%	73%	71%
Meds 'Always' Explained Before Given	300+	57%	66%	64%
Nurses 'Always' Communicated Well	300+	75%	80%	79%
Pain 'Always' Well Controlled	300+	64%	72%	71%
Room and Bathroom 'Always' Clean	300+	76%	75%	73%
Timely Help 'Always' Received	300+	62%	69%	68%
Would Definitely Recommend Hospital	300+	77%	73%	71%
Use of Medical Imaging				
Cardiac Imaging Stress Test before Surgery[1]	-	-	5.3%	5.3%
Combination Abdominal CT Scan	228	16.7%	16.4%	10.5%
Combination Brain/Sinus CT Scan[1]	-	-	2.7%	2.7%
Combination Chest CT Scan	148	8.1%	5.6%	2.7%
Follow-up Mammogram/Ultrasound	71	14.1%	7.9%	8.8%
Lumbar Spine MRI for Low Back Pain[1]	-	-	39.6%	37.2%

Texas Orthopedic Hospital

7401 South Main Street
Houston, TX 77030
Phone: 713-799-8600
URL: www.texasorthopedic.com
Type: Acute Care Hospitals
Emergency Services: Yes
Ownership: Voluntary non-profit - Other
Beds: 49

Key Personnel:
CEO/President . . . . Alice Adams
Chairman/CEO . . . . G. William Woods, MD

Measure	Cases	This Hosp.	State Avg.	U.S. Avg.
Blood Clot Prevention and Treatment				
Anticoagulation Overlap Therapy[2,7]	-	-	93%	93%
ICU Venous Thromboembolism Prophylaxis[1,2]	-	-	92%	92%
Incidence of Potentially Preventable VTE[2,7]	-	-	9%	10%
UFH with Dosages/Platelet Monitoring[2,7]	-	-	96%	97%
Venous Thromboembolism Prophylaxis[2]	144	99%	82%	85%
Warfarin Therapy Discharge Instructions[2,7]	-	-	84%	75%
Chest Pain/Possible Heart Attack Care				
Aspirin Given Within 24 Hours of Arrival[5]	-	-	94%	96%
Fibrinolytic Meds Within 30 Min. of Arrival[5]	-	-	47%	58%
Average Time to ECG (minutes)[5]	-	-	8	7
Average Time to Transfer (minutes)[5]	-	-	62	60
Children's Asthma Care				
Received Home Management Plan of Care	-	-	93%	88%
Received Reliever Medication	-	-	100%	100%
Received Systemic Corticosteroids	-	-	100%	100%
Emergency Department				
Admittance Decision Time (minutes)[2]	11	29	99	98
Head CT Results Within 45 Min. of Arrival[5]	-	-	54%	57%
Patients Who Left ER Before Being Seen	575	0%	3%	2%
Time from ER Arrival to Admit. (minutes)[2]	11	108	270	274
Time from ER Arrival to Discharge (minutes)	261	103	127	134
Time in ER Before Being Evaluated (minutes)	270	37	26	26
Time to Pain Meds for Fractures (minutes)[1]	-	-	57	57
Heart Attack Care				
Aspirin Given at Discharge[5]	-	-	99%	99%
Fibrinolytic Meds Within 30 Min. of Arrival[5]	-	-	49%	54%
PCI Within 90 Minutes of Arrival[5]	-	-	95%	96%
Statin Prescribed at Discharge[5]	-	-	98%	98%
Heart Failure Care				
ACE Inhibitor or ARB for LVSD[5]	-	-	97%	97%
Discharge Instructions Given[5]	-	-	95%	94%
Evaluation of LVS Function[5]	-	-	99%	99%
Medicare Spending				
Medicare Spending per Patient (ratio)	-	0.88	1.03	0.98
Pneumonia Care				
Appropriate Initial Antibiotic Given[5]	-	-	95%	95%
Blood Culture Timing[5]	-	-	98%	98%
Pregnancy and Delivery Care				
Newborn Deliveries Scheduled Early[2,7]	-	-	7%	6%
Preventive Care				
Immunization for Influenza[2]	361	99%	90%	90%
Immunization for Pneumonia[2]	392	97%	92%	92%
Stroke Care				
Anticoagulation Therapy for Atrial Fibrillation[5]	-	-	96%	95%
Antithrombotic Therapy Timing[5]	-	-	98%	98%
Assessed for Rehabilitation[5]	-	-	98%	97%
Discharged on Antithrombotic Therapy[5]	-	-	99%	99%
Discharged on Statin Medication[5]	-	-	95%	94%
Thrombolytic Therapy Timing[5]	-	-	68%	66%
Venous Thromboembolism Prophylaxis[5]	-	-	94%	94%
Written Stroke Educational Materials Given[5]	-	-	92%	88%
Surgical Care Improvement Project				
Appropriate Beta Blocker Usage[2]	77	100%	98%	98%
Appropriate VTP Within 24 Hours[2]	357	100%	98%	98%
Controlled Postoperative Blood Glucose[2,7]	-	-	96%	97%
Perioperative Temperature Management[2]	381	100%	100%	100%
Prophylactic Antibiotic Selection[2]	258	100%	99%	99%
Prophylactic Antibiotic Selection (Outpatient)	428	100%	98%	98%
Prophylactic Antibiotic Stopped[2]	255	99%	98%	98%
Prophylactic Antibiotic Timing[2]	258	100%	99%	99%
Prophylactic Antibiotic Timing (Outpatient)	428	100%	98%	98%
Urinary Catheter Removal[2]	138	99%	98%	97%
Survey of Patients' Hospital Experiences				
Area Around Room 'Always' Quiet at Night	300+	66%	68%	61%
Doctors 'Always' Communicated Well	300+	85%	83%	82%
Home Recovery Information Given	300+	89%	85%	85%
Hospital Given 9 or 10 on 10 Point Scale	300+	76%	73%	71%
Meds 'Always' Explained Before Given	300+	61%	66%	64%
Nurses 'Always' Communicated Well	300+	76%	80%	79%
Pain 'Always' Well Controlled	300+	71%	72%	71%
Room and Bathroom 'Always' Clean	300+	70%	75%	73%
Timely Help 'Always' Received	300+	64%	69%	68%
Would Definitely Recommend Hospital	300+	81%	73%	71%
Use of Medical Imaging				
Cardiac Imaging Stress Test before Surgery[7]	-	-	5.3%	5.3%
Combination Abdominal CT Scan[1]	-	-	16.4%	10.5%
Combination Brain/Sinus CT Scan[1]	-	-	2.7%	2.7%
Combination Chest CT Scan[1]	-	-	5.6%	2.7%
Follow-up Mammogram/Ultrasound[7]	-	-	7.9%	8.8%
Lumbar Spine MRI for Low Back Pain	172	40.1%	39.6%	37.2%

Tops Surgical Specialty Hospital

17080 Red Oak Drive
Houston, TX 77090
Phone: 281-539-2900
URL: www.tops-hospital.com
Type: Acute Care Hospitals
Emergency Services: Yes
Ownership: Physician

Measure	Cases	This Hosp.	State Avg.	U.S. Avg.
Blood Clot Prevention and Treatment				
Anticoagulation Overlap Therapy[1,2]	-	-	93%	93%
ICU Venous Thromboembolism Prophylaxis[2,7]	-	-	92%	92%
Incidence of Potentially Preventable VTE[2,7]	-	-	9%	10%
UFH with Dosages/Platelet Monitoring[1,2]	-	-	96%	97%
Venous Thromboembolism Prophylaxis[2]	30	100%	82%	85%
Warfarin Therapy Discharge Instructions[1,2]	-	-	84%	75%
Chest Pain/Possible Heart Attack Care				
Aspirin Given Within 24 Hours of Arrival[1,3]	-	-	94%	96%
Fibrinolytic Meds Within 30 Min. of Arrival[5]	-	-	47%	58%
Average Time to ECG (minutes)[1,3]	-	-	8	7
Average Time to Transfer (minutes)[5]	-	-	62	60
Children's Asthma Care				
Received Home Management Plan of Care	-	-	93%	88%
Received Reliever Medication	-	-	100%	100%
Received Systemic Corticosteroids	-	-	100%	100%
Emergency Department				
Admittance Decision Time (minutes)[1,2]	-	-	99	98
Head CT Results Within 45 Min. of Arrival[5]	-	-	54%	57%
Patients Who Left ER Before Being Seen	525	0%	3%	2%
Time from ER Arrival to Admit. (minutes)[1,2]	-	-	270	274
Time from ER Arrival to Discharge (minutes)	272	74	127	134
Time in ER Before Being Evaluated (minutes)	294	15	26	26
Time to Pain Meds for Fractures (minutes)[1]	-	-	57	57
Heart Attack Care				
Aspirin Given at Discharge[5]	-	-	99%	99%
Fibrinolytic Meds Within 30 Min. of Arrival[5]	-	-	49%	54%
PCI Within 90 Minutes of Arrival[5]	-	-	95%	96%
Statin Prescribed at Discharge[5]	-	-	98%	98%
Heart Failure Care				
ACE Inhibitor or ARB for LVSD[5]	-	-	97%	97%
Discharge Instructions Given[5]	-	-	95%	94%
Evaluation of LVS Function[5]	-	-	99%	99%
Medicare Spending				
Medicare Spending per Patient (ratio)	-	0.97	1.03	0.98
Pneumonia Care				
Appropriate Initial Antibiotic Given[5]	-	-	95%	95%
Blood Culture Timing[5]	-	-	98%	98%
Pregnancy and Delivery Care				
Newborn Deliveries Scheduled Early[7]	-	-	7%	6%
Preventive Care				
Immunization for Influenza[2]	315	96%	90%	90%
Immunization for Pneumonia[2]	391	90%	92%	92%
Stroke Care				
Anticoagulation Therapy for Atrial Fibrillation[5]	-	-	96%	95%
Antithrombotic Therapy Timing[5]	-	-	98%	98%
Assessed for Rehabilitation[5]	-	-	98%	97%
Discharged on Antithrombotic Therapy[5]	-	-	99%	99%
Discharged on Statin Medication[5]	-	-	95%	94%
Thrombolytic Therapy Timing[5]	-	-	68%	66%
Venous Thromboembolism Prophylaxis[5]	-	-	94%	94%
Written Stroke Educational Materials Given[5]	-	-	92%	88%
Surgical Care Improvement Project				
Appropriate Beta Blocker Usage	75	97%	98%	98%
Appropriate VTP Within 24 Hours	355	99%	98%	98%
Controlled Postoperative Blood Glucose[7]	-	-	96%	97%
Perioperative Temperature Management	369	100%	100%	100%
Prophylactic Antibiotic Selection	348	100%	99%	99%
Prophylactic Antibiotic Selection (Outpatient)	50	100%	98%	98%
Prophylactic Antibiotic Stopped	348	97%	98%	98%
Prophylactic Antibiotic Timing	348	98%	99%	99%
Prophylactic Antibiotic Timing (Outpatient)	50	100%	98%	98%
Urinary Catheter Removal	202	98%	98%	97%
Survey of Patients' Hospital Experiences				
Area Around Room 'Always' Quiet at Night	(a)	86%	68%	61%
Doctors 'Always' Communicated Well	(a)	90%	83%	82%
Home Recovery Information Given	(a)	89%	85%	85%
Hospital Given 9 or 10 on 10 Point Scale	(a)	82%	73%	71%
Meds 'Always' Explained Before Given	(a)	71%	66%	64%
Nurses 'Always' Communicated Well	(a)	86%	80%	79%
Pain 'Always' Well Controlled	(a)	80%	72%	71%
Room and Bathroom 'Always' Clean	(a)	83%	75%	73%
Timely Help 'Always' Received	(a)	84%	69%	68%
Would Definitely Recommend Hospital	(a)	86%	73%	71%
Use of Medical Imaging				
Cardiac Imaging Stress Test before Surgery[7]	-	-	5.3%	5.3%
Combination Abdominal CT Scan[1]	-	-	16.4%	10.5%
Combination Brain/Sinus CT Scan[1]	-	-	2.7%	2.7%
Combination Chest CT Scan[1]	-	-	5.6%	2.7%
Follow-up Mammogram/Ultrasound	2,482	4.8%	7.9%	8.8%

NOTE: Hospital profiles are in alphabetical order by state, then city, then hospital within the city; Rankings exclude hospitals with less than 25 cases except for patient surveys which excludes hospitals with less than 100 cases; (a) 100-299 cases; (1) The number of cases/patients is too few to report; (2) Data submitted were based on a sample of cases/patients; (3) Results are based on a shorter time period than required; (4) Data suppressed by CMS for one or more quarters; (5) Results are not available for this reporting period; (6) Fewer than 100 patients completed the HCAHPS survey; (7) No cases met the criteria for this measure; (8) The lower limit of the confidence interval cannot be calculated if the number of observed infections equals zero; (9) No data are available from the state/territory for this reporting period; (10) The scores shown reflect fewer than 50 completed surveys; (11) There were discrepancies in the data collection process; (12) This measure does not apply to this hospital for this reporting period; (13) Results cannot be calculated for this reporting period; (14) The results for this state are combined with nearby states to protect confidentiality; Please refer to the User's Guide for a full explanation of data.

Lumbar Spine MRI for Low Back Pain[7]	-	-	39.6%	37.2%

University General Hospital

7501 Fannin
Houston, TX 77054
Phone: 713-652-3800
URL: www.universitygeneralhospital.com
Type: Acute Care Hospitals
Emergency Services: Yes
Ownership: Proprietary
Beds: 72

Key Personnel:
Quality Assurance . . . . Misty Bass
Chief of Medical Staff . . . . Jay Davis, MD
Infection Control . . . . Pam Dieffenbach
CEO/President . . . . Kelly Riedel

Measure	Cases	This Hosp.	State Avg.	U.S. Avg.
Blood Clot Prevention and Treatment				
Anticoagulation Overlap Therapy[1,2]	-	-	93%	93%
ICU Venous Thromboembolism Prophylaxis[2]	49	76%	92%	92%
Incidence of Potentially Preventable VTE[1,2]	-	-	9%	10%
UFH with Dosages/Platelet Monitoring[2]	11	55%	96%	97%
Venous Thromboembolism Prophylaxis[2]	224	40%	82%	85%
Warfarin Therapy Discharge Instructions[1,2]	-	-	84%	75%
Chest Pain/Possible Heart Attack Care				
Aspirin Given Within 24 Hours of Arrival[5]	-	-	94%	96%
Fibrinolytic Meds Within 30 Min. of Arrival[5]	-	-	47%	58%
Average Time to ECG (minutes)[5]	-	-	8	7
Average Time to Transfer (minutes)[5]	-	-	62	60
Children's Asthma Care				
Received Home Management Plan of Care	-	-	93%	88%
Received Reliever Medication	-	-	100%	100%
Received Systemic Corticosteroids	-	-	100%	100%
Emergency Department				
Admittance Decision Time (minutes)[2]	925	79	99	98
Head CT Results Within 45 Min. of Arrival[3,7]	-	-	54%	57%
Patients Who Left ER Before Being Seen	2,914	1%	3%	2%
Time from ER Arrival to Admit. (minutes)[2]	1,122	220	270	274
Time from ER Arrival to Discharge (minutes)	1,037	173	127	134
Time in ER Before Being Evaluated (minutes)	991	46	26	26
Time to Pain Meds for Fractures (minutes)[1,3]	-	-	57	57
Heart Attack Care				
Aspirin Given at Discharge[1]	-	-	99%	99%
Fibrinolytic Meds Within 30 Min. of Arrival[7]	-	-	49%	54%
PCI Within 90 Minutes of Arrival[7]	-	-	95%	96%
Statin Prescribed at Discharge[1]	-	-	98%	98%
Heart Failure Care				
ACE Inhibitor or ARB for LVSD	13	62%	97%	97%
Discharge Instructions Given	36	50%	95%	94%
Evaluation of LVS Function	47	96%	99%	99%
Medicare Spending				
Medicare Spending per Patient (ratio)	-	1.29	1.03	0.98
Pneumonia Care				
Appropriate Initial Antibiotic Given	12	50%	95%	95%
Blood Culture Timing	21	90%	98%	98%
Pregnancy and Delivery Care				
Newborn Deliveries Scheduled Early[7]	-	-	7%	6%
Preventive Care				
Immunization for Influenza[2]	1,025	41%	90%	90%
Immunization for Pneumonia[2]	1,511	57%	92%	92%
Stroke Care				
Anticoagulation Therapy for Atrial Fibrillation[1]	-	-	96%	95%
Antithrombotic Therapy Timing	11	82%	98%	98%
Assessed for Rehabilitation[1]	-	-	98%	97%
Discharged on Antithrombotic Therapy[1]	-	-	99%	99%
Discharged on Statin Medication[1]	-	-	95%	94%
Thrombolytic Therapy Timing[1]	-	-	68%	66%
Venous Thromboembolism Prophylaxis	11	36%	94%	94%
Written Stroke Educational Materials Given[1]	-	-	92%	88%
Surgical Care Improvement Project				
Appropriate Beta Blocker Usage	38	63%	98%	98%
Appropriate VTP Within 24 Hours	134	89%	98%	98%
Controlled Postoperative Blood Glucose[7]	-	-	96%	97%
Perioperative Temperature Management	167	95%	100%	100%
Prophylactic Antibiotic Selection	70	94%	99%	99%
Prophylactic Antibiotic Selection (Outpatient)	116	93%	98%	98%
Prophylactic Antibiotic Stopped	64	88%	98%	98%
Prophylactic Antibiotic Timing	74	84%	99%	99%
Prophylactic Antibiotic Timing (Outpatient)	143	74%	98%	98%
Urinary Catheter Removal	113	77%	98%	97%
Survey of Patients' Hospital Experiences				
Area Around Room 'Always' Quiet at Night	300+	70%	68%	61%
Doctors 'Always' Communicated Well	300+	78%	83%	82%
Home Recovery Information Given	300+	82%	85%	85%
Hospital Given 9 or 10 on 10 Point Scale	300+	67%	73%	71%
Meds 'Always' Explained Before Given	300+	55%	66%	64%
Nurses 'Always' Communicated Well	300+	68%	80%	79%
Pain 'Always' Well Controlled	300+	64%	72%	71%
Room and Bathroom 'Always' Clean	300+	67%	75%	73%
Timely Help 'Always' Received	300+	52%	69%	68%
Would Definitely Recommend Hospital	300+	67%	73%	71%
Use of Medical Imaging				
Cardiac Imaging Stress Test before Surgery[1]	-	-	5.3%	5.3%
Combination Abdominal CT Scan	231	52.8%	16.4%	10.5%
Combination Brain/Sinus CT Scan[1]	-	-	2.7%	2.7%
Combination Chest CT Scan	135	31.9%	5.6%	2.7%
Follow-up Mammogram/Ultrasound	395	13.9%	7.9%	8.8%
Lumbar Spine MRI for Low Back Pain	123	39.8%	39.6%	37.2%

West Houston Medical Center

12141 Richmond Ave
Houston, TX 77082
Phone: 281-588-8080
Fax: 281-558-7619
URL: www.westhoustonmedical.com
Type: Acute Care Hospitals
Emergency Services: Yes
Ownership: Proprietary
Beds: 221

Key Personnel:
CEO . . . . Todd Caliva
Quality Assurance . . . . Sue Grochocki
Radiology. . . . . Matti Korhonen
Infection Control. . . . . Kathy Lamb
Emergency Room . . . . Lori Litzmger
Operating Room. . . . . Steven M Thomas
Anesthesiology. . . . . Frank Yang
Chief of Medical Staff. . . . . Barry L Zietz, MD

Measure	Cases	This Hosp.	State Avg.	U.S. Avg.
Blood Clot Prevention and Treatment				
Anticoagulation Overlap Therapy[2]	59	100%	93%	93%
ICU Venous Thromboembolism Prophylaxis[2]	116	99%	92%	92%
Incidence of Potentially Preventable VTE[1,2]	-	-	9%	10%
UFH with Dosages/Platelet Monitoring[1,2]	-	-	96%	97%
Venous Thromboembolism Prophylaxis[2]	370	91%	82%	85%
Warfarin Therapy Discharge Instructions[2]	46	100%	84%	75%
Chest Pain/Possible Heart Attack Care				
Aspirin Given Within 24 Hours of Arrival[1,3]	-	-	94%	96%
Fibrinolytic Meds Within 30 Min. of Arrival[5]	-	-	47%	58%
Average Time to ECG (minutes)[3,7]	-	-	8	7
Average Time to Transfer (minutes)[5]	-	-	62	60
Children's Asthma Care				
Received Home Management Plan of Care	-	-	93%	88%
Received Reliever Medication	-	-	100%	100%
Received Systemic Corticosteroids	-	-	100%	100%
Emergency Department				
Admittance Decision Time (minutes)[2]	614	128	99	98
Head CT Results Within 45 Min. of Arrival[1]	-	-	54%	57%
Patients Who Left ER Before Being Seen	51,437	2%	3%	2%
Time from ER Arrival to Admit. (minutes)[2]	618	332	270	274
Time from ER Arrival to Discharge (minutes)	475	177	127	134
Time in ER Before Being Evaluated (minutes)	531	30	26	26
Time to Pain Meds for Fractures (minutes)	165	56	57	57
Heart Attack Care				
Aspirin Given at Discharge	174	100%	99%	99%
Fibrinolytic Meds Within 30 Min. of Arrival[7]	-	-	49%	54%
PCI Within 90 Minutes of Arrival	30	97%	95%	96%
Statin Prescribed at Discharge	161	100%	98%	98%
Heart Failure Care				
ACE Inhibitor or ARB for LVSD	96	100%	97%	97%
Discharge Instructions Given	225	99%	95%	94%
Evaluation of LVS Function	274	100%	99%	99%
Medicare Spending				
Medicare Spending per Patient (ratio)	-	1.16	1.03	0.98
Pneumonia Care				
Appropriate Initial Antibiotic Given	81	98%	95%	95%
Blood Culture Timing	200	100%	98%	98%
Pregnancy and Delivery Care				
Newborn Deliveries Scheduled Early[2]	61	0%	7%	6%
Preventive Care				
Immunization for Influenza[2]	539	96%	90%	90%
Immunization for Pneumonia[2]	562	96%	92%	92%
Stroke Care				
Anticoagulation Therapy for Atrial Fibrillation	11	100%	96%	95%
Antithrombotic Therapy Timing	99	100%	98%	98%
Assessed for Rehabilitation	124	100%	98%	97%
Discharged on Antithrombotic Therapy	99	99%	99%	99%
Discharged on Statin Medication	71	100%	95%	94%
Thrombolytic Therapy Timing[1]	-	-	68%	66%
Venous Thromboembolism Prophylaxis	142	100%	94%	94%
Written Stroke Educational Materials Given	69	100%	92%	88%
Surgical Care Improvement Project				
Appropriate Beta Blocker Usage[2]	147	100%	98%	98%
Appropriate VTP Within 24 Hours[2]	305	100%	98%	98%
Controlled Postoperative Blood Glucose[2]	78	100%	96%	97%
Perioperative Temperature Management[2]	370	100%	100%	100%
Prophylactic Antibiotic Selection[2]	289	100%	99%	99%
Prophylactic Antibiotic Selection (Outpatient)	176	98%	98%	98%
Prophylactic Antibiotic Stopped[2]	267	100%	98%	98%
Prophylactic Antibiotic Timing[2]	289	100%	99%	99%
Prophylactic Antibiotic Timing (Outpatient)	177	97%	98%	98%
Urinary Catheter Removal[2]	237	100%	98%	97%
Survey of Patients' Hospital Experiences				
Area Around Room 'Always' Quiet at Night	300+	60%	68%	61%
Doctors 'Always' Communicated Well	300+	75%	83%	82%
Home Recovery Information Given	300+	81%	85%	85%
Hospital Given 9 or 10 on 10 Point Scale	300+	62%	73%	71%
Meds 'Always' Explained Before Given	300+	54%	66%	64%
Nurses 'Always' Communicated Well	300+	71%	80%	79%
Pain 'Always' Well Controlled	300+	67%	72%	71%
Room and Bathroom 'Always' Clean	300+	69%	75%	73%
Timely Help 'Always' Received	300+	53%	69%	68%
Would Definitely Recommend Hospital	300+	65%	73%	71%
Use of Medical Imaging				
Cardiac Imaging Stress Test before Surgery	126	5.6%	5.3%	5.3%
Combination Abdominal CT Scan	339	14.7%	16.4%	10.5%
Combination Brain/Sinus CT Scan[1]	-	-	2.7%	2.7%
Combination Chest CT Scan	102	1.0%	5.6%	2.7%
Follow-up Mammogram/Ultrasound	808	11.4%	7.9%	8.8%
Lumbar Spine MRI for Low Back Pain	33	48.5%	39.6%	37.2%

The Womans Hospital of Texas

7600 Fannin
Houston, TX 77054
Phone: 713-790-1234
Fax: 713-790-0469
URL: www.womenshospital.com
Type: Acute Care Hospitals
Emergency Services: Yes
Ownership: Proprietary
Beds: 275

Key Personnel:
Quality Assurance . . . . Nancy Andrews
Anesthesiology. . . . . Susan Carlyle, MD
Operating Room. . . . . Joan McComas
CEO/President. . . . . Linda Russell
Pediatric Ambulatory Care . . . . . . Don Schaffer, MD
Pediatric In-Patient Care . . . . Don Schaffer, MD
Chief of Medical Staff. . . . . Nicholas Sollene, MD
Infection Control. . . . . Elena Zaccaria

Measure	Cases	This Hosp.	State Avg.	U.S. Avg.
Blood Clot Prevention and Treatment				
Anticoagulation Overlap Therapy[1,2]	-	-	93%	93%
ICU Venous Thromboembolism Prophylaxis[1,2]	-	-	92%	92%
Incidence of Potentially Preventable VTE[1,2]	-	-	9%	10%
UFH with Dosages/Platelet Monitoring[1,2]	-	-	96%	97%
Venous Thromboembolism Prophylaxis[2]	105	91%	82%	85%
Warfarin Therapy Discharge Instructions[1,2]	-	-	84%	75%
Chest Pain/Possible Heart Attack Care				
Aspirin Given Within 24 Hours of Arrival[1,3]	-	-	94%	96%
Fibrinolytic Meds Within 30 Min. of Arrival[3,7]	-	-	47%	58%
Average Time to ECG (minutes)[1,3]	-	-	8	7

NOTE: Hospital profiles are in alphabetical order by state, then city, then hospital within the city; Rankings exclude hospitals with less than 25 cases except for patient surveys which excludes hospitals with less than 100 cases; (a) 100-299 cases; (1) The number of cases/patients is too few to report; (2) Data submitted were based on a sample of cases/patients; (3) Results are based on a shorter time period than required; (4) Data suppressed by CMS for one or more quarters; (5) Results are not available for this reporting period; (6) Fewer than 100 patients completed the HCAHPS survey; (7) No cases met the criteria for this measure; (8) The lower limit of the confidence interval cannot be calculated if the number of observed infections equals zero; (9) No data are available from the state/territory for this reporting period; (10) The scores shown reflect fewer than 50 completed surveys; (11) There were discrepancies in the data collection process; (12) This measure does not apply to this hospital for this reporting period; (13) Results cannot be calculated for this reporting period; (14) The results for this state are combined with nearby states to protect confidentiality; Please refer to the User's Guide for a full explanation of data.

Measure	Cases	This Hosp.	State Avg.	U.S. Avg.
Average Time to Transfer (minutes)[1,3]	-	-	62	60
Children's Asthma Care				
Received Home Management Plan of Care	-	-	93%	88%
Received Reliever Medication	-	-	100%	100%
Received Systemic Corticosteroids	-	-	100%	100%
Emergency Department				
Admittance Decision Time (minutes)[2]	311	0	99	98
Head CT Results Within 45 Min. of Arrival[5]	-	-	54%	57%
Patients Who Left ER Before Being Seen	3,886	0%	3%	2%
Time from ER Arrival to Admit. (minutes)[2]	311	52	270	274
Time from ER Arrival to Discharge (minutes)	437	165	127	134
Time in ER Before Being Evaluated (minutes)	456	9	26	26
Time to Pain Meds for Fractures (minutes)[1,3]	-	-	57	57
Heart Attack Care				
Aspirin Given at Discharge[5]	-	-	99%	99%
Fibrinolytic Meds Within 30 Min. of Arrival[5]	-	-	49%	54%
PCI Within 90 Minutes of Arrival[5]	-	-	95%	96%
Statin Prescribed at Discharge[5]	-	-	98%	98%
Heart Failure Care				
ACE Inhibitor or ARB for LVSD[5]	-	-	97%	97%
Discharge Instructions Given[5]	-	-	95%	94%
Evaluation of LVS Function[5]	-	-	99%	99%
Medicare Spending				
Medicare Spending per Patient (ratio)	-	0.97	1.03	0.98
Pneumonia Care				
Appropriate Initial Antibiotic Given[1]	-	-	95%	95%
Blood Culture Timing[7]	-	-	98%	98%
Pregnancy and Delivery Care				
Newborn Deliveries Scheduled Early[2]	122	2%	7%	6%
Preventive Care				
Immunization for Influenza[2]	352	66%	90%	90%
Immunization for Pneumonia[2]	44	59%	92%	92%
Stroke Care				
Anticoagulation Therapy for Atrial Fibrillation[5]	-	-	96%	95%
Antithrombotic Therapy Timing[5]	-	-	98%	98%
Assessed for Rehabilitation[5]	-	-	98%	97%
Discharged on Antithrombotic Therapy[5]	-	-	99%	99%
Discharged on Statin Medication[5]	-	-	95%	94%
Thrombolytic Therapy Timing[5]	-	-	68%	66%
Venous Thromboembolism Prophylaxis[5]	-	-	94%	94%
Written Stroke Educational Materials Given[5]	-	-	92%	88%
Surgical Care Improvement Project				
Appropriate Beta Blocker Usage[2]	19	89%	98%	98%
Appropriate VTP Within 24 Hours[2]	182	99%	98%	98%
Controlled Postoperative Blood Glucose[2,7]	-	-	96%	97%
Perioperative Temperature Management[2]	223	100%	100%	100%
Prophylactic Antibiotic Selection[2]	117	99%	99%	99%
Prophylactic Antibiotic Selection (Outpatient)	1,064	99%	98%	98%
Prophylactic Antibiotic Stopped[2]	109	100%	98%	98%
Prophylactic Antibiotic Timing[2]	116	100%	99%	99%
Prophylactic Antibiotic Timing (Outpatient)	1,064	100%	98%	98%
Urinary Catheter Removal[2]	12	100%	98%	97%
Survey of Patients' Hospital Experiences				
Area Around Room 'Always' Quiet at Night	300+	65%	68%	61%
Doctors 'Always' Communicated Well	300+	82%	83%	82%
Home Recovery Information Given	300+	85%	85%	85%
Hospital Given 9 or 10 on 10 Point Scale	300+	73%	73%	71%
Meds 'Always' Explained Before Given	300+	62%	66%	64%
Nurses 'Always' Communicated Well	300+	73%	80%	79%
Pain 'Always' Well Controlled	300+	70%	72%	71%
Room and Bathroom 'Always' Clean	300+	68%	75%	73%
Timely Help 'Always' Received	300+	56%	69%	68%
Would Definitely Recommend Hospital	300+	75%	73%	71%
Use of Medical Imaging				
Cardiac Imaging Stress Test before Surgery[7]	-	-	5.3%	5.3%
Combination Abdominal CT Scan[1]	-	-	16.4%	10.5%
Combination Brain/Sinus CT Scan[1]	-	-	2.7%	2.7%
Combination Chest CT Scan[1]	-	-	5.6%	2.7%
Follow-up Mammogram/Ultrasound	1,081	7.9%	7.9%	8.8%
Lumbar Spine MRI for Low Back Pain[7]	-	-	39.6%	37.2%

Memorial Hermann Northeast

18951 Memorial North
Humble, TX 77338
URL: www.nemch.org
Phone: 281-540-7700
Fax: 281-540-7846
Type: Acute Care Hospitals
Emergency Services: Yes
Ownership: Govt - Hospital Dist/Auth
Beds: 237

Key Personnel:
Infection Control. . . . . Kathleen Bryne, RN
Pediatric In-Patient Care . . . . Terry Buchalter
Radiology. . . . . Edwin Cacayorin
Coronary Care . . . . Faye Helms
CEO/President. . . . . Syble Missildine
Chief of Medical Staff. . . . . Angel Munoz, MD
Operating Room. . . . . Karen Pugh
Quality Assurance . . . . Lynn Sheeks

Measure	Cases	This Hosp.	State Avg.	U.S. Avg.
Blood Clot Prevention and Treatment				
Anticoagulation Overlap Therapy[2]	98	98%	93%	93%
ICU Venous Thromboembolism Prophylaxis[2]	68	100%	92%	92%
Incidence of Potentially Preventable VTE[2]	16	0%	9%	10%
UFH with Dosages/Platelet Monitoring[2]	37	100%	96%	97%
Venous Thromboembolism Prophylaxis[2]	385	91%	82%	85%
Warfarin Therapy Discharge Instructions[2]	82	76%	84%	75%
Chest Pain/Possible Heart Attack Care				
Aspirin Given Within 24 Hours of Arrival[1,3]	-	-	94%	96%
Fibrinolytic Meds Within 30 Min. of Arrival[3,7]	-	-	47%	58%
Average Time to ECG (minutes)[1,3]	-	-	8	7
Average Time to Transfer (minutes)[1,3]	-	-	62	60
Children's Asthma Care				
Received Home Management Plan of Care	-	-	93%	88%
Received Reliever Medication	-	-	100%	100%
Received Systemic Corticosteroids	-	-	100%	100%
Emergency Department				
Admittance Decision Time (minutes)[2]	656	214	99	98
Head CT Results Within 45 Min. of Arrival[1]	-	-	54%	57%
Patients Who Left ER Before Being Seen	58,680	2%	3%	2%
Time from ER Arrival to Admit. (minutes)[2]	713	454	270	274
Time from ER Arrival to Discharge (minutes)	368	217	127	134
Time in ER Before Being Evaluated (minutes)	411	41	26	26
Time to Pain Meds for Fractures (minutes)	224	74	57	57
Heart Attack Care				
Aspirin Given at Discharge[2]	210	98%	99%	99%
Fibrinolytic Meds Within 30 Min. of Arrival[2,7]	-	-	49%	54%
PCI Within 90 Minutes of Arrival[2]	33	100%	95%	96%
Statin Prescribed at Discharge[2]	207	99%	98%	98%
Heart Failure Care				
ACE Inhibitor or ARB for LVSD[2]	116	100%	97%	97%
Discharge Instructions Given[2]	283	96%	95%	94%
Evaluation of LVS Function[2]	321	100%	99%	99%
Medicare Spending				
Medicare Spending per Patient (ratio)	-	1.09	1.03	0.98
Pneumonia Care				
Appropriate Initial Antibiotic Given[2]	69	96%	95%	95%
Blood Culture Timing[2]	110	100%	98%	98%
Pregnancy and Delivery Care				
Newborn Deliveries Scheduled Early[2]	38	0%	7%	6%
Preventive Care				
Immunization for Influenza[2]	561	98%	90%	90%
Immunization for Pneumonia[2]	754	97%	92%	92%
Stroke Care				
Anticoagulation Therapy for Atrial Fibrillation	16	100%	96%	95%
Antithrombotic Therapy Timing	173	99%	98%	98%
Assessed for Rehabilitation	180	100%	98%	97%
Discharged on Antithrombotic Therapy	176	99%	99%	99%
Discharged on Statin Medication	129	98%	95%	94%
Thrombolytic Therapy Timing[1]	-	-	68%	66%
Venous Thromboembolism Prophylaxis	179	98%	94%	94%
Written Stroke Educational Materials Given	113	94%	92%	88%
Surgical Care Improvement Project				
Appropriate Beta Blocker Usage[2]	76	97%	98%	98%
Appropriate VTP Within 24 Hours[2]	229	97%	98%	98%
Controlled Postoperative Blood Glucose[2,7]	-	-	96%	97%
Perioperative Temperature Management[2]	280	100%	100%	100%
Prophylactic Antibiotic Selection[2]	129	100%	99%	99%
Prophylactic Antibiotic Selection (Outpatient)	117	100%	98%	98%
Prophylactic Antibiotic Stopped[2]	128	98%	98%	98%
Prophylactic Antibiotic Timing[2]	129	100%	99%	99%
Prophylactic Antibiotic Timing (Outpatient)	118	96%	98%	98%
Urinary Catheter Removal[2]	134	99%	98%	97%
Survey of Patients' Hospital Experiences				
Area Around Room 'Always' Quiet at Night	300+	64%	68%	61%
Doctors 'Always' Communicated Well	300+	78%	83%	82%
Home Recovery Information Given	300+	86%	85%	85%
Hospital Given 9 or 10 on 10 Point Scale	300+	71%	73%	71%
Meds 'Always' Explained Before Given	300+	63%	66%	64%
Nurses 'Always' Communicated Well	300+	80%	80%	79%
Pain 'Always' Well Controlled	300+	73%	72%	71%
Room and Bathroom 'Always' Clean	300+	68%	75%	73%
Timely Help 'Always' Received	300+	64%	69%	68%
Would Definitely Recommend Hospital	300+	73%	73%	71%
Use of Medical Imaging				
Cardiac Imaging Stress Test before Surgery[1]	-	-	5.3%	5.3%
Combination Abdominal CT Scan	625	14.1%	16.4%	10.5%
Combination Brain/Sinus CT Scan	743	1.5%	2.7%	2.7%
Combination Chest CT Scan	420	5.7%	5.6%	2.7%
Follow-up Mammogram/Ultrasound	824	8.1%	7.9%	8.8%
Lumbar Spine MRI for Low Back Pain	59	37.3%	39.6%	37.2%

Huntsville Memorial Hospital

110 Memorial Hospital Drive
Huntsville, TX 77340
Phone: 936-291-3411
Fax: 936-291-4241
E-mail: info@huntsvillememorial.com
URL: www.huntsvillememorial.com
Type: Acute Care Hospitals
Emergency Services: Yes
Ownership: Govt - Hospital Dist/Auth
Beds: 127

Key Personnel:
Emergency Room . . . . Stephen Antwi
Intensive Care Unit. . . . . Debbie Grisham
Infection Control. . . . . Deanna Hughes
Quality Assurance . . . . Phyllis Jones
Chief of Medical Staff. . . . . John Knight, MD
CEO/President. . . . . Sally Nelson
Radiology. . . . . Mobalaji Odelowo
Operating Room. . . . . Urmil Shukla

Measure	Cases	This Hosp.	State Avg.	U.S. Avg.
Blood Clot Prevention and Treatment				
Anticoagulation Overlap Therapy[2]	35	100%	93%	93%
ICU Venous Thromboembolism Prophylaxis[2]	47	85%	92%	92%
Incidence of Potentially Preventable VTE[1,2]	-	-	9%	10%
UFH with Dosages/Platelet Monitoring[1,2]	-	-	96%	97%
Venous Thromboembolism Prophylaxis[2]	378	75%	82%	85%
Warfarin Therapy Discharge Instructions[2]	23	96%	84%	75%
Chest Pain/Possible Heart Attack Care				
Aspirin Given Within 24 Hours of Arrival	118	97%	94%	96%
Fibrinolytic Meds Within 30 Min. of Arrival[1]	-	-	47%	58%
Average Time to ECG (minutes)	126	11	8	7
Average Time to Transfer (minutes)[1]	-	-	62	60
Children's Asthma Care				
Received Home Management Plan of Care	-	-	93%	88%
Received Reliever Medication	-	-	100%	100%
Received Systemic Corticosteroids	-	-	100%	100%
Emergency Department				
Admittance Decision Time (minutes)[2]	461	70	99	98
Head CT Results Within 45 Min. of Arrival	13	85%	54%	57%
Patients Who Left ER Before Being Seen	22,385	5%	3%	2%
Time from ER Arrival to Admit. (minutes)[2]	495	292	270	274
Time from ER Arrival to Discharge (minutes)	349	159	127	134
Time in ER Before Being Evaluated (minutes)	397	31	26	26
Time to Pain Meds for Fractures (minutes)	133	60	57	57
Heart Attack Care				
Aspirin Given at Discharge[1]	-	-	99%	99%
Fibrinolytic Meds Within 30 Min. of Arrival[7]	-	-	49%	54%
PCI Within 90 Minutes of Arrival[7]	-	-	95%	96%
Statin Prescribed at Discharge[1]	-	-	98%	98%
Heart Failure Care				
ACE Inhibitor or ARB for LVSD	43	95%	97%	97%
Discharge Instructions Given	125	97%	95%	94%
Evaluation of LVS Function	143	92%	99%	99%

NOTE: Hospital profiles are in alphabetical order by state, then city, then hospital within the city; Rankings exclude hospitals with less than 25 cases except for patient surveys which excludes hospitals with less than 100 cases; (a) 100-299 cases; (1) The number of cases/patients is too few to report; (2) Data submitted were based on a sample of cases/patients; (3) Results are based on a shorter time period than required; (4) Data suppressed by CMS for one or more quarters; (5) Results are not available for this reporting period; (6) Fewer than 100 patients completed the HCAHPS survey; (7) No cases met the criteria for this measure; (8) The lower limit of the confidence interval cannot be calculated if the number of observed infections equals zero; (9) No data are available from the state/territory for this reporting period; (10) The scores shown reflect fewer than 50 completed surveys; (11) There were discrepancies in the data collection process; (12) This measure does not apply to this hospital for this reporting period; (13) Results cannot be calculated for this reporting period; (14) The results for this state are combined with nearby states to protect confidentiality; Please refer to the User's Guide for a full explanation of data.

Measure	Cases	This Hosp.	State Avg.	U.S. Avg.
Medicare Spending				
Medicare Spending per Patient (ratio)	-	1.04	1.03	0.98
Pneumonia Care				
Appropriate Initial Antibiotic Given	101	96%	95%	95%
Blood Culture Timing	160	96%	98%	98%
Pregnancy and Delivery Care				
Newborn Deliveries Scheduled Early	45	4%	7%	6%
Preventive Care				
Immunization for Influenza[2]	415	100%	90%	90%
Immunization for Pneumonia[2]	483	96%	92%	92%
Stroke Care				
Anticoagulation Therapy for Atrial Fibrillation[1]	-	-	96%	95%
Antithrombotic Therapy Timing	31	97%	98%	98%
Assessed for Rehabilitation	31	94%	98%	97%
Discharged on Antithrombotic Therapy	26	96%	99%	99%
Discharged on Statin Medication	25	64%	95%	94%
Thrombolytic Therapy Timing[1]	-	-	68%	66%
Venous Thromboembolism Prophylaxis	33	70%	94%	94%
Written Stroke Educational Materials Given	16	69%	92%	88%
Surgical Care Improvement Project				
Appropriate Beta Blocker Usage	57	98%	98%	98%
Appropriate VTP Within 24 Hours	229	98%	98%	98%
Controlled Postoperative Blood Glucose[7]	-	-	96%	97%
Perioperative Temperature Management	235	100%	100%	100%
Prophylactic Antibiotic Selection	167	99%	99%	99%
Prophylactic Antibiotic Selection (Outpatient)	98	97%	98%	98%
Prophylactic Antibiotic Stopped	165	99%	98%	98%
Prophylactic Antibiotic Timing	167	96%	99%	99%
Prophylactic Antibiotic Timing (Outpatient)	98	99%	98%	98%
Urinary Catheter Removal	175	94%	98%	97%
Survey of Patients' Hospital Experiences				
Area Around Room 'Always' Quiet at Night	(a)	66%	68%	61%
Doctors 'Always' Communicated Well	(a)	86%	83%	82%
Home Recovery Information Given	(a)	80%	85%	85%
Hospital Given 9 or 10 on 10 Point Scale	(a)	60%	73%	71%
Meds 'Always' Explained Before Given	(a)	64%	66%	64%
Nurses 'Always' Communicated Well	(a)	77%	80%	79%
Pain 'Always' Well Controlled	(a)	73%	72%	71%
Room and Bathroom 'Always' Clean	(a)	73%	75%	73%
Timely Help 'Always' Received	(a)	64%	69%	68%
Would Definitely Recommend Hospital	(a)	57%	73%	71%
Use of Medical Imaging				
Cardiac Imaging Stress Test before Surgery	150	6.0%	5.3%	5.3%
Combination Abdominal CT Scan	536	12.7%	16.4%	10.5%
Combination Brain/Sinus CT Scan	646	4.3%	2.7%	2.7%
Combination Chest CT Scan	496	0.4%	5.6%	2.7%
Follow-up Mammogram/Ultrasound	715	8.7%	7.9%	8.8%
Lumbar Spine MRI for Low Back Pain	86	37.2%	39.6%	37.2%

Cook Childrens Northeast Hospital

6316 Precinct Line Rd Phone: 817-605-2500
Hurst, TX 76054
Type: Acute Care Hospitals Emergency Services: Yes
Ownership: Voluntary non-profit - Private

Measure	Cases	This Hosp.	State Avg.	U.S. Avg.
Blood Clot Prevention and Treatment				
Anticoagulation Overlap Therapy[5]	-	-	93%	93%
ICU Venous Thromboembolism Prophylaxis[5]	-	-	92%	92%
Incidence of Potentially Preventable VTE[5]	-	-	9%	10%
UFH with Dosages/Platelet Monitoring[5]	-	-	96%	97%
Venous Thromboembolism Prophylaxis[5]	-	-	82%	85%
Warfarin Therapy Discharge Instructions[5]	-	-	84%	75%
Chest Pain/Possible Heart Attack Care				
Aspirin Given Within 24 Hours of Arrival[5]	-	-	94%	96%
Fibrinolytic Meds Within 30 Min. of Arrival[5]	-	-	47%	58%
Average Time to ECG (minutes)[5]	-	-	8	7
Average Time to Transfer (minutes)[5]	-	-	62	60
Children's Asthma Care				
Received Home Management Plan of Care	-	-	93%	88%
Received Reliever Medication	-	-	100%	100%
Received Systemic Corticosteroids	-	-	100%	100%
Emergency Department				
Admittance Decision Time (minutes)[1,2]	-	-	99	98
Head CT Results Within 45 Min. of Arrival[5]	-	-	54%	57%
Patients Who Left ER Before Being Seen	3,055	1%	3%	2%
Time from ER Arrival to Admit. (minutes)[1,2]	-	-	270	274
Time from ER Arrival to Discharge (minutes)	248	100	127	134
Time in ER Before Being Evaluated (minutes)	247	25	26	26
Time to Pain Meds for Fractures (minutes)[5]	-	-	57	57
Heart Attack Care				
Aspirin Given at Discharge[5]	-	-	99%	99%
Fibrinolytic Meds Within 30 Min. of Arrival[5]	-	-	49%	54%
PCI Within 90 Minutes of Arrival[5]	-	-	95%	96%
Statin Prescribed at Discharge[5]	-	-	98%	98%
Heart Failure Care				
ACE Inhibitor or ARB for LVSD[5]	-	-	97%	97%
Discharge Instructions Given[5]	-	-	95%	94%
Evaluation of LVS Function[5]	-	-	99%	99%
Medicare Spending				
Medicare Spending per Patient (ratio)	-	-	1.03	0.98
Pneumonia Care				
Appropriate Initial Antibiotic Given[5]	-	-	95%	95%
Blood Culture Timing[5]	-	-	98%	98%
Pregnancy and Delivery Care				
Newborn Deliveries Scheduled Early[7]	-	-	7%	6%
Preventive Care				
Immunization for Influenza[1,2]	-	-	90%	90%
Immunization for Pneumonia[2,7]	-	-	92%	92%
Stroke Care				
Anticoagulation Therapy for Atrial Fibrillation[5]	-	-	96%	95%
Antithrombotic Therapy Timing[5]	-	-	98%	98%
Assessed for Rehabilitation[5]	-	-	98%	97%
Discharged on Antithrombotic Therapy[5]	-	-	99%	99%
Discharged on Statin Medication[5]	-	-	95%	94%
Thrombolytic Therapy Timing[5]	-	-	68%	66%
Venous Thromboembolism Prophylaxis[5]	-	-	94%	94%
Written Stroke Educational Materials Given[5]	-	-	92%	88%
Surgical Care Improvement Project				
Appropriate Beta Blocker Usage[5]	-	-	98%	98%
Appropriate VTP Within 24 Hours[5]	-	-	98%	98%
Controlled Postoperative Blood Glucose[5]	-	-	96%	97%
Perioperative Temperature Management[5]	-	-	100%	100%
Prophylactic Antibiotic Selection[5]	-	-	99%	99%
Prophylactic Antibiotic Selection (Outpatient)[5]	-	-	98%	98%
Prophylactic Antibiotic Stopped[5]	-	-	98%	98%
Prophylactic Antibiotic Timing[5]	-	-	99%	99%
Prophylactic Antibiotic Timing (Outpatient)[5]	-	-	98%	98%
Urinary Catheter Removal[5]	-	-	98%	97%
Survey of Patients' Hospital Experiences				
Area Around Room 'Always' Quiet at Night[1]	-	-	68%	61%
Doctors 'Always' Communicated Well[1]	-	-	83%	82%
Home Recovery Information Given[1]	-	-	85%	85%
Hospital Given 9 or 10 on 10 Point Scale[1]	-	-	73%	71%
Meds 'Always' Explained Before Given[1]	-	-	66%	64%
Nurses 'Always' Communicated Well[1]	-	-	80%	79%
Pain 'Always' Well Controlled[1]	-	-	72%	71%
Room and Bathroom 'Always' Clean[1]	-	-	75%	73%
Timely Help 'Always' Received[1]	-	-	69%	68%
Would Definitely Recommend Hospital[1]	-	-	73%	71%
Use of Medical Imaging				
Cardiac Imaging Stress Test before Surgery[7]	-	-	5.3%	5.3%
Combination Abdominal CT Scan[7]	-	-	16.4%	10.5%
Combination Brain/Sinus CT Scan[7]	-	-	2.7%	2.7%
Combination Chest CT Scan[7]	-	-	5.6%	2.7%
Follow-up Mammogram/Ultrasound[7]	-	-	7.9%	8.8%
Lumbar Spine MRI for Low Back Pain[7]	-	-	39.6%	37.2%

Baylor Medical Center at Irving

1901 N Macarthur Blvd Phone: 972-579-8100
Irving, TX 75061
URL: www.baylorhealth.com
Type: Acute Care Hospitals Emergency Services: Yes
Ownership: Voluntary non-profit - Private
Key Personnel:
CEO . . . . Joel T. Allison, FACHE

Measure	Cases	This Hosp.	State Avg.	U.S. Avg.
Blood Clot Prevention and Treatment				
Anticoagulation Overlap Therapy[2]	69	97%	93%	93%
ICU Venous Thromboembolism Prophylaxis[2]	119	97%	92%	92%
Incidence of Potentially Preventable VTE[2]	12	0%	9%	10%
UFH with Dosages/Platelet Monitoring[2]	68	100%	96%	97%
Venous Thromboembolism Prophylaxis[2]	347	97%	82%	85%
Warfarin Therapy Discharge Instructions[2]	56	96%	84%	75%
Chest Pain/Possible Heart Attack Care				
Aspirin Given Within 24 Hours of Arrival[1,3]	-	-	94%	96%
Fibrinolytic Meds Within 30 Min. of Arrival[5]	-	-	47%	58%
Average Time to ECG (minutes)[1,3]	-	-	8	7
Average Time to Transfer (minutes)[5]	-	-	62	60
Children's Asthma Care				
Received Home Management Plan of Care	-	-	93%	88%
Received Reliever Medication	-	-	100%	100%
Received Systemic Corticosteroids	-	-	100%	100%
Emergency Department				
Admittance Decision Time (minutes)[2]	672	85	99	98
Head CT Results Within 45 Min. of Arrival[1]	-	-	54%	57%
Patients Who Left ER Before Being Seen	73,987	3%	3%	2%
Time from ER Arrival to Admit. (minutes)[2]	674	304	270	274
Time from ER Arrival to Discharge (minutes)	377	203	127	134
Time in ER Before Being Evaluated (minutes)	327	16	26	26
Time to Pain Meds for Fractures (minutes)	197	38	57	57
Heart Attack Care				
Aspirin Given at Discharge	195	99%	99%	99%
Fibrinolytic Meds Within 30 Min. of Arrival[7]	-	-	49%	54%
PCI Within 90 Minutes of Arrival	39	97%	95%	96%
Statin Prescribed at Discharge	188	99%	98%	98%
Heart Failure Care				
ACE Inhibitor or ARB for LVSD	82	96%	97%	97%
Discharge Instructions Given	218	99%	95%	94%
Evaluation of LVS Function	243	100%	99%	99%
Medicare Spending				
Medicare Spending per Patient (ratio)	-	1.03	1.03	0.98
Pneumonia Care				
Appropriate Initial Antibiotic Given[2]	120	98%	95%	95%
Blood Culture Timing[2]	190	98%	98%	98%
Pregnancy and Delivery Care				
Newborn Deliveries Scheduled Early	211	2%	7%	6%
Preventive Care				
Immunization for Influenza[2]	521	97%	90%	90%
Immunization for Pneumonia[2]	597	97%	92%	92%
Stroke Care				
Anticoagulation Therapy for Atrial Fibrillation[2]	11	100%	96%	95%
Antithrombotic Therapy Timing[2]	83	100%	98%	98%
Assessed for Rehabilitation[2]	94	99%	98%	97%
Discharged on Antithrombotic Therapy[2]	84	99%	99%	99%
Discharged on Statin Medication[2]	62	98%	95%	94%
Thrombolytic Therapy Timing[1,2]	-	-	68%	66%
Venous Thromboembolism Prophylaxis[2]	97	98%	94%	94%
Written Stroke Educational Materials Given[2]	60	97%	92%	88%
Surgical Care Improvement Project				
Appropriate Beta Blocker Usage[2]	131	98%	98%	98%
Appropriate VTP Within 24 Hours[2]	404	99%	98%	98%
Controlled Postoperative Blood Glucose[2]	29	93%	96%	97%
Perioperative Temperature Management[2]	436	100%	100%	100%
Prophylactic Antibiotic Selection[2]	298	100%	99%	99%
Prophylactic Antibiotic Selection (Outpatient)	271	99%	98%	98%
Prophylactic Antibiotic Stopped[2]	292	100%	98%	98%
Prophylactic Antibiotic Timing[2]	299	100%	99%	99%
Prophylactic Antibiotic Timing (Outpatient)	271	99%	98%	98%
Urinary Catheter Removal[2]	346	98%	98%	97%
Survey of Patients' Hospital Experiences				
Area Around Room 'Always' Quiet at Night	300+	57%	68%	61%
Doctors 'Always' Communicated Well	300+	78%	83%	82%
Home Recovery Information Given	300+	83%	85%	85%
Hospital Given 9 or 10 on 10 Point Scale	300+	71%	73%	71%
Meds 'Always' Explained Before Given	300+	60%	66%	64%
Nurses 'Always' Communicated Well	300+	77%	80%	79%
Pain 'Always' Well Controlled	300+	70%	72%	71%

NOTE: Hospital profiles are in alphabetical order by state, then city, then hospital within the city; Rankings exclude hospitals with less than 25 cases except for patient surveys which excludes hospitals with less than 100 cases; (a) 100-299 cases; (1) The number of cases/patients is too few to report; (2) Data submitted were based on a sample of cases/patients; (3) Results are based on a shorter time period than required; (4) Data suppressed by CMS for one or more quarters; (5) Results are not available for this reporting period; (6) Fewer than 100 patients completed the HCAHPS survey; (7) No cases met the criteria for this measure; (8) The lower limit of the confidence interval cannot be calculated if the number of observed infections equals zero; (9) No data are available from the state/territory for this reporting period; (10) The scores shown reflect fewer than 50 completed surveys; (11) There were discrepancies in the data collection process; (12) This measure does not apply to this hospital for this reporting period; (13) Results cannot be calculated for this reporting period; (14) The results for this state are combined with nearby states to protect confidentiality; Please refer to the User's Guide for a full explanation of data.

Measure	Cases	This Hosp.	State Avg.	U.S. Avg.
Room and Bathroom 'Always' Clean	300+	71%	75%	73%
Timely Help 'Always' Received	300+	61%	69%	68%
Would Definitely Recommend Hospital	300+	72%	73%	71%
Use of Medical Imaging				
Cardiac Imaging Stress Test before Surgery	257	7.0%	5.3%	5.3%
Combination Abdominal CT Scan	726	4.3%	16.4%	10.5%
Combination Brain/Sinus CT Scan	888	1.7%	2.7%	2.7%
Combination Chest CT Scan	519	2.3%	5.6%	2.7%
Follow-up Mammogram/Ultrasound	1,914	7.8%	7.9%	8.8%
Lumbar Spine MRI for Low Back Pain	83	43.4%	39.6%	37.2%

Baylor Surgical Hospital at Las Colinas

400 West Interstate 635 Suite 101 Phone: 972-868-4000
Irving, TX 75063
URL: www.ic-sh.com
Type: Acute Care Hospitals Emergency Services: Yes
Ownership: Proprietary

Key Personnel:
Radiology. . . . . Dana Garber
Quality Assurance . . . . Sue Marco
CEO . . . . Deonna Unell
Chief of Medical Staff. . . . . Neil Williams

Measure	Cases	This Hosp.	State Avg.	U.S. Avg.
Blood Clot Prevention and Treatment				
Anticoagulation Overlap Therapy[2,7]	-	-	93%	93%
ICU Venous Thromboembolism Prophylaxis[2,7]	-	-	92%	92%
Incidence of Potentially Preventable VTE[2,7]	-	-	9%	10%
UFH with Dosages/Platelet Monitoring[2,7]	-	-	96%	97%
Venous Thromboembolism Prophylaxis[2]	45	98%	82%	85%
Warfarin Therapy Discharge Instructions[2,7]	-	-	84%	75%
Chest Pain/Possible Heart Attack Care				
Aspirin Given Within 24 Hours of Arrival[1,3]	-	-	94%	96%
Fibrinolytic Meds Within 30 Min. of Arrival[5]	-	-	47%	58%
Average Time to ECG (minutes)[1,3]	-	-	8	7
Average Time to Transfer (minutes)[5]	-	-	62	60
Children's Asthma Care				
Received Home Management Plan of Care	-	-	93%	88%
Received Reliever Medication	-	-	100%	100%
Received Systemic Corticosteroids	-	-	100%	100%
Emergency Department				
Admittance Decision Time (minutes)[1,2]	-	-	99	98
Head CT Results Within 45 Min. of Arrival[5]	-	-	54%	57%
Patients Who Left ER Before Being Seen	2,374	1%	3%	2%
Time from ER Arrival to Admit. (minutes)[1,2]	-	-	270	274
Time from ER Arrival to Discharge (minutes)	279	80	127	134
Time in ER Before Being Evaluated (minutes)	292	15	26	26
Time to Pain Meds for Fractures (minutes)[1,3]	-	-	57	57
Heart Attack Care				
Aspirin Given at Discharge[5]	-	-	99%	99%
Fibrinolytic Meds Within 30 Min. of Arrival[5]	-	-	49%	54%
PCI Within 90 Minutes of Arrival[5]	-	-	95%	96%
Statin Prescribed at Discharge[5]	-	-	98%	98%
Heart Failure Care				
ACE Inhibitor or ARB for LVSD[5]	-	-	97%	97%
Discharge Instructions Given[5]	-	-	95%	94%
Evaluation of LVS Function[5]	-	-	99%	99%
Medicare Spending				
Medicare Spending per Patient (ratio)	-	1.22	1.03	0.98
Pneumonia Care				
Appropriate Initial Antibiotic Given[5]	-	-	95%	95%
Blood Culture Timing[5]	-	-	98%	98%
Pregnancy and Delivery Care				
Newborn Deliveries Scheduled Early[7]	-	-	7%	6%
Preventive Care				
Immunization for Influenza[2]	232	96%	90%	90%
Immunization for Pneumonia[2]	156	96%	92%	92%
Stroke Care				
Anticoagulation Therapy for Atrial Fibrillation[5]	-	-	96%	95%
Antithrombotic Therapy Timing[5]	-	-	98%	98%
Assessed for Rehabilitation[5]	-	-	98%	97%
Discharged on Antithrombotic Therapy[5]	-	-	99%	99%
Discharged on Statin Medication[5]	-	-	95%	94%
Thrombolytic Therapy Timing[5]	-	-	68%	66%
Venous Thromboembolism Prophylaxis[5]	-	-	94%	94%
Written Stroke Educational Materials Given[5]	-	-	92%	88%
Surgical Care Improvement Project				
Appropriate Beta Blocker Usage	13	100%	98%	98%
Appropriate VTP Within 24 Hours	134	99%	98%	98%
Controlled Postoperative Blood Glucose[7]	-	-	96%	97%
Perioperative Temperature Management	139	100%	100%	100%
Prophylactic Antibiotic Selection	122	100%	99%	99%
Prophylactic Antibiotic Selection (Outpatient)	73	97%	98%	98%
Prophylactic Antibiotic Stopped	121	98%	98%	98%
Prophylactic Antibiotic Timing	123	98%	99%	99%
Prophylactic Antibiotic Timing (Outpatient)	73	100%	98%	98%
Urinary Catheter Removal	115	100%	98%	97%
Survey of Patients' Hospital Experiences				
Area Around Room 'Always' Quiet at Night	(a)	82%	68%	61%
Doctors 'Always' Communicated Well	(a)	87%	83%	82%
Home Recovery Information Given	(a)	89%	85%	85%
Hospital Given 9 or 10 on 10 Point Scale	(a)	81%	73%	71%
Meds 'Always' Explained Before Given	(a)	70%	66%	64%
Nurses 'Always' Communicated Well	(a)	82%	80%	79%
Pain 'Always' Well Controlled	(a)	77%	72%	71%
Room and Bathroom 'Always' Clean	(a)	88%	75%	73%
Timely Help 'Always' Received	(a)	84%	69%	68%
Would Definitely Recommend Hospital	(a)	80%	73%	71%
Use of Medical Imaging				
Cardiac Imaging Stress Test before Surgery[7]	-	-	5.3%	5.3%
Combination Abdominal CT Scan[1]	-	-	16.4%	10.5%
Combination Brain/Sinus CT Scan[1]	-	-	2.7%	2.7%
Combination Chest CT Scan[1]	-	-	5.6%	2.7%
Follow-up Mammogram/Ultrasound[7]	-	-	7.9%	8.8%
Lumbar Spine MRI for Low Back Pain[1]	-	-	39.6%	37.2%

Las Colinas Medical Center

6800 N Macarthur Blvd Phone: 972-969-2000
Irving, TX 75039 Fax: 972-969-2080
URL: www.lascolinas.com
Type: Acute Care Hospitals Emergency Services: Yes
Ownership: Voluntary non-profit - Private Beds: 70

Key Personnel:
Chief of Medical Staff. . . . . Charles W Calvert
CEO/President. . . . . Daniela C Decell
Emergency Room . . . . Alexander Kennedy, MD
Radiology. . . . . Jorge L Roman, MD
Hemotology Center . . . . Margaret C Sunderland, MD

Measure	Cases	This Hosp.	State Avg.	U.S. Avg.
Blood Clot Prevention and Treatment				
Anticoagulation Overlap Therapy[2]	36	97%	93%	93%
ICU Venous Thromboembolism Prophylaxis[2]	61	98%	92%	92%
Incidence of Potentially Preventable VTE[2,7]	-	-	9%	10%
UFH with Dosages/Platelet Monitoring[1,2]	-	-	96%	97%
Venous Thromboembolism Prophylaxis[2]	279	95%	82%	85%
Warfarin Therapy Discharge Instructions[2]	34	100%	84%	75%
Chest Pain/Possible Heart Attack Care				
Aspirin Given Within 24 Hours of Arrival[3,7]	-	-	94%	96%
Fibrinolytic Meds Within 30 Min. of Arrival[3,7]	-	-	47%	58%
Average Time to ECG (minutes)[1,3]	-	-	8	7
Average Time to Transfer (minutes)[3,7]	-	-	62	60
Children's Asthma Care				
Received Home Management Plan of Care	-	-	93%	88%
Received Reliever Medication	-	-	100%	100%
Received Systemic Corticosteroids	-	-	100%	100%
Emergency Department				
Admittance Decision Time (minutes)[2]	609	113	99	98
Head CT Results Within 45 Min. of Arrival[1]	-	-	54%	57%
Patients Who Left ER Before Being Seen	26,547	1%	3%	2%
Time from ER Arrival to Admit. (minutes)[2]	610	210	270	274
Time from ER Arrival to Discharge (minutes)	416	135	127	134
Time in ER Before Being Evaluated (minutes)	449	13	26	26
Time to Pain Meds for Fractures (minutes)	86	32	57	57
Heart Attack Care				
Aspirin Given at Discharge	87	100%	99%	99%
Fibrinolytic Meds Within 30 Min. of Arrival[7]	-	-	49%	54%
PCI Within 90 Minutes of Arrival	22	100%	95%	96%
Statin Prescribed at Discharge	76	100%	98%	98%
Heart Failure Care				
ACE Inhibitor or ARB for LVSD	36	100%	97%	97%
Discharge Instructions Given	102	100%	95%	94%
Evaluation of LVS Function	118	100%	99%	99%
Medicare Spending				
Medicare Spending per Patient (ratio)	-	1.00	1.03	0.98
Pneumonia Care				
Appropriate Initial Antibiotic Given	56	100%	95%	95%
Blood Culture Timing	101	100%	98%	98%
Pregnancy and Delivery Care				
Newborn Deliveries Scheduled Early[2]	44	0%	7%	6%
Preventive Care				
Immunization for Influenza[2]	460	100%	90%	90%
Immunization for Pneumonia[2]	407	99%	92%	92%
Stroke Care				
Anticoagulation Therapy for Atrial Fibrillation[1]	-	-	96%	95%
Antithrombotic Therapy Timing[1]	-	-	98%	98%
Assessed for Rehabilitation	13	100%	98%	97%
Discharged on Antithrombotic Therapy	13	100%	99%	99%
Discharged on Statin Medication	11	100%	95%	94%
Thrombolytic Therapy Timing[7]	-	-	68%	66%
Venous Thromboembolism Prophylaxis[1]	-	-	94%	94%
Written Stroke Educational Materials Given	11	100%	92%	88%
Surgical Care Improvement Project				
Appropriate Beta Blocker Usage[2]	55	98%	98%	98%
Appropriate VTP Within 24 Hours[2]	211	100%	98%	98%
Controlled Postoperative Blood Glucose[1,2]	-	-	96%	97%
Perioperative Temperature Management[2]	240	100%	100%	100%
Prophylactic Antibiotic Selection[2]	139	100%	99%	99%
Prophylactic Antibiotic Selection (Outpatient)	158	99%	98%	98%
Prophylactic Antibiotic Stopped[2]	133	99%	98%	98%
Prophylactic Antibiotic Timing[2]	139	100%	99%	99%
Prophylactic Antibiotic Timing (Outpatient)	158	100%	98%	98%
Urinary Catheter Removal[2]	117	100%	98%	97%
Survey of Patients' Hospital Experiences				
Area Around Room 'Always' Quiet at Night	300+	64%	68%	61%
Doctors 'Always' Communicated Well	300+	79%	83%	82%
Home Recovery Information Given	300+	86%	85%	85%
Hospital Given 9 or 10 on 10 Point Scale	300+	68%	73%	71%
Meds 'Always' Explained Before Given	300+	61%	66%	64%
Nurses 'Always' Communicated Well	300+	75%	80%	79%
Pain 'Always' Well Controlled	300+	72%	72%	71%
Room and Bathroom 'Always' Clean	300+	71%	75%	73%
Timely Help 'Always' Received	300+	59%	69%	68%
Would Definitely Recommend Hospital	300+	71%	73%	71%
Use of Medical Imaging				
Cardiac Imaging Stress Test before Surgery[1]	-	-	5.3%	5.3%
Combination Abdominal CT Scan	206	9.2%	16.4%	10.5%
Combination Brain/Sinus CT Scan[1]	-	-	2.7%	2.7%
Combination Chest CT Scan	71	5.6%	5.6%	2.7%
Follow-up Mammogram/Ultrasound	324	11.1%	7.9%	8.8%
Lumbar Spine MRI for Low Back Pain[1]	-	-	39.6%	37.2%

Faith Community Hospital

717 Magnolia St Phone: 940-567-6633
Jacksboro, TX 76458 Fax: 940-567-5714
E-mail: info@faithcommunityhospital.com
URL: www.faithcommunityhospital.com
Type: Acute Care Hospitals Emergency Services: Yes
Ownership: Govt - Hospital Dist/Auth Beds: 41

Key Personnel:
CEO/President. . . . . Frank L. Beaman
Chief of Medical Staff. . . . . Sushi B. Chokshi, MD
Cardiology. . . . . Ved Ganeshram, MD
Emergency Room . . . . Syed Jamal, MD
Infection Control. . . . . Joe Medina
Quality Assurance . . . . Jeff Miller

Measure	Cases	This Hosp.	State Avg.	U.S. Avg.
Blood Clot Prevention and Treatment				
Anticoagulation Overlap Therapy[1,2]	-	-	93%	93%
ICU Venous Thromboembolism Prophylaxis[2,7]	-	-	92%	92%
Incidence of Potentially Preventable VTE[2,7]	-	-	9%	10%
UFH with Dosages/Platelet Monitoring[1,2]	-	-	96%	97%

NOTE: Hospital profiles are in alphabetical order by state, then city, then hospital within the city; Rankings exclude hospitals with less than 25 cases except for patient surveys which excludes hospitals with less than 100 cases; (a) 100-299 cases; (1) The number of cases/patients is too few to report; (2) Data submitted were based on a sample of cases/patients; (3) Results are based on a shorter time period than required; (4) Data suppressed by CMS for one or more quarters; (5) Results are not available for this reporting period; (6) Fewer than 100 patients completed the HCAHPS survey; (7) No cases met the criteria for this measure; (8) The lower limit of the confidence interval cannot be calculated if the number of observed infections equals zero; (9) No data are available from the state/territory for this reporting period; (10) The scores shown reflect fewer than 50 completed surveys; (11) There were discrepancies in the data collection process; (12) This measure does not apply to this hospital for this reporting period; (13) Results cannot be calculated for this reporting period; (14) The results for this state are combined with nearby states to protect confidentiality; Please refer to the User's Guide for a full explanation of data.

Measure	Cases	This Hosp.	State Avg.	U.S. Avg.
Venous Thromboembolism Prophylaxis[2]	102	11%	82%	85%
Warfarin Therapy Discharge Instructions[1,2]	-	-	84%	75%
Chest Pain/Possible Heart Attack Care				
Aspirin Given Within 24 Hours of Arrival[3]	16	81%	94%	96%
Fibrinolytic Meds Within 30 Min. of Arrival[1,3]	-	-	47%	58%
Average Time to ECG (minutes)[3]	14	6	8	7
Average Time to Transfer (minutes)[3,7]	-	-	62	60
Children's Asthma Care				
Received Home Management Plan of Care	-	-	93%	88%
Received Reliever Medication	-	-	100%	100%
Received Systemic Corticosteroids	-	-	100%	100%
Emergency Department				
Admittance Decision Time (minutes)[2]	65	3	99	98
Head CT Results Within 45 Min. of Arrival[3,7]	-	-	54%	57%
Patients Who Left ER Before Being Seen	2,081	0%	3%	2%
Time from ER Arrival to Admit. (minutes)[2]	65	141	270	274
Time from ER Arrival to Discharge (minutes)	292	96	127	134
Time in ER Before Being Evaluated (minutes)	416	16	26	26
Time to Pain Meds for Fractures (minutes)[3,7]	-	-	57	57
Heart Attack Care				
Aspirin Given at Discharge[5]	-	-	99%	99%
Fibrinolytic Meds Within 30 Min. of Arrival[5]	-	-	49%	54%
PCI Within 90 Minutes of Arrival[5]	-	-	95%	96%
Statin Prescribed at Discharge[5]	-	-	98%	98%
Heart Failure Care				
ACE Inhibitor or ARB for LVSD[1,3]	-	-	97%	97%
Discharge Instructions Given[1,3]	-	-	95%	94%
Evaluation of LVS Function[1,3]	-	-	99%	99%
Medicare Spending				
Medicare Spending per Patient (ratio)	-	0.94	1.03	0.98
Pneumonia Care				
Appropriate Initial Antibiotic Given[1,2]	-	-	95%	95%
Blood Culture Timing[1,2]	-	-	98%	98%
Pregnancy and Delivery Care				
Newborn Deliveries Scheduled Early[1,2]	-	-	7%	6%
Preventive Care				
Immunization for Influenza[2]	83	82%	90%	90%
Immunization for Pneumonia[2]	109	94%	92%	92%
Stroke Care				
Anticoagulation Therapy for Atrial Fibrillation[5]	-	-	96%	95%
Antithrombotic Therapy Timing[5]	-	-	98%	98%
Assessed for Rehabilitation[5]	-	-	98%	97%
Discharged on Antithrombotic Therapy[5]	-	-	99%	99%
Discharged on Statin Medication[5]	-	-	95%	94%
Thrombolytic Therapy Timing[5]	-	-	68%	66%
Venous Thromboembolism Prophylaxis[5]	-	-	94%	94%
Written Stroke Educational Materials Given[5]	-	-	92%	88%
Surgical Care Improvement Project				
Appropriate Beta Blocker Usage[5]	-	-	98%	98%
Appropriate VTP Within 24 Hours[5]	-	-	98%	98%
Controlled Postoperative Blood Glucose[5]	-	-	96%	97%
Perioperative Temperature Management[5]	-	-	100%	100%
Prophylactic Antibiotic Selection[5]	-	-	99%	99%
Prophylactic Antibiotic Selection (Outpatient)[5]	-	-	98%	98%
Prophylactic Antibiotic Stopped[5]	-	-	98%	98%
Prophylactic Antibiotic Timing[5]	-	-	99%	99%
Prophylactic Antibiotic Timing (Outpatient)[5]	-	-	98%	98%
Urinary Catheter Removal[5]	-	-	98%	97%
Survey of Patients' Hospital Experiences				
Area Around Room 'Always' Quiet at Night[10]	<100	70%	68%	61%
Doctors 'Always' Communicated Well[10]	<100	93%	83%	82%
Home Recovery Information Given[10]	<100	92%	85%	85%
Hospital Given 9 or 10 on 10 Point Scale[10]	<100	62%	73%	71%
Meds 'Always' Explained Before Given[10]	<100	49%	66%	64%
Nurses 'Always' Communicated Well[10]	<100	84%	80%	79%
Pain 'Always' Well Controlled[10]	<100	68%	72%	71%
Room and Bathroom 'Always' Clean[10]	<100	80%	75%	73%
Timely Help 'Always' Received[10]	<100	75%	69%	68%
Would Definitely Recommend Hospital[10]	<100	61%	73%	71%
Use of Medical Imaging				
Cardiac Imaging Stress Test before Surgery[7]	-	-	5.3%	5.3%
Combination Abdominal CT Scan[1]	-	-	16.4%	10.5%
Combination Brain/Sinus CT Scan[1]	-	-	2.7%	2.7%
Combination Chest CT Scan[1]	-	-	5.6%	2.7%
Follow-up Mammogram/Ultrasound[7]	-	-	7.9%	8.8%
Lumbar Spine MRI for Low Back Pain[7]	-	-	39.6%	37.2%

East Texas Medical Center Jacksonville

501 S Ragsdale
Jacksonville, TX 75766
Phone: 903-541-5000
Fax: 903-541-5088
URL: www.etmc.org
Type: Acute Care Hospitals
Emergency Services: Yes
Ownership: Voluntary non-profit - Private
Beds: 94

Key Personnel:
Infection Control. . . . . Jana Batenar, RN
Radiology. . . . . Daniel Bennett, RT
Operating Room. . . . . Alan D Cook, RN
Chief of Medical Staff. . . . . Laurence W Cunningham, MD
CEO/President. . . . . Jack Endres
Quality Assurance . . . . Debbie McCaslin, RN

Measure	Cases	This Hosp.	State Avg.	U.S. Avg.
Blood Clot Prevention and Treatment				
Anticoagulation Overlap Therapy[1,2]	-	-	93%	93%
ICU Venous Thromboembolism Prophylaxis[2]	26	69%	92%	92%
Incidence of Potentially Preventable VTE[2,7]	-	-	9%	10%
UFH with Dosages/Platelet Monitoring[1,2]	-	-	96%	97%
Venous Thromboembolism Prophylaxis[2]	96	50%	82%	85%
Warfarin Therapy Discharge Instructions[1,2]	-	-	84%	75%
Chest Pain/Possible Heart Attack Care				
Aspirin Given Within 24 Hours of Arrival	26	96%	94%	96%
Fibrinolytic Meds Within 30 Min. of Arrival[1]	-	-	47%	58%
Average Time to ECG (minutes)	26	6	8	7
Average Time to Transfer (minutes)[1]	-	-	62	60
Children's Asthma Care				
Received Home Management Plan of Care	-	-	93%	88%
Received Reliever Medication	-	-	100%	100%
Received Systemic Corticosteroids	-	-	100%	100%
Emergency Department				
Admittance Decision Time (minutes)[2]	150	65	99	98
Head CT Results Within 45 Min. of Arrival[1]	-	-	54%	57%
Patients Who Left ER Before Being Seen	14,801	2%	3%	2%
Time from ER Arrival to Admit. (minutes)[2]	167	231	270	274
Time from ER Arrival to Discharge (minutes)	331	127	127	134
Time in ER Before Being Evaluated (minutes)	325	27	26	26
Time to Pain Meds for Fractures (minutes)	45	67	57	57
Heart Attack Care				
Aspirin Given at Discharge[1]	-	-	99%	99%
Fibrinolytic Meds Within 30 Min. of Arrival[7]	-	-	49%	54%
PCI Within 90 Minutes of Arrival[7]	-	-	95%	96%
Statin Prescribed at Discharge[1]	-	-	98%	98%
Heart Failure Care				
ACE Inhibitor or ARB for LVSD	15	93%	97%	97%
Discharge Instructions Given	35	86%	95%	94%
Evaluation of LVS Function	51	98%	99%	99%
Medicare Spending				
Medicare Spending per Patient (ratio)	-	1.07	1.03	0.98
Pneumonia Care				
Appropriate Initial Antibiotic Given	40	92%	95%	95%
Blood Culture Timing	56	98%	98%	98%
Pregnancy and Delivery Care				
Newborn Deliveries Scheduled Early	45	2%	7%	6%
Preventive Care				
Immunization for Influenza[2]	227	92%	90%	90%
Immunization for Pneumonia[2]	223	89%	92%	92%
Stroke Care				
Anticoagulation Therapy for Atrial Fibrillation[1]	-	-	96%	95%
Antithrombotic Therapy Timing[1]	-	-	98%	98%
Assessed for Rehabilitation	11	91%	98%	97%
Discharged on Antithrombotic Therapy[1]	-	-	99%	99%
Discharged on Statin Medication[1]	-	-	95%	94%
Thrombolytic Therapy Timing[1]	-	-	68%	66%
Venous Thromboembolism Prophylaxis	11	36%	94%	94%
Written Stroke Educational Materials Given[1]	-	-	92%	88%
Surgical Care Improvement Project				
Appropriate Beta Blocker Usage	33	85%	98%	98%
Appropriate VTP Within 24 Hours	84	99%	98%	98%
Controlled Postoperative Blood Glucose[7]	-	-	96%	97%
Perioperative Temperature Management	94	100%	100%	100%
Prophylactic Antibiotic Selection	65	98%	99%	99%
Prophylactic Antibiotic Selection (Outpatient)[3,7]	-	-	98%	98%
Prophylactic Antibiotic Stopped	64	97%	98%	98%
Prophylactic Antibiotic Timing	65	97%	99%	99%
Prophylactic Antibiotic Timing (Outpatient)[3,7]	-	-	98%	98%
Urinary Catheter Removal	58	91%	98%	97%
Survey of Patients' Hospital Experiences				
Area Around Room 'Always' Quiet at Night	300+	64%	68%	61%
Doctors 'Always' Communicated Well	300+	84%	83%	82%
Home Recovery Information Given	300+	87%	85%	85%
Hospital Given 9 or 10 on 10 Point Scale	300+	74%	73%	71%
Meds 'Always' Explained Before Given	300+	68%	66%	64%
Nurses 'Always' Communicated Well	300+	81%	80%	79%
Pain 'Always' Well Controlled	300+	73%	72%	71%
Room and Bathroom 'Always' Clean	300+	77%	75%	73%
Timely Help 'Always' Received	300+	69%	69%	68%
Would Definitely Recommend Hospital	300+	72%	73%	71%
Use of Medical Imaging				
Cardiac Imaging Stress Test before Surgery	95	6.3%	5.3%	5.3%
Combination Abdominal CT Scan	287	13.9%	16.4%	10.5%
Combination Brain/Sinus CT Scan	248	5.2%	2.7%	2.7%
Combination Chest CT Scan	206	13.1%	5.6%	2.7%
Follow-up Mammogram/Ultrasound	282	5.7%	7.9%	8.8%
Lumbar Spine MRI for Low Back Pain	36	50.0%	39.6%	37.2%

Mother Frances Hospital Jacksonville

2026 S Jackson Street
Jacksonville, TX 75766
Phone: 903-541-4500
URL: www.tmfhs.org
Type: Critical Access Hospitals
Emergency Services: Yes
Ownership: Voluntary non-profit - Private

Measure	Cases	This Hosp.	State Avg.	U.S. Avg.
Blood Clot Prevention and Treatment				
Anticoagulation Overlap Therapy[5]	-	-	93%	93%
ICU Venous Thromboembolism Prophylaxis[5]	-	-	92%	92%
Incidence of Potentially Preventable VTE[5]	-	-	9%	10%
UFH with Dosages/Platelet Monitoring[5]	-	-	96%	97%
Venous Thromboembolism Prophylaxis[5]	-	-	82%	85%
Warfarin Therapy Discharge Instructions[5]	-	-	84%	75%
Chest Pain/Possible Heart Attack Care				
Aspirin Given Within 24 Hours of Arrival	-	-	94%	96%
Fibrinolytic Meds Within 30 Min. of Arrival	-	-	47%	58%
Average Time to ECG (minutes)	-	-	8	7
Average Time to Transfer (minutes)	-	-	62	60
Children's Asthma Care				
Received Home Management Plan of Care	-	-	93%	88%
Received Reliever Medication	-	-	100%	100%
Received Systemic Corticosteroids	-	-	100%	100%
Emergency Department				
Admittance Decision Time (minutes)[5]	-	-	99	98
Head CT Results Within 45 Min. of Arrival	-	-	54%	57%
Patients Who Left ER Before Being Seen	-	-	3%	2%
Time from ER Arrival to Admit. (minutes)[5]	-	-	270	274
Time from ER Arrival to Discharge (minutes)	-	-	127	134
Time in ER Before Being Evaluated (minutes)	-	-	26	26
Time to Pain Meds for Fractures (minutes)	-	-	57	57
Heart Attack Care				
Aspirin Given at Discharge[1]	-	-	99%	99%
Fibrinolytic Meds Within 30 Min. of Arrival[3,7]	-	-	49%	54%
PCI Within 90 Minutes of Arrival[3,7]	-	-	95%	96%
Statin Prescribed at Discharge[3,7]	-	-	98%	98%
Heart Failure Care				
ACE Inhibitor or ARB for LVSD	22	95%	97%	97%
Discharge Instructions Given	57	98%	95%	94%
Evaluation of LVS Function	64	100%	99%	99%
Medicare Spending				
Medicare Spending per Patient (ratio)	-	-	1.03	0.98
Pneumonia Care				
Appropriate Initial Antibiotic Given	35	91%	95%	95%
Blood Culture Timing	47	100%	98%	98%

NOTE: Hospital profiles are in alphabetical order by state, then city, then hospital within the city; Rankings exclude hospitals with less than 25 cases except for patient surveys which excludes hospitals with less than 100 cases; (a) 100-299 cases; (1) The number of cases/patients is too few to report; (2) Data submitted were based on a sample of cases/patients; (3) Results are based on a shorter time period than required; (4) Data suppressed by CMS for one or more quarters; (5) Results are not available for this reporting period; (6) Fewer than 100 patients completed the HCAHPS survey; (7) No cases met the criteria for this measure; (8) The lower limit of the confidence interval cannot be calculated if the number of observed infections equals zero; (9) No data are available from the state/territory for this reporting period; (10) The scores shown reflect fewer than 50 completed surveys; (11) There were discrepancies in the data collection process; (12) This measure does not apply to this hospital for this reporting period; (13) Results cannot be calculated for this reporting period; (14) The results for this state are combined with nearby states to protect confidentiality; Please refer to the User's Guide for a full explanation of data.

Measure	Cases	This Hosp.	State Avg.	U.S. Avg.
Pregnancy and Delivery Care				
Newborn Deliveries Scheduled Early[5]	-	-	7%	6%
Preventive Care				
Immunization for Influenza[5]	-	-	90%	90%
Immunization for Pneumonia[5]	-	-	92%	92%
Stroke Care				
Anticoagulation Therapy for Atrial Fibrillation[5]	-	-	96%	95%
Antithrombotic Therapy Timing[5]	-	-	98%	98%
Assessed for Rehabilitation[5]	-	-	98%	97%
Discharged on Antithrombotic Therapy[5]	-	-	99%	99%
Discharged on Statin Medication[5]	-	-	95%	94%
Thrombolytic Therapy Timing[5]	-	-	68%	66%
Venous Thromboembolism Prophylaxis[5]	-	-	94%	94%
Written Stroke Educational Materials Given[5]	-	-	92%	88%
Surgical Care Improvement Project				
Appropriate Beta Blocker Usage[1]	-	-	98%	98%
Appropriate VTP Within 24 Hours	12	100%	98%	98%
Controlled Postoperative Blood Glucose[3,7]	-	-	96%	97%
Perioperative Temperature Management	18	100%	100%	100%
Prophylactic Antibiotic Selection	13	85%	99%	99%
Prophylactic Antibiotic Selection (Outpatient)	-	-	98%	98%
Prophylactic Antibiotic Stopped	13	100%	98%	98%
Prophylactic Antibiotic Timing	13	100%	99%	99%
Prophylactic Antibiotic Timing (Outpatient)	-	-	98%	98%
Urinary Catheter Removal[1]	-	-	98%	97%
Survey of Patients' Hospital Experiences				
Area Around Room 'Always' Quiet at Night[5]	-	-	68%	61%
Doctors 'Always' Communicated Well[5]	-	-	83%	82%
Home Recovery Information Given[5]	-	-	85%	85%
Hospital Given 9 or 10 on 10 Point Scale[5]	-	-	73%	71%
Meds 'Always' Explained Before Given[5]	-	-	66%	64%
Nurses 'Always' Communicated Well[5]	-	-	80%	79%
Pain 'Always' Well Controlled[5]	-	-	72%	71%
Room and Bathroom 'Always' Clean[5]	-	-	75%	73%
Timely Help 'Always' Received[5]	-	-	69%	68%
Would Definitely Recommend Hospital[5]	-	-	73%	71%
Use of Medical Imaging				
Cardiac Imaging Stress Test before Surgery	-	-	5.3%	5.3%
Combination Abdominal CT Scan	-	-	16.4%	10.5%
Combination Brain/Sinus CT Scan	-	-	2.7%	2.7%
Combination Chest CT Scan	-	-	5.6%	2.7%
Follow-up Mammogram/Ultrasound	-	-	7.9%	8.8%
Lumbar Spine MRI for Low Back Pain	-	-	39.6%	37.2%

Christus Jasper Memorial Hospital

1275 Marvin Hancock Drive Phone: 409-384-5461
Jasper, TX 75951 Fax: 409-384-4357
E-mail: deborah.wiegand@christushealth.org
URL: www.christusjasper.org
Type: Acute Care Hospitals Emergency Services: Yes
Ownership: Govt - Hospital Dist/Auth Beds: 81
Key Personnel:
Chief of Medical Staff . . . . Larry Brown
CEO/President . . . . George N Miller Jr

Measure	Cases	This Hosp.	State Avg.	U.S. Avg.
Blood Clot Prevention and Treatment				
Anticoagulation Overlap Therapy[1,2]	-	-	93%	93%
ICU Venous Thromboembolism Prophylaxis[2]	47	36%	92%	92%
Incidence of Potentially Preventable VTE[1,2]	-	-	9%	10%
UFH with Dosages/Platelet Monitoring[1,2]	-	-	96%	97%
Venous Thromboembolism Prophylaxis[2]	114	21%	82%	85%
Warfarin Therapy Discharge Instructions[1,2]	-	-	84%	75%
Chest Pain/Possible Heart Attack Care				
Aspirin Given Within 24 Hours of Arrival	110	96%	94%	96%
Fibrinolytic Meds Within 30 Min. of Arrival	15	67%	47%	58%
Average Time to ECG (minutes)	115	10	8	7
Average Time to Transfer (minutes)[1]	-	-	62	60
Children's Asthma Care				
Received Home Management Plan of Care	-	-	93%	88%
Received Reliever Medication	-	-	100%	100%
Received Systemic Corticosteroids	-	-	100%	100%
Emergency Department				
Admittance Decision Time (minutes)[2]	374	106	99	98
Head CT Results Within 45 Min. of Arrival	11	9%	54%	57%
Patients Who Left ER Before Being Seen	24,159	7%	3%	2%
Time from ER Arrival to Admit. (minutes)[2]	403	302	270	274
Time from ER Arrival to Discharge (minutes)	386	140	127	134
Time in ER Before Being Evaluated (minutes)	421	20	26	26
Time to Pain Meds for Fractures (minutes)	130	53	57	57
Heart Attack Care				
Aspirin Given at Discharge[1]	-	-	99%	99%
Fibrinolytic Meds Within 30 Min. of Arrival[7]	-	-	49%	54%
PCI Within 90 Minutes of Arrival[7]	-	-	95%	96%
Statin Prescribed at Discharge[1]	-	-	98%	98%
Heart Failure Care				
ACE Inhibitor or ARB for LVSD	25	84%	97%	97%
Discharge Instructions Given	59	97%	95%	94%
Evaluation of LVS Function	74	97%	99%	99%
Medicare Spending				
Medicare Spending per Patient (ratio)	-	0.99	1.03	0.98
Pneumonia Care				
Appropriate Initial Antibiotic Given	61	89%	95%	95%
Blood Culture Timing	86	92%	98%	98%
Pregnancy and Delivery Care				
Newborn Deliveries Scheduled Early[2]	19	11%	7%	6%
Preventive Care				
Immunization for Influenza[2]	258	77%	90%	90%
Immunization for Pneumonia[2]	367	88%	92%	92%
Stroke Care				
Anticoagulation Therapy for Atrial Fibrillation[1]	-	-	96%	95%
Antithrombotic Therapy Timing[1]	-	-	98%	98%
Assessed for Rehabilitation[1]	-	-	98%	97%
Discharged on Antithrombotic Therapy[1]	-	-	99%	99%
Discharged on Statin Medication[1]	-	-	95%	94%
Thrombolytic Therapy Timing[1]	-	-	68%	66%
Venous Thromboembolism Prophylaxis[1]	-	-	94%	94%
Written Stroke Educational Materials Given[1]	-	-	92%	88%
Surgical Care Improvement Project				
Appropriate Beta Blocker Usage[1]	-	-	98%	98%
Appropriate VTP Within 24 Hours[1]	-	-	98%	98%
Controlled Postoperative Blood Glucose[7]	-	-	96%	97%
Perioperative Temperature Management	11	100%	100%	100%
Prophylactic Antibiotic Selection[1]	-	-	99%	99%
Prophylactic Antibiotic Selection (Outpatient)[1]	-	-	98%	98%
Prophylactic Antibiotic Stopped[1]	-	-	98%	98%
Prophylactic Antibiotic Timing[1]	-	-	99%	99%
Prophylactic Antibiotic Timing (Outpatient)[1]	-	-	98%	98%
Urinary Catheter Removal[1]	-	-	98%	97%
Survey of Patients' Hospital Experiences				
Area Around Room 'Always' Quiet at Night	(a)	61%	68%	61%
Doctors 'Always' Communicated Well	(a)	86%	83%	82%
Home Recovery Information Given	(a)	83%	85%	85%
Hospital Given 9 or 10 on 10 Point Scale	(a)	60%	73%	71%
Meds 'Always' Explained Before Given	(a)	65%	66%	64%
Nurses 'Always' Communicated Well	(a)	76%	80%	79%
Pain 'Always' Well Controlled	(a)	70%	72%	71%
Room and Bathroom 'Always' Clean	(a)	72%	75%	73%
Timely Help 'Always' Received	(a)	69%	69%	68%
Would Definitely Recommend Hospital	(a)	56%	73%	71%
Use of Medical Imaging				
Cardiac Imaging Stress Test before Surgery[7]	-	-	5.3%	5.3%
Combination Abdominal CT Scan	373	14.5%	16.4%	10.5%
Combination Brain/Sinus CT Scan	595	0.7%	2.7%	2.7%
Combination Chest CT Scan	209	16.3%	5.6%	2.7%
Follow-up Mammogram/Ultrasound	639	12.7%	7.9%	8.8%
Lumbar Spine MRI for Low Back Pain	82	26.8%	39.6%	37.2%

South Texas Regional Medical Center

1905 Hwy 97 East Phone: 830-769-3515
Jourdanton, TX 78026 Fax: 830-769-5264
URL: www.strmc.org
Type: Acute Care Hospitals Emergency Services: Yes
Ownership: Proprietary Beds: 67
Key Personnel:
Emergency Room . . . . Stephen Cox
Quality Assurance . . . . Sandra Haley
Chief of Medical Staff . . . . Michael McFarland
CEO/President . . . . Mike Pierce
Radiology . . . . Jorge Velez

Measure	Cases	This Hosp.	State Avg.	U.S. Avg.
Blood Clot Prevention and Treatment				
Anticoagulation Overlap Therapy[1,2]	-	-	93%	93%
ICU Venous Thromboembolism Prophylaxis[2]	45	100%	92%	92%
Incidence of Potentially Preventable VTE[1,2]	-	-	9%	10%
UFH with Dosages/Platelet Monitoring[1,2]	-	-	96%	97%
Venous Thromboembolism Prophylaxis[2]	197	94%	82%	85%
Warfarin Therapy Discharge Instructions[1,2]	-	-	84%	75%
Chest Pain/Possible Heart Attack Care				
Aspirin Given Within 24 Hours of Arrival	93	100%	94%	96%
Fibrinolytic Meds Within 30 Min. of Arrival[1]	-	-	47%	58%
Average Time to ECG (minutes)	95	9	8	7
Average Time to Transfer (minutes)	12	84	62	60
Children's Asthma Care				
Received Home Management Plan of Care	-	-	93%	88%
Received Reliever Medication	-	-	100%	100%
Received Systemic Corticosteroids	-	-	100%	100%
Emergency Department				
Admittance Decision Time (minutes)[2]	351	98	99	98
Head CT Results Within 45 Min. of Arrival[1]	-	-	54%	57%
Patients Who Left ER Before Being Seen	19,758	1%	3%	2%
Time from ER Arrival to Admit. (minutes)[2]	355	280	270	274
Time from ER Arrival to Discharge (minutes)	370	118	127	134
Time in ER Before Being Evaluated (minutes)	408	25	26	26
Time to Pain Meds for Fractures (minutes)	119	58	57	57
Heart Attack Care				
Aspirin Given at Discharge[1]	-	-	99%	99%
Fibrinolytic Meds Within 30 Min. of Arrival[7]	-	-	49%	54%
PCI Within 90 Minutes of Arrival[7]	-	-	95%	96%
Statin Prescribed at Discharge[1]	-	-	98%	98%
Heart Failure Care				
ACE Inhibitor or ARB for LVSD	20	100%	97%	97%
Discharge Instructions Given	43	91%	95%	94%
Evaluation of LVS Function	51	100%	99%	99%
Medicare Spending				
Medicare Spending per Patient (ratio)	-	1.03	1.03	0.98
Pneumonia Care				
Appropriate Initial Antibiotic Given	50	98%	95%	95%
Blood Culture Timing	87	98%	98%	98%
Pregnancy and Delivery Care				
Newborn Deliveries Scheduled Early[2]	42	0%	7%	6%
Preventive Care				
Immunization for Influenza[2]	272	98%	90%	90%
Immunization for Pneumonia[2]	336	99%	92%	92%
Stroke Care				
Anticoagulation Therapy for Atrial Fibrillation[7]	-	-	96%	95%
Antithrombotic Therapy Timing	11	100%	98%	98%
Assessed for Rehabilitation[1]	-	-	98%	97%
Discharged on Antithrombotic Therapy[1]	-	-	99%	99%
Discharged on Statin Medication[1]	-	-	95%	94%
Thrombolytic Therapy Timing[7]	-	-	68%	66%
Venous Thromboembolism Prophylaxis[1]	-	-	94%	94%
Written Stroke Educational Materials Given[1]	-	-	92%	88%
Surgical Care Improvement Project				
Appropriate Beta Blocker Usage	12	92%	98%	98%
Appropriate VTP Within 24 Hours	57	98%	98%	98%
Controlled Postoperative Blood Glucose[7]	-	-	96%	97%
Perioperative Temperature Management	43	100%	100%	100%
Prophylactic Antibiotic Selection	29	100%	99%	99%
Prophylactic Antibiotic Selection (Outpatient)	33	100%	98%	98%
Prophylactic Antibiotic Stopped	29	97%	98%	98%
Prophylactic Antibiotic Timing	29	100%	99%	99%
Prophylactic Antibiotic Timing (Outpatient)	33	100%	98%	98%
Urinary Catheter Removal	40	98%	98%	97%
Survey of Patients' Hospital Experiences				
Area Around Room 'Always' Quiet at Night	(a)	64%	68%	61%
Doctors 'Always' Communicated Well	(a)	79%	83%	82%
Home Recovery Information Given	(a)	90%	85%	85%
Hospital Given 9 or 10 on 10 Point Scale	(a)	66%	73%	71%
Meds 'Always' Explained Before Given	(a)	63%	66%	64%

NOTE: Hospital profiles are in alphabetical order by state, then city, then hospital within the city; Rankings exclude hospitals with less than 25 cases except for patient surveys which excludes hospitals with less than 100 cases; (a) 100-299 cases; (1) The number of cases/patients is too few to report; (2) Data submitted were based on a sample of cases/patients; (3) Results are based on a shorter time period than required; (4) Data suppressed by CMS for one or more quarters; (5) Results are not available for this reporting period; (6) Fewer than 100 patients completed the HCAHPS survey; (7) No cases met the criteria for this measure; (8) The lower limit of the confidence interval cannot be calculated if the number of observed infections equals zero; (9) No data are available from the state/territory for this reporting period; (10) The scores shown reflect fewer than 50 completed surveys; (11) There were discrepancies in the data collection process; (12) This measure does not apply to this hospital for this reporting period; (13) Results cannot be calculated for this reporting period; (14) The results for this state are combined with nearby states to protect confidentiality; Please refer to the User's Guide for a full explanation of data.

Measure	Cases	This Hosp.	State Avg.	U.S. Avg.
Nurses 'Always' Communicated Well	(a)	76%	80%	79%
Pain 'Always' Well Controlled	(a)	68%	72%	71%
Room and Bathroom 'Always' Clean	(a)	72%	75%	73%
Timely Help 'Always' Received	(a)	59%	69%	68%
Would Definitely Recommend Hospital	(a)	63%	73%	71%
Use of Medical Imaging				
Cardiac Imaging Stress Test before Surgery	64	4.7%	5.3%	5.3%
Combination Abdominal CT Scan	324	4.6%	16.4%	10.5%
Combination Brain/Sinus CT Scan[1]	-	-	2.7%	2.7%
Combination Chest CT Scan	218	0.0%	5.6%	2.7%
Follow-up Mammogram/Ultrasound	349	13.5%	7.9%	8.8%
Lumbar Spine MRI for Low Back Pain[1]	-	-	39.6%	37.2%

Christus Saint Catherine Hospital

701 South Fry Road
Katy, TX 77450
Phone: 281-599-5700
Type: Acute Care Hospitals
Emergency Services: Yes
Ownership: Voluntary non-profit - Private
Key Personnel:
CEO/President. . . . . Jack McCabe

Measure	Cases	This Hosp.	State Avg.	U.S. Avg.
Blood Clot Prevention and Treatment				
Anticoagulation Overlap Therapy[1,2]	-	-	93%	93%
ICU Venous Thromboembolism Prophylaxis[2]	67	69%	92%	92%
Incidence of Potentially Preventable VTE[1,2]	-	-	9%	10%
UFH with Dosages/Platelet Monitoring[1,2]	-	-	96%	97%
Venous Thromboembolism Prophylaxis[2]	225	56%	82%	85%
Warfarin Therapy Discharge Instructions[1,2]	-	-	84%	75%
Chest Pain/Possible Heart Attack Care				
Aspirin Given Within 24 Hours of Arrival	17	100%	94%	96%
Fibrinolytic Meds Within 30 Min. of Arrival[3,7]	-	-	47%	58%
Average Time to ECG (minutes)	17	7	8	7
Average Time to Transfer (minutes)[3,7]	-	-	62	60
Children's Asthma Care				
Received Home Management Plan of Care	-	-	93%	88%
Received Reliever Medication	-	-	100%	100%
Received Systemic Corticosteroids	-	-	100%	100%
Emergency Department				
Admittance Decision Time (minutes)[2]	415	135	99	98
Head CT Results Within 45 Min. of Arrival	15	73%	54%	57%
Patients Who Left ER Before Being Seen	23,960	1%	3%	2%
Time from ER Arrival to Admit. (minutes)[2]	416	331	270	274
Time from ER Arrival to Discharge (minutes)	379	108	127	134
Time in ER Before Being Evaluated (minutes)	399	15	26	26
Time to Pain Meds for Fractures (minutes)	121	32	57	57
Heart Attack Care				
Aspirin Given at Discharge	24	100%	99%	99%
Fibrinolytic Meds Within 30 Min. of Arrival[7]	-	-	49%	54%
PCI Within 90 Minutes of Arrival[7]	-	-	95%	96%
Statin Prescribed at Discharge	21	100%	98%	98%
Heart Failure Care				
ACE Inhibitor or ARB for LVSD	30	100%	97%	97%
Discharge Instructions Given	85	100%	95%	94%
Evaluation of LVS Function	96	100%	99%	99%
Medicare Spending				
Medicare Spending per Patient (ratio)	-	1.03	1.03	0.98
Pneumonia Care				
Appropriate Initial Antibiotic Given	50	98%	95%	95%
Blood Culture Timing	80	96%	98%	98%
Pregnancy and Delivery Care				
Newborn Deliveries Scheduled Early[2]	32	9%	7%	6%
Preventive Care				
Immunization for Influenza[2]	354	97%	90%	90%
Immunization for Pneumonia[2]	329	91%	92%	92%
Stroke Care				
Anticoagulation Therapy for Atrial Fibrillation[1]	-	-	96%	95%
Antithrombotic Therapy Timing	14	86%	98%	98%
Assessed for Rehabilitation	15	73%	98%	97%
Discharged on Antithrombotic Therapy	14	93%	99%	99%
Discharged on Statin Medication	13	100%	95%	94%
Thrombolytic Therapy Timing[1]	-	-	68%	66%
Venous Thromboembolism Prophylaxis	15	73%	94%	94%
Written Stroke Educational Materials Given[1]	-	-	92%	88%
Surgical Care Improvement Project				
Appropriate Beta Blocker Usage	31	100%	98%	98%
Appropriate VTP Within 24 Hours	146	98%	98%	98%
Controlled Postoperative Blood Glucose[1]	-	-	96%	97%
Perioperative Temperature Management	174	100%	100%	100%
Prophylactic Antibiotic Selection	98	100%	99%	99%
Prophylactic Antibiotic Selection (Outpatient)	19	89%	98%	98%
Prophylactic Antibiotic Stopped	98	97%	98%	98%
Prophylactic Antibiotic Timing	98	99%	99%	99%
Prophylactic Antibiotic Timing (Outpatient)	20	95%	98%	98%
Urinary Catheter Removal	81	96%	98%	97%
Survey of Patients' Hospital Experiences				
Area Around Room 'Always' Quiet at Night	300+	72%	68%	61%
Doctors 'Always' Communicated Well	300+	83%	83%	82%
Home Recovery Information Given	300+	85%	85%	85%
Hospital Given 9 or 10 on 10 Point Scale	300+	75%	73%	71%
Meds 'Always' Explained Before Given	300+	63%	66%	64%
Nurses 'Always' Communicated Well	300+	77%	80%	79%
Pain 'Always' Well Controlled	300+	73%	72%	71%
Room and Bathroom 'Always' Clean	300+	77%	75%	73%
Timely Help 'Always' Received	300+	64%	69%	68%
Would Definitely Recommend Hospital	300+	77%	73%	71%
Use of Medical Imaging				
Cardiac Imaging Stress Test before Surgery	56	1.8%	5.3%	5.3%
Combination Abdominal CT Scan	253	17.8%	16.4%	10.5%
Combination Brain/Sinus CT Scan[1]	-	-	2.7%	2.7%
Combination Chest CT Scan	126	7.9%	5.6%	2.7%
Follow-up Mammogram/Ultrasound	483	6.6%	7.9%	8.8%
Lumbar Spine MRI for Low Back Pain[1]	-	-	39.6%	37.2%

Memorial Hermann Katy Hospital

23900 Katy Freeway
Katy, TX 77494
Phone: 281-392-1111
Fax: 281-644-7068
URL: www.memorialhermann.org
Type: Acute Care Hospitals
Emergency Services: Yes
Ownership: Voluntary non-profit - Private
Beds: 118
Key Personnel:
CEO/President. . . . . Scott Barbe
Infection Control. . . . . Phillis Godwin
Operating Room. . . . . Janie Mooneyhon
Radiology. . . . . Gayle S Storey
Quality Assurance . . . . Kit Zaldibar

Measure	Cases	This Hosp.	State Avg.	U.S. Avg.
Blood Clot Prevention and Treatment				
Anticoagulation Overlap Therapy[2]	52	96%	93%	93%
ICU Venous Thromboembolism Prophylaxis[2]	81	99%	92%	92%
Incidence of Potentially Preventable VTE[1,2]	-	-	9%	10%
UFH with Dosages/Platelet Monitoring[2]	16	100%	96%	97%
Venous Thromboembolism Prophylaxis[2]	322	97%	82%	85%
Warfarin Therapy Discharge Instructions[2]	31	68%	84%	75%
Chest Pain/Possible Heart Attack Care				
Aspirin Given Within 24 Hours of Arrival	67	99%	94%	96%
Fibrinolytic Meds Within 30 Min. of Arrival[7]	-	-	47%	58%
Average Time to ECG (minutes)	69	7	8	7
Average Time to Transfer (minutes)	29	46	62	60
Children's Asthma Care				
Received Home Management Plan of Care	-	-	93%	88%
Received Reliever Medication	-	-	100%	100%
Received Systemic Corticosteroids	-	-	100%	100%
Emergency Department				
Admittance Decision Time (minutes)[2]	460	73	99	98
Head CT Results Within 45 Min. of Arrival	13	62%	54%	57%
Patients Who Left ER Before Being Seen	36,447	2%	3%	2%
Time from ER Arrival to Admit. (minutes)[2]	487	259	270	274
Time from ER Arrival to Discharge (minutes)	342	188	127	134
Time in ER Before Being Evaluated (minutes)	408	30	26	26
Time to Pain Meds for Fractures (minutes)	175	73	57	57
Heart Attack Care				
Aspirin Given at Discharge	28	100%	99%	99%
Fibrinolytic Meds Within 30 Min. of Arrival[7]	-	-	49%	54%
PCI Within 90 Minutes of Arrival[7]	-	-	95%	96%
Statin Prescribed at Discharge	24	100%	98%	98%
Heart Failure Care				
ACE Inhibitor or ARB for LVSD	68	97%	97%	97%
Discharge Instructions Given	139	94%	95%	94%
Evaluation of LVS Function	177	100%	99%	99%
Medicare Spending				
Medicare Spending per Patient (ratio)	-	1.04	1.03	0.98
Pneumonia Care				
Appropriate Initial Antibiotic Given[2]	89	94%	95%	95%
Blood Culture Timing[2]	168	99%	98%	98%
Pregnancy and Delivery Care				
Newborn Deliveries Scheduled Early[2]	65	22%	7%	6%
Preventive Care				
Immunization for Influenza[2]	493	97%	90%	90%
Immunization for Pneumonia[2]	452	96%	92%	92%
Stroke Care				
Anticoagulation Therapy for Atrial Fibrillation[1]	-	-	96%	95%
Antithrombotic Therapy Timing	80	99%	98%	98%
Assessed for Rehabilitation	86	100%	98%	97%
Discharged on Antithrombotic Therapy	84	100%	99%	99%
Discharged on Statin Medication	55	98%	95%	94%
Thrombolytic Therapy Timing[1]	-	-	68%	66%
Venous Thromboembolism Prophylaxis	77	99%	94%	94%
Written Stroke Educational Materials Given	54	93%	92%	88%
Surgical Care Improvement Project				
Appropriate Beta Blocker Usage[2]	100	100%	98%	98%
Appropriate VTP Within 24 Hours[2]	405	98%	98%	98%
Controlled Postoperative Blood Glucose[2,7]	-	-	96%	97%
Perioperative Temperature Management[2]	435	100%	100%	100%
Prophylactic Antibiotic Selection[2]	280	100%	99%	99%
Prophylactic Antibiotic Selection (Outpatient)	254	99%	98%	98%
Prophylactic Antibiotic Stopped[2]	273	99%	98%	98%
Prophylactic Antibiotic Timing[2]	280	100%	99%	99%
Prophylactic Antibiotic Timing (Outpatient)	255	100%	98%	98%
Urinary Catheter Removal[2]	259	100%	98%	97%
Survey of Patients' Hospital Experiences				
Area Around Room 'Always' Quiet at Night	300+	66%	68%	61%
Doctors 'Always' Communicated Well	300+	82%	83%	82%
Home Recovery Information Given	300+	86%	85%	85%
Hospital Given 9 or 10 on 10 Point Scale	300+	76%	73%	71%
Meds 'Always' Explained Before Given	300+	64%	66%	64%
Nurses 'Always' Communicated Well	300+	78%	80%	79%
Pain 'Always' Well Controlled	300+	71%	72%	71%
Room and Bathroom 'Always' Clean	300+	75%	75%	73%
Timely Help 'Always' Received	300+	66%	69%	68%
Would Definitely Recommend Hospital	300+	79%	73%	71%
Use of Medical Imaging				
Cardiac Imaging Stress Test before Surgery[1]	-	-	5.3%	5.3%
Combination Abdominal CT Scan	788	23.6%	16.4%	10.5%
Combination Brain/Sinus CT Scan[1]	-	-	2.7%	2.7%
Combination Chest CT Scan	306	7.2%	5.6%	2.7%
Follow-up Mammogram/Ultrasound	1,289	9.4%	7.9%	8.8%
Lumbar Spine MRI for Low Back Pain	75	48.0%	39.6%	37.2%

Texas Health Presbyterian Hospital Kaufman

850 Ed Hall
Kaufman, TX 75142
Phone: 972-932-7200
Fax: 972-932-5425
URL: www.phscare.org/phk.htm
Type: Acute Care Hospitals
Emergency Services: Yes
Ownership: Voluntary non-profit - Private
Beds: 91
Key Personnel:
Chief of Medical Staff . . . . Benjamin Russel Brashear, MD
Intensive Care Unit. . . . . Shashank Dengle, MD
Infection Control. . . . . Janet Drummond
Emergency Room . . . . Michael Hueber, DO
Quality Assurance . . . . Dani Morales
Radiology. . . . . Cynthia Sherry
Operating Room. . . . . Susan Stone
CEO/President. . . . . Patsy Youngs

Measure	Cases	This Hosp.	State Avg.	U.S. Avg.
Blood Clot Prevention and Treatment				
Anticoagulation Overlap Therapy[2]	17	76%	93%	93%
ICU Venous Thromboembolism Prophylaxis[2]	29	100%	92%	92%
Incidence of Potentially Preventable VTE[2,7]	-	-	9%	10%
UFH with Dosages/Platelet Monitoring[1,2]	-	-	96%	97%
Venous Thromboembolism Prophylaxis[2]	180	97%	82%	85%

NOTE: Hospital profiles are in alphabetical order by state, then city, then hospital within the city; Rankings exclude hospitals with less than 25 cases except for patient surveys which excludes hospitals with less than 100 cases; (a) 100-299 cases; (1) The number of cases/patients is too few to report; (2) Data submitted were based on a sample of cases/patients; (3) Results are based on a shorter time period than required; (4) Data suppressed by CMS for one or more quarters; (5) Results are not available for this reporting period; (6) Fewer than 100 patients completed the HCAHPS survey; (7) No cases met the criteria for this measure; (8) The lower limit of the confidence interval cannot be calculated if the number of observed infections equals zero; (9) No data are available from the state/territory for this reporting period; (10) The scores shown reflect fewer than 50 completed surveys; (11) There were discrepancies in the data collection process; (12) This measure does not apply to this hospital for this reporting period; (13) Results cannot be calculated for this reporting period; (14) The results for this state are combined with nearby states to protect confidentiality; Please refer to the User's Guide for a full explanation of data.

Measure	Cases	This Hosp.	State Avg.	U.S. Avg.
Warfarin Therapy Discharge Instructions[2]	16	38%	84%	75%
Chest Pain/Possible Heart Attack Care				
Aspirin Given Within 24 Hours of Arrival	71	97%	94%	96%
Fibrinolytic Meds Within 30 Min. of Arrival[1]	-	-	47%	58%
Average Time to ECG (minutes)	72	6	8	7
Average Time to Transfer (minutes)[1]	-	-	62	60
Children's Asthma Care				
Received Home Management Plan of Care	-	-	93%	88%
Received Reliever Medication	-	-	100%	100%
Received Systemic Corticosteroids	-	-	100%	100%
Emergency Department				
Admittance Decision Time (minutes)[2]	298	90	99	98
Head CT Results Within 45 Min. of Arrival	13	85%	54%	57%
Patients Who Left ER Before Being Seen	27,890	2%	3%	2%
Time from ER Arrival to Admit. (minutes)[2]	314	235	270	274
Time from ER Arrival to Discharge (minutes)	400	145	127	134
Time in ER Before Being Evaluated (minutes)	442	34	26	26
Time to Pain Meds for Fractures (minutes)	105	52	57	57
Heart Attack Care				
Aspirin Given at Discharge[1]	-	-	99%	99%
Fibrinolytic Meds Within 30 Min. of Arrival[7]	-	-	49%	54%
PCI Within 90 Minutes of Arrival[7]	-	-	95%	96%
Statin Prescribed at Discharge[1]	-	-	98%	98%
Heart Failure Care				
ACE Inhibitor or ARB for LVSD	17	100%	97%	97%
Discharge Instructions Given	71	99%	95%	94%
Evaluation of LVS Function	79	100%	99%	99%
Medicare Spending				
Medicare Spending per Patient (ratio)	-	1.06	1.03	0.98
Pneumonia Care				
Appropriate Initial Antibiotic Given	74	100%	95%	95%
Blood Culture Timing	123	99%	98%	98%
Pregnancy and Delivery Care				
Newborn Deliveries Scheduled Early	22	9%	7%	6%
Preventive Care				
Immunization for Influenza[2]	317	97%	90%	90%
Immunization for Pneumonia[2]	417	97%	92%	92%
Stroke Care				
Anticoagulation Therapy for Atrial Fibrillation[1,2]	-	-	96%	95%
Antithrombotic Therapy Timing[2]	25	100%	98%	98%
Assessed for Rehabilitation[2]	25	100%	98%	97%
Discharged on Antithrombotic Therapy[2]	25	100%	99%	99%
Discharged on Statin Medication[2]	21	100%	95%	94%
Thrombolytic Therapy Timing[1,2]	-	-	68%	66%
Venous Thromboembolism Prophylaxis[2]	17	100%	94%	94%
Written Stroke Educational Materials Given[2]	13	100%	92%	88%
Surgical Care Improvement Project				
Appropriate Beta Blocker Usage[2]	32	100%	98%	98%
Appropriate VTP Within 24 Hours[2]	105	99%	98%	98%
Controlled Postoperative Blood Glucose[2,7]	-	-	96%	97%
Perioperative Temperature Management[2]	115	100%	100%	100%
Prophylactic Antibiotic Selection[2]	69	99%	99%	99%
Prophylactic Antibiotic Selection (Outpatient)[1,3]	-	-	98%	98%
Prophylactic Antibiotic Stopped[2]	68	99%	98%	98%
Prophylactic Antibiotic Timing[2]	69	100%	99%	99%
Prophylactic Antibiotic Timing (Outpatient)[1,3]	-	-	98%	98%
Urinary Catheter Removal[2]	55	98%	98%	97%
Survey of Patients' Hospital Experiences				
Area Around Room 'Always' Quiet at Night	300+	75%	68%	61%
Doctors 'Always' Communicated Well	300+	84%	83%	82%
Home Recovery Information Given	300+	85%	85%	85%
Hospital Given 9 or 10 on 10 Point Scale	300+	78%	73%	71%
Meds 'Always' Explained Before Given	300+	75%	66%	64%
Nurses 'Always' Communicated Well	300+	85%	80%	79%
Pain 'Always' Well Controlled	300+	78%	72%	71%
Room and Bathroom 'Always' Clean	300+	77%	75%	73%
Timely Help 'Always' Received	300+	74%	69%	68%
Would Definitely Recommend Hospital	300+	74%	73%	71%
Use of Medical Imaging				
Cardiac Imaging Stress Test before Surgery	200	3.0%	5.3%	5.3%
Combination Abdominal CT Scan	247	20.6%	16.4%	10.5%
Combination Brain/Sinus CT Scan	403	2.0%	2.7%	2.7%
Combination Chest CT Scan	117	39.3%	5.6%	2.7%
Follow-up Mammogram/Ultrasound	343	7.9%	7.9%	8.8%
Lumbar Spine MRI for Low Back Pain	40	40.0%	39.6%	37.2%

Otto Kaiser Memorial Hospital

3349 S Highway 181 Phone: 830-583-3401
Kenedy, TX 78119
E-mail: okmhinfo@okmh.net
URL: www.okmh.net
Type: Critical Access Hospitals Emergency Services: Yes
Ownership: Govt - Hospital Dist/Auth Beds: 25
Key Personnel:
President . . . . David Purser
CEO/President. . . . . Mary Szalwinski

Measure	Cases	This Hosp.	State Avg.	U.S. Avg.
Blood Clot Prevention and Treatment				
Anticoagulation Overlap Therapy[5]	-	-	93%	93%
ICU Venous Thromboembolism Prophylaxis[5]	-	-	92%	92%
Incidence of Potentially Preventable VTE[5]	-	-	9%	10%
UFH with Dosages/Platelet Monitoring[5]	-	-	96%	97%
Venous Thromboembolism Prophylaxis[5]	-	-	82%	85%
Warfarin Therapy Discharge Instructions[5]	-	-	84%	75%
Chest Pain/Possible Heart Attack Care				
Aspirin Given Within 24 Hours of Arrival[3]	16	94%	94%	96%
Fibrinolytic Meds Within 30 Min. of Arrival[3,7]	-	-	47%	58%
Average Time to ECG (minutes)[3]	17	5	8	7
Average Time to Transfer (minutes)[3,7]	-	-	62	60
Children's Asthma Care				
Received Home Management Plan of Care	-	-	93%	88%
Received Reliever Medication	-	-	100%	100%
Received Systemic Corticosteroids	-	-	100%	100%
Emergency Department				
Admittance Decision Time (minutes)[2]	165	32	99	98
Head CT Results Within 45 Min. of Arrival[5]	-	-	54%	57%
Patients Who Left ER Before Being Seen	9,111	1%	3%	2%
Time from ER Arrival to Admit. (minutes)[2]	200	172	270	274
Time from ER Arrival to Discharge (minutes)[5]	-	-	127	134
Time in ER Before Being Evaluated (minutes)[5]	-	-	26	26
Time to Pain Meds for Fractures (minutes)[5]	-	-	57	57
Heart Attack Care				
Aspirin Given at Discharge[5]	-	-	99%	99%
Fibrinolytic Meds Within 30 Min. of Arrival[5]	-	-	49%	54%
PCI Within 90 Minutes of Arrival[5]	-	-	95%	96%
Statin Prescribed at Discharge[5]	-	-	98%	98%
Heart Failure Care				
ACE Inhibitor or ARB for LVSD[1]	-	-	97%	97%
Discharge Instructions Given[1]	-	-	95%	94%
Evaluation of LVS Function[1]	-	-	99%	99%
Medicare Spending				
Medicare Spending per Patient (ratio)	-	-	1.03	0.98
Pneumonia Care				
Appropriate Initial Antibiotic Given[1]	-	-	95%	95%
Blood Culture Timing	20	90%	98%	98%
Pregnancy and Delivery Care				
Newborn Deliveries Scheduled Early[5]	-	-	7%	6%
Preventive Care				
Immunization for Influenza	88	90%	90%	90%
Immunization for Pneumonia[2]	202	81%	92%	92%
Stroke Care				
Anticoagulation Therapy for Atrial Fibrillation[5]	-	-	96%	95%
Antithrombotic Therapy Timing[5]	-	-	98%	98%
Assessed for Rehabilitation[5]	-	-	98%	97%
Discharged on Antithrombotic Therapy[5]	-	-	99%	99%
Discharged on Statin Medication[5]	-	-	95%	94%
Thrombolytic Therapy Timing[5]	-	-	68%	66%
Venous Thromboembolism Prophylaxis[5]	-	-	94%	94%
Written Stroke Educational Materials Given[5]	-	-	92%	88%
Surgical Care Improvement Project				
Appropriate Beta Blocker Usage[5]	-	-	98%	98%
Appropriate VTP Within 24 Hours[5]	-	-	98%	98%
Controlled Postoperative Blood Glucose[5]	-	-	96%	97%
Perioperative Temperature Management[5]	-	-	100%	100%
Prophylactic Antibiotic Selection[5]	-	-	99%	99%
Prophylactic Antibiotic Selection (Outpatient)[5]	-	-	98%	98%
Prophylactic Antibiotic Stopped[5]	-	-	98%	98%
Prophylactic Antibiotic Timing[5]	-	-	99%	99%
Prophylactic Antibiotic Timing (Outpatient)[5]	-	-	98%	98%
Urinary Catheter Removal[5]	-	-	98%	97%
Survey of Patients' Hospital Experiences				
Area Around Room 'Always' Quiet at Night[5]	-	-	68%	61%
Doctors 'Always' Communicated Well[5]	-	-	83%	82%
Home Recovery Information Given[5]	-	-	85%	85%
Hospital Given 9 or 10 on 10 Point Scale[5]	-	-	73%	71%
Meds 'Always' Explained Before Given[5]	-	-	66%	64%
Nurses 'Always' Communicated Well[5]	-	-	80%	79%
Pain 'Always' Well Controlled[5]	-	-	72%	71%
Room and Bathroom 'Always' Clean[5]	-	-	75%	73%
Timely Help 'Always' Received[5]	-	-	69%	68%
Would Definitely Recommend Hospital[5]	-	-	73%	71%
Use of Medical Imaging				
Cardiac Imaging Stress Test before Surgery[7]	-	-	5.3%	5.3%
Combination Abdominal CT Scan	183	6.6%	16.4%	10.5%
Combination Brain/Sinus CT Scan[1]	-	-	2.7%	2.7%
Combination Chest CT Scan[1]	-	-	5.6%	2.7%
Follow-up Mammogram/Ultrasound	67	19.4%	7.9%	8.8%
Lumbar Spine MRI for Low Back Pain[1]	-	-	39.6%	37.2%

Peterson Regional Medical Center

551 Hill Country Drive Phone: 830-896-4200
Kerrville, TX 78028
URL: www.petersonrmc.com
Type: Acute Care Hospitals Emergency Services: Yes
Ownership: Voluntary non-profit - Private

Measure	Cases	This Hosp.	State Avg.	U.S. Avg.
Blood Clot Prevention and Treatment				
Anticoagulation Overlap Therapy[2]	21	95%	93%	93%
ICU Venous Thromboembolism Prophylaxis[2]	93	99%	92%	92%
Incidence of Potentially Preventable VTE[1,2]	-	-	9%	10%
UFH with Dosages/Platelet Monitoring[1,2]	-	-	96%	97%
Venous Thromboembolism Prophylaxis[2]	342	100%	82%	85%
Warfarin Therapy Discharge Instructions[2]	14	93%	84%	75%
Chest Pain/Possible Heart Attack Care				
Aspirin Given Within 24 Hours of Arrival	90	100%	94%	96%
Fibrinolytic Meds Within 30 Min. of Arrival[1]	-	-	47%	58%
Average Time to ECG (minutes)	92	0	8	7
Average Time to Transfer (minutes)[1]	-	-	62	60
Children's Asthma Care				
Received Home Management Plan of Care	-	-	93%	88%
Received Reliever Medication	-	-	100%	100%
Received Systemic Corticosteroids	-	-	100%	100%
Emergency Department				
Admittance Decision Time (minutes)[2]	559	132	99	98
Head CT Results Within 45 Min. of Arrival	19	58%	54%	57%
Patients Who Left ER Before Being Seen	30,534	1%	3%	2%
Time from ER Arrival to Admit. (minutes)[2]	578	266	270	274
Time from ER Arrival to Discharge (minutes)	471	135	127	134
Time in ER Before Being Evaluated (minutes)	527	18	26	26
Time to Pain Meds for Fractures (minutes)	142	61	57	57
Heart Attack Care				
Aspirin Given at Discharge[1]	-	-	99%	99%
Fibrinolytic Meds Within 30 Min. of Arrival[7]	-	-	49%	54%
PCI Within 90 Minutes of Arrival[7]	-	-	95%	96%
Statin Prescribed at Discharge[1]	-	-	98%	98%
Heart Failure Care				
ACE Inhibitor or ARB for LVSD	41	93%	97%	97%
Discharge Instructions Given	104	95%	95%	94%
Evaluation of LVS Function	152	99%	99%	99%
Medicare Spending				
Medicare Spending per Patient (ratio)	-	1.05	1.03	0.98
Pneumonia Care				
Appropriate Initial Antibiotic Given	136	97%	95%	95%
Blood Culture Timing	224	100%	98%	98%
Pregnancy and Delivery Care				
Newborn Deliveries Scheduled Early	51	2%	7%	6%
Preventive Care				

NOTE: *Hospital profiles are in alphabetical order by state, then city, then hospital within the city; Rankings exclude hospitals with less than 25 cases except for patient surveys which excludes hospitals with less than 100 cases; (a) 100-299 cases; (1) The number of cases/patients is too few to report; (2) Data submitted were based on a sample of cases/patients; (3) Results are based on a shorter time period than required; (4) Data suppressed by CMS for one or more quarters; (5) Results are not available for this reporting period; (6) Fewer than 100 patients completed the HCAHPS survey; (7) No cases met the criteria for this measure; (8) The lower limit of the confidence interval cannot be calculated if the number of observed infections equals zero; (9) No data are available from the state/territory for this reporting period; (10) The scores shown reflect fewer than 50 completed surveys; (11) There were discrepancies in the data collection process; (12) This measure does not apply to this hospital for this reporting period; (13) Results cannot be calculated for this reporting period; (14) The results for this state are combined with nearby states to protect confidentiality; Please refer to the User's Guide for a full explanation of data.*

Measure	Cases	This Hosp.	State Avg.	U.S. Avg.
Immunization for Influenza[2]	442	97%	90%	90%
Immunization for Pneumonia[2]	632	98%	92%	92%
Stroke Care				
Anticoagulation Therapy for Atrial Fibrillation[1]	-	-	96%	95%
Antithrombotic Therapy Timing	52	98%	98%	98%
Assessed for Rehabilitation	50	98%	98%	97%
Discharged on Antithrombotic Therapy	50	100%	99%	99%
Discharged on Statin Medication	36	97%	95%	94%
Thrombolytic Therapy Timing[1]	-	-	68%	66%
Venous Thromboembolism Prophylaxis	52	100%	94%	94%
Written Stroke Educational Materials Given	28	96%	92%	88%
Surgical Care Improvement Project				
Appropriate Beta Blocker Usage	164	95%	98%	98%
Appropriate VTP Within 24 Hours	432	98%	98%	98%
Controlled Postoperative Blood Glucose[7]	-	-	96%	97%
Perioperative Temperature Management	498	100%	100%	100%
Prophylactic Antibiotic Selection	378	99%	99%	99%
Prophylactic Antibiotic Selection (Outpatient)	157	97%	98%	98%
Prophylactic Antibiotic Stopped	373	100%	98%	98%
Prophylactic Antibiotic Timing	379	99%	99%	99%
Prophylactic Antibiotic Timing (Outpatient)	157	99%	98%	98%
Urinary Catheter Removal	392	96%	98%	97%
Survey of Patients' Hospital Experiences				
Area Around Room 'Always' Quiet at Night	300+	54%	68%	61%
Doctors 'Always' Communicated Well	300+	80%	83%	82%
Home Recovery Information Given	300+	85%	85%	85%
Hospital Given 9 or 10 on 10 Point Scale	300+	69%	73%	71%
Meds 'Always' Explained Before Given	300+	62%	66%	64%
Nurses 'Always' Communicated Well	300+	75%	80%	79%
Pain 'Always' Well Controlled	300+	71%	72%	71%
Room and Bathroom 'Always' Clean	300+	69%	75%	73%
Timely Help 'Always' Received	300+	64%	69%	68%
Would Definitely Recommend Hospital	300+	70%	73%	71%
Use of Medical Imaging				
Cardiac Imaging Stress Test before Surgery	252	7.5%	5.3%	5.3%
Combination Abdominal CT Scan	902	4.4%	16.4%	10.5%
Combination Brain/Sinus CT Scan	751	1.9%	2.7%	2.7%
Combination Chest CT Scan	673	0.3%	5.6%	2.7%
Follow-up Mammogram/Ultrasound	1,560	10.8%	7.9%	8.8%
Lumbar Spine MRI for Low Back Pain	246	38.2%	39.6%	37.2%

Allegiance Specialty Hospital of Kilgore

1612 South Henderson Blvd
Kilgore, TX 75662
Phone: 903-984-3505
Fax: 903-983-4354
Type: Acute Care Hospitals
Ownership: Proprietary
Emergency Services: Yes
Beds: 60

Key Personnel:
CEO/President. . . . . Rock Bordelon
Infection Control. . . . . Melissa Lahman, RN
Quality Assurance . . . . Melissa Lehman, RN
Chief of Medical Staff. . . . . Brenda Vozza-Zeid, MD

Measure	Cases	This Hosp.	State Avg.	U.S. Avg.
Blood Clot Prevention and Treatment				
Anticoagulation Overlap Therapy[1,2]	-	-	93%	93%
ICU Venous Thromboembolism Prophylaxis[2,7]	-	-	92%	92%
Incidence of Potentially Preventable VTE[2,7]	-	-	9%	10%
UFH with Dosages/Platelet Monitoring[2,7]	-	-	96%	97%
Venous Thromboembolism Prophylaxis[2]	76	24%	82%	85%
Warfarin Therapy Discharge Instructions[2,7]	-	-	84%	75%
Chest Pain/Possible Heart Attack Care				
Aspirin Given Within 24 Hours of Arrival[5]	-	-	94%	96%
Fibrinolytic Meds Within 30 Min. of Arrival[5]	-	-	47%	58%
Average Time to ECG (minutes)[5]	-	-	8	7
Average Time to Transfer (minutes)[5]	-	-	62	60
Children's Asthma Care				
Received Home Management Plan of Care	-	-	93%	88%
Received Reliever Medication	-	-	100%	100%
Received Systemic Corticosteroids	-	-	100%	100%
Emergency Department				
Admittance Decision Time (minutes)[2,7]	-	-	99	98
Head CT Results Within 45 Min. of Arrival[5]	-	-	54%	57%
Patients Who Left ER Before Being Seen[5]	-	-	3%	2%
Time from ER Arrival to Admit. (minutes)[2,7]	-	-	270	274
Time from ER Arrival to Discharge (minutes)[5]	-	-	127	134
Time in ER Before Being Evaluated (minutes)[5]	-	-	26	26
Time to Pain Meds for Fractures (minutes)[5]	-	-	57	57
Heart Attack Care				
Aspirin Given at Discharge[5]	-	-	99%	99%
Fibrinolytic Meds Within 30 Min. of Arrival[5]	-	-	49%	54%
PCI Within 90 Minutes of Arrival[5]	-	-	95%	96%
Statin Prescribed at Discharge[5]	-	-	98%	98%
Heart Failure Care				
ACE Inhibitor or ARB for LVSD[5]	-	-	97%	97%
Discharge Instructions Given[5]	-	-	95%	94%
Evaluation of LVS Function[5]	-	-	99%	99%
Medicare Spending				
Medicare Spending per Patient (ratio)	-	1.14	1.03	0.98
Pneumonia Care				
Appropriate Initial Antibiotic Given[5]	-	-	95%	95%
Blood Culture Timing[5]	-	-	98%	98%
Pregnancy and Delivery Care				
Newborn Deliveries Scheduled Early[2,7]	-	-	7%	6%
Preventive Care				
Immunization for Influenza[2]	336	87%	90%	90%
Immunization for Pneumonia[2]	598	89%	92%	92%
Stroke Care				
Anticoagulation Therapy for Atrial Fibrillation[5]	-	-	96%	95%
Antithrombotic Therapy Timing[5]	-	-	98%	98%
Assessed for Rehabilitation[5]	-	-	98%	97%
Discharged on Antithrombotic Therapy[5]	-	-	99%	99%
Discharged on Statin Medication[5]	-	-	95%	94%
Thrombolytic Therapy Timing[5]	-	-	68%	66%
Venous Thromboembolism Prophylaxis[5]	-	-	94%	94%
Written Stroke Educational Materials Given[5]	-	-	92%	88%
Surgical Care Improvement Project				
Appropriate Beta Blocker Usage[5]	-	-	98%	98%
Appropriate VTP Within 24 Hours[5]	-	-	98%	98%
Controlled Postoperative Blood Glucose[5]	-	-	96%	97%
Perioperative Temperature Management[5]	-	-	100%	100%
Prophylactic Antibiotic Selection[5]	-	-	99%	99%
Prophylactic Antibiotic Selection (Outpatient)[5]	-	-	98%	98%
Prophylactic Antibiotic Stopped[5]	-	-	98%	98%
Prophylactic Antibiotic Timing[5]	-	-	99%	99%
Prophylactic Antibiotic Timing (Outpatient)[5]	-	-	98%	98%
Urinary Catheter Removal[5]	-	-	98%	97%
Survey of Patients' Hospital Experiences				
Area Around Room 'Always' Quiet at Night[1]	-	-	68%	61%
Doctors 'Always' Communicated Well[1]	-	-	83%	82%
Home Recovery Information Given[1]	-	-	85%	85%
Hospital Given 9 or 10 on 10 Point Scale[1]	-	-	73%	71%
Meds 'Always' Explained Before Given[1]	-	-	66%	64%
Nurses 'Always' Communicated Well[1]	-	-	80%	79%
Pain 'Always' Well Controlled[1]	-	-	72%	71%
Room and Bathroom 'Always' Clean[1]	-	-	75%	73%
Timely Help 'Always' Received[1]	-	-	69%	68%
Would Definitely Recommend Hospital[1]	-	-	73%	71%
Use of Medical Imaging				
Cardiac Imaging Stress Test before Surgery[7]	-	-	5.3%	5.3%
Combination Abdominal CT Scan[7]	-	-	16.4%	10.5%
Combination Brain/Sinus CT Scan[7]	-	-	2.7%	2.7%
Combination Chest CT Scan[7]	-	-	5.6%	2.7%
Follow-up Mammogram/Ultrasound[7]	-	-	7.9%	8.8%
Lumbar Spine MRI for Low Back Pain[7]	-	-	39.6%	37.2%

Metroplex Hospital

2201 S Clear Creek Road
Killeen, TX 76542
Phone: 254-526-7523
Fax: 254-526-3483
E-mail: dhewitt@ahcs.org
URL: www.mplex.org
Type: Acute Care Hospitals
Ownership: Voluntary non-profit - Private
Emergency Services: Yes
Beds: 213

Key Personnel:
Chief of Medical Staff. . . . . Jacquelene Adiele
Radiology. . . . . Frederick Barnett
President/CEO. . . . . Ken Finch

Measure	Cases	This Hosp.	State Avg.	U.S. Avg.
Blood Clot Prevention and Treatment				
Anticoagulation Overlap Therapy[2]	38	92%	93%	93%
ICU Venous Thromboembolism Prophylaxis[2]	103	99%	92%	92%
Incidence of Potentially Preventable VTE[1,2]	-	-	9%	10%
UFH with Dosages/Platelet Monitoring[1,2]	-	-	96%	97%
Venous Thromboembolism Prophylaxis[2]	305	97%	82%	85%
Warfarin Therapy Discharge Instructions[2]	31	97%	84%	75%
Chest Pain/Possible Heart Attack Care				
Aspirin Given Within 24 Hours of Arrival[1,3]	-	-	94%	96%
Fibrinolytic Meds Within 30 Min. of Arrival[3,7]	-	-	47%	58%
Average Time to ECG (minutes)[1,3]	-	-	8	7
Average Time to Transfer (minutes)[3,7]	-	-	62	60
Children's Asthma Care				
Received Home Management Plan of Care	-	-	93%	88%
Received Reliever Medication	-	-	100%	100%
Received Systemic Corticosteroids	-	-	100%	100%
Emergency Department				
Admittance Decision Time (minutes)[2]	459	69	99	98
Head CT Results Within 45 Min. of Arrival	11	36%	54%	57%
Patients Who Left ER Before Being Seen	51,746	5%	3%	2%
Time from ER Arrival to Admit. (minutes)[2]	461	287	270	274
Time from ER Arrival to Discharge (minutes)	346	182	127	134
Time in ER Before Being Evaluated (minutes)	383	60	26	26
Time to Pain Meds for Fractures (minutes)	191	82	57	57
Heart Attack Care				
Aspirin Given at Discharge[2]	91	99%	99%	99%
Fibrinolytic Meds Within 30 Min. of Arrival[2,7]	-	-	49%	54%
PCI Within 90 Minutes of Arrival[2]	20	85%	95%	96%
Statin Prescribed at Discharge[2]	85	100%	98%	98%
Heart Failure Care				
ACE Inhibitor or ARB for LVSD[2]	73	100%	97%	97%
Discharge Instructions Given[2]	196	100%	95%	94%
Evaluation of LVS Function[2]	230	100%	99%	99%
Medicare Spending				
Medicare Spending per Patient (ratio)	-	0.96	1.03	0.98
Pneumonia Care				
Appropriate Initial Antibiotic Given[2]	56	100%	95%	95%
Blood Culture Timing[2]	101	100%	98%	98%
Pregnancy and Delivery Care				
Newborn Deliveries Scheduled Early[2]	22	0%	7%	6%
Preventive Care				
Immunization for Influenza[2]	462	94%	90%	90%
Immunization for Pneumonia[2]	450	96%	92%	92%
Stroke Care				
Anticoagulation Therapy for Atrial Fibrillation[1,2]	-	-	96%	95%
Antithrombotic Therapy Timing[2]	47	100%	98%	98%
Assessed for Rehabilitation[2]	46	100%	98%	97%
Discharged on Antithrombotic Therapy[2]	46	100%	99%	99%
Discharged on Statin Medication[2]	34	100%	95%	94%
Thrombolytic Therapy Timing[1,2]	-	-	68%	66%
Venous Thromboembolism Prophylaxis[2]	47	100%	94%	94%
Written Stroke Educational Materials Given[2]	26	100%	92%	88%
Surgical Care Improvement Project				
Appropriate Beta Blocker Usage[2]	65	94%	98%	98%
Appropriate VTP Within 24 Hours[2]	220	100%	98%	98%
Controlled Postoperative Blood Glucose[2,7]	-	-	96%	97%
Perioperative Temperature Management[2]	249	100%	100%	100%
Prophylactic Antibiotic Selection[2]	166	98%	99%	99%
Prophylactic Antibiotic Selection (Outpatient)	130	89%	98%	98%
Prophylactic Antibiotic Stopped[2]	166	99%	98%	98%
Prophylactic Antibiotic Timing[2]	167	99%	99%	99%
Prophylactic Antibiotic Timing (Outpatient)	130	99%	98%	98%
Urinary Catheter Removal[2]	116	100%	98%	97%
Survey of Patients' Hospital Experiences				
Area Around Room 'Always' Quiet at Night[11]	300+	68%	68%	61%
Doctors 'Always' Communicated Well[11]	300+	82%	83%	82%
Home Recovery Information Given[11]	300+	88%	85%	85%
Hospital Given 9 or 10 on 10 Point Scale[11]	300+	70%	73%	71%
Meds 'Always' Explained Before Given[11]	300+	66%	66%	64%
Nurses 'Always' Communicated Well[11]	300+	80%	80%	79%
Pain 'Always' Well Controlled[11]	300+	72%	72%	71%
Room and Bathroom 'Always' Clean[11]	300+	77%	75%	73%

NOTE: Hospital profiles are in alphabetical order by state, then city, then hospital within the city; Rankings exclude hospitals with less than 25 cases except for patient surveys which excludes hospitals with less than 100 cases; (a) 100-299 cases; (1) The number of cases/patients is too few to report; (2) Data submitted were based on a sample of cases/patients; (3) Results are based on a shorter time period than required; (4) Data suppressed by CMS for one or more quarters; (5) Results are not available for this reporting period; (6) Fewer than 100 patients completed the HCAHPS survey; (7) No cases met the criteria for this measure; (8) The lower limit of the confidence interval cannot be calculated if the number of observed infections equals zero; (9) No data are available from the state/territory for this reporting period; (10) The scores shown reflect fewer than 50 completed surveys; (11) There were discrepancies in the data collection process; (12) This measure does not apply to this hospital for this reporting period; (13) Results cannot be calculated for this reporting period; (14) The results for this state are combined with nearby states to protect confidentiality; Please refer to the User's Guide for a full explanation of data.

Timely Help 'Always' Received[11]	300+	64%	69%	68%
Would Definitely Recommend Hospital[11]	300+	66%	73%	71%
Use of Medical Imaging				
Cardiac Imaging Stress Test before Surgery	196	4.1%	5.3%	5.3%
Combination Abdominal CT Scan	606	11.7%	16.4%	10.5%
Combination Brain/Sinus CT Scan	627	2.2%	2.7%	2.7%
Combination Chest CT Scan	469	8.1%	5.6%	2.7%
Follow-up Mammogram/Ultrasound	1,063	7.6%	7.9%	8.8%
Lumbar Spine MRI for Low Back Pain	241	38.2%	39.6%	37.2%

Christus Spohn Hospital Kleberg

1311 East General Cavazos Blvd
Kingsville, TX 78363
Phone: 361-595-1661
Fax: 361-595-5005
Type: Acute Care Hospitals
Emergency Services: Yes
Ownership: Voluntary non-profit - Private
Beds: 100
Key Personnel:
CEO/President. . . . . Kathy J McDonagh

Measure	Cases	This Hosp.	State Avg.	U.S. Avg.
Blood Clot Prevention and Treatment				
Anticoagulation Overlap Therapy[2]	12	92%	93%	93%
ICU Venous Thromboembolism Prophylaxis[2]	89	67%	92%	92%
Incidence of Potentially Preventable VTE[2,7]	-	-	9%	10%
UFH with Dosages/Platelet Monitoring[1,2]	-	-	96%	97%
Venous Thromboembolism Prophylaxis[2]	361	65%	82%	85%
Warfarin Therapy Discharge Instructions[2]	12	100%	84%	75%
Chest Pain/Possible Heart Attack Care				
Aspirin Given Within 24 Hours of Arrival	97	96%	94%	96%
Fibrinolytic Meds Within 30 Min. of Arrival[1]	-	-	47%	58%
Average Time to ECG (minutes)	107	16	8	7
Average Time to Transfer (minutes)	13	220	62	60
Children's Asthma Care				
Received Home Management Plan of Care	-	-	93%	88%
Received Reliever Medication	-	-	100%	100%
Received Systemic Corticosteroids	-	-	100%	100%
Emergency Department				
Admittance Decision Time (minutes)[2]	412	208	99	98
Head CT Results Within 45 Min. of Arrival	20	65%	54%	57%
Patients Who Left ER Before Being Seen	19,773	7%	3%	2%
Time from ER Arrival to Admit. (minutes)[2]	412	395	270	274
Time from ER Arrival to Discharge (minutes)	471	185	127	134
Time in ER Before Being Evaluated (minutes)	503	53	26	26
Time to Pain Meds for Fractures (minutes)	88	56	57	57
Heart Attack Care				
Aspirin Given at Discharge[1]	-	-	99%	99%
Fibrinolytic Meds Within 30 Min. of Arrival[7]	-	-	49%	54%
PCI Within 90 Minutes of Arrival[7]	-	-	95%	96%
Statin Prescribed at Discharge[1]	-	-	98%	98%
Heart Failure Care				
ACE Inhibitor or ARB for LVSD	44	68%	97%	97%
Discharge Instructions Given	160	96%	95%	94%
Evaluation of LVS Function	192	93%	99%	99%
Medicare Spending				
Medicare Spending per Patient (ratio)	-	1.00	1.03	0.98
Pneumonia Care				
Appropriate Initial Antibiotic Given[2]	90	96%	95%	95%
Blood Culture Timing[2]	92	97%	98%	98%
Pregnancy and Delivery Care				
Newborn Deliveries Scheduled Early[2]	30	23%	7%	6%
Preventive Care				
Immunization for Influenza[2]	371	91%	90%	90%
Immunization for Pneumonia[2]	487	95%	92%	92%
Stroke Care				
Anticoagulation Therapy for Atrial Fibrillation[1]	-	-	96%	95%
Antithrombotic Therapy Timing	20	95%	98%	98%
Assessed for Rehabilitation	16	88%	98%	97%
Discharged on Antithrombotic Therapy	16	88%	99%	99%
Discharged on Statin Medication	16	62%	95%	94%
Thrombolytic Therapy Timing[1]	-	-	68%	66%
Venous Thromboembolism Prophylaxis	20	80%	94%	94%
Written Stroke Educational Materials Given[1]	-	-	92%	88%
Surgical Care Improvement Project				
Appropriate Beta Blocker Usage[1]	-	-	98%	98%
Appropriate VTP Within 24 Hours	70	96%	98%	98%
Controlled Postoperative Blood Glucose[7]	-	-	96%	97%
Perioperative Temperature Management	85	100%	100%	100%
Prophylactic Antibiotic Selection	45	93%	99%	99%
Prophylactic Antibiotic Selection (Outpatient)[1]	-	-	98%	98%
Prophylactic Antibiotic Stopped	44	100%	98%	98%
Prophylactic Antibiotic Timing	45	96%	99%	99%
Prophylactic Antibiotic Timing (Outpatient)[1]	-	-	98%	98%
Urinary Catheter Removal	40	68%	98%	97%
Survey of Patients' Hospital Experiences				
Area Around Room 'Always' Quiet at Night	300+	64%	68%	61%
Doctors 'Always' Communicated Well	300+	87%	83%	82%
Home Recovery Information Given	300+	84%	85%	85%
Hospital Given 9 or 10 on 10 Point Scale	300+	62%	73%	71%
Meds 'Always' Explained Before Given	300+	65%	66%	64%
Nurses 'Always' Communicated Well	300+	78%	80%	79%
Pain 'Always' Well Controlled	300+	72%	72%	71%
Room and Bathroom 'Always' Clean	300+	73%	75%	73%
Timely Help 'Always' Received	300+	64%	69%	68%
Would Definitely Recommend Hospital	300+	58%	73%	71%
Use of Medical Imaging				
Cardiac Imaging Stress Test before Surgery[1]	-	-	5.3%	5.3%
Combination Abdominal CT Scan	257	56.0%	16.4%	10.5%
Combination Brain/Sinus CT Scan[1]	-	-	2.7%	2.7%
Combination Chest CT Scan	82	3.7%	5.6%	2.7%
Follow-up Mammogram/Ultrasound	346	6.9%	7.9%	8.8%
Lumbar Spine MRI for Low Back Pain[1]	-	-	39.6%	37.2%

Kingwood Medical Center

22999 Us Hwy 59
Kingwood, TX 77325
Phone: 281-359-7500
Fax: 281-348-8010
URL: www.kingwoodmedical.com
Type: Acute Care Hospitals
Emergency Services: Yes
Ownership: Proprietary
Beds: 155
Key Personnel:
CEO/President. . . . . Gay Nord
Chief of Medical Staff. . . . . Eugene Ogrod, MD
CEO . . . . Melinda Stephenson
Chair/CEO. . . . . Chik-Fong Wei, MD

Measure	Cases	This Hosp.	State Avg.	U.S. Avg.
Blood Clot Prevention and Treatment				
Anticoagulation Overlap Therapy[2]	96	92%	93%	93%
ICU Venous Thromboembolism Prophylaxis[2]	110	99%	92%	92%
Incidence of Potentially Preventable VTE[2]	23	0%	9%	10%
UFH with Dosages/Platelet Monitoring[2]	46	100%	96%	97%
Venous Thromboembolism Prophylaxis[2]	403	97%	82%	85%
Warfarin Therapy Discharge Instructions[2]	56	98%	84%	75%
Chest Pain/Possible Heart Attack Care				
Aspirin Given Within 24 Hours of Arrival[1,3]	-	-	94%	96%
Fibrinolytic Meds Within 30 Min. of Arrival[3,7]	-	-	47%	58%
Average Time to ECG (minutes)[1,3]	-	-	8	7
Average Time to Transfer (minutes)[3,7]	-	-	62	60
Children's Asthma Care				
Received Home Management Plan of Care	-	-	93%	88%
Received Reliever Medication	-	-	100%	100%
Received Systemic Corticosteroids	-	-	100%	100%
Emergency Department				
Admittance Decision Time (minutes)[2]	588	290	99	98
Head CT Results Within 45 Min. of Arrival[1]	-	-	54%	57%
Patients Who Left ER Before Being Seen	57,791	3%	3%	2%
Time from ER Arrival to Admit. (minutes)[2]	611	420	270	274
Time from ER Arrival to Discharge (minutes)	414	215	127	134
Time in ER Before Being Evaluated (minutes)	515	40	26	26
Time to Pain Meds for Fractures (minutes)	150	96	57	57
Heart Attack Care				
Aspirin Given at Discharge[2]	271	100%	99%	99%
Fibrinolytic Meds Within 30 Min. of Arrival[2,7]	-	-	49%	54%
PCI Within 90 Minutes of Arrival[2]	42	95%	95%	96%
Statin Prescribed at Discharge[2]	249	100%	98%	98%
Heart Failure Care				
ACE Inhibitor or ARB for LVSD	121	98%	97%	97%
Discharge Instructions Given	370	99%	95%	94%
Evaluation of LVS Function	461	100%	99%	99%
Medicare Spending				
Medicare Spending per Patient (ratio)	-	1.07	1.03	0.98
Pneumonia Care				
Appropriate Initial Antibiotic Given	194	96%	95%	95%
Blood Culture Timing	250	98%	98%	98%
Pregnancy and Delivery Care				
Newborn Deliveries Scheduled Early[2]	54	0%	7%	6%
Preventive Care				
Immunization for Influenza[2]	572	99%	90%	90%
Immunization for Pneumonia[2]	669	97%	92%	92%
Stroke Care				
Anticoagulation Therapy for Atrial Fibrillation[2]	16	100%	96%	95%
Antithrombotic Therapy Timing[2]	102	99%	98%	98%
Assessed for Rehabilitation[2]	118	100%	98%	97%
Discharged on Antithrombotic Therapy[2]	99	100%	99%	99%
Discharged on Statin Medication[2]	69	99%	95%	94%
Thrombolytic Therapy Timing[1,2]	-	-	68%	66%
Venous Thromboembolism Prophylaxis[2]	126	99%	94%	94%
Written Stroke Educational Materials Given[2]	69	100%	92%	88%
Surgical Care Improvement Project				
Appropriate Beta Blocker Usage[2]	164	100%	98%	98%
Appropriate VTP Within 24 Hours[2]	355	100%	98%	98%
Controlled Postoperative Blood Glucose[2]	95	95%	96%	97%
Perioperative Temperature Management[2]	460	100%	100%	100%
Prophylactic Antibiotic Selection[2]	302	100%	99%	99%
Prophylactic Antibiotic Selection (Outpatient)	259	100%	98%	98%
Prophylactic Antibiotic Stopped[2]	286	99%	98%	98%
Prophylactic Antibiotic Timing[2]	302	100%	99%	99%
Prophylactic Antibiotic Timing (Outpatient)	259	99%	98%	98%
Urinary Catheter Removal[2]	226	98%	98%	97%
Survey of Patients' Hospital Experiences				
Area Around Room 'Always' Quiet at Night	300+	59%	68%	61%
Doctors 'Always' Communicated Well	300+	77%	83%	82%
Home Recovery Information Given	300+	83%	85%	85%
Hospital Given 9 or 10 on 10 Point Scale	300+	64%	73%	71%
Meds 'Always' Explained Before Given	300+	57%	66%	64%
Nurses 'Always' Communicated Well	300+	72%	80%	79%
Pain 'Always' Well Controlled	300+	66%	72%	71%
Room and Bathroom 'Always' Clean	300+	67%	75%	73%
Timely Help 'Always' Received	300+	57%	69%	68%
Would Definitely Recommend Hospital	300+	67%	73%	71%
Use of Medical Imaging				
Cardiac Imaging Stress Test before Surgery	55	3.6%	5.3%	5.3%
Combination Abdominal CT Scan	571	19.1%	16.4%	10.5%
Combination Brain/Sinus CT Scan[1]	-	-	2.7%	2.7%
Combination Chest CT Scan	324	0.0%	5.6%	2.7%
Follow-up Mammogram/Ultrasound	346	5.5%	7.9%	8.8%
Lumbar Spine MRI for Low Back Pain[1]	-	-	39.6%	37.2%

Memorial Hermann Surgical Hospital Kingwood

300 Kingwood Medical Drive
Kingwood, TX 77339
Phone: 281-312-4000
Type: Acute Care Hospitals
Emergency Services: No
Ownership: Proprietary
Beds: 10
Key Personnel:
Anesthesiology. . . . . Shanaz E. Ali, MD
Radiology. . . . . Walid Khalid Adham, MD
CEO/President. . . . . Steven L Smith
Pulmonary Disease . . . . Alexander L Tiu, MD

Measure	Cases	This Hosp.	State Avg.	U.S. Avg.
Blood Clot Prevention and Treatment				
Anticoagulation Overlap Therapy[2,7]	-	-	93%	93%
ICU Venous Thromboembolism Prophylaxis[2,7]	-	-	92%	92%
Incidence of Potentially Preventable VTE[2,7]	-	-	9%	10%
UFH with Dosages/Platelet Monitoring[2,7]	-	-	96%	97%
Venous Thromboembolism Prophylaxis[2]	11	100%	82%	85%
Warfarin Therapy Discharge Instructions[2,7]	-	-	84%	75%
Chest Pain/Possible Heart Attack Care				
Aspirin Given Within 24 Hours of Arrival[1,3]	-	-	94%	96%
Fibrinolytic Meds Within 30 Min. of Arrival[3,7]	-	-	47%	58%
Average Time to ECG (minutes)[1,3]	-	-	8	7
Average Time to Transfer (minutes)[3,7]	-	-	62	60
Children's Asthma Care				
Received Home Management Plan of Care	-	-	93%	88%

NOTE: Hospital profiles are in alphabetical order by state, then city, then hospital within the city; Rankings exclude hospitals with less than 25 cases except for patient surveys which excludes hospitals with less than 100 cases; (a) 100-299 cases; (1) The number of cases/patients is too few to report; (2) Data submitted were based on a sample of cases/patients; (3) Results are based on a shorter time period than required; (4) Data suppressed by CMS for one or more quarters; (5) Results are not available for this reporting period; (6) Fewer than 100 patients completed the HCAHPS survey; (7) No cases met the criteria for this measure; (8) The lower limit of the confidence interval cannot be calculated if the number of observed infections equals zero; (9) No data are available from the state/territory for this reporting period; (10) The scores shown reflect fewer than 50 completed surveys; (11) There were discrepancies in the data collection process; (12) This measure does not apply to this hospital for this reporting period; (13) Results cannot be calculated for this reporting period; (14) The results for this state are combined with nearby states to protect confidentiality; Please refer to the User's Guide for a full explanation of data.

Measure	Cases	This Hosp.	State Avg.	U.S. Avg.
Received Reliever Medication	-	-	100%	100%
Received Systemic Corticosteroids	-	-	100%	100%
Emergency Department				
Admittance Decision Time (minutes)[7]	-	-	99	98
Head CT Results Within 45 Min. of Arrival[5]	-	-	54%	57%
Patients Who Left ER Before Being Seen	162	2%	3%	2%
Time from ER Arrival to Admit. (minutes)[7]	-	-	270	274
Time from ER Arrival to Discharge (minutes)	129	99	127	134
Time in ER Before Being Evaluated (minutes)	237	6	26	26
Time to Pain Meds for Fractures (minutes)[1,3]	-	-	57	57
Heart Attack Care				
Aspirin Given at Discharge[5]	-	-	99%	99%
Fibrinolytic Meds Within 30 Min. of Arrival[5]	-	-	49%	54%
PCI Within 90 Minutes of Arrival[5]	-	-	95%	96%
Statin Prescribed at Discharge[5]	-	-	98%	98%
Heart Failure Care				
ACE Inhibitor or ARB for LVSD[5]	-	-	97%	97%
Discharge Instructions Given[5]	-	-	95%	94%
Evaluation of LVS Function[5]	-	-	99%	99%
Medicare Spending				
Medicare Spending per Patient (ratio)	-	1.15	1.03	0.98
Pneumonia Care				
Appropriate Initial Antibiotic Given[5]	-	-	95%	95%
Blood Culture Timing[5]	-	-	98%	98%
Pregnancy and Delivery Care				
Newborn Deliveries Scheduled Early[7]	-	-	7%	6%
Preventive Care				
Immunization for Influenza	83	99%	90%	90%
Immunization for Pneumonia	80	94%	92%	92%
Stroke Care				
Anticoagulation Therapy for Atrial Fibrillation[5]	-	-	96%	95%
Antithrombotic Therapy Timing[5]	-	-	98%	98%
Assessed for Rehabilitation[5]	-	-	98%	97%
Discharged on Antithrombotic Therapy[5]	-	-	99%	99%
Discharged on Statin Medication[5]	-	-	95%	94%
Thrombolytic Therapy Timing[5]	-	-	68%	66%
Venous Thromboembolism Prophylaxis[5]	-	-	94%	94%
Written Stroke Educational Materials Given[5]	-	-	92%	88%
Surgical Care Improvement Project				
Appropriate Beta Blocker Usage	35	97%	98%	98%
Appropriate VTP Within 24 Hours	116	99%	98%	98%
Controlled Postoperative Blood Glucose[7]	-	-	96%	97%
Perioperative Temperature Management	128	100%	100%	100%
Prophylactic Antibiotic Selection	117	99%	99%	99%
Prophylactic Antibiotic Selection (Outpatient)	179	98%	98%	98%
Prophylactic Antibiotic Stopped	117	97%	98%	98%
Prophylactic Antibiotic Timing	117	100%	99%	99%
Prophylactic Antibiotic Timing (Outpatient)	179	100%	98%	98%
Urinary Catheter Removal[1]	-	-	98%	97%
Survey of Patients' Hospital Experiences				
Area Around Room 'Always' Quiet at Night[6]	<100	81%	68%	61%
Doctors 'Always' Communicated Well[6]	<100	86%	83%	82%
Home Recovery Information Given[6]	<100	87%	85%	85%
Hospital Given 9 or 10 on 10 Point Scale[6]	<100	86%	73%	71%
Meds 'Always' Explained Before Given[6]	<100	78%	66%	64%
Nurses 'Always' Communicated Well[6]	<100	86%	80%	79%
Pain 'Always' Well Controlled[6]	<100	75%	72%	71%
Room and Bathroom 'Always' Clean[6]	<100	78%	75%	73%
Timely Help 'Always' Received[6]	<100	88%	69%	68%
Would Definitely Recommend Hospital[6]	<100	87%	73%	71%
Use of Medical Imaging				
Cardiac Imaging Stress Test before Surgery[7]	-	-	5.3%	5.3%
Combination Abdominal CT Scan[7]	-	-	16.4%	10.5%
Combination Brain/Sinus CT Scan[7]	-	-	2.7%	2.7%
Combination Chest CT Scan[7]	-	-	5.6%	2.7%
Follow-up Mammogram/Ultrasound[7]	-	-	7.9%	8.8%
Lumbar Spine MRI for Low Back Pain[7]	-	-	39.6%	37.2%

Knox County Hospital

701 Se 5th Street
Knox City, TX 79529
Phone: 940-657-3535
Fax: 940-657-3005
E-mail: knoxhospital@srcaccess.net
URL: www.knoxcountytx.net
Type: Acute Care Hospitals
Emergency Services: Yes
Ownership: Govt - Hospital Dist/Auth
Beds: 14

Key Personnel:
Chief of Medical Staff.......... Shirley Barretto, MD
Quality Assurance .... Teresa A Murray
Emergency Room .... Dan Offutt
Infection Control............. Jan Rolston

Measure	Cases	This Hosp.	State Avg.	U.S. Avg.
Blood Clot Prevention and Treatment				
Anticoagulation Overlap Therapy[7]	-	-	93%	93%
ICU Venous Thromboembolism Prophylaxis[7]	-	-	92%	92%
Incidence of Potentially Preventable VTE[7]	-	-	9%	10%
UFH with Dosages/Platelet Monitoring[7]	-	-	96%	97%
Venous Thromboembolism Prophylaxis	60	18%	82%	85%
Warfarin Therapy Discharge Instructions[7]	-	-	84%	75%
Chest Pain/Possible Heart Attack Care				
Aspirin Given Within 24 Hours of Arrival[5]	-	-	94%	96%
Fibrinolytic Meds Within 30 Min. of Arrival[5]	-	-	47%	58%
Average Time to ECG (minutes)[5]	-	-	8	7
Average Time to Transfer (minutes)[5]	-	-	62	60
Children's Asthma Care				
Received Home Management Plan of Care	-	-	93%	88%
Received Reliever Medication	-	-	100%	100%
Received Systemic Corticosteroids	-	-	100%	100%
Emergency Department				
Admittance Decision Time (minutes)[2]	22	0	99	98
Head CT Results Within 45 Min. of Arrival[5]	-	-	54%	57%
Patients Who Left ER Before Being Seen	1,476	0%	3%	2%
Time from ER Arrival to Admit. (minutes)[2]	55	89	270	274
Time from ER Arrival to Discharge (minutes)	228	74	127	134
Time in ER Before Being Evaluated (minutes)	258	14	26	26
Time to Pain Meds for Fractures (minutes)[5]	-	-	57	57
Heart Attack Care				
Aspirin Given at Discharge[5]	-	-	99%	99%
Fibrinolytic Meds Within 30 Min. of Arrival[5]	-	-	49%	54%
PCI Within 90 Minutes of Arrival[5]	-	-	95%	96%
Statin Prescribed at Discharge[5]	-	-	98%	98%
Heart Failure Care				
ACE Inhibitor or ARB for LVSD[3,7]	-	-	97%	97%
Discharge Instructions Given[3,7]	-	-	95%	94%
Evaluation of LVS Function[1,3]	-	-	99%	99%
Medicare Spending				
Medicare Spending per Patient (ratio)	-	0.86	1.03	0.98
Pneumonia Care				
Appropriate Initial Antibiotic Given[1,3]	-	-	95%	95%
Blood Culture Timing[1,3]	-	-	98%	98%
Pregnancy and Delivery Care				
Newborn Deliveries Scheduled Early[7]	-	-	7%	6%
Preventive Care				
Immunization for Influenza[2]	53	68%	90%	90%
Immunization for Pneumonia[2]	86	72%	92%	92%
Stroke Care				
Anticoagulation Therapy for Atrial Fibrillation[5]	-	-	96%	95%
Antithrombotic Therapy Timing[5]	-	-	98%	98%
Assessed for Rehabilitation[5]	-	-	98%	97%
Discharged on Antithrombotic Therapy[5]	-	-	99%	99%
Discharged on Statin Medication[5]	-	-	95%	94%
Thrombolytic Therapy Timing[5]	-	-	68%	66%
Venous Thromboembolism Prophylaxis[5]	-	-	94%	94%
Written Stroke Educational Materials Given[5]	-	-	92%	88%
Surgical Care Improvement Project				
Appropriate Beta Blocker Usage[5]	-	-	98%	98%
Appropriate VTP Within 24 Hours[5]	-	-	98%	98%
Controlled Postoperative Blood Glucose[5]	-	-	96%	97%
Perioperative Temperature Management[5]	-	-	100%	100%
Prophylactic Antibiotic Selection[5]	-	-	99%	99%
Prophylactic Antibiotic Selection (Outpatient)[5]	-	-	98%	98%
Prophylactic Antibiotic Stopped[5]	-	-	98%	98%
Prophylactic Antibiotic Timing[5]	-	-	99%	99%
Prophylactic Antibiotic Timing (Outpatient)[5]	-	-	98%	98%
Urinary Catheter Removal[5]	-	-	98%	97%
Survey of Patients' Hospital Experiences				
Area Around Room 'Always' Quiet at Night[10]	<100	70%	68%	61%
Doctors 'Always' Communicated Well[10]	<100	90%	83%	82%
Home Recovery Information Given[10]	<100	63%	85%	85%
Hospital Given 9 or 10 on 10 Point Scale[10]	<100	79%	73%	71%
Meds 'Always' Explained Before Given[10]	<100	68%	66%	64%
Nurses 'Always' Communicated Well[10]	<100	88%	80%	79%
Pain 'Always' Well Controlled[10]	<100	66%	72%	71%
Room and Bathroom 'Always' Clean[10]	<100	90%	75%	73%
Timely Help 'Always' Received[10]	<100	82%	69%	68%
Would Definitely Recommend Hospital[10]	<100	71%	73%	71%
Use of Medical Imaging				
Cardiac Imaging Stress Test before Surgery[7]	-	-	5.3%	5.3%
Combination Abdominal CT Scan[1]	-	-	16.4%	10.5%
Combination Brain/Sinus CT Scan[1]	-	-	2.7%	2.7%
Combination Chest CT Scan[1]	-	-	5.6%	2.7%
Follow-up Mammogram/Ultrasound[7]	-	-	7.9%	8.8%
Lumbar Spine MRI for Low Back Pain[1]	-	-	39.6%	37.2%

Seton Medical Center Hays

6001 Kyle Pkwy
Kyle, TX 78640
Phone: 512-324-5000
URL: www.seton.net
Type: Acute Care Hospitals
Emergency Services: Yes
Ownership: Voluntary non-profit - Private
Beds: 112

Key Personnel:
President/CEO............... Robert I. Bonar, Jr., Dr. HA
President/CEO............... Jeff Cook
President/CEO............... Ken Galadish
President/CEO............... Jesus Garza
President.................... Greg W. Hartman
President/CEO............... Prathibha Varkey, MD, MPH, MBA
Quality Assurance .... Carol Wratten, MD, MBA, FACOG

Measure	Cases	This Hosp.	State Avg.	U.S. Avg.
Blood Clot Prevention and Treatment				
Anticoagulation Overlap Therapy[2]	36	100%	93%	93%
ICU Venous Thromboembolism Prophylaxis[2]	68	93%	92%	92%
Incidence of Potentially Preventable VTE[1,2]	-	-	9%	10%
UFH with Dosages/Platelet Monitoring[1,2]	-	-	96%	97%
Venous Thromboembolism Prophylaxis[2]	348	86%	82%	85%
Warfarin Therapy Discharge Instructions[2]	24	58%	84%	75%
Chest Pain/Possible Heart Attack Care				
Aspirin Given Within 24 Hours of Arrival[1,3]	-	-	94%	96%
Fibrinolytic Meds Within 30 Min. of Arrival[5]	-	-	47%	58%
Average Time to ECG (minutes)[1,3]	-	-	8	7
Average Time to Transfer (minutes)[5]	-	-	62	60
Children's Asthma Care				
Received Home Management Plan of Care	-	-	93%	88%
Received Reliever Medication	-	-	100%	100%
Received Systemic Corticosteroids	-	-	100%	100%
Emergency Department				
Admittance Decision Time (minutes)[2,7]	-	-	99	98
Head CT Results Within 45 Min. of Arrival[1]	-	-	54%	57%
Patients Who Left ER Before Being Seen	32,850	3%	3%	2%
Time from ER Arrival to Admit. (minutes)[2]	778	278	270	274
Time from ER Arrival to Discharge (minutes)	373	175	127	134
Time in ER Before Being Evaluated (minutes)	388	19	26	26
Time to Pain Meds for Fractures (minutes)	46	67	57	57
Heart Attack Care				
Aspirin Given at Discharge	146	99%	99%	99%
Fibrinolytic Meds Within 30 Min. of Arrival[7]	-	-	49%	54%
PCI Within 90 Minutes of Arrival	31	97%	95%	96%
Statin Prescribed at Discharge	142	99%	98%	98%
Heart Failure Care				
ACE Inhibitor or ARB for LVSD	46	100%	97%	97%
Discharge Instructions Given	91	93%	95%	94%
Evaluation of LVS Function	110	100%	99%	99%
Medicare Spending				
Medicare Spending per Patient (ratio)	-	1.07	1.03	0.98
Pneumonia Care				
Appropriate Initial Antibiotic Given	108	91%	95%	95%

NOTE: Hospital profiles are in alphabetical order by state, then city, then hospital within the city; Rankings exclude hospitals with less than 25 cases except for patient surveys which excludes hospitals with less than 100 cases; (a) 100-299 cases; (1) The number of cases/patients is too few to report; (2) Data submitted were based on a sample of cases/patients; (3) Results are based on a shorter time period than required; (4) Data suppressed by CMS for one or more quarters; (5) Results are not available for this reporting period; (6) Fewer than 100 patients completed the HCAHPS survey; (7) No cases met the criteria for this measure; (8) The lower limit of the confidence interval cannot be calculated if the number of observed infections equals zero; (9) No data are available from the state/territory for this reporting period; (10) The scores shown reflect fewer than 50 completed surveys; (11) There were discrepancies in the data collection process; (12) This measure does not apply to this hospital for this reporting period; (13) Results cannot be calculated for this reporting period; (14) The results for this state are combined with nearby states to protect confidentiality; Please refer to the User's Guide for a full explanation of data.

Blood Culture Timing	219	97%	98%	98%
Pregnancy and Delivery Care				
Newborn Deliveries Scheduled Early	60	0%	7%	6%
Preventive Care				
Immunization for Influenza[2]	541	94%	90%	90%
Immunization for Pneumonia[2]	648	93%	92%	92%
Stroke Care				
Anticoagulation Therapy for Atrial Fibrillation[1]	-	-	96%	95%
Antithrombotic Therapy Timing	63	95%	98%	98%
Assessed for Rehabilitation	74	92%	98%	97%
Discharged on Antithrombotic Therapy	71	100%	99%	99%
Discharged on Statin Medication	55	98%	95%	94%
Thrombolytic Therapy Timing[1]	-	-	68%	66%
Venous Thromboembolism Prophylaxis	68	91%	94%	94%
Written Stroke Educational Materials Given	47	70%	92%	88%
Surgical Care Improvement Project				
Appropriate Beta Blocker Usage	71	97%	98%	98%
Appropriate VTP Within 24 Hours	184	98%	98%	98%
Controlled Postoperative Blood Glucose	45	98%	96%	97%
Perioperative Temperature Management	215	100%	100%	100%
Prophylactic Antibiotic Selection	149	98%	99%	99%
Prophylactic Antibiotic Selection (Outpatient)	55	100%	98%	98%
Prophylactic Antibiotic Stopped	142	97%	98%	98%
Prophylactic Antibiotic Timing	149	99%	99%	99%
Prophylactic Antibiotic Timing (Outpatient)	56	98%	98%	98%
Urinary Catheter Removal	148	95%	98%	97%
Survey of Patients' Hospital Experiences				
Area Around Room 'Always' Quiet at Night	300+	65%	68%	61%
Doctors 'Always' Communicated Well	300+	80%	83%	82%
Home Recovery Information Given	300+	86%	85%	85%
Hospital Given 9 or 10 on 10 Point Scale	300+	74%	73%	71%
Meds 'Always' Explained Before Given	300+	65%	66%	64%
Nurses 'Always' Communicated Well	300+	77%	80%	79%
Pain 'Always' Well Controlled	300+	71%	72%	71%
Room and Bathroom 'Always' Clean	300+	67%	75%	73%
Timely Help 'Always' Received	300+	63%	69%	68%
Would Definitely Recommend Hospital	300+	78%	73%	71%
Use of Medical Imaging				
Cardiac Imaging Stress Test before Surgery	195	5.1%	5.3%	5.3%
Combination Abdominal CT Scan	363	2.5%	16.4%	10.5%
Combination Brain/Sinus CT Scan[1]	-	-	2.7%	2.7%
Combination Chest CT Scan	217	0.0%	5.6%	2.7%
Follow-up Mammogram/Ultrasound	88	9.1%	7.9%	8.8%
Lumbar Spine MRI for Low Back Pain[1]	-	-	39.6%	37.2%

Saint Marks Medical Center

One Saint Mark's Place
La Grange, TX 78945
Phone: 979-242-2200
URL: www.stmarksmedicalcenter.org
Type: Acute Care Hospitals
Emergency Services: Yes
Ownership: Voluntary non-profit - Private
Beds: 48

Key Personnel:
Chairman/CEO .... Joe Bailey
CEO/President............... Carol Drozd

Measure	Cases	This Hosp.	State Avg.	U.S. Avg.
Blood Clot Prevention and Treatment				
Anticoagulation Overlap Therapy[1,2]	-	-	93%	93%
ICU Venous Thromboembolism Prophylaxis[2,7]	-	-	92%	92%
Incidence of Potentially Preventable VTE[2,7]	-	-	9%	10%
UFH with Dosages/Platelet Monitoring[1,2]	-	-	96%	97%
Venous Thromboembolism Prophylaxis[2]	188	99%	82%	85%
Warfarin Therapy Discharge Instructions[1,2]	-	-	84%	75%
Chest Pain/Possible Heart Attack Care				
Aspirin Given Within 24 Hours of Arrival	72	100%	94%	96%
Fibrinolytic Meds Within 30 Min. of Arrival[1]	-	-	47%	58%
Average Time to ECG (minutes)	74	10	8	7
Average Time to Transfer (minutes)[1]	-	-	62	60
Children's Asthma Care				
Received Home Management Plan of Care	-	-	93%	88%
Received Reliever Medication	-	-	100%	100%
Received Systemic Corticosteroids	-	-	100%	100%
Emergency Department				
Admittance Decision Time (minutes)[2]	393	47	99	98
Head CT Results Within 45 Min. of Arrival[1]	-	-	54%	57%
Patients Who Left ER Before Being Seen	10,595	1%	3%	2%
Time from ER Arrival to Admit. (minutes)[2]	398	205	270	274
Time from ER Arrival to Discharge (minutes)	460	120	127	134
Time in ER Before Being Evaluated (minutes)	514	28	26	26
Time to Pain Meds for Fractures (minutes)	50	57	57	57
Heart Attack Care				
Aspirin Given at Discharge[1]	-	-	99%	99%
Fibrinolytic Meds Within 30 Min. of Arrival[1]	-	-	49%	54%
PCI Within 90 Minutes of Arrival[7]	-	-	95%	96%
Statin Prescribed at Discharge[1]	-	-	98%	98%
Heart Failure Care				
ACE Inhibitor or ARB for LVSD[1]	-	-	97%	97%
Discharge Instructions Given	30	100%	95%	94%
Evaluation of LVS Function	45	100%	99%	99%
Medicare Spending				
Medicare Spending per Patient (ratio)	-	1.06	1.03	0.98
Pneumonia Care				
Appropriate Initial Antibiotic Given	52	96%	95%	95%
Blood Culture Timing	79	100%	98%	98%
Pregnancy and Delivery Care				
Newborn Deliveries Scheduled Early	24	25%	7%	6%
Preventive Care				
Immunization for Influenza[2]	304	96%	90%	90%
Immunization for Pneumonia[2]	398	98%	92%	92%
Stroke Care				
Anticoagulation Therapy for Atrial Fibrillation[1]	-	-	96%	95%
Antithrombotic Therapy Timing	13	92%	98%	98%
Assessed for Rehabilitation	11	100%	98%	97%
Discharged on Antithrombotic Therapy[1]	-	-	99%	99%
Discharged on Statin Medication[1]	-	-	95%	94%
Thrombolytic Therapy Timing[1]	-	-	68%	66%
Venous Thromboembolism Prophylaxis	14	100%	94%	94%
Written Stroke Educational Materials Given[1]	-	-	92%	88%
Surgical Care Improvement Project				
Appropriate Beta Blocker Usage	24	100%	98%	98%
Appropriate VTP Within 24 Hours	72	100%	98%	98%
Controlled Postoperative Blood Glucose[7]	-	-	96%	97%
Perioperative Temperature Management	78	100%	100%	100%
Prophylactic Antibiotic Selection	45	100%	99%	99%
Prophylactic Antibiotic Selection (Outpatient)	18	100%	98%	98%
Prophylactic Antibiotic Stopped	41	100%	98%	98%
Prophylactic Antibiotic Timing	45	100%	99%	99%
Prophylactic Antibiotic Timing (Outpatient)	18	100%	98%	98%
Urinary Catheter Removal	21	100%	98%	97%
Survey of Patients' Hospital Experiences				
Area Around Room 'Always' Quiet at Night	(a)	63%	68%	61%
Doctors 'Always' Communicated Well	(a)	86%	83%	82%
Home Recovery Information Given	(a)	84%	85%	85%
Hospital Given 9 or 10 on 10 Point Scale	(a)	71%	73%	71%
Meds 'Always' Explained Before Given	(a)	69%	66%	64%
Nurses 'Always' Communicated Well	(a)	80%	80%	79%
Pain 'Always' Well Controlled	(a)	74%	72%	71%
Room and Bathroom 'Always' Clean	(a)	76%	75%	73%
Timely Help 'Always' Received	(a)	76%	69%	68%
Would Definitely Recommend Hospital	(a)	76%	73%	71%
Use of Medical Imaging				
Cardiac Imaging Stress Test before Surgery[1]	-	-	5.3%	5.3%
Combination Abdominal CT Scan	315	16.2%	16.4%	10.5%
Combination Brain/Sinus CT Scan[1]	-	-	2.7%	2.7%
Combination Chest CT Scan	173	11.6%	5.6%	2.7%
Follow-up Mammogram/Ultrasound	557	3.4%	7.9%	8.8%
Lumbar Spine MRI for Low Back Pain	57	42.1%	39.6%	37.2%

Brazosport Regional Health System

100 Medical Drive
Lake Jackson, TX 77566
Phone: 979-297-4411
Fax: 979-299-2861
URL: www.brazosportmemorial.com
Type: Acute Care Hospitals
Emergency Services: Yes
Ownership: Voluntary non-profit - Private
Beds: 165

Key Personnel:
Chief of Medical Staff.......... LP Bui, MD
Radiology................... Amish Dave, MD
CEO/President............... Al Guevara, Jr
Infection Control.............. Kathy Jordan
Pediatric Ambulatory Care ...... LD Lockett, MD
Pediatric In-Patient Care .... LD Lockett, MD
Intensive Care Unit............ Tina Mathews
Emergency Room .... E Tow, DO

Measure	Cases	This Hosp.	State Avg.	U.S. Avg.
Blood Clot Prevention and Treatment				
Anticoagulation Overlap Therapy[2]	13	92%	93%	93%
ICU Venous Thromboembolism Prophylaxis[2]	49	100%	92%	92%
Incidence of Potentially Preventable VTE[1,2]	-	-	9%	10%
UFH with Dosages/Platelet Monitoring[1,2]	-	-	96%	97%
Venous Thromboembolism Prophylaxis[2]	392	96%	82%	85%
Warfarin Therapy Discharge Instructions[1,2]	-	-	84%	75%
Chest Pain/Possible Heart Attack Care				
Aspirin Given Within 24 Hours of Arrival	34	100%	94%	96%
Fibrinolytic Meds Within 30 Min. of Arrival	13	54%	47%	58%
Average Time to ECG (minutes)	34	8	8	7
Average Time to Transfer (minutes)[1]	-	-	62	60
Children's Asthma Care				
Received Home Management Plan of Care	-	-	93%	88%
Received Reliever Medication	-	-	100%	100%
Received Systemic Corticosteroids	-	-	100%	100%
Emergency Department				
Admittance Decision Time (minutes)[2]	523	168	99	98
Head CT Results Within 45 Min. of Arrival	12	58%	54%	57%
Patients Who Left ER Before Being Seen	29,238	10%	3%	2%
Time from ER Arrival to Admit. (minutes)[2]	529	349	270	274
Time from ER Arrival to Discharge (minutes)	361	190	127	134
Time in ER Before Being Evaluated (minutes)	387	65	26	26
Time to Pain Meds for Fractures (minutes)	184	71	57	57
Heart Attack Care				
Aspirin Given at Discharge	46	100%	99%	99%
Fibrinolytic Meds Within 30 Min. of Arrival[1]	-	-	49%	54%
PCI Within 90 Minutes of Arrival[7]	-	-	95%	96%
Statin Prescribed at Discharge	47	100%	98%	98%
Heart Failure Care				
ACE Inhibitor or ARB for LVSD	44	95%	97%	97%
Discharge Instructions Given	141	99%	95%	94%
Evaluation of LVS Function	173	100%	99%	99%
Medicare Spending				
Medicare Spending per Patient (ratio)	-	0.96	1.03	0.98
Pneumonia Care				
Appropriate Initial Antibiotic Given[2]	71	99%	95%	95%
Blood Culture Timing[2]	164	96%	98%	98%
Pregnancy and Delivery Care				
Newborn Deliveries Scheduled Early[2]	27	7%	7%	6%
Preventive Care				
Immunization for Influenza[2]	494	88%	90%	90%
Immunization for Pneumonia[2]	550	93%	92%	92%
Stroke Care				
Anticoagulation Therapy for Atrial Fibrillation[1]	-	-	96%	95%
Antithrombotic Therapy Timing	33	100%	98%	98%
Assessed for Rehabilitation	37	97%	98%	97%
Discharged on Antithrombotic Therapy	32	100%	99%	99%
Discharged on Statin Medication	26	88%	95%	94%
Thrombolytic Therapy Timing[7]	-	-	68%	66%
Venous Thromboembolism Prophylaxis	32	97%	94%	94%
Written Stroke Educational Materials Given	30	97%	92%	88%
Surgical Care Improvement Project				
Appropriate Beta Blocker Usage	42	95%	98%	98%
Appropriate VTP Within 24 Hours	138	96%	98%	98%
Controlled Postoperative Blood Glucose[7]	-	-	96%	97%
Perioperative Temperature Management	155	100%	100%	100%
Prophylactic Antibiotic Selection	94	98%	99%	99%
Prophylactic Antibiotic Selection (Outpatient)	41	95%	98%	98%
Prophylactic Antibiotic Stopped	91	99%	98%	98%
Prophylactic Antibiotic Timing	94	99%	99%	99%
Prophylactic Antibiotic Timing (Outpatient)	44	91%	98%	98%
Urinary Catheter Removal	47	85%	98%	97%
Survey of Patients' Hospital Experiences				
Area Around Room 'Always' Quiet at Night	300+	59%	68%	61%
Doctors 'Always' Communicated Well	300+	80%	83%	82%

NOTE: Hospital profiles are in alphabetical order by state, then city, then hospital within the city; Rankings exclude hospitals with less than 25 cases except for patient surveys which excludes hospitals with less than 100 cases; (a) 100-299 cases; (1) The number of cases/patients is too few to report; (2) Data submitted were based on a sample of cases/patients; (3) Results are based on a shorter time period than required; (4) Data suppressed by CMS for one or more quarters; (5) Results are not available for this reporting period; (6) Fewer than 100 patients completed the HCAHPS survey; (7) No cases met the criteria for this measure; (8) The lower limit of the confidence interval cannot be calculated if the number of observed infections equals zero; (9) No data are available from the state/territory for this reporting period; (10) The scores shown reflect fewer than 50 completed surveys; (11) There were discrepancies in the data collection process; (12) This measure does not apply to this hospital for this reporting period; (13) Results cannot be calculated for this reporting period; (14) The results for this state are combined with nearby states to protect confidentiality; Please refer to the User's Guide for a full explanation of data.

Home Recovery Information Given	300+	83%	85%	85%
Hospital Given 9 or 10 on 10 Point Scale	300+	58%	73%	71%
Meds 'Always' Explained Before Given	300+	63%	66%	64%
Nurses 'Always' Communicated Well	300+	76%	80%	79%
Pain 'Always' Well Controlled	300+	65%	72%	71%
Room and Bathroom 'Always' Clean	300+	71%	75%	73%
Timely Help 'Always' Received	300+	61%	69%	68%
Would Definitely Recommend Hospital	300+	56%	73%	71%
Use of Medical Imaging				
Cardiac Imaging Stress Test before Surgery[1]	-	-	5.3%	5.3%
Combination Abdominal CT Scan	771	4.4%	16.4%	10.5%
Combination Brain/Sinus CT Scan	731	1.8%	2.7%	2.7%
Combination Chest CT Scan	494	3.4%	5.6%	2.7%
Follow-up Mammogram/Ultrasound	853	9.1%	7.9%	8.8%
Lumbar Spine MRI for Low Back Pain	117	44.4%	39.6%	37.2%

Lakeway Regional Medical Center

100 Medical Parkway Phone: 512-205-8102
Lakeway, TX 78734
Type: Acute Care Hospitals Emergency Services: Yes
Ownership: Proprietary

Measure	Cases	This Hosp.	State Avg.	U.S. Avg.
Blood Clot Prevention and Treatment				
Anticoagulation Overlap Therapy[2]	17	100%	93%	93%
ICU Venous Thromboembolism Prophylaxis[2]	49	84%	92%	92%
Incidence of Potentially Preventable VTE[1,2]	-	-	9%	10%
UFH with Dosages/Platelet Monitoring[1,2]	-	-	96%	97%
Venous Thromboembolism Prophylaxis[2]	87	92%	82%	85%
Warfarin Therapy Discharge Instructions[2]	16	100%	84%	75%
Chest Pain/Possible Heart Attack Care				
Aspirin Given Within 24 Hours of Arrival[5]	-	-	94%	96%
Fibrinolytic Meds Within 30 Min. of Arrival[5]	-	-	47%	58%
Average Time to ECG (minutes)[5]	-	-	8	7
Average Time to Transfer (minutes)[5]	-	-	62	60
Children's Asthma Care				
Received Home Management Plan of Care	-	-	93%	88%
Received Reliever Medication	-	-	100%	100%
Received Systemic Corticosteroids	-	-	100%	100%
Emergency Department				
Admittance Decision Time (minutes)[2,3]	245	81	99	98
Head CT Results Within 45 Min. of Arrival[3,7]	-	-	54%	57%
Patients Who Left ER Before Being Seen	5,068	0%	3%	2%
Time from ER Arrival to Admit. (minutes)[2,3]	247	225	270	274
Time from ER Arrival to Discharge (minutes)[3]	247	93	127	134
Time in ER Before Being Evaluated (minutes)[3]	270	9	26	26
Time to Pain Meds for Fractures (minutes)[3]	17	23	57	57
Heart Attack Care				
Aspirin Given at Discharge[3]	34	100%	99%	99%
Fibrinolytic Meds Within 30 Min. of Arrival[3,7]	-	-	49%	54%
PCI Within 90 Minutes of Arrival[1,3]	-	-	95%	96%
Statin Prescribed at Discharge[3]	34	88%	98%	98%
Heart Failure Care				
ACE Inhibitor or ARB for LVSD[3]	12	100%	97%	97%
Discharge Instructions Given[3]	25	56%	95%	94%
Evaluation of LVS Function[3]	29	100%	99%	99%
Medicare Spending				
Medicare Spending per Patient (ratio)	-	1.07	1.03	0.98
Pneumonia Care				
Appropriate Initial Antibiotic Given[3]	14	93%	95%	95%
Blood Culture Timing[3]	23	96%	98%	98%
Pregnancy and Delivery Care				
Newborn Deliveries Scheduled Early[2]	20	5%	7%	6%
Preventive Care				
Immunization for Influenza[2,3]	132	29%	90%	90%
Immunization for Pneumonia[2,3]	226	50%	92%	92%
Stroke Care				
Anticoagulation Therapy for Atrial Fibrillation[1]	-	-	96%	95%
Antithrombotic Therapy Timing	16	100%	98%	98%
Assessed for Rehabilitation	22	95%	98%	97%
Discharged on Antithrombotic Therapy	22	100%	99%	99%
Discharged on Statin Medication	18	100%	95%	94%
Thrombolytic Therapy Timing[1]	-	-	68%	66%
Venous Thromboembolism Prophylaxis	18	94%	94%	94%
Written Stroke Educational Materials Given	12	92%	92%	88%
Surgical Care Improvement Project				
Appropriate Beta Blocker Usage[1,3]	-	-	98%	98%
Appropriate VTP Within 24 Hours[3]	28	96%	98%	98%
Controlled Postoperative Blood Glucose[1,3]	-	-	96%	97%
Perioperative Temperature Management[3]	36	100%	100%	100%
Prophylactic Antibiotic Selection[3]	25	100%	99%	99%
Prophylactic Antibiotic Selection (Outpatient)[3]	18	100%	98%	98%
Prophylactic Antibiotic Stopped[3]	25	100%	98%	98%
Prophylactic Antibiotic Timing[3]	25	100%	99%	99%
Prophylactic Antibiotic Timing (Outpatient)[3]	18	100%	98%	98%
Urinary Catheter Removal[3]	32	91%	98%	97%
Survey of Patients' Hospital Experiences				
Area Around Room 'Always' Quiet at Night[5]	-	-	68%	61%
Doctors 'Always' Communicated Well[5]	-	-	83%	82%
Home Recovery Information Given[5]	-	-	85%	85%
Hospital Given 9 or 10 on 10 Point Scale[5]	-	-	73%	71%
Meds 'Always' Explained Before Given[5]	-	-	66%	64%
Nurses 'Always' Communicated Well[5]	-	-	80%	79%
Pain 'Always' Well Controlled[5]	-	-	72%	71%
Room and Bathroom 'Always' Clean[5]	-	-	75%	73%
Timely Help 'Always' Received[5]	-	-	69%	68%
Would Definitely Recommend Hospital[5]	-	-	73%	71%
Use of Medical Imaging				
Cardiac Imaging Stress Test before Surgery	199	5.0%	5.3%	5.3%
Combination Abdominal CT Scan	176	6.8%	16.4%	10.5%
Combination Brain/Sinus CT Scan[1]	-	-	2.7%	2.7%
Combination Chest CT Scan	89	6.7%	5.6%	2.7%
Follow-up Mammogram/Ultrasound	67	11.9%	7.9%	8.8%
Lumbar Spine MRI for Low Back Pain[1]	-	-	39.6%	37.2%

Medical Arts Hospital

2200 N Bryan Ave Phone: 806-872-2183
Lamesa, TX 79331 Fax: 806-872-0823
URL: www.medicalartshospital.org
Type: Acute Care Hospitals Emergency Services: Yes
Ownership: Govt - Hospital Dist/Auth Beds: 44

Key Personnel:
Radiology. . . . . Albert Acosta
Emergency Room . . . . Jeana Amos
Quality Assurance . . . . Mary Bond
CEO/President. . . . . Charles Butts
Chief of Medical Staff. . . . . Somchai Chong
Infection Control. . . . . Rebekah Parker
Operating Room. . . . . Rebekah Parker
Anesthesiology. . . . . William Warner, CRNA

Measure	Cases	This Hosp.	State Avg.	U.S. Avg.
Blood Clot Prevention and Treatment				
Anticoagulation Overlap Therapy[2,7]	-	-	93%	93%
ICU Venous Thromboembolism Prophylaxis[2,7]	-	-	92%	92%
Incidence of Potentially Preventable VTE[2,7]	-	-	9%	10%
UFH with Dosages/Platelet Monitoring[2,7]	-	-	96%	97%
Venous Thromboembolism Prophylaxis[2]	142	82%	82%	85%
Warfarin Therapy Discharge Instructions[2,7]	-	-	84%	75%
Chest Pain/Possible Heart Attack Care				
Aspirin Given Within 24 Hours of Arrival	38	92%	94%	96%
Fibrinolytic Meds Within 30 Min. of Arrival[1]	-	-	47%	58%
Average Time to ECG (minutes)	39	10	8	7
Average Time to Transfer (minutes)[7]	-	-	62	60
Children's Asthma Care				
Received Home Management Plan of Care	-	-	93%	88%
Received Reliever Medication	-	-	100%	100%
Received Systemic Corticosteroids	-	-	100%	100%
Emergency Department				
Admittance Decision Time (minutes)[2]	249	27	99	98
Head CT Results Within 45 Min. of Arrival[1,3]	-	-	54%	57%
Patients Who Left ER Before Being Seen	6,798	3%	3%	2%
Time from ER Arrival to Admit. (minutes)[2]	249	186	270	274
Time from ER Arrival to Discharge (minutes)	339	104	127	134
Time in ER Before Being Evaluated (minutes)	384	39	26	26
Time to Pain Meds for Fractures (minutes)	21	47	57	57
Heart Attack Care				
Aspirin Given at Discharge[5]	-	-	99%	99%
Fibrinolytic Meds Within 30 Min. of Arrival[5]	-	-	49%	54%
PCI Within 90 Minutes of Arrival[5]	-	-	95%	96%
Statin Prescribed at Discharge[5]	-	-	98%	98%
Heart Failure Care				
ACE Inhibitor or ARB for LVSD[5]	-	-	97%	97%
Discharge Instructions Given[5]	-	-	95%	94%
Evaluation of LVS Function[5]	-	-	99%	99%
Medicare Spending				
Medicare Spending per Patient (ratio)	-	0.94	1.03	0.98
Pneumonia Care				
Appropriate Initial Antibiotic Given[1,3]	-	-	95%	95%
Blood Culture Timing[3]	12	83%	98%	98%
Pregnancy and Delivery Care				
Newborn Deliveries Scheduled Early	18	56%	7%	6%
Preventive Care				
Immunization for Influenza	215	46%	90%	90%
Immunization for Pneumonia	134	75%	92%	92%
Stroke Care				
Anticoagulation Therapy for Atrial Fibrillation[5]	-	-	96%	95%
Antithrombotic Therapy Timing[5]	-	-	98%	98%
Assessed for Rehabilitation[5]	-	-	98%	97%
Discharged on Antithrombotic Therapy[5]	-	-	99%	99%
Discharged on Statin Medication[5]	-	-	95%	94%
Thrombolytic Therapy Timing[5]	-	-	68%	66%
Venous Thromboembolism Prophylaxis[5]	-	-	94%	94%
Written Stroke Educational Materials Given[5]	-	-	92%	88%
Surgical Care Improvement Project				
Appropriate Beta Blocker Usage[5]	-	-	98%	98%
Appropriate VTP Within 24 Hours[5]	-	-	98%	98%
Controlled Postoperative Blood Glucose[5]	-	-	96%	97%
Perioperative Temperature Management[5]	-	-	100%	100%
Prophylactic Antibiotic Selection[5]	-	-	99%	99%
Prophylactic Antibiotic Selection (Outpatient)[1,3]	-	-	98%	98%
Prophylactic Antibiotic Stopped[5]	-	-	98%	98%
Prophylactic Antibiotic Timing[5]	-	-	99%	99%
Prophylactic Antibiotic Timing (Outpatient)[1,3]	-	-	98%	98%
Urinary Catheter Removal[5]	-	-	98%	97%
Survey of Patients' Hospital Experiences				
Area Around Room 'Always' Quiet at Night[6]	<100	59%	68%	61%
Doctors 'Always' Communicated Well[6]	<100	83%	83%	82%
Home Recovery Information Given[6]	<100	84%	85%	85%
Hospital Given 9 or 10 on 10 Point Scale[6]	<100	75%	73%	71%
Meds 'Always' Explained Before Given[6]	<100	59%	66%	64%
Nurses 'Always' Communicated Well[6]	<100	82%	80%	79%
Pain 'Always' Well Controlled[6]	<100	71%	72%	71%
Room and Bathroom 'Always' Clean[6]	<100	79%	75%	73%
Timely Help 'Always' Received[6]	<100	71%	69%	68%
Would Definitely Recommend Hospital[6]	<100	69%	73%	71%
Use of Medical Imaging				
Cardiac Imaging Stress Test before Surgery	45	2.2%	5.3%	5.3%
Combination Abdominal CT Scan	134	11.9%	16.4%	10.5%
Combination Brain/Sinus CT Scan	115	0.0%	2.7%	2.7%
Combination Chest CT Scan	66	4.5%	5.6%	2.7%
Follow-up Mammogram/Ultrasound[7]	-	-	7.9%	8.8%
Lumbar Spine MRI for Low Back Pain[1]	-	-	39.6%	37.2%

Rollins Brook Community Hospital

608 North Key Avenue Phone: 512-556-3682
Lampasas, TX 76550 Fax: 512-556-8869
URL: www.mplex.org
Type: Critical Access Hospitals Emergency Services: Yes
Ownership: Voluntary non-profit - Church Beds: 25

Key Personnel:
CEO/President. . . . . Ernie Bovio
Radiology. . . . . Alan Cheung
Chief of Medical Staff . . . . Phillip Day, MD
Quality Assurance . . . . Kim Henry-Shahry

Measure	Cases	This Hosp.	State Avg.	U.S. Avg.
Blood Clot Prevention and Treatment				
Anticoagulation Overlap Therapy[1,2]	-	-	93%	93%
ICU Venous Thromboembolism Prophylaxis[2,7]	-	-	92%	92%
Incidence of Potentially Preventable VTE[2,7]	-	-	9%	10%
UFH with Dosages/Platelet Monitoring[1,2]	-	-	96%	97%

NOTE: Hospital profiles are in alphabetical order by state, then city, then hospital within the city; Rankings exclude hospitals with less than 25 cases except for patient surveys which excludes hospitals with less than 100 cases; (a) 100-299 cases; (1) The number of cases/patients is too few to report; (2) Data submitted were based on a sample of cases/patients; (3) Results are based on a shorter time period than required; (4) Data suppressed by CMS for one or more quarters; (5) Results are not available for this reporting period; (6) Fewer than 100 patients completed the HCAHPS survey; (7) No cases met the criteria for this measure; (8) The lower limit of the confidence interval cannot be calculated if the number of observed infections equals zero; (9) No data are available from the state/territory for this reporting period; (10) The scores shown reflect fewer than 50 completed surveys; (11) There were discrepancies in the data collection process; (12) This measure does not apply to this hospital for this reporting period; (13) Results cannot be calculated for this reporting period; (14) The results for this state are combined with nearby states to protect confidentiality; Please refer to the User's Guide for a full explanation of data.

Venous Thromboembolism Prophylaxis[2]	87	87%	82%	85%
Warfarin Therapy Discharge Instructions[1,2]	-	-	84%	75%
Chest Pain/Possible Heart Attack Care				
Aspirin Given Within 24 Hours of Arrival	41	93%	94%	96%
Fibrinolytic Meds Within 30 Min. of Arrival[7]	-	-	47%	58%
Average Time to ECG (minutes)	46	10	8	7
Average Time to Transfer (minutes)	18	76	62	60
Children's Asthma Care				
Received Home Management Plan of Care	-	-	93%	88%
Received Reliever Medication	-	-	100%	100%
Received Systemic Corticosteroids	-	-	100%	100%
Emergency Department				
Admittance Decision Time (minutes)[2]	234	59	99	98
Head CT Results Within 45 Min. of Arrival[1]	-	-	54%	57%
Patients Who Left ER Before Being Seen[5]	-	-	3%	2%
Time from ER Arrival to Admit. (minutes)[2]	319	209	270	274
Time from ER Arrival to Discharge (minutes)	341	107	127	134
Time in ER Before Being Evaluated (minutes)	299	18	26	26
Time to Pain Meds for Fractures (minutes)	63	50	57	57
Heart Attack Care				
Aspirin Given at Discharge[2,3]	-	-	99%	99%
Fibrinolytic Meds Within 30 Min. of Arrival[2,3]	-	-	49%	54%
PCI Within 90 Minutes of Arrival[2,3]	-	-	95%	96%
Statin Prescribed at Discharge[2,3]	-	-	98%	98%
Heart Failure Care				
ACE Inhibitor or ARB for LVSD[1,2]	-	-	97%	97%
Discharge Instructions Given[2]	18	94%	95%	94%
Evaluation of LVS Function[2]	25	96%	99%	99%
Medicare Spending				
Medicare Spending per Patient (ratio)	-	-	1.03	0.98
Pneumonia Care				
Appropriate Initial Antibiotic Given[2]	22	82%	95%	95%
Blood Culture Timing[1,2]	-	-	98%	98%
Pregnancy and Delivery Care				
Newborn Deliveries Scheduled Early[5]	-	-	7%	6%
Preventive Care				
Immunization for Influenza[2]	281	94%	90%	90%
Immunization for Pneumonia[2]	461	95%	92%	92%
Stroke Care				
Anticoagulation Therapy for Atrial Fibrillation[5]	-	-	96%	95%
Antithrombotic Therapy Timing[5]	-	-	98%	98%
Assessed for Rehabilitation[5]	-	-	98%	97%
Discharged on Antithrombotic Therapy[5]	-	-	99%	99%
Discharged on Statin Medication[5]	-	-	95%	94%
Thrombolytic Therapy Timing[5]	-	-	68%	66%
Venous Thromboembolism Prophylaxis[5]	-	-	94%	94%
Written Stroke Educational Materials Given[5]	-	-	92%	88%
Surgical Care Improvement Project				
Appropriate Beta Blocker Usage[1,2]	-	-	98%	98%
Appropriate VTP Within 24 Hours[1,2]	-	-	98%	98%
Controlled Postoperative Blood Glucose[2,7]	-	-	96%	97%
Perioperative Temperature Management[1,2]	-	-	100%	100%
Prophylactic Antibiotic Selection[2,7]	-	-	99%	99%
Prophylactic Antibiotic Selection (Outpatient)[5]	-	-	98%	98%
Prophylactic Antibiotic Stopped[2,7]	-	-	98%	98%
Prophylactic Antibiotic Timing[2,7]	-	-	99%	99%
Prophylactic Antibiotic Timing (Outpatient)[5]	-	-	98%	98%
Urinary Catheter Removal[1,2]	-	-	98%	97%
Survey of Patients' Hospital Experiences				
Area Around Room 'Always' Quiet at Night[11]	(a)	70%	68%	61%
Doctors 'Always' Communicated Well[11]	(a)	92%	83%	82%
Home Recovery Information Given[11]	(a)	91%	85%	85%
Hospital Given 9 or 10 on 10 Point Scale[11]	(a)	87%	73%	71%
Meds 'Always' Explained Before Given[11]	(a)	80%	66%	64%
Nurses 'Always' Communicated Well[11]	(a)	89%	80%	79%
Pain 'Always' Well Controlled[11]	(a)	83%	72%	71%
Room and Bathroom 'Always' Clean[11]	(a)	81%	75%	73%
Timely Help 'Always' Received[11]	(a)	78%	69%	68%
Would Definitely Recommend Hospital[11]	(a)	80%	73%	71%
Use of Medical Imaging				
Cardiac Imaging Stress Test before Surgery[7]	-	-	5.3%	5.3%
Combination Abdominal CT Scan	175	9.1%	16.4%	10.5%
Combination Brain/Sinus CT Scan[1]	-	-	2.7%	2.7%
Combination Chest CT Scan	108	11.1%	5.6%	2.7%
Follow-up Mammogram/Ultrasound	349	2.3%	7.9%	8.8%
Lumbar Spine MRI for Low Back Pain[1]	-	-	39.6%	37.2%

Doctors Hospital of Laredo

10700 Mcpherson Road
Laredo, TX 78041
Phone: 956-523-2000
Fax: 956-523-0444
URL: www.doctorshosplaredo.com
Type: Acute Care Hospitals
Emergency Services: Yes
Ownership: Proprietary
Beds: 180

Key Personnel:
CEO/President. . . . . Elmo Lopez

Measure	Cases	This Hosp.	State Avg.	U.S. Avg.
Blood Clot Prevention and Treatment				
Anticoagulation Overlap Therapy[2]	21	57%	93%	93%
ICU Venous Thromboembolism Prophylaxis[2]	102	88%	92%	92%
Incidence of Potentially Preventable VTE[1,2]	-	-	9%	10%
UFH with Dosages/Platelet Monitoring[1,2]	-	-	96%	97%
Venous Thromboembolism Prophylaxis[2]	400	73%	82%	85%
Warfarin Therapy Discharge Instructions[2]	18	50%	84%	75%
Chest Pain/Possible Heart Attack Care				
Aspirin Given Within 24 Hours of Arrival[1,3]	-	-	94%	96%
Fibrinolytic Meds Within 30 Min. of Arrival[3,7]	-	-	47%	58%
Average Time to ECG (minutes)[1,3]	-	-	8	7
Average Time to Transfer (minutes)[3,7]	-	-	62	60
Children's Asthma Care				
Received Home Management Plan of Care	-	-	93%	88%
Received Reliever Medication	-	-	100%	100%
Received Systemic Corticosteroids	-	-	100%	100%
Emergency Department				
Admittance Decision Time (minutes)[2]	361	138	99	98
Head CT Results Within 45 Min. of Arrival[1]	-	-	54%	57%
Patients Who Left ER Before Being Seen	29,386	2%	3%	2%
Time from ER Arrival to Admit. (minutes)[2]	370	400	270	274
Time from ER Arrival to Discharge (minutes)	363	142	127	134
Time in ER Before Being Evaluated (minutes)	397	4	26	26
Time to Pain Meds for Fractures (minutes)	158	20	57	57
Heart Attack Care				
Aspirin Given at Discharge	44	93%	99%	99%
Fibrinolytic Meds Within 30 Min. of Arrival[1]	-	-	49%	54%
PCI Within 90 Minutes of Arrival[1]	-	-	95%	96%
Statin Prescribed at Discharge	45	100%	98%	98%
Heart Failure Care				
ACE Inhibitor or ARB for LVSD	78	92%	97%	97%
Discharge Instructions Given	178	77%	95%	94%
Evaluation of LVS Function	194	99%	99%	99%
Medicare Spending				
Medicare Spending per Patient (ratio)	-	1.00	1.03	0.98
Pneumonia Care				
Appropriate Initial Antibiotic Given[2]	69	97%	95%	95%
Blood Culture Timing[2]	71	100%	98%	98%
Pregnancy and Delivery Care				
Newborn Deliveries Scheduled Early[2]	63	3%	7%	6%
Preventive Care				
Immunization for Influenza[2]	431	88%	90%	90%
Immunization for Pneumonia[2]	328	84%	92%	92%
Stroke Care				
Anticoagulation Therapy for Atrial Fibrillation[1]	-	-	96%	95%
Antithrombotic Therapy Timing	48	85%	98%	98%
Assessed for Rehabilitation	47	91%	98%	97%
Discharged on Antithrombotic Therapy	47	91%	99%	99%
Discharged on Statin Medication	37	86%	95%	94%
Thrombolytic Therapy Timing[1]	-	-	68%	66%
Venous Thromboembolism Prophylaxis	54	89%	94%	94%
Written Stroke Educational Materials Given	25	56%	92%	88%
Surgical Care Improvement Project				
Appropriate Beta Blocker Usage[2]	31	94%	98%	98%
Appropriate VTP Within 24 Hours[2]	182	93%	98%	98%
Controlled Postoperative Blood Glucose[2,7]	-	-	96%	97%
Perioperative Temperature Management[2]	219	100%	100%	100%
Prophylactic Antibiotic Selection[2]	116	99%	99%	99%
Prophylactic Antibiotic Selection (Outpatient)	119	93%	98%	98%
Prophylactic Antibiotic Stopped[2]	108	95%	98%	98%
Prophylactic Antibiotic Timing[2]	116	99%	99%	99%
Prophylactic Antibiotic Timing (Outpatient)	129	91%	98%	98%
Urinary Catheter Removal[2]	85	94%	98%	97%
Survey of Patients' Hospital Experiences				
Area Around Room 'Always' Quiet at Night	300+	67%	68%	61%
Doctors 'Always' Communicated Well	300+	82%	83%	82%
Home Recovery Information Given	300+	86%	85%	85%
Hospital Given 9 or 10 on 10 Point Scale	300+	72%	73%	71%
Meds 'Always' Explained Before Given	300+	64%	66%	64%
Nurses 'Always' Communicated Well	300+	77%	80%	79%
Pain 'Always' Well Controlled	300+	72%	72%	71%
Room and Bathroom 'Always' Clean	300+	79%	75%	73%
Timely Help 'Always' Received	300+	65%	69%	68%
Would Definitely Recommend Hospital	300+	73%	73%	71%
Use of Medical Imaging				
Cardiac Imaging Stress Test before Surgery[1]	-	-	5.3%	5.3%
Combination Abdominal CT Scan	359	15.6%	16.4%	10.5%
Combination Brain/Sinus CT Scan[1]	-	-	2.7%	2.7%
Combination Chest CT Scan	184	15.8%	5.6%	2.7%
Follow-up Mammogram/Ultrasound	443	10.4%	7.9%	8.8%
Lumbar Spine MRI for Low Back Pain	70	34.3%	39.6%	37.2%

Laredo Medical Center

1700 East Saunders
Laredo, TX 78044
Phone: 956-796-5000
URL: www.laredomedical.com
Type: Acute Care Hospitals
Emergency Services: Yes
Ownership: Voluntary non-profit - Church
Beds: 326

Key Personnel:
CEO . . . . Tim Brandt

Measure	Cases	This Hosp.	State Avg.	U.S. Avg.
Blood Clot Prevention and Treatment				
Anticoagulation Overlap Therapy[2]	34	71%	93%	93%
ICU Venous Thromboembolism Prophylaxis[2]	62	98%	92%	92%
Incidence of Potentially Preventable VTE[1,2]	-	-	9%	10%
UFH with Dosages/Platelet Monitoring[1,2]	-	-	96%	97%
Venous Thromboembolism Prophylaxis[2]	451	95%	82%	85%
Warfarin Therapy Discharge Instructions[2]	26	100%	84%	75%
Chest Pain/Possible Heart Attack Care				
Aspirin Given Within 24 Hours of Arrival[3,7]	-	-	94%	96%
Fibrinolytic Meds Within 30 Min. of Arrival[5]	-	-	47%	58%
Average Time to ECG (minutes)[3,7]	-	-	8	7
Average Time to Transfer (minutes)[5]	-	-	62	60
Children's Asthma Care				
Received Home Management Plan of Care	-	-	93%	88%
Received Reliever Medication	-	-	100%	100%
Received Systemic Corticosteroids	-	-	100%	100%
Emergency Department				
Admittance Decision Time (minutes)[2]	584	240	99	98
Head CT Results Within 45 Min. of Arrival	18	56%	54%	57%
Patients Who Left ER Before Being Seen	58,248	7%	3%	2%
Time from ER Arrival to Admit. (minutes)[2]	593	439	270	274
Time from ER Arrival to Discharge (minutes)	355	207	127	134
Time in ER Before Being Evaluated (minutes)	396	11	26	26
Time to Pain Meds for Fractures (minutes)	327	97	57	57
Heart Attack Care				
Aspirin Given at Discharge	149	100%	99%	99%
Fibrinolytic Meds Within 30 Min. of Arrival	11	91%	49%	54%
PCI Within 90 Minutes of Arrival	25	100%	95%	96%
Statin Prescribed at Discharge	145	100%	98%	98%
Heart Failure Care				
ACE Inhibitor or ARB for LVSD	117	100%	97%	97%
Discharge Instructions Given	348	100%	95%	94%
Evaluation of LVS Function	384	100%	99%	99%
Medicare Spending				
Medicare Spending per Patient (ratio)	-	0.99	1.03	0.98
Pneumonia Care				
Appropriate Initial Antibiotic Given	152	100%	95%	95%
Blood Culture Timing	341	100%	98%	98%
Pregnancy and Delivery Care				
Newborn Deliveries Scheduled Early[2]	167	0%	7%	6%
Preventive Care				

NOTE: Hospital profiles are in alphabetical order by state, then city, then hospital within the city; Rankings exclude hospitals with less than 25 cases except for patient surveys which excludes hospitals with less than 100 cases; (a) 100-299 cases; (1) The number of cases/patients is too few to report; (2) Data submitted were based on a sample of cases/patients; (3) Results are based on a shorter time period than required; (4) Data suppressed by CMS for one or more quarters; (5) Results are not available for this reporting period; (6) Fewer than 100 patients completed the HCAHPS survey; (7) No cases met the criteria for this measure; (8) The lower limit of the confidence interval cannot be calculated if the number of observed infections equals zero; (9) No data are available from the state/territory for this reporting period; (10) The scores shown reflect fewer than 50 completed surveys; (11) There were discrepancies in the data collection process; (12) This measure does not apply to this hospital for this reporting period; (13) Results cannot be calculated for this reporting period; (14) The results for this state are combined with nearby states to protect confidentiality; Please refer to the User's Guide for a full explanation of data.

Measure	Cases	This Hosp.	State Avg.	U.S. Avg.
Immunization for Influenza[2]	547	100%	90%	90%
Immunization for Pneumonia[2]	557	100%	92%	92%
Stroke Care				
Anticoagulation Therapy for Atrial Fibrillation	14	64%	96%	95%
Antithrombotic Therapy Timing	198	85%	98%	98%
Assessed for Rehabilitation	209	91%	98%	97%
Discharged on Antithrombotic Therapy	190	94%	99%	99%
Discharged on Statin Medication	138	83%	95%	94%
Thrombolytic Therapy Timing	20	35%	68%	66%
Venous Thromboembolism Prophylaxis	217	95%	94%	94%
Written Stroke Educational Materials Given	132	95%	92%	88%
Surgical Care Improvement Project				
Appropriate Beta Blocker Usage	122	98%	98%	98%
Appropriate VTP Within 24 Hours	502	100%	98%	98%
Controlled Postoperative Blood Glucose	78	97%	96%	97%
Perioperative Temperature Management	579	100%	100%	100%
Prophylactic Antibiotic Selection	397	100%	99%	99%
Prophylactic Antibiotic Selection (Outpatient)	262	99%	98%	98%
Prophylactic Antibiotic Stopped	364	99%	98%	98%
Prophylactic Antibiotic Timing	397	100%	99%	99%
Prophylactic Antibiotic Timing (Outpatient)	262	100%	98%	98%
Urinary Catheter Removal	404	100%	98%	97%
Survey of Patients' Hospital Experiences				
Area Around Room 'Always' Quiet at Night	300+	60%	68%	61%
Doctors 'Always' Communicated Well	300+	79%	83%	82%
Home Recovery Information Given	300+	81%	85%	85%
Hospital Given 9 or 10 on 10 Point Scale	300+	69%	73%	71%
Meds 'Always' Explained Before Given	300+	60%	66%	64%
Nurses 'Always' Communicated Well	300+	73%	80%	79%
Pain 'Always' Well Controlled	300+	67%	72%	71%
Room and Bathroom 'Always' Clean	300+	70%	75%	73%
Timely Help 'Always' Received	300+	55%	69%	68%
Would Definitely Recommend Hospital	300+	66%	73%	71%
Use of Medical Imaging				
Cardiac Imaging Stress Test before Surgery[1]	-	-	5.3%	5.3%
Combination Abdominal CT Scan	1,065	8.5%	16.4%	10.5%
Combination Brain/Sinus CT Scan	1,171	4.4%	2.7%	2.7%
Combination Chest CT Scan	445	5.6%	5.6%	2.7%
Follow-up Mammogram/Ultrasound	1,246	7.2%	7.9%	8.8%
Lumbar Spine MRI for Low Back Pain	101	42.6%	39.6%	37.2%

Covenant Hospital Levelland

1900 College Ave
Levelland, TX 79336
Phone: 806-894-4963
Fax: 806-894-6461
URL: www.covenanthealth.org
Type: Acute Care Hospitals
Emergency Services: Yes
Ownership: Voluntary non-profit - Church
Beds: 48

Key Personnel:
Chief of Medical Staff.......... Micheal Bailey
Emergency Room .... Charles Barton
CEO/President................ Steven L Hunter
Infection Control.............. Karen Seely
Operating Room.............. Tommie Vidalez, RN
Pediatric In-Patient Care .... Suvipa Wiri, MD

Measure	Cases	This Hosp.	State Avg.	U.S. Avg.
Blood Clot Prevention and Treatment				
Anticoagulation Overlap Therapy[1]	-	-	93%	93%
ICU Venous Thromboembolism Prophylaxis[7]	-	-	92%	92%
Incidence of Potentially Preventable VTE[7]	-	-	9%	10%
UFH with Dosages/Platelet Monitoring[1]	-	-	96%	97%
Venous Thromboembolism Prophylaxis	296	48%	82%	85%
Warfarin Therapy Discharge Instructions[1]	-	-	84%	75%
Chest Pain/Possible Heart Attack Care				
Aspirin Given Within 24 Hours of Arrival	15	93%	94%	96%
Fibrinolytic Meds Within 30 Min. of Arrival[1]	-	-	47%	58%
Average Time to ECG (minutes)	16	15	8	7
Average Time to Transfer (minutes)[1]	-	-	62	60
Children's Asthma Care				
Received Home Management Plan of Care	-	-	93%	88%
Received Reliever Medication	-	-	100%	100%
Received Systemic Corticosteroids	-	-	100%	100%
Emergency Department				
Admittance Decision Time (minutes)[2]	163	68	99	98
Head CT Results Within 45 Min. of Arrival[3,7]	-	-	54%	57%
Patients Who Left ER Before Being Seen	6,780	5%	3%	2%
Time from ER Arrival to Admit. (minutes)[2]	169	228	270	274
Time from ER Arrival to Discharge (minutes)	371	124	127	134
Time in ER Before Being Evaluated (minutes)	391	31	26	26
Time to Pain Meds for Fractures (minutes)	34	62	57	57
Heart Attack Care				
Aspirin Given at Discharge[5]	-	-	99%	99%
Fibrinolytic Meds Within 30 Min. of Arrival[5]	-	-	49%	54%
PCI Within 90 Minutes of Arrival[5]	-	-	95%	96%
Statin Prescribed at Discharge[5]	-	-	98%	98%
Heart Failure Care				
ACE Inhibitor or ARB for LVSD	12	83%	97%	97%
Discharge Instructions Given	22	100%	95%	94%
Evaluation of LVS Function	26	85%	99%	99%
Medicare Spending				
Medicare Spending per Patient (ratio)	-	0.93	1.03	0.98
Pneumonia Care				
Appropriate Initial Antibiotic Given	29	62%	95%	95%
Blood Culture Timing	19	100%	98%	98%
Pregnancy and Delivery Care				
Newborn Deliveries Scheduled Early[2]	39	5%	7%	6%
Preventive Care				
Immunization for Influenza[2]	225	55%	90%	90%
Immunization for Pneumonia[2]	204	88%	92%	92%
Stroke Care				
Anticoagulation Therapy for Atrial Fibrillation[1,3]	-	-	96%	95%
Antithrombotic Therapy Timing[1,3]	-	-	98%	98%
Assessed for Rehabilitation[1,3]	-	-	98%	97%
Discharged on Antithrombotic Therapy[1,3]	-	-	99%	99%
Discharged on Statin Medication[1,3]	-	-	95%	94%
Thrombolytic Therapy Timing[3,7]	-	-	68%	66%
Venous Thromboembolism Prophylaxis[1,3]	-	-	94%	94%
Written Stroke Educational Materials Given[1,3]	-	-	92%	88%
Surgical Care Improvement Project				
Appropriate Beta Blocker Usage[1]	-	-	98%	98%
Appropriate VTP Within 24 Hours	21	10%	98%	98%
Controlled Postoperative Blood Glucose[7]	-	-	96%	97%
Perioperative Temperature Management	27	96%	100%	100%
Prophylactic Antibiotic Selection	20	85%	99%	99%
Prophylactic Antibiotic Selection (Outpatient)[5]	-	-	98%	98%
Prophylactic Antibiotic Stopped	20	100%	98%	98%
Prophylactic Antibiotic Timing	20	100%	99%	99%
Prophylactic Antibiotic Timing (Outpatient)[5]	-	-	98%	98%
Urinary Catheter Removal[1]	-	-	98%	97%
Survey of Patients' Hospital Experiences				
Area Around Room 'Always' Quiet at Night	(a)	66%	68%	61%
Doctors 'Always' Communicated Well	(a)	89%	83%	82%
Home Recovery Information Given	(a)	86%	85%	85%
Hospital Given 9 or 10 on 10 Point Scale	(a)	75%	73%	71%
Meds 'Always' Explained Before Given	(a)	64%	66%	64%
Nurses 'Always' Communicated Well	(a)	82%	80%	79%
Pain 'Always' Well Controlled	(a)	75%	72%	71%
Room and Bathroom 'Always' Clean	(a)	74%	75%	73%
Timely Help 'Always' Received	(a)	73%	69%	68%
Would Definitely Recommend Hospital	(a)	74%	73%	71%
Use of Medical Imaging				
Cardiac Imaging Stress Test before Surgery[7]	-	-	5.3%	5.3%
Combination Abdominal CT Scan	51	33.3%	16.4%	10.5%
Combination Brain/Sinus CT Scan[1]	-	-	2.7%	2.7%
Combination Chest CT Scan[1]	-	-	5.6%	2.7%
Follow-up Mammogram/Ultrasound	209	12.0%	7.9%	8.8%
Lumbar Spine MRI for Low Back Pain[1]	-	-	39.6%	37.2%

Medical Center of Lewisville

500 West Main Street
Lewisville, TX 75057
Phone: 972-420-1000
Fax: 972-420-1805
URL: www.lewisvillemedical.com
Type: Acute Care Hospitals
Emergency Services: Yes
Ownership: Voluntary non-profit - Private
Beds: 202

Key Personnel:
Anesthesiology............... Alan Garruth, MD
CEO .... Ashley McClellan
Pediatric Ambulatory Care ...... Lynn Ogden
Pediatric In-Patient Care .... Lynn Ogden
Operating Room.............. Darlene Pletcher
Radiology.................. Lizabeth Reynol
Chief of Medical Staff.......... Barry Sanders
Infection Control............. P White

Measure	Cases	This Hosp.	State Avg.	U.S. Avg.
Blood Clot Prevention and Treatment				
Anticoagulation Overlap Therapy[2]	51	96%	93%	93%
ICU Venous Thromboembolism Prophylaxis[2]	38	97%	92%	92%
Incidence of Potentially Preventable VTE[1,2]	-	-	9%	10%
UFH with Dosages/Platelet Monitoring[2]	13	100%	96%	97%
Venous Thromboembolism Prophylaxis[2]	382	95%	82%	85%
Warfarin Therapy Discharge Instructions[2]	37	89%	84%	75%
Chest Pain/Possible Heart Attack Care				
Aspirin Given Within 24 Hours of Arrival[1,3]	-	-	94%	96%
Fibrinolytic Meds Within 30 Min. of Arrival[5]	-	-	47%	58%
Average Time to ECG (minutes)[1,3]	-	-	8	7
Average Time to Transfer (minutes)[5]	-	-	62	60
Children's Asthma Care				
Received Home Management Plan of Care	-	-	93%	88%
Received Reliever Medication	-	-	100%	100%
Received Systemic Corticosteroids	-	-	100%	100%
Emergency Department				
Admittance Decision Time (minutes)[2]	722	122	99	98
Head CT Results Within 45 Min. of Arrival	26	81%	54%	57%
Patients Who Left ER Before Being Seen	45,113	1%	3%	2%
Time from ER Arrival to Admit. (minutes)[2]	722	198	270	274
Time from ER Arrival to Discharge (minutes)	440	106	127	134
Time in ER Before Being Evaluated (minutes)	457	10	26	26
Time to Pain Meds for Fractures (minutes)	269	28	57	57
Heart Attack Care				
Aspirin Given at Discharge	143	100%	99%	99%
Fibrinolytic Meds Within 30 Min. of Arrival[7]	-	-	49%	54%
PCI Within 90 Minutes of Arrival	35	100%	95%	96%
Statin Prescribed at Discharge	140	100%	98%	98%
Heart Failure Care				
ACE Inhibitor or ARB for LVSD	57	100%	97%	97%
Discharge Instructions Given	129	99%	95%	94%
Evaluation of LVS Function	161	100%	99%	99%
Medicare Spending				
Medicare Spending per Patient (ratio)	-	1.04	1.03	0.98
Pneumonia Care				
Appropriate Initial Antibiotic Given	93	99%	95%	95%
Blood Culture Timing	197	99%	98%	98%
Pregnancy and Delivery Care				
Newborn Deliveries Scheduled Early[2]	28	7%	7%	6%
Preventive Care				
Immunization for Influenza[2]	496	99%	90%	90%
Immunization for Pneumonia[2]	542	99%	92%	92%
Stroke Care				
Anticoagulation Therapy for Atrial Fibrillation[1]	-	-	96%	95%
Antithrombotic Therapy Timing	51	98%	98%	98%
Assessed for Rehabilitation	46	100%	98%	97%
Discharged on Antithrombotic Therapy	46	100%	99%	99%
Discharged on Statin Medication	34	100%	95%	94%
Thrombolytic Therapy Timing[1]	-	-	68%	66%
Venous Thromboembolism Prophylaxis	51	100%	94%	94%
Written Stroke Educational Materials Given	32	97%	92%	88%
Surgical Care Improvement Project				
Appropriate Beta Blocker Usage[2]	102	100%	98%	98%
Appropriate VTP Within 24 Hours[2]	190	99%	98%	98%
Controlled Postoperative Blood Glucose[2]	50	94%	96%	97%
Perioperative Temperature Management[2]	290	100%	100%	100%
Prophylactic Antibiotic Selection[2]	198	99%	99%	99%
Prophylactic Antibiotic Selection (Outpatient)	43	98%	98%	98%
Prophylactic Antibiotic Stopped[2]	193	100%	98%	98%
Prophylactic Antibiotic Timing[2]	199	99%	99%	99%
Prophylactic Antibiotic Timing (Outpatient)	43	95%	98%	98%
Urinary Catheter Removal[2]	192	100%	98%	97%
Survey of Patients' Hospital Experiences				
Area Around Room 'Always' Quiet at Night	300+	63%	68%	61%
Doctors 'Always' Communicated Well	300+	79%	83%	82%
Home Recovery Information Given	300+	85%	85%	85%
Hospital Given 9 or 10 on 10 Point Scale	300+	74%	73%	71%

NOTE: Hospital profiles are in alphabetical order by state, then city, then hospital within the city; Rankings exclude hospitals with less than 25 cases except for patient surveys which excludes hospitals with less than 100 cases; (a) 100-299 cases; (1) The number of cases/patients is too few to report; (2) Data submitted were based on a sample of cases/patients; (3) Results are based on a shorter time period than required; (4) Data suppressed by CMS for one or more quarters; (5) Results are not available for this reporting period; (6) Fewer than 100 patients completed the HCAHPS survey; (7) No cases met the criteria for this measure; (8) The lower limit of the confidence interval cannot be calculated if the number of observed infections equals zero; (9) No data are available from the state/territory for this reporting period; (10) The scores shown reflect fewer than 50 completed surveys; (11) There were discrepancies in the data collection process; (12) This measure does not apply to this hospital for this reporting period; (13) Results cannot be calculated for this reporting period; (14) The results for this state are combined with nearby states to protect confidentiality; Please refer to the User's Guide for a full explanation of data.

Measure	Cases	This Hosp.	State Avg.	U.S. Avg.
Meds 'Always' Explained Before Given	300+	65%	66%	64%
Nurses 'Always' Communicated Well	300+	77%	80%	79%
Pain 'Always' Well Controlled	300+	70%	72%	71%
Room and Bathroom 'Always' Clean	300+	73%	75%	73%
Timely Help 'Always' Received	300+	64%	69%	68%
Would Definitely Recommend Hospital	300+	74%	73%	71%
Use of Medical Imaging				
Cardiac Imaging Stress Test before Surgery[1]	-	-	5.3%	5.3%
Combination Abdominal CT Scan	271	4.8%	16.4%	10.5%
Combination Brain/Sinus CT Scan[1]	-	-	2.7%	2.7%
Combination Chest CT Scan	105	1.9%	5.6%	2.7%
Follow-up Mammogram/Ultrasound	1,100	11.2%	7.9%	8.8%
Lumbar Spine MRI for Low Back Pain[1]	-	-	39.6%	37.2%

Good Shephard Medical Center - Linden

404 North Kaufman Street
Linden, TX 75563
Phone: 903-756-5561
URL: www.gsmclinden.org
Type: Critical Access Hospitals
Emergency Services: Yes
Ownership: Voluntary non-profit - Private
Key Personnel:
Operating Room. . . . . Jane Blizzard
CEO/President. . . . . John Chamberlin
Pediatric In-Patient Care . . . . Andrew Vadasz
Radiology. . . . . Pam Watkins

Measure	Cases	This Hosp.	State Avg.	U.S. Avg.
Blood Clot Prevention and Treatment				
Anticoagulation Overlap Therapy[2,7]	-	-	93%	93%
ICU Venous Thromboembolism Prophylaxis[2,7]	-	-	92%	92%
Incidence of Potentially Preventable VTE[2,7]	-	-	9%	10%
UFH with Dosages/Platelet Monitoring[2,7]	-	-	96%	97%
Venous Thromboembolism Prophylaxis[2]	114	56%	82%	85%
Warfarin Therapy Discharge Instructions[2,7]	-	-	84%	75%
Chest Pain/Possible Heart Attack Care				
Aspirin Given Within 24 Hours of Arrival	31	97%	94%	96%
Fibrinolytic Meds Within 30 Min. of Arrival[1]	-	-	47%	58%
Average Time to ECG (minutes)	34	8	8	7
Average Time to Transfer (minutes)[1]	-	-	62	60
Children's Asthma Care				
Received Home Management Plan of Care	-	-	93%	88%
Received Reliever Medication	-	-	100%	100%
Received Systemic Corticosteroids	-	-	100%	100%
Emergency Department				
Admittance Decision Time (minutes)[2]	199	30	99	98
Head CT Results Within 45 Min. of Arrival[1]	-	-	54%	57%
Patients Who Left ER Before Being Seen[5]	-	-	3%	2%
Time from ER Arrival to Admit. (minutes)[2]	213	155	270	274
Time from ER Arrival to Discharge (minutes)	357	79	127	134
Time in ER Before Being Evaluated (minutes)	424	11	26	26
Time to Pain Meds for Fractures (minutes)	35	31	57	57
Heart Attack Care				
Aspirin Given at Discharge[5]	-	-	99%	99%
Fibrinolytic Meds Within 30 Min. of Arrival[5]	-	-	49%	54%
PCI Within 90 Minutes of Arrival[5]	-	-	95%	96%
Statin Prescribed at Discharge[5]	-	-	98%	98%
Heart Failure Care				
ACE Inhibitor or ARB for LVSD[1]	-	-	97%	97%
Discharge Instructions Given	15	27%	95%	94%
Evaluation of LVS Function[3,7]	-	-	99%	99%
Medicare Spending				
Medicare Spending per Patient (ratio)	-	-	1.03	0.98
Pneumonia Care				
Appropriate Initial Antibiotic Given	37	97%	95%	95%
Blood Culture Timing	45	100%	98%	98%
Pregnancy and Delivery Care				
Newborn Deliveries Scheduled Early[3,7]	-	-	7%	6%
Preventive Care				
Immunization for Influenza[2]	205	74%	90%	90%
Immunization for Pneumonia[2]	269	83%	92%	92%
Stroke Care				
Anticoagulation Therapy for Atrial Fibrillation[5]	-	-	96%	95%
Antithrombotic Therapy Timing[5]	-	-	98%	98%
Assessed for Rehabilitation[5]	-	-	98%	97%
Discharged on Antithrombotic Therapy[5]	-	-	99%	99%
Discharged on Statin Medication[5]	-	-	95%	94%
Thrombolytic Therapy Timing[5]	-	-	68%	66%
Venous Thromboembolism Prophylaxis[5]	-	-	94%	94%
Written Stroke Educational Materials Given[5]	-	-	92%	88%
Surgical Care Improvement Project				
Appropriate Beta Blocker Usage[5]	-	-	98%	98%
Appropriate VTP Within 24 Hours[5]	-	-	98%	98%
Controlled Postoperative Blood Glucose[5]	-	-	96%	97%
Perioperative Temperature Management[5]	-	-	100%	100%
Prophylactic Antibiotic Selection[5]	-	-	99%	99%
Prophylactic Antibiotic Selection (Outpatient)[5]	-	-	98%	98%
Prophylactic Antibiotic Stopped[5]	-	-	98%	98%
Prophylactic Antibiotic Timing[5]	-	-	99%	99%
Prophylactic Antibiotic Timing (Outpatient)[5]	-	-	98%	98%
Urinary Catheter Removal[5]	-	-	98%	97%
Survey of Patients' Hospital Experiences				
Area Around Room 'Always' Quiet at Night	(a)	79%	68%	61%
Doctors 'Always' Communicated Well	(a)	85%	83%	82%
Home Recovery Information Given	(a)	79%	85%	85%
Hospital Given 9 or 10 on 10 Point Scale	(a)	70%	73%	71%
Meds 'Always' Explained Before Given	(a)	70%	66%	64%
Nurses 'Always' Communicated Well	(a)	80%	80%	79%
Pain 'Always' Well Controlled	(a)	65%	72%	71%
Room and Bathroom 'Always' Clean	(a)	78%	75%	73%
Timely Help 'Always' Received	(a)	77%	69%	68%
Would Definitely Recommend Hospital	(a)	75%	73%	71%
Use of Medical Imaging				
Cardiac Imaging Stress Test before Surgery[1]	-	-	5.3%	5.3%
Combination Abdominal CT Scan	126	4.8%	16.4%	10.5%
Combination Brain/Sinus CT Scan[1]	-	-	2.7%	2.7%
Combination Chest CT Scan	66	7.6%	5.6%	2.7%
Follow-up Mammogram/Ultrasound[1]	-	-	7.9%	8.8%
Lumbar Spine MRI for Low Back Pain[7]	-	-	39.6%	37.2%

Lamb Healthcare Center

1500 S Sunset
Littlefield, TX 79339
Phone: 806-385-6411
Fax: 806-385-3998
Type: Acute Care Hospitals
Emergency Services: Yes
Ownership: Government - Local
Beds: 75
Key Personnel:
President. . . . . Tony Barton
Radiology. . . . . Vikas Bhushan
Quality Assurance . . . . Lori Cratt
Chief of Medical Staff. . . . . Tony Hedges
Emergency Room . . . . Enricke Rodriguez, MD

Measure	Cases	This Hosp.	State Avg.	U.S. Avg.
Blood Clot Prevention and Treatment				
Anticoagulation Overlap Therapy[1]	-	-	93%	93%
ICU Venous Thromboembolism Prophylaxis[7]	-	-	92%	92%
Incidence of Potentially Preventable VTE[7]	-	-	9%	10%
UFH with Dosages/Platelet Monitoring[7]	-	-	96%	97%
Venous Thromboembolism Prophylaxis	120	5%	82%	85%
Warfarin Therapy Discharge Instructions[1]	-	-	84%	75%
Chest Pain/Possible Heart Attack Care				
Aspirin Given Within 24 Hours of Arrival[3]	14	57%	94%	96%
Fibrinolytic Meds Within 30 Min. of Arrival[3,7]	-	-	47%	58%
Average Time to ECG (minutes)[3]	15	18	8	7
Average Time to Transfer (minutes)[3,7]	-	-	62	60
Children's Asthma Care				
Received Home Management Plan of Care	-	-	93%	88%
Received Reliever Medication	-	-	100%	100%
Received Systemic Corticosteroids	-	-	100%	100%
Emergency Department				
Admittance Decision Time (minutes)	86	20	99	98
Head CT Results Within 45 Min. of Arrival[5]	-	-	54%	57%
Patients Who Left ER Before Being Seen	3,592	1%	3%	2%
Time from ER Arrival to Admit. (minutes)	132	122	270	274
Time from ER Arrival to Discharge (minutes)	223	71	127	134
Time in ER Before Being Evaluated (minutes)	230	15	26	26
Time to Pain Meds for Fractures (minutes)[1,3]	-	-	57	57
Heart Attack Care				
Aspirin Given at Discharge[3,7]	-	-	99%	99%
Fibrinolytic Meds Within 30 Min. of Arrival[3,7]	-	-	49%	54%
PCI Within 90 Minutes of Arrival[3,7]	-	-	95%	96%
Statin Prescribed at Discharge[3,7]	-	-	98%	98%
Heart Failure Care				
ACE Inhibitor or ARB for LVSD[1]	-	-	97%	97%
Discharge Instructions Given	11	27%	95%	94%
Evaluation of LVS Function	12	33%	99%	99%
Medicare Spending				
Medicare Spending per Patient (ratio)	-	0.82	1.03	0.98
Pneumonia Care				
Appropriate Initial Antibiotic Given[1]	-	-	95%	95%
Blood Culture Timing[1]	-	-	98%	98%
Pregnancy and Delivery Care				
Newborn Deliveries Scheduled Early	12	0%	7%	6%
Preventive Care				
Immunization for Influenza	148	72%	90%	90%
Immunization for Pneumonia[2]	182	75%	92%	92%
Stroke Care				
Anticoagulation Therapy for Atrial Fibrillation[3,7]	-	-	96%	95%
Antithrombotic Therapy Timing[1,3]	-	-	98%	98%
Assessed for Rehabilitation[1,3]	-	-	98%	97%
Discharged on Antithrombotic Therapy[1,3]	-	-	99%	99%
Discharged on Statin Medication[1,3]	-	-	95%	94%
Thrombolytic Therapy Timing[1,3]	-	-	68%	66%
Venous Thromboembolism Prophylaxis[1,3]	-	-	94%	94%
Written Stroke Educational Materials Given[1,3]	-	-	92%	88%
Surgical Care Improvement Project				
Appropriate Beta Blocker Usage[5]	-	-	98%	98%
Appropriate VTP Within 24 Hours[5]	-	-	98%	98%
Controlled Postoperative Blood Glucose[5]	-	-	96%	97%
Perioperative Temperature Management[5]	-	-	100%	100%
Prophylactic Antibiotic Selection[5]	-	-	99%	99%
Prophylactic Antibiotic Selection (Outpatient)[5]	-	-	98%	98%
Prophylactic Antibiotic Stopped[5]	-	-	98%	98%
Prophylactic Antibiotic Timing[5]	-	-	99%	99%
Prophylactic Antibiotic Timing (Outpatient)[5]	-	-	98%	98%
Urinary Catheter Removal[5]	-	-	98%	97%
Survey of Patients' Hospital Experiences				
Area Around Room 'Always' Quiet at Night[10]	<100	57%	68%	61%
Doctors 'Always' Communicated Well[10]	<100	83%	83%	82%
Home Recovery Information Given[10]	<100	81%	85%	85%
Hospital Given 9 or 10 on 10 Point Scale[10]	<100	62%	73%	71%
Meds 'Always' Explained Before Given[10]	<100	57%	66%	64%
Nurses 'Always' Communicated Well[10]	<100	75%	80%	79%
Pain 'Always' Well Controlled[10]	<100	60%	72%	71%
Room and Bathroom 'Always' Clean[10]	<100	74%	75%	73%
Timely Help 'Always' Received[10]	<100	62%	69%	68%
Would Definitely Recommend Hospital[10]	<100	62%	73%	71%
Use of Medical Imaging				
Cardiac Imaging Stress Test before Surgery[7]	-	-	5.3%	5.3%
Combination Abdominal CT Scan[1]	-	-	16.4%	10.5%
Combination Brain/Sinus CT Scan[1]	-	-	2.7%	2.7%
Combination Chest CT Scan[1]	-	-	5.6%	2.7%
Follow-up Mammogram/Ultrasound[7]	-	-	7.9%	8.8%
Lumbar Spine MRI for Low Back Pain[7]	-	-	39.6%	37.2%

Memorial Medical Center Livingston

1717 Hwy 59 Bypass
Livingston, TX 77351
Phone: 936-327-4381
Fax: 936-329-8730
E-mail: sfranklin@memorialhealth.com
URL: www.mymemorialhealth.org/livingston
Type: Acute Care Hospitals
Emergency Services: Yes
Ownership: Voluntary non-profit - Private
Beds: 50
Key Personnel:
CEO/President. . . . . Bryant H Krenek, Jr

Measure	Cases	This Hosp.	State Avg.	U.S. Avg.
Blood Clot Prevention and Treatment				
Anticoagulation Overlap Therapy[2]	21	76%	93%	93%
ICU Venous Thromboembolism Prophylaxis[2]	45	84%	92%	92%
Incidence of Potentially Preventable VTE[1,2]	-	-	9%	10%
UFH with Dosages/Platelet Monitoring[1,2]	-	-	96%	97%
Venous Thromboembolism Prophylaxis[2]	204	81%	82%	85%
Warfarin Therapy Discharge Instructions[2]	14	79%	84%	75%

NOTE: Hospital profiles are in alphabetical order by state, then city, then hospital within the city; Rankings exclude hospitals with less than 25 cases except for patient surveys which excludes hospitals with less than 100 cases; (a) 100-299 cases; (1) The number of cases/patients is too few to report; (2) Data submitted were based on a sample of cases/patients; (3) Results are based on a shorter time period than required; (4) Data suppressed by CMS for one or more quarters; (5) Results are not available for this reporting period; (6) Fewer than 100 patients completed the HCAHPS survey; (7) No cases met the criteria for this measure; (8) The lower limit of the confidence interval cannot be calculated if the number of observed infections equals zero; (9) No data are available from the state/territory for this reporting period; (10) The scores shown reflect fewer than 50 completed surveys; (11) There were discrepancies in the data collection process; (12) This measure does not apply to this hospital for this reporting period; (13) Results cannot be calculated for this reporting period; (14) The results for this state are combined with nearby states to protect confidentiality; Please refer to the User's Guide for a full explanation of data.

Measure	Cases	This Hosp.	State Avg.	U.S. Avg.
Chest Pain/Possible Heart Attack Care				
Aspirin Given Within 24 Hours of Arrival	160	88%	94%	96%
Fibrinolytic Meds Within 30 Min. of Arrival	59	17%	47%	58%
Average Time to ECG (minutes)	158	22	8	7
Average Time to Transfer (minutes)[1]	-	-	62	60
Children's Asthma Care				
Received Home Management Plan of Care	-	-	93%	88%
Received Reliever Medication	-	-	100%	100%
Received Systemic Corticosteroids	-	-	100%	100%
Emergency Department				
Admittance Decision Time (minutes)[2]	268	91	99	98
Head CT Results Within 45 Min. of Arrival	13	23%	54%	57%
Patients Who Left ER Before Being Seen	23,617	4%	3%	2%
Time from ER Arrival to Admit. (minutes)[2]	301	325	270	274
Time from ER Arrival to Discharge (minutes)	330	149	127	134
Time in ER Before Being Evaluated (minutes)	343	37	26	26
Time to Pain Meds for Fractures (minutes)	112	63	57	57
Heart Attack Care				
Aspirin Given at Discharge[1,2]	-	-	99%	99%
Fibrinolytic Meds Within 30 Min. of Arrival[2,7]	-	-	49%	54%
PCI Within 90 Minutes of Arrival[2,7]	-	-	95%	96%
Statin Prescribed at Discharge[1,2]	-	-	98%	98%
Heart Failure Care				
ACE Inhibitor or ARB for LVSD[2]	14	93%	97%	97%
Discharge Instructions Given[2]	56	95%	95%	94%
Evaluation of LVS Function[2]	79	97%	99%	99%
Medicare Spending				
Medicare Spending per Patient (ratio)	-	1.05	1.03	0.98
Pneumonia Care				
Appropriate Initial Antibiotic Given[2]	95	89%	95%	95%
Blood Culture Timing[2]	129	97%	98%	98%
Pregnancy and Delivery Care				
Newborn Deliveries Scheduled Early[2]	49	37%	7%	6%
Preventive Care				
Immunization for Influenza[2]	261	89%	90%	90%
Immunization for Pneumonia[2]	323	87%	92%	92%
Stroke Care				
Anticoagulation Therapy for Atrial Fibrillation[1,2]	-	-	96%	95%
Antithrombotic Therapy Timing[2]	28	100%	98%	98%
Assessed for Rehabilitation[2]	26	81%	98%	97%
Discharged on Antithrombotic Therapy[2]	26	85%	99%	99%
Discharged on Statin Medication[2]	24	79%	95%	94%
Thrombolytic Therapy Timing[2]	11	0%	68%	66%
Venous Thromboembolism Prophylaxis[2]	29	76%	94%	94%
Written Stroke Educational Materials Given[2]	15	53%	92%	88%
Surgical Care Improvement Project				
Appropriate Beta Blocker Usage[2]	40	98%	98%	98%
Appropriate VTP Within 24 Hours[2]	134	84%	98%	98%
Controlled Postoperative Blood Glucose[2,7]	-	-	96%	97%
Perioperative Temperature Management[2]	153	100%	100%	100%
Prophylactic Antibiotic Selection[2]	107	97%	99%	99%
Prophylactic Antibiotic Selection (Outpatient)[1]	-	-	98%	98%
Prophylactic Antibiotic Stopped[2]	99	95%	98%	98%
Prophylactic Antibiotic Timing[2]	107	91%	99%	99%
Prophylactic Antibiotic Timing (Outpatient)[1]	-	-	98%	98%
Urinary Catheter Removal[2]	93	96%	98%	97%
Survey of Patients' Hospital Experiences				
Area Around Room 'Always' Quiet at Night	300+	69%	68%	61%
Doctors 'Always' Communicated Well	300+	78%	83%	82%
Home Recovery Information Given	300+	87%	85%	85%
Hospital Given 9 or 10 on 10 Point Scale	300+	66%	73%	71%
Meds 'Always' Explained Before Given	300+	64%	66%	64%
Nurses 'Always' Communicated Well	300+	77%	80%	79%
Pain 'Always' Well Controlled	300+	72%	72%	71%
Room and Bathroom 'Always' Clean	300+	78%	75%	73%
Timely Help 'Always' Received	300+	64%	69%	68%
Would Definitely Recommend Hospital	300+	61%	73%	71%
Use of Medical Imaging				
Cardiac Imaging Stress Test before Surgery[1]	-	-	5.3%	5.3%
Combination Abdominal CT Scan	323	22.0%	16.4%	10.5%
Combination Brain/Sinus CT Scan[1]	-	-	2.7%	2.7%
Combination Chest CT Scan	189	28.6%	5.6%	2.7%
Follow-up Mammogram/Ultrasound	865	12.9%	7.9%	8.8%
Lumbar Spine MRI for Low Back Pain	41	41.5%	39.6%	37.2%

Scott & White Hospital - Llano

200 W Ollie
Llano, TX 78643
Phone: 325-247-5040
Fax: 325-248-2108
Type: Acute Care Hospitals
Emergency Services: Yes
Ownership: Voluntary non-profit - Private
Beds: 30

Key Personnel:
Operating Room. . . . . Debbie Coats
Chief of Medical Staff. . . . . Tiffany Gainer
Quality Assurance . . . . Linda Meridem
Hemotology Center . . . . Shannon O'Conner
CEO/President. . . . . Ernie Parisi
Radiology. . . . . DD Stiles

Measure	Cases	This Hosp.	State Avg.	U.S. Avg.
Blood Clot Prevention and Treatment				
Anticoagulation Overlap Therapy[1,2]	-	-	93%	93%
ICU Venous Thromboembolism Prophylaxis[2,7]	-	-	92%	92%
Incidence of Potentially Preventable VTE[2,7]	-	-	9%	10%
UFH with Dosages/Platelet Monitoring[2,7]	-	-	96%	97%
Venous Thromboembolism Prophylaxis[2]	132	64%	82%	85%
Warfarin Therapy Discharge Instructions[1,2]	-	-	84%	75%
Chest Pain/Possible Heart Attack Care				
Aspirin Given Within 24 Hours of Arrival	51	96%	94%	96%
Fibrinolytic Meds Within 30 Min. of Arrival[1]	-	-	47%	58%
Average Time to ECG (minutes)	50	3	8	7
Average Time to Transfer (minutes)[1]	-	-	62	60
Children's Asthma Care				
Received Home Management Plan of Care	-	-	93%	88%
Received Reliever Medication	-	-	100%	100%
Received Systemic Corticosteroids	-	-	100%	100%
Emergency Department				
Admittance Decision Time (minutes)	248	40	99	98
Head CT Results Within 45 Min. of Arrival[1]	-	-	54%	57%
Patients Who Left ER Before Being Seen	7,005	1%	3%	2%
Time from ER Arrival to Admit. (minutes)	258	183	270	274
Time from ER Arrival to Discharge (minutes)	374	106	127	134
Time in ER Before Being Evaluated (minutes)	342	11	26	26
Time to Pain Meds for Fractures (minutes)	55	51	57	57
Heart Attack Care				
Aspirin Given at Discharge[5]	-	-	99%	99%
Fibrinolytic Meds Within 30 Min. of Arrival[5]	-	-	49%	54%
PCI Within 90 Minutes of Arrival[5]	-	-	95%	96%
Statin Prescribed at Discharge[5]	-	-	98%	98%
Heart Failure Care				
ACE Inhibitor or ARB for LVSD[1]	-	-	97%	97%
Discharge Instructions Given	14	79%	95%	94%
Evaluation of LVS Function	19	100%	99%	99%
Medicare Spending				
Medicare Spending per Patient (ratio)	-	0.94	1.03	0.98
Pneumonia Care				
Appropriate Initial Antibiotic Given	27	100%	95%	95%
Blood Culture Timing	53	98%	98%	98%
Pregnancy and Delivery Care				
Newborn Deliveries Scheduled Early	23	0%	7%	6%
Preventive Care				
Immunization for Influenza	314	87%	90%	90%
Immunization for Pneumonia	346	84%	92%	92%
Stroke Care				
Anticoagulation Therapy for Atrial Fibrillation[1]	-	-	96%	95%
Antithrombotic Therapy Timing[1]	-	-	98%	98%
Assessed for Rehabilitation[1]	-	-	98%	97%
Discharged on Antithrombotic Therapy[1]	-	-	99%	99%
Discharged on Statin Medication[1]	-	-	95%	94%
Thrombolytic Therapy Timing[1]	-	-	68%	66%
Venous Thromboembolism Prophylaxis[1]	-	-	94%	94%
Written Stroke Educational Materials Given[1]	-	-	92%	88%
Surgical Care Improvement Project				
Appropriate Beta Blocker Usage[1,3]	-	-	98%	98%
Appropriate VTP Within 24 Hours[3]	14	100%	98%	98%
Controlled Postoperative Blood Glucose[3,7]	-	-	96%	97%
Perioperative Temperature Management[3]	17	100%	100%	100%
Prophylactic Antibiotic Selection[1,3]	-	-	99%	99%
Prophylactic Antibiotic Selection (Outpatient)	16	100%	98%	98%
Prophylactic Antibiotic Stopped[1,3]	-	-	98%	98%
Prophylactic Antibiotic Timing[1,3]	-	-	99%	99%
Prophylactic Antibiotic Timing (Outpatient)	16	94%	98%	98%
Urinary Catheter Removal[3]	11	100%	98%	97%
Survey of Patients' Hospital Experiences				
Area Around Room 'Always' Quiet at Night	(a)	65%	68%	61%
Doctors 'Always' Communicated Well	(a)	86%	83%	82%
Home Recovery Information Given	(a)	86%	85%	85%
Hospital Given 9 or 10 on 10 Point Scale	(a)	64%	73%	71%
Meds 'Always' Explained Before Given	(a)	71%	66%	64%
Nurses 'Always' Communicated Well	(a)	78%	80%	79%
Pain 'Always' Well Controlled	(a)	76%	72%	71%
Room and Bathroom 'Always' Clean	(a)	70%	75%	73%
Timely Help 'Always' Received	(a)	73%	69%	68%
Would Definitely Recommend Hospital	(a)	60%	73%	71%
Use of Medical Imaging				
Cardiac Imaging Stress Test before Surgery	77	2.6%	5.3%	5.3%
Combination Abdominal CT Scan	255	6.7%	16.4%	10.5%
Combination Brain/Sinus CT Scan[1]	-	-	2.7%	2.7%
Combination Chest CT Scan	201	1.0%	5.6%	2.7%
Follow-up Mammogram/Ultrasound	326	7.1%	7.9%	8.8%
Lumbar Spine MRI for Low Back Pain[1]	-	-	39.6%	37.2%

W J Mangold Memorial Hospital

320 North Main
Lockney, TX 79241
Phone: 806-652-3373
Fax: 806-652-2172
E-mail: mallen@mangold.lockney.isd.tenet.edu
URL: www.mangoldmemorial.org
Type: Critical Access Hospitals
Emergency Services: Yes
Ownership: Govt - Hospital Dist/Auth
Beds: 27

Key Personnel:
Operating Room. . . . . Angela Clay, RN
President . . . . Embre Douglas
Chief of Medical Staff . . . . Gary B Mangold, MD
Anesthesiology. . . . . Kevin L Stewart, MD
Infection Control. . . . . Trina Wilson, RN
Quality Assurance . . . . Trina Wilson, RN

Measure	Cases	This Hosp.	State Avg.	U.S. Avg.
Blood Clot Prevention and Treatment				
Anticoagulation Overlap Therapy[5]	-	-	93%	93%
ICU Venous Thromboembolism Prophylaxis[5]	-	-	92%	92%
Incidence of Potentially Preventable VTE[5]	-	-	9%	10%
UFH with Dosages/Platelet Monitoring[5]	-	-	96%	97%
Venous Thromboembolism Prophylaxis[5]	-	-	82%	85%
Warfarin Therapy Discharge Instructions[5]	-	-	84%	75%
Chest Pain/Possible Heart Attack Care				
Aspirin Given Within 24 Hours of Arrival	-	-	94%	96%
Fibrinolytic Meds Within 30 Min. of Arrival	-	-	47%	58%
Average Time to ECG (minutes)	-	-	8	7
Average Time to Transfer (minutes)	-	-	62	60
Children's Asthma Care				
Received Home Management Plan of Care	-	-	93%	88%
Received Reliever Medication	-	-	100%	100%
Received Systemic Corticosteroids	-	-	100%	100%
Emergency Department				
Admittance Decision Time (minutes)[5]	-	-	99	98
Head CT Results Within 45 Min. of Arrival	-	-	54%	57%
Patients Who Left ER Before Being Seen	-	-	3%	2%
Time from ER Arrival to Admit. (minutes)[5]	-	-	270	274
Time from ER Arrival to Discharge (minutes)	-	-	127	134
Time in ER Before Being Evaluated (minutes)	-	-	26	26
Time to Pain Meds for Fractures (minutes)	-	-	57	57
Heart Attack Care				
Aspirin Given at Discharge[5]	-	-	99%	99%
Fibrinolytic Meds Within 30 Min. of Arrival[5]	-	-	49%	54%
PCI Within 90 Minutes of Arrival[5]	-	-	95%	96%
Statin Prescribed at Discharge[5]	-	-	98%	98%
Heart Failure Care				
ACE Inhibitor or ARB for LVSD[5]	-	-	97%	97%
Discharge Instructions Given[5]	-	-	95%	94%
Evaluation of LVS Function[5]	-	-	99%	99%
Medicare Spending				
Medicare Spending per Patient (ratio)	-	-	1.03	0.98

NOTE: Hospital profiles are in alphabetical order by state, then city, then hospital within the city; Rankings exclude hospitals with less than 25 cases except for patient surveys which excludes hospitals with less than 100 cases; (a) 100-299 cases; (1) The number of cases/patients is too few to report; (2) Data submitted were based on a sample of cases/patients; (3) Results are based on a shorter time period than required; (4) Data suppressed by CMS for one or more quarters; (5) Results are not available for this reporting period; (6) Fewer than 100 patients completed the HCAHPS survey; (7) No cases met the criteria for this measure; (8) The lower limit of the confidence interval cannot be calculated if the number of observed infections equals zero; (9) No data are available from the state/territory for this reporting period; (10) The scores shown reflect fewer than 50 completed surveys; (11) There were discrepancies in the data collection process; (12) This measure does not apply to this hospital for this reporting period; (13) Results cannot be calculated for this reporting period; (14) The results for this state are combined with nearby states to protect confidentiality; Please refer to the User's Guide for a full explanation of data.

Measure	Cases	This Hosp.	State Avg.	U.S. Avg.
Pneumonia Care				
Appropriate Initial Antibiotic Given	40	88%	95%	95%
Blood Culture Timing[1]	-	-	98%	98%
Pregnancy and Delivery Care				
Newborn Deliveries Scheduled Early[5]	-	-	7%	6%
Preventive Care				
Immunization for Influenza[5]	-	-	90%	90%
Immunization for Pneumonia[5]	-	-	92%	92%
Stroke Care				
Anticoagulation Therapy for Atrial Fibrillation[5]	-	-	96%	95%
Antithrombotic Therapy Timing[5]	-	-	98%	98%
Assessed for Rehabilitation[5]	-	-	98%	97%
Discharged on Antithrombotic Therapy[5]	-	-	99%	99%
Discharged on Statin Medication[5]	-	-	95%	94%
Thrombolytic Therapy Timing[5]	-	-	68%	66%
Venous Thromboembolism Prophylaxis[5]	-	-	94%	94%
Written Stroke Educational Materials Given[5]	-	-	92%	88%
Surgical Care Improvement Project				
Appropriate Beta Blocker Usage[5]	-	-	98%	98%
Appropriate VTP Within 24 Hours[5]	-	-	98%	98%
Controlled Postoperative Blood Glucose[5]	-	-	96%	97%
Perioperative Temperature Management[5]	-	-	100%	100%
Prophylactic Antibiotic Selection[5]	-	-	99%	99%
Prophylactic Antibiotic Selection (Outpatient)	-	-	98%	98%
Prophylactic Antibiotic Stopped[5]	-	-	98%	98%
Prophylactic Antibiotic Timing[5]	-	-	99%	99%
Prophylactic Antibiotic Timing (Outpatient)	-	-	98%	98%
Urinary Catheter Removal[5]	-	-	98%	97%
Survey of Patients' Hospital Experiences				
Area Around Room 'Always' Quiet at Night	(a)	73%	68%	61%
Doctors 'Always' Communicated Well	(a)	99%	83%	82%
Home Recovery Information Given	(a)	75%	85%	85%
Hospital Given 9 or 10 on 10 Point Scale	(a)	84%	73%	71%
Meds 'Always' Explained Before Given	(a)	76%	66%	64%
Nurses 'Always' Communicated Well	(a)	92%	80%	79%
Pain 'Always' Well Controlled	(a)	80%	72%	71%
Room and Bathroom 'Always' Clean	(a)	84%	75%	73%
Timely Help 'Always' Received	(a)	85%	69%	68%
Would Definitely Recommend Hospital	(a)	83%	73%	71%
Use of Medical Imaging				
Cardiac Imaging Stress Test before Surgery	-	-	5.3%	5.3%
Combination Abdominal CT Scan	-	-	16.4%	10.5%
Combination Brain/Sinus CT Scan	-	-	2.7%	2.7%
Combination Chest CT Scan	-	-	5.6%	2.7%
Follow-up Mammogram/Ultrasound	-	-	7.9%	8.8%
Lumbar Spine MRI for Low Back Pain	-	-	39.6%	37.2%

Good Shepherd Medical Center

700 East Marshall Avenue
Longview, TX 75601
Phone: 903-315-2000
Fax: 903-315-2002
E-mail: webmaster@gsmc.org
URL: www.goodshepherdhealth.org
Type: Acute Care Hospitals
Emergency Services: Yes
Ownership: Voluntary non-profit - Private
Beds: 425

Key Personnel:

CEO/President. . . . . Edwrad Banos
Radiology. . . . . Kim Howard, MD
Chief of Medical Staff. . . . . Edna York

Measure	Cases	This Hosp.	State Avg.	U.S. Avg.
Blood Clot Prevention and Treatment				
Anticoagulation Overlap Therapy[2]	93	99%	93%	93%
ICU Venous Thromboembolism Prophylaxis[2]	61	100%	92%	92%
Incidence of Potentially Preventable VTE[1,2]	-	-	9%	10%
UFH with Dosages/Platelet Monitoring[2]	14	100%	96%	97%
Venous Thromboembolism Prophylaxis[2]	359	72%	82%	85%
Warfarin Therapy Discharge Instructions[2]	79	100%	84%	75%
Chest Pain/Possible Heart Attack Care				
Aspirin Given Within 24 Hours of Arrival[1,3]	-	-	94%	96%
Fibrinolytic Meds Within 30 Min. of Arrival[3,7]	-	-	47%	58%
Average Time to ECG (minutes)[1,3]	-	-	8	7
Average Time to Transfer (minutes)[3,7]	-	-	62	60
Children's Asthma Care				
Received Home Management Plan of Care	-	-	93%	88%
Received Reliever Medication	-	-	100%	100%
Received Systemic Corticosteroids	-	-	100%	100%
Emergency Department				
Admittance Decision Time (minutes)[2]	624	60	99	98
Head CT Results Within 45 Min. of Arrival	21	38%	54%	57%
Patients Who Left ER Before Being Seen	81,537	3%	3%	2%
Time from ER Arrival to Admit. (minutes)[2]	627	236	270	274
Time from ER Arrival to Discharge (minutes)	394	128	127	134
Time in ER Before Being Evaluated (minutes)	410	33	26	26
Time to Pain Meds for Fractures (minutes)	279	43	57	57
Heart Attack Care				
Aspirin Given at Discharge[2]	298	99%	99%	99%
Fibrinolytic Meds Within 30 Min. of Arrival[2,7]	-	-	49%	54%
PCI Within 90 Minutes of Arrival[2]	50	100%	95%	96%
Statin Prescribed at Discharge[2]	292	99%	98%	98%
Heart Failure Care				
ACE Inhibitor or ARB for LVSD[2]	115	92%	97%	97%
Discharge Instructions Given[2]	262	94%	95%	94%
Evaluation of LVS Function[2]	316	100%	99%	99%
Medicare Spending				
Medicare Spending per Patient (ratio)	-	1.00	1.03	0.98
Pneumonia Care				
Appropriate Initial Antibiotic Given[2]	106	100%	95%	95%
Blood Culture Timing[2]	195	99%	98%	98%
Pregnancy and Delivery Care				
Newborn Deliveries Scheduled Early[2]	56	2%	7%	6%
Preventive Care				
Immunization for Influenza[2]	553	94%	90%	90%
Immunization for Pneumonia[2]	691	93%	92%	92%
Stroke Care				
Anticoagulation Therapy for Atrial Fibrillation	49	96%	96%	95%
Antithrombotic Therapy Timing	287	100%	98%	98%
Assessed for Rehabilitation	359	97%	98%	97%
Discharged on Antithrombotic Therapy	326	99%	99%	99%
Discharged on Statin Medication	257	92%	95%	94%
Thrombolytic Therapy Timing	17	94%	68%	66%
Venous Thromboembolism Prophylaxis	350	98%	94%	94%
Written Stroke Educational Materials Given	193	96%	92%	88%
Surgical Care Improvement Project				
Appropriate Beta Blocker Usage[2]	183	98%	98%	98%
Appropriate VTP Within 24 Hours[2]	404	99%	98%	98%
Controlled Postoperative Blood Glucose[2]	113	93%	96%	97%
Perioperative Temperature Management[2]	499	100%	100%	100%
Prophylactic Antibiotic Selection[2]	399	99%	99%	99%
Prophylactic Antibiotic Selection (Outpatient)	466	99%	98%	98%
Prophylactic Antibiotic Stopped[2]	393	98%	98%	98%
Prophylactic Antibiotic Timing[2]	402	99%	99%	99%
Prophylactic Antibiotic Timing (Outpatient)	467	99%	98%	98%
Urinary Catheter Removal[2]	335	97%	98%	97%
Survey of Patients' Hospital Experiences				
Area Around Room 'Always' Quiet at Night	300+	70%	68%	61%
Doctors 'Always' Communicated Well	300+	82%	83%	82%
Home Recovery Information Given	300+	87%	85%	85%
Hospital Given 9 or 10 on 10 Point Scale	300+	71%	73%	71%
Meds 'Always' Explained Before Given	300+	66%	66%	64%
Nurses 'Always' Communicated Well	300+	78%	80%	79%
Pain 'Always' Well Controlled	300+	70%	72%	71%
Room and Bathroom 'Always' Clean	300+	71%	75%	73%
Timely Help 'Always' Received	300+	65%	69%	68%
Would Definitely Recommend Hospital	300+	75%	73%	71%
Use of Medical Imaging				
Cardiac Imaging Stress Test before Surgery	483	3.9%	5.3%	5.3%
Combination Abdominal CT Scan	1,299	11.0%	16.4%	10.5%
Combination Brain/Sinus CT Scan	1,309	1.1%	2.7%	2.7%
Combination Chest CT Scan	641	6.6%	5.6%	2.7%
Follow-up Mammogram/Ultrasound	2,278	7.3%	7.9%	8.8%
Lumbar Spine MRI for Low Back Pain	136	41.9%	39.6%	37.2%

Longview Regional Medical Center

2901 N Fourth St
Longview, TX 75605
Phone: 903-758-1818
Fax: 903-758-5167
URL: www.longviewregional.com
Type: Acute Care Hospitals
Emergency Services: Yes
Ownership: Proprietary
Beds: 164

Key Personnel:

Pediatrics. . . . . Kristi Bagnell, MD
Pulmonary Disease . . . . Gautam Baskaran, MD
Radiology. . . . . Scott G Bryk
CEO/President. . . . . Allyn R Harris

Measure	Cases	This Hosp.	State Avg.	U.S. Avg.
Blood Clot Prevention and Treatment				
Anticoagulation Overlap Therapy[2]	49	100%	93%	93%
ICU Venous Thromboembolism Prophylaxis[2]	91	100%	92%	92%
Incidence of Potentially Preventable VTE[1,2]	-	-	9%	10%
UFH with Dosages/Platelet Monitoring[1,2]	-	-	96%	97%
Venous Thromboembolism Prophylaxis[2]	428	96%	82%	85%
Warfarin Therapy Discharge Instructions[2]	32	100%	84%	75%
Chest Pain/Possible Heart Attack Care				
Aspirin Given Within 24 Hours of Arrival[1,3]	-	-	94%	96%
Fibrinolytic Meds Within 30 Min. of Arrival[5]	-	-	47%	58%
Average Time to ECG (minutes)[1,3]	-	-	8	7
Average Time to Transfer (minutes)[5]	-	-	62	60
Children's Asthma Care				
Received Home Management Plan of Care	-	-	93%	88%
Received Reliever Medication	-	-	100%	100%
Received Systemic Corticosteroids	-	-	100%	100%
Emergency Department				
Admittance Decision Time (minutes)[2]	465	55	99	98
Head CT Results Within 45 Min. of Arrival[1]	-	-	54%	57%
Patients Who Left ER Before Being Seen	31,728	1%	3%	2%
Time from ER Arrival to Admit. (minutes)[2]	493	234	270	274
Time from ER Arrival to Discharge (minutes)	393	141	127	134
Time in ER Before Being Evaluated (minutes)	407	15	26	26
Time to Pain Meds for Fractures (minutes)	96	56	57	57
Heart Attack Care				
Aspirin Given at Discharge	130	100%	99%	99%
Fibrinolytic Meds Within 30 Min. of Arrival[7]	-	-	49%	54%
PCI Within 90 Minutes of Arrival	23	96%	95%	96%
Statin Prescribed at Discharge	120	99%	98%	98%
Heart Failure Care				
ACE Inhibitor or ARB for LVSD	41	100%	97%	97%
Discharge Instructions Given	117	100%	95%	94%
Evaluation of LVS Function	147	100%	99%	99%
Medicare Spending				
Medicare Spending per Patient (ratio)	-	0.99	1.03	0.98
Pneumonia Care				
Appropriate Initial Antibiotic Given	99	97%	95%	95%
Blood Culture Timing	155	97%	98%	98%
Pregnancy and Delivery Care				
Newborn Deliveries Scheduled Early[2]	18	17%	7%	6%
Preventive Care				
Immunization for Influenza[2]	579	100%	90%	90%
Immunization for Pneumonia[2]	674	99%	92%	92%
Stroke Care				
Anticoagulation Therapy for Atrial Fibrillation	13	100%	96%	95%
Antithrombotic Therapy Timing	44	100%	98%	98%
Assessed for Rehabilitation	50	100%	98%	97%
Discharged on Antithrombotic Therapy	47	100%	99%	99%
Discharged on Statin Medication	29	93%	95%	94%
Thrombolytic Therapy Timing[1]	-	-	68%	66%
Venous Thromboembolism Prophylaxis	50	96%	94%	94%
Written Stroke Educational Materials Given	30	97%	92%	88%
Surgical Care Improvement Project				
Appropriate Beta Blocker Usage	259	99%	98%	98%
Appropriate VTP Within 24 Hours	526	99%	98%	98%
Controlled Postoperative Blood Glucose	111	99%	96%	97%
Perioperative Temperature Management	750	100%	100%	100%
Prophylactic Antibiotic Selection	559	98%	99%	99%
Prophylactic Antibiotic Selection (Outpatient)	386	99%	98%	98%
Prophylactic Antibiotic Stopped	536	99%	98%	98%
Prophylactic Antibiotic Timing	559	99%	99%	99%

NOTE: Hospital profiles are in alphabetical order by state, then city, then hospital within the city; Rankings exclude hospitals with less than 25 cases except for patient surveys which excludes hospitals with less than 100 cases; (a) 100-299 cases; (1) The number of cases/patients is too few to report; (2) Data submitted were based on a sample of cases/patients; (3) Results are based on a shorter time period than required; (4) Data suppressed by CMS for one or more quarters; (5) Results are not available for this reporting period; (6) Fewer than 100 patients completed the HCAHPS survey; (7) No cases met the criteria for this measure; (8) The lower limit of the confidence interval cannot be calculated if the number of observed infections equals zero; (9) No data are available from the state/territory for this reporting period; (10) The scores shown reflect fewer than 50 completed surveys; (11) There were discrepancies in the data collection process; (12) This measure does not apply to this hospital for this reporting period; (13) Results cannot be calculated for this reporting period; (14) The results for this state are combined with nearby states to protect confidentiality; Please refer to the User's Guide for a full explanation of data.

Prophylactic Antibiotic Timing (Outpatient)	387	99%	98%	98%
Urinary Catheter Removal	375	99%	98%	97%
Survey of Patients' Hospital Experiences				
Area Around Room 'Always' Quiet at Night	300+	66%	68%	61%
Doctors 'Always' Communicated Well	300+	83%	83%	82%
Home Recovery Information Given	300+	88%	85%	85%
Hospital Given 9 or 10 on 10 Point Scale	300+	73%	73%	71%
Meds 'Always' Explained Before Given	300+	64%	66%	64%
Nurses 'Always' Communicated Well	300+	78%	80%	79%
Pain 'Always' Well Controlled	300+	70%	72%	71%
Room and Bathroom 'Always' Clean	300+	77%	75%	73%
Timely Help 'Always' Received	300+	66%	69%	68%
Would Definitely Recommend Hospital	300+	75%	73%	71%
Use of Medical Imaging				
Cardiac Imaging Stress Test before Surgery	114	6.1%	5.3%	5.3%
Combination Abdominal CT Scan	584	9.1%	16.4%	10.5%
Combination Brain/Sinus CT Scan	720	0.4%	2.7%	2.7%
Combination Chest CT Scan	664	0.6%	5.6%	2.7%
Follow-up Mammogram/Ultrasound[7]	-	-	7.9%	8.8%
Lumbar Spine MRI for Low Back Pain	201	40.3%	39.6%	37.2%

Covenant Medical Center

3615 19th Street
Lubbock, TX 79410
Phone: 806-725-6000
Fax: 806-723-6289
URL: www.covenanthealth.org
Type: Acute Care Hospitals
Emergency Services: Yes
Ownership: Voluntary non-profit - Church
Beds: 920

Key Personnel:

Emergency Room . . . . Karen Baggerly
CEO/President. . . . . Steven L Hunter
Infection Control. . . . . Clark Kerr
Intensive Care Unit. . . . . Susan Sayari

Measure	Cases	This Hosp.	State Avg.	U.S. Avg.
Blood Clot Prevention and Treatment				
Anticoagulation Overlap Therapy[2]	164	94%	93%	93%
ICU Venous Thromboembolism Prophylaxis[2]	103	79%	92%	92%
Incidence of Potentially Preventable VTE[2]	48	19%	9%	10%
UFH with Dosages/Platelet Monitoring[1,2]	-	-	96%	97%
Venous Thromboembolism Prophylaxis[2]	307	71%	82%	85%
Warfarin Therapy Discharge Instructions[2]	113	89%	84%	75%
Chest Pain/Possible Heart Attack Care				
Aspirin Given Within 24 Hours of Arrival[1,3]	-	-	94%	96%
Fibrinolytic Meds Within 30 Min. of Arrival[5]	-	-	47%	58%
Average Time to ECG (minutes)[1,3]	-	-	8	7
Average Time to Transfer (minutes)[5]	-	-	62	60
Children's Asthma Care				
Received Home Management Plan of Care	-	-	93%	88%
Received Reliever Medication	-	-	100%	100%
Received Systemic Corticosteroids	-	-	100%	100%
Emergency Department				
Admittance Decision Time (minutes)[2]	586	104	99	98
Head CT Results Within 45 Min. of Arrival[1]	-	-	54%	57%
Patients Who Left ER Before Being Seen	64,104	3%	3%	2%
Time from ER Arrival to Admit. (minutes)[2]	610	278	270	274
Time from ER Arrival to Discharge (minutes)	539	159	127	134
Time in ER Before Being Evaluated (minutes)	568	27	26	26
Time to Pain Meds for Fractures (minutes)	111	91	57	57
Heart Attack Care				
Aspirin Given at Discharge	654	99%	99%	99%
Fibrinolytic Meds Within 30 Min. of Arrival[7]	-	-	49%	54%
PCI Within 90 Minutes of Arrival	48	98%	95%	96%
Statin Prescribed at Discharge	613	99%	98%	98%
Heart Failure Care				
ACE Inhibitor or ARB for LVSD	161	98%	97%	97%
Discharge Instructions Given	468	97%	95%	94%
Evaluation of LVS Function	587	99%	99%	99%
Medicare Spending				
Medicare Spending per Patient (ratio)	-	1.01	1.03	0.98
Pneumonia Care				
Appropriate Initial Antibiotic Given	314	95%	95%	95%
Blood Culture Timing	499	97%	98%	98%
Pregnancy and Delivery Care				
Newborn Deliveries Scheduled Early[2]	55	31%	7%	6%
Preventive Care				
Immunization for Influenza[2]	601	95%	90%	90%
Immunization for Pneumonia[2]	786	91%	92%	92%
Stroke Care				
Anticoagulation Therapy for Atrial Fibrillation	11	91%	96%	95%
Antithrombotic Therapy Timing	184	97%	98%	98%
Assessed for Rehabilitation	281	97%	98%	97%
Discharged on Antithrombotic Therapy	217	94%	99%	99%
Discharged on Statin Medication	171	88%	95%	94%
Thrombolytic Therapy Timing	18	61%	68%	66%
Venous Thromboembolism Prophylaxis	297	91%	94%	94%
Written Stroke Educational Materials Given	141	99%	92%	88%
Surgical Care Improvement Project				
Appropriate Beta Blocker Usage	890	96%	98%	98%
Appropriate VTP Within 24 Hours	2,285	98%	98%	98%
Controlled Postoperative Blood Glucose	255	97%	96%	97%
Perioperative Temperature Management	2,760	100%	100%	100%
Prophylactic Antibiotic Selection	1,786	98%	99%	99%
Prophylactic Antibiotic Selection (Outpatient)	744	98%	98%	98%
Prophylactic Antibiotic Stopped	1,754	95%	98%	98%
Prophylactic Antibiotic Timing	1,788	98%	99%	99%
Prophylactic Antibiotic Timing (Outpatient)	754	97%	98%	98%
Urinary Catheter Removal	1,520	96%	98%	97%
Survey of Patients' Hospital Experiences				
Area Around Room 'Always' Quiet at Night	300+	64%	68%	61%
Doctors 'Always' Communicated Well	300+	82%	83%	82%
Home Recovery Information Given	300+	87%	85%	85%
Hospital Given 9 or 10 on 10 Point Scale	300+	77%	73%	71%
Meds 'Always' Explained Before Given	300+	67%	66%	64%
Nurses 'Always' Communicated Well	300+	80%	80%	79%
Pain 'Always' Well Controlled	300+	73%	72%	71%
Room and Bathroom 'Always' Clean	300+	70%	75%	73%
Timely Help 'Always' Received	300+	68%	69%	68%
Would Definitely Recommend Hospital	300+	77%	73%	71%
Use of Medical Imaging				
Cardiac Imaging Stress Test before Surgery	225	5.8%	5.3%	5.3%
Combination Abdominal CT Scan	1,279	31.3%	16.4%	10.5%
Combination Brain/Sinus CT Scan	1,080	3.3%	2.7%	2.7%
Combination Chest CT Scan	1,088	2.6%	5.6%	2.7%
Follow-up Mammogram/Ultrasound	2,412	8.2%	7.9%	8.8%
Lumbar Spine MRI for Low Back Pain[1]	-	-	39.6%	37.2%

Grace Medical Center

2412 50th St
Lubbock, TX 79412
Phone: 806-788-4100
Fax: 806-788-4278
URL: www.highlandcommunityhospital.com
Type: Acute Care Hospitals
Emergency Services: Yes
Ownership: Proprietary
Beds: 123

Key Personnel:

Chief of Medical Staff. . . . . Weldon L Ash, MD
CEO/President. . . . . Doak Enabnit
Coronary Care . . . . Rosemary Hernandez, RN
Emergency Room . . . . Charles II, RN

Measure	Cases	This Hosp.	State Avg.	U.S. Avg.
Blood Clot Prevention and Treatment				
Anticoagulation Overlap Therapy[1]	-	-	93%	93%
ICU Venous Thromboembolism Prophylaxis	18	100%	92%	92%
Incidence of Potentially Preventable VTE[7]	-	-	9%	10%
UFH with Dosages/Platelet Monitoring[1]	-	-	96%	97%
Venous Thromboembolism Prophylaxis	232	94%	82%	85%
Warfarin Therapy Discharge Instructions[1]	-	-	84%	75%
Chest Pain/Possible Heart Attack Care				
Aspirin Given Within 24 Hours of Arrival[1]	-	-	94%	96%
Fibrinolytic Meds Within 30 Min. of Arrival[1]	-	-	47%	58%
Average Time to ECG (minutes)[1]	-	-	8	7
Average Time to Transfer (minutes)[1]	-	-	62	60
Children's Asthma Care				
Received Home Management Plan of Care	-	-	93%	88%
Received Reliever Medication	-	-	100%	100%
Received Systemic Corticosteroids	-	-	100%	100%
Emergency Department				
Admittance Decision Time (minutes)	115	55	99	98
Head CT Results Within 45 Min. of Arrival[1,3]	-	-	54%	57%
Patients Who Left ER Before Being Seen	11,305	3%	3%	2%
Time from ER Arrival to Admit. (minutes)	120	232	270	274
Time from ER Arrival to Discharge (minutes)	10,336	92	127	134
Time in ER Before Being Evaluated (minutes)	10,588	40	26	26
Time to Pain Meds for Fractures (minutes)	24	84	57	57
Heart Attack Care				
Aspirin Given at Discharge[5]	-	-	99%	99%
Fibrinolytic Meds Within 30 Min. of Arrival[5]	-	-	49%	54%
PCI Within 90 Minutes of Arrival[5]	-	-	95%	96%
Statin Prescribed at Discharge[5]	-	-	98%	98%
Heart Failure Care				
ACE Inhibitor or ARB for LVSD[7]	-	-	97%	97%
Discharge Instructions Given[1]	-	-	95%	94%
Evaluation of LVS Function[1]	-	-	99%	99%
Medicare Spending				
Medicare Spending per Patient (ratio)	-	1.01	1.03	0.98
Pneumonia Care				
Appropriate Initial Antibiotic Given	13	77%	95%	95%
Blood Culture Timing	15	100%	98%	98%
Pregnancy and Delivery Care				
Newborn Deliveries Scheduled Early[7]	-	-	7%	6%
Preventive Care				
Immunization for Influenza	456	95%	90%	90%
Immunization for Pneumonia	577	97%	92%	92%
Stroke Care				
Anticoagulation Therapy for Atrial Fibrillation[1,3]	-	-	96%	95%
Antithrombotic Therapy Timing[1,3]	-	-	98%	98%
Assessed for Rehabilitation[1,3]	-	-	98%	97%
Discharged on Antithrombotic Therapy[1,3]	-	-	99%	99%
Discharged on Statin Medication[1,3]	-	-	95%	94%
Thrombolytic Therapy Timing[3,7]	-	-	68%	66%
Venous Thromboembolism Prophylaxis[1,3]	-	-	94%	94%
Written Stroke Educational Materials Given[3,7]	-	-	92%	88%
Surgical Care Improvement Project				
Appropriate Beta Blocker Usage	77	94%	98%	98%
Appropriate VTP Within 24 Hours	309	99%	98%	98%
Controlled Postoperative Blood Glucose[7]	-	-	96%	97%
Perioperative Temperature Management	326	100%	100%	100%
Prophylactic Antibiotic Selection	268	99%	99%	99%
Prophylactic Antibiotic Selection (Outpatient)	264	98%	98%	98%
Prophylactic Antibiotic Stopped	267	97%	98%	98%
Prophylactic Antibiotic Timing	270	96%	99%	99%
Prophylactic Antibiotic Timing (Outpatient)	267	98%	98%	98%
Urinary Catheter Removal	16	100%	98%	97%
Survey of Patients' Hospital Experiences				
Area Around Room 'Always' Quiet at Night	300+	70%	68%	61%
Doctors 'Always' Communicated Well	300+	87%	83%	82%
Home Recovery Information Given	300+	88%	85%	85%
Hospital Given 9 or 10 on 10 Point Scale	300+	73%	73%	71%
Meds 'Always' Explained Before Given	300+	65%	66%	64%
Nurses 'Always' Communicated Well	300+	76%	80%	79%
Pain 'Always' Well Controlled	300+	69%	72%	71%
Room and Bathroom 'Always' Clean	300+	68%	75%	73%
Timely Help 'Always' Received	300+	68%	69%	68%
Would Definitely Recommend Hospital	300+	75%	73%	71%
Use of Medical Imaging				
Cardiac Imaging Stress Test before Surgery[1]	-	-	5.3%	5.3%
Combination Abdominal CT Scan	353	43.3%	16.4%	10.5%
Combination Brain/Sinus CT Scan	128	7.0%	2.7%	2.7%
Combination Chest CT Scan	113	25.7%	5.6%	2.7%
Follow-up Mammogram/Ultrasound	688	5.5%	7.9%	8.8%
Lumbar Spine MRI for Low Back Pain	105	44.8%	39.6%	37.2%

Lubbock Heart Hospital

4810 North Loop 289
Lubbock, TX 79416
Phone: 806-687-7777
Fax: 806-687-7778
URL: www.lubbockheart.com
Type: Acute Care Hospitals
Emergency Services: Yes
Ownership: Government - Local
Beds: 74

Key Personnel:

Chief of Medical Staff . . . . Evelyn Roney
Patient Relations . . . . Rose Shorey
CEO . . . . Roy Vinson, FACHE

NOTE: Hospital profiles are in alphabetical order by state, then city, then hospital within the city; Rankings exclude hospitals with less than 25 cases except for patient surveys which excludes hospitals with less than 100 cases; (a) 100-299 cases; (1) The number of cases/patients is too few to report; (2) Data submitted were based on a sample of cases/patients; (3) Results are based on a shorter time period than required; (4) Data suppressed by CMS for one or more quarters; (5) Results are not available for this reporting period; (6) Fewer than 100 patients completed the HCAHPS survey; (7) No cases met the criteria for this measure; (8) The lower limit of the confidence interval cannot be calculated if the number of observed infections equals zero; (9) No data are available from the state/territory for this reporting period; (10) The scores shown reflect fewer than 50 completed surveys; (11) There were discrepancies in the data collection process; (12) This measure does not apply to this hospital for this reporting period; (13) Results cannot be calculated for this reporting period; (14) The results for this state are combined with nearby states to protect confidentiality; Please refer to the User's Guide for a full explanation of data.

Measure	Cases	This Hosp.	State Avg.	U.S. Avg.
Blood Clot Prevention and Treatment				
Anticoagulation Overlap Therapy[2]	29	45%	93%	93%
ICU Venous Thromboembolism Prophylaxis[2]	79	73%	92%	92%
Incidence of Potentially Preventable VTE[1,2]	-	-	9%	10%
UFH with Dosages/Platelet Monitoring[1,2]	-	-	96%	97%
Venous Thromboembolism Prophylaxis[2]	224	58%	82%	85%
Warfarin Therapy Discharge Instructions[2]	23	83%	84%	75%
Chest Pain/Possible Heart Attack Care				
Aspirin Given Within 24 Hours of Arrival[5]	-	-	94%	96%
Fibrinolytic Meds Within 30 Min. of Arrival[5]	-	-	47%	58%
Average Time to ECG (minutes)[5]	-	-	8	7
Average Time to Transfer (minutes)[5]	-	-	62	60
Children's Asthma Care				
Received Home Management Plan of Care	-	-	93%	88%
Received Reliever Medication	-	-	100%	100%
Received Systemic Corticosteroids	-	-	100%	100%
Emergency Department				
Admittance Decision Time (minutes)[2]	100	54	99	98
Head CT Results Within 45 Min. of Arrival[5]	-	-	54%	57%
Patients Who Left ER Before Being Seen	4,597	1%	3%	2%
Time from ER Arrival to Admit. (minutes)[2]	202	134	270	274
Time from ER Arrival to Discharge (minutes)	223	119	127	134
Time in ER Before Being Evaluated (minutes)	283	16	26	26
Time to Pain Meds for Fractures (minutes)[1,3]	-	-	57	57
Heart Attack Care				
Aspirin Given at Discharge[2]	176	100%	99%	99%
Fibrinolytic Meds Within 30 Min. of Arrival[2,7]	-	-	49%	54%
PCI Within 90 Minutes of Arrival[1,2]	-	-	95%	96%
Statin Prescribed at Discharge[2]	147	86%	98%	98%
Heart Failure Care				
ACE Inhibitor or ARB for LVSD[2]	81	79%	97%	97%
Discharge Instructions Given[2]	252	92%	95%	94%
Evaluation of LVS Function[2]	275	96%	99%	99%
Medicare Spending				
Medicare Spending per Patient (ratio)	-	0.97	1.03	0.98
Pneumonia Care				
Appropriate Initial Antibiotic Given[2]	21	86%	95%	95%
Blood Culture Timing[2]	34	97%	98%	98%
Pregnancy and Delivery Care				
Newborn Deliveries Scheduled Early[7]	-	-	7%	6%
Preventive Care				
Immunization for Influenza[2]	347	84%	90%	90%
Immunization for Pneumonia[2]	553	84%	92%	92%
Stroke Care				
Anticoagulation Therapy for Atrial Fibrillation[1,2]	-	-	96%	95%
Antithrombotic Therapy Timing[2]	13	85%	98%	98%
Assessed for Rehabilitation[2]	12	50%	98%	97%
Discharged on Antithrombotic Therapy[2]	12	100%	99%	99%
Discharged on Statin Medication[1,2]	-	-	95%	94%
Thrombolytic Therapy Timing[2,7]	-	-	68%	66%
Venous Thromboembolism Prophylaxis[2]	12	67%	94%	94%
Written Stroke Educational Materials Given[1,2]	-	-	92%	88%
Surgical Care Improvement Project				
Appropriate Beta Blocker Usage[2]	146	91%	98%	98%
Appropriate VTP Within 24 Hours[2]	192	97%	98%	98%
Controlled Postoperative Blood Glucose[2]	105	86%	96%	97%
Perioperative Temperature Management[2]	241	95%	100%	100%
Prophylactic Antibiotic Selection[2]	284	98%	99%	99%
Prophylactic Antibiotic Selection (Outpatient)	273	98%	98%	98%
Prophylactic Antibiotic Stopped[2]	281	84%	98%	98%
Prophylactic Antibiotic Timing[2]	284	96%	99%	99%
Prophylactic Antibiotic Timing (Outpatient)	274	99%	98%	98%
Urinary Catheter Removal[2]	221	94%	98%	97%
Survey of Patients' Hospital Experiences				
Area Around Room 'Always' Quiet at Night	300+	68%	68%	61%
Doctors 'Always' Communicated Well	300+	83%	83%	82%
Home Recovery Information Given	300+	85%	85%	85%
Hospital Given 9 or 10 on 10 Point Scale	300+	82%	73%	71%
Meds 'Always' Explained Before Given	300+	65%	66%	64%
Nurses 'Always' Communicated Well	300+	82%	80%	79%
Pain 'Always' Well Controlled	300+	71%	72%	71%
Room and Bathroom 'Always' Clean	300+	72%	75%	73%
Timely Help 'Always' Received	300+	73%	69%	68%
Would Definitely Recommend Hospital	300+	85%	73%	71%
Use of Medical Imaging				
Cardiac Imaging Stress Test before Surgery	230	10.0%	5.3%	5.3%
Combination Abdominal CT Scan	75	34.7%	16.4%	10.5%
Combination Brain/Sinus CT Scan	225	0.9%	2.7%	2.7%
Combination Chest CT Scan	282	6.7%	5.6%	2.7%
Follow-up Mammogram/Ultrasound[7]	-	-	7.9%	8.8%
Lumbar Spine MRI for Low Back Pain[7]	-	-	39.6%	37.2%

Trustpoint Hospital

4302 Princeton
Lubbock, TX 79415
Phone: 806-749-2222
URL: www.trustpointhospital.com
Type: Acute Care Hospitals
Emergency Services: Yes
Ownership: Physician

Measure	Cases	This Hosp.	State Avg.	U.S. Avg.
Blood Clot Prevention and Treatment				
Anticoagulation Overlap Therapy[7]	-	-	93%	93%
ICU Venous Thromboembolism Prophylaxis[7]	-	-	92%	92%
Incidence of Potentially Preventable VTE[7]	-	-	9%	10%
UFH with Dosages/Platelet Monitoring[7]	-	-	96%	97%
Venous Thromboembolism Prophylaxis	184	29%	82%	85%
Warfarin Therapy Discharge Instructions[7]	-	-	84%	75%
Chest Pain/Possible Heart Attack Care				
Aspirin Given Within 24 Hours of Arrival	-	-	94%	96%
Fibrinolytic Meds Within 30 Min. of Arrival	-	-	47%	58%
Average Time to ECG (minutes)	-	-	8	7
Average Time to Transfer (minutes)	-	-	62	60
Children's Asthma Care				
Received Home Management Plan of Care	-	-	93%	88%
Received Reliever Medication	-	-	100%	100%
Received Systemic Corticosteroids	-	-	100%	100%
Emergency Department				
Admittance Decision Time (minutes)[7]	-	-	99	98
Head CT Results Within 45 Min. of Arrival	-	-	54%	57%
Patients Who Left ER Before Being Seen	-	-	3%	2%
Time from ER Arrival to Admit. (minutes)[7]	-	-	270	274
Time from ER Arrival to Discharge (minutes)	-	-	127	134
Time in ER Before Being Evaluated (minutes)	-	-	26	26
Time to Pain Meds for Fractures (minutes)	-	-	57	57
Heart Attack Care				
Aspirin Given at Discharge[5]	-	-	99%	99%
Fibrinolytic Meds Within 30 Min. of Arrival[5]	-	-	49%	54%
PCI Within 90 Minutes of Arrival[5]	-	-	95%	96%
Statin Prescribed at Discharge[5]	-	-	98%	98%
Heart Failure Care				
ACE Inhibitor or ARB for LVSD[5]	-	-	97%	97%
Discharge Instructions Given[5]	-	-	95%	94%
Evaluation of LVS Function[5]	-	-	99%	99%
Medicare Spending				
Medicare Spending per Patient (ratio)[1]	-	-	1.03	0.98
Pneumonia Care				
Appropriate Initial Antibiotic Given[5]	-	-	95%	95%
Blood Culture Timing[5]	-	-	98%	98%
Pregnancy and Delivery Care				
Newborn Deliveries Scheduled Early[7]	-	-	7%	6%
Preventive Care				
Immunization for Influenza	114	36%	90%	90%
Immunization for Pneumonia[2]	221	65%	92%	92%
Stroke Care				
Anticoagulation Therapy for Atrial Fibrillation[5]	-	-	96%	95%
Antithrombotic Therapy Timing[5]	-	-	98%	98%
Assessed for Rehabilitation[5]	-	-	98%	97%
Discharged on Antithrombotic Therapy[5]	-	-	99%	99%
Discharged on Statin Medication[5]	-	-	95%	94%
Thrombolytic Therapy Timing[5]	-	-	68%	66%
Venous Thromboembolism Prophylaxis[5]	-	-	94%	94%
Written Stroke Educational Materials Given[5]	-	-	92%	88%
Surgical Care Improvement Project				
Appropriate Beta Blocker Usage[5]	-	-	98%	98%
Appropriate VTP Within 24 Hours[5]	-	-	98%	98%
Controlled Postoperative Blood Glucose[5]	-	-	96%	97%
Perioperative Temperature Management[5]	-	-	100%	100%
Prophylactic Antibiotic Selection[5]	-	-	99%	99%
Prophylactic Antibiotic Selection (Outpatient)	-	-	98%	98%
Prophylactic Antibiotic Stopped[5]	-	-	98%	98%
Prophylactic Antibiotic Timing[5]	-	-	99%	99%
Prophylactic Antibiotic Timing (Outpatient)	-	-	98%	98%
Urinary Catheter Removal[5]	-	-	98%	97%
Survey of Patients' Hospital Experiences				
Area Around Room 'Always' Quiet at Night[1]	-	-	68%	61%
Doctors 'Always' Communicated Well[1]	-	-	83%	82%
Home Recovery Information Given[1]	-	-	85%	85%
Hospital Given 9 or 10 on 10 Point Scale[1]	-	-	73%	71%
Meds 'Always' Explained Before Given[1]	-	-	66%	64%
Nurses 'Always' Communicated Well[1]	-	-	80%	79%
Pain 'Always' Well Controlled[1]	-	-	72%	71%
Room and Bathroom 'Always' Clean[1]	-	-	75%	73%
Timely Help 'Always' Received[1]	-	-	69%	68%
Would Definitely Recommend Hospital[1]	-	-	73%	71%
Use of Medical Imaging				
Cardiac Imaging Stress Test before Surgery	-	-	5.3%	5.3%
Combination Abdominal CT Scan	-	-	16.4%	10.5%
Combination Brain/Sinus CT Scan	-	-	2.7%	2.7%
Combination Chest CT Scan	-	-	5.6%	2.7%
Follow-up Mammogram/Ultrasound	-	-	7.9%	8.8%
Lumbar Spine MRI for Low Back Pain	-	-	39.6%	37.2%

University Medical Center

602 Indiana Avenue
Lubbock, TX 79415
Phone: 806-775-8200
Fax: 806-775-9220
URL: www.teamumc.org
Type: Acute Care Hospitals
Emergency Services: Yes
Ownership: Govt - Hospital Dist/Auth
Beds: 388

Key Personnel:

CEO/President. . . . . David G Allison
Chief of Medical Staff. . . . . Sylvia Brito
Emergency Room . . . . Fred Hagedorn, MD
Infection Control. . . . . Tim Howell
Pediatric In-Patient Care . . . . Richard Lampe, MD
Anesthesiology. . . . . Gabor Racz, MD
Radiology. . . . . Glenn Roberson, MD
Operating Room. . . . . Lesa Stone

Measure	Cases	This Hosp.	State Avg.	U.S. Avg.
Blood Clot Prevention and Treatment				
Anticoagulation Overlap Therapy[2]	82	100%	93%	93%
ICU Venous Thromboembolism Prophylaxis[2]	147	95%	92%	92%
Incidence of Potentially Preventable VTE[2]	19	0%	9%	10%
UFH with Dosages/Platelet Monitoring[2]	29	100%	96%	97%
Venous Thromboembolism Prophylaxis[2]	294	90%	82%	85%
Warfarin Therapy Discharge Instructions[2]	63	94%	84%	75%
Chest Pain/Possible Heart Attack Care				
Aspirin Given Within 24 Hours of Arrival[5]	-	-	94%	96%
Fibrinolytic Meds Within 30 Min. of Arrival[5]	-	-	47%	58%
Average Time to ECG (minutes)[5]	-	-	8	7
Average Time to Transfer (minutes)[5]	-	-	62	60
Children's Asthma Care				
Received Home Management Plan of Care	-	-	93%	88%
Received Reliever Medication	-	-	100%	100%
Received Systemic Corticosteroids	-	-	100%	100%
Emergency Department				
Admittance Decision Time (minutes)[2]	546	59	99	98
Head CT Results Within 45 Min. of Arrival[1]	-	-	54%	57%
Patients Who Left ER Before Being Seen	>100k	1%	3%	2%
Time from ER Arrival to Admit. (minutes)[2]	557	258	270	274
Time from ER Arrival to Discharge (minutes)	380	180	127	134
Time in ER Before Being Evaluated (minutes)	405	41	26	26
Time to Pain Meds for Fractures (minutes)	274	68	57	57
Heart Attack Care				
Aspirin Given at Discharge	262	100%	99%	99%
Fibrinolytic Meds Within 30 Min. of Arrival[7]	-	-	49%	54%
PCI Within 90 Minutes of Arrival	59	98%	95%	96%
Statin Prescribed at Discharge	269	99%	98%	98%
Heart Failure Care				

NOTE: Hospital profiles are in alphabetical order by state, then city, then hospital within the city; Rankings exclude hospitals with less than 25 cases except for patient surveys which excludes hospitals with less than 100 cases; (a) 100-299 cases; (1) The number of cases/patients is too few to report; (2) Data submitted were based on a sample of cases/patients; (3) Results are based on a shorter time period than required; (4) Data suppressed by CMS for one or more quarters; (5) Results are not available for this reporting period; (6) Fewer than 100 patients completed the HCAHPS survey; (7) No cases met the criteria for this measure; (8) The lower limit of the confidence interval cannot be calculated if the number of observed infections equals zero; (9) No data are available from the state/territory for this reporting period; (10) The scores shown reflect fewer than 50 completed surveys; (11) There were discrepancies in the data collection process; (12) This measure does not apply to this hospital for this reporting period; (13) Results cannot be calculated for this reporting period; (14) The results for this state are combined with nearby states to protect confidentiality; Please refer to the User's Guide for a full explanation of data.

Measure	Cases	This Hosp.	State Avg.	U.S. Avg.
ACE Inhibitor or ARB for LVSD[2]	105	95%	97%	97%
Discharge Instructions Given[2]	220	99%	95%	94%
Evaluation of LVS Function[2]	262	100%	99%	99%
Medicare Spending				
Medicare Spending per Patient (ratio)	-	1.04	1.03	0.98
Pneumonia Care				
Appropriate Initial Antibiotic Given[2]	49	96%	95%	95%
Blood Culture Timing[2]	125	99%	98%	98%
Pregnancy and Delivery Care				
Newborn Deliveries Scheduled Early[2]	60	0%	7%	6%
Preventive Care				
Immunization for Influenza[2]	524	82%	90%	90%
Immunization for Pneumonia[2]	534	86%	92%	92%
Stroke Care				
Anticoagulation Therapy for Atrial Fibrillation	13	92%	96%	95%
Antithrombotic Therapy Timing	135	96%	98%	98%
Assessed for Rehabilitation	187	96%	98%	97%
Discharged on Antithrombotic Therapy	156	97%	99%	99%
Discharged on Statin Medication	132	92%	95%	94%
Thrombolytic Therapy Timing	20	85%	68%	66%
Venous Thromboembolism Prophylaxis	208	80%	94%	94%
Written Stroke Educational Materials Given	109	93%	92%	88%
Surgical Care Improvement Project				
Appropriate Beta Blocker Usage[2]	206	100%	98%	98%
Appropriate VTP Within 24 Hours[2]	381	99%	98%	98%
Controlled Postoperative Blood Glucose[2]	114	100%	96%	97%
Perioperative Temperature Management[2]	519	100%	100%	100%
Prophylactic Antibiotic Selection[2]	400	99%	99%	99%
Prophylactic Antibiotic Selection (Outpatient)	176	99%	98%	98%
Prophylactic Antibiotic Stopped[2]	381	98%	98%	98%
Prophylactic Antibiotic Timing[2]	400	100%	99%	99%
Prophylactic Antibiotic Timing (Outpatient)	176	100%	98%	98%
Urinary Catheter Removal[2]	336	99%	98%	97%
Survey of Patients' Hospital Experiences				
Area Around Room 'Always' Quiet at Night	300+	67%	68%	61%
Doctors 'Always' Communicated Well	300+	82%	83%	82%
Home Recovery Information Given	300+	84%	85%	85%
Hospital Given 9 or 10 on 10 Point Scale	300+	79%	73%	71%
Meds 'Always' Explained Before Given	300+	73%	66%	64%
Nurses 'Always' Communicated Well	300+	82%	80%	79%
Pain 'Always' Well Controlled	300+	73%	72%	71%
Room and Bathroom 'Always' Clean	300+	74%	75%	73%
Timely Help 'Always' Received	300+	70%	69%	68%
Would Definitely Recommend Hospital	300+	83%	73%	71%
Use of Medical Imaging				
Cardiac Imaging Stress Test before Surgery	529	3.2%	5.3%	5.3%
Combination Abdominal CT Scan	1,236	23.8%	16.4%	10.5%
Combination Brain/Sinus CT Scan	1,156	5.4%	2.7%	2.7%
Combination Chest CT Scan	633	21.6%	5.6%	2.7%
Follow-up Mammogram/Ultrasound	1,155	12.2%	7.9%	8.8%
Lumbar Spine MRI for Low Back Pain	176	51.7%	39.6%	37.2%

Memorial Medical Center of East Texas

1201 West Frank Street
Lufkin, TX 75901
URL: www.mymemorialhealth.org
Type: Acute Care Hospitals
Ownership: Voluntary non-profit - Private
Phone: 936-634-8111
Fax: 936-639-7004
Emergency Services: Yes
Beds: 234

Key Personnel:

Quality Assurance . . . . Tammy Butler
Radiology. . . . . Darwin Clark, MD
Operating Room. . . . . Mel Cole
Pediatric Ambulatory Care . . . . . . George Fidons, MD
Pediatric In-Patient Care . . . . George Fidons, MD
CEO/President. . . . . Bryant Krenek
Chief of Medical Staff. . . . . Jerry Robbins, MD
Emergency Room . . . . Norma Sanford

Measure	Cases	This Hosp.	State Avg.	U.S. Avg.
Blood Clot Prevention and Treatment				
Anticoagulation Overlap Therapy[2]	47	96%	93%	93%
ICU Venous Thromboembolism Prophylaxis[2]	93	90%	92%	92%
Incidence of Potentially Preventable VTE[1,2]	-	-	9%	10%
UFH with Dosages/Platelet Monitoring[2]	52	100%	96%	97%
Venous Thromboembolism Prophylaxis[2]	340	73%	82%	85%
Warfarin Therapy Discharge Instructions[2]	34	88%	84%	75%
Chest Pain/Possible Heart Attack Care				
Aspirin Given Within 24 Hours of Arrival[1,3]	-	-	94%	96%
Fibrinolytic Meds Within 30 Min. of Arrival[3,7]	-	-	47%	58%
Average Time to ECG (minutes)[1,3]	-	-	8	7
Average Time to Transfer (minutes)[3,7]	-	-	62	60
Children's Asthma Care				
Received Home Management Plan of Care	-	-	93%	88%
Received Reliever Medication	-	-	100%	100%
Received Systemic Corticosteroids	-	-	100%	100%
Emergency Department				
Admittance Decision Time (minutes)[2]	387	119	99	98
Head CT Results Within 45 Min. of Arrival[1]	-	-	54%	57%
Patients Who Left ER Before Being Seen	38,783	5%	3%	2%
Time from ER Arrival to Admit. (minutes)[2]	415	387	270	274
Time from ER Arrival to Discharge (minutes)	362	178	127	134
Time in ER Before Being Evaluated (minutes)	343	55	26	26
Time to Pain Meds for Fractures (minutes)	110	88	57	57
Heart Attack Care				
Aspirin Given at Discharge[2]	243	98%	99%	99%
Fibrinolytic Meds Within 30 Min. of Arrival[2,7]	-	-	49%	54%
PCI Within 90 Minutes of Arrival[2]	29	86%	95%	96%
Statin Prescribed at Discharge[2]	237	96%	98%	98%
Heart Failure Care				
ACE Inhibitor or ARB for LVSD[2]	92	93%	97%	97%
Discharge Instructions Given[2]	185	96%	95%	94%
Evaluation of LVS Function[2]	230	100%	99%	99%
Medicare Spending				
Medicare Spending per Patient (ratio)	-	1.02	1.03	0.98
Pneumonia Care				
Appropriate Initial Antibiotic Given[2]	71	96%	95%	95%
Blood Culture Timing[2]	100	97%	98%	98%
Pregnancy and Delivery Care				
Newborn Deliveries Scheduled Early[2]	112	23%	7%	6%
Preventive Care				
Immunization for Influenza[2]	548	93%	90%	90%
Immunization for Pneumonia[2]	773	88%	92%	92%
Stroke Care				
Anticoagulation Therapy for Atrial Fibrillation	12	83%	96%	95%
Antithrombotic Therapy Timing	116	94%	98%	98%
Assessed for Rehabilitation	143	100%	98%	97%
Discharged on Antithrombotic Therapy	130	99%	99%	99%
Discharged on Statin Medication	96	96%	95%	94%
Thrombolytic Therapy Timing	11	91%	68%	66%
Venous Thromboembolism Prophylaxis	149	97%	94%	94%
Written Stroke Educational Materials Given	63	98%	92%	88%
Surgical Care Improvement Project				
Appropriate Beta Blocker Usage[2]	136	98%	98%	98%
Appropriate VTP Within 24 Hours[2]	220	94%	98%	98%
Controlled Postoperative Blood Glucose[2]	60	90%	96%	97%
Perioperative Temperature Management[2]	295	100%	100%	100%
Prophylactic Antibiotic Selection[2]	238	95%	99%	99%
Prophylactic Antibiotic Selection (Outpatient)	219	92%	98%	98%
Prophylactic Antibiotic Stopped[2]	226	94%	98%	98%
Prophylactic Antibiotic Timing[2]	238	100%	99%	99%
Prophylactic Antibiotic Timing (Outpatient)	219	98%	98%	98%
Urinary Catheter Removal[2]	243	92%	98%	97%
Survey of Patients' Hospital Experiences				
Area Around Room 'Always' Quiet at Night	300+	69%	68%	61%
Doctors 'Always' Communicated Well	300+	82%	83%	82%
Home Recovery Information Given	300+	86%	85%	85%
Hospital Given 9 or 10 on 10 Point Scale	300+	73%	73%	71%
Meds 'Always' Explained Before Given	300+	64%	66%	64%
Nurses 'Always' Communicated Well	300+	77%	80%	79%
Pain 'Always' Well Controlled	300+	70%	72%	71%
Room and Bathroom 'Always' Clean	300+	71%	75%	73%
Timely Help 'Always' Received	300+	62%	69%	68%
Would Definitely Recommend Hospital	300+	75%	73%	71%
Use of Medical Imaging				
Cardiac Imaging Stress Test before Surgery	344	4.1%	5.3%	5.3%
Combination Abdominal CT Scan	606	59.1%	16.4%	10.5%
Combination Brain/Sinus CT Scan	760	5.0%	2.7%	2.7%
Combination Chest CT Scan	375	0.3%	5.6%	2.7%
Follow-up Mammogram/Ultrasound	1,700	7.0%	7.9%	8.8%
Lumbar Spine MRI for Low Back Pain	221	42.1%	39.6%	37.2%

Woodland Heights Medical Center

505 South John Redditt Drive
Lufkin, TX 75904
URL: www.woodlandheights.net
Type: Acute Care Hospitals
Ownership: Proprietary
Phone: 936-634-8311
Fax: 936-637-8600
Emergency Services: Yes
Beds: 146

Key Personnel:

Radiology. . . . . Glenn M Davis, MD
Pediatric Ambulatory Care . . . . . . George Fidone, MD
Pediatric In-Patient Care . . . . George Fidone, MD
Operating Room. . . . . Ruth S George, RN
CEO/President. . . . . Lance Jones
Quality Assurance . . . . Sam Price
Chief of Medical Staff. . . . . Martha Russell, MD
Infection Control. . . . . Doris Weatherford, RN

Measure	Cases	This Hosp.	State Avg.	U.S. Avg.
Blood Clot Prevention and Treatment				
Anticoagulation Overlap Therapy[2]	30	100%	93%	93%
ICU Venous Thromboembolism Prophylaxis[2]	98	100%	92%	92%
Incidence of Potentially Preventable VTE[1,2]	-	-	9%	10%
UFH with Dosages/Platelet Monitoring[2]	24	100%	96%	97%
Venous Thromboembolism Prophylaxis[2]	322	100%	82%	85%
Warfarin Therapy Discharge Instructions[2]	22	100%	84%	75%
Chest Pain/Possible Heart Attack Care				
Aspirin Given Within 24 Hours of Arrival[5]	-	-	94%	96%
Fibrinolytic Meds Within 30 Min. of Arrival[5]	-	-	47%	58%
Average Time to ECG (minutes)[5]	-	-	8	7
Average Time to Transfer (minutes)[5]	-	-	62	60
Children's Asthma Care				
Received Home Management Plan of Care	-	-	93%	88%
Received Reliever Medication	-	-	100%	100%
Received Systemic Corticosteroids	-	-	100%	100%
Emergency Department				
Admittance Decision Time (minutes)[2]	498	68	99	98
Head CT Results Within 45 Min. of Arrival[1]	-	-	54%	57%
Patients Who Left ER Before Being Seen	17,231	1%	3%	2%
Time from ER Arrival to Admit. (minutes)[2]	508	228	270	274
Time from ER Arrival to Discharge (minutes)	381	150	127	134
Time in ER Before Being Evaluated (minutes)	403	25	26	26
Time to Pain Meds for Fractures (minutes)	80	86	57	57
Heart Attack Care				
Aspirin Given at Discharge	83	100%	99%	99%
Fibrinolytic Meds Within 30 Min. of Arrival[7]	-	-	49%	54%
PCI Within 90 Minutes of Arrival[1]	-	-	95%	96%
Statin Prescribed at Discharge	76	100%	98%	98%
Heart Failure Care				
ACE Inhibitor or ARB for LVSD	53	100%	97%	97%
Discharge Instructions Given	113	98%	95%	94%
Evaluation of LVS Function	160	100%	99%	99%
Medicare Spending				
Medicare Spending per Patient (ratio)	-	0.97	1.03	0.98
Pneumonia Care				
Appropriate Initial Antibiotic Given	57	100%	95%	95%
Blood Culture Timing	92	99%	98%	98%
Pregnancy and Delivery Care				
Newborn Deliveries Scheduled Early[2]	47	0%	7%	6%
Preventive Care				
Immunization for Influenza[2]	526	100%	90%	90%
Immunization for Pneumonia[2]	666	100%	92%	92%
Stroke Care				
Anticoagulation Therapy for Atrial Fibrillation[1]	-	-	96%	95%
Antithrombotic Therapy Timing	39	100%	98%	98%
Assessed for Rehabilitation	44	100%	98%	97%
Discharged on Antithrombotic Therapy	41	100%	99%	99%
Discharged on Statin Medication	31	100%	95%	94%
Thrombolytic Therapy Timing[1]	-	-	68%	66%
Venous Thromboembolism Prophylaxis	43	100%	94%	94%
Written Stroke Educational Materials Given	25	96%	92%	88%
Surgical Care Improvement Project				
Appropriate Beta Blocker Usage	195	100%	98%	98%

NOTE: Hospital profiles are in alphabetical order by state, then city, then hospital within the city; Rankings exclude hospitals with less than 25 cases except for patient surveys which excludes hospitals with less than 100 cases; (a) 100-299 cases; (1) The number of cases/patients is too few to report; (2) Data submitted were based on a sample of cases/patients; (3) Results are based on a shorter time period than required; (4) Data suppressed by CMS for one or more quarters; (5) Results are not available for this reporting period; (6) Fewer than 100 patients completed the HCAHPS survey; (7) No cases met the criteria for this measure; (8) The lower limit of the confidence interval cannot be calculated if the number of observed infections equals zero; (9) No data are available from the state/territory for this reporting period; (10) The scores shown reflect fewer than 50 completed surveys; (11) There were discrepancies in the data collection process; (12) This measure does not apply to this hospital for this reporting period; (13) Results cannot be calculated for this reporting period; (14) The results for this state are combined with nearby states to protect confidentiality; Please refer to the User's Guide for a full explanation of data.

Measure	Cases	This Hosp.	State Avg.	U.S. Avg.
Appropriate VTP Within 24 Hours	371	100%	98%	98%
Controlled Postoperative Blood Glucose	57	91%	96%	97%
Perioperative Temperature Management	438	100%	100%	100%
Prophylactic Antibiotic Selection	245	100%	99%	99%
Prophylactic Antibiotic Selection (Outpatient)	152	100%	98%	98%
Prophylactic Antibiotic Stopped	224	100%	98%	98%
Prophylactic Antibiotic Timing	246	100%	99%	99%
Prophylactic Antibiotic Timing (Outpatient)	152	100%	98%	98%
Urinary Catheter Removal	331	100%	98%	97%
Survey of Patients' Hospital Experiences				
Area Around Room 'Always' Quiet at Night	300+	70%	68%	61%
Doctors 'Always' Communicated Well	300+	83%	83%	82%
Home Recovery Information Given	300+	87%	85%	85%
Hospital Given 9 or 10 on 10 Point Scale	300+	78%	73%	71%
Meds 'Always' Explained Before Given	300+	67%	66%	64%
Nurses 'Always' Communicated Well	300+	81%	80%	79%
Pain 'Always' Well Controlled	300+	73%	72%	71%
Room and Bathroom 'Always' Clean	300+	75%	75%	73%
Timely Help 'Always' Received	300+	74%	69%	68%
Would Definitely Recommend Hospital	300+	79%	73%	71%
Use of Medical Imaging				
Cardiac Imaging Stress Test before Surgery[1]	-	-	5.3%	5.3%
Combination Abdominal CT Scan	353	8.2%	16.4%	10.5%
Combination Brain/Sinus CT Scan	465	4.5%	2.7%	2.7%
Combination Chest CT Scan	256	0.8%	5.6%	2.7%
Follow-up Mammogram/Ultrasound	631	10.3%	7.9%	8.8%
Lumbar Spine MRI for Low Back Pain	91	47.3%	39.6%	37.2%

Seton Edgar B Davis Hospital

130 Hays Street
Luling, TX 78648
Phone: 830-875-7000
Fax: 830-875-7053
URL: www.seton.net
Type: Critical Access Hospitals
Emergency Services: Yes
Ownership: Voluntary non-profit - Private
Beds: 25

Key Personnel:
Radiology. . . . . Joshua Abramowitz
Quality Assurance . . . . James K Beckmann, Jr
Emergency Room . . . . Bertha Curtis
CEO/President. . . . . Jesus Garza

Measure	Cases	This Hosp.	State Avg.	U.S. Avg.
Blood Clot Prevention and Treatment				
Anticoagulation Overlap Therapy[5]	-	-	93%	93%
ICU Venous Thromboembolism Prophylaxis[5]	-	-	92%	92%
Incidence of Potentially Preventable VTE[5]	-	-	9%	10%
UFH with Dosages/Platelet Monitoring[5]	-	-	96%	97%
Venous Thromboembolism Prophylaxis[5]	-	-	82%	85%
Warfarin Therapy Discharge Instructions[5]	-	-	84%	75%
Chest Pain/Possible Heart Attack Care				
Aspirin Given Within 24 Hours of Arrival[5]	-	-	94%	96%
Fibrinolytic Meds Within 30 Min. of Arrival[5]	-	-	47%	58%
Average Time to ECG (minutes)[5]	-	-	8	7
Average Time to Transfer (minutes)[5]	-	-	62	60
Children's Asthma Care				
Received Home Management Plan of Care	-	-	93%	88%
Received Reliever Medication	-	-	100%	100%
Received Systemic Corticosteroids	-	-	100%	100%
Emergency Department				
Admittance Decision Time (minutes)[5]	-	-	99	98
Head CT Results Within 45 Min. of Arrival[5]	-	-	54%	57%
Patients Who Left ER Before Being Seen[5]	-	-	3%	2%
Time from ER Arrival to Admit. (minutes)[5]	-	-	270	274
Time from ER Arrival to Discharge (minutes)[5]	-	-	127	134
Time in ER Before Being Evaluated (minutes)[5]	-	-	26	26
Time to Pain Meds for Fractures (minutes)[5]	-	-	57	57
Heart Attack Care				
Aspirin Given at Discharge[7]	-	-	99%	99%
Fibrinolytic Meds Within 30 Min. of Arrival[7]	-	-	49%	54%
PCI Within 90 Minutes of Arrival[7]	-	-	95%	96%
Statin Prescribed at Discharge[7]	-	-	98%	98%
Heart Failure Care				
ACE Inhibitor or ARB for LVSD[1]	-	-	97%	97%
Discharge Instructions Given	30	100%	95%	94%
Evaluation of LVS Function	37	100%	99%	99%
Medicare Spending				
Medicare Spending per Patient (ratio)	-	-	1.03	0.98
Pneumonia Care				
Appropriate Initial Antibiotic Given	38	100%	95%	95%
Blood Culture Timing	52	98%	98%	98%
Pregnancy and Delivery Care				
Newborn Deliveries Scheduled Early[5]	-	-	7%	6%
Preventive Care				
Immunization for Influenza[5]	-	-	90%	90%
Immunization for Pneumonia[5]	-	-	92%	92%
Stroke Care				
Anticoagulation Therapy for Atrial Fibrillation[5]	-	-	96%	95%
Antithrombotic Therapy Timing[5]	-	-	98%	98%
Assessed for Rehabilitation[5]	-	-	98%	97%
Discharged on Antithrombotic Therapy[5]	-	-	99%	99%
Discharged on Statin Medication[5]	-	-	95%	94%
Thrombolytic Therapy Timing[5]	-	-	68%	66%
Venous Thromboembolism Prophylaxis[5]	-	-	94%	94%
Written Stroke Educational Materials Given[5]	-	-	92%	88%
Surgical Care Improvement Project				
Appropriate Beta Blocker Usage[3,7]	-	-	98%	98%
Appropriate VTP Within 24 Hours[1,3]	-	-	98%	98%
Controlled Postoperative Blood Glucose[5]	-	-	96%	97%
Perioperative Temperature Management[1,3]	-	-	100%	100%
Prophylactic Antibiotic Selection[1,3]	-	-	99%	99%
Prophylactic Antibiotic Selection (Outpatient)[1,3]	-	-	98%	98%
Prophylactic Antibiotic Stopped[1,3]	-	-	98%	98%
Prophylactic Antibiotic Timing[1,3]	-	-	99%	99%
Prophylactic Antibiotic Timing (Outpatient)[1,3]	-	-	98%	98%
Urinary Catheter Removal[3,7]	-	-	98%	97%
Survey of Patients' Hospital Experiences				
Area Around Room 'Always' Quiet at Night	(a)	71%	68%	61%
Doctors 'Always' Communicated Well	(a)	89%	83%	82%
Home Recovery Information Given	(a)	87%	85%	85%
Hospital Given 9 or 10 on 10 Point Scale	(a)	81%	73%	71%
Meds 'Always' Explained Before Given	(a)	76%	66%	64%
Nurses 'Always' Communicated Well	(a)	85%	80%	79%
Pain 'Always' Well Controlled	(a)	76%	72%	71%
Room and Bathroom 'Always' Clean	(a)	79%	75%	73%
Timely Help 'Always' Received	(a)	70%	69%	68%
Would Definitely Recommend Hospital	(a)	81%	73%	71%
Use of Medical Imaging				
Cardiac Imaging Stress Test before Surgery[7]	-	-	5.3%	5.3%
Combination Abdominal CT Scan	311	5.8%	16.4%	10.5%
Combination Brain/Sinus CT Scan[1]	-	-	2.7%	2.7%
Combination Chest CT Scan	228	0.4%	5.6%	2.7%
Follow-up Mammogram/Ultrasound	286	8.4%	7.9%	8.8%
Lumbar Spine MRI for Low Back Pain[1]	-	-	39.6%	37.2%

Madison Saint Joseph Health Center

100 West Cross Street
Madisonville, TX 77864
Phone: 936-348-2631
Fax: 936-348-3404
URL: www.st-joseph.org/madison
Type: Critical Access Hospitals
Emergency Services: Yes
Ownership: Voluntary non-profit - Church
Beds: 15

Key Personnel:
Operating Room. . . . . Richard D Alford
Chief of Medical Staff. . . . . Anrew Eisenderg
Emergency Room . . . . Anna McDonald
CEO/President. . . . . James W. Pope, MHHA, FACHE

Measure	Cases	This Hosp.	State Avg.	U.S. Avg.
Blood Clot Prevention and Treatment				
Anticoagulation Overlap Therapy[5]	-	-	93%	93%
ICU Venous Thromboembolism Prophylaxis[5]	-	-	92%	92%
Incidence of Potentially Preventable VTE[5]	-	-	9%	10%
UFH with Dosages/Platelet Monitoring[5]	-	-	96%	97%
Venous Thromboembolism Prophylaxis[5]	-	-	82%	85%
Warfarin Therapy Discharge Instructions[5]	-	-	84%	75%
Chest Pain/Possible Heart Attack Care				
Aspirin Given Within 24 Hours of Arrival	-	-	94%	96%
Fibrinolytic Meds Within 30 Min. of Arrival	-	-	47%	58%
Average Time to ECG (minutes)	-	-	8	7
Average Time to Transfer (minutes)	-	-	62	60
Children's Asthma Care				
Received Home Management Plan of Care	-	-	93%	88%
Received Reliever Medication	-	-	100%	100%
Received Systemic Corticosteroids	-	-	100%	100%
Emergency Department				
Admittance Decision Time (minutes)[5]	-	-	99	98
Head CT Results Within 45 Min. of Arrival	-	-	54%	57%
Patients Who Left ER Before Being Seen	-	-	3%	2%
Time from ER Arrival to Admit. (minutes)[5]	-	-	270	274
Time from ER Arrival to Discharge (minutes)	-	-	127	134
Time in ER Before Being Evaluated (minutes)	-	-	26	26
Time to Pain Meds for Fractures (minutes)	-	-	57	57
Heart Attack Care				
Aspirin Given at Discharge[5]	-	-	99%	99%
Fibrinolytic Meds Within 30 Min. of Arrival[5]	-	-	49%	54%
PCI Within 90 Minutes of Arrival[5]	-	-	95%	96%
Statin Prescribed at Discharge[5]	-	-	98%	98%
Heart Failure Care				
ACE Inhibitor or ARB for LVSD[3,7]	-	-	97%	97%
Discharge Instructions Given[1,3]	-	-	95%	94%
Evaluation of LVS Function[3]	11	100%	99%	99%
Medicare Spending				
Medicare Spending per Patient (ratio)	-	-	1.03	0.98
Pneumonia Care				
Appropriate Initial Antibiotic Given	12	100%	95%	95%
Blood Culture Timing	19	100%	98%	98%
Pregnancy and Delivery Care				
Newborn Deliveries Scheduled Early[5]	-	-	7%	6%
Preventive Care				
Immunization for Influenza[5]	-	-	90%	90%
Immunization for Pneumonia[5]	-	-	92%	92%
Stroke Care				
Anticoagulation Therapy for Atrial Fibrillation[5]	-	-	96%	95%
Antithrombotic Therapy Timing[5]	-	-	98%	98%
Assessed for Rehabilitation[5]	-	-	98%	97%
Discharged on Antithrombotic Therapy[5]	-	-	99%	99%
Discharged on Statin Medication[5]	-	-	95%	94%
Thrombolytic Therapy Timing[5]	-	-	68%	66%
Venous Thromboembolism Prophylaxis[5]	-	-	94%	94%
Written Stroke Educational Materials Given[5]	-	-	92%	88%
Surgical Care Improvement Project				
Appropriate Beta Blocker Usage[5]	-	-	98%	98%
Appropriate VTP Within 24 Hours[5]	-	-	98%	98%
Controlled Postoperative Blood Glucose[5]	-	-	96%	97%
Perioperative Temperature Management[5]	-	-	100%	100%
Prophylactic Antibiotic Selection[5]	-	-	99%	99%
Prophylactic Antibiotic Selection (Outpatient)	-	-	98%	98%
Prophylactic Antibiotic Stopped[5]	-	-	98%	98%
Prophylactic Antibiotic Timing[5]	-	-	99%	99%
Prophylactic Antibiotic Timing (Outpatient)	-	-	98%	98%
Urinary Catheter Removal[5]	-	-	98%	97%
Survey of Patients' Hospital Experiences				
Area Around Room 'Always' Quiet at Night[5]	-	-	68%	61%
Doctors 'Always' Communicated Well[5]	-	-	83%	82%
Home Recovery Information Given[5]	-	-	85%	85%
Hospital Given 9 or 10 on 10 Point Scale[5]	-	-	73%	71%
Meds 'Always' Explained Before Given[5]	-	-	66%	64%
Nurses 'Always' Communicated Well[5]	-	-	80%	79%
Pain 'Always' Well Controlled[5]	-	-	72%	71%
Room and Bathroom 'Always' Clean[5]	-	-	75%	73%
Timely Help 'Always' Received[5]	-	-	69%	68%
Would Definitely Recommend Hospital[5]	-	-	73%	71%
Use of Medical Imaging				
Cardiac Imaging Stress Test before Surgery	-	-	5.3%	5.3%
Combination Abdominal CT Scan	-	-	16.4%	10.5%
Combination Brain/Sinus CT Scan	-	-	2.7%	2.7%
Combination Chest CT Scan	-	-	5.6%	2.7%
Follow-up Mammogram/Ultrasound	-	-	7.9%	8.8%
Lumbar Spine MRI for Low Back Pain	-	-	39.6%	37.2%

NOTE: Hospital profiles are in alphabetical order by state, then city, then hospital within the city; Rankings exclude hospitals with less than 25 cases except for patient surveys which excludes hospitals with less than 100 cases; (a) 100-299 cases; (1) The number of cases/patients is too few to report; (2) Data submitted were based on a sample of cases/patients; (3) Results are based on a shorter time period than required; (4) Data suppressed by CMS for one or more quarters; (5) Results are not available for this reporting period; (6) Fewer than 100 patients completed the HCAHPS survey; (7) No cases met the criteria for this measure; (8) The lower limit of the confidence interval cannot be calculated if the number of observed infections equals zero; (9) No data are available from the state/territory for this reporting period; (10) The scores shown reflect fewer than 50 completed surveys; (11) There were discrepancies in the data collection process; (12) This measure does not apply to this hospital for this reporting period; (13) Results cannot be calculated for this reporting period; (14) The results for this state are combined with nearby states to protect confidentiality; Please refer to the User's Guide for a full explanation of data.

Methodist Mansfield Medical Center

2700 E Broad Street Phone: 682-622-2059
Mansfield, TX 76063
URL: www.methodisthealthsystem.com
Type: Acute Care Hospitals Emergency Services: Yes
Ownership: Voluntary non-profit - Private

Measure	Cases	This Hosp.	State Avg.	U.S. Avg.
Blood Clot Prevention and Treatment				
Anticoagulation Overlap Therapy[2]	85	100%	93%	93%
ICU Venous Thromboembolism Prophylaxis[2]	81	95%	92%	92%
Incidence of Potentially Preventable VTE[1,2]	-	-	9%	10%
UFH with Dosages/Platelet Monitoring[2]	27	100%	96%	97%
Venous Thromboembolism Prophylaxis[2]	401	91%	82%	85%
Warfarin Therapy Discharge Instructions[2]	69	97%	84%	75%
Chest Pain/Possible Heart Attack Care				
Aspirin Given Within 24 Hours of Arrival[1,3]	-	-	94%	96%
Fibrinolytic Meds Within 30 Min. of Arrival[3,7]	-	-	47%	58%
Average Time to ECG (minutes)[1,3]	-	-	8	7
Average Time to Transfer (minutes)[1,3]	-	-	62	60
Children's Asthma Care				
Received Home Management Plan of Care	-	-	93%	88%
Received Reliever Medication	-	-	100%	100%
Received Systemic Corticosteroids	-	-	100%	100%
Emergency Department				
Admittance Decision Time (minutes)[2]	232	150	99	98
Head CT Results Within 45 Min. of Arrival[1]	-	-	54%	57%
Patients Who Left ER Before Being Seen	52,769	3%	3%	2%
Time from ER Arrival to Admit. (minutes)[2]	239	304	270	274
Time from ER Arrival to Discharge (minutes)	385	162	127	134
Time in ER Before Being Evaluated (minutes)	405	31	26	26
Time to Pain Meds for Fractures (minutes)	251	58	57	57
Heart Attack Care				
Aspirin Given at Discharge	214	100%	99%	99%
Fibrinolytic Meds Within 30 Min. of Arrival[7]	-	-	49%	54%
PCI Within 90 Minutes of Arrival	21	100%	95%	96%
Statin Prescribed at Discharge	219	100%	98%	98%
Heart Failure Care				
ACE Inhibitor or ARB for LVSD	90	100%	97%	97%
Discharge Instructions Given	266	100%	95%	94%
Evaluation of LVS Function	311	100%	99%	99%
Medicare Spending				
Medicare Spending per Patient (ratio)	-	1.08	1.03	0.98
Pneumonia Care				
Appropriate Initial Antibiotic Given	155	100%	95%	95%
Blood Culture Timing	226	99%	98%	98%
Pregnancy and Delivery Care				
Newborn Deliveries Scheduled Early[2]	188	7%	7%	6%
Preventive Care				
Immunization for Influenza[2]	497	97%	90%	90%
Immunization for Pneumonia[2]	526	94%	92%	92%
Stroke Care				
Anticoagulation Therapy for Atrial Fibrillation[1,2]	-	-	96%	95%
Antithrombotic Therapy Timing[2]	77	100%	98%	98%
Assessed for Rehabilitation[2]	79	100%	98%	97%
Discharged on Antithrombotic Therapy[2]	77	100%	99%	99%
Discharged on Statin Medication[2]	62	100%	95%	94%
Thrombolytic Therapy Timing[1,2]	-	-	68%	66%
Venous Thromboembolism Prophylaxis[2]	72	100%	94%	94%
Written Stroke Educational Materials Given[2]	53	100%	92%	88%
Surgical Care Improvement Project				
Appropriate Beta Blocker Usage	98	100%	98%	98%
Appropriate VTP Within 24 Hours	205	100%	98%	98%
Controlled Postoperative Blood Glucose	92	99%	96%	97%
Perioperative Temperature Management	341	100%	100%	100%
Prophylactic Antibiotic Selection	218	100%	99%	99%
Prophylactic Antibiotic Selection (Outpatient)	193	99%	98%	98%
Prophylactic Antibiotic Stopped	209	100%	98%	98%
Prophylactic Antibiotic Timing	219	100%	99%	99%
Prophylactic Antibiotic Timing (Outpatient)	194	99%	98%	98%
Urinary Catheter Removal	182	100%	98%	97%
Survey of Patients' Hospital Experiences				
Area Around Room 'Always' Quiet at Night	300+	67%	68%	61%
Doctors 'Always' Communicated Well	300+	80%	83%	82%
Home Recovery Information Given	300+	83%	85%	85%
Hospital Given 9 or 10 on 10 Point Scale	300+	80%	73%	71%
Meds 'Always' Explained Before Given	300+	64%	66%	64%
Nurses 'Always' Communicated Well	300+	81%	80%	79%
Pain 'Always' Well Controlled	300+	75%	72%	71%
Room and Bathroom 'Always' Clean	300+	76%	75%	73%
Timely Help 'Always' Received	300+	65%	69%	68%
Would Definitely Recommend Hospital	300+	84%	73%	71%
Use of Medical Imaging				
Cardiac Imaging Stress Test before Surgery	174	6.9%	5.3%	5.3%
Combination Abdominal CT Scan	543	7.6%	16.4%	10.5%
Combination Brain/Sinus CT Scan	500	2.0%	2.7%	2.7%
Combination Chest CT Scan	132	13.6%	5.6%	2.7%
Follow-up Mammogram/Ultrasound	580	4.0%	7.9%	8.8%
Lumbar Spine MRI for Low Back Pain[1]	-	-	39.6%	37.2%

Falls Community Hospital & Clinic

322 Coleman Street Phone: 254-803-3561
Marlin, TX 76661 Fax: 254-883-6066
E-mail: fallshosp@aol.com
URL: www.fallshospital.org
Type: Acute Care Hospitals Emergency Services: Yes
Ownership: Voluntary non-profit - Private Beds: 44

Key Personnel:
Infection Control. . . . . Sara Chiglo, RN
Quality Assurance . . . . Sara Chiglo, RN
Chief of Medical Staff. . . . . J Scott Crockett, MD
Radiology. . . . . Jeff Johnson
Administrator . . . . Willis Reese
Hemotology Center . . . . Donna Ryan

Measure	Cases	This Hosp.	State Avg.	U.S. Avg.
Blood Clot Prevention and Treatment				
Anticoagulation Overlap Therapy[2,7]	-	-	93%	93%
ICU Venous Thromboembolism Prophylaxis[2,7]	-	-	92%	92%
Incidence of Potentially Preventable VTE[2,7]	-	-	9%	10%
UFH with Dosages/Platelet Monitoring[2,7]	-	-	96%	97%
Venous Thromboembolism Prophylaxis[2]	123	0%	82%	85%
Warfarin Therapy Discharge Instructions[2,7]	-	-	84%	75%
Chest Pain/Possible Heart Attack Care				
Aspirin Given Within 24 Hours of Arrival[5]	-	-	94%	96%
Fibrinolytic Meds Within 30 Min. of Arrival[5]	-	-	47%	58%
Average Time to ECG (minutes)[5]	-	-	8	7
Average Time to Transfer (minutes)[5]	-	-	62	60
Children's Asthma Care				
Received Home Management Plan of Care	-	-	93%	88%
Received Reliever Medication	-	-	100%	100%
Received Systemic Corticosteroids	-	-	100%	100%
Emergency Department				
Admittance Decision Time (minutes)[2]	246	1026	99	98
Head CT Results Within 45 Min. of Arrival[1,3]	-	-	54%	57%
Patients Who Left ER Before Being Seen	7,605	3%	3%	2%
Time from ER Arrival to Admit. (minutes)[2]	280	926	270	274
Time from ER Arrival to Discharge (minutes)	381	110	127	134
Time in ER Before Being Evaluated (minutes)	353	24	26	26
Time to Pain Meds for Fractures (minutes)	35	52	57	57
Heart Attack Care				
Aspirin Given at Discharge[5]	-	-	99%	99%
Fibrinolytic Meds Within 30 Min. of Arrival[5]	-	-	49%	54%
PCI Within 90 Minutes of Arrival[5]	-	-	95%	96%
Statin Prescribed at Discharge[5]	-	-	98%	98%
Heart Failure Care				
ACE Inhibitor or ARB for LVSD[1,2]	-	-	97%	97%
Discharge Instructions Given[1,2]	-	-	95%	94%
Evaluation of LVS Function[1,2]	-	-	99%	99%
Medicare Spending				
Medicare Spending per Patient (ratio)	-	1.07	1.03	0.98
Pneumonia Care				
Appropriate Initial Antibiotic Given[2]	77	44%	95%	95%
Blood Culture Timing[2]	27	78%	98%	98%
Pregnancy and Delivery Care				
Newborn Deliveries Scheduled Early[7]	-	-	7%	6%
Preventive Care				
Immunization for Influenza[2]	197	89%	90%	90%
Immunization for Pneumonia[2]	286	55%	92%	92%
Stroke Care				
Anticoagulation Therapy for Atrial Fibrillation[5]	-	-	96%	95%
Antithrombotic Therapy Timing[5]	-	-	98%	98%
Assessed for Rehabilitation[5]	-	-	98%	97%
Discharged on Antithrombotic Therapy[5]	-	-	99%	99%
Discharged on Statin Medication[5]	-	-	95%	94%
Thrombolytic Therapy Timing[5]	-	-	68%	66%
Venous Thromboembolism Prophylaxis[5]	-	-	94%	94%
Written Stroke Educational Materials Given[5]	-	-	92%	88%
Surgical Care Improvement Project				
Appropriate Beta Blocker Usage[5]	-	-	98%	98%
Appropriate VTP Within 24 Hours[5]	-	-	98%	98%
Controlled Postoperative Blood Glucose[5]	-	-	96%	97%
Perioperative Temperature Management[5]	-	-	100%	100%
Prophylactic Antibiotic Selection[5]	-	-	99%	99%
Prophylactic Antibiotic Selection (Outpatient)[5]	-	-	98%	98%
Prophylactic Antibiotic Stopped[5]	-	-	98%	98%
Prophylactic Antibiotic Timing[5]	-	-	99%	99%
Prophylactic Antibiotic Timing (Outpatient)[5]	-	-	98%	98%
Urinary Catheter Removal[5]	-	-	98%	97%
Survey of Patients' Hospital Experiences				
Area Around Room 'Always' Quiet at Night	(a)	73%	68%	61%
Doctors 'Always' Communicated Well	(a)	96%	83%	82%
Home Recovery Information Given	(a)	84%	85%	85%
Hospital Given 9 or 10 on 10 Point Scale	(a)	71%	73%	71%
Meds 'Always' Explained Before Given	(a)	78%	66%	64%
Nurses 'Always' Communicated Well	(a)	86%	80%	79%
Pain 'Always' Well Controlled	(a)	83%	72%	71%
Room and Bathroom 'Always' Clean	(a)	88%	75%	73%
Timely Help 'Always' Received	(a)	73%	69%	68%
Would Definitely Recommend Hospital	(a)	74%	73%	71%
Use of Medical Imaging				
Cardiac Imaging Stress Test before Surgery[7]	-	-	5.3%	5.3%
Combination Abdominal CT Scan	96	2.1%	16.4%	10.5%
Combination Brain/Sinus CT Scan[1]	-	-	2.7%	2.7%
Combination Chest CT Scan[1]	-	-	5.6%	2.7%
Follow-up Mammogram/Ultrasound[7]	-	-	7.9%	8.8%
Lumbar Spine MRI for Low Back Pain[1]	-	-	39.6%	37.2%

Good Shepherd Medical Center Marshall

811 S Washington Phone: 903-927-6712
Marshall, TX 75670 Fax: 903-927-6101
URL: www.marshallregional.org
Type: Acute Care Hospitals Emergency Services: Yes
Ownership: Voluntary non-profit - Private Beds: 139

Key Personnel:
Radiology. . . . . John C Campbell, MD
CEO/President. . . . . Russell J Collier
Operating Room. . . . . Susan Fenwick, RN
Quality Assurance . . . . Jim Hodges
Pediatric Ambulatory Care . . . . . . Tex Houchen, MD
Pediatric In-Patient Care . . . . . . Tex Houchen, MD
Chief of Medical Staff. . . . . Bud Siebenlist, MD
Infection Control. . . . . Tena Tiller, RN

Measure	Cases	This Hosp.	State Avg.	U.S. Avg.
Blood Clot Prevention and Treatment				
Anticoagulation Overlap Therapy[2]	17	100%	93%	93%
ICU Venous Thromboembolism Prophylaxis[2]	22	100%	92%	92%
Incidence of Potentially Preventable VTE[1,2]	-	-	9%	10%
UFH with Dosages/Platelet Monitoring[2]	11	100%	96%	97%
Venous Thromboembolism Prophylaxis[2]	281	88%	82%	85%
Warfarin Therapy Discharge Instructions[2]	26	100%	84%	75%
Chest Pain/Possible Heart Attack Care				
Aspirin Given Within 24 Hours of Arrival	105	98%	94%	96%
Fibrinolytic Meds Within 30 Min. of Arrival[7]	-	-	47%	58%
Average Time to ECG (minutes)	112	2	8	7
Average Time to Transfer (minutes)	59	129	62	60
Children's Asthma Care				
Received Home Management Plan of Care	-	-	93%	88%
Received Reliever Medication	-	-	100%	100%
Received Systemic Corticosteroids	-	-	100%	100%
Emergency Department				
Admittance Decision Time (minutes)[2]	506	66	99	98

NOTE: Hospital profiles are in alphabetical order by state, then city, then hospital within the city; Rankings exclude hospitals with less than 25 cases except for patient surveys which excludes hospitals with less than 100 cases; (a) 100-299 cases; (1) The number of cases/patients is too few to report; (2) Data submitted were based on a sample of cases/patients; (3) Results are based on a shorter time period than required; (4) Data suppressed by CMS for one or more quarters; (5) Results are not available for this reporting period; (6) Fewer than 100 patients completed the HCAHPS survey; (7) No cases met the criteria for this measure; (8) The lower limit of the confidence interval cannot be calculated if the number of observed infections equals zero; (9) No data are available from the state/territory for this reporting period; (10) The scores shown reflect fewer than 50 completed surveys; (11) There were discrepancies in the data collection process; (12) This measure does not apply to this hospital for this reporting period; (13) Results cannot be calculated for this reporting period; (14) The results for this state are combined with nearby states to protect confidentiality; Please refer to the User's Guide for a full explanation of data.

Head CT Results Within 45 Min. of Arrival	36	50%	54%	57%
Patients Who Left ER Before Being Seen	30,727	1%	3%	2%
Time from ER Arrival to Admit. (minutes)[2]	508	230	270	274
Time from ER Arrival to Discharge (minutes)	363	115	127	134
Time in ER Before Being Evaluated (minutes)	405	21	26	26
Time to Pain Meds for Fractures (minutes)	131	48	57	57
Heart Attack Care				
Aspirin Given at Discharge[1]	-	-	99%	99%
Fibrinolytic Meds Within 30 Min. of Arrival[7]	-	-	49%	54%
PCI Within 90 Minutes of Arrival[7]	-	-	95%	96%
Statin Prescribed at Discharge[1]	-	-	98%	98%
Heart Failure Care				
ACE Inhibitor or ARB for LVSD	55	98%	97%	97%
Discharge Instructions Given	97	94%	95%	94%
Evaluation of LVS Function	109	99%	99%	99%
Medicare Spending				
Medicare Spending per Patient (ratio)	-	1.01	1.03	0.98
Pneumonia Care				
Appropriate Initial Antibiotic Given	109	98%	95%	95%
Blood Culture Timing	190	98%	98%	98%
Pregnancy and Delivery Care				
Newborn Deliveries Scheduled Early	25	0%	7%	6%
Preventive Care				
Immunization for Influenza[2]	409	84%	90%	90%
Immunization for Pneumonia[2]	450	95%	92%	92%
Stroke Care				
Anticoagulation Therapy for Atrial Fibrillation[1]	-	-	96%	95%
Antithrombotic Therapy Timing	13	100%	98%	98%
Assessed for Rehabilitation	12	100%	98%	97%
Discharged on Antithrombotic Therapy	12	92%	99%	99%
Discharged on Statin Medication	11	100%	95%	94%
Thrombolytic Therapy Timing[7]	-	-	68%	66%
Venous Thromboembolism Prophylaxis	13	100%	94%	94%
Written Stroke Educational Materials Given[1]	-	-	92%	88%
Surgical Care Improvement Project				
Appropriate Beta Blocker Usage	67	100%	98%	98%
Appropriate VTP Within 24 Hours	205	96%	98%	98%
Controlled Postoperative Blood Glucose[7]	-	-	96%	97%
Perioperative Temperature Management	261	100%	100%	100%
Prophylactic Antibiotic Selection	154	99%	99%	99%
Prophylactic Antibiotic Selection (Outpatient)	27	96%	98%	98%
Prophylactic Antibiotic Stopped	152	99%	98%	98%
Prophylactic Antibiotic Timing	154	100%	99%	99%
Prophylactic Antibiotic Timing (Outpatient)	28	96%	98%	98%
Urinary Catheter Removal	130	99%	98%	97%
Survey of Patients' Hospital Experiences				
Area Around Room 'Always' Quiet at Night	300+	64%	68%	61%
Doctors 'Always' Communicated Well	300+	77%	83%	82%
Home Recovery Information Given	300+	82%	85%	85%
Hospital Given 9 or 10 on 10 Point Scale	300+	67%	73%	71%
Meds 'Always' Explained Before Given	300+	55%	66%	64%
Nurses 'Always' Communicated Well	300+	75%	80%	79%
Pain 'Always' Well Controlled	300+	65%	72%	71%
Room and Bathroom 'Always' Clean	300+	71%	75%	73%
Timely Help 'Always' Received	300+	57%	69%	68%
Would Definitely Recommend Hospital	300+	62%	73%	71%
Use of Medical Imaging				
Cardiac Imaging Stress Test before Surgery	121	4.1%	5.3%	5.3%
Combination Abdominal CT Scan	457	9.8%	16.4%	10.5%
Combination Brain/Sinus CT Scan	495	0.6%	2.7%	2.7%
Combination Chest CT Scan	267	11.6%	5.6%	2.7%
Follow-up Mammogram/Ultrasound	733	6.4%	7.9%	8.8%
Lumbar Spine MRI for Low Back Pain	60	28.3%	39.6%	37.2%

Baylor Medical Center at Mckinney

5252 West University Drive Phone: 469-742-2200
Mc Kinney, TX 75071
Type: Acute Care Hospitals Emergency Services: Yes
Ownership: Voluntary non-profit - Private

Measure	Cases	This Hosp.	State Avg.	U.S. Avg.
Blood Clot Prevention and Treatment				
Anticoagulation Overlap Therapy[2]	55	100%	93%	93%
ICU Venous Thromboembolism Prophylaxis[2]	69	100%	92%	92%
Incidence of Potentially Preventable VTE[1,2]	-	-	9%	10%
UFH with Dosages/Platelet Monitoring[2]	14	100%	96%	97%
Venous Thromboembolism Prophylaxis[2]	327	100%	82%	85%
Warfarin Therapy Discharge Instructions[2]	45	100%	84%	75%
Chest Pain/Possible Heart Attack Care				
Aspirin Given Within 24 Hours of Arrival[1,3]	-	-	94%	96%
Fibrinolytic Meds Within 30 Min. of Arrival[5]	-	-	47%	58%
Average Time to ECG (minutes)[1,3]	-	-	8	7
Average Time to Transfer (minutes)[5]	-	-	62	60
Children's Asthma Care				
Received Home Management Plan of Care	-	-	93%	88%
Received Reliever Medication	-	-	100%	100%
Received Systemic Corticosteroids	-	-	100%	100%
Emergency Department				
Admittance Decision Time (minutes)[2]	607	84	99	98
Head CT Results Within 45 Min. of Arrival[1]	-	-	54%	57%
Patients Who Left ER Before Being Seen	10,169	1%	3%	2%
Time from ER Arrival to Admit. (minutes)[2]	607	257	270	274
Time from ER Arrival to Discharge (minutes)	431	156	127	134
Time in ER Before Being Evaluated (minutes)	443	34	26	26
Time to Pain Meds for Fractures (minutes)	121	45	57	57
Heart Attack Care				
Aspirin Given at Discharge	83	100%	99%	99%
Fibrinolytic Meds Within 30 Min. of Arrival[7]	-	-	49%	54%
PCI Within 90 Minutes of Arrival	21	100%	95%	96%
Statin Prescribed at Discharge	82	98%	98%	98%
Heart Failure Care				
ACE Inhibitor or ARB for LVSD	39	100%	97%	97%
Discharge Instructions Given	113	100%	95%	94%
Evaluation of LVS Function	108	100%	99%	99%
Medicare Spending				
Medicare Spending per Patient (ratio)	-	1.02	1.03	0.98
Pneumonia Care				
Appropriate Initial Antibiotic Given	99	100%	95%	95%
Blood Culture Timing	183	99%	98%	98%
Pregnancy and Delivery Care				
Newborn Deliveries Scheduled Early	124	9%	7%	6%
Preventive Care				
Immunization for Influenza[2]	451	99%	90%	90%
Immunization for Pneumonia[2]	463	99%	92%	92%
Stroke Care				
Anticoagulation Therapy for Atrial Fibrillation[1]	-	-	96%	95%
Antithrombotic Therapy Timing	40	100%	98%	98%
Assessed for Rehabilitation	49	100%	98%	97%
Discharged on Antithrombotic Therapy	42	100%	99%	99%
Discharged on Statin Medication	36	94%	95%	94%
Thrombolytic Therapy Timing[1]	-	-	68%	66%
Venous Thromboembolism Prophylaxis	43	98%	94%	94%
Written Stroke Educational Materials Given	26	100%	92%	88%
Surgical Care Improvement Project				
Appropriate Beta Blocker Usage[2]	64	100%	98%	98%
Appropriate VTP Within 24 Hours[2]	170	99%	98%	98%
Controlled Postoperative Blood Glucose[2,7]	-	-	96%	97%
Perioperative Temperature Management[2]	198	100%	100%	100%
Prophylactic Antibiotic Selection[2]	82	100%	99%	99%
Prophylactic Antibiotic Selection (Outpatient)	165	98%	98%	98%
Prophylactic Antibiotic Stopped[2]	82	98%	98%	98%
Prophylactic Antibiotic Timing[2]	83	100%	99%	99%
Prophylactic Antibiotic Timing (Outpatient)	165	99%	98%	98%
Urinary Catheter Removal[2]	83	99%	98%	97%
Survey of Patients' Hospital Experiences				
Area Around Room 'Always' Quiet at Night	300+	64%	68%	61%
Doctors 'Always' Communicated Well	300+	81%	83%	82%
Home Recovery Information Given	300+	85%	85%	85%
Hospital Given 9 or 10 on 10 Point Scale	300+	85%	73%	71%
Meds 'Always' Explained Before Given	300+	63%	66%	64%
Nurses 'Always' Communicated Well	300+	80%	80%	79%
Pain 'Always' Well Controlled	300+	74%	72%	71%
Room and Bathroom 'Always' Clean	300+	77%	75%	73%
Timely Help 'Always' Received	300+	67%	69%	68%
Would Definitely Recommend Hospital	300+	87%	73%	71%
Use of Medical Imaging				
Cardiac Imaging Stress Test before Surgery	110	6.4%	5.3%	5.3%
Combination Abdominal CT Scan	497	6.4%	16.4%	10.5%
Combination Brain/Sinus CT Scan[1]	-	-	2.7%	2.7%
Combination Chest CT Scan	158	1.3%	5.6%	2.7%
Follow-up Mammogram/Ultrasound	325	12.9%	7.9%	8.8%
Lumbar Spine MRI for Low Back Pain[1]	-	-	39.6%	37.2%

Methodist Mckinney Hospital

8000 W Eldorado Pkwy Phone: 469-424-6400
Mc Kinney, TX 75070
Type: Acute Care Hospitals Emergency Services: Yes
Ownership: Proprietary

Measure	Cases	This Hosp.	State Avg.	U.S. Avg.
Blood Clot Prevention and Treatment				
Anticoagulation Overlap Therapy[1,2]	-	-	93%	93%
ICU Venous Thromboembolism Prophylaxis[2,7]	-	-	92%	92%
Incidence of Potentially Preventable VTE[2,7]	-	-	9%	10%
UFH with Dosages/Platelet Monitoring[2,7]	-	-	96%	97%
Venous Thromboembolism Prophylaxis[2]	30	83%	82%	85%
Warfarin Therapy Discharge Instructions[1,2]	-	-	84%	75%
Chest Pain/Possible Heart Attack Care				
Aspirin Given Within 24 Hours of Arrival[1,3]	-	-	94%	96%
Fibrinolytic Meds Within 30 Min. of Arrival[3,7]	-	-	47%	58%
Average Time to ECG (minutes)[1,3]	-	-	8	7
Average Time to Transfer (minutes)[1,3]	-	-	62	60
Children's Asthma Care				
Received Home Management Plan of Care	-	-	93%	88%
Received Reliever Medication	-	-	100%	100%
Received Systemic Corticosteroids	-	-	100%	100%
Emergency Department				
Admittance Decision Time (minutes)[2]	32	45	99	98
Head CT Results Within 45 Min. of Arrival[5]	-	-	54%	57%
Patients Who Left ER Before Being Seen	3,480	0%	3%	2%
Time from ER Arrival to Admit. (minutes)[2]	41	186	270	274
Time from ER Arrival to Discharge (minutes)	249	80	127	134
Time in ER Before Being Evaluated (minutes)	169	11	26	26
Time to Pain Meds for Fractures (minutes)[1,3]	-	-	57	57
Heart Attack Care				
Aspirin Given at Discharge[5]	-	-	99%	99%
Fibrinolytic Meds Within 30 Min. of Arrival[5]	-	-	49%	54%
PCI Within 90 Minutes of Arrival[5]	-	-	95%	96%
Statin Prescribed at Discharge[5]	-	-	98%	98%
Heart Failure Care				
ACE Inhibitor or ARB for LVSD[5]	-	-	97%	97%
Discharge Instructions Given[5]	-	-	95%	94%
Evaluation of LVS Function[5]	-	-	99%	99%
Medicare Spending				
Medicare Spending per Patient (ratio)	-	1.02	1.03	0.98
Pneumonia Care				
Appropriate Initial Antibiotic Given[1,2]	-	-	95%	95%
Blood Culture Timing[1,2]	-	-	98%	98%
Pregnancy and Delivery Care				
Newborn Deliveries Scheduled Early[7]	-	-	7%	6%
Preventive Care				
Immunization for Influenza[2]	241	48%	90%	90%
Immunization for Pneumonia[2]	268	55%	92%	92%
Stroke Care				
Anticoagulation Therapy for Atrial Fibrillation[3,7]	-	-	96%	95%
Antithrombotic Therapy Timing[1,3]	-	-	98%	98%
Assessed for Rehabilitation[1,3]	-	-	98%	97%
Discharged on Antithrombotic Therapy[1,3]	-	-	99%	99%
Discharged on Statin Medication[1,3]	-	-	95%	94%
Thrombolytic Therapy Timing[3,7]	-	-	68%	66%
Venous Thromboembolism Prophylaxis[1,3]	-	-	94%	94%
Written Stroke Educational Materials Given[1,3]	-	-	92%	88%
Surgical Care Improvement Project				
Appropriate Beta Blocker Usage[2]	69	100%	98%	98%
Appropriate VTP Within 24 Hours[2]	277	100%	98%	98%
Controlled Postoperative Blood Glucose[2,7]	-	-	96%	97%
Perioperative Temperature Management[2]	314	100%	100%	100%
Prophylactic Antibiotic Selection[2]	268	99%	99%	99%

NOTE: Hospital profiles are in alphabetical order by state, then city, then hospital within the city; Rankings exclude hospitals with less than 25 cases except for patient surveys which excludes hospitals with less than 100 cases; (a) 100-299 cases; (1) The number of cases/patients is too few to report; (2) Data submitted were based on a sample of cases/patients; (3) Results are based on a shorter time period than required; (4) Data suppressed by CMS for one or more quarters; (5) Results are not available for this reporting period; (6) Fewer than 100 patients completed the HCAHPS survey; (7) No cases met the criteria for this measure; (8) The lower limit of the confidence interval cannot be calculated if the number of observed infections equals zero; (9) No data are available from the state/territory for this reporting period; (10) The scores shown reflect fewer than 50 completed surveys; (11) There were discrepancies in the data collection process; (12) This measure does not apply to this hospital for this reporting period; (13) Results cannot be calculated for this reporting period; (14) The results for this state are combined with nearby states to protect confidentiality; Please refer to the User's Guide for a full explanation of data.

Measure	Cases	This Hosp.	State Avg.	U.S. Avg.
Prophylactic Antibiotic Selection (Outpatient)	111	85%	98%	98%
Prophylactic Antibiotic Stopped[2]	267	98%	98%	98%
Prophylactic Antibiotic Timing[2]	268	98%	99%	99%
Prophylactic Antibiotic Timing (Outpatient)	113	98%	98%	98%
Urinary Catheter Removal[2]	266	98%	98%	97%
Survey of Patients' Hospital Experiences				
Area Around Room 'Always' Quiet at Night	(a)	85%	68%	61%
Doctors 'Always' Communicated Well	(a)	86%	83%	82%
Home Recovery Information Given	(a)	88%	85%	85%
Hospital Given 9 or 10 on 10 Point Scale	(a)	77%	73%	71%
Meds 'Always' Explained Before Given	(a)	67%	66%	64%
Nurses 'Always' Communicated Well	(a)	81%	80%	79%
Pain 'Always' Well Controlled	(a)	74%	72%	71%
Room and Bathroom 'Always' Clean	(a)	79%	75%	73%
Timely Help 'Always' Received	(a)	77%	69%	68%
Would Definitely Recommend Hospital	(a)	76%	73%	71%
Use of Medical Imaging				
Cardiac Imaging Stress Test before Surgery[7]	-	-	5.3%	5.3%
Combination Abdominal CT Scan[1]	-	-	16.4%	10.5%
Combination Brain/Sinus CT Scan[1]	-	-	2.7%	2.7%
Combination Chest CT Scan[1]	-	-	5.6%	2.7%
Follow-up Mammogram/Ultrasound[1]	-	-	7.9%	8.8%
Lumbar Spine MRI for Low Back Pain[1]	-	-	39.6%	37.2%

Rio Grande Regional Hospital

101 E Ridge Rd
Mcallen, TX 78503
Phone: 956-632-6000
Fax: 956-632-6621
URL: www.riohealth.com
Type: Acute Care Hospitals
Ownership: Proprietary
Emergency Services: Yes
Beds: 320

Key Personnel:
Chief of Medical Staff . . . . Michael Jelinek
Radiology. . . . . Joe Martinez
CEO/President. . . . . Cris Rivera
Emergency Room . . . . Nanulea Sloref

Measure	Cases	This Hosp.	State Avg.	U.S. Avg.
Blood Clot Prevention and Treatment				
Anticoagulation Overlap Therapy[2]	47	100%	93%	93%
ICU Venous Thromboembolism Prophylaxis[2]	97	99%	92%	92%
Incidence of Potentially Preventable VTE[2]	12	8%	9%	10%
UFH with Dosages/Platelet Monitoring[2]	24	100%	96%	97%
Venous Thromboembolism Prophylaxis[2]	400	99%	82%	85%
Warfarin Therapy Discharge Instructions[2]	37	97%	84%	75%
Chest Pain/Possible Heart Attack Care				
Aspirin Given Within 24 Hours of Arrival[5]	-	-	94%	96%
Fibrinolytic Meds Within 30 Min. of Arrival[5]	-	-	47%	58%
Average Time to ECG (minutes)[5]	-	-	8	7
Average Time to Transfer (minutes)[5]	-	-	62	60
Children's Asthma Care				
Received Home Management Plan of Care	-	-	93%	88%
Received Reliever Medication	-	-	100%	100%
Received Systemic Corticosteroids	-	-	100%	100%
Emergency Department				
Admittance Decision Time (minutes)[2]	568	160	99	98
Head CT Results Within 45 Min. of Arrival[7]	-	-	54%	57%
Patients Who Left ER Before Being Seen	35,920	1%	3%	2%
Time from ER Arrival to Admit. (minutes)[2]	575	233	270	274
Time from ER Arrival to Discharge (minutes)	473	119	127	134
Time in ER Before Being Evaluated (minutes)	531	12	26	26
Time to Pain Meds for Fractures (minutes)	197	45	57	57
Heart Attack Care				
Aspirin Given at Discharge[2]	158	100%	99%	99%
Fibrinolytic Meds Within 30 Min. of Arrival[2,7]	-	-	49%	54%
PCI Within 90 Minutes of Arrival[2]	11	91%	95%	96%
Statin Prescribed at Discharge[2]	150	99%	98%	98%
Heart Failure Care				
ACE Inhibitor or ARB for LVSD	95	97%	97%	97%
Discharge Instructions Given	325	97%	95%	94%
Evaluation of LVS Function	385	99%	99%	99%
Medicare Spending				
Medicare Spending per Patient (ratio)	-	1.01	1.03	0.98
Pneumonia Care				
Appropriate Initial Antibiotic Given	188	98%	95%	95%
Blood Culture Timing	239	99%	98%	98%
Pregnancy and Delivery Care				
Newborn Deliveries Scheduled Early[2]	79	0%	7%	6%
Preventive Care				
Immunization for Influenza[2]	554	100%	90%	90%
Immunization for Pneumonia[2]	556	99%	92%	92%
Stroke Care				
Anticoagulation Therapy for Atrial Fibrillation[2]	11	100%	96%	95%
Antithrombotic Therapy Timing[2]	73	96%	98%	98%
Assessed for Rehabilitation[2]	95	98%	98%	97%
Discharged on Antithrombotic Therapy[2]	70	100%	99%	99%
Discharged on Statin Medication[2]	44	93%	95%	94%
Thrombolytic Therapy Timing[1,2]	-	-	68%	66%
Venous Thromboembolism Prophylaxis[2]	107	99%	94%	94%
Written Stroke Educational Materials Given[2]	70	87%	92%	88%
Surgical Care Improvement Project				
Appropriate Beta Blocker Usage[2]	119	98%	98%	98%
Appropriate VTP Within 24 Hours[2]	231	100%	98%	98%
Controlled Postoperative Blood Glucose[2]	87	99%	96%	97%
Perioperative Temperature Management[2]	312	100%	100%	100%
Prophylactic Antibiotic Selection[2]	216	100%	99%	99%
Prophylactic Antibiotic Selection (Outpatient)	95	95%	98%	98%
Prophylactic Antibiotic Stopped[2]	205	98%	98%	98%
Prophylactic Antibiotic Timing[2]	216	99%	99%	99%
Prophylactic Antibiotic Timing (Outpatient)	96	98%	98%	98%
Urinary Catheter Removal[2]	190	100%	98%	97%
Survey of Patients' Hospital Experiences				
Area Around Room 'Always' Quiet at Night	300+	63%	68%	61%
Doctors 'Always' Communicated Well	300+	79%	83%	82%
Home Recovery Information Given	300+	81%	85%	85%
Hospital Given 9 or 10 on 10 Point Scale	300+	72%	73%	71%
Meds 'Always' Explained Before Given	300+	61%	66%	64%
Nurses 'Always' Communicated Well	300+	76%	80%	79%
Pain 'Always' Well Controlled	300+	70%	72%	71%
Room and Bathroom 'Always' Clean	300+	71%	75%	73%
Timely Help 'Always' Received	300+	58%	69%	68%
Would Definitely Recommend Hospital	300+	70%	73%	71%
Use of Medical Imaging				
Cardiac Imaging Stress Test before Surgery	281	6.4%	5.3%	5.3%
Combination Abdominal CT Scan	396	3.5%	16.4%	10.5%
Combination Brain/Sinus CT Scan[1]	-	-	2.7%	2.7%
Combination Chest CT Scan	65	3.1%	5.6%	2.7%
Follow-up Mammogram/Ultrasound	568	9.3%	7.9%	8.8%
Lumbar Spine MRI for Low Back Pain[1]	-	-	39.6%	37.2%

McCamey Hospital

2500 Hwy 305 South
Mccamey, TX 79752
Phone: 432-652-8626
Fax: 432-652-4009
Type: Critical Access Hospitals
Ownership: Govt - Hospital Dist/Auth
Emergency Services: Yes
Beds: 14

Key Personnel:
Chief of Medical Staff . . . . Ramon Domingo, MD
Infection Control. . . . . Ron Freake
Anesthesiology. . . . . John Paul Loyless
Cardiology . . . . P.J. Patel, M.D
CEO . . . . Jaime J Ramirez

Measure	Cases	This Hosp.	State Avg.	U.S. Avg.
Blood Clot Prevention and Treatment				
Anticoagulation Overlap Therapy[5]	-	-	93%	93%
ICU Venous Thromboembolism Prophylaxis[5]	-	-	92%	92%
Incidence of Potentially Preventable VTE[5]	-	-	9%	10%
UFH with Dosages/Platelet Monitoring[5]	-	-	96%	97%
Venous Thromboembolism Prophylaxis[5]	-	-	82%	85%
Warfarin Therapy Discharge Instructions[5]	-	-	84%	75%
Chest Pain/Possible Heart Attack Care				
Aspirin Given Within 24 Hours of Arrival	-	-	94%	96%
Fibrinolytic Meds Within 30 Min. of Arrival	-	-	47%	58%
Average Time to ECG (minutes)	-	-	8	7
Average Time to Transfer (minutes)	-	-	62	60
Children's Asthma Care				
Received Home Management Plan of Care	-	-	93%	88%
Received Reliever Medication	-	-	100%	100%
Received Systemic Corticosteroids	-	-	100%	100%
Emergency Department				
Admittance Decision Time (minutes)[5]	-	-	99	98
Head CT Results Within 45 Min. of Arrival	-	-	54%	57%
Patients Who Left ER Before Being Seen	-	-	3%	2%
Time from ER Arrival to Admit. (minutes)[5]	-	-	270	274
Time from ER Arrival to Discharge (minutes)	-	-	127	134
Time in ER Before Being Evaluated (minutes)	-	-	26	26
Time to Pain Meds for Fractures (minutes)	-	-	57	57
Heart Attack Care				
Aspirin Given at Discharge[5]	-	-	99%	99%
Fibrinolytic Meds Within 30 Min. of Arrival[5]	-	-	49%	54%
PCI Within 90 Minutes of Arrival[5]	-	-	95%	96%
Statin Prescribed at Discharge[5]	-	-	98%	98%
Heart Failure Care				
ACE Inhibitor or ARB for LVSD[1,3]	-	-	97%	97%
Discharge Instructions Given[3,7]	-	-	95%	94%
Evaluation of LVS Function[1,3]	-	-	99%	99%
Medicare Spending				
Medicare Spending per Patient (ratio)	-	-	1.03	0.98
Pneumonia Care				
Appropriate Initial Antibiotic Given[1]	-	-	95%	95%
Blood Culture Timing[1]	-	-	98%	98%
Pregnancy and Delivery Care				
Newborn Deliveries Scheduled Early[5]	-	-	7%	6%
Preventive Care				
Immunization for Influenza[5]	-	-	90%	90%
Immunization for Pneumonia[5]	-	-	92%	92%
Stroke Care				
Anticoagulation Therapy for Atrial Fibrillation[5]	-	-	96%	95%
Antithrombotic Therapy Timing[5]	-	-	98%	98%
Assessed for Rehabilitation[5]	-	-	98%	97%
Discharged on Antithrombotic Therapy[5]	-	-	99%	99%
Discharged on Statin Medication[5]	-	-	95%	94%
Thrombolytic Therapy Timing[5]	-	-	68%	66%
Venous Thromboembolism Prophylaxis[5]	-	-	94%	94%
Written Stroke Educational Materials Given[5]	-	-	92%	88%
Surgical Care Improvement Project				
Appropriate Beta Blocker Usage[5]	-	-	98%	98%
Appropriate VTP Within 24 Hours[5]	-	-	98%	98%
Controlled Postoperative Blood Glucose[5]	-	-	96%	97%
Perioperative Temperature Management[5]	-	-	100%	100%
Prophylactic Antibiotic Selection[5]	-	-	99%	99%
Prophylactic Antibiotic Selection (Outpatient)	-	-	98%	98%
Prophylactic Antibiotic Stopped[5]	-	-	98%	98%
Prophylactic Antibiotic Timing[5]	-	-	99%	99%
Prophylactic Antibiotic Timing (Outpatient)	-	-	98%	98%
Urinary Catheter Removal[5]	-	-	98%	97%
Survey of Patients' Hospital Experiences				
Area Around Room 'Always' Quiet at Night[5]	-	-	68%	61%
Doctors 'Always' Communicated Well[5]	-	-	83%	82%
Home Recovery Information Given[5]	-	-	85%	85%
Hospital Given 9 or 10 on 10 Point Scale[5]	-	-	73%	71%
Meds 'Always' Explained Before Given[5]	-	-	66%	64%
Nurses 'Always' Communicated Well[5]	-	-	80%	79%
Pain 'Always' Well Controlled[5]	-	-	72%	71%
Room and Bathroom 'Always' Clean[5]	-	-	75%	73%
Timely Help 'Always' Received[5]	-	-	69%	68%
Would Definitely Recommend Hospital[5]	-	-	73%	71%
Use of Medical Imaging				
Cardiac Imaging Stress Test before Surgery	-	-	5.3%	5.3%
Combination Abdominal CT Scan	-	-	16.4%	10.5%
Combination Brain/Sinus CT Scan	-	-	2.7%	2.7%
Combination Chest CT Scan	-	-	5.6%	2.7%
Follow-up Mammogram/Ultrasound	-	-	7.9%	8.8%
Lumbar Spine MRI for Low Back Pain	-	-	39.6%	37.2%

Medical Center of Mckinney

4500 Medical Center Drive
Mckinney, TX 75069
Phone: 972-547-8000
Fax: 972-547-8008
URL: www.medicalcenterofmckinney.com
Type: Acute Care Hospitals
Ownership: Proprietary
Emergency Services: Yes
Beds: 259

Key Personnel:
Quality Assurance . . . . Carol Clark

NOTE: Hospital profiles are in alphabetical order by state, then city, then hospital within the city; Rankings exclude hospitals with less than 25 cases except for patient surveys which excludes hospitals with less than 100 cases; (a) 100-299 cases; (1) The number of cases/patients is too few to report; (2) Data submitted were based on a sample of cases/patients; (3) Results are based on a shorter time period than required; (4) Data suppressed by CMS for one or more quarters; (5) Results are not available for this reporting period; (6) Fewer than 100 patients completed the HCAHPS survey; (7) No cases met the criteria for this measure; (8) The lower limit of the confidence interval cannot be calculated if the number of observed infections equals zero; (9) No data are available from the state/territory for this reporting period; (10) The scores shown reflect fewer than 50 completed surveys; (11) There were discrepancies in the data collection process; (12) This measure does not apply to this hospital for this reporting period; (13) Results cannot be calculated for this reporting period; (14) The results for this state are combined with nearby states to protect confidentiality; Please refer to the User's Guide for a full explanation of data.

Emergency Room . . . . Glenda Cox
Chief of Medical Staff. . . . . Scott Donaldson, MD
CEO/President. . . . . Ernest C. Lynch III

Measure	Cases	This Hosp.	State Avg.	U.S. Avg.
Blood Clot Prevention and Treatment				
Anticoagulation Overlap Therapy[2]	65	98%	93%	93%
ICU Venous Thromboembolism Prophylaxis[2]	80	94%	92%	92%
Incidence of Potentially Preventable VTE[1,2]	-	-	9%	10%
UFH with Dosages/Platelet Monitoring[2]	29	100%	96%	97%
Venous Thromboembolism Prophylaxis[2]	362	89%	82%	85%
Warfarin Therapy Discharge Instructions[2]	53	85%	84%	75%
Chest Pain/Possible Heart Attack Care				
Aspirin Given Within 24 Hours of Arrival[5]	-	-	94%	96%
Fibrinolytic Meds Within 30 Min. of Arrival[5]	-	-	47%	58%
Average Time to ECG (minutes)[5]	-	-	8	7
Average Time to Transfer (minutes)[5]	-	-	62	60
Children's Asthma Care				
Received Home Management Plan of Care	-	-	93%	88%
Received Reliever Medication	-	-	100%	100%
Received Systemic Corticosteroids	-	-	100%	100%
Emergency Department				
Admittance Decision Time (minutes)[2]	812	147	99	98
Head CT Results Within 45 Min. of Arrival[1]	-	-	54%	57%
Patients Who Left ER Before Being Seen	32,478	2%	3%	2%
Time from ER Arrival to Admit. (minutes)[2]	817	223	270	274
Time from ER Arrival to Discharge (minutes)	406	126	127	134
Time in ER Before Being Evaluated (minutes)	460	13	26	26
Time to Pain Meds for Fractures (minutes)	102	35	57	57
Heart Attack Care				
Aspirin Given at Discharge	144	100%	99%	99%
Fibrinolytic Meds Within 30 Min. of Arrival[7]	-	-	49%	54%
PCI Within 90 Minutes of Arrival	36	100%	95%	96%
Statin Prescribed at Discharge	138	99%	98%	98%
Heart Failure Care				
ACE Inhibitor or ARB for LVSD	52	96%	97%	97%
Discharge Instructions Given	177	96%	95%	94%
Evaluation of LVS Function	236	100%	99%	99%
Medicare Spending				
Medicare Spending per Patient (ratio)	-	1.10	1.03	0.98
Pneumonia Care				
Appropriate Initial Antibiotic Given	109	95%	95%	95%
Blood Culture Timing	215	100%	98%	98%
Pregnancy and Delivery Care				
Newborn Deliveries Scheduled Early[2]	51	4%	7%	6%
Preventive Care				
Immunization for Influenza[2]	585	97%	90%	90%
Immunization for Pneumonia[2]	787	98%	92%	92%
Stroke Care				
Anticoagulation Therapy for Atrial Fibrillation[1,2]	-	-	96%	95%
Antithrombotic Therapy Timing[2]	67	99%	98%	98%
Assessed for Rehabilitation[2]	81	98%	98%	97%
Discharged on Antithrombotic Therapy[2]	68	100%	99%	99%
Discharged on Statin Medication[2]	61	98%	95%	94%
Thrombolytic Therapy Timing[1,2]	-	-	68%	66%
Venous Thromboembolism Prophylaxis[2]	85	96%	94%	94%
Written Stroke Educational Materials Given[2]	49	98%	92%	88%
Surgical Care Improvement Project				
Appropriate Beta Blocker Usage[2]	158	97%	98%	98%
Appropriate VTP Within 24 Hours[2]	282	99%	98%	98%
Controlled Postoperative Blood Glucose[2]	25	100%	96%	97%
Perioperative Temperature Management[2]	353	100%	100%	100%
Prophylactic Antibiotic Selection[2]	217	100%	99%	99%
Prophylactic Antibiotic Selection (Outpatient)	109	94%	98%	98%
Prophylactic Antibiotic Stopped[2]	203	99%	98%	98%
Prophylactic Antibiotic Timing[2]	217	100%	99%	99%
Prophylactic Antibiotic Timing (Outpatient)	109	100%	98%	98%
Urinary Catheter Removal[2]	238	100%	98%	97%
Survey of Patients' Hospital Experiences				
Area Around Room 'Always' Quiet at Night	300+	69%	68%	61%
Doctors 'Always' Communicated Well	300+	80%	83%	82%
Home Recovery Information Given	300+	86%	85%	85%
Hospital Given 9 or 10 on 10 Point Scale	300+	71%	73%	71%
Meds 'Always' Explained Before Given	300+	65%	66%	64%
Nurses 'Always' Communicated Well	300+	79%	80%	79%
Pain 'Always' Well Controlled	300+	75%	72%	71%
Room and Bathroom 'Always' Clean	300+	73%	75%	73%
Timely Help 'Always' Received	300+	69%	69%	68%
Would Definitely Recommend Hospital	300+	71%	73%	71%
Use of Medical Imaging				
Cardiac Imaging Stress Test before Surgery	64	4.7%	5.3%	5.3%
Combination Abdominal CT Scan	465	5.4%	16.4%	10.5%
Combination Brain/Sinus CT Scan	448	3.8%	2.7%	2.7%
Combination Chest CT Scan	321	2.5%	5.6%	2.7%
Follow-up Mammogram/Ultrasound	1,092	9.4%	7.9%	8.8%
Lumbar Spine MRI for Low Back Pain	46	43.5%	39.6%	37.2%

Dallas Regional Medical Center

1011 North Galloway Avenue
Mesquite, TX 75149
Phone: 214-320-7000
Fax: 972-289-9468
URL: www.dallasregionalmedicalcenter.com
Type: Acute Care Hospitals
Emergency Services: Yes
Ownership: Proprietary
Beds: 200
Key Personnel:
Radiology. . . . . Solomon Bierman
Operating Room. . . . . J Blair Biggers
Intensive Care Unit. . . . . Michelle Gann
Quality Assurance . . . . Helle Laverson
CEO . . . . Tina Pollock
Infection Control. . . . . Kim Salmon, RN
Emergency Room . . . . Penny Stillwell, RN

Measure	Cases	This Hosp.	State Avg.	U.S. Avg.
Blood Clot Prevention and Treatment				
Anticoagulation Overlap Therapy[2]	27	96%	93%	93%
ICU Venous Thromboembolism Prophylaxis[2]	94	90%	92%	92%
Incidence of Potentially Preventable VTE[1,2]	-	-	9%	10%
UFH with Dosages/Platelet Monitoring[2]	15	100%	96%	97%
Venous Thromboembolism Prophylaxis[2]	295	77%	82%	85%
Warfarin Therapy Discharge Instructions[2]	22	100%	84%	75%
Chest Pain/Possible Heart Attack Care				
Aspirin Given Within 24 Hours of Arrival[1,3]	-	-	94%	96%
Fibrinolytic Meds Within 30 Min. of Arrival[3,7]	-	-	47%	58%
Average Time to ECG (minutes)[1,3]	-	-	8	7
Average Time to Transfer (minutes)[3,7]	-	-	62	60
Children's Asthma Care				
Received Home Management Plan of Care	-	-	93%	88%
Received Reliever Medication	-	-	100%	100%
Received Systemic Corticosteroids	-	-	100%	100%
Emergency Department				
Admittance Decision Time (minutes)[2]	1,321	64	99	98
Head CT Results Within 45 Min. of Arrival[1]	-	-	54%	57%
Patients Who Left ER Before Being Seen	1,861	17%	3%	2%
Time from ER Arrival to Admit. (minutes)[2]	1,323	246	270	274
Time from ER Arrival to Discharge (minutes)	1,479	110	127	134
Time in ER Before Being Evaluated (minutes)	1,548	18	26	26
Time to Pain Meds for Fractures (minutes)	162	48	57	57
Heart Attack Care				
Aspirin Given at Discharge	110	100%	99%	99%
Fibrinolytic Meds Within 30 Min. of Arrival[7]	-	-	49%	54%
PCI Within 90 Minutes of Arrival	18	100%	95%	96%
Statin Prescribed at Discharge	111	99%	98%	98%
Heart Failure Care				
ACE Inhibitor or ARB for LVSD	64	98%	97%	97%
Discharge Instructions Given	162	96%	95%	94%
Evaluation of LVS Function	197	100%	99%	99%
Medicare Spending				
Medicare Spending per Patient (ratio)	-	1.06	1.03	0.98
Pneumonia Care				
Appropriate Initial Antibiotic Given	69	94%	95%	95%
Blood Culture Timing	144	99%	98%	98%
Pregnancy and Delivery Care				
Newborn Deliveries Scheduled Early[7]	-	-	7%	6%
Preventive Care				
Immunization for Influenza[2]	1,108	98%	90%	90%
Immunization for Pneumonia[2]	1,091	98%	92%	92%
Stroke Care				
Anticoagulation Therapy for Atrial Fibrillation[1]	-	-	96%	95%
Antithrombotic Therapy Timing	40	100%	98%	98%
Assessed for Rehabilitation	40	98%	98%	97%
Discharged on Antithrombotic Therapy	39	100%	99%	99%
Discharged on Statin Medication	29	97%	95%	94%
Thrombolytic Therapy Timing[1]	-	-	68%	66%
Venous Thromboembolism Prophylaxis	43	91%	94%	94%
Written Stroke Educational Materials Given	25	88%	92%	88%
Surgical Care Improvement Project				
Appropriate Beta Blocker Usage	65	100%	98%	98%
Appropriate VTP Within 24 Hours	207	100%	98%	98%
Controlled Postoperative Blood Glucose	18	94%	96%	97%
Perioperative Temperature Management	251	100%	100%	100%
Prophylactic Antibiotic Selection	210	98%	99%	99%
Prophylactic Antibiotic Selection (Outpatient)	88	99%	98%	98%
Prophylactic Antibiotic Stopped	209	100%	98%	98%
Prophylactic Antibiotic Timing	211	100%	99%	99%
Prophylactic Antibiotic Timing (Outpatient)	88	98%	98%	98%
Urinary Catheter Removal	196	100%	98%	97%
Survey of Patients' Hospital Experiences				
Area Around Room 'Always' Quiet at Night	300+	61%	68%	61%
Doctors 'Always' Communicated Well	300+	74%	83%	82%
Home Recovery Information Given	300+	75%	85%	85%
Hospital Given 9 or 10 on 10 Point Scale	300+	52%	73%	71%
Meds 'Always' Explained Before Given	300+	47%	66%	64%
Nurses 'Always' Communicated Well	300+	66%	80%	79%
Pain 'Always' Well Controlled	300+	65%	72%	71%
Room and Bathroom 'Always' Clean	300+	68%	75%	73%
Timely Help 'Always' Received	300+	56%	69%	68%
Would Definitely Recommend Hospital	300+	49%	73%	71%
Use of Medical Imaging				
Cardiac Imaging Stress Test before Surgery[1]	-	-	5.3%	5.3%
Combination Abdominal CT Scan	274	10.2%	16.4%	10.5%
Combination Brain/Sinus CT Scan	350	1.1%	2.7%	2.7%
Combination Chest CT Scan	104	5.8%	5.6%	2.7%
Follow-up Mammogram/Ultrasound	448	6.0%	7.9%	8.8%
Lumbar Spine MRI for Low Back Pain[1]	-	-	39.6%	37.2%

Parkview Regional Hospital

600 South Bonham Street
Mexia, TX 76667
Phone: 254-562-5332
Fax: 254-562-7532
E-mail: timpadams@aol.com
URL: www.parkviewregional.com
Type: Acute Care Hospitals
Emergency Services: Yes
Ownership: Proprietary
Beds: 59
Key Personnel:
Emergency Room . . . . Jeremy Chester
Chief of Medical Staff. . . . . Rhonda Craig
Coronary Care . . . . Mike McCarey
Chairman/CEO . . . . John Stubbs
CEO . . . . Kevin Zachary

Measure	Cases	This Hosp.	State Avg.	U.S. Avg.
Blood Clot Prevention and Treatment				
Anticoagulation Overlap Therapy[1,2]	-	-	93%	93%
ICU Venous Thromboembolism Prophylaxis[2]	11	100%	92%	92%
Incidence of Potentially Preventable VTE[2,7]	-	-	9%	10%
UFH with Dosages/Platelet Monitoring[1,2]	-	-	96%	97%
Venous Thromboembolism Prophylaxis[2]	112	88%	82%	85%
Warfarin Therapy Discharge Instructions[1,2]	-	-	84%	75%
Chest Pain/Possible Heart Attack Care				
Aspirin Given Within 24 Hours of Arrival	89	93%	94%	96%
Fibrinolytic Meds Within 30 Min. of Arrival[1]	-	-	47%	58%
Average Time to ECG (minutes)	94	8	8	7
Average Time to Transfer (minutes)[7]	-	-	62	60
Children's Asthma Care				
Received Home Management Plan of Care	-	-	93%	88%
Received Reliever Medication	-	-	100%	100%
Received Systemic Corticosteroids	-	-	100%	100%
Emergency Department				
Admittance Decision Time (minutes)[2]	445	85	99	98
Head CT Results Within 45 Min. of Arrival	11	55%	54%	57%
Patients Who Left ER Before Being Seen	9,505	1%	3%	2%
Time from ER Arrival to Admit. (minutes)[2]	445	236	270	274
Time from ER Arrival to Discharge (minutes)	347	92	127	134
Time in ER Before Being Evaluated (minutes)	408	18	26	26

NOTE: Hospital profiles are in alphabetical order by state, then city, then hospital within the city; Rankings exclude hospitals with less than 25 cases except for patient surveys which excludes hospitals with less than 100 cases; (a) 100-299 cases; (1) The number of cases/patients is too few to report; (2) Data submitted were based on a sample of cases/patients; (3) Results are based on a shorter time period than required; (4) Data suppressed by CMS for one or more quarters; (5) Results are not available for this reporting period; (6) Fewer than 100 patients completed the HCAHPS survey; (7) No cases met the criteria for this measure; (8) The lower limit of the confidence interval cannot be calculated if the number of observed infections equals zero; (9) No data are available from the state/territory for this reporting period; (10) The scores shown reflect fewer than 50 completed surveys; (11) There were discrepancies in the data collection process; (12) This measure does not apply to this hospital for this reporting period; (13) Results cannot be calculated for this reporting period; (14) The results for this state are combined with nearby states to protect confidentiality; Please refer to the User's Guide for a full explanation of data.

Measure	Cases	This Hosp.	State Avg.	U.S. Avg.
Time to Pain Meds for Fractures (minutes)	44	44	57	57
Heart Attack Care				
Aspirin Given at Discharge[3,7]	-	-	99%	99%
Fibrinolytic Meds Within 30 Min. of Arrival[3,7]	-	-	49%	54%
PCI Within 90 Minutes of Arrival[3,7]	-	-	95%	96%
Statin Prescribed at Discharge[3,7]	-	-	98%	98%
Heart Failure Care				
ACE Inhibitor or ARB for LVSD	14	79%	97%	97%
Discharge Instructions Given	31	94%	95%	94%
Evaluation of LVS Function	41	93%	99%	99%
Medicare Spending				
Medicare Spending per Patient (ratio)	-	0.95	1.03	0.98
Pneumonia Care				
Appropriate Initial Antibiotic Given	59	98%	95%	95%
Blood Culture Timing	66	91%	98%	98%
Pregnancy and Delivery Care				
Newborn Deliveries Scheduled Early[2,7]	-	-	7%	6%
Preventive Care				
Immunization for Influenza[2]	297	96%	90%	90%
Immunization for Pneumonia[2]	460	93%	92%	92%
Stroke Care				
Anticoagulation Therapy for Atrial Fibrillation[7]	-	-	96%	95%
Antithrombotic Therapy Timing[1]	-	-	98%	98%
Assessed for Rehabilitation[1]	-	-	98%	97%
Discharged on Antithrombotic Therapy[1]	-	-	99%	99%
Discharged on Statin Medication[1]	-	-	95%	94%
Thrombolytic Therapy Timing[7]	-	-	68%	66%
Venous Thromboembolism Prophylaxis[1]	-	-	94%	94%
Written Stroke Educational Materials Given[1]	-	-	92%	88%
Surgical Care Improvement Project				
Appropriate Beta Blocker Usage[1,3]	-	-	98%	98%
Appropriate VTP Within 24 Hours[1,3]	-	-	98%	98%
Controlled Postoperative Blood Glucose[3,7]	-	-	96%	97%
Perioperative Temperature Management[1,3]	-	-	100%	100%
Prophylactic Antibiotic Selection[1,3]	-	-	99%	99%
Prophylactic Antibiotic Selection (Outpatient)[1]	-	-	98%	98%
Prophylactic Antibiotic Stopped[1,3]	-	-	98%	98%
Prophylactic Antibiotic Timing[1,3]	-	-	99%	99%
Prophylactic Antibiotic Timing (Outpatient)[1]	-	-	98%	98%
Urinary Catheter Removal[1,3]	-	-	98%	97%
Survey of Patients' Hospital Experiences				
Area Around Room 'Always' Quiet at Night	(a)	75%	68%	61%
Doctors 'Always' Communicated Well	(a)	85%	83%	82%
Home Recovery Information Given	(a)	89%	85%	85%
Hospital Given 9 or 10 on 10 Point Scale	(a)	77%	73%	71%
Meds 'Always' Explained Before Given	(a)	80%	66%	64%
Nurses 'Always' Communicated Well	(a)	85%	80%	79%
Pain 'Always' Well Controlled	(a)	79%	72%	71%
Room and Bathroom 'Always' Clean	(a)	82%	75%	73%
Timely Help 'Always' Received	(a)	80%	69%	68%
Would Definitely Recommend Hospital	(a)	75%	73%	71%
Use of Medical Imaging				
Cardiac Imaging Stress Test before Surgery[1]	-	-	5.3%	5.3%
Combination Abdominal CT Scan	145	3.4%	16.4%	10.5%
Combination Brain/Sinus CT Scan[1]	-	-	2.7%	2.7%
Combination Chest CT Scan	82	0.0%	5.6%	2.7%
Follow-up Mammogram/Ultrasound	261	10.3%	7.9%	8.8%
Lumbar Spine MRI for Low Back Pain[1]	-	-	39.6%	37.2%

Midland Memorial Hospital

400 Rosalind Redfern Grover Parkway
Midland, TX 79701
Phone: 432-685-1111
Fax: 432-685-3488
E-mail: ljohnson@midland-memorial.com
URL: www.midland-memorial.com
Type: Acute Care Hospitals
Emergency Services: Yes
Ownership: Govt - Hospital Dist/Auth
Beds: 321

Key Personnel:

Pediatric Ambulatory Care . . . . . . Ronald Boren, MD
Pediatric In-Patient Care . . . . Ronald Boren, MD
Emergency Room . . . . Ann Brewington, RN
Radiology. . . . . Marlon Hughes, MD
CEO/President. . . . . Russell Meyers
Chief of Medical Staff . . . . Larry Oliver, MD
Quality Assurance . . . . Vondie Silipo, RN

Measure	Cases	This Hosp.	State Avg.	U.S. Avg.
Blood Clot Prevention and Treatment				
Anticoagulation Overlap Therapy[2]	64	98%	93%	93%
ICU Venous Thromboembolism Prophylaxis[2]	87	95%	92%	92%
Incidence of Potentially Preventable VTE[2]	11	0%	9%	10%
UFH with Dosages/Platelet Monitoring[2]	24	100%	96%	97%
Venous Thromboembolism Prophylaxis[2]	356	85%	82%	85%
Warfarin Therapy Discharge Instructions[2]	50	92%	84%	75%
Chest Pain/Possible Heart Attack Care				
Aspirin Given Within 24 Hours of Arrival[5]	-	-	94%	96%
Fibrinolytic Meds Within 30 Min. of Arrival[5]	-	-	47%	58%
Average Time to ECG (minutes)[5]	-	-	8	7
Average Time to Transfer (minutes)[5]	-	-	62	60
Children's Asthma Care				
Received Home Management Plan of Care	-	-	93%	88%
Received Reliever Medication	-	-	100%	100%
Received Systemic Corticosteroids	-	-	100%	100%
Emergency Department				
Admittance Decision Time (minutes)[2]	1,431	129	99	98
Head CT Results Within 45 Min. of Arrival[1]	-	-	54%	57%
Patients Who Left ER Before Being Seen	63,743	4%	3%	2%
Time from ER Arrival to Admit. (minutes)[2]	1,438	293	270	274
Time from ER Arrival to Discharge (minutes)	429	149	127	134
Time in ER Before Being Evaluated (minutes)	436	28	26	26
Time to Pain Meds for Fractures (minutes)	262	57	57	57
Heart Attack Care				
Aspirin Given at Discharge	223	100%	99%	99%
Fibrinolytic Meds Within 30 Min. of Arrival[7]	-	-	49%	54%
PCI Within 90 Minutes of Arrival	62	97%	95%	96%
Statin Prescribed at Discharge	227	97%	98%	98%
Heart Failure Care				
ACE Inhibitor or ARB for LVSD	113	93%	97%	97%
Discharge Instructions Given	316	98%	95%	94%
Evaluation of LVS Function	377	100%	99%	99%
Medicare Spending				
Medicare Spending per Patient (ratio)	-	1.08	1.03	0.98
Pneumonia Care				
Appropriate Initial Antibiotic Given	135	87%	95%	95%
Blood Culture Timing	202	99%	98%	98%
Pregnancy and Delivery Care				
Newborn Deliveries Scheduled Early[2]	237	13%	7%	6%
Preventive Care				
Immunization for Influenza[2]	1,259	98%	90%	90%
Immunization for Pneumonia[2]	1,854	96%	92%	92%
Stroke Care				
Anticoagulation Therapy for Atrial Fibrillation	16	94%	96%	95%
Antithrombotic Therapy Timing	111	94%	98%	98%
Assessed for Rehabilitation	133	100%	98%	97%
Discharged on Antithrombotic Therapy	127	98%	99%	99%
Discharged on Statin Medication	94	100%	95%	94%
Thrombolytic Therapy Timing	17	24%	68%	66%
Venous Thromboembolism Prophylaxis	136	96%	94%	94%
Written Stroke Educational Materials Given	73	96%	92%	88%
Surgical Care Improvement Project				
Appropriate Beta Blocker Usage	279	95%	98%	98%
Appropriate VTP Within 24 Hours	776	99%	98%	98%
Controlled Postoperative Blood Glucose	74	97%	96%	97%
Perioperative Temperature Management	968	100%	100%	100%
Prophylactic Antibiotic Selection	590	99%	99%	99%
Prophylactic Antibiotic Selection (Outpatient)	255	96%	98%	98%
Prophylactic Antibiotic Stopped	581	98%	98%	98%
Prophylactic Antibiotic Timing	590	99%	99%	99%
Prophylactic Antibiotic Timing (Outpatient)	257	98%	98%	98%
Urinary Catheter Removal	561	98%	98%	97%
Survey of Patients' Hospital Experiences				
Area Around Room 'Always' Quiet at Night	300+	60%	68%	61%
Doctors 'Always' Communicated Well	300+	77%	83%	82%
Home Recovery Information Given	300+	82%	85%	85%
Hospital Given 9 or 10 on 10 Point Scale	300+	64%	73%	71%
Meds 'Always' Explained Before Given	300+	54%	66%	64%
Nurses 'Always' Communicated Well	300+	72%	80%	79%
Pain 'Always' Well Controlled	300+	68%	72%	71%
Room and Bathroom 'Always' Clean	300+	61%	75%	73%
Timely Help 'Always' Received	300+	58%	69%	68%
Would Definitely Recommend Hospital	300+	63%	73%	71%
Use of Medical Imaging				
Cardiac Imaging Stress Test before Surgery	316	2.2%	5.3%	5.3%
Combination Abdominal CT Scan	970	11.1%	16.4%	10.5%
Combination Brain/Sinus CT Scan	605	2.1%	2.7%	2.7%
Combination Chest CT Scan	726	5.6%	5.6%	2.7%
Follow-up Mammogram/Ultrasound	2,468	8.0%	7.9%	8.8%
Lumbar Spine MRI for Low Back Pain	233	37.8%	39.6%	37.2%

Palo Pinto General Hospital

400 Southwest 25 Ave
Mineral Wells, TX 76067
Phone: 940-325-7891
Fax: 940-325-7903
URL: www.ppgh.com
Type: Acute Care Hospitals
Emergency Services: Yes
Ownership: Govt - Hospital Dist/Auth
Beds: 99

Key Personnel:

Chief of Medical Staff . . . . Mathis Adams, MD
CEO/President. . . . . Harris W Brooks
Radiology. . . . . Joe Erwin
Infection Control. . . . . Sue Lamb, RN
Quality Assurance . . . . Brenda Patton, LVN
Coronary Care . . . . Chastity Wilcox
Operating Room. . . . . Susan Woodring

Measure	Cases	This Hosp.	State Avg.	U.S. Avg.
Blood Clot Prevention and Treatment				
Anticoagulation Overlap Therapy[2]	12	83%	93%	93%
ICU Venous Thromboembolism Prophylaxis[2]	39	67%	92%	92%
Incidence of Potentially Preventable VTE[1,2]	-	-	9%	10%
UFH with Dosages/Platelet Monitoring[1,2]	-	-	96%	97%
Venous Thromboembolism Prophylaxis[2]	160	54%	82%	85%
Warfarin Therapy Discharge Instructions[1,2]	-	-	84%	75%
Chest Pain/Possible Heart Attack Care				
Aspirin Given Within 24 Hours of Arrival[3]	49	96%	94%	96%
Fibrinolytic Meds Within 30 Min. of Arrival[1,3]	-	-	47%	58%
Average Time to ECG (minutes)[3]	50	2	8	7
Average Time to Transfer (minutes)[3]	22	89	62	60
Children's Asthma Care				
Received Home Management Plan of Care	-	-	93%	88%
Received Reliever Medication	-	-	100%	100%
Received Systemic Corticosteroids	-	-	100%	100%
Emergency Department				
Admittance Decision Time (minutes)[2]	257	80	99	98
Head CT Results Within 45 Min. of Arrival	17	29%	54%	57%
Patients Who Left ER Before Being Seen	22,304	2%	3%	2%
Time from ER Arrival to Admit. (minutes)[2]	268	198	270	274
Time from ER Arrival to Discharge (minutes)	384	76	127	134
Time in ER Before Being Evaluated (minutes)	344	16	26	26
Time to Pain Meds for Fractures (minutes)	43	64	57	57
Heart Attack Care				
Aspirin Given at Discharge[1]	-	-	99%	99%
Fibrinolytic Meds Within 30 Min. of Arrival[7]	-	-	49%	54%
PCI Within 90 Minutes of Arrival[7]	-	-	95%	96%
Statin Prescribed at Discharge[1]	-	-	98%	98%
Heart Failure Care				
ACE Inhibitor or ARB for LVSD	19	100%	97%	97%
Discharge Instructions Given	38	100%	95%	94%
Evaluation of LVS Function	47	100%	99%	99%
Medicare Spending				
Medicare Spending per Patient (ratio)	-	1.06	1.03	0.98
Pneumonia Care				
Appropriate Initial Antibiotic Given	67	90%	95%	95%
Blood Culture Timing	96	98%	98%	98%
Pregnancy and Delivery Care				
Newborn Deliveries Scheduled Early[2]	27	19%	7%	6%
Preventive Care				
Immunization for Influenza[2]	253	80%	90%	90%
Immunization for Pneumonia[2]	323	86%	92%	92%
Stroke Care				
Anticoagulation Therapy for Atrial Fibrillation[1]	-	-	96%	95%
Antithrombotic Therapy Timing[1]	-	-	98%	98%
Assessed for Rehabilitation[1]	-	-	98%	97%
Discharged on Antithrombotic Therapy[1]	-	-	99%	99%

NOTE: Hospital profiles are in alphabetical order by state, then city, then hospital within the city; Rankings exclude hospitals with less than 25 cases except for patient surveys which excludes hospitals with less than 100 cases; (a) 100-299 cases; (1) The number of cases/patients is too few to report; (2) Data submitted were based on a sample of cases/patients; (3) Results are based on a shorter time period than required; (4) Data suppressed by CMS for one or more quarters; (5) Results are not available for this reporting period; (6) Fewer than 100 patients completed the HCAHPS survey; (7) No cases met the criteria for this measure; (8) The lower limit of the confidence interval cannot be calculated if the number of observed infections equals zero; (9) No data are available from the state/territory for this reporting period; (10) The scores shown reflect fewer than 50 completed surveys; (11) There were discrepancies in the data collection process; (12) This measure does not apply to this hospital for this reporting period; (13) Results cannot be calculated for this reporting period; (14) The results for this state are combined with nearby states to protect confidentiality; Please refer to the User's Guide for a full explanation of data.

Measure	Cases	This Hosp.	State Avg.	U.S. Avg.
Discharged on Statin Medication[1]	-	-	95%	94%
Thrombolytic Therapy Timing[1]	-	-	68%	66%
Venous Thromboembolism Prophylaxis[1]	-	-	94%	94%
Written Stroke Educational Materials Given[1]	-	-	92%	88%
Surgical Care Improvement Project				
Appropriate Beta Blocker Usage	14	93%	98%	98%
Appropriate VTP Within 24 Hours	75	93%	98%	98%
Controlled Postoperative Blood Glucose[7]	-	-	96%	97%
Perioperative Temperature Management	96	100%	100%	100%
Prophylactic Antibiotic Selection	65	95%	99%	99%
Prophylactic Antibiotic Selection (Outpatient)	32	97%	98%	98%
Prophylactic Antibiotic Stopped	63	100%	98%	98%
Prophylactic Antibiotic Timing	66	98%	99%	99%
Prophylactic Antibiotic Timing (Outpatient)	32	100%	98%	98%
Urinary Catheter Removal	36	97%	98%	97%
Survey of Patients' Hospital Experiences				
Area Around Room 'Always' Quiet at Night	300+	61%	68%	61%
Doctors 'Always' Communicated Well	300+	82%	83%	82%
Home Recovery Information Given	300+	89%	85%	85%
Hospital Given 9 or 10 on 10 Point Scale	300+	68%	73%	71%
Meds 'Always' Explained Before Given	300+	58%	66%	64%
Nurses 'Always' Communicated Well	300+	79%	80%	79%
Pain 'Always' Well Controlled	300+	73%	72%	71%
Room and Bathroom 'Always' Clean	300+	67%	75%	73%
Timely Help 'Always' Received	300+	72%	69%	68%
Would Definitely Recommend Hospital	300+	64%	73%	71%
Use of Medical Imaging				
Cardiac Imaging Stress Test before Surgery	210	6.7%	5.3%	5.3%
Combination Abdominal CT Scan	283	31.1%	16.4%	10.5%
Combination Brain/Sinus CT Scan	340	0.9%	2.7%	2.7%
Combination Chest CT Scan	153	7.8%	5.6%	2.7%
Follow-up Mammogram/Ultrasound	298	11.7%	7.9%	8.8%
Lumbar Spine MRI for Low Back Pain	69	44.9%	39.6%	37.2%

Mission Regional Medical Center

900 South Bryan Road
Mission, TX 78572
Phone: 956-323-9000
Fax: 956-323-9102
E-mail: mgarza@missionmc.org
URL: www.missionhospital.org
Type: Acute Care Hospitals
Emergency Services: Yes
Ownership: Voluntary non-profit - Private
Beds: 138

Key Personnel:
Chief of Medical Staff.......... Desi Canals, MD
Quality Assurance .... Carol Gruber
CEO .... Javier Iruegas, FACHE
Infection Control............. Gilbert Koschtial
Patient Relations .... Lucia Leo-Diaz, LMSW
Intensive Care Unit........... Fred Moreno
Operating Room.............. Grace Munday
Radiology.................... Vangala J Reddy

Measure	Cases	This Hosp.	State Avg.	U.S. Avg.
Blood Clot Prevention and Treatment				
Anticoagulation Overlap Therapy[2]	18	72%	93%	93%
ICU Venous Thromboembolism Prophylaxis[2]	131	93%	92%	92%
Incidence of Potentially Preventable VTE[1,2]	-	-	9%	10%
UFH with Dosages/Platelet Monitoring[1,2]	-	-	96%	97%
Venous Thromboembolism Prophylaxis[2]	339	88%	82%	85%
Warfarin Therapy Discharge Instructions[2]	13	92%	84%	75%
Chest Pain/Possible Heart Attack Care				
Aspirin Given Within 24 Hours of Arrival[1]	-	-	94%	96%
Fibrinolytic Meds Within 30 Min. of Arrival[3,7]	-	-	47%	58%
Average Time to ECG (minutes)[1]	-	-	8	7
Average Time to Transfer (minutes)[3,7]	-	-	62	60
Children's Asthma Care				
Received Home Management Plan of Care	-	-	93%	88%
Received Reliever Medication	-	-	100%	100%
Received Systemic Corticosteroids	-	-	100%	100%
Emergency Department				
Admittance Decision Time (minutes)[2]	344	93	99	98
Head CT Results Within 45 Min. of Arrival[1,3]	-	-	54%	57%
Patients Who Left ER Before Being Seen	37,723	1%	3%	2%
Time from ER Arrival to Admit. (minutes)[2]	360	294	270	274
Time from ER Arrival to Discharge (minutes)	356	164	127	134
Time in ER Before Being Evaluated (minutes)	265	31	26	26
Time to Pain Meds for Fractures (minutes)	100	51	57	57
Heart Attack Care				
Aspirin Given at Discharge	107	94%	99%	99%
Fibrinolytic Meds Within 30 Min. of Arrival[7]	-	-	49%	54%
PCI Within 90 Minutes of Arrival[1]	-	-	95%	96%
Statin Prescribed at Discharge	105	90%	98%	98%
Heart Failure Care				
ACE Inhibitor or ARB for LVSD	57	86%	97%	97%
Discharge Instructions Given	174	95%	95%	94%
Evaluation of LVS Function	218	97%	99%	99%
Medicare Spending				
Medicare Spending per Patient (ratio)	-	1.01	1.03	0.98
Pneumonia Care				
Appropriate Initial Antibiotic Given	163	96%	95%	95%
Blood Culture Timing	302	97%	98%	98%
Pregnancy and Delivery Care				
Newborn Deliveries Scheduled Early[2]	73	12%	7%	6%
Preventive Care				
Immunization for Influenza[2]	436	87%	90%	90%
Immunization for Pneumonia[2]	465	94%	92%	92%
Stroke Care				
Anticoagulation Therapy for Atrial Fibrillation[1]	-	-	96%	95%
Antithrombotic Therapy Timing	56	98%	98%	98%
Assessed for Rehabilitation	77	92%	98%	97%
Discharged on Antithrombotic Therapy	58	95%	99%	99%
Discharged on Statin Medication	46	85%	95%	94%
Thrombolytic Therapy Timing	21	0%	68%	66%
Venous Thromboembolism Prophylaxis	87	92%	94%	94%
Written Stroke Educational Materials Given	43	100%	92%	88%
Surgical Care Improvement Project				
Appropriate Beta Blocker Usage	80	94%	98%	98%
Appropriate VTP Within 24 Hours	273	95%	98%	98%
Controlled Postoperative Blood Glucose[7]	-	-	96%	97%
Perioperative Temperature Management	304	100%	100%	100%
Prophylactic Antibiotic Selection	161	98%	99%	99%
Prophylactic Antibiotic Selection (Outpatient)	27	85%	98%	98%
Prophylactic Antibiotic Stopped	141	97%	98%	98%
Prophylactic Antibiotic Timing	161	98%	99%	99%
Prophylactic Antibiotic Timing (Outpatient)	31	84%	98%	98%
Urinary Catheter Removal	70	96%	98%	97%
Survey of Patients' Hospital Experiences				
Area Around Room 'Always' Quiet at Night	300+	59%	68%	61%
Doctors 'Always' Communicated Well	300+	83%	83%	82%
Home Recovery Information Given	300+	85%	85%	85%
Hospital Given 9 or 10 on 10 Point Scale	300+	77%	73%	71%
Meds 'Always' Explained Before Given	300+	65%	66%	64%
Nurses 'Always' Communicated Well	300+	79%	80%	79%
Pain 'Always' Well Controlled	300+	73%	72%	71%
Room and Bathroom 'Always' Clean	300+	73%	75%	73%
Timely Help 'Always' Received	300+	68%	69%	68%
Would Definitely Recommend Hospital	300+	75%	73%	71%
Use of Medical Imaging				
Cardiac Imaging Stress Test before Surgery[1]	-	-	5.3%	5.3%
Combination Abdominal CT Scan	253	13.4%	16.4%	10.5%
Combination Brain/Sinus CT Scan	522	0.6%	2.7%	2.7%
Combination Chest CT Scan	105	4.8%	5.6%	2.7%
Follow-up Mammogram/Ultrasound	1,285	5.8%	7.9%	8.8%
Lumbar Spine MRI for Low Back Pain[1]	-	-	39.6%	37.2%

Ward Memorial Hospital

406 South Gary St
Monahans, TX 79756
Phone: 432-943-2511
Fax: 432-943-9415
URL: www.wardmemorial.org
Type: Critical Access Hospitals
Emergency Services: Yes
Ownership: Government - Local
Beds: 49

Key Personnel:
Operating Room............. Alberta Cartwright
Chief of Medical Staff.......... William Davison
Quality Assurance .... Kathy Dendy
Emergency Room .... Federico Gregorio
Radiology.................... Wanda Young

Measure	Cases	This Hosp.	State Avg.	U.S. Avg.
Blood Clot Prevention and Treatment				
Anticoagulation Overlap Therapy[5]	-	-	93%	93%
ICU Venous Thromboembolism Prophylaxis[5]	-	-	92%	92%
Incidence of Potentially Preventable VTE[5]	-	-	9%	10%
UFH with Dosages/Platelet Monitoring[5]	-	-	96%	97%
Venous Thromboembolism Prophylaxis[5]	-	-	82%	85%
Warfarin Therapy Discharge Instructions[5]	-	-	84%	75%
Chest Pain/Possible Heart Attack Care				
Aspirin Given Within 24 Hours of Arrival	-	-	94%	96%
Fibrinolytic Meds Within 30 Min. of Arrival	-	-	47%	58%
Average Time to ECG (minutes)	-	-	8	7
Average Time to Transfer (minutes)	-	-	62	60
Children's Asthma Care				
Received Home Management Plan of Care	-	-	93%	88%
Received Reliever Medication	-	-	100%	100%
Received Systemic Corticosteroids	-	-	100%	100%
Emergency Department				
Admittance Decision Time (minutes)[5]	-	-	99	98
Head CT Results Within 45 Min. of Arrival	-	-	54%	57%
Patients Who Left ER Before Being Seen	-	-	3%	2%
Time from ER Arrival to Admit. (minutes)[5]	-	-	270	274
Time from ER Arrival to Discharge (minutes)	-	-	127	134
Time in ER Before Being Evaluated (minutes)	-	-	26	26
Time to Pain Meds for Fractures (minutes)	-	-	57	57
Heart Attack Care				
Aspirin Given at Discharge[3,7]	-	-	99%	99%
Fibrinolytic Meds Within 30 Min. of Arrival[3,7]	-	-	49%	54%
PCI Within 90 Minutes of Arrival[3,7]	-	-	95%	96%
Statin Prescribed at Discharge[3,7]	-	-	98%	98%
Heart Failure Care				
ACE Inhibitor or ARB for LVSD[3,7]	-	-	97%	97%
Discharge Instructions Given[1,3]	-	-	95%	94%
Evaluation of LVS Function[1,3]	-	-	99%	99%
Medicare Spending				
Medicare Spending per Patient (ratio)	-	-	1.03	0.98
Pneumonia Care				
Appropriate Initial Antibiotic Given[1,3]	-	-	95%	95%
Blood Culture Timing[1,3]	-	-	98%	98%
Pregnancy and Delivery Care				
Newborn Deliveries Scheduled Early[5]	-	-	7%	6%
Preventive Care				
Immunization for Influenza[5]	-	-	90%	90%
Immunization for Pneumonia[5]	-	-	92%	92%
Stroke Care				
Anticoagulation Therapy for Atrial Fibrillation[5]	-	-	96%	95%
Antithrombotic Therapy Timing[5]	-	-	98%	98%
Assessed for Rehabilitation[5]	-	-	98%	97%
Discharged on Antithrombotic Therapy[5]	-	-	99%	99%
Discharged on Statin Medication[5]	-	-	95%	94%
Thrombolytic Therapy Timing[5]	-	-	68%	66%
Venous Thromboembolism Prophylaxis[5]	-	-	94%	94%
Written Stroke Educational Materials Given[5]	-	-	92%	88%
Surgical Care Improvement Project				
Appropriate Beta Blocker Usage[5]	-	-	98%	98%
Appropriate VTP Within 24 Hours[5]	-	-	98%	98%
Controlled Postoperative Blood Glucose[5]	-	-	96%	97%
Perioperative Temperature Management[5]	-	-	100%	100%
Prophylactic Antibiotic Selection[5]	-	-	99%	99%
Prophylactic Antibiotic Selection (Outpatient)	-	-	98%	98%
Prophylactic Antibiotic Stopped[5]	-	-	98%	98%
Prophylactic Antibiotic Timing[5]	-	-	99%	99%
Prophylactic Antibiotic Timing (Outpatient)	-	-	98%	98%
Urinary Catheter Removal[5]	-	-	98%	97%
Survey of Patients' Hospital Experiences				
Area Around Room 'Always' Quiet at Night[5]	-	-	68%	61%
Doctors 'Always' Communicated Well[5]	-	-	83%	82%
Home Recovery Information Given[5]	-	-	85%	85%
Hospital Given 9 or 10 on 10 Point Scale[5]	-	-	73%	71%
Meds 'Always' Explained Before Given[5]	-	-	66%	64%
Nurses 'Always' Communicated Well[5]	-	-	80%	79%
Pain 'Always' Well Controlled[5]	-	-	72%	71%
Room and Bathroom 'Always' Clean[5]	-	-	75%	73%
Timely Help 'Always' Received[5]	-	-	69%	68%
Would Definitely Recommend Hospital[5]	-	-	73%	71%

NOTE: Hospital profiles are in alphabetical order by state, then city, then hospital within the city; Rankings exclude hospitals with less than 25 cases except for patient surveys which excludes hospitals with less than 100 cases; (a) 100-299 cases; (1) The number of cases/patients is too few to report; (2) Data submitted were based on a sample of cases/patients; (3) Results are based on a shorter time period than required; (4) Data suppressed by CMS for one or more quarters; (5) Results are not available for this reporting period; (6) Fewer than 100 patients completed the HCAHPS survey; (7) No cases met the criteria for this measure; (8) The lower limit of the confidence interval cannot be calculated if the number of observed infections equals zero; (9) No data are available from the state/territory for this reporting period; (10) The scores shown reflect fewer than 50 completed surveys; (11) There were discrepancies in the data collection process; (12) This measure does not apply to this hospital for this reporting period; (13) Results cannot be calculated for this reporting period; (14) The results for this state are combined with nearby states to protect confidentiality; Please refer to the User's Guide for a full explanation of data.

Use of Medical Imaging				
Cardiac Imaging Stress Test before Surgery	-	-	5.3%	5.3%
Combination Abdominal CT Scan	-	-	16.4%	10.5%
Combination Brain/Sinus CT Scan	-	-	2.7%	2.7%
Combination Chest CT Scan	-	-	5.6%	2.7%
Follow-up Mammogram/Ultrasound	-	-	7.9%	8.8%
Lumbar Spine MRI for Low Back Pain	-	-	39.6%	37.2%

Cochran Memorial Hospital

205 E Grant Street Phone: 806-266-5565
Morton, TX 79346
Type: Critical Access Hospitals Emergency Services: Yes
Ownership: Govt - Hospital Dist/Auth

Measure	Cases	This Hosp.	State Avg.	U.S. Avg.
Blood Clot Prevention and Treatment				
Anticoagulation Overlap Therapy[5]	-	-	93%	93%
ICU Venous Thromboembolism Prophylaxis[5]	-	-	92%	92%
Incidence of Potentially Preventable VTE[5]	-	-	9%	10%
UFH with Dosages/Platelet Monitoring[5]	-	-	96%	97%
Venous Thromboembolism Prophylaxis[5]	-	-	82%	85%
Warfarin Therapy Discharge Instructions[5]	-	-	84%	75%
Chest Pain/Possible Heart Attack Care				
Aspirin Given Within 24 Hours of Arrival	-	-	94%	96%
Fibrinolytic Meds Within 30 Min. of Arrival	-	-	47%	58%
Average Time to ECG (minutes)	-	-	8	7
Average Time to Transfer (minutes)	-	-	62	60
Children's Asthma Care				
Received Home Management Plan of Care	-	-	93%	88%
Received Reliever Medication	-	-	100%	100%
Received Systemic Corticosteroids	-	-	100%	100%
Emergency Department				
Admittance Decision Time (minutes)[5]	-	-	99	98
Head CT Results Within 45 Min. of Arrival	-	-	54%	57%
Patients Who Left ER Before Being Seen	-	-	3%	2%
Time from ER Arrival to Admit. (minutes)[5]	-	-	270	274
Time from ER Arrival to Discharge (minutes)	-	-	127	134
Time in ER Before Being Evaluated (minutes)	-	-	26	26
Time to Pain Meds for Fractures (minutes)	-	-	57	57
Heart Attack Care				
Aspirin Given at Discharge[5]	-	-	99%	99%
Fibrinolytic Meds Within 30 Min. of Arrival[5]	-	-	49%	54%
PCI Within 90 Minutes of Arrival[5]	-	-	95%	96%
Statin Prescribed at Discharge[5]	-	-	98%	98%
Heart Failure Care				
ACE Inhibitor or ARB for LVSD[5]	-	-	97%	97%
Discharge Instructions Given[5]	-	-	95%	94%
Evaluation of LVS Function[5]	-	-	99%	99%
Medicare Spending				
Medicare Spending per Patient (ratio)	-	-	1.03	0.98
Pneumonia Care				
Appropriate Initial Antibiotic Given[5]	-	-	95%	95%
Blood Culture Timing[5]	-	-	98%	98%
Pregnancy and Delivery Care				
Newborn Deliveries Scheduled Early[5]	-	-	7%	6%
Preventive Care				
Immunization for Influenza[5]	-	-	90%	90%
Immunization for Pneumonia[5]	-	-	92%	92%
Stroke Care				
Anticoagulation Therapy for Atrial Fibrillation[5]	-	-	96%	95%
Antithrombotic Therapy Timing[5]	-	-	98%	98%
Assessed for Rehabilitation[5]	-	-	98%	97%
Discharged on Antithrombotic Therapy[5]	-	-	99%	99%
Discharged on Statin Medication[5]	-	-	95%	94%
Thrombolytic Therapy Timing[5]	-	-	68%	66%
Venous Thromboembolism Prophylaxis[5]	-	-	94%	94%
Written Stroke Educational Materials Given[5]	-	-	92%	88%
Surgical Care Improvement Project				
Appropriate Beta Blocker Usage[5]	-	-	98%	98%
Appropriate VTP Within 24 Hours[5]	-	-	98%	98%
Controlled Postoperative Blood Glucose[5]	-	-	96%	97%
Perioperative Temperature Management[5]	-	-	100%	100%
Prophylactic Antibiotic Selection[5]	-	-	99%	99%
Prophylactic Antibiotic Selection (Outpatient)	-	-	98%	98%
Prophylactic Antibiotic Stopped[5]	-	-	98%	98%
Prophylactic Antibiotic Timing[5]	-	-	99%	99%
Prophylactic Antibiotic Timing (Outpatient)	-	-	98%	98%
Urinary Catheter Removal[5]	-	-	98%	97%
Survey of Patients' Hospital Experiences				
Area Around Room 'Always' Quiet at Night[5]	-	-	68%	61%
Doctors 'Always' Communicated Well[5]	-	-	83%	82%
Home Recovery Information Given[5]	-	-	85%	85%
Hospital Given 9 or 10 on 10 Point Scale[5]	-	-	73%	71%
Meds 'Always' Explained Before Given[5]	-	-	66%	64%
Nurses 'Always' Communicated Well[5]	-	-	80%	79%
Pain 'Always' Well Controlled[5]	-	-	72%	71%
Room and Bathroom 'Always' Clean[5]	-	-	75%	73%
Timely Help 'Always' Received[5]	-	-	69%	68%
Would Definitely Recommend Hospital[5]	-	-	73%	71%
Use of Medical Imaging				
Cardiac Imaging Stress Test before Surgery	-	-	5.3%	5.3%
Combination Abdominal CT Scan	-	-	16.4%	10.5%
Combination Brain/Sinus CT Scan	-	-	2.7%	2.7%
Combination Chest CT Scan	-	-	5.6%	2.7%
Follow-up Mammogram/Ultrasound	-	-	7.9%	8.8%
Lumbar Spine MRI for Low Back Pain	-	-	39.6%	37.2%

Titus Regional Medical Center

2001 N Jefferson Phone: 903-577-6000
Mount Pleasant, TX 75455 Fax: 903-577-6027
URL: www.titusregional.com
Type: Acute Care Hospitals Emergency Services: Yes
Ownership: Govt - Hospital Dist/Auth Beds: 165

Key Personnel:
CEO . . . . John Allen
Emergency Room . . . . Peggy Helbert
CEO/President. . . . . Steve Jacobson
Chairman/CEO . . . . Rick Strudtoff

Measure	Cases	This Hosp.	State Avg.	U.S. Avg.
Blood Clot Prevention and Treatment				
Anticoagulation Overlap Therapy[2]	14	64%	93%	93%
ICU Venous Thromboembolism Prophylaxis[2]	42	81%	92%	92%
Incidence of Potentially Preventable VTE[1,2]	-	-	9%	10%
UFH with Dosages/Platelet Monitoring[1,2]	-	-	96%	97%
Venous Thromboembolism Prophylaxis[2]	118	86%	82%	85%
Warfarin Therapy Discharge Instructions[2]	11	45%	84%	75%
Chest Pain/Possible Heart Attack Care				
Aspirin Given Within 24 Hours of Arrival	77	94%	94%	96%
Fibrinolytic Meds Within 30 Min. of Arrival[1]	-	-	47%	58%
Average Time to ECG (minutes)	82	14	8	7
Average Time to Transfer (minutes)	15	88	62	60
Children's Asthma Care				
Received Home Management Plan of Care	-	-	93%	88%
Received Reliever Medication	-	-	100%	100%
Received Systemic Corticosteroids	-	-	100%	100%
Emergency Department				
Admittance Decision Time (minutes)[2]	111	62	99	98
Head CT Results Within 45 Min. of Arrival	17	76%	54%	57%
Patients Who Left ER Before Being Seen	21,681	1%	3%	2%
Time from ER Arrival to Admit. (minutes)[2]	148	226	270	274
Time from ER Arrival to Discharge (minutes)	380	105	127	134
Time in ER Before Being Evaluated (minutes)	352	26	26	26
Time to Pain Meds for Fractures (minutes)	137	57	57	57
Heart Attack Care				
Aspirin Given at Discharge[1,3]	-	-	99%	99%
Fibrinolytic Meds Within 30 Min. of Arrival[3,7]	-	-	49%	54%
PCI Within 90 Minutes of Arrival[3,7]	-	-	95%	96%
Statin Prescribed at Discharge[1,3]	-	-	98%	98%
Heart Failure Care				
ACE Inhibitor or ARB for LVSD	24	83%	97%	97%
Discharge Instructions Given	44	95%	95%	94%
Evaluation of LVS Function	63	100%	99%	99%
Medicare Spending				
Medicare Spending per Patient (ratio)	-	1.04	1.03	0.98
Pneumonia Care				
Appropriate Initial Antibiotic Given	95	95%	95%	95%
Blood Culture Timing	81	98%	98%	98%
Pregnancy and Delivery Care				
Newborn Deliveries Scheduled Early	135	6%	7%	6%
Preventive Care				
Immunization for Influenza[2]	298	81%	90%	90%
Immunization for Pneumonia[2]	241	93%	92%	92%
Stroke Care				
Anticoagulation Therapy for Atrial Fibrillation[7]	-	-	96%	95%
Antithrombotic Therapy Timing	11	91%	98%	98%
Assessed for Rehabilitation[1]	-	-	98%	97%
Discharged on Antithrombotic Therapy[1]	-	-	99%	99%
Discharged on Statin Medication[1]	-	-	95%	94%
Thrombolytic Therapy Timing[1]	-	-	68%	66%
Venous Thromboembolism Prophylaxis	12	83%	94%	94%
Written Stroke Educational Materials Given[1]	-	-	92%	88%
Surgical Care Improvement Project				
Appropriate Beta Blocker Usage	39	100%	98%	98%
Appropriate VTP Within 24 Hours	156	92%	98%	98%
Controlled Postoperative Blood Glucose[7]	-	-	96%	97%
Perioperative Temperature Management	166	100%	100%	100%
Prophylactic Antibiotic Selection	78	96%	99%	99%
Prophylactic Antibiotic Selection (Outpatient)	97	97%	98%	98%
Prophylactic Antibiotic Stopped	77	100%	98%	98%
Prophylactic Antibiotic Timing	78	99%	99%	99%
Prophylactic Antibiotic Timing (Outpatient)	97	97%	98%	98%
Urinary Catheter Removal	113	96%	98%	97%
Survey of Patients' Hospital Experiences				
Area Around Room 'Always' Quiet at Night	300+	72%	68%	61%
Doctors 'Always' Communicated Well	300+	83%	83%	82%
Home Recovery Information Given	300+	84%	85%	85%
Hospital Given 9 or 10 on 10 Point Scale	300+	68%	73%	71%
Meds 'Always' Explained Before Given	300+	66%	66%	64%
Nurses 'Always' Communicated Well	300+	81%	80%	79%
Pain 'Always' Well Controlled	300+	76%	72%	71%
Room and Bathroom 'Always' Clean	300+	77%	75%	73%
Timely Help 'Always' Received	300+	72%	69%	68%
Would Definitely Recommend Hospital	300+	66%	73%	71%
Use of Medical Imaging				
Cardiac Imaging Stress Test before Surgery	104	5.8%	5.3%	5.3%
Combination Abdominal CT Scan	473	45.2%	16.4%	10.5%
Combination Brain/Sinus CT Scan	507	2.6%	2.7%	2.7%
Combination Chest CT Scan	398	31.4%	5.6%	2.7%
Follow-up Mammogram/Ultrasound	629	21.8%	7.9%	8.8%
Lumbar Spine MRI for Low Back Pain	121	55.4%	39.6%	37.2%

East Texas Medical Center Mount Vernon

500 S State Hwy 37 Phone: 903-537-4552
Mount Vernon, TX 75457 Fax: 903-537-8100
URL: www.etmc.org
Type: Acute Care Hospitals Emergency Services: Yes
Ownership: Voluntary non-profit - Other Beds: 49

Key Personnel:
Emergency Room . . . . Nancy Bolton
Operating Room. . . . . Kathy Carr
Quality Assurance . . . . Cherry Crawley
Chief of Medical Staff . . . . Keith Gordan
Infection Control. . . . . Nilah Lahti

Measure	Cases	This Hosp.	State Avg.	U.S. Avg.
Blood Clot Prevention and Treatment				
Anticoagulation Overlap Therapy[2,7]	-	-	93%	93%
ICU Venous Thromboembolism Prophylaxis[2,7]	-	-	92%	92%
Incidence of Potentially Preventable VTE[2,7]	-	-	9%	10%
UFH with Dosages/Platelet Monitoring[2,7]	-	-	96%	97%
Venous Thromboembolism Prophylaxis[2]	120	24%	82%	85%
Warfarin Therapy Discharge Instructions[2,7]	-	-	84%	75%
Chest Pain/Possible Heart Attack Care				
Aspirin Given Within 24 Hours of Arrival[1]	-	-	94%	96%
Fibrinolytic Meds Within 30 Min. of Arrival[1,3]	-	-	47%	58%
Average Time to ECG (minutes)[1]	-	-	8	7
Average Time to Transfer (minutes)[1,3]	-	-	62	60
Children's Asthma Care				
Received Home Management Plan of Care	-	-	93%	88%
Received Reliever Medication	-	-	100%	100%

NOTE: Hospital profiles are in alphabetical order by state, then city, then hospital within the city; Rankings exclude hospitals with less than 25 cases except for patient surveys which excludes hospitals with less than 100 cases; (a) 100-299 cases; (1) The number of cases/patients is too few to report; (2) Data submitted were based on a sample of cases/patients; (3) Results are based on a shorter time period than required; (4) Data suppressed by CMS for one or more quarters; (5) Results are not available for this reporting period; (6) Fewer than 100 patients completed the HCAHPS survey; (7) No cases met the criteria for this measure; (8) The lower limit of the confidence interval cannot be calculated if the number of observed infections equals zero; (9) No data are available from the state/territory for this reporting period; (10) The scores shown reflect fewer than 50 completed surveys; (11) There were discrepancies in the data collection process; (12) This measure does not apply to this hospital for this reporting period; (13) Results cannot be calculated for this reporting period; (14) The results for this state are combined with nearby states to protect confidentiality; Please refer to the User's Guide for a full explanation of data.

Measure	Cases	This Hosp.	State Avg.	U.S. Avg.
Received Systemic Corticosteroids	-	-	100%	100%
Emergency Department				
Admittance Decision Time (minutes)[2]	130	40	99	98
Head CT Results Within 45 Min. of Arrival[1,3]	-	-	54%	57%
Patients Who Left ER Before Being Seen	3,146	1%	3%	2%
Time from ER Arrival to Admit. (minutes)[2]	148	158	270	274
Time from ER Arrival to Discharge (minutes)	266	92	127	134
Time in ER Before Being Evaluated (minutes)	322	17	26	26
Time to Pain Meds for Fractures (minutes)	13	45	57	57
Heart Attack Care				
Aspirin Given at Discharge[3,7]	-	-	99%	99%
Fibrinolytic Meds Within 30 Min. of Arrival[3,7]	-	-	49%	54%
PCI Within 90 Minutes of Arrival[3,7]	-	-	95%	96%
Statin Prescribed at Discharge[3,7]	-	-	98%	98%
Heart Failure Care				
ACE Inhibitor or ARB for LVSD[1]	-	-	97%	97%
Discharge Instructions Given	27	78%	95%	94%
Evaluation of LVS Function	42	60%	99%	99%
Medicare Spending				
Medicare Spending per Patient (ratio)	-	0.92	1.03	0.98
Pneumonia Care				
Appropriate Initial Antibiotic Given	23	74%	95%	95%
Blood Culture Timing	15	100%	98%	98%
Pregnancy and Delivery Care				
Newborn Deliveries Scheduled Early[7]	-	-	7%	6%
Preventive Care				
Immunization for Influenza[2]	241	73%	90%	90%
Immunization for Pneumonia[2]	360	81%	92%	92%
Stroke Care				
Anticoagulation Therapy for Atrial Fibrillation[1]	-	-	96%	95%
Antithrombotic Therapy Timing[1]	-	-	98%	98%
Assessed for Rehabilitation[1]	-	-	98%	97%
Discharged on Antithrombotic Therapy[1]	-	-	99%	99%
Discharged on Statin Medication[1]	-	-	95%	94%
Thrombolytic Therapy Timing[7]	-	-	68%	66%
Venous Thromboembolism Prophylaxis[1]	-	-	94%	94%
Written Stroke Educational Materials Given[7]	-	-	92%	88%
Surgical Care Improvement Project				
Appropriate Beta Blocker Usage[5]	-	-	98%	98%
Appropriate VTP Within 24 Hours[5]	-	-	98%	98%
Controlled Postoperative Blood Glucose[5]	-	-	96%	97%
Perioperative Temperature Management[5]	-	-	100%	100%
Prophylactic Antibiotic Selection[5]	-	-	99%	99%
Prophylactic Antibiotic Selection (Outpatient)[5]	-	-	98%	98%
Prophylactic Antibiotic Stopped[5]	-	-	98%	98%
Prophylactic Antibiotic Timing[5]	-	-	99%	99%
Prophylactic Antibiotic Timing (Outpatient)[5]	-	-	98%	98%
Urinary Catheter Removal[5]	-	-	98%	97%
Survey of Patients' Hospital Experiences				
Area Around Room 'Always' Quiet at Night[6]	<100	84%	68%	61%
Doctors 'Always' Communicated Well[6]	<100	96%	83%	82%
Home Recovery Information Given[6]	<100	96%	85%	85%
Hospital Given 9 or 10 on 10 Point Scale[6]	<100	84%	73%	71%
Meds 'Always' Explained Before Given[6]	<100	82%	66%	64%
Nurses 'Always' Communicated Well[6]	<100	86%	80%	79%
Pain 'Always' Well Controlled[6]	<100	76%	72%	71%
Room and Bathroom 'Always' Clean[6]	<100	79%	75%	73%
Timely Help 'Always' Received[6]	<100	86%	69%	68%
Would Definitely Recommend Hospital[6]	<100	84%	73%	71%
Use of Medical Imaging				
Cardiac Imaging Stress Test before Surgery[1]	-	-	5.3%	5.3%
Combination Abdominal CT Scan	50	0.0%	16.4%	10.5%
Combination Brain/Sinus CT Scan[1]	-	-	2.7%	2.7%
Combination Chest CT Scan[1]	-	-	5.6%	2.7%
Follow-up Mammogram/Ultrasound[7]	-	-	7.9%	8.8%
Lumbar Spine MRI for Low Back Pain[7]	-	-	39.6%	37.2%

Muleshoe Area Medical Center

708 S 1st St
Muleshoe, TX 79347
Phone: 806-272-4524
Type: Critical Access Hospitals
Emergency Services: Yes
Ownership: Govt - Hospital Dist/Auth

Measure	Cases	This Hosp.	State Avg.	U.S. Avg.
Blood Clot Prevention and Treatment				
Anticoagulation Overlap Therapy[5]	-	-	93%	93%
ICU Venous Thromboembolism Prophylaxis[5]	-	-	92%	92%
Incidence of Potentially Preventable VTE[5]	-	-	9%	10%
UFH with Dosages/Platelet Monitoring[5]	-	-	96%	97%
Venous Thromboembolism Prophylaxis[5]	-	-	82%	85%
Warfarin Therapy Discharge Instructions[5]	-	-	84%	75%
Chest Pain/Possible Heart Attack Care				
Aspirin Given Within 24 Hours of Arrival	-	-	94%	96%
Fibrinolytic Meds Within 30 Min. of Arrival	-	-	47%	58%
Average Time to ECG (minutes)	-	-	8	7
Average Time to Transfer (minutes)	-	-	62	60
Children's Asthma Care				
Received Home Management Plan of Care	-	-	93%	88%
Received Reliever Medication	-	-	100%	100%
Received Systemic Corticosteroids	-	-	100%	100%
Emergency Department				
Admittance Decision Time (minutes)[5]	-	-	99	98
Head CT Results Within 45 Min. of Arrival	-	-	54%	57%
Patients Who Left ER Before Being Seen	-	-	3%	2%
Time from ER Arrival to Admit. (minutes)[5]	-	-	270	274
Time from ER Arrival to Discharge (minutes)	-	-	127	134
Time in ER Before Being Evaluated (minutes)	-	-	26	26
Time to Pain Meds for Fractures (minutes)	-	-	57	57
Heart Attack Care				
Aspirin Given at Discharge[5]	-	-	99%	99%
Fibrinolytic Meds Within 30 Min. of Arrival[5]	-	-	49%	54%
PCI Within 90 Minutes of Arrival[5]	-	-	95%	96%
Statin Prescribed at Discharge[5]	-	-	98%	98%
Heart Failure Care				
ACE Inhibitor or ARB for LVSD[5]	-	-	97%	97%
Discharge Instructions Given[5]	-	-	95%	94%
Evaluation of LVS Function[5]	-	-	99%	99%
Medicare Spending				
Medicare Spending per Patient (ratio)	-	-	1.03	0.98
Pneumonia Care				
Appropriate Initial Antibiotic Given[1,2]	-	-	95%	95%
Blood Culture Timing[2,3]	-	-	98%	98%
Pregnancy and Delivery Care				
Newborn Deliveries Scheduled Early[5]	-	-	7%	6%
Preventive Care				
Immunization for Influenza[5]	-	-	90%	90%
Immunization for Pneumonia[5]	-	-	92%	92%
Stroke Care				
Anticoagulation Therapy for Atrial Fibrillation[5]	-	-	96%	95%
Antithrombotic Therapy Timing[5]	-	-	98%	98%
Assessed for Rehabilitation[5]	-	-	98%	97%
Discharged on Antithrombotic Therapy[5]	-	-	99%	99%
Discharged on Statin Medication[5]	-	-	95%	94%
Thrombolytic Therapy Timing[5]	-	-	68%	66%
Venous Thromboembolism Prophylaxis[5]	-	-	94%	94%
Written Stroke Educational Materials Given[5]	-	-	92%	88%
Surgical Care Improvement Project				
Appropriate Beta Blocker Usage[5]	-	-	98%	98%
Appropriate VTP Within 24 Hours[5]	-	-	98%	98%
Controlled Postoperative Blood Glucose[5]	-	-	96%	97%
Perioperative Temperature Management[5]	-	-	100%	100%
Prophylactic Antibiotic Selection[5]	-	-	99%	99%
Prophylactic Antibiotic Selection (Outpatient)	-	-	98%	98%
Prophylactic Antibiotic Stopped[5]	-	-	98%	98%
Prophylactic Antibiotic Timing[5]	-	-	99%	99%
Prophylactic Antibiotic Timing (Outpatient)	-	-	98%	98%
Urinary Catheter Removal[5]	-	-	98%	97%
Survey of Patients' Hospital Experiences				
Area Around Room 'Always' Quiet at Night[5]	-	-	68%	61%
Doctors 'Always' Communicated Well[5]	-	-	83%	82%
Home Recovery Information Given[5]	-	-	85%	85%
Hospital Given 9 or 10 on 10 Point Scale[5]	-	-	73%	71%
Meds 'Always' Explained Before Given[5]	-	-	66%	64%
Nurses 'Always' Communicated Well[5]	-	-	80%	79%
Pain 'Always' Well Controlled[5]	-	-	72%	71%
Room and Bathroom 'Always' Clean[5]	-	-	75%	73%
Timely Help 'Always' Received[5]	-	-	69%	68%
Would Definitely Recommend Hospital[5]	-	-	73%	71%
Use of Medical Imaging				
Cardiac Imaging Stress Test before Surgery	-	-	5.3%	5.3%
Combination Abdominal CT Scan	-	-	16.4%	10.5%
Combination Brain/Sinus CT Scan	-	-	2.7%	2.7%
Combination Chest CT Scan	-	-	5.6%	2.7%
Follow-up Mammogram/Ultrasound	-	-	7.9%	8.8%
Lumbar Spine MRI for Low Back Pain	-	-	39.6%	37.2%

Memorial Hospital

1204 Mound St
Nacogdoches, TX 75961
Phone: 936-564-4611
Fax: 936-568-3400
E-mail: info@nacmem.org
URL: www.nacmem.org
Type: Acute Care Hospitals
Emergency Services: Yes
Ownership: Govt - Hospital Dist/Auth
Beds: 202

Key Personnel:
Infection Control. . . . . Elenor Adams
Radiology. . . . . Mary Beth Calme
Quality Assurance . . . . Tim Hayward
Operating Room. . . . . Charles Page
Chief of Medical Staff . . . . Jeremy Scott Smith
CEO . . . . Scott Street

Measure	Cases	This Hosp.	State Avg.	U.S. Avg.
Blood Clot Prevention and Treatment				
Anticoagulation Overlap Therapy[2]	32	59%	93%	93%
ICU Venous Thromboembolism Prophylaxis[2]	131	53%	92%	92%
Incidence of Potentially Preventable VTE[1,2]	-	-	9%	10%
UFH with Dosages/Platelet Monitoring[2]	11	91%	96%	97%
Venous Thromboembolism Prophylaxis[2]	323	50%	82%	85%
Warfarin Therapy Discharge Instructions[2]	18	22%	84%	75%
Chest Pain/Possible Heart Attack Care				
Aspirin Given Within 24 Hours of Arrival[3,7]	-	-	94%	96%
Fibrinolytic Meds Within 30 Min. of Arrival[5]	-	-	47%	58%
Average Time to ECG (minutes)[3,7]	-	-	8	7
Average Time to Transfer (minutes)[5]	-	-	62	60
Children's Asthma Care				
Received Home Management Plan of Care	-	-	93%	88%
Received Reliever Medication	-	-	100%	100%
Received Systemic Corticosteroids	-	-	100%	100%
Emergency Department				
Admittance Decision Time (minutes)[2]	296	71	99	98
Head CT Results Within 45 Min. of Arrival[1]	-	-	54%	57%
Patients Who Left ER Before Being Seen	26,845	4%	3%	2%
Time from ER Arrival to Admit. (minutes)[2]	398	265	270	274
Time from ER Arrival to Discharge (minutes)	354	160	127	134
Time in ER Before Being Evaluated (minutes)	352	73	26	26
Time to Pain Meds for Fractures (minutes)	62	125	57	57
Heart Attack Care				
Aspirin Given at Discharge	78	99%	99%	99%
Fibrinolytic Meds Within 30 Min. of Arrival[7]	-	-	49%	54%
PCI Within 90 Minutes of Arrival	22	77%	95%	96%
Statin Prescribed at Discharge	76	97%	98%	98%
Heart Failure Care				
ACE Inhibitor or ARB for LVSD	47	87%	97%	97%
Discharge Instructions Given	84	80%	95%	94%
Evaluation of LVS Function	110	99%	99%	99%
Medicare Spending				
Medicare Spending per Patient (ratio)	-	1.13	1.03	0.98
Pneumonia Care				
Appropriate Initial Antibiotic Given	61	90%	95%	95%
Blood Culture Timing	100	97%	98%	98%
Pregnancy and Delivery Care				
Newborn Deliveries Scheduled Early	102	1%	7%	6%
Preventive Care				
Immunization for Influenza[2]	418	86%	90%	90%
Immunization for Pneumonia[2]	479	90%	92%	92%

NOTE: Hospital profiles are in alphabetical order by state, then city, then hospital within the city; Rankings exclude hospitals with less than 25 cases except for patient surveys which excludes hospitals with less than 100 cases; (a) 100-299 cases; (1) The number of cases/patients is too few to report; (2) Data submitted were based on a sample of cases/patients; (3) Results are based on a shorter time period than required; (4) Data suppressed by CMS for one or more quarters; (5) Results are not available for this reporting period; (6) Fewer than 100 patients completed the HCAHPS survey; (7) No cases met the criteria for this measure; (8) The lower limit of the confidence interval cannot be calculated if the number of observed infections equals zero; (9) No data are available from the state/territory for this reporting period; (10) The scores shown reflect fewer than 50 completed surveys; (11) There were discrepancies in the data collection process; (12) This measure does not apply to this hospital for this reporting period; (13) Results cannot be calculated for this reporting period; (14) The results for this state are combined with nearby states to protect confidentiality; Please refer to the User's Guide for a full explanation of data.

Measure	Cases	This Hosp.	State Avg.	U.S. Avg.
Stroke Care				
Anticoagulation Therapy for Atrial Fibrillation[1]	-	-	96%	95%
Antithrombotic Therapy Timing	46	96%	98%	98%
Assessed for Rehabilitation	52	100%	98%	97%
Discharged on Antithrombotic Therapy	44	98%	99%	99%
Discharged on Statin Medication	39	74%	95%	94%
Thrombolytic Therapy Timing[1]	-	-	68%	66%
Venous Thromboembolism Prophylaxis	57	61%	94%	94%
Written Stroke Educational Materials Given	27	4%	92%	88%
Surgical Care Improvement Project				
Appropriate Beta Blocker Usage	77	83%	98%	98%
Appropriate VTP Within 24 Hours	191	87%	98%	98%
Controlled Postoperative Blood Glucose[1]	-	-	96%	97%
Perioperative Temperature Management	246	100%	100%	100%
Prophylactic Antibiotic Selection	134	99%	99%	99%
Prophylactic Antibiotic Selection (Outpatient)	175	95%	98%	98%
Prophylactic Antibiotic Stopped	129	94%	98%	98%
Prophylactic Antibiotic Timing	134	99%	99%	99%
Prophylactic Antibiotic Timing (Outpatient)	177	93%	98%	98%
Urinary Catheter Removal	122	89%	98%	97%
Survey of Patients' Hospital Experiences				
Area Around Room 'Always' Quiet at Night	300+	62%	68%	61%
Doctors 'Always' Communicated Well	300+	81%	83%	82%
Home Recovery Information Given	300+	83%	85%	85%
Hospital Given 9 or 10 on 10 Point Scale	300+	65%	73%	71%
Meds 'Always' Explained Before Given	300+	62%	66%	64%
Nurses 'Always' Communicated Well	300+	77%	80%	79%
Pain 'Always' Well Controlled	300+	64%	72%	71%
Room and Bathroom 'Always' Clean	300+	63%	75%	73%
Timely Help 'Always' Received	300+	67%	69%	68%
Would Definitely Recommend Hospital	300+	67%	73%	71%
Use of Medical Imaging				
Cardiac Imaging Stress Test before Surgery	93	7.5%	5.3%	5.3%
Combination Abdominal CT Scan	405	11.1%	16.4%	10.5%
Combination Brain/Sinus CT Scan	473	2.1%	2.7%	2.7%
Combination Chest CT Scan	284	9.5%	5.6%	2.7%
Follow-up Mammogram/Ultrasound	957	18.0%	7.9%	8.8%
Lumbar Spine MRI for Low Back Pain	86	34.9%	39.6%	37.2%

Nacogdoches Medical Center

4920 Ne Stallings Drive — Phone: 936-569-9481
Nacogdoches, TX 75961 — Fax: 936-568-3400
URL: www.nacmedicalcenter.com
Type: Acute Care Hospitals — Emergency Services: Yes
Ownership: Voluntary non-profit - Other — Beds: 150

Measure	Cases	This Hosp.	State Avg.	U.S. Avg.
Blood Clot Prevention and Treatment				
Anticoagulation Overlap Therapy[2]	38	55%	93%	93%
ICU Venous Thromboembolism Prophylaxis[2]	90	90%	92%	92%
Incidence of Potentially Preventable VTE[1,2]	-	-	9%	10%
UFH with Dosages/Platelet Monitoring[1,2]	-	-	96%	97%
Venous Thromboembolism Prophylaxis[2]	255	83%	82%	85%
Warfarin Therapy Discharge Instructions[2]	31	97%	84%	75%
Chest Pain/Possible Heart Attack Care				
Aspirin Given Within 24 Hours of Arrival[5]	-	-	94%	96%
Fibrinolytic Meds Within 30 Min. of Arrival[5]	-	-	47%	58%
Average Time to ECG (minutes)[5]	-	-	8	7
Average Time to Transfer (minutes)[5]	-	-	62	60
Children's Asthma Care				
Received Home Management Plan of Care	-	-	93%	88%
Received Reliever Medication	-	-	100%	100%
Received Systemic Corticosteroids	-	-	100%	100%
Emergency Department				
Admittance Decision Time (minutes)[2]	471	74	99	98
Head CT Results Within 45 Min. of Arrival[1,3]	-	-	54%	57%
Patients Who Left ER Before Being Seen	790	86%	3%	2%
Time from ER Arrival to Admit. (minutes)[2]	471	256	270	274
Time from ER Arrival to Discharge (minutes)	371	143	127	134
Time in ER Before Being Evaluated (minutes)	381	29	26	26
Time to Pain Meds for Fractures (minutes)	74	76	57	57
Heart Attack Care				
Aspirin Given at Discharge	41	100%	99%	99%
Fibrinolytic Meds Within 30 Min. of Arrival[7]	-	-	49%	54%
PCI Within 90 Minutes of Arrival[1]	-	-	95%	96%
Statin Prescribed at Discharge	41	98%	98%	98%
Heart Failure Care				
ACE Inhibitor or ARB for LVSD	31	100%	97%	97%
Discharge Instructions Given	66	91%	95%	94%
Evaluation of LVS Function	84	100%	99%	99%
Medicare Spending				
Medicare Spending per Patient (ratio)	-	1.03	1.03	0.98
Pneumonia Care				
Appropriate Initial Antibiotic Given	59	97%	95%	95%
Blood Culture Timing	92	100%	98%	98%
Pregnancy and Delivery Care				
Newborn Deliveries Scheduled Early[2]	32	0%	7%	6%
Preventive Care				
Immunization for Influenza[2]	428	94%	90%	90%
Immunization for Pneumonia[2]	477	99%	92%	92%
Stroke Care				
Anticoagulation Therapy for Atrial Fibrillation[1]	-	-	96%	95%
Antithrombotic Therapy Timing	44	95%	98%	98%
Assessed for Rehabilitation	52	94%	98%	97%
Discharged on Antithrombotic Therapy	48	98%	99%	99%
Discharged on Statin Medication	39	82%	95%	94%
Thrombolytic Therapy Timing[1]	-	-	68%	66%
Venous Thromboembolism Prophylaxis	49	84%	94%	94%
Written Stroke Educational Materials Given	30	83%	92%	88%
Surgical Care Improvement Project				
Appropriate Beta Blocker Usage[2]	57	93%	98%	98%
Appropriate VTP Within 24 Hours[2]	158	94%	98%	98%
Controlled Postoperative Blood Glucose[2]	13	100%	96%	97%
Perioperative Temperature Management[2]	188	100%	100%	100%
Prophylactic Antibiotic Selection[2]	108	100%	99%	99%
Prophylactic Antibiotic Selection (Outpatient)	192	99%	98%	98%
Prophylactic Antibiotic Stopped[2]	101	99%	98%	98%
Prophylactic Antibiotic Timing[2]	108	100%	99%	99%
Prophylactic Antibiotic Timing (Outpatient)	192	99%	98%	98%
Urinary Catheter Removal[2]	94	98%	98%	97%
Survey of Patients' Hospital Experiences				
Area Around Room 'Always' Quiet at Night	300+	68%	68%	61%
Doctors 'Always' Communicated Well	300+	90%	83%	82%
Home Recovery Information Given	300+	87%	85%	85%
Hospital Given 9 or 10 on 10 Point Scale	300+	71%	73%	71%
Meds 'Always' Explained Before Given	300+	68%	66%	64%
Nurses 'Always' Communicated Well	300+	81%	80%	79%
Pain 'Always' Well Controlled	300+	74%	72%	71%
Room and Bathroom 'Always' Clean	300+	63%	75%	73%
Timely Help 'Always' Received	300+	70%	69%	68%
Would Definitely Recommend Hospital	300+	74%	73%	71%
Use of Medical Imaging				
Cardiac Imaging Stress Test before Surgery	54	1.9%	5.3%	5.3%
Combination Abdominal CT Scan	406	3.4%	16.4%	10.5%
Combination Brain/Sinus CT Scan	336	1.5%	2.7%	2.7%
Combination Chest CT Scan	270	0.0%	5.6%	2.7%
Follow-up Mammogram/Ultrasound	855	10.9%	7.9%	8.8%
Lumbar Spine MRI for Low Back Pain	105	49.5%	39.6%	37.2%

Christus Saint John Hospital

18300 Saint John Drive — Phone: 281-333-5503
Nassau Bay, TX 77058 — Fax: 281-333-8891
URL: www.christushealth.org
Type: Acute Care Hospitals — Emergency Services: Yes
Ownership: Voluntary non-profit - Private — Beds: 178

Key Personnel:

Chief of Medical Staff.......... Daniel Casso, MD
Quality Assurance .... Janet DuBois
Infection Control............. Eileen Haag
Radiology.................. Edna W McLeod
CEO/President.............. Ernie Sadau
Operating Room............. Elaine Thomson-Keith

Measure	Cases	This Hosp.	State Avg.	U.S. Avg.
Blood Clot Prevention and Treatment				
Anticoagulation Overlap Therapy[2]	33	88%	93%	93%
ICU Venous Thromboembolism Prophylaxis[2]	71	93%	92%	92%
Incidence of Potentially Preventable VTE[1,2]	-	-	9%	10%
UFH with Dosages/Platelet Monitoring[2]	11	100%	96%	97%
Venous Thromboembolism Prophylaxis[2]	330	72%	82%	85%
Warfarin Therapy Discharge Instructions[2]	22	100%	84%	75%
Chest Pain/Possible Heart Attack Care				
Aspirin Given Within 24 Hours of Arrival[1,3]	-	-	94%	96%
Fibrinolytic Meds Within 30 Min. of Arrival[5]	-	-	47%	58%
Average Time to ECG (minutes)[1,3]	-	-	8	7
Average Time to Transfer (minutes)[5]	-	-	62	60
Children's Asthma Care				
Received Home Management Plan of Care	-	-	93%	88%
Received Reliever Medication	-	-	100%	100%
Received Systemic Corticosteroids	-	-	100%	100%
Emergency Department				
Admittance Decision Time (minutes)[2]	827	174	99	98
Head CT Results Within 45 Min. of Arrival	41	78%	54%	57%
Patients Who Left ER Before Being Seen	25,910	5%	3%	2%
Time from ER Arrival to Admit. (minutes)[2]	827	341	270	274
Time from ER Arrival to Discharge (minutes)	372	166	127	134
Time in ER Before Being Evaluated (minutes)	404	24	26	26
Time to Pain Meds for Fractures (minutes)	115	64	57	57
Heart Attack Care				
Aspirin Given at Discharge	93	97%	99%	99%
Fibrinolytic Meds Within 30 Min. of Arrival[7]	-	-	49%	54%
PCI Within 90 Minutes of Arrival	20	95%	95%	96%
Statin Prescribed at Discharge	82	96%	98%	98%
Heart Failure Care				
ACE Inhibitor or ARB for LVSD	58	98%	97%	97%
Discharge Instructions Given	119	98%	95%	94%
Evaluation of LVS Function	141	100%	99%	99%
Medicare Spending				
Medicare Spending per Patient (ratio)	-	1.12	1.03	0.98
Pneumonia Care				
Appropriate Initial Antibiotic Given	117	93%	95%	95%
Blood Culture Timing	148	100%	98%	98%
Pregnancy and Delivery Care				
Newborn Deliveries Scheduled Early	69	17%	7%	6%
Preventive Care				
Immunization for Influenza[2]	551	98%	90%	90%
Immunization for Pneumonia[2]	686	98%	92%	92%
Stroke Care				
Anticoagulation Therapy for Atrial Fibrillation[1]	-	-	96%	95%
Antithrombotic Therapy Timing	28	96%	98%	98%
Assessed for Rehabilitation	25	96%	98%	97%
Discharged on Antithrombotic Therapy	24	100%	99%	99%
Discharged on Statin Medication	16	100%	95%	94%
Thrombolytic Therapy Timing[1]	-	-	68%	66%
Venous Thromboembolism Prophylaxis	29	69%	94%	94%
Written Stroke Educational Materials Given	12	67%	92%	88%
Surgical Care Improvement Project				
Appropriate Beta Blocker Usage	125	96%	98%	98%
Appropriate VTP Within 24 Hours	462	95%	98%	98%
Controlled Postoperative Blood Glucose[7]	-	-	96%	97%
Perioperative Temperature Management	518	100%	100%	100%
Prophylactic Antibiotic Selection	383	98%	99%	99%
Prophylactic Antibiotic Selection (Outpatient)	165	97%	98%	98%
Prophylactic Antibiotic Stopped	374	99%	98%	98%
Prophylactic Antibiotic Timing	383	98%	99%	99%
Prophylactic Antibiotic Timing (Outpatient)	166	97%	98%	98%
Urinary Catheter Removal	317	91%	98%	97%
Survey of Patients' Hospital Experiences				
Area Around Room 'Always' Quiet at Night	300+	58%	68%	61%
Doctors 'Always' Communicated Well	300+	74%	83%	82%
Home Recovery Information Given	300+	83%	85%	85%
Hospital Given 9 or 10 on 10 Point Scale	300+	73%	73%	71%
Meds 'Always' Explained Before Given	300+	58%	66%	64%
Nurses 'Always' Communicated Well	300+	75%	80%	79%
Pain 'Always' Well Controlled	300+	72%	72%	71%
Room and Bathroom 'Always' Clean	300+	74%	75%	73%
Timely Help 'Always' Received	300+	65%	69%	68%
Would Definitely Recommend Hospital	300+	79%	73%	71%
Use of Medical Imaging				
Cardiac Imaging Stress Test before Surgery[1]	-	-	5.3%	5.3%

NOTE: Hospital profiles are in alphabetical order by state, then city, then hospital within the city; Rankings exclude hospitals with less than 25 cases except for patient surveys which excludes hospitals with less than 100 cases; (a) 100-299 cases; (1) The number of cases/patients is too few to report; (2) Data submitted were based on a sample of cases/patients; (3) Results are based on a shorter time period than required; (4) Data suppressed by CMS for one or more quarters; (5) Results are not available for this reporting period; (6) Fewer than 100 patients completed the HCAHPS survey; (7) No cases met the criteria for this measure; (8) The lower limit of the confidence interval cannot be calculated if the number of observed infections equals zero; (9) No data are available from the state/territory for this reporting period; (10) The scores shown reflect fewer than 50 completed surveys; (11) There were discrepancies in the data collection process; (12) This measure does not apply to this hospital for this reporting period; (13) Results cannot be calculated for this reporting period; (14) The results for this state are combined with nearby states to protect confidentiality; Please refer to the User's Guide for a full explanation of data.

Measure	Cases	This Hosp.	State Avg.	U.S. Avg.
Combination Abdominal CT Scan	378	7.7%	16.4%	10.5%
Combination Brain/Sinus CT Scan[1]	-	-	2.7%	2.7%
Combination Chest CT Scan	238	0.0%	5.6%	2.7%
Follow-up Mammogram/Ultrasound	281	13.9%	7.9%	8.8%
Lumbar Spine MRI for Low Back Pain	78	30.8%	39.6%	37.2%

Grimes Saint Joseph Health Center

210 Judson St
Navasota, TX 77868
Phone: 936-825-6585
Fax: 936-825-6007
Type: Critical Access Hospitals
Emergency Services: Yes
Ownership: Voluntary non-profit - Church
Beds: 47

Key Personnel:
Radiology. . . . . Eric Alan Appelt
Chief of Medical Staff . . . . Mack Blanton
CEO/President. . . . . James W. Pope, MHHA, FACHE
Administrator . . . . Mark J. Riggins, MBA

Measure	Cases	This Hosp.	State Avg.	U.S. Avg.
Blood Clot Prevention and Treatment				
Anticoagulation Overlap Therapy[5]	-	-	93%	93%
ICU Venous Thromboembolism Prophylaxis[5]	-	-	92%	92%
Incidence of Potentially Preventable VTE[5]	-	-	9%	10%
UFH with Dosages/Platelet Monitoring[5]	-	-	96%	97%
Venous Thromboembolism Prophylaxis[5]	-	-	82%	85%
Warfarin Therapy Discharge Instructions[5]	-	-	84%	75%
Chest Pain/Possible Heart Attack Care				
Aspirin Given Within 24 Hours of Arrival	-	-	94%	96%
Fibrinolytic Meds Within 30 Min. of Arrival	-	-	47%	58%
Average Time to ECG (minutes)	-	-	8	7
Average Time to Transfer (minutes)	-	-	62	60
Children's Asthma Care				
Received Home Management Plan of Care	-	-	93%	88%
Received Reliever Medication	-	-	100%	100%
Received Systemic Corticosteroids	-	-	100%	100%
Emergency Department				
Admittance Decision Time (minutes)[5]	-	-	99	98
Head CT Results Within 45 Min. of Arrival	-	-	54%	57%
Patients Who Left ER Before Being Seen	-	-	3%	2%
Time from ER Arrival to Admit. (minutes)[5]	-	-	270	274
Time from ER Arrival to Discharge (minutes)	-	-	127	134
Time in ER Before Being Evaluated (minutes)	-	-	26	26
Time to Pain Meds for Fractures (minutes)	-	-	57	57
Heart Attack Care				
Aspirin Given at Discharge[5]	-	-	99%	99%
Fibrinolytic Meds Within 30 Min. of Arrival[5]	-	-	49%	54%
PCI Within 90 Minutes of Arrival[5]	-	-	95%	96%
Statin Prescribed at Discharge[5]	-	-	98%	98%
Heart Failure Care				
ACE Inhibitor or ARB for LVSD[1,3]	-	-	97%	97%
Discharge Instructions Given[1,3]	-	-	95%	94%
Evaluation of LVS Function[1,3]	-	-	99%	99%
Medicare Spending				
Medicare Spending per Patient (ratio)	-	-	1.03	0.98
Pneumonia Care				
Appropriate Initial Antibiotic Given[1]	-	-	95%	95%
Blood Culture Timing[1]	-	-	98%	98%
Pregnancy and Delivery Care				
Newborn Deliveries Scheduled Early[5]	-	-	7%	6%
Preventive Care				
Immunization for Influenza[5]	-	-	90%	90%
Immunization for Pneumonia[5]	-	-	92%	92%
Stroke Care				
Anticoagulation Therapy for Atrial Fibrillation[5]	-	-	96%	95%
Antithrombotic Therapy Timing[5]	-	-	98%	98%
Assessed for Rehabilitation[5]	-	-	98%	97%
Discharged on Antithrombotic Therapy[5]	-	-	99%	99%
Discharged on Statin Medication[5]	-	-	95%	94%
Thrombolytic Therapy Timing[5]	-	-	68%	66%
Venous Thromboembolism Prophylaxis[5]	-	-	94%	94%
Written Stroke Educational Materials Given[5]	-	-	92%	88%
Surgical Care Improvement Project				
Appropriate Beta Blocker Usage[5]	-	-	98%	98%
Appropriate VTP Within 24 Hours[5]	-	-	98%	98%
Controlled Postoperative Blood Glucose[5]	-	-	96%	97%
Perioperative Temperature Management[5]	-	-	100%	100%
Prophylactic Antibiotic Selection[5]	-	-	99%	99%
Prophylactic Antibiotic Selection (Outpatient)	-	-	98%	98%
Prophylactic Antibiotic Stopped[5]	-	-	98%	98%
Prophylactic Antibiotic Timing[5]	-	-	99%	99%
Prophylactic Antibiotic Timing (Outpatient)	-	-	98%	98%
Urinary Catheter Removal[5]	-	-	98%	97%
Survey of Patients' Hospital Experiences				
Area Around Room 'Always' Quiet at Night[5]	-	-	68%	61%
Doctors 'Always' Communicated Well[5]	-	-	83%	82%
Home Recovery Information Given[5]	-	-	85%	85%
Hospital Given 9 or 10 on 10 Point Scale[5]	-	-	73%	71%
Meds 'Always' Explained Before Given[5]	-	-	66%	64%
Nurses 'Always' Communicated Well[5]	-	-	80%	79%
Pain 'Always' Well Controlled[5]	-	-	72%	71%
Room and Bathroom 'Always' Clean[5]	-	-	75%	73%
Timely Help 'Always' Received[5]	-	-	69%	68%
Would Definitely Recommend Hospital[5]	-	-	73%	71%
Use of Medical Imaging				
Cardiac Imaging Stress Test before Surgery	-	-	5.3%	5.3%
Combination Abdominal CT Scan	-	-	16.4%	10.5%
Combination Brain/Sinus CT Scan	-	-	2.7%	2.7%
Combination Chest CT Scan	-	-	5.6%	2.7%
Follow-up Mammogram/Ultrasound	-	-	7.9%	8.8%
Lumbar Spine MRI for Low Back Pain	-	-	39.6%	37.2%

Nocona General Hospital

100 Park Road
Nocona, TX 76255
Phone: 940-825-3235
Fax: 940-825-3604
Type: Acute Care Hospitals
Emergency Services: Yes
Ownership: Govt - Hospital Dist/Auth
Beds: 38

Key Personnel:
Emergency Room . . . . Len Dingler, MD
Anesthesiology. . . . . Tommy Duncan, CRNA
President . . . . Charles May
Chief of Medical Staff . . . . Barbara Perry
Quality Assurance . . . . Barbara Perry
Operating Room. . . . . Bonnie Robertson, RN
Radiology. . . . . Paige Veigl

Measure	Cases	This Hosp.	State Avg.	U.S. Avg.
Blood Clot Prevention and Treatment				
Anticoagulation Overlap Therapy[2,7]	-	-	93%	93%
ICU Venous Thromboembolism Prophylaxis[2,7]	-	-	92%	92%
Incidence of Potentially Preventable VTE[2,7]	-	-	9%	10%
UFH with Dosages/Platelet Monitoring[2,7]	-	-	96%	97%
Venous Thromboembolism Prophylaxis[2]	140	22%	82%	85%
Warfarin Therapy Discharge Instructions[2,7]	-	-	84%	75%
Chest Pain/Possible Heart Attack Care				
Aspirin Given Within 24 Hours of Arrival[5]	-	-	94%	96%
Fibrinolytic Meds Within 30 Min. of Arrival[5]	-	-	47%	58%
Average Time to ECG (minutes)[5]	-	-	8	7
Average Time to Transfer (minutes)[5]	-	-	62	60
Children's Asthma Care				
Received Home Management Plan of Care	-	-	93%	88%
Received Reliever Medication	-	-	100%	100%
Received Systemic Corticosteroids	-	-	100%	100%
Emergency Department				
Admittance Decision Time (minutes)[2]	302	20	99	98
Head CT Results Within 45 Min. of Arrival[5]	-	-	54%	57%
Patients Who Left ER Before Being Seen	2,866	14%	3%	2%
Time from ER Arrival to Admit. (minutes)[2]	320	86	270	274
Time from ER Arrival to Discharge (minutes)	298	64	127	134
Time in ER Before Being Evaluated (minutes)	277	15	26	26
Time to Pain Meds for Fractures (minutes)	20	50	57	57
Heart Attack Care				
Aspirin Given at Discharge[5]	-	-	99%	99%
Fibrinolytic Meds Within 30 Min. of Arrival[5]	-	-	49%	54%
PCI Within 90 Minutes of Arrival[5]	-	-	95%	96%
Statin Prescribed at Discharge[5]	-	-	98%	98%
Heart Failure Care				
ACE Inhibitor or ARB for LVSD[1,3]	-	-	97%	97%
Discharge Instructions Given[3]	14	86%	95%	94%
Evaluation of LVS Function[3]	17	29%	99%	99%
Medicare Spending				
Medicare Spending per Patient (ratio)	-	0.96	1.03	0.98
Pneumonia Care				
Appropriate Initial Antibiotic Given[2]	35	89%	95%	95%
Blood Culture Timing[1,2]	-	-	98%	98%
Pregnancy and Delivery Care				
Newborn Deliveries Scheduled Early[7]	-	-	7%	6%
Preventive Care				
Immunization for Influenza[2]	207	84%	90%	90%
Immunization for Pneumonia[2]	265	94%	92%	92%
Stroke Care				
Anticoagulation Therapy for Atrial Fibrillation[5]	-	-	96%	95%
Antithrombotic Therapy Timing[5]	-	-	98%	98%
Assessed for Rehabilitation[5]	-	-	98%	97%
Discharged on Antithrombotic Therapy[5]	-	-	99%	99%
Discharged on Statin Medication[5]	-	-	95%	94%
Thrombolytic Therapy Timing[5]	-	-	68%	66%
Venous Thromboembolism Prophylaxis[5]	-	-	94%	94%
Written Stroke Educational Materials Given[5]	-	-	92%	88%
Surgical Care Improvement Project				
Appropriate Beta Blocker Usage[5]	-	-	98%	98%
Appropriate VTP Within 24 Hours[5]	-	-	98%	98%
Controlled Postoperative Blood Glucose[5]	-	-	96%	97%
Perioperative Temperature Management[5]	-	-	100%	100%
Prophylactic Antibiotic Selection[5]	-	-	99%	99%
Prophylactic Antibiotic Selection (Outpatient)[3,7]	-	-	98%	98%
Prophylactic Antibiotic Stopped[5]	-	-	98%	98%
Prophylactic Antibiotic Timing[5]	-	-	99%	99%
Prophylactic Antibiotic Timing (Outpatient)[1,3]	-	-	98%	98%
Urinary Catheter Removal[5]	-	-	98%	97%
Survey of Patients' Hospital Experiences				
Area Around Room 'Always' Quiet at Night[6]	<100	56%	68%	61%
Doctors 'Always' Communicated Well[6]	<100	88%	83%	82%
Home Recovery Information Given[6]	<100	66%	85%	85%
Hospital Given 9 or 10 on 10 Point Scale[6]	<100	70%	73%	71%
Meds 'Always' Explained Before Given[6]	<100	72%	66%	64%
Nurses 'Always' Communicated Well[6]	<100	80%	80%	79%
Pain 'Always' Well Controlled[6]	<100	64%	72%	71%
Room and Bathroom 'Always' Clean[6]	<100	73%	75%	73%
Timely Help 'Always' Received[6]	<100	78%	69%	68%
Would Definitely Recommend Hospital[6]	<100	62%	73%	71%
Use of Medical Imaging				
Cardiac Imaging Stress Test before Surgery[1]	-	-	5.3%	5.3%
Combination Abdominal CT Scan[1]	-	-	16.4%	10.5%
Combination Brain/Sinus CT Scan	39	0.0%	2.7%	2.7%
Combination Chest CT Scan[1]	-	-	5.6%	2.7%
Follow-up Mammogram/Ultrasound[7]	-	-	7.9%	8.8%
Lumbar Spine MRI for Low Back Pain[7]	-	-	39.6%	37.2%

North Hills Hospital

4401 Booth Calloway Road
North Richland Hills, TX 76180
Phone: 817-255-1000
Fax: 817-255-1991
URL: www.northhillshospital.com
Type: Acute Care Hospitals
Emergency Services: Yes
Ownership: Proprietary
Beds: 144

Key Personnel:
Radiology. . . . . Tilden L Childs III
Chief of Medical Staff . . . . David Haefeli, MD
CEO/President. . . . . Randolph Moresi
Emergency Room . . . . Deborah Morris
Quality Assurance . . . . Diane Richey

Measure	Cases	This Hosp.	State Avg.	U.S. Avg.
Blood Clot Prevention and Treatment				
Anticoagulation Overlap Therapy[2]	83	100%	93%	93%
ICU Venous Thromboembolism Prophylaxis[2]	80	99%	92%	92%
Incidence of Potentially Preventable VTE[2]	14	0%	9%	10%
UFH with Dosages/Platelet Monitoring[2]	14	100%	96%	97%
Venous Thromboembolism Prophylaxis[2]	340	100%	82%	85%
Warfarin Therapy Discharge Instructions[2]	62	100%	84%	75%
Chest Pain/Possible Heart Attack Care				
Aspirin Given Within 24 Hours of Arrival[1,3]	-	-	94%	96%
Fibrinolytic Meds Within 30 Min. of Arrival[5]	-	-	47%	58%
Average Time to ECG (minutes)[1,3]	-	-	8	7
Average Time to Transfer (minutes)[5]	-	-	62	60

NOTE: Hospital profiles are in alphabetical order by state, then city, then hospital within the city; Rankings exclude hospitals with less than 25 cases except for patient surveys which excludes hospitals with less than 100 cases; (a) 100-299 cases; (1) The number of cases/patients is too few to report; (2) Data submitted were based on a sample of cases/patients; (3) Results are based on a shorter time period than required; (4) Data suppressed by CMS for one or more quarters; (5) Results are not available for this reporting period; (6) Fewer than 100 patients completed the HCAHPS survey; (7) No cases met the criteria for this measure; (8) The lower limit of the confidence interval cannot be calculated if the number of observed infections equals zero; (9) No data are available from the state/territory for this reporting period; (10) The scores shown reflect fewer than 50 completed surveys; (11) There were discrepancies in the data collection process; (12) This measure does not apply to this hospital for this reporting period; (13) Results cannot be calculated for this reporting period; (14) The results for this state are combined with nearby states to protect confidentiality; Please refer to the User's Guide for a full explanation of data.

Measure	Cases	This Hosp.	State Avg.	U.S. Avg.
Children's Asthma Care				
Received Home Management Plan of Care	-	-	93%	88%
Received Reliever Medication	-	-	100%	100%
Received Systemic Corticosteroids	-	-	100%	100%
Emergency Department				
Admittance Decision Time (minutes)[2]	750	122	99	98
Head CT Results Within 45 Min. of Arrival[1]	-	-	54%	57%
Patients Who Left ER Before Being Seen	67,164	2%	3%	2%
Time from ER Arrival to Admit. (minutes)[2]	759	251	270	274
Time from ER Arrival to Discharge (minutes)	472	113	127	134
Time in ER Before Being Evaluated (minutes)	501	13	26	26
Time to Pain Meds for Fractures (minutes)	166	47	57	57
Heart Attack Care				
Aspirin Given at Discharge	201	100%	99%	99%
Fibrinolytic Meds Within 30 Min. of Arrival[7]	-	-	49%	54%
PCI Within 90 Minutes of Arrival	59	100%	95%	96%
Statin Prescribed at Discharge	199	100%	98%	98%
Heart Failure Care				
ACE Inhibitor or ARB for LVSD	84	100%	97%	97%
Discharge Instructions Given	222	100%	95%	94%
Evaluation of LVS Function	278	100%	99%	99%
Medicare Spending				
Medicare Spending per Patient (ratio)	-	1.06	1.03	0.98
Pneumonia Care				
Appropriate Initial Antibiotic Given[2]	91	98%	95%	95%
Blood Culture Timing[2]	188	99%	98%	98%
Pregnancy and Delivery Care				
Newborn Deliveries Scheduled Early[2]	32	3%	7%	6%
Preventive Care				
Immunization for Influenza[2]	553	98%	90%	90%
Immunization for Pneumonia[2]	718	99%	92%	92%
Stroke Care				
Anticoagulation Therapy for Atrial Fibrillation	17	100%	96%	95%
Antithrombotic Therapy Timing	108	100%	98%	98%
Assessed for Rehabilitation	108	100%	98%	97%
Discharged on Antithrombotic Therapy	105	100%	99%	99%
Discharged on Statin Medication	81	100%	95%	94%
Thrombolytic Therapy Timing[1]	-	-	68%	66%
Venous Thromboembolism Prophylaxis	112	100%	94%	94%
Written Stroke Educational Materials Given	58	100%	92%	88%
Surgical Care Improvement Project				
Appropriate Beta Blocker Usage[2]	152	99%	98%	98%
Appropriate VTP Within 24 Hours[2]	296	99%	98%	98%
Controlled Postoperative Blood Glucose[2]	62	97%	96%	97%
Perioperative Temperature Management[2]	437	100%	100%	100%
Prophylactic Antibiotic Selection[2]	271	100%	99%	99%
Prophylactic Antibiotic Selection (Outpatient)	253	100%	98%	98%
Prophylactic Antibiotic Stopped[2]	258	100%	98%	98%
Prophylactic Antibiotic Timing[2]	271	100%	99%	99%
Prophylactic Antibiotic Timing (Outpatient)	253	99%	98%	98%
Urinary Catheter Removal[2]	283	99%	98%	97%
Survey of Patients' Hospital Experiences				
Area Around Room 'Always' Quiet at Night	300+	64%	68%	61%
Doctors 'Always' Communicated Well	300+	77%	83%	82%
Home Recovery Information Given	300+	85%	85%	85%
Hospital Given 9 or 10 on 10 Point Scale	300+	69%	73%	71%
Meds 'Always' Explained Before Given	300+	56%	66%	64%
Nurses 'Always' Communicated Well	300+	74%	80%	79%
Pain 'Always' Well Controlled	300+	68%	72%	71%
Room and Bathroom 'Always' Clean	300+	73%	75%	73%
Timely Help 'Always' Received	300+	63%	69%	68%
Would Definitely Recommend Hospital	300+	70%	73%	71%
Use of Medical Imaging				
Cardiac Imaging Stress Test before Surgery[1]	-	-	5.3%	5.3%
Combination Abdominal CT Scan	502	3.0%	16.4%	10.5%
Combination Brain/Sinus CT Scan	617	6.2%	2.7%	2.7%
Combination Chest CT Scan	126	1.6%	5.6%	2.7%
Follow-up Mammogram/Ultrasound	534	2.6%	7.9%	8.8%
Lumbar Spine MRI for Low Back Pain[1]	-	-	39.6%	37.2%

Basin Healthcare Center

900 East 4th Street
Odessa, TX 79761
Phone: 432-425-9510
URL: www.bhcodessa.com
Type: Acute Care Hospitals
Emergency Services: Yes
Ownership: Proprietary

Measure	Cases	This Hosp.	State Avg.	U.S. Avg.
Blood Clot Prevention and Treatment				
Anticoagulation Overlap Therapy[7]	-	-	93%	93%
ICU Venous Thromboembolism Prophylaxis[7]	-	-	92%	92%
Incidence of Potentially Preventable VTE[7]	-	-	9%	10%
UFH with Dosages/Platelet Monitoring[7]	-	-	96%	97%
Venous Thromboembolism Prophylaxis	66	18%	82%	85%
Warfarin Therapy Discharge Instructions[7]	-	-	84%	75%
Chest Pain/Possible Heart Attack Care				
Aspirin Given Within 24 Hours of Arrival[1,3]	-	-	94%	96%
Fibrinolytic Meds Within 30 Min. of Arrival[3,7]	-	-	47%	58%
Average Time to ECG (minutes)[1,3]	-	-	8	7
Average Time to Transfer (minutes)[3,7]	-	-	62	60
Children's Asthma Care				
Received Home Management Plan of Care	-	-	93%	88%
Received Reliever Medication	-	-	100%	100%
Received Systemic Corticosteroids	-	-	100%	100%
Emergency Department				
Admittance Decision Time (minutes)[2]	13	70	99	98
Head CT Results Within 45 Min. of Arrival[5]	-	-	54%	57%
Patients Who Left ER Before Being Seen	2,131	0%	3%	2%
Time from ER Arrival to Admit. (minutes)[2]	14	240	270	274
Time from ER Arrival to Discharge (minutes)	387	75	127	134
Time in ER Before Being Evaluated (minutes)	403	10	26	26
Time to Pain Meds for Fractures (minutes)[1,3]	-	-	57	57
Heart Attack Care				
Aspirin Given at Discharge[3,7]	-	-	99%	99%
Fibrinolytic Meds Within 30 Min. of Arrival[3,7]	-	-	49%	54%
PCI Within 90 Minutes of Arrival[3,7]	-	-	95%	96%
Statin Prescribed at Discharge[3,7]	-	-	98%	98%
Heart Failure Care				
ACE Inhibitor or ARB for LVSD[5]	-	-	97%	97%
Discharge Instructions Given[5]	-	-	95%	94%
Evaluation of LVS Function[5]	-	-	99%	99%
Medicare Spending				
Medicare Spending per Patient (ratio)	-	0.71	1.03	0.98
Pneumonia Care				
Appropriate Initial Antibiotic Given[1]	-	-	95%	95%
Blood Culture Timing[7]	-	-	98%	98%
Pregnancy and Delivery Care				
Newborn Deliveries Scheduled Early[7]	-	-	7%	6%
Preventive Care				
Immunization for Influenza	73	93%	90%	90%
Immunization for Pneumonia[2]	36	89%	92%	92%
Stroke Care				
Anticoagulation Therapy for Atrial Fibrillation[5]	-	-	96%	95%
Antithrombotic Therapy Timing[5]	-	-	98%	98%
Assessed for Rehabilitation[5]	-	-	98%	97%
Discharged on Antithrombotic Therapy[5]	-	-	99%	99%
Discharged on Statin Medication[5]	-	-	95%	94%
Thrombolytic Therapy Timing[5]	-	-	68%	66%
Venous Thromboembolism Prophylaxis[5]	-	-	94%	94%
Written Stroke Educational Materials Given[5]	-	-	92%	88%
Surgical Care Improvement Project				
Appropriate Beta Blocker Usage[1,2]	-	-	98%	98%
Appropriate VTP Within 24 Hours[2]	20	100%	98%	98%
Controlled Postoperative Blood Glucose[2,7]	-	-	96%	97%
Perioperative Temperature Management[2]	25	100%	100%	100%
Prophylactic Antibiotic Selection[1,2]	-	-	99%	99%
Prophylactic Antibiotic Selection (Outpatient)	277	91%	98%	98%
Prophylactic Antibiotic Stopped[1,2]	-	-	98%	98%
Prophylactic Antibiotic Timing[1,2]	-	-	99%	99%
Prophylactic Antibiotic Timing (Outpatient)	279	99%	98%	98%
Urinary Catheter Removal[1,2]	-	-	98%	97%
Survey of Patients' Hospital Experiences				
Area Around Room 'Always' Quiet at Night	(a)	82%	68%	61%
Doctors 'Always' Communicated Well	(a)	84%	83%	82%
Home Recovery Information Given	(a)	85%	85%	85%
Hospital Given 9 or 10 on 10 Point Scale	(a)	74%	73%	71%
Meds 'Always' Explained Before Given	(a)	65%	66%	64%
Nurses 'Always' Communicated Well	(a)	80%	80%	79%
Pain 'Always' Well Controlled	(a)	81%	72%	71%
Room and Bathroom 'Always' Clean	(a)	75%	75%	73%
Timely Help 'Always' Received	(a)	78%	69%	68%
Would Definitely Recommend Hospital	(a)	73%	73%	71%
Use of Medical Imaging				
Cardiac Imaging Stress Test before Surgery[7]	-	-	5.3%	5.3%
Combination Abdominal CT Scan	129	29.5%	16.4%	10.5%
Combination Brain/Sinus CT Scan	35	0.0%	2.7%	2.7%
Combination Chest CT Scan[1]	-	-	5.6%	2.7%
Follow-up Mammogram/Ultrasound[7]	-	-	7.9%	8.8%
Lumbar Spine MRI for Low Back Pain	55	29.1%	39.6%	37.2%

Medical Center Hospital

500 W 4th Street
Odessa, TX 79761
Phone: 432-640-4000
Fax: 432-640-2349
URL: www.mchodessa.com
Type: Acute Care Hospitals
Emergency Services: Yes
Ownership: Govt - Hospital Dist/Auth
Beds: 307

Key Personnel:
Chief of Medical Staff.......... Bruce Becker, MD
CEO/President.............. William Bill Webster
Pediatric In-Patient Care .... Lynn McLean
Cardiac Laboratory............ Ervin Miller
Operating Room.............. Kelly Stanley
Emergency Room .... Cece Wilmes

Measure	Cases	This Hosp.	State Avg.	U.S. Avg.
Blood Clot Prevention and Treatment				
Anticoagulation Overlap Therapy[2]	124	92%	93%	93%
ICU Venous Thromboembolism Prophylaxis[2]	132	90%	92%	92%
Incidence of Potentially Preventable VTE[2]	18	6%	9%	10%
UFH with Dosages/Platelet Monitoring[2]	27	74%	96%	97%
Venous Thromboembolism Prophylaxis[2]	291	81%	82%	85%
Warfarin Therapy Discharge Instructions[2]	93	70%	84%	75%
Chest Pain/Possible Heart Attack Care				
Aspirin Given Within 24 Hours of Arrival[3,7]	-	-	94%	96%
Fibrinolytic Meds Within 30 Min. of Arrival[5]	-	-	47%	58%
Average Time to ECG (minutes)[3,7]	-	-	8	7
Average Time to Transfer (minutes)[5]	-	-	62	60
Children's Asthma Care				
Received Home Management Plan of Care	-	-	93%	88%
Received Reliever Medication	-	-	100%	100%
Received Systemic Corticosteroids	-	-	100%	100%
Emergency Department				
Admittance Decision Time (minutes)[2]	826	128	99	98
Head CT Results Within 45 Min. of Arrival[1]	-	-	54%	57%
Patients Who Left ER Before Being Seen	53,180	4%	3%	2%
Time from ER Arrival to Admit. (minutes)[2]	834	309	270	274
Time from ER Arrival to Discharge (minutes)	943	174	127	134
Time in ER Before Being Evaluated (minutes)	991	45	26	26
Time to Pain Meds for Fractures (minutes)	141	39	57	57
Heart Attack Care				
Aspirin Given at Discharge	313	98%	99%	99%
Fibrinolytic Meds Within 30 Min. of Arrival[7]	-	-	49%	54%
PCI Within 90 Minutes of Arrival	35	83%	95%	96%
Statin Prescribed at Discharge	317	98%	98%	98%
Heart Failure Care				
ACE Inhibitor or ARB for LVSD	125	93%	97%	97%
Discharge Instructions Given	273	91%	95%	94%
Evaluation of LVS Function	298	97%	99%	99%
Medicare Spending				
Medicare Spending per Patient (ratio)	-	1.02	1.03	0.98
Pneumonia Care				
Appropriate Initial Antibiotic Given	147	97%	95%	95%
Blood Culture Timing	234	98%	98%	98%
Pregnancy and Delivery Care				
Newborn Deliveries Scheduled Early[2]	48	4%	7%	6%
Preventive Care				
Immunization for Influenza[2]	748	97%	90%	90%
Immunization for Pneumonia[2]	886	97%	92%	92%

NOTE: Hospital profiles are in alphabetical order by state, then city, then hospital within the city; Rankings exclude hospitals with less than 25 cases except for patient surveys which excludes hospitals with less than 100 cases; (a) 100-299 cases; (1) The number of cases/patients is too few to report; (2) Data submitted were based on a sample of cases/patients; (3) Results are based on a shorter time period than required; (4) Data suppressed by CMS for one or more quarters; (5) Results are not available for this reporting period; (6) Fewer than 100 patients completed the HCAHPS survey; (7) No cases met the criteria for this measure; (8) The lower limit of the confidence interval cannot be calculated if the number of observed infections equals zero; (9) No data are available from the state/territory for this reporting period; (10) The scores shown reflect fewer than 50 completed surveys; (11) There were discrepancies in the data collection process; (12) This measure does not apply to this hospital for this reporting period; (13) Results cannot be calculated for this reporting period; (14) The results for this state are combined with nearby states to protect confidentiality; Please refer to the User's Guide for a full explanation of data.

Stroke Care				
Anticoagulation Therapy for Atrial Fibrillation	28	100%	96%	95%
Antithrombotic Therapy Timing	178	98%	98%	98%
Assessed for Rehabilitation	185	98%	98%	97%
Discharged on Antithrombotic Therapy	166	99%	99%	99%
Discharged on Statin Medication	119	97%	95%	94%
Thrombolytic Therapy Timing[1]	-	-	68%	66%
Venous Thromboembolism Prophylaxis	206	98%	94%	94%
Written Stroke Educational Materials Given	122	87%	92%	88%
Surgical Care Improvement Project				
Appropriate Beta Blocker Usage[2]	188	98%	98%	98%
Appropriate VTP Within 24 Hours[2]	419	99%	98%	98%
Controlled Postoperative Blood Glucose[2]	76	100%	96%	97%
Perioperative Temperature Management[2]	559	100%	100%	100%
Prophylactic Antibiotic Selection[2]	426	99%	99%	99%
Prophylactic Antibiotic Selection (Outpatient)	289	99%	98%	98%
Prophylactic Antibiotic Stopped[2]	402	96%	98%	98%
Prophylactic Antibiotic Timing[2]	426	98%	99%	99%
Prophylactic Antibiotic Timing (Outpatient)	290	99%	98%	98%
Urinary Catheter Removal[2]	433	99%	98%	97%
Survey of Patients' Hospital Experiences				
Area Around Room 'Always' Quiet at Night	300+	66%	68%	61%
Doctors 'Always' Communicated Well	300+	79%	83%	82%
Home Recovery Information Given	300+	81%	85%	85%
Hospital Given 9 or 10 on 10 Point Scale	300+	70%	73%	71%
Meds 'Always' Explained Before Given	300+	60%	66%	64%
Nurses 'Always' Communicated Well	300+	76%	80%	79%
Pain 'Always' Well Controlled	300+	71%	72%	71%
Room and Bathroom 'Always' Clean	300+	63%	75%	73%
Timely Help 'Always' Received	300+	61%	69%	68%
Would Definitely Recommend Hospital	300+	71%	73%	71%
Use of Medical Imaging				
Cardiac Imaging Stress Test before Surgery[1]	-	-	5.3%	5.3%
Combination Abdominal CT Scan	791	13.4%	16.4%	10.5%
Combination Brain/Sinus CT Scan	718	1.3%	2.7%	2.7%
Combination Chest CT Scan	341	23.2%	5.6%	2.7%
Follow-up Mammogram/Ultrasound	1,611	6.8%	7.9%	8.8%
Lumbar Spine MRI for Low Back Pain	154	33.8%	39.6%	37.2%

Odessa Regional Hospital

520 E 6th Street
Odessa, TX 79761
E-mail: achurchill@iasishealthcare.com
URL: www.odessaregionalhospital.com
Type: Acute Care Hospitals
Ownership: Proprietary

Phone: 432-582-8340
Fax: 432-582-8913
Emergency Services: Yes
Beds: 146

Key Personnel:
Chief of Medical Staff. . . . . Anne Acreman, MD
Infection Control. . . . . Micki Barnett
Intensive Care Unit. . . . . Myra DeGuzman
CEO . . . . Stacey Gerig
Quality Assurance . . . . Carol Herman
CEO/President. . . . . R Craig Preston

Measure	Cases	This Hosp.	State Avg.	U.S. Avg.
Blood Clot Prevention and Treatment				
Anticoagulation Overlap Therapy[2]	17	88%	93%	93%
ICU Venous Thromboembolism Prophylaxis[2]	99	94%	92%	92%
Incidence of Potentially Preventable VTE[1,2]	-	-	9%	10%
UFH with Dosages/Platelet Monitoring[1,2]	-	-	96%	97%
Venous Thromboembolism Prophylaxis[2]	190	94%	82%	85%
Warfarin Therapy Discharge Instructions[1,2]	-	-	84%	75%
Chest Pain/Possible Heart Attack Care				
Aspirin Given Within 24 Hours of Arrival[3,7]	-	-	94%	96%
Fibrinolytic Meds Within 30 Min. of Arrival[5]	-	-	47%	58%
Average Time to ECG (minutes)[3,7]	-	-	8	7
Average Time to Transfer (minutes)[5]	-	-	62	60
Children's Asthma Care				
Received Home Management Plan of Care	-	-	93%	88%
Received Reliever Medication	-	-	100%	100%
Received Systemic Corticosteroids	-	-	100%	100%
Emergency Department				
Admittance Decision Time (minutes)[2]	275	127	99	98
Head CT Results Within 45 Min. of Arrival[1,3]	-	-	54%	57%
Patients Who Left ER Before Being Seen	27,035	3%	3%	2%
Time from ER Arrival to Admit. (minutes)[2]	275	318	270	274
Time from ER Arrival to Discharge (minutes)	296	163	127	134
Time in ER Before Being Evaluated (minutes)	311	60	26	26
Time to Pain Meds for Fractures (minutes)	57	89	57	57
Heart Attack Care				
Aspirin Given at Discharge	172	98%	99%	99%
Fibrinolytic Meds Within 30 Min. of Arrival[7]	-	-	49%	54%
PCI Within 90 Minutes of Arrival	11	45%	95%	96%
Statin Prescribed at Discharge	148	93%	98%	98%
Heart Failure Care				
ACE Inhibitor or ARB for LVSD	37	97%	97%	97%
Discharge Instructions Given	94	86%	95%	94%
Evaluation of LVS Function	109	100%	99%	99%
Medicare Spending				
Medicare Spending per Patient (ratio)	-	1.00	1.03	0.98
Pneumonia Care				
Appropriate Initial Antibiotic Given	57	88%	95%	95%
Blood Culture Timing	80	95%	98%	98%
Pregnancy and Delivery Care				
Newborn Deliveries Scheduled Early[2]	43	19%	7%	6%
Preventive Care				
Immunization for Influenza[2]	548	98%	90%	90%
Immunization for Pneumonia[2]	374	97%	92%	92%
Stroke Care				
Anticoagulation Therapy for Atrial Fibrillation[1]	-	-	96%	95%
Antithrombotic Therapy Timing	32	100%	98%	98%
Assessed for Rehabilitation	28	89%	98%	97%
Discharged on Antithrombotic Therapy	28	96%	99%	99%
Discharged on Statin Medication	23	87%	95%	94%
Thrombolytic Therapy Timing[1]	-	-	68%	66%
Venous Thromboembolism Prophylaxis	30	77%	94%	94%
Written Stroke Educational Materials Given	14	79%	92%	88%
Surgical Care Improvement Project				
Appropriate Beta Blocker Usage	72	100%	98%	98%
Appropriate VTP Within 24 Hours	217	99%	98%	98%
Controlled Postoperative Blood Glucose	52	94%	96%	97%
Perioperative Temperature Management	268	100%	100%	100%
Prophylactic Antibiotic Selection	211	99%	99%	99%
Prophylactic Antibiotic Selection (Outpatient)	123	99%	98%	98%
Prophylactic Antibiotic Stopped	188	97%	98%	98%
Prophylactic Antibiotic Timing	211	99%	99%	99%
Prophylactic Antibiotic Timing (Outpatient)	123	99%	98%	98%
Urinary Catheter Removal	133	96%	98%	97%
Survey of Patients' Hospital Experiences				
Area Around Room 'Always' Quiet at Night	300+	63%	68%	61%
Doctors 'Always' Communicated Well	300+	80%	83%	82%
Home Recovery Information Given	300+	86%	85%	85%
Hospital Given 9 or 10 on 10 Point Scale	300+	70%	73%	71%
Meds 'Always' Explained Before Given	300+	68%	66%	64%
Nurses 'Always' Communicated Well	300+	75%	80%	79%
Pain 'Always' Well Controlled	300+	69%	72%	71%
Room and Bathroom 'Always' Clean	300+	68%	75%	73%
Timely Help 'Always' Received	300+	62%	69%	68%
Would Definitely Recommend Hospital	300+	74%	73%	71%
Use of Medical Imaging				
Cardiac Imaging Stress Test before Surgery	47	0.0%	5.3%	5.3%
Combination Abdominal CT Scan	174	17.2%	16.4%	10.5%
Combination Brain/Sinus CT Scan[1]	-	-	2.7%	2.7%
Combination Chest CT Scan[1]	-	-	5.6%	2.7%
Follow-up Mammogram/Ultrasound	912	4.5%	7.9%	8.8%
Lumbar Spine MRI for Low Back Pain[1]	-	-	39.6%	37.2%

Hamilton Hospital

901 West Hamilton
Olney, TX 76374
Type: Critical Access Hospitals
Ownership: Govt - Hospital Dist/Auth

Phone: 940-564-5521
Emergency Services: Yes

Measure	Cases	This Hosp.	State Avg.	U.S. Avg.
Blood Clot Prevention and Treatment				
Anticoagulation Overlap Therapy[5]	-	-	93%	93%
ICU Venous Thromboembolism Prophylaxis[5]	-	-	92%	92%
Incidence of Potentially Preventable VTE[5]	-	-	9%	10%
UFH with Dosages/Platelet Monitoring[5]	-	-	96%	97%
Venous Thromboembolism Prophylaxis[5]	-	-	82%	85%
Warfarin Therapy Discharge Instructions[5]	-	-	84%	75%
Chest Pain/Possible Heart Attack Care				
Aspirin Given Within 24 Hours of Arrival[1,3]	-	-	94%	96%
Fibrinolytic Meds Within 30 Min. of Arrival[1,3]	-	-	47%	58%
Average Time to ECG (minutes)[1,3]	-	-	8	7
Average Time to Transfer (minutes)[3,7]	-	-	62	60
Children's Asthma Care				
Received Home Management Plan of Care	-	-	93%	88%
Received Reliever Medication	-	-	100%	100%
Received Systemic Corticosteroids	-	-	100%	100%
Emergency Department				
Admittance Decision Time (minutes)[5]	-	-	99	98
Head CT Results Within 45 Min. of Arrival[5]	-	-	54%	57%
Patients Who Left ER Before Being Seen[5]	-	-	3%	2%
Time from ER Arrival to Admit. (minutes)[5]	-	-	270	274
Time from ER Arrival to Discharge (minutes)[5]	-	-	127	134
Time in ER Before Being Evaluated (minutes)[5]	-	-	26	26
Time to Pain Meds for Fractures (minutes)[5]	-	-	57	57
Heart Attack Care				
Aspirin Given at Discharge[5]	-	-	99%	99%
Fibrinolytic Meds Within 30 Min. of Arrival[5]	-	-	49%	54%
PCI Within 90 Minutes of Arrival[5]	-	-	95%	96%
Statin Prescribed at Discharge[5]	-	-	98%	98%
Heart Failure Care				
ACE Inhibitor or ARB for LVSD[1]	-	-	97%	97%
Discharge Instructions Given[1]	-	-	95%	94%
Evaluation of LVS Function[1]	-	-	99%	99%
Medicare Spending				
Medicare Spending per Patient (ratio)	-	-	1.03	0.98
Pneumonia Care				
Appropriate Initial Antibiotic Given	23	83%	95%	95%
Blood Culture Timing	15	87%	98%	98%
Pregnancy and Delivery Care				
Newborn Deliveries Scheduled Early[5]	-	-	7%	6%
Preventive Care				
Immunization for Influenza[5]	-	-	90%	90%
Immunization for Pneumonia[5]	-	-	92%	92%
Stroke Care				
Anticoagulation Therapy for Atrial Fibrillation[5]	-	-	96%	95%
Antithrombotic Therapy Timing[5]	-	-	98%	98%
Assessed for Rehabilitation[5]	-	-	98%	97%
Discharged on Antithrombotic Therapy[5]	-	-	99%	99%
Discharged on Statin Medication[5]	-	-	95%	94%
Thrombolytic Therapy Timing[5]	-	-	68%	66%
Venous Thromboembolism Prophylaxis[5]	-	-	94%	94%
Written Stroke Educational Materials Given[5]	-	-	92%	88%
Surgical Care Improvement Project				
Appropriate Beta Blocker Usage[5]	-	-	98%	98%
Appropriate VTP Within 24 Hours[5]	-	-	98%	98%
Controlled Postoperative Blood Glucose[5]	-	-	96%	97%
Perioperative Temperature Management[5]	-	-	100%	100%
Prophylactic Antibiotic Selection[5]	-	-	99%	99%
Prophylactic Antibiotic Selection (Outpatient)[5]	-	-	98%	98%
Prophylactic Antibiotic Stopped[5]	-	-	98%	98%
Prophylactic Antibiotic Timing[5]	-	-	99%	99%
Prophylactic Antibiotic Timing (Outpatient)[5]	-	-	98%	98%
Urinary Catheter Removal[5]	-	-	98%	97%
Survey of Patients' Hospital Experiences				
Area Around Room 'Always' Quiet at Night[5]	-	-	68%	61%
Doctors 'Always' Communicated Well[5]	-	-	83%	82%
Home Recovery Information Given[5]	-	-	85%	85%
Hospital Given 9 or 10 on 10 Point Scale[5]	-	-	73%	71%
Meds 'Always' Explained Before Given[5]	-	-	66%	64%
Nurses 'Always' Communicated Well[5]	-	-	80%	79%
Pain 'Always' Well Controlled[5]	-	-	72%	71%
Room and Bathroom 'Always' Clean[5]	-	-	75%	73%
Timely Help 'Always' Received[5]	-	-	69%	68%
Would Definitely Recommend Hospital[5]	-	-	73%	71%
Use of Medical Imaging				
Cardiac Imaging Stress Test before Surgery[7]	-	-	5.3%	5.3%

NOTE: Hospital profiles are in alphabetical order by state, then city, then hospital within the city; Rankings exclude hospitals with less than 25 cases except for patient surveys which excludes hospitals with less than 100 cases; (a) 100-299 cases; (1) The number of cases/patients is too few to report; (2) Data submitted were based on a sample of cases/patients; (3) Results are based on a shorter time period than required; (4) Data suppressed by CMS for one or more quarters; (5) Results are not available for this reporting period; (6) Fewer than 100 patients completed the HCAHPS survey; (7) No cases met the criteria for this measure; (8) The lower limit of the confidence interval cannot be calculated if the number of observed infections equals zero; (9) No data are available from the state/territory for this reporting period; (10) The scores shown reflect fewer than 50 completed surveys; (11) There were discrepancies in the data collection process; (12) This measure does not apply to this hospital for this reporting period; (13) Results cannot be calculated for this reporting period; (14) The results for this state are combined with nearby states to protect confidentiality; Please refer to the User's Guide for a full explanation of data.

Measure	Cases	This Hosp.	State Avg.	U.S. Avg.
Combination Abdominal CT Scan	93	34.4%	16.4%	10.5%
Combination Brain/Sinus CT Scan	127	0.0%	2.7%	2.7%
Combination Chest CT Scan[1]	-	-	5.6%	2.7%
Follow-up Mammogram/Ultrasound[7]	-	-	7.9%	8.8%
Lumbar Spine MRI for Low Back Pain[1]	-	-	39.6%	37.2%

Memorial Hermann Baptist Orange Hospital

608 Strickland Drive
Orange, TX 77630
Phone: 409-883-9361
Fax: 409-883-1223
URL: www.mhbh.org
Type: Acute Care Hospitals
Emergency Services: Yes
Ownership: Voluntary non-profit - Private
Beds: 199

Key Personnel:
CEO/President. . . . . Rossane Atkin
Coronary Care. . . . . Miguel Castllanos
Emergency Room . . . . Carolyn Knight, RN
Chief of Medical Staff. . . . . Steve Mazzola, MD
Operating Room. . . . . Allyson Mize
Quality Assurance . . . . Brenda Williams

Measure	Cases	This Hosp.	State Avg.	U.S. Avg.
Blood Clot Prevention and Treatment				
Anticoagulation Overlap Therapy[1,2]	-	-	93%	93%
ICU Venous Thromboembolism Prophylaxis[2]	38	82%	92%	92%
Incidence of Potentially Preventable VTE[2,7]	-	-	9%	10%
UFH with Dosages/Platelet Monitoring[1,2]	-	-	96%	97%
Venous Thromboembolism Prophylaxis[2]	129	74%	82%	85%
Warfarin Therapy Discharge Instructions[1,2]	-	-	84%	75%
Chest Pain/Possible Heart Attack Care				
Aspirin Given Within 24 Hours of Arrival	38	97%	94%	96%
Fibrinolytic Meds Within 30 Min. of Arrival[7]	-	-	47%	58%
Average Time to ECG (minutes)	37	11	8	7
Average Time to Transfer (minutes)[1]	-	-	62	60
Children's Asthma Care				
Received Home Management Plan of Care	-	-	93%	88%
Received Reliever Medication	-	-	100%	100%
Received Systemic Corticosteroids	-	-	100%	100%
Emergency Department				
Admittance Decision Time (minutes)[2]	337	110	99	98
Head CT Results Within 45 Min. of Arrival	15	87%	54%	57%
Patients Who Left ER Before Being Seen	18,697	8%	3%	2%
Time from ER Arrival to Admit. (minutes)[2]	377	350	270	274
Time from ER Arrival to Discharge (minutes)	364	159	127	134
Time in ER Before Being Evaluated (minutes)	359	52	26	26
Time to Pain Meds for Fractures (minutes)	70	75	57	57
Heart Attack Care				
Aspirin Given at Discharge[1]	-	-	99%	99%
Fibrinolytic Meds Within 30 Min. of Arrival[7]	-	-	49%	54%
PCI Within 90 Minutes of Arrival[7]	-	-	95%	96%
Statin Prescribed at Discharge[1]	-	-	98%	98%
Heart Failure Care				
ACE Inhibitor or ARB for LVSD	19	100%	97%	97%
Discharge Instructions Given	42	86%	95%	94%
Evaluation of LVS Function	48	98%	99%	99%
Medicare Spending				
Medicare Spending per Patient (ratio)	-	1.02	1.03	0.98
Pneumonia Care				
Appropriate Initial Antibiotic Given	76	96%	95%	95%
Blood Culture Timing	97	98%	98%	98%
Pregnancy and Delivery Care				
Newborn Deliveries Scheduled Early[1]	-	-	7%	6%
Preventive Care				
Immunization for Influenza[2]	257	95%	90%	90%
Immunization for Pneumonia[2]	327	99%	92%	92%
Stroke Care				
Anticoagulation Therapy for Atrial Fibrillation[3,7]	-	-	96%	95%
Antithrombotic Therapy Timing[1,3]	-	-	98%	98%
Assessed for Rehabilitation[1,3]	-	-	98%	97%
Discharged on Antithrombotic Therapy[1,3]	-	-	99%	99%
Discharged on Statin Medication[1,3]	-	-	95%	94%
Thrombolytic Therapy Timing[3,7]	-	-	68%	66%
Venous Thromboembolism Prophylaxis[1,3]	-	-	94%	94%
Written Stroke Educational Materials Given[1,3]	-	-	92%	88%
Surgical Care Improvement Project				
Appropriate Beta Blocker Usage[1]	-	-	98%	98%
Appropriate VTP Within 24 Hours	44	98%	98%	98%
Controlled Postoperative Blood Glucose[7]	-	-	96%	97%
Perioperative Temperature Management	50	100%	100%	100%
Prophylactic Antibiotic Selection	25	100%	99%	99%
Prophylactic Antibiotic Selection (Outpatient)	47	98%	98%	98%
Prophylactic Antibiotic Stopped	25	96%	98%	98%
Prophylactic Antibiotic Timing	25	100%	99%	99%
Prophylactic Antibiotic Timing (Outpatient)	48	96%	98%	98%
Urinary Catheter Removal	20	90%	98%	97%
Survey of Patients' Hospital Experiences				
Area Around Room 'Always' Quiet at Night	300+	76%	68%	61%
Doctors 'Always' Communicated Well	300+	89%	83%	82%
Home Recovery Information Given	300+	85%	85%	85%
Hospital Given 9 or 10 on 10 Point Scale	300+	73%	73%	71%
Meds 'Always' Explained Before Given	300+	74%	66%	64%
Nurses 'Always' Communicated Well	300+	84%	80%	79%
Pain 'Always' Well Controlled	300+	74%	72%	71%
Room and Bathroom 'Always' Clean	300+	72%	75%	73%
Timely Help 'Always' Received	300+	74%	69%	68%
Would Definitely Recommend Hospital	300+	69%	73%	71%
Use of Medical Imaging				
Cardiac Imaging Stress Test before Surgery[1]	-	-	5.3%	5.3%
Combination Abdominal CT Scan	377	38.5%	16.4%	10.5%
Combination Brain/Sinus CT Scan	438	6.6%	2.7%	2.7%
Combination Chest CT Scan	129	1.6%	5.6%	2.7%
Follow-up Mammogram/Ultrasound	576	5.6%	7.9%	8.8%
Lumbar Spine MRI for Low Back Pain	41	46.3%	39.6%	37.2%

Palestine Regional Medical Center

2900 S Loop 256
Palestine, TX 75801
Phone: 903-731-1000
Fax: 903-731-2217
E-mail: dprice@prhc.net
URL: www.palestineregional.com
Type: Acute Care Hospitals
Emergency Services: Yes
Ownership: Proprietary
Beds: 258

Key Personnel:
CEO/President. . . . . Randall L Hoover
Quality Assurance . . . . Deborah Howard
Infection Control. . . . . Sandra Knight
Operating Room. . . . . Cheryl Todd, RN
Intensive Care Unit. . . . . Leah Vintila

Measure	Cases	This Hosp.	State Avg.	U.S. Avg.
Blood Clot Prevention and Treatment				
Anticoagulation Overlap Therapy[2]	28	96%	93%	93%
ICU Venous Thromboembolism Prophylaxis[2]	86	99%	92%	92%
Incidence of Potentially Preventable VTE[1,2]	-	-	9%	10%
UFH with Dosages/Platelet Monitoring[2]	13	100%	96%	97%
Venous Thromboembolism Prophylaxis[2]	234	99%	82%	85%
Warfarin Therapy Discharge Instructions[2]	19	100%	84%	75%
Chest Pain/Possible Heart Attack Care				
Aspirin Given Within 24 Hours of Arrival	95	94%	94%	96%
Fibrinolytic Meds Within 30 Min. of Arrival[1]	-	-	47%	58%
Average Time to ECG (minutes)	96	2	8	7
Average Time to Transfer (minutes)[1]	-	-	62	60
Children's Asthma Care				
Received Home Management Plan of Care	-	-	93%	88%
Received Reliever Medication	-	-	100%	100%
Received Systemic Corticosteroids	-	-	100%	100%
Emergency Department				
Admittance Decision Time (minutes)[2]	372	60	99	98
Head CT Results Within 45 Min. of Arrival[1]	-	-	54%	57%
Patients Who Left ER Before Being Seen	31,689	4%	3%	2%
Time from ER Arrival to Admit. (minutes)[2]	380	193	270	274
Time from ER Arrival to Discharge (minutes)	421	108	127	134
Time in ER Before Being Evaluated (minutes)	491	18	26	26
Time to Pain Meds for Fractures (minutes)	108	52	57	57
Heart Attack Care				
Aspirin Given at Discharge	52	98%	99%	99%
Fibrinolytic Meds Within 30 Min. of Arrival[7]	-	-	49%	54%
PCI Within 90 Minutes of Arrival[1]	-	-	95%	96%
Statin Prescribed at Discharge	52	100%	98%	98%
Heart Failure Care				
ACE Inhibitor or ARB for LVSD	65	95%	97%	97%
Discharge Instructions Given	112	96%	95%	94%
Evaluation of LVS Function	144	100%	99%	99%
Medicare Spending				
Medicare Spending per Patient (ratio)	-	1.02	1.03	0.98
Pneumonia Care				
Appropriate Initial Antibiotic Given	110	94%	95%	95%
Blood Culture Timing	161	99%	98%	98%
Pregnancy and Delivery Care				
Newborn Deliveries Scheduled Early[2]	27	26%	7%	6%
Preventive Care				
Immunization for Influenza[2]	426	96%	90%	90%
Immunization for Pneumonia[2]	410	96%	92%	92%
Stroke Care				
Anticoagulation Therapy for Atrial Fibrillation[1]	-	-	96%	95%
Antithrombotic Therapy Timing	40	92%	98%	98%
Assessed for Rehabilitation	37	95%	98%	97%
Discharged on Antithrombotic Therapy	36	97%	99%	99%
Discharged on Statin Medication	26	85%	95%	94%
Thrombolytic Therapy Timing[7]	-	-	68%	66%
Venous Thromboembolism Prophylaxis	41	98%	94%	94%
Written Stroke Educational Materials Given	19	84%	92%	88%
Surgical Care Improvement Project				
Appropriate Beta Blocker Usage	73	99%	98%	98%
Appropriate VTP Within 24 Hours	226	100%	98%	98%
Controlled Postoperative Blood Glucose[7]	-	-	96%	97%
Perioperative Temperature Management	271	100%	100%	100%
Prophylactic Antibiotic Selection	37	97%	99%	99%
Prophylactic Antibiotic Selection (Outpatient)	68	100%	98%	98%
Prophylactic Antibiotic Stopped	35	100%	98%	98%
Prophylactic Antibiotic Timing	37	100%	99%	99%
Prophylactic Antibiotic Timing (Outpatient)	68	100%	98%	98%
Urinary Catheter Removal	144	100%	98%	97%
Survey of Patients' Hospital Experiences				
Area Around Room 'Always' Quiet at Night	300+	63%	68%	61%
Doctors 'Always' Communicated Well	300+	77%	83%	82%
Home Recovery Information Given	300+	83%	85%	85%
Hospital Given 9 or 10 on 10 Point Scale	300+	60%	73%	71%
Meds 'Always' Explained Before Given	300+	57%	66%	64%
Nurses 'Always' Communicated Well	300+	74%	80%	79%
Pain 'Always' Well Controlled	300+	64%	72%	71%
Room and Bathroom 'Always' Clean	300+	66%	75%	73%
Timely Help 'Always' Received	300+	58%	69%	68%
Would Definitely Recommend Hospital	300+	52%	73%	71%
Use of Medical Imaging				
Cardiac Imaging Stress Test before Surgery	63	6.3%	5.3%	5.3%
Combination Abdominal CT Scan	317	19.6%	16.4%	10.5%
Combination Brain/Sinus CT Scan	516	2.5%	2.7%	2.7%
Combination Chest CT Scan	93	34.4%	5.6%	2.7%
Follow-up Mammogram/Ultrasound	449	3.6%	7.9%	8.8%
Lumbar Spine MRI for Low Back Pain[1]	-	-	39.6%	37.2%

Pampa Regional Medical Center

1 Medical Plaza
Pampa, TX 79065
Phone: 806-665-3721
Fax: 806-665-5222
URL: www.prmctx.com
Type: Acute Care Hospitals
Emergency Services: Yes
Ownership: Proprietary
Beds: 115

Key Personnel:
Chief of Medical Staff. . . . . Laxman Bhatia, MD
Emergency Room . . . . Brenda Carter, RN
CEO . . . . Brad Morse
Quality Assurance . . . . Carol Trolinger

Measure	Cases	This Hosp.	State Avg.	U.S. Avg.
Blood Clot Prevention and Treatment				
Anticoagulation Overlap Therapy[1,2]	-	-	93%	93%
ICU Venous Thromboembolism Prophylaxis[2]	49	92%	92%	92%
Incidence of Potentially Preventable VTE[1,2]	-	-	9%	10%
UFH with Dosages/Platelet Monitoring[2,7]	-	-	96%	97%
Venous Thromboembolism Prophylaxis[2]	90	87%	82%	85%
Warfarin Therapy Discharge Instructions[1,2]	-	-	84%	75%
Chest Pain/Possible Heart Attack Care				
Aspirin Given Within 24 Hours of Arrival	21	100%	94%	96%
Fibrinolytic Meds Within 30 Min. of Arrival[1]	-	-	47%	58%
Average Time to ECG (minutes)	21	15	8	7

NOTE: Hospital profiles are in alphabetical order by state, then city, then hospital within the city; Rankings exclude hospitals with less than 25 cases except for patient surveys which excludes hospitals with less than 100 cases; (a) 100-299 cases; (1) The number of cases/patients is too few to report; (2) Data submitted were based on a sample of cases/patients; (3) Results are based on a shorter time period than required; (4) Data suppressed by CMS for one or more quarters; (5) Results are not available for this reporting period; (6) Fewer than 100 patients completed the HCAHPS survey; (7) No cases met the criteria for this measure; (8) The lower limit of the confidence interval cannot be calculated if the number of observed infections equals zero; (9) No data are available from the state/territory for this reporting period; (10) The scores shown reflect fewer than 50 completed surveys; (11) There were discrepancies in the data collection process; (12) This measure does not apply to this hospital for this reporting period; (13) Results cannot be calculated for this reporting period; (14) The results for this state are combined with nearby states to protect confidentiality; Please refer to the User's Guide for a full explanation of data.

Measure	Cases	This Hosp.	State Avg.	U.S. Avg.
Average Time to Transfer (minutes)[1]	-	-	62	60
Children's Asthma Care				
Received Home Management Plan of Care	-	-	93%	88%
Received Reliever Medication	-	-	100%	100%
Received Systemic Corticosteroids	-	-	100%	100%
Emergency Department				
Admittance Decision Time (minutes)[2]	394	71	99	98
Head CT Results Within 45 Min. of Arrival[1,3]	-	-	54%	57%
Patients Who Left ER Before Being Seen	12,671	1%	3%	2%
Time from ER Arrival to Admit. (minutes)[2]	424	222	270	274
Time from ER Arrival to Discharge (minutes)	887	105	127	134
Time in ER Before Being Evaluated (minutes)	814	24	26	26
Time to Pain Meds for Fractures (minutes)	46	59	57	57
Heart Attack Care				
Aspirin Given at Discharge	15	100%	99%	99%
Fibrinolytic Meds Within 30 Min. of Arrival[7]	-	-	49%	54%
PCI Within 90 Minutes of Arrival[1]	-	-	95%	96%
Statin Prescribed at Discharge	16	94%	98%	98%
Heart Failure Care				
ACE Inhibitor or ARB for LVSD	34	100%	97%	97%
Discharge Instructions Given	54	100%	95%	94%
Evaluation of LVS Function	71	100%	99%	99%
Medicare Spending				
Medicare Spending per Patient (ratio)	-	0.96	1.03	0.98
Pneumonia Care				
Appropriate Initial Antibiotic Given	41	98%	95%	95%
Blood Culture Timing	58	97%	98%	98%
Pregnancy and Delivery Care				
Newborn Deliveries Scheduled Early	28	0%	7%	6%
Preventive Care				
Immunization for Influenza[2]	443	100%	90%	90%
Immunization for Pneumonia[2]	480	100%	92%	92%
Stroke Care				
Anticoagulation Therapy for Atrial Fibrillation[1]	-	-	96%	95%
Antithrombotic Therapy Timing[1]	-	-	98%	98%
Assessed for Rehabilitation[1]	-	-	98%	97%
Discharged on Antithrombotic Therapy[1]	-	-	99%	99%
Discharged on Statin Medication[1]	-	-	95%	94%
Thrombolytic Therapy Timing[1]	-	-	68%	66%
Venous Thromboembolism Prophylaxis	13	92%	94%	94%
Written Stroke Educational Materials Given[1]	-	-	92%	88%
Surgical Care Improvement Project				
Appropriate Beta Blocker Usage	51	96%	98%	98%
Appropriate VTP Within 24 Hours	137	96%	98%	98%
Controlled Postoperative Blood Glucose[7]	-	-	96%	97%
Perioperative Temperature Management	168	100%	100%	100%
Prophylactic Antibiotic Selection	138	100%	99%	99%
Prophylactic Antibiotic Selection (Outpatient)	15	100%	98%	98%
Prophylactic Antibiotic Stopped	131	97%	98%	98%
Prophylactic Antibiotic Timing	138	100%	99%	99%
Prophylactic Antibiotic Timing (Outpatient)	15	100%	98%	98%
Urinary Catheter Removal	102	99%	98%	97%
Survey of Patients' Hospital Experiences				
Area Around Room 'Always' Quiet at Night	300+	63%	68%	61%
Doctors 'Always' Communicated Well	300+	80%	83%	82%
Home Recovery Information Given	300+	82%	85%	85%
Hospital Given 9 or 10 on 10 Point Scale	300+	64%	73%	71%
Meds 'Always' Explained Before Given	300+	53%	66%	64%
Nurses 'Always' Communicated Well	300+	73%	80%	79%
Pain 'Always' Well Controlled	300+	68%	72%	71%
Room and Bathroom 'Always' Clean	300+	63%	75%	73%
Timely Help 'Always' Received	300+	65%	69%	68%
Would Definitely Recommend Hospital	300+	60%	73%	71%
Use of Medical Imaging				
Cardiac Imaging Stress Test before Surgery[1]	-	-	5.3%	5.3%
Combination Abdominal CT Scan	180	29.4%	16.4%	10.5%
Combination Brain/Sinus CT Scan	244	6.1%	2.7%	2.7%
Combination Chest CT Scan	61	37.7%	5.6%	2.7%
Follow-up Mammogram/Ultrasound	155	12.9%	7.9%	8.8%
Lumbar Spine MRI for Low Back Pain[1]	-	-	39.6%	37.2%

Paris Regional Medical Center

820 Clarksville St
Paris, TX 75460
Phone: 903-785-4521
Fax: 903-737-3848
URL: www.parisregional.com
Type: Acute Care Hospitals
Emergency Services: Yes
Ownership: Proprietary
Beds: 365

Key Personnel:

Chief of Medical Staff.......... Linda Bail, DO
Infection Control.............. Mary Fitzwater
Pediatric In-Patient Care .... Kristi Graham
Quality Assurance .... Carole Grant
CEO .... Stephen Grubbs
Operating Room............. Vanessa Herron
Cardiac Laboratory............ Jamie McClahan

Measure	Cases	This Hosp.	State Avg.	U.S. Avg.
Blood Clot Prevention and Treatment				
Anticoagulation Overlap Therapy[2]	48	94%	93%	93%
ICU Venous Thromboembolism Prophylaxis[2]	72	94%	92%	92%
Incidence of Potentially Preventable VTE[1,2]	-	-	9%	10%
UFH with Dosages/Platelet Monitoring[2]	14	100%	96%	97%
Venous Thromboembolism Prophylaxis[2]	426	77%	82%	85%
Warfarin Therapy Discharge Instructions[2]	42	81%	84%	75%
Chest Pain/Possible Heart Attack Care				
Aspirin Given Within 24 Hours of Arrival[1,3]	-	-	94%	96%
Fibrinolytic Meds Within 30 Min. of Arrival[5]	-	-	47%	58%
Average Time to ECG (minutes)[1,3]	-	-	8	7
Average Time to Transfer (minutes)[5]	-	-	62	60
Children's Asthma Care				
Received Home Management Plan of Care	-	-	93%	88%
Received Reliever Medication	-	-	100%	100%
Received Systemic Corticosteroids	-	-	100%	100%
Emergency Department				
Admittance Decision Time (minutes)[2]	558	88	99	98
Head CT Results Within 45 Min. of Arrival[1]	-	-	54%	57%
Patients Who Left ER Before Being Seen	35,322	2%	3%	2%
Time from ER Arrival to Admit. (minutes)[2]	573	287	270	274
Time from ER Arrival to Discharge (minutes)	448	158	127	134
Time in ER Before Being Evaluated (minutes)	465	25	26	26
Time to Pain Meds for Fractures (minutes)	94	87	57	57
Heart Attack Care				
Aspirin Given at Discharge	151	100%	99%	99%
Fibrinolytic Meds Within 30 Min. of Arrival[7]	-	-	49%	54%
PCI Within 90 Minutes of Arrival[1]	-	-	95%	96%
Statin Prescribed at Discharge	146	99%	98%	98%
Heart Failure Care				
ACE Inhibitor or ARB for LVSD[2]	73	85%	97%	97%
Discharge Instructions Given[2]	188	95%	95%	94%
Evaluation of LVS Function[2]	240	100%	99%	99%
Medicare Spending				
Medicare Spending per Patient (ratio)	-	1.08	1.03	0.98
Pneumonia Care				
Appropriate Initial Antibiotic Given[2]	72	100%	95%	95%
Blood Culture Timing[2]	133	91%	98%	98%
Pregnancy and Delivery Care				
Newborn Deliveries Scheduled Early	120	4%	7%	6%
Preventive Care				
Immunization for Influenza[2]	524	95%	90%	90%
Immunization for Pneumonia[2]	816	96%	92%	92%
Stroke Care				
Anticoagulation Therapy for Atrial Fibrillation[1]	-	-	96%	95%
Antithrombotic Therapy Timing	50	98%	98%	98%
Assessed for Rehabilitation	50	100%	98%	97%
Discharged on Antithrombotic Therapy	47	100%	99%	99%
Discharged on Statin Medication	39	90%	95%	94%
Thrombolytic Therapy Timing[1]	-	-	68%	66%
Venous Thromboembolism Prophylaxis	50	76%	94%	94%
Written Stroke Educational Materials Given	20	75%	92%	88%
Surgical Care Improvement Project				
Appropriate Beta Blocker Usage[2]	183	97%	98%	98%
Appropriate VTP Within 24 Hours[2]	357	97%	98%	98%
Controlled Postoperative Blood Glucose[2]	115	90%	96%	97%
Perioperative Temperature Management[2]	410	100%	100%	100%
Prophylactic Antibiotic Selection[2]	387	99%	99%	99%
Prophylactic Antibiotic Selection (Outpatient)	232	97%	98%	98%
Prophylactic Antibiotic Stopped[2]	370	98%	98%	98%
Prophylactic Antibiotic Timing[2]	387	98%	99%	99%
Prophylactic Antibiotic Timing (Outpatient)	234	98%	98%	98%
Urinary Catheter Removal[2]	313	96%	98%	97%
Survey of Patients' Hospital Experiences				
Area Around Room 'Always' Quiet at Night	300+	56%	68%	61%
Doctors 'Always' Communicated Well	300+	79%	83%	82%
Home Recovery Information Given	300+	76%	85%	85%
Hospital Given 9 or 10 on 10 Point Scale	300+	50%	73%	71%
Meds 'Always' Explained Before Given	300+	56%	66%	64%
Nurses 'Always' Communicated Well	300+	72%	80%	79%
Pain 'Always' Well Controlled	300+	64%	72%	71%
Room and Bathroom 'Always' Clean	300+	64%	75%	73%
Timely Help 'Always' Received	300+	58%	69%	68%
Would Definitely Recommend Hospital	300+	50%	73%	71%
Use of Medical Imaging				
Cardiac Imaging Stress Test before Surgery	85	3.5%	5.3%	5.3%
Combination Abdominal CT Scan	398	2.3%	16.4%	10.5%
Combination Brain/Sinus CT Scan	638	1.7%	2.7%	2.7%
Combination Chest CT Scan	85	1.2%	5.6%	2.7%
Follow-up Mammogram/Ultrasound	272	14.0%	7.9%	8.8%
Lumbar Spine MRI for Low Back Pain[1]	-	-	39.6%	37.2%

Bayshore Medical Center

4000 Spencer Hwy
Pasadena, TX 77504
Phone: 713-359-1000
Fax: 713-359-1958
URL: www.bayshoremedical.com
Type: Acute Care Hospitals
Emergency Services: Yes
Ownership: Proprietary
Beds: 373

Key Personnel:

CEO/President............... Jeanna Bernard, FACHE
Infection Control.............. Janet Dougherty
Quality Assurance .... C Parker
Operating Room............. Mary Sartor
Pediatric Ambulatory Care ...... E Segura, MD
Pediatric In-Patient Care .... E Segura, MD
Chief of Medical Staff.......... Harold Walton

Measure	Cases	This Hosp.	State Avg.	U.S. Avg.
Blood Clot Prevention and Treatment				
Anticoagulation Overlap Therapy[2]	96	100%	93%	93%
ICU Venous Thromboembolism Prophylaxis[2]	121	99%	92%	92%
Incidence of Potentially Preventable VTE[2]	19	5%	9%	10%
UFH with Dosages/Platelet Monitoring[2]	42	100%	96%	97%
Venous Thromboembolism Prophylaxis[2]	395	96%	82%	85%
Warfarin Therapy Discharge Instructions[2]	75	99%	84%	75%
Chest Pain/Possible Heart Attack Care				
Aspirin Given Within 24 Hours of Arrival[1]	-	-	94%	96%
Fibrinolytic Meds Within 30 Min. of Arrival[3,7]	-	-	47%	58%
Average Time to ECG (minutes)[1]	-	-	8	7
Average Time to Transfer (minutes)[3,7]	-	-	62	60
Children's Asthma Care				
Received Home Management Plan of Care	-	-	93%	88%
Received Reliever Medication	-	-	100%	100%
Received Systemic Corticosteroids	-	-	100%	100%
Emergency Department				
Admittance Decision Time (minutes)[2]	540	131	99	98
Head CT Results Within 45 Min. of Arrival	16	44%	54%	57%
Patients Who Left ER Before Being Seen	>100k	2%	3%	2%
Time from ER Arrival to Admit. (minutes)[2]	551	308	270	274
Time from ER Arrival to Discharge (minutes)	441	148	127	134
Time in ER Before Being Evaluated (minutes)	495	15	26	26
Time to Pain Meds for Fractures (minutes)	284	55	57	57
Heart Attack Care				
Aspirin Given at Discharge	324	100%	99%	99%
Fibrinolytic Meds Within 30 Min. of Arrival[7]	-	-	49%	54%
PCI Within 90 Minutes of Arrival	50	100%	95%	96%
Statin Prescribed at Discharge	328	100%	98%	98%
Heart Failure Care				
ACE Inhibitor or ARB for LVSD	174	100%	97%	97%
Discharge Instructions Given	441	98%	95%	94%
Evaluation of LVS Function	513	100%	99%	99%
Medicare Spending				
Medicare Spending per Patient (ratio)	-	1.13	1.03	0.98
Pneumonia Care				

NOTE: Hospital profiles are in alphabetical order by state, then city, then hospital within the city; Rankings exclude hospitals with less than 25 cases except for patient surveys which excludes hospitals with less than 100 cases; (a) 100-299 cases; (1) The number of cases/patients is too few to report; (2) Data submitted were based on a sample of cases/patients; (3) Results are based on a shorter time period than required; (4) Data suppressed by CMS for one or more quarters; (5) Results are not available for this reporting period; (6) Fewer than 100 patients completed the HCAHPS survey; (7) No cases met the criteria for this measure; (8) The lower limit of the confidence interval cannot be calculated if the number of observed infections equals zero; (9) No data are available from the state/territory for this reporting period; (10) The scores shown reflect fewer than 50 completed surveys; (11) There were discrepancies in the data collection process; (12) This measure does not apply to this hospital for this reporting period; (13) Results cannot be calculated for this reporting period; (14) The results for this state are combined with nearby states to protect confidentiality; Please refer to the User's Guide for a full explanation of data.

Appropriate Initial Antibiotic Given	270	99%	95%	95%
Blood Culture Timing	425	100%	98%	98%
Pregnancy and Delivery Care				
Newborn Deliveries Scheduled Early[2]	115	2%	7%	6%
Preventive Care				
Immunization for Influenza[2]	541	97%	90%	90%
Immunization for Pneumonia[2]	567	97%	92%	92%
Stroke Care				
Anticoagulation Therapy for Atrial Fibrillation	15	100%	96%	95%
Antithrombotic Therapy Timing	194	100%	98%	98%
Assessed for Rehabilitation	211	100%	98%	97%
Discharged on Antithrombotic Therapy	195	100%	99%	99%
Discharged on Statin Medication	158	100%	95%	94%
Thrombolytic Therapy Timing	16	94%	68%	66%
Venous Thromboembolism Prophylaxis	215	99%	94%	94%
Written Stroke Educational Materials Given	138	97%	92%	88%
Surgical Care Improvement Project				
Appropriate Beta Blocker Usage[2]	119	100%	98%	98%
Appropriate VTP Within 24 Hours[2]	314	100%	98%	98%
Controlled Postoperative Blood Glucose[2]	34	97%	96%	97%
Perioperative Temperature Management[2]	424	100%	100%	100%
Prophylactic Antibiotic Selection[2]	263	99%	99%	99%
Prophylactic Antibiotic Selection (Outpatient)	138	99%	98%	98%
Prophylactic Antibiotic Stopped[2]	242	99%	98%	98%
Prophylactic Antibiotic Timing[2]	264	100%	99%	99%
Prophylactic Antibiotic Timing (Outpatient)	139	99%	98%	98%
Urinary Catheter Removal[2]	138	99%	98%	97%
Survey of Patients' Hospital Experiences				
Area Around Room 'Always' Quiet at Night	300+	58%	68%	61%
Doctors 'Always' Communicated Well	300+	76%	83%	82%
Home Recovery Information Given	300+	81%	85%	85%
Hospital Given 9 or 10 on 10 Point Scale	300+	62%	73%	71%
Meds 'Always' Explained Before Given	300+	56%	66%	64%
Nurses 'Always' Communicated Well	300+	72%	80%	79%
Pain 'Always' Well Controlled	300+	67%	72%	71%
Room and Bathroom 'Always' Clean	300+	69%	75%	73%
Timely Help 'Always' Received	300+	57%	69%	68%
Would Definitely Recommend Hospital	300+	59%	73%	71%
Use of Medical Imaging				
Cardiac Imaging Stress Test before Surgery	315	8.9%	5.3%	5.3%
Combination Abdominal CT Scan	688	10.2%	16.4%	10.5%
Combination Brain/Sinus CT Scan	746	2.4%	2.7%	2.7%
Combination Chest CT Scan	274	1.5%	5.6%	2.7%
Follow-up Mammogram/Ultrasound	517	8.3%	7.9%	8.8%
Lumbar Spine MRI for Low Back Pain[1]	-	-	39.6%	37.2%

Saint Luke's Patients Medical Center

4600 East Sam Houston Parkway South Phone: 281-487-0700
Pasadena, TX 77505
Type: Acute Care Hospitals Emergency Services: Yes
Ownership: Physician

Measure	Cases	This Hosp.	State Avg.	U.S. Avg.
Blood Clot Prevention and Treatment				
Anticoagulation Overlap Therapy[2]	40	68%	93%	93%
ICU Venous Thromboembolism Prophylaxis[2]	61	80%	92%	92%
Incidence of Potentially Preventable VTE[1,2]	-	-	9%	10%
UFH with Dosages/Platelet Monitoring[2]	21	100%	96%	97%
Venous Thromboembolism Prophylaxis[2]	392	81%	82%	85%
Warfarin Therapy Discharge Instructions[2]	26	81%	84%	75%
Chest Pain/Possible Heart Attack Care				
Aspirin Given Within 24 Hours of Arrival[1,3]	-	-	94%	96%
Fibrinolytic Meds Within 30 Min. of Arrival[3,7]	-	-	47%	58%
Average Time to ECG (minutes)[1,3]	-	-	8	7
Average Time to Transfer (minutes)[1,3]	-	-	62	60
Children's Asthma Care				
Received Home Management Plan of Care	-	-	93%	88%
Received Reliever Medication	-	-	100%	100%
Received Systemic Corticosteroids	-	-	100%	100%
Emergency Department				
Admittance Decision Time (minutes)[2]	393	180	99	98
Head CT Results Within 45 Min. of Arrival[1]	-	-	54%	57%
Patients Who Left ER Before Being Seen	15,237	5%	3%	2%
Time from ER Arrival to Admit. (minutes)[2]	441	389	270	274
Time from ER Arrival to Discharge (minutes)	443	158	127	134
Time in ER Before Being Evaluated (minutes)	419	45	26	26
Time to Pain Meds for Fractures (minutes)	54	82	57	57
Heart Attack Care				
Aspirin Given at Discharge	56	95%	99%	99%
Fibrinolytic Meds Within 30 Min. of Arrival[1]	-	-	49%	54%
PCI Within 90 Minutes of Arrival	14	79%	95%	96%
Statin Prescribed at Discharge	62	97%	98%	98%
Heart Failure Care				
ACE Inhibitor or ARB for LVSD	61	87%	97%	97%
Discharge Instructions Given	140	94%	95%	94%
Evaluation of LVS Function	186	100%	99%	99%
Medicare Spending				
Medicare Spending per Patient (ratio)	-	1.26	1.03	0.98
Pneumonia Care				
Appropriate Initial Antibiotic Given[2]	92	98%	95%	95%
Blood Culture Timing[2]	109	99%	98%	98%
Pregnancy and Delivery Care				
Newborn Deliveries Scheduled Early[7]	-	-	7%	6%
Preventive Care				
Immunization for Influenza[2]	356	99%	90%	90%
Immunization for Pneumonia[2]	541	98%	92%	92%
Stroke Care				
Anticoagulation Therapy for Atrial Fibrillation[1]	-	-	96%	95%
Antithrombotic Therapy Timing	28	96%	98%	98%
Assessed for Rehabilitation	28	96%	98%	97%
Discharged on Antithrombotic Therapy	27	93%	99%	99%
Discharged on Statin Medication	23	52%	95%	94%
Thrombolytic Therapy Timing[7]	-	-	68%	66%
Venous Thromboembolism Prophylaxis	27	89%	94%	94%
Written Stroke Educational Materials Given	13	38%	92%	88%
Surgical Care Improvement Project				
Appropriate Beta Blocker Usage[2]	104	91%	98%	98%
Appropriate VTP Within 24 Hours[2]	335	97%	98%	98%
Controlled Postoperative Blood Glucose[2,7]	-	-	96%	97%
Perioperative Temperature Management[2]	378	100%	100%	100%
Prophylactic Antibiotic Selection[2]	258	98%	99%	99%
Prophylactic Antibiotic Selection (Outpatient)	218	95%	98%	98%
Prophylactic Antibiotic Stopped[2]	253	96%	98%	98%
Prophylactic Antibiotic Timing[2]	258	99%	99%	99%
Prophylactic Antibiotic Timing (Outpatient)	218	99%	98%	98%
Urinary Catheter Removal[2]	173	98%	98%	97%
Survey of Patients' Hospital Experiences				
Area Around Room 'Always' Quiet at Night	300+	58%	68%	61%
Doctors 'Always' Communicated Well	300+	80%	83%	82%
Home Recovery Information Given	300+	81%	85%	85%
Hospital Given 9 or 10 on 10 Point Scale	300+	71%	73%	71%
Meds 'Always' Explained Before Given	300+	58%	66%	64%
Nurses 'Always' Communicated Well	300+	74%	80%	79%
Pain 'Always' Well Controlled	300+	63%	72%	71%
Room and Bathroom 'Always' Clean	300+	68%	75%	73%
Timely Help 'Always' Received	300+	64%	69%	68%
Would Definitely Recommend Hospital	300+	78%	73%	71%
Use of Medical Imaging				
Cardiac Imaging Stress Test before Surgery[1]	-	-	5.3%	5.3%
Combination Abdominal CT Scan	455	5.1%	16.4%	10.5%
Combination Brain/Sinus CT Scan[1]	-	-	2.7%	2.7%
Combination Chest CT Scan	239	0.4%	5.6%	2.7%
Follow-up Mammogram/Ultrasound	128	3.9%	7.9%	8.8%
Lumbar Spine MRI for Low Back Pain	53	41.5%	39.6%	37.2%

Surgery Specialty Hospitals of America - SE Houston

4301 B Vista Phone: 713-378-3000
Pasadena, TX 77504
Type: Acute Care Hospitals Emergency Services: Yes
Ownership: Proprietary Beds: 37
Key Personnel:
CEO/President. . . . . Farida Moeen

Measure	Cases	This Hosp.	State Avg.	U.S. Avg.
Blood Clot Prevention and Treatment				
Anticoagulation Overlap Therapy[7]	-	-	93%	93%
ICU Venous Thromboembolism Prophylaxis[7]	-	-	92%	92%
Incidence of Potentially Preventable VTE[7]	-	-	9%	10%
UFH with Dosages/Platelet Monitoring[7]	-	-	96%	97%
Venous Thromboembolism Prophylaxis	24	88%	82%	85%
Warfarin Therapy Discharge Instructions[7]	-	-	84%	75%
Chest Pain/Possible Heart Attack Care				
Aspirin Given Within 24 Hours of Arrival[5]	-	-	94%	96%
Fibrinolytic Meds Within 30 Min. of Arrival[5]	-	-	47%	58%
Average Time to ECG (minutes)[5]	-	-	8	7
Average Time to Transfer (minutes)[5]	-	-	62	60
Children's Asthma Care				
Received Home Management Plan of Care	-	-	93%	88%
Received Reliever Medication	-	-	100%	100%
Received Systemic Corticosteroids	-	-	100%	100%
Emergency Department				
Admittance Decision Time (minutes)[1,2]	-	-	99	98
Head CT Results Within 45 Min. of Arrival[5]	-	-	54%	57%
Patients Who Left ER Before Being Seen	333	0%	3%	2%
Time from ER Arrival to Admit. (minutes)[1,2]	-	-	270	274
Time from ER Arrival to Discharge (minutes)[3]	222	60	127	134
Time in ER Before Being Evaluated (minutes)[3]	227	26	26	26
Time to Pain Meds for Fractures (minutes)[5]	-	-	57	57
Heart Attack Care				
Aspirin Given at Discharge[5]	-	-	99%	99%
Fibrinolytic Meds Within 30 Min. of Arrival[5]	-	-	49%	54%
PCI Within 90 Minutes of Arrival[5]	-	-	95%	96%
Statin Prescribed at Discharge[5]	-	-	98%	98%
Heart Failure Care				
ACE Inhibitor or ARB for LVSD[5]	-	-	97%	97%
Discharge Instructions Given[5]	-	-	95%	94%
Evaluation of LVS Function[5]	-	-	99%	99%
Medicare Spending				
Medicare Spending per Patient (ratio)[1]	-	-	1.03	0.98
Pneumonia Care				
Appropriate Initial Antibiotic Given[5]	-	-	95%	95%
Blood Culture Timing[5]	-	-	98%	98%
Pregnancy and Delivery Care				
Newborn Deliveries Scheduled Early[2,7]	-	-	7%	6%
Preventive Care				
Immunization for Influenza[2]	51	98%	90%	90%
Immunization for Pneumonia[2]	38	95%	92%	92%
Stroke Care				
Anticoagulation Therapy for Atrial Fibrillation[5]	-	-	96%	95%
Antithrombotic Therapy Timing[5]	-	-	98%	98%
Assessed for Rehabilitation[5]	-	-	98%	97%
Discharged on Antithrombotic Therapy[5]	-	-	99%	99%
Discharged on Statin Medication[5]	-	-	95%	94%
Thrombolytic Therapy Timing[5]	-	-	68%	66%
Venous Thromboembolism Prophylaxis[5]	-	-	94%	94%
Written Stroke Educational Materials Given[5]	-	-	92%	88%
Surgical Care Improvement Project				
Appropriate Beta Blocker Usage[1,2]	-	-	98%	98%
Appropriate VTP Within 24 Hours[1,2]	-	-	98%	98%
Controlled Postoperative Blood Glucose[2,7]	-	-	96%	97%
Perioperative Temperature Management[1,2]	-	-	100%	100%
Prophylactic Antibiotic Selection[1,2]	-	-	99%	99%
Prophylactic Antibiotic Selection (Outpatient)[3]	22	95%	98%	98%
Prophylactic Antibiotic Stopped[1,2]	-	-	98%	98%
Prophylactic Antibiotic Timing[1,2]	-	-	99%	99%
Prophylactic Antibiotic Timing (Outpatient)[3]	22	100%	98%	98%
Urinary Catheter Removal[1,2]	-	-	98%	97%
Survey of Patients' Hospital Experiences				
Area Around Room 'Always' Quiet at Night[6]	<100	93%	68%	61%
Doctors 'Always' Communicated Well[6]	<100	97%	83%	82%
Home Recovery Information Given[6]	<100	95%	85%	85%
Hospital Given 9 or 10 on 10 Point Scale[6]	<100	93%	73%	71%
Meds 'Always' Explained Before Given[6]	<100	94%	66%	64%
Nurses 'Always' Communicated Well[6]	<100	97%	80%	79%
Pain 'Always' Well Controlled[6]	<100	97%	72%	71%
Room and Bathroom 'Always' Clean[6]	<100	91%	75%	73%
Timely Help 'Always' Received[6]	<100	99%	69%	68%
Would Definitely Recommend Hospital[6]	<100	96%	73%	71%

NOTE: Hospital profiles are in alphabetical order by state, then city, then hospital within the city; Rankings exclude hospitals with less than 25 cases except for patient surveys which excludes hospitals with less than 100 cases; (a) 100-299 cases; (1) The number of cases/patients is too few to report; (2) Data submitted were based on a sample of cases/patients; (3) Results are based on a shorter time period than required; (4) Data suppressed by CMS for one or more quarters; (5) Results are not available for this reporting period; (6) Fewer than 100 patients completed the HCAHPS survey; (7) No cases met the criteria for this measure; (8) The lower limit of the confidence interval cannot be calculated if the number of observed infections equals zero; (9) No data are available from the state/territory for this reporting period; (10) The scores shown reflect fewer than 50 completed surveys; (11) There were discrepancies in the data collection process; (12) This measure does not apply to this hospital for this reporting period; (13) Results cannot be calculated for this reporting period; (14) The results for this state are combined with nearby states to protect confidentiality; Please refer to the User's Guide for a full explanation of data.

Use of Medical Imaging				
Cardiac Imaging Stress Test before Surgery[7]	-	-	5.3%	5.3%
Combination Abdominal CT Scan[1]	-	-	16.4%	10.5%
Combination Brain/Sinus CT Scan[7]	-	-	2.7%	2.7%
Combination Chest CT Scan[7]	-	-	5.6%	2.7%
Follow-up Mammogram/Ultrasound[7]	-	-	7.9%	8.8%
Lumbar Spine MRI for Low Back Pain[7]	-	-	39.6%	37.2%

Frio Regional Hospital

200 S Ih 35   Phone: 830-334-3617
Pearsall, TX 78061   Fax: 830-334-9812
E-mail: aholmes@trhta.net
URL: www.frioregionalhospital.com
Type: Acute Care Hospitals   Emergency Services: Yes
Ownership: Voluntary non-profit - Private   Beds: 22

Key Personnel:
Chief of Medical Staff. . . . . Mauricio Escobar
Patient Relations . . . . Louisa Martinez, RN
Radiology. . . . . Pedro Taussig
CEO/President. . . . . Michael Thompson
Emergency Room . . . . Becky Waldrum

Measure	Cases	This Hosp.	State Avg.	U.S. Avg.
Blood Clot Prevention and Treatment				
Anticoagulation Overlap Therapy[2,7]	-	-	93%	93%
ICU Venous Thromboembolism Prophylaxis[2,7]	-	-	92%	92%
Incidence of Potentially Preventable VTE[2,7]	-	-	9%	10%
UFH with Dosages/Platelet Monitoring[2,7]	-	-	96%	97%
Venous Thromboembolism Prophylaxis[2]	95	49%	82%	85%
Warfarin Therapy Discharge Instructions[2,7]	-	-	84%	75%
Chest Pain/Possible Heart Attack Care				
Aspirin Given Within 24 Hours of Arrival	18	94%	94%	96%
Fibrinolytic Meds Within 30 Min. of Arrival[1]	-	-	47%	58%
Average Time to ECG (minutes)	19	5	8	7
Average Time to Transfer (minutes)[1]	-	-	62	60
Children's Asthma Care				
Received Home Management Plan of Care	-	-	93%	88%
Received Reliever Medication	-	-	100%	100%
Received Systemic Corticosteroids	-	-	100%	100%
Emergency Department				
Admittance Decision Time (minutes)[2]	44	48	99	98
Head CT Results Within 45 Min. of Arrival[1]	-	-	54%	57%
Patients Who Left ER Before Being Seen	8,384	0%	3%	2%
Time from ER Arrival to Admit. (minutes)[2]	78	200	270	274
Time from ER Arrival to Discharge (minutes)	350	104	127	134
Time in ER Before Being Evaluated (minutes)	294	30	26	26
Time to Pain Meds for Fractures (minutes)	59	49	57	57
Heart Attack Care				
Aspirin Given at Discharge[3,7]	-	-	99%	99%
Fibrinolytic Meds Within 30 Min. of Arrival[3,7]	-	-	49%	54%
PCI Within 90 Minutes of Arrival[3,7]	-	-	95%	96%
Statin Prescribed at Discharge[3,7]	-	-	98%	98%
Heart Failure Care				
ACE Inhibitor or ARB for LVSD[7]	-	-	97%	97%
Discharge Instructions Given[1]	-	-	95%	94%
Evaluation of LVS Function[1]	-	-	99%	99%
Medicare Spending				
Medicare Spending per Patient (ratio)	-	0.88	1.03	0.98
Pneumonia Care				
Appropriate Initial Antibiotic Given	17	76%	95%	95%
Blood Culture Timing	26	92%	98%	98%
Pregnancy and Delivery Care				
Newborn Deliveries Scheduled Early	18	67%	7%	6%
Preventive Care				
Immunization for Influenza	167	88%	90%	90%
Immunization for Pneumonia[2]	132	92%	92%	92%
Stroke Care				
Anticoagulation Therapy for Atrial Fibrillation[3,7]	-	-	96%	95%
Antithrombotic Therapy Timing[3,7]	-	-	98%	98%
Assessed for Rehabilitation[3,7]	-	-	98%	97%
Discharged on Antithrombotic Therapy[3,7]	-	-	99%	99%
Discharged on Statin Medication[3,7]	-	-	95%	94%
Thrombolytic Therapy Timing[3,7]	-	-	68%	66%
Venous Thromboembolism Prophylaxis[3,7]	-	-	94%	94%
Written Stroke Educational Materials Given[3,7]	-	-	92%	88%
Surgical Care Improvement Project				
Appropriate Beta Blocker Usage[5]	-	-	98%	98%
Appropriate VTP Within 24 Hours[5]	-	-	98%	98%
Controlled Postoperative Blood Glucose[5]	-	-	96%	97%
Perioperative Temperature Management[5]	-	-	100%	100%
Prophylactic Antibiotic Selection[5]	-	-	99%	99%
Prophylactic Antibiotic Selection (Outpatient)[5]	-	-	98%	98%
Prophylactic Antibiotic Stopped[5]	-	-	98%	98%
Prophylactic Antibiotic Timing[5]	-	-	99%	99%
Prophylactic Antibiotic Timing (Outpatient)[5]	-	-	98%	98%
Urinary Catheter Removal[5]	-	-	98%	97%
Survey of Patients' Hospital Experiences				
Area Around Room 'Always' Quiet at Night[10]	<100	72%	68%	61%
Doctors 'Always' Communicated Well[10]	<100	83%	83%	82%
Home Recovery Information Given[10]	<100	85%	85%	85%
Hospital Given 9 or 10 on 10 Point Scale[10]	<100	56%	73%	71%
Meds 'Always' Explained Before Given[10]	<100	33%	66%	64%
Nurses 'Always' Communicated Well[10]	<100	77%	80%	79%
Pain 'Always' Well Controlled[10]	<100	57%	72%	71%
Room and Bathroom 'Always' Clean[10]	<100	78%	75%	73%
Timely Help 'Always' Received[10]	<100	53%	69%	68%
Would Definitely Recommend Hospital[10]	<100	59%	73%	71%
Use of Medical Imaging				
Cardiac Imaging Stress Test before Surgery[7]	-	-	5.3%	5.3%
Combination Abdominal CT Scan	91	13.2%	16.4%	10.5%
Combination Brain/Sinus CT Scan[1]	-	-	2.7%	2.7%
Combination Chest CT Scan[1]	-	-	5.6%	2.7%
Follow-up Mammogram/Ultrasound	119	16.8%	7.9%	8.8%
Lumbar Spine MRI for Low Back Pain[7]	-	-	39.6%	37.2%

Reeves County Hospital District

2323 Texas Street   Phone: 432-447-3551
Pecos, TX 79772   Fax: 432-447-5434
E-mail: nsmith@trhta.net
URL: www.reevescountyhospital.com
Type: Critical Access Hospitals   Emergency Services: Yes
Ownership: Govt - Hospital Dist/Auth   Beds: 49

Key Personnel:
Operating Room. . . . . W Bang, RN
Chief of Medical Staff. . . . . WJ Bang, MD
President . . . . Leo Hung
Radiology. . . . . Alexander Kovac
CEO/President. . . . . Al LaRochelle
Infection Control. . . . . Faye Lease

Measure	Cases	This Hosp.	State Avg.	U.S. Avg.
Blood Clot Prevention and Treatment				
Anticoagulation Overlap Therapy[1,3]	-	-	93%	93%
ICU Venous Thromboembolism Prophylaxis[3,7]	-	-	92%	92%
Incidence of Potentially Preventable VTE[1,3]	-	-	9%	10%
UFH with Dosages/Platelet Monitoring[3,7]	-	-	96%	97%
Venous Thromboembolism Prophylaxis[3,7]	-	-	82%	85%
Warfarin Therapy Discharge Instructions[3,7]	-	-	84%	75%
Chest Pain/Possible Heart Attack Care				
Aspirin Given Within 24 Hours of Arrival[1,3]	-	-	94%	96%
Fibrinolytic Meds Within 30 Min. of Arrival[3,7]	-	-	47%	58%
Average Time to ECG (minutes)[1,3]	-	-	8	7
Average Time to Transfer (minutes)[1,3]	-	-	62	60
Children's Asthma Care				
Received Home Management Plan of Care	-	-	93%	88%
Received Reliever Medication	-	-	100%	100%
Received Systemic Corticosteroids	-	-	100%	100%
Emergency Department				
Admittance Decision Time (minutes)[5]	-	-	99	98
Head CT Results Within 45 Min. of Arrival[1,3]	-	-	54%	57%
Patients Who Left ER Before Being Seen[5]	-	-	3%	2%
Time from ER Arrival to Admit. (minutes)[5]	-	-	270	274
Time from ER Arrival to Discharge (minutes)[5]	-	-	127	134
Time in ER Before Being Evaluated (minutes)[5]	-	-	26	26
Time to Pain Meds for Fractures (minutes)[1,3]	-	-	57	57
Heart Attack Care				
Aspirin Given at Discharge[1,3]	-	-	99%	99%
Fibrinolytic Meds Within 30 Min. of Arrival[3,7]	-	-	49%	54%
PCI Within 90 Minutes of Arrival[3,7]	-	-	95%	96%
Statin Prescribed at Discharge[1,3]	-	-	98%	98%
Heart Failure Care				
ACE Inhibitor or ARB for LVSD[3,7]	-	-	97%	97%
Discharge Instructions Given[1,3]	-	-	95%	94%
Evaluation of LVS Function[1,3]	-	-	99%	99%
Medicare Spending				
Medicare Spending per Patient (ratio)	-	-	1.03	0.98
Pneumonia Care				
Appropriate Initial Antibiotic Given[2,3]	21	29%	95%	95%
Blood Culture Timing[2,3]	20	75%	98%	98%
Pregnancy and Delivery Care				
Newborn Deliveries Scheduled Early[5]	-	-	7%	6%
Preventive Care				
Immunization for Influenza[5]	-	-	90%	90%
Immunization for Pneumonia[5]	-	-	92%	92%
Stroke Care				
Anticoagulation Therapy for Atrial Fibrillation[5]	-	-	96%	95%
Antithrombotic Therapy Timing[5]	-	-	98%	98%
Assessed for Rehabilitation[5]	-	-	98%	97%
Discharged on Antithrombotic Therapy[5]	-	-	99%	99%
Discharged on Statin Medication[5]	-	-	95%	94%
Thrombolytic Therapy Timing[5]	-	-	68%	66%
Venous Thromboembolism Prophylaxis[5]	-	-	94%	94%
Written Stroke Educational Materials Given[5]	-	-	92%	88%
Surgical Care Improvement Project				
Appropriate Beta Blocker Usage[5]	-	-	98%	98%
Appropriate VTP Within 24 Hours[5]	-	-	98%	98%
Controlled Postoperative Blood Glucose[5]	-	-	96%	97%
Perioperative Temperature Management[5]	-	-	100%	100%
Prophylactic Antibiotic Selection[5]	-	-	99%	99%
Prophylactic Antibiotic Selection (Outpatient)[5]	-	-	98%	98%
Prophylactic Antibiotic Stopped[5]	-	-	98%	98%
Prophylactic Antibiotic Timing[5]	-	-	99%	99%
Prophylactic Antibiotic Timing (Outpatient)[5]	-	-	98%	98%
Urinary Catheter Removal[5]	-	-	98%	97%
Survey of Patients' Hospital Experiences				
Area Around Room 'Always' Quiet at Night[6]	<100	74%	68%	61%
Doctors 'Always' Communicated Well[6]	<100	90%	83%	82%
Home Recovery Information Given[6]	<100	86%	85%	85%
Hospital Given 9 or 10 on 10 Point Scale[6]	<100	69%	73%	71%
Meds 'Always' Explained Before Given[6]	<100	65%	66%	64%
Nurses 'Always' Communicated Well[6]	<100	79%	80%	79%
Pain 'Always' Well Controlled[6]	<100	74%	72%	71%
Room and Bathroom 'Always' Clean[6]	<100	77%	75%	73%
Timely Help 'Always' Received[6]	<100	68%	69%	68%
Would Definitely Recommend Hospital[6]	<100	62%	73%	71%
Use of Medical Imaging				
Cardiac Imaging Stress Test before Surgery[7]	-	-	5.3%	5.3%
Combination Abdominal CT Scan	110	8.2%	16.4%	10.5%
Combination Brain/Sinus CT Scan[1]	-	-	2.7%	2.7%
Combination Chest CT Scan[1]	-	-	5.6%	2.7%
Follow-up Mammogram/Ultrasound[7]	-	-	7.9%	8.8%
Lumbar Spine MRI for Low Back Pain[7]	-	-	39.6%	37.2%

East Texas Medical Center Pittsburg

2701 Us Hwy 271 N   Phone: 903-856-4520
Pittsburg, TX 75686   Fax: 903-856-4598
URL: www.etmc.org
Type: Critical Access Hospitals   Emergency Services: Yes
Ownership: Voluntary non-profit - Private   Beds: 49

Key Personnel:
Radiology. . . . . E Maxey Abernathy
Emergency Room . . . . Rod Caldwell
Infection Control. . . . . Clarice Hampton, RN
Operating Room. . . . . Paulia Hays, RN
Quality Assurance . . . . Lynnette Lajda
Chief of Medical Staff. . . . . Blair MacBeath, MD

Measure	Cases	This Hosp.	State Avg.	U.S. Avg.
Blood Clot Prevention and Treatment				
Anticoagulation Overlap Therapy[1,2]	-	-	93%	93%
ICU Venous Thromboembolism Prophylaxis[2,7]	-	-	92%	92%
Incidence of Potentially Preventable VTE[2,7]	-	-	9%	10%
UFH with Dosages/Platelet Monitoring[2,7]	-	-	96%	97%
Venous Thromboembolism Prophylaxis[2]	131	63%	82%	85%
Warfarin Therapy Discharge Instructions[1,2]	-	-	84%	75%

NOTE: Hospital profiles are in alphabetical order by state, then city, then hospital within the city; Rankings exclude hospitals with less than 25 cases except for patient surveys which excludes hospitals with less than 100 cases; (a) 100-299 cases; (1) The number of cases/patients is too few to report; (2) Data submitted were based on a sample of cases/patients; (3) Results are based on a shorter time period than required; (4) Data suppressed by CMS for one or more quarters; (5) Results are not available for this reporting period; (6) Fewer than 100 patients completed the HCAHPS survey; (7) No cases met the criteria for this measure; (8) The lower limit of the confidence interval cannot be calculated if the number of observed infections equals zero; (9) No data are available from the state/territory for this reporting period; (10) The scores shown reflect fewer than 50 completed surveys; (11) There were discrepancies in the data collection process; (12) This measure does not apply to this hospital for this reporting period; (13) Results cannot be calculated for this reporting period; (14) The results for this state are combined with nearby states to protect confidentiality; Please refer to the User's Guide for a full explanation of data.

Chest Pain/Possible Heart Attack Care				
Aspirin Given Within 24 Hours of Arrival	-	-	94%	96%
Fibrinolytic Meds Within 30 Min. of Arrival	-	-	47%	58%
Average Time to ECG (minutes)	-	-	8	7
Average Time to Transfer (minutes)	-	-	62	60
Children's Asthma Care				
Received Home Management Plan of Care	-	-	93%	88%
Received Reliever Medication	-	-	100%	100%
Received Systemic Corticosteroids	-	-	100%	100%
Emergency Department				
Admittance Decision Time (minutes)[2]	303	45	99	98
Head CT Results Within 45 Min. of Arrival	-	-	54%	57%
Patients Who Left ER Before Being Seen	-	-	3%	2%
Time from ER Arrival to Admit. (minutes)[2]	356	202	270	274
Time from ER Arrival to Discharge (minutes)	-	-	127	134
Time in ER Before Being Evaluated (minutes)	-	-	26	26
Time to Pain Meds for Fractures (minutes)	-	-	57	57
Heart Attack Care				
Aspirin Given at Discharge[1]	-	-	99%	99%
Fibrinolytic Meds Within 30 Min. of Arrival[7]	-	-	49%	54%
PCI Within 90 Minutes of Arrival[7]	-	-	95%	96%
Statin Prescribed at Discharge[1]	-	-	98%	98%
Heart Failure Care				
ACE Inhibitor or ARB for LVSD[2]	19	79%	97%	97%
Discharge Instructions Given[2]	54	52%	95%	94%
Evaluation of LVS Function[2]	68	82%	99%	99%
Medicare Spending				
Medicare Spending per Patient (ratio)	-	-	1.03	0.98
Pneumonia Care				
Appropriate Initial Antibiotic Given	49	80%	95%	95%
Blood Culture Timing	57	88%	98%	98%
Pregnancy and Delivery Care				
Newborn Deliveries Scheduled Early[7]	-	-	7%	6%
Preventive Care				
Immunization for Influenza[2]	299	74%	90%	90%
Immunization for Pneumonia[2]	386	85%	92%	92%
Stroke Care				
Anticoagulation Therapy for Atrial Fibrillation[1]	-	-	96%	95%
Antithrombotic Therapy Timing[1]	-	-	98%	98%
Assessed for Rehabilitation[1]	-	-	98%	97%
Discharged on Antithrombotic Therapy[1]	-	-	99%	99%
Discharged on Statin Medication[1]	-	-	95%	94%
Thrombolytic Therapy Timing[1]	-	-	68%	66%
Venous Thromboembolism Prophylaxis	12	75%	94%	94%
Written Stroke Educational Materials Given[1]	-	-	92%	88%
Surgical Care Improvement Project				
Appropriate Beta Blocker Usage[5]	-	-	98%	98%
Appropriate VTP Within 24 Hours[5]	-	-	98%	98%
Controlled Postoperative Blood Glucose[5]	-	-	96%	97%
Perioperative Temperature Management[5]	-	-	100%	100%
Prophylactic Antibiotic Selection[5]	-	-	99%	99%
Prophylactic Antibiotic Selection (Outpatient)	-	-	98%	98%
Prophylactic Antibiotic Stopped[5]	-	-	98%	98%
Prophylactic Antibiotic Timing[5]	-	-	99%	99%
Prophylactic Antibiotic Timing (Outpatient)	-	-	98%	98%
Urinary Catheter Removal[5]	-	-	98%	97%
Survey of Patients' Hospital Experiences				
Area Around Room 'Always' Quiet at Night	(a)	78%	68%	61%
Doctors 'Always' Communicated Well	(a)	91%	83%	82%
Home Recovery Information Given	(a)	89%	85%	85%
Hospital Given 9 or 10 on 10 Point Scale	(a)	81%	73%	71%
Meds 'Always' Explained Before Given	(a)	74%	66%	64%
Nurses 'Always' Communicated Well	(a)	86%	80%	79%
Pain 'Always' Well Controlled	(a)	77%	72%	71%
Room and Bathroom 'Always' Clean	(a)	84%	75%	73%
Timely Help 'Always' Received	(a)	79%	69%	68%
Would Definitely Recommend Hospital	(a)	84%	73%	71%
Use of Medical Imaging				
Cardiac Imaging Stress Test before Surgery	-	-	5.3%	5.3%
Combination Abdominal CT Scan	-	-	16.4%	10.5%
Combination Brain/Sinus CT Scan	-	-	2.7%	2.7%
Combination Chest CT Scan	-	-	5.6%	2.7%
Follow-up Mammogram/Ultrasound	-	-	7.9%	8.8%
Lumbar Spine MRI for Low Back Pain	-	-	39.6%	37.2%

Covenant Hospital Plainview

2601 Dimmitt Rd
Plainview, TX 79072
Phone: 806-296-5531
Fax: 806-293-1885
E-mail: info@covenantplainview.org
URL: www.covenantplainview.org
Type: Acute Care Hospitals
Emergency Services: Yes
Ownership: Voluntary non-profit - Private
Beds: 100
Key Personnel:
CEO/President. . . . . Steve Hunter
Chief of Medical Staff . . . . Ponnie Vering

Measure	Cases	This Hosp.	State Avg.	U.S. Avg.
Blood Clot Prevention and Treatment				
Anticoagulation Overlap Therapy[1,2]	-	-	93%	93%
ICU Venous Thromboembolism Prophylaxis[2]	34	97%	92%	92%
Incidence of Potentially Preventable VTE[2,7]	-	-	9%	10%
UFH with Dosages/Platelet Monitoring[1,2]	-	-	96%	97%
Venous Thromboembolism Prophylaxis[2]	170	91%	82%	85%
Warfarin Therapy Discharge Instructions[1,2]	-	-	84%	75%
Chest Pain/Possible Heart Attack Care				
Aspirin Given Within 24 Hours of Arrival	39	100%	94%	96%
Fibrinolytic Meds Within 30 Min. of Arrival[1,3]	-	-	47%	58%
Average Time to ECG (minutes)	42	8	8	7
Average Time to Transfer (minutes)[3]	11	195	62	60
Children's Asthma Care				
Received Home Management Plan of Care	-	-	93%	88%
Received Reliever Medication	-	-	100%	100%
Received Systemic Corticosteroids	-	-	100%	100%
Emergency Department				
Admittance Decision Time (minutes)[2]	102	54	99	98
Head CT Results Within 45 Min. of Arrival	29	21%	54%	57%
Patients Who Left ER Before Being Seen	13,838	6%	3%	2%
Time from ER Arrival to Admit. (minutes)[2]	115	208	270	274
Time from ER Arrival to Discharge (minutes)	345	135	127	134
Time in ER Before Being Evaluated (minutes)	387	37	26	26
Time to Pain Meds for Fractures (minutes)	81	64	57	57
Heart Attack Care				
Aspirin Given at Discharge[1,3]	-	-	99%	99%
Fibrinolytic Meds Within 30 Min. of Arrival[3,7]	-	-	49%	54%
PCI Within 90 Minutes of Arrival[3,7]	-	-	95%	96%
Statin Prescribed at Discharge[1,3]	-	-	98%	98%
Heart Failure Care				
ACE Inhibitor or ARB for LVSD	24	96%	97%	97%
Discharge Instructions Given	19	74%	95%	94%
Evaluation of LVS Function	25	100%	99%	99%
Medicare Spending				
Medicare Spending per Patient (ratio)	-	0.95	1.03	0.98
Pneumonia Care				
Appropriate Initial Antibiotic Given	46	93%	95%	95%
Blood Culture Timing	45	93%	98%	98%
Pregnancy and Delivery Care				
Newborn Deliveries Scheduled Early[2]	49	16%	7%	6%
Preventive Care				
Immunization for Influenza[2]	244	80%	90%	90%
Immunization for Pneumonia[2]	257	89%	92%	92%
Stroke Care				
Anticoagulation Therapy for Atrial Fibrillation[7]	-	-	96%	95%
Antithrombotic Therapy Timing[1]	-	-	98%	98%
Assessed for Rehabilitation[1]	-	-	98%	97%
Discharged on Antithrombotic Therapy[1]	-	-	99%	99%
Discharged on Statin Medication[1]	-	-	95%	94%
Thrombolytic Therapy Timing[1]	-	-	68%	66%
Venous Thromboembolism Prophylaxis[1]	-	-	94%	94%
Written Stroke Educational Materials Given[1]	-	-	92%	88%
Surgical Care Improvement Project				
Appropriate Beta Blocker Usage	24	100%	98%	98%
Appropriate VTP Within 24 Hours	155	97%	98%	98%
Controlled Postoperative Blood Glucose[7]	-	-	96%	97%
Perioperative Temperature Management	178	100%	100%	100%
Prophylactic Antibiotic Selection	72	99%	99%	99%
Prophylactic Antibiotic Selection (Outpatient)	46	96%	98%	98%
Prophylactic Antibiotic Stopped	72	100%	98%	98%
Prophylactic Antibiotic Timing	72	99%	99%	99%
Prophylactic Antibiotic Timing (Outpatient)	46	100%	98%	98%
Urinary Catheter Removal	98	98%	98%	97%
Survey of Patients' Hospital Experiences				
Area Around Room 'Always' Quiet at Night	300+	69%	68%	61%
Doctors 'Always' Communicated Well	300+	87%	83%	82%
Home Recovery Information Given	300+	85%	85%	85%
Hospital Given 9 or 10 on 10 Point Scale	300+	68%	73%	71%
Meds 'Always' Explained Before Given	300+	68%	66%	64%
Nurses 'Always' Communicated Well	300+	78%	80%	79%
Pain 'Always' Well Controlled	300+	72%	72%	71%
Room and Bathroom 'Always' Clean	300+	75%	75%	73%
Timely Help 'Always' Received	300+	69%	69%	68%
Would Definitely Recommend Hospital	300+	68%	73%	71%
Use of Medical Imaging				
Cardiac Imaging Stress Test before Surgery	80	10.0%	5.3%	5.3%
Combination Abdominal CT Scan	192	8.3%	16.4%	10.5%
Combination Brain/Sinus CT Scan	290	4.8%	2.7%	2.7%
Combination Chest CT Scan	129	3.1%	5.6%	2.7%
Follow-up Mammogram/Ultrasound[1]	-	-	7.9%	8.8%
Lumbar Spine MRI for Low Back Pain[1]	-	-	39.6%	37.2%

Baylor Regional Medical Center at Plano

4700 Alliance Boulevard
Phone: 469-814-2000
Plano, TX 75093
URL: www.baylorhealth.com
Type: Acute Care Hospitals
Emergency Services: Yes
Ownership: Voluntary non-profit - Other
Key Personnel:
CEO . . . . Joel T. Allison, FACHE
Chief of Medical Staff . . . . Irving Prengler, MD

Measure	Cases	This Hosp.	State Avg.	U.S. Avg.
Blood Clot Prevention and Treatment				
Anticoagulation Overlap Therapy[2]	73	100%	93%	93%
ICU Venous Thromboembolism Prophylaxis[2]	100	99%	92%	92%
Incidence of Potentially Preventable VTE[2]	15	7%	9%	10%
UFH with Dosages/Platelet Monitoring[2]	23	100%	96%	97%
Venous Thromboembolism Prophylaxis[2]	364	98%	82%	85%
Warfarin Therapy Discharge Instructions[2]	59	100%	84%	75%
Chest Pain/Possible Heart Attack Care				
Aspirin Given Within 24 Hours of Arrival	33	100%	94%	96%
Fibrinolytic Meds Within 30 Min. of Arrival[7]	-	-	47%	58%
Average Time to ECG (minutes)	33	8	8	7
Average Time to Transfer (minutes)[1]	-	-	62	60
Children's Asthma Care				
Received Home Management Plan of Care	-	-	93%	88%
Received Reliever Medication	-	-	100%	100%
Received Systemic Corticosteroids	-	-	100%	100%
Emergency Department				
Admittance Decision Time (minutes)[2]	494	63	99	98
Head CT Results Within 45 Min. of Arrival[1]	-	-	54%	57%
Patients Who Left ER Before Being Seen	24,455	2%	3%	2%
Time from ER Arrival to Admit. (minutes)[2]	594	210	270	274
Time from ER Arrival to Discharge (minutes)	395	152	127	134
Time in ER Before Being Evaluated (minutes)[1]	-	-	26	26
Time to Pain Meds for Fractures (minutes)	90	44	57	57
Heart Attack Care				
Aspirin Given at Discharge[1]	-	-	99%	99%
Fibrinolytic Meds Within 30 Min. of Arrival[7]	-	-	49%	54%
PCI Within 90 Minutes of Arrival[7]	-	-	95%	96%
Statin Prescribed at Discharge[1]	-	-	98%	98%
Heart Failure Care				
ACE Inhibitor or ARB for LVSD	14	100%	97%	97%
Discharge Instructions Given	57	100%	95%	94%
Evaluation of LVS Function	84	100%	99%	99%
Medicare Spending				
Medicare Spending per Patient (ratio)	-	1.09	1.03	0.98
Pneumonia Care				
Appropriate Initial Antibiotic Given	107	98%	95%	95%
Blood Culture Timing	219	99%	98%	98%
Pregnancy and Delivery Care				
Newborn Deliveries Scheduled Early[7]	-	-	7%	6%

NOTE: Hospital profiles are in alphabetical order by state, then city, then hospital within the city; Rankings exclude hospitals with less than 25 cases except for patient surveys which excludes hospitals with less than 100 cases; (a) 100-299 cases; (1) The number of cases/patients is too few to report; (2) Data submitted were based on a sample of cases/patients; (3) Results are based on a shorter time period than required; (4) Data suppressed by CMS for one or more quarters; (5) Results are not available for this reporting period; (6) Fewer than 100 patients completed the HCAHPS survey; (7) No cases met the criteria for this measure; (8) The lower limit of the confidence interval cannot be calculated if the number of observed infections equals zero; (9) No data are available from the state/territory for this reporting period; (10) The scores shown reflect fewer than 50 completed surveys; (11) There were discrepancies in the data collection process; (12) This measure does not apply to this hospital for this reporting period; (13) Results cannot be calculated for this reporting period; (14) The results for this state are combined with nearby states to protect confidentiality; Please refer to the User's Guide for a full explanation of data.

Measure	Cases	This Hosp.	State Avg.	U.S. Avg.
Preventive Care				
Immunization for Influenza[2]	597	100%	90%	90%
Immunization for Pneumonia[2]	841	99%	92%	92%
Stroke Care				
Anticoagulation Therapy for Atrial Fibrillation	14	100%	96%	95%
Antithrombotic Therapy Timing	66	98%	98%	98%
Assessed for Rehabilitation	89	98%	98%	97%
Discharged on Antithrombotic Therapy	80	99%	99%	99%
Discharged on Statin Medication	62	94%	95%	94%
Thrombolytic Therapy Timing[1]	-	-	68%	66%
Venous Thromboembolism Prophylaxis	74	100%	94%	94%
Written Stroke Educational Materials Given	55	89%	92%	88%
Surgical Care Improvement Project				
Appropriate Beta Blocker Usage[2]	136	99%	98%	98%
Appropriate VTP Within 24 Hours[2]	447	100%	98%	98%
Controlled Postoperative Blood Glucose[2,7]	-	-	96%	97%
Perioperative Temperature Management[2]	498	100%	100%	100%
Prophylactic Antibiotic Selection[2]	300	100%	99%	99%
Prophylactic Antibiotic Selection (Outpatient)	259	100%	98%	98%
Prophylactic Antibiotic Stopped[2]	277	100%	98%	98%
Prophylactic Antibiotic Timing[2]	300	100%	99%	99%
Prophylactic Antibiotic Timing (Outpatient)	259	100%	98%	98%
Urinary Catheter Removal[2]	258	100%	98%	97%
Survey of Patients' Hospital Experiences				
Area Around Room 'Always' Quiet at Night	300+	74%	68%	61%
Doctors 'Always' Communicated Well	300+	81%	83%	82%
Home Recovery Information Given	300+	86%	85%	85%
Hospital Given 9 or 10 on 10 Point Scale	300+	80%	73%	71%
Meds 'Always' Explained Before Given	300+	62%	66%	64%
Nurses 'Always' Communicated Well	300+	79%	80%	79%
Pain 'Always' Well Controlled	300+	74%	72%	71%
Room and Bathroom 'Always' Clean	300+	78%	75%	73%
Timely Help 'Always' Received	300+	67%	69%	68%
Would Definitely Recommend Hospital	300+	85%	73%	71%
Use of Medical Imaging				
Cardiac Imaging Stress Test before Surgery[1]	-	-	5.3%	5.3%
Combination Abdominal CT Scan	643	8.7%	16.4%	10.5%
Combination Brain/Sinus CT Scan	904	4.3%	2.7%	2.7%
Combination Chest CT Scan	145	9.7%	5.6%	2.7%
Follow-up Mammogram/Ultrasound	2,359	9.3%	7.9%	8.8%
Lumbar Spine MRI for Low Back Pain	74	36.5%	39.6%	37.2%

Heart Hospital Baylor Plano

1100 Allied Drive
Plano, TX 75093
Phone: 469-814-3278
URL: www.thehearthospitalbaylor.com
Type: Acute Care Hospitals
Emergency Services: Yes
Ownership: Proprietary
Beds: 116

Key Personnel:
Chief of Medical Staff.......... Trent Pettijohn, MD, PA, FACC
President.................... Mark Valentine

Measure	Cases	This Hosp.	State Avg.	U.S. Avg.
Blood Clot Prevention and Treatment				
Anticoagulation Overlap Therapy[2]	26	96%	93%	93%
ICU Venous Thromboembolism Prophylaxis[2]	254	100%	92%	92%
Incidence of Potentially Preventable VTE[1,2]	-	-	9%	10%
UFH with Dosages/Platelet Monitoring[2]	13	92%	96%	97%
Venous Thromboembolism Prophylaxis[2]	291	95%	82%	85%
Warfarin Therapy Discharge Instructions[2]	18	100%	84%	75%
Chest Pain/Possible Heart Attack Care				
Aspirin Given Within 24 Hours of Arrival[1]	-	-	94%	96%
Fibrinolytic Meds Within 30 Min. of Arrival[5]	-	-	47%	58%
Average Time to ECG (minutes)[1]	-	-	8	7
Average Time to Transfer (minutes)[5]	-	-	62	60
Children's Asthma Care				
Received Home Management Plan of Care	-	-	93%	88%
Received Reliever Medication	-	-	100%	100%
Received Systemic Corticosteroids	-	-	100%	100%
Emergency Department				
Admittance Decision Time (minutes)[2]	189	86	99	98
Head CT Results Within 45 Min. of Arrival[1]	-	-	54%	57%
Patients Who Left ER Before Being Seen	4,023	0%	3%	2%
Time from ER Arrival to Admit. (minutes)[2]	190	235	270	274
Time from ER Arrival to Discharge (minutes)	374	152	127	134
Time in ER Before Being Evaluated (minutes)	324	12	26	26
Time to Pain Meds for Fractures (minutes)[1,3]	-	-	57	57
Heart Attack Care				
Aspirin Given at Discharge	324	99%	99%	99%
Fibrinolytic Meds Within 30 Min. of Arrival[7]	-	-	49%	54%
PCI Within 90 Minutes of Arrival	24	96%	95%	96%
Statin Prescribed at Discharge	316	98%	98%	98%
Heart Failure Care				
ACE Inhibitor or ARB for LVSD	106	96%	97%	97%
Discharge Instructions Given	219	99%	95%	94%
Evaluation of LVS Function	272	100%	99%	99%
Medicare Spending				
Medicare Spending per Patient (ratio)	-	1.01	1.03	0.98
Pneumonia Care				
Appropriate Initial Antibiotic Given[1]	-	-	95%	95%
Blood Culture Timing	11	100%	98%	98%
Pregnancy and Delivery Care				
Newborn Deliveries Scheduled Early[7]	-	-	7%	6%
Preventive Care				
Immunization for Influenza[2]	395	100%	90%	90%
Immunization for Pneumonia[2]	672	99%	92%	92%
Stroke Care				
Anticoagulation Therapy for Atrial Fibrillation[1,2]	-	-	96%	95%
Antithrombotic Therapy Timing[1,2]	-	-	98%	98%
Assessed for Rehabilitation[1,2]	-	-	98%	97%
Discharged on Antithrombotic Therapy[1,2]	-	-	99%	99%
Discharged on Statin Medication[1,2]	-	-	95%	94%
Thrombolytic Therapy Timing[2,7]	-	-	68%	66%
Venous Thromboembolism Prophylaxis[1,2]	-	-	94%	94%
Written Stroke Educational Materials Given[1,2]	-	-	92%	88%
Surgical Care Improvement Project				
Appropriate Beta Blocker Usage	746	100%	98%	98%
Appropriate VTP Within 24 Hours[1]	-	-	98%	98%
Controlled Postoperative Blood Glucose	1,053	99%	96%	97%
Perioperative Temperature Management	287	100%	100%	100%
Prophylactic Antibiotic Selection	1,058	100%	99%	99%
Prophylactic Antibiotic Selection (Outpatient)	622	96%	98%	98%
Prophylactic Antibiotic Stopped	1,007	99%	98%	98%
Prophylactic Antibiotic Timing	1,058	100%	99%	99%
Prophylactic Antibiotic Timing (Outpatient)	623	99%	98%	98%
Urinary Catheter Removal	802	100%	98%	97%
Survey of Patients' Hospital Experiences				
Area Around Room 'Always' Quiet at Night	300+	80%	68%	61%
Doctors 'Always' Communicated Well	300+	87%	83%	82%
Home Recovery Information Given	300+	88%	85%	85%
Hospital Given 9 or 10 on 10 Point Scale	300+	90%	73%	71%
Meds 'Always' Explained Before Given	300+	71%	66%	64%
Nurses 'Always' Communicated Well	300+	86%	80%	79%
Pain 'Always' Well Controlled	300+	80%	72%	71%
Room and Bathroom 'Always' Clean	300+	82%	75%	73%
Timely Help 'Always' Received	300+	79%	69%	68%
Would Definitely Recommend Hospital	300+	93%	73%	71%
Use of Medical Imaging				
Cardiac Imaging Stress Test before Surgery	527	7.0%	5.3%	5.3%
Combination Abdominal CT Scan	93	2.2%	16.4%	10.5%
Combination Brain/Sinus CT Scan	162	0.6%	2.7%	2.7%
Combination Chest CT Scan	112	0.9%	5.6%	2.7%
Follow-up Mammogram/Ultrasound[7]	-	-	7.9%	8.8%
Lumbar Spine MRI for Low Back Pain[1]	-	-	39.6%	37.2%

Medical Center of Plano

3901 W 15th St
Plano, TX 75075
Phone: 972-596-6800
Fax: 972-519-1423
URL: www.medicalcenterofplano.com
Type: Acute Care Hospitals
Emergency Services: Yes
Ownership: Proprietary
Beds: 427

Key Personnel:
Chief of Medical Staff.......... Heather L Akins
Radiology.................... John Y Aryan
CEO/President............... Harvey L Fishero

Measure	Cases	This Hosp.	State Avg.	U.S. Avg.
Blood Clot Prevention and Treatment				
Anticoagulation Overlap Therapy[2]	135	100%	93%	93%
ICU Venous Thromboembolism Prophylaxis[2]	117	100%	92%	92%
Incidence of Potentially Preventable VTE[2]	47	0%	9%	10%
UFH with Dosages/Platelet Monitoring[2]	44	100%	96%	97%
Venous Thromboembolism Prophylaxis[2]	341	100%	82%	85%
Warfarin Therapy Discharge Instructions[2]	102	100%	84%	75%
Chest Pain/Possible Heart Attack Care				
Aspirin Given Within 24 Hours of Arrival[5]	-	-	94%	96%
Fibrinolytic Meds Within 30 Min. of Arrival[5]	-	-	47%	58%
Average Time to ECG (minutes)[5]	-	-	8	7
Average Time to Transfer (minutes)[5]	-	-	62	60
Children's Asthma Care				
Received Home Management Plan of Care	-	-	93%	88%
Received Reliever Medication	-	-	100%	100%
Received Systemic Corticosteroids	-	-	100%	100%
Emergency Department				
Admittance Decision Time (minutes)[2]	804	127	99	98
Head CT Results Within 45 Min. of Arrival[1,3]	-	-	54%	57%
Patients Who Left ER Before Being Seen	40,849	2%	3%	2%
Time from ER Arrival to Admit. (minutes)[2]	804	216	270	274
Time from ER Arrival to Discharge (minutes)	438	144	127	134
Time in ER Before Being Evaluated (minutes)	489	18	26	26
Time to Pain Meds for Fractures (minutes)	124	50	57	57
Heart Attack Care				
Aspirin Given at Discharge[2]	203	100%	99%	99%
Fibrinolytic Meds Within 30 Min. of Arrival[2,7]	-	-	49%	54%
PCI Within 90 Minutes of Arrival[2]	46	98%	95%	96%
Statin Prescribed at Discharge[2]	197	100%	98%	98%
Heart Failure Care				
ACE Inhibitor or ARB for LVSD[2]	80	100%	97%	97%
Discharge Instructions Given[2]	187	98%	95%	94%
Evaluation of LVS Function[2]	262	100%	99%	99%
Medicare Spending				
Medicare Spending per Patient (ratio)	-	1.13	1.03	0.98
Pneumonia Care				
Appropriate Initial Antibiotic Given[2]	75	97%	95%	95%
Blood Culture Timing[2]	118	100%	98%	98%
Pregnancy and Delivery Care				
Newborn Deliveries Scheduled Early[2]	43	2%	7%	6%
Preventive Care				
Immunization for Influenza[2]	622	100%	90%	90%
Immunization for Pneumonia[2]	649	100%	92%	92%
Stroke Care				
Anticoagulation Therapy for Atrial Fibrillation[2]	16	100%	96%	95%
Antithrombotic Therapy Timing[2]	89	98%	98%	98%
Assessed for Rehabilitation[2]	135	99%	98%	97%
Discharged on Antithrombotic Therapy[2]	110	100%	99%	99%
Discharged on Statin Medication[2]	85	99%	95%	94%
Thrombolytic Therapy Timing[2]	11	100%	68%	66%
Venous Thromboembolism Prophylaxis[2]	152	100%	94%	94%
Written Stroke Educational Materials Given[2]	70	96%	92%	88%
Surgical Care Improvement Project				
Appropriate Beta Blocker Usage[2]	195	98%	98%	98%
Appropriate VTP Within 24 Hours[2]	449	100%	98%	98%
Controlled Postoperative Blood Glucose[2]	92	97%	96%	97%
Perioperative Temperature Management[2]	517	100%	100%	100%
Prophylactic Antibiotic Selection[2]	355	100%	99%	99%
Prophylactic Antibiotic Selection (Outpatient)	277	97%	98%	98%
Prophylactic Antibiotic Stopped[2]	338	99%	98%	98%
Prophylactic Antibiotic Timing[2]	356	99%	99%	99%
Prophylactic Antibiotic Timing (Outpatient)	277	99%	98%	98%
Urinary Catheter Removal[2]	339	100%	98%	97%
Survey of Patients' Hospital Experiences				
Area Around Room 'Always' Quiet at Night	300+	61%	68%	61%
Doctors 'Always' Communicated Well	300+	78%	83%	82%
Home Recovery Information Given	300+	84%	85%	85%
Hospital Given 9 or 10 on 10 Point Scale	300+	69%	73%	71%
Meds 'Always' Explained Before Given	300+	60%	66%	64%
Nurses 'Always' Communicated Well	300+	75%	80%	79%
Pain 'Always' Well Controlled	300+	68%	72%	71%
Room and Bathroom 'Always' Clean	300+	71%	75%	73%
Timely Help 'Always' Received	300+	57%	69%	68%

NOTE: Hospital profiles are in alphabetical order by state, then city, then hospital within the city; Rankings exclude hospitals with less than 25 cases except for patient surveys which excludes hospitals with less than 100 cases; (a) 100-299 cases; (1) The number of cases/patients is too few to report; (2) Data submitted were based on a sample of cases/patients; (3) Results are based on a shorter time period than required; (4) Data suppressed by CMS for one or more quarters; (5) Results are not available for this reporting period; (6) Fewer than 100 patients completed the HCAHPS survey; (7) No cases met the criteria for this measure; (8) The lower limit of the confidence interval cannot be calculated if the number of observed infections equals zero; (9) No data are available from the state/territory for this reporting period; (10) The scores shown reflect fewer than 50 completed surveys; (11) There were discrepancies in the data collection process; (12) This measure does not apply to this hospital for this reporting period; (13) Results cannot be calculated for this reporting period; (14) The results for this state are combined with nearby states to protect confidentiality; Please refer to the User's Guide for a full explanation of data.

Would Definitely Recommend Hospital	300+	70%	73%	71%
Use of Medical Imaging				
Cardiac Imaging Stress Test before Surgery[1]	-	-	5.3%	5.3%
Combination Abdominal CT Scan	693	17.3%	16.4%	10.5%
Combination Brain/Sinus CT Scan	578	6.1%	2.7%	2.7%
Combination Chest CT Scan	434	7.4%	5.6%	2.7%
Follow-up Mammogram/Ultrasound	584	11.0%	7.9%	8.8%
Lumbar Spine MRI for Low Back Pain	54	31.5%	39.6%	37.2%

Texas Health Center for Diagnostics & Surgery

6020 W Parker Road Phone: 972-403-2700
Plano, TX 75093 Fax: 972-403-2852
URL: www.ppcds.com
Type: Acute Care Hospitals Emergency Services: Yes
Ownership: Proprietary
Key Personnel:
Operating Room. . . . . Tracey Kennedy
Anesthesiology. . . . . Sharon Martin
Imaging . . . . Mark Mendes
Chief of Medical Staff. . . . . Sarah Pinkerman
CEO/President. . . . . Larry Robertson

Measure	Cases	This Hosp.	State Avg.	U.S. Avg.
Blood Clot Prevention and Treatment				
Anticoagulation Overlap Therapy[7]	-	-	93%	93%
ICU Venous Thromboembolism Prophylaxis[7]	-	-	92%	92%
Incidence of Potentially Preventable VTE[7]	-	-	9%	10%
UFH with Dosages/Platelet Monitoring[7]	-	-	96%	97%
Venous Thromboembolism Prophylaxis	306	100%	82%	85%
Warfarin Therapy Discharge Instructions[7]	-	-	84%	75%
Chest Pain/Possible Heart Attack Care				
Aspirin Given Within 24 Hours of Arrival[5]	-	-	94%	96%
Fibrinolytic Meds Within 30 Min. of Arrival[5]	-	-	47%	58%
Average Time to ECG (minutes)[5]	-	-	8	7
Average Time to Transfer (minutes)[5]	-	-	62	60
Children's Asthma Care				
Received Home Management Plan of Care	-	-	93%	88%
Received Reliever Medication	-	-	100%	100%
Received Systemic Corticosteroids	-	-	100%	100%
Emergency Department				
Admittance Decision Time (minutes)[7]	-	-	99	98
Head CT Results Within 45 Min. of Arrival[5]	-	-	54%	57%
Patients Who Left ER Before Being Seen	92	13%	3%	2%
Time from ER Arrival to Admit. (minutes)[7]	-	-	270	274
Time from ER Arrival to Discharge (minutes)	85	122	127	134
Time in ER Before Being Evaluated (minutes)	108	20	26	26
Time to Pain Meds for Fractures (minutes)[1,3]	-	-	57	57
Heart Attack Care				
Aspirin Given at Discharge[5]	-	-	99%	99%
Fibrinolytic Meds Within 30 Min. of Arrival[5]	-	-	49%	54%
PCI Within 90 Minutes of Arrival[5]	-	-	95%	96%
Statin Prescribed at Discharge[5]	-	-	98%	98%
Heart Failure Care				
ACE Inhibitor or ARB for LVSD[5]	-	-	97%	97%
Discharge Instructions Given[5]	-	-	95%	94%
Evaluation of LVS Function[5]	-	-	99%	99%
Medicare Spending				
Medicare Spending per Patient (ratio)	-	0.93	1.03	0.98
Pneumonia Care				
Appropriate Initial Antibiotic Given[5]	-	-	95%	95%
Blood Culture Timing[5]	-	-	98%	98%
Pregnancy and Delivery Care				
Newborn Deliveries Scheduled Early[7]	-	-	7%	6%
Preventive Care				
Immunization for Influenza	311	92%	90%	90%
Immunization for Pneumonia	191	95%	92%	92%
Stroke Care				
Anticoagulation Therapy for Atrial Fibrillation[5]	-	-	96%	95%
Antithrombotic Therapy Timing[5]	-	-	98%	98%
Assessed for Rehabilitation[5]	-	-	98%	97%
Discharged on Antithrombotic Therapy[5]	-	-	99%	99%
Discharged on Statin Medication[5]	-	-	95%	94%
Thrombolytic Therapy Timing[5]	-	-	68%	66%
Venous Thromboembolism Prophylaxis[5]	-	-	94%	94%
Written Stroke Educational Materials Given[5]	-	-	92%	88%
Surgical Care Improvement Project				
Appropriate Beta Blocker Usage[1]	-	-	98%	98%
Appropriate VTP Within 24 Hours	60	100%	98%	98%
Controlled Postoperative Blood Glucose[7]	-	-	96%	97%
Perioperative Temperature Management	61	100%	100%	100%
Prophylactic Antibiotic Selection	51	96%	99%	99%
Prophylactic Antibiotic Selection (Outpatient)	436	99%	98%	98%
Prophylactic Antibiotic Stopped	49	96%	98%	98%
Prophylactic Antibiotic Timing	51	98%	99%	99%
Prophylactic Antibiotic Timing (Outpatient)	436	100%	98%	98%
Urinary Catheter Removal[7]	-	-	98%	97%
Survey of Patients' Hospital Experiences				
Area Around Room 'Always' Quiet at Night	(a)	84%	68%	61%
Doctors 'Always' Communicated Well	(a)	85%	83%	82%
Home Recovery Information Given	(a)	91%	85%	85%
Hospital Given 9 or 10 on 10 Point Scale	(a)	89%	73%	71%
Meds 'Always' Explained Before Given	(a)	73%	66%	64%
Nurses 'Always' Communicated Well	(a)	89%	80%	79%
Pain 'Always' Well Controlled	(a)	76%	72%	71%
Room and Bathroom 'Always' Clean	(a)	85%	75%	73%
Timely Help 'Always' Received	(a)	86%	69%	68%
Would Definitely Recommend Hospital	(a)	90%	73%	71%
Use of Medical Imaging				
Cardiac Imaging Stress Test before Surgery[7]	-	-	5.3%	5.3%
Combination Abdominal CT Scan	75	54.7%	16.4%	10.5%
Combination Brain/Sinus CT Scan[1]	-	-	2.7%	2.7%
Combination Chest CT Scan[1]	-	-	5.6%	2.7%
Follow-up Mammogram/Ultrasound[7]	-	-	7.9%	8.8%
Lumbar Spine MRI for Low Back Pain	179	34.6%	39.6%	37.2%

Texas Health Presbyterian Hospital Plano

6200 W Parker Rd Phone: 972-981-8000
Plano, TX 75093 Fax: 972-981-3010
URL: www.presbyplano.org
Type: Acute Care Hospitals Emergency Services: No
Ownership: Voluntary non-profit - Private Beds: 370
Key Personnel:
CEO/President. . . . . Mike Evans, RN, MS
Chief of Medical Staff. . . . . Stephen K. Hadzima, MD

Measure	Cases	This Hosp.	State Avg.	U.S. Avg.
Blood Clot Prevention and Treatment				
Anticoagulation Overlap Therapy[2]	101	86%	93%	93%
ICU Venous Thromboembolism Prophylaxis[2]	109	100%	92%	92%
Incidence of Potentially Preventable VTE[1,2]	-	-	9%	10%
UFH with Dosages/Platelet Monitoring[2]	32	100%	96%	97%
Venous Thromboembolism Prophylaxis[2]	283	86%	82%	85%
Warfarin Therapy Discharge Instructions[2]	80	68%	84%	75%
Chest Pain/Possible Heart Attack Care				
Aspirin Given Within 24 Hours of Arrival[1,3]	-	-	94%	96%
Fibrinolytic Meds Within 30 Min. of Arrival[3,7]	-	-	47%	58%
Average Time to ECG (minutes)[1,3]	-	-	8	7
Average Time to Transfer (minutes)[3,7]	-	-	62	60
Children's Asthma Care				
Received Home Management Plan of Care	-	-	93%	88%
Received Reliever Medication	-	-	100%	100%
Received Systemic Corticosteroids	-	-	100%	100%
Emergency Department				
Admittance Decision Time (minutes)[2]	274	92	99	98
Head CT Results Within 45 Min. of Arrival[1]	-	-	54%	57%
Patients Who Left ER Before Being Seen	45,716	2%	3%	2%
Time from ER Arrival to Admit. (minutes)[2]	275	260	270	274
Time from ER Arrival to Discharge (minutes)	399	156	127	134
Time in ER Before Being Evaluated (minutes)	440	24	26	26
Time to Pain Meds for Fractures (minutes)	165	62	57	57
Heart Attack Care				
Aspirin Given at Discharge	179	99%	99%	99%
Fibrinolytic Meds Within 30 Min. of Arrival[7]	-	-	49%	54%
PCI Within 90 Minutes of Arrival	32	94%	95%	96%
Statin Prescribed at Discharge	174	100%	98%	98%
Heart Failure Care				
ACE Inhibitor or ARB for LVSD	56	100%	97%	97%
Discharge Instructions Given	161	94%	95%	94%
Evaluation of LVS Function	195	100%	99%	99%
Medicare Spending				
Medicare Spending per Patient (ratio)	-	1.07	1.03	0.98
Pneumonia Care				
Appropriate Initial Antibiotic Given	151	98%	95%	95%
Blood Culture Timing	247	98%	98%	98%
Pregnancy and Delivery Care				
Newborn Deliveries Scheduled Early	369	18%	7%	6%
Preventive Care				
Immunization for Influenza[2]	537	93%	90%	90%
Immunization for Pneumonia[2]	480	92%	92%	92%
Stroke Care				
Anticoagulation Therapy for Atrial Fibrillation[2]	11	100%	96%	95%
Antithrombotic Therapy Timing[2]	80	100%	98%	98%
Assessed for Rehabilitation[2]	94	100%	98%	97%
Discharged on Antithrombotic Therapy[2]	89	100%	99%	99%
Discharged on Statin Medication[2]	63	100%	95%	94%
Thrombolytic Therapy Timing[1,2]	-	-	68%	66%
Venous Thromboembolism Prophylaxis[2]	84	98%	94%	94%
Written Stroke Educational Materials Given[2]	52	100%	92%	88%
Surgical Care Improvement Project				
Appropriate Beta Blocker Usage[2]	457	99%	98%	98%
Appropriate VTP Within 24 Hours[2]	1,643	100%	98%	98%
Controlled Postoperative Blood Glucose[2]	92	91%	96%	97%
Perioperative Temperature Management[2]	1,912	100%	100%	100%
Prophylactic Antibiotic Selection[2]	1,503	99%	99%	99%
Prophylactic Antibiotic Selection (Outpatient)	338	89%	98%	98%
Prophylactic Antibiotic Stopped[2]	1,494	100%	98%	98%
Prophylactic Antibiotic Timing[2]	1,506	98%	99%	99%
Prophylactic Antibiotic Timing (Outpatient)	349	93%	98%	98%
Urinary Catheter Removal[2]	1,426	100%	98%	97%
Survey of Patients' Hospital Experiences				
Area Around Room 'Always' Quiet at Night	300+	70%	68%	61%
Doctors 'Always' Communicated Well	300+	82%	83%	82%
Home Recovery Information Given	300+	87%	85%	85%
Hospital Given 9 or 10 on 10 Point Scale	300+	81%	73%	71%
Meds 'Always' Explained Before Given	300+	66%	66%	64%
Nurses 'Always' Communicated Well	300+	81%	80%	79%
Pain 'Always' Well Controlled	300+	75%	72%	71%
Room and Bathroom 'Always' Clean	300+	79%	75%	73%
Timely Help 'Always' Received	300+	67%	69%	68%
Would Definitely Recommend Hospital	300+	84%	73%	71%
Use of Medical Imaging				
Cardiac Imaging Stress Test before Surgery	74	4.1%	5.3%	5.3%
Combination Abdominal CT Scan	542	10.7%	16.4%	10.5%
Combination Brain/Sinus CT Scan	643	3.0%	2.7%	2.7%
Combination Chest CT Scan	247	8.5%	5.6%	2.7%
Follow-up Mammogram/Ultrasound	994	5.4%	7.9%	8.8%
Lumbar Spine MRI for Low Back Pain[1]	-	-	39.6%	37.2%

The Medical Center of Southeast Texas

2555 Jimmy Johnson Blvd Phone: 409-853-5900
Port Arthur, TX 77640 Fax: 409-853-5182
URL: www.medicalcentertexas.com
Type: Acute Care Hospitals Emergency Services: Yes
Ownership: Proprietary Beds: 224
Key Personnel:
CEO/President. . . . . Craig Desmond

Measure	Cases	This Hosp.	State Avg.	U.S. Avg.
Blood Clot Prevention and Treatment				
Anticoagulation Overlap Therapy[2]	59	80%	93%	93%
ICU Venous Thromboembolism Prophylaxis[2]	127	75%	92%	92%
Incidence of Potentially Preventable VTE[1,2]	-	-	9%	10%
UFH with Dosages/Platelet Monitoring[1,2]	-	-	96%	97%
Venous Thromboembolism Prophylaxis[2]	325	55%	82%	85%
Warfarin Therapy Discharge Instructions[2]	42	95%	84%	75%
Chest Pain/Possible Heart Attack Care				
Aspirin Given Within 24 Hours of Arrival[1,3]	-	-	94%	96%
Fibrinolytic Meds Within 30 Min. of Arrival[5]	-	-	47%	58%
Average Time to ECG (minutes)[1,3]	-	-	8	7
Average Time to Transfer (minutes)[5]	-	-	62	60
Children's Asthma Care				
Received Home Management Plan of Care	-	-	93%	88%
Received Reliever Medication	-	-	100%	100%

NOTE: Hospital profiles are in alphabetical order by state, then city, then hospital within the city; Rankings exclude hospitals with less than 25 cases except for patient surveys which excludes hospitals with less than 100 cases; (a) 100-299 cases; (1) The number of cases/patients is too few to report; (2) Data submitted were based on a sample of cases/patients; (3) Results are based on a shorter time period than required; (4) Data suppressed by CMS for one or more quarters; (5) Results are not available for this reporting period; (6) Fewer than 100 patients completed the HCAHPS survey; (7) No cases met the criteria for this measure; (8) The lower limit of the confidence interval cannot be calculated if the number of observed infections equals zero; (9) No data are available from the state/territory for this reporting period; (10) The scores shown reflect fewer than 50 completed surveys; (11) There were discrepancies in the data collection process; (12) This measure does not apply to this hospital for this reporting period; (13) Results cannot be calculated for this reporting period; (14) The results for this state are combined with nearby states to protect confidentiality; Please refer to the User's Guide for a full explanation of data.

Measure	Cases	This Hosp.	State Avg.	U.S. Avg.
Received Systemic Corticosteroids	-	-	100%	100%
Emergency Department				
Admittance Decision Time (minutes)[2]	704	119	99	98
Head CT Results Within 45 Min. of Arrival	15	60%	54%	57%
Patients Who Left ER Before Being Seen	32,006	3%	3%	2%
Time from ER Arrival to Admit. (minutes)[2]	718	354	270	274
Time from ER Arrival to Discharge (minutes)	713	193	127	134
Time in ER Before Being Evaluated (minutes)	743	64	26	26
Time to Pain Meds for Fractures (minutes)	90	88	57	57
Heart Attack Care				
Aspirin Given at Discharge	83	99%	99%	99%
Fibrinolytic Meds Within 30 Min. of Arrival[7]	-	-	49%	54%
PCI Within 90 Minutes of Arrival	14	100%	95%	96%
Statin Prescribed at Discharge	81	99%	98%	98%
Heart Failure Care				
ACE Inhibitor or ARB for LVSD	81	98%	97%	97%
Discharge Instructions Given	236	80%	95%	94%
Evaluation of LVS Function	284	100%	99%	99%
Medicare Spending				
Medicare Spending per Patient (ratio)	-	1.11	1.03	0.98
Pneumonia Care				
Appropriate Initial Antibiotic Given	117	91%	95%	95%
Blood Culture Timing	173	99%	98%	98%
Pregnancy and Delivery Care				
Newborn Deliveries Scheduled Early[2]	48	19%	7%	6%
Preventive Care				
Immunization for Influenza[2]	688	90%	90%	90%
Immunization for Pneumonia[2]	816	92%	92%	92%
Stroke Care				
Anticoagulation Therapy for Atrial Fibrillation	12	92%	96%	95%
Antithrombotic Therapy Timing	78	94%	98%	98%
Assessed for Rehabilitation	81	91%	98%	97%
Discharged on Antithrombotic Therapy	78	96%	99%	99%
Discharged on Statin Medication	61	74%	95%	94%
Thrombolytic Therapy Timing[1]	-	-	68%	66%
Venous Thromboembolism Prophylaxis	84	68%	94%	94%
Written Stroke Educational Materials Given	44	70%	92%	88%
Surgical Care Improvement Project				
Appropriate Beta Blocker Usage	156	96%	98%	98%
Appropriate VTP Within 24 Hours	390	99%	98%	98%
Controlled Postoperative Blood Glucose	67	96%	96%	97%
Perioperative Temperature Management	424	100%	100%	100%
Prophylactic Antibiotic Selection	350	99%	99%	99%
Prophylactic Antibiotic Selection (Outpatient)	145	92%	98%	98%
Prophylactic Antibiotic Stopped	325	97%	98%	98%
Prophylactic Antibiotic Timing	353	100%	99%	99%
Prophylactic Antibiotic Timing (Outpatient)	157	91%	98%	98%
Urinary Catheter Removal	302	99%	98%	97%
Survey of Patients' Hospital Experiences				
Area Around Room 'Always' Quiet at Night	300+	74%	68%	61%
Doctors 'Always' Communicated Well	300+	81%	83%	82%
Home Recovery Information Given	300+	85%	85%	85%
Hospital Given 9 or 10 on 10 Point Scale	300+	68%	73%	71%
Meds 'Always' Explained Before Given	300+	61%	66%	64%
Nurses 'Always' Communicated Well	300+	75%	80%	79%
Pain 'Always' Well Controlled	300+	67%	72%	71%
Room and Bathroom 'Always' Clean	300+	64%	75%	73%
Timely Help 'Always' Received	300+	61%	69%	68%
Would Definitely Recommend Hospital	300+	69%	73%	71%
Use of Medical Imaging				
Cardiac Imaging Stress Test before Surgery[1]	-	-	5.3%	5.3%
Combination Abdominal CT Scan	446	31.2%	16.4%	10.5%
Combination Brain/Sinus CT Scan	600	2.7%	2.7%	2.7%
Combination Chest CT Scan	163	35.6%	5.6%	2.7%
Follow-up Mammogram/Ultrasound	421	5.7%	7.9%	8.8%
Lumbar Spine MRI for Low Back Pain	61	29.5%	39.6%	37.2%

Memorial Medical Center

815 N Virginia Street Phone: 361-552-6713
Port Lavaca, TX 77979 Fax: 361-552-0312
URL: www.mmcportlavaca.com
Type: Critical Access Hospitals Emergency Services: Yes
Ownership: Government - Local Beds: 25

Key Personnel:
Coronary Care.............. Danette Bethany
Intensive Care Unit........... Danette Bethany
Quality Assurance .... Erincca Clevenger
Infection Control.............. Nadine Garner
Chief of Medical Staff.......... Jeannine Griffin, MD
CEO .... Daryn J. Kumar
Operating Room.............. Sandy Ruddick
Radiology.................. Debra Trammell

Measure	Cases	This Hosp.	State Avg.	U.S. Avg.
Blood Clot Prevention and Treatment				
Anticoagulation Overlap Therapy[5]	-	-	93%	93%
ICU Venous Thromboembolism Prophylaxis[5]	-	-	92%	92%
Incidence of Potentially Preventable VTE[5]	-	-	9%	10%
UFH with Dosages/Platelet Monitoring[5]	-	-	96%	97%
Venous Thromboembolism Prophylaxis[5]	-	-	82%	85%
Warfarin Therapy Discharge Instructions[5]	-	-	84%	75%
Chest Pain/Possible Heart Attack Care				
Aspirin Given Within 24 Hours of Arrival[1,3]	-	-	94%	96%
Fibrinolytic Meds Within 30 Min. of Arrival[5]	-	-	47%	58%
Average Time to ECG (minutes)[1,3]	-	-	8	7
Average Time to Transfer (minutes)[5]	-	-	62	60
Children's Asthma Care				
Received Home Management Plan of Care	-	-	93%	88%
Received Reliever Medication	-	-	100%	100%
Received Systemic Corticosteroids	-	-	100%	100%
Emergency Department				
Admittance Decision Time (minutes)[5]	-	-	99	98
Head CT Results Within 45 Min. of Arrival[1]	-	-	54%	57%
Patients Who Left ER Before Being Seen	38,604	1%	3%	2%
Time from ER Arrival to Admit. (minutes)[5]	-	-	270	274
Time from ER Arrival to Discharge (minutes)[5]	-	-	127	134
Time in ER Before Being Evaluated (minutes)[5]	-	-	26	26
Time to Pain Meds for Fractures (minutes)[3]	25	33	57	57
Heart Attack Care				
Aspirin Given at Discharge[3,7]	-	-	99%	99%
Fibrinolytic Meds Within 30 Min. of Arrival[3,7]	-	-	49%	54%
PCI Within 90 Minutes of Arrival[3,7]	-	-	95%	96%
Statin Prescribed at Discharge[3,7]	-	-	98%	98%
Heart Failure Care				
ACE Inhibitor or ARB for LVSD[1]	-	-	97%	97%
Discharge Instructions Given	26	100%	95%	94%
Evaluation of LVS Function	31	100%	99%	99%
Medicare Spending				
Medicare Spending per Patient (ratio)	-	-	1.03	0.98
Pneumonia Care				
Appropriate Initial Antibiotic Given	58	97%	95%	95%
Blood Culture Timing	50	100%	98%	98%
Pregnancy and Delivery Care				
Newborn Deliveries Scheduled Early[5]	-	-	7%	6%
Preventive Care				
Immunization for Influenza[5]	-	-	90%	90%
Immunization for Pneumonia[5]	-	-	92%	92%
Stroke Care				
Anticoagulation Therapy for Atrial Fibrillation[5]	-	-	96%	95%
Antithrombotic Therapy Timing[5]	-	-	98%	98%
Assessed for Rehabilitation[5]	-	-	98%	97%
Discharged on Antithrombotic Therapy[5]	-	-	99%	99%
Discharged on Statin Medication[5]	-	-	95%	94%
Thrombolytic Therapy Timing[5]	-	-	68%	66%
Venous Thromboembolism Prophylaxis[5]	-	-	94%	94%
Written Stroke Educational Materials Given[5]	-	-	92%	88%
Surgical Care Improvement Project				
Appropriate Beta Blocker Usage[7]	-	-	98%	98%
Appropriate VTP Within 24 Hours	20	100%	98%	98%
Controlled Postoperative Blood Glucose[7]	-	-	96%	97%
Perioperative Temperature Management	21	100%	100%	100%
Prophylactic Antibiotic Selection[1]	-	-	99%	99%
Prophylactic Antibiotic Selection (Outpatient)[5]	-	-	98%	98%
Prophylactic Antibiotic Stopped[1]	-	-	98%	98%
Prophylactic Antibiotic Timing[1]	-	-	99%	99%
Prophylactic Antibiotic Timing (Outpatient)[5]	-	-	98%	98%
Urinary Catheter Removal[1]	-	-	98%	97%
Survey of Patients' Hospital Experiences				
Area Around Room 'Always' Quiet at Night	(a)	67%	68%	61%
Doctors 'Always' Communicated Well	(a)	88%	83%	82%
Home Recovery Information Given	(a)	89%	85%	85%
Hospital Given 9 or 10 on 10 Point Scale	(a)	63%	73%	71%
Meds 'Always' Explained Before Given	(a)	70%	66%	64%
Nurses 'Always' Communicated Well	(a)	82%	80%	79%
Pain 'Always' Well Controlled	(a)	69%	72%	71%
Room and Bathroom 'Always' Clean	(a)	80%	75%	73%
Timely Help 'Always' Received	(a)	71%	69%	68%
Would Definitely Recommend Hospital	(a)	74%	73%	71%
Use of Medical Imaging				
Cardiac Imaging Stress Test before Surgery[1]	-	-	5.3%	5.3%
Combination Abdominal CT Scan	199	46.2%	16.4%	10.5%
Combination Brain/Sinus CT Scan[1]	-	-	2.7%	2.7%
Combination Chest CT Scan	99	57.6%	5.6%	2.7%
Follow-up Mammogram/Ultrasound	292	7.5%	7.9%	8.8%
Lumbar Spine MRI for Low Back Pain	72	56.9%	39.6%	37.2%

East Texas Medical Center Quitman

117 Winnsboro Street Phone: 903-763-4500
Quitman, TX 75783
Type: Critical Access Hospitals Emergency Services: Yes
Ownership: Voluntary non-profit - Private

Measure	Cases	This Hosp.	State Avg.	U.S. Avg.
Blood Clot Prevention and Treatment				
Anticoagulation Overlap Therapy[1,2]	-	-	93%	93%
ICU Venous Thromboembolism Prophylaxis[2,7]	-	-	92%	92%
Incidence of Potentially Preventable VTE[2,7]	-	-	9%	10%
UFH with Dosages/Platelet Monitoring[2,7]	-	-	96%	97%
Venous Thromboembolism Prophylaxis[2]	124	28%	82%	85%
Warfarin Therapy Discharge Instructions[1,2]	-	-	84%	75%
Chest Pain/Possible Heart Attack Care				
Aspirin Given Within 24 Hours of Arrival	52	92%	94%	96%
Fibrinolytic Meds Within 30 Min. of Arrival[1]	-	-	47%	58%
Average Time to ECG (minutes)	54	2	8	7
Average Time to Transfer (minutes)[1]	-	-	62	60
Children's Asthma Care				
Received Home Management Plan of Care	-	-	93%	88%
Received Reliever Medication	-	-	100%	100%
Received Systemic Corticosteroids	-	-	100%	100%
Emergency Department				
Admittance Decision Time (minutes)[2]	231	74	99	98
Head CT Results Within 45 Min. of Arrival[1]	-	-	54%	57%
Patients Who Left ER Before Being Seen	9,219	1%	3%	2%
Time from ER Arrival to Admit. (minutes)[2]	332	226	270	274
Time from ER Arrival to Discharge (minutes)	347	141	127	134
Time in ER Before Being Evaluated (minutes)	376	14	26	26
Time to Pain Meds for Fractures (minutes)	65	63	57	57
Heart Attack Care				
Aspirin Given at Discharge[1,3]	-	-	99%	99%
Fibrinolytic Meds Within 30 Min. of Arrival[3,7]	-	-	49%	54%
PCI Within 90 Minutes of Arrival[3,7]	-	-	95%	96%
Statin Prescribed at Discharge[1,3]	-	-	98%	98%
Heart Failure Care				
ACE Inhibitor or ARB for LVSD[1,2]	-	-	97%	97%
Discharge Instructions Given[2]	28	79%	95%	94%
Evaluation of LVS Function[2]	39	82%	99%	99%
Medicare Spending				
Medicare Spending per Patient (ratio)	-	-	1.03	0.98
Pneumonia Care				
Appropriate Initial Antibiotic Given	42	90%	95%	95%
Blood Culture Timing	32	91%	98%	98%
Pregnancy and Delivery Care				
Newborn Deliveries Scheduled Early[7]	-	-	7%	6%
Preventive Care				
Immunization for Influenza[2]	292	87%	90%	90%

NOTE: Hospital profiles are in alphabetical order by state, then city, then hospital within the city; Rankings exclude hospitals with less than 25 cases except for patient surveys which excludes hospitals with less than 100 cases; (a) 100-299 cases; (1) The number of cases/patients is too few to report; (2) Data submitted were based on a sample of cases/patients; (3) Results are based on a shorter time period than required; (4) Data suppressed by CMS for one or more quarters; (5) Results are not available for this reporting period; (6) Fewer than 100 patients completed the HCAHPS survey; (7) No cases met the criteria for this measure; (8) The lower limit of the confidence interval cannot be calculated if the number of observed infections equals zero; (9) No data are available from the state/territory for this reporting period; (10) The scores shown reflect fewer than 50 completed surveys; (11) There were discrepancies in the data collection process; (12) This measure does not apply to this hospital for this reporting period; (13) Results cannot be calculated for this reporting period; (14) The results for this state are combined with nearby states to protect confidentiality; Please refer to the User's Guide for a full explanation of data.

Measure	Cases	This Hosp.	State Avg.	U.S. Avg.
Immunization for Pneumonia[2]	411	91%	92%	92%
Stroke Care				
Anticoagulation Therapy for Atrial Fibrillation[1,3]	-	-	96%	95%
Antithrombotic Therapy Timing[1,3]	-	-	98%	98%
Assessed for Rehabilitation[1,3]	-	-	98%	97%
Discharged on Antithrombotic Therapy[1,3]	-	-	99%	99%
Discharged on Statin Medication[1,3]	-	-	95%	94%
Thrombolytic Therapy Timing[1,3]	-	-	68%	66%
Venous Thromboembolism Prophylaxis[1,3]	-	-	94%	94%
Written Stroke Educational Materials Given[1,3]	-	-	92%	88%
Surgical Care Improvement Project				
Appropriate Beta Blocker Usage[5]	-	-	98%	98%
Appropriate VTP Within 24 Hours[5]	-	-	98%	98%
Controlled Postoperative Blood Glucose[5]	-	-	96%	97%
Perioperative Temperature Management[5]	-	-	100%	100%
Prophylactic Antibiotic Selection[5]	-	-	99%	99%
Prophylactic Antibiotic Selection (Outpatient)[5]	-	-	98%	98%
Prophylactic Antibiotic Stopped[5]	-	-	98%	98%
Prophylactic Antibiotic Timing[5]	-	-	99%	99%
Prophylactic Antibiotic Timing (Outpatient)[5]	-	-	98%	98%
Urinary Catheter Removal[5]	-	-	98%	97%
Survey of Patients' Hospital Experiences				
Area Around Room 'Always' Quiet at Night	(a)	66%	68%	61%
Doctors 'Always' Communicated Well	(a)	91%	83%	82%
Home Recovery Information Given	(a)	91%	85%	85%
Hospital Given 9 or 10 on 10 Point Scale	(a)	79%	73%	71%
Meds 'Always' Explained Before Given	(a)	72%	66%	64%
Nurses 'Always' Communicated Well	(a)	86%	80%	79%
Pain 'Always' Well Controlled	(a)	79%	72%	71%
Room and Bathroom 'Always' Clean	(a)	82%	75%	73%
Timely Help 'Always' Received	(a)	72%	69%	68%
Would Definitely Recommend Hospital	(a)	78%	73%	71%
Use of Medical Imaging				
Cardiac Imaging Stress Test before Surgery[1]	-	-	5.3%	5.3%
Combination Abdominal CT Scan	200	6.0%	16.4%	10.5%
Combination Brain/Sinus CT Scan[1]	-	-	2.7%	2.7%
Combination Chest CT Scan	86	1.2%	5.6%	2.7%
Follow-up Mammogram/Ultrasound	222	5.0%	7.9%	8.8%
Lumbar Spine MRI for Low Back Pain[7]	-		39.6%	37.2%

Methodist Richardson Medical Center

401 W Campbell Rd
Richardson, TX 75080
Phone: 972-498-4000
Fax: 972-498-7660
E-mail: webmaster@richardsonhealth.com
URL: www.richardsonregional.com
Type: Acute Care Hospitals
Emergency Services: Yes
Ownership: Govt - Hospital Dist/Auth
Beds: 205

Key Personnel:

Radiology. . . . . John Aryan
Cardiac Laboratory. . . . . Ian Chenevert
Chief of Medical Staff. . . . . Steve Hebert, MD
President/CEO. . . . . Stephen L. Mansfield, PhD, FACHE
Coronary Care . . . . Dawn Parten
Quality Assurance . . . . Wm Pattie Sproles
Operating Room. . . . . Nancy Underwood
Infection Control. . . . . Nancy Viamonte

Measure	Cases	This Hosp.	State Avg.	U.S. Avg.
Blood Clot Prevention and Treatment				
Anticoagulation Overlap Therapy[2]	35	100%	93%	93%
ICU Venous Thromboembolism Prophylaxis[2]	66	100%	92%	92%
Incidence of Potentially Preventable VTE[1,2]	-	-	9%	10%
UFH with Dosages/Platelet Monitoring[2]	13	100%	96%	97%
Venous Thromboembolism Prophylaxis[2]	341	93%	82%	85%
Warfarin Therapy Discharge Instructions[2]	26	96%	84%	75%
Chest Pain/Possible Heart Attack Care				
Aspirin Given Within 24 Hours of Arrival[5]	-	-	94%	96%
Fibrinolytic Meds Within 30 Min. of Arrival[5]	-	-	47%	58%
Average Time to ECG (minutes)[5]	-	-	8	7
Average Time to Transfer (minutes)[5]	-	-	62	60
Children's Asthma Care				
Received Home Management Plan of Care	-	-	93%	88%
Received Reliever Medication	-	-	100%	100%
Received Systemic Corticosteroids	-	-	100%	100%
Emergency Department				
Admittance Decision Time (minutes)[2]	522	100	99	98
Head CT Results Within 45 Min. of Arrival[1,3]	-	-	54%	57%
Patients Who Left ER Before Being Seen	34,693	1%	3%	2%
Time from ER Arrival to Admit. (minutes)[2]	563	212	270	274
Time from ER Arrival to Discharge (minutes)	389	122	127	134
Time in ER Before Being Evaluated (minutes)	409	14	26	26
Time to Pain Meds for Fractures (minutes)	123	38	57	57
Heart Attack Care				
Aspirin Given at Discharge	117	100%	99%	99%
Fibrinolytic Meds Within 30 Min. of Arrival[7]	-	-	49%	54%
PCI Within 90 Minutes of Arrival	20	100%	95%	96%
Statin Prescribed at Discharge	119	99%	98%	98%
Heart Failure Care				
ACE Inhibitor or ARB for LVSD	38	100%	97%	97%
Discharge Instructions Given	88	100%	95%	94%
Evaluation of LVS Function	114	100%	99%	99%
Medicare Spending				
Medicare Spending per Patient (ratio)	-	1.19	1.03	0.98
Pneumonia Care				
Appropriate Initial Antibiotic Given[2]	80	100%	95%	95%
Blood Culture Timing[2]	130	100%	98%	98%
Pregnancy and Delivery Care				
Newborn Deliveries Scheduled Early	34	15%	7%	6%
Preventive Care				
Immunization for Influenza[2]	452	97%	90%	90%
Immunization for Pneumonia[2]	562	98%	92%	92%
Stroke Care				
Anticoagulation Therapy for Atrial Fibrillation[1]	-	-	96%	95%
Antithrombotic Therapy Timing	37	100%	98%	98%
Assessed for Rehabilitation	53	100%	98%	97%
Discharged on Antithrombotic Therapy	45	100%	99%	99%
Discharged on Statin Medication	41	100%	95%	94%
Thrombolytic Therapy Timing[1]	-	-	68%	66%
Venous Thromboembolism Prophylaxis	44	100%	94%	94%
Written Stroke Educational Materials Given	27	100%	92%	88%
Surgical Care Improvement Project				
Appropriate Beta Blocker Usage[2]	80	100%	98%	98%
Appropriate VTP Within 24 Hours[2]	255	100%	98%	98%
Controlled Postoperative Blood Glucose[2]	22	100%	96%	97%
Perioperative Temperature Management[2]	286	100%	100%	100%
Prophylactic Antibiotic Selection[2]	198	100%	99%	99%
Prophylactic Antibiotic Selection (Outpatient)	229	97%	98%	98%
Prophylactic Antibiotic Stopped[2]	196	98%	98%	98%
Prophylactic Antibiotic Timing[2]	198	99%	99%	99%
Prophylactic Antibiotic Timing (Outpatient)	232	98%	98%	98%
Urinary Catheter Removal[2]	166	100%	98%	97%
Survey of Patients' Hospital Experiences				
Area Around Room 'Always' Quiet at Night	300+	65%	68%	61%
Doctors 'Always' Communicated Well	300+	80%	83%	82%
Home Recovery Information Given	300+	83%	85%	85%
Hospital Given 9 or 10 on 10 Point Scale	300+	68%	73%	71%
Meds 'Always' Explained Before Given	300+	69%	66%	64%
Nurses 'Always' Communicated Well	300+	75%	80%	79%
Pain 'Always' Well Controlled	300+	72%	72%	71%
Room and Bathroom 'Always' Clean	300+	76%	75%	73%
Timely Help 'Always' Received	300+	65%	69%	68%
Would Definitely Recommend Hospital	300+	68%	73%	71%
Use of Medical Imaging				
Cardiac Imaging Stress Test before Surgery[1]	-	-	5.3%	5.3%
Combination Abdominal CT Scan	634	1.7%	16.4%	10.5%
Combination Brain/Sinus CT Scan[1]	-	-	2.7%	2.7%
Combination Chest CT Scan	478	1.3%	5.6%	2.7%
Follow-up Mammogram/Ultrasound	1,254	5.7%	7.9%	8.8%
Lumbar Spine MRI for Low Back Pain	62	45.2%	39.6%	37.2%

Oakbend Medical Center

1705 Jackson St
Richmond, TX 77469
Phone: 281-341-3000
Fax: 281-341-2883
URL: www.oakbendmedcenter.org
Type: Acute Care Hospitals
Emergency Services: Yes
Ownership: Govt - Hospital Dist/Auth
Beds: 185

Key Personnel:

CEO . . . . Joe Freudenberger
Administrator . . . . Sue McCarty
Hemotology Center . . . . Amirali S Popatia, MD/FACP
Chief of Medical Staff. . . . . Douglas Thibodeaux, MD

Measure	Cases	This Hosp.	State Avg.	U.S. Avg.
Blood Clot Prevention and Treatment				
Anticoagulation Overlap Therapy[2]	28	71%	93%	93%
ICU Venous Thromboembolism Prophylaxis[2]	92	92%	92%	92%
Incidence of Potentially Preventable VTE[1,2]	-	-	9%	10%
UFH with Dosages/Platelet Monitoring[1,2]	-	-	96%	97%
Venous Thromboembolism Prophylaxis[2]	294	74%	82%	85%
Warfarin Therapy Discharge Instructions[2]	16	69%	84%	75%
Chest Pain/Possible Heart Attack Care				
Aspirin Given Within 24 Hours of Arrival	32	97%	94%	96%
Fibrinolytic Meds Within 30 Min. of Arrival[7]	-	-	47%	58%
Average Time to ECG (minutes)	31	4	8	7
Average Time to Transfer (minutes)[1]	-	-	62	60
Children's Asthma Care				
Received Home Management Plan of Care	-	-	93%	88%
Received Reliever Medication	-	-	100%	100%
Received Systemic Corticosteroids	-	-	100%	100%
Emergency Department				
Admittance Decision Time (minutes)[2]	421	96	99	98
Head CT Results Within 45 Min. of Arrival[1]	-	-	54%	57%
Patients Who Left ER Before Being Seen	28,946	1%	3%	2%
Time from ER Arrival to Admit. (minutes)[2]	428	266	270	274
Time from ER Arrival to Discharge (minutes)	357	94	127	134
Time in ER Before Being Evaluated (minutes)	336	15	26	26
Time to Pain Meds for Fractures (minutes)	102	42	57	57
Heart Attack Care				
Aspirin Given at Discharge	76	93%	99%	99%
Fibrinolytic Meds Within 30 Min. of Arrival[7]	-	-	49%	54%
PCI Within 90 Minutes of Arrival	24	79%	95%	96%
Statin Prescribed at Discharge	76	97%	98%	98%
Heart Failure Care				
ACE Inhibitor or ARB for LVSD	33	91%	97%	97%
Discharge Instructions Given	85	82%	95%	94%
Evaluation of LVS Function	119	95%	99%	99%
Medicare Spending				
Medicare Spending per Patient (ratio)	-	1.17	1.03	0.98
Pneumonia Care				
Appropriate Initial Antibiotic Given	58	84%	95%	95%
Blood Culture Timing	145	98%	98%	98%
Pregnancy and Delivery Care				
Newborn Deliveries Scheduled Early	148	11%	7%	6%
Preventive Care				
Immunization for Influenza[2]	463	84%	90%	90%
Immunization for Pneumonia[2]	427	86%	92%	92%
Stroke Care				
Anticoagulation Therapy for Atrial Fibrillation[1,2]	-	-	96%	95%
Antithrombotic Therapy Timing[2]	46	100%	98%	98%
Assessed for Rehabilitation[2]	45	100%	98%	97%
Discharged on Antithrombotic Therapy[2]	44	100%	99%	99%
Discharged on Statin Medication[2]	33	97%	95%	94%
Thrombolytic Therapy Timing[1,2]	-	-	68%	66%
Venous Thromboembolism Prophylaxis[2]	48	98%	94%	94%
Written Stroke Educational Materials Given[2]	19	100%	92%	88%
Surgical Care Improvement Project				
Appropriate Beta Blocker Usage[2]	17	76%	98%	98%
Appropriate VTP Within 24 Hours[2]	128	89%	98%	98%
Controlled Postoperative Blood Glucose[2,7]	-	-	96%	97%
Perioperative Temperature Management[2]	153	100%	100%	100%
Prophylactic Antibiotic Selection[2]	89	97%	99%	99%
Prophylactic Antibiotic Selection (Outpatient)	11	100%	98%	98%
Prophylactic Antibiotic Stopped[2]	86	94%	98%	98%
Prophylactic Antibiotic Timing[2]	89	96%	99%	99%
Prophylactic Antibiotic Timing (Outpatient)	12	92%	98%	98%
Urinary Catheter Removal[2]	38	71%	98%	97%
Survey of Patients' Hospital Experiences				
Area Around Room 'Always' Quiet at Night	300+	61%	68%	61%
Doctors 'Always' Communicated Well	300+	80%	83%	82%
Home Recovery Information Given	300+	83%	85%	85%
Hospital Given 9 or 10 on 10 Point Scale	300+	68%	73%	71%

NOTE: Hospital profiles are in alphabetical order by state, then city, then hospital within the city; Rankings exclude hospitals with less than 25 cases except for patient surveys which excludes hospitals with less than 100 cases; (a) 100-299 cases; (1) The number of cases/patients is too few to report; (2) Data submitted were based on a sample of cases/patients; (3) Results are based on a shorter time period than required; (4) Data suppressed by CMS for one or more quarters; (5) Results are not available for this reporting period; (6) Fewer than 100 patients completed the HCAHPS survey; (7) No cases met the criteria for this measure; (8) The lower limit of the confidence interval cannot be calculated if the number of observed infections equals zero; (9) No data are available from the state/territory for this reporting period; (10) The scores shown reflect fewer than 50 completed surveys; (11) There were discrepancies in the data collection process; (12) This measure does not apply to this hospital for this reporting period; (13) Results cannot be calculated for this reporting period; (14) The results for this state are combined with nearby states to protect confidentiality; Please refer to the User's Guide for a full explanation of data.

Measure	Cases	This Hosp.	State Avg.	U.S. Avg.
Meds 'Always' Explained Before Given	300+	60%	66%	64%
Nurses 'Always' Communicated Well	300+	72%	80%	79%
Pain 'Always' Well Controlled	300+	69%	72%	71%
Room and Bathroom 'Always' Clean	300+	62%	75%	73%
Timely Help 'Always' Received	300+	63%	69%	68%
Would Definitely Recommend Hospital	300+	64%	73%	71%
Use of Medical Imaging				
Cardiac Imaging Stress Test before Surgery[1]	-	-	5.3%	5.3%
Combination Abdominal CT Scan	381	27.6%	16.4%	10.5%
Combination Brain/Sinus CT Scan	418	4.8%	2.7%	2.7%
Combination Chest CT Scan	178	0.0%	5.6%	2.7%
Follow-up Mammogram/Ultrasound	521	7.3%	7.9%	8.8%
Lumbar Spine MRI for Low Back Pain[1]	-	-	39.6%	37.2%

Starr County Memorial Hospital

128 N Fm Rd 3167
Rio Grande City, TX 78582
Phone: 956-487-5561
Fax: 956-487-0332
E-mail: contact@starrcountyhospital.com
URL: www.starrcountyhospital.com
Type: Acute Care Hospitals
Emergency Services: Yes
Ownership: Govt - Hospital Dist/Auth
Beds: 49

Key Personnel:
Quality Assurance . . . . Inez Hinojosa
Radiology. . . . . Juan L Lopez
CEO . . . . Thalia H Munoz
CEO/President. . . . . Thalia H Munoz
Chief of Medical Staff . . . . Porfirio Rodriguez, MD
Emergency Room . . . . Mario Segura, RN
Infection Control. . . . . Mario Segura, RN

Measure	Cases	This Hosp.	State Avg.	U.S. Avg.
Blood Clot Prevention and Treatment				
Anticoagulation Overlap Therapy[2,7]	-	-	93%	93%
ICU Venous Thromboembolism Prophylaxis[2]	84	63%	92%	92%
Incidence of Potentially Preventable VTE[2,7]	-	-	9%	10%
UFH with Dosages/Platelet Monitoring[2,7]	-	-	96%	97%
Venous Thromboembolism Prophylaxis[2]	131	50%	82%	85%
Warfarin Therapy Discharge Instructions[2,7]	-	-	84%	75%
Chest Pain/Possible Heart Attack Care				
Aspirin Given Within 24 Hours of Arrival	69	74%	94%	96%
Fibrinolytic Meds Within 30 Min. of Arrival[1]	-	-	47%	58%
Average Time to ECG (minutes)	78	23	8	7
Average Time to Transfer (minutes)[1]	-	-	62	60
Children's Asthma Care				
Received Home Management Plan of Care	-	-	93%	88%
Received Reliever Medication	-	-	100%	100%
Received Systemic Corticosteroids	-	-	100%	100%
Emergency Department				
Admittance Decision Time (minutes)[2]	431	62	99	98
Head CT Results Within 45 Min. of Arrival	27	15%	54%	57%
Patients Who Left ER Before Being Seen	11,761	15%	3%	2%
Time from ER Arrival to Admit. (minutes)[2]	542	384	270	274
Time from ER Arrival to Discharge (minutes)	393	280	127	134
Time in ER Before Being Evaluated (minutes)	602	26	26	26
Time to Pain Meds for Fractures (minutes)	60	75	57	57
Heart Attack Care				
Aspirin Given at Discharge	37	54%	99%	99%
Fibrinolytic Meds Within 30 Min. of Arrival[7]	-	-	49%	54%
PCI Within 90 Minutes of Arrival[7]	-	-	95%	96%
Statin Prescribed at Discharge	30	43%	98%	98%
Heart Failure Care				
ACE Inhibitor or ARB for LVSD[1]	-	-	97%	97%
Discharge Instructions Given	19	42%	95%	94%
Evaluation of LVS Function	22	50%	99%	99%
Medicare Spending				
Medicare Spending per Patient (ratio)	-	0.88	1.03	0.98
Pneumonia Care				
Appropriate Initial Antibiotic Given	103	89%	95%	95%
Blood Culture Timing	143	87%	98%	98%
Pregnancy and Delivery Care				
Newborn Deliveries Scheduled Early	21	33%	7%	6%
Preventive Care				
Immunization for Influenza[2]	432	75%	90%	90%
Immunization for Pneumonia[2]	525	83%	92%	92%
Stroke Care				
Anticoagulation Therapy for Atrial Fibrillation[1]	-	-	96%	95%
Antithrombotic Therapy Timing[1]	-	-	98%	98%
Assessed for Rehabilitation[1]	-	-	98%	97%
Discharged on Antithrombotic Therapy[1]	-	-	99%	99%
Discharged on Statin Medication[1]	-	-	95%	94%
Thrombolytic Therapy Timing[1]	-	-	68%	66%
Venous Thromboembolism Prophylaxis[1]	-	-	94%	94%
Written Stroke Educational Materials Given[1]	-	-	92%	88%
Surgical Care Improvement Project				
Appropriate Beta Blocker Usage[5]	-	-	98%	98%
Appropriate VTP Within 24 Hours[5]	-	-	98%	98%
Controlled Postoperative Blood Glucose[5]	-	-	96%	97%
Perioperative Temperature Management[5]	-	-	100%	100%
Prophylactic Antibiotic Selection[5]	-	-	99%	99%
Prophylactic Antibiotic Selection (Outpatient)[1,3]	-	-	98%	98%
Prophylactic Antibiotic Stopped[5]	-	-	98%	98%
Prophylactic Antibiotic Timing[5]	-	-	99%	99%
Prophylactic Antibiotic Timing (Outpatient)[1,3]	-	-	98%	98%
Urinary Catheter Removal[5]	-	-	98%	97%
Survey of Patients' Hospital Experiences				
Area Around Room 'Always' Quiet at Night	(a)	62%	68%	61%
Doctors 'Always' Communicated Well	(a)	87%	83%	82%
Home Recovery Information Given	(a)	88%	85%	85%
Hospital Given 9 or 10 on 10 Point Scale	(a)	65%	73%	71%
Meds 'Always' Explained Before Given	(a)	69%	66%	64%
Nurses 'Always' Communicated Well	(a)	82%	80%	79%
Pain 'Always' Well Controlled	(a)	73%	72%	71%
Room and Bathroom 'Always' Clean	(a)	84%	75%	73%
Timely Help 'Always' Received	(a)	68%	69%	68%
Would Definitely Recommend Hospital	(a)	63%	73%	71%
Use of Medical Imaging				
Cardiac Imaging Stress Test before Surgery[7]	-	-	5.3%	5.3%
Combination Abdominal CT Scan	78	21.8%	16.4%	10.5%
Combination Brain/Sinus CT Scan[1]	-	-	2.7%	2.7%
Combination Chest CT Scan	147	6.1%	5.6%	2.7%
Follow-up Mammogram/Ultrasound	214	8.4%	7.9%	8.8%
Lumbar Spine MRI for Low Back Pain	51	43.1%	39.6%	37.2%

Little River Healthcare

1700 Brazos
Rockdale, TX 76567
Phone: 512-446-4500
Type: Critical Access Hospitals
Emergency Services: Yes
Ownership: Proprietary

Measure	Cases	This Hosp.	State Avg.	U.S. Avg.
Blood Clot Prevention and Treatment				
Anticoagulation Overlap Therapy[5]	-	-	93%	93%
ICU Venous Thromboembolism Prophylaxis[5]	-	-	92%	92%
Incidence of Potentially Preventable VTE[5]	-	-	9%	10%
UFH with Dosages/Platelet Monitoring[5]	-	-	96%	97%
Venous Thromboembolism Prophylaxis[5]	-	-	82%	85%
Warfarin Therapy Discharge Instructions[5]	-	-	84%	75%
Chest Pain/Possible Heart Attack Care				
Aspirin Given Within 24 Hours of Arrival	-	-	94%	96%
Fibrinolytic Meds Within 30 Min. of Arrival	-	-	47%	58%
Average Time to ECG (minutes)	-	-	8	7
Average Time to Transfer (minutes)	-	-	62	60
Children's Asthma Care				
Received Home Management Plan of Care	-	-	93%	88%
Received Reliever Medication	-	-	100%	100%
Received Systemic Corticosteroids	-	-	100%	100%
Emergency Department				
Admittance Decision Time (minutes)[5]	-	-	99	98
Head CT Results Within 45 Min. of Arrival	-	-	54%	57%
Patients Who Left ER Before Being Seen	-	-	3%	2%
Time from ER Arrival to Admit. (minutes)[5]	-	-	270	274
Time from ER Arrival to Discharge (minutes)	-	-	127	134
Time in ER Before Being Evaluated (minutes)	-	-	26	26
Time to Pain Meds for Fractures (minutes)	-	-	57	57
Heart Attack Care				
Aspirin Given at Discharge[5]	-	-	99%	99%
Fibrinolytic Meds Within 30 Min. of Arrival[5]	-	-	49%	54%
PCI Within 90 Minutes of Arrival[5]	-	-	95%	96%
Statin Prescribed at Discharge[5]	-	-	98%	98%
Heart Failure Care				
ACE Inhibitor or ARB for LVSD[3,7]	-	-	97%	97%
Discharge Instructions Given[1,3]	-	-	95%	94%
Evaluation of LVS Function[1,3]	-	-	99%	99%
Medicare Spending				
Medicare Spending per Patient (ratio)	-	-	1.03	0.98
Pneumonia Care				
Appropriate Initial Antibiotic Given[5]	-	-	95%	95%
Blood Culture Timing[5]	-	-	98%	98%
Pregnancy and Delivery Care				
Newborn Deliveries Scheduled Early[5]	-	-	7%	6%
Preventive Care				
Immunization for Influenza[5]	-	-	90%	90%
Immunization for Pneumonia[5]	-	-	92%	92%
Stroke Care				
Anticoagulation Therapy for Atrial Fibrillation[5]	-	-	96%	95%
Antithrombotic Therapy Timing[5]	-	-	98%	98%
Assessed for Rehabilitation[5]	-	-	98%	97%
Discharged on Antithrombotic Therapy[5]	-	-	99%	99%
Discharged on Statin Medication[5]	-	-	95%	94%
Thrombolytic Therapy Timing[5]	-	-	68%	66%
Venous Thromboembolism Prophylaxis[5]	-	-	94%	94%
Written Stroke Educational Materials Given[5]	-	-	92%	88%
Surgical Care Improvement Project				
Appropriate Beta Blocker Usage[5]	-	-	98%	98%
Appropriate VTP Within 24 Hours[5]	-	-	98%	98%
Controlled Postoperative Blood Glucose[5]	-	-	96%	97%
Perioperative Temperature Management[5]	-	-	100%	100%
Prophylactic Antibiotic Selection[5]	-	-	99%	99%
Prophylactic Antibiotic Selection (Outpatient)	-	-	98%	98%
Prophylactic Antibiotic Stopped[5]	-	-	98%	98%
Prophylactic Antibiotic Timing[5]	-	-	99%	99%
Prophylactic Antibiotic Timing (Outpatient)	-	-	98%	98%
Urinary Catheter Removal[5]	-	-	98%	97%
Survey of Patients' Hospital Experiences				
Area Around Room 'Always' Quiet at Night[5]	-	-	68%	61%
Doctors 'Always' Communicated Well[5]	-	-	83%	82%
Home Recovery Information Given[5]	-	-	85%	85%
Hospital Given 9 or 10 on 10 Point Scale[5]	-	-	73%	71%
Meds 'Always' Explained Before Given[5]	-	-	66%	64%
Nurses 'Always' Communicated Well[5]	-	-	80%	79%
Pain 'Always' Well Controlled[5]	-	-	72%	71%
Room and Bathroom 'Always' Clean[5]	-	-	75%	73%
Timely Help 'Always' Received[5]	-	-	69%	68%
Would Definitely Recommend Hospital[5]	-	-	73%	71%
Use of Medical Imaging				
Cardiac Imaging Stress Test before Surgery	-	-	5.3%	5.3%
Combination Abdominal CT Scan	-	-	16.4%	10.5%
Combination Brain/Sinus CT Scan	-	-	2.7%	2.7%
Combination Chest CT Scan	-	-	5.6%	2.7%
Follow-up Mammogram/Ultrasound	-	-	7.9%	8.8%
Lumbar Spine MRI for Low Back Pain	-	-	39.6%	37.2%

Texas Health Presbyterian Hospital Rockwall

3150 Horizon Road
Rockwall, TX 75032
Phone: 469-698-1000
URL: www.texashealthrockwall.com
Type: Acute Care Hospitals
Emergency Services: Yes
Ownership: Physician
Beds: 50

Key Personnel:
President . . . . Ken Teel

Measure	Cases	This Hosp.	State Avg.	U.S. Avg.
Blood Clot Prevention and Treatment				
Anticoagulation Overlap Therapy[2]	36	97%	93%	93%
ICU Venous Thromboembolism Prophylaxis[2]	103	87%	92%	92%
Incidence of Potentially Preventable VTE[1,2]	-	-	9%	10%
UFH with Dosages/Platelet Monitoring[1,2]	-	-	96%	97%
Venous Thromboembolism Prophylaxis[2]	703	76%	82%	85%
Warfarin Therapy Discharge Instructions[2]	24	62%	84%	75%
Chest Pain/Possible Heart Attack Care				
Aspirin Given Within 24 Hours of Arrival	68	96%	94%	96%
Fibrinolytic Meds Within 30 Min. of Arrival[7]	-	-	47%	58%

NOTE: Hospital profiles are in alphabetical order by state, then city, then hospital within the city; Rankings exclude hospitals with less than 25 cases except for patient surveys which excludes hospitals with less than 100 cases; (a) 100-299 cases; (1) The number of cases/patients is too few to report; (2) Data submitted were based on a sample of cases/patients; (3) Results are based on a shorter time period than required; (4) Data suppressed by CMS for one or more quarters; (5) Results are not available for this reporting period; (6) Fewer than 100 patients completed the HCAHPS survey; (7) No cases met the criteria for this measure; (8) The lower limit of the confidence interval cannot be calculated if the number of observed infections equals zero; (9) No data are available from the state/territory for this reporting period; (10) The scores shown reflect fewer than 50 completed surveys; (11) There were discrepancies in the data collection process; (12) This measure does not apply to this hospital for this reporting period; (13) Results cannot be calculated for this reporting period; (14) The results for this state are combined with nearby states to protect confidentiality; Please refer to the User's Guide for a full explanation of data.

Measure	Cases	This Hosp.	State Avg.	U.S. Avg.
Average Time to ECG (minutes)	73	6	8	7
Average Time to Transfer (minutes)	13	61	62	60
Children's Asthma Care				
Received Home Management Plan of Care	-	-	93%	88%
Received Reliever Medication	-	-	100%	100%
Received Systemic Corticosteroids	-	-	100%	100%
Emergency Department				
Admittance Decision Time (minutes)[2]	438	74	99	98
Head CT Results Within 45 Min. of Arrival	16	75%	54%	57%
Patients Who Left ER Before Being Seen	25,529	2%	3%	2%
Time from ER Arrival to Admit. (minutes)[2]	449	234	270	274
Time from ER Arrival to Discharge (minutes)	443	144	127	134
Time in ER Before Being Evaluated (minutes)	455	32	26	26
Time to Pain Meds for Fractures (minutes)	164	49	57	57
Heart Attack Care				
Aspirin Given at Discharge	12	83%	99%	99%
Fibrinolytic Meds Within 30 Min. of Arrival[7]	-	-	49%	54%
PCI Within 90 Minutes of Arrival[7]	-	-	95%	96%
Statin Prescribed at Discharge	11	82%	98%	98%
Heart Failure Care				
ACE Inhibitor or ARB for LVSD	26	96%	97%	97%
Discharge Instructions Given	103	90%	95%	94%
Evaluation of LVS Function	132	99%	99%	99%
Medicare Spending				
Medicare Spending per Patient (ratio)	-	1.06	1.03	0.98
Pneumonia Care				
Appropriate Initial Antibiotic Given	137	99%	95%	95%
Blood Culture Timing	207	99%	98%	98%
Pregnancy and Delivery Care				
Newborn Deliveries Scheduled Early	85	7%	7%	6%
Preventive Care				
Immunization for Influenza[2]	426	97%	90%	90%
Immunization for Pneumonia[2]	437	96%	92%	92%
Stroke Care				
Anticoagulation Therapy for Atrial Fibrillation[1]	-	-	96%	95%
Antithrombotic Therapy Timing	25	100%	98%	98%
Assessed for Rehabilitation	29	100%	98%	97%
Discharged on Antithrombotic Therapy	29	100%	99%	99%
Discharged on Statin Medication	19	100%	95%	94%
Thrombolytic Therapy Timing[7]	-	-	68%	66%
Venous Thromboembolism Prophylaxis	25	100%	94%	94%
Written Stroke Educational Materials Given	15	100%	92%	88%
Surgical Care Improvement Project				
Appropriate Beta Blocker Usage	96	100%	98%	98%
Appropriate VTP Within 24 Hours	408	98%	98%	98%
Controlled Postoperative Blood Glucose[7]	-	-	96%	97%
Perioperative Temperature Management	422	100%	100%	100%
Prophylactic Antibiotic Selection	286	100%	99%	99%
Prophylactic Antibiotic Selection (Outpatient)	413	98%	98%	98%
Prophylactic Antibiotic Stopped	281	98%	98%	98%
Prophylactic Antibiotic Timing	287	100%	99%	99%
Prophylactic Antibiotic Timing (Outpatient)	413	100%	98%	98%
Urinary Catheter Removal	289	98%	98%	97%
Survey of Patients' Hospital Experiences				
Area Around Room 'Always' Quiet at Night	300+	65%	68%	61%
Doctors 'Always' Communicated Well	300+	78%	83%	82%
Home Recovery Information Given	300+	85%	85%	85%
Hospital Given 9 or 10 on 10 Point Scale	300+	76%	73%	71%
Meds 'Always' Explained Before Given	300+	64%	66%	64%
Nurses 'Always' Communicated Well	300+	80%	80%	79%
Pain 'Always' Well Controlled	300+	71%	72%	71%
Room and Bathroom 'Always' Clean	300+	83%	75%	73%
Timely Help 'Always' Received	300+	69%	69%	68%
Would Definitely Recommend Hospital	300+	80%	73%	71%
Use of Medical Imaging				
Cardiac Imaging Stress Test before Surgery[1]	-	-	5.3%	5.3%
Combination Abdominal CT Scan	413	12.6%	16.4%	10.5%
Combination Brain/Sinus CT Scan	426	1.9%	2.7%	2.7%
Combination Chest CT Scan	219	5.0%	5.6%	2.7%
Follow-up Mammogram/Ultrasound	331	14.5%	7.9%	8.8%
Lumbar Spine MRI for Low Back Pain	159	36.5%	39.6%	37.2%

Fisher County Hospital District

774 State Highway 70 N
Rotan, TX 79546
Phone: 325-735-2256
Fax: 325-735-2240
Type: Critical Access Hospitals
Emergency Services: Yes
Ownership: Govt - Hospital Dist/Auth
Beds: 30

Key Personnel:
Infection Control . . . . La Vona Brown
Quality Assurance . . . . La Vona Brown
Chief of Medical Staff . . . . CM Callan, MD
Emergency Room . . . . CM Callan, MD

Measure	Cases	This Hosp.	State Avg.	U.S. Avg.
Blood Clot Prevention and Treatment				
Anticoagulation Overlap Therapy[5]	-	-	93%	93%
ICU Venous Thromboembolism Prophylaxis[5]	-	-	92%	92%
Incidence of Potentially Preventable VTE[5]	-	-	9%	10%
UFH with Dosages/Platelet Monitoring[5]	-	-	96%	97%
Venous Thromboembolism Prophylaxis[5]	-	-	82%	85%
Warfarin Therapy Discharge Instructions[5]	-	-	84%	75%
Chest Pain/Possible Heart Attack Care				
Aspirin Given Within 24 Hours of Arrival	-	-	94%	96%
Fibrinolytic Meds Within 30 Min. of Arrival	-	-	47%	58%
Average Time to ECG (minutes)	-	-	8	7
Average Time to Transfer (minutes)	-	-	62	60
Children's Asthma Care				
Received Home Management Plan of Care	-	-	93%	88%
Received Reliever Medication	-	-	100%	100%
Received Systemic Corticosteroids	-	-	100%	100%
Emergency Department				
Admittance Decision Time (minutes)[5]	-	-	99	98
Head CT Results Within 45 Min. of Arrival	-	-	54%	57%
Patients Who Left ER Before Being Seen	-	-	3%	2%
Time from ER Arrival to Admit. (minutes)[5]	-	-	270	274
Time from ER Arrival to Discharge (minutes)	-	-	127	134
Time in ER Before Being Evaluated (minutes)	-	-	26	26
Time to Pain Meds for Fractures (minutes)	-	-	57	57
Heart Attack Care				
Aspirin Given at Discharge[5]	-	-	99%	99%
Fibrinolytic Meds Within 30 Min. of Arrival[5]	-	-	49%	54%
PCI Within 90 Minutes of Arrival[5]	-	-	95%	96%
Statin Prescribed at Discharge[5]	-	-	98%	98%
Heart Failure Care				
ACE Inhibitor or ARB for LVSD[5]	-	-	97%	97%
Discharge Instructions Given[5]	-	-	95%	94%
Evaluation of LVS Function[5]	-	-	99%	99%
Medicare Spending				
Medicare Spending per Patient (ratio)	-	-	1.03	0.98
Pneumonia Care				
Appropriate Initial Antibiotic Given[1,3]	-	-	95%	95%
Blood Culture Timing[1,3]	-	-	98%	98%
Pregnancy and Delivery Care				
Newborn Deliveries Scheduled Early[5]	-	-	7%	6%
Preventive Care				
Immunization for Influenza[5]	-	-	90%	90%
Immunization for Pneumonia[5]	-	-	92%	92%
Stroke Care				
Anticoagulation Therapy for Atrial Fibrillation[5]	-	-	96%	95%
Antithrombotic Therapy Timing[5]	-	-	98%	98%
Assessed for Rehabilitation[5]	-	-	98%	97%
Discharged on Antithrombotic Therapy[5]	-	-	99%	99%
Discharged on Statin Medication[5]	-	-	95%	94%
Thrombolytic Therapy Timing[5]	-	-	68%	66%
Venous Thromboembolism Prophylaxis[5]	-	-	94%	94%
Written Stroke Educational Materials Given[5]	-	-	92%	88%
Surgical Care Improvement Project				
Appropriate Beta Blocker Usage[5]	-	-	98%	98%
Appropriate VTP Within 24 Hours[5]	-	-	98%	98%
Controlled Postoperative Blood Glucose[5]	-	-	96%	97%
Perioperative Temperature Management[5]	-	-	100%	100%
Prophylactic Antibiotic Selection[5]	-	-	99%	99%
Prophylactic Antibiotic Selection (Outpatient)	-	-	98%	98%
Prophylactic Antibiotic Stopped[5]	-	-	98%	98%
Prophylactic Antibiotic Timing[5]	-	-	99%	99%
Prophylactic Antibiotic Timing (Outpatient)	-	-	98%	98%
Urinary Catheter Removal[5]	-	-	98%	97%
Survey of Patients' Hospital Experiences				
Area Around Room 'Always' Quiet at Night[5]	-	-	68%	61%
Doctors 'Always' Communicated Well[5]	-	-	83%	82%
Home Recovery Information Given[5]	-	-	85%	85%
Hospital Given 9 or 10 on 10 Point Scale[5]	-	-	73%	71%
Meds 'Always' Explained Before Given[5]	-	-	66%	64%
Nurses 'Always' Communicated Well[5]	-	-	80%	79%
Pain 'Always' Well Controlled[5]	-	-	72%	71%
Room and Bathroom 'Always' Clean[5]	-	-	75%	73%
Timely Help 'Always' Received[5]	-	-	69%	68%
Would Definitely Recommend Hospital[5]	-	-	73%	71%
Use of Medical Imaging				
Cardiac Imaging Stress Test before Surgery	-	-	5.3%	5.3%
Combination Abdominal CT Scan	-	-	16.4%	10.5%
Combination Brain/Sinus CT Scan	-	-	2.7%	2.7%
Combination Chest CT Scan	-	-	5.6%	2.7%
Follow-up Mammogram/Ultrasound	-	-	7.9%	8.8%
Lumbar Spine MRI for Low Back Pain	-	-	39.6%	37.2%

Round Rock Medical Center

2400 Round Rock Ave
Round Rock, TX 78681
Phone: 512-341-1000
Fax: 512-341-5216
URL: www.roundrockmedicalcenter.com
Type: Acute Care Hospitals
Emergency Services: Yes
Ownership: Voluntary non-profit - Other
Beds: 107

Key Personnel:
Emergency Room . . . . Arthur Boone, MD
Intensive Care Unit. . . . . Camille Compton
Chief of Medical Staff . . . . John Costanz, MD
Infection Control. . . . . Laurie Davidson
President/CEO. . . . . C. David Huffstutler
Anesthesiology. . . . . Harry Jung
Quality Assurance . . . . Dave Thomsen
Operating Room. . . . . Tom Williamson

Measure	Cases	This Hosp.	State Avg.	U.S. Avg.
Blood Clot Prevention and Treatment				
Anticoagulation Overlap Therapy[2]	48	100%	93%	93%
ICU Venous Thromboembolism Prophylaxis[2]	53	98%	92%	92%
Incidence of Potentially Preventable VTE[1,2]	-	-	9%	10%
UFH with Dosages/Platelet Monitoring[1,2]	-	-	96%	97%
Venous Thromboembolism Prophylaxis[2]	357	97%	82%	85%
Warfarin Therapy Discharge Instructions[2]	38	100%	84%	75%
Chest Pain/Possible Heart Attack Care				
Aspirin Given Within 24 Hours of Arrival[1,3]	-	-	94%	96%
Fibrinolytic Meds Within 30 Min. of Arrival[5]	-	-	47%	58%
Average Time to ECG (minutes)[1,3]	-	-	8	7
Average Time to Transfer (minutes)[5]	-	-	62	60
Children's Asthma Care				
Received Home Management Plan of Care	-	-	93%	88%
Received Reliever Medication	-	-	100%	100%
Received Systemic Corticosteroids	-	-	100%	100%
Emergency Department				
Admittance Decision Time (minutes)[2]	621	138	99	98
Head CT Results Within 45 Min. of Arrival	16	38%	54%	57%
Patients Who Left ER Before Being Seen	41,385	1%	3%	2%
Time from ER Arrival to Admit. (minutes)[2]	621	273	270	274
Time from ER Arrival to Discharge (minutes)	497	153	127	134
Time in ER Before Being Evaluated (minutes)	510	20	26	26
Time to Pain Meds for Fractures (minutes)	152	44	57	57
Heart Attack Care				
Aspirin Given at Discharge	171	100%	99%	99%
Fibrinolytic Meds Within 30 Min. of Arrival[7]	-	-	49%	54%
PCI Within 90 Minutes of Arrival	39	100%	95%	96%
Statin Prescribed at Discharge	163	100%	98%	98%
Heart Failure Care				
ACE Inhibitor or ARB for LVSD	47	100%	97%	97%
Discharge Instructions Given	120	100%	95%	94%
Evaluation of LVS Function	147	100%	99%	99%
Medicare Spending				
Medicare Spending per Patient (ratio)	-	1.05	1.03	0.98
Pneumonia Care				
Appropriate Initial Antibiotic Given	93	99%	95%	95%
Blood Culture Timing	201	100%	98%	98%

NOTE: Hospital profiles are in alphabetical order by state, then city, then hospital within the city; Rankings exclude hospitals with less than 25 cases except for patient surveys which excludes hospitals with less than 100 cases; (a) 100-299 cases; (1) The number of cases/patients is too few to report; (2) Data submitted were based on a sample of cases/patients; (3) Results are based on a shorter time period than required; (4) Data suppressed by CMS for one or more quarters; (5) Results are not available for this reporting period; (6) Fewer than 100 patients completed the HCAHPS survey; (7) No cases met the criteria for this measure; (8) The lower limit of the confidence interval cannot be calculated if the number of observed infections equals zero; (9) No data are available from the state/territory for this reporting period; (10) The scores shown reflect fewer than 50 completed surveys; (11) There were discrepancies in the data collection process; (12) This measure does not apply to this hospital for this reporting period; (13) Results cannot be calculated for this reporting period; (14) The results for this state are combined with nearby states to protect confidentiality; Please refer to the User's Guide for a full explanation of data.

Measure	Cases	This Hosp.	State Avg.	U.S. Avg.
Pregnancy and Delivery Care				
Newborn Deliveries Scheduled Early[2]	31	10%	7%	6%
Preventive Care				
Immunization for Influenza[2]	475	98%	90%	90%
Immunization for Pneumonia[2]	521	97%	92%	92%
Stroke Care				
Anticoagulation Therapy for Atrial Fibrillation	11	91%	96%	95%
Antithrombotic Therapy Timing	73	100%	98%	98%
Assessed for Rehabilitation	76	99%	98%	97%
Discharged on Antithrombotic Therapy	74	100%	99%	99%
Discharged on Statin Medication	55	96%	95%	94%
Thrombolytic Therapy Timing[1]	-	-	68%	66%
Venous Thromboembolism Prophylaxis	76	99%	94%	94%
Written Stroke Educational Materials Given	45	93%	92%	88%
Surgical Care Improvement Project				
Appropriate Beta Blocker Usage[2]	119	100%	98%	98%
Appropriate VTP Within 24 Hours[2]	339	100%	98%	98%
Controlled Postoperative Blood Glucose[2]	28	96%	96%	97%
Perioperative Temperature Management[2]	358	100%	100%	100%
Prophylactic Antibiotic Selection[2]	249	100%	99%	99%
Prophylactic Antibiotic Selection (Outpatient)	242	99%	98%	98%
Prophylactic Antibiotic Stopped[2]	246	100%	98%	98%
Prophylactic Antibiotic Timing[2]	249	100%	99%	99%
Prophylactic Antibiotic Timing (Outpatient)	242	100%	98%	98%
Urinary Catheter Removal[2]	293	99%	98%	97%
Survey of Patients' Hospital Experiences				
Area Around Room 'Always' Quiet at Night	300+	62%	68%	61%
Doctors 'Always' Communicated Well	300+	78%	83%	82%
Home Recovery Information Given	300+	88%	85%	85%
Hospital Given 9 or 10 on 10 Point Scale	300+	75%	73%	71%
Meds 'Always' Explained Before Given	300+	67%	66%	64%
Nurses 'Always' Communicated Well	300+	78%	80%	79%
Pain 'Always' Well Controlled	300+	72%	72%	71%
Room and Bathroom 'Always' Clean	300+	73%	75%	73%
Timely Help 'Always' Received	300+	68%	69%	68%
Would Definitely Recommend Hospital	300+	76%	73%	71%
Use of Medical Imaging				
Cardiac Imaging Stress Test before Surgery	247	4.5%	5.3%	5.3%
Combination Abdominal CT Scan	359	1.1%	16.4%	10.5%
Combination Brain/Sinus CT Scan[1]	-	-	2.7%	2.7%
Combination Chest CT Scan	144	0.0%	5.6%	2.7%
Follow-up Mammogram/Ultrasound	355	5.6%	7.9%	8.8%
Lumbar Spine MRI for Low Back Pain[1]	-	-	39.6%	37.2%

Scott & White Hospital - Round Rock

300 University Blvd Phone: 512-509-0100
Round Rock, TX 78664
URL: www.sw.org
Type: Acute Care Hospitals Emergency Services: Yes
Ownership: Voluntary non-profit - Private Beds: 76
Key Personnel:
Administrator . . . . Dawna Kilpatrick

Measure	Cases	This Hosp.	State Avg.	U.S. Avg.
Blood Clot Prevention and Treatment				
Anticoagulation Overlap Therapy[2]	52	96%	93%	93%
ICU Venous Thromboembolism Prophylaxis[2]	41	88%	92%	92%
Incidence of Potentially Preventable VTE[1,2]	-	-	9%	10%
UFH with Dosages/Platelet Monitoring[2]	19	100%	96%	97%
Venous Thromboembolism Prophylaxis[2]	335	93%	82%	85%
Warfarin Therapy Discharge Instructions[2]	40	78%	84%	75%
Chest Pain/Possible Heart Attack Care				
Aspirin Given Within 24 Hours of Arrival[1,3]	-	-	94%	96%
Fibrinolytic Meds Within 30 Min. of Arrival[3,7]	-	-	47%	58%
Average Time to ECG (minutes)[1,3]	-	-	8	7
Average Time to Transfer (minutes)[3,7]	-	-	62	60
Children's Asthma Care				
Received Home Management Plan of Care	-	-	93%	88%
Received Reliever Medication	-	-	100%	100%
Received Systemic Corticosteroids	-	-	100%	100%
Emergency Department				
Admittance Decision Time (minutes)[2]	493	73	99	98
Head CT Results Within 45 Min. of Arrival[1]	-	-	54%	57%
Patients Who Left ER Before Being Seen	23,016	1%	3%	2%
Time from ER Arrival to Admit. (minutes)[2]	494	198	270	274
Time from ER Arrival to Discharge (minutes)	428	90	127	134
Time in ER Before Being Evaluated (minutes)	440	19	26	26
Time to Pain Meds for Fractures (minutes)	69	62	57	57
Heart Attack Care				
Aspirin Given at Discharge	109	99%	99%	99%
Fibrinolytic Meds Within 30 Min. of Arrival[7]	-	-	49%	54%
PCI Within 90 Minutes of Arrival	19	100%	95%	96%
Statin Prescribed at Discharge	108	99%	98%	98%
Heart Failure Care				
ACE Inhibitor or ARB for LVSD	39	95%	97%	97%
Discharge Instructions Given	92	100%	95%	94%
Evaluation of LVS Function	122	100%	99%	99%
Medicare Spending				
Medicare Spending per Patient (ratio)	-	0.94	1.03	0.98
Pneumonia Care				
Appropriate Initial Antibiotic Given[2]	84	95%	95%	95%
Blood Culture Timing[2]	146	99%	98%	98%
Pregnancy and Delivery Care				
Newborn Deliveries Scheduled Early[2]	22	0%	7%	6%
Preventive Care				
Immunization for Influenza[2]	487	93%	90%	90%
Immunization for Pneumonia[2]	677	92%	92%	92%
Stroke Care				
Anticoagulation Therapy for Atrial Fibrillation[1]	-	-	96%	95%
Antithrombotic Therapy Timing	50	100%	98%	98%
Assessed for Rehabilitation	64	100%	98%	97%
Discharged on Antithrombotic Therapy	63	100%	99%	99%
Discharged on Statin Medication	46	100%	95%	94%
Thrombolytic Therapy Timing[1]	-	-	68%	66%
Venous Thromboembolism Prophylaxis	54	96%	94%	94%
Written Stroke Educational Materials Given	27	96%	92%	88%
Surgical Care Improvement Project				
Appropriate Beta Blocker Usage[2]	154	97%	98%	98%
Appropriate VTP Within 24 Hours[2]	317	97%	98%	98%
Controlled Postoperative Blood Glucose[2]	63	94%	96%	97%
Perioperative Temperature Management[2]	418	97%	100%	100%
Prophylactic Antibiotic Selection[2]	303	99%	99%	99%
Prophylactic Antibiotic Selection (Outpatient)	196	98%	98%	98%
Prophylactic Antibiotic Stopped[2]	292	98%	98%	98%
Prophylactic Antibiotic Timing[2]	304	99%	99%	99%
Prophylactic Antibiotic Timing (Outpatient)	140	96%	98%	98%
Urinary Catheter Removal[2]	267	97%	98%	97%
Survey of Patients' Hospital Experiences				
Area Around Room 'Always' Quiet at Night	300+	66%	68%	61%
Doctors 'Always' Communicated Well	300+	85%	83%	82%
Home Recovery Information Given	300+	86%	85%	85%
Hospital Given 9 or 10 on 10 Point Scale	300+	74%	73%	71%
Meds 'Always' Explained Before Given	300+	65%	66%	64%
Nurses 'Always' Communicated Well	300+	78%	80%	79%
Pain 'Always' Well Controlled	300+	70%	72%	71%
Room and Bathroom 'Always' Clean	300+	77%	75%	73%
Timely Help 'Always' Received	300+	65%	69%	68%
Would Definitely Recommend Hospital	300+	79%	73%	71%
Use of Medical Imaging				
Cardiac Imaging Stress Test before Surgery	420	5.0%	5.3%	5.3%
Combination Abdominal CT Scan	896	7.3%	16.4%	10.5%
Combination Brain/Sinus CT Scan	577	1.7%	2.7%	2.7%
Combination Chest CT Scan	521	1.3%	5.6%	2.7%
Follow-up Mammogram/Ultrasound	1,609	7.8%	7.9%	8.8%
Lumbar Spine MRI for Low Back Pain	110	34.5%	39.6%	37.2%

Seton Medical Center Williamson

201 Seton Parkway Phone: 512-324-0000
Round Rock, TX 78664
URL: www.seton.net
Type: Acute Care Hospitals Emergency Services: Yes
Ownership: Voluntary non-profit - Private Beds: 181
Key Personnel:
CEO/President . . . . Jesus Garza

Measure	Cases	This Hosp.	State Avg.	U.S. Avg.
Blood Clot Prevention and Treatment				
Anticoagulation Overlap Therapy[2]	45	96%	93%	93%
ICU Venous Thromboembolism Prophylaxis[2]	134	98%	92%	92%
Incidence of Potentially Preventable VTE[2]	15	0%	9%	10%
UFH with Dosages/Platelet Monitoring[2]	15	100%	96%	97%
Venous Thromboembolism Prophylaxis[2]	307	97%	82%	85%
Warfarin Therapy Discharge Instructions[2]	36	61%	84%	75%
Chest Pain/Possible Heart Attack Care				
Aspirin Given Within 24 Hours of Arrival[1,3]	-	-	94%	96%
Fibrinolytic Meds Within 30 Min. of Arrival[3,7]	-	-	47%	58%
Average Time to ECG (minutes)[1,3]	-	-	8	7
Average Time to Transfer (minutes)[3,7]	-	-	62	60
Children's Asthma Care				
Received Home Management Plan of Care	-	-	93%	88%
Received Reliever Medication	-	-	100%	100%
Received Systemic Corticosteroids	-	-	100%	100%
Emergency Department				
Admittance Decision Time (minutes)[2,7]	-	-	99	98
Head CT Results Within 45 Min. of Arrival[1]	-	-	54%	57%
Patients Who Left ER Before Being Seen	30,755	1%	3%	2%
Time from ER Arrival to Admit. (minutes)[2]	648	194	270	274
Time from ER Arrival to Discharge (minutes)	371	154	127	134
Time in ER Before Being Evaluated (minutes)	404	11	26	26
Time to Pain Meds for Fractures (minutes)	36	22	57	57
Heart Attack Care				
Aspirin Given at Discharge	148	100%	99%	99%
Fibrinolytic Meds Within 30 Min. of Arrival[7]	-	-	49%	54%
PCI Within 90 Minutes of Arrival	25	88%	95%	96%
Statin Prescribed at Discharge	144	99%	98%	98%
Heart Failure Care				
ACE Inhibitor or ARB for LVSD	52	98%	97%	97%
Discharge Instructions Given	137	100%	95%	94%
Evaluation of LVS Function	162	100%	99%	99%
Medicare Spending				
Medicare Spending per Patient (ratio)	-	1.09	1.03	0.98
Pneumonia Care				
Appropriate Initial Antibiotic Given	98	95%	95%	95%
Blood Culture Timing	194	98%	98%	98%
Pregnancy and Delivery Care				
Newborn Deliveries Scheduled Early	72	0%	7%	6%
Preventive Care				
Immunization for Influenza[2]	543	98%	90%	90%
Immunization for Pneumonia[2]	622	99%	92%	92%
Stroke Care				
Anticoagulation Therapy for Atrial Fibrillation[1]	-	-	96%	95%
Antithrombotic Therapy Timing	71	93%	98%	98%
Assessed for Rehabilitation	103	97%	98%	97%
Discharged on Antithrombotic Therapy	89	98%	99%	99%
Discharged on Statin Medication	57	96%	95%	94%
Thrombolytic Therapy Timing[1]	-	-	68%	66%
Venous Thromboembolism Prophylaxis	105	98%	94%	94%
Written Stroke Educational Materials Given	60	88%	92%	88%
Surgical Care Improvement Project				
Appropriate Beta Blocker Usage	87	99%	98%	98%
Appropriate VTP Within 24 Hours	231	98%	98%	98%
Controlled Postoperative Blood Glucose	59	98%	96%	97%
Perioperative Temperature Management	268	100%	100%	100%
Prophylactic Antibiotic Selection	134	98%	99%	99%
Prophylactic Antibiotic Selection (Outpatient)	184	99%	98%	98%
Prophylactic Antibiotic Stopped	128	99%	98%	98%
Prophylactic Antibiotic Timing	135	99%	99%	99%
Prophylactic Antibiotic Timing (Outpatient)	184	99%	98%	98%
Urinary Catheter Removal	190	99%	98%	97%
Survey of Patients' Hospital Experiences				
Area Around Room 'Always' Quiet at Night	300+	66%	68%	61%
Doctors 'Always' Communicated Well	300+	79%	83%	82%
Home Recovery Information Given	300+	85%	85%	85%
Hospital Given 9 or 10 on 10 Point Scale	300+	75%	73%	71%
Meds 'Always' Explained Before Given	300+	66%	66%	64%
Nurses 'Always' Communicated Well	300+	77%	80%	79%
Pain 'Always' Well Controlled	300+	69%	72%	71%
Room and Bathroom 'Always' Clean	300+	70%	75%	73%
Timely Help 'Always' Received	300+	64%	69%	68%
Would Definitely Recommend Hospital	300+	79%	73%	71%

NOTE: Hospital profiles are in alphabetical order by state, then city, then hospital within the city; Rankings exclude hospitals with less than 25 cases except for patient surveys which excludes hospitals with less than 100 cases; (a) 100-299 cases; (1) The number of cases/patients is too few to report; (2) Data submitted were based on a sample of cases/patients; (3) Results are based on a shorter time period than required; (4) Data suppressed by CMS for one or more quarters; (5) Results are not available for this reporting period; (6) Fewer than 100 patients completed the HCAHPS survey; (7) No cases met the criteria for this measure; (8) The lower limit of the confidence interval cannot be calculated if the number of observed infections equals zero; (9) No data are available from the state/territory for this reporting period; (10) The scores shown reflect fewer than 50 completed surveys; (11) There were discrepancies in the data collection process; (12) This measure does not apply to this hospital for this reporting period; (13) Results cannot be calculated for this reporting period; (14) The results for this state are combined with nearby states to protect confidentiality; Please refer to the User's Guide for a full explanation of data.

Use of Medical Imaging				
Cardiac Imaging Stress Test before Surgery	158	4.4%	5.3%	5.3%
Combination Abdominal CT Scan	264	1.5%	16.4%	10.5%
Combination Brain/Sinus CT Scan[1]	-	-	2.7%	2.7%
Combination Chest CT Scan	110	1.8%	5.6%	2.7%
Follow-up Mammogram/Ultrasound	93	9.7%	7.9%	8.8%
Lumbar Spine MRI for Low Back Pain[1]	-	-	39.6%	37.2%

Lake Pointe Medical Center

6800 Scenic Dr
Rowlett, TX 75088
Phone: 972-412-2273
Fax: 972-475-8345
URL: www.lakepointemedical.com
Type: Acute Care Hospitals
Emergency Services: Yes
Ownership: Proprietary
Beds: 99

Key Personnel:
Quality Assurance . . . . Pat Cooper
Radiology. . . . . Lucy Dossett, MD
CEO/President. . . . . John Harris
Chief of Medical Staff. . . . . David Lensch, MD
Infection Control. . . . . Maria Sparks, RN
Operating Room. . . . . Deborah Wedding, RN
Pediatric Ambulatory Care . . . . . . Pam Wieland, MD
Pediatric In-Patient Care . . . . Pam Wieland, MD

Measure	Cases	This Hosp.	State Avg.	U.S. Avg.
Blood Clot Prevention and Treatment				
Anticoagulation Overlap Therapy[2]	44	95%	93%	93%
ICU Venous Thromboembolism Prophylaxis[2]	41	100%	92%	92%
Incidence of Potentially Preventable VTE[1,2]	-	-	9%	10%
UFH with Dosages/Platelet Monitoring[1,2]	-	-	96%	97%
Venous Thromboembolism Prophylaxis[2]	347	98%	82%	85%
Warfarin Therapy Discharge Instructions[2]	28	100%	84%	75%
Chest Pain/Possible Heart Attack Care				
Aspirin Given Within 24 Hours of Arrival	30	100%	94%	96%
Fibrinolytic Meds Within 30 Min. of Arrival[7]	-	-	47%	58%
Average Time to ECG (minutes)	33	6	8	7
Average Time to Transfer (minutes)	16	43	62	60
Children's Asthma Care				
Received Home Management Plan of Care	-	-	93%	88%
Received Reliever Medication	-	-	100%	100%
Received Systemic Corticosteroids	-	-	100%	100%
Emergency Department				
Admittance Decision Time (minutes)[2]	657	77	99	98
Head CT Results Within 45 Min. of Arrival[1]	-	-	54%	57%
Patients Who Left ER Before Being Seen	29,195	1%	3%	2%
Time from ER Arrival to Admit. (minutes)[2]	671	210	270	274
Time from ER Arrival to Discharge (minutes)	443	119	127	134
Time in ER Before Being Evaluated (minutes)	460	22	26	26
Time to Pain Meds for Fractures (minutes)	156	37	57	57
Heart Attack Care				
Aspirin Given at Discharge	83	100%	99%	99%
Fibrinolytic Meds Within 30 Min. of Arrival[7]	-	-	49%	54%
PCI Within 90 Minutes of Arrival[1]	-	-	95%	96%
Statin Prescribed at Discharge	80	100%	98%	98%
Heart Failure Care				
ACE Inhibitor or ARB for LVSD	43	100%	97%	97%
Discharge Instructions Given	126	98%	95%	94%
Evaluation of LVS Function	146	99%	99%	99%
Medicare Spending				
Medicare Spending per Patient (ratio)	-	1.13	1.03	0.98
Pneumonia Care				
Appropriate Initial Antibiotic Given	105	96%	95%	95%
Blood Culture Timing	138	99%	98%	98%
Pregnancy and Delivery Care				
Newborn Deliveries Scheduled Early[2]	41	7%	7%	6%
Preventive Care				
Immunization for Influenza[2]	541	99%	90%	90%
Immunization for Pneumonia[2]	537	99%	92%	92%
Stroke Care				
Anticoagulation Therapy for Atrial Fibrillation[1]	-	-	96%	95%
Antithrombotic Therapy Timing	54	100%	98%	98%
Assessed for Rehabilitation	72	100%	98%	97%
Discharged on Antithrombotic Therapy	72	100%	99%	99%
Discharged on Statin Medication	60	100%	95%	94%
Thrombolytic Therapy Timing[1]	-	-	68%	66%
Venous Thromboembolism Prophylaxis	62	100%	94%	94%
Written Stroke Educational Materials Given	38	100%	92%	88%
Surgical Care Improvement Project				
Appropriate Beta Blocker Usage	82	98%	98%	98%
Appropriate VTP Within 24 Hours	176	100%	98%	98%
Controlled Postoperative Blood Glucose	21	76%	96%	97%
Perioperative Temperature Management	217	100%	100%	100%
Prophylactic Antibiotic Selection	118	100%	99%	99%
Prophylactic Antibiotic Selection (Outpatient)	200	99%	98%	98%
Prophylactic Antibiotic Stopped	110	99%	98%	98%
Prophylactic Antibiotic Timing	118	100%	99%	99%
Prophylactic Antibiotic Timing (Outpatient)	200	100%	98%	98%
Urinary Catheter Removal	139	99%	98%	97%
Survey of Patients' Hospital Experiences				
Area Around Room 'Always' Quiet at Night	300+	63%	68%	61%
Doctors 'Always' Communicated Well	300+	82%	83%	82%
Home Recovery Information Given	300+	83%	85%	85%
Hospital Given 9 or 10 on 10 Point Scale	300+	71%	73%	71%
Meds 'Always' Explained Before Given	300+	62%	66%	64%
Nurses 'Always' Communicated Well	300+	80%	80%	79%
Pain 'Always' Well Controlled	300+	76%	72%	71%
Room and Bathroom 'Always' Clean	300+	68%	75%	73%
Timely Help 'Always' Received	300+	66%	69%	68%
Would Definitely Recommend Hospital	300+	69%	73%	71%
Use of Medical Imaging				
Cardiac Imaging Stress Test before Surgery[1]	-	-	5.3%	5.3%
Combination Abdominal CT Scan	576	8.9%	16.4%	10.5%
Combination Brain/Sinus CT Scan[1]	-	-	2.7%	2.7%
Combination Chest CT Scan	263	0.8%	5.6%	2.7%
Follow-up Mammogram/Ultrasound	1,154	8.3%	7.9%	8.8%
Lumbar Spine MRI for Low Back Pain	134	51.5%	39.6%	37.2%

San Angelo Community Medical Center

3501 Knickerbocker Road
San Angelo, TX 76904
Phone: 325-949-9511
Fax: 325-947-6523
URL: www.sacmc.com
Type: Acute Care Hospitals
Emergency Services: Yes
Ownership: Proprietary
Beds: 168

Key Personnel:
Pediatrics. . . . . Hector Acton, MD
Radiology. . . . . John E Alexander
CEO/President. . . . . Samuel G Feazell
Intensive Care Unit. . . . . Jerry Smithwick
Quality Assurance . . . . Connie Whorton

Measure	Cases	This Hosp.	State Avg.	U.S. Avg.
Blood Clot Prevention and Treatment				
Anticoagulation Overlap Therapy[2]	19	100%	93%	93%
ICU Venous Thromboembolism Prophylaxis[2]	89	94%	92%	92%
Incidence of Potentially Preventable VTE[1,2]	-	-	9%	10%
UFH with Dosages/Platelet Monitoring[1,2]	-	-	96%	97%
Venous Thromboembolism Prophylaxis[2]	339	96%	82%	85%
Warfarin Therapy Discharge Instructions[2]	15	93%	84%	75%
Chest Pain/Possible Heart Attack Care				
Aspirin Given Within 24 Hours of Arrival[3,7]	-	-	94%	96%
Fibrinolytic Meds Within 30 Min. of Arrival[5]	-	-	47%	58%
Average Time to ECG (minutes)[3,7]	-	-	8	7
Average Time to Transfer (minutes)[5]	-	-	62	60
Children's Asthma Care				
Received Home Management Plan of Care	-	-	93%	88%
Received Reliever Medication	-	-	100%	100%
Received Systemic Corticosteroids	-	-	100%	100%
Emergency Department				
Admittance Decision Time (minutes)[2]	476	74	99	98
Head CT Results Within 45 Min. of Arrival[1]	-	-	54%	57%
Patients Who Left ER Before Being Seen	26,203	2%	3%	2%
Time from ER Arrival to Admit. (minutes)[2]	503	219	270	274
Time from ER Arrival to Discharge (minutes)	383	113	127	134
Time in ER Before Being Evaluated (minutes)	413	16	26	26
Time to Pain Meds for Fractures (minutes)	81	47	57	57
Heart Attack Care				
Aspirin Given at Discharge	90	100%	99%	99%
Fibrinolytic Meds Within 30 Min. of Arrival[7]	-	-	49%	54%
PCI Within 90 Minutes of Arrival	18	100%	95%	96%
Statin Prescribed at Discharge	86	100%	98%	98%
Heart Failure Care				
ACE Inhibitor or ARB for LVSD	25	100%	97%	97%
Discharge Instructions Given	113	98%	95%	94%
Evaluation of LVS Function	149	100%	99%	99%
Medicare Spending				
Medicare Spending per Patient (ratio)	-	1.01	1.03	0.98
Pneumonia Care				
Appropriate Initial Antibiotic Given	77	100%	95%	95%
Blood Culture Timing	110	100%	98%	98%
Pregnancy and Delivery Care				
Newborn Deliveries Scheduled Early[2]	57	4%	7%	6%
Preventive Care				
Immunization for Influenza[2]	559	97%	90%	90%
Immunization for Pneumonia[2]	592	99%	92%	92%
Stroke Care				
Anticoagulation Therapy for Atrial Fibrillation[1]	-	-	96%	95%
Antithrombotic Therapy Timing	32	100%	98%	98%
Assessed for Rehabilitation	34	100%	98%	97%
Discharged on Antithrombotic Therapy	33	100%	99%	99%
Discharged on Statin Medication	29	100%	95%	94%
Thrombolytic Therapy Timing[1]	-	-	68%	66%
Venous Thromboembolism Prophylaxis	36	100%	94%	94%
Written Stroke Educational Materials Given	19	84%	92%	88%
Surgical Care Improvement Project				
Appropriate Beta Blocker Usage	139	100%	98%	98%
Appropriate VTP Within 24 Hours	332	100%	98%	98%
Controlled Postoperative Blood Glucose	30	100%	96%	97%
Perioperative Temperature Management	458	100%	100%	100%
Prophylactic Antibiotic Selection	382	100%	99%	99%
Prophylactic Antibiotic Selection (Outpatient)	151	100%	98%	98%
Prophylactic Antibiotic Stopped	378	100%	98%	98%
Prophylactic Antibiotic Timing	383	99%	99%	99%
Prophylactic Antibiotic Timing (Outpatient)	151	100%	98%	98%
Urinary Catheter Removal	109	99%	98%	97%
Survey of Patients' Hospital Experiences				
Area Around Room 'Always' Quiet at Night	300+	65%	68%	61%
Doctors 'Always' Communicated Well	300+	83%	83%	82%
Home Recovery Information Given	300+	87%	85%	85%
Hospital Given 9 or 10 on 10 Point Scale	300+	76%	73%	71%
Meds 'Always' Explained Before Given	300+	67%	66%	64%
Nurses 'Always' Communicated Well	300+	80%	80%	79%
Pain 'Always' Well Controlled	300+	73%	72%	71%
Room and Bathroom 'Always' Clean	300+	69%	75%	73%
Timely Help 'Always' Received	300+	69%	69%	68%
Would Definitely Recommend Hospital	300+	77%	73%	71%
Use of Medical Imaging				
Cardiac Imaging Stress Test before Surgery	530	6.8%	5.3%	5.3%
Combination Abdominal CT Scan	301	3.7%	16.4%	10.5%
Combination Brain/Sinus CT Scan	401	1.7%	2.7%	2.7%
Combination Chest CT Scan	212	0.0%	5.6%	2.7%
Follow-up Mammogram/Ultrasound	1,021	4.6%	7.9%	8.8%
Lumbar Spine MRI for Low Back Pain	64	43.8%	39.6%	37.2%

Shannon Medical Center

120 East Harris Avenue
San Angelo, TX 76903
Phone: 325-653-6741
Fax: 325-657-5706
E-mail: hr@shannonhealth.org
URL: www.shannonhealth.com
Type: Acute Care Hospitals
Emergency Services: Yes
Ownership: Voluntary non-profit - Private
Beds: 400

Key Personnel:
Quality Assurance . . . . Diane Bohannan
Pediatric Ambulatory Care . . . . . . JW Herbert, MD
Pediatric In-Patient Care . . . . JW Herbert, MD
CEO/President. . . . . Bryan Horner
Chief of Medical Staff. . . . . Irv Zeitler, DO

Measure	Cases	This Hosp.	State Avg.	U.S. Avg.
Blood Clot Prevention and Treatment				
Anticoagulation Overlap Therapy[2]	64	80%	93%	93%
ICU Venous Thromboembolism Prophylaxis[2]	66	88%	92%	92%
Incidence of Potentially Preventable VTE[2]	13	0%	9%	10%
UFH with Dosages/Platelet Monitoring[2]	15	93%	96%	97%
Venous Thromboembolism Prophylaxis[2]	340	89%	82%	85%

NOTE: Hospital profiles are in alphabetical order by state, then city, then hospital within the city; Rankings exclude hospitals with less than 25 cases except for patient surveys which excludes hospitals with less than 100 cases; (a) 100-299 cases; (1) The number of cases/patients is too few to report; (2) Data submitted were based on a sample of cases/patients; (3) Results are based on a shorter time period than required; (4) Data suppressed by CMS for one or more quarters; (5) Results are not available for this reporting period; (6) Fewer than 100 patients completed the HCAHPS survey; (7) No cases met the criteria for this measure; (8) The lower limit of the confidence interval cannot be calculated if the number of observed infections equals zero; (9) No data are available from the state/territory for this reporting period; (10) The scores shown reflect fewer than 50 completed surveys; (11) There were discrepancies in the data collection process; (12) This measure does not apply to this hospital for this reporting period; (13) Results cannot be calculated for this reporting period; (14) The results for this state are combined with nearby states to protect confidentiality; Please refer to the User's Guide for a full explanation of data.

Measure	Cases	This Hosp.	State Avg.	U.S. Avg.
Warfarin Therapy Discharge Instructions[2]	51	76%	84%	75%
Chest Pain/Possible Heart Attack Care				
Aspirin Given Within 24 Hours of Arrival[1,3]	-	-	94%	96%
Fibrinolytic Meds Within 30 Min. of Arrival[5]	-	-	47%	58%
Average Time to ECG (minutes)[1,3]	-	-	8	7
Average Time to Transfer (minutes)[5]	-	-	62	60
Children's Asthma Care				
Received Home Management Plan of Care	-	-	93%	88%
Received Reliever Medication	-	-	100%	100%
Received Systemic Corticosteroids	-	-	100%	100%
Emergency Department				
Admittance Decision Time (minutes)[2]	582	80	99	98
Head CT Results Within 45 Min. of Arrival[1]	-	-	54%	57%
Patients Who Left ER Before Being Seen	55,207	2%	3%	2%
Time from ER Arrival to Admit. (minutes)[2]	703	226	270	274
Time from ER Arrival to Discharge (minutes)	417	119	127	134
Time in ER Before Being Evaluated (minutes)	432	24	26	26
Time to Pain Meds for Fractures (minutes)	150	50	57	57
Heart Attack Care				
Aspirin Given at Discharge	234	100%	99%	99%
Fibrinolytic Meds Within 30 Min. of Arrival[7]	-	-	49%	54%
PCI Within 90 Minutes of Arrival	32	97%	95%	96%
Statin Prescribed at Discharge	231	98%	98%	98%
Heart Failure Care				
ACE Inhibitor or ARB for LVSD	92	98%	97%	97%
Discharge Instructions Given	215	97%	95%	94%
Evaluation of LVS Function	256	100%	99%	99%
Medicare Spending				
Medicare Spending per Patient (ratio)	-	0.91	1.03	0.98
Pneumonia Care				
Appropriate Initial Antibiotic Given	146	99%	95%	95%
Blood Culture Timing	363	99%	98%	98%
Pregnancy and Delivery Care				
Newborn Deliveries Scheduled Early	119	1%	7%	6%
Preventive Care				
Immunization for Influenza[2]	667	90%	90%	90%
Immunization for Pneumonia[2]	746	89%	92%	92%
Stroke Care				
Anticoagulation Therapy for Atrial Fibrillation	17	100%	96%	95%
Antithrombotic Therapy Timing	140	99%	98%	98%
Assessed for Rehabilitation	160	100%	98%	97%
Discharged on Antithrombotic Therapy	140	100%	99%	99%
Discharged on Statin Medication	112	96%	95%	94%
Thrombolytic Therapy Timing[1]	-	-	68%	66%
Venous Thromboembolism Prophylaxis	178	99%	94%	94%
Written Stroke Educational Materials Given	91	98%	92%	88%
Surgical Care Improvement Project				
Appropriate Beta Blocker Usage	351	99%	98%	98%
Appropriate VTP Within 24 Hours	713	99%	98%	98%
Controlled Postoperative Blood Glucose	117	97%	96%	97%
Perioperative Temperature Management	903	100%	100%	100%
Prophylactic Antibiotic Selection	638	100%	99%	99%
Prophylactic Antibiotic Selection (Outpatient)	457	99%	98%	98%
Prophylactic Antibiotic Stopped	622	98%	98%	98%
Prophylactic Antibiotic Timing	640	100%	99%	99%
Prophylactic Antibiotic Timing (Outpatient)	460	99%	98%	98%
Urinary Catheter Removal	531	98%	98%	97%
Survey of Patients' Hospital Experiences				
Area Around Room 'Always' Quiet at Night	300+	68%	68%	61%
Doctors 'Always' Communicated Well	300+	84%	83%	82%
Home Recovery Information Given	300+	84%	85%	85%
Hospital Given 9 or 10 on 10 Point Scale	300+	75%	73%	71%
Meds 'Always' Explained Before Given	300+	67%	66%	64%
Nurses 'Always' Communicated Well	300+	81%	80%	79%
Pain 'Always' Well Controlled	300+	72%	72%	71%
Room and Bathroom 'Always' Clean	300+	75%	75%	73%
Timely Help 'Always' Received	300+	68%	69%	68%
Would Definitely Recommend Hospital	300+	78%	73%	71%
Use of Medical Imaging				
Cardiac Imaging Stress Test before Surgery	229	4.8%	5.3%	5.3%
Combination Abdominal CT Scan	523	4.2%	16.4%	10.5%
Combination Brain/Sinus CT Scan	650	2.5%	2.7%	2.7%
Combination Chest CT Scan	261	1.9%	5.6%	2.7%
Follow-up Mammogram/Ultrasound	2,113	4.6%	7.9%	8.8%
Lumbar Spine MRI for Low Back Pain	316	37.0%	39.6%	37.2%

Baptist Emergency Hospital

16088 San Pedro Phone: 210-402-4092
San Antonio, TX 78232
URL: www.baptistemergencyhospital.com
Type: Acute Care Hospitals Emergency Services: No
Ownership: Proprietary

Measure	Cases	This Hosp.	State Avg.	U.S. Avg.
Blood Clot Prevention and Treatment				
Anticoagulation Overlap Therapy[5]	-	-	93%	93%
ICU Venous Thromboembolism Prophylaxis[5]	-	-	92%	92%
Incidence of Potentially Preventable VTE[5]	-	-	9%	10%
UFH with Dosages/Platelet Monitoring[5]	-	-	96%	97%
Venous Thromboembolism Prophylaxis[5]	-	-	82%	85%
Warfarin Therapy Discharge Instructions[5]	-	-	84%	75%
Chest Pain/Possible Heart Attack Care				
Aspirin Given Within 24 Hours of Arrival[5]	-	-	94%	96%
Fibrinolytic Meds Within 30 Min. of Arrival[5]	-	-	47%	58%
Average Time to ECG (minutes)[5]	-	-	8	7
Average Time to Transfer (minutes)[5]	-	-	62	60
Children's Asthma Care				
Received Home Management Plan of Care	-	-	93%	88%
Received Reliever Medication	-	-	100%	100%
Received Systemic Corticosteroids	-	-	100%	100%
Emergency Department				
Admittance Decision Time (minutes)[5]	-	-	99	98
Head CT Results Within 45 Min. of Arrival[5]	-	-	54%	57%
Patients Who Left ER Before Being Seen	14,272	1%	3%	2%
Time from ER Arrival to Admit. (minutes)[5]	-	-	270	274
Time from ER Arrival to Discharge (minutes)[5]	-	-	127	134
Time in ER Before Being Evaluated (minutes)[5]	-	-	26	26
Time to Pain Meds for Fractures (minutes)[5]	-	-	57	57
Heart Attack Care				
Aspirin Given at Discharge[5]	-	-	99%	99%
Fibrinolytic Meds Within 30 Min. of Arrival[5]	-	-	49%	54%
PCI Within 90 Minutes of Arrival[5]	-	-	95%	96%
Statin Prescribed at Discharge[5]	-	-	98%	98%
Heart Failure Care				
ACE Inhibitor or ARB for LVSD[5]	-	-	97%	97%
Discharge Instructions Given[5]	-	-	95%	94%
Evaluation of LVS Function[5]	-	-	99%	99%
Medicare Spending				
Medicare Spending per Patient (ratio)[1]	-	-	1.03	0.98
Pneumonia Care				
Appropriate Initial Antibiotic Given[5]	-	-	95%	95%
Blood Culture Timing[5]	-	-	98%	98%
Pregnancy and Delivery Care				
Newborn Deliveries Scheduled Early[7]	-	-	7%	6%
Preventive Care				
Immunization for Influenza[5]	-	-	90%	90%
Immunization for Pneumonia[5]	-	-	92%	92%
Stroke Care				
Anticoagulation Therapy for Atrial Fibrillation[5]	-	-	96%	95%
Antithrombotic Therapy Timing[5]	-	-	98%	98%
Assessed for Rehabilitation[5]	-	-	98%	97%
Discharged on Antithrombotic Therapy[5]	-	-	99%	99%
Discharged on Statin Medication[5]	-	-	95%	94%
Thrombolytic Therapy Timing[5]	-	-	68%	66%
Venous Thromboembolism Prophylaxis[5]	-	-	94%	94%
Written Stroke Educational Materials Given[5]	-	-	92%	88%
Surgical Care Improvement Project				
Appropriate Beta Blocker Usage[5]	-	-	98%	98%
Appropriate VTP Within 24 Hours[5]	-	-	98%	98%
Controlled Postoperative Blood Glucose[5]	-	-	96%	97%
Perioperative Temperature Management[5]	-	-	100%	100%
Prophylactic Antibiotic Selection[5]	-	-	99%	99%
Prophylactic Antibiotic Selection (Outpatient)[5]	-	-	98%	98%
Prophylactic Antibiotic Stopped[5]	-	-	98%	98%
Prophylactic Antibiotic Timing[5]	-	-	99%	99%
Prophylactic Antibiotic Timing (Outpatient)[5]	-	-	98%	98%
Urinary Catheter Removal[5]	-	-	98%	97%
Survey of Patients' Hospital Experiences				
Area Around Room 'Always' Quiet at Night	(a)	92%	68%	61%
Doctors 'Always' Communicated Well	(a)	93%	83%	82%
Home Recovery Information Given	(a)	81%	85%	85%
Hospital Given 9 or 10 on 10 Point Scale	(a)	83%	73%	71%
Meds 'Always' Explained Before Given	(a)	63%	66%	64%
Nurses 'Always' Communicated Well	(a)	87%	80%	79%
Pain 'Always' Well Controlled	(a)	80%	72%	71%
Room and Bathroom 'Always' Clean	(a)	75%	75%	73%
Timely Help 'Always' Received	(a)	79%	69%	68%
Would Definitely Recommend Hospital	(a)	87%	73%	71%
Use of Medical Imaging				
Cardiac Imaging Stress Test before Surgery[7]	-	-	5.3%	5.3%
Combination Abdominal CT Scan	184	1.1%	16.4%	10.5%
Combination Brain/Sinus CT Scan[1]	-	-	2.7%	2.7%
Combination Chest CT Scan	56	0.0%	5.6%	2.7%
Follow-up Mammogram/Ultrasound[7]	-	-	7.9%	8.8%
Lumbar Spine MRI for Low Back Pain[7]	-	-	39.6%	37.2%

Baptist Medical Center

111 Dallas Street Phone: 210-297-1020
San Antonio, TX 78205 Fax: 210-297-0700
URL: www.baptisthealthsystem.org
Type: Acute Care Hospitals Emergency Services: Yes
Ownership: Proprietary Beds: 375

Key Personnel:
Coronary Care . . . . Dot Brosig
Radiology. . . . . Carla Davila
Infection Control. . . . . Claudia Doss
Quality Assurance . . . . Charles Duncan, MD
Pediatric Ambulatory Care . . . . . . Pam Flentige
Chief of Medical Staff . . . . Harry Hernandez
Operating Room. . . . . Peggy Trevor
CEO/President. . . . . Kent H Wallace

Measure	Cases	This Hosp.	State Avg.	U.S. Avg.
Blood Clot Prevention and Treatment				
Anticoagulation Overlap Therapy[2]	217	96%	93%	93%
ICU Venous Thromboembolism Prophylaxis[2]	258	99%	92%	92%
Incidence of Potentially Preventable VTE[2]	46	7%	9%	10%
UFH with Dosages/Platelet Monitoring[2]	96	98%	96%	97%
Venous Thromboembolism Prophylaxis[2]	908	77%	82%	85%
Warfarin Therapy Discharge Instructions[2]	150	91%	84%	75%
Chest Pain/Possible Heart Attack Care				
Aspirin Given Within 24 Hours of Arrival[1,3]	-	-	94%	96%
Fibrinolytic Meds Within 30 Min. of Arrival[3,7]	-	-	47%	58%
Average Time to ECG (minutes)[1,3]	-	-	8	7
Average Time to Transfer (minutes)[3,7]	-	-	62	60
Children's Asthma Care				
Received Home Management Plan of Care	268	91%	93%	88%
Received Reliever Medication	269	100%	100%	100%
Received Systemic Corticosteroids	269	100%	100%	100%
Emergency Department				
Admittance Decision Time (minutes)[2]	2,184	151	99	98
Head CT Results Within 45 Min. of Arrival	16	31%	54%	57%
Patients Who Left ER Before Being Seen	23,304	4%	3%	2%
Time from ER Arrival to Admit. (minutes)[2]	2,272	330	270	274
Time from ER Arrival to Discharge (minutes)	392	158	127	134
Time in ER Before Being Evaluated (minutes)	408	45	26	26
Time to Pain Meds for Fractures (minutes)	466	50	57	57
Heart Attack Care				
Aspirin Given at Discharge	1,141	100%	99%	99%
Fibrinolytic Meds Within 30 Min. of Arrival[7]	-	-	49%	54%
PCI Within 90 Minutes of Arrival	143	95%	95%	96%
Statin Prescribed at Discharge	1,127	99%	98%	98%
Heart Failure Care				
ACE Inhibitor or ARB for LVSD	417	100%	97%	97%
Discharge Instructions Given	1,111	95%	95%	94%
Evaluation of LVS Function	1,323	100%	99%	99%
Medicare Spending				
Medicare Spending per Patient (ratio)	-	1.04	1.03	0.98
Pneumonia Care				
Appropriate Initial Antibiotic Given	592	98%	95%	95%

NOTE: Hospital profiles are in alphabetical order by state, then city, then hospital within the city; Rankings exclude hospitals with less than 25 cases except for patient surveys which excludes hospitals with less than 100 cases; (a) 100-299 cases; (1) The number of cases/patients is too few to report; (2) Data submitted were based on a sample of cases/patients; (3) Results are based on a shorter time period than required; (4) Data suppressed by CMS for one or more quarters; (5) Results are not available for this reporting period; (6) Fewer than 100 patients completed the HCAHPS survey; (7) No cases met the criteria for this measure; (8) The lower limit of the confidence interval cannot be calculated if the number of observed infections equals zero; (9) No data are available from the state/territory for this reporting period; (10) The scores shown reflect fewer than 50 completed surveys; (11) There were discrepancies in the data collection process; (12) This measure does not apply to this hospital for this reporting period; (13) Results cannot be calculated for this reporting period; (14) The results for this state are combined with nearby states to protect confidentiality; Please refer to the User's Guide for a full explanation of data.

Measure	Cases	This Hosp.	State Avg.	U.S. Avg.
Blood Culture Timing	1,129	99%	98%	98%
Pregnancy and Delivery Care				
Newborn Deliveries Scheduled Early[2]	138	3%	7%	6%
Preventive Care				
Immunization for Influenza[2]	2,241	96%	90%	90%
Immunization for Pneumonia[2]	2,607	96%	92%	92%
Stroke Care				
Anticoagulation Therapy for Atrial Fibrillation	111	94%	96%	95%
Antithrombotic Therapy Timing	629	97%	98%	98%
Assessed for Rehabilitation	866	99%	98%	97%
Discharged on Antithrombotic Therapy	709	100%	99%	99%
Discharged on Statin Medication	552	98%	95%	94%
Thrombolytic Therapy Timing	83	94%	68%	66%
Venous Thromboembolism Prophylaxis	897	95%	94%	94%
Written Stroke Educational Materials Given	433	92%	92%	88%
Surgical Care Improvement Project				
Appropriate Beta Blocker Usage[2]	1,097	99%	98%	98%
Appropriate VTP Within 24 Hours[2]	2,615	99%	98%	98%
Controlled Postoperative Blood Glucose[2]	488	96%	96%	97%
Perioperative Temperature Management[2]	3,017	100%	100%	100%
Prophylactic Antibiotic Selection[2]	2,970	100%	99%	99%
Prophylactic Antibiotic Selection (Outpatient)	1,533	98%	98%	98%
Prophylactic Antibiotic Stopped[2]	2,868	99%	98%	98%
Prophylactic Antibiotic Timing[2]	2,971	99%	99%	99%
Prophylactic Antibiotic Timing (Outpatient)	1,543	97%	98%	98%
Urinary Catheter Removal[2]	1,685	98%	98%	97%
Survey of Patients' Hospital Experiences				
Area Around Room 'Always' Quiet at Night[11]	300+	61%	68%	61%
Doctors 'Always' Communicated Well[11]	300+	81%	83%	82%
Home Recovery Information Given[11]	300+	86%	85%	85%
Hospital Given 9 or 10 on 10 Point Scale[11]	300+	72%	73%	71%
Meds 'Always' Explained Before Given[11]	300+	61%	66%	64%
Nurses 'Always' Communicated Well[11]	300+	77%	80%	79%
Pain 'Always' Well Controlled[11]	300+	70%	72%	71%
Room and Bathroom 'Always' Clean[11]	300+	65%	75%	73%
Timely Help 'Always' Received[11]	300+	61%	69%	68%
Would Definitely Recommend Hospital[11]	300+	73%	73%	71%
Use of Medical Imaging				
Cardiac Imaging Stress Test before Surgery	726	5.2%	5.3%	5.3%
Combination Abdominal CT Scan	1,839	1.1%	16.4%	10.5%
Combination Brain/Sinus CT Scan	1,930	1.3%	2.7%	2.7%
Combination Chest CT Scan	273	4.8%	5.6%	2.7%
Follow-up Mammogram/Ultrasound[7]	-	-	7.9%	8.8%
Lumbar Spine MRI for Low Back Pain[1]	-	-	39.6%	37.2%

Christus Santa Rosa Hospital

2827 Babcock Road Phone: 210-704-2011
San Antonio, TX 78229 Fax: 210-704-3632
URL: www.christussantarosa.org
Type: Acute Care Hospitals Emergency Services: Yes
Ownership: Voluntary non-profit - Church Beds: 1,034

Key Personnel:

CEO/President. . . . . Don A Beeler
Quality Assurance . . . . Sharon Holtz
Infection Control. . . . . Nancy Mendicino
Radiology. . . . . Joaquin Mira, MD
Hemotology Center . . . . Janine Primomo
Emergency Room . . . . Prentis Vaughn, MD
Chief of Medical Staff. . . . . Richard Wayne

Measure	Cases	This Hosp.	State Avg.	U.S. Avg.
Blood Clot Prevention and Treatment				
Anticoagulation Overlap Therapy[2]	110	86%	93%	93%
ICU Venous Thromboembolism Prophylaxis[2]	149	69%	92%	92%
Incidence of Potentially Preventable VTE[2]	18	39%	9%	10%
UFH with Dosages/Platelet Monitoring[2]	40	92%	96%	97%
Venous Thromboembolism Prophylaxis[2]	712	54%	82%	85%
Warfarin Therapy Discharge Instructions[2]	69	61%	84%	75%
Chest Pain/Possible Heart Attack Care				
Aspirin Given Within 24 Hours of Arrival	57	82%	94%	96%
Fibrinolytic Meds Within 30 Min. of Arrival[7]	-	-	47%	58%
Average Time to ECG (minutes)	55	14	8	7
Average Time to Transfer (minutes)[1]	-	-	62	60
Children's Asthma Care				
Received Home Management Plan of Care	147	91%	93%	88%
Received Reliever Medication	148	100%	100%	100%
Received Systemic Corticosteroids	148	99%	100%	100%
Emergency Department				
Admittance Decision Time (minutes)[2]	648	130	99	98
Head CT Results Within 45 Min. of Arrival	40	22%	54%	57%
Patients Who Left ER Before Being Seen	>100k	3%	3%	2%
Time from ER Arrival to Admit. (minutes)[2]	648	320	270	274
Time from ER Arrival to Discharge (minutes)	1,305	134	127	134
Time in ER Before Being Evaluated (minutes)	1,385	26	26	26
Time to Pain Meds for Fractures (minutes)	533	53	57	57
Heart Attack Care				
Aspirin Given at Discharge	419	98%	99%	99%
Fibrinolytic Meds Within 30 Min. of Arrival[7]	-	-	49%	54%
PCI Within 90 Minutes of Arrival	64	91%	95%	96%
Statin Prescribed at Discharge	400	98%	98%	98%
Heart Failure Care				
ACE Inhibitor or ARB for LVSD	178	99%	97%	97%
Discharge Instructions Given	421	98%	95%	94%
Evaluation of LVS Function	524	99%	99%	99%
Medicare Spending				
Medicare Spending per Patient (ratio)	-	1.07	1.03	0.98
Pneumonia Care				
Appropriate Initial Antibiotic Given	369	97%	95%	95%
Blood Culture Timing	541	98%	98%	98%
Pregnancy and Delivery Care				
Newborn Deliveries Scheduled Early	216	13%	7%	6%
Preventive Care				
Immunization for Influenza[2]	637	89%	90%	90%
Immunization for Pneumonia[2]	864	88%	92%	92%
Stroke Care				
Anticoagulation Therapy for Atrial Fibrillation	13	92%	96%	95%
Antithrombotic Therapy Timing	129	95%	98%	98%
Assessed for Rehabilitation	142	91%	98%	97%
Discharged on Antithrombotic Therapy	127	99%	99%	99%
Discharged on Statin Medication	105	91%	95%	94%
Thrombolytic Therapy Timing	19	0%	68%	66%
Venous Thromboembolism Prophylaxis	135	58%	94%	94%
Written Stroke Educational Materials Given	74	27%	92%	88%
Surgical Care Improvement Project				
Appropriate Beta Blocker Usage	350	98%	98%	98%
Appropriate VTP Within 24 Hours	999	97%	98%	98%
Controlled Postoperative Blood Glucose	188	93%	96%	97%
Perioperative Temperature Management	1,270	100%	100%	100%
Prophylactic Antibiotic Selection	702	99%	99%	99%
Prophylactic Antibiotic Selection (Outpatient)	463	92%	98%	98%
Prophylactic Antibiotic Stopped	691	99%	98%	98%
Prophylactic Antibiotic Timing	702	99%	99%	99%
Prophylactic Antibiotic Timing (Outpatient)	469	97%	98%	98%
Urinary Catheter Removal	639	98%	98%	97%
Survey of Patients' Hospital Experiences				
Area Around Room 'Always' Quiet at Night	300+	62%	68%	61%
Doctors 'Always' Communicated Well	300+	81%	83%	82%
Home Recovery Information Given	300+	85%	85%	85%
Hospital Given 9 or 10 on 10 Point Scale	300+	71%	73%	71%
Meds 'Always' Explained Before Given	300+	61%	66%	64%
Nurses 'Always' Communicated Well	300+	78%	80%	79%
Pain 'Always' Well Controlled	300+	70%	72%	71%
Room and Bathroom 'Always' Clean	300+	70%	75%	73%
Timely Help 'Always' Received	300+	64%	69%	68%
Would Definitely Recommend Hospital	300+	73%	73%	71%
Use of Medical Imaging				
Cardiac Imaging Stress Test before Surgery	305	7.9%	5.3%	5.3%
Combination Abdominal CT Scan	1,596	5.5%	16.4%	10.5%
Combination Brain/Sinus CT Scan	1,684	2.7%	2.7%	2.7%
Combination Chest CT Scan	424	2.8%	5.6%	2.7%
Follow-up Mammogram/Ultrasound	1,931	3.2%	7.9%	8.8%
Lumbar Spine MRI for Low Back Pain	182	34.6%	39.6%	37.2%

Foundation Surgical Hospital of San Antonio

9522 Huebner Road Phone: 210-478-5400
San Antonio, TX 78240
URL: www.fshsanantonio.com
Type: Acute Care Hospitals Emergency Services: Yes
Ownership: Proprietary

Measure	Cases	This Hosp.	State Avg.	U.S. Avg.
Blood Clot Prevention and Treatment				
Anticoagulation Overlap Therapy[2,7]	-	-	93%	93%
ICU Venous Thromboembolism Prophylaxis[2,7]	-	-	92%	92%
Incidence of Potentially Preventable VTE[2,7]	-	-	9%	10%
UFH with Dosages/Platelet Monitoring[2,7]	-	-	96%	97%
Venous Thromboembolism Prophylaxis[2]	100	100%	82%	85%
Warfarin Therapy Discharge Instructions[2,7]	-	-	84%	75%
Chest Pain/Possible Heart Attack Care				
Aspirin Given Within 24 Hours of Arrival[5]	-	-	94%	96%
Fibrinolytic Meds Within 30 Min. of Arrival[5]	-	-	47%	58%
Average Time to ECG (minutes)[5]	-	-	8	7
Average Time to Transfer (minutes)[5]	-	-	62	60
Children's Asthma Care				
Received Home Management Plan of Care	-	-	93%	88%
Received Reliever Medication	-	-	100%	100%
Received Systemic Corticosteroids	-	-	100%	100%
Emergency Department				
Admittance Decision Time (minutes)[1,2]	-	-	99	98
Head CT Results Within 45 Min. of Arrival[5]	-	-	54%	57%
Patients Who Left ER Before Being Seen	186	1%	3%	2%
Time from ER Arrival to Admit. (minutes)[1,2]	-	-	270	274
Time from ER Arrival to Discharge (minutes)	230	95	127	134
Time in ER Before Being Evaluated (minutes)	200	30	26	26
Time to Pain Meds for Fractures (minutes)[5]	-	-	57	57
Heart Attack Care				
Aspirin Given at Discharge[5]	-	-	99%	99%
Fibrinolytic Meds Within 30 Min. of Arrival[5]	-	-	49%	54%
PCI Within 90 Minutes of Arrival[5]	-	-	95%	96%
Statin Prescribed at Discharge[5]	-	-	98%	98%
Heart Failure Care				
ACE Inhibitor or ARB for LVSD[5]	-	-	97%	97%
Discharge Instructions Given[5]	-	-	95%	94%
Evaluation of LVS Function[5]	-	-	99%	99%
Medicare Spending				
Medicare Spending per Patient (ratio)	-	1.19	1.03	0.98
Pneumonia Care				
Appropriate Initial Antibiotic Given[5]	-	-	95%	95%
Blood Culture Timing[5]	-	-	98%	98%
Pregnancy and Delivery Care				
Newborn Deliveries Scheduled Early[7]	-	-	7%	6%
Preventive Care				
Immunization for Influenza[2]	305	63%	90%	90%
Immunization for Pneumonia[2]	121	74%	92%	92%
Stroke Care				
Anticoagulation Therapy for Atrial Fibrillation[5]	-	-	96%	95%
Antithrombotic Therapy Timing[5]	-	-	98%	98%
Assessed for Rehabilitation[5]	-	-	98%	97%
Discharged on Antithrombotic Therapy[5]	-	-	99%	99%
Discharged on Statin Medication[5]	-	-	95%	94%
Thrombolytic Therapy Timing[5]	-	-	68%	66%
Venous Thromboembolism Prophylaxis[5]	-	-	94%	94%
Written Stroke Educational Materials Given[5]	-	-	92%	88%
Surgical Care Improvement Project				
Appropriate Beta Blocker Usage[2]	17	88%	98%	98%
Appropriate VTP Within 24 Hours[2]	119	100%	98%	98%
Controlled Postoperative Blood Glucose[2,7]	-	-	96%	97%
Perioperative Temperature Management[2]	123	100%	100%	100%
Prophylactic Antibiotic Selection[2]	37	100%	99%	99%
Prophylactic Antibiotic Selection (Outpatient)	22	91%	98%	98%
Prophylactic Antibiotic Stopped[2]	36	94%	98%	98%
Prophylactic Antibiotic Timing[2]	37	97%	99%	99%
Prophylactic Antibiotic Timing (Outpatient)	22	100%	98%	98%
Urinary Catheter Removal[2]	41	80%	98%	97%
Survey of Patients' Hospital Experiences				
Area Around Room 'Always' Quiet at Night	300+	85%	68%	61%

NOTE: Hospital profiles are in alphabetical order by state, then city, then hospital within the city; Rankings exclude hospitals with less than 25 cases except for patient surveys which excludes hospitals with less than 100 cases; (a) 100-299 cases; (1) The number of cases/patients is too few to report; (2) Data submitted were based on a sample of cases/patients; (3) Results are based on a shorter time period than required; (4) Data suppressed by CMS for one or more quarters; (5) Results are not available for this reporting period; (6) Fewer than 100 patients completed the HCAHPS survey; (7) No cases met the criteria for this measure; (8) The lower limit of the confidence interval cannot be calculated if the number of observed infections equals zero; (9) No data are available from the state/territory for this reporting period; (10) The scores shown reflect fewer than 50 completed surveys; (11) There were discrepancies in the data collection process; (12) This measure does not apply to this hospital for this reporting period; (13) Results cannot be calculated for this reporting period; (14) The results for this state are combined with nearby states to protect confidentiality; Please refer to the User's Guide for a full explanation of data.

Measure	Cases	This Hosp.	State Avg.	U.S. Avg.
Doctors 'Always' Communicated Well	300+	86%	83%	82%
Home Recovery Information Given	300+	87%	85%	85%
Hospital Given 9 or 10 on 10 Point Scale	300+	85%	73%	71%
Meds 'Always' Explained Before Given	300+	72%	66%	64%
Nurses 'Always' Communicated Well	300+	85%	80%	79%
Pain 'Always' Well Controlled	300+	77%	72%	71%
Room and Bathroom 'Always' Clean	300+	78%	75%	73%
Timely Help 'Always' Received	300+	81%	69%	68%
Would Definitely Recommend Hospital	300+	86%	73%	71%
Use of Medical Imaging				
Cardiac Imaging Stress Test before Surgery[7]	-	-	5.3%	5.3%
Combination Abdominal CT Scan[1]	-	-	16.4%	10.5%
Combination Brain/Sinus CT Scan[1]	-	-	2.7%	2.7%
Combination Chest CT Scan[7]	-	-	5.6%	2.7%
Follow-up Mammogram/Ultrasound[7]	-	-	7.9%	8.8%
Lumbar Spine MRI for Low Back Pain[7]	-	-	39.6%	37.2%

Innova Hospital San Antonio

4243 Southcross Blvd Phone: 210-368-7487
San Antonio, TX 78222
Type: Acute Care Hospitals Emergency Services: Yes
Ownership: Proprietary

Measure	Cases	This Hosp.	State Avg.	U.S. Avg.
Blood Clot Prevention and Treatment				
Anticoagulation Overlap Therapy[5]	-	-	93%	93%
ICU Venous Thromboembolism Prophylaxis[5]	-	-	92%	92%
Incidence of Potentially Preventable VTE[5]	-	-	9%	10%
UFH with Dosages/Platelet Monitoring[5]	-	-	96%	97%
Venous Thromboembolism Prophylaxis[5]	-	-	82%	85%
Warfarin Therapy Discharge Instructions[5]	-	-	84%	75%
Chest Pain/Possible Heart Attack Care				
Aspirin Given Within 24 Hours of Arrival	-	-	94%	96%
Fibrinolytic Meds Within 30 Min. of Arrival	-	-	47%	58%
Average Time to ECG (minutes)	-	-	8	7
Average Time to Transfer (minutes)	-	-	62	60
Children's Asthma Care				
Received Home Management Plan of Care	-	-	93%	88%
Received Reliever Medication	-	-	100%	100%
Received Systemic Corticosteroids	-	-	100%	100%
Emergency Department				
Admittance Decision Time (minutes)[5]	-	-	99	98
Head CT Results Within 45 Min. of Arrival	-	-	54%	57%
Patients Who Left ER Before Being Seen	-	-	3%	2%
Time from ER Arrival to Admit. (minutes)[5]	-	-	270	274
Time from ER Arrival to Discharge (minutes)	-	-	127	134
Time in ER Before Being Evaluated (minutes)	-	-	26	26
Time to Pain Meds for Fractures (minutes)	-	-	57	57
Heart Attack Care				
Aspirin Given at Discharge[5]	-	-	99%	99%
Fibrinolytic Meds Within 30 Min. of Arrival[5]	-	-	49%	54%
PCI Within 90 Minutes of Arrival[5]	-	-	95%	96%
Statin Prescribed at Discharge[5]	-	-	98%	98%
Heart Failure Care				
ACE Inhibitor or ARB for LVSD[5]	-	-	97%	97%
Discharge Instructions Given[5]	-	-	95%	94%
Evaluation of LVS Function[5]	-	-	99%	99%
Medicare Spending				
Medicare Spending per Patient (ratio)[1]	-	-	1.03	0.98
Pneumonia Care				
Appropriate Initial Antibiotic Given[5]	-	-	95%	95%
Blood Culture Timing[5]	-	-	98%	98%
Pregnancy and Delivery Care				
Newborn Deliveries Scheduled Early[5]	-	-	7%	6%
Preventive Care				
Immunization for Influenza[5]	-	-	90%	90%
Immunization for Pneumonia[5]	-	-	92%	92%
Stroke Care				
Anticoagulation Therapy for Atrial Fibrillation[5]	-	-	96%	95%
Antithrombotic Therapy Timing[5]	-	-	98%	98%
Assessed for Rehabilitation[5]	-	-	98%	97%
Discharged on Antithrombotic Therapy[5]	-	-	99%	99%
Discharged on Statin Medication[5]	-	-	95%	94%
Thrombolytic Therapy Timing[5]	-	-	68%	66%
Venous Thromboembolism Prophylaxis[5]	-	-	94%	94%
Written Stroke Educational Materials Given[5]	-	-	92%	88%
Surgical Care Improvement Project				
Appropriate Beta Blocker Usage[5]	-	-	98%	98%
Appropriate VTP Within 24 Hours[5]	-	-	98%	98%
Controlled Postoperative Blood Glucose[5]	-	-	96%	97%
Perioperative Temperature Management[5]	-	-	100%	100%
Prophylactic Antibiotic Selection[5]	-	-	99%	99%
Prophylactic Antibiotic Selection (Outpatient)	-	-	98%	98%
Prophylactic Antibiotic Stopped[5]	-	-	98%	98%
Prophylactic Antibiotic Timing[5]	-	-	99%	99%
Prophylactic Antibiotic Timing (Outpatient)	-	-	98%	98%
Urinary Catheter Removal[5]	-	-	98%	97%
Survey of Patients' Hospital Experiences				
Area Around Room 'Always' Quiet at Night[5]	-	-	68%	61%
Doctors 'Always' Communicated Well[5]	-	-	83%	82%
Home Recovery Information Given[5]	-	-	85%	85%
Hospital Given 9 or 10 on 10 Point Scale[5]	-	-	73%	71%
Meds 'Always' Explained Before Given[5]	-	-	66%	64%
Nurses 'Always' Communicated Well[5]	-	-	80%	79%
Pain 'Always' Well Controlled[5]	-	-	72%	71%
Room and Bathroom 'Always' Clean[5]	-	-	75%	73%
Timely Help 'Always' Received[5]	-	-	69%	68%
Would Definitely Recommend Hospital[5]	-	-	73%	71%
Use of Medical Imaging				
Cardiac Imaging Stress Test before Surgery	-	-	5.3%	5.3%
Combination Abdominal CT Scan	-	-	16.4%	10.5%
Combination Brain/Sinus CT Scan	-	-	2.7%	2.7%
Combination Chest CT Scan	-	-	5.6%	2.7%
Follow-up Mammogram/Ultrasound	-	-	7.9%	8.8%
Lumbar Spine MRI for Low Back Pain	-	-	39.6%	37.2%

Methodist Ambulatory Surgery Hospital NW

9150 Huebner Rd Suite 100 Phone: 210-575-5000
San Antonio, TX 78240
Type: Acute Care Hospitals Emergency Services: Yes
Ownership: Proprietary
Key Personnel:
CEO/President. . . . . Jaime Wesolowski

Measure	Cases	This Hosp.	State Avg.	U.S. Avg.
Blood Clot Prevention and Treatment				
Anticoagulation Overlap Therapy[2,7]	-	-	93%	93%
ICU Venous Thromboembolism Prophylaxis[2,7]	-	-	92%	92%
Incidence of Potentially Preventable VTE[2,7]	-	-	9%	10%
UFH with Dosages/Platelet Monitoring[2,7]	-	-	96%	97%
Venous Thromboembolism Prophylaxis[2]	43	100%	82%	85%
Warfarin Therapy Discharge Instructions[2,7]	-	-	84%	75%
Chest Pain/Possible Heart Attack Care				
Aspirin Given Within 24 Hours of Arrival[1,3]	-	-	94%	96%
Fibrinolytic Meds Within 30 Min. of Arrival[5]	-	-	47%	58%
Average Time to ECG (minutes)[1,3]	-	-	8	7
Average Time to Transfer (minutes)[5]	-	-	62	60
Children's Asthma Care				
Received Home Management Plan of Care	-	-	93%	88%
Received Reliever Medication	-	-	100%	100%
Received Systemic Corticosteroids	-	-	100%	100%
Emergency Department				
Admittance Decision Time (minutes)[1,2]	-	-	99	98
Head CT Results Within 45 Min. of Arrival[5]	-	-	54%	57%
Patients Who Left ER Before Being Seen	858	1%	3%	2%
Time from ER Arrival to Admit. (minutes)[1,2]	-	-	270	274
Time from ER Arrival to Discharge (minutes)	252	57	127	134
Time in ER Before Being Evaluated (minutes)	264	10	26	26
Time to Pain Meds for Fractures (minutes)[1,3]	-	-	57	57
Heart Attack Care				
Aspirin Given at Discharge[5]	-	-	99%	99%
Fibrinolytic Meds Within 30 Min. of Arrival[5]	-	-	49%	54%
PCI Within 90 Minutes of Arrival[5]	-	-	95%	96%
Statin Prescribed at Discharge[5]	-	-	98%	98%
Heart Failure Care				
ACE Inhibitor or ARB for LVSD[5]	-	-	97%	97%
Discharge Instructions Given[5]	-	-	95%	94%
Evaluation of LVS Function[5]	-	-	99%	99%
Medicare Spending				
Medicare Spending per Patient (ratio)	-	1.01	1.03	0.98
Pneumonia Care				
Appropriate Initial Antibiotic Given[5]	-	-	95%	95%
Blood Culture Timing[5]	-	-	98%	98%
Pregnancy and Delivery Care				
Newborn Deliveries Scheduled Early[2,7]	-	-	7%	6%
Preventive Care				
Immunization for Influenza[2]	303	99%	90%	90%
Immunization for Pneumonia[2]	342	99%	92%	92%
Stroke Care				
Anticoagulation Therapy for Atrial Fibrillation[5]	-	-	96%	95%
Antithrombotic Therapy Timing[5]	-	-	98%	98%
Assessed for Rehabilitation[5]	-	-	98%	97%
Discharged on Antithrombotic Therapy[5]	-	-	99%	99%
Discharged on Statin Medication[5]	-	-	95%	94%
Thrombolytic Therapy Timing[5]	-	-	68%	66%
Venous Thromboembolism Prophylaxis[5]	-	-	94%	94%
Written Stroke Educational Materials Given[5]	-	-	92%	88%
Surgical Care Improvement Project				
Appropriate Beta Blocker Usage[2]	38	97%	98%	98%
Appropriate VTP Within 24 Hours[2]	197	100%	98%	98%
Controlled Postoperative Blood Glucose[2,7]	-	-	96%	97%
Perioperative Temperature Management[2]	207	100%	100%	100%
Prophylactic Antibiotic Selection[2]	161	100%	99%	99%
Prophylactic Antibiotic Selection (Outpatient)	40	100%	98%	98%
Prophylactic Antibiotic Stopped[2]	157	97%	98%	98%
Prophylactic Antibiotic Timing[2]	161	100%	99%	99%
Prophylactic Antibiotic Timing (Outpatient)	40	100%	98%	98%
Urinary Catheter Removal[2]	59	100%	98%	97%
Survey of Patients' Hospital Experiences				
Area Around Room 'Always' Quiet at Night	(a)	81%	68%	61%
Doctors 'Always' Communicated Well	(a)	83%	83%	82%
Home Recovery Information Given	(a)	88%	85%	85%
Hospital Given 9 or 10 on 10 Point Scale	(a)	80%	73%	71%
Meds 'Always' Explained Before Given	(a)	70%	66%	64%
Nurses 'Always' Communicated Well	(a)	83%	80%	79%
Pain 'Always' Well Controlled	(a)	73%	72%	71%
Room and Bathroom 'Always' Clean	(a)	79%	75%	73%
Timely Help 'Always' Received	(a)	73%	69%	68%
Would Definitely Recommend Hospital	(a)	81%	73%	71%
Use of Medical Imaging				
Cardiac Imaging Stress Test before Surgery[7]	-	-	5.3%	5.3%
Combination Abdominal CT Scan[7]	-	-	16.4%	10.5%
Combination Brain/Sinus CT Scan[7]	-	-	2.7%	2.7%
Combination Chest CT Scan[7]	-	-	5.6%	2.7%
Follow-up Mammogram/Ultrasound[7]	-	-	7.9%	8.8%
Lumbar Spine MRI for Low Back Pain[7]	-	-	39.6%	37.2%

Methodist Hospital

7700 Floyd Curl Dr Phone: 210-575-4000
San Antonio, TX 78229 Fax: 210-575-0246
URL: www.mh.sahealth.com
Type: Acute Care Hospitals Emergency Services: Yes
Ownership: Proprietary Beds: 683
Key Personnel:
Operating Room. . . . . James Ashcoft
Emergency Room . . . . Ruby Jason, RN
Quality Assurance . . . . Tim Klein
Intensive Care Unit. . . . . J Pitcock
Infection Control. . . . . Cecil Robinson
CEO/President. . . . . Jaime Wesolowski

Measure	Cases	This Hosp.	State Avg.	U.S. Avg.
Blood Clot Prevention and Treatment				
Anticoagulation Overlap Therapy[2]	310	97%	93%	93%
ICU Venous Thromboembolism Prophylaxis[2]	126	99%	92%	92%
Incidence of Potentially Preventable VTE[2]	86	3%	9%	10%
UFH with Dosages/Platelet Monitoring[2]	126	100%	96%	97%
Venous Thromboembolism Prophylaxis[2]	438	94%	82%	85%
Warfarin Therapy Discharge Instructions[2]	230	97%	84%	75%
Chest Pain/Possible Heart Attack Care				
Aspirin Given Within 24 Hours of Arrival	40	98%	94%	96%

NOTE: Hospital profiles are in alphabetical order by state, then city, then hospital within the city; Rankings exclude hospitals with less than 25 cases except for patient surveys which excludes hospitals with less than 100 cases; (a) 100-299 cases; (1) The number of cases/patients is too few to report; (2) Data submitted were based on a sample of cases/patients; (3) Results are based on a shorter time period than required; (4) Data suppressed by CMS for one or more quarters; (5) Results are not available for this reporting period; (6) Fewer than 100 patients completed the HCAHPS survey; (7) No cases met the criteria for this measure; (8) The lower limit of the confidence interval cannot be calculated if the number of observed infections equals zero; (9) No data are available from the state/territory for this reporting period; (10) The scores shown reflect fewer than 50 completed surveys; (11) There were discrepancies in the data collection process; (12) This measure does not apply to this hospital for this reporting period; (13) Results cannot be calculated for this reporting period; (14) The results for this state are combined with nearby states to protect confidentiality; Please refer to the User's Guide for a full explanation of data.

Measure	Cases	This Hosp.	State Avg.	U.S. Avg.
Fibrinolytic Meds Within 30 Min. of Arrival[7]	-	-	47%	58%
Average Time to ECG (minutes)	40	4	8	7
Average Time to Transfer (minutes)[1]	-	-	62	60
Children's Asthma Care				
Received Home Management Plan of Care	523	98%	93%	88%
Received Reliever Medication	523	100%	100%	100%
Received Systemic Corticosteroids	522	100%	100%	100%
Emergency Department				
Admittance Decision Time (minutes)[2]	585	103	99	98
Head CT Results Within 45 Min. of Arrival	39	87%	54%	57%
Patients Who Left ER Before Being Seen	>100k	1%	3%	2%
Time from ER Arrival to Admit. (minutes)[2]	595	291	270	274
Time from ER Arrival to Discharge (minutes)	500	138	127	134
Time in ER Before Being Evaluated (minutes)	523	13	26	26
Time to Pain Meds for Fractures (minutes)	502	50	57	57
Heart Attack Care				
Aspirin Given at Discharge	1,317	100%	99%	99%
Fibrinolytic Meds Within 30 Min. of Arrival[7]	-	-	49%	54%
PCI Within 90 Minutes of Arrival	182	96%	95%	96%
Statin Prescribed at Discharge	1,307	100%	98%	98%
Heart Failure Care				
ACE Inhibitor or ARB for LVSD	522	99%	97%	97%
Discharge Instructions Given	1,250	96%	95%	94%
Evaluation of LVS Function	1,537	100%	99%	99%
Medicare Spending				
Medicare Spending per Patient (ratio)	-	1.04	1.03	0.98
Pneumonia Care				
Appropriate Initial Antibiotic Given	673	98%	95%	95%
Blood Culture Timing	1,244	99%	98%	98%
Pregnancy and Delivery Care				
Newborn Deliveries Scheduled Early[2]	144	1%	7%	6%
Preventive Care				
Immunization for Influenza[2]	631	98%	90%	90%
Immunization for Pneumonia[2]	671	99%	92%	92%
Stroke Care				
Anticoagulation Therapy for Atrial Fibrillation	107	99%	96%	95%
Antithrombotic Therapy Timing	640	98%	98%	98%
Assessed for Rehabilitation	835	100%	98%	97%
Discharged on Antithrombotic Therapy	666	100%	99%	99%
Discharged on Statin Medication	514	99%	95%	94%
Thrombolytic Therapy Timing	32	97%	68%	66%
Venous Thromboembolism Prophylaxis	889	100%	94%	94%
Written Stroke Educational Materials Given	412	98%	92%	88%
Surgical Care Improvement Project				
Appropriate Beta Blocker Usage[2]	393	99%	98%	98%
Appropriate VTP Within 24 Hours[2]	684	98%	98%	98%
Controlled Postoperative Blood Glucose[2]	212	98%	96%	97%
Perioperative Temperature Management[2]	907	100%	100%	100%
Prophylactic Antibiotic Selection[2]	704	99%	99%	99%
Prophylactic Antibiotic Selection (Outpatient)	1,068	100%	98%	98%
Prophylactic Antibiotic Stopped[2]	679	99%	98%	98%
Prophylactic Antibiotic Timing[2]	708	99%	99%	99%
Prophylactic Antibiotic Timing (Outpatient)	1,068	100%	98%	98%
Urinary Catheter Removal[2]	399	98%	98%	97%
Survey of Patients' Hospital Experiences				
Area Around Room 'Always' Quiet at Night	300+	61%	68%	61%
Doctors 'Always' Communicated Well	300+	80%	83%	82%
Home Recovery Information Given	300+	85%	85%	85%
Hospital Given 9 or 10 on 10 Point Scale	300+	69%	73%	71%
Meds 'Always' Explained Before Given	300+	62%	66%	64%
Nurses 'Always' Communicated Well	300+	75%	80%	79%
Pain 'Always' Well Controlled	300+	70%	72%	71%
Room and Bathroom 'Always' Clean	300+	69%	75%	73%
Timely Help 'Always' Received	300+	59%	69%	68%
Would Definitely Recommend Hospital	300+	71%	73%	71%
Use of Medical Imaging				
Cardiac Imaging Stress Test before Surgery	3,598	5.4%	5.3%	5.3%
Combination Abdominal CT Scan	2,332	6.7%	16.4%	10.5%
Combination Brain/Sinus CT Scan	2,853	3.7%	2.7%	2.7%
Combination Chest CT Scan	880	0.6%	5.6%	2.7%
Follow-up Mammogram/Ultrasound[7]	-	-	7.9%	8.8%
Lumbar Spine MRI for Low Back Pain[1]	-	-	39.6%	37.2%

Methodist Stone Oak Hospital

1139 E Sonterra Blvd
San Antonio, TX 78258
Phone: 210-638-2100
URL: www.stoneoakhealth.com
Type: Acute Care Hospitals
Ownership: Proprietary
Emergency Services: Yes
Beds: 132
Key Personnel:
CEO . . . . Dean M Alexander, FACHE

Measure	Cases	This Hosp.	State Avg.	U.S. Avg.
Blood Clot Prevention and Treatment				
Anticoagulation Overlap Therapy[2]	41	100%	93%	93%
ICU Venous Thromboembolism Prophylaxis[2]	93	100%	92%	92%
Incidence of Potentially Preventable VTE[1,2]	-	-	9%	10%
UFH with Dosages/Platelet Monitoring[2]	17	100%	96%	97%
Venous Thromboembolism Prophylaxis[2]	331	100%	82%	85%
Warfarin Therapy Discharge Instructions[2]	34	100%	84%	75%
Chest Pain/Possible Heart Attack Care				
Aspirin Given Within 24 Hours of Arrival[1,3]	-	-	94%	96%
Fibrinolytic Meds Within 30 Min. of Arrival[3,7]	-	-	47%	58%
Average Time to ECG (minutes)[1,3]	-	-	8	7
Average Time to Transfer (minutes)[3,7]	-	-	62	60
Children's Asthma Care				
Received Home Management Plan of Care	-	-	93%	88%
Received Reliever Medication	-	-	100%	100%
Received Systemic Corticosteroids	-	-	100%	100%
Emergency Department				
Admittance Decision Time (minutes)[2]	412	78	99	98
Head CT Results Within 45 Min. of Arrival[1]	-	-	54%	57%
Patients Who Left ER Before Being Seen	22,998	1%	3%	2%
Time from ER Arrival to Admit. (minutes)[2]	413	252	270	274
Time from ER Arrival to Discharge (minutes)	446	176	127	134
Time in ER Before Being Evaluated (minutes)	487	13	26	26
Time to Pain Meds for Fractures (minutes)	110	56	57	57
Heart Attack Care				
Aspirin Given at Discharge[2]	142	100%	99%	99%
Fibrinolytic Meds Within 30 Min. of Arrival[2,7]	-	-	49%	54%
PCI Within 90 Minutes of Arrival[2]	21	95%	95%	96%
Statin Prescribed at Discharge[2]	136	100%	98%	98%
Heart Failure Care				
ACE Inhibitor or ARB for LVSD[2]	22	100%	97%	97%
Discharge Instructions Given[2]	83	99%	95%	94%
Evaluation of LVS Function[2]	109	100%	99%	99%
Medicare Spending				
Medicare Spending per Patient (ratio)	-	1.07	1.03	0.98
Pneumonia Care				
Appropriate Initial Antibiotic Given[2]	65	98%	95%	95%
Blood Culture Timing[2]	92	100%	98%	98%
Pregnancy and Delivery Care				
Newborn Deliveries Scheduled Early[2]	43	2%	7%	6%
Preventive Care				
Immunization for Influenza[2]	524	100%	90%	90%
Immunization for Pneumonia[2]	528	100%	92%	92%
Stroke Care				
Anticoagulation Therapy for Atrial Fibrillation[1,2]	-	-	96%	95%
Antithrombotic Therapy Timing[2]	98	99%	98%	98%
Assessed for Rehabilitation[2]	121	100%	98%	97%
Discharged on Antithrombotic Therapy[2]	107	100%	99%	99%
Discharged on Statin Medication[2]	82	100%	95%	94%
Thrombolytic Therapy Timing[1,2]	-	-	68%	66%
Venous Thromboembolism Prophylaxis[2]	118	100%	94%	94%
Written Stroke Educational Materials Given[2]	70	99%	92%	88%
Surgical Care Improvement Project				
Appropriate Beta Blocker Usage[2]	189	98%	98%	98%
Appropriate VTP Within 24 Hours[2]	381	100%	98%	98%
Controlled Postoperative Blood Glucose[2]	83	95%	96%	97%
Perioperative Temperature Management[2]	514	100%	100%	100%
Prophylactic Antibiotic Selection[2]	380	99%	99%	99%
Prophylactic Antibiotic Selection (Outpatient)	593	99%	98%	98%
Prophylactic Antibiotic Stopped[2]	361	100%	98%	98%
Prophylactic Antibiotic Timing[2]	380	99%	99%	99%
Prophylactic Antibiotic Timing (Outpatient)	593	100%	98%	98%
Urinary Catheter Removal[2]	334	100%	98%	97%
Survey of Patients' Hospital Experiences				
Area Around Room 'Always' Quiet at Night	300+	68%	68%	61%
Doctors 'Always' Communicated Well	300+	79%	83%	82%
Home Recovery Information Given	300+	85%	85%	85%
Hospital Given 9 or 10 on 10 Point Scale	300+	73%	73%	71%
Meds 'Always' Explained Before Given	300+	59%	66%	64%
Nurses 'Always' Communicated Well	300+	74%	80%	79%
Pain 'Always' Well Controlled	300+	68%	72%	71%
Room and Bathroom 'Always' Clean	300+	75%	75%	73%
Timely Help 'Always' Received	300+	57%	69%	68%
Would Definitely Recommend Hospital	300+	74%	73%	71%
Use of Medical Imaging				
Cardiac Imaging Stress Test before Surgery	174	7.5%	5.3%	5.3%
Combination Abdominal CT Scan	352	0.6%	16.4%	10.5%
Combination Brain/Sinus CT Scan[1]	-	-	2.7%	2.7%
Combination Chest CT Scan	56	0.0%	5.6%	2.7%
Follow-up Mammogram/Ultrasound[7]	-	-	7.9%	8.8%
Lumbar Spine MRI for Low Back Pain[1]	-	-	39.6%	37.2%

Nix Health Care System

414 Navarro, Suite 600
San Antonio, TX 78205
Phone: 210-271-2188
Fax: 210-271-2023
E-mail: nmc@nixhealth.com
URL: www.nixhealth.com
Type: Acute Care Hospitals
Ownership: Proprietary
Emergency Services: Yes
Beds: 292
Key Personnel:
CEO/President. . . . . John F. Strieby

Measure	Cases	This Hosp.	State Avg.	U.S. Avg.
Blood Clot Prevention and Treatment				
Anticoagulation Overlap Therapy[2]	24	100%	93%	93%
ICU Venous Thromboembolism Prophylaxis[2]	60	75%	92%	92%
Incidence of Potentially Preventable VTE[1,2]	-	-	9%	10%
UFH with Dosages/Platelet Monitoring[1,2]	-	-	96%	97%
Venous Thromboembolism Prophylaxis[2]	258	70%	82%	85%
Warfarin Therapy Discharge Instructions[2]	13	23%	84%	75%
Chest Pain/Possible Heart Attack Care				
Aspirin Given Within 24 Hours of Arrival[5]	-	-	94%	96%
Fibrinolytic Meds Within 30 Min. of Arrival[5]	-	-	47%	58%
Average Time to ECG (minutes)[5]	-	-	8	7
Average Time to Transfer (minutes)[5]	-	-	62	60
Children's Asthma Care				
Received Home Management Plan of Care	-	-	93%	88%
Received Reliever Medication	-	-	100%	100%
Received Systemic Corticosteroids	-	-	100%	100%
Emergency Department				
Admittance Decision Time (minutes)[2]	60	68	99	98
Head CT Results Within 45 Min. of Arrival[3,7]	-	-	54%	57%
Patients Who Left ER Before Being Seen[5]	-	-	3%	2%
Time from ER Arrival to Admit. (minutes)[2]	110	212	270	274
Time from ER Arrival to Discharge (minutes)[3]	544	92	127	134
Time in ER Before Being Evaluated (minutes)[3]	511	13	26	26
Time to Pain Meds for Fractures (minutes)[3]	23	54	57	57
Heart Attack Care				
Aspirin Given at Discharge	37	100%	99%	99%
Fibrinolytic Meds Within 30 Min. of Arrival[7]	-	-	49%	54%
PCI Within 90 Minutes of Arrival[7]	-	-	95%	96%
Statin Prescribed at Discharge	35	100%	98%	98%
Heart Failure Care				
ACE Inhibitor or ARB for LVSD	22	100%	97%	97%
Discharge Instructions Given	71	90%	95%	94%
Evaluation of LVS Function	100	99%	99%	99%
Medicare Spending				
Medicare Spending per Patient (ratio)	-	1.01	1.03	0.98
Pneumonia Care				
Appropriate Initial Antibiotic Given	42	90%	95%	95%
Blood Culture Timing	43	98%	98%	98%
Pregnancy and Delivery Care				
Newborn Deliveries Scheduled Early[7]	-	-	7%	6%
Preventive Care				
Immunization for Influenza[2]	788	95%	90%	90%
Immunization for Pneumonia[2]	660	95%	92%	92%
Stroke Care				
Anticoagulation Therapy for Atrial Fibrillation[1]	-	-	96%	95%

NOTE: Hospital profiles are in alphabetical order by state, then city, then hospital within the city; Rankings exclude hospitals with less than 25 cases except for patient surveys which excludes hospitals with less than 100 cases; (a) 100-299 cases; (1) The number of cases/patients is too few to report; (2) Data submitted were based on a sample of cases/patients; (3) Results are based on a shorter time period than required; (4) Data suppressed by CMS for one or more quarters; (5) Results are not available for this reporting period; (6) Fewer than 100 patients completed the HCAHPS survey; (7) No cases met the criteria for this measure; (8) The lower limit of the confidence interval cannot be calculated if the number of observed infections equals zero; (9) No data are available from the state/territory for this reporting period; (10) The scores shown reflect fewer than 50 completed surveys; (11) There were discrepancies in the data collection process; (12) This measure does not apply to this hospital for this reporting period; (13) Results cannot be calculated for this reporting period; (14) The results for this state are combined with nearby states to protect confidentiality; Please refer to the User's Guide for a full explanation of data.

Antithrombotic Therapy Timing	25	96%	98%	98%
Assessed for Rehabilitation	23	96%	98%	97%
Discharged on Antithrombotic Therapy	22	100%	99%	99%
Discharged on Statin Medication	20	95%	95%	94%
Thrombolytic Therapy Timing[1]	-	-	68%	66%
Venous Thromboembolism Prophylaxis	28	79%	94%	94%
Written Stroke Educational Materials Given	11	0%	92%	88%
Surgical Care Improvement Project				
Appropriate Beta Blocker Usage	85	96%	98%	98%
Appropriate VTP Within 24 Hours	293	96%	98%	98%
Controlled Postoperative Blood Glucose	14	100%	96%	97%
Perioperative Temperature Management	311	100%	100%	100%
Prophylactic Antibiotic Selection	186	98%	99%	99%
Prophylactic Antibiotic Selection (Outpatient)	108	99%	98%	98%
Prophylactic Antibiotic Stopped	185	99%	98%	98%
Prophylactic Antibiotic Timing	186	99%	99%	99%
Prophylactic Antibiotic Timing (Outpatient)	108	96%	98%	98%
Urinary Catheter Removal	180	96%	98%	97%
Survey of Patients' Hospital Experiences				
Area Around Room 'Always' Quiet at Night	300+	61%	68%	61%
Doctors 'Always' Communicated Well	300+	81%	83%	82%
Home Recovery Information Given	300+	81%	85%	85%
Hospital Given 9 or 10 on 10 Point Scale	300+	71%	73%	71%
Meds 'Always' Explained Before Given	300+	63%	66%	64%
Nurses 'Always' Communicated Well	300+	74%	80%	79%
Pain 'Always' Well Controlled	300+	69%	72%	71%
Room and Bathroom 'Always' Clean	300+	76%	75%	73%
Timely Help 'Always' Received	300+	54%	69%	68%
Would Definitely Recommend Hospital	300+	70%	73%	71%
Use of Medical Imaging				
Cardiac Imaging Stress Test before Surgery	185	8.1%	5.3%	5.3%
Combination Abdominal CT Scan	227	14.1%	16.4%	10.5%
Combination Brain/Sinus CT Scan[1]	-	-	2.7%	2.7%
Combination Chest CT Scan	76	5.3%	5.6%	2.7%
Follow-up Mammogram/Ultrasound	887	7.9%	7.9%	8.8%
Lumbar Spine MRI for Low Back Pain	52	46.2%	39.6%	37.2%

San Antonio VA Medical Center

7400 Merton Minter Blvd. Phone: 210-617-5300
San Antonio, TX 78229 Fax: 210-617-5292
URL: www.vasthcs.med.va.gov
Type: Acute Care - VA Emergency Services: No
Ownership: Government Federal Beds: 1,112

Key Personnel:
Quality Assurance . . . . Gary Anziani
Radiology. Carlos Bazan, MD
Infection Control. . . . . John R Graybill
Operating Room. . . . . Pat Haney, RN
Chief of Medical Staff . . . . Geoffrey R Weiss, MD

Measure	Cases	This Hosp.	State Avg.	U.S. Avg.
Blood Clot Prevention and Treatment				
Anticoagulation Overlap Therapy	-	-	93%	93%
ICU Venous Thromboembolism Prophylaxis	-	-	92%	92%
Incidence of Potentially Preventable VTE	-	-	9%	10%
UFH with Dosages/Platelet Monitoring	-	-	96%	97%
Venous Thromboembolism Prophylaxis	-	-	82%	85%
Warfarin Therapy Discharge Instructions	-	-	84%	75%
Chest Pain/Possible Heart Attack Care				
Aspirin Given Within 24 Hours of Arrival	-	-	94%	96%
Fibrinolytic Meds Within 30 Min. of Arrival	-	-	47%	58%
Average Time to ECG (minutes)	-	-	8	7
Average Time to Transfer (minutes)	-	-	62	60
Children's Asthma Care				
Received Home Management Plan of Care	-	-	93%	88%
Received Reliever Medication	-	-	100%	100%
Received Systemic Corticosteroids	-	-	100%	100%
Emergency Department				
Admittance Decision Time (minutes)	-	-	99	98
Head CT Results Within 45 Min. of Arrival	-	-	54%	57%
Patients Who Left ER Before Being Seen	-	-	3%	2%
Time from ER Arrival to Admit. (minutes)	-	-	270	274
Time from ER Arrival to Discharge (minutes)	-	-	127	134
Time in ER Before Being Evaluated (minutes)	-	-	26	26
Time to Pain Meds for Fractures (minutes)	-	-	57	57
Heart Attack Care				
Aspirin Given at Discharge	71	100%	99%	99%
Fibrinolytic Meds Within 30 Min. of Arrival[5]	-	-	49%	54%
PCI Within 90 Minutes of Arrival[1]	-	-	95%	96%
Statin Prescribed at Discharge	69	100%	98%	98%
Heart Failure Care				
ACE Inhibitor or ARB for LVSD	101	97%	97%	97%
Discharge Instructions Given	236	100%	95%	94%
Evaluation of LVS Function	263	100%	99%	99%
Medicare Spending				
Medicare Spending per Patient (ratio)	-	-	1.03	0.98
Pneumonia Care				
Appropriate Initial Antibiotic Given	72	97%	95%	95%
Blood Culture Timing	165	98%	98%	98%
Pregnancy and Delivery Care				
Newborn Deliveries Scheduled Early	-	-	7%	6%
Preventive Care				
Immunization for Influenza[5]	-	-	90%	90%
Immunization for Pneumonia[5]	-	-	92%	92%
Stroke Care				
Anticoagulation Therapy for Atrial Fibrillation	-	-	96%	95%
Antithrombotic Therapy Timing	-	-	98%	98%
Assessed for Rehabilitation	-	-	98%	97%
Discharged on Antithrombotic Therapy	-	-	99%	99%
Discharged on Statin Medication	-	-	95%	94%
Thrombolytic Therapy Timing	-	-	68%	66%
Venous Thromboembolism Prophylaxis	-	-	94%	94%
Written Stroke Educational Materials Given	-	-	92%	88%
Surgical Care Improvement Project				
Appropriate Beta Blocker Usage[2]	182	96%	98%	98%
Appropriate VTP Within 24 Hours[2]	296	96%	98%	98%
Controlled Postoperative Blood Glucose[2]	93	97%	96%	97%
Perioperative Temperature Management[2]	314	100%	100%	100%
Prophylactic Antibiotic Selection	258	100%	99%	99%
Prophylactic Antibiotic Selection (Outpatient)	-	-	98%	98%
Prophylactic Antibiotic Stopped	249	98%	98%	98%
Prophylactic Antibiotic Timing	259	98%	99%	99%
Prophylactic Antibiotic Timing (Outpatient)	-	-	98%	98%
Urinary Catheter Removal[2]	219	100%	98%	97%
Survey of Patients' Hospital Experiences				
Area Around Room 'Always' Quiet at Night	-	-	68%	61%
Doctors 'Always' Communicated Well	-	-	83%	82%
Home Recovery Information Given	-	-	85%	85%
Hospital Given 9 or 10 on 10 Point Scale	-	-	73%	71%
Meds 'Always' Explained Before Given	-	-	66%	64%
Nurses 'Always' Communicated Well	-	-	80%	79%
Pain 'Always' Well Controlled	-	-	72%	71%
Room and Bathroom 'Always' Clean	-	-	75%	73%
Timely Help 'Always' Received	-	-	69%	68%
Would Definitely Recommend Hospital	-	-	73%	71%
Use of Medical Imaging				
Cardiac Imaging Stress Test before Surgery	-	-	5.3%	5.3%
Combination Abdominal CT Scan	-	-	16.4%	10.5%
Combination Brain/Sinus CT Scan	-	-	2.7%	2.7%
Combination Chest CT Scan	-	-	5.6%	2.7%
Follow-up Mammogram/Ultrasound	-	-	7.9%	8.8%
Lumbar Spine MRI for Low Back Pain	-	-	39.6%	37.2%

South Texas Spine & Surgical Hospital

18600 North Hardy Oak Blvd Phone: 210-404-0800
San Antonio, TX 78258
URL: www.southtexassurgical.com
Type: Acute Care Hospitals Emergency Services: Yes
Ownership: Proprietary Beds: 30

Key Personnel:
CEO/President. . . . . Chris Shoup

Measure	Cases	This Hosp.	State Avg.	U.S. Avg.
Blood Clot Prevention and Treatment				
Anticoagulation Overlap Therapy[7]	-	-	93%	93%
ICU Venous Thromboembolism Prophylaxis[7]	-	-	92%	92%
Incidence of Potentially Preventable VTE[7]	-	-	9%	10%
UFH with Dosages/Platelet Monitoring[7]	-	-	96%	97%
Venous Thromboembolism Prophylaxis	422	98%	82%	85%
Warfarin Therapy Discharge Instructions[7]	-	-	84%	75%
Chest Pain/Possible Heart Attack Care				
Aspirin Given Within 24 Hours of Arrival[5]	-	-	94%	96%
Fibrinolytic Meds Within 30 Min. of Arrival[5]	-	-	47%	58%
Average Time to ECG (minutes)[5]	-	-	8	7
Average Time to Transfer (minutes)[5]	-	-	62	60
Children's Asthma Care				
Received Home Management Plan of Care	-	-	93%	88%
Received Reliever Medication	-	-	100%	100%
Received Systemic Corticosteroids	-	-	100%	100%
Emergency Department				
Admittance Decision Time (minutes)[1]	-	-	99	98
Head CT Results Within 45 Min. of Arrival[5]	-	-	54%	57%
Patients Who Left ER Before Being Seen	166	0%	3%	2%
Time from ER Arrival to Admit. (minutes)[1]	-	-	270	274
Time from ER Arrival to Discharge (minutes)	159	95	127	134
Time in ER Before Being Evaluated (minutes)	179	15	26	26
Time to Pain Meds for Fractures (minutes)[5]	-	-	57	57
Heart Attack Care				
Aspirin Given at Discharge[5]	-	-	99%	99%
Fibrinolytic Meds Within 30 Min. of Arrival[5]	-	-	49%	54%
PCI Within 90 Minutes of Arrival[5]	-	-	95%	96%
Statin Prescribed at Discharge[5]	-	-	98%	98%
Heart Failure Care				
ACE Inhibitor or ARB for LVSD[5]	-	-	97%	97%
Discharge Instructions Given[5]	-	-	95%	94%
Evaluation of LVS Function[5]	-	-	99%	99%
Medicare Spending				
Medicare Spending per Patient (ratio)	-	0.96	1.03	0.98
Pneumonia Care				
Appropriate Initial Antibiotic Given[5]	-	-	95%	95%
Blood Culture Timing[5]	-	-	98%	98%
Pregnancy and Delivery Care				
Newborn Deliveries Scheduled Early[7]	-	-	7%	6%
Preventive Care				
Immunization for Influenza	526	97%	90%	90%
Immunization for Pneumonia	546	97%	92%	92%
Stroke Care				
Anticoagulation Therapy for Atrial Fibrillation[5]	-	-	96%	95%
Antithrombotic Therapy Timing[5]	-	-	98%	98%
Assessed for Rehabilitation[5]	-	-	98%	97%
Discharged on Antithrombotic Therapy[5]	-	-	99%	99%
Discharged on Statin Medication[5]	-	-	95%	94%
Thrombolytic Therapy Timing[5]	-	-	68%	66%
Venous Thromboembolism Prophylaxis[5]	-	-	94%	94%
Written Stroke Educational Materials Given[5]	-	-	92%	88%
Surgical Care Improvement Project				
Appropriate Beta Blocker Usage	49	100%	98%	98%
Appropriate VTP Within 24 Hours	149	100%	98%	98%
Controlled Postoperative Blood Glucose[7]	-	-	96%	97%
Perioperative Temperature Management	271	100%	100%	100%
Prophylactic Antibiotic Selection	231	100%	99%	99%
Prophylactic Antibiotic Selection (Outpatient)	360	99%	98%	98%
Prophylactic Antibiotic Stopped	231	99%	98%	98%
Prophylactic Antibiotic Timing	231	99%	99%	99%
Prophylactic Antibiotic Timing (Outpatient)	360	100%	98%	98%
Urinary Catheter Removal	124	99%	98%	97%
Survey of Patients' Hospital Experiences				
Area Around Room 'Always' Quiet at Night	300+	86%	68%	61%
Doctors 'Always' Communicated Well	300+	90%	83%	82%
Home Recovery Information Given	300+	89%	85%	85%
Hospital Given 9 or 10 on 10 Point Scale	300+	84%	73%	71%
Meds 'Always' Explained Before Given	300+	76%	66%	64%
Nurses 'Always' Communicated Well	300+	86%	80%	79%
Pain 'Always' Well Controlled	300+	80%	72%	71%
Room and Bathroom 'Always' Clean	300+	80%	75%	73%
Timely Help 'Always' Received	300+	82%	69%	68%
Would Definitely Recommend Hospital	300+	87%	73%	71%
Use of Medical Imaging				
Cardiac Imaging Stress Test before Surgery[7]	-	-	5.3%	5.3%
Combination Abdominal CT Scan[7]	-	-	16.4%	10.5%

NOTE: Hospital profiles are in alphabetical order by state, then city, then hospital within the city; Rankings exclude hospitals with less than 25 cases except for patient surveys which excludes hospitals with less than 100 cases; (a) 100-299 cases; (1) The number of cases/patients is too few to report; (2) Data submitted were based on a sample of cases/patients; (3) Results are based on a shorter time period than required; (4) Data suppressed by CMS for one or more quarters; (5) Results are not available for this reporting period; (6) Fewer than 100 patients completed the HCAHPS survey; (7) No cases met the criteria for this measure; (8) The lower limit of the confidence interval cannot be calculated if the number of observed infections equals zero; (9) No data are available from the state/territory for this reporting period; (10) The scores shown reflect fewer than 50 completed surveys; (11) There were discrepancies in the data collection process; (12) This measure does not apply to this hospital for this reporting period; (13) Results cannot be calculated for this reporting period; (14) The results for this state are combined with nearby states to protect confidentiality; Please refer to the User's Guide for a full explanation of data.

Measure	Cases	This Hosp.	State Avg.	U.S. Avg.
Combination Brain/Sinus CT Scan[7]	-	-	2.7%	2.7%
Combination Chest CT Scan[7]	-	-	5.6%	2.7%
Follow-up Mammogram/Ultrasound[7]	-	-	7.9%	8.8%
Lumbar Spine MRI for Low Back Pain[7]	-	-	39.6%	37.2%

Southwest General Hospital

7400 Barlite Blvd
San Antonio, TX 78224
Phone: 210-921-2000
Fax: 210-921-3508
E-mail: southwestgeneral@iasishealthcare.com
URL: www.swgeneralhospital.com
Type: Acute Care Hospitals
Emergency Services: Yes
Ownership: Voluntary non-profit - Private
Beds: 327

Key Personnel:
CEO/President. . . . . P. Craig Desmond
Chief of Medical Staff . . . . Damaso Oliva

Measure	Cases	This Hosp.	State Avg.	U.S. Avg.
Blood Clot Prevention and Treatment				
Anticoagulation Overlap Therapy[2]	17	100%	93%	93%
ICU Venous Thromboembolism Prophylaxis[2]	71	89%	92%	92%
Incidence of Potentially Preventable VTE[1,2]	-	-	9%	10%
UFH with Dosages/Platelet Monitoring[2]	14	100%	96%	97%
Venous Thromboembolism Prophylaxis[2]	409	75%	82%	85%
Warfarin Therapy Discharge Instructions[1,2]	-	-	84%	75%
Chest Pain/Possible Heart Attack Care				
Aspirin Given Within 24 Hours of Arrival[1,3]	-	-	94%	96%
Fibrinolytic Meds Within 30 Min. of Arrival[3,7]	-	-	47%	58%
Average Time to ECG (minutes)[1,3]	-	-	8	7
Average Time to Transfer (minutes)[3,7]	-	-	62	60
Children's Asthma Care				
Received Home Management Plan of Care	-	-	93%	88%
Received Reliever Medication	-	-	100%	100%
Received Systemic Corticosteroids	-	-	100%	100%
Emergency Department				
Admittance Decision Time (minutes)[2]	636	208	99	98
Head CT Results Within 45 Min. of Arrival[7]	-	-	54%	57%
Patients Who Left ER Before Being Seen	48,609	3%	3%	2%
Time from ER Arrival to Admit. (minutes)[2]	653	395	270	274
Time from ER Arrival to Discharge (minutes)	673	149	127	134
Time in ER Before Being Evaluated (minutes)	754	62	26	26
Time to Pain Meds for Fractures (minutes)	153	72	57	57
Heart Attack Care				
Aspirin Given at Discharge	216	92%	99%	99%
Fibrinolytic Meds Within 30 Min. of Arrival[7]	-	-	49%	54%
PCI Within 90 Minutes of Arrival	18	94%	95%	96%
Statin Prescribed at Discharge	196	96%	98%	98%
Heart Failure Care				
ACE Inhibitor or ARB for LVSD	63	97%	97%	97%
Discharge Instructions Given	177	97%	95%	94%
Evaluation of LVS Function	200	100%	99%	99%
Medicare Spending				
Medicare Spending per Patient (ratio)	-	1.04	1.03	0.98
Pneumonia Care				
Appropriate Initial Antibiotic Given	91	98%	95%	95%
Blood Culture Timing	157	99%	98%	98%
Pregnancy and Delivery Care				
Newborn Deliveries Scheduled Early[2]	56	7%	7%	6%
Preventive Care				
Immunization for Influenza[2]	601	100%	90%	90%
Immunization for Pneumonia[2]	602	100%	92%	92%
Stroke Care				
Anticoagulation Therapy for Atrial Fibrillation[1]	-	-	96%	95%
Antithrombotic Therapy Timing	53	100%	98%	98%
Assessed for Rehabilitation	56	98%	98%	97%
Discharged on Antithrombotic Therapy	54	89%	99%	99%
Discharged on Statin Medication	41	83%	95%	94%
Thrombolytic Therapy Timing[7]	-	-	68%	66%
Venous Thromboembolism Prophylaxis	55	91%	94%	94%
Written Stroke Educational Materials Given	32	100%	92%	88%
Surgical Care Improvement Project				
Appropriate Beta Blocker Usage	69	99%	98%	98%
Appropriate VTP Within 24 Hours	210	99%	98%	98%
Controlled Postoperative Blood Glucose	27	100%	96%	97%
Perioperative Temperature Management	272	100%	100%	100%
Prophylactic Antibiotic Selection	78	99%	99%	99%
Prophylactic Antibiotic Selection (Outpatient)	149	99%	98%	98%
Prophylactic Antibiotic Stopped	73	97%	98%	98%
Prophylactic Antibiotic Timing	80	99%	99%	99%
Prophylactic Antibiotic Timing (Outpatient)	149	100%	98%	98%
Urinary Catheter Removal	151	97%	98%	97%
Survey of Patients' Hospital Experiences				
Area Around Room 'Always' Quiet at Night	300+	63%	68%	61%
Doctors 'Always' Communicated Well	300+	77%	83%	82%
Home Recovery Information Given	300+	83%	85%	85%
Hospital Given 9 or 10 on 10 Point Scale	300+	60%	73%	71%
Meds 'Always' Explained Before Given	300+	58%	66%	64%
Nurses 'Always' Communicated Well	300+	71%	80%	79%
Pain 'Always' Well Controlled	300+	66%	72%	71%
Room and Bathroom 'Always' Clean	300+	62%	75%	73%
Timely Help 'Always' Received	300+	52%	69%	68%
Would Definitely Recommend Hospital	300+	59%	73%	71%
Use of Medical Imaging				
Cardiac Imaging Stress Test before Surgery[1]	-	-	5.3%	5.3%
Combination Abdominal CT Scan	196	1.5%	16.4%	10.5%
Combination Brain/Sinus CT Scan	374	4.3%	2.7%	2.7%
Combination Chest CT Scan	63	4.8%	5.6%	2.7%
Follow-up Mammogram/Ultrasound[1]	-	-	7.9%	8.8%
Lumbar Spine MRI for Low Back Pain[1]	-	-	39.6%	37.2%

University Health System

4502 Medical Dr
San Antonio, TX 78229
Phone: 210-358-4000
Fax: 210-358-4090
URL: www.universityhealthsystem.com
Type: Acute Care Hospitals
Emergency Services: Yes
Ownership: Govt - Hospital Dist/Auth
Beds: 604

Key Personnel:
Chief of Medical Staff. . . . . Bryan Alsip, MD
CEO . . . . Tim Brierty
CEO/President. . . . . George B. Hernendez, Jr., JD
Operating Room. . . . . Liz Madrid
Pediatric Ambulatory Care . . . . . . John Mangos, MD
Pediatric In-Patient Care . . . . John Mangos, MD
Radiology. . . . . Stewart R Reuter, MD
Infection Control. . . . . Becky Sanchez

Measure	Cases	This Hosp.	State Avg.	U.S. Avg.
Blood Clot Prevention and Treatment				
Anticoagulation Overlap Therapy[2]	87	98%	93%	93%
ICU Venous Thromboembolism Prophylaxis[2]	81	94%	92%	92%
Incidence of Potentially Preventable VTE[2]	42	5%	9%	10%
UFH with Dosages/Platelet Monitoring[2]	56	100%	96%	97%
Venous Thromboembolism Prophylaxis[2]	285	94%	82%	85%
Warfarin Therapy Discharge Instructions[2]	66	89%	84%	75%
Chest Pain/Possible Heart Attack Care				
Aspirin Given Within 24 Hours of Arrival[1]	-	-	94%	96%
Fibrinolytic Meds Within 30 Min. of Arrival[5]	-	-	47%	58%
Average Time to ECG (minutes)[1]	-	-	8	7
Average Time to Transfer (minutes)[5]	-	-	62	60
Children's Asthma Care				
Received Home Management Plan of Care	-	-	93%	88%
Received Reliever Medication	-	-	100%	100%
Received Systemic Corticosteroids	-	-	100%	100%
Emergency Department				
Admittance Decision Time (minutes)[2]	429	228	99	98
Head CT Results Within 45 Min. of Arrival[1]	-	-	54%	57%
Patients Who Left ER Before Being Seen	66,831	8%	3%	2%
Time from ER Arrival to Admit. (minutes)[2]	448	438	270	274
Time from ER Arrival to Discharge (minutes)	177	383	127	134
Time in ER Before Being Evaluated (minutes)	176	80	26	26
Time to Pain Meds for Fractures (minutes)	144	130	57	57
Heart Attack Care				
Aspirin Given at Discharge	168	98%	99%	99%
Fibrinolytic Meds Within 30 Min. of Arrival[7]	-	-	49%	54%
PCI Within 90 Minutes of Arrival	20	90%	95%	96%
Statin Prescribed at Discharge	165	97%	98%	98%
Heart Failure Care				
ACE Inhibitor or ARB for LVSD	131	96%	97%	97%
Discharge Instructions Given	303	90%	95%	94%
Evaluation of LVS Function	308	99%	99%	99%
Medicare Spending				
Medicare Spending per Patient (ratio)	-	0.94	1.03	0.98
Pneumonia Care				
Appropriate Initial Antibiotic Given[2]	53	81%	95%	95%
Blood Culture Timing[2]	85	74%	98%	98%
Pregnancy and Delivery Care				
Newborn Deliveries Scheduled Early[2]	30	3%	7%	6%
Preventive Care				
Immunization for Influenza[2]	530	80%	90%	90%
Immunization for Pneumonia[2]	405	79%	92%	92%
Stroke Care				
Anticoagulation Therapy for Atrial Fibrillation[1,2]	-	-	96%	95%
Antithrombotic Therapy Timing[2]	110	96%	98%	98%
Assessed for Rehabilitation[2]	172	98%	98%	97%
Discharged on Antithrombotic Therapy[2]	146	99%	99%	99%
Discharged on Statin Medication[2]	113	98%	95%	94%
Thrombolytic Therapy Timing[2]	25	88%	68%	66%
Venous Thromboembolism Prophylaxis[2]	166	99%	94%	94%
Written Stroke Educational Materials Given[2]	130	95%	92%	88%
Surgical Care Improvement Project				
Appropriate Beta Blocker Usage[2]	158	96%	98%	98%
Appropriate VTP Within 24 Hours[2]	440	95%	98%	98%
Controlled Postoperative Blood Glucose[2]	138	93%	96%	97%
Perioperative Temperature Management[2]	510	100%	100%	100%
Prophylactic Antibiotic Selection[2]	467	98%	99%	99%
Prophylactic Antibiotic Selection (Outpatient)	387	96%	98%	98%
Prophylactic Antibiotic Stopped[2]	453	95%	98%	98%
Prophylactic Antibiotic Timing[2]	468	98%	99%	99%
Prophylactic Antibiotic Timing (Outpatient)	390	96%	98%	98%
Urinary Catheter Removal[2]	261	85%	98%	97%
Survey of Patients' Hospital Experiences				
Area Around Room 'Always' Quiet at Night	300+	52%	68%	61%
Doctors 'Always' Communicated Well	300+	78%	83%	82%
Home Recovery Information Given	300+	85%	85%	85%
Hospital Given 9 or 10 on 10 Point Scale	300+	70%	73%	71%
Meds 'Always' Explained Before Given	300+	62%	66%	64%
Nurses 'Always' Communicated Well	300+	71%	80%	79%
Pain 'Always' Well Controlled	300+	68%	72%	71%
Room and Bathroom 'Always' Clean	300+	67%	75%	73%
Timely Help 'Always' Received	300+	57%	69%	68%
Would Definitely Recommend Hospital	300+	69%	73%	71%
Use of Medical Imaging				
Cardiac Imaging Stress Test before Surgery	336	4.5%	5.3%	5.3%
Combination Abdominal CT Scan	618	19.1%	16.4%	10.5%
Combination Brain/Sinus CT Scan[1]	-	-	2.7%	2.7%
Combination Chest CT Scan	484	0.4%	5.6%	2.7%
Follow-up Mammogram/Ultrasound	1,581	5.2%	7.9%	8.8%
Lumbar Spine MRI for Low Back Pain	63	39.7%	39.6%	37.2%

Central Texas Medical Center

1301 Wonder World Drive
San Marcos, TX 78666
Phone: 512-753-3690
Fax: 512-753-3598
E-mail: webmasterctmc@ahss.org
URL: www.ctmc.org
Type: Acute Care Hospitals
Emergency Services: Yes
Ownership: Voluntary non-profit - Private
Beds: 113

Key Personnel:
Intensive Care Unit. . . . . Lana Cameron, RN
Emergency Room . . . . Jennifer M Driskell, RN
CEO/President. . . . . Gary L Jepson
Quality Assurance . . . . Missi Johnson
Chief of Medical Staff . . . . Charles Matthis, MD
Operating Room. . . . . Madelyn Smith, RN
Infection Control. . . . . Faye Wright
Radiology. . . . . Gregory C de la Iglesia

Measure	Cases	This Hosp.	State Avg.	U.S. Avg.
Blood Clot Prevention and Treatment				
Anticoagulation Overlap Therapy[2]	25	88%	93%	93%
ICU Venous Thromboembolism Prophylaxis[2]	63	95%	92%	92%
Incidence of Potentially Preventable VTE[2,7]	-	-	9%	10%
UFH with Dosages/Platelet Monitoring[1,2]	-	-	96%	97%
Venous Thromboembolism Prophylaxis[2]	303	95%	82%	85%
Warfarin Therapy Discharge Instructions[2]	17	82%	84%	75%
Chest Pain/Possible Heart Attack Care				

NOTE: Hospital profiles are in alphabetical order by state, then city, then hospital within the city; Rankings exclude hospitals with less than 25 cases except for patient surveys which excludes hospitals with less than 100 cases; (a) 100-299 cases; (1) The number of cases/patients is too few to report; (2) Data submitted were based on a sample of cases/patients; (3) Results are based on a shorter time period than required; (4) Data suppressed by CMS for one or more quarters; (5) Results are not available for this reporting period; (6) Fewer than 100 patients completed the HCAHPS survey; (7) No cases met the criteria for this measure; (8) The lower limit of the confidence interval cannot be calculated if the number of observed infections equals zero; (9) No data are available from the state/territory for this reporting period; (10) The scores shown reflect fewer than 50 completed surveys; (11) There were discrepancies in the data collection process; (12) This measure does not apply to this hospital for this reporting period; (13) Results cannot be calculated for this reporting period; (14) The results for this state are combined with nearby states to protect confidentiality; Please refer to the User's Guide for a full explanation of data.

Measure	Cases	This Hosp.	State Avg.	U.S. Avg.
Aspirin Given Within 24 Hours of Arrival	31	100%	94%	96%
Fibrinolytic Meds Within 30 Min. of Arrival[7]	-	-	47%	58%
Average Time to ECG (minutes)	30	4	8	7
Average Time to Transfer (minutes)	18	50	62	60
Children's Asthma Care				
Received Home Management Plan of Care	-	-	93%	88%
Received Reliever Medication	-	-	100%	100%
Received Systemic Corticosteroids	-	-	100%	100%
Emergency Department				
Admittance Decision Time (minutes)[2]	540	105	99	98
Head CT Results Within 45 Min. of Arrival	14	86%	54%	57%
Patients Who Left ER Before Being Seen	38,953	2%	3%	2%
Time from ER Arrival to Admit. (minutes)[2]	541	308	270	274
Time from ER Arrival to Discharge (minutes)	367	136	127	134
Time in ER Before Being Evaluated (minutes)	383	12	26	26
Time to Pain Meds for Fractures (minutes)	206	52	57	57
Heart Attack Care				
Aspirin Given at Discharge[1]	-	-	99%	99%
Fibrinolytic Meds Within 30 Min. of Arrival[7]	-	-	49%	54%
PCI Within 90 Minutes of Arrival[7]	-	-	95%	96%
Statin Prescribed at Discharge[1]	-	-	98%	98%
Heart Failure Care				
ACE Inhibitor or ARB for LVSD	28	100%	97%	97%
Discharge Instructions Given	115	100%	95%	94%
Evaluation of LVS Function	154	100%	99%	99%
Medicare Spending				
Medicare Spending per Patient (ratio)	-	1.04	1.03	0.98
Pneumonia Care				
Appropriate Initial Antibiotic Given	86	99%	95%	95%
Blood Culture Timing	166	99%	98%	98%
Pregnancy and Delivery Care				
Newborn Deliveries Scheduled Early[2]	40	28%	7%	6%
Preventive Care				
Immunization for Influenza[2]	442	93%	90%	90%
Immunization for Pneumonia[2]	507	99%	92%	92%
Stroke Care				
Anticoagulation Therapy for Atrial Fibrillation[1]	-	-	96%	95%
Antithrombotic Therapy Timing	45	98%	98%	98%
Assessed for Rehabilitation	47	100%	98%	97%
Discharged on Antithrombotic Therapy	45	98%	99%	99%
Discharged on Statin Medication	39	97%	95%	94%
Thrombolytic Therapy Timing[7]	-	-	68%	66%
Venous Thromboembolism Prophylaxis	45	100%	94%	94%
Written Stroke Educational Materials Given	24	96%	92%	88%
Surgical Care Improvement Project				
Appropriate Beta Blocker Usage	38	100%	98%	98%
Appropriate VTP Within 24 Hours	167	98%	98%	98%
Controlled Postoperative Blood Glucose[7]	-	-	96%	97%
Perioperative Temperature Management	183	100%	100%	100%
Prophylactic Antibiotic Selection	77	99%	99%	99%
Prophylactic Antibiotic Selection (Outpatient)	154	99%	98%	98%
Prophylactic Antibiotic Stopped	64	100%	98%	98%
Prophylactic Antibiotic Timing	77	99%	99%	99%
Prophylactic Antibiotic Timing (Outpatient)	154	100%	98%	98%
Urinary Catheter Removal	101	98%	98%	97%
Survey of Patients' Hospital Experiences				
Area Around Room 'Always' Quiet at Night[11]	300+	65%	68%	61%
Doctors 'Always' Communicated Well[11]	300+	80%	83%	82%
Home Recovery Information Given[11]	300+	86%	85%	85%
Hospital Given 9 or 10 on 10 Point Scale[11]	300+	73%	73%	71%
Meds 'Always' Explained Before Given[11]	300+	64%	66%	64%
Nurses 'Always' Communicated Well[11]	300+	80%	80%	79%
Pain 'Always' Well Controlled[11]	300+	73%	72%	71%
Room and Bathroom 'Always' Clean[11]	300+	73%	75%	73%
Timely Help 'Always' Received[11]	300+	68%	69%	68%
Would Definitely Recommend Hospital[11]	300+	73%	73%	71%
Use of Medical Imaging				
Cardiac Imaging Stress Test before Surgery	102	7.8%	5.3%	5.3%
Combination Abdominal CT Scan	467	10.5%	16.4%	10.5%
Combination Brain/Sinus CT Scan	515	4.1%	2.7%	2.7%
Combination Chest CT Scan	182	6.6%	5.6%	2.7%
Follow-up Mammogram/Ultrasound	668	0.9%	7.9%	8.8%
Lumbar Spine MRI for Low Back Pain[1]	-	-	39.6%	37.2%

Guadalupe Regional Medical Center

1215 E Court St
Seguin, TX 78155
E-mail: fbennett@gvh.com
URL: www.gvh.com
Type: Acute Care Hospitals
Ownership: Government - Local

Phone: 830-379-2411
Fax: 830-372-1582
Emergency Services: Yes
Beds: 117

Key Personnel:
Radiology. . . . . Ken Barker
Intensive Care Unit. . . . . Margaret Beville
Operating Room. . . . . Annette Jones
Cardiac Laboratory. . . . . Steven Sokolyk, MD
Infection Control. . . . . Rhonda Unrah
Emergency Room . . . . K C Walker
Chief of Medical Staff. . . . . Steven White, MD

Measure	Cases	This Hosp.	State Avg.	U.S. Avg.
Blood Clot Prevention and Treatment				
Anticoagulation Overlap Therapy[2]	15	93%	93%	93%
ICU Venous Thromboembolism Prophylaxis[2]	59	83%	92%	92%
Incidence of Potentially Preventable VTE[1,2]	-	-	9%	10%
UFH with Dosages/Platelet Monitoring[1,2]	-	-	96%	97%
Venous Thromboembolism Prophylaxis[2]	261	78%	82%	85%
Warfarin Therapy Discharge Instructions[1,2]	-	-	84%	75%
Chest Pain/Possible Heart Attack Care				
Aspirin Given Within 24 Hours of Arrival	102	94%	94%	96%
Fibrinolytic Meds Within 30 Min. of Arrival[7]	-	-	47%	58%
Average Time to ECG (minutes)	105	9	8	7
Average Time to Transfer (minutes)[7]	-	-	62	60
Children's Asthma Care				
Received Home Management Plan of Care	-	-	93%	88%
Received Reliever Medication	-	-	100%	100%
Received Systemic Corticosteroids	-	-	100%	100%
Emergency Department				
Admittance Decision Time (minutes)[2]	371	123	99	98
Head CT Results Within 45 Min. of Arrival	33	24%	54%	57%
Patients Who Left ER Before Being Seen	36,470	1%	3%	2%
Time from ER Arrival to Admit. (minutes)[2]	379	264	270	274
Time from ER Arrival to Discharge (minutes)	345	136	127	134
Time in ER Before Being Evaluated (minutes)	382	36	26	26
Time to Pain Meds for Fractures (minutes)	86	50	57	57
Heart Attack Care				
Aspirin Given at Discharge	16	94%	99%	99%
Fibrinolytic Meds Within 30 Min. of Arrival[7]	-	-	49%	54%
PCI Within 90 Minutes of Arrival[7]	-	-	95%	96%
Statin Prescribed at Discharge	19	79%	98%	98%
Heart Failure Care				
ACE Inhibitor or ARB for LVSD	35	89%	97%	97%
Discharge Instructions Given	86	88%	95%	94%
Evaluation of LVS Function	113	96%	99%	99%
Medicare Spending				
Medicare Spending per Patient (ratio)	-	1.04	1.03	0.98
Pneumonia Care				
Appropriate Initial Antibiotic Given	64	88%	95%	95%
Blood Culture Timing	103	99%	98%	98%
Pregnancy and Delivery Care				
Newborn Deliveries Scheduled Early	103	7%	7%	6%
Preventive Care				
Immunization for Influenza[2]	370	94%	90%	90%
Immunization for Pneumonia[2]	386	95%	92%	92%
Stroke Care				
Anticoagulation Therapy for Atrial Fibrillation[1]	-	-	96%	95%
Antithrombotic Therapy Timing	17	76%	98%	98%
Assessed for Rehabilitation	23	96%	98%	97%
Discharged on Antithrombotic Therapy	23	83%	99%	99%
Discharged on Statin Medication	23	65%	95%	94%
Thrombolytic Therapy Timing[1]	-	-	68%	66%
Venous Thromboembolism Prophylaxis	17	65%	94%	94%
Written Stroke Educational Materials Given	11	73%	92%	88%
Surgical Care Improvement Project				
Appropriate Beta Blocker Usage	67	94%	98%	98%
Appropriate VTP Within 24 Hours	310	99%	98%	98%
Controlled Postoperative Blood Glucose[7]	-	-	96%	97%
Perioperative Temperature Management	353	100%	100%	100%
Prophylactic Antibiotic Selection	268	100%	99%	99%
Prophylactic Antibiotic Selection (Outpatient)	92	98%	98%	98%
Prophylactic Antibiotic Stopped	266	98%	98%	98%
Prophylactic Antibiotic Timing	269	97%	99%	99%
Prophylactic Antibiotic Timing (Outpatient)	93	92%	98%	98%
Urinary Catheter Removal	58	95%	98%	97%
Survey of Patients' Hospital Experiences				
Area Around Room 'Always' Quiet at Night	300+	75%	68%	61%
Doctors 'Always' Communicated Well	300+	84%	83%	82%
Home Recovery Information Given	300+	84%	85%	85%
Hospital Given 9 or 10 on 10 Point Scale	300+	73%	73%	71%
Meds 'Always' Explained Before Given	300+	63%	66%	64%
Nurses 'Always' Communicated Well	300+	80%	80%	79%
Pain 'Always' Well Controlled	300+	75%	72%	71%
Room and Bathroom 'Always' Clean	300+	81%	75%	73%
Timely Help 'Always' Received	300+	69%	69%	68%
Would Definitely Recommend Hospital	300+	73%	73%	71%
Use of Medical Imaging				
Cardiac Imaging Stress Test before Surgery	151	4.6%	5.3%	5.3%
Combination Abdominal CT Scan	726	10.9%	16.4%	10.5%
Combination Brain/Sinus CT Scan	550	0.4%	2.7%	2.7%
Combination Chest CT Scan	325	8.0%	5.6%	2.7%
Follow-up Mammogram/Ultrasound	716	7.3%	7.9%	8.8%
Lumbar Spine MRI for Low Back Pain	81	45.7%	39.6%	37.2%

Seymour Hospital

200 Stadium Drive
Seymour, TX 76380
Type: Acute Care Hospitals
Ownership: Govt - Hospital Dist/Auth

Phone: 940-889-5572
Fax: 940-889-3337
Emergency Services: Yes
Beds: 49

Key Personnel:
Quality Assurance . . . . Heather Greenwood, RN
CEO/President. . . . . Leslie Hardin
CEO . . . . Chris McDonnell
Chief of Medical Staff . . . . Richard Niles, MD
Chair/CEO . . . . Terry Old

Measure	Cases	This Hosp.	State Avg.	U.S. Avg.
Blood Clot Prevention and Treatment				
Anticoagulation Overlap Therapy[1,2]	-	-	93%	93%
ICU Venous Thromboembolism Prophylaxis[2,7]	-	-	92%	92%
Incidence of Potentially Preventable VTE[1,2]	-	-	9%	10%
UFH with Dosages/Platelet Monitoring[2,7]	-	-	96%	97%
Venous Thromboembolism Prophylaxis[2]	211	79%	82%	85%
Warfarin Therapy Discharge Instructions[1,2]	-	-	84%	75%
Chest Pain/Possible Heart Attack Care				
Aspirin Given Within 24 Hours of Arrival[1,3]	-	-	94%	96%
Fibrinolytic Meds Within 30 Min. of Arrival[5]	-	-	47%	58%
Average Time to ECG (minutes)[1,3]	-	-	8	7
Average Time to Transfer (minutes)[5]	-	-	62	60
Children's Asthma Care				
Received Home Management Plan of Care	-	-	93%	88%
Received Reliever Medication	-	-	100%	100%
Received Systemic Corticosteroids	-	-	100%	100%
Emergency Department				
Admittance Decision Time (minutes)	173	0	99	98
Head CT Results Within 45 Min. of Arrival[1]	-	-	54%	57%
Patients Who Left ER Before Being Seen	1,945	0%	3%	2%
Time from ER Arrival to Admit. (minutes)	180	95	270	274
Time from ER Arrival to Discharge (minutes)	328	80	127	134
Time in ER Before Being Evaluated (minutes)	311	30	26	26
Time to Pain Meds for Fractures (minutes)[1]	-	-	57	57
Heart Attack Care				
Aspirin Given at Discharge[1]	-	-	99%	99%
Fibrinolytic Meds Within 30 Min. of Arrival[7]	-	-	49%	54%
PCI Within 90 Minutes of Arrival[7]	-	-	95%	96%
Statin Prescribed at Discharge[1]	-	-	98%	98%
Heart Failure Care				
ACE Inhibitor or ARB for LVSD[7]	-	-	97%	97%
Discharge Instructions Given[1]	-	-	95%	94%
Evaluation of LVS Function[1]	-	-	99%	99%
Medicare Spending				
Medicare Spending per Patient (ratio)	-	0.93	1.03	0.98

NOTE: Hospital profiles are in alphabetical order by state, then city, then hospital within the city; Rankings exclude hospitals with less than 25 cases except for patient surveys which excludes hospitals with less than 100 cases; (a) 100-299 cases; (1) The number of cases/patients is too few to report; (2) Data submitted were based on a sample of cases/patients; (3) Results are based on a shorter time period than required; (4) Data suppressed by CMS for one or more quarters; (5) Results are not available for this reporting period; (6) Fewer than 100 patients completed the HCAHPS survey; (7) No cases met the criteria for this measure; (8) The lower limit of the confidence interval cannot be calculated if the number of observed infections equals zero; (9) No data are available from the state/territory for this reporting period; (10) The scores shown reflect fewer than 50 completed surveys; (11) There were discrepancies in the data collection process; (12) This measure does not apply to this hospital for this reporting period; (13) Results cannot be calculated for this reporting period; (14) The results for this state are combined with nearby states to protect confidentiality; Please refer to the User's Guide for a full explanation of data.

Measure	Cases	This Hosp.	State Avg.	U.S. Avg.
Pneumonia Care				
Appropriate Initial Antibiotic Given	43	84%	95%	95%
Blood Culture Timing	25	96%	98%	98%
Pregnancy and Delivery Care				
Newborn Deliveries Scheduled Early[1]	-	-	7%	6%
Preventive Care				
Immunization for Influenza	199	86%	90%	90%
Immunization for Pneumonia	250	93%	92%	92%
Stroke Care				
Anticoagulation Therapy for Atrial Fibrillation[3,7]	-	-	96%	95%
Antithrombotic Therapy Timing[1,3]	-	-	98%	98%
Assessed for Rehabilitation[1,3]	-	-	98%	97%
Discharged on Antithrombotic Therapy[1,3]	-	-	99%	99%
Discharged on Statin Medication[1,3]	-	-	95%	94%
Thrombolytic Therapy Timing[1,3]	-	-	68%	66%
Venous Thromboembolism Prophylaxis[1,3]	-	-	94%	94%
Written Stroke Educational Materials Given[3,7]	-	-	92%	88%
Surgical Care Improvement Project				
Appropriate Beta Blocker Usage[3,7]	-	-	98%	98%
Appropriate VTP Within 24 Hours[1,3]	-	-	98%	98%
Controlled Postoperative Blood Glucose[3,7]	-	-	96%	97%
Perioperative Temperature Management[1,3]	-	-	100%	100%
Prophylactic Antibiotic Selection[1,3]	-	-	99%	99%
Prophylactic Antibiotic Selection (Outpatient)[5]	-	-	98%	98%
Prophylactic Antibiotic Stopped[1,3]	-	-	98%	98%
Prophylactic Antibiotic Timing[1,3]	-	-	99%	99%
Prophylactic Antibiotic Timing (Outpatient)[5]	-	-	98%	98%
Urinary Catheter Removal[3,7]	-	-	98%	97%
Survey of Patients' Hospital Experiences				
Area Around Room 'Always' Quiet at Night[6]	<100	76%	68%	61%
Doctors 'Always' Communicated Well[6]	<100	90%	83%	82%
Home Recovery Information Given[6]	<100	87%	85%	85%
Hospital Given 9 or 10 on 10 Point Scale[6]	<100	74%	73%	71%
Meds 'Always' Explained Before Given[6]	<100	72%	66%	64%
Nurses 'Always' Communicated Well[6]	<100	82%	80%	79%
Pain 'Always' Well Controlled[6]	<100	75%	72%	71%
Room and Bathroom 'Always' Clean[6]	<100	69%	75%	73%
Timely Help 'Always' Received[6]	<100	74%	69%	68%
Would Definitely Recommend Hospital[6]	<100	70%	73%	71%
Use of Medical Imaging				
Cardiac Imaging Stress Test before Surgery[7]	-	-	5.3%	5.3%
Combination Abdominal CT Scan	54	1.9%	16.4%	10.5%
Combination Brain/Sinus CT Scan[1]	-	-	2.7%	2.7%
Combination Chest CT Scan	46	0.0%	5.6%	2.7%
Follow-up Mammogram/Ultrasound[7]	-	-	7.9%	8.8%
Lumbar Spine MRI for Low Back Pain[1]	-	-	39.6%	37.2%

Heritage Park Surgical Hospital

3601 Calais Drive Phone: 903-813-3728
Sherman, TX 75090
URL: www.heritageparksurgicalhospital.com
Type: Acute Care Hospitals Emergency Services: Yes
Ownership: Physician

Measure	Cases	This Hosp.	State Avg.	U.S. Avg.
Blood Clot Prevention and Treatment				
Anticoagulation Overlap Therapy[1]	-	-	93%	93%
ICU Venous Thromboembolism Prophylaxis[7]	-	-	92%	92%
Incidence of Potentially Preventable VTE[7]	-	-	9%	10%
UFH with Dosages/Platelet Monitoring[1]	-	-	96%	97%
Venous Thromboembolism Prophylaxis	77	49%	82%	85%
Warfarin Therapy Discharge Instructions[1]	-	-	84%	75%
Chest Pain/Possible Heart Attack Care				
Aspirin Given Within 24 Hours of Arrival[1,3]	-	-	94%	96%
Fibrinolytic Meds Within 30 Min. of Arrival[5]	-	-	47%	58%
Average Time to ECG (minutes)[1,3]	-	-	8	7
Average Time to Transfer (minutes)[5]	-	-	62	60
Children's Asthma Care				
Received Home Management Plan of Care	-	-	93%	88%
Received Reliever Medication	-	-	100%	100%
Received Systemic Corticosteroids	-	-	100%	100%
Emergency Department				
Admittance Decision Time (minutes)	23	20	99	98
Head CT Results Within 45 Min. of Arrival[5]	-	-	54%	57%
Patients Who Left ER Before Being Seen	622	0%	3%	2%
Time from ER Arrival to Admit. (minutes)	23	145	270	274
Time from ER Arrival to Discharge (minutes)	239	94	127	134
Time in ER Before Being Evaluated (minutes)	255	24	26	26
Time to Pain Meds for Fractures (minutes)[1]	-	-	57	57
Heart Attack Care				
Aspirin Given at Discharge[5]	-	-	99%	99%
Fibrinolytic Meds Within 30 Min. of Arrival[5]	-	-	49%	54%
PCI Within 90 Minutes of Arrival[5]	-	-	95%	96%
Statin Prescribed at Discharge[5]	-	-	98%	98%
Heart Failure Care				
ACE Inhibitor or ARB for LVSD[5]	-	-	97%	97%
Discharge Instructions Given[5]	-	-	95%	94%
Evaluation of LVS Function[5]	-	-	99%	99%
Medicare Spending				
Medicare Spending per Patient (ratio)	-	1.08	1.03	0.98
Pneumonia Care				
Appropriate Initial Antibiotic Given[5]	-	-	95%	95%
Blood Culture Timing[5]	-	-	98%	98%
Pregnancy and Delivery Care				
Newborn Deliveries Scheduled Early[7]	-	-	7%	6%
Preventive Care				
Immunization for Influenza	139	82%	90%	90%
Immunization for Pneumonia	121	96%	92%	92%
Stroke Care				
Anticoagulation Therapy for Atrial Fibrillation[5]	-	-	96%	95%
Antithrombotic Therapy Timing[5]	-	-	98%	98%
Assessed for Rehabilitation[5]	-	-	98%	97%
Discharged on Antithrombotic Therapy[5]	-	-	99%	99%
Discharged on Statin Medication[5]	-	-	95%	94%
Thrombolytic Therapy Timing[5]	-	-	68%	66%
Venous Thromboembolism Prophylaxis[5]	-	-	94%	94%
Written Stroke Educational Materials Given[5]	-	-	92%	88%
Surgical Care Improvement Project				
Appropriate Beta Blocker Usage	46	100%	98%	98%
Appropriate VTP Within 24 Hours	142	97%	98%	98%
Controlled Postoperative Blood Glucose[7]	-	-	96%	97%
Perioperative Temperature Management	152	100%	100%	100%
Prophylactic Antibiotic Selection	139	97%	99%	99%
Prophylactic Antibiotic Selection (Outpatient)	159	96%	98%	98%
Prophylactic Antibiotic Stopped	139	99%	98%	98%
Prophylactic Antibiotic Timing	139	97%	99%	99%
Prophylactic Antibiotic Timing (Outpatient)	164	97%	98%	98%
Urinary Catheter Removal	14	93%	98%	97%
Survey of Patients' Hospital Experiences				
Area Around Room 'Always' Quiet at Night	(a)	84%	68%	61%
Doctors 'Always' Communicated Well	(a)	88%	83%	82%
Home Recovery Information Given	(a)	94%	85%	85%
Hospital Given 9 or 10 on 10 Point Scale	(a)	89%	73%	71%
Meds 'Always' Explained Before Given	(a)	86%	66%	64%
Nurses 'Always' Communicated Well	(a)	93%	80%	79%
Pain 'Always' Well Controlled	(a)	82%	72%	71%
Room and Bathroom 'Always' Clean	(a)	82%	75%	73%
Timely Help 'Always' Received	(a)	90%	69%	68%
Would Definitely Recommend Hospital	(a)	92%	73%	71%
Use of Medical Imaging				
Cardiac Imaging Stress Test before Surgery[7]	-	-	5.3%	5.3%
Combination Abdominal CT Scan	196	75.0%	16.4%	10.5%
Combination Brain/Sinus CT Scan[1]	-	-	2.7%	2.7%
Combination Chest CT Scan[1]	-	-	5.6%	2.7%
Follow-up Mammogram/Ultrasound[7]	-	-	7.9%	8.8%
Lumbar Spine MRI for Low Back Pain	113	35.4%	39.6%	37.2%

Texas Health Presbyterian Hospital - WNJ

500 N Highland Avenue Phone: 903-870-4611
Sherman, TX 75091 Fax: 903-870-4378
URL: www.wnj.org
Type: Acute Care Hospitals Emergency Services: Yes
Ownership: Voluntary non-profit - Other Beds: 241
Key Personnel:
Cardiac Laboratory. . . . . Robert Burns
Radiology. . . . . Drew Castleberr
Quality Assurance . . . . Tracy Masson
CEO/President. . . . . K Steven Rowley
Chief of Medical Staff . . . . John Sciortino, DO
Infection Control. . . . . JoAnn Smith

Measure	Cases	This Hosp.	State Avg.	U.S. Avg.
Blood Clot Prevention and Treatment				
Anticoagulation Overlap Therapy[2]	41	100%	93%	93%
ICU Venous Thromboembolism Prophylaxis[2]	113	88%	92%	92%
Incidence of Potentially Preventable VTE[1,2]	-	-	9%	10%
UFH with Dosages/Platelet Monitoring[2]	31	100%	96%	97%
Venous Thromboembolism Prophylaxis[2]	321	67%	82%	85%
Warfarin Therapy Discharge Instructions[2]	30	90%	84%	75%
Chest Pain/Possible Heart Attack Care				
Aspirin Given Within 24 Hours of Arrival[1,3]	-	-	94%	96%
Fibrinolytic Meds Within 30 Min. of Arrival[5]	-	-	47%	58%
Average Time to ECG (minutes)[1,3]	-	-	8	7
Average Time to Transfer (minutes)[5]	-	-	62	60
Children's Asthma Care				
Received Home Management Plan of Care	-	-	93%	88%
Received Reliever Medication	-	-	100%	100%
Received Systemic Corticosteroids	-	-	100%	100%
Emergency Department				
Admittance Decision Time (minutes)[2]	672	89	99	98
Head CT Results Within 45 Min. of Arrival[1]	-	-	54%	57%
Patients Who Left ER Before Being Seen	29,700	2%	3%	2%
Time from ER Arrival to Admit. (minutes)[2]	674	262	270	274
Time from ER Arrival to Discharge (minutes)	415	121	127	134
Time in ER Before Being Evaluated (minutes)	443	31	26	26
Time to Pain Meds for Fractures (minutes)	117	79	57	57
Heart Attack Care				
Aspirin Given at Discharge	135	98%	99%	99%
Fibrinolytic Meds Within 30 Min. of Arrival[7]	-	-	49%	54%
PCI Within 90 Minutes of Arrival	12	100%	95%	96%
Statin Prescribed at Discharge	127	97%	98%	98%
Heart Failure Care				
ACE Inhibitor or ARB for LVSD	73	99%	97%	97%
Discharge Instructions Given	175	99%	95%	94%
Evaluation of LVS Function	217	99%	99%	99%
Medicare Spending				
Medicare Spending per Patient (ratio)	-	1.01	1.03	0.98
Pneumonia Care				
Appropriate Initial Antibiotic Given	86	95%	95%	95%
Blood Culture Timing	228	100%	98%	98%
Pregnancy and Delivery Care				
Newborn Deliveries Scheduled Early	34	3%	7%	6%
Preventive Care				
Immunization for Influenza[2]	576	96%	90%	90%
Immunization for Pneumonia[2]	815	99%	92%	92%
Stroke Care				
Anticoagulation Therapy for Atrial Fibrillation[1]	-	-	96%	95%
Antithrombotic Therapy Timing	49	100%	98%	98%
Assessed for Rehabilitation	59	100%	98%	97%
Discharged on Antithrombotic Therapy	49	100%	99%	99%
Discharged on Statin Medication	40	88%	95%	94%
Thrombolytic Therapy Timing[1]	-	-	68%	66%
Venous Thromboembolism Prophylaxis	61	90%	94%	94%
Written Stroke Educational Materials Given	33	97%	92%	88%
Surgical Care Improvement Project				
Appropriate Beta Blocker Usage	135	100%	98%	98%
Appropriate VTP Within 24 Hours	191	99%	98%	98%
Controlled Postoperative Blood Glucose	56	96%	96%	97%
Perioperative Temperature Management	225	100%	100%	100%
Prophylactic Antibiotic Selection	162	99%	99%	99%
Prophylactic Antibiotic Selection (Outpatient)	146	99%	98%	98%
Prophylactic Antibiotic Stopped	152	100%	98%	98%
Prophylactic Antibiotic Timing	162	99%	99%	99%
Prophylactic Antibiotic Timing (Outpatient)	146	99%	98%	98%
Urinary Catheter Removal	149	93%	98%	97%
Survey of Patients' Hospital Experiences				
Area Around Room 'Always' Quiet at Night	300+	64%	68%	61%
Doctors 'Always' Communicated Well	300+	79%	83%	82%
Home Recovery Information Given	300+	83%	85%	85%
Hospital Given 9 or 10 on 10 Point Scale	300+	64%	73%	71%

NOTE: Hospital profiles are in alphabetical order by state, then city, then hospital within the city; Rankings exclude hospitals with less than 25 cases except for patient surveys which excludes hospitals with less than 100 cases; (a) 100-299 cases; (1) The number of cases/patients is too few to report; (2) Data submitted were based on a sample of cases/patients; (3) Results are based on a shorter time period than required; (4) Data suppressed by CMS for one or more quarters; (5) Results are not available for this reporting period; (6) Fewer than 100 patients completed the HCAHPS survey; (7) No cases met the criteria for this measure; (8) The lower limit of the confidence interval cannot be calculated if the number of observed infections equals zero; (9) No data are available from the state/territory for this reporting period; (10) The scores shown reflect fewer than 50 completed surveys; (11) There were discrepancies in the data collection process; (12) This measure does not apply to this hospital for this reporting period; (13) Results cannot be calculated for this reporting period; (14) The results for this state are combined with nearby states to protect confidentiality; Please refer to the User's Guide for a full explanation of data.

Meds 'Always' Explained Before Given	300+	57%	66%	64%
Nurses 'Always' Communicated Well	300+	75%	80%	79%
Pain 'Always' Well Controlled	300+	67%	72%	71%
Room and Bathroom 'Always' Clean	300+	61%	75%	73%
Timely Help 'Always' Received	300+	63%	69%	68%
Would Definitely Recommend Hospital	300+	64%	73%	71%
Use of Medical Imaging				
Cardiac Imaging Stress Test before Surgery	512	4.9%	5.3%	5.3%
Combination Abdominal CT Scan	364	12.4%	16.4%	10.5%
Combination Brain/Sinus CT Scan	620	4.2%	2.7%	2.7%
Combination Chest CT Scan	377	14.9%	5.6%	2.7%
Follow-up Mammogram/Ultrasound	2,021	7.6%	7.9%	8.8%
Lumbar Spine MRI for Low Back Pain	71	38.0%	39.6%	37.2%

Seton Smithville Regional Hospital

800 East Highway 71 Phone: 512-237-3214
Smithville, TX 78957
URL: www.srhnet.com
Type: Acute Care Hospitals Emergency Services: Yes
Ownership: Voluntary non-profit - Private Beds: 33

Key Personnel:
President/CEO. . . . . Robert I. Bonar Jr., HA
CEO/President. . . . . Jeff Cook
President/CEO. . . . . Jesús Garza
President/CEO. . . . . Ken Gladish
President . . . . Greg W. Hartman
Operating Room. . . . . Joan Swanson
Radiology. . . . . Kelly Vitek

Measure	Cases	This Hosp.	State Avg.	U.S. Avg.
Blood Clot Prevention and Treatment				
Anticoagulation Overlap Therapy[1,2]	-	-	93%	93%
ICU Venous Thromboembolism Prophylaxis[2,7]	-	-	92%	92%
Incidence of Potentially Preventable VTE[1,2]	-	-	9%	10%
UFH with Dosages/Platelet Monitoring[2,7]	-	-	96%	97%
Venous Thromboembolism Prophylaxis[2]	130	98%	82%	85%
Warfarin Therapy Discharge Instructions[1,2]	-	-	84%	75%
Chest Pain/Possible Heart Attack Care				
Aspirin Given Within 24 Hours of Arrival	37	92%	94%	96%
Fibrinolytic Meds Within 30 Min. of Arrival[7]	-	-	47%	58%
Average Time to ECG (minutes)	37	9	8	7
Average Time to Transfer (minutes)[1]	-	-	62	60
Children's Asthma Care				
Received Home Management Plan of Care	-	-	93%	88%
Received Reliever Medication	-	-	100%	100%
Received Systemic Corticosteroids	-	-	100%	100%
Emergency Department				
Admittance Decision Time (minutes)[2]	306	61	99	98
Head CT Results Within 45 Min. of Arrival[1,3]	-	-	54%	57%
Patients Who Left ER Before Being Seen	10,758	1%	3%	2%
Time from ER Arrival to Admit. (minutes)[2]	307	183	270	274
Time from ER Arrival to Discharge (minutes)	356	94	127	134
Time in ER Before Being Evaluated (minutes)	385	21	26	26
Time to Pain Meds for Fractures (minutes)	41	29	57	57
Heart Attack Care				
Aspirin Given at Discharge[3,7]	-	-	99%	99%
Fibrinolytic Meds Within 30 Min. of Arrival[3,7]	-	-	49%	54%
PCI Within 90 Minutes of Arrival[3,7]	-	-	95%	96%
Statin Prescribed at Discharge[1,3]	-	-	98%	98%
Heart Failure Care				
ACE Inhibitor or ARB for LVSD[1]	-	-	97%	97%
Discharge Instructions Given	21	95%	95%	94%
Evaluation of LVS Function	24	100%	99%	99%
Medicare Spending				
Medicare Spending per Patient (ratio)	-	0.85	1.03	0.98
Pneumonia Care				
Appropriate Initial Antibiotic Given	21	95%	95%	95%
Blood Culture Timing	38	100%	98%	98%
Pregnancy and Delivery Care				
Newborn Deliveries Scheduled Early[7]	-	-	7%	6%
Preventive Care				
Immunization for Influenza[2]	222	95%	90%	90%
Immunization for Pneumonia[2]	301	97%	92%	92%
Stroke Care				
Anticoagulation Therapy for Atrial Fibrillation[5]	-	-	96%	95%
Antithrombotic Therapy Timing[5]	-	-	98%	98%
Assessed for Rehabilitation[5]	-	-	98%	97%
Discharged on Antithrombotic Therapy[5]	-	-	99%	99%
Discharged on Statin Medication[5]	-	-	95%	94%
Thrombolytic Therapy Timing[5]	-	-	68%	66%
Venous Thromboembolism Prophylaxis[5]	-	-	94%	94%
Written Stroke Educational Materials Given[5]	-	-	92%	88%
Surgical Care Improvement Project				
Appropriate Beta Blocker Usage[3,7]	-	-	98%	98%
Appropriate VTP Within 24 Hours[3,7]	-	-	98%	98%
Controlled Postoperative Blood Glucose[3,7]	-	-	96%	97%
Perioperative Temperature Management[1,3]	-	-	100%	100%
Prophylactic Antibiotic Selection[1,3]	-	-	99%	99%
Prophylactic Antibiotic Selection (Outpatient)[1,3]	-	-	98%	98%
Prophylactic Antibiotic Stopped[1,3]	-	-	98%	98%
Prophylactic Antibiotic Timing[1,3]	-	-	99%	99%
Prophylactic Antibiotic Timing (Outpatient)[1,3]	-	-	98%	98%
Urinary Catheter Removal[1,3]	-	-	98%	97%
Survey of Patients' Hospital Experiences				
Area Around Room 'Always' Quiet at Night[6]	<100	69%	68%	61%
Doctors 'Always' Communicated Well[6]	<100	95%	83%	82%
Home Recovery Information Given[6]	<100	90%	85%	85%
Hospital Given 9 or 10 on 10 Point Scale[6]	<100	82%	73%	71%
Meds 'Always' Explained Before Given[6]	<100	79%	66%	64%
Nurses 'Always' Communicated Well[6]	<100	88%	80%	79%
Pain 'Always' Well Controlled[6]	<100	85%	72%	71%
Room and Bathroom 'Always' Clean[6]	<100	73%	75%	73%
Timely Help 'Always' Received[6]	<100	88%	69%	68%
Would Definitely Recommend Hospital[6]	<100	80%	73%	71%
Use of Medical Imaging				
Cardiac Imaging Stress Test before Surgery[1]	-	-	5.3%	5.3%
Combination Abdominal CT Scan	266	11.7%	16.4%	10.5%
Combination Brain/Sinus CT Scan[1]	-	-	2.7%	2.7%
Combination Chest CT Scan	179	9.5%	5.6%	2.7%
Follow-up Mammogram/Ultrasound	626	11.8%	7.9%	8.8%
Lumbar Spine MRI for Low Back Pain[1]	-	-	39.6%	37.2%

Cogdell Memorial Hospital

1700 Cogdell Blvd Phone: 325-574-7437
Snyder, TX 79549 Fax: 325-574-7433
E-mail: cbrown@snydertex.com
URL: www.cogdellhospital.com
Type: Acute Care Hospitals Emergency Services: Yes
Ownership: Govt - Hospital Dist/Auth Beds: 99

Key Personnel:
Chief of Medical Staff . . . . Christy Brown
Intensive Care Unit. . . . . Cheryl Chance, RN
Operating Room. . . . . Laquita Culwell
Quality Assurance . . . . Jo Beth Hardegree, RN
Infection Control. . . . . Leslie Leucke, RN
Emergency Room . . . . Marcia Odal, MD
Chair/CEO . . . . Russell Riggan

Measure	Cases	This Hosp.	State Avg.	U.S. Avg.
Blood Clot Prevention and Treatment				
Anticoagulation Overlap Therapy[1]	-	-	93%	93%
ICU Venous Thromboembolism Prophylaxis[7]	-	-	92%	92%
Incidence of Potentially Preventable VTE[7]	-	-	9%	10%
UFH with Dosages/Platelet Monitoring[1]	-	-	96%	97%
Venous Thromboembolism Prophylaxis	220	67%	82%	85%
Warfarin Therapy Discharge Instructions[1]	-	-	84%	75%
Chest Pain/Possible Heart Attack Care				
Aspirin Given Within 24 Hours of Arrival	42	88%	94%	96%
Fibrinolytic Meds Within 30 Min. of Arrival[1]	-	-	47%	58%
Average Time to ECG (minutes)	41	10	8	7
Average Time to Transfer (minutes)[7]	-	-	62	60
Children's Asthma Care				
Received Home Management Plan of Care	-	-	93%	88%
Received Reliever Medication	-	-	100%	100%
Received Systemic Corticosteroids	-	-	100%	100%
Emergency Department				
Admittance Decision Time (minutes)	198	40	99	98
Head CT Results Within 45 Min. of Arrival[1]	-	-	54%	57%
Patients Who Left ER Before Being Seen	8,651	1%	3%	2%
Time from ER Arrival to Admit. (minutes)	202	178	270	274
Time from ER Arrival to Discharge (minutes)	319	83	127	134
Time in ER Before Being Evaluated (minutes)	400	16	26	26
Time to Pain Meds for Fractures (minutes)	35	45	57	57
Heart Attack Care				
Aspirin Given at Discharge[1,3]	-	-	99%	99%
Fibrinolytic Meds Within 30 Min. of Arrival[3,7]	-	-	49%	54%
PCI Within 90 Minutes of Arrival[3,7]	-	-	95%	96%
Statin Prescribed at Discharge[1,3]	-	-	98%	98%
Heart Failure Care				
ACE Inhibitor or ARB for LVSD[1]	-	-	97%	97%
Discharge Instructions Given	12	75%	95%	94%
Evaluation of LVS Function	16	75%	99%	99%
Medicare Spending				
Medicare Spending per Patient (ratio)	-	0.94	1.03	0.98
Pneumonia Care				
Appropriate Initial Antibiotic Given	14	57%	95%	95%
Blood Culture Timing	26	100%	98%	98%
Pregnancy and Delivery Care				
Newborn Deliveries Scheduled Early[1,2]	-	-	7%	6%
Preventive Care				
Immunization for Influenza	247	76%	90%	90%
Immunization for Pneumonia	262	72%	92%	92%
Stroke Care				
Anticoagulation Therapy for Atrial Fibrillation[7]	-	-	96%	95%
Antithrombotic Therapy Timing[1]	-	-	98%	98%
Assessed for Rehabilitation[1]	-	-	98%	97%
Discharged on Antithrombotic Therapy[1]	-	-	99%	99%
Discharged on Statin Medication[1]	-	-	95%	94%
Thrombolytic Therapy Timing[7]	-	-	68%	66%
Venous Thromboembolism Prophylaxis[1]	-	-	94%	94%
Written Stroke Educational Materials Given[1]	-	-	92%	88%
Surgical Care Improvement Project				
Appropriate Beta Blocker Usage[5]	-	-	98%	98%
Appropriate VTP Within 24 Hours[5]	-	-	98%	98%
Controlled Postoperative Blood Glucose[5]	-	-	96%	97%
Perioperative Temperature Management[5]	-	-	100%	100%
Prophylactic Antibiotic Selection[5]	-	-	99%	99%
Prophylactic Antibiotic Selection (Outpatient)	11	100%	98%	98%
Prophylactic Antibiotic Stopped[5]	-	-	98%	98%
Prophylactic Antibiotic Timing[5]	-	-	99%	99%
Prophylactic Antibiotic Timing (Outpatient)	12	92%	98%	98%
Urinary Catheter Removal[5]	-	-	98%	97%
Survey of Patients' Hospital Experiences				
Area Around Room 'Always' Quiet at Night[6]	<100	71%	68%	61%
Doctors 'Always' Communicated Well[6]	<100	82%	83%	82%
Home Recovery Information Given[6]	<100	87%	85%	85%
Hospital Given 9 or 10 on 10 Point Scale[6]	<100	61%	73%	71%
Meds 'Always' Explained Before Given[6]	<100	80%	66%	64%
Nurses 'Always' Communicated Well[6]	<100	78%	80%	79%
Pain 'Always' Well Controlled[6]	<100	68%	72%	71%
Room and Bathroom 'Always' Clean[6]	<100	79%	75%	73%
Timely Help 'Always' Received[6]	<100	68%	69%	68%
Would Definitely Recommend Hospital[6]	<100	58%	73%	71%
Use of Medical Imaging				
Cardiac Imaging Stress Test before Surgery	85	1.2%	5.3%	5.3%
Combination Abdominal CT Scan	103	35.0%	16.4%	10.5%
Combination Brain/Sinus CT Scan[1]	-	-	2.7%	2.7%
Combination Chest CT Scan[1]	-	-	5.6%	2.7%
Follow-up Mammogram/Ultrasound	167	14.4%	7.9%	8.8%
Lumbar Spine MRI for Low Back Pain[1]	-	-	39.6%	37.2%

Texas Health Harris Methodist Hospital Southlake

1545 E Southlake Blvd Phone: 817-748-8700
Southlake, TX 76092 Fax: 817-748-8787
URL: www.texashealthsouthlake.com
Type: Acute Care Hospitals Emergency Services: Yes
Ownership: Government - State Beds: 16

Key Personnel:
Operating Room. . . . . Aaronra Anderson
CEO/President. . . . . Traci Bernard, RN
Quality Assurance . . . . Sara Helin
Radiology. . . . . Anthony Romero, RT
Infection Control. . . . . Cynithia Ruddell
Chief of Medical Staff . . . . O. David Taunton, Jr., MD

NOTE: Hospital profiles are in alphabetical order by state, then city, then hospital within the city; Rankings exclude hospitals with less than 25 cases except for patient surveys which excludes hospitals with less than 100 cases; (a) 100-299 cases; (1) The number of cases/patients is too few to report; (2) Data submitted were based on a sample of cases/patients; (3) Results are based on a shorter time period than required; (4) Data suppressed by CMS for one or more quarters; (5) Results are not available for this reporting period; (6) Fewer than 100 patients completed the HCAHPS survey; (7) No cases met the criteria for this measure; (8) The lower limit of the confidence interval cannot be calculated if the number of observed infections equals zero; (9) No data are available from the state/territory for this reporting period; (10) The scores shown reflect fewer than 50 completed surveys; (11) There were discrepancies in the data collection process; (12) This measure does not apply to this hospital for this reporting period; (13) Results cannot be calculated for this reporting period; (14) The results for this state are combined with nearby states to protect confidentiality; Please refer to the User's Guide for a full explanation of data.

Measure	Cases	This Hosp.	State Avg.	U.S. Avg.
Blood Clot Prevention and Treatment				
Anticoagulation Overlap Therapy[7]	-	-	93%	93%
ICU Venous Thromboembolism Prophylaxis[7]	-	-	92%	92%
Incidence of Potentially Preventable VTE[7]	-	-	9%	10%
UFH with Dosages/Platelet Monitoring[7]	-	-	96%	97%
Venous Thromboembolism Prophylaxis	117	100%	82%	85%
Warfarin Therapy Discharge Instructions[7]	-	-	84%	75%
Chest Pain/Possible Heart Attack Care				
Aspirin Given Within 24 Hours of Arrival[3,7]	-	-	94%	96%
Fibrinolytic Meds Within 30 Min. of Arrival[5]	-	-	47%	58%
Average Time to ECG (minutes)[1,3]	-	-	8	7
Average Time to Transfer (minutes)[5]	-	-	62	60
Children's Asthma Care				
Received Home Management Plan of Care	-	-	93%	88%
Received Reliever Medication	-	-	100%	100%
Received Systemic Corticosteroids	-	-	100%	100%
Emergency Department				
Admittance Decision Time (minutes)[1,2]	-	-	99	98
Head CT Results Within 45 Min. of Arrival[5]	-	-	54%	57%
Patients Who Left ER Before Being Seen	1,943	1%	3%	2%
Time from ER Arrival to Admit. (minutes)[1,2]	-	-	270	274
Time from ER Arrival to Discharge (minutes)	250	88	127	134
Time in ER Before Being Evaluated (minutes)	275	12	26	26
Time to Pain Meds for Fractures (minutes)	13	30	57	57
Heart Attack Care				
Aspirin Given at Discharge[5]	-	-	99%	99%
Fibrinolytic Meds Within 30 Min. of Arrival[5]	-	-	49%	54%
PCI Within 90 Minutes of Arrival[5]	-	-	95%	96%
Statin Prescribed at Discharge[5]	-	-	98%	98%
Heart Failure Care				
ACE Inhibitor or ARB for LVSD[5]	-	-	97%	97%
Discharge Instructions Given[5]	-	-	95%	94%
Evaluation of LVS Function[5]	-	-	99%	99%
Medicare Spending				
Medicare Spending per Patient (ratio)	-	1.19	1.03	0.98
Pneumonia Care				
Appropriate Initial Antibiotic Given[5]	-	-	95%	95%
Blood Culture Timing[5]	-	-	98%	98%
Pregnancy and Delivery Care				
Newborn Deliveries Scheduled Early[7]	-	-	7%	6%
Preventive Care				
Immunization for Influenza[2]	354	95%	90%	90%
Immunization for Pneumonia[2]	454	96%	92%	92%
Stroke Care				
Anticoagulation Therapy for Atrial Fibrillation[5]	-	-	96%	95%
Antithrombotic Therapy Timing[5]	-	-	98%	98%
Assessed for Rehabilitation[5]	-	-	98%	97%
Discharged on Antithrombotic Therapy[5]	-	-	99%	99%
Discharged on Statin Medication[5]	-	-	95%	94%
Thrombolytic Therapy Timing[5]	-	-	68%	66%
Venous Thromboembolism Prophylaxis[5]	-	-	94%	94%
Written Stroke Educational Materials Given[5]	-	-	92%	88%
Surgical Care Improvement Project				
Appropriate Beta Blocker Usage	154	100%	98%	98%
Appropriate VTP Within 24 Hours	495	99%	98%	98%
Controlled Postoperative Blood Glucose[7]	-	-	96%	97%
Perioperative Temperature Management	546	100%	100%	100%
Prophylactic Antibiotic Selection	468	100%	99%	99%
Prophylactic Antibiotic Selection (Outpatient)	317	99%	98%	98%
Prophylactic Antibiotic Stopped	468	100%	98%	98%
Prophylactic Antibiotic Timing	468	100%	99%	99%
Prophylactic Antibiotic Timing (Outpatient)	317	100%	98%	98%
Urinary Catheter Removal	422	100%	98%	97%
Survey of Patients' Hospital Experiences				
Area Around Room 'Always' Quiet at Night	300+	89%	68%	61%
Doctors 'Always' Communicated Well	300+	89%	83%	82%
Home Recovery Information Given	300+	93%	85%	85%
Hospital Given 9 or 10 on 10 Point Scale	300+	90%	73%	71%
Meds 'Always' Explained Before Given	300+	79%	66%	64%
Nurses 'Always' Communicated Well	300+	88%	80%	79%
Pain 'Always' Well Controlled	300+	80%	72%	71%
Room and Bathroom 'Always' Clean	300+	86%	75%	73%
Timely Help 'Always' Received	300+	86%	69%	68%
Would Definitely Recommend Hospital	300+	91%	73%	71%
Use of Medical Imaging				
Cardiac Imaging Stress Test before Surgery[7]	-	-	5.3%	5.3%
Combination Abdominal CT Scan[1]	-	-	16.4%	10.5%
Combination Brain/Sinus CT Scan[1]	-	-	2.7%	2.7%
Combination Chest CT Scan[1]	-	-	5.6%	2.7%
Follow-up Mammogram/Ultrasound[7]	-	-	7.9%	8.8%
Lumbar Spine MRI for Low Back Pain	217	39.6%	39.6%	37.2%

Hansford County Hospital

707 Roland St
Spearman, TX 79081
URL: www.hchd.net
Type: Critical Access Hospitals
Ownership: Govt - Hospital Dist/Auth
Phone: 806-659-2535
Fax: 806-659-2683
Emergency Services: Yes
Beds: 112

Key Personnel:
CEO .... Jonathan Bailey
Quality Assurance .... Connie Gibson
Chief of Medical Staff .... James Wonnacott, MD

Measure	Cases	This Hosp.	State Avg.	U.S. Avg.
Blood Clot Prevention and Treatment				
Anticoagulation Overlap Therapy[5]	-	-	93%	93%
ICU Venous Thromboembolism Prophylaxis[5]	-	-	92%	92%
Incidence of Potentially Preventable VTE[5]	-	-	9%	10%
UFH with Dosages/Platelet Monitoring[5]	-	-	96%	97%
Venous Thromboembolism Prophylaxis[5]	-	-	82%	85%
Warfarin Therapy Discharge Instructions[5]	-	-	84%	75%
Chest Pain/Possible Heart Attack Care				
Aspirin Given Within 24 Hours of Arrival[1,3]	-	-	94%	96%
Fibrinolytic Meds Within 30 Min. of Arrival[1,3]	-	-	47%	58%
Average Time to ECG (minutes)[1,3]	-	-	8	7
Average Time to Transfer (minutes)[3,7]	-	-	62	60
Children's Asthma Care				
Received Home Management Plan of Care	-	-	93%	88%
Received Reliever Medication	-	-	100%	100%
Received Systemic Corticosteroids	-	-	100%	100%
Emergency Department				
Admittance Decision Time (minutes)[3]	15	8	99	98
Head CT Results Within 45 Min. of Arrival[1,3]	-	-	54%	57%
Patients Who Left ER Before Being Seen[5]	-	-	3%	2%
Time from ER Arrival to Admit. (minutes)[3]	15	164	270	274
Time from ER Arrival to Discharge (minutes)[3]	136	115	127	134
Time in ER Before Being Evaluated (minutes)[3]	149	17	26	26
Time to Pain Meds for Fractures (minutes)[1,3]	-	-	57	57
Heart Attack Care				
Aspirin Given at Discharge[3,7]	-	-	99%	99%
Fibrinolytic Meds Within 30 Min. of Arrival[3,7]	-	-	49%	54%
PCI Within 90 Minutes of Arrival[3,7]	-	-	95%	96%
Statin Prescribed at Discharge[3,7]	-	-	98%	98%
Heart Failure Care				
ACE Inhibitor or ARB for LVSD[1,3]	-	-	97%	97%
Discharge Instructions Given[1,3]	-	-	95%	94%
Evaluation of LVS Function[1,3]	-	-	99%	99%
Medicare Spending				
Medicare Spending per Patient (ratio)	-	-	1.03	0.98
Pneumonia Care				
Appropriate Initial Antibiotic Given[1,3]	-	-	95%	95%
Blood Culture Timing[1,3]	-	-	98%	98%
Pregnancy and Delivery Care				
Newborn Deliveries Scheduled Early[5]	-	-	7%	6%
Preventive Care				
Immunization for Influenza[5]	-	-	90%	90%
Immunization for Pneumonia[5]	-	-	92%	92%
Stroke Care				
Anticoagulation Therapy for Atrial Fibrillation[5]	-	-	96%	95%
Antithrombotic Therapy Timing[5]	-	-	98%	98%
Assessed for Rehabilitation[5]	-	-	98%	97%
Discharged on Antithrombotic Therapy[5]	-	-	99%	99%
Discharged on Statin Medication[5]	-	-	95%	94%
Thrombolytic Therapy Timing[5]	-	-	68%	66%
Venous Thromboembolism Prophylaxis[5]	-	-	94%	94%
Written Stroke Educational Materials Given[5]	-	-	92%	88%
Surgical Care Improvement Project				
Appropriate Beta Blocker Usage[5]	-	-	98%	98%
Appropriate VTP Within 24 Hours[5]	-	-	98%	98%
Controlled Postoperative Blood Glucose[5]	-	-	96%	97%
Perioperative Temperature Management[5]	-	-	100%	100%
Prophylactic Antibiotic Selection[5]	-	-	99%	99%
Prophylactic Antibiotic Selection (Outpatient)[5]	-	-	98%	98%
Prophylactic Antibiotic Stopped[5]	-	-	98%	98%
Prophylactic Antibiotic Timing[5]	-	-	99%	99%
Prophylactic Antibiotic Timing (Outpatient)[5]	-	-	98%	98%
Urinary Catheter Removal[5]	-	-	98%	97%
Survey of Patients' Hospital Experiences				
Area Around Room 'Always' Quiet at Night[10]	<100	78%	68%	61%
Doctors 'Always' Communicated Well[10]	<100	98%	83%	82%
Home Recovery Information Given[10]	<100	100%	85%	85%
Hospital Given 9 or 10 on 10 Point Scale[10]	<100	78%	73%	71%
Meds 'Always' Explained Before Given[10]	<100	86%	66%	64%
Nurses 'Always' Communicated Well[10]	<100	90%	80%	79%
Pain 'Always' Well Controlled[10]	<100	92%	72%	71%
Room and Bathroom 'Always' Clean[10]	<100	83%	75%	73%
Timely Help 'Always' Received[10]	<100	88%	69%	68%
Would Definitely Recommend Hospital[10]	<100	94%	73%	71%
Use of Medical Imaging				
Cardiac Imaging Stress Test before Surgery[7]	-	-	5.3%	5.3%
Combination Abdominal CT Scan	70	0.0%	16.4%	10.5%
Combination Brain/Sinus CT Scan[1]	-	-	2.7%	2.7%
Combination Chest CT Scan[1]	-	-	5.6%	2.7%
Follow-up Mammogram/Ultrasound[7]	-	-	7.9%	8.8%
Lumbar Spine MRI for Low Back Pain[1]	-	-	39.6%	37.2%

Stamford Memorial Hospital

1601 Columbia Street
Stamford, TX 79553
Type: Acute Care Hospitals
Ownership: Govt - Hospital Dist/Auth
Phone: 325-773-2725
Fax: 915-773-3781
Emergency Services: Yes
Beds: 34

Key Personnel:
CEO .... Rick DeFoore, FACHE

Measure	Cases	This Hosp.	State Avg.	U.S. Avg.
Blood Clot Prevention and Treatment				
Anticoagulation Overlap Therapy[1,2]	-	-	93%	93%
ICU Venous Thromboembolism Prophylaxis[2,7]	-	-	92%	92%
Incidence of Potentially Preventable VTE[2,7]	-	-	9%	10%
UFH with Dosages/Platelet Monitoring[2,7]	-	-	96%	97%
Venous Thromboembolism Prophylaxis[2]	148	66%	82%	85%
Warfarin Therapy Discharge Instructions[2,7]	-	-	84%	75%
Chest Pain/Possible Heart Attack Care				
Aspirin Given Within 24 Hours of Arrival[3]	15	87%	94%	96%
Fibrinolytic Meds Within 30 Min. of Arrival[1,3]	-	-	47%	58%
Average Time to ECG (minutes)[3]	14	10	8	7
Average Time to Transfer (minutes)[3,7]	-	-	62	60
Children's Asthma Care				
Received Home Management Plan of Care	-	-	93%	88%
Received Reliever Medication	-	-	100%	100%
Received Systemic Corticosteroids	-	-	100%	100%
Emergency Department				
Admittance Decision Time (minutes)	107	15	99	98
Head CT Results Within 45 Min. of Arrival[5]	-	-	54%	57%
Patients Who Left ER Before Being Seen	2,427	1%	3%	2%
Time from ER Arrival to Admit. (minutes)	134	120	270	274
Time from ER Arrival to Discharge (minutes)	285	76	127	134
Time in ER Before Being Evaluated (minutes)	257	20	26	26
Time to Pain Meds for Fractures (minutes)[1,3]	-	-	57	57
Heart Attack Care				
Aspirin Given at Discharge[5]	-	-	99%	99%
Fibrinolytic Meds Within 30 Min. of Arrival[5]	-	-	49%	54%
PCI Within 90 Minutes of Arrival[5]	-	-	95%	96%
Statin Prescribed at Discharge[5]	-	-	98%	98%
Heart Failure Care				
ACE Inhibitor or ARB for LVSD[3,7]	-	-	97%	97%
Discharge Instructions Given[1,3]	-	-	95%	94%
Evaluation of LVS Function[1,3]	-	-	99%	99%

NOTE: Hospital profiles are in alphabetical order by state, then city, then hospital within the city; Rankings exclude hospitals with less than 25 cases except for patient surveys which excludes hospitals with less than 100 cases; (a) 100-299 cases; (1) The number of cases/patients is too few to report; (2) Data submitted were based on a sample of cases/patients; (3) Results are based on a shorter time period than required; (4) Data suppressed by CMS for one or more quarters; (5) Results are not available for this reporting period; (6) Fewer than 100 patients completed the HCAHPS survey; (7) No cases met the criteria for this measure; (8) The lower limit of the confidence interval cannot be calculated if the number of observed infections equals zero; (9) No data are available from the state/territory for this reporting period; (10) The scores shown reflect fewer than 50 completed surveys; (11) There were discrepancies in the data collection process; (12) This measure does not apply to this hospital for this reporting period; (13) Results cannot be calculated for this reporting period; (14) The results for this state are combined with nearby states to protect confidentiality; Please refer to the User's Guide for a full explanation of data.

Measure	Cases	This Hosp.	State Avg.	U.S. Avg.
Medicare Spending				
Medicare Spending per Patient (ratio)	-	0.93	1.03	0.98
Pneumonia Care				
Appropriate Initial Antibiotic Given[1,3]	-	-	95%	95%
Blood Culture Timing[1,3]	-	-	98%	98%
Pregnancy and Delivery Care				
Newborn Deliveries Scheduled Early[7]	-	-	7%	6%
Preventive Care				
Immunization for Influenza	135	84%	90%	90%
Immunization for Pneumonia	184	78%	92%	92%
Stroke Care				
Anticoagulation Therapy for Atrial Fibrillation[5]	-	-	96%	95%
Antithrombotic Therapy Timing[5]	-	-	98%	98%
Assessed for Rehabilitation[5]	-	-	98%	97%
Discharged on Antithrombotic Therapy[5]	-	-	99%	99%
Discharged on Statin Medication[5]	-	-	95%	94%
Thrombolytic Therapy Timing[5]	-	-	68%	66%
Venous Thromboembolism Prophylaxis[5]	-	-	94%	94%
Written Stroke Educational Materials Given[5]	-	-	92%	88%
Surgical Care Improvement Project				
Appropriate Beta Blocker Usage[5]	-	-	98%	98%
Appropriate VTP Within 24 Hours[5]	-	-	98%	98%
Controlled Postoperative Blood Glucose[5]	-	-	96%	97%
Perioperative Temperature Management[5]	-	-	100%	100%
Prophylactic Antibiotic Selection[5]	-	-	99%	99%
Prophylactic Antibiotic Selection (Outpatient)[5]	-	-	98%	98%
Prophylactic Antibiotic Stopped[5]	-	-	98%	98%
Prophylactic Antibiotic Timing[5]	-	-	99%	99%
Prophylactic Antibiotic Timing (Outpatient)[5]	-	-	98%	98%
Urinary Catheter Removal[5]	-	-	98%	97%
Survey of Patients' Hospital Experiences				
Area Around Room 'Always' Quiet at Night[6]	<100	72%	68%	61%
Doctors 'Always' Communicated Well[6]	<100	88%	83%	82%
Home Recovery Information Given[6]	<100	81%	85%	85%
Hospital Given 9 or 10 on 10 Point Scale[6]	<100	76%	73%	71%
Meds 'Always' Explained Before Given[6]	<100	61%	66%	64%
Nurses 'Always' Communicated Well[6]	<100	83%	80%	79%
Pain 'Always' Well Controlled[6]	<100	82%	72%	71%
Room and Bathroom 'Always' Clean[6]	<100	78%	75%	73%
Timely Help 'Always' Received[6]	<100	68%	69%	68%
Would Definitely Recommend Hospital[6]	<100	73%	73%	71%
Use of Medical Imaging				
Cardiac Imaging Stress Test before Surgery[7]	-	-	5.3%	5.3%
Combination Abdominal CT Scan	71	9.9%	16.4%	10.5%
Combination Brain/Sinus CT Scan	76	0.0%	2.7%	2.7%
Combination Chest CT Scan[1]	-	-	5.6%	2.7%
Follow-up Mammogram/Ultrasound[7]	-	-	7.9%	8.8%
Lumbar Spine MRI for Low Back Pain[1]	-	-	39.6%	37.2%

Martin County Hospital District

600 E Interstate 20 | Phone: 432-756-3345
Stanton, TX 79782
Type: Critical Access Hospitals | Emergency Services: Yes
Ownership: Govt - Hospital Dist/Auth

Measure	Cases	This Hosp.	State Avg.	U.S. Avg.
Blood Clot Prevention and Treatment				
Anticoagulation Overlap Therapy[5]	-	-	93%	93%
ICU Venous Thromboembolism Prophylaxis[5]	-	-	92%	92%
Incidence of Potentially Preventable VTE[5]	-	-	9%	10%
UFH with Dosages/Platelet Monitoring[5]	-	-	96%	97%
Venous Thromboembolism Prophylaxis[5]	-	-	82%	85%
Warfarin Therapy Discharge Instructions[5]	-	-	84%	75%
Chest Pain/Possible Heart Attack Care				
Aspirin Given Within 24 Hours of Arrival	-	-	94%	96%
Fibrinolytic Meds Within 30 Min. of Arrival	-	-	47%	58%
Average Time to ECG (minutes)	-	-	8	7
Average Time to Transfer (minutes)	-	-	62	60
Children's Asthma Care				
Received Home Management Plan of Care	-	-	93%	88%
Received Reliever Medication	-	-	100%	100%
Received Systemic Corticosteroids	-	-	100%	100%
Emergency Department				
Admittance Decision Time (minutes)[1,3]	-	-	99	98
Head CT Results Within 45 Min. of Arrival	-	-	54%	57%
Patients Who Left ER Before Being Seen	-	-	3%	2%
Time from ER Arrival to Admit. (minutes)[1,3]	-	-	270	274
Time from ER Arrival to Discharge (minutes)	-	-	127	134
Time in ER Before Being Evaluated (minutes)	-	-	26	26
Time to Pain Meds for Fractures (minutes)	-	-	57	57
Heart Attack Care				
Aspirin Given at Discharge[5]	-	-	99%	99%
Fibrinolytic Meds Within 30 Min. of Arrival[5]	-	-	49%	54%
PCI Within 90 Minutes of Arrival[5]	-	-	95%	96%
Statin Prescribed at Discharge[5]	-	-	98%	98%
Heart Failure Care				
ACE Inhibitor or ARB for LVSD[5]	-	-	97%	97%
Discharge Instructions Given[5]	-	-	95%	94%
Evaluation of LVS Function[5]	-	-	99%	99%
Medicare Spending				
Medicare Spending per Patient (ratio)	-	-	1.03	0.98
Pneumonia Care				
Appropriate Initial Antibiotic Given[3,7]	-	-	95%	95%
Blood Culture Timing[3,7]	-	-	98%	98%
Pregnancy and Delivery Care				
Newborn Deliveries Scheduled Early[5]	-	-	7%	6%
Preventive Care				
Immunization for Influenza[1,3]	-	-	90%	90%
Immunization for Pneumonia[1,3]	-	-	92%	92%
Stroke Care				
Anticoagulation Therapy for Atrial Fibrillation[5]	-	-	96%	95%
Antithrombotic Therapy Timing[5]	-	-	98%	98%
Assessed for Rehabilitation[5]	-	-	98%	97%
Discharged on Antithrombotic Therapy[5]	-	-	99%	99%
Discharged on Statin Medication[5]	-	-	95%	94%
Thrombolytic Therapy Timing[5]	-	-	68%	66%
Venous Thromboembolism Prophylaxis[5]	-	-	94%	94%
Written Stroke Educational Materials Given[5]	-	-	92%	88%
Surgical Care Improvement Project				
Appropriate Beta Blocker Usage[5]	-	-	98%	98%
Appropriate VTP Within 24 Hours[5]	-	-	98%	98%
Controlled Postoperative Blood Glucose[5]	-	-	96%	97%
Perioperative Temperature Management[5]	-	-	100%	100%
Prophylactic Antibiotic Selection[5]	-	-	99%	99%
Prophylactic Antibiotic Selection (Outpatient)	-	-	98%	98%
Prophylactic Antibiotic Stopped[5]	-	-	98%	98%
Prophylactic Antibiotic Timing[5]	-	-	99%	99%
Prophylactic Antibiotic Timing (Outpatient)	-	-	98%	98%
Urinary Catheter Removal[5]	-	-	98%	97%
Survey of Patients' Hospital Experiences				
Area Around Room 'Always' Quiet at Night[5]	-	-	68%	61%
Doctors 'Always' Communicated Well[5]	-	-	83%	82%
Home Recovery Information Given[5]	-	-	85%	85%
Hospital Given 9 or 10 on 10 Point Scale[5]	-	-	73%	71%
Meds 'Always' Explained Before Given[5]	-	-	66%	64%
Nurses 'Always' Communicated Well[5]	-	-	80%	79%
Pain 'Always' Well Controlled[5]	-	-	72%	71%
Room and Bathroom 'Always' Clean[5]	-	-	75%	73%
Timely Help 'Always' Received[5]	-	-	69%	68%
Would Definitely Recommend Hospital[5]	-	-	73%	71%
Use of Medical Imaging				
Cardiac Imaging Stress Test before Surgery	-	-	5.3%	5.3%
Combination Abdominal CT Scan	-	-	16.4%	10.5%
Combination Brain/Sinus CT Scan	-	-	2.7%	2.7%
Combination Chest CT Scan	-	-	5.6%	2.7%
Follow-up Mammogram/Ultrasound	-	-	7.9%	8.8%
Lumbar Spine MRI for Low Back Pain	-	-	39.6%	37.2%

Texas Health Harris Methodist Hospital Stephenville

411 N Belknap St | Phone: 254-965-1500
Stephenville, TX 76401 | Fax: 254-965-1561
E-mail: barbaramcmahan@hmhs.com
URL: www.texashealth.org/hospitals
Type: Acute Care Hospitals | Emergency Services: Yes
Ownership: Voluntary non-profit - Private | Beds: 98

Key Personnel:

Radiology. . . . . Mark Baker
Chief of Medical Staff . . . . Karen Burroughs, MD
Emergency Room . . . . Jimmy Harris, MD
Quality Assurance . . . . Javier Montemayor
CEO/President. . . . . Deborah Paganelli
Infection Control. . . . . Laura Parker, RN
Operating Room. . . . . Doris Prim, RN

Measure	Cases	This Hosp.	State Avg.	U.S. Avg.
Blood Clot Prevention and Treatment				
Anticoagulation Overlap Therapy[2]	13	85%	93%	93%
ICU Venous Thromboembolism Prophylaxis[2]	33	97%	92%	92%
Incidence of Potentially Preventable VTE[1,2]	-	-	9%	10%
UFH with Dosages/Platelet Monitoring[1,2]	-	-	96%	97%
Venous Thromboembolism Prophylaxis[2]	132	89%	82%	85%
Warfarin Therapy Discharge Instructions[1,2]	-	-	84%	75%
Chest Pain/Possible Heart Attack Care				
Aspirin Given Within 24 Hours of Arrival	105	90%	94%	96%
Fibrinolytic Meds Within 30 Min. of Arrival[7]	-	-	47%	58%
Average Time to ECG (minutes)	111	3	8	7
Average Time to Transfer (minutes)[1]	-	-	62	60
Children's Asthma Care				
Received Home Management Plan of Care	-	-	93%	88%
Received Reliever Medication	-	-	100%	100%
Received Systemic Corticosteroids	-	-	100%	100%
Emergency Department				
Admittance Decision Time (minutes)[2]	299	49	99	98
Head CT Results Within 45 Min. of Arrival[1]	-	-	54%	57%
Patients Who Left ER Before Being Seen	18,340	2%	3%	2%
Time from ER Arrival to Admit. (minutes)[2]	300	176	270	274
Time from ER Arrival to Discharge (minutes)	414	105	127	134
Time in ER Before Being Evaluated (minutes)	442	23	26	26
Time to Pain Meds for Fractures (minutes)	52	46	57	57
Heart Attack Care				
Aspirin Given at Discharge[1]	-	-	99%	99%
Fibrinolytic Meds Within 30 Min. of Arrival[7]	-	-	49%	54%
PCI Within 90 Minutes of Arrival[7]	-	-	95%	96%
Statin Prescribed at Discharge[1]	-	-	98%	98%
Heart Failure Care				
ACE Inhibitor or ARB for LVSD	12	100%	97%	97%
Discharge Instructions Given	41	95%	95%	94%
Evaluation of LVS Function	51	100%	99%	99%
Medicare Spending				
Medicare Spending per Patient (ratio)	-	1.01	1.03	0.98
Pneumonia Care				
Appropriate Initial Antibiotic Given	45	93%	95%	95%
Blood Culture Timing	86	99%	98%	98%
Pregnancy and Delivery Care				
Newborn Deliveries Scheduled Early	31	6%	7%	6%
Preventive Care				
Immunization for Influenza[2]	285	99%	90%	90%
Immunization for Pneumonia[2]	354	98%	92%	92%
Stroke Care				
Anticoagulation Therapy for Atrial Fibrillation[1,2]	-	-	96%	95%
Antithrombotic Therapy Timing[2]	21	95%	98%	98%
Assessed for Rehabilitation[2]	19	100%	98%	97%
Discharged on Antithrombotic Therapy[2]	19	100%	99%	99%
Discharged on Statin Medication[2]	17	76%	95%	94%
Thrombolytic Therapy Timing[1,2]	-	-	68%	66%
Venous Thromboembolism Prophylaxis[2]	21	90%	94%	94%
Written Stroke Educational Materials Given[1,2]	-	-	92%	88%
Surgical Care Improvement Project				
Appropriate Beta Blocker Usage[2]	31	97%	98%	98%
Appropriate VTP Within 24 Hours[2]	150	98%	98%	98%
Controlled Postoperative Blood Glucose[2,7]	-	-	96%	97%
Perioperative Temperature Management[2]	166	100%	100%	100%
Prophylactic Antibiotic Selection[2]	131	100%	99%	99%
Prophylactic Antibiotic Selection (Outpatient)	12	100%	98%	98%
Prophylactic Antibiotic Stopped[2]	126	92%	98%	98%
Prophylactic Antibiotic Timing[2]	131	99%	99%	99%
Prophylactic Antibiotic Timing (Outpatient)	12	100%	98%	98%
Urinary Catheter Removal[2]	107	98%	98%	97%
Survey of Patients' Hospital Experiences				
Area Around Room 'Always' Quiet at Night	300+	68%	68%	61%
Doctors 'Always' Communicated Well	300+	89%	83%	82%

NOTE: Hospital profiles are in alphabetical order by state, then city, then hospital within the city; Rankings exclude hospitals with less than 25 cases except for patient surveys which excludes hospitals with less than 100 cases; (a) 100-299 cases; (1) The number of cases/patients is too few to report; (2) Data submitted were based on a sample of cases/patients; (3) Results are based on a shorter time period than required; (4) Data suppressed by CMS for one or more quarters; (5) Results are not available for this reporting period; (6) Fewer than 100 patients completed the HCAHPS survey; (7) No cases met the criteria for this measure; (8) The lower limit of the confidence interval cannot be calculated if the number of observed infections equals zero; (9) No data are available from the state/territory for this reporting period; (10) The scores shown reflect fewer than 50 completed surveys; (11) There were discrepancies in the data collection process; (12) This measure does not apply to this hospital for this reporting period; (13) Results cannot be calculated for this reporting period; (14) The results for this state are combined with nearby states to protect confidentiality; Please refer to the User's Guide for a full explanation of data.

Measure	Cases	This Hosp.	State Avg.	U.S. Avg.
Home Recovery Information Given	300+	89%	85%	85%
Hospital Given 9 or 10 on 10 Point Scale	300+	76%	73%	71%
Meds 'Always' Explained Before Given	300+	74%	66%	64%
Nurses 'Always' Communicated Well	300+	84%	80%	79%
Pain 'Always' Well Controlled	300+	76%	72%	71%
Room and Bathroom 'Always' Clean	300+	87%	75%	73%
Timely Help 'Always' Received	300+	76%	69%	68%
Would Definitely Recommend Hospital	300+	77%	73%	71%
Use of Medical Imaging				
Cardiac Imaging Stress Test before Surgery[1]	-	-	5.3%	5.3%
Combination Abdominal CT Scan	273	23.4%	16.4%	10.5%
Combination Brain/Sinus CT Scan[1]	-	-	2.7%	2.7%
Combination Chest CT Scan	170	32.4%	5.6%	2.7%
Follow-up Mammogram/Ultrasound	110	13.6%	7.9%	8.8%
Lumbar Spine MRI for Low Back Pain	62	45.2%	39.6%	37.2%

Emerus Hospital

16000 Southwest Freeway
Sugar Land, TX 77479
Phone: 281-516-0911
Type: Acute Care Hospitals
Emergency Services: Yes
Ownership: Physician

Measure	Cases	This Hosp.	State Avg.	U.S. Avg.
Blood Clot Prevention and Treatment				
Anticoagulation Overlap Therapy[5]	-	-	93%	93%
ICU Venous Thromboembolism Prophylaxis[5]	-	-	92%	92%
Incidence of Potentially Preventable VTE[5]	-	-	9%	10%
UFH with Dosages/Platelet Monitoring[5]	-	-	96%	97%
Venous Thromboembolism Prophylaxis[5]	-	-	82%	85%
Warfarin Therapy Discharge Instructions[5]	-	-	84%	75%
Chest Pain/Possible Heart Attack Care				
Aspirin Given Within 24 Hours of Arrival[5]	-	-	94%	96%
Fibrinolytic Meds Within 30 Min. of Arrival[5]	-	-	47%	58%
Average Time to ECG (minutes)[5]	-	-	8	7
Average Time to Transfer (minutes)[5]	-	-	62	60
Children's Asthma Care				
Received Home Management Plan of Care	-	-	93%	88%
Received Reliever Medication	-	-	100%	100%
Received Systemic Corticosteroids	-	-	100%	100%
Emergency Department				
Admittance Decision Time (minutes)[3]	17	54	99	98
Head CT Results Within 45 Min. of Arrival[5]	-	-	54%	57%
Patients Who Left ER Before Being Seen	7,914	1%	3%	2%
Time from ER Arrival to Admit. (minutes)[3]	17	180	270	274
Time from ER Arrival to Discharge (minutes)[3]	14	86	127	134
Time in ER Before Being Evaluated (minutes)[3]	17	22	26	26
Time to Pain Meds for Fractures (minutes)[5]	-	-	57	57
Heart Attack Care				
Aspirin Given at Discharge[5]	-	-	99%	99%
Fibrinolytic Meds Within 30 Min. of Arrival[5]	-	-	49%	54%
PCI Within 90 Minutes of Arrival[5]	-	-	95%	96%
Statin Prescribed at Discharge[5]	-	-	98%	98%
Heart Failure Care				
ACE Inhibitor or ARB for LVSD[5]	-	-	97%	97%
Discharge Instructions Given[5]	-	-	95%	94%
Evaluation of LVS Function[5]	-	-	99%	99%
Medicare Spending				
Medicare Spending per Patient (ratio)[1]	-	-	1.03	0.98
Pneumonia Care				
Appropriate Initial Antibiotic Given[5]	-	-	95%	95%
Blood Culture Timing[5]	-	-	98%	98%
Pregnancy and Delivery Care				
Newborn Deliveries Scheduled Early[7]	-	-	7%	6%
Preventive Care				
Immunization for Influenza[3]	34	0%	90%	90%
Immunization for Pneumonia[1,3]	-	-	92%	92%
Stroke Care				
Anticoagulation Therapy for Atrial Fibrillation[5]	-	-	96%	95%
Antithrombotic Therapy Timing[5]	-	-	98%	98%
Assessed for Rehabilitation[5]	-	-	98%	97%
Discharged on Antithrombotic Therapy[5]	-	-	99%	99%
Discharged on Statin Medication[5]	-	-	95%	94%
Thrombolytic Therapy Timing[5]	-	-	68%	66%
Venous Thromboembolism Prophylaxis[5]	-	-	94%	94%
Written Stroke Educational Materials Given[5]	-	-	92%	88%
Surgical Care Improvement Project				
Appropriate Beta Blocker Usage[5]	-	-	98%	98%
Appropriate VTP Within 24 Hours[5]	-	-	98%	98%
Controlled Postoperative Blood Glucose[5]	-	-	96%	97%
Perioperative Temperature Management[5]	-	-	100%	100%
Prophylactic Antibiotic Selection[5]	-	-	99%	99%
Prophylactic Antibiotic Selection (Outpatient)[5]	-	-	98%	98%
Prophylactic Antibiotic Stopped[5]	-	-	98%	98%
Prophylactic Antibiotic Timing[5]	-	-	99%	99%
Prophylactic Antibiotic Timing (Outpatient)[5]	-	-	98%	98%
Urinary Catheter Removal[5]	-	-	98%	97%
Survey of Patients' Hospital Experiences				
Area Around Room 'Always' Quiet at Night[10]	<100	67%	68%	61%
Doctors 'Always' Communicated Well[10]	<100	67%	83%	82%
Home Recovery Information Given[10]	<100	78%	85%	85%
Hospital Given 9 or 10 on 10 Point Scale[10]	<100	55%	73%	71%
Meds 'Always' Explained Before Given[10]	<100	2%	66%	64%
Nurses 'Always' Communicated Well[10]	<100	78%	80%	79%
Pain 'Always' Well Controlled[10]	<100	46%	72%	71%
Room and Bathroom 'Always' Clean[10]	<100	50%	75%	73%
Timely Help 'Always' Received[10]	<100	45%	69%	68%
Would Definitely Recommend Hospital[10]	<100	67%	73%	71%
Use of Medical Imaging				
Cardiac Imaging Stress Test before Surgery[7]	-	-	5.3%	5.3%
Combination Abdominal CT Scan	54	1.9%	16.4%	10.5%
Combination Brain/Sinus CT Scan[1]	-	-	2.7%	2.7%
Combination Chest CT Scan[1]	-	-	5.6%	2.7%
Follow-up Mammogram/Ultrasound[7]	-	-	7.9%	8.8%
Lumbar Spine MRI for Low Back Pain[7]	-	-	39.6%	37.2%

Memorial Hermann Sugar Land Hospital

17500 W Grand Parkway South
Sugar Land, TX 77479
Phone: 281-499-4800
Type: Acute Care Hospitals
Emergency Services: Yes
Ownership: Voluntary non-profit - Private

Measure	Cases	This Hosp.	State Avg.	U.S. Avg.
Blood Clot Prevention and Treatment				
Anticoagulation Overlap Therapy[2]	34	100%	93%	93%
ICU Venous Thromboembolism Prophylaxis[2]	66	95%	92%	92%
Incidence of Potentially Preventable VTE[1,2]	-	-	9%	10%
UFH with Dosages/Platelet Monitoring[1,2]	-	-	96%	97%
Venous Thromboembolism Prophylaxis[2]	311	99%	82%	85%
Warfarin Therapy Discharge Instructions[2]	29	79%	84%	75%
Chest Pain/Possible Heart Attack Care				
Aspirin Given Within 24 Hours of Arrival	55	100%	94%	96%
Fibrinolytic Meds Within 30 Min. of Arrival[7]	-	-	47%	58%
Average Time to ECG (minutes)	58	4	8	7
Average Time to Transfer (minutes)	16	54	62	60
Children's Asthma Care				
Received Home Management Plan of Care	-	-	93%	88%
Received Reliever Medication	-	-	100%	100%
Received Systemic Corticosteroids	-	-	100%	100%
Emergency Department				
Admittance Decision Time (minutes)[2]	431	74	99	98
Head CT Results Within 45 Min. of Arrival[1]	-	-	54%	57%
Patients Who Left ER Before Being Seen	25,892	1%	3%	2%
Time from ER Arrival to Admit. (minutes)[2]	453	263	270	274
Time from ER Arrival to Discharge (minutes)	371	157	127	134
Time in ER Before Being Evaluated (minutes)	419	27	26	26
Time to Pain Meds for Fractures (minutes)	141	50	57	57
Heart Attack Care				
Aspirin Given at Discharge	18	100%	99%	99%
Fibrinolytic Meds Within 30 Min. of Arrival[7]	-	-	49%	54%
PCI Within 90 Minutes of Arrival[7]	-	-	95%	96%
Statin Prescribed at Discharge	16	100%	98%	98%
Heart Failure Care				
ACE Inhibitor or ARB for LVSD	32	100%	97%	97%
Discharge Instructions Given	98	96%	95%	94%
Evaluation of LVS Function	114	100%	99%	99%
Medicare Spending				
Medicare Spending per Patient (ratio)	-	1.10	1.03	0.98
Pneumonia Care				
Appropriate Initial Antibiotic Given[2]	73	97%	95%	95%
Blood Culture Timing[2]	127	100%	98%	98%
Pregnancy and Delivery Care				
Newborn Deliveries Scheduled Early[2]	23	9%	7%	6%
Preventive Care				
Immunization for Influenza[2]	482	98%	90%	90%
Immunization for Pneumonia[2]	447	98%	92%	92%
Stroke Care				
Anticoagulation Therapy for Atrial Fibrillation[1]	-	-	96%	95%
Antithrombotic Therapy Timing	38	97%	98%	98%
Assessed for Rehabilitation	46	100%	98%	97%
Discharged on Antithrombotic Therapy	46	100%	99%	99%
Discharged on Statin Medication	36	100%	95%	94%
Thrombolytic Therapy Timing[1]	-	-	68%	66%
Venous Thromboembolism Prophylaxis	37	100%	94%	94%
Written Stroke Educational Materials Given	36	92%	92%	88%
Surgical Care Improvement Project				
Appropriate Beta Blocker Usage[2]	94	98%	98%	98%
Appropriate VTP Within 24 Hours[2]	313	98%	98%	98%
Controlled Postoperative Blood Glucose[2,7]	-	-	96%	97%
Perioperative Temperature Management[2]	350	100%	100%	100%
Prophylactic Antibiotic Selection[2]	235	99%	99%	99%
Prophylactic Antibiotic Selection (Outpatient)	118	99%	98%	98%
Prophylactic Antibiotic Stopped[2]	225	100%	98%	98%
Prophylactic Antibiotic Timing[2]	235	100%	99%	99%
Prophylactic Antibiotic Timing (Outpatient)	118	100%	98%	98%
Urinary Catheter Removal[2]	168	100%	98%	97%
Survey of Patients' Hospital Experiences				
Area Around Room 'Always' Quiet at Night	300+	69%	68%	61%
Doctors 'Always' Communicated Well	300+	82%	83%	82%
Home Recovery Information Given	300+	86%	85%	85%
Hospital Given 9 or 10 on 10 Point Scale	300+	76%	73%	71%
Meds 'Always' Explained Before Given	300+	62%	66%	64%
Nurses 'Always' Communicated Well	300+	77%	80%	79%
Pain 'Always' Well Controlled	300+	72%	72%	71%
Room and Bathroom 'Always' Clean	300+	75%	75%	73%
Timely Help 'Always' Received	300+	59%	69%	68%
Would Definitely Recommend Hospital	300+	77%	73%	71%
Use of Medical Imaging				
Cardiac Imaging Stress Test before Surgery[1]	-	-	5.3%	5.3%
Combination Abdominal CT Scan	380	10.3%	16.4%	10.5%
Combination Brain/Sinus CT Scan	335	1.2%	2.7%	2.7%
Combination Chest CT Scan	208	5.8%	5.6%	2.7%
Follow-up Mammogram/Ultrasound	853	6.7%	7.9%	8.8%
Lumbar Spine MRI for Low Back Pain	178	38.8%	39.6%	37.2%

Methodist Sugar Land Hospital

16655 Southwest Freeway
Sugar Land, TX 77479
Phone: 281-274-8000
Fax: 281-274-8361
URL: www.methodisthealth.com/sugarland
Type: Acute Care Hospitals
Emergency Services: Yes
Ownership: Voluntary non-profit - Church

Key Personnel:

Chief of Medical Staff.......... Jeffrey Jackson, MD
CEO/President.............. Chris Siebenaler
Emergency Room .... Scott Stover

Measure	Cases	This Hosp.	State Avg.	U.S. Avg.
Blood Clot Prevention and Treatment				
Anticoagulation Overlap Therapy[2]	95	100%	93%	93%
ICU Venous Thromboembolism Prophylaxis[2]	102	100%	92%	92%
Incidence of Potentially Preventable VTE[2]	18	0%	9%	10%
UFH with Dosages/Platelet Monitoring[2]	13	100%	96%	97%
Venous Thromboembolism Prophylaxis[2]	345	97%	82%	85%
Warfarin Therapy Discharge Instructions[2]	68	100%	84%	75%
Chest Pain/Possible Heart Attack Care				
Aspirin Given Within 24 Hours of Arrival[5]	-	-	94%	96%
Fibrinolytic Meds Within 30 Min. of Arrival[5]	-	-	47%	58%
Average Time to ECG (minutes)[5]	-	-	8	7
Average Time to Transfer (minutes)[5]	-	-	62	60
Children's Asthma Care				
Received Home Management Plan of Care	-	-	93%	88%

NOTE: Hospital profiles are in alphabetical order by state, then city, then hospital within the city; Rankings exclude hospitals with less than 25 cases except for patient surveys which excludes hospitals with less than 100 cases; (a) 100-299 cases; (1) The number of cases/patients is too few to report; (2) Data submitted were based on a sample of cases/patients; (3) Results are based on a shorter time period than required; (4) Data suppressed by CMS for one or more quarters; (5) Results are not available for this reporting period; (6) Fewer than 100 patients completed the HCAHPS survey; (7) No cases met the criteria for this measure; (8) The lower limit of the confidence interval cannot be calculated if the number of observed infections equals zero; (9) No data are available from the state/territory for this reporting period; (10) The scores shown reflect fewer than 50 completed surveys; (11) There were discrepancies in the data collection process; (12) This measure does not apply to this hospital for this reporting period; (13) Results cannot be calculated for this reporting period; (14) The results for this state are combined with nearby states to protect confidentiality; Please refer to the User's Guide for a full explanation of data.

Measure	Cases	This Hosp.	State Avg.	U.S. Avg.
Received Reliever Medication	-	-	100%	100%
Received Systemic Corticosteroids	-	-	100%	100%
Emergency Department				
Admittance Decision Time (minutes)[2]	330	104	99	98
Head CT Results Within 45 Min. of Arrival	12	92%	54%	57%
Patients Who Left ER Before Being Seen	38,524	4%	3%	2%
Time from ER Arrival to Admit. (minutes)[2]	397	301	270	274
Time from ER Arrival to Discharge (minutes)	353	202	127	134
Time in ER Before Being Evaluated (minutes)	424	70	26	26
Time to Pain Meds for Fractures (minutes)	144	72	57	57
Heart Attack Care				
Aspirin Given at Discharge[2]	232	100%	99%	99%
Fibrinolytic Meds Within 30 Min. of Arrival[2,7]	-	-	49%	54%
PCI Within 90 Minutes of Arrival[2]	52	100%	95%	96%
Statin Prescribed at Discharge[2]	216	100%	98%	98%
Heart Failure Care				
ACE Inhibitor or ARB for LVSD[2]	105	100%	97%	97%
Discharge Instructions Given[2]	253	100%	95%	94%
Evaluation of LVS Function[2]	325	100%	99%	99%
Medicare Spending				
Medicare Spending per Patient (ratio)	-	1.09	1.03	0.98
Pneumonia Care				
Appropriate Initial Antibiotic Given[2]	68	99%	95%	95%
Blood Culture Timing[2]	106	100%	98%	98%
Pregnancy and Delivery Care				
Newborn Deliveries Scheduled Early[2]	56	4%	7%	6%
Preventive Care				
Immunization for Influenza[2]	528	99%	90%	90%
Immunization for Pneumonia[2]	566	98%	92%	92%
Stroke Care				
Anticoagulation Therapy for Atrial Fibrillation	27	100%	96%	95%
Antithrombotic Therapy Timing	170	100%	98%	98%
Assessed for Rehabilitation	195	99%	98%	97%
Discharged on Antithrombotic Therapy	174	99%	99%	99%
Discharged on Statin Medication	136	97%	95%	94%
Thrombolytic Therapy Timing[1]	-	-	68%	66%
Venous Thromboembolism Prophylaxis	181	100%	94%	94%
Written Stroke Educational Materials Given	108	95%	92%	88%
Surgical Care Improvement Project				
Appropriate Beta Blocker Usage[2]	203	99%	98%	98%
Appropriate VTP Within 24 Hours[2]	463	100%	98%	98%
Controlled Postoperative Blood Glucose[2]	105	98%	96%	97%
Perioperative Temperature Management[2]	584	100%	100%	100%
Prophylactic Antibiotic Selection[2]	470	99%	99%	99%
Prophylactic Antibiotic Selection (Outpatient)	493	96%	98%	98%
Prophylactic Antibiotic Stopped[2]	417	99%	98%	98%
Prophylactic Antibiotic Timing[2]	470	100%	99%	99%
Prophylactic Antibiotic Timing (Outpatient)	494	98%	98%	98%
Urinary Catheter Removal[2]	339	100%	98%	97%
Survey of Patients' Hospital Experiences				
Area Around Room 'Always' Quiet at Night	300+	66%	68%	61%
Doctors 'Always' Communicated Well	300+	80%	83%	82%
Home Recovery Information Given	300+	85%	85%	85%
Hospital Given 9 or 10 on 10 Point Scale	300+	78%	73%	71%
Meds 'Always' Explained Before Given	300+	66%	66%	64%
Nurses 'Always' Communicated Well	300+	78%	80%	79%
Pain 'Always' Well Controlled	300+	71%	72%	71%
Room and Bathroom 'Always' Clean	300+	72%	75%	73%
Timely Help 'Always' Received	300+	66%	69%	68%
Would Definitely Recommend Hospital	300+	79%	73%	71%
Use of Medical Imaging				
Cardiac Imaging Stress Test before Surgery	212	8.0%	5.3%	5.3%
Combination Abdominal CT Scan	851	22.8%	16.4%	10.5%
Combination Brain/Sinus CT Scan	1,100	2.4%	2.7%	2.7%
Combination Chest CT Scan	843	2.7%	5.6%	2.7%
Follow-up Mammogram/Ultrasound	841	7.3%	7.9%	8.8%
Lumbar Spine MRI for Low Back Pain	245	33.5%	39.6%	37.2%

Saint Luke's Sugar Land Hospital

1317 Lake Pointe Parkway Phone: 281-637-7000
Sugar Land, TX 77478
URL: www.stlukessugarland.com
Type: Acute Care Hospitals Emergency Services: Yes
Ownership: Voluntary non-profit - Other Beds: 100

Measure	Cases	This Hosp.	State Avg.	U.S. Avg.
Blood Clot Prevention and Treatment				
Anticoagulation Overlap Therapy[2]	28	93%	93%	93%
ICU Venous Thromboembolism Prophylaxis[2]	75	81%	92%	92%
Incidence of Potentially Preventable VTE[1,2]	-	-	9%	10%
UFH with Dosages/Platelet Monitoring[1,2]	-	-	96%	97%
Venous Thromboembolism Prophylaxis[2]	312	77%	82%	85%
Warfarin Therapy Discharge Instructions[2]	25	72%	84%	75%
Chest Pain/Possible Heart Attack Care				
Aspirin Given Within 24 Hours of Arrival[1]	-	-	94%	96%
Fibrinolytic Meds Within 30 Min. of Arrival[3,7]	-	-	47%	58%
Average Time to ECG (minutes)[1]	-	-	8	7
Average Time to Transfer (minutes)[3,7]	-	-	62	60
Children's Asthma Care				
Received Home Management Plan of Care	-	-	93%	88%
Received Reliever Medication	-	-	100%	100%
Received Systemic Corticosteroids	-	-	100%	100%
Emergency Department				
Admittance Decision Time (minutes)[2]	479	189	99	98
Head CT Results Within 45 Min. of Arrival[1]	-	-	54%	57%
Patients Who Left ER Before Being Seen	18,633	1%	3%	2%
Time from ER Arrival to Admit. (minutes)[2]	486	357	270	274
Time from ER Arrival to Discharge (minutes)	386	177	127	134
Time in ER Before Being Evaluated (minutes)	364	73	26	26
Time to Pain Meds for Fractures (minutes)	84	62	57	57
Heart Attack Care				
Aspirin Given at Discharge	86	98%	99%	99%
Fibrinolytic Meds Within 30 Min. of Arrival[7]	-	-	49%	54%
PCI Within 90 Minutes of Arrival[1]	-	-	95%	96%
Statin Prescribed at Discharge	83	100%	98%	98%
Heart Failure Care				
ACE Inhibitor or ARB for LVSD	31	94%	97%	97%
Discharge Instructions Given	88	97%	95%	94%
Evaluation of LVS Function	107	99%	99%	99%
Medicare Spending				
Medicare Spending per Patient (ratio)	-	1.17	1.03	0.98
Pneumonia Care				
Appropriate Initial Antibiotic Given	85	98%	95%	95%
Blood Culture Timing	122	98%	98%	98%
Pregnancy and Delivery Care				
Newborn Deliveries Scheduled Early[7]	-	-	7%	6%
Preventive Care				
Immunization for Influenza[2]	341	92%	90%	90%
Immunization for Pneumonia[2]	420	93%	92%	92%
Stroke Care				
Anticoagulation Therapy for Atrial Fibrillation[1]	-	-	96%	95%
Antithrombotic Therapy Timing	30	100%	98%	98%
Assessed for Rehabilitation	37	95%	98%	97%
Discharged on Antithrombotic Therapy	33	100%	99%	99%
Discharged on Statin Medication	26	88%	95%	94%
Thrombolytic Therapy Timing[1]	-	-	68%	66%
Venous Thromboembolism Prophylaxis	36	94%	94%	94%
Written Stroke Educational Materials Given	23	26%	92%	88%
Surgical Care Improvement Project				
Appropriate Beta Blocker Usage	24	100%	98%	98%
Appropriate VTP Within 24 Hours	83	100%	98%	98%
Controlled Postoperative Blood Glucose[7]	-	-	96%	97%
Perioperative Temperature Management	92	100%	100%	100%
Prophylactic Antibiotic Selection	35	97%	99%	99%
Prophylactic Antibiotic Selection (Outpatient)	19	95%	98%	98%
Prophylactic Antibiotic Stopped	34	85%	98%	98%
Prophylactic Antibiotic Timing	35	97%	99%	99%
Prophylactic Antibiotic Timing (Outpatient)	19	100%	98%	98%
Urinary Catheter Removal	60	87%	98%	97%
Survey of Patients' Hospital Experiences				
Area Around Room 'Always' Quiet at Night	300+	70%	68%	61%
Doctors 'Always' Communicated Well	300+	80%	83%	82%
Home Recovery Information Given	300+	80%	85%	85%
Hospital Given 9 or 10 on 10 Point Scale	300+	72%	73%	71%
Meds 'Always' Explained Before Given	300+	63%	66%	64%
Nurses 'Always' Communicated Well	300+	75%	80%	79%
Pain 'Always' Well Controlled	300+	67%	72%	71%
Room and Bathroom 'Always' Clean	300+	77%	75%	73%
Timely Help 'Always' Received	300+	57%	69%	68%
Would Definitely Recommend Hospital	300+	75%	73%	71%
Use of Medical Imaging				
Cardiac Imaging Stress Test before Surgery[1]	-	-	5.3%	5.3%
Combination Abdominal CT Scan	246	7.7%	16.4%	10.5%
Combination Brain/Sinus CT Scan[1]	-	-	2.7%	2.7%
Combination Chest CT Scan	215	0.0%	5.6%	2.7%
Follow-up Mammogram/Ultrasound	84	15.5%	7.9%	8.8%
Lumbar Spine MRI for Low Back Pain[1]	-	-	39.6%	37.2%

Sugar Land Surgical Hospital

16906 Southwest Freeway Phone: 281-243-1000
Sugar Land, TX 77479
URL: www.sugarlandsurgicalhospital.com
Type: Acute Care Hospitals Emergency Services: No
Ownership: Proprietary

Measure	Cases	This Hosp.	State Avg.	U.S. Avg.
Blood Clot Prevention and Treatment				
Anticoagulation Overlap Therapy[2,7]	-	-	93%	93%
ICU Venous Thromboembolism Prophylaxis[2,7]	-	-	92%	92%
Incidence of Potentially Preventable VTE[1,2]	-	-	9%	10%
UFH with Dosages/Platelet Monitoring[2,7]	-	-	96%	97%
Venous Thromboembolism Prophylaxis[2]	30	100%	82%	85%
Warfarin Therapy Discharge Instructions[2,7]	-	-	84%	75%
Chest Pain/Possible Heart Attack Care				
Aspirin Given Within 24 Hours of Arrival[1,3]	-	-	94%	96%
Fibrinolytic Meds Within 30 Min. of Arrival[3,7]	-	-	47%	58%
Average Time to ECG (minutes)[1,3]	-	-	8	7
Average Time to Transfer (minutes)[1,3]	-	-	62	60
Children's Asthma Care				
Received Home Management Plan of Care	-	-	93%	88%
Received Reliever Medication	-	-	100%	100%
Received Systemic Corticosteroids	-	-	100%	100%
Emergency Department				
Admittance Decision Time (minutes)[1]	-	-	99	98
Head CT Results Within 45 Min. of Arrival[5]	-	-	54%	57%
Patients Who Left ER Before Being Seen	297	2%	3%	2%
Time from ER Arrival to Admit. (minutes)[1]	-	-	270	274
Time from ER Arrival to Discharge (minutes)	253	87	127	134
Time in ER Before Being Evaluated (minutes)	278	6	26	26
Time to Pain Meds for Fractures (minutes)[1,3]	-	-	57	57
Heart Attack Care				
Aspirin Given at Discharge[5]	-	-	99%	99%
Fibrinolytic Meds Within 30 Min. of Arrival[5]	-	-	49%	54%
PCI Within 90 Minutes of Arrival[5]	-	-	95%	96%
Statin Prescribed at Discharge[5]	-	-	98%	98%
Heart Failure Care				
ACE Inhibitor or ARB for LVSD[5]	-	-	97%	97%
Discharge Instructions Given[5]	-	-	95%	94%
Evaluation of LVS Function[5]	-	-	99%	99%
Medicare Spending				
Medicare Spending per Patient (ratio)	-	0.95	1.03	0.98
Pneumonia Care				
Appropriate Initial Antibiotic Given[5]	-	-	95%	95%
Blood Culture Timing[5]	-	-	98%	98%
Pregnancy and Delivery Care				
Newborn Deliveries Scheduled Early[7]	-	-	7%	6%
Preventive Care				
Immunization for Influenza	137	96%	90%	90%
Immunization for Pneumonia	152	96%	92%	92%
Stroke Care				
Anticoagulation Therapy for Atrial Fibrillation[5]	-	-	96%	95%
Antithrombotic Therapy Timing[5]	-	-	98%	98%
Assessed for Rehabilitation[5]	-	-	98%	97%
Discharged on Antithrombotic Therapy[5]	-	-	99%	99%

NOTE: Hospital profiles are in alphabetical order by state, then city, then hospital within the city; Rankings exclude hospitals with less than 25 cases except for patient surveys which excludes hospitals with less than 100 cases; (a) 100-299 cases; (1) The number of cases/patients is too few to report; (2) Data submitted were based on a sample of cases/patients; (3) Results are based on a shorter time period than required; (4) Data suppressed by CMS for one or more quarters; (5) Results are not available for this reporting period; (6) Fewer than 100 patients completed the HCAHPS survey; (7) No cases met the criteria for this measure; (8) The lower limit of the confidence interval cannot be calculated if the number of observed infections equals zero; (9) No data are available from the state/territory for this reporting period; (10) The scores shown reflect fewer than 50 completed surveys; (11) There were discrepancies in the data collection process; (12) This measure does not apply to this hospital for this reporting period; (13) Results cannot be calculated for this reporting period; (14) The results for this state are combined with nearby states to protect confidentiality; Please refer to the User's Guide for a full explanation of data.

Measure	Cases	This Hosp.	State Avg.	U.S. Avg.
Discharged on Statin Medication[5]	-	-	95%	94%
Thrombolytic Therapy Timing[5]	-	-	68%	66%
Venous Thromboembolism Prophylaxis[5]	-	-	94%	94%
Written Stroke Educational Materials Given[5]	-	-	92%	88%
Surgical Care Improvement Project				
Appropriate Beta Blocker Usage	45	98%	98%	98%
Appropriate VTP Within 24 Hours	175	100%	98%	98%
Controlled Postoperative Blood Glucose[7]	-	-	96%	97%
Perioperative Temperature Management	185	100%	100%	100%
Prophylactic Antibiotic Selection	170	100%	99%	99%
Prophylactic Antibiotic Selection (Outpatient)	133	99%	98%	98%
Prophylactic Antibiotic Stopped	169	99%	98%	98%
Prophylactic Antibiotic Timing	170	99%	99%	99%
Prophylactic Antibiotic Timing (Outpatient)	133	96%	98%	98%
Urinary Catheter Removal	122	99%	98%	97%
Survey of Patients' Hospital Experiences				
Area Around Room 'Always' Quiet at Night	(a)	89%	68%	61%
Doctors 'Always' Communicated Well	(a)	88%	83%	82%
Home Recovery Information Given	(a)	91%	85%	85%
Hospital Given 9 or 10 on 10 Point Scale	(a)	90%	73%	71%
Meds 'Always' Explained Before Given	(a)	85%	66%	64%
Nurses 'Always' Communicated Well	(a)	95%	80%	79%
Pain 'Always' Well Controlled	(a)	83%	72%	71%
Room and Bathroom 'Always' Clean	(a)	89%	75%	73%
Timely Help 'Always' Received	(a)	94%	69%	68%
Would Definitely Recommend Hospital	(a)	92%	73%	71%
Use of Medical Imaging				
Cardiac Imaging Stress Test before Surgery[7]	-	-	5.3%	5.3%
Combination Abdominal CT Scan[1]	-	-	16.4%	10.5%
Combination Brain/Sinus CT Scan[1]	-	-	2.7%	2.7%
Combination Chest CT Scan[1]	-	-	5.6%	2.7%
Follow-up Mammogram/Ultrasound[7]	-	-	7.9%	8.8%
Lumbar Spine MRI for Low Back Pain[1]	-	-	39.6%	37.2%

Hopkins County Memorial Hospital

115 Airport Rd Phone: 903-885-7671
Sulphur Springs, TX 75482
URL: www.hcmh.com
Type: Acute Care Hospitals Emergency Services: Yes
Ownership: Govt - Hospital Dist/Auth
Key Personnel:
CEO .... Michael McAndrew
Radiology.................. Thomas Varghese, M.D.

Measure	Cases	This Hosp.	State Avg.	U.S. Avg.
Blood Clot Prevention and Treatment				
Anticoagulation Overlap Therapy[2]	13	77%	93%	93%
ICU Venous Thromboembolism Prophylaxis[2]	40	68%	92%	92%
Incidence of Potentially Preventable VTE[1,2]	-	-	9%	10%
UFH with Dosages/Platelet Monitoring[1,2]	-	-	96%	97%
Venous Thromboembolism Prophylaxis[2]	230	55%	82%	85%
Warfarin Therapy Discharge Instructions[1,2]	-	-	84%	75%
Chest Pain/Possible Heart Attack Care				
Aspirin Given Within 24 Hours of Arrival	41	100%	94%	96%
Fibrinolytic Meds Within 30 Min. of Arrival[1]	-	-	47%	58%
Average Time to ECG (minutes)	43	5	8	7
Average Time to Transfer (minutes)[1]	-	-	62	60
Children's Asthma Care				
Received Home Management Plan of Care	-	-	93%	88%
Received Reliever Medication	-	-	100%	100%
Received Systemic Corticosteroids	-	-	100%	100%
Emergency Department				
Admittance Decision Time (minutes)[2]	322	56	99	98
Head CT Results Within 45 Min. of Arrival	23	43%	54%	57%
Patients Who Left ER Before Being Seen	17,631	4%	3%	2%
Time from ER Arrival to Admit. (minutes)[2]	331	196	270	274
Time from ER Arrival to Discharge (minutes)	478	116	127	134
Time in ER Before Being Evaluated (minutes)	514	25	26	26
Time to Pain Meds for Fractures (minutes)	73	56	57	57
Heart Attack Care				
Aspirin Given at Discharge	50	100%	99%	99%
Fibrinolytic Meds Within 30 Min. of Arrival[7]	-	-	49%	54%
PCI Within 90 Minutes of Arrival	12	100%	95%	96%
Statin Prescribed at Discharge	48	98%	98%	98%
Heart Failure Care				
ACE Inhibitor or ARB for LVSD	29	100%	97%	97%
Discharge Instructions Given	60	98%	95%	94%
Evaluation of LVS Function	85	99%	99%	99%
Medicare Spending				
Medicare Spending per Patient (ratio)	-	1.06	1.03	0.98
Pneumonia Care				
Appropriate Initial Antibiotic Given	121	93%	95%	95%
Blood Culture Timing	132	93%	98%	98%
Pregnancy and Delivery Care				
Newborn Deliveries Scheduled Early[2]	44	2%	7%	6%
Preventive Care				
Immunization for Influenza[2]	344	90%	90%	90%
Immunization for Pneumonia[2]	312	94%	92%	92%
Stroke Care				
Anticoagulation Therapy for Atrial Fibrillation[1]	-	-	96%	95%
Antithrombotic Therapy Timing	26	92%	98%	98%
Assessed for Rehabilitation	27	78%	98%	97%
Discharged on Antithrombotic Therapy	26	85%	99%	99%
Discharged on Statin Medication	25	72%	95%	94%
Thrombolytic Therapy Timing[1]	-	-	68%	66%
Venous Thromboembolism Prophylaxis	26	35%	94%	94%
Written Stroke Educational Materials Given	15	73%	92%	88%
Surgical Care Improvement Project				
Appropriate Beta Blocker Usage	28	86%	98%	98%
Appropriate VTP Within 24 Hours	120	88%	98%	98%
Controlled Postoperative Blood Glucose[7]	-	-	96%	97%
Perioperative Temperature Management	146	100%	100%	100%
Prophylactic Antibiotic Selection	84	92%	99%	99%
Prophylactic Antibiotic Selection (Outpatient)	132	89%	98%	98%
Prophylactic Antibiotic Stopped	83	88%	98%	98%
Prophylactic Antibiotic Timing	84	93%	99%	99%
Prophylactic Antibiotic Timing (Outpatient)	134	93%	98%	98%
Urinary Catheter Removal	44	91%	98%	97%
Survey of Patients' Hospital Experiences				
Area Around Room 'Always' Quiet at Night	300+	66%	68%	61%
Doctors 'Always' Communicated Well	300+	78%	83%	82%
Home Recovery Information Given	300+	85%	85%	85%
Hospital Given 9 or 10 on 10 Point Scale	300+	71%	73%	71%
Meds 'Always' Explained Before Given	300+	66%	66%	64%
Nurses 'Always' Communicated Well	300+	82%	80%	79%
Pain 'Always' Well Controlled	300+	72%	72%	71%
Room and Bathroom 'Always' Clean	300+	77%	75%	73%
Timely Help 'Always' Received	300+	67%	69%	68%
Would Definitely Recommend Hospital	300+	68%	73%	71%
Use of Medical Imaging				
Cardiac Imaging Stress Test before Surgery	414	3.9%	5.3%	5.3%
Combination Abdominal CT Scan	449	38.5%	16.4%	10.5%
Combination Brain/Sinus CT Scan[1]	-	-	2.7%	2.7%
Combination Chest CT Scan	220	21.4%	5.6%	2.7%
Follow-up Mammogram/Ultrasound	360	1.7%	7.9%	8.8%
Lumbar Spine MRI for Low Back Pain	67	56.7%	39.6%	37.2%

Texas Regional Medical Center at Sunnyvale

231 South Collins Road Phone: 972-892-3000
Sunnyvale, TX 75182
URL: www.texasregionalmedicalcenter.com
Type: Acute Care Hospitals Emergency Services: Yes
Ownership: Proprietary
Key Personnel:
President .... Terry Fontenot

Measure	Cases	This Hosp.	State Avg.	U.S. Avg.
Blood Clot Prevention and Treatment				
Anticoagulation Overlap Therapy[2]	30	100%	93%	93%
ICU Venous Thromboembolism Prophylaxis[2]	60	93%	92%	92%
Incidence of Potentially Preventable VTE[1,2]	-	-	9%	10%
UFH with Dosages/Platelet Monitoring[2]	16	100%	96%	97%
Venous Thromboembolism Prophylaxis[2]	358	85%	82%	85%
Warfarin Therapy Discharge Instructions[2]	23	100%	84%	75%
Chest Pain/Possible Heart Attack Care				
Aspirin Given Within 24 Hours of Arrival[1]	-	-	94%	96%
Fibrinolytic Meds Within 30 Min. of Arrival[5]	-	-	47%	58%
Average Time to ECG (minutes)[1]	-	-	8	7
Average Time to Transfer (minutes)[5]	-	-	62	60
Children's Asthma Care				
Received Home Management Plan of Care	-	-	93%	88%
Received Reliever Medication	-	-	100%	100%
Received Systemic Corticosteroids	-	-	100%	100%
Emergency Department				
Admittance Decision Time (minutes)[2]	514	80	99	98
Head CT Results Within 45 Min. of Arrival[1]	-	-	54%	57%
Patients Who Left ER Before Being Seen	30,374	10%	3%	2%
Time from ER Arrival to Admit. (minutes)[2]	514	268	270	274
Time from ER Arrival to Discharge (minutes)	337	130	127	134
Time in ER Before Being Evaluated (minutes)	381	60	26	26
Time to Pain Meds for Fractures (minutes)	182	64	57	57
Heart Attack Care				
Aspirin Given at Discharge	112	99%	99%	99%
Fibrinolytic Meds Within 30 Min. of Arrival[7]	-	-	49%	54%
PCI Within 90 Minutes of Arrival[1]	-	-	95%	96%
Statin Prescribed at Discharge	102	95%	98%	98%
Heart Failure Care				
ACE Inhibitor or ARB for LVSD[2]	57	98%	97%	97%
Discharge Instructions Given[2]	152	95%	95%	94%
Evaluation of LVS Function[2]	193	98%	99%	99%
Medicare Spending				
Medicare Spending per Patient (ratio)	-	1.16	1.03	0.98
Pneumonia Care				
Appropriate Initial Antibiotic Given	65	98%	95%	95%
Blood Culture Timing	125	98%	98%	98%
Pregnancy and Delivery Care				
Newborn Deliveries Scheduled Early[2]	31	0%	7%	6%
Preventive Care				
Immunization for Influenza[2]	443	80%	90%	90%
Immunization for Pneumonia[2]	501	95%	92%	92%
Stroke Care				
Anticoagulation Therapy for Atrial Fibrillation[1]	-	-	96%	95%
Antithrombotic Therapy Timing	46	100%	98%	98%
Assessed for Rehabilitation	43	100%	98%	97%
Discharged on Antithrombotic Therapy	43	98%	99%	99%
Discharged on Statin Medication	34	88%	95%	94%
Thrombolytic Therapy Timing[1]	-	-	68%	66%
Venous Thromboembolism Prophylaxis	47	100%	94%	94%
Written Stroke Educational Materials Given	28	86%	92%	88%
Surgical Care Improvement Project				
Appropriate Beta Blocker Usage[2]	71	100%	98%	98%
Appropriate VTP Within 24 Hours[2]	156	98%	98%	98%
Controlled Postoperative Blood Glucose[2]	24	88%	96%	97%
Perioperative Temperature Management[2]	190	100%	100%	100%
Prophylactic Antibiotic Selection[2]	168	100%	99%	99%
Prophylactic Antibiotic Selection (Outpatient)	52	92%	98%	98%
Prophylactic Antibiotic Stopped[2]	167	98%	98%	98%
Prophylactic Antibiotic Timing[2]	167	100%	99%	99%
Prophylactic Antibiotic Timing (Outpatient)	56	88%	98%	98%
Urinary Catheter Removal[2]	126	94%	98%	97%
Survey of Patients' Hospital Experiences				
Area Around Room 'Always' Quiet at Night	300+	60%	68%	61%
Doctors 'Always' Communicated Well	300+	77%	83%	82%
Home Recovery Information Given	300+	77%	85%	85%
Hospital Given 9 or 10 on 10 Point Scale	300+	71%	73%	71%
Meds 'Always' Explained Before Given	300+	62%	66%	64%
Nurses 'Always' Communicated Well	300+	77%	80%	79%
Pain 'Always' Well Controlled	300+	74%	72%	71%
Room and Bathroom 'Always' Clean	300+	73%	75%	73%
Timely Help 'Always' Received	300+	70%	69%	68%
Would Definitely Recommend Hospital	300+	74%	73%	71%
Use of Medical Imaging				
Cardiac Imaging Stress Test before Surgery	88	4.5%	5.3%	5.3%
Combination Abdominal CT Scan	278	10.1%	16.4%	10.5%
Combination Brain/Sinus CT Scan[1]	-	-	2.7%	2.7%
Combination Chest CT Scan	67	11.9%	5.6%	2.7%
Follow-up Mammogram/Ultrasound	117	17.1%	7.9%	8.8%
Lumbar Spine MRI for Low Back Pain[1]	-	-	39.6%	37.2%

NOTE: Hospital profiles are in alphabetical order by state, then city, then hospital within the city; Rankings exclude hospitals with less than 25 cases except for patient surveys which excludes hospitals with less than 100 cases; (a) 100-299 cases; (1) The number of cases/patients is too few to report; (2) Data submitted were based on a sample of cases/patients; (3) Results are based on a shorter time period than required; (4) Data suppressed by CMS for one or more quarters; (5) Results are not available for this reporting period; (6) Fewer than 100 patients completed the HCAHPS survey; (7) No cases met the criteria for this measure; (8) The lower limit of the confidence interval cannot be calculated if the number of observed infections equals zero; (9) No data are available from the state/territory for this reporting period; (10) The scores shown reflect fewer than 50 completed surveys; (11) There were discrepancies in the data collection process; (12) This measure does not apply to this hospital for this reporting period; (13) Results cannot be calculated for this reporting period; (14) The results for this state are combined with nearby states to protect confidentiality; Please refer to the User's Guide for a full explanation of data.

Sweeny Community Hospital

305 North Mckinney Phone: 979-548-3311
Sweeny, TX 77480
Type: Critical Access Hospitals Emergency Services: Yes
Ownership: Govt - Hospital Dist/Auth

Measure	Cases	This Hosp.	State Avg.	U.S. Avg.
Blood Clot Prevention and Treatment				
Anticoagulation Overlap Therapy[5]	-	-	93%	93%
ICU Venous Thromboembolism Prophylaxis[5]	-	-	92%	92%
Incidence of Potentially Preventable VTE[5]	-	-	9%	10%
UFH with Dosages/Platelet Monitoring[5]	-	-	96%	97%
Venous Thromboembolism Prophylaxis[5]	-	-	82%	85%
Warfarin Therapy Discharge Instructions[5]	-	-	84%	75%
Chest Pain/Possible Heart Attack Care				
Aspirin Given Within 24 Hours of Arrival[5]	-	-	94%	96%
Fibrinolytic Meds Within 30 Min. of Arrival[5]	-	-	47%	58%
Average Time to ECG (minutes)[5]	-	-	8	7
Average Time to Transfer (minutes)[5]	-	-	62	60
Children's Asthma Care				
Received Home Management Plan of Care	-	-	93%	88%
Received Reliever Medication	-	-	100%	100%
Received Systemic Corticosteroids	-	-	100%	100%
Emergency Department				
Admittance Decision Time (minutes)[5]	-	-	99	98
Head CT Results Within 45 Min. of Arrival[5]	-	-	54%	57%
Patients Who Left ER Before Being Seen[5]	-	-	3%	2%
Time from ER Arrival to Admit. (minutes)[5]	-	-	270	274
Time from ER Arrival to Discharge (minutes)[5]	-	-	127	134
Time in ER Before Being Evaluated (minutes)[5]	-	-	26	26
Time to Pain Meds for Fractures (minutes)[5]	-	-	57	57
Heart Attack Care				
Aspirin Given at Discharge[5]	-	-	99%	99%
Fibrinolytic Meds Within 30 Min. of Arrival[5]	-	-	49%	54%
PCI Within 90 Minutes of Arrival[5]	-	-	95%	96%
Statin Prescribed at Discharge[5]	-	-	98%	98%
Heart Failure Care				
ACE Inhibitor or ARB for LVSD[5]	-	-	97%	97%
Discharge Instructions Given[5]	-	-	95%	94%
Evaluation of LVS Function[5]	-	-	99%	99%
Medicare Spending				
Medicare Spending per Patient (ratio)	-	-	1.03	0.98
Pneumonia Care				
Appropriate Initial Antibiotic Given[5]	-	-	95%	95%
Blood Culture Timing[5]	-	-	98%	98%
Pregnancy and Delivery Care				
Newborn Deliveries Scheduled Early[5]	-	-	7%	6%
Preventive Care				
Immunization for Influenza[5]	-	-	90%	90%
Immunization for Pneumonia[5]	-	-	92%	92%
Stroke Care				
Anticoagulation Therapy for Atrial Fibrillation[5]	-	-	96%	95%
Antithrombotic Therapy Timing[5]	-	-	98%	98%
Assessed for Rehabilitation[5]	-	-	98%	97%
Discharged on Antithrombotic Therapy[5]	-	-	99%	99%
Discharged on Statin Medication[5]	-	-	95%	94%
Thrombolytic Therapy Timing[5]	-	-	68%	66%
Venous Thromboembolism Prophylaxis[5]	-	-	94%	94%
Written Stroke Educational Materials Given[5]	-	-	92%	88%
Surgical Care Improvement Project				
Appropriate Beta Blocker Usage[5]	-	-	98%	98%
Appropriate VTP Within 24 Hours[5]	-	-	98%	98%
Controlled Postoperative Blood Glucose[5]	-	-	96%	97%
Perioperative Temperature Management[5]	-	-	100%	100%
Prophylactic Antibiotic Selection[5]	-	-	99%	99%
Prophylactic Antibiotic Selection (Outpatient)[5]	-	-	98%	98%
Prophylactic Antibiotic Stopped[5]	-	-	98%	98%
Prophylactic Antibiotic Timing[5]	-	-	99%	99%
Prophylactic Antibiotic Timing (Outpatient)[5]	-	-	98%	98%
Urinary Catheter Removal[5]	-	-	98%	97%
Survey of Patients' Hospital Experiences				
Area Around Room 'Always' Quiet at Night[10]	<100	75%	68%	61%
Doctors 'Always' Communicated Well[10]	<100	62%	83%	82%
Home Recovery Information Given[10]	<100	74%	85%	85%
Hospital Given 9 or 10 on 10 Point Scale[10]	<100	66%	73%	71%
Meds 'Always' Explained Before Given[10]	<100	63%	66%	64%
Nurses 'Always' Communicated Well[10]	<100	79%	80%	79%
Pain 'Always' Well Controlled[10]	<100	58%	72%	71%
Room and Bathroom 'Always' Clean[10]	<100	60%	75%	73%
Timely Help 'Always' Received[10]	<100	72%	69%	68%
Would Definitely Recommend Hospital[10]	<100	53%	73%	71%
Use of Medical Imaging				
Cardiac Imaging Stress Test before Surgery[7]	-	-	5.3%	5.3%
Combination Abdominal CT Scan	72	6.9%	16.4%	10.5%
Combination Brain/Sinus CT Scan[1]	-	-	2.7%	2.7%
Combination Chest CT Scan	52	0.0%	5.6%	2.7%
Follow-up Mammogram/Ultrasound	91	2.2%	7.9%	8.8%
Lumbar Spine MRI for Low Back Pain[1]	-	-	39.6%	37.2%

Rolling Plains Memorial Hospital

200 E Arizona Phone: 325-235-1701
Sweetwater, TX 79556 Fax: 325-235-8705
URL: www.rpmh.net
Type: Acute Care Hospitals Emergency Services: Yes
Ownership: Govt - Hospital Dist/Auth Beds: 55
Key Personnel:
Infection Control. . . . . Dody Barnes, RN
Intensive Care Unit. . . . . Kevin Herm, RN
Emergency Room . . . . Carol Higdon, RN
Operating Room. . . . . George Jones, RN
Cardiology . . . . Larry W. Lin, MD
Surgery . . . . Lufkin R. Moses, DO
Chief of Medical Staff . . . . Mickey Williams, RN

Measure	Cases	This Hosp.	State Avg.	U.S. Avg.
Blood Clot Prevention and Treatment				
Anticoagulation Overlap Therapy[1,2]	-	-	93%	93%
ICU Venous Thromboembolism Prophylaxis[2]	53	89%	92%	92%
Incidence of Potentially Preventable VTE[2,7]	-	-	9%	10%
UFH with Dosages/Platelet Monitoring[2,7]	-	-	96%	97%
Venous Thromboembolism Prophylaxis[2]	127	94%	82%	85%
Warfarin Therapy Discharge Instructions[1,2]	-	-	84%	75%
Chest Pain/Possible Heart Attack Care				
Aspirin Given Within 24 Hours of Arrival	76	99%	94%	96%
Fibrinolytic Meds Within 30 Min. of Arrival[1]	-	-	47%	58%
Average Time to ECG (minutes)	84	15	8	7
Average Time to Transfer (minutes)[7]	-	-	62	60
Children's Asthma Care				
Received Home Management Plan of Care	-	-	93%	88%
Received Reliever Medication	-	-	100%	100%
Received Systemic Corticosteroids	-	-	100%	100%
Emergency Department				
Admittance Decision Time (minutes)[2]	236	54	99	98
Head CT Results Within 45 Min. of Arrival[1,3]	-	-	54%	57%
Patients Who Left ER Before Being Seen	12,002	1%	3%	2%
Time from ER Arrival to Admit. (minutes)[2]	236	195	270	274
Time from ER Arrival to Discharge (minutes)	324	106	127	134
Time in ER Before Being Evaluated (minutes)	375	20	26	26
Time to Pain Meds for Fractures (minutes)	43	41	57	57
Heart Attack Care				
Aspirin Given at Discharge[7]	-	-	99%	99%
Fibrinolytic Meds Within 30 Min. of Arrival[7]	-	-	49%	54%
PCI Within 90 Minutes of Arrival[7]	-	-	95%	96%
Statin Prescribed at Discharge[7]	-	-	98%	98%
Heart Failure Care				
ACE Inhibitor or ARB for LVSD	19	100%	97%	97%
Discharge Instructions Given	42	100%	95%	94%
Evaluation of LVS Function	61	100%	99%	99%
Medicare Spending				
Medicare Spending per Patient (ratio)	-	0.93	1.03	0.98
Pneumonia Care				
Appropriate Initial Antibiotic Given	52	100%	95%	95%
Blood Culture Timing	50	98%	98%	98%
Pregnancy and Delivery Care				
Newborn Deliveries Scheduled Early	31	0%	7%	6%
Preventive Care				
Immunization for Influenza[2]	279	100%	90%	90%
Immunization for Pneumonia[2]	371	100%	92%	92%
Stroke Care				
Anticoagulation Therapy for Atrial Fibrillation[1]	-	-	96%	95%
Antithrombotic Therapy Timing[1]	-	-	98%	98%
Assessed for Rehabilitation[1]	-	-	98%	97%
Discharged on Antithrombotic Therapy[1]	-	-	99%	99%
Discharged on Statin Medication[7]	-	-	95%	94%
Thrombolytic Therapy Timing[1]	-	-	68%	66%
Venous Thromboembolism Prophylaxis[1]	-	-	94%	94%
Written Stroke Educational Materials Given[7]	-	-	92%	88%
Surgical Care Improvement Project				
Appropriate Beta Blocker Usage[1,3]	-	-	98%	98%
Appropriate VTP Within 24 Hours[3]	16	100%	98%	98%
Controlled Postoperative Blood Glucose[3,7]	-	-	96%	97%
Perioperative Temperature Management[3]	17	100%	100%	100%
Prophylactic Antibiotic Selection[1,3]	-	-	99%	99%
Prophylactic Antibiotic Selection (Outpatient)[1,3]	-	-	98%	98%
Prophylactic Antibiotic Stopped[1,3]	-	-	98%	98%
Prophylactic Antibiotic Timing[1,3]	-	-	99%	99%
Prophylactic Antibiotic Timing (Outpatient)[1,3]	-	-	98%	98%
Urinary Catheter Removal[1,3]	-	-	98%	97%
Survey of Patients' Hospital Experiences				
Area Around Room 'Always' Quiet at Night	(a)	62%	68%	61%
Doctors 'Always' Communicated Well	(a)	88%	83%	82%
Home Recovery Information Given	(a)	86%	85%	85%
Hospital Given 9 or 10 on 10 Point Scale	(a)	74%	73%	71%
Meds 'Always' Explained Before Given	(a)	73%	66%	64%
Nurses 'Always' Communicated Well	(a)	84%	80%	79%
Pain 'Always' Well Controlled	(a)	72%	72%	71%
Room and Bathroom 'Always' Clean	(a)	84%	75%	73%
Timely Help 'Always' Received	(a)	77%	69%	68%
Would Definitely Recommend Hospital	(a)	75%	73%	71%
Use of Medical Imaging				
Cardiac Imaging Stress Test before Surgery	73	5.5%	5.3%	5.3%
Combination Abdominal CT Scan	133	0.0%	16.4%	10.5%
Combination Brain/Sinus CT Scan[1]	-	-	2.7%	2.7%
Combination Chest CT Scan	70	0.0%	5.6%	2.7%
Follow-up Mammogram/Ultrasound	146	13.0%	7.9%	8.8%
Lumbar Spine MRI for Low Back Pain[7]	-	-	39.6%	37.2%

Lynn County Hospital District

2600 Lockwood Street Phone: 806-998-4533
Tahoka, TX 79373
Type: Critical Access Hospitals Emergency Services: Yes
Ownership: Govt - Hospital Dist/Auth

Measure	Cases	This Hosp.	State Avg.	U.S. Avg.
Blood Clot Prevention and Treatment				
Anticoagulation Overlap Therapy[5]	-	-	93%	93%
ICU Venous Thromboembolism Prophylaxis[5]	-	-	92%	92%
Incidence of Potentially Preventable VTE[5]	-	-	9%	10%
UFH with Dosages/Platelet Monitoring[5]	-	-	96%	97%
Venous Thromboembolism Prophylaxis[5]	-	-	82%	85%
Warfarin Therapy Discharge Instructions[5]	-	-	84%	75%
Chest Pain/Possible Heart Attack Care				
Aspirin Given Within 24 Hours of Arrival[5]	-	-	94%	96%
Fibrinolytic Meds Within 30 Min. of Arrival[5]	-	-	47%	58%
Average Time to ECG (minutes)[5]	-	-	8	7
Average Time to Transfer (minutes)[5]	-	-	62	60
Children's Asthma Care				
Received Home Management Plan of Care	-	-	93%	88%
Received Reliever Medication	-	-	100%	100%
Received Systemic Corticosteroids	-	-	100%	100%
Emergency Department				
Admittance Decision Time (minutes)[5]	-	-	99	98
Head CT Results Within 45 Min. of Arrival[5]	-	-	54%	57%
Patients Who Left ER Before Being Seen	2,190	1%	3%	2%
Time from ER Arrival to Admit. (minutes)[5]	-	-	270	274
Time from ER Arrival to Discharge (minutes)[5]	-	-	127	134
Time in ER Before Being Evaluated (minutes)[5]	-	-	26	26
Time to Pain Meds for Fractures (minutes)[5]	-	-	57	57
Heart Attack Care				
Aspirin Given at Discharge[5]	-	-	99%	99%
Fibrinolytic Meds Within 30 Min. of Arrival[5]	-	-	49%	54%

NOTE: Hospital profiles are in alphabetical order by state, then city, then hospital within the city; Rankings exclude hospitals with less than 25 cases except for patient surveys which excludes hospitals with less than 100 cases; (a) 100-299 cases; (1) The number of cases/patients is too few to report; (2) Data submitted were based on a sample of cases/patients; (3) Results are based on a shorter time period than required; (4) Data suppressed by CMS for one or more quarters; (5) Results are not available for this reporting period; (6) Fewer than 100 patients completed the HCAHPS survey; (7) No cases met the criteria for this measure; (8) The lower limit of the confidence interval cannot be calculated if the number of observed infections equals zero; (9) No data are available from the state/territory for this reporting period; (10) The scores shown reflect fewer than 50 completed surveys; (11) There were discrepancies in the data collection process; (12) This measure does not apply to this hospital for this reporting period; (13) Results cannot be calculated for this reporting period; (14) The results for this state are combined with nearby states to protect confidentiality; Please refer to the User's Guide for a full explanation of data.

Measure	Cases	This Hosp.	State Avg.	U.S. Avg.
PCI Within 90 Minutes of Arrival[5]	-	-	95%	96%
Statin Prescribed at Discharge[5]	-	-	98%	98%
Heart Failure Care				
ACE Inhibitor or ARB for LVSD[5]	-	-	97%	97%
Discharge Instructions Given[5]	-	-	95%	94%
Evaluation of LVS Function[5]	-	-	99%	99%
Medicare Spending				
Medicare Spending per Patient (ratio)	-	-	1.03	0.98
Pneumonia Care				
Appropriate Initial Antibiotic Given[2,3]	-	-	95%	95%
Blood Culture Timing[2,3]	-	-	98%	98%
Pregnancy and Delivery Care				
Newborn Deliveries Scheduled Early[5]	-	-	7%	6%
Preventive Care				
Immunization for Influenza[5]	-	-	90%	90%
Immunization for Pneumonia[5]	-	-	92%	92%
Stroke Care				
Anticoagulation Therapy for Atrial Fibrillation[5]	-	-	96%	95%
Antithrombotic Therapy Timing[5]	-	-	98%	98%
Assessed for Rehabilitation[5]	-	-	98%	97%
Discharged on Antithrombotic Therapy[5]	-	-	99%	99%
Discharged on Statin Medication[5]	-	-	95%	94%
Thrombolytic Therapy Timing[5]	-	-	68%	66%
Venous Thromboembolism Prophylaxis[5]	-	-	94%	94%
Written Stroke Educational Materials Given[5]	-	-	92%	88%
Surgical Care Improvement Project				
Appropriate Beta Blocker Usage[5]	-	-	98%	98%
Appropriate VTP Within 24 Hours[5]	-	-	98%	98%
Controlled Postoperative Blood Glucose[5]	-	-	96%	97%
Perioperative Temperature Management[5]	-	-	100%	100%
Prophylactic Antibiotic Selection[5]	-	-	99%	99%
Prophylactic Antibiotic Selection (Outpatient)[5]	-	-	98%	98%
Prophylactic Antibiotic Stopped[5]	-	-	98%	98%
Prophylactic Antibiotic Timing[5]	-	-	99%	99%
Prophylactic Antibiotic Timing (Outpatient)[5]	-	-	98%	98%
Urinary Catheter Removal[5]	-	-	98%	97%
Survey of Patients' Hospital Experiences				
Area Around Room 'Always' Quiet at Night[5]	-	-	68%	61%
Doctors 'Always' Communicated Well[5]	-	-	83%	82%
Home Recovery Information Given[5]	-	-	85%	85%
Hospital Given 9 or 10 on 10 Point Scale[5]	-	-	73%	71%
Meds 'Always' Explained Before Given[5]	-	-	66%	64%
Nurses 'Always' Communicated Well[5]	-	-	80%	79%
Pain 'Always' Well Controlled[5]	-	-	72%	71%
Room and Bathroom 'Always' Clean[5]	-	-	75%	73%
Timely Help 'Always' Received[5]	-	-	69%	68%
Would Definitely Recommend Hospital[5]	-	-	73%	71%
Use of Medical Imaging				
Cardiac Imaging Stress Test before Surgery[7]	-	-	5.3%	5.3%
Combination Abdominal CT Scan[1]	-	-	16.4%	10.5%
Combination Brain/Sinus CT Scan[1]	-	-	2.7%	2.7%
Combination Chest CT Scan[1]	-	-	5.6%	2.7%
Follow-up Mammogram/Ultrasound[7]	-	-	7.9%	8.8%
Lumbar Spine MRI for Low Back Pain[7]	-	-	39.6%	37.2%

Scott & White Hospital - Taylor

305 Mallard
Taylor, TX 76574
Phone: 512-352-7611
Fax: 512-352-5166
URL: www.johnscommunityhospital.org
Type: Critical Access Hospitals
Emergency Services: Yes
Ownership: Voluntary non-profit - Private
Beds: 53

Key Personnel:
CEO/President. . . . . Ernest Balla
Pulmonology . . . . Veronica Brito, MD
Chief of Medical Staff. . . . . Pascal Gaudreault
Radiology. . . . . Sterling S Kaye, MD

Measure	Cases	This Hosp.	State Avg.	U.S. Avg.
Blood Clot Prevention and Treatment				
Anticoagulation Overlap Therapy[5]	-	-	93%	93%
ICU Venous Thromboembolism Prophylaxis[5]	-	-	92%	92%
Incidence of Potentially Preventable VTE[5]	-	-	9%	10%
UFH with Dosages/Platelet Monitoring[5]	-	-	96%	97%
Venous Thromboembolism Prophylaxis[5]	-	-	82%	85%
Warfarin Therapy Discharge Instructions[5]	-	-	84%	75%
Chest Pain/Possible Heart Attack Care				
Aspirin Given Within 24 Hours of Arrival	-	-	94%	96%
Fibrinolytic Meds Within 30 Min. of Arrival	-	-	47%	58%
Average Time to ECG (minutes)	-	-	8	7
Average Time to Transfer (minutes)	-	-	62	60
Children's Asthma Care				
Received Home Management Plan of Care	-	-	93%	88%
Received Reliever Medication	-	-	100%	100%
Received Systemic Corticosteroids	-	-	100%	100%
Emergency Department				
Admittance Decision Time (minutes)[5]	-	-	99	98
Head CT Results Within 45 Min. of Arrival	-	-	54%	57%
Patients Who Left ER Before Being Seen	-	-	3%	2%
Time from ER Arrival to Admit. (minutes)[5]	-	-	270	274
Time from ER Arrival to Discharge (minutes)	-	-	127	134
Time in ER Before Being Evaluated (minutes)	-	-	26	26
Time to Pain Meds for Fractures (minutes)	-	-	57	57
Heart Attack Care				
Aspirin Given at Discharge[5]	-	-	99%	99%
Fibrinolytic Meds Within 30 Min. of Arrival[5]	-	-	49%	54%
PCI Within 90 Minutes of Arrival[5]	-	-	95%	96%
Statin Prescribed at Discharge[5]	-	-	98%	98%
Heart Failure Care				
ACE Inhibitor or ARB for LVSD[5]	-	-	97%	97%
Discharge Instructions Given[5]	-	-	95%	94%
Evaluation of LVS Function[5]	-	-	99%	99%
Medicare Spending				
Medicare Spending per Patient (ratio)	-	-	1.03	0.98
Pneumonia Care				
Appropriate Initial Antibiotic Given[5]	-	-	95%	95%
Blood Culture Timing[5]	-	-	98%	98%
Pregnancy and Delivery Care				
Newborn Deliveries Scheduled Early[5]	-	-	7%	6%
Preventive Care				
Immunization for Influenza[5]	-	-	90%	90%
Immunization for Pneumonia[5]	-	-	92%	92%
Stroke Care				
Anticoagulation Therapy for Atrial Fibrillation[5]	-	-	96%	95%
Antithrombotic Therapy Timing[5]	-	-	98%	98%
Assessed for Rehabilitation[5]	-	-	98%	97%
Discharged on Antithrombotic Therapy[5]	-	-	99%	99%
Discharged on Statin Medication[5]	-	-	95%	94%
Thrombolytic Therapy Timing[5]	-	-	68%	66%
Venous Thromboembolism Prophylaxis[5]	-	-	94%	94%
Written Stroke Educational Materials Given[5]	-	-	92%	88%
Surgical Care Improvement Project				
Appropriate Beta Blocker Usage[5]	-	-	98%	98%
Appropriate VTP Within 24 Hours[5]	-	-	98%	98%
Controlled Postoperative Blood Glucose[5]	-	-	96%	97%
Perioperative Temperature Management[5]	-	-	100%	100%
Prophylactic Antibiotic Selection[5]	-	-	99%	99%
Prophylactic Antibiotic Selection (Outpatient)	-	-	98%	98%
Prophylactic Antibiotic Stopped[5]	-	-	98%	98%
Prophylactic Antibiotic Timing[5]	-	-	99%	99%
Prophylactic Antibiotic Timing (Outpatient)	-	-	98%	98%
Urinary Catheter Removal[5]	-	-	98%	97%
Survey of Patients' Hospital Experiences				
Area Around Room 'Always' Quiet at Night[6]	<100	65%	68%	61%
Doctors 'Always' Communicated Well[6]	<100	94%	83%	82%
Home Recovery Information Given[6]	<100	85%	85%	85%
Hospital Given 9 or 10 on 10 Point Scale[6]	<100	61%	73%	71%
Meds 'Always' Explained Before Given[6]	<100	78%	66%	64%
Nurses 'Always' Communicated Well[6]	<100	86%	80%	79%
Pain 'Always' Well Controlled[6]	<100	67%	72%	71%
Room and Bathroom 'Always' Clean[6]	<100	79%	75%	73%
Timely Help 'Always' Received[6]	<100	77%	69%	68%
Would Definitely Recommend Hospital[6]	<100	66%	73%	71%
Use of Medical Imaging				
Cardiac Imaging Stress Test before Surgery	-	-	5.3%	5.3%
Combination Abdominal CT Scan	-	-	16.4%	10.5%
Combination Brain/Sinus CT Scan	-	-	2.7%	2.7%
Combination Chest CT Scan	-	-	5.6%	2.7%
Follow-up Mammogram/Ultrasound	-	-	7.9%	8.8%
Lumbar Spine MRI for Low Back Pain	-	-	39.6%	37.2%

Scott & White Memorial Hospital

2401 31st St
Temple, TX 76508
Phone: 254-724-2111
Fax: 254-724-5579
E-mail: swhpques@swmail.sw.org
URL: www.sw.org
Type: Acute Care Hospitals
Emergency Services: Yes
Ownership: Voluntary non-profit - Private
Beds: 636

Key Personnel:
Chief of Medical Staff. . . . . Virginia Hunt
CEO/President. . . . . Alfred B Knight, MD

Measure	Cases	This Hosp.	State Avg.	U.S. Avg.
Blood Clot Prevention and Treatment				
Anticoagulation Overlap Therapy[2]	192	99%	93%	93%
ICU Venous Thromboembolism Prophylaxis[2]	85	99%	92%	92%
Incidence of Potentially Preventable VTE[2]	38	8%	9%	10%
UFH with Dosages/Platelet Monitoring[2]	144	100%	96%	97%
Venous Thromboembolism Prophylaxis[2]	326	85%	82%	85%
Warfarin Therapy Discharge Instructions[2]	152	43%	84%	75%
Chest Pain/Possible Heart Attack Care				
Aspirin Given Within 24 Hours of Arrival[1,3]	-	-	94%	96%
Fibrinolytic Meds Within 30 Min. of Arrival[5]	-	-	47%	58%
Average Time to ECG (minutes)[1,3]	-	-	8	7
Average Time to Transfer (minutes)[5]	-	-	62	60
Children's Asthma Care				
Received Home Management Plan of Care	-	-	93%	88%
Received Reliever Medication	-	-	100%	100%
Received Systemic Corticosteroids	-	-	100%	100%
Emergency Department				
Admittance Decision Time (minutes)[2]	575	84	99	98
Head CT Results Within 45 Min. of Arrival[1]	-	-	54%	57%
Patients Who Left ER Before Being Seen	78,537	1%	3%	2%
Time from ER Arrival to Admit. (minutes)[2]	580	280	270	274
Time from ER Arrival to Discharge (minutes)	417	98	127	134
Time in ER Before Being Evaluated (minutes)	429	38	26	26
Time to Pain Meds for Fractures (minutes)	142	55	57	57
Heart Attack Care				
Aspirin Given at Discharge[2]	301	100%	99%	99%
Fibrinolytic Meds Within 30 Min. of Arrival[2,7]	-	-	49%	54%
PCI Within 90 Minutes of Arrival[2]	34	91%	95%	96%
Statin Prescribed at Discharge[2]	287	100%	98%	98%
Heart Failure Care				
ACE Inhibitor or ARB for LVSD[2]	105	94%	97%	97%
Discharge Instructions Given[2]	258	100%	95%	94%
Evaluation of LVS Function[2]	324	100%	99%	99%
Medicare Spending				
Medicare Spending per Patient (ratio)	-	0.92	1.03	0.98
Pneumonia Care				
Appropriate Initial Antibiotic Given[2]	71	99%	95%	95%
Blood Culture Timing[2]	222	100%	98%	98%
Pregnancy and Delivery Care				
Newborn Deliveries Scheduled Early[2]	75	1%	7%	6%
Preventive Care				
Immunization for Influenza[2]	563	87%	90%	90%
Immunization for Pneumonia[2]	643	90%	92%	92%
Stroke Care				
Anticoagulation Therapy for Atrial Fibrillation[1,2]	-	-	96%	95%
Antithrombotic Therapy Timing[2]	92	99%	98%	98%
Assessed for Rehabilitation[2]	154	99%	98%	97%
Discharged on Antithrombotic Therapy[2]	114	100%	99%	99%
Discharged on Statin Medication[2]	88	100%	95%	94%
Thrombolytic Therapy Timing[2]	12	83%	68%	66%
Venous Thromboembolism Prophylaxis[2]	151	99%	94%	94%
Written Stroke Educational Materials Given[2]	80	95%	92%	88%
Surgical Care Improvement Project				
Appropriate Beta Blocker Usage[2]	312	98%	98%	98%
Appropriate VTP Within 24 Hours[2]	464	100%	98%	98%
Controlled Postoperative Blood Glucose[2]	148	97%	96%	97%
Perioperative Temperature Management[2]	601	100%	100%	100%
Prophylactic Antibiotic Selection[2]	506	99%	99%	99%

NOTE: Hospital profiles are in alphabetical order by state, then city, then hospital within the city; Rankings exclude hospitals with less than 25 cases except for patient surveys which excludes hospitals with less than 100 cases; (a) 100-299 cases; (1) The number of cases/patients is too few to report; (2) Data submitted were based on a sample of cases/patients; (3) Results are based on a shorter time period than required; (4) Data suppressed by CMS for one or more quarters; (5) Results are not available for this reporting period; (6) Fewer than 100 patients completed the HCAHPS survey; (7) No cases met the criteria for this measure; (8) The lower limit of the confidence interval cannot be calculated if the number of observed infections equals zero; (9) No data are available from the state/territory for this reporting period; (10) The scores shown reflect fewer than 50 completed surveys; (11) There were discrepancies in the data collection process; (12) This measure does not apply to this hospital for this reporting period; (13) Results cannot be calculated for this reporting period; (14) The results for this state are combined with nearby states to protect confidentiality; Please refer to the User's Guide for a full explanation of data.

Measure	Cases	This Hosp.	State Avg.	U.S. Avg.
Prophylactic Antibiotic Selection (Outpatient)	743	98%	98%	98%
Prophylactic Antibiotic Stopped[2]	486	99%	98%	98%
Prophylactic Antibiotic Timing[2]	508	99%	99%	99%
Prophylactic Antibiotic Timing (Outpatient)	565	98%	98%	98%
Urinary Catheter Removal[2]	263	97%	98%	97%
Survey of Patients' Hospital Experiences				
Area Around Room 'Always' Quiet at Night[11]	300+	62%	68%	61%
Doctors 'Always' Communicated Well[11]	300+	82%	83%	82%
Home Recovery Information Given[11]	300+	85%	85%	85%
Hospital Given 9 or 10 on 10 Point Scale[11]	300+	71%	73%	71%
Meds 'Always' Explained Before Given[11]	300+	63%	66%	64%
Nurses 'Always' Communicated Well[11]	300+	77%	80%	79%
Pain 'Always' Well Controlled[11]	300+	68%	72%	71%
Room and Bathroom 'Always' Clean[11]	300+	65%	75%	73%
Timely Help 'Always' Received[11]	300+	59%	69%	68%
Would Definitely Recommend Hospital[11]	300+	76%	73%	71%
Use of Medical Imaging				
Cardiac Imaging Stress Test before Surgery	902	6.5%	5.3%	5.3%
Combination Abdominal CT Scan	2,428	8.5%	16.4%	10.5%
Combination Brain/Sinus CT Scan	1,282	1.6%	2.7%	2.7%
Combination Chest CT Scan	2,047	0.1%	5.6%	2.7%
Follow-up Mammogram/Ultrasound	3,688	8.6%	7.9%	8.8%
Lumbar Spine MRI for Low Back Pain	427	41.0%	39.6%	37.2%

Temple VA Medical Center - VA Central Texas

1901 Veterans Memorial Drive
Temple, TX 76504
URL: www.centraltexas.va.gov
Type: Acute Care - VA
Ownership: Government Federal
Phone: 254-778-4811
Fax: 254-899-4007
Emergency Services: No
Beds: 1,063

Key Personnel:
Chief of Medical Staff. . . . . Everett R Jones, Jr, MD
Anesthesiology. . . . . Boo H Kim, MD
Operating Room. . . . . Joanna Roland, RN
CEO/President. . . . . Thomas C Smith, III
Infection Control. . . . . Ulf Westblom, MD

Measure	Cases	This Hosp.	State Avg.	U.S. Avg.
Blood Clot Prevention and Treatment				
Anticoagulation Overlap Therapy	-	-	93%	93%
ICU Venous Thromboembolism Prophylaxis	-	-	92%	92%
Incidence of Potentially Preventable VTE	-	-	9%	10%
UFH with Dosages/Platelet Monitoring	-	-	96%	97%
Venous Thromboembolism Prophylaxis	-	-	82%	85%
Warfarin Therapy Discharge Instructions	-	-	84%	75%
Chest Pain/Possible Heart Attack Care				
Aspirin Given Within 24 Hours of Arrival	-	-	94%	96%
Fibrinolytic Meds Within 30 Min. of Arrival	-	-	47%	58%
Average Time to ECG (minutes)	-	-	8	7
Average Time to Transfer (minutes)	-	-	62	60
Children's Asthma Care				
Received Home Management Plan of Care	-	-	93%	88%
Received Reliever Medication	-	-	100%	100%
Received Systemic Corticosteroids	-	-	100%	100%
Emergency Department				
Admittance Decision Time (minutes)	-	-	99	98
Head CT Results Within 45 Min. of Arrival	-	-	54%	57%
Patients Who Left ER Before Being Seen	-	-	3%	2%
Time from ER Arrival to Admit. (minutes)	-	-	270	274
Time from ER Arrival to Discharge (minutes)	-	-	127	134
Time in ER Before Being Evaluated (minutes)	-	-	26	26
Time to Pain Meds for Fractures (minutes)	-	-	57	57
Heart Attack Care				
Aspirin Given at Discharge	41	100%	99%	99%
Fibrinolytic Meds Within 30 Min. of Arrival[5]	-	-	49%	54%
PCI Within 90 Minutes of Arrival[5]	-	-	95%	96%
Statin Prescribed at Discharge	43	100%	98%	98%
Heart Failure Care				
ACE Inhibitor or ARB for LVSD	105	96%	97%	97%
Discharge Instructions Given	204	100%	95%	94%
Evaluation of LVS Function	222	100%	99%	99%
Medicare Spending				
Medicare Spending per Patient (ratio)	-	-	1.03	0.98
Pneumonia Care				
Appropriate Initial Antibiotic Given	64	95%	95%	95%
Blood Culture Timing	135	99%	98%	98%
Pregnancy and Delivery Care				
Newborn Deliveries Scheduled Early	-	-	7%	6%
Preventive Care				
Immunization for Influenza[5]	-	-	90%	90%
Immunization for Pneumonia[5]	-	-	92%	92%
Stroke Care				
Anticoagulation Therapy for Atrial Fibrillation	-	-	96%	95%
Antithrombotic Therapy Timing	-	-	98%	98%
Assessed for Rehabilitation	-	-	98%	97%
Discharged on Antithrombotic Therapy	-	-	99%	99%
Discharged on Statin Medication	-	-	95%	94%
Thrombolytic Therapy Timing	-	-	68%	66%
Venous Thromboembolism Prophylaxis	-	-	94%	94%
Written Stroke Educational Materials Given	-	-	92%	88%
Surgical Care Improvement Project				
Appropriate Beta Blocker Usage[2]	91	93%	98%	98%
Appropriate VTP Within 24 Hours[2]	240	100%	98%	98%
Controlled Postoperative Blood Glucose[5]	-	-	96%	97%
Perioperative Temperature Management[2]	287	100%	100%	100%
Prophylactic Antibiotic Selection	194	96%	99%	99%
Prophylactic Antibiotic Selection (Outpatient)	-	-	98%	98%
Prophylactic Antibiotic Stopped	191	98%	98%	98%
Prophylactic Antibiotic Timing	195	98%	99%	99%
Prophylactic Antibiotic Timing (Outpatient)	-	-	98%	98%
Urinary Catheter Removal[2]	180	96%	98%	97%
Survey of Patients' Hospital Experiences				
Area Around Room 'Always' Quiet at Night	-	-	68%	61%
Doctors 'Always' Communicated Well	-	-	83%	82%
Home Recovery Information Given	-	-	85%	85%
Hospital Given 9 or 10 on 10 Point Scale	-	-	73%	71%
Meds 'Always' Explained Before Given	-	-	66%	64%
Nurses 'Always' Communicated Well	-	-	80%	79%
Pain 'Always' Well Controlled	-	-	72%	71%
Room and Bathroom 'Always' Clean	-	-	75%	73%
Timely Help 'Always' Received	-	-	69%	68%
Would Definitely Recommend Hospital	-	-	73%	71%
Use of Medical Imaging				
Cardiac Imaging Stress Test before Surgery	-	-	5.3%	5.3%
Combination Abdominal CT Scan	-	-	16.4%	10.5%
Combination Brain/Sinus CT Scan	-	-	2.7%	2.7%
Combination Chest CT Scan	-	-	5.6%	2.7%
Follow-up Mammogram/Ultrasound	-	-	7.9%	8.8%
Lumbar Spine MRI for Low Back Pain	-	-	39.6%	37.2%

Christus Saint Michael Health System

2600 Saint Michael Dr
Texarkana, TX 75504
URL: www.christusstmichael.org
Type: Acute Care Hospitals
Ownership: Voluntary non-profit - Private
Phone: 903-614-1000
Fax: 903-614-2588
Emergency Services: Yes
Beds: 278

Key Personnel:
Emergency Room . . . . Claire Donohua
Radiology. . . . . Wayne East
Chief of Medical Staff. . . . . Mike Finley, MD
Quality Assurance . . . . Karey Gardner
CEO/President. . . . . Chris Karam, FACHE
Operating Room. . . . . Rae Thigpen

Measure	Cases	This Hosp.	State Avg.	U.S. Avg.
Blood Clot Prevention and Treatment				
Anticoagulation Overlap Therapy[2]	111	94%	93%	93%
ICU Venous Thromboembolism Prophylaxis[2]	97	74%	92%	92%
Incidence of Potentially Preventable VTE[2]	26	15%	9%	10%
UFH with Dosages/Platelet Monitoring[2]	16	81%	96%	97%
Venous Thromboembolism Prophylaxis[2]	380	72%	82%	85%
Warfarin Therapy Discharge Instructions[2]	76	55%	84%	75%
Chest Pain/Possible Heart Attack Care				
Aspirin Given Within 24 Hours of Arrival	22	91%	94%	96%
Fibrinolytic Meds Within 30 Min. of Arrival[3,7]	-	-	47%	58%
Average Time to ECG (minutes)	19	8	8	7
Average Time to Transfer (minutes)[3,7]	-	-	62	60
Children's Asthma Care				
Received Home Management Plan of Care	-	-	93%	88%
Received Reliever Medication	-	-	100%	100%
Received Systemic Corticosteroids	-	-	100%	100%
Emergency Department				
Admittance Decision Time (minutes)[2]	669	146	99	98
Head CT Results Within 45 Min. of Arrival	21	57%	54%	57%
Patients Who Left ER Before Being Seen	66,047	4%	3%	2%
Time from ER Arrival to Admit. (minutes)[2]	696	336	270	274
Time from ER Arrival to Discharge (minutes)	460	163	127	134
Time in ER Before Being Evaluated (minutes)	474	43	26	26
Time to Pain Meds for Fractures (minutes)	262	73	57	57
Heart Attack Care				
Aspirin Given at Discharge	315	98%	99%	99%
Fibrinolytic Meds Within 30 Min. of Arrival[7]	-	-	49%	54%
PCI Within 90 Minutes of Arrival	31	100%	95%	96%
Statin Prescribed at Discharge	300	98%	98%	98%
Heart Failure Care				
ACE Inhibitor or ARB for LVSD	186	99%	97%	97%
Discharge Instructions Given	451	92%	95%	94%
Evaluation of LVS Function	565	100%	99%	99%
Medicare Spending				
Medicare Spending per Patient (ratio)	-	1.03	1.03	0.98
Pneumonia Care				
Appropriate Initial Antibiotic Given	269	97%	95%	95%
Blood Culture Timing	383	97%	98%	98%
Pregnancy and Delivery Care				
Newborn Deliveries Scheduled Early[2]	31	10%	7%	6%
Preventive Care				
Immunization for Influenza[2]	556	94%	90%	90%
Immunization for Pneumonia[2]	709	95%	92%	92%
Stroke Care				
Anticoagulation Therapy for Atrial Fibrillation	24	96%	96%	95%
Antithrombotic Therapy Timing	163	98%	98%	98%
Assessed for Rehabilitation	182	98%	98%	97%
Discharged on Antithrombotic Therapy	171	99%	99%	99%
Discharged on Statin Medication	130	93%	95%	94%
Thrombolytic Therapy Timing	18	50%	68%	66%
Venous Thromboembolism Prophylaxis	186	95%	94%	94%
Written Stroke Educational Materials Given	78	81%	92%	88%
Surgical Care Improvement Project				
Appropriate Beta Blocker Usage[2]	354	98%	98%	98%
Appropriate VTP Within 24 Hours[2]	795	99%	98%	98%
Controlled Postoperative Blood Glucose[2]	132	96%	96%	97%
Perioperative Temperature Management[2]	1,042	100%	100%	100%
Prophylactic Antibiotic Selection[2]	794	99%	99%	99%
Prophylactic Antibiotic Selection (Outpatient)	492	98%	98%	98%
Prophylactic Antibiotic Stopped[2]	759	97%	98%	98%
Prophylactic Antibiotic Timing[2]	794	99%	99%	99%
Prophylactic Antibiotic Timing (Outpatient)	494	99%	98%	98%
Urinary Catheter Removal[2]	710	98%	98%	97%
Survey of Patients' Hospital Experiences				
Area Around Room 'Always' Quiet at Night	300+	66%	68%	61%
Doctors 'Always' Communicated Well	300+	82%	83%	82%
Home Recovery Information Given	300+	85%	85%	85%
Hospital Given 9 or 10 on 10 Point Scale	300+	74%	73%	71%
Meds 'Always' Explained Before Given	300+	67%	66%	64%
Nurses 'Always' Communicated Well	300+	81%	80%	79%
Pain 'Always' Well Controlled	300+	73%	72%	71%
Room and Bathroom 'Always' Clean	300+	75%	75%	73%
Timely Help 'Always' Received	300+	70%	69%	68%
Would Definitely Recommend Hospital	300+	77%	73%	71%
Use of Medical Imaging				
Cardiac Imaging Stress Test before Surgery	260	3.8%	5.3%	5.3%
Combination Abdominal CT Scan	1,115	18.1%	16.4%	10.5%
Combination Brain/Sinus CT Scan	1,265	1.6%	2.7%	2.7%
Combination Chest CT Scan	514	19.5%	5.6%	2.7%
Follow-up Mammogram/Ultrasound	1,606	7.0%	7.9%	8.8%
Lumbar Spine MRI for Low Back Pain	261	44.1%	39.6%	37.2%

NOTE: Hospital profiles are in alphabetical order by state, then city, then hospital within the city; Rankings exclude hospitals with less than 25 cases except for patient surveys which excludes hospitals with less than 100 cases; (a) 100-299 cases; (1) The number of cases/patients is too few to report; (2) Data submitted were based on a sample of cases/patients; (3) Results are based on a shorter time period than required; (4) Data suppressed by CMS for one or more quarters; (5) Results are not available for this reporting period; (6) Fewer than 100 patients completed the HCAHPS survey; (7) No cases met the criteria for this measure; (8) The lower limit of the confidence interval cannot be calculated if the number of observed infections equals zero; (9) No data are available from the state/territory for this reporting period; (10) The scores shown reflect fewer than 50 completed surveys; (11) There were discrepancies in the data collection process; (12) This measure does not apply to this hospital for this reporting period; (13) Results cannot be calculated for this reporting period; (14) The results for this state are combined with nearby states to protect confidentiality; Please refer to the User's Guide for a full explanation of data.

Wadley Regional Medical Center

1000 Pine Street
Texarkana, TX 75501
URL: www.wadleyhealth.com
Type: Acute Care Hospitals
Ownership: Proprietary
Phone: 903-798-8000
Fax: 903-798-8030
Emergency Services: Yes
Beds: 407

Key Personnel:
Emergency Room . . . . Cyndy Chamblee
Infection Control. . . . . Barbara Clingan
CEO/President. . . . . Thomas Gilbert
Chief of Medical Staff . . . . Stanley Knowles
Quality Assurance . . . . Kim Lewis
Operating Room. . . . . Sandra Morris

Measure	Cases	This Hosp.	State Avg.	U.S. Avg.
Blood Clot Prevention and Treatment				
Anticoagulation Overlap Therapy[2]	48	100%	93%	93%
ICU Venous Thromboembolism Prophylaxis[2]	111	98%	92%	92%
Incidence of Potentially Preventable VTE[1,2]	-	-	9%	10%
UFH with Dosages/Platelet Monitoring[1,2]	-	-	96%	97%
Venous Thromboembolism Prophylaxis[2]	405	91%	82%	85%
Warfarin Therapy Discharge Instructions[2]	36	100%	84%	75%
Chest Pain/Possible Heart Attack Care				
Aspirin Given Within 24 Hours of Arrival[1,3]	-	-	94%	96%
Fibrinolytic Meds Within 30 Min. of Arrival[5]	-	-	47%	58%
Average Time to ECG (minutes)[1,3]	-	-	8	7
Average Time to Transfer (minutes)[5]	-	-	62	60
Children's Asthma Care				
Received Home Management Plan of Care	-	-	93%	88%
Received Reliever Medication	-	-	100%	100%
Received Systemic Corticosteroids	-	-	100%	100%
Emergency Department				
Admittance Decision Time (minutes)[2]	573	151	99	98
Head CT Results Within 45 Min. of Arrival[1]	-	-	54%	57%
Patients Who Left ER Before Being Seen	44,596	3%	3%	2%
Time from ER Arrival to Admit. (minutes)[2]	597	325	270	274
Time from ER Arrival to Discharge (minutes)	461	103	127	134
Time in ER Before Being Evaluated (minutes)	474	42	26	26
Time to Pain Meds for Fractures (minutes)	115	64	57	57
Heart Attack Care				
Aspirin Given at Discharge	152	100%	99%	99%
Fibrinolytic Meds Within 30 Min. of Arrival[7]	-	-	49%	54%
PCI Within 90 Minutes of Arrival	31	84%	95%	96%
Statin Prescribed at Discharge	149	100%	98%	98%
Heart Failure Care				
ACE Inhibitor or ARB for LVSD	89	99%	97%	97%
Discharge Instructions Given	159	96%	95%	94%
Evaluation of LVS Function	204	100%	99%	99%
Medicare Spending				
Medicare Spending per Patient (ratio)	-	1.08	1.03	0.98
Pneumonia Care				
Appropriate Initial Antibiotic Given	96	96%	95%	95%
Blood Culture Timing	182	98%	98%	98%
Pregnancy and Delivery Care				
Newborn Deliveries Scheduled Early[2]	26	0%	7%	6%
Preventive Care				
Immunization for Influenza[2]	557	90%	90%	90%
Immunization for Pneumonia[2]	666	95%	92%	92%
Stroke Care				
Anticoagulation Therapy for Atrial Fibrillation	32	94%	96%	95%
Antithrombotic Therapy Timing	140	96%	98%	98%
Assessed for Rehabilitation	196	99%	98%	97%
Discharged on Antithrombotic Therapy	181	99%	99%	99%
Discharged on Statin Medication	143	95%	95%	94%
Thrombolytic Therapy Timing	23	96%	68%	66%
Venous Thromboembolism Prophylaxis	195	98%	94%	94%
Written Stroke Educational Materials Given	94	99%	92%	88%
Surgical Care Improvement Project				
Appropriate Beta Blocker Usage	192	96%	98%	98%
Appropriate VTP Within 24 Hours	422	96%	98%	98%
Controlled Postoperative Blood Glucose	68	94%	96%	97%
Perioperative Temperature Management	524	100%	100%	100%
Prophylactic Antibiotic Selection	336	99%	99%	99%
Prophylactic Antibiotic Selection (Outpatient)	347	95%	98%	98%
Prophylactic Antibiotic Stopped	325	97%	98%	98%
Prophylactic Antibiotic Timing	337	99%	99%	99%
Prophylactic Antibiotic Timing (Outpatient)	349	99%	98%	98%
Urinary Catheter Removal	364	95%	98%	97%
Survey of Patients' Hospital Experiences				
Area Around Room 'Always' Quiet at Night	300+	64%	68%	61%
Doctors 'Always' Communicated Well	300+	80%	83%	82%
Home Recovery Information Given	300+	88%	85%	85%
Hospital Given 9 or 10 on 10 Point Scale	300+	69%	73%	71%
Meds 'Always' Explained Before Given	300+	63%	66%	64%
Nurses 'Always' Communicated Well	300+	80%	80%	79%
Pain 'Always' Well Controlled	300+	70%	72%	71%
Room and Bathroom 'Always' Clean	300+	70%	75%	73%
Timely Help 'Always' Received	300+	68%	69%	68%
Would Definitely Recommend Hospital	300+	67%	73%	71%
Use of Medical Imaging				
Cardiac Imaging Stress Test before Surgery	122	7.4%	5.3%	5.3%
Combination Abdominal CT Scan	387	17.1%	16.4%	10.5%
Combination Brain/Sinus CT Scan	573	1.2%	2.7%	2.7%
Combination Chest CT Scan	174	24.7%	5.6%	2.7%
Follow-up Mammogram/Ultrasound	970	9.5%	7.9%	8.8%
Lumbar Spine MRI for Low Back Pain	108	47.2%	39.6%	37.2%

Saint Luke's Lakeside Hospital

17400 Saint Lukes Way
The Woodlands, TX 77384
URL: www.stlukeslakeside.com
Type: Acute Care Hospitals
Ownership: Voluntary non-profit - Other
Phone: 936-266-4055
Emergency Services: Yes
Beds: 30

Key Personnel:
Cardiology . . . . Vincent Aquino, MD
Chief of Medical Staff . . . . Bruce S. Lachterman, MD
Surgery . . . . Peter Shedden, MD, FACS, FRCS,
CEO . . . . Debra F Sukin

Measure	Cases	This Hosp.	State Avg.	U.S. Avg.
Blood Clot Prevention and Treatment				
Anticoagulation Overlap Therapy[1,2]	-	-	93%	93%
ICU Venous Thromboembolism Prophylaxis[1,2]	-	-	92%	92%
Incidence of Potentially Preventable VTE[2,7]	-	-	9%	10%
UFH with Dosages/Platelet Monitoring[1,2]	-	-	96%	97%
Venous Thromboembolism Prophylaxis[2]	51	98%	82%	85%
Warfarin Therapy Discharge Instructions[1,2]	-	-	84%	75%
Chest Pain/Possible Heart Attack Care				
Aspirin Given Within 24 Hours of Arrival[1]	-	-	94%	96%
Fibrinolytic Meds Within 30 Min. of Arrival[3,7]	-	-	47%	58%
Average Time to ECG (minutes)[1]	-	-	8	7
Average Time to Transfer (minutes)[1,3]	-	-	62	60
Children's Asthma Care				
Received Home Management Plan of Care	-	-	93%	88%
Received Reliever Medication	-	-	100%	100%
Received Systemic Corticosteroids	-	-	100%	100%
Emergency Department				
Admittance Decision Time (minutes)[2]	29	72	99	98
Head CT Results Within 45 Min. of Arrival[1]	-	-	54%	57%
Patients Who Left ER Before Being Seen	2,332	0%	3%	2%
Time from ER Arrival to Admit. (minutes)[2]	33	200	270	274
Time from ER Arrival to Discharge (minutes)	248	99	127	134
Time in ER Before Being Evaluated (minutes)	270	28	26	26
Time to Pain Meds for Fractures (minutes)	20	26	57	57
Heart Attack Care				
Aspirin Given at Discharge[1,3]	-	-	99%	99%
Fibrinolytic Meds Within 30 Min. of Arrival[3,7]	-	-	49%	54%
PCI Within 90 Minutes of Arrival[3,7]	-	-	95%	96%
Statin Prescribed at Discharge[1,3]	-	-	98%	98%
Heart Failure Care				
ACE Inhibitor or ARB for LVSD[1]	-	-	97%	97%
Discharge Instructions Given[1]	-	-	95%	94%
Evaluation of LVS Function[1]	-	-	99%	99%
Medicare Spending				
Medicare Spending per Patient (ratio)	-	1.11	1.03	0.98
Pneumonia Care				
Appropriate Initial Antibiotic Given[1]	-	-	95%	95%
Blood Culture Timing	11	91%	98%	98%
Pregnancy and Delivery Care				
Newborn Deliveries Scheduled Early[7]	-	-	7%	6%
Preventive Care				
Immunization for Influenza[2]	326	91%	90%	90%
Immunization for Pneumonia[2]	386	92%	92%	92%
Stroke Care				
Anticoagulation Therapy for Atrial Fibrillation[5]	-	-	96%	95%
Antithrombotic Therapy Timing[5]	-	-	98%	98%
Assessed for Rehabilitation[5]	-	-	98%	97%
Discharged on Antithrombotic Therapy[5]	-	-	99%	99%
Discharged on Statin Medication[5]	-	-	95%	94%
Thrombolytic Therapy Timing[5]	-	-	68%	66%
Venous Thromboembolism Prophylaxis[5]	-	-	94%	94%
Written Stroke Educational Materials Given[5]	-	-	92%	88%
Surgical Care Improvement Project				
Appropriate Beta Blocker Usage	138	99%	98%	98%
Appropriate VTP Within 24 Hours	361	100%	98%	98%
Controlled Postoperative Blood Glucose[7]	-	-	96%	97%
Perioperative Temperature Management	367	100%	100%	100%
Prophylactic Antibiotic Selection	349	100%	99%	99%
Prophylactic Antibiotic Selection (Outpatient)	320	100%	98%	98%
Prophylactic Antibiotic Stopped	345	100%	98%	98%
Prophylactic Antibiotic Timing	349	100%	99%	99%
Prophylactic Antibiotic Timing (Outpatient)	321	100%	98%	98%
Urinary Catheter Removal	352	99%	98%	97%
Survey of Patients' Hospital Experiences				
Area Around Room 'Always' Quiet at Night	300+	87%	68%	61%
Doctors 'Always' Communicated Well	300+	87%	83%	82%
Home Recovery Information Given	300+	88%	85%	85%
Hospital Given 9 or 10 on 10 Point Scale	300+	87%	73%	71%
Meds 'Always' Explained Before Given	300+	70%	66%	64%
Nurses 'Always' Communicated Well	300+	84%	80%	79%
Pain 'Always' Well Controlled	300+	76%	72%	71%
Room and Bathroom 'Always' Clean	300+	83%	75%	73%
Timely Help 'Always' Received	300+	81%	69%	68%
Would Definitely Recommend Hospital	300+	88%	73%	71%
Use of Medical Imaging				
Cardiac Imaging Stress Test before Surgery[1]	-	-	5.3%	5.3%
Combination Abdominal CT Scan	94	46.8%	16.4%	10.5%
Combination Brain/Sinus CT Scan	135	0.7%	2.7%	2.7%
Combination Chest CT Scan	90	14.4%	5.6%	2.7%
Follow-up Mammogram/Ultrasound[7]	-	-	7.9%	8.8%
Lumbar Spine MRI for Low Back Pain	87	34.5%	39.6%	37.2%

Saint Luke's the Woodlands Hospital

17200 Saint Luke's Way
The Woodlands, TX 77384
URL: www.stlukeswoodlands.com
Type: Acute Care Hospitals
Ownership: Voluntary non-profit - Church
Phone: 936-266-4050
Fax: 936-266-4001
Emergency Services: Yes
Beds: 86

Key Personnel:
Patient Relations . . . . Jackie Anderson, RN, MSN
Chief of Medical Staff . . . . Vincent Aquino, MD
Radiology. . . . . Matthew S Blurton
CEO/President. . . . . Debra F Sukin

Measure	Cases	This Hosp.	State Avg.	U.S. Avg.
Blood Clot Prevention and Treatment				
Anticoagulation Overlap Therapy[2]	67	75%	93%	93%
ICU Venous Thromboembolism Prophylaxis[2]	79	87%	92%	92%
Incidence of Potentially Preventable VTE[2]	11	9%	9%	10%
UFH with Dosages/Platelet Monitoring[2]	27	96%	96%	97%
Venous Thromboembolism Prophylaxis[2]	330	73%	82%	85%
Warfarin Therapy Discharge Instructions[2]	45	47%	84%	75%
Chest Pain/Possible Heart Attack Care				
Aspirin Given Within 24 Hours of Arrival[1,3]	-	-	94%	96%
Fibrinolytic Meds Within 30 Min. of Arrival[5]	-	-	47%	58%
Average Time to ECG (minutes)[1,3]	-	-	8	7
Average Time to Transfer (minutes)[5]	-	-	62	60
Children's Asthma Care				
Received Home Management Plan of Care	-	-	93%	88%
Received Reliever Medication	-	-	100%	100%
Received Systemic Corticosteroids	-	-	100%	100%
Emergency Department				
Admittance Decision Time (minutes)[2]	371	126	99	98

NOTE: Hospital profiles are in alphabetical order by state, then city, then hospital within the city; Rankings exclude hospitals with less than 25 cases except for patient surveys which excludes hospitals with less than 100 cases; (a) 100-299 cases; (1) The number of cases/patients is too few to report; (2) Data submitted were based on a sample of cases/patients; (3) Results are based on a shorter time period than required; (4) Data suppressed by CMS for one or more quarters; (5) Results are not available for this reporting period; (6) Fewer than 100 patients completed the HCAHPS survey; (7) No cases met the criteria for this measure; (8) The lower limit of the confidence interval cannot be calculated if the number of observed infections equals zero; (9) No data are available from the state/territory for this reporting period; (10) The scores shown reflect fewer than 50 completed surveys; (11) There were discrepancies in the data collection process; (12) This measure does not apply to this hospital for this reporting period; (13) Results cannot be calculated for this reporting period; (14) The results for this state are combined with nearby states to protect confidentiality; Please refer to the User's Guide for a full explanation of data.

Measure	Cases	This Hosp.	State Avg.	U.S. Avg.
Head CT Results Within 45 Min. of Arrival[1]	-	-	54%	57%
Patients Who Left ER Before Being Seen	37,967	5%	3%	2%
Time from ER Arrival to Admit. (minutes)[2]	403	365	270	274
Time from ER Arrival to Discharge (minutes)	385	192	127	134
Time in ER Before Being Evaluated (minutes)	366	84	26	26
Time to Pain Meds for Fractures (minutes)	225	60	57	57
Heart Attack Care				
Aspirin Given at Discharge	153	100%	99%	99%
Fibrinolytic Meds Within 30 Min. of Arrival[7]	-	-	49%	54%
PCI Within 90 Minutes of Arrival	27	96%	95%	96%
Statin Prescribed at Discharge	147	100%	98%	98%
Heart Failure Care				
ACE Inhibitor or ARB for LVSD	125	97%	97%	97%
Discharge Instructions Given	253	97%	95%	94%
Evaluation of LVS Function	318	100%	99%	99%
Medicare Spending				
Medicare Spending per Patient (ratio)	-	1.13	1.03	0.98
Pneumonia Care				
Appropriate Initial Antibiotic Given[2]	111	89%	95%	95%
Blood Culture Timing[2]	142	99%	98%	98%
Pregnancy and Delivery Care				
Newborn Deliveries Scheduled Early	146	18%	7%	6%
Preventive Care				
Immunization for Influenza[2]	526	94%	90%	90%
Immunization for Pneumonia[2]	602	97%	92%	92%
Stroke Care				
Anticoagulation Therapy for Atrial Fibrillation	21	95%	96%	95%
Antithrombotic Therapy Timing	112	99%	98%	98%
Assessed for Rehabilitation	163	90%	98%	97%
Discharged on Antithrombotic Therapy	133	100%	99%	99%
Discharged on Statin Medication	104	95%	95%	94%
Thrombolytic Therapy Timing	11	91%	68%	66%
Venous Thromboembolism Prophylaxis	154	90%	94%	94%
Written Stroke Educational Materials Given	104	85%	92%	88%
Surgical Care Improvement Project				
Appropriate Beta Blocker Usage[2]	232	100%	98%	98%
Appropriate VTP Within 24 Hours[2]	423	99%	98%	98%
Controlled Postoperative Blood Glucose[2]	118	96%	96%	97%
Perioperative Temperature Management[2]	531	100%	100%	100%
Prophylactic Antibiotic Selection[2]	436	100%	99%	99%
Prophylactic Antibiotic Selection (Outpatient)	310	99%	98%	98%
Prophylactic Antibiotic Stopped[2]	416	98%	98%	98%
Prophylactic Antibiotic Timing[2]	436	100%	99%	99%
Prophylactic Antibiotic Timing (Outpatient)	310	100%	98%	98%
Urinary Catheter Removal[2]	397	98%	98%	97%
Survey of Patients' Hospital Experiences				
Area Around Room 'Always' Quiet at Night	300+	61%	68%	61%
Doctors 'Always' Communicated Well	300+	79%	83%	82%
Home Recovery Information Given	300+	78%	85%	85%
Hospital Given 9 or 10 on 10 Point Scale	300+	76%	73%	71%
Meds 'Always' Explained Before Given	300+	59%	66%	64%
Nurses 'Always' Communicated Well	300+	78%	80%	79%
Pain 'Always' Well Controlled	300+	68%	72%	71%
Room and Bathroom 'Always' Clean	300+	71%	75%	73%
Timely Help 'Always' Received	300+	60%	69%	68%
Would Definitely Recommend Hospital	300+	79%	73%	71%
Use of Medical Imaging				
Cardiac Imaging Stress Test before Surgery	176	7.4%	5.3%	5.3%
Combination Abdominal CT Scan	775	17.5%	16.4%	10.5%
Combination Brain/Sinus CT Scan	586	1.4%	2.7%	2.7%
Combination Chest CT Scan	612	7.0%	5.6%	2.7%
Follow-up Mammogram/Ultrasound	634	9.0%	7.9%	8.8%
Lumbar Spine MRI for Low Back Pain[1]	-	-	39.6%	37.2%

Tomball Regional Medical Center

605 Holderrieth
Tomball, TX 77375
Phone: 281-351-1623
Fax: 281-351-4904
URL: www.tomballhospital.org
Type: Acute Care Hospitals
Emergency Services: Yes
Ownership: Govt - Hospital Dist/Auth
Beds: 205
Key Personnel:
CEO/President. . . . . Lynn L LeBouef

Measure	Cases	This Hosp.	State Avg.	U.S. Avg.
Blood Clot Prevention and Treatment				
Anticoagulation Overlap Therapy[2]	46	80%	93%	93%
ICU Venous Thromboembolism Prophylaxis[2]	107	93%	92%	92%
Incidence of Potentially Preventable VTE[1,2]	-	-	9%	10%
UFH with Dosages/Platelet Monitoring[2]	42	100%	96%	97%
Venous Thromboembolism Prophylaxis[2]	416	67%	82%	85%
Warfarin Therapy Discharge Instructions[2]	32	91%	84%	75%
Chest Pain/Possible Heart Attack Care				
Aspirin Given Within 24 Hours of Arrival[1,3]	-	-	94%	96%
Fibrinolytic Meds Within 30 Min. of Arrival[3,7]	-	-	47%	58%
Average Time to ECG (minutes)[1,3]	-	-	8	7
Average Time to Transfer (minutes)[3,7]	-	-	62	60
Children's Asthma Care				
Received Home Management Plan of Care	-	-	93%	88%
Received Reliever Medication	-	-	100%	100%
Received Systemic Corticosteroids	-	-	100%	100%
Emergency Department				
Admittance Decision Time (minutes)[2]	719	94	99	98
Head CT Results Within 45 Min. of Arrival[1]	-	-	54%	57%
Patients Who Left ER Before Being Seen	33,869	1%	3%	2%
Time from ER Arrival to Admit. (minutes)[2]	728	273	270	274
Time from ER Arrival to Discharge (minutes)	489	150	127	134
Time in ER Before Being Evaluated (minutes)	441	71	26	26
Time to Pain Meds for Fractures (minutes)	122	48	57	57
Heart Attack Care				
Aspirin Given at Discharge	145	94%	99%	99%
Fibrinolytic Meds Within 30 Min. of Arrival[7]	-	-	49%	54%
PCI Within 90 Minutes of Arrival	30	73%	95%	96%
Statin Prescribed at Discharge	140	91%	98%	98%
Heart Failure Care				
ACE Inhibitor or ARB for LVSD	88	91%	97%	97%
Discharge Instructions Given	244	87%	95%	94%
Evaluation of LVS Function	311	98%	99%	99%
Medicare Spending				
Medicare Spending per Patient (ratio)	-	1.09	1.03	0.98
Pneumonia Care				
Appropriate Initial Antibiotic Given	156	92%	95%	95%
Blood Culture Timing	225	99%	98%	98%
Pregnancy and Delivery Care				
Newborn Deliveries Scheduled Early[2]	34	6%	7%	6%
Preventive Care				
Immunization for Influenza[2]	619	84%	90%	90%
Immunization for Pneumonia[2]	819	88%	92%	92%
Stroke Care				
Anticoagulation Therapy for Atrial Fibrillation	14	93%	96%	95%
Antithrombotic Therapy Timing	95	98%	98%	98%
Assessed for Rehabilitation	105	99%	98%	97%
Discharged on Antithrombotic Therapy	101	95%	99%	99%
Discharged on Statin Medication	80	89%	95%	94%
Thrombolytic Therapy Timing[1]	-	-	68%	66%
Venous Thromboembolism Prophylaxis	108	86%	94%	94%
Written Stroke Educational Materials Given	66	77%	92%	88%
Surgical Care Improvement Project				
Appropriate Beta Blocker Usage	137	87%	98%	98%
Appropriate VTP Within 24 Hours	374	95%	98%	98%
Controlled Postoperative Blood Glucose	51	86%	96%	97%
Perioperative Temperature Management	452	99%	100%	100%
Prophylactic Antibiotic Selection	260	98%	99%	99%
Prophylactic Antibiotic Selection (Outpatient)	186	96%	98%	98%
Prophylactic Antibiotic Stopped	246	91%	98%	98%
Prophylactic Antibiotic Timing	262	99%	99%	99%
Prophylactic Antibiotic Timing (Outpatient)	198	90%	98%	98%
Urinary Catheter Removal	262	81%	98%	97%
Survey of Patients' Hospital Experiences				
Area Around Room 'Always' Quiet at Night	300+	65%	68%	61%
Doctors 'Always' Communicated Well	300+	79%	83%	82%
Home Recovery Information Given	300+	83%	85%	85%
Hospital Given 9 or 10 on 10 Point Scale	300+	66%	73%	71%
Meds 'Always' Explained Before Given	300+	59%	66%	64%
Nurses 'Always' Communicated Well	300+	75%	80%	79%
Pain 'Always' Well Controlled	300+	68%	72%	71%
Room and Bathroom 'Always' Clean	300+	65%	75%	73%
Timely Help 'Always' Received	300+	60%	69%	68%
Would Definitely Recommend Hospital	300+	68%	73%	71%
Use of Medical Imaging				
Cardiac Imaging Stress Test before Surgery	129	3.9%	5.3%	5.3%
Combination Abdominal CT Scan	718	23.0%	16.4%	10.5%
Combination Brain/Sinus CT Scan	732	2.6%	2.7%	2.7%
Combination Chest CT Scan	581	2.4%	5.6%	2.7%
Follow-up Mammogram/Ultrasound	850	14.9%	7.9%	8.8%
Lumbar Spine MRI for Low Back Pain	91	31.9%	39.6%	37.2%

East Texas Medical Center Trinity

317 Prospect Dr/po Box 3169
Trinity, TX 75862
Phone: 936-594-3541
Fax: 936-744-1182
URL: www.etmc.org
Type: Acute Care Hospitals
Emergency Services: Yes
Ownership: Voluntary non-profit - Private
Beds: 30

Measure	Cases	This Hosp.	State Avg.	U.S. Avg.
Blood Clot Prevention and Treatment				
Anticoagulation Overlap Therapy[1,2]	-	-	93%	93%
ICU Venous Thromboembolism Prophylaxis[1,2]	-	-	92%	92%
Incidence of Potentially Preventable VTE[2,7]	-	-	9%	10%
UFH with Dosages/Platelet Monitoring[2,7]	-	-	96%	97%
Venous Thromboembolism Prophylaxis[2]	266	27%	82%	85%
Warfarin Therapy Discharge Instructions[1,2]	-	-	84%	75%
Chest Pain/Possible Heart Attack Care				
Aspirin Given Within 24 Hours of Arrival[1]	-	-	94%	96%
Fibrinolytic Meds Within 30 Min. of Arrival[1,3]	-	-	47%	58%
Average Time to ECG (minutes)[1]	-	-	8	7
Average Time to Transfer (minutes)[1,3]	-	-	62	60
Children's Asthma Care				
Received Home Management Plan of Care	-	-	93%	88%
Received Reliever Medication	-	-	100%	100%
Received Systemic Corticosteroids	-	-	100%	100%
Emergency Department				
Admittance Decision Time (minutes)[2]	248	75	99	98
Head CT Results Within 45 Min. of Arrival[1]	-	-	54%	57%
Patients Who Left ER Before Being Seen	7,293	0%	3%	2%
Time from ER Arrival to Admit. (minutes)[2]	248	210	270	274
Time from ER Arrival to Discharge (minutes)	273	119	127	134
Time in ER Before Being Evaluated (minutes)	352	16	26	26
Time to Pain Meds for Fractures (minutes)	18	48	57	57
Heart Attack Care				
Aspirin Given at Discharge[5]	-	-	99%	99%
Fibrinolytic Meds Within 30 Min. of Arrival[5]	-	-	49%	54%
PCI Within 90 Minutes of Arrival[5]	-	-	95%	96%
Statin Prescribed at Discharge[5]	-	-	98%	98%
Heart Failure Care				
ACE Inhibitor or ARB for LVSD[1,2]	-	-	97%	97%
Discharge Instructions Given[2]	19	63%	95%	94%
Evaluation of LVS Function[2]	40	78%	99%	99%
Medicare Spending				
Medicare Spending per Patient (ratio)	-	1.26	1.03	0.98
Pneumonia Care				
Appropriate Initial Antibiotic Given[2]	18	94%	95%	95%
Blood Culture Timing[2]	35	89%	98%	98%
Pregnancy and Delivery Care				
Newborn Deliveries Scheduled Early[7]	-	-	7%	6%
Preventive Care				
Immunization for Influenza[2]	281	84%	90%	90%
Immunization for Pneumonia[2]	345	87%	92%	92%
Stroke Care				
Anticoagulation Therapy for Atrial Fibrillation[2,7]	-	-	96%	95%
Antithrombotic Therapy Timing[1,2]	-	-	98%	98%
Assessed for Rehabilitation[1,2]	-	-	98%	97%
Discharged on Antithrombotic Therapy[1,2]	-	-	99%	99%
Discharged on Statin Medication[1,2]	-	-	95%	94%
Thrombolytic Therapy Timing[1,2]	-	-	68%	66%
Venous Thromboembolism Prophylaxis[1,2]	-	-	94%	94%
Written Stroke Educational Materials Given[1,2]	-	-	92%	88%
Surgical Care Improvement Project				
Appropriate Beta Blocker Usage[5]	-	-	98%	98%
Appropriate VTP Within 24 Hours[5]	-	-	98%	98%

NOTE: Hospital profiles are in alphabetical order by state, then city, then hospital within the city; Rankings exclude hospitals with less than 25 cases except for patient surveys which excludes hospitals with less than 100 cases; (a) 100-299 cases; (1) The number of cases/patients is too few to report; (2) Data submitted were based on a sample of cases/patients; (3) Results are based on a shorter time period than required; (4) Data suppressed by CMS for one or more quarters; (5) Results are not available for this reporting period; (6) Fewer than 100 patients completed the HCAHPS survey; (7) No cases met the criteria for this measure; (8) The lower limit of the confidence interval cannot be calculated if the number of observed infections equals zero; (9) No data are available from the state/territory for this reporting period; (10) The scores shown reflect fewer than 50 completed surveys; (11) There were discrepancies in the data collection process; (12) This measure does not apply to this hospital for this reporting period; (13) Results cannot be calculated for this reporting period; (14) The results for this state are combined with nearby states to protect confidentiality; Please refer to the User's Guide for a full explanation of data.

Measure	Cases	This Hosp.	State Avg.	U.S. Avg.
Controlled Postoperative Blood Glucose[5]	-	-	96%	97%
Perioperative Temperature Management[5]	-	-	100%	100%
Prophylactic Antibiotic Selection[5]	-	-	99%	99%
Prophylactic Antibiotic Selection (Outpatient)[5]	-	-	98%	98%
Prophylactic Antibiotic Stopped[5]	-	-	98%	98%
Prophylactic Antibiotic Timing[5]	-	-	99%	99%
Prophylactic Antibiotic Timing (Outpatient)[5]	-	-	98%	98%
Urinary Catheter Removal[5]	-	-	98%	97%
Survey of Patients' Hospital Experiences				
Area Around Room 'Always' Quiet at Night[6]	<100	80%	68%	61%
Doctors 'Always' Communicated Well[6]	<100	83%	83%	82%
Home Recovery Information Given[6]	<100	88%	85%	85%
Hospital Given 9 or 10 on 10 Point Scale[6]	<100	77%	73%	71%
Meds 'Always' Explained Before Given[6]	<100	59%	66%	64%
Nurses 'Always' Communicated Well[6]	<100	80%	80%	79%
Pain 'Always' Well Controlled[6]	<100	76%	72%	71%
Room and Bathroom 'Always' Clean[6]	<100	87%	75%	73%
Timely Help 'Always' Received[6]	<100	76%	69%	68%
Would Definitely Recommend Hospital[6]	<100	77%	73%	71%
Use of Medical Imaging				
Cardiac Imaging Stress Test before Surgery[7]	-	-	5.3%	5.3%
Combination Abdominal CT Scan	70	1.4%	16.4%	10.5%
Combination Brain/Sinus CT Scan[1]	-	-	2.7%	2.7%
Combination Chest CT Scan[1]	-	-	5.6%	2.7%
Follow-up Mammogram/Ultrasound[7]	-	-	7.9%	8.8%
Lumbar Spine MRI for Low Back Pain[7]	-	-	39.6%	37.2%

Baylor Medical Center at Trophy Club

2850 E State Highway 114 Phone: 817-837-4600
Trophy Club, TX 76262 Fax: 817-837-4610
URL: www.tc-mc.com
Type: Acute Care Hospitals Emergency Services: Yes
Ownership: Proprietary
Key Personnel:
CEO .... Melanie Chick
Radiology.................. Tiffney Watson

Measure	Cases	This Hosp.	State Avg.	U.S. Avg.
Blood Clot Prevention and Treatment				
Anticoagulation Overlap Therapy[2,7]	-	-	93%	93%
ICU Venous Thromboembolism Prophylaxis[2,7]	-	-	92%	92%
Incidence of Potentially Preventable VTE[2,7]	-	-	9%	10%
UFH with Dosages/Platelet Monitoring[2,7]	-	-	96%	97%
Venous Thromboembolism Prophylaxis[2]	70	99%	82%	85%
Warfarin Therapy Discharge Instructions[1,2]	-	-	84%	75%
Chest Pain/Possible Heart Attack Care				
Aspirin Given Within 24 Hours of Arrival[1,3]	-	-	94%	96%
Fibrinolytic Meds Within 30 Min. of Arrival[5]	-	-	47%	58%
Average Time to ECG (minutes)[1,3]	-	-	8	7
Average Time to Transfer (minutes)[5]	-	-	62	60
Children's Asthma Care				
Received Home Management Plan of Care	-	-	93%	88%
Received Reliever Medication	-	-	100%	100%
Received Systemic Corticosteroids	-	-	100%	100%
Emergency Department				
Admittance Decision Time (minutes)[2]	32	48	99	98
Head CT Results Within 45 Min. of Arrival[1,3]	-	-	54%	57%
Patients Who Left ER Before Being Seen	2,613	1%	3%	2%
Time from ER Arrival to Admit. (minutes)[2]	33	241	270	274
Time from ER Arrival to Discharge (minutes)	258	89	127	134
Time in ER Before Being Evaluated (minutes)	267	13	26	26
Time to Pain Meds for Fractures (minutes)[1]	-	-	57	57
Heart Attack Care				
Aspirin Given at Discharge[5]	-	-	99%	99%
Fibrinolytic Meds Within 30 Min. of Arrival[5]	-	-	49%	54%
PCI Within 90 Minutes of Arrival[5]	-	-	95%	96%
Statin Prescribed at Discharge[5]	-	-	98%	98%
Heart Failure Care				
ACE Inhibitor or ARB for LVSD[5]	-	-	97%	97%
Discharge Instructions Given[5]	-	-	95%	94%
Evaluation of LVS Function[5]	-	-	99%	99%
Medicare Spending				
Medicare Spending per Patient (ratio)	-	1.45	1.03	0.98
Pneumonia Care				
Appropriate Initial Antibiotic Given[5]	-	-	95%	95%
Blood Culture Timing[5]	-	-	98%	98%
Pregnancy and Delivery Care				
Newborn Deliveries Scheduled Early[7]	-	-	7%	6%
Preventive Care				
Immunization for Influenza[2]	400	100%	90%	90%
Immunization for Pneumonia[2]	170	96%	92%	92%
Stroke Care				
Anticoagulation Therapy for Atrial Fibrillation[5]	-	-	96%	95%
Antithrombotic Therapy Timing[5]	-	-	98%	98%
Assessed for Rehabilitation[5]	-	-	98%	97%
Discharged on Antithrombotic Therapy[5]	-	-	99%	99%
Discharged on Statin Medication[5]	-	-	95%	94%
Thrombolytic Therapy Timing[5]	-	-	68%	66%
Venous Thromboembolism Prophylaxis[5]	-	-	94%	94%
Written Stroke Educational Materials Given[5]	-	-	92%	88%
Surgical Care Improvement Project				
Appropriate Beta Blocker Usage[1]	-	-	98%	98%
Appropriate VTP Within 24 Hours	67	100%	98%	98%
Controlled Postoperative Blood Glucose[7]	-	-	96%	97%
Perioperative Temperature Management	68	100%	100%	100%
Prophylactic Antibiotic Selection	52	100%	99%	99%
Prophylactic Antibiotic Selection (Outpatient)	105	99%	98%	98%
Prophylactic Antibiotic Stopped	52	96%	98%	98%
Prophylactic Antibiotic Timing	52	100%	99%	99%
Prophylactic Antibiotic Timing (Outpatient)	106	95%	98%	98%
Urinary Catheter Removal	61	100%	98%	97%
Survey of Patients' Hospital Experiences				
Area Around Room 'Always' Quiet at Night	(a)	82%	68%	61%
Doctors 'Always' Communicated Well	(a)	85%	83%	82%
Home Recovery Information Given	(a)	88%	85%	85%
Hospital Given 9 or 10 on 10 Point Scale	(a)	84%	73%	71%
Meds 'Always' Explained Before Given	(a)	69%	66%	64%
Nurses 'Always' Communicated Well	(a)	86%	80%	79%
Pain 'Always' Well Controlled	(a)	82%	72%	71%
Room and Bathroom 'Always' Clean	(a)	84%	75%	73%
Timely Help 'Always' Received	(a)	80%	69%	68%
Would Definitely Recommend Hospital	(a)	83%	73%	71%
Use of Medical Imaging				
Cardiac Imaging Stress Test before Surgery[7]	-	-	5.3%	5.3%
Combination Abdominal CT Scan[1]	-	-	16.4%	10.5%
Combination Brain/Sinus CT Scan[1]	-	-	2.7%	2.7%
Combination Chest CT Scan[1]	-	-	5.6%	2.7%
Follow-up Mammogram/Ultrasound[7]	-	-	7.9%	8.8%
Lumbar Spine MRI for Low Back Pain[1]	-	-	39.6%	37.2%

Swisher Memorial Hospital

539 Southeast 2nd Phone: 806-995-3581
Tulia, TX 79088 Fax: 806-995-8283
E-mail: info@swisherhospital.com
URL: www.swisherhospital.com
Type: Critical Access Hospitals Emergency Services: Yes
Ownership: Govt - Hospital Dist/Auth Beds: 20
Key Personnel:
CEO .... Ryan Barnard, PharmD, MBA, FA
Chief of Medical Staff.......... Cody Culwell
Radiology.................. Meredith Hochstein
Emergency Room .... Tim Stinebaugh

Measure	Cases	This Hosp.	State Avg.	U.S. Avg.
Blood Clot Prevention and Treatment				
Anticoagulation Overlap Therapy[5]	-	-	93%	93%
ICU Venous Thromboembolism Prophylaxis[5]	-	-	92%	92%
Incidence of Potentially Preventable VTE[5]	-	-	9%	10%
UFH with Dosages/Platelet Monitoring[5]	-	-	96%	97%
Venous Thromboembolism Prophylaxis[5]	-	-	82%	85%
Warfarin Therapy Discharge Instructions[5]	-	-	84%	75%
Chest Pain/Possible Heart Attack Care				
Aspirin Given Within 24 Hours of Arrival	-	-	94%	96%
Fibrinolytic Meds Within 30 Min. of Arrival	-	-	47%	58%
Average Time to ECG (minutes)	-	-	8	7
Average Time to Transfer (minutes)	-	-	62	60
Children's Asthma Care				
Received Home Management Plan of Care	-	-	93%	88%
Received Reliever Medication	-	-	100%	100%
Received Systemic Corticosteroids	-	-	100%	100%
Emergency Department				
Admittance Decision Time (minutes)[5]	-	-	99	98
Head CT Results Within 45 Min. of Arrival	-	-	54%	57%
Patients Who Left ER Before Being Seen	-	-	3%	2%
Time from ER Arrival to Admit. (minutes)[5]	-	-	270	274
Time from ER Arrival to Discharge (minutes)	-	-	127	134
Time in ER Before Being Evaluated (minutes)	-	-	26	26
Time to Pain Meds for Fractures (minutes)	-	-	57	57
Heart Attack Care				
Aspirin Given at Discharge[5]	-	-	99%	99%
Fibrinolytic Meds Within 30 Min. of Arrival[5]	-	-	49%	54%
PCI Within 90 Minutes of Arrival[5]	-	-	95%	96%
Statin Prescribed at Discharge[5]	-	-	98%	98%
Heart Failure Care				
ACE Inhibitor or ARB for LVSD[5]	-	-	97%	97%
Discharge Instructions Given[5]	-	-	95%	94%
Evaluation of LVS Function[5]	-	-	99%	99%
Medicare Spending				
Medicare Spending per Patient (ratio)	-	-	1.03	0.98
Pneumonia Care				
Appropriate Initial Antibiotic Given[5]	-	-	95%	95%
Blood Culture Timing[5]	-	-	98%	98%
Pregnancy and Delivery Care				
Newborn Deliveries Scheduled Early[5]	-	-	7%	6%
Preventive Care				
Immunization for Influenza[5]	-	-	90%	90%
Immunization for Pneumonia[5]	-	-	92%	92%
Stroke Care				
Anticoagulation Therapy for Atrial Fibrillation[5]	-	-	96%	95%
Antithrombotic Therapy Timing[5]	-	-	98%	98%
Assessed for Rehabilitation[5]	-	-	98%	97%
Discharged on Antithrombotic Therapy[5]	-	-	99%	99%
Discharged on Statin Medication[5]	-	-	95%	94%
Thrombolytic Therapy Timing[5]	-	-	68%	66%
Venous Thromboembolism Prophylaxis[5]	-	-	94%	94%
Written Stroke Educational Materials Given[5]	-	-	92%	88%
Surgical Care Improvement Project				
Appropriate Beta Blocker Usage[5]	-	-	98%	98%
Appropriate VTP Within 24 Hours[5]	-	-	98%	98%
Controlled Postoperative Blood Glucose[5]	-	-	96%	97%
Perioperative Temperature Management[5]	-	-	100%	100%
Prophylactic Antibiotic Selection[5]	-	-	99%	99%
Prophylactic Antibiotic Selection (Outpatient)	-	-	98%	98%
Prophylactic Antibiotic Stopped[5]	-	-	98%	98%
Prophylactic Antibiotic Timing[5]	-	-	99%	99%
Prophylactic Antibiotic Timing (Outpatient)	-	-	98%	98%
Urinary Catheter Removal[5]	-	-	98%	97%
Survey of Patients' Hospital Experiences				
Area Around Room 'Always' Quiet at Night[6]	<100	70%	68%	61%
Doctors 'Always' Communicated Well[6]	<100	93%	83%	82%
Home Recovery Information Given[6]	<100	84%	85%	85%
Hospital Given 9 or 10 on 10 Point Scale[6]	<100	78%	73%	71%
Meds 'Always' Explained Before Given[6]	<100	80%	66%	64%
Nurses 'Always' Communicated Well[6]	<100	88%	80%	79%
Pain 'Always' Well Controlled[6]	<100	90%	72%	71%
Room and Bathroom 'Always' Clean[6]	<100	88%	75%	73%
Timely Help 'Always' Received[6]	<100	90%	69%	68%
Would Definitely Recommend Hospital[6]	<100	81%	73%	71%
Use of Medical Imaging				
Cardiac Imaging Stress Test before Surgery	-	-	5.3%	5.3%
Combination Abdominal CT Scan	-	-	16.4%	10.5%
Combination Brain/Sinus CT Scan	-	-	2.7%	2.7%
Combination Chest CT Scan	-	-	5.6%	2.7%
Follow-up Mammogram/Ultrasound	-	-	7.9%	8.8%
Lumbar Spine MRI for Low Back Pain	-	-	39.6%	37.2%

NOTE: Hospital profiles are in alphabetical order by state, then city, then hospital within the city; Rankings exclude hospitals with less than 25 cases except for patient surveys which excludes hospitals with less than 100 cases; (a) 100-299 cases; (1) The number of cases/patients is too few to report; (2) Data submitted were based on a sample of cases/patients; (3) Results are based on a shorter time period than required; (4) Data suppressed by CMS for one or more quarters; (5) Results are not available for this reporting period; (6) Fewer than 100 patients completed the HCAHPS survey; (7) No cases met the criteria for this measure; (8) The lower limit of the confidence interval cannot be calculated if the number of observed infections equals zero; (9) No data are available from the state/territory for this reporting period; (10) The scores shown reflect fewer than 50 completed surveys; (11) There were discrepancies in the data collection process; (12) This measure does not apply to this hospital for this reporting period; (13) Results cannot be calculated for this reporting period; (14) The results for this state are combined with nearby states to protect confidentiality; Please refer to the User's Guide for a full explanation of data.

East Texas Medical Center

1000 South Beckham Street Phone: 903-597-0351
Tyler, TX 75701 Fax: 903-535-6334
URL: www.etmc.org
Type: Acute Care Hospitals Emergency Services: Yes
Ownership: Government - Local Beds: 454

Key Personnel:
Operating Room. . . . . Martha Bush
CEO/President. . . . . Elmer Ellis
Quality Assurance . . . . Bill Jennings
Infection Control. . . . . Annette Moore
Chief of Medical Staff. . . . . Bill Moore, MD
Cardiac Laboratory. . . . . John Stewart
Radiology. . . . . Bill Tobin

Measure	Cases	This Hosp.	State Avg.	U.S. Avg.
Blood Clot Prevention and Treatment				
Anticoagulation Overlap Therapy[2]	137	82%	93%	93%
ICU Venous Thromboembolism Prophylaxis[2]	102	91%	92%	92%
Incidence of Potentially Preventable VTE[2]	25	4%	9%	10%
UFH with Dosages/Platelet Monitoring[2]	31	84%	96%	97%
Venous Thromboembolism Prophylaxis[2]	271	83%	82%	85%
Warfarin Therapy Discharge Instructions[2]	105	76%	84%	75%
Chest Pain/Possible Heart Attack Care				
Aspirin Given Within 24 Hours of Arrival[1,3]	-	-	94%	96%
Fibrinolytic Meds Within 30 Min. of Arrival[3,7]	-	-	47%	58%
Average Time to ECG (minutes)[1,3]	-	-	8	7
Average Time to Transfer (minutes)[1,3]	-	-	62	60
Children's Asthma Care				
Received Home Management Plan of Care	-	-	93%	88%
Received Reliever Medication	-	-	100%	100%
Received Systemic Corticosteroids	-	-	100%	100%
Emergency Department				
Admittance Decision Time (minutes)[2]	274	140	99	98
Head CT Results Within 45 Min. of Arrival[1]	-	-	54%	57%
Patients Who Left ER Before Being Seen	66,359	7%	3%	2%
Time from ER Arrival to Admit. (minutes)[2]	288	352	270	274
Time from ER Arrival to Discharge (minutes)	351	142	127	134
Time in ER Before Being Evaluated (minutes)	368	36	26	26
Time to Pain Meds for Fractures (minutes)	218	88	57	57
Heart Attack Care				
Aspirin Given at Discharge[2]	271	100%	99%	99%
Fibrinolytic Meds Within 30 Min. of Arrival[2,7]	-	-	49%	54%
PCI Within 90 Minutes of Arrival[2]	13	100%	95%	96%
Statin Prescribed at Discharge[2]	252	100%	98%	98%
Heart Failure Care				
ACE Inhibitor or ARB for LVSD[2]	104	96%	97%	97%
Discharge Instructions Given[2]	225	95%	95%	94%
Evaluation of LVS Function[2]	296	100%	99%	99%
Medicare Spending				
Medicare Spending per Patient (ratio)	-	1.07	1.03	0.98
Pneumonia Care				
Appropriate Initial Antibiotic Given[2]	49	98%	95%	95%
Blood Culture Timing[2]	103	99%	98%	98%
Pregnancy and Delivery Care				
Newborn Deliveries Scheduled Early[2]	19	0%	7%	6%
Preventive Care				
Immunization for Influenza[2]	555	95%	90%	90%
Immunization for Pneumonia[2]	683	97%	92%	92%
Stroke Care				
Anticoagulation Therapy for Atrial Fibrillation	34	100%	96%	95%
Antithrombotic Therapy Timing	255	100%	98%	98%
Assessed for Rehabilitation	339	100%	98%	97%
Discharged on Antithrombotic Therapy	291	100%	99%	99%
Discharged on Statin Medication	214	91%	95%	94%
Thrombolytic Therapy Timing[1]	-	-	68%	66%
Venous Thromboembolism Prophylaxis	348	94%	94%	94%
Written Stroke Educational Materials Given	160	86%	92%	88%
Surgical Care Improvement Project				
Appropriate Beta Blocker Usage[2]	215	99%	98%	98%
Appropriate VTP Within 24 Hours[2]	299	100%	98%	98%
Controlled Postoperative Blood Glucose[2]	113	100%	96%	97%
Perioperative Temperature Management[2]	417	100%	100%	100%
Prophylactic Antibiotic Selection[2]	398	99%	99%	99%
Prophylactic Antibiotic Selection (Outpatient)	399	97%	98%	98%
Prophylactic Antibiotic Stopped[2]	392	98%	98%	98%
Prophylactic Antibiotic Timing[2]	398	98%	99%	99%
Prophylactic Antibiotic Timing (Outpatient)	402	95%	98%	98%
Urinary Catheter Removal[2]	336	99%	98%	97%
Survey of Patients' Hospital Experiences				
Area Around Room 'Always' Quiet at Night	300+	58%	68%	61%
Doctors 'Always' Communicated Well	300+	78%	83%	82%
Home Recovery Information Given	300+	82%	85%	85%
Hospital Given 9 or 10 on 10 Point Scale	300+	68%	73%	71%
Meds 'Always' Explained Before Given	300+	61%	66%	64%
Nurses 'Always' Communicated Well	300+	76%	80%	79%
Pain 'Always' Well Controlled	300+	70%	72%	71%
Room and Bathroom 'Always' Clean	300+	69%	75%	73%
Timely Help 'Always' Received	300+	61%	69%	68%
Would Definitely Recommend Hospital	300+	71%	73%	71%
Use of Medical Imaging				
Cardiac Imaging Stress Test before Surgery	362	5.8%	5.3%	5.3%
Combination Abdominal CT Scan	1,430	6.2%	16.4%	10.5%
Combination Brain/Sinus CT Scan	1,133	3.4%	2.7%	2.7%
Combination Chest CT Scan	1,004	0.2%	5.6%	2.7%
Follow-up Mammogram/Ultrasound	3,066	5.4%	7.9%	8.8%
Lumbar Spine MRI for Low Back Pain	202	43.1%	39.6%	37.2%

Mother Frances Hospital

800 East Dawson Phone: 903-593-8441
Tyler, TX 75701 Fax: 903-531-4067
E-mail: lukerr@trimofran.org
URL: www.tmfhs.org
Type: Acute Care Hospitals Emergency Services: Yes
Ownership: Voluntary non-profit - Church Beds: 358

Key Personnel:
Cardiac Laboratory. . . . . Linda Bowles
Coronary Care . . . . Linda Bowles
Quality Assurance . . . . Kate Bynum
Radiology. . . . . Georn Granberry
Chief of Medical Staff. . . . . Steven P. Keuer, MD
CEO/President. . . . . John McGreevy, FACHE
Pediatric In-Patient Care . . . . Bobbie Ogg
Infection Control. . . . . Sylvia Radcliffe, RN

Measure	Cases	This Hosp.	State Avg.	U.S. Avg.
Blood Clot Prevention and Treatment				
Anticoagulation Overlap Therapy[2]	134	96%	93%	93%
ICU Venous Thromboembolism Prophylaxis[2]	90	98%	92%	92%
Incidence of Potentially Preventable VTE[2]	13	0%	9%	10%
UFH with Dosages/Platelet Monitoring[2]	43	100%	96%	97%
Venous Thromboembolism Prophylaxis[2]	336	88%	82%	85%
Warfarin Therapy Discharge Instructions[2]	87	100%	84%	75%
Chest Pain/Possible Heart Attack Care				
Aspirin Given Within 24 Hours of Arrival[5]	-	-	94%	96%
Fibrinolytic Meds Within 30 Min. of Arrival[5]	-	-	47%	58%
Average Time to ECG (minutes)[5]	-	-	8	7
Average Time to Transfer (minutes)[5]	-	-	62	60
Children's Asthma Care				
Received Home Management Plan of Care	-	-	93%	88%
Received Reliever Medication	-	-	100%	100%
Received Systemic Corticosteroids	-	-	100%	100%
Emergency Department				
Admittance Decision Time (minutes)[2]	476	125	99	98
Head CT Results Within 45 Min. of Arrival[1]	-	-	54%	57%
Patients Who Left ER Before Being Seen	69,804	3%	3%	2%
Time from ER Arrival to Admit. (minutes)[2]	490	313	270	274
Time from ER Arrival to Discharge (minutes)	406	141	127	134
Time in ER Before Being Evaluated (minutes)	424	52	26	26
Time to Pain Meds for Fractures (minutes)	231	72	57	57
Heart Attack Care				
Aspirin Given at Discharge	691	99%	99%	99%
Fibrinolytic Meds Within 30 Min. of Arrival[7]	-	-	49%	54%
PCI Within 90 Minutes of Arrival	82	94%	95%	96%
Statin Prescribed at Discharge	672	97%	98%	98%
Heart Failure Care				
ACE Inhibitor or ARB for LVSD[2]	182	97%	97%	97%
Discharge Instructions Given[2]	492	99%	95%	94%
Evaluation of LVS Function[2]	625	100%	99%	99%
Medicare Spending				
Medicare Spending per Patient (ratio)	-	1.03	1.03	0.98
Pneumonia Care				
Appropriate Initial Antibiotic Given[2]	235	97%	95%	95%
Blood Culture Timing[2]	360	99%	98%	98%
Pregnancy and Delivery Care				
Newborn Deliveries Scheduled Early	207	10%	7%	6%
Preventive Care				
Immunization for Influenza[2]	564	76%	90%	90%
Immunization for Pneumonia[2]	679	82%	92%	92%
Stroke Care				
Anticoagulation Therapy for Atrial Fibrillation	37	95%	96%	95%
Antithrombotic Therapy Timing	344	98%	98%	98%
Assessed for Rehabilitation	393	98%	98%	97%
Discharged on Antithrombotic Therapy	357	98%	99%	99%
Discharged on Statin Medication	289	94%	95%	94%
Thrombolytic Therapy Timing	20	65%	68%	66%
Venous Thromboembolism Prophylaxis	400	96%	94%	94%
Written Stroke Educational Materials Given	201	99%	92%	88%
Surgical Care Improvement Project				
Appropriate Beta Blocker Usage[2]	312	98%	98%	98%
Appropriate VTP Within 24 Hours[2]	420	96%	98%	98%
Controlled Postoperative Blood Glucose[2]	196	97%	96%	97%
Perioperative Temperature Management[2]	638	100%	100%	100%
Prophylactic Antibiotic Selection[2]	559	100%	99%	99%
Prophylactic Antibiotic Selection (Outpatient)	1,220	98%	98%	98%
Prophylactic Antibiotic Stopped[2]	543	98%	98%	98%
Prophylactic Antibiotic Timing[2]	559	99%	99%	99%
Prophylactic Antibiotic Timing (Outpatient)	1,223	99%	98%	98%
Urinary Catheter Removal[2]	466	92%	98%	97%
Survey of Patients' Hospital Experiences				
Area Around Room 'Always' Quiet at Night	300+	63%	68%	61%
Doctors 'Always' Communicated Well	300+	80%	83%	82%
Home Recovery Information Given	300+	84%	85%	85%
Hospital Given 9 or 10 on 10 Point Scale	300+	74%	73%	71%
Meds 'Always' Explained Before Given	300+	63%	66%	64%
Nurses 'Always' Communicated Well	300+	77%	80%	79%
Pain 'Always' Well Controlled	300+	68%	72%	71%
Room and Bathroom 'Always' Clean	300+	70%	75%	73%
Timely Help 'Always' Received	300+	59%	69%	68%
Would Definitely Recommend Hospital	300+	79%	73%	71%
Use of Medical Imaging				
Cardiac Imaging Stress Test before Surgery	2,196	4.6%	5.3%	5.3%
Combination Abdominal CT Scan	1,640	24.8%	16.4%	10.5%
Combination Brain/Sinus CT Scan	1,406	1.9%	2.7%	2.7%
Combination Chest CT Scan	1,396	0.1%	5.6%	2.7%
Follow-up Mammogram/Ultrasound	6,818	7.0%	7.9%	8.8%
Lumbar Spine MRI for Low Back Pain	445	40.0%	39.6%	37.2%

Texas Spine & Joint Hospital

1814 Roseland Boulevard Phone: 903-525-3300
Tyler, TX 75701
URL: www.tsjh.org
Type: Acute Care Hospitals Emergency Services: Yes
Ownership: Proprietary Beds: 20

Key Personnel:
CEO/President. . . . . Tony Wahl

Measure	Cases	This Hosp.	State Avg.	U.S. Avg.
Blood Clot Prevention and Treatment				
Anticoagulation Overlap Therapy[2,7]	-	-	93%	93%
ICU Venous Thromboembolism Prophylaxis[2,7]	-	-	92%	92%
Incidence of Potentially Preventable VTE[2,7]	-	-	9%	10%
UFH with Dosages/Platelet Monitoring[2,7]	-	-	96%	97%
Venous Thromboembolism Prophylaxis[1,2]	-	-	82%	85%
Warfarin Therapy Discharge Instructions[2,7]	-	-	84%	75%
Chest Pain/Possible Heart Attack Care				
Aspirin Given Within 24 Hours of Arrival[5]	-	-	94%	96%
Fibrinolytic Meds Within 30 Min. of Arrival[5]	-	-	47%	58%
Average Time to ECG (minutes)[5]	-	-	8	7
Average Time to Transfer (minutes)[5]	-	-	62	60
Children's Asthma Care				
Received Home Management Plan of Care	-	-	93%	88%
Received Reliever Medication	-	-	100%	100%
Received Systemic Corticosteroids	-	-	100%	100%

NOTE: Hospital profiles are in alphabetical order by state, then city, then hospital within the city; Rankings exclude hospitals with less than 25 cases except for patient surveys which excludes hospitals with less than 100 cases; (a) 100-299 cases; (1) The number of cases/patients is too few to report; (2) Data submitted were based on a sample of cases/patients; (3) Results are based on a shorter time period than required; (4) Data suppressed by CMS for one or more quarters; (5) Results are not available for this reporting period; (6) Fewer than 100 patients completed the HCAHPS survey; (7) No cases met the criteria for this measure; (8) The lower limit of the confidence interval cannot be calculated if the number of observed infections equals zero; (9) No data are available from the state/territory for this reporting period; (10) The scores shown reflect fewer than 50 completed surveys; (11) There were discrepancies in the data collection process; (12) This measure does not apply to this hospital for this reporting period; (13) Results cannot be calculated for this reporting period; (14) The results for this state are combined with nearby states to protect confidentiality; Please refer to the User's Guide for a full explanation of data.

Measure	Cases	This Hosp.	State Avg.	U.S. Avg.
Emergency Department				
Admittance Decision Time (minutes)[1,2]	-	-	99	98
Head CT Results Within 45 Min. of Arrival[5]	-	-	54%	57%
Patients Who Left ER Before Being Seen	399	1%	3%	2%
Time from ER Arrival to Admit. (minutes)[1,2]	-	-	270	274
Time from ER Arrival to Discharge (minutes)	238	121	127	134
Time in ER Before Being Evaluated (minutes)	249	42	26	26
Time to Pain Meds for Fractures (minutes)[1,3]	-	-	57	57
Heart Attack Care				
Aspirin Given at Discharge[5]	-	-	99%	99%
Fibrinolytic Meds Within 30 Min. of Arrival[5]	-	-	49%	54%
PCI Within 90 Minutes of Arrival[5]	-	-	95%	96%
Statin Prescribed at Discharge[5]	-	-	98%	98%
Heart Failure Care				
ACE Inhibitor or ARB for LVSD[5]	-	-	97%	97%
Discharge Instructions Given[5]	-	-	95%	94%
Evaluation of LVS Function[5]	-	-	99%	99%
Medicare Spending				
Medicare Spending per Patient (ratio)	-	0.98	1.03	0.98
Pneumonia Care				
Appropriate Initial Antibiotic Given[2,3]	-	-	95%	95%
Blood Culture Timing[2,3]	-	-	98%	98%
Pregnancy and Delivery Care				
Newborn Deliveries Scheduled Early[7]	-	-	7%	6%
Preventive Care				
Immunization for Influenza[2]	345	75%	90%	90%
Immunization for Pneumonia[2]	494	61%	92%	92%
Stroke Care				
Anticoagulation Therapy for Atrial Fibrillation[5]	-	-	96%	95%
Antithrombotic Therapy Timing[5]	-	-	98%	98%
Assessed for Rehabilitation[5]	-	-	98%	97%
Discharged on Antithrombotic Therapy[5]	-	-	99%	99%
Discharged on Statin Medication[5]	-	-	95%	94%
Thrombolytic Therapy Timing[5]	-	-	68%	66%
Venous Thromboembolism Prophylaxis[5]	-	-	94%	94%
Written Stroke Educational Materials Given[5]	-	-	92%	88%
Surgical Care Improvement Project				
Appropriate Beta Blocker Usage[2]	72	99%	98%	98%
Appropriate VTP Within 24 Hours[2]	212	100%	98%	98%
Controlled Postoperative Blood Glucose[2,7]	-	-	96%	97%
Perioperative Temperature Management[2]	236	100%	100%	100%
Prophylactic Antibiotic Selection[2]	213	100%	99%	99%
Prophylactic Antibiotic Selection (Outpatient)	396	99%	98%	98%
Prophylactic Antibiotic Stopped[2]	213	97%	98%	98%
Prophylactic Antibiotic Timing[2]	213	100%	99%	99%
Prophylactic Antibiotic Timing (Outpatient)	396	99%	98%	98%
Urinary Catheter Removal[2]	170	99%	98%	97%
Survey of Patients' Hospital Experiences				
Area Around Room 'Always' Quiet at Night	300+	73%	68%	61%
Doctors 'Always' Communicated Well	300+	88%	83%	82%
Home Recovery Information Given	300+	90%	85%	85%
Hospital Given 9 or 10 on 10 Point Scale	300+	86%	73%	71%
Meds 'Always' Explained Before Given	300+	78%	66%	64%
Nurses 'Always' Communicated Well	300+	87%	80%	79%
Pain 'Always' Well Controlled	300+	78%	72%	71%
Room and Bathroom 'Always' Clean	300+	79%	75%	73%
Timely Help 'Always' Received	300+	83%	69%	68%
Would Definitely Recommend Hospital	300+	90%	73%	71%
Use of Medical Imaging				
Cardiac Imaging Stress Test before Surgery[7]	-	-	5.3%	5.3%
Combination Abdominal CT Scan[1]	-	-	16.4%	10.5%
Combination Brain/Sinus CT Scan	97	0.0%	2.7%	2.7%
Combination Chest CT Scan[1]	-	-	5.6%	2.7%
Follow-up Mammogram/Ultrasound[7]	-	-	7.9%	8.8%
Lumbar Spine MRI for Low Back Pain	900	35.0%	39.6%	37.2%

University of Texas Health Science Center at Tyler

11937 Us Highway 271
Tyler, TX 75708
E-mail: sally.stuart@uthct.edu
URL: www.uthct.edu
Type: Acute Care Hospitals
Ownership: Government - State
Phone: 903-877-7777
Fax: 903-877-5725
Emergency Services: Yes
Beds: 204

Key Personnel:
Chief of Medical Staff.......... Steven D Brown, MD
President.......................... Kirk A Calhoun
Operating Room.................. Steven W Cox
Quality Assurance .... Susan Cresswell
Radiology........................... David P Di Paolo
Pediatric Ambulatory Care ...... Kathryn Haar
Infection Control............... Doris Jarvis, RN
Pediatric In-Patient Care .... Teresa Serrati, RN MSN

Measure	Cases	This Hosp.	State Avg.	U.S. Avg.
Blood Clot Prevention and Treatment				
Anticoagulation Overlap Therapy[1,2]	-	-	93%	93%
ICU Venous Thromboembolism Prophylaxis[2]	56	100%	92%	92%
Incidence of Potentially Preventable VTE[1,2]	-	-	9%	10%
UFH with Dosages/Platelet Monitoring[1,2]	-	-	96%	97%
Venous Thromboembolism Prophylaxis[2]	140	95%	82%	85%
Warfarin Therapy Discharge Instructions[1,2]	-	-	84%	75%
Chest Pain/Possible Heart Attack Care				
Aspirin Given Within 24 Hours of Arrival[1]	-	-	94%	96%
Fibrinolytic Meds Within 30 Min. of Arrival[3,7]	-	-	47%	58%
Average Time to ECG (minutes)[1]	-	-	8	7
Average Time to Transfer (minutes)[1,3]	-	-	62	60
Children's Asthma Care				
Received Home Management Plan of Care	-	-	93%	88%
Received Reliever Medication	-	-	100%	100%
Received Systemic Corticosteroids	-	-	100%	100%
Emergency Department				
Admittance Decision Time (minutes)[2]	352	70	99	98
Head CT Results Within 45 Min. of Arrival[1]	-	-	54%	57%
Patients Who Left ER Before Being Seen	14,853	1%	3%	2%
Time from ER Arrival to Admit. (minutes)[2]	353	225	270	274
Time from ER Arrival to Discharge (minutes)	385	115	127	134
Time in ER Before Being Evaluated (minutes)	401	25	26	26
Time to Pain Meds for Fractures (minutes)	32	46	57	57
Heart Attack Care				
Aspirin Given at Discharge	20	95%	99%	99%
Fibrinolytic Meds Within 30 Min. of Arrival[7]	-	-	49%	54%
PCI Within 90 Minutes of Arrival[1]	-	-	95%	96%
Statin Prescribed at Discharge	17	100%	98%	98%
Heart Failure Care				
ACE Inhibitor or ARB for LVSD	18	100%	97%	97%
Discharge Instructions Given	87	99%	95%	94%
Evaluation of LVS Function	107	99%	99%	99%
Medicare Spending				
Medicare Spending per Patient (ratio)	-	0.99	1.03	0.98
Pneumonia Care				
Appropriate Initial Antibiotic Given[2]	66	98%	95%	95%
Blood Culture Timing[2]	109	98%	98%	98%
Pregnancy and Delivery Care				
Newborn Deliveries Scheduled Early[7]	-	-	7%	6%
Preventive Care				
Immunization for Influenza[2]	326	86%	90%	90%
Immunization for Pneumonia[2]	475	92%	92%	92%
Stroke Care				
Anticoagulation Therapy for Atrial Fibrillation[1]	-	-	96%	95%
Antithrombotic Therapy Timing	11	100%	98%	98%
Assessed for Rehabilitation	12	100%	98%	97%
Discharged on Antithrombotic Therapy	12	100%	99%	99%
Discharged on Statin Medication[1]	-	-	95%	94%
Thrombolytic Therapy Timing[7]	-	-	68%	66%
Venous Thromboembolism Prophylaxis	12	100%	94%	94%
Written Stroke Educational Materials Given[1]	-	-	92%	88%
Surgical Care Improvement Project				
Appropriate Beta Blocker Usage	28	96%	98%	98%
Appropriate VTP Within 24 Hours	85	94%	98%	98%
Controlled Postoperative Blood Glucose[7]	-	-	96%	97%
Perioperative Temperature Management	99	100%	100%	100%
Prophylactic Antibiotic Selection	51	100%	99%	99%
Prophylactic Antibiotic Selection (Outpatient)[1]	-	-	98%	98%
Prophylactic Antibiotic Stopped	47	100%	98%	98%
Prophylactic Antibiotic Timing	51	96%	99%	99%
Prophylactic Antibiotic Timing (Outpatient)[1]	-	-	98%	98%
Urinary Catheter Removal	63	98%	98%	97%
Survey of Patients' Hospital Experiences				
Area Around Room 'Always' Quiet at Night	(a)	61%	68%	61%
Doctors 'Always' Communicated Well	(a)	88%	83%	82%
Home Recovery Information Given	(a)	91%	85%	85%
Hospital Given 9 or 10 on 10 Point Scale	(a)	80%	73%	71%
Meds 'Always' Explained Before Given	(a)	69%	66%	64%
Nurses 'Always' Communicated Well	(a)	77%	80%	79%
Pain 'Always' Well Controlled	(a)	70%	72%	71%
Room and Bathroom 'Always' Clean	(a)	76%	75%	73%
Timely Help 'Always' Received	(a)	63%	69%	68%
Would Definitely Recommend Hospital	(a)	84%	73%	71%
Use of Medical Imaging				
Cardiac Imaging Stress Test before Surgery	179	6.7%	5.3%	5.3%
Combination Abdominal CT Scan	433	14.1%	16.4%	10.5%
Combination Brain/Sinus CT Scan	242	1.2%	2.7%	2.7%
Combination Chest CT Scan	840	0.7%	5.6%	2.7%
Follow-up Mammogram/Ultrasound	665	13.7%	7.9%	8.8%
Lumbar Spine MRI for Low Back Pain[1]	-	-	39.6%	37.2%

Uvalde Memorial Hospital

1025 Garner Field Road
Uvalde, TX 78801
URL: www.umhtx.org
Type: Acute Care Hospitals
Ownership: Govt - Hospital Dist/Auth
Phone: 830-278-6251
Fax: 830-278-8529
Emergency Services: Yes
Beds: 66

Key Personnel:
Radiology.......................... Barry Flanders
Operating Room................ G V Gaitonde
Infection Control............... Jacqueline Gillette
Cardiac Laboratory............ Linda Griffin
Intensive Care Unit............ Linda Griffin
Chief of Medical Staff.......... Dr Carl Utterback

Measure	Cases	This Hosp.	State Avg.	U.S. Avg.
Blood Clot Prevention and Treatment				
Anticoagulation Overlap Therapy[1,2]	-	-	93%	93%
ICU Venous Thromboembolism Prophylaxis[2]	186	90%	92%	92%
Incidence of Potentially Preventable VTE[2,7]	-	-	9%	10%
UFH with Dosages/Platelet Monitoring[2,7]	-	-	96%	97%
Venous Thromboembolism Prophylaxis[2]	441	80%	82%	85%
Warfarin Therapy Discharge Instructions[1,2]	-	-	84%	75%
Chest Pain/Possible Heart Attack Care				
Aspirin Given Within 24 Hours of Arrival	115	98%	94%	96%
Fibrinolytic Meds Within 30 Min. of Arrival[1]	-	-	47%	58%
Average Time to ECG (minutes)	123	8	8	7
Average Time to Transfer (minutes)[1]	-	-	62	60
Children's Asthma Care				
Received Home Management Plan of Care	-	-	93%	88%
Received Reliever Medication	-	-	100%	100%
Received Systemic Corticosteroids	-	-	100%	100%
Emergency Department				
Admittance Decision Time (minutes)[2]	613	41	99	98
Head CT Results Within 45 Min. of Arrival[1]	-	-	54%	57%
Patients Who Left ER Before Being Seen	18,378	5%	3%	2%
Time from ER Arrival to Admit. (minutes)[2]	614	222	270	274
Time from ER Arrival to Discharge (minutes)	742	151	127	134
Time in ER Before Being Evaluated (minutes)	824	29	26	26
Time to Pain Meds for Fractures (minutes)	129	81	57	57
Heart Attack Care				
Aspirin Given at Discharge[1]	-	-	99%	99%
Fibrinolytic Meds Within 30 Min. of Arrival[7]	-	-	49%	54%
PCI Within 90 Minutes of Arrival[7]	-	-	95%	96%
Statin Prescribed at Discharge[1]	-	-	98%	98%
Heart Failure Care				
ACE Inhibitor or ARB for LVSD[1]	-	-	97%	97%
Discharge Instructions Given	44	93%	95%	94%
Evaluation of LVS Function	57	96%	99%	99%
Medicare Spending				
Medicare Spending per Patient (ratio)	-	1.00	1.03	0.98

NOTE: Hospital profiles are in alphabetical order by state, then city, then hospital within the city; Rankings exclude hospitals with less than 25 cases except for patient surveys which excludes hospitals with less than 100 cases; (a) 100-299 cases; (1) The number of cases/patients is too few to report; (2) Data submitted were based on a sample of cases/patients; (3) Results are based on a shorter time period than required; (4) Data suppressed by CMS for one or more quarters; (5) Results are not available for this reporting period; (6) Fewer than 100 patients completed the HCAHPS survey; (7) No cases met the criteria for this measure; (8) The lower limit of the confidence interval cannot be calculated if the number of observed infections equals zero; (9) No data are available from the state/territory for this reporting period; (10) The scores shown reflect fewer than 50 completed surveys; (11) There were discrepancies in the data collection process; (12) This measure does not apply to this hospital for this reporting period; (13) Results cannot be calculated for this reporting period; (14) The results for this state are combined with nearby states to protect confidentiality; Please refer to the User's Guide for a full explanation of data.

Measure	Cases	This Hosp.	State Avg.	U.S. Avg.
Pneumonia Care				
Appropriate Initial Antibiotic Given	62	97%	95%	95%
Blood Culture Timing	90	94%	98%	98%
Pregnancy and Delivery Care				
Newborn Deliveries Scheduled Early	25	4%	7%	6%
Preventive Care				
Immunization for Influenza[2]	518	68%	90%	90%
Immunization for Pneumonia[2]	542	82%	92%	92%
Stroke Care				
Anticoagulation Therapy for Atrial Fibrillation[1]	-	-	96%	95%
Antithrombotic Therapy Timing	14	93%	98%	98%
Assessed for Rehabilitation	17	94%	98%	97%
Discharged on Antithrombotic Therapy	15	93%	99%	99%
Discharged on Statin Medication	15	60%	95%	94%
Thrombolytic Therapy Timing[1]	-	-	68%	66%
Venous Thromboembolism Prophylaxis	16	94%	94%	94%
Written Stroke Educational Materials Given[1]	-	-	92%	88%
Surgical Care Improvement Project				
Appropriate Beta Blocker Usage[1]	-	-	98%	98%
Appropriate VTP Within 24 Hours	42	90%	98%	98%
Controlled Postoperative Blood Glucose[7]	-	-	96%	97%
Perioperative Temperature Management	44	100%	100%	100%
Prophylactic Antibiotic Selection	28	100%	99%	99%
Prophylactic Antibiotic Selection (Outpatient)	13	92%	98%	98%
Prophylactic Antibiotic Stopped	27	96%	98%	98%
Prophylactic Antibiotic Timing	28	89%	99%	99%
Prophylactic Antibiotic Timing (Outpatient)	13	100%	98%	98%
Urinary Catheter Removal	29	97%	98%	97%
Survey of Patients' Hospital Experiences				
Area Around Room 'Always' Quiet at Night[11]	(a)	62%	68%	61%
Doctors 'Always' Communicated Well[11]	(a)	86%	83%	82%
Home Recovery Information Given[11]	(a)	91%	85%	85%
Hospital Given 9 or 10 on 10 Point Scale[11]	(a)	77%	73%	71%
Meds 'Always' Explained Before Given[11]	(a)	72%	66%	64%
Nurses 'Always' Communicated Well[11]	(a)	83%	80%	79%
Pain 'Always' Well Controlled[11]	(a)	78%	72%	71%
Room and Bathroom 'Always' Clean[11]	(a)	73%	75%	73%
Timely Help 'Always' Received[11]	(a)	74%	69%	68%
Would Definitely Recommend Hospital[11]	(a)	72%	73%	71%
Use of Medical Imaging				
Cardiac Imaging Stress Test before Surgery	65	4.6%	5.3%	5.3%
Combination Abdominal CT Scan	443	8.8%	16.4%	10.5%
Combination Brain/Sinus CT Scan	350	1.7%	2.7%	2.7%
Combination Chest CT Scan	192	10.9%	5.6%	2.7%
Follow-up Mammogram/Ultrasound	370	4.9%	7.9%	8.8%
Lumbar Spine MRI for Low Back Pain[1]	-	-	39.6%	37.2%

Wilbarger General Hospital

920 Hillcrest Dr
Vernon, TX 76384
Phone: 940-552-9351
Fax: 940-553-2981
URL: www.wghospital.com
Type: Acute Care Hospitals
Ownership: Govt - Hospital Dist/Auth
Emergency Services: Yes
Beds: 47

Key Personnel:
Radiology. . . . . Patsy Bachman
Operating Room. . . . . Tami Ferguson
Patient Relations . . . . Karen Garrett
Anesthesiology. . . . . David Hickok, CRNA
Chief of Medical Staff . . . . Randall Schaffner, MD
CEO/President. . . . . Jonathon Voelkel
Infection Control. . . . . Jackie Wilcoxson, RN

Measure	Cases	This Hosp.	State Avg.	U.S. Avg.
Blood Clot Prevention and Treatment				
Anticoagulation Overlap Therapy[1,2]	-	-	93%	93%
ICU Venous Thromboembolism Prophylaxis[1,2]	-	-	92%	92%
Incidence of Potentially Preventable VTE[1,2]	-	-	9%	10%
UFH with Dosages/Platelet Monitoring[2,7]	-	-	96%	97%
Venous Thromboembolism Prophylaxis[2]	137	49%	82%	85%
Warfarin Therapy Discharge Instructions[1,2]	-	-	84%	75%
Chest Pain/Possible Heart Attack Care				
Aspirin Given Within 24 Hours of Arrival	25	88%	94%	96%
Fibrinolytic Meds Within 30 Min. of Arrival[1]	-	-	47%	58%
Average Time to ECG (minutes)	26	14	8	7
Average Time to Transfer (minutes)[7]	-	-	62	60
Children's Asthma Care				
Received Home Management Plan of Care	-	-	93%	88%
Received Reliever Medication	-	-	100%	100%
Received Systemic Corticosteroids	-	-	100%	100%
Emergency Department				
Admittance Decision Time (minutes)[2]	210	72	99	98
Head CT Results Within 45 Min. of Arrival	14	21%	54%	57%
Patients Who Left ER Before Being Seen	7,344	2%	3%	2%
Time from ER Arrival to Admit. (minutes)[2]	246	217	270	274
Time from ER Arrival to Discharge (minutes)	494	116	127	134
Time in ER Before Being Evaluated (minutes)	504	26	26	26
Time to Pain Meds for Fractures (minutes)	26	68	57	57
Heart Attack Care				
Aspirin Given at Discharge[1,2]	-	-	99%	99%
Fibrinolytic Meds Within 30 Min. of Arrival[2,3]	-	-	49%	54%
PCI Within 90 Minutes of Arrival[2,3]	-	-	95%	96%
Statin Prescribed at Discharge[1,2]	-	-	98%	98%
Heart Failure Care				
ACE Inhibitor or ARB for LVSD[1,2]	-	-	97%	97%
Discharge Instructions Given[2]	12	42%	95%	94%
Evaluation of LVS Function[2]	16	81%	99%	99%
Medicare Spending				
Medicare Spending per Patient (ratio)	-	0.96	1.03	0.98
Pneumonia Care				
Appropriate Initial Antibiotic Given[2]	30	70%	95%	95%
Blood Culture Timing[2]	25	68%	98%	98%
Pregnancy and Delivery Care				
Newborn Deliveries Scheduled Early[7]	-	-	7%	6%
Preventive Care				
Immunization for Influenza[2]	231	76%	90%	90%
Immunization for Pneumonia[2]	308	84%	92%	92%
Stroke Care				
Anticoagulation Therapy for Atrial Fibrillation[1,3]	-	-	96%	95%
Antithrombotic Therapy Timing[1,3]	-	-	98%	98%
Assessed for Rehabilitation[1,3]	-	-	98%	97%
Discharged on Antithrombotic Therapy[1,3]	-	-	99%	99%
Discharged on Statin Medication[1,3]	-	-	95%	94%
Thrombolytic Therapy Timing[1,3]	-	-	68%	66%
Venous Thromboembolism Prophylaxis[1,3]	-	-	94%	94%
Written Stroke Educational Materials Given[1,3]	-	-	92%	88%
Surgical Care Improvement Project				
Appropriate Beta Blocker Usage[2,7]	-	-	98%	98%
Appropriate VTP Within 24 Hours[1,2]	-	-	98%	98%
Controlled Postoperative Blood Glucose[2,7]	-	-	96%	97%
Perioperative Temperature Management[1,2]	-	-	100%	100%
Prophylactic Antibiotic Selection[2,7]	-	-	99%	99%
Prophylactic Antibiotic Selection (Outpatient)[5]	-	-	98%	98%
Prophylactic Antibiotic Stopped[2,7]	-	-	98%	98%
Prophylactic Antibiotic Timing[2,7]	-	-	99%	99%
Prophylactic Antibiotic Timing (Outpatient)[5]	-	-	98%	98%
Urinary Catheter Removal[1,2]	-	-	98%	97%
Survey of Patients' Hospital Experiences				
Area Around Room 'Always' Quiet at Night[6]	<100	80%	68%	61%
Doctors 'Always' Communicated Well[6]	<100	90%	83%	82%
Home Recovery Information Given[6]	<100	94%	85%	85%
Hospital Given 9 or 10 on 10 Point Scale[6]	<100	82%	73%	71%
Meds 'Always' Explained Before Given[6]	<100	65%	66%	64%
Nurses 'Always' Communicated Well[6]	<100	88%	80%	79%
Pain 'Always' Well Controlled[6]	<100	77%	72%	71%
Room and Bathroom 'Always' Clean[6]	<100	78%	75%	73%
Timely Help 'Always' Received[6]	<100	77%	69%	68%
Would Definitely Recommend Hospital[6]	<100	66%	73%	71%
Use of Medical Imaging				
Cardiac Imaging Stress Test before Surgery[7]	-	-	5.3%	5.3%
Combination Abdominal CT Scan	179	26.8%	16.4%	10.5%
Combination Brain/Sinus CT Scan[1]	-	-	2.7%	2.7%
Combination Chest CT Scan	96	31.3%	5.6%	2.7%
Follow-up Mammogram/Ultrasound	194	8.8%	7.9%	8.8%
Lumbar Spine MRI for Low Back Pain	57	52.6%	39.6%	37.2%

Citizens Medical Center

2701 Hospital Drive
Victoria, TX 77901
Phone: 361-572-5113
Fax: 361-573-0611
E-mail: info@citizensmedicalcenter.org
URL: www.citizensmedicalcenter.org
Type: Acute Care Hospitals
Ownership: Voluntary non-profit - Other
Emergency Services: Yes
Beds: 344

Key Personnel:
Chief of Medical Staff . . . . Kurtis Krueger
Operating Room. . . . . Darlene Lewis, RN
Pediatric In-Patient Care . . . . Luciano Sarabosing
Radiology. . . . . Steven Schnicker, MD

Measure	Cases	This Hosp.	State Avg.	U.S. Avg.
Blood Clot Prevention and Treatment				
Anticoagulation Overlap Therapy[2]	37	95%	93%	93%
ICU Venous Thromboembolism Prophylaxis[2]	72	88%	92%	92%
Incidence of Potentially Preventable VTE[1,2]	-	-	9%	10%
UFH with Dosages/Platelet Monitoring[1,2]	-	-	96%	97%
Venous Thromboembolism Prophylaxis[2]	345	71%	82%	85%
Warfarin Therapy Discharge Instructions[2]	23	100%	84%	75%
Chest Pain/Possible Heart Attack Care				
Aspirin Given Within 24 Hours of Arrival[1,3]	-	-	94%	96%
Fibrinolytic Meds Within 30 Min. of Arrival[3,7]	-	-	47%	58%
Average Time to ECG (minutes)[1,3]	-	-	8	7
Average Time to Transfer (minutes)[3,7]	-	-	62	60
Children's Asthma Care				
Received Home Management Plan of Care	-	-	93%	88%
Received Reliever Medication	-	-	100%	100%
Received Systemic Corticosteroids	-	-	100%	100%
Emergency Department				
Admittance Decision Time (minutes)[2]	377	61	99	98
Head CT Results Within 45 Min. of Arrival	20	50%	54%	57%
Patients Who Left ER Before Being Seen	33,747	1%	3%	2%
Time from ER Arrival to Admit. (minutes)[2]	581	193	270	274
Time from ER Arrival to Discharge (minutes)	353	120	127	134
Time in ER Before Being Evaluated (minutes)	370	24	26	26
Time to Pain Meds for Fractures (minutes)	103	66	57	57
Heart Attack Care				
Aspirin Given at Discharge	205	100%	99%	99%
Fibrinolytic Meds Within 30 Min. of Arrival[7]	-	-	49%	54%
PCI Within 90 Minutes of Arrival	23	96%	95%	96%
Statin Prescribed at Discharge	208	97%	98%	98%
Heart Failure Care				
ACE Inhibitor or ARB for LVSD	96	91%	97%	97%
Discharge Instructions Given	229	100%	95%	94%
Evaluation of LVS Function	274	97%	99%	99%
Medicare Spending				
Medicare Spending per Patient (ratio)	-	0.99	1.03	0.98
Pneumonia Care				
Appropriate Initial Antibiotic Given	96	97%	95%	95%
Blood Culture Timing	174	98%	98%	98%
Pregnancy and Delivery Care				
Newborn Deliveries Scheduled Early[2]	45	7%	7%	6%
Preventive Care				
Immunization for Influenza[2]	553	94%	90%	90%
Immunization for Pneumonia[2]	715	92%	92%	92%
Stroke Care				
Anticoagulation Therapy for Atrial Fibrillation	13	62%	96%	95%
Antithrombotic Therapy Timing	60	95%	98%	98%
Assessed for Rehabilitation	67	96%	98%	97%
Discharged on Antithrombotic Therapy	65	91%	99%	99%
Discharged on Statin Medication	54	83%	95%	94%
Thrombolytic Therapy Timing[1]	-	-	68%	66%
Venous Thromboembolism Prophylaxis	65	92%	94%	94%
Written Stroke Educational Materials Given	38	95%	92%	88%
Surgical Care Improvement Project				
Appropriate Beta Blocker Usage	179	94%	98%	98%
Appropriate VTP Within 24 Hours	476	91%	98%	98%
Controlled Postoperative Blood Glucose	31	97%	96%	97%
Perioperative Temperature Management	548	100%	100%	100%
Prophylactic Antibiotic Selection	358	99%	99%	99%
Prophylactic Antibiotic Selection (Outpatient)	274	99%	98%	98%
Prophylactic Antibiotic Stopped	354	97%	98%	98%

NOTE: Hospital profiles are in alphabetical order by state, then city, then hospital within the city; Rankings exclude hospitals with less than 25 cases except for patient surveys which excludes hospitals with less than 100 cases; (a) 100-299 cases; (1) The number of cases/patients is too few to report; (2) Data submitted were based on a sample of cases/patients; (3) Results are based on a shorter time period than required; (4) Data suppressed by CMS for one or more quarters; (5) Results are not available for this reporting period; (6) Fewer than 100 patients completed the HCAHPS survey; (7) No cases met the criteria for this measure; (8) The lower limit of the confidence interval cannot be calculated if the number of observed infections equals zero; (9) No data are available from the state/territory for this reporting period; (10) The scores shown reflect fewer than 50 completed surveys; (11) There were discrepancies in the data collection process; (12) This measure does not apply to this hospital for this reporting period; (13) Results cannot be calculated for this reporting period; (14) The results for this state are combined with nearby states to protect confidentiality; Please refer to the User's Guide for a full explanation of data.

Measure	Cases	This Hosp.	State Avg.	U.S. Avg.
Prophylactic Antibiotic Timing	368	98%	99%	99%
Prophylactic Antibiotic Timing (Outpatient)	276	99%	98%	98%
Urinary Catheter Removal	167	88%	98%	97%
Survey of Patients' Hospital Experiences				
Area Around Room 'Always' Quiet at Night	300+	72%	68%	61%
Doctors 'Always' Communicated Well	300+	84%	83%	82%
Home Recovery Information Given	300+	80%	85%	85%
Hospital Given 9 or 10 on 10 Point Scale	300+	70%	73%	71%
Meds 'Always' Explained Before Given	300+	62%	66%	64%
Nurses 'Always' Communicated Well	300+	78%	80%	79%
Pain 'Always' Well Controlled	300+	70%	72%	71%
Room and Bathroom 'Always' Clean	300+	74%	75%	73%
Timely Help 'Always' Received	300+	65%	69%	68%
Would Definitely Recommend Hospital	300+	76%	73%	71%
Use of Medical Imaging				
Cardiac Imaging Stress Test before Surgery	437	4.8%	5.3%	5.3%
Combination Abdominal CT Scan	1,020	3.8%	16.4%	10.5%
Combination Brain/Sinus CT Scan	729	1.5%	2.7%	2.7%
Combination Chest CT Scan	824	0.5%	5.6%	2.7%
Follow-up Mammogram/Ultrasound	1,121	6.8%	7.9%	8.8%
Lumbar Spine MRI for Low Back Pain	86	33.7%	39.6%	37.2%

Detar Hospital Navarro

506 E San Antonio St
Victoria, TX 77902
URL: www.detar.com
Type: Acute Care Hospitals
Ownership: Proprietary
Phone: 361-575-7441
Fax: 361-788-6114
Emergency Services: Yes
Beds: 292

Key Personnel:
CEO/President. . . . . William R Blanchard
Operating Room. . . . . Gerri Lewis, RN
Quality Assurance . . . . Corinne Maib

Measure	Cases	This Hosp.	State Avg.	U.S. Avg.
Blood Clot Prevention and Treatment				
Anticoagulation Overlap Therapy[2]	25	100%	93%	93%
ICU Venous Thromboembolism Prophylaxis[2]	113	100%	92%	92%
Incidence of Potentially Preventable VTE[1,2]	-	-	9%	10%
UFH with Dosages/Platelet Monitoring[1,2]	-	-	96%	97%
Venous Thromboembolism Prophylaxis[2]	371	99%	82%	85%
Warfarin Therapy Discharge Instructions[2]	11	100%	84%	75%
Chest Pain/Possible Heart Attack Care				
Aspirin Given Within 24 Hours of Arrival[1,3]	-	-	94%	96%
Fibrinolytic Meds Within 30 Min. of Arrival[3,7]	-	-	47%	58%
Average Time to ECG (minutes)[1,3]	-	-	8	7
Average Time to Transfer (minutes)[3,7]	-	-	62	60
Children's Asthma Care				
Received Home Management Plan of Care	-	-	93%	88%
Received Reliever Medication	-	-	100%	100%
Received Systemic Corticosteroids	-	-	100%	100%
Emergency Department				
Admittance Decision Time (minutes)[2]	489	60	99	98
Head CT Results Within 45 Min. of Arrival[1]	-	-	54%	57%
Patients Who Left ER Before Being Seen	23,684	3%	3%	2%
Time from ER Arrival to Admit. (minutes)[2]	489	197	270	274
Time from ER Arrival to Discharge (minutes)	397	103	127	134
Time in ER Before Being Evaluated (minutes)	430	15	26	26
Time to Pain Meds for Fractures (minutes)	108	47	57	57
Heart Attack Care				
Aspirin Given at Discharge	144	100%	99%	99%
Fibrinolytic Meds Within 30 Min. of Arrival[7]	-	-	49%	54%
PCI Within 90 Minutes of Arrival	25	100%	95%	96%
Statin Prescribed at Discharge	132	99%	98%	98%
Heart Failure Care				
ACE Inhibitor or ARB for LVSD	75	100%	97%	97%
Discharge Instructions Given	183	100%	95%	94%
Evaluation of LVS Function	228	100%	99%	99%
Medicare Spending				
Medicare Spending per Patient (ratio)	-	1.01	1.03	0.98
Pneumonia Care				
Appropriate Initial Antibiotic Given	80	100%	95%	95%
Blood Culture Timing	144	100%	98%	98%
Pregnancy and Delivery Care				
Newborn Deliveries Scheduled Early[2]	56	4%	7%	6%
Preventive Care				
Immunization for Influenza[2]	552	100%	90%	90%
Immunization for Pneumonia[2]	628	100%	92%	92%
Stroke Care				
Anticoagulation Therapy for Atrial Fibrillation	16	100%	96%	95%
Antithrombotic Therapy Timing	79	100%	98%	98%
Assessed for Rehabilitation	78	100%	98%	97%
Discharged on Antithrombotic Therapy	75	100%	99%	99%
Discharged on Statin Medication	59	100%	95%	94%
Thrombolytic Therapy Timing[1]	-	-	68%	66%
Venous Thromboembolism Prophylaxis	84	100%	94%	94%
Written Stroke Educational Materials Given	41	100%	92%	88%
Surgical Care Improvement Project				
Appropriate Beta Blocker Usage	141	99%	98%	98%
Appropriate VTP Within 24 Hours	380	99%	98%	98%
Controlled Postoperative Blood Glucose	27	100%	96%	97%
Perioperative Temperature Management	417	100%	100%	100%
Prophylactic Antibiotic Selection	271	100%	99%	99%
Prophylactic Antibiotic Selection (Outpatient)	421	100%	98%	98%
Prophylactic Antibiotic Stopped	262	99%	98%	98%
Prophylactic Antibiotic Timing	271	99%	99%	99%
Prophylactic Antibiotic Timing (Outpatient)	421	100%	98%	98%
Urinary Catheter Removal	128	99%	98%	97%
Survey of Patients' Hospital Experiences				
Area Around Room 'Always' Quiet at Night	300+	68%	68%	61%
Doctors 'Always' Communicated Well	300+	82%	83%	82%
Home Recovery Information Given	300+	86%	85%	85%
Hospital Given 9 or 10 on 10 Point Scale	300+	75%	73%	71%
Meds 'Always' Explained Before Given	300+	65%	66%	64%
Nurses 'Always' Communicated Well	300+	78%	80%	79%
Pain 'Always' Well Controlled	300+	73%	72%	71%
Room and Bathroom 'Always' Clean	300+	70%	75%	73%
Timely Help 'Always' Received	300+	66%	69%	68%
Would Definitely Recommend Hospital	300+	74%	73%	71%
Use of Medical Imaging				
Cardiac Imaging Stress Test before Surgery	93	2.2%	5.3%	5.3%
Combination Abdominal CT Scan	508	15.9%	16.4%	10.5%
Combination Brain/Sinus CT Scan	527	4.2%	2.7%	2.7%
Combination Chest CT Scan	239	24.3%	5.6%	2.7%
Follow-up Mammogram/Ultrasound	672	8.0%	7.9%	8.8%
Lumbar Spine MRI for Low Back Pain	71	40.8%	39.6%	37.2%

Hillcrest Baptist Medical Center

100 Hillcrest Medical Blvd
Waco, TX 76712
E-mail: info@hillcrest.net
URL: www.hillcrest.net
Type: Acute Care Hospitals
Ownership: Voluntary non-profit - Private
Phone: 254-202-2000
Fax: 254-202-9420
Emergency Services: Yes
Beds: 393

Key Personnel:
Cardiac Laboratory. . . . . Sherwin Attai, MD
Anesthesiology. . . . . Rebecca Backstrom
Emergency Room . . . . Paul E. Chaney
Quality Assurance . . . . Shirley Davis
Chief of Medical Staff. . . . . James E Gray, MD
Radiology. . . . . Susan McJunkin
CEO/President. . . . . Glenn A Robinson
Operating Room. . . . . Becky Stewart, RN

Measure	Cases	This Hosp.	State Avg.	U.S. Avg.
Blood Clot Prevention and Treatment				
Anticoagulation Overlap Therapy[2]	34	94%	93%	93%
ICU Venous Thromboembolism Prophylaxis[2]	112	88%	92%	92%
Incidence of Potentially Preventable VTE[2]	14	0%	9%	10%
UFH with Dosages/Platelet Monitoring[2]	14	100%	96%	97%
Venous Thromboembolism Prophylaxis[2]	285	93%	82%	85%
Warfarin Therapy Discharge Instructions[2]	20	70%	84%	75%
Chest Pain/Possible Heart Attack Care				
Aspirin Given Within 24 Hours of Arrival[3]	31	97%	94%	96%
Fibrinolytic Meds Within 30 Min. of Arrival[3,7]	-	-	47%	58%
Average Time to ECG (minutes)[3]	30	14	8	7
Average Time to Transfer (minutes)[3,7]	-	-	62	60
Children's Asthma Care				
Received Home Management Plan of Care	-	-	93%	88%
Received Reliever Medication	-	-	100%	100%
Received Systemic Corticosteroids	-	-	100%	100%
Emergency Department				
Admittance Decision Time (minutes)[2]	445	106	99	98
Head CT Results Within 45 Min. of Arrival	13	54%	54%	57%
Patients Who Left ER Before Being Seen	56,609	4%	3%	2%
Time from ER Arrival to Admit. (minutes)[2]	456	324	270	274
Time from ER Arrival to Discharge (minutes)	360	158	127	134
Time in ER Before Being Evaluated (minutes)	355	42	26	26
Time to Pain Meds for Fractures (minutes)	317	66	57	57
Heart Attack Care				
Aspirin Given at Discharge	200	94%	99%	99%
Fibrinolytic Meds Within 30 Min. of Arrival[1]	-	-	49%	54%
PCI Within 90 Minutes of Arrival	14	86%	95%	96%
Statin Prescribed at Discharge	187	94%	98%	98%
Heart Failure Care				
ACE Inhibitor or ARB for LVSD	66	98%	97%	97%
Discharge Instructions Given	143	82%	95%	94%
Evaluation of LVS Function	190	99%	99%	99%
Medicare Spending				
Medicare Spending per Patient (ratio)	-	1.01	1.03	0.98
Pneumonia Care				
Appropriate Initial Antibiotic Given[2]	80	98%	95%	95%
Blood Culture Timing[2]	162	95%	98%	98%
Pregnancy and Delivery Care				
Newborn Deliveries Scheduled Early[2]	85	9%	7%	6%
Preventive Care				
Immunization for Influenza[2]	476	92%	90%	90%
Immunization for Pneumonia[2]	447	93%	92%	92%
Stroke Care				
Anticoagulation Therapy for Atrial Fibrillation[1]	-	-	96%	95%
Antithrombotic Therapy Timing	110	100%	98%	98%
Assessed for Rehabilitation	128	100%	98%	97%
Discharged on Antithrombotic Therapy	112	100%	99%	99%
Discharged on Statin Medication	93	96%	95%	94%
Thrombolytic Therapy Timing[1]	-	-	68%	66%
Venous Thromboembolism Prophylaxis	131	97%	94%	94%
Written Stroke Educational Materials Given	69	96%	92%	88%
Surgical Care Improvement Project				
Appropriate Beta Blocker Usage[2]	199	97%	98%	98%
Appropriate VTP Within 24 Hours[2]	514	99%	98%	98%
Controlled Postoperative Blood Glucose[2]	68	96%	96%	97%
Perioperative Temperature Management[2]	572	100%	100%	100%
Prophylactic Antibiotic Selection[2]	497	99%	99%	99%
Prophylactic Antibiotic Selection (Outpatient)	141	94%	98%	98%
Prophylactic Antibiotic Stopped[2]	482	99%	98%	98%
Prophylactic Antibiotic Timing[2]	498	99%	99%	99%
Prophylactic Antibiotic Timing (Outpatient)	146	96%	98%	98%
Urinary Catheter Removal[2]	356	98%	98%	97%
Survey of Patients' Hospital Experiences				
Area Around Room 'Always' Quiet at Night	300+	66%	68%	61%
Doctors 'Always' Communicated Well	300+	81%	83%	82%
Home Recovery Information Given	300+	82%	85%	85%
Hospital Given 9 or 10 on 10 Point Scale	300+	71%	73%	71%
Meds 'Always' Explained Before Given	300+	61%	66%	64%
Nurses 'Always' Communicated Well	300+	76%	80%	79%
Pain 'Always' Well Controlled	300+	70%	72%	71%
Room and Bathroom 'Always' Clean	300+	70%	75%	73%
Timely Help 'Always' Received	300+	60%	69%	68%
Would Definitely Recommend Hospital	300+	74%	73%	71%
Use of Medical Imaging				
Cardiac Imaging Stress Test before Surgery	264	3.8%	5.3%	5.3%
Combination Abdominal CT Scan	1,017	5.8%	16.4%	10.5%
Combination Brain/Sinus CT Scan	833	2.9%	2.7%	2.7%
Combination Chest CT Scan	641	1.1%	5.6%	2.7%
Follow-up Mammogram/Ultrasound	1,880	8.5%	7.9%	8.8%
Lumbar Spine MRI for Low Back Pain	91	47.3%	39.6%	37.2%

NOTE: Hospital profiles are in alphabetical order by state, then city, then hospital within the city; Rankings exclude hospitals with less than 25 cases except for patient surveys which excludes hospitals with less than 100 cases; (a) 100-299 cases; (1) The number of cases/patients is too few to report; (2) Data submitted were based on a sample of cases/patients; (3) Results are based on a shorter time period than required; (4) Data suppressed by CMS for one or more quarters; (5) Results are not available for this reporting period; (6) Fewer than 100 patients completed the HCAHPS survey; (7) No cases met the criteria for this measure; (8) The lower limit of the confidence interval cannot be calculated if the number of observed infections equals zero; (9) No data are available from the state/territory for this reporting period; (10) The scores shown reflect fewer than 50 completed surveys; (11) There were discrepancies in the data collection process; (12) This measure does not apply to this hospital for this reporting period; (13) Results cannot be calculated for this reporting period; (14) The results for this state are combined with nearby states to protect confidentiality; Please refer to the User's Guide for a full explanation of data.

Providence Health Center

6901 Medical Parkway Phone: 254-751-4000
Waco, TX 76712 Fax: 254-751-4769
URL: www.providence.net
Type: Acute Care Hospitals Emergency Services: Yes
Ownership: Voluntary non-profit - Private Beds: 214

Key Personnel:
Chief of Medical Staff.......... Brian K Becker, MD
Coronary Care.............. Jan Brown, RN
CEO/President............... Kent A Keahey
Pediatric In-Patient Care .... William Nesmith, MD
Radiology.................. Peggy Pustejovsky
Quality Assurance .... Melissa Raines, RN
Infection Control............ Melissa Rains, RN
Operating Room.............. Judy Taylor, RN

Measure	Cases	This Hosp.	State Avg.	U.S. Avg.
Blood Clot Prevention and Treatment				
Anticoagulation Overlap Therapy[2]	123	94%	93%	93%
ICU Venous Thromboembolism Prophylaxis[2]	100	84%	92%	92%
Incidence of Potentially Preventable VTE[2]	15	7%	9%	10%
UFH with Dosages/Platelet Monitoring[2]	12	92%	96%	97%
Venous Thromboembolism Prophylaxis[2]	308	74%	82%	85%
Warfarin Therapy Discharge Instructions[2]	94	76%	84%	75%
Chest Pain/Possible Heart Attack Care				
Aspirin Given Within 24 Hours of Arrival[5]	-	-	94%	96%
Fibrinolytic Meds Within 30 Min. of Arrival[5]	-	-	47%	58%
Average Time to ECG (minutes)[5]	-	-	8	7
Average Time to Transfer (minutes)[5]	-	-	62	60
Children's Asthma Care				
Received Home Management Plan of Care	-	-	93%	88%
Received Reliever Medication	-	-	100%	100%
Received Systemic Corticosteroids	-	-	100%	100%
Emergency Department				
Admittance Decision Time (minutes)[2]	671	132	99	98
Head CT Results Within 45 Min. of Arrival[1,3]	-	-	54%	57%
Patients Who Left ER Before Being Seen	86,396	3%	3%	2%
Time from ER Arrival to Admit. (minutes)[2]	683	318	270	274
Time from ER Arrival to Discharge (minutes)	362	212	127	134
Time in ER Before Being Evaluated (minutes)	353	28	26	26
Time to Pain Meds for Fractures (minutes)	31	74	57	57
Heart Attack Care				
Aspirin Given at Discharge	313	99%	99%	99%
Fibrinolytic Meds Within 30 Min. of Arrival[7]	-	-	49%	54%
PCI Within 90 Minutes of Arrival	60	93%	95%	96%
Statin Prescribed at Discharge	303	99%	98%	98%
Heart Failure Care				
ACE Inhibitor or ARB for LVSD	151	91%	97%	97%
Discharge Instructions Given	320	88%	95%	94%
Evaluation of LVS Function	411	99%	99%	99%
Medicare Spending				
Medicare Spending per Patient (ratio)	-	0.97	1.03	0.98
Pneumonia Care				
Appropriate Initial Antibiotic Given	267	96%	95%	95%
Blood Culture Timing	542	98%	98%	98%
Pregnancy and Delivery Care				
Newborn Deliveries Scheduled Early[2]	19	16%	7%	6%
Preventive Care				
Immunization for Influenza[2]	537	85%	90%	90%
Immunization for Pneumonia[2]	721	89%	92%	92%
Stroke Care				
Anticoagulation Therapy for Atrial Fibrillation	26	69%	96%	95%
Antithrombotic Therapy Timing	213	100%	98%	98%
Assessed for Rehabilitation	247	97%	98%	97%
Discharged on Antithrombotic Therapy	213	100%	99%	99%
Discharged on Statin Medication	168	94%	95%	94%
Thrombolytic Therapy Timing	14	14%	68%	66%
Venous Thromboembolism Prophylaxis	254	92%	94%	94%
Written Stroke Educational Materials Given	130	88%	92%	88%
Surgical Care Improvement Project				
Appropriate Beta Blocker Usage[2]	185	88%	98%	98%
Appropriate VTP Within 24 Hours[2]	362	96%	98%	98%
Controlled Postoperative Blood Glucose[2]	110	98%	96%	97%
Perioperative Temperature Management[2]	428	99%	100%	100%
Prophylactic Antibiotic Selection[2]	379	97%	99%	99%
Prophylactic Antibiotic Selection (Outpatient)	261	97%	98%	98%
Prophylactic Antibiotic Stopped[2]	366	97%	98%	98%
Prophylactic Antibiotic Timing[2]	381	99%	99%	99%
Prophylactic Antibiotic Timing (Outpatient)	264	94%	98%	98%
Urinary Catheter Removal[2]	221	91%	98%	97%
Survey of Patients' Hospital Experiences				
Area Around Room 'Always' Quiet at Night	300+	67%	68%	61%
Doctors 'Always' Communicated Well	300+	81%	83%	82%
Home Recovery Information Given	300+	89%	85%	85%
Hospital Given 9 or 10 on 10 Point Scale	300+	77%	73%	71%
Meds 'Always' Explained Before Given	300+	65%	66%	64%
Nurses 'Always' Communicated Well	300+	79%	80%	79%
Pain 'Always' Well Controlled	300+	73%	72%	71%
Room and Bathroom 'Always' Clean	300+	71%	75%	73%
Timely Help 'Always' Received	300+	64%	69%	68%
Would Definitely Recommend Hospital	300+	81%	73%	71%
Use of Medical Imaging				
Cardiac Imaging Stress Test before Surgery	179	3.4%	5.3%	5.3%
Combination Abdominal CT Scan	1,206	7.9%	16.4%	10.5%
Combination Brain/Sinus CT Scan	1,159	0.6%	2.7%	2.7%
Combination Chest CT Scan	736	0.3%	5.6%	2.7%
Follow-up Mammogram/Ultrasound	2,407	2.6%	7.9%	8.8%
Lumbar Spine MRI for Low Back Pain	133	45.9%	39.6%	37.2%

Baylor Medical Center at Waxahachie

1405 W Jefferson St Phone: 972-923-7000
Waxahachie, TX 75165 Fax: 972-937-5948
URL: www.bhcs.com/locations/waxahachie
Type: Acute Care Hospitals Emergency Services: Yes
Ownership: Voluntary non-profit - Other Beds: 77

Key Personnel:
Intensive Care Unit............ Brenda Dodge
Chief of Medical Staff.......... Janet Fain
CEO/President............... Jay Fox
Quality Assurance .... Phil Hall
Radiology.................. Patricia De Leon
Emergency Room .... William O'Malley, MD
Infection Control.............. Iris Wilson

Measure	Cases	This Hosp.	State Avg.	U.S. Avg.
Blood Clot Prevention and Treatment				
Anticoagulation Overlap Therapy[2]	34	94%	93%	93%
ICU Venous Thromboembolism Prophylaxis[2]	73	95%	92%	92%
Incidence of Potentially Preventable VTE[2,7]	-	-	9%	10%
UFH with Dosages/Platelet Monitoring[2]	15	100%	96%	97%
Venous Thromboembolism Prophylaxis[2]	262	94%	82%	85%
Warfarin Therapy Discharge Instructions[2]	30	100%	84%	75%
Chest Pain/Possible Heart Attack Care				
Aspirin Given Within 24 Hours of Arrival	63	98%	94%	96%
Fibrinolytic Meds Within 30 Min. of Arrival	12	42%	47%	58%
Average Time to ECG (minutes)	64	7	8	7
Average Time to Transfer (minutes)[1]	-	-	62	60
Children's Asthma Care				
Received Home Management Plan of Care	-	-	93%	88%
Received Reliever Medication	-	-	100%	100%
Received Systemic Corticosteroids	-	-	100%	100%
Emergency Department				
Admittance Decision Time (minutes)[2]	310	82	99	98
Head CT Results Within 45 Min. of Arrival	23	26%	54%	57%
Patients Who Left ER Before Being Seen	43,318	2%	3%	2%
Time from ER Arrival to Admit. (minutes)[2]	336	256	270	274
Time from ER Arrival to Discharge (minutes)	392	111	127	134
Time in ER Before Being Evaluated (minutes)	103	27	26	26
Time to Pain Meds for Fractures (minutes)	169	41	57	57
Heart Attack Care				
Aspirin Given at Discharge	11	100%	99%	99%
Fibrinolytic Meds Within 30 Min. of Arrival[7]	-	-	49%	54%
PCI Within 90 Minutes of Arrival[7]	-	-	95%	96%
Statin Prescribed at Discharge[1]	-	-	98%	98%
Heart Failure Care				
ACE Inhibitor or ARB for LVSD	66	98%	97%	97%
Discharge Instructions Given	144	99%	95%	94%
Evaluation of LVS Function	166	99%	99%	99%
Medicare Spending				
Medicare Spending per Patient (ratio)	-	1.04	1.03	0.98
Pneumonia Care				
Appropriate Initial Antibiotic Given	116	97%	95%	95%
Blood Culture Timing	151	100%	98%	98%
Pregnancy and Delivery Care				
Newborn Deliveries Scheduled Early[7]	-	-	7%	6%
Preventive Care				
Immunization for Influenza[2]	331	95%	90%	90%
Immunization for Pneumonia[2]	472	93%	92%	92%
Stroke Care				
Anticoagulation Therapy for Atrial Fibrillation[1]	-	-	96%	95%
Antithrombotic Therapy Timing	33	97%	98%	98%
Assessed for Rehabilitation	29	100%	98%	97%
Discharged on Antithrombotic Therapy	29	100%	99%	99%
Discharged on Statin Medication	24	96%	95%	94%
Thrombolytic Therapy Timing[1]	-	-	68%	66%
Venous Thromboembolism Prophylaxis	34	91%	94%	94%
Written Stroke Educational Materials Given	15	93%	92%	88%
Surgical Care Improvement Project				
Appropriate Beta Blocker Usage[2]	86	95%	98%	98%
Appropriate VTP Within 24 Hours[2]	282	99%	98%	98%
Controlled Postoperative Blood Glucose[2,7]	-	-	96%	97%
Perioperative Temperature Management[2]	294	100%	100%	100%
Prophylactic Antibiotic Selection[2]	201	100%	99%	99%
Prophylactic Antibiotic Selection (Outpatient)	14	100%	98%	98%
Prophylactic Antibiotic Stopped[2]	190	99%	98%	98%
Prophylactic Antibiotic Timing[2]	201	100%	99%	99%
Prophylactic Antibiotic Timing (Outpatient)	14	100%	98%	98%
Urinary Catheter Removal[2]	227	100%	98%	97%
Survey of Patients' Hospital Experiences				
Area Around Room 'Always' Quiet at Night	300+	71%	68%	61%
Doctors 'Always' Communicated Well	300+	76%	83%	82%
Home Recovery Information Given	300+	84%	85%	85%
Hospital Given 9 or 10 on 10 Point Scale	300+	73%	73%	71%
Meds 'Always' Explained Before Given	300+	68%	66%	64%
Nurses 'Always' Communicated Well	300+	82%	80%	79%
Pain 'Always' Well Controlled	300+	74%	72%	71%
Room and Bathroom 'Always' Clean	300+	76%	75%	73%
Timely Help 'Always' Received	300+	68%	69%	68%
Would Definitely Recommend Hospital	300+	73%	73%	71%
Use of Medical Imaging				
Cardiac Imaging Stress Test before Surgery	137	3.6%	5.3%	5.3%
Combination Abdominal CT Scan	660	3.8%	16.4%	10.5%
Combination Brain/Sinus CT Scan	699	1.6%	2.7%	2.7%
Combination Chest CT Scan	381	2.4%	5.6%	2.7%
Follow-up Mammogram/Ultrasound	1,226	8.6%	7.9%	8.8%
Lumbar Spine MRI for Low Back Pain	100	37.0%	39.6%	37.2%

Weatherford Regional Medical Center

713 E Anderson St Phone: 817-599-1190
Weatherford, TX 76086 Fax: 817-598-0326
URL: www.campbellhealth.com
Type: Acute Care Hospitals Emergency Services: Yes
Ownership: Proprietary Beds: 99

Key Personnel:
Emergency Room .... Donna Ivey, MD
Operating Room.............. Gary Jones, RN
CEO/President............... Scott M Landrum
Intensive Care Unit............ Geri Lindsey
Chief of Medical Staff.......... James B Newton, MD
Infection Control.............. Debbie Weaber
Quality Assurance .... Debbie Weaber

Measure	Cases	This Hosp.	State Avg.	U.S. Avg.
Blood Clot Prevention and Treatment				
Anticoagulation Overlap Therapy[2]	35	100%	93%	93%
ICU Venous Thromboembolism Prophylaxis[2]	100	100%	92%	92%
Incidence of Potentially Preventable VTE[1,2]	-	-	9%	10%
UFH with Dosages/Platelet Monitoring[1,2]	-	-	96%	97%
Venous Thromboembolism Prophylaxis[2]	359	98%	82%	85%
Warfarin Therapy Discharge Instructions[2]	27	100%	84%	75%
Chest Pain/Possible Heart Attack Care				
Aspirin Given Within 24 Hours of Arrival	48	100%	94%	96%
Fibrinolytic Meds Within 30 Min. of Arrival[7]	-	-	47%	58%
Average Time to ECG (minutes)	49	6	8	7
Average Time to Transfer (minutes)	18	44	62	60

NOTE: Hospital profiles are in alphabetical order by state, then city, then hospital within the city; Rankings exclude hospitals with less than 25 cases except for patient surveys which excludes hospitals with less than 100 cases; (a) 100-299 cases; (1) The number of cases/patients is too few to report; (2) Data submitted were based on a sample of cases/patients; (3) Results are based on a shorter time period than required; (4) Data suppressed by CMS for one or more quarters; (5) Results are not available for this reporting period; (6) Fewer than 100 patients completed the HCAHPS survey; (7) No cases met the criteria for this measure; (8) The lower limit of the confidence interval cannot be calculated if the number of observed infections equals zero; (9) No data are available from the state/territory for this reporting period; (10) The scores shown reflect fewer than 50 completed surveys; (11) There were discrepancies in the data collection process; (12) This measure does not apply to this hospital for this reporting period; (13) Results cannot be calculated for this reporting period; (14) The results for this state are combined with nearby states to protect confidentiality; Please refer to the User's Guide for a full explanation of data.

Measure	Cases	This Hosp.	State Avg.	U.S. Avg.
Children's Asthma Care				
Received Home Management Plan of Care	-	-	93%	88%
Received Reliever Medication	-	-	100%	100%
Received Systemic Corticosteroids	-	-	100%	100%
Emergency Department				
Admittance Decision Time (minutes)[2]	640	71	99	98
Head CT Results Within 45 Min. of Arrival[1]	-	-	54%	57%
Patients Who Left ER Before Being Seen	26,270	2%	3%	2%
Time from ER Arrival to Admit. (minutes)[2]	640	240	270	274
Time from ER Arrival to Discharge (minutes)	374	138	127	134
Time in ER Before Being Evaluated (minutes)	422	26	26	26
Time to Pain Meds for Fractures (minutes)	106	84	57	57
Heart Attack Care				
Aspirin Given at Discharge	27	100%	99%	99%
Fibrinolytic Meds Within 30 Min. of Arrival[7]	-	-	49%	54%
PCI Within 90 Minutes of Arrival[7]	-	-	95%	96%
Statin Prescribed at Discharge	24	100%	98%	98%
Heart Failure Care				
ACE Inhibitor or ARB for LVSD	30	100%	97%	97%
Discharge Instructions Given	88	100%	95%	94%
Evaluation of LVS Function	115	100%	99%	99%
Medicare Spending				
Medicare Spending per Patient (ratio)	-	1.06	1.03	0.98
Pneumonia Care				
Appropriate Initial Antibiotic Given	105	100%	95%	95%
Blood Culture Timing	213	100%	98%	98%
Pregnancy and Delivery Care				
Newborn Deliveries Scheduled Early[2]	38	5%	7%	6%
Preventive Care				
Immunization for Influenza[2]	527	100%	90%	90%
Immunization for Pneumonia[2]	647	100%	92%	92%
Stroke Care				
Anticoagulation Therapy for Atrial Fibrillation[1]	-	-	96%	95%
Antithrombotic Therapy Timing	17	100%	98%	98%
Assessed for Rehabilitation	18	100%	98%	97%
Discharged on Antithrombotic Therapy	16	100%	99%	99%
Discharged on Statin Medication	14	100%	95%	94%
Thrombolytic Therapy Timing[7]	-	-	68%	66%
Venous Thromboembolism Prophylaxis	18	100%	94%	94%
Written Stroke Educational Materials Given[1]	-	-	92%	88%
Surgical Care Improvement Project				
Appropriate Beta Blocker Usage	110	100%	98%	98%
Appropriate VTP Within 24 Hours	344	100%	98%	98%
Controlled Postoperative Blood Glucose[7]	-	-	96%	97%
Perioperative Temperature Management	367	100%	100%	100%
Prophylactic Antibiotic Selection	254	99%	99%	99%
Prophylactic Antibiotic Selection (Outpatient)	51	100%	98%	98%
Prophylactic Antibiotic Stopped	248	96%	98%	98%
Prophylactic Antibiotic Timing	254	100%	99%	99%
Prophylactic Antibiotic Timing (Outpatient)	51	100%	98%	98%
Urinary Catheter Removal	301	99%	98%	97%
Survey of Patients' Hospital Experiences				
Area Around Room 'Always' Quiet at Night	300+	71%	68%	61%
Doctors 'Always' Communicated Well	300+	79%	83%	82%
Home Recovery Information Given	300+	86%	85%	85%
Hospital Given 9 or 10 on 10 Point Scale	300+	70%	73%	71%
Meds 'Always' Explained Before Given	300+	62%	66%	64%
Nurses 'Always' Communicated Well	300+	78%	80%	79%
Pain 'Always' Well Controlled	300+	73%	72%	71%
Room and Bathroom 'Always' Clean	300+	65%	75%	73%
Timely Help 'Always' Received	300+	66%	69%	68%
Would Definitely Recommend Hospital	300+	67%	73%	71%
Use of Medical Imaging				
Cardiac Imaging Stress Test before Surgery[1]	-	-	5.3%	5.3%
Combination Abdominal CT Scan	419	9.5%	16.4%	10.5%
Combination Brain/Sinus CT Scan	526	4.4%	2.7%	2.7%
Combination Chest CT Scan	360	5.3%	5.6%	2.7%
Follow-up Mammogram/Ultrasound[7]	-	-	7.9%	8.8%
Lumbar Spine MRI for Low Back Pain	41	48.8%	39.6%	37.2%

Clear Lake Regional Medical Center

500 Medical Center Blvd
Webster, TX 77598
Phone: 281-332-2511
Fax: 281-338-3352
URL: www.clearlakermc.com
Type: Acute Care Hospitals
Emergency Services: Yes
Ownership: Proprietary
Beds: 595

Key Personnel:

Pediatric In-Patient Care . . . . Dena Drago
Quality Assurance . . . . Carol Dzierski
Chief of Medical Staff . . . . Molly Hammond, MD
CEO/President . . . . Stephen K. Jones, Jr.
Infection Control . . . . Donna Outlaw
Radiology . . . . Bill Vicinanza

Measure	Cases	This Hosp.	State Avg.	U.S. Avg.
Blood Clot Prevention and Treatment				
Anticoagulation Overlap Therapy[2]	153	99%	93%	93%
ICU Venous Thromboembolism Prophylaxis[2]	146	98%	92%	92%
Incidence of Potentially Preventable VTE[2]	20	5%	9%	10%
UFH with Dosages/Platelet Monitoring[2]	38	100%	96%	97%
Venous Thromboembolism Prophylaxis[2]	364	93%	82%	85%
Warfarin Therapy Discharge Instructions[2]	102	99%	84%	75%
Chest Pain/Possible Heart Attack Care				
Aspirin Given Within 24 Hours of Arrival	16	100%	94%	96%
Fibrinolytic Meds Within 30 Min. of Arrival[3,7]	-	-	47%	58%
Average Time to ECG (minutes)	16	4	8	7
Average Time to Transfer (minutes)[1,3]	-	-	62	60
Children's Asthma Care				
Received Home Management Plan of Care	-	-	93%	88%
Received Reliever Medication	-	-	100%	100%
Received Systemic Corticosteroids	-	-	100%	100%
Emergency Department				
Admittance Decision Time (minutes)[2]	850	107	99	98
Head CT Results Within 45 Min. of Arrival[1]	-	-	54%	57%
Patients Who Left ER Before Being Seen	76,822	1%	3%	2%
Time from ER Arrival to Admit. (minutes)[2]	859	282	270	274
Time from ER Arrival to Discharge (minutes)	499	135	127	134
Time in ER Before Being Evaluated (minutes)	545	16	26	26
Time to Pain Meds for Fractures (minutes)	459	47	57	57
Heart Attack Care				
Aspirin Given at Discharge[2]	431	100%	99%	99%
Fibrinolytic Meds Within 30 Min. of Arrival[2,7]	-	-	49%	54%
PCI Within 90 Minutes of Arrival[2]	75	96%	95%	96%
Statin Prescribed at Discharge[2]	405	100%	98%	98%
Heart Failure Care				
ACE Inhibitor or ARB for LVSD[2]	92	100%	97%	97%
Discharge Instructions Given[2]	245	98%	95%	94%
Evaluation of LVS Function[2]	310	99%	99%	99%
Medicare Spending				
Medicare Spending per Patient (ratio)	-	1.09	1.03	0.98
Pneumonia Care				
Appropriate Initial Antibiotic Given[2]	87	100%	95%	95%
Blood Culture Timing[2]	169	99%	98%	98%
Pregnancy and Delivery Care				
Newborn Deliveries Scheduled Early[2]	82	0%	7%	6%
Preventive Care				
Immunization for Influenza[2]	629	98%	90%	90%
Immunization for Pneumonia[2]	732	99%	92%	92%
Stroke Care				
Anticoagulation Therapy for Atrial Fibrillation[2]	13	100%	96%	95%
Antithrombotic Therapy Timing[2]	102	100%	98%	98%
Assessed for Rehabilitation[2]	112	97%	98%	97%
Discharged on Antithrombotic Therapy[2]	103	100%	99%	99%
Discharged on Statin Medication[2]	81	98%	95%	94%
Thrombolytic Therapy Timing[1,2]	-	-	68%	66%
Venous Thromboembolism Prophylaxis[2]	107	94%	94%	94%
Written Stroke Educational Materials Given[2]	72	94%	92%	88%
Surgical Care Improvement Project				
Appropriate Beta Blocker Usage[2]	235	97%	98%	98%
Appropriate VTP Within 24 Hours[2]	471	99%	98%	98%
Controlled Postoperative Blood Glucose[2]	118	95%	96%	97%
Perioperative Temperature Management[2]	602	100%	100%	100%
Prophylactic Antibiotic Selection[2]	429	100%	99%	99%
Prophylactic Antibiotic Selection (Outpatient)	572	100%	98%	98%
Prophylactic Antibiotic Stopped[2]	414	97%	98%	98%
Prophylactic Antibiotic Timing[2]	429	100%	99%	99%
Prophylactic Antibiotic Timing (Outpatient)	572	100%	98%	98%
Urinary Catheter Removal[2]	377	99%	98%	97%
Survey of Patients' Hospital Experiences				
Area Around Room 'Always' Quiet at Night	300+	64%	68%	61%
Doctors 'Always' Communicated Well	300+	79%	83%	82%
Home Recovery Information Given	300+	84%	85%	85%
Hospital Given 9 or 10 on 10 Point Scale	300+	66%	73%	71%
Meds 'Always' Explained Before Given	300+	62%	66%	64%
Nurses 'Always' Communicated Well	300+	76%	80%	79%
Pain 'Always' Well Controlled	300+	70%	72%	71%
Room and Bathroom 'Always' Clean	300+	70%	75%	73%
Timely Help 'Always' Received	300+	60%	69%	68%
Would Definitely Recommend Hospital	300+	67%	73%	71%
Use of Medical Imaging				
Cardiac Imaging Stress Test before Surgery	436	5.5%	5.3%	5.3%
Combination Abdominal CT Scan	1,395	5.2%	16.4%	10.5%
Combination Brain/Sinus CT Scan	1,587	3.5%	2.7%	2.7%
Combination Chest CT Scan	628	0.2%	5.6%	2.7%
Follow-up Mammogram/Ultrasound	2,599	10.1%	7.9%	8.8%
Lumbar Spine MRI for Low Back Pain	125	36.8%	39.6%	37.2%

Houston Physicians' Hospital

333 N Texas Avenue
Webster, TX 77598
Phone: 281-335-1700
URL: www.houstonphysicianshospital.com
Type: Acute Care Hospitals
Emergency Services: Yes
Ownership: Physician

Key Personnel:

CEO/President . . . . Tri Tran RN MHA/MBA

Measure	Cases	This Hosp.	State Avg.	U.S. Avg.
Blood Clot Prevention and Treatment				
Anticoagulation Overlap Therapy[7]	-	-	93%	93%
ICU Venous Thromboembolism Prophylaxis[7]	-	-	92%	92%
Incidence of Potentially Preventable VTE[1]	-	-	9%	10%
UFH with Dosages/Platelet Monitoring[7]	-	-	96%	97%
Venous Thromboembolism Prophylaxis	94	100%	82%	85%
Warfarin Therapy Discharge Instructions[7]	-	-	84%	75%
Chest Pain/Possible Heart Attack Care				
Aspirin Given Within 24 Hours of Arrival[5]	-	-	94%	96%
Fibrinolytic Meds Within 30 Min. of Arrival[5]	-	-	47%	58%
Average Time to ECG (minutes)[5]	-	-	8	7
Average Time to Transfer (minutes)[5]	-	-	62	60
Children's Asthma Care				
Received Home Management Plan of Care	-	-	93%	88%
Received Reliever Medication	-	-	100%	100%
Received Systemic Corticosteroids	-	-	100%	100%
Emergency Department				
Admittance Decision Time (minutes)	11	70	99	98
Head CT Results Within 45 Min. of Arrival[5]	-	-	54%	57%
Patients Who Left ER Before Being Seen	298	1%	3%	2%
Time from ER Arrival to Admit. (minutes)	11	180	270	274
Time from ER Arrival to Discharge (minutes)	219	93	127	134
Time in ER Before Being Evaluated (minutes)	231	18	26	26
Time to Pain Meds for Fractures (minutes)[5]	-	-	57	57
Heart Attack Care				
Aspirin Given at Discharge[5]	-	-	99%	99%
Fibrinolytic Meds Within 30 Min. of Arrival[5]	-	-	49%	54%
PCI Within 90 Minutes of Arrival[5]	-	-	95%	96%
Statin Prescribed at Discharge[5]	-	-	98%	98%
Heart Failure Care				
ACE Inhibitor or ARB for LVSD[5]	-	-	97%	97%
Discharge Instructions Given[5]	-	-	95%	94%
Evaluation of LVS Function[5]	-	-	99%	99%
Medicare Spending				
Medicare Spending per Patient (ratio)	-	1.07	1.03	0.98
Pneumonia Care				
Appropriate Initial Antibiotic Given[5]	-	-	95%	95%
Blood Culture Timing[5]	-	-	98%	98%
Pregnancy and Delivery Care				
Newborn Deliveries Scheduled Early[7]	-	-	7%	6%
Preventive Care				
Immunization for Influenza	264	92%	90%	90%

NOTE: Hospital profiles are in alphabetical order by state, then city, then hospital within the city; Rankings exclude hospitals with less than 25 cases except for patient surveys which excludes hospitals with less than 100 cases; (a) 100-299 cases; (1) The number of cases/patients is too few to report; (2) Data submitted were based on a sample of cases/patients; (3) Results are based on a shorter time period than required; (4) Data suppressed by CMS for one or more quarters; (5) Results are not available for this reporting period; (6) Fewer than 100 patients completed the HCAHPS survey; (7) No cases met the criteria for this measure; (8) The lower limit of the confidence interval cannot be calculated if the number of observed infections equals zero; (9) No data are available from the state/territory for this reporting period; (10) The scores shown reflect fewer than 50 completed surveys; (11) There were discrepancies in the data collection process; (12) This measure does not apply to this hospital for this reporting period; (13) Results cannot be calculated for this reporting period; (14) The results for this state are combined with nearby states to protect confidentiality; Please refer to the User's Guide for a full explanation of data.

Immunization for Pneumonia	262	89%	92%	92%
Stroke Care				
Anticoagulation Therapy for Atrial Fibrillation[5]	-	-	96%	95%
Antithrombotic Therapy Timing[5]	-	-	98%	98%
Assessed for Rehabilitation[5]	-	-	98%	97%
Discharged on Antithrombotic Therapy[5]	-	-	99%	99%
Discharged on Statin Medication[5]	-	-	95%	94%
Thrombolytic Therapy Timing[5]	-	-	68%	66%
Venous Thromboembolism Prophylaxis[5]	-	-	94%	94%
Written Stroke Educational Materials Given[5]	-	-	92%	88%
Surgical Care Improvement Project				
Appropriate Beta Blocker Usage	62	98%	98%	98%
Appropriate VTP Within 24 Hours	217	100%	98%	98%
Controlled Postoperative Blood Glucose[7]	-	-	96%	97%
Perioperative Temperature Management	229	100%	100%	100%
Prophylactic Antibiotic Selection	214	99%	99%	99%
Prophylactic Antibiotic Selection (Outpatient)	266	99%	98%	98%
Prophylactic Antibiotic Stopped	211	94%	98%	98%
Prophylactic Antibiotic Timing	214	100%	99%	99%
Prophylactic Antibiotic Timing (Outpatient)	266	100%	98%	98%
Urinary Catheter Removal	176	98%	98%	97%
Survey of Patients' Hospital Experiences				
Area Around Room 'Always' Quiet at Night	(a)	82%	68%	61%
Doctors 'Always' Communicated Well	(a)	87%	83%	82%
Home Recovery Information Given	(a)	88%	85%	85%
Hospital Given 9 or 10 on 10 Point Scale	(a)	85%	73%	71%
Meds 'Always' Explained Before Given	(a)	72%	66%	64%
Nurses 'Always' Communicated Well	(a)	86%	80%	79%
Pain 'Always' Well Controlled	(a)	78%	72%	71%
Room and Bathroom 'Always' Clean	(a)	78%	75%	73%
Timely Help 'Always' Received	(a)	78%	69%	68%
Would Definitely Recommend Hospital	(a)	85%	73%	71%
Use of Medical Imaging				
Cardiac Imaging Stress Test before Surgery[7]	-	-	5.3%	5.3%
Combination Abdominal CT Scan	126	59.5%	16.4%	10.5%
Combination Brain/Sinus CT Scan[1]	-	-	2.7%	2.7%
Combination Chest CT Scan[1]	-	-	5.6%	2.7%
Follow-up Mammogram/Ultrasound[7]	-	-	7.9%	8.8%
Lumbar Spine MRI for Low Back Pain	182	42.9%	39.6%	37.2%

Collingsworth General Hospital

1013 15th St
Wellington, TX 79095
Type: Critical Access Hospitals
Ownership: Proprietary
Phone: 806-447-2521
Fax: 806-447-2421
Emergency Services: Yes
Beds: 25

Key Personnel:
Chief of Medical Staff.......... Kaleem Ahmad, MD
Emergency Room .... Giovanni Baula, MD
Quality Assurance .... S Beth Calson
Infection Control.............. Laurine Gragson, RN
Administrator .... Candy Powell

Measure	Cases	This Hosp.	State Avg.	U.S. Avg.
Blood Clot Prevention and Treatment				
Anticoagulation Overlap Therapy	-	-	93%	93%
ICU Venous Thromboembolism Prophylaxis	-	-	92%	92%
Incidence of Potentially Preventable VTE	-	-	9%	10%
UFH with Dosages/Platelet Monitoring	-	-	96%	97%
Venous Thromboembolism Prophylaxis	-	-	82%	85%
Warfarin Therapy Discharge Instructions	-	-	84%	75%
Chest Pain/Possible Heart Attack Care				
Aspirin Given Within 24 Hours of Arrival[1]	-	-	94%	96%
Fibrinolytic Meds Within 30 Min. of Arrival[3,7]	-	-	47%	58%
Average Time to ECG (minutes)[1]	-	-	8	7
Average Time to Transfer (minutes)[3,7]	-	-	62	60
Children's Asthma Care				
Received Home Management Plan of Care	-	-	93%	88%
Received Reliever Medication	-	-	100%	100%
Received Systemic Corticosteroids	-	-	100%	100%
Emergency Department				
Admittance Decision Time (minutes)	-	-	99	98
Head CT Results Within 45 Min. of Arrival[5]	-	-	54%	57%
Patients Who Left ER Before Being Seen[5]	-	-	3%	2%
Time from ER Arrival to Admit. (minutes)	-	-	270	274
Time from ER Arrival to Discharge (minutes)[5]	-	-	127	134
Time in ER Before Being Evaluated (minutes)[5]	-	-	26	26
Time to Pain Meds for Fractures (minutes)[5]	-	-	57	57
Heart Attack Care				
Aspirin Given at Discharge	-	-	99%	99%
Fibrinolytic Meds Within 30 Min. of Arrival	-	-	49%	54%
PCI Within 90 Minutes of Arrival	-	-	95%	96%
Statin Prescribed at Discharge	-	-	98%	98%
Heart Failure Care				
ACE Inhibitor or ARB for LVSD	-	-	97%	97%
Discharge Instructions Given	-	-	95%	94%
Evaluation of LVS Function	-	-	99%	99%
Medicare Spending				
Medicare Spending per Patient (ratio)	-	-	1.03	0.98
Pneumonia Care				
Appropriate Initial Antibiotic Given	-	-	95%	95%
Blood Culture Timing	-	-	98%	98%
Pregnancy and Delivery Care				
Newborn Deliveries Scheduled Early	-	-	7%	6%
Preventive Care				
Immunization for Influenza	-	-	90%	90%
Immunization for Pneumonia	-	-	92%	92%
Stroke Care				
Anticoagulation Therapy for Atrial Fibrillation	-	-	96%	95%
Antithrombotic Therapy Timing	-	-	98%	98%
Assessed for Rehabilitation	-	-	98%	97%
Discharged on Antithrombotic Therapy	-	-	99%	99%
Discharged on Statin Medication	-	-	95%	94%
Thrombolytic Therapy Timing	-	-	68%	66%
Venous Thromboembolism Prophylaxis	-	-	94%	94%
Written Stroke Educational Materials Given	-	-	92%	88%
Surgical Care Improvement Project				
Appropriate Beta Blocker Usage	-	-	98%	98%
Appropriate VTP Within 24 Hours	-	-	98%	98%
Controlled Postoperative Blood Glucose	-	-	96%	97%
Perioperative Temperature Management	-	-	100%	100%
Prophylactic Antibiotic Selection	-	-	99%	99%
Prophylactic Antibiotic Selection (Outpatient)[5]	-	-	98%	98%
Prophylactic Antibiotic Stopped	-	-	98%	98%
Prophylactic Antibiotic Timing	-	-	99%	99%
Prophylactic Antibiotic Timing (Outpatient)[5]	-	-	98%	98%
Urinary Catheter Removal	-	-	98%	97%
Survey of Patients' Hospital Experiences				
Area Around Room 'Always' Quiet at Night	-	-	68%	61%
Doctors 'Always' Communicated Well	-	-	83%	82%
Home Recovery Information Given	-	-	85%	85%
Hospital Given 9 or 10 on 10 Point Scale	-	-	73%	71%
Meds 'Always' Explained Before Given	-	-	66%	64%
Nurses 'Always' Communicated Well	-	-	80%	79%
Pain 'Always' Well Controlled	-	-	72%	71%
Room and Bathroom 'Always' Clean	-	-	75%	73%
Timely Help 'Always' Received	-	-	69%	68%
Would Definitely Recommend Hospital	-	-	73%	71%
Use of Medical Imaging				
Cardiac Imaging Stress Test before Surgery[7]	-	-	5.3%	5.3%
Combination Abdominal CT Scan[1]	-	-	16.4%	10.5%
Combination Brain/Sinus CT Scan[1]	-	-	2.7%	2.7%
Combination Chest CT Scan[1]	-	-	5.6%	2.7%
Follow-up Mammogram/Ultrasound[7]	-	-	7.9%	8.8%
Lumbar Spine MRI for Low Back Pain[1]	-	-	39.6%	37.2%

Knapp Medical Center

1401 East Eight Street
Weslaco, TX 78596
E-mail: jvasquez@knappmed.org
URL: www.knappmed.org
Type: Acute Care Hospitals
Ownership: Voluntary non-profit - Private
Phone: 956-968-8567
Fax: 956-969-5132
Emergency Services: Yes
Beds: 200

Key Personnel:
Quality Assurance .... Rubin Darza
Emergency Room .... Ramiro Falas
CEO/President............... Robert W Vanderveer

Measure	Cases	This Hosp.	State Avg.	U.S. Avg.
Blood Clot Prevention and Treatment				
Anticoagulation Overlap Therapy[2]	17	88%	93%	93%
ICU Venous Thromboembolism Prophylaxis[2]	92	98%	92%	92%
Incidence of Potentially Preventable VTE[2]	12	0%	9%	10%
UFH with Dosages/Platelet Monitoring[1,2]	-	-	96%	97%
Venous Thromboembolism Prophylaxis[2]	301	90%	82%	85%
Warfarin Therapy Discharge Instructions[1,2]	-	-	84%	75%
Chest Pain/Possible Heart Attack Care				
Aspirin Given Within 24 Hours of Arrival	29	93%	94%	96%
Fibrinolytic Meds Within 30 Min. of Arrival[1]	-	-	47%	58%
Average Time to ECG (minutes)	29	15	8	7
Average Time to Transfer (minutes)	11	101	62	60
Children's Asthma Care				
Received Home Management Plan of Care	-	-	93%	88%
Received Reliever Medication	-	-	100%	100%
Received Systemic Corticosteroids	-	-	100%	100%
Emergency Department				
Admittance Decision Time (minutes)[2]	347	80	99	98
Head CT Results Within 45 Min. of Arrival	29	41%	54%	57%
Patients Who Left ER Before Being Seen	39,196	5%	3%	2%
Time from ER Arrival to Admit. (minutes)[2]	518	271	270	274
Time from ER Arrival to Discharge (minutes)	348	181	127	134
Time in ER Before Being Evaluated (minutes)	364	45	26	26
Time to Pain Meds for Fractures (minutes)	149	55	57	57
Heart Attack Care				
Aspirin Given at Discharge	29	100%	99%	99%
Fibrinolytic Meds Within 30 Min. of Arrival[1]	-	-	49%	54%
PCI Within 90 Minutes of Arrival[7]	-	-	95%	96%
Statin Prescribed at Discharge	28	89%	98%	98%
Heart Failure Care				
ACE Inhibitor or ARB for LVSD	47	98%	97%	97%
Discharge Instructions Given	201	98%	95%	94%
Evaluation of LVS Function	234	93%	99%	99%
Medicare Spending				
Medicare Spending per Patient (ratio)	-	0.98	1.03	0.98
Pneumonia Care				
Appropriate Initial Antibiotic Given	112	96%	95%	95%
Blood Culture Timing	190	95%	98%	98%
Pregnancy and Delivery Care				
Newborn Deliveries Scheduled Early[2]	47	2%	7%	6%
Preventive Care				
Immunization for Influenza[2]	411	88%	90%	90%
Immunization for Pneumonia[2]	491	92%	92%	92%
Stroke Care				
Anticoagulation Therapy for Atrial Fibrillation[1,2]	-	-	96%	95%
Antithrombotic Therapy Timing[2]	71	100%	98%	98%
Assessed for Rehabilitation[2]	81	100%	98%	97%
Discharged on Antithrombotic Therapy[2]	71	99%	99%	99%
Discharged on Statin Medication[2]	53	96%	95%	94%
Thrombolytic Therapy Timing[2]	13	62%	68%	66%
Venous Thromboembolism Prophylaxis[2]	91	99%	94%	94%
Written Stroke Educational Materials Given[2]	41	100%	92%	88%
Surgical Care Improvement Project				
Appropriate Beta Blocker Usage	88	98%	98%	98%
Appropriate VTP Within 24 Hours	369	97%	98%	98%
Controlled Postoperative Blood Glucose[7]	-	-	96%	97%
Perioperative Temperature Management	418	100%	100%	100%
Prophylactic Antibiotic Selection	294	97%	99%	99%
Prophylactic Antibiotic Selection (Outpatient)	26	96%	98%	98%
Prophylactic Antibiotic Stopped	289	99%	98%	98%
Prophylactic Antibiotic Timing	297	100%	99%	99%
Prophylactic Antibiotic Timing (Outpatient)	26	85%	98%	98%
Urinary Catheter Removal	229	100%	98%	97%
Survey of Patients' Hospital Experiences				
Area Around Room 'Always' Quiet at Night	300+	59%	68%	61%
Doctors 'Always' Communicated Well	300+	82%	83%	82%
Home Recovery Information Given	300+	84%	85%	85%
Hospital Given 9 or 10 on 10 Point Scale	300+	66%	73%	71%
Meds 'Always' Explained Before Given	300+	64%	66%	64%
Nurses 'Always' Communicated Well	300+	75%	80%	79%
Pain 'Always' Well Controlled	300+	72%	72%	71%
Room and Bathroom 'Always' Clean	300+	78%	75%	73%

NOTE: Hospital profiles are in alphabetical order by state, then city, then hospital within the city; Rankings exclude hospitals with less than 25 cases except for patient surveys which excludes hospitals with less than 100 cases; (a) 100-299 cases; (1) The number of cases/patients is too few to report; (2) Data submitted were based on a sample of cases/patients; (3) Results are based on a shorter time period than required; (4) Data suppressed by CMS for one or more quarters; (5) Results are not available for this reporting period; (6) Fewer than 100 patients completed the HCAHPS survey; (7) No cases met the criteria for this measure; (8) The lower limit of the confidence interval cannot be calculated if the number of observed infections equals zero; (9) No data are available from the state/territory for this reporting period; (10) The scores shown reflect fewer than 50 completed surveys; (11) There were discrepancies in the data collection process; (12) This measure does not apply to this hospital for this reporting period; (13) Results cannot be calculated for this reporting period; (14) The results for this state are combined with nearby states to protect confidentiality; Please refer to the User's Guide for a full explanation of data.

Measure	Cases	This Hosp.	State Avg.	U.S. Avg.
Timely Help 'Always' Received	300+	62%	69%	68%
Would Definitely Recommend Hospital	300+	63%	73%	71%
Use of Medical Imaging				
Cardiac Imaging Stress Test before Surgery	192	4.7%	5.3%	5.3%
Combination Abdominal CT Scan	630	52.1%	16.4%	10.5%
Combination Brain/Sinus CT Scan	985	2.8%	2.7%	2.7%
Combination Chest CT Scan	373	40.2%	5.6%	2.7%
Follow-up Mammogram/Ultrasound	1,313	2.4%	7.9%	8.8%
Lumbar Spine MRI for Low Back Pain	104	26.0%	39.6%	37.2%

Gulf Coast Medical Center

10141 Us 59 North
Wharton, TX 77488
URL: www.gulfcoastmedical.com
Phone: 979-532-2500
Fax: 979-282-6844
Type: Acute Care Hospitals
Ownership: Proprietary
Emergency Services: Yes
Beds: 161

Key Personnel:
Radiology. . . . . Dean Chauvin
Chief of Medical Staff . . . . Priscilla Metcalf
CEO/President. . . . . Randy Slack

Measure	Cases	This Hosp.	State Avg.	U.S. Avg.
Blood Clot Prevention and Treatment				
Anticoagulation Overlap Therapy[1,2]	-	-	93%	93%
ICU Venous Thromboembolism Prophylaxis[2]	49	86%	92%	92%
Incidence of Potentially Preventable VTE[2,7]	-	-	9%	10%
UFH with Dosages/Platelet Monitoring[1,2]	-	-	96%	97%
Venous Thromboembolism Prophylaxis[2]	55	73%	82%	85%
Warfarin Therapy Discharge Instructions[1,2]	-	-	84%	75%
Chest Pain/Possible Heart Attack Care				
Aspirin Given Within 24 Hours of Arrival	27	100%	94%	96%
Fibrinolytic Meds Within 30 Min. of Arrival[1]	-	-	47%	58%
Average Time to ECG (minutes)	28	6	8	7
Average Time to Transfer (minutes)[1]	-	-	62	60
Children's Asthma Care				
Received Home Management Plan of Care	-	-	93%	88%
Received Reliever Medication	-	-	100%	100%
Received Systemic Corticosteroids	-	-	100%	100%
Emergency Department				
Admittance Decision Time (minutes)[2]	293	58	99	98
Head CT Results Within 45 Min. of Arrival	19	11%	54%	57%
Patients Who Left ER Before Being Seen	11,481	2%	3%	2%
Time from ER Arrival to Admit. (minutes)[2]	315	236	270	274
Time from ER Arrival to Discharge (minutes)	426	116	127	134
Time in ER Before Being Evaluated (minutes)	485	24	26	26
Time to Pain Meds for Fractures (minutes)	58	55	57	57
Heart Attack Care				
Aspirin Given at Discharge[3,7]	-	-	99%	99%
Fibrinolytic Meds Within 30 Min. of Arrival[3,7]	-	-	49%	54%
PCI Within 90 Minutes of Arrival[3,7]	-	-	95%	96%
Statin Prescribed at Discharge[3,7]	-	-	98%	98%
Heart Failure Care				
ACE Inhibitor or ARB for LVSD[1]	-	-	97%	97%
Discharge Instructions Given	16	100%	95%	94%
Evaluation of LVS Function	24	100%	99%	99%
Medicare Spending				
Medicare Spending per Patient (ratio)	-	1.06	1.03	0.98
Pneumonia Care				
Appropriate Initial Antibiotic Given[2]	16	81%	95%	95%
Blood Culture Timing[2]	34	94%	98%	98%
Pregnancy and Delivery Care				
Newborn Deliveries Scheduled Early[1]	-	-	7%	6%
Preventive Care				
Immunization for Influenza[2]	245	93%	90%	90%
Immunization for Pneumonia[2]	342	91%	92%	92%
Stroke Care				
Anticoagulation Therapy for Atrial Fibrillation[1,3]	-	-	96%	95%
Antithrombotic Therapy Timing[1,3]	-	-	98%	98%
Assessed for Rehabilitation[1,3]	-	-	98%	97%
Discharged on Antithrombotic Therapy[1,3]	-	-	99%	99%
Discharged on Statin Medication[1,3]	-	-	95%	94%
Thrombolytic Therapy Timing[1,3]	-	-	68%	66%
Venous Thromboembolism Prophylaxis[1,3]	-	-	94%	94%
Written Stroke Educational Materials Given[1,3]	-	-	92%	88%
Surgical Care Improvement Project				
Appropriate Beta Blocker Usage[1]	-	-	98%	98%
Appropriate VTP Within 24 Hours	22	68%	98%	98%
Controlled Postoperative Blood Glucose[7]	-	-	96%	97%
Perioperative Temperature Management	29	100%	100%	100%
Prophylactic Antibiotic Selection[1]	-	-	99%	99%
Prophylactic Antibiotic Selection (Outpatient)[1,3]	-	-	98%	98%
Prophylactic Antibiotic Stopped[1]	-	-	98%	98%
Prophylactic Antibiotic Timing[1]	-	-	99%	99%
Prophylactic Antibiotic Timing (Outpatient)[1,3]	-	-	98%	98%
Urinary Catheter Removal	11	100%	98%	97%
Survey of Patients' Hospital Experiences				
Area Around Room 'Always' Quiet at Night[6]	<100	73%	68%	61%
Doctors 'Always' Communicated Well[6]	<100	85%	83%	82%
Home Recovery Information Given[6]	<100	82%	85%	85%
Hospital Given 9 or 10 on 10 Point Scale[6]	<100	56%	73%	71%
Meds 'Always' Explained Before Given[6]	<100	61%	66%	64%
Nurses 'Always' Communicated Well[6]	<100	73%	80%	79%
Pain 'Always' Well Controlled[6]	<100	84%	72%	71%
Room and Bathroom 'Always' Clean[6]	<100	70%	75%	73%
Timely Help 'Always' Received[6]	<100	70%	69%	68%
Would Definitely Recommend Hospital[6]	<100	60%	73%	71%
Use of Medical Imaging				
Cardiac Imaging Stress Test before Surgery[1]	-	-	5.3%	5.3%
Combination Abdominal CT Scan	105	13.3%	16.4%	10.5%
Combination Brain/Sinus CT Scan[1]	-	-	2.7%	2.7%
Combination Chest CT Scan	71	2.8%	5.6%	2.7%
Follow-up Mammogram/Ultrasound[7]	-	-	7.9%	8.8%
Lumbar Spine MRI for Low Back Pain[7]	-	-	39.6%	37.2%

Parkview Hospital

901 S. Sweetwater
Wheeler, TX 79096
Phone: 806-826-5581
Fax: 806-826-3201
E-mail: annfagan-cook@centramedia.net
URL: www.parkviewhosp.org
Type: Critical Access Hospitals
Emergency Services: Yes
Ownership: Govt - Hospital Dist/Auth

Key Personnel:
CEO/President. . . . . Ann Fagan-Cook

Measure	Cases	This Hosp.	State Avg.	U.S. Avg.
Blood Clot Prevention and Treatment				
Anticoagulation Overlap Therapy[5]	-	-	93%	93%
ICU Venous Thromboembolism Prophylaxis[5]	-	-	92%	92%
Incidence of Potentially Preventable VTE[5]	-	-	9%	10%
UFH with Dosages/Platelet Monitoring[5]	-	-	96%	97%
Venous Thromboembolism Prophylaxis[5]	-	-	82%	85%
Warfarin Therapy Discharge Instructions[5]	-	-	84%	75%
Chest Pain/Possible Heart Attack Care				
Aspirin Given Within 24 Hours of Arrival	-	-	94%	96%
Fibrinolytic Meds Within 30 Min. of Arrival	-	-	47%	58%
Average Time to ECG (minutes)	-	-	8	7
Average Time to Transfer (minutes)	-	-	62	60
Children's Asthma Care				
Received Home Management Plan of Care	-	-	93%	88%
Received Reliever Medication	-	-	100%	100%
Received Systemic Corticosteroids	-	-	100%	100%
Emergency Department				
Admittance Decision Time (minutes)[5]	-	-	99	98
Head CT Results Within 45 Min. of Arrival	-	-	54%	57%
Patients Who Left ER Before Being Seen	-	-	3%	2%
Time from ER Arrival to Admit. (minutes)[5]	-	-	270	274
Time from ER Arrival to Discharge (minutes)	-	-	127	134
Time in ER Before Being Evaluated (minutes)	-	-	26	26
Time to Pain Meds for Fractures (minutes)	-	-	57	57
Heart Attack Care				
Aspirin Given at Discharge[5]	-	-	99%	99%
Fibrinolytic Meds Within 30 Min. of Arrival[5]	-	-	49%	54%
PCI Within 90 Minutes of Arrival[5]	-	-	95%	96%
Statin Prescribed at Discharge[5]	-	-	98%	98%
Heart Failure Care				
ACE Inhibitor or ARB for LVSD[5]	-	-	97%	97%
Discharge Instructions Given[5]	-	-	95%	94%
Evaluation of LVS Function[5]	-	-	99%	99%
Medicare Spending				
Medicare Spending per Patient (ratio)	-	-	1.03	0.98
Pneumonia Care				
Appropriate Initial Antibiotic Given[1,2]	-	-	95%	95%
Blood Culture Timing[1,2]	-	-	98%	98%
Pregnancy and Delivery Care				
Newborn Deliveries Scheduled Early[5]	-	-	7%	6%
Preventive Care				
Immunization for Influenza[5]	-	-	90%	90%
Immunization for Pneumonia[5]	-	-	92%	92%
Stroke Care				
Anticoagulation Therapy for Atrial Fibrillation[5]	-	-	96%	95%
Antithrombotic Therapy Timing[5]	-	-	98%	98%
Assessed for Rehabilitation[5]	-	-	98%	97%
Discharged on Antithrombotic Therapy[5]	-	-	99%	99%
Discharged on Statin Medication[5]	-	-	95%	94%
Thrombolytic Therapy Timing[5]	-	-	68%	66%
Venous Thromboembolism Prophylaxis[5]	-	-	94%	94%
Written Stroke Educational Materials Given[5]	-	-	92%	88%
Surgical Care Improvement Project				
Appropriate Beta Blocker Usage[5]	-	-	98%	98%
Appropriate VTP Within 24 Hours[5]	-	-	98%	98%
Controlled Postoperative Blood Glucose[5]	-	-	96%	97%
Perioperative Temperature Management[5]	-	-	100%	100%
Prophylactic Antibiotic Selection[5]	-	-	99%	99%
Prophylactic Antibiotic Selection (Outpatient)	-	-	98%	98%
Prophylactic Antibiotic Stopped[5]	-	-	98%	98%
Prophylactic Antibiotic Timing[5]	-	-	99%	99%
Prophylactic Antibiotic Timing (Outpatient)	-	-	98%	98%
Urinary Catheter Removal[5]	-	-	98%	97%
Survey of Patients' Hospital Experiences				
Area Around Room 'Always' Quiet at Night[5]	-	-	68%	61%
Doctors 'Always' Communicated Well[5]	-	-	83%	82%
Home Recovery Information Given[5]	-	-	85%	85%
Hospital Given 9 or 10 on 10 Point Scale[5]	-	-	73%	71%
Meds 'Always' Explained Before Given[5]	-	-	66%	64%
Nurses 'Always' Communicated Well[5]	-	-	80%	79%
Pain 'Always' Well Controlled[5]	-	-	72%	71%
Room and Bathroom 'Always' Clean[5]	-	-	75%	73%
Timely Help 'Always' Received[5]	-	-	69%	68%
Would Definitely Recommend Hospital[5]	-	-	73%	71%
Use of Medical Imaging				
Cardiac Imaging Stress Test before Surgery	-	-	5.3%	5.3%
Combination Abdominal CT Scan	-	-	16.4%	10.5%
Combination Brain/Sinus CT Scan	-	-	2.7%	2.7%
Combination Chest CT Scan	-	-	5.6%	2.7%
Follow-up Mammogram/Ultrasound	-	-	7.9%	8.8%
Lumbar Spine MRI for Low Back Pain	-	-	39.6%	37.2%

Lake Whitney Medical Center

200 N San Jacinto Street
Whitney, TX 76692
Phone: 254-694-3165
Fax: 254-694-3299
Type: Acute Care Hospitals
Ownership: Proprietary
Emergency Services: Yes
Beds: 49

Key Personnel:
Emergency Room . . . . Jana Radle, RN
Chief of Medical Staff. . . . . Aman Ali Shah, MD
Radiology. . . . . Aman Ali Shah, MD

Measure	Cases	This Hosp.	State Avg.	U.S. Avg.
Blood Clot Prevention and Treatment				
Anticoagulation Overlap Therapy[2,7]	-	-	93%	93%
ICU Venous Thromboembolism Prophylaxis[2,7]	-	-	92%	92%
Incidence of Potentially Preventable VTE[2,7]	-	-	9%	10%
UFH with Dosages/Platelet Monitoring[2,7]	-	-	96%	97%
Venous Thromboembolism Prophylaxis[2]	98	12%	82%	85%
Warfarin Therapy Discharge Instructions[2,7]	-	-	84%	75%
Chest Pain/Possible Heart Attack Care				
Aspirin Given Within 24 Hours of Arrival[1]	-	-	94%	96%
Fibrinolytic Meds Within 30 Min. of Arrival[7]	-	-	47%	58%
Average Time to ECG (minutes)[1]	-	-	8	7
Average Time to Transfer (minutes)[1]	-	-	62	60
Children's Asthma Care				
Received Home Management Plan of Care	-	-	93%	88%

NOTE: Hospital profiles are in alphabetical order by state, then city, then hospital within the city; Rankings exclude hospitals with less than 25 cases except for patient surveys which excludes hospitals with less than 100 cases; (a) 100-299 cases; (1) The number of cases/patients is too few to report; (2) Data submitted were based on a sample of cases/patients; (3) Results are based on a shorter time period than required; (4) Data suppressed by CMS for one or more quarters; (5) Results are not available for this reporting period; (6) Fewer than 100 patients completed the HCAHPS survey; (7) No cases met the criteria for this measure; (8) The lower limit of the confidence interval cannot be calculated if the number of observed infections equals zero; (9) No data are available from the state/territory for this reporting period; (10) The scores shown reflect fewer than 50 completed surveys; (11) There were discrepancies in the data collection process; (12) This measure does not apply to this hospital for this reporting period; (13) Results cannot be calculated for this reporting period; (14) The results for this state are combined with nearby states to protect confidentiality; Please refer to the User's Guide for a full explanation of data.

Measure	Cases	This Hosp.	State Avg.	U.S. Avg.
Received Reliever Medication	-	-	100%	100%
Received Systemic Corticosteroids	-	-	100%	100%
Emergency Department				
Admittance Decision Time (minutes)[2]	289	45	99	98
Head CT Results Within 45 Min. of Arrival[1,3]	-	-	54%	57%
Patients Who Left ER Before Being Seen	3,621	3%	3%	2%
Time from ER Arrival to Admit. (minutes)[2]	325	159	270	274
Time from ER Arrival to Discharge (minutes)	214	84	127	134
Time in ER Before Being Evaluated (minutes)	191	30	26	26
Time to Pain Meds for Fractures (minutes)[1,3]	-	-	57	57
Heart Attack Care				
Aspirin Given at Discharge[1,2]	-	-	99%	99%
Fibrinolytic Meds Within 30 Min. of Arrival[2,7]	-	-	49%	54%
PCI Within 90 Minutes of Arrival[2,7]	-	-	95%	96%
Statin Prescribed at Discharge[1,2]	-	-	98%	98%
Heart Failure Care				
ACE Inhibitor or ARB for LVSD[1,3]	-	-	97%	97%
Discharge Instructions Given[3]	17	18%	95%	94%
Evaluation of LVS Function[3]	21	19%	99%	99%
Medicare Spending				
Medicare Spending per Patient (ratio)	-	0.80	1.03	0.98
Pneumonia Care				
Appropriate Initial Antibiotic Given[2]	36	75%	95%	95%
Blood Culture Timing[2]	15	93%	98%	98%
Pregnancy and Delivery Care				
Newborn Deliveries Scheduled Early[7]	-	-	7%	6%
Preventive Care				
Immunization for Influenza[2]	288	23%	90%	90%
Immunization for Pneumonia[2]	387	34%	92%	92%
Stroke Care				
Anticoagulation Therapy for Atrial Fibrillation[3,7]	-	-	96%	95%
Antithrombotic Therapy Timing[1,3]	-	-	98%	98%
Assessed for Rehabilitation[3,7]	-	-	98%	97%
Discharged on Antithrombotic Therapy[3,7]	-	-	99%	99%
Discharged on Statin Medication[3,7]	-	-	95%	94%
Thrombolytic Therapy Timing[1,3]	-	-	68%	66%
Venous Thromboembolism Prophylaxis[1,3]	-	-	94%	94%
Written Stroke Educational Materials Given[3,7]	-	-	92%	88%
Surgical Care Improvement Project				
Appropriate Beta Blocker Usage[5]	-	-	98%	98%
Appropriate VTP Within 24 Hours[5]	-	-	98%	98%
Controlled Postoperative Blood Glucose[5]	-	-	96%	97%
Perioperative Temperature Management[5]	-	-	100%	100%
Prophylactic Antibiotic Selection[5]	-	-	99%	99%
Prophylactic Antibiotic Selection (Outpatient)[5]	-	-	98%	98%
Prophylactic Antibiotic Stopped[5]	-	-	98%	98%
Prophylactic Antibiotic Timing[5]	-	-	99%	99%
Prophylactic Antibiotic Timing (Outpatient)[5]	-	-	98%	98%
Urinary Catheter Removal[5]	-	-	98%	97%
Survey of Patients' Hospital Experiences				
Area Around Room 'Always' Quiet at Night[11]	(a)	60%	68%	61%
Doctors 'Always' Communicated Well[11]	(a)	78%	83%	82%
Home Recovery Information Given[11]	(a)	72%	85%	85%
Hospital Given 9 or 10 on 10 Point Scale[11]	(a)	55%	73%	71%
Meds 'Always' Explained Before Given[11]	(a)	58%	66%	64%
Nurses 'Always' Communicated Well[11]	(a)	70%	80%	79%
Pain 'Always' Well Controlled[11]	(a)	57%	72%	71%
Room and Bathroom 'Always' Clean[11]	(a)	53%	75%	73%
Timely Help 'Always' Received[11]	(a)	65%	69%	68%
Would Definitely Recommend Hospital[11]	(a)	51%	73%	71%
Use of Medical Imaging				
Cardiac Imaging Stress Test before Surgery[7]	-	-	5.3%	5.3%
Combination Abdominal CT Scan[1]	-	-	16.4%	10.5%
Combination Brain/Sinus CT Scan	72	0.0%	2.7%	2.7%
Combination Chest CT Scan[1]	-	-	5.6%	2.7%
Follow-up Mammogram/Ultrasound[7]	-	-	7.9%	8.8%
Lumbar Spine MRI for Low Back Pain[7]	-	-	39.6%	37.2%

Kell West Regional Hospital

5402 Kell West Boulevard
Wichita Falls, TX 76310
Phone: 940-692-5888
Fax: 940-692-0915
E-mail: info@kellwest.com
URL: www.kellwest.com
Type: Acute Care Hospitals
Emergency Services: Yes
Ownership: Proprietary
Beds: 41

Key Personnel:

Cardiology . . . . Vedampattu Ganeshram, MD
Anesthesiology. . . . . James Godwin, MD
Emergency Room . . . . Joe Mendoza, MD
CEO/President. . . . . Dr Jerry Meyers
Infection Control. . . . . Catherine Padakandla, MD

Measure	Cases	This Hosp.	State Avg.	U.S. Avg.
Blood Clot Prevention and Treatment				
Anticoagulation Overlap Therapy[1]	-	-	93%	93%
ICU Venous Thromboembolism Prophylaxis	13	100%	92%	92%
Incidence of Potentially Preventable VTE[7]	-	-	9%	10%
UFH with Dosages/Platelet Monitoring[7]	-	-	96%	97%
Venous Thromboembolism Prophylaxis	344	90%	82%	85%
Warfarin Therapy Discharge Instructions[1]	-	-	84%	75%
Chest Pain/Possible Heart Attack Care				
Aspirin Given Within 24 Hours of Arrival	26	88%	94%	96%
Fibrinolytic Meds Within 30 Min. of Arrival[1]	-	-	47%	58%
Average Time to ECG (minutes)	26	32	8	7
Average Time to Transfer (minutes)[7]	-	-	62	60
Children's Asthma Care				
Received Home Management Plan of Care	-	-	93%	88%
Received Reliever Medication	-	-	100%	100%
Received Systemic Corticosteroids	-	-	100%	100%
Emergency Department				
Admittance Decision Time (minutes)	195	95	99	98
Head CT Results Within 45 Min. of Arrival[1]	-	-	54%	57%
Patients Who Left ER Before Being Seen	12,886	3%	3%	2%
Time from ER Arrival to Admit. (minutes)	196	255	270	274
Time from ER Arrival to Discharge (minutes)	915	108	127	134
Time in ER Before Being Evaluated (minutes)	959	41	26	26
Time to Pain Meds for Fractures (minutes)	88	60	57	57
Heart Attack Care				
Aspirin Given at Discharge[5]	-	-	99%	99%
Fibrinolytic Meds Within 30 Min. of Arrival[5]	-	-	49%	54%
PCI Within 90 Minutes of Arrival[5]	-	-	95%	96%
Statin Prescribed at Discharge[5]	-	-	98%	98%
Heart Failure Care				
ACE Inhibitor or ARB for LVSD[7]	-	-	97%	97%
Discharge Instructions Given[1]	-	-	95%	94%
Evaluation of LVS Function[1]	-	-	99%	99%
Medicare Spending				
Medicare Spending per Patient (ratio)	-	1.07	1.03	0.98
Pneumonia Care				
Appropriate Initial Antibiotic Given	17	94%	95%	95%
Blood Culture Timing	12	92%	98%	98%
Pregnancy and Delivery Care				
Newborn Deliveries Scheduled Early[7]	-	-	7%	6%
Preventive Care				
Immunization for Influenza	458	95%	90%	90%
Immunization for Pneumonia	567	96%	92%	92%
Stroke Care				
Anticoagulation Therapy for Atrial Fibrillation[5]	-	-	96%	95%
Antithrombotic Therapy Timing[5]	-	-	98%	98%
Assessed for Rehabilitation[5]	-	-	98%	97%
Discharged on Antithrombotic Therapy[5]	-	-	99%	99%
Discharged on Statin Medication[5]	-	-	95%	94%
Thrombolytic Therapy Timing[5]	-	-	68%	66%
Venous Thromboembolism Prophylaxis[5]	-	-	94%	94%
Written Stroke Educational Materials Given[5]	-	-	92%	88%
Surgical Care Improvement Project				
Appropriate Beta Blocker Usage	98	98%	98%	98%
Appropriate VTP Within 24 Hours	317	99%	98%	98%
Controlled Postoperative Blood Glucose[7]	-	-	96%	97%
Perioperative Temperature Management	345	99%	100%	100%
Prophylactic Antibiotic Selection	266	100%	99%	99%
Prophylactic Antibiotic Selection (Outpatient)	291	98%	98%	98%
Prophylactic Antibiotic Stopped	262	97%	98%	98%
Prophylactic Antibiotic Timing	266	99%	99%	99%
Prophylactic Antibiotic Timing (Outpatient)	290	99%	98%	98%
Urinary Catheter Removal	162	99%	98%	97%
Survey of Patients' Hospital Experiences				
Area Around Room 'Always' Quiet at Night	(a)	75%	68%	61%
Doctors 'Always' Communicated Well	(a)	88%	83%	82%
Home Recovery Information Given	(a)	88%	85%	85%
Hospital Given 9 or 10 on 10 Point Scale	(a)	78%	73%	71%
Meds 'Always' Explained Before Given	(a)	74%	66%	64%
Nurses 'Always' Communicated Well	(a)	83%	80%	79%
Pain 'Always' Well Controlled	(a)	73%	72%	71%
Room and Bathroom 'Always' Clean	(a)	82%	75%	73%
Timely Help 'Always' Received	(a)	78%	69%	68%
Would Definitely Recommend Hospital	(a)	85%	73%	71%
Use of Medical Imaging				
Cardiac Imaging Stress Test before Surgery[7]	-	-	5.3%	5.3%
Combination Abdominal CT Scan	327	26.0%	16.4%	10.5%
Combination Brain/Sinus CT Scan	202	1.0%	2.7%	2.7%
Combination Chest CT Scan	120	5.0%	5.6%	2.7%
Follow-up Mammogram/Ultrasound[7]	-	-	7.9%	8.8%
Lumbar Spine MRI for Low Back Pain[1]	-	-	39.6%	37.2%

United Regional Health Care System

1600 11th Street
Wichita Falls, TX 76301
Phone: 940-764-3055
Fax: 940-764-3996
URL: www.urhcs.org
Type: Acute Care Hospitals
Emergency Services: Yes
Ownership: Voluntary non-profit - Private
Beds: 541

Key Personnel:

Coronary Care. . . . . Pam Bradshaw, RN
CEO/President. . . . . Phyllis Cowling
Quality Assurance . . . . Lea Ann Hardy, RN
Radiology. . . . . Michael W Houck, MD
Chief of Medical Staff . . . . Scott Hoyer, MD
Infection Control. . . . . Charlene Mossman, RN
Pediatric Ambulatory Care . . . . . . Donna Ross, RN
Pediatric In-Patient Care . . . . Donna Ross, RN

Measure	Cases	This Hosp.	State Avg.	U.S. Avg.
Blood Clot Prevention and Treatment				
Anticoagulation Overlap Therapy[2]	118	97%	93%	93%
ICU Venous Thromboembolism Prophylaxis[2]	66	95%	92%	92%
Incidence of Potentially Preventable VTE[2]	16	0%	9%	10%
UFH with Dosages/Platelet Monitoring[2]	42	100%	96%	97%
Venous Thromboembolism Prophylaxis[2]	369	96%	82%	85%
Warfarin Therapy Discharge Instructions[2]	78	100%	84%	75%
Chest Pain/Possible Heart Attack Care				
Aspirin Given Within 24 Hours of Arrival[1,3]	-	-	94%	96%
Fibrinolytic Meds Within 30 Min. of Arrival[5]	-	-	47%	58%
Average Time to ECG (minutes)[1,3]	-	-	8	7
Average Time to Transfer (minutes)[5]	-	-	62	60
Children's Asthma Care				
Received Home Management Plan of Care	-	-	93%	88%
Received Reliever Medication	-	-	100%	100%
Received Systemic Corticosteroids	-	-	100%	100%
Emergency Department				
Admittance Decision Time (minutes)[2]	531	120	99	98
Head CT Results Within 45 Min. of Arrival[1]	-	-	54%	57%
Patients Who Left ER Before Being Seen	81,450	4%	3%	2%
Time from ER Arrival to Admit. (minutes)[2]	536	252	270	274
Time from ER Arrival to Discharge (minutes)	463	137	127	134
Time in ER Before Being Evaluated (minutes)	491	38	26	26
Time to Pain Meds for Fractures (minutes)	292	67	57	57
Heart Attack Care				
Aspirin Given at Discharge	319	100%	99%	99%
Fibrinolytic Meds Within 30 Min. of Arrival[1]	-	-	49%	54%
PCI Within 90 Minutes of Arrival	35	89%	95%	96%
Statin Prescribed at Discharge	319	100%	98%	98%
Heart Failure Care				
ACE Inhibitor or ARB for LVSD	155	97%	97%	97%
Discharge Instructions Given	327	98%	95%	94%
Evaluation of LVS Function	394	100%	99%	99%
Medicare Spending				
Medicare Spending per Patient (ratio)	-	1.05	1.03	0.98
Pneumonia Care				

NOTE: Hospital profiles are in alphabetical order by state, then city, then hospital within the city; Rankings exclude hospitals with less than 25 cases except for patient surveys which excludes hospitals with less than 100 cases; (a) 100-299 cases; (1) The number of cases/patients is too few to report; (2) Data submitted were based on a sample of cases/patients; (3) Results are based on a shorter time period than required; (4) Data suppressed by CMS for one or more quarters; (5) Results are not available for this reporting period; (6) Fewer than 100 patients completed the HCAHPS survey; (7) No cases met the criteria for this measure; (8) The lower limit of the confidence interval cannot be calculated if the number of observed infections equals zero; (9) No data are available from the state/territory for this reporting period; (10) The scores shown reflect fewer than 50 completed surveys; (11) There were discrepancies in the data collection process; (12) This measure does not apply to this hospital for this reporting period; (13) Results cannot be calculated for this reporting period; (14) The results for this state are combined with nearby states to protect confidentiality; Please refer to the User's Guide for a full explanation of data.

Appropriate Initial Antibiotic Given	243	96%	95%	95%
Blood Culture Timing	329	100%	98%	98%
Pregnancy and Delivery Care				
Newborn Deliveries Scheduled Early	186	13%	7%	6%
Preventive Care				
Immunization for Influenza[2]	496	97%	90%	90%
Immunization for Pneumonia[2]	611	93%	92%	92%
Stroke Care				
Anticoagulation Therapy for Atrial Fibrillation	27	100%	96%	95%
Antithrombotic Therapy Timing	194	99%	98%	98%
Assessed for Rehabilitation	249	99%	98%	97%
Discharged on Antithrombotic Therapy	222	99%	99%	99%
Discharged on Statin Medication	169	99%	95%	94%
Thrombolytic Therapy Timing	19	95%	68%	66%
Venous Thromboembolism Prophylaxis	251	99%	94%	94%
Written Stroke Educational Materials Given	126	98%	92%	88%
Surgical Care Improvement Project				
Appropriate Beta Blocker Usage	282	99%	98%	98%
Appropriate VTP Within 24 Hours	718	99%	98%	98%
Controlled Postoperative Blood Glucose	133	100%	96%	97%
Perioperative Temperature Management	806	100%	100%	100%
Prophylactic Antibiotic Selection	526	100%	99%	99%
Prophylactic Antibiotic Selection (Outpatient)	582	99%	98%	98%
Prophylactic Antibiotic Stopped	510	99%	98%	98%
Prophylactic Antibiotic Timing	532	100%	99%	99%
Prophylactic Antibiotic Timing (Outpatient)	586	98%	98%	98%
Urinary Catheter Removal	578	99%	98%	97%
Survey of Patients' Hospital Experiences				
Area Around Room 'Always' Quiet at Night	300+	68%	68%	61%
Doctors 'Always' Communicated Well	300+	80%	83%	82%
Home Recovery Information Given	300+	87%	85%	85%
Hospital Given 9 or 10 on 10 Point Scale	300+	78%	73%	71%
Meds 'Always' Explained Before Given	300+	63%	66%	64%
Nurses 'Always' Communicated Well	300+	83%	80%	79%
Pain 'Always' Well Controlled	300+	74%	72%	71%
Room and Bathroom 'Always' Clean	300+	80%	75%	73%
Timely Help 'Always' Received	300+	73%	69%	68%
Would Definitely Recommend Hospital	300+	78%	73%	71%
Use of Medical Imaging				
Cardiac Imaging Stress Test before Surgery	242	4.1%	5.3%	5.3%
Combination Abdominal CT Scan	833	9.5%	16.4%	10.5%
Combination Brain/Sinus CT Scan	1,182	1.8%	2.7%	2.7%
Combination Chest CT Scan	382	5.2%	5.6%	2.7%
Follow-up Mammogram/Ultrasound	1,462	5.1%	7.9%	8.8%
Lumbar Spine MRI for Low Back Pain	101	41.6%	39.6%	37.2%

North Runnels Hospital

7821 East Highway 153
Winters, TX 79567
Phone: 325-754-4553
Fax: 325-754-5097
E-mail: stucker@nrhd.org
URL: www.nrhd.org
Type: Critical Access Hospitals
Emergency Services: Yes
Ownership: Govt - Hospital Dist/Auth
Beds: 25

Key Personnel:
Radiology. . . . . Amy Fray-Garza
CEO/President. . . . . Sidney Tucker

Measure	Cases	This Hosp.	State Avg.	U.S. Avg.
Blood Clot Prevention and Treatment				
Anticoagulation Overlap Therapy[5]	-	-	93%	93%
ICU Venous Thromboembolism Prophylaxis[5]	-	-	92%	92%
Incidence of Potentially Preventable VTE[5]	-	-	9%	10%
UFH with Dosages/Platelet Monitoring[5]	-	-	96%	97%
Venous Thromboembolism Prophylaxis[5]	-	-	82%	85%
Warfarin Therapy Discharge Instructions[5]	-	-	84%	75%
Chest Pain/Possible Heart Attack Care				
Aspirin Given Within 24 Hours of Arrival	-	-	94%	96%
Fibrinolytic Meds Within 30 Min. of Arrival	-	-	47%	58%
Average Time to ECG (minutes)	-	-	8	7
Average Time to Transfer (minutes)	-	-	62	60
Children's Asthma Care				
Received Home Management Plan of Care	-	-	93%	88%
Received Reliever Medication	-	-	100%	100%
Received Systemic Corticosteroids	-	-	100%	100%
Emergency Department				
Admittance Decision Time (minutes)[5]	-	-	99	98
Head CT Results Within 45 Min. of Arrival	-	-	54%	57%
Patients Who Left ER Before Being Seen	-	-	3%	2%
Time from ER Arrival to Admit. (minutes)[5]	-	-	270	274
Time from ER Arrival to Discharge (minutes)	-	-	127	134
Time in ER Before Being Evaluated (minutes)	-	-	26	26
Time to Pain Meds for Fractures (minutes)	-	-	57	57
Heart Attack Care				
Aspirin Given at Discharge[5]	-	-	99%	99%
Fibrinolytic Meds Within 30 Min. of Arrival[5]	-	-	49%	54%
PCI Within 90 Minutes of Arrival[5]	-	-	95%	96%
Statin Prescribed at Discharge[5]	-	-	98%	98%
Heart Failure Care				
ACE Inhibitor or ARB for LVSD[2,3]	-	-	97%	97%
Discharge Instructions Given[1,2]	-	-	95%	94%
Evaluation of LVS Function[1,2]	-	-	99%	99%
Medicare Spending				
Medicare Spending per Patient (ratio)	-	-	1.03	0.98
Pneumonia Care				
Appropriate Initial Antibiotic Given[2,3]	-	-	95%	95%
Blood Culture Timing[2,3]	-	-	98%	98%
Pregnancy and Delivery Care				
Newborn Deliveries Scheduled Early[5]	-	-	7%	6%
Preventive Care				
Immunization for Influenza[5]	-	-	90%	90%
Immunization for Pneumonia[5]	-	-	92%	92%
Stroke Care				
Anticoagulation Therapy for Atrial Fibrillation[5]	-	-	96%	95%
Antithrombotic Therapy Timing[5]	-	-	98%	98%
Assessed for Rehabilitation[5]	-	-	98%	97%
Discharged on Antithrombotic Therapy[5]	-	-	99%	99%
Discharged on Statin Medication[5]	-	-	95%	94%
Thrombolytic Therapy Timing[5]	-	-	68%	66%
Venous Thromboembolism Prophylaxis[5]	-	-	94%	94%
Written Stroke Educational Materials Given[5]	-	-	92%	88%
Surgical Care Improvement Project				
Appropriate Beta Blocker Usage[5]	-	-	98%	98%
Appropriate VTP Within 24 Hours[5]	-	-	98%	98%
Controlled Postoperative Blood Glucose[5]	-	-	96%	97%
Perioperative Temperature Management[5]	-	-	100%	100%
Prophylactic Antibiotic Selection[5]	-	-	99%	99%
Prophylactic Antibiotic Selection (Outpatient)	-	-	98%	98%
Prophylactic Antibiotic Stopped[5]	-	-	98%	98%
Prophylactic Antibiotic Timing[5]	-	-	99%	99%
Prophylactic Antibiotic Timing (Outpatient)	-	-	98%	98%
Urinary Catheter Removal[5]	-	-	98%	97%
Survey of Patients' Hospital Experiences				
Area Around Room 'Always' Quiet at Night[5]	-	-	68%	61%
Doctors 'Always' Communicated Well[5]	-	-	83%	82%
Home Recovery Information Given[5]	-	-	85%	85%
Hospital Given 9 or 10 on 10 Point Scale[5]	-	-	73%	71%
Meds 'Always' Explained Before Given[5]	-	-	66%	64%
Nurses 'Always' Communicated Well[5]	-	-	80%	79%
Pain 'Always' Well Controlled[5]	-	-	72%	71%
Room and Bathroom 'Always' Clean[5]	-	-	75%	73%
Timely Help 'Always' Received[5]	-	-	69%	68%
Would Definitely Recommend Hospital[5]	-	-	73%	71%
Use of Medical Imaging				
Cardiac Imaging Stress Test before Surgery	-	-	5.3%	5.3%
Combination Abdominal CT Scan	-	-	16.4%	10.5%
Combination Brain/Sinus CT Scan	-	-	2.7%	2.7%
Combination Chest CT Scan	-	-	5.6%	2.7%
Follow-up Mammogram/Ultrasound	-	-	7.9%	8.8%
Lumbar Spine MRI for Low Back Pain	-	-	39.6%	37.2%

Tyler County Hospital

1100 West Bluff
Woodville, TX 75979
Phone: 409-283-8141
Fax: 409-283-6594
E-mail: jsmith@tchospital.us
URL: www.tchospital.us
Type: Acute Care Hospitals
Emergency Services: Yes
Ownership: Govt - Hospital Dist/Auth
Beds: 49

Key Personnel:
Emergency Room . . . . Louella Barr, MD
Chief of Medical Staff. . . . . James Brown, MD
CEO . . . . Sandra Gayle Wright, RN, Ed.D
Radiology. . . . . Barney Hall
Quality Assurance . . . . Jordan Wilson
Infection Control. . . . . Sondra Wilson, CNO
CEO/President. . . . . Sandra Wright, RN EdD

Measure	Cases	This Hosp.	State Avg.	U.S. Avg.
Blood Clot Prevention and Treatment				
Anticoagulation Overlap Therapy[1,2]	-	-	93%	93%
ICU Venous Thromboembolism Prophylaxis[2,7]	-	-	92%	92%
Incidence of Potentially Preventable VTE[2,7]	-	-	9%	10%
UFH with Dosages/Platelet Monitoring[2,7]	-	-	96%	97%
Venous Thromboembolism Prophylaxis[2]	352	98%	82%	85%
Warfarin Therapy Discharge Instructions[1,2]	-	-	84%	75%
Chest Pain/Possible Heart Attack Care				
Aspirin Given Within 24 Hours of Arrival	49	80%	94%	96%
Fibrinolytic Meds Within 30 Min. of Arrival[1]	-	-	47%	58%
Average Time to ECG (minutes)	50	18	8	7
Average Time to Transfer (minutes)[1]	-	-	62	60
Children's Asthma Care				
Received Home Management Plan of Care	-	-	93%	88%
Received Reliever Medication	-	-	100%	100%
Received Systemic Corticosteroids	-	-	100%	100%
Emergency Department				
Admittance Decision Time (minutes)[2]	455	45	99	98
Head CT Results Within 45 Min. of Arrival[1]	-	-	54%	57%
Patients Who Left ER Before Being Seen	10,455	1%	3%	2%
Time from ER Arrival to Admit. (minutes)[2]	480	195	270	274
Time from ER Arrival to Discharge (minutes)	343	100	127	134
Time in ER Before Being Evaluated (minutes)	380	26	26	26
Time to Pain Meds for Fractures (minutes)	49	60	57	57
Heart Attack Care				
Aspirin Given at Discharge[3,7]	-	-	99%	99%
Fibrinolytic Meds Within 30 Min. of Arrival[3,7]	-	-	49%	54%
PCI Within 90 Minutes of Arrival[3,7]	-	-	95%	96%
Statin Prescribed at Discharge[3,7]	-	-	98%	98%
Heart Failure Care				
ACE Inhibitor or ARB for LVSD	11	100%	97%	97%
Discharge Instructions Given	22	82%	95%	94%
Evaluation of LVS Function	29	100%	99%	99%
Medicare Spending				
Medicare Spending per Patient (ratio)	-	1.00	1.03	0.98
Pneumonia Care				
Appropriate Initial Antibiotic Given	28	86%	95%	95%
Blood Culture Timing	29	97%	98%	98%
Pregnancy and Delivery Care				
Newborn Deliveries Scheduled Early[7]	-	-	7%	6%
Preventive Care				
Immunization for Influenza[2]	359	57%	90%	90%
Immunization for Pneumonia[2]	508	59%	92%	92%
Stroke Care				
Anticoagulation Therapy for Atrial Fibrillation[7]	-	-	96%	95%
Antithrombotic Therapy Timing[1]	-	-	98%	98%
Assessed for Rehabilitation[1]	-	-	98%	97%
Discharged on Antithrombotic Therapy[1]	-	-	99%	99%
Discharged on Statin Medication[7]	-	-	95%	94%
Thrombolytic Therapy Timing[7]	-	-	68%	66%
Venous Thromboembolism Prophylaxis[1]	-	-	94%	94%
Written Stroke Educational Materials Given[7]	-	-	92%	88%
Surgical Care Improvement Project				
Appropriate Beta Blocker Usage[5]	-	-	98%	98%
Appropriate VTP Within 24 Hours[5]	-	-	98%	98%
Controlled Postoperative Blood Glucose[5]	-	-	96%	97%
Perioperative Temperature Management[5]	-	-	100%	100%
Prophylactic Antibiotic Selection[5]	-	-	99%	99%

NOTE: Hospital profiles are in alphabetical order by state, then city, then hospital within the city; Rankings exclude hospitals with less than 25 cases except for patient surveys which excludes hospitals with less than 100 cases; (a) 100-299 cases; (1) The number of cases/patients is too few to report; (2) Data submitted were based on a sample of cases/patients; (3) Results are based on a shorter time period than required; (4) Data suppressed by CMS for one or more quarters; (5) Results are not available for this reporting period; (6) Fewer than 100 patients completed the HCAHPS survey; (7) No cases met the criteria for this measure; (8) The lower limit of the confidence interval cannot be calculated if the number of observed infections equals zero; (9) No data are available from the state/territory for this reporting period; (10) The scores shown reflect fewer than 50 completed surveys; (11) There were discrepancies in the data collection process; (12) This measure does not apply to this hospital for this reporting period; (13) Results cannot be calculated for this reporting period; (14) The results for this state are combined with nearby states to protect confidentiality; Please refer to the User's Guide for a full explanation of data.

Measure	Cases	This Hosp.	State Avg.	U.S. Avg.
Prophylactic Antibiotic Selection (Outpatient)[5]	-	-	98%	98%
Prophylactic Antibiotic Stopped[5]	-	-	98%	98%
Prophylactic Antibiotic Timing[5]	-	-	99%	99%
Prophylactic Antibiotic Timing (Outpatient)[5]	-	-	98%	98%
Urinary Catheter Removal[5]	-	-	98%	97%
Survey of Patients' Hospital Experiences				
Area Around Room 'Always' Quiet at Night	(a)	75%	68%	61%
Doctors 'Always' Communicated Well	(a)	96%	83%	82%
Home Recovery Information Given	(a)	75%	85%	85%
Hospital Given 9 or 10 on 10 Point Scale	(a)	67%	73%	71%
Meds 'Always' Explained Before Given	(a)	82%	66%	64%
Nurses 'Always' Communicated Well	(a)	91%	80%	79%
Pain 'Always' Well Controlled	(a)	70%	72%	71%
Room and Bathroom 'Always' Clean	(a)	84%	75%	73%
Timely Help 'Always' Received	(a)	83%	69%	68%
Would Definitely Recommend Hospital	(a)	74%	73%	71%
Use of Medical Imaging				
Cardiac Imaging Stress Test before Surgery[7]	-	-	5.3%	5.3%
Combination Abdominal CT Scan	131	18.3%	16.4%	10.5%
Combination Brain/Sinus CT Scan	178	0.6%	2.7%	2.7%
Combination Chest CT Scan[1]	-	-	5.6%	2.7%
Follow-up Mammogram/Ultrasound[7]	-	-	7.9%	8.8%
Lumbar Spine MRI for Low Back Pain[7]	-	-	39.6%	37.2%

Yoakum Community Hospital

1200 Carl Ramert Drive
Yoakum, TX 77995
URL: www.yoakumhospital.org
Phone: 361-293-2321
Fax: 361-293-6172
Type: Critical Access Hospitals
Ownership: Govt - Hospital Dist/Auth
Emergency Services: Yes
Beds: 25

Key Personnel:

CEO/President. . . . . Karen Barber
Radiology. . . . . Justin Crisp, RT
Emergency Room . . . . Millie Driskell, RN
Intensive Care Unit. . . . . Millie Driskell, RN
Chief of Medical Staff. . . . . R Martin Lambert, MD
Operating Room. . . . . Shari Mikes, RN
Infection Control. . . . . Kim Mraz, RN
Quality Assurance . . . . Kim Mraz, RN

Measure	Cases	This Hosp.	State Avg.	U.S. Avg.
Blood Clot Prevention and Treatment				
Anticoagulation Overlap Therapy[5]	-	-	93%	93%
ICU Venous Thromboembolism Prophylaxis[5]	-	-	92%	92%
Incidence of Potentially Preventable VTE[5]	-	-	9%	10%
UFH with Dosages/Platelet Monitoring[5]	-	-	96%	97%
Venous Thromboembolism Prophylaxis[5]	-	-	82%	85%
Warfarin Therapy Discharge Instructions[5]	-	-	84%	75%
Chest Pain/Possible Heart Attack Care				
Aspirin Given Within 24 Hours of Arrival	-	-	94%	96%
Fibrinolytic Meds Within 30 Min. of Arrival	-	-	47%	58%
Average Time to ECG (minutes)	-	-	8	7
Average Time to Transfer (minutes)	-	-	62	60
Children's Asthma Care				
Received Home Management Plan of Care	-	-	93%	88%
Received Reliever Medication	-	-	100%	100%
Received Systemic Corticosteroids	-	-	100%	100%
Emergency Department				
Admittance Decision Time (minutes)[5]	-	-	99	98
Head CT Results Within 45 Min. of Arrival	-	-	54%	57%
Patients Who Left ER Before Being Seen	-	-	3%	2%
Time from ER Arrival to Admit. (minutes)[5]	-	-	270	274
Time from ER Arrival to Discharge (minutes)	-	-	127	134
Time in ER Before Being Evaluated (minutes)	-	-	26	26
Time to Pain Meds for Fractures (minutes)	-	-	57	57
Heart Attack Care				
Aspirin Given at Discharge[1,3]	-	-	99%	99%
Fibrinolytic Meds Within 30 Min. of Arrival[3,7]	-	-	49%	54%
PCI Within 90 Minutes of Arrival[3,7]	-	-	95%	96%
Statin Prescribed at Discharge[1,3]	-	-	98%	98%
Heart Failure Care				
ACE Inhibitor or ARB for LVSD	16	100%	97%	97%
Discharge Instructions Given	35	94%	95%	94%
Evaluation of LVS Function	61	92%	99%	99%
Medicare Spending				
Medicare Spending per Patient (ratio)	-	-	1.03	0.98
Pneumonia Care				
Appropriate Initial Antibiotic Given	20	90%	95%	95%
Blood Culture Timing	18	100%	98%	98%
Pregnancy and Delivery Care				
Newborn Deliveries Scheduled Early[5]	-	-	7%	6%
Preventive Care				
Immunization for Influenza[5]	-	-	90%	90%
Immunization for Pneumonia[5]	-	-	92%	92%
Stroke Care				
Anticoagulation Therapy for Atrial Fibrillation[5]	-	-	96%	95%
Antithrombotic Therapy Timing[5]	-	-	98%	98%
Assessed for Rehabilitation[5]	-	-	98%	97%
Discharged on Antithrombotic Therapy[5]	-	-	99%	99%
Discharged on Statin Medication[5]	-	-	95%	94%
Thrombolytic Therapy Timing[5]	-	-	68%	66%
Venous Thromboembolism Prophylaxis[5]	-	-	94%	94%
Written Stroke Educational Materials Given[5]	-	-	92%	88%
Surgical Care Improvement Project				
Appropriate Beta Blocker Usage[5]	-	-	98%	98%
Appropriate VTP Within 24 Hours[5]	-	-	98%	98%
Controlled Postoperative Blood Glucose[5]	-	-	96%	97%
Perioperative Temperature Management[5]	-	-	100%	100%
Prophylactic Antibiotic Selection[5]	-	-	99%	99%
Prophylactic Antibiotic Selection (Outpatient)	-	-	98%	98%
Prophylactic Antibiotic Stopped[5]	-	-	98%	98%
Prophylactic Antibiotic Timing[5]	-	-	99%	99%
Prophylactic Antibiotic Timing (Outpatient)	-	-	98%	98%
Urinary Catheter Removal[5]	-	-	98%	97%
Survey of Patients' Hospital Experiences				
Area Around Room 'Always' Quiet at Night	(a)	75%	68%	61%
Doctors 'Always' Communicated Well	(a)	92%	83%	82%
Home Recovery Information Given	(a)	84%	85%	85%
Hospital Given 9 or 10 on 10 Point Scale	(a)	75%	73%	71%
Meds 'Always' Explained Before Given	(a)	61%	66%	64%
Nurses 'Always' Communicated Well	(a)	86%	80%	79%
Pain 'Always' Well Controlled	(a)	84%	72%	71%
Room and Bathroom 'Always' Clean	(a)	80%	75%	73%
Timely Help 'Always' Received	(a)	83%	69%	68%
Would Definitely Recommend Hospital	(a)	72%	73%	71%
Use of Medical Imaging				
Cardiac Imaging Stress Test before Surgery	-	-	5.3%	5.3%
Combination Abdominal CT Scan	-	-	16.4%	10.5%
Combination Brain/Sinus CT Scan	-	-	2.7%	2.7%
Combination Chest CT Scan	-	-	5.6%	2.7%
Follow-up Mammogram/Ultrasound	-	-	7.9%	8.8%
Lumbar Spine MRI for Low Back Pain	-	-	39.6%	37.2%

NOTE: Hospital profiles are in alphabetical order by state, then city, then hospital within the city; Rankings exclude hospitals with less than 25 cases except for patient surveys which excludes hospitals with less than 100 cases; (a) 100-299 cases; (1) The number of cases/patients is too few to report; (2) Data submitted were based on a sample of cases/patients; (3) Results are based on a shorter time period than required; (4) Data suppressed by CMS for one or more quarters; (5) Results are not available for this reporting period; (6) Fewer than 100 patients completed the HCAHPS survey; (7) No cases met the criteria for this measure; (8) The lower limit of the confidence interval cannot be calculated if the number of observed infections equals zero; (9) No data are available from the state/territory for this reporting period; (10) The scores shown reflect fewer than 50 completed surveys; (11) There were discrepancies in the data collection process; (12) This measure does not apply to this hospital for this reporting period; (13) Results cannot be calculated for this reporting period; (14) The results for this state are combined with nearby states to protect confidentiality; Please refer to the User's Guide for a full explanation of data.

Appendix A: 30-Day Death (Mortality) Rates

What Do These Mortality Categories Show?

These categories show how hospitals' risk-adjusted 30-day death (mortality) rates for heart attack, heart failure, and pneumonia compare to the rate across the U.S., after making adjustments for how sick patients were before they were admitted to the hospital and taking into account differences in death rates that might be due to chance.

This first part of this appendix shows hospitals with 30-day risk-adjusted death (mortality) rates that are lower (better) or higher (worse) than the national rate for all three categories. Hospitals are shown to be better or worse than the U.S. national rate only if the data shows with 95% certainty, that the difference between their surgical complication rates and the U.S. national rate is not due to chance.

The second part of this appendix contains state and national summaries with the following column headers:

- **Better Than U.S. National Rate.** Hospitals in the Better Than U.S. National Rate category have risk-adjusted 30-day death (mortality) rates that are lower than the U.S. National Rate, with 95% certainty that this difference is not due to chance.
- **Worse Than U.S. National Rate.** Hospitals in the Worse Than U.S. National Rate category have risk-adjusted 30-day death (mortality) rates that are higher than the U.S. National Rate, with 95% certainty that this difference is not due to chance.
- **No Different Than U.S. National Rate.** Many hospitals in the No Different Than U.S. National Rate category have risk-adjusted 30-day death (mortality) rates that are about the same as the U.S. National Rate. Other hospitals in this category have rates that are higher or lower than the U.S. National Rate, without 95% certainty that these differences are not due to chance.
- **Number of Cases Too Small.** The number of cases is too small to classify the hospital.

Why are Death Rates for Individual Hospitals Not Shown?

Comparisons based on estimated death (mortality) rates alone can be misleading. Risk-adjusted death (mortality) rates are estimated for individual hospitals based on information taken from a particular time period. If a slightly different time period had been chosen, chances are that each hospital's results would have been somewhat different.

A range ("confidence interval" or in this case an "interval estimate") around estimates show how much variation might be due to this kind of chance. In this case, researchers are 95% confident that a hospital's death (mortality) rate fell somewhere within this specified range. The smaller the range, the more precise the estimate.

When hospitals treat a very large number of patients, chance differences will not have much effect on the overall rates. The range will be small, and the estimated death (mortality) rates will be more precise. In hospitals that treat smaller numbers of patients, however, even small chance differences could have a big impact on death (mortality) rates. The 95% confidence interval, or range, will be large, and the estimated death (mortality) rates will be less precise.

Because the number of patients treated at U.S. hospitals varies widely, the precision of hospitals' estimated death (mortality) rates also varies.

Calculation of 30-Day Risk-Standardized Mortality Rates

The 30-day death (mortality) measures are estimates of deaths from any cause within 30 days of a hospital admission, for patients hospitalized with one of several primary diagnoses. Deaths can be counted in the measures regardless of whether the patient dies while still in the hospital or after discharge. Using deaths within 30 days instead of inpatient deaths show a more consistent measurement time window because length of hospital stay varies across patients and hospitals. Also, mortality over longer time periods (such as 90 days) may have less to do with the care received in the hospital and more to do with other complicating illnesses, patients' own behavior, or care provided to patients after hospital discharge. *The Comparative Guide to American Hospitals* reports on the following 30-day mortality measures:

- 30-day death rate for heart attack (acute myocardial infarction [AMI]) patients
- 30-day death rate for heart failure (HF) patients
- 30-day death rate for pneumonia patients

Which Patients are Included

The 30-day death (mortality) measures include hospitalizations for Medicare beneficiaries aged 65 or older who were enrolled in Original Medicare (traditional fee-for-service Medicare) for the entire 12 months prior to their hospital admission. The AMI, heart failure, and pneumonia (death) mortality measures also include patients aged 65 or older who were admitted to Veteran's Health Administration (VA) hospitals. Beneficiaries enrolled in Medicare managed care plans are not included.

Where the Information Comes From

The Centers for Medicare & Medicaid Services (CMS) calculates hospital-specific 30-day mortality rates using Medicare claims and eligibility information. The AMI, HF, and pneumonia mortality measures are also calculated using VA administrative data. Using administrative data makes it possible to calculate mortality rates without having to do medical chart reviews or requiring hospitals to report additional information to CMS. Research conducted during development of the AMI, HF, and pneumonia death (mortality) measures showed that statistical models based on claims data performed well in estimating hospital mortality rates compared to models that are based on information from medical chart reviews.

Risk Adjustment

To make comparison of hospital performance equitable, the 30-day (death) mortality measures adjust for patient characteristics that may make death more likely, even if the hospital provided higher quality of care. These characteristics include the patient's age, past medical history, and other diseases or conditions (comorbidities) the patient had when admitted that are known to increase the patient's risk of dying.

Significance Testing

The statistical model used to calculate 30-day (death) mortality measures also determines how precise the estimates are, and provides the upper and lower bounds of the 95% interval estimates for each hospital's risk-adjusted mortality rates. Interval estimates, which are like confidence intervals, describe the level of uncertainty around the estimated mortality rates.

Comparing Individual Hospital Rates to the U.S. National Rate

To assign hospitals to performance categories, the hospital's interval estimate is compared to the U.S. national 30-day observed (death) mortality rate. If the 95% interval estimate includes the national observed rate for that measure, the hospital's performance is in the "No Different than U.S. National Rate" category. If the entire 95% interval estimate is below the national observed rate for that measure, then the hospital is performing "Better Than U.S. National Rate." If the entire 95% interval estimate is above the national observed rate for that measure, its performance is "WorseTthan U.S. National Rate." Hospitals with fewer than 25 eligible cases are placed into a separate category that indicates that the hospital did not have enough cases to reliably tell how well the hospital is performing.

Additional Information

For more detail on how the 30-day (death) mortality rates are calculated, visit QualityNet—Mortality Measures at www.qualitynet.org.

Hospitals whose Acute Myocardial Infarction (Heart Attack) 30-Day Mortality Rate is Better (Lower) than the U.S. National Rate

Hospital	City	State	Phone	Web Site
Advocate Lutheran General Hospital	Park Ridge	Illinois	847-723-2210	www.advocatehealth.com
Alexian Brothers Medical Center	Elk Grove Village	Illinois	847-437-5500	www.alexian.org
Arkansas Heart Hospital	Little Rock	Arkansas	501-219-7000	www.arheart.com
The Aroostook Medical Center	Presque Isle	Maine	207-768-4000	www.tamc.org
Avera Heart Hospital of South Dakota	Sioux Falls	South Dakota	605-977-7000	www.avera.org/heart-hospital
Baptist Memorial Hospital	Memphis	Tennessee	901-226-5000	www.bmhcc.org
Baptist Saint Anthony's Hospital	Amarillo	Texas	806-212-2000	www.bsahs.com
Beebe Medical Center	Lewes	Delaware	302-645-3300	www.beebemed.org
Beth Israel Deaconess Medical Center	Boston	Massachusetts	617-667-7000	www.bidmc.harvard.edu
Boca Raton Regional Hospital	Boca Raton	Florida	561-362-5002	www.brrh.com
Boone Hospital Center	Columbia	Missouri	573-815-8000	www.boone.org
Catholic Medical Center	Manchester	New Hampshire	603-668-3545	www.catholicmedicalcenter.org
Cedars - Sinai Medical Center	Los Angeles	California	310-423-5000	www.cedars-sinai.edu
Centegra Health System - Woodstock Hospital	Woodstock	Illinois	815-788-5823	www.centegra.org
Centinela Hospital Medical Center	Inglewood	California	310-673-4660	www.centinelafreeman.com
Chambersburg Hospital	Chambersburg	Pennsylvania	717-267-3000	www.summithealth.org
Champlain Valley Physicians Hospital Medical Center	Plattsburgh	New York	518-561-2000	www.cvph.org
Cypress Fairbanks Medical Center	Houston	Texas	281-897-3100	www.cyfairhospital.com
Doylestown Hospital	Doylestown	Pennsylvania	215-345-2200	www.dh.org
East Orange General Hospital	East Orange	New Jersey	973-266-4401	www.evh.org
Englewood Hospital & Medical Center	Englewood	New Jersey	201-894-3000	www.englewoodhospital.com
Evangelical Community Hospital	Lewisburg	Pennsylvania	570-522-2200	www.evanhospital.com
Firsthealth Moore Regional Hospital	Pinehurst	North Carolina	910-715-1000	www.firsthealth.org
French Hospital Medical Center	San Luis Obispo	California	805-543-5353	www.frenchmedicalcenter.org
Glendale Adventist Medical Center	Glendale	California	818-409-8202	www.glendaleadventist.com
Good Samaritan Hospital	Dayton	Ohio	937-278-2612	www.goodsamdayton.org
Hackensack University Medical Center	Hackensack	New Jersey	201-996-2000	www.humed.com
Hays Medical Center	Hays	Kansas	785-623-5000	www.haysmed.com
Henry Ford Hospital	Detroit	Michigan	313-916-2600	www.henryfordhospital.com
Holy Cross Hospital	Silver Spring	Maryland	301-754-7000	www.holycrosshealth.org
Holy Name Medical Center	Teaneck	New Jersey	201-833-3000	www.holyname.org
John T Mather Memorial Hospital of Port Jefferson	Port Jefferson	New York	631-473-1320	www.matherhospital.com
Lawrence Hospital Center	Bronxville	New York	914-787-1000	www.lawrencehealth.org
Lehigh Valley Hospital	Allentown	Pennsylvania	610-402-2273	www.lvhhn.org
Lehigh Valley Hospital - Hazleton	Hazleton	Pennsylvania	570-501-4000	www.ghha.org
Loyola Gottlieb Memorial Hospital	Melrose Park	Illinois	708-450-4924	www.gottliebhospital.org
Maimonides Medical Center	Brooklyn	New York	718-283-6000	www.maimonidesmed.org
Massachusetts General Hospital	Boston	Massachusetts	617-726-2000	www.massgeneral.org
Minneapolis VA Medical Center	Minneapolis	Minnesota	612-725-2000	www1.va.gov/minneapolis
Miriam Hospital	Providence	Rhode Island	401-793-2500	www.lifespan.org/partners/tmh
Missouri Baptist Medical Center	Town & Country	Missouri	314-996-5000	www.missouribaptistmedicalcenter.org
Montefiore Medical Center	Bronx	New York	718-920-4321	www.montefiore.org
Morristown Medical Center	Morristown	New Jersey	973-971-5450	www.morristownmemorialhospital.org
Mount Sinai Medical Center	Miami Beach	Florida	305-674-2121	www.msmc.com
Munson Medical Center	Traverse City	Michigan	231-935-5000	www.munsonhealthcare.org
New York - Presbyterian Hospital	New York	New York	212-746-4189	www.nyp.org
North Shore University Hospital	Manhasset	New York	516-562-0100	www.northshorelij.com
Northwestern Memorial Hospital	Chicago	Illinois	312-926-2000	www.nmh.org
NYU Hospitals Center	New York	New York	212-263-7300	www.med.nyu.edu
Oakwood Hospital - Dearborn	Dearborn	Michigan	313-593-7125	www.oakwood.org
Olympia Medical Center	Los Angeles	California	310-657-5900	www.olympiamc.com
Overlook Medical Center	Summit	New Jersey	908-522-2000	www.atlantichealth.org
Palisades Medical Center	North Bergen	New Jersey	201-854-5000	www.palisadesmedical.org
Presence Saint Joseph Hospital - Chicago	Chicago	Illinois	773-665-3000	www.res-health.org
Presence Saint Joseph Medical Center	Joliet	Illinois	815-725-7133	www.provena.org/stjoes
Providence Hospital & Medical Centers	Southfield	Michigan	248-849-3011	www.stjohn.org/providence
Rhode Island Hospital	Providence	Rhode Island	401-444-4000	www.rhodeislandhospital.org
Sarasota Memorial Hospital	Sarasota	Florida	941-917-9000	www.smh.com
Sherman Oaks Hospital	Sherman Oaks	California	818-981-7111	www.shermanoakshospital.com
Southcoast Hospital Group	Fall River	Massachusetts	508-679-3131	www.southcoast.org/charlton
Southside Hospital	Bay Shore	New York	631-968-3000	www.northshorelij.com
Saint Francis Hospital - Roslyn	Roslyn	New York	516-562-6000	www.stfrancisheartcenter.com
Saint Joseph Mercy Hospital	Ann Arbor	Michigan	734-712-3791	www.stjoesannarbor.or
Saint Luke's Hospital Bethlehem	Bethlehem	Pennsylvania	610-954-4000	www.slhn-lehighvalley.org
Saint Luke's Hospital	Chesterfield	Missouri	314-434-1500	www.goodhealthmatters.com

Hospital	City	State	Phone	Web Site
Saint Luke's Hospital of Kansas City	Kansas City	Missouri	816-932-2000	www.staintlukeshealthsystem.org
Saint Mary's Medical Center	Huntington	West Virginia	304-526-1234	www.st-marys.org
Saint Vincent Heart Center of Indiana	Indianapolis	Indiana	317-583-5000	www.theheartcenter.com
Trinity Rock Island	Rock Island	Illinois	309-779-5000	www.trinityqc.com
University of California Davis Medical Center	Sacramento	California	916-734-2011	www.ucdmc.ucdavis.edu
Valley Hospital	Ridgewood	New Jersey	201-447-8000	www.valleyhealth.com
Wakemed - Cary Hospital	Cary	North Carolina	919-350-2550	www.wakemed.org
Waterbury Hospital	Waterbury	Connecticut	203-573-6000	www.waterburyhospital.org
William Beaumont Hospital - Troy	Troy	Michigan	248-964-8800	www.beaumonthospitals.com
Winchester Hospital	Winchester	Massachusetts	781-729-9000	www.winchesterhospital.org
Yale-New Haven Hospital	New Haven	Connecticut	203-688-4242	www.ynhh.org
Yuma Regional Medical Center	Yuma	Arizona	928-336-7275	www.yumaregional.org

Note: Table shows hospitals nationwide whose acute myocardial infarction 30-day risk-adjusted mortality rate is better (lower) than U.S. rate of 15.2%

Hospitals whose Acute Myocardial Infarction (Heart Attack) 30-Day Mortality Rate is Worse (Higher) than the U.S. National Rate

Hospital	City	State	Phone	Web Site
Altru Hospital	Grand Forks	North Dakota	701-780-5000	www.altru.org
Baptist Health Corbin	Corbin	Kentucky	606-528-1212	www.baptistregional.com
Bronson Battle Creek Hospital	Battle Creek	Michigan	269-966-8000	www.bchealth.com
Dallas Regional Medical Center	Mesquite	Texas	214-320-7000	www.dallasregionalmedicalcenter.com
Desert Springs Hospital	Las Vegas	Nevada	702-369-7600	www.desertspringshospital.net/p12.html
Hurley Medical Center	Flint	Michigan	810-257-9000	www.hurleymc.com
Kaweah Delta Medical Center	Visalia	California	559-624-2000	www.kaweahdelta.org
Lafayette General Medical Center	Lafayette	Louisiana	337-289-7991	www.lafayettegeneral.org
Lakes Region General Hospital	Laconia	New Hampshire	603-524-3211	www.lrgh.org
Laredo Medical Center	Laredo	Texas	956-796-5000	www.laredomedical.com
Mclaren Bay Region	Bay City	Michigan	989-894-3000	www.baymed.org
National Park Medical Center	Hot Springs	Arkansas	501-321-1000	www.nationalparkmedical.com
North Hills Hospital	North Richland Hills	Texas	817-255-1000	www.northhillshospital.com
Penobscot Valley Hospital	Lincoln	Maine	207-794-3321	www.pvhhealthcare.org
Robert Wood Johnson University Hospital at Rahway	Rahway	New Jersey	732-381-4200	www.rwjuhr.com/about/history.html
Schuylkill Medical Center - East Norwegian Street	Pottsville	Pennsylvania	570-621-4000	www.schuylkillhealth.com
Saint Marys Regional Medical Center	Russellville	Arkansas	479-968-2841	www.saintmarysregional.com
University Hospital SUNY Health Science Center	Syracuse	New York	315-473-4240	www.upstate.edu
Winter Haven Hospital	Winter Haven	Florida	863-293-1121	www.winterhavenhospital.com

Note: Table shows hospitals nationwide whose acute myocardial infarction 30-day risk-adjusted mortality rate is worse (higher) than U.S. rate of 15.2%

Hospitals whose Heart Failure 30-Day Mortality Rate is Better (Lower) than the U.S. National Rate

Hospital	City	State	Phone	Web Site
Abbott Northwestern Hospital	Minneapolis	Minnesota	612-863-4509	www.abbottnorthwestern.com
Advocate Trinity Hospital	Chicago	Illinois	773-967-2000	www.advocatehealth.com/trin
Alexian Brothers Medical Center	Elk Grove Village	Illinois	847-437-5500	www.alexian.org
Atlanticare Regional Medical Center	Atlantic City	New Jersey	609-441-8020	www.atlanticare.org/acmc/index.html
Aurora Saint Lukes Medical Center	Milwaukee	Wisconsin	414-649-6000	www.aurorahealthcare.org
Banner Thunderbird Medical Center	Glendale	Arizona	602-588-5555	www.bannerhealth.com
Baptist Medical Center	San Antonio	Texas	210-297-1020	www.baptisthealthsystem.org
Bay Medical Center Sacred Heart Health System	Panama City	Florida	850-769-1511	www.baymedical.org
Bayhealth - Kent General Hospital	Dover	Delaware	302-744-7001	www.bayhealth.org/about/kent.asp
Beaumont Health System	Royal Oak	Michigan	248-898-5000	www.beaumonthospitals.com
Beth Israel Deaconess Medical Center	Boston	Massachusetts	617-667-7000	www.bidmc.harvard.edu
Beverly Hospital	Montebello	California	323-726-1222	www.beverly.org
Birmingham VA Medical Center	Birmingham	Alabama	205-933-4515	www.birmingham.va.gov
Boston Medical Center Corporation	Boston	Massachusetts	617-638-8000	www.bmc.org
Brigham & Women's Hospital	Boston	Massachusetts	617-732-5500	www.brighamandwomens.org
California Hospital Medical Center Los Angeles	Los Angeles	California	213-748-2411	www.chmcla.org
Cedars - Sinai Medical Center	Los Angeles	California	310-423-5000	www.cedars-sinai.edu
Centinela Hospital Medical Center	Inglewood	California	310-673-4660	www.centinelafreeman.com
Centrastate Medical Center	Freehold	New Jersey	732-431-2000	www.centrastate.com
Champlain Valley Physicians Hospital Medical Center	Plattsburgh	New York	518-561-2000	www.cvph.org
Charleston Area Medical Center	Charleston	West Virginia	304-388-6203	www.camc.org
Clara Maass Medical Center	Belleville	New Jersey	973-450-2002	www.sbhcs.com/hospitals
Cleveland - Wade Park VA Medical Center	Cleveland	Ohio	216-791-3800	www.cleveland.va.gov
Community Hospital	Munster	Indiana	219-836-1600	www.comhs.org/community
Conemaugh Valley Memorial Hospital	Johnstown	Pennsylvania	814-534-9000	www.conemaugh.org
Desert Valley Hospital	Victorville	California	760-241-8000	www.dvmc.com
East Orange General Hospital	East Orange	New Jersey	973-266-4401	www.evh.org
Edward Hospital	Naperville	Illinois	630-527-3000	www.edward.org
Emory University Hospital Midtown	Atlanta	Georgia	404-686-4411	www.emoryhealthcare.org
Essentia Health Saint Joseph's Medical Center	Brainerd	Minnesota	218-829-2861	www.sjmcmn.org
Excela Health Frick Hospital	Mount Pleasant	Pennsylvania	724-547-1500	www.excelahealth.org
Fairview Hospital	Cleveland	Ohio	216-476-7000	www.fairviewhospital.org
Falmouth Hospital	Falmouth	Massachusetts	508-548-5300	www.capecodhealth.com
Fawcett Memorial Hospital	Port Charlotte	Florida	941-629-1181	www.fawcetthospital.com
Firsthealth Moore Regional Hospital	Pinehurst	North Carolina	910-715-1000	www.firsthealth.org
Flagler Hospital	Saint Augustine	Florida	904-819-4426	www.flaglerhospital.com
Florida Hospital Heartland Medical Center	Sebring	Florida	863-314-4466	www.fhhd.org
Forbes Regional Hospital	Monroeville	Pennsylvania	412-858-2000	www.wpahs.org
Fort Duncan Medical Center	Eagle Pass	Texas	830-773-5321	www.fortduncanmedicalcenter.com
Fountain Valley Regional Hospital & Medical Center	Fountain Valley	California	714-966-7200	www.fountainvalleyhospital.com
Franciscan Saint James Health	Olympia Fields	Illinois	708-747-4000	www.franciscanalliance.org
Franciscan Saint Margaret Health - Hammond	Hammond	Indiana	219-932-2300	www.smmhc.com
Frederick Memorial Hospital	Frederick	Maryland	240-566-3300	www.fmh.org
Genesys Regional Medical Center - Health Park	Grand Blanc	Michigan	810-606-5000	www.genesys.org
Glendale Adventist Medical Center	Glendale	California	818-409-8202	www.glendaleadventist.com
Glendale Memorial Hospital & Health Center	Glendale	California	818-502-1900	www.glendalememorialhospital.org
Good Samaritan Hospital	Los Angeles	California	213-977-2121	www.goodsam.org
Good Shepherd Medical Center	Longview	Texas	903-315-2000	www.goodshepherdhealth.org
Grand View Hospital	Sellersville	Pennsylvania	215-453-4615	www.gvh.org
Hahnemann University Hospital	Philadelphia	Pennsylvania	215-762-7000	www.hahnemannhospital.com
Harper University Hospital	Detroit	Michigan	313-745-6211	www.harperhospital.org
Henry Ford Hospital	Detroit	Michigan	313-916-2600	www.henryfordhospital.com
Henry Ford Wyandotte Hospital	Wyandotte	Michigan	734-246-6000	www.henryfordwyandotte.com
Hillcrest Hospital	Mayfield Heights	Ohio	440-312-4500	www.hillcresthospital.org
Hollywood Presbyterian Medical Center	Los Angeles	California	213-413-3000	www.qahpmc.com
Holy Name Medical Center	Teaneck	New Jersey	201-833-3000	www.holyname.org
Houston VA Medical Center	Houston	Texas	713-794-7100	www.houston.med.va.gov
Howard County General Hospital	Columbia	Maryland	410-740-7890	www.hcgh.org
Huntington Beach Hospital	Huntington Beach	California	714-843-5000	www.hbhospital.com
Huron Valley - Sinai Hospital	Commerce Township	Michigan	248-937-3370	www.hvsh.org
Ingalls Memorial Hospital	Harvey	Illinois	708-333-2300	www.ingalls.org
Inova Fairfax Hospital	Falls Church	Virginia	703-776-3332	www.inova.org
Jersey Shore University Medical Center	Neptune	New Jersey	732-776-4900	www.meridianhealth.com
Jesse Brown VA Medical Center - VA Chicago	Chicago	Illinois	312-569-8387	www.va.gov
Kingsbrook Jewish Medical Center	Brooklyn	New York	718-604-5789	www.kingsbrook.org

Hospital	City	State	Phone	Web Site
Lawrence General Hospital	Lawrence	Massachusetts	978-683-4000	www.lawrencegeneral.org
Lehigh Valley Hospital	Allentown	Pennsylvania	610-402-2273	www.lvhhn.org
Lehigh Valley Hospital - Hazleton	Hazleton	Pennsylvania	570-501-4000	www.ghha.org
Lenox Hill Hospital	New York	New York	212-439-2345	www.lenoxhillhospital.org
Libertyhealth - Jersey City Medical Center Campus	Jersey City	New Jersey	201-915-2000	www.libertyhcs.org
Long Beach Memorial Medical Center	Long Beach	California	562-933-2000	www.memorialcare.com/long_beach
Louis A Weiss Memorial Hospital	Chicago	Illinois	773-878-8700	www.weisshospital.org
Maimonides Medical Center	Brooklyn	New York	718-283-6000	www.maimonidesmed.org
Main Line Hospital Bryn Mawr Campus	Bryn Mawr	Pennsylvania	610-526-3000	www.mainlinehealth.org
Main Line Hospital Lankenau	Wynnewood	Pennsylvania	610-645-2000	www.mainlinehealth.org/lh
Marymount Hospital	Garfield Heights	Ohio	216-581-0500	www.marymount.org
Mclaren Flint	Flint	Michigan	810-342-2000	www.mclaren.org
Medical Center of Southeastern Oklahoma	Durant	Oklahoma	405-924-3080	www.mcsohealth.com
Medstar Franklin Square Medical Center	Baltimore	Maryland	443-777-7850	www.franklinsquare.org
Medstar Good Samaritan Hospital	Baltimore	Maryland	443-444-3902	www.goodsam-md.org
Medstar Washington Hospital Center	Washington	District of Columbia	202-877-7000	www.whcenter.org
Mercy Fitzgerald Hospital	Darby	Pennsylvania	215-237-4000	www.mercyhealth.org
Mercy Hospital & Medical Center	Chicago	Illinois	312-567-2000	www.mercy-chicago.org
Mercy Medical Center	Springfield	Massachusetts	413-748-9000	www.mercycares.com
Mercy Saint Vincent Medical Center	Toledo	Ohio	419-251-3232	www.mhsnr.org
The Methodist Hospital	Houston	Texas	713-790-2221	www.methodisthealth.com
Mission Hospital Regional Medical Center	Mission Viejo	California	949-364-1400	www.mission4health.com
Missouri Baptist Medical Center	Town & Country	Missouri	314-996-5000	www.missouribaptistmedicalcenter.org
Montefiore Medical Center	Bronx	New York	718-920-4321	www.montefiore.org
Morristown Medical Center	Morristown	New Jersey	973-971-5450	www.morristownmemorialhospital.org
Mount Sinai Hospital	New York	New York	212-241-7981	www.mountsinai.org
Mountainview Hospital	Las Vegas	Nevada	702-255-5065	www.mountainview-hospital.com
New York Hospital Medical Center of Queens	Flushing	New York	718-670-1231	www.nyhq.org
New York - Presbyterian Hospital	New York	New York	212-746-4189	www.nyp.org
Newark Beth Israel Medical Center	Newark	New Jersey	973-926-7850	www.sbhcs.com
Newton - Wellesley Hospital	Newton	Massachusetts	617-243-6000	www.nwh.org
North Florida Regional Medical Center	Gainesville	Florida	352-333-4100	www.nfrmc.com
North Shore Medical Center	Salem	Massachusetts	978-741-1215	www.nsmc.partners.org
Northridge Hospital Medical Center	Northridge	California	818-885-8500	www.northridgehospital.org
Northwestern Memorial Hospital	Chicago	Illinois	312-926-2000	www.nmh.org
NYU Hospitals Center	New York	New York	212-263-7300	www.med.nyu.edu
Oakwood Hospital - Dearborn	Dearborn	Michigan	313-593-7125	www.oakwood.org
Oklahoma Heart Hospital South	Oklahoma City	Oklahoma	405-628-6000	www.okheart.com/south-campus
Olympia Medical Center	Los Angeles	California	310-657-5900	www.olympiamc.com
Oroville Hospital	Oroville	California	530-533-8500	www.orovillehospital.com
Palm Beach Gardens Medical Center	Palm Beach Gardens	Florida	561-622-1411	www.pbgmc.com
Palmetto Health Richland	Columbia	South Carolina	803-296-5678	www.palmettohealth.org
Paradise Valley Hospital	National City	California	619-470-4321	www.paradisevalleyhospital.org
Penn Presbyterian Medical Center	Philadelphia	Pennsylvania	215-662-8000	www.pennhealth.com
Pennsylvania Hospital of the Univ of PA Health Sys	Philadelphia	Pennsylvania	215-829-3000	www.pennmedicine.org/pahosp
Philadelphia VA Medical Center	Philadelphia	Pennsylvania	215-823-5857	www.philadelphia.va.gov
Portland VA Medical Center	Portland	Oregon	503-220-8262	www.va.gov/portland/index.asp
Presence Saint Joseph Hospital - Chicago	Chicago	Illinois	773-665-3000	www.res-health.org
Presence Saint Joseph Medical Center	Joliet	Illinois	815-725-7133	www.provena.org/stjoes
Presence Saints Mary & Elizabeth Medical Center	Chicago	Illinois	312-770-2000	www.reshealth.org
Providence Holy Cross Medical Center	Mission Hills	California	818-365-8051	www.providence.org
Providence Hospital	Washington	District of Columbia	202-269-7000	www.provhosp.org
Providence Hospital & Medical Centers	Southfield	Michigan	248-849-3011	www.stjohn.org/providence
Providence Little Co of Mary Medical Center Torrance	Torrance	California	310-540-7676	www.lcmhs.org
Providence Tarzana Medical Center	Tarzana	California	818-881-0800	www.encino-tarzana.com
Raritan Bay Medical Center	Perth Amboy	New Jersey	732-442-3700	www.rbmc.org
Regional Medical Center of San Jose	San Jose	California	408-259-5000	www.regionalmedicalsanjose.com
Rex Hospital	Raleigh	North Carolina	919-784-3100	www.rexhealth.com
Rio Grande Regional Hospital	Mcallen	Texas	956-632-6000	www.riohealth.com
Ronald Reagan UCLA Medical Center	Los Angeles	California	310-825-6301	www.uclahealth.org
Rush Oak Park Hospital	Oak Park	Illinois	708-383-9300	www.oakparkhospital.org
Rush University Medical Center	Chicago	Illinois	312-942-5000	www.ruch.edu
Saint Agnes Hospital	Baltimore	Maryland	410-368-2101	www.stagnes.org
Saint Francis Medical Center	Lynwood	California	310-900-8900	www.stfrancis.dochs.org
Saint Michael's Medical Center	Newark	New Jersey	973-877-5350	www.cathedralhealth.org
Saint Vincent Medical Center	Los Angeles	California	213-484-7111	www.stvincent.dochs.org
Santa Monica - UCLA Medical Center & Orthopaedic Hospital	Santa Monica	California	310-319-4000	www.healthcare.ucla.edu

Hospital	City	State	Phone	Web Site
Scottsdale Healthcare - Shea Medical Center	Scottsdale	Arizona	480-323-3009	www.shc.org
Scripps Green Hospital	La Jolla	California	858-554-3600	www.scrippshealth.org
Scripps Mercy Hospital	San Diego	California	619-294-8111	www.scrippshealth.org
Shore Medical Center	Somers Point	New Jersey	609-653-3545	www.shorememorial.org
Sinai Hospital of Baltimore	Baltimore	Maryland	410-601-5131	www.sinai-balt.com
Sinai - Grace Hospital	Detroit	Michigan	313-966-3300	www.sinaigrace.org
South Pointe Hospital	Warrensville Heights	Ohio	216-491-6000	www.southpointehospital.org
South Texas Health System	Edinburg	Texas	956-632-4000	www.edinburgregional.com
Southcoast Hospital Group	Fall River	Massachusetts	508-679-3131	www.southcoast.org/charlton
Southeastern Regional Medical Center	Lumberton	North Carolina	910-671-5000	www.srmc.org
SSM Saint Marys Health Center	Richmond Heights	Missouri	314-768-8000	www.ssmhealth.com/stmarys
Saint Alexius Medical Center	Hoffman Estates	Illinois	847-843-2000	www.alexianbrothershealth.org
Saint Catherine Hospital	East Chicago	Indiana	219-392-7004	www.comhs.org/stcatherine
Saint Elizabeth's Medical Center	Brighton	Massachusetts	617-789-3000	www.semc.org
Saint Francis Hospital & Medical Center	Hartford	Connecticut	860-714-4000	www.saintfranciscare.com
Saint Francis Hospital - Roslyn	Roslyn	New York	516-562-6000	www.stfrancisheartcenter.com
Saint John Hospital & Medical Center	Detroit	Michigan	313-343-4000	www.stjohnprovidence.org
Saint Luke's Hospital	Chesterfield	Missouri	314-434-1500	www.goodhealthmatters.com
Saint Luke's Hospital of Kansas City	Kansas City	Missouri	816-932-2000	www.staintlukeshealthsystem.org
Saint Vincent's Medical Center Southside	Jacksonville	Florida	904-296-3700	www.jaxhealth.com
Thomas Jefferson University Hospital	Philadelphia	Pennsylvania	215-955-6000	www.jeffersonhospital.org
Touro Infirmary	New Orleans	Louisiana	504-897-7011	www.touro.com
Tufts Medical Center	Boston	Massachusetts	617-636-5000	www.tuftsmedicalcenter.org
University Hospital of Brooklyn - Downstate Medical Center	Brooklyn	New York	718-270-1000	www.downstate.edu
University of Maryland Charles Regional Medical Center	La Plata	Maryland	301-609-4265	www.civista.org
University of Miami Hospital	Miami	Florida	305-325-5511	www.cedarsmedicalcenter.com
UPMC Mckeesport	Mc Keesport	Pennsylvania	412-664-2000	www.selectmedicalcorp.com
UPMC Passavant	Pittsburgh	Pennsylvania	412-367-6700	www.passavant.upmc.com
UT Southwestern University Hospital	Dallas	Texas	214-879-3758	www.utsouthwestern.edu
VA Boston Healthcare System - Jamaica Plain	Jamaica Plain	Massachusetts	617-232-9500	www.vaww.visn1.med.va.gov/boston
VA Greater Los Angeles Healthcare System	West Los Angeles	California	310-478-3711	www1.va.gov
VA New York Harbor Healthcare System	New York	New York	212-686-7500	www.nyharbor.va.gov
Valley Hospital	Ridgewood	New Jersey	201-447-8000	www.valleyhealth.com
Valley Presbyterian Hospital	Van Nuys	California	818-902-3906	www.valleypres.org
Wakemed - Raleigh Campus	Raleigh	North Carolina	919-350-8000	www.wakemed.org
Washington Adventist Hospital	Takoma Park	Maryland	301-891-5651	www.adventisthealthcare.com/wah
Waukesha Memorial Hospital	Waukesha	Wisconsin	262-928-1000	www.waukeshamemorial.org
West Haven VA Medical Center	West Haven	Connecticut	203-932-5711	www.visn1.med.va.gov/vact
Wheaton Franciscan Healthcare Saint Francis	Milwaukee	Wisconsin	414-647-5000	www.mywheaton.org
White Memorial Medical Center	Los Angeles	California	323-268-5000	www.whitememorial.com
William Beaumont Hospital - Troy	Troy	Michigan	248-964-8800	www.beaumonthospitals.com
Willis Knighton Medical Center	Shreveport	Louisiana	318-212-4000	www.wkhs.com//locations/medicalcenter.aspx
Winchester Hospital	Winchester	Massachusetts	781-729-9000	www.winchesterhospital.org
Wing Memorial Hospital & Medical Center	Palmer	Massachusetts	413-283-7651	www.winghealth.org
Yale-New Haven Hospital	New Haven	Connecticut	203-688-4242	www.ynhh.org

Note: Table shows hospitals nationwide whose heart failure 30-day risk-adjusted mortality rate is better (lower) than U.S. rate of 11.7%

Hospitals whose Heart Failure 30-Day Mortality Rate is Worse (Higher) than the U.S. National Rate

Hospital	City	State	Phone	Web Site
Abbeville General Hospital	Abbeville	Louisiana	337-893-5466	www.abgen.net
Abrom Kaplan Memorial Hospital	Kaplan	Louisiana	337-643-8300	www.compasshealthcare.com/site78.php
Albany Memorial Hospital	Albany	New York	518-471-3221	www.nehealth.com
Alegent Creighton Health Immanuel Medical Center	Omaha	Nebraska	402-572-2121	www.alegent.com
Anne Arundel Medical Center	Annapolis	Maryland	443-481-1307	www.aahs.org
Appleton Medical Center	Appleton	Wisconsin	920-731-4101	www.thedacare.org
Arkansas Methodist Medical Center	Paragould	Arkansas	870-239-7000	www.arkansasmethodist.org
Baptist Health Medical Center - North Little Rock	North Little Rock	Arkansas	501-202-3000	www.baptist-health.org
Baptist Memorial Hospital/Golden Triangle	Columbus	Mississippi	662-244-1500	www.bmhcc.org/facilities/goldentriangle
Baxter Regional Medical Center	Mountain Home	Arkansas	870-508-1000	www.baxterregional.org
Blanchard Valley Hospital	Findlay	Ohio	419-423-4500	www.bvha.org
Bolivar Medical Center	Cleveland	Mississippi	662-846-2551	www.bolivarmedical.com
Brattleboro Memorial Hospital	Brattleboro	Vermont	802-257-0341	www.bmhvt.org
Bronson Methodist Hospital	Kalamazoo	Michigan	269-341-6000	www.bronsonhealth.com
Capital Region Medical Center	Jefferson City	Missouri	573-632-5000	www.crmc.org
Carilion Roanoke Memorial Hospital	Roanoke	Virginia	540-981-7000	www.carilion.com/crmh
Carolinas Medical Center/Behaviorial Health	Charlotte	North Carolina	704-355-2000	www.carolinasmedicalcenter.org
Carroll Hospital Center	Westminster	Maryland	410-848-3000	www.carrollhospitalcenter.org
Carson Tahoe Regional Medical Center	Carson City	Nevada	775-445-8000	www.carsontahoehospital.com
Cayuga Medical Center at Ithaca	Ithaca	New York	607-274-4401	www.cayugamed.org
Central Maine Medical Center	Lewiston	Maine	207-795-0111	www.cmmc.org
Central Washington Hospital	Wenatchee	Washington	509-662-1511	www.cwhs.com
Cherokee Regional Medical Center	Cherokee	Iowa	712-225-5101	www.cherokeermc.org
Chicot Memorial Medical Center	Lake Village	Arkansas	870-265-5351	www.chicotmemorial.com
Christus Hospital	Beaumont	Texas	409-892-7171	www.christushealth.org
Citizens Baptist Medical Center	Talladega	Alabama	256-761-4542	www.bhsala.com
Citrus Memorial Hospital	Inverness	Florida	352-726-1551	www.citrusmh.com
Clarion Hospital	Clarion	Pennsylvania	814-226-9500	www.clarionhospital.org
Clovis Community Medical Center	Clovis	California	559-324-4000	www.communitymedical.org
Columbia Saint Marys Hospital Ozaukee	Mequon	Wisconsin	262-243-7300	www.columbia-stmarys.org
Community Hospital North	Indianapolis	Indiana	317-621-5335	www.ecommunity.com/north
Conway Regional Medical Center	Conway	Arkansas	501-329-3831	www.conwayregional.org
Copley Memorial Hospital	Aurora	Illinois	630-978-6200	www.rushcopley.com
Coshocton County Memorial Hospital	Coshocton	Ohio	740-622-6411	www.ccmh.com
Dekalb Regional Medical Center	Fort Payne	Alabama	256-845-3150	www.baptistmedical.org
Dominican Hospital	Santa Cruz	California	831-462-7700	www.dominicanhospital.org
Edward W Sparrow Hospital	Lansing	Michigan	517-364-1000	www.sparrow.org
Emerson Hospital	W Concord	Massachusetts	978-369-1400	www.emersonhospital.org
Fletcher Allen Hospital of Vermont	Burlington	Vermont	802-847-0000	www.fletcherallen.org
Floyd Medical Center	Rome	Georgia	706-509-6900	www.floydmed.org
Geisinger Medical Center	Danville	Pennsylvania	570-271-6211	www.geisinger.org
Geneva General Hospital	Geneva	New York	315-787-4175	www.flhealth.org
GHS Greenville Memorial Medical Center	Greenville	South Carolina	864-455-7000	www.ghs.org
Good Samaritan Hospital	Lebanon	Pennsylvania	717-270-7500	www.gshleb.org
Grossmont Hospital	La Mesa	California	619-465-0711	www.sharp.com
Hendrick Medical Center	Abilene	Texas	325-670-2000	www.ehendrick.org
Highland Hospital	Rochester	New York	585-473-2200	www.urmc.rochester.edu
Hilton Head Regional Medical Center	Hilton Head Island	South Carolina	843-681-6122	www.hiltonheadmedctr.com
Hopkins County Memorial Hospital	Sulphur Springs	Texas	903-885-7671	www.hcmh.com
Hutchinson Regional Medical Center	Hutchinson	Kansas	620-665-2001	www.hutchinsonhospital.com
Iberia General Hospital & Medical Center	New Iberia	Louisiana	337-364-0441	www.iberiamedicalcenter.com
Indiana University Health La Porte Hospital	La Porte	Indiana	219-326-1234	www.laportehealth.org
Integris Grove Hospital	Grove	Oklahoma	918-786-2243	www.integris-health.com
IU Health Goshen Hospital	Goshen	Indiana	574-364-1000	www.goshenhosp.com
Jane Phillips Medical Center	Bartlesville	Oklahoma	918-333-7200	www.jpmc.org
JFK Medical Center - A M Yelencsics Comm Hospital	Edison	New Jersey	732-321-7000	www.jfkmc.org
Johnson Memorial Hospital	Franklin	Indiana	317-736-3300	www.johnsonmemorial.org
Kadlec Regional Medical Center	Richland	Washington	509-946-4611	www.kadlecmed.org
Kootenai Medical Center	Coeur D'alene	Idaho	208-625-4001	www.kootenaihealth.org
Lake Cumberland Regional Hospital	Somerset	Kentucky	606-679-7441	www.lakecumberlandhospital.com
Lake Granbury Medical Center	Granbury	Texas	817-573-2683	www.lakegranburymedicalcenter.com
Lawrence & Memorial Hospital	New London	Connecticut	860-442-0711	www.lmhospital.org
Los Alamitos Medical Center	Los Alamitos	California	562-799-3220	www.losalamitosmedctr.com
Manatee Memorial Hospital	Bradenton	Florida	941-746-5111	www.manateememorial.com
Manchester Memorial Hospital	Manchester	Connecticut	860-647-4780	www.echn.org

Hospital	City	State	Phone	Web Site
Maury Regional Hospital	Columbia	Tennessee	931-381-1111	www.maurgregional.com
Mclaren - Greater Lansing	Lansing	Michigan	517-975-6000	www.mclaren.org
Meadville Medical Center	Meadville	Pennsylvania	814-333-5000	www.mmchs.org
Medcentral Health System Mansfield Hospital	Mansfield	Ohio	419-526-8000	www.medcentral.org
Memorial Hospital of South Bend	South Bend	Indiana	574-647-1000	www.qualityoflife.org
Mercy Health System Corp	Janesville	Wisconsin	608-756-6080	www.mercyhealthsystem.org
Mercy Hospital Springfield	Springfield	Missouri	417-820-2000	www.stjohns.com
Mercy Medical Center - Redding	Redding	California	530-225-6102	www.redding.mercy.org
Mercy Medical Center - North Iowa	Mason City	Iowa	641-428-7000	www.mercynorthiowa.com
Mountain View Regional Medical Center	Las Cruces	New Mexico	575-556-7600	www.mountainviewregional.com
Nathan Littauer Hospital	Gloversville	New York	518-725-8621	www.nlh.org
Nea Baptist Memorial Hospital	Jonesboro	Arkansas	870-972-7000	www.baptistonline.com
New Hanover Regional Medical Center	Wilmington	North Carolina	910-343-7000	www.nhrmc.org
New Milford Hospital	New Milford	Connecticut	860-355-2611	www.newmilfordhospital.org
Norman Regional Health System	Norman	Oklahoma	405-321-1700	www.normanregional.com
North Mississippi Medical Center	Tupelo	Mississippi	662-377-3000	www.nmhs.net/nmmc
North Shore University Hospital	Manhasset	New York	516-562-0100	www.northshorelij.com
Northwest Community Hospital	Arlington Heights	Illinois	847-618-1000	www.nch.org
Northwest Hospital	Seattle	Washington	206-364-0500	www.nwhospital.org
O'Connor Hospital	San Jose	California	408-947-2500	www.oconnorhospital.org
Olympic Medical Center	Port Angeles	Washington	360-417-7000	www.olympicmedical.org
Our Lady of the Lake Regional Medical Center	Baton Rouge	Louisiana	225-765-6565	www.ololrmc.com
Overton Brooks VA Medical Center - Shreveport	Shreveport	Louisiana	318-424-6037	www.va.gov/sta/guide/home.asp
Pinnacle Health Hospitals	Harrisburg	Pennsylvania	717-782-5181	www.pinnaclehealth.org
Poplar Bluff Regional Medical Center	Poplar Bluff	Missouri	573-785-7721	www.poplarbluffregional.com
Porter Regional Hospital	Valparaiso	Indiana	219-983-8300	www.portermemorial.org
Providence Alaska Medical Center	Anchorage	Alaska	907-261-3675	www.providence.org
Providence Sacred Heart Medical Center	Spokane	Washington	509-474-3040	www.shmc.org
Rideout Memorial Hospital	Marysville	California	530-749-4300	www.frhg.org
Riverview Hospital Assoc	Wisconsin Rapids	Wisconsin	715-423-6060	www.riverviewhospital.net
Sacred Heart Medical Center - Riverbend	Springfield	Oregon	541-222-7300	www.peacehealth.org/sacred-heart-riverbend
Saint Anthony Medical Center	Rockford	Illinois	815-226-2000	www.osfhealth.com
Saint Francis Medical Center	Peoria	Illinois	309-655-2000	www.osfsaintfrancis.org
Salem Hospital	Salem	Oregon	503-561-5200	www.salemhospital.org
Saline Memorial Hospital	Benton	Arkansas	501-776-6000	www.salinememorial.org
San Juan Regional Medical Center	Farmington	New Mexico	505-609-2000	www.sanjuanregional.com
Sanford Usd Medical Center	Sioux Falls	South Dakota	605-333-1000	www.sanfordhealth.org
Santa Rosa Memorial Hospital	Santa Rosa	California	707-525-5300	www.stjosephhealth.org
Sarasota Memorial Hospital	Sarasota	Florida	941-917-9000	www.smh.com
Scenic Mountain Medical Center	Big Spring	Texas	432-263-1211	www.smmccares.com
Sentara Obici Hospital	Suffolk	Virginia	757-934-4000	www.sentara.com
Saint Anthony's Hospital	Saint Petersburg	Florida	727-825-1100	www.stanthonys.com
Saint Bernards Medical Center	Jonesboro	Arkansas	870-972-4100	www.sbrmc.com
Saint Francis - Downtown	Greenville	South Carolina	864-255-1000	www.stfrancishealth.org
Saint Johns Hospital	Springfield	Illinois	217-544-6464	www.st-johns.org
Saint Joseph Regional Health Center	Bryan	Texas	979-776-3912	www.st-joseph.org/sjrhc
Saint Joseph's Mercy Health Center	Hot Springs	Arkansas	501-622-1000	www.saintjosephs.com
Saint Lucie Medical Center	Port Saint Lucie	Florida	772-335-4000	www.stluciemed.com
Saint Marys Hospital Medical Center	Green Bay	Wisconsin	920-498-4200	www.stmgb.org
Saint Marys Regional Medical Center	Russellville	Arkansas	479-968-2841	www.saintmarysregional.com
Saint Nicholas Hospital	Sheboygan	Wisconsin	920-459-8300	www.stnicholashospital.org
Saint Rose Dominican Hospitals - Rose De Lima Campus	Henderson	Nevada	702-616-5000	www.dignityhealth.org/las-vegas
Starr Regional Medical Center Athens	Athens	Tennessee	423-745-1411	www.athensrmc.com
Swedish Edmonds Hospital	Edmonds	Washington	425-640-4000	www.stevenshealthcare.org
Texas Health Harris Methodist Fort Worth	Fort Worth	Texas	817-250-2100	www.texashealth.org
The Nebraska Medical Center	Omaha	Nebraska	402-552-2040	www.nebraskamed.com
Theda Clark Medical Center	Neenah	Wisconsin	920-729-3100	www.thedacare.org
Thibodaux Regional Medical Center	Thibodaux	Louisiana	985-447-5500	www.thibodaux.com
Tulare Regional Medical Center	Tulare	California	559-688-0821	www.tdhs.org
Ukiah Valley Medical Center	Ukiah	California	707-462-3111	www.uvmc.org
Union General Hospital	Blairsville	Georgia	706-745-2111	www.uniongeneralhospital.com
United Health Services Hospitals	Johnson City	New York	607-763-6000	www.vhs.ent
United Regional Health Care System	Wichita Falls	Texas	940-764-3055	www.urhcs.org
University of Missouri Health Care	Columbia	Missouri	573-882-4141	www.missouri.edu
Utah Valley Regional Medical Center	Provo	Utah	801-373-7850	www.intermountainhealthcare.org/hospitals/uvrmc
VA Southern Arizona Healthcare System	Tucson	Arizona	520-629-1821	www.va.gov/sta/guide/home.asp
Valley Hospital	Spokane	Washington	509-924-6650	www.valleyhospital.org

Hospital	City	State	Phone	Web Site
Western Missouri Medical Center	Warrensburg	Missouri	660-747-2500	www.wmmc.com
White County Medical Center	Searcy	Arkansas	501-278-3100	www.centralarkhospital.com
Wilkes-Barre General Hospital	Wilkes-Barre	Pennsylvania	570-829-8111	www.wvhcs.org
Wyoming Medical Center	Casper	Wyoming	307-577-7201	www.wyomingmedicalcenter.com

Note: Table shows hospitals nationwide whose heart failure 30-day risk-adjusted mortality rate is worse (higher) than U.S. rate of 11.7%

Hospitals whose Pneumonia 30-Day Mortality Rate is Better (Lower) than the U.S. National Rate

Hospital	City	State	Phone	Web Site
Adventist La Grange Memorial Hospital	La Grange	Illinois	708-352-1200	www.keepingyouwell.com
Ahmc Anaheim Regional Medical Center	Anaheim	California	714-774-1450	www.memorialcare.org/anaheim
Akron General Medical Center	Akron	Ohio	330-344-6000	www.akrongeneral.org
Alhambra Hospital Medical Center	Alhambra	California	626-570-1606	www.alhambrahospital.com
Arnot Ogden Medical Center	Elmira	New York	607-737-4100	www.arnothealth.org
Augusta Health	Fishersville	Virginia	540-932-4000	www.augustamed.com
Aurora Saint Lukes Medical Center	Milwaukee	Wisconsin	414-649-6000	www.aurorahealthcare.org
Aventura Hospital & Medical Center	Aventura	Florida	305-682-7000	www.aventurahospital.com
Banner Thunderbird Medical Center	Glendale	Arizona	602-588-5555	www.bannerhealth.com
Baptist Hospital of Miami	Miami	Florida	786-596-1960	www.baptisthealth.net
Barnes-Jewish Saint Peters Hospital	Saint Peters	Missouri	636-916-9000	www.bjsph.org
Bay Medical Center Sacred Heart Health System	Panama City	Florida	850-769-1511	www.baymedical.org
Baylor Regional Medical Center at Grapevine	Grapevine	Texas	817-481-1588	www.baylorhealth.com
Beaumont Health System	Grosse Pointe	Michigan	313-343-1000	www.beaumonthospitals.com
Beaumont Health System	Royal Oak	Michigan	248-898-5000	www.beaumonthospitals.com
Benefis Hospitals	Great Falls	Montana	406-455-5000	www.benefis.org
Berkshire Medical Center	Pittsfield	Massachusetts	413-447-2000	www.berkshirehealthsystems.org
Beth Israel Deaconess Medical Center	Boston	Massachusetts	617-667-7000	www.bidmc.harvard.edu
Betsy Johnson Regional Hospital	Dunn	North Carolina	910-892-7161	www.bjrh.org
Cape Cod Hospital	Hyannis	Massachusetts	508-771-1800	www.capecodhealth.org
Casey County Hospital	Liberty	Kentucky	606-787-6275	
Cedars - Sinai Medical Center	Los Angeles	California	310-423-5000	www.cedars-sinai.edu
Centinela Hospital Medical Center	Inglewood	California	310-673-4660	www.centinelafreeman.com
Centura Health - Littleton Adventist Hospital	Littleton	Colorado	303-730-5888	www.littletonhosp.org
Christ Hospital	Cincinnati	Ohio	513-585-2000	www.thechristhospital.com
Cobre Valley Regional Medical Center	Globe	Arizona	928-425-3261	www.cvchospital.com
Community Medical Center	Toms River	New Jersey	732-557-8000	www.sbhcs.com
Corning Hospital	Corning	New York	607-937-7200	www.corninghospital.org
Cox Medical Center Branson	Branson	Missouri	417-335-7000	www.skaggs.net
Delray Medical Center	Delray Beach	Florida	561-498-4440	www.delraymedicalctr.com
Desert Valley Hospital	Victorville	California	760-241-8000	www.dvmc.com
Doctors Hospital at Renaissance	Edinburg	Texas	956-362-8677	www.dhr-rgv.com
Duke University Hospital	Durham	North Carolina	919-684-8111	www.dukehealth.org
East Valley Hospital Medical Center	Glendora	California	626-335-0231	www.eastvalleyhospital.org
Edward Hospital	Naperville	Illinois	630-527-3000	www.edward.org
Eisenhower Medical Center	Rancho Mirage	California	760-340-3911	www.emc.org
Elmhurst Memorial Hospital	Elmhurst	Illinois	630-833-1400	www.emhc.org
Englewood Hospital & Medical Center	Englewood	New Jersey	201-894-3000	www.englewoodhospital.com
Evanston Hospital	Evanston	Illinois	847-432-8000	www.enh.org
Evergreen Hospital Medical Center	Kirkland	Washington	425-899-1000	www.evergreenhospital.org
Exempla Lutheran Medical Center	Wheat Ridge	Colorado	303-425-4500	www.exemlpa.org
Falmouth Hospital	Falmouth	Massachusetts	508-548-5300	www.capecodhealth.com
Firsthealth Moore Regional Hospital	Pinehurst	North Carolina	910-715-1000	www.firsthealth.org
Flagler Hospital	Saint Augustine	Florida	904-819-4426	www.flaglerhospital.com
Forbes Regional Hospital	Monroeville	Pennsylvania	412-858-2000	www.wpahs.org
Fountain Valley Regional Hospital & Medical Center	Fountain Valley	California	714-966-7200	www.fountainvalleyhospital.com
Franklin Woods Community Hospital	Johnson City	Tennessee	423-302-1120	www.msha.com
Frederick Memorial Hospital	Frederick	Maryland	240-566-3300	www.fmh.org
Frisbie Memorial Hospital	Rochester	New Hampshire	603-332-5211	www.frisbiehospital.com
Garden Grove Hospital & Medical Center	Garden Grove	California	714-537-5160	www.gardengrovehospital.com
Garfield Medical Center	Monterey Park	California	626-573-2222	www.garfieldmedicalcenter.com
Geisinger - Bloomsburg Hospital	Bloomsburg	Pennsylvania	570-387-2100	www.tbhonline.org
Genesis Healthcare System	Zanesville	Ohio	740-454-5000	www.genesishcs.org
Genesys Regional Medical Center - Health Park	Grand Blanc	Michigan	810-606-5000	www.genesys.org
Glendale Adventist Medical Center	Glendale	California	818-409-8202	www.glendaleadventist.com
Grandview Hospital & Medical Center	Dayton	Ohio	937-723-3312	www.kmcnetwork.org
Greater Baltimore Medical Center	Baltimore	Maryland	443-849-2000	www.gbmc.org
Harper University Hospital	Detroit	Michigan	313-745-6211	www.harperhospital.org
Heartland Regional Medical Center	Saint Joseph	Missouri	816-271-6000	www.heartland-health.com
Henry Ford Macomb Hospital	Clinton Township	Michigan	586-263-2300	www.stjoe-macomb.com
Hillcrest Hospital	Mayfield Heights	Ohio	440-312-4500	www.hillcresthospital.org
Hinsdale Hospital	Hinsdale	Illinois	630-856-9000	www.keepingyouwell.com
Hollywood Presbyterian Medical Center	Los Angeles	California	213-413-3000	www.qahpmc.com
Holy Name Medical Center	Teaneck	New Jersey	201-833-3000	www.holyname.org
The Hospital of Central Connecticut	New Britain	Connecticut	860-224-5011	www.thocc.org

Hospital	City	State	Phone	Web Site
Huntington Beach Hospital	Huntington Beach	California	714-843-5000	www.hbhospital.com
Huntington Memorial Hospital	Pasadena	California	626-397-5000	www.huntingtonhospital.com
Indiana University Health	Indianapolis	Indiana	317-962-5900	www.iuhealth.org
Ingalls Memorial Hospital	Harvey	Illinois	708-333-2300	www.ingalls.org
Inova Loudoun Hospital	Leesburg	Virginia	703-858-6600	www.loudounhealthcare.org
Jersey Shore University Medical Center	Neptune	New Jersey	732-776-4900	www.meridianhealth.com
Jupiter Medical Center	Jupiter	Florida	561-747-2234	www.jupitermed.com
Kane Community Hospital	Kane	Pennsylvania	814-837-8585	www.kanehosp.com
Kingsbrook Jewish Medical Center	Brooklyn	New York	718-604-5789	www.kingsbrook.org
Lehigh Valley Hospital	Allentown	Pennsylvania	610-402-2273	www.lvhhn.org
Lehigh Valley Hospital - Hazleton	Hazleton	Pennsylvania	570-501-4000	www.ghha.org
Lehigh Valley Hospital - Muhlenberg	Bethlehem	Pennsylvania	610-402-2273	www.lvhn.org
Liberty Hospital	Liberty	Missouri	816-781-7200	www.libertyhospital.org
Los Angeles Community Hospital	Los Angeles	California	323-267-0477	www.altacorp.com
Los Robles Hospital & Medical Center	Thousand Oaks	California	805-497-2727	www.losrobleshospital.com
Maimonides Medical Center	Brooklyn	New York	718-283-6000	www.maimonidesmed.org
Mary Greeley Medical Center	Ames	Iowa	515-239-2011	www.mgmc.org
Mayo Clinic Hospital	Phoenix	Arizona	480-342-2000	www.mayoclinic.org
Medical Center of Southeastern Oklahoma	Durant	Oklahoma	405-924-3080	www.mcsohealth.com
Medical City Dallas Hospital	Dallas	Texas	972-566-6222	www.medicalcityhospital.com
Medstar Franklin Square Medical Center	Baltimore	Maryland	443-777-7850	www.franklinsquare.org
Medstar Good Samaritan Hospital	Baltimore	Maryland	443-444-3902	www.goodsam-md.org
Medstar Harbor Hospital	Baltimore	Maryland	410-350-3201	www.harborhospital.org
Memorial Mission Hospital & Asheville Surgery Center	Asheville	North Carolina	828-213-1111	www.missionhospitals.org
Mercy Memorial Hospital System	Monroe	Michigan	734-240-8400	www.mercymemorial.org
The Methodist Hospital	Houston	Texas	713-790-2221	www.methodisthealth.com
Methodist Sugar Land Hospital	Sugar Land	Texas	281-274-8000	www.methodisthealth.com/sugarland
Milford Regional Medical Center	Milford	Massachusetts	508-473-1190	www.milfordregional.org
Missouri Baptist Medical Center	Town & Country	Missouri	314-996-5000	www.missouribaptistmedicalcenter.org
Monmouth Medical Center - Southern Campus	Lakewood	New Jersey	732-363-1900	www.sbhcs.com
Montefiore Medical Center	Bronx	New York	718-920-4321	www.montefiore.org
Morristown Medical Center	Morristown	New Jersey	973-971-5450	www.morristownmemorialhospital.org
Mount Auburn Hospital	Cambridge	Massachusetts	617-492-3500	www.mountauburnhospital.org
Mount Sinai Hospital	New York	New York	212-241-7981	www.mountsinai.org
Mount Sinai Medical Center	Miami Beach	Florida	305-674-2121	www.msmc.com
New York - Presbyterian Hospital	New York	New York	212-746-4189	www.nyp.org
Newton Memorial Hospital	Newton	New Jersey	973-383-2121	www.itsyourlife.com
North Shore Medical Center	Salem	Massachusetts	978-741-1215	www.nsmc.partners.org
North Shore University Hospital	Manhasset	New York	516-562-0100	www.northshorelij.com
Northern Westchester Hospital	Mount Kisco	New York	914-666-1200	www.nwhc.net
Northwestern Memorial Hospital	Chicago	Illinois	312-926-2000	www.nmh.org
Norton Community Hospital	Norton	Virginia	703-679-8865	www.nchosp.org
NYU Hospitals Center	New York	New York	212-263-7300	www.med.nyu.edu
Oakwood Hospital - Dearborn	Dearborn	Michigan	313-593-7125	www.oakwood.org
Olympia Medical Center	Los Angeles	California	310-657-5900	www.olympiamc.com
Oroville Hospital	Oroville	California	530-533-8500	www.orovillehospital.com
Our Lady of Lourdes Medical Center	Camden	New Jersey	856-757-3500	www.lourdesnet.org
Overlook Medical Center	Summit	New Jersey	908-522-2000	www.atlantichealth.org
Owensboro Health Regional Hospital	Owensboro	Kentucky	270-688-2000	www.omhs.org
Palos Community Hospital	Palos Heights	Illinois	708-923-4000	www.paloshospital.org
Paradise Valley Hospital	National City	California	619-470-4321	www.paradisevalleyhospital.org
Park Plaza Hospital	Houston	Texas	713-527-5019	www.parkplazahospital.com
Parkland Health Center	Farmington	Missouri	573-431-6005	www.bjc.org
Piedmont Hospital	Atlanta	Georgia	404-605-5000	www.piedmonthospital.org
Portland VA Medical Center	Portland	Oregon	503-220-8262	www.va.gov/portland/index.asp
Presbyterian Intercommunity Hospital	Whittier	California	526-698-0811	www.whittierpres.com
Presence Resurrection Medical Center	Chicago	Illinois	773-774-8000	www.reshealthcare.org
Presence Saint Joseph Hospital - Chicago	Chicago	Illinois	773-665-3000	www.res-health.org
Presence Saint Joseph Medical Center	Joliet	Illinois	815-725-7133	www.provena.org/stjoes
Presence Saint Marys Hospital	Kankakee	Illinois	815-937-2490	www.provenastmarys.com
Providence Hospital & Medical Centers	Southfield	Michigan	248-849-3011	www.stjohn.org/providence
Providence Little Co of Mary Medical Center Torrance	Torrance	California	310-540-7676	www.lcmhs.org
Providence Saint Joseph Medical Center	Burbank	California	818-843-5111	www.providence.org/losangeles
Providence Tarzana Medical Center	Tarzana	California	818-881-0800	www.encino-tarzana.com
Randolph Hospital	Asheboro	North Carolina	336-625-5151	www.randolphhospital.org
Raritan Bay Medical Center	Perth Amboy	New Jersey	732-442-3700	www.rbmc.org
Reading Hospital	Reading	Pennsylvania	610-988-8000	www.readinghospital.org

Hospital	City	State	Phone	Web Site
Rex Hospital	Raleigh	North Carolina	919-784-3100	www.rexhealth.com
Rhode Island Hospital	Providence	Rhode Island	401-444-4000	www.rhodeislandhospital.org
Rio Grande Regional Hospital	Mcallen	Texas	956-632-6000	www.riohealth.com
Riverside Medical Center	Kankakee	Illinois	815-933-1671	www.riversidehealthcare.org
Riverview Medical Center	Red Bank	New Jersey	732-741-2700	www.meridianhealth.com
Robert Wood Johnson University Hospital	New Brunswick	New Jersey	732-937-8900	www.rwjuh.edu
Rockingham Memorial Hospital	Harrisonburg	Virginia	540-689-1000	www.rmhonline.com
Ronald Reagan UCLA Medical Center	Los Angeles	California	310-825-6301	www.uclahealth.org
Saint Clare's Hospital	Denville	New Jersey	973-625-6000	www.saintclares.org
Saint Francis Hospital	Tulsa	Oklahoma	918-494-2200	www.saintfrancis.com
Saint Vincent Medical Center	Los Angeles	California	213-484-7111	www.stvincent.dochs.org
San Francisco VA Medical Center	San Francisco	California	415-221-4810	www.sanfrancisco.va.gov
San Gabriel Valley Medical Center	San Gabriel	California	626-289-5454	www.sangabrielvalleymedctr.org
Santa Monica - UCLA Medical Center & Orthopaedic Hospital	Santa Monica	California	310-319-4000	www.healthcare.ucla.edu
Scott & White Hospital - Round Rock	Round Rock	Texas	512-509-0100	www.sw.org
Scott & White Memorial Hospital	Temple	Texas	254-724-2111	www.sw.org
Scripps Memorial Hospital La Jolla	La Jolla	California	858-626-4123	www.scrippshealth.org
Scripps Mercy Hospital	San Diego	California	619-294-8111	www.scrippshealth.org
Sharon Regional Health System	Sharon	Pennsylvania	724-983-3800	www.sharonregional.com
Sinai Hospital of Baltimore	Baltimore	Maryland	410-601-5131	www.sinai-balt.com
South Pointe Hospital	Warrensville Heights	Ohio	216-491-6000	www.southpointehospital.org
Southampton Hospital	Southampton	New York	516-726-8200	www.southamptonhospital.org
Southcoast Hospital Group	Fall River	Massachusetts	508-679-3131	www.southcoast.org/charlton
Southwest General Health Center	Middleburg Heights	Ohio	440-816-8000	www.swgeneral.com
Spartanburg Regional Medical Center	Spartanburg	South Carolina	864-560-6000	www.srhs.com
Spring Valley Hospital Medical Center	Las Vegas	Nevada	702-853-3000	www.springvalleyhospital.com
Saint Alexius Medical Center	Hoffman Estates	Illinois	847-843-2000	www.alexianbrothershealth.org
Saint Anthony Community Hospital	Warwick	New York	845-986-2276	www.stanthonycommunityhosp.org
Saint Luke's Hospital Bethlehem	Bethlehem	Pennsylvania	610-954-4000	www.slhn-lehighvalley.org
Saint Luke's Roosevelt Hospital	New York	New York	212-523-4000	www.wehealny.org
Saint Luke's Episcopal Hospital	Houston	Texas	832-355-1000	www.sleh.com
Saint Luke's Hospital	Cedar Rapids	Iowa	319-369-7211	www.crstlukes.com
Saint Luke's Hospital	Chesterfield	Missouri	314-434-1500	www.goodhealthmatters.com
Saint Marys Hospital	Madison	Wisconsin	608-251-6100	www.stmarysmadison.com
Saint Peter's Hospital	Albany	New York	518-525-1550	www.stpetershealthcare.org
Stafford Hospital	Stafford	Virginia	540-741-9000	www.marywashingtonhealthcare.com
Swedish Covenant Hospital	Chicago	Illinois	773-878-8200	www.swedishcovenant.org
Tomball Regional Medical Center	Tomball	Texas	281-351-1623	www.tomballhospital.org
Tri Valley Health System	Cambridge	Nebraska	308-697-3329	www.trivalleyhealth.com
Tri - City Regional Medical Center	Hawaiian Gardens	California	562-860-0401	www.tri-cityrmc.org
Trumbull Memorial Hospital	Warren	Ohio	330-841-9011	www.trumhosp.org
Tufts Medical Center	Boston	Massachusetts	617-636-5000	www.tuftsmedicalcenter.org
United Regional Medical Center	Manchester	Tennessee	931-728-3586	www.urmchealthcare.com
University Medical Center of Princeton at Plainsboro	Plainsboro	New Jersey	866-460-4776	www.princetonhcs.org
University Hospitals - Elyria Medical Center	Elyria	Ohio	440-329-7500	www.emh-healthcare.org
University of California San Diego Medical Center	San Diego	California	619-543-6222	www.health.ucsd.edu
University of Maryland Shore Medical Center at Easton	Easton	Maryland	410-822-1000	www.shorehealth.org
University of Michigan Health System	Ann Arbor	Michigan	734-764-1505	www.med.umich.edu
University of Texas Health Science Center at Tyler	Tyler	Texas	903-877-7777	www.uthct.edu
UPMC Mckeesport	Mc Keesport	Pennsylvania	412-664-2000	www.selectmedicalcorp.com
VA Boston Healthcare System - Jamaica Plain	Jamaica Plain	Massachusetts	617-232-9500	www.vaww.visn1.med.va.gov/boston
VA North Florida/South Georgia Healthcare System	Gainesville	Florida	352-376-1611	www.northflorida.va.gov
VA Sierra Nevada Healthcare System	Reno	Nevada	775-328-1263	www.reno.va.gov
Valley Hospital	Ridgewood	New Jersey	201-447-8000	www.valleyhealth.com
VHS Harlingen Hospital Company	Harlingen	Texas	956-389-1100	www.vbmc.org
Virginia Mason Medical Center	Seattle	Washington	206-223-6600	www.vmmc.org
W Palm Beach VA Medical Center	West Palm Beach	Florida	561-422-8600	www.va.gov
Waukesha Memorial Hospital	Waukesha	Wisconsin	262-928-1000	www.waukeshamemorial.org
Weirton Medical Center	Weirton	West Virginia	304-797-6000	www.weirtonmedical.com
West Anaheim Medical Center	Anaheim	California	714-827-3000	www.wamc.phcs.us
West Haven VA Medical Center	West Haven	Connecticut	203-932-5711	www.visn1.med.va.gov/vact
Wheaton Franciscan Healthcare Saint Francis	Milwaukee	Wisconsin	414-647-5000	www.mywheaton.org
White Memorial Medical Center	Los Angeles	California	323-268-5000	www.whitememorial.com
William Beaumont Hospital - Troy	Troy	Michigan	248-964-8800	www.beaumonthospitals.com
Willis Knighton Medical Center	Shreveport	Louisiana	318-212-4000	www.wkhs.com//locations/medicalcenter.aspx
Yale-New Haven Hospital	New Haven	Connecticut	203-688-4242	www.ynhh.org

Note: Table shows hospitals nationwide whose pneumonia 30-day risk-adjusted mortality rate is better (lower) than U.S. rate of 11.9%

Hospitals whose Pneumonia 30-Day Mortality Rate is Worse (Higher) than the U.S. National Rate

Hospital	City	State	Phone	Web Site
Abilene Regional Medical Center	Abilene	Texas	325-428-1000	www.abileneregional.com
Acmh Hospital	Kittanning	Pennsylvania	724-543-8404	www.acmh.org
Albemarle Hospital Authority	Elizabeth City	North Carolina	252-335-0531	www.albemarlehealth.org
Antelope Valley Hospital	Lancaster	California	661-949-5000	www.avhospital.org
Aspirus Grand View Hospital	Ironwood	Michigan	906-932-2525	www.gvhs.org
Augusta VA Medical Center	Augusta	Georgia	706-823-2201	www.va.gov
Auxilio Mutuo Hospital	Hato Rey	Puerto Rico	787-758-2000	www.auxiliopr.com
Avera Sacred Heart Hospital	Yankton	South Dakota	605-668-8000	www.avera.org/sacred-heart
Bacon County Hospital	Alma	Georgia	912-632-8961	www.baconcountyhospital.com
Baptist Memorial Hospital/Golden Triangle	Columbus	Mississippi	662-244-1500	www.bmhcc.org/facilities/goldentriangle
Baptist Memorial Hospital Union City	Union City	Tennessee	731-885-2410	www.bmhcc.org
Baxter Regional Medical Center	Mountain Home	Arkansas	870-508-1000	www.baxterregional.org
Bay Area Hospital	Coos Bay	Oregon	541-269-8111	www.bayareahospital.org
Bolivar Medical Center	Cleveland	Mississippi	662-846-2551	www.bolivarmedical.com
Bon Secours Maryview Medical Center	Portsmouth	Virginia	757-398-2200	www.bonsecourshamptonroads.com
Caldwell Medical Center	Princeton	Kentucky	270-365-0300	www.caldwellhosp.org
Cameron Regional Medical Center	Cameron	Missouri	816-632-2101	www.cameronregional.org
Carilion Roanoke Memorial Hospital	Roanoke	Virginia	540-981-7000	www.carilion.com/crmh
Carondelet Saint Joseph's Hospital	Tucson	Arizona	520-873-3000	www.carondelet.org
Carson Tahoe Regional Medical Center	Carson City	Nevada	775-445-8000	www.carsontahoehospital.com
Catawba Valley Medical Center	Hickory	North Carolina	828-326-3809	www.catawbavalleymc.org
Central Carolina Hospital	Sanford	North Carolina	919-774-2100	www.centralcarolinahosp.com
Citizens Memorial Hospital	Bolivar	Missouri	417-326-6000	www.citizensmemorial.com
Cleveland Regional Medical Center	Shelby	North Carolina	704-487-3000	www.clevelandregional.org
Community Hospital East	Indianapolis	Indiana	317-355-5411	www.ecommunity.com
Conway Regional Medical Center	Conway	Arkansas	501-329-3831	www.conwayregional.org
Coshocton County Memorial Hospital	Coshocton	Ohio	740-622-6411	www.ccmh.com
Dallas County Medical Center	Fordyce	Arkansas	870-352-6300	www.dallascountymedicalcenter.com
Dekalb Regional Medical Center	Fort Payne	Alabama	256-845-3150	www.baptistmedical.org
Delano Regional Medical Center	Delano	California	661-725-4800	www.drmc.com
Desert Springs Hospital	Las Vegas	Nevada	702-369-7600	www.desertspringshospital.net/p12.html
Doctors Medical Center	Modesto	California	209-578-1211	www.dmc-modesto.com
East Georgia Regional Medical Center	Statesboro	Georgia	912-486-1500	www.egrmc.com
East Liverpool City Hospital	East Liverpool	Ohio	330-385-7200	www.elch.org
Eastern Niagara Hospital	Lockport	New York	716-514-5700	www.enhs.org
El Centro Regional Medical Center	El Centro	California	760-339-7100	www.ecrmc.org
Eliza Coffee Memorial Hospital	Florence	Alabama	256-768-8400	www.chgroup.org
Erlanger Medical Center	Chattanooga	Tennessee	423-778-7000	www.erlanger.org
Essentia Health Saint Mary's Medical Center	Duluth	Minnesota	218-786-4000	www.smdc.org
Florida Hospital Deland	Deland	Florida	386-943-4772	www.fhdeland.org
Floyd County Memorial Hospital	Charles City	Iowa	641-228-6830	www.fcmc.us.com
Franklin General Hospital	Hampton	Iowa	641-456-5000	www.franklingeneral.com
Franklin Medical Center	Winnsboro	Louisiana	318-435-9411	www.fmc-cares.com
Fremont Area Medical Center	Fremont	Nebraska	402-721-1610	www.famc.org
Frye Regional Medical Center	Hickory	North Carolina	828-322-6070	www.fryemedctr.com
Fulton County Hospital	Salem	Arkansas	870-895-2691	www.fultoncountyhospital.org
GV (Sonny) Montgomery VA Medical Center Jackson	Jackson	Mississippi	601-362-4471	www.visn16.med.va.gov
Gadsden Regional Medical Center	Gadsden	Alabama	256-494-4000	www.gadsdenregional.com
Galesburg Cottage Hospital	Galesburg	Illinois	309-345-4555	www.cottagehospital.com
Gateway Medical Center	Clarksville	Tennessee	931-502-1000	www.todaysgateway.com
GHS Laurens County Memorial Hospital	Clinton	South Carolina	864-833-9100	www.lchcs.org
Glenwood Regional Medical Center	West Monroe	Louisiana	318-329-4600	www.grmc.com
Good Samaritan Hospital	Kearney	Nebraska	308-865-7100	www.gshs.org
Good Samaritan Hospital	Lebanon	Pennsylvania	717-270-7500	www.gshleb.org
Greenview Regional Hospital	Bowling Green	Kentucky	270-793-1000	www.greenviewhospital.com
Grossmont Hospital	La Mesa	California	619-465-0711	www.sharp.com
Halifax Health Medical Center	Daytona Beach	Florida	386-254-4000	www.halifax.org
Hammond Henry Hospital	Geneseo	Illinois	309-944-6431	www.hammondhenry.com
Harrison County Hospital	Corydon	Indiana	812-738-4251	www.hchin.org
Harrison Memorial Hospital	Cynthiana	Kentucky	859-234-2300	www.harrisonmemhosp.com
Harton Regional Medical Center	Tullahoma	Tennessee	931-393-3000	www.hartonmedicalcenter.com
Helen Keller Memorial Hospital	Sheffield	Alabama	256-386-4556	www.helenkeller.com
Helena Regional Medical Center	Helena	Arkansas	870-338-5800	www.helenaregionalmedicalcenter.com
Hemet Valley Medical Center	Hemet	California	951-652-2811	www.valleyhealthsystem.com/hemmain
Highland Hospital	Rochester	New York	585-473-2200	www.urmc.rochester.edu

Hospital	City	State	Phone	Web Site
Highlands Regional Medical Center	Sebring	Florida	863-385-6101	www.highlandsregional.com
Highline Medical Center	Burien	Washington	206-244-9970	www.hchnet.org
Hospital Pavia Santurce	Fernandez Juncos	Puerto Rico	787-727-6060	www.paviahospitalsanturce.com
Howard Memorial Hospital	Nashville	Arkansas	870-845-4400	www.howardmemorial.com
Hutchinson Regional Medical Center	Hutchinson	Kansas	620-665-2001	www.hutchinsonhospital.com
Iberia General Hospital & Medical Center	New Iberia	Louisiana	337-364-0441	www.iberiamedicalcenter.com
Indiana University Health Bloomington Hospital	Bloomington	Indiana	812-353-9555	www.bloomingtonhospital.org
Indiana University Health La Porte Hospital	La Porte	Indiana	219-326-1234	www.laportehealth.org
Inspira Medical Center Vineland	Vineland	New Jersey	856-641-6610	www.sjhs.com
Integris Grove Hospital	Grove	Oklahoma	918-786-2243	www.integris-health.com
IU Health Goshen Hospital	Goshen	Indiana	574-364-1000	www.goshenhosp.com
Jackson Hospital & Clinic	Montgomery	Alabama	334-293-8000	www.jackson.org
Jackson Memorial Hospital	Miami	Florida	305-585-1111	www.jhsmiami.org
Jacksonville Medical Center	Jacksonville	Alabama	256-782-4538	www.jmchealth.com
Jane Phillips Medical Center	Bartlesville	Oklahoma	918-333-7200	www.jpmc.org
Jeff Davis Hospital	Hazlehurst	Georgia	912-375-7781	www.jeffdavishospital.org
Jennie Stuart Medical Center	Hopkinsville	Kentucky	270-887-0100	www.jsmc.org
JFK Medical Center - A M Yelencsics Comm Hospital	Edison	New Jersey	732-321-7000	www.jfkmc.org
Keokuk Area Hospital	Keokuk	Iowa	319-524-7150	www.keokukhealthsystems.org
Lafayette General Medical Center	Lafayette	Louisiana	337-289-7991	www.lafayettegeneral.org
Lake Charles Memorial Hospital	Lake Charles	Louisiana	337-494-3200	www.lcmh.com
Lake Cumberland Regional Hospital	Somerset	Kentucky	606-679-7441	www.lakecumberlandhospital.com
Lake Granbury Medical Center	Granbury	Texas	817-573-2683	www.lakegranburymedicalcenter.com
Lexington Medical Center	West Columbia	South Carolina	803-791-2000	www.lexmed.com
Lexington VA Medical Center	Lexington	Kentucky	859-233-4511	www.lexington.va.gov
Livingston Regional Hospital	Livingston	Tennessee	931-823-5611	www.livingstonregionalhospital.com
Lompoc Valley Medical Center	Lompoc	California	805-737-3300	www.lompochospital.org
Louisville VA Medical Center	Louisville	Kentucky	502-287-4000	www.va.gov/603louisville
Madera Community Hospital	Madera	California	559-675-5555	www.maderahospital.org
Mahaska Health Partnership	Oskaloosa	Iowa	641-672-3100	www.mahaskahospital.com
Margaret Mary Community Hospital	Batesville	Indiana	812-934-6624	www.mmch.org
Marion General Hospital	Columbia	Mississippi	601-736-6303	
Marshall Medical Center South	Boaz	Alabama	256-593-8310	www.mmcenters.com/mmcsouth.php
McGehee Hospital	Mcgehee	Arkansas	870-222-5600	
Medical Center Hospital	Odessa	Texas	432-640-4000	www.mchodessa.com
Memorial Medical Center	Modesto	California	209-526-4500	www.memorialmedicalcenter.org
Memorial Healthcare	Owosso	Michigan	989-723-5211	www.memorialhealthcare.org
Memorial Hospital & Manor	Bainbridge	Georgia	229-246-3500	www.mh-m.org
Memorial Hospital of Martinsville & Henry County	Martinsville	Virginia	276-666-7200	www.martinsvillehospital.com
Memorial Hospital of South Bend	South Bend	Indiana	574-647-1000	www.qualityoflife.org
Memorial Medical Center of East Texas	Lufkin	Texas	936-634-8111	www.mymemorialhealth.org
Mercy Health - West Hospital	Cincinnati	Ohio	513-215-5000	www.e-mercy.com/west-hospital.aspx
Mercy Hospital Oklahoma City	Oklahoma City	Oklahoma	405-752-3754	www.mercyok.net/mhc
Mercy Hospital Springfield	Springfield	Missouri	417-820-2000	www.stjohns.com
Mercy Medical Center	Merced	California	209-564-5000	www.mercymercedcares.org
Mercy Medical Center	Rockville Centre	New York	516-705-2525	www.mercymedicalcenter.info
Mercy Medical Center - Mount Shasta	Mount Shasta	California	530-926-6111	www.mercymtshasta.org
Mercy Memorial Health Center	Ardmore	Oklahoma	405-223-5400	www.mercyok.com/mmhc
Methodist Healthcare Memphis Hospitals	Memphis	Tennessee	901-516-8274	www.methodisthealth.org
Mid Coast Hospital	Brunswick	Maine	207-729-0181	www.midcoasthealth.com
Midtown Medical Center	Columbus	Georgia	706-571-1000	www.columbusregional.com
Milford Hospital	Milford	Connecticut	203-876-4000	www.milfordhospital.org
Mississippi Baptist Medical Center	Jackson	Mississippi	601-968-1000	www.mbmc.org
Mizell Memorial Hospital	Opp	Alabama	334-493-3541	www.mizellmh.com
Mobile Infirmary	Mobile	Alabama	251-435-4700	www.mimc.com
Morris Hospital & Healthcare Centers	Morris	Illinois	815-942-2932	www.morrishospital.org
Mount Carmel West	Columbus	Ohio	614-234-5000	www.mountcarmelhealth.com
Multicare Good Samaritan Hospital	Puyallup	Washington	253-697-2102	www.multicare.org/goodsam
Neshoba County General Hospital	Philadelphia	Mississippi	601-663-1200	www.neshobageneral.com
New London Family Medical Center	New London	Wisconsin	920-531-2000	www.thedacare.org
North Mississippi Medical Center	Tupelo	Mississippi	662-377-3000	www.nmhs.net/nmmc
North Valley Hospital	Whitefish	Montana	406-863-3550	www.nvhosp.org
Northern Louisiana Medical Center	Ruston	Louisiana	318-254-2100	www.lincolnhealth.com
Novant Health Rowan Medical Center	Salisbury	North Carolina	704-210-5000	www.rowan.org
Novant Health Thomasville Medical Center	Thomasville	North Carolina	336-472-2000	www.thomasvillemedicalcenter.org
Och Regional Medical Center	Starkville	Mississippi	662-323-4320	www.och.org
Ohio Valley General Hospital	Mckees Rocks	Pennsylvania	412-777-6161	www.ohiovalleyhospital.org

Hospital	City	State	Phone	Web Site
Olympic Medical Center	Port Angeles	Washington	360-417-7000	www.olympicmedical.org
Orange Park Medical Center	Orange Park	Florida	904-276-8500	www.opmedical.com
Paris Regional Medical Center	Paris	Texas	903-785-4521	www.parisregional.com
Passavant Area Hospital	Jacksonville	Illinois	217-245-9551	www.passavanthospital.com
Petaluma Valley Hospital	Petaluma	California	707-778-1111	www.stjosephhealth.org
Peterson Regional Medical Center	Kerrville	Texas	830-896-4200	www.petersonrmc.com
Piedmont Medical Center	Rock Hill	South Carolina	803-329-1234	www.piedmontmedicalcenter.com
Pike Community Hospital	Waverly	Ohio	740-947-2186	www.adena.org
Pinnacle Health Hospitals	Harrisburg	Pennsylvania	717-782-5181	www.pinnaclehealth.org
Pottstown Memorial Medical Center	Pottstown	Pennsylvania	610-327-7000	www.pmmctr.org
Rappahannock General Hospital	Kilmarnock	Virginia	804-435-8000	www.rgh-hospital.com
Redlands Community Hospital	Redlands	California	909-335-5500	www.redlandshospital.com
River Parishes Hospital	Laplace	Louisiana	985-652-7000	www.riverparisheshospital.com
River Valley Medical Center	Dardanelle	Arkansas	479-229-4677	
Rockcastle County Hospital	Mount Vernon	Kentucky	606-256-2195	www.rockcastlehospital.com
Rush Foundation Hospital	Meridian	Mississippi	601-483-0011	www.rushhealthsystems.org
Rush Memorial Hospital	Rushville	Indiana	765-932-7513	www.rushmemorial.com
Russell Hospital	Alexander City	Alabama	256-329-7100	www.russellmedcenter.com
Saint Joseph Mount Sterling	Mount Sterling	Kentucky	859-498-1220	www.marychiles.org
San Gorgonio Memorial Hospital	Banning	California	951-769-2101	www.sgmh.org
San Juan VA Medical Center	San Juan	Puerto Rico	800-449-8729	www.visn8.med.va.gov/caribbean
Sentara Careplex Hospital	Hampton	Virginia	757-736-1000	www.sentara.com
Sentara Leigh Hospital	Norfolk	Virginia	757-261-6601	www.sentara.com
Sentara Obici Hospital	Suffolk	Virginia	757-934-4000	www.sentara.com
Seven Rivers Regional Medical Center	Crystal River	Florida	352-795-6560	www.srrmc.com
Shands Live Oak Regional Medical Center	Live Oak	Florida	904-362-1413	www.shands.org
Sierra View District Hospital	Porterville	California	559-784-1110	www.sierra-view.com
Skyridge Medical Center	Cleveland	Tennessee	423-339-4132	www.skyridgemedcenter.com
Somerset Medical Center	Somerville	New Jersey	908-685-2200	www.somersetmedicalcenter.com
South Central Regional Medical Center	Laurel	Mississippi	601-649-4000	www.scrmc.com
South Shore Hospital	South Weymouth	Massachusetts	781-340-8000	www.southshorehospital.org
Southampton Memorial Hospital	Franklin	Virginia	757-569-6100	www.smhfranklin.com
Southern Virginia Regional Medical Center	Emporia	Virginia	434-348-4400	www.svrmc.com
Spectrum Health - Reed City Campus	Reed City	Michigan	231-832-3271	www.spectrum-health.org
Spencer Municipal Hospital	Spencer	Iowa	712-264-8300	www.spencerhospital.org
Springfield Regional Medical Center	Springfield	Ohio	937-523-1000	www.communityhospital.com
Springs Memorial Hospital	Lancaster	South Carolina	803-286-1481	www.springsmemorial.com
Saint Anthony Regional Hospital & Nursing Home	Carroll	Iowa	712-792-3581	www.stanthonyhospital.org
Saint Anthony Shawnee Hospital	Shawnee	Oklahoma	405-273-2270	www.unityhealthcenter.com
Saint Catherine Hospital	Garden City	Kansas	620-272-2561	www.stcath-hosp.org
Saint Francis Community Hospital	Federal Way	Washington	253-944-8100	www.fhshealth.org
Saint Francis Hospital	Litchfield	Illinois	217-324-2191	www.stfrancis-litchfield.org
Saint Francis Hospital	Memphis	Tennessee	901-765-1000	www.saintfrancishosp.com
Saint Francis Hospital	Columbus	Georgia	706-596-4020	www.wecareforlife.com
Saint Francis - Downtown	Greenville	South Carolina	864-255-1000	www.stfrancishealth.org
Saint Joseph Hospital	Orange	California	714-633-9111	www.sjo.org
Saint Joseph Hospital & Health Center	Kokomo	Indiana	765-456-5300	www.stvincent.org
Saint Joseph's Hospital - Savannah	Savannah	Georgia	912-819-4100	www.sjchs.org
Saint Joseph's Medical Center of Stockton	Stockton	California	209-943-2000	www.stjospehscares.org
Saint Peter's Hospital	Helena	Montana	406-442-2480	www.stpetes.org
Saint Vincent Dunn Hospital	Bedford	Indiana	812-275-3331	www.stvincent.org/St-Vincent-Dunn
Saint Vincent's East	Birmingham	Alabama	205-838-3122	www.nolandhealth.com
Starr Regional Medical Center Athens	Athens	Tennessee	423-745-1411	www.athensrmc.com
Sumner Regional Medical Center	Gallatin	Tennessee	615-452-4210	www.mysumnermedical.com
Sunbury Community Hospital	Sunbury	Pennsylvania	570-286-3333	www.schopc.org
Sunrise Hospital & Medical Center	Las Vegas	Nevada	702-731-8000	www.sunrisehospital.com
Teche Regional Medical Center	Morgan City	Louisiana	985-384-2200	www.techeregional.com
Terrebonne General Medical Center	Houma	Louisiana	985-873-4141	www.tgmc.com
Texoma Medical Center	Denison	Texas	903-416-4000	www.texomamedicalcenter.net
Thibodaux Regional Medical Center	Thibodaux	Louisiana	985-447-5500	www.thibodaux.com
Thomas Memorial Hospital	South Charleston	West Virginia	304-766-3600	www.thomaswv.org
Trinity Medical Center	Birmingham	Alabama	205-592-1000	www.bhsala.com/montclair
Trinity Rock Island	Rock Island	Illinois	309-779-5000	www.trinityqc.com
Tuality Community Hospital	Hillsboro	Oregon	503-681-1111	www.tuality.com
Twin County Regional Hospital	Galax	Virginia	276-236-8181	www.tcrh.org
Union General Hospital	Farmerville	Louisiana	318-368-9751	www.uniongen.org
United Health Services Hospitals	Johnson City	New York	607-763-6000	www.vhs.ent

Hospital	City	State	Phone	Web Site
University Mcduffie County Regional Medical Center	Thomson	Georgia	706-595-1411	www.mrmc.org
University of Missouri Health Care	Columbia	Missouri	573-882-4141	www.missouri.edu
Upson Regional Medical Center	Thomaston	Georgia	706-647-8111	www.urmc.org
Upstate New York VA Healthcare System - Western NY	Buffalo	New York	716-862-3611	www.buffalo.va.gov
Utah Valley Regional Medical Center	Provo	Utah	801-373-7850	www.intermountainhealthcare.org/hospitals/uvrmc
VA Middle Tennessee Healthcare System	Nashville	Tennessee	615-327-5332	www.tennesseevalley.va.gov
VA Salt Lake City Healthcare - George E. Wahlen VA	Salt Lake City	Utah	801-584-1211	www1.va.gov/directory/guide/facility.asp?
Vidant Edgecombe Hospital	Tarboro	North Carolina	252-641-7700	www.vidanthealth.com/edgecombe
Vista Medical Center East	Waukegan	Illinois	847-360-4000	www.vistahealth.com
Western Plains Medical Complex	Dodge City	Kansas	620-225-8400	www.westernplainsmc.com
Wilkes-Barre General Hospital	Wilkes-Barre	Pennsylvania	570-829-8111	www.wvhcs.org
Wilson Medical Center	Wilson	North Carolina	252-399-8040	www.wilmed.org/contact.asp
Wise Regional Health System	Decatur	Texas	940-627-5921	www.wiseregional.com
Woodland Heights Medical Center	Lufkin	Texas	936-634-8311	www.woodlandheights.net
Woodland Memorial Hospital	Woodland	California	530-662-3961	www.woodlandhealthcare.org
Yakima Valley Memorial Hospital	Yakima	Washington	509-575-8000	www.yakimamemorialhospital.org
Yuma Regional Medical Center	Yuma	Arizona	928-336-7275	www.yumaregional.org

Note: Table shows hospitals nationwide whose pneumonia 30-day risk-adjusted mortality rate is worse (higher) than U.S. rate of 11.9%

Hospital Mortality from Heart Attack: State and National Summary

Area	Number of Hospitals			
	Better than U.S. National Rate[1]	Worse than U.S. National Rate[2]	No Different than U.S. National Rate[3]	Number of Cases Too Small[4]
U.S. and Territories	77	19	2579	1889
Alabama	0	0	50	50
Alaska	0	0	5	15
American Samoa	0	0	0	1
Arizona	1	0	49	19
Arkansas	1	2	30	40
California	7	1	219	103
Colorado	0	0	33	35
Connecticut	2	0	28	1
Delaware	1	0	5	1
District of Columbia	0	0	6	2
Florida	3	1	157	22
Georgia	0	0	74	65
Guam	0	0	1	0
Hawaii	0	0	12	4
Idaho	0	0	10	23
Illinois	8	0	112	61
Indiana	1	0	68	49
Iowa	0	0	35	81
Kansas	1	0	29	91
Kentucky	0	1	51	43
Louisiana	0	1	49	52
Maine	1	1	30	5
Maryland	1	0	40	6
Massachusetts	4	0	54	6
Michigan	6	3	72	49
Minnesota	1	0	36	85
Mississippi	0	0	34	50
Missouri	4	0	57	54
Montana	0	0	8	39
N. Mariana Islands	0	0	0	1
Nebraska	0	0	20	56
Nevada	0	1	18	13
New Hampshire	1	1	17	6
New Jersey	8	1	54	3
New Mexico	0	0	13	26
New York	10	1	141	31
North Carolina	2	0	83	24
North Dakota	0	1	8	32
Ohio	1	0	112	47
Oklahoma	0	0	35	71
Oregon	0	0	29	31
Pennsylvania	6	1	122	33
Puerto Rico	0	0	21	24
Rhode Island	2	0	9	0
South Carolina	0	0	42	20
South Dakota	1	0	10	40
Tennessee	1	0	66	46
Texas	2	3	189	149
Utah	0	0	16	19
Vermont	0	0	10	5
Virgin Islands	0	0	1	1
Virginia	0	0	73	9
Washington	0	0	44	40
West Virginia	1	0	29	24
Wisconsin	0	0	60	62
Wyoming	0	0	3	24

Note: (1) 30-day risk-adjusted mortality rate is better (lower) than U.S. rate of 15.2%; (2) 30-day risk-adjusted mortality rate is worse (higher) than U.S. rate of 15.2%; (3) 30-day risk-adjusted mortality rate is about the same as U.S. rate of 15.2%; (4) The number of cases is too small to classify the hospital

Hospital Mortality from Heart Failure: State and National Summary

Area	Number of Hospitals			
	Better than U.S. National Rate[1]	Worse than U.S. National Rate[2]	No Different than U.S. National Rate[3]	Number of Cases Too Small[4]
U.S. and Territories	181	139	3732	725
Alabama	1	2	89	8
Alaska	0	1	9	12
American Samoa	0	0	0	1
Arizona	2	1	57	17
Arkansas	0	11	59	7
California	30	10	246	51
Colorado	0	0	55	19
Connecticut	4	3	24	1
Delaware	1	0	6	0
District of Columbia	2	0	6	0
Florida	8	5	166	8
Georgia	1	2	126	15
Guam	0	0	1	0
Hawaii	0	0	14	5
Idaho	0	1	21	15
Illinois	16	5	156	7
Indiana	3	7	108	2
Iowa	0	2	95	21
Kansas	0	1	83	49
Kentucky	0	1	92	3
Louisiana	2	6	82	19
Maine	0	1	34	2
Maryland	9	2	35	1
Massachusetts	14	1	47	2
Michigan	12	3	106	14
Minnesota	2	0	81	48
Mississippi	0	3	77	18
Missouri	4	5	96	11
Montana	0	0	26	35
N. Mariana Islands	0	0	0	1
Nebraska	0	2	48	35
Nevada	1	2	27	5
New Hampshire	0	0	25	1
New Jersey	13	1	52	0
New Mexico	0	2	30	9
New York	13	7	156	7
North Carolina	4	3	97	8
North Dakota	0	0	24	20
Ohio	6	3	144	13
Oklahoma	2	3	84	29
Oregon	1	2	49	8
Pennsylvania	16	6	136	6
Puerto Rico	0	0	28	21
Rhode Island	0	0	11	1
South Carolina	1	3	57	2
South Dakota	0	1	26	26
Tennessee	0	2	107	7
Texas	8	8	294	62
Utah	0	1	24	17
Vermont	0	2	12	1
Virgin Islands	0	0	2	0
Virginia	1	2	79	2
Washington	0	7	58	24
West Virginia	1	0	47	6
Wisconsin	3	8	101	12
Wyoming	0	1	17	11

Note: (1) 30-day risk-adjusted mortality rate is better (lower) than U.S. rate of 11.7%; (2) 30-day risk-adjusted mortality rate is worse (higher) than U.S. rate of 11.7%; (3) 30-day risk-adjusted mortality rate is about the same as U.S. rate of 11.7%; (4) The number of cases is too small to classify the hospital

Hospital Mortality from Pneumonia: State and National Summary

Area	Number of Hospitals			
	Better than U.S. National Rate[1]	Worse than U.S. National Rate[2]	No Different than U.S. National Rate[3]	Number of Cases Too Small[4]
U.S. and Territories	203	223	4014	377
Alabama	0	13	84	4
Alaska	0	0	15	7
American Samoa	0	0	1	0
Arizona	3	2	66	10
Arkansas	0	8	66	3
California	34	19	244	45
Colorado	2	0	60	13
Connecticut	4	1	27	0
Delaware	0	0	7	0
District of Columbia	0	0	8	0
Florida	9	7	167	5
Georgia	1	11	128	3
Guam	0	0	1	0
Hawaii	0	0	14	8
Idaho	0	0	33	6
Illinois	16	7	157	4
Indiana	1	10	107	2
Iowa	2	6	105	5
Kansas	0	3	116	13
Kentucky	2	9	85	0
Louisiana	1	11	86	14
Maine	0	1	35	1
Maryland	8	0	37	1
Massachusetts	10	1	51	3
Michigan	10	3	116	6
Minnesota	1	1	112	17
Mississippi	0	10	78	10
Missouri	7	4	101	5
Montana	1	2	39	20
N. Mariana Islands	0	0	1	0
Nebraska	1	2	70	13
Nevada	3	3	24	6
New Hampshire	1	0	25	0
New Jersey	15	3	48	0
New Mexico	0	0	38	4
New York	14	6	161	4
North Carolina	6	9	94	4
North Dakota	0	0	39	5
Ohio	9	6	146	4
Oklahoma	2	5	101	11
Oregon	1	2	54	3
Pennsylvania	10	7	143	5
Puerto Rico	0	3	26	21
Rhode Island	1	0	10	1
South Carolina	1	5	55	2
South Dakota	0	1	49	6
Tennessee	2	13	96	5
Texas	13	10	306	48
Utah	0	2	33	7
Vermont	0	0	15	0
Virgin Islands	0	0	2	0
Virginia	5	10	67	5
Washington	2	5	73	9
West Virginia	1	1	51	1
Wisconsin	4	1	115	5
Wyoming	0	0	26	3

Note: (1) 30-day risk-adjusted mortality rate is better (lower) than U.S. rate of 11.9%; (2) 30-day risk-adjusted mortality rate is worse (higher) than U.S. rate of 11.9%; (3) 30-day risk-adjusted mortality rate is about the same as U.S. rate of 11.9%; (4) The number of cases is too small to classify the hospital

Appendix B: 30-Day Readmission Rates

What Do These Readmission Categories Show?

"Readmission" is when patients who have had a recent stay in the hospital go back into a hospital again. The information shows how often patients are readmitted within 30 days of discharge from a previous hospital stay for heart attack, heart failure, or pneumonia. Patients may have been readmitted back to the same hospital or to a different hospital or acute care facility. They may have been readmitted for the same condition as their recent hospital stay, or for a different reason.

This first part of this appendix shows hospitals with risk-adjusted 30-day unplanned readmission rates that are lower (better) or higher (worse) than the national rate for all three categories. Hospitals are shown to be better or worse than the U.S. national rate only if the data shows with 95% certainty, that the difference between their surgical complication rates and the U.S. national rate is not due to chance.

The second part of this appendix contains state and national summaries with the following column headers:

- **Better Than U.S. National Rate.** Hospitals in the Better Than U.S. National Rate category have risk-adjusted 30-day unplanned readmission rates that are lower than the U.S. National Rate, and with 95% certainty that this difference is not due to chance.
- **Worse Than U.S. National Rate.** Hospitals in the Worse Than U.S. National Rate category have risk-adjusted 30-day unplanned readmission rates that are higher than the U.S. National Rate, and with 95% certainty that this difference is not due to chance.
- **No Different Than U.S. National Rate.** Many hospitals in the No Different Than U.S. National Rate category have risk-adjusted 30-day unplanned readmission rates that are about the same as the U.S. National Rate. Other hospitals in this category have rates that are higher or lower than the U.S. National Rate, but without 95% certainty that these differences are not due to chance.
- **Number of Cases Too Small.** The number of cases is too small to classify the hospital..

Why are Readmission Rates for Individual Hospitals Not Shown?

Comparisons based on estimated readmission rates alone can be misleading. Risk-adjusted readmission rates are estimated for individual hospitals based on information taken from a particular time period. If a slightly different time period had been chosen, chances are that each hospital's results would have been somewhat different.

A range ("confidence interval" or in this case an "interval estimate") around estimates show how much variation might be due to this kind of chance. In this case, researchers are 95% confident that a hospital's readmission rate fell somewhere within this specified range. The smaller the range, the more precise the estimate.

When hospitals treat a very large number of patients, chance differences will not have much effect on the overall rates. The range will be small, and the estimated readmission rates will be more precise. In hospitals that treat smaller numbers of patients, however, even small chance differences could have a big impact on readmission rates. The 95% confidence interval, or range, will be large, and the estimated readmission rates will be less precise.

Because the number of patients treated at U.S. hospitals varies widely, the precision of hospitals' estimated readmission rates also varies.

Calculation of 30-Day Risk-Standardized Rates of Readmission

The 30-day readmission measures are estimates of unplanned readmission for any cause to any acute care hospital within 30 days of discharge from a hospitalization. Using unplanned readmissions within 30 days instead of over longer time periods (such as 90 days) eliminate factors outside hospitals' control such as other complicating illnesses, patients' own behavior, or care provided to patients after discharge. *The Comparative Guide to American Hospitals* reports the following 30-day readmission measures:

- 30-day unplanned readmission for heart attack (AMI) patients
- 30-day unplanned readmission for heart failure (HF) patients
- 30-day unplanned readmission for pneumonia patients
- 30-day unplanned readmission for hip/knee replacement patients
- 30-day overall rate of unplanned readmission after discharge from the hospital (hospital-wide readmission). Note: This measure includes patients admitted for internal medicine, surgery/gynecology, cardiorespiratory, cardiovascular, and neurology services. It is not a composite measure.

Which Patients are Included

The 30-day unplanned readmission measures include hospitalizations for Medicare beneficiaries aged 65 or older who were enrolled in Original Medicare (traditional fee-for-service Medicare) for the entire 12 months prior to their hospital admission (and for readmissions, for 30 days after their original admission). The AMI, heart failure, and pneumonia unplanned readmission measures also include patients aged 65 or older who were admitted to Veteran's Health Administration (VA) hospitals. Beneficiaries enrolled in Medicare managed care plans are not included. The unplanned readmission measures do not include patients who died during the index admission, or who left the hospital against medical advice.

Where the Information Comes From

The Centers for Medicare & Medicaid Services (CMS) calculates hospital-specific 30-day readmission rates using Medicare claims and eligibility information. The AMI, HF, and pneumonia readmission measures are also calculated using VA administrative data. Using administrative data makes it possible to calculate readmission rates without having to do medical chart reviews or requiring hospitals to report additional information to CMS.

Risk Adjustment

To make comparison of hospital performance equitable, the 30-day unplanned readmission measures adjust for patient characteristics that may make unplanned readmission more likely, even if the hospital provided higher quality of care. These characteristics include the patient's age, past medical history, and other diseases or conditions (comorbidities) the patient had when admitted that are known to increase the patient's risk of having an unplanned readmission.

Significance Testing

The statistical model used to calculate 30-day unplanned readmission measures also determines how precise the estimates are, and provides the upper and lower bounds of the 95% interval estimates for each hospital's readmission rates. Interval estimates, which are like confidence intervals, describe the level of uncertainty around the estimated readmission rates.

Comparing Individual Hospital Rates to the U.S. National Rate

To assign hospitals to performance categories, the hospital's interval estimate is compared to the U.S. national 30-day observed unplanned readmission rate. If the 95% interval estimate includes the national observed rate for that measure, the hospital's performance is in the "No Different than U.S. National Rate" category. If the entire 95% interval estimate is below the national observed rate for that measure, then the hospital is performing "Better Than U.S. National Rate." If the entire 95% interval estimate is above the national observed rate for that measure, its performance is "Worse Than U.S. National Rate." Hospitals with fewer than 25 eligible cases are placed into a separate category that indicates that the hospital did not have enough cases to reliably tell how well the hospital is performing.

Additional information

For more detail on how the 30-day unplanned readmission rates are calculated, please visit QualityNet—Readmission Measures at www.qualitynet.org.

Hospitals whose Acute Myocardial Infarction (Heart Attack) 30-Day Readmission Rate is Better (Lower) than the U.S. National Rate

Hospital	City	State	Phone	Web Site
Asante Rogue Regional Medical Center	Medford	Oregon	541-789-7000	www.asante.org
Aspirus Wausau Hospital	Wausau	Wisconsin	715-847-2121	www.aspirus.org
Aurora Saint Lukes Medical Center	Milwaukee	Wisconsin	414-649-6000	www.aurorahealthcare.org
Baylor Heart & Vascular Hospital	Dallas	Texas	214-820-0670	www.baylorhearthospital.com
Bellin Memorial Hospital	Green Bay	Wisconsin	920-433-3500	www.bellin.org
Central Washington Hospital	Wenatchee	Washington	509-662-1511	www.cwhs.com
Frye Regional Medical Center	Hickory	North Carolina	828-322-6070	www.fryemedctr.com
GHS Greenville Memorial Medical Center	Greenville	South Carolina	864-455-7000	www.ghs.org
Lancaster General Hospital	Lancaster	Pennsylvania	717-299-5511	www.lancastergeneral.org
Lovelace Medical Center	Albuquerque	New Mexico	505-727-8000	www.lovelace.com
Maine Medical Center	Portland	Maine	207-662-0111	www.mmc.org
Mercy Health Partners - Mercy Campus	Muskegon	Michigan	231-672-3901	www.mghp.com
Munroe Regional Medical Center	Ocala	Florida	352-351-7200	www.munroeregional.com
Parkview Regional Medical Center	Fort Wayne	Indiana	260-266-1000	www.parkview.com
Providence Sacred Heart Medical Center	Spokane	Washington	509-474-3040	www.shmc.org
Saint Joseph's Hospital of Atlanta	Atlanta	Georgia	678-843-5720	www.stjosephsatlanta.org
Sanford Medical Center Fargo	Fargo	North Dakota	701-234-2000	www.meritcare.com
Sarasota Memorial Hospital	Sarasota	Florida	941-917-9000	www.smh.com
Saint Luke's Episcopal Hospital	Houston	Texas	832-355-1000	www.sleh.com
Saint Vincent Heart Center of Indiana	Indianapolis	Indiana	317-583-5000	www.theheartcenter.com
Sutter Roseville Medical Center	Roseville	California	916-781-1000	www.sutterroseville.org
University Colo Health Memorial Hospital Central	Colorado Springs	Colorado	719-365-5000	www.memorialhospital.com
Venice Regional Medical Center - Bayfront Health	Venice	Florida	941-485-7711	www.veniceregional.com

Note: Table shows hospitals nationwide whose acute myocardial infarction 30-day readmission rate is better (lower) than U.S. rate of 18.3%

Hospitals whose Acute Myocardial Infarction (Heart Attack) 30-Day Readmission Rate is Worse (Higher) than the U.S. National Rate

Hospital	City	State	Phone	Web Site
Baxter Regional Medical Center	Mountain Home	Arkansas	870-508-1000	www.baxterregional.org
Boston Medical Center Corporation	Boston	Massachusetts	617-638-8000	www.bmc.org
Carolinas Hospital System	Florence	South Carolina	843-674-2500	www.carolinashospital.com
Centra Health	Lynchburg	Virginia	434-200-4789	www.centrahealth.com
Community Medical Center	Toms River	New Jersey	732-557-8000	www.sbhcs.com
Florida Hospital	Orlando	Florida	407-303-1976	www.floridahospital.com
Good Samaritan Regional Health Center	Mount Vernon	Illinois	618-899-1469	www.smgsi.com
Hillcrest Medical Center	Tulsa	Oklahoma	918-579-1000	www.hillcrest.com
Ingalls Memorial Hospital	Harvey	Illinois	708-333-2300	www.ingalls.org
Johnson City Medical Center	Johnson City	Tennessee	423-431-6111	www.msha.com
Kaleida Health	Buffalo	New York	716-859-8620	www.kaleidahealth.org
Lewisgale Medical Center	Salem	Virginia	540-776-4000	www.lewis-gale.com
Mercy Hospital & Medical Center	Chicago	Illinois	312-567-2000	www.mercy-chicago.org
Montefiore Medical Center	Bronx	New York	718-920-4321	www.montefiore.org
Newark Beth Israel Medical Center	Newark	New Jersey	973-926-7850	www.sbhcs.com
North Shore University Hospital	Manhasset	New York	516-562-0100	www.northshorelij.com
Northside Hospital	Saint Petersburg	Florida	813-521-5000	www.northsidehospital.com
Northwest Community Hospital	Arlington Heights	Illinois	847-618-1000	www.nch.org
Olympia Medical Center	Los Angeles	California	310-657-5900	www.olympiamc.com
Presence Saint Joseph Medical Center	Joliet	Illinois	815-725-7133	www.provena.org/stjoes
Raleigh General Hospital	Beckley	West Virginia	304-256-4100	www.raleighgeneral.com
Saint Clare's Hospital	Denville	New Jersey	973-625-6000	www.saintclares.org
Saint Michael's Medical Center	Newark	New Jersey	973-877-5350	www.cathedralhealth.org
San Juan VA Medical Center	San Juan	Puerto Rico	800-449-8729	www.visn8.med.va.gov/caribbean
Saint Joseph's Regional Medical Center	Paterson	New Jersey	973-754-2010	www.sjhmc.org
Saint Vincent's Medical Center	Bridgeport	Connecticut	203-576-5551	www.stvincents.org
Tampa VA Medical Center	Tampa	Florida	813-972-2000	www.tampa.va.gov
University Hospital - Stony Brook	Stony Brook	New York	631-444-4000	www.stonybrookmedicalcenter.org
Vidant Medical Center	Greenville	North Carolina	252-847-4100	www.uhseast.com

Note: Table shows hospitals nationwide whose acute myocardial infarction 30-day readmission rate is worse (higher) than U.S. rate of 18.3%

Hospitals whose Heart Failure 30-Day Readmission Rate is Better (Lower) than the U.S. National Rate

Hospital	City	State	Phone	Web Site
Abilene Regional Medical Center	Abilene	Texas	325-428-1000	www.abileneregional.com
Alegent Creighton Health Bergan Mercy Medical Center	Omaha	Nebraska	402-398-6060	www.alegent.com
Alpena Regional Medical Center	Alpena	Michigan	989-356-7390	www.agh.org
Asante Rogue Regional Medical Center	Medford	Oregon	541-789-7000	www.asante.org
Audrain Medical Center	Mexico	Missouri	573-582-5000	www.audrainmedicalcenter.com
Aurora Sheboygan Memorial Medical Center	Sheboygan	Wisconsin	920-451-5000	www.aurorahealthcare.org/facilities
Banner Boswell Medical Center	Sun City	Arizona	623-977-7211	www.bannerhealth.com
Banner Good Samaritan Medical Center	Phoenix	Arizona	602-239-2000	www.bannerhealth.com
Baptist Memorial Hospital	Memphis	Tennessee	901-226-5000	www.bmhcc.org
Baptist Saint Anthony's Hospital	Amarillo	Texas	806-212-2000	www.bsahs.com
Bay Medical Center Sacred Heart Health System	Panama City	Florida	850-769-1511	www.baymedical.org
Baylor All Saints Medical Center at FW	Fort Worth	Texas	817-926-2544	www.baylorhealth.com/locations/allsaints
Baylor Medical Center at Garland	Garland	Texas	972-487-5000	www.baylorhealth.com
Baylor University Medical Center	Dallas	Texas	214-820-0111	www.baylorhealth.com
Bellin Memorial Hospital	Green Bay	Wisconsin	920-433-3500	www.bellin.org
Billings Clinic Hospital	Billings	Montana	406-657-4000	www.billingsclinic.com
Boca Raton Regional Hospital	Boca Raton	Florida	561-362-5002	www.brrh.com
Boone Hospital Center	Columbia	Missouri	573-815-8000	www.boone.org
Boulder Community Hospital	Boulder	Colorado	303-440-2273	www.bch.org
Bronson Methodist Hospital	Kalamazoo	Michigan	269-341-6000	www.bronsonhealth.com
Bryan Medical Center	Lincoln	Nebraska	402-481-1111	www.bryan.org
Carolinas Medical Center/Behaviorial Health	Charlotte	North Carolina	704-355-2000	www.carolinasmedicalcenter.org
Carondelet Saint Marys Hospital	Tucson	Arizona	520-872-3000	www.carondelet.org
Catawba Valley Medical Center	Hickory	North Carolina	828-326-3809	www.catawbavalleymc.org
Cedars - Sinai Medical Center	Los Angeles	California	310-423-5000	www.cedars-sinai.edu
Central Maine Medical Center	Lewiston	Maine	207-795-0111	www.cmmc.org
Central Washington Hospital	Wenatchee	Washington	509-662-1511	www.cwhs.com
Chester County Hospital	West Chester	Pennsylvania	610-431-5000	www.cchosp.com
Christus Santa Rosa Hospital	San Antonio	Texas	210-704-2011	www.christussantarosa.org
Citrus Memorial Hospital	Inverness	Florida	352-726-1551	www.citrusmh.com
Columbia Saint Marys Hospital Ozaukee	Mequon	Wisconsin	262-243-7300	www.columbia-stmarys.org
Columbus Regional Hospital	Columbus	Indiana	812-379-4441	www.crh.org
Community Hospital of the Monterey Peninsula	Monterey	California	831-624-5311	www.chomp.org
Cox Medical Center	Springfield	Missouri	417-269-6000	www.coxhealth.com
Decatur Morgan Hospital - Decatur Campus	Decatur	Alabama	256-341-2000	www.decaturgeneral.org
Dixie Regional Medical Center	Saint George	Utah	435-251-2100	www.intermountainhealthcare.org
Dominican Hospital	Santa Cruz	California	831-462-7700	www.dominicanhospital.org
East Jefferson General Hospital	Metairie	Louisiana	504-454-4000	www.eastjeffhospital.org
Eisenhower Medical Center	Rancho Mirage	California	760-340-3911	www.emc.org
Eliza Coffee Memorial Hospital	Florence	Alabama	256-768-8400	www.chgroup.org
Elmhurst Memorial Hospital	Elmhurst	Illinois	630-833-1400	www.emhc.org
Emory University Hospital	Atlanta	Georgia	404-686-8500	www.emoryhealthcare.org
Exempla Lutheran Medical Center	Wheat Ridge	Colorado	303-425-4500	www.exemlpa.org
Fargo VA Medical Center	Fargo	North Dakota	701-232-3241	www.fargo.va.gov
Fremont Area Medical Center	Fremont	Nebraska	402-721-1610	www.famc.org
Frye Regional Medical Center	Hickory	North Carolina	828-322-6070	www.fryemedctr.com
Genesis Medical Center - Davenport	Davenport	Iowa	563-421-1000	www.genesishealth.com
GHS Greenville Memorial Medical Center	Greenville	South Carolina	864-455-7000	www.ghs.org
Hartford Hospital	Hartford	Connecticut	860-545-5000	www.harthosp.org
Hutchinson Regional Medical Center	Hutchinson	Kansas	620-665-2001	www.hutchinsonhospital.com
Integris Baptist Medical Center	Oklahoma City	Oklahoma	405-951-8110	www.integris-health.com
Intermountain Medical Center	Murray	Utah	801-507-7000	www.intermountainhealthcare.org
Iowa Methodist Medical Center	Des Moines	Iowa	515-241-6212	www.iowahealth.org
John D Archbold Memorial Hospital	Thomasville	Georgia	229-228-2880	www.archbold.org
John Muir Medical Center - Concord Campus	Concord	California	925-674-2002	www.johnmuirhealth.com
John Muir Medical Center - Walnut Creek Campus	Walnut Creek	California	925-939-3000	www.jmmdhs.com
Lancaster General Hospital	Lancaster	Pennsylvania	717-299-5511	www.lancastergeneral.org
Licking Memorial Hospital	Newark	Ohio	740-348-4000	www.lmhealth.org
Lima Memorial Health System	Lima	Ohio	419-998-4731	www.limamemorial.org
Maine Medical Center	Portland	Maine	207-662-0111	www.mmc.org
Marshalltown Medical & Surgical Center	Marshalltown	Iowa	641-754-5151	www.everydaychampions.org
Mary Hitchcock Memorial Hospital	Lebanon	New Hampshire	603-650-5000	www.dhmc.org
Mayo Clinic Health System - Eau Claire Hospital	Eau Claire	Wisconsin	715-838-3311	www.luthermidelfort.org
McKay Dee Hospital	Ogden	Utah	801-387-2800	www.intermountainhealthcare.org
Mclaren Bay Region	Bay City	Michigan	989-894-3000	www.baymed.org

Hospital	City	State	Phone	Web Site
Memorial Healthcare System	Chattanooga	Tennessee	423-495-2525	www.memorial.org
Memorial Hermann Hospital System	Houston	Texas	713-448-6796	www.memorialhermann.org
Memorial Hermann Memorial City Medical Center	Houston	Texas	713-242-3000	www.mhhs.org
Memorial Hospital of South Bend	South Bend	Indiana	574-647-1000	www.qualityoflife.org
Memorial Mission Hospital & Asheville Surgery Center	Asheville	North Carolina	828-213-1111	www.missionhospitals.org
Mercy Health Partners - Mercy Campus	Muskegon	Michigan	231-672-3901	www.mghp.com
Mercy Hospital Springfield	Springfield	Missouri	417-820-2000	www.stjohns.com
Mercy Medical Center - Redding	Redding	California	530-225-6102	www.redding.mercy.org
Methodist Charlton Medical Center	Dallas	Texas	214-947-7777	www.methodisthealthsystem.org
Methodist Hospital	San Antonio	Texas	210-575-4000	www.mh.sahealth.com
The Methodist Hospital	Houston	Texas	713-790-2221	www.methodisthealth.com
Morristown Medical Center	Morristown	New Jersey	973-971-5450	www.morristownmemorialhospital.org
Morton Plant Hospital	Clearwater	Florida	727-462-7000	www.measehospitals.com
Munson Medical Center	Traverse City	Michigan	231-935-5000	www.munsonhealthcare.org
Naples Community Hospital	Naples	Florida	239-436-5000	www.nchmd.org
New Hanover Regional Medical Center	Wilmington	North Carolina	910-343-7000	www.nhrmc.org
North Shore Medical Center	Salem	Massachusetts	978-741-1215	www.nsmc.partners.org
Northeast Georgia Medical Center	Gainesville	Georgia	770-535-3553	www.nghs.com
Oklahoma Heart Hospital	Oklahoma City	Oklahoma	405-608-3200	www.okheart.com
Owensboro Health Regional Hospital	Owensboro	Kentucky	270-688-2000	www.omhs.org
Parkview Regional Medical Center	Fort Wayne	Indiana	260-266-1000	www.parkview.com
Penn Highlands Dubois	Dubois	Pennsylvania	814-371-2200	www.drmc.org
Penn Presbyterian Medical Center	Philadelphia	Pennsylvania	215-662-8000	www.pennhealth.com
Pocono Medical Center	East Stroudsburg	Pennsylvania	570-476-3348	www.poconohealthsystem.org
Portneuf Medical Center	Pocatello	Idaho	208-239-1000	www.portmed.org
Providence Saint Peter Hospital	Olympia	Washington	360-491-9480	www.providence.org/swsa
Providence Saint Vincent Medical Center	Portland	Oregon	503-216-1234	www.providence.org
Reading Hospital	Reading	Pennsylvania	610-988-8000	www.readinghospital.org
Rex Hospital	Raleigh	North Carolina	919-784-3100	www.rexhealth.com
Roper Hospital	Charleston	South Carolina	843-724-2800	www.ropersaintfrancis.com
Sacred Heart Medical Center - Riverbend	Springfield	Oregon	541-222-7300	www.peacehealth.org/sacred-heart-riverbend
Saint Vincent Hospital	Erie	Pennsylvania	814-452-5000	www.svhs.org
Santa Rosa Memorial Hospital	Santa Rosa	California	707-525-5300	www.stjosephhealth.org
Sarasota Memorial Hospital	Sarasota	Florida	941-917-9000	www.smh.com
Scripps Green Hospital	La Jolla	California	858-554-3600	www.scrippshealth.org
Sisters of Charity Providence Hospitals	Columbia	South Carolina	803-256-5300	www.providencehospitals.com
Spartanburg Regional Medical Center	Spartanburg	South Carolina	864-560-6000	www.srhs.com
Spectrum Health - Butterworth Campus	Grand Rapids	Michigan	616-391-1774	www.spectrum-health.org
Saint Charles Medical Center - Bend	Bend	Oregon	541-382-4321	www.scmc.org
Saint Francis - Downtown	Greenville	South Carolina	864-255-1000	www.stfrancishealth.org
Saint Joseph's Hospital	Saint Paul	Minnesota	651-232-7707	www.stjosephs-stpaul.org
Saint Luke's Regional Medical Center	Boise	Idaho	208-381-2222	www.slrmc.org
Saint Vincent Hospital	Santa Fe	New Mexico	505-913-5201	www.stvin.org
Sutter Roseville Medical Center	Roseville	California	916-781-1000	www.sutterroseville.org
Tallahassee Memorial Hospital	Tallahassee	Florida	850-431-1155	www.tmh.org
Tennova Healthcare	Knoxville	Tennessee	865-545-8000	www.stmaryshealth.com
The Queens Medical Center	Honolulu	Hawaii	808-538-9011	www.queens.org
Trident Medical Center	Charleston	South Carolina	843-797-8800	www.tridenthealthsystem.com
University Colo Health Memorial Hospital Central	Colorado Springs	Colorado	719-365-5000	www.memorialhospital.com
UPMC Hamot	Erie	Pennsylvania	814-877-6000	www.hamot.org
Venice Regional Medical Center - Bayfront Health	Venice	Florida	941-485-7711	www.veniceregional.com
Virginia Hospital Center	Arlington	Virginia	703-558-5000	www.virginiahospitalcenter.com
Wesley Medical Center	Wichita	Kansas	316-962-2000	www.wesleymc.com
Williamsport Regional Medical Center	Williamsport	Pennsylvania	570-321-1000	www.susquehannahealth.org
Willis Knighton Medical Center	Shreveport	Louisiana	318-212-4000	www.wkhs.com//locations/medicalcenter.aspx

Note: Table shows hospitals nationwide whose heart failure 30-day readmission rate is better (lower) than U.S. rate of 23.0%

Hospitals whose Heart Failure 30-Day Readmission Rate is Worse (Higher) than the U.S. National Rate

Hospital	City	State	Phone	Web Site
Abbeville General Hospital	Abbeville	Louisiana	337-893-5466	www.abgen.net
Advocate Trinity Hospital	Chicago	Illinois	773-967-2000	www.advocatehealth.com/trin
Banner Baywood Medical Center	Mesa	Arizona	480-321-2000	www.bannerhealth.com
Baptist Health Medical Center - North Little Rock	North Little Rock	Arkansas	501-202-3000	www.baptist-health.org
Barnes-Jewish Hospital	Saint Louis	Missouri	314-747-3000	www.barnesjewish.org
Beaumont Health System	Royal Oak	Michigan	248-898-5000	www.beaumonthospitals.com
Beckley ARH Hospital	Beckley	West Virginia	304-255-3456	www.arh.org/beckley
Beth Israel Medical Center	New York	New York	212-420-2000	www.wehealny.org
Bolivar Medical Center	Cleveland	Mississippi	662-846-2551	www.bolivarmedical.com
Brookhaven Memorial Hospital Medical Center	Patchogue	New York	631-654-7100	www.brookhavenhospitalorg
Camden Clark Medical Center	Parkersburg	West Virginia	304-424-2111	www.ccmh.org
Capital Health System - Fuld Campus	Trenton	New Jersey	609-394-6000	www.capitalhealth.org
Capital Regional Medical Center	Tallahassee	Florida	850-656-5000	www.capitalregionalmedicalcenter.com
Carepoint Health - Bayonne Hospital Center	Bayonne	New Jersey	201-858-5000	www.bayonnemedicalcenter.org
Carepoint Health - Christ Hospital	Jersey City	New Jersey	201-795-8200	www.christhospital.org
Carepoint Health - Hoboken UMC	Hoboken	New Jersey	201-418-1004	www.bonsecoursnj.com
Carolinas Hospital System	Florence	South Carolina	843-674-2500	www.carolinashospital.com
Centegra Health System - Mc Henry Hospital	Mchenry	Illinois	815-344-5000	www.centegra.org
Chicot Memorial Medical Center	Lake Village	Arkansas	870-265-5351	www.chicotmemorial.com
Cincinnati VA Medical Center	Cincinnati	Ohio	513-861-3100	www.cincinnati.va.gov
Clinch Valley Medical Center	Richlands	Virginia	276-596-6000	www.clinchvalleymedicalcenter.com
Community Medical Center	Toms River	New Jersey	732-557-8000	www.sbhcs.com
Coney Island Hospital	Brooklyn	New York	718-616-3000	www.coneyislandhospital.com
Covenant Medical Center	Saginaw	Michigan	989-583-4000	www.covenanthealthcare.com
Crozer Chester Medical Center	Upland	Pennsylvania	610-447-2000	www.crozer.org
Culpeper Regional Hospital	Culpeper	Virginia	540-829-4100	www.culpeperhospital.com
Dallas VA Medical Center - VA North Texas	Dallas	Texas	214-742-8387	www.north-texas.med.va.gov
Danville Regional Medical Center	Danville	Virginia	434-799-2100	www.danvilleregional.org
Davis Memorial Hospital	Elkins	West Virginia	304-636-3300	www.davishealthcare.org
Detroit Receiving Hospital & University Health Center	Detroit	Michigan	313-745-3104	www.drhuhc.org
Doctors Hospital of Manteca	Manteca	California	209-823-3111	www.doctorsmanteca.com
East Georgia Regional Medical Center	Statesboro	Georgia	912-486-1500	www.egrmc.com
East Orange General Hospital	East Orange	New Jersey	973-266-4401	www.evh.org
Etmc Henderson	Henderson	Texas	903-657-7541	www.hmhtx.org
Florida Hospital	Orlando	Florida	407-303-1976	www.floridahospital.com
Flushing Hospital Medical Center	Flushing	New York	718-670-5000	www.flushinghospital.org
Forrest General Hospital	Hattiesburg	Mississippi	601-288-7000	www.forrestgeneral.com
Fountain Valley Regional Hospital & Medical Center	Fountain Valley	California	714-966-7200	www.fountainvalleyhospital.com
Franciscan Saint James Health	Olympia Fields	Illinois	708-747-4000	www.franciscanalliance.org
GV (Sonny) Montgomery VA Medical Center Jackson	Jackson	Mississippi	601-362-4471	www.visn16.med.va.gov
Georgetown Memorial Hospital	Georgetown	South Carolina	843-527-7000	www.gmhsc.com
Glenwood Regional Medical Center	West Monroe	Louisiana	318-329-4600	www.grmc.com
Griffin Hospital	Derby	Connecticut	203-732-7500	www.griffinhealth.org
Harlan Appalachian Regional Healthcare Hospital	Harlan	Kentucky	606-573-8100	www.arh.org
Harmon Memorial Hospital	Hollis	Oklahoma	580-688-3363	
Hazard ARH Regional Medical Center	Hazard	Kentucky	606-439-6600	www.arh.org/hazard
Henry Ford Hospital	Detroit	Michigan	313-916-2600	www.henryfordhospital.com
Hialeah Hospital	Hialeah	Florida	305-693-6100	www.hialeahhosp.com
Highlands Regional Medical Center	Prestonsburg	Kentucky	606-886-8511	www.hrmc.org
Hines VA Medical Center	Hines	Illinois	708-202-8387	www.visn12.med.va.gov/hines
Holy Name Medical Center	Teaneck	New Jersey	201-833-3000	www.holyname.org
Holzer Medical Center	Gallipolis	Ohio	740-446-5000	www.holzer.org
Howard University Hospital	Washington	District of Columbia	202-745-6100	www.huhosp.org
Huntington VA Medical Center	Huntington	West Virginia	304-429-0241	www.huntington.med.gov
Inspira Medical Center Woodbury	Woodbury	New Jersey	856-845-0100	www.umhospital.org
Interfaith Medical Center	Brooklyn	New York	718-613-4000	www.interfaithmedical.com
Jackson Memorial Hospital	Miami	Florida	305-585-1111	www.jhsmiami.org
Jamestown Regional Medical Center	Jamestown	Tennessee	931-879-3352	www.jamestownregional.org
Jefferson Regional Medical Center	Pittsburgh	Pennsylvania	412-469-5000	www.jeffersonregional.com
Jennings American Legion Hospital	Jennings	Louisiana	337-616-7000	www.jalh.com
Jesse Brown VA Medical Center - VA Chicago	Chicago	Illinois	312-569-8387	www.va.gov
JFK Medical Center	Atlantis	Florida	561-965-7300	www.jfkmc.com
Johns Hopkins Bayview Medical Center	Baltimore	Maryland	410-550-0123	www.hopkinsbayview.org
Jordan Hospital	Plymouth	Massachusetts	508-746-2000	www.jordanhospital.org
Kennedy University Hospital - Stratford Div	Stratford	New Jersey	856-346-6000	www.kennedyhealth.org

Hospital	City	State	Phone	Web Site
King's Daughters' Medical Center	Ashland	Kentucky	606-408-4000	www.kdmc.com
Leesburg Regional Medical Center	Leesburg	Florida	352-323-5762	www.leesburgregional.org
Lewisgale Hospital Pulaski	Pulaski	Virginia	540-994-8100	www.lewisgale.com
Libertyhealth - Jersey City Medical Center Campus	Jersey City	New Jersey	201-915-2000	www.libertyhcs.org
Lutheran Medical Center	Brooklyn	New York	718-630-8000	www.lmcmc.com
Madison River Oaks Medical Center	Canton	Mississippi	601-855-5323	www.madisonriveroaks.com
Mayo Clinic Health System - Fairmont	Fairmont	Minnesota	507-238-8101	www.fairmontmedicalcenter.org
Medical Center of Southeastern Oklahoma	Durant	Oklahoma	405-924-3080	www.mcsohealth.com
Medical Center of Trinity	Trinity	Florida	727-848-1733	www.communityhospitalnpr.com
Medstar Harbor Hospital	Baltimore	Maryland	410-350-3201	www.harborhospital.org
Memorial Hospital of Rhode Island	Pawtucket	Rhode Island	401-729-2000	www.mhriweb.org
Memorial Regional Hospital	Hollywood	Florida	954-987-2000	www.memorialregional.com
Mercy Fitzgerald Hospital	Darby	Pennsylvania	215-237-4000	www.mercyhealth.org
Mercy Hospital Saint Louis	Saint Louis	Missouri	314-569-6000	www.stjohnsmercy.org
Methodist Healthcare Memphis Hospitals	Memphis	Tennessee	901-516-8274	www.methodisthealth.org
Methodist Hospitals	Gary	Indiana	219-886-4642	www.methodisthospital.org
Metrosouth Medical Center	Blue Island	Illinois	708-597-2000	www.stfrancisblueisland.com
Midwest Regional Medical Center	Midwest City	Oklahoma	405-610-8530	www.midwestregional.com
Monmouth Medical Center - Southern Campus	Lakewood	New Jersey	732-363-1900	www.sbhcs.com
Montefiore Medical Center	Bronx	New York	718-920-4321	www.montefiore.org
Montefiore New Rochelle Hospital	New Rochelle	New York	914-632-5000	www.ssmc.org
Morton Hospital	Taunton	Massachusetts	508-828-7000	www.mortonhospital.org
Multicare Auburn Medical Center	Auburn	Washington	253-833-7711	www.armcuhs.com/p1.html
Nassau University Medical Center	East Meadow	New York	516-572-0123	www.numc.edu
New York Community Hospital of Brooklyn	Brooklyn	New York	718-692-5302	www.nych.com
New York Methodist Hospital	Brooklyn	New York	718-780-3000	www.nym.org
New York - Presbyterian Hospital	New York	New York	212-746-4189	www.nyp.org
North Carolina Baptist Hospital	Winston-Salem	North Carolina	336-716-2011	www.wfubmc.edu
North Shore Medical Center	Miami	Florida	305-835-6000	www.northshoremedical.com
North Shore University Hospital	Manhasset	New York	516-562-0100	www.northshorelij.com
Northwest Hospital Center	Randallstown	Maryland	410-521-5995	www.lifebridgehealth.org
Northwest Mississippi Regional Medical Center	Clarksdale	Mississippi	662-627-3211	www.nwmsregionalmedcenter.com
Oakwood Hospital - Dearborn	Dearborn	Michigan	313-593-7125	www.oakwood.org
Ochsner Medical Center	New Orleans	Louisiana	504-842-3000	www.ochsner.org
Olympia Medical Center	Los Angeles	California	310-657-5900	www.olympiamc.com
Orange Regional Medical Center	Middletown	New York	845-343-2424	www.ormc.org
Palisades Medical Center	North Bergen	New Jersey	201-854-5000	www.palisadesmedical.org
Palm Springs General Hospital	Hialeah	Florida	305-558-2500	www.psghosp.com
Pineville Community Hospital	Pineville	Kentucky	606-337-3051	www.pinevillehospital.com
Poplar Bluff VA Medical Center	Poplar Bluff	Missouri	573-686-4151	www.poplarbluff.va.gov
Port Huron Hospital	Port Huron	Michigan	810-987-5000	www.porthuronhospital.org
Presence Saint Joseph Medical Center	Joliet	Illinois	815-725-7133	www.provena.org/stjoes
Presence United Samaritans Medical Center	Danville	Illinois	217-443-5000	www.provena.org/usmc
Prince Georges Hospital Center	Cheverly	Maryland	301-618-2000	www.princegeorgeshospital.org
Providence VA Medical Center	Providence	Rhode Island	401-457-3042	www.visn1.med.va.gov/providence
Raritan Bay Medical Center	Perth Amboy	New Jersey	732-442-3700	www.rbmc.org
Riverview Regional Medical Center	Gadsden	Alabama	256-543-5200	www.riverviewregional.com
San Antonio VA Medical Center	San Antonio	Texas	210-617-5300	www.vasthcs.med.va.gov
San Juan VA Medical Center	San Juan	Puerto Rico	800-449-8729	www.visn8.med.va.gov/caribbean
Schuylkill Medical Center - East Norwegian Street	Pottsville	Pennsylvania	570-621-4000	www.schuylkillhealth.com
Sinai - Grace Hospital	Detroit	Michigan	313-966-3300	www.sinaigrace.org
Singing River Hospital	Pascagoula	Mississippi	228-809-5000	www.srhshealth.com
Skyridge Medical Center	Cleveland	Tennessee	423-339-4132	www.skyridgemedcenter.com
Somerset Medical Center	Somerville	New Jersey	908-685-2200	www.somersetmedicalcenter.com
South Nassau Communities Hospital	Oceanside	New York	516-632-3000	www.southnassau.org
Southcoast Hospital Group	Fall River	Massachusetts	508-679-3131	www.southcoast.org/charlton
Southeastern Regional Medical Center	Lumberton	North Carolina	910-671-5000	www.srmc.org
Southern Tennessee Medical Center	Winchester	Tennessee	931-967-8295	www.southerntennessee.com
Southside Regional Medical Center	Petersburg	Virginia	804-765-5000	www.srmconline.com
SSM Depaul Health Center	Bridgeton	Missouri	314-344-6000	www.ssmdepaul.com
SSM Saint Marys Health Center	Richmond Heights	Missouri	314-768-8000	www.ssmhealth.com/stmarys
Saint Catherine of Siena Hospital	Smithtown	New York	631-862-3000	www.stcatherines.chsli.org
Saint Francis Medical Center	Monroe	Louisiana	318-966-4000	www.stfran.com
Saint John Hospital & Medical Center	Detroit	Michigan	313-343-4000	www.stjohnprovidence.org
Saint John's Episcopal Hospital at South Shore	Far Rockaway	New York	718-869-7000	www.ehs.org
Saint John's Riverside Hospital	Yonkers	New York	914-964-4444	www.riversidehealth.org
Saint Joseph's Hospital	Tampa	Florida	813-870-4398	www.stjosephstampa.org

Hospital	City	State	Phone	Web Site
Saint Joseph's Regional Medical Center	Paterson	New Jersey	973-754-2010	www.sjhmc.org
Saint Louis - John Cochran VA Medical Center	Saint Louis	Missouri	314-652-4100	www.stlouis.va.gov
Saint Luke's Hospital Bethlehem	Bethlehem	Pennsylvania	610-954-4000	www.slhn-lehighvalley.org
Saint Luke's Roosevelt Hospital	New York	New York	212-523-4000	www.wehealny.org
Saint Mary Mercy Hospital	Livonia	Michigan	734-655-4800	www.stmarymercy.org
Saint Marys Hospital	Centralia	Illinois	618-436-6519	www.stmarys-goodsamaritan.com
Swedish Covenant Hospital	Chicago	Illinois	773-878-8200	www.swedishcovenant.org
Tampa VA Medical Center	Tampa	Florida	813-972-2000	www.tampa.va.gov
Univerity of MD Balto Washington Medical Center	Glen Burnie	Maryland	410-595-1967	www.bwmc.umms.org
University Hospital of Brooklyn - Downstate Medical Center	Brooklyn	New York	718-270-1000	www.downstate.edu
University of Miami Hospital	Miami	Florida	305-325-5511	www.cedarsmedicalcenter.com
VA Middle Tennessee Healthcare System	Nashville	Tennessee	615-327-5332	www.tennesseevalley.va.gov
VA New York Harbor Healthcare System	New York	New York	212-686-7500	www.nyharbor.va.gov
VA North Florida/South Georgia Healthcare System	Gainesville	Florida	352-376-1611	www.northflorida.va.gov
Valley Hospital	Ridgewood	New Jersey	201-447-8000	www.valleyhealth.com
W Palm Beach VA Medical Center	West Palm Beach	Florida	561-422-8600	www.va.gov
Wellmont Bristol Regional Medical Center	Bristol	Tennessee	423-844-1121	www.wellmont.org
Western Maryland Regional Medical Center	Cumberland	Maryland	240-964-8001	www.wmhs.com
Westlake Regional Hospital	Columbia	Kentucky	270-384-4753	www.westlake-healthcare.org
Whitesburg ARH Hospital	Whitesburg	Kentucky	606-633-3500	www.arh.org/whitesburg
William Beaumont Hospital - Troy	Troy	Michigan	248-964-8800	www.beaumonthospitals.com
Williamson ARH Hospital	South Williamson	Kentucky	606-237-1700	www.arh.org
Wuesthoff Medical Center Rockledge	Rockledge	Florida	321-637-2603	www.wuesthoff.org
Wyckoff Heights Medical Center	Brooklyn	New York	718-963-7272	www.wyckoffhospital.org

Note: Table shows hospitals nationwide whose heart failure 30-day readmission rate is worse (higher) than U.S. rate of 23.0%

Hospitals whose Pneumonia 30-Day Readmission Rate is Better (Lower) than the U.S. National Rate

Hospital	City	State	Phone	Web Site
Bay Medical Center Sacred Heart Health System	Panama City	Florida	850-769-1511	www.baymedical.org
Boca Raton Regional Hospital	Boca Raton	Florida	561-362-5002	www.brrh.com
Bronson Methodist Hospital	Kalamazoo	Michigan	269-341-6000	www.bronsonhealth.com
Cayuga Medical Center at Ithaca	Ithaca	New York	607-274-4401	www.cayugamed.org
Citrus Memorial Hospital	Inverness	Florida	352-726-1551	www.citrusmh.com
Eisenhower Medical Center	Rancho Mirage	California	760-340-3911	www.emc.org
Evergreen Hospital Medical Center	Kirkland	Washington	425-899-1000	www.evergreenhospital.org
Florida Hospital Waterman	Tavares	Florida	352-253-3300	www.fhwat.org
Freeman Health System - Freeman West	Joplin	Missouri	417-347-1111	www.freemanhealth.com
Kalispell Regional Medical Center	Kalispell	Montana	406-752-5111	www.krmc.org
Lake Regional Health System	Osage Beach	Missouri	573-348-8000	www.lakeregional.com
Memorial Healthcare System	Chattanooga	Tennessee	423-495-2525	www.memorial.org
Memorial Hermann Hospital System	Houston	Texas	713-448-6796	www.memorialhermann.org
Memorial Hermann Memorial City Medical Center	Houston	Texas	713-242-3000	www.mhhs.org
Memorial Medical Center of West Michigan	Ludington	Michigan	231-843-2591	www.mmcwm.com
Mercy Medical Center - Redding	Redding	California	530-225-6102	www.redding.mercy.org
Owensboro Health Regional Hospital	Owensboro	Kentucky	270-688-2000	www.omhs.org
Parkview Medical Center	Pueblo	Colorado	719-584-4000	www.parkviewmc.com
Parkview Regional Medical Center	Fort Wayne	Indiana	260-266-1000	www.parkview.com
Providence Saint Vincent Medical Center	Portland	Oregon	503-216-1234	www.providence.org
Rex Hospital	Raleigh	North Carolina	919-784-3100	www.rexhealth.com
Saint Joseph Regional Medical Center	Mishawaka	Indiana	574-335-5000	www.sjmed.com
Saint Joseph's Hospital of Atlanta	Atlanta	Georgia	678-843-5720	www.stjosephsatlanta.org
Salem Regional Medical Center	Salem	Ohio	330-332-1551	www.salemhosp.com
San Antonio Community Hospital	Upland	California	714-985-2811	www.sach.org
Sarasota Memorial Hospital	Sarasota	Florida	941-917-9000	www.smh.com
South Texas Health System	Edinburg	Texas	956-632-4000	www.edinburgregional.com
Spartanburg Regional Medical Center	Spartanburg	South Carolina	864-560-6000	www.srhs.com
Saint Edward Mercy Medical Center	Fort Smith	Arkansas	479-314-6000	www.stedwardmercy.com
Saint Francis Hospital - Roslyn	Roslyn	New York	516-562-6000	www.stfrancisheartcenter.com
Saint Francis - Downtown	Greenville	South Carolina	864-255-1000	www.stfrancishealth.org
Saint Mary's Regional Medical Center	Enid	Oklahoma	580-233-6100	www.stmarysregional.com
Saint Patrick Hospital	Missoula	Montana	406-543-7271	www.saintpatrick.org
Stormont - Vail Healthcare	Topeka	Kansas	785-354-6121	www.stormontvail.org
Virtua Memorial Hospital of Burlington County	Mount Holly	New Jersey	609-914-6200	www.virtua.org
Williamsport Regional Medical Center	Williamsport	Pennsylvania	570-321-1000	www.susquehannahealth.org
Willis Knighton Medical Center	Shreveport	Louisiana	318-212-4000	www.wkhs.com//locations/medicalcenter.aspx

Note: Table shows hospitals nationwide whose pneumonia 30-day readmission rate is better (lower) than U.S. rate of 17.6%

Hospitals whose Pneumonia 30-Day Readmission Rate is Worse (Higher) than the U.S. National Rate

Hospital	City	State	Phone	Web Site
Adena Regional Medical Center	Chillicothe	Ohio	740-779-7500	www.adena.org
Advocate Lutheran General Hospital	Park Ridge	Illinois	847-723-2210	www.advocatehealth.com
Advocate South Suburban Hospital	Hazel Crest	Illinois	708-799-8000	www.advocatehealth.com
Arnot Ogden Medical Center	Elmira	New York	607-737-4100	www.arnothealth.org
Baptist Memorial Hospital Desoto	Southaven	Mississippi	662-772-4000	www.bmhcc.org/facilities/desoto
Barnes-Jewish Hospital	Saint Louis	Missouri	314-747-3000	www.barnesjewish.org
Baxter Regional Medical Center	Mountain Home	Arkansas	870-508-1000	www.baxterregional.org
Bay Area Hospital	Coos Bay	Oregon	541-269-8111	www.bayareahospital.org
Bay Pines VA Medical Center	Bay Pines	Florida	727-398-6661	www.baypines.va.gov
Bayfront Health Punta Gorda	Punta Gorda	Florida	941-639-3131	www.charlotteregional.com
Beaumont Health System	Royal Oak	Michigan	248-898-5000	www.beaumonthospitals.com
Beckley VA Medical Center	Beckley	West Virginia	304-255-2121	www.beckley.va.gov
Beth Israel Medical Center	New York	New York	212-420-2000	www.wehealny.org
Blount Memorial Hospital	Maryville	Tennessee	865-983-7211	www.blountmemorial.org
Brandon Regional Hospital	Brandon	Florida	813-681-5551	www.brandonregionalhospital.com
Bronx VA Medical Center	Bronx	New York	718-584-9000	www.med.va.gov
Bronx - Lebanon Hospital Center	Bronx	New York	212-588-7000	www.bronx-leb.org
Brookhaven Memorial Hospital Medical Center	Patchogue	New York	631-654-7100	www.brookhavenhospitalorg
Cape Fear Valley Medical Center	Fayetteville	North Carolina	910-609-4000	www.capefearvalley.com
Casey County Hospital	Liberty	Kentucky	606-787-6275	
Chambers Memorial Hospital	Danville	Arkansas	479-495-2241	www.chambershospital.com
Cleveland Clinic	Cleveland	Ohio	216-444-2200	www.clevelandclinic.org
Cleveland - Wade Park VA Medical Center	Cleveland	Ohio	216-791-3800	www.cleveland.va.gov
Columbia MO VA Medical Center	Columbia	Missouri	573-814-6000	www.columbiamo.vc.gov
Community Hospital	Munster	Indiana	219-836-1600	www.comhs.org/community
Dallas VA Medical Center - VA North Texas	Dallas	Texas	214-742-8387	www.north-texas.med.va.gov
Davis Regional Medical Center	Statesville	North Carolina	704-873-0281	www.davisregional.com
Doctors' Community Hospital	Lanham	Maryland	301-552-8085	www.dchweb.org
East Orange General Hospital	East Orange	New Jersey	973-266-4401	www.evh.org
Florida Hospital	Orlando	Florida	407-303-1976	www.floridahospital.com
Florida Hospital Tampa	Tampa	Florida	813-615-7200	www.uch.org
Forest Hills Hospital	Forest Hills	New York	718-830-4000	www.northshorelij.com
Franklin Medical Center	Winnsboro	Louisiana	318-435-9411	www.fmc-cares.com
Garden City Hospital	Garden City	Michigan	734-421-3300	www.gchosp.org
Great River Medical Center	Blytheville	Arkansas	870-838-7300	www.greatrivermc.com
Harlan Appalachian Regional Healthcare Hospital	Harlan	Kentucky	606-573-8100	www.arh.org
Hazard ARH Regional Medical Center	Hazard	Kentucky	606-439-6600	www.arh.org/hazard
Heartland Regional Medical Center	Marion	Illinois	618-998-7000	www.heartlandregional.com
Henry Ford Hospital	Detroit	Michigan	313-916-2600	www.henryfordhospital.com
Highlands Regional Medical Center	Sebring	Florida	863-385-6101	www.highlandsregional.com
Hillcrest Hospital	Mayfield Heights	Ohio	440-312-4500	www.hillcresthospital.org
Hines VA Medical Center	Hines	Illinois	708-202-8387	www.visn12.med.va.gov/hines
Holzer Medical Center	Gallipolis	Ohio	740-446-5000	www.holzer.org
Houston VA Medical Center	Houston	Texas	713-794-7100	www.houston.med.va.gov
Howard County General Hospital	Columbia	Maryland	410-740-7890	www.hcgh.org
Huntington Hospital	Huntington	New York	631-351-2000	www.hunthosp.org
Huntington VA Medical Center	Huntington	West Virginia	304-429-0241	www.huntington.med.gov
Jackson Parish Hospital	Jonesboro	Louisiana	318-259-4435	www.jacksonparishhospital.com
Jewish Hospital & Saint Mary's Healthcare	Louisville	Kentucky	502-587-4011	www.jhhs.org
Johns Hopkins Bayview Medical Center	Baltimore	Maryland	410-550-0123	www.hopkinsbayview.org
Kennedy University Hospital - Stratford Div	Stratford	New Jersey	856-346-6000	www.kennedyhealth.org
King's Daughters' Medical Center	Ashland	Kentucky	606-408-4000	www.kdmc.com
Lake City Medical Center	Lake City	Florida	386-719-9000	www.lakecitymedical.com
Lake Health	Concord	Ohio	440-953-9600	www.lakehealth.org
Lehigh Valley Hospital - Hazleton	Hazleton	Pennsylvania	570-501-4000	www.ghha.org
Lenox Hill Hospital	New York	New York	212-439-2345	www.lenoxhillhospital.org
Little Company of Mary Hospital	Evergreen Park	Illinois	708-422-6200	www.lcmh.org
Livingston Regional Hospital	Livingston	Tennessee	931-823-5611	www.livingstonregionalhospital.com
Logan Regional Medical Center	Logan	West Virginia	304-831-1350	www.loganregionalmedicalcenter.com
Marymount Hospital	Garfield Heights	Ohio	216-581-0500	www.marymount.org
Medical Center of Southeastern Oklahoma	Durant	Oklahoma	405-924-3080	www.mcsohealth.com
Medstar Good Samaritan Hospital	Baltimore	Maryland	443-444-3902	www.goodsam-md.org
Memorial Hospital	Manchester	Kentucky	606-598-5104	www.manchestermemorial.com
Mercy Memorial Health Center	Ardmore	Oklahoma	405-223-5400	www.mercyok.com/mmhc
Metrosouth Medical Center	Blue Island	Illinois	708-597-2000	www.stfrancisblueisland.com

Hospital	City	State	Phone	Web Site
Mississippi Baptist Medical Center	Jackson	Mississippi	601-968-1000	www.mbmc.org
Monroe County Medical Center	Tompkinsville	Kentucky	270-487-9231	www.mcmccares.com
Mount Sinai Hospital	New York	New York	212-241-7981	www.mountsinai.org
Muskogee VA Medical Center	Muskogee	Oklahoma	918-577-3000	www.visn16.med.va.gov/muskogee.asp
Nassau University Medical Center	East Meadow	New York	516-572-0123	www.numc.edu
New York Hospital Medical Center of Queens	Flushing	New York	718-670-1231	www.nyhq.org
New York Methodist Hospital	Brooklyn	New York	718-780-3000	www.nym.org
North Carolina Baptist Hospital	Winston-Salem	North Carolina	336-716-2011	www.wfubmc.edu
North Oaks Medical Center	Hammond	Louisiana	985-345-2700	www.northoaks.org
Northern Westchester Hospital	Mount Kisco	New York	914-666-1200	www.nwhc.net
Northwest Hospital Center	Randallstown	Maryland	410-521-5995	www.lifebridgehealth.org
Northwestern Memorial Hospital	Chicago	Illinois	312-926-2000	www.nmh.org
Oakwood Hospital - Wayne	Wayne	Michigan	734-467-4175	www.oakwood.org
Orange Regional Medical Center	Middletown	New York	845-343-2424	www.ormc.org
Oroville Hospital	Oroville	California	530-533-8500	www.orovillehospital.com
Palos Community Hospital	Palos Heights	Illinois	708-923-4000	www.paloshospital.org
Piedmont Medical Center	Rock Hill	South Carolina	803-329-1234	www.piedmontmedicalcenter.com
Pineville Community Hospital	Pineville	Kentucky	606-337-3051	www.pinevillehospital.com
Presence United Samaritans Medical Center	Danville	Illinois	217-443-5000	www.provena.org/usmc
Princeton Community Hospital	Princeton	West Virginia	304-487-7260	www.pchonline.org
Raleigh General Hospital	Beckley	West Virginia	304-256-4100	www.raleighgeneral.com
Richmond VA Medical Center	Richmond	Virginia	804-675-5000	www.med.va.gov
Robert Packer Hospital	Sayre	Pennsylvania	570-888-6666	www.guthrie.org
Russell County Medical Center	Lebanon	Virginia	276-883-8100	www.msha.com
Saint Anne's Hospital	Fall River	Massachusetts	508-674-5600	www.saintanneshospital.org
Saint Thomas Rutherford Hospital	Murfreesboro	Tennessee	615-396-4100	www.mtmc.org
San Gabriel Valley Medical Center	San Gabriel	California	626-289-5454	www.sangabrielvalleymedctr.org
San Juan VA Medical Center	San Juan	Puerto Rico	800-449-8729	www.visn8.med.va.gov/caribbean
Santa Monica - UCLA Medical Center & Orthopaedic Hospital	Santa Monica	California	310-319-4000	www.healthcare.ucla.edu
Sentara Careplex Hospital	Hampton	Virginia	757-736-1000	www.sentara.com
Silver Cross Hospital & Medical Centers	New Lenox	Illinois	815-300-1100	www.silvercross.org
Sinai Hospital of Baltimore	Baltimore	Maryland	410-601-5131	www.sinai-balt.com
Singing River Hospital	Pascagoula	Mississippi	228-809-5000	www.srhshealth.com
Springfield Regional Medical Center	Springfield	Ohio	937-523-1000	www.communityhospital.com
Saint Anthony's Medical Center	Saint Louis	Missouri	314-525-1000	www.samcstl.org
Saint Bernard Hospital	Chicago	Illinois	773-962-3900	www.stbernardhospital.com
Saint Catherine of Siena Hospital	Smithtown	New York	631-862-3000	www.stcatherines.chsli.org
Saint Francis Hospital	Poughkeepsie	New York	845-483-5000	www.sfhhc.org
Saint Joseph's Hospital Health Center	Syracuse	New York	315-448-5111	www.sjhsyr.org
Saint Luke's Roosevelt Hospital	New York	New York	212-523-4000	www.wehealny.org
Saint Rose Dominican Hospitals - Rose De Lima Campus	Henderson	Nevada	702-616-5000	www.dignityhealth.org/las-vegas
Sumner Regional Medical Center	Gallatin	Tennessee	615-452-4210	www.mysumnermedical.com
Syracuse VA Medical Center	Syracuse	New York	315-425-4400	www1.va.gov/visns/visn02
Tampa VA Medical Center	Tampa	Florida	813-972-2000	www.tampa.va.gov
Univerity of MD Balto Washington Medical Center	Glen Burnie	Maryland	410-595-1967	www.bwmc.umms.org
University Hospital - Stony Brook	Stony Brook	New York	631-444-4000	www.stonybrookmedicalcenter.org
University Hospitals - Elyria Medical Center	Elyria	Ohio	440-329-7500	www.emh-healthcare.org
University of Alabama Hospital	Birmingham	Alabama	205-934-4011	www.health.uab.edu
University of Maryland Medical Center	Baltimore	Maryland	410-328-8667	www.umm.edu
University of Maryland Charles Regional Medical Center	La Plata	Maryland	301-609-4265	www.civista.org
Upper Valley Medical Center	Troy	Ohio	937-440-7853	www.uvmc.com
Upstate New York VA Healthcare System - Western NY	Buffalo	New York	716-862-3611	www.buffalo.va.gov
VA Central Arkansas Veterans Healthcare System	Little Rock	Arkansas	501-257-1000	www.visn16.med.va.gov
VA Maryland Healthcare System - Baltimore	Baltimore	Maryland	410-605-7016	www.maryland.va.gov
VA Middle Tennessee Healthcare System	Nashville	Tennessee	615-327-5332	www.tennesseevalley.va.gov
VA Pittsburgh Healthcare System	Pittsburgh	Pennsylvania	412-688-6100	www.pittsburg.va.gov
Vassar Brothers Medical Center	Poughkeepsie	New York	845-454-8500	www.vasserbrothers.org
Wadley Regional Medical Center	Texarkana	Texas	903-798-8000	www.wadleyhealth.com
Washington Hospital	Fremont	California	510-797-1111	www.whhs.com
Wayne Memorial Hospital	Goldsboro	North Carolina	919-736-1110	www.waynehealth.org
White County Medical Center	Searcy	Arkansas	501-278-3100	www.centralarkhospital.com
White Plains Hospital Center	White Plains	New York	914-681-0600	www.wphospital.org
William Beaumont Hospital - Troy	Troy	Michigan	248-964-8800	www.beaumonthospitals.com
Wing Memorial Hospital & Medical Center	Palmer	Massachusetts	413-283-7651	www.winghealth.org
Wyckoff Heights Medical Center	Brooklyn	New York	718-963-7272	www.wyckoffhospital.org

Note: Table shows hospitals nationwide whose pneumonia 30-day readmission rate is worse (higher) than U.S. rate of 17.6%

Hospitals whose Rate of Readmission After Hip/Knee Surgery is Better (Lower) than the U.S. National Rate

Hospital	City	State	Phone	Web Site
Arkansas Surgical Hospital	No Little Rock	Arkansas	501-748-8000	www.arksurgicalhospital.com
Blake Medical Center	Bradenton	Florida	941-792-6611	www.blakemedicalcenter.com
Boca Raton Regional Hospital	Boca Raton	Florida	561-362-5002	www.brrh.com
Christus Santa Rosa Hospital	San Antonio	Texas	210-704-2011	www.christussantarosa.org
Community Memorial Hospital	Hamilton	New York	315-824-1100	www.communitymemorial.org
Eisenhower Medical Center	Rancho Mirage	California	760-340-3911	www.emc.org
Elkhart General Hospital	Elkhart	Indiana	574-294-2621	www.egh.org
Emory University Hospital	Atlanta	Georgia	404-686-8500	www.emoryhealthcare.org
Evanston Hospital	Evanston	Illinois	847-432-8000	www.enh.org
Grace Medical Center	Lubbock	Texas	806-788-4100	www.highlandcommunityhospital.com
Heart of Florida Regional Medical Center	Davenport	Florida	863-422-4971	www.heartofflorida.com
Heartland Regional Medical Center	Saint Joseph	Missouri	816-271-6000	www.heartland-health.com
Hoag Orthopedic Institute	Irvine	California	949-727-5000	www.orthopedichospital.com
Holy Cross Hospital	Fort Lauderdale	Florida	954-771-8000	www.holy-cross.com
Hospital For Special Surgery	New York	New York	212-606-1000	www.hss.edu
Inova Mount Vernon Hospital	Alexandria	Virginia	703-664-7000	www.inova.com/inovapublic.srt/imvh/index.jsp
Kalispell Regional Medical Center	Kalispell	Montana	406-752-5111	www.krmc.org
Kansas Medical Center	Andover	Kansas	316-300-4000	www.ksmedcenter.com
Kettering Medical Center	Kettering	Ohio	937-298-4331	www.khnetwork.org
Maine Medical Center	Portland	Maine	207-662-0111	www.mmc.org
Meadville Medical Center	Meadville	Pennsylvania	814-333-5000	www.mmchs.org
Memorial Healthcare System	Chattanooga	Tennessee	423-495-2525	www.memorial.org
Memorial Mission Hospital & Asheville Surgery Center	Asheville	North Carolina	828-213-1111	www.missionhospitals.org
Mercy Medical Center - Cedar Rapids	Cedar Rapids	Iowa	319-398-6011	www.mercycare.org
Mercy Medical Center - Redding	Redding	California	530-225-6102	www.redding.mercy.org
New England Baptist Hospital	Boston	Massachusetts	617-754-5800	www.nebh.caregroup.org
Ocala Regional Medical Center	Ocala	Florida	352-401-1000	www.ocalaregional.com
Oklahoma Surgical Hospital	Tulsa	Oklahoma	918-477-5000	www.oklahomasurgicalhospital.com
Orthopaedic Hospital at Parkview North	Fort Wayne	Indiana	260-672-4050	www.parkview.com
Orthopaedic Hospital of Wisconsin	Glendale	Wisconsin	414-961-6800	www.ohow.org
Poudre Valley Hospital	Fort Collins	Colorado	970-495-7000	www.pvhs.org
Presbyterian Hospital	Albuquerque	New Mexico	505-724-8386	www.phs.org
Providence Saint John's Health Center	Santa Monica	California	310-829-5511	www.stjohns.org
Reading Hospital	Reading	Pennsylvania	610-988-8000	www.readinghospital.org
Sacred Heart Medical Center - Riverbend	Springfield	Oregon	541-222-7300	www.peacehealth.org/sacred-heart-riverbend
Saint Elizabeth Regional Medical Center	Lincoln	Nebraska	402-219-7700	www.stelizabethonline.com
Saint Joseph's Hospital of Atlanta	Atlanta	Georgia	678-843-5720	www.stjosephsatlanta.org
Saint Thomas West Hospital	Nashville	Tennessee	615-222-2111	www.stthomas.org
Salinas Valley Memorial Hospital	Salinas	California	831-757-4333	www.svmh.com
Samaritan Regional Health System	Ashland	Ohio	419-289-0491	www.samho.org
Sanford Medical Center Fargo	Fargo	North Dakota	701-234-2000	www.meritcare.com
Scottsdale Healthcare - Shea Medical Center	Scottsdale	Arizona	480-323-3009	www.shc.org
Sentara Leigh Hospital	Norfolk	Virginia	757-261-6601	www.sentara.com
Saint Joseph Hospital	Orange	California	714-633-9111	www.sjo.org
Saint Joseph Mercy Oakland	Pontiac	Michigan	248-858-3000	www.stjoesoakland.org
Sutter General Hospital	Sacramento	California	916-733-8999	www.suttermedicalcenter.org
The Orthopaedic Hospital of Lutheran Health Network	Fort Wayne	Indiana	260-435-2999	www.lutheranhealth.net
United Health Services Hospitals	Johnson City	New York	607-763-6000	www.vhs.ent
VHS Harlingen Hospital Company	Harlingen	Texas	956-389-1100	www.vbmc.org
Washington Hospital	Fremont	California	510-797-1111	www.whhs.com
Wythe County Community Hospital	Wytheville	Virginia	276-228-0200	www.wcch.org

Note: Table shows hospitals nationwide whose rate of readmission after hip/knee surgery is better (lower) than U.S. rate of 5.4%

Hospitals whose Rate of Readmission After Hip/Knee Surgery is Worse (Higher) than the U.S. National Rate

Hospital	City	State	Phone	Web Site
Abington Memorial Hospital	Abington	Pennsylvania	215-481-2000	www.amh.org
Advocate Christ Hospital & Medical Center	Oak Lawn	Illinois	708-684-8000	www.advocatehealth.com
Advocate Good Samaritan Hospital	Downers Grove	Illinois	630-275-5900	www.advocatehealth.com/gsam
Bayfront Health - Saint Petersburg	Saint Petersburg	Florida	727-823-1234	www.bayfront.org
Beaufort County Memorial Hospital	Beaufort	South Carolina	843-522-5200	www.bmhsc.org
Beaumont Health System	Royal Oak	Michigan	248-898-5000	www.beaumonthospitals.com
Centrastate Medical Center	Freehold	New Jersey	732-431-2000	www.centrastate.com
Christus Saint Michael Health System	Texarkana	Texas	903-614-1000	www.christusstmichael.org
Des Peres Hospital	Saint Louis	Missouri	314-966-9100	www.desperes hospital.com
Doctors' Community Hospital	Lanham	Maryland	301-552-8085	www.dchweb.org
Enloe Medical Center	Chico	California	530-332-7300	www.enloe.org
Froedtert Memorial Lutheran Hospital	Milwaukee	Wisconsin	414-805-3000	www.froedtert.com
Galesburg Cottage Hospital	Galesburg	Illinois	309-345-4555	www.cottagehospital.com
Grant Medical Center	Columbus	Ohio	614-566-9978	www.ohiohealth.com
Jackson County Memorial Hospital	Altus	Oklahoma	580-379-5000	www.jcmh.com
Leesburg Regional Medical Center	Leesburg	Florida	352-323-5762	www.leesburgregional.org
Mercy Hospital Saint Louis	Saint Louis	Missouri	314-569-6000	www.stjohnsmercy.org
Mercy Saint Anne Hospital	Toledo	Ohio	419-407-2663	www.mercyweb.org
Minden Medical Center	Minden	Louisiana	318-377-2321	www.mindenmedicalcenter.com
Northwestern Memorial Hospital	Chicago	Illinois	312-926-2000	www.nmh.org
Orlando Health	Orlando	Florida	321-841-5111	www.orlandoregionalmedicalcenter.org
Parkwest Medical Center	Knoxville	Tennessee	865-970-9800	www.yesparkwest.com
Penn Presbyterian Medical Center	Philadelphia	Pennsylvania	215-662-8000	www.pennhealth.com
Pennsylvania Hospital of the Univ of PA Health Sys	Philadelphia	Pennsylvania	215-829-3000	www.pennmedicine.org/pahosp
Peterson Regional Medical Center	Kerrville	Texas	830-896-4200	www.petersonrmc.com
Providence Hospital	Washington	District of Columbia	202-269-7000	www.provhosp.org
Reston Hospital Center	Reston	Virginia	703-689-9000	www.restonhospital.com
Saint Agnes Hospital	Baltimore	Maryland	410-368-2101	www.stagnes.org
Saline Memorial Hospital	Benton	Arkansas	501-776-6000	www.salinememorial.org
Shannon Medical Center	San Angelo	Texas	325-653-6741	www.shannonhealth.com
Sinai Hospital of Baltimore	Baltimore	Maryland	410-601-5131	www.sinai-balt.com
Southside Regional Medical Center	Petersburg	Virginia	804-765-5000	www.srmconline.com
Saint Joseph Regional Health Center	Bryan	Texas	979-776-3912	www.st-joseph.org/sjrhc
Saint Joseph's Hospital	Tampa	Florida	813-870-4398	www.stjosephstampa.org
Thomas Jefferson University Hospital	Philadelphia	Pennsylvania	215-955-6000	www.jeffersonhospital.org
Wellmont Holston Valley Medical Center	Kingsport	Tennessee	423-224-4000	www.wellmont.org
Woodland Heights Medical Center	Lufkin	Texas	936-634-8311	www.woodlandheights.net

Note: Table shows hospitals nationwide whose rate of readmission after hip/knee surgery is better (lower) than U.S. rate of 5.4%

Hospitals whose Rate of Readmission After Discharge From Hospital (Hospital-wide) is Better (Lower) than the U.S. National Rate

Hospital	City	State	Phone	Web Site
Abbott Northwestern Hospital	Minneapolis	Minnesota	612-863-4509	www.abbottnorthwestern.com
Alegent Creighton Health Bergan Mercy Medical Center	Omaha	Nebraska	402-398-6060	www.alegent.com
Alexian Brothers Medical Center	Elk Grove Village	Illinois	847-437-5500	www.alexian.org
Alpena Regional Medical Center	Alpena	Michigan	989-356-7390	www.agh.org
Alta Bates Summit Medical Center	Oakland	California	510-655-4000	www.altabates.com
American Fork Hospital	American Fork	Utah	801-855-3305	www.ihc.com/facility/facilityresults.jsp
Anderson Regional Medical Center	Meridian	Mississippi	601-553-6000	www.jarmc.org
Appleton Medical Center	Appleton	Wisconsin	920-731-4101	www.thedacare.org
Arkansas Surgical Hospital	No Little Rock	Arkansas	501-748-8000	www.arksurgicalhospital.com
Asante Rogue Regional Medical Center	Medford	Oregon	541-789-7000	www.asante.org
Aspirus Wausau Hospital	Wausau	Wisconsin	715-847-2121	www.aspirus.org
Athens Regional Medical Center	Athens	Georgia	706-475-7000	www.armc.org
Augusta Health	Fishersville	Virginia	540-932-4000	www.augustamed.com
Aurora Lakeland Medical Center	Elkhorn	Wisconsin	262-741-2000	www.aurorahealthcare.org/facilities
Aurora Medical Center Manitowoc County	Two Rivers	Wisconsin	920-794-5000	www.aurorahealthcare.org
Aurora Medical Center Washington County	Hartford	Wisconsin	262-673-2300	www.aurorahealthcare.org
Aurora Saint Lukes Medical Center	Milwaukee	Wisconsin	414-649-6000	www.aurorahealthcare.org
Aurora West Allis Medical Center	West Allis	Wisconsin	414-328-6000	www.aurorahealthcare.org
Avera Mckennan Hospital & University Health Center	Sioux Falls	South Dakota	605-322-8000	www.mckennan.org
Avera Queen of Peace	Mitchell	South Dakota	605-995-2000	www.averaqueenofpeace.org
Avera Saint Lukes	Aberdeen	South Dakota	605-622-5000	www.averastlukes.org
Banner Good Samaritan Medical Center	Phoenix	Arizona	602-239-2000	www.bannerhealth.com
Baptist Health Louisville	Louisville	Kentucky	502-897-8100	www.baptisteast.com
Baptist Medical Center	San Antonio	Texas	210-297-1020	www.baptisthealthsystem.org
Baptist Memorial Hospital	Memphis	Tennessee	901-226-5000	www.bmhcc.org
Baptist Saint Anthony's Hospital	Amarillo	Texas	806-212-2000	www.bsahs.com
Baylor All Saints Medical Center at FW	Fort Worth	Texas	817-926-2544	www.baylorhealth.com/locations/allsaints
Baylor Medical Center at Garland	Garland	Texas	972-487-5000	www.baylorhealth.com
Baylor Medical Center at Irving	Irving	Texas	972-579-8100	www.baylorhealth.com
Baylor Regional Medical Center at Grapevine	Grapevine	Texas	817-481-1588	www.baylorhealth.com
Baylor University Medical Center	Dallas	Texas	214-820-0111	www.baylorhealth.com
Baystate Medical Center	Springfield	Massachusetts	413-794-0000	www.baystatehealth.com
Bellin Memorial Hospital	Green Bay	Wisconsin	920-433-3500	www.bellin.org
Billings Clinic Hospital	Billings	Montana	406-657-4000	www.billingsclinic.com
Blanchard Valley Hospital	Findlay	Ohio	419-423-4500	www.bvha.org
Bon Secours Maryview Medical Center	Portsmouth	Virginia	757-398-2200	www.bonsecourshamptonroads.com
Boone Hospital Center	Columbia	Missouri	573-815-8000	www.boone.org
Borgess Medical Center	Kalamazoo	Michigan	269-226-7000	www.borgess.com
Boulder Community Hospital	Boulder	Colorado	303-440-2273	www.bch.org
Bronson Methodist Hospital	Kalamazoo	Michigan	269-341-6000	www.bronsonhealth.com
Bryan Medical Center	Lincoln	Nebraska	402-481-1111	www.bryan.org
Caldwell Memorial Hospital	Lenoir	North Carolina	828-757-5100	www.caldwellmemorial.org
California Pacific Medical Center - Pacific Campus Hospital	San Francisco	California	415-600-6000	www.cpmc.org
Cape Cod Hospital	Hyannis	Massachusetts	508-771-1800	www.capecodhealth.org
Carolinas Medical Center - Pineville	Charlotte	North Carolina	704-379-5000	www.carolinashealthcare.org
Carondelet Saint Marys Hospital	Tucson	Arizona	520-872-3000	www.carondelet.org
Carondelet Saint Joseph's Hospital	Tucson	Arizona	520-873-3000	www.carondelet.org
Carteret General Hospital	Morehead City	North Carolina	252-808-6000	www.ccgh.org
Catawba Valley Medical Center	Hickory	North Carolina	828-326-3809	www.catawbavalleymc.org
Central Dupage Hospital	Winfield	Illinois	630-682-1600	www.cdh.org
Central Vermont Medical Center	Barre	Vermont	802-371-4100	www.cvmc.hitchcock.org
Central Washington Hospital	Wenatchee	Washington	509-662-1511	www.cwhs.com
Centura Health - Penrose Saint Francis Health Services	Colorado Springs	Colorado	719-776-5000	www.centurahealth.com
Centura Health - Saint Mary Corwin Medical Center	Pueblo	Colorado	719-557-4000	www.stmarycorwin.org
Chandler Regional Medical Center	Chandler	Arizona	480-963-4561	www.chandlerregional.com
Charlotte Hungerford Hospital	Torrington	Connecticut	860-496-6666	www.charlottesweb.hungerford.org
Cheyenne Regional Medical Center	Cheyenne	Wyoming	307-634-2273	www.crmcwy.org
Christus Health Shreveport - Bossier	Shreveport	Louisiana	318-681-5000	www.christusschumpert.org
Citizens Medical Center	Victoria	Texas	361-572-5113	www.citizensmedicalcenter.org
Citrus Memorial Hospital	Inverness	Florida	352-726-1551	www.citrusmh.com
CMC - Blue Ridge	Morganton	North Carolina	828-580-5000	www.gracehcs.org
Comanche County Memorial Hospital	Lawton	Oklahoma	580-355-8620	www.memorialhealthsource.org
Community Hospital of the Monterey Peninsula	Monterey	California	831-624-5311	www.chomp.org
Community Memorial Hospital San Buenaventura	Ventura	California	805-652-5011	www.cmhhospital.org
The Corpus Christi Medical Center	Corpus Christi	Texas	361-761-1501	www.ccmedicalcenter.com

Hospital	City	State	Phone	Web Site
Covenant Medical Center	Lubbock	Texas	806-725-6000	www.covenanthealth.org
Deaconess Hospital	Oklahoma City	Oklahoma	405-604-6109	www.deaconessokc.com
Dixie Regional Medical Center	Saint George	Utah	435-251-2100	www.intermountainhealthcare.org
Doctors Hospital of Sarasota	Sarasota	Florida	941-342-1100	www.doctorsofsarasota.com
Dominican Hospital	Santa Cruz	California	831-462-7700	www.dominicanhospital.org
East Jefferson General Hospital	Metairie	Louisiana	504-454-4000	www.eastjeffhospital.org
Eastern Idaho Regional Medical Center	Idaho Falls	Idaho	208-529-6111	www.eirmc.org
Eisenhower Medical Center	Rancho Mirage	California	760-340-3911	www.emc.org
Englewood Community Hospital	Englewood	Florida	941-475-6571	www.englewoodcommunityhospital.com
Ephrata Community Hospital	Ephrata	Pennsylvania	717-733-0311	www.ephratahospital.org
Evergreen Hospital Medical Center	Kirkland	Washington	425-899-1000	www.evergreenhospital.org
Exempla Lutheran Medical Center	Wheat Ridge	Colorado	303-425-4500	www.exemlpa.org
Fairview Southdale Hospital	Edina	Minnesota	952-924-5000	www.fairview.org
Falmouth Hospital	Falmouth	Massachusetts	508-548-5300	www.capecodhealth.com
Flagler Hospital	Saint Augustine	Florida	904-819-4426	www.flaglerhospital.com
Flagstaff Medical Center	Flagstaff	Arizona	928-773-2009	www.nahealth.com
Franciscan Saint Elizabeth Health - Lafayette East	Lafayette	Indiana	765-502-4334	www.ste.org
Freeman Health System - Freeman West	Joplin	Missouri	417-347-1111	www.freemanhealth.com
Genesis Medical Center - Davenport	Davenport	Iowa	563-421-1000	www.genesishealth.com
GHS Greenville Memorial Medical Center	Greenville	South Carolina	864-455-7000	www.ghs.org
Grand View Hospital	Sellersville	Pennsylvania	215-453-4615	www.gvh.org
Greater Baltimore Medical Center	Baltimore	Maryland	443-849-2000	www.gbmc.org
Gundersen Lutheran Medical Center	La Crosse	Wisconsin	608-782-7300	www.gundluth.org
Gwinnett Medical Center	Lawrenceville	Georgia	678-312-1000	www.gwinnettmedicalcenter.org
Harlingen Medical Center	Harlingen	Texas	956-365-1000	www.harlingenmedicalcenter.com
Harrison Memorial Center	Bremerton	Washington	360-377-3911	www.harrisonmedical.org
Hill Country Memorial Hospital	Fredericksburg	Texas	830-997-4353	www.hcmbs.org
Hinsdale Hospital	Hinsdale	Illinois	630-856-9000	www.keepingyouwell.com
Hoag Memorial Hospital Presbyterian	Newport Beach	California	949-645-8600	www.hoaghospital.org
Hoag Orthopedic Institute	Irvine	California	949-727-5000	www.orthopedichospital.com
Hospital For Special Surgery	New York	New York	212-606-1000	www.hss.edu
Huguley Memorial Medical Center	Burleson	Texas	817-568-5317	www.huguley.org
Huntington Memorial Hospital	Pasadena	California	626-397-5000	www.huntingtonhospital.com
Hutchinson Regional Medical Center	Hutchinson	Kansas	620-665-2001	www.hutchinsonhospital.com
Indian River Medical Center	Vero Beach	Florida	772-567-4311	www.irmh.com
Indiana University Health Ball Memorial Hospital	Muncie	Indiana	765-747-3111	www.accesschs.org/baal-memorial-l
Indiana University Health North Hospital	Carmel	Indiana	317-688-2000	www.iuhealth.org/north
Integris Baptist Medical Center	Oklahoma City	Oklahoma	405-951-8110	www.integris-health.com
Intermountain Medical Center	Murray	Utah	801-507-7000	www.intermountainhealthcare.org
Iowa Lutheran Hospital	Des Moines	Iowa	515-263-5612	www.ihsdesmoines.org
Iowa Methodist Medical Center	Des Moines	Iowa	515-241-6212	www.iowahealth.org
IU Health West Hospital	Avon	Indiana	317-217-3000	www.iuhealth.org/west
Jane Phillips Medical Center	Bartlesville	Oklahoma	918-333-7200	www.jpmc.org
John Muir Medical Center - Walnut Creek Campus	Walnut Creek	California	925-939-3000	www.jmmdhs.com
Kalispell Regional Medical Center	Kalispell	Montana	406-752-5111	www.krmc.org
Kaweah Delta Medical Center	Visalia	California	559-624-2000	www.kaweahdelta.org
Kenmore Mercy Hospital	Kenmore	New York	716-447-6100	www.chsbuffalo.org
Kettering Medical Center	Kettering	Ohio	937-298-4331	www.khnetwork.org
Kootenai Medical Center	Coeur D'alene	Idaho	208-625-4001	www.kootenaihealth.org
Lakeview Memorial Hospital	Stillwater	Minnesota	651-439-5330	www.lakeview.org
Lancaster General Hospital	Lancaster	Pennsylvania	717-299-5511	www.lancastergeneral.org
Lawrence & Memorial Hospital	New London	Connecticut	860-442-0711	www.lmhospital.org
Lawrence Memorial Hospital	Lawrence	Kansas	785-505-6100	www.lmh.org
Lehigh Valley Hospital	Allentown	Pennsylvania	610-402-2273	www.lvhhn.org
Lexington Medical Center	West Columbia	South Carolina	803-791-2000	www.lexmed.com
Lovelace Medical Center	Albuquerque	New Mexico	505-727-8000	www.lovelace.com
Mainegeneral Medical Center	Augusta	Maine	207-872-1000	www.mainegeneral.org
Margaret R Pardee Memorial Hospital	Hendersonville	North Carolina	828-696-1000	www.pardeehospital.org
Marian Regional Medical Center	Santa Maria	California	805-739-3000	www.marinmedicalcenter.org
Marion General Hospital	Marion	Indiana	765-660-6000	www.mgh.net
Marquette General Hospital	Marquette	Michigan	906-228-9440	www.mgh.org
Marshalltown Medical & Surgical Center	Marshalltown	Iowa	641-754-5151	www.everydaychampions.org
Mary Lanning Healthcare	Hastings	Nebraska	402-463-4521	www.marylanning.org
Maui Memorial Medical Center	Wailuku	Hawaii	808-442-5101	www.mauimemorialmedical.org
Mayo Clinic Health System - Eau Claire Hospital	Eau Claire	Wisconsin	715-838-3311	www.luthermidelfort.org
Mayo Clinic Hospital	Phoenix	Arizona	480-342-2000	www.mayoclinic.org
McBride Clinic Orthopedic Hospital	Oklahoma City	Oklahoma	405-478-1717	www.mcbrideclinic.com

Hospital	City	State	Phone	Web Site
McKay Dee Hospital	Ogden	Utah	801-387-2800	www.intermountainhealthcare.org
Mclaren - Northern Michigan	Petoskey	Michigan	231-487-4000	www.northernhealth.org
The Medical Center of Aurora	Aurora	Colorado	303-695-2600	www.auroramed.com
Medical City Dallas Hospital	Dallas	Texas	972-566-6222	www.medicalcityhospital.com
Medwest Haywood	Clyde	North Carolina	828-456-7311	www.haymed.org
Memorial Healthcare System	Chattanooga	Tennessee	423-495-2525	www.memorial.org
Memorial Hermann Hospital System	Houston	Texas	713-448-6796	www.memorialhermann.org
Memorial Hermann Memorial City Medical Center	Houston	Texas	713-242-3000	www.mhhs.org
Memorial Hospital & Health Care Center	Jasper	Indiana	812-996-2345	www.mhhcc.org
Memorial Hospital of South Bend	South Bend	Indiana	574-647-1000	www.qualityoflife.org
Memorial Medical Center of West Michigan	Ludington	Michigan	231-843-2591	www.mmcwm.com
Memorial Mission Hospital & Asheville Surgery Center	Asheville	North Carolina	828-213-1111	www.missionhospitals.org
Mercy General Hospital	Sacramento	California	916-453-4545	www.mercygeneral.org
Mercy Health Partners - Mercy Campus	Muskegon	Michigan	231-672-3901	www.mghp.com
Mercy Hospital	Iowa City	Iowa	319-339-0300	www.mercyiowacity.org
Mercy Hospital	Portland	Maine	207-879-3000	www.mercyhospital.com
Mercy Hospital	Buffalo	New York	716-826-7000	www.chsbuffalo.org
Mercy Hospital - Grayling	Grayling	Michigan	989-348-5461	www.mercygrayling.munsonhealthcare.org
Mercy Hospital Northwest Arkansas	Rogers	Arkansas	479-338-8000	www.mercy4u.com
Mercy Hospital Springfield	Springfield	Missouri	417-820-2000	www.stjohns.com
Mercy Medical Center	Canton	Ohio	330-489-1001	www.thequalityhospital.com
Mercy Medical Center	Roseburg	Oregon	541-673-0611	www.mercyrose.org
Mercy Medical Center - Redding	Redding	California	530-225-6102	www.redding.mercy.org
Mercy Medical Center - Des Moines	Des Moines	Iowa	515-247-3121	www.mercydesmoines.org
Meriter Hospital	Madison	Wisconsin	608-417-6000	www.meriter.com
Methodist Hospital	San Antonio	Texas	210-575-4000	www.mh.sahealth.com
Methodist Stone Oak Hospital	San Antonio	Texas	210-638-2100	www.stoneoakhealth.com
Methodist Sugar Land Hospital	Sugar Land	Texas	281-274-8000	www.methodisthealth.com/sugarland
Midland Memorial Hospital	Midland	Texas	432-685-1111	www.midland-memorial.com
Mills - Peninsula Medical Center	Burlingame	California	650-696-5270	www.mills-peninsula.org
Morristown Medical Center	Morristown	New Jersey	973-971-5450	www.morristownmemorialhospital.org
Morton Plant Hospital	Clearwater	Florida	727-462-7000	www.measehospitals.com
The Moses H Cone Memorial Hospital	Greensboro	North Carolina	336-832-7000	www.mosescone.com
Mother Frances Hospital	Tyler	Texas	903-593-8441	www.tmfhs.org
Munroe Regional Medical Center	Ocala	Florida	352-351-7200	www.munroeregional.com
Munson Medical Center	Traverse City	Michigan	231-935-5000	www.munsonhealthcare.org
Naples Community Hospital	Naples	Florida	239-436-5000	www.nchmd.org
Nebraska Heart Hospital	Lincoln	Nebraska	402-328-3000	www.neheart.com
New England Baptist Hospital	Boston	Massachusetts	617-754-5800	www.nebh.caregroup.org
New Hanover Regional Medical Center	Wilmington	North Carolina	910-343-7000	www.nhrmc.org
Newton Medical Center	Newton	Kansas	316-804-6001	www.newtonmedicalcenter.com
Norman Regional Health System	Norman	Oklahoma	405-321-1700	www.normanregional.com
North Memorial Medical Center	Robbinsdale	Minnesota	763-520-5200	www.northmemorial.com
North Shore Medical Center	Salem	Massachusetts	978-741-1215	www.nsmc.partners.org
Northside Hospital	Atlanta	Georgia	404-851-8000	www.northside.com
Northwest Community Hospital	Arlington Heights	Illinois	847-618-1000	www.nch.org
Northwest Hospital	Seattle	Washington	206-364-0500	www.nwhospital.org
Northwest Texas Hospital	Amarillo	Texas	806-354-1110	www.nxtexashealthcare.com
Novant Health Huntersville Medical Center	Huntersville	North Carolina	704-316-4000	www.presbyterian.org
Oklahoma Heart Hospital	Oklahoma City	Oklahoma	405-608-3200	www.okheart.com
Oklahoma Surgical Hospital	Tulsa	Oklahoma	918-477-5000	www.oklahomasurgicalhospital.com
Olympic Medical Center	Port Angeles	Washington	360-417-7000	www.olympicmedical.org
Our Lady of the Lake Regional Medical Center	Baton Rouge	Louisiana	225-765-6565	www.ololrmc.com
Overlake Hospital Medical Center	Bellevue	Washington	425-688-5000	www.overlakehospital.org
Owensboro Health Regional Hospital	Owensboro	Kentucky	270-688-2000	www.omhs.org
Palmetto Health Baptist	Columbia	South Carolina	803-296-5678	www.palmettohealth.org
Palmetto Health Richland	Columbia	South Carolina	803-296-5678	www.palmettohealth.org
Park Nicollet Methodist Hospital	Saint Louis Park	Minnesota	952-993-5000	www.parknicollet.com/methodist
Parkview Medical Center	Pueblo	Colorado	719-584-4000	www.parkviewmc.com
Parkview Regional Medical Center	Fort Wayne	Indiana	260-266-1000	www.parkview.com
Peacehealth Saint Joseph Medical Center	Bellingham	Washington	360-734-5400	www.peacehealth.org
Peninsula Regional Medical Center	Salisbury	Maryland	410-543-7111	www.peninsula.org
Penn Highlands Dubois	Dubois	Pennsylvania	814-371-2200	www.drmc.org
Petaluma Valley Hospital	Petaluma	California	707-778-1111	www.stjosephhealth.org
Phelps County Regional Medical Center	Rolla	Missouri	573-458-8899	www.rollanet.org/~pcrmc
Piedmont Fayette Hospital	Fayetteville	Georgia	770-719-7071	www.fayettehospital.org
Piedmont Hospital	Atlanta	Georgia	404-605-5000	www.piedmonthospital.org

Hospital	City	State	Phone	Web Site
Plaza Medical Center of Fort Worth	Fort Worth	Texas	817-336-2100	www.plazamedicalcenter.com
Porter Regional Hospital	Valparaiso	Indiana	219-983-8300	www.portermemorial.org
Portneuf Medical Center	Pocatello	Idaho	208-239-1000	www.portmed.org
Presbyterian Hospital	Albuquerque	New Mexico	505-724-8386	www.phs.org
Presbyterian Hospital Matthews	Matthews	North Carolina	704-384-6500	www.presbyterian.org
Providence Alaska Medical Center	Anchorage	Alaska	907-261-3675	www.providence.org
Providence Holy Family Hospital	Spokane	Washington	509-482-2450	www.holy-family.org
Providence Hospital	Mobile	Alabama	251-633-1000	www.providencehospital.org
Providence Regional Medical Center Everett	Everett	Washington	425-261-2000	www.providence.org
Providence Sacred Heart Medical Center	Spokane	Washington	509-474-3040	www.shmc.org
Providence Saint John's Health Center	Santa Monica	California	310-829-5511	www.stjohns.org
Providence Saint Mary Medical Center	Walla Walla	Washington	509-522-5900	www.smmc.com
Providence Saint Peter Hospital	Olympia	Washington	360-491-9480	www.providence.org/swsa
Providence Saint Vincent Medical Center	Portland	Oregon	503-216-1234	www.providence.org
Rapid City Regional Hospital	Rapid City	South Dakota	605-719-1000	www.rcrh.org
Reading Hospital	Reading	Pennsylvania	610-988-8000	www.readinghospital.org
Reid Hospital & Health Care Services	Richmond	Indiana	765-983-3000	www.reidhosp.com
Rex Hospital	Raleigh	North Carolina	919-784-3100	www.rexhealth.com
Roper Hospital	Charleston	South Carolina	843-724-2800	www.ropersaintfrancis.com
Sacred Heart Medical Center - Riverbend	Springfield	Oregon	541-222-7300	www.peacehealth.org/sacred-heart-riverbend
Saddleback Memorial Medical Center	Laguna Hills	California	949-837-4500	www.memorialcare.org/saddleback
Saint Barnabas Medical Center	Livingston	New Jersey	973-322-5000	www.saintbarnabas.com
Saint Elizabeth Regional Medical Center	Lincoln	Nebraska	402-219-7700	www.stelizabethonline.com
Saint Joseph Regional Medical Center	Mishawaka	Indiana	574-335-5000	www.sjmed.com
Saint Joseph's Hospital of Atlanta	Atlanta	Georgia	678-843-5720	www.stjosephsatlanta.org
Saint Mary's Health Care	Grand Rapids	Michigan	616-685-5000	www.smhealthcare.org
Saint Thomas West Hospital	Nashville	Tennessee	615-222-2111	www.stthomas.org
Saint Vincent Hospital	Erie	Pennsylvania	814-452-5000	www.svhs.org
Salem Hospital	Salem	Oregon	503-561-5200	www.salemhospital.org
Salem Regional Medical Center	Salem	Ohio	330-332-1551	www.salemhosp.com
Salina Regional Health Center	Salina	Kansas	785-452-7000	www.srhc.com
Salinas Valley Memorial Hospital	Salinas	California	831-757-4333	www.svmh.com
Samaritan Albany General Hospital	Albany	Oregon	541-812-4000	www.samhealth.org/shs_facilities
Sampson Regional Medical Center	Clinton	North Carolina	910-592-8511	www.sampsonrmc.org
San Jacinto Methodist Hospital	Baytown	Texas	281-420-8600	www.methodisthealth.com/sanjacinto
Sanford Bemidji Medical Center	Bemidji	Minnesota	218-751-5430	www.nchs.com
Sanford Medical Center Fargo	Fargo	North Dakota	701-234-2000	www.meritcare.com
Sanford Usd Medical Center	Sioux Falls	South Dakota	605-333-1000	www.sanfordhealth.org
Santa Barbara Cottage Hospital	Santa Barbara	California	805-682-7111	www.cottagehealthsystem.org
Santa Rosa Memorial Hospital	Santa Rosa	California	707-525-5300	www.stjosephhealth.org
Sarasota Memorial Hospital	Sarasota	Florida	941-917-9000	www.smh.com
Saratoga Hospital	Saratoga Springs	New York	518-587-3222	www.saratogacare.org
Scottsdale Healthcare Osborn Medical Center	Scottsdale	Arizona	480-882-4000	www.shc.org
Scottsdale Healthcare - Shea Medical Center	Scottsdale	Arizona	480-323-3009	www.shc.org
Scottsdale Healthcare - Thompson Peak Hospital	Scottsdale	Arizona	480-324-7004	www.shc.org
Scripps Memorial Hospital - Encinitas	Encinitas	California	760-753-6501	www.scripps.org
Sentara Williamsburg Regional Medical Center	Williamsburg	Virginia	757-984-6000	www.sentara.com
Sequoia Hospital	Redwood City	California	650-367-5551	www.sequoiahospital.org
Seven Rivers Regional Medical Center	Crystal River	Florida	352-795-6560	www.srrmc.com
Sisters of Charity Providence Hospitals	Columbia	South Carolina	803-256-5300	www.providencehospitals.com
Sky Lakes Medical Center	Klamath Falls	Oregon	541-274-6150	www.skylakes.org
Sky Ridge Medical Center	Lone Tree	Colorado	720-225-1000	www.skyridgemedcenter.com
Sonoma Valley Hospital	Sonoma	California	707-935-5000	www.svh.com
Sonora Regional Medical Center	Sonora	California	209-532-3161	www.sonorahospital.org
South Lake Hospital	Clermont	Florida	352-394-4071	www.southlakehospital.com
Spartanburg Regional Medical Center	Spartanburg	South Carolina	864-560-6000	www.srhs.com
Spectrum Health - Butterworth Campus	Grand Rapids	Michigan	616-391-1774	www.spectrum-health.org
Saint Agnes Hospital	Fond Du Lac	Wisconsin	920-929-2300	www.agnesian.com
Saint Alexius Medical Center	Bismarck	North Dakota	701-530-7000	www.st.alexius.org
Saint Alphonsus Regional Medical Center	Boise	Idaho	208-367-2121	www.saintalphonsus.org
Saint Bernardine Medical Center	San Bernardino	California	909-881-4440	www.stbernardinemedicalcenter.com
Saint Charles Medical Center - Bend	Bend	Oregon	541-382-4321	www.scmc.org
Saint David's Medical Center	Austin	Texas	512-476-7111	www.stdavidsrehab.com
Saint Edward Mercy Medical Center	Fort Smith	Arkansas	479-314-6000	www.stedwardmercy.com
Saint Francis Hospital	Columbus	Georgia	706-596-4020	www.wecareforlife.com
Saint Francis Hospital - Roslyn	Roslyn	New York	516-562-6000	www.stfrancisheartcenter.com
Saint Francis Medical Center	Grand Island	Nebraska	308-384-4600	www.saintfrancisgi.org

Hospital	City	State	Phone	Web Site
Saint Francis - Downtown	Greenville	South Carolina	864-255-1000	www.stfrancishealth.org
Saint Joseph Hospital	Eureka	California	707-445-8121	www.stjosepheureka.org
Saint Joseph Hospital & Health Center	Kokomo	Indiana	765-456-5300	www.stvincent.org
Saint Joseph Medical Center	Reading	Pennsylvania	610-378-2300	www.sjmcberks.org
Saint Joseph Regional Medical Center	Lewiston	Idaho	208-743-2511	www.sjrmc.org
Saint Luke's Regional Medical Center	Boise	Idaho	208-381-2222	www.slrmc.org
Saint Luke's Hospital	Cedar Rapids	Iowa	319-369-7211	www.crstlukes.com
Saint Luke's Hospital	Duluth	Minnesota	218-249-5555	www.slhduluth.com
Saint Marks Hospital	Salt Lake City	Utah	801-268-7700	www.stmarkshospital.com
Saint Mary's Regional Medical Center	Enid	Oklahoma	580-233-6100	www.stmarysregional.com
Saint Marys Hospital	Madison	Wisconsin	608-251-6100	www.stmarysmadison.com
Saint Marys Hospital & Medical Center	Grand Junction	Colorado	970-298-1950	www.stmarygj.org
Saint Marys Regional Medical Center	Lewiston	Maine	207-777-8100	www.stmarysmaine.com
Saint Patrick Hospital	Missoula	Montana	406-543-7271	www.saintpatrick.org
Saint Peter's Hospital	Albany	New York	518-525-1550	www.stpetershealthcare.org
Saint Rose Dominican Hospitals - Siena Campus	Henderson	Nevada	702-616-5000	www.strosehospitals.org
Saint Vincent Heart Center of Indiana	Indianapolis	Indiana	317-583-5000	www.theheartcenter.com
Saint Vincent Hospital	Green Bay	Wisconsin	920-433-0111	www.stvincenthospital.org
Saint Vincent Hospital & Health Services	Indianapolis	Indiana	317-338-7000	www.indianapolis.stvincent.org
Sutter Auburn Faith Hospital	Auburn	California	530-888-4500	www.sutterauburnfaith.org
Sutter Roseville Medical Center	Roseville	California	916-781-1000	www.sutterroseville.org
Tallahassee Memorial Hospital	Tallahassee	Florida	850-431-1155	www.tmh.org
Tennova Healthcare	Knoxville	Tennessee	865-545-8000	www.stmaryshealth.com
Texas Health Harris Methodist Fort Worth	Fort Worth	Texas	817-250-2100	www.texashealth.org
Texas Health Presbyterian Hospital Plano	Plano	Texas	972-981-8000	www.presbyplano.org
Texas Health Presbyterian Hospital - WNJ	Sherman	Texas	903-870-4611	www.wnj.org
Texas Orthopedic Hospital	Houston	Texas	713-799-8600	www.texasorthopedic.com
The Queens Medical Center	Honolulu	Hawaii	808-538-9011	www.queens.org
The Toledo Hospital	Toledo	Ohio	419-291-7463	www.promedica.org
Touro Infirmary	New Orleans	Louisiana	504-897-7011	www.touro.com
United Hospital	Saint Paul	Minnesota	651-241-8802	www.allinahealth.org/ahs/united.nsf
University Colo Health Memorial Hospital Central	Colorado Springs	Colorado	719-365-5000	www.memorialhospital.com
University of Wisconsin Hospitals & Clinics Authority	Madison	Wisconsin	608-263-8991	www.uwhealth.org
UPMC Altoona	Altoona	Pennsylvania	814-889-2011	www.altoonaregional.org
UPMC Hamot	Erie	Pennsylvania	814-877-6000	www.hamot.org
Utah Valley Regional Medical Center	Provo	Utah	801-373-7850	www.intermountainhealthcare.org/hospitals/uvrmc
Venice Regional Medical Center - Bayfront Health	Venice	Florida	941-485-7711	www.veniceregional.com
VHS Harlingen Hospital Company	Harlingen	Texas	956-389-1100	www.vbmc.org
Via Christi Hospital Pittsburg	Pittsburg	Kansas	620-231-6100	www.via-christi.org
Via Christi Hospitals Wichita	Wichita	Kansas	316-268-5000	www.via-christi.org
Wakemed - Raleigh Campus	Raleigh	North Carolina	919-350-8000	www.wakemed.org
Wentworth - Douglass Hospital	Dover	New Hampshire	603-740-2580	www.wdhospital.com
Wesley Medical Center	Wichita	Kansas	316-962-2000	www.wesleymc.com
West Calcasieu Cameron Hospital	Sulphur	Louisiana	337-527-7034	www.wcch.com
West Shore Medical Center	Manistee	Michigan	231-398-1000	www.westshoremedcenter.org
Williamsport Regional Medical Center	Williamsport	Pennsylvania	570-321-1000	www.susquehannahealth.org
Willis Knighton Medical Center	Shreveport	Louisiana	318-212-4000	www.wkhs.com//locations/medicalcenter.aspx
Woodland Heights Medical Center	Lufkin	Texas	936-634-8311	www.woodlandheights.net
Wooster Community Hospital	Wooster	Ohio	330-263-8100	www.woosterhospital.org

Note: Table shows hospitals nationwide whose rate of readmission after discharge from hospital (hospital-wide) is better (lower) than U.S. rate of 16.0%

Hospitals whose Rate of Readmission After Discharge From Hospital (Hospital-wide) is Worse (Higher) than the U.S. National Rate

Hospital	City	State	Phone	Web Site
Adena Regional Medical Center	Chillicothe	Ohio	740-779-7500	www.adena.org
Advocate Christ Hospital & Medical Center	Oak Lawn	Illinois	708-684-8000	www.advocatehealth.com
Advocate Illinois Masonic Medical Center	Chicago	Illinois	773-975-1600	www.advocatehealth.com/immc
Advocate Trinity Hospital	Chicago	Illinois	773-967-2000	www.advocatehealth.com/trin
Albert Einstein Medical Center	Philadelphia	Pennsylvania	215-456-6090	www.einstein.edu
Anne Arundel Medical Center	Annapolis	Maryland	443-481-1307	www.aahs.org
Aria Health	Philadelphia	Pennsylvania	215-612-4129	www.ariahealth.com
Arkansas Methodist Medical Center	Paragould	Arkansas	870-239-7000	www.arkansasmethodist.org
Atlanticare Regional Medical Center	Atlantic City	New Jersey	609-441-8020	www.atlanticare.org/acmc/index.html
Aventura Hospital & Medical Center	Aventura	Florida	305-682-7000	www.aventurahospital.com
B R F Hospital Holdings	Shreveport	Louisiana	318-675-5000	www.lsumc.edu
Banner Desert Medical Center	Mesa	Arizona	480-412-3000	www.bannerhealth.com
Baptist Beaumont Hospital	Beaumont	Texas	409-212-5012	www.mhbh.org
Baptist Memorial Hospital Desoto	Southaven	Mississippi	662-772-4000	www.bmhcc.org/facilities/desoto
Barnes-Jewish Hospital	Saint Louis	Missouri	314-747-3000	www.barnesjewish.org
Baxter Regional Medical Center	Mountain Home	Arkansas	870-508-1000	www.baxterregional.org
Beaumont Health System	Grosse Pointe	Michigan	313-343-1000	www.beaumonthospitals.com
Beaumont Health System	Royal Oak	Michigan	248-898-5000	www.beaumonthospitals.com
Beckley ARH Hospital	Beckley	West Virginia	304-255-3456	www.arh.org/beckley
Bellevue Hospital Center	New York	New York	212-561-4132	www.nyc.gov/html/hhc/html/facilities/bellevue.shtml
Beth Israel Deaconess Hospital - Milton	Milton	Massachusetts	617-696-4600	www.miltonhosital.org
Beth Israel Deaconess Medical Center	Boston	Massachusetts	617-667-7000	www.bidmc.harvard.edu
Beth Israel Medical Center	New York	New York	212-420-2000	www.wehealny.org
Bluefield Regional Medical Center	Bluefield	West Virginia	304-327-1100	www.bluefield.org
Bolivar Medical Center	Cleveland	Mississippi	662-846-2551	www.bolivarmedical.com
Boston Medical Center Corporation	Boston	Massachusetts	617-638-8000	www.bmc.org
Botsford Hospital	Farmington Hills	Michigan	248-471-8000	www.botsfordsystem.org
Bridgeport Hospital	Bridgeport	Connecticut	203-384-3000	www.bridgeporthospital.com
Brigham & Women's Faulkner Hospital	Boston	Massachusetts	617-983-7000	www.brighamandwomensfaulkner.org
Brigham & Women's Hospital	Boston	Massachusetts	617-732-5500	www.brighamandwomens.org
Bronx - Lebanon Hospital Center	Bronx	New York	212-588-7000	www.bronx-leb.org
Brookdale Hospital Medical Center	Brooklyn	New York	718-240-5966	www.brookdalehospital.org
Brookhaven Memorial Hospital Medical Center	Patchogue	New York	631-654-7100	www.brookhavenhospitalorg
Brooklyn Hospital Center at Downtown Campus	Brooklyn	New York	718-250-8000	www.tbh.org
Byrd Regional Hospital	Leesville	Louisiana	337-239-9041	www.chs.net
California Hospital Medical Center Los Angeles	Los Angeles	California	213-748-2411	www.chmcla.org
Camden Clark Medical Center	Parkersburg	West Virginia	304-424-2111	www.ccmh.org
Capital Health System - Fuld Campus	Trenton	New Jersey	609-394-6000	www.capitalhealth.org
Capital Regional Medical Center	Tallahassee	Florida	850-656-5000	www.capitalregionalmedicalcenter.com
Carepoint Health - Christ Hospital	Jersey City	New Jersey	201-795-8200	www.christhospital.org
Carepoint Health - Hoboken UMC	Hoboken	New Jersey	201-418-1004	www.bonsecoursnj.com
Carolinas Hospital System	Florence	South Carolina	843-674-2500	www.carolinashospital.com
Casey County Hospital	Liberty	Kentucky	606-787-6275	
Catskill Regional Medical Center	Harris	New York	845-794-3300	www.crmcny.org
Chambers Memorial Hospital	Danville	Arkansas	479-495-2241	www.chambershospital.com
Chesapeake General Hospital	Chesapeake	Virginia	757-312-8121	www.chesapeakehealth.com
Clay County Hospital	Flora	Illinois	618-662-2131	www.claycountyhospital.org
Cleveland Clinic	Cleveland	Ohio	216-444-2200	www.clevelandclinic.org
Cleveland Clinic Hospital	Weston	Florida	954-689-5000	www.clevelandclinic.org
Clinch Valley Medical Center	Richlands	Virginia	276-596-6000	www.clinchvalleymedicalcenter.com
Coffee Regional Medical Center	Douglas	Georgia	229-384-1900	www.coffeeregional.org
Coliseum Medical Center	Macon	Georgia	478-765-4100	www.coliseumhealthsystem.com
Community Regional Medical Center	Fresno	California	559-459-6000	www.communitymedical.org
Conemaugh Valley Memorial Hospital	Johnstown	Pennsylvania	814-534-9000	www.conemaugh.org
Coney Island Hospital	Brooklyn	New York	718-616-3000	www.coneyislandhospital.com
Cooper University Hospital	Camden	New Jersey	856-342-2000	www.cooperhealth.org
Covenant Medical Center	Saginaw	Michigan	989-583-4000	www.covenanthealthcare.com
Crittenden Health System	Marion	Kentucky	270-965-5281	www.crittenden-health.org
Danville Regional Medical Center	Danville	Virginia	434-799-2100	www.danvilleregional.org
Davis Memorial Hospital	Elkins	West Virginia	304-636-3300	www.davishealthcare.org
Desert Valley Hospital	Victorville	California	760-241-8000	www.dvmc.com
Desoto Memorial Hospital	Arcadia	Florida	863-494-3535	www.dmh.org
Detroit Receiving Hospital & University Health Center	Detroit	Michigan	313-745-3104	www.drhuhc.org
Doctors Hospital	Columbus	Ohio	614-544-1000	www.columbusregional.com
Doctors Hospital of Manteca	Manteca	California	209-823-3111	www.doctorsmanteca.com

Hospital	City	State	Phone	Web Site
Drew Memorial Hospital	Monticello	Arkansas	870-367-2411	www.drewmemorial.org
Duke University Hospital	Durham	North Carolina	919-684-8111	www.dukehealth.org
Dyersburg Regional Medical Center	Dyersburg	Tennessee	731-285-2410	www.dyersburgregionalmc.com
East Georgia Regional Medical Center	Statesboro	Georgia	912-486-1500	www.egrmc.com
East Ohio Regional Hospital	Martins Ferry	Ohio	740-633-4151	www.eastohioregionalhospital.com
East Orange General Hospital	East Orange	New Jersey	973-266-4401	www.evh.org
Eastern Niagara Hospital	Lockport	New York	716-514-5700	www.enhs.org
Eastern State Hospital	Williamsburg	Virginia	757-253-5161	www.ehs.dmhmrsas.virginia.gov
Easton Hospital	Easton	Pennsylvania	610-250-4076	www.easton-hospital.com
Elmhurst Hospital Center	Elmhurst	New York	718-334-1141	www.nyc.gov
Emanuel Medical Center	Turlock	California	209-667-4200	www.emanuelmedicalcenter.org
Excela Health Frick Hospital	Mount Pleasant	Pennsylvania	724-547-1500	www.excelahealth.org
Fauquier Hospital	Warrenton	Virginia	540-316-5000	www.fauquierhospital.org
Fayette County Hospital	Vandalia	Illinois	618-283-1231	www.fayettecountyhospital.org
Fitzgibbon Hospital	Marshall	Missouri	660-886-7431	www.fitzgibbon.org
Florida Hospital	Orlando	Florida	407-303-1976	www.floridahospital.com
Flushing Hospital Medical Center	Flushing	New York	718-670-5000	www.flushinghospital.org
Forest Hills Hospital	Forest Hills	New York	718-830-4000	www.northshorelij.com
Franciscan Saint James Health	Olympia Fields	Illinois	708-747-4000	www.franciscanalliance.org
Franciscan Saint Margaret Health - Hammond	Hammond	Indiana	219-932-2300	www.smmhc.com
Franklin Hospital	Valley Stream	New York	516-256-6000	www.northshorelij.com
Frederick Memorial Hospital	Frederick	Maryland	240-566-3300	www.fmh.org
Garden City Hospital	Garden City	Michigan	734-421-3300	www.gchosp.org
Gateway Medical Center	Clarksville	Tennessee	931-502-1000	www.todaysgateway.com
Genesis Healthcare System	Zanesville	Ohio	740-454-5000	www.genesishcs.org
George Washington Univ Hospital	Washington	District of Columbia	202-716-4605	www.gwhospital.com
Glenwood Regional Medical Center	West Monroe	Louisiana	318-329-4600	www.grmc.com
Good Samaritan Hospital of Suffern	Suffern	New York	914-368-5000	www.goodsamhosp.org
Grant Medical Center	Columbus	Ohio	614-566-9978	www.ohiohealth.com
Great River Medical Center	Blytheville	Arkansas	870-838-7300	www.greatrivermc.com
Harlan Appalachian Regional Healthcare Hospital	Harlan	Kentucky	606-573-8100	www.arh.org
Harlem Hospital Center	New York	New York	212-491-8400	www.nyc.gov/hhc
Harper University Hospital	Detroit	Michigan	313-745-6211	www.harperhospital.org
Harris Hospital	Newport	Arkansas	870-523-8911	www.harrishospital.com
Harton Regional Medical Center	Tullahoma	Tennessee	931-393-3000	www.hartonmedicalcenter.com
Hazard ARH Regional Medical Center	Hazard	Kentucky	606-439-6600	www.arh.org/hazard
Health Alliance Hospital Broadway Campus	Kingston	New York	914-331-3131	www.kingstonregionalhealth.org
Henry Ford Hospital	Detroit	Michigan	313-916-2600	www.henryfordhospital.com
Hialeah Hospital	Hialeah	Florida	305-693-6100	www.hialeahhosp.com
Highlands Regional Medical Center	Prestonsburg	Kentucky	606-886-8511	www.hrmc.org
Hollywood Presbyterian Medical Center	Los Angeles	California	213-413-3000	www.qahpmc.com
Holy Cross Hospital	Chicago	Illinois	773-471-8000	www.holycrosshospital.org
Holzer Medical Center	Gallipolis	Ohio	740-446-5000	www.holzer.org
Hospital of Univ of Pennsylvania	Philadelphia	Pennsylvania	215-662-3227	www.upenn.edu
Howard University Hospital	Washington	District of Columbia	202-745-6100	www.huhosp.org
Hudson Valley Hospital Center	Cortlandt Manor	New York	914-734-3611	www.hvhc.org
Illinois Valley Community Hospital	Peru	Illinois	815-223-3300	www.ivch.org
Ingalls Memorial Hospital	Harvey	Illinois	708-333-2300	www.ingalls.org
Jackson Memorial Hospital	Miami	Florida	305-585-1111	www.jhsmiami.org
Jackson Parish Hospital	Jonesboro	Louisiana	318-259-4435	www.jacksonparishhospital.com
Jackson Park Hospital	Chicago	Illinois	773-947-7500	www.jacksonparkhospital.org
Jacobi Medical Center	Bronx	New York	718-918-5000	www.ci.nyc.ny.us/html/hhc
Jamaica Hospital Medical Center	Jamaica	New York	718-262-6000	www.jamaicahospital.org
Jane Todd Crawford Hospital	Greensburg	Kentucky	270-932-4211	
Jeanes Hospital	Philadelphia	Pennsylvania	215-728-2000	www.jeanes.com
Jennie Stuart Medical Center	Hopkinsville	Kentucky	270-887-0100	www.jsmc.org
Jennings American Legion Hospital	Jennings	Louisiana	337-616-7000	www.jalh.com
JFK Medical Center	Atlantis	Florida	561-965-7300	www.jfkmc.com
JFK Medical Center - A M Yelencsics Comm Hospital	Edison	New Jersey	732-321-7000	www.jfkmc.org
John H Stroger Jr Hospital	Chicago	Illinois	312-864-6000	www.cookcountygov.com
Johns Hopkins Bayview Medical Center	Baltimore	Maryland	410-550-0123	www.hopkinsbayview.org
The Johns Hopkins Hospital	Baltimore	Maryland	410-955-9540	www.jhmi.edu
Johnson City Medical Center	Johnson City	Tennessee	423-431-6111	www.msha.com
Kendall Regional Medical Center	Miami	Florida	305-223-3000	www.kendallmed.com
Kennedy University Hospital - Stratford Div	Stratford	New Jersey	856-346-6000	www.kennedyhealth.org
Kent County Memorial Hospital	Warwick	Rhode Island	401-737-7000	www.kentri.org
Kentucky River Medical Center	Jackson	Kentucky	606-666-6000	www.kentuckyrivermc.com

Hospital	City	State	Phone	Web Site
King's Daughters' Medical Center	Ashland	Kentucky	606-408-4000	www.kdmc.com
Kings County Hospital Center	Brooklyn	New York	718-245-3901	www.nyc.gov/html/hhc/html/facilities/kings.shtml
Kingsbrook Jewish Medical Center	Brooklyn	New York	718-604-5789	www.kingsbrook.org
Knox County Hospital	Barbourville	Kentucky	606-546-4175	www.knoxcohospital.com
Lahey Hospital & Medical Center - Burlington	Burlington	Massachusetts	781-744-5100	www.lahey.org
Lake Pointe Medical Center	Rowlett	Texas	972-412-2273	www.lakepointemedical.com
Lake Wales Medical Center	Lake Wales	Florida	863-676-1433	www.lakewalesmedicalcenter.com
Larkin Community Hospital	South Miami	Florida	305-284-7500	www.larkinhospital.com
Laurel Regional Medical Center	Laurel	Maryland	301-725-4300	www.laurelregionalhospital.org
Lawrence Hospital Center	Bronxville	New York	914-787-1000	www.lawrencehealth.org
Leesburg Regional Medical Center	Leesburg	Florida	352-323-5762	www.leesburgregional.org
Lenox Hill Hospital	New York	New York	212-439-2345	www.lenoxhillhospital.org
Lewisgale Hospital Pulaski	Pulaski	Virginia	540-994-8100	www.lewisgale.com
Libertyhealth - Jersey City Medical Center Campus	Jersey City	New Jersey	201-915-2000	www.libertyhcs.org
Lincoln Medical & Mental Health Center	Bronx	New York	718-579-5000	www.nyc.gov/html/hhc/lincoln
Little Company of Mary Hospital	Evergreen Park	Illinois	708-422-6200	www.lcmh.org
Long Island Jewish Medical Center	New Hyde Park	New York	718-470-7000	www.northshorelij.com
Lowell General Hospital	Lowell	Massachusetts	978-937-6000	www.lowellgeneral.org
Loyola University Medical Center	Maywood	Illinois	708-216-9000	www.lumc.edu
Lutheran Medical Center	Brooklyn	New York	718-630-8000	www.lmcmc.com
Maimonides Medical Center	Brooklyn	New York	718-283-6000	www.maimonidesmed.org
Mary Immaculate Hospital	Newport News	Virginia	757-886-6000	www.bonsecourshamptonroad.com
Medical Center of Southeastern Oklahoma	Durant	Oklahoma	405-924-3080	www.mcsohealth.com
Medical College of Georgia Hospitals & Clinics	Augusta	Georgia	706-721-6569	www.mcghealth.org
Medical College of Virginia Hospitals	Richmond	Virginia	804-828-0938	www.vcuhealth.org
Medstar Good Samaritan Hospital	Baltimore	Maryland	443-444-3902	www.goodsam-md.org
Medstar Montgomery Medical Center	Olney	Maryland	301-774-8882	www.montgomerygeneral.com
Memorial Hospital	Manchester	Kentucky	606-598-5104	www.manchestermemorial.com
Memorial Hospital	Nacogdoches	Texas	936-564-4611	www.nacmem.org
Memorial Hospital of Gardena	Gardena	California	310-532-4200	www.avantihospitals.com
Memorial Hospital of Salem County	Salem	New Jersey	856-935-1000	www.mhshealth.com
Memorial Hospital of Stilwell	Stilwell	Oklahoma	918-696-3101	www.stilwellmemorialhospital.com
Memorial Regional Hospital	Hollywood	Florida	954-987-2000	www.memorialregional.com
Mercy Fitzgerald Hospital	Darby	Pennsylvania	215-237-4000	www.mercyhealth.org
Mercy Hospital & Medical Center	Chicago	Illinois	312-567-2000	www.mercy-chicago.org
Mercy Hospital Anderson	Cincinnati	Ohio	513-624-4006	www.e-mercy.com/mercy-hospital-anderson.aspx
Mercy Hospital Fairfield	Fairfield	Ohio	513-870-7197	www.e-mercy.com/mercy-hospital-fairfield.aspx
Mercy Hospital Jefferson	Crystal City	Missouri	636-933-1000	www.jeffersonmemorial.org
Mercy Medical Center	Baltimore	Maryland	410-332-9237	www.mdmercy.com
Mercy Regional Medical Center	Ville Platte	Louisiana	337-363-5684	www.vpmc.com
Methodist Hospital	Henderson	Kentucky	270-827-7700	www.methodisthospital.net
Methodist Hospitals	Gary	Indiana	219-886-4642	www.methodisthospital.org
Metrosouth Medical Center	Blue Island	Illinois	708-597-2000	www.stfrancisblueisland.com
Middlesboro Appalachian Regional Healthcare Hospital	Middlesboro	Kentucky	606-242-1101	www.arh.org/middlesboro
Midwest Regional Medical Center	Midwest City	Oklahoma	405-610-8530	www.midwestregional.com
Milford Regional Medical Center	Milford	Massachusetts	508-473-1190	www.milfordregional.org
Miriam Hospital	Providence	Rhode Island	401-793-2500	www.lifespan.org/partners/tmh
Mission Regional Medical Center	Mission	Texas	956-323-9000	www.missionhospital.org
Monmouth Medical Center - Southern Campus	Lakewood	New Jersey	732-363-1900	www.sbhcs.com
Monroe County Medical Center	Tompkinsville	Kentucky	270-487-9231	www.mcmccares.com
Montefiore Medical Center	Bronx	New York	718-920-4321	www.montefiore.org
Montefiore New Rochelle Hospital	New Rochelle	New York	914-632-5000	www.ssmc.org
Morgan County ARH Hospital	West Liberty	Kentucky	606-743-3186	www.arh.org/morgan
Morton Hospital	Taunton	Massachusetts	508-828-7000	www.mortonhospital.org
Mountainview Hospital	Las Vegas	Nevada	702-255-5065	www.mountainview-hospital.com
Musc Medical Center	Charleston	South Carolina	843-792-2300	www.musc.edu
Nacogdoches Medical Center	Nacogdoches	Texas	936-569-9481	www.nacmedicalcenter.com
Nassau University Medical Center	East Meadow	New York	516-572-0123	www.numc.edu
Natchez Community Hospital	Natchez	Mississippi	601-445-6205	www.natchezcommunityhospital.com
Nazareth Hospital	Philadelphia	Pennsylvania	215-335-6000	www.nazarethhospital.org
New York Community Hospital of Brooklyn	Brooklyn	New York	718-692-5302	www.nych.com
New York Hospital Medical Center of Queens	Flushing	New York	718-670-1231	www.nyhq.org
New York Methodist Hospital	Brooklyn	New York	718-780-3000	www.nym.org
New York - Presbyterian Hospital	New York	New York	212-746-4189	www.nyp.org
Newark Beth Israel Medical Center	Newark	New Jersey	973-926-7850	www.sbhcs.com
North Oaks Medical Center	Hammond	Louisiana	985-345-2700	www.northoaks.org
North Shore University Hospital	Manhasset	New York	516-562-0100	www.northshorelij.com

Hospital	City	State	Phone	Web Site
Northside Hospital	Saint Petersburg	Florida	813-521-5000	www.northsidehospital.com
Northwest Hospital Center	Randallstown	Maryland	410-521-5995	www.lifebridgehealth.org
Northwest Mississippi Regional Medical Center	Clarksdale	Mississippi	662-627-3211	www.nwmsregionalmedcenter.com
Northwestern Memorial Hospital	Chicago	Illinois	312-926-2000	www.nmh.org
Norwegian - American Hospital	Chicago	Illinois	773-292-8200	www.nahospital.org
Nyack Hospital	Nyack	New York	845-348-2000	www.nyackhospital.org
NYU Hospitals Center	New York	New York	212-263-7300	www.med.nyu.edu
Oakwood Hospital - Dearborn	Dearborn	Michigan	313-593-7125	www.oakwood.org
Oakwood Hospital - Taylor	Taylor	Michigan	313-295-5253	www.oakwod.org
Oakwood Hospital - Wayne	Wayne	Michigan	734-467-4175	www.oakwood.org
Ohio State University Hospitals	Columbus	Ohio	614-293-9700	www.jamesline.com
Olympia Medical Center	Los Angeles	California	310-657-5900	www.olympiamc.com
Orange Regional Medical Center	Middletown	New York	845-343-2424	www.ormc.org
Oroville Hospital	Oroville	California	530-533-8500	www.orovillehospital.com
Osceola Regional Medical Center	Kissimmee	Florida	407-846-2266	www.osceolaregional.com
Pacifica Hospital of the Valley	Sun Valley	California	818-767-3310	www.pacificahospital.com
Palisades Medical Center	North Bergen	New Jersey	201-854-5000	www.palisadesmedical.org
Palm Springs General Hospital	Hialeah	Florida	305-558-2500	www.psghosp.com
Palmetto General Hospital	Hialeah	Florida	305-823-5000	www.palmettogeneral.com
Palms West Hospital	Loxahatchee	Florida	561-753-4245	www.palmswesthospital.com
Peacehealth Southwest Medical Center	Vancouver	Washington	360-256-2000	www.swmedicalcenter.org
Peconic Bay Medical Center	Riverhead	New York	631-548-6000	www.pbmedicalcenter.org
Pekin Memorial Hospital	Pekin	Illinois	309-347-1151	www.pekinhospital.org
Pennsylvania Hospital of the Univ of PA Health Sys	Philadelphia	Pennsylvania	215-829-3000	www.pennmedicine.org/pahosp
Perry Community Hospital	Linden	Tennessee	931-589-2121	
Pineville Community Hospital	Pineville	Kentucky	606-337-3051	www.pinevillehospital.com
Poplar Bluff Regional Medical Center	Poplar Bluff	Missouri	573-785-7721	www.poplarbluffregional.com
Pottstown Memorial Medical Center	Pottstown	Pennsylvania	610-327-7000	www.pmmctr.org
Presence Saint Francis Hospital	Evanston	Illinois	847-316-4000	www.reshealth.org
Presence Saint Joseph Hospital - Chicago	Chicago	Illinois	773-665-3000	www.res-health.org
Presence Saint Joseph Medical Center	Joliet	Illinois	815-725-7133	www.provena.org/stjoes
Presence Saints Mary & Elizabeth Medical Center	Chicago	Illinois	312-770-2000	www.reshealth.org
Presence Saint Marys Hospital	Kankakee	Illinois	815-937-2490	www.provenastmarys.com
Presence United Samaritans Medical Center	Danville	Illinois	217-443-5000	www.provena.org/usmc
Providence Hospital	Washington	District of Columbia	202-269-7000	www.provhosp.org
Providence Hospital & Medical Centers	Southfield	Michigan	248-849-3011	www.stjohn.org/providence
Queens Hospital Center	Jamaica	New York	718-883-3000	www.nyc.gov/html/hhc/qhn/home.html
Raleigh General Hospital	Beckley	West Virginia	304-256-4100	www.raleighgeneral.com
Raritan Bay Medical Center	Perth Amboy	New Jersey	732-442-3700	www.rbmc.org
Reston Hospital Center	Reston	Virginia	703-689-9000	www.restonhospital.com
Rhode Island Hospital	Providence	Rhode Island	401-444-4000	www.rhodeislandhospital.org
Richmond University Medical Center	Staten Island	New York	718-818-1234	www.rumcsi.org
Riverside Methodist Hospital	Columbus	Ohio	614-566-5000	www.ohiohealth.com
Robert Packer Hospital	Sayre	Pennsylvania	570-888-6666	www.guthrie.org
Robert Wood Johnson University Hospital	New Brunswick	New Jersey	732-937-8900	www.rwjuh.edu
Ronald Reagan UCLA Medical Center	Los Angeles	California	310-825-6301	www.uclahealth.org
Roseland Community Hospital	Chicago	Illinois	773-995-3000	www.roselandhospital.org
Roxborough Memorial Hospital	Philadelphia	Pennsylvania	215-483-9900	www.roxboroughmemorial.com
Rush University Medical Center	Chicago	Illinois	312-942-5000	www.ruch.edu
Saint Francis Hospital	Tulsa	Oklahoma	918-494-2200	www.saintfrancis.com
Saint Francis Medical Center	Peoria	Illinois	309-655-2000	www.osfsaintfrancis.org
Saint Michael's Medical Center	Newark	New Jersey	973-877-5350	www.cathedralhealth.org
Saint Peter's University Hospital	New Brunswick	New Jersey	732-745-8600	www.saintpetersuh.com
Saint Thomas Rutherford Hospital	Murfreesboro	Tennessee	615-396-4100	www.mtmc.org
Saline Memorial Hospital	Benton	Arkansas	501-776-6000	www.salinememorial.org
San Joaquin Community Hospital	Bakersfield	California	661-395-3000	www.sanjoaquinhospital.org
San Luke's Memorial Hospital	Ponce	Puerto Rico	787-844-2080	www.ssepr.com/hospital_sanlucas.html
Sandhills Regional Medical Center	Hamlet	North Carolina	910-958-2361	www.hma-corp.com
Santa Monica - UCLA Medical Center & Orthopaedic Hospital	Santa Monica	California	310-319-4000	www.healthcare.ucla.edu
Scotland Memorial Hospital	Laurinburg	North Carolina	910-291-7000	www.scotlandhealth.org
Silver Cross Hospital & Medical Centers	New Lenox	Illinois	815-300-1100	www.silvercross.org
Sinai Hospital of Baltimore	Baltimore	Maryland	410-601-5131	www.sinai-balt.com
Sinai - Grace Hospital	Detroit	Michigan	313-966-3300	www.sinaigrace.org
Singing River Hospital	Pascagoula	Mississippi	228-809-5000	www.srhshealth.com
South Nassau Communities Hospital	Oceanside	New York	516-632-3000	www.southnassau.org
South Shore Hospital	Chicago	Illinois	773-768-0810	www.southshorehospital.com
Southern Tennessee Medical Center	Winchester	Tennessee	931-967-8295	www.southerntennessee.com

Hospital	City	State	Phone	Web Site
Southern Virginia Regional Medical Center	Emporia	Virginia	434-348-4400	www.svrmc.com
Southwest Healthcare System	Murrieta	California	951-696-6000	www.ivrmc-rsmc.com
Saint Anthony's Medical Center	Saint Louis	Missouri	314-525-1000	www.samcstl.org
Saint Barnabas Hospital	Bronx	New York	212-960-9000	www.stbarnabashospital.org
Saint Bernard Hospital	Chicago	Illinois	773-962-3900	www.stbernardhospital.com
Saint Catherine of Siena Hospital	Smithtown	New York	631-862-3000	www.stcatherines.chsli.org
Saint Claire Regional Medical Center	Morehead	Kentucky	606-783-6500	www.st-claire.org
Saint Elizabeth Hospital	Belleville	Illinois	618-234-2120	www.steliz.org
Saint Elizabeth's Medical Center	Brighton	Massachusetts	617-789-3000	www.semc.org
Saint Francis Hospital	Poughkeepsie	New York	845-483-5000	www.sfhhc.org
Saint John Hospital & Medical Center	Detroit	Michigan	313-343-4000	www.stjohnprovidence.org
Saint John Macomb - Oakland Hospital - Macomb Center	Warren	Michigan	586-573-5000	www.stjohn.org
Saint John's Episcopal Hospital at South Shore	Far Rockaway	New York	718-869-7000	www.ehs.org
Saint John's Riverside Hospital	Yonkers	New York	914-964-4444	www.riversidehealth.org
Saint Joseph Health Services of RI	North Providence	Rhode Island	401-456-3000	www.fatimahospital.com
Saint Joseph Mercy Oakland	Pontiac	Michigan	248-858-3000	www.stjoesoakland.org
Saint Joseph Regional Health Center	Bryan	Texas	979-776-3912	www.st-joseph.org/sjrhc
Saint Joseph's Hospital	Philadelphia	Pennsylvania	215-787-2000	www.nphs.com
Saint Joseph's Medical Center	Yonkers	New York	914-378-7000	www.saintjosephs.org
Saint Joseph's Regional Medical Center	Paterson	New Jersey	973-754-2010	www.sjhmc.org
Saint Louis University Hospital	Saint Louis	Missouri	314-577-8000	www.slucare.edu/clinical
Saint Luke's Roosevelt Hospital	New York	New York	212-523-4000	www.wehealny.org
Saint Luke's Episcopal Hospital	Houston	Texas	832-355-1000	www.sleh.com
Saint Mary Medical Center	Hobart	Indiana	219-942-0551	www.comhs.org/stmary
Saint Mary Mercy Hospital	Livonia	Michigan	734-655-4800	www.stmarymercy.org
Saint Mary's of Michigan Medical Center	Saginaw	Michigan	989-776-8000	www.stmarysofmichigan.org
Saint Marys Hospital	Centralia	Illinois	618-436-6519	www.stmarys-goodsamaritan.com
Saint Rose Hospital	Hayward	California	510-782-6200	www.strosehospital.org
Saint Vincent Hospital	Worcester	Massachusetts	508-363-5000	www.stvincenthospital.com
Saint Vincent's Medical Center	Bridgeport	Connecticut	203-576-5551	www.stvincents.org
Saint Vincent's Medical Center	Jacksonville	Florida	904-308-7300	www.jaxhealth.com
Staten Island University Hospital	Staten Island	New York	718-226-9000	www.siuh.edu
Stephens County Hospital	Toccoa	Georgia	706-282-4250	www.stephenscountyhospital.com
Strong Memorial Hospital	Rochester	New York	585-275-2121	www.urmc.rochester.edu
Summa Health System Barberton Hospital	Barberton	Ohio	330-615-3000	www.barbhosp.com
Sumner Regional Medical Center	Gallatin	Tennessee	615-452-4210	www.mysumnermedical.com
Sunrise Hospital & Medical Center	Las Vegas	Nevada	702-731-8000	www.sunrisehospital.com
Swedish Covenant Hospital	Chicago	Illinois	773-878-8200	www.swedishcovenant.org
Temple University Hospital	Philadelphia	Pennsylvania	215-707-2000	www.tuh.templehealth.org
The University of Chicago Medical Center	Chicago	Illinois	773-702-1000	www.uchospitals.edu
Thomas Jefferson University Hospital	Philadelphia	Pennsylvania	215-955-6000	www.jeffersonhospital.org
Thorek Memorial Hospital	Chicago	Illinois	312-525-6780	www.thorek.org
Trinitas Regional Medical Center	Elizabeth	New Jersey	908-994-5000	www.trinitashospital.org
Tristar Summit Medical Center	Hermitage	Tennessee	615-316-3000	www.summitmedctr.com
Tufts Medical Center	Boston	Massachusetts	617-636-5000	www.tuftsmedicalcenter.org
Tulane Medical Center	New Orleans	Louisiana	504-988-1900	www.tuhc.com
UAMS Medical Center	Little Rock	Arkansas	501-686-5000	www.uams.edu/medcenter
UF Health Shands Hospital	Gainesville	Florida	352-265-8000	www.shands.org
Umass Memorial Medical Center	Worcester	Massachusetts	508-334-1000	www.umassmemorial.org
Union Hospital	Terre Haute	Indiana	812-238-7606	www.uhhg.org
University Health Care/University Hospitals & Clinics	Salt Lake City	Utah	801-581-2121	www.healthcare.utah.edu
University Hospital	Newark	New Jersey	973-972-5658	www.theuniversityhospital.com
University Hospital - Stony Brook	Stony Brook	New York	631-444-4000	www.stonybrookmedicalcenter.org
University Hospital of Brooklyn - Downstate Medical Center	Brooklyn	New York	718-270-1000	www.downstate.edu
University Hospitals - Elyria Medical Center	Elyria	Ohio	440-329-7500	www.emh-healthcare.org
University Hospitals Ahuja Medical Center	Beachwood	Ohio	216-767-8793	www.uhhospitals.org/ahuja
University Hospitals Case Medical Center	Cleveland	Ohio	216-844-1000	www.uhhs.com
University of Alabama Hospital	Birmingham	Alabama	205-934-4011	www.health.uab.edu
University of Arizona Medical Center	Tucson	Arizona	520-694-0111	www.azumc.com
University of Cincinnati Medical Center	Cincinnati	Ohio	513-584-1000	www.universityhospitalcincinnati.com
University of Illinois Hospital	Chicago	Illinois	312-996-3900	www.uic.edu
University of Iowa Hospital & Clinics	Iowa City	Iowa	319-356-1616	www.uihealthcare.com
University of Kentucky Hospital	Lexington	Kentucky	859-323-5000	www.uhealthcare.uky.edu
University of Louisville Hospital	Louisville	Kentucky	502-562-3000	www.uoflhealthcare.org
University of Maryland Medical Center	Baltimore	Maryland	410-328-8667	www.umm.edu
University of Maryland Medical Center Midtown Campus	Baltimore	Maryland	410-225-8996	www.marylandgeneral.org
University of Miami Hospital	Miami	Florida	305-325-5511	www.cedarsmedicalcenter.com

Hospital	City	State	Phone	Web Site
University of Michigan Health System	Ann Arbor	Michigan	734-764-1505	www.med.umich.edu
University of North Carolina Hospital	Chapel Hill	North Carolina	919-966-4131	www.unchealthcare.org
University of Texas Medical Branch Galveston	Galveston	Texas	409-772-1011	www.utmb.edu
University of Virginia Medical Center	Charlottesville	Virginia	800-251-3627	www.uvahealth.com
UPMC Presbyterian Shadyside	Pittsburgh	Pennsylvania	412-647-8788	www.upmc.edu
Valley Hospital	Ridgewood	New Jersey	201-447-8000	www.valleyhealth.com
Valley Hospital Medical Center	Las Vegas	Nevada	702-388-4000	www.valleyhealthsystem.org
Vanderbilt University Hospital	Nashville	Tennessee	615-322-3454	www.mc.vanderbilt.edu
Vassar Brothers Medical Center	Poughkeepsie	New York	845-454-8500	www.vasserbrothers.org
Vidant Medical Center	Greenville	North Carolina	252-847-4100	www.uhseast.com
Vidant Roanoke Chowan Hospital	Ahoskie	North Carolina	252-209-3000	www.uhseast.com
Washington Hospital	Fremont	California	510-797-1111	www.whhs.com
Wellmont Bristol Regional Medical Center	Bristol	Tennessee	423-844-1121	www.wellmont.org
Wellmont Holston Valley Medical Center	Kingsport	Tennessee	423-224-4000	www.wellmont.org
Wesley Medical Center	Hattiesburg	Mississippi	601-268-8000	www.wesley.com
West Chester Hospital	West Chester	Ohio	513-298-3000	www.westchesterhospital.uchealth.com
West River Regional Medical Center	Hettinger	North Dakota	701-567-4561	www.wrhs.com
West Virginia University Hospitals	Morgantown	West Virginia	304-598-4000	www.wvuh.com
Westchester General Hospital	Miami	Florida	305-263-9270	www.westchestergeneralhospital.com
Westchester Medical Center	Valhalla	New York	914-285-7017	www.wcmc.com
Western Arizona Regional Medical Center	Bullhead City	Arizona	928-763-2273	www.warmc.com
Western Maryland Regional Medical Center	Cumberland	Maryland	240-964-8001	www.wmhs.com
White County Medical Center	Searcy	Arkansas	501-278-3100	www.centralarkhospital.com
White River Medical Center	Batesville	Arkansas	870-262-1200	www.wrmc.com
William Beaumont Hospital - Troy	Troy	Michigan	248-964-8800	www.beaumonthospitals.com
Williamson ARH Hospital	South Williamson	Kentucky	606-237-1700	www.arh.org
Williamson Memorial Hospital	Williamson	West Virginia	304-235-2500	www.hmawmh.com
Winter Haven Hospital	Winter Haven	Florida	863-293-1121	www.winterhavenhospital.com
Wyckoff Heights Medical Center	Brooklyn	New York	718-963-7272	www.wyckoffhospital.org
Yale-New Haven Hospital	New Haven	Connecticut	203-688-4242	www.ynhh.org

Note: Table shows hospitals nationwide whose rate of readmission after discharge from hospital (hospital-wide) is better (lower) than U.S. rate of 16.0%

Hospital Heart Attack Readmission Rates: State and National Summary

Area	Number of Hospitals			
	Better than U.S. National Rate[1]	Worse than U.S. National Rate[2]	No Different than U.S. National Rate[3]	Number of Cases Too Small[4]
U.S. and Territories	23	29	2327	2085
Alabama	0	0	39	58
Alaska	0	0	5	14
American Samoa	0	0	0	1
Arizona	0	0	47	21
Arkansas	0	1	27	46
California	1	1	201	122
Colorado	1	0	32	33
Connecticut	0	1	27	3
Delaware	0	0	6	1
District of Columbia	0	0	6	2
Florida	3	3	144	32
Georgia	1	0	64	72
Guam	0	0	1	0
Hawaii	0	0	11	5
Idaho	0	0	9	23
Illinois	0	5	103	71
Indiana	2	0	61	54
Iowa	0	0	27	82
Kansas	0	0	27	82
Kentucky	0	0	40	55
Louisiana	0	0	44	56
Maine	1	0	21	15
Maryland	0	0	39	7
Massachusetts	0	1	52	10
Michigan	1	0	76	51
Minnesota	0	0	31	89
Mississippi	0	0	30	49
Missouri	0	0	53	59
Montana	0	0	8	35
N. Mariana Islands	0	0	1	0
Nebraska	0	0	19	53
Nevada	0	0	18	14
New Hampshire	0	0	15	10
New Jersey	0	5	55	6
New Mexico	1	0	11	26
New York	0	4	132	45
North Carolina	1	1	67	40
North Dakota	1	0	7	33
Ohio	0	0	96	61
Oklahoma	0	1	31	67
Oregon	1	0	23	36
Pennsylvania	1	0	120	41
Puerto Rico	0	1	12	32
Rhode Island	0	0	11	0
South Carolina	1	1	36	22
South Dakota	0	0	9	38
Tennessee	0	1	56	55
Texas	2	0	176	153
Utah	0	0	14	20
Vermont	0	0	8	7
Virgin Islands	0	0	1	1
Virginia	0	2	62	17
Washington	2	0	40	40
West Virginia	0	1	24	28
Wisconsin	3	0	50	68
Wyoming	0	0	2	24

Note: (1) 30-day readmission rate is better (lower) than U.S. rate of 18.3%; (2) 30-day readmission rate is worse (higher) than U.S. rate of 18.3%; (3) 30-day readmission rate is about the same as U.S. rate of 18.3%; (4) The number of cases is too small to classify the hospital

Hospital Heart Failure Readmission Rates: State and National Summary

Area	Number of Hospitals			
	Better than U.S. National Rate[1]	Worse than U.S. National Rate[2]	No Different than U.S. National Rate[3]	Number of Cases Too Small[4]
U.S. and Territories	120	159	3876	631
Alabama	2	1	92	6
Alaska	0	0	12	10
American Samoa	0	0	0	1
Arizona	3	1	60	14
Arkansas	0	3	71	3
California	10	3	280	46
Colorado	3	0	54	17
Connecticut	1	2	29	0
Delaware	0	0	7	0
District of Columbia	0	1	7	0
Florida	8	16	157	6
Georgia	3	1	129	11
Guam	0	0	1	0
Hawaii	1	0	13	5
Idaho	2	0	20	16
Illinois	1	10	168	5
Indiana	3	1	113	3
Iowa	3	0	97	18
Kansas	2	0	85	46
Kentucky	1	8	86	1
Louisiana	2	5	86	16
Maine	2	0	33	2
Maryland	0	6	40	1
Massachusetts	1	3	59	1
Michigan	6	10	108	11
Minnesota	1	1	86	43
Mississippi	0	6	77	13
Missouri	4	6	101	6
Montana	1	0	30	29
N. Mariana Islands	0	0	0	1
Nebraska	3	0	47	35
Nevada	0	0	30	5
New Hampshire	1	0	24	1
New Jersey	1	16	49	1
New Mexico	1	0	32	9
New York	0	22	156	5
North Carolina	6	2	97	8
North Dakota	1	0	24	19
Ohio	2	2	153	10
Oklahoma	2	3	87	25
Oregon	4	0	51	5
Pennsylvania	9	5	144	6
Puerto Rico	0	1	28	20
Rhode Island	0	2	9	1
South Carolina	6	2	53	2
South Dakota	0	0	29	26
Tennessee	3	6	102	4
Texas	11	3	308	52
Utah	3	0	22	17
Vermont	0	0	14	1
Virgin Islands	0	0	2	0
Virginia	1	5	76	2
Washington	2	1	64	21
West Virginia	0	5	45	4
Wisconsin	4	0	111	10
Wyoming	0	0	18	11

Note: (1) 30-day readmission rate is better (lower) than U.S. rate of 23.0%; (2) 30-day readmission rate is worse (higher) than U.S. rate of 23.0%; (3) 30-day readmission rate is about the same as U.S. rate of 23.0%; (4) The number of cases is too small to classify the hospital

Hospital Pneumonia Readmission Rates: State and National Summary

Area	Number of Hospitals			
	Better than U.S. National Rate[1]	Worse than U.S. National Rate[2]	No Different than U.S. National Rate[3]	Number of Cases Too Small[4]
U.S. and Territories	37	135	4285	376
Alabama	0	1	96	5
Alaska	0	0	15	6
American Samoa	0	0	1	0
Arizona	0	0	72	9
Arkansas	1	5	68	3
California	3	5	290	46
Colorado	1	0	62	12
Connecticut	0	1	31	0
Delaware	0	0	7	0
District of Columbia	0	0	8	0
Florida	5	8	170	5
Georgia	1	0	138	4
Guam	0	0	1	0
Hawaii	0	0	14	8
Idaho	0	0	33	7
Illinois	0	11	169	5
Indiana	2	1	115	2
Iowa	0	0	113	5
Kansas	1	0	118	13
Kentucky	1	8	87	0
Louisiana	1	3	95	13
Maine	0	0	36	1
Maryland	0	11	34	1
Massachusetts	0	2	62	1
Michigan	2	5	122	6
Minnesota	0	0	112	19
Mississippi	0	3	87	8
Missouri	2	3	107	6
Montana	2	0	40	20
N. Mariana Islands	0	0	1	0
Nebraska	0	0	77	9
Nevada	0	1	29	6
New Hampshire	0	0	26	0
New Jersey	1	2	63	2
New Mexico	0	0	39	3
New York	2	24	154	5
North Carolina	1	4	104	5
North Dakota	0	0	40	4
Ohio	1	11	149	6
Oklahoma	1	3	103	12
Oregon	1	1	55	3
Pennsylvania	1	3	157	4
Puerto Rico	0	1	26	23
Rhode Island	0	0	11	1
South Carolina	2	1	58	2
South Dakota	0	0	51	5
Tennessee	1	5	105	5
Texas	3	4	325	49
Utah	0	0	37	5
Vermont	0	0	15	0
Virgin Islands	0	0	2	0
Virginia	0	3	79	7
Washington	1	0	81	7
West Virginia	0	5	48	1
Wisconsin	0	0	120	5
Wyoming	0	0	27	2

Note: (1) 30-day readmission rate is better (lower) than U.S. rate of 17.6%; (2) 30-day readmission rate is worse (higher) than U.S. rate of 17.6%; (3) 30-day readmission rate is about the same as U.S. rate of 17.6%; (4) The number of cases is too small to classify the hospital

Hospital Readmission Rate After Hip/Knee Surgery: State and National Summary

Area	Number of Hospitals			
	Better than U.S. National Rate[1]	Worse than U.S. National Rate[2]	No Different than U.S. National Rate[3]	Number of Cases Too Small[4]
U.S. and Territories	51	38	2738	665
Alabama	0	0	52	9
Alaska	0	0	8	0
American Samoa	0	0	0	0
Arizona	1	0	48	7
Arkansas	1	1	28	7
California	8	1	199	90
Colorado	1	0	49	6
Connecticut	0	1	28	0
Delaware	0	0	5	1
District of Columbia	0	1	4	2
Florida	5	4	138	15
Georgia	2	0	77	15
Guam	0	0	0	0
Hawaii	0	0	8	6
Idaho	0	0	23	5
Illinois	1	4	110	24
Indiana	3	0	78	29
Iowa	1	0	47	17
Kansas	1	0	42	12
Kentucky	0	0	42	19
Louisiana	0	1	59	15
Maine	1	0	25	6
Maryland	0	3	40	2
Massachusetts	1	0	55	5
Michigan	1	1	96	18
Minnesota	0	0	67	16
Mississippi	0	0	29	7
Missouri	1	2	64	13
Montana	1	0	19	6
N. Mariana Islands	0	0	0	0
Nebraska	1	0	31	13
Nevada	0	0	23	2
New Hampshire	0	0	22	4
New Jersey	0	1	54	7
New Mexico	1	0	21	3
New York	3	0	119	30
North Carolina	1	0	82	6
North Dakota	1	0	7	1
Ohio	2	2	133	20
Oklahoma	1	1	45	19
Oregon	1	0	39	10
Pennsylvania	2	4	123	29
Puerto Rico	0	0	8	28
Rhode Island	0	0	9	1
South Carolina	0	1	40	13
South Dakota	0	0	17	1
Tennessee	2	2	53	19
Texas	3	5	204	51
Utah	0	0	26	6
Vermont	0	0	12	1
Virgin Islands	0	0	1	0
Virginia	3	2	55	9
Washington	0	0	53	9
West Virginia	0	0	26	6
Wisconsin	1	1	82	21
Wyoming	0	0	13	4

Note: (1) 30-day readmission rate is better (lower) than U.S. rate of 5.4%; (2) 30-day readmission rate is worse (higher) than U.S. rate of 5.4%; (3) 30-day readmission rate is about the same as U.S. rate of 5.4%; (4) The number of cases is too small to classify the hospital

Hospital Readmission Rate After Discharge From Hospital (Hospital-wide): State and National Summary

Area	Number of Hospitals			
	Better than U.S. National Rate[1]	Worse than U.S. National Rate[2]	No Different than U.S. National Rate[3]	Number of Cases Too Small[4]
U.S. and Territories	316	369	3966	158
Alabama	1	1	92	3
Alaska	1	0	20	1
American Samoa	0	0	1	0
Arizona	9	3	64	5
Arkansas	3	11	60	0
California	29	17	283	10
Colorado	9	0	63	3
Connecticut	2	4	25	0
Delaware	0	0	6	0
District of Columbia	0	3	4	0
Florida	13	23	143	2
Georgia	7	5	129	1
Guam	0	0	1	0
Hawaii	2	0	13	6
Idaho	6	0	32	2
Illinois	4	37	137	1
Indiana	14	4	104	2
Iowa	7	1	106	2
Kansas	7	0	125	6
Kentucky	2	20	72	0
Louisiana	6	8	102	9
Maine	3	0	32	1
Maryland	3	14	28	0
Massachusetts	5	13	46	0
Michigan	12	20	93	6
Minnesota	8	0	119	4
Mississippi	1	6	86	5
Missouri	4	6	100	2
Montana	3	0	50	8
N. Mariana Islands	0	0	0	1
Nebraska	6	0	79	4
Nevada	1	3	28	3
New Hampshire	1	0	25	0
New Jersey	2	21	41	0
New Mexico	2	0	38	2
New York	6	57	110	4
North Carolina	15	6	88	2
North Dakota	2	1	38	2
Ohio	6	17	141	7
Oklahoma	9	4	106	6
Oregon	8	0	48	2
Pennsylvania	11	17	134	7
Puerto Rico	0	1	47	4
Rhode Island	0	4	7	0
South Carolina	8	2	52	0
South Dakota	5	0	52	2
Tennessee	4	12	96	1
Texas	31	8	341	20
Utah	6	1	34	2
Vermont	1	0	13	0
Virgin Islands	0	0	2	0
Virginia	3	11	66	4
Washington	12	1	71	2
West Virginia	0	7	42	1
Wisconsin	15	0	107	1
Wyoming	1	0	24	2

Note: (1) 30-day readmission rate is better (lower) than U.S. rate of 16.0%; (2) 30-day readmission rate is worse (higher) than U.S. rate of 16.0%; (3) 30-day readmission rate is about the same as U.S. rate of 16.0%; (4) The number of cases is too small to classify the hospital

Appendix C: Surgical Complication Rates

What Do These Surgical Complication Measures Show?

This appendix shows how hospitals' surgical complication rates compare to the rate across the U.S. The categories are:

- A Wound That Splits Open After Surgery on the Abdomen or Pelvis
- Accidental Cuts and Tears From Medical Treatment
- Collapsed Lung Due to Medical Treatment
- Deaths Among Patients With Serious Treatable Complications After Surgery
- Rate of Complications for Hip/Knee Replacement Patients
- Serious Blood Clots After Surgery
- Serious Complications (see below for details)

This first part of this appendix shows hospitals with surgical complication rates that are lower (better) or higher (worse) than the national rate for all categories. Hospitals are shown to be better or worse than the U.S. national rate only if the data shows with 95% certainty, the difference between their surgical complication rates and the U.S. national rate is not due to chance.

The second part of this appendix contains state and national summaries with the following column headers:

- **Better Than U.S. National Rate.** Hospitals in the Better Than U.S. National Rate category have surgical complication rates that are lower than the U.S. National Rate, with 95% certainty that this difference is not due to chance.
- **Worse Than U.S. National Rate.** Hospitals in the Worse Than U.S. National Rate category have surgical complication rates that are higher than the U.S. National Rate, with 95% certainty that this difference is not due to chance.
- **No Different Than U.S. National Rate.** Many hospitals in the No Different Than U.S. National Rate category have surgical complication rates that are about the same as the U.S. National Rate. Other hospitals in this category have rates that are higher or lower than the U.S. National Rate, without 95% certainty that these differences are not due to chance.
- **Number of Cases Too Small.** The number of cases is too small to classify the hospital.

Serious Complications

Measures of serious complications are drawn from the Agency for Healthcare Research and Quality (AHRQ) Patient Safety Indicators (PSIs). The overall score for serious complications is based on how often adult patients had certain serious, but potentially preventable, complications related to medical or surgical inpatient hospital care. This composite or summary measure is based on the following measures:

- Collapsed lung that results from medical treatment (Iatrogenic pneumothorax, adult)
- Blood clots, in the lung or a large vein, after surgery (Postoperative Pulmonary Embolism or Deep Vein Thrombosis Rate)
- A wound that splits open after surgery (Postoperative wound dehiscence)
- Accidental cuts and tears (Accidental puncture or laceration)
- Pressure sores (Pressure ulcers)
- Infections from a large venous catheters (Central venous catheter-related blood stream infection rate)
- Broken hip from a fall after surgery (Postoperative hip fracture rate)
- Blood stream infection after surgery (Postoperative sepsis)

Which Patients are Included

The Serious Complications measure applies only to Medicare beneficiaries enrolled in Original Medicare (traditional fee-for-service (FFS) Medicare) who were discharged from a hospital that was paid through the inpatient prospective payment system (IPPS) after the beneficiary had an inpatient stay. Non-Medicare patients and beneficiaries enrolled in Medicare managed care plans are also excluded from the data.

Where the Information Comes From

The Centers for Medicare & Medicaid Services (CMS) calculates the indicators of patient safety data from the claims hospitals submit for Medicare beneficiaries enrolled in Original Medicare(traditional FFS Medicare). The rate for each PSI is calculated by dividing the actual number of outcomes at each hospital by the number of eligible discharges for that measure at each hospital, multiplied by 1,000. The composite value reported on Hospital Compare is the weighted averages of the component indicators. PSI data are only calculated for hospitals that are paid through the IPPS, which excludes Critical Access hospitals (CAHs), long-term care hospitals (LTCHs), Maryland waiver hospitals, cancer hospitals, children's inpatient facilities, rural health clinics, federally qualified health centers, inpatient psychiatric hospitals, inpatient rehabilitation facilities, Veterans Administration/ Department of Defense hospitals, and religious, non-medical health care institutions.

Risk Adjustment

The measures of serious complications reported are risk adjusted to account for differences in hospital patients' characteristics. In addition, the rates reported are "smoothed" to reflect the fact that measures for small hospitals are measured less accurately (i.e., are less reliable) than for larger hospitals.

Comparing Individual Hospital Rates to Benchmarks

For the composite measure, CMS assigns comparative performance categories. If the interval estimate includes and/or overlaps with the national composite value, the hospital's performance is in the "no different than U.S. national rate" category. If the entire interval estimate is below the national composite value, then the hospital is performing "better than U.S. national rate." If the entire interval estimate is above the national composite value, it is "worse than U.S. national rate."

Additional Information

For more detail on Serious Complications measures (AHRQ Patient Safety Indicators) visit the Agency for Healthcare Research and Quality (AHRQ) Patient Safety Indicator Resources Web site at www.qualityindicators.ahrq.gov.

Hospitals whose Surgical Complication Rate is Better (Lower) than the U.S. National Rate

Measure: A Wound That Splits Open After Surgery on the Abdomen or Pelvis

Hospital	City	State	Phone	Web Site
No hospitals met this criteria.				

Note: Table shows hospitals nationwide whose surgical complication rate is better (lower) than U.S. rate of 0.92%

Hospitals whose Surgical Complication Rate is Worse (Higher) than the U.S. National Rate

Measure: A Wound That Splits Open After Surgery on the Abdomen or Pelvis

Hospital	City	State	Phone	Web Site
Aurora Lakeland Medical Center	Elkhorn	Wisconsin	262-741-2000	www.aurorahealthcare.org/facilities
Banner Thunderbird Medical Center	Glendale	Arizona	602-588-5555	www.bannerhealth.com
Beaumont Health System	Royal Oak	Michigan	248-898-5000	www.beaumonthospitals.com
Bronson Methodist Hospital	Kalamazoo	Michigan	269-341-6000	www.bronsonhealth.com
Central Carolina Hospital	Sanford	North Carolina	919-774-2100	www.centralcarolinahosp.com
Cjw Medical Center	Richmond	Virginia	804-330-2001	www.hcavirginia.com
Eastern Idaho Regional Medical Center	Idaho Falls	Idaho	208-529-6111	www.eirmc.org
Erlanger Medical Center	Chattanooga	Tennessee	423-778-7000	www.erlanger.org
Exeter Hospital	Exeter	New Hampshire	603-778-7311	www.exeterhospital.com
Fairfield Medical Center	Lancaster	Ohio	740-687-8009	www.fmchealth.org
Florida Hospital Deland	Deland	Florida	386-943-4772	www.fhdeland.org
Florida Hospital Fish Memorial	Orange City	Florida	386-917-5000	www.fhfishmemorial.org
Frye Regional Medical Center	Hickory	North Carolina	828-322-6070	www.fryemedctr.com
Genesys Regional Medical Center - Health Park	Grand Blanc	Michigan	810-606-5000	www.genesys.org
Good Samaritan Hospital	San Jose	California	408-559-2011	www.goodsamsj.org
Health Alliance Hospital Broadway Campus	Kingston	New York	914-331-3131	www.kingstonregionalhealth.org
Inspira Medical Center Woodbury	Woodbury	New Jersey	856-845-0100	www.umhospital.org
Lake Cumberland Regional Hospital	Somerset	Kentucky	606-679-7441	www.lakecumberlandhospital.com
Lake Regional Health System	Osage Beach	Missouri	573-348-8000	www.lakeregional.com
Lakeland Hospital - Saint Joseph	Saint Joseph	Michigan	269-983-8300	www.lakelandhealth.org
Longmont United Hospital	Longmont	Colorado	303-651-5111	www.luhcares.org
Maine Medical Center	Portland	Maine	207-662-0111	www.mmc.org
Mayo Clinic Hospital Rochester	Rochester	Minnesota	507-255-5123	www.mayoclinic.org/saintmaryshospital
The Medical Center of Aurora	Aurora	Colorado	303-695-2600	www.auroramed.com
Medstar Washington Hospital Center	Washington	District of Columbia	202-877-7000	www.whcenter.org
Memorial Health Univ Medical Center	Savannah	Georgia	912-350-8000	www.memorialhealth.com
Mercy Saint Anne Hospital	Toledo	Ohio	419-407-2663	www.mercyweb.org
Miami Valley Hospital	Dayton	Ohio	937-208-8000	www.miamivalleyhospital.com
Mountainview Hospital	Las Vegas	Nevada	702-255-5065	www.mountainview-hospital.com
Norton Hospitals	Louisville	Kentucky	502-629-6560	www.nortonhealthcare.com
Pali Momi Medical Center	Aiea	Hawaii	808-486-6000	www.kapiolani.org
Pottstown Memorial Medical Center	Pottstown	Pennsylvania	610-327-7000	www.pmmctr.org
Robert Wood Johnson University Hospital at Rahway	Rahway	New Jersey	732-381-4200	www.rwjuhr.com/about/history.html
Southeast Georgia Health System - Brunswick Campus	Brunswick	Georgia	912-466-7000	www.sghs.org
Spring Valley Hospital Medical Center	Las Vegas	Nevada	702-853-3000	www.springvalleyhospital.com
Saint Joseph Regional Health Center	Bryan	Texas	979-776-3912	www.st-joseph.org/sjrhc
Saint Luke's Episcopal Hospital	Houston	Texas	832-355-1000	www.sleh.com
Touro Infirmary	New Orleans	Louisiana	504-897-7011	www.touro.com
University of Wisconsin Hospitals & Clinics Authority	Madison	Wisconsin	608-263-8991	www.uwhealth.org
UNM Hospital	Albuquerque	New Mexico	505-272-2111	www.hospitals.unm.edu/unmh
Wayne Memorial Hospital	Honesdale	Pennsylvania	570-253-8100	www.wmh.org

Note: Table shows hospitals nationwide whose surgical complication rate is worse (higher) than U.S. rate of 0.92%

Hospitals whose Surgical Complication Rate is Better (Lower) than the U.S. National Rate

Measure: Accidental Cuts and Tears From Medical Treatment

Hospital	City	State	Phone	Web Site
Advocate Christ Hospital & Medical Center	Oak Lawn	Illinois	708-684-8000	www.advocatehealth.com
Advocate Good Samaritan Hospital	Downers Grove	Illinois	630-275-5900	www.advocatehealth.com/gsam
Advocate Lutheran General Hospital	Park Ridge	Illinois	847-723-2210	www.advocatehealth.com
Arkansas Heart Hospital	Little Rock	Arkansas	501-219-7000	www.arheart.com
Asante Rogue Regional Medical Center	Medford	Oregon	541-789-7000	www.asante.org
Atlanticare Regional Medical Center	Atlantic City	New Jersey	609-441-8020	www.atlanticare.org/acmc/index.html
Aventura Hospital & Medical Center	Aventura	Florida	305-682-7000	www.aventurahospital.com
Baptist Beaumont Hospital	Beaumont	Texas	409-212-5012	www.mhbh.org
Baystate Medical Center	Springfield	Massachusetts	413-794-0000	www.baystatehealth.com
Bethesda Hospital East	Boynton Beach	Florida	561-737-7733	www.bethesdahealthcare.com
Cape Regional Medical Center	Cape May Ct House	New Jersey	609-463-2000	www.caperegional.com
Cedars - Sinai Medical Center	Los Angeles	California	310-423-5000	www.cedars-sinai.edu
Central Dupage Hospital	Winfield	Illinois	630-682-1600	www.cdh.org
Christiana Care Health Services	Newark	Delaware	302-733-1000	www.christianacare.org
Christus Spohn Hospital Corpus Christi	Corpus Christi	Texas	361-902-4103	www.christusspohn.org
Clear Lake Regional Medical Center	Webster	Texas	281-332-2511	www.clearlakermc.com
Community Medical Center	Toms River	New Jersey	732-557-8000	www.sbhcs.com
Delray Medical Center	Delray Beach	Florida	561-498-4440	www.delraymedicalctr.com
Duke University Hospital	Durham	North Carolina	919-684-8111	www.dukehealth.org
Englewood Hospital & Medical Center	Englewood	New Jersey	201-894-3000	www.englewoodhospital.com
Florida Hospital	Orlando	Florida	407-303-1976	www.floridahospital.com
Floyd Medical Center	Rome	Georgia	706-509-6900	www.floydmed.org
Glendale Adventist Medical Center	Glendale	California	818-409-8202	www.glendaleadventist.com
Good Samaritan Hospital Medical Center	West Islip	New York	631-376-3000	www.good-samaritan-hospital.org
Good Samaritan Medical Center	Brockton	Massachusetts	508-427-3000	www.goodsamaritanmedical.org
Indiana University Health	Indianapolis	Indiana	317-962-5900	www.iuhealth.org
Integris Baptist Medical Center	Oklahoma City	Oklahoma	405-951-8110	www.integris-health.com
Integris Southwest Medical Center	Oklahoma City	Oklahoma	405-636-7000	www.integris-health.com
Jackson - Madison County General Hospital	Jackson	Tennessee	731-541-5000	www.wth.org
Lakeland Regional Medical Center	Lakeland	Florida	863-687-1100	www.lrmc.com
Laredo Medical Center	Laredo	Texas	956-796-5000	www.laredomedical.com
Lovelace Medical Center	Albuquerque	New Mexico	505-727-8000	www.lovelace.com
Marietta Memorial Hospital	Marietta	Ohio	740-374-1400	www.mmhospital.org
Marion General Hospital	Marion	Ohio	740-383-8400	www.mariongeneral.com
Mayo Clinic	Jacksonville	Florida	904-953-2000	www.mayoclinic.org/jacksonville
Mayo Clinic Hospital	Phoenix	Arizona	480-342-2000	www.mayoclinic.org
Mayo Clinic Hospital Rochester	Rochester	Minnesota	507-255-5123	www.mayoclinic.org/saintmaryshospital
Mayo Clinic Methodist- Hospital	Rochester	Minnesota	507-266-7890	www.mayoclinic.org/methodisthospital
Mclaren Bay Region	Bay City	Michigan	989-894-3000	www.baymed.org
Memorial Healthcare System	Chattanooga	Tennessee	423-495-2525	www.memorial.org
Memorial Hermann Hospital System	Houston	Texas	713-448-6796	www.memorialhermann.org
Memorial Hermann Memorial City Medical Center	Houston	Texas	713-242-3000	www.mhhs.org
Memorial Hermann Texas Medical Center	Houston	Texas	713-704-3700	www.mhhs.org
Memorial Hospital	Belleville	Illinois	618-233-7750	www.memhosp.com
Memorial Regional Hospital	Hollywood	Florida	954-987-2000	www.memorialregional.com
Mercy Hospital Fairfield	Fairfield	Ohio	513-870-7197	www.e-mercy.com/mercy-hospital-fairfield.aspx
Methodist Hospital	San Antonio	Texas	210-575-4000	www.mh.sahealth.com
The Methodist Hospital	Houston	Texas	713-790-2221	www.methodisthealth.com
Methodist Willowbrook Hospital	Houston	Texas	281-477-1000	www.houstonmethodist.org/willowbrook-hospital
Mississippi Baptist Medical Center	Jackson	Mississippi	601-968-1000	www.mbmc.org
Munroe Regional Medical Center	Ocala	Florida	352-351-7200	www.munroeregional.com
North Florida Regional Medical Center	Gainesville	Florida	352-333-4100	www.nfrmc.com
Northwestern Memorial Hospital	Chicago	Illinois	312-926-2000	www.nmh.org
Ocala Regional Medical Center	Ocala	Florida	352-401-1000	www.ocalaregional.com
Our Lady of Lourdes Medical Center	Camden	New Jersey	856-757-3500	www.lourdesnet.org
Overlook Medical Center	Summit	New Jersey	908-522-2000	www.atlantichealth.org
Palos Community Hospital	Palos Heights	Illinois	708-923-4000	www.paloshospital.org
Presence Resurrection Medical Center	Chicago	Illinois	773-774-8000	www.reshealthcare.org
Presence Saint Joseph Medical Center	Joliet	Illinois	815-725-7133	www.provena.org/stjoes
Providence Little Co of Mary Medical Center Torrance	Torrance	California	310-540-7676	www.lcmhs.org
Providence Tarzana Medical Center	Tarzana	California	818-881-0800	www.encino-tarzana.com
Roper Hospital	Charleston	South Carolina	843-724-2800	www.ropersaintfrancis.com
Saint Thomas West Hospital	Nashville	Tennessee	615-222-2111	www.stthomas.org
Scripps Memorial Hospital La Jolla	La Jolla	California	858-626-4123	www.scrippshealth.org

Hospital	City	State	Phone	Web Site
Sentara Careplex Hospital	Hampton	Virginia	757-736-1000	www.sentara.com
Sentara Leigh Hospital	Norfolk	Virginia	757-261-6601	www.sentara.com
Sentara Norfolk General Hospital	Norfolk	Virginia	757-388-3000	www.sentara.com
Sentara Virginia Beach General Hospital	Virginia Beach	Virginia	757-395-8000	www.sentara.com
Shasta Regional Medical Center	Redding	California	530-244-5454	www.shastaregional.com
South Shore Hospital	South Weymouth	Massachusetts	781-340-8000	www.southshorehospital.org
Saint Francis Hospital	Columbus	Georgia	706-596-4020	www.wecareforlife.com
Saint Francis Hospital - Roslyn	Roslyn	New York	516-562-6000	www.stfrancisheartcenter.com
Saint John Medical Center	Tulsa	Oklahoma	918-744-3606	www.sjmc.org
Saint John's Riverside Hospital	Yonkers	New York	914-964-4444	www.riversidehealth.org
Saint Luke's Episcopal Hospital	Houston	Texas	832-355-1000	www.sleh.com
Saint Mary Medical Center	Langhorne	Pennsylvania	215-750-2003	www.stmaryhealthcare.org
Saint Mary Mercy Hospital	Livonia	Michigan	734-655-4800	www.stmarymercy.org
Saint Vincent Heart Center of Indiana	Indianapolis	Indiana	317-583-5000	www.theheartcenter.com
Staten Island University Hospital	Staten Island	New York	718-226-9000	www.siuh.edu
Sutter General Hospital	Sacramento	California	916-733-8999	www.suttermedicalcenter.org
Swedish Covenant Hospital	Chicago	Illinois	773-878-8200	www.swedishcovenant.org
Tennova Healthcare	Knoxville	Tennessee	865-545-8000	www.stmaryshealth.com
The Nebraska Medical Center	Omaha	Nebraska	402-552-2040	www.nebraskamed.com
Tuomey Healthcare System	Sumter	South Carolina	803-774-8900	www.tuomey.com
UF Health Shands Hospital	Gainesville	Florida	352-265-8000	www.shands.org
United Hospital Center	Bridgeport	West Virginia	681-342-1000	www.uhcwv.org
University of Kentucky Hospital	Lexington	Kentucky	859-323-5000	www.uhealthcare.uky.edu
University of Michigan Health System	Ann Arbor	Michigan	734-764-1505	www.med.umich.edu
Valley Hospital	Ridgewood	New Jersey	201-447-8000	www.valleyhealth.com
Vanderbilt University Hospital	Nashville	Tennessee	615-322-3454	www.mc.vanderbilt.edu
Virtua West Jersey Hospitals Berlin	Berlin	New Jersey	856-322-3200	www.virtua.org
Williamsport Regional Medical Center	Williamsport	Pennsylvania	570-321-1000	www.susquehannahealth.org
Winchester Medical Center	Winchester	Virginia	540-536-8000	www.valleyhealthlink.com
Winthrop - University Hospital	Mineola	New York	516-663-0333	www.winthrop.org

Note: Table shows hospitals nationwide whose surgical complication rate is better (lower) than U.S. rate of 1.83%

Hospitals whose Surgical Complication Rate is Worse (Higher) than the U.S. National Rate

Measure: Accidental Cuts and Tears From Medical Treatment

Hospital	City	State	Phone	Web Site
Adena Regional Medical Center	Chillicothe	Ohio	740-779-7500	www.adena.org
Adirondack Medical Center	Saranac Lake	New York	518-891-4141	www.amccares.org
Aiken Regional Medical Center	Aiken	South Carolina	803-641-5900	www.aikenregional.com
Alaska Native Medical Center	Anchorage	Alaska	907-563-2662	www.anmc.org
Appleton Medical Center	Appleton	Wisconsin	920-731-4101	www.thedacare.org
Atlanta Medical Center	Atlanta	Georgia	404-265-4000	www.atlantamedcenter.com
B R F Hospital Holdings	Shreveport	Louisiana	318-675-5000	www.lsumc.edu
Baptist Saint Anthony's Hospital	Amarillo	Texas	806-212-2000	www.bsahs.com
Barnes-Jewish Hospital	Saint Louis	Missouri	314-747-3000	www.barnesjewish.org
Baylor University Medical Center	Dallas	Texas	214-820-0111	www.baylorhealth.com
Beth Israel Deaconess Medical Center	Boston	Massachusetts	617-667-7000	www.bidmc.harvard.edu
Blessing Hospital	Quincy	Illinois	217-223-5811	www.blessinghealthsystem.org
Borgess Medical Center	Kalamazoo	Michigan	269-226-7000	www.borgess.com
Boston Medical Center Corporation	Boston	Massachusetts	617-638-8000	www.bmc.org
Bridgeport Hospital	Bridgeport	Connecticut	203-384-3000	www.bridgeporthospital.com
Carney Hospital	Boston	Massachusetts	617-506-2000	www.caritascarney.org
Caromont Regional Medical Center	Gastonia	North Carolina	704-834-4891	www.caromont.org
Catholic Medical Center	Manchester	New Hampshire	603-668-3545	www.catholicmedicalcenter.org
Centra Health	Lynchburg	Virginia	434-200-4789	www.centrahealth.com
Central Texas Medical Center	San Marcos	Texas	512-753-3690	www.ctmc.org
Centrastate Medical Center	Freehold	New Jersey	732-431-2000	www.centrastate.com
Cheshire Medical Center	Keene	New Hampshire	603-354-5400	www.cheshire-med.com
Chilton Medical Center	Pompton Plains	New Jersey	973-831-5000	www.chiltonmemorial.org
Clearview Regional Medical Center	Monroe	Georgia	770-267-1792	www.clearviewregionalmedicalcenter.com
Cleveland Clinic	Cleveland	Ohio	216-444-2200	www.clevelandclinic.org
Clovis Community Medical Center	Clovis	California	559-324-4000	www.communitymedical.org
Community Regional Medical Center	Fresno	California	559-459-6000	www.communitymedical.org
Covenant Hospital Plainview	Plainview	Texas	806-296-5531	www.covenantplainview.org
Crestwood Medical Center	Huntsville	Alabama	256-882-3100	www.crestwoodmedcenter.com
Crossgates River Oaks Hospital	Brandon	Mississippi	601-825-2811	www.rankinmedcenter.com
Crouse Hospital	Syracuse	New York	315-470-7449	www.crouse.org
Dameron Hospital	Stockton	California	209-944-5550	www.dameronhospital.org
Deaconess Hospital	Spokane	Washington	509-473-5800	www.deaconessmedicalcenter.org
Deaconess Hospital	Evansville	Indiana	812-450-5000	www.deaconess.com
Desert Regional Medical Center	Palm Springs	California	760-323-6511	www.desertmedctr.com
Eisenhower Medical Center	Rancho Mirage	California	760-340-3911	www.emc.org
El Camino Hospital	Mountain View	California	650-940-7000	www.elcaminohospital.org
Eliza Coffee Memorial Hospital	Florence	Alabama	256-768-8400	www.chgroup.org
Emory University Hospital Midtown	Atlanta	Georgia	404-686-4411	www.emoryhealthcare.org
Faith Regional Health Services	Norfolk	Nebraska	402-371-4880	www.frhs.org
Firsthealth Moore Regional Hospital	Pinehurst	North Carolina	910-715-1000	www.firsthealth.org
Geisinger Medical Center	Danville	Pennsylvania	570-271-6211	www.geisinger.org
Geisinger Wyoming Valley Medical Center	Wilkes Barre	Pennsylvania	570-826-7300	www.geisinger.org
Gila Regional Medical Center	Silver City	New Mexico	575-538-4000	www.grmc.org
Good Samaritan Hospital	San Jose	California	408-559-2011	www.goodsamsj.org
Good Samaritan Hospital	Dayton	Ohio	937-278-2612	www.goodsamdayton.org
Good Shepherd Medical Center Marshall	Marshall	Texas	903-927-6712	www.marshallregional.org
Grady Memorial Hospital	Atlanta	Georgia	404-616-4252	www.gradyhealthsystem.org
Grinnell Regional Medical Center	Grinnell	Iowa	641-236-7511	www.grmc.us
Grossmont Hospital	La Mesa	California	619-465-0711	www.sharp.com
Harborview Medical Center	Seattle	Washington	206-731-3000	www.harborview.org
Hennepin County Medical Center	Minneapolis	Minnesota	612-873-3000	www.hcmc.org
Henrico Doctors' Hospital	Richmond	Virginia	804-289-4500	www.henricodoctors.com
Heritage Valley Beaver	Beaver	Pennsylvania	412-728-7000	www.heritagevalley.org
The Indiana Heart Hospital	Indianapolis	Indiana	317-621-8063	www.hearthospital.com
Inspira Medical Center Vineland	Vineland	New Jersey	856-641-6610	www.sjhs.com
Intermountain Medical Center	Murray	Utah	801-507-7000	www.intermountainhealthcare.org
Jewish Hospital & Saint Mary's Healthcare	Louisville	Kentucky	502-587-4011	www.jhhs.org
John Dempsey Hospital	Farmington	Connecticut	860-679-1145	www.uconnhealth.orgorwww.uchc.edu
JPS Health Network	Fort Worth	Texas	817-921-3431	www.jpshealthnet.org
Jupiter Medical Center	Jupiter	Florida	561-747-2234	www.jupitermed.com
Kadlec Regional Medical Center	Richland	Washington	509-946-4611	www.kadlecmed.org
Kaiser Foundation Hospital - Fontana	Fontana	California	909-427-5500	www.kaiserpermanente.com
Kaweah Delta Medical Center	Visalia	California	559-624-2000	www.kaweahdelta.org

Hospital	City	State	Phone	Web Site
Keck Hospital of USC	Los Angeles	California	323-442-8656	www.uscuh.com
Kingman Regional Medical Center	Kingman	Arizona	928-757-2101	www.azkrmc.com
Kuakini Medical Center	Honolulu	Hawaii	808-536-2236	www.kuakini.org
LDS Hospital	Salt Lake City	Utah	801-408-1100	www.intermountainhealthcare.org
Lourdes Hospital	Paducah	Kentucky	270-444-2444	www.ehealthconnection.com
Magee Womens Hospital of UPMC Health System	Pittsburgh	Pennsylvania	412-641-4010	www.magee.edu
Maine Medical Center	Portland	Maine	207-662-0111	www.mmc.org
Manchester Memorial Hospital	Manchester	Connecticut	860-647-4780	www.echn.org
Marin General Hospital	Greenbrae	California	415-925-7900	www.maringeneral.com
Mary Hitchcock Memorial Hospital	Lebanon	New Hampshire	603-650-5000	www.dhmc.org
Mat-Su Regional Medical Center	Palmer	Alaska	907-746-8600	www.matsuregional.com
Mayo Clinic Health System - Mankato	Mankato	Minnesota	507-625-4031	www.isj-mhs.org
Mayo Clinic Health System - Eau Claire Hospital	Eau Claire	Wisconsin	715-838-3311	www.luthermidelfort.org
McKay Dee Hospital	Ogden	Utah	801-387-2800	www.intermountainhealthcare.org
Medical College of Virginia Hospitals	Richmond	Virginia	804-828-0938	www.vcuhealth.org
Medical West	Bessemer	Alabama	205-481-7000	www.uab.edu
Medstar Washington Hospital Center	Washington	District of Columbia	202-877-7000	www.whcenter.org
Memorial Medical Center	Modesto	California	209-526-4500	www.memorialmedicalcenter.org
Memorial Health Univ Medical Center	Savannah	Georgia	912-350-8000	www.memorialhealth.com
Memorial Hospital	York	Pennsylvania	717-843-8623	www.mhyork.org
Memorial Hospital & Health Care Center	Jasper	Indiana	812-996-2345	www.mhhcc.org
Memorial Hospital of Carbondale	Carbondale	Illinois	618-549-0721	www.sih.net
Memorial Medical Center	Springfield	Illinois	217-788-3000	www.memorialmedical.com
Mercy General Hospital	Sacramento	California	916-453-4545	www.mercygeneral.org
Mercy Health Hackley Campus	Muskegon	Michigan	231-726-3511	www.hackley.org
Mercy Hospital - Cadillac	Cadillac	Michigan	231-876-7200	www.mercycadillac.munsonhealthcare.org
Mercy Medical Center - Des Moines	Des Moines	Iowa	515-247-3121	www.mercydesmoines.org
Mercy Memorial Health Center	Ardmore	Oklahoma	405-223-5400	www.mercyok.com/mmhc
Methodist Hospital of Sacramento	Sacramento	California	916-423-6010	www.methodistsacramento.org
Methodist Jennie Edmundson	Council Bluffs	Iowa	712-396-6000	www.bestcare.org
Metro Health Hospital	Wyoming	Michigan	616-252-7200	www.metrohealth.net
Metrohealth System	Cleveland	Ohio	216-778-7089	www.metrohealth.org
Miami Valley Hospital	Dayton	Ohio	937-208-8000	www.miamivalleyhospital.com
Milton S Hershey Medical Center	Hershey	Pennsylvania	717-531-8521	www.hmc.psu.edu
Montrose Memorial Hospital	Montrose	Colorado	970-249-2211	www.montrosehospital.com
Morton Plant Hospital	Clearwater	Florida	727-462-7000	www.measehospitals.com
Mount Sinai Hospital	New York	New York	212-241-7981	www.mountsinai.org
Muhlenberg Community Hospital	Greenville	Kentucky	270-338-8000	www.mchky.org
Multicare Good Samaritan Hospital	Puyallup	Washington	253-697-2102	www.multicare.org/goodsam
Musc Medical Center	Charleston	South Carolina	843-792-2300	www.musc.edu
Nash General Hospital	Rocky Mount	North Carolina	252-443-8000	www.nhcs.org
New Hanover Regional Medical Center	Wilmington	North Carolina	910-343-7000	www.nhrmc.org
Newport Hospital	Newport	Rhode Island	401-846-6400	www.newporthospital.org
Northwest Medical Center	Tucson	Arizona	520-742-9000	www.northwestmedicalcenter.com
Novant Health Presbyterian Medical Center	Charlotte	North Carolina	704-384-4000	www.presbyterian.org
O U Medical Center	Oklahoma City	Oklahoma	405-271-5911	www.oumedcenter.com
OHSU Hospital & Clinics	Portland	Oregon	503-494-4036	www.ohsu.edu
Oklahoma State University Medical Center	Tulsa	Oklahoma	918-587-2561	www.tulsaregional.com
Our Lady of the Lake Regional Medical Center	Baton Rouge	Louisiana	225-765-6565	www.ololrmc.com
Overland Park Regional Medical Center	Overland Park	Kansas	913-541-5301	www.oprmc.com
Parkview Medical Center	Pueblo	Colorado	719-584-4000	www.parkviewmc.com
Peacehealth Saint Joseph Medical Center	Bellingham	Washington	360-734-5400	www.peacehealth.org
Phelps County Regional Medical Center	Rolla	Missouri	573-458-8899	www.rollanet.org/~pcrmc
Physicians Regional Medical Center - Pine Ridge	Naples	Florida	239-348-4000	www.physiciansregional.com
Pinnacle Health Hospitals	Harrisburg	Pennsylvania	717-782-5181	www.pinnaclehealth.org
Providence Holy Cross Medical Center	Mission Hills	California	818-365-8051	www.providence.org
Providence Sacred Heart Medical Center	Spokane	Washington	509-474-3040	www.shmc.org
Rhode Island Hospital	Providence	Rhode Island	401-444-4000	www.rhodeislandhospital.org
Ridgeview Medical Center	Waconia	Minnesota	952-442-2191	www.ridgeviewmedical.org
Riverview Hospital Assoc	Wisconsin Rapids	Wisconsin	715-423-6060	www.riverviewhospital.net
Ronald Reagan UCLA Medical Center	Los Angeles	California	310-825-6301	www.uclahealth.org
Rush University Medical Center	Chicago	Illinois	312-942-5000	www.ruch.edu
Russellville Hospital	Russellville	Alabama	256-332-1611	www.russellvillehospital.com
Sacred Heart Hospital	Eau Claire	Wisconsin	715-717-4121	www.sacredhearteauclaire.org
Saint Anthony Medical Center	Rockford	Illinois	815-226-2000	www.osfhealth.com
Saint Francis Medical Center	Peoria	Illinois	309-655-2000	www.osfsaintfrancis.org
Saint Joseph's Hospital of Atlanta	Atlanta	Georgia	678-843-5720	www.stjosephsatlanta.org

Hospital	City	State	Phone	Web Site
Saint Mary's Health Care	Grand Rapids	Michigan	616-685-5000	www.smhealthcare.org
Saint Mary's Regional Medical Center	Reno	Nevada	775-770-3000	www.saintmarysreno.com
Salem Hospital	Salem	Oregon	503-561-5200	www.salemhospital.org
Salina Regional Health Center	Salina	Kansas	785-452-7000	www.srhc.com
Sanford Usd Medical Center	Sioux Falls	South Dakota	605-333-1000	www.sanfordhealth.org
Santiam Memorial Hospital	Stayton	Oregon	503-769-2175	www.santiamhospital.com
Sarasota Memorial Hospital	Sarasota	Florida	941-917-9000	www.smh.com
Seton Medical Center Austin	Austin	Texas	512-324-1000	www.seton.net
Sharp Memorial Hospital	San Diego	California	858-939-3400	www.sharp.com/memorial
Sky Ridge Medical Center	Lone Tree	Colorado	720-225-1000	www.skyridgemedcenter.com
Slidell Memorial Hospital	Slidell	Louisiana	985-643-2200	www.slidelmemorial.org
Southeast Alabama Medical Center	Dothan	Alabama	334-793-8701	www.samc.org
Southwestern Vermont Medical Center	Bennington	Vermont	802-442-6361	www.svhealthcare.org
Spectrum Health - Butterworth Campus	Grand Rapids	Michigan	616-391-1774	www.spectrum-health.org
Springhill Medical Center	Mobile	Alabama	251-344-9630	www.springhillmedicalcenter.com
Saint Elizabeth Health Center	Youngstown	Ohio	330-746-7211	www.hmhs.org
Saint Elizabeth Medical Center	Utica	New York	315-798-8100	www.stemc.org
Saint Francis Health Center	Topeka	Kansas	785-295-8000	www.stfrancistopeka.org
Saint Francis - Downtown	Greenville	South Carolina	864-255-1000	www.stfrancishealth.org
Saint Helena Hospital	Saint Helena	California	707-963-3611	www.sthelenahospital.org
Saint Joseph Medical Center	Tacoma	Washington	253-627-4101	www.fhshealth.org
Saint Joseph Mercy Hospital	Ann Arbor	Michigan	734-712-3791	www.stjoesannarbor.or
Saint Joseph's Hospital & Medical Center	Phoenix	Arizona	602-406-3000	www.stjosephs-phx.org
Saint Louis University Hospital	Saint Louis	Missouri	314-577-8000	www.slucare.edu/clinical
Saint Luke's Hospital Bethlehem	Bethlehem	Pennsylvania	610-954-4000	www.slhn-lehighvalley.org
Saint Luke's Hospital	Chesterfield	Missouri	314-434-1500	www.goodhealthmatters.com
Saint Luke's Hospital of Kansas City	Kansas City	Missouri	816-932-2000	www.staintlukeshealthsystem.org
Saint Marys Hospital	Madison	Wisconsin	608-251-6100	www.stmarysmadison.com
Stanford Hospital	Stanford	California	650-723-5708	www.stanfordhospital.com
Swedish Medical Center	Seattle	Washington	206-386-6000	www.swedish.org
Swedish Medical Center - Cherry Hill	Seattle	Washington	206-320-2000	www.swedish.org
Tacoma General Allenmore Hospital	Tacoma	Washington	253-403-1000	www.multicare.org
Tampa General Hospital	Tampa	Florida	813-844-7000	www.tgh.org
Heart Hospital Baylor Plano	Plano	Texas	469-814-3278	www.thehearthospitalbaylor.com
Theda Clark Medical Center	Neenah	Wisconsin	920-729-3100	www.thedacare.org
Thomas Hospital	Fairhope	Alabama	251-928-2375	www.thomashospital.com
Town & Country Hospital	Tampa	Florida	813-882-7159	www.townandcountryhospital.com
Trinity Hospitals	Minot	North Dakota	701-857-5000	www.trinityhealth.org
Trinity Medical Center	Birmingham	Alabama	205-592-1000	www.bhsala.com/montclair
Trinity Rock Island	Rock Island	Illinois	309-779-5000	www.trinityqc.com
Trumbull Memorial Hospital	Warren	Ohio	330-841-9011	www.trumhosp.org
Tulane Medical Center	New Orleans	Louisiana	504-988-1900	www.tuhc.com
UF Health Jacksonville	Jacksonville	Florida	904-244-0411	www.shandsjacksonville.org
UMC of Southern Nevada	Las Vegas	Nevada	702-383-2000	www.umc-cares.org
University Colo Health Memorial Hospital Central	Colorado Springs	Colorado	719-365-5000	www.memorialhospital.com
University Health Care/University Hospitals & Clinics	Salt Lake City	Utah	801-581-2121	www.healthcare.utah.edu
University Health System	San Antonio	Texas	210-358-4000	www.universityhealthsystem.com
University of California Davis Medical Center	Sacramento	California	916-734-2011	www.ucdmc.ucdavis.edu
University of Cincinnati Medical Center	Cincinnati	Ohio	513-584-1000	www.universityhospitalcincinnati.com
University of Colorado Hospital	Aurora	Colorado	720-848-0000	www.uch.edu
University of Kansas Hospital	Kansas City	Kansas	913-588-7332	www.kumc.edu
University of Miami Hospital	Miami	Florida	305-325-5511	www.cedarsmedicalcenter.com
University of Minnesota Medical Center - Fairview	Minneapolis	Minnesota	612-273-3000	www.uofmmedicalcenter.org
University of Toledo Medical Center	Toledo	Ohio	419-383-3407	www.utmc.utoledo.edu
University of Wisconsin Hospitals & Clinics Authority	Madison	Wisconsin	608-263-8991	www.uwhealth.org
UPMC Hamot	Erie	Pennsylvania	814-877-6000	www.hamot.org
UPMC Passavant	Pittsburgh	Pennsylvania	412-367-6700	www.passavant.upmc.com
UPMC Presbyterian Shadyside	Pittsburgh	Pennsylvania	412-647-8788	www.upmc.edu
UT Southwestern University Hospital	Dallas	Texas	214-879-3758	www.utsouthwestern.edu
Utah Valley Regional Medical Center	Provo	Utah	801-373-7850	www.intermountainhealthcare.org/hospitals/uvrmc
Ventura County Medical Center	Ventura	California	805-652-6075	www.vchca.org
Vidant Medical Center	Greenville	North Carolina	252-847-4100	www.uhseast.com
Virginia Mason Medical Center	Seattle	Washington	206-223-6600	www.vmmc.org
Waukesha Memorial Hospital	Waukesha	Wisconsin	262-928-1000	www.waukeshamemorial.org
Wesley Medical Center	Hattiesburg	Mississippi	601-268-8000	www.wesley.com
West Virginia University Hospitals	Morgantown	West Virginia	304-598-4000	www.wvuh.com
Wheaton Franciscan Saint Joseph	Milwaukee	Wisconsin	414-447-2000	www.wfhealthcare.org

Hospital	City	State	Phone	Web Site
Winchester Hospital	Winchester	Massachusetts	781-729-9000	www.winchesterhospital.org
Women & Infants Hospital of Rhode Island	Providence	Rhode Island	401-274-1100	www.womenandinfants.com
The Women's Hospital	Newburgh	Indiana	812-842-4200	www.deaconess.com
Yavapai Regional Medical Center	Prescott	Arizona	928-771-5676	www.yrmc.org

Note: Table shows hospitals nationwide whose surgical complication rate is worse (higher) than U.S. rate of 1.83%

Hospitals whose Surgical Complication Rate is Better (Lower) than the U.S. National Rate

Measure: Collapsed Lung Due to Medical Treatment

Hospital	City	State	Phone	Web Site
Centinela Hospital Medical Center	Inglewood	California	310-673-4660	www.centinelafreeman.com
Centra Health	Lynchburg	Virginia	434-200-4789	www.centrahealth.com
Community Medical Center	Toms River	New Jersey	732-557-8000	www.sbhcs.com
Evanston Hospital	Evanston	Illinois	847-432-8000	www.enh.org
New York - Presbyterian Hospital	New York	New York	212-746-4189	www.nyp.org
Norton Hospitals	Louisville	Kentucky	502-629-6560	www.nortonhealthcare.com
Spectrum Health - Butterworth Campus	Grand Rapids	Michigan	616-391-1774	www.spectrum-health.org
Virtua West Jersey Hospitals Berlin	Berlin	New Jersey	856-322-3200	www.virtua.org
Willis Knighton Medical Center	Shreveport	Louisiana	318-212-4000	www.wkhs.com//locations/medicalcenter.aspx

Note: Table shows hospitals nationwide whose surgical complication rate is better (lower) than U.S. rate of 0.32%

Hospitals whose Surgical Complication Rate is Worse (Higher) than the U.S. National Rate

Measure: Collapsed Lung Due to Medical Treatment

Hospital	City	State	Phone	Web Site
Abilene Regional Medical Center	Abilene	Texas	325-428-1000	www.abileneregional.com
Banner Heart Hospital	Mesa	Arizona	480-854-5050	www.bannerhealth.com
Baylor Medical Center at Garland	Garland	Texas	972-487-5000	www.baylorhealth.com
Baylor Regional Medical Center at Grapevine	Grapevine	Texas	817-481-1588	www.baylorhealth.com
Bert Fish Medical Center	New Smyrna Beach	Florida	386-424-5000	www.bertfish.com
Beth Israel Deaconess Medical Center	Boston	Massachusetts	617-667-7000	www.bidmc.harvard.edu
Bryan Medical Center	Lincoln	Nebraska	402-481-1111	www.bryan.org
Capital Region Medical Center	Jefferson City	Missouri	573-632-5000	www.crmc.org
Carolinas Medical Center - Union	Monroe	North Carolina	704-283-3100	www.carolinashealthcare.org/cmc-union
Champlain Valley Physicians Hospital Medical Center	Plattsburgh	New York	518-561-2000	www.cvph.org
Community Regional Medical Center	Fresno	California	559-459-6000	www.communitymedical.org
Des Peres Hospital	Saint Louis	Missouri	314-966-9100	www.desperesshospital.com
Feather River Hospital	Paradise	California	530-877-9361	www.frhosp.org
Florida Hospital	Orlando	Florida	407-303-1976	www.floridahospital.com
Hays Medical Center	Hays	Kansas	785-623-5000	www.haysmed.com
Inova Fairfax Hospital	Falls Church	Virginia	703-776-3332	www.inova.org
Kansas Medical Center	Andover	Kansas	316-300-4000	www.ksmedcenter.com
Largo Medical Center	Largo	Florida	727-588-5200	www.largomedical.com
Lawrence Memorial Hospital	Lawrence	Kansas	785-505-6100	www.lmh.org
Loma Linda University Medical Center	Loma Linda	California	909-558-4000	www.llumc.edu
Madera Community Hospital	Madera	California	559-675-5555	www.maderahospital.org
Maine Medical Center	Portland	Maine	207-662-0111	www.mmc.org
Massachusetts General Hospital	Boston	Massachusetts	617-726-2000	www.massgeneral.org
Mclaren - Northern Michigan	Petoskey	Michigan	231-487-4000	www.northernhealth.org
Medical West	Bessemer	Alabama	205-481-7000	www.uab.edu
Midmichigan Medical Center - Midland	Midland	Michigan	989-839-3000	www.midmichigan.org
Mills - Peninsula Medical Center	Burlingame	California	650-696-5270	www.mills-peninsula.org
Norman Regional Health System	Norman	Oklahoma	405-321-1700	www.normanregional.com
Northwest Texas Hospital	Amarillo	Texas	806-354-1110	www.nxtexashealthcare.com
NYU Hospitals Center	New York	New York	212-263-7300	www.med.nyu.edu
Orange Regional Medical Center	Middletown	New York	845-343-2424	www.ormc.org
Orlando Health	Orlando	Florida	321-841-5111	www.orlandoregionalmedicalcenter.org
Parkridge Medical Center	Chattanooga	Tennessee	423-894-4220	www.tristarhealth.com
Piedmont Hospital	Atlanta	Georgia	404-605-5000	www.piedmonthospital.org
Pikeville Medical Center	Pikeville	Kentucky	606-218-3500	www.pikevillehospital.org
Providence Health Center	Waco	Texas	254-751-4000	www.providence.net
Providence Saint Vincent Medical Center	Portland	Oregon	503-216-1234	www.providence.org
Ronald Reagan UCLA Medical Center	Los Angeles	California	310-825-6301	www.uclahealth.org
Saint Francis Medical Center	Peoria	Illinois	309-655-2000	www.osfsaintfrancis.org
Saint Joseph Hospital	Lexington	Kentucky	859-313-1000	www.sjhlex.org
Saint Joseph's Hospital of Atlanta	Atlanta	Georgia	678-843-5720	www.stjosephsatlanta.org
Sanford Medical Center Fargo	Fargo	North Dakota	701-234-2000	www.meritcare.com
Self Regional Healthcare	Greenwood	South Carolina	864-227-4111	www.selfregional.org
Sentara Norfolk General Hospital	Norfolk	Virginia	757-388-3000	www.sentara.com
Sharp Memorial Hospital	San Diego	California	858-939-3400	www.sharp.com/memorial
Silver Cross Hospital & Medical Centers	New Lenox	Illinois	815-300-1100	www.silvercross.org
SSM Depaul Health Center	Bridgeton	Missouri	314-344-6000	www.ssmdepaul.com
Saint Bernards Medical Center	Jonesboro	Arkansas	870-972-4100	www.sbrmc.com
Saint John Medical Center	Tulsa	Oklahoma	918-744-3606	www.sjmc.org
Saint John's Episcopal Hospital at South Shore	Far Rockaway	New York	718-869-7000	www.ehs.org
Saint Luke's Hospital of Kansas City	Kansas City	Missouri	816-932-2000	www.saintlukeshealthsystem.org
Saint Tammany Parish Hospital	Covington	Louisiana	985-898-4000	www.stph.org
Sturdy Memorial Hospital	Attleboro	Massachusetts	508-222-5200	www.sturdymemorial.org
Theda Clark Medical Center	Neenah	Wisconsin	920-729-3100	www.thedacare.org
UMC of Southern Nevada	Las Vegas	Nevada	702-383-2000	www.umc-cares.org
University Medical Center of El Paso	El Paso	Texas	915-521-7602	www.thomasoncares.org
University of Alabama Hospital	Birmingham	Alabama	205-934-4011	www.health.uab.edu
University of Toledo Medical Center	Toledo	Ohio	419-383-3407	www.utmc.utoledo.edu
UPMC Presbyterian Shadyside	Pittsburgh	Pennsylvania	412-647-8788	www.upmc.edu
Williamsport Regional Medical Center	Williamsport	Pennsylvania	570-321-1000	www.susquehannahealth.org

Note: Table shows hospitals nationwide whose surgical complication rate is worse (higher) than U.S. rate of 0.32%

Hospitals whose Surgical Complication Rate is Better (Lower) than the U.S. National Rate

Measure: Deaths Among Patients With Serious Treatable Complications After Surgery

Hospital	City	State	Phone	Web Site
Advocate Lutheran General Hospital	Park Ridge	Illinois	847-723-2210	www.advocatehealth.com
Alexian Brothers Medical Center	Elk Grove Village	Illinois	847-437-5500	www.alexian.org
Aurora West Allis Medical Center	West Allis	Wisconsin	414-328-6000	www.aurorahealthcare.org
Banner Thunderbird Medical Center	Glendale	Arizona	602-588-5555	www.bannerhealth.com
Baptist Saint Anthony's Hospital	Amarillo	Texas	806-212-2000	www.bsahs.com
Bayfront Health Punta Gorda	Punta Gorda	Florida	941-639-3131	www.charlotteregional.com
Delray Medical Center	Delray Beach	Florida	561-498-4440	www.delraymedicalctr.com
Emory University Hospital	Atlanta	Georgia	404-686-8500	www.emoryhealthcare.org
Evanston Hospital	Evanston	Illinois	847-432-8000	www.enh.org
Fawcett Memorial Hospital	Port Charlotte	Florida	941-629-1181	www.fawcetthospital.com
Franciscan Saint Francis Health - Indianapolis	Indianapolis	Indiana	317-865-5001	www.stfrancishospitals.org
Gwinnett Medical Center	Lawrenceville	Georgia	678-312-1000	www.gwinnettmedicalcenter.org
Hackensack University Medical Center	Hackensack	New Jersey	201-996-2000	www.humed.com
Henry Ford Wyandotte Hospital	Wyandotte	Michigan	734-246-6000	www.henryfordwyandotte.com
Hinsdale Hospital	Hinsdale	Illinois	630-856-9000	www.keepingyouwell.com
Hospital For Special Surgery	New York	New York	212-606-1000	www.hss.edu
JFK Medical Center	Atlantis	Florida	561-965-7300	www.jfkmc.com
JFK Medical Center - A M Yelencsics Comm Hospital	Edison	New Jersey	732-321-7000	www.jfkmc.org
Los Robles Hospital & Medical Center	Thousand Oaks	California	805-497-2727	www.losrobleshospital.com
Martin Medical Center	Stuart	Florida	772-287-5200	www.mmhs.com
Mayo Clinic Hospital	Phoenix	Arizona	480-342-2000	www.mayoclinic.org
Mayo Clinic Methodist- Hospital	Rochester	Minnesota	507-266-7890	www.mayoclinic.org/methodisthospital
Mclaren Flint	Flint	Michigan	810-342-2000	www.mclaren.org
Memorial Hermann Memorial City Medical Center	Houston	Texas	713-242-3000	www.mhhs.org
Missouri Baptist Medical Center	Town & Country	Missouri	314-996-5000	www.missouribaptistmedicalcenter.org
Mother Frances Hospital	Tyler	Texas	903-593-8441	www.tmfhs.org
North Colorado Medical Center	Greeley	Colorado	970-352-4121	www.bannerhealth.com
North Kansas City Hospital	North Kansas City	Missouri	816-691-2000	www.nkch.org
Northwestern Memorial Hospital	Chicago	Illinois	312-926-2000	www.nmh.org
NYU Hospitals Center	New York	New York	212-263-7300	www.med.nyu.edu
OHSU Hospital & Clinics	Portland	Oregon	503-494-4036	www.ohsu.edu
Palm Beach Gardens Medical Center	Palm Beach Gardens	Florida	561-622-1411	www.pbgmc.com
Palos Community Hospital	Palos Heights	Illinois	708-923-4000	www.paloshospital.org
Providence Hospital & Medical Centers	Southfield	Michigan	248-849-3011	www.stjohn.org/providence
Saint Alexius Medical Center	Hoffman Estates	Illinois	847-843-2000	www.alexianbrothershealth.org
Saint Alexius Medical Center	Bismarck	North Dakota	701-530-7000	www.st.alexius.org
Saint David's Medical Center	Austin	Texas	512-476-7111	www.stdavidsrehab.com
Saint Elizabeth Health Center	Youngstown	Ohio	330-746-7211	www.hmhs.org
Saint John Macomb - Oakland Hospital - Macomb Center	Warren	Michigan	586-573-5000	www.stjohn.org
Saint Joseph's Hospital & Medical Center	Phoenix	Arizona	602-406-3000	www.stjosephs-phx.org
Saint Luke's Hospital	Cedar Rapids	Iowa	319-369-7211	www.crstlukes.com
Heart Hospital Baylor Plano	Plano	Texas	469-814-3278	www.thehearthospitalbaylor.com
University of Wisconsin Hospitals & Clinics Authority	Madison	Wisconsin	608-263-8991	www.uwhealth.org

Note: Table shows hospitals nationwide whose surgical complication rate is better (lower) than U.S. rate of 110.25%

Hospitals whose Surgical Complication Rate is Worse (Higher) than the U.S. National Rate

Measure: Deaths Among Patients With Serious Treatable Complications After Surgery

Hospital	City	State	Phone	Web Site
Baptist Health Medical Center - Little Rock	Little Rock	Arkansas	501-202-2000	www.baptist-health.com
Baptist Medical Center	San Antonio	Texas	210-297-1020	www.baptisthealthsystem.org
Carolinas Hospital System	Florence	South Carolina	843-674-2500	www.carolinashospital.com
Carolinas Medical Center/Behaviorial Health	Charlotte	North Carolina	704-355-2000	www.carolinasmedicalcenter.org
Christian Hospital Northeast - Northwest	Saint Louis	Missouri	314-653-5000	www.christianhospital.org
Christiana Care Health Services	Newark	Delaware	302-733-1000	www.christianacare.org
Community Regional Medical Center	Fresno	California	559-459-6000	www.communitymedical.org
Conway Medical Center	Conway	South Carolina	843-347-8037	www.conwayhospital.com
Cooper University Hospital	Camden	New Jersey	856-342-2000	www.cooperhealth.org
Cullman Regional Medical Center	Cullman	Alabama	256-737-2000	www.crmchospital.com
Doctors Hospital	Augusta	Georgia	706-651-6008	www.doctors-hospital.net
Doctors Medical Center	Modesto	California	209-578-1211	www.dmc-modesto.com
Duke University Hospital	Durham	North Carolina	919-684-8111	www.dukehealth.org
East Texas Medical Center	Tyler	Texas	903-597-0351	www.etmc.org
Erlanger Medical Center	Chattanooga	Tennessee	423-778-7000	www.erlanger.org
Fairbanks Memorial Hospital	Fairbanks	Alaska	907-452-8181	www.bannerhealth.com
Fletcher Allen Hospital of Vermont	Burlington	Vermont	802-847-0000	www.fletcherallen.org
Florida Hospital Tampa	Tampa	Florida	813-615-7200	www.uch.org
Good Samaritan Hospital Medical Center	West Islip	New York	631-376-3000	www.good-samaritan-hospital.org
Halifax Health Medical Center	Daytona Beach	Florida	386-254-4000	www.halifax.org
Health Alliance Hospital Broadway Campus	Kingston	New York	914-331-3131	www.kingstonregionalhealth.org
Hillcrest Medical Center	Tulsa	Oklahoma	918-579-1000	www.hillcrest.com
Integris Baptist Medical Center	Oklahoma City	Oklahoma	405-951-8110	www.integris-health.com
Jewish Hospital & Saint Mary's Healthcare	Louisville	Kentucky	502-587-4011	www.jhhs.org
Kaleida Health	Buffalo	New York	716-859-8620	www.kaleidahealth.org
Lake Cumberland Regional Hospital	Somerset	Kentucky	606-679-7441	www.lakecumberlandhospital.com
Lakeland Regional Medical Center	Lakeland	Florida	863-687-1100	www.lrmc.com
Magnolia Regional Health Center	Corinth	Mississippi	662-293-7660	www.mrhc.org
Marian Regional Medical Center	Santa Maria	California	805-739-3000	www.marinmedicalcenter.org
Mary Hitchcock Memorial Hospital	Lebanon	New Hampshire	603-650-5000	www.dhmc.org
Medical Center of Central Georgia	Macon	Georgia	478-633-6805	www.mccg.org
Medical Center of Plano	Plano	Texas	972-596-6800	www.medicalcenterofplano.com
Medical College of Georgia Hospitals & Clinics	Augusta	Georgia	706-721-6569	www.mcghealth.org
Methodist Healthcare Memphis Hospitals	Memphis	Tennessee	901-516-8274	www.methodisthealth.org
Milton S Hershey Medical Center	Hershey	Pennsylvania	717-531-8521	www.hmc.psu.edu
Mobile Infirmary	Mobile	Alabama	251-435-4700	www.mimc.com
Nazareth Hospital	Philadelphia	Pennsylvania	215-335-6000	www.nazarethhospital.org
North Carolina Baptist Hospital	Winston-Salem	North Carolina	336-716-2011	www.wfubmc.edu
North Mississippi Medical Center	Tupelo	Mississippi	662-377-3000	www.nmhs.net/nmmc
Northeast Alabama Regional Medical Center	Anniston	Alabama	256-235-5121	www.rmccares.org
Oklahoma State University Medical Center	Tulsa	Oklahoma	918-587-2561	www.tulsaregional.com
Phoebe Putney Memorial Hospital	Albany	Georgia	229-312-4068	www.phoebeputney.com
Renown Regional Medical Center	Reno	Nevada	775-982-4100	www.renown.org
Riverside Methodist Hospital	Columbus	Ohio	614-566-5000	www.ohiohealth.com
Robert Wood Johnson University Hospital	New Brunswick	New Jersey	732-937-8900	www.rwjuh.edu
Robert Wood Johnson University Hospital - Hamilton	Hamilton	New Jersey	609-586-7900	www.rwjhamilton.org
Saint Francis Medical Center	Peoria	Illinois	309-655-2000	www.osfsaintfrancis.org
Sentara Norfolk General Hospital	Norfolk	Virginia	757-388-3000	www.sentara.com
Saint John Medical Center	Tulsa	Oklahoma	918-744-3606	www.sjmc.org
Saint Joseph's Hospital - Savannah	Savannah	Georgia	912-819-4100	www.sjchs.org
Saint Luke's Episcopal Hospital	Houston	Texas	832-355-1000	www.sleh.com
Saint Mary's Medical Center	Huntington	West Virginia	304-526-1234	www.st-marys.org
Saint Vincent's East	Birmingham	Alabama	205-838-3122	www.nolandhealth.com
Strong Memorial Hospital	Rochester	New York	585-275-2121	www.urmc.rochester.edu
Sunrise Hospital & Medical Center	Las Vegas	Nevada	702-731-8000	www.sunrisehospital.com
Tampa General Hospital	Tampa	Florida	813-844-7000	www.tgh.org
Trident Medical Center	Charleston	South Carolina	843-797-8800	www.tridenthealthsystem.com
UF Health Shands Hospital	Gainesville	Florida	352-265-8000	www.shands.org
Umass Memorial Medical Center	Worcester	Massachusetts	508-334-1000	www.umassmemorial.org
University Hospital	Newark	New Jersey	973-972-5658	www.theuniversityhospital.com
University Medical Center	Lubbock	Texas	806-775-8200	www.teamumc.org
University of Alabama Hospital	Birmingham	Alabama	205-934-4011	www.health.uab.edu
University of Kentucky Hospital	Lexington	Kentucky	859-323-5000	www.uhealthcare.uky.edu
University of Mississippi Medical Center	Jackson	Mississippi	601-984-4100	www.umc.edu

Hospital	City	State	Phone	Web Site
University of South Alabama Medical Center	Mobile	Alabama	251-471-7110	www.southalabama.edu/usamc
Vidant Medical Center	Greenville	North Carolina	252-847-4100	www.uhseast.com
Virtua West Jersey Hospitals Berlin	Berlin	New Jersey	856-322-3200	www.virtua.org

Note: Table shows hospitals nationwide whose surgical complication rate is worse (higher) than U.S. rate of 110.25%

Hospitals whose Surgical Complication Rate is Better (Lower) than the U.S. National Rate

Measure: Rate of Complications for Hip/Knee Replacement Patients

Hospital	City	State	Phone	Web Site
Arkansas Surgical Hospital	No Little Rock	Arkansas	501-748-8000	www.arksurgicalhospital.com
Baptist Health Louisville	Louisville	Kentucky	502-897-8100	www.baptisteast.com
Barnes-Jewish Hospital	Saint Louis	Missouri	314-747-3000	www.barnesjewish.org
Beaumont Health System	Royal Oak	Michigan	248-898-5000	www.beaumonthospitals.com
Boone Hospital Center	Columbia	Missouri	573-815-8000	www.boone.org
Bronson Methodist Hospital	Kalamazoo	Michigan	269-341-6000	www.bronsonhealth.com
Cape Cod Hospital	Hyannis	Massachusetts	508-771-1800	www.capecodhealth.org
Carilion Roanoke Memorial Hospital	Roanoke	Virginia	540-981-7000	www.carilion.com/crmh
Covenant Medical Center	Lubbock	Texas	806-725-6000	www.covenanthealth.org
Crittenton Hospital Medical Center	Rochester	Michigan	248-652-5000	www.crittenton.com
Delray Medical Center	Delray Beach	Florida	561-498-4440	www.delraymedicalctr.com
Doctors Hospital at Renaissance	Edinburg	Texas	956-362-8677	www.dhr-rgv.com
Florida Hospital Memorial Medical Center	Daytona Beach	Florida	386-676-6000	www.fhmd.com
Franciscan Saint Elizabeth Health - Lafayette East	Lafayette	Indiana	765-502-4334	www.ste.org
Heart of Florida Regional Medical Center	Davenport	Florida	863-422-4971	www.heartofflorida.com
Heartland Regional Medical Center	Saint Joseph	Missouri	816-271-6000	www.heartland-health.com
Hoag Orthopedic Institute	Irvine	California	949-727-5000	www.orthopedichospital.com
Holy Cross Hospital	Fort Lauderdale	Florida	954-771-8000	www.holy-cross.com
Hospital For Special Surgery	New York	New York	212-606-1000	www.hss.edu
Indian River Medical Center	Vero Beach	Florida	772-567-4311	www.irmh.com
Indiana Orthopaedic Hospital	Indianapolis	Indiana	317-956-1000	www.indianaorthopaedichospital.com
Jupiter Medical Center	Jupiter	Florida	561-747-2234	www.jupitermed.com
Kansas Medical Center	Andover	Kansas	316-300-4000	www.ksmedcenter.com
Kansas Surgery & Recovery Center	Wichita	Kansas	316-634-0090	www.ksrc.org
Maine Medical Center	Portland	Maine	207-662-0111	www.mmc.org
Mayo Clinic Methodist- Hospital	Rochester	Minnesota	507-266-7890	www.mayoclinic.org/methodisthospital
Mclaren - Greater Lansing	Lansing	Michigan	517-975-6000	www.mclaren.org
Memorial Healthcare System	Chattanooga	Tennessee	423-495-2525	www.memorial.org
Memorial Mission Hospital & Asheville Surgery Center	Asheville	North Carolina	828-213-1111	www.missionhospitals.org
Mississippi Baptist Medical Center	Jackson	Mississippi	601-968-1000	www.mbmc.org
Nebraska Orthopaedic Hospital	Omaha	Nebraska	402-609-1600	www.neorthohospital.com
New England Baptist Hospital	Boston	Massachusetts	617-754-5800	www.nebh.caregroup.org
North Mississippi Medical Center	Tupelo	Mississippi	662-377-3000	www.nmhs.net/nmmc
Ocala Regional Medical Center	Ocala	Florida	352-401-1000	www.ocalaregional.com
Oklahoma Surgical Hospital	Tulsa	Oklahoma	918-477-5000	www.oklahomasurgicalhospital.com
Olathe Medical Center	Olathe	Kansas	913-791-4200	www.ohsi.com
Orthopaedic Hospital at Parkview North	Fort Wayne	Indiana	260-672-4050	www.parkview.com
Plaza Medical Center of Fort Worth	Fort Worth	Texas	817-336-2100	www.plazamedicalcenter.com
Poudre Valley Hospital	Fort Collins	Colorado	970-495-7000	www.pvhs.org
Proctor Hospital	Peoria	Illinois	309-691-1000	www.proctor.org
Providence Saint John's Health Center	Santa Monica	California	310-829-5511	www.stjohns.org
Quail Creek Surgical Hospital	Amarillo	Texas	806-354-6100	www.physurg.com
Riverside Medical Center	Kankakee	Illinois	815-933-1671	www.riversidehealthcare.org
Roper Hospital	Charleston	South Carolina	843-724-2800	www.ropersaintfrancis.com
Sacred Heart Hospital	Pensacola	Florida	850-416-7000	www.sacred-heart.org
Saint Elizabeth Regional Medical Center	Lincoln	Nebraska	402-219-7700	www.stelizabethonline.com
Saint Joseph Regional Medical Center	Mishawaka	Indiana	574-335-5000	www.sjmed.com
Saint Joseph's Hospital of Atlanta	Atlanta	Georgia	678-843-5720	www.stjosephsatlanta.org
Saint Thomas Midtown Hospital	Nashville	Tennessee	615-284-5555	www.baptisthospital.com
Samaritan Regional Health System	Ashland	Ohio	419-289-0491	www.samho.org
Sanford Medical Center Bismarck	Bismarck	North Dakota	701-323-6000	www.medcenterone.com
Sentara Leigh Hospital	Norfolk	Virginia	757-261-6601	www.sentara.com
Seton Medical Center Austin	Austin	Texas	512-324-1000	www.seton.net
South Nassau Communities Hospital	Oceanside	New York	516-632-3000	www.southnassau.org
Southside Hospital	Bay Shore	New York	631-968-3000	www.northshorelij.com
Southwest General Health Center	Middleburg Heights	Ohio	440-816-8000	www.swgeneral.com
Saint Francis Hospital & Medical Center	Hartford	Connecticut	860-714-4000	www.saintfranciscare.com
Saint Helena Hospital	Saint Helena	California	707-963-3611	www.sthelenahospital.org
Saint Joseph Hospital	Orange	California	714-633-9111	www.sjo.org
Saint Joseph Mercy Oakland	Pontiac	Michigan	248-858-3000	www.stjoesoakland.org
Saint Joseph's Hospital - Savannah	Savannah	Georgia	912-819-4100	www.sjchs.org
Saint Peter's Hospital	Albany	New York	518-525-1550	www.stpetershealthcare.org
Saint Vincent's Medical Center	Jacksonville	Florida	904-308-7300	www.jaxhealth.com
Sutter General Hospital	Sacramento	California	916-733-8999	www.suttermedicalcenter.org

Hospital	City	State	Phone	Web Site
Tampa General Hospital	Tampa	Florida	813-844-7000	www.tgh.org
Texas Health Presbyterian Hospital Dallas	Dallas	Texas	214-345-6789	www.texashealth.org
Torrance Memorial Medical Center	Torrance	California	310-325-9110	www.torrancememorial.org
Valley Medical Center	Renton	Washington	425-228-3450	www.valleymed.org
VHS Harlingen Hospital Company	Harlingen	Texas	956-389-1100	www.vbmc.org
Washington Hospital	Fremont	California	510-797-1111	www.whhs.com
Western Maryland Regional Medical Center	Cumberland	Maryland	240-964-8001	www.wmhs.com
William Beaumont Hospital - Troy	Troy	Michigan	248-964-8800	www.beaumonthospitals.com
Yavapai Regional Medical Center	Prescott	Arizona	928-771-5676	www.yrmc.org

Note: Table shows hospitals nationwide whose surgical complication rate is better (lower) than U.S. rate of 3.4%

Hospitals whose Surgical Complication Rate is Worse (Higher) than the U.S. National Rate

Measure: Rate of Complications for Hip/Knee Replacement Patients

Hospital	City	State	Phone	Web Site
Alegent Health Mercy Hospital	Council Bluffs	Iowa	712-328-5000	www.alegent.com/mercy
Atrium Medical Center	Franklin	Ohio	513-420-5102	www.atriummedcenter.org
Baptist Memorial Hospital	Memphis	Tennessee	901-226-5000	www.bmhcc.org
Baptist Saint Anthony's Hospital	Amarillo	Texas	806-212-2000	www.bsahs.com
Beaumont Health System	Grosse Pointe	Michigan	313-343-1000	www.beaumonthospitals.com
Bridgeport Hospital	Bridgeport	Connecticut	203-384-3000	www.bridgeporthospital.com
Carolinas Medical Center - Northeast	Concord	North Carolina	704-783-3000	www.northeastmedical.org
Central Maine Medical Center	Lewiston	Maine	207-795-0111	www.cmmc.org
Community Memorial Hospital San Buenaventura	Ventura	California	805-652-5011	www.cmhhospital.org
D C H Regional Medical Center	Tuscaloosa	Alabama	205-759-7111	www.dchsystem.com
Decatur Morgan Hospital - Decatur Campus	Decatur	Alabama	256-341-2000	www.decaturgeneral.org
Defiance Regional Medical Center	Defiance	Ohio	419-783-6955	www.promedica.org/defiance
Doctors Medical Center	Modesto	California	209-578-1211	www.dmc-modesto.com
East Ohio Regional Hospital	Martins Ferry	Ohio	740-633-4151	www.eastohioregionalhospital.com
Floyd Medical Center	Rome	Georgia	706-509-6900	www.floydmed.org
Froedtert Memorial Lutheran Hospital	Milwaukee	Wisconsin	414-805-3000	www.froedtert.com
Gadsden Regional Medical Center	Gadsden	Alabama	256-494-4000	www.gadsdenregional.com
Genesis Medical Center - Davenport	Davenport	Iowa	563-421-1000	www.genesishealth.com
Genesys Regional Medical Center - Health Park	Grand Blanc	Michigan	810-606-5000	www.genesys.org
Grant Medical Center	Columbus	Ohio	614-566-9978	www.ohiohealth.com
Henry County Medical Center	Paris	Tennessee	731-642-1220	www.hcmc-tn.org
Houston Orthopedic & Spine Hospital	Bellaire	Texas	713-622-2262	www.foundationsurgicalhospital.com
Johnson City Medical Center	Johnson City	Tennessee	423-431-6111	www.msha.com
Lancaster General Hospital	Lancaster	Pennsylvania	717-299-5511	www.lancastergeneral.org
Louis A Weiss Memorial Hospital	Chicago	Illinois	773-878-8700	www.weisshospital.org
The Medical Center of Aurora	Aurora	Colorado	303-695-2600	www.auroramed.com
Mercy Health System Corp	Janesville	Wisconsin	608-756-6080	www.mercyhealthsystem.org
Mercy Saint Anne Hospital	Toledo	Ohio	419-407-2663	www.mercyweb.org
Mountain View Hospital	Payson	Utah	801-465-7100	www.mvhpayson.com
North Colorado Medical Center	Greeley	Colorado	970-352-4121	www.bannerhealth.com
North Kansas City Hospital	North Kansas City	Missouri	816-691-2000	www.nkch.org
Northwestern Memorial Hospital	Chicago	Illinois	312-926-2000	www.nmh.org
Novant Health Rowan Medical Center	Salisbury	North Carolina	704-210-5000	www.rowan.org
NYU Hospitals Center	New York	New York	212-263-7300	www.med.nyu.edu
Onslow Memorial Hospital	Jacksonville	North Carolina	910-577-2345	www.onslowmemorial.org
Overland Park Regional Medical Center	Overland Park	Kansas	913-541-5301	www.oprmc.com
Park Ridge Health	Hendersonville	North Carolina	828-684-8501	www.parkridgehospital.org
Pennsylvania Hospital of the Univ of PA Health Sys	Philadelphia	Pennsylvania	215-829-3000	www.pennmedicine.org/pahosp
Peterson Regional Medical Center	Kerrville	Texas	830-896-4200	www.petersonrmc.com
Pinnacle Health Hospitals	Harrisburg	Pennsylvania	717-782-5181	www.pinnaclehealth.org
Poplar Bluff Regional Medical Center	Poplar Bluff	Missouri	573-785-7721	www.poplarbluffregional.com
Reston Hospital Center	Reston	Virginia	703-689-9000	www.restonhospital.com
Riddle Memorial Hospital	Media	Pennsylvania	610-566-9400	www.riddlehospital.org
Saint Michael's Medical Center	Newark	New Jersey	973-877-5350	www.cathedralhealth.org
Shady Grove Adventist Hospital	Rockville	Maryland	240-826-6517	www.adventisthealthcare.com/sgah
Shannon Medical Center	San Angelo	Texas	325-653-6741	www.shannonhealth.com
South Central Regional Medical Center	Laurel	Mississippi	601-649-4000	www.scrmc.com
South Lake Hospital	Clermont	Florida	352-394-4071	www.southlakehospital.com
Southside Regional Medical Center	Petersburg	Virginia	804-765-5000	www.srmconline.com
Spring Valley Hospital Medical Center	Las Vegas	Nevada	702-853-3000	www.springvalleyhospital.com
Saint Alexius Medical Center	Hoffman Estates	Illinois	847-843-2000	www.alexianbrothershealth.org
Saint Anthony Hospital	Oklahoma City	Oklahoma	405-272-7000	www.saintsok.com
Saint Catherine of Siena Hospital	Smithtown	New York	631-862-3000	www.stcatherines.chsli.org
Saint Clair Memorial Hospital	Pittsburgh	Pennsylvania	412-942-6209	www.stclair.org
Saint Elizabeth Hospital	Appleton	Wisconsin	920-738-2000	www.affinityhealth.org
Saint Luke's Hospital Bethlehem	Bethlehem	Pennsylvania	610-954-4000	www.slhn-lehighvalley.org
Saint Marys Hospital	Madison	Wisconsin	608-251-6100	www.stmarysmadison.com
Saint Vincent Anderson Regional Hospital	Anderson	Indiana	765-646-8373	www.stjohnshealthsystem.org
Saint Vincent Healthcare	Billings	Montana	406-657-7000	www.svh-mt.org
Saint Vincent's Medical Center	Bridgeport	Connecticut	203-576-5551	www.stvincents.org
Sutter Auburn Faith Hospital	Auburn	California	530-888-4500	www.sutterauburnfaith.org
Sutter Solano Medical Center	Vallejo	California	707-554-5280	www.suttersolano.org
Swedish Medical Center	Englewood	Colorado	303-788-5000	www.swedishhospital.com/default.asp
Trinity Medical Center	Birmingham	Alabama	205-592-1000	www.bhsala.com/montclair

Hospital	City	State	Phone	Web Site
University of Kansas Hospital	Kansas City	Kansas	913-588-7332	www.kumc.edu
University of Toledo Medical Center	Toledo	Ohio	419-383-3407	www.utmc.utoledo.edu
Wentworth - Douglass Hospital	Dover	New Hampshire	603-740-2580	www.wdhospital.com
White River Medical Center	Batesville	Arkansas	870-262-1200	www.wrmc.com

Note: Table shows hospitals nationwide whose surgical complication rate is worse (higher) than U.S. rate of 3.4%

Hospitals whose Surgical Complication Rate is Better (Lower) than the U.S. National Rate

Measure: Serious Blood Clots After Surgery

Hospital	City	State	Phone	Web Site
Abbott Northwestern Hospital	Minneapolis	Minnesota	612-863-4509	www.abbottnorthwestern.com
Advocate Condell Medical Center	Libertyville	Illinois	847-990-5200	www.condell.org
Allegiance Health	Jackson	Michigan	517-788-4800	www.footehealth.org
Arkansas Heart Hospital	Little Rock	Arkansas	501-219-7000	www.arheart.com
Asante Rogue Regional Medical Center	Medford	Oregon	541-789-7000	www.asante.org
Aurora Saint Lukes Medical Center	Milwaukee	Wisconsin	414-649-6000	www.aurorahealthcare.org
Avera Mckennan Hospital & University Health Center	Sioux Falls	South Dakota	605-322-8000	www.mckennan.org
Avera Saint Lukes	Aberdeen	South Dakota	605-622-5000	www.averastlukes.org
Bakersfield Memorial Hospital	Bakersfield	California	661-327-1792	www.bakersfieldmemorial.org
Banner Baywood Medical Center	Mesa	Arizona	480-321-2000	www.bannerhealth.com
Banner Good Samaritan Medical Center	Phoenix	Arizona	602-239-2000	www.bannerhealth.com
Baptist Beaumont Hospital	Beaumont	Texas	409-212-5012	www.mhbh.org
Baptist Health Lexington	Lexington	Kentucky	859-260-6104	www.centralbap.com
Baptist Health Louisville	Louisville	Kentucky	502-897-8100	www.baptisteast.com
Baptist Health Medical Center - Little Rock	Little Rock	Arkansas	501-202-2000	www.baptist-health.com
Baystate Medical Center	Springfield	Massachusetts	413-794-0000	www.baystatehealth.com
Benefis Hospitals	Great Falls	Montana	406-455-5000	www.benefis.org
Berkshire Medical Center	Pittsfield	Massachusetts	413-447-2000	www.berkshirehealthsystems.org
Billings Clinic Hospital	Billings	Montana	406-657-4000	www.billingsclinic.com
Camden Clark Medical Center	Parkersburg	West Virginia	304-424-2111	www.ccmh.org
Cape Cod Hospital	Hyannis	Massachusetts	508-771-1800	www.capecodhealth.org
Carilion New River Valley Medical Center	Christiansburg	Virginia	540-731-2000	www.carilion.com
Carolinas Medical Center/Behaviorial Health	Charlotte	North Carolina	704-355-2000	www.carolinasmedicalcenter.org
Caromont Regional Medical Center	Gastonia	North Carolina	704-834-4891	www.caromont.org
Carson Tahoe Regional Medical Center	Carson City	Nevada	775-445-8000	www.carsontahoehospital.com
Centra Health	Lynchburg	Virginia	434-200-4789	www.centrahealth.com
Central Maine Medical Center	Lewiston	Maine	207-795-0111	www.cmmc.org
Charlotte Hungerford Hospital	Torrington	Connecticut	860-496-6666	www.charlottesweb.hungerford.org
Comanche County Memorial Hospital	Lawton	Oklahoma	580-355-8620	www.memorialhealthsource.org
Community Hospital North	Indianapolis	Indiana	317-621-5335	www.ecommunity.com/north
Community Medical Center	Toms River	New Jersey	732-557-8000	www.sbhcs.com
Cox Medical Center	Springfield	Missouri	417-269-6000	www.coxhealth.com
Doctors Hospital of Sarasota	Sarasota	Florida	941-342-1100	www.doctorsofsarasota.com
Duke University Hospital	Durham	North Carolina	919-684-8111	www.dukehealth.org
Eastern Idaho Regional Medical Center	Idaho Falls	Idaho	208-529-6111	www.eirmc.org
Eisenhower Medical Center	Rancho Mirage	California	760-340-3911	www.emc.org
El Camino Hospital	Mountain View	California	650-940-7000	www.elcaminohospital.org
Elkhart General Hospital	Elkhart	Indiana	574-294-2621	www.egh.org
Essentia Health - Fargo	Fargo	North Dakota	701-364-8000	www.dakotaclinic.com
Exeter Hospital	Exeter	New Hampshire	603-778-7311	www.exeterhospital.com
Flagstaff Medical Center	Flagstaff	Arizona	928-773-2009	www.nahealth.com
Fort Sanders Regional Medical Center	Knoxville	Tennessee	865-541-1101	www.fsregional.com
Franciscan Saint Elizabeth Health - Lafayette East	Lafayette	Indiana	765-502-4334	www.ste.org
Geisinger - Community Medical Center	Scranton	Pennsylvania	570-969-8240	www.cmchealthsys.org
Genesis Medical Center - Davenport	Davenport	Iowa	563-421-1000	www.genesishealth.com
Glens Falls Hospital	Glens Falls	New York	518-926-1000	www.glensfallshospital.org
Good Samaritan Regional Medical Center	Corvallis	Oregon	541-768-5111	www.samhealth.org/shs_facilities
Gundersen Lutheran Medical Center	La Crosse	Wisconsin	608-782-7300	www.gundluth.org
Harrison Memorial Center	Bremerton	Washington	360-377-3911	www.harrisonmedical.org
Hays Medical Center	Hays	Kansas	785-623-5000	www.haysmed.com
Heartland Regional Medical Center	Saint Joseph	Missouri	816-271-6000	www.heartland-health.com
Hendrick Medical Center	Abilene	Texas	325-670-2000	www.ehendrick.org
Holy Cross Hospital	Fort Lauderdale	Florida	954-771-8000	www.holy-cross.com
Indiana University Health Bloomington Hospital	Bloomington	Indiana	812-353-9555	www.bloomingtonhospital.org
Indiana University Health North Hospital	Carmel	Indiana	317-688-2000	www.iuhealth.org/north
Inova Mount Vernon Hospital	Alexandria	Virginia	703-664-7000	www.inova.com/inovapublic.srt/imvh/index.jsp
Integris Baptist Medical Center	Oklahoma City	Oklahoma	405-951-8110	www.integris-health.com
Jackson Hospital & Clinic	Montgomery	Alabama	334-293-8000	www.jackson.org
Jackson - Madison County General Hospital	Jackson	Tennessee	731-541-5000	www.wth.org
John Muir Medical Center - Concord Campus	Concord	California	925-674-2002	www.johnmuirhealth.com
John Muir Medical Center - Walnut Creek Campus	Walnut Creek	California	925-939-3000	www.jmmdhs.com
Kalispell Regional Medical Center	Kalispell	Montana	406-752-5111	www.krmc.org
Kootenai Medical Center	Coeur D'alene	Idaho	208-625-4001	www.kootenaihealth.org
Lakeland Hospital - Saint Joseph	Saint Joseph	Michigan	269-983-8300	www.lakelandhealth.org

Hospital	City	State	Phone	Web Site
Marian Regional Medical Center	Santa Maria	California	805-739-3000	www.marinmedicalcenter.org
Mary Washington Hospital	Fredericksburg	Virginia	540-741-1100	www.medicorp.org
Maury Regional Hospital	Columbia	Tennessee	931-381-1111	www.maurgregional.com
Mayo Clinic Methodist- Hospital	Rochester	Minnesota	507-266-7890	www.mayoclinic.org/methodisthospital
Mcleod Regional Medical Center - Pee Dee	Florence	South Carolina	843-777-2900	www.mcleodhealth.org
Medical Center of Central Georgia	Macon	Georgia	478-633-6805	www.mccg.org
Memorial Healthcare System	Chattanooga	Tennessee	423-495-2525	www.memorial.org
Memorial Hospital at Gulfport	Gulfport	Mississippi	228-867-4000	www.gulfportmemorial.com
Memorial Hospital of Carbondale	Carbondale	Illinois	618-549-0721	www.sih.net
Memorial Mission Hospital & Asheville Surgery Center	Asheville	North Carolina	828-213-1111	www.missionhospitals.org
Mercy Hospital	Coon Rapids	Minnesota	763-236-8205	www.allinamercy.org
Mercy Medical Center - Cedar Rapids	Cedar Rapids	Iowa	319-398-6011	www.mercycare.org
Mercy Medical Center - Redding	Redding	California	530-225-6102	www.redding.mercy.org
Mercy Medical Center - North Iowa	Mason City	Iowa	641-428-7000	www.mercynorthiowa.com
Methodist Hospital	San Antonio	Texas	210-575-4000	www.mh.sahealth.com
Methodist Medical Center of Oak Ridge	Oak Ridge	Tennessee	865-835-1000	www.mmcoakridge.com
Mother Frances Hospital	Tyler	Texas	903-593-8441	www.tmfhs.org
Munson Medical Center	Traverse City	Michigan	231-935-5000	www.munsonhealthcare.org
New England Baptist Hospital	Boston	Massachusetts	617-754-5800	www.nebh.caregroup.org
Novant Health Charlotte Orthopedic Hospital	Charlotte	North Carolina	704-316-2000	www.presbyterian.org
NW Arkansas Hospitals	Springdale	Arkansas	479-751-5711	www.northwesthealth.org
Ochsner Medical Center	New Orleans	Louisiana	504-842-3000	www.ochsner.org
Oklahoma Heart Hospital	Oklahoma City	Oklahoma	405-608-3200	www.okheart.com
Olathe Medical Center	Olathe	Kansas	913-791-4200	www.ohsi.com
Parker Adventist Hospital	Parker	Colorado	303-269-4000	www.parkerhospital.org
Parkview Medical Center	Pueblo	Colorado	719-584-4000	www.parkviewmc.com
Parkview Regional Medical Center	Fort Wayne	Indiana	260-266-1000	www.parkview.com
Parkwest Medical Center	Knoxville	Tennessee	865-970-9800	www.yesparkwest.com
Peacehealth Saint Joseph Medical Center	Bellingham	Washington	360-734-5400	www.peacehealth.org
Peconic Bay Medical Center	Riverhead	New York	631-548-6000	www.pbmedicalcenter.org
Presence Covenant Medical Center	Urbana	Illinois	217-337-2000	www.provena.org/covenant
Providence Sacred Heart Medical Center	Spokane	Washington	509-474-3040	www.shmc.org
Providence Saint John's Health Center	Santa Monica	California	310-829-5511	www.stjohns.org
Providence Saint Joseph Medical Center	Burbank	California	818-843-5111	www.providence.org/losangeles
Regional Medical Center Bayonet Point	Hudson	Florida	727-819-2929	www.mchealth.comorwww.heartoftampa.com
Riverview Medical Center	Red Bank	New Jersey	732-741-2700	www.meridianhealth.com
Sacred Heart Medical Center - Riverbend	Springfield	Oregon	541-222-7300	www.peacehealth.org/sacred-heart-riverbend
Saint Francis Medical Center	Cape Girardeau	Missouri	573-331-3000	www.sfmc.net
Saint Joseph Hospital	Lexington	Kentucky	859-313-1000	www.sjhlex.org
Saint Joseph Regional Medical Center	Mishawaka	Indiana	574-335-5000	www.sjmed.com
Saint Mary's Health Care	Grand Rapids	Michigan	616-685-5000	www.smhealthcare.org
Saint Thomas West Hospital	Nashville	Tennessee	615-222-2111	www.stthomas.org
Salinas Valley Memorial Hospital	Salinas	California	831-757-4333	www.svmh.com
San Jacinto Methodist Hospital	Baytown	Texas	281-420-8600	www.methodisthealth.com/sanjacinto
Sanford Medical Center Fargo	Fargo	North Dakota	701-234-2000	www.meritcare.com
Sanford Usd Medical Center	Sioux Falls	South Dakota	605-333-1000	www.sanfordhealth.org
Sarasota Memorial Hospital	Sarasota	Florida	941-917-9000	www.smh.com
Scott & White Memorial Hospital	Temple	Texas	254-724-2111	www.sw.org
Seton Medical Center Austin	Austin	Texas	512-324-1000	www.seton.net
Shannon Medical Center	San Angelo	Texas	325-653-6741	www.shannonhealth.com
Shasta Regional Medical Center	Redding	California	530-244-5454	www.shastaregional.com
South Georgia Medical Center	Valdosta	Georgia	229-333-1020	www.sgmc.org
Saint Charles Medical Center - Bend	Bend	Oregon	541-382-4321	www.scmc.org
Saint Cloud Hospital	Saint Cloud	Minnesota	320-251-2700	www.centracare.com
Saint David's Medical Center	Austin	Texas	512-476-7111	www.stdavidsrehab.com
Saint Elizabeth Medical Center	Lakeside Park	Kentucky	859-292-2000	www.stelizabeth.com
Saint Helena Hospital	Saint Helena	California	707-963-3611	www.sthelenahospital.org
Saint Joseph Hospital	Orange	California	714-633-9111	www.sjo.org
Saint Joseph Mercy Oakland	Pontiac	Michigan	248-858-3000	www.stjoesoakland.org
Saint Joseph's Hospital Health Center	Syracuse	New York	315-448-5111	www.sjhsyr.org
Saint Joseph's Medical Center of Stockton	Stockton	California	209-943-2000	www.stjospehscares.org
Saint Luke's Hospital	Cedar Rapids	Iowa	319-369-7211	www.crstlukes.com
Saint Mary's Regional Medical Center	Enid	Oklahoma	580-233-6100	www.stmarysregional.com
Saint Marys Hospital	Madison	Wisconsin	608-251-6100	www.stmarysmadison.com
Saint Patrick Hospital	Missoula	Montana	406-543-7271	www.saintpatrick.org
Saint Vincent Healthcare	Billings	Montana	406-657-7000	www.svh-mt.org
Saint Vincent Hospital	Santa Fe	New Mexico	505-913-5201	www.stvin.org

Hospital	City	State	Phone	Web Site
Saint Vincent Hospital & Health Services	Indianapolis	Indiana	317-338-7000	www.indianapolis.stvincent.org
Saint Vincent's Medical Center	Jacksonville	Florida	904-308-7300	www.jaxhealth.com
Sutter General Hospital	Sacramento	California	916-733-8999	www.suttermedicalcenter.org
Swedish American Hospital	Rockford	Illinois	815-968-4400	www.swedishamerican.org
Swedish Medical Center	Seattle	Washington	206-386-6000	www.swedish.org
Tallahassee Memorial Hospital	Tallahassee	Florida	850-431-1155	www.tmh.org
Texas Health Harris Methodist Hurst - Euless - Bedford	Bedford	Texas	817-848-4000	www.texashealth.org
Thibodaux Regional Medical Center	Thibodaux	Louisiana	985-447-5500	www.thibodaux.com
Trinity Rock Island	Rock Island	Illinois	309-779-5000	www.trinityqc.com
United Regional Health Care System	Wichita Falls	Texas	940-764-3055	www.urhcs.org
University Health Care/University Hospitals & Clinics	Salt Lake City	Utah	801-581-2121	www.healthcare.utah.edu
University Medical Center	Lubbock	Texas	806-775-8200	www.teamumc.org
University of Washington Medical Center	Seattle	Washington	206-598-3300	www.washington.edu/medical/uwmc
Vanderbilt University Hospital	Nashville	Tennessee	615-322-3454	www.mc.vanderbilt.edu
VHS Harlingen Hospital Company	Harlingen	Texas	956-389-1100	www.vbmc.org
Via Christi Hospitals Wichita	Wichita	Kansas	316-268-5000	www.via-christi.org
Virginia Mason Medical Center	Seattle	Washington	206-223-6600	www.vmmc.org
Wakemed - Raleigh Campus	Raleigh	North Carolina	919-350-8000	www.wakemed.org
Washington Hospital	Fremont	California	510-797-1111	www.whhs.com
Wesley Medical Center	Wichita	Kansas	316-962-2000	www.wesleymc.com
Winchester Medical Center	Winchester	Virginia	540-536-8000	www.valleyhealthlink.com
Winter Haven Hospital	Winter Haven	Florida	863-293-1121	www.winterhavenhospital.com
Wyoming Medical Center	Casper	Wyoming	307-577-7201	www.wyomingmedicalcenter.com
Yakima Valley Memorial Hospital	Yakima	Washington	509-575-8000	www.yakimamemorialhospital.org

Note: Table shows hospitals nationwide whose surgical complication rate is better (lower) than U.S. rate of 4.14%

Hospitals whose Surgical Complication Rate is Worse (Higher) than the U.S. National Rate

Measure: Serious Blood Clots After Surgery

Hospital	City	State	Phone	Web Site
Advocate Good Samaritan Hospital	Downers Grove	Illinois	630-275-5900	www.advocatehealth.com/gsam
Advocate Illinois Masonic Medical Center	Chicago	Illinois	773-975-1600	www.advocatehealth.com/immc
Advocate Lutheran General Hospital	Park Ridge	Illinois	847-723-2210	www.advocatehealth.com
Albert Einstein Medical Center	Philadelphia	Pennsylvania	215-456-6090	www.einstein.edu
Alegent Health Mercy Hospital	Council Bluffs	Iowa	712-328-5000	www.alegent.com/mercy
Alexian Brothers Medical Center	Elk Grove Village	Illinois	847-437-5500	www.alexian.org
Aultman Hospital	Canton	Ohio	330-452-9911	www.aultman.com
B R F Hospital Holdings	Shreveport	Louisiana	318-675-5000	www.lsumc.edu
Baptist Memorial Hospital Desoto	Southaven	Mississippi	662-772-4000	www.bmhcc.org/facilities/desoto
Barnes-Jewish Hospital	Saint Louis	Missouri	314-747-3000	www.barnesjewish.org
Beaumont Health System	Grosse Pointe	Michigan	313-343-1000	www.beaumonthospitals.com
Beaumont Health System	Royal Oak	Michigan	248-898-5000	www.beaumonthospitals.com
Bon Secours Saint Francis Medical Center	Midlothian	Virginia	804-594-7400	www.richmond.bonsecours.com
Bridgeport Hospital	Bridgeport	Connecticut	203-384-3000	www.bridgeporthospital.com
Brigham & Women's Hospital	Boston	Massachusetts	617-732-5500	www.brighamandwomens.org
Brookdale Hospital Medical Center	Brooklyn	New York	718-240-5966	www.brookdalehospital.org
Brookwood Medical Center	Birmingham	Alabama	205-877-1000	www.bwmc.com
Cape Coral Hospital	Cape Coral	Florida	239-574-2323	www.leememorial.org
Carilion Roanoke Memorial Hospital	Roanoke	Virginia	540-981-7000	www.carilion.com/crmh
Cedars - Sinai Medical Center	Los Angeles	California	310-423-5000	www.cedars-sinai.edu
Centennial Medical Center	Frisco	Texas	972-963-3333	www.centennialmedcenter.com
Charleston Area Medical Center	Charleston	West Virginia	304-388-6203	www.camc.org
Christian Hospital Northeast - Northwest	Saint Louis	Missouri	314-653-5000	www.christianhospital.org
Christiana Care Health Services	Newark	Delaware	302-733-1000	www.christianacare.org
Christus Saint Frances Cabrini Hospital	Alexandria	Louisiana	318-487-1122	www.cabrini.org
Christus Saint Michael Health System	Texarkana	Texas	903-614-1000	www.christusstmichael.org
Cleveland Clinic	Cleveland	Ohio	216-444-2200	www.clevelandclinic.org
Conemaugh Valley Memorial Hospital	Johnstown	Pennsylvania	814-534-9000	www.conemaugh.org
Coney Island Hospital	Brooklyn	New York	718-616-3000	www.coneyislandhospital.com
Cooper University Hospital	Camden	New Jersey	856-342-2000	www.cooperhealth.org
Crouse Hospital	Syracuse	New York	315-470-7449	www.crouse.org
D C H Regional Medical Center	Tuscaloosa	Alabama	205-759-7111	www.dchsystem.com
Danbury Hospital	Danbury	Connecticut	203-797-7000	www.danburyhospital.com
Delnor Community Hospital	Geneva	Illinois	630-208-3000	www.delnor.com
Doctors Hospital	Augusta	Georgia	706-651-6008	www.doctors-hospital.net
Doctors Hospital	Coral Gables	Florida	305-666-2111	www.baptisthealth.net
Edward Hospital	Naperville	Illinois	630-527-3000	www.edward.org
El Paso Specialty Hospital	El Paso	Texas	915-544-3636	www.elpasospecialtyhospital.com
Emory University Hospital Midtown	Atlanta	Georgia	404-686-4411	www.emoryhealthcare.org
Evanston Hospital	Evanston	Illinois	847-432-8000	www.enh.org
Flagler Hospital	Saint Augustine	Florida	904-819-4426	www.flaglerhospital.com
Florida Hospital	Orlando	Florida	407-303-1976	www.floridahospital.com
Franciscan Saint Margaret Health - Hammond	Hammond	Indiana	219-932-2300	www.smmhc.com
Geisinger Medical Center	Danville	Pennsylvania	570-271-6211	www.geisinger.org
Genesys Regional Medical Center - Health Park	Grand Blanc	Michigan	810-606-5000	www.genesys.org
Glen Cove Hospital	Glen Cove	New York	516-674-7300	www.northshorelij.com
Grady Memorial Hospital	Atlanta	Georgia	404-616-4252	www.gradyhealthsystem.org
Grand View Hospital	Sellersville	Pennsylvania	215-453-4615	www.gvh.org
Gulf Coast Medical Center Lee Memorial Health System	Fort Myers	Florida	239-768-5000	www.leememorial.org
Hackensack University Medical Center	Hackensack	New Jersey	201-996-2000	www.humed.com
Hackettstown Regional Medical Center	Hackettstown	New Jersey	908-852-5100	www.hrmcnj.org
Hahnemann University Hospital	Philadelphia	Pennsylvania	215-762-7000	www.hahnemannhospital.com
Harris Health System	Houston	Texas	713-566-6417	www.hchdonline.com
Hartford Hospital	Hartford	Connecticut	860-545-5000	www.harthosp.org
Henry Ford Hospital	Detroit	Michigan	313-916-2600	www.henryfordhospital.com
Henry Ford West Bloomfield Hospital	W Bloomfield	Michigan	248-325-1000	www.henryford.com
Henry Ford Wyandotte Hospital	Wyandotte	Michigan	734-246-6000	www.henryfordwyandotte.com
Heritage Valley Beaver	Beaver	Pennsylvania	412-728-7000	www.heritagevalley.org
Heritage Valley Sewickley	Sewickley	Pennsylvania	412-741-6600	www.heritagevalley.org
Hillcrest Hospital	Mayfield Heights	Ohio	440-312-4500	www.hillcresthospital.org
Holmes Regional Medical Center	Melbourne	Florida	321-434-7000	www.healthfirst.org
Holy Name Medical Center	Teaneck	New Jersey	201-833-3000	www.holyname.org
Hospital of Univ of Pennsylvania	Philadelphia	Pennsylvania	215-662-3227	www.upenn.edu
Huntington Memorial Hospital	Pasadena	California	626-397-5000	www.huntingtonhospital.com

Hospital	City	State	Phone	Web Site
Hurley Medical Center	Flint	Michigan	810-257-9000	www.hurleymc.com
Ingalls Memorial Hospital	Harvey	Illinois	708-333-2300	www.ingalls.org
Intermountain Medical Center	Murray	Utah	801-507-7000	www.intermountainhealthcare.org
Jackson Memorial Hospital	Miami	Florida	305-585-1111	www.jhsmiami.org
Jeanes Hospital	Philadelphia	Pennsylvania	215-728-2000	www.jeanes.com
JFK Medical Center	Atlantis	Florida	561-965-7300	www.jfkmc.com
JFK Medical Center - A M Yelencsics Comm Hospital	Edison	New Jersey	732-321-7000	www.jfkmc.org
John H Stroger Jr Hospital	Chicago	Illinois	312-864-6000	www.cookcountygov.com
JPS Health Network	Fort Worth	Texas	817-921-3431	www.jpshealthnet.org
Jupiter Medical Center	Jupiter	Florida	561-747-2234	www.jupitermed.com
Lancaster General Hospital	Lancaster	Pennsylvania	717-299-5511	www.lancastergeneral.org
Lee Memorial Hospital	Fort Myers	Florida	239-332-1111	www.leememorial.org
Legacy Emanuel Medical Center	Portland	Oregon	503-413-2200	www.legacyhealth.org
Lehigh Valley Hospital	Allentown	Pennsylvania	610-402-2273	www.lvhhn.org
Lehigh Valley Hospital - Muhlenberg	Bethlehem	Pennsylvania	610-402-2273	www.lvhn.org
Lenox Hill Hospital	New York	New York	212-439-2345	www.lenoxhillhospital.org
Little Company of Mary Hospital	Evergreen Park	Illinois	708-422-6200	www.lcmh.org
Louis A Weiss Memorial Hospital	Chicago	Illinois	773-878-8700	www.weisshospital.org
Lourdes Hospital	Paducah	Kentucky	270-444-2444	www.ehealthconnection.com
Lovelace Medical Center	Albuquerque	New Mexico	505-727-8000	www.lovelace.com
Loyola University Medical Center	Maywood	Illinois	708-216-9000	www.lumc.edu
Magee Womens Hospital of UPMC Health System	Pittsburgh	Pennsylvania	412-641-4010	www.magee.edu
Maimonides Medical Center	Brooklyn	New York	718-283-6000	www.maimonidesmed.org
Marin General Hospital	Greenbrae	California	415-925-7900	www.maringeneral.com
Mary Hitchcock Memorial Hospital	Lebanon	New Hampshire	603-650-5000	www.dhmc.org
Marymount Hospital	Garfield Heights	Ohio	216-581-0500	www.marymount.org
Mclaren Flint	Flint	Michigan	810-342-2000	www.mclaren.org
The Medical Center of Aurora	Aurora	Colorado	303-695-2600	www.auroramed.com
Medical Center of Mckinney	Mckinney	Texas	972-547-8000	www.medicalcenterofmckinney.com
Medical Center of Plano	Plano	Texas	972-596-6800	www.medicalcenterofplano.com
Medstar Georgetown University Hospital	Washington	District of Columbia	202-784-3000	www.georgetownuniversityhospital.org
Memorial Healthcare	Owosso	Michigan	989-723-5211	www.memorialhealthcare.org
Memorial Hermann Texas Medical Center	Houston	Texas	713-704-3700	www.mhhs.org
Memorial Hospital Jacksonville	Jacksonville	Florida	904-399-6111	www.memorialhospitaljax.com
Memorial Medical Center	Las Cruces	New Mexico	575-522-8641	www.mmclc.org
Menorah Medical Center	Overland Park	Kansas	913-498-6773	www.menorahmedicalcenter.com
Mercy Fitzgerald Hospital	Darby	Pennsylvania	215-237-4000	www.mercyhealth.org
Mercy Hospital Springfield	Springfield	Missouri	417-820-2000	www.stjohns.com
Mercy Saint Vincent Medical Center	Toledo	Ohio	419-251-3232	www.mhsnr.org
Miami Valley Hospital	Dayton	Ohio	937-208-8000	www.miamivalleyhospital.com
Midwest Orthopedic Specialty Hospital	Franklin	Wisconsin	414-817-5800	www.mymosh.com
Milton S Hershey Medical Center	Hershey	Pennsylvania	717-531-8521	www.hmc.psu.edu
Ministry Saint Josephs Hospital	Marshfield	Wisconsin	715-387-7850	www.stjosephs-marshfield.org
Mobile Infirmary	Mobile	Alabama	251-435-4700	www.mimc.com
Montefiore Medical Center	Bronx	New York	718-920-4321	www.montefiore.org
Morristown Medical Center	Morristown	New Jersey	973-971-5450	www.morristownmemorialhospital.org
Naples Community Hospital	Naples	Florida	239-436-5000	www.nchmd.org
Nason Hospital	Roaring Spring	Pennsylvania	814-224-2141	www.nasonhospital.com
Nathan Littauer Hospital	Gloversville	New York	518-725-8621	www.nlh.org
Newark Beth Israel Medical Center	Newark	New Jersey	973-926-7850	www.sbhcs.com
North Shore University Hospital	Manhasset	New York	516-562-0100	www.northshorelij.com
North Suburban Medical Center	Thornton	Colorado	303-451-7800	www.northsuburban.com
Northside Hospital	Atlanta	Georgia	404-851-8000	www.northside.com
Northwestern Memorial Hospital	Chicago	Illinois	312-926-2000	www.nmh.org
Novant Health Rowan Medical Center	Salisbury	North Carolina	704-210-5000	www.rowan.org
NYU Hospitals Center	New York	New York	212-263-7300	www.med.nyu.edu
O U Medical Center	Oklahoma City	Oklahoma	405-271-5911	www.oumedcenter.com
Oakwood Hospital - Southshore	Trenton	Michigan	734-671-3800	www.oakwood.org/oakwood-hospital-southshore
Och Regional Medical Center	Starkville	Mississippi	662-323-4320	www.och.org
OHSU Hospital & Clinics	Portland	Oregon	503-494-4036	www.ohsu.edu
Orlando Health	Orlando	Florida	321-841-5111	www.orlandoregionalmedicalcenter.org
Our Lady of the Lake Regional Medical Center	Baton Rouge	Louisiana	225-765-6565	www.ololrmc.com
Overlook Medical Center	Summit	New Jersey	908-522-2000	www.atlantichealth.org
Owensboro Health Regional Hospital	Owensboro	Kentucky	270-688-2000	www.omhs.org
Palmetto General Hospital	Hialeah	Florida	305-823-5000	www.palmettogeneral.com
Parkland Health & Hospital System	Dallas	Texas	214-590-8000	www.parklandhospital.com
Pennsylvania Hospital of the Univ of PA Health Sys	Philadelphia	Pennsylvania	215-829-3000	www.pennmedicine.org/pahosp
Piedmont Hospital	Atlanta	Georgia	404-605-5000	www.piedmonthospital.org

Hospital	City	State	Phone	Web Site
Pinnacle Health Hospitals	Harrisburg	Pennsylvania	717-782-5181	www.pinnaclehealth.org
Plainview Hospital	Plainview	New York	516-719-3000	www.nslij.com
Pratt Regional Medical Center	Pratt	Kansas	620-450-1160	www.prmc.org
Proctor Hospital	Peoria	Illinois	309-691-1000	www.proctor.org
Providence Hospital & Medical Centers	Southfield	Michigan	248-849-3011	www.stjohn.org/providence
Providence Memorial Hospital	El Paso	Texas	915-577-6011	www.sphn.com
Raleigh General Hospital	Beckley	West Virginia	304-256-4100	www.raleighgeneral.com
Regional Medical Center at Memphis	Memphis	Tennessee	901-545-7928	www.the-med.org
Riddle Memorial Hospital	Media	Pennsylvania	610-566-9400	www.riddlehospital.org
Robert Wood Johnson University Hospital	New Brunswick	New Jersey	732-937-8900	www.rwjuh.edu
Rose Medical Center	Denver	Colorado	303-320-2121	www.rosemed.com
Saint Barnabas Medical Center	Livingston	New Jersey	973-322-5000	www.saintbarnabas.com
Saint Peter's University Hospital	New Brunswick	New Jersey	732-745-8600	www.saintpetersuh.com
Saratoga Hospital	Saratoga Springs	New York	518-587-3222	www.saratogacare.org
Scripps Memorial Hospital La Jolla	La Jolla	California	858-626-4123	www.scrippshealth.org
Scripps Mercy Hospital	San Diego	California	619-294-8111	www.scrippshealth.org
Sentara Norfolk General Hospital	Norfolk	Virginia	757-388-3000	www.sentara.com
Sharp Memorial Hospital	San Diego	California	858-939-3400	www.sharp.com/memorial
Sierra Medical Center	El Paso	Texas	915-747-4000	www.sphn.com
Sinai - Grace Hospital	Detroit	Michigan	313-966-3300	www.sinaigrace.org
Somerset Medical Center	Somerville	New Jersey	908-685-2200	www.somersetmedicalcenter.com
South Lake Hospital	Clermont	Florida	352-394-4071	www.southlakehospital.com
Saint Alphonsus Regional Medical Center	Boise	Idaho	208-367-2121	www.saintalphonsus.org
Saint Anthonys Memorial Hospital	Effingham	Illinois	217-342-2121	www.stanthonyshospital.org
Saint Catherine of Siena Hospital	Smithtown	New York	631-862-3000	www.stcatherines.chsli.org
Saint Clare Hospital	Lakewood	Washington	253-588-1711	www.fhshealth.org
Saint Elizabeth Hospital	Belleville	Illinois	618-234-2120	www.steliz.org
Saint John's Episcopal Hospital at South Shore	Far Rockaway	New York	718-869-7000	www.ehs.org
Saint Joseph Hospital	Nashua	New Hampshire	603-882-3000	www.stjosephhospital.com
Saint Joseph Medical Center	Tacoma	Washington	253-627-4101	www.fhshealth.org
Saint Louis University Hospital	Saint Louis	Missouri	314-577-8000	www.slucare.edu/clinical
Saint Luke's Hospital Bethlehem	Bethlehem	Pennsylvania	610-954-4000	www.slhn-lehighvalley.org
Saint Luke's Roosevelt Hospital	New York	New York	212-523-4000	www.wehealny.org
Saint Luke's Warren Hospital	Phillipsburg	New Jersey	908-859-6700	www.warrenhospital.org
Saint Luke's Episcopal Hospital	Houston	Texas	832-355-1000	www.sleh.com
Saint Luke's Hospital	Chesterfield	Missouri	314-434-1500	www.goodhealthmatters.com
Saint Mary's Medical Center	West Palm Beach	Florida	561-840-6202	www.stmarysmc.com
Saint Mary's of Michigan Medical Center	Saginaw	Michigan	989-776-8000	www.stmarysofmichigan.org
Saint Vincent Hospital	Worcester	Massachusetts	508-363-5000	www.stvincenthospital.com
Staten Island University Hospital	Staten Island	New York	718-226-9000	www.siuh.edu
Summa Health Systems Hospitals	Akron	Ohio	330-375-3000	www.summahealth.org
Swedish Medical Center	Englewood	Colorado	303-788-5000	www.swedishhospital.com/default.asp
Tampa General Hospital	Tampa	Florida	813-844-7000	www.tgh.org
Temple University Hospital	Philadelphia	Pennsylvania	215-707-2000	www.tuh.templehealth.org
Carle Foundation Hospital	Urbana	Illinois	217-383-3311	www.carle.com
The University of Chicago Medical Center	Chicago	Illinois	773-702-1000	www.uchospitals.edu
Thomas Jefferson University Hospital	Philadelphia	Pennsylvania	215-955-6000	www.jeffersonhospital.org
Tri - City Medical Center	Oceanside	California	760-724-8411	www.tricitymed.org
Tucson Medical Center	Tucson	Arizona	520-327-5461	www.tmcaz.com
University Hospital	Augusta	Georgia	706-722-9011	www.universityhealth.org
University Hospital	Newark	New Jersey	973-972-5658	www.theuniversityhospital.com
University Hospital - Stony Brook	Stony Brook	New York	631-444-4000	www.stonybrookmedicalcenter.org
University Hospital SUNY Health Science Center	Syracuse	New York	315-473-4240	www.upstate.edu
University of California Davis Medical Center	Sacramento	California	916-734-2011	www.ucdmc.ucdavis.edu
University of Cincinnati Medical Center	Cincinnati	Ohio	513-584-1000	www.universityhospitalcincinnati.com
University of Illinois Hospital	Chicago	Illinois	312-996-3900	www.uic.edu
University of Miami Hospital	Miami	Florida	305-325-5511	www.cedarsmedicalcenter.com
University of Mississippi Medical Center	Jackson	Mississippi	601-984-4100	www.umc.edu
University of North Carolina Hospital	Chapel Hill	North Carolina	919-966-4131	www.unchealthcare.org
University of Tn Memorial Hospital	Knoxville	Tennessee	865-544-9000	www.utmedicalcenter.org
University of Toledo Medical Center	Toledo	Ohio	419-383-3407	www.utmc.utoledo.edu
University of Virginia Medical Center	Charlottesville	Virginia	800-251-3627	www.uvahealth.com
UPMC Presbyterian Shadyside	Pittsburgh	Pennsylvania	412-647-8788	www.upmc.edu
Valley Hospital	Ridgewood	New Jersey	201-447-8000	www.valleyhealth.com
Westchester Medical Center	Valhalla	New York	914-285-7017	www.wcmc.com
Wyckoff Heights Medical Center	Brooklyn	New York	718-963-7272	www.wyckoffhospital.org
Yale-New Haven Hospital	New Haven	Connecticut	203-688-4242	www.ynhh.org

Note: Table shows hospitals nationwide whose surgical complication rate is worse (higher) than U.S. rate of 4.14%

Hospitals whose Surgical Complication Rate is Better (Lower) than the U.S. National Rate

Measure: Serious Complications

Hospital	City	State	Phone	Web Site
Advocate Christ Hospital & Medical Center	Oak Lawn	Illinois	708-684-8000	www.advocatehealth.com
Allegiance Health	Jackson	Michigan	517-788-4800	www.footehealth.org
Anmed Health	Anderson	South Carolina	864-261-1109	www.anmed.com
Arkansas Heart Hospital	Little Rock	Arkansas	501-219-7000	www.arheart.com
Asante Rogue Regional Medical Center	Medford	Oregon	541-789-7000	www.asante.org
Atlanticare Regional Medical Center	Atlantic City	New Jersey	609-441-8020	www.atlanticare.org/acmc/index.html
Avera Mckennan Hospital & University Health Center	Sioux Falls	South Dakota	605-322-8000	www.mckennan.org
Baptist Beaumont Hospital	Beaumont	Texas	409-212-5012	www.mhbh.org
Baptist Health Lexington	Lexington	Kentucky	859-260-6104	www.centralbap.com
Baptist Health Louisville	Louisville	Kentucky	502-897-8100	www.baptisteast.com
Baystate Medical Center	Springfield	Massachusetts	413-794-0000	www.baystatehealth.com
Bethesda Hospital East	Boynton Beach	Florida	561-737-7733	www.bethesdahealthcare.com
Bethesda North	Cincinnati	Ohio	513-865-1241	www.trihealth.com
Billings Clinic Hospital	Billings	Montana	406-657-4000	www.billingsclinic.com
Carolina East Medical Center	New Bern	North Carolina	252-633-8640	www.cravenhealthcare.org
Carson Tahoe Regional Medical Center	Carson City	Nevada	775-445-8000	www.carsontahoehospital.com
Centinela Hospital Medical Center	Inglewood	California	310-673-4660	www.centinelafreeman.com
Central Dupage Hospital	Winfield	Illinois	630-682-1600	www.cdh.org
Christus Hospital	Beaumont	Texas	409-892-7171	www.christushealth.org
Christus Spohn Hospital Corpus Christi	Corpus Christi	Texas	361-902-4103	www.christusspohn.org
Community Hospital	Munster	Indiana	219-836-1600	www.comhs.org/community
Community Medical Center	Toms River	New Jersey	732-557-8000	www.sbhcs.com
Conway Regional Medical Center	Conway	Arkansas	501-329-3831	www.conwayregional.org
Cox Medical Center	Springfield	Missouri	417-269-6000	www.coxhealth.com
Delray Medical Center	Delray Beach	Florida	561-498-4440	www.delraymedicalctr.com
Duke University Hospital	Durham	North Carolina	919-684-8111	www.dukehealth.org
East Texas Medical Center	Tyler	Texas	903-597-0351	www.etmc.org
Englewood Hospital & Medical Center	Englewood	New Jersey	201-894-3000	www.englewoodhospital.com
Exeter Hospital	Exeter	New Hampshire	603-778-7311	www.exeterhospital.com
Floyd Medical Center	Rome	Georgia	706-509-6900	www.floydmed.org
Floyd Memorial Hospital & Health Services	New Albany	Indiana	812-949-5500	www.floydmedical.org
Genesis Medical Center - Davenport	Davenport	Iowa	563-421-1000	www.genesishealth.com
Glens Falls Hospital	Glens Falls	New York	518-926-1000	www.glensfallshospital.org
Heartland Regional Medical Center	Saint Joseph	Missouri	816-271-6000	www.heartland-health.com
Holy Cross Hospital	Fort Lauderdale	Florida	954-771-8000	www.holy-cross.com
Indiana University Health	Indianapolis	Indiana	317-962-5900	www.iuhealth.org
Indiana University Health Arnett Hospital	Lafayette	Indiana	765-448-8000	www.iuhealth.org/arnett
Integris Baptist Medical Center	Oklahoma City	Oklahoma	405-951-8110	www.integris-health.com
Integris Southwest Medical Center	Oklahoma City	Oklahoma	405-636-7000	www.integris-health.com
Jackson - Madison County General Hospital	Jackson	Tennessee	731-541-5000	www.wth.org
John Muir Medical Center - Concord Campus	Concord	California	925-674-2002	www.johnmuirhealth.com
Lakeland Hospital - Saint Joseph	Saint Joseph	Michigan	269-983-8300	www.lakelandhealth.org
Laredo Medical Center	Laredo	Texas	956-796-5000	www.laredomedical.com
Lehigh Valley Hospital - Hazleton	Hazleton	Pennsylvania	570-501-4000	www.ghha.org
Marietta Memorial Hospital	Marietta	Ohio	740-374-1400	www.mmhospital.org
Mary Washington Hospital	Fredericksburg	Virginia	540-741-1100	www.medicorp.org
Mayo Clinic	Jacksonville	Florida	904-953-2000	www.mayoclinic.org/jacksonville
Mayo Clinic Hospital	Phoenix	Arizona	480-342-2000	www.mayoclinic.org
Mayo Clinic Methodist- Hospital	Rochester	Minnesota	507-266-7890	www.mayoclinic.org/methodisthospital
Mclaren Bay Region	Bay City	Michigan	989-894-3000	www.baymed.org
Mcleod Regional Medical Center - Pee Dee	Florence	South Carolina	843-777-2900	www.mcleodhealth.org
Medcentral Health System Mansfield Hospital	Mansfield	Ohio	419-526-8000	www.medcentral.org
Memorial Healthcare System	Chattanooga	Tennessee	423-495-2525	www.memorial.org
Memorial Hermann Hospital System	Houston	Texas	713-448-6796	www.memorialhermann.org
Memorial Mission Hospital & Asheville Surgery Center	Asheville	North Carolina	828-213-1111	www.missionhospitals.org
Mercy Medical Center - Cedar Rapids	Cedar Rapids	Iowa	319-398-6011	www.mercycare.org
Methodist Hospital	San Antonio	Texas	210-575-4000	www.mh.sahealth.com
Methodist Medical Center of Illinois	Peoria	Illinois	309-672-5522	www.mmci.org
Methodist Willowbrook Hospital	Houston	Texas	281-477-1000	www.houstonmethodist.org/willowbrook-hospital
Metrowest Medical Center	Framingham	Massachusetts	508-383-1000	www.mwmc.com
Mississippi Baptist Medical Center	Jackson	Mississippi	601-968-1000	www.mbmc.org
Monongalia County General Hospital	Morgantown	West Virginia	304-598-1200	www.mongeneral.com
Mother Frances Hospital	Tyler	Texas	903-593-8441	www.tmfhs.org
Munroe Regional Medical Center	Ocala	Florida	352-351-7200	www.munroeregional.com

Hospital	City	State	Phone	Web Site
Munson Medical Center	Traverse City	Michigan	231-935-5000	www.munsonhealthcare.org
Nebraska Heart Hospital	Lincoln	Nebraska	402-328-3000	www.neheart.com
New York Community Hospital of Brooklyn	Brooklyn	New York	718-692-5302	www.nych.com
North Mississippi Medical Center	Tupelo	Mississippi	662-377-3000	www.nmhs.net/nmmc
Oklahoma Heart Hospital	Oklahoma City	Oklahoma	405-608-3200	www.okheart.com
Our Lady of Lourdes Medical Center	Camden	New Jersey	856-757-3500	www.lourdesnet.org
Palos Community Hospital	Palos Heights	Illinois	708-923-4000	www.paloshospital.org
Parkview Regional Medical Center	Fort Wayne	Indiana	260-266-1000	www.parkview.com
Parkwest Medical Center	Knoxville	Tennessee	865-970-9800	www.yesparkwest.com
Pomona Valley Hospital Medical Center	Pomona	California	909-865-9500	www.pvhmc.com
Presence Saint Joseph Medical Center	Joliet	Illinois	815-725-7133	www.provena.org/stjoes
Providence Little Co of Mary Medical Center Torrance	Torrance	California	310-540-7676	www.lcmhs.org
Providence Saint Joseph Medical Center	Burbank	California	818-843-5111	www.providence.org/losangeles
Redmond Regional Medical Center	Rome	Georgia	706-802-3012	www.redmondregional.com
Regional Medical Center Bayonet Point	Hudson	Florida	727-819-2929	www.mchealth.comorwww.heartoftampa.com
Roper Hospital	Charleston	South Carolina	843-724-2800	www.ropersaintfrancis.com
Saint Thomas West Hospital	Nashville	Tennessee	615-222-2111	www.stthomas.org
Sentara Careplex Hospital	Hampton	Virginia	757-736-1000	www.sentara.com
Sentara Leigh Hospital	Norfolk	Virginia	757-261-6601	www.sentara.com
Shasta Regional Medical Center	Redding	California	530-244-5454	www.shastaregional.com
Southcoast Hospital Group	Fall River	Massachusetts	508-679-3131	www.southcoast.org/charlton
Saint Elizabeth Medical Center	Lakeside Park	Kentucky	859-292-2000	www.stelizabeth.com
Saint Francis Hospital	Columbus	Georgia	706-596-4020	www.wecareforlife.com
Saint Francis Hospital - Roslyn	Roslyn	New York	516-562-6000	www.stfrancisheartcenter.com
Saint Luke's Hospital	Cedar Rapids	Iowa	319-369-7211	www.crstlukes.com
Saint Mary Medical Center	Langhorne	Pennsylvania	215-750-2003	www.stmaryhealthcare.org
Saint Mary Mercy Hospital	Livonia	Michigan	734-655-4800	www.stmarymercy.org
Saint Vincent Heart Center of Indiana	Indianapolis	Indiana	317-583-5000	www.theheartcenter.com
Saint Vincent Hospital & Health Services	Indianapolis	Indiana	317-338-7000	www.indianapolis.stvincent.org
Saint Vincent's Medical Center	Jacksonville	Florida	904-308-7300	www.jaxhealth.com
Sutter General Hospital	Sacramento	California	916-733-8999	www.suttermedicalcenter.org
Texas Health Harris Methodist Hurst - Euless - Bedford	Bedford	Texas	817-848-4000	www.texashealth.org
Thibodaux Regional Medical Center	Thibodaux	Louisiana	985-447-5500	www.thibodaux.com
Tuomey Healthcare System	Sumter	South Carolina	803-774-8900	www.tuomey.com
United Hospital Center	Bridgeport	West Virginia	681-342-1000	www.uhcwv.org
University Hospitals - Elyria Medical Center	Elyria	Ohio	440-329-7500	www.emh-healthcare.org
University of Michigan Health System	Ann Arbor	Michigan	734-764-1505	www.med.umich.edu
UPMC Altoona	Altoona	Pennsylvania	814-889-2011	www.altoonaregional.org
Vanderbilt University Hospital	Nashville	Tennessee	615-322-3454	www.mc.vanderbilt.edu
Virtua West Jersey Hospitals Berlin	Berlin	New Jersey	856-322-3200	www.virtua.org
Washington Hospital	Fremont	California	510-797-1111	www.whhs.com
Williamsport Regional Medical Center	Williamsport	Pennsylvania	570-321-1000	www.susquehannahealth.org
Willis Knighton Bossier Health Center	Bossier City	Louisiana	318-212-7000	www.wkhs.com/locations/bossier.aspx
Winchester Medical Center	Winchester	Virginia	540-536-8000	www.valleyhealthlink.com

Note: Table shows hospitals nationwide whose surgical complication rate is better (lower) than U.S. rate of 0.61%

Hospitals whose Surgical Complication Rate is Worse (Higher) than the U.S. National Rate

Measure: Serious Complications

Hospital	City	State	Phone	Web Site
Adirondack Medical Center	Saranac Lake	New York	518-891-4141	www.amccares.org
Appleton Medical Center	Appleton	Wisconsin	920-731-4101	www.thedacare.org
Aurora Medical Center Kenosha	Kenosha	Wisconsin	262-948-5600	www.aurorahealthcare.org
B R F Hospital Holdings	Shreveport	Louisiana	318-675-5000	www.lsumc.edu
Baptist Memorial Hospital Desoto	Southaven	Mississippi	662-772-4000	www.bmhcc.org/facilities/desoto
Baptist Saint Anthony's Hospital	Amarillo	Texas	806-212-2000	www.bsahs.com
Barnes-Jewish Hospital	Saint Louis	Missouri	314-747-3000	www.barnesjewish.org
Baylor University Medical Center	Dallas	Texas	214-820-0111	www.baylorhealth.com
Beaumont Health System	Royal Oak	Michigan	248-898-5000	www.beaumonthospitals.com
Beth Israel Deaconess Medical Center	Boston	Massachusetts	617-667-7000	www.bidmc.harvard.edu
Blessing Hospital	Quincy	Illinois	217-223-5811	www.blessinghealthsystem.org
Boston Medical Center Corporation	Boston	Massachusetts	617-638-8000	www.bmc.org
Bridgeport Hospital	Bridgeport	Connecticut	203-384-3000	www.bridgeporthospital.com
Brigham & Women's Hospital	Boston	Massachusetts	617-732-5500	www.brighamandwomens.org
Cape Coral Hospital	Cape Coral	Florida	239-574-2323	www.leememorial.org
Carilion Roanoke Memorial Hospital	Roanoke	Virginia	540-981-7000	www.carilion.com/crmh
Centennial Medical Center	Frisco	Texas	972-963-3333	www.centennialmedcenter.com
Central Texas Medical Center	San Marcos	Texas	512-753-3690	www.ctmc.org
Charleston Area Medical Center	Charleston	West Virginia	304-388-6203	www.camc.org
Chilton Medical Center	Pompton Plains	New Jersey	973-831-5000	www.chiltonmemorial.org
Christus Saint Frances Cabrini Hospital	Alexandria	Louisiana	318-487-1122	www.cabrini.org
Clearview Regional Medical Center	Monroe	Georgia	770-267-1792	www.clearviewregionalmedicalcenter.com
Cleveland Clinic	Cleveland	Ohio	216-444-2200	www.clevelandclinic.org
Clovis Community Medical Center	Clovis	California	559-324-4000	www.communitymedical.org
Community Regional Medical Center	Fresno	California	559-459-6000	www.communitymedical.org
Conemaugh Valley Memorial Hospital	Johnstown	Pennsylvania	814-534-9000	www.conemaugh.org
Cooper University Hospital	Camden	New Jersey	856-342-2000	www.cooperhealth.org
Crouse Hospital	Syracuse	New York	315-470-7449	www.crouse.org
Dameron Hospital	Stockton	California	209-944-5550	www.dameronhospital.org
Deaconess Hospital	Spokane	Washington	509-473-5800	www.deaconessmedicalcenter.org
Emory University Hospital Midtown	Atlanta	Georgia	404-686-4411	www.emoryhealthcare.org
Evanston Hospital	Evanston	Illinois	847-432-8000	www.enh.org
Firsthealth Moore Regional Hospital	Pinehurst	North Carolina	910-715-1000	www.firsthealth.org
Geisinger Medical Center	Danville	Pennsylvania	570-271-6211	www.geisinger.org
Geisinger Wyoming Valley Medical Center	Wilkes Barre	Pennsylvania	570-826-7300	www.geisinger.org
Genesys Regional Medical Center - Health Park	Grand Blanc	Michigan	810-606-5000	www.genesys.org
Gila Regional Medical Center	Silver City	New Mexico	575-538-4000	www.grmc.org
Good Samaritan Hospital	San Jose	California	408-559-2011	www.goodsamsj.org
Good Shepherd Medical Center Marshall	Marshall	Texas	903-927-6712	www.marshallregional.org
Grady Memorial Hospital	Atlanta	Georgia	404-616-4252	www.gradyhealthsystem.org
Grand View Hospital	Sellersville	Pennsylvania	215-453-4615	www.gvh.org
Grossmont Hospital	La Mesa	California	619-465-0711	www.sharp.com
Gulf Coast Medical Center Lee Memorial Health System	Fort Myers	Florida	239-768-5000	www.leememorial.org
Hackettstown Regional Medical Center	Hackettstown	New Jersey	908-852-5100	www.hrmcnj.org
Hahnemann University Hospital	Philadelphia	Pennsylvania	215-762-7000	www.hahnemannhospital.com
Harborview Medical Center	Seattle	Washington	206-731-3000	www.harborview.org
Hartford Hospital	Hartford	Connecticut	860-545-5000	www.harthosp.org
Hennepin County Medical Center	Minneapolis	Minnesota	612-873-3000	www.hcmc.org
Henry Ford Hospital	Detroit	Michigan	313-916-2600	www.henryfordhospital.com
Henry Ford West Bloomfield Hospital	W Bloomfield	Michigan	248-325-1000	www.henryford.com
Heritage Valley Beaver	Beaver	Pennsylvania	412-728-7000	www.heritagevalley.org
Holy Cross Hospital	Taos	New Mexico	575-758-8883	www.taoshospital.org
Hospital of Univ of Pennsylvania	Philadelphia	Pennsylvania	215-662-3227	www.upenn.edu
Huntington Memorial Hospital	Pasadena	California	626-397-5000	www.huntingtonhospital.com
Inova Fairfax Hospital	Falls Church	Virginia	703-776-3332	www.inova.org
Inspira Medical Center Vineland	Vineland	New Jersey	856-641-6610	www.sjhs.com
Intermountain Medical Center	Murray	Utah	801-507-7000	www.intermountainhealthcare.org
Jackson Memorial Hospital	Miami	Florida	305-585-1111	www.jhsmiami.org
JFK Medical Center - A M Yelencsics Comm Hospital	Edison	New Jersey	732-321-7000	www.jfkmc.org
John Dempsey Hospital	Farmington	Connecticut	860-679-1145	www.uconnhealth.orgorwww.uchc.edu
JPS Health Network	Fort Worth	Texas	817-921-3431	www.jpshealthnet.org
Kaweah Delta Medical Center	Visalia	California	559-624-2000	www.kaweahdelta.org
Keck Hospital of USC	Los Angeles	California	323-442-8656	www.uscuh.com
Lancaster General Hospital	Lancaster	Pennsylvania	717-299-5511	www.lancastergeneral.org

Hospital	City	State	Phone	Web Site
LDS Hospital	Salt Lake City	Utah	801-408-1100	www.intermountainhealthcare.org
Lee Memorial Hospital	Fort Myers	Florida	239-332-1111	www.leememorial.org
Lenox Hill Hospital	New York	New York	212-439-2345	www.lenoxhillhospital.org
Lourdes Hospital	Paducah	Kentucky	270-444-2444	www.ehealthconnection.com
Lower Keys Medical Center	Key West	Florida	305-294-5531	www.lkmc.com
Loyola University Medical Center	Maywood	Illinois	708-216-9000	www.lumc.edu
Magee Womens Hospital of UPMC Health System	Pittsburgh	Pennsylvania	412-641-4010	www.magee.edu
Maine Medical Center	Portland	Maine	207-662-0111	www.mmc.org
Marin General Hospital	Greenbrae	California	415-925-7900	www.maringeneral.com
Mary Hitchcock Memorial Hospital	Lebanon	New Hampshire	603-650-5000	www.dhmc.org
Mayo Clinic Health System - Mankato	Mankato	Minnesota	507-625-4031	www.isj-mhs.org
McKay Dee Hospital	Ogden	Utah	801-387-2800	www.intermountainhealthcare.org
The Medical Center of Aurora	Aurora	Colorado	303-695-2600	www.auroramed.com
Medical Center of Plano	Plano	Texas	972-596-6800	www.medicalcenterofplano.com
Medical College of Virginia Hospitals	Richmond	Virginia	804-828-0938	www.vcuhealth.org
Medical West	Bessemer	Alabama	205-481-7000	www.uab.edu
Medstar Georgetown University Hospital	Washington	District of Columbia	202-784-3000	www.georgetownuniversityhospital.org
Medstar Washington Hospital Center	Washington	District of Columbia	202-877-7000	www.whcenter.org
Memorial Medical Center	Modesto	California	209-526-4500	www.memorialmedicalcenter.org
Memorial Hospital Jacksonville	Jacksonville	Florida	904-399-6111	www.memorialhospitaljax.com
Memorial Medical Center	Springfield	Illinois	217-788-3000	www.memorialmedical.com
Menorah Medical Center	Overland Park	Kansas	913-498-6773	www.menorahmedicalcenter.com
Mercy Hospital - Cadillac	Cadillac	Michigan	231-876-7200	www.mercycadillac.munsonhealthcare.org
Mercy Memorial Health Center	Ardmore	Oklahoma	405-223-5400	www.mercyok.com/mmhc
Mercy Saint Vincent Medical Center	Toledo	Ohio	419-251-3232	www.mhsnr.org
Metrohealth System	Cleveland	Ohio	216-778-7089	www.metrohealth.org
Miami Valley Hospital	Dayton	Ohio	937-208-8000	www.miamivalleyhospital.com
Milton S Hershey Medical Center	Hershey	Pennsylvania	717-531-8521	www.hmc.psu.edu
Ministry Saint Josephs Hospital	Marshfield	Wisconsin	715-387-7850	www.stjosephs-marshfield.org
Montefiore Medical Center	Bronx	New York	718-920-4321	www.montefiore.org
Newark Beth Israel Medical Center	Newark	New Jersey	973-926-7850	www.sbhcs.com
North Shore University Hospital	Manhasset	New York	516-562-0100	www.northshorelij.com
North Suburban Medical Center	Thornton	Colorado	303-451-7800	www.northsuburban.com
Novant Health Presbyterian Medical Center	Charlotte	North Carolina	704-384-4000	www.presbyterian.org
NYU Hospitals Center	New York	New York	212-263-7300	www.med.nyu.edu
O U Medical Center	Oklahoma City	Oklahoma	405-271-5911	www.oumedcenter.com
OHSU Hospital & Clinics	Portland	Oregon	503-494-4036	www.ohsu.edu
Our Lady of the Lake Regional Medical Center	Baton Rouge	Louisiana	225-765-6565	www.ololrmc.com
Overland Park Regional Medical Center	Overland Park	Kansas	913-541-5301	www.oprmc.com
Parkland Health & Hospital System	Dallas	Texas	214-590-8000	www.parklandhospital.com
Parkview Medical Center	Pueblo	Colorado	719-584-4000	www.parkviewmc.com
Piedmont Hospital	Atlanta	Georgia	404-605-5000	www.piedmonthospital.org
Pinnacle Health Hospitals	Harrisburg	Pennsylvania	717-782-5181	www.pinnaclehealth.org
Plainview Hospital	Plainview	New York	516-719-3000	www.nslij.com
Providence Holy Cross Medical Center	Mission Hills	California	818-365-8051	www.providence.org
Providence Sacred Heart Medical Center	Spokane	Washington	509-474-3040	www.shmc.org
Rhode Island Hospital	Providence	Rhode Island	401-444-4000	www.rhodeislandhospital.org
Ridgeview Medical Center	Waconia	Minnesota	952-442-2191	www.ridgeviewmedical.org
Robert Wood Johnson University Hospital	New Brunswick	New Jersey	732-937-8900	www.rwjuh.edu
Ronald Reagan UCLA Medical Center	Los Angeles	California	310-825-6301	www.uclahealth.org
Rose Medical Center	Denver	Colorado	303-320-2121	www.rosemed.com
Rush University Medical Center	Chicago	Illinois	312-942-5000	www.ruch.edu
Sacred Heart Hospital	Eau Claire	Wisconsin	715-717-4121	www.sacredhearteauclaire.org
Saint Anthony Medical Center	Rockford	Illinois	815-226-2000	www.osfhealth.com
Saint Barnabas Medical Center	Livingston	New Jersey	973-322-5000	www.saintbarnabas.com
Saint Francis Medical Center	Peoria	Illinois	309-655-2000	www.osfsaintfrancis.org
Saint Mary's Health Care	Grand Rapids	Michigan	616-685-5000	www.smhealthcare.org
Santa Clara Valley Medical Center	San Jose	California	408-885-5000	www.sccgov.org
Saratoga Hospital	Saratoga Springs	New York	518-587-3222	www.saratogacare.org
Sentara Norfolk General Hospital	Norfolk	Virginia	757-388-3000	www.sentara.com
Sharp Memorial Hospital	San Diego	California	858-939-3400	www.sharp.com/memorial
Sierra Medical Center	El Paso	Texas	915-747-4000	www.sphn.com
Sinai - Grace Hospital	Detroit	Michigan	313-966-3300	www.sinaigrace.org
Somerset Medical Center	Somerville	New Jersey	908-685-2200	www.somersetmedicalcenter.com
Springhill Medical Center	Mobile	Alabama	251-344-9630	www.springhillmedicalcenter.com
Saint Alphonsus Regional Medical Center	Boise	Idaho	208-367-2121	www.saintalphonsus.org
Saint Clare Hospital	Lakewood	Washington	253-588-1711	www.fhshealth.org

Hospital	City	State	Phone	Web Site
Saint Elizabeth Health Center	Youngstown	Ohio	330-746-7211	www.hmhs.org
Saint Joseph Medical Center	Tacoma	Washington	253-627-4101	www.fhshealth.org
Saint Joseph Mercy Hospital	Ann Arbor	Michigan	734-712-3791	www.stjoesannarbor.or
Saint Joseph's Hospital & Medical Center	Phoenix	Arizona	602-406-3000	www.stjosephs-phx.org
Saint Louis University Hospital	Saint Louis	Missouri	314-577-8000	www.slucare.edu/clinical
Saint Luke's Hospital Bethlehem	Bethlehem	Pennsylvania	610-954-4000	www.slhn-lehighvalley.org
Saint Luke's Episcopal Hospital	Houston	Texas	832-355-1000	www.sleh.com
Saint Luke's Hospital	Chesterfield	Missouri	314-434-1500	www.goodhealthmatters.com
Saint Luke's Hospital of Kansas City	Kansas City	Missouri	816-932-2000	www.staintlukeshealthsystem.org
Stamford Hospital	Stamford	Connecticut	203-276-1000	www.stamhealth.org
Summa Health Systems Hospitals	Akron	Ohio	330-375-3000	www.summahealth.org
Sunrise Hospital & Medical Center	Las Vegas	Nevada	702-731-8000	www.sunrisehospital.com
Swedish Medical Center	Englewood	Colorado	303-788-5000	www.swedishhospital.com/default.asp
Swedish Medical Center - Cherry Hill	Seattle	Washington	206-320-2000	www.swedish.org
Tampa General Hospital	Tampa	Florida	813-844-7000	www.tgh.org
The University of Chicago Medical Center	Chicago	Illinois	773-702-1000	www.uchospitals.edu
Theda Clark Medical Center	Neenah	Wisconsin	920-729-3100	www.thedacare.org
Thomas Hospital	Fairhope	Alabama	251-928-2375	www.thomashospital.com
Thomas Jefferson University Hospital	Philadelphia	Pennsylvania	215-955-6000	www.jeffersonhospital.org
Trinity Hospitals	Minot	North Dakota	701-857-5000	www.trinityhealth.org
Trinity Medical Center	Birmingham	Alabama	205-592-1000	www.bhsala.com/montclair
Tucson Medical Center	Tucson	Arizona	520-327-5461	www.tmcaz.com
Tulane Medical Center	New Orleans	Louisiana	504-988-1900	www.tuhc.com
UF Health Jacksonville	Jacksonville	Florida	904-244-0411	www.shandsjacksonville.org
UMC of Southern Nevada	Las Vegas	Nevada	702-383-2000	www.umc-cares.org
University Colo Health Memorial Hospital Central	Colorado Springs	Colorado	719-365-5000	www.memorialhospital.com
University Health System	San Antonio	Texas	210-358-4000	www.universityhealthsystem.com
University Hospital - Stony Brook	Stony Brook	New York	631-444-4000	www.stonybrookmedicalcenter.org
University Hospital SUNY Health Science Center	Syracuse	New York	315-473-4240	www.upstate.edu
University Medical Center of El Paso	El Paso	Texas	915-521-7602	www.thomasoncares.org
University of Alabama Hospital	Birmingham	Alabama	205-934-4011	www.health.uab.edu
University of California Davis Medical Center	Sacramento	California	916-734-2011	www.ucdmc.ucdavis.edu
University of Cincinnati Medical Center	Cincinnati	Ohio	513-584-1000	www.universityhospitalcincinnati.com
University of Illinois Hospital	Chicago	Illinois	312-996-3900	www.uic.edu
University of Kansas Hospital	Kansas City	Kansas	913-588-7332	www.kumc.edu
University of Miami Hospital	Miami	Florida	305-325-5511	www.cedarsmedicalcenter.com
University of Mississippi Medical Center	Jackson	Mississippi	601-984-4100	www.umc.edu
University of Toledo Medical Center	Toledo	Ohio	419-383-3407	www.utmc.utoledo.edu
UPMC Hamot	Erie	Pennsylvania	814-877-6000	www.hamot.org
UPMC Passavant	Pittsburgh	Pennsylvania	412-367-6700	www.passavant.upmc.com
UPMC Presbyterian Shadyside	Pittsburgh	Pennsylvania	412-647-8788	www.upmc.edu
UT Southwestern University Hospital	Dallas	Texas	214-879-3758	www.utsouthwestern.edu
Utah Valley Regional Medical Center	Provo	Utah	801-373-7850	www.intermountainhealthcare.org/hospitals/uvrmc
Valley Hospital	Ridgewood	New Jersey	201-447-8000	www.valleyhealth.com
Vidant Medical Center	Greenville	North Carolina	252-847-4100	www.uhseast.com
Waukesha Memorial Hospital	Waukesha	Wisconsin	262-928-1000	www.waukeshamemorial.org
Wesley Medical Center	Hattiesburg	Mississippi	601-268-8000	www.wesley.com
West Virginia University Hospitals	Morgantown	West Virginia	304-598-4000	www.wvuh.com
Wheaton Franciscan Saint Joseph	Milwaukee	Wisconsin	414-447-2000	www.wfhealthcare.org
Yale-New Haven Hospital	New Haven	Connecticut	203-688-4242	www.ynhh.org

Note: Table shows hospitals nationwide whose surgical complication rate is worse (higher) than U.S. rate of 0.61%

Surgical Complication Rate: State and National Summary

Measure: A Wound That Splits Open After Surgery on the Abdomen or Pelvis

Area	Number of Hospitals			
	Better than U.S. National Rate[1]	Worse than U.S. National Rate[2]	No Different than U.S. National Rate[3]	Number of Cases Too Small[4]
U.S. and Territories	0	42	2703	391
Alabama	0	0	58	18
Alaska	0	0	8	0
American Samoa	n/a	n/a	n/a	n/a
Arizona	0	1	49	9
Arkansas	0	0	35	9
California	0	2	245	49
Colorado	0	2	37	4
Connecticut	0	0	29	0
Delaware	0	0	6	0
District of Columbia	0	1	6	0
Florida	0	2	157	3
Georgia	0	2	83	15
Guam	n/a	n/a	n/a	n/a
Hawaii	0	1	11	2
Idaho	0	1	10	1
Illinois	0	0	122	3
Indiana	0	0	72	11
Iowa	0	0	30	4
Kansas	0	0	39	11
Kentucky	0	2	51	10
Louisiana	0	1	62	17
Maine	0	1	18	1
Maryland	n/a	n/a	n/a	n/a
Massachusetts	0	0	57	1
Michigan	0	4	80	6
Minnesota	0	1	40	9
Mississippi	0	0	37	7
Missouri	0	1	61	10
Montana	0	0	11	1
N. Mariana Islands	n/a	n/a	n/a	n/a
Nebraska	0	0	19	0
Nevada	0	2	19	0
New Hampshire	0	1	12	0
New Jersey	0	2	59	3
New Mexico	0	1	22	3
New York	0	1	146	9
North Carolina	0	2	79	4
North Dakota	0	0	6	0
Ohio	0	3	117	7
Oklahoma	0	0	47	21
Oregon	0	0	32	0
Pennsylvania	0	2	128	14
Puerto Rico	n/a	n/a	n/a	n/a
Rhode Island	0	0	11	0
South Carolina	0	0	49	4
South Dakota	0	0	10	7
Tennessee	0	1	66	22
Texas	0	2	205	55
Utah	0	0	23	4
Vermont	0	0	6	0
Virgin Islands	n/a	n/a	n/a	n/a
Virginia	0	1	64	7
Washington	0	0	46	2
West Virginia	0	0	28	3
Wisconsin	0	2	58	4
Wyoming	0	0	9	2

Note: (1) Surgical complication rate is better (lower) than U.S. rate of 0.92%; (2) Surgical complication rate is worse (higher) than U.S. rate of 0.92%; (3) Surgical complication rate is about the same as U.S. rate of 0.92%; (4) The number of cases is too small to classify the hospital; n/a not available

Surgical Complication Rate: State and National Summary

Measure: Accidental Cuts and Tears From Medical Treatment

Area	Number of Hospitals			
	Better than U.S. National Rate[1]	Worse than U.S. National Rate[2]	No Different than U.S. National Rate[3]	Number of Cases Too Small[4]
U.S. and Territories	95	203	3133	42
Alabama	0	8	89	0
Alaska	0	2	7	0
American Samoa	n/a	n/a	n/a	n/a
Arizona	1	4	61	1
Arkansas	1	0	45	0
California	7	22	280	1
Colorado	0	5	40	1
Connecticut	0	4	27	1
Delaware	1	0	5	0
District of Columbia	0	1	6	0
Florida	11	8	151	1
Georgia	2	6	100	0
Guam	n/a	n/a	n/a	n/a
Hawaii	0	1	13	0
Idaho	0	0	13	1
Illinois	10	7	111	1
Indiana	2	4	83	1
Iowa	0	3	31	0
Kansas	0	4	52	0
Kentucky	1	3	61	0
Louisiana	0	4	88	6
Maine	0	1	19	0
Maryland	n/a	n/a	n/a	n/a
Massachusetts	3	4	54	0
Michigan	3	7	85	0
Minnesota	2	4	46	0
Mississippi	1	2	61	3
Missouri	0	5	71	2
Montana	0	0	13	0
N. Mariana Islands	n/a	n/a	n/a	n/a
Nebraska	1	1	21	1
Nevada	0	2	22	0
New Hampshire	0	3	10	0
New Jersey	8	3	54	1
New Mexico	1	1	31	0
New York	5	4	158	2
North Carolina	1	6	82	0
North Dakota	0	1	6	0
Ohio	3	9	126	3
Oklahoma	3	3	83	2
Oregon	1	3	29	0
Pennsylvania	2	11	140	3
Puerto Rico	n/a	n/a	n/a	n/a
Rhode Island	0	3	8	0
South Carolina	2	3	52	0
South Dakota	0	1	20	0
Tennessee	5	0	92	0
Texas	11	10	301	7
Utah	0	5	26	1
Vermont	0	1	5	0
Virgin Islands	n/a	n/a	n/a	n/a
Virginia	5	3	70	2
Washington	0	11	37	0
West Virginia	1	1	29	0
Wisconsin	0	9	57	0
Wyoming	0	0	11	0

Note: (1) Surgical complication rate is better (lower) than U.S. rate of 1.83%; (2) Surgical complication rate is worse (higher) than U.S. rate of 1.83%; (3) Surgical complication rate is about the same as U.S. rate of 1.83%; (4) The number of cases is too small to classify the hospital; n/a not available

Surgical Complication Rate: State and National Summary

Measure: Collapsed Lung Due to Medical Treatment

Area	Number of Hospitals			
	Better than U.S. National Rate[1]	Worse than U.S. National Rate[2]	No Different than U.S. National Rate[3]	Number of Cases Too Small[4]
U.S. and Territories	9	60	3366	38
Alabama	0	2	95	0
Alaska	0	0	9	0
American Samoa	n/a	n/a	n/a	n/a
Arizona	0	1	65	1
Arkansas	0	1	45	0
California	1	7	302	0
Colorado	0	0	45	1
Connecticut	0	0	31	1
Delaware	0	0	6	0
District of Columbia	0	0	7	0
Florida	0	4	166	1
Georgia	0	2	106	0
Guam	n/a	n/a	n/a	n/a
Hawaii	0	0	14	0
Idaho	0	0	13	1
Illinois	1	2	125	1
Indiana	0	0	89	1
Iowa	0	0	34	0
Kansas	0	3	52	1
Kentucky	1	2	62	0
Louisiana	1	1	92	4
Maine	0	1	19	0
Maryland	n/a	n/a	n/a	n/a
Massachusetts	0	3	58	0
Michigan	1	2	92	0
Minnesota	0	0	52	0
Mississippi	0	0	64	3
Missouri	0	4	72	2
Montana	0	0	13	0
N. Mariana Islands	n/a	n/a	n/a	n/a
Nebraska	0	1	23	0
Nevada	0	1	23	0
New Hampshire	0	0	13	0
New Jersey	2	0	63	1
New Mexico	0	0	33	0
New York	1	4	162	2
North Carolina	0	1	88	0
North Dakota	0	1	6	0
Ohio	0	1	136	4
Oklahoma	0	2	88	1
Oregon	0	1	32	0
Pennsylvania	0	2	152	2
Puerto Rico	n/a	n/a	n/a	n/a
Rhode Island	0	0	11	0
South Carolina	0	1	56	0
South Dakota	0	0	21	0
Tennessee	0	1	96	0
Texas	0	6	316	7
Utah	0	0	31	1
Vermont	0	0	6	0
Virgin Islands	n/a	n/a	n/a	n/a
Virginia	1	2	75	2
Washington	0	0	48	0
West Virginia	0	0	31	0
Wisconsin	0	1	65	0
Wyoming	0	0	11	0

Note: (1) Surgical complication rate is better (lower) than U.S. rate of 0.32%; (2) Surgical complication rate is worse (higher) than U.S. rate of 0.32%; (3) Surgical complication rate is about the same as U.S. rate of 0.32%; (4) The number of cases is too small to classify the hospital; n/a not available

Surgical Complication Rate: State and National Summary

Measure: Deaths Among Patients With Serious Treatable Complications After Surgery

Area	Number of Hospitals			
	Better than U.S. National Rate[1]	Worse than U.S. National Rate[2]	No Different than U.S. National Rate[3]	Number of Cases Too Small[4]
U.S. and Territories	43	70	1831	1058
Alabama	0	6	33	29
Alaska	0	1	4	3
American Samoa	n/a	n/a	n/a	n/a
Arizona	3	0	39	15
Arkansas	0	1	20	17
California	1	3	164	116
Colorado	1	0	27	14
Connecticut	0	0	22	7
Delaware	0	1	4	1
District of Columbia	0	0	6	1
Florida	6	5	124	26
Georgia	2	5	50	41
Guam	n/a	n/a	n/a	n/a
Hawaii	0	0	5	9
Idaho	0	0	8	4
Illinois	7	1	87	29
Indiana	1	0	54	29
Iowa	1	0	22	10
Kansas	0	0	25	23
Kentucky	0	3	31	25
Louisiana	0	0	38	28
Maine	0	0	9	11
Maryland	n/a	n/a	n/a	n/a
Massachusetts	0	1	42	15
Michigan	4	0	56	28
Minnesota	1	0	23	24
Mississippi	0	3	20	16
Missouri	2	1	44	23
Montana	0	0	9	2
N. Mariana Islands	n/a	n/a	n/a	n/a
Nebraska	0	0	17	5
Nevada	0	2	14	5
New Hampshire	0	1	10	2
New Jersey	2	5	50	7
New Mexico	0	0	10	14
New York	2	4	91	58
North Carolina	0	4	57	25
North Dakota	1	0	5	0
Ohio	1	1	84	37
Oklahoma	0	4	27	27
Oregon	1	0	17	14
Pennsylvania	0	2	80	60
Puerto Rico	n/a	n/a	n/a	n/a
Rhode Island	0	0	7	4
South Carolina	0	3	29	21
South Dakota	0	0	6	9
Tennessee	0	2	45	30
Texas	5	5	147	81
Utah	0	0	16	11
Vermont	0	1	3	2
Virgin Islands	n/a	n/a	n/a	n/a
Virginia	0	1	46	21
Washington	0	0	40	6
West Virginia	0	1	19	8
Wisconsin	2	0	39	25
Wyoming	0	0	2	9

Note: (1) Surgical complication rate is better (lower) than U.S. rate of 110.25%; (2) Surgical complication rate is worse (higher) than U.S. rate of 110.25%; (3) Surgical complication rate is about the same as U.S. rate of 110.25%; (4) The number of cases is too small to classify the hospital; n/a not available

Surgical Complication Rate: State and National Summary

Measure: Rate of Complications for Hip/Knee Replacement Patients

Area	Number of Hospitals			
	Better than U.S. National Rate[1]	Worse than U.S. National Rate[2]	No Different than U.S. National Rate[3]	Number of Cases Too Small[4]
U.S. and Territories	75	68	2655	687
Alabama	0	4	46	11
Alaska	0	0	7	1
American Samoa	0	0	0	0
Arizona	1	0	48	6
Arkansas	1	1	28	7
California	7	4	196	89
Colorado	1	3	46	6
Connecticut	1	2	26	0
Delaware	0	0	5	1
District of Columbia	0	0	5	2
Florida	11	1	134	16
Georgia	2	1	76	15
Guam	0	0	0	0
Hawaii	0	0	8	6
Idaho	0	0	23	5
Illinois	2	3	108	25
Indiana	4	1	73	32
Iowa	0	2	46	17
Kansas	3	2	37	13
Kentucky	1	0	41	19
Louisiana	0	0	59	16
Maine	1	1	24	5
Maryland	2	1	41	1
Massachusetts	2	0	54	5
Michigan	6	2	88	20
Minnesota	1	0	65	17
Mississippi	2	1	24	9
Missouri	3	2	61	14
Montana	0	1	19	6
N. Mariana Islands	0	0	0	0
Nebraska	2	0	30	13
Nevada	0	1	22	2
New Hampshire	0	1	21	4
New Jersey	0	1	53	9
New Mexico	0	0	22	2
New York	4	2	116	30
North Carolina	1	4	77	8
North Dakota	1	0	7	1
Ohio	2	6	128	21
Oklahoma	1	1	46	18
Oregon	0	0	40	10
Pennsylvania	0	6	123	27
Puerto Rico	0	0	8	27
Rhode Island	0	0	9	1
South Carolina	1	0	39	14
South Dakota	0	0	16	2
Tennessee	2	3	50	21
Texas	7	4	198	54
Utah	0	1	25	6
Vermont	0	0	12	1
Virgin Islands	0	0	1	0
Virginia	2	2	54	11
Washington	1	0	52	9
West Virginia	0	0	26	6
Wisconsin	0	4	79	22
Wyoming	0	0	13	4

Note: (1) Surgical complication rate is better (lower) than U.S. rate of 3.4%; (2) Surgical complication rate is worse (higher) than U.S. rate of 3.4%; (3) Surgical complication rate is about the same as U.S. rate of 3.4%; (4) The number of cases is too small to classify the hospital; n/a not available

Surgical Complication Rate: State and National Summary

Measure: Serious Blood Clots After Surgery

Area	Number of Hospitals			
	Better than U.S. National Rate[1]	Worse than U.S. National Rate[2]	No Different than U.S. National Rate[3]	Number of Cases Too Small[4]
U.S. and Territories	155	203	2846	114
Alabama	1	3	72	5
Alaska	0	0	8	1
American Samoa	n/a	n/a	n/a	n/a
Arizona	3	1	58	1
Arkansas	3	0	41	2
California	16	8	274	5
Colorado	2	4	38	0
Connecticut	1	5	23	0
Delaware	0	1	5	0
District of Columbia	0	1	6	0
Florida	7	18	138	2
Georgia	2	6	92	4
Guam	n/a	n/a	n/a	n/a
Hawaii	0	0	14	0
Idaho	2	1	10	1
Illinois	5	20	100	2
Indiana	8	1	79	1
Iowa	4	1	29	0
Kansas	4	2	46	3
Kentucky	4	2	57	2
Louisiana	2	3	80	7
Maine	1	0	19	0
Maryland	n/a	n/a	n/a	n/a
Massachusetts	4	2	52	2
Michigan	5	13	74	0
Minnesota	4	0	47	0
Mississippi	1	3	39	9
Missouri	3	5	62	5
Montana	5	0	7	1
N. Mariana Islands	n/a	n/a	n/a	n/a
Nebraska	0	0	23	0
Nevada	1	0	20	0
New Hampshire	1	2	10	0
New Jersey	2	15	47	1
New Mexico	1	2	23	3
New York	3	21	133	5
North Carolina	6	2	79	0
North Dakota	2	0	4	0
Ohio	0	9	122	4
Oklahoma	4	1	68	11
Oregon	4	2	26	1
Pennsylvania	1	23	127	2
Puerto Rico	n/a	n/a	n/a	n/a
Rhode Island	0	0	11	0
South Carolina	1	0	54	2
South Dakota	3	0	15	1
Tennessee	8	2	77	5
Texas	13	12	257	23
Utah	1	1	27	1
Vermont	0	0	6	0
Virgin Islands	n/a	n/a	n/a	n/a
Virginia	5	4	62	1
Washington	7	2	39	0
West Virginia	1	2	28	0
Wisconsin	3	2	61	0
Wyoming	1	0	10	0

Note: (1) Surgical complication rate is better (lower) than U.S. rate of 4.14%; (2) Surgical complication rate is worse (higher) than U.S. rate of 4.14%; (3) Surgical complication rate is about the same as U.S. rate of 4.14%; (4) The number of cases is too small to classify the hospital; n/a not available

Surgical Complication Rate: State and National Summary

Measure: Serious Complications

Area	Number of Hospitals			
	Better than U.S. National Rate[1]	Worse than U.S. National Rate[2]	No Different than U.S. National Rate[3]	Number of Cases Too Small[4]
U.S. and Territories	108	182	3184	0
Alabama	0	5	92	0
Alaska	0	0	9	0
American Samoa	n/a	n/a	n/a	n/a
Arizona	1	2	64	0
Arkansas	2	0	44	0
California	8	15	287	0
Colorado	0	6	40	0
Connecticut	0	6	26	0
Delaware	0	0	6	0
District of Columbia	0	2	5	0
Florida	7	9	155	0
Georgia	3	4	101	0
Guam	n/a	n/a	n/a	n/a
Hawaii	0	0	14	0
Idaho	0	1	13	0
Illinois	5	9	115	0
Indiana	7	0	83	0
Iowa	3	0	31	0
Kansas	0	3	53	0
Kentucky	3	1	61	0
Louisiana	2	4	92	0
Maine	0	1	19	0
Maryland	n/a	n/a	n/a	n/a
Massachusetts	3	3	55	0
Michigan	6	8	81	0
Minnesota	1	3	48	0
Mississippi	2	3	62	0
Missouri	2	4	72	0
Montana	1	0	12	0
N. Mariana Islands	n/a	n/a	n/a	n/a
Nebraska	1	0	23	0
Nevada	1	2	21	0
New Hampshire	1	1	11	0
New Jersey	5	10	51	0
New Mexico	0	2	31	0
New York	3	10	157	0
North Carolina	3	3	83	0
North Dakota	0	1	6	0
Ohio	4	8	129	0
Oklahoma	3	2	86	0
Oregon	1	1	31	0
Pennsylvania	4	16	136	0
Puerto Rico	n/a	n/a	n/a	n/a
Rhode Island	0	1	10	0
South Carolina	4	0	53	0
South Dakota	1	0	20	0
Tennessee	5	0	92	0
Texas	10	13	306	0
Utah	0	4	28	0
Vermont	0	0	6	0
Virgin Islands	n/a	n/a	n/a	n/a
Virginia	4	4	72	0
Washington	0	6	42	0
West Virginia	2	2	27	0
Wisconsin	0	7	59	0
Wyoming	0	0	11	0

Note: (1) Surgical complication rate is better (lower) than U.S. rate of 0.61%; (2) Surgical complication rate is worse (higher) than U.S. rate of 0.61%; (3) Surgical complication rate is about the same as U.S. rate of 0.61%; (4) The number of cases is too small to classify the hospital; n/a not available

Appendix D: Best Hospitals by Selected Category

What Do These Tables Show?

This appendix shows the best hospitals nationwide based on their average scores in 11 categories. The categories are:

- Blood Clot Prevention and Treatment
- Children's Asthma Care
- Emergency Department Care
- Heart Care
- Pneumonia Care
- Preventative Care
- Stroke Care
- Surgical Care
- Patient's Hospital Experiences
- Use of Medical Imaging
- Lowest Medicare Spending per Beneficiary

How Were the Hospitals Selected?

Hospitals were selected for inclusion in three ways:

- Hospitals that achieved a perfect 100% average score in all qualified measures in a given category.
- Hospitals that were in the top 5% of hospitals based on their average score in a given category.
- Hospitals whose Medicare spending ratios fell below a certain threshold.

How Were Average Scores Calculated?

The average score for any given category was calculated by averaging the scores of the individual measures that made up that category. In some instances, not all measures were included in the average score calculation. A meaure was omitted if: 1) data was not available 2) the measure did not meet the 25 case threshold for inclusion (except Patient's Hospital Experiences in which the threshold was 100 or more completed surveys). Note that the Pregnancy Care category did not have enough information available to calculate an average score.

Best Hospitals for Blood Clot Prevention and Treatment

Hospital	City	State	Phone	Web Site
Baptist Hospital of Miami	Miami	Florida	786-596-1960	www.baptisthealth.net
Berkshire Medical Center	Pittsfield	Massachusetts	413-447-2000	www.berkshirehealthsystems.org
Blanchard Valley Hospital	Findlay	Ohio	419-423-4500	www.bvha.org
Boca Raton Regional Hospital	Boca Raton	Florida	561-362-5002	www.brrh.com
Brandon Regional Hospital	Brandon	Florida	813-681-5551	www.brandonregionalhospital.com
Capital Regional Medical Center	Tallahassee	Florida	850-656-5000	www.capitalregionalmedicalcenter.com
Centerpoint Medical Center	Independence	Missouri	816-698-7000	www.centerpointmedical.com
Community Hospital of the Monterey Peninsula	Monterey	California	831-624-5311	www.chomp.org
Delray Medical Center	Delray Beach	Florida	561-498-4440	www.delraymedicalctr.com
Doctors' Community Hospital	Lanham	Maryland	301-552-8085	www.dchweb.org
Fairview Southdale Hospital	Edina	Minnesota	952-924-5000	www.fairview.org
Flushing Hospital Medical Center	Flushing	New York	718-670-5000	www.flushinghospital.org
Fort Sanders Regional Medical Center	Knoxville	Tennessee	865-541-1101	www.fsregional.com
Henrico Doctors' Hospital	Richmond	Virginia	804-289-4500	www.henricodoctors.com
Heritage Valley Beaver	Beaver	Pennsylvania	412-728-7000	www.heritagevalley.org
Heritage Valley Sewickley	Sewickley	Pennsylvania	412-741-6600	www.heritagevalley.org
John Randolph Medical Center	Hopewell	Virginia	804-541-1600	www.johnrandolphmed.com
Kaiser Foundation Hospital - Roseville	Roseville	California	916-784-4000	www.kaiserpermanente.org/roseville
Kendall Regional Medical Center	Miami	Florida	305-223-3000	www.kendallmed.com
Lewisgale Medical Center	Salem	Virginia	540-776-4000	www.lewis-gale.com
Lovelace Medical Center	Albuquerque	New Mexico	505-727-8000	www.lovelace.com
Mclaren Lapeer Region	Lapeer	Michigan	810-667-5500	www.lapeerregional.org
The Medical Center of Aurora	Aurora	Colorado	303-695-2600	www.auroramed.com
Medical Center of Plano	Plano	Texas	972-596-6800	www.medicalcenterofplano.com
Memorial Hospital Pembroke	Pembroke Pines	Florida	954-962-9650	www.memorialpembroke.com\
Memorial Hospital West	Pembroke Pines	Florida	954-436-5000	www.memorialwest.com
Memorial Regional Hospital	Hollywood	Florida	954-987-2000	www.memorialregional.com
Mercy Hospital of Folsom	Folsom	California	916-983-7400	www.mercyfolsom.org
Mercy Memorial Hospital System	Monroe	Michigan	734-240-8400	www.mercymemorial.org
Methodist Dallas Medical Center	Dallas	Texas	214-947-2879	www.mhd.com
Mountain View Regional Medical Center	Las Cruces	New Mexico	575-556-7600	www.mountainviewregional.com
Nazareth Hospital	Philadelphia	Pennsylvania	215-335-6000	www.nazarethhospital.org
North Florida Regional Medical Center	Gainesville	Florida	352-333-4100	www.nfrmc.com
Northside Hospital	Atlanta	Georgia	404-851-8000	www.northside.com
Northside Hospital Cherokee	Canton	Georgia	770-720-5298	www.northside.com/cherokee
Northside Hospital Forsyth	Cumming	Georgia	404-851-8700	www.gbhcs.org
Novant Health Forsyth Medical Center	Winston-Salem	North Carolina	336-718-5000	www.forsythmedicalcenter.org
Oak Hill Hospital	Brooksville	Florida	352-596-6632	www.oakhillhospital.com
Orange Park Medical Center	Orange Park	Florida	904-276-8500	www.opmedical.com
Overland Park Regional Medical Center	Overland Park	Kansas	913-541-5301	www.oprmc.com
Rapides Regional Medical Center	Alexandria	Louisiana	318-769-3000	www.rapidesregional.com
Regional Medical Center Bayonet Point	Hudson	Florida	727-819-2929	www.mchealth.comorwww.heartoftampa.com
Riverside Medical Center	Kankakee	Illinois	815-933-1671	www.riversidehealthcare.org
Rockdale Medical Center	Conyers	Georgia	770-918-3000	www.rockdalehospital.org
Rose Medical Center	Denver	Colorado	303-320-2121	www.rosemed.com
Saint Clares Hospital of Weston	Weston	Wisconsin	715-393-3000	www.ministryhealth.org
Saint Lucie Medical Center	Port Saint Lucie	Florida	772-335-4000	www.stluciemed.com
Saint Mary Medical Center	Hobart	Indiana	219-942-0551	www.comhs.org/stmary
Saint Mary's Medical Center	West Palm Beach	Florida	561-840-6202	www.stmarysmc.com
Saint Mary's Medical Center	Blue Springs	Missouri	816-228-5900	www.stmaryskc.com
Saint Vincent's Medical Center Southside	Jacksonville	Florida	904-296-3700	www.jaxhealth.com
Sisters of Charity Hospital	Buffalo	New York	716-862-1000	www.chsbuffalo.org
South Miami Hospital	South Miami	Florida	786-662-4000	www.baptisthealth.net
Southern Hills Hospital & Medical Center	Las Vegas	Nevada	702-880-2100	www.southernhillshospital.com
Springs Memorial Hospital	Lancaster	South Carolina	803-286-1481	www.springsmemorial.com
Summa Western Reserve Hospital	Cuyahoga Falls	Ohio	330-971-7000	www.westernreservehospital.org
Texoma Medical Center	Denison	Texas	903-416-4000	www.texomamedicalcenter.net
Trinity Medical Center	Birmingham	Alabama	205-592-1000	www.bhsala.com/montclair
Tulane Medical Center	New Orleans	Louisiana	504-988-1900	www.tuhc.com
United Hospital Center	Bridgeport	West Virginia	681-342-1000	www.uhcwv.org
University Medical Center of El Paso	El Paso	Texas	915-521-7602	www.thomasoncares.org
UPMC Horizon	Greenville	Pennsylvania	724-588-2100	www.upmc.com
UPMC Mckeesport	Mc Keesport	Pennsylvania	412-664-2000	www.selectmedicalcorp.com
Venice Regional Medical Center - Bayfront Health	Venice	Florida	941-485-7711	www.veniceregional.com
Vista Medical Center East	Waukegan	Illinois	847-360-4000	www.vistahealth.com

Hospital	City	State	Phone	Web Site
Wesley Medical Center	Wichita	Kansas	316-962-2000	www.wesleymc.com
West Georgia Medical Center	Lagrange	Georgia	706-882-1411	www.wghealth.org
West Virginia University Hospitals	Morgantown	West Virginia	304-598-4000	www.wvuh.com

Note: The hospitals shown above represent the top 5% of the 1,268 hospitals nationwide for which an average score was calculated. Average scores were calculated for hospitals with qualifying data (25 cases or more) in at least 5 of 6 measures in the Blood Clot Prevention and Treatment category.

Best Hospitals for Children's Asthma Care

Hospital	City	State	Phone	Web Site
Carroll Hospital Center	Westminster	Maryland	410-848-3000	www.carrollhospitalcenter.org
Cleveland Clinic	Cleveland	Ohio	216-444-2200	www.clevelandclinic.org
Lawnwood Regional Medical Center & Heart Institute	Fort Pierce	Florida	772-461-4000	www.lawnwoodmed.com
Memorial Regional Hospital	Hollywood	Florida	954-987-2000	www.memorialregional.com
Renown Regional Medical Center	Reno	Nevada	775-982-4100	www.renown.org

Note: The hospitals shown above represent the top 5% of the 90 hospitals nationwide for which an average score was calculated. Average scores were calculated for hospitals with qualifying data (25 cases or more) in all three measures in the Children's Asthma category.

Best Hospitals for Emergency Department Care

Hospital	City	State	Phone	Web Site
Abraham Lincoln Memorial Hospital	Lincoln	Illinois	217-732-2161	www.almh.org
Albemarle Hospital Authority	Elizabeth City	North Carolina	252-335-0531	www.albemarlehealth.org
Alliance Community Hospital	Alliance	Ohio	330-596-7527	www.achosp.org
Ashtabula County Medical Center	Ashtabula	Ohio	440-997-2262	www.acmchealth.org
Aspirus Wausau Hospital	Wausau	Wisconsin	715-847-2121	www.aspirus.org
Aurora Medical Center	Summit	Wisconsin	262-434-1000	www.aurorahealthcare.org
Avera Sacred Heart Hospital	Yankton	South Dakota	605-668-8000	www.avera.org/sacred-heart
Avera Saint Mary's Hospital	Pierre	South Dakota	605-224-3100	www.st-marys.com
Avoyelles Hospital	Marksville	Louisiana	318-253-8611	www.avoyelleshospital.com
Bates County Memorial Hospital	Butler	Missouri	660-200-7000	www.bcmhospital.com
Bear River Valley Hospital	Tremonton	Utah	435-207-4708	www.intermountainhealthcare.org
Bellevue Hospital	Bellevue	Ohio	419-483-4040	www.bellevuehospital.com
Bluffton Hospital	Bluffton	Ohio	419-358-9010	www.bvhealthsystem.org
Bourbon Community Hospital	Paris	Kentucky	859-987-3600	www.bourbonhospital.com
Brigham City Community Hospital	Brigham City	Utah	435-734-9471	www.brighamcityhospital.com
Brookings Hospital	Brookings	South Dakota	605-696-7701	www.brookingshospital.org
Cache Valley Speciality Hospital	North Logan	Utah	435-713-9700	www.cachevalleyhospital.com
Cameron Regional Medical Center	Cameron	Missouri	816-632-2101	www.cameronregional.org
Carson City Hospital	Carson City	Michigan	989-584-3131	www.carsoncityhospital.com
Cogdell Memorial Hospital	Snyder	Texas	325-574-7437	www.cogdellhospital.com
Colorado Plains Medical Center	Fort Morgan	Colorado	970-867-3391	www.coloradoplainsmedicalcenter.com
Crossroads Community Hospital	Mount Vernon	Illinois	618-244-5500	www.crossroadscommnityhospital.com
Custer Regional Hospital	Custer	South Dakota	605-673-2229	www.rcrh.org/facilities
Dauterive Hospital	New Iberia	Louisiana	337-365-7311	www.dauterivehospital.com
Daviess Community Hospital	Washington	Indiana	812-254-2760	www.dchosp.org
Decatur County Memorial Hospital	Greensburg	Indiana	812-663-4331	www.dcmh.net
Detroit Receiving Hospital & University Health Center	Detroit	Michigan	313-745-3104	www.drhuhc.org
Dupont Hospital	Fort Wayne	Indiana	260-416-3000	www.theduponthospital.com
East Cooper Medical Center	Mount Pleasant	South Carolina	843-881-0100	www.eastcoopermedctr.com
El Paso Specialty Hospital	El Paso	Texas	915-544-3636	www.elpasospecialtyhospital.com
Encino Hospital Medical Center	Encino	California	818-995-5000	www.encino-tarzana.com
Englewood Community Hospital	Englewood	Florida	941-475-6571	www.englewoodcommunityhospital.com
Evanston Regional Hospital	Evanston	Wyoming	307-789-3636	www.evanstonregionalhospital.com
Excela Health Frick Hospital	Mount Pleasant	Pennsylvania	724-547-1500	www.excelahealth.org
Fairmont General Hospital	Fairmont	West Virginia	304-367-7100	www.fghi.com
Fort Hamilton Hughes Memorial Hospital	Hamilton	Ohio	513-867-2000	www.forthamiltonhospital.com
Fremont Area Medical Center	Fremont	Nebraska	402-721-1610	www.famc.org
Genesis Medical Center - Dewitt	Dewitt	Iowa	563-659-4200	www.genesishealth.com
Good Samaritan Health Center	Merrill	Wisconsin	715-536-5511	www.ministryhealth.org/GSHC/home.nws
Good Samaritan Hospital	Kearney	Nebraska	308-865-7100	www.gshs.org
Graham Hospital Association	Canton	Illinois	309-647-5240	www.grahamhospital.org
Great Bend Regional Hospital	Great Bend	Kansas	620-792-8833	www.greatbendsurgical.com
Grove City Medical Center	Grove City	Pennsylvania	724-450-7000	www.uchpa.org
Hamilton General Hospital	Hamilton	Texas	254-386-3151	www.hamiltonhospital.org
Harrington Memorial Hospital	Southbridge	Massachusetts	508-765-9771	www.harringtonhospital.org
Harris Hospital	Newport	Arkansas	870-523-8911	www.harrishospital.com
Heber Valley Medical Center	Heber City	Utah	435-654-2500	www.intermountainhealthcare.org
Henderson County Community Hospital	Lexington	Tennessee	731-968-1801	www.hendersoncchospital.com
Hill Regional Hospital	Hillsboro	Texas	254-580-8500	www.hillregionalhospital.com
Hillside Hospital	Pulaski	Tennessee	931-363-7531	www.hillsidehospital.com
Holdenville Hospital Authority	Holdenville	Oklahoma	405-379-4200	
The Hospital at Westlake Medical Center	Austin	Texas	512-327-0000	www.westlakemedical.com
Hutchinson Health	Hutchinson	Minnesota	320-234-5000	www.hahc-hmc.com
Illinois Valley Community Hospital	Peru	Illinois	815-223-3300	www.ivch.org
Integris Blackwell Regional Hospital	Blackwell	Oklahoma	580-363-2311	www.integrisblackwell.com
Integris Health Edmond	Edmond	Oklahoma	405-657-3000	www.integrisok.com/integris-health-edmond-ok
Integris Marshall County Medical Center	Madill	Oklahoma	580-795-3384	www.integris-health.com/integris
Iroquois Memorial Hospital	Watseka	Illinois	815-432-5201	www.iroquoismemorial.com
Kansas Medical Center	Andover	Kansas	316-300-4000	www.ksmedcenter.com
Lafayette Regional Health Center	Lexington	Missouri	660-259-2203	www.lafayetteregionalhealthcenter.com
Lake Region Healthcare Corporation	Fergus Falls	Minnesota	218-736-8000	www.lrhc.org
Lakeland Community Hospital	Haleyville	Alabama	205-485-7117	www.lifepointhospitals.com
Lakeland Regional Medical Center	Lakeland	Florida	863-687-1100	www.lrmc.com
Lander Regional Hospital	Lander	Wyoming	307-332-4420	www.landerhospital.com
Lawrence Medical Center	Moulton	Alabama	256-974-2200	www.lawrencemedicalcenter.com

Hospital	City	State	Phone	Web Site
Livingston Regional Hospital	Livingston	Tennessee	931-823-5611	www.livingstonregionalhospital.com
Madison Memorial Hospital	Rexburg	Idaho	208-359-6900	www.madisonhospital.org
Maple Grove Hospital	Maple Grove	Minnesota	763-581-1000	www.maplegrove.org
Mary Greeley Medical Center	Ames	Iowa	515-239-2011	www.mgmc.org
Mary Lanning Healthcare	Hastings	Nebraska	402-463-4521	www.marylanning.org
Mayo Clinic Health System - Fairmont	Fairmont	Minnesota	507-238-8101	www.fairmontmedicalcenter.org
McBride Clinic Orthopedic Hospital	Oklahoma City	Oklahoma	405-478-1717	www.mcbrideclinic.com
McCullough - Hyde Memorial Hospital	Oxford	Ohio	513-523-2111	www.mhmh.org
McDonough District Hospital	Macomb	Illinois	309-833-4101	www.mdh.org
Mercer County Joint Township Community Hospital	Coldwater	Ohio	419-678-4843	www.mercer-health.com
Mercy Health System Corp	Janesville	Wisconsin	608-756-6080	www.mercyhealthsystem.org
Mercy Medical Center	Roseburg	Oregon	541-673-0611	www.mercyrose.org
Mercy Medical Center - Dubuque	Dubuque	Iowa	563-589-8000	www.mercydubuque.com
Mercy Regional Medical Center	Ville Platte	Louisiana	337-363-5684	www.vpmc.com
Meriter Hospital	Madison	Wisconsin	608-417-6000	www.meriter.com
Mesa View Regional Hospital	Mesquite	Nevada	702-346-8040	www.mesaviewhospital.com
Minden Medical Center	Minden	Louisiana	318-377-2321	www.mindenmedicalcenter.com
Ministry Saint Michaels Hospital of Stevens Point	Stevens Point	Wisconsin	715-346-5000	www.saintmichaelshospital.org
Moore County Hospital District	Dumas	Texas	806-935-7171	www.mchd.net
Mount Pleasant Hospital	Mount Pleasant	South Carolina	843-724-2954	www.rsfh.com
Mountain View Hospital	Payson	Utah	801-465-7100	www.mvhpayson.com
Neshoba County General Hospital	Philadelphia	Mississippi	601-663-1200	www.neshobageneral.com
Nevada Regional Medical Center	Nevada	Missouri	417-667-3355	www.nrmchealth.com
Ottawa Regional Hospital & Healthcare Center	Ottawa	Illinois	815-433-3100	www.community-hospital.org
Park City Medical Center	Park City	Utah	435-658-7000	www.intermountainhealthcare.org
Parkview Lagrange Hospital	Lagrange	Indiana	260-463-9000	www.parkview.com
Ponca City Medical Center	Ponca City	Oklahoma	580-765-3321	www.poncamedcenter.com
Portage Health	Hancock	Michigan	906-483-1000	www.portagehealth.org
Prairie Lakes Hospital	Watertown	South Dakota	605-882-7000	www.prairielakes.com
Presbyterian Saint Lukes Medical Center	Denver	Colorado	303-839-6000	www.pslmc.com
Proctor Hospital	Peoria	Illinois	309-691-1000	www.proctor.org
Providence Seaside Hospital	Seaside	Oregon	503-717-7000	www.providence.org/northcoast
Pushmataha County - Town of Antlers Hospital Authority	Antlers	Oklahoma	580-298-3341	www.pushhospital.com
Riverview Regional Medical Center	Carthage	Tennessee	615-735-9815	www.sumner.org
Rockcastle County Hospital	Mount Vernon	Kentucky	606-256-2195	www.rockcastlehospital.com
Sagewest Health Care	Riverton	Wyoming	307-856-4161	www.riverton-hospital.com
Saint Charles Parish Hospital	Luling	Louisiana	985-785-6242	www.stch.net
Saint Clare Hospital Health Services	Baraboo	Wisconsin	608-356-1400	www.stclare.com
Saint Elizabeth Grant	Williamstown	Kentucky	859-824-8240	www.stelizabeth.com
Saint Elizabeth Hospital	Appleton	Wisconsin	920-738-2000	www.affinityhealth.org
Saint James Healthcare	Butte	Montana	406-723-2500	www.stjameshealthcare.org
Saint James Hospital	Pontiac	Illinois	815-842-2828	www.osfsaintjames.org
Saint John Hospital	Leavenworth	Kansas	913-596-3930	www.providence-health.org
Saint Johns Medical Center	Jackson	Wyoming	307-733-3636	www.tetonhospital.org
Saint Margarets Hospital	Spring Valley	Illinois	815-664-1176	www.aboutsmh.org
Saint Marys Hospital	Madison	Wisconsin	608-251-6100	www.stmarysmadison.com
Saint Marys Hospital Superior	Superior	Wisconsin	715-817-7000	www.smdc.org
Saint Marys Janesville Hospital	Janesville	Wisconsin	608-373-8000	www.stmarysjanesville.com
Samaritan Albany General Hospital	Albany	Oregon	541-812-4000	www.samhealth.org/shs_facilities
Sanford Medical Center Bismarck	Bismarck	North Dakota	701-323-6000	www.medcenterone.com
Sanford Worthington Medical Center	Worthington	Minnesota	507-372-2941	www.worthingtonhospital.com
Santa Ynez Valley Cottage Hospital	Solvang	California	805-688-6431	www.cottagehealthsystem.org
Seton Smithville Regional Hospital	Smithville	Texas	512-237-3214	www.srhnet.com
Share Memorial Hospital	Alva	Oklahoma	580-327-2800	www.smcok.com
Shelby Memorial Hospital	Shelbyville	Illinois	217-774-3961	www.mysmh.org
Silverton Hospital	Silverton	Oregon	503-873-1500	www.silvertonhospital.org
Smyth County Community Hospital	Marion	Virginia	276-378-1000	www.scchosp.org
South Central Kansas Medical Center	Arkansas City	Kansas	620-442-2500	www.sckrmc.com
Spearfish Regional Hospital	Spearfish	South Dakota	605-644-4000	www.rcrh.org
Spencer Municipal Hospital	Spencer	Iowa	712-264-8300	www.spencerhospital.org
Springhill Medical Center	Springhill	Louisiana	318-539-1000	www.smccare.com
Stephens Memorial Hospital	Breckenridge	Texas	254-559-2241	www.smhtx.com
Stonewall Jackson Memorial Hospital	Weston	West Virginia	304-269-8080	www.stonewallhospital.com
Swedish Issaquah	Issaquah	Washington	425-313-4000	www.swedish.org/locations/issaquah-campus
Swedish Medical Center	Seattle	Washington	206-386-6000	www.swedish.org
Taylorville Memorial Hospital	Taylorville	Illinois	217-824-3331	www.svmh.org
Toppenish Community Hospital	Toppenish	Washington	509-865-1520	www.hma-corp.com

Hospital	City	State	Phone	Web Site
Tristar Ashland City Medical Center	Ashland City	Tennessee	615-792-3030	www.centennialashlandcity.com
UPMC Bedford Memorial	Everett	Pennsylvania	814-623-6161	www.upmc.com
UPMC Northwest	Seneca	Pennsylvania	814-676-7600	www.northwest.upmc.com
Valley West Community Hospital	Sandwich	Illinois	815-786-8484	www.snd.softfarm.com/sandhosp
Via Christi Hospital Wichita Saint Teresa	Wichita	Kansas	316-796-7800	www.via-christi.org
Walla Walla General Hospital	Walla Walla	Washington	509-525-0480	www.wwgh.com
Winn Parish Medical Center	Winnfield	Louisiana	318-648-3000	www.winnparishmedical.com
Winona Health Services	Winona	Minnesota	507-454-3650	www.winonahealth.org
Woodward Regional Hospital	Woodward	Oklahoma	580-254-8492	www.woodwardhospital.com
Yampa Valley Medical Center	Steamboat Springs	Colorado	970-879-1322	www.yvmc.org
York Hospital	York	Maine	207-363-4321	www.yorkhospital.com

Note: The hospitals shown above represent the top 5% of the 2,872 hospitals nationwide for which an average score was calculated. Average scores were calculated for hospitals with qualifying data (25 cases or more) in at least 6 of 7 measures in the Emergency Department Care category.

Best Hospitals for Heart Care

Hospital	City	State	Phone	Web Site
Advocate Good Shepherd Hospital	Barrington	Illinois	847-381-9600	www.advocatehealth.com
Advocate Illinois Masonic Medical Center	Chicago	Illinois	773-975-1600	www.advocatehealth.com/immc
Alegent Creighton Health Immanuel Medical Center	Omaha	Nebraska	402-572-2121	www.alegent.com
Arkansas Heart Hospital	Little Rock	Arkansas	501-219-7000	www.arheart.com
Baptist Hospital of Miami	Miami	Florida	786-596-1960	www.baptisthealth.net
Baylor Heart & Vascular Hospital	Dallas	Texas	214-820-0670	www.baylorhearthospital.com
Beaumont Health System	Grosse Pointe	Michigan	313-343-1000	www.beaumonthospitals.com
Blanchard Valley Hospital	Findlay	Ohio	419-423-4500	www.bvha.org
Boca Raton Regional Hospital	Boca Raton	Florida	561-362-5002	www.brrh.com
Brooklyn Hospital Center at Downtown Campus	Brooklyn	New York	718-250-8000	www.tbh.org
Broward Health North	Pompano Beach	Florida	954-786-6950	www.browardhealth.org
Calvert Memorial Hospital	Prince Frederick	Maryland	410-535-8239	www.calverthospital.com
Carepoint Health - Bayonne Hospital Center	Bayonne	New Jersey	201-858-5000	www.bayonnemedicalcenter.org
Cedars - Sinai Medical Center	Los Angeles	California	310-423-5000	www.cedars-sinai.edu
Centinela Hospital Medical Center	Inglewood	California	310-673-4660	www.centinelafreeman.com
Decatur Memorial Hospital	Decatur	Illinois	217-877-8121	www.dmhcares.org
Dekalb Regional Medical Center	Fort Payne	Alabama	256-845-3150	www.baptistmedical.org
Delray Medical Center	Delray Beach	Florida	561-498-4440	www.delraymedicalctr.com
Doctors Hospital	Augusta	Georgia	706-651-6008	www.doctors-hospital.net
Doctors Hospital	Columbus	Ohio	614-544-1000	www.columbusregional.com
Eastern Idaho Regional Medical Center	Idaho Falls	Idaho	208-529-6111	www.eirmc.org
Fairview Southdale Hospital	Edina	Minnesota	952-924-5000	www.fairview.org
Florida Hospital North Pinellas	Tarpon Springs	Florida	727-942-5000	www.hemh.com
Fort Sanders Regional Medical Center	Knoxville	Tennessee	865-541-1101	www.fsregional.com
Gateway Regional Medical Center	Granite City	Illinois	618-798-3175	www.sehs.com
Good Samaritan Hospital Medical Center	West Islip	New York	631-376-3000	www.good-samaritan-hospital.org
Good Samaritan Hospital of Suffern	Suffern	New York	914-368-5000	www.goodsamhosp.org
Hackettstown Regional Medical Center	Hackettstown	New Jersey	908-852-5100	www.hrmcnj.org
Health Central	Ocoee	Florida	407-296-1820	www.health-central.org
High Point Regional Hospital	High Point	North Carolina	336-878-6000	www.highpointregional.com
Holy Name Medical Center	Teaneck	New Jersey	201-833-3000	www.holyname.org
Homestead Hospital	Homestead	Florida	786-243-8000	www.baptisthealth.net
Hospital De La Concepcion	San German	Puerto Rico	787-892-1860	www.hospitalconcepcion.org
Hospital of Univ of Pennsylvania	Philadelphia	Pennsylvania	215-662-3227	www.upenn.edu
Hudson Valley Hospital Center	Cortlandt Manor	New York	914-734-3611	www.hvhc.org
Indiana University Health Bloomington Hospital	Bloomington	Indiana	812-353-9555	www.bloomingtonhospital.org
Ingalls Memorial Hospital	Harvey	Illinois	708-333-2300	www.ingalls.org
Jamaica Hospital Medical Center	Jamaica	New York	718-262-6000	www.jamaicahospital.org
JFK Medical Center	Atlantis	Florida	561-965-7300	www.jfkmc.com
John Dempsey Hospital	Farmington	Connecticut	860-679-1145	www.uconnhealth.orgorwww.uchc.edu
Kaiser Foundation Hospital	Honolulu	Hawaii	808-432-0000	www.kaiserpermanente.com
Kaiser Foundation Hospital - Fremont/Hayward	Hayward	California	510-784-4000	www.kaiserpermanente.org
Kaiser Foundation Hospital - Manteca	Manteca	California	209-825-3700	www.healthy.kaiserpermanente.org
Kaiser Foundation Hospital - Orange Co-Anaheim	Anaheim	California	714-644-2000	www.healthy.kaiserpermanente.org
Kaiser Foundation Hospital - Redwood City	Redwood City	California	650-299-2000	www.seiu-uhw.org/aboutuhw
Kaiser Foundation Hospital - Sacramento	Sacramento	California	916-973-5000	www.kaiserpermanente.org
Kaiser Foundation Hospital - Santa Clara	Santa Clara	California	408-236-6400	www.members.kaiserpermanente.org
Kaiser Foundation Hospital - South Bay	Harbor City	California	310-517-6441	www.kaiserpermanente.org
Kaiser Foundation Hospital - South San Francisco	South San Francisco	California	650-742-3200	www.healthy.kaiserpermanente.org
Kaiser Foundation Hospital South Sacramento	Sacramento	California	916-688-2000	www.mydoctor.kaiserpermanente.org
Kansas Medical Center	Andover	Kansas	316-300-4000	www.ksmedcenter.com
Keck Hospital of USC	Los Angeles	California	323-442-8656	www.uscuh.com
La Palma Intercommunity Hospital	La Palma	California	714-670-7400	www.lapalmaintercommunityhospital.com
Lakeview Hospital	Bountiful	Utah	801-299-2211	www.lakeviewhospital.com
Lakeview Regional Medical Center	Covington	Louisiana	985-867-4443	www.lakeviewregional.com
Laredo Medical Center	Laredo	Texas	956-796-5000	www.laredomedical.com
Las Colinas Medical Center	Irving	Texas	972-969-2000	www.lascolinas.com
Lawnwood Regional Medical Center & Heart Institute	Fort Pierce	Florida	772-461-4000	www.lawnwoodmed.com
Lawrence Memorial Hospital	Lawrence	Kansas	785-505-6100	www.lmh.org
Lewisgale Medical Center	Salem	Virginia	540-776-4000	www.lewis-gale.com
Loyola University Medical Center	Maywood	Illinois	708-216-9000	www.lumc.edu
Manatee Memorial Hospital	Bradenton	Florida	941-746-5111	www.manateememorial.com
Mary Greeley Medical Center	Ames	Iowa	515-239-2011	www.mgmc.org
Medical Center of Arlington	Arlington	Texas	817-465-3241	www.medicalcenterarlington.com
Medical Center of Trinity	Trinity	Florida	727-848-1733	www.communityhospitalnpr.com

Hospital	City	State	Phone	Web Site
Memorial Regional Hospital	Hollywood	Florida	954-987-2000	www.memorialregional.com
Mercy Fitzgerald Hospital	Darby	Pennsylvania	215-237-4000	www.mercyhealth.org
Methodist Mansfield Medical Center	Mansfield	Texas	682-622-2059	www.methodisthealthsystem.com
Methodist Sugar Land Hospital	Sugar Land	Texas	281-274-8000	www.methodisthealth.com/sugarland
Metropolitan Hospital of Miami	Miami	Florida	305-264-1000	www.pahnet.org
Mid Coast Hospital	Brunswick	Maine	207-729-0181	www.midcoasthealth.com
Newark Beth Israel Medical Center	Newark	New Jersey	973-926-7850	www.sbhcs.com
North Florida Regional Medical Center	Gainesville	Florida	352-333-4100	www.nfrmc.com
North Hills Hospital	North Richland Hills	Texas	817-255-1000	www.northhillshospital.com
North Okaloosa Medical Center	Crestview	Florida	850-689-8100	www.northokaloosa.com
North Suburban Medical Center	Thornton	Colorado	303-451-7800	www.northsuburban.com
Novant Health Forsyth Medical Center	Winston-Salem	North Carolina	336-718-5000	www.forsythmedicalcenter.org
NYU Hospitals Center	New York	New York	212-263-7300	www.med.nyu.edu
Ocala Regional Medical Center	Ocala	Florida	352-401-1000	www.ocalaregional.com
Orange Park Medical Center	Orange Park	Florida	904-276-8500	www.opmedical.com
Palms West Hospital	Loxahatchee	Florida	561-753-4245	www.palmswesthospital.com
Paradise Valley Hospital	Phoenix	Arizona	602-923-5000	www.paradisevalleyhospital.com
Paradise Valley Hospital	National City	California	619-470-4321	www.paradisevalleyhospital.org
Parma Community General Hospital	Parma	Ohio	440-743-3000	www.parmahopsital.org
Penn Presbyterian Medical Center	Philadelphia	Pennsylvania	215-662-8000	www.pennhealth.com
Phelps Memorial Hospital Assn	Sleepy Hollow	New York	914-366-3000	www.phelpshospital.org
Pikeville Medical Center	Pikeville	Kentucky	606-218-3500	www.pikevillehospital.org
Plaza Medical Center of Fort Worth	Fort Worth	Texas	817-336-2100	www.plazamedicalcenter.com
Porter Regional Hospital	Valparaiso	Indiana	219-983-8300	www.portermemorial.org
Portsmouth Regional Hospital	Portsmouth	New Hampshire	603-436-5110	www.portsmouthhospital.com
Presbyterian Community Hospital	San Juan	Puerto Rico	787-721-2160	www.presbypr.com
Providence Memorial Hospital	El Paso	Texas	915-577-6011	www.sphn.com
Riverside Community Hospital	Riverside	California	951-788-3000	www.rchc.org
Riverside Methodist Hospital	Columbus	Ohio	614-566-5000	www.ohiohealth.com
Riverview Regional Medical Center	Gadsden	Alabama	256-543-5200	www.riverviewregional.com
Roper Hospital	Charleston	South Carolina	843-724-2800	www.ropersaintfrancis.com
Rose Medical Center	Denver	Colorado	303-320-2121	www.rosemed.com
Round Rock Medical Center	Round Rock	Texas	512-341-1000	www.roundrockmedicalcenter.com
Saint Anthony Hospital	Oklahoma City	Oklahoma	405-272-7000	www.saintsok.com
Saint John's Riverside Hospital	Yonkers	New York	914-964-4444	www.riversidehealth.org
Saint Luke's Magic Valley Rmc	Twin Falls	Idaho	208-814-1000	www.stlukesonline.org/magic_valley
Saint Mary Medical Center	Hobart	Indiana	219-942-0551	www.comhs.org/stmary
Saint Mary Medical Center	Langhorne	Pennsylvania	215-750-2003	www.stmaryhealthcare.org
Saint Mary's Health Center	Jefferson City	Missouri	573-761-7000	www.stmarys-jeffcity.com
Saint Mary's Hospital - Passaic	Passaic	New Jersey	973-365-4300	www.smh-nj.com
Sanford Medical Center Bismarck	Bismarck	North Dakota	701-323-6000	www.medcenterone.com
Scripps Green Hospital	La Jolla	California	858-554-3600	www.scrippshealth.org
Scripps Memorial Hospital La Jolla	La Jolla	California	858-626-4123	www.scrippshealth.org
Sebastian River Medical Center	Sebastian	Florida	772-589-3187	www.srmcenter.com
Sentara Norfolk General Hospital	Norfolk	Virginia	757-388-3000	www.sentara.com
Shady Grove Adventist Hospital	Rockville	Maryland	240-826-6517	www.adventisthealthcare.com/sgah
Sistema Integrados De Salud Del Sur Oeste	Mayaguez	Puerto Rico	787-652-9200	
Southern Hills Hospital & Medical Center	Las Vegas	Nevada	702-880-2100	www.southernhillshospital.com
Spotsylvania Regional Medical Center	Fredericksburg	Virginia	540-498-4000	www.spotsrmc.com
SSM Depaul Health Center	Bridgeton	Missouri	314-344-6000	www.ssmdepaul.com
SSM Saint Marys Health Center	Richmond Heights	Missouri	314-768-8000	www.ssmhealth.com/stmarys
Sutter Medical Center of Santa Rosa	Santa Rosa	California	707-576-4000	www.suttersantarosa.org
University Hospital	Newark	New Jersey	973-972-5658	www.theuniversityhospital.com
University of South Alabama Medical Center	Mobile	Alabama	251-471-7110	www.southalabama.edu/usamc
Venice Regional Medical Center - Bayfront Health	Venice	Florida	941-485-7711	www.veniceregional.com
Vista Medical Center East	Waukegan	Illinois	847-360-4000	www.vistahealth.com
Walker Baptist Medical Center	Jasper	Alabama	205-387-4000	www.bhsala.com/walker
Wellmont Bristol Regional Medical Center	Bristol	Tennessee	423-844-1121	www.wellmont.org
Wesley Medical Center	Wichita	Kansas	316-962-2000	www.wesleymc.com
West Florida Hospital	Pensacola	Florida	850-494-4000	www.westfloridahospital.com
West Virginia University Hospitals	Morgantown	West Virginia	304-598-4000	www.wvuh.com
Wichita VA Medical Center	Wichita	Kansas	316-685-2221	www.wichita.va.gov

Note: The 127 hospitals shown above all achieved a perfect 100% average score. Average scores were calculated for hospitals with qualifying data (25 cases or more) in at least 5 of 11 measures in the following categories: Chest Pain/Possible Heart Attack; Heart Attack; Heart Failure. A total of 2,234 hospitals nationwide were considered.

Best Hospitals for Pneumonia Care

Hospital	City	State	Phone	Web Site
Abilene Regional Medical Center	Abilene	Texas	325-428-1000	www.abileneregional.com
Advocate Christ Hospital & Medical Center	Oak Lawn	Illinois	708-684-8000	www.advocatehealth.com
Advocate Illinois Masonic Medical Center	Chicago	Illinois	773-975-1600	www.advocatehealth.com/immc
Alaska Regional Hospital	Anchorage	Alaska	907-276-1131	www.alaskaregional.com
Alegent Creighton Health Creighton University Med	Omaha	Nebraska	402-449-4000	www.creightonhospital.com
Alegent Creighton Health Midlands Hospital	Papillion	Nebraska	402-593-3000	www.alegent.com
Allegheny General Hospital	Pittsburgh	Pennsylvania	412-359-3131	www.allhealth.edu
Asante Ashland Community Hospital	Ashland	Oregon	541-201-4001	www.ashlandhospital.org
Asante Rogue Regional Medical Center	Medford	Oregon	541-789-7000	www.asante.org
Ashtabula County Medical Center	Ashtabula	Ohio	440-997-2262	www.acmchealth.org
Aurora Baycare Medical Center	Green Bay	Wisconsin	920-288-8000	www.aurorabaycare.com
Aurora West Allis Medical Center	West Allis	Wisconsin	414-328-6000	www.aurorahealthcare.org
Aventura Hospital & Medical Center	Aventura	Florida	305-682-7000	www.aventurahospital.com
Avera Marshall Regional Medical Center	Marshall	Minnesota	507-537-9661	www.averamarshall.org
Baptist Hospital of Miami	Miami	Florida	786-596-1960	www.baptisthealth.net
Baptist Memorial Hospital Huntingdon	Huntingdon	Tennessee	731-986-4461	www.bmhcc.org
Baptist Memorial Hospital North Mississippi	Oxford	Mississippi	662-232-8100	www.baptistonline.org/facilities/oxford
Baptist Memorial Hospital Union City	Union City	Tennessee	731-885-2410	www.bmhcc.org
Beaumont Health System	Grosse Pointe	Michigan	313-343-1000	www.beaumonthospitals.com
Bellevue Medical Center	Bellevue	Nebraska	402-763-3600	www.bellevuemed.com
Berkshire Medical Center	Pittsfield	Massachusetts	413-447-2000	www.berkshirehealthsystems.org
Big Bend Regional Medical Center	Alpine	Texas	432-837-3447	www.bigbendhealthcare.com
Bolivar Medical Center	Cleveland	Mississippi	662-846-2551	www.bolivarmedical.com
Bon Secours Memorial Regional Medical Center	Mechanicsville	Virginia	804-764-6000	www.bonsecours.com
Bonner General Hospital	Sandpoint	Idaho	208-263-1441	www.bonnergeneral.org
Brigham & Women's Faulkner Hospital	Boston	Massachusetts	617-983-7000	www.brighamandwomensfaulkner.org
Broadlawns Medical Center	Des Moines	Iowa	515-282-2200	www.broadlawns.org
Brookings Hospital	Brookings	South Dakota	605-696-7701	www.brookingshospital.org
Broward Health North	Pompano Beach	Florida	954-786-6950	www.browardhealth.org
Buchanan General Hospital	Grundy	Virginia	276-935-1000	www.bgh.org
Bucyrus Community Hospital	Bucyrus	Ohio	419-562-4677	www.bchonline.org
California Pacific Medical Center - Pacific Campus Hospital	San Francisco	California	415-600-6000	www.cpmc.org
California Pacific Medical Center - Saint Luke's Campus	San Francisco	California	415-641-6562	www.stlukes.sf.org
Carepoint Health - Bayonne Hospital Center	Bayonne	New Jersey	201-858-5000	www.bayonnemedicalcenter.org
Carney Hospital	Boston	Massachusetts	617-506-2000	www.caritascarney.org
Carolinas Hospital System	Florence	South Carolina	843-674-2500	www.carolinashospital.com
Centinela Hospital Medical Center	Inglewood	California	310-673-4660	www.centinelafreeman.com
Central Peninsula General Hospital	Soldotna	Alaska	907-262-4404	www.cpgh.org
Chatuge Regional Hospital	Hiawassee	Georgia	706-896-2222	www.chatugeregionalhospital.org
Coffee Regional Medical Center	Douglas	Georgia	229-384-1900	www.coffeeregional.org
Conroe Regional Medical Center	Conroe	Texas	936-539-1111	www.conroeregional.com
Coosa Valley Medical Center	Sylacauga	Alabama	256-249-5000	www.cvhealth.net
Coral Gables Hospital	Coral Gables	Florida	305-445-8461	www.coralgableshospital.com
The Corpus Christi Medical Center	Corpus Christi	Texas	361-761-1501	www.ccmedicalcenter.com
Davis Hospital & Medical Center	Layton	Utah	801-807-1000	www.davishospital.com
Delray Medical Center	Delray Beach	Florida	561-498-4440	www.delraymedicalctr.com
Detar Hospital Navarro	Victoria	Texas	361-575-7441	www.detar.com
Detroit (John D. Dingell) VA Medical Center	Detroit	Michigan	313-576-1000	www.detroit.va.gov
Doctors Hospital	Augusta	Georgia	706-651-6008	www.doctors-hospital.net
Dominican Hospital	Santa Cruz	California	831-462-7700	www.dominicanhospital.org
Down East Community Hospital	Machias	Maine	207-255-3356	www.dech.org
Dupont Hospital	Fort Wayne	Indiana	260-416-3000	www.theduponthospital.com
East Texas Medical Center - Gilmer	Gilmer	Texas	903-841-7100	www.etmc.org
Eastern Idaho Regional Medical Center	Idaho Falls	Idaho	208-529-6111	www.eirmc.org
El Camino Hospital	Mountain View	California	650-940-7000	www.elcaminohospital.org
Encino Hospital Medical Center	Encino	California	818-995-5000	www.encino-tarzana.com
Englewood Community Hospital	Englewood	Florida	941-475-6571	www.englewoodcommunityhospital.com
Excela Health Latrobe Hospital	Latrobe	Pennsylvania	724-537-1000	www.excelahealth.org
Faith Regional Health Services	Norfolk	Nebraska	402-371-4880	www.frhs.org
Falmouth Hospital	Falmouth	Massachusetts	508-548-5300	www.capecodhealth.com
Fannin Regional Hospital	Blue Ridge	Georgia	706-632-3711	www.fanninregionalhospital.com
Fawcett Memorial Hospital	Port Charlotte	Florida	941-629-1181	www.fawcetthospital.com
Florida Hospital North Pinellas	Tarpon Springs	Florida	727-942-5000	www.hemh.com
Flowers Hospital	Dothan	Alabama	334-793-5000	www.flowershospital.com
Forest Hills Hospital	Forest Hills	New York	718-830-4000	www.northshorelij.com

Hospital	City	State	Phone	Web Site
Fostoria Community Hospital	Fostoria	Ohio	419-435-7734	www.promedica.org
Franciscan Saint Anthony Health - Michigan City	Michigan City	Indiana	219-879-8511	www.samhc.org
Franciscan Saint Elizabeth Health - Lafayette East	Lafayette	Indiana	765-502-4334	www.ste.org
Frankfort Regional Medical Center	Frankfort	Kentucky	502-875-5240	www.frankfortregional.com
Garden Grove Hospital & Medical Center	Garden Grove	California	714-537-5160	www.gardengrovehospital.com
Garden Park Medical Center	Gulfport	Mississippi	228-575-7000	www.gardenparkmedical.com
Genesis Medical Center - Davenport	Davenport	Iowa	563-421-1000	www.genesishealth.com
Georgetown Memorial Hospital	Georgetown	South Carolina	843-527-7000	www.gmhsc.com
Good Samaritan Hospital Medical Center	West Islip	New York	631-376-3000	www.good-samaritan-hospital.org
Greene Memorial Hospital	Xenia	Ohio	937-352-2000	www.ketteringhealth.org/greene
Hackensack - Umc Mountainside	Montclair	New Jersey	973-429-6000	www.mountainsidenow.org
Hackettstown Regional Medical Center	Hackettstown	New Jersey	908-852-5100	www.hrmcnj.org
Hammond Henry Hospital	Geneseo	Illinois	309-944-6431	www.hammondhenry.com
Hardin Memorial Hospital	Kenton	Ohio	419-673-0761	www.hardinmemorial.org
Harlingen Medical Center	Harlingen	Texas	956-365-1000	www.harlingenmedicalcenter.com
Heart of Lancaster Regional Medical Center	Lititz	Pennsylvania	717-625-5000	www.heartoflancaster.com
Helena Regional Medical Center	Helena	Arkansas	870-338-5800	www.helenaregionalmedicalcenter.com
Henderson County Community Hospital	Lexington	Tennessee	731-968-1801	www.hendersoncchospital.com
Holy Family Memorial	Manitowoc	Wisconsin	920-320-2011	www.hfmhealth.org
Hospital Pavia Santurce	Fernandez Juncos	Puerto Rico	787-727-6060	www.paviahospitalsanturce.com
Howard Memorial Hospital	Nashville	Arkansas	870-845-4400	www.howardmemorial.com
Huntington Beach Hospital	Huntington Beach	California	714-843-5000	www.hbhospital.com
Hutchinson Health	Hutchinson	Minnesota	320-234-5000	www.hahc-hmc.com
Ingalls Memorial Hospital	Harvey	Illinois	708-333-2300	www.ingalls.org
Intermountain Medical Center	Murray	Utah	801-507-7000	www.intermountainhealthcare.org
Jackson Hospital & Clinic	Montgomery	Alabama	334-293-8000	www.jackson.org
Jamaica Hospital Medical Center	Jamaica	New York	718-262-6000	www.jamaicahospital.org
Jay Hospital	Jay	Florida	850-675-4532	www.bhcpns.org
Jefferson Medical Center	Ranson	West Virginia	304-728-1600	www.jeffmem.com
Jennings American Legion Hospital	Jennings	Louisiana	337-616-7000	www.jalh.com
JFK Medical Center	Atlantis	Florida	561-965-7300	www.jfkmc.com
The Johns Hopkins Hospital	Baltimore	Maryland	410-955-9540	www.jhmi.edu
Kaiser Foundation Hospital - Orange Co-Anaheim	Anaheim	California	714-644-2000	www.healthy.kaiserpermanente.org
Kaiser Foundation Hospital - San Jose	San Jose	California	408-972-7000	www.mydoctor.kaiserpermanente.org
Kaiser Foundation Hospital - Santa Clara	Santa Clara	California	408-236-6400	www.members.kaiserpermanente.org
Kendall Regional Medical Center	Miami	Florida	305-223-3000	www.kendallmed.com
Kenmore Mercy Hospital	Kenmore	New York	716-447-6100	www.chsbuffalo.org
Kennewick General Hospital	Kennewick	Washington	509-586-6111	www.kennewickgeneral.com
Lake City Medical Center	Lake City	Florida	386-719-9000	www.lakecitymedical.com
Lake Forest Hospital	Lake Forest	Illinois	847-234-5600	www.lakeforesthospital.com
Lake Wales Medical Center	Lake Wales	Florida	863-676-1433	www.lakewalesmedicalcenter.com
Lakeview Medical Center	Rice Lake	Wisconsin	715-234-1515	www.lakeviewmedical.com
Lakeview Regional Medical Center	Covington	Louisiana	985-867-4443	www.lakeviewregional.com
Lancaster Regional Medical Center	Lancaster	Pennsylvania	717-291-8123	www.lancasterregional.com
Laredo Medical Center	Laredo	Texas	956-796-5000	www.laredomedical.com
Largo Medical Center	Largo	Florida	727-588-5200	www.largomedical.com
Las Colinas Medical Center	Irving	Texas	972-969-2000	www.lascolinas.com
Lawnwood Regional Medical Center & Heart Institute	Fort Pierce	Florida	772-461-4000	www.lawnwoodmed.com
Lawrence Memorial Hospital	Walnut Ridge	Arkansas	870-886-1200	www.lawrencehealth.net
Lee's Summit Medical Center	Lees Summit	Missouri	816-282-5000	www.leessummithospital.com
Lehigh Regional Medical Center	Lehigh Acres	Florida	239-369-2101	www.lehighregional.com
Lewisgale Hospital Montgomery	Blacksburg	Virginia	540-951-1111	www.mrhospital.com
Lewisgale Medical Center	Salem	Virginia	540-776-4000	www.lewis-gale.com
Libertyhealth - Jersey City Medical Center Campus	Jersey City	New Jersey	201-915-2000	www.libertyhcs.org
Little Company of Mary Hospital	Evergreen Park	Illinois	708-422-6200	www.lcmh.org
Littleton Regional Healthcare	Littleton	New Hampshire	603-444-9000	www.littletonhospital.org
Lock Haven Hospital	Lock Haven	Pennsylvania	570-893-5000	www.lockhavenhospital.com
Lucas County Health Center	Chariton	Iowa	641-774-3000	www.lchcia.com
Marin General Hospital	Greenbrae	California	415-925-7900	www.maringeneral.com
Mary Greeley Medical Center	Ames	Iowa	515-239-2011	www.mgmc.org
Maryvale Hospital	Phoenix	Arizona	623-848-5000	www.maryvalehospital.com
Mat-Su Regional Medical Center	Palmer	Alaska	907-746-8600	www.matsuregional.com
Mayo Clinic Health System - Fairmont	Fairmont	Minnesota	507-238-8101	www.fairmontmedicalcenter.org
Mayo Clinic Health System - Northland	Barron	Wisconsin	715-537-3186	www.luthermidelfortnorthland.org
McKenzie Regional Hospital	Mc Kenzie	Tennessee	731-352-5344	www.mckenzieregionalhospital.com
Mease Hospital Dunedin	Dunedin	Florida	727-733-1111	www.measehospitals.com
Medical Center of Arlington	Arlington	Texas	817-465-3241	www.medicalcenterarlington.com

Hospital	City	State	Phone	Web Site
Medical Center of Trinity	Trinity	Florida	727-848-1733	www.communityhospitalnpr.com
Medical City Dallas Hospital	Dallas	Texas	972-566-6222	www.medicalcityhospital.com
Medwest Swain	Bryson City	North Carolina	828-488-2155	www.westcarehealth.org
Memorial Healthcare System	Chattanooga	Tennessee	423-495-2525	www.memorial.org
Memorial Hospital Los Banos	Los Banos	California	209-826-0591	www.memoriallosbanos.org
Memorial Hospital Pembroke	Pembroke Pines	Florida	954-962-9650	www.memorialpembroke.com\
Memorial Hospital West	Pembroke Pines	Florida	954-436-5000	www.memorialwest.com
Memorial Regional Hospital	Hollywood	Florida	954-987-2000	www.memorialregional.com
Menorah Medical Center	Overland Park	Kansas	913-498-6773	www.menorahmedicalcenter.com
Mercy General Hospital	Sacramento	California	916-453-4545	www.mercygeneral.org
Mercy Hospital - Fort Scott	Fort Scott	Kansas	620-223-7057	www.mercy.net
Mercy Hospital of Defiance	Defiance	Ohio	419-782-8444	www.mercyweb.org/mercy_defiance.aspx
Mercy Medical Center	Springfield	Massachusetts	413-748-9000	www.mercycares.com
Mercy Regional Health Center	Manhattan	Kansas	785-776-2831	www.mercyregional.org
Methodist Medical Center of Oak Ridge	Oak Ridge	Tennessee	865-835-1000	www.mmcoakridge.com
Methodist Richardson Medical Center	Richardson	Texas	972-498-4000	www.richardsonregional.com
Metroplex Hospital	Killeen	Texas	254-526-7523	www.mplex.org
Minden Medical Center	Minden	Louisiana	318-377-2321	www.mindenmedicalcenter.com
Ministry Sacred Heart Hospital	Tomahawk	Wisconsin	715-453-7700	www.ministryhealth.org
Ministry Saint Marys Hospital	Rhinelander	Wisconsin	715-361-2000	www.ministryhealth.org
Ministry Saint Michaels Hospital of Stevens Point	Stevens Point	Wisconsin	715-346-5000	www.saintmichaelshospital.org
Moberly Regional Medical Center	Moberly	Missouri	660-263-8400	www.moberlyhospital.com
Monmouth Medical Center - Southern Campus	Lakewood	New Jersey	732-363-1900	www.sbhcs.com
Mount Pleasant Hospital	Mount Pleasant	South Carolina	843-724-2954	www.rsfh.com
Mountain Home VA Medical Center	Mountain Home	Tennessee	423-926-1171	www.mountainhome.va.gov
Mountain View Hospital	Payson	Utah	801-465-7100	www.mvhpayson.com
Mountain View Regional Medical Center	Las Cruces	New Mexico	575-556-7600	www.mountainviewregional.com
Myrtue Medical Center	Harlan	Iowa	712-755-5161	www.shelbycohealth.com
New Ulm Medical Center	New Ulm	Minnesota	507-233-1000	www.newulmmedicalcenter.com
New York Community Hospital of Brooklyn	Brooklyn	New York	718-692-5302	www.nych.com
Noble Hospital	Westfield	Massachusetts	413-568-2811	www.noblehospital.org
North Austin Medical Center	Austin	Texas	512-901-1000	www.cornerstonehealthcaregroup.com
North Florida Regional Medical Center	Gainesville	Florida	352-333-4100	www.nfrmc.com
North Shore Medical Center	Miami	Florida	305-835-6000	www.northshoremedical.com
North Suburban Medical Center	Thornton	Colorado	303-451-7800	www.northsuburban.com
Northeast Regional Medical Center	Kirksville	Missouri	660-785-1000	www.nermc.com
Northern Westchester Hospital	Mount Kisco	New York	914-666-1200	www.nwhc.net
Northside Hospital	Saint Petersburg	Florida	813-521-5000	www.northsidehospital.com
Northside Hospital	Atlanta	Georgia	404-851-8000	www.northside.com
Northside Hospital Cherokee	Canton	Georgia	770-720-5298	www.northside.com/cherokee
Norwalk Hospital Association	Norwalk	Connecticut	203-852-2000	www.norwalkhosp.org
Novant Health Forsyth Medical Center	Winston-Salem	North Carolina	336-718-5000	www.forsythmedicalcenter.org
Novant Health Franklin Medical Center	Louisburg	North Carolina	919-496-5131	www.franklinregionalmedicalctr.com
Novant Health Huntersville Medical Center	Huntersville	North Carolina	704-316-4000	www.presbyterian.org
Novant Health Thomasville Medical Center	Thomasville	North Carolina	336-472-2000	www.thomasvillemedicalcenter.org
Oak Hill Hospital	Brooksville	Florida	352-596-6632	www.oakhillhospital.com
Oaklawn Hospital	Marshall	Michigan	269-781-4271	www.oaklawnhospital.org
OHSU Hospital & Clinics	Portland	Oregon	503-494-4036	www.ohsu.edu
Oklahoma State University Medical Center	Tulsa	Oklahoma	918-587-2561	www.tulsaregional.com
Orange Park Medical Center	Orange Park	Florida	904-276-8500	www.opmedical.com
Overton Brooks VA Medical Center - Shreveport	Shreveport	Louisiana	318-424-6037	www.va.gov/sta/guide/home.asp
Palm Bay Hospital	Palm Bay	Florida	321-434-8000	www.health-first.org
Parkway Regional Hospital	Fulton	Kentucky	270-472-2522	www.parkwayregionalhospital.com
Piggott Community Hospital	Piggott	Arkansas	870-598-3881	www.piggottcommunityhospital.com
Plateau Medical Center	Oak Hill	West Virginia	304-469-8600	www.plateaumedicalcenter.com
Pleasant Valley Hospital	Point Pleasant	West Virginia	304-675-4340	www.pvalley.org
Pomerene Hospital	Millersburg	Ohio	330-674-1015	www.pomerenehospital.org
Portsmouth Regional Hospital	Portsmouth	New Hampshire	603-436-5110	www.portsmouthhospital.com
Promedica Herrick Hospital	Tecumseh	Michigan	517-424-3000	www.promedica.org/herrick
Putnam General Hospital	Eatonton	Georgia	706-485-2711	www.putnamgeneral.com
Rapides Regional Medical Center	Alexandria	Louisiana	318-769-3000	www.rapidesregional.com
Raulerson Hospital	Okeechobee	Florida	863-763-2151	www.raulersonhospital.com
Regional Hospital of Jackson	Jackson	Tennessee	731-661-2000	www.regionalhospitaljackson.com
Regional Medical Center of San Jose	San Jose	California	408-259-5000	www.regionalmedicalsanjose.com
Renown South Meadows Medical Center	Reno	Nevada	775-982-7000	www.renown.org
River Parishes Hospital	Laplace	Louisiana	985-652-7000	www.riverparisheshospital.com
Riverview Medical Center	Red Bank	New Jersey	732-741-2700	www.meridianhealth.com

Hospital	City	State	Phone	Web Site
Rockford Memorial Hospital	Rockford	Illinois	815-968-6861	www.rhsnet.org
Roper Hospital	Charleston	South Carolina	843-724-2800	www.ropersaintfrancis.com
Rose Medical Center	Denver	Colorado	303-320-2121	www.rosemed.com
Roxborough Memorial Hospital	Philadelphia	Pennsylvania	215-483-9900	www.roxboroughmemorial.com
Saint Anthony Hospital	Chicago	Illinois	773-521-1710	www.cath-health.org
Saint Anthony Shawnee Hospital	Shawnee	Oklahoma	405-273-2270	www.unityhealthcenter.com
Saint Anthony's Health Center	Alton	Illinois	618-465-2571	www.sahc.org
Saint Barnabas Medical Center	Livingston	New Jersey	973-322-5000	www.saintbarnabas.com
Saint Catherine Hospital	East Chicago	Indiana	219-392-7004	www.comhs.org/stcatherine
Saint Clare Hospital Health Services	Baraboo	Wisconsin	608-356-1400	www.stclare.com
Saint Clares Hospital of Weston	Weston	Wisconsin	715-393-3000	www.ministryhealth.org
Saint Francis Hospital	Escanaba	Michigan	906-786-3311	www.osfstfrancis.or
Saint Francis Medical Center	Trenton	New Jersey	609-599-5000	www.stfrancismedical.com
Saint James Hospital	Pontiac	Illinois	815-842-2828	www.osfsaintjames.org
Saint Joseph Hospital	Fort Wayne	Indiana	260-425-3000	www.stjoehospital.com
Saint Joseph Hospital & Health Center	Kokomo	Indiana	765-456-5300	www.stvincent.org
Saint Joseph Mercy Port Huron	Port Huron	Michigan	810-985-1510	www.mercyporthuron.com
Saint Joseph Regional Medical Center - Plymouth	Plymouth	Indiana	574-948-4000	www.sjmed.com
Saint Joseph's Hospital	Breese	Illinois	618-526-4511	www.stjoebreese.com
Saint Joseph's Mercy Health Center	Hot Springs	Arkansas	501-622-1000	www.saintjosephs.com
Saint Louise Regional Hospital	Gilroy	California	408-848-2000	www.saintlouiseregionalhospital.org
Saint Lucie Medical Center	Port Saint Lucie	Florida	772-335-4000	www.stluciemed.com
Saint Luke's Magic Valley Rmc	Twin Falls	Idaho	208-814-1000	www.stlukesonline.org/magic_valley
Saint Luke's Quakertown Hospital	Quakertown	Pennsylvania	215-538-4500	www.slhn-lehighvalley.com
Saint Margarets Hospital	Spring Valley	Illinois	815-664-1176	www.aboutsmh.org
Saint Mary Medical Center	Hobart	Indiana	219-942-0551	www.comhs.org/stmary
Saint Mary's Good Samaritan Hospital	Greensboro	Georgia	706-453-7331	www.stmarysgoodsam.org
Saint Vincent Anderson Regional Hospital	Anderson	Indiana	765-646-8373	www.stjohnshealthsystem.org
Saint Vincent's Birmingham	Birmingham	Alabama	205-939-7000	www.stv.org
Saint Vincent's East	Birmingham	Alabama	205-838-3122	www.nolandhealth.com
Saint Vincent's Medical Center Southside	Jacksonville	Florida	904-296-3700	www.jaxhealth.com
Samaritan Hospital	Moses Lake	Washington	509-765-5606	www.samaritanhealthcare.com
San Angelo Community Medical Center	San Angelo	Texas	325-949-9511	www.sacmc.com
Scripps Mercy Hospital	San Diego	California	619-294-8111	www.scrippshealth.org
Sebastian River Medical Center	Sebastian	Florida	772-589-3187	www.srmcenter.com
Seton Highland Lakes	Burnet	Texas	512-715-3000	www.seton.net
Shands Lake Shore Regional Medical Center	Lake City	Florida	386-292-8000	www.shands.org
Sharp Coronado Hospital & Healthcare Center	Coronado	California	619-435-6251	www.sharp.com/coronado
Shasta Regional Medical Center	Redding	California	530-244-5454	www.shastaregional.com
Sibley Memorial Hospital	Washington	District of Columbia	202-537-4680	www.sibley.org
Signature Healthcare Brockton Hospital	Brockton	Massachusetts	508-941-7000	www.brocktonhospital.com
Silverton Hospital	Silverton	Oregon	503-873-1500	www.silvertonhospital.org
Singing River Hospital	Pascagoula	Mississippi	228-809-5000	www.srhshealth.com
Sisters of Charity Hospital	Buffalo	New York	716-862-1000	www.chsbuffalo.org
South Miami Hospital	South Miami	Florida	786-662-4000	www.baptisthealth.net
Southern Nh Medical Center	Nashua	New Hampshire	603-577-2000	www.snhmc.org
Sparks Regional Medical Center	Fort Smith	Arkansas	501-441-4000	www.sparks.org
Spokane VA Medical Center	Spokane	Washington	509-434-7000	www.spokane.med.va.gov
Spotsylvania Regional Medical Center	Fredericksburg	Virginia	540-498-4000	www.spotsrmc.com
Stafford Hospital	Stafford	Virginia	540-741-9000	www.marywashingtonhealthcare.com
Staten Island University Hospital	Staten Island	New York	718-226-9000	www.siuh.edu
Summit Medical Center	Van Buren	Arkansas	479-471-4300	www.summitmc.net
Sutter Medical Center of Santa Rosa	Santa Rosa	California	707-576-4000	www.suttersantarosa.org
Sycamore Medical Center	Miamisburg	Ohio	937-384-8776	www.khnetwork.org/sycamore
Takoma Regional Hospital	Greeneville	Tennessee	423-639-3151	www.takoma.org
Texas Health Arlington Memorial Hospital	Arlington	Texas	817-548-6100	www.texashealth.org
Texas Health Harris Methodist Hospital Alliance	Fort Worth	Texas	682-212-2004	www.texashealth.org/alliance
Texoma Medical Center	Denison	Texas	903-416-4000	www.texomamedicalcenter.net
Thorek Memorial Hospital	Chicago	Illinois	312-525-6780	www.thorek.org
Three Rivers Medical Center	Louisa	Kentucky	606-638-9451	www.threeriversmedicalcenter.com
Togus VA Medical Center	Augusta	Maine	207-623-8411	www.maine.va.gov
Transylvania Regional Hospital	Brevard	North Carolina	828-883-5302	www.tchospital.org
Trinity Medical Center	Birmingham	Alabama	205-592-1000	www.bhsala.com/montclair
Tristar Hendersonville Medical Center	Hendersonville	Tennessee	615-338-1000	www.hendersonvillemedicalcenter.com
Tristar Southern Hills Medical Center	Nashville	Tennessee	615-781-4000	www.southernhills.com
Tristar Stonecrest Medical Center	Smyrna	Tennessee	615-768-2000	www.stonecrestmedical.com
Tucson Medical Center	Tucson	Arizona	520-327-5461	www.tmcaz.com

Hospital	City	State	Phone	Web Site
Twin Cities Hospital	Niceville	Florida	850-678-4131	www.tchealthcare.com
UH Geauga Medical Center	Chardon	Ohio	440-269-6000	www.uhgeauga.org
UHHS Memorial Hospital of Geneva	Geneva	Ohio	440-466-1141	www.uhhospitals.org/geneva
University of Maryland Medical Center	Baltimore	Maryland	410-328-8667	www.umm.edu
University of Miami Hospital	Miami	Florida	305-325-5511	www.cedarsmedicalcenter.com
UPMC Mckeesport	Mc Keesport	Pennsylvania	412-664-2000	www.selectmedicalcorp.com
VA Pittsburgh Healthcare System	Pittsburgh	Pennsylvania	412-688-6100	www.pittsburg.va.gov
Valley West Community Hospital	Sandwich	Illinois	815-786-8484	www.snd.softfarm.com/sandhosp
Venice Regional Medical Center - Bayfront Health	Venice	Florida	941-485-7711	www.veniceregional.com
Viera Hospital	Melbourne	Florida	321-434-9000	www.health-first.org
Waupun Memorial Hospital	Waupun	Wisconsin	920-324-6530	www.agnesian.com
Wayne County Hospital	Monticello	Kentucky	606-348-9343	www.waynehospital.org
Weatherford Regional Medical Center	Weatherford	Texas	817-599-1190	www.campbellhealth.com
Wesley Medical Center	Wichita	Kansas	316-962-2000	www.wesleymc.com
West Palm Hospital	West Palm Beach	Florida	561-844-6141	www.columbiahospital.com
Western Pennsylvania Hospital	Pittsburgh	Pennsylvania	412-578-5000	www.wpahs.org/wph/contact/index.html
White County Medical Center	Searcy	Arkansas	501-278-3100	www.centralarkhospital.com
Wichita VA Medical Center	Wichita	Kansas	316-685-2221	www.wichita.va.gov
Wilcox Memorial Hospital	Lihue	Hawaii	808-245-1103	www.wilcoxhealth.org
William Beaumont Hospital - Troy	Troy	Michigan	248-964-8800	www.beaumonthospitals.com
Williamsport Regional Medical Center	Williamsport	Pennsylvania	570-321-1000	www.susquehannahealth.org
Woodward Regional Hospital	Woodward	Oklahoma	580-254-8492	www.woodwardhospital.com

Note: The 288 hospitals shown above all achieved a perfect 100% average score. Average scores were calculated for hospitals with qualifying data (25 cases or more) in both measures in the Pneumonia Care category. A total of 3,347 hospitals nationwide were considered.

Best Hospitals for Preventative Care

Hospital	City	State	Phone	Web Site
Abilene Regional Medical Center	Abilene	Texas	325-428-1000	www.abileneregional.com
Adena Regional Medical Center	Chillicothe	Ohio	740-779-7500	www.adena.org
Alton Memorial Hospital	Alton	Illinois	618-463-7300	www.altonmemorialhospital.org
Arizona Spine & Joint Hospital	Mesa	Arizona	480-832-4770	www.azspineandjoint.com
Atrium Medical Center	Franklin	Ohio	513-420-5102	www.atriummedcenter.org
Avera Heart Hospital of South Dakota	Sioux Falls	South Dakota	605-977-7000	www.avera.org/heart-hospital
Bailey Medical Center	Owasso	Oklahoma	918-376-8000	www.baileymedicalcenter.com
Baptist Hospital of Miami	Miami	Florida	786-596-1960	www.baptisthealth.net
Baptist Memorial Hospital Huntingdon	Huntingdon	Tennessee	731-986-4461	www.bmhcc.org
Barstow Community Hospital	Barstow	California	760-256-1761	www.barstowhospital.com
Belton Regional Medical Center	Belton	Missouri	816-348-1236	www.beltonregionalmedicalcenter.com
Biloxi Regional Medical Center	Biloxi	Mississippi	228-436-1104	www.hmabrmc.com
Broward Health North	Pompano Beach	Florida	954-786-6950	www.browardhealth.org
Byrd Regional Hospital	Leesville	Louisiana	337-239-9041	www.chs.net
Calhoun Health Services	Calhoun City	Mississippi	662-628-6611	www.nmhs.net
Carepoint Health - Bayonne Hospital Center	Bayonne	New Jersey	201-858-5000	www.bayonnemedicalcenter.org
Carrington Health Center	Carrington	North Dakota	701-652-3141	www.carringtonhealthcenter.net
Centerpoint Medical Center	Independence	Missouri	816-698-7000	www.centerpointmedical.com
Centinela Hospital Medical Center	Inglewood	California	310-673-4660	www.centinelafreeman.com
Central Mississippi Medical Center	Jackson	Mississippi	601-376-1000	www.centralmississippimedicalcenter.com
Chesterfield General Hospital	Cheraw	South Carolina	843-537-7881	www.chesterfieldgeneral.com
Clay County Hospital	Flora	Illinois	618-662-2131	www.claycountyhospital.org
Coosa Valley Medical Center	Sylacauga	Alabama	256-249-5000	www.cvhealth.net
Coral Gables Hospital	Coral Gables	Florida	305-445-8461	www.coralgableshospital.com
The Corpus Christi Medical Center	Corpus Christi	Texas	361-761-1501	www.ccmedicalcenter.com
Cypress Pointe Hospital East	Slidell	Louisiana	504-690-8200	
Delray Medical Center	Delray Beach	Florida	561-498-4440	www.delraymedicalctr.com
Detar Hospital Navarro	Victoria	Texas	361-575-7441	www.detar.com
Dyersburg Regional Medical Center	Dyersburg	Tennessee	731-285-2410	www.dyersburgregionalmc.com
Encino Hospital Medical Center	Encino	California	818-995-5000	www.encino-tarzana.com
Fannin Regional Hospital	Blue Ridge	Georgia	706-632-3711	www.fanninregionalhospital.com
Flowers Hospital	Dothan	Alabama	334-793-5000	www.flowershospital.com
Garden Grove Hospital & Medical Center	Garden Grove	California	714-537-5160	www.gardengrovehospital.com
Garden Park Medical Center	Gulfport	Mississippi	228-575-7000	www.gardenparkmedical.com
Greenbrier Valley Medical Center	Ronceverte	West Virginia	304-647-4411	www.gvmc.com
Hedrick Medical Center	Chillicothe	Missouri	660-646-1480	www.saintlukeshealthsystem.org
Helena Regional Medical Center	Helena	Arkansas	870-338-5800	www.helenaregionalmedicalcenter.com
Henderson County Community Hospital	Lexington	Tennessee	731-968-1801	www.hendersoncchospital.com
Henry County Memorial Hospital	New Castle	Indiana	765-521-0890	www.hcmhcares.org
Heritage Medical Center	Shelbyville	Tennessee	931-685-5433	www.heritagemedicalcenter.com
Highlands Regional Medical Center	Sebring	Florida	863-385-6101	www.highlandsregional.com
Holy Name Medical Center	Teaneck	New Jersey	201-833-3000	www.holyname.org
The Hospital at Westlake Medical Center	Austin	Texas	512-327-0000	www.westlakemedical.com
Huntington Beach Hospital	Huntington Beach	California	714-843-5000	www.hbhospital.com
Indiana University Health Blackford Hospital	Hartford City	Indiana	765-348-0300	www.accesschs.org
Ingalls Memorial Hospital	Harvey	Illinois	708-333-2300	www.ingalls.org
Integris Mayes County Medical Center	Pryor	Oklahoma	918-825-1600	www.integris-health.com
Jeff Davis Hospital	Hazlehurst	Georgia	912-375-7781	www.jeffdavishospital.org
JFK Medical Center	Atlantis	Florida	561-965-7300	www.jfkmc.com
John Randolph Medical Center	Hopewell	Virginia	804-541-1600	www.johnrandolphmed.com
Kansas Medical Center	Andover	Kansas	316-300-4000	www.ksmedcenter.com
Kentucky River Medical Center	Jackson	Kentucky	606-666-6000	www.kentuckyrivermc.com
L V Stabler Memorial Hospital	Greenville	Alabama	334-382-2200	www.lvstabler.com
Lafayette Regional Health Center	Lexington	Missouri	660-259-2203	www.lafayetteregionalhealthcenter.com
Lakeview Regional Medical Center	Covington	Louisiana	985-867-4443	www.lakeviewregional.com
Laredo Medical Center	Laredo	Texas	956-796-5000	www.laredomedical.com
Lawnwood Regional Medical Center & Heart Institute	Fort Pierce	Florida	772-461-4000	www.lawnwoodmed.com
Lehigh Regional Medical Center	Lehigh Acres	Florida	239-369-2101	www.lehighregional.com
Lehigh Valley Hospital - Hazleton	Hazleton	Pennsylvania	570-501-4000	www.ghha.org
Lewisgale Medical Center	Salem	Virginia	540-776-4000	www.lewis-gale.com
Livingston Regional Hospital	Livingston	Tennessee	931-823-5611	www.livingstonregionalhospital.com
Logan Regional Medical Center	Logan	West Virginia	304-831-1350	www.loganregionalmedicalcenter.com
McNairy Regional Hospital	Selmer	Tennessee	731-645-3221	www.mcnairyregionalhospital.com
Medical Center of Plano	Plano	Texas	972-596-6800	www.medicalcenterofplano.com
Medical Center of Southeastern Oklahoma	Durant	Oklahoma	405-924-3080	www.mcsohealth.com

Hospital	City	State	Phone	Web Site
Medical Center South Arkansas	El Dorado	Arkansas	870-863-2000	www.themedcenter.net
Memorial Hospital Los Banos	Los Banos	California	209-826-0591	www.memoriallosbanos.org
Memorial Hospital Pembroke	Pembroke Pines	Florida	954-962-9650	www.memorialpembroke.com\
Memorial Hospital West	Pembroke Pines	Florida	954-436-5000	www.memorialwest.com
Menorah Medical Center	Overland Park	Kansas	913-498-6773	www.menorahmedicalcenter.com
Methodist Stone Oak Hospital	San Antonio	Texas	210-638-2100	www.stoneoakhealth.com
Mills - Peninsula Medical Center	Burlingame	California	650-696-5270	www.mills-peninsula.org
Mimbres Memorial Hospital	Deming	New Mexico	575-546-5803	www.mimbresmemorial.com
Minden Medical Center	Minden	Louisiana	318-377-2321	www.mindenmedicalcenter.com
Moberly Regional Medical Center	Moberly	Missouri	660-263-8400	www.moberlyhospital.com
Mount Desert Island Hospital	Bar Harbor	Maine	207-288-5081	www.mdihospital.com
Mountain View Hospital	Idaho Falls	Idaho	208-557-2899	www.mountainviewhospital.org
Mountain View Regional Medical Center	Las Cruces	New Mexico	575-556-7600	www.mountainviewregional.com
Newberry County Memorial Hospital	Newberry	South Carolina	803-405-7145	www.newberryhospital.org
North Carolina Specialty Hospital	Durham	North Carolina	919-956-9300	www.ncspecialty.com
Northeast Regional Medical Center	Kirksville	Missouri	660-785-1000	www.nermc.com
Northern Louisiana Medical Center	Ruston	Louisiana	318-254-2100	www.lincolnhealth.com
Northern Maine Medical Center	Fort Kent	Maine	207-834-3195	www.nmmc.org
Ocala Regional Medical Center	Ocala	Florida	352-401-1000	www.ocalaregional.com
Oconee Regional Medical Center	Milledgeville	Georgia	478-454-3550	www.oconeeregional.com
Oklahoma Heart Hospital South	Oklahoma City	Oklahoma	405-628-6000	www.okheart.com/south-campus
Oklahoma Surgical Hospital	Tulsa	Oklahoma	918-477-5000	www.oklahomasurgicalhospital.com
Orange Park Medical Center	Orange Park	Florida	904-276-8500	www.opmedical.com
Palm Springs General Hospital	Hialeah	Florida	305-558-2500	www.psghosp.com
Pampa Regional Medical Center	Pampa	Texas	806-665-3721	www.prmctx.com
Parkway Regional Hospital	Fulton	Kentucky	270-472-2522	www.parkwayregionalhospital.com
Person Memorial Hospital	Roxboro	North Carolina	336-599-2121	www.personhospital.com
Ponca City Medical Center	Ponca City	Oklahoma	580-765-3321	www.poncamedcenter.com
Rapides Regional Medical Center	Alexandria	Louisiana	318-769-3000	www.rapidesregional.com
Raulerson Hospital	Okeechobee	Florida	863-763-2151	www.raulersonhospital.com
Regional Hospital of Jackson	Jackson	Tennessee	731-661-2000	www.regionalhospitaljackson.com
Regional Medical Center Bayonet Point	Hudson	Florida	727-819-2929	www.mchealth.comorwww.heartoftampa.com
The Regional Medical Center of Acadiana	Lafayette	Louisiana	337-981-2949	www.medicalcentersw.com
Renown South Meadows Medical Center	Reno	Nevada	775-982-7000	www.renown.org
Research Medical Center	Kansas City	Missouri	816-276-4000	www.researchmedicalcenter.com
Riverview Medical Center	Red Bank	New Jersey	732-741-2700	www.meridianhealth.com
Riverview Regional Medical Center	Gadsden	Alabama	256-543-5200	www.riverviewregional.com
Rolling Plains Memorial Hospital	Sweetwater	Texas	325-235-1701	www.rpmh.net
Rush University Medical Center	Chicago	Illinois	312-942-5000	www.ruch.edu
Russellville Hospital	Russellville	Alabama	256-332-1611	www.russellvillehospital.com
Saint Elizabeth Florence	Florence	Kentucky	859-212-5220	www.stlukehospitals.com
Saint Elizabeth Ft Thomas	Fort Thomas	Kentucky	859-572-3100	www.cardinalhill.org
Saint Elizabeth Grant	Williamstown	Kentucky	859-824-8240	www.stelizabeth.com
Saint Elizabeth Medical Center	Lakeside Park	Kentucky	859-292-2000	www.stelizabeth.com
Saint James Mercy Hospital	Hornell	New York	607-324-8000	www.stjamesmercy.org
Saint Joseph Hospital & Health Center	Kokomo	Indiana	765-456-5300	www.stvincent.org
Saint Luke's Miners Memorial Hospital	Coaldale	Pennsylvania	570-645-2131	www.slhn-lehighvalley.org
Saint Mary's Health Center	Jefferson City	Missouri	573-761-7000	www.stmarys-jeffcity.com
Sebastian River Medical Center	Sebastian	Florida	772-589-3187	www.srmcenter.com
Sherman Oaks Hospital	Sherman Oaks	California	818-981-7111	www.shermanoakshospital.com
Skagit Valley Hospital	Mount Vernon	Washington	360-424-4111	www.skagitvalleyhospital.org
Sonoma Developmental Center	Eldridge	California	707-938-6393	www.dds.ca.gov/sonoma/index.cfm
South Baldwin Regional Medical Center	Foley	Alabama	251-949-3400	www.southbaldwinrmc.com
South Bay Hospital	Sun City Center	Florida	813-634-3301	www.southbayhospital.com
Southwest General Hospital	San Antonio	Texas	210-921-2000	www.swgeneralhospital.com
Stones River Hospital & Dekalb Community Hospital	Smithville	Tennessee	615-215-5000	www.dekalb-hospital.com
Stormont - Vail Healthcare	Topeka	Kansas	785-354-6121	www.stormontvail.org
Temple Community Hospital	Los Angeles	California	213-382-7252	www.templecommunityhospital.com
Terre Haute Regional Hospital	Terre Haute	Indiana	812-232-0021	www.regionalhospital.com
Texas Health Harris Methodist Hospital Azle	Azle	Texas	817-444-8700	www.hmhs.org
Tomah Memorial Hospital	Tomah	Wisconsin	608-372-2181	www.tomahhospital.org
Trinity Hospital of Augusta	Augusta	Georgia	706-481-7000	www.trinityofaugusta.com
Trinity Medical Center	Birmingham	Alabama	205-592-1000	www.bhsala.com/montclair
Twin Cities Hospital	Niceville	Florida	850-678-4131	www.tchealthcare.com
Tyrone Hospital	Tyrone	Pennsylvania	814-684-1255	www.tyronehospital.org
UPMC East	Monroeville	Pennsylvania	412-357-3000	www.upmc.com
Valley West Community Hospital	Sandwich	Illinois	815-786-8484	www.snd.softfarm.com/sandhosp

Hospital	City	State	Phone	Web Site
Vaughan Regional Medical Center Parkway Campus	Selma	Alabama	334-418-4100	www.vaughanregional.com
Vista Medical Center East	Waukegan	Illinois	847-360-4000	www.vistahealth.com
Walker Baptist Medical Center	Jasper	Alabama	205-387-4000	www.bhsala.com/walker
Weatherford Regional Medical Center	Weatherford	Texas	817-599-1190	www.campbellhealth.com
West Anaheim Medical Center	Anaheim	California	714-827-3000	www.wamc.phcs.us
West Kendall Baptist Hospital	Miami	Florida	786-467-2011	www.baptisthealth.net
West Palm Hospital	West Palm Beach	Florida	561-844-6141	www.columbiahospital.com
West Virginia University Hospitals	Morgantown	West Virginia	304-598-4000	www.wvuh.com
Western Arizona Regional Medical Center	Bullhead City	Arizona	928-763-2273	www.warmc.com
Westside Regional Medical Center	Plantation	Florida	954-473-6600	www.westsidehospital.com
Woodland Heights Medical Center	Lufkin	Texas	936-634-8311	www.woodlandheights.net
Woodward Regional Hospital	Woodward	Oklahoma	580-254-8492	www.woodwardhospital.com

Note: The 144 hospitals shown above all achieved a perfect 100% average score. Average scores were calculated for hospitals with qualifying data (25 cases or more) in both measures in the Preventative Care category. A total of 3,674 hospitals nationwide were considered.

Best Hospitals for Stroke Care

Hospital	City	State	Phone	Web Site
Baptist Hospital of Miami	Miami	Florida	786-596-1960	www.baptisthealth.net
Bellevue Medical Center	Bellevue	Nebraska	402-763-3600	www.bellevuemed.com
Blanchard Valley Hospital	Findlay	Ohio	419-423-4500	www.bvha.org
Boca Raton Regional Hospital	Boca Raton	Florida	561-362-5002	www.brrh.com
Bronx - Lebanon Hospital Center	Bronx	New York	212-588-7000	www.bronx-leb.org
Brookdale Hospital Medical Center	Brooklyn	New York	718-240-5966	www.brookdalehospital.org
Cabell Huntington Hospital	Huntington	West Virginia	304-526-2000	www.cabellhuntington.org
Capital Health Medical Center - Hopewell	Pennington	New Jersey	609-303-4000	www.capitalhealth.org
Capital Regional Medical Center	Tallahassee	Florida	850-656-5000	www.capitalregionalmedicalcenter.com
Caromont Regional Medical Center	Gastonia	North Carolina	704-834-4891	www.caromont.org
Catawba Valley Medical Center	Hickory	North Carolina	828-326-3809	www.catawbavalleymc.org
Central Carolina Hospital	Sanford	North Carolina	919-774-2100	www.centralcarolinahosp.com
Cjw Medical Center	Richmond	Virginia	804-330-2001	www.hcavirginia.com
Cleveland Clinic Hospital	Weston	Florida	954-689-5000	www.clevelandclinic.org
Cox Medical Center Branson	Branson	Missouri	417-335-7000	www.skaggs.net
Delray Medical Center	Delray Beach	Florida	561-498-4440	www.delraymedicalctr.com
Detar Hospital Navarro	Victoria	Texas	361-575-7441	www.detar.com
Doctors Hospital	Augusta	Georgia	706-651-6008	www.doctors-hospital.net
Falmouth Hospital	Falmouth	Massachusetts	508-548-5300	www.capecodhealth.com
Fawcett Memorial Hospital	Port Charlotte	Florida	941-629-1181	www.fawcetthospital.com
Forest Hills Hospital	Forest Hills	New York	718-830-4000	www.northshorelij.com
Fort Walton Beach Medical Center	Fort Walton Beach	Florida	850-862-1111	www.fwbmedicalcenter.com
Good Samaritan Hospital Medical Center	West Islip	New York	631-376-3000	www.good-samaritan-hospital.org
Grant Medical Center	Columbus	Ohio	614-566-9978	www.ohiohealth.com
Heartland Regional Medical Center	Saint Joseph	Missouri	816-271-6000	www.heartland-health.com
Holland Community Hospital	Holland	Michigan	616-392-5141	www.hoho.org
Homestead Hospital	Homestead	Florida	786-243-8000	www.baptisthealth.net
John Randolph Medical Center	Hopewell	Virginia	804-541-1600	www.johnrandolphmed.com
Kaiser Foundation Hospital - Redwood City	Redwood City	California	650-299-2000	www.seiu-uhw.org/aboutuhw
Kaiser Foundation Hospital - San Diego	San Diego	California	619-528-5000	www.members.kaiserpermanente.org
Kaiser Foundation Hospital - South Bay	Harbor City	California	310-517-6441	www.kaiserpermanente.org
Kaiser Foundation Hospital - South San Francisco	South San Francisco	California	650-742-3200	www.healthy.kaiserpermanente.org
Lake Pointe Medical Center	Rowlett	Texas	972-412-2273	www.lakepointemedical.com
Lakeview Regional Medical Center	Covington	Louisiana	985-867-4443	www.lakeviewregional.com
Lawnwood Regional Medical Center & Heart Institute	Fort Pierce	Florida	772-461-4000	www.lawnwoodmed.com
Lewisgale Medical Center	Salem	Virginia	540-776-4000	www.lewis-gale.com
Libertyhealth - Jersey City Medical Center Campus	Jersey City	New Jersey	201-915-2000	www.libertyhcs.org
Los Alamitos Medical Center	Los Alamitos	California	562-799-3220	www.losalamitosmedctr.com
Lovelace Medical Center	Albuquerque	New Mexico	505-727-8000	www.lovelace.com
Main Line Hospital Paoli	Paoli	Pennsylvania	610-648-1000	www.mainlinehealth.org
Marshall Medical Center	Placerville	California	530-622-1441	www.marshallmedical.org
Mary Immaculate Hospital	Newport News	Virginia	757-886-6000	www.bonsecourshamptonroad.com
Maui Memorial Medical Center	Wailuku	Hawaii	808-442-5101	www.mauimemorialmedical.org
Memorial Hospital Pembroke	Pembroke Pines	Florida	954-962-9650	www.memorialpembroke.com\
Memorial Hospital West	Pembroke Pines	Florida	954-436-5000	www.memorialwest.com
Mercy Hospital	Bakersfield	California	661-632-5000	www.mercybakersfield.org
Methodist Dallas Medical Center	Dallas	Texas	214-947-2879	www.mhd.com
Methodist Hospital of Southern California	Arcadia	California	626-445-4441	www.methodisthospital.org
Methodist Mansfield Medical Center	Mansfield	Texas	682-622-2059	www.methodisthealthsystem.com
Methodist Medical Center of Oak Ridge	Oak Ridge	Tennessee	865-835-1000	www.mmcoakridge.com
Methodist Richardson Medical Center	Richardson	Texas	972-498-4000	www.richardsonregional.com
Methodist Stone Oak Hospital	San Antonio	Texas	210-638-2100	www.stoneoakhealth.com
Metroplex Hospital	Killeen	Texas	254-526-7523	www.mplex.org
Mills - Peninsula Medical Center	Burlingame	California	650-696-5270	www.mills-peninsula.org
Monmouth Medical Center - Southern Campus	Lakewood	New Jersey	732-363-1900	www.sbhcs.com
Morristown Hamblen Hospital Association	Morristown	Tennessee	423-586-4231	www.mhhs1.org
Newton - Wellesley Hospital	Newton	Massachusetts	617-243-6000	www.nwh.org
North Austin Medical Center	Austin	Texas	512-901-1000	www.cornerstonehealthcaregroup.com
North Cypress Medical Center	Cypress	Texas	281-890-0203	www.ncmc-hospital.com
North Hills Hospital	North Richland Hills	Texas	817-255-1000	www.northhillshospital.com
Northside Hospital	Saint Petersburg	Florida	813-521-5000	www.northsidehospital.com
Northwest Community Hospital	Arlington Heights	Illinois	847-618-1000	www.nch.org
Novant Health Forsyth Medical Center	Winston-Salem	North Carolina	336-718-5000	www.forsythmedicalcenter.org
Novant Health Thomasville Medical Center	Thomasville	North Carolina	336-472-2000	www.thomasvillemedicalcenter.org
Oak Hill Hospital	Brooksville	Florida	352-596-6632	www.oakhillhospital.com

Hospital	City	State	Phone	Web Site
Pali Momi Medical Center	Aiea	Hawaii	808-486-6000	www.kapiolani.org
Palms of Pasadena Hospital	Saint Petersburg	Florida	727-381-1000	www.palmspasadena.com
Pikeville Medical Center	Pikeville	Kentucky	606-218-3500	www.pikevillehospital.org
Portsmouth Regional Hospital	Portsmouth	New Hampshire	603-436-5110	www.portsmouthhospital.com
Presence Saints Mary & Elizabeth Medical Center	Chicago	Illinois	312-770-2000	www.reshealth.org
Reston Hospital Center	Reston	Virginia	703-689-9000	www.restonhospital.com
Richmond University Medical Center	Staten Island	New York	718-818-1234	www.rumcsi.org
Saint Catherine of Siena Hospital	Smithtown	New York	631-862-3000	www.stcatherines.chsli.org
Saint Clair Memorial Hospital	Pittsburgh	Pennsylvania	412-942-6209	www.stclair.org
Saint Joseph Medical Center	Kansas City	Missouri	816-942-4000	www.stjosehkc.com
Saint Mary's Medical Center	San Francisco	California	415-668-1000	www.stmarysmedicalcenter.org
Salinas Valley Memorial Hospital	Salinas	California	831-757-4333	www.svmh.com
San Gabriel Valley Medical Center	San Gabriel	California	626-289-5454	www.sangabrielvalleymedctr.org
San Ramon Regional Medical Center	San Ramon	California	925-275-9200	www.sanramonmedctr.com
Scripps Memorial Hospital La Jolla	La Jolla	California	858-626-4123	www.scrippshealth.org
Sebastian River Medical Center	Sebastian	Florida	772-589-3187	www.srmcenter.com
Shasta Regional Medical Center	Redding	California	530-244-5454	www.shastaregional.com
Sherman Hospital	Elgin	Illinois	847-742-9800	www.shermanhealth.com
Sierra Nevada Memorial Hospital	Grass Valley	California	530-274-6000	www.snmh.org
South Baldwin Regional Medical Center	Foley	Alabama	251-949-3400	www.southbaldwinrmc.com
South Bay Hospital	Sun City Center	Florida	813-634-3301	www.southbayhospital.com
South Miami Hospital	South Miami	Florida	786-662-4000	www.baptisthealth.net
South Pointe Hospital	Warrensville Heights	Ohio	216-491-6000	www.southpointehospital.org
Southern Nh Medical Center	Nashua	New Hampshire	603-577-2000	www.snhmc.org
Sparks Regional Medical Center	Fort Smith	Arkansas	501-441-4000	www.sparks.org
Springs Memorial Hospital	Lancaster	South Carolina	803-286-1481	www.springsmemorial.com
Sunrise Hospital & Medical Center	Las Vegas	Nevada	702-731-8000	www.sunrisehospital.com
Sutter Auburn Faith Hospital	Auburn	California	530-888-4500	www.sutterauburnfaith.org
Temple Community Hospital	Los Angeles	California	213-382-7252	www.templecommunityhospital.com
Texas Health Harris Methodist Hurst - Euless - Bedford	Bedford	Texas	817-848-4000	www.texashealth.org
Texas Health Presbyterian Hospital Plano	Plano	Texas	972-981-8000	www.presbyplano.org
Texoma Medical Center	Denison	Texas	903-416-4000	www.texomamedicalcenter.net
Thibodaux Regional Medical Center	Thibodaux	Louisiana	985-447-5500	www.thibodaux.com
Trinity Medical Center	Birmingham	Alabama	205-592-1000	www.bhsala.com/montclair
University Hospitals Case Medical Center	Cleveland	Ohio	216-844-1000	www.uhhs.com
University of Kentucky Hospital	Lexington	Kentucky	859-323-5000	www.uhealthcare.uky.edu
UPMC East	Monroeville	Pennsylvania	412-357-3000	www.upmc.com
Vaughan Regional Medical Center Parkway Campus	Selma	Alabama	334-418-4100	www.vaughanregional.com
Vista Medical Center East	Waukegan	Illinois	847-360-4000	www.vistahealth.com
Wellmont Bristol Regional Medical Center	Bristol	Tennessee	423-844-1121	www.wellmont.org
Wesley Medical Center	Wichita	Kansas	316-962-2000	www.wesleymc.com
West Florida Hospital	Pensacola	Florida	850-494-4000	www.westfloridahospital.com
West Houston Medical Center	Houston	Texas	281-588-8080	www.westhoustonmedical.com
Wilcox Memorial Hospital	Lihue	Hawaii	808-245-1103	www.wilcoxhealth.org

Note: The hospitals shown above represent the top 5% of the 1,762 hospitals nationwide for which an average score was calculated. Average scores were calculated for hospitals with qualifying data (25 cases or more) in at least 6 of 11 measures in the Stroke Care category.

Best Hospitals for Surgical Care

Hospital	City	State	Phone	Web Site
Arizona Orthopedic & Surgical Speciality Hospital	Chandler	Arizona	480-603-9000	www.azosh.com
Avera Queen of Peace	Mitchell	South Dakota	605-995-2000	www.averaqueenofpeace.org
Baptist Health Corbin	Corbin	Kentucky	606-528-1212	www.baptistregional.com
Baptist Memorial Hospital Union City	Union City	Tennessee	731-885-2410	www.bmhcc.org
Baptist Memorial Hospital Union County	New Albany	Mississippi	662-538-7631	www.baptistonline.org
Baylor Medical Center at Uptown	Dallas	Texas	214-443-3000	www.bmcuptown.com
Baylor Regional Medical Center at Plano	Plano	Texas	469-814-2000	www.baylorhealth.com
Belton Regional Medical Center	Belton	Missouri	816-348-1236	www.beltonregionalmedicalcenter.com
Boca Raton Regional Hospital	Boca Raton	Florida	561-362-5002	www.brrh.com
Broward Health Coral Springs	Coral Springs	Florida	954-344-3000	www.coralspringsmedicalcenter.org
Broward Health Imperial Point	Fort Lauderdale	Florida	954-776-8500	www.nbhd.org
Broward Health Medical Center	Fort Lauderdale	Florida	954-355-4400	www.browardhealth.org
Carolinas Medical Center - Pineville	Charlotte	North Carolina	704-379-5000	www.carolinashealthcare.org
Caromont Regional Medical Center	Gastonia	North Carolina	704-834-4891	www.caromont.org
Dauterive Hospital	New Iberia	Louisiana	337-365-7311	www.dauterivehospital.com
Doctors Hospital	Augusta	Georgia	706-651-6008	www.doctors-hospital.net
Dupont Hospital	Fort Wayne	Indiana	260-416-3000	www.theduponthospital.com
East Alabama Medical Center	Opelika	Alabama	334-749-3411	www.eamc.org
Englewood Community Hospital	Englewood	Florida	941-475-6571	www.englewoodcommunityhospital.com
Exempla Good Samaritan Medical Center	Lafayette	Colorado	303-689-4000	www.exempla.org
Fairview Park Hospital	Dublin	Georgia	478-274-3100	www.fairviewparkhospital.com
Fannin Regional Hospital	Blue Ridge	Georgia	706-632-3711	www.fanninregionalhospital.com
Flowers Hospital	Dothan	Alabama	334-793-5000	www.flowershospital.com
Fort Walton Beach Medical Center	Fort Walton Beach	Florida	850-862-1111	www.fwbmedicalcenter.com
Garden Park Medical Center	Gulfport	Mississippi	228-575-7000	www.gardenparkmedical.com
GHS Patewood Memorial Hospital	Greenville	South Carolina	864-797-1000	www.ghs.org
Holland Community Hospital	Holland	Michigan	616-392-5141	www.hoho.org
Ingalls Memorial Hospital	Harvey	Illinois	708-333-2300	www.ingalls.org
Institute For Orthopaedic Surgery	Lima	Ohio	419-224-7586	www.ioshospital.com
Jefferson Regional Medical Center	Pine Bluff	Arkansas	870-541-7100	www.jrmc.org
JFK Medical Center	Atlantis	Florida	561-965-7300	www.jfkmc.com
Jupiter Medical Center	Jupiter	Florida	561-747-2234	www.jupitermed.com
Kansas Medical Center	Andover	Kansas	316-300-4000	www.ksmedcenter.com
Lake City Medical Center	Lake City	Florida	386-719-9000	www.lakecitymedical.com
Lawnwood Regional Medical Center & Heart Institute	Fort Pierce	Florida	772-461-4000	www.lawnwoodmed.com
Lee's Summit Medical Center	Lees Summit	Missouri	816-282-5000	www.leessummithospital.com
Lewisgale Hospital Montgomery	Blacksburg	Virginia	540-951-1111	www.mrhospital.com
Magee Womens Hospital of UPMC Health System	Pittsburgh	Pennsylvania	412-641-4010	www.magee.edu
Margaret R Pardee Memorial Hospital	Hendersonville	North Carolina	828-696-1000	www.pardeehospital.org
Marion General Hospital	Marion	Ohio	740-383-8400	www.mariongeneral.com
Mary Greeley Medical Center	Ames	Iowa	515-239-2011	www.mgmc.org
McKenzie - Willamette Medical Center	Springfield	Oregon	541-726-4400	www.mckweb.com
Medical Center Enterprise	Enterprise	Alabama	334-347-0584	www.mcehospital.com
Memorial Hospital Pembroke	Pembroke Pines	Florida	954-962-9650	www.memorialpembroke.com\
Memorial Hospital West	Pembroke Pines	Florida	954-436-5000	www.memorialwest.com
Memorial Regional Hospital	Hollywood	Florida	954-987-2000	www.memorialregional.com
Mercy Medical Center	Roseburg	Oregon	541-673-0611	www.mercyrose.org
Methodist Dallas Medical Center	Dallas	Texas	214-947-2879	www.mhd.com
Methodist Mansfield Medical Center	Mansfield	Texas	682-622-2059	www.methodisthealthsystem.com
Mountain View Regional Medical Center	Las Cruces	New Mexico	575-556-7600	www.mountainviewregional.com
Mountainview Hospital	Las Vegas	Nevada	702-255-5065	www.mountainview-hospital.com
North Carolina Specialty Hospital	Durham	North Carolina	919-956-9300	www.ncspecialty.com
North Central Surgical Center	Dallas	Texas	214-265-2810	www.northcentral-sc.com
North Florida Regional Medical Center	Gainesville	Florida	352-333-4100	www.nfrmc.com
North Mississippi Medical Center	Tupelo	Mississippi	662-377-3000	www.nmhs.net/nmmc
North Suburban Medical Center	Thornton	Colorado	303-451-7800	www.northsuburban.com
Northern Westchester Hospital	Mount Kisco	New York	914-666-1200	www.nwhc.net
Northside Hospital	Atlanta	Georgia	404-851-8000	www.northside.com
Northside Hospital Cherokee	Canton	Georgia	770-720-5298	www.northside.com/cherokee
Northside Hospital Forsyth	Cumming	Georgia	404-851-8700	www.gbhcs.org
Northwest Medical Center	Margate	Florida	954-974-0400	www.northwestmed.com
Novant Health Charlotte Orthopedic Hospital	Charlotte	North Carolina	704-316-2000	www.presbyterian.org
Novant Health Forsyth Medical Center	Winston-Salem	North Carolina	336-718-5000	www.forsythmedicalcenter.org
Novant Health Park Hospital	Winston-Salem	North Carolina	336-718-0600	www.novanthealth.org
Novant Health Rowan Medical Center	Salisbury	North Carolina	704-210-5000	www.rowan.org

Hospital	City	State	Phone	Web Site
Ocala Regional Medical Center	Ocala	Florida	352-401-1000	www.ocalaregional.com
Oklahoma Surgical Hospital	Tulsa	Oklahoma	918-477-5000	www.oklahomasurgicalhospital.com
Orange Park Medical Center	Orange Park	Florida	904-276-8500	www.opmedical.com
The Orthopaedic Hospital of Lutheran Health Network	Fort Wayne	Indiana	260-435-2999	www.lutheranhealth.net
Orthopaedic Hospital of Wisconsin	Glendale	Wisconsin	414-961-6800	www.ohow.org
Oss Orthopaedic Hospital	York	Pennsylvania	717-718-2000	www.osshealth.com
Pinnacle Health Hospitals	Harrisburg	Pennsylvania	717-782-5181	www.pinnaclehealth.org
Portsmouth Regional Hospital	Portsmouth	New Hampshire	603-436-5110	www.portsmouthhospital.com
Quail Creek Surgical Hospital	Amarillo	Texas	806-354-6100	www.physurg.com
Rapides Regional Medical Center	Alexandria	Louisiana	318-769-3000	www.rapidesregional.com
Raulerson Hospital	Okeechobee	Florida	863-763-2151	www.raulersonhospital.com
Regional Hospital of Jackson	Jackson	Tennessee	731-661-2000	www.regionalhospitaljackson.com
The Regional Medical Center of Acadiana	Lafayette	Louisiana	337-981-2949	www.medicalcentersw.com
Renown South Meadows Medical Center	Reno	Nevada	775-982-7000	www.renown.org
Reston Hospital Center	Reston	Virginia	703-689-9000	www.restonhospital.com
River Oaks Hospital	Flowood	Mississippi	601-936-2390	www.riveroakshospital.org
Rose Medical Center	Denver	Colorado	303-320-2121	www.rosemed.com
Saint Anthony's Health Center	Alton	Illinois	618-465-2571	www.sahc.org
Saint Charles Hospital	Port Jefferson	New York	631-474-6000	www.stcharles.org
Saint Elizabeth Florence	Florence	Kentucky	859-212-5220	www.stlukehospitals.com
Saint Elizabeth Medical Center	Lakeside Park	Kentucky	859-292-2000	www.stelizabeth.com
Saint Francis Regional Medical Center	Shakopee	Minnesota	952-403-3000	www.stfrancis-shakopee.com
Saint Lucie Medical Center	Port Saint Lucie	Florida	772-335-4000	www.stluciemed.com
Saint Luke's Lakeside Hospital	The Woodlands	Texas	936-266-4055	www.stlukeslakeside.com
Saint Luke's South Hospital	Overland Park	Kansas	913-317-7904	www.saintlukeshealthsystem.org
Saint Mary Medical Center	Hobart	Indiana	219-942-0551	www.comhs.org/stmary
Saint Vincent Healthcare	Billings	Montana	406-657-7000	www.svh-mt.org
Saint Vincent's Medical Center Southside	Jacksonville	Florida	904-296-3700	www.jaxhealth.com
San Angelo Community Medical Center	San Angelo	Texas	325-949-9511	www.sacmc.com
Scripps Green Hospital	La Jolla	California	858-554-3600	www.scrippshealth.org
Scripps Memorial Hospital - Encinitas	Encinitas	California	760-753-6501	www.scripps.org
Sebastian River Medical Center	Sebastian	Florida	772-589-3187	www.srmcenter.com
South Baldwin Regional Medical Center	Foley	Alabama	251-949-3400	www.southbaldwinrmc.com
South Miami Hospital	South Miami	Florida	786-662-4000	www.baptisthealth.net
South Nassau Communities Hospital	Oceanside	New York	516-632-3000	www.southnassau.org
Sparks Regional Medical Center	Fort Smith	Arkansas	501-441-4000	www.sparks.org
Springs Memorial Hospital	Lancaster	South Carolina	803-286-1481	www.springsmemorial.com
Strong Memorial Hospital	Rochester	New York	585-275-2121	www.urmc.rochester.edu
Tanner Medical Center - Carrollton	Carrollton	Georgia	770-836-9580	www.tanner.org
Texas Health Harris Methodist Hospital Southlake	Southlake	Texas	817-748-8700	www.texashealthsouthlake.com
Texas Orthopedic Hospital	Houston	Texas	713-799-8600	www.texasorthopedic.com
Trinity Medical Center	Birmingham	Alabama	205-592-1000	www.bhsala.com/montclair
Twin Cities Hospital	Niceville	Florida	850-678-4131	www.tchealthcare.com
UH Geauga Medical Center	Chardon	Ohio	440-269-6000	www.uhgeauga.org
UPMC East	Monroeville	Pennsylvania	412-357-3000	www.upmc.com
Venice Regional Medical Center - Bayfront Health	Venice	Florida	941-485-7711	www.veniceregional.com
Walker Baptist Medical Center	Jasper	Alabama	205-387-4000	www.bhsala.com/walker
West Florida Hospital	Pensacola	Florida	850-494-4000	www.westfloridahospital.com
West Georgia Medical Center	Lagrange	Georgia	706-882-1411	www.wghealth.org
West Kendall Baptist Hospital	Miami	Florida	786-467-2011	www.baptisthealth.net
West Palm Hospital	West Palm Beach	Florida	561-844-6141	www.columbiahospital.com

Note: The hospitals shown above represent the top 5% of the 2,338 hospitals nationwide for which an average score was calculated. Average scores were calculated for hospitals with qualifying data (25 cases or more) in at least 9 of 10 measures in the Surgical Care Improvment Project category.

Best Hospitals in Terms of Patient's Hospital Experiences

Hospital	City	State	Phone	Web Site
Abbeville Area Medical Center	Abbeville	South Carolina	864-366-5011	www.abbevilleareamc.com
Advanced Surgical Hospital	Washington	Pennsylvania	724-884-0710	www.ashospital.net
Animas Surgical Hospital	Durango	Colorado	970-247-3537	www.animassorgical.com
Arizona Orthopedic & Surgical Speciality Hospital	Chandler	Arizona	480-603-9000	www.azosh.com
Arkansas Heart Hospital	Little Rock	Arkansas	501-219-7000	www.arheart.com
Arkansas Surgical Hospital	No Little Rock	Arkansas	501-748-8000	www.arksurgicalhospital.com
Avera Heart Hospital of South Dakota	Sioux Falls	South Dakota	605-977-7000	www.avera.org/heart-hospital
Avera Saint Anthony's Hospital	O' Neill	Nebraska	402-336-2611	www.avera-sta.org
Baptist Emergency Hospital	San Antonio	Texas	210-402-4092	www.baptistemergencyhospital.com
Barton County Memorial Hospital	Lamar	Missouri	417-682-6081	www.bcmh.net
Baylor Heart & Vascular Hospital	Dallas	Texas	214-820-0670	www.baylorhearthospital.com
Baylor Medical Center at Frisco	Frisco	Texas	214-618-2000	www.bmcf.com
Baylor Medical Center at Trophy Club	Trophy Club	Texas	817-837-4600	www.tc-mc.com
Baylor Medical Center at Uptown	Dallas	Texas	214-443-3000	www.bmcuptown.com
Baylor Orthopedic & Spine Hospital at Arlington	Arlington	Texas	817-549-2364	www.baylorarlington.com
Baylor Surgical Hospital at Las Colinas	Irving	Texas	972-868-4000	www.ic-sh.com
Bear River Valley Hospital	Tremonton	Utah	435-207-4708	www.intermountainhealthcare.org
Bigfork Valley Hospital	Bigfork	Minnesota	218-743-3177	www.bigforkvalley.org
Black Hills Surgical Hospital	Rapid City	South Dakota	605-721-4700	www.bhsh.com
Black River Memorial Hospital	Black River Falls	Wisconsin	715-284-5361	www.brmh.net
Blue Hill Memorial Hospital	Blue Hill	Maine	207-374-2836	www.bhmh.org/default.html
Bluffton Hospital	Bluffton	Ohio	419-358-9010	www.bvhealthsystem.org
Boone County Health Center	Albion	Nebraska	402-395-2191	www.boonecohealth.org
Brodstone Memorial Hospital	Superior	Nebraska	402-879-3281	www.brodstonehospital.org
Bucks County Specialty Hospital	Bensalem	Pennsylvania	215-244-7400	www.bcshospital.com
Caldwell Memorial Hospital	Columbia	Louisiana	318-649-6111	
Central Louisiana Surgical Hospital	Alexandria	Louisiana	318-449-6400	www.clshospital.com
Chickasaw Nation Medical Center	Ada	Oklahoma	580-436-3980	www.chickasaw.net
Choctaw Nation Healthcare	Talihina	Oklahoma	918-567-7000	www.choctawnationhealth.com
Citizens Medical Center	Columbia	Louisiana	318-649-6106	www.citizensmedcenter.com
Clinton County Hospital	Albany	Kentucky	606-387-6421	www.clintoncountyhospital.com
Columbia Center	Mequon	Wisconsin	262-243-7408	www.columbiacenter.org
Community Hospital	Torrington	Wyoming	307-532-4181	www.bannerhealth.com
Community Medical Center	Falls City	Nebraska	402-245-2428	www.hhs.state.ne.us/index.htm
Community Memorial Hospital	Hicksville	Ohio	419-542-6692	www.cmhosp.com
Coordinated Health Orthopedic Hospital	Bethlehem	Pennsylvania	610-691-4300	www.coordinatedhealth.com
Cypress Pointe Surgical Hospital	Hammond	Louisiana	985-510-6200	www.cpsh.org
Dakota Plains Surgical Center	Aberdeen	South Dakota	605-225-3300	www.orthopediccenterofthedakotas.com
Doctors Hospital at Deer Creek	Leesville	Louisiana	337-392-5088	www.dhdc.md
East Texas Medical Center - Gilmer	Gilmer	Texas	903-841-7100	www.etmc.org
East Texas Medical Center Pittsburg	Pittsburg	Texas	903-856-4520	www.etmc.org
Electra Memorial Hospital	Electra	Texas	940-495-3981	www.electrahospital.com
Fairview Hospital	Great Barrington	Massachusetts	413-528-0790	www.berkshirehealthsystems.com
Fairway Medical Center	Covington	Louisiana	985-801-3010	www.fairwaymedical.com
Fayette Medical Center	Fayette	Alabama	205-932-5966	www.dchsystem.com
First Care Health Center	Park River	North Dakota	701-284-7500	www.firstcarehc.com
Floyd County Memorial Hospital	Charles City	Iowa	641-228-6830	www.fcmc.us.com
Fostoria Community Hospital	Fostoria	Ohio	419-435-7734	www.promedica.org
Foundation Surgical Hospital of San Antonio	San Antonio	Texas	210-478-5400	www.fshsanantonio.com
Fresno Surgical Hospital	Fresno	California	559-431-8000	www.fresnosurgerycenter.com
GHS Patewood Memorial Hospital	Greenville	South Carolina	864-797-1000	www.ghs.org
Glacial Ridge Hospital	Glenwood	Minnesota	320-634-2208	www.glacialridge.org
Grant Regional Health Center	Lancaster	Wisconsin	608-723-2143	www.grantregional.com
Great Falls Clinic Medical Center	Great Falls	Montana	406-216-8000	www.gfclinic.com
Green Clinic Surgical Hospital	Ruston	Louisiana	318-232-7700	www.green-clinic.com
Grundy County Memorial Hospital	Grundy Center	Iowa	319-824-5421	www.grundyhospital.com
H B Magruder Memorial Hospital	Port Clinton	Ohio	419-734-3131	www.magruderhospital.com
Heart Hospital Baylor Plano	Plano	Texas	469-814-3278	www.thehearthospitalbaylor.com
Heart Hospital of Lafayette	Lafayette	Louisiana	337-521-1000	www.hearthospitaloflafayette.com
Heritage Park Surgical Hospital	Sherman	Texas	903-813-3728	www.heritageparksurgicalhospital.com
Hill Country Memorial Hospital	Fredericksburg	Texas	830-997-4353	www.hcmbs.org
Hillsboro Area Hospital	Hillsboro	Illinois	217-532-6111	www.hillsboroareahospital.org
Hoag Orthopedic Institute	Irvine	California	949-727-5000	www.orthopedichospital.com
Houston Orthopedic & Spine Hospital	Bellaire	Texas	713-622-2262	www.foundationsurgicalhospital.com
Houston Physicians' Hospital	Webster	Texas	281-335-1700	www.houstonphysicianshospital.com

Hospital	City	State	Phone	Web Site
Indiana Orthopaedic Hospital	Indianapolis	Indiana	317-956-1000	www.indianaorthopaedichospital.com
Institute For Orthopaedic Surgery	Lima	Ohio	419-224-7586	www.ioshospital.com
Integris Health Edmond	Edmond	Oklahoma	405-657-3000	www.integrisok.com/integris-health-edmond-ok
Jefferson County Health Center	Fairfield	Iowa	641-472-4111	www.jchospital.org
Kansas City Orthopaedic Institute	Leawood	Kansas	913-319-7633	www.kcoi.com
Kentuckiana Medical Center	Clarksville	Indiana	812-280-3300	www.kentuckianamedcen.com
King's Daughters Medical Center - Brookhaven	Brookhaven	Mississippi	601-833-6011	www.kdmc.org
Lady of the Sea General Hospital	Cut Off	Louisiana	985-632-6401	www.losgh.org
Lafayette Surgical Specialty Hospital	Lafayette	Louisiana	337-769-4100	www.lafayettesurgical.com
Lakeview Memorial Hospital	Stillwater	Minnesota	651-439-5330	www.lakeview.org
Lawrence County Hospital	Monticello	Mississippi	601-587-4051	www.smrmc.com/index.php
Lincoln Surgical Hospital	Lincoln	Nebraska	402-484-9090	www.lincolnsurgery.com
Mackinac Straits Hospital & Health Center	Saint Ignace	Michigan	906-643-8585	www.mackinacstraitshealth.org
Manhattan Surgical Hospital	Manhattan	Kansas	785-776-5100	www.manhattansurgical.com
Mariners Hospital	Tavernier	Florida	305-434-3000	www.baptisthealth.net
Marion Regional Medical Center	Hamilton	Alabama	205-921-6200	www.nmhs.net
Mayo Clinic Hospital	Phoenix	Arizona	480-342-2000	www.mayoclinic.org
McBride Clinic Orthopedic Hospital	Oklahoma City	Oklahoma	405-478-1717	www.mcbrideclinic.com
Menlo Park Surgical Hospital	Menlo Park	California	650-324-8500	www.pamf.org/mpsh
Mercy Willard Hospital	Willard	Ohio	419-964-5000	www.mercyweb.org/mercy_willard.aspx
Miami County Medical Center	Paola	Kansas	913-557-4385	www.olathehealth.org
Mid - Valley Hospital	Peckville	Pennsylvania	570-383-5000	
Midwest Orthopedic Specialty Hospital	Franklin	Wisconsin	414-817-5800	www.mymosh.com
Midwest Surgical Hospital	Omaha	Nebraska	402-399-1900	www.mwsurgicalhospital.com
Millinocket Regional Hospital	Millinocket	Maine	207-723-5161	www.mrhme.org
Ministry Door County Medical Center	Sturgeon Bay	Wisconsin	920-743-5566	www.doorcountymemorial.org
Mount Carmel New Albany Surgical Hospital	New Albany	Ohio	614-775-6600	www.mountcarmelhealth.com
Mount Desert Island Hospital	Bar Harbor	Maine	207-288-5081	www.mdihospital.com
Mountain View Regional Hospital	Casper	Wyoming	307-995-8100	www.monroehospital.com
Nebraska Orthopaedic Hospital	Omaha	Nebraska	402-609-1600	www.neorthohospital.com
The Neuromedical Center Hospital	Baton Rouge	Louisiana	225-763-9900	www.theneuromedicalcenter.com
North Carolina Specialty Hospital	Durham	North Carolina	919-956-9300	www.ncspecialty.com
North Central Surgical Center	Dallas	Texas	214-265-2810	www.northcentral-sc.com
Northside Medical Center	Columbus	Georgia	706-494-2100	www.hughstonsports.com
Northwest Hills Surgical Hospital	Austin	Texas	512-346-1994	www.scasurgery.com
Northwest Specialty Hospital	Post Falls	Idaho	208-262-2300	www.northwestspecialtyhospital.com
Northwest Surgical Hospital	Oklahoma City	Oklahoma	404-848-1918	www.nwsurgicalokc.com
Oak Leaf Surgical Hospital	Eau Claire	Wisconsin	715-831-8130	www.oakleafsurgical.com
Ogallala Community Hospital	Ogallala	Nebraska	308-284-4011	www.bannerhealth.com
Oklahoma Center for Orthopaedic & Multi-Spec	Oklahoma City	Oklahoma	405-602-6500	www.ocomhospital.com
Oklahoma Heart Hospital	Oklahoma City	Oklahoma	405-608-3200	www.okheart.com
Oklahoma Heart Hospital South	Oklahoma City	Oklahoma	405-628-6000	www.okheart.com/south-campus
Oklahoma Spine Hospital	Oklahoma City	Oklahoma	405-749-2700	www.oklahomaspine.com
Oklahoma Surgical Hospital	Tulsa	Oklahoma	918-477-5000	www.oklahomasurgicalhospital.com
Orange City Area Health System	Orange City	Iowa	712-737-4984	www.ochealthsystem.org
Orthopaedic Hospital of Wisconsin	Glendale	Wisconsin	414-961-6800	www.ohow.org
OSF Holy Family Medical Center	Monmouth	Illinois	309-734-3141	www.cmchospital.com
Oss Orthopaedic Hospital	York	Pennsylvania	717-718-2000	www.osshealth.com
Ouachita Community Hospital	West Monroe	Louisiana	318-322-1339	www.ouachitahospital.com
P & S Surgical Hospital	Monroe	Louisiana	318-388-4040	www.pssurgery.com
Patients' Hospital of Redding	Redding	California	530-225-8700	www.patientshospital.com
Pella Regional Health Center	Pella	Iowa	641-628-3150	www.pellahealth.org
Pender Community Hospital	Pender	Nebraska	402-385-3083	www.pendercommunityhospital.com
Physician's Care Surgical Hospital	Royersford	Pennsylvania	610-495-4793	www.phycarehospital.com
The Physicians Centre	Bryan	Texas	979-731-3100	www.thephysicianscentre.com
Physicians Medical Center	Houma	Louisiana	985-853-1390	www.physicianshouma.com
Physicians' Medical Center	New Albany	Indiana	812-206-7660	www.pmcdev.interactivemedialab.com
Physicians' Specialty Hospital	Fayetteville	Arkansas	479-571-7002	www.pshfay.com
Quail Creek Surgical Hospital	Amarillo	Texas	806-354-6100	www.physurg.com
Richland Parish Hospital - Delhi	Delhi	Louisiana	318-878-5171	www.delhihospital.com
River Falls Area Hospital	River Falls	Wisconsin	715-307-6000	www.allina.com
Rochelle Community Hospital	Rochelle	Illinois	815-562-2181	www.rcha.net
Rockcastle County Hospital	Mount Vernon	Kentucky	606-256-2195	www.rockcastlehospital.com
Rollins Brook Community Hospital	Lampasas	Texas	512-556-3682	www.mplex.org
Sacred Heart Hospital on the Gulf	Port Saint Joe	Florida	850-229-5600	www.sacred-heart.org/gulf
Saint Joseph Memorial Hospital	Murphysboro	Illinois	618-684-3156	www.sih.net
Saint Joseph's Hospital	Breese	Illinois	618-526-4511	www.stjoebreese.com

Hospital	City	State	Phone	Web Site
Saint Luke's Lakeside Hospital	The Woodlands	Texas	936-266-4055	www.stlukeslakeside.com
Saint Luke's Wood River Medical Center	Ketchum	Idaho	208-727-8800	www.stlukesonline.org/wood_river
Saint Thomas Hospital for Spinal Surgery	Nashville	Tennessee	615-515-8200	www.hospitalforspinalsurgery.com
Salina Surgical Hospital	Salina	Kansas	785-827-0610	www.salinasurgical.com
Sanford Luverne Medical Center	Luverne	Minnesota	507-283-2321	www.sanfordluverne.org
Sauk Prairie Hospital	Prairie Du Sac	Wisconsin	608-643-3311	www.spmh.org
Sharp Coronado Hospital & Healthcare Center	Coronado	California	619-435-6251	www.sharp.com/coronado
Sioux Falls Specialty Hospital	Sioux Falls	South Dakota	605-334-6730	www.sfsurgical.com
Siouxland Surgery Center	Dakota Dunes	South Dakota	605-232-3332	www.siouxlandsurg.com
South Texas Spine & Surgical Hospital	San Antonio	Texas	210-404-0800	www.southtexassurgical.com
South Texas Surgical Hospital	Corpus Christi	Texas	361-993-2000	www.nshinc.com
Southern Surgical Hospital	Slidell	Louisiana	985-641-0600	www.sshla.com
Southwestern Regional Medical Center	Tulsa	Oklahoma	918-496-5000	www.cancercenter.com/southwestern
Specialists Hospital Shreveport	Shreveport	Louisiana	318-213-3800	www.specialistshospitalshreveport.com
Stanislaus Surgical Hospital	Modesto	California	209-572-2700	www.stanislaussurgical.com
Stewart Memorial Community Hospital	Lake City	Iowa	712-464-3171	www.stewartmemorial.org
Stoughton Hospital	Stoughton	Wisconsin	608-873-6611	www.stoughtonhospital.com
Sugar Land Surgical Hospital	Sugar Land	Texas	281-243-1000	www.sugarlandsurgicalhospital.com
Surgical Hospital at Southwoods	Youngstown	Ohio	330-758-1954	www.surgeryatsouthwoods.com
Surgical Institute of Reading	Wyomissing	Pennsylvania	717-999-9999	www.sireading.com
Surgical Specialty Center at Coordinated Health	Allentown	Pennsylvania	610-871-9110	www.coordinatedhealth.com
Surgical Specialty Center of Baton Rouge	Baton Rouge	Louisiana	225-408-5730	www.sscbr.com
Sutter Surgical Hospital - North Valley	Yuba City	California	530-749-5700	www.suttersurgicalhospitalnorthvalley.org
Texas Health Center for Diagnostics & Surgery	Plano	Texas	972-403-2700	www.ppcds.com
Texas Health Harris Methodist Hospital Southlake	Southlake	Texas	817-748-8700	www.texashealthsouthlake.com
Texas Institute for Surgery at Presbyterian Hospital	Dallas	Texas	214-647-5300	www.texasinstituteforsurgery.org
Texas Spine & Joint Hospital	Tyler	Texas	903-525-3300	www.tsjh.org
Tishomingo Health Services	Iuka	Mississippi	662-423-6051	www.nmhs.net/iuka
Tops Surgical Specialty Hospital	Houston	Texas	281-539-2900	www.tops-hospital.com
Treasure Valley Hospital	Boise	Idaho	208-373-5000	www.treasurevalleyhospital.com
Tulsa Spine & Specialty Hospital	Tulsa	Oklahoma	918-388-5701	www.tulsaspinehospital.com
United Regional Medical Center	Manchester	Tennessee	931-728-3586	www.urmchealthcare.com
University Hospitals Conneaut Medical Center	Conneaut	Ohio	440-593-1131	www.uhhospitals.org/conneaut
Upland Hills Health	Dodgeville	Wisconsin	608-930-8000	www.uplandhillshealth.org
USMD Hospital at Arlington	Arlington	Texas	817-472-3400	www.usmdhospital.com
USMD Hospital at Fort Worth	Fort Worth	Texas	817-433-9100	www.usmdfortworth.com
Vernon Memorial Hospital	Viroqua	Wisconsin	608-637-2101	www.vmh.org
Vidant Bertie Hospital	Windsor	North Carolina	252-794-6600	www.vidanthealth.com/bertie
W J Mangold Memorial Hospital	Lockney	Texas	806-652-3373	www.mangoldmemorial.org
Wellspan Surgery & Rehabilitation Hospital	York	Pennsylvania	717-812-6100	www.wellspan.org
West Kendall Baptist Hospital	Miami	Florida	786-467-2011	www.baptisthealth.net
Westlake Regional Hospital	Columbia	Kentucky	270-384-4753	www.westlake-healthcare.org
Whitman Hospital & Medical Center	Colfax	Washington	509-397-3435	www.whitmanhospital.com
Wright Memorial Hospital	Trenton	Missouri	660-359-5621	www.saintlukeshealthsystem.org
York Hospital	York	Maine	207-363-4321	www.yorkhospital.com

Note: The hospitals shown above represent the top 5% of the 3,591 hospitals nationwide for which an average score was calculated. Average scores were calculated for hospitals with qualifying data (100 completed surveys or more) in all ten measures in the Survey of Patient's Hospital Experiences category.

Best Hospitals in Terms of Use of Medical Imaging

Hospital	City	State	Phone	Web Site
Alameda Hospital	Alameda	California	510-522-3700	www.alamedahospital.org
Bartlett Regional Hospital	Juneau	Alaska	907-796-8900	www.bartletthospital.org
Caldwell Memorial Hospital	Lenoir	North Carolina	828-757-5100	www.caldwellmemorial.org
Capital Regional Medical Center	Tallahassee	Florida	850-656-5000	www.capitalregionalmedicalcenter.com
Carroll County Memorial Hospital	Carrollton	Kentucky	502-732-4321	www.ccmhosp.com
Centrastate Medical Center	Freehold	New Jersey	732-431-2000	www.centrastate.com
Chandler Regional Medical Center	Chandler	Arizona	480-963-4561	www.chandlerregional.com
Chinese Hospital	San Francisco	California	415-982-2400	www.chinesehospital-sf.org
Community Regional Medical Center	Fresno	California	559-459-6000	www.communitymedical.org
Conemaugh Valley Memorial Hospital	Johnstown	Pennsylvania	814-534-9000	www.conemaugh.org
Deaconess Hospital	Spokane	Washington	509-473-5800	www.deaconessmedicalcenter.org
Doctors Medical Center	Modesto	California	209-578-1211	www.dmc-modesto.com
Doctors Medical Center - San Pablo	San Pablo	California	510-970-5000	www.doctorsmedicalcenter.org
Dominican Hospital	Santa Cruz	California	831-462-7700	www.dominicanhospital.org
Emanuel Medical Center	Turlock	California	209-667-4200	www.emanuelmedicalcenter.org
Enloe Medical Center	Chico	California	530-332-7300	www.enloe.org
Evergreen Hospital Medical Center	Kirkland	Washington	425-899-1000	www.evergreenhospital.org
Exempla Saint Joseph Hospital	Denver	Colorado	303-837-7111	www.exempla.org
Fairview Hospital	Cleveland	Ohio	216-476-7000	www.fairviewhospital.org
Fairview Park Hospital	Dublin	Georgia	478-274-3100	www.fairviewparkhospital.com
Glens Falls Hospital	Glens Falls	New York	518-926-1000	www.glensfallshospital.org
Good Samaritan Hospital	San Jose	California	408-559-2011	www.goodsamsj.org
Halifax Health Medical Center	Daytona Beach	Florida	386-254-4000	www.halifax.org
Harrison Memorial Center	Bremerton	Washington	360-377-3911	www.harrisonmedical.org
Hartford Hospital	Hartford	Connecticut	860-545-5000	www.harthosp.org
Healthalliance Hospitals	Leominster	Massachusetts	978-466-2000	www.healthalliance.com
Heart Hospital Baylor Plano	Plano	Texas	469-814-3278	www.thehearthospitalbaylor.com
Holy Redeemer Hospital & Medical Center	Meadowbrook	Pennsylvania	215-947-3000	www.holyredeemer.com
Huntington Hospital	Huntington	New York	631-351-2000	www.hunthosp.org
Huntington Memorial Hospital	Pasadena	California	626-397-5000	www.huntingtonhospital.com
Indiana University Health White Memorial Hospital	Monticello	Indiana	574-583-7111	www.whitecmh.org
Inova Fairfax Hospital	Falls Church	Virginia	703-776-3332	www.inova.org
Jefferson Medical Center	Ranson	West Virginia	304-728-1600	www.jeffmem.com
Johnson Memorial Hospital	Stafford Springs	Connecticut	860-684-4251	www.johnsonhealthnetwork.com
Lake City Medical Center	Lake City	Florida	386-719-9000	www.lakecitymedical.com
Lake Regional Health System	Osage Beach	Missouri	573-348-8000	www.lakeregional.com
Lakewood Regional Medical Center	Lakewood	California	562-602-6751	www.lakewoodregional.com
Lasalle General Hospital	Jena	Louisiana	318-992-9200	www.lasallegeneralhospital.com
Little Falls Hospital	Little Falls	New York	315-823-5261	www.lfhny.org
Long Island Jewish Medical Center	New Hyde Park	New York	718-470-7000	www.northshorelij.com
Lourdes Medical Center of Burlington County	Willingboro	New Jersey	609-835-2900	www.lourdesnet.org/lourdes
Lovelace Medical Center	Albuquerque	New Mexico	505-727-8000	www.lovelace.com
Lowell General Hospital	Lowell	Massachusetts	978-937-6000	www.lowellgeneral.org
Mainegeneral Medical Center	Augusta	Maine	207-872-1000	www.mainegeneral.org
Maria Parham Medical Center	Henderson	North Carolina	252-438-4143	www.mphosp.org
Marin General Hospital	Greenbrae	California	415-925-7900	www.maringeneral.com
Mary Greeley Medical Center	Ames	Iowa	515-239-2011	www.mgmc.org
Mary Washington Hospital	Fredericksburg	Virginia	540-741-1100	www.medicorp.org
Maui Memorial Medical Center	Wailuku	Hawaii	808-442-5101	www.mauimemorialmedical.org
Mayo Clinic Health System - Albert Lea	Albert Lea	Minnesota	507-373-2384	www.mayoclinichealthsystem.org
McKenzie - Willamette Medical Center	Springfield	Oregon	541-726-4400	www.mckweb.com
Medstar Franklin Square Medical Center	Baltimore	Maryland	443-777-7850	www.franklinsquare.org
Medstar Southern Maryland Hospital Center	Clinton	Maryland	301-868-8000	www.medstarhealth.org
Memorial Medical Center	Modesto	California	209-526-4500	www.memorialmedicalcenter.org
Mercy General Hospital	Sacramento	California	916-453-4545	www.mercygeneral.org
Mercy Gilbert Medical Center	Gilbert	Arizona	480-728-8327	www.dignityhealth.org/mercygilbert
Mercy Hospital	Coon Rapids	Minnesota	763-236-8205	www.allinamercy.org
Mercy Medical Center - Clinton	Clinton	Iowa	563-244-5555	www.mercyclinton.com
Mercy Medical Center - Redding	Redding	California	530-225-6102	www.redding.mercy.org
Mercy San Juan Medical Center	Carmichael	California	916-537-5000	www.mercysanjuan.org
Mercy Willard Hospital	Willard	Ohio	419-964-5000	www.mercyweb.org/mercy_willard.aspx
Methodist Hospital of Sacramento	Sacramento	California	916-423-6010	www.methodistsacramento.org
Methodist Hospital of Southern California	Arcadia	California	626-445-4441	www.methodisthospital.org
Metrosouth Medical Center	Blue Island	Illinois	708-597-2000	www.stfrancisblueisland.com
Miriam Hospital	Providence	Rhode Island	401-793-2500	www.lifespan.org/partners/tmh

Hospital	City	State	Phone	Web Site
Nashoba Valley Medical Center	Ayer	Massachusetts	978-784-9000	www.nashobamed.com
Newton Memorial Hospital	Newton	New Jersey	973-383-2121	www.itsyourlife.com
North Florida Regional Medical Center	Gainesville	Florida	352-333-4100	www.nfrmc.com
Northbay Medical Center	Fairfield	California	707-646-5000	www.northbay.org
Ocala Regional Medical Center	Ocala	Florida	352-401-1000	www.ocalaregional.com
Page Memorial Hospital	Luray	Virginia	540-743-4561	www.pagememorialhospital.org
Palomar Health Downtown Campus	Escondido	California	760-739-3000	www.pph.org
Paris Regional Medical Center	Paris	Texas	903-785-4521	www.parisregional.com
Peacehealth Saint Joseph Medical Center	Bellingham	Washington	360-734-5400	www.peacehealth.org
Penobscot Bay Medical Center	Rockport	Maine	207-596-8000	www.nehealth.org
PIH Hospital - Downey	Downey	California	526-904-5000	www.drmci.org
Pomerado Hospital	Poway	California	858-485-6511	www.pph.org
Providence Sacred Heart Medical Center	Spokane	Washington	509-474-3040	www.shmc.org
Regional Medical Center of San Jose	San Jose	California	408-259-5000	www.regionalmedicalsanjose.com
Riverview Hospital Assoc	Wisconsin Rapids	Wisconsin	715-423-6060	www.riverviewhospital.net
Robert Wood Johnson University Hospital	New Brunswick	New Jersey	732-937-8900	www.rwjuh.edu
Saint Alphonsus Medical Center - Ontario	Ontario	Oregon	541-881-7000	www.holyrosary-ontario.org
Saint Alphonsus Regional Medical Center	Boise	Idaho	208-367-2121	www.saintalphonsus.org
Saint David's Medical Center	Austin	Texas	512-476-7111	www.stdavidsrehab.com
Saint Joseph Mercy Port Huron	Port Huron	Michigan	810-985-1510	www.mercyporthuron.com
Saint Joseph's Hospital Health Center	Syracuse	New York	315-448-5111	www.sjhsyr.org
Saint Mary's Hospital - Troy	Troy	New York	518-272-5000	www.setonhealth.org
Saint Marys Hospital	Waterbury	Connecticut	203-574-6000	www.stmh.org
Saint Thomas Rutherford Hospital	Murfreesboro	Tennessee	615-396-4100	www.mtmc.org
Salinas Valley Memorial Hospital	Salinas	California	831-757-4333	www.svmh.com
Santa Rosa Memorial Hospital	Santa Rosa	California	707-525-5300	www.stjosephhealth.org
Santiam Memorial Hospital	Stayton	Oregon	503-769-2175	www.santiamhospital.com
Scottsdale Healthcare - Thompson Peak Hospital	Scottsdale	Arizona	480-324-7004	www.shc.org
Scottsdale Healthcare Osborn Medical Center	Scottsdale	Arizona	480-882-4000	www.shc.org
Shady Grove Adventist Hospital	Rockville	Maryland	240-826-6517	www.adventisthealthcare.com/sgah
Sharp Chula Vista Medical Center	Chula Vista	California	619-502-5800	www.sharp.com
Southwest Regional Medical Center	Georgetown	Ohio	513-378-7800	www.browncountygeneralhospital.com
Stafford Hospital	Stafford	Virginia	540-741-9000	www.marywashingtonhealthcare.com
Sutter Delta Medical Center	Antioch	California	925-779-7200	www.sutterdelta.org
Sutter General Hospital	Sacramento	California	916-733-8999	www.suttermedicalcenter.org
Sutter Roseville Medical Center	Roseville	California	916-781-1000	www.sutterroseville.org
Swedish Edmonds Hospital	Edmonds	Washington	425-640-4000	www.stevenshealthcare.org
Tallahassee Memorial Hospital	Tallahassee	Florida	850-431-1155	www.tmh.org
Texas Health Presbyterian Hospital Dallas	Dallas	Texas	214-345-6789	www.texashealth.org
Trinity Rock Island	Rock Island	Illinois	309-779-5000	www.trinityqc.com
Union Hospital Clinton	Clinton	Indiana	765-832-1234	www.unionhospitalhealthgroup.org/wcch
University Medical Center at Brackenridge	Austin	Texas	512-324-7000	www.seton.net/locations/brackenridge
University Medical Center of Princeton at Plainsboro	Plainsboro	New Jersey	866-460-4776	www.princetonhcs.org
Valley Hospital	Spokane	Washington	509-924-6650	www.valleyhospital.org
Vidant Duplin Hospital	Kenansville	North Carolina	910-296-0941	www.dgh.org
Virtua Memorial Hospital of Burlington County	Mount Holly	New Jersey	609-914-6200	www.virtua.org
Warren Memorial Hospital	Front Royal	Virginia	703-636-0300	www.valleyhealthlink.com
Waterbury Hospital	Waterbury	Connecticut	203-573-6000	www.waterburyhospital.org
Watsonville Community Hospital	Watsonville	California	831-724-4741	www.watsonvillehospital.com
West Hills Hospital & Medical Center	West Hills	California	818-676-4100	www.westhillshospital.com
West Valley Medical Center	Caldwell	Idaho	208-459-4641	www.westvalleymedctr.com
Wooster Community Hospital	Wooster	Ohio	330-263-8100	www.woosterhospital.org

Note: The hospitals shown above represent the top 5% of the 2,308 hospitals nationwide for which an average score was calculated. Average scores were calculated for hospitals with qualifying data (25 cases or more) in at least 4 of 5 measures in the Use of Medical Imaging category. The measure, Follow-up Mammogram/Ultrasound, was not included in the average score.

Hospitals with the Lowest Medicare Spending per Beneficiary

Hospital	City	State	Phone	Web Site
Basin Healthcare Center	Odessa	Texas	432-425-9510	www.bhcodessa.com
Beaver Valley Hospital	Beaver	Utah	435-438-7102	
Bob Wilson Memorial Grant County Hospital	Ulysses	Kansas	620-356-1266	www.bwmgch.com
Brighton Hospital	Brighton	Michigan	810-227-1211	www.stjohn.org/brighton
Cherokee Indian Hospital Authority	Cherokee	North Carolina	704-497-9163	
Chinle Comprehensive Health Care Facility	Chinle	Arizona	928-674-7001	
Crownpoint Healthcare Facility	Crownpoint	New Mexico	505-786-5291	www.ihs.gov
Dhhs Usphs Indian Health Services	San Fidel	New Mexico	505-552-5300	www.ihs.gov
Eastern State Hospital	Williamsburg	Virginia	757-253-5161	www.ehs.dmhmrsas.virginia.gov
Epic Medical Center	Eufaula	Oklahoma	918-689-2535	
Fort Defiance Indian Hospital	Fort Defiance	Arizona	928-729-8000	www.home.navajo.his.gov
Gallup Indian Medical Center	Gallup	New Mexico	505-722-1000	www.ihs.gov/facilitiesservices
Guadalupe County Hospital	Santa Rosa	New Mexico	575-472-3417	
Harmon Memorial Hospital	Hollis	Oklahoma	580-688-3363	
Ira Davenport Memorial Hospital	Bath	New York	607-776-8500	www.davenportandtaylor.org
Kaiser Foundation Hospital - Antioch	Antioch	California	925-813-6500	www.kaiserpermanente.org
Kaiser Foundation Hospital - Fresno	Fresno	California	559-448-4500	www.kaiserpermanente.org
Kaiser Foundation Hospital - San Diego	San Diego	California	619-528-5000	www.members.kaiserpermanente.org
Kaiser Foundation Hospital - San Francisco	San Francisco	California	415-833-2646	www.permanente.net
Kaiser Foundation Hospital - South San Francisco	South San Francisco	California	650-742-3200	www.healthy.kaiserpermanente.org
Kaiser Foundation Hospital - Vacaville	Vacaville	California	707-624-4000	www.kaiserpermanente.org
Kaiser Sunnyside Medical Center	Clackamas	Oregon	503-571-2880	www.members.kaiserpermanente.org
Keefe Memorial Hospital	Cheyenne Wells	Colorado	719-767-5661	
Laguna Honda Hospital & Rehabilitation Center	San Francisco	California	415-759-2300	www.dph.sf.ca.us/chn/lagunahondahosp
Lewis County General Hospital	Lowville	New York	315-376-5200	www.lcgh.net
Memorial Hospital of Texas County	Guymon	Oklahoma	580-338-6515	www.mhtcguymon.org
Morton County Hospital	Elkhart	Kansas	620-697-2141	www.mchswecare.com
Mount Edgecumbe Hospital	Sitka	Alaska	907-966-2411	www.searhc.org
Newman Memorial Hospital	Shattuck	Oklahoma	580-938-2551	
P H S Indian Hospital at Belcourt - Quentin N Burdick	Belcourt	North Dakota	701-477-6111	
P H S Indian Hospital at Browning - Blackfeet	Browning	Montana	406-338-6157	www.ihs.gov
Phoenix Indian Medical Center	Phoenix	Arizona	602-263-1200	www.ihs.gov
PHS Indian Hospital at Pine Ridge	Pine Ridge	South Dakota	605-867-5131	www.ihs.gov
PHS Indian Hospital at Rosebud	Rosebud	South Dakota	605-747-2231	www.ihs.gov
Provident Hospital of Chicago	Chicago	Illinois	312-572-2000	www.providentfoundation.org
Red Lake Hospital	Redlake	Minnesota	218-679-3912	
Sacred Heart University District	Eugene	Oregon	541-686-7300	www.peacehealth.org
Sonoma Developmental Center	Eldridge	California	707-938-6393	www.dds.ca.gov/sonoma/index.cfm
South Lyon Medical Center	Yerington	Nevada	775-781-3761	
Tuba City Regional Health Care Corporation	Tuba City	Arizona	928-283-2501	www.tcrhcc.org
USPHS Lawton Indian Hospital	Lawton	Oklahoma	580-354-5000	
Valley Forge Medical Center & Hospital	Norristown	Pennsylvania	215-539-8500	www.vfmc.net
Wayne Medical Center	Waynesboro	Tennessee	931-722-5411	
Whiteriver PHS Indian Hospital	Whiteriver	Arizona	928-338-4911	
Whitfield Medical Surgical Hospital	Whitfield	Mississippi	601-351-8001	
Yalobusha General Hospital	Water Valley	Mississippi	662-473-1411	
Yukon Kuskokwim Delta Regional Hospital	Bethel	Alaska	907-543-6300	www.ykhc.org
Zuni Comprehensive Community Health Center	Zuni	New Mexico	505-782-4431	www.ihs.gov

Note: These 48 hospitals had an average ratio of 0.75 or less in the Medicare Spending per Beneficiary category. A total of 3,229 hospitals had medicare spending data available.

Appendix E: Glossary

Accreditation
An evaluative process in which a healthcare organization undergoes an examination of its policies, procedures and performance by an external private sector organization ("accrediting body") to ensure that it is meeting predetermined criteria. It usually involves both on- and off-site surveys. Also see the terms American Osteopathic Association, The Joint Commission, and Medicare-Certified Hospitals.

Acute Care—VA Medical Center
The Veterans Health Administration (VA) Medical Centers deliver inpatient hospital care and related services for surgery and short-term health conditions, as well as comprehensive primary, specialty and long-term care. The VA's medical benefits package is available to Veterans (including Reservists and National Guard) who served on active duty and meet eligibility requirements. Other groups can also be eligible. For more information, visit the U.S. Department of Veterans Affairs.

Acute care hospital
A hospital that provides inpatient medical care and other related services for surgery, acute medical conditions or injuries (usually for a short-term illness or condition).

Acute myocardial infarction (AMI)
See Heart Attack.

American Hospital Association (AHA)
The national organization that represents and serves all types of hospitals, health care networks, and their patients and communities. AHA takes part in national health policy development, legislative and regulatory debates, and legal matters. It also provides education for health care leaders and is a source of information on health care issues and trends.

American Osteopathic Association (AOA)
A member association representing approximately 52,000 osteopathic physicians (D.O.s). The AOA serves as the primary certifying body for D.O.s, and is the accrediting agency for all osteopathic medical colleges and health care facilities. The AOA writes a performance report on each hospital that it checks. You can call or write to AOA to find out a hospital's level of accreditation.

Angioplasty
In angioplasty, a catheter is used to insert a balloon that is inflated to open a blocked blood vessel. Percutaneous transluminal coronary angioplasty (PTCA) is one of several procedures used to open a blocked blood vessel, known collectively as a percutaneous coronary intervention (PCI).

Angiotensin converting enzyme (ACE) inhibitor
A drug used to treat heart attacks, heart failure, or a decreased function of the left heart. It stops production of a hormone that can narrow blood vessels, which helps reduce the pressure in the heart and lower blood pressure.

Angiotensin receptor blocker (ARB)
A drug used to treat patients with heart failure and a decreased function of the left heart. ARBs block the action of a hormone that can narrow blood vessels. This helps reduce the pressure in the heart and lower blood pressure.

Antibiotic
Drugs used to fight bacteria in the body.

ASA Physical Status Classification
Assessment by the anesthesiologist of the patient's preoperative physical condition using the American Society of Anesthesiologists' (ASA) Classification of Physical Status.

Asthma
A chronic lung condition that causes problems getting air in and out of the lungs. Children with asthma may experience wheezing, coughing, chest tightness and trouble breathing.

Atherectomy
A procedure where a blade or laser on a catheter cuts through and removes blockages in blood vessels. It is one of several procedures used to open a blocked blood vessel (known as a Percutaneous Coronary Intervention or PCI).

Beta blocker
A type of drug that is used to lower blood pressure, treat chest pain (angina) and heart failure, and to help prevent a heart attack. Beta blockers relieve the stress on the heart by slowing the heart rate and reducing the force with which the heart muscles contract to pump blood. They also help keep blood vessels from constricting in the heart, brain, and body.

Blood clot
Blood clots are clumps that occur when blood hardens from a liquid to a solid. A blood clot can partly or completely block the flow of blood in a blood vessel.

Blood culture
A blood test that shows if there are bacteria in the blood and what type of bacteria exist. It helps your doctor decide which antibiotic to use to treat a bacterial infection.

Blood thinners
Blood thinners reduce the risk of heart attack and stroke by reducing the formation of blood clots in arteries and veins. There are two main types of blood thinners-anticoagulants, such as heparin or warfarin (also called Coumadin) and antiplatelet drugs, such as aspirin.

Cardiac surgery registry
A registry collects and analyzes information on certain medical topics, conditions, or procedures for hospitals or other providers. The registry then provides the hospitals or providers with information to help them improve the care they provide. A cardiac surgery registry is one example of a registry in which hospitals or providers that perform cardiac surgery can participate.

Centers for Medicare & Medicaid Services (CMS)
The federal agency that runs the Medicare program for the elderly aged and disabled. In addition, CMS works with the states to run the Medicaid program for low-income individuals. CMS works to make sure that the people in these programs are able to get high quality health care.

Centers for Medicare & Medicaid Services (CMS) National Surgical Quality Pilot
In September of 2011, CMS engaged the American College of Surgeons (ACS) to publically report surgical outcome measures on the Hospital Compare website. Hospitals volunteering in this multispecialty surgical registry are provided with nationally validated, risk-adjusted, outcomes-based surgical quality measures. Hospitals report for one or any combination of three surgical measures—elderly surgical outcomes, colectomy outcomes, and lower-extremity bypass outcomes—collected through participation in the American College of Surgeons National Surgical Quality Improvement Program (ACS NSQIP®), a nationally validated, risk-adjusted, outcomes-based program to measure and improve the quality of surgical care in the private sector.

Certification (Medicare-certified)
State government agencies inspect health care providers, including hospitals, nursing homes, dialysis facilities and home health agencies, as well as other health care providers. These providers are certified if they pass inspection. Being certified is not the same as being accredited. Medicare or Medicaid only pays for care provided by certified or accredited providers.

Cesarean section (C-section)
A cesarean section (C-section) is the delivery of a baby through a surgical opening in the mother's lower belly area. A C-section delivery is done when it is not possible or safe for the mother to deliver the baby through the vagina.

Children's hospital
A hospital with a majority of its inpatients under the age of 18, which participates and is paid in the Medicare program as a children's hospital.

Chronic illness
An illness that persists over a long period of time.

Comorbidities
Two or more diseases that are present at the same time.

Critical access hospital (CAH)
A small facility that provides outpatient services, as well as inpatient services on a limited basis, to people in rural areas.

Computerized tomography (CT) scan
An imaging test that uses multiple x-rays to produce detailed pictures of the inside of the body (bones, organs, and other body parts).

Department of Health And Human Services (DHHS)
A federal agency that administers programs for protecting the health of all Americans, including Medicare, Medicaid, and the Children's Health Insurance Program (CHIP).

Diastolic pressure
The lowest pressure in the artery, occurring when the heart is filling with blood. In a blood pressure reading, the diastolic pressure is the second number recorded.

Elective delivery
An elective delivery is a delivery performed for a nonmedical reason. Some nonmedical reasons include wanting to schedule the birth of the baby on a specific date, living far away from the hospital, or discomfort in the last weeks of pregnancy.

Fibrinolysis, fibrinolytic drugs
Fibrinolytic drugs are "clot-busting" drugs that can help dissolve blood clots in blood vessels and improve blood flow to your heart. They are important for treating heart attacks. If you have a heart attack, your doctor may give you a fibrinolytic drug, perform a percutaneous coronary intervention (PCI), or both.

Heart attack
A heart attack, also called an acute myocardial infarction (AMI), happens when one of the heart's arteries becomes blocked and the supply of blood and oxygen to part of the heart muscle is slowed or stopped. When the heart muscle doesn't get the oxygen and nutrients it needs, the affected heart tissue may die.

Heart failure
In heart failure, the heart cannot pump enough blood through the body. The heart cannot fill with enough blood or pump with enough force, or both. Heart failure develops over time as the pumping action of the heart gets weaker. It can affect the right, the left, or both sides of the heart. Heart failure does not mean that the heart has stopped working or is about to stop working.

Hemorrhagic stroke
A hemorrhagic stroke occurs when a blood vessel in part of the brain becomes weak and bursts open, causing blood to leak into the brain. Some people have defects in the blood vessels of the brain that make this more likely.

Heparin injection
Heparin is a type of anticoagulant or "blood thinner," and is used to prevent blood clots from forming in people who have certain medical conditions or who are undergoing certain medical procedures that increase the chance that clots will form. Heparin is also used to stop the growth of clots that have already formed in the blood vessels.

Index admission
An index admission is the admission with a principal diagnosis of a specified condition that meets the inclusion and exclusion criteria for the measure.

Influenza
A serious and sometimes deadly lung infection that can spread quickly in a community. Symptoms include fever-often a high temperature of more than 102° Fahrenheit (38.9° Celsius), headache, muscle aches and pains, chills, cough and chest pain when you take a breath ("pleuritic chest pain"). Although most people recover from the illness, the Centers for Disease Control and Prevention (the CDC) estimates that in the United States more than 200,000 people are hospitalized and about 36,000 people die from the flu and its complications every year.

Influenza vaccination ("Flu Shot")
The main way to keep from getting flu is to get a yearly flu vaccination. Learn more about the flu from the Centers for Disease Control and Prevention (CDC). Hospitals should check to make sure that pneumonia patients get a flu shot during flu season to protect them from another lung infection and to help prevent the spread of influenza in the community.

Inpatient hospital services
Services you get when you're admitted to a hospital, including bed and board, nursing services, diagnostic or therapeutic services, and medical or surgical services.

International Classification of Diseases, Ninth Revision, Clinical Modification (ICD-9-CM)
The classification used to code and classify mortality data from death certificates.

Ischemic stroke
Ischemic stroke occurs when a blood vessel that supplies blood to the brain is blocked by a blood clot. Ischemic strokes may be caused by clogged arteries. Fat, cholesterol, and other substances collect on the artery walls, forming a sticky substance called plaque.

Left ventricular function assessment
A test to check how well the heart is pumping.

Long-term care hospital
Acute care hospitals that provide treatment for patients who stay, on average, more than 25 days. Most patients are transferred from an intensive or critical care unit. These hospitals provide services like comprehensive rehabilitation, respiratory therapy, head trauma treatment, and pain management.

Magnetic resonance imaging (MRI)
An imaging test that uses powerful magnets and radio waves to create pictures of the body. It does not use radiation (x-rays).

Measurement
The process of collecting data to assess performance conducted at a single point in time or repeated over time.

Medicaid
A joint federal and state program that helps with medical costs for some people with low incomes and limited resources. Medicaid programs vary from state to state, but most health care costs are covered if you qualify for both Medicare and Medicaid.

Medical imaging
Tests that create images of various parts of the body to screen for or diagnose medical conditions. Examples of medical imaging include CT Scans, MRIs, and mammograms.

Medicare Advantage Plan (Part C)
A type of Medicare health plan offered by a private company that contracts with Medicare to provide you with all your Part A and Part B benefits. Medicare Advantage Plans include Health Maintenance Organizations (HMOs), Preferred Provider Organizations (PPOs), Private Fee-for-Service Plans, Special Needs Plans, and Medicare Medical Savings Account Plans. If you're enrolled in a Medicare Advantage Plan, Medicare services are covered through the plan and aren't paid for under Original Medicare. Most Medicare Advantage Plans offer prescription drug coverage.

Medicare health plan
A plan offered by a private company that contracts with Medicare to provide Part A and Part B benefits to people with Medicare who enroll in the plan. Medicare health plans include all Medicare Advantage Plans, Medicare Cost Plans, Demonstration/Pilot Programs, and Programs of All-inclusive Care for the Elderly (PACE).

Medicare Severity-Diagnosis Related Group (MS-DRG)
The Medicare Severity - Diagnosis Related Groups (MS-DRGs) are payment groups designed for the Medicare population. Patients who have similar clinical characteristics and similar costs are assigned to an MS-DRG. The MS-DRG will be linked to a fixed payment amount based on the average cost of patients in the group. Patients can be assigned to an MS-DRG based on their diagnosis, surgical procedures, age and other information. Hospitals provide this information on their bills and Medicare uses this information to decide how much the hospitals should be paid. There may be some groups of MS-DRGs that are based on complications or comorbidities (CCs) or major complications or comorbidities (MCCs). Complications are new problems that are the result of a procedure, treatment, or illness.

Medicare-certified hospital
In order to receive any payment from either the Medicare or Medicaid programs, a hospital must meet a set of basic standards for quality of care, called "conditions of participation." Medicare-certified hospitals are reviewed periodically (every three years), either by their State Survey Agency or a CMS-approved national accreditation organization, to assure that they are continuing to provide services of acceptable quality. Accreditation is optional, but most short-term acute hospitals in the United States choose to be Medicare-certified based on accreditation by a CMS approved national accreditation organization. There are currently three CMS-approved national hospital accreditation organizations: the American Osteopathic Association/health care Facilities Accreditation Program (AOA/HFAP), Det Norske Veritas Healthcare (DNV Healthcare), and The Joint Commission (TJC).

Number of completed surveys
The "number of completed surveys" is the total number of patients who completed a survey. When at least 300 patients have completed the survey for a hospital, we can be more confident that the survey results are fully representative of patients' experiences at that hospital and are reliable for assessing the hospital's performance. However, smaller hospitals could sample all of their HCAHPS-eligible discharges but, because of their small size, still have fewer than 300 completed surveys.

Original Medicare
Original Medicare is fee-for-service coverage under which the government pays your health care providers directly for your Part A and/or Part B benefits.

Osteopathic doctor
A licensed physician who can do surgery and prescribe drugs who has training in manipulative therapy. Also called a Doctor of Osteopathy (DO).

Outpatient hospital care
Medical or surgical care you get from a hospital when your doctor hasn't written an order to admit you to the hospital as an inpatient. Outpatient hospital care may include emergency department services, observation services, outpatient surgery, lab tests, or X-rays. Your care may be considered outpatient hospital care even if you spend the night at the hospital.

Outpatient Prospective Payment System (OPPS)
Under the Outpatient Prospective Payment System (OPPS), hospitals are paid a set amount of money (called the payment rate) to provide certain outpatient services to people with Medicare.

Oxygenation assessment
Test that measures the amount of oxygen in your blood to see if you need oxygen therapy.

Patient discharge
Patients are considered "discharged" from a hospital when they are released to go home or to another health care setting, or when they die during the hospital stay.

Percutaneous coronary interventions (PCI)
The procedures called percutaneous coronary interventions (PCI), such as angioplasty and atherectomy are among those that are the most effective for opening blocked blood vessels that cause heart attacks. Doctors may perform a PCI, or give certain drugs to open the blockage, and in some cases, they may do both.

Plan of care
A written plan of care created with your physician and hospital staff. It tells what services you will get to reach and keep your best physical, mental, and social wellbeing. The hospital staff keeps your doctor up-to-date on how you are doing and updates your care plan as needed.

Pneumonia
An inflammation of the lungs caused by a viral or bacterial infection. This fills your lungs with mucus and lowers the oxygen level in your blood. Symptoms can include fever, fatigue, difficulty breathing, chills, a "wet" cough, and chest pain. For more on pneumonia, visit MedlinePlus

Pneumonia (pneumococcal) vaccination
Vaccine given to prevent pneumonia, estimated to protect against 80% of bacteria causing pneumonia.

Provider
A doctor, hospital, health care professional or health care facility.

Psychiatric hospital
A facility that provides inpatient psychiatric services for the diagnosis and treatment of mental illness on a 24-hour basis, by or under the supervision of a physician.

Quality
Quality health care is how well a doctor, hospital, health plan, or other provider of health care, keeps its patients healthy or treats them when they are sick. Good quality health care means doing the right thing at the right time, in the right way, for the right person and getting the best possible results.

Quality assurance
The process of looking at how well a medical service is provided. The process may include formally reviewing health care given to a person, or group of persons, locating the problem, correcting the problem, and then checking to see if what was done worked.

Quality Improvement Organizations (QIOs)
A group of practicing doctors and other health care experts paid by the federal government to check and improve the care given to people with Medicare.

Ratio
The amount of one thing compared to the amount of another, such as the number of combination CT scans done compared to the number of all CT scans done.

Readmissions
Patients who are admitted to the hospital for treatment of medical problems sometimes get other serious injuries, complications, or conditions, and may even die. Some patients may experience problems soon after they are discharged and need to be admitted to the hospital again. These events can often be prevented if hospitals follow best practices for treating patients.

Registry
A registry collects and analyzes information on certain medical topics, conditions, or procedures for hospitals or other providers. The registry then provides the hospitals or providers with information to help them improve the care they provide. Examples of registries in which hospitals can participate include: a multispecialty surgical registry , a nursing care registry, and a stroke care registry.

Rehabilitation hospital
A hospital that specializes in improving or restoring a patient's functional ability through therapies. Sometimes called a post-acute hospital.

Reliever medications
Relievers are medications that relax the bands of muscle surrounding the airways and are used to quickly make breathing easier.

Risk-adjusted
"Risk-adjusted" means that the measure calculations take into account how sick patients were when they went in for their initial hospital stay. When rates are risk-adjusted, it means that hospitals that usually take care of sicker patients won't have a worse rate just because their patients were sicker when they arrived at the hospital. When rates are risk-adjusted, it helps make comparisons fair and meaningful.

Risk-adjusted 30-day death (mortality) rates
The 30-day Risk-Adjusted Death (Mortality) Rates are produced using a complex statistical model, that relies on Medicare claims and enrollment information. The model predicts patient deaths for any cause within 30 days of hospital admission for heart attack or heart failure, whether the patients die while still in the hospital or after discharge. Thirty-day mortality is used because this is the time period when deaths are most likely to be related to the care patients received in the hospital. Deaths that occur outside the hospital within 30 days are included along with deaths that occur in the hospital, because some hospitals discharge patients sooner than others.

Screening mammogram
A medical procedure to check for breast cancer before you or a doctor may be able to find it manually.

Stent
A small wire tube inserted in a blood vessel by a catheter to hold open a blocked blood vessel. This is one of several procedures called a percutaneous coronary intervention (PCI) that are used to open a blocked blood vessel.

Structural measures
A structural measure reflects the environment in which providers care for patients, such as whether or not a hospital uses an electronic health record.

Survey of patients' experiences
A national, standardized survey of hospital patients about their experiences during a recent inpatient hospital stay. This is also referred to as HCAHPS (Hospital Consumer Assessment of Healthcare Providers and Systems).

Survey response rate
Tells what percentage of patients who were asked to complete the survey actually did complete it. In general, the higher this response rate percentage, the more confident we can be that the survey results for a hospital are representative of patients' experiences at that hospital and are reliable for assessing the hospital's performance.

Systemic corticosteroid
Inflammation-reducing, anti-allergic medications that affect the body as a whole.

Teaching hospital
Hospitals that train residents in approved medical, osteopathic, dental or podiatry residency programs.

The Joint Commission (JC)
An independent, not-for-profit organization that accredits and certifies a large number of health care organizations and programs in the United States. The Joint Commission's hospital accreditation program has held deeming authority since the inception of the Medicare program in 1965. The Joint Commission's mission is to continuously improve health care for the public, in collaboration with other stakeholders, by evaluating health care organizations and inspiring them to excel in providing safe and effective care of the highest quality and value.

Thrombolytic therapy
Thrombolytic therapy is the use of drugs to break up or dissolve blood clots, which are the main cause of both heart attacks and stroke.

Treatment
Something done to help with a health problem. For example, giving certain drugs and performing surgery are treatments.

Treatment options

The choices you have when there is more than one way to treat your health problem.

Venous thromboembolism (VTE)

Venous thromboembolism (VTE) is a term that includes both deep vein thrombosis and pulmonary embolism. A deep vein thrombosis (DVT) is a blood clot that forms in a vein deep in the body. A pulmonary embolism (PE) is a loose blood clot that travels to an artery in the lungs and can block blood flow.

Warfarin

A medication used to prevent blood clots from forming or growing larger in your blood and blood vessels.

Source: Medicare.gov

Regional Hospital Profile Index

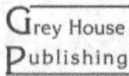

2014 Title List

Visit **www.GreyHouse.com** for Product Information, Table of Contents and Sample Pages

General Reference

America's College Museums
American Environmental Leaders: From Colonial Times to the Present
An African Biographical Dictionary
An Encyclopedia of Human Rights in the United States
Constitutional Amendments
Encyclopedia of African-American Writing
Encyclopedia of the Continental Congress
Encyclopedia of Gun Control & Gun Rights
Encyclopedia of Invasions & Conquests
Encyclopedia of Prisoners of War & Internment
Encyclopedia of Religion & Law in America
Encyclopedia of Rural America
Encyclopedia of the United States Cabinet, 1789-2010
Encyclopedia of War Journalism
Encyclopedia of Warrior Peoples & Fighting Groups
From Suffrage to the Senate: America's Political Women
Nations of the World
Political Corruption in America
Speakers of the House of Representatives, 1789-2009
The Environmental Debate: A Documentary History
The Evolution Wars: A Guide to the Debates
The Religious Right: A Reference Handbook
The Value of a Dollar: 1860-2009
The Value of a Dollar: Colonial Era
This is Who We Were: A Companion to the 1940 Census
This is Who We Were: The 1920s
This is Who We Were: The 1950s
This is Who We Were: The 1960s
US Land & Natural Resource Policy
Working Americans 1770-1869 Vol. IX: Revolutionary War to the Civil War
Working Americans 1880-1999 Vol. I: The Working Class
Working Americans 1880-1999 Vol. II: The Middle Class
Working Americans 1880-1999 Vol. III: The Upper Class
Working Americans 1880-1999 Vol. IV: Their Children
Working Americans 1880-2003 Vol. V: At War
Working Americans 1880-2005 Vol. VI: Women at Work
Working Americans 1880-2006 Vol. VII: Social Movements
Working Americans 1880-2007 Vol. VIII: Immigrants
Working Americans 1880-2009 Vol. X: Sports & Recreation
Working Americans 1880-2010 Vol. XI: Inventors & Entrepreneurs
Working Americans 1880-2011 Vol. XII: Our History through Music
Working Americans 1880-2012 Vol. XIII: Education & Educators
World Cultural Leaders of the 20th & 21st Centuries

Business Information

Complete Television, Radio & Cable Industry Directory
Directory of Business Information Resources
Directory of Mail Order Catalogs
Directory of Venture Capital & Private Equity Firms
Environmental Resource Handbook
Food & Beverage Market Place
Grey House Homeland Security Directory
Grey House Performing Arts Directory
Hudson's Washington News Media Contacts Directory
New York State Directory
Sports Market Place Directory

Education Information

Charter School Movement
Comparative Guide to American Elementary & Secondary Schools
Complete Learning Disabilities Directory
Educators Resource Directory
Special Education

Health Information

Comparative Guide to American Hospitals
Complete Directory for Pediatric Disorders
Complete Directory for People with Chronic Illness
Complete Directory for People with Disabilities
Complete Mental Health Directory
Diabetes in America: A Geographic & Demographic Analysis
Directory of Health Care Group Purchasing Organizations
Directory of Hospital Personnel
HMO/PPO Directory
Medical Device Register
Older Americans Information Directory

Statistics & Demographics

America's Top-Rated Cities
America's Top-Rated Small Towns & Cities
America's Top-Rated Smaller Cities
American Tally
Ancestry & Ethnicity in America
Comparative Guide to American Hospitals
Comparative Guide to American Suburbs
Profiles of America
Profiles of... Series – State Handbooks
The Hispanic Databook
Weather America

Financial Ratings Series

TheStreet.com Ratings Guide to Bond & Money Market Mutual Funds
TheStreet.com Ratings Guide to Common Stocks
TheStreet.com Ratings Guide to Exchange-Traded Funds
TheStreet.com Ratings Guide to Stock Mutual Funds
TheStreet.com Ratings Ultimate Guided Tour of Stock Investing
Weiss Ratings Consumer Guides
Weiss Ratings Guide to Banks & Thrifts
Weiss Ratings Guide to Credit Unions
Weiss Ratings Guide to Health Insurers
Weiss Ratings Guide to Life & Annuity Insurers
Weiss Ratings Guide to Property & Casualty Insurers

Bowker's Books In Print® Titles

Books In Print®
Books In Print® Supplement
American Book Publishing Record® Annual
American Book Publishing Record® Monthly
Books Out Loud™
Bowker's Complete Video Directory™
Children's Books In Print®
El-Hi Textbooks & Serials In Print®
Forthcoming Books®
Law Books & Serials In Print™
Medical & Health Care Books In Print™
Publishers, Distributors & Wholesalers of the US™
Subject Guide to Books In Print®
Subject Guide to Children's Books In Print®

Canadian General Reference

Associations Canada
Canadian Almanac & Directory
Canadian Environmental Resource Guide
Canadian Parliamentary Guide
Financial Services Canada
Governments Canada
Health Services Canada
Libraries Canada
Major Canadian Cities
The History of Canada

Grey House Publishing | Salem Press | H.W. Wilson
4919 Route, 22 PO Box 56, Amenia NY 12501-0056

2014 Title List

Visit **www.SalemPress.com** for Product Information, Table of Contents and Sample Pages

Literature

American Ethnic Writers
Critical Insights: Authors
Critical Insights: New Literary Collection Bundles
Critical Insights: Themes
Critical Insights: Works
Critical Survey of Drama
Critical Survey of Graphic Novels: Heroes & Super Heroes
Critical Survey of Graphic Novels: History, Theme & Technique
Critical Survey of Graphic Novels: Independents & Underground Classics
Critical Survey of Graphic Novels: Manga
Critical Survey of Long Fiction
Critical Survey of Mystery & Detective Fiction
Critical Survey of Mythology and Folklore: Heroes and Heroines
Critical Survey of Mythology and Folklore: Love, Sexuality & Desire
Critical Survey of Mythology and Folklore: World Mythology
Critical Survey of Poetry
Critical Survey of Poetry: American Poetry
Critical Survey of Poetry: British, Irish & Commonwealth Poets
Critical Survey of Poetry: European Poets
Critical Survey of Poetry: European Poets
Critical Survey of Poetry: Topical Essays
Critical Survey of Poetry: World Poets
Critical Survey of Science Fiction & Fantasy Literature
Critical Survey of Shakespeare's Sonnets
Critical Survey of Short Fiction
Critical Survey of Short Fiction: American Writers
Critical Survey of Short Fiction: British, Irish & Commonwealth Poets
Critical Survey of Short Fiction: European Writers
Critical Survey of Short Fiction: Topical Essays
Critical Survey of Short Fiction: World Writers
Cyclopedia of Literary Characters
Introduction to Literary Context: American Post-Modernist Novels
Introduction to Literary Context: American Short Fiction
Introduction to Literary Context: English Literature
Introduction to Literary Context: World Literature
Magill's Literary Annual 2014
Magill's Survey of American Literature
Magill's Survey of World Literature
Masterplots
Masterplots II: African American Literature
Masterplots II: Christian Literature
Masterplots II: Drama Series
Masterplots II: Short Story Series
Notable African American Writers
Notable American Novelists
Notable Playwrights
Short Story Writers

Science, Careers & Mathematics

Applied Science
Applied Science: Engineering & Mathematics
Applied Science: Science & Medicine
Applied Science: Technology
Biomes and Ecosystems
Careers in Chemistry
Careers in Communications & Media
Careers in Healthcare
Careers in Hospitality & Tourism
Careers in Law & Criminology
Careers in Physics
Computer Technology Inventors
Contemporary Biographies in Chemistry
Contemporary Biographies in Communications & Media
Contemporary Biographies in Healthcare
Contemporary Biographies in Hospitality & Tourism
Contemporary Biographies in Law & Criminology
Contemporary Biographies in Physics
Earth Science
Earth Science: Earth Materials & Resources
Earth Science: Earth's Surface and History
Earth Science: Physics & Chemistry of the Earth
Earth Science: Weather, Water & Atmosphere
Encyclopedia of Energy
Encyclopedia of Environmental Issues
Encyclopedia of Global Resources
Encyclopedia of Global Warming
Encyclopedia of Mathematics and Society
Encyclopedia of the Ancient World
Forensic Science
Internet Innovators
Introduction to Chemistry
Magill's Encyclopedia of Science: Animal Life
Magill's Encyclopedia of Science: Plant life
Magill's Medical Guide
Notable Natural Disasters
Solar System

Health

Addictions & Substance Abuse
Cancer
Complementary & Alternative Medicine
Genetics & Inherited Conditions
Infectious Diseases & Conditions
Magill's Medical Guide
Psychology & Mental Health
Psychology Basics

2014 Title List

Visit www.SalemPress.com for Product Information, Table of Contents and Sample Pages

History and Social Science

A 2000s in America
50 States
African American History
Agriculture in History (check)
American First Ladies
American Heroes
American Indian Tribes
American Presidents
American Villains
Ancient Greece
Bill of Rights, The
Cold War, The
Defining Documents: American Revolution 1754-1805
Defining Documents: Civil War 1860-1865
Defining Documents: Emergence of Modern America, 1868-1918
Defining Documents: Exploration & Colonial America 1492-1755
Defining Documents: Manifest Destiny 1803-1860
Defining Documents: Reconstruction, 1865-1880
Defining Documents: The 1920s
Defining Documents: The 1930s
Defining Documents: World War I
Eighties in America
Encyclopedia of American Immigration
Fifties in America
Forties in America
Great Athletes
Great Events from History: 17th Century
Great Events from History: 18th Century
Great Events from History: 19th Century
Great Events from History: 20th Century, 1901-1940
Great Events from History: 20th Century, 1941-1970
Great Events from History: 20th Century, 1971-200
Great Events from History: Ancient World
Great Events from History: Middle Ages
Great Events from History: Modern Scandals
Great Events from History: Renaissance & Early Modern Era
Great Lives from History: 17th Century
Great Lives from History: 18th Century
Great Lives from History: 19th Century
Great Lives from History: 20th Century
Great Lives from History: African Americans
Great Lives from History: Ancient World
Great Lives from History: Asian & Pacific Islander Americans
Great Lives from History: Incredibly Wealthy
Great Lives from History: Inventors & Inventions
Great Lives from History: Jewish Americans
Great Lives from History: Latinos
Great Lives from History: Middle Ages
Great Lives from History: Notorious Lives
Great Lives from History: Renaissance & Early Modern Era
Great Lives from History: Scientists & Science
Historical Encyclopedia of American Business
Immigration in U.S. History
Magill's Guide to Military History
Milestone Documents in African American History
Milestone Documents in American History
Milestone Documents in World History
Milestone Documents of American Leaders
Milestone Documents of World Religions
Musicians & Composers 20th Century
Nineties in America
Seventies in America
Sixties in America
Survey of American Industry and Careers
Thirties in America
Twenties in America
U.S. Court Cases
U.S. Laws, Acts, and Treaties
U.S. Legal System
U.S. Supreme Court
United States at War
USA in Space
Weapons and Warfare
World Conflicts: Asia and the Middle East

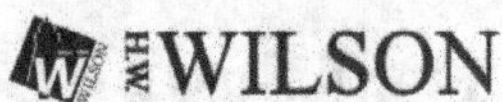
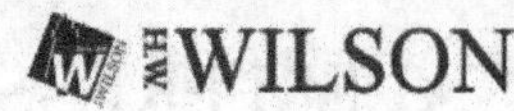

2014 Title List

Visit **www.HwWilsonInPrint.com** for Product Information, Table of Contents and Sample Pages

Current Biography

Current Biography Cumulative Index 1946-2013
Current Biography Magazine
Current Biography Yearbook-2004
Current Biography Yearbook-2005
Current Biography Yearbook-2006
Current Biography Yearbook-2007
Current Biography Yearbook-2008
Current Biography Yearbook-2009
Current Biography Yearbook-2010
Current Biography Yearbook-2011
Current Biography Yearbook-2012
Current Biography Yearbook-2013
Current Biography Yearbook-2014

Core Collections

Senior High Core Collection
Middle & Junior High School Core
Children's Core Collection
Fiction Core Collection
Public Library Core Collection: Nonfiction

Sears List

Sears List of Subject Headings
Sears: Lista de Encabezamientos de Materia

The Reference Shelf

Aging in America
Revisiting Gender
The U.S. National Debate Topic, 2014/2015
Embracing New Paradigms in education
Marijuana Reform
Representative American Speeches 2013-2014
Reality Television
The Business of Food
The Future of U.S. Economic Relations: Mexico, Cuba, and Venezuela
Sports in America
Global Climate Change
Representative American Speeches, 2012-2013
Conspiracy Theories
The Arab Spring
U.S. National Debate Topic: Transportation Infrastructure
Families: Traditional and New Structures
Faith & Science
Representative American Speeches 2011-2012
Social Networking
Dinosaurs
Space Exploration & Development
U.S. Infrastructure
Politics of the Ocean
Representative American Speeches 2010-2011
Robotics
The News and its Future
American Military Presence Overseas
Russia
Graphic Novels and Comic Books
Representative American Speeches 2009-2010

Readers' Guide

Readers Guide to Periodicals Literature
Abridged Readers' Guide to Periodical Literature
Short Story Index

Indexes

Short Story Index
Index to Legal Periodicals & Books

Facts About Series

Facts About the Presidents, Eighth Edition
Facts About China
Facts About the 20th Century
Facts About American Immigration
Facts About World's Languages

Nobel Prize Winners

Nobel Prize Winners, 2002-2013

World Authors

World Authors 2000-2005
World Authors 2006-2013

Famous First Facts

Famous First Facts, Seventh Edition
Famous First Facts About American Politics
Famous First Facts About Sports
Famous First Facts About the Environment
Famous First Facts, International Edition

American Book of Days

The American Book of Days, Fifth Edition
The International Book of Days

Junior Authors & Illustrators

Tenth Book of Junior Authors & Illustrations

Monographs

The Barnhart Dictionary of Etymology
Celebrate the World
Indexing from A to Z
Radical Change: Books for Youth in a Digital Age
The Poetry Break
Guide to the Ancient World

Wilson Chronology

Wilson Chronology of Asia and the Pacific
Wilson Chronology of Human Rights
Wilson Chronology of Ideas
Wilson Chronology of the Arts
Wilson Chronology of the World's Religions
Wilson Chronology of Women's Achievements

Book Review Digest

Book Review Digest, 2014

Grey House Publishing | Salem Press | H.W. Wilson
4919 Route, 22 PO Box 56, Amenia NY 12501-0056

LINDENHURST MEMORIAL LIBRARY
3 1801 00550 8605

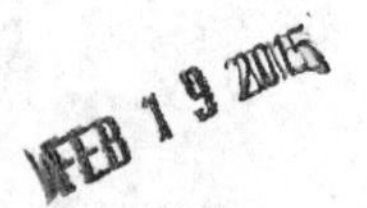

FEB 1 9 2015